JN249509

JP XVIII

THE JAPANESE PHARMACOPOEIA

EIGHTEENTH EDITION

〈I〉

Official from June 7, 2021

English Version

PMRJ

PHARMACEUTICAL AND MEDICAL DEVICE
REGULATORY SCIENCE SOCIETY OF JAPAN

Published 2022 by

PHARMACEUTICAL AND MEDICAL DEVICE
REGULATORY SCIENCE SOCIETY OF JAPAN

2-12-15, Shibuya, Shibuya-ku, Tokyo, 150-0002 JAPAN

Distributed by

YAKUJI NIPPO, LTD.

1, Kanda Izumicho, Chiyoda-ku, Tokyo, 101-8648 JAPAN

Notice: This *English Version* of the Japanese Pharmacopoeia is published for the convenience of users unfamiliar with the Japanese language. When and if any discrepancy arises between the Japanese original and its English translation, the former is authentic.

ISBN978-4-8408-1589-5 C3047

Printed in Japan

JP XVIII
TOTAL CONTENTS

I

II

The Ministry of Health, Labour and Welfare Ministerial Notification No. 220

Pursuant to Paragraph 1, Article 41 of Act on Securing Quality, Efficacy and Safety of Products Including Pharmaceuticals and Medical Devices (Law No. 145, 1960), this notification stated that the Japanese Pharmacopoeia was revised as follows*.

TAMURA Norihisa
The Minister of Health, Labour and Welfare

June 7, 2021

Japanese Pharmacopoeia

Pursuant to Paragraph 1, Article 41 of Act on Securing Quality, Efficacy and Safety of Products Including Pharmaceuticals and Medical Devices (Law No. 145, 1960), the Japanese Pharmacopoeia was revised as follows.

(The text referred to by the term ''as follows'' are omitted here. All of the revised Japanese Pharmacopoeia in accordance with this notification are made available for public exhibition at the Pharmaceutical Evaluation Division, Pharmaceutical Safety and Environmental Health Bureau, Ministry of Health, Labour and Welfare, at each Regional Bureau of Health and Welfare, and at each Prefectural Office in Japan).

Supplementary Provisions

(Effective Date)

Article 1 This Notification is applied from the date of the notification. (referred to as the ''notification date'' in the next and third articles)

(Transitional measures)

Article 2 In the case of drugs which are listed in the Japanese Pharmacopoeia (hereinafter referred to as ''previous Pharmacopoeia'') and have been approved as of the notification date as prescribed under Paragraph 1, Article 14 of Act on Securing Quality, Efficacy and Safety of Products Including Pharmaceuticals and Medical Devices [including drugs the Minister of Health, Labour and Welfare specifies (the Ministry of Health and Welfare Ministerial Notification No. 104, 1994) as of the day before the notification date as those exempted from marketing approval pursuant to Paragraph 1, Article 14 of the same law (hereinafter referred to as ''drugs exempted from approval'')], the Name and Standards established in the previous Pharmacopoeia (limited to part of the Name and Standards for the drugs concerned) may be accepted to conform to the Name and Standards established in the revised Japanese Pharmacopoeia (hereinafter referred to as ''new Pharmacopoeia'') (limited to part of the Name and Standards for the drugs concerned) in accordance with this notification before and on December 31, 2022.

Article 3 In the case of drugs which are listed in the new Pharmacopoeia (excluding those listed in the previous Pharmacopoeia) and have been approved as of the notification date as prescribed under the Paragraph 1, Article 14 of the same law (including those exempted from approval), they may be accepted as those being not listed in the new Pharmacopoeia before and on December 31, 2022.

Article 4 In the case of drugs which are listed in the new Pharmacopoeia, their commonly used names established in the previous Pharmacopoeia may be accepted to conform to the Name established in the new Pharmacopoeia before and on June 30, 2024.

Article 5 In the case of drugs which are listed in the new Pharmacopoeia, the previous provisions are applied before and on June 30, 2024, regardless of the Paragraph 34 of General Notices.

*The term ''as follows'' here indicates the contents of the Japanese Pharmacopoeia Eighteenth Edition from General Notice to Ultraviolet-Visible Reference Spectra (pp. 1 – 2587).

CONTENTS

PREFACE

The Japanese Pharmacopoeia (JP) is an official document that defines the specifications, criteria and standard test methods necessary to properly assure the quality of medicines in Japan.

Paragraph 2, Article 41 of the Law on Securing Quality, Efficacy and Safety of Products including Pharmaceuticals and Medical Devices stipulates that full-fledged JP revisions shall be presented at least every 10 years. Since the JP 9th edition, full-fledged revisions have been made every 5 years. In addition to the full-fledged revisions, a supplement has been promulgated twice in every 5 years since the JP 12th edition as well as partial revisions have been made as necessary to take account of recent progress of science and in the interests of international harmonization.

The 17th Edition of the JP was promulgated by Ministerial Notification No. 64 of the Ministry of Health, Labour and Welfare (MHLW) on March 7, 2016.

In July 2016, the Committee on JP established the basic principles for the preparation of the JP 18th Edition, setting out the roles and characteristics of the JP, the definite measures for the revision, and the date of the revision.

At the Committee, the five basic principles of JP, which we refer to as the "five pillars", were established as follows: 1) Including all drugs which are important from the viewpoint of health care and medical treatment; 2) Making qualitative improvement by introducing the latest science and technology; 3) Promoting further internationalization in response to globalization of drug market; 4) Making prompt partial revision as necessary and facilitating smooth administrative operation; and 5) Ensuring transparency regarding the revision, and disseminating the JP to the public. It was agreed that the Committee on JP should make efforts, on the basis of these principles, to ensure that the JP is used more effectively in the fields of health care and medical treatment by taking appropriate measurements, including getting the understanding and cooperation of other parties concerned.

It was agreed that the JP should provide an official standard, being required to assure the quality of medicines in Japan in response to the progress of science and technology and medical demands at the time. It should define the standards for specifications, as well as the methods of testing to assure overall quality of all drugs in principle, and it should have a role in clarifying the criteria for quality assurance of drugs that are recognized to be essential for public health and medical treatment. The JP has been prepared with the aid of the knowledge and experience of many professionals in the pharmaceutical field. Therefore, the JP should have the characteristics of an official standard, which might be widely used by all parties concerned, and it should play an appropriate role of providing information and understanding about the quality of drugs to the public. Moreover, as a pharmaceutical quality standard, it should contribute promoting and maintaining of advancedness as well as international consistency and harmonization of technical requirements in the international community. It was also agreed that JP articles should cover drugs, which are important from the viewpoint of health care and medical treatment, clinical performance or merits and frequency of use, as soon as possible after they reach the market.

The target date for the publication of the JP 18th Edition (the Japanese edition) was set as April 2021.

JP drafts are discussed in the following committees that were established in the Pharmaceuticals and Medical Devices Agency: Expert Committee; Sub-expert Committee; Sub-committee on Manufacturing Process-related Matters; Committee on Chemicals; Committee on Antibiotics; Committee on Biologicals; Committee on Crude Drugs; Committee on Pharmaceutical Excipients; Committee on Physico-Chemical Methods; Committee on Drug Formulation; Committee on Physical Methods; Committee on Biological Methods; Committee on Nomenclature for Pharmaceuticals; Committee on International Harmonization; and Committee on Reference Standards.

In the Committee on JP, Mitsuru Hashida took the role of chairman from April 2016 to June 2021.

In accordance with the above principles, the committees initiated deliberations on selection of articles and on revisions for General Notices, General Rules for Crude Drugs, General Rules for Preparations, General Tests, Monographs and so on.

Draft revisions covering subjects in General Rules for Preparations, General Tests and Monographs, for which discussions were finished between August 2015 and March 2017, were prepared for a supplement to the JP 17. The draft revisions were examined by the Committee on JP in April 2017, followed by the Pharmaceutical Affairs and Food Sanitation Council (PAFSC) in June 2017, and then submitted to the Minister of Health, Labour and Welfare.

The supplement was named "Supplement I to the JP 17th Edition", promulgated on December 1, 2017 by Ministerial Notification No. 348 of MHLW, and became effective.

Numbers of discussions in the committees to prepare the supplement drafts were as follows: Expert Committee (8); Sub-committee on Manufacturing Process-related Matters (9); Committee on Chemicals (20); Committee on Antibiotics (5); Committee on Biologicals (8); Committee on Crude Drugs (17); Committee on Pharmaceutical Excipients (10); Committee on Physico-Chemical Methods (14, including working group); Committee on Drug Formulation (27, including working group); Committee on Physical Methods (8); Committee on Biological Methods (6); Committee on Nomenclature for Pharmaceuticals (7); Committee on International Harmonization (6); and Committee on Reference Standards (4).

It should be noted that in the preparation of the drafts for the supplement, generous cooperation was given by the Pharmaceutical Technology Committee of the Osaka Pharmaceutical Manufacturers Association, the Pharmacopeia and CMC Committee of the Pharmaceutical Manufacturers' Association of Tokyo, the Tokyo Crude Drugs Association, the International Pharmaceutical Excipients Council Japan, the Home Medicine Association of Japan, the Japan Kampo Medicines Manufacturers Association, the Japan Flavor and Fragrance Materials Association, the Japan Medicinal Plant Federation, the Japan Pharmaceutical Manufacturers Association, the Federation of Pharmaceutical Manufacturers' Association of Japan, the Parenteral Drug Association Japan Chapter, the Japan Reagent Association, the Japan Oilseed Processors Association, the Japan Analytical Instruments Manufacturers' Association, and the Asian Society of Innovative Packaging Technology.

In consequence of this revision, the JP 17th Edition carries 1977 articles, owing to the addition of 32 articles and the deletion of 17 articles.

Draft revisions covering subjects in General Notices, General Rules for Preparations, General Tests and Monographs, for which discussions were finished between April 2017 and November 2018, were prepared for a supplement to the JP 17. The draft revisions were examined by the Committee on JP in January 2019, followed by the PAFSC in March 2019, and then submitted to the Minister of Health, Labour and Welfare.

The supplement was named "Supplement II to the JP 17th Edition", promulgated on June 28, 2019 by Ministerial Notification No. 49 of MHLW, and became effective.

Numbers of discussions in the committees to prepare the supplement drafts were as follows: Expert Committee (11, including working group); Subcommittee on Manufacturing Process-related Matters (6); Committee on Chemicals (18); Committee on Antibiotics (3); Committee on Biologicals (7); Committee on Crude Drugs (15); Committee on Pharmaceutical Excipients (10); Committee on Physico-Chemical Methods (11, including working group); Committee on Drug Formulation (19, including working group); Committee on Physical Methods (7); Committee on Biological Methods (6); Committee on Nomenclature for Pharmaceuticals (5); and Committee on International Harmonization (4).

It should be noted that in the preparation of the drafts for the supplement, generous cooperation was given by the Pharmaceutical Technology Committee of the Kansai Pharmaceutical Industries Association, the Pharmacopeia and CMC Committee of the Pharmaceutical Manufacturers' Association of Tokyo, the Tokyo Crude Drugs Association, the International Pharmaceutical Excipients Council Japan, the Home Medicine Association of Japan, the Japan Kampo Medicines Manufacturers Association, the Japan Flavor and Fragrance Materials Association, the Japan Medicinal Plant Federation, the Japan Pharmaceutical Manufacturers Association, the Federation of Pharmaceutical Manufacturers' Association of Japan, the Parenteral Drug Association Japan Chapter, the Japan Reagent Association, the Japan Oilseed Processors Association, the Japan Analytical Instruments Manufacturers' Association, and the Asian Society of Innovative Packaging Technology.

In consequence of this revision, the JP 17th Edition carries 2008 articles, owing to the addition of 34 articles and the deletion of 3 articles.

Draft revisions covering subjects in General Notices, General Rules for Crude Drugs, General Rules for Preparations, General Tests and Monographs, for which discussions were finished between December 2018 and August 2020, were prepared for a supplement to the JP 18. The draft revisions were examined by the Committee on JP in October 2020, followed by the PAFSC in December 2020, and then submitted to the Minister of Health, Labour and Welfare.

Numbers of discussions in the committees to prepare the revision drafts were as follows: Expert Committee (12, including working group); Committee on Chemicals (19); Committee on Antibiotics (3); Committee on Biologicals (8); Committee on Crude Drugs (14); Committee on Pharmaceutical Excipients (10, including working group); Committee on Physico-Chemical Methods (7); Committee on Drug Formulation (20, including working group); Committee on Physical Methods (7); Committee on Biological Methods (7); Committee on Nomenclature for Pharmaceuticals (6); Committee on International Harmonization (7); and Committee on Reference Standards (7, including working group).

It should be noted that in the preparation of the revision drafts, generous cooperation was given by the

Pharmaceutical Technology Committee of the Kansai Pharmaceutical Industries Association, the Pharmacopeia and CMC Committee of the Pharmaceutical Manufacturers' Association of Tokyo, the Tokyo Crude Drugs Association, the International Pharmaceutical Excipients Council Japan, the Home Medicine Association of Japan, the Japan Kampo Medicines Manufacturers Association, the Japan Flavor and Fragrance Materials Association, the Japan Medicinal Plant Federation, the Japan Pharmaceutical Manufacturers Association, the Federation of Pharmaceutical Manufacturers' Association of Japan, the Parenteral Drug Association Japan Chapter, the Japan Reagent Association, the Japan Oilseed Processors Association, the Japan Analytical Instruments Manufacturers' Association, and the Asian Society of Innovative Packaging Technology.

In consequence of this revision, the JP 18th Edition carries 2033 articles, owing to the addition of 33 articles and the deletion of 8 articles.

The principles of description and the salient points of the revision in this volume are as follows:

1. The JP 18th Edition comprises the following items, in order: Notification of MHLW; Contents; Preface; General Notices; General Rules for Crude Drugs; General Rules for Preparations; General Tests, Processes and Apparatus; Official Monographs; then followed by Infrared Reference Spectra and Ultraviolet-visible Reference Spectra; General Information; Table of Standard Atomic Weights as an appendix; and a Cumulative Index.

2. The articles in Official Monographs, Infrared Reference Spectra and Ultraviolet-visible Reference Spectra are respectively placed in alphabetical order in principle.

3. The following items in each monograph are put in the order shown below, except that unnecessary items are omitted depending on the nature of the drug:

(1) English title
(2) Commonly used name(s)
(3) Latin title (only for crude drugs)
(4) Title in Japanese
(5) Structural formula or empirical formula
(6) Molecular formula and molecular mass
(7) Chemical name
(8) Chemical Abstracts Service (CAS) Registry Number
(9) Origin
(10) Limits of the content of the ingredient(s) and/or the unit of potency
(11) Labeling requirements
(12) Method of preparation
(13) Manufacture
(14) Description
(15) Identification tests
(16) Specific physical and/or chemical values
(17) Purity tests
(18) Potential adulteration
(19) Loss on drying or Ignition, or Water
(20) Residue on ignition, Total ash or Acid-insoluble ash
(21) Tests being required for pharmaceutical preparations
(22) Other special tests
(23) Assay
(24) Containers and storage
(25) Shelf life
(26) Others

4. In each monograph, the following physical and chemical values representing the properties and quality of the drug are given in the order indicated below, except that unnecessary items are omitted depending on the nature of drug:

(1) Alcohol number
(2) Absorbance
(3) Congealing point
(4) Refractive index
(5) Osmolar ratio
(6) Optical rotation
(7) Constituent amino acids
(8) Viscosity
(9) pH
(10) Content ratio of the active ingredients
(11) Specific gravity
(12) Boiling point
(13) Melting point
(14) Acid value
(15) Saponification value
(16) Ester value
(17) Hydroxyl value
(18) Iodine value

5. Identification tests comprise the following items, which are generally put in the order given below:

(1) Coloration reactions
(2) Precipitation reactions
(3) Decomposition reactions
(4) Derivatives
(5) Infrared and/or ultraviolet-visible absorption spectrometry
(6) Nuclear magnetic resonance spectrometry
(7) Chromatography
(8) Special reactions
(9) Cations
(10) Anions

6. Purity tests comprise the following items, which are generally put in the order given below, except that unnecessary items are omitted depending on the nature of drug:

(1) Color

(2) Odor
(3) Clarity and/or color of solution
(4) Acidity or alkalinity
(5) Acidity
(6) Alkalinity
(7) Chloride
(8) Sulfate
(9) Sulfite
(10) Nitrate
(11) Nitrite
(12) Carbonate
(13) Bromide
(14) Iodide
(15) Soluble halide
(16) Thiocyanate
(17) Selenium
(18) Cationic salts
(19) Ammonium
(20) Heavy metals
(21) Iron
(22) Manganese
(23) Chromium
(24) Bismuth
(25) Tin
(26) Aluminum
(27) Zinc
(28) Cadmium
(29) Mercury
(30) Copper
(31) Lead
(32) Silver
(33) Alkaline earth metals
(34) Arsenic
(35) Free phosphoric acid
(36) Foreign matters
(37) Related substances
(38) Isomer
(39) Enantiomer
(40) Diastereomer
(41) Polymer
(42) Residual solvent
(43) Other impurities
(44) Residue on evaporation
(45) Readily carbonizable substances

7. The following paragraph was newly added to General Notices:

(1) Paragraph 34: The provision for elemental impurities based on ICH Q3D ''Guideline for Elemental Impurities'' was added.

8. The following paragraph of General Notices was revised:

(1) Paragraph 8: Atomic masses adopted in the Japanese Pharmacopoeia were determined to conform to the table of ''Atomic Weights of the Elements 2015'' (IUPAC), however, the atomic masses of the elements whose atomic weight is indicated with an interval in the 2015 table were determined to conform to the table of ''Atomic Weights of the Elements 2007'' (IUPAC).

9. The following item was newly added to General Tests, Processes and Apparatus:

(1) 2.05 Size-Exclusion Chromatography

10. The following items in General Tests, Processes and Apparatus were revised:

(1) Preamble
(2) 2.46 Residual Solvents
(3) 2.48 Water Determination
(4) 2.51 Conductivity Measurement
(5) 2.52 Thermal Analysis
(6) 2.66 Elemental Impurities
(7) 4.06 Sterility Test
(8) 5.01 Crude Drugs Test
(9) 9.01 Reference Standards
(10) 9.41 Reagents, Test Solutions
(11) 9.62 Measuring Instruments, Appliances

11. The following Reference Standards were added:

Bicalutamide RS
Cabergoline RS
Celecoxib RS
Eribulin Mesilate RS
Eribulin Mesilate Related Substance C for System Suitability RS
Ethyl Loflazepate RS
Fenofibrate RS
Gefitinib RS
Glucagon RS
Rilmazafone Hydrochloride RS
Rosuvastatin Calcium RS
Saccharin RS
Timolol Maleate RS
Triazolam RS

12. The following Reference Standard was revised in Japanese title:

Saccharin Sodium RS

13. The following Reference Standards were deleted from the list of ''9.01 (2) The reference standards which are prepared by National Institute of Infectious Diseases'' and added to the list of ''9.01 (1) The reference standards which are prepared by those who have been registered to prepare them by the Minister of Health, Labour and Welfare, according to the Ministerial ordinance established by the Minister separately'':

Cefepime Dihydrochloride RS
Cefotiam Hydrochloride RS
Ceftriaxone Sodium RS
Clarithromycin RS
Epirubicin Hydrochloride RS

Minocycline Hydrochloride RS
Piperacillin RS
Roxithromycin RS
Sulbactam RS
Tazobactam RS
Vancomycin Hydrochloride RS

14. The following substances were newly added to the Official Monographs:

Bicalutamide
Cabergoline
Celecoxib
Cloperastine Fendizoate
Cloperastine Fendizoate Tablets
Copovidone
Dorzolamide Hydrochloride and Timolol Maleate Ophthalmic Solution
Eribulin Mesilate
Ethyl Loflazepate
Ethyl Loflazepate Tablets
Fenofibrate
Fenofibrate Tablets
Fludiazepam Tablets
Gefitinib
Glucagon (Genetical Recombination)
Heparin Sodium Lock Solution
Heparin Sodium Solution for Dialysis
Irinotecan Hydrochloride Injection
Methotrexate for Injection
Miglitol Tablets
Phenobarbital Tablets
Pitavastatin Calcium Orally Disintegrating Tablets
Rilmazafone Hydrochloride Hydrate
Rilmazafone Hydrochloride Tablets
Rosuvastatin Calcium
Rosuvastatin Calcium Tablets
Silodosin Orally Disintegrating Tablets
Telmisartan and Amlodipine Besilate Tablets
Triazolam
Zopiclone
Zopiclone Tablets
Byakkokaninjinto Extract
Unseiin Extract

15. The following monographs were revised:

Aprindine Hydrochloride
Azathioprine Tablets
Bepotastine Besilate
Bleomycin Hydrochloride
Bleomycin Sulfate
Calcitonin Salmon
Calcium Folinate Hydrate
Calcium Paraaminosalicylate Hydrate
Carmellose Calcium
Carmellose Sodium
Croscarmellose Sodium
Cefoperazone Sodium
Celmoleukin (Genetical Recombination)
Clinofibrate
Clopidogrel Sulfate
Colistin Sodium Methanesulfonate
Dihydroergotoxine Mesilate
Dimorpholamine
Diphenhydramine
Diphenhydramine Hydrochloride
Distigmine Bromide
Dorzolamide Hydrochloride
Enviomycin Sulfate
Epoetin Alfa (Genetical Recombination)
Epoetin Beta (Genetical Recombination)
Ergometrine Maleate
Ethambutol Hydrochloride
Ethyl Aminobenzoate
Filgrastim (Genetical Recombination)
Fradiomycin Sulfate
Gelatin
Purified Gelatin
Gentamicin Sulfate
Glucose Injection
Human Menopausal Gonadotrophin
Heparin Calcium
Heparin Sodium
Low Substituted Hydroxypropylcellulose
Hypromellose
Insulin Human (Genetical Recombination)
Insulin Aspart (Genetical Recombination)
Insulin Glargine (Genetical Recombination)
Kallidinogenase
Kitasamycin Acetate
Kitasamycin Tartrate
Anhydrous Lactose
Lactose Hydrate
Lauromacrogol
Lenograstim (Genetical Recombination)
Levofloxacin Hydrate
Levofloxacin Fine Granules
Levofloxacin Injection
Levofloxacin Tablets
Lysozyme Hydrochloride
Methylcellulose
Methylergometrine Maleate
Mexiletine Hydrochloride
Montelukast Sodium
Nafamostat Mesilate
Nartograstim (Genetical Recombination)
Norgestrel and Ethinylestradiol Tablets
Olmesartan Medoxomil
Oxybuprocaine Hydrochloride
Oxygen
Oxytocin
Paroxetine Hydrochloride Hydrate
Pitavastatin Calcium Hydrate
Pitavastatin Calcium Tablets

Polymixin B Sulfate
Povidone
Povidone-Iodine
Protamine Sulfate
Pullulan
Saccharin
Saccharin Sodium Hydrate
Scopolamine Butylbromide
Scopolamine Hydrobromide Hydrate
Purified Shellac
White Shellac
Silodosin
Silodosin Tablets
Sodium Lauryl Sulfate
Wheat Starch
Sucrose
Teceleukin (Genetical Recombination)
Tetracaine Hydrochloride
Valaciclovir Hydrochloride
Valsartan
Vasopressin Injection
Voriconazole
Voriconazole for Injection
Alpinia Officinarum Rhizome
Asiasarum Root
Asparagus Root
Atractylodes Lancea Rhizome
Bearberry Leaf
Belladonna Root
Bupleurum Root
Cardamon
Cinnamon Bark
Cinnamon Oil
Clove
Powdered Clove
Cnidium Rhizome
Powdered Cnidium Rhizome
Coptis Rhizome
Powdered Coptis Rhizome
Cornus Fruit
Curcuma Rhizome
Dioscorea Rhizome
Ephedra Herb
Euodia Fruit
Gardenia Fruit
Powdered Gardenia Fruit
Glycyrrhiza
Goreisan Extract
Goshuyuto Extract
Hangekobokuto Extract
Houttuynia Herb
Imperata Rhizome
Ipecac Syrup
Powdered Japanese Gentian
Japanese Zanthoxylum Peel
Powdered Japanese Zanthoxylum Peel
Jujube Seed
Kamikihito Extract
Kamishoyosan Extract
Keishibukuryogan Extract
Lilium Bulb
Lycium Fruit
Magnolia Bark
Powdered Magnolia Bark
Mentha Oil
Moutan Bark
Powdered Moutan Bark
Nelumbo Seed
Notopterygium
Nuphar Rhizome
Nutmeg
Nux Vomica
Nux Vomica Extract Powder
Orengedokuto Extract
Perilla Herb
Peucedanum Root
Phellodendron Bark
Powdered Phellodendron Bark
Plantago Herb
Plantago Seed
Pogostemon Herb
Polyporus Sclerotium
Powdered Polyporus Sclerotium
Poria Sclerotium
Powdered Poria Sclerotium
Pueraria Root
Quercus Bark
Ryokeijutsukanto Extract
Saffron
Salvia Miltiorrhiza Root
Sappan Wood
Scopolia Rhizome
Scopolia Extract Powder
Scopolia Extract and Ethyl Aminobenzoate Powder
Sophora Root
Powdered Sophora Root
Toad Cake
Tokakujokito Extract
Trichosanthes Root
Uncaria Hook

16. A part or all of the commonly used names were deleted from the following monographs (chemical drugs, etc):

Acebutolol Hydrochloride
Acetazolamide
Acetylcholine Chloride for Injection
Acetylcysteine
Aclarubicin Hydrochloride
Acrinol Hydrate
Adrenaline Injection
Adrenaline Solution
Afloqualone

Aldioxa
Aldioxa Granules
Aldioxa Tablets
Alimemazine Tartrate
Alprenolol Hydrochloride
Alprostadil
Alprostadil Alfadex
Aluminum Potassium Sulfate Hydrate
Amantadine Hydrochloride
Ambenonium Chloride
Amikacin Sulfate
Amikacin Sulfate for Injection
Amikacin Sulfate Injection
Aminophylline Hydrate
Amiodarone Hydrochloride
Amiodarone Hydrochloride Tablets
Amitriptyline Hydrochloride
Amitriptyline Hydrochloride Tablets
Amlodipine Besilate
Amlodipine Besilate Tablets
Amosulalol Hydrochloride
Amosulalol Hydrochloride Tablets
Amoxicillin Hydrate
Anhydrous Ampicillin
Ampicillin Hydrate
Ampicillin Sodium
Aprindine Hydrochloride
Aprindine Hydrochloride Capsules
Arbekacin Sulfate
Arbekacin Sulfate Injection
Argatroban Hydrate
L-Arginine Hydrochloride
L-Arginine Hydrochloride Injection
Arotinolol Hydrochloride
Arsenic Trioxide
Aspoxicillin Hydrate
Atropine Sulfate Hydrate
Atropine Sulfate Injection
Azelastine Hydrochloride
Azelastine Hydrochloride Granules
Bacampicillin Hydrochloride
Beclometasone Dipropionate
Bekanamycin Sulfate
Benidipine Hydrochloride
Benidipine Hydrochloride Tablets
Benserazide Hydrochloride
Benzalkonium Chloride
Benzalkonium Chloride Concentrated Solution 50
Benzalkonium Chloride Solution
Benzethonium Chloride
Benzethonium Chloride Solution
Benzylpenicillin Benzathine Hydrate
Benzylpenicillin Potassium
Berberine Chloride Hydrate
Betahistine Mesilate
Betahistine Mesilate Tablets
Betamethasone Dipropionate
Betamethasone Sodium Phosphate
Betamethasone Valerate
Betamethasone Valerate and Gentamicin Sulfate Cream
Betamethasone Valerate and Gentamicin Sulfate Ointment
Betaxolol Hydrochloride
Bethanechol Chloride
Bifonazole
Biperiden Hydrochloride
Bismuth Subgallate
Bisoprolol Fumarate
Bisoprolol Fumarate Tablets
Bleomycin Hydrochloride
Bleomycin Sulfate
Freeze-dried Botulism Antitoxin, Equine
Bromhexine Hydrochloride
Bromocriptine Mesilate
Bufetolol Hydrochloride
Buformin Hydrochloride
Buformin Hydrochloride Delayed-release Tablets
Buformin Hydrochloride Tablets
Bunazosin Hydrochloride
Bupivacaine Hydrochloride Hydrate
Buprenorphine Hydrochloride
Butenafine Hydrochloride
Butenafine Hydrochloride Cream
Butenafine Hydrochloride Solution
Butenafine Hydrochloride Spray
Butropium Bromide
Caffeine and Sodium Benzoate
Caffeine Hydrate
Calcitonin Salmon
Precipitated Calcium Carbonate Fine Granules
Precipitated Calcium Carbonate Tablets
Calcium Chloride Hydrate
Calcium Folinate Hydrate
Calcium Gluconate Hydrate
Calcium Hydroxide
Calcium Lactate Hydrate
Calcium Levofolinate Hydrate
Calcium Oxide
Calcium Paraaminosalicylate Hydrate
Dibasic Calcium Phosphate Hydrate
Monobasic Calcium Phosphate Hydrate
Calcium Sodium Edetate Hydrate
Camostat Mesilate
Carbazochrome Sodium Sulfonate Hydrate
Carbidopa Hydrate
Carbon Dioxide
Carteolol Hydrochloride
Cefadroxil for Syrup
Cefalexin for Syrup
Cefatrizine Propylene Glycolate for Syrup
Cefcapene Pivoxil Hydrochloride Hydrate

Cefcapene Pivoxil Hydrochloride Fine Granules
Cefcapene Pivoxil Hydrochloride Tablets
Cefditoren Pivoxil
Cefditoren Pivoxil Fine Granules
Cefditoren Pivoxil Tablets
Cefepime Dihydrochloride Hydrate
Cefepime Dihydrochloride for Injection
Cefixime Hydrate
Cefmenoxime Hydrochloride
Cefminox Sodium Hydrate
Cefotiam Hydrochloride
Cefotiam Hydrochloride for Injection
Cefozopran Hydrochloride
Cefozopran Hydrochloride for Injection
Cefpirome Sulfate
Cefpodoxime Proxetil
Cefpodoxime Proxetil for Syrup
Cefroxadine Hydrate
Cefroxadine for Syrup
Ceftazidime Hydrate
Cefteram Pivoxil
Cefteram Pivoxil Fine Granules
Cefteram Pivoxil Tablets
Ceftibuten Hydrate
Ceftriaxone Sodium Hydrate
Cefuroxime Axetil
Cetirizine Hydrochloride
Cetirizine Hydrochloride Tablets
Cetotiamine Hydrochloride Hydrate
Cetraxate Hydrochloride
Chloramphenicol Sodium Succinate
Chlorhexidine Gluconate Solution
Chlorhexidine Hydrochloride
Chlormadinone Acetate
Chlorphenesin Carbamate
Chlorphenesin Carbamate Tablets
Chlorpheniramine Maleate
Chlorpheniramine Maleate Injection
Chlorpheniramine Maleate Powder
Chlorpheniramine Maleate Tablets
d-Chlorpheniramine Maleate
Chlorpromazine Hydrochloride
Chlorpromazine Hydrochloride Injection
Chlorpromazine Hydrochloride Tablets
Cibenzoline Succinate
Cibenzoline Succinate Tablets
Ciclosporin
Cilazapril Hydrate
Ciprofloxacin Hydrochloride Hydrate
Citric Acid Hydrate
Clebopride Malate
Clemastine Fumarate
Clindamycin Hydrochloride
Clindamycin Hydrochloride Capsules
Clindamycin Phosphate
Clindamycin Phosphate Injection
Clobetasol Propionate
Clocapramine Hydrochloride Hydrate
Clofedanol Hydrochloride
Clomifene Citrate
Clomifene Citrate Tablets
Clomipramine Hydrochloride
Clonidine Hydrochloride
Cloperastine Hydrochloride
Cloxacillin Sodium Hydrate
Cocaine Hydrochloride
Codeine Phosphate Hydrate
1% Codeine Phosphate Powder
10% Codeine Phosphate Powder
Codeine Phosphate Tablets
Colestimide
Colistin Sulfate
Cortisone Acetate
Croconazole Hydrochloride
Cyclopentolate Hydrochloride
Cyclophosphamide Hydrate
Cyproheptadine Hydrochloride Hydrate
Dantrolene Sodium Hydrate
Daunorubicin Hydrochloride
Deferoxamine Mesilate
Dehydrocholic Acid Injection
Demethylchlortetracycline Hydrochloride
Dextran Sulfate Sodium Sulfur 5
Dextran Sulfate Sodium Sulfur 18
Dextromethorphan Hydrobromide Hydrate
Dibekacin Sulfate
Dibekacin Sulfate Ophthalmic Solution
Dibucaine Hydrochloride
Dicloxacillin Sodium Hydrate
Diethylcarbamazine Citrate
Diethylcarbamazine Citrate Tablets
Difenidol Hydrochloride
Diflorasone Diacetate
Diflucortolone Valerate
Dihydrocodeine Phosphate
1% Dihydrocodeine Phosphate Powder
10% Dihydrocodeine Phosphate Powder
Dihydroergotamine Mesilate
Dihydroergotoxine Mesilate
Dilazep Hydrochloride Hydrate
Diltiazem Hydrochloride
Dimemorfan Phosphate
Dinoprost
Diphenhydramine Hydrochloride
Diphenhydramine and Bromovalerylurea Powder
Freeze-dried Diphtheria Antitoxin, Equine
Distigmine Bromide
Distigmine Bromide Tablets
Dobutamine Hydrochloride
Donepezil Hydrochloride
Donepezil Hydrochloride Fine Granules
Donepezil Hydrochloride Tablets

Dopamine Hydrochloride
Dopamine Hydrochloride Injection
Doxapram Hydrochloride Hydrate
Doxazosin Mesilate
Doxazosin Mesilate Tablets
Doxorubicin Hydrochloride
Doxorubicin Hydrochloride for Injection
Doxycycline Hydrochloride Hydrate
Doxycycline Hydrochloride Tablets
Ecabet Sodium Hydrate
Emedastine Fumarate
Enalapril Maleate
Enalapril Maleate Tablets
Enviomycin Sulfate
Eperisone Hydrochloride
Ephedrine Hydrochloride
Ephedrine Hydrochloride Injection
10% Ephedrine Hydrochloride Powder
Ephedrine Hydrochloride Tablets
Epirizole
Epirubicin Hydrochloride
Ergocalciferol
Ergometrine Maleate
Ergometrine Maleate Injection
Ergometrine Maleate Tablets
Ergotamine Tartrate
Erythromycin Ethylsuccinate
Erythromycin Lactobionate
Erythromycin Stearate
Estradiol Benzoate
Estradiol Benzoate Injection (Aqueous Suspension)
Ethambutol Hydrochloride
Ethenzamide
Ethyl L-Cysteine Hydrochloride
Ethylmorphine Hydrochloride Hydrate
Etilefrine Hydrochloride
Etilefrine Hydrochloride Tablets
Faropenem Sodium Hydrate
Fentanyl Citrate
Ferrous Sulfate Hydrate
Fexofenadine Hydrochloride
Flavoxate Hydrochloride
Flecainide Acetate
Flecainide Acetate Tablets
Fludrocortisone Acetate
Flurazepam Hydrochloride
Fluvoxamine Maleate
Fluvoxamine Maleate Tablets
Formoterol Fumarate Hydrate
Fosfomycin Calcium Hydrate
Fradiomycin Sulfate
Fursultiamine Hydrochloride
Gabexate Mesilate
β-Galactosidase (Aspergillus)
β-Galactosidase (Penicillium)
Gentamicin Sulfate
Gentamicin Sulfate Ophthalmic Solution
Glutathione
Glyceryl Monostearate
Glycine
Gonadorelin Acetate
Guaifenesin
Guanabenz Acetate
Freeze-dried Habu Antivenom, Equine
L-Histidine Hydrochloride Hydrate
Homatropine Hydrobromide
Homochlorcyclizine Hydrochloride
Hydralazine Hydrochloride
Hydralazine Hydrochloride for Injection
Hydralazine Hydrochloride Powder
Hydralazine Hydrochloride Tablets
Hydrocortisone Acetate
Hydrocortisone Butyrate
Hydrocortisone Sodium Phosphate
Hydrocortisone Sodium Succinate
Hydrocortisone Succinate
Hydrocotarnine Hydrochloride Hydrate
Hydroxocobalamin Acetate
Hydroxyzine Hydrochloride
Hydroxyzine Pamoate
Hypromellose
Hypromellose Acetate Succinate
Hypromellose Phthalate
Idarubicin Hydrochloride
Idarubicin Hydrochloride for Injection
Ifenprodil Tartrate
Ifenprodil Tartrate Fine Granules
Ifenprodil Tartrate Tablets
Imidapril Hydrochloride
Imidapril Hydrochloride Tablets
Imipenem Hydrate
Imipramine Hydrochloride
Imipramine Hydrochloride Tablets
Insulin Human (Genetical Recombination)
Insulin Human (Genetical Recombination) Injection
Ipratropium Bromide Hydrate
Irsogladine Maleate
Irsogladine Maleate Fine Granules
Irsogladine Maleate Tablets
Isepamicin Sulfate
Isepamicin Sulfate Injection
l-Isoprenaline Hydrochloride
Isosorbide Dinitrate
Isosorbide Dinitrate Tablets
Isosorbide Mononitrate 70%/Lactose 30%
Isoxsuprine Hydrochloride
Isoxsuprine Hydrochloride Tablets
Josamycin Propionate
Kainic Acid Hydrate
Kanamycin Monosulfate
Kanamycin Sulfate
Ketamine Hydrochloride

Ketoconazole Solution
Ketotifen Fumarate
Kitasamycin
Kitasamycin Acetate
Kitasamycin Tartrate
Labetalol Hydrochloride
Labetalol Hydrochloride Tablets
Lactose Hydrate
Lauromacrogol
Lenampicillin Hydrochloride
Levallorphan Tartrate
Levallorphan Tartrate Injection
Levofloxacin Hydrate
Levomepromazine Maleate
Levothyroxine Sodium Hydrate
Lidocaine Injection
Limaprost Alfadex
Lincomycin Hydrochloride Hydrate
Lincomycin Hydrochloride Injection
Lisinopril Hydrate
Lobenzarit Sodium
Loxoprofen Sodium Hydrate
L-Lysine Acetate
L-Lysine Hydrochloride
Lysozyme Hydrochloride
Magnesium Sulfate Hydrate
Maltose Hydrate
Freeze-dried Mamushi Antivenom, Equine
Manidipine Hydrochloride
Manidipine Hydrochloride Tablets
D-Mannitol
D-Mannitol Injection
Maprotiline Hydrochloride
Meclofenoxate Hydrochloride
Mefloquine Hydrochloride
Mepenzolate Bromide
Mepivacaine Hydrochloride
Mepivacaine Hydrochloride Injection
Mercaptopurine Hydrate
Meropenem Hydrate
Metenolone Acetate
Metenolone Enanthate
Metenolone Enanthate Injection
Metformin Hydrochloride
Metformin Hydrochloride Tablets
Methylbenactyzium Bromide
Methyldopa Hydrate
dl-Methylephedrine Hydrochloride
10% *dl*-Methylephedrine Hydrochloride Powder
Methylergometrine Maleate
Methylergometrine Maleate Tablets
Metoprolol Tartrate
Metoprolol Tartrate Tablets
Mexiletine Hydrochloride
Miconazole Nitrate
Micronomicin Sulfate
Midecamycin Acetate
Minocycline Hydrochloride
Minocycline Hydrochloride for Injection
Minocycline Hydrochloride Tablets
Morphine Hydrochloride Hydrate
Morphine Hydrochloride Injection
Morphine Hydrochloride Tablets
Morphine and Atropine Injection
Morphine Sulfate Hydrate
Mosapride Citrate Hydrate
Mosapride Citrate Powder
Mosapride Citrate Tablets
Mupirocin Calcium Hydrate
Nafamostat Mesilate
Naloxone Hydrochloride
Naphazoline Hydrochloride
Naphazoline Nitrate
Neostigmine Methylsulfate
Neostigmine Methylsulfate Injection
Nicardipine Hydrochloride
Nicardipine Hydrochloride Injection
Noradrenaline Injection
Noscapine
Noscapine Hydrochloride Hydrate
Olopatadine Hydrochloride
Olopatadine Hydrochloride Tablets
Opium Alkaloids Hydrochlorides
Opium Alkaloids Hydrochlorides Injection
Opium Alkaloids and Atropine Injection
Opium Alkaloids and Scopolamine Injection
Weak Opium Alkaloids and Scopolamine Injection
Orciprenaline Sulfate
Oxapium Iodide
Oxprenolol Hydrochloride
Oxybuprocaine Hydrochloride
Oxycodone Hydrochloride Hydrate
Compound Oxycodone Injection
Compound Oxycodone and Atropine Injection
Oxytetracycline Hydrochloride
Pancuronium Bromide
Papaverine Hydrochloride
Papaverine Hydrochloride Injection
Paroxetine Hydrochloride Hydrate
Pentoxyverine Citrate
Peplomycin Sulfate
Peplomycin Sulfate for Injection
Perphenazine Maleate
Perphenazine Maleate Tablets
Pethidine Hydrochloride
Pethidine Hydrochloride Injection
10% Phenobarbital Powder
Phenol
Phenol and Zinc Oxide Liniment
Phenylephrine Hydrochloride
Phenytoin
Phenytoin Powder

Phenytoin Tablets
Phenytoin Sodium for Injection
Phytonadione
Pilocarpine Hydrochloride
Pilocarpine Hydrochloride Tablets
Pioglitazone Hydrochloride
Pioglitazone Hydrochloride Tablets
Pipemidic Acid Hydrate
Piperazine Phosphate Hydrate
Piperazine Phosphate Tablets
Pirenzepine Hydrochloride Hydrate
Pitavastatin Calcium Hydrate
Pivmecillinam Hydrochloride
Pivmecillinam Hydrochloride Tablets
Polymixin B Sulfate
Polyoxyl 40 Stearate
Povidone
Prasterone Sodium Sulfate Hydrate
Prazosin Hydrochloride
Prednisolone Acetate
Prednisolone Sodium Phosphate
Prednisolone Succinate
Prednisolone Sodium Succinate for Injection
Procainamide Hydrochloride
Procainamide Hydrochloride Injection
Procainamide Hydrochloride Tablets
Procaine Hydrochloride
Procaine Hydrochloride Injection
Procarbazine Hydrochloride
Procaterol Hydrochloride Hydrate
Prochlorperazine Maleate
Prochlorperazine Maleate Tablets
Promethazine Hydrochloride
Propafenone Hydrochloride
Propafenone Hydrochloride Tablets
Propantheline Bromide
Propiverine Hydrochloride
Propiverine Hydrochloride Tablets
Propranolol Hydrochloride
Propranolol Hydrochloride Tablets
Protamine Sulfate
Protamine Sulfate Injection
Protirelin Tartrate Hydrate
Pyridostigmine Bromide
Pyridoxal Phosphate Hydrate
Pyridoxine Hydrochloride
Pyridoxine Hydrochloride Injection
Quinapril Hydrochloride
Quinapril Hydrochloride Tablets
Quinidine Sulfate Hydrate
Quinine Hydrochloride Hydrate
Quinine Sulfate Hydrate
Ranitidine Hydrochloride
0.1% Reserpine Powder
Retinol Acetate
Retinol Palmitate
Riboflavin Butyrate
Riboflavin Sodium Phosphate
Riboflavin Sodium Phosphate Injection
Ribostamycin Sulfate
Ritodrine Hydrochloride
Ritodrine Hydrochloride Tablets
Roxatidine Acetate Hydrochloride
Roxatidine Acetate Hydrochloride Extended-release Capsules
Roxatidine Acetate Hydrochloride Extended-release Tablets
Roxatidine Acetate Hydrochloride for Injection
Saccharin Sodium Hydrate
Salbutamol Sulfate
Sarpogrelate Hydrochloride
Sarpogrelate Hydrochloride Fine Granules
Sarpogrelate Hydrochloride Tablets
Scopolamine Butylbromide
Scopolamine Hydrobromide Hydrate
Freeze-dried Smallpox Vaccine
Sodium Acetate Hydrate
Sodium Bisulfite
Sodium Carbonate Hydrate
Isotonic Sodium Chloride Solution
Sodium Citrate Hydrate
Disodium Edetate Hydrate
Dibasic Sodium Phosphate Hydrate
Sodium Picosulfate Hydrate
Sodium Starch Glycolate
Dried Sodium Sulfite
Sodium Thiosulfate Hydrate
Sorbitan Sesquioleate
D-Sorbitol
D-Sorbitol Solution
Spectinomycin Hydrochloride Hydrate
Spiramycin Acetate
Corn Starch
Potato Starch
Rice Starch
Wheat Starch
Streptomycin Sulfate
Streptomycin Sulfate for Injection
Sucralfate Hydrate
Sulfamethoxazole
Sulfamonomethoxine Hydrate
Sulpyrine Hydrate
Sultamicillin Tosilate Hydrate
Sultamicillin Tosilate Tablets
Suxamethonium Chloride Hydrate
Suxamethonium Chloride Injection
Suxamethonium Chloride for Injection
Tacalcitol Hydrate
Talampicillin Hydrochloride
Taltirelin Hydrate
Tamoxifen Citrate
Tamsulosin Hydrochloride

Tamsulosin Hydrochloride Extended-release Tablets
Temocapril Hydrochloride
Temocapril Hydrochloride Tablets
Terbinafine Hydrochloride
Terbinafine Hydrochloride Cream
Terbinafine Hydrochloride Solution
Terbinafine Hydrochloride Spray
Terbinafine Hydrochloride Tablets
Terbutaline Sulfate
Testosterone Enanthate
Testosterone Enanthate Injection
Testosterone Propionate
Testosterone Propionate Injection
Tetracaine Hydrochloride
Tetracycline Hydrochloride
Thiamine Chloride Hydrochloride
Thiamine Chloride Hydrochloride Injection
Thiamine Chloride Hydrochloride Powder
Thiamine Nitrate
L-Threonine
Tiapride Hydrochloride
Tiapride Hydrochloride Tablets
Tiaramide Hydrochloride
Tiaramide Hydrochloride Tablets
Ticlopidine Hydrochloride
Timepidium Bromide Hydrate
Timolol Maleate
Tipepidine Hibenzate
Tipepidine Hibenzate Tablets
Tizanidine Hydrochloride
Tocopherol
Tocopherol Acetate
Tocopherol Calcium Succinate
Tocopherol Nicotinate
Todralazine Hydrochloride Hydrate
Tolnaftate
Tolnaftate Solution
Tolperisone Hydrochloride
Tosufloxacin Tosilate Hydrate
Tosufloxacin Tosilate Tablets
Trehalose Hydrate
Trichomycin
Triclofos Sodium
Triclofos Sodium Syrup
Trihexyphenidyl Hydrochloride
Trihexyphenidyl Hydrochloride Tablets
Trimebutine Maleate
Trimetazidine Hydrochloride
Trimetazidine Hydrochloride Tablets
Trimetoquinol Hydrochloride Hydrate
Tulobuterol Hydrochloride
L-Tyrosine
Ursodeoxycholic Acid
Ursodeoxycholic Acid Granules
Ursodeoxycholic Acid Tablets
Valaciclovir Hydrochloride Tablets
Vancomycin Hydrochloride
Vancomycin Hydrochloride for Injection
Verapamil Hydrochloride
Verapamil Hydrochloride Tablets
Vinblastine Sulfate
Vinblastine Sulfate for Injection
Vincristine Sulfate
Zinc Sulfate Hydrate
Zolpidem Tartrate
Zolpidem Tartrate Tablets

17. The following monographs were deleted:
Cholera Vaccine
Diphtheria-Tetanus Combined Toxoid
Gas Gangrene Antitoxin, Equine
Japanese Encephalitis Vaccine
Freeze-dried Japanese Encephalitis Vaccine
Methylrosanilinium Chloride
Live Oral Poliomyelitis Vaccine
Weil's Disease and Akiyami Combined Vaccine

18. The following articles were newly added to Ultraviolet-visible Reference Spectra:
Bicalutamide
Cabergoline
Celecoxib
Cloperastine Fendizoate
Ethyl Loflazepate
Fenofibrate
Gefitinib
Rilmazafone Hydrochloride Hydrate
Rosuvastatin Calcium
Triazolam
Zopiclone

19. The following articles were newly added to Infrared Reference Spectra:
Bicalutamide
Cabergoline
Celecoxib
Cloperastine Fendizoate
Copovidone
Ethyl Loflazepate
Fenofibrate
Gefitinib
Rilmazafone Hydrochloride Hydrate
Rosuvastatin Calcium
Sodium Lauryl Sulfate
Triazolam
Zopiclone

Those who were engaged in the preparation of JP 18 are as follows:
ABE Misato
ABE Yasuhiro
AITA Youhei
AKAO Kenichi
ARATO Teruyo

ARIMOTO Keiko
ARUGA Naoki
ASAI Yumi
ASAMA Hiroshi
ASHIZAWA Kazuhide
ASO Shinichiro
ASO Yukio
DEMIZU Yosuke
EMURA Makoto
FUCHINO Hiroyuki
FUJII Hirosato
FUJII Makiko
FUJII Norikazu
FUJIMOTO Yuzo
FUKAMI Toshiro
FUKASAWA Masayoshi
FUKAZAWA Hidesuke
FUKUDA Shinji
FUKUHARA Kiyoshi
FURUICHI Harumi
FURUKAWA Hiromitsu
GODA Yukihiro
GOTO Takashi
GOTO Tamami
HAISHIMA Yuji
HAKAMATA Hideki
HAKAMATSUKA Takashi
HANADA Kentaro
HANAJIRI Ruri
HARAZONO Akira
HASEGAWA Atsuhiro
HASHIDA Mitsuru*
HASHII Noritaka
HATANO Rika
HAYAKAWA Masako
HAYASHI Ai
HAYASHI Akira
HAYASHI Yoshinori
HIGANO Taro
HIGUCHI Yasuhiko
HIRAI Kenichi
HIYAMA Yukio
HORI Masatoshi
HYUGA Masashi
ICHINOSE Koji
IGOSHI Nobukazu
IIMORI Jumpei
IKARASHI Yoshiaki
IKEDO Shingo
IKEGAMI Kazuhiko
IMAMOTO Tsuyoshi
INOUE Takayuki
ISHIDA Masato
ISHII Akiko
ITAI Shigeru
ITO Michiho
ITO Ryoichi
ITO Yuji
IZUTANI Yusuke
IZUTSU Kenichi
KAIDA Naoki
KAMMOTO Toshihiro
KANEBAKO Makoto
KATAYAMA Hirohito
KATO Kumiko
KATORI Noriko
KAWAHARA Nobuo
KAWAI Tamotsu
KAWAMATA Tomomi
KAWANISHI Toru
KAWANO Noriaki
KAWARASAKI Yoshihiko
KAWASAKI Nana
KIJIMA Keiji
KIKUCHI Yutaka
KIKUCHI Yuuichi
KIMURA Noritaka
KISHIMOTO Yasuhiro
KITADA Mitsukazu
KITAJIMA Akihito
KITTAKA Atsushi
KIUCHI Fumiyuki
KOBAYASHI Takashi
KOCHI Rika
KOHAMA Ai
KOHITA Hideki
KOIDE Tatsuo
KOJIMA Takashi
KOKUBO Hiroyasu
KOMATSU Katsuko
KONDA Toshifumi
KONDO Seizo
KUBOSAKI Atsutaka
KUBOTA Kiyoshi
KUMASAKA Kenichi
KURIHARA Masaaki
KUROIWA Yuki
KUSUNOKI Hideki
MAEKAWA Keiko
MAKIURA Toshinobu
MARUYAMA Takuro
MASADA Sayaka
MATSUMOTO Kazuhiro
MATSUMOTO Makoto
MATSUMURA Hajime
MATSUURA Tadashi
MIKAMI Eiichi
MISAWA Takashi
MITSUHASHI Takao
MIYATA Naoki
MIYAZAKI Takashi
MIYAZAKI Tamaki

MIZUNO Takeshi
MORI Mitsuo
MORIBE Kunikazu
MORIMOTO Seiki
MORIMOTO Takashi
MORISAKI Takahito
MORITA Osamu
MORIYASU Takako
MURABAYASHI Mika
MURAI Toshimi
MUROI Masashi
NAKA Nobuyuki
NAKAGAWA Hidehiko
NAKAGAWA Shinsaku
NAKAGAWA Tsutomu
NAKAGAWA Yukari
NAKAI Toru
NAKAJIMA Emi
NAKAKO Mayumi
NAKANO Tatsuya
NAKASHIMA Tatsumi
NANAURA Mitsuo
NASU Masao
NISHIHARA Yutaka
NISHIKAWA Noriaki
NISHIMURA Masahiro
NOGUCHI Shuji
OBA Sumiaki
OBARA Sakae
OCHIAI Masaki
OGAWA Toru
OGURA Yasumitsu
OGURI Kazuki
OHGAMI Yasutaka
OHTA Shigeru
OKUBO Tsuneo
OKUDA Akihiro
OKUDA Haruhiro
OMURA Koichi
ONO Makoto
ONODA Hiroshi
OSUMI Yuko
OTSUKA Masami
OUCHI Tadashi
SAITO Hideyuki
SAITO Yoshiro
SAKAI Eiji
SAKAMOTO Tomoaki**
SANTA Tomofumi
SASAKI Hiroshi
SASAKI Kunio
SASAKI Satoshi
SASAKI Yuko
SASAOKI Kazumichi
SATO Hiroyasu
SATO Koji
SATO Kyoko
SATO Norihisa
SEGAWA Masashi
SEKIGAWA Fujio
SEKIGUCHI Michiko
SHIBATA Hiroko
SHIBAYAMA Keigo
SHIBAZAKI Keiko
SHIDA Shizuka
SHIMADA Yasuo
SHIMAZAWA Rumiko
SHIMIZU Masaro
SHIMOKAWA Sayuri
SHINOHARA Katsuaki
SHIRATORI Makoto
SHIROTA Osamu
SHODA Takuji
SUDO Hirotaka
SUDO Keiichi
SUGAI Motoyuki
SUGIMOTO Chishio
SUGIMOTO Naoki
SUZUKI Mikio
SUZUKI Noriyuki
SUZUKI Ryoji
SUZUKI Shigeo
SUZUKI Tomoyuki
TACHIBANA Katsumi
TADA Minoru
TADAKI Shinichi
TAGUCHI Nobuo
TAKAHASHI Yoshikazu
TAKAI Yoshiaki
TAKANO Akihito
TAKAO Masaki
TAKEBAYASHI Kenji
TAKEDA Osami
TAKEDA Tomoko
TAKEUCHI Hirohumi
TAKEUCHI Hisashi
TANABE Toyoshige
TANAKA Masakazu
TANAKA Satoshi
TANAKA Setsuko
TANAKA Tomohide
TANIMOTO Tsuyoshi
TAOKA Yukako
TERABAYASHI Susumu
TERADA Katsuhide
TERAOKA Reiko
TOKUMOTO Hiroko
TOKUNAGA Hiroshi
TOKUOKA Shogo
TOMIOKA Kiyoshi
TOMITSUKA Hiroyuki
TOYODA Taichi

TSUDA Shigeki
TSUDA Tsubasa
UCHIDA Eriko
UCHIYAMA Nahoko
UETAKE Atsuhiro
USHIRODA Osamu
WADA Yoshio
WATANABE Takumi
YAMADA Rumiko
YAMADA Yuko
YAMAGUCHI Shigeharu
YAMAGUCHI Tetsuji
YAMAJI Hiroki
YAMAMOTO Eiichi
YAMAMOTO Keiji
YAMAMOTO Tosuke
YAMAMOTO Yutaka
YAMASHITA Chikamasa
YAMAUCHI Hitoshi
YAMAZAKI Takeshi
YASUHARA Masato
YASUO Shiho
YOMOTA Chikako
YONEDA Sachiyo
YONEMOCHI Etsuo
YOSHIDA Hiroyuki
YOSHIDA Naoya

*: Chairman, the Committee on JP
**: Acting Chairman, the Committee on JP

The Japanese Pharmacopoeia

EIGHTEENTH EDITION

GENERAL NOTICES

1. The official name of this pharmacopoeia is 第十八改正日本薬局方, and may be abbreviated as 日局十八, 日局18, JP XVIII or JP 18.

2. The English name of this pharmacopoeia is The Japanese Pharmacopoeia, Eighteenth Edition.

3. Among drugs, the Japanese Pharmacopoeia Drugs (the JP Drugs) are those specified in the monographs. The title names and the commonly used names adopted in the monograph should be used as official names. In the drug monograph, in addition to English name, chemical name or Latin name can be mentioned in the title, as appropriate.

4. Crude Drugs and their related products are placed together in ''Crude Drugs and Related Drugs'' in the posterior part of the Official Monographs. These include: Extracts, Powders, Tinctures, Syrups, Spirits, Fluidextracts or Suppositories containing Crude Drugs as the active ingredient, and combination preparations containing Crude Drugs as the principal active ingredient.

5. The JP Drugs are to be tested according to the provisions given in the pertinent monographs, General Notices, General Rules for Crude Drugs, General Rules for Preparations, and General Tests for their conformity to the Japanese Pharmacopoeia. However, the headings of ''Description'' and in addition ''Containers and storage'' and ''Shelf life'' in the monographs on preparations are given for information, and should not be taken as indicating standards for conformity. Nevertheless, Containers under ''Containers and storage'' in the monograph on preparations containing crude drugs as main active ingredients are the standards for conformity.

6. In principle, unless otherwise specified, animals used for preparing the JP Drugs or their source materials must be healthy.

7. In this English version, the JP Drugs described in the monographs begin with a capital letter.

8. The molecular formulas or constitution formulas in parentheses ( ) after the name of drugs or chemicals designate chemically pure substances. Atomic masses adopted in the Japanese Pharmacopoeia conform to the table of ''Atomic Weights of the Elements 2015'' (IUPAC)-Standard Atomic Weights 2017 (Atomic Weights Subcommittee of the Chemical Society of Japan). However, the atomic masses of the elements whose atomic weight is indicated with an interval in the 2015 table conform to the table of ''Atomic Weights of the Elements 2007'' (IUPAC)-Standard Atomic Weights 2010 (Atomic Weights Subcommittee of the Chemical Society of Japan).

Molecular masses are indicated to two decimal places rounded from three decimals.

9. The following abbreviations are used for the principal units.

meter	m
centimeter	cm
millimeter	mm
micrometer	μm
nanometer	nm
kilogram	kg
gram	g
milligram	mg
microgram	μg
nanogram	ng
picogram	pg
Celsius degree	°C
mole	mol
millimole	mmol
square centimeter	cm^2
liter	L
milliliter	mL
microliter	μL
megahertz	MHz
per centimeter	cm^{-1}
newton	N
kilopascal	kPa
pascal	Pa
pascal second	Pa·s
millipascal second	mPa·s
square millimeter per second	mm^2/s
lux	lx
mole per liter	mol/L
millimole per liter	mmol/L
mass per cent	%
mass parts per million	ppm
mass parts per billion	ppb
volume per cent	vol%
volume parts per million	vol ppm
mass per volume per cent	w/v%
microsiemens per centimeter	$\mu S \cdot cm^{-1}$
endotoxin unit	EU
colony forming unit	CFU

Note: ''ppm'' used in the Nuclear Magnetic Resonance Spectroscopy indicates the chemical shift, and ''w/v%'' is used in the formula or composition of preparations.

10. The unit used for expressing the potency of the JP Drugs is recognized as the quantity of drug.

Usually it is expressed by a definite quantity of a definite standard substance which shows a definite biological activity, and differs according to each drug. The units are determined, in principle, by comparison with each reference standard by means of biological methods. The term ''Unit'' used for the JP articles indicates the unit defined in the Japanese Pharmacopoeia.

11. The statement ''Being specified separately.'' in the monographs means that the tests are to be specified when the drugs are granted approval based on the Law on Securing Quality, Efficacy and Safety of Products including Pharmaceuticals and Medical Devices.

12. From the point of view of quality assurance, requirements that should be noted on manufacturing processes, if appropriate in addition to the specifications, are shown in the heading ''Manufacture'' in monograph. It may contain requirements regarding control of materials, manufacturing processes and intermediates, and requirements regarding tests in process and omission of tests for the release. The fulfilment of requirements mentioned in this heading are confirmed based on the information obtained during the establishment of manufacturing method at the development stage, the control of manufacturing processes, or the tests for the release. Also even in the case of absence of the heading ''Manufacture'' in monograph, it is important to note appropriate controls of materials, manufacturing processes and intermediates in individual drugs.

13. When an assurance that a product is of the JP Drug quality is obtained consistently from data derived from the manufacturing process validation studies, and from the records of appropriate manufacturing process control and of the test results of the quality control, the performance of some test items in the monograph at release on a product may be omitted as occasion demands. Moreover, the quality evaluation of final products (drug substances and drug products) based on in-process data including in-process testing results and monitoring data on process parameters can replace specifications and test methods in the monograph or performing the test methods, if appropriate.

14. The test methods specified in the Japanese Pharmacopoeia can be replaced by alternative methods which give better accuracy and precision. However, where a difference in test results is suspected, only the result obtained by the procedure given in the Pharmacopoeia is effective for the final judgment.

15. The details of the biological test methods may be changed insofar as they do not affect the essential qualities of the test.

16. The temperature for the tests or storage is described, in principle, in specific figures. However, the following expressions may be used instead.

Standard temperature, ordinary temperature, room temperature, and lukewarm are defined as 20°C, 15 - 25°C, 1 - 30°C, and 30 - 40°C, respectively. A cold place, unless otherwise specified, shall be a place having a temperature of 1 - 15°C.

The temperature of cold water, lukewarm water, warm water, and hot water are defined as not exceeding 10°C, 30 - 40°C, 60 - 70°C, and about 100°C, respectively.

The term ''heated solvent'' or ''hot solvent'' means a solvent heated almost to the boiling point of the solvent, and the term ''warmed solvent'' or ''warm solvent'' usually means a solvent heated to a temperature between 60°C and 70°C. The term ''heat on or in a water bath'' indicates, unless otherwise specified, heating with a boiling water bath or a steam bath at about 100°C.

Cold extraction and warm extraction are usually performed at temperatures of 15 - 25°C and 35 - 45°C, respectively.

17. To measure the number of drops, a dropping device which delivers 20 drops of water weighing 0.90 - 1.10 g at 20°C shall be used.

18. The term ''in vacuum'' indicates, unless otherwise specified, a pressure not exceeding 2.0 kPa.

19. The acidity or alkalinity of a solution, unless otherwise specified, is determined by blue or red litmus papers. To indicate these properties more precisely, pH values are used.

20. The terms in Table 1 are used to express the degree of cutting of Crude Drugs or fineness of powder Drugs.

Table 1

Sieve No.	4	6.5	8.6	18	50	100	200
Nominal Designation of sieve	4750 μm	2800 μm	2000 μm	850 μm	300 μm	150 μm	75 μm
Names of the drugs which pass through the respective sieves	Coarse cutting	Moderately fine cutting	Fine cutting	Coarse powder	Moderately fine powder	Fine powder	Very fine powder

21. The water to be used in the tests of drugs shall be the water suitable for performing the relevant test, such as the water not containing any substance that would interfere with the test.

22. As for wording ''solution of a solute'', where the name of the solvent is not stated, the term ''solution'' indicates a solution in water.

23. For solution an expression such as ''(1 in 3)'', ''(1 in 10)'', or ''(1 in 100)'' means that 1 g of a solid is dissolved in, or 1 mL of a liquid is diluted with the solvent to make the total volume of 3 mL, 10 mL or 100 mL, respectively. For the liquid mixture an expression such as ''(10:1)'' or ''(5:3:1)'' means that the respective numbers of parts, by volume, of the designated liquids are to be mixed.

24. The term "weigh accurately" means to weigh down to the degree of 0.1 mg, 10 μg, 1 μg or 0.1 μg by taking into account the purpose of the test and using a relevant weighing device. The term "weigh exactly" means to weigh to the given decimal places.

25. A value of "n" figures in a test of the JP Drugs shall be obtained by rounding off a value of "n + 1" figures.

26. Unless otherwise specified, all tests of the JP Drugs shall be performed at the ordinary temperature and observations of the results shall follow immediately after the operations. However, the judgment for a test which is affected by temperature should be based on the conditions at the standard temperature.

27. The terms "immediately"/"at once" used in the test of the JP Drugs mean that the procedure is to be performed within 30 seconds after the preceding procedure.

28. In the section under the heading Description, the term "white" is used to indicate white or practically white, and "colorless" is colorless or practically colorless. Unless otherwise specified, the test of color is carried out by placing 1 g of a solid drug on a sheet of white paper or in a watch glass placed on white paper. A liquid drug is put into a colorless test tube of 15-mm internal diameter and is observed in front of a white background through a layer of 30 mm. For the test of clarity of liquid drugs the same procedure is applied with either a black or white background. For the observation of fluorescence of a liquid drug, only a black background shall be used.

29. In the section under the heading Description, the term "odorless" is used to indicate odorless or practically odorless. Unless otherwise specified, the test of odor shall be carried out by placing 1 g of a solid drug or 1 mL of a liquid drug in a beaker.

30. In the section under the heading Description, solubilities are expressed by the terms in Table 2. Unless otherwise specified, solubility means the degree of dissolution of the JP Drugs, previously powdered in the case of a solid drug, within 30 minutes in a solvent at 20 ± 5°C, by vigorous shaking for 30 seconds each time at 5-minute intervals.

Table 2

Descriptive term	Volume of solvent required for dissolving 1 g or 1 mL of solute
Very soluble	Less than 1 mL
Freely soluble	From 1 mL to less than 10 mL
Soluble	From 10 mL to less than 30 mL
Sparingly soluble	From 30 mL to less than 100 mL
Slightly soluble	From 100 mL to less than 1000 mL
Very slightly soluble	From 1000 mL to less than 10000 mL
Practically insoluble, or insoluble	10000 mL and over

31. In the test of a drug, the term "dissolve" or "miscible" indicates that it dissolves in, or mixes in arbitrary proportion with the solvent to form a clear solution or mixture. Insoluble materials other than the drug including fibers should not be detected or practically invisible, if any.

32. Identification is the test to identify the active ingredient(s) of the drug based upon its specific property.

33. Purity is the test to detect impurities/contaminants in drugs, and it, as well as other requirements in each monograph, specifies the purity of the drug usually by limiting the kind/nature and quantity of the impurities/contaminants. The impurities/contaminants subject to the purity test are those supposed to generate/contaminate during the manufacturing process or storage, including hazardous agents such as heavy metals, arsenic, etc. If any foreign substances are used or supposed to be added, it is necessary to perform tests to detect or limit the presence of such substances.

34. In principle, the JP Drug Products are controlled appropriately according to the direction under Elemental Impurities of the General Tests. When elemental impurities in the drug products are appropriately controlled in accordance with the direction, it is not necessary to perform the tests on elemental impurities such as heavy metals and arsenic specified in the monographs including, but not limited to, those of drug products, drug substances and excipients.

35. In principle, unless specified in the monograph, the JP Drugs are controlled appropriately according to the direction under Residual Solvents of the general tests.

36. Concerning harmful substances reported as intentionally contaminated to drugs, the control requirement for the presence or absence of contamination is described in the heading "Potential adulteration" in the monograph, as necessary. These substances are controlled by tests on materials, manufacturing processes, intermediates, or final products. The necessity and frequency of the tests are specified separately on individual drugs depending on the control strategy established as part of quality risk management.

37. The term "constant mass" in drying or ignition, unless otherwise specified, means that the mass difference after an additional 1 hour of drying or ignition is not more than 0.10% of the preceding mass of the dried substance or ignited residue. For Crude Drugs, the difference is not more than 0.25%. However, when the difference does not exceed 0.5 mg in a chemical balance, 50 μg in a semi-microbalance, or 5 μg in a microbalance, the constant mass has been attained.

38. Assay is the test to determine the composition, the content of the active ingredients, and the potency unit of medicine by physical, chemical or biological procedures.

39. In stating the appropriate quantities to be taken for assay, the use of the word "about" indicates a quantity within 10% of the specified mass. The word "dry" in respect of the sample indicates drying under the same conditions, as described in Loss on drying in the monograph.

40. For the content of an ingredient determined by Assay in the monographs, if it is expressed simply as "not less than a certain percentage" without indicating its upper limit, 101.0% is understood as the upper limit.

41. Sterility means a condition when no target microorganism is detected by the specified method. Sterilization means a process whereby killing or removal of all living microorganisms in an object to be sterilized is accomplished. Aseptic technique is controlled technique to maintain the aseptic condition.

42. The container is the device which holds the JP Drugs. The stopper or cap, etc., is considered as part of the container. The containers have no physical and chemical reactivity affecting the specified description and quality of the contents.

43. A well-closed container protects the contents from extraneous solids and from loss of the drug under ordinary or customary conditions of handling, shipment, and storage.

Where a well-closed container is specified, it may be replaced by a tight container.

44. A tight container protects the contents from extraneous solids or liquids, from loss of the contents, and from efflorescence, deliquescence, or evaporation under ordinary or customary conditions of handling, shipment, and storage.

Where a tight container is specified, it may be replaced by a hermetic container.

45. A hermetic container is impervious to air or any other gas under ordinary or customary conditions of handling, shipment, and storage.

46. The term "light-resistant" means that it can prevent transmittance of light affecting in the specified properties and quality of the contents and protect the contained medicament from the light under ordinary or customary conditions of handling, shipment, and storage.

47. For the JP Drugs, the contents or potency in terms of units of the active ingredient(s) in the monographs have to be shown on the immediate container or wrapping of them.

48. The origin, numerical value or physical properties of the JP Drugs, being stipulated by the special labeling requirements in the monographs, have to be shown on the immediate container or wrapping of them.

49. The harmonized General Tests and Monographs among the Japanese Pharmacopoeia, the European Pharmacopoeia and the United States Pharmacopeia are preceded by the statement as such.

The parts of the text, being not harmonized, are surrounded by the symbols (◆ ◆ or ◇ ◇).

—Abbreviations—

CS: Colorimetric Stock Solution

RS: Reference Standard

TS: Test Solution

VS: Refer to a solution listed in Standard Solutions for Volumetric Analysis <*9.21*>.

The JP Drugs are to be tested according to the provisions given in the pertinent monographs, General Notices, General Rules for Crude Drugs, General Rules for Preparations, and General Tests for their conformity to the Japanese Pharmacopoeia. (See the General Notices 5.)

GENERAL RULES FOR CRUDE DRUGS

1. Crude drugs in the monographs include medicinal parts obtained from plants or animals, cell inclusions and secretes separated from the origins, their extracts, and minerals. General Rules for Crude Drugs and Crude Drugs Test are applicable to the following:

Acacia, Achyranthes Root, Agar, Akebia Stem, Alisma Tuber, Aloe, Alpinia Officinarum Rhizome, Aluminum Silicate Hydrate with Silicon Dioxide, Amomum Seed, Anemarrhena Rhizome, Angelica Dahurica Root, Apricot Kernel, Aralia Rhizome, Areca, Artemisia Capillaris Flower, Artemisia Leaf, Asiasarum Root, Asparagus Root, Astragalus Root, Atractylodes Lancea Rhizome, Atractylodes Rhizome, Bear Bile, Bearberry Leaf, Belladonna Root, Benincasa Seed, Benzoin, Bitter Cardamon, Bitter Orange Peel, Brown Rice, Bupleurum Root, Burdock Fruit, Calumba, Capsicum, Cardamon, Cassia Seed, Catalpa Fruit, Cherry Bark, Chrysanthemum Flower, Cimicifuga Rhizome, Cinnamon Bark, Cistanche Herb, Citrus Unshiu Peel, Clematis Root, Clove, Cnidium Monnieri Fruit, Cnidium Rhizome, Codonopsis Root, Coix Seed, Condurango, Coptis Rhizome, Cornus Fruit, Corydalis Tuber, Crataegus Fruit, Curcuma Rhizome, Cyperus Rhizome, Digenea, Dioscorea Rhizome, Dolichos Seed, Eleutherococcus Senticosus Rhizome, Ephedra Herb, Epimedium Herb, Eucommia Bark, Euodia Fruit, Fennel, Forsythia Fruit, Fritillaria Bulb, Gambir, Gardenia Fruit, Gastrodia Tuber, Gentian, Geranium Herb, Ginger, Ginseng, Glehnia Root and Rhizome, Glycyrrhiza, Gypsum, Hedysarum Root, Hemp Fruit, Honey, Houttuynia Herb, Immature Orange, Imperata Rhizome, Ipecac, Japanese Angelica Root, Japanese Gentian, Japanese Valerian, Japanese Zanthoxylum Peal, Jujube, Jujube Seed, Koi, Leonurus Herb, Lilium Bulb, Lindera Root, Lithospermum Root, Longan Aril, Longgu, Lonicera Leaf and Stem, Loquat Leaf, Lycium Bark, Lycium Fruit, Magnolia Bark, Magnolia Flower, Mallotus Bark, Malt, Mentha Herb, Moutan Bark, Mulberry Bark, Nelumbo Seed, Notopterygium, Nuphar Rhizome, Nutmeg, Nux Vomica, Ophiopogon Root, Oriental Bezoar, Oyster Shell, Panax Japonicus Rhizome, Peach Kernel, Peony Root, Perilla Herb, Peucedanum Root, Pharbitis Seed, Phellodendron Bark, Picrasma Wood, Pinellia Tuber, Plantago Herb, Plantago Seed, Platycodon Root, Pogostemon Herb, Polygala Root, Polygonatum Rhizome, Polygonum Root, Polyporus Sclerotium, Poria Sclerotium, Powdered Acacia, Powdered Agar, Powdered Alisma Tuber, Powdered Aloe, Powdered Amomum Seed, Powdered Atractylodes Lancea Rhizome, Powdered Atractylodes Rhizome, Powdered Calumba, Powdered Capsicum, Powdered Cinnamon Bark, Powdered Clove, Powdered Cnidium Rhizome, Powdered Coix Seed, Powdered Coptis Rhizome, Powdered Corydalis Tuber, Powdered Cyperus Rhizome, Powdered Dioscorea Rhizome, Powdered Fennel, Powdered Gambir, Powdered Gardenia Fruit, Powdered Gentian, Powdered Geranium Herb, Powdered Ginger, Powdered Ginseng, Powdered Glycyrrhiza, Powdered Ipecac, Powdered Japanese Angelica Root, Powdered Japanese Gentian, Powdered Japanese Valerian, Powdered Longgu, Powdered Magnolia Bark, Powdered Moutan Bark, Powdered Oyster Shell, Powdered Panax Japonicus Rhizome, Powdered Peach Kernel, Powdered Peony Root, Powdered Phellodendron Bark, Powdered Picrasma Wood, Powdered Platycodon Root, Powdered Polygala Root, Powdered Polyporus Sclerotium, Powdered Poria Sclerotium, Powdered Processed Aconite Root, Powdered Rhubarb, Powdered Rose Fruit, Powdered Scutellaria Root, Powdered Senega, Powdered Senna Leaf, Powdered Smilax Rhizome, Powdered Sophora Root, Powdered Sweet Hydrangea Leaf, Powdered Swertia Herb, Powdered Tragacanth, Powdered Turmeric, Powdered Zanthoxylum Fruit, Prepared Glycyrrhiza, Processed Aconite Root, Processed Ginger, Prunella Spike, Pueraria Root, Quercus Bark, Red Ginseng, Rehmannia Root, Rhubarb, Rose Fruit, Rosin, Royal Jelly, Safflower, Saffron, Salvia Miltiorrhiza Root, Saposhnikovia Root and Rhizome, Sappan Wood, Saussurea Root, Schisandra Fruit, Schizonepeta Spike, Scopolia Rhizome, Scutellaria Root, Senega, Senna Leaf, Sesame, Sinomenium Stem and Rhizome, Smilax Rhizome, Sophora Root, Sweet Hydrangea Leaf, Swertia Herb, Toad Cake, Tragacanth, Tribulus Fruit, Trichosanthes Root, Turmeric, Uncaria Hook.

2. Crude drugs are usually used in the forms of whole crude drugs, cut crude drugs or powdered crude drugs.

Whole crude drugs are the medicinal parts or their ingredients prepared by drying and/or simple processes, as specified in the monographs.

Cut crude drugs are small pieces or small blocks prepared by cutting or crushing of the whole crude drugs, and also coarse, moderately fine or fine cutting of the crude drugs in whole, and, unless otherwise specified, are required to conform to the specifications of the whole crude drugs used as original materials.

Powdered crude drugs are coarse, moderately fine, fine or very fine powder prepared from the whole crude drugs or the cut crude drugs; usually powdered crude drugs as fine powder are specified in the monographs.

3. Unless otherwise specified, crude drugs are used in dried form. The drying is usually carried out at a temperature not exceeding 60°C.

4. The origin of crude drugs is to serve as the acceptance criteria. Such statements as 'other species of the same genus' and 'allied plants' or 'allied animals' appearing in the origin of crude drugs usually indicate plants or animals which may be used as materials for crude drugs containing the same effective constituents.

5. Description in each monograph for crude drugs covers the crude drug derived from its typical original plant or animal and includes statements of characteristic properties of the crude drug, which are all to serve as the evaluation criteria as well as the aspects obtained by microscopic observation. As for the color, odor and solubility, apply correspondingly to the prescription of the General Notices, except the odor which is to serve as the acceptance criteria. The taste is to serve as the acceptance criteria.

6. Powdered crude drugs, otherwise specified, may be mixed with diluents so as to attain proper content and potency.

7. Powdered crude drugs do not contain fragments of tissues, cells, cell inclusions or other foreign matter alien to the original crude drugs or cut crude drugs.

8. Crude drugs are as free as possible from contaminants and other impurities due to molds, insects and other animals and from other foreign matters, and are required to be kept in a clean and hygienic state.

9. Crude drugs are preserved under protection from moisture and insect damage, unless otherwise specified. In order to avoid insect damage, suitable fumigants may be used to preserve crude drugs, provided that the fumigants are so readily volatilized as to be harmless at the usual dosage of the crude drugs, and such fumigants that may affect the therapeutic efficacy of the crude drugs or interfere with the testing are precluded.

10. Crude drugs are preserved in well-closed containers unless otherwise specified.

GENERAL RULES FOR PREPARATIONS

[1] General Notices for Preparations

(1) General Notices for Preparations present general rules for pharmaceutical dosage forms.

(2) In [3] Monographs for Preparations, dosage forms are classified mainly by administration routes and application sites, and furthermore are subdivided according to their forms, functions and characteristics.

Those preparations containing mainly crude drugs as active raw materials are described under [4] Monographs for Preparations Related to Crude Drugs.

(3) In Monographs for Preparations and Monographs for Preparations Related to Crude Drugs, dosage forms, which are generally or widely used, are described. However, any other appropriate dosage forms may be used where appropriate. For example, a dosage form suitable for a particular application may be designated by combining an administration route and a name of a dosage form listed in these chapters.

(4) In these monographs, preparation characteristics are specified for the dosage forms. The preparation characteristics are confirmed by appropriate tests.

(5) In the case of preparations, functions that control the release rate of active substance(s) may be added for the purpose of controlling the onset and duration of therapeutic effects and/or decreasing adverse or side effects. The preparations modified in release rate must have an appropriate function of controlled release for the intended use. The added functional modification must generally be displayed on the pack insert and on the direct container or packaging of these preparations.

(6) Pharmaceutical excipients are substances other than active substances contained in preparations, and they are used to increase the utility of the active substance(s) and preparation, to make formulation process easier, to keep the product quality, to improve the usability, and so forth. Suitable excipients may be added for these purposes. The excipients to be used, however, must be pharmacologically inactive and harmless in the administered amount and must not interfere with the therapeutic efficacy of the preparations.

(7) Purified water to be used for preparations is Purified Water or Purified Water in Containers, and water for injection is Water for Injection or Water for Injection in Containers.

Vegetable oils to be used for preparations are usually edible oils listed in the Pharmacopoeia. When starch is called for, unless otherwise specified, any kind of starch listed in the Pharmacopoeia may be used.

In addition, ethanol specified in vol% is prepared by adding Purified Water or Water for Injection to ethanol at the specified vol%.

(8) Sterile preparations are preparations verified to be aseptic. There are terminal sterilization and aseptic technique as basic manufacturing process of sterile preparations.

Terminal sterilization is a process to sterilize preparations after filling in a container. In this process microbial lethality after sterilization is quantitatively measured or evaluated, and this process is performed under the condition where the sterility assurance level of 10^{-6} or less is ensured by using suitable biological indicators.

Aseptic technique is a process for appropriate control of a risk of microbial contamination, and is a manufacturing process of preparations using a series of aseptic processes with sterile raw materials or after filtration sterilization.

This technique generally requires the presterilization of all equipments and materials used, and this process is performed under the condition to give a defined sterility assurance level in the clean areas where microbial and particulate levels are adequately maintained by using appropriate techniques.

(9) Even non-sterile preparations should be prepared with precautions to prevent contamination and growth of microorganisms, and the test of Microbiological Examination of Non-sterile Products *<4.05>* or Microbial Limit Test for Crude Drugs and Preparations containing Crude Drugs as Main Ingredient *<5.02>* is applied to them, if necessary.

(10) The test for Content Uniformity under the Uniformity of Dosage Units and the Dissolution Test are not intended to apply to the crude drug component of preparations which are prepared using crude drugs or preparations related to crude drugs as raw materials.

(11) Unless otherwise specified, preserve preparations at room temperature. Store them in light-resistant containers or packaging, if light affects the quality of the preparation.

[2] General Notices for Packaging of Preparations

(1) General notices for packaging of preparations describe the basic items on a principle and the packaging suitability for packaging of preparations using container and wrapper.

(2) Principle of packaging of preparations

In the development phase of preparations, it is important for the packaging of preparations to fully evaluate its suitability for maintaining the specified quality of preparations over the shelf life. Based on the evaluation of the packaging suitability depending on the characteristics of the preparation, items such as specification and test methods of finished products, in-process tests and evaluation of the materials used for packaging and the like to control the quality appropriately are established. The properness of the established requirements can be verified conclusively by the stability studies of finished products.

For the change of the packaging, it is necessary to examine the items described above.

It is necessary to perform the appropriate test to confirm that the unintended changes of the packaging exert no influence to the quality of finished product.

(3) Packaging suitability

Packaging suitability includes the components of Protection of preparation, Compatibility of preparation and package, Safety of the materials used for package, and additional Performance at the time of administration.

Depending on the characteristics of preparation, the package should have functions such as of moisture-proofness, light-resistance, barrier property for gases and microorganisms, and protection against the shock that might occur at the time of transportation, and the like (Protection).

The package should be composed of the shape and material that do not cause physical and chemical interaction with the preparation (Compatibility).

It should be composed of the materials which leaching and migrating quantity of the constituents and impurities to preparations are sufficiently low from the point of view of safety (Safety).

The packaging performance shall include not merely the protection of preparations but also the improvement of patient compliance, ease of use, etc. Functions of ensuring safety of patients such as a prevention of accidental ingestion and improvement of safety of medical staffs should also be included (Performance).

The packaging suitability is examined based on the test methods listed in the General Tests and appropriate techniques depending on the dosage form and the characteristics of the preparation. Items for appropriate quality control are established based on the test methods and the like used for packaging suitability.

For designing of the packaging of injections, the packaging suitability is examined by appropriate selection from Test for Glass Containers for Injections <*7.01*>, Test Methods for Plastic Containers <*7.02*>, Test for Rubber Closure for Aqueous Infusions <*7.03*>, a container integrity test, a light stability test, the descriptions in Monographs, and the like. Items for appropriate quality control are established based on the adopted techniques for the packaging suitability.

[3] Monographs for Preparations

(1) In the Monographs for Preparations, the definitions of dosage forms, manufacturing methods, test methods, containers and packaging, and storage are described.

(2) The descriptions of the test methods in these monographs are fundamental requirements, and the manufacturing methods represent commonly used methods.

(3) Preparation in single-dose package means a preparation packaged for single-dose use.

1. Preparations for Oral Administration

(1) Immediate-release dosage forms are preparations showing a release pattern of active substance(s) that is not intentionally modified and is generally dependent on the intrinsic solubility of the active substance.

(2) Modified-release dosage forms are preparations showing a release pattern of active substance(s) that is suitably modified for the desired purpose by means of a specific formulation design and/or manufacturing method. Modified-release dosage forms include delayed-release and extended-release preparations.

(i) Delayed-release preparations

Delayed-release preparations are designed to release the bulk of the active substance(s) not in stomach but mainly in small intestine, in order to prevent degradation or decomposition of the active substance(s) in stomach or to decrease the irritation of the active substance(s) on stomach. Delayed-release preparations are generally coated with an acid-insoluble enteric film. Delayed-release preparations are included in a group of modified-release dosage forms that delay the start to release active substance(s).

(ii) Extended-release preparations

Extended-release preparations are designed to control the release rate and release period of active substance(s) and to restrict the release to appropriate sites in the gastrointestinal tracts in order to decrease the dosing frequency and/or to reduce adverse or side effects. Extended-release preparations are generally prepared by using suitable agents that prolong the release of the active substance(s).

(3) Oral dosage forms such as capsules, granules and tablets can be coated with appropriate coating agents, such as sugars, sugar alcohols, or polymers, for the purpose of enabling the ingestion easy or of preventing degradation of the active substance(s).

1-1. Tablets

(1) Tablets are solid preparations having a desired shape and size, intended for oral administration. Orally Disintegrating Tablets, Chewable Tablets, Effervescent Tablets, Dispersible Tablets and Soluble Tablets are included in this category.

(2) Tablets are usually prepared by the following procedures. Delayed-release or extended-release tablets can be prepared by appropriate methods.

(i) Mix homogeneously active substance(s) and excipients such as diluents, binders and disintegrators, granulate with water or a binder solution by a suitable method, mix with a lubricant, and then compress into a desired shape and size.

(ii) Mix homogeneously active substance(s) and excipients such as diluents, binders, and disintegrators, and then directly compress with a lubricant, or compress after adding active substance(s) and a lubricant to granules previously prepared from excipients and then mixing homogeneously.

(iii) Mix homogeneously active substance(s) and excipients such as diluents and binders, moisten with a solvent, form into a certain shape and size or mold the mixed mass into a certain shape and size, and then dry by a suitable method.

(iv) Plain Tablets are usually prepared according to (i), (ii) or (iii).

(v) Film-coated Tablets can be prepared, usually, by coating Plain Tablets with thin films using suitable film coating agents such as polymers.

(vi) Sugar-coated Tablets can be prepared, usually, by coating Plain Tablets using suitable coating agents including sugars or sugar alcohols.

(vii) Multiple-layer Tablets can be prepared by compressing granules of different compositions to form layered tablets by a suitable method.

(viii) Pressure-coated Tablets can be prepared by compressing granules to cover inner core tablets with different compositions.

(3) Unless otherwise specified, Tablets meet the requirements of Uniformity of Dosage Units ⟨*6.02*⟩.

(4) Unless otherwise specified, Tablets meet the requirements of Dissolution Test ⟨*6.10*⟩ or Disintegration Test ⟨*6.09*⟩. For Effervescent tablets from which active substance(s) are dissolved before use and Soluble tablets, these tests are not required.

(5) Well-closed containers are usually used for the preparations. For preparations susceptible to degradation by moisture, a moisture-proof container or packaging may be used.

1-1-1. Orally Disintegrating Tablets/Orodispersible Tablets

(1) Orally Disintegrating Tablets are tablets which are quickly dissolved or disintegrated in the oral cavity.

(2) Orally Disintegrating Tablets shows an appropriate disintegration.

1-1-2. Chewable Tablets

(1) Chewable Tablets are tablets which are administered by chewing.

(2) Chewable Tablets must be in shape and size avoiding danger of suffocation.

1-1-3. Effervescent Tablets

(1) Effervescent Tablets are tablets which are quickly dissolved or dispersed with bubbles in water.

(2) Effervescent tablets are usually prepared using suitable acidic substances and carbonates or hydrogen carbonates.

1-1-4. Dispersible Tablets

(1) Dispersible Tablets are tablets which are administered after having been dispersed in water.

1-1-5. Soluble Tablets

(1) Soluble Tablets are tablets which are administered after having been dissolved in water.

1-2. Capsules

(1) Capsules are preparations enclosed in capsules or wrapped with capsule bases, intended for oral administration. Capsules are classified into Hard Capsules and Soft Capsules.

(2) Capsules are usually prepared by the following methods. Delayed-release or extended-release capsules can be prepared by a suitable method. Coloring agents, preservatives, etc. may be added to the capsule bases.

(i) Hard Capsules: A homogeneous mixture of active substance(s) with diluents and other suitable excipients, or granules or formed masses prepared by a suitable method, are filled into capsule shells as they are or after slight compression.

(ii) Soft Capsules: Active substance(s) and suitable excipients (including solvents) are mixed, enclosed by a suitable capsule base such as gelatin plasticized by addition of glycerin, D-sorbitol, etc. and molded in a suitable shape and size.

(3) Unless otherwise specified, Capsules meet the requirements of Uniformity of Dosage Units ⟨*6.02*⟩.

(4) Unless otherwise specified, Capsules meet the requirements of Dissolution Test ⟨*6.10*⟩ or Disintegration Test ⟨*6.09*⟩.

(5) Well-closed containers are usually used for

The JP Drugs are to be tested according to the provisions given in the pertinent monographs, General Notices, General Rules for Crude Drugs, General Rules for Preparations, and General Tests for their conformity to the Japanese Pharmacopoeia. (See the General Notices 5.)

Capsules. For Capsules susceptible to degradation by moisture, a moisture-proof container or packaging may be used.

1-3. Granules

(1) Granules are preparations prepared by granulation, intended for oral administration. Effervescent Granules are included in this category.

(2) Granules are usually prepared by the following methods. Granules can be coated using suitable coating agents if necessary. Extended-release or delayed-release granules can also be prepared by a suitable method.

(i) To powdery active substance(s) add diluents, binders, disintegrators, or other suitable excipients, mix to homogenize, and granulate by a suitable method.

(ii) To previously granulated active substance(s) add excipients such as diluents, and mix to homogenize.

(iii) To previously granulated active substance(s) add excipients such as diluents, and granulate by a suitable method.

(3) Among Granules, the preparations may be referred to as ''Fine Granules'' if, when Particle Size Distribution Test for Preparations <*6.03*> is performed, all granules pass through a No. 18 (850 μm) sieve, and not more than 10% of which remain on a No. 30 (500 μm) sieve.

(4) Unless otherwise specified, the Granules in single-dose packages meet the requirements of Uniformity of Dosage Units <*6.02*>.

(5) Unless otherwise specified, Granules comply with Dissolution Test <*6.10*> or Disintegration Test <*6.09*>. However, this provision is not to be applied to Effervescent granules, which are dissolved before use, and Disintegration Test <*6.09*> is not required for the Granules not more than 10% of which remain on a No. 30 (500 μm) sieve when the test is performed as directed under Particle Size Distribution Test for Preparations <*6.03*>.

(6) Among Granules, the particulate preparations may be referred to as ''Powders'' if, when the Particle Size Distribution Test for Preparations <*6.03*> is performed, all granules pass through a No. 18 (850 μm) sieve, and not more than 5% remain on a No. 30 (500 μm) sieve.

(7) Well-closed containers are usually used for Granules. For the preparations susceptible to degradation by moisture, a moisture-proof container or packaging may be used.

1-3-1. Effervescent Granules

(1) Effervescent granules are granules which are quickly dissolved or dispersed with bubbles in water.

(2) Effervescent granules are usually prepared using suitable acidic substances and carbonates or hydrogen carbonates.

1-4. Powders

(1) Powders are preparations in powder form, intended for oral administration.

(2) Powders are usually prepared by homogeneously mixing active substance(s) with diluents or other suitable excipients.

(3) Unless otherwise specified, the Powders in single-dose packages meet the requirements of Uniformity of Dosage Units <*6.02*>.

(4) Unless otherwise specified, Powders meet the requirements of Dissolution Test <*6.10*>.

(5) Well-closed containers are usually used for Powders. For the preparations susceptible to degradation by moisture, a moisture-proof container or packaging may be used.

1-5. Liquids and Solutions for Oral Administration

(1) Liquids and Solutions for Oral Administration are preparations in liquid form or flowable and viscous gelatinous state, intended for oral administration. Elixirs, Suspensions, Emulsions and Lemonades are included in this category.

(2) Liquids and Solutions for Oral Administration are usually prepared by dissolving, emulsifying or suspending active substance(s) in Purified Water together with excipients, and by filtering if necessary.

(3) For Liquids and Solutions for Oral Administration which are apt to deteriorate, prepare before use.

(4) Unless otherwise specified, the preparations in single-dose packages meet the requirement of Uniformity of Dosage Units <*6.02*>.

(5) Tight containers are usually used for Liquids and Solutions for Oral Administration. For the preparations susceptible to degradation by evaporation of water, a low-moisture-permeability container or packaging may be used.

1-5-1. Elixirs

(1) Elixirs are clear, sweetened and aromatic liquid preparations, containing ethanol, intended for oral administration.

(2) Elixirs are usually prepared by dissolving solid active substance(s) or their extractives in ethanol and Purified Water, adding aromatic agents and sucrose, other sugars or sweetening agents, and clarifying by filtration or other procedure.

1-5-2. Suspensions

(1) Suspensions are liquid preparations of active substance(s) suspended finely and homogeneously in a vehicle, intended for oral administration.

(2) Suspensions are usually prepared by adding suspending agent or other suitable excipients and Purified Water or oil to solid active substance(s), and suspending homogeneously as the whole by a suitable

method.

(3) Mix homogeneously before use, if necessary.

(4) Unless otherwise specified, Suspensions meet the requirements of Dissolution Test <*6.10*>.

1-5-3. Emulsions

(1) Emulsions are liquid preparations of active substance(s) emulsified finely and homogeneously in a liquid vehicle, intended for oral administration.

(2) Emulsions are usually prepared by adding emulsifying agents and Purified Water to liquid active substance(s), and emulsifying finely and homogeneously by a suitable method.

(3) Mix homogeneously before use, where necessary.

1-5-4. Lemonades

(1) Lemonades are sweet and sour, clear liquid preparations, intended for oral administration.

1-6. Syrups

(1) Syrups are viscous liquid or solid preparations containing sugars or sweetening agents, intended for oral administration. Preparations for Syrups are included in this category.

(2) Syrups are usually prepared by dissolving, mixing, suspending or emulsifying active substance(s) in a solution of sucrose, other sugars or sweetening agents, or in Simple Syrup. Where necessary, the mixture is boiled, and filtered while hot.

(3) For Syrups which are apt to deteriorate, prepare before use.

(4) Unless otherwise specified, Syrups in single-dose packages meet the requirements of Uniformity of Dosage Units <*6.02*>.

(5) Unless otherwise specified, Syrups in which active substance(s) is suspended meet the requirements of Dissolution Test <*6.10*>.

(6) Tight containers are usually used for Syrups. For the preparations susceptible to degradation by evaporation of water, a low-moisture-permeability container or packaging may be used.

1-6-1. Preparations for Syrups

(1) Preparations for Syrups are preparations in form of granules or powders, which become syrups by adding water. They may be termed "Dry Syrups".

(2) Preparations for Syrup are usually prepared with sugars or sweetening agents as directed under 1-3. Granules or 1-4. Powders.

(3) Preparations for Syrups are usually to be used after having been dissolved or suspended in water.

(4) Unless otherwise specified, the Preparations for Syrups other than preparations which are to be used after having been dissolved meet the requirements of Dissolution Test <*6.10*> or Disintegration Test <*6.09*>. However, Disintegration Test <*6.09*> is not required for the Preparations, if, when the Particle Size Distribution Test for Preparations <*6.03*> is performed, not more than 10% of the total amount remains on a No. 30 (500 μm) sieve.

(5) Well-closed containers are usually used for Preparations for Syrups. For the Preparations for Syrups susceptible to degradation by moisture, a moisture-proof container or packaging may be used.

1-7. Jellies for Oral Administration

(1) Jellies for Oral Administration are non-flowable gelatinous preparations having a certain shape and size, intended for oral administration.

(2) Jellies for oral application are usually prepared by mixing active substance(s) with suitable excipients and polymer gel base, gelatinizing and forming into a certain shape and size by a suitable method.

(3) Unless otherwise specified, Jellies for Oral Administration meet the requirements of Uniformity of Dosage Units <*6.02*>.

(4) Unless otherwise specified, Jellies for Oral Administration meet the requirements of Dissolution Test <*6.10*> or show an appropriate disintegration.

(5) Tight containers are usually used for Jellies for Oral Administration. For the preparations susceptible to degradation by evaporation of water, a low-moisture-permeability container or packaging may be used.

1-8. Films for Oral Administration

(1) Films for Oral Administration are preparations in film form, intended for oral administration.

(2) Films for Oral Administration are usually prepared by spreading to dry a solution, composed of active substance(s) and a mixture of water-soluble polymer and other additives as a base, or by melting the mixture of active substances(s) and the base to form. Layers different in additive compositions may be stacked in appropriate manner to form the films.

(3) Unless otherwise specified, Films for Oral Administration meet the requirement of Uniformity of Dosage Units <*6.02*>.

(4) Unless otherwise specified, Films for Oral Administration meet the requirement of Dissolution Test <*6.10*> or show an appropriate disintegration.

(5) Well-closed containers are usually used for Films for Oral Administration. For the preparations susceptible to degradation by moisture, a moisture-proof container or packaging may be used.

1-8-1. Orally Disintegrating Films

(1) Orally Disintegrating Films are films which are quickly dissolved or disintegrated in the oral cavity.

(2) Orally Disintegrating Films show an appropriate disintegration.

2. Preparations for Oro-mucosal Application

2-1. Tablets for Oro-mucosal Application

(1) Tablets for Oro-mucosal Application are solid

preparations having a certain form, intended for oral cavity application.

Troches/Lozenges, Sublingual Tablets, Buccal Tablets, Mucoadhesive Tablets and Medicated Chewing Gums are included in this category.

(2) Tablets for Oro-mucosal Application are prepared as directed under 1-1. Tablets.

(3) Unless otherwise specified, Tablets for Oro-mucosal Application meet the requirements of Uniformity of Dosage Units <*6.02*>.

(4) Tablets for Oro-mucosal Application have an appropriate dissolution or disintegration.

(5) Well-closed containers are usually used for Tablets for Oro-mucosal Application. For the preparations susceptible to degradation by moisture, a moisture-proof container or packaging may be used.

2-1-1. Troches/Lozenges

(1) Troches/Lozenges are tablets for oro-mucosal application, which are gradually dissolved or disintegrated in the mouth, and are intended for application locally to the oral cavity or the throat.

(2) Troches/Lozenges must be in shape and size avoiding danger of suffocation.

2-1-2. Sublingual Tablets

(1) Sublingual Tablets are tablets for oro-mucosal application, from which active substance(s) are quickly dissolved sublingually and absorbed via the oral mucosa.

2-1-3. Buccal Tablets

(1) Buccal Tablets are tablets for oro-mucosal application, from which the active substance(s) are dissolved gradually between the cheek and teeth, and absorbed via the oral mucosa.

2-1-4. Mucoadhesive Tablets

(1) Mucoadhesive Tablets are tablets for oro-mucosal application that are applied by adhesion to the oral mucosa.

(2) Mucoadhesive Tablets are usually prepared by using hydrophilic polymers to form hydrogel.

2-1-5. Medicated Chewing Gums

(1) Medicated Chewing Gums are tablets for oro-mucosal application, releasing active substance(s) by chewing.

(2) Medicated Chewing Gums are usually prepared using suitable gum bases such as vegetable resin, thermoplastic resin and elastomer.

2-2. Liquids and Solutions for Oro-mucosal Application

(1) Liquids and Solutions for Oro-mucosal Application are preparations in liquid form or flowable and viscous gelatinous state, intended for oral cavity application.

(2) Liquids and Solutions for Oro-mucosal Application are usually prepared by mixing active substance(s) with suitable excipients and Purified Water or suitable vehicles to dissolve homogenously or to emulsify or suspend, and by filtering if necessary.

(3) For Liquids and Solutions for Oro-mucosal Application which are apt to deteriorate, prepare before use.

(4) Unless otherwise specified, the preparations in single-dose packages meet the requirement of the Uniformity of Dosage Units <*6.02*>.

(5) Tight containers are usually used for Liquids and Solutions for Oro-mucosal Application. For the preparations susceptible to degradation by evaporation of water, a low-moisture-permeability container or packaging may be used.

2-2-1. Preparations for Gargles

(1) Preparations for Gargles are liquid preparations intended to apply locally to the oral and throat cavities. Solid type preparations to be dissolved in water before use are also included in this category.

(2) Solid type preparations to be dissolved in water before use are prepared as directed under 1-1. Tablets or 1-3. Granules.

2-3. Sprays for Oro-mucosal Application

(1) Sprays for Oro-mucosal Application are preparations that are applied active substance(s) by spraying into the oral cavity in mist, powder, foam or paste forms.

(2) Sprays for Oro-mucosal Application are usually prepared by the following methods:

(i) Dissolve or suspend active substance(s) and suitable excipients in a solvent, filter, where necessary, and fill into a container together with liquefied or compressed gas.

(ii) Dissolve or suspend active substance(s) and suitable excipients in a solvent, fill into a container, and fit with a pump for spraying.

(3) Unless otherwise specified, metered-dose types among Sprays for Oro-mucosal Application have an appropriate uniformity of delivered dose.

(4) Tight containers or pressure-resistant containers are usually used for Sprays for Oro-mucosal Application.

2-4. Semi-solid Preparations for Oro-mucosal Application

(1) Semi-solid Preparations for Oro-mucosal Application are preparations in cream, gel or ointment forms, intended for application to the oral mucosa.

(2) Semi-solid Preparations for Oro-mucosal Application are usually prepared by emulsifying active substance(s) together with excipients using "Purified Water" and oil component such as petrolatum, or by homogenizing active substance(s) together with suitable excipients using polymer gel or oil and fats as the base.

(i) Creams for oro-mucosal application are prepared as directed under 11-5. Creams.

(ii) Gels for oro-mucosal application are prepared as directed under 11-6. Gels.

(iii) Ointments for oro-mucosal application are prepared as directed under 11-4. Ointments.

For Semi-solid Preparations for Oro-mucosal Application which are apt to deteriorate, prepare before use.

(3) Sufficient amounts of suitable preservatives to prevent the growth of microorganisms may be added for Semi-solid Preparations for Oro-mucosal Application filled in multiple-dose containers.

(4) Semi-solid Preparations for Oro-mucosal Application have a suitable viscosity to apply to the oral mucosa.

(5) Tight containers are usually used for Semi-solid Preparations for Oro-mucosal Application. For the preparations susceptible to degradation by evaporation of water, a low-moisture-permeability container or packaging may be used.

3. Preparations for Injection

3-1. Injections

(1) Injections are sterile preparations to be administered directly into the body through skin, muscle or blood vessel, usually in form of a solution, a suspension or an emulsion of active substance(s), or of a solid that contains active substance(s) to be dissolved or suspended before use.

Parenteral Infusions, Implants/Pellets, Prolonged-Release Injections and Liposome Injections are included in this category.

(2) Injections in solution, suspension or emulsion form are usually prepared by the following methods.

(i) Dissolve, suspend or emulsify active substance(s) with or without excipients in Water for Injection or an aqueous or nonaqueous vehicle homogeneously, fill into containers for injection, seal, and sterilize.

(ii) Dissolve, suspend or emulsify active substance(s) with or without excipients in Water for Injection or an aqueous or nonaqueous vehicle, and filtrate aseptically, or prepare aseptically a homogeneous liquid, fill into containers for injection, and seal.

Every care should be taken to prevent contamination with microorganisms. The overall processes of preparing injections, from the preparation of active solution to the sterilization, should be completed as rapidly as possible, taking into consideration the composition of the injection and the storage conditions. The concentration of active substance(s) expressed in % represents w/v%.

Injections that are to be dissolved or suspended before use and are designated in the name as ''for injection'' may be accompanied by a suitable vehicle to dissolve or suspend the supplied preparation (hereinafter referred to as ''vehicle attached to preparation'').

(3) Injections may be prepared as Freeze-dried Injections or Powders for Injections to prevent degradation or deactivation of the active substance(s) in solution.

(i) Freeze-dried Injections

Freeze-dried Injections are usually prepared by dissolving active substance(s) with or without excipients such as diluents in Water for Injection, sterilizing the solution by aseptic filtration, filling the filtrate directly into individual containers for injection and being freeze-dried, or dividing the filtrate in special containers, being freeze-dried and transferred into individual containers for injection.

(ii) Powders for Injections

Powders for injections are usually prepared by filtrating aseptically a solution of active substance(s), obtaining powders by crystallization from the solution or mixing additionally the powders with sterilized excipients, and filling the powders into individual containers for injections.

(4) To prevent errors in the preparation with vehicles attached or administration of injections, or bacterial or foreign matter contamination, or for the purpose of urgent use, prefilled syringes or cartridges may be prepared.

(i) Prefilled Syringes for Injections

Prefilled Syringes for injections are usually prepared by dissolving, suspending or emulsifying active substance(s) with or without excipients in a vehicle, and filling into syringes.

(ii) Cartridges for Injections

Cartridges for Injections are usually prepared by dissolving, suspending or emulsifying active substance(s) with or without excipients in a vehicle, and filling into cartridges.

The cartridges are used by fixing in an injection device for exclusive use.

(5) Vehicles used in Injections or attached to preparations must be harmless in the amounts usually administered and must not interfere with the therapeutic efficacy of the active substance(s).

The vehicles are classified into the following two groups. They should meet each requirement.

(i) Aqueous vehicles: As the vehicle of aqueous injections, Water for Injection is usually used. Isotonic Sodium Chloride Solution, Ringer's Solution, or other suitable aqueous solutions may be used instead.

Unless otherwise specified, these aqueous vehicles, other than those exclusively for intracutaneous, subcutaneous or intramuscular administration, meet the requirements of Bacterial Endotoxins Test <*4.01*>.

When the Bacterial Endotoxins Test <*4.01*> is not

applicable to aqueous vehicles, the Pyrogen Test <*4.04*> may be applied instead.

(ii) Non-aqueous vehicles: Vegetable oils are usually used as vehicles for oily injections. These oils, unless otherwise specified, are clear at 10°C, the acid value is not more than 0.56, the saponification value is between 185 and 200, and the iodine value falls between 79 and 137. They meet the requirements of Mineral Oil Test <*1.05*>.

Organic vehicles miscible with water, such as ethanol, are usually used as vehicles for hydrophilic injections.

(6) Unless otherwise specified, any coloring agent must not be added solely for the purpose of coloring the preparations.

(7) Sodium chloride or other excipients may be added to aqueous injections to adjust them isotonic to blood or other body fluids. Acids or alkalis may be added to adjust the pH.

(8) Injections supplied in multiple-dose containers may be added sufficient amounts of suitable preservatives to prevent the growth of microorganisms.

(9) Unless otherwise specified, Injections and vehicles attached to preparations other than those used exclusively for intracutaneous, subcutaneous or intramuscular administration meet the requirements of Bacterial Endotoxins Test <*4.01*>. In the case where the Bacterial Endotoxins Test <*4.01*> is not applicable, Pyrogen Test <*4.04*> may be applied instead.

(10) Unless otherwise specified, Injections and vehicles attached to preparations meet the requirements of Sterility Test <*4.06*>.

(11) Containers of Injections are colorless and meet the requirements of Test for Glass Containers for Injections <*7.01*>. Where specified in individual monographs, these containers may be replaced by colored containers meeting the requirements of Test for Glass Containers for Injections <*7.01*> or by plastic containers for aqueous injections meeting the requirements of Test Methods for Plastic Containers <*7.02*>.

(12) Unless otherwise specified, rubber closures used for glass containers of 100 mL or more of aqueous infusions meet the requirements of Test for Rubber Closure for Aqueous Infusions <*7.03*>.

(13) Unless otherwise specified, Injections and vehicles attached to preparations meet the requirements of Foreign Insoluble Matter Test for Injections <*6.06*>.

(14) Unless otherwise specified, Injections and vehicles attached to preparations meet the requirements of Insoluble Particulate Matter Test for Injections <*6.07*> or Insoluble Particulate Matter Test for Therapeutic Protein Injections <*6.17*>.

(15) Unless otherwise specified, the actual volume of Injections meets the requirements of Test for Extractable Volume of Parenteral Preparations <*6.05*>.

(16) Unless otherwise specified, Injections to be dissolved or suspended before use meet the requirements of Uniformity of Dosage Units <*6.02*>.

(17) Among the suspensions for injection in unit-dose containers, the preparations that could impair the uniform dispersion upon standing have an appropriate uniformity.

(18) Suspensions for injection are usually not to be injected into the blood vessels or spinal cord, and emulsions for injection are not to be injected into the spinal cord.

(19) The maximum size of particles observed in suspensions for injection is usually not larger than 150 μm, and that of particles in emulsions for injection is usually not larger than 7 μm.

(20) The following information, unless otherwise specified, must be written on the package leaflet, or the container or wrapper.

(i) In cases where the vehicle is not specified, the name of the employed vehicle, with the exception of Water for Injection, sodium chloride solution not exceeding 0.9 w/v% and those vehicles in which acids or alkalis are used in order to adjust the pH.

(ii) In case of vehicle attached to preparation, the name of the vehicle, content volume, ingredients and quantities or ratios, and a statement of the presence of the vehicle on the outer container or outer wrapper.

(iii) Name and quantity of stabilizers, preservatives, and diluents if added. In the case where nitrogen or carbon dioxide is filled in the container to replace the air inside, a statement of this replacement is not required.

(21) For ampoules or other containers of 2 mL or less, the designations "injection", "for injection" and "aqueous suspension for injection" may be replaced by "inj.", "for inj." and "aq. susp. for inj.", respectively.

For ampoules or other containers of more than 2 mL and not exceeding 10 mL, made of glass or similar materials, the designations "injection", "for injection" and "aqueous suspension for injection" may be abbreviated in the same way as above, when the information is printed directly on the surface of ampoules or containers.

(22) Hermetic containers or tight containers which are able to prevent microbial contamination are usually used for the preparations. For the preparations susceptible to degradation by evaporation of water, a low-moisture-permeability container or packaging may be used.

3-1-1. Parenteral Infusions

(1) Parenteral Infusions are usually injections of not less than 100 mL, intended for intravenous administration.

(2) Parenteral Infusions are mainly administered for the purpose of water supply, correction of electro-

lyte abnormality and nutritional support, and they are also used by mixing with other injections for treatments by continual infusion.

3-1-2. Implants/Pellets

(1) Implants/Pellets are solid or gel-like form injections, intended for subcutaneous or intramuscular administration by means of an implant device or operative treatment, for the purpose of releasing active substance(s) for a long period of time.

(2) Implants/Pellets are usually prepared in a form of pellet, microsphere or gel using biodegradable polymers.

(3) Unless otherwise specified, Implants/Pellets meet the requirements of Uniformity of Dosage Units *<6.02>*.

(4) Implants/Pellets have an appropriate function of controlled release.

(5) Foreign Insoluble Matter Test for Injections, Insoluble Particulate Matter for Injections and Test for Extractable Volume of Parenteral Preparations are not required for Implants/Pellets.

3-1-3. Prolonged Release Injections

(1) Prolonged Release Injections are injections to be used for intramuscular administration, for the purpose of releasing active substance(s) for a long period of time.

(2) Prolonged Release Injections are usually prepared by dissolving or suspending active substance(s) in a non-aqueous vehicle such as vegetable oil, or by suspending microspheres prepared with biodegradable polymers.

(3) Prolonged Release Injections have an appropriate function of controlled release.

3-1-4. Liposome Injections

(1) Liposome Injections are injections to be used for intravenous administration, which are intended for improvement of in vivo stability, delivery to a target region and control of release, of active substance(s).

(2) Liposome Injections are usually prepared by using amphipathic lipid, etc. to make aqueous injections or freeze-dried injections in which closed microvesicles composed of a lipid bilayer membrane are dispersed.

(3) Liposome Injections have an appropriate function of controlled release.

(4) Liposome Injections have an appropriate particle size.

4. Preparations for Dialysis

4-1. Dialysis Agents

(1) Dialysis Agents are preparations in liquid, or in solid which are to be dissolved before use, intended for peritoneal dialysis or hemodialysis.

They are classified into Peritoneal dialysis agents and Hemodialysis agents.

(2) Unless otherwise specified, Dialysis Agents meet the requirements of Bacterial Endotoxins Test *<4.01>*.

(3) The solid preparations which are to be dissolved before use among Dialysis agents have an appropriate uniformity of dosage units.

4-1-1. Peritoneal Dialysis Agents

(1) Peritoneal Dialysis Agents are sterile dialysis agents, intended to be used for peritoneal dialysis.

(2) Peritoneal Dialysis Agents are usually prepared by dissolving active substance(s) with suitable excipients in a vehicle to make a certain volume, or by filling active substance(s) combined with suitable excipients in a container, and sealing it. Sterilize if necessary. Every care should be taken to prevent microbial contamination. The overall processes from preparation to sterilization for preparing the agents should be completed as rapidly as possible, taking into consideration the composition of the agents and the storage conditions. The concentration of Peritoneal dialysis agents expressed in % represents w/v%. In the case of solid preparations which are dissolved before use, prepare as directed under 1-1. Tablets or 1-3. Granules.

(3) If necessary, pH adjusting agents, isotonic agents or other excipients may be added.

(4) Unless otherwise specified, the vehicle used for Peritoneal dialysis agents is Water for Injection.

(5) Unless otherwise specified, Peritoneal Dialysis Agents meet the requirements of Sterility Test *<4.06>*.

(6) Unless otherwise specified, Peritoneal Dialysis Agents meet the requirements of 4. Parenteral infusions under Test for Extractable Volume of Parenteral Preparations *<6.05>*. The mass (g) of content may convert to the volume (mL) by dividing by the density.

(7) Unless otherwise specified, Peritoneal Dialysis Agents meet the requirements of Foreign Insoluble Matter Test for Injections *<6.06>*.

(8) Unless otherwise specified, Peritoneal Dialysis Agents meet the requirements of Insoluble Particulate Matter Test for Injections *<6.07>*.

(9) Colorless containers meeting the requirements of Test for Glass Containers for Injections *<7.01>* are used for Peritoneal Dialysis Agents. Where specified otherwise, the colored containers meeting the requirements of Test for Glass Containers for Injections *<7.01>* or the plastic containers for aqueous injections meeting the requirements of Test Methods for Plastic Containers *<7.02>* may be used.

(10) Unless otherwise specified, the rubber closures of the containers meet the requirements of Test for Rubber Closure for Aqueous Infusions *<7.03>*.

(11) Hermetic containers, or tight containers which are able to prevent microbial contamination are usually used for Peritoneal Dialysis Agents. For the preparations susceptible to degradation by evaporation of water, a low-moisture-permeability container

or packaging may be used.

4-1-2. Hemodialysis Agents

(1) Hemodialysis agents are dialysis agents to be used for hemodialysis.

(2) Hemodialysis Agents are usually prepared by dissolving active substance(s) with excipients in a vehicle to make a certain volume, or by filling active substance(s) with excipient(s) in a container. In the case of the solid preparations to be dissolved before use, prepare as directed under 1-1. Tablets or 1-3. Granules.

(3) If necessary, pH adjusting agents, isotonic agents or other excipients may be added.

(4) Unless otherwise specified, the vehicle used for Hemodialysis agents is Water for Injection or water suitable for dialysis.

(5) Tight containers which are able to prevent microbial contamination are usually used for Hemodialysis Agents. For the preparations susceptible to degradation by evaporation of water, a low-moisture-permeability container or packaging may be used.

5. Preparations for Inhalation

5-1. Inhalations

(1) Inhalations are preparations intended for administration as aerosols to the bronchial tubes or lung.

Inhalations are classified into Dry Powder Inhalers, Inhalation Liquid Preparations and Metered-dose Inhalers.

(2) For administration of Inhalations, suitable devices or apparatus are used, or they are placed in containers which have an appropriate function of inhalation device.

5-1-1. Dry Powder Inhalers

(1) Dry Powder Inhalers are preparations which deliver a constant respiratory intake, intended for administration as solid particle aerosols.

(2) Dry Powder Inhalers are usually prepared by pulverizing active substance(s) into fine particles. Where necessary, lactose or other suitable excipients are added to make homogenous mixture.

(3) Metered-dose types among Dry Powder Inhalers meet the requirements of Uniformity of Delivered Dose for Inhalations <*6.14*>, unless otherwise specified.

(4) Dry Powder Inhalers meet the requirements of Aerodynamic Particle Size Measurement for Inhalations <*6.15*>, unless otherwise specified.

(5) Well-closed containers are usually used for Dry Powder Inhalers. For the preparations susceptible to degradation by moisture, a moisture-proof container or packaging may be used.

5-1-2. Inhalation Liquids and Solutions

(1) Inhalation Liquid Preparations are liquid inhalations which are administered by an inhalation device such as operating nebulizers.

(2) Inhalation Liquid Preparations are usually prepared by mixing active substance(s) with a vehicle and suitable isotonic agents and/or pH adjusting agents to make a solution or suspension, and by filtering where necessary.

(3) Sufficient amounts of suitable preservatives may be added to Inhalation Liquid Preparations to prevent the growth of microorganisms.

(4) Tight containers are usually used for Inhalation Liquid Preparations. For the preparations susceptible to degradation by evaporation of water, a low-moisture-permeability container or packaging may be used.

5-1-3. Metered-dose Inhalers

(1) Metered-dose Inhalers are preparations which deliver a constant dose of active substance(s) from the container together with propellant filled in.

(2) Metered-dose Inhalers are usually prepared by dissolving active substance(s) with a suitable dispersing agents and stabilizers in a vehicle to make a solution or suspension, and by filling in pressure-resistant containers together with liquid propellant, and setting metering valves.

(3) Metered-dose Inhalers meet the requirements of Uniformity of Delivered Dose for Inhalations <*6.14*>, unless otherwise specified.

(4) Metered-dose Inhalers meet the requirements of Aerodynamic Particle Size Measurement for Inhalations <*6.15*>, unless otherwise specified.

(5) Pressure-resistant and hermetic containers are usually used for Metered-dose Inhalers.

6. Preparations for Ophthalmic Application

6-1. Ophthalmic Liquids and Solutions

(1) Ophthalmic Liquids and Solutions are sterile preparations of liquid, or solid to be dissolved or suspended before use, intended for application to the conjunctival sac or other ocular tissues.

(2) Ophthalmic Liquids and Solutions are usually prepared by dissolving, suspending active substance(s) in a vehicle after adding excipients to make a constant volume, or mixing active substance(s) and excipients, and filling into containers. The overall processes, from preparation to sterilization, should be completed with sufficient care to prevent microbial contamination as rapidly as possible, taking into consideration the composition of the preparations and the storage conditions. The concentration of active substance expressed in % represents w/v%.

Ophthalmic Liquids and Solutions to be dissolved or suspended before use and designated in the name as ''for ophthalmic application'' may be accompanied by a vehicle for dissolving or suspending the preparation (hereinafter referred to as ''vehicle attached to preparation'').

(3) Vehicles to prepare Ophthalmic Liquids and Solutions or vehicle attached to the preparations must

be harmless in the amounts usually administered and must not interfere with the therapeutic efficacy of the active substance(s).

Vehicles for Ophthalmic Liquids and Solutions are classified into the following two groups.

(i) Aqueous vehicles: As the vehicles for the aqueous preparations Purified Water or suitable aqueous vehicles are used. For vehicles attached to the preparations sterilized Purified Water or sterilized aqueous vehicles are used.

(ii) Non-aqueous vehicles: As the vehicles for the non-aqueous preparations vegetable oils are usually used. Suitable organic solvents may be also used as the non-aqueous vehicles.

(4) Unless otherwise specified, any coloring agents must not be added solely for the purpose of coloring Ophthalmic Liquids and Solutions or vehicles attached to the preparations.

(5) Sodium chloride or other excipients may be added to Ophthalmic Liquids and Solutions to adjust them isotonic to lacrimal fluid. Acids or alkalis may be also added to adjust the pH.

(6) Unless otherwise specified, Ophthalmic Liquids and Solutions and vehicles attached to the preparations meet the requirements of Sterility Test <*4.06*>.

(7) Sufficient amounts of appropriate preservatives to prevent the growth of microorganisms may be added to the preparations filled in multiple dose containers.

(8) Unless otherwise specified, Ophthalmic Liquids and Solutions prepared in aqueous solutions or the vehicles attached to the preparations meet the requirements of Foreign Insoluble Matter Test for Ophthalmic Solutions <*6.11*>.

(9) Unless otherwise specified, Ophthalmic Liquids and Solutions and the vehicles attached to the preparations meet the requirements of Insoluble Particulate Matter Test for Ophthalmic Solutions <*6.08*>.

(10) The maximum particle size observed in Ophthalmic suspensions is usually not larger than 75 μm.

(11) Transparent tight containers, which do not disturb the test of Foreign Insoluble Matter Test for Ophthalmic Solutions <*6.11*>, are usually used for Ophthalmic Liquids and Solutions. For the preparations susceptible to degradation by evaporation of water, a low-moisture-permeability container or packaging may be used.

6-2. Ophthalmic Ointments

(1) Ophthalmic Ointments are sterile preparations of semi-solid, intended for application to the conjunctival sac or other ocular tissues.

(2) Ophthalmic Ointments are usually prepared by mixing homogeneously solution of or finely powdered active substance(s) with petrolatum or other bases, and filling into containers. The overall processes, from preparation to sterilization, should be completed with sufficient care to prevent microbial contamination as rapidly as possible, taking into consideration the composition of the preparations and the storage conditions.

(3) Sufficient amounts of suitable preservatives may be added to Ophthalmic Ointments filled in multiple dose containers to prevent the growth of microorganisms.

(4) Unless otherwise specified, Ophthalmic Ointments meet the requirements of Sterility Test <*4.06*>, and unless otherwise specified, the test is carried out by the Membrane filtration method.

(5) Unless otherwise specified, Ophthalmic Ointments meet the requirements of Test for Metal Particles in Ophthalmic Ointments <*6.01*>.

(6) The maximum particle size of active substance(s) in Ophthalmic Ointments is usually not larger than 75 μm.

(7) Ophthalmic Ointments have a suitable viscosity for applying to the ocular tissues.

(8) Tight containers which are able to prevent microbial contamination are usually used for Ophthalmic Ointments. For the preparations susceptible to degradation by evaporation of water, a low-moisture-permeability container or packaging may be used.

7. Preparations for Otic Application

7-1. Ear Preparations

(1) Ear Preparations are liquid, semi-solid, or solid preparations which are to be dissolved or suspended before use, intended for application to the external or internal ear.

(2) Ear Preparations are usually prepared by filling in containers with liquids in which active substance(s) and excipients are dissolved or suspended in a vehicle to make a constant volume, or with powders in which active substance(s) and excipients are mixed. The overall processes, from preparation to sterilization, should be completed with sufficient care to prevent microbial contamination as rapidly as possible, taking into consideration the composition of the preparations and the storage conditions. The concentration of active substance of Ear Preparations expressed in % represents w/v%.

In the case where the sterile preparations are prepared, proceed as directed under 6-1. Ophthalmic Liquids and Solutions.

Ear Preparations which are to be dissolved or suspended before use and designated in the name as ''for otic preparation'' may be accompanied by a vehicle to dissolve or suspend (hereinafter referred to as ''vehicle attached to preparation'').

(3) Vehicles used for Ear Preparations or the vehicle attached to the preparation are classified into the following two groups.

(i) Aqueous vehicles: As the vehicles for the aqueous preparations or the vehicles attached to the preparations, Purified Water or suitable aqueous vehicles are used. For the sterile preparations, Sterilized Purified Water or suitable sterilized aqueous vehicles are used as the vehicle attached to the preparations.

(ii) Non-aqueous vehicles: As the vehicles for the non-aqueous preparations vegetable oils are usually used. Suitable organic solvents may be also used as non-aqueous vehicles.

(4) Unless otherwise specified, any coloring agents must not be added solely for the purpose of coloring Ear Preparations or vehicle attached to the preparations.

(5) Sufficient amounts of suitable preservatives to prevent the growth of microorganisms may be added to the preparations filled in multiple dose containers.

(6) Unless otherwise specified, sterile Ear preparations and the vehicles attached to the sterile preparations meet the requirements of Sterility Test *<4.06>*.

(7) Tight containers are usually used for Ear Preparations. For the preparations susceptible to degradation by evaporation of water, a low-moisture-permeability container or packaging may be used.

8. Preparations for Nasal Application

8-1. Nasal Preparations

(1) Nasal Preparations are preparations intended for application to the nasal cavities or nasal mucous membrane.

Nasal preparations are classified into Nasal dry powder inhalers and Nasal Liquid Preparations.

(2) Where necessary, Nasal Preparations are sprayed for inhalation by using a suitable atomizing device such as spray-pump.

(3) Unless otherwise specified, metered-dose type preparations among Nasal Preparations show the appropriate uniformity of delivered dose.

8-1-1. Nasal Dry Powder Inhalers

(1) Nasal Dry Powder Inhalers are fine powdered preparations, intended for application to the nasal cavities.

(2) Nasal Dry Powder Inhalers are usually prepared by pulverizing active substance(s) into moderately fine particles, or by mixing homogeneously with excipients where necessary.

(3) Well-closed containers are usually used for Nasal Dry Powder Inhalers. For the preparations susceptible to degradation by moisture, a moisture-proof container or packaging may be used.

8-1-2. Nasal Liquids and Solutions

(1) Nasal Liquids and Solutions are liquid preparations, or solid preparations to be dissolved or suspended before use, intended for application to the nasal cavities.

(2) Nasal Liquids and Solutions are usually prepared by dissolving or suspending active substance(s) in a vehicle together with excipients, and filtering where necessary. Isotonic agents and/or pH adjusting agents may be used.

(3) Nasal Liquids and Solutions, which are to be dissolved or suspended before use and designated in the name as "for nasal application", may be accompanied by a vehicle to dissolve or suspend.

(4) Sufficient amounts of suitable preservatives to prevent the growth of microorganisms may be added to the preparations filled in multiple dose containers.

(5) Tight containers are usually used for Nasal Liquids and Solutions. For the preparations susceptible to degradation by evaporation of water, a low-moisture-permeability container or packaging may be used.

9. Preparations for Rectal Application

9-1. Suppositories for Rectal Application

(1) Suppositories for Rectal Application are semi-solid preparations of a desired shape and size, intended for intrarectal application, which release active substance(s) by melting at body temperature or dissolving or dispersing gradually in the secretions.

(2) Suppositories for Rectal Application are usually prepared by mixing homogenously active substance(s) and excipients such as dispersing agents and emulsifying agents, dissolving or suspending uniformly in a base which is liquefied by warming, filling a constant volume of the resultant material into containers, and molding it into a shape and size. Lipophilic bases or hydrophilic bases are usually used.

(3) Suppositories for Rectal Application are usually a conical- or spindle-shaped.

(4) Unless otherwise specified, Suppositories for Rectal Application meet the requirements of Uniformity of Dosage Units *<6.02>*.

(5) Suppositories for Rectal Application show an appropriate release. Release of Suppositories for Rectal Application prepared using a lipophilic base can be evaluated by melting behavior of suppositories in place of release of active substances. When the melting behavior of Suppositories for Rectal Application is measured according to Method 2 under Melting Point Determination *<2.60>* unless otherwise specified, it shows an appropriate melting temperature.

(6) Well-closed containers are usually used for Suppositories for Rectal Application. For the preparations susceptible to degradation by moisture, a moisture-proof container or packaging may be used.

9-2. Semi-solid Preparations for Rectal Application

(1) Semi-solid Preparations for Rectal Application are preparations which are in a form of cream, gel or ointment intended for application to around or inside

of the anus.

(2) Semi-solid Preparations for Rectal Application are usually prepared by emulsifying active substance(s) with excipients in Purified Water and oil component such as vaseline, or by homogenously mixing active substance(s) and excipients in a base of polymer gel or grease.

(i) Creams for rectal application: Prepare as directed under 11-5. Creams.

(ii) Gels for rectal application: Prepare as directed under 11-6. Gels.

(iii) Ointments for rectal application: Prepare as directed under 11-4. Ointments.

For the preparations which are apt to deteriorate, prepare before use.

(3) Sufficient amounts of suitable preservatives to prevent the growth of microorganisms may be added to the Preparations filled in multiple dose containers.

(4) Semi-solid Preparations for Rectal Application have a suitable viscosity for applying to the rectum.

(5) Tight containers are usually used for Semi-solid Preparations for Rectal Application. For the preparations susceptible to degradation by evaporation of water, a low-moisture-permeability container or packaging may be used.

9-3. Enemas for Rectal Application

(1) Enemas for Rectal Application are preparations in liquid form or viscous and gelatinous state, intended for application via the anus.

(2) Enemas for Rectal Application are usually prepared by dissolving or suspending active substance(s) in Purified Water or a suitable aqueous vehicle to make a given volume, and filling in containers. Dispersing agents, stabilizers and/or pH adjusting agents may be used.

(3) Tight containers are usually used for Enemas for Rectal Application. For the preparations susceptible to degradation by evaporation of water, a low-moisture-permeability container or packaging may be used.

10. Preparations for Vaginal Application

10-1. Tablets for Vaginal Use

(1) Tablets for Vaginal Use are solid preparations of a desired shape and size, intended for application to the vagina, which release active substance(s) by dissolving or dispersing gradually in the secretions.

(2) Tablets for Vaginal Use are usually prepared as directed under 1-1. Tablets.

(3) Unless otherwise specified, Tablets for Vaginal Use meet the requirements of Uniformity of Dosage Units <*6.02*>.

(4) Tablets for Vaginal Use show an appropriate release.

(5) Well-closed containers are usually used for Tablets for Vaginal Use. For the preparations susceptible to degradation by moisture, a moisture-proof container or packaging may be used.

10-2. Suppositories for Vaginal Use

(1) Suppositories for Vaginal Use are semi-solid preparations of a desired shape and size, intended for application to the vagina, which release active substance(s) by melting at body temperature or by dissolving or dispersing gradually in the secretions.

(2) Suppositories for Vaginal Use are prepared according to 9-1. Suppositories for Rectal Application.

(3) Suppositories for Vaginal Use are usually spherical or ovoid shaped.

(4) Unless otherwise specified, Suppositories for Vaginal Use meet the requirements of Uniformity of Dosage Units <*6.02*>.

(5) Suppositories for Vaginal Use show an appropriate release. Release of Suppositories for Vaginal Use prepared using a lipophilic base can be evaluated by melting behavior of suppositories in place of release of active substances. When the melting behavior of Suppositories for Vaginal Use is measured according to Method 2 under Melting Point Determination <*2.60*> unless otherwise specified, it shows an appropriate melting temperature.

(6) Well-closed containers are usually used for Suppositories for Vaginal Use. For the preparations susceptible to degradation by moisture, a moisture-proof container or packaging may be used.

11. Preparations for Cutaneous Application

(1) Preparations for Cutaneous Application also include Transdermal Systems which are intended for percutaneous absorption to deliver active substance(s) to the systemic circulation through the skin. The release rate of active substance(s) from Transdermal Systems is generally appropriately controlled.

11-1. Solid Preparations for Cutaneous Application

(1) Solid Preparations for Cutaneous Application are solid preparations intended for application to the skin (including scalp) or nails. Powders for Cutaneous Application are included in this category.

(2) Unless otherwise specified, Solid Preparations for Cutaneous Application in single-dose packages meet the requirements of Uniformity of Dosage Units <*6.02*>.

(3) Well-closed containers are usually used for Solid Preparations for Cutaneous Application. For the preparations susceptible to degradation by moisture, a moisture-proof container or packaging may be used.

11-1-1. Powders for Cutaneous Application

(1) Powders for Cutaneous Application are powdery solid preparations intended for external application.

(2) Powders for Cutaneous Application are usually prepared by mixing homogeneously active substance(s) and excipients such as diluents and pulverizing the mixture.

11-2. Liquids and Solutions for Cutaneous Application

(1) Liquids and Solutions for Cutaneous Application are liquid preparations intended for application to the skin (including scalp) or nails. Liniments and Lotions are included in this category.

(2) Liquids and Solutions for Cutaneous Application are usually prepared by mixing active substance(s) and excipients in a vehicle, and filtering if necessary.

For the preparations which are apt to deteriorate, prepare before use.

(3) Unless otherwise specified, Liquids and Solutions for Cutaneous Application in single-dose packages such as Transdermal Systems meet the requirements of Uniformity of Dosage Units <*6.02*>.

(4) Tight containers are usually used for Liquids and Solutions for Cutaneous Application. For the preparations susceptible to degradation by evaporation of water, a low-moisture-permeability container or packaging may be used.

11-2-1. Liniments

(1) Liniments are liquid or muddy preparations intended for external application to the skin by rubbing.

11-2-2. Lotions

(1) Lotions are external liquids in which active substance(s) are dissolved, emulsified or finely dispersed in an aqueous vehicle.

(2) Lotions are usually prepared by dissolving, suspending or emulsifying active substance(s) in Purified Water with excipients and making homogeneous as a whole.

(3) Lotions in which the components have separated out during storage may be used after mixing to re-homogenize them, provided that the active substance(s) has not deteriorated.

11-3. Sprays for Cutaneous Application

(1) Sprays for Cutaneous Application are preparations intended for spraying active substance(s) onto the skin in mists, powders, foams or paste state.

Sprays for Cutaneous Application are classified into Aerosols for Cutaneous Application and Pump Sprays for Cutaneous Application.

(2) Sprays for Cutaneous Application are usually prepared by dissolving or suspending active substance(s) in a vehicle, filtering where necessary, and filling in containers.

(3) Unless otherwise specified, metered-dose type sprays show an appropriate uniformity of delivered dose.

11-3-1. Aerosols for Cutaneous Application

(1) Aerosols for Cutaneous Application are sprays which atomize active substance(s) together with liquefied or compressed gas filled in containers.

(2) Aerosols for Cutaneous Application are usually prepared by dissolving or suspending active substance(s) in a vehicle, filling with liquefied propellants in pressure-resistant containers, and setting a continuous spray valve. If necessary, dispersing agents and stabilizers may be used.

(3) Pressure-resistant containers are usually used for Aerosols for Cutaneous Application.

11-3-2. Pump Sprays for Cutaneous Application

(1) Pump Sprays for Cutaneous Application are sprays which atomize active substance(s) in containers by pumping.

(2) Pump Sprays for Cutaneous Application are usually prepared by dissolving or suspending active substance(s) with excipients in a vehicle, filling in containers and setting pumps to the containers.

(3) Tight containers are usually used for Pump Sprays for Cutaneous Application. For the preparations susceptible to degradation by evaporation of water, a low-moisture-permeability container or packaging may be used.

11-4. Ointments

(1) Ointments are semi-solid preparations to be applied to the skin, which dissolve or disperse active substance(s) in a base. There are two types, hydrophobic ointments and hydrophilic ointments.

(2) Hydrophobic ointments are usually prepared by warming to melt hydrophobic bases such as fatty oils, waxes or paraffin, adding and mixing active substance(s) in the bases to be dissolved or dispersed, and kneading the whole to make homogeneous.

Hydrophilic ointments are usually prepared by warming to melt hydrophilic bases such as macrogol, adding and mixing active substance(s) in the bases, and kneading the whole to make homogeneous.

For Ointments which are apt to deteriorate, prepare before use.

(3) Ointments have a suitable viscosity for application to the skin.

(4) Tight containers are usually used for Ointments. For the preparations susceptible to degradation by evaporation of water, a low-moisture-permeability container or packaging may be used.

11-5. Creams

(1) Creams are semi-solid preparations to be applied to the skin, which are in the form of oil-in-water or water-in-oil emulsions. Hydrophobic preparations in the form of water-in-oil emulsions may be termed "Oily creams".

(2) Creams are usually prepared by mixing homogenously and emulsifying an oil-phase compo-

nent and a water-phase component, both warmed, of which either one contains the active substance(s). These components have the following constituents.

Oil-phase component: Vaseline, fatty alcohols, etc., with or without emulsifying agent(s) or other suitable excipients.

Water-phase component: Purified Water with or without emulsifying agent(s) or other suitable excipients.

For Creams which are apt to deteriorate, prepare before use.

(3) Creams have a suitable viscosity for applying to the skin.

(4) Tight containers are usually used for Creams. For the preparations susceptible to degradation by evaporation of water, a low-moisture-permeability container or packaging may be used.

11-6. Gels

(1) Gels are gelatinous preparations intended for application to the skin.

There are Aqueous Gels and Oily Gels.

(2) Gels are usually prepared by the following methods.

(i) Aqueous Gels: To active substance(s) add polymers, other excipients and Purified Water, dissolve or suspend, and gelatinize by warming and cooling or by adding a gelatinizing agents.

(ii) Oily Gels: To active substance(s) add liquid oily bases such as glycols, fatty alcohols and other excipients, and mix.

(3) Gels have a suitable viscosity for application to the skin.

(4) Tight containers are usually used for Gels. For the preparations susceptible to degradation by evaporation of water, a low-moisture-permeability container or packaging may be used.

11-7. Patches

(1) Patches are preparations intended to be attached on the skin.

Patches are classified into Tapes/Plasters and Cataplasms/Gel Patches.

(2) Patches are usually prepared by mixing active substance(s) homogeneously with a base such as a polymer or a mixture of polymers, spreading on a backing layer or liner, and cutting into a given size. Percutaneous absorption type preparations may be prepared by using a release rate-controlling membrane. Where necessary, adhesive agents or penetration enhancers may be used.

(3) Unless otherwise specified, Patches of Transdermal Systems meet the requirements of Uniformity of Dosage Units <*6.02*>.

(4) Unless otherwise specified, Patches meet the requirement of Methods of Adhesion Testing <*6.12*>.

(5) Unless otherwise specified, Patches meet the requirement of Release Test for Preparations for Cutaneous Application <*6.13*>.

11-7-1. Tapes

(1) Tapes are patches which are prepared with bases containing practically no water.

Plasters are included in this category.

(2) Tapes are usually prepared by mixing homogeneously active substance(s) with or without excipients and a base of non water-soluble natural or synthetic polymers such as resins, plastics or rubber, and spreading on a cloth or spreading and sealing on a cloth or plastic film, cutting into a given size. The preparations may be also prepared by filling a mixture of active substance(s) and a base with or without other excipients in releasers composed with a release-controlling film, supporter and liner.

(3) Well-closed containers are usually used for Tapes. For the preparations susceptible to degradation by moisture, a moisture-proof container or packaging may be used.

11-7-2. Cataplasms/Gel Patches

(1) Cataplasms/Gel Patches are patches using water containing bases.

(2) Cataplasms/Gel patches are usually prepared by mixing active substance(s), Purified Water, and Glycerin or other liquid materials, or by mixing and kneading natural or synthetic polymers, which are soluble in water or absorbent of water, with Purified Water, adding active substance(s), mixing the whole homogeneously, spreading on a cloth or film, and cutting into a given size.

(3) Tight containers are usually used for Cataplasms/Gel Patches. For the preparations susceptible to degradation by evaporation of water, a low-moisture-permeability container or packaging may be used.

[4] Monographs for Preparations Related to Crude Drugs

Preparations Related to Crude Drugs

(1) Preparations related to crude drugs are preparations mainly derived from crude drugs. Extracts, Pills, Spirits, Infusions and Decoctions, Teabags, Tinctures, Aromatic Waters, and Fluidextracts are included in this category.

Definitions, methods of preparations, test methods, containers and packaging, and storage of these preparations are described in this chapter.

(2) The descriptions of the test methods and the containers and packaging in this chapter are fundamental requirements, and the preparation methods represent commonly used methods.

1. Extracts

(1) Extracts are preparations, prepared by concentrating extractives of crude drugs. There are following two kinds of extracts.

(i) Viscous extracts

(ii) Dry extracts

(2) Unless otherwise specified, Extracts are usually prepared as follows.

(i) Crude drugs, pulverized to suitable sizes, are extracted for a certain period of time with suitable solvents by means of cold extraction or warm extraction, or by percolation as directed in (ii) of (2) under 6. Tinctures. The extractive is filtered, and the filtrate is concentrated or dried by a suitable method to make a millet jelly-like consistency for the viscous extracts, or to make crushable solid masses, granules or powder for the dry extracts.

Extracts, which are specified the content of active substance(s), are prepared by assaying active substance(s) in a portion of sample and adjusting, if necessary, to specified strength with suitable diluents.

(ii) Weigh crude drugs, pulverized to suitable sizes, according to the prescription and heat for a certain period of time after adding 10 - 20 times amount of water. After separating the solid and liquid by centrifugation, the extractive is concentrated or dried by a suitable method to make a millet jelly-like consistency for the viscous extracts, or to make crushable solid masses, granules or powder for the dry extracts.

(3) Extracts have order and taste derived from the crud drugs used.

(4) Unless otherwise specified, Extracts meet the requirements of Heavy Metals Limit Test <*1.07*> when the test solution and the control solution are prepared as follows.

Test solution: Ignite 0.30 g of Extracts to ash, add 3 mL of dilute hydrochloric acid, warm, and filter. Wash the residue with two 5-mL portions of water. Neutralize the combined filtrate and washings (indicator: a drop of phenolphthalein TS) by adding ammonia TS until the color of the solution changes to pale red, filter where necessary, and add 2 mL of dilute acetic acid and water to make 50 mL.

Control solution: Proceed with 3 mL of dilute hydrochloric acid in the same manner as directed in the preparation of the test solution, and add 3.0 mL of Standard Lead Solution and water to make 50 mL.

(5) Tight containers are used for these preparations.

2. Pills

(1) Pills are spherical preparations, intended for oral administration.

(2) Pills are usually prepared by mixing drug substance(s) uniformly with diluents, binders, disintegrators or other suitable excipient(s) and rolling into spherical form by a suitable method. They may be coated with a coating agent by a suitable method.

(3) Unless otherwise specified, Pills comply with Disintegration Test <*6.09*>.

(4) Well-closed or tight containers are usually used for these preparations.

3. Spirits

(1) Spirits are fluid preparations, usually prepared by dissolving volatile drug substance(s) in ethanol or in a mixture of ethanol and water.

(2) Spirits should be stored remote from fire.

(3) Tight containers are used for these preparations.

4. Infusions and Decoctions

(1) Infusions and Decoctions are fluid preparations, usually obtained by macerating crude drugs in water.

(2) Infusions and Decoctions are usually prepared by the following method.

Cut crude drugs into a size as directed below, and transfer suitable amounts to an infusion or decoction apparatus.

Leaves, flowers and whole plants: Coarse cutting
Woods, stems, barks, roots and rhizomes
: Moderately fine cutting
Seeds and fruits: Fine cutting

(i) Infusions: Usually, damp 50 g of crude drugs with 50 mL of water for about 15 minutes, pour 900 mL of hot water to them, and heat for 5 minutes with several stirrings. Filter through a cloth after cooling.

(ii) Decoctions: Usually, heat one-day dose of crude drugs with 400 - 600 mL of water until to lose about a half amount of added water spending more than 30 minutes, and filter through a cloth while warm.

Prepare Infusions or Decoctions when used.

(3) These preparations have odor and taste derived from the crude drugs used.

(4) Tight containers are usually used for these preparations.

5. Teabags

(1) Teabags are preparations, usually packed one-day dose or one dose of crude drugs cut into a size of between coarse powder and coarse cutting in paper or cloth bags.

(2) Teabags are usually used according to the preparation method as directed under 4. Infusions and Decoctions.

(3) Well-closed or tight containers are usually used for these preparations.

6. Tinctures

(1) Tinctures are liquid preparations, usually prepared by extracting crude drugs with ethanol or with a mixture of ethanol and purified water.

(2) Unless otherwise specified, Tinctures are usually prepared from coarse powder or fine cuttings of crude drugs by means of either maceration or percolation as described below.

(i) Maceration: Place crude drugs in a suitable container, and add an amount of a solvent, equivalent to the same volume or about three-fourths of the volume of the crude drugs. Stopper container, and allow the container to stand for about 5 days or until the soluble constituents have satisfactorily dissolved at room temperature with occasional stirring. Separate the solid and liquid by centrifugation or other suitable methods. In the case where about three-fourths volume of the solvent is added, wash the residue with a suitable amount of the solvent, and squeeze the residue, if necessary. Combine the extract and washings, and add sufficient solvent to make up the volume. In the case where the total volume of the solvent is added, sufficient amounts of the solvent may be added to make up for reduced amount, if necessary. Allow the mixture to stand for about 2 days, and obtain a clear liquid by decantation or filtration.

(ii) Percolation: Pour solvent in small portions to crude drugs placed in a container, and mix well to moisten the crude drugs. Stopper container, and allow it to stand for about 2 hours at room temperature. Pack the contents as tightly as possible in an appropriate percolator, open the lower opening, and slowly pour sufficient solvent to cover the crude drugs. When the percolate begins to drip, close the opening, and allow the mixture to stand for 2 to 3 days at room temperature. Then, open the opening, and allow the percolate to drip at a rate of 1 to 3 mL per minute. Add an appropriate quantity of the solvent to the percolator, and continue to percolate until the desired volume has passed. Mix thoroughly, allow standing for 2 days, and obtain a clear liquid by decantation or filtration. The time of standing and the flow rate may be varied depending on the kind and amount of crude drugs to be percolated.

Tinctures, prepared by either of the above methods and specified the content of marker constituent or ethanol, are prepared by assaying the content using a portion of the sample and adjusting the content with a sufficient amount of the percolate or solvent as required on the basis of the result of the assay.

(3) Tinctures should be stored remote from fire.

(4) Tight containers are used for these preparations.

7. Aromatic Waters

(1) Aromatic Waters are clear liquid preparations, saturated essential oils or other volatile substances in water.

(2) Unless otherwise specified, Aromatic Waters are usually prepared by the following process.

Shake thoroughly for 15 minutes 2 mL of an essential oil or 2 g of a volatile substance with 1000 mL of lukewarm purified water, set the mixture aside for 12 hours or longer, filter through moistened filter paper, and add purified water to make 1000 mL. Alternatively, incorporate thoroughly 2 mL of an essential oil or 2 g of a volatile substance with sufficient talc, refined siliceous earth or pulped filter-paper, add 1000 mL of purified water, agitate thoroughly for 10 minutes, and then filter the mixture. To obtain a clear filtrate repeat the filtration if necessary, and add sufficient purified water passed through the filter paper to make 1000 mL.

(3) Aromatic Waters have odor and taste derived from the essential oils or volatile substances used.

(4) Tight containers are used for these preparations.

8. Fluidextracts

(1) Fluidextracts are liquid percolates of crude drugs, usually prepared so that each mL contains soluble constituents from 1 g of the crude drugs. Where the content is specified, it takes precedence.

(2) Unless otherwise specified, Fluidextracts are usually prepared from coarse powder or fine cutting of crude drugs by either of following maceration or percolation.

(i) Maceration: Place a certain amount of crude drugs in a suitable vessel, add a solvent to cover the crude drugs, close the vessel, and allow the vessel to stand at room temperature with occasional stirring for about 5 days or until the soluble constituents have satisfactorily dissolved. Separate the solid and liquid by centrifugation or other suitable method. Usually, reserve a volume of the liquid equivalent to about three-fourths of the total volume, and use it as the first liquid. Wash the residue with appropriate amount of the solvent, combine the washings and the remaining of the first liquid, concentrate if necessary, mix with the first liquid, and use it as solution (A). To the solution (A) add the solvent, if necessary, to make equal amount of the mass of the crude drugs. Allow the mixture to stand for about 2 days, and collect a clear liquid by decantation or filtration.

(ii) Percolation: Mix well 1000 g of the crude drugs with the first solvent to moisten them, close the container, and allow it to stand for about 2 hours at room temperature. Transfer the content to a suitable percolator, stuff it as tightly as possible, open the lower opening of the percolator, and slowly pour the second solvent to cover the crude drugs. Close the lower opening when the solvent begins to drop, and allow the mixture to stand for 2 to 3 days at room temperature. Open the lower opening, and allow the percolate to run out at the rate of 0.5 to 1.0 mL per minute.

Set aside the first 850 mL of the percolate as the first percolate. Add the second solvent to the percolator, then drip the percolate, and use it as the second percolate.

The period of standing and the flow rate during percolation may be varied depending on the kind and the amount of crude drugs used. The flow rate is usually regulated as follows, depending on the using amount of crude drugs.

Mass of crude drug	Volume of solution running per minute
Not more than 1000 g	0.5 – 1.0 mL
Not more than 3000 g	1.0 – 2.0 mL
Not more than 10000 g	2.0 – 4.0 mL

Concentrate the second percolate, taking care not to lose the volatile substances of the crude drug, mix with the first percolate, and use it as solution (A). To the solution (A) add the second solvent to make 1000 mL, and allow the mixture to stand for about 2 days. Decant the supernatant liquid or filter the liquid to obtain a clear solution.

Fluidextracts for which the content of marker constituent or ethanol is specified are obtained by adjusting the content with a sufficient amount of the second solvent as required on the basis of the result of the assay made with a portion of the solution (A).

(3) Fluidextracts have odor and taste derived from the crude drugs used.

(4) Unless otherwise specified, Fluidextracts meet the requirements of Heavy Metals Limit Test <*1.07*> when the test solution and the control solution are prepared as follows.

Test solution: Ignite 1.0 g of Fluidextracts to ash, add 3 mL of dilute hydrochloric acid, warm, and filter. Wash the residue with two 5-mL portions of water. Neutralize the combined filtrate and washings (indicator: a drop of phenolphthalein TS) by adding ammonia TS until the color of the solution changes to pale red, filter if necessary, and add 2 mL of the dilute acetic acid and water to make 50 mL.

Control solution: Proceed with 3 mL of dilute hydrochloric acid in the same manner as directed in the preparation of the test solution, and add 3.0 mL of Standard Lead Solution and water to make 50 mL.

(5) Tight containers are used for these preparations.

GENERAL TESTS, PROCESSES AND APPARATUS

General Tests, Processes and Apparatus includes common methods for tests, useful test methods for quality recognition of drugs and other articles related to them.

The number of each test method is a category number given individually according to its content.

1. Chemical Methods
2. Physical Methods
3. Powder Property Determinations
4. Biological Tests/Biochemical Tests/Microbial Tests
5. Tests for Crude Drugs
6. Tests for Preparations
7. Tests for Containers and Packaging Materials
8. Others*
9. Reference Standards; Standard Solutions; Reagents, Test Solutions; Measuring Instruments, Appliances, etc.

* At present there are no methods in this section.

The number in blackets (< >) appeared in monograph indicates the number corresponding to the general test method.

1. Chemical Methods

1.01 Alcohol Number Determination

Alcohol Number Determination represents the number of milliliters of ethanol at 15°C obtained from 10 mL of tincture or other preparations containing ethanol by the following procedures.

1. Method 1 Distilling method

This is a method to determine the Alcohol Number by reading the number of milliliters of ethanol distillate at 15°C obtained from 10 mL of a sample measured at 15°C by the following procedures.

1.1. Apparatus

Use hard glass apparatus as illustrated in Fig. 1.01-1. Ground glass may be used for the joints.

1.2. Reagent

Alkaline phenolphthalein solution: To 1 g of phenolphthalein add 7 mL of sodium hydroxide TS and water to make 100 mL.

1.3. Procedure

Transfer 10 mL of the sample preparation, accurately measured at 15 ± 2°C, to the distilling flask A, add 5 mL of water and boiling chips. Distil ethanol carefully into the glass-stoppered, volumetric cylinder D.

By reference to Table 1.01-1, a suitable volume of distillate (mL) should be collected, according to the content of ethanol in the sample preparation.

Prevent bumping during distillation by rendering the sample strongly acidic with phosphoric acid or sulfuric acid, or by adding a small amount of paraffin, beeswax or silicone resin before starting the distillation.

When the samples contain the following substances, carry out pretreatment as follows before distillation.

Table 1.01-1

Ethanol content in the sample (vol%)	Distillate to be collected (mL)
more than 80	13
80 – 70	12
70 – 60	11
60 – 50	10
50 – 40	9
40 – 30	8
less than 30	7

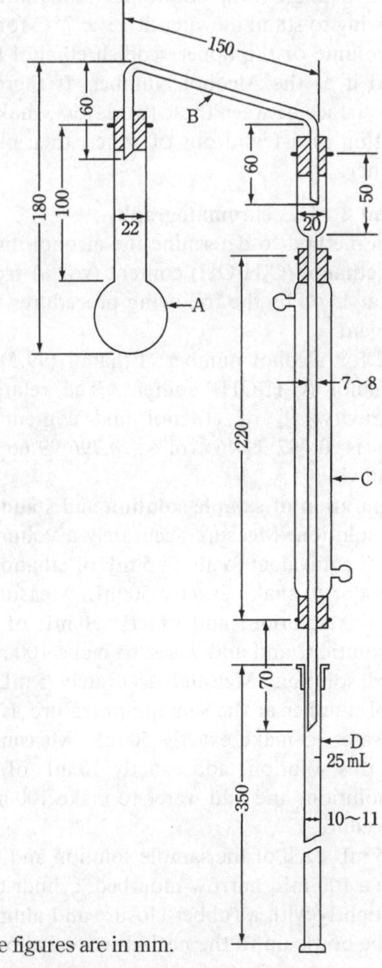

The figures are in mm.

A: Distilling flask (50 mL)
B: Delivery tube
C: Condenser
D: Glass-stoppered volumetric cylinder (25 mL, graduated in 0.1 mL)

Fig. 1.01-1

(i) Glycerin: Add sufficient water to the sample so that the residue in the distilling flask, after distillation, contains at least 50% of water.

(ii) Iodine: Decolorize the sample with zinc powder.

(iii) Volatile substances: Preparations containing appreciable proportions of essential oil, chloroform, diethyl ether or camphor require treatment as follows. Mix 10 mL of the sample, accurately measured, with 10 mL of saturated sodium chloride solution in a separator, add 10 mL of petroleum benzin, and shake. Collect the separated aqueous layer. The petroleum benzin layer was extracted with two 5 mL portions of saturated sodium chloride solution. Combine the aqueous layers, and distill. According to the ethanol content in the sample, collect a volume of distillate 2 to 3 mL more than that shown in the above Table.

(iv) Other substances: Render preparations containing free ammonia slightly acidic with dilute sulfuric acid. If volatile acids are present, render the preparation slightly alkaline with sodium hydroxide TS, and if the preparations contain soap along with volatile substances, decompose the soap with an excess of dilute sulfuric acid before the extraction with petroleum benzin in the treatment described in (iii).

To the distillate add 4 to 6 g of potassium carbonate and 1 to 2 drops of alkaline phenolphthalein solution, and shake vigorously. If the aqueous layer shows no white turbidity, agitate the distillate with additional potassium carbonate. After allowing to stand in water at 15 ± 2°C for 30 minutes, read the volume of the upper reddish ethanol layer in mL, and regard it as the Alcohol Number. If there is no clear boundary surface between these two layers, shake vigorously after addition of a few drops of water, then observe in the same manner.

2. Method 2 Gas chromatography

This is a method to determine the alcohol number by determining ethanol (C_2H_5OH) content (vol%) from a sample measured at 15°C by the following procedures.

2.1. Reagent

Ethanol for alcohol number: Ethanol (99.5) with determined ethanol (C_2H_5OH) content. The relation between specific gravity d^{15}_{15} of ethanol and content of ethanol (C_2H_5OH) is 0.797:99.46 vol%, 0.796:99.66 vol%, and 0.795:99.86 vol%.

2.2. Preparation of sample solution and standard solution

Sample solution: Measure accurately a volume of sample at 15 ± 2°C equivalent to about 5 mL of ethanol (C_2H_5OH), and add water to make exactly 50 mL. Measure accurately 25 mL of this solution, add exactly 10 mL of the internal standard solution, and add water to make 100 mL.

Standard solution: Measure accurately 5 mL of ethanol for alcohol number at the same temperature as the sample, and add water to make exactly 50 mL. Measure accurately 25 mL of this solution, add exactly 10 mL of the internal standard solution, and add water to make 100 mL.

2.3. Procedure

Place 25 mL each of the sample solution and the standard solution in a 100-mL, narrow-mouthed, cylindrical glass bottle sealed tightly with a rubber closure and aluminum band, immerse the bottle up to the neck in water, allowed to stand at room temperature for more than 1 hour in a room with little change in temperature, shake gently so as not to splash the solution on the closure, and allow to stand for 30 minutes. Perform the test with 1 mL each of the gas in the bottle with a syringe according to the Gas Chromatography <*2.02*> under the following conditions, and calculate the ratios, Q_T and Q_S, of the peak height of ethanol to that of the internal standard.

$$\text{Alcohol number} = \frac{Q_T}{Q_S} \times \frac{5\ (\text{mL})}{\text{a volume (mL) of sample}} \times \frac{\text{ethanol } (C_2H_5OH) \text{ content (vol\%) of ethanol for alcohol number}}{9.406}$$

Internal standard solution—A solution of acetonitrile (3 in 50).

Operating conditions—

Detector: A hydrogen flame-ionization detector.

Column: A glass tube about 3 mm in inside diameter and about 1.5 m in length, packed with 150- to 180-μm porous ethylvinylbenzene-divinylbenzene copolymer (mean pore size: 0.0075 μm, 500 – 600 m^2/g) for gas chromatography.

Column temperature: A constant temperature between 105°C and 115°C.

Carrier gas: Nitrogen.

Flow rate: Adjust so that the retention time of ethanol is 5 to 10 minutes.

Selection of column: Proceed with 1 mL of the gas obtained from the standard solution in the bottle under the above operating conditions, and calculate the resolution. Use a column giving elution of ethanol and the internal standard in this order with the resolution between these peaks being not less than 2.0.

1.02 Ammonium Limit Test

Ammonium Limit Test is a limit test for ammonium salt contained in drugs.

In each monograph, the permissible limit for ammonium (as NH_4^+) is described in terms of percentage (%) in parentheses.

1. Apparatus

Use a distilling apparatus for ammonium limit test as illustrated in Fig. 1.02-1. For the distillation under reduced pressure, use the apparatus shown in Fig. 1.02-2. Either apparatus are composed of hard glass, and ground-glass joints may be used. All rubber parts used in the apparatus should be boiled for 10 to 30 minutes in sodium hydroxide TS and for 30 to 60 minutes in water, and finally washed thoroughly with water before use.

2. Procedure

2.1. Preparation of test solution and control solution

Unless otherwise specified, test solutions and control solution are prepared as directed in the following.

Place an amount of the sample, directed in the monograph, in the distilling flask A. Add 140 mL of water and 2 g of magnesium oxide, and connect the distillation apparatus. To the receiver (measuring cylinder) F add 20 mL of boric acid solution (1 in 200) as an absorbing solution, and immerse the lower end of the condenser. Adjust the heating to give a rate of 5 to 7 mL per minute of distillate, and distill until the distillate measures 60 mL. Remove the receiver from the lower end of the condenser, rinsing the end part with a small quantity of water, add sufficient water to make 100 mL and designate it as the test solution.

For the distillation under reduced pressure, take the amount of sample specified in the monograph to the vacuum distillation flask L, add 70 mL of water and 1 g of magnesium oxide, and connect to the apparatus (Fig. 1.02-2). To the receiver M add 20 mL of a solution of boric acid (1 in 200) as absorbing liquid, put the end of the branch tube of

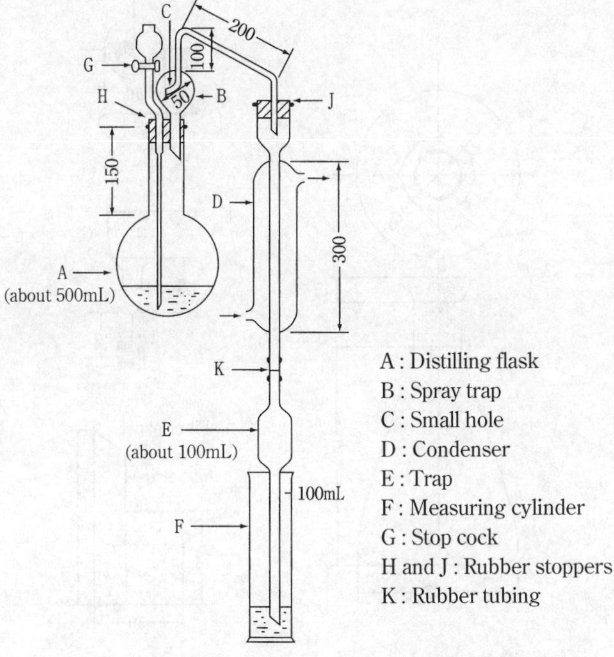

Fig. 1.02-1 Distilling apparatus for ammonium limit test

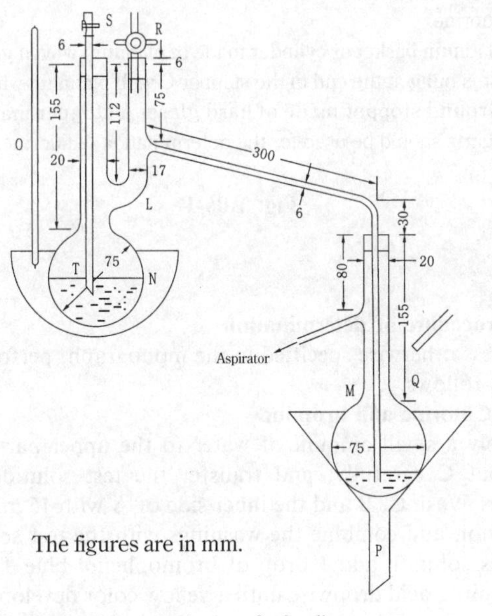

Fig. 1.02-2 Vacuum distilling apparatus for ammonium limit test

the distillation flask L in the absorbing liquid, and keep at 60°C using a water bath or alternative equipment. Adjust the reduced pressure to get the distillate at a rate of 1 to 2 mL per minute, and continue the distillation until to get 30 mL of the distillate. Cool the receiver M with running water during the distillation. Get off the end of the branch tube from surface of the absorbing liquid, rinse in the end with a small amount of water, then add water to the liquid to make 100 mL, and perform the test using this solution as the test solution.

Place a volume of Standard Ammonium Solution, directed in the monograph, in the distilling flask A or the vacuum distillation flask L, proceed as for the preparation of the test solution, and designate it as the control solution.

2.2. Test of the test solution and the control solution

Unless otherwise specified, proceed as directed in the following.

Place 30 mL each of the test solution and the control solution in Nessler tubes, add 6.0 mL of phenol-sodium pentacyanonitrosylferrate (III) TS to each solution, and mix. Then add 4 mL of sodium hypochlorite-sodium hydroxide TS and water to make 50 mL, mix, and allow to stand for 60 minutes. Compare the color of both solutions against a white background by viewing downward or transversely: the color developed in the test solution is not more intense than that of the control solution.

1.03 Chloride Limit Test

Chloride Limit Test is a limit test for chloride contained in drugs.

In each monograph, the permissible limit for chloride (as Cl) is described in terms of percentage (%) in parentheses.

1. Procedure

Unless otherwise specified, transfer the quantity of the sample, directed in the monograph, to a Nessler tube, and dissolve it in a proper volume of water to make 40 mL. Add 6 mL of dilute nitric acid and water to make 50 mL, and use this solution as the test solution. Transfer the volume of 0.01 mol/L hydrochloric acid VS, directed in the monograph, to another Nessler tube, add 6 mL of dilute nitric acid and water to make 50 mL, and use this solution as the control solution. When the test solution is not clear, filter both solutions by using the same procedure.

Add 1 mL of silver nitrate TS to the test solution and to the control solution, mix well, and allow to stand for 5 minutes protecting from light. Compare the opalescence developed in both solutions against a black background by viewing downward or transversely.

The opalescence developed in the test solution is not more than that of the control solution.

1.04 Flame Coloration Test

Flame Coloration Test is a method to detect an element, by means of the property that the element changes the colorless flame of a Bunsen burner to its characteristic color.

(1) Salt of metal—The platinum wire used for this test is about 0.8 mm in diameter, and the end part of it is straight. In the case of a solid sample, make the sample into a gruel by adding a small quantity of hydrochloric acid, apply a little of the gruel to the 5-mm end of the platinum wire, and test by putting the end part in a colorless flame, keeping the platinum wire horizontal. In the case of a liquid sample, immerse the end of the platinum wire into the sample to about 5 mm in length, remove from the sample gently, and perform the test in the same manner as for the solid sample.

(2) Halide—Cut a copper net, 0.25 mm in opening and 0.174 mm in wire diameter, into a strip 1.5 cm in width and 5 cm in length, and wind in round one end of a copper wire. Heat the copper net strongly in the colorless flame of Bunsen burner until the flame no longer shows a green or blue color, and then cool it. Repeat this procedure several times, and coat the net completely with cupric oxide. After cooling, unless otherwise specified, apply about 1 mg of the sample to the copper net, ignite, and burn it. Repeat this procedure three times, and then test by putting the copper net in the colorless flame.

The description, "Flame coloration persists", in a monograph, indicates that the reaction persists for 4 seconds.

1.05 Mineral Oil Test

Mineral Oil Test is a method to test mineral oil in nonaqueous solvents for injections and for eye drops.

1. Procedure

Pour 10 mL of the sample into a 100-mL flask, and add 15 mL of sodium hydroxide solution (1 in 6) and 30 mL of ethanol (95). Put a short-stemmed, small funnel on the neck of the flask, and heat on a water bath to make clear, with frequent shaking. Then transfer the solution to a shallow porcelain dish, evaporate the ethanol on a water bath, add 100 mL of water to the residue, and heat on a water bath: no turbidity is produced in the solution.

1.06 Oxygen Flask Combustion Method

Oxygen Flask Combustion Method is a method for the identification or the determination of halogens or sulfur produced by combusting organic compounds, which contain chlorine, bromine, iodine, fluorine or sulfur, in a flask filled with oxygen.

1. Apparatus

Use the apparatus shown in Fig. 1.06-1.

2. Preparation of test solution and blank solution

Unless otherwise specified, prepare them by the following method.

2.1. Preparation of sample

(i) For solid samples: Place the quantity of the sample specified in the monograph on the center of the filter illustrated in the figure, weigh accurately, wrap the sample carefully along the dotted line without scattering, and place the parcel in a platinum basket or cylinder B, leaving its fuse-strip on the outside.

(ii) For liquid samples: Roll a suitable amount of absorbent cotton with filter paper, 50 mm in length and 5 mm in width, so that the end part of the paper is left to a length of about 20 mm as a fuse-strip, and place the parcel in a platinum basket or cylinder B. Place the sample in a suitable glass tube, weigh accurately, and moisten the cotton with the quantity of the sample specified in the monograph, bringing the edge of the sample in contact with the cotton.

2.2. Method of combustion

Place the absorbing liquid specified in the monograph in flask A, fill it with oxygen, moisten the ground part of the stopper C with water, then ignite the fuse-strip, immediately transfer it to the flask, and keep the flask airtight until the combustion is completed. Shake the flask occasionally until the white smoke in A vanishes completely, allow to stand for 15 to 30 minutes, and designate the resulting solution as the test solution. Prepare the blank solution in the same manner, without sample.

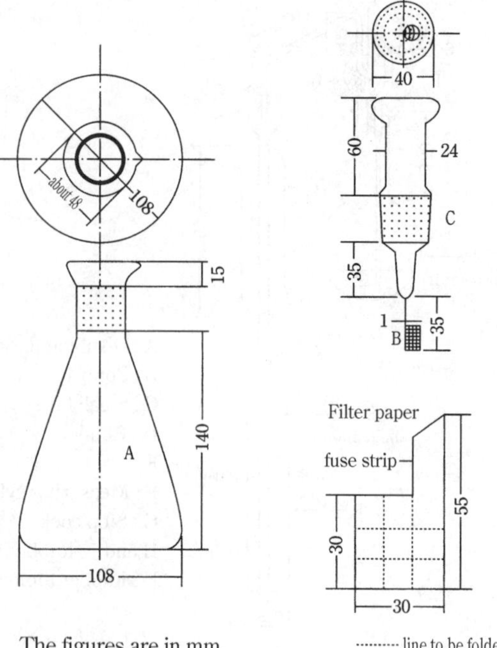

A: Colorless, thick-walled (about 2 mm), 500-mL hard glass flask, the upper part of which is made like a saucer. A flask made of quartz should be used for the determination of fluorine.

B: Platinum basket or cylinder made of platinum woven gauge. (It is hung at the end of the stopper C with platinum wire).

C: Ground stopper made of hard glass. A stopper made of quartz should be used for the determination of fluorine.

Fig. 1.06-1

3. Procedure of determination

Unless otherwise specified in the monograph, perform the test as follows.

3.1. Chlorine and bromine

Apply a small amount of water to the upper part of A, pull out C carefully, and transfer the test solution to a beaker. Wash C, B and the inner side of A with 15 mL of 2-propanol, and combine the washings with the test solution. To this solution add 1 drop of bromophenol blue TS, add dilute nitric acid dropwise until a yellow color develops, then add 25 mL of 2-propanol, and titrate <*2.50*> with 0.005 mol/L silver nitrate VS according to the potentiometric titration. Perform the test with the blank solution in the same manner, and make any necessary correction.

Each mL of 0.005 mol/L silver nitrate VS
= 0.1773 mg of Cl

Each mL of 0.005 mol/L silver nitrate VS
= 0.3995 mg of Br

3.2. Iodine

Apply a small amount of water to the upper part of A, pull out C carefully, add 2 drops of hydrazine monohydrate to the test solution, put C on A, and decolorize the solution by vigorous shaking. Transfer the content of A to a beaker, wash C, B and the inner side of A with 25 mL of 2-propanol, and transfer the washings to the above beaker. To this solution add 1 drop of bromophenol blue TS, then add dilute nitric acid dropwise until a yellow color develops, and titrate <*2.50*> with 0.005 mol/L silver nitrate VS according to the potentiometric titration. Perform the test with the blank solution in the same manner, and make any necessary correction.

Each mL of 0.005 mol/L silver nitrate VS
= 0.6345 mg of I

3.3. Fluorine

Apply a small amount of water to the upper part of A, pull out C carefully, transfer the test solution and the blank solution to 50 mL volumetric flasks separately, wash C, B and the inner side of A with water, add the washings and water to make 50 mL, and use these solutions as the test solution and the correction solution. Pipet the test solution (V mL) equivalent to about 30 μg of fluorine, V mL of the correction solution and 5 mL of standard fluorine solution, transfer to 50-mL volumetric flasks separately, add 30 mL of a mixture of alizarin complexone TS, acetic acid-potassium acetate buffer solution (pH 4.3) and cerium (III) nitrate TS (1:1:1), add water to make 50 mL, and allow to stand for 1 hour. Perform the test with these solutions as directed under Ultraviolet-visible Spectrophotometry *<2.24>*, using a blank prepared with 5 mL of water in the same manner. Determine the absorbances, A_T, A_C and A_S, of the subsequent solutions of the test solution, the correction solution and the standard solution at 600 nm.

Amount (mg) of fluorine (F) in the test solution
= amount (mg) of fluorine in 5 mL of

$$\text{the standard solution} \times \frac{A_T - A_C}{A_S} \times \frac{50}{V}$$

Standard Fluorine Solution: Dry sodium fluoride (standard reagent) in a platinum crucible between 500°C and 550°C for 1 hour, cool it in a desiccator (silica gel), weigh accurately about 66.3 mg of it, and dissolve in water to make exactly 500 mL. Pipet 10 mL of this solution, and dilute with sufficient water to make exactly 100 mL.

3.4. Sulfur

Apply a small amount of water to the upper part of A, pull out C carefully, and wash C, B and the inner side of A with 15 mL of methanol. To this solution add 40 mL of methanol, then add exactly 25 mL of 0.005 mol/L barium perchlorate VS, allow to stand for 10 minutes, add 0.15 mL of arsenazo III TS with a measuring pipet, and titrate *<2.50>* with 0.005 mol/L sulfuric acid VS. Perform the test with the blank solution in the same manner.

Each mL of 0.005 mol/L barium perchlorate VS
= 0.1604 mg of S

1.07 Heavy Metals Limit Test

Heavy Metals Limit Test is a limit test of the quantity of heavy metals contained as impurities in drugs. The heavy metals are the metallic inclusions that are darkened with sodium sulfide TS in acidic solution, as their quantity is expressed in terms of the quantity of lead (Pb).

In each monograph, the permissible limit for heavy metals (as Pb) is described in terms of ppm in parentheses.

1. Preparation of test solutions and control solutions

Unless otherwise specified, test solutions and control solutions are prepared as directed in the following:

1.1. Method 1

Place an amount of the sample, directed in the monograph, in a Nessler tube. Dissolve in water to make 40 mL. Add 2 mL of dilute acetic acid and water to make 50 mL, and designate it as the test solution.

The control solution is prepared by placing the volume of Standard Lead Solution directed in the monograph in a Nessler tube, and adding 2 mL of dilute acetic acid and water to make 50 mL.

1.2. Method 2

Place an amount of the sample, directed in the monograph, in a quartz or porcelain crucible, cover loosely with a lid, and carbonize by gentle ignition. After cooling, add 2 mL of nitric acid and 5 drops of sulfuric acid, heat cautiously until white fumes are no longer evolved, and incinerate by ignition between 500°C and 600°C. Cool, add 2 mL of hydrochloric acid, evaporate to dryness on a water bath, moisten the residue with 3 drops of hydrochloric acid, add 10 mL of hot water, and warm for 2 minutes. Then add 1 drop of phenolphthalein TS, add ammonia TS dropwise until the solution develops a pale red color, add 2 mL of dilute acetic acid, filter if necessary, and wash with 10 mL of water. Transfer the filtrate and washings to a Nessler tube, and add water to make 50 mL. Designate it as the test solution.

The control solution is prepared as follows: Evaporate a mixture of 2 mL of nitric acid, 5 drops of sulfuric acid and 2 mL of hydrochloric acid on a water bath, further evaporate to dryness on a sand bath, and moisten the residue with 3 drops of hydrochloric acid. Hereinafter, proceed as directed in the test solution, then add the volume of Standard Lead Solution directed in the monograph and water to make 50 mL.

1.3. Method 3

Place an amount of the sample, directed in the monograph, in a quartz or porcelain crucible, heat cautiously, gently at first, and then incinerate by ignition between 500°C and 600°C. After cooling, add 1 mL of aqua regia, evaporate to dryness on a water bath, moisten the residue with 3 drops of hydrochloric acid, add 10 mL of hot water, and warm for 2 minutes. Add 1 drop of phenolphthalein TS, add ammonia TS dropwise until the solution develops a pale red color, add 2 mL of dilute acetic acid, filter if necessary, wash with 10 mL of water, transfer the filtrate and washings to a Nessler tube, and add water to make 50 mL. Designate it as the test solution.

The control solution is prepared as follows: Evaporate 1 mL of aqua regia to dryness on a water bath. Hereinafter, proceed as directed for the test solution, and add the volume of Standard Lead Solution directed in the monograph and water to make 50 mL.

1.4. Method 4

Place an amount of the sample, directed in the monograph, in a platinum or porcelain crucible, mix with 10 mL of a solution of magnesium nitrate hexahydrate in ethanol (95) (1 in 10), fire the ethanol to burn, and carbonize by gradual heating. Cool, add 1 mL of sulfuric acid, heat carefully, and incinerate by ignition between 500°C and 600°C. If a carbonized substance remains, moisten with a small amount of sulfuric acid, and incinerate by ignition. Cool, dissolve the residue in 3 mL of hydrochloric acid, evaporate on a water bath to dryness, wet the residue with 3 drops of hydrochloric acid, add 10 mL of water, and dissolve by warming. Add 1 drop of phenolphthalein TS, add ammonia TS dropwise until a pale red color develops, then add 2 mL of dilute acetic acid, filter if necessary, wash with 10 mL of water, transfer the filtrate and the washing to a Nessler tube, add water to make 50 mL, and use this solution as the test solution.

The control solution is prepared as follows: Take 10 mL of a solution of magnesium nitrate hexahydrate in ethanol

(95) (1 in 10), and fire the ethanol to burn. Cool, add 1 mL of sulfuric acid, heat carefully, and ignite between 500°C and 600°C. Cool, and add 3 mL of hydrochloric acid. Hereinafter, proceed as directed in the test solution, then add the volume of Standard Lead Solution directed in the monograph and water to make 50 mL.

2. Procedure

Add 1 drop of sodium sulfide TS to each of the test solution and the control solution, mix thoroughly, and allow to stand for 5 minutes. Then compare the colors of both solutions by viewing the tubes downward or transversely against a white background. The test solution has no more color than the control solution.

1.08 Nitrogen Determination (Semimicro-Kjeldahl Method)

Nitrogen Determination is a method to determine nitrogen in an organic substance in which the nitrogen is converted into ammonia nitrogen by thermal decomposition of the organic substance with sulfuric acid, and the ammonia liberated by alkali and trapped by distillation with steam is determined by titration.

1. Apparatus

Use the apparatus illustrated in Fig. 1.08-1. It is thoroughly constructed of hard glass, and ground glass surfaces may be used for joints. All rubber parts used in the apparatus should be boiled for 10 to 30 minutes in sodium hydroxide TS and for 30 to 60 minutes in water, and finally washed thoroughly with water before use.

Alternatively, apparatus can be used in which some of the procedures, such as digestion of organic substances, distillation of the liberated ammonia, and endpoint detection methods in titrimetry (e.g., potentiometric titration or titration by colorimeter) are automated.

2. System suitability

If an automated apparatus is used, it is necessary to confirm periodically the suitability of the apparatus according to the following method:

Weigh accurately about 1.7 g of amidosulfuric acid (standard reagent), previously dried in a desiccator (in vacuum, silica gel) for about 48 hours, dissolve in water to make exactly 200 mL. Pipet 2 mL of this solution, and transfer to a digestion flask. When the test is performed as directed in the instrumental manual the nitrogen content (%) in amidosulfuric acid should be determined between 14.2% and 14.6%.

3. Reagents, Test Solutions

Decomposition accelerator: Unless otherwise specified, use 1 g of a powdered mixture of 10 g of potassium sulfate and 1 g of cupper (II) sulfate pentahydrate. The composition and amount of the digestion accelerator may be modified if it is confirmed that the modified one give almost the same results using the sample as those obtained from the conventional catalyst.

4. Procedure

Unless otherwise specified, proceed by the following method. Weigh accurately or pipet a quantity of the sample corresponding to 2 to 3 mg of nitrogen (N:14.01), and place in the Kjeldahl flask A. Add the decomposition accelerator and wash down any adhering sample from the neck of the flask with a small quantity of water. Add 7 mL of sulfuric acid, allowing it to flow down the inside wall of the flask.

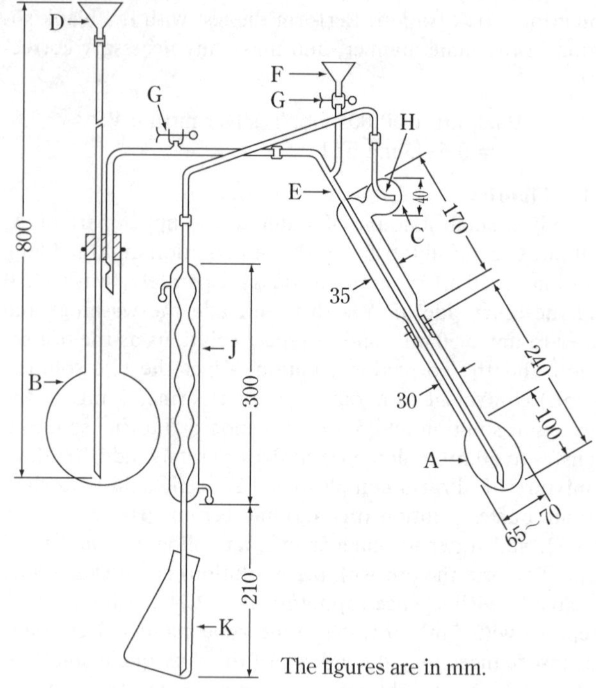

A: Kjeldahl flask
B: Steam generator, containing water, to which 2 to 3 drops of sulfuric acid and fragments of boiling tips for preventing bumping have been added
C: Spray trap
D: Water supply funnel
E: Steam tube
F: Funnel for addition of alkali solution to flask A
G: Rubber tubing with a clamp
H: A small hole having a diameter approximately equal to that of the delivery tube
J: Condenser, the lower end of which is beveled
K: Absorption flask

Fig. 1.08-1

Then, while shaking the flask, add cautiously 1 mL of hydrogen peroxide (30) drop by drop along the inside wall of the flask. Heat the flask gradually, then heat so strong that the vapor of sulfuric acid is condensed at the neck of the flask, until the solution changes through a blue and clear to a vivid green and clear, and the inside wall of the flask is free from a carbonaceous material. If necessary, add a small quantity of hydrogen peroxide (30) after cooling, and heat again. After cooling, add cautiously 20 mL of water, cool the solution, and connect the flask to the distillation apparatus (Fig. 1.08-1) washed beforehand by passing steam through it. To the absorption flask K add 15 mL of boric acid solution (1 in 25), 3 drops of bromocresol green-methyl red TS and sufficient water to immerse the lower end of the condenser tube J. Add 30 mL of sodium hydroxide solution (2 in 5) through the funnel F, rinse cautiously the funnel with 10 mL of water, close the clamp attached to the rubber tubing G, then begin the distillation with stream, and continue until the distillate measures 80 to 100 mL. Remove the absorption flask from the lower end of the condenser tube J, rinsing the end part with a small quantity of water, and titrate <*2.50*> the distillate with 0.005 mol/L sulfuric acid VS until the color of the solution changes from green through pale grayish blue to pale grayish red-purple. Perform a blank determination in the same manner, and make any necessary correction.

Each mL of 0.005 mol/L sulfuric acid VS
= 0.1401 mg of N

If an automated apparatus is used, proceed as directed in the instrumental procedure.

1.09 Qualitative Tests

Qualitative Tests are applied to the identification of drugs and are done generally with quantities of 2 to 5 mL of the test solution.

Acetate

(1) When warmed with diluted sulfuric acid (1 in 2), acetates evolve the odor of acetic acid.

(2) When an acetate is warmed with sulfuric acid and a small quantity of ethanol (95), the odor of ethyl acetate is evolved.

(3) Neutral solutions of acetates produce a red-brown color with iron (III) chloride TS, and a red-brown precipitate when boiled. The precipitate dissolves and the color of the solution changes to yellow upon addition of hydrochloric acid.

Aluminum salt

(1) Solutions of aluminum salts, when treated with ammonium chloride TS and ammonia TS, yield a gelatinous, white precipitate which does not dissolve in an excess of ammonia TS.

(2) Solutions of aluminum salts, when treated with sodium hydroxide TS, yield a gelatinous, white precipitate which dissolves in an excess of the reagent.

(3) Solutions of aluminum salts, when treated with sodium sulfide TS, yield a gelatinous, white precipitate which dissolves in an excess of the reagent.

(4) Add ammonia TS to solutions of aluminum salts until a gelatinous, white precipitate is produced. The color of the precipitate changes to red upon addition of 5 drops of alizarin red S TS.

Ammonium salt

When heated with an excess of sodium hydroxide TS, ammonium salts evolve the odor of ammonia. This gas changes moistened red litmus paper to blue.

Antimony salt, primary

(1) When primary antimony salts are dissolved in a slight excess of hydrochloric acid for the test and then diluted with water, a white turbidity is produced. The mixture produces an orange precipitate upon addition of 1 to 2 drops of sodium sulfide TS. When the precipitate is separated, and sodium sulfide TS is added to one portion of the precipitate and sodium hydroxide TS is added to another portion, it dissolves in either of these reagents.

(2) Add water to acidic solutions of primary antimony salts in hydrochloric acid until a small quantity of precipitate is produced, and then add sodium thiosulfate TS: the precipitate dissolves. A red precipitate is reproduced when the solution is heated.

Aromatic amines, primary

Acidic solutions of primary aromatic amines, when cooled in ice, mixed with 3 drops of sodium nitrite TS under agitation, allowed to stand for 2 minutes, mixed well with 1 mL of ammonium amidosulfate TS, allowed to stand for 1 minute, and then mixed with 1 mL of *N*,*N*-diethyl-*N*′-1-naphtylethylenediamine oxalate TS, exhibit a red-purple color.

Arsenate

(1) Neutral solutions of arsenates produce no precipitate with 1 to 2 drops of sodium sulfide TS, but produce a yellow precipitate with hydrochloric acid subsequently added. The separated precipitate dissolves in ammonium carbonate TS.

(2) Neutral solutions of arsenates produce a dark red-brown precipitate with silver nitrate TS. When dilute nitric acid is added to one portion of the suspension, and ammonia TS is added to another portion, the precipitate dissolves in either of these reagents.

(3) Neutral or ammonia alkaline solutions of arsenates produce with magnesia TS a white, crystalline precipitate, which dissolves by addition of dilute hydrochloric acid.

Arsenite

(1) Acidic solutions of arsenites in hydrochloric acid produce a yellow precipitate with 1 to 2 drops of sodium sulfide TS. When hydrochloric acid is added to one portion of the separated precipitate, it does not dissolve. When ammonium carbonate TS is added to another portion, the precipitate dissolves.

(2) Slightly alkaline solutions of arsenites produce a yellow-white precipitate with silver nitrate TS. When ammonia TS is added to one portion of the suspension, and dilute nitric acid is added to another portion, the precipitate dissolves in either of these reagents.

(3) Slightly alkaline solutions of arsenites produce a green precipitate with copper (II) sulfate TS. When the separated precipitate is boiled with sodium hydroxide TS, it changes to red-brown.

Barium salt

(1) When Flame Coloration Test (1) <*1.04*> is applied to barium salts, a persistent yellow-green color develops.

(2) Solutions of barium salts produce with dilute sulfuric acid a white precipitate, which does not dissolve upon addition of dilute nitric acid.

(3) Acidic solutions of barium salts in acetic acid produce a yellow precipitate with potassium chromate TS. The precipitate dissolves by addition of dilute nitric acid.

Benzoate

(1) Concentrated solutions of benzoates produce a white, crystalline precipitate with dilute hydrochloric acid. The separated precipitate, washed with cold water and dried, melts between 120°C and 124°C <*2.60*>.

(2) Neutral solutions of benzoates produce a light yellow-red precipitate upon dropwise addition of iron (III) chloride TS. The precipitate changes to white on subsequent addition of dilute hydrochloric acid.

Bicarbonate

(1) Bicarbonates effervesce upon addition of dilute hydrochloric acid, generating a gas, which produces a white precipitate immediately, when passed into calcium hydroxide TS (common with carbonates).

(2) Solutions of bicarbonates produce no precipitate with magnesium sulfate TS, but produce a white precipitate when boiled subsequently.

(3) Cold solutions of bicarbonates remain unchanged or exhibits only a slightly red color upon addition of 1 drop of phenolphthalein TS (discrimination from carbonates).

Bismuth salt

(1) Bismuth salts, dissolved in a slight excess of hydrochloric acid, yield a white turbidity upon dilution with water. A dark brown precipitate is produced with 1 to 2 drops of sodium sulfide TS subsequently added.

(2) Acidic solutions of bismuth salts in hydrochloric acid exhibit a yellow color upon addition of thiourea TS.

(3) Solution of bismuth salts in dilute nitric acid or in dilute sulfuric acid yield with potassium iodide TS a black precipitate, which dissolves in an excess of the reagent to give an orange-colored solution.

Borate

(1) When ignite a mixture of a borate with sulfuric acid and methanol, it burns with a green flame.

(2) Turmeric paper, when moistened with acidic solutions of borates in hydrochloric acid and dried by warming, exhibits a red color, which changes to blue with ammonia TS added dropwise.

Bromate

(1) Acidic solutions of bromates in nitric acid yield with 2 to 3 drops of silver nitrate TS a white, crystalline precipitate, which dissolves upon heating. When 1 drop of sodium nitrite TS is added to this solution, a light yellow precipitate is produced.

(2) Acidic solutions of bromates in nitric acid exhibit a yellow to red-brown color upon addition of 5 to 6 drops of sodium nitrite TS. When 1 mL of chloroform is added to the mixture and shaken, the chloroform layer exhibits a yellow to red-brown color.

Bromide

(1) Solutions of bromides yield a light yellow precipitate with silver nitrate TS. Upon addition of dilute nitric acid to a portion of the separated precipitate, it does not dissolve. When ammonia solution (28) is added to another portion and shaken, the separated solution yields a white turbidity upon acidifying with dilute nitric acid.

(2) Solutions of bromides exhibit a yellow-brown color with chlorine TS. The mixture is separated into 2 portions. When one portion is shaken with chloroform, the chloroform layer exhibits a yellow-brown to red-brown color. When phenol is added to the other portion, a white precipitate is produced.

Calcium salt

(1) When Flame Coloration Test (1) <*1.04*> is applied to calcium salts, a yellow-red color develops.

(2) Solutions of calcium salts yield a white precipitate with ammonium carbonate TS.

(3) Solutions of calcium salts yield a white precipitate with ammonium oxalate TS. The separated precipitate does not dissolve in dilute acetic acid, but dissolves in dilute hydrochloric acid.

(4) Neutral solutions of calcium salts produce no precipitate, when mixed with 10 drops of potassium chromate TS and heated (discrimination from strontium salts).

Carbonate

(1) Carbonates effervesce upon addition of dilute hydrochloric acid, generating a gas, which produces a white precipitate immediately, when passed into calcium hydroxide TS (common with bicarbonates).

(2) Solutions of carbonates yield with magnesium sulfate TS a white precipitate, which dissolves by addition of dilute acetic acid.

(3) Cold solutions of carbonates exhibit a red color with 1 drop of phenolphthalein TS (discrimination from bicarbonates).

Ceric salt

(1) When a cerous salt is mixed with 2.5 times its mass of lead (IV) oxide, nitric acid is added and the solution is boiled, it exhibits a yellow color.

(2) Solutions of cerous salts yield a yellow to red-brown precipitate upon addition of hydrogen peroxide TS and ammonia TS.

Chlorate

(1) Solutions of chlorates yield no precipitate with silver nitrate TS. When 2 to 3 drops of sodium nitrite TS and dilute nitric acid are added to the mixture, a white precipitate is produced gradually, which dissolves by addition of ammonia TS.

(2) When indigocarmine TS is added dropwise to neutral solutions of chlorates until a light blue color appears, and the mixture is acidified with dilute sulfuric acid, the blue color vanishes promptly upon subsequent dropwise addition of sodium hydrogensulfite TS.

Chloride

(1) Solutions of chlorides evolve an odor of chlorine, when mixed with sulfuric acid and potassium permanganate, and heated. The gas evolved turns moistened potassium iodide starch paper blue.

(2) Solutions of chlorides yield a white precipitate with silver nitrate TS. When dilute nitric acid is added to a portion of the separated precipitate, it does not dissolve. When an excess of ammonia TS is added to another portion, the precipitate dissolves.

Chromate

(1) Solutions of chromates exhibit a yellow color.

(2) Solutions of chromates produce a yellow precipitate with lead (II) acetate TS. When acetic acid (31) is added to a portion of the suspension, the precipitate does not dissolve. When dilute nitric acid is added to another portion, the precipitate dissolves.

(3) When acidic solutions of chromates in sulfuric acid are mixed with an equal volume of ethyl acetate and 1 to 2 drops of hydrogen peroxide TS, shaken immediately and allowed to stand, the ethyl acetate layer exhibits a blue color.

Citrate

(1) When 20 mL of a mixture of pyridine and acetic anhydride (3:1) is added to 1 or 2 drops of a solution of citrate, and the solution is allowed to stand for 2 to 3 minutes, a red-brown color develops.

(2) Neutral solutions of citrates, when mixed with an equal volume of dilute sulfuric acid and two-thirds volume of potassium permanganate TS, heated until the color of permanganate is discharged, and then treated dropwise with bromine TS to one-tenth of total volume, yield a white precipitate.

(3) Neutral solutions of citrates, when boiled with an excess of calcium chloride TS, yield a white crystalline precipitate. When sodium hydroxide TS is added to a portion of the separated precipitate, it does not dissolve. When dilute hydrochloric acid is added to another portion, the precipitate dissolves.

Cupric salt

(1) When a well polished iron plate is immersed in acidic solutions of cupric salts in hydrochloric acid, a red metallic film appears on its surface.

(2) Solutions of cupric salts produce a light blue precipitate with a small quantity of ammonia TS. The precipitate dissolves in an excess of the reagent, yielding a deep blue-colored solution.

(3) Solutions of cupric salts yield a red-brown precipitate with potassium hexacyanoferrate (II) TS. When dilute nitric acid is added to a portion of the suspension, the precipitate does not dissolve. When ammonia TS is added to another portion, the precipitate dissolves, yielding a deep blue-colored solution.

(4) Solutions of cupric salts produce a black precipitate with sodium sulfide TS. When dilute hydrochloric acid, dilute sulfuric acid or sodium hydroxide TS is added to a portion of the separated precipitate, it does not dissolve. When hot dilute nitric acid is added to another portion, the precipitate dissolves.

Cyanide

(1) Solutions of cyanides yield a white precipitate with an excess of silver nitrate TS. When dilute nitric acid is added to a portion of the separated precipitate, it does not dissolve. When ammonia TS is added to another portion, the precipitate dissolves.

(2) Solutions of cyanides yield a blue precipitate, when mixed by shaking with 2 to 3 drops of iron (II) sulfate TS, 2 to 3 drops of dilute iron (III) chloride TS and 1 mL of sodium hydroxide TS, and then acidified with dilute sulfuric acid.

Dichromate

(1) Solutions of dichromates exhibit a yellow-red color.

(2) Solutions of dichromates produce a yellow precipitate with lead (II) acetate TS. When acetic acid (31) is added to one portion of the suspension, the precipitate dose not dissolve. When dilute nitric acid is added to another portion, the precipitate dissolves.

(3) When acidic solutions of dichromates in sulfuric acid are mixed with an equal volume of ethyl acetate and with 1 to 2 drops of hydrogen peroxide TS, shaken immediately and allowed to stand, the ethyl acetate layer exhibits a blue color.

Ferric salt

(1) Slightly acidic solutions of ferric salts yield with potassium hexacyanoferrate (II) TS a blue precipitate, which does not dissolve in dilute hydrochloric acid subsequently added.

(2) Solutions of ferric salts yield with sodium hydroxide TS a gelatinous, red-brown precipitate, which changes to black upon addition of sodium sulfide TS. The separated precipitate dissolves in dilute hydrochloric acid, yielding a white turbidity.

(3) Slightly acidic solutions of ferric salts exhibit a purple color with 5-sulfosalicylic acid TS.

Ferricyanide

(1) Solutions of ferricyanides exhibit a yellow color.

(2) Solutions of ferricyanides yield with iron (II) sulfate TS a blue precipitate, which does not dissolve in dilute hydrochloric acid subsequently added.

Ferrocyanide

(1) Solutions of ferrocyanides yield with iron (III) chloride TS a blue precipitate, which does not dissolve in dilute hydrochloric acid subsequently added.

(2) Solutions of ferrocyanides yield with copper (II) sulfate TS a red-brown precipitate, which does not dissolve in dilute hydrochloric acid subsequently added.

Ferrous salt

(1) Slightly acidic solutions of ferrous salts yield with potassium hexacyanoferrate (III) TS a blue precipitate, which does not dissolve in dilute hydrochloric acid subsequently added.

(2) Solutions of ferrous salts yield with sodium hydroxide TS a grayish green, gelatinous precipitate, which changes to black with sodium sulfide TS. The separated precipitate dissolves in dilute hydrochloric acid.

(3) Neutral or slightly acidic solutions of ferrous salts exhibit an deep red color upon dropwise addition of a solution of 1,10-phenanthroline monohydrate in ethanol (95) (1 in 50).

Fluoride

(1) When solutions of fluorides are heated with chromic acid-sulfuric acid TS, the inside of the test tube is not moistened uniformly.

(2) Neutral or slightly acidic solutions of fluorides exhibit a blue-purple color after standing with 1.5 mL of a mixture of alizarin complexone TS, acetic acid-potassium acetate buffer solution (pH 4.3) and cerium (III) nitrate TS (1:1:1).

Glycerophosphate

(1) Solutions of glycerophosphates remain unaffected by addition of calcium chloride TS, but yield a precipitate when boiled.

(2) Solutions of glycerophosphates yield no precipitate with hexaammonium heptamolybdate TS in the cold, but yield a yellow precipitate when boiled for a long time.

(3) When glycerophosphates are mixed with an equal mass of powdered potassium hydrogen sulfate and heated gently over a free flame, the pungent odor of acrolein is evolved.

Iodide

(1) Solutions of iodides yield a yellow precipitate with silver nitrate TS. When dilute nitric acid is added to one portion of the suspension, and ammonia solution (28) to another portion, the precipitates do not dissolve in either of these reagents.

(2) Acidic solutions of iodides exhibit a yellow-brown color with 1 to 2 drops of sodium nitrite TS and then yield a black-purple precipitate. The solutions exhibit a deep blue color with starch TS subsequently added.

Lactate

Acidic solutions of lactates in sulfuric acid, when heated with potassium permanganate TS, evolve the odor of acetaldehyde.

Lead salt

(1) Solutions of lead salts yield a white precipitate with dilute sulfuric acid. When dilute nitric acid is added to a portion of the separated precipitate, it does not dissolve. When sodium hydroxide TS is added to another portion and warmed, or when ammonium acetate TS is added to another portion, the precipitate dissolves.

(2) Solutions of lead salts yield with sodium hydroxide TS a white precipitate, which dissolves in an excess of sodium hydroxide TS, and yields a black precipitate upon subsequent addition of sodium sulfide TS.

(3) Acidic solutions of lead salts in dilute acetic acid yield with potassium chromate TS a yellow precipitate, which does not dissolve in ammonia TS but dissolves in sodium hydroxide TS subsequently added.

Lithium salt

(1) When Flame Coloratuion Test (1) *<1.04>* is applied to lithium salts, a persistent red color develops.

(2) Solutions of lithium salts yield with disodium hydrogenphosphate TS a white precipitate, which dissolves upon subsequent addition of dilute hydrochloric acid.

(3) Solutions of lithium salts yield no precipitate with dilute sulfuric acid (discrimination from strontium salts).

Magnesium salt

(1) Solutions of magnesium salts yield upon warming with ammonium carbonate TS a white precipitate, which dissolves in ammonium chloride TS. A white, crystalline precipitate is reproduced by subsequent addition of disodium hydrogenphosphate TS.

(2) Solutions of magnesium salts yield with sodium hydroxide TS a white, gelatinous precipitate. When iodine TS is added to one portion of the suspension, the precipitate develops a dark-brown color. When excess sodium hydroxide TS is added to another portion, the precipitate does not dissolve.

Manganese salt

(1) Solutions of manganese salts yield a white precipitate with ammonia TS. When silver nitrate TS is added to a portion of the suspension, the precipitate changes to black. When another portion is allowed to stand, the upper part of the precipitate exhibits a brownish color.

(2) Acidic solutions of manganese salts in dilute nitric acid exhibit a purple-red color with a small quantity of powdered bismuth sodium trioxide.

Mercuric salt

(1) A copper plate is immersed in solutions of mercuric salts, allowed to stand, taken out, and then washed with water. The plate becomes bright and silvery white in appearance, when rubbed with paper or cloth (common with mercurous salts).

(2) Solutions of mercuric salts yield with a small quantity of sodium sulfide TS a black precipitate, which dissolves in an excess of the reagent. The black precipitate is reproduced by subsequent addition of ammonium chloride TS.

(3) When potassium iodide TS is added dropwise to neutral solutions of mercuric salts, a red precipitate is produced. The precipitate dissolves in an excess of the reagent.

(4) Acidic solutions of mercuric salts in hydrochloric acid yield with a small quantity of tin (II) chloride TS a white precipitate, which changes to grayish black upon addition of an excess of the reagent.

Mercurous salt

(1) A copper plate is immersed in solutions of mercurous salts, allowed to stand, taken out, and then washed with water. The plate becomes bright and silvery white in appearance, when rubbed with paper or cloth (common with mercuric salts).

(2) Mercurous salts or their solutions exhibit a black color with sodium hydroxide TS.

(3) Solutions of mercurous salts yield a white precipitate with dilute hydrochloric acid. The separated precipitate changes to black upon addition of ammonia TS.

(4) Solutions of mercurous salts yield with potassium iodide TS a yellow precipitate, which changes to green, when allowed to stand, and changes again to black upon subsequent addition of an excess of the reagent.

Mesilate

(1) To mesilates add twice its mass of sodium hydroxide, heat gently to melt, and continue heating for 20 to 30 seconds. After cooling, add a little amount of water, then add dilute hydrochloric acid, and warm: the gas evolved changes moistened potassium iodate-starch paper to blue.

(2) To mesilates add threefold its mass of sodium nitrate and anhydrous sodium carbonate, mix, and heat gradually. After cooling, dissolve the residue in diluted hydrochloric acid (1 in 5), and filter if necessary. The filtrate yields a white precipitate upon addition of barium chloride TS.

Nitrate

(1) Solutions of nitrates, when mixed with an equal volume of sulfuric acid, the mixture is cooled, and iron (II) sulfate TS is superimposed, a dark brown ring is produced at the junction of the two liquids.

(2) Solutions of nitrates exhibit a blue color with diphenylamine TS.

(3) When potassium permanganate TS is added to acidic solutions of nitrates in sulfuric acid, the red-purple color of the reagent does not fade (discrimination from nitrites).

Nitrite

(1) Solutions of nitrites, when acidified with dilute sulfuric acid, evolve a yellow-brown gas with a characteristic odor. The solutions exhibit a dark brown color upon addition of a small quantity of iron (II) sulfate crystals.

(2) Solutions of nitrites, when 2 to 3 drops of potassium iodide TS and dilute sulfuric acid are added dropwise, exhibit a yellow-brown color, and then yield a black-purple precipitate. When the mixture is shaken with 2 mL of chloroform, the chloroform layer exhibits a purple color.

(3) Solutions of nitrites, when mixed with thiourea TS and acidified with dilute sulfuric acid, and iron (III) chloride TS is added dropwise, exhibit a dark red color. When the mixture is shaken with 2 mL of diethyl ether, the diethyl ether layer exhibits a red color.

Oxalate

(1) When potassium permanganate TS is added dropwise to warm acidic solutions of oxalates in sulfuric acid, the reagent is decolorized.

(2) Solutions of oxalates yield a white precipitate with calcium chloride TS. The separated precipitate does not dissolve in dilute acetic acid but dissolves upon subsequent addition of dilute hydrochloric acid.

Permanganate

(1) Solutions of permanganates exhibit a red-purple color.

(2) When an excess of hydrogen peroxide TS is added to acidic solutions of permanganates in sulfuric acid, the solutions effervesce and decolorize permanganates.

(3) Acidic solutions of permanganates in sulfuric acid are decolorized, when an excess of oxalic acid TS is added and heated.

Peroxide

(1) Solutions of peroxides are mixed with an equal volume of ethyl acetate and 1 to 2 drops of potassium dichromate TS, and then acidified with dilute sulfuric acid. When the mixture is shaken immediately and allowed to stand, the ethyl acetate layer exhibits a blue color.

(2) Acidic solutions of peroxides in sulfuric acid decolorize dropwise added potassium permanganate TS, and effervesce to evolve a gas.

Phosphate (Orthophosphate)

(1) Neutral solutions of phosphates yield with silver nitrate TS a yellow precipitate, which dissolves upon addition of dilute nitric acid or ammonia TS.

(2) Acidic solutions in dilute nitric acid of phosphates yield a yellow precipitate with hexaammonium heptamolybdate TS on warming. The precipitate dissolves upon subsequent addition of sodium hydroxide TS or ammonia TS.

(3) Neutral or ammonia-alkaline solutions of phosphates yield with magnesia TS a white, crystalline precipitate, which dissolves upon subsequent addition of dilute hydrochloric acid.

Potassium salt

(1) When Flame Coloration Test (1) <*1.04*> is applied to potassium salts, a pale purple color develops. When it gives a yellow color, a red-purple color can be seen through cobalt glass.

(2) Neutral solutions of potassium salts yield a white, crystalline precipitate with sodium hydrogen tartrate TS. The formation of the precipitate is accelerated by rubbing the inside wall of the test tube with a glass rod. The separated precipitate dissolves upon addition of any of ammonia TS, sodium hydroxide TS or sodium carbonate TS.

(3) Acidic solutions of potassium salts in acetic acid (31) yield a yellow precipitate with sodium hexanitrocobaltate (III) TS.

(4) Potassium salts do not evolve the odor of ammonia, when an excess of sodium hydroxide TS is added and warmed (discrimination from ammonium salts).

Salicylate

(1) Salicylates evolve the odor of phenol, when an excess of soda-lime is added and heated.

(2) Concentrated solutions of salicylates yield a white, crystalline precipitate with dilute hydrochloric acid. The separated precipitate, washed well with cold water and dried, melts <*2.60*> at about 159°C.

(3) Neutral solutions of salicylates exhibit with 5 to 6 drops of dilute iron (III) chloride TS a red color, which changes to purple and then fades when dilute hydrochloric acid is added dropwise.

Silver salt

(1) Solutions of silver salts yield a white precipitate with dilute hydrochloric acid. When dilute nitric acid is added subsequently to a portion of the suspension, the precipitate does not dissolve. When an excess of ammonia TS is added to another portion, the precipitate dissolves.

(2) Solutions of silver salts yield with potassium chromate TS a red precipitate, which dissolves upon addition of dilute nitric acid.

(3) Solutions of silver salts yield a grayish brown precipitate with ammonia TS added dropwise. When ammonia TS is added dropwise until the precipitate dissolves, then 1 to 2 drops of formaldehyde solution are added and warmed, a mirror of metallic silver is deposited on the inside wall of the container.

Sodium salt

(1) When Flame Coloration Test (1) <*1.04*> is applied to sodium salts, a yellow color develops.

(2) Concentrated, neutral or slightly alkaline solutions of sodium salts yield a white, crystalline precipitate with potassium hexahydroxoantimonate (V) TS. The formation of the precipitate is accelerated by rubbing the inside wall of the test tube with a glass rod.

Stannic salt

(1) When the outside bottom of a test tube containing water is moistened with acidic solutions of stannic salts in hydrochloric acid and is placed in a nonluminous flame of a Bunsen burner, a blue flame mantle is seen around the bottom of the test tube (common with stannous salts).

(2) When granular zinc is immersed in acidic solutions of stannic salts in hydrochloric acid, a spongy, gray substance is deposited on the surface of the granules (common with stannous salts).

(3) Add iron powder to acidic solutions of stannic salts in hydrochloric acid, allow to stand, and then filter. When iodine-starch TS is added dropwise to the filtrate, the color of the test solution disappears.

(4) Acidic solutions of stannic salts in hydrochloric acid, to which ammonia TS is added dropwise until a small quantity of precipitate is produced, yield a light yellow precipitate with 2 to 3 drops of sodium sulfide TS. The separated precipitate dissolves upon addition of sodium sulfide TS and light yellow precipitate is reproduced by subsequent addition of hydrochloric acid.

Stannous salt

(1) When the outside bottom of a test tube containing water is moistened with acidic solutions of stannous salts in hydrochloric acid and is placed in a nonluminous flame of a Bunsen burner, a blue flame mantle is seen around the bottom of the test tube (common with stannic salts).

(2) When granular zinc is immersed in acidic solutions of stannous salts in hydrochloric acid, a spongy, gray substance is deposited on the surface of the granules (common with stannic salts).

(3) When iodine-starch TS is added dropwise to solutions of stannous salts, the color of the test solution disappears.

(4) Acidic solutions of stannous salts in hydrochloric acid, to which ammonia TS is added dropwise until a small quantity of precipitate is produced, yield a dark brown precipitate with 2 to 3 drops of sodium sulfide TS. When sodium sulfide TS is added to a portion of the separated precipitate, it does not dissolve. When ammonium polysulfide TS is added to another portion, the precipitate dissolves.

Sulfate

(1) Solutions of sulfates yield with barium chloride TS a white precipitate, which does not dissolve upon addition of dilute nitric acid.

(2) Neutral solutions of sulfates yield with lead (II) acetate TS a white precipitate, which dissolves upon subsequent addition of ammonium acetate TS.

(3) When an equal volume of dilute hydrochloric acid is added, solutions of sulfates yield no white turbidity (discrimination from thiosulfates), and do not evolve the odor of sulfur dioxide (discrimination from sulfites).

Sulfide

(1) Most kinds of sulfides evolve the odor of hydrogen sulfide with dilute hydrochloric acid. This gas blackens lead (II) acetate paper moistened with water.

Sulfite and Bisulfite

(1) When iodine TS is added dropwise to acidic solutions of sulfites or bisulfites in acetic acid (31), the color of the reagent fades.

(2) When an equal volume of dilute hydrochloric acid is added, solutions of sulfites or bisulfites evolve the odor of sulfur dioxide but yield no turbidity (discrimination from thiosulfates). The solutions yield immediately with 1 drop of sodium sulfide TS a white turbidity, which changes gradually to a pale yellow precipitate.

Tartrate

(1) Neutral tartrate solutions yield a white precipitate with silver nitrate TS. When nitric acid is added to a portion of the separated precipitate, it dissolves. When ammonia TS is added to another portion and warmed, the precipitate dissolves and metallic silver is deposited gradually on the inside wall of the test tube, forming a mirror.

(2) Solutions of tartrates exhibit a red-purple to purple color, when 2 drops of acetic acid (31), 1 drop of iron (II) sulfate TS, 2 to 3 drops of hydrogen peroxide TS and an excess of sodium hydroxide TS are added.

(3) When a solution, prepared by mixing 2 to 3 drops of a solution of resorcinol (1 in 50) and 2 to 3 drops of a solution of potassium bromide (1 in 10) with 5 mL of sulfuric acid, is added to 2 to 3 drops of solutions of tartrates, and then heated for 5 to 10 minutes on a water bath, a deep blue color is produced. The solution exhibits a red to red-orange color when poured to 3 mL of water after cooling.

Thiocyanate

(1) Solutions of thiocyanates yield a white precipitate with an excess of silver nitrate TS. When dilute nitric acid is added to a portion of the suspension, the precipitate does not dissolve. When ammonia solution (28) is added to another portion, the precipitate dissolves.

(2) Solutions of thiocyanates produce with iron (III) chloride TS a red color, which is not decolored by addition of hydrochloric acid.

Thiosulfate

(1) When iodine TS is added dropwise to acidic solutions of thiosulfates in acetic acid (31), the color of the reagent fades.

(2) When an equal volume of dilute hydrochloric acid is added, solutions of thiosulfates evolve the odor of sulfur dioxide, and yield gradually a white turbidity, which changes to yellow on standing.

(3) Solutions of thiosulfates yield with an excess of silver nitrate TS a white precipitate, which changes to black on standing.

Zinc salt

(1) Neutral to alkaline solutions of zinc salts yield a whitish precipitate with ammonium sulfide TS or sodium sulfide TS. The separated precipitate does not dissolve in dilute acetic acid but dissolves upon subsequent addition of dilute hydrochloric acid.

(2) Solutions of zinc salts yield a white precipitate with potassium hexacyanoferrate (II) TS. When dilute hydrochloric acid is added to a portion of the suspension, the precipitate does not dissolve. When sodium hydroxide TS is added to another portion, the precipitate dissolves.

(3) Neutral to weakly acidic solutions of zinc salts yield a white precipitate, when 1 or 2 drops of pyridine and 1 mL of potassium thiocyanate TS are added.

1.10 Iron Limit Test

Iron Limit Test is a limit test for iron contained in drugs. The limit is expressed in term of iron (Fe).

In each monograph, the permissible limit for iron (as Fe) is described in terms of ppm in parentheses.

1. Preparation of test solutions and control solutions

Unless otherwise specified, test solutions and control solutions are prepared as follows:

1.1. Method 1

Weigh the amount of sample specified in individual monograph, add 30 mL of acetic acid-sodium acetate buffer solution for iron limit test (pH 4.5), dissolve by warming if necessary, and designate this solution as the test solution.

Prepare the control solution as follows: To the amount of Standard Iron Solution specified in individual monograph add 30 mL of acetic acid-sodium acetate buffer solution for iron limit test (pH 4.5).

1.2. Method 2

Weigh the amount of sample specified in individual monograph, add 10 mL of dilute hydrochloric acid, and dissolve by warming if necessary. Dissolve 0.5 g of L-tartaric acid, and add one drop of phenolphthalein TS. Add ammonia TS dropwise until the solution develops a pale red color. Add 20 mL of acetic acid-sodium acetate buffer solution for iron limit test (pH 4.5) and designate this solution as the test solution.

Prepare the control solution as follows: To the amount of Standard Iron Solution specified in individual monograph add 10 mL of dilute hydrochloric acid, and proceed as directed for the test solution.

1.3. Method 3

Place the amount of sample specified in individual monograph in a crucible, moisten with a small amount of sulfuric acid, heat cautiously and gently at first, and then incinerate by ignition. After cooling, add 1 mL of diluted hydrochloric acid (2 in 3) and 0.5 mL of diluted nitric acid (1 in 3), evaporate on a water bath to dryness, and to the residue add 0.5 mL of diluted hydrochloric acid (2 in 3) and 10 mL of water. After dissolving by warming, add 30 mL of acetic acid-sodium acetate buffer solution for iron limit test (pH 4.5), and designate this solution as the test solution.

Prepare the control solution as follows: Transfer the amount of Standard Iron Solution specified in individual monograph to a crucible, and add 1 mL of diluted hydrochloric acid (2 in 3) and 0.5 mL of diluted nitric acid (1 in 3), evaporate on a water bath to dryness, and proceed as directed for the test solution.

In this procedure, use a quartz or porcelain crucible, which is immersed in boiling dilute hydrochloric acid for 1 hour and washed thoroughly with water and dried.

2. Procedure

Unless otherwise specified, proceed as follows:

2.1. Method A

Transfer the test solution and the control solution to separate Nessler tubes, to each add 2 mL of a solution of L-ascorbic acid (1 in 100), mix well, and allow to stand for 30 minutes. Add 1 mL of a solution of α, α'-dipyridyl in ethanol (95) (1 in 200), add water to make 50 mL, and allow to stand for 30 minutes. Then compare the colors developed in both solutions against a white background. The test solution has no more color than the control solution.

2.2. Method B

Dissolve 0.2 g of L-ascorbic acid in the test solution and the control solution, and allow to stand for 30 minutes. Add 1 mL of a solution of α, α'-dipyridyl in ethanol (95) (1 in 200), and allow to stand for 30 minutes. Then add 2 mL of a solution of 2,4,6-trinitrophenol (3 in 1000) and 20 mL of 1,2-dichloroethane, shake vigorously, collect the 1,2-dichloroethane layer, and filter through a pledget of absorbent cotton in a funnel on which 5 g of anhydrous sodium sulfate is placed if necessary. Then compare the colors developed in both solutions against a white background. The test solution has no more color than the control solution.

1.11 Arsenic Limit Test

Arsenic Limit Test is a limit test for arsenic contained in drugs. The limit is expressed in terms of arsenic trioxide (As_2O_3).

In each monograph, the permissible limit for arsenic (as As_2O_3) is described in terms of ppm in parentheses.

1. Apparatus

Use the apparatus illustrated in Fig. 1.11-1.

Place glass wool F in the exit tube B up to about 30 mm in height, moisten the glass wool uniformly with a mixture of an equal volume of lead (II) acetate TS and water, and apply gentle suction to the lower end to remove the excess of the mixture. Insert the tube vertically into the center of the rubber stopper H, and attach the tube to the generator bottle A

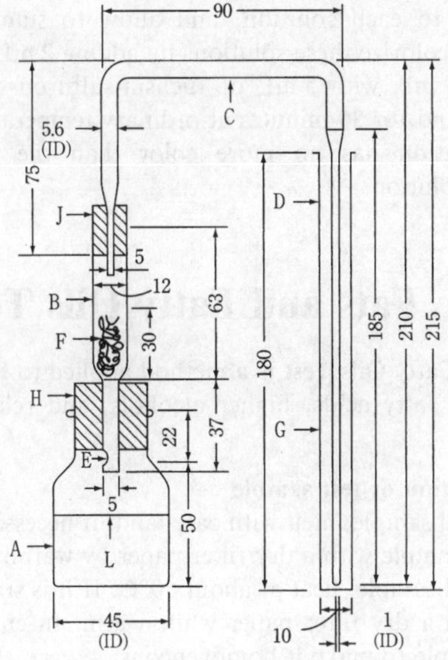

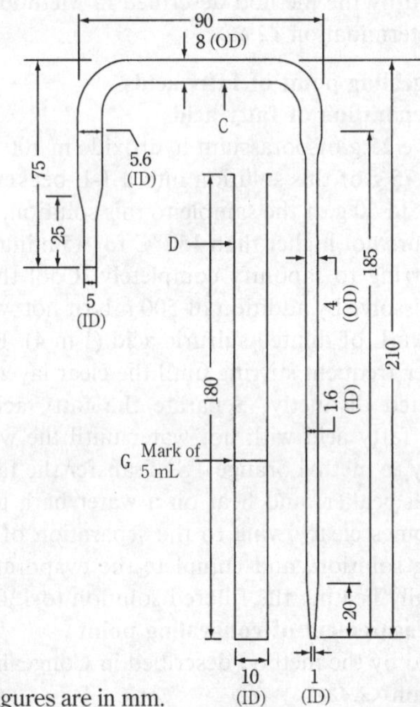

The figures are in mm.

A: Generator bottle (capacity up to the shoulder: approximately 70 mL)
B: Exit tube
C: Glass tube (inside diameter: 5.6 mm, the tip of the part to be inserted in the absorber tube D is drawn out to 1 mm in diameter)
D: Absorber tube (inside diameter: 10 mm)
E: Small perforation
F: Glass wool (about 0.2 g)
G: Mark of 5 mL
H and J: Rubber stoppers
L: Mark of 40 mL

Fig. 1.11-1 Arsenic limit test apparatus

so that the small perforation E in the lower end of B extends slightly below. At the upper end of B, attach the rubber stopper J to hold the tube C vertically. Make the lower end to the exit tube of C level with that of the rubber stopper J.

2. Preparation of the test solution

Unless otherwise specified, proceed as directed in the following.

2.1. Method 1

Weigh the amount of the sample directed in the monograph, add 5 mL of water, dissolve by heating if necessary, and designate the solution as the test solution.

2.2. Method 2

Weigh the amount of the sample directed in the monograph, add 5 mL of water, and add 1 mL of sulfuric acid except in the cases that the samples are inorganic acids. Add 10 mL of sulfurous acid solution, transfer to a small beaker, and evaporate the mixture on a water bath until it is free from sulfurous acid and is reduced to about 2 mL in volume. Dilute with water to make 5 mL, and designate it as the test solution.

2.3. Method 3

Weigh the amount of the sample directed in the monograph, and place it in a crucible of platinum, quartz or porcelain. Add 10 mL of a solution of magnesium nitrate hexahydrate in ethanol (95) (1 in 50), ignite the ethanol, and heat gradually to incinerate. If carbonized material still remains by this procedure, moisten with a small quantity of nitric acid, and ignite again to incinerate. After cooling, add 3 mL of hydrochloric acid, heat on a water bath to dissolve the residue, and designate it as the test solution.

2.4. Method 4

Weigh the amount of the sample directed in the monograph, and place it in a crucible of platinum, quartz or porcelain. Add 10 mL of a solution of magnesium nitrate hexahydrate in ethanol (95) (1 in 10), burn the ethanol, heat gradually, and ignite to incinerate. If carbonized material still remains by this procedure, moisten with a small quantity of nitric acid, and ignite again to incinerate in the same manner. After cooling, add 3 mL of hydrochloric acid, heat on a water bath to dissolve the residue, and designate it as the test solution.

2.5. Method 5

Weigh the amount of the sample directed in the monograph, add 10 mL of *N,N*-dimethylformamide, dissolve by heating if necessary, and designate the solution as the test solution.

3. Test solutions

(i) Absorbing solution for hydrogen arsenide: Dissolve 0.50 g of silver *N,N*-diethyldithiocarbamate in pyridine to make 100 mL. Preserve this solution in a glass-stoppered bottle protected from light, in a cold place.

(ii) Standard Arsenic Stock Solution: Weigh exactly 0.100 g of finely powdered arsenic trioxide dried at 105°C for 4 hours, and add 5 mL of sodium hydroxide solution (1 in 5) to dissolve. Add dilute sulfuric acid to neutralize, add further 10 mL of dilute sulfuric acid, add freshly boiled and cooled water to make exactly 1000 mL, and preserve in a glass-stoppered bottle.

(iii) Standard Arsenic Solution: Pipet 10 mL of Standard Arsenic Stock Solution, add 10 mL of dilute sulfuric acid, and add freshly boiled and cooled water to make exactly 1000 mL. Each mL of the solution contains 1 μg of arsenic trioxide (As_2O_3). Prepare Standard Arsenic Solution just before use.

In the case where the preparation of Standard Arsenic Stock Solution is difficult, Certified Standard Arsenic Solution may be used to prepare Standard Arsenic Solution as follows: Pipet 15 mL of Certified Standard Arsenic Solution, add 1 mL of dilute sulfuric acid, and add freshly boiled and cooled water to make exactly 100 mL. Pipet 5 mL of this solution, add 1 mL of dilute sulfuric acid, and add freshly boiled and cooled water to make exactly 100 mL. Prepare just before use.

(iv) Certified Standard Arsenic Solution: JCSS Arsenic Standard Solution (100 mg/L) Each mL of this solution contains 0.1 mg of arsenic (A_S).

JCSS (Japan Calibration Service System) is a registration system of calibration service.

4. Procedure

Unless otherwise specified, proceed using apparatus shown in Fig. 1.11-1. Carry out the preparation of the standard color at the same time.

Place the test solution in the generator bottle A and, if necessary, wash down the solution in the bottle with a small quantity of water. Add 1 drop of methyl orange TS, and after neutralizing with ammonia TS, ammonia solution (28) or dilute hydrochloric acid, add 5 mL of diluted hydrochloric acid (1 in 2) and 5 mL of potassium iodide TS, and allow to stand for 2 to 3 minutes. Add 5 mL of acidic tin (II) chloride TS, and allow to stand for 10 minutes. Then add water to make 40 mL, add 2 g of zinc for arsenic analysis, and immediately connect the rubber stopper H fitted with B and C with the generator bottle A. Transfer 5 mL of the absorbing solution for hydrogen arsenide to the absorber tube D, insert the tip of C to the bottom of the absorber tube D, then immerse the generator bottle A up to the shoulder in water maintained at 25°C, and allow to stand for 1 hour. Disconnect the absorber tube, add pyridine to make 5 mL, if necessary, and observe the color of the absorbing solution: the color produced is not more intense than the standard color.

Preparation of standard color: Measure accurately 2 mL of Standard Arsenic Solution in the generator bottle A. Add 5 mL of diluted hydrochloric acid (1 in 2) and 5 mL of potassium iodide TS, and allow to stand for 2 to 3 minutes. Add 5 mL of acidic tin (II) chloride TS, allow to stand at room temperature for 10 minutes, and then proceed as directed above. The color produced corresponds to 2 μg of arsenic trioxide (As_2O_3) and is used as the standard.

5. Note

Apparatus, reagents and test solutions used in the test should contain little or no arsenic. If necessary, perform a blank determination.

1.12 Methanol Test

Methanol Test is a method to determine methanol adhering in ethanol.

1. Reagents

(i) Standard Methanol Solution—To 1.0 g of methanol, accurately measured, add water to make exactly 1000 mL. To 5 mL of this solution, exactly measured, add 2.5 mL of methanol-free ethanol and water to make exactly 50 mL.

(ii) Solution A—To 75 mL of phosphoric acid add water to make 500 mL, then dissolve 15 g of potassium permanganate in this solution.

(iii) Solution B—Add sulfuric acid carefully to an equal volume of water, cool, and dissolve 25 g of oxalic acid dihydrate in 500 mL of this dilute sulfuric acid.

2. Procedure

Pipet 1 mL of the sample, and add water to make exactly 20 mL. Use this solution as the sample solution. Transfer 5 mL each of the sample solution and the Standard Methanol Solution, accurately measured, to test tubes, add 2 mL of Solution A to each solution, and allow to stand for 15 minutes. Decolorize these solutions by adding 2 mL of Solution B, and mix with 5 mL of fuchsin-sulfurous acid TS. Allow to stand for 30 minutes at ordinary temperature. The sample solution has no more color than the Standard Methanol Solution.

1.13 Fats and Fatty Oils Test

Fats and Fatty Oils Test is a method applied to fats, fatty oils, waxes, fatty acids, higher alcohols, and related substances.

1. Preparation of test sample

For a solid sample, melt with care, and, if necessary, filter the melted sample with a dry filter paper by warming. For a turbid liquid sample, heat at about 50°C. If it is still turbid, filter it with a dry filter paper while warm. In either case, mix the sample to make it homogeneous.

2. Melting point

Proceed by the method described in Method 2 of Melting Point Determination <*2.60*>.

3. Congealing point of fatty acids

3.1. Preparation of fatty acids

Dissolve 25 g of potassium hydroxide in 100 g of glycerin. Transfer 75 g of this solution into a 1-L beaker, and heat at 150°C. Add 50 g of the sample to this solution, and heat at a temperature not higher than 150°C for 15 minutes under frequent stirring to saponify completely. Cool the solution to 100°C, dissolve by addition of 500 mL of hot water, and add slowly 50 mL of diluted sulfuric acid (1 in 4). Heat the solution under frequent stirring until the clear layer of fatty acid is separated distinctly. Separate the fatty acid layer, and wash the fatty acid with hot water until the washing shows no acidity to methyl orange TS. Transfer the fatty acid layer to a small beaker, and heat on a water bath until the fatty acid becomes clear owing to the separation of water. Filter the warm solution, and complete the evaporation of water by carefully heating the filtered solution to 130°C.

3.2. Measurement of congealing point

Proceed by the method described in Congealing Point Determination <*2.42*>.

4. Specific gravity

4.1. Liquid sample at ordinary temperature

Proceed by the method described in Determination of Specific Gravity and Density <*2.56*>.

4.2. Solid sample at ordinary temperature

Unless otherwise specified, fill a pycnometer with water at 20°C. Weigh accurately the pycnometer, and, after discarding the water and drying, weigh accurately the empty pycnometer. Then, fill the pycnometer with the melted sample to about three-fourths of the depth, and allow to stand at a temperature a little higher than the melting temperature of the sample for 1 hour to drive off the air in the sample. After keeping at the specified temperature, weigh accurately the pycnometer. Fill up the pycnometer with water over the sample at 20°C, and weigh accurately again.

The other procedure is the same as described in Method 1 of Determination of Specific Gravity and Density <*2.56*>.

$$d = \frac{M_1 - M}{(M_2 - M) - (M_3 - M_1)}$$

M: Mass (g) of the empty pycnometer
M_1: Mass (g) of the pycnometer filled with the sample

Table 1.13-1

Acid value	Amount (g) of sample
Less than 5	20
5 to 15	10
15 to 30	5
30 to 100	2.5
More than 100	1.0

M_2: Mass (g) of the pycnometer filled with water
M_3: Mass (g) of the pycnometer filled with the sample and water

5. Acid value

The acid value is the number of milligrams of potassium hydroxide (KOH) required to neutralize the free acids in 1 g of sample.

5.1. Procedure

Unless otherwise specified, weigh accurately the amount of sample shown in Table 1.13-1, according to the expected acid value of the sample, in a glass-stoppered, 250-mL flask, add 100 mL of a mixture of diethyl ether and ethanol (95) (1:1 or 2:1) as the solvent, and dissolve the sample by warming, if necessary. Then, add a few drops of phenolphthalein TS, and titrate <*2.50*> with 0.1 mol/L potassium hydroxide-ethanol VS until the solution develops a light red color which persists for 30 seconds. If the sample solutions are turbid at lower temperature, titration should be done while warm. To the solvent used add phenolphthalein TS as an indicator, and add 0.1 mol/L potassium hydroxide-ethanol VS before use, until the solvent remains light red for 30 seconds.

$$\text{Acid value} = \frac{\begin{array}{c}\text{consumed volume (mL) of 0.1 mol/L} \\ \text{potassium hydroxide-ethanol VS}\end{array} \times 5.611}{\text{amount (g) of sample}}$$

6. Saponification value

The saponification value is the number of milligrams of potassium hydroxide (KOH) required to saponify the esters and to neutralize the free acids in 1 g of the sample.

6.1. Procedure

Unless otherwise specified, weigh accurately 1 to 2 g of the sample, transfer to a 200-mL flask, and add exactly 25 mL of 0.5 mol/L potassium hydroxide-ethanol VS. Attach a short reflux condenser or an air condenser 750 mm in length and 6 mm in diameter to the neck of the flask, and heat gently in a water bath for 1 hour with frequent shaking. Cool the solution, add 1 mL of phenolphthalein TS, and titrate <*2.50*> immediately the excess potassium hydroxide with 0.5 mol/L hydrochloric acid VS. If the sample solution is turbid at lower temperature, titration should be done while warm. Perform a blank determination in the same manner.

$$\text{Saponification value} = \frac{(a - b) \times 28.05}{\text{amount (g) of sample}}$$

a: Volume (mL) of 0.5 mol/L hydrochloric acid VS consumed in the blank determination
b: Volume (mL) of 0.5 mol/L hydrochloric acid VS consumed for titration of the sample

7. Ester value

The ester value is the number of milligrams of potassium hydroxide (KOH) required to saponify the esters in 1 g of sample.

7.1. Procedure

Unless otherwise specified, designate the difference between the saponification value and the acid value determined as the ester value.

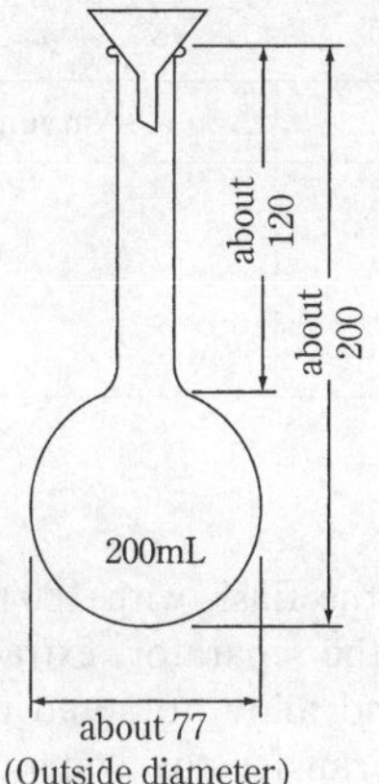

Fig. 1.13-1 Hydroxyl value determination flask

8. Hydroxyl value

The hydroxyl value is the number of milligrams of potassium hydroxide (KOH) required to neutralize acetic acid combined with hydroxyl groups, when 1 g of the sample is acetylated by the following procedure.

8.1. Procedure

Place about 1 g of the sample, weighed accurately, in a 200-mL round-bottom flask (shown in Fig. 1.13-1), and add exactly 5 mL of pyridine-acetic anhydride TS. Place a small funnel on the neck of the flask, and heat by immersing the flask up to 1 cm from the bottom in an oil bath between 95°C and 100°C. Put a thick, round paper with a round hole on the joint of the neck of the flask to protect the neck from the heat of the oil bath. After heating for 1 hour, take the flask from the oil bath, and cool by standing. Add 1 mL of water to the flask, and shake to decompose acetic anhydride. Heat the flask in the oil bath for 10 minutes again. After cooling, wash the funnel and neck with 5 mL of neutralized ethanol down into the flask, and titrate <*2.50*> with 0.5 mol/L potassium hydroxide-ethanol VS (indicator: 1 mL of phenolphthalein TS). Perform a blank determination in the same manner.

$$\text{Hydroxyl value} = \frac{(a - b) \times 28.05}{\text{amount (g) of sample}} + \text{acid value}$$

a: Volume (mL) of 0.5 mol/L potassium hydroxide-ethanol VS consumed in the blank determination
b: Volume (mL) of 0.5 mol/L potassium hydroxide-ethanol VS consumed for titration of the sample

9. Unsaponifiable matter

Unsaponifiable matter is calculated as the difference between the amount of materials, which are unsaponifiable by the procedure described below, soluble in diethyl ether and insoluble in water, and the amount of fatty acids expressed in terms of the amount of oleic acid. Its limit is expressed as a percentage in the monograph.

9.1. Procedure

Transfer about 5 g of the sample, accurately weighed, to a 250-mL flask. Add 50 mL of potassium hydroxide-ethanol TS, attach a reflux condenser to the flask, boil gently on a water bath for 1 hour with frequent shaking, and then transfer to the first separator. Wash the flask with 100 mL of warm water, and transfer the washing to the separator. Further, add 50 mL of water to the separator, and cool to room

Table 1.13-2

Iodine value	Amount (g) of sample
Less than 30	1.0
30 to 50	0.6
50 to 100	0.3
More than 100	0.2

temperature. Wash the flask with 100 mL of diethyl ether, add the washing to the separator, extract by vigorous shaking for 1 minute, and allow to stand until both layers are separated clearly. Transfer the water layer to the second separator, add 50 mL of diethyl ether, shake, and allow to stand in the same manner. Transfer the water layer in the second separator to the third separator, add 50 mL of diethyl ether, and extract by shaking again in the same manner. Combine the diethyl ether extracts in the second and third separators into the first separator, wash each separator with a small amount of diethyl ether, and combine the washings into the first separator. Wash the combined extracts in the first separator with 30 mL portions of water successively, until the washing does not develop a light red color with 2 drops of phenolphthalein TS. Add a small amount of anhydrous sodium sulfate to the diethyl ether extracts, and allow to stand for 1 hour. Filter the diethyl ether extracts with dry filter paper, and collect the filtrates into a tared flask. Wash well the first separator with diethyl ether, and add the washing to the flask through the above filter paper. After evaporation of the filtrate and washing almost to dryness on a water bath, add 3 mL of acetone, and evaporate again to dryness on a water bath. Complete the drying between 70°C and 80°C under reduced pressure (about 2.67 kPa) for 30 minutes, allow to stand for cooling in a desiccator (reduced pressure, silica gel) for 30 minutes, and then weigh. After weighing, add 2 mL of diethyl ether and 10 mL of neutralized ethanol, and dissolve the residue by shaking well. Add a few drops of phenolphthalein TS, and titrate <*2.50*> the remaining fatty acids in the residue with 0.1 mol/L potassium hydroxide-ethanol VS until the solution develops a light red color which persists for 30 seconds.

$$\text{Unsaponifiable matter (\%)} = \frac{a - (b \times 0.0282)}{\text{amount (g) of sample}} \times 100$$

a: Amount (g) of the extracts
b: Volume (mL) of 0.1 mol/L potassium hydroxide-ethanol VS consumed for titration

10. Iodine value

The iodine value, when measured under the following conditions, is the number of grams of iodine (I), representing the corresponding amount of halogen, which combines with 100 g of sample.

10.1. Procedure

Unless otherwise specified, weigh accurately the amount of sample shown in Table 1.13-2, according to the expected iodine value of the sample, in a small glass container. In a 500-mL glass-stoppered flask place the container containing the sample, add 20 mL of cyclohexane to dissolve the sample, then add exactly 25 mL of Wijs' TS, and mix well. Stopper the flask, and allow to stand, protecting against light, between 20°C and 30°C for 30 minutes (when the expected iodine value is more than 100, for 1 hour) with occasional shaking. Add 20 mL of potassium iodide solution (1 in 10) and 100 mL of water, and shake. Then, titrate <*2.50*> the liberated iodine with 0.1 mol/L sodium thiosulfate VS (indicator: 1 mL of starch TS). Perform a blank determination in the same manner.

$$\text{Iodine value} = \frac{(a - b) \times 1.269}{\text{amount (g) of sample}}$$

a: Volume (mL) of 0.1 mol/L sodium thiosulfate VS consumed in the blank determination
b: Volume (mL) of 0.1 mol/L sodium thiosulfate VS consumed for titration of the sample

1.14 Sulfate Limit Test

Sulfate Limit Test is a limit test for sulfate contained in drugs.

In each monograph, the permissible limit for sulfate (as SO_4) is described in terms of percentage (%) in parentheses.

1. Procedure

Unless otherwise specified, transfer the quantity of the sample, directed in the monograph, to a Nessler tube, dissolve it in sufficient water, and add water to make 40 mL. Add 1 mL of dilute hydrochloric acid and water to make 50 mL, and use this solution as the test solution. Transfer the volume of 0.005 mol/L sulfuric acid VS, directed in the monograph, to another Nessler tube, add 1 mL of dilute hydrochloric acid and water to make 50 mL, and use this solution as the control solution. When the test solution is not clear, filter both solutions according to the same procedure.

Add 2 mL of barium chloride TS to the test solution and to the control solution, mix well, and allow to stand for 10 minutes. Compare the white turbidity produced in both solutions against a black background by viewing downward or transversely.

The turbidity produced in the test solution is not thicker than that of the control solution.

1.15 Readily Carbonizable Substances Test

Readily Carbonizable Substances Test is a method to examine the minute impurities contained in drugs, which are readily colored by addition of sulfuric acid.

1. Procedure

Before use, wash the Nessler tubes thoroughly with sulfuric acid for readily carbonizable substances. Unless otherwise specified, proceed as follows. When the sample is solid, place 5 mL of sulfuric acid for readily carbonizable substances in a Nessler tube, to which add a quantity of the finely powdered sample, little by little, as directed in the monograph, and dissolve it completely by stirring with a glass rod. When the sample is liquid, transfer a volume of the sample, as directed in the monograph, to a Nessler tube, add 5 mL of sulfuric acid for readily carbonizable substances, and mix by shaking. If the temperature of the content of the tube rises, cool the content; maintain it at the standard temperature, if the reaction may be affected by the temperature. Allow to stand for 15 minutes, and compare the color of the liquid with that of the matching fluid in the Nessler tube specified in the monograph, by viewing transversely against a white background.

2. Physical Methods

Chromatography

2.01 Liquid Chromatography

Liquid Chromatography is a method to develop a mixture injected into a column prepared with a suitable stationary phase by passing a liquid as a mobile phase through the column, in order to separate the mixture into its components by making use of the difference of retention capacity against the stationary phase, and to determine the components. This method can be applied to a liquid or soluble sample, and is used for identification, purity test, and quantitative determination.

A mixture injected into the column is distributed between the mobile phase and the stationary phase with a characteristic ratio (k) for each component.

$$k = \frac{\text{amount of compound in the stationary phase}}{\text{amount of compound in the mobile phase}}$$

The ratio k represents the mass distribution ratio in liquid chromatography.

Since the relation given below exists among the ratio (k), the time for which the mobile phase is passed through the column (t_0: time measured from the time of injection of a compound with $k = 0$ to the time of elution at the peak maximum), and the retention time (t_R: time measured from the time of injection of a compound to be determined to the time of elution at the peak maximum), the retention time for a compound on a column has a characteristic value under fixed chromatographic conditions.

$$t_R = (1 + k)\, t_0$$

1. Apparatus

Basically, the apparatus required for the liquid chromatographic procedure consists of a pumping system for the mobile phase, a sample injection port, a column, a detector and a recorder. A mobile phase component regulator, a thermostat for the column, a pumping system for reaction reagents and a chemical reaction chamber are also used, if necessary. The pumping system serves to deliver the mobile phase and the reagents into the column and connecting tube at a constant flow rate. The sample injection port is used to deliver a quantity of the sample to the apparatus with high reproducibility. The column is a tube with a smooth interior, made of inert metal, etc., in which a packing material for liquid chromatography is uniformly packed. A column with a stationary phase chemically bound on the inside wall instead of the column packed with the packing material may be used. The detector is used to detect a property of the samples which is different from that of the mobile phase, and may be an ultraviolet or visible spectrophotometer, fluorometric detector, differential refractometer, electrochemical detector, chemiluminescence detector, electric conductivity detector, mass spectrophotometer, etc. The output signal is usually proportional to the concentration of samples at amounts of less than a few μg. The recorder is used to record the output signals of the detector. As required, a data processor may be used as the recorder to record or output the chromatogram, retention times or amounts of the components. The mobile phase component regulator is used to vary the ratio of the mobile phase components in a stepwise or gradient fashion.

2. Procedure

Fix the detector, column and mobile phase to the apparatus, and adjust the flow rate and the column temperature to the values described in the operating conditions specified in the individual monograph. Inject a volume of the sample solution or the standard solution specified in the individual monograph with the sample injector into the column through the sample injection port. The separated components are detected by the detector, and recorded by the recorder as a chromatogram. If the components to be analyzed have no readily detectable physical properties such as absorbance or fluorescence, the detection is achieved by changing the components to suitable derivatives. Usually, the derivatization is performed as a pre- or post-column labeling.

3. Identification and purity test

When Liquid Chromatography is used for identification of a component of a sample, it is performed by confirming identity of the retention time of the component and that of an authentic specimen, or by confirming that the peak shape of the component is unchanged after mixing the sample with an authentic specimen. If a detector which is able to obtain chemical structural information of the component at the same time is used, highly specific identification can be achieved by confirming identity of the chemical structure of the component and that of an authentic specimen, in addition to the identity of their retention times.

When Liquid Chromatography is used for purity test, it is generally performed by comparing the peak area of target impurity from the sample solution with that of the main component from a standard solution, which is prepared by diluting the sample solution to a concentration corresponding to the specified limit of the impurity, or by calculating target impurity content using the peak area percentage method. Unless otherwise specified, if a sample is separated into isomers in the chromatogram, the isomer ratio is calculated by using the peak area percentage method.

The peak area percentage method is a method to calculate the proportion of the components from the ratio of the peak area of each component to the sum of the peak areas of every peak recorded in the chromatogram. In order to obtain accurate results in evaluating the proportion of the components, it is necessary to correct the area of each component based on its correction factor to the principal component.

4. Assay

4.1. Internal standard method

In the internal standard method, choose a stable compound as an internal standard which shows a retention time close to that of the compound to be assayed, and whose peak is well separated from all other peaks in the chromatogram. Prepare several kinds of standard solutions containing a fixed amount of the internal standard and several graded amounts of the authentic specimen specified in the individual monograph. Based on the chromatogram obtained by injection of a fixed volume of individual standard solutions, calculate the ratio of peak area or peak height of the authentic specimen to that of the internal standard, and prepare a calibration curve by plotting these ratios on the ordinate against the amount of the authentic specimen or the ratio of the amount of the authentic specimen to that of the internal standard on the abscissa. The calibration curve is usually obtained as a straight line passing through the origin. Then, prepare a sample solution containing the internal standard in the same amount as in the standard solutions used for the preparation of the calibration curve according to the method specified in the individual monograph, perform the liquid chromatography under the same operating conditions as for the preparation of the calibration curve, calculate the ratio of the peak area or peak height of the objective compound to that of the internal standard, and read the amount of the compound from the calibration curve.

In an individual monograph, generally one of the standard solutions with a concentration within the linear range of the calibration curve and a sample solution with a concentration close to that of the standard solution are prepared, and the chromatography is performed with these solutions under fixed conditions to determine the amount of the objective compound.

4.2. Absolute calibration curve method

Prepare standard solutions with several graded amounts of the authentic specimen, and inject accurately a fixed volume of these standard solutions. With the chromatogram obtained, prepare a calibration curve by plotting the peak areas or peak heights on the ordinate against the amount of the authentic specimen on the abscissa. The calibration curve is generally obtained as a straight line passing through the origin. Then, prepare a sample solution according to the method specified in the individual monograph, perform the liquid chromatography under the same conditions as for the preparation of the calibration curve, measure the peak area or peak height of the objective compound, and read the amount of the compound from the calibration curve.

In an individual monograph, generally one of the standard solutions with a concentration within the linear range of the calibration curve and a sample solution with a concentration close to that of the standard solution are prepared, and the chromatography is performed with these solutions under a fixed condition to obtain the amount of the component. In this method, all procedures, such as the injection procedure, must be carried out under a strictly constant condition.

5. Method for peak measuring

Generally, the following methods are used.

5.1. Peak height measuring method

(i) Peak height method: Measure the distance between the maximum of the peak and the intersecting point of a perpendicular line from the maximum of the peak to the horizontal axis of recording paper with a tangent linking the baselines on both sides of the peak.

(ii) Automatic peak height method: Measure the signals from the detector as the peak height using a data processing system.

5.2. Peak area measuring method

(i) Width at half-height method: Multiply the peak width at the half-height by the peak height.

(ii) Automatic integration method: Measure the signals from the detector as the peak area using a data processing system.

6. System suitability

System suitability testing is an integral part of test methods using chromatography, and is used to ensure that the performance of the chromatographic systems used is as suitable for the analysis of the drug as was at the time when the verification of the test method was performed using the system. System suitability testing should be carried out at every series of drug analysis. The test procedures and acceptance criteria of system suitability testing must be prescribed in the test method of drugs. The results of drug analyses are not acceptable unless the requirements of system suitability have been met.

In system suitability testing of the chromatographic systems, the evaluation of "System performance" and "System repeatability" is usually required. For quantitative purity tests, the evaluation of "Test for required detectability" may also be required.

6.1. Test for required detectability

For purity tests, when it is confirmed that the target impurity is distinctly detected at the concentration of its specification limit, it is considered verified that the system used has adequate performance to achieve its intended use.

For quantitative purity tests, "Test for required detectability" is usually required, and in order to confirm, in some degree, the linearity of response near its specification limit, the range of expected response to the injection of a certain volume of target impurity solution at the concentration of its specification limit should be prescribed. For limit test, "Test for required detectability" is not required, if the test is performed by comparing the response from sample solution with that from standard solution at the concentration of its specification limit. "Test for required detectability" is also not required, if it is confirmed that the impurity can be detected at its specification limit by the evaluation of "System repeatability" or some other procedure.

6.2. System performance

When it is confirmed that the specificity for determining the test ingredient is ensured, it is considered verified that the system used has adequate performance to achieve its intended use.

In assay, "System performance" should be defined by the resolution between the test ingredient and a target substance to be separated (a closely eluting compound is preferable), and when appropriate, by their order of elution. In purity tests, both the resolution and the order of elution between the test ingredient and a target substance to be separated (a closely eluting compound is preferable) should be prescribed. In addition, if necessary, the symmetry factor of the test ingredient should be prescribed together with them. However, if there is no suitable target substance to be separated, it is acceptable to define "System performance" using the number of theoretical plates and the symmetry factor of the test ingredient.

6.3. System repeatability

When it is confirmed that the degree of variation (precision) of the response of the test ingredient is at a level that meets the requirement of "System repeatability", it is considered verified that the system used has adequate performance to achieve its intended use.

The allowable limit of "System repeatability" is normally defined as the relative standard deviation (*RSD*) of the response of the test ingredient in replicate injections of standard solution. It is acceptable to confirm the repeatability of the system not only by replicate injections of standard solution before sample injections, but also by divided injections of standard solution before and after sample injections, or by interspersed injections of standard solution among sample injections.

In principle, total number of replicate injections should be 6. However, in the case that a long time is necessary for one analysis, such as the analysis using the gradient method, or the analysis of samples containing late eluting components, it may be acceptable to decrease the number of replicate injections by adopting new allowable limit of "System repeatability" which can guarantee a level of "System repeatability" equivalent to that at 6 replicate injections.

The allowable limit of "System repeatability" should be set at an appropriate level based on the data when suitability of the method for the evaluation of quality of the drug was verified, and the precision necessary for the quality test.

7. Point to consider on changing the operating conditions

Among the operating conditions specified in the individual monograph, inside diameter and length of the column, particle size of the packing material (pore size in the case of monolithic columns), column temperature, composition ratio of the mobile phase, composition of buffer solutions in the mobile phase, pH of the mobile phase, concentration of ion-pair forming agents in the mobile phase, ionic strength of the mobile phase, flow rate of the mobile phase, number and timing of mobile phase composition changes in gradient program, flow rate of mobile phase in gradient program, composition and flow rate of derivatizing reagents, and reaction time and chamber temperature in chemical reaction may be modified within the ranges in which the liquid chromatographic system used conforms to the requirements of system suitability.

8. Terminology

(i) **SN ratio:** It is defined by the following formula.

$$S/N = \frac{2H}{h}$$

H: Peak height of the target ingredient peak from the baseline

h: Width of background noise of the chromatogram of sample solution or solvent blank around the peak of the target ingredient

The baseline and background noise are measured over a range 20 times of peak width at the center point of peak height of the target ingredient. When a solvent blank is used, measure over almost the same range as mentioned above around the point where the target ingredient elutes.

(ii) **Symmetry factor:** It shows the degree of symmetry of a peak in the chromatogram, and is defined as S in the following equation.

$$S = \frac{W_{0.05\,h}}{2f}$$

$W_{0.05\,h}$: Width of the peak at one-twentieth of the peak height

f: Distance between the perpendicular from the peak maximum and the leading edge of the peak at one-twentieth of the peak height

Where $W_{0.05\,h}$ and f have the same unit.

(iii) **Relative standard deviation:** Generally, it is defined as RSD (%) in the following equation.

$$\mathrm{RSD}\ (\%) = \frac{100}{\overline{X}} \times \sqrt{\frac{\sum_{i=1}^{n}(x_i - \overline{X})^2}{n-1}}$$

x_i: Observed value

$\overline{X}$: Mean of observed values

n: Number of replicate measurements

(iv) **Complete separation of peak**: It means that the resolution between two peaks is not less than 1.5. It is also called as "baseline separation".

(v) **Peak-valley ratio:** It indicates the degree of separation between 2 peaks on a chromatogram when baseline separation cannot be attained, and is defined as p/v by the following formula.

$$p/v = \frac{H_p}{H_v}$$

H_p: peak height from the baseline of the minor peak

H_v: height from the baseline of the lowest point (peak valley) of the curve between major and minor peaks

(vi) **Separation factor:** It shows the relation between the retention times of peaks in the chromatogram, and is defined as α in the following equation.

$$\alpha = \frac{t_{R2} - t_0}{t_{R1} - t_0}$$

t_{R1}, t_{R2}: Retention times of two compounds used for the resolution measurement ($t_{R1} < t_{R2}$)

t_0: Time of passage of the mobile phase through the column (time measured from the time of injection of a compound with $k = 0$ to the time of elution at the peak maximum)

The separation factor (α) indicates thermodynamic difference in partition of two compounds. It is basically the ratio of their partition equilibrium coefficients or of their mass-distribution ratios, and is obtained from the chromatogram as the ratio of the retention times of the two compounds.

(vii) **Resolution:** It shows the relation between the retention time and the peak width of peaks in the chromatogram, and is defined as R_S in the following equation.

$$R_S = 1.18 \times \frac{t_{R2} - t_{R1}}{W_{0.5\,h1} + W_{0.5\,h2}}$$

t_{R1}, t_{R2}: Retention times of two compounds used for the measurement of resolution ($t_{R1} < t_{R2}$)

$W_{0.5\,h1}$, $W_{0.5\,h2}$: Peak widths at half peak height

Where t_{R1}, t_{R2}, $W_{0.5\,h1}$ and $W_{0.5\,h2}$ have the same unit.

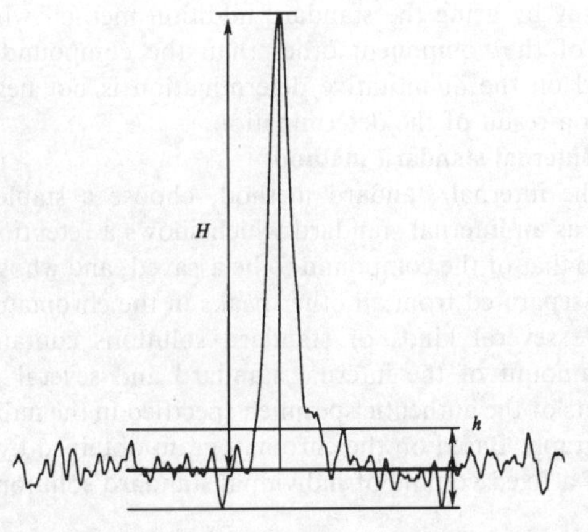

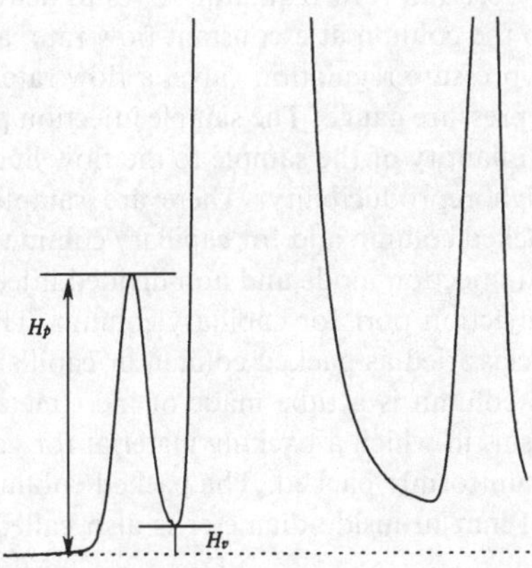

(viii) **Number of theoretical plates:** It indicates the extent of band broadening of a compound in the column, and is generally defined as N in the following equation.

$$N = 5.54 \times \frac{t_R{}^2}{W_{0.5\,h}{}^2}$$

t_R: Retention time of compound
$W_{0.5\,h}$: Width of the peak at half peak height

Where t_R and $W_{0.5\,h}$ have the same unit

9. Note

Avoid the use of authentic specimens, internal standards, reagents or solvents containing substances that may interfere with the determination.

2.02 Gas Chromatography

Gas Chromatography is a method to develop a mixture injected into a column prepared with a suitable stationary phase by passing a gas (carrier gas) as a mobile phase through the column, in order to separate the mixture into its components by making use of the difference of retention capacity against the stationary phase, and to determine the components. This method can be applied to a gaseous or vaporizable sample, and is used for identification, purity test, and quantitative determination.

A mixture injected into the column is distributed between the mobile phase and the stationary phase with a characteristic ratio (k) for each component.

$$k = \frac{\text{amount of compound in the stationary phase}}{\text{amount of compound in the mobile phase}}$$

Since the relation given below exists among the ratio (k), the time for which the mobile phase is passed through the column (t_0: time measured from the time of injection of a compound with $k = 0$ to the time of elution at the peak maximum), and the retention time (t_R: time measured from the time of injection of a compound to be determined to the time of elution at the peak maximum), the retention time for a compound on a column has a characteristic value under fixed chromatographic conditions.

$$t_R = (1 + k)\, t_0$$

1. Apparatus

Basically, the apparatus required for the gas chromatographic procedure consists of a carrier gas-introducing port and flow regulator, a sample injection port, a column, a column oven, a detector and a recorder. Gas introducing port and flow regulator for a combustion gas, a burning supporting gas and an accessory gas and sample injection port for headspace are also used, if necessary. The carrier gas-introducing port and flow regulator serves to deliver the carrier gas into the column at a constant flow rate, and usually consist of a pressure regulation valve, a flow rate regulation valve and a pressure gauge. The sample injection port is used to deliver a quantity of the sample to the flow line of carrier gas with high reproducibility. There are sample injection ports for packed column and for capillary column. There are both divided injection mode and non-divided injection mode to sample injection port for capillary column. The columns are usually classified as packed column or capillary column. The packed column is a tube made of inert metal, glass or synthetic resin, in which a packing material for gas chromatography is uniformly packed. The packed column with not more than 1 mm in inside diameter is also called a packed capillary column (micro packed column). A capillary column is a tube made of inert metal, glass, quartz or synthetic resin, whose inside wall is bound chemically with stationary phase for gas chromatography. The column oven has the setting capacity for a column with required length and the temperature regulation system for keeping the constant column temperature. The detector is used to detect a component separated on the column, and may be an alkaline thermal ionization detector, a flame photometry detector, mass spectrophotometer, hydrogen flame-ionization detector, an electron capture detector, a thermal conductivity detector, etc. The recorder is used to record the output signals of the detector.

2. Procedure

Unless otherwise specified, proceed by the following method. Fix the detector, column and carrier gas to the apparatus, and adjust the flow rate and the column temperature to the values described in the operating conditions specified in the individual monograph. Inject a volume of the sample solution or the standard solution specified in the individual monograph with the sample injector into the column system through the sample injection port. The separated components are detected by the detector, and recorded by the recorder as a chromatogram.

3. Identification and purity test

Identification of a component of a sample is performed by confirming identity of the retention time of the component and that of an authentic specimen, or by confirming that the peak shape of the component is unchanged after mixing the sample with an authentic specimen.

In general, the purity of the sample is determined by comparing the peak area of target impurity from the sample solution with that of the main component from a standard solution, which is prepared by diluting the sample solution to a concentration corresponding to the specified limit of the impurity, or by calculating target impurity content using the peak area percentage method. Unless otherwise specified, if a sample is separated into isomers in the chromatogram, the isomer ratio is calculated by using the peak area percentage method.

The peak area percentage method is a method to calculate the proportion of the components from the ratio of the peak area of each component to the sum of the peak areas of every peak recorded in the chromatogram. In order to obtain accurate results in evaluating the proportion of the components, it is necessary to correct the area of each component based on its response factor to the principal component.

4. Assay

In general, perform the assay by using the internal standard method. The absolute calibration curve method is used when a suitable internal standard is not available. Perform the assay by using the standard addition method when the effect of the component other than the compound to be assayed on the quantitative determination is not negligible against a result of the determination.

4.1. Internal standard method

In the internal standard method, choose a stable compound as an internal standard which shows a retention time close to that of the compound to be assayed, and whose peak is well separated from all other peaks in the chromatogram. Prepare several kinds of standard solutions containing a fixed amount of the internal standard and several graded amounts of the authentic specimen specified in the individual monograph. Based on the chromatogram obtained by injection of a fixed volume of individual standard solutions, calculate the ratio of peak area or peak height of the authentic specimen to that of the internal standard, and prepare a calibration curve by plotting these ratios on the ordinate against the amount of the authentic specimen or the ratio of the amount of the authentic specimen to that of the internal standard on the abscissa. The calibration curve is usually obtained as a straight line passing through the origin. Then, prepare a sample solution containing the internal standard in the same amount as in the standard solutions used for the preparation of the calibration curve according to the method specified in the individual monograph, perform the gas chromatography under the same operating conditions as for the preparation of the calibration curve, calculate the ratio of the peak area or peak height of the objective compound to that of the internal standard, and read the amount of the compound from the calibration curve.

In an individual monograph, generally one of the standard solutions with a concentration within the linear range of the calibration curve and a sample solution with a concentration close to that of the standard solution are prepared, and the chromatography is performed with these solutions under fixed conditions to determine the amount of the objective compound.

4.2. Absolute calibration curve method

Prepare standard solutions with several graded amounts of the authentic specimen, and inject accurately a fixed volume of these standard solutions. With the chromatogram obtained, prepare a calibration curve by plotting the peak areas or peak heights on the ordinate against the amount of the authentic specimen on the abscissa. The calibration curve is generally obtained as a straight line passing through the origin. Then, prepare a sample solution according to the method specified in the individual monograph, perform the gas chromatography under the same conditions as for the preparation of the calibration curve, measure the peak area or peak height of the objective compound, and read the amount of the compound from the calibration curve.

In an individual monograph, generally one of the standard solutions with a concentration within the linear range of the calibration curve and a sample solution with a concentration close to that of the standard solution are prepared, and the chromatography is performed with these solutions under a fixed condition to obtain the amount of the component. In this method, all procedures, such as the injection procedure, must be carried out under a strictly constant condition.

4.3. Standard addition method

Pipet a fixed volume of more than 4 sample solutions, add exactly the standard solution so that stepwise increasing amounts of the object compound are contained in the solutions except 1 sample solution, diluted exactly each solution with and without standard solution to a definite volume, and use each solution as the sample solution. Based on the chromatogram obtained by exact injection of a fixed volume of individual sample solutions, measure the peak area or peak height of individual sample solutions. Calculate the concentration of standard objective compound added into each sample solution, plot the amounts (concentration) of added standard object compound on the abscissa and the peak area or peak height on the ordinate on the graph, extend the calibration curve obtained by linking the plots, and determine the amount of object compound to be assayed from the distance between the origin and the intersecting point of the calibration curve with the abscissa. This method is available only in the case that the calibration curve is a straight line, and passes through the origin when the absolute calibration curve method is employed. In this method, all procedures must be carried out under a strictly constant condition.

5. Method for peak measuring

Generally, the following methods are used.

5.1. Peak height measuring method

(i) Peak height method: Measure the distance between the maximum of the peak and the intersecting point of a perpendicular line from the maximum of the peak to the horizontal axis of recording paper with a tangent linking the baselines on either side of the peak.

(ii) Automatic peak height method: Measure the signals from the detector as the peak height using a data processing system.

5.2. Peak area measuring method

(i) Width at half-height method: Multiply the peak width at the half-height by the peak height.

(ii) Automatic integration method: Measure the signals from the detector as the peak area using a data processing system.

6. System suitability

Refer to "System suitability" described under 2.01 Liquid Chromatography.

7. Point to consider in changing the operating conditions

Among the operating conditions specified in the individual monograph, inside diameter and length of column, particle size of packing material, concentration or thickness of stationary phase, column temperature, temperature-rising rate, kind and flow rate of carrier gas, and split ratio may be modified within the ranges in which the gas chromatographic system used conforms to the requirements of system suitability. Headspace sample injection device and its operating conditions may be also modified, provided that they give equivalent or more accuracy and precision.

8. Terminology

The definition of terms described under 2.01 Liquid Chromatography shall apply in 2.02 Gas Chromatography.

9. Note

Avoid the use of authentic specimens, internal standards, reagents or solvents containing substances that may interfere with the determination.

2.03 Thin-layer Chromatography

Thin-layer Chromatography is a method to separate each ingredient by developing a mixture in a mobile phase, using a thin-layer made of a suitable stationary phase, and is applied for identification, purity test, etc. of substances.

1. Preparation of thin-layer plate

Generally, proceed by the following method.

A smooth and uniformly thick glass plate having a size of 50 mm × 200 mm or 200 mm × 200 mm is used for preparing a thin-layer plate. Using a suitable apparatus, apply a water suspension of powdered solid substance for the stationary phase, directed in the monograph, on one side of the glass plate to make a uniform layer of 0.2 to 0.3 mm in thickness. After air-drying, dry further by heating at a fixed temperature between 105°C and 120°C for 30 to 60 minutes. A suitable plastic plate may be used instead of the glass plate. Preserve the dried plate with protection from moisture.

2. Procedure

Unless otherwise specified, proceed by the following method.

Designate a line about 20 mm distant from the bottom of

the thin-layer plate as the starting line, spot 2 to 6 mm in diameter the directed volumes of the sample solution or the standard solution in the monograph using micropipets at points on this line, separated by more than 10 mm, and air-dry. Unless otherwise specified, attach the filter paper along with the inside wall of the container, and wet the filter paper with the developing solvent. In the container, the developing solvent is placed up to about 10 mm in height from the bottom beforehand, seal the container closely, and allow it to stand for 1 hour at ordinary temperature. Place the plate in the container, avoiding contact with the inside wall, and seal the container. Develop it at ordinary temperature.

When the solvent front has ascended from the starting line to the distance directed in the monograph, remove the plate from the container. Immediately put a mark at the solvent front. After air-drying, observe the location, color, etc., of each spot by the method specified in the monograph. Calculate the Rf value by using the following equation:

$$Rf = \frac{\text{distance from the starting line to the center of the spot}}{\text{distance from the starting line to the solvent front}}$$

2.04 Amino Acid Analysis of Proteins

Amino acid analysis of proteins refers to the methodology used to determine the amino acid composition or content of proteins, peptides, and other pharmaceutical preparations. Amino acid analysis can be used to quantify protein and peptides, to determine the identity of proteins or peptides based on their amino acid composition, to support protein and peptide structure analysis, to evaluate fragmentation strategies for peptide mapping, and to detect atypical amino acids that might be present in a protein or peptide. It is necessary to hydrolyze a protein/peptide to its individual amino acid constituents before amino acid analysis. Following protein/peptide hydrolysis, the amino acid analysis procedure can be the same as that practiced for free amino acids in other pharmaceutical preparations. The amino acid constituents of the test sample are typically derivatized for analysis.

1. Hydrolysis of Protein and Peptide

Acid hydrolysis at 110°C for 24 hours using 6 mol/L hydrochloric acid containing phenol (Method 1) is the most common method for hydrolyzing protein and samples. The result should be analyzed carefully because several amino acids are chemically modified during the acid hydrolysis and thus not recovered quantitatively. Tryptophan is destroyed; serine and threonine are partially destroyed; methionine might undergo oxidation; and cysteine is typically recovered as cystine (but cystine recovery is usually poor because of partial destruction or reduction to cysteine). Peptide bonds involving isoleucine and valine are partially cleaved; and asparagine and glutamine are deamidated, resulting in aspartic acid and glutamic acid, respectively.

The hydrolysis techniques, Methods 2 to 11, are used to address these concerns. Some of the hydrolysis techniques, Methods 4 to 11, may cause modifications of cysteine, methionine, asparagines and glutamine to other amino acids. Therefore, the benefits of using a given hydrolysis technique are weighed against the concerns with the technique and are tested adequately before employing a method other than acid hydrolysis by Method 1.

(i) Method 1: Hydrolysis using hydrochloric acid containing phenol (liquid phase hydrolysis, vapor phase hydrolysis)

Prevention of tryptophan oxidation

(ii) Method 2: Mercaptoethanesulfonic acid hydrolysis (vapor phase hydrolysis)

(iii) Method 3: Hydrolysis using hydrochloric acid containing thioglycolic acid (vapor phase hydrolysis)

Cysteine-cystine and methionine oxidation

(iv) Method 4: Hydrolysis by Method 1 or Method 2 after oxidation with performic acid

Cysteine-cystine oxidation

(v) Method 5: Hydrolysis using hydrochloric acid containing sodium azide (liquid phase hydrolysis)

(vi) Method 6: Hydrolysis using hydrochloric acid containing dimethylsulfoxide (vapor phase hydrolysis)

Cysteine-cystine reduction and alkylation

(vii) Method 7: Hydrochloric acid hydrolysis after a vapor phase pyridylethylation reaction

(viii) Method 8: Hydrochloric acid hydrolysis after a liquid phase pyridylethylation reaction

(ix) Method 9: Hydrochloric acid hydrolysis after a liquid phase carboxymethylation reaction

Conversion of cysteine-cystine to mixed disulfide

(x) Method 10: Hydrochloric acid hydrolysis after a reaction with dithiodiglycolic acid or dithiodipropionic acid

Derivatization of asparagine and glutamine

(xi) Method 11: Hydrochloric acid hydrolysis after reaction with bis(1,1-trifuoroacetoxy) iodobenzene

A time-course study is often employed to analyze the starting concentration of amino acids that are partially destroyed or slow to cleave. An acceptable alternative to the time-course study is to subject an amino acid calibration standard to the same hydrolysis conditions as the test sample. This technique will allow the analyst to account for some residue destruction.

Microwave acid hydrolysis has been used and is rapid but requires special equipment as well as special precautions. Complete proteolysis, using a mixture of proteases, has been used but can be complicated, requires the proper controls, and is typically more applicable to peptides than proteins.

2. Methodologies of Amino Acid Analysis

The amino acid analysis techniques include the postcolumn derivatization for detection (Methods 1 to 2) after the separation of the free amino acids by ion-exchange chromatography and the precolumn derivatization of the free amino acids (Methods 2 to 7) followed by reversed-phase HPLC.

(i) Method l: Ninhydrin

(ii) Method 2: *o*-Phthalaldehyde (OPA)

(iii) Method 3: Phenylisothiocyanate (PITC)

(iv) Method 4: 6-Aminoquinolyl-*N*-hydroxysuccinimidyl carbamate (AQC)

(v) Method 5: (Dimethylamino)azobenzenesulfonyl chloride (DABS-Cl)

(vi) Method 6: 9-Fluorenylmethyl chloroformate (FMOC-Cl)

(vii) Method 7: 7-Fluoro-4-nitrobenzo-2-oxa-1,3-diazole (NBD-F)

Among these methods, ion-exchange chromatography with postcolumn ninhydrin derivertization is one of the most common methods employed for quantitative amino acid analysis. The choice of any one technique often depends on the sensitivity required from the assay. Instruments and reagents for these procedures are available commercially. Furthermore, many modifications of these methodologies exist with different reagent preparations, reaction procedures, chromatographic systems, etc. Specific parameters may vary according to the exact equipment and procedure used.

2.05 Size-Exclusion Chromatography

Size-exclusion chromatography is a separation technique of liquid chromatography, which separates molecules in solution based on their size. It is used for the determination of the molecular mass of high-molecular mass compounds such as polysaccharides, nucleic acids, proteins and chemically synthesized polymers, determination of the molecular mass distribution, purity tests and so on. A method using an aqueous solvent as the mobile phase for water-soluble high-molecular compounds is also called gel filtration chromatography. A method using an organic solvent as the mobile phase is also called gel permeation chromatography. This chapter describes procedures using an aqueous solvent as the mobile phase. The principle of the separation is the same when using an organic solvent as the mobile phase.

1. Principle of separation

Components to be tested are separated according to the easiness of entry into the pores of the packing material of the column. Molecules larger than the pores move rapidly through the spaces between the particles of the packing material without entering the pores, and elute at the position of the retention volume of an unretained compound (V_0) of the column. Molecules smaller than the pores enter into the pores depending on their sizes, and smaller molecules elute later because they enter deeper into the pores. All molecules smaller than a certain size elute at the position of a completely permeated compound, or the total mobile phase volume (V_t). The elution position of a molecule will be influenced not only by molecular mass but also by the structure of the molecule, solvent, interaction between the molecule and the packing material, etc.

2. Apparatus and measurement conditions

Usually follow Liquid Chromatography <*2.01*>. A porous packing material is used for a column. As packing materials, silica particles whose surface are coated with hydrophilic modification, or cross-linked hydrophilic polymers are used. Since measurable molecular mass range differs depending on the pore size of a packing material and its distribution, select an appropriate column. In order to expand the measurable molecular mass range, a column may be connected with another column having the different target molecular mass range. For a mobile phase, a buffer solution etc. is used. It is important to select appropriately a mobile phase to suppress interaction other than the principle of size exclusion between a packing material and a component to be tested. Adjustment of pH, addition of salt, etc. may be useful to suppress electrostatic interaction between a packing material and a component to be tested, and addition of an organic solvent (methanol, acetonitrile, etc.) may be useful to suppress hydrophobic interaction. The flow rate of a mobile phase, column temperature, sample injection volume, and the concentration of a sample solution should be set appropriately because they affect the separation. As a detector, an ultraviolet-visible spectrophotometer, a differential refractometer, a static light scattering detector, an evaporative light scattering detector, etc. are used. Usually, the molecular mass of a component to be tested is determined by comparing the elution position with molecular mass standards, but when using a static light scattering detector, the molecular mass of molecules in an eluate can be obtained directly.

3. Procedure

Follow Liquid Chromatography <*2.01*>.

4. Measurement of molecular mass

When determining molecular mass, average molecular mass or molecular mass distribution by size exclusion chromatography, measure a sample solution and molecular mass standard solutions prepared using appropriate molecular mass standards under the same test conditions, and determine as follows, unless otherwise specified. The molecular mass standards should have the similar physical properties as a component to be tested. The obtained molecular mass value depends on the molecular mass standards used and analysis conditions.

4.1. Molecular mass of a monodisperse component

A molecular mass calibration curve is prepared by plotting the relationship of retention volume (or retention time) and the logarithmic value of molecular mass labelled on molecular mass standards. The molecular mass will be determined from the molecular mass calibration curve for the retention volume (or retention time) obtained from the chromatogram of a sample solution. Usually, the molecular mass of a component to be tested should be within the range of the molecular mass calibration curve.

4.2. Average molecular mass of a polydisperse component

A molecular mass calibration curve is prepared from chromatograms obtained from molecular mass standard solutions. A chromatogram obtained from a sample solution is divided, and the molecular mass of each eluted fraction is obtained from the molecular mass calibration curve. The concentration or amount of the component in each fraction is determined, and the number-average molecular mass (M_n), mass-average molecular mass (M_w) and dispersity (d) of the sample are calculated by the following equations.

The dispersity may be an indicator of the width of molecular mass distribution.

$$M_n = \frac{\sum M_i N_i}{\sum N_i} = \frac{\sum C_i}{\sum \frac{C_i}{M_i}} = \frac{1}{\sum \frac{w_i}{M_i}}$$

$$M_w = \frac{\sum M_i^2 N_i}{\sum M_i N_i} = \frac{\sum C_i M_i}{\sum C_i} = \sum w_i M_i,$$

$$d = \frac{M_w}{M_n}$$

M_i: Molecular mass of i-th fraction
C_i: Concentration of i-th fraction
N_i: Number of molecules in i-th fraction
w_i: Mass fraction of i-th fraction $\left(w_i = \frac{M_i N_i}{\sum M_i N_i} = \frac{C_i}{\sum C_i} \right)$

4.3. Molecular mass distribution

As a distribution curve showing molecular mass distribution, an integral molecular mass distribution curve plotting the logarithmic value of molecular mass on the abscissa and the integral value of mass fraction on the ordinate, and a differential molecular mass distribution curve plotting the logarithmic value of molecular mass on the abscissa and the slope of the integral molecular mass distribution curve determined at each molecular mass on the ordinate, are used.

Specifications for molecular mass distribution can be shown in a form depending on the purpose, such as mass average molecular mass, dispersity, mass fractions of molecules in a specific molecular mass range.

5. Points to consider on system suitability and changes in operating conditions

Liquid Chromatography <*2.01*> is applied to points to consider on specifications of system suitability and changes in operating conditions.

Spectroscopic Methods

2.21 Nuclear Magnetic Resonance Spectroscopy

Nuclear Magnetic Resonance (NMR) Spectroscopy is based on the phenomenon that specific radio frequency radiation is absorbed by magnetic nuclei in a sample placed in a magnetic field; target nuclei are ^{1}H, ^{13}C, ^{15}N, ^{19}F, ^{31}P, etc. These nuclei have intrinsic spin angular momentum, of which the magnitude is given by $I\ (I + 1)/\mathrm{h}/2\pi$, where I is the spin quantum number and is integral or half-integral ($I = 1/2$ for ^{1}H and ^{13}C). When the magnetic nuclei are placed in a magnetic field, they are oriented in $2I + 1$ possible orientations corresponding to $2I + 1$ equally spaced energy levels (two energy levels for ^{1}H and ^{13}C). The transition between two successive quantized energy levels corresponding to adjacent orientations can be induced by electromagnetic radiation with a suitable frequency. The precise relation between the field strength and the resonant frequency ν is given by

$$\nu = \gamma \cdot \frac{H_0}{2\pi}$$

where H_0 is the strength of the applied external magnetic field and γ is the gyromagnetic ratio, a constant characterizing a particular isotope. The absorption of radiation (NMR signal) can occur only when the irradiating radio frequency satisfies the resonance condition. Since the absorption coefficient (the transition probability) does not depend on the environment in which the nuclei are located, the intensity is basically proportional to the number of nuclei. The excess spins shifted to the higher energy levels by the transition process return to the thermal equilibrium state at various rates determined by a characteristic time constant (known as the relaxation time).

A nucleus is shielded from the applied magnetic field by the electrons belonging to its own atom and to the molecule. Therefore nuclei in different environments are shielded to different extents and resonate at different frequencies. The difference in resonance frequencies is defined as chemical shift (δ), which is independent of the strength of the magnetic field, and is given by

$$\delta = \frac{\nu_S - \nu_R}{\nu_R} + \delta_R$$

where,

ν_S: The resonance frequency of the observed signal,

ν_R: The resonance frequency of the reference signal,

δ_R: The chemical shift of the reference signal (in the case of the value not being 0).

The chemical shifts are normally expressed in ppm, a dimensionless unit, by assuming the chemical shift of the reference compound as 0 ppm. When the chemical shift of the reference compound is not assumed to be 0 ppm, chemical shifts of samples are corrected accordingly.

In addition to the shielding due to electrons, the nucleus is subjected to effects due to the spin orientations of other magnetic nuclei through chemical bonds, resulting in an additional splitting of the signal. The spacing between two adjacent components of the signal is known as the spin-spin coupling constant (J). Coupling constants are measured in hertz and are independent of the strength of the external magnetic field. The increased number of interacting nuclei will make the multiplet pattern more complex.

From the NMR spectrum the following four parameters can be obtained: chemical shift, spin-spin coupling constant, resonance intensity (intensities of ^{1}H are proportional to the number of nuclei and those of ^{13}C and others are susceptible to the nuclear Overhauser effect (NOE) and relaxation) and relaxation time. These parameters are useful for structural determination, identification and quantitative analysis of molecules. Spin decoupling, NOE, and two-dimensional NMR techniques are also available for structural analysis.

1. Spectrometer

There are two types of spectrometers.

1.1. Fourier transform NMR (FT-NMR) spectrometers (Fig. 2.21-1)

Target nuclei are simultaneously excited in all frequency range of the nuclei by means of an intense radio frequency pulse. The FID (free induction decay) after the pulse is detected, which is a time domain signal, is converted to a frequency domain spectrum by Fourier transformation. Number of data points suitable for the spectral range, flip angle, acquisition time, delay time and number of scans should be set appropriately.

Recently FT-NMR is commonly used because of its high sensitivity and various advanced applications.

1.2. Continuous wave NMR (CW-NMR) spectrometers (Fig. 2.21-2)

In the case of the CW method, a spectrum is obtained by sweeping the radio frequency or magnetic field continuously over the frequency range of the nuclei being observed.

2. Measurement

For NMR measurements, the sensitivity and resolution of the instrument must be adjusted to the optimum levels. The excitation and observation of magnetization are provided by using coils. The coils need the optimization to the Larmor frequency of the targeted nuclear spin called as ''Tuning'' and sensitivity setting called as ''Matching''. An additional operation is to apply an electronic current to plural shim coils wrapping the sample and/or a correction current for optimization of resolution. This is necessary for adjusting unevenness of spatial strength in the static magnetic field around the sample. After optimizing the sensitivity and resolution of NMR instrument using ethylbenzene, 1,2-

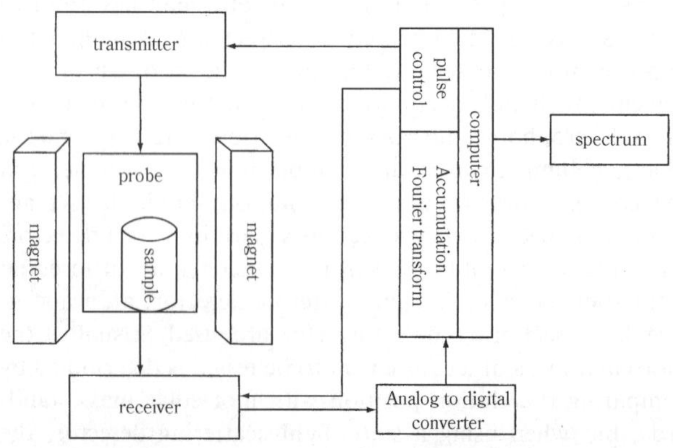

Fig. 2.21-1 FT-NMR spectrometer

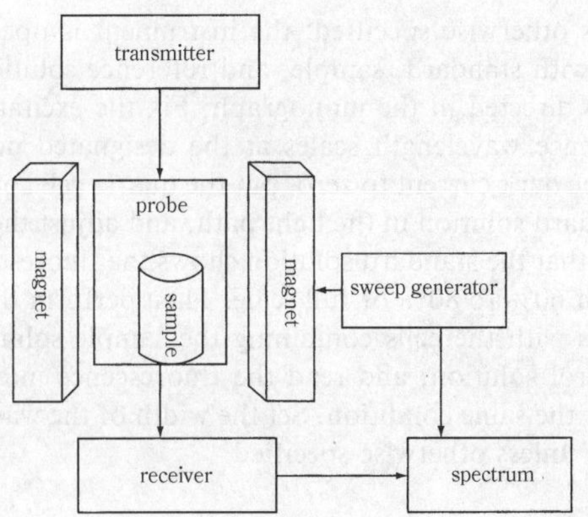

Fig. 2.21-2 CW-NMR spectrometer

dichlorobenzene, etc. dissolved in an appropriate deuterated NMR solvent, spectrum is usually measured by the following method.

An NMR tube should be prepared for internal reference method (a solution which is the sample and a drop of the reference compound dissolved in a suitable solvent is directly transferred into the NMR tube) or external reference method (a sealed capillary tube containing the reference compound is inserted into the NMR tube with the sample solution). The measurement should be conducted by setting the NMR tube into the NMR probe. The sample solutions should be completely homogeneous. In particular, solid contaminants should be removed in order to obtain good spectra.

Various deuterated NMR solvents are commonly used for NMR measurement and the following points should be considered in selecting an appropriate solvent: (i) The solvent signals do not overlap with the sample signals. (ii) The sample must be soluble in the solvent selected. (iii) The solvent does not react with the sample. Furthermore, it should be noted that chemical shifts can depend upon the solvent employed, sample concentration and deuterium ion concentration, and that viscous solutions usually give rather broad, poorly resolved spectra.

For the reference standards use the reagents for nuclear magnetic resonance spectroscopy. For ^{1}H and ^{13}C spectra, tetramethylsilane (TMS) is usually used as the reference compound for samples dissolved in organic solvents. For samples dissolved in deuterium oxide, sodium 2,2-dimethyl-2-silapentane-5-sulfonate (DSS) or sodium 3-(trimethylsilyl)propionate (TSP) is used. For other nuclei, nitromethane, trichlorofluoromethane and phosphoric acid are used as reference compounds for ^{15}N, ^{19}F and ^{31}P, respectively. Furthermore, chemical shifts of residual protons in deuterated solvents and ^{13}C in the solvent instead of a reference compound can be used for ^{1}H and ^{13}C NMR.

3. Record of apparatus and measurement conditions

Type of instrument, frequency, solvent, temperature, sample concentration, reference compound, experimental technique, etc. should be recorded to allow appropriate comparison of spectra, because NMR spectra depend on the measurement conditions.

4. Identification

The sample solution is prepared and tested by the method directed in each monograph. Usually in the case of ^{1}H NMR, the sample is identified by the following method.

4.1. Identification by the use of chemical shift, signal multiplicity and signal relative intensity

When chemical shifts, multiplicities and relative intensities of signals are defined, the sample can be identified as being the same substance when all chemical shifts, multiplicities and relative intensities are the same as those prescribed in principle. However, when NMR spectra of the same sample are measured in the different magnitude of magnetic field, it should be noted that the multiplicities of signals sometimes are not identical. This is due to the difference in resolution ability among instruments and the relative relation between the size of spin-spin coupling and the difference in resonance frequency of spin-spin coupled nuclei. Therefore, the multiplicities of signals should be evaluated, considering the magnitude of magnetic field of NMR instrument.

4.2. Identification by the use of a Reference Standard

Measurement conditions should be the same as those used in the case of the Reference Standard. When the spectra of a sample and the Reference Standard exhibit the same multiplicities and relative intensities of signal at the same chemical shifts, the sample can be identified as being the same substance as the Reference Standard.

5. Experimental techniques of ^{1}H and ^{13}C NMR spectroscopy

NMR spectroscopy includes one-, two- and multi-dimensional techniques, which are used for various purposes.

Spin decoupling, and NOE are available in one-dimensional ^{1}H NMR spectroscopy. Spin decoupling can assign coupling correlations. NOE (nuclear Overhauser effect) can show correlations among spatially proximal protons, and provide information about configuration or conformation.

In one-dimensional ^{1}H NMR spectroscopy, the peak intensity in a fully relaxed spectrum of a compound is directly proportional to the number of ^{1}H nuclei, when NMR instrument and experimental conditions are optimized for quantitative analysis. Accordingly, high-reliable purity, content etc. based on molar amount (mol) can be determined by using the internal reference materials having traceability to International System of Units (SI). This measurement method is called quantitative ^{1}H NMR.

Broadband decoupling, INEPT and DEPT are usually applied in one-dimensional ^{13}C spectroscopy. The broadband decoupling technique simplifies a spectrum and achieves enhancement of sensitivity. INEPT (insensitive nuclei enhanced by polarization transfer) and DEPT (distortionless enhancement of polarization transfer) enhance the sensitivity of ^{13}C by means of polarization transfer from directly bonded ^{1}H with a large magnetic moment. They can be applied to identify primary, secondary, tertiary or quaternary carbon.

Two-dimensional spectroscopy can observe all correlation peaks between nuclei through spin-spin coupling or NOE in a single experiment, and there are many techniques for homonuclear and heteronuclear measurements. Representative techniques are described below.

(i) COSY (2D correlation spectroscopy), TOCSY (total correlation spectroscopy), HOHAHA (homonuclear Hartmann-Hahn spectroscopy): Correlation between protons through scalar spin-spin coupling is obtained and intramolecular connectivities of hydrogen atoms are revealed.

(ii) NOESY (2D nuclear Overhauser enhancement and exchange spectroscopy): NOE is measured by a two-dimensional technique. Approximate distances between spatially proximate hydrogen atoms are obtained to analyze the three-dimensional structure.

(iii) INADEQUATE (incredible natural abundance double quantum transfer experiment): Although this technique is insensitive because it involves double quantum transfer by ^{13}C-^{13}C scalar coupling in a sample with natural isotopic abundance, the connectivities of all neighboring ^{13}C nuclei can be obtained to analyze the carbon skeleton.

(iv) HMQC (heteronuclear multiple quantum coherence): This technique observes correlations between ^{1}H and ^{13}C with direct spin-spin coupling using ^{1}H detection and reveals intramolecular chemical bonds between hydrogen and carbon atoms.

(v) HMBC (heteronuclear multiple bond connectivity): This technique observes correlations between ^{1}H and ^{13}C with long range spin-spin coupling using ^{1}H detection and reveals intramolecular connectivities of hydrogen and carbon atoms.

There are many other techniques such as 2D J-resolved spectroscopy, DQF-COSY (double quantum filtered COSY), HSQC (heteronuclear single quantum coherence) and DOSY (diffusion ordered spectroscopy). Furthermore, multidimensional NMR techniques are used to analyze macromolecules.

2.22 Fluorometry

Fluorometry is a method to measure the intensity of fluorescence emitted from a solution of fluorescent substance irradiated with an exciting light in a certain wavelength range. This method is also applied to the phosphorescent substances.

Fluorescence intensity F in a dilute solution is proportional to the concentration c in mol per liter of the solution and the pathlength l of light through the solution in centimeter.

$$F = kI_0\phi\varepsilon cl$$

k: Constant

I_0: Intensity of exciting light

ϕ: Quantum yield of fluorescence or phosphorescence

$$\text{Quantum yield of fluorescence or phosphorescence} = \frac{\text{number of quanta as fluorescence or phosphorescence}}{\text{number of quanta absorbed}}$$

ε: Molar extinction coefficient of the substance at the excitation wavelength

1. Apparatus

Spectrofluorometer is usually used. Generally, a xenon lamp, laser, an alkaline halide lamp, etc. which provide stable exciting light are used as the light source. Usually, a nonfluorescent quartz cell (1 cm × 1 cm) with four transparent sides is used as the container for sample solution.

2. Procedure

Excitation spectrum is obtained by measuring fluorescence intensities of sample solution with varying excitation wavelengths at a fixed emission wavelength (in the vicinity of the fluorescence maximum) and drawing a curve showing the relationship between the excitation wavelength and the fluorescence intensity. Fluorescence spectrum is obtained by measuring fluorescence intensities of sample solution with varying emission wavelengths at a fixed excitation wavelength (in the vicinity of the excitation maximum) and drawing the same curve as described for the excitation spectrum. If necessary, the spectra are corrected with regard to the optical characteristics of the apparatus.

The fluorescence intensity is usually measured at the excitation and the emission wavelengths in the vicinity of excitation and emission maxima of the fluorescent substance. The fluorescence intensity is expressed as a value relative to that of a standard solution, because it is readily affected even by a slight change in the condition for the measurement.

Unless otherwise specified, the instrument is operated as follows with standard, sample, and reference solutions prepared as directed in the monograph: Fix the excitation and fluorescence wavelength scales at the designated positions, adjust the dark current to zero, put the quartz cell containing the standard solution in the light path, and adjust the instrument so that the standard solution shows the fluorescence intensity of 60% to 80% of full scale. Then perform the measurements with the cells containing the sample solution and the control solution, and read the fluorescence intensity as % under the same condition. Set the width of the wavelength properly unless otherwise specified.

3. Note

The fluorescence intensity is readily affected by the concentration, temperature and pH of the solution, and nature and purity of solvents or reagents used.

2.23 Atomic Absorption Spectrophotometry

Atomic Absorption Spectrophotometry is a method to determine the amount or the concentration of an element in a sample specimen being examined, by utilizing the phenomenon that atoms being in the ground state absorb the light of specific wavelength, characteristic of the respective atom, when the light passes through an atomic vapor layer of the element to be determined.

1. Apparatus

Usually, the apparatus consists of a light source, a sample atomizer, a spectroscope, a photometer and a recording system. Some are equipped with a background compensation system. As a light source, usually a hollow cathode lamp specified for each element is used and sometimes a discharge lamp is also used. There are three types of sample atomizer: the flame type, the electrothermal type, and the cold-vapor type. The first one is composed of a burner and a gas-flow regulator, the second one is composed of an electric furnace and a power source, and the third one is composed of a mercury generator and an absorption cell. The third one is further classified into two subtypes, which differ in the atomizing method for mercury containing-compounds: one utilizes chemical reduction-vaporization and the other utilizes a thermal reduction-vaporization method.

For the selection of an appropriate analytical wavelength in a spectroscope, a grating for light diffraction or an interference filter can be used. A recording system is composed of a display and a recording device. A background compensation system is employed for the correction of atmospheric effects on the measuring system. Several principles can be utilized for background compensation, using continuous spectrum sources, the Zeeman splitted spectrum, the nonresonance spectrum, or self-inversion phenomena.

Another special options such as a hydride generator and a heating cell, can also be used for analyzing such as selenium. As a hydride generator, a batch method and/or a continuous flow method can be applied. While as a heating cell, there are two kinds of cell: one for heating by flame and the other for heating by electric furnace.

2. Procedure

Unless otherwise specified, proceed by any of the following methods.

2.1. Flame type

Fit the specific light source to the lamp housing and switch on the instrument. After lighting the lamp and selecting the analytical wavelength specified in the monograph, set an appropriate electric current and slit-width. Next, a mixture of a combustible gas and a supporting gas is ignited and the gas flow rate and/or pressure should be adjusted to optimum conditions. The zero adjustment of the detecting system must be done through nebulizing the blank solvent into the flame. After setting up the measuring system, the sample solution prepared by the specified procedure is introduced into the flame and the light absorption at the characteristic wavelength of the element to be determined is measured.

2.2. Electrothermal type

Fit the specific light source to the lamp housing and switch on the instrument. After lighting the lamp and selecting the analytical wavelength specified in the monograph, set an appropriate electric current and slit-width. Further, set an electric furnace to the appropriate temperature, electric current, and heating program, as directed separately in the monograph. When a suitable amount of sample is injected into the heated furnace with an appropriate stream of inert gas, the sample is dried and ashed, simultaneously with atomization of the metallic compound included in the specimen. The atomic absorption specified is observed and the intensity of absorption is measured. Details of the sample preparation method are provided separately in the monograph.

2.3. Cold vapor type

Fit the mercury lamp to the lamp housing and switch on the instrument. After lighting the lamp and selecting the analytical wavelength specified in the monograph, set an appropriate electric current and a slit-width. In the chemical atomization-vaporization method, a mercury containing compound in the sample solution, prepared by the specified procedure, is chemically reduced to metallic mercury by adding a proper reducing reagent to the closed vessel and the generated mercury is vaporized and introduced into the absorption cell with a flow of inert gas. In the thermal atomization-vaporization method, the sample specimen on a quartz dish is heated electrically and the generated atomic mercury is vaporized and introduced into the absorption cell with a flow of inert gas. Thus, in both methods, the generated atomic mercury is carried into the absorption cell as cold vapor and the intensity of the characteristic atomic absorption of mercury is measured.

3. Determination

Usually, proceed by any of the following methods. In the determination, the possibility of interference for various reasons and the background effect must be considered and avoided if possible.

3.1. Calibration curve method

Prepare standard solutions at more than 3 concentration levels, measure the specific absorption due to these standard solutions, and prepare the calibration curve of the atomic absorption against the concentration. Then measure the atomic absorption due to the sample specimen, in which the concentration of the element to be determined should be adjusted to be within the concentration range of the standard solutions, and determine the amount or the concentration of the element to be examined using the calibration curve.

3.2. Standard addition method

To equal volumes of more than 3 sample solutions, prepared as directed in the monograph, add a measured quantity of the standard solutions to produce a series of solutions containing increasing amounts of the element to be examined, and further add a solvent to make up a constant volume. Measure the atomic absorption for the respective solutions, and plot the obtained values on a graph with the added amount or the concentration on the abscissa and the absorbance on the ordinate. Extrapolate the linear plot obtained by linking the data points, and determine the amount or the concentration of the element to be examined from the distance between the origin and the point where the plot intersects with the abscissa. This method is available only when the calibration curve obtained by Method (1) is confirmed to be linear and to pass through the origin.

3.3. Internal standard method

Prepare a series of standard solutions of the element to be determined, each containing a definite amount of the internal standard element directed in the monograph. For these standard solutions, measure the atomic absorption due to the standard element and the internal standard element separately at the respective wavelengths under the same operating conditions, and obtain the ratio of absorbance by the standard element to that by the internal standard element. Prepare a calibration curve for the element to be determined, with the amount or the concentration of the standard element on the abscissa and the above-mentioned ratio of the absorbance on the ordinate. Then prepare sample solutions, adding the same amount of the internal standard element as contained in the standard solutions. Measure the ratio of the absorbance due to the element to be determined to that due to the internal standard element under the same conditions as employed for preparing the calibration curve, and determine the amount or the concentration of the element being examined by using the calibration curve.

4. Note

Reagents, test solutions, and gases used in this test should not interfere in any process of the measurement.

2.24 Ultraviolet-visible Spectrophotometry

Ultraviolet-visible Spectrophotometry is a method to measure the degree of absorption of light between the wavelengths of 200 nm and 800 nm by substances for the tests of their identity and purity, and for assay. When an atomic absorption spectrophotometer is used for these purposes, proceed as directed under Atomic Absorption Spectrophotometry <*2.23*>. When monochromatic light passes through a substance in the solution, the ratio of transmitted light intensity I to incident light intensity I_0 is called transmittance t; transmittance expressed in the percentage is called percent transmission T, and common logarithm of the reciprocal of transmittance is called absorbance A.

$$t = \frac{I}{I_0} \qquad T = \frac{I}{I_0} \times 100 = 100t \qquad A = \log \frac{I_0}{I}$$

The absorbance A is proportional to the concentration c of a substance in the solution and the length l of the layer of the solution through which light passes.

$$A = kcl \quad (k\text{: constant})$$

The constant, calculated on the basis that l is 1 cm and c is 1 mol/L, is called molar absorption coefficient ε. The molar absorption coefficient at the wavelength of maximum absorption is expressed as ε_{max}.

When a light beam passes through a substance in the solution, the absorbance by the sample differs depending on the wavelength of the light. So, an absorption spectrum is obtained by determining the absorbances of a light beam at various wavelengths and by graphically plotting the relation between absorbance and wavelength. From the absorption spectrum, it is possible to determine the wavelength of maximum absorption λ_{max} and that of minimum absorption λ_{min}.

The absorption spectrum of a substance in the solution is characteristic, depending on its chemical structure. Therefore, it is possible to identify a substance by comparing the spectrum of a sample within the specified wavelength range with the Reference Spectrum or the spectrum of Reference Standard, by determining the wavelengths of maximum absorption, or by measuring the ratio of absorbances at two specified wavelengths. For the purpose of assay, the absorbance by a sample solution with a certain concentration is measured at the wavelength of the maximum absorption λ_{max} and compared it with the absorbance of a standard solution with a certain concentration.

1. Apparatus and adjustment

A spectrophotometer or a photoelectric photometer is used for the measurement of absorbance.

After adjusting the spectrophotometer or photoelectric photometer based on the operation manual of the apparatus, it should be confirmed that the wavelength and the transmission rate meet the specifications of the tests described below.

The calibration of wavelength should be carried out as follows. Using an optical filter for wavelength calibration, measure the transmission rate in the vicinity of the standard wavelength value shown in the test results form, under the test conditions given in the test results form attached to each of the filters. When performing a test to determine the wavelength which shows minimal transmission rate, the difference between the measured wavelength and the standard wavelength value should be within ± 0.5 nm. When the measurement is repeated three times, each value obtained should be within the mean ± 0.2 nm. It is also possible to carry out the test using a deuterium discharge lamp at bright line wavelengths of 486.00 nm and 656.10 nm. In the case of these tests, the difference between the measured wavelength and the wavelength of the bright line should be within ± 0.3 nm. When the measurement is repeated three times, each value obtained should be within the mean ± 0.2 nm.

The calibration of transmission rate or absorbance should be carried out as follows. Using an optical filter for transmission rate calibration, determine the transmission rate at the standard wavelength value under the test conditions given in the test results form attached to each of the filters. The difference between the measured transmission rate and the standard transmission rate value should be within the range of from 1% larger of the upper limit to 1% smaller of the lower limit for the relative accuracy shown in the test results form. When the measurement is repeated three times, each absorbance obtained (or calculated from the transmission rate) should be within the mean ± 0.002 when the absorbance is not more than 0.500, and within the mean ± 0.004 when the absorbance is more than 0.500. In addition, it will be desirable to confirm the linearity of transmission rate at the same wavelength using several optical filters for calibration of transmission rate with different transmission rates.

2. Procedure

After adjusting the apparatus as directed in the Apparatus and adjustment, select and set the light source, detector, mode of measurement, measuring wavelength or wavelength range, spectrum width and scanning speed.

Subsequently, allow the apparatus to stand for a certain time to confirm its stability. Then, usually adjust the apparatus so that the transmittance is 0% at measuring wavelength or over measuring wavelength range after shutting the sample side of light path. Then open the shutter and adjust the transmittance to 100% (the absorbance is zero). Adjusting the transmittance to 100% is usually done by putting cells containing the control solution in both light paths. For the control solution, unless otherwise specified, blank solvent is used.

Then perform the measurement with the cell containing the sample solution, and read the absorbance at measuring wavelength, or measure the spectrum over measuring wavelength range. Unless otherwise specified, a cell with a path length of 1 cm, made of quartz for ultraviolet range and of quartz or glass for visible range, is used. Special consideration is needed with the absorption of solvents in the ultraviolet range; use a solvent which does not disturb accurate measurement.

3. Specific absorbance

In the Japanese Pharmacopoeia, the absorbance, calculated on the basis that l is 1 cm and c (concentration of a medicament) is 1 w/v%, is called specific absorbance, and is expressed as $E^{1\%}_{1\,\mathrm{cm}}$.

$$E^{1\%}_{1\,\mathrm{cm}} = \frac{A}{c \times l}$$

l: Length of the layer of the solution (cm)
A: Absorbance value
c: Concentration of the sample in the solution (w/v%)

The description of, for example, "$E^{1\%}_{1\,\mathrm{cm}}$ (241 nm): 500 – 530 (after drying, 2 mg, methanol, 200 mL)" in the monograph, indicates that observed $E^{1\%}_{1\,\mathrm{cm}}$ value is between 500 and 530, when the test is performed in the following manner: The sample is dried under the conditions specified in the Test for Loss on Drying, and about 2 mg of the sample is weighed accurately with a microbalance, and dissolved in methanol to make exactly 200 mL, then the absorbance of the solution is measured as directed in the Procedure at a wavelength of 241 nm using a cell with a path length of 1 cm.

4. Identification

Prepare the sample solution as directed in the monograph, and test as directed in the Procedure. Usually, the test is performed by a single method or in a combination of a few methods in the following methods using the absorbance or absorption spectrum obtained from the sample solution. Subtle differences in the absorption spectrum arising from differences in the apparatus used may be neglected.

4.1. Identification using Reference Spectrum

When the absorption spectrum obtained from the sample solution exhibits similar intensities of absorption at the same wavelengths as those of the Reference Spectrum, the identity of the sample and the reference may be confirmed. In this case, the range of the wavelength to be compared is the range shown on the Reference Spectrum.

Reference spectrum: Reference spectra are specified under the Ultraviolet-visual Reference Spectra, which are used as the reference for the test of identification specified in the monograph.

4.2. Identification using Reference Standard

When the absorption spectrum obtained from the sample solution exhibits similar intensities of absorption at the same wavelengths as those of the spectrum obtained from the Reference Standard, the identity of the sample and the reference may be confirmed. In this case, the range of the wavelength to be compared is the range shown on the Reference Spectrum. When the relevant Reference Spectrum is not available, the range is that specified in the monograph.

4.3. Identification using absorption wavelength

When maximum absorption wavelengths of the spectrum obtained from the sample solution match the wavelengths specified in the monograph, the identity of the substance may be confirmed. In this case, the range of the wavelength to be compared is the range shown on the Reference Spectrum.

4.4. Identification using the ratio of the absorbances obtained at two or more wavelengths

When the ratios of absorbances at the specified wavelengths in the spectrum obtained from the sample solution meet the specifications in the monograph, the identity of the substance may be confirmed.

5. Assay

Prepare the control solution, the sample solution and the standard solution as directed in the monograph, measure the absorbances of the sample solution and the standard solution according to the method described in the Procedure, and determine the amount of the substance to be assayed in the sample by comparing the absorbances.

2.25 Infrared Spectrophotometry

Infrared Spectrophotometry is a method of measurement of the extent, at various wave numbers, of absorption of infrared radiation when it passes through a layer of a substance. In the graphic representation of infrared spectra, the plot usually shows units of wave numbers as the abscissa and units of transmittance or absorbance as the ordinate. Wave number and transmittance or absorbance at each absorption maximum may be read graphically on an absorption spectrum and/or obtained by a data-processor. Since the wave number and the respective intensity of an absorption maximum depend on the chemical structure of a substance, this measurement can be used to identify or determine a substance.

1. Instrument and adjustment

Several models of dispersive infrared spectrophotometers or Fourier-transform infrared spectrophotometers are available.

The instruments, adjusted according to the instruction manual of each individual instrument, should comply with the following test for resolving power, transmittance reproducibility and wave number reproducibility. When the spectrum of a polystyrene film about 0.04 mm thick is recorded, the depth of the trough from the maximum absorption at about 2850 cm^{-1} to the minimum at about 2870 cm^{-1} should be not less than 18% transmittance and that from the maximum at about 1583 cm^{-1} to the minimum at about 1589 cm^{-1} should be not less than 12% transmittance.

The wave number (cm^{-1}) scale is usually calibrated by the use of several characteristic absorption wave numbers (cm^{-1}) of a polystyrene film shown below. The number in parentheses indicates the permissible range.

3060.0 (±1.5) 2849.5 (±1.5) 1942.9 (±1.5)
1601.2 (±1.0) 1583.0 (±1.0) 1154.5 (±1.0)
1028.3 (±1.0)

When the dispersive infrared spectrophotometer is used, the permissible range of the absorption wave numbers at 1601.2 cm^{-1} and at 1028.3 cm^{-1} should be both within ±2.0 cm^{-1}.

As the repeatability of transmittance and wave number, the difference of transmittance should be within 0.5% when the spectrum of a polystyrene film is measured twice at several wave numbers from 3000 to 1000 cm^{-1}, and the difference of wave number should be within 5 cm^{-1} at about 3000 cm^{-1} and within 1 cm^{-1} at about 1000 cm^{-1}.

2. Preparation of samples and measurement

Unless otherwise specified, when it is directed to perform the test "after drying the sample", use a sample dried under the conditions specified in the monograph. Prepare the specimen for the measurement according to one of the following procedures. Because the amount of specimen or mixture described is as an example and that depends on the measurement conditions, prepare it so that the transmittance of most of the absorption bands is in the range of 5% to 80%. If the sample is a salt it should be noted that the salt exchange can be occurred between added potassium bromide or potassium chloride. As a general rule in the disk method or the diffuse reflectance method, potassium chloride is used for a hydrochloride sample. For other salts, correspondence such as to try the paste method is needed.

Single crystals of sodium chloride, potassium bromide, etc. are available for the optical plate.

Generally, the reference cell or material is placed in the reference beam for double-beam instruments, while for single-beam instruments, it is placed in the same optical path in place of the specimen and measured separately under the same operating conditions. The composition and preparation of the reference depend on the sample preparation methods, and sometimes the background absorption of the atmosphere can be utilized.

Unless otherwise specified in the monograph, the spectrum is usually recorded between 4000 cm^{-1} and 400 cm^{-1}. The spectrum should be scanned using the same instrumental conditions as were used to ensure compliance with the requirements for the resolving power and for the precision of wave number scale and of wave numbers.

2.1. Potassium bromide disk or potassium chloride disk method

Powder 1 to 2 mg of a solid sample in an agate mortar, triturate rapidly with 0.10 to 0.20 g of potassium bromide for infrared spectrophotometry or potassium chloride for infrared spectrophotometry with precautions against moisture absorption, and compress the mixture with a press in a suitable die (disk-forming container) to make the sample disk. Adjust the amount of sample, potassium bromide or potassium chloride according to the size of the disk. Prepare a potassium bromide reference disk or a potassium chloride reference disk in the same manner as the sample disk. If necessary to obtain a transparent disk, press the mixture under reduced pressure not exceeding 0.67 kPa in a die with pressure applied to the die of 50 to 100 kN (5000 – 10,000 kg) per cm^2 for 5 to 8 minutes.

2.2. Solution method

Place the sample solution prepared by the method directed in each monograph in a fixed cell for liquid, and usually measure the spectrum against the reference solvent used for preparing the sample solution. The solvent used in this method should not show any interaction or chemical reaction with the specimen to be examined and should not damage the optical plate. The thickness of the fixed cell is usually 0.1 mm or 0.5 mm.

2.3. Paste method

Powder 5 to 10 mg of a solid specimen in an agate mortar, and, unless otherwise specified, triturate the specimen with 1 to 2 drops of liquid paraffin to give a homogeneous paste. After spreading the paste to make a thin film in the center of an optical plate, place the plate upon another optical plate with precautions against intrusion of air, bubbles in the film, and examine its absorption spectrum.

2.4. Liquid film method

Examine 1 to 2 drops of a liquid specimen as a thin film held between two optical plates. When the absorption intensity is not sufficient, place spacers of aluminum foil, etc., between the two optical plates to make a thicker liquid film.

2.5. Film method

Examine a thin film just as it is or a prepared thin film as directed in each monograph.

2.6. Gas sampling method

Put a sample gas in a gas cell previously evacuated under the pressure directed in the monograph, and examine its absorption spectrum. The path length of the gas cell is usually 5 cm or 10 cm, but, if necessary, may exceed 1 m.

2.7. ATR method

Place a specimen in close contact with an attenuated total reflectance (ATR) prism, and examine its reflectance spectrum.

2.8. Diffuse reflectance method

Powder 1 to 3 mg of a solid specimen into a fine powder of not more than about 50 μm particle size in an agate mortar, and triturate rapidly with 0.05 to 0.10 g of potassium bromide for infrared spectrophotometry or potassium chloride for infrared spectrophotometry with precautions against moisture absorption. Place the mixture in a sample cup, and examine its reflectance spectrum.

3. Identification

When the spectrum of a specimen and the Reference Spectrum of the substance expected to be found or the spectrum of the Reference Standard exhibit similar intensities of absorption at the same wave numbers, the specimen can be identified as being the substance expected to be found. Furthermore, when several specific absorption wave numbers are specified in the monograph, the identification of a specimen with the substance expected to be found can be confirmed by the appearance of absorption bands at the specified wave numbers.

3.1. Identification by the use of a Reference Standard

When the spectra of a specimen and the Reference Standard exhibit similar intensities of absorption at the same wave numbers, the specimen can be identified as being the same substance as the Reference Standard. When a sample treatment method for a solid specimen is indicated in the monograph in the case of nonconformity of the spectrum with that of the Reference Standard, treat the specimen being examined and the Reference Standard in the same manner as directed in the monograph, then repeat the measurement.

3.2. Identification by the use of a Reference Spectrum

When the spectra of a specimen and the Reference Spectrum exhibit similar intensities of absorption at the same wave numbers, the specimen can be identified as being the same substance associated with the Reference Spectrum. When a sample treatment method for a solid specimen is indicated in the monograph in the case of nonconformity of the spectrum with the Reference Spectrum, treat the specimen being examined as directed in the monograph, then repeat the measurement. Infrared Reference Spectra, in the range between 4000 cm^{-1} and 400 cm^{-1}, are shown in the section "Infrared Reference Spectra" for the monographs requiring the identification test by Infrared Spectrophotometry, except for monographs in which "Identification by absorption wave number" is specified.

3.3. Identification by the use of absorption wave number

When several specific absorption wave numbers of the substance being examined are specified in the monograph, a specimen can be identified as being the same substance as the expected substance by confirmation of clear appearance of the absorption bands at all the specified wave numbers.

2.26 Raman Spectroscopy

Raman spectroscopy is a vibrational spectroscopic technique, which evaluates a sample to be examined qualitatively or quantitatively by analyzing a spectrum obtained by dispersing very weak scattered light, having different wavelengths from irradiation light, generated when the sample is irradiated with the light. Raman scattering is observed when the polarizability of molecules changes with the vibration of chemical bonds of molecules in a sample.

Raman spectroscopy generally uses monochromatic laser light as excitation light. When the laser light is irradiated to the sample to be examined, the molecules in the sample is excited and the light with the same wavelength of the irradiation light, known as Rayleigh scattering, is scattered. The scattered light detected in the shorter wavelength side than the Rayleigh scattering is referred to as anti-Stokes scattering. The scattered light detected in the longer wavelength side than the Rayleigh scattering is referred to as Stokes scattering. Generally Stokes scattering with strong Raman scattering intensity is used for analysis. Raman spectra are usually indicated by Raman shift on the horizontal axis and Raman scattering intensity on the vertical axis.

Raman spectroscopy is capable of measuring samples (solid, semi-solid, liquid, gas, etc.) rapidly and nondestructively without pre-treatment. Application of Raman spectroscopy in the pharmaceutical field includes qualitative or quantitative evaluation of the active pharmaceutical ingredients and additives in drug substances or drug products. Raman spectroscopy can also be used for the evaluation of the physical conditions of substances, such as crystal form and crystallinity. Raman micro-spectroscopy can also be used for the evaluation of the distributions of active pharmaceutical ingredients and additives in the drug products. Furthermore, using an optical fiber probe enables it to measure the spectra of samples at a location remote from the equipment body without sampling, so that it can be used to perform pharmaceutical manufacturing process control online (or in-line).

1. Apparatus

Raman spectrometers are composed of a light source unit, a sample unit, a spectrometry unit, a detector unit, a signal processing unit, a data processing unit and a display-record-output unit. Raman spectrometers are classified into dispersive Raman spectrometers and Fourier transform Raman spectrometers according to their spectroscopic systems.

1.1. Light source

The laser which stably emits monochromatic light as excitation light to samples is used for the light source. The lasers include gas lasers such as a He-Ne laser and solid state lasers, and select a laser with wavelengths and output power according to the purpose. Pay attention to safety standards relating to a laser, when this test is performed.

1.2. Sample unit

The sample unit is composed of an optical system for collecting Raman scattering light generated by irradiation of excitation light and a sample cell. Combination of these take the form of a sample chamber, while there are apparatuses with no sample chamber, such as optical fiber probes and portable Raman spectrometers that can be carried. Representative sample chambers are macroscopic sample chambers and microscopic sample chambers. The components of these optical systems are different, respectively.

1.3. Monochromator and detector

Many dispersive Raman spectrometers use an optical filter to eliminate excitation light and use a single monochromator combined with a multichannel detector, since the configuration is simple and high sensitivity can be obtained. Detectors include multiple elements detectors and single element detectors, and general dispersive Raman spectrometers use a multiple elements detector such as a CCD detector.

Fourier transform (FT) Raman spectrometers obtain spectra by Fourier transformation of interference waveforms using an interferometer. FT-Raman spectrometers are mainly used for near infrared Raman measurement.

2. Methods Used for Measurement

The Raman spectroscopy is applicable to solid samples having a complicated shape in addition to gas/solution samples inside a glass sample cell being transparent in the visible region, using mainly light in the visible region as excitation light. In the view of the size of a measurement region and Raman scattering efficiency, an optimum optical system is selected according to the sample. The excitation wavelength, the measurement mode of the apparatus, etc. are selected and set.

2.1. Macroscopic measurement

Since the macroscopic sample chamber has a high degree of freedom in the scattering configuration, samples can be measured irrespective of solid, liquid, gas, size and shape. It is also applicable to Raman measurement under low temperature, high temperature and high pressure which require the setting of a large sample cell. Usually, in the macroscopic sample chamber three configurations: forward scattering (transmission), 90° scattering and back scattering configurations, can be usable and an appropriate scattering configuration can be selected depending on a sample.

2.2. Microscopic measurement

The microscopic sample chamber is based on an optical microscope and applicable to local analysis. In the optical system of the microscopic sample chamber a microscope objective lens works simultaneously as an excitation light converging lens and a Raman scattering light condensing lens.

Mapping measurement repeats local measurements by moving a sample or laser light position to generate a Raman image showing the two or three dimensional distribution of Raman scattering intensity. Raman images are made by using various spectral information such as a ratio of the intensity of two bands.

2.3. Probe measurement

The optical fiber probe is the collective term of the apparatus of which sample section is separated from a Raman spectrometer body by using an optical fiber and is applicable to *in situ* measurement and on-line (or in-line) measurement.

2.4. Measurement by portable apparatus

The portable Raman spectrometer is possible to carry and perform analysis using Raman spectroscopy outside of laboratory. Main application of this apparatus is judgement on acceptance of pharmaceutical materials. It is used for rather simple measurement.

2.5. Points to note in measurement

Note the following points for solid, liquid and suspended samples.

(i) Measurement of solid sample: There is a possibility that the filling status, the difference in the particle diameter and the roughness of the surface of the sample could affect the scattering intensity. When measuring a crystalline sample, be careful about the effect of crystal shape. There is also a possibility that the light transparency of the sample affect the spectrum intensity. When a sample is physically and chemically inhomogeneous, it might be recommended to enlarge the spot size of laser irradiation, measure plural samples, measure the plural points of the same sample or crush the sample to homogenize.

(ii) Measurement of liquid sample: It is possible to subtract the spectrum of the solvent if there is no interaction between the solvent and the sample. When there are insoluble matters in solution, remove the matters using a filter before measurement not to obtain the Raman scattering of the matters. When a sample shows high reactivity by laser irradiation in solution, measure the sample by stirring carefully not to irradiate the same place.

(iii) Measurement of suspended sample: A suspended sample may settle, so be careful about the positioning of laser irradiation. For samples that are prone to settle, devising measurement such as optimizing the irradiation time and stirring might be helpful. When the Raman scattering of a suspended sample is weak, it is also possible to subtract the spectrum of the solvent likewise the case of measurement of a liquid sample.

3. Factors that affect spectrum

When Raman spectroscopy is applied, note the following items as factors affecting spectra.

3.1. Temperature of sample

Sample heating by laser irradiation can cause a variety of effects, such as physical form change (melting and burning) and polymorph transform. Since the chance of sample heating is increased when the spot size of laser irradiation at a sample is squeezed, be careful not to damage the sample when microscopic measurement is carried out. To prevent the sample overheating, a variety of methods can be employed such as suppressing laser output, irradiating a laser without focusing and cooling a sample.

3.2. Sample characteristics

Since Raman signals are very weak, the fluorescence of a sample itself and minute impurities may interfere with Raman scattering light. Fluorescence can be reduced by choosing an excitation light source with a longer wavelength, however it should be noted that it generally decreases the intensity of the Raman scattering. Photobleaching resulted by laser irradiation before measurement, appropriate irradiation time and accumulation count may mitigate the fluorescence.

When measuring a colored sample, select the wavelength of an excitation laser depending on the absorption characteristics of the sample. When measuring a sample in a container such as, a cell for measurement, a bag or a bottle, take careful note of the spectral characteristics derived from the container in addition to the sample.

4. Control of apparatus performance

Estimate the accuracy of the wave number of Raman shift after adjusting a Raman spectrometer. Measure Raman spectra using an excitation laser utilized for actual measurement and an appropriate standard substance. Polystyrene is an example.

In the cases of 2.1., 2.2. and 2.3., make correction using at least three wave numbers among the below peak wave numbers (cm^{-1}) obtained from the spectrum of polystyrene. The number in parentheses indicates the permissible range.

620.9 (± 1.5)
1001.4 (± 1.5)
1031.8 (± 1.5)
1602.3 (± 1.5)
3054.3 (± 3.0) (Note: 3054.3 cm^{-1} cannot be measured

depending on an excitation wavelength.)

In the case of 2.4., make correction in the same manner using at least three wave numbers among the below peak wave numbers (cm^{-1}).

620.9 (± 2.5)
1001.4 (± 2.0)
1031.8 (± 2.0)
1602.3 (± 3.0)

Other substance such as cyclohexane can be used as a standard substance, if it is validated.

5. Qualitative and quantitative analysis

5.1. Qualitative analysis

As Raman spectroscopy observe the vibrational energy of a molecule and can obtain a characteristic spectrum depending on the structure of a substance to be analyzed, qualitative analysis based on chemical structural information can be performed.

When the Raman spectra of a sample and the Reference Standard of a substance to be identified are compared and both spectra exhibit similar scattering intensities at the same Raman shifts, the identity of those can be confirmed.

When a sample treatment method for a solid sample is indicated in the monograph in the case of nonconformity of the scattering spectrum with that of the Reference Standard, treat the sample and the Reference Standard under the condition as directed in the monograph, then repeat the measurement.

When the characteristic scattering wave numbers of a substance to be identified are specified in the monograph, the clear appearance of the scattering of a sample at all the specified scattering wave numbers can confirm the identity of the sample with the substance to be identified.

Raman spectroscopy is also applicable to the process control of drug substances or drug products by using a score obtained from a Raman spectrum by a chemometric methodology such as principal component analysis, and characteristic peak wave numbers of the substance to be examined, as indices. Chemometrics usually means mathematical technique and statistic technique for quantization and informatization of chemical data.

5.2. Quantitative analysis

The concentrations of components of a sample to be analyzed can be calculated by calibration curves plotting the relationship between scattering intensity at a specified wave number and concentration.

In the case where the composition of components of a sample is complicated, the concentrations of components in the sample can also be calculated by developing a calibration model about a spectrum measured using an existing standard sample by a chemometric methodology and applying the model to the spectrum of the sample to be examined. Chemometric methodologies for obtaining a calibration model include multiple regression analysis method and PLS (Partial least squares) regression analysis method.

The variation of peak intensity at around the reference values of wave numbers using a standard sample, polystyrene etc. used in 4., is preferable to be within ± 10% compared to that obtained in the last measurement.

Other Physical Methods

2.41 Loss on Drying Test

Loss on Drying Test is a method to measure the loss in mass of the sample, when dried under the conditions specified in each monograph. This method is applied to determine the amount of water, all or a part of water of crystallization, or volatile matter in the sample, which is removed during the drying.

The description, for example, "not more than 1.0% (1 g, 105°C, 4 hours)" in a monograph, indicates that the loss in mass is not more than 10 mg per 1 g of the substance in the test in which about 1 g of the substance is accurately weighed and dried at 105°C for 4 hours, and "not more than 0.5% (1 g, in vacuum, phosphorus (V) oxide, 4 hours)," indicates that the loss in mass is not more than 5 mg per 1 g of the substance in the test in which about 1 g of the substance is accurately weighed, transferred into a desiccator (phosphorus (V) oxide), and dried in vacuum for 4 hours.

1. Procedure

Weigh accurately a weighing bottle that has been dried for 30 minutes according to the method specified in the monograph. Take the sample within the range of ±10% of the amount directed in the monograph, transfer into the weighing bottle, and, unless otherwise specified, spread the sample so that the layer is not thicker than 5 mm, then weigh it accurately. Place the loaded bottle in a drying chamber, and dry under the conditions specified in the monograph. When the size of the sample is large, convert it to small particles having a size not larger than 2 mm in diameter by quick crushing, and use the crushed sample for the test. After drying, remove from the drying chamber, and reweigh accurately. When the sample is dried by heating, the temperature is within the range of ±2°C of that directed in the monograph, and, after drying the bottle, the sample is allowed to cool in a desiccator (silica gel) before weighing.

If the sample melts at a temperature lower than that specified in the monograph, expose the sample for 1 to 2 hours to a temperature between 5°C and 10°C below the melting temperature, dry under the conditions specified in the monograph. Use a desiccant specified in the monograph, and renew frequently.

2.42 Congealing Point Determination

The congealing point is the temperature measured by the following method.

1. Apparatus

Use the apparatus illustrated in Fig. 2.42-1.

2. Procedure

Transfer the sample into sample container B up to the marked line C. When the sample is solid, melt the sample by heating to a temperature not higher than 20°C above the expected congealing point, and transfer to B. Fill the glass or plastic bath D with water at a temperature about 5°C below the expected congealing point. When the sample is liquid at room temperature, fill bath D with water at a temperature between 10°C and 15°C lower than the expected congealing point.

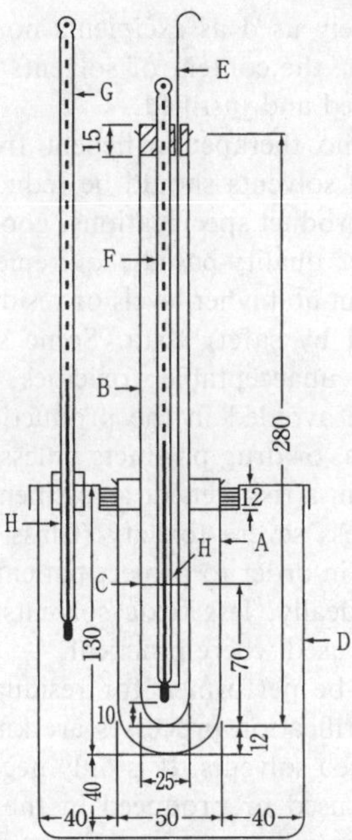

The figures are in mm.

A: Cylinder made of glass (the tube is painted with silicone oil on both sides of the wall to prevent clouding).
B: Sample container (a hard glass test tube, which is painted with silicone oil to prevent clouding, except at the region of the wall in contact with the sample; insert it into cylinder A, and fix with cork stopper).
C: A marked line.
D: Bath made of glass or plastics.
E: Stirring rod made of glass or stainless steel (3 mm in diameter, the lower end part of it is bent to make a loop, about 18 mm in diameter).
F: Thermometer with an immersion line.
G: Thermometer with an immersion line or a total immersion thermometer.
H: Immersion line

Fig. 2.42-1

Insert the sample container B containing the sample into cylinder A. Adjust the immersion line H of thermometer F to the same level of the meniscus of the sample. After cooling the sample to about 5°C above the expected congealing point, move vertically the stirrer E at the rate of about 60 to 80 strokes per minute, and observe the thermometer readings at 30-second intervals. The temperature falls gradually. Discontinue stirring, when an appreciable amount of crystals has formed and the temperature is constant or has begun to rise. Usually, read the maximum temperature (reading of F), that is constant for a while after a rise of temperature. If no rise of temperature occurs, read the temperature that is constant for a while. The average of not less than four consecutive readings that lie within a range of 0.2°C constitutes the congealing point.

3. Note

If a state of super cooling is anticipated, rub the inner wall of bath B or put a small fragment of the solid sample into bath B for promoting the congealment, when the temperature approaches near the expected congealing point.

2.43 Loss on Ignition Test

Loss on Ignition Test is a method to measure the loss in mass when the sample is ignited under the conditions specified in each monograph. This method is usually applied to inorganic drugs which lose a part of the components or impurities during ignition.

The description, for example, "40.0 – 52.0% (1 g, 450 – 550°C, 3 hours)" in a monograph, indicates that the loss in mass is 400 to 520 mg per g of the substance in the test in which about 1 g of the substance is weighed accurately and ignited between 450°C and 550°C for 3 hours.

1. Procedure

Previously ignite a crucible or a dish of platinum, quartz or porcelain to constant mass, at the temperature directed in the monograph, and weigh accurately after cooling.

Take the sample within the range of ± 10% of the amount directed in the monograph, transfer into the above ignited container, and weigh it accurately. Ignite under the conditions directed in the monograph, and, after cooling, reweigh accurately. Use a desiccator (silica gel) for the cooling.

2.44 Residue on Ignition Test

This test is harmonized with the European Pharmacopoeia and the U. S. Pharmacopeia.

The parts of the text that are not harmonized are marked with symbols (◆ ◆).

Information on the harmonization with the European Pharmacopoeia and the U.S. Pharmacopeia is available on the website of the Pharmaceuticals and Medical Devices Agency.

◆The Residue on Ignition Test is a method to measure the amount of residual substance not volatilized from a sample when the sample is ignited in the presence of sulfuric acid according to the procedure described below. This test is usually used for determining the content of inorganic impurities in an organic substance.

The description, for example, "not more than 0.1% (1 g)", in a monograph, indicates that the mass of the residue is not more than 1 mg per 1 g of the substance in the test in which about 1 g of the substance is weighed accurately and ignited by the procedure described below, and "after drying" indicates that the sample is tested after being dried under the conditions specified in the test for Loss on drying.◆

1. Procedure

Ignite a suitable crucible (for example, silica, platinum, quartz or porcelain) at 600 ± 50°C for 30 minutes, cool the crucible in a desiccator (silica gel or other suitable desiccant) and weigh it accurately.

Take the amount of test sample specified in the individual monograph in the crucible and weigh the crucible accurately.

Moisten the sample with a small amount (usually 1 mL) of sulfuric acid, then heat gently at a temperature as low as practicable until the sample is thoroughly charred. After cooling, moisten the residue with a small amount (usually 1 mL) of sulfuric acid, heat gently until white fumes are no longer evolved, and ignite at 600 ± 50°C until the residue is completely incinerated. Ensure that flames are not produced at any time during the procedure. Cool the crucible in a desiccator (silica gel or other suitable desiccant), weigh accurately and calculate the percentage of residue.

Unless otherwise specified, if the amount of the residue so obtained exceeds the limit specified in the individual monograph, repeat the moistening with sulfuric acid, heating and ignition as before, using a 30-minute ignition period, until two consecutive weighings of the residue do not differ by more than 0.5 mg or until the percentage of residue complies with the limit in the individual monograph.

2.45 Refractive Index Determination

Refractive Index Determination is a method to measure the refractive index of the sample to air. Generally, when light proceeds from one medium into another, the direction is changed at the boundary surface. This phenomenon is called refraction. When light passes from the first isotropic medium into the second, the ratio of the sine of the angle of incidence, i, to that of the angle of refraction, r, is constant with regard to these two media and has no relation to the angle of incidence. This ratio is called the refractive index of the second medium with respect to the first, or the relative refractive index, n.

$$n = \frac{\sin i}{\sin r}$$

The refractive index obtained when the first medium is a vacuum is called the absolute refractive index, N, of the second medium.

In isotropic substances, the refractive index is a characteristic constant at a definite wavelength, temperature, and pressure. Therefore, this measurement is applied to purity test of substances, or to determination of the composition of homogeneous mixtures of two substances.

The measurement is usually carried out at 20°C, and the D line of the sodium spectrum is used for irradiation. This value is expressed as n_D^{20}.

1. Procedure

For the measurement of refractive index, usually the Abbé refractometer is used at a temperature in the range of ±0.2°C of that directed in the monograph. Use of the Abbé refractometer permits direct reading of n_D under incandescent light, with a measurable range from 1.3 to 1.7, and an attainable precision of 0.0002.

2.46 Residual Solvents

The chapter of residual solvents describes the control, identification and quantification of organic solvents remaining in drug substances, excipients and drug products.

I. Control of residual solvents

1. Introduction

Residual solvents in pharmaceuticals (except for crude drugs and their preparations) are defined here as organic volatile chemicals that are used or produced in the manufacture of drug substances or excipients, or in the preparation of drug products. The solvents are not completely removed by practical manufacturing techniques. Appropriate selection of the solvent for the synthesis of drug substance may enhance the yield, or determine characteristics such as crystal form, purity, and solubility. Therefore, the solvent may sometimes be a critical parameter in the synthetic process. The test method described in this chapter does not address solvents deliberately used as excipients nor does it address solvates. However, the content of solvents in such products should be evaluated and justified.

Since there is no therapeutic benefit from residual solvents, all residual solvents should be reduced to the extent possible to meet product specifications, good manufacturing practices, or other quality-based requirements. Drug products should contain no higher levels of residual solvents than can be supported by safety data. Some solvents that are known to cause unacceptable toxicities (Class 1, Table 2.46-1) should be avoided in the production of drug substances, excipients, or drug products unless their use can be strongly justified in a risk-benefit assessment. Some solvents associated with less severe toxicity (Class 2, Table 2.46-2) should be limited in order to protect patients from potential adverse effects. Ideally, less toxic solvents (Class 3, Table 2.46-3) should be used where practical.

Testing should be performed for residual solvents when production or purification processes are known to result in the presence of such solvents. It is only necessary to test for solvents that are used or produced in the manufacture or purification of drug substances, excipients, or drug products. Although manufacturers may choose to test the drug product, a cumulative method may be used to calculate the residual solvent levels in the drug product from the levels in the ingredients used to produce the drug product. If the calculation results in a level equal to or below that recommended in this chapter, no testing of the drug product for residual solvents needs to be considered. If, however, the calculated level is above the recommended level, the drug product should be tested to ascertain whether the formulation process has reduced the relevant solvent level to within the acceptable amount. Drug product should also be tested if a solvent is used during its manufacture.

The limit applies to all dosage forms and routes of administration. Higher levels of residual solvents may be acceptable in certain cases such as short term (30 days or less) or topical application. Justification for these levels should be made on a case-by-case basis.

2. General principles

2.1. Classification of residual solvents by risk assessment

The term "PDE" (Permitted Daily Exposure) is defined in this chapter as a pharmaceutically acceptable daily intake of residual solvents. Residual solvents regulated in this chapter were evaluated for their possible risk to human health and placed into one of three classes as follows:

(i) Class 1 solvents: Solvents to be avoided in the manufacture of pharmaceuticals

Known human carcinogens, strongly suspected human carcinogens, and environmental hazards. Class 1 solvents are listed in Table 2.46-1.

(ii) Class 2 solvents: Solvents to be limited in pharmaceuticals

Non-genotoxic animal carcinogens or possible causative agents of other irreversible toxicity such as neurotoxicity or teratogenicity. Solvents suspected of other significant but reversible toxicities. Class 2 solvents are listed in Table 2.46-2.

(iii) Class 3 solvents: Solvents with low toxic potential

Solvents with low toxic potential to human; no health-based exposure limit is needed. Class 3 solvents are listed in Table 2.46-3 and have PDEs of 50 mg or more per day.

2.2. Option for describing limits of Class 2 solvents

Two options are available when setting limits for Class 2 solvents.

2.2.1. Option 1

The concentration limits in ppm can be calculated using equation (1) below by assuming a product mass of 10 g administered daily.

$$\text{Concentration limit (ppm)} = \frac{1000 \times PDE}{\text{dose}} \quad (1)$$

Here, PDE is given in terms of mg per day and dose is given in g per day.

These limits are considered acceptable for all drug substances, excipients, or drug products. Therefore, this option may be applied if the daily dose is not known or fixed. If all excipients and drug substances in a formulation meet the limits given in Option 1, then these components may be used in any proportion. No further calculation is necessary provided the daily dose does not exceed 10 g. Products that are administered in doses greater than 10 g per day should be considered under Option 2.

2.2.2. Option 2

It is not considered necessary for each component of the drug product to comply with the limits given in Option 1. The PDE in terms of mg per day as stated in Table 2.46-2 can be used with the known maximum daily dose and equation (1) above to determine the concentration of residual solvent allowed in drug product. Such limits are considered acceptable provided that it has been demonstrated that the residual solvent has been reduced to the practical minimum. The limits should be realistic in relation to analytical precision, manufacturing capability, reasonable variation in the manufacturing process, and the limits should reflect contemporary manufacturing standards.

Option 2 may be applied by adding the amounts of a residual solvent present in each of the components of the drug product. The sum of the amounts of solvent per day should be less than that given by the PDE.

3. Analytical procedures

Residual solvents are typically determined using chromatographic techniques such as gas chromatography. If only Class 3 solvents are present, a nonspecific method such as loss on drying may be used. The analytical method should be validated adequately.

4. Reporting levels of residual solvents

Manufacturers of drug products need certain information about the content of residual solvents in excipients or drug substances. The following statements are given as examples of the required information.

(i) Only Class 3 solvents are likely to be present. Loss on drying is not more than 0.5%.

(ii) Only Class 2 solvents are likely to be present. Name the Class 2 solvents that are present. All are not more than the Option 1 limit.

(iii) Only Class 2 solvents and Class 3 solvents are likely to be present. Residual Class 2 solvents are not more than the Option 1 limit and residual Class 3 solvents are not more than 0.5%.

If Class 1 solvents are likely to be present, they should be identified and quantified. "Likely to be present" refers to the solvents that were used in the final manufacturing step and to the solvents that were used in earlier manufacturing steps and not always possible to be excluded even in a validated process.

If solvents of Class 2 or Class 3 are present at greater than their Option 1 limits or 0.5%, respectively, they should be identified and quantified.

5. Limits of residual solvents

5.1. Solvents to be avoided in manufacture of pharmaceuticals

Solvents in Class 1 should not be employed in the manufacture of drug substances, excipients, and drug products because of their unacceptable toxicity or their deleterious environmental effect. However, if their use is unavoidable in order to produce a drug product with a significant therapeutic advance, then their levels should be restricted as shown in Table 2.46-1, unless otherwise justified. 1,1,1-Trichloroethane is included in Table 2.46-1 because it is an environmental hazard. The stated limit of 1500 ppm shown in Table 2.46-1 is based on the assessment of the safety data.

Table 2.46-1 Class 1 solvents (solvents that should be avoided in the manufacture of pharmaceuticals)

Solvent	Concentration Limit (ppm)	Concern
Benzene	2	Carcinogen
Carbon tetrachloride	4	Toxic and environmental hazard
1,2-Dichloroethane	5	Toxic
1,1-Dichloroethene	8	Toxic
1,1,1-Trichloroethane	1500	Environmental hazard

Table 2.46-2 Class 2 solvents (residual amount should be limited in pharmaceuticals)

Solvent	PDE (mg/day)	Concentration limit (ppm)
Acetonitrile	4.1	410
Chlorobenzene	3.6	360
Chloroform	0.6	60
Cumene	0.7	70
Cyclohexane	38.8	3880
1,2-Dichloroethene	18.7	1870
Dichloromethane	6.0	600
1,2-Dimethoxyethane	1.0	100
N,N-Dimethylacetamide	10.9	1090
N,N-Dimethylformamide	8.8	880
1,4-Dioxane	3.8	380
2-Ethoxyethanol	1.6	160
Ethylene glycol	6.2	620
Formamide	2.2	220
Hexane	2.9	290
Methanol	30.0	3000
2-Methoxyethanol	0.5	50
Methyl butyl ketone	0.5	50
Methylcyclohexane	11.8	1180
Methyl isobutyl ketone	45	4500
N-Methylpyrrolidone	5.3	530
Nitromethane	0.5	50
Pyridine	2.0	200
Sulfolane	1.6	160
Tetrahydrofuran	7.2	720
Tetralin	1.0	100
Toluene	8.9	890
1,1,2-Trichloroethene	0.8	80
Xylene*	21.7	2170

* Usually 60% *m*-xylene, 14% *p*-xylene, 9% *o*-xylene with 17% ethylbenzene

5.2. Solvents to be limited in pharmaceuticals

Solvents in Table 2.46-2 should be limited in drug products because of their inherent toxicities.

PDEs are given to the nearest 0.1 mg per day, and concentrations are given to the nearest 10 ppm. The stated values do not reflect the necessary analytical precision of determination. Precision should be determined as part of the validation of the method.

5.3. Solvents with low toxic potential

Solvents in Class 3 shown in Table 2.46-3 may be regarded as less toxic and of lower risk to human health. Class 3 includes no solvent known as a human health hazard at levels normally accepted in pharmaceuticals. The amounts of these residual solvents of 50 mg per day or less (corresponding to 5000 ppm or 0.5% under Option 1) would be acceptable without justification. Higher amounts may also be acceptable provided they are realistic in relation to manufacturing capability and good manufacturing practice.

5.4 Solvents for which no adequate toxicological data was found

The following solvents (Table 2.46-4) may also be related to the manufacturer of drug substances, excipients, or drug products. However, no adequate toxicological data on which to base a PDE was found. Manufacturers should supply justification for residual levels of these solvents in drug products.

II. Identification and quantification of residual solvents

Whenever possible, the substance under test needs to be dissolved to release the residual solvent. Because drug products, as well as active ingredients and excipients are treated, it may be acceptable that in some cases, some of the components of formulations will not dissolve completely. In those cases, the drug product may first need to be pulverized into a fine powder so that any residual solvent that may be present can be released. This operation should be performed as fast as possible to prevent the loss of volatile solvents during the procedure.

Table 2.46-3 Class 3 solvents (limited by GMP or other quality-based requirements in pharmaceuticals)

Acetic acid	Heptane
Acetone	Isobutyl acetate
Anisole	Isopropyl acetate
1-Butanol	Methyl acetate
2-Butanol	3-Methyl-1-butanol
n-Butyl acetate	Methyl ethyl ketone
tert-Butyl methyl ether	2-Methyl-1-propanol
Dimethylsulfoxide	Pentane
Ethanol	1-Pentanol
Ethyl acetate	1-Propanol
Diethyl ether	2-Propanol
Ethyl formate	Propyl acetate
Formic acid	Triethylamine

Table 2.46-4 Solvents for which no adequate toxicological data were found

1,1-Diethoxypropane	Methyl isopropyl ketone
1,1-Dimethoxymethane	Methyltetrahydrofuran
2,2-Dimethoxypropane	Petroleum ether
Isooctane	Trichloroacetic acid
Isopropyl ether	Trifluoroacetic acid

In the operating conditions of gas chromatography and headspace described below, parameters to be set and their description may be different depending on the apparatus. When setting these conditions, it is necessary to change them according to the apparatus used, if it is confirmed that they meet the system suitability.

In addition to the reagents specified to be used for the test, those that meet the purpose of the test can be used.

1. Class 1 and Class 2 residual solvents

The following procedures are useful to identify and quantify residual solvents when the information regarding which solvents are likely to be present in the material is not available. When the information about the presence of specific residual solvents is available, it is not necessary to perform Procedure A and Procedure B, and only Procedure C or other appropriate procedure is needed to quantify the amount of residual solvents.

A flow chart for the identification of residual solvents and the application of limit and quantitative tests is shown in Fig. 2.46-1.

1.1. Water-soluble articles

1.1.1. Procedure A

The test is performed by gas chromatography <*2.02*> according to the following conditions.

Class 1 standard stock solution: To about 9 mL of dimethylsulfoxide add exactly 1 mL of Residual Solvents Class 1 RS, and add water to make exactly 100 mL. Pipet 1 mL of this solution in a volumetric flask, previously filled with about 50 mL of water and add water to make exactly 100 mL. Pipet 10 mL of this solution in a volumetric flask,

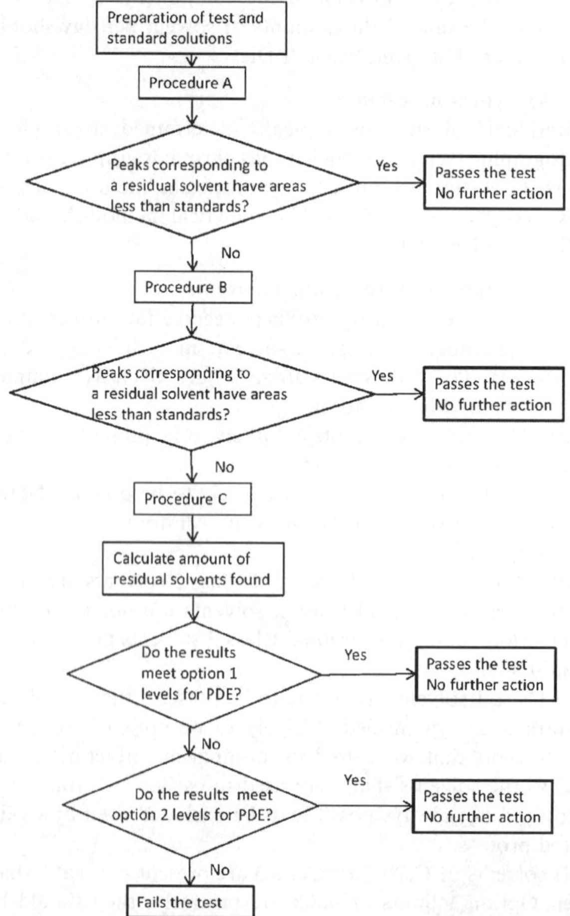

Fig. 2.46-1 Flow chart for the identification of residual solvents and the application of limit and qualification tests

previously filled with about 50 mL of water and add water to make exactly 100 mL.

Class 1 standard solution: Pipet 1 mL of Class 1 standard stock solution in an appropriate head space vial containing exactly 5 mL of water, stopper, cap, and shake.

Class 2 standard stock solution A: Pipet 1 mL of Residual Solvents Class 2A RS, add water to make exactly 100 mL.

Class 2 standard stock solution B: Pipet 1 mL of Residual Solvents Class 2B RS, add water to make exactly 100 mL.

Class 2 standard stock solution C: Pipet 1 mL of Residual Solvents Class 2C RS, add water to make exactly 100 mL.

Class 2 standard solution A: Pipet 1 mL of Class 2 standard stock solution A in an appropriate headspace vial, add exactly 5 mL of water, stopper, cap, and shake.

Class 2 standard solution B: Pipet 5 mL of Class 2 standard stock solution B in an appropriate headspace vial, add exactly 1 mL of water, stopper, cap, and shake.

Class 2 standard solution C: Pipet 1 mL of Class 2 standard stock solution C in an appropriate headspace vial, add exactly 5 mL of water, stopper, cap, and shake.

Test stock solution: Dissolve 0.25 g of the article under test in water, and add water to make exactly 25 mL.

Test solution: Pipet 5 mL of the test stock solution in an appropriate headspace vial, add exactly 1 mL of water, and stopper, cap, and shake.

Class 1 system suitability solution: Pipet 1 mL of Class 1 standard stock solution in an appropriate headspace vial, add exactly 5 mL of the test stock solution, and stopper, cap, and shake.

Operating conditions—

Detector: A hydrogen flame-ionization detector.

Column: A fused silica column (or a wide-bore column) 0.32 mm (or 0.53 mm) in inside diameter and 30 m in length, coated with 6% cyanopropylphenyl-94% dimethyl silicon polymer for gas chromatography in 1.8 μm (or 3.0 μm) thickness.

Column temperature: Maintain the temperature at 40°C for 20 minutes after injection, raise to 240°C at a rate of 10°C per minute, and maintain at 240°C for 20 minutes.

Injection port temperature: 140°C.

Detector temperature: 250°C.

Carrier gas: Nitrogen or Helium.

Flow rate: About 35 cm per second.

Split ratio: 1:5. (Note: The split ratio can be modified in order to optimize sensitivity.)

System suitability—

Test for required detectability: When the procedure is run with Class 1 standard solution and Class 1 system suitability solution under the above operating conditions, the SN ratio of the peak of 1,1,1-trichloroethane obtained with Class 1 standard solution is not less than 5, and the SN ratio of each peak obtained with Class 1 system suitability solution is not less than 3, respectively.

System performance: When the procedure is run with Class 2 standard solution A or the solution for system suitability under the above operating conditions, the resolution between acetonitrile and dichloromethane is not less than 1.0. Pipet 1 mL of a solution of Residual Solvents for System Suitability RS (1 in 100) in an appropriate headspace vial, add exactly 5 mL of water, stopper, cap, mix, and use this solution as the solution for system suitability.

System repeatability: When the test is repeated 6 times with Class 1 standard solution under the above operating conditions, the relative standard deviation of each peak area is not more than 15%.

Separately inject (following one of the headspace operating parameter sets described in Table 2.46-5) equal volumes of headspace (about 1.0 mL) of Class 1 standard solution, Class 2 standard solution A, Class 2 standard solution B, Class 2 standard solution C and the test solution into the chromatograph, record the chromatograms, and measure the responses for the major peaks. If a peak response of any peak, other than a peak for 1,1,1-trichloroethane, in the test solution is greater than or equal to a corresponding peak in either Class 1 standard solution, Class 2 standard solution A, Class 2 standard solution B or Class 2 standard solution C, or a peak response of 1,1,1-trichloroethane is greater than or equal to 150 times the peak response corresponding to 1,1,1-trichloroethane in Class 1 standard solution, proceed to Procedure B to verify the identity of the peak; otherwise the article meets the requirements of this test.

1.1.2. Procedure B

The test is performed by gas chromatography <2.02> according to the following conditions.

Class 1 standard stock solution, Class 1 standard solution, Class 1 system suitability solution, Class 2 standard stock solutions A, B and C, Class 2 standard solutions A, B and C, test stock solution and test solution: Prepare as directed for Procedure A.

Operating conditions—

Detector: A hydrogen flame-ionization detector.

Column: A fused silica column (or a wide-bore column) 0.32 mm (or 0.53 mm) in inside diameter and 30 m in length, coated with polyethylene glycol for gas chromatography in 0.25 μm thickness.

Column temperature: Maintain the temperature at 50°C for 20 minutes after injection, raise to 165°C at a rate of 6°C per minute, and maintain at 165°C for 20 minutes.

Injection port temperature: 140°C.

Detector temperature: 250°C.

Carrier gas: Nitrogen or Helium.

Flow rate: About 35 cm per second.

Split ratio: 1:5. (Note: The split ratio can be modified in order to optimize sensitivity.)

System suitability—

Test for required detectability: When the procedure is run with Class 1 standard solution and Class 1 system suitability solution under the above operating conditions, the SN ratio of the peak of benzene obtained with Class 1 standard solution is not less than 5, and the SN ratio of each peak obtained with Class 1 system suitability solution is not less than 3, respectively.

System performance: When the procedure is run with Class 2 standard solution A or the solution for system suitability under the above operating conditions, the resolution between acetonitrile and *cis*-1,2-dichloroethene is not less than 1.0. Pipet 1 mL of a solution of Residual Solvents for System Suitability RS (1 in 100) in an appropriate headspace vial, add exactly 5 mL of water, stopper, cap, mix, and use this solution as the solution for system suitability.

System repeatability: When the test is repeated 6 times with Class 1 standard solution under the above operating conditions, the relative standard deviation of each peak area is not more than 15%.

Separately inject (following one of the headspace operating parameter sets described in Table 2.46-5) equal volumes of headspace (about 1.0 mL) of Class 1 standard solution, Class 2 standard solution A, Class 2 standard solution B, Class 2 standard solution C and the test solution into the chromatograph, record the chromatograms, and measure the responses for the major peaks. If the peak response(s) of the peak(s) in the test solution is/are greater than or equal to a corresponding peak(s) in either Class 1 standard solution, Class 2 standard solution A, Class 2 standard solution B or

Class 2 standard solution C, proceed to Procedure C to quantify the peak(s); otherwise, the article meets the requirements of this test.

1.1.3. Procedure C

The test is performed by gas chromatography <*2.02*> according to the following conditions.

Class 1 standard stock solution, Class 1 standard solution, Class 2 standard stock solution A, Class 2 standard solution A, Class 2 standard stock solution C, Class 2 standard solution C and Class 1 system suitability solution: Prepare as directed for Procedure A.

Standard stock solution (Note: Prepare a separate standard stock solution for each peak identified and verified by Procedures A and B. For Class 1 solvents other than 1,1,1-trichloroethane, prepare the first dilution as directed for the first dilution under Class 1 standard stock solution in Procedure A.): Transfer an accurately measured volume of each individual solvent corresponding to each residual solvent peak identified and verified by Procedures A and B to a suitable container, and dilute quantitatively, and stepwise if necessary, with water to obtain a solution having a final concentration of 1/20 of the value stated in Table 2.46-1 or Table 2.46-2.

Standard solution: Pipet 1 mL of the standard stock solution in an appropriate headspace vial, add exactly 5 mL of water, stopper, cap, and shake.

Test stock solution: Weigh accurately about 0.25 g of the article under test, dissolve in water, and add water to make exactly 25 mL.

Test solution: Pipet 5 mL of the test stock solution in an appropriate headspace vial, add exactly 1 mL of water, stopper, cap, and shake.

Spiked test solution (Note: prepare a separate spiked test solution for each peak identified and verified by Procedure A and B): Pipet 5 mL of the test stock solution in an appropriate headspace vial, add exactly 1 mL of the standard stock solution, stopper, cap, and shake.

Operating conditions and system suitability fundamentally follow the procedure A. Test for required detectability is unnecessary, and use Standard solution instead of Class 1 standard solution for system repeatability. If the results of the chromatography from Procedure A are found to be inferior to those found with Procedure B, the operating conditions from Procedure B may be substituted.

Perform the test (following one of the headspace operating parameters described in Table 2.46-5) with equal volumes of about 1.0 mL each of the standard solution, test solution, and spiked test solution, and measure the peak areas for the major peaks. Calculate the amount of each residual solvent found in the article under test by the formula:

$$\text{Amount of residual solvent (ppm)} = 5\,(C/M)\{A_T/(A_S - A_T)\}$$

C: Concentration (μg/mL) of the appropriate Reference Standard in the standard stock solution

M: Amount (g) of the article under test taken to prepare the test stock solution

A_T: Peak responses of each residual solvent obtained from the test solution

A_S: Peak responses of each residual solvent obtained from the spiked test solution

1.2. Water-insoluble articles

1.2.1. Procedure A

The test is performed by gas chromatography <*2.02*> according to the following conditions. Dimethylsulfoxide may be substituted as an alternative solvent to *N,N*-dimethylformamide.

Class 1 standard stock solution: To about 80 mL of *N,N*-dimethylformamide add 1 mL of Residual Solvents Class 1 RS, and add *N,N*-dimethylformamide to make exactly 100 mL. Pipet 1 mL of this solution in a volumetric flask, previously filled with about 80 mL of *N,N*-dimethylformamide and add *N,N*-dimethylformamide to make exactly 100 mL (this solution is the intermediate diluent prepared from Residual Solvents Class 1 RS and use it for preparation of Class 1 system suitability solution). Pipet 1 mL of this solution, and add *N,N*-dimethylformamide to make exactly 10 mL.

Class 1 standard solution: Pipet 1 mL of Class 1 standard stock solution in an appropriate head space vial containing exactly 5 mL of water, stopper, cap, and shake.

Class 2 standard stock solution A: Pipet 1 mL of Residual Solvents Class 2A RS, dissolve in about 80 mL of *N,N*-dimethylformamide, and add *N,N*-dimethylformamide to make exactly 100 mL.

Class 2 standard stock solution B: Pipet 0.5 mL of Residual Solvents Class 2B RS, add *N,N*-dimethylformamide to make exactly 10 mL.

Class 2 standard stock solution C: Pipet 1 mL of Residual Solvents Class 2C RS, dissolve in about 80 mL of *N,N*-dimethylformamide, and add *N,N*-dimethylformamide to make exactly 100 mL.

Class 2 standard solution A: Pipet 1 mL of Class 2 standard stock solution A in an appropriate headspace vial, add exactly 5 mL of water, stopper, cap, and shake.

Class 2 standard solution B: Pipet 1 mL of Class 2 standard stock solution B in an appropriate headspace vial, add exactly 5 mL of water, stopper, cap, and shake.

Class 2 standard solution C: Pipet 1 mL of Class 2 standard stock solution C in an appropriate headspace vial, add exactly 5 mL of water, stopper, cap, and shake.

Test stock solution: Dissolve 0.5 g of the article under test in *N,N*-dimethylformamide, and add *N,N*-dimethylformamide to make exactly 10 mL.

Test solution: Pipet 1 mL of the test stock solution in an appropriate headspace vial, add exactly 5 mL of water, stopper, cap, and shake.

Class 1 system suitability solution: Pipet 5 mL of the test stock solution and 0.5 mL of the intermediate dilution prepared from Residual Solvents Class 1 RS, and mix. Pipet 1 mL of this solution in an appropriate headspace vial, add exactly 5 mL of water, stopper, cap, and shake.

Operating conditions—

Detector: A hydrogen flame-ionization detector.

Column: A wide-bore column 0.53 mm in inside diameter and 30 m in length, coated with 6% cyanopropylphenyl-94% dimethyl silicon polymer for gas chromatography in 3.0 μm thickness.

Column temperature: Maintain the temperature at 40°C for 20 minutes after injection, raise to 240°C at a rate of 10°C per minute, and maintain at 240°C for 20 minutes.

Injection port temperature: 140°C.

Detector temperature: 250°C.

Carrier gas: Helium.

Flow rate: About 35 cm per second.

Split ratio: 1:3. (Note: The split ratio can be modified in order to optimize sensitivity.)

System suitability—

Test for required detectability: When the procedure is run with Class 1 standard solution and Class 1 system suitability solution under the above operating conditions, the SN ratio of the peak of 1,1,1-trichloroethane obtained with Class 1 standard solution is not less than 5, and the SN ratio of each peak obtained with Class 1 system suitability solution is not less than 3, respectively.

System performance: When the procedure is run with Class 2 standard solution A or the solution for system suitability under the above operating conditions, the resolution between acetonitrile and dichloromethane is not less than 1.0. Pipet 1 mL of the *N*,*N*-dimethylformamide solution of Residual Solvents for System Suitability RS (1 in 100) in an appropriate headspace vial, add exactly 5 mL of water, stopper, cap, and shake, and use this solution as the solution for system suitability.

System repeatability: When the test is repeated 6 times with Class 1 standard solution under the above operating conditions, the relative standard deviation of each peak areas is not more than 15%.

Separately inject (use headspace operating parameters in column 3 of Table 2.46-5) equal volumes of headspace (about 1.0 mL) of Class 1 standard solution, Class 2 standard solution A, Class 2 standard solution B, Class 2 standard solution C, and the test solution into the chromatograph, record the chromatograms, and measure the responses for the major peaks. If a peak response of any peak, other than a peak for 1,1,1-trichloroethane, in the test solution is greater than or equal to a corresponding peak in either Class 1 standard solution, Class 2 standard solution A, Class 2 standard solution B or Class 2 standard solution C, or a peak response of 1,1,1-trichloroethane is greater than or equal to 150 times the peak response corresponding to 1,1,1-trichloroethane in Class 1 standard solution, proceed to Procedure B to verify the identity of the peak; otherwise, the article meets the requirements of this test.

1.2.2. Procedure B

The test is performed by gas chromatography <*2.02*> according to the following conditions.

Class 1 standard stock solution, Class 1 standard solution, Class 1 system suitability solution, Class 2 standard stock solutions A, B and C, Class 2 standard solutions A, B and C, test stock solution, and test solution: Proceed as directed for Procedure A.

Proceed as directed for Procedure B under Water-soluble articles with a split ratio of 1:3. (Note: The split ratio can be modified in order to optimize sensitivity.) The solution for system suitability: Proceed as directed for Procedure A.

Separately inject (use headspace operating parameters in Table 2.46-5) equal volumes of headspace (about 1.0 mL) of Class 1 standard solution, Class 2 standard solution A, Class 2 standard solution B, Class 2 standard solution C and the test solution into the chromatograph, record the chromatograms, and measure the responses for the major peaks. If the peak response(s) of the peak(s) in the test solution is/are greater than or equal to a corresponding peak(s) in either Class 1 standard solution, Class 2 standard solution A, Class 2 standard solution B or Class 2 standard solution C, proceed to Procedure C to quantify the peak; otherwise, the article meets the requirements of this test.

1.2.3 Procedure C

The test is performed by gas chromatography <*2.02*> according to the following conditions.

Class 1 standard stock solution, Class 1 standard solution, Class 1 system suitability solution, Class 2 standard stock solution A, Class 2 standard solution A, Class 2 standard stock solution C and Class 2 standard solution C: Proceed as directed for Procedure A.

Standard stock solution (Note: Prepare a separate standard stock solution for each peak identified and verified by Procedures A and B. For Class 1 solvents other than 1,1,1-trichloroethane, prepare the first dilution as directed for the first dilution under Class 1 standard stock solution in Procedure A.): Transfer an accurately measured volume of each individual solvent corresponding to each residual solvent peak identified and verified by Procedures A and B to a suitable container, and dilute quantitatively, and stepwise if necessary, with water to obtain a solution having a final concentration of 1/20 of the value stated in Table 2.46-1 or Table 2.46-2.

Standard solution: Pipet 1 mL of the standard stock solution in an appropriate headspace vial, add exactly 5 mL of water, stopper, cap, and shake.

Test stock solution: Weigh accurately about 0.5 g of the article under test, and add *N*,*N*-dimethylformamide to make exactly 10 mL.

Test solution: Pipet 1 mL of test stock solution in an appropriate headspace vial, add exactly 5 mL of water, stopper, cap, and shake.

Spiked test solution (Note: prepare a separate spiked test solution for each peak identified and verified by Procedure A and B): Pipet 1 mL of test stock solution in an appropriate headspace vial, add exactly 4 mL of water, stopper, cap, and shake.

Operating conditions and system suitability fundamentally follow the procedure A. Test for required detectability is unnecessary, and use Standard solution instead of Class 1 standard solution for system repeatability. If the results of the chromatography from Procedure A are found to be inferior to those found with Procedure B, the operating conditions from Procedure B may be substituted.

Perform the test (use headspace operating parameters in Table 2.46-5) with about 1.0 mL each of the standard solution, test solution, and spiked test solution, and measure the responses for the major peaks. Calculate the amount of each residual solvent found in the article under test by the formula:

$$\text{Amount of residual solvent (ppm)} = 10\,(C/M)\{A_T/(A_S - A_T)\}$$

C: Concentration (μg/mL) of the appropriate Reference Standard in the standard stock solution

M: Amount (g) of the article under test taken to prepare the test stock solution

A_T: Peak responses of each residual solvent obtained from the test solution

A_S: Peak responses of each residual solvent obtained from

Table 2.46-5 Headspace operating parameters

	Headspace Operating Parameter Sets		
	1	2	3
Equilibration temperature (°C)	80	105	80
Equilibration time (min.)	60	45	45
Transfer-line temperature (°C)	85	110	105
Syringe temperature (°C)	80 - 90	105 - 115	80 - 90
Carrier gas: nitrogen or helium at an appropriate pressure			
Pressurization time (s)	≧ 60	≧ 60	≧ 60
Injection volume (mL)*	1	1	1

* Or follow the instrument manufacture's recommendations, as long as the method criteria are met. Injecting less than 1 mL is allowed as long as adequate sensitivity is achieved.

the spiked test solution

1.3. Headspace operating parameters and other considerations

Examples of headspace operating parameters are shown in Table 2.46-5.

These test methods describe the analytical methods using the headspace gas chromatography. The following Class 2 residual solvents are not readily detected by the headspace injection conditions because of the low sensitivity: 2-ethoxyethanol, ethylene glycol, formamide, 2-methoxyethanol, *N*-methylpyrrolidone, and sulfolane. Other appropriate validated procedures are to be employed for the quantification of these residual solvents. In the headspace methods, *N,N*-dimethylformamide and *N,N*-dimethylacetoamide are often used as solvents. As not only 6 solvents described above but these two solvents are not included in Residual Solvents Class 2A RS, Residual Solvents Class 2B RS and/or Residual Solvents Class 2C RS, appropriate validated procedures are to be employed for these residual solvents as necessary.

2. Class 3 residual solvents

Perform the test according to 1. Otherwise, an appropriate validated procedure is to be employed. Prepare appropriately standard solutions, etc. according to the residual solvent under test.

If only Class 3 solvents are present, the level of residual solvents may be determined by Loss on Drying <*2.41*>. However, when the value of the loss on drying is more than 0.5%, or other solvents exist, the individual Class 3 residual solvent or solvents present in the article under test should be identified using the procedures as described above or other appropriate procedure, and quantified as necessary.

3. Reference Standards

(i) Residual Solvents Class 1 RS (A mixture of benzene, carbon tetrachloride, 1,2-dichloroethane, 1,1-dichloroethene and 1,1,1-trichloroethane)

(ii) Residual Solvents Class 2A RS (A mixture of acetonitrile, chlorobenzene, cumene, cyclohexane, 1,2-dichloroethene (*cis*-1,2-dichloroethene, *trans*-1,2-dichloroethene), dichloromethane, 1,4-dioxane, methanol, methylcyclohexane, tetrahydrofuran, toluene and xylene (*m*-xylene, *p*-xylene, *o*-xylene, ethylbenzene))

(iii) Residual Solvents Class 2B RS (A mixture of chloroform, 1,2-dimethoxyethane, hexane, methyl butyl ketone, nitromethane, pyridine, tetralin and 1,1,2-trichloroethene)

(iv) Residual Solvents Class 2C RS (Methyl isobutyl ketone)

(v) Residual Solvents for System Suitability RS (A mixture of acetonitrile, *cis*-1,2-dichloroethene and dichloromethane)

2.47 Osmolarity Determination

Osmolarity Determination is a method for measuring the osmotic concentration of the sample solution from the extent of the freezing-point depression.

When a solution and a pure solvent are separated by a semipermeable membrane, through which the solvent can pass freely, but the solute cannot, a part of the solvent passes into the solution compartment through the membrane. The pressure difference produced between the two compartments concomitantly with the solvent migration through the membrane, is defined as the osmotic pressure Π (Pa). The osmotic pressure is a physical quantity depending on the total of the molecular species present, including neutral molecules and ions, and does not depend on the kind of solute. A solution property, such as osmotic pressure, freezing-point depression, boiling-point elevation etc., which depends not on the kind of solute, but on the total number of all molecular species, is called a colligative property of a solution.

The osmotic pressure of a polymer solution can be measured directly as the hydrostatic pressure difference between two compartments separated by a semipermeable membrane, such as a cellulose membrane. However, this is not applicable to a solution containing low molecular species, which can pass through a semipermeable membrane. Though the osmotic pressure of such a solution cannot be measured directly, the direction and extent of solvent migration through biological membranes can be predicted from the total number of all molecular species present when the solution is placed under physiological conditions. Other colligative properties of a solution such as freezing-point depression, boiling-point elevation, vapor-pressure depression, etc. can be directly obtained by observing changes of temperature and/or pressure, etc. These solution properties depend on the total number of ionic and neutral species in the solution in the same way as the osmotic pressure, and the molecular particle concentration is defined as the osmotic concentration. The osmotic concentration can be defined in two ways, one being mass-based concentration (osmolality, mol/kg) and the other, volume-based concentration (osmolarity, mol/L). In practice, the latter is more convenient.

Unless otherwise specified, the freezing-point depression method is used for measuring the osmotic concentration. The method is based on the linear dependency of the freezing-point depression ΔT (°C) upon the osmolality m (mol/kg), as expressed in the following equation,

$$\Delta T = K \cdot m$$

In this equation, K is the molal freezing-point depression constant, and it is known to be 1.86°C kg/mol for water. Since the constant K is defined on the basis of molarity, the molar osmotic concentration can be obtained from the above equation. In the dilute osmotic concentration range, osmolality m (mol/kg) can be assumed to be numerically equal to osmolarity c (mol/L). Thus, the conventional osmolarity (mol/L) and the unit of osmole (Osm) are adopted in this test method. One Osm means that the Avogadro number (6.022×10^{23}/mol) of species is contained in 1 L of solution. Usually the osmotic concentration is expressed as the submultiple milliosmole (mOsm, mosmol/L) in the Pharmacopoeia.

1. Apparatus

Usually, the osmotic concentration of a solution can be obtained by measuring the extent of the freezing-point depression. The apparatus (osmometer) is composed of a sample cell for a fixed volume of sample solution and a cell holder, a cooling unit and bath with a temperature regulator, and a thermistor for detecting temperature.

2. Procedure

A fixed volume of the test solution is introduced into the sample cell, as indicated for the individual apparatus.

The apparatus must first be calibrated by the two-point calibration method by using osmolal standard solutions. For the calibration, select two different standard solutions just covering the expected osmolar concentration of a sample solution. Other than the indicated osmolal standard solutions in the Table 2.47-1, water can also be used as a standard solution (0 mOsm) for measuring low osmolar sample solutions (0 – 100 mOsm). Next, after washing the sample cell

Table 2.47-1

Standard solution for osmometer calibration (milliosmoles)	Amount of sodium chloride (g)
100	0.309
200	0.626
300	0.946
400	1.270
500	1.593
700	2.238
1000	3.223

and the thermistor as indicated for the individual apparatus, measure the degree of the freezing-point depression caused by a sample solution. Using the above-mentioned relation of osmolar concentration m and ΔT, the osmolarity of a sample solution can be obtained, and it is assumed to be numerically equal to the osmolarity.

In the case of higher osmolar solutions over 1000 mOsm, dilute the sample with water and prepare n'/n times diluted sample solution (n in n'). Measure the osmolarity of the diluted solution, as described above. In this case, it is necessary to state that the calculated osmolarity for the sample (see below) is an apparent osmolarity obtained by the dilution method. When the determination is performed using n'/n times diluted solution, the dilution number should be selected so that the osmolar concentration is near but not exceeding 1000 mOsm, and dilute in one step.

In the case of solid samples, such as freeze-dried medicines, prepare a sample solution by dissolving the solid using the indicated solution for dissolution.

3. Suitability of the apparatus

After the calibration of the apparatus, a suitability test must be done by repeating the measurement of osmolarity for one of the standard solutions not less than 6 times. In performing the test, it is advisable that the osmolarity of a sample solution and the selected standard solution are similar to each other. In this test, the repeatability of measured values and the deviation of the average from the indicated value should be less than 2.0% and 3.0%, respectively. When the requirement is not met, calibrate the apparatus again by the two-point calibration method, and repeat the test.

4. Preparation of the osmolar standard solutions

Weigh exactly an amount indicated in Table 2.47-1 of sodium chloride (standard reagent), previously dried between 500°C and 650°C for 40 to 50 minutes and allowed to cool in a desiccator (silica gel). Dissolve the weighed sodium chloride in exactly 100 g of water to make the corresponding osmolar standard solution.

5. Osmolar ratio

In this test method the osmolar ratio is defined as the ratio of osmolarity of a sample solution to that of the isotonic sodium chloride solution. The ratio can be used as a measure of isotonicity of sample solution. Since the osmolarity of the isotonic sodium chloride solution (NaCl 0.900 g/100 mL) c_S (mOsm) is assumed to be constant (286 mOsm), the osmolar ratio of a sample solution, of which the osmolarity is c_T (mOsm), can be calculated by means of the following equation,

$$\text{Osmolar ratio} = c_T/c_S$$

c_S: 286 mOsm

When the measurement is done by the dilution method, because the sample has an osmolarity over 1000 mOsm, the apparent osmolarity of the sample solution c_T can be calculated as $n'/n \cdot c'_T = c_T$, in which n'/n is the dilution number and c'_T is the measured osmolarity for the diluted solution. In this calculation, a linear relation between osmolarity and solute concentration is assumed. The dilution must be made in one step. Thus when the dilution measurement is performed, the dilution number is stated as (n in n').

2.48 Water Determination (Karl Fischer Method)

Water Determination determines water content in sample materials, utilizing the fact that water reacts with iodine and sulfur dioxide quantitatively in the presence of a lower alcohol such as methanol, and an organic base such as pyridine (Karl Fischer reaction). The reaction proceeds in the manner shown in the following equation:

$$I_2 + SO_2 + 3C_5H_5N + CH_3OH + H_2O \rightarrow 2(C_5H_5N^+H)I^- + (C_5H_5N^+H)^-OSO_2OCH_3$$

In this measurement there are two methods different in iodine-providing principle (the volumetric titration method and the coulometric titration method). In the volumetric titration method, iodine is previously dissolved in a reagent for water determination, and water content is determined by measuring the amount of iodine consumed as a result of reaction with water. In the coulometric titration method, iodine is produced by electrolysis of iodide ion in an anolyte solution for water determination. Based on the quantitative reaction of the generated iodine with water, the water content in a sample specimen can be indirectly determined by measuring the quantity of electricity which is required for the production of iodine during the titration.

$$2I^- \rightarrow I_2 + 2e^-$$

1. Volumetric titration

1.1. Apparatus

Generally, the apparatus consists of automatic burettes, a titration flask, a stirrer, and equipment for amperometric titration at constant voltage or potentiometric titration at constant current. Karl Fischer TS for water determination is extremely hygroscopic, so the overall equipment for titration should be designed to be protected from the entry of water. Desiccants such as silica gel or calcium chloride for water determination can be used.

1.2. Reagents

1.2.1. Solvents for water determination

As a solvent for water determination, use principally methanol for water determination. Other solvents, including ethylene glycol for water determination, chloroform for water determination, diethylene glycol monoethyl ether for water determination, propylene carbonate for water determination, and formamide for water determination, or a mixture of these solvents can be used, taking solubility of a sample specimen and interference of a sample specimen with the Karl Fischer reaction into account.

1.2.2. Base for water determination

Use pyridine for water determination, imidazole for water determination, and 2-methylaminopyridine for water determination, for example.

1.2.3. Preparation and standardization of Karl Fischer TS for water determination

(1) Preparation

Use an appropriately prepared Karl Fischer TS for water

determination. For example, dissolve 63 g of iodine in 100 mL of pyridine for water determination, and cool the solution in an ice bath. Pass dried sulfur dioxide gas through this solution until the mass increase of the solution reaches 32 g. Then make up to 500 mL by adding methanol for water determination, and use this solution as Karl Fischer TS for water determination. Karl Fischer TS for water determination can be prepared with other appropriate solvents for water determination and bases for water determination.

Store Karl Fischer TS for water determination in tightly stoppered bottles in a cold place, protecting it from light and moisture, and allow to stand for more than 24 hours before use.

(2) Standardization

When water is titrated with Karl Fischer TS for water determination, the equivalent amount of water per unit volume of Karl Fischer TS for water determination, factor f (mg/mL), change over time with slight moisture. Standardize before use.

According to the procedure described in section 1.3. Procedure, take a suitable quantity of methanol for water determination in a dried titration flask, and titrate the solvent with a Karl Fischer TS for water determination to make the inside of the flask anhydrous. Then, weigh 5 to 30 mg of water accurately and put it in the titration flask quickly, and titrate the water dissolved in the solvent with a Karl Fischer TS for water determination to the end point, under vigorous stirring. When the quantity of titrant is V (mL), calculate the factor, f (mg/mL), of the Karl Fischer TS for water determination by using the following equation:

$$f(\text{mg/mL}) = M/V$$

M: Amount (mg) of water taken

V: Volume (mL) of Karl Fischer TS for water determination consumed for titration of water

1.2.4. Preparation and standardization of standard water-methanol solution

Prepare and standardize the standard water-methanol solution as follows, beforehand.

(1) Preparation

Take 500 mL of methanol for water determination in a dried 1000-mL volumetric flask, add 2.0 mL of water, and adjust with the methanol for water determination to make 1000 mL. The standard water-methanol solution is preserved in a cold place, protecting it from light and moisture.

(2) Standardization

Take a suitable quantity of methanol for water determination in a dried titration flask, and titrate the water contaminated with Karl Fischer TS for water determination to make the content of the flask anhydrous. Then, add exactly 10 mL of Karl Fischer TS for water determination to this solution in the flask, titrate it with the prepared standard water-methanol solution to the end point, and measure the quantity of titrant, V (mL). Calculate the factor of the standard water-methanol solution, f' (mg/mL), by using the following equation:

$$f'(\text{mg/mL}) = (f \times 10)/V$$

f: Factor (mg/mL) of Karl Fischer TS for water determination

10: Volume (mL) of Karl Fischer TS for water determination taken

V: Volume (mL) of titrant of the standard water-methanol solution

1.3. Procedure

As a rule, the titration of water with a Karl Fischer TS for water determination should be performed at the same temperature as that at which the standardization was done, with protection from moisture.

Immerse a pair of platinum electrodes (or double platinum electrode) in a solution to be titrated, add a Karl Fischer TS for water determination while applying a constant small voltage between the two electrodes, and measure the changed small current (μA) (Amperometric titration at constant voltage). When the current stops changing and persists for a certain time (usually, longer than 30 seconds), this electric state is designated as the end point of the titration.

Otherwise, apply a definite current between two platinum electrodes, and add Karl Fischer TS for water determination. The variable potential (mV) is measured (Potentiometric titration at constant current).

Unless otherwise specified, the titration of water with Karl Fischer TS for water determination should be performed by either direct titration or back titration.

1.3.1. Direct titration

Unless otherwise specified, proceed by the following method.

Take a suitable quantity of the solvent for water determination in a dried titration flask, and titrate the water contaminated with Karl Fischer TS for water determination to the end point to make the content of the flask anhydrous. Weigh accurately M (mg) of sample specimen containing 5 to 30 mg of water, transfer it quickly into the titration flask, dissolve by stirring, titrate the solution to be examined with Karl Fischer TS for water determination to the end point under vigorous stirring, and measure the quantity of titrant, V (mL). In the case of an insoluble sample specimen, powder the sample quickly, weigh accurately M (mg) of the sample containing 5 to 30 mg of water, and transfer it quickly into the titration vessel, stir the mixture, protecting it from moisture, and perform the titration under vigorous stirring.

Though the titration procedure should be performed under atmospheric conditions at low humidity, if the effect of atmospheric moisture cannot be avoided, for instance, if a long time is required for extraction and titration of water, a blank test must be done and the data must be corrected, as necessary.

$$\text{Water content (\%)} = \{(V \times f)/M\} \times 100$$

M: Amount (mg) of the sample taken

V: Volume (mL) of titrant of Karl Fischer TS for water determination consumed for titration

f: Factor (mg/mL) of Karl Fischer TS for water determination

1.3.2. Back titration

Unless otherwise specified, proceed by the following method.

Take a suitable quantity of the solvent for water determination in the dried titration vessel, and titrate the water contaminated with Karl Fischer TS for water determination to the end point to make the content of the flask anhydrous. Weigh accurately M (mg) of sample specimen having 5 to 30 mg of water, transfer the sample quickly into the titration vessel, dissolve it in the solution by stirring, add an excessive and definite volume, V' (mL), of Karl Fischer TS for water determination, and then titrate the solution with the standard water-methanol solution to the end point under vigorous stirring, and measure the quantity of titrant, V (mL). In the case of an insoluble sample specimen, powder the sample quickly, weigh accurately the mass, M (mg), transfer it quickly into the titration vessel, and add an excessive and definite volume, V' (mL), of Karl Fischer TS for water determination. After stirring, with protection from moisture, perform the titration under vigorous stirring. Calculate the water content (%) in the sample by using the following equation:

$$\text{Water content (\%)} = [\{(V' \times f) - (V \times f')\}/M] \times 100$$

M: Amount (mg) of the sample taken
V: Volume (mL) of titrant of the standard water-methanol solution
V': Excessive and definite volume (mL) of Karl Fischer TS for water determination
f: Factor (mg/mL) of Karl Fischer TS for water determination
f': Factor (mg/mL) of the standard water-methanol solution

1.4. Suitability of determination

Perform an appropriate suitability test for determination to verify the validity of devices and reagent systems for the volumetric titration method, before changing operating conditions, or periodically, as necessary. These conditions include device components such as electrodes and types of solvents and test solutions for water determination.

Perform a suitability test for determination, for example, for a sample containing 5 to 30 mg of water, as shown in the following procedure.

First, determine the water content in the sample, using the established devices and reagent systems. Then, add water or a solution containing a known quantity of water, equivalent to 50 to 100% of the water content determined in the sample, into the same titration flask, and determine the water. A solution containing a known quantity of water can be obtained by purchasing a certified, traceable, commercially available standard solution. Repeat these procedures 5 times and calculate each recovery, r (%), for each addition by using the following equation:

$$r\ (\%) = (M_2/M_1) \times 100$$

M_1: Amount (mg) of water added
M_2: Amount (mg) of water determined

Plot the cumulative amount of water added on the x-axis, and the sum of the amount of water that is initially determined, M, and the cumulative amount of water that is determined after adding water or a solution containing a known amount of water on the y-axis. Determine the gradient, b, and the intercept on the y-axis, a, of the regression line obtained, and the intercept on the x-axis of the extrapolated regression line, d, and calculate the percentage errors, e_1 (%) and e_2 (%), by using the following equation:

$$e_1\ (\%) = \{(a - M)/M\} \times 100$$
$$e_2\ (\%) = \{(|d| - M)/M\} \times 100$$

a: Intercept on the y-axis of the regression line (mg H_2O)
d: Intercept on the x-axis of the regression line (mg H_2O)
M: Water content measured in the sample (mg H_2O)

When the following criteria are met, the devices and reagent systems evaluated are appropriate water determination systems for the sample.

- When the mean water recovery, R (%) is calculated based on the water recovery, r (%), the R is between 97.5% and 102.5%.
- $|e_1|$ and $|e_2|$ are not more than 2.5%.
- b is between 0.975 and 1.025.

2. Coulometric titration

2.1. Apparatus

Usually, the apparatus used for coulometric titration is comprised of a titration flask equipped with an electrolytic cell for iodine production, a stirrer, and a potentiometric titration system at constant current. The electrolytic cell for iodine production is composed of an anode and a cathode, separated by a diaphragm. The anode is immersed in the anolyte solution for water determination and the cathode is immersed in the catholyte solution for water determination. Both electrodes are usually made of platinum-mesh.

Because both the anolyte and the catholyte solutions for water determination are strongly hygroscopic, the titration system should be designed to be protected from water. Desiccants such as silica gel or calcium chloride for water determination can be used.

2.2. Preparation of anolyte and catholyte solutions for water determination

Unless otherwise specified, an anolyte solution for water determination and a catholyte solution for water determination are prepared using solutions having composition described below.

Anolyte solution for water determination—A mixture of iodine, sulfur dioxide, or imidazole for water determination {or 1,3-di(4-pyridyl)propane, diethanolamine, or alternative bases}, and an organic solvent, such as methanol for water determination

Catholyte solution for water determination—A mixture of an inorganic or organic salt, such as lithium chloride, choline chloride, or diethanolamine hydrochloride, and an organic solvent, such as methanol for water determination

2.3. Procedure

Take a suitable volume of an anolyte solution for water determination in a titration vessel, immerse in this solution a pair of platinum electrodes (or a double platinum electrode). Separately, immerse an electrolytic cell for iodine production filled with a catholyte solution for water determination in the anolyte. Switch on the electrolytic system and make the content of the titration vessel anhydrous. Next weigh accurately M (mg) of a sample specimen containing 0.2 to 5 mg of water, add it quickly to the vessel, dissolve by stirring, perform the titration to the end point under vigorous stirring, and calculate the quantity of electricity, C (C) {electric current (A) × time (s)} required for production of iodine during the titration.

Calculate the water content (%) in the sample based on the quantity of electricity, C (C), required for production of iodine and the amount, M (mg), of the sample taken, by using the following equation:

$$\text{Water content (\%)} = \{C/(10.71 \times M)\} \times 100$$

M: Amount (mg) of the sample taken
C: Quantity of electricity (C) required for production of iodine
10.71: Quantity of electricity (C/mg) corresponding to 1 mg of water (H_2O)

When a sample specimen cannot be dissolved in the anolyte, powder it quickly, with protection from atmospheric moisture, and add an accurately weighed amount, M (mg), of the sample estimated to contain 0.2 to 5 mg of water to the vessel. After stirring the mixture, with protection from atmospheric moisture, perform the titration under vigorous stirring, and proceed in the same manner.

Though the titration procedure should be performed under atmospheric conditions at low humidity, if the effect of atmospheric moisture cannot be avoided, for instance, if a long time is required for extraction and titration of water, a blank test must be done and the data must be corrected, as necessary.

2.4. Suitability of determination

Perform a suitability test for appropriate determination and verify the validity of devices and reagents systems for the coulometric titration method, before changing operating conditions, or periodically, as necessary. These conditions include device components such as electrodes and types of solvents and test solutions for water determination.

Perform a water recovery test, for example, using water or a solution containing known quantity of water before and after determination of water content in the sample. A solution containing a known quantity of water can be obtained by purchasing a certified, traceable, commercially available standard solution. Add water or a solution containing a known quantity of water, containing about 1000 μg or about 100 μg of water, which is closer to the expected quantity of water in the sample, perform the coulometric titration for water content, and calculate the recovery.

The devices and reagent systems are assessed as appropriate for the sample if the added water is 1000 μg and the recovery is between 97.5% and 102.5% or if the added water is 100 μg and the recovery is between 90.0% and 110.0%.

3. Utilization of water vaporizer and suitability of determination

In the case of a sample which is insoluble in a solvent or interferes with the Karl Fischer reaction, water in the sample can be heated by a water vaporizer, and introduced into the titration vessel, by using a stream of nitrogen gas as a career.

Suitability of determination using a water vaporizer can be assessed by, for example, the quantity of water determined in another method as the theoretical quantity of water for an appropriate substance or a stable hydrate. An appropriate quantity close to the theoretical quantity of water of the substance needs to be detected under appropriate conditions (including temperature, time, and amount of sample) based on the instructions of the devices.

2.49 Optical Rotation Determination

1. Principle

Generally, the vibrations of light take place on planes perpendicular to the direction of the beam. In case of the ordinary light, the directions of the planes are unrestricted, while in case of the plane polarized light, commonly called as polarized light, the vibrations take place on only one plane that includes the advancing direction of the beam. And it is called that these beams have plane of polarization. Some drugs in the liquid state or in solution have a property of rotating the plane of the polarized light either to the right or to the left. This property is referred to as optical activity or optical rotation, and is inherently related to the chemical constitution of the substance.

The optical rotation is a degree of rotation of polarized plane, caused by the optically active substance or its solution, and it is measured by the polarimeter. The optical rotation is proportional to the length of the polarimeter tube, and is also related to the solution concentration, the temperature and the measurement wavelength. The character of the rotation is indicated by the direction of the rotation, when facing to the advancing direction of the polarized light. Thus in case of rotation to the right, it is called dextrorotatory and expressed by placing plus sign (+), while in case of rotation to the left, it is called levorotatory and expressed by placing minus sign (−) before the figure of the angular rotation. For example, +20° means 20° of rotation to the right, while −20° means 20° of rotation to the left.

The optical rotation α_x^t (°) means degree of rotation of the plate of polarization, when it is measured at t°C by using specific monochromatic light x (expressed by wavelength of light source or the specific beam name).

2. Apparatus and measurement

Polarimeter consists of a light source, a polarizer, a polarimeter tube and an analyzer. The measurement is generally performed at 20°C or 25°C, using a 100-mm tube and the D line of sodium lamp as the light source. The bright line spectrum of mercury lamp can be used as the monochromatic light source.

If a light beam close to the sodium D line can be obtained by the use of an appropriate interference filter, a continuous beam such as of xenon lamp may be used alternatively.

2.1. Verification for accuracy of apparatus

Accuracy of the scale of the apparatus is verified by measuring the optical rotation of a solution of sucrose for optical rotation if the reading indicates the value of its known specific optical rotation. For daily verification an optical rotation known quartz plate may be used for this purpose.

3. Characteristic evaluation by optical rotation

Generally, when the optical rotation is settled as the specification to express the quality characteristic of a drug, Specific optical rotation $[\alpha]_x^t$ (°), *i.e.*, the optical rotation equivalent of 1 g/mL in sample concentration and 1 mm in path length of sample solution, is used. For the evaluation of the quality characteristic of drugs such as crude drugs, when it is not possible to determine the concentration of an optically active drug, the optical rotation α_x^t (°) is used as the specification or to specify the amount of optically active impurities.

The specific optical rotation and the optical rotation can also be used for the description, purity and assay of drugs.

The specific optical rotation, $[\alpha]_x^t$, is calculated from the measured rotation angle of the polarization plane, α_x^t, by the following equation. Though, the degree (°) is expediently used as the unit of the specific optical rotation in the pharmaceutical monographs, accurately it is stated as (°·mm^{-1}·(g/mL)$^{-1}$).

$$[\alpha]_x^t = \frac{\alpha}{lc} \times 100$$

t: The temperature (°C) of measurement.

x: The wavelength (nm) of the specific monochromatic light. In the case of the sodium D line, it is described as D.

α: The angle, in degrees, of rotation of the plane of the polarized light.

l: The thickness of the layer of sample solution, *i.e.*, the length of the polarimeter tube (mm).

c: Drug concentration in g/mL. When an intact liquid drug is used for the direct measurement without dilution by an appropriate solvent, c equals to its density (g/mL). However, unless otherwise specified, the specific gravity may be used instead of the density.

The description in the monograph, for example, "$[\alpha]_D^{20}$: −33.0 − −36.0° (after drying, 1 g, water, 20 mL, 100 mm)," means the measured specific optical rotation $[\alpha]_D^{20}$ should be in the range of −33.0° and −36.0°, when 1 g of accurately weighed sample dried under the conditions, specified in the test item of Loss on drying, is taken, and dissolved in water to make exactly 20 mL, then put in the polarimeter tube of 100 mm length, of which temperature is kept at 20°C. And the description "α_D^{20}: −33.0 − −36.0°

(100 mm)'' means the measured optical rotation, α_D^{20}, should be in the range of −33.0° and −36.0°, when sample or a solution of sample is put in the tube of 100 mm length, at 20°C.

2.50 Endpoint Detection Methods in Titrimetry

Titrimetry is a method or a procedure for volumetric analysis, which is usually classified into acid-base titration (neutralization titration or pH titration), precipitation titration, complexation titration, oxidation-reduction titration, etc., according to the kind of reaction or the nature of the phenomenon occurring between the titrate and the titrant (standard solution for volumetric analysis). Furthermore, titration performed in a nonaqueous solvent is generally called nonaqueous titration, which is frequently used for volumetric analysis of weak acids, weak bases, and their salts. The endpoint in titrimetry can be detected by color changes of indicators and/or by changes of electrical signals such as electrical potential or electrical current.

The indicator method is one of the endpoint detection methods in titrimetry. In this method the color of an indicator dye, dissolved in the titrate, changes dramatically in the vicinity of the equivalence point due to its physico-chemical character, and this property is used for visual endpoint detection. Selection of an indicator and specification of the color change induced in the respective titration system, should be described in the individual monograph. An appropriate indicator should change color clearly, in response to a slight change in physico-chemical properties of the titrate, such as pH, etc., in the vicinity of the equivalence point.

Regarding the electrical endpoint detection methods, there are an electrical potential method and an electrical current method, which are called potentiometric and amperometric titration methods, respectively. They are generically named electrometric titration. In the potentiometric titration method, the endpoint of a titration is usually determined to be the point at which the differential potential change becomes maximum or minimum as a function of the quantity of titrant added. In the amperometric titration method, unless otherwise specified, a bi-amperometric titration method is used, and the endpoint is determined by following the change of microcurrent during the course of a titration. Furthermore, the quantity of electricity (electrical current × time) is often used as another electrochemical signal to follow a chemical reaction, as described in Coulometric Titration under Water Determination <*2.48*>.

The composition of a titration system, such as amount of specimen, solvent, standard solution for volumetric analysis, endpoint detection method, equivalent amount of substance to be examined (mg)/standard solution (mL), should be specified in the individual monograph. Standardization of the standard solution and titration of a specimen are recommended to be done at the same temperature. When there is a marked difference in the temperatures at which the former and the latter are performed, it is necessary to make an appropriate correction for the volume change of the standard solution due to the temperature difference.

1. Indicator Method

Weigh an amount of a specimen in a flask or a suitable vessel as directed in the monograph or in ''*Standard Solutions for Volumetric Analysis*'', and add a specified quantity of solvent to dissolve the specimen. After adding a defined indicator to the solution to prepare the titrate, titrate by adding a standard solution for volumetric analysis by using a buret. In the vicinity of the endpoint, observe the color change induced by the cautious addition of 0.1 mL or less of the titrant. Calculate the quantity of titrant added from the readings on the scale of the buret used for the titration at the starting point and at the endpoint at which the specified color change appears, as directed in the individual monograph or in the ''*Standard Solutions for Volumetric Analysis*''. Although addition of the volumetric standard solution by buret is usually done manually, an automatic buret can also be used.

Unless otherwise specified, perform a blank determination according to the following method, and make any necessary correction.

Measure a specified quantity of solvent, as directed in the monograph or in the ''*Standard Solutions for Volumetric Analysis*'', and titrate as directed. The required quantity of the standard solution added to reach a specified color change, is assumed to be the blank quantity for the titration system. However, when the blank quantity is too small to evaluate accurately, the quantity can be assumed to be zero.

2. Electrical Endpoint Detection Methods

2.1. Potentiometric titration

2.1.1. Apparatus

The apparatus consists of a beaker to contain the specimen, a buret for adding a standard solution, an indicator electrode and a reference electrode, a potentiometer for measuring potential difference between the electrodes or an adequate pH meter, a recorder, and a stirrer for gentle stirring of the solution to be examined. Separately, an automatic titration apparatus assembled from suitable units and/or parts, including a data processing system, can also be used.

In this titration method, unless otherwise specified, indicator electrodes designated in Table 2.50-1 are used according to the kind of titration. As a reference electrode, usually a silver-silver chloride electrode is used. Besides the single indicator electrodes as seen in Table 2.50-1, a combined refer-

Table 2.50-1 Kind of titration and indicator electrode

Kind of titration	Indicator electrode
Acid-base titration (Neutralization titration, pH titration)	Glass electrode
Precipitation titration (Titration of halogen ion by silver nitrate)	Silver electrode. A silver-silver chloride electrode is used as a reference electrode, which is connected with the titrate by a salt bridge of saturated potassium nitrate solution.
Oxidation-reduction titration (Diazo titration, etc.)	Platinum electrode
Complexation titration (Chelometric titration)	Mercury-mercury chloride (II) electrode
Nonaqueous titration (Perchloric acid titration, Tetramethylammonium hydroxide titration)	Glass electrode

ence electrode and indicator electrode can also be used.

When the potentiometric titration is carried out by the pH measurement method, the pH meter should be adjusted according to the pH Determination <*2.54*>.

2.1.2. Procedure

Weigh a defined amount of a specimen in a beaker, and add an indicated quantity of solvent to dissolve the specimen, as directed in the monograph. After the potential difference E (mV) or the pH value of the solvent to be used for titration has reached a stable value, immerse both reference and indicator electrodes, which have previously been washed with the solvent being used, in the solution to be examined, and titrate with a standard solution for volumetric analysis with gentle stirring of the solution. During the titration, the tip of the buret should be dipped into the solution, to be examined. The endpoint of titration is determined by following the variation of the potential difference between two electrodes as a function of the quantity of titrant added. In the vicinity of the endpoint, the amounts of a titrant added should be 0.1 mL or less for adequate titrimetry. Plot the obtained potential values along the ordinate and the quantity of a titrant added V (mL) along the abscissa to draw a titration curve, and obtain the endpoint from the maximum or the minimum value of $\Delta E/\Delta V$ or from the value of electromotive force or pH corresponding to the equivalence point.

Unless otherwise specified, the decision of the endpoint in this method is usually made by either of the following methods.

(i) Drawing method

Usually, draw two parallel tangent lines with a slope of about 45° to the obtained titration curve. Next, draw a 3rd parallel line at the same distance from the previously drawn two parallel lines, and decide the intersection point of this line with the titration curve. Further, from the intersection point, draw a vertical line to the abscissa, and read the quantity of titrant added as the endpoint of the titration.

Separately, the endpoint of the titration can also be obtained from the maximum or the minimum of the differential titration curve ($\Delta E/\Delta V$ vs. V).

(ii) Automatic detection method

In the case of potentiometric titration using an automatic titration system, the endpoint can be determined by following the respective instrumental indications. The endpoint is decided either by following the variation of the differential potential change or the absolute potential difference as a function of the quantity of titrant added: in the former case the quantity given by the maximum or the minimum of the differential values, and in the latter the quantity given by the indicator reaching the endpoint potential previously set for the individual titration system, are assumed to be the endpoint volumes, respectively.

2.2. Amperometric titration

2.2.1. Apparatus

The apparatus consists of a beaker for holding a specimen, a buret for adding a standard solution for volumetric analysis, two small platinum plates or wires of the same shape as the indicator electrode, a device to load direct current microvoltage between two electrodes, a microammeter to measure the indicator current between the two electrodes, a recorder, and a stirrer which can gently stir the solution in a beaker. Separately, an automatic titration apparatus assembled from suitable units and/or parts, including a data processing system, can also be used.

2.2.2. Procedure

Weigh a defined amount of a specimen in a beaker, and add an indicated quantity of solvent to dissolve the specimen, as directed in the individual monograph. Next, after washing the two indicator electrodes with water, immerse both electrodes in the solution to be examined, apply a constant voltage suitable for measurement across two electrodes by using an appropriate device, and titrate the solution with a standard solution for volumetric analysis. During the titration, the tip of the buret should be dipped into the solution to be examined. The endpoint of titration is determined by following the changes of microcurrent between the two electrodes as a function of the quantity of titrant added. In the vicinity of the endpoint, the amounts of the titrant added should be 0.1 mL or less for adequate titrimetry. Plot the obtained current values along the ordinate and the quantity of the titrant added V (mL) along the abscissa to draw a titration curve, and usually take the inflection point of the titration curve (the point of intersection given by the extrapolation of two straight lines before and after the inflection) as the endpoint in amperometric titration.

The blank test in this titration is usually performed as follows: Take a volume of the solvent specified in the individual monograph or in the "Standard Solution for Volumetric Analysis", and use this as the sample solution. Determine the amount of the volumetric standard solution needed for giving the endpoint, and use this volume as the blank. If this volume is too small to determine accurately, the blank may be considered as 0 (mL).

Unless otherwise specified, the endpoint in this titration is decided by either of the following methods.

(i) Drawing method

Usually, extrapolate the two straight lines before and after the inflection, and obtain the inflection point of the titration curve. Next, read the quantity of titrant added at the inflection point, and assume this point to be the endpoint.

(ii) Automatic detection method

In the case of amperometric titration using an automatic titration system, the endpoint can be determined by following the instrumental indications. The endpoint is decided by following the variation of the indicator current during the course of a titration, and the quantity of titrant added is assumed to be that at which the current has reached the endpoint current set previously for the individual titration system.

When atmospheric carbon dioxide or oxygen is expected to influence the titration, a beaker with a lid should be used, and the procedure should be carried out in a stream of an inert gas, such as nitrogen gas. Further, when a specimen is expected to be influenced by light, use a light-resistant container to avoid exposure of the specimen to direct sunlight.

2.51 Conductivity Measurement

This test is harmonized with the European Pharmacopoeia and the U. S. Pharmacopeia.

The parts of the text that are not harmonized among the targeted texts for the harmonization are marked with symbols (◆ ◆), and the texts that are uniquely specified by the JP other than the targeted texts for the harmonization are marked with symbols (◇ ◇).

Information on the harmonization with the European Pharmacopoeia and the U.S. Pharmacopeia is available on the website of the Pharmaceuticals and Medical Devices Agency.

This chapter provides information on how to apply electrical conductivity measurements (hereafter referred to as "conductivity") of fluid solutions, including pure fluids.

This chapter is intended for fluid applications when conductivity is used to measure, monitor, or control chemical dispensing, chemical purity, ionic concentration, and other applications where the ionic character of the fluid needs to be known or controlled.

Applications include, but are not limited to, solutions that may be used in clean-in-place, chromatography detection, ionic solution preparations, end point detection, dosing, fermentation, and buffer production.

In some cases, conductivity measurements can be extended to pure organic fluids such as alcohols and glycols where a weak conductivity signal exists, and the signal can be significantly increased if the organics become contaminated with water or salts.

Conductivity is the measurement of the ability of a fluid to conduct electricity via its chemical ions. The ability of any ion to electrically conduct is directly related to its ion mobility. Conductivity is directly proportional to the concentrations of ions in the fluid, according to Equation (1):

$$\kappa = 1000 \sum_{i}^{all\ ions} C_i \cdot \lambda_i \qquad (1)$$

κ = conductivity (S/cm)
C_i = concentration of chemical ion i (mol/L)
λ_i = specific molar conductance of ion i ($S \cdot cm^2/mol$)

Although the SI unit S/m is the appropriate SI unit for conductivity, historically the unit S/cm has been selected by industry as the accepted unit.

On the basis of Equation (1), conductivity is not ion selective because it responds to all ions. Furthermore, the specific molar conductance of each ion is different. As a result, unless the percentage composition of ions of the solution is limited and known, the precise concentrations of ionic species cannot be determined from conductivity measurements.

However, for examples such as a solution of a single salt or acid or base, such as a caustic solution used in cleaning, the precise concentration can be directly determined. Despite the lack of ionic specificity, conductivity is a valuable laboratory and process tool for measurement and control of total ionic content because it is proportional to the sum of the concentrations of all ionic species (anions and cations) for diluted solutions as described in Equation (1). At higher concentrations, conductivity measurements are not perfectly linear with concentration. Conductivity measurements cannot be applied to solids or gases, but they can be applied to the condensate of gases.

Another variable that influences conductivity measurements is the fluid temperature. As the fluid temperature increases, the ion conductance increases, making this physicochemical phenomenon the predominant reason for the temperature-compensation requirement when testing conductive fluids.

The conductivity, κ, is proportional to the conductance, G (S), of a fluid between two electrodes (Equation (2)):

$$\kappa = G \times (d/A) = G \times K \qquad (2)$$

κ = conductivity (S/cm)
G = conductance (S)
d = distance between the electrodes (cm)
A = area of the conducting electrodes (cm^2)
K = cell constant (cm^{-1}), which also equals the ratio of d/A

The resistivity ρ ($\Omega \cdot cm$) of the fluid is, by definition, the reciprocal of the conductivity (Equation (3)):

$$\rho = 1/\kappa = 1/(G \times K) = R/K \qquad (3)$$

ρ = resistivity ($\Omega \cdot cm$)
κ = conductivity (S/cm)
G = conductance (S)
K = cell constant (cm^{-1})
R = resistance (Ω), which is the reciprocal of the conductance, G

1. Apparatus

An electrical conductivity measurement consists of the determination of resistance of the fluid between and around the electrodes of the conductivity sensor. To achieve this measurement, the primary instrumentation is the resistance-measuring circuit and the conductivity sensor, and they are usually connected by a cable when the sensor and the user interface are separated.

The resistance measurement is made by applying an alternating current (AC, meaning the flow of electric charge periodically reverses direction) voltage (or current) to the electrodes, measuring the current (or voltage), and calculating the resistance according to Ohm's Law. The alternating source is used to prevent the polarization (collection of ions) at the electrodes. Depending on the instrument, the measuring frequency of the measuring system adjusts automatically according to the measuring conditions of the instrument, and there may be multiple resistance-measuring circuits embedded in the measuring system. The resistance-measurement circuit may be embedded in the transmitter or in the sensor.

The conductivity sensor consists of at least two electrical conductors of a fixed size and geometry, separated by an electrical insulator. The electrodes, insulator, and any other wetted materials should be constructed of materials that are unreactive to fluids with which they may come into contact. Also, the sensor construction should withstand the environmental conditions (process or ambient temperature, pressure, cleaning applications) that it would be subjected to.

Most conductivity sensors have temperature devices such as a platinum resistance temperature device (RTD) or negative temperature coefficient (NTC) thermistor embedded inside the sensor, although external temperature measurement is possible. The purpose of the temperature measurement is for temperature compensation of the conductivity measurement.

2. Cell Constant Determination

The purpose of the sensor's cell constant is to normalize the conductance (or resistance) measurement for the geometrical construction of the two electrodes.

The cell constant is determined by immersing the conductivity sensor in a solution of known conductivity.

Solutions of known conductivity can be obtained by preparation of specific mixtures according to national authoritative sources or procurement of commercially available certified and traceable standard solutions.

These recipes or certified solutions can range from 5 to 200,000 μS/cm, depending on the level of accuracy desired. Alternatively the cell constant is determined by comparison to other reference conductivity measuring systems (also available as an accredited calibration service). [Note—Conductivity measurements are not perfectly linear with concentration.]

The measured cell constant of the conductivity sensor must be within 5% of the nominal value indicated by the sensor certificate, unless otherwise prescribed.

Modern conductivity sensors normally do not change their cell constant over their lifetime. If a change of the cell constant is detected during calibration, a cleaning of the sensor is appropriate according to the manufacturer's recommendations. Following that, the calibration procedure should be repeated. Sometimes "memory effects" appear, particularly when changing from high to low concentrations if the sensor is not well flushed.

3. Calibration of Temperature

In addition to verifying the sensor's cell constant, the embedded temperature device (or external temperature device) should be appropriately calibrated for the application to apply the temperature compensation algorithm accurately. The temperature accuracy that is required depends on the criticality of the temperature to the application. An accuracy of ± 1°C typically suffices.

4. Calibration of Measurement Electronics

The measurement circuit of the system is fundamentally an AC resistance measuring device. Appropriate verification and/or calibration of the measuring circuit is required for measurement systems with signal transfer via analog cable. This is accomplished by disconnecting the measuring circuit from the sensor's electrodes, attaching traceable resistors of known value with the cable of the measurement system to the measuring circuit, and verifying that the measured resistance agrees with the resistor value to an acceptable level. A typical acceptance criterion for the resistance accuracy is $<2\%$ of the reading at resistances $>100\ \Omega$, and increasing to 5% at lower resistances. However, the application criticality should ultimately determine the desired accuracy.

For conductivity systems that cannot have the resistance-measuring circuit disconnected from the electrodes (e.g., measurement circuit and electrodes in one mutual housing), it may be difficult to directly adjust or verify the circuit accuracy, depending on the sensor design. An alternative method of verifying the measurement system integrity is a system calibration according to the procedures for the cell constant determination for each measuring circuit that is intended to be used.

If verification/calibration of the sensor's cell constant, temperature device, and measuring circuit are done at the same service interval, the measuring circuit should be verified first, the temperature device next, and the cell constant last. Because all of these parameters are typically very stable due to modern electronics and stable sensor construction, frequent calibration (such as daily) is not usually required. Comparison to qualified reference systems is also a proper means of calibration. Calibration is performed at appropriate intervals as defined in the quality management system.

5. Temperature Compensation

Because the conductivity of a fluid is temperature dependent, temperature compensation of the conductivity measurement is necessary unless otherwise prescribed. An appropriate temperature compensation algorithm will ensure that changes in the conductivity measurement can be ascribed to concentration changes and not temperature changes. Conductivity measurements are normally referenced to 25°C. A common form of linear temperature compensation uses Equation (4):

$$\kappa_{25} = \frac{\kappa_T}{[1 + \alpha(T - 25)]} \qquad (4)$$

κ_{25} = conductivity compensated to 25°C
κ_T = conductivity at T
α = temperature coefficient of the conductivity
T = measured temperature

A temperature coefficient of 2.1% per 1°C is commonly used for many salt solutions. Most salt-based solutions have linear compensation factors ranging from 1.9% to 2.2% per 1°C. Depending on the fluid samples, other forms of temperature compensation may be appropriate. ◇Non-linear temperature compensation will carry out temperature compensation using preprogrammed data in the instrument. Non-linear temperature compensation data for a variety of solutions is widely available, e.g. for natural waters, and for ultrapure water with traces of ammonia.◇

In cases of very low conductivity ($<10\ \mu$S/cm), such as purified water for cleaning/rinsing purpose, two compensations need to be made. One is for the intrinsic conductivity of water, and the other is for the other ionic species in water. These compensations are normally combined and embedded in the microprocessor-controlled conductivity measurement systems. This is not supplied in all conductivity measurement technologies.

6. Conductivity Measurement of Fluids

For off-line batch measurements, rinse the cleaned sensor with the fluid to be measured. Then immerse the sensor in the fluid to be measured, and record the temperature and the temperature-compensated conductivity as required. Be sure that the position of the sensor in the container does not affect the conductivity measurement, because the container walls can affect the measurement for some electrode designs.

For continuous on-line or in-line measurements, install the cleaned sensor into the pipe, tank, or other containment vessel, and flush, if necessary. Make sure proper installation procedures are applied to prevent bubbles or particles from collecting between the electrodes. Be sure that the position of the sensor in the pipe or tank does not affect the conductivity measurement, because the nearby surfaces can affect the measurement for some electrode designs.

Record the temperature and the temperature-compensated conductivity as required.

For all batch or continuous measurements, ensure that the wetted components of the sensor are compatible with the fluid and the temperature to be measured.

2.52 Thermal Analysis

This test is harmonized with the European Pharmacopoeia and the U.S. Pharmacopeia.

The corresponding part of the attributes/provisions which are agreed as non-harmonized within the scope of the harmonization is marked with symbols (◆ ◆), and the corresponding parts which are agreed as the JP local requirement other than the scope of the harmonization are marked with symbols (◇ ◇).

Information on the harmonization with the European Pharmacopoeia and the U.S. Pharmacopeia is available on the website of the Pharmaceuticals and Medical Devices Agency.

Thermal analysis is a group of techniques in which the variation of a physical property of a substance is measured as a function of temperature. The most commonly used techniques are those which measure changes of mass or changes in energy of a sample of a substance.

These techniques have different applications:
—determination of phase changes,
—determination of changes in chemical composition,
—determination of purity.

◇Among the below methods, Thermogravimetry can be used as an alternative method for "Loss on Drying <2.41>" or "Water Determination <2.48>". However, it must be confirmed beforehand that no volatile component except for water is included in the test specimen when Thermogravimetry is used as an alternative method for "Water Determination".◇

1. Thermogravimetry

Thermogravimetry (TG) or Thermogravimetric Analysis (TGA) is a technique in which the mass of a sample of a substance is recorded as a function of temperature according to a controlled temperature programme.

1.1. Instrument

The essential components of a thermobalance are a device for heating or cooling the substance according to a given temperature program, a sample holder in a controlled atmosphere, an electrobalance and an electronic output of the signal to a recorder or a computer.

1.2. Temperature calibration

The temperature sensor close to or in contact with the sample is calibrated using the Curie temperature of a ferromagnetic substance such as nickel. In the case of an instrument capable of simultaneously conducting TG/TGA and Differential Thermal Analysis (DTA), the same certified reference materials as those for Differential Scanning Calorimetry (DSC) and DTA may be used, such as indium for thermal analysis, tin for thermal analysis and/or zinc (standard reagent).

1.3. Calibration of the electrobalance

Place an appropriate quantity of ◆Calcium Oxalate Monohydrate for Calibration of Apparatus RS or ◆a suitable certified reference material in the sample holder and record the mass. Set the heating rate according to the manufacturer's instructions (e.g. 5°C/min) and start the temperature increase. Record the thermogravimetric curve as a graph with temperature, or time, on the abscissa, increasing from left to right, and mass on the ordinate, decreasing downwards. Stop the temperature increase at about 250°C. Measure the difference on the graph between the initial and final mass-temperature plateaux, or mass-time plateaux, which corresponds to the loss of mass. The declared loss of mass for the certified reference material is stated on the label.

1.4. Method

Apply the same procedure to the substance to be examined, using the conditions prescribed in the monograph. Calculate the loss of mass of the substance to be examined from the difference measured in the graph obtained. Express the loss of mass as $\Delta m/m$ (%). If the instrument is in frequent use, carry out temperature calibration regularly. Otherwise, carry out such checks before each measurement.

Since the conditions are critical, the following parameters are noted for each measurement: pressure or flow rate, composition of the gas, mass of the sample, heating rate, temperature range, sample pre-treatment including any isothermal period.

2. Differential Scanning Calorimetry

Differential Scanning Calorimetry (DSC) is a technique that can be used to demonstrate the energy phenomena produced during heating (or cooling) of a substance (or a mixture of substances) and to determine the changes in enthalpy and specific heat and the temperatures at which these occur.

The technique is used to determine the difference in heat flow (with reference to the temperature) evolved or absorbed by the test sample compared with the reference cell, as a function of the temperature. Two types of DSC instruments are available, those using power compensation to maintain a null temperature difference between sample and reference and those that apply a constant rate of heating and detect temperature differential as a difference in heat flow between sample and reference.

2.1. Instrument

The instrument for the power compensation DSC consists of a furnace containing a sample holder with a reference cell and a test cell. The instrument for the heat flow DSC consists of a furnace containing a single cell with a sample holder for the reference crucible and the test crucible.

A temperature-programming device, thermal detector(s) and a recording system which can be connected to a computer are attached. The measurements are carried out under a controlled atmosphere.

2.2. Calibration of the instrument

Calibrate the instrument for temperature and enthalpy change, using suitable certified materials or reference standards.

2.2.1. Temperature calibration

It can be performed using certified reference materials having an intrinsic thermal property, such as melting point of pure metals or organic substances, or phase transition point of crystalline inorganic salts or oxides. Melting points of indium for thermal analysis, tin for thermal analysis and/or zinc (standard reagent) are usually employed for calibration.

2.2.2. Heat-quantity calibration

For accurate estimation of a quantity of heat change (enthalpic change) of a test sample, caused by a certain physical change accompanying a temperature change, it is necessary to calibrate the instrument using suitable certified reference materials. Similarly to temperature calibration, heat-quantity calibration may be performed using suitable certified reference materials showing a known definite enthalpic change caused by physical changes, such as melting of pure metals and/or organic substances, or phase transition of crystalline inorganic salts. Heats of fusion of indium for thermal analysis, tin for thermal analysis and/or zinc (standard reagent) are usually employed for calibration.

2.3. Operating procedure

Weigh in a suitable crucible an appropriate quantity of the substance to be examined; place it in the sample holder. Place an empty crucible in the reference holder. Set the initial and final temperatures, and the heating rate according to the operating conditions prescribed in the monograph.

Begin the analysis and record the differential scanning calorimetric curve, with the temperature or time on the abscissa (values increasing from left to right) and the energy change on the ordinate (specify whether the change is endothermic or exothermic).

The temperature at which the phenomenon occurs (the onset temperature) corresponds to the intersection (A) of the extension of the baseline with the tangent at the point of greatest slope (inflexion point) of the curve (see Fig. 2.52-1). The end of the thermal phenomenon is indicated by the peak of the curve.

The enthalpy of the phenomenon is proportional to the

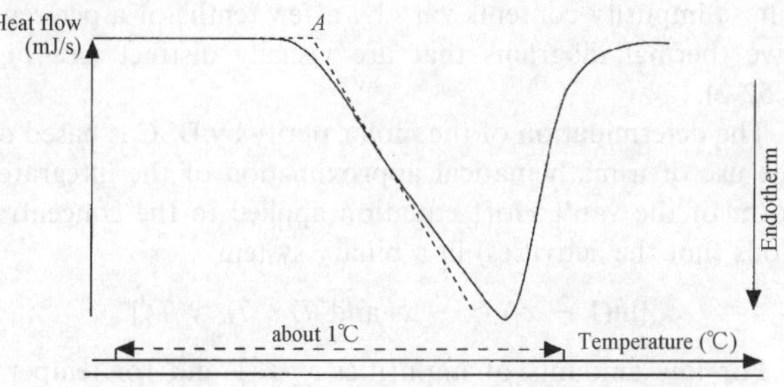

Fig. 2.52-1 Thermogram

Table 2.52-1

solid-solid transition	Allotropy-polymorphism desolvation amorphous-crystalline
solid-liquid transition	Melting glass transition
solid-gas transition	sublimation
liquid-solid transition	freezing recrystallisation glass transition
liquid-gas transition	evaporation

area under the curve limited by the baseline; the proportionality factor is determined from the measurement of the heat of fusion of a known substance (e.g., indium for thermal analysis) under the same operating conditions.

Each thermogram may be accompanied by the following data: conditions employed, record of last calibration, mass of the sample and identification (including thermal history), container, atmosphere (identity, flow rate, pressure), direction and rate of temperature change, instrument and recorder sensitivity.

2.4. Applications

2.4.1. Phase changes

Determination of the temperature, heat capacity change and enthalpy of phase changes undergone by a substance as a function of temperature. The transitions that may be observed include those shown in Table 2.52-1.

2.4.2. Changes in chemical composition

Measurement of heat and temperatures of reaction under given experimental conditions, so that, for example, the kinetics of decomposition or of desolvation can be determined.

2.4.3. Application to phase diagrams

Establishment of phase diagrams for solid mixtures. The establishment of a phase diagram may be an important step in the preformulation and optimization of the freeze-drying process.

2.4.4. Determination of purity

The measurements of the fraction of substance melted at a temperature and the heat of fusion by DSC enable the impurity content of a substance to be determined from a single thermal diagram, requiring the use of only a few milligrams of sample with no need for repeated accurate measurements of the true temperature.

In theory, the melting of an entirely crystalline, pure substance at constant pressure is characterized by a heat of fusion ΔH_f in an infinitely narrow range, corresponding to the melting point T_0. A broadening of this range is a sensitive indicator of impurities. Hence, samples of the same substance, whose impurity contents vary by a few tenths of a per cent, give thermal diagrams that are visually distinct (see Fig. 2.52-2).

The determination of the molar purity by DSC is based on the use of a mathematical approximation of the integrated form of the van't Hoff equation applied to the concentrations (not the activities) in a binary system.

$$[\ln(1 - x_2) \approx - x_2 \text{ and } T \times T_0 \approx T_0^2]$$

For low amounts of impurities $x_2 \ll 1$ and for temperatures close to the melting point T_0 the equation can be written as follows, in which T and x_2 are variables:

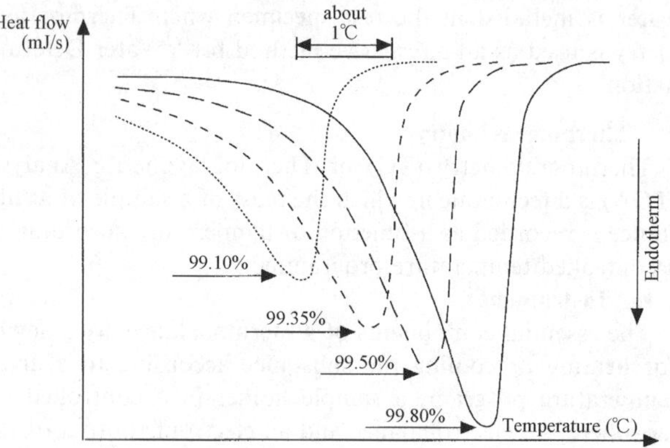

Fig. 2.52-2 Thermal diagrams according to purity

$$T = T_0 - \frac{RT_0^2}{\Delta H_f} \times x_2 \qquad (1)$$

T: temperature of the sample, in kelvins,

T_0: melting point of the chemically pure substance, in kelvins,

R: gas constant for ideal gases, in joules-kelvin^{-1}·mole^{-1},

ΔH_f: molar heat of fusion of the pure substance, in joules·mole^{-1},

x_2: mole fraction of the impurity i.e. the number of molecules of the impurity divided by the total number of molecules in the liquid phase (or molten phase) at temperature T (expressed in kelvins),

Hence, the determination of purity by DSC is limited to the detection of impurities forming a eutectic mixture with the principal compound and present at a mole fraction of typically less than 2 per cent in the substance to be examined.

This method cannot be applied to:

—amorphous substances,

—solvates or polymorphic compounds that are unstable within the experimental temperature range,

—impurities forming solid solutions with the principal substance,

—impurities that are insoluble in the liquid phase or in the melt of the principal substance.

During the heating of the substance to be examined, the impurity melts completely at the eutectic temperature. Above this temperature, the solid phase contains only the pure substance. As the temperature increases progressively from the eutectic temperature to the melting point of the pure substance, the mole fraction of impurity in the liquid decreases, since the quantity of liquefied pure substance increases. For all temperatures above the eutectic point:

$$x_2 = \frac{1}{F} \times x_2^* \qquad (2)$$

F: molten fraction of the analyzed sample,

x_2^*: mole fraction of the impurity in the analyzed sample.

When the entire sample has melted, $F = 1$ and $x_2 = x_2^*$. If equation (2) is combined with equation (1), the following equation is obtained:

$$T = T_0 - \frac{RT_0^2}{\Delta H_f} \times \frac{1}{F} \times x_2^*$$

The value of the heat of fusion of the pure substance is obtained by integrating the melting peak. The melting point T_0 of the pure substance is extrapolated from the plot of temperature T, expressed in kelvins versus $1/F$. The slope α of the curve, obtained after linearization, if necessary, corresponding to $RT_0^2x_2^*/\Delta H_f$ allows x_2^* to be evaluated. The fraction x_2^* multiplied by 100 gives the mole fraction in per cent for the total eutectic impurities.

2.53 Viscosity Determination

Viscosity Determination is a method to determine the viscosity of liquid samples using a viscometer.

When a liquid moves in a definite direction, and the liquid velocity has a gradient with respect to the direction rectangular to that of flow, a force of internal friction is generated along both sides of a hypothetical plane parallel to the movement. This flow property of a liquid is expressed in terms of viscosity. The internal friction per unit area on the parallel plane is called slip stress or shear stress, and the velocity gradient with respect to the direction rectangular to that of flow is called slip velocity or shear velocity. A liquid of which the slip velocity is proportional to its slip stress is called a Newtonian liquid. The proportionality constant, η, is a characteristic of a liquid at a certain temperature and is called viscosity. The viscosity is expressed in the unit of Pascal second (Pa·s), and usually milli-Pascal second (mPa·s).

A liquid whose slip velocity is not proportional to its slip stress is called a non-Newtonian liquid. Since the viscosity for a sample of a non-Newtonian liquid changes with its slip velocity, the viscosity measured at a certain slip velocity is called an apparent viscosity. In that case, the value of slip stress divided by the corresponding slip velocity is called an apparent viscosity. Thus, the relationship between apparent viscosity and slip velocity will permit characterization of the flow properties of a given non-Newtonian liquid.

The value of the viscosity, η, divided by the density, ρ, at the same temperature is defined as a kinematic viscosity, ν, which is expressed in the unit of meters squared per second (m^2/s), and usually millimeters squared per second (mm^2/s).

The viscosity of a liquid is determined either by the following *Method I* or *Method II*.

1. Method I Viscosity measurement by capillary tube viscometer

For measuring the viscosity of a Newtonian liquid, a capillary tube viscometer is usually used, in which the downflowing time of a liquid, t (s), required for a definite volume of the liquid to flow through a capillary tube is measured and the kinematic viscosity, ν, is calculated according to the following equation.

$$\nu = Kt$$

Further, the viscosity, η, is calculated from the next equation:

$$\eta = \nu\rho = Kt\rho$$

where ρ (g/mL) is the density of the liquid measured at the same temperature, t (°C).

The parameter K (mm^2/s^2) represents the viscometer constant and is previously determined by using the *Standard Liquids for Calibrating Viscometers* with known kinematic viscosity. In the case of a liquid having a similar viscosity to water, water itself can be used as a reference standard liquid for the calibration. The kinematic viscosity of water is 1.0038 mm^2/s at 20°C. In the cases of liquids having a slightly higher viscosity than water, the *Standard Liquids for Calibrating Viscometers* should be used for the calibration.

The intrinsic viscosity, $[\eta]$ (dL/g), of a polymer solution is obtained by plotting the relation of viscosity versus concentration and extrapolating the obtained straight line to zero concentration. Intrinsic viscosity shows the degree of molecular expansion of a polymer substance in a given solvent (sample solution) and is also a measure of the average molecular mass of the polymer substance.

The downflowing time t (s) for a polymer solution, whose concentration is c (g/dL), and t_0 (s) for the solvent used for dissolving the polymer, are measured by using the same viscometer, and then the intrinsic viscosity of a given polymer substance, $[\eta]$, is calculated according to the following equation:

$$[\eta] = \lim_{c \to 0} \frac{\left(\frac{t}{t_0}\right) - 1}{c} \quad \text{or} \quad [\eta] = \lim_{c \to 0} \frac{\ln \frac{t}{t_0}}{c}$$

When the concentration dependency of $\{(t/t_0) - 1\}/c$ is not large, the value of $\{(t/t_0) - 1\}/c$ at a concentration directed in the respective monograph can be assumed to be the intrinsic viscosity for a given substance.

Unless otherwise specified, the viscosity of a sample solution is measured with the following apparatus and procedure.

1.1. Apparatus

For measurement of the kinematic viscosity in the range of 1 to 100,000 mm^2/s, the Ubbelohde-type viscometer illustrated in Fig. 2.53-1 can be used. The approximate relations between kinematic viscosity range and inside diameter of the capillary tube suitable for the measurement of various liquids with different viscosity, are given in Table 2.53-1. Although a capillary tube viscometer other than the Ubbelohde-type one specified in Table 2.53-1 can also be used, a viscometer should be selected in which the downflowing time, t (s), of a sample solution to be determined would be between 200 s and 1000 s.

1.2. Procedure

Place a sample solution in a viscometer from the upper

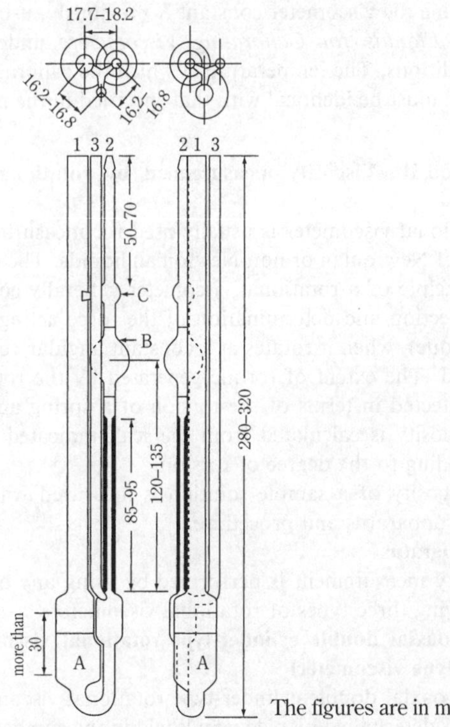

Fig. 2.53-1 Ubbelohde-type viscometer

Table 2.53-1 Specifications of the Ubbelohde-type viscometer

Viscometer constant K (mm^2/s^2)	Inner diameter of capillary tube (mm) Permissible tolerance ±10%	Volume of bulb B (mL) Permissible tolerance ±10%	Measuring range of kinematic viscosity (mm^2/s)
0.005	0.46	3.0	1 - 5
0.01	0.58	4.0	2 - 10
0.03	0.73	4.0	6 - 30
0.05	0.88	4.0	10 - 50
0.1	1.03	4.0	20 - 100
0.3	1.36	4.0	60 - 300
0.5	1.55	4.0	100 - 500
1.0	1.83	4.0	200 - 1,000
3.0	2.43	4.0	600 - 3,000
5.0	2.75	4.0	1,000 - 5,000
10.0	3.27	4.0	2,000 - 10,000
30.0	4.32	4.0	6,000 - 30,000
50.0	5.20	5.0	10,000 - 50,000
100	6.25	5.0	20,000 - 100,000

end of *tube 1*, so that the meniscus of the solution is at a level between the two marked lines of *bulb A*. Place the viscometer vertically in a thermostatted bath maintained at a specified temperature within 0.1°C, until *bulb C* is fully immersed, and let it stand for about 20 minutes to attain the specified temperature. Close *tube 3* with a finger and pull the sample solution up to the middle part of *bulb C* by gentle suction from the top of *tube 2*, taking care not to introduce any bubbles into *tube 2*, and stop the suction. Open the end of *tube 3*, and immediately close the end of *tube 2*. After confirming that the liquid column is cut off at the lowest end of the capillary tube, open the end of *tube 2* to make the sample solution flow down through the capillary tube. Record the time, t (s), required for the meniscus of the sample solution to fall from the upper to the lower marked line of *bulb B*.

Determine the viscometer constant K previously, using the *Standard Liquids for Calibrating Viscometers* under the same conditions. The temperature at which the calibration is conducted must be identical with that specified in the monograph.

2. Method II Viscosity measurement by rotational viscometer

A rotational viscometer is usually used for measuring the viscosity of Newtonian or non-Newtonian liquids. The measuring principle of a rotational viscometer generally consists in the detection and determination of the force acting on a rotor (torque), when it rotates at a constant angular velocity in a liquid. The extent of torque generated by the rotation can be detected in terms of the torsion of a spring and the liquid viscosity is calculated from the scale-indicated value corresponding to the degree of torsion.

The viscosity of a sample solution is measured with the following apparatus and procedure.

2.1. Apparatus

Viscosity measurement is performed by using any one of the following three types of rotational viscometers.

2.1.1. Coaxial double cylinder-type rotational viscometer (Couette type viscometer)

In the coaxial double cylinder-type rotational viscometer, viscosity is determined by placing a liquid in the gap between the inner and the outer cylinders, which share the same cen-

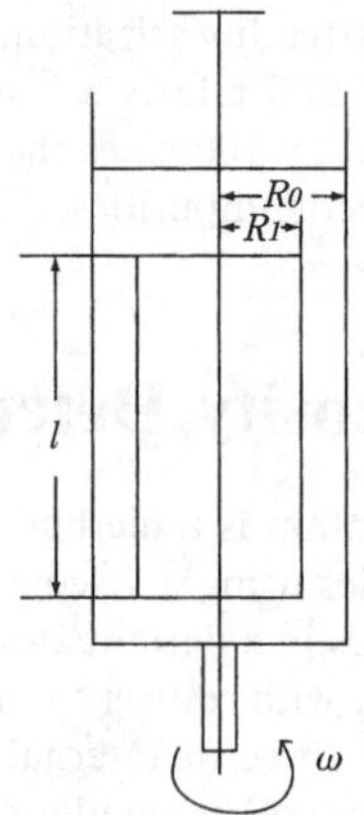

Fig. 2.53-2a Coaxial double cylinder-type rotational viscometer

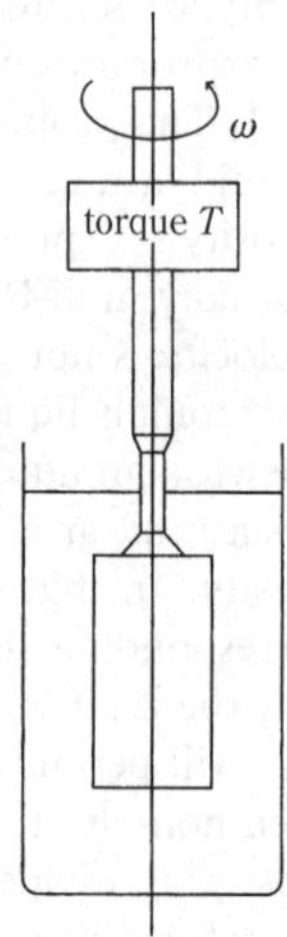

Fig. 2.53-2b Single cylinder-type rotational viscometer

tral axis and rotate separately, and the generated torque acting on one cylinder surface when the other cylinder is rotated, and the corresponding angular velocity, are measured.

As shown in Fig. 2.53-2a, the inner cylinder is hung by a wire whose twist constant is designated as k. In Fig. 2.53-2a, half the outer diameter of the inner cylinder and inner diameter of the outer cylinder are designated as R_i and R_o, respectively, and the length of the inner cylinder immersed in a liquid is designated as l. When a liquid is introduced into the gap between the two cylinders, and the outer cylinder is made to rotate at a constant angular velocity, ω, the inner cylinder is also forced to rotate due to the viscosity of the liquid. Consequently, torque, T, is generated by the forced rotation in a viscous liquid, and in the steady state the torque is balanced by the torsion of the wire, as indicated by the degree of rotation θ. Then, the relationship can be expressed by $T = k\theta$ and the viscosity of a liquid, η, is determined from the following equation by measuring the relationship between ω and θ. Conversely, viscosity measurement can also be performed by rotating the inner cylinder, and the same relationship holds.

$$\eta = \frac{100T}{4\pi l\omega}\left[\frac{1}{R_i^2} - \frac{1}{R_o^2}\right]$$

η: Viscosity of a liquid (mPa·s)
π: Circumference/diameter ratio
l: Length of the inner cylinder (cm)
ω: Angular velocity (rad/s)

T: Torque acting on cylinder surface (10^{-7} N·m)
R_i: 1/2 of outer diameter of the inner cylinder (cm)
R_o: 1/2 of inner diameter of the outer cylinder (cm)

2.1.2. Single cylinder-type rotational viscometer (Brookfield type viscometer)

In the single cylinder-type rotational viscometer, viscosity is determined by measuring the torque acting on the cylinder surface when the cylinder immersed in a liquid is rotated at a given angular velocity. Use an apparatus of the type illustrated in Fig. 2.53-2b. If the apparatus constant K_B is previously determined experimentally by using the *Standard Liquids for Calibrating Viscometers*, the viscosity of a liquid, η, can be obtained from the following equation.

$$\eta = K_B \frac{T}{\omega}$$

where, η: viscosity of a liquid (mPa·s)
K_B: Apparatus constant of viscometer (rad/cm^3)
ω: Angular velocity (rad/s)
T: Torque acting on cylinder surface (10^{-7} N·m)

2.1.3. Cone-flat plate-type rotational viscometer (Cone-plate type viscometer)

In the cone-flat plate-type rotational viscometer, viscosity is determined by placing a liquid in the gap between a flat disc and a cone with a large vertical angle sharing the same rotational axis, and the torque and the corresponding angular velocity are measured, when either the disc or the cone is rotated in a viscous liquid.

As shown in Fig. 2.53-2c, a liquid is introduced to fill the gap between a flat disc and a cone forming an angle α(rad). When either the flat disc or the cone is rotated at a constant angular velocity or a constant torque, the torque acting on the disc or cone surface rotated by the viscous flow and the corresponding angular velocity in the steady state, are measured. The viscosity of the liquid, η, can be calculated from the following equation.

$$\eta = \frac{3\alpha}{2\pi R^3} \cdot \frac{100T}{\omega}$$

η: Viscosity of a liquid (mPa·s)
π: Circumference/diameter ratio
R: Radius of cone (cm)
α: Angle between flat disc and cone (rad)
ω: Angular velocity (rad/s)
T: Torque acting on flat disc or cone surface (10^{-7} N·m)

2.2. Procedure

Set up the viscometer so that its rotational axis is perpendicular to the horizontal plane. Place a sufficient quantity of a sample solution in the viscometer, and allow the measuring system to stand until a specified temperature is attained, as directed in the monograph. Where it is desired to measure the viscosity within a precision of 1%, measuring temperature should be controlled within 0.1°C. Next, after confirming that the sample solution is at the designated temperature, start operating the rotational viscometer. After the forced rotation induced by the viscous flow has reached a steady state and the indicated value on the scale, which corresponds to the rotational frequency or the torque, has become constant, read the value on the scale. Then, calculate the viscosity η by using the respective equation appropriate to the type of viscometer being used. Determination or confirmation of the apparatus constant should be conducted beforehand by using the *Standard Liquids for Calibrating Viscometers*, and the validation of the apparatus and operating procedure should also be performed by using those standard liquids.

In the case of a non-Newtonian liquid, repeat the procedure for measuring the viscosity of the liquid with variation of the rotation velocity or torque from one measurement to another. From a series of such viscosity measurements, the relationship between the slip velocity and the slip stress of a non-Newtonian liquid, *i.e.*, the flow characteristics of a non-Newtonian liquid, can be obtained.

Calibration of a rotational viscometer is conducted by using water and the *Standard Liquids for Calibrating Viscometers*. These standard liquids are used for the determination or confirmation of the apparatus constant of the rotational viscometer. They are also used for periodic recalibration of the viscometer to confirm maintenance of a specified precision.

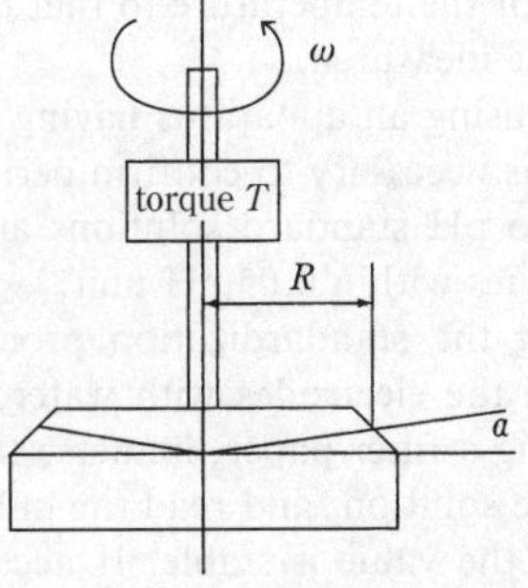

Fig. 2.53-2c Cone-flat plate-type rotational viscometer

2.54 pH Determination

pH is defined as the reciprocal of the common logarithm of hydrogen ion activity, which is the product of hydrogen ion concentration and the activity coefficient. Conventionally it is used as a scale of hydrogen ion concentration of a sample solution.

pH of a sample solution is expressed by the following equation in relation to the pH of a standard solution (pHs), and can be measured by a pH meter using a glass electrode.

$$\text{pH} = \text{pHs} + \frac{E - E_s}{2.3026\,RT/F}$$

pHs: pH value of a pH standard solution.
E: Electromotive force (volt) induced on the following galvanic cell composed of a glass electrode and suitable reference electrode in a sample solution:

Glass electrode | sample solution | reference electrode

E_s: Electromotive force (volt) induced on the following galvanic cell composed of a glass electrode and suitable reference electrode in a pH standard solution:

Glass electrode | standard pH solution | reference electrode

R: Gas constant
T: Absolute temperature
F: Faraday's constant

The value of 2.3026 RT/F (V) in the above equation means the degree of electromotive force (V) per one pH unit and it is dependent on the temperature as shown in Table 2.54-1:

1. pH Standard solution

The pH standard solutions are used as a standard of pH,

Table 2.54-1 Temperature dependency of the electromotive force (V)

Temperature of solution (°C)	2.3026 RT/F (V)	Temperature of solution (°C)	2.3026 RT/F (V)
5	0.05519	35	0.06114
10	0.05618	40	0.06213
15	0.05717	45	0.06313
20	0.05817	50	0.06412
25	0.05916	55	0.06511
30	0.06015	60	0.06610

Table 2.54-2 pH values of six pH standard solutions

Temper-ature (°C)	Oxalate pH standard solution	Phthalate pH standard solution	Phosphate pH standard solution	Borate pH standard solution	Carbonate pH standard solution	Calcium hydroxide pH standard solution
0	1.67	4.01	6.98	9.46	10.32	13.43
5	1.67	4.01	6.95	9.39	10.25	13.21
10	1.67	4.00	6.92	9.33	10.18	13.00
15	1.67	4.00	6.90	9.27	10.12	12.81
20	1.68	4.00	6.88	9.22	10.07	12.63
25	1.68	4.01	6.86	9.18	10.02	12.45
30	1.69	4.01	6.85	9.14	9.97	12.30
35	1.69	4.02	6.84	9.10	9.93	12.14
40	1.70	4.03	6.84	9.07		11.99
50	1.71	4.06	6.83	9.01		11.70
60	1.73	4.10	6.84	8.96		11.45

for standardization of a pH meter. To prepare the pH standard solutions, use distilled water or water with a conductivity not more than 2 μS·cm^{-1} (25°C) and an organic carbon not more than 0.50 mg/L, boiled for not less than 15 minutes and cooled in a container fitted with a carbon dioxide-absorbing tube (soda lime). Next, prepare individually 6 kinds of pH standard solutions shown in Table 2.54-2.

Store the pH standard solutions in hard glass or polyethylene bottles. For storage of alkaline pH standard solutions, it is preferable to use a bottle fitted with a carbon dioxide-absorbing tube. Since the pH may change gradually during storage over a long period, it is necessary to ascertain whether the expected pH value is held or not by comparison with newly prepared standard, when the solution is used after long storage.

(i) Oxalate pH standard solution—Pulverize potassium trihydrogen dioxalate dihydrate for pH determination, and dry in a desiccator (silica gel). Weigh 12.71 g (0.05 mole) of it accurately, and dissolve in water to make exactly 1000 mL.

(ii) Phthalate pH standard solution—Pulverize potassium hydrogen phthalate for pH determination, and dry at 110°C to constant mass. Weigh 10.21 g (0.05 mole) of it accurately, and dissolve in water to make exactly 1000 mL.

(iii) Phosphate pH standard solution—Pulverize potassium dihydrogen phosphate for pH determination and disodium hydrogen phosphate for pH determination, and dry at 110°C to constant mass. Weigh 3.40 g (0.025 mole) of potassium dihydrogen phosphate and 3.55 g (0.025 mole) of disodium hydrogen phosphate accurately, and dissolve in water to make exactly 1000 mL.

(iv) Borate pH standard solution—Allow sodium tetraborate for pH determination to stand in a desiccator (saturated sodium bromide aqueous solution) until it reaches constant mass. Weigh 3.81 g (0.01 mole) of it accurately, and dissolve in water to make exactly 1000 mL.

(v) Carbonate pH standard solution—Dry sodium hydrogen carbonate for pH determination in a desiccator (silica gel) to constant mass, and weigh 2.10 g (0.025 mole) of it accurately. Dry sodium carbonate for pH determination between 300°C and 500°C to constant mass, and weigh 2.65 g (0.025 mole) of it accurately. Dissolve both reagents in water to make exactly 1000 mL.

(vi) Calcium hydroxide pH standard solution—Reduce calcium hydroxide for pH determination to a fine powder, transfer 5 g to a flask, add 1000 mL of water, shake well, and allow the solution to become saturated at a temperature between 23°C and 27°C. Then filter the supernatant at the same temperature and use the clear filtrate (about 0.02 mol/L).

The pH values of these pH standard solutions at various temperatures are shown in the Table 2.54-2. pH values at an arbitrary temperature not indicated in Table 2.54-2 can be calculated by the interpolation method.

2. Apparatus

A pH meter generally consists of an electrode system of a glass electrode and a reference electrode, an amplifier and an indicating unit for controlling the apparatus and for displaying the measured value of electromotive force. The indicating unit is usually fitted with dials for zero and span (sensitivity) adjustment. Sometimes a temperature compensation dial is included.

The reproducibility of a pH meter should be within 0.05 pH unit, when measurements for an arbitrary pH standard solution are repeated five times, following the procedure described below. After each measurement it is necessary to wash the detecting unit well with water.

3. Procedure

Immerse the glass electrode previously in water for more than several hours. Start the measurement after confirming stable running of the apparatus. Rinse well the detecting unit with water, and remove the remaining water gently with a piece of filter paper.

To standardize the pH meter, two pH standard solutions are usually used as follows. Immerse the detection unit in the phosphate pH standard solution and adjust the indicated pH to the pH value shown in the *Table*. Next, immerse the detection system in the second pH standard solution, which should be selected so that the expected pH of the sample solution to be determined is between the pH values of the two pH standard solutions, and measure the pH under the same conditions as used for the first pH standard solution. Adjust the indicated pH to the defined pH value using the span adjustment dial, when the observed pH is not identical with that tabulated. Repeat the above standardization procedure until both pH standard solutions give observed pH values within 0.05 pH unit of the tabulated value without further adjustments. When a pH meter is fitted with a temperature compensation dial, the standardization procedure is done after the setting of the temperature to that of the pH standard solution to be measured.

In the case of using an apparatus having an auto-calibration function, it is necessary to confirm periodically that the pH values of two pH standard solutions are identical with the tabulated values within 0.05 pH unit.

After finishing the standardization procedure described above, rinse well the electrodes with water, remove the attached water using a filter paper, immerse the electrode system in the sample solution, and read the indicated pH value after confirming the value is stable. If necessary, a sample solution can be agitated gently.

In the pH determination, the temperature of a sample solution must be controlled to be the same as that of the pH standard solutions with which the pH meter was standardized (within 2°C). When a sample solution is alkaline, the measurement should be done in a vessel with a cover and if necessary, in a stream of inert gas such as nitrogen. Furthermore for a strongly alkaline solution above pH 11 containing alkali metal ions, an alkali error may be induced in the pH measurement. Thus, in such a case, an electrode with less alkali error should be used and an appropriate correction should be applied to the measured value.

4. Note

Construction and treatment in detail are different for different pH meters.

2.55 Vitamin A Assay

Vitamin A Assay is a method to determine vitamin A in Retinol Acetate, Retinol Palmitate, Vitamin A Oil, Cod Liver Oil and other preparations. Method 1 is for the assay of synthetic vitamin A esters, using the ultraviolet-visible spectrophotometry (Method 1-1) or the liquid chromatography (Method 1-2). Method 2 is for the assay of vitamin A of natural origin, containing many geometrical isomers, using the ultraviolet-visible spectrophotometry to determine vitamin A as vitamin A alcohol obtained by saponification in an alkaline solution and extraction.

One Vitamin A Unit (equal to 1 vitamin A I.U.) is equivalent to 0.300 μg of vitamin A (all-*trans* vitamin A alcohol).

1. Procedure

All procedures should be carried out quickly and care should be taken as far as possible to avoid exposure to light, air, oxidants, oxidizing catalysts (e.g. copper, iron), acids and heat. If necessary, light-resistant vessels may be used.

Generally, for synthetic vitamin A esters apply Method 1-1 or Method 1-2, but if the assay conditions required for Method 1-1 are not suitable, apply Method 2.

1.1. Method 1-1

Weigh accurately about 0.1 g of the sample, and dissolve in 2-propanol for vitamin A assay to make exactly 50 mL. Dilute this solution with 2-propanol for vitamin A assay to make a solution so that each mL contains 10 to 15 vitamin A Units, and use this solution as the sample solution. Determine the absorption spectrum of the sample solution between 220 nm and 400 nm as directed under Ultraviolet-visible Spectrophotometry <*2.24*> to obtain the wavelength of the maximum absorption and the absorbances at 300 nm, 310 nm, 320 nm, 326 nm, 330 nm, 340 nm and 350 nm. When the maximum absorption lies between 325 nm and 328 nm, and the ratios, $A_{\lambda i}/A_{326}$, of each absorbance, $A_{\lambda i}$, at 300 nm, 310 nm, 320 nm, 330 nm, 340 nm and 350 nm to the absorbance, A_{326}, at 326 nm are within the range of ± 0.030 of the values in the Table 2.55-1, the potency of vitamin A in Units per g of the sample is calculated from the following equation.

$$\text{Units of vitamin A in 1 g} = \frac{A_{326}}{M} \times \frac{V}{100} \times 1900$$

A_{326}: Absorbance at 326 nm
V: Total volume (mL) of the sample solution
M: Amount (g) of sample in V mL of the sample solution
1900: Conversion factor from specific absorbance of retinol ester to IU (Unit/g)

This method is applied to drugs or preparations containing vitamin A esters (retinol acetate or retinol palmitate) as the main component. However, when the wavelength of maximum absorption does not lie between 325 nm and 328 nm, or when the absorbance ratio $A_{\lambda i}/A_{326}$ is not within the range of ± 0.030 of the values in Table 2.55-1, apply Method 2.

Table 2.55-1 Absorbance ratio, $A_{\lambda i}/A_{326}$, of retinol acetate and retinol palmitate

λ_i (nm)	$A_{\lambda i}/A_{326}$	
	Retinol acetate	Retinol palmitate
300	0.578	0.590
310	0.815	0.825
320	0.948	0.950
330	0.972	0.981
340	0.786	0.795
350	0.523	0.527

1.2. Method 1-2

Proceed with an appropriate amount of sample as directed under Liquid Chromatography <*2.01*>.

For the assay of retinol acetate and retinol palmitate use Retinol Acetate Reference Standard and Retinol Palmitate Reference Standard, respectively, and fix appropriately the operating procedure, the operating conditions and the system suitability based on the characteristics of the substance to be tested and the species and amount of coexisting substances.

1.3. Method 2

Unless otherwise specified, weigh accurately a sample containing not less than 500 Units of vitamin A, and not more than 1 g of fat, transfer to a flask, and add 30 mL of aldehyde-free ethanol and 1 mL of a solution of pyrogallol in ethanol (95) (1 in 10). Then add 3 mL of a solution of potassium hydroxide (9 in 10), attach a reflux condenser, and heat on a water bath for 30 minutes to saponify. Cool quickly to ordinary temperature, add 30 mL of water, transfer to a separator A, wash the flask with 10 mL of water and then 40 mL of diethyl ether, transfer the washings to the separator A, shake well, and allow to stand. Transfer the water layer so obtained to a separator B, wash the flask with 30 mL of diethyl ether, add the washing to the separator B, and extract by shaking. Transfer the water layer to a flask, add the diethyl ether layer to the separator A, transfer the water layer in the flask to the separator B, add 30 mL of diethyl ether, and extract by shaking. Transfer the diethyl ether layer so obtained to the separator A, add 10 mL of water, allow the separator A to stand after gentle turning upside-down 2 or 3 times, and remove the water layer. Wash the content of the separator A with three 50-mL portions of water with increasingly vigorous shaking as the washing proceeds. Further wash with 50-mL portions of water until the washing no longer shows a pink color with phenolphthalein TS, and allow to stand for 10 minutes. Remove remaining water as far as possible, transfer the diethyl ether to an Erlenmeyer flask, wash the separator with two 10-mL portions of diethyl ether, add the washings to the flask, add 5 g of anhydrous sodium sulfate to the flask, mix by shaking, and transfer the diethyl ether to a round-bottomed flask by decantation. Wash the remaining sodium sulfate in the flask with two or more 10-mL portions of diethyl ether, and transfer the washings to the flask. Evaporate the diethyl ether in a water bath at 45°C while swirling the flask, using an aspirator, to about 1 mL, immediately add an exactly measured amount of 2-propanol for vitamin A assay to make a solution containing 6 to 10 vitamin A Units per mL, and designate the solution as the sample solution. Determine the absorbances, A_{310} at 310 nm, A_{325} at 325 nm, and A_{334} at 334 nm, of the sample solution as directed under Ultraviolet-visible Spectrophotometry.

Units of vitamin A in 1 g of the sample

$$= \frac{A_{325}}{M} \times \frac{V}{100} \times f \times 1830$$

$$f = 6.815 - 2.555 \times \frac{A_{310}}{A_{325}} - 4.260 \times \frac{A_{334}}{A_{325}}$$

A_{325}: Absorbance at 325 nm
V: Total volume (mL) of the sample solution
M: Amount (g) of sample in V mL of the sample solution
f: Correction factor
1830: Conversion factor from specific absorbance of retinol alcohol to IU (Unit/g)

2.56 Determination of Specific Gravity and Density

The density ρ (g/mL or g/cm^3) means the mass per unit volume, and the relative density means the ratio of the mass of a sample specimen to that of an equal volume of a standard substance. The relative density is also called the specific gravity.

The specific gravity, $d_t^{t'}$, means the ratio of the mass of the sample specimen at t'°C to that of an equal volume of water (H_2O) at t°C . Unless otherwise specified, the measurement is to be performed by Method 1, Method 2 or Method 4. When the specified value is accompanied with the term "about" in the monograph, Method 3 is also available.

1. Method 1. Measurement using a pycnometer

A pycnometer is a glass vessel with a capacity of usually 10 mL to 100 mL, having a ground-glass stopper fitted with a thermometer, and a side inlet-tube with a marked line and a ground-glass cap.

Weigh a pycnometer, previously cleaned and dried, to determine its mass M. Remove the stopper and the cap. Fill the pycnometer with the sample solution, keeping them at a slightly lower temperature by 1°C to 3°C than the specified temperature t'°C, and stopper them, taking care not to leave bubbles. Raise the temperature gradually, and when the thermometer shows the specified temperature, remove the portion of the sample solution above the marked line through the side tube, cap the side tube, and wipe the outside surface thoroughly. Measure the mass M_1 of the pycnometer filled with the sample solution. Perform the same procedure, using the same pycnometer containing water, and note the mass M_2 at the specified temperature t°C. The specific gravity $d_t^{t'}$ can be calculated by use of the following equation.

$$d_t^{t'} = \frac{M_1 - M}{M_2 - M}$$

Further, when measurements for a sample solution and water are performed at the same temperature (t°C = t'°C), the density of the sample solution at the temperature t'°C ($\rho_T^{t'}$) can be calculated from the measured specific gravity $d_{t'}^{t'}$ and the density of water at the temperature t'°C ($\rho_{S1}^{t'}$) indicated in Table 2.56-1 by using the following equation.

$$\rho_T^{t'} = \rho_{S1}^{t'} d_{t'}^{t'}$$

Table 2.56-1 Density of water

Temp. °C	Density g/mL	Temp. °C	Density g/mL	Temp. °C	Density g/mL	Temp. °C	Density g/mL
0	0.999 84						
1	0.999 90	11	0.999 61	21	0.997 99	31	0.995 34
2	0.999 94	12	0.999 50	22	0.997 77	32	0.995 03
3	0.999 96	13	0.999 38	23	0.997 54	33	0.994 70
4	0.999 97	14	0.999 24	24	0.997 30	34	0.994 37
5	0.999 96	15	0.999 10	25	0.997 04	35	0.994 03
6	0.999 94	16	0.998 94	26	0.996 78	36	0.993 68
7	0.999 90	17	0.998 77	27	0.996 51	37	0.993 33
8	0.999 85	18	0.998 60	28	0.996 23	38	0.992 97
9	0.999 78	19	0.998 41	29	0.995 94	39	0.992 59
10	0.999 70	20	0.998 20	30	0.995 65	40	0.992 22

* In this Table, although the unit of density is represented by g/mL in order to harmonize with the unit expression in the text, it should be expressed in g/cm^3 seriously.

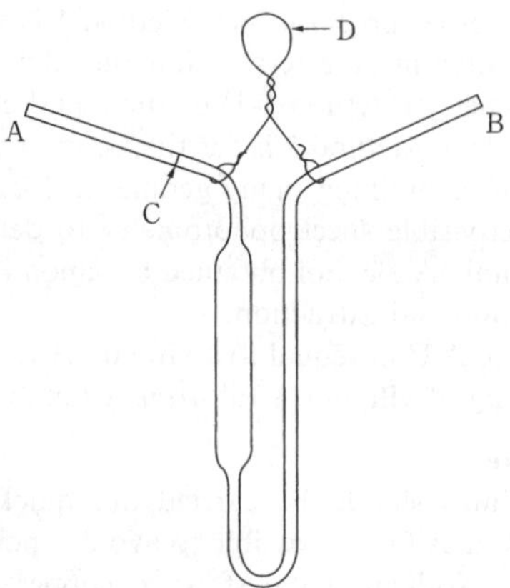

Fig. 2.56-1 Sprengel-Ostwald pycnometer

2. Method 2. Measurement using a Sprengel-Ostwald pycnometer

A Sprengel-Ostwald pycnometer is a glass vessel with a capacity of usually 1 mL to 10 mL. As shown in Fig. 2.56-1, both ends are thick-walled fine tubes (inside diameter: 1 - 1.5 mm, outside diameter: 3 - 4 mm), one of which, tube A, has a line C marked on it. Determine the mass of a pycnometer, M, previously cleaned and dried, by hanging it on the arm of a chemical balance with a platinum or aluminum wire D. Immerse the fine tube B in the sample solution, which is at a lower temperature by 3°C to 5°C than the specified temperature t'°C. Attach rubber tubing or a ground-glass tube to the end of A, and suck up the sample solution until the meniscus is above the marked line C, taking care to prevent bubble formation. Immerse the pycnometer in a water bath kept at the specified temperature t'°C for about 15 minutes, and then, by attaching a piece of filter paper to the end of B, adjust the level of the sample solution to the marked line C. Take the pycnometer out of the water bath, wipe thoroughly the outside surface and determine the mass M_1. By use of the same pycnometer, perform the same procedure for the standard solution of water. Weigh the pycnometer containing water at the specified temperature t°C, and note the mass M_2. Calculate the specific gravity $d_t^{t'}$, according to the equation described in Method 1.

Further, when measurements of specific gravity for a sample solution and water are performed at the same temperature (t'°C = t°C), the density of sample solution at temperature t'°C can be calculated by using the equation described in Method 1.

3. **Method 3. Measurement using a hydrometer**

Clean a hydrometer with ethanol (95) or diethyl ether. Stir the sample well with a glass rod, and float the hydrometer in the well. When the temperature is adjusted to the specified temperature t'°C and the hydrometer comes to a standstill, read the specific gravity $d_{t}^{t'}$ or the density $\rho_{T}^{t'}$ at the upper brim of the meniscus. Here the temperature t°C indicates the temperature at which the hydrometer is calibrated. If specific instructions for reading the meniscus are supplied with the hydrometer, the reading must be in accordance with the instructions.

Further, when measurement of the specific gravity for a sample solution is performed at the same temperature (t'°C = t°C), at which the hydrometer is calibrated, the density of a sample solution at t'°C, $\rho_{T}^{t'}$, can be calculated by using the specific gravity $d_{t}^{t'}$ and the equation shown in Method 1.

4. **Method 4. Measurement using an oscillator-type density meter**

Density measurement with an oscillator-type density meter is a method for obtaining the density of liquid or gas by measuring the intrinsic vibration period T (s) of a glass tube cell filled with sample specimen. When a glass tube containing a sample is vibrated, it undergoes a vibration with an intrinsic vibration period T in proportion to the mass of the sample specimen. If the volume of the vibrating part of the sample cell is fixed, the relation of the square of intrinsic oscillation period and density of the sample specimen shall be linear.

Before measuring a sample density, the respective intrinsic oscillation periods T_{S1} and T_{S2} for two reference substances (density: ρ_{S1}, ρ_{S2}) must be measured at a specified temperature t'°C, and the cell constant $K_{t'}$ ($g \cdot cm^{-3} s^{-2}$) must be determined by using the following equation.

$$K_{t'} = \frac{\rho_{S1}^{t'} - \rho_{S2}^{t'}}{T_{S1}^{2} - T_{S2}^{2}}$$

Usually, water and dried air are chosen as reference substances. Here the density of water at t'°C, $\rho_{S1}^{t'}$, is taken from Table 2.56-1, and that of dried air $\rho_{S2}^{t'}$ is calculated by using the following equation, where the pressure of dried air is at p kPa.

$$\rho_{S2}^{t'} = 0.0012932 \times \{273.15/(273.15 + t')\} \times (p/101.325)$$

Next, introduce a sample specimen into a sample cell having a cell constant $K_{t'}$, the intrinsic vibration period, T_{T}, for the sample under the same operation conditions as employed for the reference substances. The density of a sample specimen at t'°C, $\rho_{T}^{t'}$, is calculated by use of the following equation, by introducing the intrinsic oscillation period T_{S1} and the density of water at a specified temperature t'°C, $\rho_{S1}^{t'}$, into the equation.

$$\rho_{T}^{t'} = \rho_{S1}^{t'} + K_{t'}\,(T_{T}^{2} - T_{S1}^{2})$$

Further, the specific gravity of a sample specimen $d_{t}^{t'}$ against water at a temperature t°C can be obtained by using the equation below, by introducing the density of water at a temperature t°C, ρ_{S1}^{t}, indicated in Table 2.56-1.

$$d_{t}^{t'} = \frac{\rho_{T}^{t'}}{\rho_{S1}^{t}}$$

4.1. **Apparatus**

An oscillator-type density meter is usually composed of a glass tube cell of about 1 mL capacity, the curved end of which is fixed to the vibration plate, an oscillator which applies an initial vibration to the cell, a detector for measuring the intrinsic vibration period, and a temperature controlling system.

A schematic illustration of the apparatus is depicted in Fig. 2.56-2.

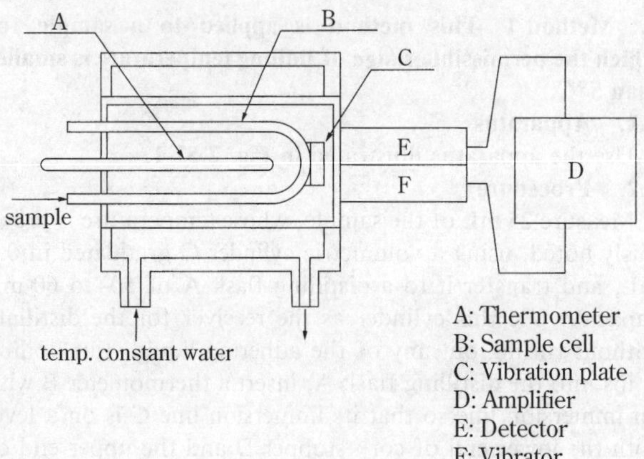

Fig. 2.56-2 Oscillator-type density meter

4.2. **Procedure**

A sample cell, water, and a sample specimen are previously adjusted to a specified temperature t'°C. Wash the sample cell with water or an appropriate solvent, and dry it thoroughly with a flow of dried air. Stop the flow of dried air, confirm that the temperature is at the specified value, and then measure the intrinsic oscillation period T_{S2} given by the dried air. Separately, the atmospheric pressure p (kPa) must be measured at the time and place of the examination. Next, introduce water into the sample cell and measure the intrinsic oscillation period T_{S1} given by water. Using these values of the intrinsic oscillation period and the atmospheric pressure, the sample cell constant $K_{t'}$ can be determined by use of the above-mentioned equation.

Next, introduce a sample specimen into the glass cell, confirm the specified temperature, and measure the intrinsic oscillation period T_{T} given by the sample specimen. Using the intrinsic oscillation periods for water and the sample specimen, the density of water $\rho_{S1}^{t'}$, and the cell constant $K_{t'}$, the density of the sample specimen $\rho_{T}^{t'}$ can be obtained by use of the above equation. If necessary, the specific gravity of the sample specimen $d_{t}^{t'}$ against water at a temperature t°C, can be calculated by using the density of water ρ_{S1}^{t} shown in Table 2.56-1.

In this measurement, avoid the occurrence of bubble formation in the sample cell, when a sample specimen or water is introduced into the cell.

2.57 Boiling Point and Distilling Range Test

The boiling point and distilling range are determined by Method 1 or Method 2 as described herein, unless otherwise specified. Boiling point is the temperature shown between when the first 5 drops of distillate leave the tip of the condenser and when the last liquid evaporates from the bottom of the flask. Distilling range test is done to determine the volume of the distillate which has been collected in the range of temperature directed in the monograph.

1. Method 1 This method is applied to a sample for which the permissible range of boiling temperature is smaller than 5°C.

1.1. Apparatus

Use the apparatus illustrated in Fig. 2.57-1.

1.2. Procedure

Measure 25 mL of the sample, whose temperature is previously noted, using a volumetric cylinder G graduated in 0.1 mL, and transfer it to a distilling flask A of 50- to 60-mL capacity. Use this cylinder as the receiver for the distillate without rinsing out any of the adhering liquid. Put boiling chips into the distilling flask A, insert a thermometer B with an immersion line so that its immersion line C is on a level with the lower end of cork stopper D and the upper end of its mercury bulb is located in the center of the delivery tube, and connect condenser E with the distilling flask A and adapter F with the condenser E. Insert the open end of F into the mouth of cylinder G (receiver) so that air can pass through slightly. Use a hood with a height sufficient to shield A, and heat A with a suitable heat source. When direct flame is applied as the heat source, put A on a hole of a fire-resistant, heat-insulating board [a board consisting of a fire-resistant, heat-insulating material, 150 mm square and about 6 mm thick (or a wire gauge of 150 mm square bonded to fire-resistant, heat-insulation materials in about 6 mm thickness), having an its center a round hole 30 mm in diameter].

Unless otherwise specified, distil the liquid sample by the application of heat, at a rate of 4 to 5 mL per minute of distillate in the case of liquids whose boiling temperature to be determined is lower than 200°C and at a rate of 3 to 4 mL per minute in the case of liquids whose boiling temperature is 200°C or over, and read the boiling point. For the distilling range test, bring the temperature of distillate to the temperature at which the volume was originally measured, and measure the volume of distillate.

Liquids that begin to distil below 80°C are cooled to between 10°C and 15°C before measuring the volume, and the receiving cylinder is kept immersed in ice up to a point 25 mm from the top during the distillation.

Correct the observed temperature for any variation in the barometric pressure from the normal (101.3 kPa), by allowing 0.1 degree for each 0.36 kPa of variation, adding if the pressure is lower, or subtracting if higher than 101.3 kPa.

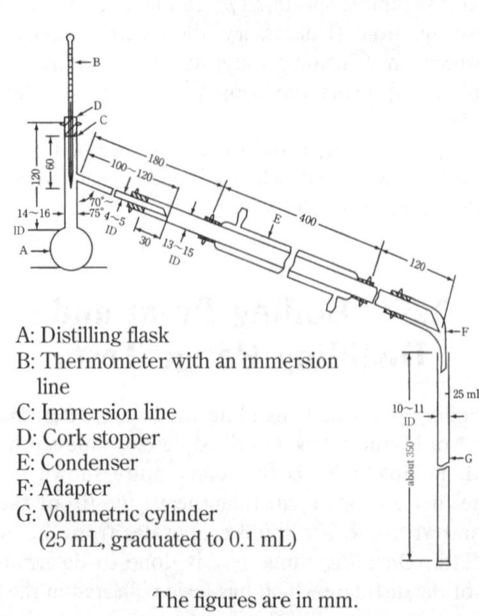

A: Distilling flask
B: Thermometer with an immersion line
C: Immersion line
D: Cork stopper
E: Condenser
F: Adapter
G: Volumetric cylinder (25 mL, graduated to 0.1 mL)

The figures are in mm.

Fig. 2.57-1

2. Method 2 This method is applied to the sample for which the permissible range of boiling temperature is 5°C or more.

2.1. Apparatus

The same apparatus as described in Method 1 is used. However, use a 200-mL distilling flask A with a neck 18 to 24 mm in inside diameter having a delivery tube 5 to 6 mm in inside diameter. The fire-resistant, heat-insulating board used for direct flame heating should have in its center a round hole 50 mm in diameter.

2.2. Procedure

Measure 100 mL of the sample, whose temperature is previously noted, using a volumetric cylinder graduated in 1 mL, and carry out the distillation in the same manner as in Method 1.

2.58 X-Ray Powder Diffraction Method

This test is harmonized with the European Pharmacopoeia and the U.S. Pharmacopeia.

The parts of the text that are not harmonized are marked with symbols (◆ ◆).

Information on the harmonization with the European Pharmacopoeia and the U.S. Pharmacopeia is available on the website of the Pharmaceuticals and Medical Devices Agency.

◆X-Ray Powder Diffraction Method is a method for measuring characteristic X-ray diffraction angles and intensities from randomly oriented powder crystallites irradiated by a monochromated X-ray beam.◆

Every crystalline phase of a given substance produces a characteristic X-ray diffraction pattern. Diffraction patterns can be obtained from a randomly oriented crystalline powder composed of crystallites or crystal fragments of finite size. Essentially 3 types of information can be derived from a powder diffraction pattern: angular position of diffraction lines (depending on geometry and size of the unit cell); intensities of diffraction lines (depending mainly on atom type and arrangement, and particle orientation within the sample); and diffraction line profiles (depending on instrumental resolution, crystallite size, strain and specimen thickness).

Experiments giving angular positions and intensities of lines can be used for applications such as qualitative phase analysis (for example, identification of crystalline phases) and quantitative phase analysis of crystalline materials. An estimate of the amorphous and crystalline fractions*(1)* can also be made. The X-ray powder diffraction (XRPD) method provides an advantage over other means of analysis in that it is usually non-destructive in nature (specimen preparation is usually limited to grinding to ensure a randomly oriented sample). XRPD investigations can also be carried out under *in situ* conditions on specimens exposed to non-ambient conditions, such as low or high temperature and humidity.

1. Principle

X-ray diffraction results from the interaction between X-rays and electron clouds of atoms. Depending on the atomic arrangement, interferences arise from the scattered X-rays. These interferences are constructive when the path difference between 2 diffracted X-ray waves differs by an integral num-

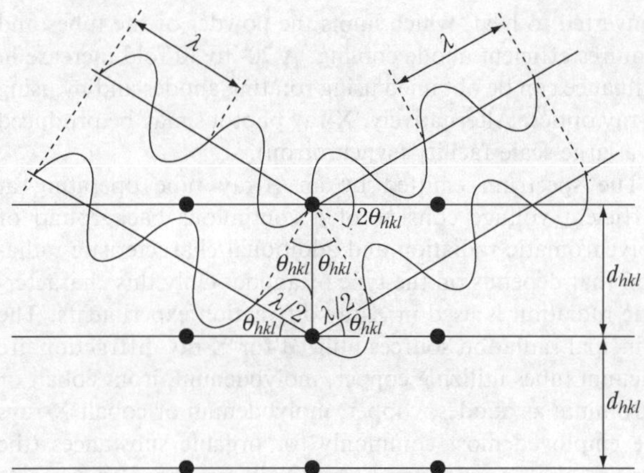

Fig. 2.58-1 Diffraction of X-rays by a crystal according to Bragg's law

ber of wavelengths. This selective condition is described by the Bragg equation, also called Bragg's law (see Fig. 2.58-1)

$$2d_{hkl}\sin\theta_{hkl} = n\lambda$$

The wavelength λ of the X-rays is of the same order of magnitude as the distance between successive crystal lattice planes, or d_{hkl} (also called 'd-spacings'). θ_{hkl} is the angle between the incident ray and the family of lattice planes, and $\sin\theta_{hkl}$ is inversely proportional to the distance between successive crystal planes or d-spacings.

The direction and spacing of the planes with reference to the unit cell axes are defined by the Miller indices $\{hkl\}$. These indices are the reciprocals, reduced to the next-lower integer, of the intercepts that a plane makes with the unit cell axes. The unit cell dimensions are given by the spacings, a, b and c and the angles between them, α, β and γ. The interplanar spacing for a specified set of parallel hkl planes is denoted by d_{hkl}. Each such family of planes may show higher orders of diffraction where the d values for the related families of planes, nh, nk, nl are diminished by the factor $1/n$ (n being an integer: 2,3,4, etc.). Every set of planes throughout a crystal has a corresponding Bragg diffraction angle, θ_{hkl}, associated with it (for a specific wavelength λ).

A powder specimen is assumed to be polycrystalline so that at any angle θ_{hkl} there are always crystallites in an orientation allowing diffraction according to Bragg's law(2). For a given X-ray wavelength, the positions of the diffraction peaks (also referred to as 'lines', 'reflections' or 'Bragg reflections') are characteristic of the crystal lattice (d-spacings), their theoretical intensities depend on the crystallographic unit cell content (nature and positions of atoms), and the line profiles on the perfection and extent of the crystal lattice. Under these conditions the diffraction peak has a finite intensity arising from atomic arrangement, type of atoms, thermal motion and structural imperfections, as well as from instrument characteristics. The intensity is dependent upon many factors such as structure factor, temperature factor, crystallinity, polarization factor, multiplicity and Lorentz factor. The main characteristics of diffraction line profiles are 2θ position, peak height, peak area and shape (characterized by, for example, peak width or asymmetry, analytical function, empirical representation). An example of the type of powder patterns obtained for 5 different solid phases of a substance are shown in Fig. 2.58-2.

In addition to the diffraction peaks, an X-ray diffraction experiment also generates a more-or-less uniform background, upon which the peaks are superimposed. Besides

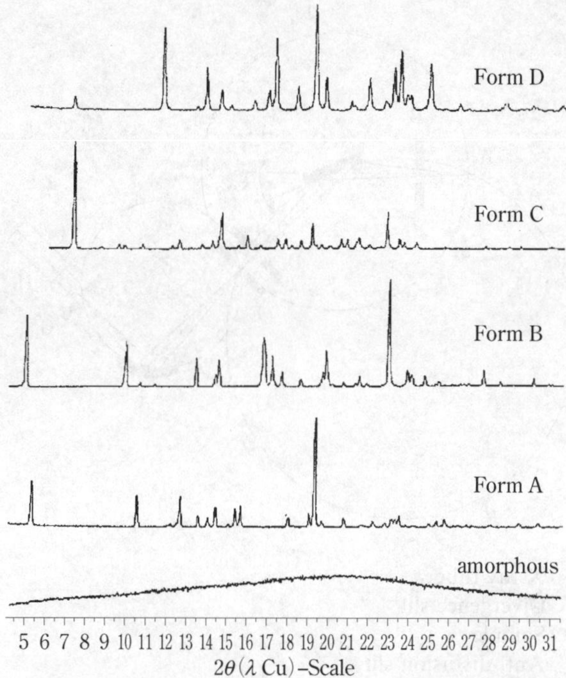

Fig. 2.58-2 X-ray powder diffraction patterns collected for 5 different solid phases of a substance (the intensities are normalized)

specimen preparation, other factors contribute to the background, for instance the sample holder, diffuse scattering from air and equipment, other instrumental parameters such as detector noise, general radiation from the X-ray tube, etc. The peak to background ratio can be increased by minimizing background and by choosing prolonged exposure times.

2. Instrument

2.1. Instrument set-up

X-ray diffraction experiments are usually performed using powder diffractometers or powder cameras. A powder diffractometer generally comprises 5 main parts: an X-ray source; incident beam optics, which may perform monochromatization, filtering, collimation and/or focusing of the beam; a goniometer; diffraction beam optics, which may perform monochromatization, filtering, collimation and focusing or parallelising of the beam; and a detector. Data collection and data processing systems are also required and are generally included in current diffraction measurement equipment.

Depending on the type of analysis to be performed (phase identification, quantitative analysis, lattice parameters determination, etc.), different XRPD instrument configurations and performance levels are required. The simplest instruments used to measure powder patterns are powder cameras. Replacement of photographic film as the detection method by photon detectors has led to the design of diffractometers in which the geometric arrangement of the optics is not truly focusing but parafocusing, such as in the Bragg-Brentano geometry. The Bragg-Brentano parafocusing configuration is currently the most widely used and is therefore briefly described here.

A given instrument may provide a horizontal or vertical $\theta/2\theta$ geometry or a vertical θ/θ geometry. For both geometries, the incident X-ray beam forms an angle θ with the specimen surface plane and the diffracted X-ray beam forms an angle 2θ with the direction of the incident X-ray beam (an

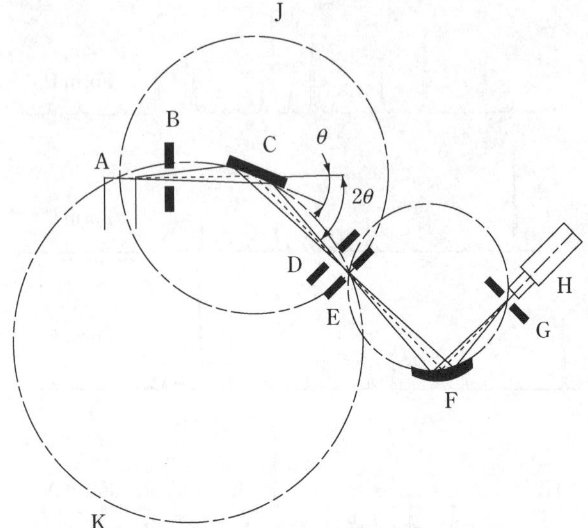

A. X-ray tube
B. Divergence slit
C. Sample
D. Anti-diffusion slit
E. Receiving slit
F. Monochromator
G. Detector receiving slit
H. Detector
J. Diffractometer circle
K. Focusing circle

Fig. 2.58-3 Geometric arrangement of the Bragg-Brentano parafocusing geometry

angle θ with the specimen surface plane). The basic geometric arrangement represented in Fig. 2.58-3. The divergent beam of radiation from the X-ray tube (the so-called 'primary beam') passes through the parallel plate collimators and a divergence slit assembly and illuminates the flat surface of the specimen. All the rays diffracted by suitably oriented crystallites in the specimen at an angle 2θ converge to a line at the receiving slit. A second set of parallel plate collimators and a scatter slit may be placed either behind or before the receiving slit. The axes of the line focus and of the receiving slit are at equal distances from the axis of the goniometer. The X-ray quanta are counted by a radiation detector, usually a scintillation counter, a sealed-gas proportional counter, or a position-sensitive solid-state detector such as imaging plate or CCD detector. The receiving slit assembly and the detector are coupled together and move tangentially to the focusing circle. For $\theta/2\theta$ scans the goniometer rotates the specimen about the same axis as that of the detector, but at half the rotational speed, in $\theta/2\theta$ motion. The surface of the specimen thus remains tangential to the focusing circle. The parallel plate collimator limits the axial divergence of the beam and hence partially controls the shape of the diffracted line profile.

A diffractometer may also be used in transmission mode. The advantage with this technology is to lessen the effects due to preferred orientation. A capillary of about 0.5 – 2 mm thickness can also be used for small sample amounts.

2.2. X-ray radiation

In the laboratory, X-rays are obtained by bombarding a metal anode with electrons emitted by the thermionic effect and accelerated in a strong electric field (using a high-voltage generator). Most of the kinetic energy of the electrons is converted to heat, which limits the powder of the tubes and requires efficient anode cooling. A 20- to 30-fold increase in brilliance can be obtained using rotating anodes and by using X-ray optics. Alternatively, X-ray photons may be produced in a large-scale facility (synchrotron).

The spectrum emitted by an X-ray tube operating at sufficient voltage consists of a continuous background of polychromatic radiation and additional characteristic radiation that depends on the type of anode. Only this characteristic radiation is used in X-ray diffraction experiments. The principal radiation sources utilized for X-ray diffraction are vacuum tubes utilizing copper, molybdenum, iron, cobalt or chromium as anodes; copper, molybdenum or cobalt X-rays are employed most commonly for organic substances (the use of cobalt anodes can be especially preferred to separate distinct X-ray lines). The choice of radiation to be used depends on the absorption characteristics of the specimen and possible fluorescence by atoms present in the specimen. The wavelengths used in powder diffraction generally correspond to the K_α radiation from the anode. Consequently, it is advantageous to make the X-ray beam 'monochromatic' by eliminating all the other components of the emission spectrum. This can be partly obtained using K_β filters, i.e. metal filters selected as having an absorption edge between the K_α and K_β wavelengths emitted by the tube.

Such a filter is usually inserted between the X-ray tube and the specimen. Another, more-and-more-commonly used way to obtain a monochromatic X-ray beam is via a large monochromator crystal (usually referred to as a 'monochromator'). This crystal is placed before or behind the specimen and diffracts the different characteristic peaks of the X-ray beam (i.e. K_α and K_β) at different angels, so that only one of them may be selected to enter into the detector. It is even possible to separate $K_{\alpha 1}$ and $K_{\alpha 2}$ radiations by using a specialized monochromator. Unfortunately, the gain in getting a monochromatic beam by using a filter or a monochromator is counteracted by a loss in intensity. Another way of separating K_α and K_β wavelengths is by using curved X-rays mirrors that can simultaneously monochromate and focus or parallelize the X-ray beam.

2.3. Radiation protection

Exposure of any part of the human body to X-rays can be injurious to health. It is therefore essential that whenever X-ray equipment is used, adequate precautions are taken to protect the operator and any other person in the vicinity. Recommended practice for radiation protection as well as limits for the levels of X-radiation exposure are those established by national legislation in each country. If there are no official regulations or recommendations in a country, the latest recommendations of the International Commission on Radiological Protection should be applied.

3. Specimen preparation and mounting

The preparation of the powdered material and mounting of the specimen in a suitable holder are critical steps in many analytical methods, and are particularly so for X-ray powder diffraction analysis, since they can greatly affect the quality of the data to be collected[(3)]. The main sources of error due to specimen preparation and mounting are briefly discussed here for instruments in Bragg-Brentano parafocusing geometry.

3.1. Specimen preparation

In general, the morphology of many crystalline particles tends to give a specimen that exhibits some degree of preferred orientation in the specimen holder. This is particularly evident for needle-like or plate-like crystals when size reduction yields finer needles or platelets. Preferred orientation in the specimen influences the intensities of various reflections, so that some are more intense and others are less intense, compared to what would be expected from a completely random specimen. Several techniques can be employed to improve randomness in the orientation of crystallites (and therefore to minimize preferred orientation), but further reduction of particle size is often the best and simplest approach. The optimum number of crystallites depends on the diffractometer geometry, the required resolution and the specimen attenuation of the X-ray beam. In some cases, particle sizes as large as 50 μm will provide satisfactory results in phase identification. However, excessive milling (crystallite sizes less than approximately 0.5 μm) may cause line broadening and significant changes to the sample itself such as:

(i) specimen contamination by particles abraded from the milling instruments (mortar, pestle, balls, etc.);
(ii) reduced degree of crystallinity;
(iii) solid-state transition to another polymorph;
(iv) chemical decomposition;
(v) introduction of internal stress;
(vi) solid-state reactions.

Therefore, it is advisable to compare the diffraction pattern of the non-ground specimen with that corresponding to a specimen of smaller particle size (e.g. a milled specimen). If the X-ray powder diffraction pattern obtained is of adequate quality considering its intended use, then grinding may not be required. It should be noted that if a sample contains more than one phase and if sieving is used to isolate particles to a specific size, the initial composition may be altered.

4. Control of the instrument performance

Goniometers and the corresponding incident and diffracted X-ray beam optics have many mechanical parts that need adjustment. The degree of alignment or misalignment directly influences the quality of the results of an XRPD investigation. Therefore, the different components of the diffractometer must be carefully adjusted (optical and mechanical systems, etc.) to adequately minimize systematic errors, while optimizing the intensities received by the detector. The search for maximum intensity and maximum resolution is always antagonistic when aligning a diffractometer. Hence, the best compromise must be sought whilst performing the alignment procedure. There are many different configurations and each supplier's equipment requires specific alignment procedures.

The overall diffractometer performance must be tested and monitored periodically using suitable certified reference materials. Depending on the type of analysis, other well-defined reference materials may also be employed, although the use of certified reference materials is preferred.

5. Qualitative phase analysis (Identification of phases)

The identification of the phase composition of an unknown sample by XRPD is usually based on the visual or computer-assisted comparison of a portion of its X-ray diffraction powder pattern to the experimental or calculated pattern of a reference material. Ideally, these reference patterns are collected on well-characterized single-phase specimens. This approach makes it possible in most cases to identify a crystalline substance by its 2θ diffraction angles or d-spacings and by its relative intensities. The computer-aided comparison of the diffraction pattern of the unknown sample to the comparison data can be based either on a more-or-less extended 2θ-range of the whole diffraction pattern or on a set of reduced data derived from the pattern. For example, the list of d-spacings and normalized intensities I_{norm}, a so-called (d, I_{norm})-list extracted from the pattern, is the crystallographic fingerprint of the material, and can be compared to (d, I_{norm})-lists of single-phase samples complied in databases.

For most organic crystals, when using CuK_α radiation, it is appropriate to record the diffraction pattern in a 2θ-range from as near 0° as possible to at least 40°. The agreement in the 2θ-diffraction angles between specimen and reference is within 0.2° for the same crystal form, while relative intensities between specimen and reference may vary considerably due to preferred orientation effects. By their very nature, variable hydrates and solvates are recognized to have varying unit cell dimensions and as such shifting occurs in peak positions of the measured XRPD patterns for these materials. In these unique materials, variance in 2-θ positions of greater than 0.2° is not unexpected. As such, peak position variances such as 0.2° are not applicable to these materials. For other types of samples (e.g. inorganic salts), it may be necessary to extend the 2θ-region scanned to well beyond 40°. It is generally sufficient to scan past the 10 strongest reflections identified in single phase X-ray powder diffraction database files.

It is sometimes difficult or even impossible to identify phases in the following cases:

(i) non-crystallized or amorphous substances;
(ii) the components to be identified are present in low mass fractions of the analyte amounts (generally less than 10 per cent m/m);
(iii) pronounced preferred orientation effects;
(iv) the phase has not been filed in the database used;
(v) formation of solid solutions;
(vi) presence of disordered structures that alter the unit cell;
(vii) the specimen comprises too many phases;
(viii) presence of lattice deformations;
(ix) structural similarity of different phases.

6. Quantitative phase analysis

If the sample under investigation is a mixture of 2 or more known phases, of which not more than 1 is amorphous, the percentage (by volume or by mass) of each crystalline phase and of the amorphous phase can, in many cases, be determined. Quantitative phase analysis can be based on the integrated intensities, on the peak heights of several individual diffraction lines[4], or on the full pattern. These integrated intensities, peak heights or full-pattern data points are compared to the corresponding values of reference materials. These reference materials shall be single-phase or a mixture of known phases. The difficulties encountered during quantitative analysis are due to specimen preparation (the accuracy and precision of the results require in particular homogeneity of all phases and a suitable particle size distribution in each phase) and to matrix effects. In favorable cases, amounts of crystalline phases as small as 10 per cent may be determined in solid matrices.

6.1. Polymorphic samples

For a sample composed of 2 polymorphic phases a and b, the following expression may be used to quantify the fraction F_a of phase a:

$$F_a = \frac{1}{1 + K\,(I_b/I_a)}$$

The fraction is derived by measuring the intensity ratio between the 2 phases, knowing the value of the constant K. K is the ratio of the absolute intensities of the 2 pure polymorphic phases I_{oa}/I_{ob}. Its value can be determined by measuring standard samples.

6.2. Methods using a standard

The most commonly used methods for quantitative analysis are:

–the 'external standard method';

–the 'internal standard method';

–the 'spiking method' (often also called the 'standard addition method').

The 'external standard method' is the most general method and consists of comparing the X-ray diffraction pattern of the mixture, or the respective line intensities, with those measured in a reference mixture or with the theoretical intensities of a structural model, if it is fully known.

To limit errors due to matrix effects, an internal reference material with crystallite size and X-ray absorption coefficient comparable to those of the components of the sample, and with a diffraction pattern that does not overlap at all that of the sample to be analyzed, can be used. A known quantity of this reference material is added to the sample to be analyzed and to each of the reference mixtures. Under these conditions, a linear relationship between line intensity and concentration exists. This application, called the 'internal standard method', requires a precise measurement of diffraction intensities.

In the 'spiking method' (or 'standard addition method'), some of the pure phase a is added to the mixture containing the unknown concentration of a. Multiple additions are made to prepare an intensity-versus-concentration plot in which the negative x intercept is the concentration of the phase a in the original sample.

7. Estimate of the amorphous and crystalline fractions

In a mixture of crystalline and amorphous phases, the crystalline and amorphous fractions can be estimated in several ways. The choice of the method used depends on the nature of the sample:

(i) if the sample consists of crystalline fractions and an amorphous fraction of different chemical compositions, the amounts of each of the individual crystalline phases may be estimated using appropriate standard substances as described above; the amorphous fraction is then deduced indirectly by subtraction;

(ii) if the sample consists of one amorphous and one crystalline fraction, either as a 1-phase or a 2-phase mixture, with the same elemental composition, the amount of the crystalline phase ('the degree of crystallinity') can be estimated by measuring 3 areas of the diffractogram:

A = total area of the peaks arising from diffraction from the crystalline fraction of the sample:

B = total area below area A;

C = background area (due to air scattering, fluorescence, equipment, etc.)

When these areas have been measured, the degree of crystallinity can be roughly estimated using the following formula:

$$\% \text{ crystallinity} = 100A/(A + B - C)$$

It is noteworthy that this method does not yield absolute degree-of-crystallinity values and hence is generally used for comparative purposes only. More sophisticated methods are also available, such as the Ruland method.

8. Single crystal structure

In general, the determination of crystal structures is performed from X-ray diffraction data obtained using single crystals. However, crystal structure analysis of organic crystals is a challenging task, since the lattice parameters are comparatively large, the symmetry is low and the scattering properties are normally very low. For any given crystalline form of a substance, knowledge of the crystal structure allows the calculation of the corresponding XRPD pattern, thereby providing a 'preferred-orientation-free' reference XRPD pattern, which may be used for phase identification.

(1) There are many other applications of the X-ray powder diffraction technique that can be applied to crystalline pharmaceutical substances such as: determination of crystal structures, refinement of crystal structures, determination of crystallographic purity of crystalline phases, characterization of crystallographic texture, etc. These applications are not described in this chapter.

(2) An 'ideal' powder for diffraction experiments consists of a large number of small, randomly oriented spherical crystallites (coherently diffracting crystalline domains). If this number is sufficiently large, there are always enough crystallites in any diffracting orientation to give reproducible diffraction patterns.

(3) Similarly, changes in the specimen can occur during data collection in the case of a non-equilibrium specimen (temperature, humidity).

(4) If the crystal structures of all components are known, the Rietveld method can be used to quantify them with good accuracy. If the crystal structures of the components care not known, the Pawley or least squares methods can be used.

2.59 Test for Total Organic Carbon

Test for Total Organic Carbon is a method for measuring the amount of organic carbon, which forms organic compounds, in water. Normally, organic carbon can be oxidized to carbon dioxide by a dry decomposition method, where organic compounds are oxidized by combustion, or by a wet decomposition method, where organic compounds are oxidized by applying ultraviolet rays or by adding oxidizing agent. The amount of carbon dioxide generated in the decomposition process is measured using an appropriate method such as infrared gas analysis, electric conductivity measurement, or resistivity measurement. The amount of organic carbon in water can be calculated from the amount of carbon dioxide measured in one of the above methods.

There are two types of carbon in water: organic carbon and inorganic carbon. For measuring the amount of organic carbon, two approaches can be taken. One method is to measure the amount of total carbon in water, then to subtract the amount of inorganic carbon from that of total carbon. The other method is to remove inorganic carbon from the test water, then to measure the amount of remaining organic carbon.

1. Instrument

The instrument consists of a sample injection port, a decomposition device, a carbon dioxide separation block, a detector, and a data processor or a recorder. The instrument should be capable of measuring the amount of organic carbon down to 0.050 mg/L.

The sample injection port is designed to be able to accept a specific amount of sample injected by a microsyringe or other appropriate sampling devices. The decomposition device for the dry decomposition method consists of a combustion tube and an electric furnace to heat the sample. Both devices are adjusted to operate at specified temperatures. The decomposition device for the wet decomposition method consists of an oxidizing reaction box, an ultraviolet ray lamp, a decomposition aid injector, and a heater. The decomposition device for either method should be capable of generating not less than 0.450 mg/L of organic carbon when using a solution of 0.806 mg/L sodium dodecylbenzenesulfonate as the sample. The carbon dioxide separation block removes water from carbon dioxide formed in the decomposition process or separates carbon dioxide from the decomposed gas. An infrared gas analyzer, electric conductivity meter or specific resistance meter is used as the detector which converts the concentration of carbon dioxide into electric signal. The data processor calculates the concentration of the total organic carbon in the sample based on the electric signal converted by the detector. The recorder records the electric signal intensity converted by the detector.

2. Reagents and standard solutions

(i) Water used for measuring organic carbon (water for measurement): This water is used for preparing standard solutions or decomposition aid or for rinsing the instrument. The amount of organic carbon in this water, when collected into a sample container, should be not more than 0.250 mg/L.

(ii) Standard potassium hydrogen phthalate solution: The concentration of this standard solution is determined as specified for the instrument. Dry potassium hydrogen phthalate (standard reagent) at 105°C for 4 hours, and allow it to cool in a desiccator (silica gel). Weigh accurately a prescribed amount of dried potassium hydrogen phthalate, and dissolve it in the water for measurement to prepare the standard solution.

(iii) Standard solution for measuring inorganic carbon: The concentration of this standard solution is determined as specified for the instrument. Dry sodium hydrogen carbonate in a desiccator (sulfuric acid) for not less than 18 hours. Dry sodium carbonate decahydrate separately between 500°C and 600°C for 30 minutes, and allow to cool in a desiccator (silica gel). Weigh accurately prescribed amounts of these compounds so that the ratio of their carbon content is 1:1, and dissolve them in the water for measurement to prepare the standard solution.

(iv) Decomposition aid: Dissolve a prescribed amount of potassium peroxodisulfate or other substances that can be used for the same purpose, in the water for measurement up to the concentration as specified for the instrument.

(v) Gas for removing inorganic carbon or carrier gas: Nitrogen, oxygen, or other gases that can be used for the same purpose.

(vi) Acid for removing inorganic carbon: Dilute hydrochloric acid, phosphoric acid or other acids that can be used for the same purpose, with the water for measurement down to the concentration as specified for the instrument.

3. Apparatus

(i) Sample container and reagent container: Use a container made of the material which does not release organic carbon from its surface, such as hard glass. Soak the container before use in a mixture of diluted hydrogen peroxide solution (1 in 3) and dilute nitric acid (1:1), and wash well with the water for measurement.

(ii) Microsyringe: Wash a microsyringe with a mixture of a solution of sodium hydroxide (1 in 20) and ethanol (99.5) (1:1), or diluted hydrochloric acid (1 in 4), and rinse well with the water for measurement.

4. Procedure

Employ an analytical method suitable for the instrument used. Calibrate the instruments using the standard potassium hydrogen phthalate solution with the test procedure specified for the instrument.

It is recommended that this instrument be incorporated into the manufacturing line of the water to be tested.

Otherwise, this test should be performed in a clean circumstance where the use of organic solvents or other substances that may affect the result of this test is prohibited, using a large sample container to collect a large volume of the water to be tested. The measurement should be done immediately after the sample collection.

4.1. Measurement of organic carbon by subtracting inorganic carbon from total carbon

According to the test procedure specified for the instrument used, inject a suitable volume of the sample for measuring the expected amount of total carbon into the instrument from sample injection port, and decompose organic and inorganic carbon in the sample. Detect the generated carbon dioxide with the detector, and calculate the amount of total carbon in the sample using a data processor or a recorder. Change the setting of the instrument for measuring inorganic carbon exclusively, and measure the amount of inorganic carbon in the same manner as total carbon. The amount of organic carbon can be obtained by subtracting the amount of inorganic carbon from that of total carbon.

4.2. Measurement of organic carbon after removing inorganic carbon

Remove inorganic carbon by adding the acid for removing inorganic carbon to the sample, followed by bubbling the gas for removing inorganic carbon (e.g. nitrogen) into the sample. According to the test procedure specified for the instrument used, inject a suitable volume of the sample for measuring the expected amount of organic carbon into the instrument from sample injection port, and decompose the sample. Detect the generated carbon dioxide with the detector, and calculate the amount of organic carbon in the sample using a data processor or a recorder.

For the instrument where the removal of inorganic carbon is performed in the instrument, first inject a suitable volume of the sample for measuring the expected amount of organic carbon into the instrument from sample injection port, according to the test procedure specified for the instrument used. Then, remove inorganic carbon by adding the acid for removing inorganic carbon to the sample in the decomposition device, followed by bubbling the gas for removing inorganic carbon into the sample. Decompose organic carbon, detect the generated carbon dioxide with the detector, and calculate the amount of organic carbon using a data processor or a recorder.

2.60 Melting Point Determination

The melting point is defined to be the temperature at which a crystalline substance melts during heating, when the solid phase and the liquid phase are in an equilibrium. However, in this Pharmacopoeia it is conventionally defined to be the temperature at which the remaining solid sample melts completely when it is subjected to continuous heating and the change of the sample state that accompanies heating is accurately observed. Since a pure substance has an intrinsic melting point, it is used for the identification and/or confirmation of a substance and also as an indicator of the purity of a substance.

The melting point is determined by either of the following methods: Method 1 is applied to those substances of which the purity is comparably high and which can be pulverized, Method 2 to those substances which are insoluble in water and can not be readily pulverized, and Method 3 to petrolatums.

Unless otherwise specified, measurement is performed by Method 1.

1. Method 1

This method is applied to those substances of which the purity is comparably high and which can be pulverized.

1.1. Apparatus

Use the apparatus illustrated in the Fig. 2.60-1.

Alternatively, apparatus in which some of the procedures, such as stirring, heating, and cooling are automated, can be used.

(i) Bath fluid: Usually use clear silicone oil having a viscosity of 50 to 100 mm^2/s at an ordinary temperature.

(ii) Thermometer with an immersion line: There are six types of thermometers, Type 1—Type 6, which are specified by an appropriate measuring temperature range. For melting points lower than 50°C, use a thermometer Type 1; for 40°C to 100°C, Type 2; for 90°C to 150°C, Type 3; for 140°C to 200°C, Type 4; for 190°C to 250°C, Type 5; for 240°C to 320°C, Type 6.

(iii) Capillary tube: Use a hard glass capillary tube 120 mm long, 0.8 to 1.2 mm in inner diameter and 0.2 to 0.3 mm thick, with one end closed.

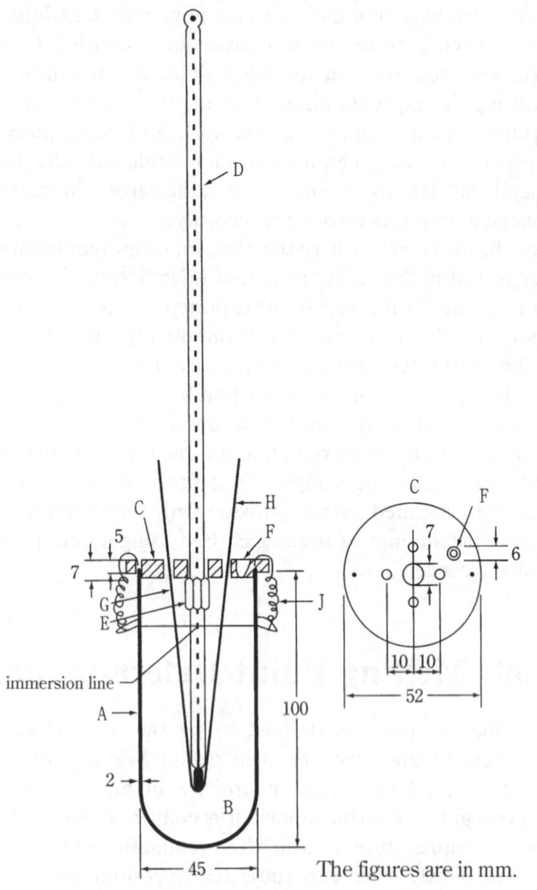

Fig. 2.60-1 Melting point determination apparatus

1.2. Procedure

Pulverize the sample to a fine powder, and, unless otherwise specified, dry in a desiccator (silica gel) for 24 hours. When it is specified to do the test after drying, dry the sample under the conditions specified in the monograph before measurement. Place the sample in a dried capillary tube H, and pack it tightly so as to form a layer about 2.5 - 3.5 mm high by dropping the capillary repeatedly, with the closed end of H down, through a glass tube, about 70 cm long, held vertically on a glass or porous plate.

Heat the bath fluid B until the temperature rises to about 10°C below the expected melting point, place the thermometer D in the bath with the immersion line at the same level as the meniscus of the bath fluid, and insert capillary tube H into a coil spring G so that the packed sample is placed in a position corresponding to the center of the mercury bulb of the thermometer D. Continue heating to raise the temperature at a rate of approximately 3°C per minute until the temperature rises to 5°C below the expected melting point, then carefully regulate the rate of temperature increase to 1°C per minute.

Read the thermometer indication of the instantaneous temperature at which the sample liquefies completely and no solid is detectable in the capillary, and designate the indicated temperature as the melting point of the sample specimen.

1.2.1. System suitability test

Confirmation of the system suitability of the apparatus should be done periodically by using Reference Standards for Apparatus Suitability. The Reference Standard is prepared for the suitability test of the apparatus when it is used with Type 2—Type 5 thermometers, and consists of 6 highly purified substances: acetanilide, acetophenetidine, caffeine, sulfanilamide, sulfapyridine, and vanillin. The label shows the certified melting points of the respective substances (the end point of the melting change), MP_f.

After selecting one of the thermometers and the appropriate Melting Point Standard based upon the expected melting point of a sample specimen, perform a melting point measurement of the selected Reference Standard, according to the above procedure. When the value of the obtained melting point of the Reference Standard is within $MP_f \pm 0.5$°C in the case of vanillin and acetanilide, within $MP_f \pm 0.8$°C in the case of acetophenetidine and sulfanilamide, and within $MP_f \pm 1.0$°C in the case of sulfapyridine and caffeine, the apparatus is assumed to be suitable.

The above-mentioned measurement is repeated 3 times and the average is determined to be the melting point of the Reference Standard tested. When the above suitability test criteria are not met in a certain melting point measurement system of an apparatus and a Reference Standard, do the test again, after checking the packing of the sample specimen into the capillary tube, the locations and positioning of the thermometer and the capillary tube, the heating and stirring of the bath fluid, and the control of the temperature increasing rate. When a melting point measurement system does not meet the suitability test criteria again after checking these measuring conditions, the thermometer with an immersion line should be calibrated again or replaced with a new one.

2. Method 2

This method is applied to substances such as fats, fatty acids, paraffins or waxes.

2.1. Apparatus

Instead of the apparatus specified in Method 1, use a water-containing beaker as a bath fluid and a heating vessel. In this measurement, total immersion mercury-filled thermometers can also be used in place of the thermometer with an immersion line. Furthermore, the capillary tube should be the same as specified in Method 1, except that both ends of the tube are open.

2.2. Procedure

Carefully melt the sample at as low a temperature as possible, and, taking care to prevent bubbles, introduce it into a capillary tube to a height of about 10 mm. Allow the capillary containing the sample to stand for 24 hours at below 10°C, or for at least 1 hour in contact with ice, holding the capillary so that the sample can not flow out. Then attach the capillary to the thermometer by means of a rubber band so that the absorbed sample is located at a position corresponding to the center of the mercury bulb. Adjust the capillary tube in a water-containing beaker to such a position that the lower edge of the sample is located 30 mm below the water surface. Heat the beaker with constant stirring until the temperature rises to 5°C below the expected melting point. Then regulate the rate of temperature increase to 1°C per minute. The temperature at which the sample begins floating in the capillary is taken as the melting point of the sample specimen.

3. Method 3

This method is applied to petrolatums.

3.1. Apparatus

Instead of the apparatus specified in Method 1, use a water-containing beaker as a bath fluid and a heating vessel. In this measurement, total immersion mercury-filled thermometers can also be used in place of the thermometer with an immersion line.

3.2. Procedure

Melt the sample slowly by heating, with thorough stirring, until the temperature reaches 90 – 92°C. Discontinue the heating, and allow the sample to cool to 8 – 10°C above the expected melting point. Chill the bulb of the thermometer to 5°C, wipe and dry, and, while still cold, stick half of the thermometer bulb into the melted sample. Withdraw it immediately, hold vertically, cool until the attached sample becomes turbid, then dip the sample-bearing bulb for 5 minutes in water having a temperature below 16°C. Next, fix the thermometer securely in a test tube by means of a cork stopper so that the lower end is located 15 mm above the bottom. Suspend the test tube in a water-containing beaker held at a temperature about 16°C, and raise the temperature of the water bath to 30°C at a rate of 2°C per minute, then continue heating carefully at a rate of 1°C per minute until it reaches the melting point. Read the thermometer indication of the instantaneous temperature at which the first drop of the sample leaves the thermometer. If the variations between three repeated determinations are not more than 1°C, take the average of the three as the melting point. If any variation is greater than 1°C, make two additional measurements, and take the average of the five as the melting point.

2.61 Turbidity Measurement

Turbidity measurement is used to determine the turbidity (degree of opalescence) for the decision whether the article to be examined complies with the clarity requirement stated in the Purity.

As a rule, the visual method is specified for the requirement in individual monograph.

1. Visual method

This is used to determine the degree of opalescence with white (or faintly-colored) fine particles. So the degree of opalescence of a colored sample is liable to be determined lower that it is difficult to compare the degree correctly without using similarly colored reference suspension.

1.1. Reference suspensions

Pipet 5 mL, 10 mL, 30 mL and 50 mL of formazin opalescence standard solution, dilute them separately to exactly 100 mL with water, and use these solutions so obtained as Reference suspensions I, II, III and IV, respectively. Shake before use. Degrees of opalescence of Reference suspensions I, II, III and IV are equivalent to 3 NTU, 6 NTU, 18 NTU and 30 NTU, respectively.

1.2. Procedure

Place sufficient of the test solution, water or the solvent to prepare the test solution and, where necessary, newly prepared Reference suspensions in separate flat-bottomed test tubes, 15 – 25 mm in inside diameter and of colorless and transparent, to a depth of 40 mm, and compare the contents of the tubes against a black background by viewing in diffused light down the vertical axes of the tubes. The diffused light must be such that Reference suspension I can be readily distinguished from water, and that Reference suspension II can readily be distinguished from Reference suspension I.

In this test Reference suspensions are used when the clarity of the test solution is obscurely and it is not easy to determine that its degree of opalescence is similar or not similar to water or to the solvent used to prepare the test solution.

1.3. Interpretation

A liquid is considered "clear" when its clarity is the same as that of water or of the solvent used to prepare the liquid or its turbidity is not more pronounced than that of Reference suspension I. If the turbidity of the liquid is more than that of Reference suspension I, consider as follows: When the turbidity is more than that of Reference suspension I but not more than that of Reference suspension II, express "it is not more than Reference suspension II". In the same way, when the turbidity is more than that of Reference suspension II but not more than that of Reference suspension III, express "it is not more than Reference suspension III", and when the turbidity is more than that of Reference suspension III but not more than that of Reference suspension IV, express "it is not more than Reference suspension IV". When the turbidity is more than that of Reference suspension IV, express "it is more than Reference suspension IV".

1.4. Reagent solutions

Formazin opalescence standard solution: To exactly 3 mL of formazin stock suspension add water to make exactly 200 mL. Use within 24 hours after preparation. Shake thoroughly before use. Degrees of opalescence of this standard solution is equivalent to 60 NTU.

2. Photoelectric photometry

The turbidity can also be estimated by instrumental measurement of the light absorbed or scattered on account of submicroscopic optical density inhomogeneities of opalescent solutions and suspensions. The photoelectric photometry is able to provide more objective determination than the visual method. Though they can determine the turbidity by measuring the scattered or transmitted light, the measuring system and light source must be specified in individual test method, and for the comparison of observed data, the same measuring system and light source should be used.

In each case, the linear relationship between turbidity and concentration must be demonstrated by constructing a calibration curve using at least 4 concentrations. For colored samples, the turbidity value is liable to be estimated lower because of attenuating both incident and scattered lights due to the absorption by the color, and the transmission-dispersion method is principally used.

2.1. Turbidimetry

When a light passes through a turbid liquid the transmitted light is decreased by scattering with the particles dispersed in the liquid. A linear relationship is observed between turbidity and concentration when the particles with a constant size are uniformly dispersed, the size is small and the suspension is not higher concentration. The turbidity can be measured by Ultraviolet-visual Spectrophotometry <2.24> using spectrophotometer or photoelectric photometer. The turbidity of the sample in higher concentration can also be measured, however, it is susceptible to the color of the sample, and the measurement is usually performed at around 660 nm to avoid possible disturbance occurred from the absorption by the color.

2.2. Nephelometry

When a suspension is viewed at right angles to the direction of the incident light, it appears opalescent due to the refraction of light from the particles of the suspension (Tyndall effect). A certain portion of the light entering a turbid liquid is transmitted, another portion is absorbed and the remaining portion is scattered by the suspended particles. The scattered light measuring method shows the linear relationship between the nephelometric turbidity units (NTU) values and relative detector signals in a low turbidity range. As the degree of turbidity increases, not all the particles are exposed to the incident light and the scattered radiation of other particles is hindered on its way to the detector.

2.3. Ratio Turbidimetry

This method measures both scattered and transmitted light values at the same time, and the turbidity is determined from the ratio of the scattered light value to the transmitted light value. This procedure compensates for the light that is diminished by the color of the sample and eliminates the influence of the color. When the measurement is performed by using an integrating sphere, it is particularly called the integrating sphere method, which measures the total transmitted light value as well as the scattered light value occurred with the suspended particles, and the turbidity can be determined from the ratio of them.

2.4. Application of photoelectric photometry for monograph requirements

The turbidity of the test solution, determined by the photoelectric photometry, can be used as an indicating standard for the conformity to the clarity requirements by converting into NTU by using turbidity known reference solutions such as Reference suspensions I - IV, if needed, and water or the solvent used. In an automatically compensable apparatus being calibrated with turbidity known reference solutions, the measuring result is given in NTU and it can be compared directly with required specified value.

NTU is often used as the unit in the turbidity determinations. It is the unit used in the case when the turbidity is estimated by the instrument which measures the $90 \pm 30°$ scattered light against the incident light intensity, using tungsten lamp, and in the case the estimation is performed by the instrument which measures the $90 \pm 2.5°$ scattered light against the incident light intensity using 860 nm infrared light, FNU is used as the unit. FNU is equivalent to NTU at a range of smaller measurements (less than 40 NTU). For the unit of formazin concentration, FTU is also used, which is defined as a suspension of 1 mg formazin in 1L of purified water is 1 FTU.

2.62 Mass Spectrometry

Mass spectrometry (MS) is a method to separate and detect the ions generated from the ionization of molecules according to their m/z values, and it is used for the identification and purity test of the substances. The m/z value is the dimensionless parameter obtained from dividing the relative mass (m) of the ion (the ratio of the mass of the ion to the unified atomic mass unit) by the charge number (z) of the ion. The unified atomic mass unit is defined as one-twelfth of the mass of a ^{12}C atom in its ground state, and it is used to express masses of atoms, molecules and ions. The result of measurement is shown as the mass spectrum in which the m/z values of the ions and the relative intensities of the signals corresponding to the ions are shown on the x-axis and the y-axis, respectively.

The precise mass of a molecule or an ion consisting of only a single isotope (usually, the isotope with the greatest natural abundance) of each element comprising a sample molecule is referred to as the ''monoisotopic mass.'' Usually not only a monoisotopic ion but also its isotopic ions are seen in the mass spectrum. The molecular mass of the sample substance can be determined from the m/z value of the molecular ion. When the fragment ions are observed, the molecular structure of the sample substance can be estimated and confirmed based on the masses of the fragment ions and the mass differences among the molecular ion and the fragment ions. In tandem mass spectrometry (MS/MS), the product ions, generated by the dissociation of the selected precursor ion with m/z value, are used for the mass spectrometry. The structural estimation and confirmation of the precursor ion can be performed using the m/z value of the product ion observed in the measurement. The schematic diagram of the MS and the MS/MS is shown in Fig. 2.62-1.

1. Mass Spectrometer

A mass spectrometer usually consists of a sample introduction unit, an ionization unit (ion source), a mass analyzer, a detector and data processor, and an exhaust system to maintain the mass analyzer under high vacuum (Fig. 2.62-1).

1.1. Sample Introduction

For the introduction of the sample into the ion source, the following methods are used; Direct infusion method, in which solution samples are injected into the ion source by using a syringe pump or capillary tip, for example; Direct inlet method, in which a liquid or solid sample is placed in a glass tube or other appropriate vessel and introduced into

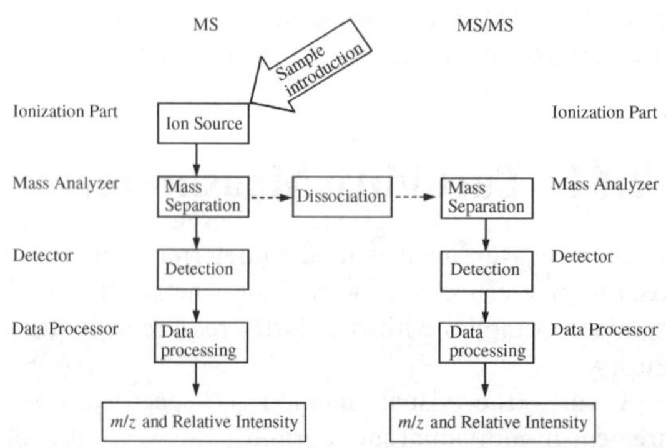

Fig. 2.62-1 Schematic diagram of mass spectrometry (MS) and tandem mass spectrometry (MS/MS)

the vicinity of the electron beams or reactant ion atmosphere of the ion source. In addition, the method, in which each component separated by the chromatographic technique such as gas chromatography or liquid chromatography and capillary electrophoresis is introduced into the ion source successively, is also used.

1.2. Ion Source

When the sample substances are introduced into the mass spectrometer, ions with a positive or negative charge are generated from the substance in the ion source. There are various ionization methods in mass spectrometry, and it is important to select the most suitable ionization method according to the polarity and molecular mass of the sample substance to be measured and the purpose of the measurement. Typical ionization methods are as follows.

1.2.1. Electron Ionization (EI) Method

In the EI method, the vaporized sample molecule (M) is ionized by receiving the energy of thermal electrons (usually, 70 eV), and the molecular ion ($M^{+\cdot}$) and fragment ions with the structural information of the sample molecule are generated. This method is suitable for ionizing nonpolar molecules such as volatile or gaseous samples with low molecular mass up to approximately 1000. It is used for the identification of substances using a data library or other source, because mass spectra with reproducible fragmentation patterns can be obtained by this method.

1.2.2. Chemical Ionization (CI) Method

In the CI method, the vaporized sample molecules are ionized through ion/molecule reactant with reaction ions generated from reagent gases such as methane, isobutane and ammonia. When a reagent gas is introduced into the ionization chamber, protonated ions of the molecules $[M + H]^+$, deprotonated ions of the molecules $[M - H]^-$ or reactant ion adducts of the molecules are generated. Since the ions generated by the CI method have internal energy values that are much lower than those obtained by the EI method, the fragmentation of sample molecules hardly occurs.

1.2.3. Electrospray Ionization (ESI) Method

When the sample solution is sprayed through a capillary with a tip to which high voltage is applied, atomized charged droplets are produced. Subsequently, the sample molecules will be ionized when the charge density of the droplets increases, accompanied by the evaporation of the solvent; $[M + H]^+$, $[M - H]^-$, or alkali metal ion adduct of the molecules is thus generated. This method is used for the ionization of sample substances from those with low molecular mass and relatively high polarity to those with high molecular mass. The ESI method can also be applied for the measurement of biopolymers such as peptides, proteins and polysaccharides, because the method makes it easy to generate multiply-charged ions such as $[M + nH]^{n+}$ and $[M - nH]^{n-}$.

1.2.4. Atmospheric Pressure Chemical Ionization (APCI) Method

In the APCI method, the sample solution is sprayed and vaporized by passing through a heated capillary using nitrogen as the carrier, and the corona discharge is induced at the time with a high-voltage needle electrode, and the solvent molecules are thus ionized. The sample molecules will be ionized through the ion/molecule reaction with the solvent ions, and $[M + H]^+$, $[M - H]^-$, or alkali metal ion adduct of the molecules will be generated. This method is suitable for ionizing nonpolar to highly polar compounds with a molecular mass up to approximately 1500.

1.2.5. Matrix-assisted Laser Desorption/Ionization (MALDI) Method

When a mixture of the sample and a matrix such as α-cyano-4-hydroxycinnamic acid or sinapinic acid is irradiated with a pulsed laser, the sample molecules will be vaporized quickly and ionized, accompanied by the electronic excitation of the matrix. At that time, the proton transfer occurs between the matrix and the sample molecules, and $[M + H]^+$, $[M - H]^-$, or alkali metal ion adduct of the molecules is generated. With the MALDI method, it is possible to ionize the compounds from low molecular mass of several hundreds to high molecular mass of several hundred thousand by selecting the appropriate matrix. Since the amount of the sample required for the measurement is very small, this method is used for the ionization of samples of biological origin such as peptides and proteins.

1.2.6. Other Ionization Methods

Various other ionization methods have been developed, including the field ionization (FI) method, the field desorption (FD) method, the fast atom bombardment (FAB) method, the secondary ion mass spectrometry (SIMS) method, the atmospheric pressure photoionization (APPI) method, and an ionization method in which the volatile substances on the material surface can be directly ionized using the ionization by the collision reaction with helium in the excited state in the open space.

1.2.7. Sample Introduction Method and Ionization Method

Each ionization technique is closely related to the sample introduction methods. In the case of the gas chromatography mass spectrometry (GC-MS), vaporized substances separated by a capillary column are directly introduced into a high-vacuum ion source and ionized by the EI method or CI method, for example. In the case of liquid chromatography mass spectrometry (LC-MS), the liquid phase containing sample substances separated by the LC column is sprayed under atmospheric pressure, and the sample substances are ionized by an ionization method described above at the interface to introduce the ions to the high-vacuum mass analyzer. At that time, it is necessary to ensure that the mobile phase to be used has an appropriate composition for both the column separation and the ionization. In the case of capillary electrophoresis mass spectrometry, the flow rate is usually adjusted by adding an appropriate solution to the electrolyte at the end of the capillary, and the sample substance is ionized by the ESI method or other ionization method.

1.3. Mass Analyzers

In a mass analyzer, the ions generated in the ion source are separated according to their m/z values. As a result, the mass and the relative abundance of the ions derived from the samples to be analyzed can be measured. The following mass analyzers are commonly used for MS.

1.3.1. Quadrupole (Q) Analyzer

The quadrupole (Q) analyzer has four rod electrodes set parallel to each other, to which high-frequency alternating current voltage is applied and on which direct current voltage is superimposed. The ions that enter this space oscillate according to their m/z values, and only ions with a specific m/z value have a stable trajectory and will be able to pass through the space. The ions with different m/z values can also become able to pass through the analyzer with a change in the applied voltage, and thereby the mass spectrum can be obtained. The mass resolving power of a Q analyzer is generally low, but Q analyzers are widely used for the qualitative and quantitative analyses as general-purpose equipment, since they have a relatively wide dynamic range and simple composition that can be downsized.

1.3.2. Ion-trap (IT) Analyzers

An ion-trap (IT) analyzer is made of an electric field or magnetic field or a combination of field, and is used to trap the ions in a space. The three most commonly used IT analyzers are as follows.

1.3.2.1. Paul Ion-trap

The Paul ion-trap is a synonym for quadrupole ion-trap (QIT). Although it is similar to the quadrupole analyzer in principle, it is able to trap ions stably by using ring electrodes and end-capped electrodes instead of rod electrodes. The trapped ions are discharged into the detector according to their m/z values by a scan of the high-frequency voltage, and thereby the mass spectrum can be obtained. This method is frequently used for qualitative analyses such as structure analysis because multiple-stage mass spectrometry (MS^n) can be achieved by using only one analyzer. The instrument with the sensitivity and dynamic range improved by using four electrodes with a hyperbolic surface is referred to as a linear ion-trap (LIT) analyzer.

1.3.2.2. Kingdon Trap

In the Kingdon trap analyzer, ions are trapped while rotating around a spindle-shaped electrode. The image current induced by the ions oscillating according to their m/z values is measured. The mass spectrum is obtained by Fourier-transforming the measured waveform data on the time axis to those on the frequency axis. This analyzer is used for qualitative analyses such as structure analyses because it has extremely high mass resolving power and mass accuracy.

1.3.2.3. Penning Ion-trap

The Penning ion-trap is used for Fourier transform-ion cyclotron resonance (FT-ICR). The ions that enter into the strong magnetic field formed by a superconducting magnet show cyclotron movement due to the effect of the Lorenz force. Here, the angular frequency (ω) can be expressed by the following equation.

$$\omega = qB/m$$

where m is the mass in atomic mass units of the ion, q is the electric charge of the ion, and B is the magnetic flux density. When the high-frequency electric field with this frequency is applied to the magnetic field, the ions move along the spiral orbital. These rotating ion groups induce the electric current, which changes periodically according to its respective m/z value in the detecting electrode. The mass spectrum can be obtained by Fourier-transforming the signals measured above and further converting the frequencies to the m/z values. The Penning ion-trap is used for precise structural studies in combination with various dissociation techniques for precursor ions, since an FT-ICR analyzer has extremely high mass resolving power and mass accuracy.

1.3.3. Time-of-flight (TOF) Analyzer

In the time-of-flight (TOF) analyzer, the ions are separated based on the difference of the flight times necessary for reaching the detector. For the ions with the mass m accelerated by the constant voltage V, the time t necessary for the ions to fly a distance L and reach the detector can be expressed by the following equation.

$$t = \sqrt{m/z} \times \frac{L}{\sqrt{2eV}}$$

The time of flight t is proportional to the square root of the m/z value, and consequently, the ions with smaller mass reach the detector faster. In the reflector mode in which the ions are reflected by the reflectron with the electrodes arranged side by side, high mass resolving power can be obtained by bringing the distribution of the kinetic energy of the ions into focus and doubling the flight distance of the ions. TOF analyzers are used for the analyses of high-molecular-mass compounds such as proteins in combination with the MALDI method and other techniques, since the mass range measurable by this method does not have a margin, theoretically. It is also frequently used for the qualitative analyses of low-molecular-mass substances, since it has high mass resolving power.

1.3.4. Magnetic Sector Analyzer

The ions that enter a magnetic sector analyzer are deflected by the Lorenz force of the magnetic field perpendicular to the ion current. At that time, ions with different m/z values (with the velocity v) fly into the magnetic field with different radii of curvature r according to the following equation.

$$r = \frac{mv}{qB}$$

Only ions with a specific m/z value are able to pass through the slit placed on the path of the ions. The mass spectrum can be obtained by scanning the magnetic flux density B, and introducing the ions with different m/z values passed through the slit into the detector in order. A magnetic sector analyzer is usually used as a double-focusing-type instrument in which the electric sector is combined with the magnetic sector, and the analyzer is used for both qualitative and quantitative analyses, since it has high mass resolving power and is also highly quantitative.

1.4. Detectors

Ions that have passed through a mass analyzer are usually transduced to the electric signal by releasing the electrons at the detector. The following detectors are in current use. In Fourier-transform-type instruments, the electric current induced by the movement of the ions at the detector is identified with a detection electrode.

1.4.1. Secondary Electron Multiplier (SEM)

A secondary electron multiplier (SEM) has a multistage arrangement of electrodes called dynodes. The secondary electrons emitted by the collision of the ions that enter the multiplier to the first dynode are sequentially multiplied, and finally transduced to the electric signal and recorded. This multiplying effect of the secondary electrons enables the detection of small amounts of ions.

1.4.2. Channel Electron Multiplier (CEM)

A channel electron multiplier (CEM) has a pipe-shaped channel configuration, and the secondary electrons are emitted by the collision of the ions that entered the multiplier to the inner wall of the channel. Multiple amplification is achieved by repeating this process at every opposite side of the inner wall. A CEM is simpler compared to SEMs, and with a CEM it is possible to downsize.

1.4.3. Microchannel Plate (MCP)

A microchannel plate (MCP) has a configuration in which many very small CEMs are accumulated to form a detector. It is used for the detector of TOF-type instruments, since an MCP has a wide ion-receiving surface, and the time dispersion of the secondary electrons is small because of the very thin structure of the MCP.

1.4.4. Faraday Cup (FC)

A Faraday cup (FC) is a simple detector that receives the charge of the ions that have entered an ion detector, and it transduces the charge to the electric current. It has a cup-shaped configuration so that the secondary electrons emitted from the ions can be captured.

2. Tandem Mass Spectrometers

Tandem mass spectrometry (TMS) is a technique in which precursor ions are selected from the fragment ions of the sample substance at the first-stage mass analyzer, and the product ions generated by dissociating the precursor ions are separated and detected at the second-stage mass analyzer. TMS is used for (1) the structural estimation and confirmation of fragment ions, and (2) specific and high sensitive analyses. There are two categories of TMS: TMA in space, and TMS in time.

With TMS in space, the selection of the precursor ions, the dissociation of the precursor ions, and the separation of the product ions are conducted at the first-stage mass analyzer, the intermediate region, and the second stage mass analyzer, respectively. With TMS in time, the selection/dissociation/separation of the ions are conducted at the different time zones in the same mass analyzer. TMS in space includes the triple quadrupole-type, quadrupole/time-of-flight-type, and time-of-flight/time of flight-type mass analyzers. The latter includes the ion-trap type mass analyzer, with which multiple-stage mass spectrometry (MS^n) can be performed by repeating the selection and dissociation of the precursor ions and the separation of the product ions multiple times.

2.1. Dissociation of Precursor Ions

2.1.1. Collision-induced Dissociation (CID)

In this dissociation method, a part or all of the collision energy is converted to the internal energy of the ions by the collision of the accelerated ions with the neutral collision gases (He, Ar, N_2, etc.), and subsequently the ions obtaining excess internal energy are excited and dissociated.

2.1.2. Post-source Decay (PSD)

In the MALDI method, the ions generated at the ionization source are dissociated during the interval between leaving the accelerating region and reaching the detector, due to the excess internal energy of the ions themselves or the collision with the residual gas. PSD is used for MS/MS using a reflectron time-of-flight mass spectrometer.

2.1.3. Others

Other dissociation methods are electron capture dissociation, electron transfer dissociation, infrared multiphoton dissociation, and surface-induced dissociation.

2.2. Constitutions of Principal Tandem Mass Spectrometers

2.2.1. Triple Quadrupole Mass Spectrometer (Q-q-Q)

A triple quadrupole mass spectrometer (Q-q-Q) has a configuration in which three quadrupoles are tandemly connected so that the first quadrupole is used for the selection of the precursor ions, the second quadrupole is used as the collision chamber for the dissociation of the precursor ions, and the third quadrupole is used for the mass separation of the product ions. Various scanning methods can be employed, and this type of spectrometer is frequently used for quantitative analyses in particular.

2.2.2. Quadrupole Time-of-flight Mass Spectrometer (Q-TOF)

A quadrupole time-of-flight mass spectrometer (Q-TOF) has a configuration in which the third quadrupole in the Q-q-Q is replaced with a TOF mass analyzer. The precursor ions are selected at the first quadrupole, and the separation of generated ions is conducted by the orthogonal-type TOF. Measurement with high sensitivity and high resolution is possible.

2.2.3. Time-of-flight Time-of-flight Mass Spectrometer (TOF-TOF)

A time-of-flight time-of-flight mass spectrometer (TOF-TOF) consists of a TOF analyzer in which the precursor ions are selected, the collision chamber, and a TOF analyzer in which the mass separation of the product ions is performed. It is used for MALDI-TOF-TOF mass spectrometry.

2.2.4. Other Mass Spectrometers

The mass spectrometers other than those described above are the four-sector mass spectrometer with the configuration in which two double-focusing instruments are connected, and the LIT-Kingdon trap and QIT-TOF, in which an in-time-type mass analyzer is used.

3. Methods Used for Measurement

3.1. Mass Spectrometry

The following measurement methods are used with mass spectrometry. An outline of the data obtained by each method is also described.

3.1.1. Total Ion Monitoring (TIM)

Total ion monitoring (TIM) is also known as the full-scan mode. It is the technique in which the mass spectrometer is operated so that all ions within the selected m/z range are detected and recorded, and the integrated value of the amounts of ions observed in each scanning is called the total ion current (TIC).

The chromatogram in which the total ion current obtained from the mass spectrum measured in LC-MS and GC-MS is plotted against the retention time is called the total ion current chromatogram (TICC), and the chromatogram in which the relative intensity at the specific m/z value is expressed as the function of time is called the extracted ion chromatogram (EIC).

3.1.2. Selected Ion Monitoring (SIM)

In selected ion monitoring (SIM), the mass spectrometer is operated so that only the ions with a specific m/z value are continuously detected and recorded instead of measuring the mass spectrum. SIM is used for the assay and high-sensitivity detection of sample substances in LC-MS and GC-MS.

3.2. Tandem Mass Spectrometry (TMS)

The following methods are used for measurements using TMS. An outline of the data obtained by each method is also described.

3.2.1. Product Ion Analysis

Product ion analysis is used to detect the product ions generated from the precursor ions with a selected m/z value, and with this method the sample's qualitative information can be obtained.

3.2.2. Precursor Ion Scan

Precursor ion scan is a method for scanning the precursor ions from which the product ions with a specific m/z value are generated by dissociation, and it is used for the specific detection of a substance with a specified substructure in the sample.

3.2.3. Constant Neutral Loss Scan

In constant neutral loss scan, the precursor ions that undergo the loss of specified mass (desorption of neutral species) due to dissociation are scanned. This method is used for the specific detection of substances with a specified substructure in the sample.

3.2.4. Selected Reaction Monitoring (SRM)

Selected reaction monitoring (SRM) detects product ions with a specific m/z value generated by the dissociation of the precursor ions with a specified m/z value, and it is used for the quantitative detection of trace amounts of substances present in a complex matrix. Although this method is similar to SIM, the specificity is improved by using the product ions generated from the precursor ions for the detection.

4. Application to Various Tests

In pharmaceutical analyses, mass spectrometry is used for the identification and purity tests of molecules as a specific detection method based on the mass and the structural information of the molecules.

4.1. Optimization of Instruments

In mass spectrometry, in order to obtain a good shape, sensitivity, and mass accuracy of the ion peak it is necessary to pre-optimize the measurement parameters of each component unit of the instrument by using an appropriate standard material in accord with the ionization method and mass range.

4.1.1. Tuning

The shape, sensitivity, and relative intensity of the ion peak detected are optimized by adjusting the parameters such as the gas pressure, temperature, and voltage of the ion source, mass analyzer, and detector. The various parameters of the ion source affect the generation of ion species, the species transported to the mass analyzer, and the relative intensity. The parameters related to the mass analyzer influence the peak width, mass accuracy, resolving power, and sensitivity, and the detector parameters affect the signal intensity and system sensitivity.

4.1.2. Calibration

The mass calibration of a mass spectrometer is carried out based on the mass of standard material. The reproducibility of the measurement mass values is affected by the electrical variation of the instrument, the surface cleanliness of each component unit such as the ion source, and the room temperature. There are the external and internal standard techniques for mass calibration. The number of points for the calibration differs according to the type of mass spectrometer.

4.1.3. Mass Resolving Power

The ability to separate two adjacent ion peaks from each other is referred to as the mass resolving power. Higher mass resolving power capacitates to separate and detect the ion peaks with a small mass difference. In magnetic-sector mass spectrometry, the mass resolving power R is calculated by the following equation when two peaks with the mass of M and $M + \Delta M$ overlap each other to 10% of either peak height.

$$R = M/\Delta M$$

When an instrument other than a magnetic-sector mass spectrometer is used, such as a quadrupole mass spectrometer or a time-of-flight mass spectrometer, the mass resolving power can usually be calculated by the method using peak width at half-height. When the width of the ion peak with the mass of m is Δm, the mass resolving power is calculated by $R = m/\Delta m$, and is discriminated from that of the magnetic-sector mass spectrometer.

4.2. Test for Identification

The identification of a test substance using mass spectrometry is usually performed by the confirmation of the mass of the test substance molecule. The test should be performed after confirming in advance that the measurement value is within the range specified in the monograph using the standard solutions defined in the monograph, or the specified ion can be detected. According to the mass resolving power of the instrument and the mass of the test substance molecule, the mass of the test substance molecule obtained from mass spectrometry can be adjusted to the monoisotopic mass or the average mass.

In general, the mass of the molecule consisting of only principle isotopes should be obtained from the monoisotopic peak. However, when the monoisotopic peak cannot be identified because, for example, the molecular mass is high or the resolution is not sufficient, the average mass should be calculated from the weighted average of the peak. When samples with high molecular mass such as proteins are analyzed by ESI/MS, the average mass should be calculated by the deconvolution technique, because the ESI mass spectra would show a series of multiply-charged ions with different charge states. It may be combined with the detection of the fragment ions or the product ions generated from the test substance molecule, which includes characteristic partial structural information.

4.3. Purity test

The purity test of a test substance using mass spectrometry is usually performed in combination with a separation technique such as chromatography using a standard solution with a concentration corresponding to the specified limit of the impurity in the sample. The peak responses of the molecular ions or the characteristic fragment ions and product ions generated from the specified impurity in the sample solution should be compared with those of the ions generated from the substance in the standard solution. To obtain more precise values, the method in which the stable isotope-labeled compound of the analyte is added to the sample solution as the internal standard is also important. When the test is performed using mass spectrometry in combination with, for example, chromatography, a system suitability test should also be required in accord with the chromatography.

2.63 Inductively Coupled Plasma-Atomic Emission Spectrometry and Inductively Coupled Plasma-Mass Spectrometry

Inductively coupled plasma-atomic emission spectrometry (ICP-AES) and inductively coupled plasma-mass spectrometry (ICP-MS) are elemental analysis methods in which inductively coupled plasma (ICP) is used as the excitation source or the ion source.

ICP is an excitation source composed of high-temperature argon plasma with intense thermal energy, which is formed by the inductive coupling method. The atoms contained in the sample solution are excited when the solution is sprayed into the plasma. ICP-AES is the method used to measure the atomic emission spectrum of the light emitted from the plasma at the time and to identify and analyze the contents of elements contained in the sample by determining the wavelength and intensity of its spectral lines. Since ICP is also a good ionization source, the atoms in the sample solution are ionized when the solution is sprayed into the plasma. ICP-MS is the method used to measure the mass spectrum of the element ions generated by ICP at the time by separating the element ions into those with each m/z value and counting the intensities of ion peaks using a mass spectrometer as the detector.

When intense energy is added to an atom from the outside, the peripheral electrons of the atom would transit to an excited state by absorbing certain energy. The electron in the excited state would release the absorbed energy as the light when it returns to its ground state. The light released at the time has a frequency ν (or wavelength λ) characteristic of each element. When h is Planck's constant and c is the velocity of light, the energy ΔE of the released light is expressed by the following equation.

$$\Delta E = h\nu = hc/\lambda$$

Since there are many excited states with various energy levels to which peripheral electrons might transit, many emission lines with various levels of energy can generate from one element, although some lines are strong and others are weak. However, there is only a limited number of emission lines observed in the ultraviolet/visible region and with enough sensitivity for the qualitative and quantitative analyses of each element. Since each element exhibits its own spectral line with a characteristic frequency (or wavelength) in the atomic emission spectrum, the elements contained in the sample solution can be identified by determining the wavelengths of spectral lines in the spectrum. Quantitative analyses of the elements in the sample solution can also be performed by determining the intensity of the spectral line characteristic of each element. The elemental analysis method using this principle is ICP-AES.

ICP-MS is the elemental analysis method alternative to optical analysis methods such as atomic absorption spectrometry and ICP-AES. In ICP-MS, the element ions generated by the ICP are separated into those with each m/z value and the intensities of the separated ions are counted with a mass spectrometer. Compared to ICP-AES, ICP-MS is higher sensitive, and with it an isotope analysis can be performed.

ICP-AES and ICP-MS are both excellent trace analysis methods specific for the inorganic impurities or coexisting elements in drug substances and drug products. Therefore, using these methods, qualitative and quantitative analyses can be performed not only for alkaline/alkaline-earth metals and heavy metals, but also for many elements for which adequate control is required to ensure the safety of pharmaceutical products. It would be useful for the quality assurance of drug substances to apply these methods to the profile analyses of inorganic elements contained in the substances, because these methods enable the simultaneous analysis of many elements.

1. Instruments

1.1. Instrument Configuration of ICP-AES

An ICP-AES is composed of an excitation source, a sample introduction system, a light emission unit, a spectroscope, a photometer and a data processor.

The excitation source consists of a high-frequency power generator, a control circuit to supply and control the electric energy to the light emission unit, and a gas source. The sample introduction system, the main components of which are a nebulizer and a spray chamber, is used for introducing sample solutions to the light emission unit after nebulizing the solutions.

The main components of the light emission unit, in which the elements containing in the sample solution are atomized and excited to induce light emission, are a torch and a high-frequency induction coil. The torch has a triple tube structure, and the sample solution is introduced through the central tube. Argon gas is used to form the plasma and to transport the sample solution. For the observation method of the light emitted from the light emission unit, there are two viewing modes: the lateral viewing mode in which the radial light of the plasma is observed, and the axial viewing mode in which the central light of the plasma is observed.

The spectroscope separates the light from the light emission unit to the spectral lines, and is composed of optical devices such as a light-converging system and diffraction grating. There are two types of spectrometers: wavelength-scanning spectrometers (monochromators) and simultaneously measuring spectrometers (polychromators) of the wavelength-fixed type. In addition, it is necessary to form a vacuum or to substitute the air in the chamber of the photometer with argon or nitrogen gas, when it is required to measure the spectral lines of the vacuum ultraviolet region (190 nm or shorter).

The photometer, which consists of a detector and a signal processing system, transduces the light energy of incident light to the electric signal proportional to the intensity of the light. For the detector, a photomultiplier or a semiconductor detector is used.

The data processor is used to process the data obtained by the measurements, and it displays the calibration curves and measurement results.

1.2. Instrument Configuration of ICP-MS

An ICP-MS system is composed of an excitation source, a sample introduction system, an ionization port, an interface, an ion lens, a mass analyzer, an ion detector and a data processor.

The excitation source, sample introduction system and ionization port have the same configuration as their counterparts in an ICP-AES system.

The interface is the boundary component for introducing the ions generated by the plasma under atmospheric pressure into a high-vacuum mass analyzer, and is composed of the sampling cone and skimmer cone.

The ion lens brings the ions introduced via the interface into focus and helps introduce the focused ions into the mass analyzer efficiently.

For the mass analyzer, a common choice is a quadrupole mass analyzer. The interference caused by the polyatomic ions described later can be suppressed by placing a collision/reaction cell within the vacuum region before the mass analyzer, and introducing a gas such as hydrogen, helium, ammonia or methane into the cell.

The ion detector transduces the energy of the ions that reached the detector to an electric signal which is amplified by the multiplier. The data processor is used to process the data of the electric signal from the ion detector, and to display the calibration curves and measurement results, etc.

2. Pretreatment of Sample

When the samples to be analyzed are organic compounds such as pharmaceutical drug substances, they are usually digested and ashed by the dry ash method or the wet digestion method, and the sample solutions for ICP-AES or ICP-MS are prepared by dissolving the residues in small quantities of nitric acid or hydrochloric acid. When a sample is difficult to digest in the usual manner, the sample can be sealed in a closed, pressurized container and digested using microwave digestion equipment. Although liquid samples containing small amounts of organic solvents can be introduced directly into an ICP-AES or ICP-MS instrument without pretreatment, another alternative is introducing oxygen as the option gas to prevent the build-up of carbon generated from the solvent onto the torch and the interface by contributing to the incineration of organic solvents.

3. Operation of ICP-AES

The operation of an ICP-AES system is as follows. The argon plasma is formed by setting the argon gas flow at the specified rate and turning the high-frequency power source on. After confirmation that the state of the plasma is stable, a quantity of the sample solution or the standard solution prepared by the method prescribed in the monograph is introduced into the instrument via the sample injection port, and the emission intensity of the analytical line specified for the element is measured. When it is necessary to perform a test for the confirmation or identification of some elements, the emission spectrum in the wavelength range in which analytical lines specified for the elements that appear is measured.

3.1. Performance Evaluations of Spectrometers

Since each spectrometer requires its own calibration method that accords with its properties, a wavelength calibration must be performed according to the procedure indicated by the manufacturer.

For expressing the wavelength-resolving power of a spectrometer, the half height width of the analytical line in the emission spectrum of a specified element is usually defined in the form of "not more than xxx nm (a constant value)." The following emission lines, from the line with a low wavelength to that with a high wavelength, are usually selected for the above purpose: arsenic (As: 193.696 nm), manganese (Mn: 257.610 nm), copper (Cu: 324.754 nm) and barium (Ba: 455.403 nm).

3.2. Optimization of Operating Conditions

The operating conditions usually adopted are as follows. The operating conditions of the instrument should be optimized after stabilizing the state of the plasma by warming up the instrument for 15 - 30 min. The operating parameters should usually be set as follows: high frequency power, 0.8 - 1.4 kW; argon gas flow rate, 10 - 18 L/min for the coolant gas (plasma gas), 0 - 2 L/min for the auxiliary gas, and 0.5 - 2 L/min for the carrier gas. In the lateral viewing mode, the point for measuring the light emitted from the plasma should be set within the range of 10 - 25 mm from the top edge of the induction coil, and the aspiration rate of the sample solution should be set at 0.5 - 2 mL/min. In the axial viewing mode, the optical axis should be adjusted so that the maximum value can be obtained for the intensity of emission line measured. The integration time should be set within the range of one to several tens of seconds, taking the stability of the intensity of the emission line measured into account. When a test using an ICP-AES system is defined in a JP monograph, the operating conditions such as the analytical line (nm), high-frequency power (kW), and argon gas flow rate (L/min) should be prescribed in the monograph. However, it is necessary to optimize the operating conditions individually for each instrument and for each viewing mode used for the measurement.

3.3. Interference and Its Suppression or Correction

In the term ICP-AES, the word "interference" is used as a general term that indicates the influence of the coexisting components or matrix on the measurement results. Various interferences are roughly classified as either non-spectral interference (such as physical interference and ionization interference) or spectral interference. Their effects can be eliminated or reduced by applying the appropriate suppression or correction methods for the measurement.

Physical interference means that the measurement results are influenced by the difference between the spray efficiencies of the sample solution and the standard solution used for its calibration in the light emission unit, when the physical properties (such as viscosity, density and surface tension) of the solutions differ. The effective methods for eliminating or reducing this type of physical influence are as follows. The sample solution should be diluted to the level at which such interference will not occur; the properties between the sample solution and the standard solution used for its calibration should be matched as much as possible (matrix-matching method); and the internal standard method (intensity ratio method) or the standard addition method should be used.

Ionization interference indicates the influence due to the change in the ionization rate caused by the increase of electron density in the plasma, which is induced by a large number of electrons generated from the elements coexisting in the sample solution at a high concentration. The suppression or correction method against the ionization interference is essentially the same as the method used in the case of physical interference. The measurement conditions with low ionization interference can also be set by the selection and adjustment of the observation method of emitted light, the height for viewing, high-frequency power and carrier gas flow rate, and so on.

Spectral interference is the phenomenon which influences the analytical results of the sample by overlapping the various emission lines and/or the light with a continuous spectrum with the analytical line of the analyte element. To avoid this type of interference, it is necessary to select another analytical line which will not suffer from the spectral interference. However, when no suitable analytical lines can be found, it is necessary to carry out the correction of the spectral interference. In addition, when the pretreatment of the organic samples is not sufficient, the molecular band spectra (NO, OH, NH, CH, etc.) derived from nitrogen, oxygen, hydrogen and carbon remaining in the sample solution might appear at the wavelength close to the analytical line of the analyte element, and could interfere with the analysis.

4. Operation of ICP-MS

In the operation of an ICP-MS system, after the confirmation that the state of the plasma is stable, the optimization of the instrument is performed and the system's suitability is confirmed. A quantity of the sample solution or the standard solution prepared by the method prescribed in the monograph is introduced, and the ion count numbers of the signal at the *m/z* value specified for the analyte element are determined. When it is necessary to perform a test for the confirmation or identification of some elements, the mass spectrum in the *m/z* value range specified for the analyte elements is measured.

4.1. Performance Evaluation of Mass Spectrometer

The performance evaluation items for mass spectrometers are the mass accuracy and the mass resolving power. The mass accuracy should be adjusted by matching the *m/z* value of the mass axis of the mass analyzer to that of the standard element in the standard solution for the optimization specified in the operating conditions section of the monograph. With quadrupole mass spectrometers, it is preferable that the mass accuracy be within ± 0.2. For the mass resolving power, it is preferable that the peak width at 10% of the peak height in the observed ion peak is not more than 0.9.

4.2. Optimization of Operating Conditions

When a limit test or a quantitative test is performed, the sensitivity, background and generation ratio of oxide ions and doubly charged ions defined below should be optimized previously to assure that the performance of the instrument is suitable. For the optimization of operating conditions, the solutions of the elements which represent the low mass number elements, intermediate mass number elements and high mass number elements and are unlikely to be contaminated from the environment (e.g., ^{7}Li, ^{9}Be, ^{59}Co, ^{89}Y, ^{115}In, ^{140}Ce, ^{205}Tl and ^{209}Bi) are usually used as the standard solutions after adjusting to adequate concentrations.

The sensitivity is evaluated by the ion count numbers per second of integration time (cps). When a limit test or quantitative test is performed, it is preferable to have the sensitivity of several tens of thousands cps per 1 μg/L (ppb) for each element with a low mass number, intermediate mass number or high mass number.

For the background, it is preferable to be not more than 10 cps, when the measurement is performed at the *m/z* value at which no elements exist naturally (e.g., *m/z* value of 4, 8 or 220).

For the generation ratio of oxide ions and doubly charged ions, the count numbers of oxide ions (e.g., ^{140}Ce: $^{140}Ce^{16}O^{+}$, *m/z* 156), doubly charged ions ($^{140}Ce^{2+}$, *m/z* 70) and monovalent ions ($^{140}Ce^+$, m/z 140) should be measured, and the generation ratios are calculated by dividing the ion count number of the oxide ions and doubly charged ions by that of the monovalent ions. It is preferable that the generation ratio of oxide ions (i.e., $^{140}Ce^{16}O^+/^{140}Ce^+$) is not more than 0.03 and that of doubly charged ions (i.e., $^{140}Ce^{2+}/^{140}Ce^+$) is not more than 0.05.

4.3. Interferences and their Suppression or Correction

In measurements using ICP-MS, attention must be paid to spectral interference and non-spectral interference.

Spectral interference includes isobaric interference and the interference caused by overlapping the mass spectrum of the analyte element with those of polyatomic ions or doubly charged ions. Isobaric interference is the interference by the isobaric element with the atomic mass adjacent to that of the analyte element, for example, the overlap of ^{40}Ar with ^{40}Ca and ^{204}Hg with ^{204}Pb. Since argon plasma is used as the ionization source, the polyatomic ions such as $^{40}Ar^{16}O$, $^{40}Ar^{16}O^1H$, $^{40}Ar_2$ might be generated, and they would interfere with the measurements of ^{56}Fe, ^{57}Fe and ^{80}Se, respectively. When an instrument equipped with a collision/reaction cell is used, these polyatomic ions can be decreased in the cell. Doubly charged ions are the ions exhibiting their ion peaks at 1/2 the m/z value of the corresponding monovalent ions, and the interference might occur when the element with an isotope with the mass number twice that of the analyte element might be present in the sample solution.

Non-spectral interference includes not only the physical interference and the ionization interference as in the case of the ICP-AES, but also the matrix interference unique to ICP-MS. Matrix interference is the phenomenon in which the ion count numbers of every analyte element generally decrease when large amounts of other elements might coexist in the sample solution. This tendency becomes more significant when the mass number of a co-existing element is larger and its concentration is higher, and when the mass number of the analyte element is smaller. The extent of non-spectral interference can be estimated based on the recovery rate obtained by adding a known amount of the analyte element to the unknown sample. When it is found that the recovery rate is low and the reliability of the analysis is not assured, the correction should be carried out by using the internal standard method or the standard addition method. For ICP-MS in particular, the influence of non-spectral interference can be reduced by using the isotope dilution method.

5. System Suitability

When a limit test or quantitative test is performed using these methods, it is necessary to confirm that the performance of the instrument is suitable by carrying out a system suitability test as defined below in advance of the limit test or quantitative test.

5.1. Evaluation for Required Detectability and Linearity

In an evaluation of an ICP-MS system for the required detectability and linearity, a solution is prepared in which the analyte element is not contained and the standard solution with the concentration of the specification limit of the analyte element, and these solutions are used as the blank solution and the solution for the system suitability test, respectively. The spectra obtained with these solutions are measured according to the test conditions optimized individually for each instrument, and it must be confirmed whether the emission line (or ion peak) of the analyte element is clearly observed at the specified wavelength (or m/z value) in the solution for system suitability test when compared with the blank solution. In this regard, the limit of the analyte element should be specified at the concentration of more than the quantitation limit (10σ). The test for required detectability is not required in the assay.

For the evaluation of linearity, it should be confirmed that the correlation coefficient of the calibration curve prepared by the procedure described in the section below, "6.2. Quantitative Analysis" is not less than 0.99. The confirmation of linearity is not required in quantitative analyses in the section 6.1. or when isotope dilution in the section 6.2. is performed.

5.2. Evaluation for System Repeatability

Unless otherwise specified, when the test is repeated six times using the solution with the lowest concentration among those used for plotting the calibration curve according to the test conditions optimized individually for each instrument, it should be confirmed that the relative standard deviation of the observed values for the emission intensity (or ion count number) of the analyte element is not more than the specified value (e.g., not more than 3% for an assay, and not more than 5% for a purity test).

6. Qualitative and Quantitative Analyses

6.1. Qualitative Analyses

In ICP-AES, when the wavelengths and relative emission intensities of multiple emission lines from the sample solution conform to those of the emission lines from the elements contained in the standard solution, the presence of the elements can be confirmed. In addition, the library of ICP-emission spectra attached to each instrument or the wavelength table of the spectra can also be used instead of the standard solution. Since the mass number region covering all the elements can be scanned in a short time in ICP-MS, the elements contained in the sample solution can be analyzed qualitatively based on the m/z value of the ion peak in the mass spectrum obtained from the sample solution.

It would be feasible to list the metal catalysts and inorganic elements that might be contained in the sample as impurities, and for some elements (such as arsenic and lead) it might be necessary to monitor them in a routine manner from the point of view of safety, and to carry out the profile of these inorganic impurities as a part of the manufacturing controls for a drug substance. In addition, the standard solution of each element should be prepared at an appropriate concentration considering the acceptance limit of each element to be specified separately.

6.2. Quantitative Analyses

The quantitative analysis of an inorganic element in the sample solution is usually performed by one of the following methods based on the emission intensity or ion count numbers obtained by the integration of measurement data in a specified time.

(i) Calibration curve method: Prepare standard solutions for plotting a calibration curve with different concentrations (four or more) of the analyte element. Using these standard solutions, the emission intensities at the analytical line specified for the analyte element by ICP-AES or the ion count numbers at the m/z value specified for the analysis of the element by ICP-MS are measured. The data obtained are then plotted against the concentrations, and this plot is used as the calibration curve. The concentration of the analyte element in the sample solution is determined by using this calibration curve.

(ii) Internal standard method: Prepare standard solutions for plotting a calibration curve with a fixed concentration of the internal standard element and different concentrations (four or more) of the analyte element. Using these standard solutions, the ratios of the emission intensities (or ion count numbers) of the analyte element to those of the internal standard element are determined. The data obtained are plotted against the concentrations, and this plot is used as the calibration curve. The internal standard element is also added to the sample solution, so that the concentration of internal standard element in the solution becomes the same as that in the standard solution. The concentration of the analyte element in the sample solution is determined by using the calibration curve plotted above.

Before this method is applied, it is necessary to verify that the internal standard element to be added is not contained in the sample solution. If the internal standard element to be added is present in the sample solution, it is necessary to verify that the contaminated amount of standard element is negligible compared to the amount to be added. In addition, in ICP-AES, the following requirements are to be met for the internal standard element: the changes in the emission intensity due to the measurement conditions and properties of the solution should be similar to those of the analyte element, and the emission line which does not cause spectral interference to the analytical line of the analyte element should be selected for the analysis. In contrast, in ICP-MS, it is preferable to select an internal standard element which does not cause spectral interference to the analyte element and has the ionization efficiency and mass number equivalent to the analyte element.

(iii) Standard addition method: Take 4 portions or more of the sample solution with the same volume, and prepare the following solutions; the solution in which the analyte element is not added; the standard solutions for plotting calibration curve in which the analyte element is added at different concentrations (3 or more). Measure the emission intensities at the specified analytical line or the ion count numbers at the specified m/z value for these solutions. Plot the obtained data against the concentrations calculated from the added amount of the analyte element. Calibrate the concentration of the analyte element in the sample solution from the absolute value of the horizontal axis (concentration)-intercept of the regression line.

In ICP-AES, this method is useful for the correction of non-spectral interference caused by coexisting substances in the sample solution, and it is applicable only to the cases in which spectral interference does not exist, or the background and the spectral interference are exactly corrected and the relationship between the emission intensity and the concentration shows good linearity. In ICP-MS, this method is useful for the correction of non-spectral interference caused by coexisting substances in the sample solution, and it is applicable only to the cases in which the spectral interference is exactly corrected and the relationship between the ion count number and the concentration shows good linearity down to the low concentration region.

(iv) Isotope dilution method: Isotope dilution method is applicable only to the ICP-MS. The concentration of the analyte element is determined from the change of the isotope composition ratio of the element by adding a substance containing a concentrated isotope with a known isotope composition that is different from the natural composition to the sample solution. It is applicable only to the element which has two or more stable isotopes naturally and is able to perform the isotope analysis. It is the feature of this method that the analytical precision is high and is not influenced by non-spectral interference, because the quantitation can be performed only by adding an adequate amount of a substance containing a concentrated isotope and measuring the isotope composition ratio of the sample solution.

7. Note

Water and reagents and the standard solutions used in this test are as follows.

(i) For water, water for an ICP analysis should be used. It should be verified prior to the test that the impurities contained in the water do not interfere with the analysis of the analyte element. Here, the water for an ICP analysis has the electric conductivity of 1 μS·cm^{-1} or less (25°C).

(ii) Reagents that are suitable for ICP analyses and are of high quality should be used.

(iii) For argon gas, either liquefied argon or compressed argon gas with the purity of 99.99 vol% or higher should be used.

(iv) For the standard solutions, they should be prepared by diluting the Standard Solution (e.g., the Standard Solution defined in the JP, or a standard solution with a concentration certified by a public institution or scientific organization) to the specified concentration using the water for ICP analysis. However, in cases in which interference with the analysis might occur, it is preferable to match the properties of the standard solution to those of the sample solution.

(v) When a standard solution containing multiple elements is prepared, a combination of the test solutions and elements should be selected so that precipitation and/or mutual interference does not occur.

2.64 Glycosylation Analysis of Glycoprotein

Glycosylation analysis is a method to confirm the consistency of the oligosaccharides attached to glycoprotein drug. The main types of oligosaccharides observed in glycoprotein drug are N-linked oligosaccharides, which are attached to asparagine residue, and O-linked oligosaccharides, which are attached to serine or threonine residues. Oligosaccharides have a diverse variety in structure, and attached oligosaccharides may be heterogeneous even in same glycoprotein and at same attachment site. Glycoprotein generally consists of a mixture of heterogeneous molecules (glycoforms), which differ only in glycosylation. Some oligosaccharides of glycoprotein may involve in stabilization of glycoprotein structure, prevention of enzymatic degradation, modulation of the biological activities, clearance from the bloodstream, intake into the cell, and immunogenicity. Since the oligosaccharide structures and their heterogeneity in the recombinant glycoproteins may change depending on the cell lines, culture conditions, etc., it is important to ensure consistency of the glycosylation for ensurement of the efficacy and safety of glycoprotein drug. Methods to evaluate the glycosylation of glycoprotein are classified into 1) analysis of released monosaccharides obtained after degradation of glycoprotein (monosaccharide analysis), 2) analysis of released oligosaccharides obtained from the glycoprotein (oligosaccharide analysis/oligosaccharide profiling), 3) analysis of glycopeptides obtained after proteolytic treatment of the glycoprotein (glycopeptide analysis), and 4) analysis of intact glycoprotein (glycoform analysis). In the setting specification for glycosylation analysis, methods should be properly selected and used alone or in combination, in consideration of the structural characteristics in the oligosaccharides, which affect efficacy and safety of the substance being tested.

1. Monosaccharide analysis

Monosaccharide analysis is a method to provide the information of the identity and contents of monosaccharides, which constitute the oligosaccharides attached to the glycoprotein drugs, etc. The kind of the monosaccharides that constitute oligosaccharide is limited. Typically, amino sugars, such as *N*-acetyl glucosamine and *N*-acetyl galactosamine, neutral sugars, such as galactose, mannose, glucose and fucose, and sialic acids, such as *N*-acetyl neuraminic acid and *N*-glycolyl neuraminic acid, may be analyzed. Monosaccharide analysis consist of releasing monosaccharides from the glycoprotein and quantitative analysis of released monosaccharides. Monosaccharide analysis is generally performed after isolation and purification of the glycoprotein using appropriate methods, because excipients and salts can interfere the analysis.

1.1. Release of monosaccharides

1.1.1. Neutral and amino sugars

Neutral and amino sugars are generally released by acid hydrolysis. The hydrolysis rate is dependent on the identity of monosaccharide and linkage, and the degradation rate of released monosaccharide is different between the individual monosaccharides. Thus, the conditions of acid hydrolysis should be optimized in order to release and recover the monosaccharides with high efficiency. Standard materials of neutral and amino sugars should be treated as tested samples.

1.1.2. Sialic acids

Sialic acids are released by mild acid hydrolysis or sialidase digestion, because they are labile. In general, sialidases with broad substrate specificity, such as those from *Arthrobacter ureafaciens* or *Clostridium perfringens* may be used.

1.2. Quantitative analysis of monosaccharides

Released monosaccharides are quantitatively analyzed by several methods, including high-pH anion-exchange chromatography/pulsed amperometric detection as underivatized monosaccharides, and liquid chromatography with fluorometric or UV detection after derivatization. Content of each monosaccharide is determined by internal standard method or absolute calibration method. For derivatization of neutral and amino sugar, 2-aminobenzoic acid, 2-aminopyridine, ethyl 4-aminobenzoate, 3-methyl-1-phenyl-5-pyrazolone may be used. For derivatization of sialic acid, 1,2-diamino-4,5-methylenedioxybenzene, or 1,2 phenylenediamine can be used. Analysis of derivatized monosaccharides can be performed by reversed-phase chromatography or anion-exchange chromatography with formation of borate complexes, etc. The analytical results are typically expressed as molar ratio of individual monosaccharide to glycoprotein, and then confirmed to be within the specified criteria.

2. Oligosaccharide analysis/Oligosaccharide profiling

Oligosaccharide analysis is a method to confirm consistency of the oligosaccharide identities, structures and distribution. Oligosaccharides attached to glycoprotein are released by enzymatic or chemical treatments, and then the released oligosaccharides were analyzed using liquid chromatography *<2.01>*, capillary electrophoresis, mass spectrometry *<2.62>* and in combination of them as underivatized or derivatized for the purpose of improvement in sensitivity and separation. The analytical results were obtained as chromatogram, electropherogram or mass spectrum, respectively, and they are referred to as oligosaccharide profile which provides oligosaccharide identities and distribution. If oligosaccharide profiling is performed after decreasing heterogeneity by exoglycosidase digestions for insufficient resolutions due to high oligosaccharide heterogeneity, the relationship of oligosaccharide structures to the efficacy and safety of the therapeutic glycoprotein are considered, and enzymes should be selected so that structures to be evaluated are not lost.

2.1. Release and purification of oligosaccharides

Enzymatic or chemical treatment are used for releasing oligosaccharides from the glycoprotein. N-linked oligosaccharides are released by peptide N-glycosidase digestion or hydrazinolysis, and O-linked oligosaccharides are released by alkaline β-elimination, hydrazine degradation, and endo O-glycanase. Because releasing efficacy may be affected by identity of protein, glycosylation sites and oligosaccharide structure, releasing conditions should be optimized for each glycoprotein. Careful attention should be taken to the possibility of structural changes in oligosaccharides, such as loss of sialic acids, anomerization at reducing end residues, and successive degradation from reducing end (peeling reaction).

There are several methods to recover the oligosaccharides from the reaction mixtures after releasing, including depletion of protein by ice-cold ethanol precipitation and then extraction from the supernatant, and solid phase extraction using a media, which oligosaccharides have adsorption to, etc. Reproducibility of oligosaccharide recovery should be evaluated, and it should be confirmed that recovery does not differ between oligosaccharides.

2.2. Analysis of released oligosaccharides

Derivatization of released oligosaccharides is usually carried out by reacting aldehyde group at reducing end with derivatizing agent. Given that oligosaccharide react with derivatizing agent stoichiometrically, relative peak responses may suggest molar ratios of the oligosaccharides attached to the glycoprotein. It should be confirmed that derivatizing method has sufficient reaction yield and reproducibility, and that structural changes during derivatization, such as loss of sialic acid residues, are at minimum. If needed, excessive reagents are removed or derivatized oligosaccharides are purified not to affect the test results. It should be confirmed that oligosaccharide profile does not change due to different recovery rates. Test methods should be appropriately selected considering structures and distribution of oligosaccharides which affect efficacy and safety.

Oligosaccharide profile obtained from the product under test is compared with that of reference material, treated in the same conditions, and then it is confirmed that peaks of oligosaccharides that is considered important for efficacy and safety are comparable from the view point of peak position and peak response by visual inspection. Otherwise, relative abundance of each oligosaccharide is calculated as a percentage of the total peak response or as a relative peak response, and then it is confirmed to be within the specified range.

2.2.1. Liquid chromatography *<2.01>*

Oligosaccharides derivatized with a tag, such as 2-aminobenzamide, 2-aminobenzoic acid, 2-aminopyridine, or others, may be separated by chromatography based on hydrophilic interaction, reversed-phase, ion-exchange, or mix mode of them, and then detected using fluorometric detector. Underivatized oligosaccharides may be analyzed using high-pH anion-exchange chromatography/pulsed amperometric detection. Analytical methods should be selected and optimized according to the characteristics of the oligosaccharides to be tested.

2.2.2. Capillary electrophoresis

Derivatizing agents with multiple negative charges, such as 8-aminopyrene-1,3,6-trisulfonic acid, are often used for analysis of lower sialylated oligosaccharides, to reduce the time required for analysis. Derivatizing agents with low negative charge, such as 2-aminobenzoic acid may be used for analysis of highly sialylated oligosaccharides in order to achieve the separation based on the number of sialylation. Electrolyte buffer containing borate may be used for adding negative charge and increasing resolution by forming oligosaccharide-borate complex. Derivatized oligosaccharides are separated by capillary zone electrophoresis using appropriate electrolyte buffer, and then detected using laser-induced fluorometric detector, etc. In general, capillary is used with the inner wall surface modified using neutral polymers covalently or dynamically in order to prevent electroosmotic flow. pH and compositions of the electrolyte are selected so that good separation is achieved.

2.2.3. Mass spectrometry <*2.62*>

Derivatized or underivatized oligosaccharides may be analyzed by mass spectrometer, where they are ionized by soft ionization techniques, such as electrospray ionization or matrix-assisted laser desorption/ionization, then separated based on m/z values, and detected. Both of positive and negative ion mode are available. Because ionization efficiency of oligosaccharides depends on their structures, ionization polarity should be selected according to the characteristics of the oligosaccharides. Mass spectrometry coupled with liquid chromatography or capillary electrophoresis provides not only elution time or migration time but also information of molecular mass, and allow us more specific oligosaccharide profiling. It is noted that the reproducibility of oligosaccharide profile obtained by mass spectrometry is lower than liquid chromatography and capillary electrophoresis, and that sialic acid residues in the sialo-oligosaccharides tend to be lost in positive ion mode. Mass spectrometry should be used with consideration of the characteristics of oligosaccharides responsible for efficacy and safety.

3. Glycopeptide analysis

Glycopeptide analysis is a method to provide the information about site-specific glycosylation properties, such as the degree of occupancy, oligosaccharide structures and heterogeneity. If particular oligosaccharides at specific sites affect biological activity or pharmacokinetics, glycopeptide analysis should be performed. Glycoprotein is digested by specific protease, and resultant mixture of glycopeptides and peptides are subjected to liquid chromatography coupled with mass spectrometer, and mass spectra of the glycopeptides are obtained. Glycopeptide ion is assigned based on masses of peptides and information of product ions obtained by tandem mass spectrometry or multiple-stage mass spectrometry. Glycopeptides may be fractionated by liquid chromatography, and then glycopeptides are subjected to mass spectrometry by offline coupling, or oligosaccharides released from glycopeptides were subjected to oligosaccharide analysis/oligosaccharide profiling using liquid chromatography or capillary electrophoresis.

4. Glycoform analysis of glycoprotein

Glycoform analysis is a method to confirm overall glycosylation characteristics and their consistency as glycoprotein. It is desirable to obtain the glycoform profiles to reflect oligosaccharide structures that play a role in efficacy and safety of the glycoprotein. If the degree of sialylation significantly contributes to the efficacy of the glycoprotein, isoelectric focusing, capillary isoelectric focusing, capillary zone electrophoresis, or ion-exchange chromatography, etc, may be performed to provide the charge-based glycoform profiles. Mass spectrometry provides the glycoform profiles based on molecular mass. Size-exclusion chromatography, capillary gel electrophoresis and SDS-PAGE may be useful for confirmation of the glycosylation status of a protein. Glycoform profile of the product under test is confirmed that peak position and response are comparable with that of similarly treated standard material, or that the distribution of glycoform is within the specified ranges. If glycoprotein has high molecular mass and/or many glycosylation sites, it may be difficult to separate each glycoform peak adequately. Separation and reproducibility of glycoform profile should be evaluated during method development.

2.65 Methods for Color Matching

Methods for Color Matching are applied to the purity test where the color of a test solution is examined by comparing with a matching fluid for color.

1. Matching fluids for color

Matching fluids for color A to T are prepared by measuring exactly the volume of three colorimetric stock solutions and water as directed in Table 2.65-1 with a buret or a pipet graduated to less than 0.1 mL, and mixing. Store the solutions in glass-stoppered bottles.

For each of the matching fluids of B-series (B1 to B9), BY-series (BY1 to BY7), Y-series (Y1 to Y7), GY-series (GY1 to GY7) and R-series (R1 to R7), the primary matching solutions for individual color are prepared first by mixing the three colorimetric stock solutions as directed in Table 2.65-2, then mix the primary matching solution for corresponding color as directed in Table 2.65-3 to prepare desired matching fluid for color.

2. Procedure

Compare a test solution with a matching fluid for color specified in monograph according to the following manners, and confirm that the test solution has no more color than the specified matching fluid for color.

When the matching fluids for color A to T are used, unless otherwise specified, place the test solution and the matching fluid for color in Nessler tubes, and view transversely against a white background.

When the matching fluids for color of B-series, BY-series, Y-series, GY-series or R-series are used, compare the color by the following two methods, and state the used method number in the monograph. A solution is *colourless* if it has the appearance of water or the solvent or is not more intensely coloured than matching solution B9.

Method 1: Place separately 2.0 mL each of a test solution and a reference liquid such as water, solvent or the matching fluid for color specified in the monograph in clear and colorless glass test tubes, 12 mm in outside diameter, and compare the color by viewing transversely against a white background under scattering light.

Method 2: Place separately a test solution and a reference liquid such as water, solvent or the matching fluid for color specified in the monograph in clear and colorless flat-bottom test tubes, 15 - 25 mm in internal diameter, so that the depth of the layer is 40 mm, and compare the color by viewing vertically against a white background under scattering light.

3. Colorimetric stock solutions

Cobalt (II) Chloride CS: Dissolve 65 g of cobalt (II) chloride hexahydrate in 25 mL of hydrochloric acid and water to make 1000 mL. Pipet 10 mL of this solution, add water to make exactly 250 mL. Pipet 25 mL of the solution, add 75 mL of water and 50 mg of murexide-sodium chloride indicator, and add dropwise diluted ammonia solution (28) (1 in 10) until the color of the solution changes from red-purple to orange-yellow. Titrate <*2.50*> with 0.01 mol/L disodium dihydrogen ethylenediamine tetraacetate VS until the color of

Table 2.65-1 Composition of matching fluids for color A to T

Matching fluid for color	Cobalt (II) Chloride CS (mL)	Iron (III) Chloride CS (mL)	Copper (II) Sulfate CS (mL)	Water (mL)
A	0.1	0.4	0.1	4.4
B	0.3	0.9	0.3	3.5
C	0.1	0.6	0.1	4.2
D	0.3	0.6	0.4	3.7
E	0.4	1.2	0.3	3.1
F	0.3	1.2	—	3.5
G	0.5	1.2	0.2	3.1
H	0.2	1.5	—	3.3
I	0.4	2.2	0.1	2.3
J	0.4	3.5	0.1	1.0
K	0.5	4.5	—	—
L	0.8	3.8	0.1	0.3
M	0.1	2.0	0.1	2.8
N	—	4.9	0.1	—
O	0.1	4.8	0.1	—
P	0.2	0.4	0.1	4.3
Q	0.2	0.3	0.1	4.4
R	0.3	0.4	0.2	4.1
S	0.2	0.1	—	4.7
T	0.5	0.5	0.4	3.6

Table 2.65-2 Primary matching solutions for color used for preparation of a series of matching fluids for color (B-series, BY-series, Y-series, GY-series, R-series)

Primary matching solutions for individual color	Volumes to mix (mL)			
	Iron (III) Chloride CS	Cobalt (II) Chloride CS	Copper (II) Sulfate CS	Diluted dilute hydrochloric acid 1 in 10
Brown primary matching solution	3.0	3.0	2.4	1.6
Brownish yellow primary matching solution	2.4	1.0	0.4	6.2
Yellow primary matching solution	2.4	0.6	0.0	7.0
Greenish yellow primary matching solution	9.6	0.2	0.2	0.0
Red primary matching solution	1.0	2.0	0.0	7.0

the solution changes from yellow to red-purple, after the addition of 0.2 mL of diluted ammonia solution (28) (1 in 10) near the end-point.

Each mL of 0.01 mol/L disodium dihydrogen ethylenediamine tetraacetate VS
= 2.379 mg of $CoCl_2.6H_2O$

According to the titrated value, add diluted hydrochloric acid (1 in 40) to make a solution containing 59.5 mg of

Table 2.65-3 Compositions of a series of matching fluids for color (B-series, BY-series, Y-series, GY-series, R-series)

Matching fluid for color	Volumes to mix (mL)	
	Primary matching solutions for individual color	Diluted dilute hydrochloric acid 1 in 10
	Brown primary matching solution	
B1	75.0	25.0
B2	50.0	50.0
B3	37.5	62.5
B4	25.0	75.0
B5	12.5	87.5
B6	5.0	95.0
B7	2.5	97.5
B8	1.5	98.5
B9	1.0	99.0
	Brownish yellow primary matching solution	
BY1	100.0	0.0
BY2	75.0	25.0
BY3	50.0	50.0
BY4	25.0	75.0
BY5	12.5	87.5
BY6	5.0	95.0
BY7	2.5	97.5
	Yellow primary matching solution	
Y1	100.0	0.0
Y2	75.0	25.0
Y3	50.0	50.0
Y4	25.0	75.0
Y5	12.5	87.5
Y6	5.0	95.0
Y7	2.5	97.5
	Greenish yellow primary matching solution	
GY1	25.0	75.0
GY2	15.0	85.0
GY3	8.5	91.5
GY4	5.0	95.0
GY5	3.0	97.0
GY6	1.5	98.5
GY7	0.75	99.25
	Red primary matching solution	
R1	100.0	0.0
R2	75.0	25.0
R3	50.0	50.0
R4	37.5	62.5
R5	25.0	75.0
R6	12.5	87.5
R7	5.0	95.0

cobalt (II) chloride hexahydrate ($CoCl_2.6H_2O$: 237.93) in each mL, and use. Store the solution in a glass-stoppered bottle.

Copper (II) Sulfate CS: Dissolve 65 g of copper (II) sulfate pentahydrate in 25 mL of hydrochloric acid and water to make 1000 mL. Pipet 10 mL of this solution, and add water to make exactly 250 mL. Pipet 25 mL of this solution, add 75 mL of water, 10 mL of a solution of ammonium chloride (3 in 50), 2 mL of diluted ammonia solution (28) (1 in 10) and 50 mg of murexide-sodium chloride indicator. Titrate

⟨2.50⟩ with 0.01 mol/L disodium dihydrogen ethylenediamine tetraacetate VS until the color of the solution changes from green to purple.

Each mL of 0.01 mol/L disodium dihydrogen ethylenediamine tetraacetate VS
= 2.497 mg of $CuSO_4.5H_2O$

According to the titrated value, add diluted hydrochloric acid (1 in 40) to make a solution containing 62.4 mg of copper (II) sulfate pentahydrate ($CuSO_4.5H_2O$: 249.69) in each mL, and use. Store the solution in a glass-stoppered bottle.

Iron (III) Chloride CS: Dissolve 55 g of iron (III) chloride hexahydrate in 25 mL of hydrochloric acid and water to make 1000 mL. Pipet 10 mL of this solution in an iodine flask, add 15 mL of water and 3 g of potassium iodide, stopper tightly, and allow to stand in a dark place for 15 minutes. Add 100 mL of water to the mixture, and titrate *⟨2.50⟩* the liberated iodine with 0.1 mol/L sodium thiosulfate VS (indicator: 1 mL of starch TS).

Each mL of 0.1 mol/L sodium thiosulfate VS
= 27.03 mg of $FeCl_3.6H_2O$

According to the titrated value, add diluted hydrochloric According to the titrated value, add diluted hydrochloric acid (1 in 40) to make a solution containing 45.0 mg of iron (III) chloride hexahydrate ($FeCl_3.6H_2O$: 270.30) in each mL, and use. Store the solution in a glass-stoppered bottle.

2.66 Elemental Impurities

I. Control of Elemental Impurities in Drug Products

1. Introduction

Elemental impurities in drug products may arise from several sources; they may be residues intentionally added such as catalysts in the synthetic process of drug substances, impurities from natural products contained in drug substances and excipients, etc., which are components of the drug product, and contaminants from manufacturing equipment and container/closure systems. The amounts of these impurities in drug products should be controlled within acceptable limits, except when they are stipulated in monographs.

The permitted daily exposures (PDEs) of elemental impurities are established to protect the health of all patients based on the evaluation of the toxic data of elemental impurities, and more strict limits are not needed if elemental impurities in drug products do not exceed the PDEs. In some cases, lower level of elemental impurities may be warranted when it is known that elemental impurities have been shown to have an impact on the quality attributes of the drug product (e.g., element catalyzed degradation of drug substances).

Elemental impurities in drug products are assessed and controlled based on a risk management approach.

2. Scope

The control of elemental impurities applies to drug products. It also applies to drug products containing purified proteins and peptides (including proteins and peptides produced from genetic recombinant or non-recombinant origins), their derivatives, and drug products which they are components (e.g., conjugates) are within the scope of this chapter, as are drug products containing synthetic peptides, polynucleotides, and oligosaccharides.

It does not apply to crude drugs, radiopharmaceuticals, vaccines, cell metabolites, DNA products, allergenic extracts, cells, whole blood, cellar blood components, plasma, blood plasma protein fraction preparations, blood preparations, dialysate solutions not intended for systematic circulation, and drug products based on genes (gene therapy), cells (cell therapy) and tissues (tissue engineering). Also, it does not apply to elements that are intentionally included in the drug product for therapeutic benefit.

3. The PDEs for Elemental Impurities for Oral, Parenteral and Inhalation Routes of Administration, and Element Classification

The PDEs of elemental impurities established for preparations for oral, parenteral and inhalation routes of administration are shown in Table 2.66-1. If the PDEs for the other administration route are necessary, generally consider the oral PDE as a starting point in the establishment, and assess if the elemental impurity is expected to have local effects when administered by the intended route of administration.

Parenteral drug products with maximum daily volumes up to 2 L may use the maximum daily volume to calculate permissible concentrations from PDEs. For products whose daily volumes or general clinical practice may exceed 2 L (e.g., saline, dextrose, total parenteral nutrition, solutions for irrigation), a 2-L volume may be used to calculate permissible concentrations from PDEs.

As shown in Table 2.66-1, elemental impurities are divided into three classes based on their toxicity (PDE) and likelihood of occurrence in the drug product. The likelihood of occurrence is derived from several factors, such as probability of use in pharmaceutical processes, elemental impurities in materials used in pharmaceutical processes, the observed natural abundance and environmental distribution of the

Table 2.66-1 PDEs for Elemental Impurities

Element	Class	Oral PDE (μg/day)	Parenteral PDE (μg/day)	Inhalation PDE (μg/day)
Cd	1	5	2	3
Pb	1	5	5	5
As	1	15	15	2
Hg	1	30	3	1
Co	2A	50	5	3
V	2A	100	10	1
Ni	2A	200	20	5
Tl	2B	8	8	8
Au	2B	100	100	1
Pd	2B	100	10	1
Ir	2B	100	10	1
Os	2B	100	10	1
Rh	2B	100	10	1
Ru	2B	100	10	1
Se	2B	150	80	130
Ag	2B	150	10	7
Pt	2B	100	10	1
Li	3	550	250	25
Sb	3	1200	90	20
Ba	3	1400	700	300
Mo	3	3000	1500	10
Cu	3	3000	300	30
Sn	3	6000	600	60
Cr	3	11000	1100	3

element.

Class 1: The elements, As, Cd, Hg, and Pb, are classified as this category and are human toxicant elements. As these elements are limited in the manufacture of pharmaceuticals, they are rarely used. Their presence in drug products usually comes from used materials such as mined excipients. These four elements require evaluation during the risk assessment, across all sources and routes of administration having possibility of contamination. Testing may be applied when the risk assessment identifies further control necessary to ensure that the PDE will be met, however it is not necessary for all components to determine for Class 1 elemental impurities.

Class 2: Elemental impurities classified as Class 2 have lower toxicity than the elements in Class 1, and are route-dependent human toxicants. These elements are further divided in 2A and 2B based on their relative likelihood of occurrence in the drug product. The class 2A elements are Co, Ni and V, which are known to exist naturally. These elements have relatively high probability of occurrence in drug products, and thus require evaluation during the risk assessment, across all potential sources and routes of administration. Because the Class 2B elements have the low probability of their existence in natural, they may be excluded from the risk assessment unless they are intentionally added during the manufacture of drug substances, excipients or other components of the drug product. The elemental impurities in Class 2B include Ag, Au, Ir, Os, Pd, Pt, Rh, Ru, Se and Tl.

Class 3: The elements in this class have relatively low toxicities by the oral route of administration, and their oral PDEs are more than 500 μg/day. For oral routes of administration, unless these elements are intentionally added, they do not need to be considered during the risk assessment. For parenteral and inhalation products, the potential for inclusion of these elemental impurities should be evaluated even in the case where they are not intentionally added, unless the route specific PDE is above 500 μg/day. The elements in this class include Ba, Cr, Cu, Li, Mo, Sb and Sn.

4. Risk Assessment and Control of Elemental Impurities

The technique of quality risk management should be considered in controls for elemental impurities in drug products, and the risk assessment should be based on scientific knowledge and principles. The risk assessment would be focused on assessing the levels of elemental impurities in a drug product in relation to the PDEs. Useful information for this risk assessment includes measured data of drug products and components, measured data and the risk assessment result supplied by drug substance and/or excipient manufacturers, and/or data available in published literature, but is not limited to them.

The risk assessment should be performed depending on the level of risk, and do not always require a formal risk management process. The use of informal risk management processes may also be considered acceptable.

4.1. General Principles

The risk assessment process consists of the following three steps.

1) Identify known and potential sources of elemental impurities that may find their way into the drug product.

2) Evaluate the presence of a particular elemental impurity in the drug product by determining the observed or predicted level of the impurity and comparing with the established PDE.

3) Summarize the risk assessment, and identify if controls built into the process are sufficient. Identify additional controls to be considered to limit elemental impurities in the drug product.

In many cases, the steps are considered simultaneously. The risk assessment may be iterated to develop a final approach to ensure the elemental impurities do not exceed the PDE certainly.

4.2. Sources of Elemental Impurities

In considering the production of a drug product, there are broad categories of potential sources of elemental impurities.

• Residual impurities resulting from elements intentionally added (e.g., metal catalysts) in the formation of the drug substance, excipients or other components. The risk assessment of the drug substance should be studied about the potential for inclusion of elemental impurities in the drug product.

• Elemental impurities that are not intentionally added and are potentially present in the drug substance, water or excipients used in the preparation of the drug product.

• Elemental impurities that are potentially introduced into the drug substance and/or drug product from manufacturing equipment.

• Elemental impurities that have the potential to be leached into the drug substance and drug product from container closure systems.

During the risk assessment, the potential contributions from each of these sources should be considered to determine the overall contribution of elemental impurities to the drug product.

4.3. Identification of Potential Elemental Impurities

Potential elemental impurities derived from intentionally added catalysts and inorganic reagents: If any element is intentionally added, it should be considered in the risk assessment.

Potential elemental impurities that may be present in drug substances and/or excipients: While not intentionally added, some elemental impurities may be present in some drug substances and/or excipients. The possibility for inclusion of these elements in the drug product should be reflected in the risk assessment.

Potential elemental impurities derived from manufacturing equipment: The contribution of elemental impurities from this source may be limited and the subset of elemental impurities that should be considered in the risk assessment will depend on the manufacturing equipment used in the production of the drug product. The specific elemental impurities of concern should be assessed based on the knowledge of the composition of the components of the manufacturing equipment that come in contact with components of the drug product. The risk assessment of this source of elemental impurities is one that can potentially be utilized for many drug products using similar process trains or processes.

In general, the processes used to prepare a given drug substance are considerably more aggressive than processes used in preparing the drug product when assessed relative to the potential to leach or remove elemental impurities from manufacturing equipment. Contributions of elemental impurities from drug product processing equipment would be expected to be lower than contributions observed for the drug substance. However, when this is not the case based on process knowledge or understanding, the potential for incorporation of elemental impurities from the drug product manufacturing equipment in the risk assessment (e.g., hot melt extrusion) should be considered.

Elemental impurities leached from container closure systems: The identification of potential elemental impurities that may be introduced from container closure systems should be based on a scientific understanding of likely interactions between a particular drug product type and its packaging. When a review of the materials of construction demonstrates that the container closure system does not contain elemental impurities, no additional risk assessment needs to be performed. It is recognized that the probability of elemental leaching into solid dosage forms is minimal and does not require further consideration in the risk assessment. For liquid and semi-solid dosage forms there is a higher probability that elemental impurities could leach from the container closure system during the shelf-life of the drug product. Studies to understand potential leachables from the container closure system (after washing, sterilization, irradiation, etc.) should be performed.

Factors that should be considered (for liquid and semi-solid dosage forms) are shown as follows, but are not limited.

- Hydrophilicity/hydrophobicity, Ionic content, pH, Temperature (cold chain vs room temperature and processing conditions), Contact surface area, Container/material composition, Terminal sterilization, Packaging process, Material sterilization, Duration of storage

Table 2.66-2 provides recommendations for inclusion of elemental impurities in the risk assessment. This table can be applied to all sources of elemental impurities in the drug product.

4.4. Evaluation

As the potential elemental impurity identification process is concluded, there are following two possible outcomes.

Table 2.66-2 Elements to be Considered in the Risk Assessment

Element	Class	If intentionally added (all routes)	If not intentionally added		
			Oral	Parenteral	Inhalation
Cd	1	○	○	○	○
Pb	1	○	○	○	○
As	1	○	○	○	○
Hg	1	○	○	○	○
Co	2A	○	○	○	○
V	2A	○	○	○	○
Ni	2A	○	○	○	○
Tl	2B	○	×	×	×
Au	2B	○	×	×	×
Pd	2B	○	×	×	×
Ir	2B	○	×	×	×
Os	2B	○	×	×	×
Rh	2B	○	×	×	×
Ru	2B	○	×	×	×
Se	2B	○	×	×	×
Ag	2B	○	×	×	×
Pt	2B	○	×	×	×
Li	3	○	×	○	○
Sb	3	○	×	○	○
Ba	3	○	×	×	○
Mo	3	○	×	×	○
Cu	3	○	×	○	○
Sn	3	○	×	×	○
Cr	3	○	×	×	○

○: necessary ×: unnecessary

1) The risk assessment process does not identify any potential elemental impurities.

2) The risk assessment process identifies one or more potential elemental impurities. For any elemental impurities identified in the process, the risk assessment should consider if there are multiple sources of the identified elemental impurity or impurities.

During the risk assessment, a number of factors that can influence the level of the potential elemental impurity in the drug product should be considered.

4.5. Summary of Risk Assessment Process

The risk assessment is summarized by reviewing relevant product or component specific data combined with information and knowledge gained across products or processes to identify the significant probable elemental impurities that may be observed in the drug product.

The significance of the observed or predicted level of the elemental impurity should be considered in relation to the PDE of the elemental impurity. As a measure of the significance of the observed elemental impurity level, a control threshold is defined as a level that is 30% of the established PDE in the drug product. The control threshold may be used to determine if additional controls may be required.

If the total elemental impurity level from all sources in the drug product is expected to be consistently less than 30% of the PDE, then additional controls are not required, provided adequate controls on elemental impurities are demonstrated by the appropriate assessment of the data.

If the risk assessment fails to demonstrate that an elemental impurity level is consistently less than the control threshold, controls should be established to ensure that the elemental impurity level does not exceed the PDE in the drug product.

The variability of the level of an elemental impurity should be factored into the application of the control threshold to drug products. Sources of variability may include the following.

- Variability of the analytical method
- Variability of the elemental impurity level in the specific sources
- Variability of the elemental impurity level in the drug product

For some components that have inherent variability (e.g., mined excipients), more data may be needed to apply the control threshold.

5. Converting between PDEs and Concentration Limits

The PDEs reported in μg per day (μg/day) give the maximum permitted quantity of each element that may be contained in the maximum daily dose of a drug product. Because the PDE reflects total exposure from the drug product, it is useful to convert the PDE into concentrations as a tool in evaluating elemental impurities in drug products or their components. Any of the following options may be selectable as long as the resulting permitted concentrations assure that the drug product does not exceed the PDEs. In the choice of a specific option the daily dose of the drug product needs to be determined or assumed.

Option 1: Common permitted concentration limits of elements across drug product components for drug products with daily doses of not more than 10 g: This option is not intended to imply that all elements are present at the same concentration, but rather provides a simplified approach to the calculations. The option assumes the daily dose of the drug product is 10 g or less, and that elemental impurities identified in the risk assessment (the target elements) are present in all components of the drug product. Using Equation (1) below and a daily dose of 10 g of drug product, this option calculates a common permissible target elemental concentration for each component in the drug product.

$$\text{Concentration } (\mu\text{g/g}) = \frac{PDE\ (\mu\text{g/day})}{\text{daily dose of drug product (g/day)}} \quad (1)$$

This approach, for each target element, allows determination of a fixed common maximum concentration in µg per g in each component.

The permitted concentrations are provided in Table 2.66-3.

If all the components in a drug product do not exceed the Option 1 permitted concentrations for all target elements identified in the risk assessment, then all these components may be used in any proportion in the drug product. If the permitted concentrations in Table 2.66-3 are not applied, Options 2a, 2b, or 3 should be followed.

Option 2a: Common permitted concentration limits of elements across drug product components for a drug product with a specified daily dose: This option is similar to Option 1, except that the drug daily dose is not assumed to be 10 g. The common permitted concentration of each element is determined using Equation (1) and the actual maximum daily dose. This approach, for each target element, allows determination of a fixed common maximum concentration in µg per g in each component based on the actual daily dose provided. If all components in a drug product do not exceed the Option 2a permitted concentrations for all target elements identified in the risk assessment, then all these components may be used in any proportion in the drug product.

Option 2b: Permitted concentration limits of elements in individual components of a drug product with a specified daily dose: Permitted concentrations based on the distribution of elements in the components (e.g., higher concentrations in components with the presence of an element in question) may be set. For each element identified as potentially present in the components of the drug product, the maximum expected mass of the elemental impurity in the final drug product can be calculated by multiplying the mass of each component material times the permitted concentration pre-established in each material and summing over all components in the drug product, as described in Equation (2). The total mass of the elemental impurity in the drug product should comply with the PDEs unless justified according to other relevant sections of this general information. If the risk assessment has determined that a specific element is not a potential impurity in a specific component, there is no need to establish a quantitative result for that element in that component. This approach allows that the maximum permitted concentration of an element in certain components of the drug product may be higher than the Option 1 or Option 2a limit, but this should then be compensated by lower allowable concentrations in the other components of the drug product. Equation (2) may be used to demonstrate that component-specific limits for each element in each component of a drug product assure that the PDE will be met.

$$PDE\ (\mu\text{g/day}) \geqq \sum_{k=1}^{N} C_k \cdot M_k \quad (2)$$

k = an index for each of N components in the drug product

C_k = permitted concentration of the elemental impurity in component k (µg/g)

M_k = mass of component k in the maximum daily dose of the drug product (g)

Option 3: Finished Product Analysis: The concentration of each element may be measured in the final drug product. Equation (1) may be used with the maximum total daily dose of the drug product to calculate a maximum permitted concentration of the elemental impurity.

Table 2.66-3 Permitted Concentrations of Elemental Impurities for Option 1

Element	Class	Oral Concentration (µg/g)	Parenteral Concentration (µg/g)	Inhalation Concentration (µg/g)
Cd	1	0.5	0.2	0.3
Pb	1	0.5	0.5	0.5
As	1	1.5	1.5	0.2
Hg	1	3	0.3	0.1
Co	2A	5	0.5	0.3
V	2A	10	1	0.1
Ni	2A	20	2	0.5
Tl	2B	0.8	0.8	0.8
Au	2B	10	10	0.1
Pd	2B	10	1	0.1
Ir	2B	10	1	0.1
Os	2B	10	1	0.1
Rh	2B	10	1	0.1
Ru	2B	10	1	0.1
Se	2B	15	8	13
Ag	2B	15	1	0.7
Pt	2B	10	1	0.1
Li	3	55	25	2.5
Sb	3	120	9	2
Ba	3	140	70	30
Mo	3	300	150	1
Cu	3	300	30	3
Sn	3	600	60	6
Cr	3	1100	110	0.3

6. Speciation and Other Considerations

Speciation is defined as the distribution of elements among chemical species based on the difference of molecular structure including ionic element, molecules, or complexes, reflecting isotopic composition, electronic or oxidation state. When the toxicities of different species of the same element are known to be different, the PDE has been established using the toxicity information on the species expected to be in the drug product.

When elemental impurity measurements are used in the risk assessment, total elemental impurity levels in drug products may be used to assess compliance with the PDEs. The identification of speciation is not particularly expected, however such information could be used to justify lower or higher levels when the identified species is more or less toxic, respectively, than the species used for the calculation of the PDEs.

When total elemental impurity levels in components are used in the risk assessment, providing information on release of an elemental impurity from the component in which it is found is not expected. However, such information could be used to justify levels higher than those based on the total elemental impurity content of the drug product.

7. Analytical Procedures

The determination of elemental impurities should be conducted using appropriate procedures suitable for their intended purposes. Unless otherwise justified, the test should be specific for each elemental impurity identified for control during the risk assessment. The following II. Elemental Impurities-Procedures or suitable alternative procedures (analytical procedures) for determining levels of elemental impurities should be used.

8. Lifecycle Management

If changes to the drug product or components have the potential to change the elemental impurity content of the drug product, the risk assessment, including established controls for elemental impurities, should be re-evaluated. Such changes could include changes in synthetic routes, excipient suppliers, raw materials, processes, equipment, container closure systems or facilities.

II. Elemental Impurities—Procedures

Procedures of Elemental Impurities are methods to control elemental impurities contained in drug products and their components, etc. This chapter describes two analytical procedures (Procedures 1 and 2) and validation criteria for the evaluation of the levels of elemental impurities. The chapter permits the use of any procedure that meets the validation criteria specified in this chapter. As the chemical composition of the considered substances and the specification limits for the element(s) of interest vary considerably, it is difficult to describe all suitable sample preparation and measurement methods. By means of validation studies, analysts will confirm that the analytical procedure is suitable for use on specified material. It is not necessary to cross validate against either procedure 1 or 2 provided that requirements for procedure validation are met. As elemental impurities may be ubiquitous and have the potential to be present in trace amounts therefore special precautions may be necessary to avoid sample contamination. (Note: Methods such as atomic absorption spectrometry other than methods described in this chapter, if validated, can also be used without cross validation against analytical procedure 1 or 2.)

1. Sample Preparation

Forms of sample preparation include Neat, Direct aqueous solution, Direct organic solution, and Indirect solution. The selection of the appropriate sample preparation depends on the material under test and is the responsibility of the analyst. When a sample preparation is not indicated in the monograph, an analyst may use any appropriately validated sample preparation procedure, including but not limited to procedures described below. In cases where spiking of a material under test is necessary to provide an acceptable signal intensity, the blank should be spiked with the same *Target elements*, and where possible, using the same spiking solution. The material or mixture under test must be spiked before any sample preparation steps are performed. Standard solutions may contain multiple *Target elements*. (Note: If intended for a quantitative test, appropriate material handling procedures should be followed e.g. volatile liquids should be pipetted, viscous liquids should be weighed.)

Neat: Used for liquids or analytical procedures that allow the examination of unsolvated samples.

Direct aqueous solution: Used when the sample is soluble in an aqueous solvent.

Direct organic solution: Used when the sample is soluble in an organic solvent.

Indirect solution: Generally, an indirect solution is obtained when a material is not directly soluble in aqueous or organic solvents. Total metal extraction is the preferred sample preparation approach to obtain an *indirect solution*. Digest the sample using the *Closed vessel digestion* procedure provided below or one similar to it.

Closed vessel digestion: This sample preparation procedure is designed for samples that must be digested in a *Concentrated acid* using a closed vessel digestion apparatus. *Closed vessel digestion* minimizes the loss of volatile impurities. The choice of a *Concentrated acid* depends on the sample matrix. The use of any of the *Concentrated acids* may be appropriate, but each introduces inherent safety risks. Therefore, appropriate safety precautions should be used at all times. (Note: Weights and volumes provided may be adjusted to meet the requirements of the digestion apparatus used.)

An example procedure that has been shown to have broad applicability is the following. Dehydrate and predigest 0.5 g of material under test in 5 mL of freshly prepared *Concentrated acid*. Allow to sit loosely covered for 30 min in a fume hood. Add an additional 10 mL of *Concentrated acid*, and digest, using a closed vessel technique, until digestion or extraction results in a clear solution. Repeat, if necessary, by adding an additional 5 mL of *Concentrated acid*. (Note: Where *closed vessel digestion* is necessary, follow the manufacturer's recommended procedures to ensure safe use.)

Clear solutions are expected in the validation. In those cases where a clear solution cannot be obtained, appropriate studies should ensure that the recovery is suitable for the intended use.

Reagents: All reagents used for the preparation of sample and standard solutions should be sufficiently pure for the intended purpose.

2. Analytical Procedures 1 and 2

System standardization and suitability evaluation using applicable reference materials should be performed for each analytical sequence.

2.1. Procedure and Detection Technique

Procedure 1 can be used for elemental impurities generally amenable to detection by inductively coupled plasma-atomic (optical) emission spectroscopy (ICP-AES or ICP-OES). *Procedure 2* can be used for elemental impurities generally amenable to detection by inductively coupled plasma-mass spectrometry (ICP-MS). Before initial use, the analyst should verify that the procedure is appropriate for the instrument and sample used (procedural verification) by meeting the procedure validation requirements below.

2.2. Procedure 1: ICP-OES

Standard solution 1: 1.5*J* of the *Target element(s)* in a *Matrix matched solution*.

Standard solution 2: 0.5*J* of the *Target element(s)* in a *Matrix matched solution*.

Sample stock solution: Proceed as directed in 1. *Sample Preparation* above. Allow the sample to cool, if necessary. For mercury determination, add an appropriate stabilizer, if necessary.

Sample solution: Dilute the *Sample stock solution* with an appropriate solvent to obtain a final concentration of the *Target element(s)* within the calibrated range.

Blank: *Matrix matched solution*.

Elemental spectrometric system

Mode: ICP.

Detector: Optical detection system.

Rinse: Diluent used.

Standardization: *Standard solution 1*, *Standard solution 2*, and *Blank*.

System suitability Sample: Standard solution of the *Target element(s)* in a *Matrix matched solution* at a concentration within the calibrated range.

Suitability requirements

Short term Instrumental Stability: Compare results obtained from *System suitability sample* before and after the analysis of the *Sample solution*.

Suitability criteria: NMT 20% deviation between both samples for each *Target element*. (Note: If samples are high in mineral content, rinse the system well in order to minimize carryover and check it by measuring a blank solution before introducing the *System Suitability Sample*.)

Analysis: Analyze according to manufacturer's suggestion for programs and wavelength. Calculate and report results on the basis of the original sample size. [Note: Appropriate measures must be taken to correct for matrix-induced interferences (e.g., wavelength overlaps).]

2.3. Procedure 2: ICP–MS

Standard solution 1: 1.5*J* of the *Target element(s)* in a *Matrix matched solution*.

Standard solution 2: 0.5*J* of the *Target element(s)* in a *Matrix matched solution*.

Sample stock solution: Proceed as directed in 1. *Sample Preparation* above. Allow the sample to cool, if necessary. For mercury determination, add an appropriate stabilizer, if necessary.

Sample solution: Dilute the *Sample stock solution* with an appropriate solvent to obtain a final concentration of the *Target element(s)* within the calibrated range.

Blank: *Matrix matched solution*.

Elemental spectrometric system

Mode: ICP. [Note: An instrument with a cooled spray chamber is recommended. (A collision cell or reaction cell may also be beneficial.)]

Detector: Mass spectrometer.

Rinse: Diluent used.

Standardization: *Standard solution 1*, *Standard solution 2*, and *Blank*.

System suitability Sample: Standard solution of the *Target element(s)* in a *Matrix matched solution* at a concentration within the calibrated range.

Suitability requirements

Short term Instrumental Stability: Compare results obtained from *system suitability sample* before and after the analysis of the *Sample solution*.

Suitability criteria: NMT 20% deviation between both samples for each *Target element*. (Note: If samples are high in mineral content, rinse the system well in order to minimize carryover and check it by measuring a blank before introducing the *System suitability sample*.)

Analysis: Analyze according to the manufacturer's suggestions for program and *m/z*. Calculate and report results based on the original sample size. [Note: Appropriate measures must be taken to correct for matrix-induced interferences (e.g., argon chloride interference with arsenic determinations).]

3. Requirements for Procedure Validation

All procedures must be validated and shown to be acceptable, in accordance with the validation requirements described below. The level of validation necessary to ensure that a procedure is acceptable depends on whether a limit test or a quantitative determination is used. Any procedure that has been validated and meets the acceptance criteria that follow is considered to be suitable for use. If appropriate, the validation method and criteria may be changed according to the purpose of evaluating the levels of the content of elemental impurities. They may differ from the requirements to meet the system suitability criteria described in Inductively Coupled Plasma-Atomic Emission Spectrometry and Inductively Coupled Plasma-Mass Spectrometry <*2.63*>.

3.1. Procedures for Limits Tests

The following section defines the validation parameters for the acceptability of limit tests. Meeting these requirements must be demonstrated experimentally using an appropriate system suitability test and reference materials. The suitability of the method must be determined by conducting studies with the material or mixture under test spiked with known concentrations of each *Target element* of interest at the appropriate *Target concentration*.

3.1.1. Detectability

Standard solution: A preparation of reference materials for the *Target element(s)* at 1.0*J* in a *Matrix matched solution*.

Spiked sample solution 1: Prepare a solution of the sample under test, spiked with appropriate reference materials for the *Target element(s)* at the *Target concentration*, solubilized or digested as described in *Sample Preparation*.

Spiked sample solution 2: Prepare a solution of the sample under test, spiked with appropriate reference materials for the *Target element(s)* at 80% of the *Target concentration*, solubilized or digested as described in *Sample Preparation*.

Unspiked sample solution: A sample of material under test, solubilized or digested in the same manner as the spiked *Sample solutions*.

Acceptance criteria

Non-instrumental procedures: *Spiked sample solution 1* provides a signal or intensity equivalent to or greater than that of the *Standard solution*. *Spiked sample solution 2* must provide a signal or intensity less than that of *Spiked sample solution 1*. (Note: The signal from each *Spiked sample solution* is NLT the *Unspiked sample solution* determination.)

Instrumental procedures: The average value of the three replicate measurements of *Spiked sample solution 1* is within ± 15% of the average value obtained for the replicate measurements of the *Standard solution*. The average value of the replicate measurements of *Spiked sample solution 2* must provide a signal intensity or value less than that of the *Standard solution*. (Note: Correct the values obtained for each of the spiked solutions using the *Unspiked sample solution*.)

3.1.2. Specificity

The procedure must be able to unequivocally assess each *Target element* in the presence of components that may be expected to be present, including other *Target element*s, and matrix components.

3.1.3. Precision, only for Instrumental Methods (Repeatability)

Sample solutions: Six independent samples of the material under test, spiked with appropriate reference materials for the *Target elements* at the *Target concentration*.

Acceptance criteria

Relative standard deviation: NMT 20% for each *Target element*

3.2. Procedures for Quantitative Tests

The following section defines the validation parameters for the acceptability of procedures for quantitative tests. Meeting these requirements must be demonstrated experimentally, using an appropriate system suitability test and reference materials.

3.2.1. Accuracy

Standard solutions: Prepare solutions containing the *Target element(s)* at three concentrations ranging from 0.5 to 1.5 of *J*, using appropriate reference materials, in a *Matrix matched solution* and *blank*.

Test samples: Prepare samples of the material under test spiked with appropriate reference materials for the *Target element(s)* before any sample preparation steps (digestion or solubilization) at 3 concentrations ranging from 50% to

150% of the *Target concentration*. The concentrations of the added reference materials after the preparation of the samples range from 0.5 to 1.5 of *J*, and should contain at least three different concentrations.

Acceptance criteria

Spike recovery: 70%–150% for the mean of three replicate preparations at each concentration

3.2.2. Precision

Repeatability

Test samples: Six independent samples of material under test (taken from the same lot) spiked with appropriate reference materials for the *Target element(s)* at the *Target concentration*. Or at least 9 determinations (e.g., 3 replicates of 3 concentrations) covering the specified range.

Acceptance criteria

Relative standard deviation: NMT 20% (n = 6) for each *Target element*

Intermediate precision (ruggedness)

Perform the *Repeatability* analysis again at least once either on a different day, with a different instrumentation, with a different analyst, or a combination thereof. Combine the results of this analysis with the *Repeatability* analysis so the total number of samples is at least 12.

Acceptance criteria

Relative standard deviation: NMT 25% (n = 12) for each *Target element*

3.2.3. Specificity

The procedure must be able to unequivocally assess each *Target element* in the presence of components that may be expected to be present, including other *Target elements*, and matrix components.

3.2.4. Range and Linearity

Demonstrated by meeting the *Accuracy* requirement.

3.2.5. Limit of Quantification

LOQ of 50% of *J* is confirmed when the accuracy acceptance criteria for the corresponding spiked solution is met. Acceptance criterion: the LOQ is less than or equal to 50% of *J*.

4. Glossary

(i) Concentrated acid: Concentrated ultra-pure nitric, sulfuric, hydrochloric, or hydrofluoric acids or any other acid or mixture of acids that is demonstrated suitable.

(ii) Matrix matched solution: Solutions having the same solvent composition as the *Sample solution*. In the case of an aqueous solution, *Matrix matched solution* would indicate that the same acids, acid concentrations and mercury stabilizer are used in both preparations.

(iii) Target elements: Elements whose levels in the drug product must be controlled within acceptable limits.

(iv) Target limit or Target concentration: The acceptance value for the elemental impurity being evaluated. Exceeding the *Target limit* indicates that a material under test exceeds the acceptable value. *Target limits* in the final drug product can be approximated by dividing the *PDEs* by the maximum daily dose. When evaluating the significance of elemental impurity levels, it is possible to set the *Target limits* to the values obtained by dividing 30% of *PDEs* by the maximum daily dose. Furthermore, when the permitted concentration limit of each element in the individual components of the drug product is set, it can be set as the *Target concentration*.

(v) *J*: The concentration (w/v) of the *Target element(s)* at the *Target limit*, appropriately diluted to the working range of the instrument. If a dilution is not necessary, *J* is equal to the *Target concentration*. For example, if the target elements are lead and arsenic for an analysis of an oral solid drug product with a daily dose of 10 g/day using inductively coupled plasma-mass spectrometry (ICP-MS), the target limit for these elements would be 0.5 μg/g and 1.5 μg/g. However, in both cases, the linear dynamic range of the ICP-MS is known to extend from 0.01 ng/mL to 0.1 μg/mL for these elements. Therefore, a dilution factor of at least 1:100 is required to ensure that the analysis occurs in the linear dynamic range of the instrument. *J* would thus equal 5 ng/mL and 15 ng/mL for lead and arsenic, respectively.

(vi) Appropriate reference materials: In principle, where *appropriate reference materials* are specified in the chapter, certified reference materials (CRM) from a national metrology institute (NMI), or reference materials that are traceable to the CRM of an NMI should be used.

(vii) Cross validate: Verification whether or not the same result can be obtained from the corresponding analyses for the same sample.

3. Powder Property Determinations

3.01 Determination of Bulk and Tapped Densities

This test is harmonized with the European Pharmacopoeia and the U.S. Pharmacopeia.

The parts of the text that are not harmonized are marked with symbols (◆ ◆).

Information on the harmonization with the European Pharmacopoeia and the U.S. Pharmacopeia is available on the website of the Pharmaceuticals and Medical Devices Agency.

◆Determination of Bulk and Tapped Densities is a method to determine the bulk densities of powdered drugs under loose and tapped packing conditions respectively. Loose packing is defined as the state obtained by pouring a powder sample into a vessel without any consolidation, and tapped packing is defined as the state obtained when the vessel containing the powder sample is to be repeatedly dropped a specified distance at a constant drop rate until the apparent volume of sample in the vessel becomes almost constant.◆

1. Bulk density

The bulk density of a powder is the ratio of the mass of an untapped powder sample and its volume including the contribution of the interparticulate void volume. Hence, the bulk density depends on both the density of powder particles and the spatial arrangement of particles in the powder bed. The bulk density is expressed in grams per milliliter (g/mL) although the international unit is kilogram per cubic meter (1 g/mL = 1000 kg/m^3) because the measurements are made using cylinders. It may also be expressed in grams per cubic centimeter (g/cm^3).

The bulking properties of a powder are dependent upon the preparation, treatment and storage of the sample, i.e. how it was handled. The particles can be packed to have a range of bulk densities and, moreover, the slightest disturbance of the powder bed may result in a changed bulk density. Thus, the bulk density of a powder is often very difficult to measure with good reproducibility and, in reporting the results, it is essential to specify how the determination was made.

The bulk density of a powder is determined by measuring the volume of a known mass of powder sample, that may have been passed through a sieve into a graduated cylinder (Method 1), or by measuring the mass of a known volume of powder that has been passed through a volumeter into a cup (Method 2) or a measuring vessel (Method 3). Method 1 and Method 3 are favoured.

1.1. Method 1: Measurement in a graduated cylinder

1.1.1. Procedure

Pass a quantity of powder sufficient to complete the test through a sieve with apertures greater than or equal to 1.0 mm, if necessary, to break up agglomerates that may have formed during storage; this must be done gently to avoid changing the nature of the material. Into a dry graduated cylinder of 250 mL (readable to 2 mL), gently introduce, without compacting, approximately 100 g of the test sample (m) weighed with 0.1 per cent accuracy. Carefully level the powder without compacting, if necessary, and read the unsettled apparent volume (V_0) to the nearest graduated unit. Calculate the bulk density in g per mL by the formula m/V_0. Generally, replicate determinations are desirable for the determination of this property.

If the powder density is too low or too high, such that the test sample has an untapped apparent volume of either more than 250 mL or less than 150 mL, it is not possible to use 100 g of powder sample. Therefore, a different amount of powder has to be selected as test sample, such that its untapped apparent volume is 150 mL to 250 mL (apparent volume greater than or equal to 60 per cent of the total volume of the cylinder); the mass of the test sample is specified in the expression of results.

For test samples having an apparent volume between 50 mL and 100 mL, a 100 mL cylinder readable to 1 mL can be used; the volume of the cylinder is specified in the expression of results.

1.2. Method 2: Measurement in a volumeter

1.2.1. Apparatus

The apparatus (Fig. 3.01-1) consists of a top funnel fitted with a 1.0 mm sieve. The funnel is mounted over a baffle box containing four glass baffle plates over which the powder slides and bounces as it passes. At the bottom of the baffle box is a funnel that collects the powder and allows it to pour into a cup mounted directly below it. The cup may be cylindrical (25.00 ± 0.05 mL volume with an inside diameter of 30.00 ± 2.00 mm) or cubical (16.39 ± 0.20 mL volume with inside dimensions of 25.400 ± 0.076 mm).

1.2.2. Procedure

Allow an excess of powder to flow through the apparatus into the sample receiving cup until it overflows, using a minimum of 25 cm^3 of powder with the cubical cup and 35 cm^3 of powder with the cylindrical cup. Carefully, scrape excess powder from the top of the cup by smoothly moving the edge of the blade of a spatula perpendicular to and in contact with the top surface of the cup, taking care to keep the spatula perpendicular to prevent packing or removal of powder from the cup. Remove any material from the side of the cup and determine the mass (m) of the powder to the nearest 0.1 per cent. Calculate the bulk density in g per mL by the formula m/V_0 in which V_0 is the volume of the cup and record the average of 3 determinations using 3 different powder samples.

1.3. Method 3: Measurement in a vessel

1.3.1. Apparatus

The apparatus consists of a 100 mL cylindrical vessel of stainless steel with dimensions as specified in Fig. 3.01-2.

1.3.2. Procedure

Pass a quantity of powder sufficient to complete the test through a 1.0 mm sieve, if necessary, to break up agglomerates that may have formed during storage and allow the obtained sample to flow freely into the measuring vessel until it overflows. Carefully scrape the excess powder from the top of the vessel as described for Method 2. Determine the mass (m_0) of the powder to the nearest 0.1 per cent by subtraction of the previously determined mass of the empty measuring vessel. Calculate the bulk density (g/mL) by the formula $m_0/100$ and record the average of 3 determinations using 3 different powder samples.

2. Tapped density

The tapped density is an increased bulk density attained after mechanically tapping a container containing the powder sample.

The tapped density is obtained by mechanically tapping a graduated measuring cylinder or vessel containing the powder sample. After observing the initial powder volume or mass, the measuring cylinder or vessel is mechanically tapped, and volume or mass readings are taken until little further volume or mass change is observed. The mechanical tapping is achieved by raising the cylinder or vessel and allowing it to drop, under its own mass, a specified distance by either of 3 methods as described below. Devices that rotate the cylinder or vessel during tapping may be preferred to minimize any possible separation of the mass during tapping down.

2.1. Method 1

2.1.1. Apparatus

The apparatus (Fig. 3.01-3) consists of the following:

(i) a 250 mL graduated cylinder (readable to 2 mL) with a mass of 220 ± 44 g,

(ii) a settling apparatus capable of producing, in 1 min, either nominally 250 ± 15 taps from a height of 3 ± 0.2 mm, or nominally 300 ± 15 taps from a height of 14 ± 2 mm. The support for the graduated cylinder, with its holder, has a mass of 450 ± 10 g.

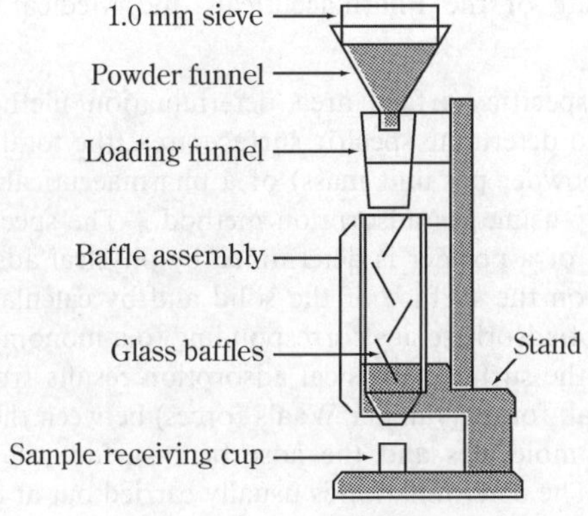

Fig. 3.01-1 Volumeter

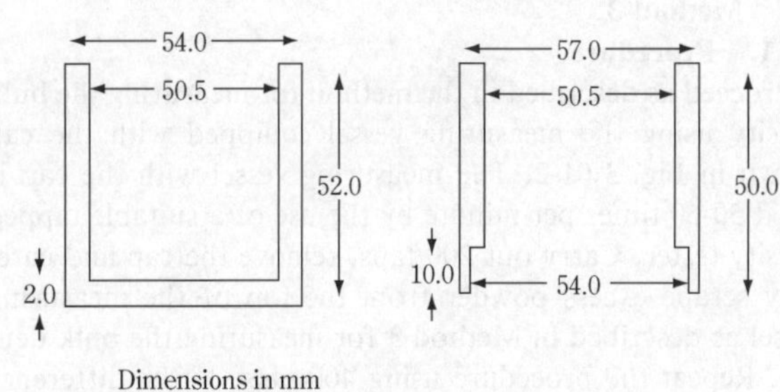

Fig. 3.01-2 Measuring vessel (left) and cap (right)

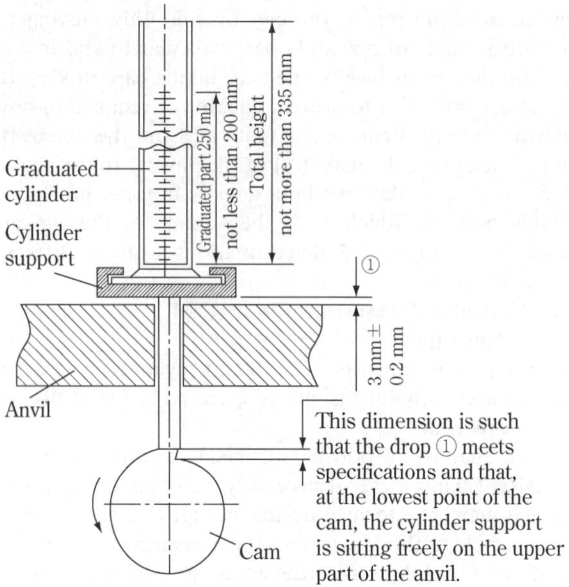

Fig. 3.01-3 Tapping apparatus

2.1.2. Procedure

Proceed as described above for the determination of the bulk volume (V_0).

Secure the cylinder in the holder. Carry out 10, 500 and 1250 taps on the same powder sample and read the corresponding volumes V_{10}, V_{500} and V_{1250} to the nearest graduated unit. If the difference between V_{500} and V_{1250} is less than or equal to 2 mL, V_{1250} is the tapped volume. If the difference between V_{500} and V_{1250} exceeds 2 mL, repeat in increments such as 1250 taps, until the difference between succeeding measurements is less than or equal to 2 mL. Fewer taps may be appropriate for some powders, when validated. Calculate the tapped density (g/mL) using the formula m/V_f in which V_f is the final tapped volume. Generally, replicate determinations are desirable for the determination of this property. Specify the drop height with the results.

If it is not possible to use a 100 g test sample, use a reduced amount and a suitable 100 mL graduated cylinder (readable to 1 mL) weighing 130 ± 16 g and mounted on a holder weighing 240 ± 12 g. If the difference between V_{500} and V_{1250} is less than or equal to 1 mL, V_{1250} is the tapped volume. If the difference between V_{500} and V_{1250} exceeds 1 mL, repeat in increments such as 1250 taps, until the difference between succeeding measurements is less than or equal to 1 mL. The modified test conditions are specified in the expression of the results.

2.2. Method 2

2.2.1. Procedure

Proceed as directed under Method 1 except that the mechanical tester provides a fixed drop of 3 ± 0.2 mm at a nominal rate of 250 taps per minute.

2.3. Method 3

2.3.1. Procedure

Proceed as described in the method for measuring the bulk density using the measuring vessel equipped with the cap shown in Fig. 3.01-2. The measuring vessel with the cap is lifted 50-60 times per minute by the use of a suitable tapped density tester. Carry out 200 taps, remove the cap and carefully scrape excess powder from the top of the measuring vessel as described in Method 3 for measuring the bulk density. Repeat the procedure using 400 taps. If the difference between the 2 masses obtained after 200 and 400 taps exceeds 2 per cent, carry out a test using 200 additional taps until the difference between succeeding measurements is less than 2 per cent. Calculate the tapped density (g/mL) using the formula $m_f/100$ where m_f is the mass of powder in the measuring vessel. Record the average of 3 determinations using 3 different powder samples. The test conditions including tapping height are specified in the expression of the results.

3. Measures of powder compressibility

Because the interparticulate interactions influencing the bulking properties of a powder are also the interactions that interfere with powder flow, a comparison of the bulk and tapped densities can give a measure of the relative importance of these interactions in a given powder. Such a comparison is often used as an index of the ability of the powder to flow, for example the Compressibility Index or the Hausner Ratio.

The Compressibility Index and Hausner Ratio are measures of the propensity of a powder to be compressed as described above. As such, they are measures of the powder ability to settle and they permit an assessment of the relative importance of interparticulate interactions. In a free-flowing powder, such interactions are less significant, and the bulk and tapped densities will be closer in value. For poorer flowing materials, there are frequently greater interparticulate interactions, and a greater difference between the bulk and tapped densities will be observed. These differences are reflected in the Compressibility Index and the Hausner Ratio.

Compressibility Index:

$$100\ (V_0 - V_f)/V_0$$

V_0: Unsettled apparent volume
V_f: Final tapped volume

Hauser Ratio:

$$V_0/V_f$$

Depending on the material, the compressibility index can be determined using V_{10} instead of V_0. If V_{10} is used, it is clearly stated in the results.

3.02 Specific Surface Area by Gas Adsorption

This test is harmonized with the European Pharmacopoeia and the U. S. Pharmacopeia.

The parts of the text that are not harmonized are marked with symbols (◆ ◆).

Information on the harmonization with the European Pharmacopoeia and the U.S. Pharmacopeia is available on the website of the Pharmaceuticals and Medical Devices Agency.

◆The specific surface area determination method is a method to determine specific surface area (the total surface area of powder per unit mass) of a pharmaceutical powder sample by using gas adsorption method.◆ The specific surface area of a powder is determined by physical adsorption of a gas on the surface of the solid and by calculating the amount of adsorbate gas corresponding to a monomolecular layer on the surface. Physical adsorption results from relatively weak forces (van der Waals forces) between the adsorbate gas molecules and the adsorbent surface of the test powder. The determination is usually carried out at the temperature of liquid nitrogen. The amount of gas adsorbed can be measured by a volumetric or continuous flow procedure.

1. Measurements

1.1. Multi-point measurement

When the gas is physically adsorbed by the powder sample, the following relationship (Brunauer, Emmett and Teller (BET) adsorption isotherm) holds when the relative pressure (P/P_0) is in the range of 0.05 to 0.30 for pressure P of the adsorbate gas in equilibrium for the volume of gas adsorbed, V_a.

$$1/[V_a\{(P_0/P) - 1\}] = \{(C - 1)/V_mC\} \times (P/P_0) + (1/V_mC) \quad (1)$$

P: Partial vapour pressure of adsorbate gas in equilibrium with the surface at -195.8°C (b.p. of liquid nitrogen), in pascals

P_0: Saturated pressure of adsorbate gas, in pascals

V_a: Volume of gas adsorbed at standard temperature and pressure (STP) [0°C and atmospheric pressure (1.013×10^5 Pa)], in milliliters

V_m: Volume of gas adsorbed at STP to produce an apparent monolayer on the sample surface, in milliliters

C: Dimensionless constant that is related to the enthalpy of adsorption of adsorbate gas on the powder sample

A value of V_a is measured at each of not less than 3 values of P/P_0. Then the BET value, $1/[V_a\{(P_0/P) - 1\}]$, is plotted against P/P_0 according to equation (1). This plot should yield a straight line usually in the approximate relative pressure range 0.05 to 0.3. The data are considered acceptable if the correlation coefficient, r, of the linear regression is not less than 0.9975; that is, r^2 is not less than 0.995. From the resulting linear plot, the slope, which is equal to $(C - 1)/V_mC$, and the intercept, which is equal to $1/(V_mC)$, are evaluated by linear regression analysis. From these values, V_m is calculated as 1/(*slope* + *intercept*), while C is calculated as (*slope*/*intercept*) + 1. From the value of V_m so determined, the specific surface area, S, in m^2g^{-1}, is calculated by the equation:

$$S = (V_mNa)/(m \times 22{,}400) \quad (2)$$

N: Avogadro constant (6.022×10^{23} mol^{-1}),

a: Effective cross-sectional area of one adsorbate molecule, in square meters (0.162×10^{-18} m^2 for nitrogen and 0.195×10^{-18} m^2 for krypton)

m: Mass of test powder, in grams

22,400: Volume, in milliliters, occupied by one mole of the adsorbate gas at STP allowing for minor departures from the ideal

A minimum of 3 data points is required. Additional measurements may be carried out, especially when non-linearity is obtained at a P/P_0 value close to 0.3. Because non-linearity is often obtained at a P/P_0 value below 0.05, values in this region are not recommended. The test for linearity, the treatment of the data, and the calculation of the specific surface area of the sample are described above.

1.2. Single-point measurement

Normally, at least 3 measurements of V_a each at different values of P/P_0 are required for the determination of specific surface area by the dynamic flow gas adsorption technique (*Method I*) or by volumetric gas adsorption (*Method II*). However, under certain circumstances described below, it may be acceptable to determine the specific surface area of a powder from a single value of V_a measured at a single value of P/P_0 such as 0.300 (corresponding to 0.300 mole of nitrogen or 0.001038 mole fraction of krypton), using the following equation for calculating V_m:

$$V_m = V_a\{1 - (P/P_0)\} \quad (3)$$

The single-point method may be employed directly for a series of powder samples of a given material for which the material constant C is much greater than unity. These circumstances may be verified by comparing values of specific surface area determined by the single-point method with that determined by the multiple-point method for the series of powder samples. Close similarity between the single-point values and multiple-point values suggests that $1/C$ approaches zero. The single-point method may be employed indirectly for a series of very similar powder samples of a given material for which the material constant C is not infinite but may be assumed to be invariant. Under these circumstances, the error associated with the single-point method can be reduced or eliminated by using the multiple-point method to evaluate C for one of the samples of the series from the BET plot, from which C is calculated as (1 + *slope*/*intercept*). Then V_m is calculated from the single value of V_a measured at a single value of P/P_0 by the equation:

$$V_m = V_a\{(P_0/P) - 1\}[(1/C) + \{(C - 1)/C\} \times (P/P_0)] \quad (4)$$

2. Sample preparation

Before the specific surface area of the sample can be determined, it is necessary to remove gases and vapors that may have become physically adsorbed onto the surface during storage and handling. If outgassing is not achieved, the specific surface area may be reduced or may be variable because some parts of surface area are covered with molecules of the previously adsorbed gases or vapors. The outgassing conditions are critical for obtaining the required precision and accuracy of specific surface area measurements on pharmaceuticals because of the sensitivity of the surface of the materials. The outgassing conditions must be demonstrated to yield reproducible BET plots, a constant weight of test powder, and no detectable physical or chemical changes in the test powder.

The outgassing conditions defined by the temperature, pressure and time should be so chosen that the original surface of the solid is reproduced as closely as possible.

Outgassing of many substances is often achieved by applying a vacuum, by purging the sample in a flowing stream of a non-reactive, dry gas, or by applying a desorption-adsorption cycling method. In either case, elevated temperatures are sometimes applied to increase the rate at which the contaminants leave the surface. Caution should be exercised when outgassing powder samples using elevated temperatures to avoid affecting the nature of the surface and the integrity of the sample.

If heating is employed, the recommended temperature and time of outgassing are as low as possible to achieve reproducible measurement of specific surface area in an acceptable time. For outgassing sensitive samples, other outgassing methods such as the desorption-adsorption cycling method may be employed.

The standard technique is the adsorption of nitrogen at liquid nitrogen temperature.

For powders of low specific surface area (<0.2 m^{2}g^{-1}) the proportion adsorbed is low. In such cases the use of krypton at liquid nitrogen temperature is preferred because the low vapor pressure exerted by this gas greatly reduces error. All gases used must be free from moisture.

Accurately weigh a quantity of the test powder such that the total surface of the sample is at least 1 m^2 when the adsorbate is nitrogen and 0.5 m^2 when the adsorbate is krypton. Lower quantities of sample may be used after appropriate validation.

Because the amount of gas adsorbed under a given pressure tends to increase on decreasing the temperature, adsorp-

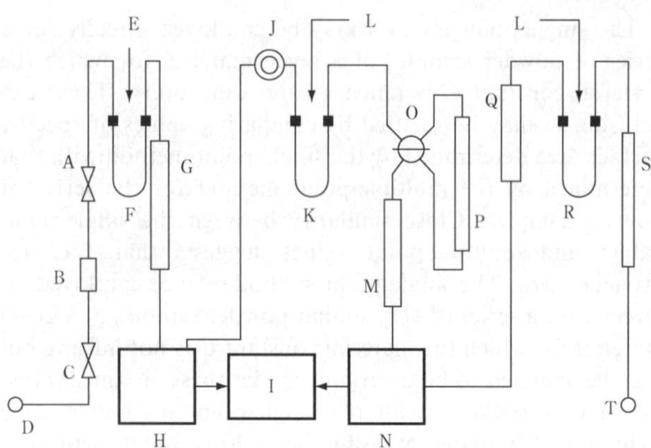

Fig. 3.02-1 Schematic diagram of the dynamic flow method apparatus

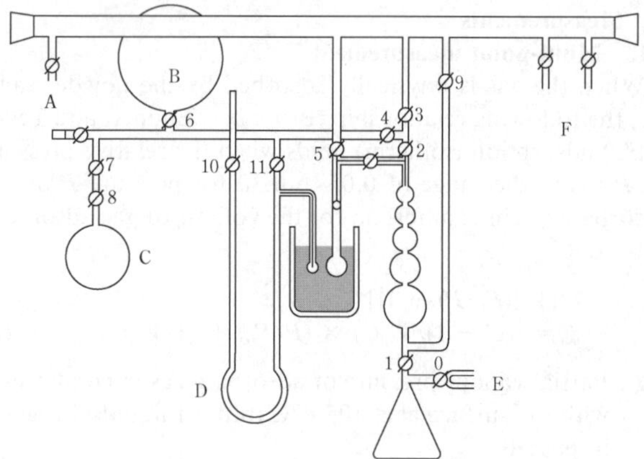

Fig. 3.02-2 Schematic diagram of the volumetric method apparatus

tion measurements are usually made at a low temperature. Measurement is performed at −195.8°C, the boiling point of liquid nitrogen.

Adsorption of gas should be measured either by Method I or Method II.

3. Methods

3.1. Method 1: The dynamic flow method

In the dynamic flow method (see Fig. 3.02-1), the recommended adsorbate gas is dry nitrogen or krypton, while helium is employed as a diluent gas, which is not adsorbed under the recommended conditions. A minimum of 3 mixtures of the appropriate adsorbate gas with helium are required within the P/P_0 range 0.05 to 0.30.

The gas detector-integrator should provide a signal that is approximately proportional to the volume of the gas passing through it under defined conditions of temperature and pressure. For this purpose, a thermal conductivity detector with an electronic integrator is one among various suitable types. A minimum of 3 data points within the recommended range of 0.05 to 0.30 for P/P_0 is to be determined.

A known mixture of the gases, usually nitrogen and helium, is passed through a thermal conductivity cell, through the sample again through the thermal conductivity cell and then to a recording potentiometer. Immerse the sample cell in liquid nitrogen, then the sample adsorbs nitrogen from the mobile phase. This unbalances the thermal conductivity cell, and a pulse is generated on a recorder chart.

Remove from the coolant; this gives a desorption peak equal in area and in the opposite direction to the adsorption peak.

Since this is better defined than the adsorption peak, it is the one used for the determination.

To effect the calibration, inject a known quantity of adsorbate into the system, sufficient to give a peak of similar magnitude to the desorption peak and obtain the proportion of gas volume per unit peak area.

Use a nitrogen/helium mixture for a single-point determination and several such mixtures or premixing 2 streams of gas for a multiple-point determination. Calculation is essentially the same as for the volumetric method.

3.2. Method 2: The volumetric method

In the volumetric method (see Fig. 3.02-2), the recommended adsorbate gas is nitrogen is admitted into the evacuated space above the previously outgassed powder sample to give a defined equilibrium pressure, P, of the gas. The use of a diluent gas, such as helium, is therefore unnecessary, although helium may be employed for other purposes, such as to measure the dead volume.

Since only pure adsorbate gas, instead of a gas mixture, is employed, interfering effects of thermal diffusion are avoided in this method.

Admit a small amount of dry nitrogen into the sample tube to prevent contamination of the clean surface, remove the sample tube, insert the stopper, and weigh it. Calculate the weight of the sample. Attach the sample tube to the volumetric apparatus. Cautiously evacuate the sample down to the specified pressure (e.g. between 2 Pa and 10 Pa). Alternately, some instruments operate by evacuating to a defined rate of pressure change (e.g. less than 13 Pa/30 s) and holding for a defined period of time before commencing the next step.

If the principle of operation of the instrument requires the determination of the dead volume in the sample tube, for example, by the admission of a non-adsorbed gas, such as helium, this procedure is carried out at this point, followed by evacuation of the sample. The determination of dead volume may be avoided using difference measurements, that is, by means of reference and sample tubes connected by a differential transducer.

Raise a Dewar vessel containing liquid nitrogen at −195.8°C up to a defined point on the sample cell. Admit a sufficient volume of adsorbate gas to give the lowest desired relative pressure. Measure the volume adsorbed, V_a. For multipoint measurements, repeat the measurement of V_a at successively higher P/P_0 values. When nitrogen is used as the adsorbate gas, P/P_0 values of 0.10, 0.20, and 0.30 are often suitable.

4. Reference materials

Periodically verify the functioning of the apparatus using appropriate reference materials of known surface area, such as α-alumina for specific surface area determination, which should have a specific surface area similar to that of the sample to be examined.

3.03 Powder Particle Density Determination

This test is harmonized with the European Pharmacopoeia and the U.S. Pharmacopoeia.

The parts of the test that are not harmonized are marked with symbols (◆ ◆).

Information on the harmonization with the European Pharmacopoeia and the U.S. Pharmacopeia is available on the website of the Pharmaceuticals and Medical Devices Agency.

Powder Particle Density Determination is ◆a method to determine particle density of powdered pharmaceutical drugs or raw materials of drugs◆, and generally performed using a gas displacement pycnometer. The gas pycnometric density is determined by measuring the volume occupied by a known mass of powder which is equivalent to the volume of gas displaced by the powder using a gas displacement pycnometer. In gas pycnometric density measurements, the volume determined excludes the volume occupied by open pores; however, it includes the volume occupied by sealed pores or pores inaccessible to the gas. Usually, helium is used as a test gas due to its high diffusivity into small open pores. If gases other than helium are used, different values would be obtained, since the penetration of the gas is dependent on the size of the pore as well as the cross-sectional area of the gas.

The measured density is a volume weighted average of the densities of individual powder particles. It is called the particle density, distinct from the true density of solid or the bulk density of powder. The density of solids is expressed in grams per cubic centimeter (g/cm^3), although the international unit is the kilogram per cubic meter (1 g/cm^3 = 1000 kg/m^3).

1. Apparatus

The schematic diagram of particle density apparatus for gas displacement pycnometric measurement is shown in Fig. 3.03-1. The apparatus consists of a test cell in which the sample is placed, an expansion cell and a manometer (M). The test cell, with an empty cell volume (V_c), is connected through a valve (A) to an expansion cell, with a volume (V_r).

Generally, helium is used as the measurement gas. The apparatus has to be equipped with a system capable of pressuring the test cell to the defined pressure (P) through the manometer.

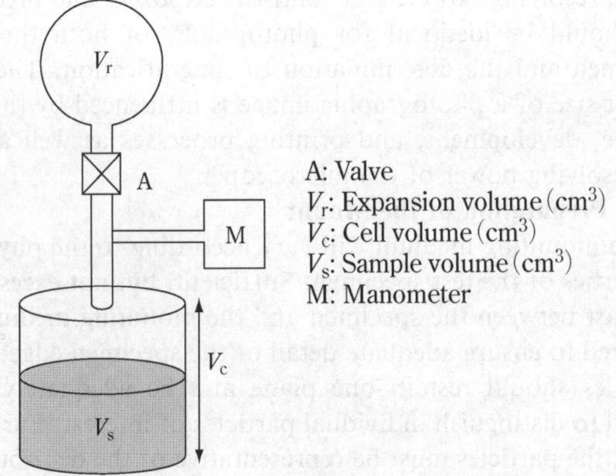

Fig. 3.03-1 Schematic diagram of a gas pycnometer

2. Calibration of apparatus

The volumes of the test cell (V_c) and the expansion cell (V_r) must be accurately determined to the nearest 0.001 cm^3, and to assure accuracy of the results of volume obtained, calibration of the apparatus is carried out as follows using a calibration ball of known volume for particle density measurement.

The final pressures (P_f) are determined for the initial empty test cell followed by the test cell placed with the calibration ball for particle density measurement in accordance with the procedures, and Vc and V_r are calculated using the equation described in the section of Procedure. Calculation can be made taking into account that the sample volume (V_s) is zero in the first run.

3. Procedure

The gas pycnometric density measurement is performed at a temperature between 15°C and 30°C and must not vary by more than 2°C during the course of measurement.

Volatile contaminants in the powder are removed by degassing the powder under a constant purge of helium prior to the measurement. Occasionally, powders may have to be degassed under vacuum. Because volatiles may be evolved during the measurement, weighing of the sample is done after the pycnometric measurement of volume.

Weigh the mass of the test cell and record it. After weighing out the amount of the sample as described in the individual monograph and placing it in the test cell, seal the cell in the pycnometer.

Open the valve (A) which connects the expansion cell with the test cell, confirm with the manometer (M) that the pressure inside the system is stable, and then read the system reference pressure (P_r). Secondly, close the valve that connects to the two cells, and introduce the measurement gas into the test cell to achieve positive pressure. Confirm with the manometer that the pressure inside the system is stable, and then read the initial pressure (P_i). Open the valve to connect the test cell with the expansion cell. After confirming that the indicator of the manometer is stable, read the final pressure (P_f), and calculate the sample volume (V_s) with the following equation.

$$V_s = V_c - \frac{V_r}{\dfrac{P_i - P_r}{P_f - P_r} - 1}$$

V_r: Expansion volume (cm^3)
V_c: Cell volume (cm^3)
V_s: Sample volume (cm^3)
P_i: Initial pressure (kPa)
P_f: Final pressure (kPa)
P_r: System reference pressure (kPa)

Repeat the measurement sequence for the same powder sample until consecutive measurements of the sample volume agree to within 0.2%, and calculate the mean of sample volumes (V_s). Finally, unload the test cell, weigh the mass of the test cell, and calculate the final sample mass (m) by deducting the empty cell mass from the test cell mass. The powder particle density ρ is calculated by the following equation:

$$\rho = m/V_s$$

ρ: Powder particle density in g/cm^3,
m: Final sample mass in g,
V_s: Sample volume in cm^3

If the pycnometer differs in operation or construction

from the one shown in Fig. 3.03-1, follow the instructions of the manufacturer of the pycnometer. The sample conditioning is indicated with the results. For example, indicate whether the sample was tested as is or dried under specific conditions such as those described for loss on drying.

3.04 Particle Size Determination

This test is harmonized with the European Pharmacopoeia and the U.S. Pharmacopeia.

The parts of the text that are not harmonized are marked with symbols (◆ ◆).

Information on the harmonization with the European Pharmacopoeia and the U.S. Pharmacopeia is available on the website of the Pharmaceuticals and Medical Devices Agency.

◆Particle Size Determination is a method to determine directly or indirectly morphological appearance, shape, size and its distribution of powdered pharmaceutical drugs and excipients to examine their micromeritic properties. Optical microscopy and analytical sieving method may be used depending on the measuring purpose and the properties of test specimen.◆

1. Method 1. Optical Microscopy

◆The optical microscopy is used to observe the morphological appearance and shape of individual particle either directly with the naked eye or by using a microscopic photograph, in order to measure the particle size. The particle size distribution can also be determined by this method. It is also possible with this method to measure the size of the individual particle even when different kinds of particles mingle if they are optically distinguishable. Data processing techniques, such as image analysis, can be useful for determining the particle size distribution.◆

This method for particle characterization can generally be applied to particles 1 μm and greater. The lower limit is imposed by the resolving power of the microscope. The upper limit is less definite and is determined by the increased difficulty associated with the characterization of larger particles. Various alternative techniques are available for particle characterization outside the applicable range of optical microscopy. Optical microscopy is particularly useful for characterizing particles that are not spherical. This method may also serve as a base for the calibration of faster and more routine methods that may be developed.

1.1. Apparatus

Use a microscope that is stable and protected from vibration. The microscope magnification (product of the objective magnification, ocular magnification, and additional magnifying components) must be sufficient to allow adequate characterization of the smallest particles to be classified in the test specimen. The greatest numerical aperture of the objective should be sought for each magnification range. Polarizing filters may be used in conjunction with suitable analyzers and retardation plates. Color filters of relatively narrow spectral transmission should be used with achromatic objectives and are preferable with apochromats and are required for appropriate color rendition in photomicrography. Condensers corrected for at least spherical aberration should be used in the microscope substage and with the lamp. The numerical aperture of the substage condenser should match that of the objective under the condition of use; this is affected by the actual aperture of the condenser diaphragm and the presence of immersion oils.

1.1.1. Adjustment

The precise alignment of all elements of the optical system and proper focusing are essential. The focusing of the elements should be done in accordance with the recommendations of the microscope manufacturer. Critical axial alignment is recommended.

1.1.1.1. Illumination

A requirement for good illumination is a uniform and adjustable intensity of light over the entire field of view; Kohler illumination is preferred. With colored particles, choose the color of the filters used so as to control the contrast and detail of the image.

1.1.1.2. Visual Characterization

The magnification and numerical aperture should be sufficiently high to allow adequate resolution of the images of the particles to be characterized. Determine the actual magnification using a calibrated stage micrometer to calibrate an ocular micrometer. Errors can be minimized if the magnification is sufficient that the image of the particle is at least 10 ocular divisions. Each objective must be calibrated separately. To calibrate the ocular scale, the stage micrometer scale and the ocular scale should be aligned. In this way, a precise determination of the distance between ocular stage divisions can be made.

◆When the particle size is measured, an ocular micrometer is inserted at the position of the ocular diaphragm, and a calibrated stage micrometer is placed at the center of the microscope stage and fixed in place. The ocular is attached to the lens barrel and adjusted to the focus point of the stage micrometer scale. Then, the distance between the scales of the two micrometers is determined, and the sample size equivalent 1 division of the ocular scale is calculated using the following formula:

The particle size equivalent 1 division on the ocular scale (μm) = Length on the stage micrometer (μm)/Number of scale divisions on the ocular micrometer

The stage micrometer is removed and the test specimen is placed on the microscope stage. After adjusting the focus, the particle sizes are determined from the number of scale divisions read through the ocular.◆

Several different magnifications may be necessary to characterize materials having a wide particle size distribution.

1.1.1.3. Photographic Characterization

If particle size is to be determined by photographic methods, take care to ensure that the object is sharply focused at the plane of the photographic emulsion. Determine the actual magnification by photographing a calibrated stage micrometer, using photographic film of sufficient speed, resolving power, and contrast. Exposure and processing should be identical for photographs of both the test specimen and the determination of magnification. The apparent size of a photographic image is influenced by the exposure, development, and printing processes as well as by the resolving power of the microscope.

1.2. Preparation of the Mount

The mounting medium will vary according to the physical properties of the test specimen. Sufficient, but not excessive, contrast between the specimen and the mounting medium is required to ensure adequate detail of the specimen edge. The particles should rest in one plane and be adequately dispersed to distinguish individual particles of interest. Furthermore, the particles must be representative of the distribution of sizes in the material and must not be altered during preparation of the mount. Care should be taken to ensure that this important requirement is met. Selection of the mounting medium must include a consideration of the analyte solubility.

1.3. Characterization

1.3.1. Crystallinity Characterization

The crystallinity of a material may be characterized to determine compliance with the crystallinity requirement where stated in the individual monograph of a drug substance. Unless otherwise specified in the individual monograph, mount a few particles of the specimen in mineral oil on a clean glass slide. Examine the mixture using a polarizing microscope: the particles show birefringence (interference colors) and extinction positions when the microscope stage is revolved.

1.3.2. Limit Test of Particle Size by Microscopy

Weigh a suitable quantity of the powder to be examined (for example, 10 to 100 mg), and suspend it in 10 mL of a suitable medium in which the powder does not dissolve, adding, if necessary, a wetting agent. A homogeneous suspension of particles can be maintained by suspending the particles in a medium of similar or matching density and by providing adequate agitation. Introduce a portion of the homogeneous suspension into a suitable counting cell, and scan under a microscope an area corresponding to not less than 10 μg of the powder to be examined. Count all the particles having a maximum dimension greater than the prescribed size limit. The size limit and the permitted number of particles exceeding the limit are defined for each substance.

1.3.3. Particle Size Characterization

The measurement of particle size varies in complexity depending on the shape of the particle and the number of particles characterized must be sufficient to insure an acceptable level of uncertainty in the measured parameters[1]. For spherical particles, size is defined by the diameter. For irregular particles, a variety of definitions of particle size exist. In general, for irregularly shaped particles, characterization of particle size must also include information on the type of diameter measured as well as information on particle shape. Several commonly used measurements of particle size are defined below (see Fig. 3.04-1).

(i) Feret's Diameter: The distance between imaginary parallel lines tangent to a randomly oriented particle and perpendicular to the ocular scale.

(ii) Martin's Diameter: The diameter of the particle at the point that divides a randomly oriented particle into two equal projected areas.

(iii) Projected area Diameter: The diameter of a circle that has the same projected are as the particle.

(iv) Length: The longest dimension from edge to edge of a particle oriented parallel to the ocular scale.

(v) Width: The longest dimension of the particle measured at right angles to the length.

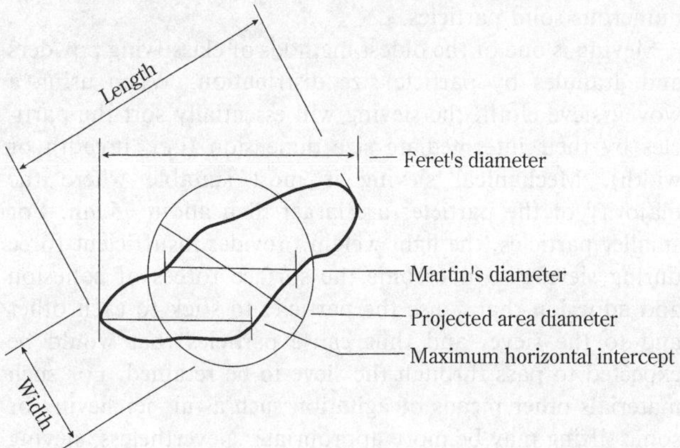

Fig. 3.04-1 Commonly used measurements of particle size

1.3.4. Particle Shape Characterization

For irregularly shaped particles, characterization of particle size must also include information on particle shape. The homogeneity of the powder should be checked using appropriate magnification. The following defines some commonly used descriptors of particle shape (see Fig. 3.04-2).

(i) Acicular: Slender, needle-like particle of similar width and thickness.

(ii) Columnar: Long, thin particle with a width and thickness that are greater than those of an acicular particle.

(iii) Flake: Thin, flat particle of similar length and width.

(iv) Plate: Flat particles of similar length and width but with greater thickness than flakes.

(v) Lath: Long, thin, and blade-like particle.

(vi) Equant: Particles of similar length, width, and thickness; both cubical and spherical particles are included.

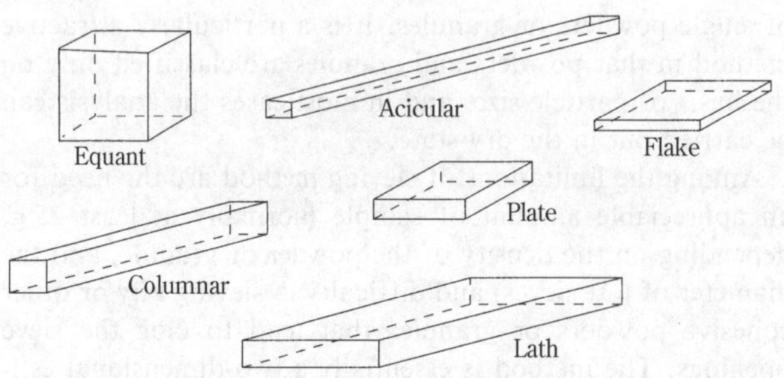

Fig. 3.04-2 Commonly used descriptions of particle shape

1.3.5. General Observations

A particle is generally considered to be the smallest discrete unit. A particle may be a liquid or semisolid droplet; a single crystal or polycrystalline; amorphous or an agglomerate. Particles may be associated.

This degree of association may be described by the following terms.

(i) Lamellar: Stacked plates.

(ii) Aggregate: Mass of adhered particles.

(iii) Agglomerate: Fused or cemented particles.

(iv) Conglomerate: Mixture of two or more types of particles.

(v) Spherulite: Radial cluster.

(vi) Drusy: Particle covered with tiny particles.

Particle condition may be described by the following terms.

(i) Edges: Angular, rounded, smooth, sharp, fractured.

(ii) Optical: Color (using proper color balancing filters), transparent, translucent, opaque.

(iii) Defects: Occlusions, inclusions.

Surface characteristics may be described by the following terms.

(i) Cracked: Partial split, break, or fissure.

(ii) Smooth: Free of irregularities, roughness, or projections.

(iii) Porous: Having openings or passageways.

(iv) Rough: Bumpy, uneven, not smooth.

(v) Pitted: Small indentations.

2. Method 2. Analytical Sieving Method

◆The analytical sieving method is a method to estimate the particle size distribution of powdered pharmaceutical drugs by sieving. The particle size determined by this method is shown as the size of a minimum sieve opening through which the particle passes. ''Powder'' here means a gathering of numerous solid particles.◆

Sieving is one of the oldest methods of classifying powders and granules by particle size distribution. When using a woven sieve cloth, the sieving will essentially sort the particles by their intermediate size dimension (i.e., breadth or width). Mechanical sieving is most suitable where the majority of the particles are larger than about 75 μm. For smaller particles, the light weight provides insufficient force during sieving to overcome the surface forces of cohesion and adhesion that cause the particles to stick to each other and to the sieve, and thus cause particles that would be expected to pass through the sieve to be retained. For such materials other means of agitation such as air-jet sieving or sonic sifting may be more appropriate. Nevertheless, sieving can sometimes be used for some powders or granules having median particle sizes smaller than 75 μm where the method can be validated. In pharmaceutical terms, sieving is usually the method of choice for classification of the coarser grades of single powders or granules. It is a particularly attractive method in that powders and granules are classified only on the basis of particle size, and in most cases the analysis can be carried out in the dry state.

Among the limitations of sieving method are the need for an appreciable amount of sample (normally at least 25 g, depending on the density of the powder or granule, and the diameter of test sieves) and difficulty in sieving oily or other cohesive powders or granules that tend to clog the sieve openings. The method is essentially a two-dimensional estimate of size because passage through the sieve aperture is frequently more dependent on maximum width and thickness than on length.

This method is intended for estimation of the total particle size distribution of a single material. It is not intended for determination of the proportion of particles passing or retained on one or two sieves.

Estimate the particle size distribution as described under *Dry Sieving Method*, unless otherwise specified in the individual monograph. Where difficulty is experienced in reaching the endpoint (i.e., material does not readily pass through the sieves) or when it is necessary to use the finer end of the sieving range (below 75 μm), serious consideration should be given to the use of an alternative particle-sizing method.

Sieving should be carried out under conditions that do not cause the test sample to gain or lose moisture. The relative humidity of the environment in which the sieving is carried out should be controlled to prevent moisture uptake or loss by the sample. In the absence of evidence to the contrary, analytical test sieving is normally carried at ambient humidity. Any special conditions that apply to a particular material should be detailed in the individual monograph.

Principles of Analytical Sieving: Analytical test sieves are constructed from a woven-wire mesh, which is of simple weave that is assumed to give nearly square apertures and is sealed into the base of an open cylindrical container. The basic analytical method involves stacking the sieves on top of one another in ascending degrees of coarseness, and then placing the test powder on the top sieve.

The nest of sieves is subjected to a standardized period of agitation, and then the weight of material retained on each sieve is accurately determined. The test gives the weight percentage of powder in each sieve size range.

This sieving process for estimating the particle size distribution of a single pharmaceutical powder is generally intended for use where at least 80% of the particles are larger than 75 μm. The size parameter involved in determining particle size distribution by analytical sieving is the length of the size of the minimum square aperture through which the particle will pass.

2.1. Procedure

2.1.1. Test Sieves

Test sieves suitable for pharmacopoeial tests conform to the most current edition of International Organisation for Standardization (ISO) Specification ISO 3310-1; Test sieves—Technical requirements and testing (see Table 3.04-1).

Unless otherwise specified in the monograph, use those ISO sieves listed in the Table 3.04-1 as recommended in the particular region.

Sieves are selected to cover the entire range of particle sizes present in the test specimen. A nest of sieves having a $\sqrt{2}$ progression of the area of the sieve openings is recommended. The nest of sieves is assembled with the coarsest screen at the top and the finest at the bottom. Use micrometers or millimeters in denoting test sieve openings. [Note—Mesh numbers are provided in the table for conversion purposes only.] Test sieves are made from stainless steel or, less preferably, from brass or other suitable non-reactive wire.

2.1.1.1. Calibration of test sieves

Calibration and recalibration of test sieves is in accordance with the most current edition of ISO 3310-1[2]. Sieves should be carefully examined for gross distortions and fractures, especially at their screen frame joints, before use. Sieves may be calibrated optically to estimate the average opening size, and opening variability, of the sieve mesh. Alternatively, for the evaluation of the effective opening of test sieves in the size range of 212 to 850 μm, Standard Glass Spheres are available. Unless otherwise specified in the individual monograph, perform the sieve analysis at controlled room temperature and at ambient relative humidity.

2.1.1.2. Cleaning Test Sieves

Ideally, test sieves should be cleaned using only an air jet or a liquid stream. If some apertures remain blocked by test particles, careful gentle brushing may be used as a last resort.

2.1.2. Test Specimen

If the test specimen weight is not given in the monograph for a particular material, use a test specimen having a weight between 25 and 100 g, depending on the bulk density of the material, and test sieves having a 200 mm diameter. For 76 mm sieves the amount of material that can be accommodated is approximately 1/7th that which can be accommodated on a 200 mm sieve. Determine the most appropriate weight for a given material by test sieving accurately weighed specimens of different weights, such as 25, 50, and 100 g, for the same time period on a mechanical shaker. [Note—If the test results are similar for the 25-g and 50-g specimens, but the 100-g specimen shows a lower percentage through the finest sieve, the 100-g specimen size is too large.] Where only a specimen of 10 to 25 g is available, smaller diameter test sieves conforming to the same mesh specifications may be substituted, but the endpoint must be re-determined. The use of test samples having a smaller mass (e.g. down to 5 g) may be needed. For materials with low apparent particle density, or for materials mainly comprising particles with a highly iso-diametrical shape, specimen weights below 5 g for a 200 mm screen may be necessary to avoid excessive blocking of the sieve. During validation of a particular sieve analysis method, it is expected that the problem of sieve blocking will have been addressed.

If the test material is prone to picking up or losing significant amounts of water with varying humidity, the test must be carried out in an appropriately controlled environ-

Table 3.04-1. Sizes of standard sieve series in range of interest

ISO Nominal Aperture			US Sieve No.	Recommended USP Sieves (microns)	European Sieve No.	Japan Sieve No.
Principal sizes	Supplementary sizes					
R 20/3	R 20	R 40/3				
11.20 mm	11.20 mm	11.20 mm			11200	
	10.00 mm					
		9.50 mm				
	9.00 mm					
8.00 mm	8.00 mm	8.00 mm				
	7.10 mm					
		6.70 mm				
	6.30 mm					
5.60 mm	5.60 mm	5.60 mm			5600	3.5
	5.00 mm					
		4.75 mm				4
	4.50 mm					
4.00 mm	4.00 mm	4.00 mm	5	4000	4000	4.7
	3.55 mm					
		3.35 mm	6			5.5
	3.15 mm					
2.80 mm	2.80 mm	2.80 mm	7	2800	2800	6.5
	2.50 mm					
		2.36 mm	8			7.5
	2.24 mm					
2.00 mm	2.00 mm	2.00 mm	10	2000	2000	8.6
	1.80 mm					
		1.70 mm	12			10
	1.60 mm					
1.40 mm	1.40 mm	1.40 mm	14	1400	1400	12
	1.25 mm					
		1.18 mm	16			14
	1.12 mm					
1.00 mm	1.00 mm	1.00 mm	18	1000	1000	16
	900 µm					
		850 µm	20			18
	800 µm					
710 µm	710 µm	710 µm	25	710	710	22
	630 µm					
		600 µm	30			26
	560 µm					
500 µm	500 µm	500 µm	35	500	500	30
	450 µm					
		425 µm	40			36
	400 µm					
355 µm	355 µm	355 µm	45	355	355	42
	315 µm					
		300 µm	50			50
	280 µm					
250 µm	250 µm	250 µm	60	250	250	60
	224 µm					
		212 µm	70			70
	200 µm					
180 µm	180 µm	180 µm	80	180	180	83
	160 µm					
		150 µm	100			100
	140 µm					
125 µm	125 µm	125 µm	120	125	125	119
	112 µm					
		106 µm	140			140
	100 µm					
90 µm	90 µm	90 µm	170	90	90	166
	80 µm					
		75 µm	200			200
	71 µm					
63 µm	63 µm	63 µm	230	63	63	235
	56 µm					
		53 µm	270			282
	50 µm					
45 µm	45 µm	45 µm	325	45	45	330
	40 µm					
		38 µm			38	391

ment. Similarly, if the test material is known to develop an electrostatic charge, careful observation must be made to ensure that such charging is not influencing the analysis. An antistatic agent, such as colloidal silicon dioxide and/or aluminum oxide, may be added at a 0.5 percent (m/m) level to minimize this effect. If both of the above effects cannot be eliminated, an alternative particle-sizing technique must be selected.

2.1.3. Agitation Methods

Several different sieve and powder agitation devices are commercially available, all of which may be used to perform sieve analyses. However, the different methods of agitation may give different results for sieve analyses and endpoint determinations because of the different types and magnitude of the forces acting on the individual particles under test. Methods using mechanical agitation or electromagnetic agitation, and that can induce either a vertical oscillation or a horizontal circular motion, or tapping or a combination of both tapping and horizontal circular motion are available. Entrainment of the particles in an air stream may also be used. The results must indicate which agitation method was used and the agitation parameters used (if they can be varied), since changes in the agitation conditions will give different results for the sieve analysis and endpoint determinations, and may be sufficiently different to give a failing result under some circumstances.

2.1.4. Endpoint Determination

The test sieving analysis is complete when the weight on any of the test sieves does not change by more than 5% or 0.1 g (10% in the case of 76 mm sieves) of the previous weight on that sieve. If less than 5% of the total specimen weight is present on a given sieve, the endpoint for that sieve is increased to a weight change of not more than 20% of the previous weight on that sieve.

If more than 50% of the total specimen weight is found on any one sieve, unless this is indicated in the monograph, the test should be repeated, but with the addition to the sieve nest of a coarser sieve intermediate between that carrying the excessive weight and the next coarsest sieve in the original nest, i.e., addition of the ISO series sieve omitted from the nest of sieves.

2.2. Sieving Methods

2.2.1. Mechanical Agitation (Dry Sieving Method)

Tare each test sieve to the nearest 0.1 g. Place an accurately weighed quantity of test specimen on the top (coarsest) sieve, and place the lid. Agitate the nest of sieves for 5 minutes. Then carefully remove each from the nest without loss of material. Reweigh each sieve, and determine the weight of material on each sieve. Determine the weight of material in the collecting pan in a similar manner. Reassemble the nest of sieves, and agitate for 5 minutes. Remove and weigh each sieve as previously described. Repeat these steps until the endpoint criteria are met (see *Endpoint Determination* under *Test Sieves*). Upon completion of the analysis, reconcile the weights of material. Total losses must not exceed 5% of the weight of the original test specimen.

Repeat the analysis with a fresh specimen, but using a single sieving time equal to that of the combined times used above. Confirm that this sieving time conforms to the requirements for endpoint determination. When this endpoint has been validated for a specific material, then a single fixed time of sieving may be used for future analyses, providing the particle size distribution falls within normal variation.

If there is evidence that the particles retained on any sieve are aggregates rather than single particles, the use of mechanical dry sieving is unlikely to give good reproducibility, a different particle size analysis method should be used.

2.2.2. Air Entrainment Methods (Air Jet and Sonic Shifter Sieving)

Different types of commercial equipment that use a moving air current are available for sieving. A system that uses a single sieve at a time is referred to as *air jet* sieving. It uses the same general sieving methodology as that described under the *Dry Sieving Method*, but with a standardized air jet replacing the normal agitation mechanism. It requires sequential analyses on individual sieves starting with the finest sieve to obtain a particle size distribution. Air jet sieving often includes the use of finer test sieves than used in ordinary dry sieving. This technique is more suitable where only oversize or undersize fractions are needed.

In the *sonic sifting* method, a nest of sieves is used, and the test specimen is carried in a vertically oscillating column of air that lifts the specimen and then carries it back against the mesh openings at a given number of pulses per minute. It may be necessary to lower the sample amount to 5 g, when sonic shifting is employed.

The air jet sieving and sonic sieving methods may be useful for powders or granules when mechanical sieving techniques are incapable of giving a meaningful analysis.

These methods are highly dependent upon proper dispersion of the powder in the air current. This requirement may be hard to achieve if the method is used at the lower end of the sieving range (i.e., below 75 μm), when the particles tend to be more cohesive, and especially if there is any tendency for the material to develop an electrostatic charge. For the above reasons endpoint determination is particularly critical, and it is very important to confirm that the oversize material comprises single particles and is not composed of aggregates.

2.3. Interpretation

The raw data must include the weight of test specimen, the total sieving time, and the precise sieving methodology and the set values for any variable parameters, in addition to the weights retained on the individual sieves and in the pan. It may be convenient to convert the raw data into a cumulative weight distribution, and if it is desired to express the distribution in terms of a cumulative weight undersize, the range of sieves used should include a sieve through which all the material passes. If there is evidence on any of the test sieves that the material remaining on it is composed of aggregates formed during the sieving process, the analysis is invalid.

[1)]Additional information on particle size measurement, sample size, and data analysis is available, for example, in ISO 9276.

[2)]International Organization for Standardization (ISO) Specification ISO 3310-1; Test sieves-Technical requirements and testing

3.05 Water-Solid Interactions: Determination of Sorption-Desorption Isotherms and of Water Activity

This test is harmonized with the European Pharmacopoeia and the U.S. Pharmacopeia.

The parts of the text that are not harmonized are marked with symbols (◆ ◆).

Information on the harmonization with the European Pharmacopoeia and the U.S. Pharmacopeia is available on the website of the Pharmaceuticals and Medical Devices Agency.

◆The powder of drug as drug substances or preparations

often contacts with water during the production process or storage. For the assessment of the water-solid interactions, determinations of sorption-desorption isotherms and water activity are used. Water is interacted physically with solid in two ways, by an adsorption onto the surface of solid or an absorption permeating into the solid. In the case where both the adsorption and absorption are occurred, the term ''sorption'' is usually used.◆

1. Determination of Sorption-Desorption Isotherms

1.1 Principle

The tendency to take up water vapour is best assessed by measuring sorption or desorption as a function of relative humidity, at constant temperature, and under conditions where sorption or desorption is essentially occurring independently of time, i.e. equilibrium. Relative humidity, RH, is defined by the following equation:

$$\mathrm{RH} = (P_c/P_0) \times 100$$

P_c: pressure of water vapour in the system;
P_0: saturation pressure of water vapour under the same conditions.

The ratio P_c/P_0 is referred to as the relative pressure. Sorption or water uptake is best assessed by starting with dried samples and subjecting them to a known relative humidity. Desorption is studied by beginning with a system already containing sorbed water and reducing the relative humidity. As the name indicates, the sorption-desorption isotherm is valid only for the reference temperature, hence a special isotherm exists for each temperature. Ordinarily, at equilibrium, moisture content at a particular relative humidity must be the same, whether determined from sorption or desorption measurements. However, it is common to see sorption-desorption hysteresis.

1.2 Methods

Samples may be stored in chambers at various relative humidities. The mass gained or lost for each sample is then measured. The major advantage of this method is convenience, while the major disadvantages are the slow rate of reaching constant mass, particularly at high relative humidities, and the error introduced in opening and closing the chamber for weighing. Dynamic gravimetric water sorption systems allow the on-line weighing of a sample in a controlled system to assess the interaction of the material with moisture at various programmable levels of relative humidity at a constant temperature. The major benefit of a controlled system is that isothermal conditions can be more reliably established and that the dynamic response of the sample to changing conditions can be monitored. Data points for the determination of the sorption isotherm (e.g. from 0% to approximately 95% RH, non condensing) are only taken after a sufficiently constant signal indicates that the sample has reached equilibrium at a given level of humidity. In some cases (e.g. deliquescence), the maximum time may be restricted although the equilibrium level is not reached. The apparatus must adequately control the temperature to ensure a good baseline stability as well as accurate control of the relative humidity generation. The required relative humidities can be generated, e.g. by accurately mixing dry and saturated vapour gas with flow controllers. The electrostatic behaviour of the powder must also be considered. The verification of the temperature and the relative humidity (controlled with, for example, a certified hygrometer, certified salt solutions or deliquescence points of certified salts over an adequate range), must be consistent with the instrument specification. The balance must provide a sufficient mass resolution and long term stability.

It is also possible to measure amounts of water uptake not detectable gravimetrically using volumetric techniques. In the case of adsorption, to improve sensitivity, one can increase the specific surface area of the sample by reducing particle size or by using larger samples to increase the total area. It is important, however, that such comminution of the solid does not alter the surface structure of the solid or render it more amorphous or otherwise less ordered in crystallinity. For absorption, where water uptake is independent of specific surface area, only increasing sample size will help. Increasing sample size, however, will increase the time to establish some type of equilibrium. To establish accurate values, it is important to get desolvation of the sample as thoroughly as possible. Higher temperatures and lower pressures (vacuum) facilitate this process; however, one must be aware of any adverse effects this might have on the solid such as dehydration, chemical degradation or sublimation. Using higher temperatures to induce desorption, as in a thermogravimetric apparatus, likewise must be carefully carried out because of these possible pitfalls.

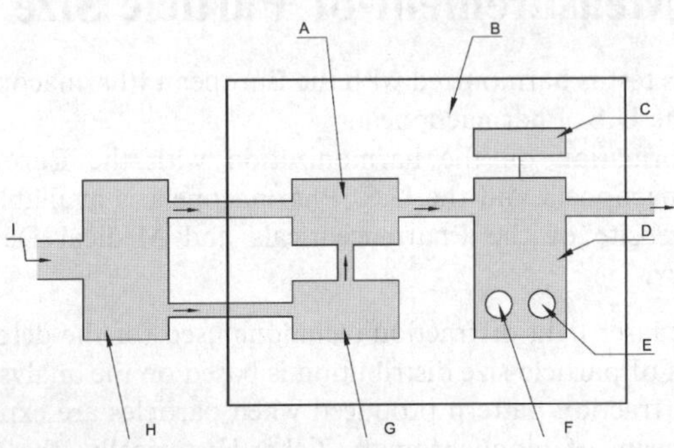

A. Humidity controller
B. Temperature controlled chamber
C. Balance module
D. Humidity regulated module
E. Reference
F. Sample
G. Vapour humidifier
H. Flow control module
I. Dry gas

Fig. 3.05-1 Example of an apparatus for the determination of the water sorption (other designs are possible)

1.3. Report and interpretation of the data

Sorption data are usually reported as a graph of the apparent mass change in per cent of the mass of the dry sample as a function of relative humidity or time. Sorption isotherms are reported both in tabular form and as a graph. The measurement method must be traceable with the data.

Adsorption-desorption hysteresis can be interpreted, for example, in terms of the porosity of the sample, its state of agglomeration (capillary condensation), the formation of hydrates, polymorphic change, or liquefying of the sample. Certain types of systems, particularly those with microporous solids and amorphous solids, are capable of sorbing large amounts of water vapour. Here, the amount of water associated with the solid as relative humidity is decreased, is greater than the amount that originally sorbed as the relative humidity was increased. For microporous solids, vapour adsorption-desorption hysteresis is an equilibrium phenomenon associated with the process of capillary condensation. This takes place because of the high degree of irregular curvature of the micropores and the fact that they ''fill'' (adsorption) and ''empty'' (desorption) under different equilibrium conditions. For non-porous solids capable of absorbing water, hysteresis occurs because of a change in the degree of vapour-solid interaction due to a change in the equilibrium state of the solid, e.g. conformation of polymer chains, or because the time scale for structural equilibrium is longer than the time scale for water desorption. In measuring sorption-desorption isotherms, it is therefore important to establish that something close to an equilibrium state has been reached. Particularly with hydrophilic polymers at high relative humidities, the establishment of water sorption or desorption values independent of time is quite difficult, since one is usually dealing with a polymer plasticised into its "fluid" state, where the solid is undergoing significant change.

In the case of crystal hydrate formation, the plot of water uptake versus pressure or relative humidity will in these cases exhibit a sharp increase in uptake at a particular pressure and the amount of water taken up will usually exhibit a stoichiometric mole: mole ratio of water to solid. In some cases, however, crystal hydrates will not appear to undergo a phase change or the anhydrous form will appear amorphous. Consequently, water sorption or desorption may appear more like that seen with adsorption processes. X-ray crystallographic analysis and thermal analysis are particularly useful for the study of such systems.

For situations where water vapour adsorption occurs predominantly, it is very helpful to measure the specific surface area of the solid by an independent method and to express adsorption as mass of water sorbed per unit area of solid surface. This can be very useful in assessing the possible importance of water sorption in affecting solid properties. For example, 0.5% *m/m* uptake of water could hardly cover the bare surface of 100 m^2/g, while for 1.0 m^2/g this amounts to 100 times more surface coverage. In the case of pharmaceutical solids which have a specific surface area in the range of 0.01 m^2/g to 10 m^2/g, what appears to be low water content could represent a significant amount of water for the available surface. Since the "dry surface area" is not a factor in absorption, sorption of water with amorphous or partially amorphous solids can be expressed on the basis of unit mass corrected for crystallinity, when the crystal form does not sorb significant amounts of water relative to the amorphous regions.

2. Determination of the Water Activity

2.1. Principle

Water activity, A_w, is the ratio of vapour pressure of water in the product (P) to saturation pressure of water vapour (P_0) at the same temperature. It is numerically equal to 1/100 of the relative humidity (RH) generated by the product in a closed system. RH can be calculated from direct measurements of partial vapour pressure or dew point, or from indirect measurement by sensors whose physical or electric characteristics are altered by the RH to which they are exposed. Ignoring activity coefficients, the relationship between A_w and equilibrium relative humidity (ERH) are represented by the following equations:

$$A_w = P/P_0$$
$$\text{ERH}\ (\%) = A_w \times 100$$

2.2. Method

The water activity is determined by placing the sample in a small airtight cup inside which the equilibrium between the water in the solid and the headspace can be established. The volume of the headspace must be small in relation to the sample volume in order not to change the sorption state of sample during the test. The equilibration as a thermodynamic process takes time but may be accelerated by forced circulation within the cell. The acquired water activity value is only valid for the simultaneously determined temperature. This requires a precise temperature-measuring device as part of the equipment. Furthermore, the probe must be thermally insulated to guarantee a constant temperature during the test. The sensor measuring the humidity of the headspace air above the sample is a key component. Theoretically, all types of hygrometers can be used, but for analytical purposes miniaturization and robustness are a precondition. The A_w measurement may be conducted using the dew point/chilled mirror method[1]. A polished, chilled mirror is used as a condensing surface. The cooling system is electronically linked to a photoelectric cell into which light is reflected from the condensing mirror. An air stream, in equilibrium with the test sample, is directed at the mirror which cools until condensation occurs on the mirror. The temperature at which this condensation begins is the dew point from which the ERH is determined. Commercially available instruments using the dew point/chilled mirror method or other technologies need to be evaluated for suitability, validated, and calibrated when used to make water activity determinations.

These instruments are typically calibrated over an adequate range, for example, using some saturated salt solutions at 25°C such as those listed in Table 3.05-1.

Table 3.05-1 Standard saturated salt solutions

Saturated salt solutions at 25°C	ERH (%)	A_w
Potassium sulphate (K_2SO_4)	97.3	0.973
Barium chloride ($BaCl_2$)	90.2	0.902
Sodium chloride (NaCl)	75.3	0.753
Magnesium nitrate ($Mg(NO_3)_2$)	52.9	0.529
Magnesium chloride ($MgCl_2$)	32.8	0.328
Lithium chloride (LiCl)	11.2	0.112

1) AOAC International Official Method 978.18.

3.06 Laser Diffraction Measurement of Particle Size

This test is harmonized with the European Pharmacopoeia and the U.S. Pharmacopoeia.

Information on the harmonization with the European Pharmacopoeia and the U.S. Pharmacopeia is available on the website of the Pharmaceuticals and Medical Devices Agency.

The laser light diffraction technique used for the determination of particle-size distribution is based on the analysis of the diffraction pattern produced when particles are exposed to a beam of monochromatic light. Historically, the early laser diffraction instruments only used scattering at small angles. However, the technique has since been broadened to include laser light scattering in a wider range and application of the Mie theory, in addition to the Fraunhofer approximation and anomalous diffraction.

The technique cannot distinguish between scattering by primary particles and scattering by clusters of primary particles, i.e. by agglomerates or aggregates. As most particulate samples contain agglomerates or aggregates and as the focus of interest is generally on the size distribution of primary particles, the clusters are usually dispersed into primary particles before measurement.

For non-spherical particles, an equivalent sphere-size distribution is obtained because the technique assumes spherical particles in its optical model. The resulting particle-size distribution may differ from those obtained by methods based on other physical principles (e.g. sedimentation, sieving).

This chapter provides guidance for the measurement of size distributions of particles in different dispersed systems, for example, powders, sprays, aerosols, suspensions, emulsions, and gas bubbles in liquids, through analysis of their angular light-scattering patterns. It does not address specific requirements of particle-size measurement of specific products. This technique complies with ISO13320-1 (1999) and 9276-1 (1998).

1. Instrument

The instrument is located in an environment where it is not affected by electrical noise, mechanical vibrations, temperature fluctuations, humidity or direct bright light. An example of a set-up of a laser light diffraction instrument is given in Fig. 3.06-1. Other equipment may be used.

The instrument comprises a laser light source, beam processing optics, a sample measurement region (or cell), a Fourier lens, and a multi-element detector for measuring the scattered light pattern. A data system is also required for deconvolution of the scattering data into a volumetric size distribution and associated data analysis and reporting.

The particles can enter the laser beam in 2 positions. In the conventional case the particles enter the parallel beam before the collecting lens and within its working distance. In so-called reversed Fourier optics the particles enter behind the collecting lens and thus, in a converging beam. The advantage of the conventional set-up is that a reasonable path length for the sample is allowed within the working distance of the lens. The second set-up allows only small path lengths but enables measurement of scattered light at larger angles, which is useful when submicron particles are present.

The interaction of the incident light beam and the ensemble of dispersed particles results in a scattering pattern with different light intensities at various angles. The total angular intensity distribution, consisting of both direct and scattered light, is then focused onto a multi-element detector by a lens or a series of lenses. These lenses create a scattering pattern that, within limits, does not depend on the location of the particles in the light beam. Hence, the continuous angular intensity distribution is converted into a discrete spatial intensity distribution on a set of detector elements.

It is assumed that the measured scattering pattern of the particle ensemble is identical to the sum of the patterns from all individual single scattering particles presented in random relative positions. Note that only a limited angular range of scattered light is collected by the lens(es) and, therefore, by the detector.

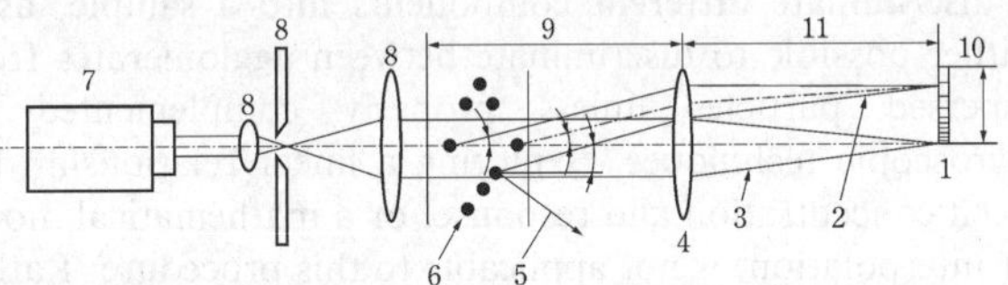

1. Obscuration detector
2. Scattered beam
3. Direct beam
4. Fourier lens
5. Scattered light not collected by lens (4)
6. Particle ensemble
7. Light source laser
8. Beam processing unit
9. Working distance of lens (4)
10. Multi-element detector
11. Focal distance of lens (4)

Fig. 3.06-1 Example of a set-up of a laser light diffraction instrument

2. Development of the method

The measurement of particle size by laser diffraction can give reproducible data, even in the sub-micron region, provided the instrument used and the sample tested are carefully controlled to limit variability of the test conditions (e.g. dispersion medium, method of preparation of the sample dispersion).

Traditionally, the measurement of particle size using laser diffraction has been limited to particles in the range of approximately 0.1 μm to 3 mm. Because of recent advances in lens and equipment design, newer instruments are capable of exceeding this range routinely. With the validation report the user demonstrates the applicability of the method for its intended use.

2.1. Sampling

The sampling technique must be adequate to obtain a representative sample of a suitable volume for the particle size measurement. Sample splitting techniques such as rotating riffler or the cone and quartering method may be applied.

2.2. Evaluation of the dispersion procedure

Inspect the sample to be analyzed, visually or with the aid of a microscope, to estimate its size range and particle shape. The dispersion procedure must be adjusted to the purpose of the measurement. The purpose may be such that it is preferable to deagglomerate clusters into primary particles as far as possible, or it may be desirable to retain clusters as intact as possible. In this sense, the particles of interest may be either primary particles or clusters.

For the development of a method it is highly advisable to check that comminution of the particles does not occur, and conversely, that dispersion of particles or clusters is satisfactory. This can usually be done by changing the dispersing energy and monitoring the change of the particle-size distribution. The measured size distribution must not change significantly when the sample is well dispersed and the particles are neither fragile nor soluble. Moreover, if the manufacturing process (e.g. crystallization, milling) of the material has changed, the applicability of the method must by verified (e.g. by microscopic comparison).

Sprays, aerosols and gas bubbles in a liquid should be measured directly, provided that their concentration is adequate, because sampling or dilution generally alters the particle-size distribution.

In other cases (such as emulsions, pastes and powders), representative samples may be dispersed in suitable liquids. Dispersing aids (wetting agents, stabilizers) and/or mechanical forces (e.g. agitation, sonication) are often applied for deagglomeration or deaggregation of clusters and stabilization of the dispersion. For these liquid dispersions, a recirculating system is most commonly used, consisting of an optical measuring cell, a dispersion bath usually equipped with stirrer and ultrasonic elements, a pump, and tubing. Non-recirculating, stirred cells are useful when only small amounts of a sample are available or when special dispersion liquids are used.

Dry powders can also be converted into aerosols through the use of suitable dry powder dispersers, which apply mechanical force for deagglomeration or deaggregation. Generally, the dispersers use the energy of compressed gas or the differential pressure of a vacuum to disperse the particles to an aerosol, which is blown through the measuring zone, usually into the inlet of a vacuum unit that collects the particles. However, for free flowing, coarser particles or granules the effect of gravity may be sufficient to disperse the particles adequately.

If the maximum particle size of the sample exceeds the measuring range of the instrument, the material that is too coarse can be removed by sieving and the mass and percentage of removed material are reported. However, after presieving, note that the sample is no longer representative, unless otherwise proven.

2.3. Optimization of the liquid dispersion

Liquids, surfactants, and dispersing aids used to disperse powders must:

(i) be transparent at the laser wavelength and practically free from air bubbles or particles;

(ii) have a refractive index that differs from that of the test material;

(iii) be non-solvent of the test material (pure liquid or pre-filtered, saturated solution);

(iv) not alter the size of the test materials (e.g. by solubility, solubility enhancement, or recrystallization effects);

(v) favor easy formation and stability of the dispersion;

(vi) be compatible with the materials used in the instrument (such as O-rings, gaskets, tubing, etc.);

(vii) possess a suitable viscosity to facilitate recirculation, stirring and filtration.

Surfactants and/or dispersing aids are often used to wet the particles and to stabilize the dispersion. For weak acids and weak bases, buffering of the dispersing medium at low or high pH respectively can assist in identifying a suitable dispersant.

A preliminary check of the dispersion quality can be performed by visual or microscopic inspection. It is also possible to take fractional samples out of a well-mixed stock dispersion. Such stock dispersions are formed by adding a liquid to the sample while mixing it with, for example, a glass rod, a spatula or a vortex mixer. Care must be taken to ensure the transfer of a representative sample and that settling of larger particles does not occur. Therefore a sample paste is prepared or sampling is carried out quickly from a suspension maintained under agitation.

2.4. Optimization of the gas dispersion

For sprays and dry powder dispersions, a compressed gas free from oil, water and particles may be used. To remove such materials from the compressed gas, a dryer with a filter can be used. Any vacuum unit should be located away from the measurement zone, so that its output does not disturb the measurement.

2.5. Determination of the concentration range

In order to produce an acceptable SN ratio in the detector, the particle concentration in the dispersion must exceed a minimum level. Likewise, it must be below a maximum level in order to avoid multiple scattering. The concentration range is influenced by the width of the laser beam, the path length of the measurement zone, the optical properties of the particles, and the sensitivity of the detector elements.

In view of the above, measurements must be performed at different particle concentrations to determine the appropriate concentration range for any typical sample of material. (Note: in different instruments, particle concentrations are usually represented by differently scaled and differently named numbers, e.g. obscuration, optical concentration, proportional number of total mass).

2.6. Determination of the measuring time

The time of measurement, the reading time of the detector and the acquisition frequency is determined experimentally in accordance with the required precision. Generally, the time for measurement permits a large number of detector scans or sweeps at short time intervals.

2.7. Selection of an appropriate optical model

Most instruments use either the Fraunhofer or the Mie theory, though other approximation theories are sometimes applied for calculation of the scattering matrix. The choice of the theoretical model depends on the intended application and the different assumptions (size, absorbance, refractive index, roughness, crystal orientation, mixture, etc.) made for the test material. If the refractive index values (real and imaginary parts for the used wavelength) are not exactly known, then the Fraunhofer approximation or the Mie theory with a realistic estimate of the refractive index can be used. The former has the advantages that it is simple and it does not need refractive index values; the latter usually provides less-biased particle-size distributions for small particles. For instance, if the Fraunhofer model is used for samples containing an appreciable amount of small, transparent particles, a significantly large amount of small particles may be calculated. In order to obtain traceable results, it is essential to document the refractive index values used, since small differences in the values assumed for the real and imaginary part of the complex refractive index may cause significant differences in the resulting particle-size distributions. Small values of the imaginary part of the refractive index (about $0.01 - 0.1i$) are often applied to allow the correction of the absorbance for the surface roughness of the particles. It should be noted, in general, that the optical properties of the substance to be tested, as well as the structure (e.g. shape, surface roughness and porosity) bear upon the final result.

2.8. Validation

Typically, the validity of a procedure may be assessed by the evaluation of its specificity, linearity, range, accuracy, precision and robustness. In particle-size analysis by laser light diffraction, specificity as defined by ICH (Validation of Analytical Procedures) is not applicable as it is not possible to discriminate different components into a sample, as is neither possible to discriminate between agglomerates from dispersed particles unless properly complemented by microscopic techniques. Exploring a linear relationship between concentration and response, or a mathematical model for interpolation, is not applicable to this procedure. Rather than evaluating linearity, this method requires the definition of a concentration range within which the result of the measurements does not vary significantly. Concentrations below that range produce an error due to a poor SN ratio, while concentrations above that range produce an error due to multiple scattering. The range depends mostly in the instrument hardware. Accuracy should be confirmed through an appropriate instrument qualification and comparison with microscopy, while precision may be assessed by means of a repeatability determination.

The attainable repeatability of the method mainly depends on the characteristics of the material (milled/not milled, robust/fragile, width of its size distribution, etc.), whereas the required repeatability depends on the purpose of the measurement. Mandatory limits cannot be specified in this chapter, as repeatabilities (different sample preparations) may vary appreciably from one substance to another. However, it is good practice to aim at acceptance criteria for repeatability such as RSD (%) ≦ 10% [$n=6$] for any central value of the distribution (e.g. for x_{50}). Values at the sides of the distribution (e.g. x_{10} and x_{90}) are oriented towards less stringent acceptance criteria such as RSD ≦ 15% [$n=6$]. Below 10 μm, these values must be doubled. Robustness may be tested during the selection and optimization of the dispersion media and forces. The change of the dispersing energy may be monitored by the change in the particle-size distribution.

3. Measurement

A representative sample, dispersed at an adequate concentration in a suitable liquid or gas, is passed through a beam of monochromatic light, usually a laser. The light scattered by the particles at various angles is measured by a multi-element detector. Numerical values representing the scattering pattern are then recorded for analysis. These scattering pattern values are then transformed, using an appropriate optical model and mathematical procedure, to yield the proportion of total volume to a discrete number of size classes, forming a volumetric particle-size distribution.

3.1. Precautions

(i) never look into the direct path of the laser beam or its reflections;

(ii) earth all instrument components to prevent ignition of solvents or dust explosions;

(iii) check the instrument set-up (e.g. warm-up, required measuring range and lens, appropriate working distance, position of the detector, no direct bright daylight);

(iv) in the case of wet dispersions, avoid air bubbles, evaporation of liquid, schlieren or other inhomogeneities in the dispersion; similarly, avoid improper mass-flow from the disperser or turbulent air-flow in the case of dry dispersions; such effects can cause erroneous particle-size distributions.

3.2. Measurement of the light scattering of dispersed sample(s)

After proper alignment of the optical part of the instrument, a blank measurement of the particle-free dispersion medium must be performed using the same method as that used for the measurement of the sample. The background signal must be below an appropriate threshold. The detector data are saved in order to substract them later from the data obtained with the sample. The sample dispersion is measured according to the developed method.

For each detector element, an average signal is calculated, sometimes together with its standard deviation. The magnitude of the signal from each detector element depends upon the detection area, the light intensity and the quantum efficiency. The co-ordinates (size and position) of the detector elements together with the focal distance of the lens determine the range of scattering angles for each element. Most instruments also measure the intensity of the central (unscattered) laser beam. The ratio of the intensity of a dispersed sample to that in its absence (the blank measurement) indicates the proportion of scattered light and hence the particle concentration.

3.3. Conversion of scattering pattern into particle-size distribution

This deconvolution step is the inverse of the calculation of a scattering pattern for a given particle-size distribution. The assumption of spherical particle shape is particularly important as most algorithms use the mathematical solution for scattering from spherical particles. Furthermore, the measured data always contain some random and systematic errors, which may vitiate the size distributions. Several mathematical procedures have been developed for use in the available instruments. They contain some weighting of deviations between measured and calculated scattering patterns (e.g. least squares), some constraints (e.g. non-negativity for amounts of particles), and/or some smoothing of the size distribution curve.

The algorithms used are specific to each maker and model of equipment, and are proprietary. The differences in the algorithms between different instruments may give rise to differences in the calculated particle-size distributions.

3.4. Replicates

The number of replicate measurements (with individual sample preparations) to be performed, depends on the required measurement precision. It is recommended to set this number in a substance-specific method.

4. Reporting of results

The particle-size distribution data are usually reported as cumulative undersize distribution and/or as density distribution by volume. The symbol x is used to denote the particle size, which in turn is defined as the diameter of a volume-equivalent sphere. $Q_3(x)$ denotes the volume fraction undersize at the particle size x. In a graphical representation, x is plotted on the abscissa and the dependent variable $Q_3(x)$ on the ordinate. Most common characteristic values are calculated from the particle-size distribution by interpolation. The particle sizes at the undersize values of 10%, 50%, and 90% (denoted as x_{10}, x_{50}, and x_{90} respectively) are frequently used. x_{50} is also known as the median particle size. It is recognized that the symbol d is also widely used to designate the particle size, thus the symbol x may be replaced by d.

Moreover, sufficient information must be documented about the sample, the sample preparation, the dispersion conditions, and the cell type. As the results depend on the particular instrument, data analysis program, and optical model used, these details must also be documented.

5. Control of the instrument performance

Use the instrument according to the manufacturer's instructions and carry out the prescribed qualifications at an appropriate frequency, according to the use of the instrument and substances to be tested.

5.1. Calibration

Laser diffraction systems, although assuming idealized properties of the particles, are based on first principles of laser light scattering. Thus, calibration in the strict sense is not required. However, it is still necessary to confirm that the instrument is operating correctly. This can be undertaken using any certified reference material that is acceptable in industrial practice. The entire measurement procedure is examined, including sample collection, sample dispersion, sample transport through the measuring zone, measurement, and the deconvolution procedure. It is essential that the total operational procedure is fully described.

The preferred certified reference materials consist of spherical particles of a known distribution. They must be certified as to the mass-percentage size distribution by an absolute technique, if available, and used in conjunction with an agreed, detailed operation procedure. It is essential that the real and imaginary parts of the complex refractive index of the material are indicated if the Mie theory is applied in data analysis. The representation of the particle-size distribution by volume will equal that of the distribution by mass, provided that the density of the particles is the same for all size fractions.

The response of a laser diffraction instrument is considered to meet the requirements if the mean value of x_{50} from at least 3 independent measurements does not deviate by more than 3% from the certified range of values of the certified reference material. The mean values for x_{10} and x_{90} must not deviate by more than 5% from the certified range of values. Below 10 μm, these values must be doubled.

Although the use of materials consisting of spherical particles is preferable, non-spherical particles may also be employed. Preferably, these particles have certified or typical values from laser diffraction analysis performed according to an agreed, detailed operating procedure. The use of reference values from methods other than laser diffraction may cause a significant bias. The reason for this bias is that the different principles inherent in the various methods may lead to different sphere-equivalent diameters for the same non-spherical particle.

Although the use of certified reference materials is preferred, other well-defined reference materials may also be employed. They consist of substances of typical composition and particle-size distribution for a specified class of substances. Their particle-size distribution has proven to be stable over time. The results must comply with previously determined data, with the same precision and bias as for the certified reference material.

5.2. Qualification of the system

In addition to the calibration, the performance of the instrument must be qualified at regular time intervals or as frequently as appropriate. This can be undertaken using any suitable reference material as mentioned in the previous paragraph.

The qualification of the system is based on the concept that the equipment, electronics, software and analytical operations constitute an integral system, which can be evaluated as an entity. Thus the entire measurement procedure is examined, including sample collection, sample dispersion, sample transport through the measuring zone, and the measurement and deconvolution procedure. It is essential that the total operational procedure is fully described.

In general, unless otherwise specified in the individual monograph, the response of a laser diffraction instrument is considered to meet the requirements if the x_{50} value does not deviate by more than 10% from the range of values of the reference material. If optionally the values at the sides of the distribution are evaluated (e.g. x_{10} and x_{90}), then these values must not deviate by more than 15% from the certified range of values. Below 10 μm, these values must be doubled. For calibration of the instrument stricter requirements are laid down in 5.1. Calibration.

4. Biological Tests/Biochemical Tests/Microbial Tests

4.01 Bacterial Endotoxins Test

This test is harmonized with the European Pharmacopoeia and the U.S. Pharmacopeia.

Information on the harmonization with the European Pharmacopoeia and the U.S. Pharmacopeia is available on the website of the Pharmaceuticals and Medical Devices Agency.

Bacterial Endotoxins Test is a test to detect or quantify bacterial endotoxins of gram-negative bacterial origin using an amoebocyte lysate prepared from blood corpuscle extracts of horseshoe crab (*Limulus polyphemus* or *Tachypleus tridentatus*). There are two types of techniques for this test: the gel-clot techniques, which are based on gel formation by the reaction of the lysate TS with endotoxins, and the photometric techniques, which are based on endotoxin-induced optical changes of the lysate TS. The latter include turbidimetric techniques, which are based on the change in lysate TS turbidity during gel formation, and chromogenic techniques, which are based on the development of color after cleavage of a synthetic peptide-chromogen complex.

Proceed by any one of these techniques for the test. In the event of doubt or dispute, the final decision is made based on the limit test of the gel-clot techniques, unless otherwise indicated.

The test is carried out in a manner that avoids endotoxin contamination.

1. Apparatus

Depyrogenate all glassware and other heat-stable materials in a hot-air oven using a validated process. Commonly used minimum time and temperature settings are 30 minutes at 250°C. If employing plastic apparatus, such as multi-well plates and tips for micropipettes, use only that which has been shown to be free of detectable endotoxin and which does not interfere with the test.

2. Preparation of Solutions

2.1. Standard Endotoxin Stock Solution

Prepare Standard Endotoxin Stock Solution by dissolving Japanese Pharmacopoeia Endotoxin Reference Standard that has been calibrated to the current WHO International Standard for Endotoxin, using water for bacterial endotoxins test (BET). Endotoxin is expressed in Endotoxin Units (EU). One EU is equal to one International Unit (IU) of endotoxin.

2.2. Standard Endotoxin Solution

After mixing Standard Endotoxin Stock Solution thoroughly, prepare appropriate serial dilutions of Standard Endotoxin Solution, using water for BET. Use dilutions as soon as possible to avoid loss of activity by adsorption.

2.3. Sample Solutions

Unless otherwise specified, prepare sample solutions by dissolving or diluting drugs, using water for BET. By the sample, an aqueous solution other than water for BET may be used to dissolve or dilute. If necessary, adjust the pH of the sample solution so that the pH of the mixture of the lysate TS and sample solution falls within the specified pH range for the lysate to be used. The pH of the sample solution may be in the range of 6.0 to 8.0. For adjustment of pH, acid, base or a suitable buffer solution may be used. The acid and base are prepared from their concentrated solutions or solids using water for BET, and then stored in containers free of detectable endotoxin. The buffer solutions must be validated to be free of detectable endotoxin and interfering factors.

3. Determination of Maximum Valid Dilution

The Maximum Valid Dilution (MVD) is the maximum allowable dilution of a sample solution at which the endotoxin limit can be determined.

Determine the MVD from the following equation:

MVD
= (Endotoxin limit × Concentration of sample solution)/λ

Endotoxin limit:

The endotoxin limit for injections, defined on the basis of dose, equals K/M, where K is a threshold pyrogenic dose of endotoxin per kg body mass (EU/kg), and M is equal to the maximum bolus dose of product per kg body mass. When the product is to be injected at frequent intervals or infused continuously, M is the maximum total dose administered in a single hour period.

Concentration of sample solution:

mg/mL in the case of endotoxin limit specified by mass (EU/mg)

mEq/mL in the case of endotoxin limit specified by equivalent (EU/mEq)

Units/mL in the case of endotoxin limit specified by biological unit (EU/Unit)

mL/mL in the case of endotoxin limit specified by volume (EU/mL)

λ: the labeled lysate reagent sensitivity in the gel-clot techniques (EU/mL) or the lowest point used (EU/mL) in the standard regression curve of the turbidimetric or chromogenic techniques

4. Gel-clot techniques

The gel-clot techniques detect or quantify endotoxins based on clotting of the lysate TS in the presence of endotoxin.

To ensure both the precision and validity of the test, perform the tests for confirming the labeled lysate reagent sensitivity (4.1.1.) and for interfering factors (4.1.2.) as described under Preparatory testing (4.1.).

4.1. Preparatory testing

4.1.1. Test for confirmation of labeled lysate reagent sensitivity

The labeled sensitivity of lysate is defined as the lowest concentration of endotoxin that is needed to cause the lysate TS to clot under the conditions specified for the lysate to be used.

The test for confirmation of the labeled lysate sensitivity is to be carried out when each new lot of lysate is used or when there is any change in the experimental conditions which may affect the outcome of the test.

Prepare standard solutions having four concentrations equivalent to 2 λ, λ, 0.5 λ and 0.25 λ by diluting the Standard Endotoxin Stock Solution with water for BET. Mix a volume of the lysate TS with an equal volume of one of the standard solutions (usually, 0.1 mL aliquots) in each test tube. When single test vials or ampoules containing lyophilized lysate are used, add solutions directly to the vial or ampoule.

Keep the tubes (or containers such as vials or ampoules) containing the reaction mixture usually at 37 ± 1°C for 60 ± 2 minutes, avoiding vibration. To test the integrity of the gel after incubation, invert each tube or container through approximately 180° in one smooth motion. If a firm gel has formed that remains in place upon inversion, record the result as positive. A result is negative if either a firm gel is not formed, or if a fragile gel has formed but flows out upon inversion.

Making the standard solutions of four concentrations one set, test four replicates of the set.

The test is valid when 0.25 λ of the standard solution shows a negative result in each set of tests. If the test is not valid, repeat the test after verifying the test conditions.

The endpoint is the last positive test in the series of decreasing concentrations of endotoxin. Calculate the geometric mean endpoint concentration of the four replicate series using the following formula:

$$\text{Geometric Mean Endpoint Concentration} = \text{antilog}\,(\Sigma e/f)$$

Σe: The sum of the log endpoint concentrations of the dilution series used

f: The number of replicates

If the geometric mean endpoint concentration is not less than 0.5 λ and not more than 2.0 λ, the labeled sensitivity is confirmed, and is used in tests performed with this lysate.

Table 4.01-1

Solution	Endotoxin Concentration/ Solution to which endotoxin is added	Diluent	Dilution factor	Endotoxin concentration	Number of replicates
A*1	0/Sample solution	—	—	—	4
B*2	2λ/Sample solution	Sample solution	1 2 4 8	2λ 1λ 0.5λ 0.25λ	4
C*3	2λ/Water for BET	Water for BET	1 2 4 8	2λ 1λ 0.5λ 0.25λ	2
D*4	0/Water for BET	—	—	—	2

*1 Negative control. Sample solution only.

*2 Sample solutions added with standard endotoxin (for testing interfering factors).

*3 Standard endotoxin solutions for confirmation of the labeled lysate reagent sensitivity.

*4 Negative control. Water for BET only.

4.1.2. Test for interfering factors

This test is performed to check for the presence of enhancing or inhibiting factors for the reaction in sample solutions.

Prepare the solutions A, B, C and D according to Table 4.01-1, and test solutions A and B and solutions C and D in quadruplicate and in duplicate, respectively. Concerning the incubation temperature, incubation time, and procedure for the confirmation of gel formation, follow the procedure described in 4.1.1.

The geometric mean endpoint concentrations of B and C solutions are determined by using the formula described in 4.1.1.

This test must be repeated when there is any change in the experimental conditions which may affect the outcome of the test.

The test is valid if solutions A and D show no reaction and the result for solution C confirms the labeled sensitivity.

If the geometric mean endpoint concentration of solution B is not less than 0.5 λ and not greater than 2.0 λ, the sample solution being examined does not contain interfering factors and complies with the test for interfering factors. Otherwise the sample solution interferes with the test.

If the sample under test does not comply with the test at a dilution less than the MVD, repeat the test using a greater dilution, not exceeding the MVD. The use of a more sensitive lysate permits a greater dilution of the sample to be examined. Furthermore, interference of the sample solution or diluted sample solution may be eliminated by suitable treatment, such as filtration, neutralization, dialysis or heat treatment. To establish that the treatment chosen effectively eliminates interference without loss of endotoxins, perform the assay described above using the preparation to be examined to which Standard Endotoxin has been added and which has then been submitted to the chosen treatment.

4.2. Limit test

This method tests whether or not a sample contains endotoxins greater than the endotoxin limit specified in the individual monograph based on the gel formation in the presence of endotoxins at a concentration of more than the labeled lysate sensitivity.

4.2.1. Procedure

Prepare solutions A, B, C and D according to Table

Table 4.01-2

Solution	Endotoxin concentration/Solution to which endotoxin is added	Number of replicates
A*1	0/Sample solution	2
B*2	2λ/Sample solution	2
C*3	2λ/Water for BET	2
D*4	0/Water for BET	2

*1 Sample solution for the limit test. The solution may be diluted not to exceed the MVD.
*2 Positive control. Sample solution at the same dilution as solution A, containing standard endotoxin at a concentration of 2λ.
*3 Positive control. Standard endotoxin solution containing standard endotoxin concentration of 2λ.
*4 Negative control. Water for BET only.

Table 4.01-3

Solution	Endotoxin concentration/ Solution to which endotoxin is added	Diluent	Dilution factor	Endotoxin concentration	Number of replicates
A*1	0/Sample solution	Water for BET	1 2 4 8	— — — —	2
B*2	2λ/Sample solution	—	1	2λ	2
C*3	2λ/Water for BET	Water for BET	1 2 4 8	2λ 1λ 0.5λ 0.25λ	2
D*4	0/Water for BET	—	—	—	2

*1 Sample solutions for the Quantitative test. The dilution range of the dilution series may be changed as appropriate, but not exceeding the MVD.
*2 Positive control. Sample solution at the same dilution as the solution A diluted at the lowest dilution factor, containing standard endotoxin at a concentration of 2λ.
*3 Standard endotoxin solutions for confirmation of the labeled lysate sensitivity.
*4 Negative control. Water for BET only.

4.01-2. Making these four solutions one set, test two replicates of the set. In preparing solutions A and B, use the sample solutions complying with 4.1.2.

Concerning the test conditions including the incubation temperature, incubation time, and procedure for the confirmation of gel formation, follow the procedure under 4.1.1.

4.2.2. Interpretation

The test is valid when both replicates of solutions B and C are positive and those of solution D are negative.

When a negative result is found for both replicates of solution A, the sample complies with the Bacterial Endotoxins Test.

When a positive result is found for both replicates of solution A, the sample does not comply with the test.

When a positive result is found for one replicate of solution A and a negative result is found for the other, repeat the test. In the repeat test, the sample complies with the test if a negative result is found for both replicates of solution A. The sample does not comply with the test if a positive result is found for one or both replicates of solution A.

However, if the sample does not comply with the test at a dilution less than the MVD, the test may be repeated using a greater dilution, not exceeding the MVD.

4.3. Quantitative Test

This method measures endotoxin concentrations of samples by determining an endpoint of gel formation.

4.3.1. Procedure

Prepare solutions A, B, C and D according to Table 4.01-3. Making these four solutions one set, test two replicates of the set. When preparing solutions A and B, use sample solutions complying with 4.1.2. Concerning the test conditions, follow the procedure described in 4.1.1.

4.3.2. Calculation and interpretation

The test is valid when the following three conditions are met: (a) both replicates of the negative control solution D are negative, (b) both replicates of the positive product control solution B are positive and (c) the geometric mean endpoint concentration of solution C is in the range of 0.5 λ to 2 λ.

The endpoint is defined as the maximum dilution showing the last positive test in the dilution series of solution A, and the endotoxin concentration of the sample solution is calculated by multiplying the endpoint dilution factor by λ.

If none of the dilutions of solution A is positive, report the endotoxin concentration of the sample solution as less than $\lambda \times$ the lowest dilution factor of the sample solution.

If all dilutions are positive, the endotoxin concentration of the sample solution is reported as equal to or greater than the greatest dilution factor of solution A multiplied by λ.

Calculate the endotoxin concentration (in EU/mL, EU/mg, EU/mEq or EU/Unit) of the sample based on the endotoxin concentration of the sample solution. The sample complies with the Bacterial Endotoxins Test if the endotoxin concentration of the sample in both replicates meets the requirement for the endotoxin limit (in EU/mL, EU/mg, EU/mEq or EU/Unit) specified in the individual monograph.

5. Photometric quantitative techniques

5.1. Turbidimetric technique

This technique measures the endotoxin concentrations of samples based on the measurement of turbidity change accompanying gel formation of the lysate TS. This technique is classified as either endpoint-turbidimetric or kinetic-turbidimetric.

The endpoint-turbidimetric technique is based on the quantitative relationship between the concentration of endotoxins and the turbidity of the reaction mixture at a specified reaction time.

The kinetic-turbidimetric technique is based on the quantitative relationship between the concentration of endotoxins and either the time needed to reach a predetermined turbidity of the reaction mixture or the rate of turbidity development.

The test is usually carried out at 37 ± 1°C, and turbidity is expressed in terms of either absorbance or transmission.

5.2. Chromogenic technique

This technique measures the endotoxin concentrations of sample solutions based on the measurement of chromophore released from a synthetic chromogenic substrate by the reaction of endotoxins with the lysate TS. This technique is classified as either endpoint-chromogenic or kinetic-chromogenic.

The endpoint-chromogenic technique is based on the quantitative relationship between the concentration of endotoxins and the release of chromophore at the end of an incubation period.

The kinetic-chromogenic technique is based on the quantitative relationship between the concentration of endotoxins and either the time needed to reach a predetermined absorbance (or transmittance) of the reaction mixture or the rate of color development.

The test is usually carried out at 37 ± 1°C.

5.3. Preparatory testing

To assure the precision and validity of the turbidimetric or chromogenic techniques, perform both Test for assurance of criteria for the standard curve (5.3.1.) and Test for interfering factors (5.3.2.), as indicated below.

5.3.1. Test for assurance of criteria for the standard curve

The test is to be carried out when each new lot of lysate reagent is used or when there is any change in the experimental conditions which may affect the outcome of the test.

Using the Standard Endotoxin Solution, prepare at least three endotoxin concentrations to generate the standard curve within the range of endotoxin concentrations indicated by the instructions for the lysate reagent used. Perform the test using at least three replicates of each standard endotoxin concentration according to the optimal conditions for the lysate reagent used (with regard to volume ratios, incubation time, temperature, pH, etc.).

If the desired range is greater than two logs, additional standards should be included to bracket each log increase in the range of the standard curve.

If the absolute value of the correlation coefficient, $|r|$, is greater than or equal to 0.980 for the range of endotoxin concentrations set up, the criteria for the standard curve are valid and the curve complies with the test.

If the standard curve does not comply with the test, repeat the test after verifying the test conditions.

5.3.2. Test for interfering factors

Prepare solutions A, B, C and D according to Table 4.01-4. Perform the test on these solutions following the optimal conditions for the lysate reagent used (with regard to volume of sample solution and lysate TS, volume ratio of sample solution to lysate TS, incubation time, etc.).

The test for interfering factors must be repeated when any condition changes, which is likely to influence the result of the test.

The test is valid when the following conditions are met.

1: The absolute value of the correlation coefficient of the standard curve generated using solution C is greater than or equal to 0.980.

2: The result with solution D does not exceed the limit of the blank value required in the description of the lysate employed, or it is less than the endotoxin detection limit of the lysate employed.

Calculate the recovery of the endotoxin added to solution B from the concentration found in solution B after subtracting the endotoxin concentration found in solution A. When the recovery of the endotoxin added to solution B is within 50% to 200%, the sample solution under test is considered to be free of interfering factors and the solution complies with the test.

When the endotoxin recovery is out of the specified range, the sample solution under test is considered to contain interfering factors. If the sample under test does not comply with the test, repeat the test using a greater dilution, not exceeding the MVD. Furthermore, interference of the sample solution or diluted sample solution not to exceed the MVD may be eliminated by suitable treatment, such as filtration, neutralization, dialysis or heat treatment. To establish that the treatment chosen effectively eliminates interference without loss of endotoxins, perform the assay described above using the preparation to be examined to which Standard Endotoxin has been added and which has then been submitted to the chosen treatment.

5.4. Quantitative test

5.4.1. Procedure

Prepare solutions A, B, C and D according to Table 4.01-4, and follow the procedure described in 5.3.2.

Table 4.01-4

Solution	Endotoxin concentration	Solution to which endotoxin is added	Number of test tubes or wells
A*1	0	Sample solution	Not less than 2
B*2	Middle concentration of the standard curve	Sample solution	Not less than 2
C*3	At least 3 concentrations	Water for BET	Each not less than 2
D*4	0	Water for BET	Not less than 2

*1 Sample solution only (for assaying endotoxin concentration in the sample solution). The sample solution may be diluted not to exceed the MVD.

*2 Sample solution at the same dilution as solution A, containing added standard endotoxin at a concentration equal to or near the middle of the standard curve.

*3 Standard endotoxin solutions at the concentrations used in 5.3.1. (for the standard curve).

*4 Negative control. Water for BET only.

5.4.2. Calculation of endotoxin concentration

Calculate the mean endotoxin concentration of solution A using the standard curve generated with solution C. The test is valid when all the following requirements are met.

1: The absolute value of the correlation coefficient of the standard curve generated using solution C is greater than or equal to 0.980.

2: The endotoxin recovery, calculated from the concentration found in solution B after subtracting the concentration of endotoxin found in solution A, is within the range of 50% to 200%.

3: The result with solution D does not exceed the limit of the blank value required in the description of the lysate employed, or it is less than the endotoxin detection limit of the lysate employed.

5.4.3. Interpretation

The sample complies with the Bacterial Endotoxins Test if the endotoxin concentration of the sample calculated from the mean endotoxin concentration of solution A meets the requirement of the endotoxin limit (in EU/mL, EU/mg, EU/mEq or EU/Unit) specified in the individual monograph.

4.02 Microbial Assay for Antibiotics

Microbial Assay for Antibiotics is a method to determine the antimicrobial potency of antibiotics based on their antimicrobial activities. There are three methods for this test: the cylinder-plate, perforated plate, and turbidimetric methods. The former two are based on the measurement of the size of the zones of microbial growth inhibition in a nutrient agar medium, and the turbidimetric method is based on the measurement of the inhibition of turbidity development in a fluid medium with microbial growth. Unless otherwise specified in the individual monograph, tests specified to be carried out by the cylinder-plate method may be conducted under the same test conditions using the perforated plate method instead. If necessary, first sterilize water, isotonic sodium chloride solution, buffer solutions, reagents, test solutions and essential parts of measuring instruments and appliances to be used for the test. In performing the test, precautions must be taken to prevent biohazard.

1. Cylinder-plate method

The cylinder-plate method is a method to determine the

antimicrobial potency of the antibiotic to be tested, and is based on the measurement of the size of the zone of growth inhibition of a test organism by the use of cylinder-agar plates.

1.1. Test organisms

Use the test organism specified in the individual monograph.

1.2. Culture media

Unless otherwise specified, use media with the following compositions. When 'peptone' is indicated as an ingredient of a medium, either meat peptone or casein peptone is applicable. Use sodium hydroxide TS or 1 mol/L hydrochloric acid TS to adjust the pH of the medium to obtain the specified value after sterilization. In the case of the medium for *Bacillus subtilis* ATCC 6633, adjust the pH using ammonia TS, potassium hydroxide TS or 1 mol/L hydrochloric acid TS. A different medium to the one specified for each test organism may be used if it has both a similar composition and an equal or better growth efficiency of the test organism in comparison with the specified medium. Unless otherwise specified, sterilize the media to be used in an autoclave.

(1) Agar media for seed and base layer

1) Media for test organism *Bacillus subtilis* ATCC 6633

i.
Peptone	5.0 g
Meat extract	3.0 g
Agar	15.0 g
Water	1000 mL

Mix all the ingredients, and sterilize. Adjust the pH of the solution so that it will be 7.8 to 8.0 after sterilization.

ii.
Peptone	5.0 g
Meat extract	3.0 g
Trisodium citrate dihydrate	10.0 g
Agar	15.0 g
Water	1000 mL

Mix all the ingredients, and sterilize. Adjust the pH of the solution so that it will be 6.5 to 6.6 after sterilization.

2) Medium for test organism *Saccharomyces cerevisiae* ATCC 9763

Glucose	10.0 g
Peptone	9.4 g
Meat extract	2.4 g
Yeast extract	4.7 g
Sodium chloride	10.0 g
Agar	15.0 g
Water	1000 mL

Mix all the ingredients, and sterilize. Adjust the pH of the solution so that it will be 6.0 to 6.2 after sterilization.

3) Media for other organisms

i.
Glucose	1.0 g
Peptone	6.0 g
Meat extract	1.5 g
Yeast extract	3.0 g
Agar	15.0 g
Water	1000 mL

Mix all the ingredients, and sterilize. Adjust the pH of the solution so that it will be 6.5 to 6.6 after sterilization.

ii.
Glucose	1.0 g
Meat peptone	6.0 g
Casein peptone	4.0 g
Meat extract	1.5 g
Yeast extract	3.0 g
Agar	15.0 g
Water	1000 mL

Mix all the ingredients, and sterilize. Adjust the pH of the solution so that it will be 6.5 to 6.6 after sterilization.

iii.
Peptone	10.0 g
Meat extract	5.0 g
Sodium chloride	2.5 g
Agar	15.0 g
Water	1000 mL

Mix all the ingredients, and sterilize. Adjust the pH of the solution so that it will be 6.5 to 6.6 after sterilization.

(2) Agar media for transferring test organisms

1) Medium for test organism *Saccharomyces cerevisiae* ATCC 9763

Glucose	15.0 g
Peptone	5.0 g
Yeast extract	2.0 g
Magnesium sulfate heptahydrate	0.5 g
Potassium dihydrogen phosphate	1.0 g
Agar	15.0 g
Water	1000 mL

Mix all the ingredients, and sterilize. Adjust the pH of the solution so that it will be 6.0 to 6.2 after sterilization.

2) Media for other organisms

i.
Glucose	1.0 g
Meat peptone	6.0 g
Casein peptone	4.0 g
Meat extract	1.5 g
Yeast extract	3.0 g
Agar	15.0 g
Water	1000 mL

Mix all the ingredients, and sterilize. Adjust the pH of the solution so that it will be 6.5 to 6.6 after sterilization.

ii.
Peptone	10.0 g
Meat extract	5.0 g
Sodium chloride	2.5 g
Agar	15.0 g
Water	1000 mL

Mix all the ingredients, and sterilize. Adjust the pH of the solution so that it will be 6.5 to 6.6 after sterilization.

1.3. Preparation of agar slant or plate media

Unless otherwise specified, dispense approximately 9 mL of melted agar medium in each test tube (approximately 16 mm in inside diameter), and make them as slant media, or dispense approximately 20 mL of melted agar medium in each Petri dish (approximately 90 mm in inside diameter), and make them as plate media.

1.4. Preparation of stock suspensions of test spores or organisms

Unless otherwise specified, prepare stock suspensions of test spore or organism cultures as follows. Check the aspects of the test spores or organisms as occasion demands.

(i) Preparation of a stock spore suspension of test organism *Bacillus subtilis* ATCC 6633

Inoculate the test organism onto the slant or plate of the agar medium which was prepared for transferring the test organisms specified in 1.2. (2) 2) i. Incubate at 32 to 37°C for 16 to 24 hours. Inoculate the subcultured test organism onto a suitable volume of slant or plate of the agar medium (described above), which was prepared for transferring the test organisms specified in 1.2. (2) 2) ii. Then incubate at 32 to 37°C for not less than 1 week to prepare spores. Suspend the spores in isotonic sodium chloride solution, heat at 65°C for 30 minutes, and then centrifuge. Wash the spore sediment three times with isotonic sodium chloride solution by means of centrifugation. Re-suspend the spore sediment in water or isotonic sodium chloride solution, and heat again at 65°C for 30 minutes to prepare the stock spore suspension. The concentration of the test organism is confirmed with the turbidity or absorbance, as occasion demands. Store the stock spore suspension at a temperature not exceeding 5°C, and use within 6 months. If the stock spore suspension shows a clear and definite zone of growth inhibition in an antibiotics potency test using adequate antibiotics, it may be used for further 6 months.

(ii) Preparation of a stock suspension of the test organism *Saccharomyces cerevisiae* ATCC 9763

Inoculate test organism onto the slant or plate agar medium which has been prepared for transferring test organism specified in 1.2. (2) 1). Incubate at 25 to 26°C for 40 to 48 hours. The subculture should be performed at least three times. Inoculate the subcultured test organism onto another slant or plate of the agar medium (described above), and incubate at 25 to 26°C for 40 to 48 hours. Scrape away and suspend the resulting growth from the agar surface in isotonic sodium chloride solution, and use this as a stock suspension of the test organism. The concentration of the test organism is confirmed with the turbidity or absorbance, as occasion demands. Store the stock suspensions of the test organisms at a temperature not exceeding 5°C, and use within 30 days.

(iii) Preparation of a stock suspension of other test organisms

Inoculate the test organism onto the slant or the plate of the agar medium which has been prepared for transferring the test organisms specified in 1.2. (2) 2) i. Incubate the inoculated slant at 32 to 37°C for 16 to 24 hours. The subculture should be performed at least three times. Inoculate the subcultured test organism onto another slant or plate agar medium (described above), and incubate the slant at 32 to 37 °C for 16 to 24 hours. Scrape away and suspend the resulting growth from the agar surface in isotonic sodium chloride solution, and use this as a stock suspension of the test organism. The concentration of the test organism is confirmed with the turbidity or absorbance, as occasion demands. Store the stock suspensions of the test organisms at a temperature not exceeding 5°C, and use within 5 days.

1.5. Preparation of agar base layer plates

Unless otherwise specified, dispense 20 mL of the melted agar medium for the base layer into each Petri dish, and in the case of a large dish, dispense a quantity of the agar medium to form a uniform layer 2 to 3 mm thick. Distribute the agar evenly in each dish on a flat, level surface, and allow it to harden.

1.6. Preparation of seeded agar layers

Unless otherwise specified, determine the volume of the stock suspension of the spore or the test organism with which the employed standard solution shows a clear and definite zone of growth inhibition. Prepare the seeded agar layer by mixing thoroughly the previously determined volume of stock suspension of spore or test organism with agar medium for the seed layer kept at 48 to 51°C. Usually, the rate of a stock spore suspension and a stock suspension of the test organism to add to the agar medium for the seed layer are 0.1 to 1.0 vol% and 0.5 to 2.0 vol%, respectively.

1.7. Preparation of cylinder-agar plates

Dispense 4 to 6 mL of the seeded agar layer, which is specified in the individual monograph, on an agar base layer plate in a Petri dish. In the case of large dishes, dispense a quantity of the agar medium to form a uniform layer 1.5 to 2.5 mm thick, and spread evenly over the surface before hardening. After coagulating the agar, allow the plate to stand under a clean atmosphere to exhale moisture vapor of the inside of Petri or large dishes and water on the agar surface. Place 4 cylinders on an agar plate in a Petri dish so that the individual cylinders are equidistant from the center of the plate and equally spaced from one another (the cylinders are set on the circumference of a circle of 25 to 28 mm radius). When large dish plates are used, place cylinders on each plate according to the method of preparation for Petri dish agar plates. A set of 4 cylinders on each large dish plate is considered to be equivalent to one Petri dish plate. Use stainless steel cylinders with the following dimensions: outside diameter 7.9 to 8.1 mm; inside diameter 5.9 to 6.1 mm; length 9.9 to 10.1 mm. The cylinders should not interfere with the test. Prepare the cylinder-agar plates before use.

1.8. Standard solutions

Use both a standard solution of high concentration and one of low concentration, as specified in the individual monograph. Unless otherwise specified, prepare the standard solutions before use.

1.9. Sample solutions

Use both a sample solution of high concentration and one of low concentration, as specified in the individual monograph. Unless otherwise specified, prepare the sample solutions before use.

1.10. Procedure

Unless otherwise specified, use 5 cylinder-agar plates as one assay set when Petri dishes are employed. When large dishes are employed, the number of cylinders for one assay set should be equal to that defined when using Petri dishes. Apply the standard solution of high concentration and that of low concentration to a pair of cylinders set opposite each other on each plate. Apply the high and low concentration sample solutions to the remaining 2 cylinders. The same volume of these solutions must be added to each cylinder. Incubate the plates at 32 to 37°C for 16 to 20 hours. Using a suitable measuring tool, measure the diameters of circular inhibition zones with a precision that can discriminate differences of at least 0.25 mm. Each procedure should be performed quickly under clean laboratory conditions.

1.11. Estimation of potency

The following correlation between the potency (*P*) of solution in a cylinder and the diameter (*d*) of zone of inhibition is established.

$$d = \alpha \log P + \beta$$

where, α and β are constants.

If necessary, ascertain the values in the above equation.

Based on this equation, estimate the potency of the sample solutions by application of the following equation:

Amount (potency) of sample
$= A \times$ Potency of S_H per mL $\times$ Dilution factor of U_H

where:

$$\log A = \frac{IV}{W}$$

$I = \log$ (potency of S_H/potency of S_L)
$V = \Sigma U_H + \Sigma U_L - \Sigma S_H - \Sigma S_L$
$W = \Sigma U_H + \Sigma S_H - \Sigma U_L - \Sigma S_L$

The sum of the diameter (mm) of the inhibitory zone measured in each plate is designated as follows:

for standard solution of high concentration (S_H) = ΣS_H
for standard solution of low concentration (S_L) = ΣS_L
for sample solution of high concentration (U_H) = ΣU_H
for sample solution of low concentration (U_L) = ΣU_L

2. Perforated plate method

The perforated plate method is a method to determine the antimicrobial potency of an antibiotic, based on the measurement of the size of the zone of growth inhibition of a test organism by the use of perforated agar plates.

This method is carried out by the use of perforated agar plates in lieu of cylinder-agar plates used in Cylinder-plate method.

Proceed as directed below, but comply with the requirements of Cylinder-plate method, such as test organisms, media, preparation of agar slant or plate media, preparation of stock suspensions of spores or test organisms, preparation of agar base layer plates, preparation of seeded agar layers, standard solutions, sample solutions, and estimation of potency.

2.1. Preparation of perforated agar plates

Dispense 4 to 6 mL of the seeded agar layer specified in the individual monograph on each agar base layer plate of the Petri dish. In the case of large dishes, dispense a quantity of the agar medium to form a uniform layer 1.5 to 2.5 mm thick, and spread evenly over the surface before hardening. After coagulating the agar, allow the plate to stand under a clean atmosphere to exhale moisture vapor of the inside of Petri or large dishes and water on the agar surface. Using a suitable tool, prepare 4 circular cavities having a diameter of 7.9 to 8.1 mm on a Petri dish agar plate so that the individual cavities are equidistant from the center of the plate. The cavities spaced equally from one another on the circumference of a circle with radius 25 to 28 mm, and are deep enough to reach the bottom of dish. When large dish plates are used, prepare the circular cavities on each plate according to the method of preparation for Petri dish agar plates. A set of 4 cavities on each large dish plate is considered to be equivalent to one Petri dish plate. Prepare the perforated agar plates before use.

2.2. Procedure

Unless otherwise specified, use 5 perforated agar plates as one assay set when Petri dishes are employed. When large dishes are employed, the number of cavities for one assay set should be equal to that defined when using Petri dishes. Apply the high and low concentration standard solutions to a pair of cavities prepared opposite each other on each plate, and apply the high and low concentration sample solutions to the remaining 2 cavities. The same volume of these solutions must be added to each cavity. Incubate the plates at 32 to 37°C for 16 to 20 hours. Using a suitable measuring tool, measure the diameters of the circular inhibition zones with a precision that can discriminate differences of at least 0.25 mm. Each procedure should be performed quickly under clean laboratory conditions.

3. Turbidimetric method

The turbidimetric method is a method to determine the antimicrobial potency of an antibiotic, based on the measurement of the inhibition of growth of a microbial culture in a fluid medium. The inhibition of growth of a test organism is photometrically measured as changes in turbidity of the microbial culture.

3.1. Test organisms

Use the test organism specified in the individual monograph.

3.2. Culture media

Unless otherwise specified, use media with the following compositions. When peptone is indicated as an ingredient of a medium, either meat peptone or casein peptone is applicable. Use sodium hydroxide TS or 1 mol/L hydrochloric acid TS to adjust the pH of the medium to obtain the specified value after sterilization. A different medium to the one specified for each test organism may be used if it has both a similar composition and an equal or better growth efficiency of the test organism in comparison with the specified medium. Unless otherwise specified, sterilize the media to be used in an autoclave.

(1) Agar media for transferring test organisms

Glucose	1.0 g
Peptone	6.0 g
Meat extract	1.5 g
Yeast extract	3.0 g
Sodium chloride	2.5 g
Agar	15.0 g
Water	1000 mL

Mix all the ingredients, and sterilize. Adjust the pH of the solution so that it will be 6.5 to 6.6 after sterilization.

(2) Liquid media for suspending test organisms

Glucose	1.0 g
Peptone	5.0 g
Meat extract	1.5 g
Yeast extract	1.5 g
Sodium chloride	3.5 g
Potassium dihydrogen phosphate	1.32 g
Disodium hydrogen phosphate*	3.0 g
Water	1000 mL

Mix all the ingredients, and sterilize. Adjust the pH of the solution so that it will be 7.0 to 7.1 after sterilization.

*Dipotassium hydrogen phosphate (3.68 g) may be used in lieu of disodium hydrogen phosphate (3.0 g).

3.3. Preparation of agar slant or plate media

Unless otherwise specified, proceed as directed in Preparation of agar slant or plate media under Cylinder-plate method.

3.4. Preparation of stock suspensions of test organisms

Unless otherwise specified, inoculate the test organism onto the slant or plate of the agar medium which was prepared for transferring the specified test organism. Incubate the inoculated medium at 32 to 37°C for 16 to 24 hours. The subculture should be performed at least three times. Check the aspects of the test spores or organisms as occasion demands. Inoculate the subcultured test organism onto another slant or plate of the agar medium (described above), and incubate the slant at 32 to 37°C for 16 to 24 hours. After incubation, suspend the test organism in the liquid medium for suspending the test organism, and use as the suspension of the test organism. The concentration of the test organism is confirmed with the turbidity or absorbance, as occasion demands.

3.5. Standard solutions

Use the standard solutions specified in the individual monograph. Unless otherwise specified, prepare the standard solutions before use.

3.6. Sample solutions

Use the sample solutions specified in the individual monograph. Unless otherwise specified, prepare the sample solutions before use.

3.7. Procedure

Unless otherwise specified, proceed as follows:

Distribute 1.0 mL of each concentration of the standard solution, the sample solution, and water used as a control, into each set composed of 3 test tubes (about 14 mm in inside diameter and about 13 cm in length). Add 9.0 mL of the suspension of the test organism to each tube, and then incubate in a water bath maintained at 35 to 37°C for 3 to 4 hours. After incubation, add 0.5 mL of dilute formaldehyde (1 in 3) to each tube, and read each transmittance or absorbance at a wavelength of 530 nm.

3.8. Estimation of potency

Average the transmittance or absorbance values of each concentration of the standard solution, the sample solution and water used as a control, respectively. Generate the standard curve based on the average values of transmittance or absorbance of each concentration of the standard solution, and estimate the potency of the sample solution from its average value of transmittance or absorbance using the obtained standard curve.

If the standard dilutions of five concentrations in geometric progression are used, calculate the L and H values from the following equations. Plot point L and point H on graph paper and construct a straight line for the standard curve.

$$L = \frac{3a + 2b + c - e}{5}$$

$$H = \frac{3e + 2d + c - a}{5}$$

where:

L: Calculated value of transmittance or absorbance for the lowest concentration of the standard curve.

H: Calculated value of transmittance or absorbance for the highest concentration of the standard curve.

a, b, c, d, e: Average transmittance or absorbance values for each standard dilution, where a is the value from the lowest concentration standard solution, b, c and d are the values from each geometrically increased concentration standard solution, respectively, and e is the value from the highest concentration standard solution.

4.03 Digestion Test

Digestion Test is a test to measure the activity of digestive enzymes, as crude materials or preparations, on starch, protein and fat.

1. Assay for Starch Digestive Activity

The assay for starch digestive activity is performed through the measurement of starch saccharifying activity, dextrinizing activity, and liquefying activity.

1.1. Measurement of starch saccharifying activity

The starch saccharifying activity can be obtained by measuring an increase of reducing activity owing to the hydrolysis of the glucoside linkages when amylase acts on the starch. Under the conditions described in Procedure, one starch saccharifying activity unit is the amount of enzyme that catalyzes the increase of reducing activity equivalent to 1 mg of glucose per minute.

1.1.1. Preparation of Sample Solution

Dissolve the sample in an appropriate amount of water, or a buffer or salts solution specified in the monograph so that the reducing activity increases in proportion to the concentration of the sample solution, when measuring under the conditions described in Procedure. The concentration is normally 0.4 to 0.8 starch saccharifying activity unit/mL. Filter if necessary.

1.1.2. Preparation of Substrate Solution

Use potato starch TS for measuring the starch digestive activity. If necessary, add 10 mL of buffer or salts solution specified in the monograph, instead of 10 mL of 1 mol/L acetic acid-sodium acetate buffer solution (pH 5.0).

1.1.3. Procedure

Pipet 10 mL of the substrate solution, stand at 37 ± 0.5°C for 10 minutes, add exactly 1 mL of the sample solution, and shake immediately. Allow this solution to stand at 37 ± 0.5°C for exactly 10 minutes, add exactly 2 mL of alkaline tartrate solution of the Fehling's TS for amylolytic activity test, and shake immediately. Then, add exactly 2 mL of copper solution of the Fehling's TS for amylolytic activity test, shake gently, heat the solution in a water bath for exactly 15 minutes, and then immediately cool to below 25°C. Then, add exactly 2 mL of concentrated potassium iodide TS and 2 mL of diluted sulfuric acid (1 in 6), and titrate <*2.50*> the released iodine with 0.05 mol/L sodium thiosulfate VS to the disappearance of the blue color produced by addition of 1 to 2 drops of soluble starch TS (a mL). Separately, pipet 10 mL of water instead of the substrate solution and titrate <*2.50*> in the same manner (b mL).

$$\text{Starch saccharifying activity (unit/g)} = \text{amount (mg) of glucose} \times \frac{1}{10} \times \frac{1}{M}$$

$$\text{Amount (mg) of glucose} = (b - a) \times 1.6$$

M: Amount (g) of sample in 1 mL of sample solution

1.2. Measurement of starch dextrinizing activity

The starch dextrinizing activity can be obtained by measuring a decrease in starch coloration by iodine resulting from hydrolysis of the straight chain component (amylose) in starch when amylase acts on the starch. Under the conditions described in Procedure, one starch dextrinizing activity unit is the amount of enzyme required to reduce the coloration of potato starch by iodine by 10% per minute.

1.2.1. Preparation of Sample Solution

Dissolve the sample in an appropriate amount of water or a buffer or salts solution specified in the monograph so that the coloration of starch by iodine decreases in proportion to the concentration of the sample solution, when measuring under the conditions described in Procedure. The concentration is normally 0.2 to 0.5 starch dextrinizing activity unit/mL. Filter if necessary.

1.2.2. Preparation of Substrate Solution

Prepare the substrate solution in the same manner as the substrate solution in the measurement of starch saccharifying activity.

1.2.3. Procedure

Pipet 10 mL of the substrate solution, stand at 37 ± 0.5°C for 10 minutes, add exactly 1 mL of the sample solution, and shake immediately. Allow this solution to stand at 37 ± 0.5°C for exactly 10 minutes. Pipet 1 mL of this solution, add it to 10 mL of 0.1 mol/L hydrochloric acid TS, and shake immediately. Pipet 0.5 mL of this solution, add exactly 10 mL of 0.0002 mol/L iodine TS, and shake. Determine the absorbance A_T of this solution at the wavelength of 660 nm as directed under Ultraviolet-visible Spectrophotometry <*2.24*>. Separately, using 1 mL of water instead of the sample solution, determine the absorbance A_B in the same manner.

$$\text{Starch dextrinizing activity (unit/g)} = \frac{(A_B - A_T)}{A_B} \times \frac{1}{M}$$

M: Amount (g) of sample in 1 mL of sample solution

1.3. Measurement of starch liquefying activity

The starch liquefying activity can be obtained by measuring a decrease in the viscosity of starch solution resulting from the hydrolysis of molecules when amylase acts on the starch. Under the conditions described in Procedure, one starch liquefying activity unit is the amount of enzyme required to reduce the viscosity of the substrate solution equivalent to 1 g of potato starch from 200% to 100% of that of the 50% sucrose standard solution.

1.3.1. Preparation of Sample Solution

Dissolve the sample in an appropriate amount of water, or a buffer or salts solution specified in the monograph so that the viscosity decreases in proportion to the concentration of the sample solution, when measuring under the conditions described in Procedure. The concentration is normally 0.15

to 0.25 starch liquefying activity unit/mL. Filter if necessary.

1.3.2. Preparation of Substrate Solution

Weigh accurately about 1 g of potato starch, and measure the loss on drying at 105°C for 2 hours. Weigh exactly potato starch equivalent to 15.00 g calculated on the dried basis, add 300 mL of water, then add gradually 25 mL of 2 mol/L sodium hydroxide TS under thorough shaking, until the mixture forms a paste. Heat the mixture in a water bath for 10 minutes, shaking it occasionally. After cooling, neutralize the mixture with 2 mol/L hydrochloric acid TS, and add 50 mL of the buffer solution specified in the monograph and water to make exactly 500 g. Prepare before use.

1.3.3. Preparation of 50% Standard Sucrose Solution

Dissolve 50.0 g of sucrose in 50.0 mL of water.

1.3.4. Procedure

Put 50 mL of the 50% standard sucrose solution in a 100-mL conical flask, and allow it to stand in a thermostat at 37 ± 0.5°C for 15 minutes. Fix a viscometer shown in Fig. 4.03-1 so that its lower end almost touches the bottom of the flask and that the water in the thermostat circulates around the outer cylinder of the viscometer. After slowly pulling up the 50% standard sucrose solution by suction to the middle of the upper bulb of the viscometer, let it flow down by gravity, measuring the time taken for the solution to fall from the upper to the lower indicators (t_1 seconds). Take exactly 50 g of the substrate solution in another 100-mL conical flask, and stand it in another thermostat at 37 ± 0.5°C for 20 minutes. Add exactly 1 mL of the sample solution to it, and shake the flask immediately. Fix a viscometer vertically so that its lower end almost touches the bottom of the flask and that the water in the thermostat circulates around the outer cylinder of the viscometer. Occasionally pull the reaction solution up by suction to the middle of the upper bulb slowly, then let it flow down by gravity, measuring the time taken for the solution to fall from the upper to the lower indicators (t seconds). Repeat this operation until t becomes shorter than t_1. At each measurement, record the time (T' seconds) from the moment that the sample solution is added to the moment that the solution surface in the flask passes the upper indicator. ($T' + t/2$) is the reaction time (T) corresponding to t. Draw a curve for both t and T. Obtain T_1 and T_2 that correspond to t_1 and ($2 \times t_1$) by interpolation.

$$\text{Starch liquefying activity (unit/g)} = \frac{60}{(T_1 - T_2)} \times \frac{1.5}{M}$$

M: Amount (g) of sample in 1 mL of sample solution

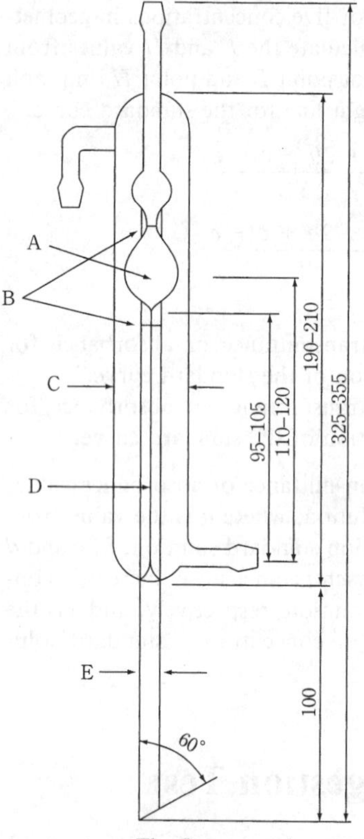

A: Bulb volume: 5 mL
B: Indicators
C: Outside diameter: 30 mm
D: Capillary inside diameter: 1.25–1.30 mm
E: Outside diameter: 8 mm
The figures are in mm.

Fig. 4.03-1

2. Assay for Protein Digestive Activity

The protein digestive activity can be obtained by the colorimetric measurement, making use of Folin's reaction, of the amount of acid-soluble low-molecular products, which is increased owing to the hydrolysis of the peptide linkages when protease acts on casein. One protein digestive activity unit is the amount of enzymes that produces Folin's TS-colorable substance equivalent to 1 μg of tyrosine per minute under the conditions described in Procedure.

2.1. Preparation of Sample Solution

Dissolve the sample in an appropriate amount of water, or a buffer or salts solution specified in the monograph so that the amount of non-protein, Folin's TS-colorable substances increase in proportion to the concentration of the sample solution, when measuring under the conditions described in Procedure. The concentration is normally 15 to 30 protein digestive activity unit/mL.

2.2. Tyrosine Calibration Curve

Weigh exactly 50 mg of Tyrosine for Digestion Test RS, previously dried at 105°C for 3 hours, and dissolve in 0.2 mol/L hydrochloric acid TS to make exactly 50 mL. Pipet 1 mL, 2 mL, 3 mL and 4 mL of this solution separately, and add 0.2 mol/L hydrochloric acid TS to each solution to make exactly 100 mL. Pipet 2 mL of each solution, and add exactly 5 mL of 0.55 mol/L sodium carbonate TS and 1 mL of diluted Folin's TS (1 in 3) to each solution, shake immediately, then stand them at 37 ± 0.5°C for 30 minutes. Determine the absorbances, A_1, A_2, A_3 and A_4, of these solutions at 660 nm as directed under Ultraviolet-visible Spectrophotometry <*2.24*>, using a solution prepared with exactly 2 mL of 0.2 mol/L hydrochloric acid TS in the same manner as the blank. Then, draw a calibration curve with the absorbances, A_1, A_2, A_3 and A_4 as the ordinate, and with the amount (μg) of tyrosine in 2 mL of each solution as the abscissa. Obtain the amount (μg) of tyrosine for the absorbance difference of 1.

2.3. Preparation of Substrate Solution

(i) Substrate solution 1: Weigh accurately about 1 g of milk casein, and measure the loss on drying at 105°C for 2 hours. Weigh exactly an amount of milk casein equivalent to 1.20 g calculated on the dried basis, add 12 mL of lactic acid TS and 150 mL of water, and warm to dissolve in a water bath. After cooling in running water, adjust to the pH specified in the monograph with 1 mol/L hydrochloric acid TS or sodium hydroxide TS, and add water to make exactly 200 mL. Prepare before use.

(ii) Substrate solution 2: Weigh accurately about 1 g of milk casein, and measure the loss on drying at 105°C for 2 hours. Weigh exactly an amount of milk casein equivalent to 1.20 g calculated on the dried basis, add 160 mL of 0.05 mol/L disodium hydrogenphosphate TS, and warm to dissolve in a water bath. After cooling in running water, adjust to the pH specified in the monograph with the 1 mol/L hydrochloric acid TS or sodium hydroxide TS, and add water to make exactly 200 mL. Prepare before use.

2.4. Preparation of Precipitation Reagent

(i) Trichloroacetic acid TS A: Dissolve 7.20 g of trichloroacetic acid in water to make 100 mL.

(ii) Trichloroacetic acid TS B: Dissolve 1.80 g of trichloroacetic acid, 1.80 g of anhydrous sodium acetate and 5.5 mL of 6 mol/L acetic acid TS in water to make 100 mL.

2.5. Procedure

Pipet 5 mL of the substrate solution specified in the monograph, stand at 37 ± 0.5°C for 10 minutes, add exactly 1 mL of the sample solution, and shake immediately. After standing this solution at 37 ± 0.5°C for exactly 10 minutes, add exactly 5 mL of trichloroacetic acid TS A or B as specified in the monograph, shake, stand it at 37 ± 0.5°C for 30 minutes, and then filter. Discard the first 3 mL of the filtrate, exactly measure the subsequent 2 mL of the filtrate, add exactly 5 mL of 0.55 mol/L sodium carbonate TS and 1 mL of diluted Folin's TS (1 in 3) to the solution, shake well, and stand it at 37 ± 0.5°C for 30 minutes. Determine the absorbance A_T of this solution at 660 nm as directed under Ultraviolet-visible Spectrophotometry <2.24>, using water as the blank. Separately, pipet 1 mL of the sample solution, add exactly 5 mL of trichloroacetic acid TS A or B to the solution as specified in the monograph, and shake. To this solution add exactly 5 mL of the substrate solution specified in the monograph, shake immediately, and stand it at 37 ± 0.5°C for 30 minutes. Follow the same procedure for the sample solution, and determine the absorbance A_B at 660 nm.

Protein digestive activity (unit/g)

$$= (A_T - A_B) \times F \times \frac{11}{2} \times \frac{1}{10} \times \frac{1}{M}$$

M: Amount (g) of sample in 1 mL of sample solution

F: Amount (μg) of tyrosine for absorbance 1 determined from Tyrosine Calibration Curve

3. Assay for Fat Digestive Activity

The fat digestive activity can be obtained by back titration of the amount of fatty acid produced from the hydrolysis of the ester linkage, when lipase acts on olive oil. One fat digestive activity unit is the amount of enzymes that produces 1 μmole of fatty acid per minute under the conditions described in Procedure.

3.1. Preparation of Sample Solution

Dissolve or suspend the sample in an appropriate amount of cold water, or a buffer or salts solution specified in the monograph so that the amount of fatty acid increases in proportion to the concentration of the sample solution, when measuring under the conditions described in Procedure. The concentration is normally 1 to 5 fat digestive activity unit/mL.

3.2. Preparation of Substrate Solution

Take 200 to 300 mL of a mixture of emulsifier and olive oil (3:1) in a blender (see Fig. 4.03-2), and emulsify it at 12,000 to 16,000 revolutions per minute for 10 minutes, while cooling the solution to a temperature below 10°C. Stand this solution in a cool place for 1 hour, and make sure before use that the oil does not separate.

3.3. Preparation of Emulsifier

Dissolve 20 g of polyvinyl alcohol specified in the monograph in 800 mL of water by heating between 75°C and 80°C for 1 hour while stirring. After cooling, filter the solution if necessary, and add water to make exactly 1000 mL.

3.4. Procedure

Pipet 5 mL of the substrate solution and 4 mL of the buffer solution specified in the monograph, transfer them to

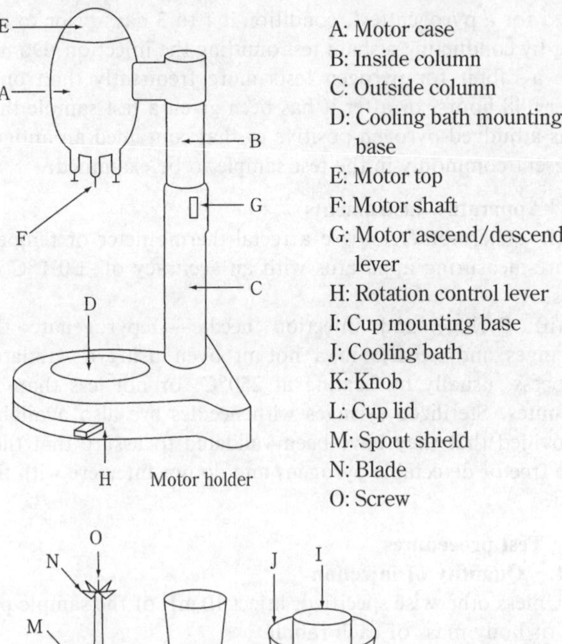

Fig. 4.03-2 Blender

a conical flask, and shake. After standing the mixture at 37 ± 0.5°C for 10 minutes, add exactly 1 mL of the sample solution, and shake immediately. Stand this solution at 37 ± 0.5°C for exactly 20 minutes, add 10 mL of a mixture of ethanol (95) and acetone (1:1), and shake. Then add exactly 10 mL of 0.05 mol/L sodium hydroxide VS, add 10 mL of a mixture of ethanol (95) and acetone (1:1), and shake. Titrate <2.50> the excess sodium hydroxide with 0.05 mol/L hydrochloric acid VS (b mL) (indicator: 2 to 3 drops of phenolphthalein TS). Separately, pipet 5 mL of the substrate solution and 4 mL of buffer solution specified in the monograph, transfer them to a conical flask, and shake. After standing it at 37 ± 0.5°C for 10 minutes, add 10 mL of a mixture of ethanol (95) and acetone (1:1), then add exactly 1 mL of the sample solution, and shake. Add exactly 10 mL of 0.05 mol/L sodium hydroxide VS, and titrate <2.50> in the same manner (a mL).

Fat digestive activity (unit/g)

$$= 50 \times (a - b) \times \frac{1}{20} \times \frac{1}{M}$$

M: Amount (g) of sample in 1 mL of sample solution

4.04 Pyrogen Test

Pyrogen Test is a method to test the existence of pyrogens by using rabbits.

1. Test animals

Use healthy mature rabbits, each weighing not less than 1.5 kg, which have not lost body mass when kept on a constant diet for not less than one week. House the rabbits individually in an area free from disturbances likely to excite them. Keep the temperature of the area constant between 20°C and 27°C for at least 48 hours before and throughout the test. Before using a rabbit that has not previously been used for a pyrogen test, condition it 1 to 3 days prior to the test by conducting a sham test omitting the injection. Do not use a rabbit for pyrogen tests more frequently than once every 48 hours, or after it has been given a test sample that was adjudged pyrogen-positive or that contained an antigen present commonly in the test sample to be examined.

2. Apparatus, instruments

(i) Thermometer—Use a rectal thermometer or temperature-measuring apparatus with an accuracy of ±0.1°C or less.

(ii) Syringe and injection needle—Depyrogenate the syringes and needles in a hot-air oven using a validated process, usually by heating at 250°C for not less than 30 minutes. Sterilized syringes with needles are also available provided that they have been validated to assure that they are free of detectable pyrogens and do not interfere with the test.

3. Test procedures

3.1. Quantity of injection

Unless otherwise specified, inject 10 mL of the sample per kg of body mass of each rabbit.

3.2. Procedure

Perform the test in a separate area at an environmental temperature similar to that of the room wherein the animals were housed and free from disturbances likely to excite them. Withhold food from the rabbits for several hours before the first record of the temperature and throughout the testing period. The test animals are usually restrained with loosely fitting neck stocks that allow the rabbits to assume a natural resting posture. Determine the temperature of each rabbit by inserting the thermometer or temperature-measuring probe into the rectum of the test animal to a constant depth within the range of 60 mm to 90 mm. The "control temperature" of each rabbit is the mean of two temperature readings recorded for that rabbit at an interval of 30 min in the 40 min immediately preceding the injection of the sample to be examined. Rabbits showing a temperature variation greater than 0.2°C between the two successive temperature readings or rabbits having an initial temperature higher than 39.8°C are withdrawn from the test.

Warm the test solution to a temperature of 37 ± 2°C before injection, and inject the solution slowly into the marginal vein of the ear of each rabbit over a period not exceeding 10 min. Hypotonic test sample may be made isotonic by the addition of pyrogen-free sodium chloride. Record the temperature of each rabbit during a period of 3 hours after the injection, taking the measurements at intervals of not more than 30 min. The difference between the control temperature and the maximum temperature of each rabbit is taken to be the rise in body temperature. Consider any temperature decreases as zero rise.

4. Interpretation of results

The test is carried out on a group of three rabbits and the result is judged on the basis of the sum of the three temperature rises. Repeat if necessary on further groups of three rabbits to a total of three groups, depending on the results obtained. If the summed response of the first group does not exceed 1.3°C, the sample is judged to be pyrogen-negative. If the summed response exceeds 2.5°C, the sample is judged to be pyrogen-positive. If the summed response exceeds 1.3°C but does not exceed 2.5°C, repeat the test on another group of three rabbits. If the summed response of the first and second group does not exceed 3.0°C, the sample is judged to be pyrogen-negative. If the summed response of the 6 rabbits exceeds 4.2°C, the sample is judged to be pyrogen-positive. If the summed response exceeds 3.0°C but does not exceed 4.2°C, repeat the test on one more group of three rabbits. If the summed response of the 9 rabbits does not exceed 5.0°C, the sample is judged to be pyrogen-negative. If the summed response exceeds 5.0°C, the sample is judged to be pyrogen-positive.

When the test sample is judged to be pyrogen-negative, the sample passes the pyrogen test.

4.05 Microbiological Examination of Non-sterile Products

This chapter includes microbial enumeration tests and tests for specified micro-organisms. For the test, use a mixture of several portions selected at random from the bulk or from the contents of a sufficient number of containers. If test specimens are diluted with fluid medium, the test should be performed quickly. In performing the test, precautions must be taken to prevent biohazard.

I. Microbiological Examination of Non-sterile Products: Microbial Enumeration Tests

These tests are harmonized with the European Pharmacopoeia and the U.S. Pharmacopeia.

Information on the harmonization with the European Pharmacopoeia and the U.S. Pharmacopeia is available on the website of the Pharmaceuticals and Medical Devices Agency.

The tests described hereafter will allow quantitative enumeration of mesophilic bacteria and fungi which may grow under aerobic conditions.

The tests are designed primarily to determine whether a substance or preparation complies with an established specification for microbiological quality. When used for such purposes follow the instructions given below, including the number of samples to be taken and interpret the results as stated below.

The methods are not applicable to products containing viable micro-organisms as active ingredients.

Alternative microbiological procedures, including automated methods, may be used, provided that their equivalence to the Pharmacopoeial method has been demonstrated.

1. General Procedures

Carry out the determination under conditions designed to avoid extrinsic microbial contamination of the product to be examined. The precautions taken to avoid contamination must be such that they do not affect any micro-organisms which are to be revealed in the test.

If the product to be examined has antimicrobial activity, this is insofar as possible removed or neutralized. If inactivators are used for this purpose their efficacy and their absence of toxicity for micro-organisms must be demonstrated.

If surface-active substances are used for sample preparation, their absence of toxicity for micro-organisms and their compatibility with inactivators used must be demonstrated.

2. Enumeration Methods

Use the membrane filtration method, or the plate-count methods, as prescribed. The most probable number (MPN) method is generally the least accurate method for microbial counts, however, for certain product groups with very low bioburden, it may be the most appropriate method.

The choice of a method is based on factors such as the nature of the product and the required limit of micro-organisms. The method chosen must allow testing of a sufficient

Table 4.05-I-1 Preparation and use of test micro-organisms

Micro-organism	Preparation of test strain	Growth promotion		Suitability of counting method in the presence of the product	
		Total aerobic microbial count	Total yeasts and moulds count	Total aerobic microbial count	Total yeasts and moulds count
Staphylococcus aureus such as ATCC 6538, NCIMB 9518, CIP 4.83 or NBRC 13276	*Casein soya bean digest agar* or *casein soya bean digest broth* 30 – 35°C 18 – 24 hours	*Casein soya bean digest agar* and *casein soya bean digest broth* ≦100 CFU 30 – 35°C ≦3 days		*Casein soya bean digest agar*/MPN *casein soya bean digest broth* ≦100 CFU 30 – 35°C ≦3 days	
Pseudomonas aeruginosa such as ATCC 9027, NCIMB 8626, CIP 82.118 or NBRC 13275	*Casein soya bean digest agar* or *casein soya bean digest broth* 30 – 35°C 18 – 24 hours	*Casein soya bean digest agar* and *casein soya bean digest broth* ≦100 CFU 30 – 35°C ≦3 days		*Casein soya bean digest agar*/MPN *casein soya bean digest broth* ≦100 CFU 30 – 35°C ≦3 days	
Bacillus subtilis such as ATCC 6633, NCIMB 8054, CIP 52.62 or NBRC 3134	*Casein soya bean digest agar* or *casein soya bean digest broth* 30 – 35°C 18 – 24 hours	*Casein soya bean digest agar* and *casein soya bean digest broth* ≦100 CFU 30 – 35°C ≦3 days		*Casein soya bean digest agar*/MPN *casein soya bean digest broth* ≦100 CFU 30 – 35°C ≦3 days	
Candida albicans such as ATCC 10231, NCPF 3179, IP 48.72 or NBRC 1594	*Sabouraud-dextrose agar* or *Sabouraud-dextrose broth* 20 – 25°C 2 – 3 days	*Casein soya bean digest agar* ≦100 CFU 30 – 35°C ≦5 days	*Sabouraud-dextrose agar* ≦100 CFU 20 – 25°C ≦5 days	*Casein soya bean digest agar* ≦100 CFU 30 – 35°C ≦5 days MPN: not applicable	*Sabouraud-dextrose agar* ≦100 CFU 20 – 25°C ≦5 days
Aspergillus brasiliensis such as ATCC 16404, IMI 149007, IP 1431.83 or NBRC 9455	*Sabouraud-dextrose agar* or *potato-dextrose agar* 20 – 25°C 5 – 7 days, or until good sporulation is achieved	*Casein soya bean digest agar* ≦100 CFU 30 – 35°C ≦5 days	*Sabouraud-dextrose agar* ≦100 CFU 20 – 25°C ≦5 days	*Casein soya bean digest agar* ≦100 CFU 30 – 35°C ≦5 days MPN: not applicable	*Sabouraud-dextrose agar* ≦100 CFU 20 – 25°C ≦5 days

sample size to judge compliance with the specification. The suitability of the chosen method must be established.

3. Growth Promotion Test, Suitability of the Counting Method and Negative Controls

The ability of the test to detect micro-organisms in the presence of product to be tested must be established.

Suitability must be confirmed if a change in testing performance, or the product, which may affect the outcome of the test is introduced.

3.1. Preparation of test strains

Use standardised stable suspensions of test strains or prepare as stated below. Seed lot culture maintenance techniques (seed-lot systems) are used so that the viable micro-organisms used for inoculation are not more than 5 passages removed from the original master seed-lot. Grow each of the bacterial and fungal test strains separately as described in Table 4.05-I-1.

Use *buffered sodium chloride-peptone solution pH 7.0* or *phosphate buffer solution pH 7.2* to make test suspensions; to suspend *Aspergillus brasiliensis* spores, 0.05 per cent of polysorbate 80 may be added to the buffer. Use the suspensions within 2 hours or within 24 hours if stored at 2 – 8°C. As an alternative to preparing and then diluting a fresh suspension of vegetative cells of *Aspergillus brasiliensis* or *Bacillus subtilis*, a stable spore suspension is prepared and then an appropriate volume of the spore suspension is used for test inoculation. The stable spore suspension may be maintained at 2 – 8°C for a validated period of time.

3.2. Negative control

To verify testing conditions, a negative control is performed using the chosen diluent in place of the test preparation. There must be no growth of micro-organisms. A negative control is also performed when testing the products as described under 4. Testing of Products. A failed negative control requires an investigation.

3.3. Growth promotion of the media

Test each batch of ready-prepared medium and each batch of medium, prepared either from dehydrated medium or from the ingredients described.

Table 4.05-I-2 Common neutralizing agents for interfering substances

Interfering substance	Potential neutralizing method
Glutaraldehyde, Mercurials	Sodium hydrogen sulfite (Sodium bisulfite)
Phenolics, Alcohol, Aldehydes, Sorbate	Dilution
Aldehydes	Glycine
Quaternary Ammonium Compounds (QACs), Parahydroxybenzoates (Parabens), Bis-biguanides	Lecithin
QAC, Iodine, Parabens	Polysorbate
Mercurials	Thioglycollate
Mercurials, Halogens, Aldehydes	Thiosulfate
EDTA (edetate)	Mg or Ca ions

Inoculate portions/plates of *casein soya bean digest broth* and *casein soya bean digest agar* with a small number (not more than 100 CFU) of the micro-organisms indicated in Table 4.05-I-1, using a separate portion/plate of medium for each. Inoculate plates of *Sabouraud-dextrose agar* with a small number (not more than 100 CFU) of the micro-organisms indicated in Table 4.05-I-1, using a separate plate of medium for each. Incubate in the conditions described in Table 4.05-I-1.

For solid media, growth obtained must not differ by a factor greater than 2 from the calculated value for a standardized inoculum. For a freshly prepared inoculum, growth of the micro-organisms comparable to that previously obtained with a previously tested and approved batch of medium occurs. Liquid media are suitable if clearly visible growth of the micro-organisms comparable to that previously obtained with a previously tested and approved batch of medium occurs.

3.4. Suitability of the counting method in the presence of product

3.4.1. Preparation of the sample

The method for sample preparation depends on the physical characteristics of the product to be tested. If none of the procedures described below can be demonstrated to be satisfactory, an alternative procedure must be developed.

(i) Water-soluble products: Dissolve or dilute (usually a 1 in 10 dilution is prepared) the product to be examined in *buffered sodium chloride-peptone solution pH 7.0*, *phosphate buffer solution pH 7.2* or *casein soya bean digest broth*. If necessary adjust to pH 6 – 8. Further dilutions, where necessary, are prepared with the same diluent.

(ii) Non-fatty products insoluble in water: Suspend the product to be examined (usually a 1 in 10 dilution is prepared) in *buffered sodium chloride-peptone solution pH 7.0*, *phosphate buffer solution pH 7.2* or *casein soya bean digest broth*. A surface-active agent such as 1 g/L of polysorbate 80 may be added to assist the suspension of poorly wettable substances. If necessary adjust to pH 6 – 8. Further dilutions, where necessary, are prepared with the same diluent.

(iii) Fatty products: Dissolve in isopropyl myristate, sterilised by filtration or mix the product to be examined with the minimum necessary quantity of sterile polysorbate 80 or another non-inhibitory sterile surface-active reagent, heated if necessary to not more than 40°C, or in exceptional cases to not more than 45°C. Mix carefully and if necessary maintain the temperature in a water-bath. Add sufficient of the pre-warmed chosen diluent to make a 1 in 10 dilution of the original product. Mix carefully whilst maintaining the temperature for the shortest time necessary for the formation of an emulsion. Further serial tenfold dilutions may be prepared using the chosen diluent containing a suitable concentration of sterile polysorbate 80 or another non-inhibitory sterile surface-active reagent.

(iv) Fluids or solids in aerosol form: Aseptically transfer the product into a membrane filter apparatus or a sterile container for further sampling. Use either the total contents or a defined number of metered doses from each of the containers tested.

(v) Transdermal patches: Remove the protective cover sheets ("release liner") of the transdermal patches and place them, adhesive side upwards, on sterile glass or plastic trays. Cover the adhesive surface with sterile porous material, for example sterile gauze, to prevent the patches from sticking together, and transfer the patches to a suitable volume of the chosen diluent containing inactivators such as polysorbate 80 and/or lecithin. Shake the preparation vigorously for at least 30 minutes.

3.4.2. Inoculation and dilution

Add to the sample prepared as described above (3.4.1.) and to a control (with no test material included) a sufficient volume of the microbial suspension to obtain an inoculum of not more than 100 CFU. The volume of the suspension of the inoculum should not exceed 1 per cent of the volume of diluted product.

To demonstrate acceptable microbial recovery from the product, the lowest possible dilution factor of the prepared sample must be used for the test. Where this is not possible due to antimicrobial activity or poor solubility, further appropriate protocols must be developed. If inhibition of growth by the sample cannot otherwise be avoided, the aliquot of the microbial suspension may be added after neutralization, dilution or filtration.

3.4.3. Neutralization/removal of antimicrobial activity

The number of micro-organisms recovered from the prepared sample diluted as described in 3.4.2. and incubated following the procedure described in 3.4.4., is compared to the number of micro-organisms recovered from the control preparation.

If growth is inhibited (reduction by a factor greater than 2), then modify the procedure for the particular enumeration test to ensure the validity of the results. Modification of the procedure may include, for example, (1) an increase in the volume of the diluent or culture medium, (2) incorporation of a specific or general neutralizing agents into the diluent,

(3) membrane filtration or (4) a combination of the above measures.

Neutralizing agents. Neutralizing agents may be used to neutralize the activity of antimicrobial agents (Table 4.05-I-2). They may be added to the chosen diluent or the medium preferably before sterilization. If used, their efficacy and their absence of toxicity for micro-organisms must be demonstrated by carrying out a blank with neutralizer and without product.

If no suitable neutralizing method can be found, it can be assumed that the failure to isolate the inoculated organism is attributable to the microbicidal activity of the product. This information serves to indicate that the article is not likely to be contaminated with the given species of the micro-organism. However, it is possible that the product only inhibits some of the micro-organisms specified herein, but does not inhibit others not included amongst the test strains or for which the latter are not representative. Then, perform the test with the highest dilution factor compatible with microbial growth and the specific acceptance criterion.

3.4.4. Recovery of micro-organism in the presence of product

For each of the micro-organisms listed in Table 4.05-I-1, separate tests are performed. Only micro-organisms of the added test strain are counted.

3.4.4.1. Membrane filtration

Use membrane filters having a nominal pore size not greater than 0.45 μm. The type of filter material is chosen in such a way that the bacteria-retaining efficiency is not affected by the components of the sample to be investigated. For each of the micro-organisms listed in Table 4.05-I-1, one membrane filter is used.

Transfer a suitable amount of the sample prepared as described under 3.4.1. to 3.4.3. (preferably representing 1 g of the product, or less if large numbers of CFU are expected) to the membrane filter, filter immediately and rinse the membrane filter with an appropriate volume of diluent.

For the determination of total aerobic microbial count (TAMC), transfer the membrane filter to the surface of *casein soya bean digest agar*. For the determination of total combined yeasts/moulds count (TYMC) transfer the membrane to the surface of *Sabouraud-dextrose agar*. Incubate the plates as indicated in Table 4.05-I-1. Perform the counting.

3.4.4.2. Plate-count methods

Perform plate-count methods at least in duplicate for each medium and use the mean count of the result.

(i) Pour-plate method: For Petri dishes 9 cm in diameter, add to the dish 1 mL of the sample prepared as described under 3.4.1. to 3.4.3. and 15 - 20 mL of *casein soya bean digest agar* or *Sabouraud-dextrose agar*, both media being at not more than 45°C. If larger Petri dishes are used, the amount of agar medium is increased accordingly. For each of the micro-organisms listed in Table 4.05-I-1, at least 2 Petri dishes are used.

Incubate the plates as indicated in Table 4.05-I-1. Take the arithmetic mean of the counts per medium and calculate the number of CFU in the original inoculum.

(ii) Surface-spread method: For Petri dishes 9 cm in diameter, add 15 - 20 mL of *casein soya bean digest agar* or *Sabouraud-dextrose agar* at about 45°C to each Petri dish and allow to solidify. If larger Petri dishes are used, the volume of the agar is increased accordingly. Dry the plates, for example in a laminar-air-flow cabinet or in an incubator. For each of the micro-organisms listed in Table 4.05-I-1, at least 2 Petri dishes are used. Spread a measured volume of not less than 0.1 mL of the sample prepared as described under 3.4.1. to 3.4.3. over the surface of the medium. Incubate and count as prescribed under 3.4.4.2. (i).

3.4.4.3. Most-probable-number (MPN) method

The precision and accuracy of the MPN method is less than that of the membrane filtration method or the plate-count method. Unreliable results are obtained particularly for the enumeration of moulds. For these reasons the MPN method is reserved for the enumeration of TAMC in situations where no other method is available. If the use of the method is justified, proceed as follows.

Prepare a series of at least 3 serial tenfold dilutions of the product as described under 3.4.1. to 3.4.3.. From each level of dilution, 3 aliquots of 1 g or 1 mL are used to inoculate 3 tubes with 9 - 10 mL of *casein soya bean digest broth*. If necessary a surface-active agent such as polysorbate 80, or an inactivator of antimicrobial agents may be added to the medium. Thus, if 3 levels of dilution are prepared 9 tubes are inoculated.

Incubate all tubes at 30 - 35°C for not more than 3 days. If reading of the results is difficult or uncertain owing to the nature of the product to be examined, subculture in the same broth, or *casein soya bean digest agar*, for 1 - 2 days at the same temperature and use these results. Determine the most probable number of micro-organisms per gram or millilitre of the product to be examined from Table 4.05-I-3.

3.5. Results and interpretation

When verifying the suitability of the membrane filtration method or the plate-count method, a mean count of any of the test organisms not differing by a factor greater than 2 from the value of the control defined in 3.4.2. in the absence of the product must be obtained. When verifying the suitability of the MPN method the calculated value from the inoculum must be within 95 per cent confidence limits of the results obtained with the control.

If the above criteria cannot be met for one or more of the organisms tested with any of the described methods, the method and test conditions that come closest to the criteria are used to test the product.

4. Testing of Products

4.1. Amount used for the test

Unless otherwise prescribed, use 10 g or 10 mL of the product to be examined taken with the precautions referred to above. For fluids or solids in aerosol form, sample 10 containers. For transdermal patches, sample 10 patches.

The amount to be tested may be reduced for active substances that will be formulated in the following conditions: the amount per dosage unit (e.g. tablet, capsule, injection) is less than or equal to 1 mg or the amount per gram or millilitre (for preparations not presented in dose units) is less than 1 mg. In these cases, the amount of sample to be tested is not less than the amount present in 10 dosage units or 10 g or 10 mL of the product.

For materials used as active substances where sample quantity is limited or batch size is extremely small (i.e. less than 1000 mL or 1000 g), the amount tested shall be 1 per cent of the batch unless a lesser amount is prescribed or justified and authorised.

For products where the total number of entities in a batch is less than 200 (e.g. samples used in clinical trials), the sample size may be reduced to 2 units, or 1 unit if the size is less than 100.

Select the sample(s) at random from the bulk material or from the available containers of the preparation. To obtain the required quantity, mix the contents of a sufficient number of containers to provide the sample.

Table 4.05-I-3 Most-probable-number values of micro-organisms

Observed combinations of numbers of tubes showing growth in each set			MPN per g or per mL of product	95 per cent confidence limits
Number of g or mL of product per tube				
0.1	0.01	0.001		
0	0	0	Less than 3	0 – 9.4
0	0	1	3	0.1 – 9.5
0	1	0	3	0.1 – 10
0	1	1	6.1	1.2 – 17
0	2	0	6.2	1.2 – 17
0	3	0	9.4	3.5 – 35
1	0	0	3.6	0.2 – 17
1	0	1	7.2	1.2 – 17
1	0	2	11	4 – 35
1	1	0	7.4	1.3 – 20
1	1	1	11	4 – 35
1	2	0	11	4 – 35
1	2	1	15	5 – 38
1	3	0	16	5 – 38
2	0	0	9.2	1.5 – 35
2	0	1	14	4 – 35
2	0	2	20	5 – 38
2	1	0	15	4 – 38
2	1	1	20	5 – 38
2	1	2	27	9 – 94
2	2	0	21	5 – 40
2	2	1	28	9 – 94
2	2	2	35	9 – 94
2	3	0	29	9 – 94
2	3	1	36	9 – 94
3	0	0	23	5 – 94
3	0	1	38	9 – 104
3	0	2	64	16 – 181
3	1	0	43	9 – 181
3	1	1	75	17 – 199
3	1	2	120	30 – 360
3	1	3	160	30 – 380
3	2	0	93	18 – 360
3	2	1	150	30 – 380
3	2	2	210	30 – 400
3	2	3	290	90 – 990
3	3	0	240	40 – 990
3	3	1	460	90 – 1980
3	3	2	1100	200 – 4000
3	3	3	More than 1100	

4.2. Examination of the product

4.2.1. Membrane filtration

Use a filtration apparatus designed to allow the transfer of the filter to the medium. Prepare the sample using a method that has been shown suitable as described in section 3 and transfer the appropriate amount to each of 2 membrane filters and filter immediately. Wash each filter following the procedure shown to be suitable.

For the determination of TAMC, transfer one of the membrane filters to the surface of *casein soya bean digest agar*. For the determination of TYMC, transfer the other membrane to the surface of *Sabouraud-dextrose agar*. Incubate the plate of *casein soya bean digest agar* at 30 – 35°C for 3 – 5 days and the plate of *Sabouraud-dextrose agar* at

20 - 25°C for 5 - 7 days. Calculate the number of CFU per gram or per millilitre of product.

When examining transdermal patches, filter 10 per cent of the volume of the preparation described under 3.4.1. separately through each of 2 sterile filter membranes. Transfer one membrane to *casein soya bean digest agar* for TAMC and the other membrane to *Sabouraud-dextrose agar* for TYMC.

4.2.2. Plate-count methods

(i) Pour-plate method: Prepare the sample using a method that has been shown to be suitable as described in section 3. Prepare for each medium at least 2 Petri dishes for each level of dilution. Incubate the plates of *casein soya bean digest agar* at 30 - 35°C for 3 - 5 days and the plates of *Sabouraud-dextrose agar* at 20 - 25°C for 5 - 7 days. Select the plates corresponding to a given dilution and showing the highest number of colonies less than 250 for TAMC and 50 for TYMC. Take the arithmetic mean per culture medium of the counts and calculate the number of CFU per gram or per millilitre of product.

(ii) Surface-spread method: Prepare the sample using a method that has been shown to be suitable as described in section 3. Prepare at least 2 Petri dishes for each medium and each level of dilution. For incubation and calculation of the number of CFU proceed as described for the pour-plate method.

4.2.3. Most-probable-number method

Prepare and dilute the sample using a method that has been shown to be suitable as described in section 3. Incubate all tubes for 3 - 5 days at 30 - 35°C. Subculture if necessary, using the procedure shown to be suitable. Record for each level of dilution the number of tubes showing microbial growth. Determine the most probable number of micro-organisms per gram or millilitre of the product to be examined from Table 4.05-I-3.

4.3. Interpretation of the results

The total aerobic microbial count (TAMC) is considered to be equal to the number of CFU found using *casein soya bean digest agar*; if colonies of fungi are detected on this medium, they are counted as part of TAMC. The total combined yeasts/mould count (TYMC) is considered to be equal to the number of CFU found using *Sabouraud-dextrose agar*; if colonies of bacteria are detected on this medium, they are counted as part of TYMC. When the TYMC is expected to exceed the acceptance criterion due to the bacterial growth, *Sabouraud-dextrose agar* containing antibiotics may be used. If the count is carried out by the MPN method the calculated value is the TAMC.

When an acceptance criterion for microbiological quality is prescribed it is interpreted as follows:

– 10^1 CFU: maximum acceptable count = 20,

– 10^2 CFU: maximum acceptable count = 200,

– 10^3 CFU: maximum acceptable count = 2000,

and so forth.

The recommended solutions and media are described in II. *Tests for specified micro-organisms.*

II. Microbiological Examination of Non-sterile Products: Tests for Specified Micro-organisms

These tests are harmonized with the European Pharmacopoeia and the U.S. Pharmacopeia.

Information on the harmonization with the European Pharmacopoeia and the U.S. Pharmacopeia is available on the website of the Pharmaceuticals and Medical Devices Agency.

The tests described hereafter will allow determination of the absence or limited occurrence of specified micro-organisms which may be detected under the conditions described.

The tests are designed primarily to determine whether a substance or preparation complies with an established specification for microbiological quality. When used for such purposes follow the instructions given below, including the number of samples to be taken and interpret the results as stated below.

Alternative microbiological procedures, including automated methods may be used, provided that their equivalence to the Pharmacopoeial method has been demonstrated.

1. General Procedures

The preparation of samples is carried out as described in I. *Microbial enumeration tests.*

If the product to be examined has antimicrobial activity, this is insofar as possible removed or neutralized as described in I. *Microbial enumeration tests.*

If surface-active substances are used for sample preparation, their absence of toxicity for micro-organisms and their compatibility with inactivators used must be demonstrated as described in I. *Microbial enumeration tests.*

2. Growth Promoting and Inhibitory Properties of the Media, Suitability of the Test and Negative Controls

The ability of the test to detect micro-organisms in the presence of the product to be tested must be established. Suitability must be confirmed if a change in testing performance, or the product, which may affect the outcome of the test is introduced.

2.1. Preparation of test strains

Use standardized stable suspensions of test strains or prepare as stated below. Seed lot culture maintenance techniques (seed-lot systems) are used so that the viable micro-organisms used for inoculation are not more than 5 passages removed from the original master seed-lot.

2.1.1. Aerobic micro-organisms

Grow each of the bacterial test strains separately in containers containing *casein soya bean digest broth* or on *casein soya bean digest agar* at 30 - 35°C for 18 - 24 hours. Grow the test strain for *Candida albicans* separately on *Sabouraud-dextrose agar* or in *Sabouraud-dextrose broth* at 20 - 25°C for 2–3 days.

Staphylococcus aureus such as ATCC 6538, NCIMB 9518, CIP 4.83 or NBRC 13276,

Pseudomonas aeruginosa such as ATCC 9027, NCIMB 8626, CIP 82.118 or NBRC 13275,

Escherichia coli such as ATCC 8739, NCIMB 8545, CIP 53.126 or NBRC 3972,

Salmonella enterica subsp. *enterica* serovar Typhimurium such as ATCC 14028

or, as an alternative,

Salmonella enterica subsp. *enterica* serovar Abony such as NBRC 100797, NCTC 6017 or CIP 80.39,

Candida albicans such as ATCC 10231, NCPF 3179, IP 48.72 or NBRC 1594.

Use *buffered sodium chloride-peptone solution pH 7.0* or *phosphate buffer solution pH 7.2* to make test suspensions. Use the suspensions within 2 hours or within 24 hours if stored at 2 - 8°C.

2.1.2. Clostridia

Use *Clostridium sporogenes* such as ATCC 11437 (NBRC 14293, NCIMB 12343, CIP 100651) or ATCC 19404 (NCTC 532 or CIP 79.3). Grow the clostridial test strain under anaerobic conditions in *reinforced medium for Clostridia* at 30 - 35°C for 24 - 48 hours. As an alternative to preparing and then diluting down a fresh suspension of vegetative cells of *Cl. sporogenes*, a stable spore suspension is used for test inoculation. The stable spore suspension may be maintained at 2 - 8°C for a validated period.

2.2. Negative control

To verify testing conditions a negative control is performed using the chosen diluent in place of the test preparation. There must be no growth of micro-organisms. A negative control is also performed when testing the products as described under 3. A failed negative control required an investigation.

2.3. Growth promotion and inhibitory properties of the media

Test each batch of ready-prepared medium and each batch of medium prepared either from dehydrated medium or from ingredients.

Verify suitable properties of relevant media as described in Table 4.05-II-1.

(i) Test for growth promoting properties, liquid media: inoculate a portion of the appropriate medium with a small number (not more than 100 CFU) of the appropriate micro-organism. Incubate at the specified temperature for not more than the shortest period of time specified in the test. Clearly visible growth of the micro-organism comparable to that previously obtained with a previously tested and approved batch of medium occurs.

(ii) Test for growth promoting properties, solid media: perform surface-spread method, inoculating each plate with a small number (not more than 100 CFU) of the appropriate micro-organism. Incubate at the specified temperature for not more than the shortest period of time specified in the test. Growth of the micro-organism comparable to that previously obtained with a previously tested and approved batch of medium occurs.

(iii) Test for inhibitory properties, liquid or solid media: inoculate the appropriate medium with at least 100 CFU of the appropriate micro-organism. Incubate at the specified temperature for not less than the longest period of time specified in the test. No growth of the test micro-organism occurs.

(iv) Test for indicative properties: perform surface-spread method, inoculating each plate with a small number (not more than 100 CFU) of the appropriate micro-organism. Incubate at the specified temperature for a period of time within the range specified in the test. Colonies are comparable in appearance and indication reactions to those previously obtained with a previously tested and approved batch of medium.

2.4. Suitability of the test method

For each product to be tested perform sample preparation as described in the relevant paragraph in section 3. Add each test strain at the time of mixing, in the prescribed growth medium. Inoculate the test strains individually. Use a number of micro-organisms equivalent to not more than 100 CFU in the inoculated test preparation.

Perform the test as described in the relevant paragraph in section 3 using the shortest incubation period prescribed.

The specified micro-organisms must be detected with the indication reactions as described in section 3.

Any antimicrobial activity of the product necessitates a modification of the test procedure (see 3.4.3. of I. *Microbial enumeration tests*).

If for a given product the antimicrobial activity with respect to a micro-organism for which testing is prescribed cannot be neutralized, then it is to be assumed that the inhibited micro-organism will not be present in the product.

3. Testing of Products

3.1. Bile-tolerant gram-negative bacteria

3.1.1. Sample preparation and pre-incubation

Prepare a sample using a 1 in 10 dilution of not less than 1 g of the product to be examined as described in I. *Microbial enumeration tests*, but using *casein soya bean digest broth* as the chosen diluent, mix and incubate at 20 - 25°C for a time sufficient to resuscitate the bacteria but not sufficient to encourage multiplication of the organisms (usually 2 hours but not more than 5 hours).

3.1.2. Test for absence

Unless otherwise prescribed use the volume corresponding to 1 g of the product, as prepared in 3.1.1. to inoculate *enterobacteria enrichment broth-Mossel*. Incubate at 30 - 35°C for 24 - 48 hours. Subculture on plates of *violet red bile glucose agar*. Incubate at 30 - 35°C for 18 - 24 hours.

The product complies with the test if there is no growth of colonies.

3.1.3. Quantitative test

3.1.3.1. Selection and subculture

Inoculate suitable quantities of *enterobacteria enrichment broth-Mossel* with the preparation as described under 3.1.1. and/or dilutions of it containing respectively 0.1 g, 0.01 g and 0.001 g (or 0.1 mL, 0.01 mL and 0.001 mL) of the product to be examined. Incubate at 30 - 35°C for 24 - 48 hours. Subculture each of the cultures on a plate of *violet red bile glucose agar*. Incubate at 30 - 35°C for 18 - 24 hours.

3.1.3.2. Interpretation

Growth of colonies constitutes a positive result. Note the smallest quantity of the product that gives a positive result and the largest quantity that gives a negative result. Determine from Table 4.05-II-2 the probable number of bacteria.

3.2. *Escherichia coli*

3.2.1. Sample preparation and pre-incubation

Prepare a sample using a 1 in 10 dilution of not less than 1 g of the product to be examined as described in I. *Microbial enumeration tests* and use 10 mL or the quantity corresponding to 1 g or 1 mL to inoculate a suitable amount (determined as described under 2.4.) of *casein soya bean digest broth*, mix and incubate at 30 - 35°C for 18 - 24 hours.

3.2.2. Selection and subculture

Shake the container, transfer 1 mL of *casein soya bean digest broth* to 100 mL of *MacConkey broth* and incubate at 42 - 44°C for 24 - 48 hours. Subculture on a plate of *MacConkey agar* at 30 - 35°C for 18 - 72 hours.

3.2.3. Interpretation

Growth of colonies indicates the possible presence of *E. coli*. This is confirmed by identification tests.

The product complies with the test if no colonies are present or if the identification tests are negative.

3.3. *Salmonella*

3.3.1. Sample preparation and pre-incubation

Prepare the product to be examined as described in I. *Microbial enumeration tests* and use the quantity corresponding to not less than 10 g or 10 mL to inoculate a suitable amount (determined as described under 2.4.) of *casein soya bean digest broth*, mix and incubate at 30 - 35°C for 18 - 24 hours.

3.3.2. Selection and subculture

Transfer 0.1 mL of *casein soya bean digest broth* to 10 mL of *Rappaport Vassiliadis Salmonella enrichment broth* and incubate at 30 - 35°C for 18 - 24 hours. Subculture on plates of *xylose, lysine, deoxycholate agar*. Incubate at 30 - 35°C for 18 - 48 hours.

Table 4.05-II-1 Growth promoting, inhibitory and indicative properties of media

Medium	Property	Test strains
Test for bile-tolerant gram-negative bacteria		
Enterobacteria enrichment broth-Mossel	Growth promoting	*E. coli* *P. aeruginosa*
	Inhibitory	*S. aureus*
Violet red bile glucose agar	Growth promoting + Indicative	*E. coli* *P. aeruginosa*
Test for *Escherichia coli*		
MacConkey broth	Growth promoting	*E. coli*
	Inhibitory	*S. aureus*
MacConkey agar	Growth promoting + Indicative	*E. coli*
Test for *Salmonella*		
Rappaport Vassiliadis Salmonella enrichment broth	Growth promoting	*Salmonella enterica* subsp. *enterica* serovar Typhimurium or *Salmonella enterica* subsp. *enterica* serovar Abony
	Inhibitory	*S. aureus*
Xylose, lysine, deoxycholate agar	Growth promoting + Indicative	*Salmonella enterica* subsp. *enterica* serovar Typhimurium or *Salmonella enterica* subsp. *enterica* serovar Abony
Test for *Pseudomonas aeruginosa*		
Cetrimide agar	Growth promoting	*P. aeruginosa*
	Inhibitory	*E. coli*
Test for *Staphylococcus aureus*		
Mannitol salt agar	Growth promoting + Indicative	*S. aureus*
	Inhibitory	*E. coli*
Test for Clostridia		
Reinforced medium for Clostridia	Growth promoting	*Cl. sporogenes*
Columbia agar	Growth promoting	*Cl. sporogenes*
Test for *Candida albicans*		
Sabouraud-dextrose broth	Growth promoting	*C. albicans*
Sabouraud-dextrose agar	Growth promoting + Indicative	*C. albicans*

3.3.3. Interpretation

The possible presence of *Salmonella* is indicated by the growth of well-developed, red colonies, with or without black centres. This is confirmed by identification tests.

The product complies with the test if colonies of the types described are not present or if the confirmatory identification tests are negative.

3.4. ***Pseudomonas aeruginosa***

3.4.1. Sample preparation and pre-incubation

Prepare a sample using a 1 in 10 dilution of not less than 1 g of the product to be examined as described in I. *Microbial enumeration tests* and use 10 mL or the quantity corresponding to 1 g or 1 mL to inoculate a suitable amount (determined as described under 2.4.) of *casein soya bean digest broth* and mix. When testing transdermal patches, filter the volume of sample corresponding to 1 patch of the preparation described in I. *Microbial enumeration tests* (3.4.1.) through a sterile filter membrane and place in 100 mL of *casein soya bean digest broth*. Incubate at 30 – 35°C for 18 – 24 hours.

3.4.2. Selection and subculture

Subculture on a plate of *cetrimide agar* and incubate at

Table 4.05-II-2 Interpretation of results

Results for each quantity of product			Probable number of bacteria per gram or mL of product
0.1 g or 0.1 mL	**0.01 g or 0.01 mL**	**0.001 g or 0.001 mL**	
+	+	+	more than 10^3
+	+	−	less than 10^3 and more than 10^2
+	−	−	less than 10^2 and more than 10
−	−	−	less than 10

30 - 35°C for 18 - 72 hours.

3.4.3. Interpretation

Growth of colonies indicates the possible presence of *P. aeruginosa*. This is confirmed by identification tests.

The product complies with the test if colonies are not present or if the confirmatory identification tests are negative.

3.5. ***Staphylococcus aureus***

3.5.1. Sample preparation and pre-incubation

Prepare a sample using a 1 in 10 dilution of not less than 1 g of the product to be examined as described in I. *Microbial enumeration tests* and use 10 mL or the quantity corresponding to 1 g or 1 mL to inoculate a suitable amount (determined as described under 2.4.) of *casein soya bean digest broth* and homogenise. When testing transdermal patches, filter the volume of sample corresponding to 1 patch of the preparation described in I. *Microbial enumeration tests* (3.4.1.) through a sterile filter membrane and place in 100 mL of *casein soya bean digest broth*. Incubate at 30 - 35°C for 18 - 24 hours.

3.5.2. Selection and subculture

Subculture on a plate of *mannitol salt agar* and incubate at 30 - 35°C for 18 - 72 hours.

3.5.3. Interpretation

The possible presence of *S. aureus* is indicated by the growth of yellow/white colonies surrounded by a yellow zone. This is confirmed by identification tests.

The product complies with the test if colonies of the types described are not present or if the confirmatory identification tests are negative.

3.6. ***Clostridia***

3.6.1. Sample preparation and heat treatment

Prepare a sample using a 1 in 10 dilution (with a minimum total volume of 20 mL) of not less than 2 g or 2 mL of the product to be examined as described in I. *Microbial enumeration tests*. Divide the sample into two portions of at least 10 mL. Heat 1 portion at 80°C for 10 minutes and cool rapidly. Do not heat the other portion.

3.6.2. Selection and subculture

Use 10 mL or the quantity corresponding to 1 g or 1 mL of the product to be examined of both portions to inoculate suitable amounts (determined as described under 2.4.) of *reinforced medium for Clostridia*. Incubate under anaerobic conditions at 30 - 35°C for 48 hours. After incubation, make subcultures from each tube on *Columbia agar* and incubate under anaerobic conditions at 30 - 35°C for 48 - 72 hours.

3.6.3. Interpretation

The occurrence of anaerobic growth of rods (with or without endospores) giving a negative catalase reaction indicates the presence of Clostridia. This is confirmed by identification tests.

The product complies with the test if colonies of the types described are not present or if the confirmatory identification tests are negative.

3.7. ***Candida albicans***

3.7.1. Sample preparation and pre-incubation

Prepare the product to be examined as described in I. *Microbial enumeration tests* and use 10 mL or the quantity corresponding to not less than 1 g or 1 mL to inoculate 100 mL of *Sabouraud-dextrose broth* and mix. Incubate at 30 - 35°C for 3-5 days.

3.7.2. Selection and subculture

Subculture on a plate of *Sabouraud-dextrose agar* and incubate at 30 - 35°C for 24 - 48 hours.

3.7.3. Interpretation

Growth of white colonies may indicate the presence of *C. albicans*. This is confirmed by identification tests.

The product complies with the test if such colonies are not present or if the confirmatory identification tests are negative.

The following section is given for information.

4. Recommended Solutions and Culture Media

The following solutions and culture media have been found satisfactory for the purposes for which they are prescribed in the test for microbial contamination in the Pharmacopoeia. Other media may be used provided that their suitability can be demonstrated.

(i) *Phosphate buffer solution pH 7.2*

Prepare a mixture of water and stock buffer solution (800:1 V/V) and sterilize.

Stock buffer solution. Transfer 34 g of potassium dihydrogen phosphate to a 1000 mL volumetric flask, dissolve in 500 mL of purified water, adjust to pH 7.2 to ±0.2 with sodium hydroxide, add purified water to volume and mix. Dispense in containers and sterilize. Store at a temperature of 2 - 8°C.

(ii) *Buffered sodium chloride-peptone solution pH 7.0*

Potassium dihydrogen phosphate	3.6 g
Disodium hydrogen phosphate dihydrate	7.2 g
	(equivalent to 0.067 mol phosphate)
Sodium chloride	4.3 g
Peptone (meat or casein)	1.0 g
Water	1000 mL

Sterilize in an autoclave using a validated cycle.

(iii) *Casein soya bean digest broth*

Pancreatic digest of casein	17.0 g
Papaic digest of soya bean	3.0 g
Sodium chloride	5.0 g
Dipotassium hydrogen phosphate	2.5 g
Glucose monohydrate	2.5 g
Purified water	1000 mL

Adjust the pH so that after sterilization it is 7.3 ± 0.2 at 25°C. Sterilize in an autoclave using a validated cycle.

(iv) *Casein soya bean digest agar*

Pancreatic digest of casein	15.0 g
Papaic digest of soya bean	5.0 g
Sodium chloride	5.0 g
Agar	15.0 g
Purified water	1000 mL

Adjust the pH so that after sterilization it is 7.3 ± 0.2 at 25°C. Sterilize in an autoclave using a validated cycle.

(v) *Sabouraud-dextrose agar*

Dextrose	40.0 g
Mixture of peptic digest of animal tissue and pancreatic digest of casein (1:1)	10.0 g
Agar	15.0 g
Purified water	1000 mL

Adjust the pH so that after sterilization it is 5.6 ± 0.2 at 25°C. Sterilize in an autoclave using a validated cycle.

(vi) *Potato dextrose agar*

Infusion from potatoes	200 g
Dextrose	20.0 g
Agar	15.0 g
Purified water	1000 mL

Adjust the pH so that after sterilization it is 5.6 ± 0.2 at 25°C. Sterilize in an autoclave using a validated cycle.

(vii) *Sabouraud-dextrose broth*

Dextrose	20.0 g
Mixture of peptic digest of animal tissue and pancreatic digest of casein (1:1)	10.0 g
Purified water	1000 mL

Adjust the pH so that after sterilization it is 5.6 ± 0.2 at 25°C. Sterilize in an autoclave using a validated cycle.

(viii) *Enterobacteria enrichment broth-Mossel*

Pancreatic digest of gelatin	10.0 g
Glucose monohydrate	5.0 g
Dehydrated ox bile	20.0 g
Potassium dihydrogen phosphate	2.0 g
Disodium hydrogen phosphate dihydrate	8.0 g
Brilliant green	15 mg
Purified water	1000 mL

Adjust the pH so that after heating it is 7.2 ± 0.2 at 25°C. Heat at 100°C for 30 minutes and cool immediately.

(ix) *Violet red bile glucose agar*

Yeast extract	3.0 g
Pancreatic digest of gelatin	7.0 g
Bile salts	1.5 g
Sodium chloride	5.0 g
Glucose monohydrate	10.0 g
Agar	15.0 g
Neutral red	30 mg
Crystal violet	2 mg
Purified water	1000 mL

Adjust the pH so that after heating it is 7.4 ± 0.2 at 25°C. Heat to boiling; do not heat in an autoclave.

(x) *MacConkey broth*

Pancreatic digest of gelatin	20.0 g
Lactose monohydrate	10.0 g
Dehydrated ox bile	5.0 g
Bromocresol purple	10 mg
Purified water	1000 mL

Adjust the pH so that after sterilization it is 7.3 ± 0.2 at 25°C. Sterilize in an autoclave using a validated cycle.

(xi) *MacConkey agar*

Pancreatic digest of gelatin	17.0 g
Peptones (meat and casein)	3.0 g
Lactose monohydrate	10.0 g
Sodium chloride	5.0 g
Bile salts	1.5 g
Agar	13.5 g
Neutral red	30 mg
Crystal violet	1 mg
Purified water	1000 mL

Adjust the pH so that after sterilization it is 7.1 ± 0.2 at 25°C. Boil for 1 minute with constant shaking then sterilize in an autoclave using a validated cycle.

(xii) *Rappaport Vassiliadis Salmonella Enrichment broth*

Soya peptone	4.5 g
Magnesium chloride hexahydrate	29.0 g
Sodium chloride	8.0 g
Dipotassium hydrogen phosphate	0.4 g
Potassium dihydrogen phosphate	0.6 g
Malachite green	36 mg
Purified water	1000 mL

Dissolve, warming slightly. Sterilize in an autoclave using a validated cycle, at a temperature not exceeding 115°C. The pH is to be 5.2 ± 0.2 at 25°C after heating and autoclaving.

(xiii) *Xylose, lysine, deoxycholate agar*

Xylose	3.5 g
L-Lysine	5.0 g
Lactose monohydrate	7.5 g
Sucrose	7.5 g
Sodium chloride	5.0 g
Yeast extract	3.0 g
Phenol red	80 mg
Agar	13.5 g
Sodium desoxycholate	2.5 g
Sodium thiosulfate	6.8 g
Ammonium iron (III) citrate	0.8 g
Purified water	1000 mL

Adjust the pH so that after heating it is 7.4 ± 0.2 at 25°C. Heat to boiling, cool to 50°C and pour into Petri dishes. Do not heat in an autoclave.

(xiv) *Cetrimide agar*

Pancreatic digest of gelatin	20.0 g
Magnesium chloride	1.4 g
Dipotassium sulfate	10.0 g
Cetrimide	0.3 g
Agar	13.6 g
Purified water	1000 mL
Glycerol	10.0 mL

Heat to boiling for 1 minute with shaking. Adjust the pH so that after sterilization it is 7.2 ± 0.2 at 25°C. Sterilize in an autoclave using a validated cycle.

(xv) *Mannitol salt agar*

Pancreatic digest of casein	5.0 g
Peptic digest of animal tissue	5.0 g
Beef extract	1.0 g
D-Mannitol	10.0 g
Sodium chloride	75.0 g
Agar	15.0 g
Phenol red	25 mg
Purified water	1000 mL

Heat to boiling for 1 minute with shaking. Adjust the pH so that after sterilization it is 7.4 ± 0.2 at 25°C. Sterilize in an autoclave using a validated cycle.

(xvi) *Reinforced medium for Clostridia*

Beef extract	10.0 g
Peptone	10.0 g
Yeast extract	3.0 g
Soluble starch	1.0 g
Glucose monohydrate	5.0 g
Cysteine hydrochloride	0.5 g
Sodium chloride	5.0 g
Sodium acetate	3.0 g
Agar	0.5 g
Purified water	1000 mL

Hydrate the agar, dissolve by heating to boiling with continuous stirring. If necessary, adjust the pH so that after sterilization it is about 6.8 ± 0.2 at 25°C. Sterilize in an autoclave using a validated cycle.

(xvii) *Columbia agar*

Pancreatic digest of casein	10.0 g
Meat peptic digest	5.0 g
Heart pancreatic digest	3.0 g
Yeast extract	5.0 g
Maize starch	1.0 g
Sodium chloride	5.0 g
Agar, according to gelling power	10.0 g to 15.0 g
Purified water	1000 mL

Hydrate the agar, dissolve by heating to boiling with continuous stirring. If necessary, adjust the pH so that after sterilization it is 7.3 ± 0.2 at 25°C. Sterilize in an autoclave using a validated cycle. Allow to cool to 45 - 50°C; add, where necessary, gentamicin sulfate corresponding to 20 mg of gentamicin base and pour into Petri dishes.

4.06 Sterility Test

This test is harmonized with the European Pharmacopoeia and the U.S. Pharmacopeia.

The corresponding part of the attributes/provisions which are agreed as non-harmonized within the scope of the harmonization is marked with symbols (◆ ◆), and the corresponding parts which are agreed as the JP local requirement other than the scope of the harmonization are marked with symbols (◇ ◇).

Information on the harmonization with the European Pharmacopoeia and the U.S. Pharmacopeia is available on the website of the Pharmaceuticals and Medical Devices Agency.

The test is applied to substances, preparations or articles which, according to the Pharmacopoeia, are required to be sterile. However, a satisfactory result only indicates that no contaminating micro-organism has been found in the sample examined in the conditions of the test.

1. Precautions against microbial contamination

The test for sterility is carried out under aseptic conditions. In order to achieve such conditions, the test environment has to be adapted to the way in which the sterility test is performed. The precautions taken to avoid contamination are such that they do not affect any micro-organisms which are to be revealed in the test. The working conditions in which the tests are performed are monitored regularly by appropriate sampling of the working area and by carrying out appropriate controls.

2. Culture media and incubation temperatures

Media for the test may be prepared as described below, or equivalent commercial media may be used provided that they comply with the growth promotion test.

The following culture media have been found to be suitable for the test for sterility. Fluid thioglycollate medium is primarily intended for the culture of anaerobic bacteria; however, it will also detect aerobic bacteria. Soya-bean casein digest medium is suitable for the culture of both fungi and aerobic bacteria.

(i) Fluid thioglycollate medium

L-Cystine	0.5 g
Agar	0.75 g
Sodium chloride	2.5 g
Glucose monohydrate/anhydrous	5.5/5.0 g
Yeast extract (water-soluble)	5.0 g
Pancreatic digest of casein	15.0 g
Sodium thioglycollate or	0.5 g
Thioglycolic acid	0.3 mL
Resazurin sodium solution (1 in 1000), freshly prepared	1.0 mL
Water	1000 mL

(pH after sterilization 7.1 ± 0.2)

Mix the L-cystine, agar, sodium chloride, glucose, water-soluble yeast extract and pancreatic digest of casein with water, and heat until solution is effected. Dissolve the sodium thioglycollate or thioglycollic acid in the solution and, if necessary, add sodium hydroxide TS so that, after sterilization, the solution will have a pH of 7.1 ± 0.2. If filtration is necessary, heat the solution again without boiling and filter while hot through moistened filter paper. Add the resazurin sodium solution (1 in 1000), mix and place the medium in suitable vessels which provide a ratio of surface to depth of medium such that not more than the upper half of the medium has undergone a color change indicative of oxygen uptake at the end of the incubation period. Sterilize using a validated process. If the medium is stored, store at a temperature between 2°C and 25°C in a sterile, tight container. If more than the upper one-third of the medium has acquired a pink color, the medium may be restored once by heating the containers in a water-bath or in free-flowing steam until the pink color disappears and cooling quickly, taking care to prevent the introduction of non-sterile air into the container. Do not use the medium for a longer storage period than has been validated.

Fluid thioglycollate medium is to be incubated at 30 - 35°C. For products containing a mercurial preservative that cannot be tested by the membrane-filtration method, fluid thioglycollate medium incubated at 20 - 25°C may be used instead of soya-bean casein digest medium provided that it has been validated as described in growth promotion test.

Where prescribed or justified and authorized, the following alternative thioglycollate medium might be used. Prepare a mixture having the same composition as that of the fluid thioglycollate medium, but omitting the agar and the resazurin sodium solution (1 in 1000), sterilize as directed above. The pH after sterilization is 7.1 ± 0.2. Heat in a water bath prior to use and incubate at 30 - 35°C under anaerobic conditions.

(ii) Soya-bean casein digest medium

Pancreatic digest of casein	17.0 g
Papaic digest of soya-bean meal	3.0 g
Sodium chloride	5.0 g
Dipotassium hydrogen phosphate	2.5 g
Glucose monohydrate/anhydrous	2.5/2.3 g
Water	1000 mL

(pH after sterilization 7.3 ± 0.2)

Dissolve the solids in water, warming slightly to effect solution. Cool the solution to room temperature. Add sodium

Table 4.06-1. Strains of the test micro-organisms suitable for use in the Growth Promotion Test and the Method suitability Test

Aerobic bacteria *Staphylococcus aureus*	ATCC 6538, CIP 4.83, NCTC 10788, NCIMB 9518, NBRC 13276
Bacillus subtilis	ATCC 6633, CIP 52.62, NCIMB 8054, NBRC 3134
Pseudomonas aeruginosa	ATCC 9027, NCIMB 8626, CIP 82.118, NBRC 13275
Anaerobic bacterium *Clostridium sporogenes*	ATCC 19404, CIP 79.3, NCTC 532 or ATCC 11437, NBRC 14293
Fungi *Candida albicans*	ATCC 10231, IP 48.72, NCPF 3179, NBRC 1594
Aspergillus brasiliensis	ATCC 16404, IP 1431.83, IMI 149007, NBRC 9455

hydroxide TS, if necessary, so that after sterilization the solution will have a pH of 7.3 ± 0.2. Filter, if necessary, to clarify, distribute into suitable vessels and sterilize using a validated process. Store at a temperature between 2°C and 25°C in a sterile tight container, unless it is intended for immediate use. Do not use the medium for a longer storage period than has been validated.

Soya-bean casein digest medium is to be incubated at 20 – 25°C.

3. Suitability of the culture medium

The media used comply with the following tests, carried out before or in parallel with the test on the product to be examined.

3.1. Sterility

Incubate portions of the media for 14 days. No growth of micro-organisms occurs.

3.2. Growth promotion test of aerobes, anaerobes and fungi

Test each batch of ready-prepared medium and each batch of medium prepared either from dehydrated medium or from ingredients. Suitable strains of micro-organisms are indicated in Table 4.06-1.

Inoculate portions of fluid thioglycollate medium with a small number (not more than 100 CFU) of the following micro-organisms, using a separate portion of medium for each of the following species of micro-organism:
Clostridium sporogenes,
Pseudomonas aeruginosa,
Staphylococcus aureus.

Inoculate portions of soya-bean casein digest medium with a small number (not more than 100 CFU) of the following micro-organisms, using a separate portion of medium for each of the following species of micro-organism:
Aspergillus brasiliensis,
Bacillus subtilis,
Candida albicans.

Incubate for not more than 3 days in the case of bacteria and not more than 5 days in the case of fungi.

Seed lot culture maintenance techniques (seed-lot systems) are used so that the viable micro-organisms used for inoculation are not more than five passages removed from the original master seed-lot.

The media are suitable if a clearly visible growth of the micro-organisms occurs.

4. Method suitability test

Carry out a test as described below under 5. Test for sterility of the product to be examined using exactly the same methods except for the following modifications.

(i) Membrane filtration: After transferring the content of the container or containers to be tested to the membrane add an inoculum of a small number of viable micro-organisms (not more than 100 CFU) to the final portion of sterile diluent used to rinse the filter.

(ii) Direct inoculation: After transferring the contents of the container or containers to be tested to the culture medium add an inoculum of a small number of viable micro-organisms (not more than 100 CFU) to the medium.

In both cases use the same micro-organisms as those described above under 3.2. Growth promotion test of aerobes, anaerobes and fungi. Perform a growth promotion test as a positive control. Incubate all the containers containing medium for not more than 5 days.

If clearly visible growth of micro-organisms is obtained after the incubation, visually comparable to that in the control vessel without product, either the product possesses no antimicrobial activity under the conditions of the test or such activity has been satisfactorily eliminated. The test for sterility may then be carried out without further modification.

If clearly visible growth is not obtained in the presence of the product to be tested, visually comparable to that in the control vessels without product, the product possesses antimicrobial activity that has not been satisfactorily eliminated under the conditions of the test. Modify the conditions in order to eliminate the antimicrobial activity and repeat the method suitability test.

This method suitability is performed:

a) when the test for sterility has to be carried out on a new product;
b) whenever there is a change in the experimental conditions of the test.

The method suitability may be performed simultaneously with the Test for sterility of the product to be examined.

5. Test for sterility of the product to be examined

The test may be carried out using the technique of membrane filtration or by direct inoculation of the culture media with the product to be examined. Appropriate negative controls are included. The technique of membrane filtration is used whenever the nature of the product permits, that is, for filterable aqueous preparations, for alcoholic or oily preparations and for preparations miscible with or soluble in aqueous or oily solvents provided these solvents do not have an antimicrobial effect in the conditions of the test.

5.1. Membrane filtration

Use membrane filters having a nominal pore size not greater than 0.45 μm whose effectiveness to retain micro-organisms has been established. Cellulose nitrate filters, for example, are used for aqueous, oily and weakly alcoholic solutions and cellulose acetate filters, for example, for strongly alcoholic solutions. Specially adapted filters may be needed for certain products, e.g. for antibiotics.

The technique described below assumes that membranes about 50 mm in diameter will be used. If filters of a different diameter are used the volumes of the dilutions and the washings should be adjusted accordingly. The filtration apparatus and membrane are sterilized by appropriate means. The apparatus is designed so that the solution to be examined can be introduced and filtered under aseptic conditions; it permits the aseptic removal of the membrane for transfer to the

Table 4.06-2. Minimum quantity to be used for each medium

Quantity per container	Minimum quantity to be used for each medium unless otherwise justified and authorized
Liquids	
—Less than 1 mL:	The whole contents of each container
—1 – 40 mL:	Half the contents of each container but not less than 1 mL
—Greater than 40 mL and not greater than 100 mL	20 mL
—Greater than 100 mL:	10% of the contents of the container but not less than 20 mL
Antibiotic liquids	1 mL
Insoluble preparations, creams and ointments to be suspended or emulsified	Use the contents of each container to provide not less than 200 mg
Solids	
—Less than 50 mg	The whole contents of each container
—50 mg or more but less than 300 mg	Half the contents of each container but not less than 50 mg
—300 mg – 5 g	150 mg
—Greater than 5 g	500 mg

medium or it is suitable for carrying out the incubation after adding the medium to the apparatus itself.

(i) Aqueous solutions: If appropriate, transfer a small quantity of a suitable, sterile diluent such as a 1 g/L neutral solution of meat or casein peptone pH 7.1 ± 0.2 onto the membrane in the apparatus and filter. The diluent may contain suitable neutralizing substances and/or appropriate inactivating substances for example in the case of antibiotics.

Transfer the contents of the container or containers to be tested to the membrane or membranes, if necessary after diluting to the volume used in the method suitability test with the chosen sterile diluent but in any case using not less than the quantities of the product to be examined prescribed in Table 4.06-2. Filter immediately. If the product has antimicrobial properties, wash the membrane not less than three times by filtering through it each time the volume of the chosen sterile diluent used in the method suitability test. Do not exceed a washing cycle of 5 times 100 mL per filter, even if during method suitability it has been demonstrated that such a cycle does not fully eliminate the antimicrobial activity. Transfer the whole membrane to the culture medium or cut it aseptically into two equal parts and transfer one half to each of two suitable media. Use the same volume of each medium as in the method suitability test. Alternatively, transfer the medium onto the membrane in the apparatus. Incubate the media for not less than 14 days.

(ii) Soluble solids: Use for each medium not less than the quantity prescribed in Table 4.06-2 of the product dissolved in a suitable solvent such as the solvent provided with the preparation, water for injection, saline or a 1 g/L neutral solution of meat or casein peptone and proceed with the test as described above for aqueous solutions using a membrane appropriate to the chosen solvent.

(iii) Oils and oily solutions: Use for each medium not less than the quantity of the product prescribed in Table 4.06-2. Oils and oily solutions of sufficiently low viscosity may be filtered without dilution through a dry membrane. Viscous oils may be diluted as necessary with a suitable sterile diluent such as isopropyl myristate shown not to have antimicrobial activity in the conditions of the test. Allow the oil to penetrate the membrane by its own weight then filter, applying the pressure or suction gradually. Wash the membrane at least three times by filtering through it each time about 100 mL of a suitable sterile solution such as 1 g/L neutral meat or casein peptone containing a suitable emulsifying agent at a concentration shown to be appropriate in the method suitability of the test, for example polysorbate 80 at a concentration of 10 g/L. Transfer the membrane or membranes to the culture medium or media or vice versa as described above for aqueous solutions, and incubate at the same temperatures and for the same times.

(iv) Ointments and creams: Use for each medium not less than the quantities of the product prescribed in Table 4.06-2. Ointments in a fatty base and emulsions of the water-in-oil type may be diluted to 1 per cent in isopropyl myristate as described above, by heating, if necessary, to not more than 40°C. In exceptional cases it may be necessary to heat to not more than 44°C. Filter as rapidly as possible and proceed as described above for oils and oily solutions.

5.2. Direct inoculation of the culture medium

Transfer the quantity of the preparation to be examined prescribed in Table 4.06-2 directly into the culture medium so that the volume of the product is not more than 10 per cent of the volume of the medium, unless otherwise prescribed. If the product to be examined has antimicrobial activity, carry out the test after neutralizing this with a suitable neutralizing substance or by dilution in a sufficient quantity of culture medium. When it is necessary to use a large volume of the product it may be preferable to use a concentrated culture medium prepared in such a way that it takes account of the subsequent dilution. Where appropriate the concentrated medium may be added directly to the product in its container.

(i) Oily liquids: Use media to which have been added a suitable emulsifying agent at a concentration shown to be appropriate in the method suitability of the test, for example polysorbate 80 at a concentration of 10 g/L.

(ii) Ointments and creams: Prepare by diluting to about 1 in 10 by emulsifying with the chosen emulsifying agent in a suitable sterile diluent such as a 1 g/L neutral solution of meat or casein peptone. Transfer the diluted product to a medium not containing an emulsifying agent.

Incubate the inoculated media for not less than 14 days. Observe the cultures several times during the incubation period. Shake cultures containing oily products gently each day. However when fluid thioglycollate medium is used for the detection of anaerobic micro-organisms keep shaking or mixing to a minimum in order to maintain anaerobic conditions.

6. Observation and interpretation of results

At intervals during the incubation period and at its conclusion, examine the media for macroscopic evidence of microbial growth. If the material being tested renders the medium turbid so that the presence or absence of microbial growth cannot be readily determined by visual examination, 14 days after the beginning of incubation transfer portions (each not less than 1 mL) of the medium to fresh vessels of the same medium and then incubate the original and transfer vessels for not less than 4 days.

If no evidence of microbial growth is found, the product to be examined complies with the test for sterility. If evi-

Table 4.06-3. Minimum number of items to be tested

Number of items in the batch*	Minimum number of items to be tested for each medium, unless otherwise justified and authorized**
Parenteral preparations	
—Not more than 100 containers	10% or 4 containers whichever is the greater
—More than 100 but not more than 500 containers	10 containers
—More than 500 containers	2% or 20 containers ◇(10 containers for parenterals with a nominal volume of 100 mL or more)◇ whichever is the less
Ophthalmic and other non-injectable preparations	
—Not more than 200 containers	5% or 2 containers whichever is the greater
—More than 200 containers	10 containers
—If the product is presented in the form of single-dose containers, apply the scheme shown above for preparations for parenteral use	
Bulk solid products	
—Up to 4 containers	Each container
—More than 4 containers but not more than 50 containers	20% or 4 containers whichever is the greater
—More than 50 containers	2% or 10 containers whichever is the greater

* If the batch size is not known, use the maximum number of items prescribed.

** If the contents of one container are enough to inoculate the two media, this column gives the number of containers needed for both the media together.

dence of microbial growth is found the product to be examined does not comply with the test for sterility, unless it can be clearly demonstrated that the test was invalid for causes unrelated to the product to be examined. The test may be considered invalid only if one or more of the following conditions are fulfilled:

(i) the data of the microbiological monitoring of the sterility testing facility show a fault;

(ii) a review of the testing procedure used during the test in question reveals a fault;

(iii) microbial growth is found in the negative controls;

(iv) after determination of the identity of the microorganisms isolated from the test, the growth of this species or these species may be ascribed unequivocally to faults with respect to the material and/or the technique used in conducting the sterility test procedure.

If the test is declared to be invalid it is repeated with the same number of units as in the original test. If no evidence of microbial growth is found in the repeat test the product examined complies with the test for sterility. If microbial growth is found in the repeat test the product examined does not comply with the test for sterility.

7. Application of the test to parenteral preparations, ophthalmic and other non-injectable preparations required to comply with the test for sterility

When using the technique of membrane filtration, use, whenever possible, the whole contents of the container, but not less than the quantities indicated in Table 4.06-2, diluting where necessary to about 100 mL with a suitable sterile solution, such as 1 g/L neutral meat or casein peptone.

When using the technique of direct inoculation of media, use the quantities shown in Table 4.06-2, unless otherwise justified and authorized. The tests for bacterial and fungal sterility are carried out on the same sample of the product to be examined. When the volume or the quantity in a single container is insufficient to carry out the tests, the contents of two or more containers are used to inoculate the different media.

8. Minimum number of items to be tested

The minimum number of items to be tested in relation to the size of the batch is given in Table 4.06-3.

5. Tests for Crude Drugs

5.01 Crude Drugs Test

Crude Drugs Test is applied to the crude drugs mentioned in the General Rules for Crude Drugs.

1. Sampling

Unless otherwise specified, sample should be taken by the following methods. If necessary, preserve the samples in tight containers.

(i) When crude drugs to be sampled are small-sized, cut or powdered, 50 to 250 g of sample should be taken after mixing thoroughly.

(ii) When crude drugs to be sampled are large-sized, 250 to 500 g of sample should be taken after mixing thoroughly.

(iii) When the mass of each single piece of the crude drugs is not less than 100 g, not less than 5 pieces should be taken for a sample, or not less than 500 g of the sample should be taken after cutting to a suitable size and mixing thoroughly.

2. Preparation of the test sample for analysis

Preparations are to be made by mixing the sample well. Powdered drugs should be used as they are, and in the case of unpowdered drugs, unless otherwise specified, grind the sample into powder. If the sample cannot be ground into powder, reduce it as finely as possible, spread it out in a thin layer, and withdraw a typical portion for analysis. If necessary, preserve the test sample in a tight container.

3. Microscopic examination

3.1. Apparatus

Use an optical microscope with objectives of 10 and 40 magnifications, and an ocular of 10 magnifications.

3.2. Preparation for microscopic examination

(i) Section: To a section on a slide glass add 1 to 2 drops of a mounting agent, and put a cover glass on it, taking precaution against inclusion of bubbles. Usually use a section 10 to 20 μm in thickness.

(ii) Powder: Place about 1 mg of powdered sample on a slide glass, apply 1 to 2 drops of a swelling agent, stir well with a small rod preventing inclusion of bubbles, and allow to stand for a while to swell the sample. Apply 1 drop of the mounting agent, and put a cover glass on it so that the tissue sections spread evenly without overlapping each other, taking precaution against inclusion of bubbles. In the case where the tissue sections are opaque, place about 1 mg of powdered sample on a slide glass, apply 1 to 2 drops of chloral hydrate TS, heat to make the tissues clear while stirring with a small glass rod to prevent boiling. After cooling, apply 1 drop of mounting agent, and put a cover glass on it in the same manner as above.

Unless otherwise specified, use a mixture of water and glycerin (1:1) or a mixture of water, ethanol (95) and glycerin (1:1:1) as the mounting agent and swelling agent.

3.3. Observation of components in the Description

In each monograph, description is usually given of the outer portion and the inner portion of a section in this order, followed by a specification of cell contents. Observation should be made in the same order. In the case of a powdered sample, description is given of a characteristic component or a matter present in large amount, rarely existing matter, and cell contents in this order. Observation should be made in the same order.

4. Purity

4.1 Heavy metals

There are two ways to specify the heavy metals, one is to specify with the total amount of heavy metals and the other is with individual amount of particular metal(s). Heavy metals for crude drugs are usually specified with the total amount of heavy metals according to Heavy Metals Limit Test <*1.07*> described in monographs. However, rarely there is the case where the test cannot be carried out due to getting turbid or such of the test solution. In these cases, the acceptance can be evaluated by determining individual amount of particular metal(s) using Atomic Absorption Spectrophotometry <*2.23*> or Inductively Coupled Plasma-Atomic Emission Spectrometry and Inductively Coupled Plasma-Mass Spectrometry <*2.63*>.

4.2. Foreign matter

Unless otherwise specified, weigh 25 to 500 g of the sample, spread out in a thin layer, and separate the foreign matter by inspecting with the naked eye or with the use of a magnifying glass of 10 magnifications. Weigh, and determine the percentage of foreign matter.

4.3. Total BHC's and total DDT's

Sodium chloride, anhydrous sodium sulfate and synthetic magnesium silicate for column chromatography used in this procedure are used after drying by heating at about 130°C for more than 12 hours and cooling in a desiccator (silica gel). Chromatographic column is prepared as follows: Place 20 g of synthetic magnesium silicate for column chromatography in a 200-mL flask, add 50 mL of hexane for Purity of crude drug, shake vigorously, and immediately pour the mixture into a chromatographic tube about 2 cm in inside diameter and about 30 cm in length. Drip until the depth of hexane layer at the upper part is about 5 cm, introduce 8 g of anhydrous sodium sulfate from the top, and further drip until a small quantity of hexane is left at the upper part.

Weigh accurately about 5 g of pulverized sample, place in a glass-stoppered centrifuge tube, add 30 mL of a mixture of acetone for Purity of crude drug and water (5:2), stopper tightly, shake for 15 minutes, centrifuge, and separate the supernatant liquid. Repeat the same procedure twice with the residue using two 30-mL portions of the mixture of acetone for Purity of crude drug and water (5:2). Combine all the supernatant liquids, and concentrate under low pressure (in vacuo) at a temperature not higher than 40°C until the order of acetone is faint. Transfer the concentrated solution to a separator containing 100 mL of sodium chloride TS, and shake twice with two 50-mL portions of hexane for Purity of crude drug for 5 minutes each. Combine the hexane layers, transfer to a separator containing 50 mL of sodium chloride TS, and shake for 5 minutes. Take the hexane layer, dry with 30 g of anhydrous sodium sulfate, and filter. Wash the residue on the filter paper with 20 mL of hexane for Purity of crude drug. Combine the filtrate and the washings, and concentrate under low pressure (in vacuo) at a temperature not higher than 40°C to about 5 mL. Transfer this solution to the chromatographic column and allow to pass with 300 mL of a mixture of hexane for Purity of crude drug and diethyl ether for Purity of crude drug (17:3) at a rate of not more than 5 mL per minute. After concentrating the eluate under low pressure (vacuo) at a temperature not higher than 40°C, add hexane for Purity of crude drug to make exactly 5 mL. Transfer this solution to a glass-stoppered test tube, add 1 mL of sulfuric acid, and shake carefully. Take 4 mL of the upper layer, transfer to a separate glass-stoppered test tube, add 2 mL of water, and shake gently. Take 3 mL of the upper layer so obtained, transfer to a glass-stoppered centrifuge tube, dry with 1 g of anhydrous sodium sulfate, centrifuge, and use the supernatant liquid as the sample solution. Separately, weigh accurately about 10 mg each of α-BHC, β-BHC, γ-BHC, δ-BHC, *o,p′*-DDT, *p,p′*-DDT, *p,p′*-DDD and *p,p′*-DDE, dissolve in 5 mL of acetone for Purity of crude drug, and add hexane for Purity of crude drug to make exactly 100 mL. Pipet 10 mL of this solution, and add hexane for Purity of crude drug to make exactly 100 mL. Pipet 1 mL of this solution, add hexane for Purity of crude drug to make exactly 100 mL, and use this solution as the standard solution. Perform the test with 1 μL each of the sample solution and the standard solution as directed under Gas Chromatography <*2.02*> according to the following conditions, and determine the peak areas corresponding to α-BHC, β-BHC, γ-BHC, δ-BHC, *o,p′*-DDT, *p,p′*-DDT, *p,p′*-DDD and *p,p′*-DDE, A_{TA} and A_{SA}; A_{TB} and A_{SB}; A_{TC} and A_{SC}; A_{TD} and A_{SD}; A_{TE} and A_{SE}; A_{TF} and A_{SF}; A_{TG} and A_{SG}; A_{TH} and A_{SH}. Calculate the content of each of α-BHC, β-BHC, γ-BHC, δ-BHC, *o,p′*-DDT, *p,p′*-DDT, *p,p′*-DDD and *p,p′*-DDE by means of the following equations.

Content (ppm) of α-BHC

$$= \frac{\text{amount (g) of } \alpha - \text{BHC}}{M} \times \frac{A_{TA}}{A_{SA}} \times 50$$

Content (ppm) of β-BHC

$$= \frac{\text{amount (g) of } \beta - \text{BHC}}{M} \times \frac{A_{TB}}{A_{SB}} \times 50$$

Content (ppm) of γ-BHC

$$= \frac{\text{amount (g) of } \gamma - \text{BHC}}{M} \times \frac{A_{TC}}{A_{SC}} \times 50$$

Content (ppm) of δ-BHC

$$= \frac{\text{amount (g) of } \delta - \text{BHC}}{M} \times \frac{A_{TD}}{A_{SD}} \times 50$$

Content (ppm) of *o,p′*-DDT

$$= \frac{\text{amount (g) of } o,p' - \text{DDT}}{M} \times \frac{A_{TE}}{A_{SE}} \times 50$$

Content (ppm) of *p,p′*-DDT

$$= \frac{\text{amount (g) of } p,p' - \text{DDT}}{M} \times \frac{A_{TF}}{A_{SF}} \times 50$$

Content (ppm) of p,p'- DDD

$$= \frac{\text{amount (g) of } p,p' - \text{DDD}}{M} \times \frac{A_{TG}}{A_{SG}} \times 50$$

Content (ppm) of p,p'-DDE

$$= \frac{\text{amount (g) of } p,p' - \text{DDE}}{M} \times \frac{A_{TH}}{A_{SH}} \times 50$$

M: Amount (g) of pulverized sample

Content (ppm) of total BHC's
= content (ppm) of α-BHC + content (ppm) of β-BHC + content (ppm) of γ-BHC + content (ppm) of δ-BHC

Content (ppm) of total DDT's
= content (ppm) of o,p'-DDT + content (ppm) of p,p'-DDT + content (ppm) of p,p'-DDD + content (ppm) of p,p'-DDE

Operating conditions—

Detector: An electron capture detector.

Sample injection system: A splitless injection system.

Column: A fused silica capillary column about 0.3 mm in inside diameter and about 30 m in length, coated the inside wall with 7% cyanopropyl-7% phenylmethylsilicone polymer for gas chromatography in a thickness of 0.25 to 1.0 μm.

Column temperature: Maintain the temperature at 60°C for 2 minutes after injection, program to increase the temperature at a rate of 10°C per minute to 200°C, and then program to increase the temperature at a rate of 2°C per minute to 260°C.

Carrier gas: Helium.

Flow rate: Adjust so that the retention times of the objective compounds are between 10 and 30 minutes.

System suitability—

Test for required detectability: To exactly 1 mL of the standard solution add hexane for Purity of crude drug to make exactly 10 mL. Confirm that the peak area of each objective compound obtained with 1 μL of this solution is equivalent to 5 to 15% of that of corresponding compound with 1 μL of the standard solution.

System performance: When the procedure is run with 1 μL of the standard solution under the above operating conditions, the peaks of the object compounds separate completely each other.

System repeatability: Repeat the test 6 times with 1 μL of the standard solution under the above operating conditions, the relative standard deviation of the peak area of each object compound is not more than 10%.

5. Loss on drying

Unless otherwise specified, transfer 2 to 6 g of the test sample for analysis to a tared weighing bottle, and weigh accurately. Dry at 105°C for 5 hours, allow to cool in a desiccator (silica gel), and weigh accurately. Continue the drying at 105°C, and weigh accurately at 1-hour intervals. When the mass of the sample becomes constant, the loss of mass represents the percentage of loss on drying (%). When the period of time for drying is specified, weigh accurately after drying for the period of time specified, and determine the loss on drying (%).

6. Total ash

Ignite previously a crucible of platinum, quartz or porcelain between 500°C and 550°C for 1 hour. Cool, and weigh accurately the crucible. Unless otherwise specified, weigh accurately 2 to 4 g of the test sample for analysis in this crucible, take off the lid or keep it open a little if necessary, heat the crucible at a low temperature at first, then gradually heat to a temperature between 500°C and 550°C, ignite to incinerate the residue for more than 4 hours until no carbonized substance remains in the ash, cool, and weigh accurately the ash. Incinerate repeatedly to constant mass, cool, weigh accurately, and determine the amount (%) of total ash. If a carbonized substance remains and a constant mass cannot be obtained in the above-mentioned method, extract the charred mass with hot water, collect the insoluble residue on filter paper for quantitative analysis, and incinerate the residue and filter paper until no carbonized substance remains in the ash. Then add the filtrate, evaporate it to dryness, and incinerate. Cool, weigh accurately, and determine the mass (%) of the total ash. If a carbon-free ash cannot be obtained even in this way, moisten the ash with a small amount of ethanol (95), break up the ash with a glass rod, wash the rod with a small amount of ethanol (95), evaporate carefully, and determine the mass of the total ash as described above. A desiccator (silica gel) is used for cooling.

7. Acid-insoluble ash

Add carefully 25 mL of dilute hydrochloric acid to the total ash, boil gently for 5 minutes, collect the insoluble matter on filter paper for quantitative analysis, and wash thoroughly with hot water. Dry the residue together with the filter paper, and ignite to incinerate in a tared crucible of platinum, quartz or porcelain for 3 hours. Cool in a desiccator (silica gel), weigh, and determine the amount (%) of acid-insoluble ash. When the amount determined exceeds the limit specified, incinerate repeatedly to a constant mass.

8. Extract content

The test for the extract content in crude drugs is performed as directed in the following methods:

8.1. Dilute ethanol-soluble extract

Unless otherwise specified, weigh accurately about 2.3 g of the sample for analysis, extract with 70 mL of dilute ethanol in a suitable flask with occasional shaking for 5 hours, and allow to stand for 16 to 20 hours. Filter, and wash the flask and residue with small portions of dilute ethanol until the filtrate measures 100 mL. Evaporate a 50 mL aliquot of the filtrate to dryness, dry at 105°C for 4 hours, and cool in a desiccator (silica gel). Weigh accurately the amount, multiply it by 2, and determine the amount of dilute ethanol-soluble extract. Calculate the extract content (%) with respect to the amount of the sample on the dried basis, obtained under the loss on drying.

8.2. Water-soluble extract

Proceed as directed in 8.1., using water instead of dilute ethanol, weigh accurately the amount, multiply by 2, and determine the amount of water-soluble extract. Calculate the extract content (%) with respect to the amount of the sample on the dried basis, obtained under the loss on drying.

8.3. Diethyl ether-soluble extract

Unless otherwise specified, dry the test sample for analysis in a desiccator (silica gel) for 48 hours, weigh accurately about 2 g of it, and place in a suitable flask. Add 70 mL of diethyl ether, attach a reflux condenser to the flask, and boil gently on a water bath for 4 hours. Cool, filter, and wash the flask and the residue with small portions of diethyl ether until the filtrate measures 100 mL. Evaporate a 50 mL aliquot of the filtrate to dryness on a water bath, dry in a desiccator (silica gel) for 24 hours, weigh accurately the amount, multiply it by 2, determine the amount of diethyl ether-soluble extract, and calculate the extract content (%).

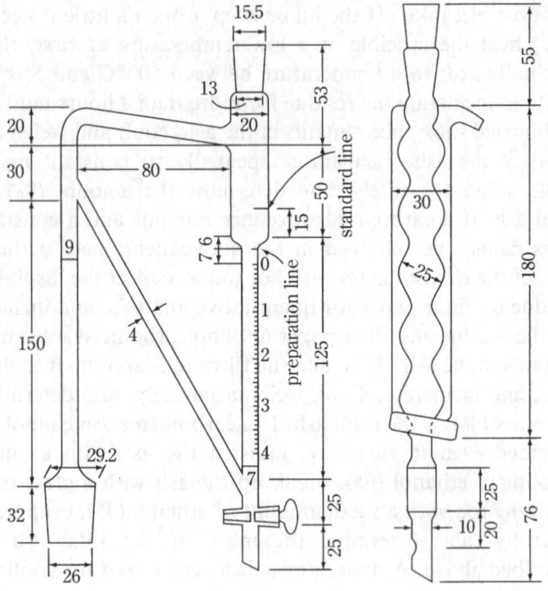

The figures are in mm.

Fig. 5.01-1 **Fig. 5.01-2**

9. Essential oil content

The test of essential oil content in crude drugs is performed as directed in the following method.

9.1. Essential oil determination

Weigh the quantity of the test sample for analysis directed in the monograph in a 1-L hard glass-stoppered flask, and add from 5 to 10 times as much water as the drug. Set up an apparatus for essential oil determination (Fig. 5.01-1), inserting a reflux condenser (Fig. 5.01-2) in the upper mouth of it, and heat the content of the flask in an oil bath between 130°C and 150°C to boiling. The graduated tube of the apparatus is to be previously filled with water to the standard line, and 2.0 mL of xylene is added to the graduated tube. Unless otherwise specified, continue boiling for 5 hours, allow to stand for some time, and open the stopper of the apparatus. Draw off the water slowly until the surface of the oil layer corresponds to the preparation line, and allow it to stand for more than 1 hour at ordinary temperature. Then lower the surface of the oil layer to the zero line, and read the volume (mL) of the oil at ordinary temperature. Subtract the volume (mL) of xylene from the volume of the total oil.

10. Assay of Marker Compounds for the Assay of Crude Drugs and Extracts of Kampo Formulations Utilizing Nuclear Magnetic Resonance (NMR) Spectroscopy

10.1. Principle of Quantitative Analytical Technique Utilizing Nuclear Magnetic Resonance (NMR) Spectroscopy

The spectra obtained by proton nuclear magnetic resonance (^{1}H-NMR) spectroscopy after dissolving the substance to be measured in a solvent, are frequently used as a powerful analytical method for determining the chemical structure of the substance from the following reasons: the resonance signals appear at different chemical shifts depending on the chemical structure of the substance measured; the signals are split by spin-spin interactions through chemical bonds mainly depending on the number of ^{1}H bonded to adjacent carbon atoms; the signal intensities (areas) are proportional to the number of ^{1}H resonating at the same frequency; etc.

In the ^{1}H-NMR spectra, the proton nuclei (^{1}Hs) in different chemical environments within the same molecule are observed as the separate signals having different chemical shifts depending on their resonance frequencies. Accordingly, we can compare the intensities of 2 signals having different chemical shifts each other. The intensity of the signal S_i would be given by the following equation (1);

$$S_i \propto N_i \frac{m}{VM} p \sin\beta \frac{1 - e^{-T_r/T_{1i}}}{1 - e^{-T_r/T_{1i}} \cos\beta} M_0 \quad (1)$$

where N_i is the number of resonating ^{1}H which gives the signal, V is the volume of the sample solution, m is the mass of the sample, M is the molecular mass of the substance measured, p is the purity of the sample, β is the excitation pulse angle, T_{1i} is the spin-lattice relaxation time of ^{1}H which gives the signal, T_r is the repetition time, M_0 is the equilibrium magnetization and the subscript i indicates the independent signal. The relaxation time of a ^{1}H is different depending on the environments of the ^{1}Hs. Since the sensitivity of NMR is not so good, the signal-to-noise ratio (SN ratio) of signals should generally be improved by measuring it repeatedly and averaging noises. When the NMR measurement is performed under the condition with the repetition time T_r sufficiently longer than the longest T_1 among the T_1s of the signals observed for the analyte compound, the condition of $1 - e^{-T_r/T_1} \approx 1$ for all of the signals of the analyte compounds would be satisfied and quantitative analysis utilizing NMR (quantitative NMR) can be performed. On the other hand, when NMR is used for the structural determination, priority is given to improve detection sensitivity, and the condition for increasing the SN ratio of signals by using repeated measurements is usually used. Under this condition, since the repetition time is not long enough to ensure quantitative NMR, the proportion of signal intensity to the number of each equivalent ^{1}H nuclei in the measured molecule is not obtained precisely. However, when NMR is measured under the conditions which ensure quantitative performance, the signal intensity ratio proportional to each number of equivalent molecule is obtained.

When the intensity of two signals having different chemical shifts in the same molecule are compared under the quantitative conditions which ensure quantitative performance, the following equation (2) is obtained and the signal intensities S_i and S_j are found to be proportional to the number of resonating ^{1}Hs.

$$\frac{S_i}{S_j} = \frac{N_i}{N_j} \quad (2)$$

This proportionality between the signal area and number of resonating ^{1}H can be applied to the signals from 2 different molecules. In this case, since it is considered that the excitation pulse angle and the volume of the sample solution used for the measurement can be kept constant independent of the substance measured, the following equation (3), in which the observed signal area S is proportional only to the purity, molecular mass and mass used for the measurement of analyte compound, can be obtained. (a and s indicate the signals of the analyte compound and a reference substance (internal standard), respectively.)

$$P_a = \frac{S_a}{S_s} \frac{N_s}{N_a} \frac{M_a}{M_s} \frac{m_s}{m_a} P_s \quad (3)$$

Although there are some prerequisites to be met, such that each molecule should not interact (such as react) with other molecules in the solution and the molecule should have separate signals at different chemical shifts from others, we will be able to evaluate the purity of the analyte compound by measuring its ^{1}H-NMR under the conditions which ensure quantitative performance, if we have a standard material with known purity and use it as an internal standard for the measurement. In other words, if a standard material whose molecular mass and accurate purity are known would be provided as the superior standard, we can evaluate the purity of the substances coexisting in the solution of the standard material by measuring ^{1}H-NMR of the solution. In this case, when traceability of the measurement to the International System of Units (SI) is guaranteed for the standard material, purity of the analyte compound can be calculated indirectly as the SI traceable value by using the standard material as the superior standard. In such a measurement, it is necessary to dissolve the sample and the standard material in a solution. Thus, it is practically important for precise evaluation of the purity of analyte compound that both of the sample and the standard material should be weighed accurately, and dissolved in a solvent for NMR measurement.

10.2. Supply of Reference Standard and Software for Quantitative NMR

Quantitative determination based on the aforementioned principle is called quantitative NMR (qNMR). From among certified reference materials supplied from public institutions (NMIJ CRM), those with SI traceable pricing have been marketed as reference standard for qNMR. Easy-to-use solid-state compounds include 1,4-bis(trimethylsilyl)benzene-d_4 (1,4-BTMSB-d_4), methanol, and dimethylsulfoxide for organic solvent use and 3-(trimethylsilyl)-1-propanesulfonic acid-d_6-sodium salt (DSS-d_6), maleic acid and dimethyl sulfone for aquatic use which both exhibit a sharp peak for specific chemical shifts in ^{1}H-NMR. In addition, such measurement software capable of performing qNMR easier is also supplied by NMR manufacturers.

10.3. Marker Compounds for Assay and Reference Substances for Quantitative Analysis of Crude Drugs and Extracts of Kampo Formulations in the JP

If it is possible to price a reagent used as a quantitative index component in a crude medicine with a correct content using qNMR based on the above-mentioned principle, it also becomes possible to use the reagent as a reference substance for analysis with assured metrological traceability. According to a result of a validation experiment, in case of a compound with molecular mass of around 300 to be measured, it is possible to perform pricing at an ordinary laboratory level by using about 10 mg of the compound for the measurement while ensuring two significant figures even if including errors between used devices. As content of quantitative index component in a crude medicine is just a few percent at most in general and the minimum unit of regulation values is 0.1%, two significant figures is believed to be enough to ensure the accuracy of the content of reference substances for quantitative analysis in consideration of variation for each crude medicine as a natural substance.

Such reagents priced with SI traceable quantitative value (degree of purity) by qNMR that have been defined in a paragraph for reagents and test solutions are available as Japanese Pharmacopoeia reagents for quantitative analysis. Further, in cases where a reagent priced by qNMR is used as a reference substance for quantitative analysis such as HPLC and involved in a calculation of quantitative value of subject compound after converting degree of purity (%) of the priced reagent, it becomes possible to use the resulting quantitative value as a SI traceable value. In addition, in cases where a reagent priced by qNMR is used as a reference material for a quantitative analysis based on HPLC, condition of the quantitative analysis is based on an assumption that no impurity is recognized at any peak of a component of the reagent to be quantified, which is required to be confirmed separately by a device such as photodiode array detector or mass spectrometer.

10.4. Precautions for Performing qNMR

In order to perform qNMR, such device is required that is capable of gated decoupling for ^{13}C-NMR with higher accuracy in a magnetic field with a resonance frequency of at least 400 MHz or higher for ^{1}H-NMR in consideration of resolution required for separation of impurities from peaks and even detection sensitivity as well. Further, it is also required to perform measurement under the condition that receiving sensitivity of the receiver is appropriate with optimally adjusted probe tuning and shim.

In terms of reagents for quantification for which qNMR is performed, amounts of reagents and reference standard for qNMR to be taken are defined in paragraph 9.41 Reagents, Test Solutions. As high accuracy is required for weighing both of them, it is required to take the amounts by the minimum weight of the balance or higher. Defined amounts to be taken for both of them are those described as validated realistic minimum amounts using an ultramicrobalance. Therefore, in cases where both of them are completely dissolved, SN ratio of spectrum is improved when measured after increasing the amounts while keeping the quantitative ratio, resulting in measurements with higher accuracy in most cases. Even though SN ratio is even more improved when a measurement is performed by integrating as many times as possible resulting in a measurement result with higher accuracy, it is required to consider stability of the magnetic field and the devices if the measurement lasts more than a few hours. Sensitivity is also improved, albeit a little, by using deuterated solvent with higher deuteration rate. In some cases, impurity signals may be detected on a spectrum which have not been observed before, by further improving SN ratio. In cases where any existence of signal derived from such impurities has been made clear, the range of chemical shift where such signal exists should not be integrated. In addition, as signals of small amount of impurities have been observed also in deuterated solvent for NMR measurement or 1,4-BTMSB-d_4 or DSS-d_6 as reference standard for qNMR, it is important to recognize the range of these impurities signals before qNMR measurement. Moreover, qNMR measurement should be performed immediately after sample preparation, since impurity signals have been confirmed to increase albeit a little by little if samples are kept in the solvent for measurement for long hours. Even though it is not necessary to measure NMR under qNMR condition for confirming impurity signals, it is easier to distinguish them from satellite signals by performing a measurement under the condition of decoupling of ^{13}C nuclei without spinning. While 1,4-BTMSB-d_4 and DSS-d_6, which are used for qNMR as reference standard for qNMR, have chemical shift values at around 0.2 ppm and 0.1 ppm respectively when tetramethylsilane (in organic solvent) or DSS (in deuterated water) is used as the reference for chemical shifts (δ), chemical shifts of other signals are indicated by regarding the chemical shifts of these reference standard for qNMR as 0 ppm for convenience when measuring qNMR.

The SN ratio of a signal used in NMR is calculated using the formula of signal intensity/(2 × noise intensity), and this noise intensity is the root-mean-square value of individual noise intensities in the noise area.

5.02 Microbial Limit Test for Crude Drugs and Preparations containing Crude Drugs as Main Ingredient

Microbial limit test for crude drugs and preparations containing crude drugs as main ingredient (crude drug preparations) includes microbial enumeration tests and tests for specified micro-organisms. For the test, use a mixture of several portions selected at random from the bulk or from the contents of a sufficient number of containers. If test specimens are diluted with fluid medium, the test should be performed quickly. In performing the test, precautions must be taken to prevent biohazard.

I. Total Viable Aerobic Count

The tests described hereafter will allow quantitative enumeration of mesophilic bacteria and fungi which may grow under aerobic conditions.

The tests are designed primarily to determine whether a substance or preparation complies with an established specification for microbiological quality. When used for such purposes follow the instructions given below, including the number of samples to be taken and interpret the results as stated below.

Alternative microbiological procedures, including rapid methods, may be used, provided that they give a result equal to or better than that of the Pharmacopoeial methods.

1. General Procedures

Carry out the determination under conditions designed to avoid extrinsic microbial contamination of the product to be examined. The precautions taken to avoid contamination must be such that they do not affect any micro-organisms which are to be revealed in the test.

If the product to be examined has antimicrobial activity, this is insofar as possible removed or neutralised. If inactivators are used for this purpose their efficacy and their absence of toxicity for micro-organisms must be demonstrated.

If surface-active substances are used for sample preparation, their absence of toxicity for micro-organisms and their compatibility with inactivators used must be demonstrated.

2. Enumeration Methods

The choice of a method is based on factors such as the nature of the product and the required limit of micro-organisms. The method chosen must allow testing of a sufficient sample size to judge compliance with the specification. The suitability of the chosen method must be established.

3. Growth Promotion Test, Suitability of the Counting Method and Negative Controls

The ability of the test to detect micro-organisms in the presence of product to be tested must be established.

Suitability must be confirmed if a change in testing performance, or the product, which may affect the outcome of the test is introduced.

3.1. Preparation of test strains

Use standardised stable suspensions of test strains or prepare as stated below.

Seed lot culture maintenance techniques (seed-lot systems) are used so that the viable micro-organisms used for inoculation are not more than 5 passages removed from the original master seed-lot. Grow each of the bacterial and fungal test strains separately as described in Table 5.02-I-1.

Use Buffered Sodium Chloride-Peptone Solution (pH 7.0) or Phosphate Buffer (pH 7.2) to make test suspensions; to suspend *Aspergillus brasiliensis* spores, 0.05% of polysorbate 80 may be added to the buffer. Use the suspensions within 2 h or within 24 h if stored at 2 – 8°C. As an alternative to preparing and then diluting a fresh suspension of vegetative cells of *Aspergillus brasiliensis* or *Bacillus subtilis*, a stable spore suspension is prepared and then an appropriate volume of the spore suspension is used for test inoculation. The stable spore suspension may be maintained at 2 – 8°C for a validated period of time.

3.2. Negative control

To verify testing conditions, a negative control is performed using the chosen diluent in place of the test preparation. There must be no growth of micro-organisms. A negative control is also performed when testing the products as described under 4. Testing of Products. A failed negative control requires an investigation.

3.3. Growth promotion of the media

Test each batch of ready-prepared medium and each batch of medium, prepared either from dehydrated medium or from the ingredients described.

Inoculate portions/plates of Fluid Soybean-Casein Digest Medium and Soybean-Casein Digest Agar Medium with a small number (not more than 100 CFU) of the microorganisms indicated in Table 5.02-I-1, using a separate portion/plate of medium for each. Inoculate plates of Sabouraud Glucose Agar Medium with a small number (not more than 100 CFU) of the micro-organisms indicated in Table 5.02-I-1, using a separate plate of medium for each. Incubate in the conditions described in Table 5.02-I-1.

For solid media, growth obtained must not differ by a factor greater than 2 from the calculated value for a standardized inoculum. For a freshly prepared inoculum, growth of the micro-organisms comparable to that previously obtained with a previously tested and approved batch of medium occurs.

Liquid media are suitable if clearly visible growth of the micro-organisms comparable to that previously obtained with a previously tested and approved batch of medium occurs.

3.4. Suitability of the counting method in the presence of product

3.4.1. Preparation of the sample

The method for sample preparation depends on the physical characteristics of the product to be tested. If none of the procedures described below can be demonstrated to be satisfactory, an alternative procedure must be developed.

Buffered Sodium Chloride-Peptone Solution (pH 7.0), Phosphate Buffer (pH 7.2) or Fluid Soybean-Casein Digest Medium is used to suspend or dilute the test specimen. Unless otherwise specified, usually take 10 g or 10 mL of the test specimen, and suspend or dissolve it in 90 mL of the buffer or fluid medium specified. A test specimen as a suspension must be shaken for 10 minutes. If necessary, for the product to be tested which recovery rate of microorganisms is low, repeat the same method and use this as the test fluid. A different quantity or volume may be used if the nature of the test specimen requires it. A surface-active agent such as 1 g/L of polysorbate 80 may be added to assist the suspension of poorly wettable substances. If necessary adjust to pH 6 – 8. Further dilutions, where necessary, are prepared with the same diluent.

3.4.2. Inoculation and dilution

Add to the sample prepared as described above (3.4.1.) and to a control (with no test material included) a sufficient volume of the microbial suspension to obtain an inoculum of not more than 100 CFU. The volume of the suspension of

Table 5.02-I-1 Preparation and use of test micro-organisms

Micro-organism	Preparation of test strain	Growth promotion		Suitability of counting method in the presence of the product	
		Total aerobic microbial count	Total yeasts and moulds count	Total aerobic microbial count	Total yeasts and moulds count
Staphylococcus aureus such as ATCC 6538, NCIMB 9518, CIP 4.83 or NBRC 13276	Soybean-Casein Digest Agar Medium or Fluid Soybean-Casein Digest Medium 30 – 35°C 18 – 24 h	Soybean-Casein Digest Agar Medium* and Fluid Soybean-Casein Digest Medium ≦ 100 CFU 30 – 35°C ≦ 3 days		Soybean-Casein Digest Agar Medium/MPN Fluid Soybean-Casein Digest Medium ≦ 100 CFU 30 – 35°C ≦ 5 days	
Pseudomonas aeruginosa such as ATCC 9027, NCIMB 8626, CIP 82.118 or NBRC 13275	Soybean-Casein Digest Agar Medium or Fluid Soybean-Casein Digest Medium 30 – 35°C 18 – 24 h	Soybean-Casein Digest Agar Medium* and Fluid Soybean-Casein Digest Medium ≦ 100 CFU 30 – 35°C ≦ 3 days		Soybean-Casein Digest Agar Medium/MPN Fluid Soybean-Casein Digest Medium ≦ 100 CFU 30 – 35°C ≦ 5 days	
Bacillus subtilis such as ATCC 6633, NCIMB 8054, CIP 52.62 or NBRC 3134	Soybean-Casein Digest Agar Medium or Fluid Soybean-Casein Digest Medium 30 – 35°C 18 – 24 h	Soybean-Casein Digest Agar Medium* and Fluid Soybean-Casein Digest Medium ≦ 100 CFU 30 – 35°C ≦ 3 days		Soybean-Casein Digest Agar Medium/MPN Fluid Soybean-Casein Digest Medium ≦ 100 CFU 30 – 35°C ≦ 5 days	
Candida albicans such as ATCC 10231, NCPF 3179, IP 48.72 or NBRC 1594	Sabouraud Glucose Agar Medium or Fluid Sabouraud Glucose Medium 20 – 25°C 2 – 3 days	Soybean-Casein Digest Agar Medium* ≦ 100 CFU 30 – 35°C ≦ 5 days	Sabouraud Glucose Agar Medium with antibiotics ≦ 100 CFU 20 – 25°C ≦ 5 days	Soybean-Casein Digest Agar Medium ≦ 100 CFU 30 – 35°C ≦ 5 days MPN: not applicable	Sabouraud Glucose Agar Medium with antibiotics ≦ 100 CFU 20 – 25°C ≦ 5 days
Aspergillus brasiliensis such as ATCC 16404, IMI 149007, IP 1431.83 or NBRC 9455	Sabouraud Glucose Agar Medium or Potato Dextrose Agar Medium 20 – 25°C 5 – 7 days, or until good sporulation is achieved	Soybean-Casein Digest Agar Medium* ≦ 100 CFU 30 – 35°C ≦ 5 days	Sabouraud Glucose Agar Medium with antibiotics ≦ 100 CFU 20 – 25°C ≦ 5 days	Soybean-Casein Digest Agar Medium ≦ 100 CFU 30 – 35°C ≦ 5 days MPN: not applicable	Sabouraud Glucose Agar Medium with antibiotics ≦ 100 CFU 20 – 25°C ≦ 5 days

* In the case where TTC TS or amphotericin B TS is added, check with the media with these additives. When amphotericin B TS is added, the check for *C. albicans* and *A. brasiliensis* is not required.

the inoculum should not exceed 1 per cent of the volume of diluted product.

To demonstrate acceptable microbial recovery from the product, the lowest possible dilution factor of the prepared sample must be used for the test. Where this is not possible due to antimicrobial activity or poor solubility, further appropriate protocols must be developed.

If inhibition of growth by the sample cannot otherwise be avoided, the aliquot of the microbial suspension may be added after neutralization, dilution or filtration.

3.4.3. Neutralization/removal of antimicrobial activity

The number of micro-organisms recovered from the prepared sample diluted as described in 3.4.2. and incubated following the procedure described in 3.4.4., is compared to the number of micro-organisms recovered from the control preparation.

If growth is inhibited (reduction by a factor greater than 2), then modify the procedure for the particular enumeration test to ensure the validity of the results. Modification of the procedure may include, for example, (1) an increase in the volume of the diluent or culture medium, (2) incorporation of a specific or general neutralizing agents into the diluent, (3) membrane filtration or (4) a combination of the above measures.

Neutralizing agents—Neutralizing agents may be used to neutralize the activity of antimicrobial agents. They may be added to the chosen diluent or the medium preferably before sterilization. If used, their efficacy and their absence of toxicity for micro-organisms must be demonstrated by carrying out a blank with neutralizing agents, without product.

If no suitable neutralizing method can be found, it can be assumed that the failure to isolate the inoculated organism is attributable to the microbicidal activity of the product. This information serves to indicate that the article is not likely to be contaminated with the given species of the micro-organism. However, it is possible that the product only inhibits some of the micro-organisms specified herein, but does not inhibit others not included amongst the test strains or for which the latter are not representative. Then, perform the test with the highest dilution factor compatible with microbial growth and the specific acceptance criterion.

3.4.4. Recovery of micro-organism in the presence of product

For each of the micro-organisms listed in Table 5.02-I-1, separate tests are performed. Only micro-organisms of the added test strain are counted.

3.4.4.1. Membrane filtration method

Use membrane filters having a nominal pore size not greater than 0.45 μm. The type of filter material is chosen in such a way that the bacteria-retaining efficiency is not affected by the components of the sample to be investigated. For each of the micro-organisms listed in Table 5.02-I-1, one membrane filter is used.

Transfer a suitable amount of the sample prepared as described under 3.4.1. to 3.4.3. (preferably representing 1 g of the product, or less if large numbers of CFU are expected) to the membrane filter, filter immediately and rinse the membrane filter with an appropriate volume of diluent.

For the determination of total aerobic microbial count (TAMC), transfer the membrane filter to the surface of Soybean-Casein Digest Agar Medium. For the determination of total combined yeasts/moulds count (TYMC) transfer the membrane to the surface of Sabouraud Glucose Agar Medium with antibiotics. For Soybean-Casein Digest Agar Medium that is suffused with fungi or when the TAMC is expected to exceed the acceptance criterion due to the fungus growth, amphotericin B TS as an antimycotic may be added to the agar. Incubate the plates as indicated in Table 5.02-I-1. Perform the counting.

3.4.4.2. Plate-count methods

Perform plate-count methods at least in duplicate for each medium and use the mean count of the result.

(i) Pour-plate method: For Petri dishes 9 cm in diameter, add to the dish 1 mL of the sample prepared as described under 3.4.1. to 3.4.3. and 15 - 20 mL of Soybean-Casein Digest Agar Medium or Sabouraud Glucose Agar Medium with antibiotics, both media being warmed at not more than 45°C. For Soybean-Casein Digest Agar Medium, TTC TS may be added to distinct the colonies from the fragments of crude drugs existed in specimens, and when the agar medium is suffused with fungi or the TAMC is expected to exceed the acceptance criterion due to the fungus growth, amphotericin B TS as an antimycotic may be added to the medium. In the case of Sabouraud Glucose Agar Medium with antibiotics that is suffused with fungi, Rose Bengal TS may be added. If larger Petri dishes are used, the amount of agar medium is increased accordingly. For each of the micro-organisms listed in Table 5.02-I-1, at least 2 Petri dishes are used.

Incubate the plates as indicated in Table 5.02-I-1. Take the arithmetic mean of the counts per medium and calculate the number of CFU in the original inoculum.

(ii) Surface-spread method: For Petri dishes 9 cm in diameter, add 15 - 20 mL of Soybean-Casein Digest Agar Medium or Sabouraud Glucose Agar Medium with antibiotics at about 45°C to each Petri dish and allow to solidify. Dry the plates, for example in a laminar-air-flow cabinet or in an incubator. The test solutions to be added to the agar medium are the same as described in (i) Pour-plate method. If larger Petri dishes are used, the volume of the agar is increased accordingly. For each of the micro-organisms listed in Table 5.02-I-1, at least 2 Petri dishes are used. Spread a measured volume of not less than 0.1 mL of the sample prepared as described under 3.4.1. to 3.4.3. over the surface of the medium. Incubate and count as prescribed under 3.4.4.2. (i).

3.4.4.3. Most-probable-number (MPN) method

The precision and accuracy of the MPN method is less than that of the membrane filtration method or the plate-count method. Unreliable results are obtained particularly for the enumeration of moulds. For these reasons the MPN method is reserved for the enumeration of TAMC in situations where no other method is available. If the use of the method is justified, proceed as follows.

Prepare a series of at least 3 serial tenfold dilutions of the product as described under 3.4.1. to 3.4.3. From each level of dilution, 3 aliquots of 1 g or 1 mL are used to inoculate 3 tubes with 9 - 10 mL of Fluid Soybean-Casein Digest Medium. If necessary a surface-active agent such as polysorbate 80, or an inactivator of antimicrobial agents may be added to the medium. Thus, if 3 levels of dilution are prepared 9 tubes are inoculated.

Incubate all tubes at 30 - 35°C for not more than 3 days. If reading of the results is difficult or uncertain owing to the nature of the product to be examined, subculture in the same broth, or Soybean-Casein Digest Agar Medium, for 1 - 2 days at the same temperature and use these results. Determine the most probable number of micro-organisms per gram or millilitre of the product to be examined from Table 5.02-I-2.

3.5. Results and interpretation

When verifying the suitability of the membrane filtration method or the plate-count method, a mean count of any of the test organisms not differing by a factor greater than 2 from the value of the control defined in 3.4.2. in the absence of the product must be obtained. When verifying the suitability of the MPN method the calculated value from the inoculum must be within 95 per cent confidence limits of the results obtained with the control.

If the above criteria cannot be met for one or more of the organisms tested with any of the described methods, the method and test conditions that come closest to the criteria are used to test the product.

4. Testing of Products

4.1. Sampling and preparation of the test specimens

Select the sample(s) at random from the bulk material or from the available containers of the preparation. To obtain the required quantity, mix the contents of a sufficient number of containers to provide the sample.

Unless otherwise specified, samples should be taken by the following methods.

(i) When crude drugs to be sampled are small-sized, cut or powdered, 50 to 250 g of sample should be taken after mixing thoroughly.

(ii) When crude drugs to be sampled are large-sized, 250 to 500 g of sample should be taken after mixing thoroughly and cutting.

(iii) When the mass of each single piece of the crude drug is not less than 100 g, not less than 5 pieces should be taken for a sample, or not less than 500 g of the sample should be taken after cutting to a suitable size and mixing thoroughly. If necessary, cut more for use.

(iv) When crude drugs to be sampled are in the form of a solution or a preparation, the sample should be taken after mixing thoroughly.

4.2. Examination of the product

4.2.1. Membrane filtration method

Use a filtration apparatus designed to allow the transfer of the filter to the medium.

Prepare the sample using a method that has been shown suitable as described in section 3 and transfer the appropriate amount to each of 2 membrane filters and filter immediately. Wash each filter following the procedure shown to be suitable.

For the determination of TAMC, transfer one of the membrane filters to the surface of Soybean-Casein Digest Agar Medium. For the determination of TYMC, transfer the other membrane to the surface of Sabouraud Glucose Agar Medium with antibiotics. Incubate the plate of Soybean-Casein Digest Agar Medium at 30 - 35°C for 5 - 7 days and the plate of Sabouraud Glucose Agar Medium with antibiotics at 20 - 25°C for 5 - 7 days.

Calculate the number of CFU per gram or per millilitre of product.

4.2.2. Plate-count methods

(i) Pour-plate method: Prepare the sample using a method that has been shown to be suitable as described in section 3. Prepare for each medium at least 2 Petri dishes for each level of dilution. Incubate the plates of Soybean-Casein Digest Agar Medium at 30 - 35°C for 5 - 7 days and the plates of Sabouraud Glucose Agar Medium with antibiotics at 20 - 25°C for 5 - 7 days. Select the plates corresponding to a given dilution and showing the highest number of colonies less than 250 for TAMC and 50 for TYMC. Take the arithmetic mean per culture medium of the counts and calculate the number of CFU per gram or per millilitre of product.

(ii) Surface-spread method: Prepare the sample using a method that has been shown to be suitable as described in section 3. Prepare at least 2 Petri dishes for each medium and each level of dilution. For incubation and calculation of the number of CFU proceed as described for the pour-plate method.

4.2.3. Most-probable-number method

Prepare and dilute the sample using a method that has been shown to be suitable as described in section 3. Incubate all tubes for 3 - 5 days at 30 - 35°C. Subculture if necessary, using the procedure shown to be suitable. Record for each level of dilution the number of tubes showing microbial growth.

Determine the most probable number of micro-organisms per gram or millilitre of the product to be examined from Table 5.02-I-2.

4.3. Interpretation of the results

The total aerobic microbial count (TAMC) is considered to be equal to the number of CFU found using Soybean-Casein Digest Agar Medium; if colonies of fungi are detected on this medium, they are counted as part of TAMC. The total combined yeasts/mould count (TYMC) is considered to be equal to the number of CFU found using Sabouraud Glucose Agar Medium with antibiotics; if colonies of bacteria

Table 5.02-I-2 Most-probable-number values of micro-organisms

Observed combinations of numbers of tubes showing growth in each set			MPN per g or mL of product	95 percent confidence limits
Number of g or mL of product per tube				
0.1	0.01	0.001		
0	0	0	< 3	0 - 9.4
0	0	1	3	0.1 - 9.5
0	1	0	3	0.1 - 10
0	1	1	6.1	1.2 - 17
0	2	0	6.2	1.2 - 17
0	3	0	9.4	3.5 - 35
1	0	0	3.6	0.2 - 17
1	0	1	7.2	1.2 - 17
1	0	2	11	4 - 35
1	1	0	7.4	1.3 - 20
1	1	1	11	4 - 35
1	2	0	11	4 - 35
1	2	1	15	5 - 38
1	3	0	16	5 - 38
2	0	0	9.2	1.5 - 35
2	0	1	14	4 - 35
2	0	2	20	5 - 38
2	1	0	15	4 - 38
2	1	1	20	5 - 38
2	1	2	27	9 - 94
2	2	0	21	5 - 40
2	2	1	28	9 - 94
2	2	2	35	9 - 94
2	3	0	29	9 - 94
2	3	1	36	9 - 94
3	0	0	23	5 - 94
3	0	1	38	9 - 104
3	0	2	64	16 - 181
3	1	0	43	9 - 181
3	1	1	75	17 - 199
3	1	2	120	30 - 360
3	1	3	160	30 - 380
3	2	0	93	18 - 360
3	2	1	150	30 - 380
3	2	2	210	30 - 400
3	2	3	290	90 - 990
3	3	0	240	40 - 990
3	3	1	460	90 - 1980
3	3	2	1100	200 - 4000
3	3	3	> 1100	

are detected on this medium, they are counted as part of TYMC. In the case here the bacterial growth is expected not to give any affection to the interpretation of the result, Sabouraud Glucose Agar Medium containing no antibiotics may be used. If the count is carried out by the MPN method the calculated value is the TAMC.

The recommended solutions and media are described in "II. Tests for Specified Micro-organisms".

II. Tests for Specified Micro-organisms

The tests described hereafter will allow determination of the absence of, or limited occurrence of specified micro-organisms which may be detected under the conditions described.

The tests are designed primarily to determine whether a substance or preparation complies with an established specification for microbiological quality. When used for such purposes follow the instructions given below, including the number of samples to be taken and interpret the results as stated below.

Alternative microbiological procedures, including rapid methods, may be used, provided that they give a result equal to or better than that of the Pharmacopoeial methods.

1. General Procedures

The preparation of samples is carried out as described in I. Total Viable Aerobic Count.

If the product to be examined has antimicrobial activity, this is insofar as possible removed or neutralized as described in I. Total viable aerobic count.

If surface-active substances are used for sample preparation, their absence of toxicity for micro-organisms and their compatibility with inactivators used must be demonstrated as described in I. Total Viable Aerobic Count.

For the scarce crude drugs and those products, the quantity of sample or the volume of medium may be adjusted accordingly based on a risk estimation.

2. Growth Promoting and Inhibitory Properties of the Media, Suitability of the Test and Negative Controls

The ability of the test to detect micro-organisms in the presence of the product to be tested must be established. Suitability must be confirmed if a change in testing performance, or the product, which may affect the outcome of the test is introduced.

2.1. Preparation of test strains

Use standardised stable suspensions of test strains or prepare as stated below. Seed lot culture maintenance techniques (seed-lot systems) are used so that the viable micro-organisms used for inoculation are not more than 5 passages removed from the original master seed-lot.

Grow each of the bacterial test strains separately in containers containing Fluid Soybean-Casein Digest Medium or on Soybean-Casein Digest Agar Medium at 30 - 35°C for 18 - 24 hours.

Staphylococcus aureus such as ATCC 6538, NCIMB 9518, CIP 4.83 or NBRC 13276,

Pseudomonas aeruginosa such as ATCC 9027, NCIMB 8626, CIP 82.118 or NBRC 13275,

Escherichia coli such as ATCC 8739, NCIMB 8545, CIP 53.126 or NBRC 3972,

Salmonella enterica subsp. *enterica* serovar Typhimurium such as ATCC 14028

or, as an alternative,

Salmonella enterica subsp. *enterica* serovar Abony such as NBRC 100797, NCTC 6017 or CIP 80.39,

Use Buffered Sodium Chloride-Peptone Solution (pH 7.0) or Phosphate Buffer (pH 7.2) to make test suspensions. Use the suspensions within 2 hours or within 24 hours if stored at 2 - 8°C.

Table 5.02-II-1 Growth promoting, inhibitory and indicative properties of media

Medium	Property	Test strains
Test for bile-tolerant gram-negative bacteria		
Enterobacteria enrichment broth-Mossel	Growth promoting	*E. coli* *P. aeruginosa*
	Inhibitory	*S. aureus*
VRB (Violet/Red/Bile) Agar with glucose	Growth promoting + Indicative	*E. coli* *P. aeruginosa*
Test for *Escherichia coli*		
Fluid MacConkey Broth Medium	Growth promoting	*E. coli*
	Inhibitory	*S. aureus*
MacConkey Agar Medium	Growth promoting + Indicative	*E. coli*
Enzyme substrate medium for *E. coli*	Growth promoting + Indicative	*E. coli*
Test for *Salmonella*		
Fluid Rappaport Vassiliadis Salmonella Enrichment Broth Medium	Growth promoting	*Salmonella enterica* subsp. *enterica* serovar Typhimurium or *Salmonella enterica* subsp. *enterica* serovar Abony
	Inhibitory	*S. aureus*
XLD (Xylose-Lysine-Deoxycholate) Agar Medium	Growth promoting + Indicative	*Salmonella enterica* subsp. *enterica* serovar Typhimurium or *Salmonella enterica* subsp. *enterica* serovar Abony
Enzyme substrate medium for *Salmonella*	Growth promoting + Indicative	*Salmonella enterica* subsp. *enterica* serovar Typhimurium or *Salmonella enterica* subsp. *enterica* serovar Abony
Test for *Staphylococcus aureus*		
Fluid Soybean-Casein Digest Medium with 7.5% Sodium Chloride	Growth promoting	*S. aureus*
Vogel-Johnson Agar Medium	Growth promoting + Indicative	*S. aureus*
	Inhibitory	*E. coli*
Baird-Parker Agar Medium	Growth promoting + Indicative	*S. aureus*
	Inhibitory	*E. coli*
Mannitol Salt Agar Medium	Growth promoting + Indicative	*S. aureus*
	Inhibitory	*E. coli*

2.2. Negative control

To verify testing conditions a negative control is performed using the chosen diluent in place of the test preparation. There must be no growth of micro-organisms. A failed negative control required an investigation. A negative control is also performed when testing the products as described under 3. Testing of Products.

2.3. Growth promotion and inhibitory properties of the media

Test each batch of ready-prepared medium and each batch of medium prepared either from dehydrated medium or from ingredients.

Verify suitable properties of relevant media as described in Table 5.02-II-1.

(i) Test for growth promoting properties, liquid media: inoculate a portion of the appropriate medium with a small number (not more than 100 CFU) of the appropriate micro-organism. Incubate at the specified temperature for not more than the shortest period of time specified in the test. Clearly visible growth of the micro-organism comparable to that previously obtained with a previously tested and approved batch of medium occurs.

(ii) Test for growth promoting properties, solid media: perform surface-spread method, inoculating each plate with a small number (not more than 100 CFU) of the appropriate micro-organism. Incubate at the specified temperature for not more than the shortest period of time specified in the test. Growth of the micro-organism comparable to that previously obtained with a previously tested and approved batch of medium occurs.

(iii) Test for inhibitory properties, liquid or solid media: inoculate the appropriate medium with at least 100 CFU of the appropriate micro-organism. Incubate at the specified temperature for not less than the longest period of time specified in the test. No growth of the test micro-organism occurs.

(iv) Test for indicative properties, solid media: perform surface-spread method, inoculating each plate with a small number (not more than 100 CFU) of the appropriate micro-organism. Incubate at the specified temperature for a period of time within the range specified in the test. Colonies are comparable in indication reactions to those previously obtained with a previously tested and approved batch of medium.

(v) Test for indicative properties, liquid media: inoculate a portion of the appropriate medium with a small number (not more than 100 CFU) of the appropriate micro-organism. Incubate at the specified temperature for a period of time within the range specified in the test. Colonies are comparable in indication reactions to those previously obtained with a previously tested and approved batch of medium.

2.4. Suitability of the test method

For each product to be tested perform sample preparation as described in the relevant paragraph in section 3. Add each test strain at the time of mixing, in the prescribed growth medium. Inoculate the test strains individually. Use a number of micro-organisms equivalent to not more than 100 CFU in the inoculated test preparation.

Perform the test as described in the relevant paragraph in section 3 using the shortest incubation period prescribed.

The specified micro-organisms must be detected with the indication reactions as described in section 3.

Any antimicrobial activity of the product necessitates a modification of the test procedure (see 3.4.3. of I. Total Viable Aerobic Count).

If for a given product the antimicrobial activity with respect to a micro-organism for which testing is prescribed cannot be neutralised, then it is to be assumed that the inhibited micro-organism will not be present in the product.

Table 5.02-II-2 Interpretation of results

Results for each quantity of product				Probable number of bacteria per gram or mL of product
0.1 g or 0.1 mL	**0.01 g or 0.01 mL**	**0.001 g or 0.001 mL**	**0.0001 g or 0.0001 mL**	
+	+	+	+	more than 10^4
+	+	+	−	less than 10^4 and more than 10^3
+	+	−	−	less than 10^3 and more than 10^2
+	−	−	−	less than 10^2 and more than 10
−	−	−	−	less than 10

3. Testing of Products

3.1. Bile-tolerant gram-negative bacteria

3.1.1. Sample preparation and pre-incubation

Prepare a sample using a 1 in 10 dilution of not less than 1 g of the product to be examined as described in I. Total viable aerobic count, but using Fluid Soybean-Casein Digest Medium as the chosen diluent, mix and incubate at 20 – 25°C for a time sufficient to resuscitate the bacteria but not sufficient to encourage multiplication of the organisms (usually 2 hours but not more than 5 hours).

3.1.2. Selection and subculture

Inoculate to a suitable amount of Fluid Enterobacteria Enrichment Broth Mossel Medium successive three dilutions which are chosen according to an objective acceptable limit from four dilutions of the sample preparation described under 3.1.1. and/or the dilutions of it, containing respectively 0.1 g, 0.01 g, 0.001 g and 0.0001 g (or 0.1 mL, 0.01 mL, 0.001 mL and 0.0001 mL) of the product to be examined. Incubate at 30 – 35°C for 24 – 48 hours. Subculture each of the cultures on a plate of VRB (Violet/Red/Bile) Agar with glucose. Incubate at 30 – 35°C for 18 – 24 hours.

3.1.3. Interpretation

Generally, growth of colonies constitutes a positive result. Note the smallest quantity of the product that gives a positive result and the largest quantity that gives a negative result. Determine from Table 5.02-II-2 the probable number of bile-tolerant gram-negative bacteria.

3.2. Escherichia coli

3.2.1. Qualitative test

3.2.1.1. Sample preparation and pre-incubation

Prepare a sample using a 1 in 10 dilution of not less than 1 g of the product to be examined as described in "I. Total viable aerobic count" and use 10 mL or the quantity corresponding to 1 g or 1 mL to inoculate a suitable amount (determined as described under 2.4.) of Fluid Soybean-Casein Digest Medium, mix and incubate at 30 – 35°C for 18 – 24 hours.

3.2.1.2. Selection and subculture

Shake the container, transfer 1 mL of Fluid Soybean-Casein Digest Medium to 10 mL of Fluid MacConkey Broth Medium and incubate at 44 ± 0.5°C for 24 – 48 hours. Subculture on a plate of MacConkey Agar Medium at 30 – 35°C for 18 – 72 hours. An appropriate enzyme substrate medium for *E. coli* such as CHE Agar Medium or ESC Medium may be used instead of MacConkey Agar Medium. When such enzyme substrate media are used, incubate under the conditions indicated for each medium.

3.2.1.3. Interpretation

Growth of brick-red colonies surrounded by a reddish precipitation line on MacConkey Agar Medium or of colonies showing aspects or responses corresponding to *E. coli* on an enzyme substrate medium for *E. coli* indicates the possible presence of *E. coli*. This is confirmed by identification tests.

The product complies with the test if no colonies showing such aspects or responses are present or if the identification tests are negative.

3.2.2. Quantitative test

3.2.2.1. Sample preparation and pre-incubation

Inoculate to a suitable amount (determined as described under 2.4) of Fluid Soybean-Casein Digest Medium three amounts of a 1 in 10 dilution, prepared as directed in I. Total Viable Aerobic Count, respectively equivalent to 0.1 g, 0.01 g and 0.001 g (or 0.1 mL, 0.01 mL and 0.001 mL) of the product to be examined, mix, and incubate at 30 - 35°C for 18 - 24 hours.

3.2.2.2. Selection and subculture

Shake the container, transfer 1 mL of Fluid Soybean-Casein Digest Medium to 10 mL of Fluid MacConkey Broth Medium and incubate at 44 ± 0.5°C for 24 - 48 hours. Subculture on a plate of MacConkey Agar Medium at 30 - 35°C for 18 - 72 hours. An appropriate enzyme substrate medium for *E. coli* such as CHE Agar Medium or ESC Medium may be used instead of MacConkey Agar Medium. When such enzyme substrate media are used, incubate under the conditions indicated for each medium.

3.2.2.3. Interpretation

Growth of brick-red colonies surrounded by a reddish precipitation line on MacConkey Agar Medium or of colonies showing aspects or responses corresponding to *E. coli* on an enzyme substrate medium for *E. coli* indicates the possible presence of *E. coli*. This is confirmed by identification tests.

Note the smallest quantity of the product that gives a positive result and the largest quantity that gives a negative result, and determine the probable number of *E. coli* from Table 5.02-II-3.

3.3. Salmonella

3.3.1. Sample preparation and pre-incubation

Inoculate 10 g or 10 mL of the product to be examined to a suitable amount (determined as described under 2.4.) of Fluid Soybean-Casein Digest Medium, mix and incubate at 30 - 35°C for 18 - 24 hours.

3.3.2. Selection and subculture

Inoculate 0.1 mL of Fluid Soybean-Casein Digest Medium to 10 mL of Fluid Rappaport Vassiliadis Salmonella Enrichment Broth Medium and incubate at 42 ± 0.5°C for 18 - 24 hours. Transfer on plates of XLD (Xylose-Lysine-Desoxycholate) Agar Medium, and incubate at 30 - 35°C for 18 - 48 hours. An appropriate enzyme substrate medium such as CHS Agar Medium or ES II Agar Medium may be used instead of XLD Agar Medium. When such enzyme substrate media are used, incubate under the conditions indicated for each medium.

3.3.3. Interpretation

The possible presence of *Salmonella* is indicated by the growth of well-developed, red colonies, with or without black centers or of colonies showing aspects or responses corresponding to *Salmonella*. This is confirmed by identification tests.

The product complies with the test if colonies of the types described are not present or if the confirmatory identification tests are negative.

Table 5.02-II-3 Interpretation of results

Results for each quantity of product			Probable number of microorganisms per gram or mL
0.1 g or 0.1 mL	0.01 g or 0.01 mL	0.001 g or 0.001 mL	
+	+	+	more than 10^3
+	+	−	less than 10^3 and more than 10^2
+	−	−	less than 10^2 and more than 10
−	−	−	less than 10

Table 5.02-II-4 Morphologic characteristics of *Staphylococcus aureus* on selective agar media

Medium	Colonial characteristic
Vogel-Johnson Agar Medium	Black surrounded by a yellow zone
Baird-Parker Agar Medium	Black, shiny, surrounded by a clear zone
Mannitol-Salt Agar Medium	Yellow colonies surrounded by a yellow zone

The following section is given for information.

3.4. Staphylococcus aureus

3.4.1. Sample preparation and pre-incubation

Prepare a sample using a 1 in 10 dilution of not less than 1 g of the product to be examined as described in I. Total Viable Aerobic Count and use 10 mL or the quantity corresponding to 1 g or 1 mL to inoculate a suitable amount (determined as described under 2.4.) of Fluid Soybean-Casein Digest Medium and homogenise.

Incubate at 30 - 35°C for 24 - 48 hours.

3.4.2. Selection and enrichment subculture

To 9 mL of Fluid Soybean-Casein Digest Medium with 7.5% Sodium Chloride add 1 mL of Fluid Soybean-Casein Digest Medium and incubate at 30 - 35°C for 24 - 48 hours.

3.4.3. Selection and subculture

If the growth is apparent, take a portion of the culture fluid by means of an inoculating loop and streak it on the surface of either Vogel-Johnson Agar Medium, Baird-Parker Agar Medium or Mannitol-Salt Agar Medium, and incubate at 30 - 35°C for 24 - 48 hours.

3.4.4. Interpretation

The product complies with the test if colonies of the characteristics described in Table 5.02-II-4 are not present or if the confirmatory identification tests are negative.

4. Recommended Solutions, Culture Media and Test Solutions

The following solutions, culture media and test solutions have been found satisfactory for the purposes for which they are prescribed in the test for microbial contamination in the Pharmacopoeia. Other media may be used provided that their suitability can be demonstrated.

(i) Phosphate Buffer (pH 7.2)

Prepare a mixture of water and stock buffer solution (800:1 *V/V*) and sterilize.

Stock buffer solution: Transfer 34 g of potassium dihydrogen phosphate to a 1000 mL volumetric flask, dissolve in 500 mL of water, adjust to pH 7.0 to 7.4 with sodium hydroxide TS, add water to volume and mix. Dispense in containers and sterilize. Store at a temperature of 2 – 8°C.

(ii) Buffered Sodium Chloride-Peptone Solution (pH 7.0)

Potassium dihydrogen phosphate	3.6 g
Disodium hydrogen phosphate dihydrate	7.2 g
(equivalent to 0.067 mol phosphate)	
Sodium chloride	4.3 g
Peptone (meat or casein)	1.0 g
Water	1000 mL

Sterilize in an autoclave using a validated cycle.

(iii) Fluid Soybean-Casein Digest Medium

Casein peptone	17.0 g
Soybean peptone	3.0 g
Sodium chloride	5.0 g
Dipotassium hydrogen phosphate	2.5 g
Glucose monohydrate	2.5 g
Water	1000 mL

Adjust the pH so that after sterilization it is 7.1 – 7.5 at 25°C. Sterilize in an autoclave using a validated cycle.

(iv) Soybean-Casein Digest Agar Medium

Casein peptone	15.0 g
Soybean peptone	5.0 g
Sodium chloride	5.0 g
Agar	15.0 g
Water	1000 mL

Adjust the pH so that after sterilization it is 7.1 – 7.5 at 25°C. Sterilize in an autoclave using a validated cycle.

(v) Sabouraud Glucose Agar Medium

Glucose	40.0 g
Peptones (animal tissue and casein 1:1)	10.0 g
Agar	15.0 g
Water	1000 mL

Adjust the pH so that after sterilization it is 5.4 – 5.8 at 25°C. Sterilize in an autoclave using a validated cycle. Just prior to use, add 0.10 g of benzylpenicillin potassium and 0.10 g of tetracycline per liter of medium as sterile solutions or, alternatively, add 50 mg of chloramphenicol per liter of medium.

(vi) Potato Dextrose Agar Medium

Infusion from potatoes	200 g
Glucose	20.0 g
Agar	15.0 g
Water	1000 mL

Adjust the pH so that after sterilization it is 5.4 – 5.8 at 25°C. Sterilize in an autoclave using a validated cycle.

(vii) Fluid Sabouraud Glucose Medium

Glucose	20.0 g
Peptones (animal tissue and casein 1:1)	10.0 g
Water	1000 mL

Adjust the pH so that after sterilization it is 5.4 – 5.8 at 25°C. Sterilize in an autoclave using a validated cycle.

(viii) Fluid Enterobacteria Enrichment Broth Mossel Medium

Gelatin peptone	10.0 g
Glucose monohydrate	5.0 g
Bile salts	20.0 g
Potassium dihydrogen phosphate	2.0 g
Disodium hydrogen phosphate dihydrate	8.0 g
Brilliant green	15 mg
Water	1000 mL

Adjust the pH so that after heating it is 7.0 – 7.4 at 25°C. Heat at 100°C for 30 min and cool immediately.

(ix) VRB (Violet/Red/Bile) Agar with glucose

Yeast extract	3.0 g
Gelatin peptone	7.0 g
Bile salts	1.5 g
Sodium chloride	5.0 g
Glucose monohydrate	10.0 g
Agar	15.0 g
Neutral red	30 mg
Crystal violet	2 mg
Water	1000 mL

Adjust the pH so that after heating it is 7.2 – 7.6 at 25°C. Heat to boiling; do not heat in autoclave.

(x) Fluid MacConkey Broth Medium

Gelatin peptone	20.0 g
Lactose monohydrate	10.0 g
Dehydrated ox bile	5.0 g
Bromocresol purple	10 mg
Water	1000 mL

Adjust the pH so that after sterilization it is 7.1 – 7.5 at 25°C. Sterilize in an autoclave using a validated cycle.

(xi) MacConkey Agar Medium

Gelatin peptone	17.0 g
Peptones (meat and casein)	3.0 g
Lactose monohydrate	10.0 g
Sodium chloride	5.0 g
Bile salts	1.5 g
Agar	13.5 g
Neutral red	30 mg
Crystal violet	1 mg
Water	1000 mL

Adjust the pH so that after sterilization it is 6.9 – 7.3 at 25°C. Boil for 1 min with constant shaking then sterilize in an autoclave using a validated cycle.

(xii) Fluid Rappaport Vassiliadis Salmonella Enrichment Medium

Soya peptone	4.5 g
Magnesium chloride hexahydrate	29.0 g
Sodium chloride	8.0 g
Dipotassium hydrogen phosphate	0.4 g
Potassium dihydrogen phosphate	0.6 g
Malachite green	36 mg
Water	1000 mL

Dissolve, warming slightly. Sterilize in an autoclave using a validated cycle, at a temperature not exceeding 115°C. The pH is to be 5.0 – 5.4 at 25°C after heating and autoclaving.

(xiii) XLD (Xylose-Lysine-Desoxycholate) Agar Medium

Xylose	3.5 g
L-Lysine	5.0 g
Lactose monohydrate	7.5 g
Sucrose	7.5 g
Sodium chloride	5.0 g
Yeast extract	3.0 g
Phenol red	80 mg
Agar	13.5 g
Sodium desoxycholate	2.5 g
Sodium thiosulfate	6.8 g
Ammonium iron (III) citrate	0.8 g
Water	1000 mL

Adjust the pH so that after heating it is 7.2 – 7.6 at 25°C. Heat to boiling, cool to 50°C and pour into Petri dishes. Do not heat in autoclave.

(xiv) Fluid Soybean-Casein Digest Medium with 7.5% Sodium Chloride

Pancreatic digest of casein 17.0 g
Soybean peptone 3.0 g
Sodium chloride 75.0 g
Dipotassium hydrogen phosphate 2.5 g
Glucose monohydrate 2.5 g
Water 1000 mL

To (iii) Fluid Soybean-Casein Digest Medium (containing 5.0 g of sodium chloride) add 70.0 g of sodium chloride, mix, and adjust the pH so that after sterilization it is 7.1 - 7.5 at 25°C. Sterilize in an autoclave using a validated cycle.

(xv) Vogel-Johnson Agar Medium

Casein peptone 10.0 g
Yeast extract 5.0 g
D-Mannitol 10.0 g
Dipotassium hydrogen phosphate 5.0 g
Lithium chloride 5.0 g
Glycine 10.0 g
Phenol red 25 mg
Agar 16.0 g
Water 1000 mL

Mix all the components and boil for 1 min to resolve. Adjust the pH so that after sterilization it is 7.0 - 7.4. After sterilization in an autoclave using a validated cycle, cool to 45 - 50°C, add 20 mL of a sterile solution of potassium tellurite (1 in 100), and mix.

(xvi) Baird-Parker Agar Medium

Pancreatic digest of casein 10.0 g
Meat extract 5.0 g
Yeast extract 1.0 g
Lithium chloride 5.0 g
Glycine 12.0 g
Sodium pyruvate 10.0 g
Agar 20.0 g
Water 950 mL

Mix all the components and boil for 1 min with frequent agitation. Adjust the pH so that after sterilization it is 6.6 - 7.0. After sterilization in an autoclave using a validated cycle, cool to 45 - 50°C, add 10 mL of a sterile solution of potassium tellurite (1 in 100) and 50 mL of egg-yolk emulsion, mix gently, and pour into Petri dishes. The egg-yolk emulsion is prepared by mixing egg-yolk and sterile saline in a ratio of about 30% to 70%.

(xvii) Mannitol Salt Agar Medium

Casein peptone 5.0 g
Animal tissue peptone 5.0 g
Beef extract 1.0 g
D-Mannitol 10.0 g
Sodium chloride 75.0 g
Agar 15.0 g
Phenol red 25 mg
Water 1000 mL

Heat to boiling for 1 min with shaking. Adjust the pH so that after sterilization it is 7.2 - 7.6 at 25°C. Sterilize in an autoclave using a validated cycle.

Enzyme substrate media for *Escherichia coli*

Use the media shown below as examples and that have been validated their capabilities.

(xviii) CHE Ager Medium

Casein peptone 5.0 g
A mixture of yeast extract and meat extract 3.3 g
A mixture of selecting agent and particular enzyme substrate 9.0 g
Sodium chloride 5.0 g
Ager 15.0 g
Water 1000 mL

Adjust the pH so that after heating it is 5.8 - 6.2 at 25°C. Sterilize in an autoclave using a validated cycle, or heat to boiling, cool to 50°C and pour into Petri dishes.

(xix) ESC Medium

Peptone 5.0 g
Potassium nitrate 1.0 g
Sodium chloride 5.0 g
Sodium lauryl sulfate 0.1 g
Sodium pyruvate 1.0 g
Isopropyl-β-thiogalactopyranoside 0.1 g
Potassium dihydrogen phosphate 1.0 g
Dipotassium hydrogen phosphate 4.0 g
5-Bromo-4-chloro-3-indolyl-β-D-galactopyranoside 0.1 g
4-Methylumbelliferyl-β-D-glucuronide 0.1 g
Water 1000 mL

Adjust the pH so that after sterilization it is 6.9 - 7.3 at 25°C. Sterilize in an autoclave using a validated cycle.

Enzyme substrate media for *Salmonella*

Use the media shown below as examples and that have been validated their capabilities.

(xx) CHS Agar Medium

Peptone 5.0 g
Yeast extract 2.0 g
Sodium chloride 0.8 g
Other salts 7.2 g
A mixture of selecting agent and particular enzyme substrate 4.9 g
Ager 15.0 g
Water 1000 mL

Adjust the pH so that after heating it is 7.4 - 7.8 at 25°C. Heat to boiling, cool to 50°C and pour into Petri dishes. Do not heat in autoclave.

(xxi) ESII Agar Medium

Peptone 10.0 g
Yeast extract 1.0 g
Sodium chloride 5.0 g
Disodium hydrogen phosphate 1.0 g
Sodium thiosulfate 1.0 g
Sodium deoxycholate 1.0 g
D-Mannitol 15.0 g
Neutral red 30 mg
Synthetic enzyme substract 0.45 g
Novobiocin 0.02 g
Ager 15.0 g
Water 1000 mL

Adjust the pH so that after sterilization it is 6.9 - 7.3 at 25°C. Sterilize in an autoclave using a validated cycle. Cool to 50°C and pour into Petri dishes.

(xxii) Amphotericin B TS: Dissolve 22.5 mg of amphotericin B powder in 9 mL of sterile purified water.

Amphotericin B powder: Amphotericin B that is added sodium deoxycholate, sterilized by γ-ray.

(xxiii) Rose bengal TS: Dissolve 1 g of rose bengal in water to make 100 mL.

(xxiv) TTC TS: Dissolve 0.8 g of 2,3,5-triphenyl-2*H*-tetrazolium chloride in water to make 100 mL, divide into small tubes, and sterilize in an autoclave using a validated cycle. Store protected from light.

Preparation method

(i) Ager medium with TTC: Just prior to use, add 2.5 to 5 mL of TTC TS per liter (20 to 40 mg/L) of sterile ager medium and mix.

(ii) Ager medium with amphotericin B: Just prior to use, add 2 mL of amphotericin B TS per liter (5 mg/L) of ager medium previously sterilized in an autoclave using a validated cycle, and mix.

(iii) Ager medium with rose bengal: Add 5 mL of rose bengal TS per liter (50 mg/L) of agar medium, mix, and sterilize in an autoclave using a validated cycle.

6. Tests for Preparations

6.01 Test for Metal Particles in Ophthalmic Ointments

Test of Metal Particles in Ophthalmic Ointments is a method to test the existence of foreign metal particles in the ophthalmic ointments described in General Rules for Preparations.

1. Preparation of test sample

The test should be carried out in a clean place. Take 10 ophthalmic ointments to be tested, and extrude 5 g each of their contents into separate flat-bottomed petri dishes 60 mm in diameter. Cover the dishes, and heat between 85°C and 110°C for 2 hours to dissolve bases completely. Allow the samples to cool to room temperature without agitation to solidify the contents. When the amount of the content is less than 5 g, extrude the contents as completely as practicable, and proceed in the same manner as described above.

2. Procedure

Invert each dish on the stage of a suitable microscope previously adjusted to provide not less than 40 times magnifications and equipped with an eyepiece micrometer disk. Each dish is illuminated from above 45° relative to the plane of the dish. Examine the entire bottom of each dish for metal particles, and record the total number of particles, measuring 50 μm or more in any dimension.

Note: Use petri dishes with a clean bottom and free from foams and scratches, and if possible, the walls are at right angles with the bottom.

3. Evaluation

The preparation complies with the test if the total number of metal particles of a size equal to or greater than 50 μm found in 10 units tested, is not more than 50, and also the number of dishes containing more than 8 particles is not more than 1. If this requirement is not met, repeat the test with a further 20 units in the same manner, and if the total number of the particles found in the total of 30 units is not more than 150, and also the number of dishes containing more than 8 particles is not more than 3, the preparation complies with the test.

6.02 Uniformity of Dosage Units

This test is harmonized with the European Pharmacopoeia and the U.S. Pharmacopeia.

The corresponding part of the attributes/provisions which are agreed as non-harmonized within the scope of the harmonization is marked with symbols (◆ ◆), and the corresponding parts which are agreed as the JP local requirement other than the scope of the harmonization are marked with symbols (◇ ◇).

Information on the harmonization with the European Pharmacopoeia and the U.S. Pharmacopeia is available on the website of the Pharmaceuticals and Medical Devices Agency.

The term "Uniformity of dosage unit" is defined as the degree of uniformity in the amount of the drug substance among dosage units. Therefore, the requirements of this chapter apply to each drug substance being comprised in dosage units containing one or more drug substances, unless otherwise specified elsewhere in this Pharmacopoeia.

To ensure the consistency of dosage units, each unit in a batch should have a drug substance content within a narrow range around the label claim. Dosage forms such as tablets, capsules, packets of powders or granules, ampoules, contain a single dose or a part of a dose of a drug substance in each dosage unit. The Uniformity of Dosage Units specification is not intended to apply to solutions, suspensions, emulsions, or gels in unit-dose containers intended for external, cutaneous administration.

The uniformity of dosage units can be demonstrated by either of two methods, *Content uniformity* or *Mass variation* (see Table 6.02-1). The test for *Content Uniformity* of preparations presented in dosage units is based on the assay of the individual contents of drug substance(s) of a number of dosage units to determine whether the individual contents are within the limits set. The *Content Uniformity* method may be applied in all cases.

The test for *Mass Variation* is applicable for the following dosage forms:

(i) solutions enclosed in unit-dose containers and into soft capsules ◇in which all components are perfectly dissolved◇;

(ii) solids (including powders, granules and sterile solids) that are packaged in single-dose packages and contain no active or inactive added substances;

(iii) solids (including sterile solids) that are packaged in single-dose packages, with or without active or inactive added substances, that have been prepared from true solutions ◇in which all components are perfectly dissolved◇ and freeze-dried in the final packages and are labeled to indicate this method of preparation; and

(iv) hard capsules, uncoated tablets, or film-coated tablets, containing 25 mg or more of a drug substance comprising 25% or more, by weight, of the dosage unit or, in the case of hard capsules, the capsule contents, ◇or in the case of film-coated tablets, the pre-coated tablets,◇ except that uniformity of other drug substances present in lesser proportions is demonstrated by meeting *Content Uniformity* requirements.

The test for *Content Uniformity* is required for all dosage forms not meeting the above conditions for the *Mass Variation* test. Alternatively, products listed in item (iv) above that do not meet the 25 mg/25% threshold limit may be tested for uniformity of dosage units by *Mass Variation* instead of the *Content Uniformity* test if the concentration relative standard deviation (RSD) of the drug substance in the final dosage units is not more than 2%, based on process validation data and development data, and if there has been regulatory approval of such a change. The concentration RSD is the RSD of the concentration per dosage unit (w/w or w/v), where concentration per dosage unit equals the assay result per dosage unit divided by the individual dosage unit weight. See the RSD formula in Table 6.02-2.

1. Content Uniformity

Select not less than 30 units, and proceed as follows for the dosage form designated.

Where different procedures are used for assay of the

Table 6.02-1 Application of Content Uniformity (CU) and Mass Variation (MV) Test for dosage forms

Dosage Forms	Type	Sub-type	Dose and ratio of drug substance	
			≥ 25 mg & ≥ 25%	< 25 mg or < 25%
Tablets	uncoated		MV	CU
	coated	Film	MV	CU
		Others	CU	CU
Capsules	hard		MV	CU
	soft	Sus., eml., gel	CU	CU
		Solutions	MV	MV
Solids in single-dose packages ◇(divided forms, lyophilized forms, et al.)◇	Single component		MV	MV
	Multiple components	Freeze-dried from solutions in final container	MV	MV
		Others	CU	CU
Solutions ◇(perfectly dissolved)◇ enclosed in unit-dose containers			MV	MV
Others—Among the preparations not classified as the above dosage forms in this table, suppositories, percutaneous absorption type preparations (patches), semi-solid dosage forms intended for application of active pharmaceutical ingredients to the skin for the purpose of systemic action, and the like.			CU	CU

Sus.: suspension; eml.: emulsion;

preparation and for the content uniformity test, it may be necessary to establish a correction factor to be applied to the results of the latter.

(i) Solid dosage forms: Assay 10 units individually using an appropriate analytical method. Calculate the acceptance value (see Table 6.02-2).

(ii) Liquid or Semi-Solid dosage forms: Assay 10 units individually using an appropriate analytical method. Carry out the assay on the amount of well-mixed material that is removed from an individual container in conditions of normal use and express the results as delivered dose. Calculate the acceptance value (see Table 6.02-2).

1.1. Calculation of Acceptance Value

Calculate the acceptance value by the formula:

$$|M - \bar{X}| + ks,$$

in which the terms are as defined in Table 6.02-2.

2. Mass Variation

◇*Mass Variation* is carried out based on the assumption that the concentration (mass of drug substance per mass of dosage unit) is uniform in a lot.◇

Carry out an assay for the drug substance(s) on a representative sample of the batch using an appropriate analytical method. This value is result A, expressed as % of label claim (see *Calculation of the Acceptance Value*). Select not less than 30 dosage units, and proceed as follows for the dosage form designated.

(i) Uncoated or Film-coated Tablets: Accurately weigh 10 tablets individually. Calculate the content, expressed as % of label claim, of each tablet from the mass of the individual tablets and the result of the assay. Calculate the acceptance value.

(ii) Hard Capsules: Accurately weigh 10 capsules individually, taking care to preserve the identity of each capsule. Remove the contents of each capsule by suitable means. Accurately weigh the emptied shells individually, and calculate for each capsule the net mass of its contents by subtracting the mass of the shell from the respective gross mass. Calculate the drug substance content of each capsule from the mass of the individual capsules and the result of the assay. Calculate the acceptance value.

(iii) Soft Capsules: Accurately weigh the 10 intact capsules individually to obtain their gross masses, taking care to preserve the identity of each capsule. Then cut open the capsules by means of a suitable clean, dry cutting instrument such as scissors or a sharp open blade, and remove the contents by washing with a suitable solvent. Allow the occluded solvent to evaporate from the shells at room temperature over a period of about 30 minutes, taking precautions to avoid uptake or loss of moisture. Weigh the individual shells, and calculate the net contents. Calculate the drug substance content in each capsule from the mass of product removed from the individual capsules and the result of the assay. Calculate the acceptance value.

(iv) Solid dosage forms other than tablets and capsules: Proceed as directed for *Hard Capsules*, treating each dosage unit as described therein. Calculate the acceptance value.

(v) Liquid dosage forms: Accurately weigh the amount of liquid that is removed from each of 10 individual containers in conditions of normal use. If necessary, compute the equivalent volume after determining the density. Calculate the drug substance content in each container from the mass of product removed from the individual containers and the result of the assay. Calculate the acceptance value.

2.1. Calculation of Acceptance Value

Calculate the acceptance value as shown in *Content Uniformity*, except that ◇the value of $\bar{X}$ is replaced with A,

Table 6.02-2

Variable	Definition	Conditions	Value
$\overline{X}$	Mean of individual contents ($x_1, x_2, \ldots, x_n$) expressed as a percentage of the label claim		
$x_1, x_2, \ldots, x_n$	Individual contents of the dosage units tested, expressed as a percentage of the label claim		
n	Sample size (number of dosage units in a sample)		
k	Acceptability constant	If n = 10, then	2.4
		If n = 30, then	2.0
s	Sample standard deviation		$\sqrt{\dfrac{\sum_{i=1}^{n}(x_i - \overline{X})^2}{n-1}}$
RSD	Relative standard deviation (the sample standard deviation expressed as a percentage of the mean)		$\dfrac{100s}{\overline{X}}$
M (case 1)	Reference value	If 98.5% $\leqq \overline{X} \leqq$ 101.5%, then	$M = \overline{X}$ ($AV = ks$)
To be applied when $T \leqq 101.5$		If $\overline{X}$ < 98.5%, then	M = 98.5% ($AV = 98.5 - \overline{X} + ks$)
		If $\overline{X}$ > 101.5%, then	M = 101.5% ($AV = \overline{X} - 101.5 + ks$)
M (case 2)	Reference value	If 98.5% $\leqq \overline{X} \leqq T$, then	$M = \overline{X}$ ($AV = ks$)
To be applied when $T > 101.5$		If $\overline{X}$ < 98.5%, then	M = 98.5% ($AV = 98.5 - \overline{X} + ks$)
		If $\overline{X} > T$, then	$M = T$% ($AV = \overline{X} - T + ks$)
Acceptance Value (AV)			General formula: $\lvert M - \overline{X}\rvert + ks$ [Calculations are specified above for the different cases.]
$L1$	Maximum allowed acceptance value		$L1$ = 15.0 unless otherwise specified.
$L2$	Maximum allowed range for deviation of each dosage unit tested from the calculated value of M	On the low side, no dosage unit result can be less than 0.75M while on the high side, no dosage unit result can be greater than 1.25M (This is based on an $L2$ value of 25.0.)	$L2$ = 25.0 unless otherwise specified.
T	Target content per dosage unit at time of manufacture, expressed as the percentage of the label claim. Unless otherwise stated, T is 100.0%, or T is the manufacturer's approved target content per dosage unit.		

and that◇ the individual contents of the dosage units are replaced with the individual estimated contents defined below.

$x_1, x_2 \ldots x_n$: individual estimated contents of the dosage units tested

$$x_i = w_i \times \frac{A}{\overline{W}}$$

$w_1, w_2 \ldots w_n$: Individual masses of the dosage units tested

A: Content of drug substance (% of label claim) obtained using an appropriate analytical method

$\overline{W}$: Mean of individual masses ($w_1, w_2 \ldots w_n$)

3. Criteria

Apply the following criteria, unless otherwise specified.

(i) Solid, Semi-Solid and Liquid dosage forms: The requirements for dosage uniformity are met if the acceptance value of the first 10 dosage units is less than or equal to $L1$%. If the acceptance value is greater than $L1$%, test the next 20 dosage units and calculate the acceptance value. The requirements are met if the final acceptance value of the 30 dosage units is less than or equal to $L1$% and no individual content of the dosage unit is less than $(1 - L2 \times 0.01)M$ nor more than $(1 + L2 \times 0.01)M$ in *Calculation of Acceptance Value* under *Content Uniformity* or under *Mass Variation*. Unless otherwise specified, $L1$ is 15.0 and $L2$ is 25.0.

6.03 Particle Size Distribution Test for Preparations

Particle Size Distribution Test for Preparations is a method to determine the particle size distribution of preparations described in General Rules for Preparations.

1. Procedure

The test is performed employing No. 18 (850 μm) and No. 30 (500 μm) sieves with the inside diameter of 75 mm.

Weigh accurately 10.0 g of sample to be tested, and place on the uppermost sieve which is placed on the other sieves described above and a close-fitting receiving pan and is covered with a lid. Shake the sieves in a horizontal direction for 3 minutes, and tap slightly at intervals. Weigh the amount remaining on each sieve and in the receiving pan.

6.04 Test for Acid-neutralizing Capacity of Gastrointestinal Medicines

Test for Acid-neutralizing Capacity of Gastrointestinal Medicines is a test to determine the acid-neutralizing capacity of a medicine, as a crude material or preparation, which reacts with the stomach acid and exercises an acid control action in the stomach. When performing the test according to the following procedure, the acid-neutralizing capacity of a crude material is expressed in terms of the amount (mL) of 0.1 mol/L hydrochloric acid VS consumed per g of the material, and that of a preparation is expressed by the amount (mL) of 0.1 mol/L hydrochloric acid VS consumed per dose per day (when the daily dose varies, the minimum dose is used).

1. Preparation of sample

A crude material and a solid preparation which conforms to Powders in the General Rules for Preparations: may be used, without any treatment, as the sample. Preparations in dose-unit packages: weigh accurately the content of not less than 20 packages, calculate the average mass of the content for a daily dose, mix uniformly, and use the mixture as the sample. Granules in dose-unit packages and other solid preparations which do not conform to Powders in the General Rules for Preparations: weigh accurately the content of not less than 20 packages, calculate the average mass of the content for a daily dose, powder it, and use as the sample. Granules not in dose-unit packages and other solid preparations which do not conform to Powders in the General Rules for Preparations: take not less than 20 doses, powder it, and use as the sample. Capsules and tablets: take not less than 20 doses, weigh accurately, calculate the average mass for a daily dose, powder it, and use as the sample. Liquid preparations: shake well, and use as the sample.

2. Procedure

Take an amount of the sample so that 'a' in the equation falls between 20 mL and 30 mL, and perform the test.

Accurately weigh the sample of the crude material or preparation, and place it in a glass-stoppered 200-mL flask. Add exactly 100 mL of 0.1 mol/L hydrochloric acid VS, stopper tightly, shake at 37 ± 2°C for 1 hour, and filter. Take precaution against gas to be generated on the addition of 0.1 mol/L hydrochloric acid VS, and stopper tightly. After cooling, filter the solution again, if necessary. Pipet 50 mL of the filtrate, and titrate *<2.50>* the excess hydrochloric acid with 0.1 mol/L sodium hydroxide VS (pH Determination *<2.54>*, end point: pH 3.5). Perform a blank determination in the same manner.

For liquid preparations, pipet the sample in a 100-mL volumetric flask, add water to make 45 mL, then add exactly 50 mL of 0.2 mol/L hydrochloric acid VS while shaking. Add water again to make the solution 100 mL. Transfer the solution to a glass-stoppered 200-mL flask, wash the residue with 20.0 mL of water, stopper tightly, shake at 37 ± 2°C for 1 hour, and filter. Pipet 60 mL of the filtrate, and titrate *<2.50>* the excess hydrochloric acid with 0.1 mol/L sodium hydroxide VS (pH Determination *<2.54>*, end point: pH 3.5). Perform a blank determination in the same manner.

Acid-neutralizing capacity (amount of 0.1 mol/L hydrochloric acid VS consumed per g or daily dose) (mL)

$$= (b - a) \times 2 \times (t/s)$$

a: Amount (mL) of 0.1 mol/L sodium hydroxide VS consumed

b: Amount (mL) of 0.1 mol/L sodium hydroxide VS consumed in the blank determination

t: 1000 mg of crude material, or daily dose of preparation (in mg of solid preparation, mL of liquid preparation)

s: Amount of the sample taken (in mg of crude material and solid preparation, mL of liquid preparation)

6.05 Test for Extractable Volume of Parenteral Preparations

This test is harmonized with the European Pharmacopoeia and the U.S. Pharmacopeia.

The parts of the text that are not harmonized are marked with symbols (◆ ◆).

Information on the harmonization with the European Pharmacopoeia and the U.S. Pharmacopeia is available on the website of the Pharmaceuticals and Medical Devices Agency.

◆Test for Extractable Volume of Parenteral Preparations is performed to confirm that a slightly excess volume is filled for the nominal volume to be withdrawn. Injections may be supplied in single-dose containers such as ampoules or plastic bags, or in multi-dose containers filled with a volume of injection which is sufficient to permit administration of the nominal volume declared on the label. The excess volume is determined by the characteristics of the product.◆

Suspensions and emulsions must be shaken before withdrawal of the contents and before the determination of the density. Oily and viscous preparations may be warmed according to the instructions on the label, if necessary, and thoroughly shaken immediately before removing the contents. The contents are then cooled to 20 – 25°C before measuring the volume.

1. Single-dose containers

Select one container if the volume is 10 mL or more, 3 containers if the nominal volume is more than 3 mL and less than 10 mL, or 5 containers if the nominal volume is 3 mL or less. Take up individually the total contents of each container selected into a dry syringe of a capacity not exceeding three times the volume to be measured, and fitted with a 21-gage needle not less than 2.5 cm in length. Expel any air bubbles from the syringe and needle, then discharge the contents of the syringe without emptying the needle into a standardised dry cylinder (graduated to contain rather than to deliver the designated volumes) of such size that the volume to be measured occupies at least 40% of its graduated volume. Alternatively, the volume of the contents in milliliters may be calculated as the mass in grams divided by the density.

For containers with a nominal volume of 2 mL or less the contents of a sufficient number of containers may be pooled to obtain the volume required for the measurement provided that a separate, dry syringe assembly is used for each container. The contents of containers holding 10 mL or more may be determined by opening them and emptying the contents directly into the graduated cylinder or tared beaker.

The volume is not less than the nominal volume in case of containers examined individually, or, in case of containers with a nominal volume of 2 mL or less, is not less than the sum of the nominal volumes of the containers taken collectively.

2. Multi-dose containers

For injections in multidose containers labeled to yield a specific number of doses of a stated volume, select one container and proceed as directed for single-dose containers using the same number of separate syringe assemblies as the number of doses specified. The volume is such that each syringe delivers not less than the stated dose.

3. Cartridges and pre-filled syringes

Select one container if the volume is 10 mL or more, 3 containers if the nominal volume is more than 3 mL and less than 10 mL, or 5 containers if the nominal volume is 3 mL or less. If necessary, fit the containers with the accessories required for their use (needle, piston, syringe) and transfer the entire contents of each container without emptying the needle into a dry tared beaker by slowly and constantly depressing the piston. Determine the volume in milliliters calculated as the mass in grams divided by the density.

The volume measured for each of the containers is not less than the nominal volume.

4. Parenteral infusions

Select one container. Transfer the contents into a dry measuring cylinder of such a capacity that the volume to be determined occupies at least 40% of the nominal volume of the cylinder. Measure the volume transferred.

The volume is not less than the nominal volume.

6.06 Foreign Insoluble Matter Test for Injections

Foreign Insoluble Matter Test for Injections is a test method to examine foreign insoluble matters in injections.

1. Method 1.

This method is applied to either injections in solution, suspension or emulsion, and vehicles for solid injections to be dissolved or suspended before use.

Clean the exterior of containers, and inspect against both a white and a black background for 5 seconds each time with the unaided eyes at a position of light intensity of 2000 to 3750 lx under a white light source: Injections or vehicles must be free from readily detectable foreign insoluble matters. As to Injections in plastic containers for aqueous injections, the inspection should be performed with the unaided eyes at a position of light intensity of approximately 8000 to 10,000 lx, with a white light source at appropriate distances above and below the container. The inspection time should be extended accordingly if the inspection is not easy.

2. Method 2.

This method is applied to solid injections to be dissolved or suspended before use.

Clean the exterior of containers, and dissolve or suspend the contents with vehicles attached to the preparations or with Water for Injection carefully, avoiding any contamination with extraneous foreign substances. The solution thus constituted must be free from foreign insoluble matters that is clearly detectable when inspected against both a white and a black background for 5 seconds each time with the unaided eyes at a position of light intensity of 2000 to 3750 lx under a white light source. The inspection time should be extended accordingly if the inspection is not easy.

6.07 Insoluble Particulate Matter Test for Injections

This test is harmonized with the European Pharmacopoeia and the U.S. Pharmacopeia.

The parts of the text that are not harmonized are marked with symbols (◆ ◆).

Information on the harmonization with the European Pharmacopoeia and the U.S. Pharmacopeia is available on the website of the Pharmaceuticals and Medical Devices Agency.

Insoluble particulate matters in injections and parenteral infusions consist of extraneous, mobile undissolved particles, other than gas bubbles, that are unintentionally present in the solutions.

For the determination of particulate contamination, 2 procedures, Method 1 (Light Obscuration Particle Count Test) and Method 2 (Microscopic Particle Count Test), are specified hereinafter. When examining injections and parenteral infusions for sub-visible particles, Method 1 is preferably applied. However, it may be necessary to test some preparations by Method 1 followed by Method 2 to reach a conclusion on conformance to the requirements.

Not all parenteral preparations can be examined for sub-visible particles by one or both of these methods. When Method 1 is not applicable, e.g. in case of preparations having reduced clarity or increased viscosity, the test should be carried out according to Method 2. Emulsions, colloids, and liposomal preparations are examples. Similarly, products that produce air or gas bubbles when drawn into the sensor may also require microscopic particle count testing. If the viscosity of the preparation to be tested is sufficiently high so as to preclude its examination by either test method, a quantitative dilution with an appropriate diluent may be made to decrease viscosity, as necessary, to allow the analysis to be performed.

The results obtained in examining a discrete unit or group of units for particulate contamination cannot be extrapolated with certainty to other units that remain untested. Thus, statistically sound sampling plans must be developed if valid inferences are to be drawn from observed data to characterise the level of particulate contamination in a large group of units.

1. Method 1. Light Obscuration Particle Count Test

1.1. Apparatus

Use a suitable apparatus based on the principle of light blockage which allows an automatic determination of the size of particles and the number of particles according to size. ◆It is necessary to perform calibration, as well as to demonstrate the sample volume accuracy, sample flow rate, particle size response curve, sensor resolution, and counting accuracy, at least once a year.◆

◆1.1.1. Calibration

Particles to be used for calibration should be subject to particle size sensitivity measurement, using spherical polystyrene particles having at least 5, 10 and 25 μm in diameter (PSL particles) in mono-dispersed suspension. The PSL particles should have either a domestic or international traceability in terms of length, with a level of uncertainly at not greater than 3%. The particles to be used for calibration should be dispersed in *particle-free water*.

1.1.1.1. Manual method

The particle size response of the system to be applied should be determined using at least 3 channels for threshold-voltage setting, according to the half counting method of window moving type. The threshold-voltage window should be ±20% of the measuring particle size. After measuring the sensitivity of response for the designated particle size, the size response curve is prepared by the method indicated by the manufacturer from particle-response measuring point, and threshold-voltage of 5, 10 and 25 μm of the apparatus is obtained.

1.1.1.2. Electronic method

In the use of multichannel peak height analyzer, the particle size response is measured by half-count method of moving window system same as the manual method, and the particle size response curve is prepared by the method designated by the instrument manufacturer, then, the threshold-voltage of 5, 10 and 25 μm of the apparatus is obtained. In this case, the instrument manufacturer or the user should validate the obtainability of the same result as that of the manual method.

1.1.1.3. Automated method

The particle size response curve of the apparatus may be obtained by using the software developed by the user or supplied by the instrument manufacturer, whereas the manufacturer or the user should validate the obtainability of the same result as that of the manual method.

1.1.2. Sample volume accuracy

Sample volume accuracy should fall within 5% of the measuring value in case the decrease of test solution is measured by the mass method after measuring the test solution of 10 mL.

1.1.3. Sample flow rate

The flow rate of the sample indicated into the sensor should be calculated from the observed sample volume and time, and should be conformed within the range of the manufacturer's specification for sensor used.

1.1.4. Sensor

There is a possibility of changes of particle size resolution and counting rate of particle-detecting sensor in each sensor by assembling accuracy and parts accuracy even in the same type sensor. The threshold accuracy also needs to be confirmed. Testing should accordingly be performed for each of particle size resolution, accuracy in counting and in threshold setting, using Particle Count Reference Standard Suspension (PSL spheres having mean diameter of approximately 10 μm, of a concentration at 1000 particles/mL ±10%, not more than 5% of CV value).

During measurement, stirring should be made for assuring the uniformity in sample concentration.

1.1.4.1. Sensor resolution (Particle size resolution of apparatus)

Measurement should be made by either one of the following methods. The difference between the threshold of particle size counting 16% and 84% of the total counts and the test-particle size should be within 10%, whereas, electronic method and automated method should be both validated for obtaining the same result as that of the manual method.

(i) Manual method to obtain the spread of histogram prepared from the counting value of the apparatus.

(ii) Electronic method to obtain the spread of histogram of the classification of system-responding signal by using the multichannel peak height analyzer.

(iii) Automated method to obtain the spread of histogram of responsive signal of the test-particle by using the software prepared by the manufacturer or the user.

1.1.4.2. Particle counting accuracy

Data obtained by counting particles of 5 μm and greater should be 763 to 1155 particles per mL.

1.1.4.3. Threshold accuracy

Particle size calculated from a threshold corresponding to 50% counts for particles of 5 μm and greater should fall within ±5% of the mean diameter of the test particles.◆

1.2. General precautions

The test is carried out under conditions limiting particulate contamination, preferably in a laminar-flow cabinet.

Very carefully wash the glassware and filtration equipment used, except for the membrane filters, with a warm detergent solution and rinse with abundant amounts of water to remove all traces of detergent. Immediately before use, rinse the equipment from top to bottom, outside and then inside, with *particle-free water*.

Take care not to introduce air bubbles into the preparation to be examined, especially when fractions of the preparation are being transferred to the container in which the determination is to be carried out.

In order to check that the environment is suitable for the test, that the glassware is properly cleaned and that the water to be used is particle-free, the following test is carried out: determine the particulate contamination of 5 samples of *particle-free water*, each of 5 mL, according to the method described below. If the number of particles of 10 μm or greater size exceeds 25 for the combined 25 mL, the precautions taken for the test are not sufficient. The preparatory steps must be repeated until the environment, glassware and water are suitable for the test.

1.3. Method

Mix the contents of the sample by slowly inverting the container 20 times successively. If necessary, cautiously remove the sealing closure. Clean the outer surfaces of the container opening using a jet of *particle-free water* and remove the closure, avoiding any contamination of the contents. Eliminate gas bubbles by appropriate measures such as allowing to stand for 2 minutes or sonicating.

For large-volume parenterals or for small-volume parenterals having a volume of 25 mL or more, single units are tested. For small-volume parenterals less than 25 mL in volume, the contents of 10 or more units are combined in a cleaned container to obtain a volume of not less than 25 mL; where justified and authorised, the test solution may be prepared by mixing the contents of a suitable number of vials and diluting to 25 mL with *particle-free water* or with an appropriate solvent without contamination of particles when *particle-free water* is not suitable.

Powders for parenteral use are reconstituted with *particle-free water* or with an appropriate solvent without contamination of particles when *particle-free water* is not suitable.

The number of test specimens must be adequate to provide a statistically sound assessment. For large-volume parenterals or for small-volume parenterals having a volume of 25 mL or more, fewer than 10 units may be tested, based on an appropriate sampling plan.

Remove 4 portions, each of not less than 5 mL, and count the number of particles equal to or greater than 10 μm and 25 μm. Disregard the result obtained for the first portion, and calculate the mean number of particles for the preparation to be examined.

1.4. Evaluation

If the average number of particles exceeds the limits, test the preparation by Method 2 (Microscopic Particle Count

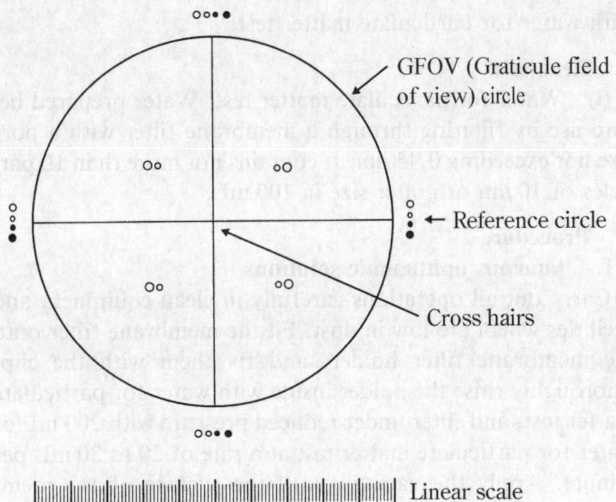

Fig. 6.07-1 Circular diameter graticule

Test).

Test 1.A—Solutions for injection supplied in containers with a nominal content of ◆equal to or◆ more than 100 mL

The preparation complies with the test if the average number of particles present in the units tested does not exceed 25 per milliliter equal to or greater than 10 μm and does not exceed 3 per milliliter equal to or greater than 25 μm.

Test 1.B—Solutions for injection supplied in containers with a nominal content of less than 100 mL

The preparation complies with the test if the average number of particles present in the units tested does not exceed 6000 per container equal to or greater than 10 μm and does not exceed 600 per container equal to or greater than 25 μm.

2. Method 2. Microscopic Particle Count Test

2.1. Apparatus

Use a suitable binocular microscope, filter assembly for retaining particulate contamination and membrane filter for examination.

The microscope is equipped with an ocular micrometer calibrated with an objective micrometer, a mechanical stage capable of holding and traversing the entire filtration area of the membrane filter, two suitable illuminators to provide episcopic illumination in addition to oblique illumination, and is adjusted to 100 ± 10 magnifications. The ocular micrometer is a circular diameter graticule (see Fig. 6.07-1) and consists of a large circle divided by crosshairs into quadrants, transparent and black reference circles 10 μm and 25 μm in diameter at 100 magnifications, and a linear scale graduated in 10 μm increments. It is calibrated using a stage micrometer that is certified by either a domestic or international standard institution. A relative error of the linear scale of the graticule within ± 2% is acceptable. The large circle is designated the graticule field of view (GFOV).

Two illuminators are required. One is an episcopic brightfield illuminator internal to the microscope, the other is an external, focussable auxiliary illuminator adjustable to give reflected oblique illumination at an angle of 10° to 20°.

The filter assembly for retaining particulate contamination consists of a filter holder made of glass or other suitable material, and is equipped with a vacuum source and a suitable membrane filter.

The membrane filter is of suitable size, black or dark gray in color, non-gridded or gridded, and 1.0 μm or finer in nominal pore size.

2.2. General precautions

The test is carried out under conditions limiting particulate contamination, preferably in a laminar-flow cabinet.

Very carefully wash the glassware and filter assembly used, except for the membrane filter, with a warm detergent solution and rinse with abundant amounts of water to remove all traces of detergent. Immediately before use, rinse both sides of the membrane filter and the equipment from top to bottom, outside and then inside, with *particle-free water*.

In order to check that the environment is suitable for the test, that the glassware and the membrane filter are properly cleaned and that the water to be used is particle-free, the following test is carried out: determine the particulate contamination of a 50 mL volume of *particle-free water* according to the method described below. If more than 20 particles 10 μm or larger in size or if more than 5 particles 25 μm or larger in size are present within the filtration area, the precautions taken for the test are not sufficient. The preparatory steps must be repeated until the environment, glassware, membrane filter and water are suitable for the test.

2.3. Method

Mix the contents of the samples by slowly inverting the container 20 times successively. If necessary, cautiously remove the sealing closure. Clean the outer surfaces of the container opening using a jet of *particle-free water* and remove the closure, avoiding any contamination of the contents.

For large-volume parenterals, single units are tested. For small-volume parenterals less than 25 mL in volume, the contents of 10 or more units is combined in a cleaned container; where justified and authorised, the test solution may be prepared by mixing the contents of a suitable number of vials and diluting to 25 mL with *particle-free water* or with an appropriate solvent without contamination of particles when *particle-free water* is not suitable. Small-volume parenterals having a volume of 25 mL or more may be tested individually.

Powders for parenteral use are constituted with *particle-free water* or with an appropriate solvent without contamination of particles when *particle-free water* is not suitable.

The number of test specimens must be adequate to provide a statistically sound assessment. For large-volume parenterals or for small-volume parenterals having a volume of 25 mL or more, fewer than 10 units may be tested, based on an appropriate sampling plan.

Wet the inside of the filter holder fitted with the membrane filter with several milliliter of *particle-free water*. Transfer to the filtration funnel the total volume of a solution pool or of a single unit, and apply vacuum. If needed add stepwise a portion of the solution until the entire volume is filtered. After the last addition of solution, begin rinsing the inner walls of the filter holder by using a jet of *particle-free water*. Maintain the vacuum until the surface of the membrane filter is free from liquid. Place the filter in a petri dish and allow the filter to air-dry with the cover slightly ajar. After the filter has been dried, place the petri dish on the stage of the microscope, scan the entire membrane filter under the reflected light from the illuminating device, and count the number of particles that are equal to or greater than 10 μm and the number of particles that are equal to or greater than 25 μm. Alternatively, partial filter count and determination of the total filter count by calculation is allowed. Calculate the mean number of particles for the preparation to be examined.

The particle sizing process with the use of the circular diameter graticule is carried out by transforming mentally the image of each particle into a circle and then comparing it to the 10 μm and 25 μm graticule reference circles. Thereby the particles are not moved from their initial locations within the graticule field of view and are not superimposed on the reference circles for comparison. The inner diameter of the transparent graticule reference circles is used to size white and transparent particles, while dark particles are sized by using the outer diameter of the black opaque graticule reference circles.

In performing the microscopic particle count test (Method 2) do not attempt to size or enumerate amorphous, semi-liquid, or otherwise morphologically indistinct materials that have the appearance of a stain or discoloration on the membrane filter. These materials show little or no surface relief and present a gelatinous or film-like appearance. In such cases the interpretation of enumeration may be aided by testing a sample of the solution by Method 1.

2.4. Evaluation

Test 2.A—Solutions for injection supplied in containers with a nominal content of ◆equal to or◆ more than 100 mL
The preparation complies with the test if the average number of particles present in the units tested does not exceed 12 per milliliter equal to or greater than 10 μm and does not exceed 2 per milliliter equal to or greater than 25 μm.

Test 2.B—Solutions for injection supplied in containers with a nominal content of less than 100 mL
The preparation complies with the test if the average number of particles present in the units tested does not exceed 3000 per container equal to or greater than 10 μm and does not exceed 300 per container equal to or greater than 25 μm.

◆3. Reagents

Particle-free water: The filtered water through a membrane filter with a pore size not exceeding 0.45 μm, containing not more than 5 particles of 10 μm or greater size, and not more than 2 particles of 25 μm or greater size in 10 mL of the insoluble particle number measured by the light obscuration particle counter.◆

6.08 Insoluble Particulate Matter Test for Ophthalmic Solutions

Insoluble Particulate Matter Test for Ophthalmic Solutions is to examine for the size and the number of insoluble particulate matter in Ophthalmic Solutions.

1. Apparatus

Use a microscope, filter assembly for retaining insoluble particulate matter and membrane filter for determination.

(i) Microscope: The microscope is equipped with an ocular micrometer calibrated with an objective micrometer, a mobile stage and an illuminator, and is adjusted to 100 magnifications.

(ii) Filter assembly for retaining insoluble particulate matter: The filter assembly for retaining insoluble particulate matter consists of a filter holder made of glass or a proper material uncapable of causing any trouble in testing, and a clip. The unit is capable of fitting with a membrane filter 25 mm or 13 mm in diameter and can be used under reduced pressure.

(iii) Membrane filter for testing: The membrane filter is white in color, 25 mm or 13 mm in diameter, not more than 10 μm in nominal pore size and is imprinted with about 3 mm grid marks. Upon preliminary testing, the insoluble particulate matter equal to or greater than 25 μm in size should not be found on the filter. When necessary, wash the filter with water for particulate matter test.

2. Reagents

(i) Water for particulate matter test: Water prepared before use by filtering through a membrane filter with a pore size not exceeding 0.45 μm. It contains not more than 10 particles of 10 μm or grater size in 100 mL.

3. Procedure

3.1. Aqueous ophthalmic solutions

Carry out all operations carefully in clean equipment and facilities which are low in dust. Fit the membrane filter onto the membrane filter holder, and fix them with the clip. Thoroughly rinse the holder inside with water for particulate matter test, and filter under reduced pressure with 200 mL of water for particulate matter test at a rate of 20 to 30 mL per minute. Apply the vacuum until the surface of the membrane filter is free from water, and remove the membrane filter. Place the filter in a flat-bottomed petri dish with the cover slightly ajar, and dry the filter fully at a temperature not exceeding 50°C. After the filter has been dried, place the petri dish on the stage of the microscope. Under a down-light from an illuminating device, adjust the grid of the membrane filter to the coordinate axes of the microscope, adjust the microscope so as to get the best view of the insoluble particulate matter, then count the number of particles that are equal to or greater than 150 μm within the effective filtering area of the filter, moving the mobile stage, and ascertain that the number is not more than 1. In this case the particle is sized on the longest axis.

Fit another membrane filter to the filtration device, and fix them with the clip, then wet the inside of the filter holder with several mL of water for particulate matter test. Clean the outer surface of the container, and mix the sample solution gently by inverting the container several times. Remove the cap, clean the outer surface of the nozzle, and pour the sample solution into a measuring cylinder which has been rinsed well with water for particulate matter test. Repeat the process to prepare 25 mL of the test solution. Pour the test solution into the filter holder along the inner wall of the holder. Apply the vacuum and filter mildly so as to keep the solution always on the filter. As for viscous sample solution, dilute suitably with water for particulate matter test or suitable diluent and then filter as described above. When the amount of the solution on the filter becomes small, add 30 mL of water for particulate matter test or suitable diluent in such manner as to wash the inner wall of the filter holder. Repeat the process 3 times with 30 mL of the water for particulate matter test. Apply the vacuum gently until the surface of the membrane filter is free from water. Place the filter in a petri dish, and dry the filter at a temperature below 50°C with the cover slightly ajar. After the filter has been dried, place the petri dish on the stage of the microscope, and count the number of particles which are equal to or larger than 300 μm within the effective filtering area of the filter according to the same procedure of the microscope as described above. In this case the particle is sized on the longest axis.

3.2. Ophthalmic solutions which are dissolved before use

Proceed as directed in Aqueous Ophthalmic Solutions after dissolving the sample with the constituted solution.

3.3. Suspension type ophthalmic solutions

Proceed as directed in Aqueous Ophthalmic Solutions. Take 25 mL of the sample in a vessel, which has been rinsed well with water for particulate matter test, add a suitable amount of a suspension-solubilizing solvent or an adequate solvent, shake to dissolve the suspending particles, and use this solution as the sample solution.

Use a membrane filter which is not affected by the solvent to be used.

3.4. Ophthalmic solutions contained in a single-dose container

Proceed as directed in Aqueous Ophthalmic Solutions, using 10 samples for the test. A 13-mm diameter membrane filter and a 4-mm diameter filter holder for retaining insoluble particulate matter are used.

4. Evaluation

The preparation complies with the test if the calculated number per mL of insoluble particles of a size equal to or greater than 300 μm is not more than 1.

6.09 Disintegration Test

This test is harmonized with the European Pharmacopoeia and the U.S. Pharmacopeia.

The parts of the text that are not harmonized are marked with symbols (◆ ◆).

Information on the harmonization with the European Pharmacopoeia and the U.S. Pharmacopeia is available on the website of the Pharmaceuticals and Medical Devices Agency.

Disintegration Test is provided to determine whether tablets, capsules, ◆granules, dry syrups or pills◆ disintegrate within the prescribed time when placed in a liquid medium at the experimental conditions presented below.

For the purposes of this test, disintegration does not imply complete solution of the unit or even of its active constituent.

1. Apparatus

The apparatus consists of a basket-rack assembly, a 1000-mL, low-form beaker, 138 to 160 mm in height and having an inside diameter of 97 to 115 mm for the immersion fluid, a thermostatic arrangement for heating the fluid between 35° and 39°, and a device for raising and lowering the basket in the immersion fluid at a constant frequency rate between 29 and 32 cycles per minute through a distance of not less than 53 mm and not more than 57 mm. The volume of the fluid in the vessel is such that at the highest point of the upward stroke the wire mesh remains at least 15 mm below the surface of the fluid and descends to not less than 25 mm from the bottom of the vessel on the downward stroke. At no time should the top of the basket-rack assembly become submerged. The time required for the upward stroke is equal to the time required for the downward stroke, and the change in stroke direction is a smooth transition, rather than an abrupt reversal of motion. The basket-rack assembly moves vertically along its axis. There is no appreciable horizontal motion or movement of the axis from the vertical.

(i) Basket-rack assembly: The basket-rack assembly consists of six open-ended transparent tubes, each 77.5 ± 2.5 mm long and having an inside diameter of 20.7 to 23 mm and a wall 1.0 to 2.8 mm thick; the tubes are held in a vertical position by two plates, each 88 to 92 mm in diameter and 5 to 8.5 mm in thickness, with six holes, each 22 to 26 mm in diameter, equidistant from the center of the plate and equally spaced from one another. Attached to the under surface of the lower plate is a woven stainless steel wire cloth, which has a plain square weave with 1.8- to 2.2-mm apertures and with a wire diameter of 0.57 to 0.66 mm. The parts of the apparatus are assembled and rigidly held by means of three bolts passing through the two plates. A suitable means is provided to suspend the basket-rack assembly from the raising and lowering device using a point on its axis. The basket-rack assembly conforms to the dimensions found in Fig. 6.09-1. The design of the basket-rack assembly may be varied somewhat provided the specifications for the glass tubes and the screen mesh size are maintained: ◆for example, in order to secure the glass tubes and the upper and the lower plastic plates in position at the top or the bottom, an acid-resistant metal plate, 88 – 92 mm in diameter and 0.5 – 1 mm in thickness, having 6 perforations, each about 22 to 26 mm in diameter, may be used which coincide with those of the upper plastic plate and upper open ends of the glass tubes.◆

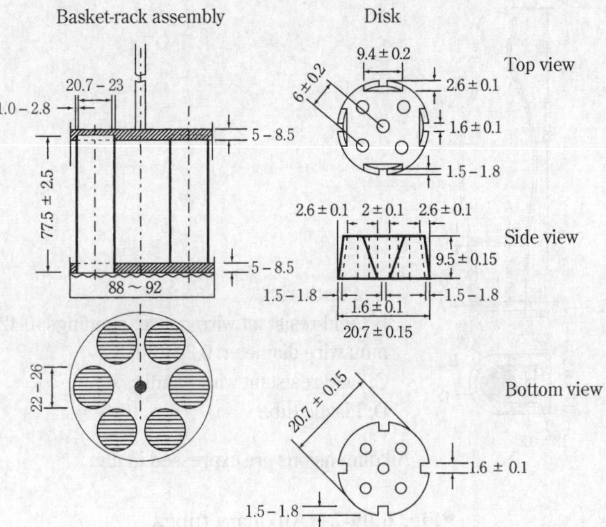

Fig. 6.09-1 Disintegration apparatus

(ii) Disks: The use of disks is permitted only where specified or allowed. Each tube is provided with a cylindrical disk 9.5 ± 0.15 mm thick and 20.7 ± 0.15 mm in diameter. The disk is made of a suitable, transparent plastic material having a specific gravity of between 1.18 and 1.20. Five parallel 2 ± 0.1 mm holes extend between the ends of the cylinder. One of the holes is centered on the cylindrical axis. The other holes are centered 6 ± 0.2 mm from the axis on imaginary lines perpendicular to the axis and parallel to each other. Four identical trapezoidal-shaped planes are cut into the wall of the cylinder, nearly perpendicular to the ends of the cylinder. The trapezoidal shape is symmetrical; its parallel sides coincide with the ends of the cylinder and are parallel to an imaginary line connecting the centers of two adjacent holes 6 mm from the cylindrical axis. The parallel side of the trapezoid on the bottom of the cylinder has a length of 1.6 ± 0.1 mm, and its bottom edges lie at a depth of 1.5 – 1.8 mm from the cylinder's circumference. The parallel side of the trapezoid on the top of the cylinder has a length of 9.4 ± 0.2 mm, and its center lies at a depth of 2.6 ± 0.1 mm from the cylinder's circumference. All surfaces of the disk are smooth. If the use of disks is specified, add a disk to each tube, and operate the apparatus as directed under Procedure. The disks conform to dimensions found in Fig. 6.09-1. The use of automatic detection employing modified disks is permitted where the use of disks is specified or allowed. Such disks must comply with the requirements for density and dimension given in this chapter.

◆(iii) Auxiliary tube: The auxiliary tube, as illustrated in Fig. 6.09-2, consists of a plastic tube D, 12 ± 0.2 mm in in-

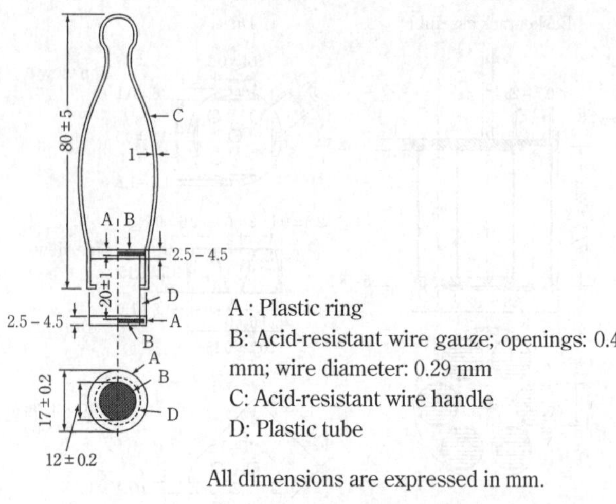

◆**Fig. 6.09-2** Auxiliary tube◆

side diameter, 17 ± 0.2 mm in outside diameter, 20 ± 1 mm in length, having both outside ends screw-cut, and two plastic rings A, each 12 ± 0.2 mm in inside diameter, 17 ± 0.2 mm in outside diameter, 2.5 - 4.5 mm in length, having one inside end screw-cut. Acid-resistant woven wire gauze having 0.42-mm openings and 0.29-mm wire diameter is placed in each plastic ring and the rings are attached by screws to each end of the plastic tube. The distance between two wire gauzes is 20 ± 1 mm. A handle of an acid-resistant wire, 1 mm in diameter and 80 ± 5 mm in length, is attached to the mid portion of the plastic tube. The auxiliary tube is used for the test of granules and capsules containing enteric coated granules.◆

2. Procedure

2.1. Immediate-release preparations

In case of tablets, capsules ◆and pills (except for pills containing crude drugs),◆ place 1 dosage unit in each of the six tubes of the basket, and if prescribed add a disk. ◆Unless otherwise specified, operate the apparatus, using water as the immersion fluid,◆ maintained at 37 ± 2°C as the immersion fluid. ◆Unless otherwise specified, carry out the test for 20 minutes for capsules, 30 minutes for plain tablets, and 60 minutes for coated tablets and pills.◆ Lift the basket from the fluid, and observe the dosage units. ◆Complete disintegration is defined as that state in which any residue of the unit, except fragments of insoluble coating or capsule shell, remaining on the screen of the test apparatus or adhering to the lower surface of the disks, if used, is a soft mass having no palpably firm core.◆ The test is met if all of the dosage units have disintegrated completely. If 1 or 2 dosage units fail to disintegrate, repeat the test on 12 additional dosage units. The test is met if not less than 16 of the total of 18 dosage units tested are disintegrated.

◆For pills containing crude drugs, carry out the test for 60 minutes in the same manner, using 1st fluid for disintegration test as the immersion fluid. When any residue of the unit is observed, carry out the test successively for 60 minutes, using 2nd fluid for disintegration test.◆

◆In case of granules and dry syrups, shake preparations on a No. 30 (500 μm) sieve as directed in Particle Size Distribution Test for Preparations <*6.03*>, transfer 0.10 g of the residue on the sieve to each of the 6 auxiliary tubes, secure the 6 tubes to the bottom of the basket tightly, and operate the apparatus, using water as the immersion fluid, maintained at 37 ± 2°C as the immesion fluid, unless otherwise specified. Observe the samples after 30 minutes of operation for plain granules and after 60 minutes for coated granules, unless otherwise specified. Complete disintegration is defined as that state in which any residue of the granules, except fragments of insoluble coating in the auxiliary tube, is a soft mass having no palpably firm core. The test is met if all of 6 samples in the auxiliary tubes have disintegrated completely. If 1 or 2 samples fail to disintegrate, repeat the test on 12 additional samples. The test is met if not less than 16 of the total of 18 samples tested are disintegrated.◆

◆**2.2. Enteric coated preparations**

Unless otherwise specified, perform the following two tests, (a) the test with 1st fluid for disintegration test and (b) the test with the 2nd fluid for disintegration test, separately.

2.2.1. Enteric coated tablets and capsules

(i) The test with 1st fluid for disintegration test: Carry out the test for 120 minutes, using 1st fluid for disintegration test according to the procedure described in immediate release preparations. Disintegration is defined as that state in which the tablet or capsule is broken or the enteric coating film is ruptured or broken. The test is met if none of six dosage units is disintegrated. If 1 or 2 dosage units are disintegrated, repeat the test on additional 12 dosage units. The test is met if not less than 16 of the total of 18 dosage units tested are not disintegrated.

(ii) The test with 2nd fluid for disintegration test: According to the procedure described in immediate-release preparations, carry out the test with new dosage units for 60 minutes, using 2nd fluid for disintegration test and determine if the test is met or not.

2.2.2. Enteric coated granules and capsules containing the enteric coated granules

Shake granules or contents taken out from capsules on a No. 30 (500 μm) sieve as directed in Particle Size Distribution Test for Preparations <*6.03*>, transfer 0.10 g of the residue on the sieve to each of the 6 auxiliary tubes, secure the 6 tubes to the bottom of the basket tightly, and operate the apparatus, using the 1st and 2nd fluids for disintegration test.

(i) The test with 1st fluid for disintegration test: According to the procedure described in immediate-release preparations, carry out the test for 60 minutes, using 1st fluid for disintegration test. The test is met if particles fallen from the openings of the wire gauze number not more than 15.

(ii) The test with 2nd fluid for disintegration test: According to the procedure described in immediate-release preparations, carry out the test with new samples for 30 minutes, using 2nd fluid for disintegration test and determine if test is met or not.◆

6.10 Dissolution Test

This test is harmonized with the European Pharmacopoeia and the U.S. Pharmacopeia.

The parts of the text that are not harmonized are marked with symbols (◆ ◆).

Information on the harmonization with the European Pharmacopoeia and the U.S. Pharmacopeia is available on the website of the Pharmaceuticals and Medical Devices Agency.

Dissolution Test is provided to determine compliance with the dissolution requirements for dosage forms administered orally. ◆This test also aims at preventing significant bioinequivalence.◆ In this test, a dosage unit is defined as 1 tablet or 1 capsule or the amount specified equivalent to minimum dose.

1. Apparatus

1.1. Apparatus for Basket Method (Apparatus 1)

The assembly consists of the following: a vessel, which may be covered, made of glass or other inert, transparent material*[1]; a motor; a drive shaft; and a cylindrical basket. The vessel is partially immersed in a suitable water bath of any convenient size or heated by a suitable device such as a heating jacket. The water bath or heating device permits holding the temperature inside the vessel at 37 ± 0.5°C during the test and keeping the bath fluid in constant, smooth motion. No part of the assembly, including the environment in which the assembly is placed, contributes significant motion, agitation, or vibration beyond that due to the smoothly rotating stirring element. Make the apparatus to permit observation of the specimen and stirring element during the test. The vessel is cylindrical, with a hemispherical bottom and a capacity of 1 liter. Its height is 160 mm to 210 mm and its inside diameter is 98 mm to 106 mm. Its sides are flanged at the top. Use a fitted cover to retard evaporation.*[2] The shaft is positioned so that its axis is not more than 2 mm at any point from the vertical axis of the vessel and rotates smoothly and without significant wobble that could affect the results. Adjust a speed-regulating device to maintain the shaft rotation speed at a specified rate, within ± 4%.

Shaft and basket components of the stirring element shown in Fig. 6.10-1 are fabricated of stainless steel (SUS316) or other inert material. A basket having a gold coating of about 0.0001 inch (2.5 μm) thick may be used. The dosage unit is placed in a dry basket at the beginning of each test. The distance between the inside bottom of the vessel and the bottom of the basket is maintained at 25 ± 2 mm during the test.

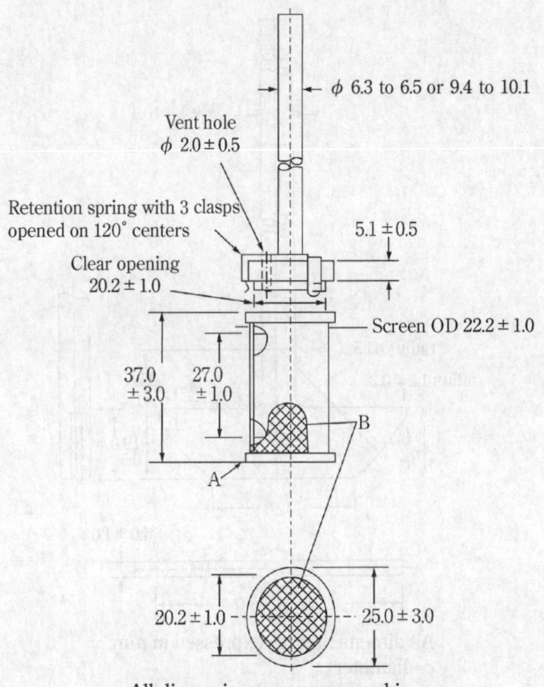

A: Note–Maximum allowable runout at "A" is ±1.0 mm when the part is rotated on center line axis with basket mounted.

B: Screen with welded seam, 0.22–0.31 mm wire diameter with wire openings of 0.36–0.44 mm [Note–After welding, the screen may be slightly altered.]

Fig. 6.10-1 Apparatus 1, Basket stirring element

1.2. Apparatus for Paddle Method (Apparatus 2)

Use the assembly from Apparatus 1, except that a paddle formed from a blade and a shaft is used as the stirring element. The shaft is positioned so that its axis is not more than 2 mm from the vertical axis of the vessel, at any point, and rotates smoothly without significant wobble that could affect the results. The vertical center line of the blade passes through the axis of the shaft so that the bottom of the blade is flush with the bottom of the shaft. The paddle conforms to the specifications shown in Fig. 6.10-2. The distance of 25 ± 2 mm between the bottom of the blade and the inside bottom of the vessel is maintained during the test. The metallic or suitably inert, rigid blade and shaft comprise a single entity. A suitable two-part detachable design may be used provided the assembly remains firmly engaged during the test. The paddle blade and shaft may be coated with a suitable coating so as to make them inert. The dosage unit is ◆usually◆ allowed to sink to the bottom of the vessel before rotation of the blade is started. A small, loose piece of nonreactive material, such as not more than a few turns of wire helix or such one shown in Fig. 6.10-2a, may be attached to the dosage unit that would otherwise float. Other validated sinker devices may also be used. ◆If the use of sinker is specified, unless otherwise specified, use the sinker device shown in Fig. 6.10-2a.◆

1.3. Apparatus for Flow-Through Cell Method (Apparatus 3)

The assembly consists of a reservoir and a pump for the dissolution medium; a flow-through cell; a water bath that maintains the dissolution medium at 37 ± 0.5°C. Use the cell size specified in the individual monograph.

The pump forces the dissolution medium upwards through the flow-through cell. The pump has a delivery range between 4 and 16 mL per minute, with standard flow rates of 4, 8, and 16 mL per minute. It must deliver a constant flow (±5% of the nominal flow rate); the flow profile should be sinusoidal with a pulsation of 120 ± 10 pulses per minute. A pump without the pulsation may also be used. Dissolution test procedure using the flow-through cell must be characterized with respect to rate and any pulsation.

The flow-through cell (see Figures 6.10-3 and 6.10-4), of transparent and inert material, is mounted vertically with a filter system (specified in the individual monograph) that prevents escape of undissolved particles from the top of the cell; standard cell diameters are 12 and 22.6 mm; the bottom cone is usually filled with small glass beads of about 1-mm diameter with one bead of about 5 mm positioned at the apex to protect the fluid entry tube; a tablet holder (see Figures 6.10-3 and 6.10-4) is available for positioning of special dosage forms. The cell is immersed in a water bath, and the temperature is maintained at 37 ± 0.5°C.

The apparatus uses a clamp mechanism of two O-rings to assemble the cell. The pump is separated from the dissolution unit in order to shield the latter against any vibrations originating from the pump. The position of the pump should not be on a level higher than the reservoir flasks. Tube connections are as short as possible. Use suitably inert tubing, such as polytef, with about 1.6-mm inner diameter and inert flanged-end connections.

2. Apparatus Suitability

The determination of suitability of a test assembly to perform dissolution testing must include conformance to the dimensions and tolerances of the apparatus as given above. In addition, critical test parameters that have to be monitored periodically during use include volume and tempera-

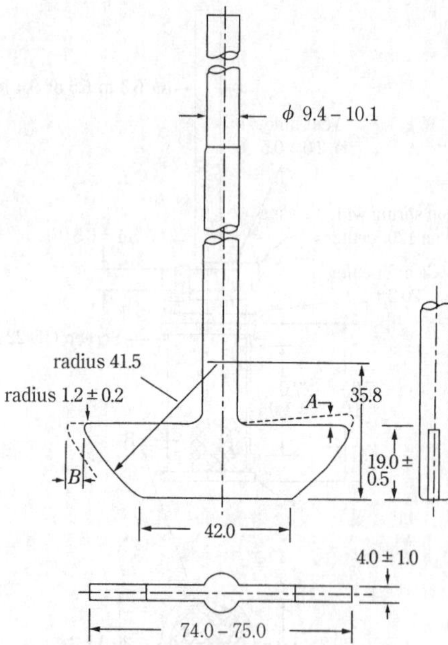

All dimensions are expressed in mm.
φ=diameter

Notes:
(1) A and B dimensions are not to vary more than 0.5 mm when part is rotated on centering axis.
(2) Tolerances are ±1.0 mm unless otherwise stated.

Fig. 6.10-2 Apparatus 2, Paddle stirring element

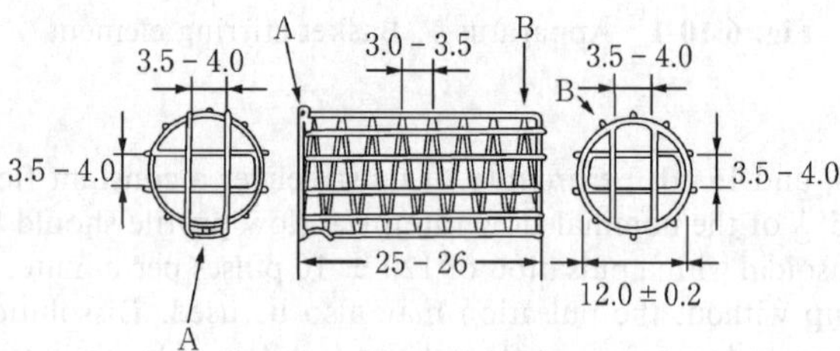

All dimensions are expressed in mm.

A: Acid-resistant wire clasp
B: Acid-resistant wire support

Fig. 6.10-2a Alternative sinker

ture of the dissolution medium, rotation speed (Basket Method and Paddle Method), and flow rate of medium (Flow-Through Cell Method).

Determine the acceptable performance of the dissolution test assembly periodically.

3. Procedure

3.1. Basket Method or Paddle Method

3.1.1. Immediate-release Dosage Forms

(i) Procedure: Place the stated volume of the dissolution medium (±1%) in the vessel of the specified apparatus, assemble the apparatus, equilibrate the dissolution medium to 37 ± 0.5°C, and remove the thermometer. Place 1 dosage unit in the apparatus, taking care to exclude air bubbles from the surface of the dosage unit, and immediately operate the apparatus at the specified rate. Within the time interval specified, or at each of the times stated, withdraw a specimen from a zone midway between the surface of the Dissolution Medium and the top of the rotating basket or

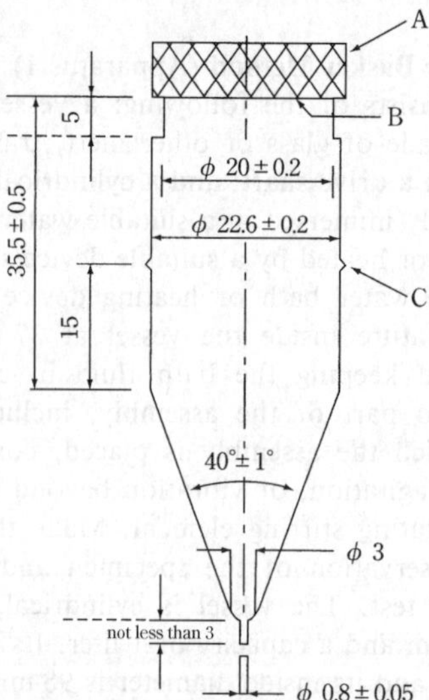

A: Filter chamber
B: No. 36 sieve (0.425 mm) or wire gauze (d: 0.2 mm, w: 0.45 mm)
C: Score for the sample holder

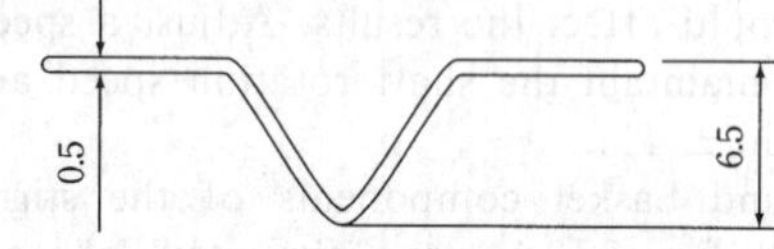

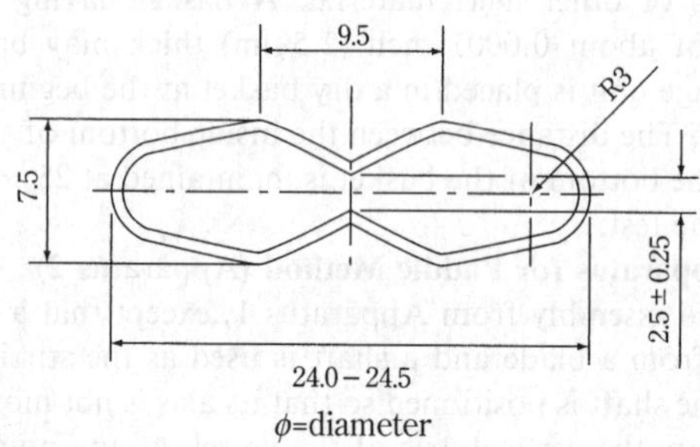

Fig. 6.10-3 Apparatus 3
Large cell for tablets and capsules (top); tablet holder for the large cell (bottom)
(All dimensions are expressed in mm unless otherwise noted.)

blade, not less than 10 mm from the vessel wall. [NOTE—Where multiple sampling times are specified, replace the aliquots withdrawn for analysis with equal volumes of fresh Dissolution Medium at 37°C or, where it can be shown that replacement of the medium is not necessary, correct for the volume change in the calculation. Keep the vessel covered for the duration of the test, and verify the temperature of the mixture under test at suitable times.] Perform the analysis using an indicated assay method.*3 Repeat the test with additional dosage units.

If automated equipment is used for sampling or the apparatus is otherwise modified, verification that the modified apparatus will produce results equivalent to those obtained with the standard apparatus described in this chapter, is necessary.

(ii) Dissolution Medium: An appropriate dissolution medium is used. The volume specified refers to measurements mode between 20°C and 25°C. If the dissolution medium is a buffered solution, adjust the solution so that its pH is within 0.05 unit of the specified pH. [NOTE—Dissolved gases can cause bubbles to form, which may change the results of the test. If dissolved gases influence the dissolution

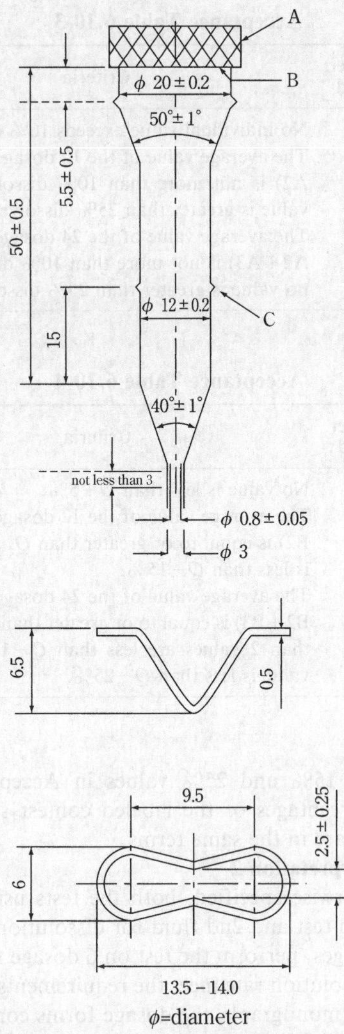

Fig. 6.10-4 Apparatus 3
Small cell for tablets and capsules (top); tablet holder for the small cell (bottom)
(All dimensions are expressed in mm unless otherwise noted.)

results, remove dissolved gases prior testing.*4]

(iii) Time: Where a single time specification is given, the test may be concluded in a shorter period if the requirement for minimum amount dissolved is met. Specimens are to be withdrawn only at the stated times, within a tolerance of ±2%.

3.1.2. Extended-release Dosage Forms

(i) Procedure: Proceed as described for Immediate-Release Dosage Forms.

(ii) Dissolution Medium: Proceed as directed under Immediate-Release Dosage Forms.

(iii) Time: The test-time points, generally three, are expressed in hours.

3.1.3. Delayed-release Dosage Forms

(i) ◆Procedure: Unless otherwise specified, proceed the acid stage test and buffer stage test separately as described for Immediate-Release Dosage Forms.◆

(ii) ◆Dissolution Medium: Acid stage: Unless 1st fluid for dissolution test is used, proceed as directed under Immediate-Release Dosage Forms. Buffer stage: Unless 2nd fluid for dissolution test is used, proceed as directed under Immediate-Release Dosage Forms.◆

(iii) ◆Time: Acid stage: Generally, test time is 2 hours for tablets and capsules, and 1 hour for granules. Buffer stage: The same as directed under Immediate-Release Dosage Forms.◆ All test times stated are to be observed within a tolerance of ±2%, unless otherwise specified.

3.2. Flow-Through Cell Method

3.2.1. Immediate-release Dosage Forms

(i) Procedure: Place the glass beads into the cell specified in the individual monograph. Place 1 dosage unit on top of the beads or, if specified, on a wire carrier. Assemble the filter head and fix the parts together by means of a suitable clamping device. Introduce by the pump the dissolution medium warmed to 37 ± 0.5°C through the bottom of the cell to obtain the flow rate specified and measured with an accuracy of 5%. Collect the eluate by fractions at each of the times stated. Perform the analysis as directed. Repeat the test with additional dosage units.

(ii) Dissolution Medium: Proceed as directed under Immediate-Release Dosage Forms under Basket Method and Paddle Method.

(iii) Time: Proceed as directed under Immediate-Release Dosage Forms under Basket Method and Paddle Method.

3.2.2. Extended-release Dosage Forms

(i) Procedure: Proceed as described for Immediate-Release Dosage Forms under Flow-Through Cell Method.

(ii) Dissolution Medium: Proceed as described for Immediate-Release under Flow-Through Cell Method.

(iii) Time: The test-time points, generally three, are expressed in hours.

4. Interpretation

4.1. Immediate-release Dosage Forms

◆Follow Interpretation 1 when the value Q is specified in the individual monograph, otherwise follow Interpretation 2.◆

4.1.1. Interpretation 1

Unless otherwise specified, the requirements are met if the quantities of active ingredient dissolved from the dosage units tested conform to Acceptance Table 6.10-1. Continue testing through the three stages unless the results conform at either S1 or S2. The quantity, Q, ◆is the specified amount of dissolved active ingredient,◆ expressed as a percentage of the labeled content of the dosage unit; the 5%, 15%, and 25% values in the Acceptance Tables are percentage of the labeled content so that three values and Q are in the same terms.

4.1.2. ◆Interpretation 2

Unless otherwise specified, perform the test on 6 dosage forms: if the individual dissolution rate meet the requirements specified in the individual monograph, the dosage forms conform to the test. When individual dissolution rates of 1 or 2 dosage forms fail to meet the requirements, repeat the test on another 6 dosage forms: if individual dissolution rates of not less than 10 dosage forms out of 12 meet the requirements, the dosage forms conform to the test.◆

4.2. Extended-release Dosage Forms

4.2.1. ◆Interpretation 1◆

Unless otherwise specified, the requirements are met if the quantities of active ingredient dissolved from the dosage units tested conform to Acceptance Table 6.10-2. Continue testing through the three levels unless the results conform at either L1 or L2. Limits on the amounts of active ingredient dissolved are expressed in terms of the percentage of labeled content. The limits embrace each value of Q_i, the amount dissolved at each specified fractional dosing interval. Where more than one range is specified, the acceptance criteria apply individually to each range.

4.2.2. ◆Interpretation 2

Unless otherwise specified, perform the test on 6 dosage forms: if the individual dissolution rate meet the require-

Acceptance Table 6.10-1

Stage	Number Tested	Acceptance Criteria
S1	6	Each value is not less than $Q+5\%$.
S2	6	Average value of the 12 dosage units (S1+S2) is equal to or greater than Q, and no value is less than $Q-15\%$.
S3	12	Average value of the 24 dosage units (S1+S2+S3) is equal to or greater than Q, not more than 2 values are less than $Q-15\%$, and no value is less than $Q-25\%$.

Acceptance Table 6.10-2

Level	Number Tested	Criteria
L1	6	No individual value lies outside each of the stated ranges and no individual value is less than the stated amount at the final test time.
L2	6	The average value of the 12 dosage units (L1+L2) lies within each of the stated ranges and is not less than the stated amount at the final test time; no value is more than 10% of labeled content outside each of the stated ranges; and no value is more than 10% of labeled content below the stated amount at the final test time.
L3	12	The average value of the 24 dosage units (L1+L2+L3) lies within each of the stated ranges, and is not less than the stated amount at the final test time; not more than 2 of the 24 values are more than 10% of labeled content outside each of the stated ranges; not more than 2 of the 24 values are more than 10% of labeled content below the stated amount at the final test time; and no value is more than 20% of labeled content outside each of the stated ranges or more than 20% of labeled content below the stated amount at the final test time.

ments specified in the individual monograph, the dosage forms conform to the test. When individual dissolution rates of 1 or 2 dosage forms fail to meet the requirements, repeat the test on another 6 dosage forms: if individual dissolution rates of not less than 10 dosage forms out of 12 meet the requirements, the dosage forms conform to the test. Where more than one range is specified, the acceptance criteria apply individually to each range.◆

4.3. Delayed-release Dosage Forms

◆Follow Interpretation 1 when the value Q is specified in the test using 2nd fluid for dissolution test in the individual monograph, otherwise follow Interpretation 2.

4.3.1. Interpretation 1

(i) Test using 1st fluid for dissolution test: Unless otherwise specified, the requirements of this portion of the test are met if the quantities, based on the percentage of the labeled content, of active ingredient dissolved from the units tested conform to Acceptance Table 6.10-3. Continue testing through the three levels unless the result conforms at A2.◆

(ii) ◆Test using 2nd fluid for dissolution test◆: Unless otherwise specified, the requirements are met if the quantities of active ingredient dissolved from the units tested conform to Acceptance Table 6.10-4. Continue testing through the three levels unless the results of both stages conform at an earlier level. The value of Q in Acceptance Table 6.10-4 is the amount ◆specified in monograph◆ of active ingredient dissolved, expressed as a percentage of the labeled content.

Acceptance Table 6.10-3

Level	Number Tested	Criteria
A1	6	No individual value exceeds 10% dissolved.
A2	6	The average value of the 12 dosage units (A1+A2) is not more than 10% dissolved, and no value is greater than 25% dissolved.
A3	12	The average value of the 24 dosage units (A1+A2+A3) is not more than 10% dissolved, and no value is greater than 25% dissolved.

Acceptance Table 6.10-4

Level	Number Tested	Criteria
B1	6	No value is less than $Q+5\%$.
B2	6	The average value of the 12 dosage units (B1+B2) is equal to or greater than Q, and no value is less than $Q-15\%$.
B3	12	The average value of the 24 dosage units (B1+B2+B3) is equal to or greater than Q, not more than 2 values are less than $Q-15\%$, and no value is less than $Q-25\%$.

The 5% and 15% and 25% values in Acceptance Table 6.10-4 are percentages of the labeled contest so that these values and Q are in the same terms.

4.3.2. ◆Interpretation 2

Unless otherwise specified, both the tests using 1st fluid for dissolution test and 2nd fluid for dissolution test in acid and buffer stages, perform the test on 6 dosage forms: if the individual dissolution rate meet the requirements specified in the individual monograph, the dosage forms conform to the test. When individual dissolution rates of 1 or 2 dosage forms fail to meet the requirements, repeat the test on another 6 dosage forms: if individual dissolution rates of not less than 10 dosage forms out of 12 meet the requirements, the dosage forms conform to the test.◆

*1The materials should not sorb, react, or interfere with the specimen being tested.

*2If a cover is used, it provides sufficient openings to allow ready insertion of the thermometer and withdrawal of specimens.

*3Test specimens are filtered immediately upon sampling unless filtration is demonstrated to be unnecessary. Use an inert filter that does not cause adsorption of the ingredient or contain extractable substances that would interfere with the analysis.

*4One method of deaeration is as follows: Heat the medium, while stirring gently, to about 41°C, immediately filter under vacuum using a filter having a porosity of 0.45 μm or less, with vigorous stirring, and continue stirring under vacuum for about 5 minutes. Other validated deaeration techniques for removal of dissolved gases may be used.

6.11 Foreign Insoluble Matter Test for Ophthalmic Liquids and Solutions

Foreign Insoluble Matter Test for Ophthalmic Liquids and Solutions is a test method to examine foreign insoluble matters in ophthalmic liquids and solutions.

When inspect with the unaided eyes at a position of luminous intensity of 3000 – 5000 lx under a white light source after cleaning the exterior of containers, Ophthalmic Solutions must be clear and free from readily detectable foreign insoluble matters.

6.12 Methods of Adhesion Testing

These are testing methods to measure the adhesion of patches. The methods include peel adhesion testing, inclined ball tack testing, rolling ball tack testing, and probe tack testing

The tests are conducted at 24°C ± 2°C unless otherwise specified. However, if the acceptable range of 24°C ± 2°C temperature cannot be maintained, set a range as close to that as possible.

1. Preparation of samples

The following method will be followed to prepare samples unless otherwise specified. Use a package, such as an aluminum material that is not affected by humidity for the sample, and allow it to stand at 24°C ± 2°C for over 12 hours. The sample can be cut to an appropriate size as needed. Furthermore, visually confirm that dust is not adhered to the adhesive side of the sample, take care not to touch the sample with bare hands, and prevent foreign matter from adhering to it.

2. Cleaning method for testing instruments

To clean the testing plates, balls, and probe for adhesion testing, use cleaning solvents such as acetone, 2-butanone, ethanol (99.5), ethyl acetate, heptane, water, and methanol. Utilize soft cloth, such as gauze, absorbent cotton, or waste cloth, that does not generate lint or dust during use, is absorbent, and free from additives that dissolve in cleaning solvents. Apply a cleaning solvent on a clean cloth, wipe the surfaces of the instruments, and repeat wiping with a new cloth until dry. Repeat this step until the instruments are determined clean by visual observation. Lastly, apply acetone, 2-butanone, or another appropriate solvent on a cloth, wipe the surfaces of the instruments, and repeat wiping with a new cloth until dry. Use the cleaned instruments for testing within 10 hours. Take care not to touch the surfaces with fingers, and preserve them without damaging or contaminating. Do not use any instrument if it is dirty, discolored, or has a number of scratches. With respect to new testing plates, balls, and probe, wipe well using cloth soaked with a cleaning solvent, and additionally, clean with the method described above before use.

3. Measurement methods

3.1. Peel adhesion testing

The peel adhesion test measures the force required to remove (peel away) the sample adhered to the testing plate at a 180 or 90-degree angle.

3.1.1. Equipment

The equipment consists of an application device and a tensile tester. The application device (Figures of equipment 6.12-1a and 6.12-1b) is structured in such a way that only the mass of the roller is applied to the sample as pressure when the sample is crimped. The roller should be made of steel or equivalent covered with the rubber for crimping rollers whose material is prescribed in the Japanese Industrial Standard Z 0237:2009 (a diameter of 85 ± 2.5 mm, a width of 45 ± 1.5 mm, a thickness of about 6 mm). In addition, the shape must be exactly cylindrical, and without irregularities on the surface. Set the mass of the roller to 2000 ± 100 g or 1000 ± 50 g.

With regard to the testing plate for adhesion testing, the plate prescribed in the Japanese Industrial Standard Z 0237:2009 or equivalent should be used unless otherwise specified.

Use a tensile tester with a relative pointing error of ± 1.0 %. The representation of measurements may be any one of the analog type, digital type, digital recording system, and chart recording system.

3.1.2. Operation procedures

Prepare the sample in such a way that it has a chucking allowance on one end, and adhere it to the testing plate using the application device after exposing the adhesive side within 5 minutes. Loosen the sample in holding the chucking allowance on the testing plate so that the testing plate will not come into contact with the sample prior to adhesion. Adhere the sample to the testing plate while crimping along the long side direction with the roller. This will prevent air from entering between the sample and the testing plate. If air enters, do not use the sample. Crimping should be done under constant load either at the rate of approximately 10 mm per second back and forth two times or at the rate of approximately 5 mm per second back and forth once. After crimping the sample with the roller, perform a peel adhesion test at the prescribed time (for example, 30 ± 10 minutes). Use a 2 kg crimping roller for a sample with a width of 17 mm or larger, and a 1 kg crimping roller for a sample with a width under 17 mm.

3.1.2.1. 180-degree peel test

Prepare an upper chuck and a lower chuck at the top and the bottom of the tensile tester as parts to secure the testing plate and the sample. Figure 6.12-2a shows an example of measuring instruments for 180-degree peel tests. When peeling the sample, hold the chucking allowance and fold back to a 180-degree angle so that it overlaps the backside of the sample. Secure one end of the testing plate to the lower chuck and the chucking allowance to the upper chuck of the tensile tester. Next, run the tensile tester at the tension rate of 5.0 ± 0.2 mm per second and start measuring. Ignore the measurements for the first 25% of the sample length. After that, average the measurements of adhesion for the 50% of the length peeled from the testing plate, which will be the value of the peel adhesion test. Express the unit in N/cm.

3.1.2.2. 90-degree peel test

Figure 6.12-2b provides an example of measuring instruments for 90-degree peel tests. Except for securing the

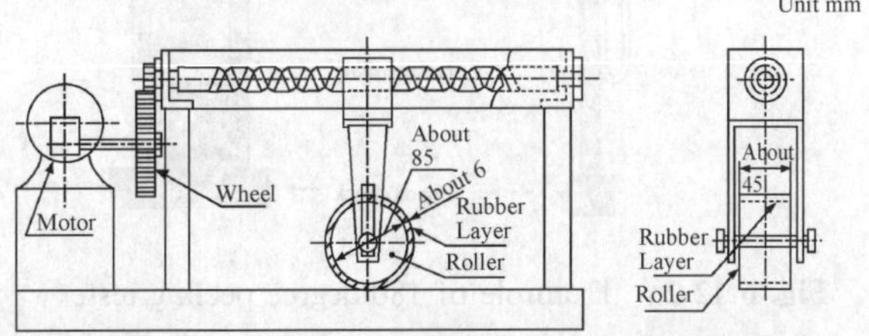

Fig. 6.12-1a Example of the automatic application device

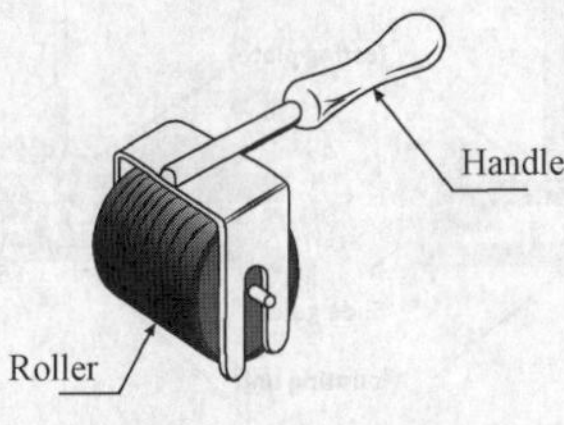

Fig. 6.12-1b Example of the manual application device

chucking allowance to the upper chuck and folding back the sample to a 90-degree angle, perform the test in the same manner as the 180-degree peel test.

3.2. Inclined ball tack testing

In the inclined ball tack test, balls are rolled down a ramp, and the largest size of the ball that stops is determined.

3.2.1. Equipment

3.2.1.1. Ball rolling device

Use a ramp with an inclined plane of 300 mm or longer having an inclination angle of 30 degrees. An example is given in Figure 6.12-3.

3.2.1.2. Balls

Use No. 2 to No. 32 balls for adhesion testing. SUJ2, a high carbon content chromium bearing steel material specified in Japanese Industrial Standard G 4805:2008, should be used for the material of the balls for adhesion testing. As for precision, use hard balls for rolling bearing in Grade 40 or above prescribed in Japanese Industrial Standard B 1501:2009. Table 6.12-1 shows the numbers and sizes of balls.

3.2.2. Operation procedures

Secure the ball-rolling device horizontally on the stand using a level. The sample must be larger than 10 mm in width and 70 mm in length unless otherwise specified. Fix the sample in the prescribed position on the ramp with the adhesive side up, and attach paper for the runway to the upper end of the sample. Set the length of the runway to 100 mm. When fixing the sample, take care that it will not be off the plate, wrinkled, or bent; if the edge of the sample is curved and off the plate, stick the part to the plate with another adhesive tape. Then, leave the adhesive face between 50 mm and 100 mm in length at the center, and cover the lower end with an appropriate piece of paper. As for the paper to cover the upper and lower ends of the adhesive side, use that of an appropriate material so that the ball can roll down without slipping.

Roll the balls down from the top of the ramp, and the number (No.) of the largest ball that stops on the adhesive face will be the value of the inclined ball tack test.

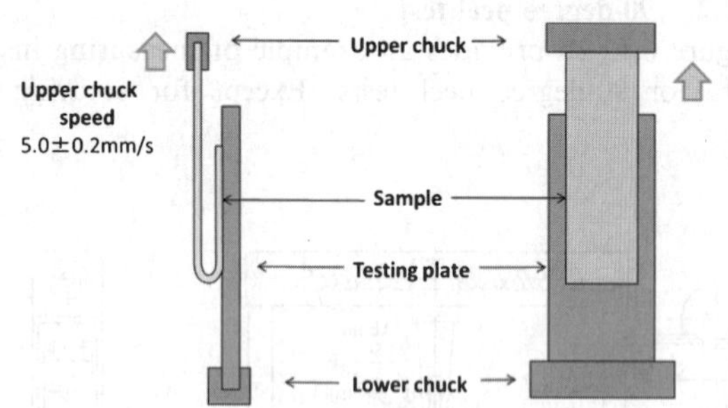

Fig. 6.12-2a Example of 180-degree peeling tester

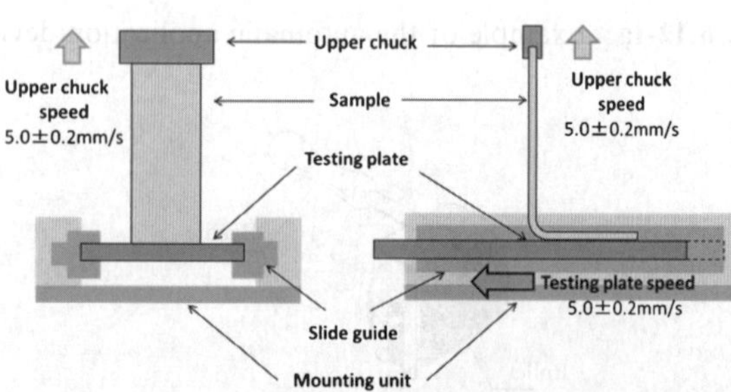

Fig. 6.12-2b Example of 90-degree peeling tester

3.3. Rolling ball tack testing

In the rolling ball tack test, a ball of specified size is rolled down a ramp from the start position, and the distance to the position at which the ball stops is measured.

3.3.1. Equipment

3.3.1.1. Ball-rolling device

The ball-rolling device has an inclination angle of 21.5 degrees, and Figure 6.12-4 shows an example.

3.3.1.2. Balls

Use No. 14 balls (a diameter of 7/16 inch) for adhesion testing as noted in 3.2.1.2 unless otherwise specified.

3.3.2. Operation procedures

Secure the sample on the smooth, hard, and flat plate with another adhesive tape, etc. When fixing the sample, take care that it will not be off the plate, wrinkled, or bent; if the edge of the sample is curved and off the plate, stick the part to the plate with another adhesive tape. Secure the ball rolling device horizontally on the stand with the sample using a level. Roll the ball down from the start position.

Measure the distance when the ball stopped on the adhesive face. Measure the length between the end of the inclined plane and the midpoint at which the adhesive is in contact with the ball, which will be the value of the rolling ball tack test. Express the unit in mm.

Table 6.12-1 Types of steel ball
Diameter (mm) is a reference level

No.	Diameter (inch)	Diameter (mm)	No.	Diameter (inch)	Diameter (mm)
1	1/32	0.8	17	17/32	13.5
2	1/16	1.6	18	9/16	14.3
3	3/32	2.4	19	19/32	15.1
4	1/8	3.2	20	5/8	15.9
5	5/32	4.0	21	21/32	16.7
6	3/16	4.8	22	11/16	17.5
7	7/32	5.6	23	23/32	18.3
8	1/4	6.4	24	3/4	19.1
9	9/32	7.1	25	25/32	19.8
10	5/16	7.9	26	13/16	20.6
11	11/32	8.7	27	27/32	21.4
12	3/8	9.5	28	7/8	22.2
13	13/32	10.3	29	29/32	23.0
14	7/16	11.1	30	15/16	23.8
15	15/32	11.9	31	31/32	24.6
16	1/2	12.7	32	1	25.4

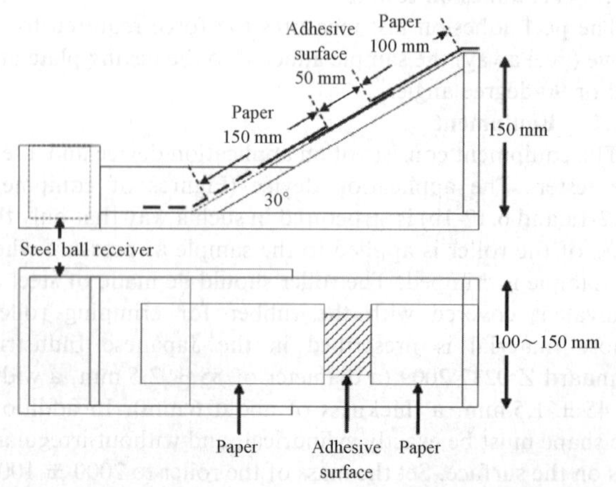

Fig. 6.12-3 Example of inclined ball tack tester

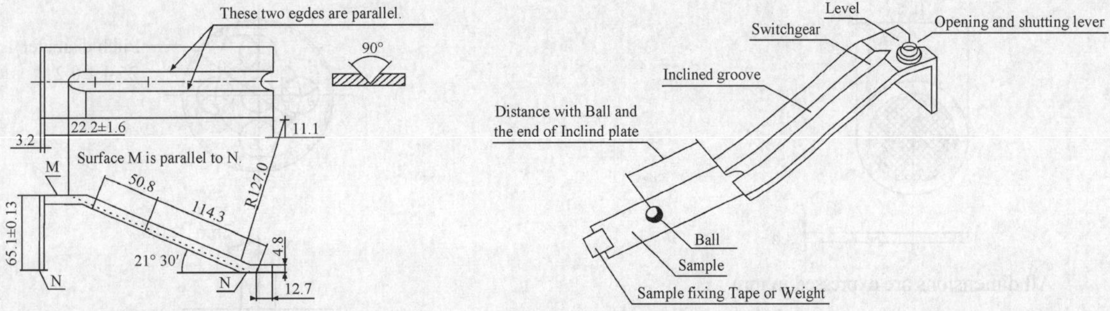

Fig. 6.12-4 Example of rolling ball tack tester
(All dimensions are expressed in mm unless otherwise noted.)

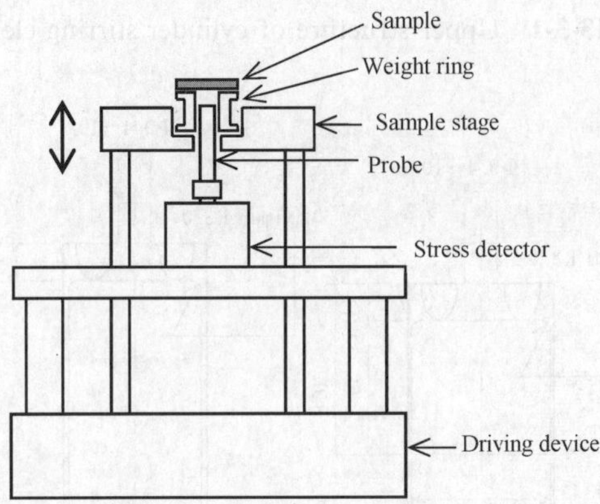

Fig. 6.12-5 Example of probe tack tester

3.4. Probe tack testing

The probe tack test measures the force required for peeling a prescribed cylindrical probe after bringing the probe into contact with the adhesive side of a patch briefly.

3.4.1. Equipment

The equipment consists of a probe, a sample stage, and a stress detector, and has a mechanism to give constant load for a certain period of time by a weight ring. As for the material of the probe for adhesion testing, use SUS304 with the root-mean-square value (*Rq*) of 250 to 500 nm for surface roughness, and a diameter of 5 mm unless otherwise specified. Furthermore, the equipment has a feature that can control the speed so that the probe's contact with the adhesive side of the patch and peeling will be done at a constant rate. An example of device that applies a load by weight rings is provided in Figure 6.12-5. A device without weight rings may also be used.

3.4.2. Operation procedures

Adhere the sample to the weight ring ensuring that there is no slack and place on the sample stage. Next, bring the probe into contact with the adhesive side of the sample at the rate of 10 ± 0.01 mm per second, and maintain for 1.0 ± 0.1 seconds with the contact load of 0.98 ± 0.01 N/cm^2 unless otherwise specified. Immediately after that, peel the probe vertically from the adhesive face at the rate of 10 ± 0.01 mm per second. Measure the maximum load required for peeling, which will be the value of the probe tack test. Express the unit in N/cm^2.

6.13 Release Test for Preparations for Cutaneous Application

This chapter describes the method to measure release profiles of active ingredients from preparations for cutaneous application and is provided to determine compliance of the preparations with drug-release requirements. Since the relation between efficacy and release profile depends on each characteristic of these preparations, this release test is an effective method for a quality control of each preparation. Particularly, for transdermal absorption type pharmaceutical preparations, it is necessary to maintain an appropriate control on the release profiles of active ingredients.

1. Paddle over disk method

1.1. Apparatus

Use the assembly for the paddle method (Apparatus 2) described under Dissolution Test <*6.10*> and, addition to the paddle and vessel, a stainless steel (SUS316) disk consisting of a screen with a wire opening of 125 μm is used to sink samples on the bottom of the vessel. If necessary, other device which is similar to Fig. 6.13-1 with a different size or shape may be used. Other appropriate devices instead of the disk may be used as long as they are chemically inert and do not interfere with the analysis. The disk attached with a sample is installed parallel to the bottom of the paddle blade. The distance between the bottom of the paddle blade and the surface of the disk is 25 ± 2 mm, unless otherwise specified in individual monograph (Fig. 6.13-2).

Additionally, apparatus suitability and handling of dissolution medium, etc., are in principle proceed as directed under Dissolution Test <*6.10*>.

1.2. Procedure

Prior to set a disk, place the prescribed volume of the dissolution medium in the vessel and maintain the temperature of the medium at 32 ± 0.5°C. Fix the sample on a disk as the release surface facing up in a suitable manner by using a double-sided adhesive tape or the like. When a function of the sample is not compromised by cutting, an appropriate and exactly measured piece of the sample may be cut and used for the test. If necessary, a porous membrane may be attached to the release surface for suppressing a shape change of the preparation. The characteristics of the membrane used such as hydrophobicity or hydrophilicity and the pore size must be stated in the test method. When a membrane is used, it is applied so that no air bubbles occur between the membrane and the release surface.

Install the disk at the bottom of the vessel as that the release surface of the sample is set upwards, and paralleled

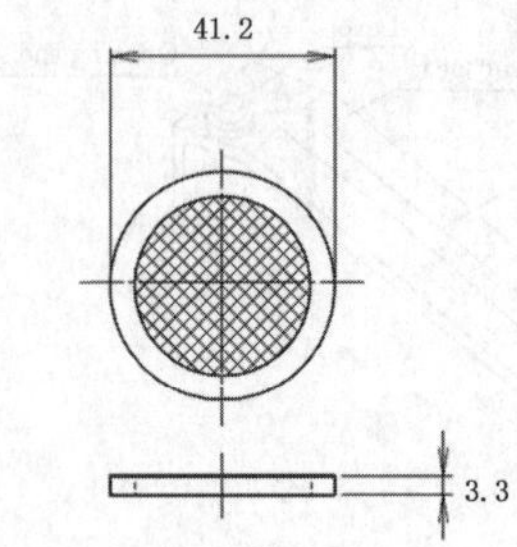

All dimensions are expressed in mm.

Fig. 6.13-1 Paddle over disk

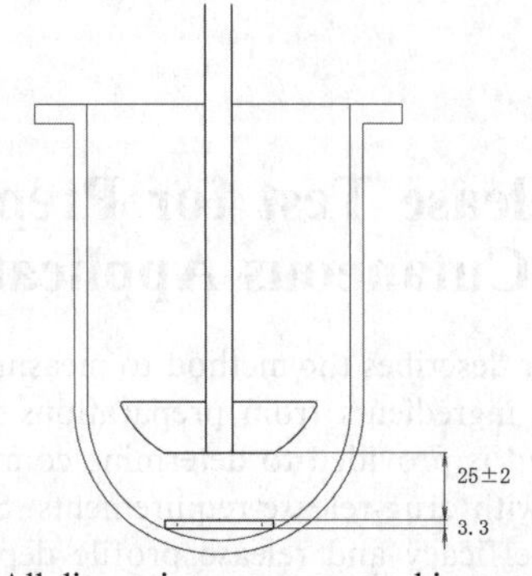

All dimensions are expressed in mm.

Fig. 6.13-2 Paddle and vessel

to the bottom of the paddle blade and to the surface of the dissolution medium. Immediately after the installation, rotate the paddle at the specified rate, and then at the specified interval or time, withdraw a specimen from the zone midway between the surface of the dissolution medium and the top of the paddle blade, not less than 10 mm from the vessel wall. (Note: Where multiple sampling times are specified, replace the aliquots withdrawn for analysis with equal volumes of fresh dissolution medium of 32°C or, where replacement of the medium is not necessary, correct for the volume change in the calculation. Keep the vessel covered for the duration of the test, and verify the temperature of the mixture under test at suitable intervals.) Perform the assay of the released active ingredients using the specified analytical method.

In the case where a different device in shape and material from that in Fig. 6.13-2 is used for sinking a sample with almost the same procedure stated, the method can be considered as the paddle over disk method, however, it needs to state the information about the used device.

2. Cylinder method

2.1. Apparatus

Use the vessel of the apparatus for the Paddle Method (Apparatus 2) described in Dissolution Test <*6.10*>, and use a stainless steel cylinder stirring element shown in Fig. 6.13-3-1 and Fig. 6.13-3-2 instead of a paddle. The cylinder is fabricated of chemically inert material such as stainless steel (SUS316), and the surface of the cylinder is electrolytically-polished. The cylinder whose size is adjusted to the same size as Fig. 6.13-3-2 (B) by equipping with an additional cylindrical device to the cylinder of Fig. 6.13-3-2 (A) can be used. The distance between the inside bottom of the vessel and the lower side of the cylinder is maintained at 25 ± 2 mm. Additionally, apparatus suitability and handling of dissolution

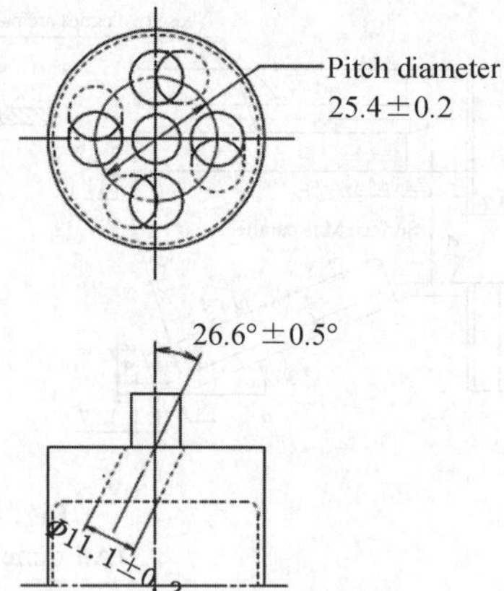

All dimensions are expressed in mm.

Fig. 6.13-3-1 Upper structure of cylinder stirring element

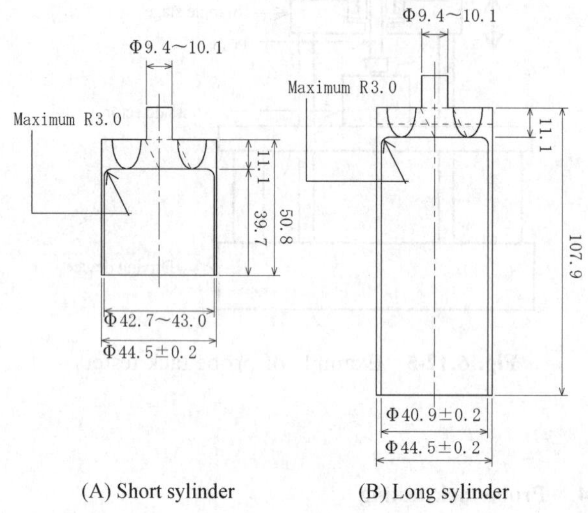

All dimensions are expressed in mm.

Fig. 6.13-3-2 Cylinder stirring element

medium, etc., are performed as directed under Dissolution Test <*6.10*>.

2.2. Procedure

Place the prescribed volume of the dissolution medium in the vessel and maintain the temperature of the medium to 32 ± 0.5°C. Remove the protective liner from the sample and fix the sample on the cylinder as the release surface being outside by a suitable method using a double-sided adhesive tape or the like. If necessary, a porous membrane may be attached to the release surface. The characteristics of the membrane used such as hydrophobicity or hydrophilicity and the pore size must be stated in the test method.

Install the cylinder in the dissolution test apparatus, and immediately after the installation, rotate the cylinder at the specified rate. At the specified interval or time, withdraw a specimen from the zone midway between the surface of the dissolution medium and the bottom of the cylinder, not less than 10 mm from the vessel wall. (Note: Where multiple sampling times are specified, replace the aliquots withdrawn for analysis with equal volumes of fresh dissolution medium of 32°C or, where replacement of the medium is not necessary, correct for the volume change in the calculation. Keep the vessel covered for the duration of the test, and verify the

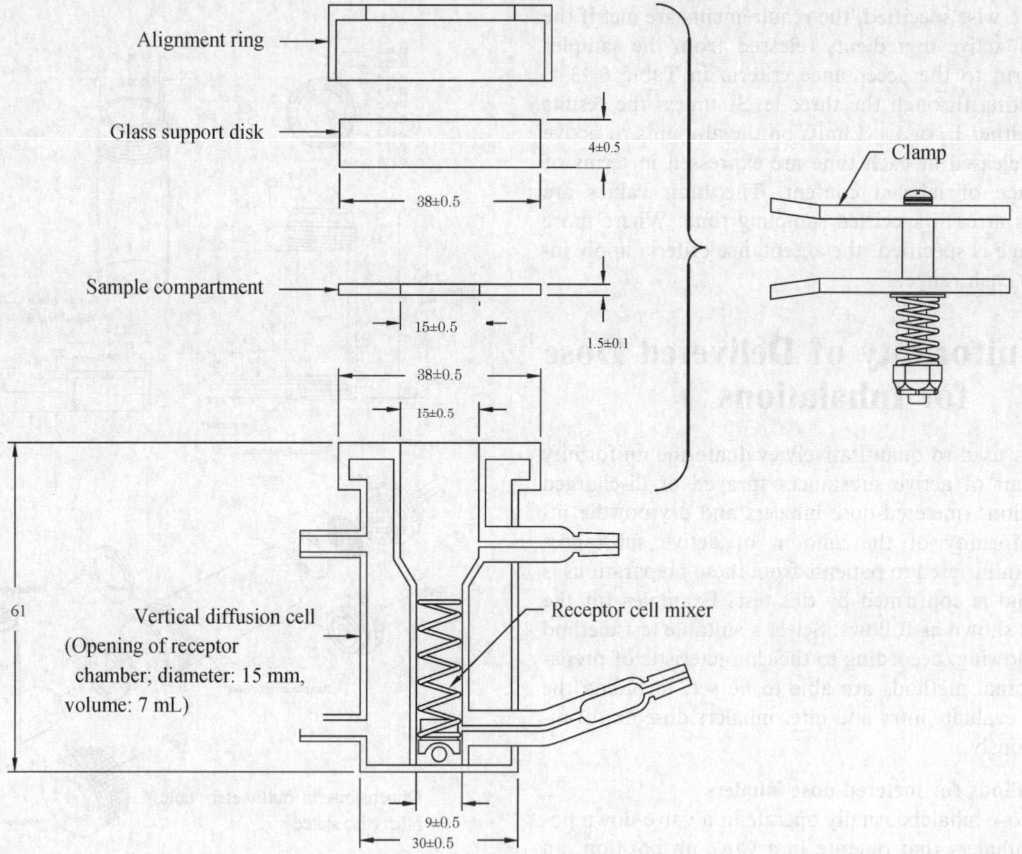

All dimensions are expressed in mm.

Fig. 6.13-4 Vertical diffusion cell

temperature of the mixture under test at appropriate intervals.) Perform the assay of the released active ingredients on each sample using the specified analytical method.

3. Vertical diffusion cell method

3.1. Apparatus

The assembly is composed of a vertical diffusion cell separated to two chambers and the chambers are fixed by a clamp. An example of the vertical diffusion cell is shown in Fig. 6.13-4. These cells are made of chemically inert materials such as glass or plastic, which do not interfere with the analysis.

3.2. Procedure

Place the prescribed volume of the dissolution medium in the receptor chamber with a rotator and maintain the medium temperature at 32 ± 1.0°C. If necessary, a porous membrane may be attached to the release surface. The characteristics of the membrane used such as hydrophobicity or hydrophilicity and the pore size must be stated. Place the sample evenly in the donor side and immediately rotate the rotator at a constant rate by a magnetic stirrer. At the specified intervals or time, withdraw a specimen. Take care not to enter bubble in the dissolution medium at the sampling. Perform the assay of the released active ingredients using the specified analytical method. Repeat the test with additional sample in the same manner.

4. Dissolution medium

Usually an arbitrary buffer in the range of pH 5 to 7 (ion strength is about 0.05) may be used as a dissolution medium. If necessary, addition of surfactant, change of the pH or ion strength may be allowed. Water, a mixture of water and alcohol, organic solvents, etc., may be used where they do not affect the shape of the samples. The volume of the dissolution medium used in the test is 200 mL, 500 mL or 900 mL, though in the case of 200 mL, a special vessel and mini-paddle should be used.

5. Interpretation

The specified range of quantities released from a sample at each sampling time is described in the individual monograph.

Table 6.13-1 Acceptance criteria

Level	Number tested	Acceptance criteria
L_1	6	No individual value lies outside each of the stated ranges (including the limit values).
L_2	6	The average value of the 12 samples (L_1 + L_2) lies within each of the stated ranges (including the limit values) and no individual value is more than 10% of labeled content outside each of the stated ranges.
L_3	12	The average value of the 24 samples (L_1 + L_2 + L_3) lies within each of the stated ranges (including the limit values), and not more than 2 of the 24 values are more than 10% of labeled content outside each of the stated ranges and no value is more than 20 % of labeled content outside each of the stated ranges.

Unless otherwise specified, the requirements are met if the quantities of active ingredients released from the samples tested conform to the acceptance criteria in Table 6.13-1. Continue testing through the three levels unless the results conform at either L_1 or L_2. Limits on the amounts of active ingredients released at each time are expressed in terms of the percentage of labeled content. The limit values are release ratios at each specified sampling time. Where more than one range is specified, the acceptance criteria apply individually to each range.

6.14 Uniformity of Delivered Dose for Inhalations

This test is used to quantitatively evaluate the uniformity of the amount of active substances sprayed or discharged from inhalations (metered-dose inhalers and dry powder inhalers). Uniformity of the amount of active substances which are administered to patients from these preparations is necessary, and is confirmed by this test. Examples for the evaluation is shown as follows. Select a suitable test method from the following, according to the characteristic of preparations. Original methods are able to be set, including the test that can evaluate intra and inter-inhalers dose uniformity simultaneously.

1. Test methods for metered-dose inhalers

Metered-dose inhalers usually operate in a valve-down position. For inhalers that operate in a valve-up position, an equivalent test is applied using methods that ensure the complete collection of the delivered dose.

The dose collection apparatus must be capable of quantitatively capturing the delivered dose.

The following apparatus (Fig. 6.14-1) and procedure may be used.

The apparatus consists of a filter-support base with an open-mesh filter-support, such as a stainless steel screen, a collection tube that is clamped or screwed to the filter-support base, and a mouthpiece adapter to ensure an airtight seal between the collection tube and the mouthpiece. Use a mouthpiece adapter that ensures that the front face of the inhaler's mouthpiece is flush with the front face or the 2.5 mm indented shoulder of the sample collection tube, as appropriate. The vacuum connector is connected to a system comprising a vacuum source and a flow regulator. The source is adjusted to draw air through the complete assembly, including the filter and the inhaler to be tested, at 28.3 L per minute (±5%). Air should be drawn continuously through the apparatus to avoid loss of the active substance into the atmosphere. The filter-support base is designed to accommodate 25 mm diameter filter disks. The filter disk and other materials used in the construction of the apparatus must be compatible with the active substance and solvents that are used to extract the active substance from the filter. One end of the collection tube is designed to hold the filter disk tightly against the filter-support base. When assembled, the joints between the components of the apparatus are airtight so that when a vacuum is applied to the base of the filter, all of the air drawn through the collection tube passes through the inhaler.

1.1. Test method 1: evaluation of intra-inhaler dose uniformity

Take one inhaler, and perform the test. Unless otherwise prescribed in the instructions to the patient, shake the inhaler for 5 seconds and discharge one delivery to waste. Discharge the inverted inhaler into the apparatus, depressing the valve for a sufficient time to ensure complete discharge. Repeat the procedure until the number of deliveries that constitute the minimum recommended dose have been sampled. Quantitatively collect the contents of the apparatus and determine the amount of active substance as the delivered dose.

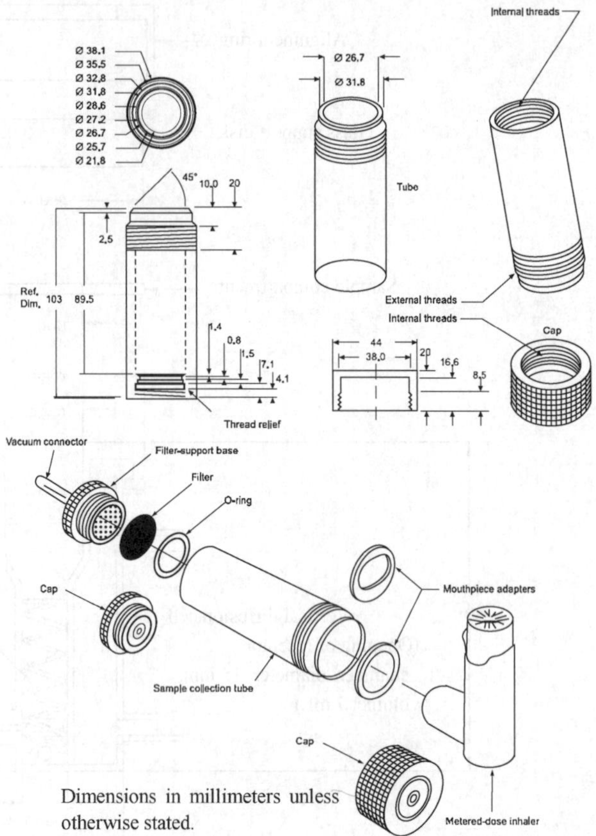

Fig. 6.14-1 Dose collection apparatus for metered-dose inhalers

Repeat the procedure for a further 2 doses.

Discharge the inhaler to waste, waiting not less than 5 seconds between actuations, until $(n/2) + 1$ deliveries remain, where n is the number of deliveries stated on the label. Collect 4 doses using the procedure described above.

Discharge the inhaler to waste, waiting not less than 5 seconds between actuations, until 3 doses remain. Collect these 3 doses using the procedure described above. Determine 10 delivered doses per one inhaler, i.e., 3 doses at the beginning, 4 doses at the middle and 3 doses at the end by the above process.

For preparations containing more than one active substance, carry out the test for uniformity of delivered dose for each active substance.

The mean of the delivered doses or the delivered dose stated on the label is used as the limit for judgement.

The preparation complies with the test if 9 out of 10 results lie between 75% and 125% of the limit and all lie between 65% and 135% of the limit. If 2 or 3 values lie outside the limits of 75 to 125%, repeat the test for 2 more inhalers, and obtain 30 values as the total. Not more than 3 of the 30 values lie outside the limits of 75 to 125% and no value lies outside the limits of 65 to 135%.

In justified cases, these ranges may be extended. But no value should be less than 50% or more than 150% of the limit.

The mean value must be within 85 to 115% of the label claim for delivered dose.

Table 6.14-1 Specifications of the apparatus described in Fig. 6.14-2

Code	Component	Description
A	Sample collection tube	Dimensions of 34.85 mm internal diameter × 12 cm length
B	Filter	47 mm glass fiber filter
C	Connector	Internal diameter ≧ 8 mm (e.g., short metal coupling, with low-diameter branch to P3)
D	Vacuum tubing	A length of suitable tubing having an internal diameter ≧ 8 mm and an internal volume of 25 ± 5 mL.
E	Two-way solenoid valve	A 2-way, 2-port solenoid valve having a minimum airflow resistance orifice with internal diameter ≧ 8 mm and an opening time ≦ 100 ms
F	Vacuum pump	Pump must be capable of drawing the required flow rate through the assembled apparatus with the dry powder inhaler in the mouthpiece adapter. Connect the pump to the 2-way solenoid valve using short and/or wide (≧ 10 mm internal diameter) vacuum tubing and connectors to minimize pump capacity requirements.
G	Timer	Timer capable of driving the solenoid valve for the required time period.
P1	Pressure tap	2.2 mm internal diameter, 3.1 mm outer diameter, flush with internal surface of the sample collection tube, centered and burr-free, 59 mm from its inlet. The pressure tap P1 must never be open to the atmosphere. Differential pressure to the atmosphere is measured at P1.
P2, P3	Pressure measurements	Absolute pressure
H	Flow control valve	Adjustable regulating valve with maximum Cv ≧ 1.

1.2. Test method 2: evaluation of inter-inhaler dose uniformity

Take one inhaler, and perform the test. Unless otherwise prescribed in the instructions to the patient, shake the inhaler for 5 seconds and discharge one delivery to waste. Discharge the inverted inhaler into the apparatus, depressing the valve for a sufficient time to ensure complete discharge. Repeat the procedure until the number of deliveries that constitute the minimum recommended dose have been sampled. Quantitatively collect the contents of the apparatus and determine the amount of active substance as the delivered dose.

Repeat the procedure for a further 9 inhalers. Determine 10 delivered doses, each 1 dose at the beginning for 10 inhalers, by the above process.

For preparations containing more than one active substance, carry out the test for uniformity of delivered dose for each active substance.

The mean of the delivered doses or the delivered dose stated on the label is used as the limit for judgement.

The preparation complies with the test if 9 out of 10 results lie between 75% and 125% of the limit and all lie between 65% and 135% of the limit. If 2 or 3 values lie outside the limits of 75 to 125%, repeat the above procedure for 20 more inhalers, and obtain 30 values as the total. Not more than 3 of the 30 values lie outside the limits of 75 to 125% and no value lies outside the limits of 65 to 135%.

In justified cases, these ranges may be extended. But no value should be less than 50% or more than 150% of the limit.

The mean value must be within 85 to 115% of the label claim for delivered dose.

2. Test method for dry powder inhalers

The dose collection apparatus must be capable of quantitatively capturing the delivered dose. A dose collection apparatus similar to that described for the valuation of metered-dose inhalers may be used provided that the dimensions of the tube and the filter can accommodate the measured flow rate. A suitable tube is defined in Table 6.14-1. Connect the tube to a flow system according to the scheme specified in Table 6.14-1 and Fig. 6.14-2.

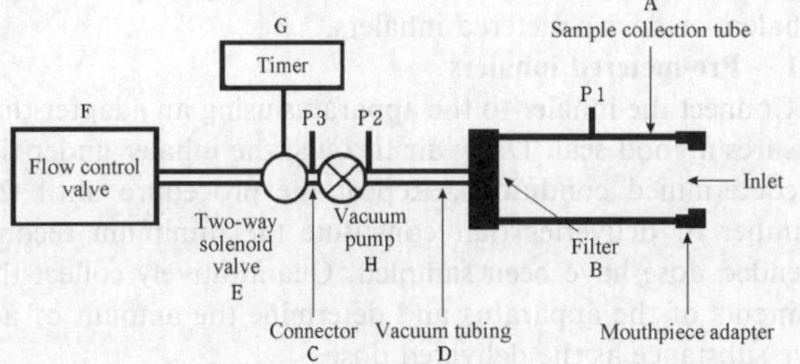

Fig. 6.14-2 Apparatus suitable for measuring the uniformity of delivered dose for dry powder inhalers

Unless otherwise specified, determine the test flow rate and duration using the dose collection tube, the associated flow system, a suitable differential pressure meter and a suitable volumetric flowmeter, calibrated for the flow leaving the meter, according to the following procedure.

Prepare the inhaler for use according to the instructions to the patient and connect it to the inlet of the apparatus using a mouthpiece adapter to ensure an airtight seal. Use a mouthpiece adapter that ensures that the front face of the inhaler mouthpiece is flush with the front face of the sample collection tube. Connect one port of a differential pressure meter to the pressure reading point P1 in Fig. 6.14-2, and let the other be open to the atmosphere. Switch on the pump, open the 2-way solenoid valve and adjust the flow control valve until the pressure drop across the inhaler is 4.0 kPa (40.8 cm H_2O) as indicated by the differential pressure meter. Remove the inhaler from the mouthpiece adapter and, without touching the flow control valve, connect a flowmeter to the inlet of the sampling apparatus. Use a flowmeter calibrated for the volumetric flow leaving the meter, or calculate the volumetric flow leaving the meter (Q_{out}) using the ideal gas law. For a meter calibrated for the entering volumetric flow (Q_{in}), use the following expression.

$$Q_{out} = \frac{Q_{in} \times P_0}{P_0 - \Delta P}$$

P_0: atmospheric pressure
ΔP: pressure drop over the meter

If the flow rate is above 100 L per minute, adjust the flow control valve to obtain a flow rate of 100 L per minute (±5%). Note the volumetric airflow rate exiting the meter and define this as the test flow rate, $Q_{out'}$, in L per minute. Define the test flow duration, T, in seconds so that a volume of 4 L of air is drawn from the mouthpiece of the inhaler at the test flow rate, $Q_{out'}$. Ensure that critical flow occurs in the flow control valve by the following procedure: with the inhaler in place and the test flow rate $Q_{out'}$, measure the absolute pressure on both sides of the control valve (pressure reading points P2 and P3 in Fig. 6.14-2); a ratio P3/P2 of less than or equal to 0.5 indicates critical flow; switch to a more powerful pump and re-measure the test flow rate if critical flow is not indicated.

Dry powder inhalers contain two types of inhalers, pre-metered inhalers where powders for one emission are pre-dispensed in capsules or other suitable dosage forms and device-metered inhalers where powders for one emission are metered within the inhalers. Perform the test by the following methods depending on each function of the pre-metered inhalers or device-metered inhalers.

2.1. Pre-metered inhalers

Connect the inhaler to the apparatus using an adapter that ensures a good seal. Draw air through the inhaler under the predetermined conditions. Repeat the procedure until the number of deliveries that constitute the minimum recommended dose have been sampled. Quantitatively collect the contents of the apparatus and determine the amount of active substance as the delivered dose.

Repeat the procedure for a further 9 doses. The sampling procedure to obtain 10 values of delivered doses is prescribed individually in considering the discharge mechanism of each preparation.

For preparations containing more than one active substance, carry out the test for uniformity of delivered dose for each active substance.

The mean of the delivered doses or the delivered dose stated on the label is used as the limit for judgement.

The preparation complies with the test if 9 out of 10 results lie between 75% and 125% of the limit and all lie between 65% and 135% of the limit. If 2 or 3 values lie outside the limits of 75 to 125%, repeat the above procedure for 20 more delivered doses, and obtain 30 values as the total. Not more than 3 of the 30 values lie outside the limits of 75 to 125% and no value lies outside the limits of 65 to 135%.

In justified cases, these ranges may be extended. But no value should be less than 50% or more than 150% of the limit.

The mean value must be within 85 to 115% of the label claim for delivered dose.

2.2. Device-metered inhalers

2.2.1. Test method 1: evaluation of intra-inhaler dose uniformity

Take one inhaler, and perform the test. Connect the inhaler to the apparatus using an adapter that ensures a good seal. Draw air through the inhaler under the predetermined conditions. Repeat the procedure until the number of deliveries that constitute the minimum recommended dose have been sampled. Quantitatively collect the contents of the apparatus and determine the amount of active substance as the delivered dose.

Repeat the procedure for a further 2 doses.

Discharge the inhaler to waste until $(n/2) + 1$ deliveries remain, where n is the number of deliveries stated on the label. If necessary, store the inhaler to discharge electrostatic charges. Collect 4 doses using the procedure described above.

Discharge the inhaler to waste until 3 doses remain. If necessary, store the inhaler to discharge electrostatic charges. Collect 3 doses using the procedure described above. Determine 10 delivered doses per one inhaler, i.e., 3 doses at the beginning, 4 doses at the middle and 3 doses at the end by the above process.

For preparations containing more than one active substance, carry out the test for uniformity of delivered dose for each active substance.

The mean of the delivered doses or the delivered dose stated on the label is used as the limit for judgement.

The preparation complies with the test if 9 out of 10 results lie between 75% and 125% of the limit and all lie between 65% and 135% of the limit. If 2 or 3 values lie outside the limits of 75 to 125%, repeat the test for 2 more inhalers, and obtain 30 values as the total. Not more than 3 of the 30 values lie outside the limits of 75 to 125% and no value lies outside the limits of 65 to 135%.

In justified cases, these ranges may be extended. But no value should be less than 50% or more than 150% of the limit.

The mean value must be within 85 to 115% of the label claim for delivered dose.

2.2.2. Test method 2: evaluation of inter-inhaler dose uniformity

Take one inhaler, and perform the test. Connect the inhaler to the apparatus using an adapter that ensures a good seal. Draw air through the inhaler under the predetermined conditions. Repeat the procedure until the number of deliveries that constitute the minimum recommended dose have been sampled. Quantitatively collect the contents of the apparatus and determine the amount of active substance as the delivered dose.

Repeat the procedure for a further 9 inhalers. Determine 10 delivered doses, each 1 dose at the beginning for 10 inhalers, by the above process.

For preparations containing more than one active substance, carry out the test for uniformity of delivered dose for each active substance.

The mean of the delivered doses or the delivered dose stated on the label is used as the limit for judgement.

The preparation complies with the test if 9 out of 10 results lie between 75% and 125% of the limit and all lie between 65% and 135% of the limit. If 2 or 3 values lie outside the limits of 75 to 125%, repeat the above procedure for 20 more inhalers, and obtain 30 values as the total. Not more than 3 of the 30 values lie outside the limits of 75 to 125% and no value lies outside the limits of 65 to 135%.

In justified cases, these ranges may be extended. But no value should be less than 50% or more than 150% of the limit.

The mean value must be within 85 to 115% of the label claim for delivered dose.

6.15 Aerodynamic Particle Size Measurement for Inhalations

This test is used to evaluate the fine particle characteristics of the aerosol clouds generated by preparations for inhalation, and is performed using one of the following apparatuses and test procedures. If justified, modified equipment or test procedure may be used.

1. Stage mensuration

The most reliable calibration for the separation characteristic of each impaction stage is performed in terms of the relationship between the stage collection efficiency and the aerodynamic diameter of particles and droplets passing through it as an aerosol.

Calibration is usually performed by examination of the jet nozzle dimensions, the spatial arrangement of the jet nozzle and its collection part, and the airflow rate passing through it.

Because jet nozzles can corrode and wear over time, the critical dimensions of each stage must be measured on a regular basis to confirm them being within required ranges.

Only apparatuses that conform to specifications are used for aerodynamic particle size measurement for inhalations. An alternate validated and justified method of mensuration may be used.

2. Re-entrainment

When using the apparatuses 2 and 3, the selected technique should seek to minimize particle re-entrainment (from an upper to a lower impaction stage) where this may affect the amounts of drug collected. For example, minimizing the number of sampled doses and coating the particle collection surfaces are used to minimize particle re-entrainment. Glycerol, silicone oil or similar high viscosity liquid are used to coat particle collection surfaces. Plate coating must be part of method validation and may be omitted where it is demonstrated that the aerodynamic particle size is not influenced by the coating.

3. Inter-stage drug losses (wall losses)

Wall losses should be considered in method development and validation. If the wall losses affect the recovery rate (mass balance) of drugs, they should be controlled. Wall losses will be dependent upon a number of factors including the impactor type, operating conditions, formulation type and discharged amount to an impactor. How the wall loss is reflected within the calculation of the aerodynamic diameter of particles should be judged based up on the level and variability of the wall loss. For example, in cases where wall losses are low or have a low level of variability, the aerodynamic particle size is calculated by the assay of the drug recovered from the collection plate. In cases where wall losses are high or variable, it may be necessary to collect the wall loss drug separately and take it into account for calculation of the aerodynamic particle size.

4. Recovery rate of drugs (mass balance)

In addition to the size distribution, good analytical practice dictates that a mass balance be performed in order to confirm that the amount of the drug discharged from the inhaler, which is collected in the mouthpiece adapter and the apparatus, is within an acceptable range around the expected value. The total mass of drug collected in all of the components of the mouthpiece adapter and the apparatus divided by the minimum recommended dose described in the dosage and administration is not less than 75% and not more than 125% of the average delivered dose determined under Uniformity of Delivered Dose for Inhalations <*6.14*>. This mass balance is necessary to ensure that the test results of particle size distributions are valid.

5. Measurement of fine particle dose and particle size distribution

5.1. Multi-stage liquid impinger method (Apparatus 1)

The apparatus used for the multi-stage liquid impinger method (apparatus 1) is shown in Fig. 6.15-1. The apparatus 1 consists of impaction stages 1 (pre-separator), 2, 3 and 4 and an integral filter stage (stage 5), see Figures 6.15-1 to 6.15-3. An impaction stage comprises an upper horizontal metal partition wall (B) through which a metal inlet jet tube (A) with its collection plate (D) is protruding. A glass cylinder (E) with sampling port (F) forms the vertical wall of the stage, and the stage is connected to the next lower stage by the tube (H) through a lower horizontal metal partition wall (G). The tube into stage 4 (U) ends in a multi-jet arrangement. The collection plate (D) is secured in a metal frame (J) which is fastened by two wires (K) to a sleeve (L) secured on the jet tube. The horizontal face of the collection plate is perpendicular to the axis of the jet tube and centrally aligned. The upper surface of the collection plate is slightly raised above the edge of the metal frame. A recess around the perimeter of the horizontal partition wall guides the position of the glass cylinder. The glass cylinders are sealed against the horizontal partition walls with gaskets (M) and clamped together by six bolts (N). The sampling ports are sealed by stoppers. The bottom-side (back) of the lower partition wall of stage 4 has a concentrical protrusion fitted with a rubber O-ring (P) which seals against the edge of a filter placed in the filter holder. The filter holder (R) is constructed as a basin with a concentrical recess in which a perforated filter support (S) is flush fitted. The filter holder is dimensioned for 76 mm diameter filters. The assembly of impac-

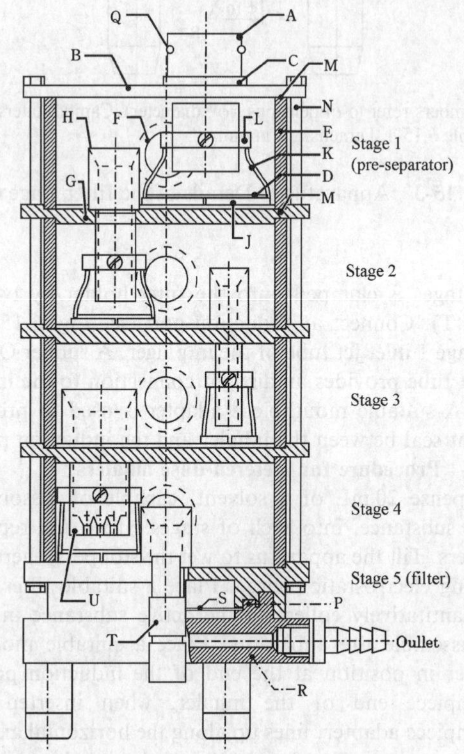

Capital letters refer to Table 6.15-1.

Fig. 6.15-1 Multi-stage liquid impinger (Apparatus 1)

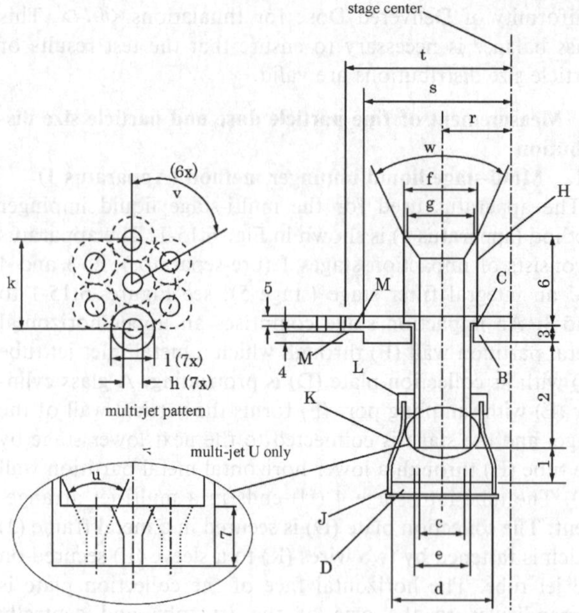

Inserts show end of multi-jet tube U leading to stage 4.
Numbers and lowercase letters refer to Table 6.15-2 and capital letters refer to Table 6.15-1.

Fig. 6.15-2 Apparatus 1: Details of jet tube and collection plate

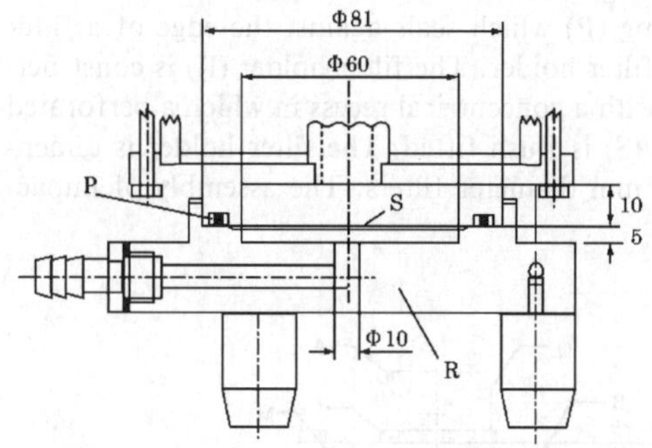

Numbers refer to dimensions (ϕ : diameter). Capital letters refer to Table 6.15-1. Dimensions in mm.

Fig. 6.15-3 Apparatus 1: Details of the filter stage (stage 5)

tion stages is clamped onto the filter holder by two snaplocks (T). Connect an induction port (see Fig. 6.15-4) onto the stage 1 inlet jet tube of the impinger. A rubber O-ring on the jet tube provides an airtight connection to the induction port. A suitable mouthpiece adapter is used to provide an airtight seal between the inhaler and the induction port.

5.1.1. Procedure for metered-dose inhalers

Dispense 20 mL of a solvent, capable of dissolving the active substance, into each of stages 1 to 4 and replace the stoppers. Tilt the apparatus to wet the stoppers, thereby neutralizing electrostatic charge. Place a suitable filter capable of quantitatively collecting the active substance in stage 5 and assemble the apparatus. Place a suitable mouthpiece adapter in position at the end of the induction port. The mouthpiece end of the inhaler, when inserted to the mouthpiece adapter, lines up along the horizontal axis of the induction port. The front face of the inhaler mouthpiece must be flush with the front face of the induction port. When attached to the mouthpiece adapter, the inhaler is positioned in the same orientation as intended for use. Con-

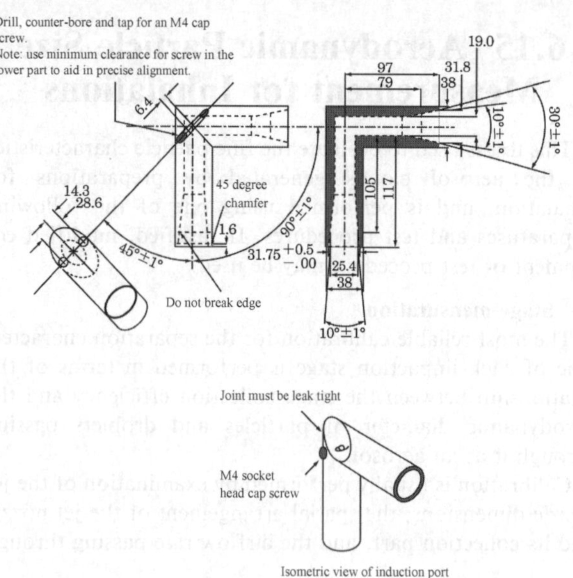

Dimensions in mm unless otherwise stated.

Note

(1) Material may be aluminium, stainless steel or other suitable material.

(2) Machine from 38 mm bar stock.

(3) Bore 19 mm hole through bar.

(4) Cut tube to exact 45° as shown.

(5) The inner bores and tapers should be smooth – surface roughness Ra approx. 0.4 μm.

(6) Mill joining cads of stock to provide a liquid tight leak-free seal.

(7) Set up a holding fixture for aligning the inner 19 mm bore and for drilling and tapping M4 × 0.7 threads. There must be virtually no mismatch of the inner bores in the miter joint.

Fig. 6.15-4 Induction port

nect a suitable vacuum pump to the outlet of the apparatus and adjust the air flow through the apparatus, as measured at the inlet to the induction port, to 30 L per minute (±5%). Switch off the pump.

Unless otherwise prescribed in the patient instructions, shake the inhaler for 5 seconds and discharge one delivery to waste. Switch on the pump to the apparatus, locate the mouthpiece end of the inhaler in the adapter and discharge the inhaler into the apparatus, actuating the inhaler for a sufficient time to ensure complete discharge. Wait for 5 seconds before removing the assembled inhaler from the adapter. Repeat the procedure. The number of discharges should be minimized and typically would not be greater than 10. The number of discharges is sufficient to ensure an accurate and precise determination of the fine particle dose. After the final discharge, wait for 5 seconds and then switch off the pump.

Dismantle the filter stage of the apparatus. Carefully remove the filter and extract the active substance into an aliquot of the solvent. Remove the induction port and mouthpiece adapter from the apparatus and extract the active substance into an aliquot of the solvent. If necessary, rinse the inside of the inlet jet tube to stage 1 with the solvent, allowing the solvent to flow into the stage. Extract the active substance from the inner walls and the collection plate of each of the 4 upper stages of the apparatus into the solution in the respective stage by carefully tilting and rotating the apparatus, observing that no liquid transfer occurs be-

Table 6.15-1 Component specification for apparatus 1 in Figures 6.15-1, 2 and 3

Code*	Item	Description	Dimensions**
A, H	Jet tube	Metal tube screwed onto partition wall sealed by gasket (C), polished inner surface	see Fig. 6.15-2
B, G	Partition wall	Circular metal plate —diameter —thickness	 120 see Fig. 6.15-2
C	Gasket	e.g. polytetrafluoroethylene	to fit jet tube
D	Collection plate	Porosity 0 sintered-glass disk —diameter	 see Fig. 6.15-2
E	Glass cylinder	Plane polished cut glass tube —height, including gaskets —outer diameter —wall thickness —sampling port (F) diameter —stopper in sampling port	 46 100 3.5 18 ISO24/25
J	Metal frame	L-profiled circular frame with slit —inner diameter —height —thickness of horizontal section —thickness of vertical section	 to fit collection plate 4 0.5 2
K	Wire	Steel wire interconnecting metal frame and sleeve (2 for each frame) —diameter	 1
L	Sleeve	Metal sleeve secured on jet tube by screw —inner diameter —height —thickness	 to fit jet tube 6 5
M	Gasket	e.g. silicone	to fit glass cylinder
N	Bolt	Metal bolt with nut (6 pairs) —length —diameter	 205 4
P	O-ring	Rubber O-ring —diameter × thickness	 66.34 × 2.62
Q	O-ring	Rubber O-ring —diameter × thickness	 29.1 × 1.6
R	Filter holder	Metal housing with stand and outlet	see Fig. 6.15-3
S	Filter support	Perforated sheet metal —diameter —hole diameter —distance between holes (center-points)	 65 3 4
T	Snap-locks		
U	Multi-jet tube	Jet tube (H) ending in multi-jet arrangement	see Fig. 6.15-2

* Refers to Fig. 6.15-1.

** Measures in mm with tolerances according to JIS B 0405 unless otherwise stated.

Table 6.15-2 Dimensions(1) of jet tube with collection plate of apparatus 1

Type	Code(2)	Stage 1	Stage 2	Stage 3	Stage 4	Filter (Stage 5)
Distance (Length)	1	9.5 (− .0 + .5)	5.5 (− .0 + .5)	4.0 (− .0 + .5)	6.0 (− .0 + .5)	n.a.
Distance (Length)	2	26	31	33	30.5	0
Distance (Length)	3	8	5	5	5	5
Distance (Length)	4	3	3	3	3	n.a.
Distance (Length)	5	0	3	3	3	3
Distance (Length)	6(3)	20	25	25	25	25
Distance (Length)	7	n.a.	n.a.	n.a.	8.5	n.a.
Diameter	c	25	14	8.0 (± .1)	21	14
Diameter	d	50	30	20	30	n.a.
Diameter	e	27.9	16.5	10.5	23.9	n.a.
Diameter	f	31.75 (− .0 + .5)	22	14	31	22
Diameter	g	25.4	21	13	30	21
Diameter	h	n.a.	n.a.	n.a	2.70 (± .5)	n.a.
Diameter	l	n.a.	n.a.	n.a	6.3	n.a.
Diameter	k	n.a.	n.a.	n.a	12.6	n.a.
Radius(4)	r	16	22	27	28.5	0
Radius	s	46	46	46	46	n.a.
Radius	t	n.a.	50	50	50	50
Angle	w	10°	53°	53°	53°	53°
Angle	u	n.a.	n.a.	n.a.	45°	n.a.
Angle	v	n.a.	n.a.	n.a.	60°	n.a.

(1) Measures in mm with tolerances according to JIS B 0405 unless otherwise stated.
(2) Refer to Fig. 6.15-2
(3) Including gasket
(4) Relative centerline of stage compartment
n.a.: not applicable

tween the stages.

Using a suitable method of analysis, determine the amount of active substance contained in each of the aliquots of solvent. Calculate the fine particle dose (see 6. Calculations).

5.1.2. Procedure for dry powder inhalers

Place a suitable low resistance filter capable of quantitatively collecting the active substance in stage 5 and assemble the apparatus. Connect the apparatus to a flow system according to the scheme specified in Fig. 6.15-5 and Table 6.15-3. Unless otherwise prescribed, conduct the test at the flow rate, Q_{out}, used in Uniformity of Delivered Dose for Inhalations <6.14>, drawing 4 L of air from the mouthpiece of the inhaler and through the apparatus.

Connect a flowmeter to the induction port. Use a flowmeter calibrated for the volumetric flow leaving the meter, or calculate the volumetric flow leaving the meter (Q_{out}) using the ideal gas law. For a meter calibrated for the entering volumetric flow (Q_{in}), use the following expression:

$$Q_{out} = \frac{Q_{in} \times P_0}{P_0 - \Delta P}$$

P_0: atmospheric pressure
ΔP: pressure drop over the meter

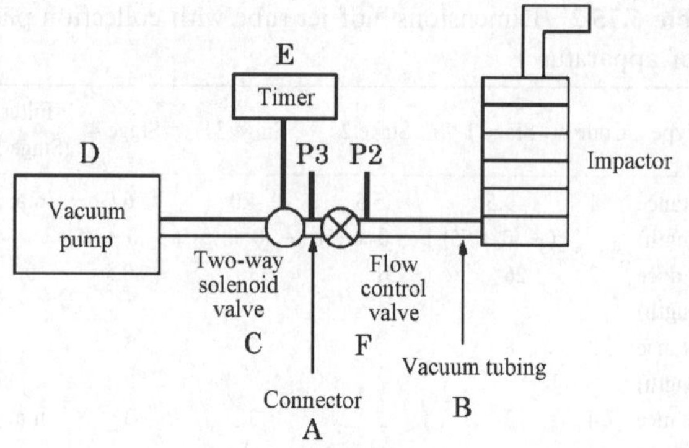

Capital letters refer to Table 6.15-3.

Fig. 6.15-5 Experimental set-up for testing dry powder inhalers

Adjust the flow control valve to achieve steady flow through the system at the required rate, Q_{out} ($\pm 5\%$). Ensure that critical flow occurs in the flow control valve by the following procedure. Switch off the pump.

With the inhaler in place and the test flow rate established, measure the absolute pressure on both sides of the control valve (pressure reading points P2 and P3 in Fig. 6.15-5). A ratio *P3/P2* of less than or equal to 0.5 indicates critical flow. Switch to a more powerful pump and re-measure the test flow rate if critical flow is not indicated.

Dispense 20 mL of a solvent, capable of dissolving the active substance, into each of the 4 upper stages of the apparatus and replace the stoppers. Tilt the apparatus to wet the stoppers, thereby neutralizing electrostatic charge. Place a suitable mouthpiece adapter in position at the end of the induction port. The mouthpiece end of the inhaler, when inserted to the mouthpiece adapter, lines up along the horizontal axis of the induction port. The front face of the inhaler mouthpiece must be flush with the front face of the induction port. When attached to the mouthpiece adapter, the inhaler is positioned in the same orientation as intended for use.

Prepare the dry powder inhaler for use according to the patient instructions. With the pump running and the 2-way solenoid valve closed, locate the mouthpiece of the inhaler in the mouthpiece adapter. Discharge the powder into the apparatus by opening the valve for the required time, T ($\pm 5\%$). Repeat the discharge procedure. The number of discharges should be minimized and typically would not be greater than 10. The number of discharges is sufficient to ensure an accurate and precise determination of fine particle dose.

Dismantle the filter stage of the apparatus. Carefully remove the filter and extract the active substance into an aliquot of the solvent. Remove the induction port and mouthpiece adapter from the apparatus and extract the active substance into an aliquot of the solvent. If necessary, rinse the inside of the inlet jet tube to stage 1 with the solvent, allowing the solvent to flow into the stage. Extract the active substance from the inner walls and the collection plate of each of the 4 upper stages of the apparatus into the solution in the respective stage by carefully tilting and rotating the apparatus, observing that no liquid transfer occurs between the stages.

Using a suitable method of analysis, determine the amount of active substance contained in each of the aliquots of solvent. Calculate the fine particle dose (see 6. Calculations).

Table 6.15-3 Component specification for Fig. 6.15-5

Code*	Item	Description
A	Connector	ID ≧ 8 mm, e.g., short metal coupling, with low-diameter branch to P3.
B	Vacuum tubing	A length of suitable tubing having an ID ≧ 8 mm and an internal volume of 25 ± 5 mL.
C	Two-way solenoid valve	A 2-way, 2-port solenoid valve having a minimum airflow resistance orifice with ID ≧ 8 mm and an opening time ≦ 100 ms.
D	Vacuum pump	Pump must be capable of drawing the required flow rate through the assembled apparatus with the inhaler in the mouthpiece adapter, or equivalent. Connect the pump to the 2-way solenoid valve using short and/or wide (ID ≧ 10 mm) vacuum tubing and connectors to minimize pump capacity requirements.
E	Timer	Timer capable to drive the 2-way solenoid valve for the required duration, or equivalent.
P2, P3	Pressure measurements	Determine under steady-state flow condition with an absolute pressure transducer.
F	Flow control valve	Adjustable regulating valve with maximum C_v ≧ 1.

* Refer to Fig. 6.15-5.
ID: inner diameter

5.2. Andersen cascade impactor method (Apparatus 2)

The apparatus used for Andersen cascade impactor method (apparatus 2) is shown in Fig. 6.15-6. The apparatus 2 consists of 8 stages together with a final filter. Material of construction may be aluminium, stainless steel or other suitable material. The stages are clamped together and sealed with O-rings. Critical dimensions of apparatus 2 are provided in Table 6.15-4. In use, some occlusions and wear of nozzles will occur. In-use mensuration tolerances need to be justified.

The configuration used for metered-dose inhalers is shown in Fig. 6.15-6. The entry cone (see Fig. 6.15-7b) of the impactor is connected to an induction port (see Fig. 6.15-4). A suitable mouthpiece adapter is used to provide an airtight seal between the inhaler and the induction port.

In the configuration for dry powder inhalers, a pre-separator is placed above the top stage to collect large masses of non-respirable powder. The top of the pre-separator shown in Fig. 6.15-7a is used to adapt the pre-separator to the induction port. To accommodate high flow rates through the impactor, the outlet nipple, used to connect the impactor to the vacuum system, is enlarged to have an internal diameter greater than or equal to 8 mm.

5.2.1. Procedure for metered-dose inhalers

Assemble the Andersen cascade impactor with a suitable filter in place. Ensure that the system is airtight by a suitable method. Place a suitable mouthpiece adapter in position at the end of the induction port. The mouthpiece end of the inhaler, when inserted to the mouthpiece adapter, lines up along the horizontal axis of the induction port. The front face of the inhaler mouthpiece must be flush with the front face of the induction port. When attached to the mouthpiece adapter, the inhaler unit is positioned in the same orientation as the intended use. Connect a suitable pump to the outlet of the apparatus and adjust the air flow through the apparatus,

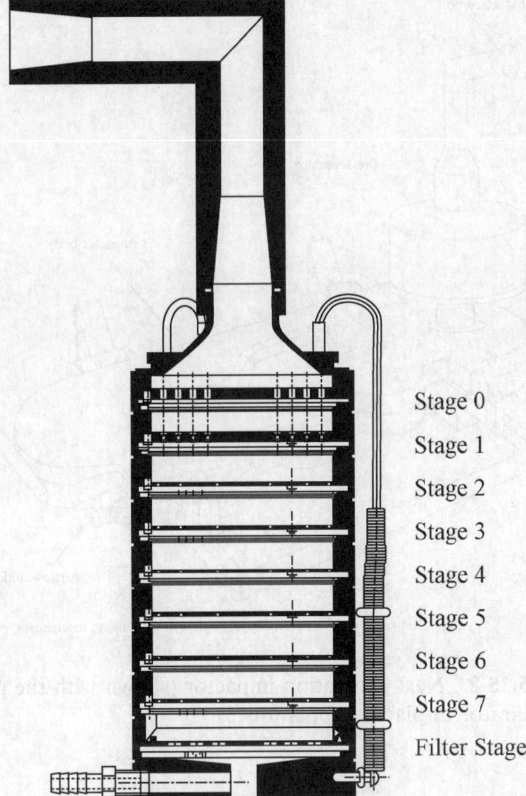

Fig. 6.15-6 Andersen cascade impactor used for metered-dose inhalers (Apparatus 2)

Table 6.15-4 Critical dimensions for apparatus 2

Description	Number of nozzle	Dimension (mm)
Stage 0 nozzle diameter	96	2.55 ± 0.025
Stage 1 nozzle diameter	96	1.89 ± 0.025
Stage 2 nozzle diameter	400	0.914 ± 0.0127
Stage 3 nozzle diameter	400	0.711 ± 0.0127
Stage 4 nozzle diameter	400	0.533 ± 0.0127
Stage 5 nozzle diameter	400	0.343 ± 0.0127
Stage 6 nozzle diameter	400	0.254 ± 0.0127
Stage 7 nozzle diameter	201	0.254 ± 0.0127

as measured at the inlet to the induction port, to 28.3 L per minute (±5%). Switch off the pump.

Unless otherwise prescribed in the patient instructions, shake the inhaler for 5 seconds and discharge one delivery to waste. Switch on the pump to the apparatus, locate the mouthpiece end of the inhaler in the adapter and discharge the inhaler into the apparatus, actuating the inhaler for a sufficient time to ensure complete discharge. Wait for 5 seconds before removing the assembled inhaler from the adapter. Repeat the procedure. The number of discharges should be minimized and typically would not be greater than 10. The number of discharges is sufficient to ensure an accurate and precise determination of the fine particle dose. After the final discharge, wait for 5 seconds and then switch off the pump.

Dismantle the apparatus. Carefully remove the filter and extract the active substance into an aliquot of the solvent. Remove the induction port and mouthpiece adapter from the

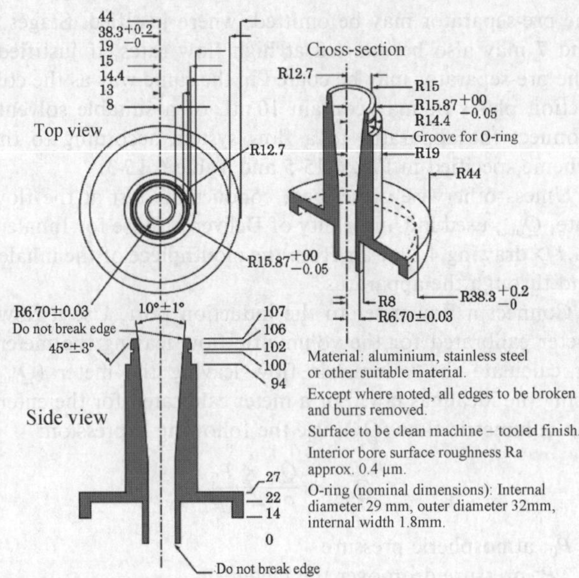

Fig. 6.15-7a Expanded view of top for the Andersen pre-separator adapted to the induction port

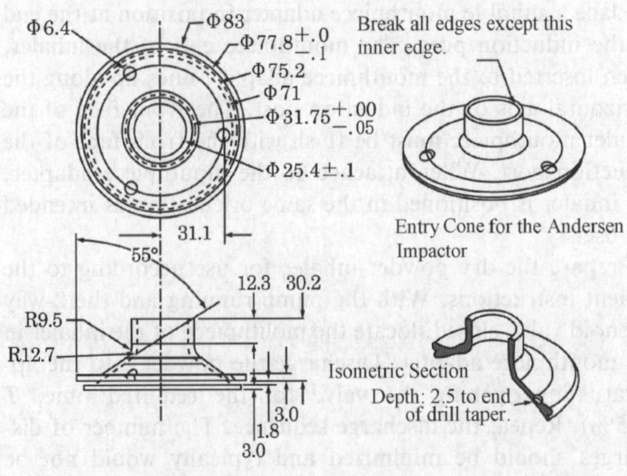

Material may be aluminum, stainless steel, or other suitable material. Surface roughness (Ra) should be approximately 0.4 μm. Dimensions in mm unless otherwise stated.

Fig. 6.15-7b Expanded view of the entry cone for mounting induction port on the Andersen cascade impactor without pre-separator.

apparatus and extract the active substance into an aliquot of the solvent. Extract the active substance from the inner walls and the collection plate of each of the stages of the apparatus into aliquots of the solvent.

Using a suitable method of analysis, determine the amount of active substance contained in each of the aliquots of solvent. Calculate the fine particle dose (see 6. Calculations).

5.2.2. Procedure for dry powder inhalers

The aerodynamic cut-off diameters of the individual stages of this apparatus are currently not well-established at flow rates other than 28.3 L per minute. Users must justify and validate the use of the impactor in the chosen conditions, when flow rates different from 28.3 L per minute are selected.

Assemble the Andersen cascade impactor with the pre-separator and a suitable filter in place and ensure that the system is airtight. Depending on the product characteristics, the pre-separator may be omitted, where justified. Stages 6 and 7 may also be omitted at high flow rates, if justified. The pre-separator may be coated in the same way as the collection plates or may contain 10 mL of a suitable solvent. Connect the apparatus to a flow system according to the scheme specified in Fig. 6.15-5 and Table 6.15-3.

Unless otherwise prescribed, conduct the test at the flow rate, Q_{out}, used in Uniformity of Delivered Dose for Inhalers <*6.14*> drawing 4 L of air from the mouthpiece of the inhaler and through the apparatus.

Connect a flowmeter to the induction port. Use a flowmeter calibrated for the volumetric flow leaving the meter, or calculate the volumetric flow leaving the meter (Q_{out}) using the ideal gas law. For a meter calibrated for the entering volumetric flow (Q_{in}), use the following expression:

$$Q_{out} = \frac{Q_{in} \times P_0}{P_0 - \Delta P}$$

P_0: atmospheric pressure
ΔP: pressure drop over the meter

Adjust the flow control valve to achieve steady flow through the system at the required rate, Q_{out} ($\pm 5\%$). Ensure that critical flow occurs in the flow control valve by the procedure described in 5.1.2. Procedure for dry powder inhalers. Switch off the pump.

Place a suitable mouthpiece adapter in position at the end of the induction port. The mouthpiece end of the inhaler, when inserted to the mouthpiece adapter, lines up along the horizontal axis of the induction port. The front face of the inhaler mouthpiece must be flush with the front face of the induction port. When attached to the mouthpiece adapter, the inhaler is positioned in the same orientation as intended for use.

Prepare the dry powder inhaler for use according to the patient instructions. With the pump running and the 2-way solenoid valve closed, locate the mouthpiece of the inhaler in the mouthpiece adapter. Discharge the powder into the apparatus by opening the valve for the required time, T ($\pm 5\%$). Repeat the discharge sequence. The number of discharges should be minimized and typically would not be greater than 10. The number of discharges is sufficient to ensure an accurate and precise determination of fine particle dose.

Dismantle the apparatus. Carefully remove the filter and extract the active substance into an aliquot of the solvent. Remove the pre-separator, induction port and mouthpiece adapter from the apparatus and extract the active substance into an aliquot of the solvent. Extract the active substance from the inner walls and the collection plate of each of the stages of the apparatus into the solvent.

Using a suitable method of analysis, determine the amount of active substance contained in each of the aliquots of solvent. Calculate the fine particle dose (see 6. Calculations).

5.3. Next generation impactor method (Apparatus 3)

The apparatus used for next generation impactor method (apparatus 3) is shown in Fig. 6.15-8. The apparatus 3 is a cascade impactor with 7 stages and a micro-orifice collector (MOC). Over the flow rate range of 30 to 100 L per minute the 50%-collection efficiency cut-off diameters (D_{50} values) range between 0.24 μm and 11.7 μm, evenly spaced on a logarithmic scale. In this flow range, there are always at least 5 stages with D_{50} values between 0.5 μm and 6.5 μm. The collection efficiency curves for each stage are sharp and minimize overlap between stages.

Material of construction may be aluminium, stainless steel or other suitable material.

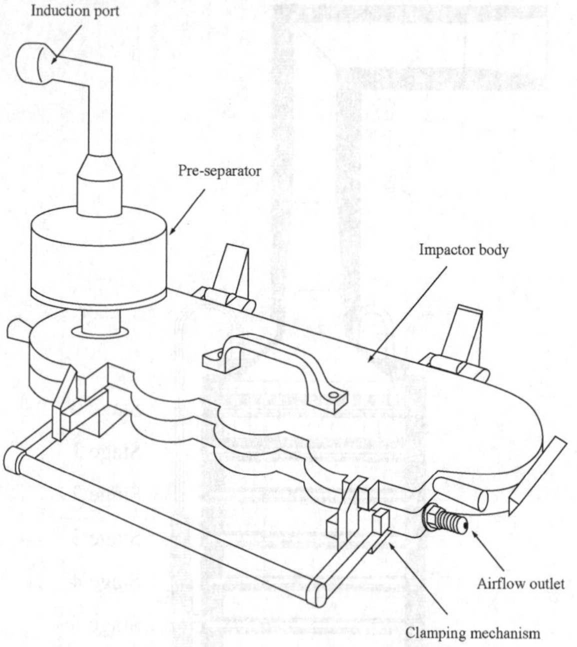

Fig. 6.15-8 Next generation impactor (shown with the pre-separator in place) (Apparatus 3)

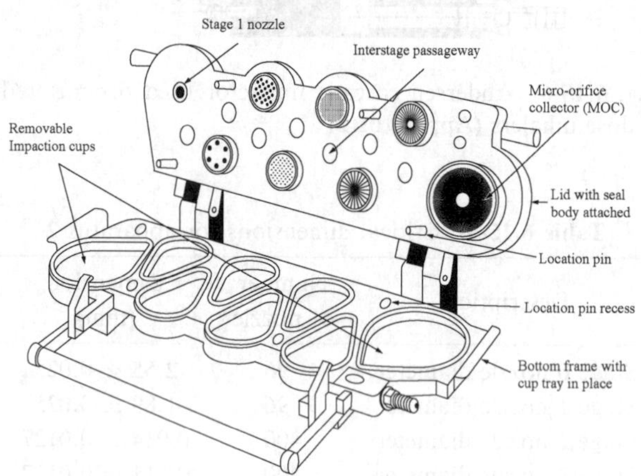

Fig. 6.15-9 Apparatus 3 showing component parts

The impactor configuration has removable impaction cups with all the cups in one plane (Figures 6.15-8 to 6.15-11). There are three main sections to the impactor; the bottom frame that holds the impaction cups, the seal body that holds the jets and the lid that contains the interstage passageways (Figures 6.15-8 and 6.15-9). Multiple nozzles are used at all but the first stage (Fig. 6.15-10). The flow passes through the impactor in a saw-tooth pattern.

Critical dimensions are provided in Table 6.15-5.

In routine operation, the seal body and lid are held together as a single assembly. The impaction cups are accessible when this assembly is opened at the end of an inhaler test. The cups are held in a support tray, so that all cups can be removed from the impactor simultaneously by lifting out the tray.

An induction port with internal dimensions defined in Fig. 6.15-4 connects to the impactor inlet. A pre-separator can be added when required, typically with dry powder inhalers, and connects between the induction port and the impactor. A suitable mouthpiece adapter is used to provide an airtight seal between the inhaler and the induction port.

Table 6.15-5 Critical dimensions for apparatus 3

Description	Dimension (mm)
Pre-separator (dimension a—see Fig. 6.15-12)	12.8 ± 0.05
Stage 1* nozzle diameter	14.3 ± 0.05
Stage 2* nozzle diameter	4.88 ± 0.04
Stage 3* nozzle diameter	2.185 ± 0.02
Stage 4* nozzle diameter	1.207 ± 0.01
Stage 5* nozzle diameter	0.608 ± 0.01
Stage 6* nozzle diameter	0.323 ± 0.01
Stage 7* nozzle diameter	0.206 ± 0.01
MOC*	aprox. 0.070
Cup depth (dimension b—see Fig. 6.15-11)	14.625 ± 0.10
Collection cup surface roughness (Ra)	0.5 to 2 μm
Stage 1 nozzle to seal body distance** —dimension c	0 ± 1.18
Stage 2 nozzle to seal body distance** —dimension c	5.236 ± 0.736
Stage 3 nozzle to seal body distance** —dimension c	8.445 ± 0.410
Stage 4 nozzle to seal body distance** —dimension c	11.379 ± 0.237
Stage 5 nozzle to seal body distance** —dimension c	13.176 ± 0.341
Stage 6 nozzle to seal body distance** —dimension c	13.999 ± 0.071
Stage 7 nozzle to seal body distance** —dimension c	14.000 ± 0.071
MOC nozzle to seal body distance** —dimension c	14.429 to 14.571

* See Fig. 6.15-10
** See Fig. 6.15-11

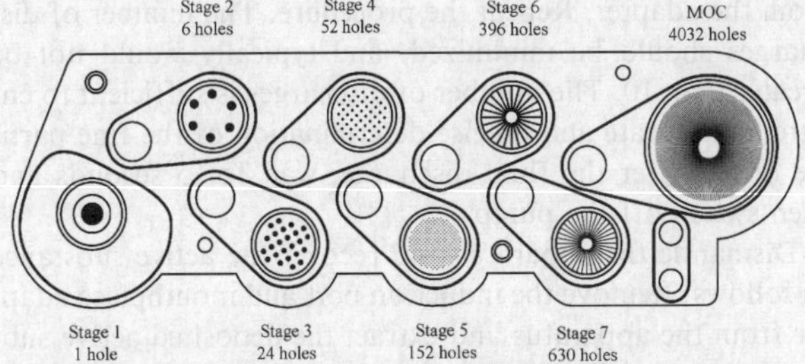

Fig. 6.15-10 Apparatus 3: nozzle configuration

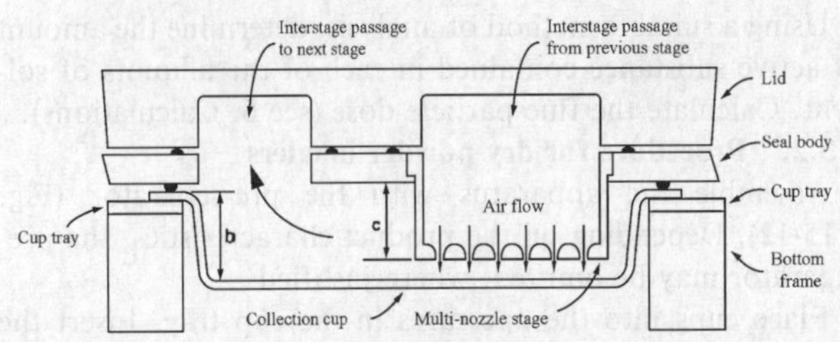

Fig. 6.15-11 Apparatus 3: configuration of interstage passageways

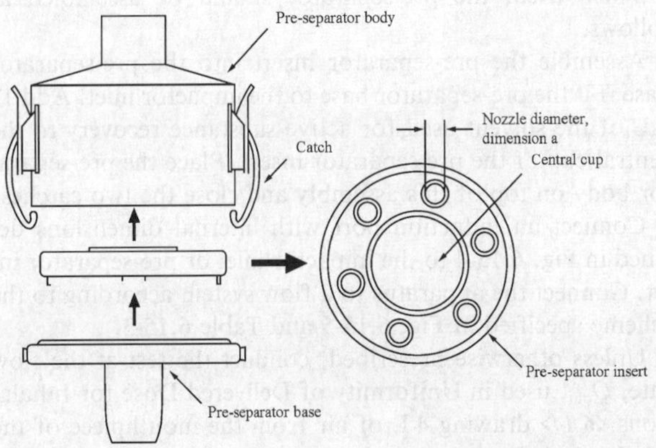

Fig. 6.15-12 Apparatus 3: pre-separator configuration

Apparatus 3 contains a terminal MOC that for most preparations will eliminate the need for a final filter as determined by method validation. The MOC is a collection plate with nominally 4032 holes, each approximately 70 μm in diameter. Most particles not captured on stage 7 of the impactor will be captured on the cup surface below the MOC. For impactors operated at 60 L per minute, the MOC is capable of collecting 80% of 0.14 μm particles. For preparations with a significant fraction of particles not captured by the MOC, there is an optional filter holder that can replace the MOC or be placed downstream of the MOC (a glass fiber filter is suitable).

5.3.1. Procedure for metered-dose inhalers

Place cups into the apertures in the cup tray. Insert the cup tray into the bottom frame, and lower into place. Close the impactor lid with the seal body attached and operate the handle to lock the impactor together so that the system is airtight.

Connect an induction port with internal dimensions defined in Fig. 6.15-4 to the impactor inlet. Place a suitable mouthpiece adapter in position at the end of the induction port. The mouthpiece end of the inhaler to the mouthpiece adapter, when inserted, lines up along the horizontal axis of the induction port. The front face of the inhaler mouthpiece must be flush with the front face of the induction port. When attached to the mouthpiece adapter, the inhaler is positioned in the same orientation as intended for use. Connect a suitable pump to the outlet of the apparatus and adjust the air flow through the apparatus, as measured at the inlet to the induction port, to 30 L per minute (±5%). Switch off the pump.

Unless otherwise prescribed in the patient instructions, shake the inhaler for 5 seconds and discharge one delivery to waste. Switch on the pump to the apparatus, locate the mouthpiece end of the inhaler in the adapter and discharge the inhaler into the apparatus, actuating the inhaler for a sufficient time to ensure a complete discharge.

Wait for 5 seconds before removing the assembled inhaler

from the adapter. Repeat the procedure. The number of discharges should be minimized, and typically would not be greater than 10. The number of discharges is sufficient to ensure an accurate and precise determination of the fine particle dose. After the final discharge, wait for 5 seconds and then switch off the pump.

Dismantle the apparatus and recover the active substance as follows. Remove the induction port and mouthpiece adapter from the apparatus and extract the deposited active substance into an aliquot of the solvent. Open the impactor by releasing the handle and lifting the lid. Remove the cup tray, with the collection cups, and extract the active substance in each cup into an aliquot of the solvent.

Using a suitable method of analysis, determine the amount of active substance contained in each of the aliquots of solvent. Calculate the fine particle dose (see 6. Calculations).

5.3.2. Procedure for dry powder inhalers

Assemble the apparatus with the pre-separator (Fig. 6.15-12). Depending on the product characteristics, the pre-separator may be omitted, where justified.

Place cups into the apertures in the cup tray. Insert the cup tray into the bottom frame, and lower into place. Close the impactor lid with the seal body attached and operate the handle to lock the impactor together so that the system is airtight.

When used, the pre-separator should be assembled as follows.

Assemble the pre-separator insert into the pre-separator base. Fit the pre-separator base to the impactor inlet. Add 15 mL of the solvent used for active substance recovery to the central cup of the pre-separator insert. Place the pre-separator body on top of this assembly and close the two catches.

Connect an induction port with internal dimensions defined in Fig. 6.15-4 to the impactor inlet or pre-separator inlet. Connect the apparatus to a flow system according to the scheme specified in Fig. 6.15-5 and Table 6.15-3.

Unless otherwise prescribed, conduct the test at the flow rate, Q_{out}, used in Uniformity of Delivered Dose for Inhalations <*6.14*> drawing 4 L of air from the mouthpiece of the inhaler and through the apparatus. Connect a flowmeter to the induction port. Use a flowmeter calibrated for the volumetric flow leaving the meter, or calculate the volumetric flow leaving the meter (Q_{out}) using the ideal gas law. For a meter calibrated for the entering volumetric flow (Q_{in}), use the following expression:

$$Q_{out} = \frac{Q_{in} \times P_0}{P_0 - \Delta P}$$

P_0: atmospheric pressure

ΔP: pressure drop over the meter

Adjust the flow control valve to achieve steady flow through the system at the required rate, Q_{out} ($\pm 5\%$). Ensure that critical flow occurs in the flow control valve by the procedure described in 5.1.2. Procedure for dry powder inhalers. Switch off the pump.

Place a suitable mouthpiece adapter in position at the end of the induction port. The mouthpiece end of the inhaler, when inserted to the mouthpiece adapter, lines up along the horizontal axis of the induction port. The front face of the inhaler mouthpiece must be flush with the front face of the induction port. When attached to the mouthpiece adapter, the inhaler is positioned in the same orientation as intended for use.

Prepare the dry powder inhaler for use according to the patient instructions. With the pump running and the 2-way solenoid valve closed, locate the mouthpiece of the inhaler in the mouthpiece adapter. Discharge the powder into the apparatus by opening the valve for the required time, T ($\pm 5\%$). Repeat the discharge sequence. The number of discharges should be minimized and typically would not be greater than 10. The number of discharges is sufficient to ensure an accurate and precise determination of fine particle dose.

Dismantle the apparatus and recover the active substance as follows.

Remove the induction port and mouthpiece adapter from the pre-separator, when used, and extract the deposited active substance into an aliquot of the solvent. When used, remove the pre-separator from the impactor, being careful to avoid spilling the cup liquid into the impactor. Recover the active substance from the pre-separator.

Open the impactor by releasing the handle and lifting the

Table 6.15-6 Calculations for Apparatus 1

Cut-off diameter (μm)	Mass of active substance deposited on stage per discharge	Cumulative mass of active substance per discharge	Cumulative fraction of active substance (%)
$d_4 = 1.7 \times q$	Mass from filter stage (m_5*)	$c_4 = m_5$	$f_4 = (c_4/c) \times 100$
$d_3 = 3.1 \times q$	Mass from stage 4 (m_4)	$c_3 = c_4 + m_4$	$f_3 = (c_3/c) \times 100$
$d_2 = 6.8 \times q$	Mass from stage 3 (m_3)	$c_2 = c_3 + m_3$	$f_2 = (c_2/c) \times 100$
	Mass from stage 2 (m_2)	$c = c_2 + m_2$	100

* Stage 5 is the filter stage.

$q = \sqrt{(60/Q)}$, Q: the test flow rate in L per minute (Q_{out} for dry powder inhalers).

Table 6.15-7 Calculations for Apparatus 2 when used at a flow rate of 28.3 L per minute

Cut-off diameter (μm)	Mass of active substance deposited on stage per discharge	Cumulative mass of active substance per discharge	Cumulative fraction of active substance (%)
$d_7 = 0.4$	Mass from filter stage (m_8)	$c_7 = m_8$	$f_7 = (c_7/c) \times 100$
$d_6 = 0.7$	Mass from stage 7 (m_7)	$c_6 = c_7 + m_7$	$f_6 = (c_6/c) \times 100$
$d_5 = 1.1$	Mass from stage 6 (m_6)	$c_5 = c_6 + m_6$	$f_5 = (c_5/c) \times 100$
$d_4 = 2.1$	Mass from stage 5 (m_5)	$c_4 = c_5 + m_5$	$f_4 = (c_4/c) \times 100$
$d_3 = 3.3$	Mass from stage 4 (m_4)	$c_3 = c_4 + m_4$	$f_3 = (c_3/c) \times 100$
$d_2 = 4.7$	Mass from stage 3 (m_3)	$c_2 = c_3 + m_3$	$f_2 = (c_2/c) \times 100$
$d_1 = 5.8$	Mass from stage 2 (m_2)	$c_1 = c_2 + m_2$	$f_1 = (c_1/c) \times 100$
$d_0 = 9.0$	Mass from stage 1 (m_1)	$c_0 = c_1 + m_1$	$f_0 = (c_0/c) \times 100$
	Mass from stage 0 (m_0)	$c = c_0 + m_0$	100

Table 6.15-8 Calculations for Apparatus 3

Cut-off diameter (μm)	x	Mass of active substance deposited on stage per discharge	Cumulative mass of active substance per discharge	Cumulative fraction of active substance (%)
$d_7 = 0.34 \times q$	0.67	Mass from MOC or terminal filter (m_8)	$c_7 = m_8$	$F_7 = (c_7/c) \times 100$
$d_6 = 0.55 \times q$	0.60	Mass from stage 7 (m_7)	$c_6 = c_7 + m_7$	$F_6 = (c_6/c) \times 100$
$d_5 = 0.94 \times q$	0.53	Mass from stage 6 (m_6)	$c_5 = c_6 + m_6$	$F_5 = (c_5/c) \times 100$
$d_4 = 1.66 \times q$	0.47	Mass from stage 5 (m_5)	$c_4 = c_5 + m_5$	$F_4 = (c_4/c) \times 100$
$d_3 = 2.82 \times q$	0.50	Mass from stage 4 (m_4)	$c_3 = c_4 + m_4$	$F_3 = (c_3/c) \times 100$
$d_2 = 4.46 \times q$	0.52	Mass from stage 3 (m_3)	$c_2 = c_3 + m_3$	$F_2 = (c_2/c) \times 100$
$d_1 = 8.06 \times q$	0.54	Mass from stage 2 (m_2)	$c_1 = c_2 + m_2$	$F_1 = (c_1/c) \times 100$
		Mass from stage 1 (m_1)	$c = c_1 + m_1$	100

$q = (60/Q)^x$, Q: the test flow rate in L per minute, x: listed in the table

lid. Remove the cup tray, with the collection cups, and extract the active substance in each cup into an aliquot of the solvent.

Using a suitable method of analysis, determine the amount of active substance contained in each of the aliquots of solvent. Calculate the fine particle dose (see 6. Calculations).

6. Calculations

From the analysis of the solutions, calculate the mass of active substance deposited on each stage per discharge and the mass of active substance per discharge deposited in the induction port, mouthpiece adapter and when used, the pre-separator.

Starting at the collection site (filter or MOC) close to the airflow outlet of the apparatus, derive a table of cumulative mass versus cut-off diameter of the respective stage (see Table 6.15-6 for Apparatus 1, Table 6.15-7 for Apparatus 2, Table 6.15-8 for Apparatus 3). Calculate the Fine Particle Dose (FPD) by interpolation of the mass of the active substance less than or equal to 5 μm. Or it is possible to calculate the FPD as the mass of the active substance deposited on the stages corresponding to the cut-off diameter of 5 μm and less.

If necessary, and where appropriate (e.g., where there is a log-normal distribution), determine values for the Mass Median Aerodynamic Diameter (MMAD) and Geometric Standard Deviation (GSD) from the cumulative fraction of active substance versus cut-off diameter (see Tables 6.15-6 to 6.15-8). Appropriate computational methods may also be used.

6.16 Rheological Measurements for Semi-solid Preparations

Rheological measurements for semi-solid preparations are methods to measure fluidity and deformation by adding force to semi-solid preparations such as Semi-solid Preparations for Oro-mucosal Application, Ophthalmic Ointments, Ointments, Creams and Gels.

There are two methods: spreadability test and penetrometry.

These methods are more practical to determine rheological properties of semi-solid preparations, though Method II Viscosity measurement by rotational viscometer under Viscosity Determination <2.53> can evaluate precisely rheological properties of semi-solids.

1. Spreadability test

Spreadability test is a method for measuring flowability of semi-solid preparations using a spread meter (also known as a parallel plate viscometer).

A spread meter measures a spreading diameter etc. of a sample by observing the characteristic of the concentric spreading over time when the sample is sandwiched between two parallel plates [glass (or plastic) plate and fixed plate] placed horizontally and pushed outward with the own weight of the glass plate.

Generally there is a reciprocal relationship between fluidity as an index of flowability and viscosity, however flowability measured by this method does not necessarily correlate with apparent viscosity (mPa·s) measured by viscosity determination.

This method targets relatively soft preparations in particular among semi-solid preparations.

1.1. Apparatus

An example of spread meters is shown in Fig. 6.16-1.

There are two parallel plates placed horizontally. The fixed plate installed in the lower part has engraved scales at 1 mm intervals to measure the distance from the center and has a cylindrical hole (0.5 mL) at the center for inserting a sample.

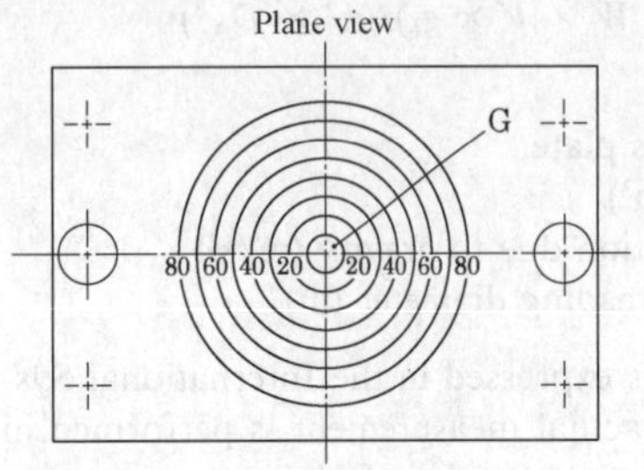

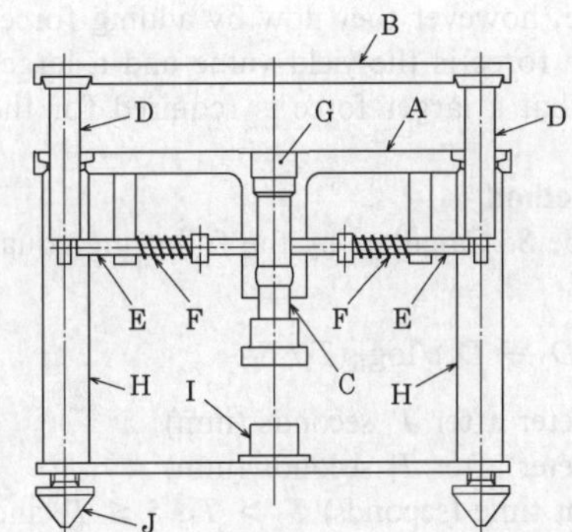

Fig. 6.16-1 Example of spread meter

The weight-loading glass plate positioned in the upper part is made of transparent glass or acrylate resin etc. and has a mass of 115 g. The glass plate is supported by rods. Pushing the piston up raise the bottom of the hole to push the sample above the fixed plate. In connection with it the glass plate falls (20 mm, commonly) and the sample spreads concentrically on the fixed plate with the own weight of the glass plate. Measuring the extent of the spread provides the flowability of the sample.

1.2. Procedure and measurement conditions

Before measurement remove a glass plate from an apparatus and clean the glass plate, a fixed plate and a specimen hole. Fill a sample in the specimen hole at the center of the fixed plate and flatten the sample by a spatula etc. so that the upper face of the sample is flush with the fixed plate and become flat. Wipe the sample protruded off. Make sure that the apparatus is horizontal by a level and install the glass plate to the support rod. Push the piston up and start time measurement simultaneously. Measure the spread of the sample on the fixed plate by the scale in mm unit over time and record them.

A constant temperature is needed during measurement and it is preferable to perform the measurement in the room controlled at 25 ± 2°C.

Bring the temperature of samples equal to that of the measurement environment by allowing them to stand in the measurement environment.

1.3. Analysis

Characteristics of flowability obtained with the measurement using a spread meter are expressed as spread meter diameter D and spread meter yield value YV in the case of the single-point method and as spread meter slope S and spread meter intercept IC in the case of the multi-point method. They are calculated by the following methods, respectively.

1.3.1. Single-point method

(i) Spread meter diameter D: Expressed as the spreading diameter (mm) after the specified time (usually, 60 seconds).

A larger spreading diameter indicates higher flowability.

(ii) Spread meter yield value YV: Calculate by the following equation.

$$YV = (4.8 \times W \times V \times g_n)/(\pi^2 \times D_\infty{}^5)$$

YV: Yield value (Pa)
W: Mass (kg) of glass plate
V: Sample volume (m^3)
g_n: Standard acceleration due to gravity (m/s^2)
D_∞: Maximum of spreading diameter (m)

The above equation is expressed in the International System of Units, however actual measurement is performed in the Centimeter-Gram-Second System of Units.

Many semi-solid preparations have no flowability when leave them as they are, however they flow by adding force. The limit value of the force is the yield value and a larger yield value indicates that a larger force is required for the flow of a sample.

1.3.2. Multi-point method

(i) Spread meter slope S: Calculate by the following equation.

$$S = (D_2 - D_1)/\log_{10}(T_2/T_1)$$

D_1: Spreading diameter after T_1 seconds (mm)
D_2: Spreading diameter after T_2 seconds (mm)
T_1, T_2: Measurement time (seconds) $T_2 > T_1$, $5 \leqq T_1$ and $T_2 \leqq 100$, $\Delta T = (T_2 - T_1) > 40$

In general, plot the spreading diameter measured each time on a semi-logarithmic graph to obtain an almost straight line connecting each point. Spread meter slope S corresponds to its slope.

A larger S indicates a larger flow of a sample.

(ii) Spread meter intercept IC: Plot logarithms of times (T_1, T_2) as abscissa against spreading diameters (D_1, D_2) as ordinate and draw a line connecting these two points. Obtain the intersection point ($T = 1$) of this extension line and the ordinate axis as spread meter IC.

A larger IC indicates higher flowability of a sample.

2. Penetrometry

Penetrometry is a method for measuring hardness or softness of semi-solid preparations using a penetrometer.

A penetrometer is an apparatus for measuring the distance traveled by a cone penetrant inside a sample and the consistency is expressed as ten times of the value measured in units of 0.1 mm. A smaller value indicates a harder sample.

This method targets relatively hard preparations in particular among semi-solid preparations.

2.1. Apparatus

2.1.1. Penetrometer

An example of penetrometers is shown in Fig. 6.16-2.

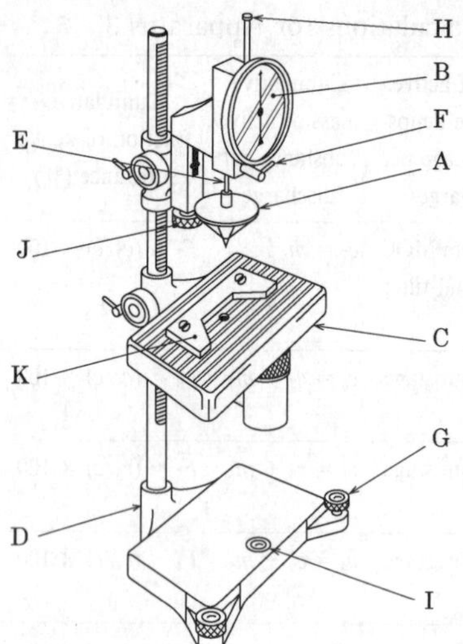

A: Cone
B: Dial gage
C: Sample stage
D: Support base
E: Holder
F: Metal clamping tool
G: Screw for horizontal control
H: Rack for measurement
I: Level
J: Fine adjustment knob
K: Centering tool

Fig. 6.16-2 Example of penetrometer

Adjust a penetrometer so that the position of the tip of a prescribed cone touches the surface of a sample filled in a sample container, penetrate the cone into the sample with its own weight for a certain time and calculate the consistency from the depth measured in units of 0.1 mm.

Adjust exactly the cone part or the sample stage of the penetrometer so that the position of the tip of the cone touches the horizontal surface of the sample keeping the reading of the dial gage zero. Adjust the cone in advance so that the cone falls more than 62 mm smoothly when released from the state fixed to the penetrometer and the top of the cone does not hit the bottom of the sample container after the fall. The penetrometer must be equipped with a screw for horizontal control and a level to maintain a cone holder being vertical.

2.1.2. Cone

A standard cone is a conical body made of magnesium or other suitable metal, which has a removable hardened steel needle. Fig. 6.16-3 shows the specifications of the standard cone.

The upper end of a holder is equipped with a stopper and the lower end is devised to connect a cone. The inner struc-

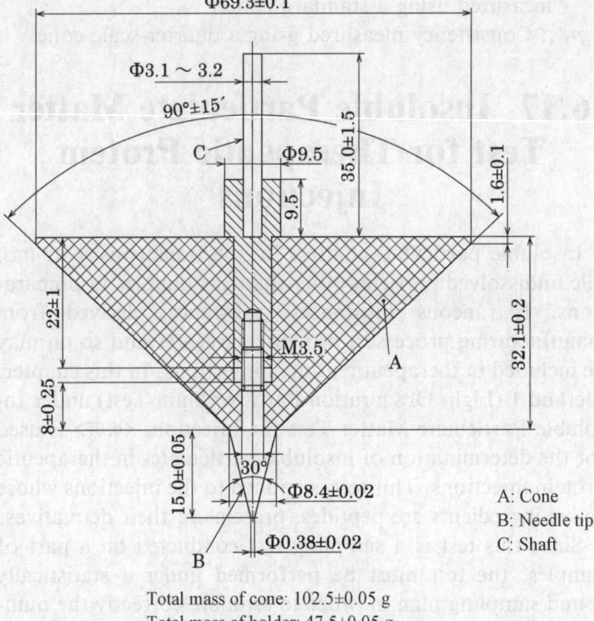

Fig. 6.16-3 Standard cone

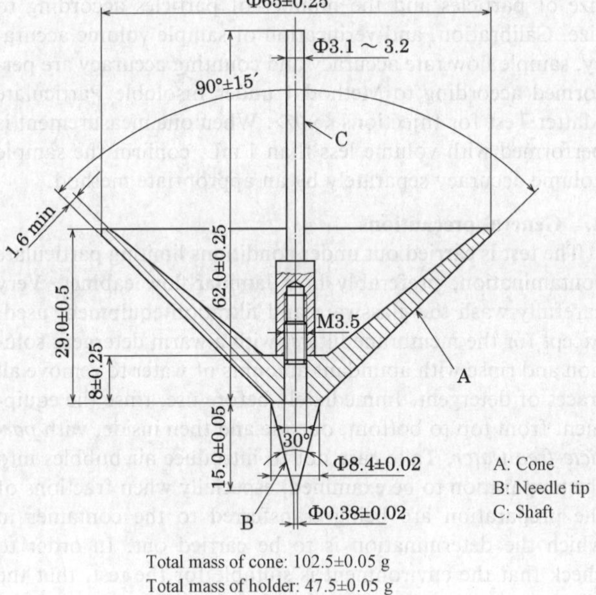

Fig. 6.16-4 Optional cone

ture of the cone may be changed in order to conform to the prescribed mass as far as there is no change in shape and mass distribution of the cone. The outer surface of the cone must be without scratches and smooth enough.

Fig. 6.16-4, 6.16-5 and 6.16-6 show the specifications of an optional cone, a half-scale cone and a quarter-scale cone. The half-scale and quarter-scale cones are the prescribed cones that are scaled down to a half and a quarter of the standard cone or the optional cone.

Select a suitable cone based on the sample volume and the consistency of a preparation to be tested and convert the measured consistency to the value equivalent to that measured using a standard cone.

An optional cone may be used to measure the sample having a consistency of not more than 400. Use a half-scale cone or a quarter-scale cone, when a sample has a consistency of

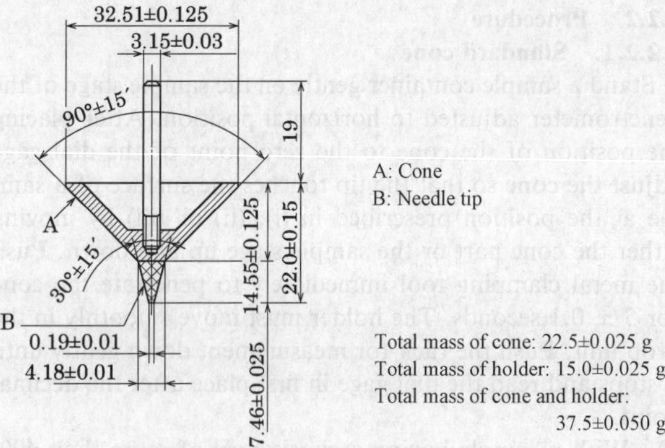

Fig. 6.16-5 Half-scale cone

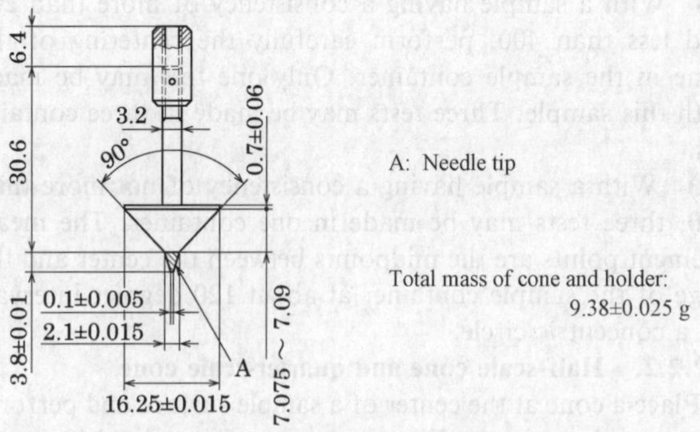

Fig. 6.16-6 Quarter-scale cone

175 to 385 and a standard cone is not available because of small sample amounts.

2.2. Procedure and measurement conditions

2.2.1. Sample preparation

Stand a prepared empty container and a container with a lid containing a necessary amount of a sample in a water bath at 25°C and bring the temperature of the sample at 25 ± 0.5°C. Transfer the sample in the container with a lid to the empty container at a time, if possible. Remove air bubbles mixed in the sample in the sample container by a suitable method and fill the container with an excessive amount of the sample using a spatula again. Be careful not to stir the sample and not to make vacant space inside the sample in this procedure. Flatten the surface of the sample by removal of the excessive sample by moving a spatula, of which surface is inclined about 45 degrees in the direction of the movement, along the upper edge of the container. Hereafter do not touch the surface of the sample before measurement. Perform the test promptly to keep the temperature of the sample evenly at 25 ± 0.5°C.

The consistency of soft samples is affected by the container diameter. With soft samples having a consistency of not less than 265, use a container with an inside diameter of 76.2 mm (a half-scale cone: 38.1 mm, a quarter-scale cone: 19.0 mm). The consistency of relatively hard samples having a consistency of not more than 265 is hardly affected by the container diameter when using a container with an inside diameter of not less than 76.2 mm.

The amount of sample required for the test depends on the sizes of the sample container and the cone, and the procedure specified according to the consistency.

2.2.2. Procedure

2.2.2.1. Standard cone

Stand a sample container gently on the sample stage of the penetrometer adjusted to horizontal position. After placing the position of the cone to the zero point of the dial gage adjust the cone so that the tip touches the surface of a sample at the position prescribed in (i), (ii) or (iii) by moving either the cone part or the sample stage up and down. Push the metal clamping tool immediately to penetrate the cone for 5 ± 0.1 seconds. The holder must move smoothly in the drop unit. Push the rack for measurement down gently until it stops and read the dial gage in first place after the decimal point.

(i) With a sample having a consistency of more than 400, only one test may be made in one container by placing the center of the sample container within 0.3 mm from the needle tip. Three tests may be made in three containers.

(ii) With a sample having a consistency of more than 200 and less than 400, perform carefully the centering of the cone in the sample container. Only one test may be made with this sample. Three tests may be made in three containers.

(iii) With a sample having a consistency of not more than 200, three tests may be made in one container. The measurement points are the midpoints between the center and the edge of the sample container at about 120 degrees intervals on a concentric circle.

2.2.2.2. Half-scale cone and quarter-scale cone

Place a cone at the center of a sample surface and perform a penetration pretest. The pretest may be omitted if an approximate value of consistency is known. Perform the measurement of consistency according to the procedure in 2.2.2.1. and place the position of the tip according to the following (i) or (ii).

(i) With a sample having a consistency of more than 97 when using a half-scale cone or more than 47 when using a quarter-scale cone, only one test may be made in one container by placing carefully the needle tip at the center of the sample container. Three tests may be made in three containers.

(ii) With a sample having a consistency of not more than 97 when using a half-scale cone or not more than 47 when using a quarter-scale cone, three tests may be made in one sample container. The measurement points are the midpoints between the center and the edge of the sample container at about 120 degrees intervals on a concentric circle so that the cone does not collide with the edge of the sample container and the measurement position of previous tests.

2.3. Analysis

2.3.1. Conversion of consistency measured using a half-scale or quarter-scale cone

Convert the consistency obtained using a half-scale or quarter-scale cone to the value equivalent to that obtained using a standard cone by the following equation.

2.3.1.1. Conversion of consistency obtained using a half-scale cone

$$P = 2p_{1/2} + 5$$

P: Consistency converted to the value equivalent to that measured using the standard cone

$p_{1/2}$: Consistency measured using a half-scale cone

2.3.1.2. Conversion of consistency obtained using a quarter-scale cone

$$P = 3.75p_{1/4} + 24$$

P: Consistency converted to the value equivalent to that measured using a standard cone

$p_{1/4}$: Consistency measured using a quarter-scale cone

6.17 Insoluble Particulate Matter Test for Therapeutic Protein Injections

Insoluble particulate matters in injections consist of mobile undissolved particles other than gas bubbles in preparations. Extraneous substances, substances derived from manufacturing processes, protein aggregates and so on may be included in therapeutic protein injections. In this chapter, Method 1 (Light Obscuration Particle Count Test) under Insoluble Particulate Matter Test for Injections <*6.07*> is used for the determination of insoluble particulates in therapeutic protein injections. This test is applied to the injections whose active ingredients are peptides, proteins or their derivatives.

Since this test is a sampling test conducted on a part of samples, the test must be performed under a statistically sound sampling plan in order to estimate correctly the number of particles in the population.

1. Apparatus

Use a suitable apparatus based on the principle of light blockage which allows an automatic determination of the size of particles and the number of particles according to size. Calibration, and verification of sample volume accuracy, sample flow rate accuracy and counting accuracy are performed according to Method 1 under Insoluble Particulate Matter Test for Injections <*6.07*>. When one measurement is performed with volume less than 1 mL, confirm the sample volume accuracy separately by an appropriate method.

2. General precautions

The test is carried out under conditions limiting particulate contamination, preferably in a laminar-flow cabinet. Very carefully wash the glassware and filtration equipment used, except for the membrane filters, with a warm detergent solution and rinse with abundant amounts of water to remove all traces of detergent. Immediately before use, rinse the equipment from top to bottom, outside and then inside, with *particle-free water*. Take care not to introduce air bubbles into the preparation to be examined, especially when fractions of the preparation are being transferred to the container in which the determination is to be carried out. In order to check that the environment is suitable for the test, that the glassware is properly cleaned and that the number of particles in the *particle-free water* to be used is within specifications, the following test is carried out using 5 mL of the *particle-free water*. When one measurement is performed with volume less than 1 mL, 1 mL of *particle-free water* may be used. Determine the particulate contamination of 5 samples of *particle-free water*. If the number of particles of 10 μm or greater size exceeds 1 per 1 mL, the precautions taken for the test are not sufficient. In this case, the preparatory steps must be repeated until the environment, filtration equipment glassware and *particle-free water* are suitable for the test.

3. Method

Treat a protein solution in an appropriate manner because of its tendency to generate air bubbles. In the case of an injection to be dissolved before use, use a specified solvent. When solvent is not specified, dissolve in *particle-free water* or use other suitable solvent comparable to *particle-free water*. Mix the contents of the sample gently and thoroughly by an appropriate procedure such as swirling the container slowly. If the container is sealed, cautiously remove the sealing closure. Clean the outer surfaces of the container opening using a jet of *particle-free water* and remove the closure, avoiding any contamination at the contents. For elimination of air bubbles, it is recommended to allow a container to stand under ambient pressure or reduced pressure. Other procedures are applicable if confirmed to be appropriate. Sonicating is not appropriate because it may aggregate or denature proteins. If necessary, after degassing, mix the contents gently and thoroughly by swirling slowly the container so as not to introduce air bubbles, and use it for the test. The measurement volume is 1 to 5 mL. The measurement volume can be reduced to 0.2 mL when the validity of the reduction is confirmed in considering the property of the sample and the tare volume of the apparatus. Set the volume necessary for the test in consideration of counting 4 portions.

In the case of injections where the volume necessary for the test can be obtained from one container, individual containers are tested. For injections with insufficient volume, combine the contents of several containers in one clean container to obtain the necessary volume after mixing the contents of containers gently and thoroughly. Where justified, the volume necessary for the test may be prepared by diluting the test solution with *particle-free water* or an appropriate solvent comparable to *particle-free water*. The validity of the dilution procedure and the solvent used for the dilution is confirmed by, for example, demonstrating consistent result regardless of the dilution. The number of test specimens must be adequate to provide a statistically sound assessment.

Take 4 portions and count the number of particles equal to or greater than 10 μm and 25 μm. Disregard the result obtained for the first portion, and calculate the mean number of particles for the preparation to be examined.

4. Evaluation

The preparation complies with the test if the average number of particles meets the following requirement.

A—Solutions for injection supplied in containers with a nominal content of equal to or more than 100 mL.

The average number of particles of equal to or greater than 10 μm does not exceed 25 per mL and that of particles of equal to or greater than 25 μm does not exceed 3 per mL.

B—Solutions for injection supplied in containers with a nominal content of less than 100 mL.

The average number of particles of equal to or greater than 10 μm does not exceed 6000 per container and that of particles of equal to or greater than 25 μm does not exceed 600 per container.

7. Tests for Containers and Packing Materials

7.01 Test for Glass Containers for Injections

The glass containers for injections do not interact physically or chemically with the contained medicament to alter any property or quality, can protect the contained medicament from the invasion of microbes by means of perfect sealing or other suitable process, and meet the following requirements. The surface-treated container for aqueous infusion is made from glass which meets the requirements for the soluble alkali test for a container not to be fused under method 1.

(1) The containers are colorless or light brown and transparent, and have no bubbles which interfere the test of Foreign Insoluble Matter Test for Injections <*6.06*>.

(2) Multiple-dose containers are closed by rubber stoppers or any other suitable stoppers. The stoppers permit penetration of an injection needle without detachment of fragments, and upon withdrawal of the needle, they reclose the containers immediately to prevent external contamination, and also do not interact physically or chemically with the contained medicaments.

Containers intended for aqueous infusions are closed by rubber stoppers meeting the requirements of the test for Rubber Closure for Aqueous Infusions <*7.03*>.

(3) Soluble alkali test—The testing methods may be divided into the following two methods according to the type of container or the dosage form of the medicament.

(i) Method 1: This method is applied to containers to be fused, or containers not to be fused except containers for aqueous infusions with a capacity exceeding 100 mL.

Rinse thoroughly the inside and outside of the containers to be tested with water, dry, and roughly crush, if necessary. Transfer 30 to 40 g of the glass to a steel mortar, and crush. Sieve the crushed glass through a No. 12 (1400 μm) sieve. Transfer the portion retained on the sieve again to the steel mortar, and repeat this crushing procedure until 2/3 of the amount of powdered glass has passed through a No. 12 (1400 μm) sieve. Combine all portions of the glass powder passed through a No. 12 (1400 μm) sieve, shake the sieve in a horizontal direction for 5 minutes with slight tapping at intervals using No. 18 (850 μm) and No. 50 (300 μm) sieves. Transfer 7 g of the powder, which has passed through a No. 18 (850 μm) sieve but not through a No. 50 (300 μm) sieve to a No. 50 (300 μm) sieve, immerse it in a suitable container filled with water, and wash the contents with gentle shaking for 1 minute. Rinse again with ethanol (95) for 1 minute, dry the washed glass powder at 100°C for 30 minutes, and allow to cool in a desiccator (silica gel). Transfer exactly 5.0 g of the powder thus prepared to a 200-mL conical flask of hard glass, add 50 mL of water, and gently shake the flask so that the powder disperses on the bottom of the flask evenly. Cover the flask with a small beaker of hard glass or a watch glass of hard glass, then heat it in boiling water for 2 hours, and immediately cool to room temperature. Decant the water from the flask into a 250-mL conical flask of hard glass, wash well the residual powdered glass with three 20-mL portions of water, and add the washings to the decanted water. Add 5 drops of bromocresol green-methyl red TS and titrate <*2.50*> with 0.01 mol/L sulfuric acid VS until the color of the solution changes from green through pale grayish blue to pale grayish red-purple. Perform a blank determination in the same manner, and make any necessary correction.

The quantity of 0.01 mol/L sulfuric acid VS consumed does not exceed the following quantity, according to the type of containers.

Containers to be fused	0.30 mL
Containers not to be fused (including injection syringes used as containers)	2.00 mL

(ii) Method 2: This method is applied to containers not to be fused for aqueous infusions with a capacity exceeding 100 mL.

Rinse thoroughly the inside and outside of the containers to be tested with water, and dry. Add a volume of water equivalent to 90% of the actual capacity of the container, cover it with a small beaker of hard glass or close tightly with a suitable stopper, heat in an autoclave at 121°C for 1 hour, and allow to stand until the temperature falls to room temperature. Pipet 100 mL of this solution, and transfer to a 250-mL conical flask of hard glass. Add 5 drops of bromocresol green-methyl red TS, and titrate *<2.50>* with 0.01 mol/L sulfuric acid VS until the color of the solution changes from green through pale grayish blue to pale grayish red-purple. Pipet 100 mL of water, transfer to a 250-mL conical flask of hard glass, perform a blank determination in the same manner, and make any necessary correction. The quantity of 0.01 mol/L sulfuric acid VS consumed does not exceed 0.10 mL.

(4) Soluble iron test for light-resistant containers—Rinse thoroughly five or more light-resistant containers to be tested with water, and dry at 105°C for 30 minutes. Pour a volume of 0.01 mol/L hydrochloric acid VS corresponding to the labeled volume of the container into individual containers, and fuse them. In the case of containers not to be fused, cover them with small beakers of hard glass or watch glasses of hard glass. Heat them at 105°C for 1 hour. After cooling, prepare the test solution with 40 mL of this solution according to Method 1 of Iron Limit Test *<1.10>*, and perform the test according to Method B. Prepare the control solution with 2.0 mL of the Standard Iron Solution.

(5) Light transmission test for light-resistant containers—Cut five light-resistant containers to be tested, prepare test pieces with surfaces as flat as possible, and clean the surfaces. Fix a test piece in a cell-holder of a spectrophotometer to allow the light pass through the center of the test piece perpendicularly to its surface. Measure the light transmittance of the test piece with reference to air between 290 nm and 450 nm and also between 590 nm and 610 nm at intervals of 20 nm each. The percent transmissions obtained between 290 nm and 450 nm are not more than 50% and that between 590 nm and 610 nm are not less than 60%. In the case of containers not to be fused having a wall thickness not less than 1.0 mm, the percent transmissions between 590 nm and 610 nm are not less than 45%.

7.02 Test Methods for Plastic Containers

Test methods for plastic containers may be used for designing and assuring quality of plastic containers. Not all tests described here will be necessary in any phases for any containers. On the other hand, the set does not include sufficient numbers and kinds of tests needed for any design verification and quality assurance of any containers. Additional tests may be considered if necessary.

It is not allowable for plastic containers for aqueous injections to interact with the pharmaceutical contained therein resulting in the deterioration of its efficacy, safety or stability, and to contaminate with microorganisms. They should meet the requirements prescribed in 2. Requirements for Plastic Containers for Aqueous Injections.

1. Test methods

1.1. Combustion tests

1.1.1. Residue on ignition

Weigh accurately about 5 g of cut pieces of the container and perform the test according to Residue on Ignition *<2.44>*.

1.1.2. Heavy metals

Place an appropriate amount of cut pieces of the container in a porcelain crucible, and perform the test according to Method 2 of Heavy Metals Limit Test *<1.07>*. Prepare the control solution with 2.0 mL of Standard Lead Solution.

1.1.3. Lead

1.1.3.1. Method 1

Place 2.0 g of cut pieces of a container in a crucible of platinum or quartz, moisten with 2 mL of sulfuric acid, heat slowly to dryness, then heat to combustion at between 450°C and 500°C. Repeat this procedure, if necessary. After cooling, moisten the residue with water, add 2 to 4 mL of hydrochloric acid, evaporate to dryness on a water bath, then add 1 to 5 mL of hydrochloric acid, and warm to dissolve. Then add 0.5 to 1 mL of a mixture of a solution of citric acid monohydrate (1 in 2) and hydrochloric acid (1:1), and add 0.5 to 1 mL of a warmed solution of ammonium acetate (2 in 5). Filter through a glass filter (G3) if insoluble matter remains. To the obtained filtrate add 10 mL of a solution of diammonium hydrogen citrate (1 in 4), 2 drops of bromothymol blue TS and ammonia TS until the color of the solution changes from yellow to green. Then add 10 mL of a solution of ammonium sulfate (2 in 5) and water to make 100 mL. Add 20 mL of a solution of sodium *N,N*-diethyldithiocarbamate trihydrate (1 in 20) to this solution, mix, allow to stand for a few minutes, then add 20.0 mL of 4-methyl-2-pentanone, and shake vigorously. Allow to stand to separate the 4-methyl-2-pentanone layer, filter if necessary, and use the layer as the sample solution.

Separately, to 2.0 mL of Standard Lead Solution add water to make exactly 10 mL. To 1.0 mL of this solution add 10 mL of a solution of diammonium hydrogen citrate (1 in 4) and 2 drops of bromothymol blue TS, then proceed in the same manner as for the sample solution, and use the solution so obtained as the standard solution.

Perform the test with the sample solution and standard solution according to Atomic Absorption Spectrophotometry *<2.23>* under the following conditions, and determine the concentration of lead in the sample solution.

Gas: Combustible gas—Acetylene or hydrogen.
Supporting gas—Air.
Lamp: Lead hollow-cathode lamp.
Wavelength: 283.3 nm.

1.1.3.2. Method 2

Cut a container into pieces smaller than 5-mm square, take 2.0 g of the pieces into a glass beaker, add 50 mL of 2-butanone and 0.1 mL of nitric acid, and warm to dissolve. To this solution add 96 mL of methanol gradually to precipitate a resinous substance, and filter by suction.

Wash the beaker and the resinous substance with 12 mL of methanol followed by 12 mL of water, combine the washings and the filtrate, and concentrate to about 10 mL under reduced pressure. Transfer into a separator, add 10 mL of ethyl acetate and 10 mL of water, shake vigorously, and allow to stand to separate the water layer. Evaporate the water layer to dryness, add 5 mL of hydrochloric acid to the residue, and warm to dissolve. Then add 1 mL of a mixture of a solution of citric acid monohydrate (1 in 2) and hydrochloric acid (1:1), and add 1 mL of a warmed solution of ammonium acetate (2 in 5). Filter through a glass filter (G3) if insoluble matter remains. To the solution so obtained add 10 mL of a solution of diammonium hydrogen citrate (1 in 4) and 2 drops of bromothymol blue TS, and then add ammonia TS until the color of the solution changes from yellow to green. Further add 10 mL of a solution of ammonium sulfate (2 in 5) and water to make 100 mL. Add 20 mL of a solution of sodium *N,N*-diethyldithiocarbamate trihydrate (1 in 20) to this solution, mix, allow to stand for a few minutes, then add 20.0 mL of 4-methyl-2-pentanone, and shake vigorously. Allow to stand to separate the 4-methyl-2-pentanone layer, filter the layer if necessary, and use the layer as the sample solution.

Separately, pipet 5 mL of Standard Lead Solution, add water to make exactly 50 mL, and to 2.0 mL of this solution add 10 mL of a solution of diammonium hydrogen citrate (1 in 4) and 2 drops of bromothymol blue TS, then proceed in the same manner as for the sample solution, and use the solution so obtained as the standard solution. Perform the test with the sample solution and standard solution according to Atomic Absorption Spectrophotometry <*2.23*> under the conditions described in Method 1, and determine the concentration of lead in the sample solution.

1.1.4. Cadmium

1.1.4.1. Method 1

To 2.0 mL of Standard Cadmium Solution add 10 mL of a solution of diammonium hydrogen citrate (1 in 4) and 2 drops of bromothymol blue TS, and proceed in the same manner as for the sample solution in "1.1.3.1. Method 1", and use the solution so obtained as the standard solution. Perform the test with the sample solution obtained in "1.1.3.1. Method 1" and the standard solution according to Atomic Absorption Spectrophotometry <*2.23*> under the following conditions, and determine the concentration of cadmium in the sample solution.

Gas: Combustible gas—Acetylene or hydrogen.
  Supporting gas—Air.

Lamp: Cadmium hollow-cathode lamp.

Wavelength: 228.8 nm.

1.1.4.2. Method 2

To 2.0 mL of Standard Cadmium Solution add 10 mL of a solution of diammonium hydrogen citrate (1 in 4) and 2 drops of bromothymol blue TS, and proceed in the same manner as for the sample solution in "1.1.3.2. Method 2", and use the solution so obtained as the standard solution. Perform the test with the sample solution obtained in "1.1.3.2. Method 2" and the standard solution according to Atomic Absorption Spectrophotometry <*2.23*> under the conditions described in "1.1.4.1. Method 1", and determine the concentration of cadmium in the sample solution.

1.1.5. Tin

Cut a container into pieces smaller than 5-mm square, place 5.0 g of the pieces in a Kjeldahl flask, add 30 mL of a mixture of sulfuric acid and nitric acid (1:1), and decompose by gentle heating in a muffle furnace, occasionally adding dropwise a mixture of sulfuric acid and nitric acid (1:1) until the content changes to a clear, brown solution. Then heat until the color of the solution changes to a clear, light yellow, and heat to slowly concentrate to practical dryness. After cooling, dissolve the residue in 5 mL of hydrochloric acid by warming, and after cooling, add water to make exactly 10 mL. Pipet 5 mL of this solution into a 25-mL volumetric flask (A). Transfer the remaining solution to a 25-mL beaker (B) by washing out with 10 mL of water, add 2 drops of bromocresol green TS, neutralize with diluted ammonia solution (28) (1 in 2), and measure the volume consumed for neutralization as *a* mL. To the volumetric flask, A, add potassium permanganate TS dropwise until a slight pale red color develops, and add a small amount of L-ascorbic acid to decolorize. Add 1.5 mL of 1 mol/L hydrochloric acid TS, 5 mL of a solution of citric acid monohydrate (1 in 10), *a* mL of diluted ammonia solution (28) (1 in 2), 2.5 mL of polyvinyl alcohol TS, 5.0 mL of phenylfluorone-ethanol TS and water to make 25 mL. Shake well, then allow to stand for about 20 minutes, and use this solution as the sample solution.

Separately, pipet 1.0 mL of Standard Tin Solution, add 5 mL of water, add potassium permanganate TS dropwise until a slight pale red color develops, proceed in the same manner as for the sample solution, and use this solution as the standard solution.

Determine the absorbances of the sample solution and the standard solution according to Ultraviolet-visible Spectrophotometry <*2.24*> at 510 nm, using water as the blank.

1.2. Extractable substances

Cut the container at homogeneous regions of low curvature and preferably the same thickness, gather pieces to make a total surface area of about 1200 cm² when the thickness is 0.5 mm or less, or about 600 cm² when the thickness is greater than 0.5 mm, and subdivide in general into strips approximately 0.5 cm in width and 5 cm in length. Wash them with water, and dry at room temperature. Place these strips in a 300-mL hard glass vessel, add exactly 200 mL of water, and seal the opening with a suitable stopper. After heating the vessel in an autoclave at 121°C for 1 hour, take out the vessel, allow to stand until the temperature falls to room temperature, and use the content as the test solution.

For containers made of composite plastics, the extraction may be performed by filling a labeled volume of water in the container. In this case, it is necessary to record the ratio of the volume of water used and the inside area of the container.

When containers are deformed at 121°C, the extraction may be performed at the highest temperature which does not cause deformation among the following conditions: at 100 ± 2°C for 2 ± 0.2 hours, at 70 ± 2°C for 24 ± 2 hours, at 50 ± 2°C for 72 ± 2 hours or at 37 ± 1°C for 72 ± 2 hours.

Prepare the blank solution with water in the same manner. For containers made of composite plastics, water is used as the blank solution.

Perform the following tests with the test solution and the blank solution:

(i) Foaming test: Place 5 mL of the test solution in a glass-stoppered test tube about 15 mm in inside diameter and about 200 mm in length, shake vigorously for 3 minutes, and measure the time needed for almost complete disappearance of the foam thus generated.

(ii) pH <*2.54*>: To 20 mL each of the test solution and the blank solution add 1.0 mL of a solution of potassium chloride (1 in 1000), and obtain the difference in the reading of pH between these solutions.

(iii) Potassium permanganate-reducing substances: Place 20.0 mL of the test solution in a glass-stoppered conical flask, add 20.0 mL of 0.002 mol/L potassium permanganate VS and 1 mL of dilute sulfuric acid, and boil for 3 minutes. After cooling, add 0.10 g of potassium iodide, stopper tightly, shake, then allow to stand for 10 minutes, and titrate <*2.50*> with 0.01 mol/L sodium thiosulfate VS (indicator: 5 drops of starch TS). Perform the test in the same manner, using 20.0 mL of the blank solution, and obtain the difference of the consumption of 0.002 mol/L potassium permanganate VS between these solutions.

(iv) UV spectrum: Read the maximum absorbances between 220 nm and 240 nm and between 241 nm and 350 nm of the test solution against the blank solution as directed under Ultraviolet-visible Spectrophotometry <*2.24*>.

(v) Residue on evaporation: Evaporate 20 mL of the test solution on a water bath to dryness, and weigh the residue after drying at 105°C for 1 hour.

1.3. Test for fine particles

1.3.1. Test procedure

Rinse thoroughly the inside and outside of containers to be tested with water for particle matter test, fill the container with the labeled volume of water for particulate matter test or 0.9 w/v% sodium chloride solution, adjust the amount of air in the container to about 50 mL per 500 mL of the labeled volume, put tight stopper to the container, and heat it at 121°C for 25 minutes in an autoclave. After allowing to cool for 2 hours, take out the container from the autoclave, and then allow to stand at ordinary temperature for about 24 hours. If the containers are deformed at 121°C, employ a suitable temperature-time combination as directed under 1.2. Extractable substances. Clean the outside of the container, mix by turning upside-down 5 or 6 times, insert immediately a clean needle of filterless infusion set into the container through the rubber closure of the container, take the effluent from the container while mixing gently in a clean container for measurement, and use it as the test solution.

Counting of the fine particles must be performed in dustless, clean facilities or apparatus, using a light-shielded automatic fine particle counter. The sensor of the counter to be used must be able to count fine particles of 1.5 μm or more in diameter. The volume to be measured is 10 mL. Adjust the counter before measurement. For calibration of the diameter and number of particles, the standard particles for calibration of the light-shielded automatic fine particle counter should be used in suspension in water for particulate matter test or 0.9 w/v% sodium chloride solution.

Count five times the numbers of particles with diameters of 5 - 10 μm, 10 - 25 μm and more than 25 μm while stirring the test solution, and calculate the average particle numbers of four counts, excluding the first, as the number of particles in 1.0 mL of the test solution.

1.3.2. Reagent

Water for particulate matter test and 0.9 w/v% sodium chloride solution to be used for the tests should not contain more than 0.5 particles of 5 - 10 μm in size per 1.0 mL.

1.4. Transparency test

1.4.1. Method 1

This method can only be applied to containers which have a smooth and not embossed surface and rather low curvature.

Cut the container at homogeneous regions of low curvature and preferably the same thickness to make 5 pieces of about 0.9 × 4 cm in size, immerse each piece in a cell for determination of the ultraviolet spectrum filled with water, and determine the transmittance at 450 nm as directed under Ultraviolet-visible Spectrophotometry <*2.24*> using a cell filled with water as a blank.

1.4.2. Method 2

Sensory test—This method can be applied to containers which have a rough or embossed surface. It can also be applied to testing of the transparency of containers in case where the turbidity of their pharmaceutical contents must be checked.

1.4.2.1. Test solutions

(i) Formazin standard suspension: To 15 mL of formazin stock suspension add water to make 1000 mL. Use within 24 hours of preparation. Shake thoroughly before use.

(ii) Reference suspension: To 50 mL of Formazin standard suspension add water to make 100 mL.

1.4.2.2. Test procedures

(i) with control: Take two of containers to be tested, and fill one of them with the labeled volume of the reference suspension and the other with the same volume of water. Show these two containers to five subjects, separately, ask which one seems to be more turbid, and calculate the rate of correct answers.

(ii) without control: Take six of containers to be tested, put number to each of them, and fill three of them with the labeled volume of the reference suspension and the others with the same volume of water. Show each one of these containers at random order to five subjects, separately, ask if it is turbid or not, and calculate the percentage of the answer judged as "turbid" (100 X/15, X: number of containers judged as "turbid") for reference suspension-filled containers group and water-filled containers group, respectively.

1.5. Water vapor permeability test

1.5.1. Method 1

This test method is applicable to containers for aqueous injection. Fill the container with the labeled volume of water. After closing it hermetically, accurately weigh the container and record the value. Store the container at 65 ± 5% relative humidity and a temperature of 20 ± 2°C for 14 days, and then accurately weigh the container again and record the value. Calculate the mass loss during storage.

1.5.2. Method 2

This test method is provided for evaluating moisture permeability of containers for hygroscopic drugs. Unless otherwise specified, perform the test according to the following procedure.

1.5.2.1. Desiccant

Place a quantity of calcium chloride for water determination in a shallow container, taking care to exclude any fine powder, then dry at 110°C for 1 hour, and cool in a desiccator.

1.5.2.2. Procedure

Select 12 containers, clean their surfaces with a dry cloth, and close and open each container 30 times in the same manner. Ten among the 12 containers are used as "test containers" and the remaining two, as "control containers". A torque for closing screw-capped containers is specified in Table 7.02-1. Add desiccant to 10 of the containers, designated test containers, filling each to within 13 mm of the closure if the container volume is 20 mL or more, or filling each to two-thirds of capacity if the container volume is less than 20 mL. If the interior of the container is more than 63 mm in depth, an inert filler or spacer may be placed in the bottom to minimize the total mass of the container and

Table 7.02-1 Torque applicable to screw-type container

Closure Diameter (mm)	Torque (N·cm)
8	59
10	60
13	88
15	59 - 98
18	78 - 118
20	88 - 137
22	98 - 157
24	118 - 206
28	137 - 235
30	147 - 265
33	167 - 284
38	196 - 294
43	196 - 304
48	216 - 343
53	235 - 402
58	265 - 451
63	284 - 490
66	294 - 510
70	314 - 569
83	363 - 735
86	451 - 735
89	451 - 794
100	510 - 794
110	510 - 794
120	618 - 1069
132	677 - 1069

desiccant; the layer of desiccant in such a container shall be not less than 5 cm in depth. Close each container immediately after adding desiccant, applying the torque designated in the table. To each of the control containers, add a sufficient number of glass beads to attain a mass approximately equal to that of each of the test containers, and close, applying the torque designated in the table. Record the mass of the individual containers so prepared to the nearest 0.1 mg if the container volume is less than 20 mL, to the nearest 1 mg if the container volume is 20 mL or more but less than 200 mL, or to the nearest 10 mg if the container volume is 200 mL or more, and store the containers at 75 ± 3% relative humidity and a temperature of 20 ± 2°C.

After 14 days, record the mass of the individual containers in the same manner. Completely fill 5 empty containers with water or a non-compressible, free-flowing solid such as fine glass beads, to the level indicated by the closure surface when in place. Transfer the contents of each to a graduated cylinder, and determine the average container volume, in mL. Calculate the rate of moisture permeability, in mg per day per liter, by use of the formula:

$$(1000/14V)\ [(T_f - T_i) - (C_f - C_i)]$$

V: Average volume (mL)

$T_f - T_i$: Difference between the final and initial masses of each test container (mg)

$C_f - C_i$: Average of the differences between the final and initial masses of the two controls (mg)

1.6. Leakage test

Fill a container with a solution of fluorescein sodium (1 in 1000), stopper tightly, place filter papers on and under the container, and apply a pressure of 6.9 N (0.7 kg)/cm² at 20°C for 10 minutes. Judge the leakiness by observing the color of the paper.

1.7. Cytotoxicity test

The following test methods are designed to detect cytotoxic substances in plastic materials by evaluating the cytotoxicity of the culture medium extracts from plastic containers for pharmaceutical products. Other appropriate standard methods of cytotoxicity testing may be used for the evaluation, if appropriate. However, the final decision shall be made based upon the test methods given here, if the test results obtained according to the other methods are questionable. Other than those of the culture medium, reagents and test solutions being specified for the test may be used if they meet for the purpose of the test.

1.7.1. Cell lines

The recommended cell lines are L929 cells (ATCC. CCL1) and V79 cells (JCRB0603). In addition, other established cell lines may be used when it is confirmed that they form well-defined colonies reproducibly, with characteristics comparable to those of L929 cells and V79 cells.

1.7.2. Culture medium

(i) Medium for L929 cells: To Eagle's minimum essential medium add fetal calf serum (FCS) to make 10 vol% FCS.

(ii) Medium for V79 cells: M05 medium prepared by adding 10 mL each of nonessential amino acid TS and 100 mmol/L sodium pyruvate TS to 1000 mL of Eagle's minimum essential medium, then adding fetal calf serum (FCS) to make 5 vol% FCS. Medium for L929 cells may be used instead if it gives equivalent sensitivity.

1.7.3. Reference materials and control substances

(i) Negative reference material: high-density polyethylene film

(ii) Positive reference material (A): polyurethane film containing 0.1% zinc diethyldithiocarbamate

(iii) Positive reference material (B): polyurethane film containing 0.25% zinc dibutyldithiocarbamate

(iv) Control substances: zinc diethyldithiocarbamate or zinc dibutyldithiocarbamate

1.7.4. Test procedure

(i) Sample preparation: When the material of the container consists of a single homogeneous layer, subdivide the cut pieces of a container into pieces of the size of approximately 2 × 15 mm and subject the pieces to the test. When the material of the container has multiple layers, prepare cut pieces with a surface area of one side of 2.5 cm² and subject the pieces to the test without subdividing them into smaller pieces.

(ii) Preparation of sample solutions: Transfer an appropriate amount of the sample to a screw-capped glass bottle or a sterile disposable centrifuge tube. Cap the bottle or tube loosely and cover the cap with clean aluminum foil. Sterilize the bottle or tube by autoclaving at 121°C for 15 minutes. When the material of the sample is not resistant to heat during autoclaving, gas sterilization with ethylene oxide (EO) may be used. In the case of EO sterilization, sufficient aeration should be achieved to avoid an additional toxic effect of residual EO in the test results. To the bottle or tube add the culture medium in a proportion of 1 mL per 2.5 cm² (one side) or 10 mL per 1 g of the sample, loosely cap the bottle or tube, and allow to stand in an incubator maintaining 5% carbon dioxide at 37°C for 24 hours. Transfer the culture medium extract, which is designated 100% sample solution, to a sterilized screw-capped glass bottle or a sterile disposable centrifuge tube. Dilute the 100% sample solution with fresh culture medium using a dilution factor of two to prepare serial dilutions having extract concentrations of 50%, 25%, 12.5%, 6.25%, 3.13% and so on.

(iii) Preparation of cell suspension: Remove the culture medium from the maintained cell culture vessel (flask or dish), and add gently a suitable volume of phosphate buffer solution for cytotoxicity test. Rinse the cells by gentle rotation of the slanted cell culture vessel two or three times, and discard the phosphate buffer solution. Add a sufficient volume of trypsin solution to cover the cell layer. Cap the vessel and place in an incubator maintaining 5% carbon dioxide at 37°C for 1 to 2 minutes. After confirming detachment of the cell layer from the bottom surface of the vessel by using a microscope and by gently tapping of the vessel, add an appropriate volume of the fresh culture medium and gently pipet the cells completely out of the vessel. Transfer the pipetted cell suspension into a sterile disposable centrifuge tube and centrifuge. Discard the supernatant liquid, resuspend the cells in an appropriate volume of flesh phosphate buffer solution for cytotoxicity test by pipetting, and centrifuge the tube again. Discard the supernatant liquid, and add an appropriate volume of fresh culture medium to the tube. Resuspend the cells by gentle pipetting and make a homogeneous cell suspension. Determine the cell concentration using a hemocytometer.

(iv) Cytotoxicity test: Dilute the cell suspension prepared according to procedure (iii) with culture medium to adjust the cell concentration to 100 cells/mL. Place a 0.5 mL aliquot of the diluted cell suspension on each well of a sterile disposable multiple well plate (24 wells). Incubate the plate in the incubator maintaining 5% carbon dioxide at 37°C for 4 - 24 hours to attach the cells to the bottom surface of the well. Discard the medium from each well, and add a 0.5 mL aliquot of the prepared sample solutions having various concentrations or fresh medium to at least 3 wells each. Place the plate immediately in the incubator and incubate the plate for the appropriate period: 7 - 9 days for L929 cells; 6 - 7 days for V79 cells. After the incubation, discard the medium from the plate, add an appropriate volume of methanol or dilute formaldehyde TS to each well and allow the plate to stand for about 30 minutes to fix the cells. Discard the methanol or dilute formaldehyde TS from each well and add an appropriate volume of dilute Giemsa's TS to each well. After ensuring good staining of the colonies, discard the stain solution from the wells, wash with water, dry, and count the number of colonies in each well. Calculate a mean number of colonies for each concentration of the sample solution, and divide the mean by the mean number of colonies for the fresh medium to obtain the relative plating efficiency (%) for each extract concentration of the sample solution. Plot the extract concentration (%) of the sample solution on a logarithmic scale and the relative plating efficiency on an ordinary scale on semilogarithmic graph paper to obtain a colony formation inhibition curve of the container. Read the 50% inhibition concentration, IC_{50} (%), at which the colony number is half that in the control group, from the inhibition curve.

It is recommended to check the sensitivity and the reproducibility of the test system by the use of suitable reference materials or control substances in the test system, if necessary.

2. Requirements for plastic containers for aqueous injections

2.1. Polyethylene or polypropylene containers for aqueous injections

The containers are made of polyethylene or polypropylene and free from any adhesive.

(1) Transparency—The containers have a transmittance of not less than 55%, when tested as directed in "1.4.1. Method 1". When "1.4.1. Method 1" can not be applied, test according to "1.4.2.2. (ii) Method 2B". In this case, the rate that the water-containing container is judged as "being turbid" is not more than 20%, and the rate that the reference suspension-containing container is judged as "being turbid" is not less than 80%.

(2) Appearance—The containers do not have strips, cracks, bubbles, or other faults which cause difficulties in practical use.

(3) Water vapor permeability—Proceed as directed in "1.5.1. Method 1". The loss of mass is not more than 0.20%.

(4) Heavy metals *<1.07>*—The test solution has no more color than the control solution when the amount of the sample taken is 1.0 g.

(5) Lead—Perform the test as directed in "1.1.3.1. Method 1". The absorbance of the sample solution is not more than that of the standard solution.

(6) Cadmium—Perform the test as directed in "1.1.4.1. Method 1". The absorbance of the sample solution is not more than that of the standard solution.

(7) Residue on ignition *<2.44>*—Not more than 0.1% (5 g).

(8) Extractable substances—

(i) Foaming test: the foam formed almost disappears within 3 minutes.

(ii) pH: the difference in the reading of pH between the test solution and the blank solution is not more than 1.5.

(iii) Potassium permanganate-reducing substances: The difference in the consumption of 0.002 mol/L potassium permanganate VS between the test solution and the blank solution is not more than 1.0 mL.

(iv) UV spectrum: The maximum absorbance between 220 nm and 240 nm is not more than 0.08, and that between 241 nm and 350 nm is not more than 0.05.

(v) Residue on evaporation: Not more than 1.0 mg.

(9) Cytotoxicity—IC_{50} (%) is not less than 90%. The result obtained by the other standard methods is negative.

2.2. Polyvinyl chloride containers for aqueous injections

The containers are composed of homopolymer of vinyl chloride, free from any adhesive, and the plasticizer added to the material should be only di(2-ethylhexyl)phthalate. The containers may be covered with easily removable material to prevent the permeation of water vapor. In this case, perform the water vapor permeability test on the covered containers.

(1) Thickness—Measure the thickness of a container at five different locations. The difference between the maximum and minimum values of thickness is 0.05 mm or less.

(2) Transparency—Proceed as directed in (1) under "2.1. Polyethylene or polypropylene containers for aqueous injections".

(3) Appearance—Proceed as directed in (2) under "2.1. Polyethylene or polypropylene containers for aqueous injections".

(4) Leakage—Proceed with the test according to "1.6. Leakage test". The solution contained does not leak.

(5) Flexibility—Insert the spike needle for infusion through a rubber closure of the container used in (4) Leakage. The contained solution is almost completely discharged without displacement by air.

(6) Water vapor permeability—Proceed as directed in (3) under "2.1. Polyethylene or polypropylene containers for aqueous injections".

(7) Heavy metals *<1.07>*—The test solution has no more color than the control solution when the amount of the sample taken is 1.0 g.

(8) Lead—Perform the test as directed in "1.1.3.2. Method 2". The absorbance of the sample solution is not more than that of the standard solution.

(9) Cadmium—Perform the test as directed in "1.1.4.2. Method 2". The absorbance of the sample solution is not more than that of the standard solution.

(10) Tin—The absorbance of the sample solution is not more than that of the standard solution.

(11) Vinyl chloride—Wash cut pieces of a container with water, wipe them thoroughly with a filter paper, subdivide them into pieces smaller than 5 mm square, and put 0.5 g of them into a 20-mL vial. Add 2.5 mL of *N,N*-dimethylacetoamide to the vial to dissolve the sample pieces, put a tight stopper on the vial, and use the solution in the vial as the sample solution. If the sample is hardly soluble, allow to stand the vial at room temperature for a night, put a tight stopper on the vial, and use the liquid part in the vial as the sample solution. Separately, to a 20-mL vial add 2.5 mL of *N,N*-dimethylacetoamide, add 50 μL of Standard Vinyl Chloride Solution, previously cooled with dry ice-methanol, put a tight stopper on the vial, and use the solution in the vial as the standard solution.

After heating the vials containing sample solution and standard solution at 90°C for 1 hour, perform the test with 0.5 mL each of vapor phases in these vials as directed under Gas Chromatography *<2.02>* according to the following conditions: the peak area of vinyl chloride obtained from the sample solution is not larger than that from the standard solution.

Operating conditions—

Detector: A hydrogen flame-ionization detector.

Column: A fused silicate column 0.25 mm in inside diameter and 25 m in length, coated the inside surface with porous styrene-divinylbenzene copolymer for gas chromatography the inside surface in 3 μm thickness.

Column temperature: Maintain at 50°C for 2 minutes

after injection, then rise to 120°C at a rate of 10°C per minute, then rise to 250°C at a rate of 20°C per minute, and keep at 250°C for 10 minutes.

Injection port temperature: A constant temperature of about 200°C.

Detector temperature: A constant temperature of about 250°C.

Carrier gas: Nitrogen or helium.

Flow rate: Adjust so that the retention time of vinyl chloride is about 7 minutes.

Split ratio: 1:5.

System suitability—

System performance: When the procedure is run with 0.5 mL of the vapor phase of the standard solution under the above operating conditions, vinyl chloride and ethanol are eluted in this order with the resolution between these peaks being not less than 3.0.

System repeatability: When the test is repeated 6 times under the above operating conditions with 0.5 mL of the vapor phase of the standard solution heated at 90°C for 1 hour, the relative standard deviation of the peak area of vinyl chloride is not more than 5.0%.

(12) Fine particles—The number of fine particles in 1.0 mL of the test solution is not more than 100 of 5 to 10 μm, not more than 10 of 10 to 25 μm and not more than 1 of 25 μm or more.

(13) Residue on ignition *<2.44>*—Not more than 0.1% (5 g).

(14) Extractable substances—Proceed as directed in (8) under "2.1. Polyethylene or polypropylene containers for aqueous injections".

(15) Cytotoxicity—Proceed as directed in (9) under "2.1. Polyethylene or polypropylene containers for aqueous injections".

2.3. Plastic containers for aqueous injections being not described above

The containers meet the following specifications and other necessary specifications for their materials with regard to heavy metals, residue on ignition and extractable substances, etc.

(1) Transparency—Proceed as directed in (1) under "2.1. Polyethylene or polypropylene containers for aqueous injections".

(2) Appearance—Proceed as directed in (2) under "2.1. Polyethylene or polypropylene containers for aqueous injections".

(3) Vapor permeability—Proceed as directed in (3) under "2.1. Polyethylene or polypropylene containers for aqueous injections".

(4) Cytotoxicity—Proceed as directed in (9) under "2.1. Polyethylene or polypropylene containers for aqueous injections".

7.03 Test for Rubber Closure for Aqueous Infusions

The rubber closure for aqueous infusions means a rubber closure (containing material coated or laminated with the stuff like plastics) used for a container for aqueous infusion having a capacity of 100 mL or more. The rubber closure when in use does not interact physically or chemically with the contained medicament to alter any property or quality, does not permit the invasion of microbes, does not disturb the use of the contained infusion, and meets the following requirements.

1. Cadmium

Wash the rubber closures with water, dry at room temperature, cut into minute pieces, mix well, place 2.0 g of them in a crucible of platinum or quartz, moisten them with 2 mL of sulfuric acid, heat gradually to dryness, and ignite between 450°C and 500°C until the residue is incinerated. When incineration was insufficient, moisten the residue with 1 mL of sulfuric acid, heat to dryness, and ignite again. Repeat the above-mentioned procedure if necessary. Cool the crucible, moisten the residue with water, add 2 to 4 mL of hydrochloric acid, heat on a water bath to dryness, add 1 to 5 mL of hydrochloric acid, and dissolve by heating. Then add 0.5 to 1 mL of a mixture of a solution of citric acid monohydrate (1 in 2) and hydrochloric acid (1:1) and 0.5 to 1 mL of a warmed solution of ammonium acetate (2 in 5). When any insoluble residue remains, filter through a glass filter. To the solution thus obtained add 10 mL of a solution of diammonium hydrogen citrate (1 in 4), 2 drops of bromothymol blue TS and ammonia TS until the color of the solution changes from yellow to green. Then add 10 mL of ammonium sulfate solution (2 in 5) and water to make 100 mL. Next, add 20 mL of a solution of sodium *N,N*-diethyldithiocarbamate trihydrate (1 in 20), mix, allow to stand for a few minutes, add 20 mL of 4-methyl-2-pentanone, and mix by vigorous shaking. Allow to stand to separate the 4-methyl-2-pentanone layer from the solution, filter if necessary, and use as the sample solution. On the other hand, to exactly 10 mL of Standard Cadmium Solution add 10 mL of a solution of diammonium hydrogen citrate (1 in 4) and 2 drops of bromothymol blue TS, proceed in the same manner as for the sample solution, and use this solution as the standard solution. Perform the tests according to Atomic Absorption Spectrophotometry *<2.23>* under the following conditions, using the sample solution and the standard solution. The absorbance of the sample solution is not more than that of the standard solution.

Gas: Combustible gas—Acetylene or hydrogen.

Supporting gas—Air.

Lamp: Cadmium hollow-cathode lamp.

Wavelength: 228.8 nm.

2. Lead

To exactly 1 mL of the Standard Lead Solution add 10 mL of a solution of diammonium hydrogen citrate (1 in 4) and 2 drops of bromothymol blue TS, proceed as directed for the sample solution under **1**, and use this solution as the standard solution. Perform the tests according to Atomic Absorption Spectrophotometry *<2.23>* under the following conditions, using the sample solution and the standard solution obtained in **1**. The absorbance of the sample solution is not more than that of the standard solution.

Gas: Combustible gas—Acetylene or hydrogen.

Supporting gas—Air.

Lamp: Lead hollow-cathode lamp.

Wavelength: 283.3 nm.

3. Extractable substances

Wash the rubber closures with water, and dry at room temperature. Place an amount of them, equivalent to about 150 cm^2 in surface area, in a glass vessel, add 2 mL of water per cm^2 of the sample, stopper adequately, heat at 121°C for 1 hour in an autoclave, take out the glass vessel, allow to cool to room temperature, then remove immediately the rubber closures, and use the remaining solution as the test solution. Prepare the blank solution with water in the same manner. Perform the following tests with the test solution and the blank solution.

3.1. Description

The test solution is clear and colorless. Read the transmittance of the test solution at 430 nm and 650 nm (10 mm), using the blank solution as the blank. Both of them are not less than 99.0%.

3.2. pH *<2.54>*

To 20 mL each of the test solution and the blank solution add 1 mL each of potassium chloride solution, prepared by dissolving 1.0 g of potassium chloride in water to make 1000 mL. The difference of pH between the two solutions is not more than 1.0.

3.3. Zinc

To exactly 10 mL of the test solution add diluted dilute nitric acid (1 in 3) to make exactly 20 mL, and use this solution as the sample solution. Further, to exactly 1 mL of Standard Zinc Solution for atomic absorption spectrophotometry add diluted nitric acid (1 in 3) to make exactly 20 mL, and use this solution as the standard solution. Perform the tests according to Atomic Absorption Spectrophotometry *<2.23>*, using these solutions, under the following conditions. The absorbance of the sample solution is not more than that of the standard solution.

Gas: Combustible gas—Acetylene.
 Supporting gas—Air.
Lamp: Zinc hollow-cathode lamp.
Wavelength: 213.9 nm.

3.4. Potassium Permanganate-reducing substances

Measure 100 mL of the test solution in a glass-stoppered conical flask, add 10 mL of 0.002 mol/L potassium permanganate VS, then add 5 mL of dilute sulfuric acid, and boil for 3 minutes. After cooling, add 0.10 g of potassium iodide, stopper, mix by shaking, then allow to stand for 10 minutes, and titrate *<2.50>* with 0.01 mol/L sodium thiosulfate VS (indicator: 5 drops of starch TS). Perform the blank test in the same manner, using 100 mL of the blank solution. The difference in mL of 0.002 mol/L potassium permanganate VS required between the tests is not more than 2.0 mL.

3.5. Residue on evaporation

Measure 100 mL of the test solution, evaporate on a water bath to dryness, and dry the residue at 105°C for 1 hour. The mass of the residue is not more than 2.0 mg.

3.6. UV spectrum

Read the absorbance of the test solution between 220 nm and 350 nm against the blank solution as directed under Ultraviolet-visible Spectrophotometry *<2.24>*: it is not more than 0.20.

4. Cytotoxicity test

The following test methods are designed to detect cytotoxic substances in rubber materials by evaluating the cytotoxicity of the culture medium extracts from rubber closure for aqueous infusion. Other appropriate standard methods of cytotoxicity testing may be used for the evaluation, if appropriate. However, the final decision shall be made based upon the test methods given here, if the test results obtained according to the other methods are questionable. Other than those of the culture medium, reagents and test solutions being specified for the test may be used if they meet for the purpose of the test.

4.1. Cell lines

The recommended cell lines are L929 cells (ATCC. CCL1) and V79 cells (JCRB0603). In addition, other established cell lines may be used when it is confirmed that they form well-defined colonies reproducibly, with characteristics comparable to those of L929 cells and V79 cells.

4.2. Culture medium

(i) Medium for L929 cells: To Eagle's minimum essential medium add fetal calf serum (FCS) to make 10 vol% FCS.

(ii) Medium for V79 cells: M05 medium prepared by adding 10 mL each of nonessential amino acid TS and 100 mmol/L sodium pyruvate TS to 1000 mL of Eagle's minimum essential medium, then adding fetal calf serum (FCS) to make 5 vol% FCS. Medium for L929 cells may be used instead if it gives equivalent sensitivity.

4.3. Reference materials and control substances

(i) Negative reference material: Highdensity polyethylene film

(ii) Positive reference material (A): Polyurethane film containing 0.1% zinc diethyldithiocarbamate

(iii) Positive reference material (B): Polyurethane film containing 0.25% zinc dibutyldithiocarbamate

(iv) Control substances: Zinc diethyldithiocarbamate (reagent grade) or zinc dibutyldithiocarbamate

4.4. Test procedure

(i) Sample preparation: Rubber closure is subjected to the test without cutting into pieces. Reference material is divided into pieces of approximately 2 × 15 mm and subjected to the test.

(ii) Preparation of sample solutions: Transfer an appropriate amount of the sample to a screw-capped glass bottle or a sterile disposable centrifuge tube. Cap the bottle or tube loosely and cover the cap with clean aluminum foil. Sterilize the bottle or tube by autoclaving at 121°C for 15 minutes. When the material of the sample is not resistant to heat during autoclaving, gas sterilization with ethylene oxide (EO) may be used. In the case of EO sterilization, sufficient aeration should be achieved to avoid an additional toxic effect of residual EO in the test results. To the bottle or tube add the culture medium in a proportion of 60 cm^2 surface area or 10 mL per 1 g of the sample, loosely cap the bottle or tube, and allow to stand in an incubator maintaining 5% carbon dioxide at 37°C for 24 hours. To the reference material add 10 mL of the culture medium per 1 g and extract in the same manner. Transfer the culture medium extract, which is designated 100% sample solution, to a sterilized screw-capped glass bottle or a sterile disposable centrifuge tube. Dilute the 100% sample solution with fresh culture medium using a dilution factor of two to prepare serial dilutions having extract concentrations of 50%, 25%, 12.5%, 6.25%, 3.13% and so on.

(iii) Preparation of cell suspension: Remove the culture medium from the maintained cell culture vessel (flask or dish), and add gently a suitable volume of phosphate buffer solution for cytotoxicity test. Rinse the cells by gentle rotation of the slanted cell culture vessel two or three times, and discard the phosphate buffer solution. Add a sufficient volume of trypsin solution to cover the cell layer. Cap the vessel and place in an incubator maintaining 5% carbon dioxide at 37°C for 1 to 2 minutes. After confirming detachment of the cell layer from the bottom surface of the vessel by using a microscope and by gently tapping of the vessel, add an appropriate volume of the fresh culture medium and gently pipet the cells completely out of the vessel. Transfer the pipetted cell suspension into a sterile disposable centrifuge tube and centrifuge. Discard the supernatant liquid, resuspend the cells in an appropriate volume of flesh phosphate buffer solution for cytotoxicity test by pipetting, and centrifuge the tube again. Discard the supernatant liquid, and add an appropriate volume of fresh culture medium to the vessel. Resuspend the cells by gentle pipetting and make a homogeneous cell suspension. Determine the cell concentration using a hemocytometer.

(iv) Cytotoxicity test: Dilute the cell suspension prepared according to procedure (iii) with culture medium to adjust the cell concentration to 100 cells/mL. Place a 0.5 mL aliquot of the diluted cell suspension on each well of a sterile disposable multiple well plate (24 wells). Incubate the plate in the incubator maintaining 5% carbon dioxide at 37°C for 4 – 24 hours to attach the cells to the bottom surface of the well. Discard the medium from each well, and add a 0.5 mL aliquot of the prepared sample solutions having various concentration or fresh medium to at least 3 wells each. Place the plate immediately in the incubator and incubate the plate for the appropriate period: 7 – 9 days for L929 cells; 6 – 7 days for V79 cells. After the incubation, discard the medium from the plate, add an appropriate volume of methanol or dilute formaldehyde TS to each well and allow the plate to stand for about 30 minutes to fix the cells. Discard the methanol or dilute formaldehyde TS from each well and add an appropriate volume of dilute Giemsa's TS to each well. After ensuring good staining of the colonies, discard the stain solution from the wells, wash with water, dry, and count the number of colonies in each well. Calculate a mean number of colonies for each concentration of the sample solution, and divide the mean by the mean number of colonies for the fresh medium to obtain the relative plating efficiency (%) for each extract concentration of the sample solution. Plot the extract concentration (%) of the sample solution on a logarithmic scale and the relative plating efficiency on an ordinary scale on semilogarithmic graph paper to obtain a colony formation inhibition curve of the rubber closure. Read the 50% inhibition concentration, IC_{50} (%), at which the colony number is half that in the negative control group, from the inhibition curve.

It is recommended to check the sensitivity and the reproducibility of the test system by the use of suitable reference materials or control substances in the test system, if necessary.

4.5. Interpretation

IC_{50} (%) is not less than 90%.

5. Acute systemic toxicity

This test is performed when the sample solution does not meet the requirements of the cytotoxicity test.

The sample solution meets the requirements, when examined under the following conditions against the blank solution.

5.1. Preparation of the sample solution and the blank solution

Wash the rubber closures with water and Water for Injection successively, and dry under clean conditions at room temperature avoiding contamination. Transfer the rubber closures to a glass container. Add isotonic sodium chloride solution of 10 times the mass of the test material, stopper adequately, heat in an autoclave at 121°C for 1 hour, take out the glass container, and allow to cool to room temperature. The solution thus obtained is used as the sample solution. The blank solution is prepared in the same manner.

5.2. Test procedures

(i) Test animals: Use healthy male or female mice of inbred strain or from a closed colony, weighing 17 to 25 g.

(ii) Procedure: Separate the animals into two groups of 5 mice, and inject intravenously 50 mL each of the solutions per kg body mass. From the viewpoint of animal rights, it is recommended to start the test with small size animal groups first, such as with 3 animals, and then add 2 animals to each group if the acceptable result was obtained.

5.3. Interpretation

Observe the animals for 72 hours after injection: During the observation period, none of the animals treated with the sample solution show any weight loss, abnormality or death.

9. Reference Standards; Standard Solutions; Reagents, Test Solutions; Measuring Instruments, Appliances, etc.

Reference Standards

9.01 Reference Standards

Generally, reference standards are standard materials used for quality tests of pharmaceuticals, prepared to constant quality, assured its level of quality by official organization, and supplied officially. The Japanese Pharmacopoeia Reference Standards are reference standards used for the tests of drugs specified in the Japanese Pharmacopoeia and for the General Tests. Besides, standard materials are substances employed as the standard for measuring chemical, physical and biological characteristics in a quantitative and qualitative manner, and also used for calibration and checking accuracy of apparatus for the tests of pharmaceuticals.

The Japanese Pharmacopoeia Reference Standards are used for Assay, Identification, Purity, calibration of apparatus and system suitability in monographs and in the General Tests. The application and usage of The Japanese Pharmacopoeia Reference Standards are directed in monographs and in the General Tests.

The Japanese Pharmacopoeia Reference Standards are as follows:

(1) The reference standards which are prepared by those who have been registered to prepare them by the Minister of Health, Labour and Welfare, according to the Ministerial ordinance established by the Minister separately.

Acetaminophen RS
Acetanilide for Apparatus Suitability RS
Acetophenetidine for Apparatus Suitability RS
Aciclovir RS
Adrenaline Bitartrate for Purity RS
Alendronate Sodium RS
Alprostadil RS
p-Aminobenzoyl Glutamic Acid for Purity RS
Amitriptyline Hydrochloride RS
Amlexanox RS
Amlodipine Besilate RS
Ampicillin RS
Anhydrous Lactose for Identification RS
Ascorbic Acid RS
Aspirin RS
Atorvastatin Calcium RS
Atropine Sulfate RS
Auranofin RS
Azathioprine RS
Azithromycin RS
Baclofen RS
Baicalin RS
Beclometasone Dipropionate RS
Berberine Chloride RS
Betamethasone RS
Betamethasone Sodium Phosphate RS
Betamethasone Valerate RS
Bicalutamide RS

Bisacodyl RS
Bromfenac Sodium RS
Butyl Parahydroxybenzoate RS
Cabergoline RS
Caffeine RS
Caffeine for Apparatus Suitability RS
Calcitonin Salmon RS
Calcium Folinate RS
Calcium Oxalate Monohydrate for Calibration of Apparatus RS
Calcium Pantothenate RS
Camostat Mesilate RS
d-Camphor RS
dl-Camphor RS
Carbidopa RS
Carboplatin RS
L-Carnosine RS
Cefazolin RS
Cefepime Dihydrochloride RS
Cefmetazole RS
Cefotiam Hydrochloride RS
Ceftriaxone Sodium RS
Celecoxib RS
Cellacefate for Identification RS
Cetotiamine Hydrochloride RS
Chlordiazepoxide RS
Chlormadinone Acetate RS
Chlorpheniramine Maleate RS
Cholecalciferol RS
Ciclosporin RS
Cilnidipine RS
Cilostazol RS
Ciprofloxacin RS
Cisplatin RS
Citicoline RS
Clarithromycin RS
Clobetasol Propionate RS
Clofibrate RS
Clomifene Citrate RS
Clopidogrel Sulfate RS
Cortisone Acetate RS
Cyanocobalamin RS
Danazol RS
Deferoxamine Mesilate RS
Deslanoside RS
Dexamethasone RS
Diethylcarbamazine Citrate RS
Diflorasone Diacetate RS
Diflucortolone Valerate RS
Digoxin RS
Dihydroergotoxine Mesilate RS
Dobutamine Hydrochloride RS
Docetaxel RS
Donepezil Hydrochloride RS
Doripenem RS
Dorzolamide Hydrochloride RS
Doxazosin Mesilate RS
Edrophonium Chloride RS
Elcatonin RS
Enalapril Maleate RS
Endotoxin RS
Entacapone RS
Entacapone Related Substance A for System Suitability RS
Epalrestat RS
Epirubicin Hydrochloride RS
Epitiostanol RS
Eplerenone RS
Epoetin Alfa RS
Epoetin Beta RS
Ergocalciferol RS
Ergometrine Maleate RS
Eribulin Mesilate RS
Eribulin Mesilate Related Substance C for System Suitability RS
Estradiol Benzoate RS
Estriol RS
Ethenzamide RS
Ethinylestradiol RS
Ethyl Aminobenzoate RS
Ethyl Icosapentate RS
Ethyl Loflazepate RS
Ethyl Parahydroxybenzoate RS
Etoposide RS
Fenofibrate RS
Fexofenadine Hydrochloride RS
Filgrastim RS
Fludrocortisone Acetate RS
Fluocinolone Acetonide RS
Fluocinonide RS
Fluorometholone RS
Flutamide RS
Fluvoxamine Maleate RS
Folic Acid RS
Fradiomycin Sulfate RS
Furosemide RS
Fursultiamine Hydrochloride RS
Gabexate Mesilate RS
Gatifloxacin RS
Gefarnate RS
Gefitinib RS
Ginsenoside Rb_1 RS
Ginsenoside Rg_1 RS
Gitoxin for Purity RS
Glimepiride RS
Glucagon RS
Glucose RS
D-Glucuronolactone RS
Glycyrrhizic Acid RS
Gonadorelin Acetate RS
Guaifenesin RS
Heparin Sodium RS
Heparin Sodium for Identification RS
Low-molecular Mass Heparin RS
High-molecular Mass Urokinase RS
Human Chorionic Gonadotrophin RS
Human Menopausal Gonadotrophin RS
Hydrochlorothiazide RS
Hydrocortisone RS
Hydrocortisone Acetate RS
Hydrocortisone Sodium Phosphate RS
Hydrocortisone Succinate RS
Hydroxyethylcellulose for Identification RS
Idoxuridine RS
Imipramine Hydrochloride RS
Indapamide RS
Indometacin RS
Insulin Aspart RS
Insulin Glargine RS
Insulin Human RS
Interleukin-2 RS
Ipriflavone RS
Isoflurane RS
Isomalt RS

Kallidinogenase RS
Lactose for Identification RS
Lactulose RS
Lanoconazole RS
Lansoprazole RS
Lenograstim RS
Leuprorelin Acetate RS
Limaprost RS
Losartan Potassium RS
Loxoprofen RS
Lysozyme RS
Maltose RS
Manidipine Hydrochloride RS
D-Mannitol RS
Mecobalamin RS
Medroxyprogesterone Acetate RS
Menatetrenone RS
Meropenem RS
Mestranol RS
Methotrexate RS
Methoxsalen RS
Methyldopa RS
Methylergometrine Maleate RS
Methyl Parahydroxybenzoate RS
Methylprednisolone Succinate RS
Methyltestosterone RS
Metildigoxin RS
Mexiletine Hydrochloride RS
Microcrystalline Cellulose for Identification RS
Miglitol RS
Minocycline Hydrochloride RS
Mitiglinide Calcium RS
Mizoribine RS
Montelukast Dicyclohexylamine RS
Montelukast Racemate for System Suitability RS
Montelukast for System Suitability RS
Montelukast Sodium for Identification RS
Nabumetone RS
Nartograstim RS
Nateglinide RS
Neostigmine Methylsulfate RS
Nicotinamide RS
Nicotinic Acid RS
Nilvadipine RS
Nizatidine RS
Noradrenaline Bitartrate RS
Norgestrel RS
Olmesartan Medoxomil RS
Over-sulfated Chondroitin Sulfate for System Suitability RS
Oxytocin RS
Ozagrel Sodium RS
Paeoniflorin RS
Paroxetine Hydrochloride RS
Pazufloxacin Mesilate RS
Pemirolast Potassium RS
Pentobarbital RS
Perphenazine RS
Phytonadione RS
Pioglitazone Hydrochloride RS
Piperacillin RS
Pitavastatin Methylbenzylamine RS
Potassium Sucrose Octasulfate RS
Povidone for Identification RS
Pranlukast RS
Pravastatin 1,1,3,3-Tetramethylbutylammonium RS
Prazosin Hydrochloride RS
Prednisolone RS
Prednisolone Acetate RS
Prednisolone Succinate RS
Primidone RS
Probenecid RS
Probucol RS
Prochlorperazine Maleate RS
Progesterone RS
Propiverine Hydrochloride RS
Propyl Parahydroxybenzoate RS
Puerarin RS
Pyridoxal Phosphate RS
Pyridoxine Hydrochloride RS
Quetiapine Fumarate RS
Rabeprazole Sodium RS
Ranitidine Hydrochloride RS
Reserpine RS
Residual Solvents Class 1 RS
Residual Solvents Class 2A RS
Residual Solvents Class 2B RS
Residual Solvents Class 2C RS
Residual Solvents for System Suitability RS
Retinol Acetate RS
Retinol Palmitate RS
Ribavirin RS
Riboflavin RS
Rilmazafone Hydrochloride RS
Risedronic Acid RS
Ritodrine Hydrochloride RS
Rosuvastatin Calcium RS
Roxatidine Acetate Hydrochloride RS
Roxithromycin RS
Saccharated Pepsin RS
Saccharin RS
Saccharin Sodium RS
Sarpogrelate Hydrochloride RS
Scopolamine Hydrobromide RS
Sennoside A RS
Sennoside B RS
Sevoflurane RS
Silodosin RS
Simvastatin RS
Sitagliptin Phosphate RS
Sitagliptin Phosphate for System Suitability RS
Sivelestat RS
Spironolactone RS
Sulbactam RS
Sulfadiazine Silver RS
Sulfanilamide for Apparatus Suitability RS
Sulfapyridine for Apparatus Suitability RS
Swertiamarin RS
Tacalcitol RS
Tacrolimus RS
Tazobactam RS
Teprenone RS
Testosterone Propionate RS
Thiamine Chloride Hydrochloride RS
Thiamylal RS
Thrombin RS
Timolol Maleate RS
Tocopherol RS
Tocopherol Acetate RS
Tocopherol Nicotinate RS
Tocopherol Succinate RS
Tolbutamide RS
Tolnaftate RS
Tosufloxacin Tosilate RS

Tranexamic Acid RS
Trehalose RS
Triamcinolone RS
Triamcinolone Acetonide RS
Triazolam RS
Trichlormethiazide RS
Trihexyphenidyl Hydrochloride RS
Troxipide RS
Tyrosine for Digestion Test RS
Ubidecarenone RS
Ulinastatin RS
Valaciclovir Hydrochloride RS
Valsartan RS
Vancomycin Hydrochloride RS
Vanillin for Apparatus Suitability RS
Vasopressin RS
Vinblastine Sulfate RS
Vincristine Sulfate RS
Voriconazole RS
Warfarin Potassium RS
Zidovudine RS
Zonisamide RS

(2) The reference standards which are prepared by National Institute of Infectious Diseases.

Aclarubicin RS
Actinomycin D RS
Amikacin Sulfate RS
Amoxicillin RS
Amphotericin B RS
Arbekacin Sulfate RS
Aspoxicillin RS
Aztreonam RS
Bacampicillin Hydrochloride RS
Bacitracin RS
Bekanamycin Sulfate RS
Benzylpenicillin Potassium RS
Bleomycin A_2 Hydrochloride RS
Carumonam Sodium RS
Cefaclor RS
Cefadroxil RS
Cefalexin RS
Cefalotin Sodium RS
Cefatrizine Propylene Glycolate RS
Cefbuperazone RS
Cefcapene Pivoxil Hydrochloride RS
Cefdinir RS
Cefditoren Pivoxil RS
Cefixime RS
Cefmenoxime Hydrochloride RS
Cefminox Sodium RS
Cefodizime Sodium RS
Cefoperazone RS
Cefotaxime RS
Cefotetan RS
Cefotiam Hexetil Hydrochloride RS
Cefozopran Hydrochloride RS
Cefpiramide RS
Cefpirome Sulfate RS
Cefpodoxime Proxetil RS
Cefroxadine RS
Cefsulodin Sodium RS
Ceftazidime RS
Cefteram Pivoxil Mesitylene Sulfonate RS
Ceftibuten Hydrochloride RS
Ceftizoxime RS
Cefuroxime Axetil RS
Chloramphenicol RS
Chloramphenicol Palmitate RS
Chloramphenicol Succinate RS
Ciclacillin RS
Clindamycin Hydrochloride RS
Clindamycin Phosphate RS
Cloxacillin Sodium RS
Colistin Sodium Methanesulfonate RS
Colistin Sulfate RS
Cycloserine RS
Daunorubicin Hydrochloride RS
Demethylchlortetracycline Hydrochloride RS
Dibekacin Sulfate RS
Dicloxacillin Sodium RS
Diethanolammonium Fusidate RS
Doxorubicin Hydrochloride RS
Doxycycline Hydrochloride RS
Enviomycin Sulfate RS
Erythromycin RS
Faropenem Sodium RS
Flomoxef Triethylammonium RS
Fosfomycin Phenethylammonium RS
Gentamicin Sulfate RS
Idarubicin Hydrochloride RS
Imipenem RS
Interferon Alfa RS
Isepamicin Sulfate RS
Josamycin RS
Josamycin Propionate RS
Kanamycin Monosulfate RS
Latamoxef Ammonium RS
Lenampicillin Hydrochloride RS
Leucomycin A_5 RS
Lincomycin Hydrochloride RS
Lithium Clavulanate RS
Micronomicin Sulfate RS
Midecamycin RS
Midecamycin Acetate RS
Mitomycin C RS
Mupirocin Lithium RS
Nystatin RS
Oxytetracycline Hydrochloride RS
Panipenem RS
Peplomycin Sulfate RS
Phenethicillin Potassium RS
Pimaricin RS
Pirarubicin RS
Pivmecillinam Hydrochloride RS
Polymixin B Sulfate RS
Pyrrolnitrin RS
Ribostamycin Sulfate RS
Rifampicin RS
Spectinomycin Hydrochloride RS
Spiramycin II Acetate RS
Streptomycin Sulfate RS
Sulbenicillin Sodium RS
Sultamicillin Tosilate RS
Talampicillin Hydrochloride RS
Teicoplanin RS
Tetracycline Hydrochloride RS
Tobramycin RS
Trichomycin RS

Standard Solutions

9.21 Standard Solutions for Volumetric Analysis

Standard Solutions for Volumetric Analysis are the solutions of reagent with an accurately known concentration, mainly used for the volumetric analysis.

They are prepared to a specified molar concentration. A 1 molar solution is a solution which contains exactly 1 mole of a specified substance in each 1000 mL of the solution and is designated as 1 mol/L.

If necessary, these solutions are diluted to other specified molar concentrations and the diluted solutions are also used as standard solutions. For example, 0.1 mol/L solution is obtained by diluting 1 mol/L solution 10 times by volume.

Unless otherwise directed, standard solutions for volumetric analysis should be stored in colorless or light-resistant, glass-stoppered bottles.

Preparation and Standardization

A volumetric standard solution is prepared according to one of the following methods. The degree of difference from a specified concentration n (mol/L) is expressed as a factor (molar concentration coefficient) f. Usually, standard solutions are prepared so that the factor is in the range of 0.970 – 1.030. The determination procedure of the factor is called standardization of the standard solution.

(1) Weigh accurately a quantity equivalent to about 1 mole or its multiple or a fractional mole number of the pure substance, and dissolve it in the specified solvent to make exactly 1000 mL to prepare a standard solution having a concentration close to the specified molarity n (mol/L). In this case, the factor f of the standard solution is obtained by dividing the mass of the pure substance taken (g) by the molecular mass of the substance (g) and the specified molarity number n.

When a pure substance is not obtainable, it is permissible to use a highly purified substance whose purity has been exactly determined and certified.

(2) In the case where a pure substance or a highly purified substance is not obtainable, weigh a quantity equivalent to about 1 mole or its multiple or a fractional mole number of the substance specified for each standard solution and dissolve it in the specified solvent to make about 1000 mL to prepare a standard solution having a concentration close to the specified molarity n (mol/L). The factor f of this solution is determined by applying the standardization procedure described for the respective standard solution. The procedure is classified into direct and indirect methods, as follows:

a) Direct method

Weigh accurately a standard reagent or an indicated substance specified for each standard solution, dissolve it in the specified solvent, then titrate with the prepared standard solution to be standardized, and determine the factor f by applying the following equation.

$$f = \frac{1000m}{VMn}$$

M: Molecular mass equivalent to 1 mole of the standard reagent or the specified substance (g)

m: Mass of the standard reagent or the specified substance taken (g)

V: Volume of the prepared standard solution consumed for the titration (mL)

n: Arithmetical mole number of the specified molar concentration of the standard solution to be standardized (e.g. n = 0.02 for 0.02 mol/L standard solution)

b) Indirect method

When an appropriate standard reagent is not available, titrate a defined volume V_2 (mL) of a standard solution to be standardized with the specified standard solution having a known factor (f_1), and calculate the factor (f_2) by applying the following equation.

$$f_2 = \frac{V_1 \times f_1}{V_2}$$

f_1: Factor of the titrating standard solution having a known factor

f_2: Factor of the prepared standard solution to be standardized

V_1: Volume of the titrating standard solution consumed (mL)

V_2: Volume of the prepared standard solution taken (mL)

(3) Standard solutions may be prepared by diluting exactly an accurately measured volume of a standard solution having a known factor, according to the specified dilution procedure. During this dilution procedure, the original factor of the standard solution is assumed to remain constant.

Ammonium Iron (II) Sulfate, 0.1 mol/L

1000 mL of this solution contains 39.214 g of ammonium iron (II) sulfate hexahydrate [$Fe(NH_4)_2(SO_4)_2.6H_2O$: 392.14].

Preparation—Dissolve 40 g of ammonium iron (II) sulfate hexahydrate in a cooled mixture of 30 mL of sulfuric acid and 300 mL of water, dilute with water to make 1000 mL, and standardize the solution as follows:

Standardization—Measure exactly 25 mL of the prepared ammonium iron (II) sulfate solution, and add 25 mL of water and 5 mL of phosphoric acid. Titrate <*2.50*> the solution with 0.02 mol/L potassium permanganate VS. Calculate the molarity factor.

Note: Prepare before use.

Ammonium Iron (II) Sulfate, 0.02 mol/L

1000 mL of this solution contains 7.843 g of ammonium iron (II) sulfate hexahydrate [$Fe(NH_4)_2(SO_4)_2.6H_2O$: 392.14].

Preparation—Before use, dilute 0.1 mol/L ammonium Iron (II) sulfate VS with diluted sulfuric acid (3 in 100) to make exactly 5 times the initial volume.

Ammonium Iron (III) Sulfate, 0.1 mol/L

1000 mL of this solution contains 48.22 g of ammonium iron (III) sulfate dodecahydrate [$FeNH_4(SO_4)_2.12H_2O$: 482.19].

Preparation—Dissolve 49 g of ammonium iron (III) sulfate dodecahydrate in a cooled mixture of 6 mL of sulfuric acid and 300 mL of water, add water to make 1000 mL, and standardize the solution as follows:

Standardization—Measure exactly 25 mL of the prepared ammonium iron (III) sulfate solution into an iodine flask, add 5 mL of hydrochloric acid, and shake the mixture. Dissolve 2 g of potassium iodide, and stopper the flask. After allowing the mixture to stand for 10 minutes, add 50 mL of water, and titrate <*2.50*> the liberated iodine with 0.1 mol/L sodium thiosulfate VS. When the solution assumes a light yellow color as the end point is approached, add 3 mL of starch TS. Continue the titration, until the blue color disappears. Perform a blank determination, make any necessary correction, and calculate the molarity factor.

Note: Store protected from light. This solution, if stored for a long period of time, should be restandardized.

Ammonium Thiocyanate, 0.1 mol/L

1000 mL of this solution contains 7.612 g of ammonium thiocyanate (NH_4SCN: 76.12).

Preparation—Dissolve 8 g of ammonium thiocyanate in water to make 1000 mL, and standardize the solution as follows:

Standardization—Measure exactly 25 mL of the 0.1 mol/L silver nitrate VS, and add 50 mL of water, 2 mL of nitric acid and 2 mL of ammonium iron (III) sulfate TS. Titrate <*2.50*> the solution with the prepared ammonium thiocyanate solution to the first appearance of a persistent red-brown color with shaking. Calculate the molarity factor.

Note: Store protected from light.

Ammonium Thiocyanate, 0.02 mol/L

1000 mL of this solution contains 1.5224 g of ammonium thiocyanate (NH_4SCN: 76.12).

Preparation—Before use, dilute 0.1 mol/L ammonium thiocyanate VS with water to make exactly 5 times the initial volume.

Barium chloride, 0.1 mol/L

1000 mL of this solution contains 24.426 g of barium chloride dihydrate ($BaCl_2.2H_2O$: 244.26).

Preparation—Dissolve 24.5 g of barium chloride dihydrate in water to make 1000 mL, and standardize the solution as follows:

Standardization—Measure exactly 20 mL of the prepared solution, add 3 mL of hydrochloric acid, and warm the mixture. Add 40 mL of diluted sulfuric acid (1 in 130), previously warmed, heat the mixture on a water bath for 30 minutes, and allow it to stand overnight. Filter the mixture, wash the precipitate on the filter paper with water until the last washing shows no turbidity with silver nitrate TS, transfer the precipitate together with the filter paper to a tared crucible, and then heat strongly to ashes. After cooling, add 2 drops of sulfuric acid, and heat again at about 700°C for 2 hours. After cooling, weigh accurately the mass of the residue, and calculate the molarity factor as barium sulfate ($BaSO_4$).

Each mL of 0.1 mol/L barium chloride VS
= 23.34 mg of $BaSO_4$

Barium Chloride, 0.02 mol/L

1000 mL of this solution contains 4.885 g of barium chloride dihydrate ($BaCl_2.2H_2O$: 244.26).

Preparation—Dissolve 4.9 g of barium chloride dihydrate in water to make 1000 mL, and standardize the solution as follows:

Standardization—Measure exactly 100 mL of the prepared barium chloride solution, add 3 mL of hydrochloric acid, and warm the mixture. Add 40 mL of diluted sulfuric acid (1 in 130), warmed previously, heat the mixture on a water bath for 30 minutes, and allow to stand overnight. Filter the mixture, wash the collected precipitate of filter paper with water until the last washing shows no turbidity with silver nitrate TS, transfer the precipitate together with the filter paper to a tared crucible, and then heat strongly to ashes. After cooling, add 2 drops of sulfuric acid, and heat strongly again at about 700°C for 2 hours. After cooling, weigh accurately the residue as barium sulfate ($BaSO_4$), and calculate the molarity factor.

Each mL of 0.02 mol/L barium chloride VS
= 4.668 mg of $BaSO_4$

Barium Chloride, 0.01 mol/L

1000 mL of this solution contains 2.4426 g of barium chloride dihydrate ($BaCl_2.2H_2O$: 244.26).

Preparation—Before use, dilute 0.02 mol/L barium chloride VS with water to make exactly twice the initial volume.

Barium Perchlorate, 0.005 mol/L

1000 mL of this solution contains 1.6812 g of barium perchlorate [$Ba(ClO_4)_2$: 336.23].

Preparation—Dissolve 1.7 g of barium perchlorate in 200 mL of water, dilute with 2-propanol to make 1000 mL, and standardize the solution as follows:

Standardization—Measure exactly 20 mL of the prepared barium perchlorate solution, add 55 mL of methanol and 0.15 mL of arsenazo III TS. Titrate <*2.50*> the solution with 0.005 mol/L sulfuric acid VS until its purple color changes through red-purple to red. Calculate the molarity factor.

Benzethonium chloride, 0.004 mol/L

1000 mL of this solution contains 1.7923 g of benzethonium chloride ($C_{27}H_{42}ClNO_2$: 448.08).

Preparation—Dissolve 1.792 g of benzethonium chloride for assay, previously dried at 105°C for 4 hours, in water to make exactly 1000 mL, and standardize the solution as follows:

Standardization—Pipet 10 mL of the prepared benzethonium chloride solution, adjust to pH between 2.6 and 3.4 by adding dropwise diluted dilute hydrochloric acid (1 in 2), add 1 drop of methyl orange TS, and titrate <*2.50*> with 0.02 mol/L sodium tetraphenylboron VS until the color of the solution becomes red. Calculate the molarity factor.

Each mL of 0.02 mol/L sodium tetraphenylboron VS
= 8.962 mg of $C_{27}H_{42}ClNO_2$

Bismuth Nitrate, 0.01 mol/L

1000 mL of this solution contains 4.851 g of bismuth nitrate pentahydrate [$Bi(NO_3)_3.5H_2O$: 485.07].

Preparation—Dissolve 4.86 g of bismuth nitrate pentahydrate in 60 mL of dilute nitric acid, add water to make 1000 mL, and standardize the solution as follows:

Standardization—Measure exactly 25 mL of the prepared bismuth nitrate solution, add 50 mL of water and 1 drop of xylenol orange TS, and titrate <*2.50*> the solution with 0.01 mol/L disodium dihydrogen ethylenediamine tetraacetate VS until the red color changes to yellow. Calculate the molarity factor.

Bromine, 0.05 mol/L

1000 mL of this solution contains 7.990 g of bromine (Br: 79.90).

Preparation—Dissolve 2.8 g of potassium bromate and 15 g of potassium bromide in water to make 1000 mL, and standardize the solution as follows:

Standardization—Measure exactly 25 mL of the prepared solution into an iodine flask. Add 120 mL of water, quickly add 5 mL of hydrochloric acid, stopper the flask immediately, and shake it gently. Then add 5 mL of potassium iodide TS, re-stopper immediately, shake the mixture gently, and allow to stand for 5 minutes. Titrate <*2.50*> the liberated iodine with 0.1 mol/L sodium thiosulfate VS. When the solution assumes a light yellow color as the end point is approached, add 3 mL of starch TS. Continue the titration, until the blue color disappears. Perform a blank determination, make any necessary correction, and calculate the molarity factor.

Ceric Ammonium Sulfate, 0.1 mol/L

See cerium (IV) tetraammonium sulfate, 0.1 mol/L.

Ceric Ammonium Sulfate, 0.01 mol/L

See cerium (IV) tetraammonium sulfate, 0.01 mol/L.

Cerium (IV) Sulfate, 0.1 mol/L

1000 mL of this solution contains 40.43 g of cerium (IV) sulfate tetrahydrate [$Ce(SO_4)_2.4H_2O$: 404.30].

Preparation—Dissolve 40.43 g of cerium sulfate (IV) tetrahydrate in 550 mL of diluted sulfuric acid (1 in 11). After cooling, add water to make 1000 mL, and standardize the solution as follows:

Standardization—Weigh accurately about 0.2 g of sodium oxalate (standard reagent), previously dried between 150°C and 200°C for 1 to 1.5 hours, and allow to cool in a desiccator (silica gel), and dissolve in 75 mL of water. Add a mixture of 5 mL of water and 2 mL of sulfuric acid with stirring, add 10 mL of hydrochloric acid, and warm to 70 - 75°C. Titrate *<2.50>* the solution with 0.1 mol/L cerium (IV) sulfate VS until the solution shows a persistent pale yellow color, and calculate the molarity factor.

Each mL of 0.1 mol/L cerium sulfate (IV) VS
= 6.700 mg of $Na_2C_2O_4$

Cerium (IV) Tetraammonium Sulfate, 0.1 mol/L

1000 mL of this solution contains 63.26 g of cerium (IV) tetraammonium sulfate dihydrate [$Ce(NH_4)_4(SO_4)_4.2H_2O$: 632.55].

Preparation—Dissolve 64 g of cerium (VI) tetraammonium sulfate dihydrate in 0.5 mol/L sulfuric acid VS to make 1000 mL, allow to stand for 24 hours, filter the solution through a glass filter (G3 or G4), if necessary, and standardize the solution as follows:

Standardization—Measure exactly 25 mL of the prepared cerium (IV) tetraammonium sulfate solution into an iodine flask. Add 20 mL of water and 20 mL of dilute sulfuric acid, then dissolve 1 g of potassium iodide in the mixture. Immediately titrate *<2.50>* the solution with 0.1 mol/L sodium thiosulfate VS. When the solution assumes a light yellow color as the end point is approached, add 3 mL of starch TS. Continue the titration, until the blue color disappears. Perform a blank determination, make any necessary correction, and calculate the molarity factor.

Note: Store protected from light. This solution, if stored for a long period of time, should be restandardized.

Cerium (IV) Tetraammonium Sulfate, 0.01 mol/L

1000 mL of this solution contains 6.326 g of cerium (IV) tetraammonium sulfate dihydrate [$Ce(NH_4)_4(SO_4)_4.2H_2O$: 632.55].

Preparation—Before use, dilute 0.1 mol/L cerium (IV) tetraammonium sulfate VS with 0.5 mol/L sulfuric acid VS to make exactly 10 times the initial volume.

Copper (II) Nitrate, 0.1 mol/L

1000 mL of this solution contains 24.16 g of copper (II) nitrate trihydrate [$Cu(NO_3)_2.3H_2O$: 241.60].

Preparation—Dissolve 24.2 g of copper (II) nitrate trihydrate in water to make 1000 mL, and standardize the solution as follows:

Standardization—Measure exactly 10 mL of the prepared 0.1 mol/L copper (II) nitrate, and add 1 mL of sodium nitrate solution (9 in 20), 20 mL of acetic acid-ammonium acetate buffer solution, pH 4.8, and 70 mL of water. Titrate *<2.50>* with 0.05 mol/L disodium dihydrogen ethylenediamine tetraacetate VS using a copper electrode as the indicator electrode, a complex type silver-silver chloride electrode as the reference electrode, and potassium chloride solution (1 in 4) as the inner solution.

Disodium Dihydrogen Ethylenediamine Tetraacetate, 0.1 mol/L

1000 mL of this solution contains 37.224 g of disodium dihydrogen ethylenediamine tetraacetate dehydrate ($C_{10}H_{14}N_2Na_2O_8.2H_2O$: 372.24).

Preparation—Dissolve 38 g of disodium dihydrogen ethylenediamine tetraacetate dihydrate in water to make 1000 mL, and standardize the solution as follows:

Standardization—Wash zinc (standard reagent) with dilute hydrochloric acid, water and then acetone, dry at 110°C for 5 minutes, and allow to cool in a desiccator (silica gel). Weigh accurately about 1.3 g of this zinc, add 20 mL of dilute hydrochloric acid and 8 drops of bromine TS, and dissolve it by gentle warming. Expel any excess of bromine by boiling, and add water to make exactly 200 mL. Pipet 25 mL of this solution, and neutralize with sodium hydroxide solution (1 in 50). Add 5 mL of ammonia-ammonium chloride buffer solution, pH 10.7, and 0.04 g of eriochrome black T-sodium chloride indicator. Titrate *<2.50>* the solution with the prepared disodium dihydrogen ethylenediamine tetraacetate solution until the red-purple color changes to blue-purple. Calculate the molarity factor.

Each mL of 0.1 mol/L disodium dihydrogen
ethylenediamine tetraacetate VS
= 6.538 mg of Zn

Note: Store in polyethylene bottles.

Disodium Dihydrogen Ethylenediamine Tetraacetate, 0.05 mol/L

1000 mL of this solution contains 18.612 g of disodium dihydrogen ethylenediamine tetraacetate dehydrate ($C_{10}H_{14}N_2Na_2O_8.2H_2O$: 372.24).

Preparation—Dissolve 19 g of disodium dihydrogen ethylenediamine tetraacetate dihydrate in water to make 1000 mL, and standardize the solution as follows:

Standardization—Wash zinc (standard reagent) with dilute hydrochloric acid, water and then acetone, dry at 110°C for 5 minutes, and allow to cool in a desiccator (silica gel). Weigh accurately about 0.8 g of this zinc, add 12 mL of dilute hydrochloric acid and 5 drops of bromine TS, and dissolve it by gentle warming. Expel any excess of bromine by boiling, and add water to make exactly 200 mL. Measure exactly 20 mL of this solution, and neutralize with sodium hydroxide solution (1 in 50). Add 5 mL of ammonia-ammonium chloride buffer solution, pH 10.7, and 0.04 g of eriochrome black T-sodium chloride indicator. Titrate *<2.50>* the solution with the prepared disodium dihydrogen ethylenediamine tetraacetate solution until the red-purple color changes to blue-purple. Calculate the molarity factor.

Each mL of 0.05 mol/L disodium dihydrogen
ethylenediamine tetraacetate VS
= 3.269 mg of Zn

Note: Store in polyethylene bottles.

Disodium Dihydrogen Ethylenediamine Tetraacetate, 0.02 mol/L

1000 mL of this solution contains 7.445 g of disodium

dihydrogen ethylenediamine tetraacetate dihydrate ($C_{10}H_{14}N_2Na_2O_8.2H_2O$: 372.24).

Preparation—Dissolve 7.5 g of disodium dihydrogen ethylenediamine tetraacetate dihydrate in water to make 1000 mL, and standardize the solution as follows:

Standardization—Proceed as directed for standardization under 0.05 mol/L disodium dihydrogen ethylenediamine tetraacetate VS, but weigh accurately 0.3 g of zinc (standard reagent), previously washed with dilute hydrochloric acid, with water and with acetone, and cooled in a desiccator (silica gel) after drying at 110°C for 5 minutes, and add 5 mL of dilute hydrochloric acid and 5 drops of bromine TS.

Each mL of 0.02 mol/L disodium dihydrogen ethylenediamine tetraacetate VS
= 1.308 mg of Zn

Note: Store in polyethylene bottles.

Disodium Dihydrogen Ethylenediamine Tetraacetate, 0.01 mol/L

1000 mL of this solution contains 3.7224 g of disodium dihydrogen ethylenediamine tetraacetate dihydrate ($C_{10}H_{14}N_2Na_2O_8.2H_2O$: 372.24).

Preparation—Before use, dilute 0.02 mol/L disodium dihydrogen ethylenediamine tetraacetate VS with water to make exactly twice the initial volume.

Disodium Dihydrogen Ethylenediamine Tetraacetate, 0.001 mol/L

1000 mL of this solution contains 0.37224 g of disodium dihydrogen ethylenediamine tetraacetate dihydrate ($C_{10}H_{14}N_2Na_2O_8.2H_2O$: 372.24).

Preparation—Before use, dilute 0.01 mol/L disodium dihydrogen ethylenediamine tetraacetate VS with water to make exactly 10 times the initial volume.

Ferric Ammonium Sulfate, 0.1 mol/L

See Ammonium Iron (III) Sulfate, 0.1 mol/L.

Ferrous Ammonium Sulfate, 0.1 mol/L

See Ammonium Iron (II) Sulfate, 0.1 mol/L.

Ferrous Ammonium Sulfate, 0.02 mol/L

See Ammonium Iron (II) Sulfate, 0.02 mol/L.

Hydrochloric Acid, 2 mol/L

1000 mL of this solution contains 72.92 g of hydrochloric acid (HCl: 36.46).

Preparation—Dilute 180 mL of hydrochloric acid with water to make 1000 mL, and standardize the solution as follows:

Standardization—Proceed as directed for standardization under 1 mol/L hydrochloric acid VS, but weigh about 1.5 g of sodium carbonate (standard reagent) accurately, and dissolve in 100 mL of water.

Each mL of 2 mol/L hydrochloric acid VS
= 106.0 mg of Na_2CO_3

Hydrochloric Acid, 1 mol/L

1000 mL of this solution contains 36.461 g of hydrochloric acid (HCl: 36.46).

Preparation—Dilute 90 mL of hydrochloric acid with water to make 1000 mL, and standardize the solution as follows:

Standardization—Weigh accurately about 0.8 g of sodium carbonate (standard reagent), previously heated between 500°C and 650°C for 40 to 50 minutes and allowed to cool in a desiccator (silica gel). Dissolve it in 50 mL of water, and titrate <*2.50*> with the prepared hydrochloric acid to calculate the molarity factor (Indicator method: 3 drops of methyl red TS; or potentiometric titration). In the indicator method, when the end-point is approached, boil the content carefully, stopper the flask loosely, allow to cool, and continue the titration until the color of the solution changes to persistent orange to orange-red. In the potentiometric titration, titrate with vigorous stirring, without boiling.

Each mL of 1 mol/L hydrochloric acid VS
= 53.00 mg of Na_2CO_3

Hydrochloric Acid, 0.5 mol/L

1000 mL of this solution contains 18.230 g of hydrochloric acid (HCl: 36.46).

Preparation—Dilute 45 mL of hydrochloric acid with water to make 1000 mL, and standardize the solution as follows:

Standardization—Proceed as directed for standardization under 1 mol/L hydrochloric acid VS, but weigh accurately about 0.4 g of sodium carbonate (standard reagent), and dissolve in 50 mL of water.

Each mL of 0.5 mol/L hydrochloric acid VS
= 26.50 mg of Na_2CO_3

Hydrochloric Acid, 0.2 mol/L

1000 mL of this solution contains 7.292 g of hydrochloric acid (HCl: 36.46).

Preparation—Dilute 18 mL of hydrochloric acid with water to make 1000 mL, and standardize the solution as follows:

Standardization—Proceed as directed for standardization under 1 mol/L hydrochloric acid VS, but weigh accurately about 0.15 g of sodium carbonate (standard reagent), and dissolve in 30 mL of water.

Each mL of 0.2 mol/L hydrochloric acid VS
= 10.60 mg of Na_2CO_3

Hydrochloric Acid, 0.1 mol/L

1000 mL of this solution contains 3.6461 g of hydrochloric acid (HCl: 36.46).

Preparation—Before use, dilute 0.2 mol/L hydrochloric acid VS with water to make exactly twice the initial volume.

Each mL of 0.1 mol/L hydrochloric acid VS
= 5.300 mg of Na_2CO_3

Hydrochloric Acid, 0.05 mol/L

1000 mL of this solution contains 1.8230 g of hydrochloric acid (HCl: 36.46).

Preparation—Before use, dilute 0.2 mol/L hydrochloric acid VS with water to make exactly 4 times the initial volume.

Hydrochloric Acid, 0.02 mol/L

1000 mL of this solution contains 0.7292 g of hydrochloric acid (HCl: 36.46).

Preparation—Before use, dilute 0.2 mol/L hydrochloric acid VS with water to make exactly 10 times the initial volume.

Hydrochloric Acid, 0.01 mol/L

1000 mL of this solution contains 0.36461 g of hydrochloric acid (HCl: 36.46).

Preparation—Before use, dilute 0.2 mol/L hydrochloric

acid VS with water to make exactly 20 times the initial volume.

Hydrochloric Acid, 0.001 mol/L

1000 mL of this solution contains 0.036461 g of hydrochloric acid (HCl: 36.46).

Preparation—Before use, dilute 0.2 mol/L hydrochloric acid VS with water to make exactly 200 times the initial volume.

Iodine, 0.05 mol/L

1000 mL of this solution contains 12.690 g of iodine (I: 126.90).

Preparation—Dissolve 13 g of iodine in 100 mL of a solution of potassium iodide (2 in 5), add 1 mL of dilute hydrochloric acid and water to make 1000 mL, and standardize the solution as follows:

Standardization—Measure exactly 15 mL of the iodine solution, and titrate *<2.50>* with 0.1 mol/L sodium thiosulfate VS (Indicator method: starch TS; or potentiometric titration: platinum electrode). In the indicator method, when the solution assumes a light yellow color as the end point is approached, add 3 mL of starch TS, and continue the titration until the blue color disappears. Calculate the molarity factor.

Note: Store protected from light. This solution, if stored for a long period, should be restandardized before use.

Iodine, 0.025 mol/L

1000 mL of this solution contains 6.345 g of iodine (I:126.90).

Preparation—Before use, dilute 0.05 mol/L iodine VS with water to make exactly twice the initial volume.

Iodine, 0.01 mol/L

1000 mL of this solution contains 2.5381 g of iodine (I: 126.90).

Preparation—Before use, dilute 0.05 mol/L iodine VS with water to make exactly 5 times the initial volume.

Iodine, 0.005 mol/L

1000 mL of this solution contains 1.2690 g of iodine (I: 126.90).

Preparation—Before use, dilute 0.05 mol/L iodine VS with water to make exactly 10 times the initial volume.

Iodine, 0.002 mol/L

1000 mL of this solution contains 0.5076 g of iodine (I: 126.90).

Preparation—Before use, dilute 0.05 mol/L iodine VS with water to make exactly 25 times the initial volume.

Magnesium Chloride, 0.05 mol/L

1000 mL of this solution contains 10.165 g of magnesium chloride hexahydrate ($MgCl_2.6H_2O$: 203.30).

Preparation—Dissolve 10.2 g of magnesium chloride hexahydrate in freshly boiled and cooled water to make 1000 mL, and standardize the solution as follows:

Standardization—Measure exactly 25 mL of the prepared magnesium chloride solution. Add 50 mL of water, 3 mL of pH 10.7 ammonia-ammonium chloride buffer solution and 0.04 g of eriochrome black T-sodium chloride indicator, and titrate *<2.50>* with 0.05 mol/L disodium dihydrogen ethylenediamine tetraacetate VS until the red-purple color of the solution changes to blue-purple. Calculate the molarity factor.

Magnesium Chloride, 0.01 mol/L

1000 mL of this solution contains 2.0330 g of magnesium chloride hexahydrate ($MgCl_2.6H_2O$: 203.30).

Preparation—Before use, dilute 0.05 mol/L magnesium chloride VS with water to make exactly 5 times the initial volume.

Oxalic Acid, 0.05 mol/L

1000 mL of this solution contains 6.303 g of oxalic acid ($C_2H_2O_4.2H_2O$: 126.07).

Preparation—Dissolve 6.3 g of oxalic acid dihydrate in water to make 1000 mL, and standardize the solution as follows:

Standardization—Measure exactly 25 mL of the prepared oxalic acid solution in a 500-mL conical flask, and add 200 mL of diluted sulfuric acid (1 in 20), previously boiled for 10 to 15 minutes and then cooled to 27 ± 3°C. Transfer freshly standardized 0.02 mol/L potassium permanganate VS to a burette. Add quickly 22 mL of the 0.02 mol/L potassium permanganate VS to the oxalic acid solution from the burette under gentle stirring, and allow to stand until the red color of the mixture disappears. Heat the solution up to between 55°C and 60°C, and complete the titration *<2.50>* by adding 0.02 mol/L potassium permanganate VS until a light red color persists for 30 seconds. Add the last 0.5 to 1 mL dropwise, being particularly careful to allow the solution to become decolorized before the next drop is added. Calculate the molarity factor.

Note: Store protected from light.

Oxalic Acid, 0.005 mol/L

1000 mL of this solution contains 0.6303 g of oxalic acid dihydrate ($C_2H_2O_4.2H_2O$: 126.07).

Preparation—Before use, dilute 0.05 mol/L oxalic acid VS with water to make exactly 10 times the initial volume.

Perchloric Acid, 0.1 mol/L

1000 mL of this solution contains 10.046 g of perchloric acid ($HClO_4$: 100.46).

Preparation—Add slowly 8.7 mL of perchloric acid to 1000 mL of acetic acid (100) while keeping the temperature at about 20°C. Allow the mixture to stand for about 1 hour. Perform quickly the test as directed under Water Determination with 3.0 mL of the mixture, and designate the water content as A (g/dL). To the rest mixture add slowly [(A − 0.03) × 52.2] mL of acetic anhydride with shaking at about 20°C. Allow the solution to stand for 24 hours, and standardize it as follows:

Standardization—Weigh accurately about 0.3 g of potassium hydrogen phthalate (standard reagent), previously dried at 105°C for 4 hours and allowed to cool in a desiccator (silica gel). Dissolve it in 50 mL of acetic acid (100), and titrate *<2.50>* the solution with the prepared perchloric acid solution (Indicator method: 3 drops of crystal violet TS; or potentiometric titration). In the indicator method, titrate until the solution acquires a blue color. Perform a blank determination, make any necessary correction, and calculate the molarity factor.

Each mL of 0.1 mol/L perchloric acid VS
= 20.42 mg of $KHC_6H_4(COO)_2$

Note: Store protected from moisture.

Perchloric Acid, 0.05 mol/L

1000 mL of this solution contains 5.023 g of perchloric acid ($HClO_4$: 100.46).

Preparation—Before use, dilute 0.1 mol/L perchloric acid

VS with acetic acid for nonaqueous titration to make exactly twice the initial volume. Perform quickly the test as directed under Water Determination with 8.0 mL of acetic acid for nonaqueous titration, and designate the water content as A (g/dL). If A is not less than 0.03, add [(A − 0.03) × 52.2] mL of acetic anhydride to 1000 mL of acetic acid for nonaqueous titration, and use it for the preparation.

Perchloric Acid, 0.02 mol/L

1000 mL of this solution contains 2.0092 g of perchloric acid ($HClO_4$: 100.46).

Preparation—Before use, dilute 0.1 mol/L perchloric acid VS with acetic acid for nonaqueous titration to make exactly 5 times the initial volume. Perform quickly the test as directed under Water Determination with 8.0 mL of acetic acid for nonaqueous titration, and designate the water content as A (g/dL). If A is not less than 0.03, add [(A − 0.03) × 52.2] mL of acetic anhydride to 1000 mL of acetic acid for nonaqueous titration, and use it for the preparation.

Perchloric Acid-1,4-Dioxane, 0.1 mol/L

1000 mL of this solution contains 10.046 g of perchloric acid ($HClO_4$: 100.46).

Preparation—Dilute 8.5 mL of perchloric acid with 1,4-dioxane to make 1000 mL, and standardize the solution as follows:

Standardization—Weigh accurately about 0.5 g of potassium hydrogen phthalate (standard reagent), previously dried at 105°C for 4 hours and allowed to cool in a desiccator (silica gel). Dissolve it in 80 mL of acetic acid for nonaqueous titration, and add 3 drops of crystal violet TS. Titrate <*2.50*> the solution with the prepared perchloric acid-1,4-dioxane solution until it acquires a blue color. Perform a blank determination, make any necessary correction, and calculate the molarity factor.

Each mL of 0.1 mol/L perchloric acid-1,4-dioxane VS
= 20.42 mg of $KHC_6H_4(COO)_2$

Note: Store in a cold place, protected from moisture.

Perchloric Acid-1,4-Dioxane, 0.05 mol/L

1000 mL of this solution contains 5.023 g of perchloric acid ($HClO_4$: 100.46).

Preparation—Before use, dilute 0.1 mol/L perchloric acid-1,4-dioxane VS with 1,4-dioxane to make exactly twice the initial volume.

Perchloric Acid-1,4-Dioxane, 0.004 mol/L

1000 mL of this solution contains 0.4018 g of perchloric acid ($HClO_4$: 100.46).

Preparation—Before use, dilute 0.1 mol/L perchloric acid-1,4-dioxane VS with 1,4-dioxane to make exactly 25 times the initial volume.

Potassium Bichromate, 1/60 mol/L

See Potassium Dichromate, 1/60 mol/L.

Potassium Bromate, 1/60 mol/L

1000 mL of this solution contains 2.7833 g of potassium bromate ($KBrO_3$: 167.00).

Preparation—Dissolve 2.8 g of potassium bromate in water to make 1000 mL, and standardize the solution as follows:

Standardization—Measure exactly 25 mL of the prepared potassium bromate solution into an iodine flask. Add 2 g of potassium iodide and 5 mL of dilute sulfuric acid, stopper the flask, and allow the solution to stand for 5 minutes. Add 100 mL of water, and titrate <*2.50*> the liberated iodine with 0.1 mol/L sodium thiosulfate VS. When the solution assumes a light yellow color as the end point is approached, add 3 mL of starch TS. Continue the titration until the blue color disappears. Perform a blank determination, make any necessary correction, and calculate the molarity factor.

Potassium Dichromate, 1/60 mol/L

1000 mL of this solution contains 4.903 g of potassium dichromate ($K_2Cr_2O_7$: 294.18).

Preparation—Weigh accurately about 4.903 g of potassium dichromate (standard reagent), previously powdered, dried between 100°C and 110°C for 3 to 4 hours and allowed to cool in a desiccator (silica gel), dissolve it in water to make exactly 1000 mL, and calculate the molarity factor.

Potassium Ferricyanide, 0.1 mol/L

See Potassium Hexacyanoferrate (III), 0.1 mol/L.

Potassium Ferricyanide, 0.05 mol/L

See Potassium Hexacyanoferrate (III), 0.05 mol/L.

Potassium Hexacyanoferrate (III), 0.1 mol/L

1000 mL of this solution contains 32.924 g of potassium hexacyanoferrate (III) [$K_3Fe(CN)_6$: 329.24].

Preparation—Dissolve 33 g of potassium hexacyanoferrate (III) in water to make 1000 mL, and standardize the solution as follows:

Standardization—Measure exactly 25 mL of the prepared potassium hexacyanoferrate (III) solution into an iodine flask. Add 2 g of potassium iodide and 10 mL of dilute hydrochloric acid, stopper the flask, and allow to stand for 15 minutes. Add 15 mL of zinc sulfate TS, and titrate <*2.50*> the liberated iodine with 0.1 mol/L sodium thiosulfate VS. When the solution assumes a light yellow color as the end point is approached, add 3 mL of starch TS. Continue the titration, until the blue color disappears. Perform a blank determination, make any necessary correction, and calculate the molarity factor.

Note: Store protected from light. This solution, if stored for a long period, should be restandardized.

Potassium Hexacyanoferrate (III), 0.05 mol/L

1000 mL of this solution contains 16.462 g of potassium hexacyanoferrate (III) [$K_3Fe(CN)_6$: 329.24].

Preparation—Before use, dilute 0.1 mol/L potassium hexacyanoferrate (III) VS with water to make exactly twice the initial volume.

Potassium Hydroxide, 1 mol/L

1000 mL of this solution contains 56.11 g of potassium hydroxide (KOH: 56.11).

Preparation—Dissolve 65 g of potassium hydroxide in 950 mL of water. Add a freshly prepared, saturated solution of barium hydroxide octahydrate until no more precipitate is produced. Shake the mixture thoroughly, and allow it to stand for 24 hours in a tightly stoppered bottle. Decant the supernatant liquid or filter the solution through a glass filter (G3 or G4), and standardize the solution as follows:

Standardization—Weigh accurately about 2.5 g of amidosulfuric acid (standard reagent), previously dried in a desiccator (in vacuum, silica gel) for about 48 hours. Dissolve it in 25 mL of freshly boiled and cooled water, and add 2 drops of bromothymol blue TS. Titrate <*2.50*> the solution with the prepared potassium hydroxide solution until it acquires a green color. Calculate the molarity factor.

Each mL of 1 mol/L potassium hydroxide VS
= 97.09 mg of $HOSO_2NH_2$

Note: Store in tightly stoppered bottles or in containers provided with a carbon dioxide-absorbing tube (soda-lime). This solution, if stored for a long period, should be restandardized.

Potassium Hydroxide, 0.5 mol/L

1000 mL of this solution contains 28.053 g of potassium hydroxide (KOH: 56.11).

Preparation—Weigh 32 g of potassium hydroxide, proceed as directed for preparation under 1 mol/L potassium hydroxide VS, and standardize the solution as follows:

Standardization—Proceed as directed for standardization under 1 mol/L potassium hydroxide VS, but weigh accurately about 1.3 g of amidosulfuric acid (standard reagent).

Each mL of 0.5 mol/L potassium hydroxide VS
= 48.55 mg of $HOSO_2NH_2$

Note: Store as directed under 1 mol/L potassium hydroxide VS. This solution, if stored for a long period, should be restandardized.

Potassium Hydroxide, 0.1 mol/L

1000 mL of this solution contains 5.611 g of potassium hydroxide (KOH: 56.11).

Preparation—Weigh 6.5 g of potassium hydroxide, proceed as directed for preparation under 1 mol/L potassium hydroxide VS, and standardize the solution as follows:

Standardization—Proceed as directed for standardization under 1 mol/L potassium hydroxide VS, but weigh accurately about 0.25 g of amidosulfuric acid (standard reagent).

Each mL of 0.1 mol/L potassium hydroxide VS
= 9.709 mg of $HOSO_2NH_2$

Note: Store as directed under 1 mol/L potassium hydroxide VS. This solution, if stored for a long period, should be restandardized.

Potassium Hydroxide-Ethanol, 0.5 mol/L

1000 mL of this solution contains 28.053 g of potassium hydroxide (KOH: 56.11).

Preparation—Dissolve 35 g of potassium hydroxide in 20 mL of water, and add aldehyde-free ethanol to make 1000 mL. Allow the solution to stand for 24 hours in a tightly stoppered bottle. Then quickly decant the supernatant liquid, and standardize the solution as follows:

Standardization—Measure exactly 15 mL of 0.25 mol/L sulfuric acid VS, add 50 mL of water, and titrate with the prepared potassium hydroxide-ethanol solution to calculate the molarity factor (Indicator method: 2 drops of phenolphthalein TS; or potentiometric titration). In the indicator method, titrate <*2.50*> until the solution acquires a light red color.

Note: Store in tightly stoppered bottles, protected from light. Standardize before use.

Potassium Hydroxide-Ethanol, 0.1 mol/L

1000 mL of this solution contains 5.611 g of potassium hydroxide (KOH: 56.11).

Preparation—Weigh 7 g of potassium hydroxide, proceed as directed for preparation under 0.5 mol/L potassium hydroxide-ethanol VS, and standardize the solution as follows:

Standardization—Proceed as directed for standardization under 0.5 mol/L potassium hydroxide-ethanol VS, but measure exactly 15 mL of 0.05 mol/L sulfuric acid VS.

Note: Store as directed under 0.5 mol/L potassium hydroxide-ethanol VS. Standardize before use.

Potassium Iodate, 0.05 mol/L

1000 mL of this solution contains 10.700 g of potassium iodate (KIO_3: 214.00).

Preparation—Weigh accurately about 10.700 g of potassium iodate (standard reagent), previously dried between 120°C and 140°C for 1.5 to 2 hours and allowed to cool in a desiccator (silica gel), and dissolve it in water to make exactly 1000 mL. Calculate the molarity factor.

Potassium Iodate, 1/60 mol/L

1000 mL of this solution contains 3.567 g of potassium iodate (KIO_3: 214.00).

Preparation—Weigh accurately about 3.567 g of potassium iodate (standard reagent), previously dried between 120°C and 140°C for 2 hours and allowed to cool in a desiccator (silica gel), and dissolve it in water to make exactly 1000 mL. Calculate the molarity factor.

Potassium Iodate, 1/1200 mol/L

1000 mL of this solution contains 0.17833 g of potassium iodate (KIO_3: 214.00).

Preparation—Weigh accurately about 0.17833 g of potassium iodate, previously dried between 120°C and 140°C for 1.5 to 2 hours and allowed to cool in a desiccator (silica gel), and dissolve it in water to make exactly 1000 mL. Calculate the molarity factor.

Potassium Permanganate, 0.02 mol/L

1000 mL of this solution contains 3.1607 g of potassium permanganate ($KMnO_4$: 158.03).

Preparation—Dissolve 3.2 g of potassium permanganate in water to make 1000 mL, and boil the solution for 15 minutes. Allow the solution to stand for at least 48 hours in a tightly stoppered flask, and filter it through a glass filter (G3 or G4). Standardize the solution as follows:

Standardization—Weigh accurately about 0.3 g of sodium oxalate (standard reagent), previously dried between 150°C and 200°C for 1 to 1.5 hours and allowed to cool in a desiccator (silica gel), transfer it to a 500 mL conical flask, dissolve in 30 mL of water, add 250 mL of diluted sulfuric acid (1 in 20), and warm the mixture between 30°C and 35°C. Transfer the prepared potassium permanganate solution to a buret, add quickly 40 mL of the solution under gentle stirring from the buret, and allow to stand until the red color of the mixture disappears. Warm the solution between 55°C and 60°C, and complete the titration <*2.50*> with the potassium permanganate solution until a light red color persists for 30 seconds. Add the last 0.5 to 1 mL dropwise before the end point, being particularly careful to allow the solution to be decolorized before the next drop is added. Calculate the molarity factor.

Each mL of 0.02 mol/L potassium permanganate VS
= 6.700 mg of $Na_2C_2O_4$

Note: Store protected from light. This solution, if stored for a long period, should be restandardized.

Potassium Permanganate, 0.002 mol/L

1000 mL of this solution contains 0.31607 g of potassium permanganate ($KMnO_4$: 158.03).

Preparation—Before use, dilute 0.02 mol/L potassium permanganate VS with water to make exactly 10 times the initial volume.

Silver Nitrate, 0.1 mol/L

1000 mL of this solution contains 16.987 g of silver nitrate ($AgNO_3$: 169.87).

Preparation—Dissolve 17.0 g of silver nitrate in water to make 1000 mL, and standardize the solution as follows:

Standardization—Weigh accurately about 80 mg of sodium chloride (standard reagent), previously dried between 500°C and 650°C for 40 to 50 minutes and allowed to cool in a desiccator (silica gel), dissolve it in 50 mL of water, and titrate <*2.50*> under vigorous stirring with the prepared silver nitrate solution to calculate the molarity factor (Indicator method: 3 drops of fluorescein sodium TS; or potentiometric titration: silver electrode). In the indicator method, titrate until the color of the solution changes from yellow-green to orange through yellow.

Each mL of 0.1 mol/L silver nitrate VS
= 5.844 mg of NaCl

Note: Store protected from light.

Silver Nitrate, 0.02 mol/L

1000 mL of this solution contains 3.3974 g of silver nitrate ($AgNO_3$: 169.87).

Preparation—Before use, dilute 0.1 mol/L silver nitrate VS with water to make exactly 5 times the initial volume.

Silver Nitrate, 0.01 mol/L

1000 mL of this solution contains 1.6987 g of silver nitrate ($AgNO_3$: 169.87).

Preparation—Before use, dilute 0.1 mol/L silver nitrate VS with water to make exactly 10 times the initial volume.

Silver Nitrate, 0.005 mol/L

1000 mL of this solution contains 0.8494 g of silver nitrate ($AgNO_3$: 169.87).

Preparation—Before use, dilute 0.1 mol/L silver nitrate VS with water to make exactly 20 times the initial volume.

Silver Nitrate, 0.001 mol/L

1000 mL of this solution contains 0.16987 g of silver nitrate ($AgNO_3$: 169.87).

Preparation—Dilute 0.1 mol/L silver nitrate VS with water to make exactly 100 times of the initial volume before use.

Sodium Acetate, 0.1 mol/L

1000 mL of this solution contains 8.203 g of sodium acetate (CH_3COONa: 82.03).

Preparation—Dissolve 8.20 g of anhydrous sodium acetate in acetic acid (100) to make 1000 mL, and standardize the solution as follows:

Standardization—Pipet 25 mL of the prepared sodium acetate solution, add 50 mL of acetic acid (100) and 1 mL of *p*-naphtholbenzeine TS, and titrate <*2.50*> with 0.1 mol/L perchloric acid VS until a yellow-brown color changes through yellow to green. Perform a blank determination, make any necessary correction, and calculate the molarity factor.

Sodium Hydroxide, 1 mol/L

1000 mL of this solution contains 39.997 g of sodium hydroxide (NaOH: 40.00).

Preparation—Dissolve 42 g of sodium hydroxide in 950 mL of water. Add a freshly prepared, saturated solution of barium hydroxide octahydrate until no more precipitate is produced. Mix well the mixture, and allow to stand for 24 hours in a tightly stoppered bottle. Decant the supernatant liquid or filter the solution through a glass filter (G3 or G4), and standardize the solution as follows:

Standardization—Weigh accurately about 1.5 g of amidosulfuric acid (standard reagent), previously dried in a desiccator (in vacuum, silica gel) for about 48 hours. Dissolve it in 25 mL of freshly boiled and cooled water, and titrate <*2.50*> the solution with the prepared sodium hydroxide solution to calculate the molarity factor (Indicator method: 2 drops of bromothymol blue TS; or potentiometric titration). In the indicator method, titrate until the solution acquires a green color.

Each mL of 1 mol/L sodium hydroxide VS
= 97.09 mg of $HOSO_2NH_2$

Note: Store in tightly stoppered bottles or in containers provided with a carbon dioxide-absorbing tube (soda lime). This solution, if stored for a long period, should be restandardized.

Sodium Hydroxide, 0.5 mol/L

1000 mL of this solution contains 19.999 g of sodium hydroxide (NaOH: 40.00).

Preparation—Weigh 22 g of sodium hydroxide, proceed as directed for preparation under 1 mol/L sodium hydroxide VS, and standardize the solution as follows:

Standardization—Proceed as directed for standardization under 1 mol/L sodium hydroxide VS, but weigh accurately about 0.7 g of amidosulfuric acid (standard reagent).

Each mL of 0.5 mol/L sodium hydroxide VS
= 48.55 mg of $HOSO_2NH_2$

Note: Store as directed under 1 mol/L sodium hydroxide VS. This solution, if stored for a long period, should be restandardized.

Sodium Hydroxide, 0.2 mol/L

1000 mL of this solution contains 7.999 g of sodium hydroxide (NaOH: 40.00).

Preparation—Weigh 9 g of sodium hydroxide, proceed as directed for preparation under 1 mol/L sodium hydroxide VS, and standardize the solution as follows:

Standardization—Proceed as directed for standardization under 1 mol/L sodium hydroxide VS, but weigh accurately about 0.3 g of amidosulfuric acid (standard reagent).

Each mL of 0.2 mol/L sodium hydroxide VS
= 19.42 mg of $HOSO_2NH_2$

Note: Store as directed under 1 mol/L sodium hydroxide VS. This solution, if stored for a long period, should be restandardized.

Sodium Hydroxide, 0.1 mol/L

1000 mL of this solution contains 3.9997 g of sodium hydroxide (NaOH: 40.00).

Preparation—Weigh 4.5 g of sodium hydroxide, proceed as directed for preparation under 1 mol/L sodium hydroxide VS, and standardize the solution as follows.

Standardization—Proceed as directed for standardization under 1 mol/L sodium hydroxide VS, but weigh accurately about 0.15 g of amidosulfuric acid (standard reagent).

Each mL of 0.1 mol/L sodium hydroxide VS
= 9.709 mg of $HOSO_2NH_2$

Note: Store as directed under 1 mol/L sodium hydroxide VS. This solution, if stored for a long period, should be restandardized.

Sodium Hydroxide, 0.05 mol/L

1000 mL of this solution contains 1.9999 g of sodium hydroxide (NaOH: 40.00).

Preparation—Before use, dilute 0.1 mol/L sodium hydroxide VS with freshly boiled and cooled water to make exactly twice the initial volume.

Sodium Hydroxide, 0.02 mol/L

1000 mL of this solution contains 0.7999 g of sodium hydroxide (NaOH: 40.00).

Preparation—Before use, dilute 0.1 mol/L sodium hydroxide VS with freshly boiled and cooled water to make exactly 5 times the initial volume.

Sodium Hydroxide, 0.01 mol/L

1000 mL of this solution contains 0.39997 g of sodium hydroxide (NaOH: 40.00).

Preparation—Before use, dilute 0.1 mol/L sodium hydroxide VS with freshly boiled and cooled water to make exactly 10 times the initial volume.

Sodium Hydroxide-Ethanol, 0.025 mol/L

1000 mL of this solution contains 1.000 g of sodium hydroxide (NaOH: 40.00).

Preparation—Dissolve 2.1 g of sodium hydroxide in 100 mL of ethanol (99.5), stopper tightly, and allow to stand for a night. To 50 mL of the supernatant liquid add 650 mL of ethanol (99.5) and freshly boiled and cooled water to make 1000 mL, and standardize the solution as follows:

Standardization—Weigh accurately about 25 mg of amidosulfuric acid (standard reagent), previously dried in a desiccator (in vacuum, silica gel) for 48 hours. Dissolve in 30 mL of diluted ethanol (99.5) with fleshly boiled and cooled water (7 in 10), and titrate <*2.50*> with the prepared sodium hydroxide-ethanol to calculate the molarity factor (potentiometric titration).

Each mL of 0.025 mol/L sodium hydroxide-ethanol VS
= 2.427 mg of $HOSO_2NH_2$

Note: Store in light-resistant, well-stoppered bottles. The standardization should be performed before using.

Sodium Lauryl Sulfate, 0.01 mol/L

1000 mL of this solution contains 2.8838 g of sodium lauryl sulfate ($C_{12}H_{25}NaO_4S$: 288.38).

Preparation—Dissolve 2.9 g of sodium lauryl sulfate in water to make 1000 mL, and standardize the solution as follows:

Standardization—Weigh accurately about 0.3 g of papaverine hydrochloride for assay, previously dried, and dissolve in water to make exactly 100 mL. Pipet 10 mL of this solution into a glass-stoppered conical flask, add 5 mL each of water and dilute sulfuric acid and 60 mL of dichloromethane, then add 5 to 6 drops of a solution of methyl yellow in dichloromethane (1 in 500) as indicator, and titrate <*2.50*>, while vigorous shaking, with the sodium lauryl sulfate solution prepared above, using a buret with a minimum graduation of 0.02 mL. End point is reached when the color of the dichloromethane layer changes from yellow to orange-red after dropwise addition of the sodium lauryl sulfate solution, vigorous shaking and standing for a while.

Each mL of 0.01 mol/L sodium lauryl sulfate VS
= 3.759 mg of $C_{20}H_{21}NO_4.HCl$

Sodium Methoxide, 0.1 mol/L

1000 mL of this solution contains 5.402 g of sodium methoxide (CH_3ONa: 54.02).

Preparation—Add little by little 2.5 g of freshly cut sodium pieces to 150 mL of methanol cooled in ice-water. After the sodium has dissolved, add benzene to make 1000 mL, and standardize the solution as follows:

Standardization—Weigh accurately about 0.3 g of benzoic acid, previously dried for 24 hours in a desiccator (silica gel), dissolve it in 80 mL of *N,N*-dimethylformamide, and add 3 drops of thymol blue-*N,N*-dimethylformamide TS. Titrate <*2.50*> the solution with the prepared sodium methoxide solution until a blue color appears. Perform a blank determination, make any necessary correction, and calculate the molarity factor.

Each mL of 0.1 mol/L sodium methoxide VS
= 12.21 mg of C_6H_5COOH

Note: Store in a cold place, protected from moisture. Standardize before use.

Sodium Methoxide-Dioxane, 0.1 mol/L

See Sodium Methoxide-1,4-Dioxane, 0.1 mol/L.

Sodium Methoxide-1,4-Dioxane, 0.1 mol/L

1000 mL of this solution contains 5.402 g of sodium methoxide (CH_3ONa: 54.02).

Preparation—Add little by little 2.5 g of freshly cut sodium pieces to 150 mL of methanol cooled in ice-water. After the sodium has dissolved, add 1,4-dioxane to make 1000 mL, and standardize the solution as follows:

Standardization—Weigh accurately about 0.3 g of benzoic acid, previously dried in a desiccator (silica gel) for 24 hours, dissolve it in 80 mL of *N,N*-dimethylformamide, and add 3 drops of thymol blue-*N,N*-dimethylformamide TS. Titrate <*2.50*> the solution with the prepared sodium methoxide-1,4-dioxane solution until a blue color appears. Perform a blank determination, make any necessary correction, and calculate the molarity factor.

Each mL of 0.1 mol/L sodium methoxide-1,4-dioxane VS
= 12.21 mg of C_6H_5COOH

Note: Store in a cold place, protected from moisture. Standardize before use.

Sodium Nitrite, 0.1 mol/L

1000 mL of this solution contains 6.900 g of sodium nitrite ($NaNO_2$: 69.00).

Preparation—Dissolve 7.2 g of sodium nitrite in water to make 1000 mL, and standardize the solution as follows:

Standardization—Weigh accurately about 0.44 g of sulfanilamide for titration of diazotization, previously dried at 105°C for 3 hours and allowed to cool in a desiccator (silica gel), dissolve in 10 mL of hydrochloric acid, 40 mL of water and 10 mL of a solution of potassium bromide (3 in 10), cool below 15°C, and titrate with the prepared sodium nitrite solution as directed in the potentiometric titration or amperometric titration under Endpoint Detection Methods in Titrimetry <*2.50*>. Calculate the molarity factor.

Each mL of 0.1 mol/L sodium nitrite VS
= 17.22 mg of $H_2NC_6H_4SO_2NH_2$

Note: Store protected from light. This solution, if stored for a long period, should be restandardized.

Sodium Oxalate, 0.005 mol/L

1000 mL of this solution contains 0.6700 g of sodium oxalate ($Na_2C_2O_4$: 134.00).

Preparation—Weigh accurately about 0.6700 g of sodium

oxalate (standard reagent), previously dried between 150°C and 200°C for 2 hours and allowed to cool in a desiccator (silica gel), dissolve it in water to make exactly 1000 mL, and calculate the molarity factor.

Sodium Tetraphenylborate, 0.02 mol/L

1000 mL of this solution contains 6.844 g of sodium tetraphenylborate [$NaB(C_6H_5)_4$: 342.22].

Preparation—Dissolve 7.0 g of sodium tetraphenylborate in water to make 1000 mL, and standardize the solution as follows:

Standardization—Weigh 0.5 g of potassium hydrogen phthalate (standard reagent), dissolve it in 100 mL of water, add 2 mL of acetic acid (31), and warm to 50°C in a water bath. Add slowly 50 mL of the prepared sodium tetraphenylborate solution under stirring from a buret, then cool the mixture quickly, and allow to stand for 1 hour at room temperature. Transfer the precipitate to a tared glass filter (G4), wash with three 5 mL portions of potassium tetraphenylborate TS, dry at 105°C for 1 hour, and weigh accurately the glass filter. Calculate the molarity factor from the mass of potassium tetraphenylborate [$KB(C_6H_5)_4$: 358.32].

Each mL of 0.02 mol/L sodium tetraphenylborate VS
= 7.166 mg of $KB(C_6H_5)_4$

Note: Prepare before use.

Sodium Tetraphenylboron, 0.02 mol/L

See Sodium Tetraphenylborate, 0.02 mol/L.

Sodium Thiosulfate, 0.1 mol/L

1000 mL of this solution contains 24.818 g of sodium thiosulfate pentahydrate ($Na_2S_2O_3.5H_2O$: 248.18).

Preparation—Dissolve 25 g of sodium thiosulfate and 0.2 g of anhydrous sodium carbonate in freshly boiled and cooled water to make 1000 mL, allow to stand for 24 hours, and standardize the solution as follows:

Standardization—Weigh accurately about 50 mg of potassium iodate (standard reagent), previously dried between 120°C and 140°C for 1.5 to 2 hours and allowed to cool in a desiccator (silica gel), and transfer to an iodine flask. Dissolve it in 25 mL of water, add 2 g of potassium iodide and 10 mL of dilute sulfuric acid, and stopper the flask. After allowing the mixture to stand for 10 minutes, add 100 mL of water, and titrate <*2.50*> the liberated iodine with the prepared sodium thiosulfate solution (Indicator method; or potentiometric titration: platinum electrode). In the indicator method, when the solution assumes a light yellow color as the end point is approached, add 3 mL of starch TS. Continue the titration, until the blue color disappears. Perform a blank determination, make any necessary correction, and calculate the molarity factor.

Each mL of 0.1 mol/L sodium thiosulfate VS
= 3.567 mg of KIO_3

Note: This solution, if stored for a long period, should be restandardized.

Sodium Thiosulfate, 0.05 mol/L

1000 mL of this solution contains 12.409 g of sodium thiosulfate pentahydrate ($Na_2S_2O_3.5H_2O$: 248.18).

Preparation—Before use, dilute 0.1 mol/L sodium thiosulfate VS with freshly boiled and cooled water to make exactly 2 times the initial volume.

Sodium Thiosulfate, 0.02 mol/L

1000 mL of this solution contains 4.964 g of sodium thiosulfate pentahydrate ($Na_2S_2O_3.5H_2O$: 248.18).

Preparation—Before use, dilute 0.1 mol/L sodium thiosulfate VS with freshly boiled and cooled water to make exactly 5 times the initial volume.

Sodium Thiosulfate, 0.01 mol/L

1000 mL of this solution contains 2.4818 g of sodium thiosulfate pentahydrate ($Na_2S_2O_3.5H_2O$: 248.18).

Preparation—Before use, dilute 0.1 mol/L sodium thiosulfate VS with freshly boiled and cooled water to make exactly 10 times the initial volume.

Sodium Thiosulfate, 0.005 mol/L

1000 mL of this solution contains 1.2409 g of sodium thiosulfate pentahydrate ($Na_2S_2O_3.5H_2O$: 248.18).

Preparation—Before use, dilute 0.1 mol/L sodium thiosulfate VS with freshly boiled and cooled water to make exactly 20 times the initial volume.

Sodium Thiosulfate, 0.002 mol/L

1000 mL of this solution contains 0.4964 g of sodium thiosulfate pentahydrate ($Na_2S_2O_3.5H_2O$: 248.18).

Preparation—Before use, dilute 0.1 mol/L sodium thiosulfate VS with freshly boiled and cooled water to make exactly 50 times the initial volume.

Sulfuric Acid, 0.5 mol/L

1000 mL of this solution contains 49.04 g of sulfuric acid (H_2SO_4: 98.08).

Preparation—Add slowly, under stirring, 30 mL of sulfuric acid to 1000 mL of water, allow to cool, and standardize the solution as follows:

Standardization—Weigh accurately about 0.8 g of sodium carbonate (standard reagent), previously heated between 500°C and 650°C for 40 to 50 minutes and allowed to cool in a desiccator (silica gel). Dissolve it in 50 mL of water, and titrate <*2.50*> the solution with the prepared sulfuric acid (Indicator method: 3 drops of methyl red TS; or potentiometric titration). In the indicator method, when the end point is approached, boil the solution carefully, stopper the flask loosely, allow to cool, and continue the titration, until the color of the solution changes to persistent orange to orange-red. Calculate the molarity factor. In the potentiometric titration, titrate with vigorous stirring without boiling.

Each mL of 0.5 mol/L sulfuric acid VS
= 53.00 mg of Na_2CO_3

Sulfuric Acid, 0.25 mol/L

1000 mL of this solution contains 24.520 g of sulfuric acid (H_2SO_4: 98.08).

Preparation—Add slowly, under stirring, 15 mL of sulfuric acid to 1000 mL of water, allow to cool, and standardize the solution as follows:

Standardization—Proceed as directed for standardization under 0.5 mol/L sulfuric acid VS, but weigh accurately about 0.4 g of sodium carbonate (standard reagent), and dissolve in 50 mL of water.

Each mL of 0.25 mol/L sulfuric acid VS
= 26.50 mg of Na_2CO_3

Sulfuric Acid, 0.1 mol/L

1000 mL of this solution contains 9.808 g of sulfuric acid (H_2SO_4: 98.08).

Preparation—Add slowly, under stirring, 6 mL of sulfuric acid to 1000 mL of water, allow to cool, and standardize the solution as follows:

Standardization—Proceed as directed for standardization under 0.5 mol/L sulfuric acid VS, but weigh accurately about 0.15 g of sodium carbonate (standard reagent), and dissolve in 50 mL of water.

Each mL of 0.1 mol/L sulfuric acid VS
= 10.60 mg of Na_2CO_3

Sulfuric Acid, 0.05 mol/L

1000 mL of this solution contains 4.904 g of sulfuric acid (H_2SO_4: 98.08).

Preparation—Add slowly, under stirring, 3 mL of sulfuric acid to 1000 mL of water, allow to cool, and standardize the solution as follows:

Standardization—Proceed as directed for standardization under 0.5 mol/L sulfuric acid VS, but weigh accurately about 80 mg of sodium carbonate (standard reagent), and dissolve in 30 mL of water.

Each mL of 0.05 mol/L sulfuric acid VS
= 5.300 mg of Na_2CO_3

Sulfuric Acid, 0.025 mol/L

1000 mL of this solution contains 2.4520 g of sulfuric acid (H_2SO_4: 98.08).

Preparation—Before use, dilute 0.05 mol/L sulfuric acid VS with water to make exactly twice the initial volume.

Sulfuric Acid, 0.02 mol/L

1000 mL of this solution contains 1.9616 g of sulfuric acid (H_2SO_4: 98.08).

Preparation—Before use, dilute 0.05 mol/L sulfuric acid VS with water to make exactly 2.5 times the initial volume.

Sulfuric Acid, 0.01 mol/L

1000 mL of this solution contains 0.9808 g of sulfuric acid (H_2SO_4: 98.08).

Preparation—Before use, dilute 0.05 mol/L sulfuric acid VS with water to make exactly 5 times the initial volume.

Sulfuric Acid, 0.005 mol/L

1000 mL of this solution contains 0.4904 g of sulfuric acid (H_2SO_4: 98.08).

Preparation—Before use, dilute 0.05 mol/L sulfuric acid VS with water to make exactly 10 times the initial volume.

Surfuric Acid, 0.0005 mol/L

1000 mL of this solution contains 0.04904 g of sulfuric acid (H_2SO_4: 98.08).

Preparation—Before use, dilute 0.05 mol/L sulfuric acid VS with water to make exactly 100 times the initial volume.

Tetrabutylammonium Hydroxide, 0.1 mol/L

1000 mL of this solution contains 25.947 g of tetrabutyl ammonium hydroxide [$(C_4H_9)_4NOH$: 259.47].

Preparation—Before use, dilute a volume of 10% tetrabutylammonium hydroxide-methanol TS, equivalent to 26.0 g of tetrabutylammonium hydroxide, with 2-propanol to make 1000 mL, and standardize the solution as follows:

Standardization—Weigh accurately about 0.3 g of benzoic acid, previously dried in a desiccator (silica gel) for 24 hours, dissolve it in 50 mL of acetone, and titrate <2.50> the solution with the prepared tetrabutylammonium hydroxide solution (potentiometric titration). Perform a blank determination in the same manner and make necessary corrections.

Each mL of 0.1 mol/L tetrabutylammonium hydroxide VS
= 12.21 mg of C_6H_5COOH

Note: Store in tightly stoppered bottles. This solution, if stored for a long period, should be restandardized.

Tetramethylammonium Hydroxide, 0.2 mol/L

1000 mL of this solution contains 18.231 g of tetramethylammonium hydroxide [$(CH_3)_4NOH$: 91.15].

Preparation—Before use, dilute a volume of tetramethylammonium hydroxide-methanol TS, equivalent to 18.4 g of tetramethylammonium hydroxide, with water to make 1000 mL, and standardize the solution as follows:

Standardization—Weigh accurately about 0.4 g of benzoic acid, previously dried in a desiccator (silica gel) for 24 hours, dissolve it in 60 mL of *N,N*-dimethylformamide, and titrate <2.50> the solution with the prepared 0.2 mol/L tetramethyl ammonium hydroxide solution (Indicator method: 3 drops of thymol blue-*N,N*-dimethylformamide TS; or potentiometric titration). In the indicator method, titrate until a blue color is produced. Perform a blank determination in the same manner, make any necessary correction, and calculate the molarity factor.

Each mL of 0.2 mol/L tetramethylammonium hydroxide VS
= 24.42 mg of C_6H_5COOH

Note: Store in tightly stoppered bottles. This solution, if stored for a long period, should be restandardized.

Tetramethylammonium Hydroxide, 0.1 mol/L

1000 mL of this solution contains 9.115 g of tetramethylammonium hydroxide [$(CH_3)_4NOH$: 91.15].

Preparation—Before use, dilute a volume of tetramethylammonium hydroxide-methanol TS, equivalent to 9.2 g of tetramethylammonium hydroxide, with water to make 1000 mL, and standardize the solution as follows:

Standardization—Proceed as directed for standardization under 0.2 mol/L tetramethylammonium hydroxide VS. Weigh accurately about 0.2 g of benzoic acid and titrate <2.50>.

Each mL of 0.1 mol/L tetramethylammonium hydroxide VS
= 12.21 mg of C_6H_5COOH

Note: Store in tightly stoppered bottles. This solution, if stored for a long period, should be restandardized.

Tetramethylammonium Hydroxide, 0.02 mol/L

1000 mL of this solution contains 1.8231 g of tetramethylammonium hydroxide [$(CH_3)_4NOH$: 91.15].

Preparation—Before use, dilute 0.1 mol/L tetramethylammonium hydroxide VS with freshly boiled and cooled water to make exactly 5 times the initial volume.

Tetramethylammonium Hydroxide-Methanol, 0.1 mol/L

1000 mL of this solution contains 9.115 g of tetramethylammonium hydroxide [$(CH_3)_4NOH$: 91.15].

Preparation—Before use, dilute a volume of tetramethylammonium hydroxide-methanol TS, equivalent to 9.2 g of tetramethylammonium hydroxide, with methanol to make 1000 mL, and standardize the solution as follows:

Standardization—Proceed as directed for standardization under 0.1 mol/L tetramethylammonium hydroxide VS.

Note: Store in tightly stoppered bottles. This solution, if stored for a long period, should be restandardized.

Titanium (III) Chloride, 0.1 mol/L

1000 mL of this solution contains 15.423 g of titanium (III) chloride ($TiCl_3$: 154.23).

Preparation—Add 75 mL of hydrochloric acid to 75 mL of titanium (III) chloride (20), and dilute with freshly boiled and cooled water to make 1000 mL. Transfer the solution into a buret provided with a reservoir protected from light, replace the air with hydrogen, and allow to stand for 48 hours. Before use, standardize the solution as follows:

Standardization—Weigh 3 g of ammonium iron (II) sulfate hexahydrate in a wide-mouthed, 500 mL conical flask. Passing carbon dioxide through the flask, dissolve it in 50 mL of freshly boiled and cooled water, and add 25 mL of diluted sulfuric acid (27 in 100). Rapidly add exactly 40 mL of 0.02 mol/L potassium permanganate VS to the mixture, while passing carbon dioxide through the flask. Titrate <*2.50*> with the prepared titanium (III) chloride solution until the calculated end point is approached, then add 5 g of ammonium thiocyanate immediately, and continue the titration with the prepared titanium (III) chloride solution until the color of the solution disappears. Perform a blank determination. Calculate the molarity factor.

Note: Store after the air has been displaced with hydrogen.

Titanium Trichloride, 0.1 mol/L

See Titanium (III) Chloride, 0.1 mol/L.

Zinc, 0.1 mol/L

1000 mL of this solution contains 6.538 g of zinc (Zn: 65.38).

Preparation—To 6.538 g of zinc (standard reagent), previously washed with dilute hydrochloric acid, with water and then acetone, and cooled in a desiccator (silica gel) after drying at 110°C for 5 minutes, add 80 mL of dilute hydrochloric acid and 2.5 mL of bromine TS, dissolve by gentle warming, evaporate excess bromine by boiling, and add water to make exactly 1000 mL.

Zinc Acetate, 0.05 mol/L

1000 mL of this solution contains 10.975 g of zinc acetate dihydrate [$Zn(CH_3COO)_2.2H_2O$: 219.50].

Preparation—Dissolve 11.1 g of zinc acetate dihydrate in 40 mL of water and 4 mL of dilute acetic acid, add water to make 1000 mL, and standardize the solution as follows:

Standardization—Measure exactly 20 mL of 0.05 mol/L disodium dihydrogen ethylenediamine tetraacetate VS, and add 50 mL of water, 3 mL of ammonia-ammonium chloride buffer solution, pH 10.7, and 0.04 g of eriochrome black T-sodium chloride reagent. Titrate <*2.50*> the solution with the prepared zinc acetate solution, until the blue color changes to blue-purple. Calculate the molarity factor.

Zinc Acetate, 0.02 mol/L

1000 mL of this solution contains 4.390 g of zinc acetate dihydrate [$Zn(CH_3COO)_2.2H_2O$: 219.50].

Preparation—Dissolve 4.43 g of zinc acetate dihydrate in 20 mL of water and 2 mL of dilute acetic acid, add water to make 1000 mL, and standardize the solution as follows:

Standardization—Proceed as directed for standardization under 0.05 mol/L zinc acetate VS, but measure exactly 20 mL of 0.02 mol/L disodium dihydrogen ethylenediamine tetraacetate VS.

Zinc Sulfate, 0.1 mol/L

1000 mL of this solution contains 28.755 g of zinc sulfate heptahydrate ($ZnSO_4.7H_2O$: 287.55).

Preparation—Dissolve 28.8 g of zinc sulfate heptahydrate in water to make 1000 mL, and standardize the solution as follows:

Standardization—Pipet 25 mL of the prepared zinc sulfate solution, add 5 mL of ammonia-ammonium chloride buffer solution, pH 10.7, and 0.04 g of eriochrome black T-sodium chloride indicator, and titrate <*2.50*> with 0.1 mol/L disodium dihydrogen ethylenediamine tetraacetate VS until the color of the solution changes from red-purple to blue-purple. Calculate the molarity factor.

Zinc sulfate, 0.05 mol/L

1000 mL of this solution contains 14.378 g of zinc sulfate heptahydrate ($ZnSO_4.7H_2O$: 287.55).

Preparation—Before use, dilute 0.1 mol/L zinc sulfate VS with water to make exactly twice the initial volume.

Zinc sulfate, 0.02 mol/L

1000 mL of this solution contains 5.7510 g of zinc sulfate heptahydrate ($ZnSO_4.7H_2O$: 287.55).

Preparation—Before use, dilute 0.1 mol/L zinc sulfate VS with water to make exactly 5 times the initial volume.

9.22 Standard Solutions

Standard Solutions are used as the standard for the comparison in a text of the Pharmacopoeia.

Borate pH Standard Solution See pH Determination <*2.54*>.

Calcium Hydroxide pH Standard Solution See pH Determination <*2.54*>.

Carbonate pH Standard Solution See pH Determination <*2.54*>.

Certified Standard Arsenic Solution See Arsenic Limit Test <*1.11*>.

Formazin stock suspension To 25 mL of hexamethylenetetramine TS add 25 mL of hydrazinium sulfate TS, mix, and use after allowing to stand at room temperature for 24 hours. Store in a glass container free from surface defects. Use within 2 months. Shake thoroughly before use. The turbidity of this suspension is equivalent to 4000 NTU.

Oxalate pH Standard Solution See pH Determination <*2.54*>.

pH Standard Solution, Borate See pH Determination <*2.54*>.

pH Standard Solution, Calcium Hydroxide See pH Determination <*2.54*>.

pH Standard Solution, Carbonate See pH Determination <*2.54*>.

pH Standard Solution, Oxalate See pH Determination <*2.54*>.

pH Standard Solution, Phosphate See pH Determination <*2.54*>.

pH Standard Solution, Phthalate See pH Determination <*2.54*>.

Phosphate pH Standard Solution See pH Determination <*2.54*>.

Phthalate pH Standard Solution See pH Determination

<2.54>.

Standard Aluminum Solution for Atomic Absorption Spectrophotometry To exactly 10 mL of Standard Aluminum Stock Solution add water to make exactly 100 mL. Prepare before use. Each mL of this solution contains 0.100 mg of aluminum (Al).

Standard Aluminum Stock Solution Weigh 1.0 g of aluminum, add 60 mL of diluted hydrochloric acid (1 in 2), dissolve by heating, cool, add water to make 1000 mL. Pipet 10 mL of this solution, add 30 mL of water and 5 mL of acetic acid-ammonium acetate buffer solution, pH 3.0, and adjust the pH to about 3 with ammonia TS added dropwise. Then, add 0.5 mL of Cu-PAN TS, and titrate *<2.50>* with 0.01 mol/L disodium dihydrogen ethylenediamine tetraacetate VS while boiling until the color of the solution changes from red to yellow lasting for more than 1 minute. Perform a brank determination in the same manner, and make any necessary correction.

Each mL of 0.01 mol/L disodium dihydrogen ethylenediamine tetraacetate VS
= 0.2698 mg of Al

Standard Ammonium Solution Dissolve 2.97 g of ammonium chloride, exactly weighed, in water for ammonium limit test to make exactly 1000 mL. Measure exactly 10 mL of this solution, and add water for ammonium limit test to make exactly 1000 mL. Each mL of this solution contains 0.01 mg of ammonium (NH_4^+).

Standard Arsenic Solution See Arsenic Limit Test *<1.11>*.

Standard Arsenic Stock Solution See Arsenic Limit Test *<1.11>*.

Standard Boron Solution Weigh exactly 0.286 g of boric acid, previously dried in a desiccator (silica gel) to constant mass, and dissolve in water to make exactly 1000 mL. Pipet 10 mL of this solution, and add water to make exactly 1000 mL. Each mL of this solution contains 0.5 μg of boron (B).

Standard Cadmium Solution Measure exactly 10 mL of Standard Cadmium Stock Solution, and add diluted nitric acid (1 in 3) to make exactly 1000 mL. Pipet 10 mL of this solution, and add diluted nitric acid (1 in 3) to make 100 mL. Each mL of this solution contains 0.001 mg of cadmium (Cd). Prepare before use.

Standard Cadmium Stock Solution Dissolve 1.000 g of cadmium ground metal, exactly weighed, in 100 mL of dilute nitric acid by gentle heating, cool, and add dilute nitric acid to make exactly 1000 mL.

Standard Calcium Solution Weigh exactly 0.250 g of calcium carbonate, add 5 mL of dilute hydrochloric acid and 25 mL of water, and dissolve by heating. After cooling, add water to make exactly 1000 mL. Each mL of this solution contains 0.1 mg of calcium (Ca).

Standard Calcium Solution for Atomic Absorption Spectrophotometry Weigh accurately 0.250 g of calcium carbonate, and add 1 mol/L hydrochloric acid TS to make exactly 100 mL. Each mL of this solution contains 1.00 mg of calcium (Ca).

Standard Chloride Solution Pipet 10 mL of Standard Chloride Stock Solution, add water to make exactly 1000 mL. Prepare before use. Each mL of this solution contains 5 μg of chloride (Cl).

Standard Chloride Stock Solution Weigh accurately 0.842 g of sodium chloride, previously dried at 130°C for 2 hours, and dissolve in water to make exactly 1000 mL.

Standard Chromium Solution for Atomic Absorption Spectrophotometry Weigh exactly 0.283 g of potassium dichromate (standard reagent), dissolve in water to make exactly 1000 mL. Each mL contains 0.10 mg of chromium (Cr).

Standard Copper Solution Pipet 10 mL of Standard Copper Stock Solution, and dilute with water to make exactly 1000 mL. Each mL of this solution contains 0.01 mg of copper (Cu). Prepare before use.

Standard Copper Stock Solution Weigh exactly 1.000 g of copper (standard reagent), add 100 mL of dilute nitric acid, and dissolve by heating. After cooling, add water to make exactly 1000 mL.

Standard Cyanide Solution Measure exactly a volume of Standard Cyanide Stock Solution, equivalent to 10 mg of cyanide (CN), add 100 mL of sodium hydroxide TS and water to make exactly 1000 mL. Each mL of this solution contains 0.01 mg of cyanide (CN). Prepare before use.

Standard Cyanide Stock Solution Dissolve 2.5 g of potassium cyanide in water to make exactly 1000 mL. Measure exactly 100 mL of this solution, add 0.5 mL of 4-dimethylaminobenzylidene rhodanine TS, and titrate *<2.50>* with 0.1 mol/L silver nitrate VS until the solution shows a red color.

Each mL of 0.1 mol/L silver nitrate VS
= 5.204 mg of CN

Standard Fluorine Solution See Oxygen Flask Combustion Method *<1.06>*.

Standard Glyoxal Solution Dilute Standard Glyoxal Stock Solution to 10 times with ethanol (99.5). Prepare before use. Each mL of this solution contains 2 μg of glyoxal ($C_2H_2O_2$).

Standard Glyoxal Stock Solution Transfer a quantity of 40% glyoxal TS, equivalent to 0.200 g of glyoxal, in a 100-mL volumetric flask, and dilute to 100 mL with ethanol (99.5). Dilute to 100-fold with ethanol (99.5) before use. Each mL of this solution contains 20 μg of glyoxal ($C_2H_2O_2$).

Standard Gold Solution for Atomic Absorption Spectrophotometry To 25 mL of Standard Gold Stock Solution, exactly measured, add water to make exactly 1000 mL. Each mL of this solution contains 0.025 mg of gold (Au).

Standard Gold Stock Solution Dissolve 0.209 g of hydrogen tetrachloroaurate (III) tetrahydrate, exactly weighed, in 2 mL of aqua regia, heat on a water bath for 10 minutes, and add 1 mol/L hydrochloric acid TS to make exactly 100 mL. Each mL of this solution contains 1.00 mg of gold (Au).

Standard Hydrogen Peroxide Stock Solution To an amount of hydrogen peroxide (30) add water to make a solution so that each mL contains 0.30 g of hydrogen peroxide (H_2O_2:34.01). Pipet 1 mL of this solution, add water to make exactly 10 mL, pipet 1 mL of this solution, transfer it to a flask containing 10 mL of water and 10 mL of dilute sulfuric acid, and titrate *<2.50>* with 0.02 mol/L potassium permanganate VS until the color of the solution changes to slightly red. Perform a blank determination in the same manner, and make any necessary correction.

Each mL of 0.02 mol/L potassium permanganate VS
= 1.701 mg of H_2O_2

Standard Hydrogen Peroxide Solution To exactly 10 mL of Standard Hydrogen Peroxide Stock Solution add water to make exactly 100 mL. Prepare before use. Each mL contains 30 mg of hydrogen peroxide (H_2O_2:34.01).

Standard Iron Solution Weigh exactly 86.3 mg of ammonium iron (III) sulfate dodecahydrate, dissolve in 100 mL of water, and add 5 mL of dilute hydrochloric acid and water to make exactly 1000 mL. Each mL of this solution contains 0.01 mg of iron (Fe).

Standard Iron Solution for Atomic Absorption Spectrophotometry To exactly 5 mL of Standard Iron Stock Solution add water to make exactly 200 mL. Prepare before use. Each mL of this solution contains 0.250 mg of iron (Fe).

Standard Iron Solution (2) for Atomic Absorption Spectrophotometry To exactly 2 mL of Standard Iron Stock Solution add water to make exactly 250 mL. Pipet 10 mL of this solution, add water to make exactly 100 mL. Prepare before use. Each mL contains 8 μg of iron (Fe).

Standard Iron Stock Solution Dissolve exactly 4.840 g of iron (III) chloride hexahydrate in diluted hydrochloric acid (9 in 25) to make exactly 100 mL.

Standard Lead Solution Measure exactly 10 mL of Standard Lead Stock Solution, and add water to make exactly 100 mL. Each mL of this solution contains 0.01 mg of lead (Pb). Prepare before use.

Standard Lead Stock Solution Weigh exactly 159.8 mg of lead (II) nitrate, dissolve in 10 mL of dilute nitric acid, and add water to make exactly 1000 mL. Prepare and store this solution using glass containers, free from soluble lead salts.

Standard Liquids for Calibrating Viscosimeters [JIS, Standard Liquids for Calibrating Viscosimeters (Z 8809)]

Standard Magnesium Solution for Atomic Absorption Spectrophotometry To exactly 1 mL of Standard Magnesium Stock Solution add water to make exactly 100 mL. Prepare before use. Each mL of this solution contains 0.0100 mg of magnesium (Mg).

Standard Magnesium Stock Solution Dissolve exactly 8.365 g of magnesium chloride hexahydrate in 2 mol/L hydrochloric acid TS to make exactly 1000 mL.

Standard Mercury Solution Weigh exactly 13.5 mg of mercury (II) chloride, previously dried for 6 hours in a desiccator (silica gel), dissolve in 10 mL of dilute nitric acid, and add water to make exactly 1000 mL. Pipet 10 mL of this solution, and add 10 mL of dilute nitric acid and water to make exactly 1000 mL. Each mL of this solution contains 0.1 μg of mercury (Hg). Prepare before use.

Standard Methanol Solution See Methanol Test *<1.12>*.

Standard Nickel Solution Dissolve 6.73 g of ammonium nickel (II) sulfate hexahydrate, exactly weighed, in water to make exactly 1000 mL. Pipet 5 mL of this solution, add water to make exactly 1000 mL. Each mL of this solution contains 0.005 mg of nickel (Ni).

Standard Nickel Solution for Atomic Absorption Spectrophotometry To exactly 10 mL of Standard Nickel Stock Solution add water to make exactly 1000 mL. Prepare before use. Each mL of this solution contains 0.01 mg of nickel (Ni).

Standard Nickel Stock Solution Dissolve exactly 4.48 g of nickel (II) sulfate hexahydrate in water to make exactly 1000 mL.

Standard Nitric Acid Solution Weigh exactly 72.2 mg of potassium nitrate, dissolve in water to make exactly 1000 mL. Each mL of this solution contains 0.01 mg of nitrogen (N).

Standard Palladium Solution for ICP Analysis Standard solution specified by the Measurement Law. Each mL of this solution contains 1 mg of palladium (Pd).

Standard Phosphoric Acid Solution Weigh exactly 0.358 g of potassium dihydrogen phosphate, previously dried to constant mass in a desiccator (silica gel), and add 10 mL of diluted sulfuric acid (3 in 10) and water to make exactly 1000 mL. Pipet 10 mL of this solution, and add water to make exactly 100 mL. Each mL of this solution contains 0.025 mg of phosphoric acid (as PO_4).

Standard Potassium Stock Solution Weigh exactly 9.534 g of potassium chloride, previously dried at 130°C for 2 hours, and dissolve in water to make exactly 1000 mL. Each mL of this solution contains 5.00 mg of potassium (K).

Standard Selenium Solution To exactly 1 mL of Standard Selenium Stock Solution add water to make exactly 1000 mL. Prepare before use. It contains 1.0 μg of selenium (Se) per mL.

Standard Selenium Stock Solution Dissolve exactly 1.405 g of selenium dioxide in 0.1 mol/L nitric acid to make exactly 1000 mL.

Standard Silver Solution for Atomic Absorption Spectrophotometry Measure exactly 10 mL of Standard Silver Stock Solution, and add water to make exactly 1000 mL. Each mL of this solution contains 0.01 mg of silver (Ag). Prepare before use.

Standard Silver Stock Solution Dissolve 1.575 g of silver nitrate, exactly weighed, in water to make exactly 1000 mL. Each mL of this solution contains 1.00 mg of silver (Ag).

Standard Sodium Dodecylbenzene Sulfonate Solution Weigh exactly 1.000 g of sodium dodecylbenzene sulfonate, and dissolve in water to make exactly 1000 mL. Pipet 10 mL of this solution, and add water to make exactly 1000 mL. Each mL of this solution contains 0.01 mg of sodium dodecylbenzene sulfonate [$CH_3(CH_2)_{11}C_6H_4SO_3Na$].

Standard Sodium Stock Solution Weigh exactly 2.542 g of sodium chloride (standard reagent), previously dried at 130°C for 2 hours, and dissolve in water to make exactly 1000 mL. Each mL of this solution contains 1.00 mg of sodium (Na).

Standard Sulfite Solution Dissolve exactly 3.150 g of anhydrous sodium sulfite in freshly prepared distilled water to make exactly 100 mL. Pipet 0.5 mL of this solution, add freshly prepared distilled water to make exactly 100 mL. Each mL of this solution contains 80 μg of sulfur dioxide (SO_2). Prepare before use.

Standard Tin Solution Weigh exactly 0.250 g of tin, and dissolve in 10 mL of sulfuric acid by heating. After cooling, transfer this solution with 400 mL of diluted hydrochloric acid (1 in 5) to a 500-mL volumetric flask, and add diluted hydrochloric acid (1 in 5) to make 500 mL. Pipet 10 mL of this solution, and add diluted hydrochloric acid (1 in 5) to make exactly 1000 mL. Each mL of this solution contains 0.005 mg of tin (Sn). Prepare before use.

Standard Vinyl Chloride Solution Transfer about 190 mL of ethanol for gas chromatography into a 200-mL volumetric flask, and stopper with a silicone rubber stopper. Cooling this volumetric flask in a methanol-dry ice bath, inject 0.20 g of vinyl chloride, previously liquidized, through the silicone rubber stopper, and then inject ethanol for gas chromatography, previously cooled in a methanol-dry ice bath, through the silicone rubber stopper to make 200 mL. Pipet 1 mL of this solution, add ethanol for gas chromatography, cooled previously in a methanol-dry ice bath to make exactly 100 mL. Preserve in a hermetic container, at a temperature not exceeding −20°C. This solution contains 10 μg of vinyl chloride per mL.

Standard Water-Methanol Solution See Water Determination *<2.48>*.

Standard Zinc Solution Measure exactly 25 mL of Standard Zinc Stock Solution, and add water to make exactly 1000 mL. Prepare before use. Each mL of this solution contains 0.025 mg of zinc (Zn).

Standard Zinc Solution for Atomic Absorption Spectrophotometry To exactly 10 mL of Standard Zinc Stock Solution add water to make exactly 1000 mL. Prepare before use. Each mL of this solution contains 0.01 mg of zinc (Zn).

Standard Zinc Stock Solution Dissolve exactly 1.000 g of zinc (standard reagent), in 100 mL of water and 5 mL of hydrochloric acid with the aid of gentle heating, cool, and add water to make exactly 1000 mL.

9.23 Matching Fluids for Color

Refer to Color Comparison Tests *<2.65>*.

Reagents, Test Solutions, etc.

9.41 Reagents, Test Solutions

Reagents are the substances used in the tests of the Pharmacopoeia. The reagents that are described as "Standard reagent for volumetric analysis", "Special class", "First class", "For water determination", etc. in square brackets meet the corresponding requirements of the Japan Industrial Standards (JIS). The tests for them are performed according to the test methods of JIS. The reagents that are described as "Certified reference material" are those noted a certificate on the basis of JIS Q 0030 and guaranteed the traceability of the international system of units. These reference materials are provided by the Metrology Management Center, National Institute of Advanced Industrial Science and Technology (AIST) and manufacturers of the certified reference materials. In the case where the reagent name in the Pharmacopoeia differs from that of JIS, the JIS name is given in the brackets. The reagents for which a monograph's title is given in the brackets meet the requirements of the corresponding monograph. In the case of the reagents that are described merely as test items, the corresponding test method of the Pharmacopoeia is applied.

Test Solutions are the solutions prepared for use in the tests of the Pharmacopoeia.

Acemetacin $C_{21}H_{18}ClNO_6$ [Same as the namesake monograph]

Acemetacin for assay $C_{21}H_{18}ClNO_6$ [Same as the monograph Acemetacin. When dried, it contains not less than 99.5% of acemetacin ($C_{21}H_{18}ClNO_6$) meeting the following additional specifications.]

Purity Related substances—Dissolve 40 mg of acemetacin for assay in 10 mL of methanol, and use this solution as the sample solution. Pipet 1 mL of this solution, and add methanol to make exactly 10 mL. Pipet 1 mL of this solution, add methanol to make exactly 20 mL, and use this solution as the standard solution. Perform the test with exactly 10 μL each of the sample solution and standard solution as directed under Liquid Chromatography *<2.01>* according to the following conditions. Determine each peak area of both solutions by the automatic integration method: the area of each peak other than acemetacin obtained from the sample solution is not larger than 1/2 times the peak area of acemetacin from the standard solution, and the total area of the peaks other than acemetacin from the sample solution is not larger than the peak area of acemetacin from the standard solution.

Operating conditions

Detector, column, column temperature, mobile phase, and flow rate: Proceed as directed in the operating conditions in the Assay under Acemetacin Tablets.

Time span of measurement: About 4 times as long as the retention time of Acemetacin.

System Suitability

Test for required detectability: Pipet 1 mL of the standard solution, and add methanol to make exactly 20 mL. Confirm that the peak area of acemetacin obtained with 10 μL of this solution is equivalent to 3 to 7% of that with 10 μL of the standard solution.

System performance: Dissolve 75 mg of acemetacin and 75 mg of indometacin in 50 mL of methanol. To 4 mL of this solution add 1 mL of a solution of hexyl parahydroxybenzoate in methanol (1 in 250), and add methanol to make 50 mL. When the procedure is run with 10 μL of this solution under the above operating conditions, acemetacin, indometacin and hexyl parahydroxybenzoate are eluted in this order with the resolutions between the peaks of acemetacin and indometacin and between the peaks of indometacin and hexyl parahydroxybenzoate being not less than 3, respectively.

System repeatability: When the test is repeated 6 times with 10 μL of the standard solution under the above operating conditions, the relative standard deviation of the peak area of acemetacin is not more than 1.5%.

Acenaphthene $C_{12}H_{10}$ White to pale yellow-white, crystals or crystalline powder, having a characteristic aroma. Freely soluble in diethyl ether and in chloroform, soluble in acetonitrile, sparingly soluble in methanol, and practically insoluble in water.

Identification—Determine the infrared absorption spectrum of acenaphthene according to the paste method under Infrared Spectrophotometry *〈2.25〉*: it exhibits absorption at the wave numbers of about 1605 cm^{-1}, 840 cm^{-1}, 785 cm^{-1} and 750 cm^{-1}.

Melting point 〈2.60〉: 93 - 96°C

Purity—Dissolve 0.1 g of acenaphthene in 5 mL of chloroform, and use this solution as the sample solution. Perform the test with 2 μL of the sample solution as directed under Gas Chromatography *〈2.02〉* according to the following conditions. Determine each peak area by the automatic integration method, and calculate the amount of acenaphthene by the area percentage method: it is not less than 98.0 %.

Operating conditions

Detector: A hydrogen flame-ionization detector.

Column: A glass column about 3 mm in inside diameter and about 2 m in length, packed with 150 to 180 μm siliceous earth for gas chromatography coated with 10% of polyethylene glycol 20 M for gas chromatography.

Column temperature: A constant temperature of about 210°C.

Carrier gas: Nitrogen.

Flow rate: Adjust so that the retention time of acenaphthene is about 8 minutes.

Detection sensitivity: Adjust the detection sensitivity so that the peak height of acenaphthene obtained with 2 μL of the solution prepared by adding chloroform to 1.0 mL of the sample solution to make 100 mL is 5 to 15% of the full scale.

Time span of measurement: About 3 times as long as the retention time of acenaphthene, beginning after the solvent peak.

Residue on ignition 〈2.44〉—Not more than 0.1% (1 g).

Acetal $C_6H_{14}O_2$ A clear and colorless, volatile liquid. Miscible with water and with ethanol (95).

Refractive index 〈2.45〉 n_D^{20}: about 1.382

Specific gravity 〈2.56〉 d_{20}^{20}: about 0.824

Boiling point 〈2.57〉: about 103°C

Acetaldehyde CH_3CHO [K 8030, First class]

Acetaldehyde ammonia trimer trihydrate $(C_2H_5N)_3.3H_2O$ Colorless or white to pale yellow, crystals or powder.

Content: not less than 95.0%. Assay—Weigh accurately about 0.9 g of acetaldehyde ammonia trimer trihydrate, dissolve in 50 mL of water, and titrate *〈2.50〉* with 1 mol/L hydrochloric acid VS (potentiometric titration).

Each mL of 1 mol/L hydrochloric acid VS
= 61.08 mg of $(C_2H_5N)_3.3H_2O$

Acetaldehyde for assay CH_3CHO Distil 100 mL of acetaldehyde under reduced pressure, discard the first 20 mL of the distillate, and use the subsequent distillate. Prepare before use.

Acetaldehyde for gas chromatography CH_3CHO A clear and colorless, flammable liquid. Miscible with water and with ethanol (95).

Refractive index 〈2.45〉 n_D^{20}: about 1.332

Specific gravity 〈2.56〉 d_{20}^{20}: about 0.788

Boiling point 〈2.57〉: about 21°C

Acetaminophen $C_8H_9NO_2$ [Same as the namesake monograph]

Acetanilide C_8H_9NO White, crystals or crystalline powder.

Melting point 〈2.60〉: 114 - 117°C

***o*-Acetanisidide** $C_9H_{11}NO_2$ White to light brown, crystals or crystalline powder. Freely soluble in acetonitrile and in ethanol (99.5), and slightly soluble in water. Melting point: 86 - 89°C

***p*-Acetanisidide** $C_9H_{11}NO_2$ White to purplish white, crystals or crystalline powder, having a characteristic odor. It is freely soluble in acetonitrile and in ethanol (95), and very slightly soluble in water.

Melting point 〈2.60〉: 126 - 132°C

Content: not less than 98.0%. Assay—Dissolve 0.1 g of *p*-acetanisidide in 5 mL of ethanol (95). Perform the test with 2 μL of this solution as directed under Gas Chromatography *〈2.02〉* according to the following conditions, and determine the area of each peak by the automatic integration method.

$$\text{Content (\%)} = \frac{\text{peak area of } p\text{-acetanisidide}}{\text{total of all peak areas}} \times 100$$

Operating conditions

Detector: A hydrogen flame-ionization detector.

Column: A glass tube 3 mm in inside diameter and 2 m in length, packed with acid-treated and silanized siliceous earth for gas chromatography coated with alkylene glycol phthalate ester for gas chromatography in 1% (177–250 μm in particle diameter).

Column temperature: A constant temperature of about 210°C.

Carrier gas: Nitrogen.

Flow rate: Adjust to a constant flow rate of between 30 mL and 50 mL per minute and so that the retention time of *p*-acetanisidide is between 11 minutes and 14 minutes.

Time span of measurement: About 3 times as long as the retention time of *p*-acetanisidide, beginning after the solvent peak.

Acetate buffer solution (pH 3.5) Dissolve 50 g of ammonium acetate in 100 mL of 6 mol/L hydrochloric acid TS, adjust to pH 3.5 with ammonia TS or 6 mol/L hydrochloric acid TS, if necessary, and add water to make 200 mL.

0.05 mol/L Acetate buffer solution (pH 4.0) To 3.0 mL of acetic acid (100) add 900 mL of water, adjust to pH 4.0 with sodium hydroxide TS, and add water to make 1000 mL.

Acetate buffer solution (pH 4.5) Dissolve 63 g of anhydrous sodium acetate in a suitable amount of water, add 90 mL of acetic acid (100) and water to make 1000 mL.

0.01 mol/L Acetate buffer solution (pH 5.0) Dissolve 770 g of ammonium acetate in 900 mL of water, add acetic acid (31) to adjust the pH to 5.0, and then add water to make 1000 mL.

Acetate buffer solution (pH 5.4) To 5.78 mL of acetic acid (100) add water to make 1000 mL (solution A). Dissolve 8.2 g of anhydrous sodium acetate in water to make 1000 mL (solution B). Mix 176 mL of the solution A and 824 mL of the solution B, and adjust, if necessary, the pH to 5.4 with the solution A or the solution B.

Acetate buffer solution (pH 5.5) Dissolve 2.72 g of sodium acetate trihydrate in water to make 1000 mL, and adjust the pH to 5.5 with diluted acetic acid (100) (3 in 2500).

0.02 mL/L Acetate buffer solution (pH 6.0) Dissolve 1.76 g of sodium chloride in 4 mL of 1 mol/L acetic acid-sodium acetate buffer solution (pH 6.0), and add water to make 200 mL.

Acetic acid See acetic acid (31).

Acetic acid (31) Dilute 31.0 g of acetic acid (100) with water to make 100 mL (5 mol/L).

Acetic acid (100) CH_3COOH [K 8355, Acetic Acid, Special class]

Acetic acid-ammonium acetate buffer solution (pH 3.0) Add acetic acid (31) to ammonium acetate TS, and adjust the pH to 3.0.

Acetic acid-ammonium acetate buffer solution (pH 4.5) Dissolve 77 g of ammonium acetate in 200 mL of water, adjust the pH to 4.5 by adding acetic acid (100), and add water to make 1000 mL.

Acetic acid-ammonium acetate buffer solution (pH 4.8) Dissolve 77 g of ammonium acetate in about 200 mL of water, and add 57 mL of acetic acid (100) and water to make 1000 mL.

Acetic acid buffer solution containing 0.1% bovine serum albumin Dissolve 0.1 g of bovine serum albumin in sodium acetate trihydrate solution (1 in 100) to make exactly 100 mL, and adjust the pH to 4.0 with 1 mol/L hydrochloric acid TS.

Acetic acid, dilute Dilute 6 g of acetic acid (100) with water to make 100 mL (1 mol/L).

Acetic acid for nonaqueous titration CH_3COOH [K 8355, Special class. meeting with following requirement.]

Purity Acetic anhydride—Dissolve 1.0 g of aniline in acetic acid for nonaqueous titration to make 100 mL, and use this solution as the sample solution. Pipet 25 mL of the sample solution, titrate <*2.50*> with 0.1 mol/L perchloric acid VS, and designate the consumed volume as A (mL). A is not less than 26 mL. Pipet 25 mL of the sample solution, add 75 mL of acetic acid for nonaqueous titration, and titrate <*2.50*> with 0.1 mol/L perchloric acid VS, and designate the consumed volume as B (mL) (potentiometric titration). $A - B$ is not more than 0.1 (mL) (not more than 0.001 g/dL).

Acetic acid, glacial See acetic acid (100).

Acetic acid-potassium acetate buffer solution (pH 4.3) Dissolve 14 g of potassium acetate in 20.5 mL of acetic acid (100), and add water to make 1000 mL.

Acetic acid-sodium acetate buffer solution (pH 4.0) Dissolve 5.44 g of sodium acetate trihydrate in 900 mL of water, adjust the pH 4.0 with acetic acid (100), and add water to make 1000 mL.

0.05 mol/L Acetic acid-sodium acetate buffer solution (pH 4.0) To 3.0 g of acetic acid (100) add water to make 1000 mL. Adjust to pH 4.0 with a solution prepared by dissolving 3.4 g of sodium acetate trihydrate in water to make 500 mL.

0.1 mol/L Acetic acid-sodium acetate buffer solution (pH 4.0) Dissolve 13.61 g of sodium acetate trihydrate in 750 mL of water, adjust the pH to 4.0 with acetic acid (100), and add water to make 1000 mL.

Acetic acid-sodium acetate buffer solution (pH 4.5) To 80 mL of sodium acetate TS add 120 mL of dilute acetic acid and water to make 1000 mL.

Acetic acid-sodium acetate buffer solution (pH 4.5), for iron limit test Dissolve 75.4 mL of acetic acid (100) and 111 g of sodium acetate trihydrate in 1000 mL of water.

0.05 mol/L Acetic acid-sodium acetate buffer solution (pH 4.6) Dissolve 6.6 g of sodium acetate trihydrate in 900 mL of water, and add 3 mL of acetic acid and water to make 1000 mL.

Acetic acid-sodium acetate buffer solution (pH 4.7) Dissolve 27.2 g of sodium acetate trihydrate in 900 mL of water, adjust the pH to 4.7 by adding acetic acid (100) dropwise, and add water to make 1000 mL.

Acetic acid-sodium acetate buffer solution (pH 5.0) To 140 mL of sodium acetate TS add 60 mL of dilute acetic acid and water to make 1000 mL.

1 mol/L Acetic acid-sodium acetate buffer solution (pH 5.0) To sodium acetate TS add dilute acetic acid, and adjust the pH to 5.0.

Acetic acid-sodium acetate buffer solution (pH 5.5) Dissolve 20 g of sodium acetate trihydrate in 80 mL of water, adjust the pH to 5.5 by adding acetic acid (100) dropwise, and add water to make 100 mL.

Acetic acid-sodium acetate buffer solution (pH 5.6) Dissolve 12 g of sodium acetate trihydrate in 0.66 mL of acetic acid (100) and water to make 100 mL.

1 mol/L Acetic acid-sodium acetate buffer solution (pH 6.0) Adjust the pH of sodium acetate TS to 6.0 with dilute acetic acid.

Acetic acid-sodium acetate TS Mix 17 mL of 1 mol/L sodium hydroxide VS with 40 mL of dilute acetic acid, and add water to make 100 mL.

Acetic acid-sodium acetate TS (pH 7.0) Dissolve 4.53 g of sodium acetate trihydrate in water to make 100 mL, and adjust the pH to 7.0 with diluted acetic acid (100) (1 in 50).

0.02 mol/L Acetic acid-sodium acetate TS Dissolve 2.74 g of sodium acetate trihydrate in a suitable amount of water, and add 2 mL of acetic acid (100) and water to make 1000 mL.

0.25 mol/L Acetic acid TS To 3 g of acetic acid (100) add water to make 200 mL.

2 mol/L Acetic acid TS To 12 g of acetic acid (100) add water to make 100 mL.

6 mol/L Acetic acid TS Dilute 36 g of acetic acid (100) with water to make 100 mL.

Acetic acid-sulfuric acid TS To 5 mL of acetic acid (100) add cautiously 5 mL of sulfuric acid while cooling in an ice bath, and mix.

Acetic anhydride $(CH_3CO)_2O$ [K 8886, Special class]

Acetic anhydride-pyridine TS Place 25 g of acetic anhydride in a 100 mL volumetric flask, add pyridine to make 100 mL, and mix well. Preserve in light-resistant containers, protected from air. This solution may be used even if it becomes colored during storage.

Acetone CH_3COCH_3 [K 8034, Special class]

Acetone for nonaqueous titration Add potassium permanganate to acetone in small portions, and shake. When the mixture keeps its purple color after standing for 2 to 3 days, distil, and dehydrate with freshly ignited anhydrous potassium carbonate. Distil by using a fractionating column under protection from moisture, and collect the fraction distilling at 56°C.

Acetone for purity of crude drug CH_3COCH_3 [K 8034, Acetone, Special class] Use acetone meeting the following additional specification. Evaporate 300.0 mL of acetone to be tested in vacuum at a temperature not higher than 40°C, add the acetone to make exactly 1 mL, and use this solution as the sample solution. Separately, dissolve 2.0 mg of γ-BHC in hexane for purity of crude drug to make exactly 100 mL. Pipet 1 mL of this solution, and add hexane for purity of crude drug to make exactly 100 mL. Further pipet 2 mL of this solution, add hexane for purity of crude drug to make exactly 100 mL, and use this solution as the standard solution (1). Perform the test with exactly 1 μL each of the sample solution and standard solution (1) as directed under Gas Chromatography <*2.02*> according to the following operating conditions, and determine each peak area by the automatic integration method: the total area of peaks other than the solvent peak obtained from the sample solution is not larger than the peak area of γ-BHC from the standard solution (1).
Operating conditions
Proceed the operating conditions in 4.3. under Crude Drugs Test <*5.01*> except time span of measurement.
Time span of measurement: About three times as long as the retention time of γ-BHC, beginning after the solvent peak.
System suitability
Proceed the system suitability in 4.3. under Crude Drugs Test <*5.01*> except test for required detectability.
Test for required detectability: Pipet 1 mL of the standard solution (1), add hexane for purity of crude drug to make exactly 20 mL, and use this solution as the standard solution (2). Adjust the detection sensitivity so that the peak area of γ-BHC obtained from 1 μL of the standard solution (2) can be measured by the automatic integration method, and the peak height of γ-BHC from 1 μL of the standard solution (1) is about 20% of the full scale.

Acetonitrile CH_3CN [K 8032, Special class]

Acetonitrile for liquid chromatography CH_3CN Colorless and clear liquid. Miscible with water.
Purity Ultraviolet light absorbing substances—Determine the absorbances of acetonitrile for liquid chromatography at the following wavelengths as directed under Ultraviolet-visible Spectrophotometry <*2.24*>, using water as the control: not more than 0.07 at 200 nm, not more than 0.046 at 210 nm, not more than 0.027 at 220 nm, not more than 0.014 at 230 nm and not more than 0.009 at 240 nm.

Acetrizoic acid $C_9H_6I_3NO_3$ White powder.
Purity Related substances—Dissolve 60 mg of acetrizoic acid in a solution of meglumine (3 in 1000) to make 100 mL. To 10 mL of this solution add water to make 100 mL, and use this solution as the sample solution. Proceed the test with 5 μL of the sample solution as directed in the Assay under Meglumine Sodium Amidotrizoate Injection: any peaks other than the principal peak are not observed.

Acetylacetone $CH_3COCH_2COCH_3$ [K 8027, Special class]

Acetylacetone TS Dissolve 150 g of ammonium acetate in a sufficient quantity of water, and add 3 mL of acetic acid (100), 2 mL of acetylacetone and water to make 1000 mL. Prepare before use.

Acetyl chloride CH_3COCl A clear and colorless liquid.

Acetylene See dissolved acetylene.

***N*-Acetylgalactosamine** $C_8H_{15}NO_6$ White, crystals or crystalline powder.
Content: not less than 98.0%. Assay – Dissolve 36 mg of *N*-acetylgalactosamine in 1 mL of water. Perform the test with 15 μL of this solution as directed under Liquid Chromatography <*2.01*> according to the following conditions. Determine each peak area by the automatic integration method, and calculate their amounts by the area percentage method.
Operating conditions
Detector: A differential refractometer (Detector temperature: a constant temperature of about 40°C).
Column: A stainless steel column 8 mm in inside diameter and 30 cm in length, packed with styrene-divinylbenzene copolymer for liquid chromatography (7 μm in particle diameter).
Column temperature: A constant temperature of about 80°C.
Mobile phase: Water.
Flow rate: 0.5 mL per minute.
Time span of measurement: About 3 times as long as the retention time of *N*-acetylgalactosamine.

***N*-Acetylneuraminic acid** $C_{11}H_{19}NO_9$ White, crystals or crystalline powder.
Content: not less than 98.0%. Assay—Dissolve 30 mg of *N*-acetylneuraminic acid in 1 mL of the mobile phase. Perform the test with 15 μL of this solution as directed under Liquid Chromatography <*2.01*> according to the following conditions. Determine each peak area by the automatic integration method, and calculate their amounts by the area percentage method.
Operating conditions
Detector: A differential refractometer (detector temperature: a constant temperature of about 40°C).
Column: A stainless steel column 8 mm in inside diameter and 30 cm in length, packed with styrene-divinylbenzene copolymer for liquid chromatography (6 μm in particle diameter).
Column temperature: A constant temperature of about 50°C.
Mobile phase: 10 mmol/L perchloric acid.
Flow rate: 0.5 mL per minute.
Time span of measurement: About 3 times as long as the retention time of *N*-acetylneuraminic acid.

***N*-Acetylneuraminic acid for epoetin alfa** $C_{11}H_{19}NO_9$ White needle crystalline powder.

0.4 mmol/L *N*-Acetylneuraminic acid TS Weigh accurately about 15.5 mg of *N*-acetylneuraminic acid for epoetin alfa, dissolve in water to make exactly 50 mL. To exactly *V* mL of this solution add water to make exactly 100 mL.

$$V\,(\text{mL}) = 309.3 \times 2/\text{amount (mg) of } N\text{-acetylneuraminic acid taken}$$

Achyranthes root for thin-layer chromatography A heat-dried, pulverized root of *Achyranthes fauriei* H. Léveillé et Vaniot (*Amaranthaceae*) meeting the following additional specifications.

Identification (1) To 2 g of pulverized achyranthes root for thin-layer chromatography add 10 mL of water, shake for 10 minutes, add 5 mL of 1-butanol, shake for 10 minutes, centrifuge, and use the supernatant liquid as the sample solution. Separately, dissolve 1 mg of chikusetsusaponin IV for thin-layer chromatography in 1 mL of methanol, and use this solution as the standard solution. Perform the test with these solutions as directed under Thin-layer Chromatography <2.03>. Spot 10 μL each of the sample solution and standard solution on a plate of silica gel for thin-layer chromatography. Develop the plate with a mixture of ethyl acetate, water and formic acid (5:1:1) to a distance of about 10 cm, and air-dry the plate. Spray evenly dilute sulfuric acid on the plate, and heat the plate at 105°C for 10 minutes: the standard solution shows a deep purplish red spot at around *R*f value of 0.35, and the sample solution shows spots equivalent to those described below:

*R*f value	Color and shape of the spot
Around 0	A weak spot, black
Around 0.1	A weak spot, strong purplish red
Around 0.2	A weak, tailing spot, strong purplish red
Around 0.25	A strong spot, deep purplish red
Around 0.35	A leading spot, deep purplish red
Around 0.45	A weak spot, dull yellow
Around 0.5	A weak spot, grayish purplish red
Around 0.75	A weak spot, grayish red
Around 0.9	A weak spot, dull red

(2) Perform the test with the sample solution and standard solution obtained under (1) as directed in the method under (1), except using a mixture of 1-propanol, ethyl acetate and water (4:4:3) as the developing solvent: the standard solution shows a deep purplish red spot at around *R*f value of 0.45, and the sample solution shows spots equivalent to those described below:

*R*f value	Color and shape of the spot
Around 0.25	A weak spot, strongly purplish red
Around 0.25 - 0.3	A leading spot or two strong spots, strongly purplish red
Around 0.35	A deep purplish red spot
Around 0.4	A weak spot, dull red
Around 0.42	A dark red spot
Around 0.45	A weak spot, grayish red
Around 0.65	A weak spot, dull greenish yellow
Around 0.7	A weak spot, grayish red
Around 0.85	A weak spot, grayish red
Around 0.95	A weak spot, dull yellow-red

Acidic ferric chloride TS See iron (III) chloride TS, acidic.

Acidic potassium chloride TS See potassium chloride TS, acidic.

Acidic potassium permanganate TS See potassium permanganate TS, acidic.

Acidic stannous chloride TS See tin (II) chloride TS, acidic.

Acid-treated gelatin See gelatin, acid-treated.

Aconitine for purity $C_{34}H_{47}NO_{11}$ White, crystals or crystalline powder. Sparingly soluble in acetonitrile and in ethanol (99.5), slightly soluble in diethyl ether, and practically insoluble in water. Melting point: about 185°C (with decomposition).

Identification—Determine the infrared absorption spectrum of aconitine for purity as directed in the potassium bromide disk method under Infrared Spectrophotometry <2.25>: it exhibits absorption at the wave numbers of about 3500 cm^{-1}, 1718 cm^{-1}, 1278 cm^{-1}, 1111 cm^{-1}, 1097 cm^{-1} and 717 cm^{-1}.

Absorbance <2.24> $E^{1\%}_{1\,cm}$ (230 nm): 211 - 243 [5 mg, ethanol (99.5), 200 mL].

Purity Related substances—(1) Dissolve 5.0 mg of aconitine for purity in 2 mL of acetonitrile, and use this solution as the sample solution. Pipet 1 mL of the sample solution, add acetonitrile to make exactly 50 mL, and use this solution as the standard solution. Perform the test with these solutions as directed under Thin-layer Chromatography <2.03>. Spot 20 μL each of the sample solution and standard solution on a plate of silica gel for thin-layer chromatography, and proceed the test as directed in the Identification in Processed Aconite Root: the spot other than the principal spot obtained from the sample solution is not more intense than the spot from the standard solution.

(2) Dissolve 5.0 mg of aconitine for purity in 5 mL of acetonitrile, and use this solution as the sample solution. Pipet 1 mL of the sample solution, add acetonitrile to make exactly 50 mL, and use this solution as the standard solution. Perform the test with exactly 10 μL each of the sample solution and standard solution as directed under Liquid Chromatography <2.01> according to the following conditions, and determine each peak area by the automatic integration method: the total area of the peaks other than aconitine obtained from the sample solution is not larger than the peak area of aconitine from the standard solution.

Operating conditions

Detector, column, and column temperature: Proceed as directed in the operating conditions in the Purity (3) under Processed Aconitine Root.

Mobile phase: A mixture of phosphate buffer solution for processed aconite root and tetrahydrofuran (9:1).

Flow rate: Adjust so that the retention time of aconitine is about 26 minutes.

Time span of measurement: About 3 times as long as the retention time of aconitine, beginning after the solvent peak.

System suitability

Test for required detectability: Pipet 1 mL of the standard solution, and add acetonitrile to make exactly 20 mL. Confirm that the peak area of aconitine obtained with 10 μL of this solution is equivalent to 3.5 to 6.5% of that with 10 μL of the standard solution.

System performance: Dissolve 1 mg each of aconitine for purity, hypaconitine for purity and mesaconitine for purity, and 8 mg of jesaconitine for purity in 200 mL of acetonitrile. When the procedure is run with 10 μL of this solution under the above operating conditions, mesaconitine, hypaconitine, aconitine and jesaconitine are eluted in this order, and each resolution between these peaks is not less than 1.5, respectively.

System repeatability: When the test is repeated 6 times with 10 μL of the standard solution under the above operating conditions, the relative standard deviation of the peak area of aconitine is not more than 1.5%.

Water <2.48>: not more than 1.0% (5 mg, coulometric

titration).

Aconitum diester alkaloids standard solution for purity It is a solution containing 10 mg of aconitine for purity, 10 mg of jesaconitine for purity, 30 mg of hypaconitine for purity and 20 mg of mesaconitine for purity in 1000 mL of a mixture of phosphate buffer solution for processed aconite root and acetonitrile (1:1). When proceed the test with 20 μL of this solution as directed in the Purity (3) under Processed Aconite Root at the detection wavelength 231 nm, the peaks of aconitine, jesaconitine, hypaconitine and mesaconitine are observed, and the ratio of their peak heights is about 10:1:35:30. When proceed the test at the detection wavelength 254 nm, the peaks of aconitine, jesaconitine, hypaconitine and mesaconitine are observed, and the ratio of their peak heights is about 2:8:7:6.

Aconitum monoester alkaloids standard TS for assay Weigh accurately about 20 mg of benzoylmesaconine hydrochloride for assay (separately, determine the water), about 10 mg of benzoylhypaconine hydrochloride for assay (separately, determine the water) and about 20 mg of 14-anisoylaconine hydrochloride for assay (separately, determine the water), dissolve in a mixture of phosphate buffer solution for processed aconite root and tetrahydrofuran (183:17) to make exactly 1000 mL. Perform the test with 20 μL of this solution as directed in the Purity under benzoylmesaconine hydrochloride for assay: the peaks of benzoylmesaconine, benzoylhypaconine and 14-anisoylaconine appear with a peak area ratio of about 2:1:2.

Aconitum monoester alkaloids standard TS for component determination See aconitum monoester alkaloids standard TS for assay.

Acrinol See acrinol hydrate.

Acrinol hydrate $C_{15}H_{15}N_3O.C_3H_6O_3.H_2O$ [Same as the namesake monograph]

Acrylamide $CH_2CHCONH_2$ White or pale yellow crystalline powder.

Melting point <*2.60*>: 83 – 87°C

Content: not less than 97.0%.

Acteoside for thin-layer chromatography See Verbascoside for thin-layer chromatography.

Activated alumina Aluminum oxide with specially strong adsorptive activity.

Activated charcoal [Same as the monograph Medicinal Carbon]

Activated thromboplastin-time assay reagent It is prepared by lyophilization of phospholipid (0.4 mg/mL) which is suspended in 1 mL of a solution of *N*-2-Hydroxyethylpiperazine-*N*′-2-ethanesulfonic acid (61 in 5000), mixed with both silica-gel (4.3 mg/mL) and dextran after the extraction and purification from rabbit brain. Activated thromboplastin-time: 25 – 45 seconds (as assayed with human normal plasma).

Activated thromboplastin-time assay TS Dissolve an aliquot of activated thromboplastin-time assay reagent equivalent to 0.4 mg of phospholipid in 1 mL of water.

Adipic acid $C_4H_8(COOH)_2$ White, crystals or crystalline powder. Freely soluble in ethanol (95), and sparingly soluble in water.

Melting point <*2.60*>: 151 – 154°C

Content: not less than 98.0%. Assay—Weigh accurately about 1 g of adipic acid, and dissolve in 100 mL of water by warming, cool, and titrate <*2.50*> with 1 mol/L sodium hydroxide VS (indicator: 2 drops of phenolphthalein TS).

Each mL of 1 mol/L sodium hydroxide VS
= 73.07 mg of $C_6H_{10}O_4$

Agar [K 8263, Special class, or same as the monograph Agar or Agar Powder. Loss on drying is not more than 15%.]

Agar medium, ordinary See ordinary agar medium.

Agar slant Dispense portions of about 10 mL of ordinary agar medium into test tubes, and sterilize by autoclaving. Before the medium congeals, allow to stand in a slanting position, and solidify. When the coagulating water is lost, reprepare by dissolving with the aid of heat.

Ajmaline for assay $C_{20}H_{26}N_2O_2$ [Same as the monograph Ajmaline. When dried, it contains not less than 99.0% of ajmaline ($C_{20}H_{26}N_2O_2$).]

Alacepril $C_{20}H_{26}N_2O_5S$ [Same as the namesake monograph]

Alacepril for assay $C_{20}H_{26}N_2O_5S$ [Same as the monograph Alacepril. When dried, it contains not less than 99.0% of alacepril ($C_{20}H_{26}N_2O_5S$).]

β-Alanine $C_3H_7NO_2$ Colorless crystals or a white crystalline powder. Freely soluble in water, very slightly soluble in methanol, and practically insoluble in ethanol (99.5) and in diethyl ether.

Purity Related substances—Dissolve 5.0 mg of β-Alanine in 10 mL of diluted methanol (4 in 5), and use this solution as the sample solution. Pipet 1 mL of the sample solution, add diluted methanol (4 in 5) to make exactly 100 mL, and use this solution as the standard solution. Perform the test with these solutions as directed under Thin-layer Chromatography <*2.03*>. Spot 2 μL each of the sample solution and standard solution on a plate of silica gel for thin-layer chromatography. Develop the plate with a mixture of 1-butanol, water and acetic acid (100) (5:2:2) to a distance of about 8 cm, and air-dry the plate. Spray evenly a solution of ninhydrin in acetone (1 in 50) on the plate, and heat the plate at 80°C for 5 minutes: the spot other than the principal spot obtained from the sample solution is not more intense than the spot from the standard solution.

L-Alanine $C_3H_7NO_2$ [K 9101, Special class]

Albiflorin $C_{23}H_{28}O_{11}$ White powder having no odor. Freely soluble in water, in methanol and in ethanol (99.5).

Identification—Determine the absorption spectrum of a solution of albiflorin in diluted methanol (1 in 2) (1 in 100,000) as directed under Ultraviolet-visible Spectrophotometry <*2.24*>: it exhibits a maximum between 230 nm and 234 nm.

Purity (1) Related substances 1—Dissolve 1 mg of albiflorin in 1 mL of methanol, and perform the test with 10 μL of this solution as directed in the Identification (2) under Peony Root: any spot other than the principal spot with an *R*f value of about 0.2 does not appear.

(2) Related substances 2—Dissolve 1 mg of albiflorin in 10 mL of diluted methanol (1 in 2), and use this solution as the sample solution. Perform the test with 10 μL of the sample solution as directed in the Assay under Peony Root: when measure the peak areas for 2 times the retention time of paeoniflorin, the total area of the peaks other than albiflorin obtained from the sample solution is not larger than 1/10 times the total area of the peaks other than the solvent peak.

Albumin TS Carefully separate the white from the yolk of a fresh hen's egg. Shake the white with 100 mL of water until the mixture is thoroughly mixed, and filter. Prepare before use.

Alcian blue 8 GX $C_{56}H_{68}Cl_{14}CuN_{16}S_4$ Dark blue-purple powder.

Alcian blue staining solution Dissolve 0.5 g of alcian blue 8 GX in 100 mL of diluted acetic acid (100) (3 in 100).

Aldehyde dehydrogenase Each mg contains not less than 2 enzyme activity units. White powder.

Assay—Dissolve about 20 mg of aldehyde dehydrogenase, accurately weighed, in 1 mL of water, add ice-cold solution of bovine serum albumin (1 in 100) to make exactly 200 mL, and use this solution as the sample solution. In a spectrophotometric cell, place 2.50 mL of pyrophosphate buffer solution (pH 9.0), 0.20 mL of a solution prepared by dissolving 20.0 mg of β-nicotinamide adenine dinucleotide (β-NAD) in water to make exactly 1 mL, 0.10 mL of a pyrazole solution (17 in 2500) and 0.10 mL of the sample solution, stir, stopper tightly, and allow to stand at 25 ± 1°C for 2 minutes. To this solution add 0.01 mL of an acetaldehyde solution (3 in 1000), stir, stopper tightly, determine every 30 seconds the absorbance at 340 nm as directed under Ultraviolet-visible Spectrophotometry <2.24>, and calculate a change (ΔA) in absorbance per minute starting from the spot where the relation of time and absorbance is shown with a straight line. One enzyme activity unit means an amount of enzyme which oxidizes 1 μmol of acetaldehyde per minute when the test is conducted under the conditions of the Procedure.

Enzyme activity unit (unit/mg) of aldehyde dehydrogenase

$$= \frac{2.91 \times \Delta A \times 200}{6.3 \times M \times 0.10 \times 1000}$$

M: Amount (g) of aldehyde dehydrogenase taken

Aldehyde dehydrogenase TS Dissolve an amount equivalent to 70 aldehyde dehydrogenase units in 10 mL of water. Prepare before use.

Aldehyde-free ethanol See ethanol, aldehyde-free.

Aldioxa for assay $C_4H_7AlN_4O_5$ [Same as the monograph Aldioxa. When dried, it contains not less than 67.3% and not more than 71.0% of allantoin ($C_4H_6N_4O_3$) and not less than 11.6% and not more than 12.5% of aluminum (Al).]

Alendronate sodium hydrate $C_4H_{12}NNaO_7P_2.3H_2O$ [Same as the namesake monograph]

Alisma tuber triterpenes TS for identification Dissolve 1 mg of alisol A for thin-layer chromatography, 1 mg of alisol B and 1 mg of alisol B monoacetate in 5 mL of methanol.

Alisol A for thin-layer chromatography $C_{30}H_{50}O_5$ A white to pale yellow powder. Very soluble in methanol, freely soluble in ethanol (99.5), and practically insoluble in water.

Optical rotation <2.49> $[\alpha]^{20}_{D}$: +86 – +106° (5 mg previously dried on silica gel for 24 hours, methanol, 1 mL, 50 mm).

Purity Related substances—Dissolve 1 mg of alisol A for thin-layer chromatography in 1 mL of methanol. Proceed the test with 5 μL of this solution as directed in the Identification (6) under Saireito Extract: no spot appears other than the principal spot of around Rf value of 0.3.

Alisol B $C_{30}H_{48}O_4$ White, crystals or crystalline powder. Freely soluble in methanol and in ethanol (99.5), and practically insoluble in water.

Identification Determine the infrared absorption spectrum of alisol B as directed in the potassium bromide disk method under Infrared Spectrophotometry <2.25>: it exhibits absorption at the wave numbers of about 1704 cm^{-1}, 1458 cm^{-1} and 1244 cm^{-1}.

Purity Related substances—Dissolve 1 mg of alisol B in 1 mL of methanol, and use this solution as the sample solution. To exactly 0.5 mL of the sample solution add methanol to make exactly 25 mL, and use this solution as the standard solution. Perform the test with these solutions as directed under Thin-layer Chromatography <2.03>. Spot 2 μL each of the sample solution and standard solution on a plate of silica gel for thin-layer chromatography. Develop the plate with a mixture of ethyl acetate, hexane and acetic acid (100) (10:10:3) to a distance of about 7 cm, and air-dry the plate. Spray evenly vanillin-sulfuric acid-ethanol TS for spraying on the plate, and heat the plate at 105°C for 5 minutes: the spot other than the principal spot which appears at an Rf value of about 0.4 obtained from the sample solution is not more intense than the spot from the standard solution.

Alisol B monoacetate $C_{32}H_{50}O_5$ White, crystals or crystalline powder. Freely soluble in methanol and in ethanol (99.5), and practically insoluble in water.

Identification Determine the infrared absorption spectrum of alisol B monoacetate as directed in the potassium bromide disk method under Infrared Spectrophotometry <2.25>: it exhibits absorption at the wave numbers of about 3480 cm^{-1}, 1743 cm^{-1}, 1704 cm^{-1} and 1232 cm^{-1}.

Purity Related substances—Dissolve 1 mg of alisol B monoacetate in 1mL of methanol, and use this solution as the sample solution. To exactly 0.5 mL of the sample solution add methanol to make exactly 25 mL, and use this solution as the standard solution. Perform the test with these solutions as directed under Thin-layer Chromatography <2.03>. Spot 2 μL each of the sample solution and standard solution on a plate of silica gel for thin-layer chromatography. Develop the plate with a mixture of ethyl acetate, hexane and acetic acid (100) (10:10:3) to a distance of about 7 cm, and air-dry the plate. Spray evenly vanillin-sulfuric acid-ethanol TS for spraying on the plate, and heat the plate at 105°C for 5 minutes: the spot other than the principal spot which appears at an Rf value of about 0.5 obtained from the sample solution is not more intense than the spot from the standard solution.

Alizarin complexone $C_{19}H_{15}NO_8$ (1,2-Dihydroxyanthraquino-3-ylmethylamine-N,N-diacetate) A yellow-brown powder. Soluble in ammonia TS, and practically insoluble in water, in ethanol (95) and in diethyl ether.

Sensitivity—Dissolve 0.1 g of alizarin complexone by adding 2 drops of ammonia solution (28), 2 drops of ammonium acetate TS and 20 mL of water. To 10 mL of this solution add acetic acid-potassium acetate buffer solution (pH 4.3) to make 100 mL. Place 1 drop of this solution on a white spot plate, add 1 drop of a solution of sodium fluoride (1 in 100,000) and 1 drop of cerium (III) nitrate TS, stir, and observe under scattered light after 1 minute: a blue-purple color is produced, and the color of the control solution is red-purple. Use a solution prepared in the same manner, to which 1 drop of water is added in place of a solution of sodium fluoride, as the control solution.

Alizarin complexone TS Dissolve 0.390 g of alizarin complexone in 20 mL of a freshly prepared solution of sodium hydroxide (1 in 50), then add 800 mL of water and 0.2 g of sodium acetate trihydrate, and dissolve. Adjust the pH to 4 to 5 with 1 mol/L hydrochloric acid VS, and add water to make 1000 mL.

Alizarin red S $C_{14}H_7NaO_7S$ [K 8057, Special class]

Alizarin red S TS Dissolve 0.1 g of alizarin red S in water to make 100 mL, and filter if necessary.

Alizarin S See alizarin red S.

Alizarin S TS See alizarin red S TS.

Alizarin yellow GG $C_{13}H_8N_3NaO_5$ [K 8056, Special class]

Alizarin yellow GG-thymolphthalein TS Mix 10 mL of alizarin GG TS with 20 mL of thymolphthalein TS.

Alizarin yellow GG TS Dissolve 0.1 g of alizarin yellow GG in 100 mL of ethanol (95), and filter if necessary.

Alkali copper TS Dissolve 70.6 g of disodium hydrogen phosphate dodecahydrate, 40.0 g of potassium sodium tartrate tetrahydrate and 180.0 g of anhydrous sodium sulfate in 600 mL of water, and add 20 mL of a solution of sodium hydroxide (1 in 5). To this mixture add, with stirring, 100 mL of a solution of copper (II) sulfate pentahydrate (2 in 25), 33.3 mL of 0.05 mol/L potassium iodate VS and water to make 1000 mL.

Alkaline blue tetrazolium TS See blue tetrazolium TS, alkaline.

Alkaline copper solution See alkaline copper TS for protein content determination.

Alkaline copper sulfate TS See copper (II) sulfate TS, alkaline.

Alkaline copper TS Dissolve 2 g of anhydrous sodium carbonate in 100 ml of dilute sodium hydroxide TS. To 50 mL of this solution add 1 mL of a mixture of a solution of copper (II) sulfate pentahydrate (1 in 100) and a solution of potassium tartrate (1 in 50) (1:1), and mix.

Alkaline copper TS for protein content determination Dissolve 0.8 g of sodium hydroxide in water to make 100 mL. Dissolve 4 g of anhydrous sodium carbonate in this solution to make solution A. Combine 1 mL of copper (II) sulfate pentahydrate solution (1 in 50) and 1 mL of sodium tartrate dihydrate solution (1 in 25) to make solution B. Mix 50 mL of solution A and 1 mL of solution B. Prepare at the time of use.

Alkaline copper TS (2) Dissolve 20 g of anhydrous sodium carbonate in dilute sodium hydroxide TS to make 1000 mL, and use this solution as solution A. Dissolve 0.5 g of copper (II) sulfate pentahydrate in potassium sodium tartarate tetrahydrate solution (1 in 100) to make 100 mL, and use this solution as solution B. To 50 mL of solution A add 1 mL of solution B. Prepare before use.

Alkaline 1,3-dinitrobenzen TS See 1,3-dinitrobenzene TS, alkaline.

Alkaline *m*-dinitrobenzene TS See 1,3-dinitrobenzene TS, alkaline.

Alkaline glycerin TS To 200 g of glycerin add water to make 235 g, and add 142.5 mL of sodium hydroxide TS and 47.5 mL of water.

Alkaline hydroxylamine TS See hydroxylamine TS, alkaline.

Alkaline phenolphthalein TS See Alcohol Number Determination *<1.01>*.

Alkaline phosphatase See phosphatase, alkaline.

Alkaline phosphatase TS See phosphatase TS, alkaline.

Alkaline picric acid TS See 2,4,6-trinitrophenol TS, alkaline.

Alkaline 1.6% potassium periodate-0.2% potassium permanganate TS See 1.6% potassium periodate-0.2% potassium permanganate TS, alkaline.

Alkaline 2,4,6-trinitrophenol TS See 2,4,6-trinitrophenol TS, alkaline.

Alkaline potassium ferricyanide TS See potassium hexacyanoferrate (III) TS, alkaline.

Alkylene glycol phthalate ester for gas chromatography Prepared for gas chromatography.

Allantoin for thin-layer chromatography $C_4H_6N_4O_3$ A white, crystalline powder or powder. Slightly soluble in water, and practically insoluble in methanol and in ethanol (99.5).

Identification Determine the infrared absorption spectrum of the substance to be examined as directed in the potassium bromide disk method under Infrared Spectrophotometry *<2.25>*: it exhibits absorption at the wave numbers of about 3440 cm^{-1}, 3340 cm^{-1}, 1721 cm^{-1}, 1532 cm^{-1} and 1061 cm^{-1}.

Purity Related substances—Dissolve 2 mg of the substance to be examined in 1 mL of water by warming, and add 2 mL of methanol. Perform the test with 5 μL of this solution as directed in the Identification (3) under Dioscorea Rhizome: no spot is observed except the principal spot with an *Rf* value of about 0.5.

Allopurinol $C_5H_4N_4O$ [Same as the namesake monograph]

Allopurinol for assay $C_5H_4N_4O$ [Same as the monograph Allopurinol. When dried, it contains not less than 99.0% of allopurinol ($C_5H_4N_4O$).]

Alminoprofen for assay $C_{13}H_{17}NO_2$ [Same as the monograph Alminoprofen. When dried, it contains not less than 99.5% of alminoprofen ($C_{13}H_{17}NO_2$).]

Alternative thioglycolate medium See Sterility Test *<4.06>*.

Aluminon $C_{22}H_{23}N_3O_9$ [K 8011, Special class]

Aluminon TS Dissolve 0.1 g of aluminon in water to make 100 mL, and allow this solution to stand for 24 hours.

Aluminum Al [K 8069, Special class]

Aluminum chloride See aluminum (III) chloride hexahydrate.

Aluminum chloride TS See Aluminum (III) chloride TS.

Aluminum (III) chloride TS Dissolve 64.7 g of aluminum (III) chloride hexahydrate in 71 mL of water, add 0.5 g of activated charcoal, then shake for 10 minutes, and filter. Adjust the pH of the filtrate to 1.5 with a solution of sodium hydroxide (1 in 100) with stirring, and filter if necessary.

Aluminum (III) chloride hexahydrate $AlCl_3.6H_2O$ [K 8114, Special class]

Aluminum oxide Al_2O_3 White crystals, crystalline powder, or powder. Boiling point: about 3000°C. Melting point:

about 2000°C.

Aluminum potassium sulfate dodecahydrate $AlK(SO_4)_2.12H_2O$ [K 8255, Special class]

6-Amidino-2-naphthol methanesulfonate $C_{11}H_{10}N_2O.CH_4O_3S$ A white to pale yellow crystalline powder. Melting point: about 233°C (with decomposition).

Purity—A solution obtained by dissolving 0.5 g of 6-amidino-2-naphthol methanesulfonate in 10 mL of methanol is clear.

Amidosulfuric acid (standard reagent) $HOSO_2NH_2$ In addition to JIS K 8005 standard reagent for volumetric analysis, certified reference material which can be used for volumetric analysis may be used.

Amidotrizoic acid for assay $C_{11}H_9I_3N_2O_4$ [Same as the monograph Amidotrizoic Acid. It contains not less than 99.0% of amidotrizoic acid ($C_{11}H_9I_3N_2O_4$), calculated on the dried basis.]

***p*-Aminoacetophenone** See 4-aminoacetophenone.

***p*-Aminoacetophenone TS** See 4-aminoacetophenone TS.

4-Aminoacetophenone $H_2NC_6H_4COCH_3$ Light yellow, crystals or crystalline powder, having a characteristic odor.

Melting point <2.60>: 105 – 108°C

4-Aminoacetophenone TS Dissolve 0.100 g of 4-aminoacetophenone in methanol to make exactly 100 mL.

4-Aminoantipyrine $C_{11}H_{13}N_3O$ [K 8048, Special class]

4-Aminoantipyrine hydrochloride $C_{11}H_{13}N_3O.HCl$ Light yellow crystalline powder. It dissolves in water. Melting point: 232 – 238°C (decomposition).

Purity Clarity of solution—Dissolve 1 g of 4-aminoantipyrine hydrochloride in 25 mL of water: the solution is almost clear.

Content: 100.6 – 108.5%. Assay—Weigh accurately about 0.5 g of 4-aminoantipyrine hydrochloride, dissolve in 50 mL of water, and, if necessary, neutralize with 0.1 mol/L sodium hydroxide VS (indicator: red litmus paper). Add 4 drops of dichlorofluorescein TS, and titrate <2.50> with 0.1 mol/L silver nitrate VS.

Each mL of 0.1 mol/L silver nitrate VS
= 23.97 mg of $C_{11}H_{13}N_3O.HCl$

4-Aminoantipyrine hydrochloride TS Dissolve 1 g of 4-aminoantipyrine hydrochloride in water to make 50 mL.

4-Aminoantipyrine TS Dissolve 0.1 g of 4-aminoantipyrine in 30 mL of water, add 10 mL of a solution of sodium carbonate decahydrate (1 in 5), 2 mL of sodium hydroxide TS and water to make 100 mL. Prepare before use.

2-Aminobenzimidazole $C_7H_7N_3$ White to light yellow, crystals or crystalline powder. Melting point: about 231°C (with decomposition).

Aminobenzoate derivatization TS To 0.28 g of ethyl aminobenzoate add 600 μL of methanol, warm at about 50°C to dissolve, and add 170 μL of acetic acid and 145 μL of borane-pyridine complex.

***p*-Aminobenzoic acid** See 4-aminobenzoic acid.

3-Aminobenzoic acid $C_7H_7NO_2$ White crystals.

Melting point <2.60>: About 174°C

4-Aminobenzoic acid $H_2NC_6H_4COOH$ White to very pale yellow crystalline powder.

Purity Clarity of solution—Dissolve 0.1 g of 4-aminobenzoic acid in 10 mL of ethanol (95): the solution is clear.

2-Amino-1-butanol $CH_3CH_2CH(NH_2)CH_2OH$ Clear, colorless to light yellow liquid. Miscible with water and with methanol.

Refractive index <2.45> n_D^{20}: 1.450 – 1.455

Specific gravity <2.56> d_{20}^{20}: 0.944 – 0.950

Purity Related substances—Weigh 50 mg of 2-amino-1-butanol, and mix with exactly 10 mL of methanol. Perform the test with 2 μL of this solution as directed in the Purity (4) under Ethambutol Hydrochloride: any spot other than the principal spot at the *R*f value of about 0.3 does not appear.

4-Aminobutylic acid $H_2NCH_2CH_2CH_2COOH$ White, crystals or crystalline powder. Melting point: about 200°C (with decomposition).

***ε*-Aminocaproic acid** $C_6H_{13}NO_2$ White, crystals or crystalline powder, having no odor or slightly a characteristic odor. Freely soluble in water and in acetic acid (100), slightly soluble in methanol, and practically insoluble in ethanol. Melting point: about 200°C (with decomposition).

Identification—Determine the infrared absorption spectrum of ε-aminocaproic acid as directed in the potassium bromide disk method under Infrared Spectrophotometry <2.25>: it exhibits absorption at the wave numbers of about 1564 cm^{-1}, 1541 cm^{-1}, 1391 cm^{-1} and 1269 cm^{-1}.

4-Amino-6-chlorobenzene-1,3-disulfonamide $C_6H_8ClN_3O_4S_2$ White, crystals or crystalline powder.

Identification—Determine the infrared absorption spectrum of 4-amino-6-chlorobenzene-1,3-disulfonamide as directed in the potassium bromide disk method under Infrared Spectrophotometry <2.25>: it exhibits absorption at the wave numbers of about 3380 cm^{-1}, 3250 cm^{-1}, 1638 cm^{-1}, 1597 cm^{-1}, 1544 cm^{-1} and 1324 cm^{-1}.

Storage—Preserve in tight containers.

2-Amino-5-chlorobenzophenone for thin-layer chromatography $C_{13}H_{10}ClNO$ Yellow crystalline powder.

Melting point <2.60>: 97 – 101°C

Purity Related substances—Dissolve 10 mg of 2-amino-5-chlorobenzophenone for thin-layer chromatography in methanol to make exactly 200 mL, and perform the test with this solution as directed in the purity (2) under Chlordiazepoxide: any spot other than the principal spot at the *R*f value about 0.7 does not appear.

4-Amino-*N*,*N*-diethylaniline sulfate monohydrate $H_2NC_6H_4N(C_2H_5)_2.H_2SO_4.H_2O$ White to slightly colored powder. It dissolves in water.

Melting point <2.60>: 173 – 176°C

Residue on ignition <2.44>: not more than 0.1% (1 g).

4-Amino-*N*,*N*-diethylaniline sulfate TS Dissolve 0.2 g of 4-amino-*N*,*N*-diethylaniline sulfate monohydrate in water to make 100 mL. Prepare before use, protected from light.

2-Aminoethanethiol hydrochloride $H_2NCH_2CH_2SH.HCl$ White, crystal or granule.

Melting point <2.60>: 65 – 71°C

2-Aminoethanol $H_2NCH_2CH_2OH$ [K 8109, Special class]

3-(2-Aminoethyl)indole $C_{10}H_{12}N_2$ Yellow-brown crystals.

Melting point <2.60>: about 118°C.

***N*-Aminohexamethyleneimine** $(CH_2)_6NNH_2$ Clear, colorless to pale yellow liquid.

Refraction index <2.45> n_D^{20}: 1.482 – 1.487
Specific gravity <2.56> d_{20}^{20}: 0.936 – 0.942

2-Amino-2-hydroxymethyl-1,3-propanediol $C_4H_{11}NO_3$ [K 9704, Special class]

2-Amino-2-hydroxymethyl-1,3-propanediol hydrochloride $C_4H_{11}NO_3.HCl$ White, crystals or crystalline powder

4-(Aminomethyl)benzoic acid $C_8H_9NO_2$ A white powder.

Purity—Dissolve 10 mg of 4-(aminomethyl)benzoic acid in 100 mL of water, and use this as the sample solution. Pipet 1 mL of the sample solution, add water to make exactly 20 mL, and use this solution as the standard solution. Perform the test with exactly 20 μL each of the sample solution and standard solution as directed under Liquid Chromatography <2.01> according to the operating conditions as directed in the Purity (5) under Tranexamic Acid, and determine each peak area by the automatic integration method: each area of the peak other than 4-(aminomethyl)benzoic acid obtained from the sample solution is not larger than the peak area of 4-(aminomethyl)benzoic acid from the standard solution.

1-Amino-2-methylnaphthalene $C_{11}H_{11}N$ Pale yellow to pale brown, masses or liquid.

2-Aminomethylpiperidine $C_6H_{14}N$ A colorless or light yellow, clear liquid, having an amine like characteristic odor.

Identification—Determine the infrared absorption spectrum as directed in the liquid film method under Infrared Spectrophotometry <2.25>: it exhibits absorption at the wave numbers of about 3280 cm^{-1}, 1600 cm^{-1}, 1440 cm^{-1}, 1120 cm^{-1} and 840 cm^{-1}.

Purity Related substances—Perform the test with 0.8 μL of 2-aminomethylpiperidine as directed under Gas Chromatography <2.02>. Determine each peak area by the automatic integration method, and calculate these amounts by the area percentage method: the total amount of the peaks other than 2-aminomethylpiperidine is not more than 1.5%.

Operating conditions

Detector: A hydrogen flame-ionization detector.

Column: A glass column 3 mm in inside diameter and 2 m in length, packed with siliceous earth for gas chromatography (150 – 180 μm) coated with 10% of polyethylene glycol 20M for gas chromatography and 2% of potassium hydroxide.

Column temperature: 100°C at beginning, and raise to 200°C at a rate of 10°C per minute after injection.

Carrier gas: Nitrogen.

Flow rate: Adjust so that the retention time of 2-aminomethylpiperidine is about 5 minutes.

Time span of measurement: About 2 times as long as the retention time of 2-aminomethylpiperidine.

1-Amino-2-naphthol-4-sulfonic acid $C_{10}H_9NO_4S$ [K 8050, Special class]

1-Amino-2-naphthol-4-sulfonic acid TS Mix thoroughly 5 g of anhydrous sodium sulfite, 94.3 g of sodium bisulfite and 0.7 g of 1-amino-2-naphthol-4-sulfonic acid. Before use, dissolve 1.5 g of this mixture in water to make 10 mL.

***m*-Aminophenol** See 3-aminophenol.

2-Aminophenol C_6H_7NO Pale yellow-brown crystals. Soluble in ethanol (99.5), and sparingly soluble in water.

Melting point <2.60>: About 172°C

3-Aminophenol $H_2NC_6H_4OH$ White, crystals or crystalline powder.

Melting point <2.60>: 121 – 125°C

Content: not less than 97.0%. Assay—Weigh accurately about 0.2 g, dissolve in 50 mL of acetic acid for nonaqueous titration, and titrate <2.50> with 0.1 mol/L perchloric acid VS (potentiometric titration). Perform a blank determination in the same manner, and make any necessary correction.

Each mL of 0.1 mol/L perchloric acid VS
= 10.91 mg of $H_2NC_6H_4OH$

4-Aminophenol C_6H_7NO A white to yellowish white crystalline powder. Soluble in ethanol (99.5), and sparingly soluble in water.

Melting point <2.60>: About 186°C

***p*-Aminophenol hydrochloride** See 4-aminophenol hydrochloride.

4-Aminophenol hydrochloride $HOC_6H_4NH_2.HCl$ White to pale colored crystals. Freely soluble in water and in ethanol (95). Melting point: about 306°C (with decomposition).

Content: not less than 99.0%. Assay—Weigh accurately about 0.17 g of 4-aminophenol hydrochloride, dissolve in 50 mL of acetic acid for nonaqueous titration and 5 mL of mercury (II) acetate TS for nonaqueous titration, and titrate <2.50> with 0.1 mol/L perchloric acid-1,4-dioxane VS (indicator: 1 mL of *p*-naphtholbenzeine TS). Perform a blank determination in the same manner, and make any necessary correction.

Each mL of 0.1 mol/L perchloric acid-1,4-dioxane VS
= 14.56 mg of C_6H_8NOCl

Storage—Preserve in tight, light-resistant containers.

Aminopropylsilanized silica gel for pretreatment Prepared for pretreatment.

Aminopyrine $C_{13}H_{17}N_3O$ White to pale yellow, crystals or crystalline powder.

Melting point <2.60>: 107 – 109°C

6-Aminoquinolyl-*N*-hydroxysuccinimidyl carbamate $C_{14}H_{11}N_3O_4$ Prepared for biochemistry or amino acid analysis.

L-2-Aminosuberic acid $C_8H_{15}NO_4$ White, crystals or crystalline powder. Odorless.

Optical rotation <2.49> $[\alpha]_D^{20}$: +19.1 – +20.1° (after drying, 0.1 g, 5 mol/L hydrochloric acid TS, 100 mm).

Loss on drying <2.41>: not more than 0.3% (1 g, 105°C, 2 hours).

Assay—Weigh accurately about 0.3 g of L-2-aminosuberic acid, previously dried, add exactly 6 mL of formic acid to dissolve, then add exactly 50 mL of acetic acid (100), and titrate <2.50> with 0.1 mol/L perchloric acid VS (potentiometric titration). Perform a blank determination in the same manner, and make any necessary correction.

Each mL of 0.1 mol/L perchloric acid VS
= 18.92 mg of $C_8H_{15}NO_4$

Amiodarone hydrochloride for assay $C_{25}H_{29}I_2NO_3.HCl$ [Same as the monograph Amiodarone Hydrochloride. When dried, it contains not less than 99.5% of amiodarone hydrochloride ($C_{25}H_{29}I_2NO_3.HCl$).]

Ammonia-ammonium acetate buffer solution (pH 8.0) To ammonium acetate TS add ammonia TS dropwise to adjust the pH to 8.0.

Ammonia-ammonium acetate buffer solution (pH 8.5) Dissolve 50 g of ammonium acetate in 800 mL of water and 200 mL of ethanol (95), and add ammonia solution (28) to adjust the pH to 8.5.

Ammonia-ammonium chloride buffer solution (pH 8.0) Dissolve 1.07 g of ammonium chloride in water to make 100 mL, and adjust the pH to 8.0 by adding diluted ammonia TS (1 in 30).

Ammonia-ammonium chloride buffer solution (pH 10.0) Dissolve 70 g of ammonium chloride in water, add 100 mL of ammonia solution (28), dilute with water to make 1000 mL, and add ammonia solution (28) dropwise to adjust the pH to 10.0.

Ammonia-ammonium chloride buffer solution (pH 10.7) Dissolve 67.5 g of ammonium chloride in water, add 570 mL of ammonia solution (28), and dilute with water to make 1000 mL.

Ammonia-ammonium chloride buffer solution (pH 11.0) Dissolve 53.5 g of ammonium chloride in water, add 480 mL of ammonia solution (28), and dilute with water to make 1000 mL.

Ammonia copper TS To 0.5 g of cupric carbonate monohydrate add 10 mL of water, triturate, and add 10 mL of ammonia solution (28).

Ammonia-ethanol TS To 20 mL of ammonia solution (28) add 100 mL of ethanol (99.5).

Ammonia gas NH_3 Prepare by heating ammonia solution (28).

Ammonia-saturated 1-butanol TS To 100 mL of 1-butanol add 60 mL of diluted ammonia solution (28) (1 in 100), shake vigorously for 10 minutes, and allow to stand. Use the upper layer.

Ammonia solution (28) NH_3 [K 8085, Ammonia Water, Special class, Density: about 0.90 g/mL, Content: 28 – 30%]

Ammonia TS To 400 mL of ammonia solution (28) add water to make 1000 mL (10%).

1 mol/L Ammonia TS To 65 mL of ammonia solution (28) add water to make 1000 mL.

13.5 mol/L Ammonia TS To exactly 9 mL of water add ammonia solution (28) to make exactly 50 mL.

Ammonia water See ammonia TS.

1 mol/L Ammonia water See 1 mol/L ammonia TS.

13.5 mol/L Ammonia water See 13.5 mol/L ammonia TS.

Ammonia water, strong See ammonia solution (28).

Ammonium acetate CH_3COONH_4 [K 8359, Special class]

Ammonium acetate TS Dissolve 10 g of ammonium acetate in water to make 100 mL.

0.5 mol/L Ammonium acetate TS Dissolve 38.5 g of ammonium acetate in water to make 1000 mL.

Ammonium amidosulfate $NH_4OSO_2NH_2$ [K 8588, Special class]

Ammonium amidosulfate TS Dissolve 1 g of ammonium amidosulfate in water to make 40 mL.

Ammonium amminetrichloroplatinate for liquid chromatography $Cl_3H_7N_2Pt$ To 20 g of cisplatin add 600 mL of 6 mol/L hydrochloric acid TS, and heat under a reflux condenser for 4 – 6 hours to boil while stirring. After cooling, evaporate the solvent, and dry the orange residue at room temperature under reduced pressure. To the residue so obtained add 300 mL of methanol, and heat at about 50°C to dissolve. Filter, separate insoluble yellow solids, and wash the solids with 10 mL of methanol. Combine the filtrate and the washing, heat at about 50°C, and add slowly 100 mL of ethyl acetate while stirring. Cool the mixture to room temperature avoiding exposure to light, and allow to stand at −10°C for 1 hour. Filter the mixture to take off the formed crystals, wash the crystals with 100 mL of acetone, combine the washing to the filtrate, and evaporate to dryness to obtain orange crystals. If necessary, repeat the purification procedure described above to take off the insoluble crystals. To the orange crystals obtained add 300 to 500 mL of a mixture of acetone and methanol (5:1), and heat at about 50°C while stirring to dissolve. Filter while hot to take off the insoluble crystals, wash the crystals with the mixture, and combine the filtrate and washing. Repeat the procedure several times, and evaporate to dryness. Suspense the crystals so obtained in 50 mL of acetone, filter, wash the crystals with 20 mL of acetone, and dry the crystals at room temperature under reduced pressure. It is a yellow-brown crystalline powder.

Identification—Determine the infrared absorption spectrum of the substance to be examined, previously dried at 80°C for 3 hours, as directed in the potassium bromide disk method under Infrared Spectrophotometry <2.25>: it exhibits absorption at the wave numbers of about 3480 cm^{-1}, 3220 cm^{-1}, 1622 cm^{-1}, 1408 cm^{-1} and 1321 cm^{-1}.

Purity Related substances—Cisplatin Conduct this procedure using light-resistant vessels. Dissolve 10 mg in *N,N*-dimethylformamide to make exactly 10 mL, and use this solution as the sample solution. Separately, dissolve 10 mg of Cisplatin in *N,N*-dimethylformamide to make exactly 50 mL. Pipet 5 mL of this solution, add *N,N*-dimethylformamide to make exactly 20 mL, and use this solution as the standard solution. Perform the test with exactly 40 μL each of the sample solution and standard solution as directed under Liquid Chromatography <2.01> according to the following conditions, and determine the peak area of cisplatin by the automatic integration method: the peak area obtained from the sample solution is not larger than that from the standard solution.

Operating conditions

Proceed as directed in the operating conditions in the Assay under Cisplatin.

System suitability

System performance: When the procedure is run with 40 μL of the standard solution under the above operating conditions, the number of theoretical plates and the symmetry factor of the peak of cisplatin are not less than 2500 and not more than 2.0, respectively.

System repeatability: When the test is repeated 6 times with 40 μL of the standard solution under the above operating conditions, the relative standard deviation of the peak area of cisplatin is not more than 5.0%.

Ammonium aurintricarboxylate See aluminon.

Ammonium carbonate [K 8613, Special class]

Ammonium carbonate TS Dissolve 20 g of ammonium carbonate in 20 mL of ammonia TS and water to make 100 mL.

Ammonium chloride NH_4Cl [K 8116, Special class]

Ammonium chloride-ammonia TS To ammonia solution

(28) add an equal volume of water, and saturate this solution with ammonium chloride.

Ammonium chloride buffer solution (pH 10) Dissolve 5.4 g of ammonium chloride in water, and add 21 mL of ammonia solution (28) and water to make 100 mL.

Ammonium chloride TS Dissolve 10.5 g of ammonium chloride in water to make 100 mL (2 mol/L).

Ammonium citrate See diammonium hydrogen citrate.

Ammonium dihydrogenphosphate $NH_4H_2PO_4$ [K 9006, Special class]

0.02 mol/L Ammonium dihydrogenphosphate TS Dissolve 2.30 g of ammonium dihydrogen phosphate in water to make 1000 mL.

Ammonium formate $HCOONH_4$ Colorless crystals. Very soluble in water.

Melting point <2.60>: 116 – 119°C

0.05 mol/L Ammonium formate buffer solution (pH 4.0) Dissolve 3.15 g of ammonium formate in 750 mL of water, adjust to pH 4.0 with formic acid, and add water to make 1000 mL.

Ammonium hydrogen carbonate NH_4HCO_3 White or semi-transparency, crystals, crystalline powder or masses, having an ammonia odor.

0.1 mol/L Ammonium hydrogen carbonate TS Dissolve 7.9 g of ammonium hydrogen carbonate in 500 mL of water. Adjust to pH 10.3 with 5 mol/L sodium hydroxide TS, and add water to make 1000 mL.

Ammonium iron (II) sulfate hexahydrate $FeSO_4(NH_4)_2SO_4.6H_2O$ [K 8979, Special class]

Ammonium iron (III) citrate [Same as the monograph Ferric Ammonium Citrate in the Japanese Standards of Food Additives]

Ammonium iron (III) sulfate dodecahydrate $FeNH_4(SO_4)_2.12H_2O$ [K 8982, Special class]

Ammonium iron (III) sulfate TS Dissolve 8 g of ammonium iron (III) sulfate dodecahydrate in water to make 100 mL.

Ammonium iron (III) sulfate TS, acidic Dissolve 20 g of ammonium iron (III) sulfate dodecahydrate in a suitable amount of water, add 9.4 mL of sulfuric acid, and add water to make 100 mL.

Ammonium iron (III) sulfate TS, dilute To 2 mL of ammonium iron (III) sulfate TS add 1 mL of 1 mol/L hydrochloric acid TS and water to make 100 mL.

Ammonium molybdate See hexaammonium heptamolybdate tetrahydrate.

Ammonium molybdate-sulfuric acid TS See hexaammonium heptamolybdate-sulfuric acid TS

Ammonium molybdate TS See hexaammonium heptamolybdate TS.

Ammonium nickel (II) sulfate See ammonium nickel (II) sulfate hexahydrate.

Ammonium nickel (II) sulfate hexahydrate $(NH_4)_2Ni(SO_4)_2.6H_2O$ Green, crystals or crystalline powder.

Identification—(1) Dissolve 1 g of ammonium nickel (II) sulfate hexahydrate in 20 mL of water, and use this solution as the sample solution. To 5 mL of the sample solution add 1 mL of barium chloride TS: a white precipitate is produced.

(2) To 5 mL of the sample solution obtained in (1) add 5 mL of 8 mol/L sodium hydroxide TS: a green precipitate is formed, and the liquid evolves ammonia on heating.

(3) To 5 mL of the sample solution obtained in (1) add 1 mL each of ammonia TS and dimethylglyoxime TS: a red precipitate is formed.

Content: not less than 99.0%. Assay—Weigh accurately about 1 g of ammonium nickel (II) sulfate hexahydrate, add 100 mL of water and 5 mL of ammonium chloride TS, then add exactly 20 mL of 0.1 mol/L disodium dihydrogen ethylenediamine tetraacetate VS, warm to 50 – 60°C, add 10 mL of diluted ammonia solution (28) (1 in 2), and titrate with 0.1 mol/L disodium dihydrogen ethylenediamine tetraacetate VS until the color of the solution is changed from green to blue-purple (indicator: 50 mg of murexide-sodium chloride indicator).

Each mL of disodium dihydrogen ethylenediamine tetraacetate VS
$= 39.50$ mg of $(NH_4)_2Ni(SO_4)_2.6H_2O$

Ammonium nitrate NH_4NO_3 [K 8545, Special class]

Ammonium oxalate See ammonium oxalate monohydrate.

Ammonium oxalate monohydrate $(NH_4)_2C_2O_4.H_2O$ [K 8521, Special class]

Ammonium oxalate TS Dissolve 3.5 g of ammonium oxalate monohydrate in water to make 100 mL (0.25 mol/L).

Ammonium peroxodisulfate $(NH_4)_2S_2O_8$ [K 8252, Special class]

10% Ammonium peroxodisulfate TS Dissolve 1 g of ammonium peroxodisulfate in water to make 10 mL.

Ammonium persulfate See ammonium peroxodisulfate.

Ammonium polysulfide TS $(NH_4)_2S_n$ [K 8943, Ammonium Sulfide Solution (yellow), $(NH_4)_2S_x$, First class]

Ammonium pyrrolidinedithiocarbamate $C_5H_{12}N_2S_2$ A white or light yellow, crystalline powder. Sparingly soluble in water, and very slightly soluble in ethanol (95).

Storage—Preserve in a light-resistant glass container, at 2 – 10°C.

Ammonium sodium hydrogenphosphate tetrahydrate $NaNH_4HPO_4.4H_2O$ [K 9013, Special class]

Ammonium sulfamate See ammonium amidosulfate.

Ammonium sulfamate TS See ammonium amidosulfate TS.

Ammonium sulfate $(NH_4)_2SO_4$ [K 8960, Special class]

Ammonium sulfate TS Dissolve 39.6 g of ammonium sulfate in 70 mL of water, adjust to pH 8.0 with sodium hydroxide TS, and add water to make 100 mL (3 mol/L).

Ammonium sulfate buffer solution Dissolve 264 g of ammonium sulfate in 1000 mL of water, add 1000 mL of 0.5 mol/L sulfuric acid TS, shake, and filter. The pH of this solution is about 1.

Ammonium sulfide TS $(NH_4)_2S$ [K 8943, Ammonium Sulfide Solution, (colorless), First class] Store in small, well-filled containers, protected from light.

Ammonium tartrate See L-ammonium tartrate.

L-Ammonium tartrate $C_4H_{12}N_2O_6$ [K 8534, (+) Ammonium tartrate, Special class]

Ammonium thiocyanate NH_4SCN [K 9000, Special class]

Ammonium thiocyanate-cobalt (II) nitrate TS Dissolve 17.4 g of ammonium thiocyanate and 2.8 g of cobalt (II) nitrate hexahydrate in water to make 100 mL.

Ammonium thiocyanate TS Dissolve 8 g of ammonium thiocyanate in water to make 100 mL (1 mol/L).

Ammonium trifluoromethanesulfonate White, crystals or crystalline powder.

Identification—Determine the infrared absorption spectrum of ammonium trifluoromethanesulfonate as directed in the ATR method under Infrared Spectrophotometry <*2.25*>: it exhibits absorption at the wave numbers of about 3190 cm^{-1}, 3090 cm^{-1}, 1227 cm^{-1}, 1164 cm^{-1}, and 1032 cm^{-1}.

Ammonium vanadate See ammonium vanadate (V).

Ammonium vanadate (V) NH_4VO_3 [K 8747, Special class]

Amosulalol hydrochloride for assay $C_{18}H_{24}N_2O_5S.HCl$ [Same as the monograph Amosulalol Hydrochloride. It contains not less than 99.0% of amosulalol hydrochloride ($C_{18}H_{24}N_2O_5S.HCl$), calculated on the anhydrous basis.]

Amoxicillin See amoxicillin hydrate.

Amoxicillin hydrate $C_{16}H_{19}N_3O_5S.3H_2O$ [Same as the namesake monograph]

Amphoteric electrolyte solution for pH 3 to 10 Extremely pale yellow liquid. Mixture consisting of multiple types of molecules, buffer capacity is 0.35 mmol/pH-mL. Forms a pH gradient over a pH range of 3 to 10 when mixed with polyacrylamide gel and placed in an electric field.

Amphoteric electrolyte solution for pH 6 to 9 Forms a pH gradient over a pH range of 6 to 9 when mixed with polyacrylamide gel and placed in an electric field. Prepare by diluting a 0.35 mmol/pH-mL buffer capacity solution about 20-fold with water. Almost colorless.

Amphoteric electrolyte solution for pH 8 to 10.5 Extremely pale yellow liquid. Mixture consisting of multiple types of molecules, buffer capacity is 0.35 mmol/pH-mL. Forms a pH gradient over a pH range of 8 to 10.5 when mixed with polyacrylamide gel and placed in an electric field.

Ampiroxicam for assay $C_{20}H_{21}N_3O_7S$ [Same as the monograph Ampiroxicam]

Amygdalin for assay $C_{20}H_{27}NO_{11}$ Amygdalin for thin-layer chromatography. However, it meets the following requirements:

Absorbance <*2.24*> $E^{1\%}_{1\,cm}$ (263 nm): 5.2 – 5.8 [20 mg, methanol, 20 mL; separately determine the water <*2.48*> (5 mg, coulometric titration) and calculate on the anhydrous basis].

Purity Related substances—Dissolve 5 mg of amygdalin for assay in 10 mL of the mobile phase, and use this solution as the sample solution. Pipet 1 mL of the sample solution, add the mobile phase to make exactly 100 mL, and use this solution as the standard solution. Perform the test with exactly 10 μL each of the sample solution and standard solution as directed under Liquid Chromatography <*2.01*> according to the following conditions, and determine each peak area by the automatic integration method: the total area of the peaks other than amygdalin obtanied from the sample solution is not larger than the peak area of amygdalin from the standard solution.

Operating conditions

Detector, column, column temperature, mobile phase, and flow rate: Proceed as directed in the operating conditions in the Assay (3) under Keishibukuryogan Extract.

Time span of measurement: About 3 times as long as the retention time of amygdalin.

System suitability

System performance and system repeatability: Proceed as directed in the system suitability in the Assay (3) under Keishibukuryogan Extract.

Test for required detectability: Pipet 1 mL of the standard solution, and add the mobile phase to make exactly 20 mL. Confirm that the peak area of amygdalin obtained with 10 μL of this solution is equivalent to 3.5 to 6.5% of that with 10 μL of the standard solution.

Amygdalin for component determination See amygdalin for assay.

Amygdalin for thin-layer chromatography $C_{20}H_{27}NO_{11}$ A white, odorless powder. Soluble in water, sparingly soluble in methanol, and practically insoluble in ethanol (99.5).

Identification—Determine the absorption spectrum of a solution of amygdalin for thin-layer chromatography in methanol (1 in 1000) as directed under Ultraviolet-visible Spectrophotometry <*2.24*>: it exhibits maxima between 250 nm and 254 nm, between 255 nm and 259 nm, between 261 nm and 265 nm, and between 267 nm and 271 nm.

Purity Related substances—Dissolve 5 mg of amygdalin for thin-layer chromatography in 2 mL of methanol, and use this solution as the sample solution. Pipet 1 mL of the sample solution, add methanol to make exactly 100 mL, and use this solution as the standard solution. Perform the test with 10 μL each of the sample solution and standard solution as directed in the Identification under Peach Kernel: any spot other than the principal spot at the *R*f value of about 0.3 obtained from the sample solution is not more intense than the spot from the standard solution.

***n*-Amyl alcohol** $CH_3(CH_2)_4OH$ Clear, colorless liquid, having a characteristic odor. Sparingly soluble in water, and miscible with ethanol (95) and with diethyl ether.

Refractive index <*2.45*> n^{20}_D: 1.409 – 1.411

Specific gravity <*2.56*> d^{20}_4: 0.810 – 0.820

Distilling range <*2.57*>: 135 – 140°C, not less than 95 vol%.

***t*-Amyl alcohol** $(CH_3)_2C(OH)CH_2CH_3$ Clear, colorless liquid, having a characteristic odor. Miscible with *t*-butyl alcohol and with 2-butanone, and freely soluble in water.

Specific gravity <*2.56*> d^{20}_{20}: 0.808 – 0.815

Purity Acid and ester—To 20 mL of *t*-amyl alcohol add 20 mL of ethanol (95) and 5.0 mL of 0.1 mol/L sodium hydroxide VS, and heat gently under a reflux condenser in a water bath for 10 minutes. Cool, add 2 drops of phenolphthalein TS, and titrate <*2.50*> with 0.1 mol/L hydrochloric acid VS. Perform a blank determination in the same manner: not more than 1.25 mL of 0.1 mol/L sodium hydroxide VS is consumed.

Nonvolatile residue—Evaporate 50 mL of *t*-amyl alcohol, and dry at 105°C for 1 hour: the residue is not more than 1.6 mg.

Distilling range <*2.57*>: 100 – 103°C, not less than 95 vol%.

***tert*-Amyl alcohol** See *t*-amyl alcohol.

Amyl alcohol, iso See 3-methyl-1-butanol.

Anemarrhena rhizome [Same as the namesake monograph]

Anesthetic ether See ether, anesthetic.

Anhydrous caffeine See caffeine, anhydrous.

Anhydrous cupric sulfate See copper (II) sulfate.

Anhydrous dibasic sodium phosphate See disodium hydrogen phosphate, anhydrous.

Anhydrous dibasic sodium phosphate for pH determination See disodium hydrogen phosphate for pH determination.

Anhydrous hydrazine for amino acid analysis Prepared for amino acid analysis.

Anhydrous lactose $C_{12}H_{22}O_{11}$ [Same as the monograph Anhydrous Lactose]

Anhydrous potassium carbonate See potassium carbonate.

Anhydrous sodium acetate See sodium acetate, anhydrous.

Anhydrous sodium carbonate See sodium carbonate, anhydrous.

Anhydrous sodium sulfate See sodium sulfate, anhydrous.

Anhydrous sodium sulfite See sodium sulfite, anhydrous.

Aniline $C_6H_5NH_2$ [K 8042, Special class]

Aniline sulfate $(C_6H_5NH_2)_2.H_2SO_4$ White to gray-white crystalline powder.

Purity Clarity and color of solution—Dissolve 1.0 g of aniline sulfate in 50 mL of water: the solution is clear and colorless.

Animal tissue peptone See peptone, animal tissue.

***p*-Anisaldehyde** See 4-methoxybenzaldehyde.

***p*-Anisaldehyde-acetic acid TS** See 4-methoxybenzaldehyde-acetic acid TS.

***p*-Anisaldehyde-sulfuric acid TS** See 4-methoxybenzaldehyde-sulfuric acid TS.

Anisole C_7H_8O A colorless liquid. Boiling point: about 155°C.

Specific gravity <2.56> d_{20}^{20}: 0.995 – 1.001

14-Anisoylaconine hydrochloride for assay $C_{33}H_{47}NO_{11}.HCl$ White, crystalline powder or powder. Freely soluble in methanol, sparingly soluble in water and in ethanol (99.5). Melting point: about 210°C (with decomposition).

Absorbance <2.24> $E_{1\,cm}^{1\%}$ (258 nm): 276 – 294 (5 mg calculated on the anhydrous basis, methanol, 200 mL).

Purity (1) Related substances—To 1.0 mg of 14-anisoylaconine hydrochloride for assay add exactly 1 mL of ethanol (99.5). Perform the test with 5 μL of this solution as directed in the Identification under Processed Aconite Root: any spot other than the principle spot with an *Rf* value of about 0.5 does not appear.

(2) Related substances—Dissolve 5.0 mg of 14-anisoylaconine hydrochloride for assay in 5 mL of the mobile phase, and use this solution as the sample solution. Pipet 1 mL of the sample solution, add the mobile phase to make exactly 50 mL, and use this solution as the standard solution. Perform the test with exactly 20 μL each of the sample solution and standard solution as directed under Liquid Chromatography <*2.01*> according to the following conditions. Determine each peak area of both solutions by the automatic integration method: the total area of the peaks other than 14-anisoylaconine obtained from the sample solution is not larger than the peak area of 14-anisoylaconine from the standard solution.

Operating conditions

Column, column temperature, mobile phase and flow rate: Proceed as directed in the operating conditions in the Assay (3) under Goshajinkigan Extract.

Detector: An ultraviolet absorption photometer (wavelength: 245 nm).

Time span of measurement: About 4 times as long as the retention time of 14-anisoylaconine.

System suitability

Test for required detectability: Pipet 1 mL of the standard solution, and add the mobile phase to make exactly 20 mL. Confirm that the peak area of 14-anisoylaconine obtained with 20 μL of this solution is equivalent to 3.5 to 6.5% of that with 20 μL of the standard solution.

System performance: When the procedure is run with 20 μL of aconitum monoester alkaloids standard TS for assay under the above operating conditions, benzoylmesaconine, benzoylhypaconine and 14-anisoylaconine are eluted in this order with the resolution between these peaks being not less than 4, respectively.

System repeatability: When the test is repeated 6 times with 20 μL of aconitum monoester alkaloids standard TS for assay under the above operating conditions, the relative standard deviations of the peak areas of benzoylmesaconine, benzoylhypaconine and 14-anisoylaconine are not more than 1.5%, respectively.

14-Anisoylaconine hydrochloride for component determination See 14-anisoylaconine hydrochloride for assay.

Anode solution A for water determination Dissolve 100 g of diethanolamine in 900 mL of a mixture of methanol for water determination and chloroform for water determination (1:1), pass dried sulfur dioxide gas through this solution while cooling until the mass increase of the solution reaches 64 g. Then add 20 g of iodine, and add water until the color of the solution changes from brown to yellow. To 600 mL of this solution add 400 mL of chloroform for water determination.

Anthrone $C_{14}H_{10}O$ Light yellow, crystals or crystalline powder.

Melting point <2.60>: 154 – 160°C

Storage—Preserve in a light-resistant tight container.

Anthrone TS Dissolve 35 mg of anthrone in 100 mL of sulfuric acid.

Anti-A type antibody for blood typing Conforms to the requirements of antibody for blood typing.

Anti-B type antibody for blood typing Conforms to the requirements of antibody for blood typing.

Anti-bradykinin antibody A colorless to light brown, clear solution prepared by dissolving rabbit origin anti-bradykinin antibody in 0.04 mol/L phosphate buffer solution (pH 7.0) containing 1 mg/mL of bovine serum albumin.

Performance test—To a suitable amount of anti-bradykinin antibody to be tested add 0.04 mol/L phosphate buffer solution (pH 7.0) containing 1 mg/mL bovine serum albumin to make a 1 vol% solution. Perform the test with 0.1

mL of this solution as directed in the Purity (2) under Kallidinogenase, and determine the absorbances at 490 - 492 nm, A_1 and A_2, of the standard solution (1) and the standard solution (7): the value, $A_2 - A_1$, is not less than 1.

Anti-bradykinin antibody TS To 0.15 mL of anti-bradykinin antibody, 15 mg of bovine serum albumin, 2.97 mg of sodium dihydrogen phosphate dihydrate, 13.5 mg of disodium hydrogen phosphate dodecahydrate and 13.5 mg of sodium chloride add water to make 15 mL, and lyophilize. Dissolve this in 15 mL of water. Prepare before use.

Anti-interferon alfa antiserum Antiserum prepared by immunizing rabbits with interferon alfa, which is capable of reacting specifically with interferon alfa to neutralize 10,000 Units or more of interferon alfa in 1 mL.

Antimony (III) chloride $SbCl_3$ [K 8400, Special class]

Antimony (III) chloride TS Wash chloroform with an equal volume of water twice or three times, add freshly ignited and cooled potassium carbonate, and allow to stand overnight in a well-closed container protected from light. Separate the chloroform layer, and distil it, preferably with protection from light. With this chloroform, wash the surface of antimony (III) chloride until the rinsing solution becomes clear, add the chloroform to this antimony (III) chloride to make a saturated solution, and place in light-resistant, glass-stoppered bottles. Prepare before use.

Antimony trichloride See antimony (III) chloride.

Antimony trichloride TS See antimony (III) chloride TS.

Antipyrine $C_{11}H_{12}N_2O$ [Same as the namesake monograph]

Anti-thrombin III A white powder.
Water <2.48>: not more than 5%.
Content: not less than 80% and not more than 130% of the labeled amount.

Anti-thrombin III TS Dissolve 10 unit of anti-thrombin III in 10 mL of water.

Anti-ulinastatin rabbit serum Antiserum obtained by immunizing rabbits with Ulinastatin, with an antibody titer of 16 times or more. Preserve at below −20°C.

Anti-urokinase serum Take Urokinase containing not less than 140,000 Unit per mg of protein, dissolve in isotonic sodium chloride solution to make a solution containing 1 mg of protein per mL, and emulsify with an equal volume of Freund's complete adjuvant. Inject intracutaneously three 2-mL portions of the emulsion to a healthy rabbit weighed between 2.5 kg and 3.0 kg in a week interval. Collect the blood from the rabbit at 7 to 10 days after the last injection, and prepare the anti-serum.

Performance test—Dissolve 1.0 g of agar in 100 mL of boric acid-sodium hydroxide buffer solution (pH 8.4) by warming, and pour the solution into a Petri dish to make a depth of about 2 mm. After cooling, bore three of a pair-well 2.5 mm in diameter with a space of 6 mm each other. In one of the wells of each pair-well, place 10 μL of anti-urokinase serum, and in each another well, place 10 μL of a solution of Urokinase containing 30,000 Units per mL in isotonic sodium chloride solution, 10 μL of human serum and 10 μL of human urine, respectively, and allow to stand overnight: a precipitin line appears between anti-urokinase serum and urokinase, and not appears between anti-urokinase serum and human serum or human urine.

α-Apooxytetracycline $C_{22}H_{22}N_2O_8$ Yellow-brown to green powder.
Melting point <2.60>: 200 - 205°C

β-Apooxytetracycline $C_{22}H_{22}N_2O_8$ Yellow-brown to brown powder.
Purity Related substances—Dissolve 8 mg of β-apooxytetracycline in 5 mL of 0.01 mol/L sodium hydroxide TS, add 0.01 mol/L hydrochloric acid TS to make 100 mL, and use this solution as the sample solution. Proceed the test with 20 μL of the sample solution as directed in the Purity (2) under Oxytetracycline Hydrochloride, determine each peak area by the automatic integration method, and calculate the amounts of them by the area percentage method: the total amount of the peaks other than β-apooxytetracycline is not more than 10%.

Aprindine hydrochloride for assay $C_{22}H_{30}N_2.HCl$ [Same as the monograph Aprindine Hydrochloride. When dried, it contains not less than 99.5% of aprindine hydrochloride ($C_{22}H_{30}N_2.HCl$).]

Aprotinin A clear and colorless liquid containing aprotinin extracted from the lung or parotid gland of a healthy cattle. The pH is between 5.0 and 7.0.
Content: not less than 15,000 KIE Units and not more than 25,000 KIE Units of aprotinin per mL. Assay—(i) Trypsin solution: Weigh an amount of crystalline trypsin equivalent to about 250 FIP Units of trypsin according to the labeled FIP Units, and dissolve in 0.001 mol/L hydrochloric acid TS to make exactly 10 mL. Prepare before use, and preserve in ice.
(ii) Sample solution: To a suitable quantity of aprotinin add sodium tetraborate-calcium chloride buffer solution (pH 8.0) so that each mL contains 800 KIE Units of aprotinin, and use this solution as the sample solution.
(iii) Apparatus: Use a glass bottle as a reaction reservoir, 20 mm in inside diameter and 50 mm in height, stopper with a rubber stopper equipped with a glass/silver-silver chloride electrode for pH determination, a nitrogen-induction tube and an exhaust port. Fix the reaction reservoir in a thermostat, and keep the temperature of the bath at 25 ± 0.1°C by means of a precise thermoregulator.
(iv) Procedure: To 5.0 mL of N-α-benzoyl-L-arginine ethyl ester TS add 45.0 mL of sodium tetraborate-calcium chloride buffer solution (pH 8.0), and use this solution as the substrate solution. Pipet 1 mL of the trypsin solution, add sodium tetraborate-calcium chloride buffer solution (pH 8.0) to make exactly 10 mL, and use this solution as the test solution I. Transfer 10.0 mL of the substrate solution to the reaction reservoir, adjust the pH of the solution to 8.00 by adding dropwise 0.1 mol/L sodium hydroxide VS while stirring and passing a current of nitrogen, add exactly 1 mL of the test solution I previously allowed to stand at 25 ± 0.1°C for 10 minutes, then immediately add dropwise 0.1 mol/L sodium hydroxide VS by a 50-μL micropipet (minimum graduation of 1 μL), while stirring, to keep the reaction solution at pH 8.00, and read the amount of 0.1 mol/L sodium hydroxide VS consumed and the reaction time when the pH reached 8.00. Continue this procedure up to 6 minutes. Separately, pipet 2 mL of the trypsin solution and 1 mL of the sample solution, add sodium tetraborate-calcium chloride buffer solution (pH 8.0) to make exactly 10 mL, and use this solution as the test solution II. Transfer 10.0 mL of the substrate solution to the reaction reservoir, adjust the pH of the solution to 8.00, while stirring and passing a current of nitrogen, add exactly 1 mL of the test solution II, previously allowed to stand at 25 ± 0.1°C for 10 minutes, and proceed in the same manner. Separately, transfer 10.0 mL of the sub-

strate solution to the reaction reservoir, adjust the pH of the solution to 8.00, while stirring and passing a current of nitrogen, add 1.0 mL of sodium tetraborate-calcium chloride buffer solution (pH 8.0), previously allowed to stand at 25 ± 0.1°C for 10 minutes, and perform a blank determination in the same manner.

(v) Calculation: Plot the amount of consumption (μL) of 0.1 mol/L sodium hydroxide VS against the reaction time (minutes), select linear reaction times, t_1 and t_2, designate the corresponding consumption amount of 0.1 mol/L sodium hydroxide VS as v_1 and v_2, respectively, and designate μmol of sodium hydroxide consumed per minute as D.

$$D\ (\mu\text{mol NaOH/minute}) = \frac{v_2 - v_1}{t_2 - t_1} \times \frac{1}{10}$$

KIE Units per mL of aprotinin

$$= \frac{2\,(D_A - D_0) - (D_B - D_0)}{L} \times n \times 32.5$$

L: Amount (mL) of the sample solution added to the test solution II

n: Dilution coefficient of aprotinin

D_A: μmol of sodium hydroxide consumed in 1 minute when the test solution I is used

D_B: μmol of sodium hydroxide consumed in 1 minute when the test solution II is used

D_0: μmol of sodium hydroxide consumed in 1 minute when the solution for blank determination is used

32.5: Equivalent coefficient for calculation of KIE Units from FIP Units

One KIE Unit means an amount of aprotinin making a reduction of 50% off the potency of 2 Units of kallidinogenase at pH 8.0 and room temperature for 2 hours.

Storage—Preserve in a light-resistant, hermetic containers and in a cold place.

Aprotinin TS Measure an appropriate amount of aprotinin, and dissolve in 0.05 mol/L phosphate buffer solution (pH 7.0) to prepare a solution containing 50 KIE Units per mL.

Aqua regia Add 1 volume of nitric acid to 3 volumes of hydrochloric acid. Prepare before use.

L-Arabinose $C_5H_{10}O_5$ A white crystalline powder.

Optical rotation <2.49> $[\alpha]_D^{20}$: +103.0 – +105.5° Weigh accurately about 5 g of L-arabinose, previously dried at 105°C for 2 hours, dissolve in 30 mL of water, add 0.4 mL of ammonia TS, and add water to make exactly 50 mL. Allow to stand for 1 hour, and determine using a 100-mm cell.

Melting point <2.60>: 155 – 160°C

Arbutin for assay $C_{12}H_{16}O_7$ Use arbutin for thin-layer chromatography meeting the following additional specifications.

Absorbance <2.24> $E^{1\%}_{1\,\text{cm}}$ (280 nm): 70 – 76 [4 mg, previously dried in a desiccator (in vacuum, silica gel) for 12 hours, water, 100 mL].

Purity Related substances—Dissolve 40 mg of arbutin for assay in 100 mL of water, and use this solution as the sample solution. Pipet 1 mL of the sample solution, add water to make exactly 100 mL, and use this solution as the standard solution (1). Perform the test with exactly 10 μL each of the sample solution and standard solution (1) as directed under Liquid Chromatography <2.01> according to the following conditions, and determine each peak area of the both solutions by the automatic integration method: the total area of the peaks other than arbutin from the sample solution is not larger than the peak area of arbutin from the standard solution (1).

Operating conditions

Proceed as directed in the operating conditions in the Assay under Bearberry Leaf except time span of measurement and test for required detectability.

Time span of measurement: About 3 times as long as the retention time of arbutin, beginning after the solvent peak.

System suitability

Test for required detectability: Pipet 1 mL of the standard solution (1), add water to make exactly 20 mL, and use this solution as the standard solution (2). Adjust the detection sensitivity so that the peak area of arbutin obtained with 10 μL of the standard solution (2) can be measured by the automatic integration method and the peak height of arbutin with 10 μL of the standard solution (1) is about 20% of the full scale.

Arbutin for component determination See arbutin for assay.

Arbutin for thin-layer chromatography $C_{12}H_{16}O_7$ Colorless to white, crystals or crystalline powder, and odorless. Freely soluble in water, soluble in methanol, sparingly soluble in ethanol (95), and practically insoluble in ethyl acetate and in chloroform.

Melting point <2.60>: 199 – 201°C

Purity Related substances—Dissolve 1.0 mg of arbutin for thin-layer chromatography in exactly 1 mL of a mixture of ethanol (95) and water (7:3). Perform the test with 20 μL of this solution as directed in the Identification (2) under Bearberry Leaf: any spot other than the principal spot with an *R*f value of about 0.4 does not appear.

Arecoline hydrobromide for thin-layer chromatography $C_8H_{13}NO_2.HBr$ White crystals. Freely soluble in water, soluble in methanol, and practically insoluble in diethyl ether.

Melting point <2.60>: 169 – 171°C

Purity Related substances—Dissolve 5 mg of arecoline hydrobromide for thin-layer chromatography in exactly 1 mL of methanol. Perform the test with 10 μL of this solution as directed in the Identification under Areca: any spot other than the principal spot at the *R*f value of about 0.6 does not appear.

L-Arginine $C_6H_{14}N_4O_2$ White, crystals or crystalline powder. It has a characteristic odor.

Optical rotation <2.49> $[\alpha]_D^{20}$: +26.9 – +27.9° (After drying, 4 g, 6 mol/L hydrochloric acid TS, 50 mL, 200 mm).

Loss on drying <2.41>: not more than 0.50% (1 g, 105°C, 3 hours).

Content: not less than 98.0% and not more than 102.0%. Assay—Weigh accurately about 0.15 g of L-arginine, previously dried, dissolve in 3 mL of formic acid, add 50 mL of acetic acid (100), and titrate <2.50> with 0.1 mol/L perchloric acid VS until the color of the solution changes to green through yellow (indicator: 10 drops of *p*-naphtholbenzein TS). Perform a blank determination in the same manner, and make any necessary correction.

Each mL of 0.1 mol/L perchloric acid VS
= 8.710 mg of $C_6H_{14}N_4O_2$

L-Arginine hydrochloride $C_6H_{14}N_4O_2.HCl$ [Same as the namesake monograph]

Argon Ar [K 1105, First class]

Aristolochic acid I for crude drugs purity test $C_{17}H_{11}NO_7$ Yellow crystalline powder. Melting point: about 280°C (with decomposition).

Absorbance <2.24> $E^{1\%}_{1\,cm}$ (318 nm): 384 - 424 (1 mg, methanol, 100 mL).

Purity Related substances—Dissolve 1.0 mg of aristolochic acid I for crude drugs purity test in 100 mL of diluted methanol (3 in 4), and use this solution as the sample solution. Pipet 1 mL of the sample solution, add diluted methanol (3 in 4) to make exactly 100 mL, and use this solution as the standard solution. Perform the test with exactly 10 μL each of the sample solution and standard solution as directed under Liquid Chromatography <2.01> according to the following conditions, and determine each peak area by the automatic integration method: the total area of the peaks other than aristolochic acid I obtained from the sample solution is not larger than the peak area of aristolochic acid I from the standard solution.

Operating conditions

Detector, column, column temperature, mobile phase, and flow rate: Proceed as directed in the operating conditions in the Purity (5) under Asiasarum Root.

Time span of measurement: About 3 times as long as the retention time of aristolochic acid I, beginning after the solvent peak.

System suitability

Proceed as directed in the system suitability in the Purity (5) under Asiasarum Root.

Arsenazo III $C_{22}H_{18}As_2N_4O_{14}S_2$ [K 9524, Special class]

Arsenazo III TS Dissolve 0.1 g of arsenazo III in water to make 50 mL.

Arsenic-free zinc See zinc for arsenic analysis.

Arsenic trioxide As_2O_3 [K 8044, Diarsenic trioxide, Special class]

Arsenic trioxide TS Add 1 g of arsenic trioxide to 30 mL of a solution of sodium hydroxide (1 in 40), dissolve by heating, cool, and add gently acetic acid (100) to make 100 mL.

Arsenic (III) trioxide See arsenic trioxide.

Arsenic (III) trioxide TS See arsenic trioxide TS.

Artemisia·argyi for purity test Powder of the leaf and twig of *Artemisia argyi* H. Léveillé et Vaniot (*Compositae*).

Identification—To 0.5 g of artemisia·argyi for purity test add 5 mL of a mixture of methanol and water (3:2), shake for 10 minutes, centrifuge, and use the supernatant liquid as the sample solution. Perform the test with the sample solution as directed under Thin-layer Chromatography <2.03>. Spot 10 μL of the sample solution on a plate of octadecylsilanized silica gel for thin-layer chromatography. Develop the plate with a mixture of methanol and water (4:1) to a distance of about 7 cm, and air-dry the plate. Spray evenly dilute sulfuric acid on the plate, heat the plate at 105°C for 5 minutes, and examine under ultraviolet light (main wavelength: 365 nm): two green fluorescent spots appear at *Rf* values of about 0.3 and about 0.4 (eupatilin and jaceosidin).

Asarinin for thin-layer chromatography $C_{20}H_{18}O_6$ White, crystals or crystalline powder. Slightly soluble in methanol and in ethanol (99.5), and practically insoluble in water. Melting point: 118 - 122°C.

Identification—Determine the absorption spectrum of a solution in methanol (3 in 200,000) as directed under Ultraviolet-visible Spectrophotometry <2.24>: it exhibits maxima between 234 nm and 238 nm, and between 285 nm and 289 nm.

Purity Related substances—Dissolve 1 mg of asarinin for thin-layer chromatography in 1 mL of methanol, and perform the test with 1 μL of this solution as directed in the Identification (7) under Shoseiryuto Extract: no spot other than the principal spot at an *Rf* value of about 0.4 appears.

(*E*)-Asarone $C_{12}H_{16}O_3$ White powder. Freely soluble in methanol and in ethanol (99.5) and practically insoluble in water. Melting point: about 60°C.

Identification—Determine the infrared absorption spectrum of (*E*)-asarone as directed in the potassium bromide disk method under Infrared Spectrophotometry <2.25>, it exhibits absorption at the wave numbers of about 2990 cm^{-1}, 2940 cm^{-1}, 2830 cm^{-1}, 1609 cm^{-1}, 1519 cm^{-1}, 1469 cm^{-1}, 1203 cm^{-1}, 1030 cm^{-1}, 970 cm^{-1} and 860 cm^{-1}.

Purity Related substances—Dissolve 2 mg of (*E*)-asarone in 10 mL of methanol, and use this solution as the sample solution. Perform the test with 10 μL of the sample solution as directed under Liquid Chromatography <2.01> according to the following conditions, determine the area of each peak by the automatic integration method, and calculate the amount by the area percentage method: the total amount of the peaks other than (*E*)-asarone is not larger than 10%.

Operating conditions

Detector: An ultraviolet absorption photometer (wavelength: 230 nm).

Column: A stainless steel column 4.6 mm in inside diameter and 15 cm in length, packed with octadecylsilanized silica gel for liquid chromatography (5 μm in particle diameter).

Column temperature: A constant temperature of about 40°C.

Mobile phase: A mixture of water and acetonitrile (13:7).

Flow rate: 1.0 mL per minute.

Time span of measurement: About 3 times as long as the retention time of (*E*)-asarone, beginning after the solvent peak.

System suitability

System performance: Dissolve 1 mg of (*E*)-asarone and 1 mg of perillaldehyde for thin-layer chromatography in 50 mL of methanol. When the procedure is run with 10 μL of this solution under the above operating conditions, perillaldehyde and (*E*)-asarone are eluted in this order with the resolutions between the peaks being not less than 1.5.

Ascorbic acid See L-ascorbic acid.

L-Ascorbic acid $C_6H_8O_6$ [K 9502, L(+)-Ascorbic Acid, Special class]

Ascorbic acid for iron limit test See L-ascorbic acid.

0.012 g/dL L-Ascorbic acid-hydrochloric acid TS Dissolve 15 mg of L-ascorbic acid in 25 mL of methanol, add carefully 100 mL of hydrochloric acid, and mix. Prepare before use.

0.02 g/dL L-Ascorbic acid-hydrochloric acid TS Dissolve 25 mg of L-ascorbic acid in 25 mL of methanol, add carefully 100 mL of hydrochloric acid, and mix. Prepare before use.

0.05 g/dL L-Ascorbic acid-hydrochloric acid TS Dissolve 50 mg of L-ascorbic acid in 30 mL of methanol, add carefully hydrochloric acid to make 100 mL. Prepare before use.

L-Asparagine monohydrate $C_4H_8N_2O_3.H_2O$ [K8021, Special class]

DL-Aspartic acid $C_4H_7NO_4$ A white crystalline powder that is sparingly soluble in water. Melting point: 270 to

271°C.

L-Aspartic acid $C_4H_7NO_4$ [K 9045, Special class]

Aspartic acid See L-aspartic acid.

Aspirin $C_9H_8O_4$ [Same as the namesake monograph]

Astragaloside IV for thin-layer chromatography $C_{41}H_{68}O_{14}$ A white powder. Sparingly soluble in methanol, very slightly soluble in ethanol (99.5), and practically insoluble in water.

Optical rotation <2.49> $[\alpha]_D^{20}$: +19 – +26° (10 mg dried with silica gel for 24 hours, methanol, 2 mL, 50 mm).

Purity Related substances—Dissolve 1 mg of astragaloside IV for thin-layer chromatography in 1 mL of methanol. Proceed the test with 5 μL of this solution as directed in the Identification (4) under Hochuekkito Extract: no spot appears other than the principal spot of around *Rf* value of 0.4.

Atractylenolide III for assay $C_{15}H_{20}O_3$ Use atractylenolide III for thin-layer chromatography. It meets the following additional specifications.

Absorbance <2.24> $E^{1\%}_{1\,cm}$ (219 nm): 446 – 481 (5 mg, methanol, 500 mL).

Purity Related substances—Dissolve 5 mg of atractylenolide III for assay in 50 mL of methanol, and use this solution as the sample solution. To exactly 1 mL of the sample solution add methanol to make exactly 100 mL, and use this solution as the standard solution. Perform the test with exactly 10 μL each of the sample solution and standard solution as directed under Liquid Chromatography <2.01> according to the following conditions, and determine each peak area by the automatic integration method: the total area of the peaks other than atractylenolide III obtained from the sample solution is not larger than the peak area of atractylenolide III from the standard solution.

Operating conditions

Column, column temperature and mobile phase: Proceed as directed in the operating conditions in the Assay (3) under Tokishakuyakusan Extract.

Detector: An ultraviolet absorption photometer (wavelength: 220 nm).

Flow rate: Adjust so that the retention time of atractylenolide III is about 11 minutes.

Time span of measurement: About 5 times as long as the retention time of atractylenolide III, beginning after the solvent peak.

System suitability

Test for required detectability: To exactly 1 mL of the standard solution add methanol to make exactly 20 mL. Confirm that the peak area of atractylenolide III obtained with 10 μL of this solution is equivalent to 3.5 to 6.5% of that with 10 μL of the standard solution.

System performance: When the procedure is run with 10 μL of the standard solution under the above operating conditions, the number of theoretical plates and the symmetry factor of the peak of atractylenolide III are not less than 5000 and not more than 1.5, respectively.

System repeatability: When the test is repeated 6 times with 10 μL of the standard solution under the above operating conditions, the relative standard deviation of the peak area of atractylenolide III is not more than 1.5%.

Atractylenolide III for thin-layer chromatography $C_{15}H_{20}O_3$ White, crystals or crystalline powder. Freely soluble in methanol, soluble in ethanol (99.5), and practically insoluble in water. Melting point: 193 – 196°C.

Identification—(1) Determine the absorption spectrum of a solution of atractylenolide III for thin-layer chromatography in methanol (1 in 100,000) as directed under Ultraviolet-visible Spectrophotometry <2.24>: it exhibits a maximum between 217 nm and 221 nm.

(2) Determine the infrared absorption spectrum of atractylenolide III for thin-layer chromatography as directed in the potassium bromide disk method under Infrared Spectrophotometry <2.25>: it exhibits absorption at the wave numbers of about 3350 cm^{-1}, 1742 cm^{-1}, 1641 cm^{-1} and 1384 cm^{-1}.

Purity Related substances—Dissolve 2 mg of atractylenolide III for thin-layer chromatography in 2 mL of methanol, and use this solution as the sample solution. Pipet 1 mL of the sample solution, add methanol to make exactly 50 mL, and use this solution as the standard solution. Perform the test with these solutions as directed under Thin-layer Chromatography <2.03>. Proceed the test with 5 μL each of the sample solution and standard solution as directed in the Identification (3) under Tokishakuyakusan Extract: the spot other than the principal spot with an *Rf* value of about 0.5 obtained from the sample solution is not more intense than the spot from the standard solution.

Atractylodin for assay $C_{13}H_{10}O$ White to pale yellow-crystals. Freely soluble in methanol and in ethanol (99.5), and practically insoluble in water. Melting point: about 54°C.

Identification—Conduct this procedure without exposure to light, using light-resistant vessels. Determine the absorption spectrum of a solution of atractylodin for assay in methanol (1 in 250,000) as directed under Ultraviolet-visible Spectrophotometry <2.24>: it exhibits maxima between 256 nm and 260 nm, between 270 nm and 274 nm, between 332 nm and 336 nm and between 352 nm and 356 nm.

Absorbance <2.24> $E^{1\%}_{1\,cm}$ (272 nm): 763 – 819 (2 mg, methanol, 250 mL). Conduct this procedure without exposure to light, using light-resistant vessels.

Purity Related substances—

(i) Conduct this procedure without exposure to light, using light-resistant vessels. Dissolve 2 mg of atractylodin for assay in 2 mL of methanol, and use this solution as the sample solution. To exactly 1 mL of the sample solution add methanol to make exactly 100 mL, and use this solution as the standard solution. Perform the test with these solutions as directed under Thin-layer Chromatography <2.03>. Spot 10 μL each of the sample solution and standard solution on a plate of silica gel for thin-layer chromatography and immediately develop the plate with a mixture of hexane and acetone (7:1) to a distance of about 10 cm, and air-dry the plate. Spray evenly vanillin-sulfuric acid-ethanol TS for splaying on the plate, and heat the plate at 105°C for 5 minutes: the spot other than the principle spot which appears at an *Rf* value of about 0.4 obtained from the sample solution is not more intense than the spot from the standard solution.

(ii) Conduct this procedure without exposure to light, using light-resistant vessels. Dissolve 5 mg of atractylodin for assay in 250 mL of methanol, and use this solution as the sample solution. To exactly 1 mL of the sample solution add methanol to make exactly 100 mL, and use this solution as the standard solution. Perform the test with exactly 20 μL each of the sample solution and standard solution as directed under Liquid Chromatography <2.01> according to the following conditions, and determine each peak area by the automatic integration method: the total area of the peaks other than atractylodin obtained from the sample solution is not larger than the peak area of atractylodin from the standard solution.

Operating conditions

Detector, column, column temperature and mobile phase: Proceed as directed in the operating conditions in the Assay (4) under Tokishakuyakusan Extract.

Flow rate: Adjust so that the retention time of atractylodin is about 13 minutes.

Time span of measurement: About 5 times as long as the retention time of atractylodin, beginning after the solvent peak.

System suitability

Test for required detectability: To exactly 1 mL of the standard solution add methanol to make exactly 20 mL. Confirm that the peak area of atractylodin obtained with 20 μL of this solution is equivalent to 3.5 to 6.5% of that with 20 μL of the standard solution.

System performance: Put a suitable amount of the standard solution in a colorless vessel, and expose to ultraviolet light (main wavelength: 365 nm) for about 1 minute. When the procedure is run with 20 μL of this solution under the above operating conditions, a peak of an isomer is found in addition to the peak of atractylodin, and the isomer and atractylodin are eluted in this order with the resolution between these peaks being not less than 1.5.

System repeatability: When the test is repeated 6 times with 20 μL of the standard solution under the above operating conditions, the relative standard deviation of the peak area of atractylodin is not more than 1.5%.

Atractylodin TS for assay Conduct this procedure without exposure to light, using light-resistant vessels. Weigh accurately about 5 mg of atractylodin for assay, and dissolve in methanol to make exactly 1000 mL.

Atropine sulfate See atropine sulfate hydrate.

Atropine sulfate for assay See atropine sulfate hydrate for assay.

Atropine sulfate for thin-layer chromatography See atropine sulfate hydrate for thin-layer chromatography.

Atropine sulfate hydrate $(C_{17}H_{23}NO_3)_2.H_2SO_4.H_2O$ [Same as the namesake monograph]

Atropine sulfate hydrate for assay $(C_{17}H_{23}NO_3)_2.H_2SO_4.H_2O$ [Same as the monograph Atropine Sulfate Hydrate. When dried, it contains not less than 99.0% of atropine sulfate $[(C_{17}H_{23}NO_3)_2.H_2SO_4]$.]

Atropine sulfate hydrate for thin-layer chromatography $(C_{17}H_{23}NO_3)_2.H_2SO_4.H_2O$ Use atropine sulfate hydrate for assay meeting the following additional specification. To about 50 mg of the substance to be examined, dissolve in ethanol (95) to make 10 mL, and use this solution as the sample solution. Perform the test with the sample solution as directed under Thin-layer Chromatography <2.03>. Spot 50 μL of the sample solution on a plate of silica gel for thin-layer chromatography, develop the plate with a mixture of chloroform and diethylamine (9:1) to a distance of about 10 cm, air-dry the plate, and spray evenly hydrogen hexachloroplatinate (IV)-potassium iodide TS on the plate: any spot other than the principle spot at the *R*f value of about 0.4 does not appear.

A-type erythrocyte suspension Prepare a suspension containing 1 vol% of erythrocyte separated from human A-type blood in isotonic sodium chloride solution.

Avidin-biotin TS To 15 mL of phosphate-buffered sodium chloride TS add 2 drops each of avidin TS and biotinylated peroxidase TS, and mix.

Azelastine hydrochloride for assay $C_{22}H_{24}ClN_3O.HCl$ [Same as the monograph Azelastine Hydrochloride]

Azelnidipine for assay $C_{33}H_{34}N_4O_6$ [Same as the monograph Azelnidipine. When dried, it contains not less than 99.5% of azelnidipine ($C_{33}H_{34}N_4O_6$).]

2,2′-Azinobis(3-ethylbenzothiazoline-6-sulfonic acid) diammonium salt $C_{18}H_{16}N_4O_6S_4.(NH_4)_2$ A bluish green crystalline powder.

Melting point <2.60>: about 330°C (with decomposition).

2,2′-Azinobis(3-ethylbenzothiazoline-6-sulfonic acid) diammonium salt TS Dissolve 5.3 g of citric acid monohydrate in water to make 500 mL. To this solution add a solution prepared by dissolving 7.1 g of anhydrous disodium hydrogen phosphate in water to make 500 mL to adjust to pH 4.3. To 20 mL of this solution add 15 mg of 2,2′-azinobis(3-ethylbenzothiazoline-6-sulfonic acid) diammonium salt. To this solution add 14 μL of hydrogen peroxide TS before use.

Azosemide for assay $C_{12}H_{11}ClN_6O_2S_2$ [Same as the monograph Azosemide]

Baicalein for resolution check $C_{15}H_{10}O_5$ Yellow, crystals or crystalline powder. Slightly soluble in methanol and in ethanol (99.5), and practically insoluble in water.

Identification—Determine the absorption spectrum of a solution of baicalein for resolution check in methanol (1 in 200,000) as directed under Ultraviolet-visible Spectrophotometry <2.24>: it exhibits maxima between 213 nm and 217 nm, between 273 nm and 277 nm, and between 321 nm and 325 nm.

Purity Related substances—Dissolve 1 mg of baicalein for resolution check in 50 mL of methanol, and use this solution as the sample solution. Perform the test with 10 μL of the sample solution as directed under Liquid Chromatography <2.01> according to the following conditions: the total area of the peaks other than baicalein obtained from the sample solution is not larger than 1/10 times the total area of all peaks other than the solvent peak.

Operating conditions

Detector, column, column temperature, mobile phase, and flow rate: Proceed as directed in the operating conditions in the Assay (4) i) under Saikokeishito Extract.

Time span of measurement: About 2 times as long as the retention time of baicalein.

System Suitability

System performance: When the procedure is run with 10 μL of the sample solution under the above operating conditions, the number of theoretical plates and the symmetry factor of the peak of baicalein are not less than 5000 and not more than 1.5, respectively.

System repeatability: When the test is repeated 6 times with 10 μL of the sample solution under the above operating conditions, the relative standard deviation of the peak area of baicalein is not more than 1.5%.

Baicalin for thin-layer chromatography $C_{21}H_{18}O_{11}$ Light yellow, crystals or powder. Slightly soluble in methanol and in ethanol (99.5), and practically insoluble in water.

Identification Determine the infrared absorption spectrum of baicalin to be examined as directed in the potassium bromide disk method under Infrared Spectrophotometry <2.25>: it exhibits absorption at the wave numbers of about 3390 cm^{-1}, 1662 cm^{-1}, 1492 cm^{-1}, 1068 cm^{-1} and 685 cm^{-1}.

Purity Related substance—Dissolve 1 mg of baicalin to be examined in exactly 1 mL of methanol. Perform the test with 10 μL of this solution as directed in the Identification

(2) under Scutellaria Root: any spot other than the principal spot with an *Rf* value of about 0.4 does not appear.

Baicalin hydrate for thin-layer chromatography See baicalin for thin-layer chromatography.

Balsam Canada balsam for microscopy. Before use, dilute to a suitable concentration with xylene.

Bamethan sulfate $(C_{12}H_{19}NO_2)_2.H_2SO_4$ [Same as the namesake monograph]

Barbaloin for assay $C_{21}H_{22}O_9$ Use barbaloin for thin-layer chromatography meeting the following additional specifications.

Absorbance <2.24> $E^{1\%}_{1\,cm}$ (360 nm): 260 – 290 [10 mg dried in a desiccator (in vacuum, phosphorus (V) oxide) for not less than 24 hours, methanol, 500 mL].

Purity Related substances—Dissolve 10 mg of barbaloin for assay in 10 mL of methanol, and use this solution as the sample solution. Pipet 1 mL of the sample solution, add methanol to make exactly 100 mL, and use this solution as the standard solution (1). Perform the test with exactly 20 μL each of the sample solution and standard solution (1) as directed under Liquid Chromatography <2.01> according to the following conditions, and determine each peak area by the automatic integration method: the total area of the peaks other than barbaloin obtained from the sample solution is not larger than the peak area of barbaloin from the standard solution (1).

Operating conditions

Proceed the operating conditions in the Assay under Aloe except detector and time span of measurement.

Detector: An ultraviolet absorption photometer (wavelength: 300 nm).

Time span of measurement: About 3 times as long as the retention time of barbaloin, beginning after the solvent peak.

System suitability

Test for required detectability: Pipet 1 mL of the standard solution (1), add methanol to make exactly 20 mL, and use this solution as the standard solution (2). Adjust the detection sensitivity so that the peak area of barbaloin obtained with 20 μL of the standard solution (2) can be measured by the automatic integration method and the peak height of barbaloin with 20 μL of the standard solution (1) is about 20 % of the full scale.

Barbaloin for component determination See barbaloin for assay.

Barbaloin for thin-layer chromatography $C_{21}H_{22}O_9$ Light yellow crystalline powder. Freely soluble in methanol, practically insoluble in water.

Melting point <2.60>: 148°C

Purity Related substances—Dissolve 1.0 mg of barbaloin for thin-layer chromatography in exactly 1 mL of methanol. Perform the test with 20 μL of this solution as directed in the Identification (2) under Aloe: any spot other than the principal spot at the *Rf* value of about 0.3 does not appear.

Barbital $C_8H_{12}N_2O_3$ [Same as the namesake monograph]

Barbital buffer solution Dissolve 15 g of barbital sodium in 700 mL of water, adjust the pH to 7.6 with dilute hydrochloric acid, and filter.

Barbital sodium $C_8H_{11}N_2NaO_3$ White, odorless, crystals or crystalline powder, having a bitter taste. Freely soluble in water, slightly soluble in ethanol (95), and practically insoluble in diethyl ether.

pH <2.54>—The pH of a solution of 1.0 g of barbital sodium in 200 mL of water is between 9.9 and 10.3.

Loss on drying <2.41>: not more than 1.0% (1 g, 105°C, 4 hours).

Content: not less than 98.5%. Assay—Weigh accurately about 0.5 g of barbital sodium, previously dried, transfer to a separator, dissolve in 20 mL of water, add 5 mL of ethanol (95) and 10 mL of dilute hydrochloric acid, and extract with 50 mL of chloroform. Then extract with three 25-mL portions of chloroform, combine the total extract, wash with two 5-mL portions of water, and extract the washings with two 10-mL portions of chloroform. Combine the chloroform extracts, and filter into a conical flask. Wash the filter paper with three 5-mL portions of chloroform, combine the filtrate and the washings, add 10 mL of ethanol (95), and titrate <2.50> with 0.1 mol/L potassium hydroxide-ethanol VS until the color of the solution changes from yellow to purple through light purple (indicator: 2 mL of alizarin yellow GG-thymolphthalein TS). Perform a blank determination in the same manner, and make any necessary correction.

Each mL of 0.1 mol/L potassium hydroxide-ethanol VS
= 20.62 mg of $C_8H_{11}N_2NaO_3$

Barium chloride See barium chloride dihydrate.

Barium chloride dihydrate $BaCl_2.2H_2O$ [K 8155, Special class]

Barium chloride TS Dissolve 12 g of barium chloride dihydrate in water to make 100 mL (0.5 mol/L).

Barium hydroxide See barium hydroxide octahydrate.

Barium hydroxide octahydrate $Ba(OH)_2.8H_2O$ [K 8577, Special class] Store in tightly stoppered containers.

Barium hydroxide TS Saturate barium hydroxide octahydrate in freshly boiled and cooled water (0.25 mol/L). Prepare before use.

Barium nitrate $Ba(NO_3)_2$ [K 8565, Special class]

Barium nitrate TS Dissolve 6.5 g of barium nitrate in water to make 100 mL (0.25 mol/L).

Barium oxide BaO A white to yellow-white or grayish white powder.

Identification (1) Dissolve 0.5 g of barium oxide in 15 mL of water and 5 mL of hydrochloric acid, and add 10 mL of dilute sulfuric acid: white precipitates appear.

(2) Perform the test with barium oxide as directed under Flame Coloration Test <1.04> (1): a green color appears.

Barium perchlorate $Ba(ClO_4)_2$ [K 9551, Special class]

Becanamycin sulfate $C_{18}H_{37}N_5O_{10}.xH_2SO_4$ [Same as the namesake monograph]

Beclometasone dipropionate $C_{28}H_{37}ClO_7$ [Same as the namesake monograph]

Benidipine hydrochloride $C_{28}H_{31}N_3O_6.HCl$ [Same as the namesake monograph]

Benidipine hydrochloride for assay $C_{28}H_{31}N_3O_6.HCl$ [Same as the monograph Benidipine Hydrochloride. When dried, it contains not less than 99.5% of benidipine hydrochloride ($C_{28}H_{31}N_3O_6.HCl$)]

Benzaldehyde C_6H_5CHO [K 8857, First class]

Benzalkonium chloride [Same as the namesake monograph]

Benzalphthalide $C_{15}H_{10}O_2$ Yellow crystalline powder. Melting point: 99 - 102°C.

Benz[a]anthracene $C_{18}H_{12}$ White to yellow, crystalline powder or powder. Practically insoluble in water, in methanol and in ethanol (99.5). Melting point: 158 - 163°C.

Identification Perform the test with benz[a]anthracene as directed in the Purity: the mass spectrum of the main peak shows a molecular ion peak (*m/z* 228) and a fragment ion peak (*m/z* 114).

Purity Related substances—Dissolve 3.0 mg of benz[a]anthracene in methanol to make 100 mL, and use the sample solution as the sample solution. Perform the test with 1 µL of this solution as directed under Gas Chromatography <2.02> according to the following conditions, and determine each peak area by the automatic integration method. Calculate the amounts of these peaks by the area percentage method: the total amount of the peaks other than benz[a]anthracene is not more than 2.0%.

Operating conditions

Detector: A mass spectrophotometer (EI).

Mass scan range: 15.00 - 300.00.

Time of measurement: 12 - 30 minutes.

Column: A fused silica column 0.25 mm in inside diameter and 30 m in length, coated inside with 5% diphenyl-95% dimethylpolysiloxane for gas chromatography in thickness of 0.25 - 0.5 µm.

Column temperature: Inject at a constant temperature of about 45°C, raise the temperature to 240°C at a rate of 40°C per minute, maintain at 240°C for 5 minutes, raise to 300°C at a rate of 4°C per minute, raise to 320°C at a rate of 10°C per minute, and maintain at 320°C for 3 minutes.

Injection port temperature: At a constant temperature of about 250°C.

Interface temperature: At a constant temperature of 300°C.

Carrier gas: Helium.

Flow rate: Adjust so that the retention time of benz[a]anthracene is about 15 minutes.

Splitless.

System suitability

Test for required detectability: Pipet 1 mL of the sample solution, and add methanol to make exactly 10 mL. Confirm that the peak area of benz[a]anthracene obtained with 1 µL of this solution is equivalent to 5 to 15% of that with 1 µL of the standard solution.

Benzene C_6H_6 [K 8858, Special class]

Benzethonium chloride for assay $C_{27}H_{42}ClNO_2$ [Same as the monograph Benzethonium Chloride. When dried, it contains not less than 99.0% of benzethonium chloride ($C_{27}H_{42}ClNO_2$).]

Benzoic acid C_6H_5COOH [K 8073, Special class]

Benzoin $C_6H_5CH(OH)COC_6H_5$ White to pale yellow, crystals or powder.

Melting point <2.60>: 132 - 137°C

Benzophenone $C_6H_5COC_6H_5$ Colorless crystals, having a characteristic odor.

Melting point <2.60>: 48 - 50°C

Benzo[a]pyrene $C_{20}H_{12}$ Light yellow to green-yellow, crystalline powder or powder. Practically insoluble in water, in methanol and in ethanol (99.5). Melting point: 176 - 181°C.

Identification—Perform the test with benzo[a]pyrene as directed in the Purity: the mass spectrum of the main peak shows a molecular ion peak (*m/z* 252) and a fragment ion peak (*m/z* 125).

Purity Related substances—Dissolve 3.0 mg of benzo[a]pyrene in methanol to make 100 mL, and use this solution as the sample solution. Perform the test with 1 µL of the sample solution as directed under Gas Chromatography <2.02> under the following conditions, and determine each peak area by the automatic integration method. Calculate the amounts of these peaks by the area percentage method: the total amount of the peaks other than benzo[a]pyrene is not more than 3.0%.

Operating conditions

Detector: A mass spectrophotometer (EI).

Mass scan range: 15.00 - 300.00.

Time of measurement: 12 - 30 minutes.

Column: A fused silica column 0.25 mm in inside diameter and 30 m in length, coated inside with 5% diphenyl-95% dimethylpolysiloxane for gas chromatography in thickness of 0.25–0.5 µm.

Column temperature: Inject at a constant temperature of about 45°C, raise the temperature to 240°C at a rate of 40°C per minute, maintain at 240°C for 5 minutes, raise to 300°C at a rate of 4°C per minute, raise to 320°C at a rate of 10°C per minute, and maintain at 320°C for 3 minutes.

Injection port temperature: A constant temperature of about 250°C.

Interface temperature: A constant temperature of about 300°C.

Carrier gas: Helium.

Flow rate: Adjust so that the retention time of benzo[a]pyrene is about 22 minutes.

Splitless.

System suitability

Test for required detectability: Pipet 1 mL of the sample solution, add methanol to make exactly 10 mL. Confirm that the peak area of benzo[a]pyrene obtained with 1 µL of this solution is equivalent to 5 to 15% of that with 1 µL of the sample solution.

***p*-Benzoquinone** $C_6H_4O_2$ Yellow to yellow-brown, crystals or crystalline powder, having a pungent odor. Soluble in ethanol (95) and in diethyl ether, slightly soluble in water. It is gradually changed to a black-brown color by light.

Melting point <2.60>: 111 - 116°C

Content: not less than 98.0%. Assay—Weigh accurately about 0.1 g of *p*-benzoquinone, place in an iodine bottle, add exactly 25 mL of water and 25 mL of diluted sulfuric acid (1 in 15), dissolve 3 g of potassium iodide by shaking, and titrate <2.50> with 0.1 mol/L sodium thiosulfate VS (indicator: 3 mL of starch TS). Perform a blank determination in the same manner.

Each mL of 0.1 mol/L sodium thiosulfate VS
= 5.405 mg of $C_6H_4O_2$

***p*-Benzoquinone TS** Dissolve 1 g of *p*-benzoquinone in 5 mL of acetic acid (100), and add ethanol (95) to make 100 mL.

***N*-α-Benzoyl-L-arginine ethyl ester hydrochloride** $C_{15}H_{22}N_4O_3.HCl$ White, crystals or crystalline powder. Freely soluble in water and in ethanol (95), and slightly soluble in diethyl ether.

Optical rotation <2.49> $[\alpha]_D^{20}$: −15.5 - −17.0° (2.5 g, water, 50 mL, 100 mm).

Melting point <2.60>: 129 - 133°C

Purity (1) Clarity and color of solution—Dissolve 0.1 g

of *N*-α-benzoyl-L-arginine ethyl ester hydrochloride in 20 mL of water: the solution is clear and colorless.

(2) Related substances—Weigh 0.10 g of *N*-α-benzoyl-L-arginine ethyl ester hydrochloride, dissolve in 6 mL of water, add 4 mL of hydrochloric acid, heat in a boiling water bath for 5 minutes to decompose, and use this solution as the sample solution. Perform the test with the sample solution as directed under Paper Chromatography. Spot 5 μL of the sample solution on a chromatographic filter paper. Develop with a mixture of water, acetic acid (100) and 1-butanol (5:4:1) to a distance of about 30 cm, and air-dry the paper. Spray evenly a solution of ninhydrin in acetone (1 in 50) upon the paper, and heat at 90°C for 10 minutes: only one purple spot appears.

Content: not less than 99.0%. Assay—Weigh accurately about 0.6 g of *N*-α-benzoyl-L-arginine ethyl ester hydrochloride, dissolve in 50 mL of water, neutralize with 0.1 mol/L sodium hydroxide VS, if necessary, and titrate <*2.50*> with 0.1 mol/L silver nitrate VS (indicator: 4 drops of dichlorofluorescein TS).

Each mL of 0.1 mol/L silver nitrate VS
= 34.28 mg of $C_{15}H_{22}N_4O_3$.HCl

***N*-α-Benzoyl-L-arginine ethyl ester TS** Dissolve 70 mg of *N*-α-benzoyl-L-arginine ethyl ester hydrochloride in freshly boiled and cooled water to make exactly 10 mL.

***N*-α-Benzoyl-L-arginine-4-nitroanilide hydrochloride** $C_{19}H_{22}N_6O_4$.HCl Light yellow crystalline powder.

Optical rotation <*2.49*> $[\alpha]_D^{20}$: +45.5 – +48.0° (after drying, 0.5 g, *N,N*-dimethylformamide, 25 mL, 100 mm).

Purity Related substances—Dissolve 0.20 g of *N*-α-benzoyl-L-arginine-4-nitroanilide hydrochloride in 10 mL of *N,N*-dimethylformamide, and use this solution as the sample solution. Perform the test with the sample solution as directed under Thin-layer Chromatography <*2.03*>. Spot 10 μL of the sample solution on a plate of silica gel for thin-layer chromatography, develop the plate with a mixture of 1-butanol, water and acetic acid (100) (4:1:1) to a distance of about 10 cm, and air-dry the plate. Exposure the plate to a vapor of iodine: only one spot appears.

***N*-α-Benzoyl-L-arginine-4-nitroanilide TS** Dissolve 0.1 g of *N*-α-benzoyl-L-arginine-4-nitroanilide hydrochloride in water to make 100 mL.

Benzoyl chloride C_6H_5COCl A clear and colorless fuming liquid. Specific gravity: about 1.2 g/mL.

Identification—Determine the infrared absorption spectrum of benzoyl chloride as directed in the liquid film method as directed under Infrared Spectrophotometry <*2.25*>: it exhibits absorption at the wave numbers of about 1775 cm^{-1}, 1596 cm^{-1}, 1450 cm^{-1}, 1307 cm^{-1}, 1206 cm^{-1}, 873 cm^{-1}, 776 cm^{-1} and 671 cm^{-1}.

Benzoylhypaconine hydrochloride for assay $C_{31}H_{43}NO_9$.HCl White, crystals or crystalline powder. Freely soluble in methanol, soluble in water, and sparingly soluble in ethanol (99.5). Melting point: about 230°C (with decomposition).

Absorbance <*2.24*> $E_{1\,cm}^{1\%}$ (230 nm): 225 – 240 (5 mg calculated on the anhydrous basis, methanol, 200 mL).

Purity (1) Related substances—To 1.0 mg of benzoylhypaconine hydrochloride for assay add exactly 1 mL of ethanol (99.5). Perform the test with 5 μL of this solution as directed in the Identification under Processed Aconite Root: no spot other than the principal spot with an *Rf* value of about 0.5 appears.

(2) Related substance—Dissolve 5.0 mg of benzoylhypaconine hydrochloride for assay in 5 mL of the mobile phase, and use this solution as the sample solution. Pipet 1 mL of the sample solution, add the mobile phase to make exactly 50 mL, and use this solution as the standard solution. Perform the test with exactly 20 μL each of the sample solution and standard solution as directed under Liquid Chromatography <*2.01*> according to the following conditions. Determine each peak area of both solutions by the automatic integration method: the total area of the peaks other than benzoylhypaconine obtained from the sample solution is not larger than the peak area of benzoylhypaconine from the standard solution.

Operating conditions

Column, column temperature, mobile phase and flow rate: Proceed as directed in the operating conditions in the Assay (3) under Goshajinkigan Extract.

Detector: An ultraviolet absorption photometer (wavelength: 245 nm).

Time span of measurement: About 5 times as long as the retention time of benzoylhypaconine.

System suitability

Test for required detectability: Pipet 1 mL of the standard solution, and add the mobile phase to make exactly 20 mL. Confirm that the peak area of benzoylhypaconine obtained with 20 μL of this solution is equivalent to 3.5 to 6.5% of that with 20 μL of the standard solution.

System performance: When the procedure is run with 20 μL of aconitum monoester alkaloids standard TS for assay under the above operating conditions, benzoylmesaconine, benzoylhypaconine and 14-anisoylaconine are eluted in this order with the resolution between these peaks being not less than 4, respectively.

System repeatability: When the test is repeated 6 times with 20 μL of aconitum monoester alkaloids standard TS for assay under the above operating conditions, the relative standard deviations of the peak areas of benzoylmesaconine, benzoylhypaconine and 14-anisoylaconine are not more than 1.5%, respectively.

Benzoylhypaconine hydrochloride for component determination See benzoylhypaconine hydrochloride for assay.

***N*-Benzoyl-L-isoleucyl-L-glutamyl(γ-OR)-glycyl-L-arginyl-*p*-nitroanilide hydrochloride** An equal amount mixture of two components, R = H and R = CH_3. A white powder. Slightly soluble in water.

Absorbance <*2.24*> $E_{1\,cm}^{1\%}$ (316 nm): 166 – 184 (10 mg, water, 300 mL).

Benzoylmesaconine hydrochloride for assay $C_{31}H_{43}NO_{10}$.HCl Benzoylmesaconine hydrochloride for thin-layer chromatography meeting the following additional specifications.

Purity Related substances—Dissolve 5.0 mg of benzoylmesaconine hydrochloride for assay in 5 mL of the mobile phase, and use this solution as the sample solution. Pipet 1 mL of the sample solution, add the mobile phase to make exactly 50 mL, and use this solution as the standard solution. Perform the test with exactly 20 μL each of the sample solution and standard solution as directed under Liquid Chromatography <*2.01*> according to the following conditions. Determine each peak area of both solutions by the automatic integration method: the total area of the peaks other than benzoylmesaconine obtained from the sample solution is not larger than the peak area of benzoylmesaconine from the standard solution.

Operating conditions

Column, column temperature, mobile phase and flow

rate: Proceed as directed in the operating conditions in the Assay (3) under Goshajinkigan Extract.

Detector: An ultraviolet absorption photometer (wavelength: 245 nm).

Time span of measurement: About 6 times as long as the retention time of benzoylmesaconine.

System suitability

Test for required detectability: Pipet 1 mL of the standard solution, and add the mobile phase to make exactly 20 mL. Confirm that the peak area of benzoylmesaconine obtained with 20 μL of this solution is equivalent to 3.5 to 6.5% of that with 20 μL of the standard solution.

System performance: When the procedure is run with 20 μL of aconitum monoester alkaloids standard TS for assay under the above operating conditions, benzoylmesaconine, benzoylhypaconine and 14-anisoylaconine are eluted in this order with the resolution between these peaks being not less than 4, respectively.

System repeatability: When the test is repeated 6 times with 20 μL of aconitum monoester alkaloids standard TS for assay under the above operating conditions, the relative standard deviations of the peak areas of benzoylmesaconine, benzoylhypaconine and 14-anisoylaconine are not more than 1.5%, respectively.

Benzoylmesaconine hydrochloride for component determination See benzoylmesaconine hydrochloride for assay.

Benzoylmesaconine hydrochloride for thin-layer chromatography $C_{31}H_{43}NO_{10}.HCl$ White, crystals or crystalline powder. Soluble in water and in ethanol (99.5) and sparingly soluble in methanol. Melting point: about 250°C (with decomposition).

Absorbance <2.24> $E^{1\%}_{1\,cm}$ (230 nm): 217 – 231 (5 mg calculated on the anhydrous basis, methanol, 200 mL).

Purity Related substances—Dissolve 1.0 mg of benzoylmesaconine hydrochloride for thin-layer chromatography in exactly 1 mL of ethanol (99.5). Perform the test with 5 μL of this solution as directed in the Identification under Processed Aconite Root: no spot other than the principal spot with an *R*f value of about 0.4 appears.

Benzoyl peroxide, 25% water containing $(C_6H_5CO)_2O_2$ White, moist, crystals or powder. Soluble in chloroform and in diethyl ether, and very slightly soluble in water and in ethanol (95). Melting point: 103 – 106°C (dried substance) (with decomposition).

Loss on drying <2.41>: not more than 30% (0.1 g, in vacuum, silica gel, constant mass).

Benzyl alcohol $C_6H_5CH_2OH$ Clear and colorless liquid, having a characteristic odor.

Specific gravity <2.56> d^{20}_{20}: 1.045 – 1.050.

Storage—Preserve in a light-resistant tight container.

Benzyl benzoate $C_6H_5COOCH_2C_6H_5$ A colorless oily liquid. Congealing point: about 18°C. Boiling point: about 323°C.

Specific gravity <2.56> d^{20}_{20}: 1.118 – 1.123.

Storage—Preserve in a light-resistant tight container.

Benzyl parahydroxybenzoate $C_{14}H_{12}O_3$ White, fine crystals or crystalline powder. Freely soluble in ethanol (95), and very slightly soluble in water.

Melting point <2.60>: 109 – 112°C

Residue on ignition <2.44>: not more than 0.1%.

Content: not less than 99.0%. Assay—Weigh accurately about 1 g of benzyl parahydroxybenzoate, add exactly 20 mL of 1 mol/L sodium hydroxide VS, heat at about 70°C for 1 hour, and immediately cool in ice. Titrate *<2.50>* the excess sodium hydroxide with 0.5 mol/L sulfuric acid VS up to the second equivalent point (potentiometric titration). Perform a blank determination in the same manner.

Each mL of 1 mol/L sodium hydroxide VS
= 228.2 mg of $C_{14}H_{12}O_3$

Benzylpenicillin benzathine See benzylpenicillin benzathine hydrate.

Benzylpenicillin benzathine hydrate $(C_{16}H_{18}N_2O_4S)_2.C_{16}H_{20}N_2.4H_2O$ [Same as the namesake monograph]

Benzylpenicillin potassium $C_{16}H_{17}KN_2O_4S$ [Same as the namesake monograph]

Benzyl *p*-hydroxybenzoate See benzyl parahydroxybenzoate.

***p*-Benzylphenol** $C_6H_5CH_2C_6H_4OH$ White to pale yellow-white, crystals or crystalline powder.

Melting point <2.60>: 80 – 85°C

Bepotastine besilate for assay $C_{21}H_{25}ClN_2O_3.C_6H_6O_3S$ [Same as the monograph Bepotastine Besilate. However, it contains not less than 99.5% of bepotastine besilate ($C_{21}H_{25}ClN_2O_3.C_6H_6O_3S$), calculated on the anhydrous and residual solvent-free basis.]

Beraprost sodium $C_{24}H_{29}NaO_5$ [Same as the namesake monograph]

Beraprost sodium for assay $C_{24}H_{29}NaO_5$ [Same as the monograph Beraprost Sodium. When dried it contains not less than 99.0% of beraprost sodium ($C_{24}H_{29}NaO_5$).]

Berberine chloride See berberine chloride hydrate.

Berberine chloride for thin-layer chromatography See berberine chloride hydrate for thin-layer chromatography.

Berberine chloride hydrate $C_{20}H_{18}ClNO_4.xH_2O$ [Same as the namesake monograph]

Berberine chloride hydrate for thin-layer chromatography $C_{20}H_{18}ClNO_4.xH_2O$ [Same as the monograph Berberine Chloride Hydrate] or berberine chloride hydrate meeting the following requirements. Yellow, crystals or crystalline powder. Sparingly soluble in methanol, slightly soluble in ethanol (99.5), and very slightly soluble in water.

Identification Determine the absorption spectrum of a solution of the substance to be examined (1 in 100,000) as directed under Ultraviolet-visible Spectrophotometry *<2.24>*: it exhibits maxima between 226 nm and 230 nm, between 261 nm and 265 nm, and between 342 nm and 346 nm.

Purity Related substances—Dissolve 10 mg of the substance to be examined in 10 mL of methanol, and use this solution as the sample solution. Pipet 1 mL of the sample solution, add methanol to make exactly 100 mL, and use this solution as the standard solution. Perform the test with 10 μL each of the sample solution and standard solution as directed in the Identification (2) under Phellodendron Bark: any spot other than the principal spot with an *R*f value of about 0.3 obtained from the sample solution is not more intense than the spot from the standard solution.

Bergenin for thin-layer chromatography $C_{14}H_{16}O_9$ White, crystals or crystalline powder. Freely soluble in methanol, slightly soluble in ethanol (99.5), very slightly soluble in water, and practically insoluble in diethyl ether.

Identification—Determine the absorption spectrum of a solution of bergenin for thin-layer chromatography in methanol (1 in 50,000) as directed under Ultraviolet-visible Spectrophotometry <2.24>: it exhibits maxima between 217 nm and 221 nm, and between 273 nm and 277 nm, and a minimum between 241 nm and 245 nm.

Purity Related substances—Dissolve 1.0 mg of bergenin for thin-layer chromatography in 1 mL of methanol. Perform the test with 20 μL of this solution as directed in the Identification under Mallotus Bark: no spot other than the principal spot at the *Rf* value of about 0.5 appears.

Betahistine mesilate $C_8H_{12}N_2.2CH_4O_3S$ [Same as the namesake monograph]

Betahistine mesilate for assay $C_8H_{12}N_2.2CH_4O_3S$ [Same as the monograph Betahistine Mesilate. When dried, it contains not less than 99.0% of betahistine mesilate ($C_8H_{12}N_2.2CH_4O_3S$).]

Betamipron $C_{10}H_{11}NO_3$ [Same as the namesake monograph]

Betamipron for assay $C_{10}H_{11}NO_3$ [Same as the monograph Betamipron. It contains not less than 99.5% of betamipron ($C_{10}H_{11}NO_3$), calculated on the anhydrous basis.]

Bezafibrate for assay $C_{19}H_{20}ClNO_4$ [Same as the monograph Bezafibrate. When dried it contains not less than 99.0% of bezafibrate ($C_{19}H_{20}ClNO_4$).]

BGLB Dissolve 10 g of peptone and 10 g of lactose monohydrate in 500 mL of water, add 200 mL of fresh ox bile or a solution prepared by dissolving 20 g of dried ox bile powder in 200 mL of water and adjusted the pH to between 7.0 and 7.5, then add water to make 975 mL, and again adjust to pH 7.4. Then add 13.3 mL of a solution of brilliant green (1 in 1000) and water to make 1000 mL in total volume, and filter through absorbent cotton. Dispense 10 mL portions of the filtrate into tubes for fermentation, and sterilize by autoclaving at 121°C for not more than 20 minutes, then cool quickly, or sterilize fractionally on each of three successive days for 30 minutes at 100°C.

α-BHC (α-Hexachlorocyclohexane) $C_6H_6Cl_6$

Melting point <2.60>: 157 – 159°C

Purity Related substances—Dissolve 10 mg of α-BHC in 5 mL of acetone for purity of crude drug, and add hexane for purity of crude drug to make exactly 100 mL. Pipet 1 mL of this solution, add hexane for purity of crude drug to make exactly 100 mL, and use this solution as the sample solution. Pipet 1 mL of the sample solution, add hexane for purity of crude drug to make exactly 100 mL, and use this solution as the standard solution (1). Perform the test with exactly 1 μL each of the sample solution and standard solution (1) as directed under Gas Chromatography <2.02> according to the following conditions, and measure each peak area from these solutions by the automatic integration method: the total area of the peaks other than α-BHC obtained from the sample solution is not larger than the peak area of α-BHC from the standard solution (1).

Operating conditions

Proceed the operating conditions in 4. Purity 4.3. under Crude Drugs Test <5.01> except detection sensitivity and time span of measurement.

Detection sensitivity: Pipet 1 mL of the standard solution (1), add hexane for purity of crude drug to make exactly 20 mL, and use this solution as standard solution (2). Adjust the detection sensitivity so that the peak area of α-BHC obtained with 1 μL of the standard solution (2) can be measured by the automatic integration method, and the peak height of α-BHC with 1 μL of the standard solution (1) is about 20% of the full scale.

Time span of measurement: About twice as long as the retention time of α-BHC, beginning after the solvent peak.

β-BHC (β-Hexachlorocyclohexane) $C_6H_6Cl_6$

Melting point <2.60>: 308 – 310°C

Purity Related substances—Proceed as directed in the Purity under α-BHC using the following standard solution (1).

Standard solution (1): Pipet 2 mL of the sample solution, and add hexane for purity of crude drug to make exactly 100 mL.

γ-BHC (γ-Hexachlorocyclohexane) $C_6H_6Cl_6$

Melting point <2.60>: 112 – 114°C

Purity Related substances—Proceed as directed in the Purity under α-BHC.

δ-BHC (δ-Hexachlorocyclohexane) $C_6H_6Cl_6$

Melting point <2.60>: 137 – 140°C

Purity Related substances—Proceed as directed in the Purity under α-BHC using the following standard solution (1).

Standard solution (1): Pipet 5 mL of the sample solution, and add hexane for purity of crude drug to make exactly 100 mL.

Bifonazole $C_{22}H_{18}N_2$ [Same as the namesake monograph]

Bile salts See Microbial Limit Test for Crude Drugs <5.02>.

Bilirubin for assay $C_{33}H_{36}N_4O_6$ A red-orange powder. Very slightly soluble in dimethyl sulfoxide, and practically insoluble in water and in ethanol (99.5).

Identification—Determine the infrared absorption spectrum of bilirubin for assay as directed in the ATR method under Infrared Spectrophotometry <2.25>: it exhibits absorption at the wave numbers of about 3400 cm^{-1}, 2910 cm^{-1}, 1686 cm^{-1} and 1643 cm^{-1}.

Absorbance <2.24> $E^{1\%}_{1\,cm}$ (453 nm): 970 – 1134 (1 mg, dimethyl sulfoxide, 200 mL). Conduct this procedure without exposure to light, using light-resistant vessels.

Purity Related substances—Conduct this procedure without exposure to light, using light-resistant vessels. The following sample solution and standard solution should be prepared before use. Dissolve 5 mg of bilirubin for assay in 50 mL of a warmed mixture of dimethyl sulfoxide and acetic acid (100) (9:1), cool and use this solution as the sample solution. Pipet 1 mL of the sample solution, add a mixture of dimethyl sulfoxide and acetic acid (100) (9:1) to make exactly 50 mL, and use this solution as the standard solution. Perform the test with exactly 10 μL each of the sample solution and standard solution as directed under Liquid Chromatography <2.01> according to the following conditions, and determine each peak area by the automatic integration method: the total area of the peaks other than bilirubin obtained from the sample solution is not larger than the peak area of bilirubin from the standard solution.

Operating conditions

Detector, column, column temperature, mobile phase and flow rate: Proceed as directed in the operating conditions in the Assay under Oriental Bezoar.

Time span of measurement: About 3 times as long as the retention time of bilirubin, beginning after the solvent peak.

System suitability

System performance and system repeatability: Proceed as directed in the system suitability in the Assay under Oriental Bezoar.

Biotin-labeled elderberry lectin A solution of elderberry lectin labeled with biotin, dissolved in appropriate buffer solution.

2-(4-Biphenylyl)propionic acid $C_{15}H_{14}O_2$ Light yellow-white powder.

Melting point <2.60>: 145 - 148°C

Purity—Dissolve 1 mg of 2-(4-biphenylyl) propionic acid in a mixture of water and acetonitrile (11:9) to make 50 mL. Perform the test with 20 μL of this solution as directed under Liquid Chromatography <2.01> according to the operating conditions of the Related substances in the Purity (3) under Flurbiprofen. Determine each peak area of the solution in about twice as long as the retention time of the main peak by the automatic integration method, and calculate the amount of 2-(4-biphenylyl)propionic acid by the area percentage method: it is not less than 98.0%.

Content: not less than 98.0%. Assay—Weigh accurately about 0.5 g of 2-(4-biphenilyl)propionic acid, previously dried in vacuum over silica gel for 4 hours, dissolve in 50 mL of ethanol (95), and titrate <2.50> with 0.1 mol/L sodium hydroxide VS (indicator: 3 drops of phenolphthalein TS). Perform a blank determination in the same manner, and make any necessary correction.

Each mL of 0.1 mol/L sodium hydroxide VS
= 22.63 mg of $C_{15}H_{14}O_2$

2,2′-Bipyridyl $C_{10}H_8N_2$ [K 8486, Special class]

Bis(*cis*-3,3,5-trimethylcyclohexyl) phthalate $C_6H_4[COOC_6H_8(CH_3)_3]_2$ White crystalline powder.

Melting point <2.60>: 91 - 94°C

Bisdemethoxycurcumin $C_{19}H_{16}O_4$ Yellow to orange crystalline powder. Sparingly soluble in methanol, slightly soluble in ethanol (99.5), and practically insoluble in water. Melting point: 213 - 217°C.

Identification—Determine the absorption spectrum of a solution of bisdemethoxycurcumin in methanol (1 in 400,000) as directed under Ultraviolet-visible Spectrophotometry <2.24>: it exhibits a maximum between 413 nm and 417 nm.

Purity Related substances—(1) Dissolve 4 mg of bisdemethoxycurcumin in 2 mL of methanol, and use this solution as the sample solution. Pipet 1 mL of the sample solution, add methanol to make exactly 20 mL, and use this solution as the standard solution. Perform the test with these solutions as directed under Thin-layer Chromatography <2.03>. Spot 5 μL each of the sample solution and standard solution on a plate of silica gel for thin-layer chromatography. Develop the plate with a mixture of dichloromethane and methanol (19:1) to a distance of about 10 cm, and air-dry the plate. Examine under ultraviolet light (main wavelength: 365 nm): the spots other than the principal spot at *R*f value of about 0.3 obtained from the sample solution are not more intense than the spot from the standard solution.

(2) Dissolve 1.0 mg of bisdemethoxycurcumin in 5 mL of methanol, and use this solution as the sample solution. Pipet 1 mL of the sample solution, add methanol to make exactly 20 mL, and use this solution as the standard solution. Perform the test with exactly 10 μL each of the sample solution and standard solution as directed under Liquid Chromatography <2.01> according to the following conditions. Determine each peak area from both solutions by the automatic integration method: the total area of the peaks other than bisdemethoxycurcumin obtained from the sample solution is not larger than the peak area of bisdemethoxycurcumin from the standard solution.

Operating conditions

Column, column temperature, mobile phase and flow rate: Proceed as directed in the operating conditions in the Assay under Turmeric.

Detector: A visible absorption photometer (wavelength: 422 nm).

Time span of measurement: About 4 times as long as the retention time of bisdemethoxycurcumin, beginning after the solvent peak.

System suitability

System performance and system repeatability: Proceed as directed in the system suitability in the Assay under Turmeric.

Test for required detectability: Pipet 1 mL of the standard solution, and add methanol to make exactly 20 mL. Confirm that the peak area of bisdemethoxycurcumin obtained with 10 μL of this solution is equivalent to 3.5 to 6.5% of that with 10 μL of the standard solution.

4,4′-Bis(diethylamino)benzophenone $[(C_2H_5)_2NC_6H_4]_2CO$ Light yellow crystals.

Content: not less than 98%. Assay—Weigh accurately 0.25 g of 4,4′-bis(diethylamino)benzophenone, dissolve in 50 mL of acetic acid (100), and titrate <2.50> with 0.1 mol/L perchloric acid VS (potentiometric titration). Perform a blank titration in the same manner, and make any necessary correction.

Each mL of 0.1 mol/L perchloric acid VS
= 16.22 mg of $C_{21}H_{28}N_2O$

***N,N′*-Bis[2-hydroxy-1-(hydroxymethyl)ethyl]-5-hydroxyacetylamino-2,4,6-triiodoisophthalamide** $C_{16}H_{20}I_3N_3O_8$ White crystalline powder.

Identification (1) Heat 0.1 g of *N,N′*-bis[2-hydroxy-1-(hydroxymethyl)ethyl]-5-hydroxyacetylamino-2,4,6-triiodoisophthalamide over free flame: a purple colored gas evolves.

(2) Determine the infrared absorption spectrum of *N,N′*-bis[2-hydroxy-1-(hydroxymethyl)ethyl]-5-hydroxyacetylamino-2,4,6-triiodoisophthalamide as directed in the potassium bromide disk method under Infrared Spectrophotometry <2.25>: it exhibits absorption at the wave numbers of about 3390 cm^{-1}, 3230 cm^{-1}, 2880 cm^{-1}, 1637 cm^{-1}, 1540 cm^{-1}, 1356 cm^{-1} and 1053 cm^{-1}.

Purity—Dissolve 0.10 g of *N,N′*-bis[2-hydroxy-1-(hydroxymethyl)ethyl]-5-hydroxyacetylamino-2,4,6-triiodoisophthalamide in 10 mL of water, and use this solution as the sample solution. Pipet 1 mL of the sample solution, add water to make exactly 100 mL, and use this solution as the standard solution. Perform the test with exactly 20 μL each of the sample solution and standard solution as directed under Liquid Chromatography <2.01> according to the following conditions. Determine each peak area of both solutions by automatic integration method: the total area of the peaks other than *N,N′*-bis[2-hydroxy-1-(hydroxymethyl)ethyl]-5-hydroxyacetylamino-2,4,6-triiodoisophthalamide obtained from the sample solution is not larger than 3 times of the peak area of *N,N′*-bis[2-hydroxy-1-(hydroxymethyl)ethyl]-5-hydroxyacetylamino-2,4,6-triiodoisophthalamide from the standard solution.

Operating conditions

Proceed as directed in the operating conditions in the Purity (6) under Iopamidol.

System suitability

Proceed as directed in the system suitability in the Purity (6) under Iopamidol.

Bismuth nitrate See bismuth nitrate pentahydrate.

Bismuth nitrate pentahydrate $Bi(NO_3)_3.5H_2O$ [K 8566, Special class]

Bismuth nitrate-potassium iodide TS Dissolve 0.35 g of bismuth nitrate pentahydrate in 4 mL of acetic acid (100) and 16 mL of water (solution A). Dissolve 8 g of potassium iodide in 20 mL of water (solution B). To 20 mL of a mixture of solution A and solution B (1:1) add 80 mL of dilute sulfuric acid and 0.2 mL of hydrogen peroxide (30). Prepare before use.

Bismuth nitrate TS Dissolve 5.0 g of bismuth nitrate pentahydrate in acetic acid (100) to make 100 mL.

Bismuth potassium iodide TS Dissolve 10 g of L-tartaric acid in 40 mL of water, add 0.85 g of bismuth subnitrate, shake for 1 hour, add 20 mL of a solution of potassium iodide (2 in 5), shake thoroughly, allow to stand for 24 hours, and filter (solution A). Separately, dissolve 10 g of L-tartaric acid in 50 mL of water, add 5 mL of solution A, and preserve in a light-resistant, glass-stoppered bottle.

Bismuth sodium trioxide $NaBiO_3$ A yellow-brown powder.

Identification—(1) To 10 mg of bismuth sodium trioxide add 5 mL of a solution of manganese (II) nitrate hexahydrate (4 in 125) and 1 mL of diluted nitric acid (1 in 3), and shake vigorously for 10 seconds: a red-purple color is developed.

(2) Dissolve 10 mg of bismuth sodium trioxide in 2 mL of diluted hydrochloric acid (1 in 2): this solution responds to Qualitative Tests <*1.09*> (1) for sodium salt.

Bismuth subnitrate [Same as the namesake monograph]

Bismuth subnitrate TS Dissolve 10 g of L-tartaric acid in 40 mL of water, add 0.85 g of bismuth subnitrate, stir for 1 hour, then add 20 mL of a solution of potassium iodide (2 in 5), and shake well. After standing for 24 hours, filter, and preserve the filtrate in a light-resistant bottle.

Bismuth sulfite indicator Prepared for microbial test.

Bisoprolol fumarate for assay $(C_{18}H_{31}NO_4)_2.C_4H_4O_4$ [Same as the monograph Bisoprolol Fumarate. However, when dried, it contains not less than 99.0% of bisoprolol fumarate [$(C_{18}H_{31}NO_4)_2.C_4H_4O_4$]. Also, when performing the Purity (2) under Bisoprolol Fumarate, the total area of the peaks other than bisoprolol obtained from the sample solution is not larger than 1/5 times the peak area of bisoprolol from the standard solution].

Purify as follows if needed.

Purification method—Dissolve, with heating, 2 g of Bisoprolol Fumarate in 200 mL of ethyl acetate, add 0.5 g of activated carbon, shake well, and filter using a glass filter (G4). Place the filtrate in ice water for 2 hours while occasional shaking. Collect the crystals that precipitate out using a glass filter (G3). Dry the crystals obtained in vacuum at 80°C for 5 hours using phosphorus (V) oxide as a desiccant.

Bis-(1-phenyl-3-methyl-5-pyrazolone) $C_{20}H_{18}N_4O_2$ White to pale yellow, crystals or crystalline powder. It dissolves in mineral acids and in alkali hydroxides, and it does not dissolve in water, in ammonia TS, or in organic solvents. Melting point: not below 300°C.

Residue on ignition <*2.44*>: not more than 0.1%.

Nitrogen content <*1.08*>: 15.5 - 16.5%

Bis(1,1-trifluoroacetoxy)iodobenzene $C_{10}H_5F_6IO_4$ Prepared for amino acid analysis or biochemistry.

Bis-trimethyl silyl acetamide $CH_3CON[Si(CH_3)_3]_2$ Colorless liquid.

Refractive index <*2.45*> n_D^{20}: 1.414 - 1.418

Specific gravity <*2.56*> d_{20}^{20}: 0.825 - 0.835

Boiling point <*2.57*>: 71 - 73°C

1,4-Bis(trimethylsilyl)benzene-d_4 for nuclear magnetic resonance spectroscopy See 1,4-BTMSB-d_4 for nuclear magnetic resonance spectroscopy.

Bitter orange peel [Same as the namesake monograph]

Block buffer solution Dissolve 4 g of blocking agent in 100 mL of water, and add 100 mL of 0.01 mol/L phosphate buffer-sodium chloride TS (pH 7.4).

Blocking agent Powder whose main ingredient is bovine-derived lactoprotein. For immunological research purposes.

Blocking TS for epoetin alfa Used for Western blotting.

Blocking TS for nartograstim test Dissolve 1.0 g of bovine serum albumin in phosphate-buffered sodium chloride TS to make 100 mL.

Blood agar medium Sterilize 950 mL of heart infusion agar medium under increased pressure. Allow the media to cool to about 50°C, add 50 mL of horse or sheep defibrinated blood, dispense in sterilized Petri dishes, and make them as plate media.

1% blood suspension Wash a defibrinated animal blood in isotonic solution, and make it into suspension to contain 1 vol%. Prepare before use.

Blotting TS Dissolve 5.81 g of 2-amino-2-hydroxymethyl-1,3-propanediol, 2.93 of glycine and 0.38 g of sodium lauryl sulfate in a suitable amount of water, add 200 mL of methanol, and add water to make 1000 mL.

Blue tetrazolium $C_{40}H_{32}Cl_2N_8O_2$ Light yellow crystals. Freely soluble in methanol, in ethanol (95) and in chloroform, slightly soluble in water, and practically insoluble in acetone and in ether. Melting point: about 245°C (with decomposition).

Absorbance <*2.24*> $E_{1\,cm}^{1\%}$ (252 nm): not less than 826 (methanol).

Blue tetrazolium TS, alkaline To 1 volume of a solution of blue tetrazolium in methanol (1 in 200) add 3 volumes of a solution of sodium hydroxide in methanol (3 in 25). Prepare before use.

Borane-pyridine complex C_5H_8BN

Content: not less than 80%. Assay—Accurately weigh about 30 mg of borane-pyridine complex, dissolve in 40 mL of 0.05 mol/L iodide solution, add 10 mL of diluted sulfuric acid (1 in 6), and titrate <*2.50*> with 0.1 mol/L sodium thiosulfate VS (indicator: starch TS). Perform a blank determination in the same manner, and make any necessary correction.

Each mL of 0.1 mol/L sodium thiosulfate VS
= 1.549 mg of C_5H_8BN

Borate-hydrochloric acid buffer solution (pH 9.0) Dissolve 19.0 g of sodium tetraborate decahydrate in 900 mL of water, adjust the pH to exactly 9.0 with 1 mol/L hydrochloric acid TS, and add water to make 1000 mL.

Borax See sodium tetraborate decahydrate.

Boric acid H_3BO_3 [K 8863, Special class]

Boric acid-magnesium chloride buffer solution (pH 9.0) Dissolve 3.1 g of boric acid in 210 mL of dilute sodium hydroxide TS, and add 10 mL of a solution of magnesium chloride hexahydrate (1 in 50) and water to make 1000 mL. Adjust the pH to 9.0, if necessary.

Boric acid-methanol buffer solution Weigh exactly 2.1 g of boric acid, dissolve in 28 mL of sodium hydroxide TS, and dilute with water to exactly 100 mL. Mix equal volumes of this solution and methanol, and shake.

Boric acid-potassium chloride-sodium hydroxide buffer solution (pH 9.0) To 50 mL of 0.2 mol/L boric acid-0.2 mol/L potassium chloride TS for buffer solution add 21.30 mL of 0.2 mol/L sodium hydroxide VS and water to make 200 mL.

Boric acid-potassium chloride-sodium hydroxide buffer solution (pH 9.2) To 50 mL of 0.2 mol/L boric acid-0.2 mol/L potassium chloride TS for buffer solution add 26.70 mL of 0.2 mol/L sodium hydroxide VS and water to make 200 mL.

Boric acid-potassium chloride-sodium hydroxide buffer solution (pH 9.6) To 50 mL of 0.2 mol/L boric acid-0.2 mol/L potassium chloride TS for buffer solution add 36.85 mL of 0.2 mol/L sodium hydroxide VS and water to make 200 mL.

Boric acid-potassium chloride-sodium hydroxide buffer solution (pH 10.0) To 50 mL of 0.2 mol/L boric acid-0.2 mol/L potassium chloride TS for buffer solution add 43.90 mL of 0.2 mol/L sodium hydroxide VS and water to make 200 mL.

0.2 mol/L Boric acid-0.2 mol/L potassium chloride TS for buffer solution Dissolve 12.376 g of boric acid and 14.911 g of potassium chloride in water to make 1000 mL.

Boric acid-sodium hydroxide buffer solution (pH 8.4) Dissolve 24.736 g of boric acid in 0.1 mol/L sodium hydroxide VS to make exactly 1000 mL.

Borneol acetate $C_{12}H_{20}O_2$ A white to pale brown solid, or colorless to pale brown, clear liquid. Very soluble in methanol and in ethanol (99.5), and practically insoluble in water.

Identification Determine the infrared absorption spectrum of borneol acetate as directed in the liquid film method under Infrared Spectrophotometry <2.25>: it exhibits absorption at the wave numbers of about 2950 cm^{-1}, 1736 cm^{-1}, 1454 cm^{-1} and 1248 cm^{-1}.

Purity Related substances—Dissolve 50 mg of borneol acetate in 5 mL of methanol, and use this solution as the sample solution. Pipet 1 mL of the sample solution, add methanol to make exactly 20 mL, and use this solution as the standard solution. Perform the test with these solutions as directed under Thin-layer Chromatography <2.03>. Spot 5 μL each of the sample solution and standard solution on a plate of silica gel for thin-layer chromatography. Develop the plate with a mixture of hexane, diethyl ether and methanol (15:5:1) to a distance of about 7 cm, and air-dry the plate. Spray evenly 4-methoxybenzaldehyde-sulfuric acid TS on the plate, and heat at 105°C for 10 minutes: the spot at an *R*f value of about 0.7 obtained from the sample solution is not more intense than the spot from the standard solution.

Boron trifluoride BF_3 Colorless gas, having an irritating odor.

Boiling point <2.57>: −100.3°C
Melting point <2.60>: −127.1°C

Boron trifluoride-methanol TS A solution containing 14 g/dL of boron trifluoride (BF_3: 67.81) in methanol.

Bovine activated blood coagulation factor X A protein obtained from bovine plasma. It has an activity to decompose prothrombin specifically and limitedly and produce thrombin. It does not contain thrombin and plasmin. It contains not less than 500 Units per mg protein. One unit indicates an amount of the factor X which hydrolyzes 1 μmol of *N*-benzoyl-L-isoleucyl-L-glutamyl(γ-OR)-glycyl-L-arginyl-*p*-nitroanilide in 1 minute at 25°C.

Bovine serum Serum obtained from blood of bovine. Interleukin-2 dependent cell growth suppression substance is removed by heat at 56°C for 30 minutes before use

Bovine serum albumin Obtained from cattle serum as Cohn's fifth fraction. Contains not less than 95% of albumin.

Bovine serum albumin for assay White or pale yellow, crystals or crystalline powder.

Take about 50 mg of bovine serum albumin containing 99 % or more albumin in glass ampoules and put them in the desiccator, whose humidity is adjusted to 31%RH at 25°C with calcium chloride-saturated solution, for 2 weeks, and then take out and seal them immediately.

Protein content: not less than 88%. Assay—Weigh accurately about 0.1 g of bovine serum albumin for assay, dissolve in water, and add water to make exactly 20 mL. Put exactly 3 mL of the solution in the Kjeldahl flask, and determine protein content following Nitrogen Determination <1.08>.

Each mL of 0.005 mol/L sulfuric acid VS
= 0.8754 mg protein

Storage—Store at 4°C or lower.

Bovine serum albumin for gel filtration molecular mass marker Albumin obtained from bovine serum. For gel filtration chromatography.

Bovine serum albumin for test of ulinastatin White crystalline powder obtained from bovine serum by a purification method which does not denature albumin and other serum proteins. It contains not less than 99% of albumin.

0.1% Bovine serum albumin-acetate buffer solution Dissolve 0.1 g of bovine serum albumin in a solution of sodium acetate trihydrate (1 in 100) to make exactly 100 mL, and adjust to pH 4.0 with 1 mol/L hydrochloric acid TS.

Bovine serum albumin-isotonic sodium chloride solution Dissolve 0.1 g of bovine serum albumin in 100 mL of isotonic sodium chloride solution. Prepare before use.

1 w/v% Bovine serum albumin-phosphate buffer-sodium chloride TS Dissolve 1 g of bovine serum albumin in 100 mL of 0.01 mol/L phosphate buffer-sodium chloride TS (pH 7.4).

0.1 w/v% Bovine serum albumin-sodium chloride-phosphate buffer solution Dissolve 8.0 g of sodium chloride, 0.2 g of potassium chloride, 1.15 g of anhydrous disodium hydrogen phosphate and 0.2 g of potassium dihydrogen phosphate in water to make 1000 mL. To this solution add a solution of bovine serum albumin dissolved 1.0 g in 10 mL of water.

Bovine serum albumin-sodium chloride-phosphate buffer solution (pH 7.2) Dissolve 10.75 g of disodium hydrogen phosphate dodecahydrate, 7.6 g of sodium chloride and 1.0 g of bovine serum albumin in water to make 1000 mL. Adjust to pH 7.2 with dilute sodium hydroxide TS or diluted phosphoric acid (1 in 10) before use.

Bovine serum albumin TS for nartograstim test Dissolve 0.5 g of bovine serum albumin and 0.5 mL of polysorbate 20 in phosphate-buffered sodium chloride TS to make 500 mL.

Bovine serum albumin TS for secretin Dissolve 0.1 g of bovine serum albumin, 0.1 g of L-cysteine hydrochloride monohydrate, 0.8 g of L-alanine, 0.01 g of citric acid monohydrate, 0.14 g of disodium hydrogen phosphate dodecahydrate and 0.45 g of sodium chloride in 100 mL of water for injection.

Bovine serum albumin TS for Secretin RS Dissolve 0.1 g of bovine serum albumin, 0.8 g of L-alanine, 0.01 g of citric acid monohydrate, 0.14 g of disodium hydrogen phosphate dodecahydrate and 0.45 g of sodium chloride in 100 mL of water for injection.

Bradykinin $C_{50}H_{73}N_{15}O_{11}$ A white powder. Freely soluble in water and in acetic acid (31), and practically insoluble in diethyl ether.

Optical rotation <2.49> $[\alpha]_D^{20}$: −80 − −90° (15 mg, water, 5 mL, 100 mm).

Purity Related substances—Dissolve 2.0 mg of bradykinin in 0.2 mL of water, and use this solution as the sample solution. Perform the test with the sample solution as directed under Thin-layer Chromatography <*2.03*>. Spot 5 μL of the sample solution on a plate of cellulose for thin-layer chromatography. Develop the plate with a mixture of 1-butanol, water, pyridine and acetic acid (31) (15:12:10:3) to a distance of about 10 cm, and dry the plate at 60°C. Spray evenly a solution of ninhydrin in 1-butanol (1 in 1000) on the plate, and heat at 60°C for 30 to 60 minutes: any spot other than the principal spot arisen from bradykinin does not appear.

Brilliant green $C_{27}H_{34}N_2O_4S$ Fine, glistening, yellow crystals. It dissolves in water and in ethanol (95). The wavelength of absorption maximum: 623 nm.

Bromine Br [K 8529, Special class]

Bromine-acetic acid TS Dissolve 10 g of sodium acetate trihydrate in acetic acid (100) to make 100 mL, add 5 mL of bromine, and shake.

Storage—Preserve in light-resistant containers, preferably in a cold place.

Bromine-carbon tetrachloride TS To 0.1 g of bromine add carbon tetrachloride to make 100 mL, and to 2 mL of this solution add carbon tetrachloride to make 100 mL. Prepare before use.

Bromine-cyclohexane TS Dissolve 0.1 g of bromine in cyclohexane to make 100 mL. To 2 mL of this solution add cyclohexane to make 10 mL. Prepare before use.

Bromine-sodium hydroxide TS To 100 mL of a solution of sodium hydroxide (3 in 100) add 0.2 mL of bromine. Prepare before use.

Bromine TS Prepare by saturating water with bromine as follows: Transfer 2 to 3 mL of bromine to a glass-stoppered bottle, the stopper of which should be lubricated with petrolatum, add 100 mL of cold water, insert the stopper, and shake.

Storage—Preserve in light-resistant containers, preferably in a cold place.

Bromocresol green $C_{21}H_{14}Br_4O_5S$ [K 8840, Special class]

Bromocresol green-crystal violet TS Dissolve 0.3 g of bromocresol green and 75 mg of crystal violet in 2 mL of ethanol (95), and dilute with acetone to make 100 mL.

Bromocresol green-methyl red TS Dissolve 0.15 g of bromocresol green and 0.1 g of methyl red in 180 mL of ethanol (99.5), and add water to make 200 mL.

Bromocresol green-sodium hydroxide-acetic acid-sodium acetate TS To 0.25 g of bromocresol green add 15 mL of water and 5 mL of dilute sodium hydroxide TS, then add a small quantity of acetic acid-sodium acetate buffer solution (pH 4.5), dissolve while shaking, and add acetic acid-sodium acetate buffer solution (pH 4.5) to make 500 mL. Wash 250 mL of this solution with two 100-mL portions of dichloromethane. Filter if necessary.

Bromocresol green-sodium hydroxide-ethanol TS Dissolve 50 mg of bromocresol green in 0.72 mL of 0.1 mol/L sodium hydroxide VS and 20 mL of ethanol (95), and add water to make 100 mL.

Test for sensitivity—To 0.2 mL of the bromocresol green-sodium hydroxide-ethanol TS add 100 mL of freshly boiled and cool water: the solution is blue, and not more than 0.2 mL of 0.02 mol/L hydrochloric acid VS is required to change the color of this solution to yellow.

Color change: pH 3.6 (yellow) to pH 5.2 (blue).

Bromocresol green-sodium hydroxide TS Triturate 0.2 g of bromocresol green with 2.8 mL of 0.1 mol/L sodium hydroxide VS in a mortar, add water to make 200 mL, and filter if necessary.

Bromocresol green TS Dissolve 50 mg of bromocresol green in 100 mL of ethanol (95), and filter if necessary.

Bromocresol purple $C_{21}H_{16}Br_2O_5S$ [K 8841, Special class]

Bromocresol purple-dipotassium hydrogenphosphate-citric acid TS Mix 30 mL of bromocresol purple-sodium hydroxide TS and 30 mL of dipotassium hydrogen phosphate-citric acid buffer solution (pH 5.3), and wash with three 60-mL portions of chloroform.

Bromocresol purple-sodium hydroxide TS Triturate 0.4 g of bromocresol purple with 6.3 mL of dilute sodium hydroxide TS in a mortar, add water to make 250 mL, and filter if necessary.

Bromocresol purple TS Dissolve 50 mg of bromocresol purple in 100 mL of ethanol (95), and filter if necessary.

Bromophenol blue $C_{19}H_{10}Br_4O_5S$ [K 8844, Special class]

Bromophenol blue-potassium hydrogen phthalate TS Dissolve 0.1 g of bromophenol blue in potassium hydrogen phthalate buffer solution (pH 4.6) to make 100 mL.

Bromophenol blue TS Dissolve 0.1 g of bromophenol blue in 100 mL of dilute ethanol, and filter if necessary.

0.05% Bromophenol blue TS Dissolve 10 mg of bromophenol blue in water to make 20 mL.

Bromophenol blue TS, dilute Dissolve 50 mg of bromophenol blue in 100 mL of ethanol (99.5). Prepare before use.

Bromophenol blue TS (pH 7.0) Mix 10 mL of bromophenol blue TS and 10 mL of ethanol (95), and adjust the pH to 7.0 with diluted dilute sodium hydroxide TS (1 in 10).

***N*-Bromosuccinimide** $C_4H_4BrNO_2$ [K 9553, Special class]

***N*-Bromosuccinimide TS** Dissolve 1 g of *N*-bromosuccinimide in 1000 mL of water.

Bromothymol blue $C_{27}H_{28}Br_2O_5S$ [K 8842, Special class]

Bromothymol blue TS Dissolve 0.1 g of bromothymol blue in 100 mL of dilute ethanol, and filter if necessary.

Bromothymol blue-sodium hydroxide TS To 0.2 g of powdered bromothymol blue add 5 mL of dilute sodium hydroxide TS and a small quantity of water, dissolve by shaking in a water bath at 50°C, then add water to make 100 mL.

Bromothymol blue-sodium hydroxide-ethanol TS Dissolve 50 mg of bromothymol blue in 4 mL of diluted 0.2 mol/L sodium hydroxide TS (1 in 10) and 20 mL of ethanol (95), and add water to make 100 mL.

Bromovalerylurea $C_6H_{11}BrN_2O_2$ [Same as the namesake monograph]

Brotizolam for assay $C_{15}H_{10}BrClN_4S$ [Same as the monograph Brotizolam. When dried, it contains not less than 99.0% of brotizolam ($C_{15}H_{10}BrClN_4S$).]

Brucine See brucine *n*-hydrate.

Brucine dihydrate See brucine *n*-hydrate.

Brucine *n*-hydrate $C_{23}H_{26}N_2O_4.nH_2O$ [K 8832, Special class]

1,4-BTMSB-d_4 for nuclear magnetic resonance spectroscopy $C_{12}H_{18}D_4Si_2$ 1,4-Bis(trimethylsilyl)benzene-d_4 that the traceability to the international unit system was secured.

B-type erythrocyte suspension Prepare a suspension containing 1 vol% of erythrocyte separated from human B-type blood in isotonic sodium chloride solution.

Bucillamine $C_7H_{13}NO_3S_2$ [Same as the namesake monograph]

Bucillamine for assay $C_7H_{13}NO_3S_2$ [Same as the monograph Bucillamine. However, when dried, it contains not less than 99.0% of bucillamine ($C_7H_{13}NO_3S_2$). Furthermore, it conforms to the following test.]

Purity Related substances—Dissolve 60 mg of bucillamine for assay in 20 mL of a mixture of water and methanol (1:1) and use this solution as the sample solution. Pipet 1 mL of the sample solution, add the mixture of water and methanol (1:1) to make exactly 100 mL, and use this solution as the standard solution. When the test is performed according to the Purity (3) under Bucillamine, the total area of the peaks other than bucillamine obtained from the sample solution is not larger than the peak area of bucillamine from the standard solution.

Bufalin for assay $C_{24}H_{34}O_4.xH_2O$ White, odorless crystalline powder.

Absorbance <2.24> $E^{1\%}_{1\,cm}$ (300 nm): 143 – 153 (10 mg, methanol, 250 mL). Use the sample dried in a desiccator (silica gel) for 24 hours for the test.

Purity Related substances—Dissolve 40 mg of bufalin for assay in 5 mL of chloroform and use this solution as the sample solution. Pipet 1 mL of the sample solution, add chloroform to make exactly 100 mL, and use this solution as the standard solution. Perform the test with these solutions as directed under Thin-layer Chromatography <2.03>. Spot 5 μL each of the sample solution and standard solution on a plate of silica gel for thin-layer chromatography. Develop the plate with a mixture of cyclohexane, acetone and chloroform (4:3:3) to a distance of about 14 cm, and air-dry. Spray evenly sulfuric acid, and heat at 100°C for 2 to 3 minutes: any spot other than the principal spot obtained from the sample solution is not larger and not more intense than the spot from the standard solution.

Content: not less than 99.0%. Assay—Weigh accurately about 10 mg of bufalin for assay, previously dried in a desiccator (silica gel) for 24 hours, dissolve in methanol to make exactly 10 mL, and use this solution as the sample solution. Perform the test with 20 μL of the sample solution as directed under Liquid Chromatography <2.01> according to the following conditions. Determine the peak area by the automatic integration method, and calculate the amount of bufalin by the area percentage method.

Operating conditions

Detector: An ultraviolet absorption photometer (wavelength: 300 nm).

Column: A stainless steel column 4 to 6 mm in inside diameter and 15 to 30 cm in length, packed with octadecylsilanized silica gel for liquid chromatography (5 to 10 μm in particle diameter).

Column temperature: A constant temperature of about 40°C.

Mobile phase: A mixture of water and acetonitrile (1:1).

Flow rate: Adjust so that the retention time of bufalin is about 6 minutes.

Time span of measutrement: About twice as long as the retention time of bufalin, beginning after the solvent peak.

System suitability

Test for required detectability: Pipet 1 mL of the sample solution, add methanol to make exactly 100 mL, and use this solution as the standard solution (1). Pipet 1 mL of the standard solution (1), add methanol to make exactly 20 mL, and use this solution as the standard solution (2). Adjust the detection sensitivity so that the peak area of bufalin obtained with 20 μL of the standard solution (2) can be measured by the automatic integration method and the peak height of bufalin with 20 μL of the standard solution (1) is about 20% of the full scale.

System performance: Dissolve 10 mg each of bufalin for assay, cinobufagin for assay and resibufogenin for assay in methanol to make 200 mL. When the procedure is run with 20 μL of this solution under the above operating conditions, bufalin, cinobufagin and resibufogenin are eluted in this order with the resolutions between these peaks being not less than 1.5, respectively.

Bufalin for component determination See bufalin for assay.

Buffer solution for celmoleukin Combine 12.5 mL of 0.5 mol/L tris buffer solution (pH 6.8), 10 mL of sodium lauryl sulfate solution (1→10), 10 mL of glycerin, and 17.5 mL of water, shake, then add 5 mg of bromophenol blue to dissolve.

Storage—Store in a cool place, shielded from light.

Buffer solution for enzyme digestion Dissolve 0.30 g of urea in a mixture of 100 μL of 2-amino-2-hydroxymethyl-1,3-propanediol solution containing 6.06 g in 100 mL of water, 100 μL of 2-amino-2-hydroxymethyl-1,3-propanediol hydrochloride solution containing 7.88 g in 100 mL of water, 100 μL of methylamine hydrochloride solution containing 2.70 g in 100 mL of water, 50 μL of dithiothreitol in solution containing 30.9 mg in 1 mL of water and 420 μL of water.

Buffer solution for epoetin alfa sample Dissolve 1.2 g of 2-amino-2-hydroxymethyl-1,3-propanediol and 3.2 g of sodium lauryl sulfate in a suitable amount of water, adjust to pH 6.8 with 6 mol/L hydrochloric acid TS, 1 mol/L hydrochloric acid TS or 0.1 mol/L hydrochloric acid TS, add

32 mg of bromophenol blue and 16 mL of glycerin, and add water to make 40 mL. Before use, dissolve 50 mg of dithiothreitol in 10 mL of this solution.

Buffer solution for filgrastim sample Dissolve 1.2 g of 2-amino-2-hydroxymethyl-1,3-propanediol and 3.2 g of sodium lauryl sulfate in a suitable amount of water, adjust to pH 6.8 with 6 mol/L hydrochloric acid TS, 1 mol/L hydrochloric acid TS or 0.1 mol/L hydrochloric acid TS, add 32 mg of bromophenol blue and 16 mL of glycerin, and add water to make 40 mL.

Buffer solution for nartograstim sample Mix 0.8 mL of sodium lauryl sulfate solution (1 in 10), 0.5 mL of 0.5 mol/L tris buffer solution (pH 6.8), 0.4 mL of glycerin and 0.1 mL of bromophenol blue solution (1 in 200). Prepare before use.

Buffer solution for SDS polyacrylamide gel electrophoresis Dissolve 3.0 g of 2-amino-2-hydroxymethyl-1,3-propanediol, 14.4 g of glycine and 1.0 g of sodium lauryl sulfate in water to make 1000 mL.

Buformin hydrochloride for assay $C_6H_{15}N_5.HCl$ [Same as the monograph Buformin Hydrochloride. When dried, it contains not less than 99.5% of buformin hydrochloride ($C_6H_{15}N_5.HCl$).]

***n*-Butanol** See 1-butanol.

***sec*-Butanol** See 2-butanol.

1-Butanol $CH_3(CH_2)_2CH_2OH$ [K 8810, Special class]

2-Butanol $CH_3CH_2CH(OH)CH_3$ [K 8812, Special class]

2-Butanone $CH_3COC_2H_5$ [K 8900, Special class]

Butenafine hydrochloride for assay $C_{23}H_{27}N.HCl$ [Same as the monograph Butenafine Hydrochloride]

***N-t*-Butoxycarbonyl-L-glutamic acid-α-phenyl ester** $C_{16}H_{21}NO_6$ White powder.

Melting point <*2.60*>: 95–104°C

Purity Related substances—Dissolve 10 mg of *N-t*-butoxycarbonyl-L-glutamic acid-α-phenyl ester in 5 mL of dilute ethanol, and use this solution as the sample solution. Pipet 1 mL of the sample solution, add dilute ethanol to make exactly 50 mL, and use this solution as the standard solution. Perform the test with these solutions as directed under Thin-layer Chromatography <*2.03*>. Spot 10 μL each of the sample solution and standard solution on three plates of silica gel with fluorescent indicator for thin-layer chromatography. Develop the first plate with a mixture of chloroform, ethyl acetate and acetic acid (100) (25:25:1), the second plate with a mixture of benzene, 1,4-dioxane and acetic acid (100) (95:25:4), and the third plate with a mixture of chloroform, methanol and acetic acid (100) (45:4:1) to a distance of about 12 cm, and air-dry these plates. Examine under ultraviolet light (main wavelength: 254 nm): the spots other than the principal spot obtained from the sample solution are not more intense than the spot from the standard solution in all plates.

Butyl acetate $CH_3COOCH_2CH_2CH_2CH_3$ [K 8377, Special class]

***n*-Butyl acetate** See butyl acetate

***t*-Butyl alcohol** $(CH_3)_3COH$ A crystalline solid, having a characteristic odor. A colorless liquid at above an ordinary temperature. Specific gravity d^{20}_{20}: about 0.78; Boiling point: about 83°C; Melting point: about 25°C.

Identification—Determine the infrared absorption spectrum as directed in the liquid film method as directed under Infrared Spectrophotometry <*2.25*>: it exhibits absorption at the wave numbers of about 3370 cm^{-1}, 2970 cm^{-1}, 1471 cm^{-1}, 1202 cm^{-1}, 1022 cm^{-1}, 913 cm^{-1} and 749 cm^{-1}.

***n*-Butylamine** $CH_3CH_2CH_2CH_2NH_2$ A colorless liquid, having an amine-like, characteristic odor. Miscible with water, with ethanol (95) and with diethyl ether. The solution in water shows alkalinity and rapidly absorbs carbon dioxide from the air.

Specific gravity <*2.56*> d^{20}_{20}: 0.740 – 0.747

Distilling range <*2.57*>: 76.5 – 79°C, not less than 96 vol%.

Butyl benzoate $C_6H_5COOCH_2CH_2CH_2CH_3$ A clear and colorless liquid.

Refractive index <*2.45*> n^{20}_{D}: 1.495 – 1.500

Specific gravity <*2.56*> d^{20}_{20}: 1.006 – 1.015

***n*-Butylboronic acid** $C_4H_{11}BO_2$ White flakes.

Melting point <*2.60*>: 90 – 92°C

***n*-Butyl chloride** See 1-chlorobutane.

***n*-Butyl formate** $HCOO(CH_2)_3CH_3$ Clear and colorless liquid, having a characteristic odor.

Specific gravity <*2.56*> d^{20}_{20}: 0.884 – 0.904

***tert*-Butyl methyl ether** $(CH_3)_3COCH_3$ Clear colorless liquid, having a specific odor.

Refractive index <*2.45*> n^{20}_{D}: 1.3689

Specific gravity <*2.56*> d^{20}_{4}: 0.7404

Butyl parahydroxybenzoate $HOC_6H_4COOCH_2CH_2CH_2CH_3$ [Same as the namesake monograph]

Butyl parahydroxybenzoate for resolution check $C_{11}H_{14}O_3$ Colorless crystals or a white crystalline powder. Very soluble in methanol, freely soluble in ethanol (95) and in acetone, and practically insoluble in water. Melting point: 68 – 71°C.

Identification—Determine the infrared absorption spectrum of butyl parahydroxybenzoate for resolution check as directed in the potassium bromide disk method under Infrared Spectrophotometry <*2.25*>, and compare the spectrum with the Reference Spectrum of Butyl Parahydroxybenzoate or the spectrum of Butyl Parahydroxybenzoate RS: both spectra exhibit similar intensities of absorption at the same wave numbers.

Purity Related substances—Dissolve 50 mg of butyl parahydroxybenzoate for resolution check in 2.5 mL of methanol, and add the mobile phase to make 50 mL. To 10 mL of this solution add the mobile phase to make 100 mL, and use this solution as the sample solution. Pipet 1 mL of the sample solution, add the mobile phase to make exactly 10 mL, and use this solution as the standard solution. Perform the test with exactly 10 μL each of the sample solution and standard solution as directed under Liquid Chromatography <*2.01*> according to the following conditions. Determine each peak area by the automatic integration method: total area of the peaks other than butyl parahydroxybenzoate obtained from the sample solution is not larger than the peak area of butyl parahydroxybenzoate from the standard solution.

Operating conditions

Detector, column, column temperature, mobile phase, and flow rate: Proceed as directed in the operating conditions in the Assay under Butyl Parahydroxybenzoate.

Time span of measurement: About 1.5 times as long as the retention time of butyl parahydroxybenzoate.

System suitability

Test for required detectability: Pipet 1 mL of the standard solution, and add methanol to make exactly 20 mL. Confirm that the peak area of butyl parahydroxybenzoate obtained with 10 μL of this solution is equivalent to 3.5 to 6.5% of that with 10 μL of the standard solution.

System performance: When the procedure is run with 10 μL of the standard solution under the above operating conditions, the number of theoretical plates and the symmetry factor of the peak of butyl parahydroxybenzoate are not less than 2500 and not more than 2.0, respectively.

System repeatability: When the test is repeated 6 times with 10 μL of the standard solution under the above operating conditions, the relative standard deviation of the peak area of butyl parahydroxybenzoate is not more than 5.0%.

Butyrolactone $C_4H_6O_2$ Clear, colorless to practically colorless liquid.

Specific gravity <2.56> d_4^{25}: 1.128 – 1.135

Boiling point <2.57>: 198 – 208°C

Cadmium acetate See cadmium acetate dihydrate.

Cadmium acetate dihydrate $Cd(CH_3COO)_2.2H_2O$ White, crystals or crystalline powder.

Identification—(1) Dissolve 0.2 g of cadmium acetate dihydrate in 20 mL of water, and use this solution as the sample solution. To 10 mL of the sample solution add 2 mL of iron (III) chloride TS: a red-brown color is produced.

(2) To 10 mL of the sample solution obtained in (1) add 1 mL of sodium sulfide TS: a yellow precipitate is produced.

Cadmium ground metal Cd [H 2113, First class]

Cadmium-ninhydrin TS Dissolve 50 mg of cadmium acetate dihydrate in 5 mL of water and 1 mL of acetic acid (100), add 2-butanone to make 50 mL, and dissolve 0.1 g of ninhydrin in this solution. Prepare before use.

Cadralazine for assay $C_{12}H_{21}N_5O_3$ [Same as the monograph Cadralazine. When dried, it contains not less than 99.0% of cadralazine ($C_{12}H_{21}N_5O_3$).]

Caffeine See caffeine hydrate.

Caffeine hydrate $C_8H_{10}N_4O_2.H_2O$ [Same as the namesake monograph]

Caffeine, anhydrous $C_8H_{10}N_4O_2$ [Same as the monograph Anhydrous Caffeine]

Calcium acetate monohydrate $(CH_3COO)_2Ca.H_2O$ [K 8364, Special class]

Calcium carbonate $CaCO_3$ [K 8617, Special class]

Calcium carbonate for assay $CaCO_3$ [Same as the monograph Precipitated Calcium Carbonate. When dried, it contains not less than 99.0% of calcium carbonate ($CaCO_3$).]

Calcium chloride See calcium chloride dihydrate.

Calcium chloride dihydrate $CaCl_2.2H_2O$ [K 8122, Special class]

Calcium chloride dihydrate for assay See calcium chloride hydrate for assay.

Calcium chloride for drying $CaCl_2$ [K 8124, For drying]

Calcium chloride hydrate for assay $CaCl_2.2H_2O$ [Same as the monograph, Calcium Chloride Hydrate. It contains not less than 99.0% of calcium chloride hydrate ($CaCl_2.2H_2O$).]

Calcium chloride for water determination $CaCl_2$ [K 8125, For water determination]

Calcium chloride TS Dissolve 7.5 g of calcium chloride dihydrate in water to make 100 mL (0.5 mol/L).

Calcium gluconate for thin-layer chromatography See calcium gluconate hydrate for thin-layer chromatography.

Calcium gluconate hydrate for thin-layer chromatography [Same as the monograph Calcium Gluconate Hydrate. When the test is performed as directed in the Identification (1) under Calcium Gluconate Hydrate, any spot other than the principal spot at the *Rf* value of about 0.4 does not appear.]

Calcium hydroxide $Ca(OH)_2$ [K 8575, Special class]

Calcium hydroxide for pH determination Calcium hydroxide prepared for pH determination.

Calcium hydroxide pH standard solution See pH Determination <2.54>.

Calcium hydroxide TS To 3 g of calcium hydroxide add 1000 mL of cold distilled water, and occasionally shake the mixture vigorously for 1 hour. Allow to stand, and use the supernatant liquid (0.04 mol/L).

Calcium nitrate See calcium nitrate tetrahydrate.

Calcium nitrate tetrahydrate $Ca(NO_3)_2.4H_2O$ [K 8549, Special class]

Calcium oxide CaO [K 8410, Special class]

Calcium pantothenate $C_{18}H_{32}CaN_2O_{10}$ [Same as the namesake monograph]

Calcium paraaminosalicylate hydrate for assay $C_7H_5CaNO_3.3\frac{1}{2}H_2O$ [Same as the monograph Calcium Paraaminosalicylate Hydrate. It contains not less than 99.0% of calcium paraaminosalicylate ($C_7H_5CaNO_3$), calculated on the anhydrous basis.]

Camphor $C_{10}H_{16}O$ [Same as the monograph *d*-Camphor or *dl*-Camphor]

***d*-Camphorsulfonic acid** $C_{10}H_{16}O_4S$ White, crystals or crystalline powder, having a characteristic odor. Very soluble in water, and soluble in chloroform.

Purity Clarity and color of solution—Dissolve 1.0 g of *d*-camphorsulfonic acid in 10 mL of water: the solution is clear and colorless or pale yellow.

Loss on drying <2.41>: not more than 2.0% (1 g, 105°C, 5 hours).

Content: not less than 99.0%, calculated on the dried basis. Assay—Weigh accurately about 4 g of *d*-camphorsulfonic acid, dissolve in 50 mL of water, and titrate <2.50> with 1 mol/L sodium hydroxide VS (indicator: 3 drops of methyl red TS). Perform a blank determination in the same manner, and make any necessary correction.

Each mL of 1 mol/L sodium hydroxide VS
= 232.3 mg of $C_{10}H_{16}O_4S$

Candesartan cilexetil $C_{33}H_{34}N_6O_6$ [Same as the namesake monograph]

Candesartan cilexetil for assay $C_{33}H_{34}N_6O_6$ [Same as the monograph Candesartan Cilexetil. It contains not less than 99.5% of candesartan cilexetil ($C_{33}H_{34}N_6O_6$), calculated on the anhydrous basis, and when performed the test as directed in the Purity (2) under Candesartan Cilexetil, the total area of the peaks other than candesartan cilexetil obtained from the sample solution is not larger than 1/2 times the peak area of candesartan cilexetil from the standard solution.]

Caprylic acid $CH_3(CH_2)_6COOH$ A clear and colorless, oily liquid, having a slight unpleasant odor. Freely soluble in ethanol (95) and in chloroform, and very slightly soluble in water.

Refractive index <2.45> n_D^{20}: 1.426 – 1.430

Specific gravity <2.56> d_4^{20}: 0.908 – 0.912

Distilling range <2.57>: 238 – 242°C, not less than 95 vol%.

(*E*)-Capsaicin for assay $C_{18}H_{27}NO_3$ Use (*E*)-capsaicin for thin-layer chromatography meeting the following additional specifications.

Absorbance <2.24> $E_{1cm}^{1\%}$ (281 nm): 97 – 105 (10 mg, methanol, 200 mL). Use the sample dried in a desiccator (in vacuum, phosphorus (V) oxide, 40°C) for 5 hours for the test.

Purity Related substances—Dissolve 10 mg of (*E*)-capsaicin for assay in 50 mL of methanol, and use this solution as the sample solution. Pipet 1 mL of the sample solution, add methanol to make exactly 100 mL, and use this solution as the standard solution. Perform the test with exactly 20 μL each of the sample solution and standard solution as directed under Liquid Chromatography <2.01> according to the following conditions, and determine each peak area from these solutions by the automatic integration method: the total area of the peaks other than capsaicin obtained from the sample solution is not larger than the peak area of capsaicin from the standard solution.

Operating conditions

Detector, column, column temperature, mobile phase, and flow rate: Proceed as directed in the operating conditions in the Assay under Capsicum.

Time span of measurement: About 3 times as long as the retention time of capsaicin, beginning after the solvent peak.

System suitability

System performance and system repeatability: Proceed the system suitability in the Assay under Capsicum.

Test for required detectability: Pipet 1 mL of the standard solution, and add methanol to make exactly 20 mL. Confirm that the peak area of capsaicin obtained with 20 μL of this solution is equivalent to 3.5 to 6.5% of that with 20 μL of the standard solution.

(*E*)-Capsaicin for component determination See (*E*)-capsaicin for assay.

Capsaicin for thin-layer chromatography See (*E*)-capsaicin for thin-layer chromatography.

(*E*)-Capsaicin for thin-layer chromatography $C_{18}H_{27}NO_3$ White crystals, having a strong irritative odor. Very soluble in methanol, freely soluble in ethanol (95) and in diethyl ether, and practically insoluble in water.

Melting point <2.60>: 65 – 70°C

Purity Related substances—Dissolve 20 mg of (*E*)-capsaicin for thin-layer chromatography in 2 mL of methanol, and use this solution as the sample solution. Pipet 1 mL of the sample solution, add methanol to make exactly 100 mL, and use this solution as the standard solution. Perform the test with 10 μL each of the sample solution and standard solution as directed in the Identification under Capsicum: any spot other than the principal spot at an *Rf* value of about 0.5 obtained from the sample solution is not more intense than the spot from the standard solution.

Carbazochrome $C_{10}H_{12}N_4O_3$ Yellow-red to red, crystals or crystalline powder. Melting point: about 222°C (with decomposition).

Content: not less than 98.0%. Assay—Dissolve about 0.2 g of carbazochrome, weighed accurately, in 20 mL of acetic acid (100) by heating, add 80 mL of acetic anhydride, cool, and titrate <2.50> with 0.1 mol/L perchloric acid VS (potentiometric titration). Perform a blank determination in the same manner, and make any necessary correction.

Each mL of 0.1 mol/L perchloric acid VS
= 23.62 mg of $C_{10}H_{12}N_4O_3$

Carbazochrome sodium sulfonate for component determination See carbazochrome sodium sulfonate trihydrate.

Carbazochrome sodium sulfonate trihydrate
$C_{10}H_{11}N_4NaO_5S.3H_2O$ [Same as the monograph Carbazochrome Sodium Sulfonate Hydrate. It contains not less than 99.0% of carbazochrome sodium sulfonate ($C_{10}H_{11}N_4NaO_5S$), calculated on the anhydrous basis, and meets the following additional requirement.]

Water <2.48>: 14.0 – 15.0%.

Carbazole $C_{12}H_9N$ White to nearly white foliaceous or plate-like crystals or crystalline powder. Freely soluble in pyridine and in acetone, slightly soluble in ethanol (99.5), and practically insoluble in water. It readily sublimes when heated.

Melting point <2.60>: 243 – 245°C

Purity Clarity and color of solution—To 0.5 g of carbazole add 20 mL of ethanol (99.5), and dissolve by warming: the solution is clear.

Residue on ignition: Not more than 0.1% (1 g).

Carbazole TS Dissolve 0.125 g of carbazole in ethanol (99.5) to make 100 mL.

L-Carbocisteine for assay $C_5H_9NO_4S$ [Same as the monograph L-Carbocisteine. When dried, it contains not less than 99.0% of L-carbocisteine ($C_5H_9NO_4S$).]

0.1 mol/L Carbonate buffer solution (pH 9.6) Dissolve 3.18 g of anhydrous sodium carbonate and 5.88 g of sodium hydrogen carbonate in water to make 1000 mL.

Carbon dioxide CO_2 [Same as the namesake monograph]

Carbon disulfide CS_2 [K 8732, Special class]
Preserve in tightly stoppered containers in a dark, cold place, remote from fire.

Carbonic anhydrase White powder. Derived from bovine RBC. Molecular weight about 29,000.

Carbon monoxide CO A toxic, colorless gas. Prepare by passing the gas generated by reacting formic acid with sulfuric acid through a layer of sodium hydroxide TS. Carbon monoxide from a metal cylinder may be used.

Carbon tetrachloride CCl_4 [K 8459, Special class]

Carboplatin $C_6H_{12}N_2O_4Pt$ [Same as the namesake monograph]

Carvedilol for assay $C_{24}H_{26}N_2O_4$ [Same as the monograph Carvedilol]

Casein, milk A white to light yellow, powder or grain.

Identification—Determine the infrared absorption spectrum as directed in the potassium bromide disk method as directed under Infrared Spectrophotometry <2.25>: it exhibits absorption at the wave numbers of about 1650 cm^{-1}, 1540 cm^{-1} and 1250 cm^{-1}.

Casein (milk origin) See casein, milk.

Casein peptone See peptone, casein.

Castor oil [Same as the namesake monograph]

Catechol $C_6H_4(OH)_2$ White crystals.
Melting point <*2.60*>: 104 - 107°C
Storage—Preserve in a light-resistant tight container.

Cefadroxil $C_{16}H_{17}N_3O_5S$ [Same as the namesake monograph]

Cefatrizine propylene glycolate $C_{18}H_{18}N_6O_5S_2.C_3H_8O_2$ [Same as the namesake monograph]

Cefcapene pivoxil hydrochloride hydrate $C_{23}H_{29}N_5O_8S_2.HCl.H_2O$ [Same as the namesake monograph]

Cefdinir lactam ring-cleavage lactones $C_{14}H_{15}N_5O_6S_2$ A mixture of 4 diastereoisomers. A white to yellow powder.
Identification—Determine the infrared absorption spectrum of cefdinir lactam ring-cleavage lactones as directed in the paste method under Infrared Spectrophotometry <*2.25*>: it exhibits absorption at the wave numbers of about 1743 cm^{-1}, 1330 cm^{-1}, 1163 cm^{-1} and 1047 cm^{-1}.
Content: not less than 90%. Assay—Dissolve about 5 mg of cefdinir lactam ring-cleavage lactones in 5 mL of 0.1 mol/L phosphate buffer solution (pH 7.0), and use this solution as the sample solution. Perform the test with 5 µL of the sample solution as directed in the operating conditions of the Purity (2) under Cefdinir, and determine the areas of each peak by the automatic integration method. Calculate the percent of the total peak area of 4 cefdinir lactam ring-cleavage lactones to the total area of all peaks.

Cell suspension solution for teceleukin Centrifuge for 5 minutes at 1000 rpm culture medium of NK-7 cells that have been cultured statically for 2 to 4 hours. Remove the supernatant by aspiration, and add potency measuring medium for teceleukin to a cell concentration of 2 to 4 × 10^5 cells/mL.

Celmoleukin for liquid chromatography $C_{693}H_{1118}N_{178}O_{203}S_7$ [Same as the monograph Celmoleukin (Genetical Recombination). However, contains 0.5 to 1.5 mg of protein per mL, polymers amount for 0.5% or less, and conforms to the following test].
Identification (1) When the amino acid sequence is investigated using the Edman technique and liquid chromatography, the amino acids are detected in the following sequence: alanine, proline, threonine, serine, serine, serine, threonine, lysine, lysine, threonine, glutamine, leucine, glutamine, leucine, and glutamic acid. Also, based on the results of the protein content determination test, place an amount of celmoleukin equivalent to about 0.3 mg in a hydrolysis tube, evaporate to dryness under vacuum, and then add 100 µL of hydrazine anhydride for amino acid sequence analysis. Reduce the internal pressure of the hydrolysis tube by heating at about 100°C for 6 hours. After evaporating to dryness under vacuum, add 250 µL of water to dissolve the residue. To this solution add 200 µL of benzaldehyde, shake occasionally, leave for one hour, centrifuge, and remove the aqueous layer. Add 250 µL of water to the benzaldehyde layer, shake, centrifuge, combine the aqueous layers, and evaporate to dryness under vacuum. Threonine is detected when amino acid analysis is conducted using the postcolumn technique with ninhydrin on a solution of the residue dissolved by adding 100 µL of 0.02 mol/L hydrochloric acid TS.
(2) Add 1 mL of protein digestive enzyme TS to 1 mL of celmoleukin for liquid chromatography, shake, and leave at 37°C for 18 to 24 hours. Pipet 1 mL of this solution and add 25 µL of trifluoroacetic acid (1 in 10). To another 1 mL, add 10 µL of 2-mercaptoethanol, leave at 37°C for 30 minutes, and then add 25 µL of trifluoroacetic acid (1 in 10). Perform the test with these two solutions separately as directed in the operating conditions of the Identification (1) under Celmoleukin (Genetical Recombination). Repeatedly pipet the celmoleukin derived peak fraction that elutes and when the test is performed according to Celmoleukin (Genetical Recombination), Constituent amino acids, except for the lysines in positions 9 and 49 from the amino terminal amino acid, a peptide estimated from the complete primary structure is detected.

Cephaeline hydrobromate $C_{28}H_{38}N_2O_4.2HBr$ A white or light-yellow crystalline powder.
Purity—Dissolve 10 mg of cephaeline hydrobromate in 10 mL of the mobile phase, and use this solution as the sample solution. Pipet 1 mL of the sample solution, add the mobile phase to make exactly 10 mL, and use this solution as the standard solution. Perform the test with exactly 10 µL each of the sample solution and standard solution as directed in the Assay under Ipecac: when measure the peak areas for 2 times the retention time of emetine, the total area of the peaks other than cephaeline obtained from the sample solution is not larger than the peak area of cephaeline from the standard solution.

Ceric ammonium sulfate See cerium (IV) tetraammonium sulfate dihydrate.

Ceric ammonium sulfate-phosphoric acid TS See cerium (IV) tetraammonium sulfate-phosphoric acid TS.

Ceric ammonium sulfate TS See cerium (IV) tetraammonium sulfate TS.

Cerium (III) nitrate hexahydrate $Ce(NO_3)_3.6H_2O$ A colorless or light yellow crystalline powder. It dissolves in water.
Purity (1) Chloride <*1.03*>: not more than 0.036%.
(2) Sulfate <*1.14*>: not more than 0.120%.
Content: not less than 98.0%. Assay—To about 1.5 g of cerium (III) nitrate hexahydrate, accurately weighed, add 5 mL of sulfuric acid, and heat it until white fumes are evolved vigorously. After cooling, add 200 mL of water, 0.5 mL of 0.1 mol/L silver nitrate VS, dissolve 5 g of ammonium peroxodisulfate, dissolve, and boil it for 15 minutes. After cooling, add 2 drops of 1,10-phenanthroline TS, and titrate <*2.50*> with 0.1 mol/L ammonium iron (II) sulfate VS until the pale blue color of the solution changes to red.

Each mL of 0.1 mol/L ammonium iron (II) sulfate VS
= 43.42 mg of $Ce(NO_3)_3.6H_2O$

Cerium (III) nitrate TS Dissolve 0.44 g of cerium (III) nitrate hexahydrate in water to make 1000 mL.

Cerium (IV) diammonium nitrate $Ce(NH_4)_2(NO_3)_6$ [K 8556, Diammonium cerium (IV) nitrate, Special class]

Cerium (IV) diammonium nitrate TS Dissolve 6.25 g of cerium (IV) diammonium nitrate in 160 mL of diluted dilute nitric acid (9 in 50). Use within 3 days.

Cerium (IV) sulfate tetrahydrate $Ce(SO_4)_2 \cdot 4H_2O$ [K 8976, Special class]

Cerium (IV) tetraammonium sulfate dihydrate $Ce(SO_4)_2.2(NH_4)_2SO_4.2H_2O$ [K 8977, Tetraammonium cerium (IV) sulfate dihydrate, Special class]

Cerium (IV) tetraammonium sulfate-phosphoric acid TS Dissolve 0.1 g of cerium (IV) tetraammonium sulfate dihydrate in diluted phosphoric acid (4 in 5) to make 100 mL.

Cerium (IV) tetraammonium sulfate TS Dissolve 6.8 g of cerium (IV) tetraammonium sulfate dihydrate in diluted sulfuric acid (3 in 100) to make 100 mL.

Cerous nitrate See cerium (III) nitrate hexahydrate.

Cerous nitrate TS See cerium (III) nitrate TS.

Cesium chloride CsCl White, crystals or crystalline powder. Very soluble in water, and freely soluble in ethanol (99.5).

Loss on drying <2.41>: Not more than 1.0% (1 g, 110°C, 2 hours).

Content: not less than 99.0%. Assay—Weigh accurately about 0.5 g, previously dried, and dissolve in water to make exactly 200 mL. Pipet 20 mL of this solution, add 30 mL of water, and titrate <2.50> with 0.1 mol/L silver nitrate VS (indicator: fluorescein sodium TS).

Each mL of 0.1 mol/L silver nitrate VS
= 16.84 mg of CsCl

Cesium chloride TS To 25.34 g of cesium chloride add water to make 1000 mL.

Cetanol [Same as the namesake monograph]

Cetirizine hydrochloride for assay $C_{21}H_{25}ClN_2O_3.2HCl$ [Same as the monograph Cetirizine Hydrochloride. When dried, it contains not less than 99.5% of cetirizine hydrochloride ($C_{21}H_{25}ClN_2O_3.2HCl$).]

Cetrimide $C_{17}H_{38}BrN$ White to pale yellow-white powder, having a faint, characteristic odor.

Purity Clarity of solution—Dissolve 1.0 g of cetrimide in 5 mL of water: the solution is clear.

Content: not less than 96.0%. Assay—Weigh accurately about 2 g of cetrimide, previously dried, and dissolve in water to make exactly 100 mL. Pipet 25 mL of this solution into a separator, add 25 mL of chloroform, 10 mL of 0.1 mol/L sodium hydroxide VS and 10 mL of a freshly prepared solution of potassium iodide (1 in 20), shake well, allow to stand, and remove the chloroform layer. Wash the solution with three 10-mL portions of chloroform, take the water layer, and add 40 mL of hydrochloric acid. After cooling, titrate with 0.05 mol/L potassium iodide VS until the deep brown color of the solution almost disappears, add 2 mL of chloroform, and titrate <2.50> again until the red-purple color of the chloroform layer disappears. The end point is reached when the red-purple color of the chloroform layer no more reappears within 5 minutes after the chloroform layer is decolorized. Perform a blank determination with 20 mL of water, 10 mL of a solution of potassium iodide (1 in 20) and 40 mL of hydrochloric acid.

Each mL of 0.05 mol/L potassium iodate VS
= 33.64 mg of $C_{17}H_{38}BrN$

Cetylpyridinium chloride monohydrate $C_{21}H_{38}ClN.H_2O$ White, powder or crystals. Odorless or having slightly a characteristic odor.

Melting point <2.60>: 80 – 84°C

Water <2.48>: 4.5 – 5.5%

Residue on ignition <2.44>: Not more than 0.2% (1 g).

Content: 99.0 – 102.0%, calculated on the anhydrous basis. Assay—Weigh accurately about 0.2 g of cetylpyridinium chloride monohydrate, dissolve in 75 mL of water, add 10 mL of chloroform, 0.4 mL of bromophenol blue solution (1 in 2000) and 5 mL of freshly prepared sodium hydrogen carbonate solution (21 in 5000), and titrate <2.50> with 0.02 mol/L sodium tetraphenylboron VS until the blue color in the chloroform layer disappears by vigorous shaking after adding 1 drop of the titrant.

Each mL of 0.02 mol/L sodium tetraphenylboron VS
= 6.800 mg of $C_{21}H_{38}ClN$

Chenodeoxycholic acid for thin-layer chromatography $C_{24}H_{40}O_4$ White, crystals or crystalline powder. Very soluble in methanol and in acetic acid (100), freely soluble in ethanol (95), soluble in acetone, sparingly soluble in ethyl acetate, slightly soluble in chloroform, and practically insoluble in water. Melting point: about 119°C (recrystallize from ethyl acetate).

Purity Related substances—Dissolve 25 mg of chenodeoxycholic acid for thin-layer chromatography in a mixture of chloroform and ethanol (95) (9:1) to make exactly 250 mL and use this solution as the sample solution. Perform the test with this solution as directed under the Thin-layer Chromatography <2.03>. Spot 10 μL of the sample solution on a plate of silica gel for thin-layer chromatography. Develop the plate with a mixture of chloroform, acetone and acetic acid (100) (7:2:1) to a distance of about 10 cm, and air-dry the plate. Dry the plate at 120°C for 30 minutes, spray evenly a solution of phosphomolybdic acid *n*-hydrate in ethanol (95) (1 in 5) immediately, and heat at 120°C for 2 or 3 minutes: any spot other than the principal spot at the *Rf* value of about 0.4 does not appear.

Content: not less than 98.0%. Assay—Weigh accurately about 0.5 g of chenodeoxycholic acid for thin-layer chromatography, previously dried under reduced pressure (phosphorus (V) oxide) at 80°C for 4 hours, and dissolve in 40 mL of neutralized ethanol and 20 mL of water. Add 2 drops of phenolphthalein TS, and titrate <2.50> with 0.1 mol/L sodium hydroxide VS. Near the end point add 100 mL of freshly boiled and cooled water, and titrate again.

Each mL of 0.1 mol/L sodium hydroxide VS
= 39.26 mg of $C_{24}H_{40}O_4$

0.5 vol% Chicken erythrocyte suspension Centrifuge the blood taken from healthy chicken, discard the supernatant liquid. To the residue add 0.01 mol/L phosphate buffer solution to make 45 mL, suspend the cells, and centrifuge. Discard the supernatant liquid, and repeat the same procedure 3 times more. Suspend 5 mL of the middle layer of the residue so obtained in 40 mL of 0.01 mol/L phosphate buffer solution, and centrifuge. Discard the supernatant liquid, suspend 3 mL of the middle layer of the residue in 10 mL of 0.01 mol/L phosphate buffer solution, and centrifuge. Discard the supernatant liquid, and suspend 2 mL of the middle layer of the residue in 18 mL of 0.01 mol/L phosphate buffer solution. To 10 mL of this solution add 190 mL of 0.01 mol/L phosphate buffer solution, and stir to suspend.

Chikusetsusaponin IV for thin-layer chromatography $C_{47}H_{74}O_{18}$ White crystalline powder. Freely soluble in methanol and in ethanol (95), and practically insoluble in diethyl ether. Melting point: about 215°C (with decomposition).

Purity Related substances—Dissolve 2 mg of chikusetsusaponin IV for thin-layer chromatography in 1 mL of methanol, and perform the test with 5 μL of this solution as directed in the Identification under Panax Japonicus Rhizome: any spot other than the principal spot with an *Rf* value of about 0.4 does not appear.

Chloral hydrate $C_2H_3Cl_3O_2$ [Same as the namesake

monograph]

Chloral hydrate TS Dissolve 5 g of chloral hydrate in 3 mL of water.

Chloramine See sodium toluensulfonchloramide trihydrate.

Chloramine TS See sodium toluensulfonchloramide TS.

Chloramphenicol $C_{11}H_{12}Cl_2N_2O_5$ [Same as the monograph Chloramphenicol]

Chlorauric acid See hydrogen tetrachloroaurate (III) tetrahydrate.

Chlorauric acid TS See hydrogen tetrachloroaurate (III) tetrahydrate TS.

Chlordiazepoxide $C_{16}H_{14}ClN_3O$ [Same as the namesake monograph]

Chlordiazepoxide for assay $C_{16}H_{14}ClN_3O$ [Same as the monograph Chlordiazepoxide. When dried, it contains not less than 99.0% of $C_{16}H_{14}ClN_3O$.]

Chlorhexidine hydrochloride $C_{22}H_{30}Cl_2N_{10}.2HCl$ [Same as the namesake monograph]

Chlorinated lime [Same as the namesake monograph]

Chlorinated lime TS Triturate 1 g of chlorinated lime with 9 mL of water, and filter. Prepare before use.

Chlorine Cl_2 A yellow-green gas, having a suffocating odor. It is heavier than air, and dissolves in water. Prepare from chlorinated lime with hydrochloric acid. Chlorine from a metal cylinder may be used.

Chlorine TS Use a saturated solution of chlorine in water. Preserve this solution in fully filled, light-resistant, glass-stoppered bottles, preferably in a cold place. In the case where the preparation of the saturated solution of chlorine is difficult, a ready-to-use aqueous solution of chlorine may be used by considering adjustment of conditions such as amount of the solution used in a test tube while noting the difference from the saturated concentration.

Chloroacetic acid $C_2H_3ClO_2$ [K 8899, Special class]

***p*-Chloroaniline** See 4-chloroaniline

4-Chloroaniline $H_2NC_6H_4Cl$ White, crystals or crystalline powder. Freely soluble in ethanol (95) and in acetone, and soluble in hot water.

Melting point <2.60>: 70 – 72°C

Residue on ignition <2.44>: not more than 0.1% (1 g).

4-Chlorobenzenediazonium TS Dissolve 0.5 g of 4-chloroaniline in 1.5 mL of hydrochloric acid, and add water to make 100 mL. To 10 mL of this solution add 10 mL of sodium nitrite TS and 5 mL of acetone. Prepare before use.

***p*-Chlorobenzene sulfonamide** See 4-chlorobenzene sulfonamide.

4-Chlorobenzene sulfonamide $ClC_6H_4SO_2NH_2$ White to pale yellow, odorless, crystalline powder. Dissolves in acetone.

Purity Related substances—Dissolve 0.60 g of 4-chlorobenzene sulfonamide in acetone to make exactly 300 mL, and perform the test with 5 μL of this solution as directed in the Purity (5) under Chlorpropamide: any spot other than the principal spot at the *R*f value of about 0.5 does not appear.

***p*-Chlorobenzoic acid** See 4-chlorobenzoic acid.

4-Chlorobenzoic acid ClC_6H_4COOH White, crystals or powder. Sparingly soluble in ethanol (95), slightly soluble in chloroform, and practically insoluble in water.

Melting point <2.60>: 238 – 242°C

Content: not less than 99.0%. Assay—Weigh accurately about 0.3 g of 4-chlorobenzoic acid, dissolve in 30 mL of neutralized ethanol, and titrate <2.50> with 0.1 mol/L sodium hydroxide VS (indicator: 2 drops of phenolphthalein TS).

Each mL of 0.1 mol/L sodium hydroxide VS
= 15.66 mg of $C_7H_5ClO_2$

4-Chlorobenzophenone $C_{13}H_9ClO$ A white, crystalline powder or powder.

Identification—Determine the absorption spectrum of a solution of 4-chlorobenzophenone in ethanol (99.5) (3 in 50,000) as directed under Ultraviolet-visible Spectrophotometry <2.24>: it exhibits a maximum between 256 nm and 260 nm.

Melting point <2.60>: 73 – 78°C

Content: not less than 98.0%.

Assay—Dissolve 1 g of 4-chlorobenzophenon in acetone to make 10 mL, and use this solution as the sample solution. Perform the test with 1 μL of the sample solution as directed under Gas Chromatography <2.02> according to the following conditions. Determine each peak area by the automatic integration method, and calculate the amount of 4-chlorobenzophenone by the area percentage method.

Operating conditions

Detector: A hydrogen flame-ionization detector.

Column: A fused silica column 0.25 mm in inside diameter and 30 m in length, coated with dimethylpolysiloxane for gas chromatography in thickness of 0.25 μm.

Column temperature: A constant temperature of about 220°C.

Injection port temperature: 270°C.

Detector temperature: 250°C.

Carrier gas: Helium.

Flow rate: 1.33 mL per minute.

Split ratio: 1:100.

Time span of measurement: About 3 times as long as the retention time of 4-chlorobenzophenon.

System suitability

System performance: To 1 mL of the sample solution add acetone to make 10 mL. When the procedure is run with 1 μL of this solution under the above operating conditions, the number of theoretical plates and the symmetry factor of the peak of 4-chlorobenzophenone are not less than 50,000 and not more than 1.2, respectively.

System repeatability: To 1 mL of the sample solution add acetone to make 10 mL. When the test is repeated 6 times with 1 μL of this solution under the above operating conditions, the relative standard deviation of the peak area of 4-chlorobenzophenone is not more than 2.0%.

1-Chlorobutane $CH_3(CH_2)_3Cl$ Clear and colorless liquid, miscible with ethanol (95) and with diethyl ether, practically insoluble in water.

Refractive index <2.45> n_D^{20}: 1.401 – 1.045

Specific gravity <2.56> d_{20}^{20}: 0.884 – 0.890

Boiling point <2.57>: about 78°C

Chlorobutanol $C_4H_7Cl_3O$ [Same as the namesake monograph]

1-Chloro-2,4-dinitrobenzene $C_6H_3(NO_2)_2Cl$ Light yellow, crystals or crystalline powder.

Melting point <2.60>: 50 – 54°C

Storage—Preserve in a light-resistant tight container.

3′-Chloro-3′-deoxythymidine for liquid chromatography $C_{10}H_{13}N_2O_4Cl$ Occurs as a white powder.

Purity—Dissolve 10 mg of 3′-chloro-3′-deoxythymidine for liquid chromatography in the mobile phase to make 100 mL. Perform the test with 10 μL of this solution as directed in the Purity **(3)** under Zidovudine: a peak is not observed at the retention time for zidovudine.

(2-Chloroethyl) diethylamine hydrochloride $C_6H_{14}ClN.HCl$ White powder.

Content: not less than 95.0%. Assay—Weigh accurately about 0.2 g of (2-chloroethyl)diethylamine hydrochloride, previously dried at 45°C for 3 hours under reduced pressure, and dissolve in 15 mL of acetic acid (100). To this solution add 10 mL of a mixture of acetic acid (100) and mercury (II) acetate TS for nonaqueous titration (5:3), and titrate *<2.50>* with 0.1 mol/L perchloric acid VS (potentiometric titration). Perform a blank determination in the same manner, and make any necessary correction.

Each mL of 0.1 mol/L perchloric acid VS
= 17.21 mg of $C_6H_{14}ClN.HCl$

Chloroform $CHCl_3$ [K 8322, Special class]

Chloroform, ethanol-free Mix 20 mL of chloroform with 20 mL of water, gently shake for 3 minutes, separate the chloroform layer, wash the layer again with two 20-mL portions of water, and filter it through dry filter paper. To the filtrate add 5 g of anhydrous sodium sulfate, shake for 5 minutes, allow the mixture to stand for 2 hours, and filter through dry filter paper. Prepare before use.

Chloroform for water determination To 1000 mL of chloroform add 30 g of synthetic zeolite for drying, stopper tightly, allow to stand for about 8 hours with occasional gentle shaking, then allow to stand for about 16 hours, and collect the clear layer of chloroform. Preserve the chloroform, protecting it from moisture. The water content of this chloroform should not be more than 0.1 mg per mL.

Chlorogenic acid for thin-layer chromatography See (*E*)-chlorogenic acid for thin-layer chromatography.

(*E*)-Chlorogenic acid for thin-layer chromatography $C_{16}H_{18}O_9$ A white powder. Freely soluble in methanol and in ethanol (99.5), and sparingly soluble in water. Melting point: about 205°C (with decomposition).

Purity Related substances—Dissolve 1.0 mg of (*E*)-chlorogenic acid for thin-layer chromatography in 2 mL of methanol, and use this solution as the sample solution. Perform the test with the sample solution as directed under Thin-layer Chromatography *<2.03>*. Spot 10 μL of the sample solution on a plate of silica gel for thin-layer chromatography, develop the plate with a mixture of ethyl acetate, water and formic acid (6:1:1) to a distance of about 10 cm, and air-dry the plate. Examine under ultraviolet light (main wavelength: 365 nm): no spot other than the principal spot with an *R*f value of about 0.5 appears.

***p*-Chlorophenol** See 4-Chlorophenol.

4-Chlorophenol ClC_6H_4OH Colorless or pale red, crystals or crystalline mass, having a characteristic odor. Very soluble in ethanol (95), in chloroform, in diethyl ether and in glycerin, and sparingly soluble in water. Melting point: about 43°C.

Content: not less than 99.0%. Assay—Weigh accurately about 0.2 g of 4-chlorophenol, and dissolve in water to make 100 mL. Measure exactly 25 mL of this solution into an iodine flask, add exactly 20 mL of 0.05 mol/L bromine VS and then 5 mL of hydrochloric acid, stopper immediately, shake occasionally for 30 minutes, and allow to stand for 15 minutes. Add 5 mL of a solution of potassium iodide (1 in 5), stopper immediately, shake well, and titrate *<2.50>* with 0.1 mol/L sodium thiosulfate VS (indicator: 1 mL of starch TS). Perform a blank determination in the same manner.

Each mL of 0.05 mol/L bromine VS
= 3.214 mg of C_6H_5ClO

Storage—Preserve in tight, light-resistant containers.

(2-Chlorophenyl)-diphenylmethanol for thin-layer chromatography $C_{19}H_{15}ClO$ To 5 g of clotrimazole add 300 mL of 0.2 mol/L hydrochloric acid TS, boil for 30 minutes, cool, and extract with 100 mL of diethyl ether. Wash the diethyl ether extract with two 10 mL portions of 0.2 mol/L hydrochloric acid TS, then with two 10-mL portions of water. Shake the diethyl ether extract with 5 g of anhydrous sodium sulfate, and filter. Evaporate the diethyl ether of the filtrate, dissolve the residue in 200 mL of methanol by warming, and filter. Warm the filtrate, and add gradually 100 mL of water by stirring. Cool in an ice bath, filter the separated crystals, and dry in a desiccator (phosphorus (V) oxide) for 24 hours. A white crystalline powder. Very soluble in dichloromethane, freely soluble in diethyl ether, soluble in methanol, and practically insoluble in water.

Melting point <2.60>: 92 – 95°C

Purity Related substances—Dissolve 10 mg of (2-chlorophenyl)-diphenylmethanol for thin-layer chromatography in dichloromethane to make exactly 20 mL, and perform the test with 10 μL of this solution as directed in the Purity (7) under Clotrimazole: any spot other than the principal spot does not appear.

Chloroplatinic acid See hydrogen hexachloroplatinate (IV) hexahydrate.

Chloroplatinic acid-potassium iodide TS See hydrogen hexachloroplatinate (IV)-potassium iodide TS.

Chloroplatinic acid TS See hydrogen hexachloroplatinate (IV) TS.

3-Chloro-1,2-propanediol $C_3H_7ClO_2$ A clear and colorless viscous liquid.

Purity Dissolve 0.20 g of 3-chloro-1,2-propanediol in 100 mL of diethyl ether, and use this solution as the sample solution. Pipet 1 mL of the sample solution, add diethyl ether to make exactly 100 mL, and use this solution as the standard solution. Perform the test with exactly 5 μL each of the sample solution and standard solution as directed under Gas Chromatography *<2.02>* according to the following conditions, and determine each peak area by the automatic integration method: the total area of the peaks other than 3-chloro-1,2-propanediol obtained from the sample solution is not larger than 2 times the peak area from the standard solution.

Operating conditions

Proceed as directed in the operating conditions in the Purity (6) under Iohexol except the time span of measurement.

Time span of measurement: About 5 times as long as the retention time of 3-chloro-1,2-propanediol, beginning after the solvent peak.

System suitability

System performance and system repeatability: Proceed as directed in the system suitability in the Purity (6) under Iohexol.

Test for required detectability: To exactly 5 mL of the standard solution add diethyl ether to make exactly 20 mL. Confirm that the peak area of 3-chloro-1,2-propanediol obtained with 5 μL of this solution is equivalent to 20 to 30% of that with 5 μL of the standard solution.

Chlorotrimethylsilane $(CH_3)_3SiCl$ A colorless or practically colorless liquid, having a pungent odor. Evolves fumes in a damp atmosphere. Very soluble in diethyl ether, and reactable with water or with ethanol. Boiling point: about 58°C.

Chlorphenesin carbamate for assay $C_{10}H_{12}ClNO_4$ [Same as the monograph Chlorphenesin Carbamate. When dried, it contains not less than 99.0% of chlorphenesin carbamate ($C_{10}H_{12}ClNO_4$).]

Chlorpheniramine maleate $C_{16}H_{19}ClN_2.C_4H_4O_4$ [Same as the namesake monograph]

Chlorpromazine hydrochloride for assay $C_{17}H_{19}ClN_2S.HCl$ [Same as the monograph Chlorpromazine Hydrochloride]

Chlorpropamide for assay $C_{10}H_{13}ClN_2O_3S$ [Same as the monograph Chlorpropamide. When dried, it contains not less than 99.0% of chlorpropamide ($C_{10}H_{13}ClN_2O_3S$).]

Cholesterol $C_{27}H_{46}OH$ [Same as the namesake monograph]

Cholesterol benzoate $C_{34}H_{50}O_2$ White crystalline powder. Melting point: 145 - 152°C.

Cholic acid for thin-layer chromatography $C_{24}H_{40}O_5$ White, crystals or crystalline powder. Soluble in acetic acid (100), sparingly soluble in acetone and in ethanol (95), and very slightly soluble in water. Melting point: about 198°C.

Purity Related substances—Dissolve 25 mg of cholic acid for thin-layer chromatography in acetone to make exactly 250 mL and use this solution as the sample solution. Perform the test with the sample solution as directed under the Thin-layer Chromatography <*2.03*>. Spot 10 μL of the sample solution on a plate of silica gel for thin-layer chromatography. Develop the plate with a mixture of chloroform, acetone and acetic acid (100) (7:2:1) to a distance of about 10 cm, and air-dry the plate. Dry the plate at 120°C for 30 minutes, spray evenly a solution of phosphomolybdic acid *n*-hydrate in ethanol (95) (1 in 5) immediately, and heat at 120°C for 2 or 3 minutes: any spot other than the principal spot, having *R*f value of about 0.1, does not appear.

Content: not less than 98.0%. Assay—Weigh accurately about 0.5 g of cholic acid for thin-layer chromatography, previously dried at 80°C for 4 hours (in vacuum, phosphorous (V) oxide), dissolve in 40 mL of neutralized ethanol and 20 mL of water, add 2 drops of phenolphthalein TS, and titrate with 0.1 mol/L sodium hydroxide VS until immediately before the end-point has been reached. Then add 100 mL of freshly boiled and cooled water, and continue the titration <*2.50*>. Perform a blank determination in the same manner, and make any necessary correction.

Each mL of 0.1 mol/L sodium hydroxide VS
= 40.86 mg of $C_{24}H_{40}O_5$

Choline chloride $[(CH_3)_3NCH_2CH_2OH]Cl$ White crystalline powder.

Melting point <*2.60*>: 303 - 305°C (with decomposition).

Water <*2.48*>: less than 0.1%.

Chromic acid-sulfuric acid TS Saturate chromium (VI) oxide in sulfuric acid.

Chromium trioxide See chromium (VI) oxide.

Chromium trioxide TS See chromium (VI) oxide TS.

Chromium (VI) oxide CrO_3 A dark red-purple thin needle-shaped or inner prism-like crystals, or light masses.

Identification—To 5 mL of a solution (1 in 50) add 0.2 mL of lead (II) acetate TS: yellow precipitates appear, which do not dissolve on the addition of acetic acid.

Chromium (VI) oxide TS Dissolve 3 g of chromium (VI) oxide in water to make 100 mL.

Chromogenic synthetic substrate Equal amount mixture of *N*-benzoyl-L-isoleucyl-L-glutamyl-glycyl-L-arginyl-*p*-nitroanilid hydrochloride and *N*-benzoyl-L-isoleucyl-γ-methoxy glutamyl-glycyl-L-arginyl-*p*-nitroanilid hydrochloride. White to pale yellow, masses or powder. It is slightly soluble in water.

Identification—Perform the test with the solution of chromogenic synthetic substrate (1 in 30,000) as directed under Ultraviolet-visible Spectrophotometry <*2.24*>: the absorption maximum at about 316 nm is observed.

Purity Free 4-nitroaniline: not more than 0.5%.

Loss on drying <*2.41*>: not more than 5% (0.2 g, reduced pressure (0.3 kPa), calcium chloride, 30 to 40°C, 18 hours).

Content: not less than 95% and not more than 105% of the labeled amount.

Chromophore TS for teceleukin Mix 0.1 mL of diluted hydrogen peroxide (30) (1 in 20) with 10 mL of 0.2 mol/L citric acid buffer (pH 3.8) containing 0.2 mmol/L 3,3′,5,5′-tetramethylbenzidine dihydrochloride dihydrate, and use immediately.

Chromotropic acid See disodium chromotropate dihydrate.

Chromotropic acid TS Dissolve 50 mg of disodium chromotropate dihydrate in the solution prepared by cautiously adding 68 mL of sulfuric acid to 30 mL of water, cooling, then adding water to make 100 mL. Preserve in light-resistant containers.

Chromotropic acid TS, concentrated Suspend 0.5 g of disodium chromotropate dihydrate in 50 mL of sulfuric acid, centrifuge, and use the supernatant liquid. Prepare before use.

α-Chymotrypsin A slightly yellowish white lyophilized powder. It contains not less than 350 U per mg of α-chymotrypsin.

Chymotrypsinogen for gel filtration molecular mass marker A chymotrypsinogen obtained from bovine spleen. For gel filtration chromatography.

Cibenzoline succinate for assay $C_{18}H_{18}N_2.C_4H_6O_4$ [Same as the monograph Cibenzoline Succinate. When dried, it contains not less than 99.0% of cibenzoline succinate ($C_{18}H_{18}N_2.C_4H_6O_4$) and meets the following requirement.]

Purity Related substances—Dissolve 0.10 g of cibenzoline succinate for assay in 2 mL of methanol, and use this solution as the sample solution. Pipet 1 mL of the sample solution, and add methanol to make exactly 100 mL. To exactly 1 mL of this solution add methanol to make exactly 10 mL, and use this solution as the standard solution. Perform the test with these solutions as directed under Thin-layer Chromatography <*2.03*>. Spot 10 μL each of the sample solution and standard solution on a plate of silica gel with fluorescent indicator for thin-layer chromatography. Develop the plate with a mixture of ethyl acetate, methanol and ammonia solution (28) (20:3:2) to a distance of about 10 cm, air-dry the plate, and dry at 80°C for 30 minutes. After cooling, examine under ultraviolet light (main wavelength: 254 nm): the spot other than the principal spot obtained with the sample solution is not more intense than the spot with the standard solution. On standing the plate for 30 minutes in the tank saturated with iodine vapor, the spot other than the principal spot with the sample solution is not more intense than the spot with the standard solution.

Cilastatin ammonium for assay $C_{16}H_{29}N_3O_5S$: 375.48 A white crystalline powder.

Purity Related substances—Dissolve 40 mg of the substance to be examined in 25 mL of water, and use this solution as the sample solution. Pipet 3 mL of the sample solution, add water to make exactly 100 mL, and use this solution as the standard solution. Perform the test with exactly 20 μL each of the sample solution and standard solution as directed under Liquid Chromatography <2.01> according to the following conditions, and determine the each peak area by the automatic integration method. Separately, perform the test with 20 μL of water in the same manner to correct any variance of the peak area caused the variation of the baseline: the total area of the peaks other than cilastatin obtained from the sample solution is not larger than 1/6 times the peak area of cilastatin from the standard solution.

Operating conditions

Detector: An ultraviolet absorption photometer (wavelength: 210 nm).

Column: A stainless steel column 4.6 mm in inside diameter and 25 cm in length, packed with octadecylsilanized silica gel for liquid chromatography (5 μm in particle diameter).

Column temperature: A constant temperature of about 50°C.

Mobile phase A: A mixture of diluted phosphoric acid (1 in 1000) and acetonitrile (7:3).

Mobile phase B: Diluted phosphoric acid (1 in 1000).

Flowing of mobile phase: Control the gradient by mixing the mobile phases A and B as directed in the following table.

Time after injection of sample (min)	Mobile phase A (vol%)	Mobile phase B (vol%)
0 – 30	15 → 100	85 → 0
30 – 40	100	100

Flow rate: 2.0 mL per minute.

Time span of measurement: 40 minutes.

System suitability

Test for required detectability: To exactly 1 mL of the standard solution add water to make exactly 30 mL. Confirm that the peak area of cilastatin obtained with 20 μL of this solution is equivalent to 2.3 to 4.5% of that with 20 μL of the standard solution.

System performance: When the procedure is run with 20 μL of the standard solution under the above operating conditions: the retention time of cilastatin is about 20 minutes, and the number of theoretical plates and the symmetry factor of the peak of cilastatin are not less than 10,000 and not more than 2.5, respectively.

System repeatability: When the test is repeated 3 times with 20 μL of the standard solution under the above operating conditions, the relative standard deviation of the peak area of cilastatin is not more than 3.0%.

Residual solvent—Weigh accurately about 1 g of cilastatin ammonium for assay, dissolve in water to make exactly 100 mL, and use this solution as the sample solution. Separately, weigh accurately about 0.10 g of ethanol (99.5), add water to make exactly 100 mL, and use this solution as the standard solution. Perform the test with exactly 1 μL each of the sample solution and standard solution as directed under Gas Chromatography <2.02> according to the following conditions. Determine the peak areas, A_T and A_S, of ethanol in each solution, and calculate the amount of ethanol (C_2H_5OH): not more than 0.5%.

$$\text{Amount (\%) of ethanol } (C_2H_5OH) = M_S/M_T \times A_T/A_S \times 100$$

M_S: Amount (mg) of ethanol (99.5) taken

M_T: Amount (mg) of cilastatine ammonium for assay taken

Operating conditions

Detector: A hydrogen flame-ionization detector.

Column: A fused silica column 0.5 mm in inside diameter and 30 m in length, coated the inside with 5% diphenyl-95% dimethylpolysiloxane for gas chromatography in thickness of 5 μm.

Column temperature: Inject the sample at a constant temperature of about 50°C, maintain for 150 seconds, then raise to 70°C at the rate of 8°C per minute, and maintain for 30 seconds.

Carrier gas: Helium.

Flow rate: Adjust so that the retention time of ethanol is about 1 minute.

Split ratio: 5:1.

System suitability

Test for required detectability: To exactly 1 mL of the standard solution add water to make exactly 10 mL, and designate this the solution for system suitability test. To exactly 1 mL of the solution for system suitability test add water to make exactly 10 mL. Confirm that the peak area of ethanol obtained with 1 μL of this solution is equivalent to 7 to 13% of that with 1 μL of the solution for system suitability test.

System performance: When the procedure is run with 1 μL of the standard solution under the above operating conditions, the number of theoretical plates and the symmetry factor of the peak of ethanol are not less than 1500 and not more than 3.0, respectively.

System repeatability: When the test is repeated 6 times with 1 μL of the standard solution under the above operating conditions, the relative standard deviation of the peak area of ethanol is not more than 2.0%.

Water <2.48>: not more than 0.5% (0.5 g, volumetric titration, direct titration).

Residue on ignition <2.44>: not more than 0.5% (1 g).

Content: not less than 99.0% of cilastatin ammonium ($C_{16}H_{29}N_3O_5S$), calculated on the anhydrous and ethanol-free basis. Assay—Weigh accurately about 0.5 g of cilastatin ammonium for assay, dissolve in 30 mL of methanol, and add 5 mL of water. Adjust to pH 3.0 with 0.1 mol/L hydrochloric acid TS, and titrate <2.50> with 0.1 mol/L sodium hydroxide VS from the first equivalence point to the second equivalence point (potentiometric titration).

$$\text{Each mL of 0.1 mol/L sodium hydroxide VS} = 37.55 \text{ mg of } C_{16}H_{29}N_3O_5S$$

Cilazapril See cilazapril hydrate.

Cilazapril for assay See cilazapril hydrate for assay.

Cilazapril hydrate $C_{22}H_{31}N_3O_5.H_2O$ [Same as the namesake monograph]

Cilazapril hydrate for assay $C_{22}H_{31}N_3O_5.H_2O$ [Same as the monograph Cilazapril Hydrate. It contains not less than 99.0% of cilazapril ($C_{22}H_{31}N_3O_5$), calculated on the anhydrous basis.]

Cinchonidine $C_{19}H_{22}N_2O$ White, crystals or crystalline powder. Soluble in methanol, in ethanol (95) and in chloroform, sparingly soluble in diethyl ether, and practically insoluble in water. A solution of cinchonidine in ethanol (95) (1 in 100) is levorotatory. Melting point: about 207°C.

Content: not less than 98.0%. Assay—Weigh accurately about 0.3 g of cinchonidine, dissolve in 20 mL of acetic acid (100), add 80 mL of acetic anhydride, and titrate <*2.50*> with 0.1 mol/L perchloric acid VS (indicator: 3 drops of crystal violet). Perform a blank determination in the same manner, and make any necessary correction.

Each mL of 0.1 mol/L perchloric acid VS
= 14.72 mg of $C_{19}H_{22}N_2O$

Cinchonine $C_{19}H_{22}N_2O$ White, crystals or powder.

Identification—Dissolve 1 g of cinochonine in 20 mL of diluted hydrochloric acid (1 in 4), and add 2 mL of potassium hexacyanoferrate (II) TS: yellow precipitates appear, which are dissolved by heating, and crystals are formed after allowing to cool.

Purity Cinchonidine and quinine—To 1 g of cinchonine add 30 mL of water, add diluted hydrochloric acid (2 in 3) dropwise until the substance to be tested dissolves, and neutralize with ammonia TS. To this solution add 10 mL of a solution of sodium tartrate dihydrate (1 in 2), boil, and allow to stand for 1 hour: no precipitates appear.

Content: not less than 98.0%. Assay—Weigh accurately about 0.3 g of cinchonine, dissolve in 50 mL of acetic acid (100), and titrate <*2.50*> with 0.1 mol/L perchloric acid VS (potentiometric titration). Perform a blank determination in the same manner, and make any necessary correction.

Each mL of 0.1 mol/L perchloric acid VS
= 14.72 mg of $C_{19}H_{22}N_2O$

Cineol for assay $C_{10}H_{18}O$ Clear and colorless liquid, having a characteristic aroma.

Refractive index <*2.45*> n_D^{20}: 1.457 – 1.459

Specific gravity <*2.56*> d_{20}^{20}: 0.920 – 0.930

Purity Related substances—Dissolve 0.10 g of cineol for assay in 25 mL of hexane and use this solution as the sample solution. Perform the test with 2 μL of the sample solution as directed under Gas Chromatography <*2.02*> according to the following conditions. Determine each peak area by the automatic integration method and calculate the amount of them by the area percentage method: the total amount of the peaks other than cineol is not more than 1.0%.

Operating conditions

Proceed in the operating conditions in the Assay under Eucalyptus Oil except test for time span of measurement.

Time span of measurement: About 3 times as long as the retention time of cineol, beginning after the solvent peak.

System suitability

Test for required detectability: To 1 mL of the sample solution add hexane to make 100 mL. Adjust so that the peak height of cineol obtained with 2 μL of this solution is 40 to 60% of the full scale.

Cinnamaldehyde for thin-layer chromatography See (*E*)-cinnamaldehyde for thin-layer chromatography.

(*E*)-Cinnamaldehyde for thin-layer chromatography C_9H_8O A colorless or light yellow liquid, having a characteristic aromatic odor. Very soluble in methanol and in ethanol (99.5), and practically insoluble in water.

Absorbance <*2.24*> $E_{1\,cm}^{1\%}$ (285 nm): 1679 – 1943 (5 mg, methanol, 2000 mL).

Purity Related substances—Dissolve 10 mg of (*E*)-cinnamaldehyde for thin-layer chromatography in 2 mL of methanol. Perform the test with 1 μL of this solution as directed in the Identification (3) under Kakkonto Extract: no spot other than the principal spot at an *Rf* value of about 0.4 appears.

Cinnamic acid $C_9H_8O_2$ White crystalline powder, having a characteristic odor.

Melting point <*2.60*>: 132 – 135°C

(*E*)-Cinnamic acid for assay $C_9H_8O_2$ Use (*E*)-cinnamic acid for thin-layer chromatography meeting the following additional specifications. Its content is corrected based on the amount (%) of (*E*)-cinnamic acid obtained in the Assay.

Unity of peak—Conduct this procedure without exposure to light, using light-resistant vessels. Dissolve 1 mg of (*E*)-cinnamic acid for assay in 50 mL of the mobile phase, and use this solution as the sample solution. Perform the test with 10 μL of the sample solution as directed under Liquid Chromatography <*2.01*> according to the following conditions, and compare the absorption spectra of at least 3 points including the top of (*E*)-cinnamic acid peak and around the two middle peak heights of before and after the top: no difference in form is observed between their spectra.

Operating conditions

Column, column temperature, mobile phase, and flow rate: Proceed as directed in the operating conditions in the Assay (1) under Ryokeijutsukanto Extract.

Detector: A photodiode array detector (wavelength: 273 nm, spctrum range of measurement: 220 – 400 nm).

System suitability

System performance: Proceed as directed in the system suitability in the Assay (1) under Ryokeijutsukanto Extract.

Assay—Weigh accurately 5 mg of (*E*)-cinnamic acid for assay and 1 mg of 1,4-BTMSB-d_4 for nuclear magnetic resonance spectroscopy using an ultramicrobalance, dissolve both in 1 mL of deuterated chloroform for nuclear magnetic resonance spectroscopy, and use this solution as the sample solution. Transfer the sample solution into an NMR tube 5 mm in outer diameter, measure ^{1}H-NMR as directed under Nuclear Magnetic Resonance Spectroscopy <*2.21*> and Crude Drugs Test <*5.01*> according to the following conditions, using 1,4-BTMSB-d_4 for nuclear magnetic resonance spectroscopy as the reference standard for qNMR. Calculate the resonance intensity *A* (equivalent to 1 hydrogen) of the signal around δ 6.20 ppm assuming the signal of the reference standard for qNMR as δ 0 ppm.

Amount (%) of (*E*)-cinnamic acid ($C_9H_8O_2$)
$= M_S \times I \times P/(M \times N) \times 0.6541$

M: Amount (mg) of (*E*)-cinnamic acid for assay 2 taken

M_S: Amount (mg) of 1,4-BTMSB-d_4 for nuclear magnetic resonance spectroscopy taken

I: Signal resonance intensity *A* based on the signal resonance intensity of 1,4-BTMSB-d_4 for nuclear magnetic resonance spectroscopy as 18.000

N: Number of the hydrogen derived from *A*

P: Purity (%) of 1,4-BTMSB-d_4 for nuclear magnetic resonance spectroscopy

Operating conditions

Apparatus: A nuclear magnetic resonance spectrometer having ^{1}H resonance frequency of not less than 400 MHz.

Target nucleus: ^1H.

Digital resolution: 0.25 Hz or lower.

Measuring spectrum range: 20 ppm or upper, including between −5 ppm and 15 ppm.

Spinning: off.

Pulse angle: 90°.

^{13}C decoupling: on.

Delay time: Repeating pulse waiting time not less than 60 seconds.

Integrating times: 8 or more times.

Dummy scanning: 2 or more times.

Measuring temperature: A constant temperature between 20°C and 30°C.

System suitability

Test for required detectability: When the procedure is run with the sample solution under the above operating conditions, the SN ratio of the signal of around δ 6.20 ppm is not less than 100.

System performance: When the procedure is run with the sample solution under the above operating conditions, the signal of around δ 6.20 ppm is no overlapped with any obvious signal of foreign substance.

System repeatability: When the test is repeated 6 times with the sample solution under the above operating conditions, the relative standard deviation of the ratio of the resonance intensity A to that of the reference standard for qNMR is not more than 1.0%.

(*E*)-Cinnamic acid for thin-layer chromatography $C_9H_8O_2$ White, crystals or crystalline powder, having a characteristic aromatic odor. Freely soluble in methanol and in ethanol (99.5), and practically insoluble in water.

Absorbance <2.24> $E^{1\%}_{1\,cm}$ (273 nm): 1307 – 1547 (5 mg dried with silica gel for 24 hours, methanol, 1000 mL).

Melting point <2.60>: 132 – 136°C

Purity Related substances—Conduct this procedure without exposure to light, using light-resistant vessels. Dissolve 10 mg of (*E*)-cinnamic acid for thin-layer chromatography in 5 mL of methanol, and use this solution as the sample solution. Pipet 1 mL of the sample solution, add methanol to make exactly 100 mL, and use this solution as the standard solution. Proceed the test with 10 μL each of the sample solution and standard solution as directed in the Identification (1) under Ryokeijutsukanto Extract: the spot other than the principal spot at an Rf value of about 0.5 obtained from the sample solution is not more intense than the spot from the standard solution.

(*E*)-Cinnamic acid for component determination See (*E*)-cinnamic acid for assay.

Cinobufagin for assay $C_{26}H_{34}O_6$ A white crystalline powder. It is odorless.

Absorbance <2.24> $E^{1\%}_{1\,cm}$ (295 nm): 125 – 137 (10 mg, methanol, 250 mL). Use the sample dried in a desiccator (silica gel) for 24 hours for the test.

Purity Related substances—Proceed with 40 mg of cinobufagin for assay as directed in the Purity under bufalin for assay.

Content: not less than 98.0%. Assay—Weigh accurately about 10 mg of cinobufagin for assay, previously dried in a desiccator (silica gel) for 24 hours, dissolve in methanol to make exactly 10 mL, and use this solution as the sample solution. Perform the test with 20 μL of the sample solution as directed under Liquid Chromatography <2.01> according to the following conditions. Determine each peak area by the automatic integration method and calculate the amount of cinobufagin by the area percentage method.

Operating conditions

Detector: An ultraviolet absorption photometer (wavelength: 295 nm).

Column: A stainless steel column 4 to 6 mm in inside diameter and 15 to 30 cm in length, packed with octadecylsilanized silica gel for liquid chromatography (5 to 10 μm in particle diameter).

Column temperature: A constant temperature of about 40°C.

Mobile phase: A mixture of water and acetonitrile (1:1).

Flow rate: Adjust so that the retention time of cinobufagin is about 7 minutes.

Time span of measurement: About twice as long as the retention time of cinobufagin, beginning after the solvent peak.

System suitability

Test for required detectability: Pipet 1 mL of the sample solution, add methanol to make exactly 100 mL, and use this solution as the standard solution (1). Pipet 1 mL of the standard solution (1), add methanol to make exactly 20 mL, and use this solution as the standard solution (2). Adjust the detection sensitivity so that the peak area of cinobufagin obtained with 20 μL of the standard solution (2) can be measured by the automatic integration method and the peak height of cinobufagin with 20 μL of the standard solution (1) is about 20% of the full scale.

System performance: Dissolve 10 mg each of cinobufagin for assay, bufalin for assay and resibufogenin for assay in 200 mL of methanol. When the procedure is run with 20 μL of this solution under the above operating conditions, bufalin, cinobufagin and resibufogenin are eluted in this order, and each resolution between these peaks is not less than 1.5, respectively.

Cinobufagin for component determination See cinobufagin for assay.

Cinoxacin for assay $C_{12}H_{10}N_2O_5$ [Same as the monograph Cinoxacin. When dried, it contains not less than 99.0% of cinoxacin ($C_{12}H_{10}N_2O_5$).]

Cisplatin $Cl_2H_6N_2Pt$ [Same as the namesake monograph]

0.05 mol/L Citrate buffer solution (pH 6.6) Dissolve 147 g of trisodium citrate dihydrate in 2000 mL of water, add 3.6 g of citric acid monohydrate to dissolve, and add water to make 10 L. To this solution add 0.1 mol/L sodium citrate TS or 0.1 mol/L citric acid TS to adjust the pH to 6.6.

Citric acid See citric acid monohydrate.

Citric acid-acetic acid TS To 1 g of citric acid monohydrate add 90 mL of acetic anhydride and 10 mL of acetic acid (100), and dissolve under shaking.

Citric acid-acetic anhydride TS To 1 g of citric acid monohydrate add 50 mL of acetic anhydride, and dissolve by heating. Prepare before use.

Citric acid monohydrate $C_6H_8O_7.H_2O$ [K 8283, or same as the monograph Citric Acid Hydrate]

Citric acid-phosphate-acetonitrile TS Dissolve 2.1 g of citric acid monohydrate, 13.4 g of dipotassium hydrogen phosphate and 3.1 g of potassium dihydrogen phosphate in 1000 mL of a mixture of water and acetonitrile (3:1).

0.01 mol/L Citric acid TS Dissolve 2.1 g of citric acid monohydrate in water to make 1000 mL.

0.1 mol/L Citric acid TS Dissolve 21 g of citric acid monohydrate in water to make 1000 mL.

1 mol/L Citric acid TS for buffer solution Dissolve 210.14 g of citric acid monohydrate in water to make 1000 mL.

Clofibrate $C_{12}H_{15}ClO_3$ [Same as the namesake monograph]

Clomipramine hydrochloride for assay $C_{19}H_{23}ClN_2.HCl$ [Same as the monograph Clomipramine Hydrochloride. When dried, it contains not less than 99.0% of clomipramine hydrochloride ($C_{19}H_{23}ClN_2.HCl$).]

Clonazepam for assay $C_{15}H_{10}ClN_3O_3$ [Same as the monograph Clonazepam]

32D Clone3 cells A cloned cell line established by culturing mouse bone marrow origin 32D cell line in the presence of G-CSF.

Cloperastine fendizoate for assay $C_{20}H_{24}ClNO.C_{20}H_{14}O_4$ [Same as the monograph Cloperastine Fendizoate]

Clorazepate dipotassium for assay $C_{16}H_{10}ClKN_2O_3.KOH$ [Same as the monograph Clorazepate Dipotassium. When dried it contains not less than 99.0% of clorazepate dipotassium ($C_{16}H_{10}ClKN_2O_3.KOH$).]

Clotiazepam for assay $C_{16}H_{15}ClN_2OS$ [Same as the monograph Clotiazepam. When dried, it contains not less than 99.0% of clotiazepam ($C_{16}H_{15}ClN_2OS$).]

Clotrimazole $C_{22}H_{17}ClN_2$ [Same as the namesake monograph]

Cloxazolam $C_{17}H_{14}Cl_2N_2O_2$ [Same as the namesake monograph]

Cobalt (II) chloride-ethanol TS Dissolve 0.5 g of cobalt (II) chloride hexahydrate, previously dried at 105°C for 2 hours, in ethanol (99.5) to make 100 mL.

Cobalt (II) chloride hexahydrate $CoCl_2.6H_2O$ [K 8129, Special class]

Cobalt (II) chloride TS Dissolve 2 g of cobalt (II) chloride hexahydrate in 1 mL of hydrochloric acid and water to make 100 mL (0.08 mol/L).

Cobalt (II) nitrate hexahydrate $Co(NO_3)_2.6H_2O$ [K 8552, Special class]

Cobaltous chloride See cobalt (II) chloride hexahydrate.

Cobaltous nitrate See cobalt (II) nitrate hexahydrate.

Codeine phosphate for assay See codeine phosphate hydrate for assay.

Codeine phosphate hydrate for assay $C_{18}H_{21}NO_3.H_3PO_4.½H_2O$ [Same as the monograph Codeine Phosphate Hydrate. It contains not less than 99.0% of codeine phosphate ($C_{18}H_{21}NO_3.H_3PO_4$), calculated on the anhydrous basis.]

Collodion Clear, colorless, viscous liquid, having a diethyl ether-like odor.

pH ⟨*2.54*⟩: 5.0–8.0

Stir 5 g of collodion while warming, add 10 mL of water gradually, and dry at 110°C after evaporating to dryness: mass of the residue is 0.250–0.275 g.

Concentrated chromotropic acid TS See chromotropic acid, concentrated.

Concentrated diazobenzenesulfonic acid TS See diazobenzenesulfonic acid TS, concentrated.

Concentrated potassium iodide TS See potassium idide TS, concentrated.

Congo red $C_{32}H_{22}N_6Na_2O_6S_2$ [K 8352, Special class]

Congo red TS Dissolve 0.5 g of congo red in 100 mL of a mixture of water and ethanol (95) (9:1).

Coomassie brilliant blue G-250 $C_{47}H_{48}N_3NaO_7S_2$ A deep violet powder. A solution in ethanol (99.5) (1 in 100,000) exhibits an absorption maxima at a wavelength of 608 nm.

Coomassie brilliant blue R-250 $C_{45}H_{44}N_3NaO_7S_2$ Deep blue-purple powder. Odorless.

Content: not less than 50%.

Coomassie brilliant blue TS for interferon alfa Dissolve 20 mg of Coomassie brilliant blue G-250 in diluted perchloric acid (43 in 1000) to make 100 mL, and filter. Determine the absorbance of the filtrate at 465 nm as directed under Ultraviolet-visible Spectrophotometry ⟨*2.24*⟩, and add Coomassie brilliant blue G-250 or diluted perchloric acid (43 in 1000) so that the absorbance is 1.3 – 1.5.

Coomassie staining TS Dissolve 125 mg of Coomassie brilliant blue R-250 in 100 mL of a mixture of water, methanol and acetic acid (100) (5:4:1), and filter.

Copper Cu [K 8660, Special class]

Copper (standard reagent) Cu In addition to JIS K 8005 standard reagent for volumetric analysis, certified reference material which can be used for volumetric analysis may be used.

Copper (II) acetate monohydrate $Cu(CH_3COO)_2.H_2O$ Blue-green, crystals or crystalline powder.

Identification—(1) Dissolve 1 g of copper (II) acetate monohydrate in 10 mL of diluted sulfuric acid (1 in 2), and heat: the odor of acetic acid is perceptible.

(2) Dissolve 0.1 g of copper (II) acetate monohydrate in 20 mL of water, and add 3 mL of ammonia solution (28): a dark blue color is developed.

Copper (II) acetate TS, strong Dissolve 13.3 g of copper (II) acetate monohydrate in a mixture of 195 mL of water and 5 mL of acetic acid.

Copper (II) chloride-acetone TS Dissolve 0.3 g of copper (II) chloride dihydrate in acetone to make 10 mL.

Copper (II) chloride dihydrate $CuCl_2.2H_2O$ [K 8145, Special class]

Copper (II) citrate TS Dissolve 25 g of copper (II) sulfate pentahydrate, 50 g of citric acid monohydrate and 144 g of anhydrous sodium carbonate in water to make 1000 mL.

Copper (II) disodium ethylenediamine tetraacetate tetrahydrate $C_{10}H_{12}CuN_2Na_2O_8.4H_2O$ A blue powder.

pH ⟨*2.54*⟩: 7.0 – 9.0

Purity Clarity and color of solution—Add 0.10 g of copper (II) disodium ethylenediamine tetraacetate tetrahydrate to 10 mL of freshly boiled and cooled water: the solution is blue in color and clear.

Content: not less than 98.0%. Assay—Weigh accurately about 0.45 g of copper (II) disodium ethylenediamine tetraacetate tetrahydrate, and add water to make exactly 100 mL. Pipet 10 mL of this solution, adjust the pH of the mixture to about 1.5 by adding 100 mL of water and dilute nitric acid, then add 5 mL of a solution of 1,10-phenanthroline monohydrate in methanol (1 in 20), and titrate <*2.50*> with 0.01 mol/L bismuth nitrate VS until the color of the solution changes from yellow to red (indicator: 2 drops of xylenol orange TS).

Each mL of 0.01 mol/L bismuth nitrate VS
= 4.698 mg of $C_{10}H_{12}CuN_2Na_2O_8.4H_2O$

Copper (II) hydroxide $Cu(OH)_2$ Light blue powder. Practically insoluble in water.

Content: not less than 95.0% as $Cu(OH)_2$. Assay—Weigh accurately about 0.6 g of Copper (II) hydroxide, and dissolve in 3 mL of hydrochloric acid and water to make exactly 500 mL. Pipet 25 mL of this solution, add 75 mL of water, 10 mL of a solution of ammonium chloride (3 in 50), 3 mL of diluted ammonia solution (28) (1 in 10) and 0.05 g of murexide-sodium chloride indicator, and titrate <*2.50*> with 0.01 mol/L disodium dihydrogen ethylenediamine tetraacetate VS until the color of the liquid is changed from yellow-green to red-purple.

Each mL of 0.01 mol/L disodium dihydrogen
ethylenediamine tetraacetate VS
= 0.9756 mg of $Cu(OH)_2$

Copper (II) nitrate trihydrate $Cu(NO_3)_2.3H_2O$ Blue, crystals or crystalline powder. Very soluble in water, and freely soluble in ethanol (99.5).

Identification (1) A solution of copper (II) nitrate trihydrate (1 in 10) responds to Qualitative Tests <*1.09*> (2) for cupric salt.

(2) A solution of copper (II) nitrate trihydrate (1 in 10) responds to Qualitative Tests <*1.09*> (1) for nitrate.

Purity (1) Iron—Weigh accurately 5.0 g of copper (II) nitrate trihydrate, add 10 mL of a mixture of water and nitric acid (2:1), add water to make exactly 100 mL, and use this solution as the sample stock solution. Pipet 20 mL of the sample stock solution, add water to make exactly 100 mL, and use this solution as the sample solution. Separately, pipet 20 mL of the sample stock solution, add exactly 3 mL of Standard Iron Solution add water to make exactly 100 mL, and use this solution as the standard solution. Perform the test with the sample solution and standard solution as directed under Atomic Absorption Spectrophotometry <*2.23*> according to the following conditions, and determine the absorbances, A_T and A_S, of the sample solution and standard solution: A_T is not greater than ($A_S - A_T$) (not more than 0.003%).

Gas: Combustible gas—Acetylene.
Supporting gas—Air.
Lamp: Iron hollow-cathode lamp.
Wavelength: 248.3 nm.

(2) Zinc—Use the sample solution in (1) as the sample solution. Separately, pipet 20 mL of the sample stock solution in (1), add exactly 5 mL of a solution, prepared by adding water to exactly 4 mL of Standard Zinc Solution to make exactly 10 mL, add water to make exactly 100 mL, and use this solution as the standard solution. Perform the test with the sample solution and standard solution as directed under Atomic Absorption Spectrophotometry <*2.23*> according to the following conditions, and determine the absorbances, A_T and A_S, of the sample solution and standard solution: A_T is not greater than ($A_S - A_T$) (not more than 0.005%).

Gas: Combustible gas—Acetylene.
Supporting gas—Air.
Lamp: Zinc hollow-cathode lamp.
Wavelength: 213.9 nm.

(3) Calcium—Use the sample solution in (1) as the sample solution. Separately, pipet 20 mL of the sample stock solution in (1), add exactly 5 mL of a solution, prepared by adding water to exactly 1 mL of Standard Calcium Solution to make exactly 10 mL, add water to make exactly 100 mL, and use this solution as the standard solution. Perform the test with the sample solution and standard solution as directed under Atomic Absorption Spectrophotometry <*2.23*> according to the following conditions, and determine the absorbances, A_T and A_S, of the sample solution and standard solution: A_T is not greater than ($A_S - A_T$) (not more than 0.005%).

Gas: Combustible gas—Acetylene.
Supporting gas—Air or nitrous oxide.
Lamp: Calcium hollow-cathode lamp.
Wavelength: 422.7 nm.

(4) Nickel—Use the sample solution in (1) as the sample solution. Separately, pipet 20 mL of the sample stock solution in (1), add exactly 4 mL of Standard Nickel Solution and water to make exactly 100 mL, and use this solution as the standard solution. Perform the test with the sample solution and standard solution as directed under Atomic Absorption Spectrophotometry <*2.23*> according to the following conditions, and determine the absorbances, A_T and A_S, of the sample solution and standard solution: A_T is not greater than ($A_S - A_T$) (not more than 0.002%).

Gas: Combustible gas—Acetylene.
Supporting gas—Air.
Lamp: Nickel hollow-cathode lamp.
Wavelength: 232.0 nm.

Content—Not less than 77.0% and not more than 80.0% as $Cu(NO_3)_2$. Assay—Weigh accurately about 0.6 g of copper (II) nitrate trihydrate, dissolve in water to make exactly 250 mL. Pipet 25 mL of this solution, add 75 mL of water, 6 mL of ammonium chloride solution (1 in 10), and 1 mL of a mixture of water and ammonia solution (28) (10:1), and titrate <*2.50*> with 0.01 mol/L disodium dihydrogen ethylenediamine tetraacetate VS until the color of the solution is changed from green to red-purple (indicator: 50 mg of murexide-sodium chloride indicator).

Each mL of 0.01 mol/L disodium dihydrogen
ethylenediamine tetraacetate VS
= 1.876 mg of $Cu(NO_3)_2$

Copper (II) sulfate $CuSO_4$ [K 8984, First class]

Copper (II) sulfate pentahydrate $CuSO_4.5H_2O$ [K 8983, Special class]

Copper (II) sulfate-pyridine TS Dissolve 4 g of copper (II) sulfate pentahydrate in 90 mL of water, then add 30 mL of pyridine. Prepare before use.

Copper (II) sulfate TS Dissolve 12.5 g of copper (II) sulfate pentahydrate in water to make 100 mL (0.5 mol/L).

Copper (II) sulfate TS, alkaline Dissolve 150 g of potassium bicarbonate, 101.4 g of potassium carbonate and 6.93 g of copper (II) sulfate pentahydrate in water to make 1000 mL.

Coptisine chloride for thin-layer chromatography $C_{19}H_{14}NO_4Cl$ Orange-red, crystals or crystalline powder. Slightly soluble in methanol, and very slightly soluble in water and in ethanol (99.5). Melting point: about 260°C (with decomposition).

Identification Determine the absorption spectrum of a solution of coptisine chloride for thin-layer chromatography (1 in 100,000) as directed under Ultraviolet-visible Spectrophotometry <*2.24*>: it exhibits maxima between 237 nm and

241 nm, between 264 nm and 268 nm, between 354 nm and 358 nm, and between 452 nm and 462 nm.

Purity Related substances—Dissolve 1 mg of coptisine chloride for thin-layer chromatography in 2 mL of methanol, and use this solution as the sample solution. Pipet 1 mL of the sample solution, add methanol to make exactly 20 mL, and use this solution as the standard solution. Perform the test with these solutions as directed under Thin-layer Chromatography <2.03>. Spot 1 μL each of the sample solution and standard solution on a plate of silica gel for thin-layer chromatography, develop the plate with a mixture of methanol, ammonium acetate solution (3 in 10) and acetic acid (100) (20:1:1) to a distance of about 10 cm, and air-dry the plate. Examine under ultraviolet light (main wavelength: 365 nm): the spot other than the principal spot at an *Rf* value of about 0.4 obtained from the sample solution is not more intense than the spot from the standard solution.

Corn oil [Same as the namesake monograph]

Cortisone acetate $C_{23}H_{30}O_6$ [Same as the namesake monograph]

Cottonseed oil A refined, nonvolatile fatty oil obtained from the seed of plants of *Gossypium hirsutum* Linné (*Gossypium*) or of other similar species. A pale yellow, odorless, oily liquid. Miscible with chloroform, with diethyl ether, and with hexane and with carbon disulfide. Slightly soluble in ethanol (95).

Refractive index <2.45> n_D^{20}: 1.472 – 1.474
Specific gravity <2.56> d_{25}^{25}: 0.915 – 0.921
Acid value <1.13>: not more than 0.5.
Saponification value <1.13>: 190 – 198
Iodine value <1.13>: 103 – 116

Cresol $CH_3C_6H_4(OH)$ [Same as the namesake monograph]

***m*-Cresol** $CH_3C_6H_4(OH)$ [K 8305, Special class]

***p*-Cresol** C_7H_8O [K 8306, Special class]

Cresol red $C_{21}H_{18}O_5S$ [K 8308, Special class]

Cresol red TS Dissolve 0.1 g of cresol red in 100 mL of ethanol (95), and filter if necessary.

Crystalline trypsin To trypsin obtained from bovine pancreas add an appropriate amount of trichloroacetic acid to precipitate the trypsin, and recrystallize in ethanol (95). White to yellow-white, crystals or powder. It is odorless. Freely soluble in water and in sodium tetraborate-calcium chloride buffer solution (pH 8.0).

Content: not less than 45 FIP Units of trypsin per mg. Assay—(i) Sample solution: Weigh accurately an appropriate amount of crystalline trypsin, dissolve in 0.001 mol/L hydrochloric acid TS to prepare a solution containing 50 FIP Units per mL, and use this solution as the sample solution. Prepare before use, and preserve in ice.
(ii) Apparatus: Use a glass bottle as a reaction reservoir, 20 mm in inside diameter and 50 mm in height, stopper with a rubber stopper equipped with a glass/silver-silver chloride electrode for pH determination, a nitrogen-induction tube and an exhaust port. Fix the reaction reservoir in a thermostat, and keep the temperature of the both at 25 ± 0.1°C by means of a precise thermoregulator.
(iii) Procedure: Pipet 1.0 mL of *N*-α-benzoyl-L-arginine ethyl ester TS, transfer to the reaction reservoir, and add 9.0 mL of sodium tetraborate-calcium chloride buffer solution (pH 8.0). Allow to stand in the thermostat for 10 minutes to make the temperature of the contents reach to 25 ± 0.1°C, adjust the pH of the solution to 8.00 by adding dropwise 0.1 mol/L sodium hydroxide VS while stirring and passing a current of nitrogen, add 0.05 mL of the sample solution previously allowed to stand at 25 ± 0.1°C, then immediately add dropwise 0.1 mol/L sodium hydroxide VS by a 50 μL-micropipet (minimum graduation of 1 μL) while stirring, to keep the reaction solution at pH 8.00, and read the amount of 0.1 mol/L sodium hydroxide VS consumed and the reaction time when the pH reached 8.00. Continue this procedure up to 8 minutes. Separately, transfer 10 mL of sodium tetraborate-calcium chloride buffer solution (pH 8.0), and perform a blank determination in the same manner.
(iv) Calculation: Plot the amount of consumption (μL) of 0.1 mol/L sodium hydroxide VS against the reaction time (minutes), select linear reaction times, t_1 and t_2, designate the corresponding consumption amount of 0.1 mol/L sodium hydroxide VS as v_1 and v_2, respectively, and designate μmol of sodium hydroxide consumed per minute as *D* (FIP Unit).

$$D\ (\mu\text{mol NaOH/min}) = \frac{v_2 - v_1}{t_2 - t_1} \times \frac{1}{10}$$

FIP Units per mL of crystalline trypsin

$$= \frac{(D_I - D_0) \times T}{L \times M}$$

D_1: μmol of sodium hydroxide consumed in 1 minute when the sample solution is used
D_0: μmol of sodium hydroxide consumed in 1 minute when the solution for blank determination is used
M: Amount (mg) of crystalline trypsin taken
L: Amount (mL) of the sample solution put in the reaction reservoir
T: Total volume (mL) of the sample solution

One FIP Unit is an amount of enzyme which decomposes 1 μmol of *N*-α-benzoyl-L-arginine ethyl ester per minute under the conditions described in the Assay.

Storage—Preserve in a cold place.

Crystalline trypsin for ulinastatin assay A proteolytic enzyme prepared from bovine pancreas. White to light yellow crystalline powder. Odorless. Sparingly soluble in water, and dissolves in 0.001 mol/L hydrochloric acid TS.

Content: not less than 3200 trypsin Units per mg. Assay—(i) Sample solution: Weigh accurately about 20 mg of crystalline trypsin for ulinastatin assay, and dissolve in 0.001 mol/L hydrochloric acid TS so that each mL of the solution contains about 3000 trypsin Units. Dilute this solution with 0.001 mol/L hydrochloric acid TS so that each mL of the solution contains about 40 trypsin Units, and use this solution as the sample solution.
(ii) Diluent: Dissolve 4.54 g of potassium dihydrogen phosphate in water to make exactly 500 mL (Solution I). Dissolve 4.73 g of anhydrous disodium hydrogen phosphate in water to make exactly 500 mL (Solution II). To 80 mL of Solution II add a suitable amount of Solution I to adjust to pH 7.6.
(iii) Substrate solution: Dissolve 85.7 mg of *N*-α-benzoyl-L-arginine ethyl ester hydrochloride in water to make exactly 100 mL, and use this solution as the substrate stock solution. Pipet 10 mL of the substrate stock solution, add the diluent to make exactly 100 mL, and use this solution as the substrate solution. The absorbance of the substrate solution determined at 253 nm as directed under Ultraviolet-visible Spectrophotometry <2.24> using water as the blank is between 0.575 and 0.585. If the absorbance of the substrate solution is not in this range, adjust with the diluent or the substrate stock solution.
(iv) Procedure: Pipet 3 mL of the substrate solution, previ-

ously warmed at 25 ± 0.1°C, into a 1-cm quartz cell, add exactly 0.2 mL of the sample solution, and start the determination of the absorbance change at 253 nm for 5 minutes at 25 ± 0.1°C using a solution prepared by adding exactly 0.2 mL of 0.001 mol/L hydrochloric acid TS to exactly 3 mL of the substrate solution as the blank. Determine the difference of the absorbance change per minute, A, when the difference has been constant for at least 3 minutes.
(v) Calculation: Trypsin Units per mg is obtained by use of the following equation. One trypsin Unit is an amount of the enzyme which gives 0.003 change in absorbance per minute under the conditions described above.

$$\text{Trypsin Units per mg} = \frac{A}{0.003 \times M}$$

M: Amount (mg) of the substance to be assayed in 0.2 mL of the sample solution

Storage—Preserve in a cold place.

Crystal violet $C_{25}H_{30}ClN_3.9H_2O$ [K 8294, Special class]

Crystal violet TS Dissolve 0.1 g of crystal violet 10 mL of acetic acid (100).

Culture medium for celmoleukin Take a specified amount of RPMI-1640 powdered medium, add water to dissolve, and add *N*-2-hydroxyethylpiperazine-*N′*-2-ethansulfonic acid as a buffering agent to a concentration of 0.025 mol/L. To 1000 mL of this solution add 0.1 g (potency) of streptomycin sulfate, 100,000 units of potassium benzylpenicillin, and 2 g of sodium hydrogen carbonate, adjust the pH to 7.1 to 7.2 with sodium hydroxide TS, and then sterilize by filtration. To this solution add fetal calf serum heated at 56°C for 30 minutes to 20 vol%.

Cu-PAN Prepare by mixing 1 g of 1-(2-pyridylazo)-2-naphthol (free acid) with 11.1 g of copper (II) disodium ethylenediamine tetraacetate tetrahydrate. A grayish orange-yellow, grayish red-brown or light grayish purple powder.

Absorbance—Dissolve 0.50 g of Cu-PAN in diluted 1,4-dioxane (1 in 2) to make exactly 50 mL. Pipet 1 mL of this solution, add methanol to make exactly 100 mL. Read the absorbance of this solution at 470 nm as directed under Ultraviolet-visible Spectrophotometry <2.24>, using water as the blank solution: the absorbance is not less than 0.48.

Purity Clarity and color of solution—Dissolve 0.50 g of Cu-PAN in 50 mL of diluted 1,4-dioxane (1 in 2): the solution is clear and yellow-brown.

Cu-PAN TS Dissolve 1 g of Cu-PAN in 100 mL of diluted 1,4-dioxane (1 in 2).

Cupferron $C_6H_9N_3O_2$ [K 8289, Special class]

Cupferron TS Dissolve 6 g of cupferron in water to make 100 mL. Prepare before use.

Cupric acetate See copper (II) acetate monohydrate.

Cupric acetate TS, strong See copper (II) acetate monohydrate TS, strong.

Cupric carbonate See cupric carbonate monohydrate.

Cupric carbonate monohydrate $CuCO_3.Cu(OH)_2.H_2O$ A blue to blue-green powder. It is insoluble in water, and dissolves foamingly in dilute acid. It dissolves in ammonia TS and shows a deep blue color.

Purity (1) Chloride <1.03>: not more than 0.036%.
(2) Sulfate <1.14>: not more than 0.120%.
(3) Iron—Dissolve 5.0 g of cupric carbonate monohydrate in excess ammonia TS and filter. Wash the residue with ammonia TS, dissolve in dilute hydrochloric acid, add excess ammonia TS and filter. Wash the residue with ammonia TS, and dry to constant mass: the residue is not more than 10 mg.

Cupric chloride See copper (II) chloride dihydrate.

Cupric chloride-acetone TS See copper (II) chloride-acetone TS.

Cupric sulfate See copper (II) sulfate pentahydrate.

Cupric sulfate, anhydrous See copper (II) sulfate (anhydrous).

Cupric sulfate-pyridine TS See copper (II) sulfate-pyridine TS.

Cupric sulfate TS, alkaline See copper (II) sulfate TS, alkaline.

Cupric sulfate TS See copper (II) sulfate TS.

1 mol/L Cupriethylenediamine TS Put 100 g of copper (II) hydroxide in a 1-L thick-walled bottle marked a 500-mL line, and add water to make 500 mL. Connect the bottle with a liquid introducing funnel, a nitrogen introducing glass tube and a gas removing glass tube. Adjust so that the lower end of the nitrogen introducing tube is located at about 1.3 cm above of the bottom of the bottle. Introduce the nitrogen for about 3 hours to replacing the inside gas by adjusting the pressure (about 14 kPa) to get a mild bubbling. Then add gradually 160 mL of ethylenediamine TS through the funnel while introducing the nitrogen and cooling the bottle with the running water, and replace the funnel with a glass rod to close tightly. After introducing the nitrogen for further 10 minutes, replace the gas removing tube with a glass rod to close tightly. Keep the inside pressure with the nitrogen to about 14 kPa. After allowing the bottle to stand for about 16 hours while occasional shaking, filter the content if necessary using a glass-filter under reducing pressure, and reserve under nitrogen atmosphere. The concentration of copper (II) ion of this solution is about 1.3 mol/L. Determine the concentration of ethylenediamine of this solution X (mol/L) and copper (II) ion Y (mol/L) by the following Assays, and adjust to that X is 1.96–2.04, Y is 0.98–1.02 and X/Y is 1.96–2.04 by adding water, copper (II) hydroxide or ethylenediamine TS, then determine X and Y again in the same manner, and use this solution as the test solution.

Assay (1) Ethylenediamine—Pipet 1 mL (V_1) of the solution to be assayed, add 60 mL of water, and titrate <2.50> with 0.1 mol/L hydrochloric acid VS (pH Determination <2.54>; End point is about pH 8.4).

$$X = \frac{N_1 a}{V_1}$$

X: Concentration of ethylenediamine (mol/L)
a: Volume of 0.1 mol/L hydrochloric acid VS consumed for the titration (mL)
N_1: Concentration of 0.1 mol/L hydrochloric acid VS (mol/L)

(2) Copper (II) ion—Pipet 2 mL (V_2) of the solution to be assayed, add 20 mL of water, about 3 g of potassium iodide and 50 mL of 2 mol/L sulfuric acid TS, shake for 5 minutes, and titrate <2.50> the liberated iodine with 0.1 mol/L sodium thiosulfate VS. When the solution turns light yellow at near the end point add 3 mL of starch TS and 10 mL of a solution of ammonium thiocyanate (1 in 5), and then titrate until the blue color disappears.

$$Y = \frac{N_2 b}{V_2}$$

Y: Concentration of copper (II) ion (mol/L)
b: Volume of 0.1 mol/L sodium thiosulfate VS consumed for the titration (mL)
N_2: Concentration of 0.1 mol/L sodium thiosulfate VS (mol/L)

Curcumin $C_{21}H_{20}O_6$ A reddish yellow crystalline powder.

Melting point <*2.60*>: 180 – 183°C

Storage—Preserve in a light-resistant tight container.

Curcumin TS Dissolve 0.125 g of curcumin in acetic acid (100) to make 100 mL. Prepare before use.

Curcumin for assay $C_{21}H_{20}O_6$ Yellow to orange crystalline powder. Slightly soluble in methanol, very slightly soluble in ethanol (99.5), and practically insoluble in water.

Absorbance <*2.24*> $E^{1\%}_{1\,cm}$ (422 nm): 1460 – 1700 [dried in a desiccator (in vacuum, silica gel for 24 hours), 2.5 mg, methanol, 1000 mL.]

Melting point <*2.60*>: 180 – 184°C

Purity Related substances—(1) Dissolve 4 mg of curcumin for assay in 2 mL of methanol, and use this solution as the sample solution. Pipet 1 mL of this solution, add methanol to make exactly 50 mL, and use this solution as the standard solution. Perform the test with these solutions as directed under Thin-layer chromatography <*2.03*>. Spot 5 μL each of the sample solution and standard solution on a plate of silica gel for thin-layer chromatography. Develop the plate with a mixture of dichloromethane and methanol (19:1) to a distance of about 10 cm, and air-dry the plate. Examine under ultraviolet light (main wavelength: 365 nm): the spots other than the principal spot at the *R*f value of about 0.5 obtained from the sample solution are not more intense than the spot from the standard solution.

(2) Dissolve 1.0 mg of curcumin for assay in 5 mL of methanol, and use this solution as the sample solution. Pipet 1 mL of the sample solution, add methanol to make exactly 50 mL, and use this solution as the standard solution. Perform the test with exactly 10 μL each of the sample solution and standard solution as directed under Liquid Chromatography <*2.01*> according to the following conditions. Determine each peak from both solutions by the automatic integration method: the total area of the peaks other than curcumin obtained from the sample solution is not larger than the peak area of curcumin from the standard solution.

Operating conditions

Column, column temperature, mobile phase and flow rate: Proceed as directed in the operating conditions in the Assay under Turmeric.

Detector: A visible absorption photometer (wavelength: 422 nm).

Time span of measurement: About 4 times as long as the retention time of curcumin, beginning after the solvent peak.

System suitability

System performance and system repeatability: Proceed as directed in the system suitability in the Assay under Turmeric.

Test for required detectability: Pipet 1 mL of the standard solution, add methanol to make exactly 20 mL. Confirm that the peak area of curcumin obtained with 10 μL of this solution is equivalent to 3.5 to 6.5% of that with 10 μL of the standard solution.

Curcumin for component determination See curcumin for assay.

Cyanoacetic acid $C_3H_3NO_2$ White to light yellow crystals. Very soluble in water.

Content: not less than 99%. Assay—Weigh accurately about 300 mg of cyanoacetic acid, add 25 mL of water and 25 mL of ethanol (95) to dissolve, and titrate <*2.50*> with 0.1 mol/L sodium hydroxide VS (potentiometric titration). Perform a blank determination in the same manner, and make any necessary correction.

Each mL of 0.1 mol/L sodium hydroxide VS
= 85.06 mg of $C_3H_3NO_2$

Cyanocobalamin $C_{63}H_{88}CoN_{14}O_{14}P$ [Same as the namesake monograph]

Cyanogen bromide TS To 100 mL of ice-cold water add 1 mL of bromine, shake vigorously, and add ice-cold potassium cyanide TS dropwise until the color of bromine just disappears. Prepare this test solution in a draft chamber before use.

On handling this solution, be careful not to inhale its vapors, which are very toxic.

1-Cyanoguanidine $NH_2C(NH)NHCN$ A white crystalline powder. Freely soluble in water.

Melting point <*2.60*>: 209 – 212°C

Loss on drying <*2.41*>: not more than 0.1% (1 g, 105°C, 3 hours).

Nitrogen content <*1.08*>: 66.0 – 67.3% (after drying).

Cyanopropylmethylphenylsilicone for gas chromatography Prepared for gas chromatography.

6% Cyanopropylphenyl-94% dimethyl silicone polymer for gas chromatography Prepared for gas chromatography.

6% Cyanopropyl-6% phenyl-methyl silicone polymer for gas chromatography Prepared for gas chromatography.

7% Cyanopropyl-7% phenyl-methyl silicone polymer for gas chromatography Prepared for gas chromatography.

Cycloartenyl ferulate for thin-layer chromatography $C_{40}H_{58}O_4$ A white to light brown, crystalline powder or powder. Soluble in acetone, slightly soluble in acetonitrile, and practically insoluble in water and in methanol. Melting point: about 155°C.

Identification (1) Determine the absorption spectrum of a solution of cycloartenyl ferulate for thin-layer chromatography in heptane (1 in 50,000) as directed under Ultraviolet-visible Spectrophotometry <*2.24*>: it exhibits maxima between 229 nm and 233 nm, between 289 nm and 293 nm, and between 313 nm and 317 nm.

(2) Determine the infrared absorption spectrum of cycloartenyl ferulate for thin-layer chromatography as directed in the potassium bromide disk method under Infrared Spectrophotometry <*2.25*>: it exhibits absorption at the wave numbers of about 2940 cm^{-1}, 1691 cm^{-1}, 1511 cm^{-1} and 1270 cm^{-1}.

Purity Related substances—Dissolve 2.0 mg of cycloartenyl ferulate for thin-layer chromatography in 2 mL of acetone, and use this solution as the sample solution. Pipet 1 mL of the sample solution, add methanol to make exactly 100 mL, and use this solution as the standard solution. Perform the test with 5 μL each of the sample solution and standard solution as directed in the Identification under Brown Rice: the spot other than the principle spot at an *R*f value of about 0.4, obtained from the sample solution is not more intense than the spot from the standard solution.

Cyclobutanecarboxylic acid $C_5H_8O_2$ A clear and colorless liquid. Congealing point: −7.5°C.

1,1-Cyclobutanedicarboxylic acid $C_6H_8O_4$ White crystals.

Melting point <*2.60*>: 159 – 163°C

Purity Related substances—Dissolve 20 mg of 1,1-cyclobutanedicarboxylic acid in 100 mL of the mobile phase used in the Purity (1) under Carboplatin, and use this solution as the sample solution. Perform the test with 25 μL of the sample solution as directed in the Purity (1) under Carboplatin. Determine each peak area by the automatic integration method, and calculate their amounts by the area percentage method: the total amount of the peaks other than 1,1-cyclobutanedicarboxylic acid is not more than 2%. However, the time span of measurement for this calculation is about 2 times as long as the retention time of 1,1-cyclobutanedicarboxylic acid, beginning after the solvent peak.

Content: not less than 99.0%. Assay—Dissolve about 30 mg of 1,1-cyclobutanedicarboxylic acid, accurately weighed, in 50 mL of water, and titrate <*2.50*> with 0.1 mol/L sodium hydroxide VS (potentiometric titration). Perform the blank determination in the same manner, and make any necessary correction.

Each mL of 0.1 mol/L sodium hydroxide VS
= 7.207 mg of $C_6H_8O_4$

Cyclohexane C_6H_{12} [K 8464, Special class]

Cyclohexylamine $C_6H_{11}NH_2$ A clear and colorless liquid, having a characteristic amine-like odor. Miscible with water, with *N,N*-dimethylformamide and with acetone.

Purity Related substances—Use cyclohexylamine as the sample solution. Separately, pipet 1 mL of cyclohexylamine, add hexane to make exactly 100 mL, and use this solution as the standard solution. Perform the test as directed in Thin-layer Chromatography <*2.03*>. Spot 5 μL each of the sample solution and standard solution on a plate of silica gel for thin-layer chromatography, develop the plate with a mixture of ethyl acetate, methanol, ammonia water (28) and cyclohexane (6:2:1:1) to a distance of about 10 cm, and air-dry the plate. Allow the plate to stand in iodine vapor: the spot other than the principal spot obtained from the sample solution is not more intense than the spot from the standard solution.

Cyclohexylmethanol $C_7H_{14}O$ A liquid having slight camphor odor. Soluble in ethanol (99.5).

Refractive index <*2.45*> n_D^{20}: about 1.464

Bioling point <*2.57*>: about 185°C.

Cyclophosphamide hydrate for assay
$C_7H_{15}Cl_2N_2O_2P.H_2O$ [Same as the monograph Cyclophosphamide Hydrate. It contains not less than 99.0% of cyclophosphamide hydrate ($C_7H_{15}Cl_2N_2O_2P.H_2O$).]

Cyclosporine U $C_{81}H_{109}N_{11}O_{12}$ White powder.

Optical rotation <*2.49*> $[\alpha]_D^{20}$: about −190°C (0.1 g, methonol, 20 mL 100 mm).

L-Cysteic acid $C_3H_7NO_5S$ White powder.

Optical rotation <*2.49*> $[\alpha]_D^{20}$: +7.5 – +9.0° (1.5 g, water, 20 mL, 100 mm).

Melting point <*2.60*>: about 260°C.

L-Cysteine hydrochloride See L-cysteine hydrochloride monohydrate.

L-Cysteine hydrochloride monohydrate
$HSCH_2CH(NH_2)COOH.HCl.H_2O$ [K 8470, Special class]

L-Cystine $HOOCCH(NH_2)CH_2SSCH_2CH(NH_2)COOH$ [K 9048, L(−)-Cystine, Special class]

Cytochrome c An oxidase (molecular weight: 8000 – 13,000) derived from bovine cardiac muscle.

Cytosine $C_4H_5N_3O$ White, crystalline powder or powder.

Absorbance <*2.24*> $E_{1\,cm}^{1\%}$ (276 nm): not less than 800 (after drying, 40 mg, 10,000 mL of 0.1 mol/L hydrochloric acid TS).

Dacuronium bromide for thin-layer chromatography
$C_{33}H_{58}Br_2N_2O_3$ White crystalline powder. Very soluble in water, freely soluble in ethanol (95), and practically insoluble in acetic anhydride. Hygroscopic.

Identification—Determine the infrared absorption spectrum of dacuronium bromide for thin-layer chromatography as directed in the potassium bromide disk method under Infrared Spectrophotometry <*2.25*>: it exhibits absorptions at the wave numbers at about 2940 cm^{-1}, 1737 cm^{-1}, 1630 cm^{-1}, 1373 cm^{-1}, 1233 cm^{-1} and 1031 cm^{-1}.

Purity Related substances—Dissolve 10 mg of dacuronium bromide for thin-layer chromatography in 2 mL of ethanol (95), and use this solution as the sample solution. Pipet 1 mL of the sample solution, add ethanol (95) to make exactly 100 mL, and use this solution as the standard solution. Perform the test with 10 μL each of the sample solution and standard solution as directed in the Purity (2) Related substances under Pancuronium Bromide: the spots other than the principal spot obtained from the sample solution do not show more intense color than the spot from the standard solution.

Water <*2.48*>: not more than 1.0% (1 g, volumetric titration, direct titration).

Content: not less than 98.0%, calculated on the anhydrous basis. Assay—Weigh accurately about 0.2 g of dacuronium bromide for thin-layer chromatography, dissolve in 50 mL of acetic anhydride by warming, and titrate <*2.50*> with 0.1 mol/L perchloric acid VS (potentiometric titration). Perform a blank determination in the same manner, and make any necessary correction.

Each mL of 0.1 mol/L perchloric acid VS
= 34.53 mg of $C_{33}H_{58}Br_2N_2O_3$

***p,p'*-DDD (2,2-Bis(4-chlorophenyl)-1,1-dichloroethane)**
$C_{14}H_{10}Cl_4$

Melting point <*2.60*>: 108 – 110°C

Purity Related substances—Dissolve 10 mg of *p,p'*-DDD in hexane for purity of crude drug to make exactly 100 mL, pipet 1 mL of this solution, add hexane for purity of crude drug to make exactly 100 mL, and use this solution as the sample solution. Pipet 2 mL of the sample solution, add hexane for purity of crude drug to make exactly 100 mL, and use this solution as the standard solution (1). Perform the test with exactly 1 μL each of the sample solution and standard solution (1) as directed under Gas Chromatography <*2.02*> according to the following conditions, and measure each peak area from these solutions by the automatic integration method: the total peak area other than *p,p'*-DDD obtained from the sample solution is not larger than the peak area of *p,p'*-DDD from the standard solution (1).

Operating conditions

Proceed the operating conditions in the Purity 4.3. under Crude Drugs Test <*5.01*> except detection sensitivity and time span of measurement.

Detection sensitivity: Pipet 1 mL of the standard solution (1), add hexane for purity of crude drug to make exactly 20 mL, and use this solution as the standard solution (2). Adjust the detection sensitivity so that the peak area of *p,p′*-DDD obtained with 1 μL of the standard solution (2) can be measured by the automatic integration method, and the peak height of *p,p′*-DDD with 1 μL of the standard solution (1) is about 20% of the full scale.

Time span of measurement: About twice as long as the retention time of *p,p′*-DDD, beginning after the solvent peak.

***p,p′*-DDE (2,2-Bis(4-chlorophenyl)-1,1-dichloroethylene)** $C_{14}H_8Cl_4$
Melting point <2.60>: 88 – 90°C
Purity Related substances—Proceed as directed in the Purity of *p,p′*-DDD using the following standard solution (1).

Standard solution (1): Pipet 1 mL of the sample solution, and add hexane for purity of crude drug to make exactly 100 mL.

***o,p′*-DDT (1,1,1-Trichloro-2-(2-chlorophenyl)-2-(4-chlorophenyl)ethane)** $C_{14}H_9Cl_5$
Melting point <2.60>: 73 – 75°C
Purity Related substances—Proceed as directed in the Purity of *p,p′*-DDD.

***p,p′*-DDT (1,1,1-Trichloro-2,2-bis(4-chlorophenyl) ethane)** $C_{14}H_9Cl_5$
Melting point <2.60>: 108 – 110°C
Purity Related substances—Proceed as directed in the Purity of *p,p′*-DDD using the following standard solution (1).

Standard solution (1): Pipet 1 mL of the sample solution, and add hexane for purity of crude drug to make exactly 100 mL.

Decolorized fuchsin TS Add 1 g of fuchsin in 100 mL of water, heat at about 50°C, then cool with occasional shaking. After standing for 48 hours, mix and filter. To 4 mL of the filtration add 6 mL of hydrochloric acid and water to make 100 mL. Use after standing for at least 1 hour. Prepare before use.

***n*-Decyl trimethylammonium bromide** $C_{13}H_{30}NBr$ White powder. Melting point: about 232°C (with decomposition).

Content: not less than 99%. Assay—Weigh accurately about 0.5 g of *n*-decyl trimethylammonuim bromide, dissolve in 50 mL of water, and titrate <2.50> with 0.1 mol/L silver nitrate VS (indicator: 1 mL of potassium chromate TS). Perform a blank determination in the same manner, and make any necessary correction.

Each mL of 0.1 mol/L silver nitrate VS
= 28.03 mg of $C_{13}H_{30}NBr$

0.005 mol/L *n*-Decyl trimethylammonium bromide TS Dissolve 6.94 g of potassium dihydrogen phosphate, 3.22 g of disodium hydrogen phosphate dodecahydrate and 1.40 g of *n*-decyl trimethylammonium bromide in water to make 1000 mL.

Defibrinated blood of rabbit Transfer 100 mL of blood obtained from rabbit to a flask, put in about 20 glass balls 8 mm in diameter, shake for 5 minutes gently, and filter through gauze. Prepare before use.

Dehydrated ethanol See ethanol (99.5).

Dehydrated ether See diethyl ether, dehydrated.

Dehydrated pyridine See pyridine, dehydrated.

Dehydrocorydaline nitrate for assay $C_{22}H_{24}N_2O_7$ Yellow, crystals or crystalline powder. It is sparingly soluble in methanol, and slightly soluble in water and in ethanol (99.5).
Melting point: about 240°C (with decomposition).

Absorbance <2.24> $E^{1\%}_{1\,cm}$ (333 nm): 577 – 642 (3 mg, water, 500 mL). Use the sample dried in a desiccator (silica gel) for not less than 1 hour for the test.

Purity (1) Related substances 1—Dissolve 5.0 mg of dehydrocorydaline nitrate for assay in 1 mL of a mixture of water and methanol (1:1), and use this solution as the sample solution. Pipet 0.5 mL of the sample solution, add a mixture of water and methanol (1:1) to make exactly 50 mL, and use this solution as the standard solution. Perform the test with these solutions as directed under Thin-layer Chromatography <2.03>. Spot 5 μL each of the sample solution and standard solution on a plate of silica gel for thin-layer chromatography. Develop immediately with a mixture of methanol, a solution of ammonium acetate (3 in 10) and acetic acid (100) (20:1:1) to a distance of about 10 cm, and air-dry the plate. Spray Dragendorff's TS for spraying on the plate, air-dry, and spray sodium nitrite TS: the spots other than the principal spot obtained from the sample solution are not more intense than the spot from the standard solution.

(2) Related substances 2—Dissolve 5.0 mg of dehydrocorydaline nitrate for assay in 10 mL of the mobile phase, and use this solution as the sample solution. Pipet 1 mL of the sample solution, add the mobile phase to make exactly 100 mL, and use this solution as the standard solution. Perform the test with exactly 5 μL each of the sample solution and standard solution as directed under Liquid Chromatography <2.01> according to the following conditions, and determine each peak area from these solutions by the automatic integration method: the total area of peaks other than dehydrocorydaline obtained from the sample solution is not larger than the peak area of dehydrocorydaline from the standard solution.

Operating conditions

Column, column temperature, mobile phase, and flow rate: Proceed as directed in the operating conditions in the Assay under Corydalis Tuber.

Detector: An ultraviolet absorption photometer (wavelength: 230 nm).

Time span of measurement: About 3 times as long as the retention time of dehydrocorydaline, beginning after the peak of nitric acid.

System suitability

System performance and system repeatability: Proceed as directed in the system suitability in the Assay under Corydalis Tuber.

Test for required detectability: To exactly 1 mL of the standard solution add the mobile phase to make exactly 20 mL. Confirm that the peak area of dehydrocorydaline obtained with 5 μL of this solution is equivalent to 3.5 to 6.5% of that with 5 μL of the standard solution.

Dehydrocorydaline nitrate for component determination See dehydrocorydaline nitrate for assay.

Dehydrocorydaline nitrate for thin-layer chromatography $C_{22}H_{24}N_2O_7$ Yellow, crystals or crystalline powder. Sparingly soluble in methanol, and slightly soluble in water and in ethanol (99.5). Melting point: about 240°C (with decomposition).

Purity Related substances—Dissolve 5.0 mg of dehydrocorydaline nitrate for thin-layer chromatography in 1 mL of a mixture of water and methanol (1:1), and use this solution as the sample solution. Pipet 0.5 mL of the sample solution, add a mixture of water and methanol (1:1) to make exactly

50 mL, and use this solution as the standard solution. Perform the test with these solutions as directed under Thin-layer Chromatography <2.03>. Spot 5 μL each of the sample solution and standard solution on a plate of silica gel for thin-layer chromatography. Develop immediately with a mixture of methanol, a solution of ammonium acetate (3 in 10) and acetic acid (100) (20:1:1) to a distance of about 10 cm, and air-dry the plate. Examine under ultraviolet light (main wavelength: 365 nm) and then spray Dragendorff's TS on the plate: the spot other than the principal spot obtained from the sample solution is not more intense than the spot obtained from the standard solution in either case.

Demethoxycurcumin $C_{20}H_{18}O_5$ Yellow to orange, crystalline powder or powder. Sparingly soluble in methanol and in ethanol (99.5), and practically insoluble in water. Melting point: 166 - 170°C.

Identification Determine the absorption spectrum of a solution of demethoxycurcumin in methanol (1 in 400,000) as directed under Ultraviolet-visible Spectrophotometry <2.24>: it exhibits a maximum between 416 nm and 420 nm.

Purity Related substances—(1) Dissolve 4 mg of demethoxycurcumin in 2 mL of methanol, and use this solution as the sample solution. Pipet 1 mL of this solution, add methanol to make exactly 20 mL, and use this solution as the standard solution. Perform the test as directed under Thin-layer Chromatography <2.03>. Spot 5 μL each of the sample solution and standard solution on a plate of silica gel for thin-layer chromatography. Develop the plate with a mixture of dichloromethane and methanol (19:1) to a distance of about 10 cm, and air-dry the plate. Examine under ultraviolet light (main wavelength: 365 nm): the spots other than the principal spot at the *R*f value of about 0.3 obtained from the sample solution are not more intense than the spot from the standard solution.

(2) Dissolve 1.0 mg of demethoxycurcumin in 5 mL of methanol, and use this solution as the sample solution. Pipet 1 mL of the sample solution, add methanol to make exactly 20 mL, and use this solution as the standard solution. Perform the test with exactly 10 μL each of the sample solution and standard solution as directed under Liquid Chromatography <2.01> according to the following conditions. Determine each peak area from both solutions by the automatic integration method: the total area of the peaks other than demethoxycurcumin obtained from the sample solution is not larger than the peak area of demethoxycurcumin from the standard solution.

Operating conditions

Column, column temperature, mobile phase and flow rate: Proceed as directed in the operating conditions in the Assay under Turmeric.

Detector: A visible absorption photometer (wavelength: 422 nm).

Time span of measurement: About 4 times as long as the retention time of demethoxycurcumin, beginning after the solvent peak.

System suitability

System performance and system repeatability: Proceed as directed in the system suitability in the Assay under Turmeric.

Test for required detectability: Pipet 1 mL of the standard solution, and add methanol to make exactly 20 mL. Confirm that the peak area of demethoxycurcumin obtained with 10 μL of this solution is equivalent to 3.5 to 6.5% of that with 10 μL of the standard solution.

***N*-Demethylerythromycin** $C_{36}H_{65}NO_{13}$ White to light yellow-white powder.

***N*-Demethylroxithromycin** $C_{40}H_{74}N_2O_{15}$ White powder.

Identification—Determine the infrared absorption spectrum of a solution of the substance to be tested in chloroform (1 in 20) as directed in the solution method under Infrared Spectrophotometry <2.25> using a 0.1-mm cell made of potassium bromide: it exhibits absorption at the wave numbers of about 3600 cm^{-1}, 3520 cm^{-1}, 3450 cm^{-1}, 3340 cm^{-1}, 1730 cm^{-1} and 1627 cm^{-1}.

Deoxycholic acid for thin-layer chromatography $C_{24}H_{40}O_4$ A white powder. Soluble in methanol and in ethanol (99.5), and practically insoluble in water. Melting point: about 175°C (with decomposition).

Identification—Determine the infrared absorption spectrum of deoxycholic acid for thin-layer chromatography as directed in the potassium bromide disk method under Infrared Spectrophotometry <2.25>: it exhibits absorption at the wave numbers of about 2930 cm^{-1}, 1716 cm^{-1}, 1447 cm^{-1} and 1042 cm^{-1}.

Purity Related substances—Dissolve 20 mg of deoxycholic acid for thin-layer chromatography in 10 mL of methanol, and use this solution as the sample solution. Pipet 1 mL of the sample solution, add methanol to make exactly 100 mL, and use this solution as the standard solution. Perform the test with these solutions as directed under Thin-Layer Chromatography <2.03>. Perform the test with 5 μL each of the sample solution and standard solution as directed in the Identification under Oriental Bezoar: the spots other than the principal spot at an *Rf* value of about 0.5 obtained from the sample solution are not more intense than the spot from the standard solution.

2′-Deoxyuridine for liquid chromatography $C_9H_{12}N_2O_5$ White crystalline powder.

Melting point <2.60>: 162 - 166°C

Purity—Dissolve 3.0 mg of 2′-deoxyuridine for liquid chromatography in diluted methanol (1 in 25) to make 50 mL. Perform the test with 10 μL of this solution as directed under Liquid Chromatography <2.01> according to the operating conditions in the Purity under Idoxuridine Ophthalmic Solution. Determine each peak area by the automatic integration method to the range about twice the retention time of 2′-deoxyuridine, and calculate the amount of 2′-deoxyuridine by the area percentage method: it shows a purity of not less than 98.5%.

Content: not less than 98.5%. Assay—Weigh accurately about 5 mg of 2′-deoxyuridine for liquid chromatography, previously dried in vacuum at 60°C for 3 hours, and dissolve in water to make exactly 250 mL. Pipet 10 mL of this solution, dilute with water to make exactly 20 mL. Perform the test with this solution as directed under Ultraviolet-visible Spectrophotometry <2.24>, and determine absorbance *A* at the maximum wavelength at about 262 nm.

$$\text{Amount (mg) of deoxyuridine } (C_9H_{12}N_2O_5) = \frac{A}{447} \times 5000$$

Dermatan sulfate Dermatan sulfate is mucopolysaccharide purified from the skin and small intestines of pigs by alkaline extraction, followed by digestion with protease and fractionation by alcohol. When cellulose acetate membrane electrophoresis of dermatan sulfate is performed and the membrane is stained in a toluidine blue O solution (1 in 200), a single band appears.

Operation conditions of cellulose acetate membrane electrophoresis—

Cellulose acetate membrane: 6 cm in width and 10 cm in length.

Mobile phase: Dissolve 52.85 g of calcium acetate monohydrate in water to make 1000 mL.

Run time: 3 hours (1.0 mA/cm).

Deuterated acetone for nuclear magnetic resonance spectroscopy CD_3COCD_3 Prepared for nuclear magnetic resonance spectroscopy.

Deuterated dimethylsulfoxide for nuclear magnetic resonance spectroscopy $(CD_3)_2SO$ Prepared for nuclear magnetic resonance spectroscopy.

Deuterated formic acid for nuclear magnetic resonance spectroscopy DCOOD Prepared for nuclear magnetic resonance spectroscopy.

Deuterated hydrochloric acid for nuclear magnetic resonance spectroscopy DCl Prepared for nuclear magnetic resonance spectroscopy.

Deuterated methanol for nuclear magnetic resonance spectroscopy CD_3OD Prepared for nuclear magnetic resonance spectroscopy.

Deuterated NMR solvents Prepared for nuclear magnetic resonance spectroscopy. For example: deuterated dimethylsulfoxide [$(CD_3)_2SO$], deuterated pyridine (C_5D_5N), deuterochloroform ($CDCl_3$), heavy water (D_2O), etc.

Deuterated pyridine for nuclear magnetic resonance spectroscopy C_5D_5N Prepared for nuclear magnetic resonance spectroscopy.

Deuterochloroform for nuclear magnetic resonance spectroscopy $CDCl_3$ Prepared for nuclear magnetic resonance spectroscopy.

Devarda's alloy [K 8653, For Nitrogen analysis]

Diacetyl $CH_3COCOCH_3$ A yellow to yellow-green, clear liquid, having a strong, pungent odor. Miscible with ethanol (95) and with diethyl ether, and freely soluble in water.

Congealing point <2.42>: −2.0 – −5.5°C

Refractive index <2.45> n_D^{20}: 1.390 – 1.398

Specific gravity <2.56> d_{20}^{20}: 0.98 – 1.00

Boiling point <2.57>: 85 – 91°C

Purity Clarity of solution—Dissolve 1.0 g of diacetyl in 10 mL of water: the solution is clear.

Content: not less than 95.0%. Assay—Weigh accurately about 0.4 g of diacetyl, add exactly 75 mL of hydroxylamine TS, and heat on a water bath for 1 hour under a reflux condenser. After cooling, titrate <2.50> the excess hydroxylamine with 0.5 mol/L hydrochloric acid VS until the color of the solution changes from blue to yellow-green through green (indicator: 3 drops of bromophenol blue TS). Perform a blank determination in the same manner, and make any necessary correction.

Each mL of 0.5 mol/L hydrochloric acid VS
= 21.52 mg of $C_4H_6O_2$

Diacetyl TS Dissolve 1 mL of diacetyl in water to make 100 mL, and dilute 5 mL of this solution with water to make 100 mL. Prepare before use.

3,3′-Diaminobenzidine tetrahydrochloride $C_{12}H_{14}N_4.4HCl$ Occurs as white to yellowish brown, needle-shaped crystals, and is soluble in water.

2,3-Diaminonaphthalene $C_{10}H_{10}N_2$ Light yellow-brown, crystals or powder. Slightly soluble in ethanol (95) and in diethyl ether, and practically insoluble in water.

Melting point <2.60>: 193 – 198°C

Sensitivity—Pipet separately 40 mL each of the selenium standard solution and diluted nitric acid (1 in 60) as the blank solution into beakers, and to these solutions add ammonia solution (28) to adjust the pH to between 1.8 and 2.2. Dissolve 0.2 g of hydroxylammonium chloride in each of these solutions under gentle shaking, add 5 mL of 2,3-diaminonaphthalene TS, mix by shaking, and allow to stand for 100 minutes. Transfer these solutions to separators separately, rinse the beakers with 10 mL of water, add these rinsings to the separators, extract each with 5.0 mL of cyclohexane by thorough shaking for 2 minutes, and centrifuge the cyclohexane layers to remove moisture. When the absorbance at 378 nm of cyclohexane extract obtained from selenium standard solution for sensitivity is determined using the solution obtained from the blank solution as the reference solution as directed under Ultraviolet-visible Spectrophotometry <2.24>, it is not less than 0.08.

Selenium standard solution for sensitivity—Weigh accurately 40 mg of selenium, dissolve in 100 mL of diluted nitric acid (1 in 2), by heating on water bath if necessary, and add water to make exactly 1000 mL. Pipet 5 mL of this solution, and add water to make exactly 200 mL. Pipet 2 mL of this solution, and add diluted nitric acid (1 in 60) to make exactly 50 mL. Prepare before use. This solution contains 0.04 μg of selenium (Se) per mL.

2,4-Diaminophenol dihydrochloride $C_6H_8N_2O.2HCl$ Pale yellow-brown to grayish yellow-green crystalline powder. Freely soluble in water, slightly soluble in ethanol (95), and practically insoluble in diethyl ether.

Purity Clarity of solution—Dissolve 1.0 g of 2,4-diaminophenol dihydrochloride in 20 mL of water: the solution is clear or a slight turbidity is produced.

Loss on drying <2.41>: not more than 0.5% (1 g, 105°C, 3 hours).

Residue on ignition <2.44>: not more than 0.5% (1 g).

Content: not less than 98.0%. Assay—Weigh accurately about 0.2 g of 2,4-diaminophenol dihydrochloride, dissolve in 50 mL of water, and titrate <2.50> with 0.1 mol/L silver nitrate VS (potentiometric titration). Perform a blank determination in the same manner, and make any necessary correction.

Each mL of 0.1 mol/L silver nitrate VS
= 9.853 mg of $C_6H_8N_2O.2HCl$

2,4-Diaminophenol dihydrochloride TS Dissolve 1 g of 2,4-diaminophenol dihydrochloride and 20 g of sodium bisulfite in 100 mL of water, and filter, if necessary.

2,4-Diaminophenol hydrochloride See 2,4-diaminophenol dihydrochloride.

2,4-Diaminophenol hydrochloride TS See 2,4-diaminophenol dihydrochloride TS.

Diammonium hydrogen citrate $C_6H_{14}N_2O_7$ [K 8284, Special class]

Diammonium hydrogen phosphate $(NH_4)_2HPO_4$ [K 9016, Special class]

Diazepam for assay $C_{16}H_{13}ClN_2O$ [Same as the monograph, Diazepam. When dried, it contains not less than 99.0% of diazepam ($C_{16}H_{13}ClN_2O$), and meets the additional following requirement.]

Purity Related substance—Dissolve 50 mg of diazepam

for assay in 10 mL of water, add methanol to make 100 mL, and use this solution as the sample solution. Pipet 1 mL of the sample solution, and add methanol to make exactly 100 mL. Pipet 2 mL of this solution, add methanol to make exactly 20 mL, and use this solution as the standard solution. Perform the test with exactly 10 μL each of the sample solution and standard solution as directed under Liquid Chromatography <*2.01*> according to the following conditions, and determine each peak area by the automatic integration method: the area of the peak other than diazepam obtained from the sample solution is not larger than the peak area of diazepam from the standard solution.

Operating conditions

Detector, column, column temperature, mobile phase, and flow rate: Proceed as directed in the operating conditions in the Assay under Diazepam Tablets.

Time span of measurement: About 4.5 times as long as the retention time of diazepam, beginning after the solvent peak.

System suitability

System performance: When the procedure is run with 10 μL of the standard solution under the above operating conditions, the number of theoretical plates and the symmetry factor of the peak of diazepam are not less than 5000 and not more than 1.5, respectively.

System repeatability: When the test is repeated 6 times with 10 μL of the standard solution under the above operating conditions, the relative standard deviation of the peak area of diazepam is not more than 2.0%.

Diazobenzenesulfonic acid TS Weigh 0.9 g of sulfanilic acid, previously dried at 105°C for 3 hours, dissolve it in 10 mL of dilute hydrochloric acid by heating, and add water to make 100 mL. To 3.0 mL of this solution add 2.5 mL of sodium nitrite TS, and allow to stand for 5 minutes while cooling with ice. Then add 5 mL of sodium nitrite TS and water to make 100 mL, and allow to stand in ice water for 15 minutes. Prepare before use.

Diazobenzenesulfonic acid TS, concentrated Weigh 0.2 g of sulfanilic acid, previously dried at 105°C for 3 hours, dissolve it in 20 mL of 1 mol/L hydrochloric acid TS by warming. Cool this solution with ice, and add 2.2 mL of a solution of sodium nitrite (1 in 25) dropwise under stirring. Allow to stand in ice water for 10 minutes, and add 1 mL of a solution of sulfamic acid (1 in 20). Prepare before use.

Diazo TS Weigh accurately 0.9 g of sulfanilic acid, add 0.9 mL of hydrochloric acid and 20 mL of water, and dissolve by heating. After cooling, filter, and dilute the filtrate with water to make exactly 100 mL. Pipet 1.5 mL of this solution, cool in an ice bath, and add exactly 1 mL of sodium nitrite solution (1 in 20) dropwise, while shaking. Cool in an ice bath for 10 minutes, add cold water to make exactly 50 mL. Store in a cold place, and use within 8 hours.

Dibasic ammonium phosphate See diammonium hydrogen phosphate.

Dibasic potassium phosphate See dipotassium hydrogen phosphate.

Dibasic potassium phosphate-citric acid buffer solution (pH 5.3) See dipotassium hydrogen phosphate-citric acid buffer solution (pH 5.3).

1 mol/L Dibasic potassium phosphate TS for buffer solution See 1 mol/L dipotassium hydrogen phosphate TS for buffer solution.

Dibasic sodium ammonium phosphate See ammonium sodium hydrogen phosphate tetrahydrate.

Dibasic sodium phosphate See disodium hydrogen phosphate dodecahydrate.

Dibasic sodium phosphate, anhydrous See disodium hydrogen phosphate.

Dibasic sodium phosphate, anhydrous, for pH determination See disodium hydrogen phosphate for pH determination.

Dibasic sodium phosphate-citric acid buffer solution (pH 4.5) See disodium hydrogen phosphate-citric acid buffer solution (pH 4.5).

Dibasic sodium phosphate-citric acid buffer solution (pH 5.4) See disodium hydrogen phosphate-citric acid buffer solution (pH 5.4).

Dibasic sodium phosphate-citric acid buffer solution (pH 6.0) See disodium hydrogen phosphate-citric acid buffer solution (pH 6.0).

Dibasic sodium phosphate TS See disodium hydrogen phosphate TS.

0.05 mol/L Dibasic sodium phosphate TS See 0.05 mol/L disodium hydrogen phosphate TS.

0.5 mol/L Dibasic sodium phosphate TS See 0.5 mol/L disodium hydrogen phosphate TS.

Dibekacin sulfate $C_{18}H_{37}N_5O_8.xH_2SO_4$ [Same as the namesake monograph]

Dibenz[*a,h*]anthracene $C_{22}H_{14}$ Very pale yellow to green-yellow, crystalline powder or powder. Practically insoluble in water, in methanol and in ethanol (99.5). Melting point: 265 – 270°C.

Identification Perform the test with dibenz[*a,h*]anthracene as directed in the Purity: the mass spectrum of the main peak shows a molecular ion peak (*m/z* 278) and a fragment ion peak (*m/z* 139).

Purity Related substances—Dissolve 3.0 mg of dibenz[*a,h*]anthracene in methanol to make 100 mL, and use this solution as the sample solution. Perform the test with 1 μL of the sample solution as directed under Gas Chromatography <*2.02*> according to the following conditions, and determine each peak area by the automatic integration method. Calculate the amounts of these peaks by the area percentage method: the total amount of the peaks other than dibenz[*a,h*]anthracene is not more than 7.0%.

Operating conditions

Detector: A mass spectrophotometer (EI).

Mass scan range: 15.00 – 300.00.

Time of measurement: 12 – 30 minutes.

Column: A fused silica column 0.25 mm in inside diameter and 30 m in length, coated inside with 5% diphenyl-95% dimethylpolysiloxane for gas chromatography in thickness of 0.25 – 0.5 μm.

Column temperature: Inject at a constant temperature of about 45°C, raise the temperature to 240°C at a rate of 40°C per minute, maintain at 240°C for 5 minutes, raise to 300°C at a rate of 4°C per minute, raise to 320°C at a rate of 10°C per minute, and maintain at 320°C for 3 minutes.

Injection port temperature: A constant temperature of about 250°C.

Interface temperature: A constant temperature of about 300°C.

Carrier gas: Helium.

Flow rate: Adjust so that the reaction time of the peak of dibenz[*a,h*]anthracene is about 27 minutes.

Splitless.

System suitability

Test for required detectability: Pipet 1 mL of the sample solution, and add methanol to make exactly 10 mL. Confirm that the peak area of dibenz[*a,h*]anthracene obtained with 1 μL of this solution is equivalent to 5 to 15% of that with 1 μL of the standard solution.

Dibenzyl $C_{14}H_{14}$ White crystals, freely soluble in diethyl ether, soluble in methanol and in ethanol (95), and practically insoluble in water.

Melting point <*2.60*> 50 – 54°C

Purity Related substances—Dissolve 32 mg of dibenzyl in methanol to make exactly 50 mL, and use this solution as the sample solution. Perform the test with 20 μL of the sample solution as directed under Liquid Chromatography <*2.01*> according to the operating conditions in the Assay under Vinblastine Sulfate for Injection: any peak other than dibenzyl does not appear. Adjust the detection sensitivity so that the peak height of dibenzyl obtained from 20 μL of the solution prepared by adding methanol to 10 mL of the sample solution to make 20 mL, is 3 to 5 cm, and the time span of measurement is about 1.2 times as long as the retention time of dibenzyl after the solvent peak.

***N,N'*-Dibenzylethylenediamine diacetate** $C_{16}H_{20}N_2.2C_2H_4O_2$ A white to slightly pale yellow crystalline powder.

Identification—Determine the infrared absorption spectrum of the substance to be examined as directed in the potassium bromide disk method under Infrared Spectrophotometry <*2.25*>: it exhibits absorption at the wave numbers of about 1530 cm^{-1}, 1490 cm^{-1}, 1460 cm^{-1}, 1400 cm^{-1} and 1290 cm^{-1}.

Content: not less than 99.0%. Assay—Weigh accurately about 25 mg of *N,N'*-dibenzylethylenediamine diacetate, dissolve in 25 mL of methanol, and add a solution containing 1.02 g of disodium hydrogen phosphate, anhydrous and 6.80 g of potassium dihydrogen phosphate in 1000 mL of water to make exactly 50 mL. Pipet 5 mL of this solution, add a mixture of the solution containing 1.02 g of anhydrous disodium hydrogen phosphate and 6.80 g of potassium dihydrogen phosphate in 1000 mL of water and methanol (1:1) to make exactly 20 mL, and use this solution as the sample solution. Separately, weigh accurately about 8 mg of acetic acid (100), add 25 mL of methanol, and add the solution containing 1.02 g of anhydrous disodium hydrogen phosphate and 6.80 g of potassium dihydrogen phosphate in 1000 mL of water to make exactly 50 mL. Pipet 5 mL of this solution, add a mixture of the solution containing 1.02 g of disodium hydrogen phosphate, anhydrous and 6.80 g of potassium dihydrogen phosphate in 1000 mL of water and methanol (1:1) to make exactly 20 mL, and use this solution as the control solution. Perform the test with exactly 20 μL each of the sample solution and control solution as directed under Liquid Chromatography <*2.01*> according to the following conditions, and determine each peak area by the automatic integration method. After making correction for the peak areas based on the valiance of the base-line and the peak of acetic acid on the chromatogram obtained with the sample solution, calculate the amount of *N,N'*-dibenzylethylenediamine by the area percentage method.

Operating conditions

Detector: An ultraviolet absorption photometer (wavelength: 220 nm).

Column: A stainless steel column 4.6 mm in inside diameter and 25 cm in length, packed with octadecylsilanized silica gel for liquid chromatography (5 μm in particle diameter).

Column temperature: A constant temperature of about 40°C.

Mobile phase: A mixture of water, methanol and 0.25 mol/L potassium dihydrogen phosphate TS (pH 3.5) (11:7:2).

Flow rate: Adjust so that the retention time of *N,N'*-dibenzylethylenediamine is about 4 minutes.

Time span of measurement: About 5 times as long as the retention time of *N,N'*-dibenzylethylenediamine.

System suitability

System performance: Dissolve an amount of benzylpenicillin benzathine, equivalent to about 85,000 Units, in 25 mL of methanol, add a solution containing 1.02 g of anhydrous disodium hydrogen phosphate and 6.80 g of potassium dihydrogen phosphate in 1000 mL of water to make exactly 50 mL. Pipet 5 mL of this solution, add a mixture of the solution containing 1.02 g of anhydrous disodium hydrogen phosphate and 6.80 g of potassium dihydrogen phosphate in 1000 mL of water and methanol (1:1) to make exactly 20 mL. When the procedure is run with 20 μL of this solution under the above operating conditions, *N,N'*-dibenzylethylenediamine and benzylpenicillin are eluted in this order with the resolution between these peaks being not less than 20.

System repeatability: When the test is repeated 6 times with 20 μL of the standard solution under the above operating conditions, the relative standard deviation of the peak area of *N,N'*-dibenzylethylenediamine is not more than 2.0%.

2,6-Dibromo-*N*-chloro-1,4-benzoquinone monoimine $C_6H_2Br_2ClNO$ [K 8491, Special class]

2,6-Dibromo-*N*-chloro-1,4-benzoquinone monoimine TS Dissolve 0.5 g of 2,6-dibromo-*N*-chloro-1,4-benzoquinone monoimine in methanol to make 100 mL.

2,6-Dibromo-*N*-chloro-1,4-benzoquinone monoimine TS, dilute Dissolve 0.2 g of 2,6-dibromo-*N*-chloro-1,4-benzoquinone monoimine in methanol to make 100 mL.

2,6-Dibromoquinone chlorimide See 2,6-dibromo-*N*-chloro-1, 4-benzoquinone monoimine.

2,6-Dibromoquinone chlorimide TS See 2,6-dibromo-*N*-chloro-1, 4-benzoquinone monoimine TS.

Dibucaine hydrochloride $C_{20}H_{29}N_3O_2.HCl$ [Same as the namesake monograph]

Dibutylamine $C_8H_{19}N$ Colorless, clear liquid.

Refractive index <*2.45*> n_D^{20} 1.415 – 1.419

Density <*2.56*> (20°C): 0.756 – 0.761 g/mL

Di-*n*-butyl ether $(C_4H_9)_2O$ Clear, colorless, water-nonmiscible liquid.

Specific gravity <*2.56*> d_4^{20}: 0.768 – 0.771

Di-*n*-butyl phthalate $C_6H_4(COOC_4H_9)_2$ Clear, colorless liquid.

Purity Related substances—Dissolve 0.5 g of di-*n*-butyl phthalate in 50 mL of methanol, and use this solution as the sample solution. Perform the test with 10 μL of the sample solution as directed in the Assay under Nicardipine Hydrochloride Injection, and determine the peak area by the automatic integration method. Calculate the amount of di-*n*-butyl phthalate by the area percentage method: the amount of di-*n*-butyl phthalate is not less than 98.0%, and no peak appears at the same position as nicardipine. Adjust the detection sensitivity so that the peak height of di-*n*-butyl phthalate obtained from 10 μL of the sample solution is 50 to 100% of the full scale, and measure about 2 times as long as the retention time of di-*n*-butyl phthalate, beginning after the solvent peak.

3,4-Dichloroaniline $C_6H_5Cl_2N$ A white to brown solid.
Melting point ⟨*2.60*⟩: 69 – 75°C

1,2-Dichlorobenzene $C_6H_4Cl_2$ A colorless liquid.
Specific gravity ⟨*2.56*⟩ d_4^{20}: 1.306
Boiling point ⟨*2.57*⟩: 180 – 181°C

1,2-Dichloroethane $ClCH_2CH_2Cl$ [K 8465, Special class]

Dichlorofluorescein $C_{20}H_{10}Cl_2O_5$ Orange to red-brown powder.
Identification (1) Dissolve 0.1 g in 10 mL of sodium hydroxide TS: the solution is an orange-red color, and red-orange precipitates appear by the addition of 10 mL of dilute hydrochloric acid.
(2) Dissolve 0.1 g in 10 mL of sodium hydroxide TS, and add 40 mL of water: a green-yellow fluorescence is exhibited.

Dichlorofluorescein TS Dissolve 0.1 g of dichlorofluorescein in 60 mL of ethanol (95), add 2.5 mL of 0.1 mol/L sodium hydroxide VS, and dilute with water to make 100 mL.

2,6-Dichloroindophenol sodium dihydrate $C_{12}H_6Cl_2NNaO_2.2H_2O$ [K 8469, Special class]

2,6-Dichloroindophenol sodium TS Add 0.1 g of 2,6-dichloroindophenol sodium dihydrate to 100 mL of water, warm, and filter. Use within 3 days.

2,6-Dichloroindophenol sodium TS for titration See the monograph Ascorbic Acid Powder.

2,6-Dichloroindophenol sodium-sodium acetate TS Mix equal volumes of 2,6-dichloroindophenol sodium dihydrate solution (1 in 20) and acetic acid-sodium acetate TS (pH 7.0). Prepare before use.

Dichloromethane CH_2Cl_2 [K 8161, Special class]

2,6-Dichlorophenol $C_6H_4Cl_2O$ White to purplish white crystals.
Melting point ⟨*2.60*⟩: 65 – 67°C

2,6-Dichlorophenol-indophenol sodium See 2,6-dichloroindophenol sodium dihydrate.

2,6-Dichlorophenol-indophenol sodium TS See 2,6-dichloroindophenol sodium TS.

2,6-Dichlorophenol-indophenol sodium TS for titration See 2,6-dichloroindophenol sodium TS for titration.

Diclofenac sodium $C_{14}H_{10}Cl_2NNaO_2$ [Same as the namesake monograph]

Diclofenac sodium for assay $C_{14}H_{10}Cl_2NNaO_2$ [Same as the monograph Diclofenac Sodium. When dried, it contains not less than 99.0% of diclofenac sodium ($C_{14}H_{10}Cl_2NNaO_2$).]

Dicyclohexyl $C_{12}H_{22}$
Specific gravity ⟨*2.56*⟩ d_{20}^{20}: about 0.864
Boiling point ⟨*2.57*⟩: about 227°C
Melting point ⟨*2.60*⟩: about 4°C

***N,N′*-Dicyclohexylcarbodiimide** $C_{13}H_{22}N_2$ Colorless or white, crystals or crystalline mass. Dissolves in ethanol (95), but decomposes in water to produce a white precipitate.
Melting point ⟨*2.60*⟩: 35 – 36°C

***N,N′*-Dicyclohexylcarbodiimide-dehydrated ethanol TS** See *N,N′*-dicyclohexylcarbodiimide-ethanol TS.

***N,N′*-Dicyclohexylcarbodiimide-ethanol TS** Dissolve 6 g of *N,N′*-dicyclohexylcarbodiimide in ethanol (99.5) to make 100 mL.
Storage—Preserve in tight containers, in a cold place.

Dicyclohexyl phthalate $C_6H_4(COOC_6H_{11})_2$ A white, crystalline powder.
Melting point ⟨*2.60*⟩: 63 – 66°C
Purity Clarity and color of solution—Dissolve 1.0 g of dicyclohexyl phthalate in 20 mL of ethanol (95): the solution is clear and colorless.

Dicyclohexylurea $C_6H_{11}NHCONHC_6H_{11}$ A white crystalline powder, having no odor.
Purity Related substances—Dissolve 50 mg of dicyclohexylurea in methanol to make 100 mL. Pipet 10 mL of this solution, and add methanol to make 100 mL. Pipet 20 mL of this solution, add 10 mL of 0.5 mol/L sodium hydroxide TS, shake, then add 5 mL of diluted hydrochloric acid (1 in 10), shake, and use this solution as the sample solution. Perform the test with 50 μL of the sample solution as directed under Liquid Chromatography ⟨*2.01*⟩ according to the following conditions, determine the area of each peak by the automatic integration method, and calculate the amount by the area percentage method: the total amount of the peaks other than dicyclohexylurea is not more than 3.0%.
Operating conditions
Detector, column, column temperature, mobile phase, and flow rate: Proceed as directed in the operating conditions in the Purity (4) (ii) under Acetohexamide.
Time span of measurement: About 5 times as long as the retention time of dicyclohexylurea, beginning after the solvent peak.
System suitability
System performance, and system repeatability: Proceed as directed in the system suitability in the Purity (4) (ii) under Acetohexamide.
Test for required detectability: To exactly 5 mL of the standard solution add water to make exactly 200 mL. Confirm that the peak area of dicyclohexylurea obtained with 50 μL of this solution is equivalent to 1.8 to 3.3% of that with 50 μL of the standard solution.

Diethanolamine $C_4H_{11}NO_2$ Colorless viscous liquid.
Melting point ⟨*2.60*⟩: 27 – 30°C
Water ⟨*2.48*⟩: less than 0.1%.

Diethanolamine hydrochloride See 2,2′-iminodiethanol hydrochloride.

Diethylamine $(C_2H_5)_2NH$ A clear, colorless liquid, having an amine-like odor. Miscible with water and with ethanol (95). The solution in water is alkaline, and readily absorbs carbon dioxide in air.
Specific gravity ⟨*2.56*⟩ d_4^{10}: 0.702 – 0.708
Distilling range ⟨*2.57*⟩: 54 – 58°C; not less than 96 vol%.
Content: not less than 99.0%. Assay—Weigh accurately about 1.5 g of diethylamine in a flask containing exactly 30 mL of 0.5 mol/L sulfuric acid VS, and titrate ⟨*2.50*⟩ the excess of sulfuric acid with 1 mol/L sodium hydroxide VS (indicator: 2 drops of methyl red TS). Perform a blank determination in the same manner.

Each mL of 0.5 mol/L sulfuric acid VS
= 73.14 mg of $(C_2H_5)_2NH$

Diethylene glycol $HO(CH_2CH_2O)_2H$ Colorless and odorless liquid. Miscible with water and with ethanol (95).

Specific gravity <2.56> d_{20}^{20}: 1.118 – 1.120

Diethylene glycol adipate for gas chromatography Prepared for gas chromatography.

Diethylene glycol dimethyl ether $(CH_3OCH_2CH_2)_2O$ Clear and colorless liquid, miscible with water.

Specific gravity <2.56> d_4^{20}: 0.940 – 0.950

Distilling range <2.57>: 158 – 160°C, not less than 95 vol%.

Diethylene glycol monoethyl ether [2-(2-ethoxyethoxy) ethanol] $C_2H_5(OCH_2CH_2)_2OH$ Clear, colorless liquid, of which boiling point is about 203°C. Miscible with water.

Refractive index <2.45> n_D^{20}: 1.425 – 1.429

Specific gravity <2.56> d_{20}^{20}: 0.990 – 0.995

Acid (as CH_3COOH*)*: less than 0.01%.

Diethylene glycol monoethyl ether for water determination To 1000 mL of diethylene glycol monoethyl ether add 30 g of synthetic zeolite for drying, stopper tightly, allow to stand for about 8 hours with occasional gentle shaking, then allow to stand for about 16 hours, and collect the clear layer of diethylene glycol monoethyl ether. Preserve this protecting it from moisture. The water content of this diethylene glycol monoethyl ether should not be more than 0.3 mg per mL.

Diethylene glycol succinate ester for gas chromatography Prepared for gas chromatography.

Diethylene glycol succinate polyester for gas chromatography Prepared for gas chromatography.

Diethyl ether $C_2H_5OC_2H_5$ [K 8103, Special class]

Diethyl ether, dehydrated $C_2H_5OC_2H_5$ [K 8103, Special class. The water content is not more than 0.01%.]

Diethyl ether for purity of crude drug $C_2H_5OC_2H_5$ [K 8103, Special class] Use diethyl ether meeting the following additional specification. Evaporate 300.0 mL of diethyl ether for purity of crude drug in vacuum at a temperature not higher than 40°C, add the diethyl ether to make exactly 1 mL, and use this solution as the sample solution. Separately, dissolve 2.0 mg of γ-BHC in hexane for purity of crude drug to make exactly 100 mL. Pipet 1 mL of this solution, and add hexane for purity of crude drug to make exactly 100 mL. Pipet 2 mL of this solution, add hexane for purity of crude drug to make exactly 100 mL, and use this solution as the standard solution (1). Perform the test with exactly 1 μL each of the sample solution and standard solution (1) as directed under Gas Chromatography <2.02> according to the following conditions, and determine each peak area by the automatic integration method: the total area of peaks other than the solvent peak obtained from the sample solution is not larger than the peak area of γ-BHC from the standard solution (1).

Operating conditions

Proceed the operating conditions in the 4. Purity 4.3. under the Crude Drugs Test <5.01> except time span of measurement.

Time span of measurement: About three times as long as the retention time of γ-BHC, beginning after the peak of solvent.

Test for required detectability: Pipet 1 mL of the standard solution (1), add hexane for purity of crude drug to make exactly 20 mL, and use this solution as the standard solution (2). Adjust the detection sensitivity so that the peak area of γ-BHC obtained from 1 μL of the standard solution (2) can be measured by the automatic integration method, and the peak height of γ-BHC from 1 μL of the standard solution (1) is about 20% of the full scale.

***N,N*-Diethyl-*N'*-1-naphthylethylenediamine oxalate** $C_{18}H_{24}N_2O_4$ A white crystalline powder.

Identification—Determine the infrared absorption spectrum as directed in the potassium bromide disk method under Infrared Spectrophotometry <2.25>: it exhibits absorption at the wave numbers of about 3340 cm^{-1}, 2940 cm^{-1}, 1581 cm^{-1}, 1536 cm^{-1}, 1412 cm^{-1}, 789 cm^{-1}, 774 cm^{-1} and 721 cm^{-1}.

Purity Clarity of solution—To 0.1 g of *N,N*-diethyl-*N'*-1-naphthylethylenediamine oxalate add 20 mL of water, and dissolve by warming: the solution is clear.

***N,N*-Diethyl-*N'*-1-naphthylethylenediamine oxalate-acetone TS** Dissolve 1 g of *N,N*-diethyl-*N'*-1-naphthylethylenediamine oxalate in 100 mL of a mixture of acetone and water (1:1). Prepare before use.

***N,N*-Diethyl-*N'*-1-naphthylethylenediamine oxalate TS** Dissolve 1 g of *N,N*-diethyl-*N'*-1-naphthylethylenediamine oxalate in water to make 1000 mL.

Diethyl phthalate $C_6H_4(COOC_2H_5)_2$ A colorless, clear liquid.

Refractive index <2.45> n_D^{20}: 1.500 – 1.505

Diethyl terephthalate $C_6H_4(COOC_2H_5)_2$ White to pale brownish white, crystalline or mass.

Melting point <2.60>: 44 – 46°C

Content: not less than 99%. Assay—Dissolve 0.1 g of diethyl terephthalate in 10 mL of methanol. Perform the test with 2 μL of this solution as directed under Gas Chromatography <2.02> according to the following conditions, and determine the area of each peak by the automatic integration method.

$$\text{Content (\%)} = \frac{\text{peak area of diethyl terephthalate}}{\text{total of all peak areas}} \times 100$$

Operating conditions

Detector: A hydrogen flame-ionization detector.

Column: A glass tube 4 mm in inside diameter and 2 m in length, packed with siliceous earth for gas chromatography, 177- to 250- μm in particle diameter, coated with methylsilicone polymer for gas chromatography at the ratio of 10%.

Column temperature: A constant temperature of about 200°C.

Carrier gas: Helium.

Flow rate: Adjust so that the retention time of diethyl terephthalate is between 6 and 7 minutes.

Time span of measurement: About 5 times as long as the retention time of diethyl terephthalate, beginning after the solvent peak.

Difenidol hydrochloride $C_{21}H_{27}NO.HCl$ [Same as the namesake monograph]

4,4'-Difluorobenzophenone $C_{13}H_8F_2O$ A white crystalline powder.

Melting point <2.60>: 106 – 109°C

Digitonin $C_{56}H_{92}O_{29}$ White to whitish, crystals or crystalline powder.

Optical rotation <2.49> $[\alpha]_D^{20}$: −47 – −50° (2 g dried at 105°C for 2 hours, diluted acetic acid (100) (3 in 4), 50 mL, 100 mm).

Sensitivity—Dissolve 0.5 g of digitonin in 20 mL of ethanol (95) by warming, and add ethanol (95) to make 50 mL. To 0.5 mL of this solution add 10 mL of a solution of cholesterol in ethanol (95) (1 in 5000), cool to 10°C, and allow to stand for 30 minutes while vigorous shaking occasionally: A precipitate is produced.

Digoxin $C_{41}H_{64}O_{14}$ [Same as the namesake monograph]

Dihydrocodeine phosphate for assay $C_{18}H_{23}NO_3.H_3PO_4$ [Same as the monograph Dihydrocodeine Phosphate. It contains not less than 99.0% of dihydrocodeine phosphate ($C_{18}H_{23}NO_3.H_3PO_4$), calculated on the dried basis.]

Dihydroergocristine mesilate for thin-layer chromatography $C_{35}H_{41}N_5O_5.CH_4O_3S$ A pale yellowish white powder. Freely soluble in methanol, in ethanol (95) and in chloroform, sparingly soluble in water. Melting point: about 190°C (with decomposition).

Purity Related substances—Dissolve 6 mg of dihydroergocristine mesilate for thin-layer chromatography in exact 100 mL of a mixture of chloroform and methanol (9:1), and perform the test with 5 µL of this solution as directed in the Purity (3) under Dihydroergotoxine Mesilate: any spot other than the principal spot at the *R*f value around 0.4 does not appear.

1-[(2*R*,5*S*)-2,5-Dihydro-5-(hydroxymethyl)-2-furyl] thymine for thin-layer chromatography $C_{10}H_{12}N_2O_4$ Occurs as a white powder.

Purity—Dissolve 0.1 g of 1-[(2*R*,5*S*)-2,5-dihydro-5-(hydroxymethyl)-2-furyl]thymine for thin-layer chromatography in 100 mL of methanol and perform the test as directed in the Purity **(2)** under Zidovudine: spots other than the principal spot with an *R*f value of about 0.23 are not observed.

3,4-Dihydro-6-hydroxy-2(1*H*)-quinolinone $C_9H_9NO_2$ A white to light brown, powder or granule. Melting point: about 240°C (with decomposition).

Identification—Determine the infrared absorption spectrum as directed in the potassium bromide disk method under Infrared Spectrophotometry <*2.25*>: it exhibits absorption at the wave numbers of about 3210 cm^{-1}, 1649 cm^{-1}, 1502 cm^{-1}, 1252 cm^{-1} and 816 cm^{-1}.

2,4-Dihydroxybenzoic acid $C_7H_6O_4$ White to pale brown powder.

Purity Clarity of solution—Dissolve 1.0 g of 2,4-dihydroxybenzoic acid in 20 mL of ethanol (95): the solution is clear.

Content: not less than 95%. Assay—Weigh accurately about 1 g of 2,4-dihydroxybenzoic acid, dissolve in 50 mL of ethanol (95) and 50 mL of water, and titrate <*2.50*> with 0.1 mol/L sodium hydroxide VS.

Each mL of 0.1 mol/L sodium hydroxide VS
= 15.41 mg of $C_7H_6O_4$

1,3-Dihydroxynaphthalene $C_{10}H_6(OH)_2$ Crystals or purple-brown powder. Freely soluble in water and in ethanol (95).

Melting point <*2.60*>: about 125°C

2,7-Dihydroxynaphthalene $C_{10}H_6(OH)_2$

Purity: not less than 97.0%.

2,7-Dihydroxynaphthalene TS Dissolve 0.10 g of 2,7-dihydroxynaphthalene in 1000 mL of sulfuric acid, and allow to stand until the yellow color initially developed disappears. If the solution is blackened notably, prepare freshly.

Diisopropylamine $[(CH_3)_2CH]_2NH$ Colorless, clear liquid, having an amine-like odor. Miscible with water and with ethanol (95). The solution in water is alkaline.

Refractive index <*2.45*> n_D^{20}: 1.391 - 1.394

Specific gravity <*2.56*> d_{20}^{20}: 0.715 - 0.722

Diisopropyl 1,3-dithiolan-2-ylidenemalonate $C_{12}H_{18}O_4S_2$ White crystals.

Identification—Determine the absorption spectrum of a solution of diisopropyl 1,3-dithiolan-2-ylidenemalonate in methanol (1 in 125,000) as directed under Ultraviolet-visible Spectrophotometry <*2.24*>: it exhibits a maximum between 304 nm and 308 nm.

Melting point <*2.60*>: 54 - 57°C

Diltiazem hydrochloride $C_{22}H_{26}N_2O_4S.HCl$ [Same as the namesake monograph]

Diltiazem hydrochloride for assay $C_{22}H_{26}N_2O_4S.HCl$ [Same as the monograph Diltiazem Hydrochloride. However, when dried, it contains not less than 99.0% of diltiazem hydrochloride ($C_{22}H_{26}N_2O_4S.HCl$).]

Dilute acetic acid See acetic acid, dilute.

Dilute ammonium iron (III) sulfate TS See ammonium iron (III) sulfate TS, dilute.

Dilute bismuth subnitrate-potassium iodide TS for spraying Dissolve 10 g of L-tartaric acid in 50 mL of water, and add 5 mL of bismuth subnitrate TS.

Dilute bromophenol blue TS See bromophenol blue TS, dilute.

Dilute 2,6-Dibromo-*N*-chloro-1,4-benzoquinone monoamine TS See 2,6-dibromo-*N*-chloro-1,4-benzoquinone monoamine TS, dilute.

Dilute *p*-dimethylaminobenzaldehyde-ferric chloride TS See 4-dimethylaminobenzaldehyde-iron (III) chloride TS, dilute.

Dilute 4-dimethylaminobenzaldehyde-iron (III) chloride TS See 4-dimethylaminobenzaldehyde-iron (III) chloride TS, dilute.

Diluted ethanol See ethanol, diluted.

Dilute ethanol See ethanol, dilute.

Dilute ferric ammonium sulfate TS See ammonium iron (III) sulfate TS, dilute.

Dilute ferric chloride TS See iron (III) chloride TS, dilute.

Dilute Folin's TS See folin's TS, dilute.

Dilute formaldehyde TS See formaldehyde TS, dilute.

Dilute Giemsa's TS See Giemsa's TS, dilute.

Dilute hydrochloric acid See hydrochloric acid, dilute.

Dilute hydrogen peroxide TS See hydrogen peroxide TS, dilute.

Dilute iodine TS See iodine TS, dilute.

Dilute iron-phenol TS See iron-phenol TS, dilute.

Dilute lead subacetate TS See lead subacetate TS, dilute.

Dilute methyl red TS See methyl red TS, dilute.

Dilute nitric acid See nitric acid, dilute.

Dilute phenolphthalein TS See phenolphthalein TS, dilute.

Dilute phenol red TS See phenol red TS, dilute.

Dilute potassium hydroxide-ethanol TS See potassium hydroxide-ethanol TS, dilute.

Dilute sodium hydroxide TS See sodium hydroxide TS, dilute.

Dilute sodium pentacyanonitrosylferrate (III)-potassium hexacyanoferrate (III) TS See sodium pentacyanonitrosylferrate (III)-potassium hexacyanoferrate (III) TS, dilute.

Dilute sulfuric acid See sulfuric acid, dilute.

Dilute thymol blue TS See thymol blue TS, dilute.

Dilute vanadium pentoxide TS See vanadium (V) oxide TS, dilute.

Dilution fluid for particle counter A fluid used for blood dilution.

Dimedon $C_8H_{12}O_2$ White to pale yellow crystalline powder.

Melting point <*2.60*>: 145 – 149°C

Dimenhydrinate for assay $C_{17}H_{21}NO.C_7H_7ClN_4O_2$ [Same as the monograph Dimenhydrinate. When dried, it contains not less than 53.8% and not more than 54.9% of diphenhydramine ($C_{17}H_{21}NO$) and not less than 45.2% and not more than 46.1% of 8-chlorotheophylline ($C_7H_7ClN_4O_2$).]

Dimethoxymethane $C_3H_8O_2$ Colorless, clear and volatile liquid. Miscible with methanol, with ethanol (95) and with diethyl ether.

***N,N*-Dimethylacetamide** $CH_3CON(CH_3)_2$ Clear and colorless liquid.

Specific gravity <*2.56*> *d*: 0.938 – 0.945 (Method 3).

Boiling point <*2.57*>: 163 – 165°C

Purity—Perform the test with 3 μL of *N,N*-dimethylacetamide as directed under Gas Chromatography <*2.02*> according to the following conditions, determine each peak area by the automatic integration method, and calculate the amount of *N,N*-dimethylacetamide by the area percentage method: not less than 98.0%.

Operating conditions

Detector: A hydrogen flame-ionization detector.

Column: A fused silica column 0.25 mm in inside diameter and 30 m in length, coated the inside surface 0.5 μm in thickness with polyethylene glycol 20 M for gas chromatography.

Column temperature: The sample is injected at a constant temperature of about 70°C, maintain this temperature for 1 minute, then raise to 200°C at a rate of 10°C per minute, and maintain at 200°C for 3 minutes.

Carrier gas: Helium.

Flow rate (linear velocity): About 30 cm per second.

Time span of measurement: About 2 times as long as the retention time of *N,N*-dimethylacetamide.

System suitability

Test for required detectability: To exactly 1.0 g of *N,N*-dimethylacetamide add acetone to make exactly 100 mL. Pipet 5 mL of this solution, and add acetone to make exactly 50 mL. Confirm that the peak area of *N,N*-dimethylacetamide obtained with 3 μL of this solution is equivalent to 40 to 60% of the full-scale.

System repeatability: When the test is repeated with 3 μL of *N,N*-dimethylacetamide under the above operating conditions, the relative standard deviation of the peak area of *N,N*-dimethylacetamide is not more than 2.0%.

Water <*2.48*>: not more than 0.2% (0.1 g, Coulometric titration).

Dimethylamine $(CH_3)_2NH$ Colorless, clear liquid, having amine-like, characteristic odor. It is miscible with water and with ethanol (99.5). It is alkaline.

Specific gravity <*2.56*> d_{20}^{20}: 0.85 – 0.93

Content: 38.0 – 45.0%. Assay—Weigh accurately about 1 g of dimethylamine, transfer to a flask containing exactly 20 mL of 0.5 mol/L sulfuric acid VS, and titrate <*2.50*> the excess sulfuric acid with 1 mol/L sodium hydroxide VS (indicator: 2 drops of methyl red TS). Perform a blank determination in the same manner.

Each mL of 0.5 mol/L sulfuric acid VS
= 45.08 mg of $(CH_3)_2NH$

2,6-Dimethylaniline $C_8H_{11}N$ A clear liquid. Soluble in ethanol (95), and sparingly soluble in water. Specific gravity d_{20}^{20}: about 0.98.

4-Dimethylaminoantipyrine $C_{13}H_{17}N_3O$ Colorless to white crystals, or a white crystalline powder.

Purity Related substances—Proceed the test with 5 μL of a solution of 4-dimethylaminoantipyrine (1 in 2000) as directed in the Assay under Cefpiramide Sodium, determine each peak area in a range of about 2 times as long as the retention time of 4-dimethylaminoantipyrine, beginning after the solvent peak by the automatic integration method, and calculate the total amount of the peaks other than 4-dimethylaminoantipyrine by the area percentage method: not more than 1.0%.

(Dimethylamino)azobenzenesulfonyl chloride $C_{14}H_{14}ClN_3O_2S$ Prepared for amino acid analysis or biochemistry.

***p*-Dimethylaminobenzaldehyde** See 4-dimethylaminobenzaldehyde.

4-Dimethylaminobenzaldehyde $(CH_3)_2NC_6H_4CHO$ [K 8496, *p*-Dimethylaminobenzaldehyde, Special class]

***p*-Dimethylaminobenzaldehyde-ferric chloride TS** See 4-dimethylaminobenzaldehyde-iron (III) chloride TS.

***p*-Dimethylaminobenzaldehyde-ferric chloride TS, dilute** See 4-dimethylaminobenzaldehyde-iron (III) chloride TS, dilute.

***p*-Dimethylaminobenzaldehyde-hydrochloric acid TS** See 4-dimethylaminobenzaldehyde-hydrochloric acid TS.

4-Dimethylaminobenzaldehyde-hydrochloric acid TS Dissolve 1.0 g of 4-dimethylaminobenzaldehyde in 50 mL of hydrochloric acid while cooling, and add 50 mL of ethanol (95).

4-Dimethylaminobenzaldehyde-hydrochloric acid-acetic acid TS Dissolve 8 g of 4-dimethylaminobenzaldehyde in 50 mL of a mixture of acetic acid (100) and hydrochloric acid (19:1). Prepare before use.

4-Dimethylaminobenzaldehyde-iron (III) chloride TS Dissolve 0.125 g of 4-dimethylaminobenzaldehyde in a cold mixture of 65 mL of sulfuric acid and 35 mL of water, then add 0.05 mL of iron (III) chloride TS. Use within 7 days.

4-Dimethylaminobenzaldehyde-iron (III) chloride TS, dilute To 80 mL of water add carefully 100 mL of 4-dimethylaminobenzaldehyde-iron (III) chloride TS and 0.15 mL of iron (III) chloride TS, while cooling with ice.

***p*-Dimethylaminobenzaldehyde TS** See 4-dimethylaminobenzaldehyde TS.

4-Dimethylaminobenzaldehyde TS Dissolve 10 g of 4-dimethylaminobenzaldehyde in a cold mixture of 90 mL of sulfuric acid and 10 mL of water. Prepare before use.

***p*-Dimethylaminobenzaldehyde TS for spraying** See 4-dimethylaminobenzaldehyde TS for spraying.

4-Dimethylaminobenzaldehyde TS for spraying Dissolve 1.0 g of 4-dimethylaminobenzaldehyde in 20 mL of dilute sulfuric acid. Prepare before use.

***p*-Dimethylaminobenzylidene rhodanine** See 4-dimethylaminobenzylidene rhodanine.

4-Dimethylaminobenzylidene rhodanine $C_{12}H_{12}N_2OS_2$ [K 8495, Special class]

***p*-Dimethylaminobenzylidene rhodanine TS** See 4-dimethylaminobenzylidene rhodanine TS.

4-Dimethylaminobenzylidene rhodanine TS Dissolve 20 mg of 4-dimethylaminobenzylidene rhodanine in acetone to make 100 mL.

***p*-Dimethylaminocinnamaldehyde** See 4-dimethylaminocinnamaldehyde.

4-Dimethylaminocinnamaldehyde $C_{11}H_{13}NO$ Orange, crystals or crystalline powder, having a characteristic odor. Freely soluble in dilute hydrochloric acid, sparingly soluble in ethanol (95) and in diethyl ether, and practically insoluble in water.

Melting point ⟨*2.60*⟩: 140 – 142°C

Purity Clarity of solution—Dissolve 0.20 g of 4-dimethylaminocinnamaldehyde in 20 mL of ethanol (95): the solution is clear.

Loss on drying ⟨*2.41*⟩: not more than 0.5% (1 g, 105°C, 2 hours).

Residue on ignition ⟨*2.44*⟩: not more than 0.1% (1 g).

Nitrogen content ⟨*1.08*⟩: 7.8 – 8.1% (105°C, 2 hours, after drying).

***p*-Dimethylaminocinnamaldehyde TS** See 4-dimethylaminocinnamaldehyde TS.

4-Dimethylaminocinnamaldehyde TS Before use, add 1 mL of acetic acid (100) to 10 mL of a solution of 4-dimethylaminocinnamaldehyde in ethanol (95) (1 in 2000).

Dimethylaminophenol $(CH_3)_2NC_6H_4OH$ Dark purple, crystals or crystalline mass.

Melting point ⟨*2.60*⟩: 85°C

Dimethylaniline See *N,N*-dimethylaniline.

***N,N*-Dimethylaniline** $C_6H_5N(CH_3)_2$ Colorless or light yellow liquid, having a characteristic odor.

Specific gravity ⟨*2.56*⟩ d^{20}_{20}: 0.955 – 0.960

Distilling range ⟨*2.57*⟩: 192 – 195°C, not less than 95 vol%.

Dimethylformamide See *N,N*-dimethylformamide.

***N,N*-Dimethylformamide** $HCON(CH_3)_2$ [K 8500, Special class]

***N,N*-Dimethylformamide for liquid chromatography** $HCON(CH_3)_2$ [K 8500, *N,N*-Dimethylformamide, Special class] Read absorbance as directed under Ultraviolet-visible Spectrophotometry ⟨*2.24*⟩ (in a 1-cm cell, using water as the blank): the absorbance is not more than 0.60 at 270 nm, not more than 0.15 at 280 nm, and not more than 0.05 at 300 nm.

Dimethylglyoxime $C_4H_8N_2O_2$ [K 8498, Special class]

Dimethylglyoxime-thiosemicarbazide TS Solution A: Dissolve 0.5 g of dimethylglyoxime in hydrochloric acid to make 100 mL. Prepare before use. Solution B: Dissolve 0.1 g of thiosemicarbazide in 50 mL of water with the aid of warming if necessary, and add diluted hydrochloric acid (1 in 2) to make 100 mL. Prepare before use.

Mix 10 mL each of solution A and solution B, add diluted hydrochloric acid (1 in 2) to make 100 mL, and allow the mixture to stand for 1 hour. Use within 24 hours.

Dimethylglyoxime TS Dissolve 1 g of dimethylglyoxime in ethanol (95) to make 100 mL.

Dimethyl malonate $C_5H_8O_4$ Clear, colorless or pale yellow liquid.

Specific gravity ⟨*2.56*⟩ d^{20}_{4}: 1.152 – 1.162

Water ⟨*2.48*⟩: not more than 0.3%.

Residue on ignition ⟨*2.44*⟩: not more than 0.1%.

***N,N*-Dimethyl-*n*-octylamine** $C_{10}H_{23}N$ Colorless liquid.

Refractive index ⟨*2.45*⟩ n^{20}_{D}: 1.424

***N,N*-Dimethyl-*p*-phenylenediammonium dichloride** $H_2NC_6H_4N(CH_3)_2.2HCl$ [K 8193, *N,N*-Dimethyl-*p*-phenyl enediammonium dichloride, Special class]

***N,N*-Dimethyl-*p*-phenylenediammonium hydrochloride** See *N,N*-dimethyl-*p*-phenylenediamine dichloride.

Dimethyl phthalate $C_{10}H_{10}O_4$ A colorless, clear liquid, having a slight aroma.

Refractive index ⟨*2.45*⟩ n^{20}_{D}: 1.513 – 1.517

Specific gravity ⟨*2.56*⟩ d^{20}_{20}: 1.191 – 1.196

Dimethylpolysiloxane for gas chromatography Prepared for gas chromatography.

Dimethylsulfoxide $(CH_3)_2SO$ [K 9702, Special class]

Dimethylsulfoxide for ultraviolet-visible spectrophotometry $(CH_3)_2SO$ Colorless crystals or clear colorless liquid, having a characteristic odor. It is highly hygroscopic.

Congealing point ⟨*2.42*⟩: not less than 18.3°C.

Purity—Read absorbance of dimethylsulfoxide for ultraviolet-visible spectrophotometry, immediately after saturating with nitrogen, using water as the blank as directed under Ultraviolet-visible Spectrophotometry ⟨*2.24*⟩: its value is not more than 0.20 at 270 nm, not more than 0.09 at 275 nm, not more than 0.06 at 280 nm, and not more than 0.015 at 300 nm. It exhibits no characteristic absorption between 260 nm and 350 nm.

Water ⟨*2.48*⟩: not more than 0.1%.

2,6-Dimethyl-4-(2-nitrosophenyl)3,5-pyridinedicarboxylic acid dimethyl ester for thin-layer chromatography $C_{17}H_{16}N_2O_5$ Irradiate xenon light at 50,000 lx of illumination for 8 hours to a methanol solution of nifedipine (1 in 100), and evaporate the methanol on a water bath. Recrystallize the residue 4 times from 1-propanol, and dry in a desiccator (in vacuum, phosphorus pentoxide). Pale blue crystals. Very soluble in chloroform, freely soluble in acetone, and practically insoluble in water.

Melting point ⟨*2.60*⟩: 93 – 95°C

Content: not less than 99.0%. Assay—Weigh accurately about 0.4 g of 2,6-dimethyl-4-(2-nitrosophenyl)-3,5-pyridinedicarboxylic acid dimethyl ester for thin-layer chromatography, dissolve in 70 mL of acetic acid (100), and titrate ⟨*2.50*⟩ with 0.1 mol/L perchloric acid VS (potentiometric titration). Perform a blank determination in the same manner, and make any necessary correction.

Each mL of 0.1 mol/L perchloric acid VS
= 32.83 mg of $C_{17}H_{16}N_2O_5$

3-(4,5-Dimethylthiazole-2-yl)-2,5-diphenyl-2*H*-tetrazolium bromide $C_{18}H_{16}BrN_5S$ Yellow crystals. Melting point:

about 195°C (with decomposition).

3-(4,5-Dimethylthiazole-2-yl)-2,5-diphenyl-2*H*-tetrazolium bromide TS Dissolve 5 g of 3-(4,5-dimethylthiazole-2-yl)-2,5-diphenyl-2*H*-tetrazolium bromide in phosphate-buffered sodium chloride TS to make 1000 mL.

Dimidium bromide $C_{20}H_{18}BrN_3$ Red to dark brown, crystalline powder or powder.

Identification—(1) Determine the infrared absorption spectrum of dimidium bromide as directed in the potassium bromide disk method under Infrared Spectrophotometry <*2.25*>: it exhibits absorption at the wave numbers of about 3300 cm^{-1}, 1619 cm^{-1}, 1489 cm^{-1}, 1470 cm^{-1}, 1422 cm^{-1} and 1316 cm^{-1}.

(2) A solution of dimidium bromide (1 in 1000) responds to Qualitative Tests <*1.09*> (1) for bromide.

Dimidium bromide-patent blue TS Dissolve each 0.5 g of dimidium bromide and 0.25 g of patent blue in 30 mL of a warmed mixture of water and ethanol (99.5) (9:1), combine the solutions, and add a mixture of water and ethanol (99.5) (9:1) to make 250 mL. To 20 mL of this solution add 270 mL of diluted sulfuric acid (7 in 675) and water to make 500 mL.

Storage—Preserve in light-resistant containers.

Dimorpholamine for assay $C_{20}H_{38}N_4O_4$ [Same as the monograph Dimorpholamine. When dried, it contains not less than 99.0% of dimorpholamine ($C_{20}H_{38}N_4O_4$).]

2,2′-dinaphthylether $C_{20}H_{14}O$ White crystals.

Melting point <*2.60*>: 102 – 107°C

***m*-Dinitrobenzene** See 1,3-dinitrobenzene.

1,2-Dinitrobenzene $C_6H_4(NO_2)_2$ Occurs as yellowish white to brownish yellow, crystals or a crystalline powder.

Identification—Determine the infrared absorption spectrum of 1,2-dinitrobenzene as directed in the paste method under Infrared Spectrophotometry <*2.25*>: it exhibits absorption at the wave numbers of about 3100 cm^{-1}, 1585 cm^{-1}, 1526 cm^{-1}, 1352 cm^{-1}, and 793 cm^{-1}.

Melting point <*2.60*>: 116 – 119°C

1,3-Dinitrobenzene $C_6H_4(NO_2)_2$ Light yellow to reddish-yellow, crystals or crystalline powder.

Melting point <*2.60*>: 88 – 92°C.

Storage—Preserve in a light-resistant tight container.

***m*-Dinitrobenzene TS** See 1,3-dinitrobenzene TS.

1,3-Dinitrobenzene TS Dissolve 1 g of 1,3-dinitrobenzene in 100 mL of ethanol (95). Prepare before use.

***m*-Dinitrobenzene TS, alkaline** See 1,3-dinitrobenzene TS, alkaline.

1,3-Dinitrobenzene TS, alkaline Mix 1 mL of tetramethylammonium hydroxide and 140 mL of ethanol (99.5), titrate a part of the mixture with 0.01 mol/L hydrochloric acid VS (indicator: methyl red TS), and dilute the remainder with ethanol (99.5) to give a 0.008 mol/L solution. Before use, mix 40 mL of this solution with 60 mL of a solution of 1,3-dinitrobenzene in benzene (1 in 20).

2,4-Dinitrochlorobenzene See 1-chloro-2, 4-dinitrobenzene.

2,4-Dinitrofluorobenzene See 1-fluoro-2, 4-dinitrobenzene.

2,4-Dinitrophenol $C_6H_3OH(NO_2)_2$ Yellow, crystals or crystalline powder.

Melting point <*2.60*>: 110 – 114°C

2,4-Dinitrophenol TS Dissolve 0.5 g of 2,4-dinitrophenol in 100 mL of ethanol (95).

2,4-Dinitrophenylhydrazine $(NO_2)_2C_6H_3NHNH_2$ [K 8480, Special class]

2,4-Dinitrophenylhydrazine-diethylene glycol dimethyl ether TS Dissolve 3 g of 2,4-dinitrophenylhydrazine in 100 mL of diethylene glycol dimethyl ether while heating, cool, and filter if necessary.

2,4-Dinitrophenylhydrazine-ethanol TS Dissolve 1.5 g of 2,4-dinitrophenylhydrazine in a cold mixture of 10 mL of sulfuric acid and 10 mL of water, then add a mixture of 1 volume of aldehyde-free ethanol and 3 volumes of water to make 100 mL, and filter if necessary.

2,4-Dinitrophenylhydrazine TS Dissolve 1.5 g of 2,4-dinitrophenylhydrazine in a cold mixture of 10 mL of sulfuric acid and 10 mL of water, then add water to make 100 mL, and filter if necessary.

Dinonyl phthalate $C_6H_4(COOC_9H_{19})_2$ Colorless to pale yellow, clear liquid.

Specific gravity <*2.56*> d^{20}_{20}: 0.967 – 0.987

Acid value <*1.13*>: not more than 2.

Dioxane See 1,4-dioxane.

1,4-Dioxane $C_4H_8O_2$ [K 8461, Special class]

Diphenhydramine $C_{17}H_{21}NO$ [Same as the namesake monograph]

Diphenhydramine tannate [Same as the namesake monograph]

Diphenyl $C_{12}H_{10}$ White, crystals or crystalline powder, having a characteristic odor. Freely soluble in acetone and in diethyl ether, soluble in ethanol (95), and practically insoluble in water.

Melting point <*2.60*>: 68 – 72°C

Purity—Dissolve 0.10 g of diphenyl in 5 mL of acetone and use this solution as the sample solution. Perform the test with 2 μL of the sample solution as directed under Gas Chromatography <*2.02*> according to the following conditions. Determine each peak area by the automatic integration method and calculate the amount of diphenyl by the area percentage method: it shows the purity of not less than 98.0%.

Operating conditions

Detector: A hydrogen flame-ionization detector.

Column: A glass tube about 3 mm in inside diameter and about 2 m in length, packed with 150 to 180 μm mesh siliceous earth for gas chromatography coated with 10% of polyethylene glycol 20 M for thin-layer chromatography.

Column temperature: A constant temperature of about 180°C.

Carrier gas: Nitrogen.

Flow rate: Adjust so that the retention time of diphenyl is about 8 minutes.

Detection sensitivity: Adjust the detection sensitivity so that the peak height of diphenyl obtained with 2 μL of the solution prepared by adding acetone to 1.0 mL of the sample solution to make 100 mL, is 5 to 15% of the full scale.

Time span of measurement: About 3 times as long as the retention time of diphenyl, beginning after the solvent peak.

Diphenylamine $(C_6H_5)_2NH$ [K 8487, Special class]

Diphenylamine-acetic acid TS Dissolve 1.5 g of diphenylamine in 1.5 mL of sulfuric acid and acetic acid (100) to make 100 mL.

Diphenylamine-acetic acid (100) TS See diphenylamine-acetic acid TS.

Diphenylamine TS Dissolve 1 g of diphenylamine in 100 mL of sulfuric acid. Use the colorless solution.

9,10-Diphenylanthracene $C_{26}H_{18}$ Yellow crystalline powder. Soluble in diethyl ether, and practically insoluble in water.

Melting point <*2.60*>: about 248°C

1,4-Diphenylbenzene $C_{18}H_{14}$ White scaly crystals, having a slight aromatic odor. It is freely soluble in ethanol (99.5), and slightly soluble in water.

Identification—Determine the infrared absorption spectrum as directed in the potassium bromide disk method under Infrared Spectrophotometry <*2.25*>: it exhibits absorption at the wave numbers of about 3050 cm^{-1}, 3020 cm^{-1}, 1585 cm^{-1}, 1565 cm^{-1}, 1476 cm^{-1}, 1450 cm^{-1}, 995 cm^{-1}, 834 cm^{-1}, 740 cm^{-1} and 680 cm^{-1}.

Diphenylcarbazide See 1,5-diphenylcarbonohydrazide.

Diphenylcarbazide TS See 1,5-diphenylcarbonohydrazide TS.

Diphenylcarbazone $C_6H_5N_2CON_2H_2C_6H_5$ A yellowish-red crystalline powder.

Identification—Determine the infrared absorption spectrum of diphenylcarbazone as directed in the potassium bromide disk method as directed under Infrared Spectrophotometry <*2.25*>: it exhibits absorption at the wave numbers of about 1708 cm^{-1}, 1602 cm^{-1}, 1497 cm^{-1}, 1124 cm^{-1}, 986 cm^{-1}, 748 cm^{-1} and 692 cm^{-1}.

Storage—Preserve in a light-resistant tight container.

Diphenylcarbazone TS Dissolve 1 g of diphenylcarbazone in ethanol (95) to make 1000 mL.

1,5-Diphenylcarbonohydrazide $C_{13}H_{14}N_4O$ [K 8488, Special class]

1,5-Diphenylcarbonohydrazide TS Dissolve 0.2 g of 1,5-diphenylcarbonohydrazide in 100 mL of a mixture of ethanol (95) and acetic acid (100) (9:1).

5% Diphenyl-95% dimethylpolysiloxane for gas chromatography Prepared for gas chromatography.

Diphenyl ether $C_{12}H_{10}O$ Colorless crystals, having a geranium-like aroma. Dissolves in ethanol (95) and in diethyl ether, and practically insoluble in water.

Specific gravity <*2.56*> d_{25}^{25}: 1.072 – 1.075

Boiling point <*2.57*>: 254 – 259°C

Melting point <*2.60*>: 28°C

Diphenyl imidazole $C_{15}H_{12}N_2$ White, crystals or crystalline powder, freely soluble in acetic acid (100), and sparingly soluble in methanol.

Melting point <*2.60*>: 234 – 238°C

Loss on drying <*2.41*>: not more than 0.5% (0.5 g, 105°C, 3 hours).

Content: not less than 99.0%. Assay—Dissolve about 0.3 g of diphenyl imidazole, previously dried and weighed accurately, in 70 mL of acetic acid (100), and titrate <*2.50*> with 0.1 mol/L perchloric acid VS (indicator: 2 drops of crystal violet TS).

Each mL of 0.1 mol/L perchloric acid VS
= 22.03 mg of $C_{15}H_{12}N_2$

Diphenyl phthalate $C_6H_4(COOC_6H_5)_2$ White crystalline powder.

Melting point <*2.60*>: 71 – 76°C

Purity Related substances—Dissolve 60 mg of diphenyl phthalate in 50 mL of chloroform and use this solution as the sample solution. Perform the test with 10 μL of the sample solution as directed in the Assay under Tolnaftate Solution: any peak other than the principal peak at the retention time of about 8 minutes and the peak of the solvent does not appear. Adjust the detection sensitivity so that the peak height of diphenyl phthalate obtained from 10 μL of the sample solution is 50 to 100% of the full scale, and the time span of measurement is about twice as long as the retention time of diphenyl phthalate, beginning after the solvent peak.

1,1-Diphenyl-4-pyperidino-1-butene hydrochloride for thin-layer chromatography $C_{21}H_{25}N.HCl$ To 1 g of diphenidol hydrochloride add 30 mL of 1 mol/L hydrochloric acid TS, and heat under a reflux condenser for 1 hour. After cooling, extract twice with 30 mL-portions of chloroform, combine the chloroform extracts, wash twice with 10 mL portions of water, and evaporate chloroform under reduced pressure. Recrystallize the residue from a mixture of diethyl ether and ethanol (95) (3:1), and dry in a desiccator (in vacuum, silica gel) for 2 hours. White crystals or crystalline powder.

Absorbance <*2.24*> $E_{1\,cm}^{1\%}$ (250 nm): 386 – 446 (10 mg, water, 1000 mL).

Melting point <*2.60*>: 176 – 180°C

Content: not less than 99.0%. Assay—Dissolve about 0.2 g of 1,1-diphenyl-4-pyperidino-1-butene hydrochloride for thin-layer chromatography, previously weighed accurately, in 20 mL of acetic acid (100), add 20 mL of acetic anhydride, and titrate <*2.50*> with 0.05 mol/L perchloric acid VS (potentiometric titration). Perform a blank determination in the same manner, and make any necessary correction.

Each mL of 0.05 mol/L perchloric acid VS
= 16.39 mg of $C_{21}H_{25}N.HCl$

Diphenyl sulfone for assay $C_{12}H_{10}O_2S$ White, crystals or crystalline powder. It dissolves in dimethylsulfoxide.

It is used after correcting with the amount of diphenyl sulfone obtained in the Assay.

Identification—Proceed as directed in the Assay: it exhibits a triplet-like signal equivalent to 4 protons around δ 7.65 ppm, triplet-like signals equivalent to 2 protons around δ 7.73 ppm, and doublet-like signals equivalent to 4 protons around δ 7.99 ppm.

Unity of peak—Dissolve 10 mg of diphenyl sulfone for assay in 100 mL of methanol. To 10 mL of this solution add methanol to make 100 mL, and use this solution as the sample solution. Perform the test with 10 μL of the sample solution as directed under Liquid Chromatography <*2.01*> according to the following conditions, and compare the absorption spectra of at least 3 points including the top of diphenyl sulfone peak and around the two middle peak heights of before and after the top: no difference in form is observed between their spectra.

Operating conditions

Column, column temperature, mobile phase, and flow rate: Proceed as directed in the operating conditions in the Assay under Perilla Herb.

Detector: A photodiode array detector (wavelength: 234 nm, spectrum range of measurement: 220 – 400 nm).

System suitability

System performance: Proceed as directed in the system suitability in the Assay under Perilla Herb.

The unity of peak is unnecessary if the content (%) of diphenyl sulfone ($C_{12}H_{10}O_2S$) is between 99.5% and 100.5%.

Assay—Weigh accurately 5 mg of diphenyl sulfone for assay and 1 mg of DSS-d_6 for nuclear magnetic resonance spectroscopy using an ultramicrobalance, dissolve in 2 mL of deuterated dimethyl sulfoxide for nuclear magnetic resonance spectroscopy, and use this solution as the sample solution. Transfer the sample solution into an NMR tube 5 mm in outer diameter, measure ^{1}H-NMR as directed under Nuclear Magnetic Resonance Spectroscopy <2.21> and Crude Drugs Test <5.01> according to the following conditions, using DSS-d_6 for nuclear magnetic resonance spectroscopy as the reference standard for qNMR. Calculate the resonance intensities, A_1 (equivalent to 6 hydrogens) and A_2 (equivalent to 4 hydrogens), of the signals around δ 7.64 – 7.74 ppm and δ 7.98 – 8.01 ppm assuming the signal of the reference standard for qNMR as δ 0 ppm.

$$\text{Amount (\%) of diphenyl sulfone } (C_{12}H_{10}O_2S) = M_S \times I \times P/(M \times N) \times 0.9729$$

M: Amount (mg) of diphenyl sulfone for assay taken
M_S: Amount (mg) of DSS-d_6 for nuclear magnetic resonance spectroscopy taken
I: Sum of the signal resonance intensities, A_1 and A_2, based on the signal resonance intensity of DSS-d_6 for nuclear magnetic resonance spectroscopy as 9.000
N: Sum of numbers of the hydrogen derived from A_1 and A_2
P: Purity (%) of DSS-d_6 for nuclear magnetic resonance spectroscopy

Operating conditions
Apparatus: An apparatus of nuclear magnetic resonance spectrom measurement having ^{1}H resonance frequency of not less than 400 MHz.
Target nucleus: ^{1}H.
Digital resolution: 0.25 Hz or lower.
Measuring spectrum range: 20 ppm or upper, including between −5 ppm and 15 ppm.
Spinning: off.
Pulse angle: 90°.
^{13}C decoupling: on.
Delay time: Repeating pulse waiting time not less than 60 seconds.
Integrating times: 8 or more times.
Dummy scanning: 2 or more times.
Measuring temperature: A constant temperature between 20°C and 30°C.
System suitability
Test for required detectability: When the procedure is run with the sample solution under the above operating conditions, the SN ratio of each signal around δ 7.64 – 7.74 ppm and δ 7.98 – 8.01 ppm is not less than 100.
System performance: When the procedure is run with the sample solution under the above operating conditions, the signals around δ 7.64 – 7.74 ppm and δ 7.98 – 8.01 ppm are not overlapped with any signal of obvious foreign substances, and the ratios of the resonance intensities, $(A_1/6)/(A_2/4)$, of each signal around δ 7.64 – 7.74 ppm and δ 7.98 – 8.01 ppm are between 0.99 and 1.01, respectively.
System repeatability: When the test is repeated 6 times with the sample solution under the above operating conditions, the relative standard deviation of the ratio of the resonance intensity, A_1 or A_2 to that of the reference standard for qNMR are not more than 1.0%.

Dipicolinic acid $C_7H_5NO_4$ White powder.
Identification—Determine the infrared absorption spectrum of dipicolinic acid as directed in the potassium bromide disk method under Infrared Spectrophotometry <2.25>: it exhibits absorption at the wave numbers of about 2630 cm^{-1}, 1701 cm^{-1}, 1576 cm^{-1}, 1416 cm^{-1}, 1300 cm^{-1} and 1267 cm^{-1}.
Purity Clarity and color of solution—Dissolve by warming 0.5 g of dipicolinic acid in 20 mL of ethanol (99.5), and cool: a clear, colorless liquid.
Content: Not less than 98.0%. *Assay*—Weigh accurately about 0.1 g of dipicolinic acid, add 25 mL of ethanol (99.5), dissolve by warning, cool, then titrate <2.50> with 0.1 mol/L sodium hydroxide VS (indicator: 2 drops of phenolphthalein TS). Perform a blank determination in the same manner, and make any necessary correction.

Each mL of 0.1 mol/L sodium hydroxide VS
= 8.356 mg of $C_7H_5O_4N$

Dipotassium hydrogen phosphate K_2HPO_4 [K 9017, Special class]

Dipotassium hydrogen phosphate-citric acid buffer solution (pH 5.3) Mix 100 mL of 1 mol/L dipotassium hydrogen phosphate TS for buffer solution and 38 mL of 1 mol/L citric acid TS for buffer solution, and add water to make 200 mL.

1 mol/L Dipotassium hydrogen phosphate TS for buffer solution Dissolve 174.18 g of dipotassium hydrogen phosphate in water to make 1000 mL.

Dipotassium tetraborate tetrahydrate $K_2B_4O_7.4H_2O$ White, crystalline powder or powder. Slightly soluble in ethanol (99.5).

Diprophylline $C_{10}H_{14}N_4O_4$ A white, powder or grain. Freely soluble in water, and slightly soluble in ethanol (95).
Identification—Determine the infrared absorption spectrum of the substance to be examined, previously dried at 105°C for 4 hours, as directed in the potassium bromide disk method under Infrared Spectrophotometry <2.25>: it exhibits absorption at the wave numbers of about 3460 cm^{-1}, 3330 cm^{-1}, 1651 cm^{-1}, 1242 cm^{-1}, 1059 cm^{-1} and 1035 cm^{-1}.

α,α′-Dipyridyl See 2,2′-bipyridyl.

Disodium chromotropate dihydrate $C_{10}H_6Na_2O_8S_2.2H_2O$ [K 8316, Special class] Preserve in light-resistant containers.

Disodium dihydrogen ethylenediamine tetraacetate dihydrate $C_{10}H_{14}N_2Na_2O_8.2H_2O$ [K 8107, Special class]

0.4 mol/L Disodium dihydrogen ethylenediamine tetraacetate TS (pH 8.5) Dissolve 148.9 g of disodium dihydrogen ethylenediamine tetraacetate dihydrate in about 800 mL of water, adjust to pH 8.5 with 8 mol/L sodium hydroxide TS, and add water to make 1000 mL.

0.04 mol/L Disodium dihydrogen ethylenediamine tetraacetate TS Dissolve 14.890 g of disodium dihydrogen ethylenediamine tetraacetate dihydrate in water to make 1000 mL.

0.1 mol/L Disodium dihydrogen ethylenediamine tetraacetate TS Dissolve 37.2 g of disodium dihydrogen ethylenediamine tetraacetate dihydrate in water to make 1000 mL.

Disodium ethylenediaminetetraacetate See disodium dihydrogen ethylenediamine tetraacetate dihydrate.

Disodium ethylenediaminetetraacetate copper See copper (II) disodium ethylenediamine tetraacetate tetrahydrate.

0.1 mol/L Disodium ethylenediaminetetraacetate TS See 0.1 mol/L disodium dihydrogen ethylenediamine tetraacetate TS.

Disodium hydrogen phosphate, anhydrous Na_2HPO_4 [K 9020, Special class]

Disodium hydrogen phosphate-citric acid buffer solution (pH 3.0) Dissolve 35.8 g of disodium hydrogen phosphate dodecahydrate in water to make 500 mL. To this solution add a solution of citric acid monohydrate (21 in 1000) to adjust the pH to 3.0.

Disodium hydrogen phosphate-citric acid buffer solution (pH 4.5) Dissolve 21.02 g of citric acid monohydrate in water to make 1000 mL, and adjust the pH to 4.5 with a solution prepared by dissolving 35.82 g of disodium hydrogenphosphate dodecahydrate in water to make 1000 mL.

Disodium hydrogen phosphate-citric acid buffer solution (pH 5.0) Dissolve 7.1 g of anhydrous disodium hydrogen phosphate in water to make 1000 mL, and adjust to pH 5.0 with a solution prepared by dissolving 5.25 g of citric acid monohydrate in water to make 1000 mL.

Disodium hydrogen phosphate-citric acid buffer solution (pH 5.4) Dissolve 1.05 g of citric acid monohydrate and 2.92 g of disodium hydrogen phosphate dodecahydrate in 200 mL of water, and adjust to pH 5.4 with phosphoric acid or sodium hydroxide TS, if necessary.

Disodium hydrogen phosphate-citric acid buffer solution (pH 5.5) To 1000 mL of 0.05 mol/L disodium hydrogen phosphate TS add an amount of a solution, prepared by dissolving 5.25 g of citric acid monohydrate in water to make 1000 mL, to adjust to pH 5.5.

Disodium hydrogen phosphate-citric acid buffer solution (pH 6.0) Dissolve 71.6 g of disodium hydrogen phosphate dodecahydrate in water to make 1000 mL. To this solution add a solution, prepared by dissolving 21.0 g of citric acid monohydrate in water to make 1000 mL, until the pH becomes 6.0 (ratio of volume: about 63:37).

0.05 mol/L Disodium hydrogen phosphate-citric acid buffer solution (pH 6.0) To 1000 mL of 0.05 mol/L disodium hydrogen phosphate TS add a solution prepared by dissolving 5.25 g of citric acid monohydrate in water to make 1000 mL to adjust pH 6.0.

Disodium hydrogen phosphate-citric acid buffer solution (pH 6.8) To 1000 mL of 0.05 mol/L disodium hydrogen phosphate TS add a solution prepared by dissolving 5.25 g of citric acid monohydrate in water to make 1000 mL to adjust the pH to 6.8.

Disodium hydrogen phosphate-citric acid buffer solution (pH 7.2) Dissolve 7.1 g of anhydrous disodium hydrogen phosphate in water to make 1000 mL. Adjust this solution to pH 7.2 with a solution prepared by dissolving 5.3 g of citric acid monohydrate in water to make 1000 mL.

Disodium hydrogen phosphate-citric acid buffer solution (pH 7.5) To 1000 mL of 0.05 mol/L disodium hydrogen phosphate TS add a solution prepared by dissolving 5.25 g of citric acid monohydrate in water to make 1000 mL to adjust the pH to 7.5.

Disodium hydrogen phosphate-citric acid buffer solution (pH 8.2) Dissolve 20.7 g of anhydrous disodium hydrogen phosphate, 7.38 g of citric acid monohydrate, and 0.535 g of sodium dihydrogen phosphate dihydrate in 400 mL of water, adjust to pH 8.2 with a solution of sodium hydroxide (1 in 2), and add water to make 500 mL.

Disodium hydrogen phosphate-citric acid buffer solution for penicillium origin *β*-galactosidase (pH 4.5) Dissolve 71.6 g of disodium hydrogen phosphate dodecahydrate in water to make 1000 mL, and adjust the pH to 4.5 with a solution prepared by dissolving 21.0 g of citric acid monohydrate in water to make 1000 mL (volume ratio: about 44:56).

Disodium hydrogen phosphate dodecahydrate $Na_2HPO_4.12H_2O$ [K 9019, Special class]

Disodium hydrogen phosphate for pH determination Na_2HPO_4 [K 9020, for pH determination]

Disodium hydrogen phosphate TS Dissolve 12 g of disodium hydrogen phosphate dodecahydrate in water to make 100 mL (0.3 mol/L).

0.05 mol/L Disodium hydrogen phosphate TS Dissolve 7.098 g of anhydrous disodium hydrogen phosphate in water to make 1000 mL.

0.5 mol/L Disodium hydrogen phosphate TS Dissolve 70.982 g of anhydrous disodium hydrogen phosphate in water to make 1000 mL.

Disodium 1-nitroso-2-naphthol-3,6-disulfonate $C_{10}H_5NNa_2O_8S_2$ Yellow, crystals or crystalline powder.

Identification—Determine the infrared absorption spectrum as directed in the potassium bromide disk method as directed under Infrared Spectrophotometry <*2.25*>: it exhibits absorption at the wave numbers of about 3400 cm^{-1}, 1639 cm^{-1}, 1451 cm^{-1}, 1270 cm^{-1}, 1231 cm^{-1}, 1173 cm^{-1}, 1049 cm^{-1}, 848 cm^{-1} and 662 cm^{-1}.

Storage—Preserve in a light-resistant tight container.

Dissolved acetylene C_2H_2 [K 1902]

Distigmine bromide for assay $C_{22}H_{32}Br_2N_4O_4$ [Same as the monograph Distigmine Bromide. It contains not less than 99.0% of distigmine bromide ($C_{22}H_{32}Br_2N_4O_4$), calculated on the anhydrous basis.]

Distilled water for injection [Use the water prescribed by the monographs of Water for Injection or Sterile Water for Injection in Containers. Prepared by distillation. It is not necessary to check the conformity to all the specification items of the monograph, if it is confirmed that the water to be used is suitable for the purpose of relevant test.]

2,6-Di-*tert*-butylcresol $[(CH_3)_3C]_2C_6H_2(CH_3)OH$ A white crystalline powder. Freely soluble in ethanol (95).

Melting point <*2.60*>: 69 – 71°C

Residue on ignition <*2.44*>: not more than 0.05%.

2,6-Di-*tert*-butylcresol TS Dissolve 0.1 g of 2,6-di-*tert*-butylcresol in ethanol (95) to make 10 mL.

2,6-Di-*tert*-butyl-*p*-cresol See 2,6-di-*tert*-butylcresol.

2,6-Di-*tert*-butyl-*p*-cresol TS See 2,6-di-*tert*-butylcresol TS.

1,3-Di (4-pyridyl) propane $C_{13}H_{14}N_2$ A light yellow powder.

Melting point <*2.60*>: 61 – 62°C

Water <*2.48*>: less than 0.1%.

1,1′-[3,3′-Dithiobis(2-methyl-1-oxopropyl)]-L-diproline $C_{18}H_{28}N_2O_6S_2$ White, crystals or crystalline powder. Sparingly soluble in methanol, and practically insoluble in water.

Identification—Determine the infrared absorption spectrum of 1,1′-[3,3′-dithiobis(2-methyl-1-oxopropyl)]-L-diproline according to potassium bromide disk method under Infrared Spectrophotometry <*2.25*>: it exhibits absorption at the wave numbers of about 2960 cm^{-1}, 1750 cm^{-1}, 1720 cm^{-1}, 1600 cm^{-1}, 1480 cm^{-1}, 1450 cm^{-1} and 1185 cm^{-1}.

Purity Related substances—Dissolve 0.10 g of 1,1′-[3,3′-dithiobis (2-methyl-1-oxopropyl)]-L-diproline in exactly 10 mL of methanol. Perform the test with this solution as directed in the Purity (3) under Captopril: any spot other than the principal spot at the *R*f value of about 0.2 does not appear.

Content: not less than 99.0%. Assay—Weigh accurately about 0.3 g of 1,1′-[3,3′-dithiobis (2-methyl-1-oxopropyl)]-L-diproline, dissolve in 20 mL of methanol, add 50 mL of water, and titrate <*2.50*> with 0.1 mol/L sodium hydroxide VS until the color of the solution changes from yellow through blue-green to blue (indicator: 3 drops of bromothymol blue TS). Perform a blank determination in the same manner, and make any necessary correction.

Each mL of 0.1 mol/L sodium hydroxide VS
= 21.63 mg of $C_{18}H_{28}N_2O_6S_2$

Dithiodiglycolic acid $C_4H_6O_4S_2$ Prepared for biochemistry or amino acid analysis.

Dithiodipropionic acid $C_6H_{10}O_4S_2$ Prepared for biochemistry or amino acid analysis.

Dithiothreitol $C_4H_{10}O_2S_2$ Crystals.
Melting point <*2.60*>: about 42°C

Dithizone $C_6H_5NHNHCSN:NC_6H_5$ [K 8490, Special class]

Dithizone solution for extraction Dissolve 30 mg of dithizone in 1000 mL of chloroform, and add 5 mL of ethanol (95), and store. Before use, shake a suitable volume of the solution with one-half of its volume of diluted nitric acid (1 in 100), and use the chloroform layer after discarding the water layer.

Dithizone TS Dissolve 25 mg of dithizone in ethanol (95) to make 100 mL. Prepare before use.

DNA standard stock solution for interferon alfa (NAMALWA) To 1 × 10^9 Namalwa cells add 0.1 mL of proteinase K solution and 20 mL of *N*-lauroyl sarcosine sodium TS, lyse the cells by gentle stirring at 50 ± 1°C for 3 hours, add 20 mL of water-saturated phenol, and stir gently at room temperature for 3 hours. Add 10 mL of a mixture of chloroform and 3-methyl-l-butanol (24:1), centrifuge, and discard the lower layer. Add 20 mL of water-saturated phenol to the upper layer, stir gently at room temperature for 2 hours, and centrifuge. Collect the lower layer, dialyze for 24 hours against dialysis buffer A, add ribonuclease A and ribonuclease T_1 so that each mL of the inner solution obtained contains 25 μg of ribonuclease A and 25 units of ribonuclease T_1, and stir gently at 37 ± 1°C for 3 hours. Add sodium lauryl sulfate solution (1 in 10) and proteinase K solution so that each mL contains 5 mg of sodium lauryl sulfate and 50 μg of proteinase K, and stir gently at 50 ± 1°C for 2 hours. Add an equal volume of phenol-saturated TE buffer solution, stir gently at room temperature for 2 hours, and centrifuge. After removing the lower layer, repeat the same operation. Collect the upper layer, and dialyze for 10 hours against dialysis buffer B, then change the external solution to dialysis buffer C, and dialyze for 24 hours. Collect the inner solution, add 0.1 volume of acetic acid-sodium acetate buffer solution (pH 5.2) and 2.2 volume of ethanol (99.5), and stir gently. Collect the DNA precipitated by winding on a glass rod, wash with diluted ethanol (7 in 10), dry in vacuum, dissolve the residue in 4 mL of TE buffer solution, and use this solution as the standard DNA. Dilute with water so that each mL contains exactly 40 ng of DNA following the specific absorbance of double-stranded DNA, $E^{1\%}_{1\,cm}$ (260 nm), is 200.

Docetaxel hydrate $C_{43}H_{53}NO_{14}.3H_2O$ [Same as the namesake monograph]

Dopamine hydrochloride for assay $C_8H_{11}NO_2.HCl$ [Same as the monograph Dopamine hydrochloride. When dried, it contains not less than 99.0% of dopamine hydrochloride ($C_8H_{11}NO_2.HCl$).]

Doxepin hydrochloride $C_{19}H_{21}NO.HCl$ White, crystals or crystalline powder. Melting point: 185 - 191°C.

Doxifluridine $C_9H_{11}FN_2O_5$ [Same as the namesake monograph]

Doxifluridine for assay $C_9H_{11}FN_2O_5$ [Same as the monograph Doxifluridine. When dried, it contains not less than 99.5% of doxifluridine ($C_9H_{11}FN_2O_5$).]

Doxorubicin hydrochloride $C_{27}H_{29}NO_{11}.HCl$ [Same as the namesake monograph]

Dragendorff's TS Dissolve 0.85 g of bismuth subnitrate in 10 mL of acetic acid (100) and 40 mL of water with vigorous shaking (solution A). Dissolve 8 g of potassium iodide in 20 mL of water (solution B). Immediately before use, mix equal volumes of solution A, solution B and acetic acid (100). Store solution A and solution B in light-resistant containers.

Dragendorff's TS for spraying Add 20 mL of diluted acetic acid (31) (1 in 5) to 4 mL of a mixture of equal volumes of solution A and solution B of Dragendorff's TS. Prepare before use.

Dried human normal plasma powder Freeze-dried normal plasma obtained from healthy human.

Dried sodium carbonate Na_2CO_3 [Same as the namesake monograph]

Droxidopa for assay $C_9H_{11}NO_5$ [Same as the monograph Droxidopa. When dried, it contains not less than 99.5% of droxidopa ($C_9H_{11}NO_5$).]

DSS-d_6 for nuclear magnetic resonance spectroscopy $C_6H_9D_6NaO_3SSi$ Sodium 3-(trimethylsilyl)-1-propanesulfonate-d_6 that the traceability to the International System of Units has been secured.

Dydrogesterone for assay $C_{21}H_{28}O_2$ [Same as the monograph Dydrogesterone. When dried, it contains not less than 99.0% of dydrogesterone ($C_{21}H_{28}O_2$).]

Eagle's minimum essential medium Dissolve 6.80 g of sodium chloride, 400 mg of potassium chloride, 115 mg of anhydrous sodium dihydrogen phosphate, 93.5 mg (as anhydrous) of magnesium sulfate, 200 mg (as anhydrous) of calcium chloride, 1.00 g of glucose, 126 mg of L-arginine hydrochloride, 73.0 mg of L-lysine hydrochloride, 31.4 mg of L-cysteine hydrochloride monohydrate, 36.0 mg of L-tyrosine, 42.0 mg of L-histidine hydrochloride monohydrate, 52.0 mg of L-isoleucine, 52.0 mg of L-leucine, 15.0 mg of methionine, 32.0 mg of phenylalanine, 48.0 mg of L-threonine, 10.0 mg of L-tryptophan, 46.0 mg of L-valine, 75.0 mg of succinic acid, 100 mg of sodium succinate hexahydrate, 1.8 mg of choline bitartrate, 1.0 mg of folic acid, 2.0 mg of myoinositol, 1.0 mg of nicotinamide, 1.0 mg of calcium D-pantothenate, 1.0 mg of pyridoxal hydrochloride, 0.1 mg of riboflavin, 1.0 mg of thiamine chloride hydrochloride, 20 μg of biotin and 6.0 mg of phenol red in 1000 mL of water, heat in an autoclave at 121°C for 15 minutes and cool to room temperature, then add separately sterilized 22 mL of 10% sodium hydrogen carbonate TS and 10 mL of glutamine TS.

Eagle's minimum essential medium containing bovine serum To Eagle's minimum essential medium add an adequate amount of bovine serum.

Ebastine for assay $C_{32}H_{39}NO_2$ [Same as the monograph Ebastine. When dried, it contains not less than 99.5% of ebastine ($C_{32}H_{39}NO_2$).]

Ecabet sodium hydrate for assay $C_{20}H_{27}NaO_5S.5H_2O$ [Same as the monograph Ecabet Sodium Hydrate. It contains not less than 99.5% of ecabet sodium ($C_{20}H_{27}NaO_5S$), calculated on the anhydrous basis.]

E. coli protein Process E. coli cells (*E. coli* N4830/pTB281) retaining a plasmid deficient in the celmoleukin gene according to the celmoleukin purification process in the following order; (i) extraction, (ii) butylated vinyl polymer hydrophobic column chromatography, (iii) carboxymethylated vinyl polymer ion-exchange column chromatography, and (iv) sulfopropyl-polymer ion-exchange chromatography, and during process (iv) collect the fractions corresponding to the celmoleukin elution position. Dialyze the fractions obtained in (iv) against 0.01 mol/L acetate buffer solution (pH 5.0), and take the dialysis solution as E.coli protein.

Description—Clear and colorless solution.

Identification—When the absorption spectrum is determined as directed under Ultraviolet-visible Spectrophotometry <2.24>, an absorption maximum is observed in the region of 278 nm.

Protein content: When determining the protein content using the Assay (1) under Celmoleukin (Genetical Recombination), the protein content per mL is 0.1 to 0.5 mg.

E. coli protein stock solution A solution obtained by culturing a bacteria that contains a plasmid lacking the teceleukin gene but is otherwise exactly identical to the teceleukin-producing E. coli strain in every function except teceleukin production, and then purified using a purification technique that is more simple than that for teceleukin. Determine the amount of protein by Bradford method using bovine serum albumin as the standard substance. Store shielded from light at −70°C.

Edaravone for assay $C_{10}H_{10}N_2O$ [Same as the monograph Edaravone. When dried, it contains not less than 99.5% of edaravone ($C_{10}H_{10}N_2O$).]

Egg albumin for gel filtration molecular mass marker Obtained from chicken egg white, for gel filtration chromatography.

Elderberry lectin It is a lectin derived from the Japan or Western elderberry, specifically recognizes a sugar chain with sialic acid is bound to end by α-2, 6 linkage.

Elderberry lectin TS Dilute biotin-labeled elderberry lectin with 0.01 mol/L tris buffer solution-sodium chloride TS (pH 7.4) so that the concentration is 10 μg/mL. Prepare before use.

Eleutheroside B for liquid chromatography $C_{17}H_{24}O_9$ A white crystalline powder. Sparingly soluble in methanol, slightly soluble in water, and very slightly soluble in ethanol (99.5). Melting point: 190 - 194°C.

Identification—Determine the absorption spectrum of a solution of eleutheroside B for liquid chromatography in methanol (1 in 200,000) as directed under Ultraviolet-visible Spectrophotometry <2.24>: it exhibits a maximum between 263 nm and 267 nm.

Purity Related substances—Dissolve 1.0 mg of eleutheroside B for liquid chromatography in 10 mL of the mobile phase, and use this solution as the sample solution. Pipet 1 mL of the sample solution, add the mobile phase to make exactly 50 mL, and use this solution as the standard solution. Perform the test with exactly 10 μL each of the sample solution and standard solution as directed under Liquid Chromatography <2.01> according to the following conditions. Determine each peak area by the automatic integration method: the total area of the peaks other than eleutheroside B obtained from the sample solution is not larger than the peak area of eleutheroside B from the standard solution.

Operating conditions

Detector, column, column temperature, mobile phase, and flow rate: Proceed as directed in the operating conditions in the Identification under Eleutherococcus Senticosus Rhizome.

Time span of measurement: About 3 times as long as the retention time of eleutheroside B, beginning after the solvent peak.

System suitability

System performance: Proceed as directed in the system suitability in the Identification under Eleutherococcus Senticosus Rhizome.

Test for required detectability: To exactly 1 mL of the standard solution add the mobile phase to make exactly 20 mL. Confirm that the peak area of eleutheroside B obtained with 10 μL of this solution is equivalent to 3.5 to 6.5% of that with 10 μL of the standard solution.

EMB plate medium Melt eosin methylene blue agar medium by heating, and cool to about 50°C. Transfer about 20 mL of this medium to a Petri dish, and solidify horizontally. Place the dish with the cover slightly opened in the incubator to evaporate the inner vapor and water on the plate.

Emedastine fumarate for assay $C_{17}H_{26}N_4O.2C_4H_4O_4$ [Same as the monograph Emedastine Fumarate. When dried it contains not less than 99.5% of emedastine fumarate ($C_{17}H_{26}N_4O.2C_4H_4O_4$).]

Emetine hydrochloride for assay $C_{29}H_{40}N_2O_4.2HCl$ A white or light-yellow crystalline powder. Soluble in water.

Absorbance <2.24> $E^{1\%}_{1\,cm}$ (283 nm): 116 - 127 (10 mg, diluted methanol (1 in 2), 400 mL). [after drying in a desiccator (in vacuum, phosphorus (V) oxide, 50°C) for 5 hours].

Melting point <2.60>: about 250°C [with decomposition, after drying in a desiccator (in vacuum, phosphorus (V) oxide, 50°C) for 5 hours].

Purity Related substances—Dissolve 10 mg of emetine hydrochloride for assay in 10 mL of the mobile phase, and use this solution as the sample solution. Pipet 1 mL of the sample solution, add the mobile phase to make exactly 100 mL, and use this solution as the standard solution. Perform the test with exactly 10 μL each of the sample solution and standard solution as directed under Liquid Chromatography <2.01> according to the following conditions. Determine the peak areas from both solutions by the automatic integration method: the total area of peaks other than emetine obtained from the sample solution is not larger than the peak of emetine from the standard solution.

Operating conditions

Detector, column, column temperature, mobile phase, and flow rate: Proceed as directed in the operating conditions in the Assay under Ipecac.

Time span of measurement: About 3 times as long as the retention time of emetine.

System suitability

System performance and System repeatability: Proceed as directed in the system suitability in the Assay under Ipecac.

Test for required detectability: Pipet 1 mL of the standard solution, add the mobile phase to make exactly 20 mL. Confirm that the peak area of emetine obtained with 10 μL of this solution is equivalent to 3.5 to 6.5% of that with 10 μL of the standard solution.

Emetime hydrochloride for component determination See emetine hydrochloride for assay.

Emorfazone for assay $C_{11}H_{17}N_3O_3$ [Same as the monograph Emorfazone. When dried, it contains not less than 99.0% of emorfazone ($C_{11}H_{17}N_3O_3$).]

Enalapril maleate $C_{20}H_{28}N_2O_5.C_4H_4O_4$ [Same as the namesake monograph]

Endo's medium Melt 1000 mL of the ordinary agar medium by heating in a water bath, and adjust the pH to between 7.5 and 7.8. Add 10 g of lactose monohydrate previously dissolved in a small quantity of water, mix thoroughly, and add 1 mL of fuchsin-ethanol TS. After cooling to about 50°C, add dropwise a freshly prepared solution of sodium sulfite heptahydrate (1 in 10) until a light red color develops owing to reducing fuchsin, requiring about 10 to 15 mL of a solution of sodium sulfite heptahydrate (1 in 10). Dispense the mixture, and sterilize fractionally on each of three successive days for 15 minutes at 100°C.

Endo's plate medium Melt Endo's medium by heating, and cool to about 50°C. Transfer about 20 mL of this medium to a Petri dish, and solidify horizontally. Place the dishes with the cover slightly opened in the incubator to evaporate the inner vapor and water on the surface of the agar.

Enflurane $C_3H_2ClF_5O$ [Same as the namesake monograph]

Enzyme TS The supernatant liquid is obtained as follows: To 0.3 g of an enzyme preparation potent in amylolytic and phosphorolytic activities, obtained from *Aspergillus oryzae*, add 10 mL of water and 0.5 mL of 0.1 mol/L hydrochloric acid TS, mix vigorously for a few minutes, and centrifuge. Prepare before use.

Enzyme TS for glucagon Dissolve 2 mg of α-chymotrypsin in 1 mL of 0.1 mol/L ammonium hydrogen carbonate TS.

Eosin See eosin Y.

Eosin Y $C_{20}H_6Br_4Na_2O_5$ Red, masses or powder.

Identification—To 10 mL of a solution (1 in 1000) add 1 drop of hydrochloric acid: yellow-red precipitates appear.

Eosin methylene blue agar medium Dissolve by boiling 10 g of casein peptone, 2 g of dipotassium hydrogenphosphate and 25 to 30 g of agar in about 900 mL of water. To this mixture add 10 g of lactose monohydrate, 20 mL of a solution of eosin Y(1 in 50), 13 mL of a solution of methylene blue (1 in 200) and warm water to make 1000 mL. Mix thoroughly, dispense, sterilize by autoclaving at 121°C for not more than 20 minutes, and cool quickly by immersing in cold water, or sterilize fractionally on each of three successive days for 30 minutes at 100°C.

Ephedrine hydrochloride $C_{10}H_{15}NO.HCl$ [Same as the namesake monograph]

Ephedrine hydrochloride for assay See ephedrine hydrochloride.

Ephedrine hydrochloride for assay of crude drugs $C_{10}H_{15}NO.HCl$ Ephedrine hydrochloride for assay or the substance that complies with the following requirements.

White, crystals or crystalline powder. Freely soluble in water, and soluble in ethanol (95).

Identification—Determine the infrared absorption spectrum of ephedrine hydrochloride for assay of crude drugs, previously dried, as directed in the potassium chloride disk method under Infrared Spectrophotometry <2.25>, and compare the spectrum with the Reference Spectrum of Ephedrine Hydrochloride: both spectra exhibit similar intensities of absorption at the same wave numbers.

Optical rotation <2.49> $[\alpha]_D^{20}$: −33.0 – −36.0° (after drying, 0.1 g, water, 2 mL, 100 mm).

Melting point <2.60>: 218 – 222°C

Purity Related substances—Dissolve 10 mg of ephedrine hydrochloride for assay of crude drugs in 10 mL of the mobile phase, and use this solution as the sample solution. Pipet 1 mL of the sample solution, add the mobile phase to make exactly 100 mL, and use this solution as the standard solution. Perform the test with exactly 10 μL each of the sample solution and standard solution as directed under Liquid Chromatography <2.01> according to the following conditions. Determine each peak area by the automatic integration method: the total area of the peaks other than ephedrine obtained from the sample solution is not larger than the peak area of ephedrine from the standard solution.

Operating conditions

Detector, column, column temperature, mobile phase, and flow rate: Proceed as directed in the operating conditions in the Assay under Ephedra Herb.

Time span of measurement: About 3 times as long as the retention time of ephedrine, beginning after the solvent peak.

System suitability

System performance and system repeatability: Proceed as directed in the system suitability in the Assay under Ephedra Herb.

Test for required detectability: Pipet 1 mL of the standard solution, and add the mobile phase to make exactly 20 mL. Confirm that the peak area of ephedrine obtained with 10 μL of this solution is equivalent to 3.5 to 6.5% of that with 10 μL of the standard solution.

Loss on drying <2.41>: Not more than 0.5% (0.1 g, 105°C, 3 hours).

6-Epidoxycycline hydrochloride $C_{22}H_{24}N_2O_8.HCl$ Yellow to dark yellow, crystals or crystalline powder.

Purity Related substances—Dissolve 20 mg of 6-epidoxycycline hydrochloride in 25 mL of 0.01 mol/L hydrochloric acid TS, and use this solution as the sample solution. Proceed the test with 20 μL of the sample solution as directed in the Purity (2) under Doxycycline Hydrochloride Hydrate, determine each peak area by the automatic integration method, and calculate the amounts of them by the area percentage method: the total area of the peaks other than 6-epidoxycycline is not more than 10%.

4-Epioxytetracycline $C_{22}H_{24}N_2O_9$ Green-brown to brown powder.

Purity Related substances—Dissolve 20 mg of 4-epioxytetracycline in 25 mL of 0.01 mol/L hydrochloric acid TS, and use this solution as the sample solution. Proceed the test with 20 μL of the sample solution as directed in the Purity (2) under Oxytetracycline Hydrochloride, determine each peak area by the automatic integration method, and calculate the amounts of them by the area percentage method: the total amount of the peaks other than 4-epioxytetracycline is not more than 10%.

Eriochrome black T $C_{20}H_{12}N_3NaO_7S$ [K 8736, Special class]

Eriochrome black T-sodium chloride indicator Mix 0.1 g of eriochrome black T and 10 g of sodium chloride, and triturate until the mixture becomes homogeneous.

Eriochrome black T TS Dissolve 0.3 g of eriochrome black T and 2 g of hydroxylammonium chloride in methanol to make 50 mL. Use within 1 week. Preserve in light-resistant containers.

Erythromycin B $C_{37}H_{67}NO_{12}$ White to light yellow-white powder.

Purity Related substances—Dissolve 10 mg of erythromycin B in 1 mL of methanol, add a mixture of phosphate buffer solution (pH 7.0) and methanol (15:1) to make 5 mL, and use this solution as the sample solution. Pipet 1 mL of the sample solution, add a mixture of phosphate buffer solution (pH 7.0) and methanol (15:1) to make exactly 20 mL, and use this solution as the standard solution. Proceed with exactly 100 μL each of the sample solution and standard solution as directed in the Purity (3) under Erythromycin, and determine each peak area from the solutions by the automatic integration method: the total of areas of the peaks other than erythromycin B obtained from the sample solution is not more than the peak area of erythromycin B from the standard solution.

Erythromycin C $C_{36}H_{65}NO_{13}$ White to light yellow-white powder.

Purity Related substances—Dissolve 10 mg of erythromycin C in 1 mL of methanol, add a mixture of phosphate buffer solution (pH 7.0) and methanol (15:1) to make 5 mL, and use this solution as the sample solution. Pipet 1 mL of the sample solution, add a mixture of phosphate buffer solution (pH 7.0) and methanol (15:1) to make exactly 20 mL, and use this solution as the standard solution. Proceed with exactly 100 μL each of the sample solution and standard solution as directed in the Purity (3) under Erythromycin, and determine each peak area from the solutions by the automatic integration method: the total of areas of the peaks other than erythromycin C obtained from the sample solution is not more than the peak area of erythromycin C from the standard solution.

Essential oil Same as the essential oil under the monograph.

Etacrynic acid for assay $C_{13}H_{12}Cl_2O_4$ [Same as the monograph Etacrynic acid. When dried, it contains not less than 99.0% of etacrynic acid ($C_{13}H_{12}Cl_2O_4$).]

Ethanol See ethanol (95).

Ethanol (95) C_2H_5OH [K 8102, Special class]

Ethanol (95), methanol-free Perform the test for methanol, by using this methanol-free ethanol (95) in place of the standard solution, as directed in Methanol Test <*1.12*>: it is practically colorless.

Ethanol (99.5) C_2H_5OH [K 8101, Special class]

Ethanol (99.5) for liquid chromatography C_2H_5OH A clear, colorless liquid, miscible with water.

Purity Ultraviolet absorbing substance—Perform the test as directed under Ultraviolet-visible Spectrophotometry <*2.24*> using water as the blank: the absorbances at 210 nm, at 220 nm, at 230 nm, at 240 nm, at 254 nm and at 260 nm are not more than 0.70, 0.40, 0.20, 0.10, 0.02 and 0.01, respectively.

Ethanol, aldehyde-free Transfer 1000 mL of ethanol (95) to a glass-stoppered bottle, add the solution prepared by dissolving 2.5 g of lead (II) acetate trihydrate in 5 mL of water, and mix thoroughly. In a separate container, dissolve 5 g of potassium hydroxide in 25 mL of warm ethanol (95), cool, and add this solution gently, without stirring, to the first solution. After 1 hour, shake this mixture vigorously, allow to stand overnight, decant the supernatant liquid, and distil the ethanol.

Ethanol, dehydrated See ethanol (99.5).

Ethanol, dilute To 1 volume of ethanol (95) add 1 volume of water.

Ethanol, diluted Prepare by diluting ethanol (99.5).

Ethanol for alcohol number determination See Alcohol Number Determination <*1.01*>.

Ethanol for disinfection [Same as the namesake monograph]

Ethanol for gas chromatography Use ethanol prepared by distilling ethanol (99.5) with iron (II) sulfate heptahydrate. Preserve in containers, in which the air has been displaced with nitrogen, in a dark, cold place.

Ethanol-free chloroform See chloroform, ethanol-free.

Ethanol-isotonic sodium chloride solution To 1 volume of ethanol (95) add 19 volumes of isotonic sodium chloride solution.

Ethanol, methanol-free See ethanol (95), methanol-free.

Ethanol, neutralized To a suitable quantity of ethanol (95) add 2 to 3 drops of phenolphthalein TS, then add 0.01 mol/L or 0.1 mol/L sodium hydroxide VS until a light red color develops. Prepare before use.

Ethenzamide $C_9H_{11}NO_2$ [Same as the namesake monograph].

Ether See diethyl ether.

Ether, anesthetic $C_2H_5OC_2H_5$ [Same as the namesake monograph]

Ether, dehydrated See diethyl ether, dehydrated.

Ether for purity of crude drug See diethyl ether for purity of crude drug.

Ethinylestradiol $C_{20}H_{24}O_2$ [Same as the namesake monograph]

4′-Ethoxyacetophenone $C_2H_5OC_6H_4COCH_3$ White crystals.

Melting point <*2.60*>: 37 – 39°C

3-Ethoxy-4-hydroxybenzaldehyde $C_9H_{10}O_3$ White to pale yellow-white crystalline. Freely soluble in ethanol (95), and slightly soluble in water.

Melting point <*2.60*>: 76 – 78°C

Content: not less than 98.0%. Assay—Weigh accurately about 0.3 g of 3-ethoxy-4-hydroxybenzaldehyde, previously dried in a desiccator (phosphorous (V) oxide) for 4 hours, dissolve in 50 mL of *N*,*N*-dimethylformamide, and titrate <*2.50*> with 0.1 mol/L sodium methoxide VS (indicator: thymol blue TS).

Each mL of 0.1 mol/L sodium methoxide VS
= 16.62 mg of $C_9H_{10}O_3$

***p*-Ethoxyphenol** See 4-ethoxyphenol.

4-Ethoxyphenol $C_8H_{10}O_2$ White to light yellow-brown, crystals or crystalline powder. Freely soluble in ethanol (95), and very slightly soluble in water.

Melting point <2.60>: 62 – 68°C

Purity—Dissolve 0.5 g of 4-Ethoxyphenol in 5 mL of ethanol (95), and use this solution as the sample solution. Perform the test with 1 μL of the sample solution as directed under Gas Chromatography <2.02> according to the following conditions. Measure each peak area by the automatic integration method and calculate the amount of substance other than 4-ethoxyphenol by the area percentage method: it is not more than 2.0%.

Operating conditions

Detector: Thermal conductivity detector.

Column: A glass column about 3 mm in inside diameter and about 2 m in length, packed with 180 to 250 μm siliceous earth for gas chromatography coated with methylsilicone polymer for gas chromatography.

Column temperature: A constant temperature of about 150°C.

Carrier gas: Helium.

Flow rate: Adjust so that the retention time of 4-ethoxyphenol is about 5 minutes.

Detection sensitivity: Adjust the detection sensitivity so that the peak height of 4-ethoxyphenol obtained with μL of the sample solution is not less than 50% of the full scale.

Time span of measurement: 3 times as long as the retention time of 4-ethoxyphenol, beginning after the solvent peak.

Ethyl acetate $CH_3COOC_2H_5$ [K 8361, Special class]

Ethylamine hydrochloride $C_2H_5NH_2.HCl$ White to light yellow-brown, crystals or crystalline powder, having a deliquescency.

Ethyl aminobenzoate $C_9H_{11}NO_2$ [Same as the namesake monograph]

Ethylbenzene $C_6H_5C_2H_5$ A colorless liquid. Freely soluble in ethanol (99.5) and in acetone, and practically insoluble in water.

Specific gravity <2.56> d_4^{20}: 0.862 – 0.872

Boiling point <2.57>: about 135°C

Ethyl benzoate $C_6H_5COOC_2H_5$ Clear, colorless liquid.

Refractive index <2.45> n_D^{20}: 1.502 – 1.507

Specific gravity <2.56> d_{20}^{20}: 1.045 – 1.053

Ethyl *n*-caprylate $C_{10}H_{20}O_2$ Clear and colorless to almost colorless liquid.

Specific gravity <2.56> d_{20}^{20}: 0.864 – 0.871

Purity Related substances—Dissolve 0.10 g of ethyl *n*-caprylate in 10 mL of dichloromethane and use this solution as the sample solution. Pipet 1 mL of the sample solution, add dichloromethane to make exactly 100 mL, and use this solution as the standard solution (1). Perform the test with exactly 5 μL each of the sample solution and standard solution (1) as directed under Gas Chromatography <2.02> according to the following conditions, and determine each peak area from these solutions by the automatic integration method: the total peak areas other than ethyl *n*-caprylate obtained from the sample solution is not larger than the peak area of ethyl *n*-caprylate from the standard solution (1).

Operating conditions

Proceed the operating conditions in the Assay under Mentha Oil except time span of measurement.

Time span of measurement: 3 times as long as the retention time of ethyl *n*-caprylate, beginning after the solvent peak.

System suitability

Test for required detectability: Pipet 1 mL of the standard solution (1), add dichloromethane to make exactly 20 mL, and use this solution as the standard solution (2). Adjust the detection sensitivity so that the peak area of ethyl *n*-caprylate obtained with 5 μL of the standard solution (2) can be measured by the automatic integration method and the peak height of ethyl *n*-caprylate with 5 μL of the standard solution (1) is about 20% of the full scale.

Ethyl carbamate $H_2NCOOC_2H_5$ White, crystals or powder.

Melting point <2.60>: 48 – 50°C

Purity Clarity of solution—Dissolve 5 g of ethyl carbamate in 20 mL of water: the solution is clear.

Ethyl cyanoacetate $NCCH_2COOC_2H_5$ Colorless or light yellow, clear liquid, having an aromatic odor. Specific gravity d_{20}^{20}: about 1.08.

Identification—To 0.5 mL of a solution of ethyl cyanoacetate in ethanol (99.5) (1 in 10,000) add a mixture of 1 mL of a solution of quinhydrone in diluted ethanol (99.5) (1 in 2) (1 in 20,000) and 1 drop of ammonia solution (28): a light blue color develops.

Ethylenediamine $C_2H_8N_2$ [Same as the namesake monograph]

Ethylenediamine TS Dissolve 70 g of ethylenediamine in 30 g of water.

Ethylene glycol $HOCH_2CH_2OH$ [K 8105, Special class]

Ethylene glycol for water determination Distil ethylene glycol, and collect the fraction distilling between 195°C and 198°C. The water content is not more than 1.0 mg per mL.

Ethylene oxide A colorless flammable gas. Use ethylene oxide from a metal cylinder.

Boiling point <2.57>: 9 – 12°C

Ethyl formate $HCOOC_2H_5$ A clear and colorless liquid. Miscible with ethanol (95) and with acetone, and soluble in water.

Identification—Determine the infrared absorption spectrum of ethyl formate as directed in the liquid film method under Infrared Spectrophotometry <2.25>: it exhibits absorption at the wave numbers of about 2980 cm^{-1}, 2930 cm^{-1}, 1718 cm^{-1}, 1470 cm^{-1}, 1449 cm^{-1}, 1387 cm^{-1}, 1302 cm^{-1}, 1181 cm^{-1}, 1004 cm^{-1}, 840 cm^{-1} and 747 cm^{-1}.

Purity—(1) Perform the test with 1 μL of ethyl formate as directed under Gas Chromatography <2.02> according to the following conditions, determine each peak area by the automatic integration method, and calculate the amount of ethyl formate by the area percentage method: not less than 97.0%.

Operating conditions

Detector: A thermal conductivity detector.

Column: A fused silica column 0.25 mm in inside diameter and 30 m in length, coated the inside surface with a layer about 0.25 μm thick of polyethylene glycol 20M for gas chromatography.

Column temperature: Maintain at 50°C for 1 minute after injecting sample, raise the temperature to 150°C at the rate of 10°C per minute, and maintain at 150°C for 1 minute.

Carrier gas: Helium.

Flow rate: 41 cm per second.
Split ratio: 1:110.
Time span of measurement: About 5 times as long as the retention time of ethyl formate.

(2) Acid (as formic acid) Dissolve 0.5 g of potassium iodate and 5 g of potassium iodide in 50 mL of water, and add 2 g of ethyl formate. After allowing to stand for 10 minutes, add 2 drops of starch TS and 1.30 mL of 0.1 mol/L sodium thiosulfate VS: the solution is colorless (not more than 0.3%).

Water <*2.48*>: not more than 0.5% (1 g, coulometric titration).

2-Ethylhexyl parahydroxybenzoate $C_{15}H_{22}O_3$ Pale yellow, clear viscous liquid. Miscible with methanol (99.5). Practically insoluble in water.

Content: not less than 98.0%. Assay—Weigh accurately about 1 g of 2-ethylhexyl parahydroxybenzoate, add exactly 20 mL of 1 mol/L sodium hydroxide VS, heat at about 70°C for 1 hour, and immediately cool in ice. Titrate <*2.50*> the excess sodium hydroxide with 0.5 mol/L sulfuric acid VS up to the second equivalent point (potentiometric titration). Perform a blank determination in the same manner.

Each mL of 1 mol/L sodium hydroxide VS
= 250.3 mg of $C_{15}H_{22}O_3$

Ethyl iodide See iodoethane.

***N*-Ethylmaleimide** $C_6H_7NO_2$ White crystals, having a pungent, characteristic odor. Freely soluble in ethanol (95), and slightly soluble in water.

Melting point <*2.60*>: 43 – 46°C

Purity Clarity and color of solution—Dissolve 1 g of *N*-ethylmaleimide in 20 mL of ethanol (95): the solution is clear and colorless.

Content: not less than 99.0%. Assay—Dissolve about 0.1 g of *N*-ethylmaleimide, accurately weighed, in 20 mL of ethanol (95), add exactly 20 mL of 0.1 mol/L sodium hydroxide VS, and titrate <*2.50*> with 0.1 mol/L hydrochloric acid VS (indicator: 2 drops of phenolphthalein TS). Perform a blank determination in the same manner.

Each mL of 0.1 mol/L sodium hydroxide VS
= 12.51 mg of $C_6H_7NO_2$

***N*-Ethylmorpholine** $C_6H_{13}NO$ A colorless to yellow-brown liquid.

Refractive index <*2.45*> n_D^{20}: 1.439 – 1.443

Specific gravity <*2.56*> d_4^{20}: 0.908 – 0.916

Ethyl parahydroxybenzoate $HOC_6H_4COOC_2H_5$ [Same as the namesake monograph]

2-Ethyl-2-phenylmalondiamide $C_{11}H_{14}O_2N_2$ White, odorless crystals. Soluble in ethanol (95), and very slightly soluble in water. Melting point: about 120°C (with decomposition).

Purity Related substances—To 5.0 mg of 2-ethyl-2-phenylmalondiamide add 4 mL of pyridine and 1 mL of bis-trimethylsilylacetamide, shake thoroughly, and heat at 100°C for 5 minutes. After cooling, add pyridine to make exactly 10 mL, and use this solution as the sample solution. Perform the test with 2 μL of the sample solution as directed under Gas Chromatography <*2.02*> according to the operating conditions in the Purity (3) under Primidone: any peak other than the peaks of 2-ethyl-2-phenylmalondiamide and the solvent does not appear. Adjust the detection sensitivity so that the peak height of 2-ethyl-2-phenylmalondiamide obtained from 2 μL of the sample solution is about 80% of the full scale, and the time span of measurement is about twice as long as the retention time of 2-ethyl-2-phenylmalondiamide, beginning after the solvent peak.

Ethyl propionate $CH_3CH_2COOC_2H_5$ Colorless, clear liquid.

Specific gravity <*2.56*> d_4^{20}: 0.890 – 0.892

Etidronate disodium for assay $C_2H_6Na_2O_7P_2$ [Same as the monograph Etidronate Disodium. When dried, it contains not less than 99.0% of etidronate disodium ($C_2H_6Na_2O_7P_2$).]

Etilefrine hydrochloride $C_{10}H_{15}NO_2.HCl$ [Same as the namesake monograph]

Etilefrine hydrochloride for assay $C_{10}H_{15}NO_2.HCl$ [Same as the monograph Etilefrine Hydrochloride. When dried, it contains not less than 99.0% of etilefrine hydrochloride ($C_{10}H_{15}NO_2.HCl$).]

Etizolam for assay $C_{17}H_{15}ClN_4S$ [Same as the monograph Etizolam. When dried, it contains not less than 99.0% of etizolam ($C_{17}H_{15}ClN_4S$).]

Eugenol for thin-layer chromatography $C_{10}H_{12}O_2$ Colorless to yellow, clear liquid, having a characteristic odor. Miscible with methanol and with ethanol (99.5), and slightly soluble in water.

Identification—Determine the absorption spectrum of a solution of eugenol for thin-layer chromatography in methanol (1 in 100,000) as directed under Ultraviolet-visible Spectrophotometry <*2.24*>: it exhibits maxima between 227 nm and 231 nm, and between 280 nm and 284 nm.

Purity Related substances—Dissolve 5 mg of eugenol for thin-layer chromatography in 1 mL of methanol. Perform the test with 1 μL of this solution as directed in the Identification under Clove: any spot other than the principal spot with an *Rf* value of about 0.4 does not appear.

Euodia fruit [Same as the namesake monograph]

Evodiamine for assay $C_{19}H_{17}N_3O$ White to light yellow, crystals or crystalline powder. Very slightly soluble in methanol and in ethanol (99.5), and practically insoluble in water. Correct the content based on the amount (%) obtained in the Assay.

Identification—Measure ^{1}H-NMR as directed in the Assay: When the signal of the reference standard for qNMR as δ 0 ppm, it exhibits a double doublet-like signal equivalent to one proton around δ 2.82 ppm, signals equivalent to four protons which includes a singlet signal around δ 2.91 ppm and a multiplet signal around δ 2.90 ppm – δ 2.98 ppm, a double triplet-like signal equivalent to one proton around δ 3.23 ppm, a double doublet-like signal equivalent to one proton around δ 4.66 ppm, a singlet signal equivalent to one proton around δ 6.16 ppm, a triplet-like signal equivalent to one proton around δ 7.00 ppm, a triplet-like signal equivalent to one proton around δ 7.05 ppm, a doublet-like signal equivalent to one proton around δ 7.08 ppm, a triplet-like signal equivalent to one proton around δ 7.14 ppm, a doublet-like signal equivalent to one proton around δ 7.39 ppm, a doublet-like signal equivalent to one proton around δ 7.51 ppm, a multiplet signal equivalent to one proton around δ 7.52 ppm and a double doublet-like signal equivalent to one proton around δ 7.83 ppm.

Unity of peak—Dissolve 1 mg of evodiamine for assay in 20 mL of methanol, and use this solution as the sample solution. Perform the test with 10 μL of the sample solution as directed under Liquid Chromatography <*2.01*> according to the following conditions, and compare the absorption spectra of at least 3 points including the top of evodiamine peak and around the two middle peak heights of before and after the top: no difference in form is observed among their spectra.

Operating conditions

Column, column temperature, mobile phase and flow rate: Proceed as directed in the operating conditions in the Assay (1) under Goshuyuto Extract.

Detector: A photodiode array detector (wavelength: 282 nm: spectrum range of measurement: 220 – 400 nm).

System suitability

System performance: When the procedure is run with 10 μL of the sample solution under the above operating conditions, the number of theoretical plates and the symmetry factor of the peak of evodiamine are not less than 5000 and not more than 1.5, respectively.

Assay—Weigh accurately 5 mg of evodiamine for assay and 1 mg of DSS-d_6 for nuclear magnetic resonance spectroscopy using an ultramicrobalance, dissolve them in 1 mL of deuterated dimethylsulfoxide for nuclear magnetic resonance spectroscopy, and use this solution as the sample solution. Transfer the sample solution into an NMR tube 5 mm in outer diameter, and measure ^{1}H-NMR as directed under Nuclear Magnetic Resonance Spectroscopy <2.21> and Crude Drugs Test <5.01> according to the following conditions, using DSS-d_6 for nuclear magnetic resonance spectroscopy as the reference standard for qNMR. Calculate the resonance intensity A (equivalent to 1 hydrogen) of the signal around δ 6.16 ppm assuming the signal of the reference standard for qNMR as δ 0 ppm.

$$\text{Amount (\%) of evodiamine } (C_{19}H_{17}N_3O) = M_S \times I \times P/(M \times N) \times 1.3521$$

M: Amount (mg) of evodiamine for assay taken

M_S: Amount (mg) of DSS-d_6 for nuclear magnetic resonance spectroscopy taken

I: Signal resonance intensity A based on the signal resonance intensity of DSS-d_6 for nuclear magnetic resonance spectroscopy as 9.000

N: Number of the hydrogen derived from A

P: Purity (%) of DSS-d_6 for nuclear magnetic resonance spectroscopy

Operating conditions

Apparatus: A nuclear magnetic resonance spectrometer having ^{1}H resonance frequency of not less than 400 MHz.

Target nucleus: ^{1}H.

Digital resolution: 0.25 Hz or lower.

Measuring spectrum range: 20 ppm or upper, including between −5 ppm and 15 ppm.

Spinning: off.

Pulse angle: 90°.

^{13}C decoupling: on.

Delay time: Repeating pulse waiting time not less than 60 seconds.

Integrating times: 8 or more times.

Dummy scanning: 2 or more times.

Measuring temperature: A constant temperature between 20°C and 30°C.

System suitability

Test for required detectability: When the procedure is run with the sample solution under the above operating conditions, the SN ratio of the signal around δ 6.16 ppm is not less than 100.

System performance: When the procedure is run with the sample solution under the above operating conditions, the signal around δ 6.16 ppm is not overlapped with any signal of obvious foreign substance.

System repeatability: When the test is repeated 6 times with the sample solution under the above operating conditions, the relative standard deviation of the ratio of the resonance intensity A to that of the reference standard for qNMR is not more than 1.0%.

Factor IIa A lyophilized factor IIa purified from human plasma. A white to pale yellow powder. It contains not less than 2000 IU per mg of protein.

Factor Xa It is prepared from lyophilization of Factor Xa which has been prepared from bovine plasma. White or pale yellow, masses or powder.

Purity Clarity and color of solution—Dissolve 71 n*kat*$_{s\text{-}2222}$ of it in 10 mL water; the solution is clear and colorless or pale yellow.

Content: not less than 75% and not more than 125% of the label.

Factor Xa TS Dissolve 71 n*kat*$_{s\text{-}2222}$ of factor Xa in 10 mL of water.

Famotidine for assay $C_8H_{15}N_7O_2S_3$ [Same as the monograph Famotidine. When dried, it contains not less than 99.0% of famotidine ($C_8H_{15}N_7O_2S_3$), and when proceed as directed in the Purity (3), the total related substance is not more than 0.4%.]

Fatty acid methyl esters mixture TS Dissolve 0.50 g of a mixture of methyl myristate for gas chromatography, methyl palmitate for gas chromatography, methyl palmitoleate for gas chromatography, methyl stearate for gas chromatography, methyl oleate for gas chromatography, methyl linoleate for gas chromatography and methyl linolenate for gas chromatography, corresponding to the composition of Polysorbate 80, in heptane to make 50.0 mL.

Fatty oil Same as the fatty oil under the monograph.

FBS-IMDM Dissolve an amount of the powder for 1 L of Iscove's modified Dulbecco's powder medium, 0.1 g of kanamycin sulfate (not less than 600 μg potency/mg), 3.0 g of sodium hydrogen carbonate and 36 μL of 2-mercapto ethanol solution (1 in 10) in water to make 1000 mL, and sterilize by filtration. To this solution add fetal calf serum, previously heated at 56°C for 30 minutes, so that the concentration of the serum is 10 vol%.

Fehling's TS The copper solution—Dissolve 34.66 g of copper (II) sulfate pentahydrate in water to make 500 mL. Keep this solution in a glass-stoppered bottles in well-filled.

The alkaline tartrate solution—Dissolve 173 g of potassium sodium tartrate tetrahydrate and 50 g of sodium hydroxide in water to make 500 mL. Preserve this solution in a polyethylene container.

Before use, mix equal volumes of both solutions.

Fehling's TS for amylolytic activity test The copper solution—Dissolve 34.660 g of copper (II) sulfate pentahydrate, accurately weighed, in water to make exactly 500 mL. Preserve this solution in well-filled, glass-stoppered bottles.

The alkaline tartrate solution—Dissolve 173 g of potassium sodium tartrate tetrahydrate and 50 g of sodium hydroxide in water to make exactly 500 mL. Preserve this solution in polyethylene containers.

Before use, mix exactly equal volumes of both solutions.

Felbinac for assay $C_{14}H_{12}O_2$ [Same as the monograph Felbinac. When dried, it contains not less than 99.0% of felbinac ($C_{14}H_{12}O_2$).]

Felodipine for assay $C_{18}H_{19}Cl_2NO_4$ [Same as the monograph Felodipine. It contains not less than 99.5% of ferodipine ($C_{18}H_{19}Cl_2NO_4$), calculated on the dried basis.]

Ferric ammonium citrate See ammonium iron (III) citrate.

Ferric ammonium sulfate See ammonium iron (III) sulfate dodecahydrate.

Ferric ammonium sulfate TS See ammonium iron (III) sulfate TS.

Ferric ammonium sulfate TS, dilute See ammonium iron (III) sulfate TS, dilute.

Ferric chloride See iron (III) chloride hexahydrate.

Ferric chloride-acetic acid TS See iron (III) chloride-acetic acid TS.

Ferric chloride-iodine TS See iron (III) chloride-iodine TS.

Ferric chloride-methanol TS See iron (III) chloride-methanol TS.

Ferric chloride-pyridine TS, anhydrous See iron (III) chloride-pyridine TS, anhydrous.

Ferric chloride TS See iron (III) chloride TS.

Ferric chloride TS, acidic See iron (III) chloride TS, acidic.

Ferric chloride TS, dilute See iron (III) chloride TS, dilute.

Ferric nitrate See iron (III) nitrate enneahydrate.

Ferric nitrate TS See iron (III) nitrate TS.

Ferric perchlorate See iron (III) perchlorate hexahydrate.

Ferric perchlorate-dehydrated ethanol TS See iron (III) perchlorate-ethanol TS.

Ferric salicylate TS See Iron salicylate TS

Ferric sulfate See iron (III) sulfate *n*-hydrate.

Ferric sulfate TS See iron (III) sulfate TS.

Ferrous ammonium sulfate See ammonium iron (II) sulfate hexahydrate.

Ferrous sulfate See iron (II) sulfate heptahydrate.

Ferrous sulfate TS See iron (II) sulfate TS.

Ferrous sulfide See iron (II) sulfide.

Ferrous tartrate TS See iron (II) tartrate TS.

Ferrous thiocyanate TS See iron (II) thiocyanate TS.

Ferrous trisodium pentacyanoamine TS See iron (II) trisodium pentacyanoamine TS.

(*E*)-Ferulic acid $C_{10}H_{10}O_4$ White to light yellow, crystals or crystalline powder. Freely soluble in methanol, soluble in ethanol (99.5), and practically insoluble in water. Melting point: 173 – 176°C.

Identification—Determine the absorption spectrum of a solution in methanol (1 in 200,000) as directed under Ultraviolet-visible Spectrophotometry <*2.24*>: it exhibits maxima between 215 nm and 219 nm, between 231 nm and 235 nm, and between 318 nm and 322 nm.

Purity Related substances—Conduct this procedure without exposure to light, using light-resistant vessels. Dissolve 1 mg of (*E*)-ferulic acid in 1 mL of methanol, and use this solution as the sample solution. Perform the test with the sample solution as directed under Thin-layer Chromatography <*2.03*>. Spot 2 μL of the sample solution on a plate of silica gel for thin-layer chromatography. Develop the plate with a mixture of ethyl acetate, acetone and water (20:12:3) to a distance of about 7 cm, and air-dry the plate. Spray evenly dilute sulfuric acid on the plate, and heat the plate at 105°C for 5 minutes. Examine under ultraviolet light (main wavelength: 365 nm): no spot appears other than the principle spot at the *Rf* value of about 0.6.

(*E*)-Ferulic acid for assay $C_{10}H_{10}O_4$ Use (*E*)-Ferulic acid. It meets the requirements of the following 1) (*E*)-ferulic acid for assay 1 or 2) (*E*)-ferulic acid for assay 2 (Purity value by qNMR). The former is used after drying in a desiccator (silica gel) for 24 hours, and latter is used with correction for its amount based on the result obtained in the Assay.

1) (*E*)-Ferulic acid for assay 1

Absorbance <*2.24*> $E^{1\%}_{1\,cm}$ (320 nm): 878 – 969 (5 mg, methanol, 1000 mL).

Purity Related substances—Conduct this procedure without exposure to light, using light-resistant vessels. Dissolve 5 mg of (*E*)-ferulic acid for assay 1 in 10 mL of a mixture of water and methanol (1:1), and use this solution as the sample solution. Pipet 1 mL of the sample solution, add a mixture of water and methanol (1:1) to make exactly 100 mL, and use this solution as the standard solution. Perform the test with exactly 10 μL each of the sample solution and standard solution as directed under Liquid Chromatography <*2.01*> according to the following conditions, and determine each peak area by the automatic integration method: the total area of the peaks other than (*E*)-ferulic acid obtained from the sample solution is not larger than the peak area of (*E*)-ferulic acid from the standard solution.

Operating conditions

Detector, column, column temperature, mobile phase and flow rate: Proceed as directed in the operating conditions in the Assay (1) under Tokishakuyakusan Extract.

Time span of measurement: About 6 times as long as the retention time of (*E*)-ferulic acid, beginning after the solvent peak.

System suitability

Test for required detectability: Pipet 1 mL of the standard solution, and add a mixture of water and methanol (1:1) to make exactly 20 mL. Confirm that the peak area of (*E*)-ferulic acid obtained with 10 μL of this solution is equivalent to 3.5 to 6.5% of that with 10 μL of the standard solution.

System performance: When the procedure is run with 10 μL of the standard solution under the above operating conditions, the number of theoretical plates and the symmetry factor of the peak of (*E*)-ferulic acid are not less than 5000 and not more than 1.5, respectively.

System repeatability: When the test is repeated 6 times with 10 μL of the standard solution under the above operating conditions, the relative standard deviation of the peak area of (*E*)-ferulic acid is not more than 1.5%.

2) (*E*)-Ferulic acid for assay 2 (Purity value by quantitative NMR)

Unity of peak—Conduct this procedure without exposure to light, using light-resistant vessels. Dissolve 5 mg of (*E*)-ferulic acid for assay 2 in 10 mL of a mixture of water and methanol (1:1), and use this solution as the sample solution. Perform the test with 10 μL of the sample solution as directed under Liquid Chromatography <*2.01*> according to the following conditions, and compare the absorption spectra of at least 3 points including the top of (*E*)-ferulic acid peak and around the two middle peak heights of before and after the top: no difference in form is observed among their spectra.

Operating conditions

Column, column temperature, mobile phase and flow rate: Proceed as directed in the operating conditions in the Assay (1) under Tokishakuyakusan Extract.

Detector: A photodiode array detector (wavelength: 320 nm, spectrum range of measurement: 220 – 400 nm).

System suitability

System performance: When the procedure is run with 10 μL of the sample solution under the above operating conditions, the number of theoretical plates and the symmetry factor of the peak of (*E*)-ferulic acid are not less than 5000 and not more than 1.5, respectively.

Assay—Weigh accurately 5 mg of (*E*)-ferulic acid for assay 2 and 1 mg of 1,4-BTMSB-d_4 for nuclear magnetic resonance spectroscopy using an ultramicrobalance, dissolve in 1 mL of deuterated methanol for nuclear magnetic resonance spectroscopy, and use this solution as the sample solution. Transfer the sample solution into an NMR tube 5 mm in outer diameter, and measure ^{1}H-NMR as directed under Nuclear Magnetic Resonance Spectroscopy <*2.21*> and Crude Drugs Test <*5.01*> according to the following conditions, using 1,4-BTMSB-d_4 for nuclear magnetic resonance spectroscopy as the reference standard for qNMR. Calculate the resonance intensity *A* (equivalent to 1 hydrogen) of the signal around δ 6.06 ppm assuming the signal of the reference standard for qNMR as δ 0 ppm.

$$\text{Amount (\%) of } (E)\text{-ferulic acid } (C_{10}H_{10}O_4) = M_S \times I \times P/(M \times N) \times 0.8573$$

M: Amount (mg) of (*E*)-ferulic acid for assay 2 taken

M_S: Amount (mg) of 1,4-BTMSB-d_4 for nuclear magnetic resonance spectroscopy taken

I: Signal resonance intensity *A* based on the signal resonance intensity of 1,4-BTMSB-d_4 for nuclear magnetic resonance spectroscopy as 18.000

N: Number of hydrogen derived from *A*

P: Purity (%) of 1,4-BTMSB-d_4 for nuclear magnetic resonance spectroscopy

Operating conditions

Apparatus: A nuclear magnetic resonance spectrometer having ^{1}H resonance frequency of not less than 400 MHz.

Target nucleus: ^{1}H.

Digital resolution: 0.25 Hz or lower.

Measuring spectrum range: 20 ppm or upper, including between − 5 ppm and 15 ppm.

Spinning: off.

Pulse angle: 90°.

^{13}C decoupling: on.

Delay time: Repeating pulse waiting time not less than 60 seconds.

Integrating times: 8 or more times.

Dummy scanning: 2 or more times.

Measuring temperature: A constant temperature between 20°C and 30°C.

System suitability

Test for required detectability: When the procedure is run with the sample solution under the above operating conditions, the SN ratio of the signal around δ 6.06 ppm is not less than 100.

System performance: When the procedure is run with the sample solution under the above operating conditions, the signal around δ 6.06 ppm is not overlapped with any signal of obvious foreign substances.

System repeatability: When the test is repeated 6 times with the sample solution under the above operating conditions, the relative standard deviation of the ratio of the resonance intensity *A* to that of the reference standard for qNMR is not more than 1.0%.

Fetal calf serum Serum obtained from fetal calves. Interleukin-2 dependent cell growth suppression substance is removed by heat at 56°C for 30 min before use.

Fibrinogen Fibrinogen is prepared from human or bovine blood by fractional precipitation with ethanol or ammonium sulfate. It may contain citrate, oxalate and sodium chloride. A white amorphous solid. Add 1 mL of isotonic sodium chloride solution to 10 mg of fibrinogen. It, when warmed to 37°C, dissolves with a slight turbidity, and clots on the subsequent addition of 1 unit of thrombin.

1st Fluid for disintegration test See 1st fluid for dissolution test.

1st Fluid for dissolution test Dissolve 2.0 g of sodium chloride in 7.0 mL of hydrochloric acid and water to make 1000 mL. It is clear and colorless, and has a pH of about 1.2.

Fixed oil Same as the vegetable oils under the monograph.

FL cell Established cell strain derived from normal human amnion. Subculture the cells in Eagle's minimum essential medium containing bovine serum.

Flecainide acetate $C_{17}H_{20}F_6N_2O_3.C_2H_4O_2$ [Same as the namesake monograph]

Flecainide acetate for assay $C_{17}H_{20}F_6N_2O_3.C_2H_4O_2$ [Same as the monograph Flecainide Acetate. When dried, it contains not less than 99.0% of flecainide acetate ($C_{17}H_{20}F_6N_2O_3.C_2H_4O_2$). Additionally, when perform the test as directed in the Purity (3), the sample solution does not show the spot corresponding to the spot obtained from the standard solution, and when perform the test as directed in the Purity (4), the total area of the peaks other than flecainide obtained from the sample solution is not larger than the peak area of flecainide from the standard solution.]

Flopropione $C_9H_{10}O_4$ [Same as the namesake monograph]

Flopropione for assay $C_9H_{10}O_4$ [Same as the monograph Flopropione. It contains not less than 99.0% of flopropione ($C_9H_{10}O_4$), calculated on the anhydrous basis.]

Fluconazole for assay $C_{13}H_{12}F_2N_6O$ [Same as the monograph Fluconazole]

Fludiazepam for assay $C_{16}H_{12}ClFN_2O$ [Same as the monograph Fludiazepam. It meets the following additional requirements.]

Purity Related substances—Dissolve 25 mg of fludiazepam for assay in 50 mL of a mixture of acetonitrile and water (3:2), and use this solution as the sample solution. Pipet 5 mL of the sample solution, add a mixture of acetonitrile and water (3:2) to make exactly 50 mL. Pipet 2.5 mL of this solution, add a mixture of acetonitrile and water (3:2) to make exactly 50 mL, and use this solution as the standard solution. Perform the test with exactly 20 μL each of the sample solution and standard solution as directed under Liquid Chromatography <*2.01*> according to the following conditions, and determine each peak area by the automatic integration method: the area of the peak other than fludiazepam obtained from the sample solution is not larger than 2/5 times the peak area of fludiazepam from the standard solution, and the total area of the peaks other than fludiazepam from the sample solution is not larger than the peak area of fludiazepam from the standard solution.

Operating conditions

Detector, column, column temperature, mobile phase and flow rate: Proceed as directed in the operating conditions in the Assay under Fludiazepam Tablets.

Time span of measurement: About 4 times as long as the retention time of fludiazepam, beginning after the solvent peak.

System suitability

Test for required detectability: Pipet 1 mL of the standard solution, and add a mixture of acetonitrile and water (3:2) to make exactly 10 mL. Confirm that the peak area of fludiazepam obtained with 20 μL of this solution is equivalent to 7 to 13% of that with 20 μL of the standard solution.

System performance: When the procedure is run with 20 μL of the standard solution under the above operating conditions, the number of theoretical plates and the symmetry factor of the peak of fludiazepam are not less than 6000 and not more than 2.0, respectively.

System repeatability: When the test is repeated 6 times with 20 μL of the standard solution under the above operating conditions, the relative standard deviation of the peak area of fludiazepam is not more than 2.0%.

Fluid thioglycolate medium See the Sterility Test *<4.06>*.

Fluocinolone acetonide $C_{24}H_{30}F_2O_6$ [Same as the namesake monograph]

9-Fluorenylmethyl chloroformate $C_{15}H_{11}ClO_2$ White, crystals or crystalline powder.

Melting point <2.60>: 60 – 63°C

9-Fluorenylmethyl chloroformate $C_{15}H_{11}ClO_2$ Prepared for amino acid analysis or biochemistry.

Fluorescamine $C_{17}H_{10}O_4$ A white powder.

Fluorescein $C_{20}H_{12}O_5$ An yellowish red powder.

Identification—Determine the infrared absorption spectrum as directed in the potassium bromide disk method under Infrared Spectrophotometry *<2.25>*: it exhibits absorption at the wave numbers of about 1597 cm^{-1}, 1466 cm^{-1}, 1389 cm^{-1}, 1317 cm^{-1}, 1264 cm^{-1}, 1247 cm^{-1}, 1213 cm^{-1}, 1114 cm^{-1} and 849 cm^{-1}.

Fluorescein sodium $C_{20}H_{10}Na_2O_5$ [Same as the namesake monograph].

Fluorescein sodium TS Dissolve 0.2 g of fluorescein sodium in water to make 100 mL.

Fluorescence TS Mix 400 μL of sodium dithionite solution containing 6.27 g in 200 mL of water, 210 μL of 2-mercaptoethanol, 321 μL of acetic acid (100), 400 μL of 1,2-diamino-4,5-methylenedioxybenzene solution containing 31.1 mg in 1.0 mL of water and 2669 μL of water. Prepare before use.

4-Fluorobenzoic acid $C_7H_5FO_2$ White, crystals or crystalline powder.

Identification—Determine the infrared absorption spectrum as directed in the potassium bromide disk method under Infrared Spectrophotometry *<2.25>*: it exhibits absorption at the wave numbers of about 1684 cm^{-1}, 1606 cm^{-1} and 1231 cm^{-1}.

Melting point <2.60>: 182 – 188°C

1-Fluoro-2,4-dinitrobenzene $C_6H_3(NO_2)_2F$ Light yellow, liquid or crystalline masses. Melting point: about 25°C.

Identification—Determine the infrared absorption spectrum as directed in the liquid film method as directed under Infrared Spectrophotometry *<2.25>*: it exhibits absorption at the wave numbers of about 3110 cm^{-1}, 1617 cm^{-1}, 1538 cm^{-1}, 1345 cm^{-1}, 1262 cm^{-1} and 743 cm^{-1}.

Storage—Preserve in a light-resistant tight container.

Fluorogenic substrate TS A solution containing oxidation-reduction indicator.

7-Fluoro-4-nitrobenzo-2-oxa-1,3-diazole $C_6H_2FN_3O_3$ Prepared for amino acid analysis or biochemistry.

Fluoroquinolonic acid for thin-layer chromatography $C_{13}H_9ClFNO_3$ A white to light brown powder.

Purity Perform the test with 8 μL of a solution of fluoroquinolonic acid for thin-layer chromatography in acetonitrile (1 in 1250) as directed under Liquid Chromatography *<2.01>* according to the following conditions, determine each peak area by the automatic integration method, and calculate the amount of them by the area percentage method: the amount of the peak of fluoroquinolonic acid is not less than 98.0%.

Operating conditions

Detector: An ultraviolet absorption photometer (wavelength: 263 nm).

Column: A stainless steel column 4 mm in inside diameter and 12.5 cm in length, packed with octadecylsilanized silica gel for liquid chromatography (5 μm in particle diameter).

Column temperature: A constant temperature of about 40°C.

Mobile phase A: Diluted phosphoric acid (1 in 500).

Mobile phase B: Methanol.

Flow of mobile phase: Control the gradient by mixing the mobile phases A and B as directed in the following table.

Time after injection of sample (min)	Mobile phase A (vol%)	Mobile phase B (vol%)
0 – 5.5	60 → 55	40 → 45
5.5 – 14	55 → 25	45 → 75
14 – 15	25 → 15	75 → 85

Flow rate: 1.5 mL per minute (the retention time of fluoroquinolonic acid is about 8 minutes).

Time span of measurement: For 15 minutes after injection, beginning after the solvent peak.

System suitability

System performance: When perform the test with 8 μL of a solution of fluoroquinolonic acid for thin-layer chromatography in acetonitrile (1 in 1250) according to the above operating conditions, the number of theoretical plates and the symmetry factor of the peak of fluoroquinolonic acid are not less than 10,000 and not more than 1.5, respectively.

Flurazepam for assay $C_{21}H_{23}ClFN_3O$ [Same as the monograph Flurazepam. When dried, it contains not less than 99.3%of flurazepam ($C_{21}H_{23}ClFN_3O$).]

Flutoprazepam for assay $C_{19}H_{16}ClFN_2O$ [Same as the monograph Flutoprazepam. When dried, it contains not less than 99.5% of flutoprazepam ($C_{19}H_{16}ClFN_2O$).]

Folic acid $C_{19}H_{19}N_7O_6$ [Same as the namesake monograph]

Folin's TS Place 20 g of sodium tungstate (VI) dihydrate, 5 g of disodium molybdate (VI) dihydrate and about

140 mL of water in a 300-mL volumetric flask, add 10 mL of diluted phosphoric acid (17 in 20) and 20 mL of hydrochloric acid, and boil gently using a reflux condenser with ground-glass joints for 10 hours. To the mixture add 30 g of lithium sulfate monohydrate and 10 mL of water, and then add a very small quantity of bromine to change the deep green color of the solution to yellow. Remove the excess bromine by boiling for 15 minutes without a condenser, and cool. Add water to make 200 mL, and filter through a glass filter. Store it free from dust. Use this solution as the stock solution, and dilute with water to the directed concentration before use.

Folin's TS, dilute Titrate <2.50> Folin's TS with 0.1 mol/L sodium hydroxide VS (indicator: phenolphthalein TS), and determine the acid concentration. Prepare by adding water to Folin's TS so the acid concentration is 1 mol/L.

Formaldehyde solution HCHO [K 8872, Special class]

Formaldehyde solution-sulfuric acid TS Add 1 drop of formaldehyde solution to 1 mL of sulfuric acid. Prepare before use.

Formaldehyde solution TS To 0.5 mL of formaldehyde solution add water to make 100 mL.

Formaldehyde TS, dilute Dilute formaldehyde solution to 10 times its volume with water.

Formalin See formaldehyde solution.

Formalin TS See formaldehyde solution TS.

Formalin-sulfuric acid TS See formaldehyde solution-sulfuric acid TS.

Formamide $HCONH_2$ [K 8873, Special class]

Formamide for water determination $HCONH_2$ [K 8873, Special class; water content per g of formamide for water determination should be not more than 1 mg.]

Formazin opalescence standard solution To 15 mL of formazin stock suspension add water to make 1000 mL. Use within 24 hours after preparation. Shake thoroughly before use.

Formic acid HCOOH [K 8264, Special class, specific gravity: not less than 1.21].

2-Formylbenzoic acid $CHOC_6H_4COOH$ White crystals. Melting point: 97 – 99°C.

Content: not less than 99.0%. Assay—Weigh accurately about 0.3 g of 2-formylbenzoic acid, previously dried (in vacuum, phosphorus (V) oxide, 3 hours), dissolve in 50 mL of freshly boiled and cooled water, and titrate <2.50> with 0.1 mol/L sodium hydroxide VS (indicator: 3 drops of phenol red TS).

Each mL of 0.1 mol/L sodium hydroxide VS
= 15.01 mg of $C_8H_6O_3$

Forsythia fruit [Same as the namesake monograph.]

Freund's complete adjuvant A suspension of 5 mg of mycobacteria of *Corynebacterium butyricum*, killed by heating, in 10 mL of a mixture of mineral oil and arlacel A (17:3).

Fructose $C_6H_{12}O_6$ [Same as the namesake monograph]

Fructose for thin-layer chromatography $C_6H_{12}O_6$ Colorless to white, crystals or crystalline powder. Very soluble in water, and sparingly soluble in ethanol (99.5). It is deliquescence with the atmospheric moisture.

Optical rotation <2.49> $[\alpha]_D^{20}$: −88 – −94° (1 g, diluted ammonia solution (28) (1 in 1000), 100 mL, 100 mm. Previously, dried over silica gel as the desiccant for 3 hours).

Purity Related substances—Dissolve 2 mg of Fructose for thin-layer chromatography in 1 mL of a mixture of water and methanol (1:1), and use this solution as the sample solution. Perform the test with the sample solution as directed under Thin-layer chromatography <2.03>. Spot 2 μL of the sample solution on a plate of silica gel for thin-layer chromatography. Develop the plate with a mixture of 2-propanol, water and methanol (3:2:2) to a distance of about 7 cm, and air-dry the plate. Spray evenly 1,3-naphthalenediol TS to the plate, and heat the plate at 105°C for 10 minutes: any spot other than the principle spot with an *R*f value of about 0.6 does not appear.

Fuchsin A lustrous, green, crystalline powder or mass, slightly soluble in water and in ethanol (95).

Loss on drying <2.41>: 17.5 – 20.0% (1 g, 105°C, 4 hours).

Residue on ignition <2.44>: not more than 0.1% (1 g).

Fuchsin-ethanol TS Dissolve 11 g of fuchsin in 100 mL of ethanol (95).

Fuchsin-sulfurous acid TS Dissolve 0.2 g of fuchsin in 120 mL of hot water, and allow the solution to cool. Add a solution prepared by dissolving 2 g of anhydrous sodium sulfite in 20 mL of water, then add 2 mL of hydrochloric acid and water to make 200 mL, and allow to stand for at least 1 hour. Prepare before use.

Fudosteine for assay $C_6H_{13}NO_3S$ [Same as the monograph Fudosteine]

Fumaric acid for thin-layer chromatography $C_4H_4O_4$ White, crystalline powder, odorless, and has a characteristic acid taste.

Purity—Perform the test as directed in the Identification (5) under Clemastine Fumarate: any spot other than the principal spot at the *R*f value of about 0.8 does not appear.

Fuming nitric acid See nitric acid, fuming.

Fuming sulfuric acid See sulfuric acid, fuming.

Furfural $C_5H_4O_2$ A clear, colorless liquid.

Specific gravity <2.56> d_{20}^{20}: 1.160 – 1.165

Distilling range <2.57>: 160 – 163°C, not less than 95 vol%.

D-Galactosamine hydrochloride $C_6H_{13}NO_5.HCl$ White powder. Melting point: about 180°C (with decomposition).

Optical rotation <2.49> $[\alpha]_D^{20}$: +90 – +97° (1 g, water, 100 mL, 100 mm).

Galactose See D-galactose.

D-Galactose $C_6H_{12}O_6$ White, crystals, granules or powder.

Identification—Determine the infrared absorption spectrum as directed in the potassium bromide disk method under Infrared Spectrophotometry <2.25>: it exhibits absorption at the wave numbers of about 3390 cm^{-1}, 3210 cm^{-1}, 3140 cm^{-1}, 1151 cm^{-1}, 1068 cm^{-1}, 956 cm^{-1}, 836 cm^{-1}, 765 cm^{-1} and 660 cm^{-1}.

Optical rotation <2.49> $[\alpha]_D^{20}$: +79 – +82° (2.5 g after drying for 18 hours in a desiccator (silica gel), diluted ammonia solution (28) (1 in 300), 25 mL, 100 mm).

Gallic acid See gallic acid monohydrate.

Gallic acid monohydrate $C_6H_2(OH)_3COOH.H_2O$ White to pale yellow-white, crystals or powder.

Melting point <*2.60*>: about 260°C (with decomposition).

Gelatin [Same as the monograph Gelatin. It is the gelling grade.]

Gelatin, acid-treated [Same as the monograph Gelatin. It is the gelling grade and its isoelectric point is at pH between 7.0 and 9.0]

Gelatin peptone See peptone, gelatin.

Gelatin-phosphate buffer solution Dissolve 13.6 g of potassium dihydrogen phosphate, 15.6 g of sodium dihydrogen phosphate dihydrate and 1.0 g of sodium azide in water to make 1000 mL, adjust the pH to 3.0 with diluted phosphoric acid (1 in 75) (solution A). Dissolve 5.0 g of acid-treated gelatin in 400 mL of the solution A by warming, after cooling, adjust the pH to 3.0 with diluted phosphoric acid (1 in 75), and add the solution A to make 1000 mL.

Gelatin-phosphate buffer solution (pH 7.0) Dissolve 1.15 g of sodium dihydrogen phosphate dihydrate, 5.96 g of disodium hydrogen phosphate dodecahydrate and 5.4 g of sodium chloride in 500 mL of water. Dissolve 1.2 g of gelatin to this solution by heating, and after cooling add water to make 600 mL.

Gelatin-phosphate buffer solution (pH 7.4) To 50 mL of 0.2 mol/L potassium dihydrogen phosphate TS for buffer solution add 39.50 mL of 0.2 mol/L sodium hydroxide TS and 50 mL of water. Dissolve 0.2 g of gelatin to this solution by heating, then after cooling adjust to pH 7.4 with 0.2 mol/L sodium hydroxide TS, and add water to make 200 mL.

Gelatin-tris buffer solution Dissolve 6.06 g of 2-amino-2-hydroxymethyl-1,3-propanediol and 2.22 g of sodium chloride in 700 mL of water. Separately, dissolve 10 g of acid-treated gelatin in 200 mL of water by warming. After cooling, mix these solutions, and adjust the pH to 8.8 with dilute hydrochloric acid, and add water to make 1000 mL.

Gelatin-tris buffer solution (pH 8.0) Dissolve 40 g of 2-amino-2-hydroxymethyl-1,3-propanediol and 5.4 g of sodium chloride in 500 mL of water. To this solution add 1.2 g of gelatin to dissolve by heating, adjust to pH 8.0 with dilute hydrochloric acid after cooling, and add water to make 600 mL.

Gelatin TS Dissolve 1 g of gelatin in 50 mL of water by gentle heating, and filter if necessary. Prepare before use.

Geniposide for assay $C_{17}H_{24}O_{10}$ Use geniposide for thin-layer chromatography meeting the following additional specifications. Correct the content based on the amount (%) obtained in the Assay.

Unity of peak—Dissolve 5 mg of geniposide for assay in 50 mL of diluted methanol (1 in 2). To 1 mL of this solution add diluted methanol (1 in 2) to make 100 mL, and use this solution as the sample solution. Perform the test with 10 μL of the sample solution as directed under Liquid Chromatography <*2.01*> according to the following conditions, and compare the absorption spectra of at least 3 points including the top of geniposide peak and around the two middle peak heights of before and after the top: no difference in form is observed between their spectra.

Operating conditions

Column, column temperature, mobile phase, and flow rate: Proceed as directed in the operating conditions in the Assay under Gardenia Fruit.

Detector: A photodiode array detector (wavelength: 240 nm, spectrum range of measurement: 220 – 400 nm).

System suitability

System performance: Proceed as directed in the system suitability in the Assay under Gardenia Fruit.

Assay—Weigh accurately 10 mg of geniposide for assay and 1 mg of 1,4-BTMSB-d_4 for nuclear magnetic resonance spectroscopy using an ultramicrobalance, dissolve in 1 mL of deuterated methanol for nuclear magnetic resonance spectroscopy, and use this solution as the sample solution. Transfer the sample solution into an NMR tube 5 mm in outer diameter, measure ^{1}H-NMR as directed under Nuclear Magnetic Resonance Spectroscopy <*2.21*> and Crude Drugs Test <*5.01*> according to the following conditions, using 1,4-BTMSB-d_4 for nuclear magnetic resonance spectroscopy as the reference standard for qNMR. Calculate the resonance intensities, A_1 (equivalent to 1 hydrogen) and A_2 (equivalent to 1 hydrogen), of the signals around δ 3.93 ppm and δ 4.06 ppm assuming the signal of the reference standard for qNMR as δ 0 ppm.

$$\text{Amount (\%) of geniposide } (C_{17}H_{24}O_{10}) = M_S \times I \times P/(M \times N) \times 1.7147$$

M: Amount (mg) of geniposide for assay taken

M_S: Amount (mg) of 1,4-BTMSB-d_4 for nuclear magnetic resonance spectroscopy taken

I: Sum of the signal resonance intensities, A_1 and A_2, based on the signal resonance intensity of 1,4-BTMSB-d_4 for nuclear magnetic resonance spectroscopy as 18.000

N: Sum of number of the hydrogen derived from A_1 and A_2

P: Purity (%) of 1,4-BTMSB-d_4 for nuclear magnetic resonance spectroscopy

Operating conditions

Apparatus: An apparatus of nuclear magnetic resonance spectrum measurement having ^{1}H resonance frequency of not less than 400 MHz.

Target nucleus: ^{1}H.

Digital resolution: 0.25 Hz or lower.

Measuring spectrum range: 20 ppm or upper, including between −5 ppm and 15 ppm.

Spinning: off.

Pulse angle: 90°.

^{13}C decoupling: on.

Delay time: Repeating pulse waiting time not less than 60 seconds.

Integrating times: 8 or more times.

Dummy scanning: 2 or more times.

Measuring temperature: A constant temperature between 20°C and 30°C.

System suitability

Test for required detectability: When the procedure is run with the sample solution under the above operating conditions, the SN ratio of the two signals around δ 3.93 ppm and δ 4.06 ppm is not less than 100.

System performance: When the procedure is run with the sample solution under the above operating conditions, the two signals of around δ 3.93 ppm and δ 4.06 ppm are not overlapped with any signal of obvious foreign substance, and the ratios of the resonance intensities, A_1/A_2, of each signal around δ 3.93 ppm and δ 4.06 ppm are between 0.99 and 1.01, respectively.

System repeatability: When the test is repeated 6 times with the sample solution under the above operating conditions, the relative standard deviation of the ratio of the resonance intensity, A_1 or A_2, to that of the reference standard for qNMR is not more than 1.0%.

Geniposide for component determination See geniposide for assay.

Geniposide for thin-layer chromatography $C_{17}H_{24}O_{10}$ White, crystals or crystalline powder. Freely soluble in water and in methanol, and soluble in ethanol (99.5). Melting point: about 160°C.

Purity Related substances—Dissolve 1.0 mg of geniposide for thin-layer chromatography in exactly 1 mL of methanol, and perform the test with 20 μL of this solution as directed in the Identification (2) under Gardenia Fruit: no spot other than the principal spot at an *R*f value of about 0.3 is observed.

Gentamicin B $C_{19}H_{38}N_4O_{10}$ White to pale yellow-white powder. Very soluble in water, and practically insoluble in ethanol (95).

Content: not less than 80.0%. Assay—Dissolve a suitable amount of gentamicin B in 0.05 mol/L sulfuric acid TS to make the solution containing 0.1 mg of gentamicin B per mL, and use this solution as the sample solution. Perform the test with 5 μL of the sample solution as directed under Liquid Chromatography <2.01> according to the following conditions, and determine each peak area by the automatic integration method. Calculate the amount of gentamicin B by the area percentage method.

Operating conditions

Apparatus, detector, column, column temperature, reaction coil, mobile phase, reagent, reaction temperature, flow rate of the mobile phase, and flow rate of the reagent: Proceed as directed in the operating conditions in the Assay under Isepamicin Sulfate.

Time span of measurement: About 3 times as long as the retention time of gentamicin B.

System suitability

Proceed as directed in the system suitability in the Assay under Isepamicin Sulfate.

Gentiopicroside for thin-layer chromatography $C_{16}H_{20}O_9$ A white powder. Freely soluble in water and in methanol, and practically insoluble in diethyl ether. Melting point: about 110°C (with decomposition).

Purity Related substances—Dissolve 10 mg of gentiopicroside for thin-layer chromatography in 2 mL of methanol, and use this solution as the sample solution. Pipet 1 mL of the sample solution, and methanol to make exactly 100 mL, and use this solution as the standard solution. Perform the test with 10 μL each of the sample solution and standard solution as directed in the Identification (2) under Gentian: the spots other than the principal spot at the *R*f value of about 0.4 from the sample solution are not more intense than the spot from the standard solution.

Gentisic acid $C_7H_6O_4$ Light yellow crystals.

Melting point <2.60>: About 200°C

Giemsa's TS Dissolve 3 g of azure II-eosin Y and 0.8 g of azure II in 250 g of glycerin by warming to 60°C. After cooling, add 250 g of methanol, and mix well. Allow to stand for 24 hours, and filter. Store in tightly stoppered bottles.

Azure II-eosin Y is prepared by coupling eosin Y to azure II. Azure II is the mixture of equal quantities of methylene azure (azure I), prepared by oxidizing methylene blue, and methylene blue.

Giemsa's TS, dilute Dilute Giemsa's TS to about 50 times its volume with a solution prepared by dissolving 4.54 g of potassium dihydrogen phosphate and 4.75 g of anhydrous disodium hydrogen phosphate in water to make 1000 mL, and filter with a filter paper. Prepare before use.

[6]-Gingerol for assay $C_{17}H_{26}O_4$ [6]-Gingerol for thin-layer chromatography. It meets the requirements of the following 1) [6]-Gingerol for assay 1 or 2) [6]-Gingerol for assay 2 (Purity value by quantitative NMR). The latter is used with correction for its amount based on the result obtained in the Assay 2.

1) [6]-Gingerol for assay 1

Absorbance <2.24> $E^{1\%}_{1\,\mathrm{cm}}$ (281 nm): 101 – 112 [7 mg, ethanol (99.5), 200 mL].

Purity Related substances—Dissolve 5 mg of [6]-gingerol for assay 1 in 5 mL of methanol, and use this solution as the sample solution. Pipet 1 mL of the sample solution, add methanol to make exactly 50 mL, and use this solution as the standard solution. Perform the test with exactly 10 μL each of the sample solution and standard solution as directed under Liquid Chromatography <2.01> according to the following conditions, and determine each peak area by the automatic integration method: the total area of the peaks other than [6]-gingerol obtained from the sample solution is not larger than the peak area of [6]-gingerol obtained from the standard solution.

Operating conditions

Detector, column, column temperature, mobile phase and flow rate: Proceed as directed in the operating conditions in the Assay (3) under Hangekobokuto Extract.

Time span of measurement: About 6 times as long as the retention time of [6]-gingerol.

System suitability

System performance: Proceed as directed in the system suitability in the Assay (3) under Hangekobokuto Extract.

Test for required detectability: Pipet 1 mL of the standard solution, and add methanol to make exactly 20 mL. Confirm that the peak area of [6]-gingerol obtained with 10 μL of this solution is equivalent to 3.5 to 6.5% of that with 10 μL of the standard solution.

System repeatability: When the test is repeated 6 times with 10 μL of the standard solution under the above operating conditions, the relative standard deviation of the peak area of [6]-gingerol is not more than 1.5%.

2) [6]-Gingerol for assay 2 (Purity value by quantitative NMR)

Unity of peak—Dissolve 5 mg of [6]-gingerol for assay 2 in 5 mL of methanol, and use this solution as the sample solution. Perform the test with 10 μL of the sample solution as directed under Liquid Chromatography <2.01> according to the following conditions, and compare the absorption spectra of at least 3 points including the top of [6]-gingerol peak and around the two middle peak heights of before and after the top: no difference in form is observed among their spectra.

Operating conditions

Column, column temperature, mobile phase, and flow rate: Proceed as directed in the operating conditions in the Assay (3) under Hangekobokuto Extract.

Detector: A photodiode array detector (wavelength: 282 nm, measuring range of spectrum: 220 – 400 nm).

System suitability

System performance: Proceed as directed in the system suitability in the Assay (3) under Hangekobokuto Extract.

Assay—Weigh accurately 5 mg of [6]-gingerol for assay 2 and 1 mg of 1,4-BTMSB-d_4 for nuclear magnetic resonance spectroscopy using an ultramicrobalance, dissolve both in 1 mL of deuterated methanol for nuclear magnetic resonance spectroscopy, and use this solution as the sample solution. Transfer the sample solution into an NMR tube 5 mm in outer diameter, and measure ^{1}H-NMR as directed under Nuclear Magnetic Resonance Spectroscopy <*2.21*> and Crude Drugs Test <*5.01*> according to the following conditions, using 1,4-BTMSB-d_4 for nuclear magnetic resonance spectroscopy as the reference standard for qNMR. Calculate the resonance intensities, A_1 (equivalent to 3 hydrogens) and A_2 (equivalent to 1 hydrogen), of the signals around δ 3.56 ppm and δ 6.52 ppm assuming the signal of the reference standard for qNMR as δ 0 ppm.

Amount (%) of [6]-gingerol ($C_{17}H_{26}O_4$)
$= M_S \times I \times P/(M \times N) \times 1.2997$

M: Amount (mg) of [6]-gingerol for assay 2 taken
M_S: Amount (mg) of 1,4-BTMSB-d_4 for nuclear magnetic resonance spectroscopy taken
I: Sum of the signal resonance intensities, A_1 and A_2, based on the signal resonance intensity of 1,4-BTMSB-d_4 for nuclear magnetic resonance spectroscopy as 18.000
N: Sum of the numbers of the hydrogen derived from A_1 and A_2
P: Purity (%) of 1,4-BTMSB-d_4 for nuclear magnetic resonance spectroscopy

Operating conditions
Apparatus: A nuclear magnetic resonance spectrometer having ^{1}H resonance frequency of not less than 400 MHz.
Target nucleus: ^{1}H.
Digital resolution: 0.25 Hz or lower.
Measuring spectrum range: 20 ppm or upper, including between −5 ppm and 15 ppm.
Spinning: off.
Pulse angle: 90°.
^{13}C decoupling: on.
Delay time: Repeating pulse waiting time not less than 60 seconds.
Integrating times: 8 or more times.
Dummy scanning: 2 or more times.
Measuring temperature: A constant temperature between 20°C and 30°C.
System suitability
Test for required detectability: When the procedure is run with the sample solution under the above operating conditions, the SN ratio of each signal around δ 3.56 ppm and δ 6.52 ppm is not less than 100.
System performance: When the procedure is run with the sample solution under the above operating conditions, the signals around δ 3.56 ppm and δ 6.52 ppm are not overlapped with any signal of obvious foreign substance, and the ratio of the resonance intensities, $(A_1/3)/A_2$, of each signal around δ 3.56 ppm and δ 6.52 ppm is between 0.99 and 1.01.
System repeatability: When the test is repeated 6 times with the sample solution under the above operating conditions, the relative standard deviation of the ratio of the resonance intensity, A_1 or A_2, to that of the reference standard for qNMR is not more than 1.0%.

[6]-Gingerol for component determination See [6]-gingerol for assay.

[6]-Gingerol for thin-layer chromatography $C_{17}H_{26}O_4$ A yellow-white to yellow, liquid or solid. Freely soluble in methanol and in ethanol (99.5), and practically insoluble in water.

Identification—Determine the absorption spectrum of a solution of [6]-gingerol for thin-layer chromatography in ethanol (99.5) (7 in 200,000) as directed under Ultraviolet-visible Spectrophotometry <*2.24*>: it exhibits a maximum between 279 nm and 283 nm.

Purity Related substances—Dissolve 1.0 mg of [6]-gingerol for thin-layer chromatography in exactly 2 mL of methanol. Perform the test with 10 μL of this solution as directed in the Identification under Ginger: any spot other than the principal spot at the *Rf* value of about 0.3 does not appear.

Ginsenoside Rb$_1$ for thin-layer chromatography $C_{54}H_{92}O_{23}$ A white powder. Freely soluble in water and in methanol, and sparingly soluble in ethanol (99.5). It is hygroscopic.

Identification Determine the infrared absorption spectrum of ginsenoside Rb$_1$ for thin-layer chromatography as directed in the potassium bromide disk method under Infrared Spectrophotometry <*2.25*>: it exhibits absorption at the wave numbers of about 3390 cm^{-1}, 1650 cm^{-1}, 1077cm^{-1} and 1038 cm^{-1}.

Purity Related substances—Dissolve 2 mg of ginsenoside Rb$_1$ for thin-layer chromatography in 1 mL of methanol, and use this solution as the sample solution. Pipet 0.5 mL of the sample solution, add methanol to make exactly 25 mL, and use this solution as the standard solution. Perform the test with 2 μL each of the sample solution and standard solution as directed in the Identification (2) under Ginseng by developing the plate without entirely drying after applying the solutions: any spot other than the principal spot with an *Rf* value of about 0.3 obtained from the sample solution is not more intense than the spot from the standard solution.

Ginsenoside Rc $C_{53}H_{90}O_{22}$ A white crystalline powder. It is odorless.

Purity—Dissolve 1 mg of ginsenoside Rc in diluted methanol (3 in 5) to make 10 mL. Perform the test with 10 μL of this solution as directed under Liquid Chromatography <*2.01*> according to the conditions directed in the Assay (2) under Ginseng until ginsenoside Rc is eluted: the total area of the peaks other than ginsenoside Rc and solvent peak is not larger than 1/10 times the total peak area excluding the peak area of the solvent.

Ginsenoside Re $C_{48}H_{82}O_{18}$ A white crystalline powder. It is odorless.

Purity—Dissolve 1.0 mg of ginsenoside Re in diluted methanol (3 in 5) to make 10 mL. Perform the test with 10 μL of this solution as directed under Liquid Chromatography <*2.01*> according to the conditions directed in the Assay (1) under Ginseng until ginsenoside Re is eluted: the total area of the peaks other than ginsenoside Re and solvent peak is not larger than 1/10 times the total peak area excluding the peak area of the solvent.

Ginsenoside Rg$_1$ for thin-layer chromatography $C_{42}H_{72}O_{14}$ A white, powder or crystalline powder. Very soluble in methanol and in ethanol (99.5), and soluble in water. It is hygroscopic.

Identification Determine the infrared absorption spectrum of ginsenoside Rg$_1$ for thin-layer chromatography as directed in the potassium bromide disk method under Infrared Spectrophotometry <*2.25*>: it exhibits absorption at the wave numbers of about 3390 cm^{-1}, 1642 cm^{-1}, 1075 cm^{-1} and 1032 cm^{-1}.

Purity Related substances—Dissolve 2 mg of ginsenoside Rg$_1$ for thin-layer chromatography in 1 mL of methanol, and use this as the sample solution. Pipet 0.5 mL of the sample solution, add methanol to make exactly 25 mL, and use as the standard solution. Perform the test with 2 μL each of the sample solution and standard solution as directed in the Identification (2) under Ginseng by developing the plate without entirely drying after applying the solutions: any spot other than the principal spot with an *R*f value of about 0.5 obtained from the sample solution is not more intense than the spot from the standard solution.

Glacial acetic acid See acetic acid (100).

Glacial acetic acid for nonaqueous titration See acetic acid for nonaqueous titration.

Glacial acetic acid-sulfuric acid TS See acetic acid sulfuric acid TS.

γ-Globulin A plasma protein obtained from human serum as Cohn's II and III fractions. White crystalline powder. It contains not less than 98% of γ-globulin in the total protein.

D-Glucosamine hydrochloride $C_6H_{13}NO_5.HCl$ White, crystals or crystalline powder.

Content: not less than 98%. Assay—Dissolve about 0.4 g of D-glucosamine hydrochloride, accurately weighed, in 50 mL of water, add 5 mL of diluted nitric acid (1 in 3), and titrate <*2.50*> with 0.1 mol/L silver nitrate VS (potentiometric titration).

Each mL of 0.1 mol/L silver nitrate VS
= 21.56 mg of $C_6H_{13}NO_5.HCl$

Glucose $C_6H_{12}O_6$ [Same as the namesake monograph]

Glucose detection TS Dissolve 1600 units of glucose oxidase, 16 mg of 4-aminoantipyrine, 145 units of peroxidase and 0.27 g of *p*-hydroxybenzoic acid in tris buffer solution (pH 7.0) to make 200 mL.

Glucose detection TS for penicillium origin β-galactosidase Dissolve glucose oxidase (not less than 500 units), peroxidase (not less than 50 units), 10 mg of 4-aminoantipyrine and 0.1 g of phenol in phosphate buffer (pH 7.2) to make 100 mL.

Glucose oxidase Obtained from *Aspergillus niger*. White powder. It is freely soluble in water. It contains about 200 Units per mg. One unit indicates an amount of the enzyme which produces 1 μmol of D-glucono-δ-lactone in 1 minute at 25°C and pH 7.0 from glucose used as the substrate.

Glucose TS Dissolve 30 g of glucose in water to make 100 mL. Prepare as directed under Injections.

4′-*O*-Glucosyl-5-*O*-methylvisamminol for thin-layer chromatography $C_{22}H_{28}O_{10}$ White, crystals or crystalline powder. Freely soluble in methanol and in ethanol (99.5), and sparingly soluble in water.

Identification—Determine the absorption spectrum of a solution of 4′-*O*-glucosyl-5-*O*-methylvisamminol for thin-layer chromatography in ethanol (99.5) (1 in 50,000) as directed under Ultraviolet-visible Spectrophotometry <*2.24*>: it exhibits a maximum between 286 nm and 290 nm.

Purity Related substances—Dissolve 1 mg of 4′-*O*-glucosyl-5-*O*-methylvisamminol for thin-layer chromatography in 1 mL of methanol. Perform the test with 5 μL of this solution directed in the Identification under Saposhnikovia Root and Rhizome: no spots other than the principal spot at around *R*f value of 0.3 appears.

L-Glutamic acid $HOOC(CH_2)_2CH(NH_2)COOH$ [K 9047, Special class]

L-Glutamine $H_2NCO(CH_2)_2CH(NH_2)COOH$ [K 9103, L(+)-glutamine, Special class]

Glutamine TS Dissolve 2.92 g of L-glutamine in water to make 100 mL, and sterilize by filtration through a membrane filter with a pore size not exceeding 0.22 μm.

7-(Glutarylglycyl-L-arginylamino)-4-methylcoumarin $C_{23}H_{30}N_6O_7$ White powder. It is freely soluble in acetic acid (100), sparingly soluble in dimethylsulfoxide, and practically insoluble in water.

Absorbance <*2.24*> $E^{1\%}_{1\,cm}$ (325 nm): 310 – 350 [2 mg, diluted acetic acid (100) (1 in 500), 200 mL].

Optical rotation <*2.49*> $[\alpha]^{20}_{D}$: −50 – −60° [0.1 g, diluted acetic acid (100) (1 in 2), 10 mL, 100 mm].

Purity Related substances—Prepare the sample solution by dissolving 5 mg of 7-(glutarylglycyl-L-arginylamino)-4-methylcoumarin in 0.5 mL of acetic acid (100), and perform the test as directed under Thin-layer Chromatography <*2.03*>. Spot 5 μL of the sample solution on a plate of silica gel for thin-layer chromatography. Develop the plate with a mixture of 1-butanol, water, pyridine and acetic acid (100) (15:12:10:3) to a distance of about 10 cm, air-dry the plate, and dry more at 80°C for 30 minutes. After cooling, allow the plate to stand for 30 minutes in a box filled with iodine vapors: any observable spot other than the principal spot at the *R*f value of about 0.6 does not appear.

7-(Glutarylglycyl-L-arginylamino)-4-methylcoumarin TS Dissolve 5 mg of 7-(glutarylglycyl-L-arginylamino)-4-methylcoumarin in 0.5 to 1 mL of acetic acid (100), lyophilize, dissolve this in 1 mL of dimethylsulfoxide, and use this solution as solution A. Dissolve 30.0 g of 2-amino-2-hydroxymethyl-1,3-propanediol and 14.6 g of sodium chloride in 400 mL of water, adjust the pH to 8.5 with dilute hydrochloric acid, add water to make 500 mL, and use this solution as solution B. Mix 1 mL of the solution A and 500 mL of the solution B before use.

Glutathione $C_{10}H_{17}N_3O_6S$ [Same as the namesake monograph]

Glycerin $C_3H_8O_3$ [K 8295, Glycerol, Special class, or same as the monograph Concentrated Glycerin]

85% Glycerin $C_3H_8O_3$ [Same as the monograph Glycerin]

Glycerin for gas chromatography $C_3H_8O_3$ [K 8295, Special class or for gas chromatography] When perform the test as directed in the Purity (11) under Concentrated Glycerin, it does not show any peak at the retention times corresponding to ethylene glycol and diethylene glycol.

Glycine H_2NCH_2COOH [K 8291, Special class]

Glycolic acid $C_2H_4O_3$ *Purity*: not less than 98.0%.

***N*-Glycolylneuraminic acid** $C_{11}H_{19}NO_{10}$ White needle crystalline powder.

0.1 mmol/L *N*-Glycolylneuraminic acid TS Weigh accurately about 16.5 mg of *N*-glycolylneuraminic acid, and dissolve in water to make exactly 50 mL. To exactly *V* mL of this solution add water to make exactly 100 mL.

V (mL) = 325.3 × 0.5/amount (mg) of
N-glycolylneuraminic acid taken

Glycyrrhizic acid monoammonium salt for resolution check See monoammonium glycyrrhizinate for solution check

Glycyrrhizic acid for thin-layer chromatography $C_{42}H_{62}O_{16}$ White, crystals or crystalline powder. Freely soluble in ethanol (99.5), and practically insoluble in water.

Identification Determine the infrared absorption spectrum of glycyrrhizic acid for thin-layer chromatography as directed in the potassium bromide disk method under Infrared Spectrophotometry <*2.25*>: it exhibits absorption at the wave numbers of about 3420 cm^{-1}, 1722 cm^{-1}, 1654 cm^{-1} and 1389 cm^{-1}.

Purity Related substances—Dissolve 4 mg of glycyrrhizic acid for thin-layer chromatography in 2 mL of ethanol (99.5), and use this solution as the sample solution. Pipet 1 mL of the sample solution, add ethanol (99.5) to make exactly 100 mL, and use this solution as the standard solution. Perform the test with 10 μL each of the sample solution and standard solution as directed in the Identification under Glycyrrhiza: the spots other than the principal spot with an *R*f value of about 0.3 obtained from the sample solution are not more intense than the spot from the standard solution.

40% glyoxal TS *Content:* 38 – 42%. Assay—Put 1.000 g of 40% glyoxal TS in a glass-stoppered flask, add 20 mL of a solution of hydroxylammonium chloride (7 in 100) and 50 mL of water. Stopper tightly, allow to stand for 30 minutes, titrate <*2.50*> with 1 mol/L sodium hydroxide VS (indicator: 1.0 mL of methyl red-methylene blue TS). Perform a blank determination in the same manner, and make any necessary correction.

Each mL of 1 mol/L sodium hydroxide VS
= 29.02 mg of $C_2H_2O_2$

Goat anti-ECP antibody Combine 1 volume of ECP standard substance (equivalent to about 1 mg of protein) and 1 volume of Freund's complete adjuvant, and immunize goats subcutaneously in the back region with this solution 5 times at 2 week intervals. Harvest blood on the 10th day after completing the immunization to obtain goat antiserum. Goat anti-ECP antibody is obtained by preparing an immobilized ECP column in which ECP standard substance is bound to sepharose 4B and then purifying by affinity column chromatography.

Description: Clear and colorless solution.

Identification: When sodium lauryl sulfate-supplemented polyacrylamide gel electrophoresis is conducted under non-reducing conditions, the molecular weight of the major band is within the range of 1.30×10^5 to 1.70×10^5.

Protein content: When determining the protein content using Assay (1) under Celmoleukin (Genetical Recombination), the protein content per mL is 0.2 to 1.0 mg.

Goat anti-ECP antibody TS Dilute goat anti-ECP antibody with 0.1 mol/L carbonate buffer solution (pH 9.6) to prepare a solution containing 50 μg protein per mL.

Griess-Romijn's nitric acid reagent Triturate thoroughly 1 g of 1-naphthylamine, 10 g of sulfanilic acid and 1.5 g of zinc dust in a mortar.

Storage—Preserve in tight, light-resistant containers.

Griess-Romijn's nitrous acid reagent Triturate thoroughly 1 g of 1-naphthylamine, 10 g of sulfanilic acid and 89 g of tartaric acid in a mortar.

Storage—Preserve in tight, light-resistant containers.

Guaiacol $CH_3OC_6H_4OH$ Clear, colorless to yellow, liquid or colorless crystals, having a characteristic aroma. Sparingly soluble in water, and miscible with ethanol (95), with chloroform and with diethyl ether. Melting point: about 28°C.

Purity—Perform the test with 0.5 μL of guaiacol as directed under Gas Chromatography <*2.02*> according to the following conditions. Determine each peak area by the automatic integration method, and calculate the amount of guaiacol by the area percentage method:It showed the purity of not less than 99.0%.

Operating conditions

Detector: A hydrogen flame-ionization detector

Column: A glass column about 3 mm in inside diameter and about 2 m in length, packed with siliceous earth for gas chromatography, 150- to 180-μm in particle diameter, coated with polyethylene glycol 20 M at the ratio of 20%.

Column temperature: A constant temperature of about 200°C.

Carrier gas: Nitrogen.

Flow rate: Adjust so that the retention time of guaiacol is 4 to 6 minutes.

Detection sensitivity: Adjust the detection sensitivity so that the peak height of guaiacol obtained with 0.5 μL of guaiacol is about 90% of the full scale.

Time span of measurement: About 3 times as long as the retention time of guaiacol.

Guaiacol for assay $C_7H_8O_2$ Colorless to yellow clear liquid or colorless crystals with a characteristic, aromatic odor. Miscible with methanol and with ethanol (99.5), and sparingly soluble in water. Congealing point: 25 – 30°C.

Identification—Determine the infrared absorption spectrum of guaiacol for assay as directed in the ATR method under Infrared Spectrophotometry <*2.25*>: it exhibits absorption at the wave numbers of about 1595 cm^{-1}, 1497 cm^{-1}, 1443 cm^{-1}, 1358 cm^{-1}, 1255 cm^{-1}, 1205 cm^{-1}, 1108 cm^{-1}, 1037 cm^{-1}, 1020 cm^{-1}, 916 cm^{-1}, 833 cm^{-1}, and 738 cm^{-1}.

Purity Related substances—Perform the test with 0.5 μL of guaiacol for assay as directed under Gas Chromatography <*2.02*> according to the following conditions. Determine each peak area by the automatic integration method: the total area of the peaks other than the peak of guaiacol is not more than 2.0%.

Operating conditions

Detector: A hydrogen flame-ionization detector.

Column: A fused silica column 0.25 mm in inside diameter and 60 m in length, coated inside with polymethylsiloxane for gas chromatography in 0.25 to 0.5 μm in thickness.

Column temperature: Raise the temperature from 100°C to 130°C at a rate of 5°C per minute, raise to 140°C at a rate of 2°C per minute, raise to 200°C at a rate of 15°C per minute, and maintain at 200°C for 2 minutes.

Injection port temperature: 200°C.

Detector temperature: 250°C.

Carrier gas: Helium.

Flow rate: Adjust so that the retention time of guaiacol is about 8 minutes.

Split ratio: 1:50.

System suitability

Test for required detectability: Weigh accurately about 70 mg of guaiacol for assay, add methanol to make exactly 100 mL, and use this solution as the solution for system suitability test. Confirm that the peak area of guaiacol obtained from 1 μL of the solution for system suitability test is equivalent to 0.08 to 0.16% of that of guaiacol obtained when 0.5 μL of guaiacol for assay is injected.

System performance: When the procedure is run with 1 μL of the solution for system suitability test under the above operating conditions, the number of theoretical plates and the symmetry factor of the peak of guaiacol are not less than 200,000 and not more than 1.5, respectively.

System repeatability: When the test is repeated 6 times with 1 μL of the solution for system suitability test under the above operating conditions, the relative standard deviation of the peak area of guaiacol is not more than 2.0%.

Guaifenesin $C_{10}H_{14}O_4$ [Same as the namesake monograph]

Guanine $C_5H_5N_5O$ White to pale yellow-white powder.

Absorbance <*2.24*> Weigh accurately about 10 mg of guanine, dissolve in 20 mL of dilute sodium hydroxide TS, and add 2 mL of 1 mol/L hydrochloric acid TS and 0.1 mol/L hydrochloric acid TS to make exactly 1000 mL. Determine the absorbances, $E^{1\%}_{1\%}$, of this solution at 248 nm and 273 nm: they are between 710 and 770, and between 460 and 500, respectively.

Loss on drying <*2.41*>: Not more than 1.5% (0.5 g, 105°C, 4 hours).

Haloperidol for assay $C_{21}H_{23}ClFNO_2$ [Same as the monograph Haloperidol]

Hanus' TS Dissolve 20 g of iodine monobromide in 1000 mL of acetic acid (100).

Storage—Preserve in light-resistant, glass-stoppered bottles, in a cold place.

Heart infusion agar medium Prepared for biochemical tests.

Heavy hydrogenated solvent for nuclear magnetic resonance spectroscopy Prepared for nuclear magnetic resonance spectroscopy. Heavy hydrogenated chloroform ($CDCl_3$), heavy hydrogenated dimethyl sulfoxide [$(CD_3)_2SO$], heavy water (D_2O), and heavy hydrogenated pyridine (C_5D_5N) are available.

Heavy water for nuclear magnetic resonance spectroscopy D_2O Prepared for nuclear magnetic resonance spectroscopy.

Helium He Not less than 99.995 vol%.

Hematoxylin $C_{16}H_{14}O_6.xH_2O$ White or light yellow to brownish, crystals or crystalline powder. It is soluble in hot water and in ethanol (95), and sparingly soluble in cold water.

Residue on ignition <*2.44*>: not more than 0.1% (1 g).

Hematoxylin TS Dissolve 1 g of hematoxylin in 12 mL of ethanol (99.5). Dissolve 20 g of aluminum potassium sulfate 12-water in 200 mL of warm water, cool, and filter. After 24 hours, mix these two prepared solutions. Allow to stand for 8 hours in a wide-mouthed bottle without using a stopper, and filter.

Heparin sodium [Same as the namesake monograph]

HEPES buffer solution (pH 7.5) Dissolve 2.38 g of *N*-2-hydroxyethylpiperazine-*N'*-2-ethanesulfonic acid in 90 mL of water, adjust to pH 7.5 with diluted 6 mol/L sodium hydroxide TS (5 in 6), and add water to make 100 mL.

Heptafluorobutylic acid $C_4HF_7O_2$ A clear and colorless liquid.

Content: Not less than 98.0%. Assay—Take 30 mL of water in a glass-stoppered flask, weigh accurately the mass of the flask, add about 4.3 g of heptafluorobutylic acid, and weigh accurately the mass of this flask. Then, add 40 mL of water, and titrate <*2.50*> with 1 mol/L sodium hydroxide VS (indicator: 2 drops of phenolphthalein TS).

Each mL of 1 mol/L sodium hydroxide VS
= 214.0 mg of $C_4HF_7O_2$

Heptane $CH_3(CH_2)_5CH_3$ [K 9701, Special class]

Heptane for liquid chromatography C_7H_{16} Clear and colorless solution.

Purity Ultraviolet-absorbing substances—Perform the test as directed under Ultraviolet-visible Spectrophotometry <*2.24*>, and determine the absorbances of heptane for liquid chromatography at 210 nm, 220 nm, 230 nm and 240 nm, using water as the control solution: the absorbance is not more than 0.35, not more than 0.15, not more than 0.05 and not more than 0.03, respectively.

Heptyl parahydroxybenzoate $C_{14}H_{20}O_3$ White, crystals or crystalline powder.

Melting point <*2.60*>: 45 – 50°C

Content: Not less than 98.0% Assay—Weigh accurately about 3.5 g of heptyl parahydroxybenzoate, dissolve in 50 mL of diluted *N*,*N*-dimethylformamide (4 in 5), and titrate <*2.50*> with 1 mol/L sodium hydroxide VS (potentiometric titration). Perform a blank determination in the same manner, and make any necessary correction.

Each mL of 1 mol/L sodium hydroxide VS
= 236.3 mg of $C_{14}H_{20}O_3$

Hesperidin for assay $C_{28}H_{34}O_{15}$ Hesperidin for thin-layer chromatography. It meets the following requirement.

Optical rotation <*2.49*> $[\alpha]^{20}_D$: −100 – −120° (5 mg dried with silica gel for 24 hours, methanol, 50 mL, 100 mm).

Purity Related substances—Dissolve 2 mg of hesperidin for assay in 10 mL of methanol, and use this solution as the sample solution. Pipet 1 mL of the sample solution, add the mobile phase to make exactly 100 mL, and use this solution as the standard solution. Perform the test with exactly 10 μL each of the sample solution and standard solution as directed under Liquid Chromatography <*2.01*> according to the following conditions, and determine each peak area by the automatic integration method: the total area of the peaks other than hesperidin and the solvent obtained from the sample solution is not larger than the peak area of hesperidin from the standard solution.

Operating conditions

Detector, column, column temperature, mobile phase, and flow rate: Proceed as directed in the operating conditions in the Assay (1) under Hochuekkito Extract.

Time span of measurement: About 6 times as long as the retention time of hesperidin.

System suitability

System performance, and system repeatability: Proceed as directed in the system suitability in the Assay (1) under Hochuekkito Extract.

Test for required detectability: To exactly 1 mL of the standard solution add the mobile phase to make exactly 20 mL. Confirm that the peak area of hesperidin obtained with 10 μL of this solution is equivalent to 3.5 to 6.5% of that with 10 μL of the standard solution.

Hesperidin for component determination See hesperidin for assay.

Hesperidin for thin-layer chromatography $C_{28}H_{34}O_{15}$ A white to light brown-yellow, crystalline powder or powder. Very slightly soluble in methanol and in ethanol (99.5), and practically insoluble in water. Melting point: about 245°C (with decomposition).

Absorbance <*2.24*> $E^{1\%}_{1\,cm}$ (284 nm): 310 – 340 (8 mg dried in a desiccator (silica gel) for 24 hours, methanol, 500 mL).

Purity Related substances—Dissolve 1 mg of hesperidin for thin-layer chromatography in 2 mL of methanol. Perform the test with 20 μL of this solution as directed in the Identification (6) under Hochuekkito Extract: no spot other than the principle spot of around *R*f value of 0.3 appears.

Hexaammonium heptamolybdate-cerium (IV) sulfate TS Dissolve 2.5 g of hexaammonium heptamolybdate tetrahydrate and 1.0 g of cerium (IV) sulfate tetrahydrate in diluted sulfuric acid (3 in 50) to make 100 mL. Prepare before use.

Hexaammonium heptamolybdate-sulfuric acid TS Dissolve 1.0 g of hexaammonium heptamolybdate tetrahydrate in diluted sulfuric acid (3 in 20) to make 40 mL. Prepare before use.

Hexaammonium heptamolybdate tetrahydrate $(NH_4)_6Mo_7O_{24}.4H_2O$ [K 8905, Special class]

Hexaammonium heptamolybdate TS dissolve 21.2 g of hexaammonium heptamolybdate tetrahydrate in water to make 200 mL (10%). Prepare before use.

1,1,1,3,3,3-Hexamethyldisilazane $(CH_3)_3SiNHSi(CH_3)_3$ A colorless or practically colorless, liquid. Very soluble in diethyl ether, and reactable with water or with ethanol. Boiling point: about 125°C.

Hexamethylenetetramine $(CH_2)_6N_4$ [K 8847, Special class]

Hexamethylenetetramine TS Dissolve exactly 2.5 g of hexamethylenetetramine in exactly 25 mL of water.

Hexamine See hexamethylenetetramine.

Hexane C_6H_{14} [K 8848, Special class]

Hexane for liquid chromatography C_6H_{14} Colorless, clear liquid. Miscible with ethanol (95), with diethyl ether, with chloroform and with benzene.

Boiling point: about 69°C.

Purity (1) Ultraviolet absorptive substances—Read the absorbances of hexane for liquid chromatography as directed under Ultraviolet-visible Spectrophotometry <*2.24*>, using water as the blank: not more than 0.3 at the wavelength of 210 nm, and not more than 0.01 between 250 nm and 400 nm.

(2) Peroxide—To a mixture of 100 mL of water and 25 mL of dilute sulfuric acid add 25 mL of a solution of potassium iodide (1 in 10) and 20 g of hexane for liquid chromatography. Stopper tightly, shake, and allow to stand in a dark place for 15 minutes. Titrate <*2.50*> this solution, while shaking well, with 0.01 mol/L sodium thiosulfate VS (indicator: 1 mL of starch TS). Perform a blank determination in the same manner, and make any necessary correction (not more than 0.0005%).

***n*-Hexane for liquid chromatography** See hexane for liquid chromatography.

Hexane for purity of crude drug C_6H_{14} [K 8848, Special class] Use hexane meeting the following additional specification. Evaporate 300.0 mL of hexane for purity of crude drug in vacuum at a temperature not higher than 40°C, add the hexane to make exactly 1 mL, and use this solution as the sample solution. Separately, dissolve 2.0 mg of γ-BHC in hexane to make exactly 100 mL. Pipet 1 mL of this solution, and add hexane to make exactly 100 mL. Further pipet 2 mL of this solution, add hexane to make exactly 100 mL, and use this solution as the standard solution I. Perform the test with exactly 1 μL each of the sample solution and standard solution I as directed under Gas Chromatography <*2.02*> according to the following conditions, and determine each peak area by the automatic integration method: the total area of the peaks other than the solvent peak obtained from the sample solution is not larger than the peak area of γ-BHC from the standard solution I.

Operating conditions

Proceed the operating conditions in 4.3. under Crude Drugs Test <*5.01*> except the time span of measurement.

Time span of measurement: About three times as long as the retention time of γ-BHC, beginning after the solvent peak.

System suitability

Test for required detectability: Pipet 1 mL of the standard solution I, add hexane to make exactly 20 mL, and use this solution as the standard solution II. Adjust the detection sensitivity so that the peak area of γ-BHC obtained with 1 μL of the standard solution II can be measured by the automatic integration method, and the peak height of γ-BHC with 1 μL of the standard solution I is about 20% of the full scale.

Hexane for ultraviolet-visible spectrophotometry C_6H_{14} [K 8848, Special class]. When determining the absorbance of hexane for ultraviolet-visible spectrophotometry as directed under Ultraviolet-visible Spectrophotometry <*2.24*>, using water as the blank solution, its value is not more than 0.10 at 220 nm and not more than 0.02 at 260 nm, and it has no characteristic absorption between 260 nm and 350 nm.

***n*-Hexane for ultraviolet-visible spectrophotometry** See hexane for ultraviolet-visible spectrophotometry.

1-Hexanol $C_6H_{14}O$ A clear and colorless liquid.

Specific gravity d^{20}_{20}: 0.816 – 0.821

Boiling point 156 – 158°C.

Hexyl parahydroxybenzoate $C_{13}H_{18}O_3$ White, crystals or crystalline powder.

Melting point <*2.60*>: 49 – 53°C

Content: not less than 98.0%. Assay—Weigh accurately about 0.3 g of hexyl parahydroxybenzoate, dissolve in 50 mL of diluted *N,N*-dimethylformamide (4 in 5), and titrate <*2.50*> with 0.1 mol/L sodium hydroxide VS (potentiometric titration). Perform a blank determination in the same manner, and make any necessary correction.

Each mL of 0.1 mol/L sodium hydroxide VS
= 22.23 mg of $C_{13}H_{18}O_3$

High-density polyethylene film Prepared for cytotoxicity test. It does not show cytotoxicity.

Hirsutine See hirsutine for thin-layer chromatography.

Hirsutine for assay $C_{22}H_{28}N_2O_3$ Hirsutine for thin-layer chromatography. It meets the following requirements.

Absorbance <*2.24*>: $E^{1\%}_{1\,\mathrm{cm}}$ (245 nm): 354 – 389 (5 mg calculated on the anhydrous basis, a mixture of methanol and dilute acetic acid (7:3), 500 mL).

Purity Related substances—Dissolve 5 mg of hirsutine for assay in 100 mL of a mixture of methanol and dilute acetic acid (7:3), use this solution as the sample solution. Pipet 1 mL of the sample solution, add a mixture of methanol and dilute acetic acid (7:3) to make exactly 50 mL, and use this solution as the standard solution. Perform the test with exactly 20 μL each of the sample solution and standard solution as directed under Liquid-chromatography <*2.01*> according to the following conditions. Determine each peak area by the automatic integration method: the total area of the peaks other than hirsutine obtained from the sample solution is not larger than the peak area of hirsutine from the standard solution.

Operating conditions

Detector, column, column temperature, mobile phase, and flow rate: Proceed as directed in the operating conditions in the Assay under Uncaria Hook.

Time span of measurement: About 1.5 times as long as the retention time of hirsutine, beginning after the solvent peak.
System suitability

System performance: Proceed as directed in the system suitability in the Assay under Uncaria Hook.

Test for required detectability: Pipet 1 mL of the standard solution, add a mixture of methanol and dilute acetic acid (7:3) to make exactly 20 mL. Confirm that the peak area of hirsutine obtained with 20 μL of this solution is equivalent to 3.5 to 6.5% of that with 20 μL of the standard solution.

System repeatability: When the test is repeated 6 times with 20 μL of the standard solution under the above operating conditions, the relative standard deviation of the peak area of hirsutine is not more than 1.5%.

Hirsutine for thin-layer chromatography $C_{22}H_{28}N_2O_3$ A white or light orange, crystalline or powder. Very soluble in methanol, freely soluble in ethanol (99.5), and practically insoluble in water. Melting point: about 105°C.

Identification—Determine the absorption spectrum of a solution of hirsutine for thin-layer chromatography in a mixture of methanol and dilute acetic acid (7:3) (1 in 100,000) as directed under Ultraviolet-visible Spectrophotometry <*2.24*>: it exhibits a maximum between 287 nm and 291 nm.

Purity Related substances—Dissolve 1.0 mg of hirsutine for thin-layer chromatography in 1 mL of methanol, and use this solution as the sample solution. Perform the test with this solution as directed under Thin-layer Chromatography <*2.03*>. Spot 10 μL of the sample solution on a plate of silica gel with fluorescent indicator for thin-layer chromatography. Develop the plate with a mixture of 1-butanol, water and acetic acid (100) (7:2:1) to a distance of about 10 cm, and air-dry the plate. Examine under ultraviolet light (main wavelength: 254 nm): no spot other than the principal spot at around *R*f value of 0.55 appears.

L-Histidine $C_6H_9N_3O_2$ [Same as the namesake monograph]

L-Histidine hydrochloride See L-histidine hydrochloride monohydrate.

L-Histidine hydrochloride monohydrate $C_6H_9N_3O_2.HCl.H_2O$ [K 9050, Special class]

Homatropine hydrobromide $C_{16}H_{21}NO_3.HBr$ [Same as the namesake monograph]

Honokiol $C_{18}H_{18}O_2$ Odorless white, crystals or crystalline powder.

Purity—Dissolve 1 mg of honokiol in the mobile phase to make 10 mL, and use this solution as the sample solution. Perform the Liquid Chromatography <*2.01*> with 10 μL of the sample solution as directed in the Assay under Magnolia Bark: when measure the peak areas for 2 times as long as the retention time of magnolol, the total area of peaks other than honokiol obtained from the sample solution is not larger than 1/10 times the total area of the peaks other than the solvent peak.

Horseradish peroxidase An oxidase (Molecular weight: about 40,000) derived from horseradish.

Horse serum Collect the blood from horse in a flask, coagulate, and allow to stand at room temperature until the serum is separated. Transfer the separated serum in glass containers, and preserve at −20°C.

Human anti-thrombin A serine protease inhibitor obtained from healthy human plasma. A protein that inhibits activities of activated blood coagulation factor II (thrombin) and activated blood coagulation factor X. It contains not less than 6 IU per mg of protein.

Human antithrombin III Serine protease inhibition factor obtained from normal plasma of health human. It is a protein, which inhibits the activities of thrombin and activated blood coagulation factor X. It contains not less than 300 Units per mg protein. One unit indicates an amount of the antithrombin III which inhibits 1 unit of thrombin at 25°C under the existence of heparin.

Human chorionic gonadotrophin TS Weigh accurately a suitable amount of Human Chorionic Gonadotrophin according to the labeled amount, and dissolve in bovine serum albumin-sodium chloride-phosphate buffer solution (pH 7.2) so that each 1.0 mL contains 80 human chorionic gonadotrophin Units.

Human insulin desamido substance-containing TS Dissolve 1.5 mg of Insulin Human in 1 mL of 0.01 mol/L hydrochloric acid TS, allow to stand at 25°C for 3 days, and when the procedure is run with this solution according to the conditions as directed in the Purity (1) under Insulin Human (Genetical Recombination), the solution contains about 5% of the desamido substance.

Human insulin dimer-containing TS Allow to stand Insulin Human (Genetical Recombination) at 25°C for 10 days or more, and dissolve 4 mg of this in 1 mL of 0.01 mol/L hydrochloric acid TS.

Human normal plasma Dissolve an amount of dried human normal plasma powder, equivalent to 1 mL of the normal plasma of human, in 1 mL of water. Store between 2°C and 10°C, and use within one week.

Human serum albumin for assay White to light yellow powder. Albumin content is at least 99%. Convert to the dehydrate using the following water determination method.

Water <*2.48*>: (0.2 g, volumetric titration, direct titration). However, in a dehydration solvent, use a mixture of pyridine for water determination and ethylene glycol for water determination (5:1).

Hyaluronic acid $(C_{14}H_{21}NO_{11})_n$ A white powder.

Hyaluronidase Obtained from *Streptomyces albogriseolus*. A lyophilized white powder.

Content: Not less than 100 units of hyaluronidase per ampule.

Assay (i) Sample solution: Dissolve the content of 1 ampoule by adding exactly 2 mL of cold water. Dilute this solution with cold water so that each mL contains exactly 1.3 to 3.8 units of hyaluronidase. Prepare before use, and store in a cold place.

(ii) Substrate solution: To exactly 50 mg of hyaluronic acid add 40 mL of 0.02 mol/L acetate buffer solution (pH 6.0), stir for 5 hours to dissolve, and add 0.02 mol/L acetate buffer solution (pH 6.0) to make exactly 50 mL.

(iii) 4-Dimethylaminobenzaldehyde solution: To a mixture of 0.6 mL of water and 11.9 mL of hydrochloric acid add acetic acid to make exactly 100 mL, and dissolve 10.0 g of 4-dimethylaminobenzaldehyde in this solution. To exactly 1 mL of this solution add exactly 9 mL of acetic acid. Prepare before use.

(iv) Borate solution: Dissolve 4.95 g of boric acid in 40 mL of water, adjust to pH 9.1 with potassium hydroxide TS, and add water to make 100 mL.

(v) Procedure: Pipet 0.5 mL of substrate solution, warm at 60 ± 0.5°C for 10 minutes, add exactly 0.5 mL of sample solution, and shake immediately. After allowing this solution to stand at 60 ± 0.5°C for exactly 30 minutes, add exactly 0.2 mL of borate solution, shake, heat the vessel covered with a marble in a water bath for exactly 3 minutes, and cool the vessel with running water. Then, add exactly 3 mL of 4-dimethylaminobenzaldehyde solution, shake, and allow to stand at 37 ± 0.5°C for exactly 20 minutes. Determine the absorbance, A_1, at 585 nm of this solution as directed under Ultraviolet-visible Spectrophotometry <2.24>, using water as the blank. Separately, pipet 0.5 mL of substrate solution, allow to stand at 60 ± 0.5°C for 40 minutes, add exactly 0.2 mL of borate solution, and shake. Add exactly 0.5 mL of sample solution, and shake immediately. Heat the vessel covered with a marble in a water bath for exactly 3 minutes, and cool the vessel with running water. Then, proceed in the same manner as above, and determine the absorbance, A_0, of this solution.

(vi) Calculation: Calculate the enzyme activity in 1 ampoule by the following equation, where 1 unit means the amount of enzyme which decreases 50% in absorbance at 660 nm of hyaluronic acid in 30 minutes at 60°C and pH 6.0.

$$\text{Hyaluronidase unit in 1 ampoule} = (A_1 - A_0) \times D_m \times 3.2 \times 4$$

D_m: Dilution factor for sample solution
3.2: Conversion factor to turbidity reduction unit

Hydralazine hydrochloride $C_8H_8N_4.HCl$ [Same as the namesake monograph]

Hydralazine hydrochloride for assay $C_8H_8N_4.HCl$ [Same as the monograph Hydralazine Hydrochloride. When dried, it contains not less than 99.0% of hydralazine hydrochloride ($C_8H_8N_4.HCl$).]

Hydrazine monohydrate $NH_2NH_2.H_2O$ Colorless liquid, having a characteristic odor.

Hydrazine sulfate See hydrazinium sulfate.

Hydrazinium sulfate $N_2H_6SO_4$ [K 8992, Special class]

Hydrazinium sulfate TS Dissolve exactly 1.0 g of hydrazinium sulfate in exactly 100 mL of water. Use after standing for 4 – 6 hours.

Hydriodic acid HI [K 8917, Special class]

Hydrobromic acid HBr [K 8509, Special class]

Hydrochloric acid HCl [K 8180, Special class]

Hydrochloric acid-ammonium acetate buffer solution (pH 3.5) Dissolve 25 g of ammonium acetate in 45 mL of 6 mol/L hydrochloric acid TS, and add water to make 100 mL.

Hydrochloric acid, dilute Dilute 23.6 mL of hydrochloric acid with water to make 100 mL (10%).

Hydrochloric acid-ethanol TS Dilute 23.6 mL of hydrochloric acid with ethanol (95) to make 100 mL.

0.01 mol/L Hydrochloric acid-methanol TS To 20 mL of 0.5 mol/L hydrochloric acid TS add methanol to make 1000 mL.

0.05 mol/L Hydrochloric acid-methanol TS To 100 mL of 0.5 mol/L hydrochloric acid add methanol to make 1000 mL.

Hydrochloric acid-2-propanol TS Add 0.33 mL of hydrochloric acid to 100 mL of 2-propanol, mix, and store in a dark and cool place.

Hydrochloric acid-potassium chloride buffer solution (pH 2.0) To 10.0 mL of 0.2 mol/L hydrochloric acid VS add 88.0 mL of 0.2 mol/L potassium chloride TS, adjust the pH to 2.0 ± 0.1 with 0.2 mol/L hydrochloric acid VS or 0.2 mol/L potassium chloride TS, then add water to make 200 mL.

Hydrochloric acid, purified Add 0.3 g of potassium permanganate to 1000 mL of diluted hydrochloric acid (1 in 2), distil, discard the first 250 mL of the distillate, and collect the following 500 mL of the distillate.

0.001 mol/L Hydrochloric acid TS Dilute 10 mL of 0.1 mol/L hydrochloric acid TS with water to make 1000 mL.

0.01 mol/L Hydrochloric acid TS Dilute 100 mL of 0.1 mol/L hydrochloric acid TS with water to make 1000 mL.

0.02 mol/L Hydrochloric acid TS Dilute 100 mL of 0.2 mol/L hydrochloric acid TS with water to make 1000 mL.

0.05 mol/L Hydrochloric acid TS Dilute 100 mL of 0.5 mol/L hydrochloric acid TS with water to make 1000 mL.

0.1 mol/L Hydrochloric acid TS Dilute 100 mL of 1 mol/L hydrochloric acid TS with water to make 1000 mL.

0.2 mol/L Hydrochloric acid TS Dilute 18 mL of hydrochloric acid with water to make 1000 mL.

0.5 mol/L Hydrochloric acid TS Dilute 45 mL of hydrochloric acid with water to make 1000 mL.

1 mol/L Hydrochloric acid TS Dilute 90 mL of hydrochloric acid with water to make 1000 mL.

2 mol/L Hydrochloric acid TS Dilute 180 mL of hydrochloric acid with water to make 1000 mL.

3 mol/L Hydrochloric acid TS Dilute 270 mL of hydrochloric acid with water to make 1000 mL.

5 mol/L Hydrochloric acid TS Dilute 450 mL of hydrochloric acid with water to make 1000 mL.

6 mol/L Hydrochloric acid TS Dilute 540 mL of hydrochloric acid with water to make 1000 mL.

7.5 mol/L Hydrochloric acid TS Dilute 675 mL of hydrochloric acid with water to make 1000 mL.

10 mol/L Hydrochloric acid TS Dilute 900 mL of hydrochloric acid with water to make 1000 mL.

6 mol/L Hydrochloric acid TS for amino acid automatic analysis Contains 19 – 21% hydrogen chloride (HCl: 36.46) for amino acid automatic analysis (constant boiling hydrochloric acid).

Hydrochlorothiazide $C_7H_8ClN_3O_4S_2$ [Same as the namesake monograph]

Hydrocortisone $C_{21}H_{30}O_5$ [Same as the namesake monograph]

Hydrocortisone acetate $C_{23}H_{32}O_6$ [Same as the namesake monograph]

Hydrocotarnine hydrochloride for assay See hydrocotarnine hydrochloride hydrate for assay.

Hydrocotarnine hydrochloride hydrate for assay $C_{12}H_{15}NO_3.HCl.H_2O$ [Same as the monograph Hydrocotarnine Hydrochloride Hydrate. When dried, it contains not less than 99.0% of hydrocotarnine hydrochloride ($C_{12}H_{15}NO_3.HCl$).]

Hydrofluoric acid HF [K 8819, Special class] It contains not less than 46.0% of HF.

Hydrogen H_2 [K 0512, Standard substance, Third class] It contains not less than 99.99% of H_2.

Hydrogen chloride-ethanol TS Pass dry hydrogen chloride, which is generated by slowly adding 100 mL of sulfuric acid dropwise to 100 mL of hydrochloric acid and dried by washing with sulfuric acid, through 75 g of ethanol (99.5) cooled in an ice bath until the increase in mass has reached 25 g. Prepare before use.

Hydrogen hexachloroplatinate (IV) hexahydrate $H_2PtCl_6.6H_2O$ [K 8153, Special class]

Hydrogen hexachloroplatinate (IV)-potassium iodide TS To 3 mL of hydrogen hexachloroplatinate (IV) TS add 97 mL of water and 100 mL of a solution of potassium iodide (3 in 50). Prepare before use.

Hydrogen hexachloroplatinate (IV) TS Dissolve 2.6 g of hydrogen hexachloroplatinate (IV) hexahydrate in water to make 20 mL (0.125 mol/L).

Hydrogen peroxide (30) H_2O_2 [K 8230, Hydrogen peroxide, Special class, Concentration: 30.0 - 35.5%.]

Hydrogen peroxide-sodium hydroxide TS To a mixture of water and hydrogen peroxide (30) (9:1) add 3 drops of bromophenol blue TS, and then add 0.01 mol/L sodium hydroxide TS until a purple-blue color develops. Prepare before use.

Hydrogen peroxide TS Dilute 1 volume of hydrogen peroxide (30) with 9 volumes of water. Prepare before use (3%).

Hydrogen peroxide TS, dilute Dilute 1 mL of hydrogen peroxide (30) with 500 mL of water, and dilute 5 mL of this solution with water to make 100 mL. Prepare before use.

Hydrogen peroxide water, strong See hydrogen peroxide (30).

Hydrogen sulfide H_2S Colorless, poisonous gas, heavier than air. It dissolves in water. Prepare by treating iron (II) sulfide with dilute sulfuric acid or dilute hydrochloric acid. Other sulfides yielding hydrogen sulfide with dilute acids may be used.

Hydrogen sulfide TS A saturated solution of hydrogen sulfide. Prepare by passing hydrogen sulfide into cold water.

Storage—Preserve in well-filled, light-resistant bottles, in a dark, cold place.

Hydrogen tetrachloroaurate (III) tetrahydrate $HAuCl_4.4H_2O$ [K 8127, Special class]

Hydrogen tetrachloroaurate (III) TS Dissolve 1 g of hydrogen tetrachloroaurate (III) tetrahydrate in 35 mL of water.

Hydroquinone $C_6H_4(OH)_2$ [K 8738, Special class]

Hydroxocobalamin acetate $C_{62}H_{89}CoN_{13}O_{15}P.C_2H_4O_2$ Dark red, crystals or powder.

Loss on drying <2.41>: not more than 12% (50 mg, in vacuum not exceeding 0.67 kPa, phosphorus (V) oxide, 100°C, 6 hours).

Content: not less than 98.0%. Assay—Proceed as directed in the Assay under Hydroxocobalamin Acetate.

***m*-Hydroxyacetophenone** $C_8H_8O_2$ White to light yellow-white crystalline powder.

Melting point <2.60>: about 96°C

Purity Related substances—Perform the test with 10 μL of a solution of *m*-hydroxyacetophenone in 0.1 mol/L phosphate buffer solution (pH 4.5) (1 in 15,000) as directed in the Assay under Cefalexin: Any obstructive peaks for determination of cefalexin are not observed.

***p*-Hydroxyacetophenone** $C_8H_8O_2$ White to pale yellow, crystals or crystalline powder. It is freely soluble in methanol.

Melting point <2.60>: 107 - 111°C

Purity—Weigh 1 mg of *p*-hydroxyacetophenone, add methanol and dissolve to make exactly 10 mL, and use this solution as the sample solution. Perform the test with 20 μL of the sample solution as directed under Liquid Chromatography <2.01> according to the Assay under Peony Root: the total area of the peaks other than *p*-hydroxyacetophenone obtained from the sample solution is not larger than the total area of the peaks other than the solvent peak.

3-Hydroxybenzoic acid HOC_6H_4COOH White, crystals or crystalline powder.

Identification—Determine the infrared absorption spectrum according to the paste method under Infrared Spectrophotometry <2.25>: it exhibits absorption at the wave numbers of about 3300 cm^{-1}, 1690 cm^{-1}, 1600 cm^{-1}, 1307 cm^{-1}, 1232 cm^{-1} and 760 cm^{-1}.

Melting point <2.60>: 203 - 206°C

Purity Clarity of solution—Dissolve 1.0 g of 3-hydroxybenzoic acid in 20 mL of methanol: the solution is clear.

Content: not less than 99.0%. Assay—Weigh accurately about 0.2 g of 3-hydroxybenzoic acid, dissolve in 20 mL of diluted ethanol (95) (1 in 2), and titrate <2.50> with 0.1 mol/L sodium hydroxide VS (indicator: 3 drops of cresol red TS) until the color of the solution changes from yellow to dark orange-red. Perform a blank determination in the same manner, and make any necessary correction.

Each mL of 0.1 mol/L sodium hydroxide VS
= 13.81 mg of $C_7H_6O_3$

***p*-Hydroxybenzoic acid** See parahydroxybenzoic acid.

10-Hydroxy-2-(*E*)-decenoic acid for assay $C_{10}H_{18}O_3$ 10-hydroxy-2-(*E*)-decenoic acid for thin-layer chromatography. It meets the requirement of the following 1) 10-Hydroxy-2-(*E*)-decenoic acid for assay 1 or 2) 10-Hydroxy-2-(*E*)-decenoic acid for assay 2 (Purity value by quantitative NMR). The latter is used with correction for its amount based on the result obtained in the Assay.

1) 10-Hydroxy-2-(*E*)-decenoic acid for assay 1

Purity Related substances—Dissolve 10 mg of 10-hydroxy-2-(*E*)-decenoic acid for assay 1 in 100 mL of methanol, and use this solution as the sample solution. Pipet 1 mL of the sample solution, add methanol to make exactly 100 mL, and use this solution as the standard solution. Perform the test with exactly 10 μL each of the sample solution and standard solution as directed under Liquid Chromatography <2.01> according to the following conditions. Determine each peak area by the automatic integration method: the total area of the peaks other than 10-hydroxy-2-(*E*)-decenoic acid obtained from the sample solution is not larger than the peak area of 10-hydroxy-2-(*E*)-decenoic acid from the standard solution.

Operating conditions

Detector, column, column temperature, mobile phase and flow rate: Proceed as directed in the operating conditions in the Assay under Royal Jelly.

Time span of measurement: About 4 times as long as the retention time of 10-hydroxy-2-(*E*)-decenoic acid, beginning after the solvent peak.

System suitability

Test for required detectability: Pipet 1 mL of the standard solution, and add methanol to make exactly 20 mL. Confirm that the peak area of 10-hydroxy-2-(*E*)-decenoic acid obtained with 10 μL of this solution is equivalent to 3.5 to 6.5% of that with 10 μL of the standard solution.

System performance: Dissolve 1 mg of propyl parahydroxybenzoate for resolution check in 10 mL of the sample solution. When the procedure is run with 10 μL of this solution under the above operating conditions, 10-hydroxy-2-(*E*)-decenoic acid and propyl parahydroxybenzoate are eluted in this order with the resolution between these peaks being not less than 1.5.

System repeatability: When the test is repeated 6 times with 10 μL of the standard solution under the above operating conditions, the relative standard deviation of the peak area of 10-hydroxy-2-(*E*)-decenoic acid is not more than 1.5%.

2) 10-Hydroxy-2-(*E*)-decenoic acid for assay 2 (Purity value by quantitative NMR)

Unity of peak—Dissolve 1 mg of 10-hydroxy-2-(*E*)-decenoic acid for assay 2 in 50 mL of methanol, and use this solution as the sample solution. Perform the test with 10 μL of the sample solution as directed under Liquid Chromatography <*2.01*> according to the following conditions, and compare the absorption spectra of at least 3 points including the top of 10-hydroxy-2-(*E*)-decenoic acid peak and around the two middle peak heights of before and after the top: no difference in form is observed among their spectra.

Operating conditions

Column, column temperature, mobile phase, and flow rate: Proceed as directed in the operating conditions in the Assay under Royal Jelly.

Detector: A photodiode array detector (wavelength: 215 nm: spectrum range of measurement: 200 – 400 nm).

System suitability

System performance: Dissolve 1 mg each of 10-hydroxy-2-(*E*)-decenoic acid for assay 2 and propyl parahydroxybenzoate for resolution check in methanol to make 50 mL. When the procedure is run with 10 μL of this solution under the above operating conditions, 10-hydroxy-2-(*E*)-decenoic acid and propyl parahydroxybenzoate are eluted in this order with the resolution between these peaks being not less than 1.5.

Assay—Weigh accurately 5 mg of 10-hydroxy-2-(*E*)-decenoic acid for assay 2 and 1 mg of 1,4-BTMSB-d_4 for nuclear magnetic resonance spectroscopy using an ultramicrobalance, dissolve in 1 mL of deuterated methanol for nuclear magnetic resonance spectroscopy, and use this solution as the sample solution. Transfer the sample solution into an NMR tube 5 mm in outer diameter, and measure ^{1}H-NMR as directed under Nuclear Magnetic Resonance Spectroscopy <*2.21*> and Crude Drugs Test <*5.01*> according to the following conditions, using 1,4-BTMSB-d_4 for nuclear magnetic resonance spectroscopy as the reference standard for qNMR. Calculate the resonance intensities, A_1 (equivalent to 1 hydrogen) and A_2 (equivalent to 1 hydrogen), of the signals around δ 5.54 ppm and δ 6.70 ppm assuming the signal of the reference standard for qNMR as δ 0 ppm.

Amount (%) of 10-hydroxy-2-(*E*)-decenoic acid ($C_{10}H_{18}O_3$)
$= M_S \times I \times P/(M \times N) \times 0.8223$

M: Amount (mg) of 10-hydroxy-2-(*E*)-decenoic acid for assay 2 taken

M_S: Amount (mg) of 1,4-BTMSB-d_4 for nuclear magnetic resonance spectroscopy taken

I: Sum of the signal resonance intensities, A_1 and A_2, based on the signal resonance intensity of 1,4-BTMSB-d_4 for nuclear magnetic resonance spectroscopy as 18.000

N: Sum of the numbers of the hydrogen derived from A_1 and A_2

P: Purity (%) of 1,4-BTMSB-d_4 for nuclear magnetic resonance spectroscopy

Operating conditions

Apparatus: A nuclear magnetic resonance spectrometer having ^{1}H resonance frequency of not less than 400 MHz.

Target nucleus: ^{1}H.

Digital resolution: 0.25 Hz or lower.

Measuring spectrum range: 20 ppm or upper, including between −5 ppm and 15 ppm.

Spinning: off.

Pulse angle: 90°.

^{13}C decoupling: on.

Delay time: Repeating pulse waiting time not less than 60 seconds.

Integrating times: 8 or more times.

Dummy scanning: 2 or more times.

Measuring temperature: A constant temperature between 20°C and 30°C.

System suitability

Test for required detectability: When the procedure is run with the sample solution under the above operating conditions, the SN ratio of each signal around δ 5.54 ppm and δ 6.70 ppm is not less than 100.

System performance: When the procedure is run with the sample solution under the above operating conditions, the signals around δ 5.54 ppm and δ 6.70 ppm are not overlapped with any signal of obvious foreign substances, and the ratio of the resonance intensities, A_1/A_2, of each signal around δ 5.54 ppm and δ 6.70 ppm is between 0.99 and 1.01.

System repeatability: When the test is repeated 6 times with the sample solution under the above operating conditions, the relative standard deviations of the ratios of the resonance intensity, A_1 or A_2, to that of the reference standard for qNMR are not more than 1.0%.

10-Hydroxy-2-(*E*)-decenoic acid for component determination See 10-hydroxy-2-(*E*)-decenoic acid for assay.

10-Hydroxy-2-(*E*)-decenoic acid for thin-layer chromatography $C_{10}H_{18}O_3$ White crystalline powder. Very soluble in methanol, freely soluble in ethanol (99.5), soluble in diethyl ether, and slightly soluble in water.

Identification—Determine the absorption spectrum of a solution of 10-hydroxy-2-(*E*)-decenoic acid for thin-layer chromatography in ethanol (99.5) (1 in 125,000) as directed under Ultraviolet-visible Spectrophotometry <*2.24*>: it exhibits a maximum between 206 nm and 210 nm.

Melting point <*2.60*>: 63 – 66°C

Purity Related substances—Dissolve 5.0 mg of 10-hydroxy-2-(*E*)-decenoic acid for thin-layer chromatography in 1 mL of diethyl ether. Perform the test with 20 μL of this solution as directed in the Identification under Royal Jelly: no spot other than the principal spot at around *Rf* value of 0.5 appears.

***d*-3-Hydroxy-*cis*-2,3-dihydro-5-[2-(dimethylamino)ethyl]-2-(4-methoxyphenyl)-1,5-benzothiazepine-4(5*H*)-one hydrochloride** $C_{20}H_{24}N_2O_3S.HCl$ To 9 g of diltiazem hydrochloride add 50 mL of ethanol (99.5), and dissolve by heating at 80°C. To this solution add slowly 50 mL of a solution of potassium hydroxide in ethanol (99.5) (33 in 500) dropwise, and heat for 4 hours with stirring. Cool in an ice bath, filter, and evaporate the filtrate to dryness. Dissolve the residue in ethanol (99.5), add slowly a solution of hydrochloric acid in ethanol (99.5) (59 in 250) to make acidic, and filter. Add diethyl ether slowly to the filtrate, and filter the crystals produced. To the crystals add ethanol (99.5), heat to dissolve, add 0.5 g of activated charcoal, allow to stand, and filter. After cooling the filtrate in an ice-methanol bath, filter the crystals formed, and wash with diethyl ether. Further, add ethanol (99.5) to the crystals, and heat to dissolve. After cooling, filter the crystals produced, and dry under reduced pressure. White, crystals or crystalline powder, having a slight, characteristic odor.

Purity—Dissolve 50 mg of *d*-3-hydroxy-*cis*-2,3-dihydro-5-[2-(dimethylamino)ethyl]-2-(4-methoxyphenyl)-1,5-benzothiazepine-4-(5*H*)-one hydrochloride in chloroform to make exactly 10 mL, and use this solution as the sample solution. Perform the test with the sample solution as directed under Thin-layer Chromatography <*2.03*>. Spot 20 μL of the sample solution on a plate of silica gel for thin-layer chromatography. Develop the plate with a mixture of ethanol (99.5), chloroform, water and acetic acid (100) (12:10:3:1) to a distance of about 13 cm, and air-dry the plate. Spray evenly iodine TS on the plate: any spot other than the principal spot does not appear.

Water <*2.48*>: not more than 1.0% (0.5 g).

Content: not less than 99.0%, calculated on the anhydrous basis. Assay—Weigh accurately about 0.5 g of *d*-3-hydroxy-*cis*-2,3-dihydro-5-[2-(dimethylamino)ethyl]-2-(4-methoxyphenyl)-1,5-benzothiazepine-4-(5*H*)-one hydrochloride, dissolve in 2.0 mL of formic acid, add 60 mL of acetic anhydride, and titrate <*2.50*> with 0.1 mol/L perchloric acid VS (potentiometric titration). Perform a blank determination in the same manner, and make any necessary correction.

Each mL of 0.1 mol/L perchloric acid VS
= 40.89 mg of $C_{20}H_{24}N_2O_3S.HCl$

***d*-3-Hydroxy-*cis*-2,3-dihydro-5-[2-(dimethylamino)ethyl]-2-(*p*-methoxyphenyl)-1,5-benzothiazepine-4 (5H)-one hydrochloride** See *d*-3-hydroxy-*cis*-2,3-dihydro-5-[2-(dimethylamino)ethyl]-2-(4-methoxyphenyl)-1,5-benzothiazepine-4 (5*H*)-one hydrochloride.

***N*-(2-Hydroxyethyl)isonicotinamide nitric ester** $C_8H_9N_3O_4$ A white crystalline powder.

Identification—Determine the infrared absorption spectrum of *N*-(2-hydroxyethyl)isonicotinamide nitric ester as directed in the potassium bromide disk method under Infrared Spectrophotometry <*2.25*>: it exhibits absorption at the wave numbers of about 3270 cm^{-1}, 1653 cm^{-1}, 1546 cm^{-1} and 1283 cm^{-1}.

***N*-2-Hydroxyethylpiperazine-*N′*-2-ethanesulfonic acid** $C_8H_{18}N_2O_4S$ White crystalline powder.

Purity Clarity and color of solution—Dissolve 11.9 g of *N*-2-hydroxyethylpiperazine-*N′*-2-ethanesulfonic acid in 50 mL of water: the solution is clear and colorless.

Content: not less than 99.0%. Assay—Weigh accurately about 1 g of *N*-2-hydroxyethylpiperazine-*N′*-2-ethanesulfonic acid, dissolve in 60 mL of water, and titrate <*2.50*> with 0.5 mol/L sodium hydroxide VS (Potentiometric titration).

Each mL of 0.5 mol/L sodium hydroxide VS
= 119.2 mg of $C_8H_{18}N_2O_4S$

1-(2-Hydroxyethyl)-1*H*-tetrazol-5-thiol $C_3H_6N_4OS$ White, crystals or powder.

Melting point <*2.60*>: 136 – 141°C

Purity Related substances—Dissolve 0.10 g of 1-(2-hydroxyethyl)-1*H*-tetrazol-5-thiol in 1 mL of water, and use this solution as the sample solution. Pipet 0.5 mL of the sample solution, add water to make exactly 25 mL, and use this solution as the standard solution. Perform the test with these solutions as directed under Thin-layer Chromatography <*2.03*>. Spot 1 μL each of the sample solution and standard solution on a plate of silica gel with fluorescent indicator for thin-layer chromatography, develop with a mixture of ethyl acetate, water, methanol and formic acid (60:10:7:6) to a distance of about 10 cm, and air-dry the plate. Examine under ultraviolet light (main wavelength: 254 nm): the spot other than the principal spot obtained from the sample solution is not more intense than the spot from the standard solution.

2-Hydroxy-1-(2-hydroxy-4-sulfo-1-naphthylazo)-3-naphthoic acid $C_{21}H_{14}N_2O_7S$ [K 8776, Special class]

4-Hydroxyisophthalic acid $HOC_6H_3(COOH)_2$ White, crystals or powder.

Content: not less than 98.0%. Assay—Weigh accurately about 0.14 g of 4-hydroxyisophthalic acid, dissolve in 50 mL of ethanol (95), and titrate <*2.50*> with 0.1 mol/L sodium hydroxide VS (potentiometric titration). Perform a blank determination in the same manner, and make any necessary correction.

Each mL of 0.1 mol/L sodium hydroxide VS
= 9.107 mg of $C_8H_6O_5$

Hydroxylamine hydrochloride See hydroxylammonium chloride.

Hydroxylamine hydrochloride-ferric chloride TS See hydroxylammonium chloride-iron (III) chloride TS.

Hydroxylamine hydrochloride TS See hydroxylammonium chloride TS.

Hydroxylamine perchlorate $NH_2OH.HClO_4$ Hygroscopic, white crystals. Dissolves in water and in ethanol (95).

Melting point <*2.60*>: 87.5 – 90°C

Hydroxylamine perchlorate-dehydrated ethanol TS See hydroxylamine perchlorate-ethanol TS.

Hydroxylamine perchlorate-ethanol TS Dilute 2.99 mL of hydroxylamine perchlorate TS with ethanol (99.5) to make 100 mL.

Storage—Preserve in tight containers, in a cold place.

Hydroxylamine perchlorate TS An ethanol (99.5) solution which contains 13.4% of hydroxylamine perchlorate.

Storage—Preserve in tight containers, in a cold place.

Hydroxylamine TS Dissolve 10 g of hydroxylammonium chloride in 20 mL of water, and add ethanol (95) to make 200 mL. To this solution add, with stirring, 150 mL of 0.5 mol/L potassium hydroxide-ethanol VS, and filter. Prepare before use.

Hydroxylamine TS, alkaline Mix equal volumes of a solution of hydroxylammonium chloride in methanol (7 in 100) and a solution of sodium hydroxide in methanol (3 in 25), and filter. Prepare before use.

Hydroxylamine hydrochloride TS (pH 3.1) See hydroxylammonium chloride TS (pH 3.1).

Hydroxylammonium chloride $NH_2OH.HCl$ [K 8201, Special class]

Hydroxylammonium chloride-ethanol TS Dissolve 34.8 g of hydroxylammonium chloride in water to make 100 mL, and use this solution as Solution A. Dissolve 10.3 g of sodium acetate trihydrate and 86.5 g of sodium hydroxide in water to make 1000 mL, and use this solution as Solution B.

Mix 1 volume of Solution A, 1 volume of Solution B and 4 volumes of ethanol (95).

Hydroxylammonium chloride-iron (III) chloride TS Acidify 100 mL of a solution of iron (III) chloride hexahydrate in ethanol (95) (1 in 200) with hydrochloric acid, and dissolve 1 g of hydroxylammonium chloride in the solution.

Hydroxylammonium chloride TS Dissolve 20 g of hydroxylammonium chloride in water to make 65 mL, transfer it to a separator, add 2 to 3 drops of thymol blue TS, then add ammonia solution (28) until the solution exhibits a yellow color. Shake well after adding 10 mL of a solution of sodium *N*,*N*-diethyldithiocarbamate trihydrate (1 in 25), allow to stand for 5 minutes, and extract this solution with 10 to 15 mL portions of chloroform. Repeat the extraction until 5 mL of the extract does not exhibit a yellow color, upon adding 5 drops of a solution of copper (II) sulfate pentahydrate (1 in 100) and shaking it. Add 1 to 2 drops of thymol blue TS, add dropwise dilute hydrochloric acid to this aqueous solution until it exhibits a red color, then add water to make 100 mL.

Hydroxylammonium chloride TS (pH 3.1) Dissolve 6.9 g of hydroxylammonium chloride in 80 mL of water, adjust the pH to 3.1 by adding dilute sodium hydroxide TS, and add water to make 100 mL.

4-Hydroxy-3-methoxybenzyl nonylic acid amide $C_{17}H_{27}NO_3$ A white crystalline powder, having a faint, characteristic odor.

Purity Related substances—Dissolve 10 mg of 4-Hydroxy-3-methoxybenzyl nonylic acid amide in 50 mL of methanol, and use this solution as the sample solution. Pipet 1 mL of the sample solution, add methanol to make exactly 20 mL, and use this solution as the standard solution. Perform the test with exactly 20 μL each of the sample solution and standard solution as directed in the Assay under Capsicum: when measure the peak areas 2 times as long as the retention time of capsaicin, the total area of the peaks other than 4-hydroxy-3-methoxybenzyl nonylic acid amide from the sample solution is not larger than the peak area of 4-hydroxy-3-methoxybenzyl nonylic acid amide from the standard solution.

3-(3-Hydroxy-4-methoxyphenyl)-2-(*E*)-propenoic acid See (*E*)-isoferulic acid.

3-(3-Hydroxy-4-methoxyphenyl)-2-(*E*)-propenoic acid-(*E*)-ferulic acid TS for thin-layer chromatography See (*E*)-isoferulic acid-(*E*)-ferulic acid TS for thin-layer chromatography.

2-[4-(2-Hydroxymethyl)-1-piperazinyl] propanesulfonic acid $C_8H_{18}N_2O_4S$ A white crystalline powder.

Residue on ignition <2.44>: not more than 0.1%.

Content: not less than 99%.

***N*-(3-Hydroxyphenyl)acetamide** $C_8H_9NO_2$ White to pale yellow-white crystals. It is freely soluble in ethanol (95), and sparingly soluble in water.

Melting point <2.60>: 146 – 149°C

Purity (1) Clarity and color of solution—Dissolve 0.5 g of *N*-(3-hydroxyphenyl)acetamide in 50 mL of water: the solution is clear and colorless.

(2) Related substances—Dissolve 0.1 g of *N*-(3-hydroxyphenyl)acetamide in 1000 mL of water. Pipet 10 mL of this solution, add 6.5 mL of acetonitrile and water to make exactly 50 mL, and use this solution as the sample solution. Perform the test with 10 μL of the sample solution as directed in the Assay under Aspoxicillin Hydrate: any peak other than those of *N*-(3-hydroxyphenyl)acetamide and the solvent does not appear.

3-(*p*-Hydroxyphenyl)propionic acid $C_9H_{10}O_3$ White to light yellow-brown, crystals or crystalline powder, having a faint, characteristic odor.

Content: not less than 99.0%. Assay—Weigh accurately about 0.2 g of 3-(*p*-hydroxyphenyl)propionic acid, previously dried (in vacuum, 60°C, 4 hours), dissolve in 5 mL of methanol, add 45 mL of water, and titrate <2.50> with 0.1 mol/L sodium hydroxide VS (indicator: 5 drops of bromothymol blue TS).

Each mL of 0.1 mol/L sodium hydroxide VS
= 16.62 mg of $C_9H_{10}O_3$

Hyodeoxycholic acid for thin-layer chromatography $C_{24}H_{40}O_4$ White to pale brown, crystalline powder or powder. Freely soluble in methanol an in ethanol (99.5), and practically insoluble in water.

Identification—Determine the infrared absorption spectrum of hyodeoxycholic acid for thin-layer chromatography as directed in the potassium bromide disk method under Infrared Spectrophotometry <2.25>: it exhibits absorption at the wave numbers of about 2940 cm^{-1}, 2840 cm^{-1}, 1740 cm^{-1}, 1460 cm^{-1}, 1340 cm^{-1}, 1200 cm^{-1}, 1160 cm^{-1}, 1040 cm^{-1} and 600 cm^{-1}.

Optical rotation <2.49> $[\alpha]_D^{20}$: +7 – +10° (0.4 g, ethanol (99.5), 20 mL, 100 mm).

Melting point <2.60>: 198 – 205°C

Purity Related substances—Dissolve 20 mg of hyodeoxycholic acid for thin-layer chromatography in 1 mL of methanol, and use this solution as the sample solution. Pipet 0.2 mL of the sample solution, add methanol to make exactly 10 mL, and use this solution as the standard solution. Perform the test with these solutions as directed under Thin-layer Chromatography <2.03>. Spot 5 μL each of the sample solution and standard solution on a plate of silica gel for thin-layer chromatography. Develop the plate with a mixture of chloroform, acetone and acetic acid (100) (7:2:1) to a distance of about 10 cm, and air-dry the plate. Splay evenly dilute sulfuric acid on the plate, and heat the plate at 105°C for 10 minutes: the spots other than the principal spot at the *Rf* value of about 0.3 obtained from the sample solution are not more intense than the spot from the standard solution.

Hypaconitine for purity $C_{33}H_{45}NO_{10}$ White, crystals or crystalline powder. Soluble in acetonitrile, sparingly soluble in ethanol (99.5) and in diethyl ether, and practically insoluble in water. Melting point: about 175°C (with decomposition).

Identification—Determine the infrared absorption spectrum of hypaconitine for purity as directed in the potassium bromide disk method under Infrared Spectrophotometry <2.25>: it exhibits absorption at the wave numbers of about 3500 cm^{-1}, 1728 cm^{-1}, 1712 cm^{-1}, 1278 cm^{-1}, 1118 cm^{-1}, 1099 cm^{-1} and 714 cm^{-1}.

Absorbance <2.24> $E^{1\%}_{1\,cm}$ (230 nm): 217 – 252 [5 mg, ethanol (99.5), 200 mL].

Purity Related substances—(1) Dissolve 5.0 mg of hypaconitine for purity in 2 mL of acetonitrile, and use as the sample solution. Pipet 1 mL of the sample solution, add acetonitrile to make exactly 50 mL, and use as the standard solution. Perform the test with these solutions as directed under Thin-layer Chromatography <2.03>. Spot 20 μL each of the sample solution and standard solution on a plate of silica gel for thin-layer chromatography, and proceed the test as directed in the Identification in Processed Aconite Root: the spot other than the principal spot obtained from the sample solution is not more intense than the spot from the standard solution.

(2) Dissolve 5.0 mg of hypaconitine for purity in 5 mL of acetonitrile, and use as the sample solution. Pipet 1 mL of the sample solution, add acetonitrile to make exactly 50 mL, and use as the standard solution. Perform the test with exactly 10 μL each of the sample solution and standard solution as directed under Liquid Chromatography *<2.01>* according to the following conditions, and determine each peak area by the automatic integration method: the total area of the peaks other than hypaconitine obtained from the sample solution is not larger than the peak area of hypaconitine from the standard solution.

Operating conditions

Detector, column, and column temperature: Proceed as directed in the operating conditions in the Purity (3) under Processed Aconite Root.

Mobile phase: A mixture of phosphate buffer solution for processed aconite root and tetrahydrofuran (9:1).

Flow rate: Adjust so that the retention time of hypaconitine is about 23 minutes.

Time span of measurement: About 3 times as long as the retention time of hypaconitine, beginning after the solvent peak.

System suitability

Test for required detectability: Pipet 1 mL of the standard solution, and add acetonitrile to make exactly 20 mL. Confirm that the peak area of hypaconitine obtained with 10 μL of this solution is equivalent to 3.5 to 6.5% of that with 10 μL of the standard solution.

System performance: Dissolve 1 mg each of hypaconitine for purity, aconitine for purity and mesaconitine for purity, and 8 mg of jesaconitine for purity in 200 mL of acetonitrile. When the procedure is run with 10 μL of this solution under the above operating conditions, mesaconitine, hypaconitine, aconitine and jesaconitine are eluted in this order, and each resolution between these peaks is not less than 1.5, respectively.

System repeatability: When the test is repeated 6 times with 10 μL of the standard solution under the above operating conditions, the relative standard deviation of the peak area of hypaconitine is not more than 1.5%.

Water <2.48>: not more than 1.0% (5 mg, coulometric titration).

Hyperoside for thin-layer chromatography $C_{21}H_{20}O_{12}$ Yellow, crystals or crystalline powder. Slightly soluble in methanol, very slightly soluble in ethanol (99.5), and practically insoluble in water. Melting point: about 220°C (with decomposition).

Identification—Determine the absorption spectrum of a solution of hyperoside for thin-layer chromatography in methanol (1 in 100,000) as directed under Ultraviolet-visible Spectrophotometry *<2.24>*: it exhibits a maximum between 255 nm and 259 nm.

Purity Related substances—Dissolve 1 mg of hyperoside for thin-layer chromatography in 20 mL of methanol. Perform the test with 10 μL of this solution as directed in the Identification 2) under Crataegus Fruit: any spot other than the principal spot of around *Rf* value of 0.5 does not appear.

Hypophosphorus acid See phosphinic acid.

Hypoxanthine $C_5H_4N_4O$ White, crystals or crystalline powder. Freely soluble in ammonia TS, sparingly soluble in dilute hydrochloric acid and in hot water, very slightly soluble in water, and practically insoluble in methanol.

Purity Related substances—Dissolve 5.0 mg of hypoxanthine in 100 mL of a solution of ammonia solution (28) in methanol (1 in 10) to make exactly 100 mL. Proceed with this solution as directed in the Purity (4) under Mercaptopurine Hydrate: any spot other than the principal spot at the *Rf* value of about 0.2 does not appear.

Content: not less than 97.0% and not more than 103.0%. Assay—Weigh accurately about 0.15 g of hypoxanthine, previously dried at 105°C for 3 hours, and dissolve in phosphate buffer solution (pH 7.0) to make exactly 1000 mL. Pipet 10 mL of this solution, and dilute with phosphate buffer solution (pH 7.0) to make exactly 250 mL. Read the absorbance *A* of this solution at the wavelength of 250 nm as directed under Ultraviolet-visible Spectrophotometry *<2.24>*.

Amount (mg) of hypoxanthine ($C_5H_4N_4O$)

$$= \frac{A}{779} \times 250{,}000$$

Ibuprofen $C_{13}H_{18}O_2$ [Same as the namesake monograph]

Ibuprofen piconol $C_{19}H_{23}NO_2$ [Same as the namesake monograph]

Ibuprofen piconol for assay $C_{19}H_{23}NO_2$ [Same as the monograph Ibuprofen Piconol. It contains not less than 99.0% of ibuprofen piconol ($C_{19}H_{23}NO_2$), calculated on the anhydrous basis, and meets the following additional requirement.]

Purity Related substances—Dissolve 0.15 g of ibuprofen piconol for assay in the mobile phase to make 100 mL. To 10 mL of this solution add the mobile phase to make 30 mL, and use this as the sample solution. Pipet 1 mL of the sample solution, add the mobile phase to make exactly 100 mL, and use this solution as the standard solution. Perform the test with exactly 5 μL each of the sample solution and standard solution as directed under Liquid Chromatography *<2.01>* according to the following conditions, and determine the peak areas by the automatic integration method: the total area of the peaks other than ibuprofen piconol obtained from the sample solution is not larger than the peak area of ibuprofen piconol from the standard solution.

Operating conditions

Detector, column, column temperature, mobile phase, and flow rate: Perform as directed in the operating conditions in the Assay under Ibuprofen Piconol Ointment.

Time span of measurement: About 2 times as long as the retention time of ibuprofen piconol.

System suitability

Test for required detectability: To exactly 1 mL of the standard solution add the mobile phase to make exactly 20 mL. Confirm that the peak area of ibuprofen piconol obtained with 5 μL of this solution is equivalent to 3.5 to 6.5% of that with 5 μL of the standard solution.

System performance: When the procedure is run with 5 μL of the standard solution under the above operating conditions, the number of theoretical plates and the symmetry factor of the peak of ibuprofen piconol are not less than 5000 and not more than 1.3, respectively.

System repeatability: When the test is repeated 6 times with 5 μL of the standard solution under the above operating conditions, the relative standard deviation of the peak area of ibuprofen piconol is not more than 2.0%.

Icariin for thin-layer chromatography $C_{33}H_{40}O_{15}$ Light yellow crystals. Very slightly soluble in methanol and in ethanol (99.5), and practically insoluble in water. Melting point: about 234°C (with decomposition).

Purity Related substances—Dissolve 1.0 mg of icariin

for thin-layer chromatography in 1 mL of methanol. Perform the test with 10 μL of this solution as directed in the Identification under Epimedium Herb: no spot other than the principal spot at an *Rf* value of about 0.4 appears.

Ifenprodil tartrate for assay $(C_{21}H_{27}NO_2)_2.C_4H_6O_6$ [Same as the monograph Ifenprodil Tartrate. It contains not less than 99.5% of ifenprodil tartrate $[(C_{21}H_{27}NO_2)_2.C_4H_6O_6]$, calculated on the anhydrous basis, and meets the following additional requirement.]

Purity Related substances—Dissolve 20 mg of ifenprodil tartrate for assay in 200 mL of the mobile phase A, and use this solution as the sample solution. Pipet 1 mL of the sample solution, add the mobile phase A to make exactly 100 mL, and use this solution as the standard solution. Perform the test with exactly 20 μL each of the sample solution and standard solution as directed under Liquid Chromatography *<2.01>* according to the following conditions. Determine each peak area by the automatic integration method: the total area of the peaks other than ifenprodil obtained from the sample solution is not larger than 1/2 times the peak area of ifenprodil from the standard solution. For the area of the peak, having the relative retention time of about 0.55 to ifenprodil, multiply the correction factor, 7.1.

Operating conditions

Detector, column, column temperature, and flow rate: Proceed as directed in the operating conditions in the Assay under Ifenprodil Tartrate Fine Granules.

Mobile phase A: Dissolve 6.8 g of potassium dihydrogen phosphate in 900 mL of water, adjust to pH 6.5 with potassium hydroxide TS, and add water to make 1000 mL. To 420 mL of this solution, add 320 mL of methanol for liquid chromatography and 260 mL of acetonitrile for liquid chromatography.

Mobile phase B: Methanol for liquid chromatography.

Flowing of mobile phase: Control the gradient by mixing the mobile phases A and B as directed in the following table.

Time after injection of sample (min)	Mobile phase A (vol%)	Mobile phase B (vol%)
0.0 - 15.0	100	0
15.0 - 15.1	100 → 0	0 → 100
15.1 - 35.0	0	100

Time span of measurement: For 35 minutes after injection of the sample solution.

System suitability

Test for required detectability: Pipet 1 mL of the standard solution, add the mobile phase A to make exactly 10 mL. Confirm that the peak area of ifenprodil obtained with 20 μL of this solution is equivalent to 7 to 13% of that with the standard solution.

System performance: When the procedure is run with 20 μL of the standard solution under the above operating conditions, the number of theoretical plates and the symmetry factor of the peak of ifenprodil are not less than 3500 and not more than 2.0, respectively.

System repeatability: When the test is repeated 6 times with 20 μL of the standard solution under the above operating conditions, the relative standard deviation of the peak area of ifenprodil is not more than 2.0%.

Imidapril hydrochloride $C_{20}H_{27}N_3O_6.HCl$ [Same as the namesake monograph]

Imidapril hydrochloride for assay $C_{20}H_{27}N_3O_6.HCl$ [Same as the monograph Imidapril Hydrochloride. When dried, it contains not less than 99.0% of imidapril hydrochloride $(C_{20}H_{27}N_3O_6.HCl)$.]

Imidazole $C_3H_4N_2$ White crystalline powder. Very soluble in water and in methanol.

Absorbance <2.24> $E^{1\%}_{1\,cm}$ (313 nm): not more than 0.031 (8 g, water, 100 mL).

Melting point <2.60>: 89 - 92°C

Imidazole for thin-layer chromatography $C_3H_4N_2$ White crystalline powder. Very soluble in water and in methanol, and freely soluble in ethyl acetate and in dichloromethane.

Melting point <2.60>: 89 - 92°C

Purity Related substances—Dissolve 10 mg of imidazole for thin-layer chromatography in exactly 20 mL of dichloromethane, and proceed with this solution as directed in the Purity (6) under Clotrimazole: any spot other than the principal spot does not appear.

Imidazole for water determination Imidazole for thin-layer chromatography. Water content per g of imidazole for water determination should not be more than 1 mg.

Imidazole hydrobromide $C_3H_4N_2.HBr$ White to pale yellow crystals. Melting point: about 221°C.

Imidazole TS Dissolve 8.25 g of imidazole in 65 mL of water, adjust the pH to 6.8 with 5 mol/L hydrochloric acid TS, and add water to make 100 mL.

Iminodibenzyl $C_{14}H_{13}N$ White to light brown, crystals or crystalline powder, having a slight, characteristic odor.

Melting point <2.60>: 104 - 110°C

Purity (1) Clarity of solution—Dissolve 1.0 g of iminodibenzyl in 20 mL of methanol by heating on a water bath: the solution is clear.

(2) Related substances—Proceed as directed in the Purity (6) under Carbamazepine: any spot other than the principal spot at the *Rf* value of about 0.9 does not appear.

Nitrogen <1.08>: 6.8 - 7.3%.

2,2′-Iminodiethanol hydrochloride $C_4H_{11}NO_2.HCl$ A light yellow liquid.

Refractive index <2.45> n^{20}_{D}: 1.515 - 1.519

Specific gravity <2.56> d^{20}_{20}: 1.259 - 1.263

Water <2.48>: less than 0.1%.

Imipramine hydrochloride $C_{19}H_{24}N_2.HCl$ [Same as the namesake monograph]

Immature orange [Same as the namesake monograph]

Indigo carmine $C_{16}H_8N_2Na_2O_8S_2$ [K 8092, Special class]

Indigo carmine TS Dissolve 0.20 g of indigo carmine in water to make 100 mL. Use within 60 days.

2,3-Indolinedione $C_8H_5NO_2$ [K 8089, Special class]

Indometacin $C_{19}H_{16}ClNO_4$ [Same as the namesake monograph]

Insulin human [Same as the monograph Insulin Human (Genetical Recombination)]

Interleukin-2 dependent mouse natural killer cell NKC3 Fractionate using discontinuous concentration gradient method cells obtained by removing adhesive cells and phagocytic cells from C3H/He mouse spleen cells. Then, cultivate in soft agar containing interleukin-2 the cell fraction with potent NK activity and obtain the colonies. From among the cell lines obtained, one of the cell lines dependent on interleukin-2 that grows in liquid medium and serially subcultured in liquid medium containing interleukin-2 is identified as NKC3.

Iodine I [K 8920, Special class]

Iodine bromide (II) TS Dissolve 20 g of iodine monobromide in acetic acid (100) to make 1000 mL. Store protected from light.

Iodine for assay I [Same as the monograph Iodine]

Iodine monobromide IBr Black-brown, crystals or masses. It dissolves in water, in ethanol (95), in acetic acid (100), in diethyl ether and in carbon disulfide.

Melting point <2.60>: 37 – 43°C

Storage—Preserve in light-resistant glass containers, in a cold place.

Iodine-starch TS To 100 mL of starch TS add 3 mL of dilute iodine TS.

Iodine trichloride ICl_3 [K 8403, Special class]

Iodine TS Dissolve 14 g of iodine in 100 mL of a solution of potassium iodide (2 in 5), add 1 mL of dilute hydrochloric acid, and dilute with water to make 1000 mL (0.05 mol/L).

Storage—Preserve in light-resistant containers.

Iodine TS, dilute To 1 volume of iodine TS add 4 volumes of water.

0.0002 mol/L Iodine TS Measure exactly 1 mL of 0.5 mol/L iodine TS, add water to make exactly 250 mL, pipet 10 mL of the solution, and add water to make exactly 100 mL. Prepare before use.

0.5 mol/L Iodine TS To 12.7 g of iodine and 25 g of potassium iodide add 10 mL of water, triturate, and add water to make 100 mL.

Iodoacetic acid ICH_2COOH White or practically white crystals.

Iodoethane C_2H_5I A colorless or a dark-brown, clear liquid, having diethyl ether-like odor.

Distilling range <2.57>: 71.0 – 72.5°C, not less than 94 vol%.

Iodoethane for assay C_2H_5I Colorless to pale yellow liquid, turning brown on exposure to air and light. Miscible with ethanol (95). Specific gravity d^{20}_{20}: about 1.95; Boiling point: about 72°C.

Refractive index <2.45> n^{20}_D: 1.509 – 1.515.

Content: not less than 99.0%. Assay—Proceed as directed in the Assay under isopropyl iodide for assay.

Each mL of 0.1 mol/L silver nitrate VS
= 15.60 mg of C_2H_5I

Storage—Preserve in tight, light-resistant containers.

Iodomethane CH_3I [K 8919, Special class]

Iodomethane for assay CH_3I Colorless to dark brown, clear liquid. On exposure to light, it liberates iodine and becomes brown. Miscible with ethanol (95) and with diethyl ether, and sparingly soluble in water. Use the distillate obtained between 42.2°C and 42.6°C.

Specific gravity <2.56> d^{25}_{25}: 2.27 – 2.28.

Purity—Perform the test with 1 μL of iodomethane for assay as directed under Gas Chromatography <2.02> according to the operating conditions in the Assay under Hypromellose. Measure each peak area by the automatic integration method, and calculate the amount of iodomethane by the area percentage method: it shows the purity of not less than 99.8%. Adjust the detection sensitivity so that the peak height of iodomethane from 1 μL of iodomethane for assay is about 80% of the full scale.

Content: not less than 98.0%. Assay—Proceed as directed in the Assay under isopropyl iodide for assay.

Each mL of 0.1 mol/L silver nitrate VS
= 14.19 mg of CH_3I

5-Iodouracil for liquid chromatography $C_4H_3IN_2O_2$ White crystalline powder. Melting point: about 275°C (with decomposition).

Purity—Dissolve 3 mg of 5-iodouracil for liquid chromatography in diluted methanol (1 in 25) to make 10 mL. Perform the test with 10 μL of this solution as directed under Liquid Chromatography <2.01>, according to the operating conditions in the Purity under Idoxuridine Ophthalmic Solution. Determine each peak area by the automatic integration method over a time span of twice as long as the retention time of the principal peak, and calculate the amount of 5-iodouracil by the area percentage method: It shows the purity of not less than 98.5%.

Content: not less than 98.5%. Assay—Weigh accurately about 5 mg of 5-iodouracil for liquid chromatography, previously dried at 60°C for 3 hours under reduced pressure, dissolve in water to make exactly 250 mL. Perform the test with this solution as directed under Ultraviolet-visible Spectrophotometry <2.24>, and determine the absorbance A at the wavelength of maximum absorption at about 282 nm.

$$\text{Amount (mg) of 5-iodouracil } (C_4H_3IN_2O_2) = \frac{A}{265} \times 2500$$

Iopamidol for assay $C_{17}H_{22}I_3N_3O_8$ [Same as the monograph Iopamidol]

Iotalamic acid for assay $C_{11}H_9I_3N_2O_4$ [Same as the monograph Iotalamic Acid]

Irbesartan for assay $C_{25}H_{28}N_6O$ [Same as the monograph Irbesartan]

Irinotecan hydrochloride hydrate for assay $C_{33}H_{38}N_4O_6.HCl.3H_2O$ [Same as the monograph Irinotecan Hydrochloride Hydrate]

Iron Fe Iron in the forms of strips, sheets, granules or wires. Fe: not less than 97.7%. It is attracted by a magnet.

Iron (II) sulfate heptahydrate $FeSO_4.7H_2O$ [K 8978, Special class]

Iron (II) sulfate TS Dissolve 8 g of iron (II) sulfate heptahydrate in 100 mL of freshly boiled and cooled water. Prepare before use.

Iron (II) sulfide FeS [K 8948, for hydrogen sulfide development]

Iron (II) tartrate TS Dissolve 1 g of iron (II) sulfate heptahydrate, 2 g of potassium sodium tartrate tetrahydrate and 0.1 g of sodium hydrogen sulfite in water to make 100 mL.

Iron (II) thiocyanate TS Add 3 mL of dilute sulfuric acid to 35 mL of water, and remove the dissolved oxygen by boiling the solution. Dissolve 1 g of iron (II) sulfate heptahydrate in this hot solution, cool, and then dissolve 0.5 g of potassium thiocyanate. When the solution is pale red in color, decolorize by adding reduced iron, separate the excess of reduced iron by decanting, and preserve the solution with protection from oxygen. Do not use a solution showing a pale red color.

Iron (II) trisodium pentacyanoamine TS To 1.0 g of sodium pentacyanonitrosylferrate (III) dihydrate add 3.2 mL of ammonia TS, shake, stopper closely, and allow to stand in a refrigerator overnight. Add this solution to 10 mL of ethanol (99.5), filter a yellow colored precipitate by suction, wash with dehydrated diethyl ether, dry, and preserve in a desiccator. Before using, dissolve in water to make a solution of 1.0 mg/mL, and store in a refrigerator. Use within 7 days after preparation.

Iron (III) chloride-acetic acid TS Dissolve 0.1 g of iron (III) chloride hexahydrate in diluted acetic acid (31) (3 in 100) to make 100 mL.

Iron (III) chloride-amidosulfuric acid TS Dissolve 10 g of iron (III) chloride hexahydrate and 16 g of amidosulfuric acid (standard reagent) in water to make 1000 mL.

Iron (III) chloride hexahydrate $FeCl_3.6H_2O$ [K 8142, Special class]

Iron (III) chloride-iodine TS Dissolve 5 g of iron (III) chloride hexahydrate and 2 g of iodine in a mixture of 50 mL of acetone and 50 mL of a solution of L-tartaric acid (1 in 5).

Iron (III) chloride-methanol TS Dissolve 1 g of iron (III) chloride hexahydrate in methanol to make 100 mL.

Iron (III) chloride-potassium hexacyanoferrate (III) TS Dissolve 0.1 g of potassium hexacyanoferrate (III) in 20 mL of iron (III) chloride TS. Prepare before use.

Iron (III) chloride-pyridine TS, anhydrous Heat gradually 1.7 g of iron (III) chloride hexahydrate by direct application of flame, melt, and solidify. After cooling, dissolve the residue in 100 mL of chloroform, add 8 mL of pyridine, and filter.

Iron (III) chloride TS Dissolve 9 g of iron (III) chloride hexahydrate in water to make 100 mL (0.33 mol/L).

Iron (III) chloride TS, acidic To 60 mL of acetic acid (100) add 5 mL of sulfuric acid and 1 mL of iron (III) chloride hexahydrate TS.

Iron (III) chloride TS, dilute Dilute 2 mL of iron (III) chloride TS with water to make 100 mL. Prepare before use.

Iron (III) nitrate enneahydrate $Fe(NO_3)_3.9H_2O$ [K 8559, Special class]

Iron (III) nitrate TS Dissolve 1 g of iron (III) nitrate enneahydrate in hydrochloric acid-potassium chloride buffer solution (pH 2.0) to make 300 mL.

Iron (III) perchlorate-ethanol TS Dissolve 0.8 g of iron (III) perchlorate hexahydrate in perchloric acid-ethanol TS to make 100 mL.

Storage—Preserve in tight containers, in a cold place.

Iron (III) perchlorate hexahydrate $Fe(ClO_4)_3.6H_2O$ Hygroscopic, light purple crystals, and a solution in ethanol (99.5) (1 in 125) is clear and orange in color.

Iron (III) sulfate *n*-hydrate $Fe_2(SO_4)_3.xH_2O$ [K 8981, Special class]

Iron (III) sulfate TS Dissolve 50 g of iron (III) sulfate *n*-hydrate in an excess of water, and add 200 mL of sulfuric acid and water to make 1000 mL.

Iron-phenol TS Dissolve 1.054 g of ammonium iron (II) sulfate hexahydrate in 20 mL of water, add 1 mL of sulfuric acid and 1 mL of hydrogen peroxide (30), heat until effervescence ceases, and dilute with water to make 50 mL. To 3 volumes of this solution contained in a volumetric flask add sulfuric acid, with cooling, to make 100 volumes, yielding the iron-sulfuric acid solution. Purify phenol by distillation, discarding the first 10% and the last 5%, and collect the distillate, with exclusion of moisture, in a dry, tared, glass-stoppered flask of about twice the volume of the phenol. Stopper the flask, solidify the phenol in an ice bath, breaking the top crust with a glass rod to ensure complete crystallization, and after drying, weigh the flask. To the glass-stoppered flask add 1.13 times the mass of phenol of the iron-sulfuric acid solution, insert the stopper in the flask, and allow to stand, without cooling but with occasional shaking, until the phenol is liquefied, then shake the mixture vigorously. Allow to stand in a dark place for 16 to 24 hours. To the mixture add diluted sulfuric acid (10 in 21) equivalent to 23.5% of its mass, mix well, transfer to dry glass-stoppered bottles, and preserve in a dark place, with protection from atmospheric moisture. Use within 6 months.

Iron-phenol TS, dilute To 10 mL of iron-phenol TS add 4.5 mL of water. Prepare before use.

Iron powder Fe A lusterless, gray to grayish black powder, being attracted by a magnet.

Identification—To 1 mL of a solution of iron powder in hydrochloric acid (1 in 50) add water to make 15 mL, and add 0.1 mL of potassium hexacyanoferrate (III) TS: a blue color appears.

Iron salicylate TS Dissolve 0.1 g of ammonium iron (III) sulfate dodecahydrate in 50 mL of diluted sulfuric acid (1 in 250), and add water to make 100 mL. Measure 20 mL of this solution, and add 10 mL of a solution of sodium salicylate (23 in 2000), 4 mL of dilute acetic acid, 16 mL of sodium acetate TS and water to make 100 mL. Prepare before use.

Irsogladine maleate $C_9H_7Cl_2N_5.C_4H_4O_4$ [Same as the namesake monograph]

Irsogladine maleate for assay $C_9H_7Cl_2N_5.C_4H_4O_4$ [Same as the monograph Irsogladine Maleate. When dried, it contains not less than 99.5% of irsogladine maleate ($C_9H_7Cl_2N_5.C_4H_4O_4$).]

Isatin See 2,3-indolinedione.

Iscove's modified Dulbecco's fluid medium for filgrastim A fluid medium for cell culture, containing 0.165 g of anhydrous calcium chloride, 97.67 mg of anhydrous magnesium sulfate, 0.330 g of potassium chloride, 76 μg of potassium nitrate, 4.5 g of sodium chloride, 0.125 g of sodium dihydrogen phosphate monohydrate, 17.3 μg of sodium selenite pentahydrate, 30 mg of glycine, 25 mg of L-alanine, 84 mg of L-arginine hydrochloride, 25 mg of L-asparagine, 30 mg of L-aspartic acid, 91.4 mg of L-cystine dihydrochloride, 75 mg of L-glutamic acid, 0.584 g of L-glutamine, 42 mg of L-histidine hydrochloride monohydrate, 0.105 g of L-isoleucine, 0.105 g of L-leucine, 0.146 g of L-lysine hydrochloride, 30 mg of L-methionine, 66 mg of L-phenylalanine, 40 mg of L-proline, 42 mg of L-serine, 95 mg of L-threonine, 16 mg of L-tryptophan, 0.104 g of disodium L-tyrosine, 94 mg of L-valine, 13 μg of biotin, 4 mg of choline chloride, 4 mg of calcium D-pantothenate, 4 mg of folic acid, 4 mg of nicotinic acid amide, 4 mg of pyridoxal hydrochloride, 0.4 mg of riboflavin, 4 mg of thiamine hydrochloride, 13 μg of cyanocobalamin, 7.2 mg of myoinositol, 4.5 g of glucose, 5.958 g of *N*-2-hydroxyethylpiperazine-*N'*-2-ethanesulfonic acid, 15 mg of phenol red, 0.110 g of sodium pyruvate and 3.024 g of sodium hydrogen carbonate in 1 L.

Iscove's modified Dulbecco's powder medium A powder to make fluid medium for cell culture, containing 0.165 g of anhydrous calcium chloride, 97.67 mg of anhydrous magnesium sulfate, 0.330 g of potassium chloride, 76 μg of potassium nitrate, 4.5 g of sodium chloride, 0.125 g of sodium dihydrogen phosphate monohydrate, 17.3 μg of sodium selenite pentahydrate, 30 mg of glycin, 25 mg of L-alanine, 84 mg of L-arginine hydrochloride, 25 mg of L-asparagine, 30 mg of L-aspartic acid, 91.4 mg of L-cystine dihydrochloride, 75 mg of L-glutamic acid, 0.584 g of L-glutamine, 42 mg of L-histidine hydrochloride monohydrate, 0.105 g of L-isoleucine, 0.105 g of L-leucine, 0.146 g of L-lysine hydrochloride, 30 mg of L-methionine, 66 mg of phenylalanine, 40 mg of L-proline, 42 mg of L-serine, 95 mg of L-threonine, 16 mg of L-tryptophan, 0.104 g of disodium L-tyrosine, 94 mg of L-valine, 13 μg of biotin, 4 mg of choline chloride, 4 mg of calcium D-pantothenate, 4 mg of folic acid, 4 mg of nicotinic acid amide, 4 mg of pyridoxal hydrochloride, 0.4 mg of riboflavin, 4 mg of thiamine hydrochloride, 13 μg of cyanocobalamin, 7.2 mg of myoinositol, 4.5 g of glucose, 5.958 g of *N*-2-hydroxyethylpiperazine-*N*-2-ethanesulfonate, 15 mg of phenol red and 0.110 g of sodium pyruvate in each L.

Isoamyl acetate See 3-methylbutyl acetate.

Isoamyl alcohol See 3-methyl-1-butanol.

Isoamyl benzoate $C_{12}H_{16}O_2$
Specific gravity <2.56> d_4^{15}: 0.993
Boiling point <2.57>: 260 – 262°C

Isoamyl parahydroxybenzoate $C_{12}H_{16}O_3$ White crystalline powder, having a faint characteristic odor.

It is very soluble in acetonitrile, in ethanol (95), in acetone and in diethyl ether, and practically insoluble in water.
Melting point <2.60>: 62 – 64°C

Isobutanol See 2-methyl-1-propanol.

Isobutyl parahydroxybenzoate $C_{11}H_{14}O_3$ Colorless crystals or white crystalline powder. Freely soluble in ethanol (95), and practically insoluble in water.
Melting point <2.60>: 74 – 78°C
Residue on ignition <2.44>: not more than 0.1%.
Content: not less than 99.0%. Assay—Weigh accurately about 1 g of isobutyl parahydroxybenzoate, add exactly 20 mL of 1 mol/L sodium hydroxide VS, heat at about 70°C for 1 hour, and immediately cool in ice. Titrate <2.50> the excess sodium hydroxide with 0.5 mol/L sulfuric acid VS up to the second equivalent point (potentiometric titration). Perform a blank determination in the same manner.

Each mL of 1 mol/L sodium hydroxide VS
= 194.2 mg of $C_{11}H_{14}O_3$

Isobutyl salicylate $C_{11}H_{14}O_3$ Colorless, clear liquid, having a characteristic odor.
Refractive index <2.45> n_D^{20}: 1.506 – 1.511
Specific gravity <2.56> d_4^{20}: 1.068 – 1.073
Boiling point <2.57>: 260 – 262°C
Purity—Perform the test with 1 μL of isobutyl salicylate as directed under Gas Chromatography <2.02> according to the following conditions. Determine each peak area by the automatic integration method, and calculate the amount of isobutyl salicylate by the area percentage method: It shows the purity of not less than 97.0%.
Operating conditions

Detector: A thermal conductivity detector.

Column: A column about 3 mm in inside diameter and about 2 m in length, packed with siliceous earth for gas chromatography, 180 to 250 μm in particle diameter, coated with polyehylene glycol 20 M for gas chromatography at the ratio of 10%.

Column temperature: A constant temperature of about 220°C.

Carrier gas: Helium.

Flow rate: About 20 mL per minute.

Detection sensitivity: Adjust the detection sensitivity so that the peak height of isobutyl salicylate obtained from 1 μL of the isobutyl salicylate is about 60 to 80% of the full scale.

Time span of measurement: About 3 times as long as the retention time of isobutyl salicylate.

(*E*)-Isoferulic acid $C_{10}H_{10}O_4$ White to light yellow, crystals or crystalline powder. Sparingly soluble in methanol and in ethanol (99.5), and practically insoluble in water. Melting point: about 230°C (with decomposition).

Identification—Determine the absorption spectrum of a solution of (*E*)-isoferulic acid in methanol (1 in 200,000) as directed under Ultraviolet-visible Spectrophotometry <2.24>: it exhibits maxima between 215 nm and 219 nm, between 238 nm and 242 nm, between 290 nm and 294 nm, and between 319 nm and 323 nm.

Purity Related substances—Conduct this procedure without exposure to light, using light-resistant vessels. Dissolve 1 mg of (*E*)-isoferulic acid in 1 mL of methanol, and use this solution as the sample solution. Perform the test with the sample solution as directed under Thin-layer Chromatography <2.03>. Spot 2 μL of the sample solution on a plate of silica gel for thin-layer chromatography. Develop the plate with a mixture of ethyl acetate, acetone and water (20:12:3) to a distance of about 7 cm, and air-dry the plate. Spray evenly sulfuric acid on the plate, heat the plate at 105°C for 5 minutes, and examine under ultraviolet light (main wavelength: 365 nm): no spot other than the principal spot at an *Rf* value of about 0.6 appears.

(*E*)-Isoferulic acid-(*E*)-ferulic acid TS for thin-layer chromatography Dissolve 1 mg each of (*E*)-isoferulic acid and (*E*)-ferulic acid in 2 mL of methanol.

Isoelectric point markers for teceleukin Dissolve 0.02 to 0.05 mg of cytochrome C, trypsinogen, lentil-lectin basic band, lentil-lectin middle band, lentil-lectin acidic band, horse myoglobin basic band, horse myoglobin acidic band, human carbonic anhydrase B, bovine carbonic anhydrase B, and β-lactoglobulin A, in 0.1 mL of saccharose solution (3 in 10).

L-Isoleucine $C_6H_{13}NO_2$ [Same as the namesake monograph]

L-Isoleucine for assay $C_6H_{13}NO_2$ [Same as the monograph L-Isoleucine. When dried, it contains not less than 99.0% of L-isoleucine ($C_6H_{13}NO_2$).]

Isomalt $C_{12}H_{24}O_{11}$ White, powder or grain. Very soluble in water, and practically insoluble in ethanol (99.5).

Isoniazid $C_6H_7N_3O$ [Same as the namesake monograph]

Isoniazid for assay $C_6H_7N_3O$ [Same as the monograph Isoniazid. When dried, it contains not less than 99.0% of isoniazid ($C_6H_7N_3O$).]

Isoniazid TS Dissolve 0.1 g of isoniazid for assay in a mixture of 50 mL of methanol and 0.12 mL of hydrochloric acid, and add methanol to make 200 mL.

Isonicotinic acid White, crystals or powder. Melting

point: about 315°C (decomposition).

Isonicotinic acid amide $C_6H_6N_2O$ White, crystals or crystalline powder.

Melting point <*2.60*>: 155 – 158°C

Purity Clarity of solution—Dissolve 1.0 g of the substance to be tested in 20 mL of methanol: the solution is clear.

Content: not less than 99.0%. Assay—Weigh accurately about 0.3 g of isonicotinic acid amide, previously dried, and dissolve in 20 mL of acetic acid (100) by heating. After cooling, add 100 mL of benzene, and titrate <*2.50*> with 0.1 mol/L perchloric acid VS until the color of the solution changes from purple to blue-green (indicator: 3 drops of crystal violet TS). Perform a blank determination in the same manner, and make any necessary correction.

Each mL of 0.1 mol/L perchloric acid VS
= 11.21 mg of $C_6H_6N_2O$

Isooctane See octane, iso.

Isopromethazine hydrochloride for thin-layer chromatography $C_{17}H_{20}N_2S.HCl$ White crystalline powder. Odorless. Freely soluble in water, in ethanol (95) and in chloroform, and practically insoluble in diethyl ether.

Melting point <*2.60*>: 186 – 195°C

Purity Related substances—Dissolve 5.0 mg of isopromethazine hydrochloride for thin-layer chromatography in exactly 25 mL of ethanol (95), and perform the test with this solution as directed in the Purity (3) under Promethazine Hydrochloride: any spot other than the principal spot at the *R*f value of about 0.65 does not appear.

Isopropanol See 2-propanol.

Isopropanol for liquid chromatography See 2-propanol for liquid chromatography.

Isopropylamine See propylamine, iso.

Isopropylamine-ethanol TS To 20 mL of isopropylamine add ethanol (99.5) to make 100 mL. Prepare before use.

Isopropyl *p*-aminobenzoate See isopropyl 4-aminobenzoate.

Isopropyl 4-aminobenzoate $H_2NC_6H_4COOCH(CH_3)_2$ Pale brown crystals.

Melting point <*2.60*>: 83 – 86°C

Isopropyl benzoate $C_6H_5COOCH(CH_3)_2$ A clear, colorless liquid, having a characteristic odor.

Refractive index <*2.45*> n_D^{20}: 1.490 – 1.498

Specific gravity <*2.56*> d_{20}^{20}: 1.008 – 1.016

Isopropylether See propylether, iso.

Isopropyl *p*-hydroxybenzoate See isopropyl parahydroxybenzoate.

Isopropyl iodide for assay C_3H_7I Colorless, clear liquid. On exposure to light it liberates iodine and becomes brown. Miscible with ethanol (95), with diethyl ether and with petroleum benzin, and not miscible with water. Use the distillate obtained between 89.0°C and 89.5°C.

Specific gravity <*2.56*> d_4^{20}: 1.700 – 1.710

Purity—Perform the test with 1 μL of isopropyl iodide for assay as directed under Gas Chromatography <*2.02*> according to the operating conditions in the Assay under Hypromellose. Measure each peak area by the automatic integration method, and calculate the amount of isopropyl iodide by the area percentage method: It shows the purity of not less than 99.8%. Adjust the detection sensitivity so that the peak height of isopropyl iodide from 1 μL of isopropyl iodide for assay is about 80% of the full scale.

Content: not less than 98.0%. Assay—Transfer 10 mL of ethanol (95) into a brown volumetric flask, weigh accurately, add 1 mL of isopropyl iodide for assay, and weigh accurately again. Add ethanol (95) to make exactly 100 mL, pipet 20 mL of this solution into the second brown volumetric flask, add exactly 50 mL of 0.1 mol/L silver nitrate VS and then 2 mL of nitric acid, stopper, shake occasionally for 2 hours in a dark place, and allow to stand overnight in a dark place. Shake occasionally for 2 hours, add water to make exactly 100 mL, and filter through dry filter paper. Discard the first 20 mL of the filtrate, pipet the next 50 mL, and titrate <*2.50*> the excess silver nitrate with 0.1 mol/L ammonium thiocyanate VS (indicator: 2 mL of ammonium iron (III) sulfate TS). Perform a blank determination in the same manner.

Each mL of 0.1 mol/L silver nitrate VS
= 17.00 mg of C_3H_7I

Isopropyl myristate $C_{17}H_{34}O_2$ Colorless, clear, oily liquid, and odorless. Congeals at about 5°C. Soluble in 90% alcohol, miscible with many organic solvents and with solid oils, and insoluble in water, in glycerin and in propylene glycol.

Refractive index <*2.45*> n_D^{20}: 1.432 – 1.436

Specific gravity <*2.56*> d_{20}^{20}: 0.846 – 0.854

Acid value <*1.13*>: not more than 1.

Saponification value <*1.13*>: 202 – 212

Iodine value <*1.13*>: not more than 1.

Residue on ignition <*2.44*>: not more than 0.1% (1 g).

Isopropyl myristate for sterility test $C_{17}H_{34}O_2$ Transfer 100 mL of isopropyl myristate into a centrifuge tube, add 100 mL of twice-distilled water, and shake vigorously for 10 minutes. Then centrifuge at a rate of 1800 revolutions per minute for 20 minutes, separate the supernatant liquid (isopropyl myristate layer), and determine the pH of the residual water layer: not less than 5.5.

Treat isopropyl myristate which meets the requirements of pH determination as follows: 500 mL of isopropyl myristate, which has met the requirements of pH determination, is percolated through a 15-cm high layer of activated alumina filled in a glass column 20 mm in diameter and 20 cm in length with a slightly positive pressure in order to facilitate adequate flow, and then sterilized by filtration.

Isopropyl parahydroxybenzoate $C_{10}H_{12}O_3$ Colorless fine crystals, or white crystalline powder. Freely soluble in ethanol (95), and very slightly soluble in water.

Melting point <*2.60*>: 84 – 86°C

Residue on ignition <*2.44*>: not more than 0.1%.

Content: not less than 99.0%. Assay—Weigh accurately about 1 g of isopropyl parahydroxybenzoate, add exactly 20 mL of 1 mol/L sodium hydroxide VS, heat at about 70°C for 1 hour, and immediately cool in ice. Titrate <*2.50*> the excess sodium hydroxide with 0.5 mol/L sulfuric acid VS up to the second equivalent point (potentiometric titration). Perform a blank determination in the same manner.

Each mL of 1 mol/L sodium hydroxide VS
= 180.2 mg of $C_{10}H_{12}O_3$

4-Isopropylphenol $C_9H_{12}O$ White to reddish yellow, crystals or crystalline powder.

Melting point <*2.60*>: 59 – 63°C

Isosorbide dinitrate for assay $C_6H_8N_2O_8$ [Same as the monograph Isosorbide Dinitrate. It contains not less than

99.0% of isosorbide dinitrate ($C_6H_8N_2O_8$), calculated on the anhydrous basis, meeting the following additional specifications.]

Purity Related substances—Dissolve 50 mg of isosorbide dinitrate for assay in 50 mL of a mixture of water and methanol (1:1), and use this solution as the sample solution. Pipet 1 mL of this solution, add a mixture of water and methanol (1:1) to make exactly 200 mL, and use this solution as the standard solution. Perform the test with exactly 10 μL each of the sample solution and standard solution as directed under Liquid Chromatography *<2.01>* according to the following conditions, and determine each peak area of both solutions by the automatic integration method: the total area of the peaks other than the peak of isosorbide dinitrate obtained from the sample solution is not larger than the peak area of isosorbide dinitrate from the standard solution.

Operating conditions

Detector, column, column temperature, mobile phase and flow rate: Proceed as directed in the operating conditions in the Assay under Isosorbide Dinitrate Tablets.

Time span of measurement: About 2 times as long as the retention time of isosorbide dinitrate, beginning after the solvent peak.

System suitability

Test for required detectability: Pipet 5 mL of the standard solution, and add a mixture of water and methanol (1:1) to make exactly 50 mL. Confirm that the peak area of isosorbide dinitrate obtained with 10 μL of this solution is equivalent to 7 to 13% of that with 10 μL of the standard solution.

System performance: When the procedure is run with 10 μL of the standard solution under the above operating conditions, the number of theoretical plates and the symmetry factor of the peak of isosorbide dinitrate are not less than 3000 and not more than 1.5, respectively.

System repeatability: When the test is repeated 6 times with 10 μL of the standard solution under the above operating conditions, the relative standard deviation of the peak area of isosorbide dinitrate is not more than 2.0%.

Isosorbide mononitrate for assay $C_6H_9NO_6$ Odorless white crystals.

Method of purification: To Isosorbide Mononitrate 70%/Lactose 30% add not less than 3-fold volume of ethyl acetate, shake vigorously, filter through a membrane filter with a pore size not exceeding 0.5 μm, and evaporate the filtrate to dryness on a water bath under reduced pressure. Recrystallize the residue from a mixture of hexane and ethyl acetate (3:2), and dry under reduced pressure on silica gel for 4 hours.

Identification—Determine the infrared absorption spectrum of isosorbide mononitrate for assay, previously dried, as directed in the potassium bromide disk method under Infrared Spectrophotometry *<2.25>*: it exhibits absorption at the wave numbers of between 3210 cm^{-1} and 3230 cm^{-1}, and about 1651 cm^{-1}, 1635 cm^{-1}, 1282 cm^{-1}, 1093 cm^{-1} and 852 cm^{-1}.

Optical rotation <2.49> $[\alpha]_D^{20}$: +171 – +176° (after drying, 1 g, ethanol (95), 100 mL, 100 mm).

Melting point <2.60>: 89 – 92°C

Purity Related substances—Dissolve 50 mg of isosorbide mononitrate for assay in 5 mL of water, and use this solution as the sample solution. Pipet 1 mL of the sample solution, add water to make exactly 100 mL. Pipet 5 mL of this solution, add water to make exactly 50 mL, and use this solution as the standard solution. Perform the test with exactly 10 μL each of the sample solution and standard solution as directed under Liquid Chromatography *<2.01>* according to the following conditions. Determine each peak area by the automatic integration method: the area of the peak other than isosorbide mononitrate obtained from the sample solution is not larger than the peak area of isosorbide mononitrate from the standard solution, and the total area of the peaks other than isosorbide mononitrate from the sample solution is not larger than 2 times the peak area of isosorbide mononitrate from the standard solution. For the area of the peak, having a relative retention time of about 4.5 to isosorbide mononitrate, multiply its correction factor, 0.62.

Operating conditions

Detector, column, column temperature, mobile phase, and flow rate: Proceed as directed in the operating conditions in the Assay under Isosorbide Mononitrate 70%/Lactose 30%.

Time span of measurement: About 5 times as long as the retention time of isosorbide mononitrate, beginning after the solvent peak.

System suitability

System performance: When the procedure is run with 10 μL of the standard solution under the above operating conditions, the number of theoretical plates and the symmetry factor of the peak of isosorbide mononitrate are not less than 2000 and not more than 1.5, respectively.

System repeatability: When the test is repeated 6 times with 10 μL of the standard solution under the above operating conditions, the relative standard deviation of the peak area of isosorbide mononitrate is not more than 2.0%.

Loss on drying <2.41>: not more than 0.5% (1 g, in vacuum, silica gel, 4 hours).

Content: not less than 99.0%. Assay—Weigh accurately about 0.2 g of previously dried isosorbide mononitrate for assay, put in a Kjeldahl flask, dissolve in 10 mL of water, add 3 g of Devarda's alloy and 40 mL of water, and set the flask on the apparatus as shown in the figure under Nitrogen Determination *<1.08>*. Put exactly 25 mL of 0.05 mol/L sulfuric acid VS and 5 drops of bromocresol green-methyl red TS in an absorption flask, and set to the apparatus to immerse the lower end of the condenser. Add 15 mL of sodium hydroxide solution (1 in 2) through the funnel, rinse cautiously the funnel with 20 ml of water, immediately close the clamp attached to the rubber tubing, then begin the distillation with steam, and continue until the distillate measures about 100 mL. Remove the absorption flask from the lower end of the condenser, rinse the end part of the condenser with a small quantity of water, and titrate *<2.50>* with 0.1 mol/L sodium hydroxide VS until the color of the solution changes from red to light blue-green through a light red-purple. Perform a blank determination in the same manner.

Each mL of 0.05 mol/L sulfuric acid VS
= 19.11 mg of $C_6H_9NO_6$

Isotonic sodium chloride solution [Same as the namesake monograph]

Isoxsuprine hydrochloride for assay $C_{18}H_{23}NO_3.HCl$ [Same as the monograph Isoxsuprine Hydrochloride]

Japanese acid clay Natural hydrous aluminum silicate, grayish white powder, having a particle size of about 75 μm.

Loss on drying <2.41>: not more than 10% (1 g, 105°C, 4 hours).

Water adsorbing capacity: not less than 2.5%. Weigh accurately about 10 g of Japanese acid clay in weighing bottle, allow to stand for 24 hours with cover in a chamber, in which humidity is maintained to 80% by means of sulfuric acid (specific gravity 1.19), reweigh, and determine the increase of mass of the sample.

Japanese zanthoxylum peel [Same as the namesake monograph]

Jesaconitine for purity $C_{35}H_{49}NO_{12}$ A white powder. Freely soluble in acetonitrile, in ethanol (99.5) and in diethyl ether, and practically insoluble in water.

Identification—Determine the infrared absorption spectrum of jesaconitine for purity as directed in the potassium bromide disk method under Infrared Spectrophotometry <2.25>: it exhibits absorption at the wave numbers of about 3500 cm^{-1}, 1715 cm^{-1}, 1607 cm^{-1}, 1281 cm^{-1}, 1259 cm^{-1}, 1099 cm^{-1} and 772 cm^{-1}.

Absorbance <2.24> $E^{1\%}_{1\,cm}$ (258 nm): 270 – 291 [5 mg, ethanol (99.5), 200 mL].

Purity Related substances—(1) Dissolve 5.0 mg of jesaconitine for purity in 2 mL of acetonitrile, and use this solution as the sample solution. Pipet 1 mL of the sample solution, add acetonitrile to make exactly 50 mL, and use this solution as the standard solution. Perform the test with these solutions as directed under Thin-layer Chromatography <2.03>. Spot 20 μL each of the sample solution and standard solution on a plate of silica gel for thin-layer chromatography, and proceed the test as directed in the Identification in Processed Aconite Root: the spot other than the principal spot obtained from the sample solution is not more intense than the spot from the standard solution.

(2) Dissolve 5.0 mg of jesaconitine for purity in 5 mL of acetonitrile, and use this solution as the sample solution. Pipet 1 mL of the sample solution, add acetonitrile to make exactly 50 mL, and use this solution as the standard solution. Perform the test with exactly 10 μL each of the sample solution and standard solution as directed under Liquid Chromatography <2.01> according to the following conditions, and determine each peak area by the automatic integration method: the total area of the peaks other than jesaconitine obtained from the sample solution is not larger than the peak area of jesaconitine from the standard solution.

Operating conditions

Detector, column, and column temperature: Proceed as directed in the operating conditions in the Purity under Processed Aconite Root.

Mobile phase: A mixture of phosphate buffer solution for processed aconite root and tetrahydrofuran (9:1).

Flow rate: Adjust so that the retention time of jesaconitine is about 36 minutes.

Time span of measurement: About 3 times as long as the retention time of jesaconitine, beginning after the solvent peak.

System suitability

Test for required detectability: Pipet 1 mL of the standard solution, and add acetonitrile to make exactly 20 mL. Confirm that the peak area of jesaconitine obtained with 10 μL of this solution is equivalent to 3.5 to 6.5% of that with 10 μL of the standard solution.

System performance: Dissolve 1 mg of jesaconitine for purity and 5 mg each of aconitine for purity, hypaconitine for purity and mesaconitine for purity in 200 mL of acetonitrile. When the procedure is run with 10 μL of this solution under the above operating conditions, mesaconitine, hypaconitine, aconitine and jesaconitine are eluted in this order, and each resolution between these peaks is not less than 1.5, respectively.

System repeatability: When the test is repeated 6 times with 10 μL of the standard solution under the above operating conditions, the relative standard deviation of the peak area of jesaconitine is not more than 1.5%.

Water <2.48>: not more than 1.0% (5 mg, coulometric titration).

Josamycin $C_{42}H_{69}NO_{15}$ [Same as the namesake monograph]

Josamycin propionate $C_{45}H_{73}NO_{16}$ [Same as the namesake monograph]

Kainic acid See kainic acid hydrate.

Kainic acid for assay See kainic acid hydrate.

Kainic acid hydrate $C_{10}H_{15}NO_4.H_2O$ [Same as the namesake monograph]

Kainic acid hydrate for assay See kainic acid hydrate.

Kanamycin sulfate $C_{18}H_{36}N_4O_{11}.xH_2SO_4$ [Same as the namesake monograph]

Karl Fischer TS for water determination See Water Determination <2.48>.

Kerosene It is mainly a mixture of hydrocarbons in the methane series, and a colorless, clear liquid, having not a disagreeable, characteristic odor.

Specific gravity <2.56>: about 0.80

Distilling range <2.57>: 180 – 300°C

Ketoconazole $C_{26}H_{28}Cl_2N_4O_4$ [Same as the namesake monograph]

Ketoconazole for assay $C_{26}H_{28}Cl_2N_4O_4$ [Same as the monograph Ketoconazole. When dried, it contains not less than 99.5% of ketoconazole ($C_{26}H_{28}Cl_2N_4O_4$).]

Kininogen Produced by purifying from bovine plasma. Dissolve an appropriate amount of kininogen in 0.02 mol/L phosphate buffer solution (pH 8.0) so that 10 mL of the solution contains 1 mg of kininogen, and use this solution as the sample solution. Perform the following tests with the sample solution: it meets the requirement of each test.

(i) Immediately after the sample solution is prepared, add 0.1 mL of a solution of trichloroacetic acid (1 in 5) to 0.5 mL of the sample solution, shake, and centrifuge. To 0.5 mL of the supernatant liquid add 0.5 mL of gelatin-tris buffer solution (pH 8.0), and shake. To 0.1 mL of this solution add 1.9 mL of trichloroacetic acid-gelatin-tris buffer solution. Proceed with 0.1 mL of this solution as directed in the Purity (2) under Kallidinogenase, and determine the amount of kinin: kinin is not detected.

(ii) Warm 0.5 mL of the sample solution at 30 ± 0.5°C for 20 minutes, and proceed as directed in (i): kinin is not detected.

(iii) Perform the test with 0.5 mL of the sample solution as directed in the Purity (2) under Kallidinogenase: the decomposition of bradykinin is not observed.

(iv) To 0.5 mL of the sample solution add 0.5 mL of 0.02 mol/L phosphate buffer solution (pH 8.0) containing 500 μg of crystalline trypsin, previously warmed at 30 ± 0.5°C for 5 minutes, warm this solution at 30 ± 0.5°C for 5 minutes, add 0.2 mL of a solution of trichloroacetic acid (1 in 5), and shake. Then boil for 3 minutes, cool in ice immediately, and centrifuge. To 0.5 mL of the supernatant liquid add 0.5 mL of gelatin-tris buffer solution (pH 8.0), and shake. To 0.1 mL of this solution add 0.9 mL of trichloroacetic acid-gelatin-tris buffer solution. To 0.1 mL of this solution add trichloroacetic acid-gelatin-tris buffer solution to make 20 mL, then proceed as directed in (i), and determine the amount, B_K, of kinin per well. Calculate the kinin-releasing activity per mg by the following equation: not less than 10 μg bradykinin equivalent per mg.

Kinin-releasing activity per mg (μg bradykinin equivalent/mg) = $B_K \times 0.96$

Kininogen TS Dissolve a sufficient quantity of kininogen in 0.02 mol/L phosphate buffer solution (pH 8.0) to prepare a solution having an ability in each mL to release kinin corresponding to not less than 1 μg of bradykinin.

Labetalol hydrochloride $C_{19}H_{24}N_2O_3.HCl$ [Same as the namesake monograph]

Labetalol hydrochloride for assay $C_{19}H_{24}N_2O_3.HCl$ [Same as the monograph Labetalol Hydrochloride. However, when dried, it contains not less than 99.0% of labetalol hydrochloride ($C_{19}H_{24}N_2O_3.HCl$).]

Lactic acid $CH_3CH(OH)COOH$ [K 8726, Special class]

Lactic acid TS Dissolve 12.0 g of lactic acid in water to make 100 mL.

α-Lactoalbumin White powder. Derived from milk. Molecular weight of about 14,200.

Lactobionic acid $C_{12}H_{22}O_{12}$ Colorless crystals or white crystalline powder.

Melting point <2.60>: 113 – 118°C

Purity—Dissolve 0.10 g of lactobionic acid in 10 mL of a mixture of methanol and water (3:2), and perform the test with 10 μL of this solution as directed in the Identification (2) under Erythromycin Lactobionate: the spot other than the principal spot is not found.

β-Lactoglobulin Prepare from milk. White to light yellow powder.

Nitrogen content <1.08>: not less than 14% (calculated on the dried basis).

Lactose See lactose monohydrate.

α-Lactose and β-lactose mixture (1:1) Use a mixture of lactose monohydrate and anhydrous lactose (3:5).

Lactose broth After adding lactose monohydrate to ordinary broth in the ratio of 0.5%, add about 12 mL of bromothymol blue-sodium hydroxide TS to 1000 mL of the medium. Then dispense portions of about 10 mL into tubes for fermentation, and sterilize fractionally on each of three successive days for 15 to 30 minutes at 100°C by using an autoclave, or sterilize by autoclaving for not more than 20 minutes at 121°C, and cool quickly by immersing in cold water.

Lactose broth, three times concentrated Add lactose monohydrate to ordinary broth prepared by using 330 mL in place of 1000 mL of water in the ratio of 1.5%, and prepare according to the method of preparation under lactose broth, with 25 mL portions in tubes for fermentation.

Lactose broth, twice concentrated Add lactose monohydrate to ordinary broth prepared by using 500 mL in place of 1000 mL of water in the ratio of 1.0% and prepare according to the method of preparation under lactose broth.

Lactose monohydrate $C_{12}H_{22}O_{11}.H_2O$ [Same as the monograph Lactose].

Lactose substrate TS Dissolve 6.0 g of lactose monohydrate in disodium hydrogen phosphate-citric acid buffer solution (pH 4.5) to make 100 mL.

Lactose substrate TS for β-galactosidase (penicillium) Dissolve 6.0 g of lactose monohydrate in diluted disodium hydrogen phosphate-citric acid buffer solution (pH 4.5) (1 in 10) to make 100 mL.

Lafutidine for assay $C_{22}H_{29}N_3O_4S$ [Same as the monograph Lafutidine. When dried, it contains not less than 99.5% of lafutidine ($C_{22}H_{29}N_3O_4S$).]

Lanoconazole $C_{14}H_{10}ClN_3S_2$ [Same as the namesake monograph]

Lanthanum-alizarin complexone TS To 1 mL of ammonia water (28) add 10 mL of water. To 4 mL of this solution add 4 mL of a solution of ammonium acetate (1 in 5) and 192 mg of alizarin complexone, and label this solution as alizarin complexone stock solution. Dissolve 41 g of sodium acetate trihydrate in 400 mL of water, and add 24 mL of acetic acid (100). To this solution add the total volume of the alizarin complexone stock solution, add 400 mL of acetone, and label this solution as alizarin complexone solution. To 10 mL of diluted hydrochloric acid (1 in 6) add 163 mg of lanthanum (III) oxide, heat to dissolve, and label this solution as lanthanum (III) oxide solution. To the alizarin complexone solution add the lanthanum (III) oxide solution, and mix. After cooling, adjust to pH 4.7 with acetic acid (100) or ammonia water (28), and add water to make 1000 mL. Prepare before use.

Lanthanum chloride TS To 58.65 g of lanthanum (III) oxide add 100 mL of hydrochloric acid, and boil. After cooling, add water to make 1000 mL.

Lanthanum (III) oxide La_2O_3 White crystals.

Loss on ignition <2.43>: not more than 0.5% (1 g, 1000°C, 1 hour).

Lauromacrogol [Same as the namesake monograph]

Lead acetate See lead (II) acetate trihydrate.

Lead acetate TS See lead (II) acetate TS.

Lead dioxide See lead (IV) oxide.

Lead monoxide See lead (II) oxide.

Lead nitrate See lead (II) nitrate.

Lead subacetate TS Place the yellowish mixture, obtained by triturating 3 g of lead (II) acetate trihydrate and 1 g of lead (II) oxide with 0.5 mL of water, in a beaker, and heat on a water bath, covering with a watch glass, until it shows a homogeneous, white to reddish white color. Then add 9.5 mL of hot water in small portions, cover it again with a watch glass, and set it aside. Decant the supernatant liquid, and adjust the specific gravity to 1.23 to 1.24 (15°C) by adding water.

Storage—Preserve in tightly stoppered bottles.

Lead subacetate TS, dilute To 2 mL of lead subacetate TS add freshly boiled and cooled water to make 100 mL. Prepare before use.

Lead (II) acetate trihydrate $Pb(CH_3COO)_2.3H_2O$ [K 8374, Special class]

Lead (II) acetate TS To 9.5 g of lead (II) acetate trihydrate add freshly boiled and cooled water to make 100 mL.

Storage—Preserve in tightly stoppered bottles (0.25 mol/L).

Lead (II) nitrate $Pb(NO_3)_2$ [K 8563, Special class]

Lead (II) oxide PbO [K 8090, Special class]

Lead (IV) oxide PbO_2 A dark brown to black-brown, powder or granules.

Identification—A supernatant liquid of a solution of lead (IV) oxide in dilute acetic acid (1 in 100) responds to Qualitative Tests <*1.09*> (3) for lead salt.

Lecithin A pale yellow to yellow-brawn, powder or grains, having a characteristic odor.
It is emulsified with water. Hygroscopic.

L-Leucine $C_6H_{13}NO_2$ [Same as the namesake monograph]

L-Leucine for assay $C_6H_{13}NO_2$ [Same as the monograph L-Leucine. When dried, it contains not less than 99.0% of L-leucine ($C_6H_{13}NO_2$).]

Levallorphan tartrate for assay $C_{19}H_{25}NO.C_4H_6O_6$ [Same as the monograph Levallorphan Tartrate. When dried, it contains not less than 99.0% of levallorphan tartrate ($C_{19}H_{25}NO.C_4H_6O_6$).]

Levofloxacin hydrate for assay $C_{18}H_{20}FN_3O_4.½H_2O$ [Same as the monograph Levofloxacin Hydrate]

Levothyroxine sodium See levothyroxine sodium hydrate.

Levothyroxine sodium for thin-layer chromatography See levothyroxine sodium hydrate for thin-layer chromatography.

Levothyroxine sodium hydrate $C_{15}H_{10}I_4NNaO_4.xH_2O$ [Same as the namesake monograph]

Levothyroxine sodium hydrate for thin-layer chromatography $C_{15}H_{10}I_4NNaO_4.xH_2O$ [Same as the monograph Levothyroxine Sodium Hydrate. Proceed the test as directed in the Purity (3) under Levothyroxine Sodium Hydrate: any spot other than the principal spot at the *Rf* value of about 0.26 does not appear.]

Lidocaine for assay $C_{14}H_{22}N_2O$ [same as the monograph Lidocaine]

(*Z*)-Ligustilide for thin-layer chromatography $C_{12}H_{14}O_2$ A clear, yellow-grown liquid, having a characteristic odor. Miscible with methanol and with ethanol (99.5), and practically insoluble in water.
Identification—Determine the absorption spectrum of a solution in methanol (1 in 100,000) as directed under Ultraviolet-visible Spectrophotometry <*2.24*>: it exhibits a maximum between 320 nm and 324 nm.
Purity Related substances—Dissolve 1 mg of (*Z*)-ligustilide for thin-layer chromatography in 10 mL of methanol. Proceed the test with 1 μL of this solution as directed in the Identification (5) under Hochuekkito Extract: no spot other than the principle spot of around *Rf* value of 0.6 appears.

(*Z*)-Ligustilide TS for thin-layer chromatography Dissolve 1 mg of (*Z*)-ligustilide for thin-layer chromatography in 10 mL of methanol.

Limonene $C_{10}H_{16}$ Clear and colorless liquid, having a characteristic aroma and a bitter taste.
Refractive index <*2.45*> n_D^{20}: 1.472 – 1.474
Specific gravity <*2.56*> d_{20}^{20}: 0.841 – 0.846
Purity Related substances—Dissolve 0.1 g of limonene in 25 mL of hexane and use this solution as the sample solution. Perform the test with 2 μL of the sample solution as directed under Gas Chromatography <*2.02*> according to the following conditions. Determine each peak area by the automatic integration method and calculate the amount of them by the area percentage method: the total amount of the peaks other than limonene is not more than 3.0%.
Operating conditions
Proceed the operating conditions in the Assay under Eucalyptus Oil except test for time span of measurement.
Time span of measurement: About 3 times as long as the retention time of limonene, beginning after the solvent peak.
System suitability
Test for required detectability: To 1 mL of the sample solution add hexane to make 100 mL. Adjust so that the peak height of limonene obtained with 2 μL of this solution is 40 to 60% of the full scale.

Limonin for thin-layer chromatography $C_{26}H_{30}O_8$ White, crystals or crystalline powder. Slightly soluble in methanol and in ethyl acetate, and practically insoluble in water and in ethanol (99.5). Melting point: about 290°C.
Identification Determine the infrared absorption spectrum as directed in the potassium bromide disk method under Infrared-visible Spectrophotometry <*2.25*>: it exhibits absorption at the wave numbers of about 1759 cm^{-1}, 1709 cm^{-1}, 1166 cm^{-1}, 798 cm^{-1} and 601 cm^{-1}.
Purity Related substances—Dissolve 1 mg of limonin for thin-layer chromatography in 1 mL of ethyl acetate, and perform the test with 1 μL of this solution as directed in the Identification (2) under Orengedokuto Extract: no spot other than the principal spot at an *Rf* value of about 0.4 appears.

Liothyronine sodium $C_{15}H_{11}I_3NNaO_4$ [Same as the namesake monograph]

Liothyronine sodium for thin-layer chromatography $C_{15}H_{11}I_3NNaO_4$ [Same as the monograph Liothyronine Sodium. Proceed as directed for the Identification (1) under Liothyronine Sodium Tablets: any spot other than the principal spot at the *Rf* value of about 0.3 to 0.4 does not appear.]

Liquid paraffin See paraffin, liquid.

Liquiritin for thin-layer chromatography $C_{21}H_{22}O_9$ White, crystals or crystalline powder. Sparingly soluble in methanol, slightly soluble in ethanol (99.5), and practically insoluble in water. Melting point: about 210°C (with decomposition).
Identification—Determine the absorption spectrum of a solution of liquiritin for thin-layer chromatography in diluted methanol (1 in 2) (1 in 100,000) as directed under Ultraviolet-visible Spectrophotometry <*2.24*>: it exhibits maxima between 215 nm and 219 nm, and between 275 nm and 279 nm.
Purity Related substances—Dissolve 1.0 mg of liquiritin for thin-layer chromatography in 1 mL of methanol, and perform the test with 1 μL of this solution as directed in the Identification (5) under Kakkonto Extract: no spot other than the principal spot with an *Rf* value of about 0.4 appears.

Lisinopril See lisinopril hydrate.

Lisinopril for assay See lisinopril hydrate for assay.

Lisinopril hydrate $C_{21}H_{31}N_3O_5.2H_2O$ [Same as the namesake monograph]

Lisinopril hydrate for assay $C_{21}H_{31}N_3O_5.2H_2O$ [Same as the monograph Lisinopril Hydrate. It contains not less than 99.5% of lisinopril ($C_{21}H_{31}N_3O_5$: 405.49), calculated on the anhydrous basis.]

Lithium acetate dihydrate $CH_3COOLi.2H_2O$ Colorless crystals.
Dilute acetic acid insoluble substances—To 40.0 g of lithi-

um acetate dihydrate add 45 mL of water, heat in a water bath to dissolve, cool, then dissolve in dilute acetic acid, and filter by suction. Wash the filter with water, dry the filter at 105 ± 2°C for 1 hour, and weigh the mass of the residue after cooling: not more than 0.0025%.

Content: not less than 97.0%. Assay—Weigh accurately 0.3 g of lithium acetate dihydrate, add exactly 50 mL of acetic acid (100) and exactly 5 mL of acetic anhydride, dissolve by heating in a water bath, and titrate *<2.50>* with 0.1 mol/L perchloric acid VS after cooling (potentiometric titration). Perform a blank determination in the same manner, and make any necessary correction.

Each mL of 0.1 mol/L perchloric acid VS
= 10.20 mg of $CH_3COOLi.2H_2O$

Lithium bromide LiBr White, crystals or crystalline powder. It is hygroscopic.

Purity (1) Chloride *<1.03>*: not more than 0.1%.

(2) Sulfate *<1.14>*: not more than 0.01%.

Lithium chloride LiCl White, crystals or masses.

Identification—Perform the test as directed under Flame Coloration Test *<1.04>* (1): a persistent red color appears.

Lithium hydroxide monohydrate $LiOH.H_2O$ White, crystals or crystalline powder, having a hygroscopicity.

Lithium perchlorate $LiClO_4$ White, crystals or crystalline powder.

Content: not less than 98%. Assay—Accurately weigh about 0.2 g of lithium perchlorate, dissolve in 30 mL of water. Transfer the solution to a chromatographic column, prepared by pouring about 25 mL of strongly acidic ion-exchange resin (H type) for column chromatography into a chromatographic tube about 11 mm in inside diameter and about 300 mm in height (after adding 200 mL of 1 mol/L hydrochloride TS and flowing at a flow rate of 3 - 4 mL per minute, wash the chromatographic column with water until the color of the rinse water changes to yellowish red when adding methyl orange TS to the eluate), and flow at a flow rate of 3 - 4 mL per minute. Then, wash the column with about 30 mL of water at a flow rate of 3 – 4 mL per minute 5 times. Combine the rinse water and the eluate, and titrate *<2.50>* with 0.1 mol/L sodium hydroxide VS (indicator: 3 drops of bromothymol blue TS). Perform a blank determination, and make any necessary correction.

Each mL of 0.1 mol/L sodium hydroxide VS
= 10.64 mg of $LiClO_4$

Lithium sulfate See lithium sulfate monohydrate.

Lithium sulfate monohydrate $Li_2SO_4.H_2O$ [K 8994, Special class]

Lithocholic acid for thin-layer chromatography
$C_{24}H_{40}O_3$ White, crystals or crystalline powder. Soluble in ethanol (95), in acetic acid (100) and in acetone, slightly soluble in chloroform, and practically insoluble in water. Melting point: about 186°C.

Purity Related substances—Dissolve 25 mg of lithocholic acid for thin-layer chromatography in a mixture of chloroform and ethanol (95) (9:1) to make exactly 25 mL. Dilute 1.0 mL of this solution with a mixture of chloroform and ethanol (95) (9:1) to make exactly 100 mL. Perform the test with 10 µL of this solution as directed in the Purity (4) under Ursodeoxycholic Acid: any spot other than the principal spot with the *Rf* value of about 0.7 does not appear.

Content: 98.0%. Assay—Weigh accurately about 0.5 g of lithocholic acid for thin-layer chromatography, previously dried at 80°C for 4 hours under reduced pressure (phosphorus (V) oxide), dissolve in 40 mL of neutralized ethanol and 20 mL of water. Add 2 drops of phenolphthalein TS, titrate *<2.50>* with 0.1 mol/L sodium hydroxide VS, add 100 mL of freshly boiled and cooled water near the end point, and continue the titration.

Each mL of 0.1 mol/L sodium hydroxide VS
= 37.66 mg of $C_{24}H_{40}H_3$

Locke-Ringer's TS

Sodium chloride	9.0 g
Potassium chloride	0.42 g
Calcium chloride dihydrate	0.24 g
Magnesium chloride hexahydrate	0.2 g
Sodium hydrogen carbonate	0.5 g
Dextrose	0.5 g
Water, freshly distilled with a hard-glass apparatus	a sufficient quantity
To make	1000 mL

Prepare before use. The constituents except dextrose and sodium hydrogen carbonate can be made up in concentrated stock solutions, stored in a dark place, and diluted before use.

Loganin for assay $C_{17}H_{26}O_{10}$ Loganin for thin-layer chromatography. It meets the requirement of the following 1) Loganin for assay 1 or 2) Loganin for assay 2 (Purity value by qNMR). The former is used after drying in a desiccator (silica gel) for 24 hours, and the latter is used with correction for its amount based on the result obtained in the Assay.

1) Loganin for assay 1

Absorbance *<2.24>* $E^{1\%}_{1cm}$ (235 nm): 275 - 303 [5 mg after drying in a desiccator (silica gel) for 24 hours, methanol, 500 mL]

Purity Related substances—Dissolve 2 mg of loganin for assay 1 in 5 mL of the mobile phase, and use this solution as the sample solution. Pipet 1 mL of the sample solution, add the mobile phase to make exactly 100 mL, and use this solution as the standard solution. Perform the test with exactly 10 µL each of the sample solution and standard solution as directed under Liquid Chromatography *<2.01>* according to the following conditions, and determine each peak area by the automatic integration method: the total area of the peaks other than loganin obtained from the sample solution is not larger than the peak area of loganin from the standard solution.

Operating conditions

Detector, column, column temperature, mobile phase and flow rate: Proceed as directed in the operating conditions in the Assay (1) under Goshajinkigan Extract.

Time span of measurement: About 3 times as long as the retention time of loganin.

System suitability

System performance and system repeatability: Proceed as directed in the system suitability in the Assay (1) under Goshajinkigan Extract.

Test for required detectability: Pipet 1 mL of the standard solution, and add the mobile phase to make exactly 20 mL. Confirm that the peak area of loganin obtained with 10 µL of this solution is equivalent to 3.5 to 6.5% of that with 10 µL of the standard solution.

2) Loganin for assay 2 (Purity value by qNMR)

Unity of peak—Dissolve 2 mg of loganin for assay 2 in 5 mL of the mobile phase, and use this solution as the sample solution. Perform the test with 10 μL of the sample solution as directed under Liquid Chromatography <2.01> according to the following conditions, and compare the absorption spectra of at least 3 points including the top of loganin peak and around the two middle peak heights of before and after the top: no difference in form is observed among their spectra.

Operating conditions

Column, column temperature, mobile phase, and flow rate: Proceed as directed in the operating conditions in the Assay (1) under Goshajinkigan Extract.

Detector: A photodiode array detector (wavelength: 238 nm, spectrum range of measurement: 220 – 400 nm).

System suitability

System performance: Proceed as directed in the system suitability in the Assay (1) under Goshajinkigan Extract.

Assay—Weigh accurately 5 mg of loganin for assay 2 and 1 mg of 1,4-BTMSB-d_4 for nuclear magnetic resonance spectroscopy using an ultramicrobalance, dissolve in 1 mL of deuterated methanol for nuclear magnetic resonance spectroscopy, and use this solution as the sample solution. Transfer the sample solution into an NMR tube 5 mm in outer diameter, and measure ^{1}H-NMR as directed under Nuclear Magnetic Resonance Spectroscopy <2.21> and Crude Drugs Test <5.01> according to the following conditions, using 1,4-BTMSB-d_4 for nuclear magnetic resonance spectroscopy as the reference standard for qNMR. Calculate the resonance intensity A (equivalent to 1 hydrogen) of the signal around δ 7.14 ppm assuming the signal of the reference standard for qNMR as δ 0 ppm.

$$\text{Amount (\%) of loganin } (C_{17}H_{26}O_{10}) = M_S \times I \times P/(M \times N) \times 1.7235$$

M: Amount (mg) of loganin for assay 2 taken

M_S: Amount (mg) of 1,4-BTMSB-d_4 for nuclear magnetic resonance spectroscopy taken

I: Signal resonance intensity A based on the signal resonance intensity of 1,4-BTMSB-d_4 for nuclear magnetic resonance spectroscopy as 18.000

N: Number of the hydrogen derived from A

P: Purity (%) of 1,4-BTMSB-d_4 for nuclear magnetic resonance spectroscopy

Operating conditions

Apparatus: A nuclear magnetic resonance spectrometer having ^{1}H resonance frequency of not less than 400 MHz.

Target nucleus: ^{1}H.

Digital resolution: 0.25 Hz or lower.

Measuring spectrum range: 20 ppm or upper, including between −5 ppm and 15 ppm.

Spinning: off.

Pulse angle: 90°.

^{13}C decoupling: on.

Delay time: Repeating pulse waiting time not less than 60 seconds.

Integrating times: 8 or more times.

Dummy scanning: 2 or more times.

Measuring temperature: A constant temperature between 20°C and 30°C.

System suitability

Test for required detectability: When the procedure is run with the sample solution under the above operating conditions, the SN ratio of each signal around δ 5.02 ppm and δ 7.14 ppm is not less than 100.

System performance: When the procedure is run with the sample solution under the above operating conditions, the two signals around δ 5.02 ppm and δ 7.14 ppm are not overlapped with any signal of obvious foreign substance. Furthermore, when determined the resonance intensities A_1 and A, both equivalent to 1 hydrogen, of each signal around δ 5.02 ppm and δ 7.14 ppm, the ratio of them, A_1/A, is between 0.99 and 1.01.

System repeatability: When the test is repeated 6 times with the sample solution under the above operating conditions, the relative standard deviation of the ratio of the resonance intensity A to that of the reference standard for qNMR is not more than 1.0%.

Loganin for component determination See loganin for assay.

Loganin for thin-layer chromatography $C_{17}H_{26}O_{10}$ White, crystals or crystalline powder. Soluble in water, sparingly soluble in methanol, and very slightly soluble in ethanol (99.5). Melting point: 221 – 227°C.

Purity Related substances—Dissolve 1.0 mg of loganin for thin-layer chromatography in 2 mL of methanol. Perform the test with 10 μL of this solution as directed in the Identification under Cornus Fruit: any spot other than the principal spot at the Rf value of about 0.4 does not appear.

Losartan potassium $C_{22}H_{22}ClKN_6O$ [Same as the namesake monograph]

Lovastatin $C_{24}H_{36}O_5$ White, crystals or crystalline powder. Soluble in acetonitrile and in methanol, sparingly soluble in ethanol (99.5), and practically insoluble in water.

Optical rotation <2.49> $[\alpha]_D^{20}$: +325 – +340° (50 mg calculated on the dried basis, acetonitrile, 10 mL, 100 mm).

Loss on drying <2.41>: Not more than 1.0% (1 g, under reduced pressure not exceeding 0.67 kPa, 60°C, 3 hours).

Low-molecular mass heparin for calculation of molecular mass.

It is a low-molecular mass heparin with a disaccharide unit prepared, and display the molecular mass distribution between 600 and more than 10,000. When the average of molecular mass of Low-molecular mass heparin international standard is determined as a reference with this, the difference compared as a reference with the Low-molecular mass heparin international standard is not less than 5%.

Luteolin for thin-layer chromatography $C_{15}H_{10}O_6$ Light yellow to yellow-brown crystalline powder. Slightly soluble in methanol and in ethanol (99.5), and practically insoluble in water. Melting point: about 310°C (with decomposition).

Purity Related substances—Dissolve 1.0 mg of luteolin for thin-layer chromatography in 1 mL of methanol. Proceed the test with 10 μL of this solution as directed in the Identification under Chrysanthemum Flower: any spot other than the principal spot at an Rf value of about 0.7 does not appear.

Lysate reagent A lyophilized product obtained from amebocyte lysate of horseshoe crab (*Limulus polyphemus* or *Tachypleus tridentatus*). Amebocyte lysate preparations which do not react to β-glucans are available: they are prepared by removing the G factor reacting to β-glucans from amebocyte lysate or by inhibiting the G factor reacting system of amebocyte lysate.

Lysate TS Dissolve a lysate reagent in water for bacterial endotoxins test, or in a suitable buffer, by gentle stirring.

Lysil endopeptidase White, powder or masses. An exotoxin produced by *Achromobacter*. Molecular weight:

27,500.

L-Lysine hydrochloride $C_6H_{14}N_2O_2.HCl$ [Same as the namesake monograph]

Lysyl endopeptidase A protease obtained from *Lysobacter enzymogenes*. It contains about 150 units per mg, where 1 unit is an enzyme amount which hydrolyzes 1 μmol of tosyl-glycyl-prolyl-lysine-4-nitroanilide acetate per minute at pH 7.7 and 25°C.

Macrogol 600 $HOCH_2(CH_2OCH_2)_nCH_2OH$, n = 11 – 13 Clear, colorless, viscous liquid or a white, petrolatum-like solid, having a faint, characteristic odor. Very soluble in water, in ethanol (95), in acetone and in macrogol 400, soluble in diethyl ether, and practically insoluble in petroleum benzine. Congealing point: 18 – 23°C.

Average molecular mass: When perform the test as directed in the Average molecular mass test under Macrogol 400, it is between 570 and 630.

Magnesia TS Dissolve 5.5 g of magnesium chloride hexahydrate and 7 g of ammonium chloride in 65 mL of water, add 35 mL of ammonia TS, allow the mixture to stand for a few days in tightly stoppered bottles, and filter. If the solution is not clear, filter before use.

Magnesium Mg [K 8875, Special class]

Magnesium chloride See magnesium chloride hexahydrate.

Magnesium chloride hexahydrate $MgCl_2.6H_2O$ [K 8159, Special class]

Magnesium nitrate See magnesium nitrate hexahydrate.

Magnesium nitrate hexahydrate $Mg(NO_3)_2.6H_2O$ [K 8567, Special class]

Magnesium oxide MgO [K 8432, Special class]

Magnesium powder Mg [K 8876, Special class]

Magnesium sulfate See magnesium sulfate heptahydrate.

Magnesium sulfate heptahydrate $MgSO_4.7H_2O$ [K 8995, Special class]

Magnesium sulfate TS Dissolve 12 g of magnesium sulfate heptahydrate in water to make 100 mL (0.5 mol/L).

Magnoflorine iodide for assay $C_{20}H_{24}INO_4$ White to light yellowish white, crystals or crystalline powder. Slightly soluble in water and in methanol, and very slightly soluble in ethanol (99.5). Melting point: about 250°C (with decomposition).

It is used after correcting with the amount of magnoflorine iodide obtained in the Assay.

Identification (1) Determine the absorption spectrum of a solution of magnoflorine iodide for assay in methanol (1 in 200,000) as directed under Ultraviolet-visible Spectrophotometry <*2.24*>: it exhibits a maximum between 221 nm and 225 nm.

(2) Determine the infrared absorption spectrum of magnoflorine iodide for assay as directed in the potassium bromide disk method under Infrared Spectrophotometry <*2.25*>: it exhibits absorption at the wave numbers of about 3170 cm^{-1}, 3000 cm^{-1}, 2840 cm^{-1}, 1459 cm^{-1}, 1231 cm^{-1}, 1122 cm^{-1} and 833 cm^{-1}.

Absorbance <*2.24*> $E^{1\%}_{1\,cm}$ (223 nm): 1066 – 1132 (5 mg, methanol, 1000 mL).

Purity Related substances—Dissolve 5 mg of magnoflorine iodide for assay in 2 mL of a mixture of water and methanol (1:1), and use this solution as the sample solution. Pipet 1 mL of the sample solution, add a mixture of water and methanol (1:1) to make exactly 100 mL, and use this solution as the standard solution. Perform the test with these solutions as directed under Thin-layer Chromatography <*2.03*>. Spot 10 μL each of the sample solution and standard solution on a plate of silica gel for thin-layer chromatography. Develop the plate with a mixture of ethyl acetate, acetone, water and formic acid (5:3:1:1) to a distance of about 7 cm, and air-dry the plate. Spray evenly Dragendorff's TS for spraying on the plate, air-dry the plate, and spray evenly sodium nitrite TS: the spot other than the principal spot at the *Rf* value of about 0.3 obtained from the sample solution is not more intense than the spot from the standard solution.

Unity of peak: Dissolve 5 mg of magnoflorine iodide for assay in 10 mL of a mixture of water and methanol (1:1), and use this solution as the sample solution. Perform the test with 10 μL of the sample solution as directed under Liquid Chromatography <*2.01*> according to the following conditions, and compare the absorption spectra of at least 3 points including the top of magnoflorine peak and around the two middle peak heights of before and after the top: no difference is observed in the shape between their spectra.

Operating conditions

Column, column temperature, and mobile phase: Proceed as directed in the operating conditions in the Assay (4) under Kakkontokasenkyushin'i Extract.

Detector: A photodiode array detector (wavelength: 303 nm; spectrum range of measurement: 220 – 400 nm).

Flow rate: Adjust so that the retention time of magnoflorine is about 20 minutes.

System suitability

System performance: To 1 mL of the sample solution add a mixture of water and methanol (1:1) to make 100 mL. When the procedure is run with 10 μL of this solution under the above operating conditions, the number of theoretical plates and the symmetry factor of the peak of magnoflorine are not less than 5000 and not more than 1.5, respectively.

System repeatability: To 1 mL of the sample solution add a mixture of water and methanol (1:1) to make 100 mL. When the test is repeated 6 times with 10 μL of this solution under the above operating conditions, the relative standard deviation of the peak area of magnoflorine is not more than 1.5%.

Assay—Weigh accurately 5 mg of magnoflorine iodide for assay and 1 mg of DSS-d_6 for nuclear magnetic resonance spectroscopy using an ultramicrobalance, dissolve in 1 mL of deuterated dimethylsulfoxide for nuclear magnetic resonance spectroscopy, and use this solution as the sample solution. Transfer the sample solution into an NMR tube 5 mm in outer diameter, and measure ^{1}H-NMR spectrum as directed under Nuclear Magnetic Resonance Spectroscopy <*2.21*> and Crude Drugs Test <*5.01*> according to the following conditions, using DSS-d_6 for nuclear magnetic resonance spectroscopy as the reference standard for qNMR. Calculate the signal integrated intensity A (equivalent to 3 hydrogen) around δ 6.94 – δ 7.05 ppm [the integrated intensities A_1 (equivalent to 2 hydrogen) and A_2 (equivalent to 1 hydrogen) of the signals around δ 6.96 ppm and δ 7.04 ppm], assuming the signal of the reference standard for qNMR as δ 0 ppm.

$$\text{Amount (\%) of magnoflorine iodide } (C_{20}H_{24}INO_4) = M_S \times I \times P/(M \times N) \times 2.0918$$

M: Amount (mg) of magnoflorine iodide for assay taken

M_S: Amount (mg) of DSS-d_6 for nuclear magnetic resonance spectroscopy taken

I: The signal integrated intensity *A* based on the signal integrated intensity of DSS-d_6 for nuclear magnetic resonance spectroscopy as 9.000

N: Number of hydrogen derived from *A*

P: Purity (%) of DSS-d_6 for nuclear magnetic resonance spectroscopy

Operating conditions

Apparatus: A nuclear magnetic resonance spectroscopy apparatus having ^{1}H resonance frequency of not less than 400 MHz.

Target nucleus: ^{1}H.

Digital resolution: 0.25 Hz or lower.

Measuring spectrum width: 20 ppm or upper, including between −5 ppm and 15 ppm.

Spinning: off.

Pulse angle: 90°.

^{13}C decoupling: on.

Delay time: Repeating pulse waiting time 60 seconds or longer.

Integrating times: 8 or more times.

Dummy scanning: 2 or more times.

Measuring temperature: A constant temperature of 20 – 30°C.

System suitability

Test for required detectability: When the procedure is run with the sample solution under the above operating conditions, the SN ratio of the signal around δ 6.94 – δ 7.05 ppm is not less than 100.

System performance: When the procedure is run with the sample solution under the above operating conditions, the two signals of around δ 6.96 – δ 7.04 ppm are not overlapped with any signal of obvious foreign substance, and the ratio of the integrated intensity of each signal $(A_1/2)/A_2$ is between 0.99 and 1.01.

System repeatability: When the test is repeated 6 times with the sample solution under the above operating conditions, the relative standard deviation of the ratio of the integrated intensity *A* to that of the reference standard for qNMR is not more than 1.0%.

Magnolia flower [Same as the namesake monograph]

Magnolol for assay $C_{18}H_{18}O_2$ Use magnolol for thin-layer chromatography meeting the following additional specifications. Correct the content based on the amount (%) obtained in the Assay.

Unity of peak—Dissolve 5 mg of magnolol for assay in 10 mL of the mobile phase. To 1 mL of this solution add the mobile phase to make 100 mL, and use this solution as the sample solution. Perform the test with 10 μL of the sample solution as directed under Liquid Chromatography *<2.01>* according to the following conditions, and compare the absorption spectra of at least 3 points including the top of magnolol peak and around the two middle peak heights of before and after the top: no difference in form is observed between their spectra.

Operating conditions

Column, column temperature, mobile phase, and flow rate: Proceed as directed in the operating conditions in the Assay under Magnolia Bark.

Detector: A photodiode array detector (wavelength: 289 nm, spectrum range of measurement: 220 – 400 nm).

System suitability

System performance: Proceed as directed in the system suitability in the Assay under Magnolia Bark.

Assay—Weigh accurately 5 mg of magnolol for assay and 1 mg of 1,4-BTMSB-d_4 for nuclear magnetic resonance spectroscopy using an ultramicrobalance, dissolve in 1 mL of deuterated chloroform for nuclear magnetic resonance spectroscopy, and use this solution as the sample solution. Transfer the sample solution into an NMR tube 5 mm in outer diameter, measure ^{1}H-NMR as directed under Nuclear Magnetic Resonance Spectroscopy *<2.21>* and Crude Drugs Test *<5.01>* according to the following conditions, using 1,4-BTMSB-d_4 for nuclear magnetic resonance spectroscopy as the reference standard for qNMR. Calculate the resonance intensities, A_1 (equivalent to 2 hydrogen) and A_2 (equivalent to 2 hydrogen), of the signals around δ 6.70 ppm and δ 6.81 ppm assuming the signal of the reference standard for qNMR as δ 0 ppm.

$$\text{Amount (\%) of magnolol } (C_{18}H_{18}O_2) = M_S \times I \times P/(M \times N) \times 1.1758$$

M: Amount (mg) of magnolol for assay taken

M_S: Amount (mg) of 1,4-BTMSB-d_4 for nuclear magnetic resonance spectroscopy taken

I: Sum of the signal resonance intensities, A_1 and A_2, based on the signal resonance intensity of 1,4-BTMSB-d_4 for nuclear magnetic resonance spectroscopy as 18.000

N: Sum of numbers of the hydrogen derived from A_1 and A_2

P: Purity (%) of 1,4-BTMSB-d_4 for nuclear magnetic resonance spectroscopy

Operating conditions

Apparatus: An apparatus of nuclear magnetic resonance spectrum measurement having ^{1}H resonance frequency of not less than 400 MHz.

Target nucleus: ^{1}H.

Digital resolution: 0.25 Hz or lower.

Measuring spectrum range: 20 ppm or upper, including between −5 ppm and 15 ppm.

Spinning: off.

Pulse angle: 90°.

^{13}C decoupling: on.

Delay time: Repeating pulse waiting time not less than 60 seconds.

Integrating times: 8 or more times.

Dummy scanning: 2 or more times.

Measuring temperature: A constant temperature between 20°C and 30°C.

System suitability

Test for required detectability: When the procedure is run with the sample solution under the above operating conditions, the SN ratio of the two signals of around δ 6.70 ppm and δ 6.81 ppm is not less than 100.

System performance: When the procedure is run with the sample solution under the above operating conditions, the two signals of around δ 6.70 ppm and δ 6.81 ppm are not overlapped with any signal of obvious foreign substance, and the ratios of the resonance intensities, A_1/A_2, of each signal around δ 6.70 ppm and δ 6.81 ppm are between 0.99 and 1.01, respectively.

System repeatability: When the test is repeated 6 times with the sample solution under the above operating conditions, the relative standard deviation of the ratio of the resonance intensity, A_1 or A_2, to that of the reference standard for qNMR is not more than 1.0%.

Magnolol for component determination See magnolol for assay.

Magnolol for thin-layer chromatography $C_{18}H_{18}O_2$ Odorless, white, crystals or crystalline powder. Freely soluble in methanol and in ethanol (99.5), and practically insoluble in water. Melting point: about 102°C.

Identification—Determine the absorption spectrum of a solution of magnolol for thin-layer chromatography in methanol (1 in 50,000) as directed under Ultraviolet-visible Spectrophotometry <*2.24*>: it exhibits a maximum between 287 nm and 291 nm.

Purity Related substances—Dissolve 1.0 mg of magnolol for thin-layer chromatography in 1 mL of methanol, and use this solution as the sample solution. Perform the test with the sample solution as directed under Thin-layer Chromatography <*2.03*>. Spot 10 μL of the sample solution on a plate of silica gel with fluorescent indicator for thin-layer chromatography, develop the plate with a mixture of hexane, acetone and acetic acid (100) (20:15:1) to a distance of about 10 cm, and air-dry the plate. Examine under ultraviolet light (main wavelength: 254 nm): any spot other than the principal spot of around *R*f value of 0.5 does not appear.

Malachite green See malachite green oxalate.

Malachite green oxalate $C_{52}H_{54}N_4O_{12}$ [K 8878, Malachite green (oxalate), Special class]

Maleic acid $C_4H_4O_4$ A white crystalline powder.

Identification—Determine the infrared absorption spectrum of maleic acid as directed in the potassium bromide disk method as directed under Infrared Spectrophotometry <*2.25*>: it exhibits absorption at the wave numbers of about 1706 cm^{-1}, 1637 cm^{-1}, 1587 cm^{-1}, 1567 cm^{-1}, 1436 cm^{-1}, 1263 cm^{-1}, 876 cm^{-1} and 786 cm^{-1}.

4-(*N*-Maleimidomethyl)cyclohexane-1-carboxylic acid *N*-succinimidyl ester $C_{16}H_{18}N_2O_2$ Colorless crystals, which is decomposed by acid or alkali.

Maltitol $C_{12}H_{24}O_{11}$ A white crystalline powder. Very soluble in water, and practically insoluble in ethanol (99.5).

Maltose See maltose monohydrate.

Maltose monohydrate $C_{12}H_{22}O_{11}.H_2O$ [Same as the namesake monograph].

Maltotriose $C_{18}H_{32}O_{16}$ A white powder.

Identification—Determine the infrared absorption spectrum of maltotriose as directed in the potassium bromide disk method under Infrared Spectrophotometry <*2.25*>: it exhibits absorption at the wave numbers of about 3420 cm^{-1}, 1420 cm^{-1}, 1153 cm^{-1} and 1024 cm^{-1}.

Manganese dioxide MnO_2 Black to black-brown, masses or powder.

Identification—To 0.5 g of monganese dioxide add 20 mL of water and 3 mL of hydrochloric acid, and 3 mL of hydrogen peroxide (30). Alkalinize the solution with ammonia solution (28) while cooling, and add 25 mL of hydrogen sulfide TS: pale red precipitates appear.

Manganese (II) nitrate hexahydrate $Mn(NO_3)_2.6H_2O$ [K 8568, Special class]

Mangiferin for assay $C_{19}H_{18}O_{11}$ Yellow crystals or crystalline powder. It is practically insoluble in water or ethanol (99.5).It is used after correcting with the amount (%) of mangiferin obtained in the Assay.

Identification—Measure ^{1}H-NMR as directed in the Assay: When the signal of the reference standard for qNMR as δ 0 ppm, it exhibits a multiple signal equivalent to one proton around δ 3.15 ppm, a multiple signal equivalent to one proton around δ 3.19 ppm, a multiple signal equivalent to one proton around δ 3.22 ppm, a multiple signal equivalent to one proton around δ 3.43 ppm, a doublet-like signal equivalent to one proton around δ 3.71 ppm, a triplet-like signal equivalent to one proton around δ 4.07 ppm, a doublet-like signal equivalent to one proton around δ 4.61 ppm, a single signal equivalent to one proton around δ 6.40 ppm, a single signal equivalent to one proton around δ 6.89 ppm, and a single signal equivalent to one proton around δ 7.40 ppm.

Unity of peak—Dissolve 1 mg of mangiferin for assay in 20 mL of diluted methanol (1 in 2) and use this solution as the sample solution. Perform the test with 10 μL of the sample solution as directed under Liquid Chromatography <*2.01*> according to the following conditions, and compare the absorption spectra of at least 3 points including the top of mangiferin peak and around the two middle peak heights of before and after the top: no difference in form is observed between their spectra.

Operating conditions

Column, column temperature, mobile phase, and flow rate: Proceed as directed in the operating conditions in the Assay (1) under Byakkokaninjinto Extract.

Detector: A photodiode array detector (wavelength: 367 nm, spectrum range of measurement: 220 – 400 nm).

System suitability

System performance: When the procedure is run with 10 μL of the sample solution under the above operating conditions, the number of theoretical plates and the symmetry factor of the peak of mangiferin are not less than 5000 and not more than 1.5, respectively.

Assay—Weigh accurately 5 mg of mangiferin for assay and 1 mg of DSS-d_6 for nuclear magnetic resonance spectroscopy using an ultramicrobalance, dissolve in 1 mL of deuterated dimethylsulfoxide for nuclear magnetic resonance spectroscopy, and use this solution as the sample solution. Transfer the sample solution into an NMR tube 5 mm in outer diameter, measure ^{1}H-NMR as directed under Nuclear Magnetic Resonance Spectroscopy <*2.21*> and Crude Drugs Test <*5.01*> according to the following conditions, using DSS-d_6 for nuclear magnetic resonance spectroscopy as the reference standard for qNMR. Calculate the resonance intensities, A_1 (equivalent to 1 hydeogen), A_2 (equivalent to 1 hydeogen), and A_2 (equivalent to 1 hydeogen), of the signals around δ 6.40 ppm, δ 6.89 ppm, and δ 7.40 ppm assuming the signal of the reference standard for qNMR as δ 0 ppm.

$$\text{Amount (\%) of mangiferin } (C_{19}H_{18}O_{11}) = M_S \times I \times P/(M \times N) \times 1.8824$$

M: Amount (mg) of mangiferin for assay taken

M_S: Amount (mg) of DSS-d_6 for nuclear magnetic resonance spectroscopy taken

I: Sum of the signal resonance intensities, A_1, A_2 and A_3, based on the signal resonance intensity of DSS-d_6 for nuclear magnetic resonance spectroscopy as 9.000

N: Sum of numbers of the hydeogen derived from A_1, A_2 and A_3

P: Purity (%) of DSS-d_6 for nuclear magnetic resonance spectroscopy

Operating conditions

Apparatus: An apparatus of nuclear magnetic resonance spectrum measurement having ^{1}H resonance frequency of not less than 400 MHz.

Target nucleus: ^{1}H.

Digital resolution: 0.25 Hz or lower.

Measuring spectrum range: 20 ppm or upper, including between −5 ppm and 15 ppm.

Spinning: off.

Pulse angle: 90°.
^{13}C decoupling: on.
Delay time: Repeating pulse waiting time not less than 60 seconds.
Integrating times: 8 or more times.
Dummy scanning: 2 or more times.
Measuring temperature: A constant temperature between 20°C and 30°C.

System suitability

Test for required detectability: When the procedure is run with the sample solution under the above operating conditions, the SN ratio of each signal around δ 6.40 ppm, δ 6.89 ppm, and δ 7.40 ppm is not less than 100.

System performance: When the procedure is run with the sample solution under the above operating conditions, the three signals around δ 6.40 ppm, δ 6.89 ppm, and δ 7.40 ppm are not overlapped with any signal of obvious foreign substance, and the ratios of the resonance intensities, A_1/A_2, A_1/A_3, and A_2/A_3, of each signal around δ 6.40 ppm, δ 6.89 ppm, and δ 7.40 ppm are between 0.99 and 1.01, respectively.

System repeatability: When the test is repeated 6 times with the sample solution under the above operating conditions, the relative standard deviation of the ratio of the resonance intensity, A_1 or A_2 or A_3, to that of the reference standard for qNMR is not more than 1.0%.

Manninotriose for thin-layer chromatography $C_{18}H_{32}O_{16}$ A white powder. Very soluble in water, and practically insoluble in ethanol (99.5). It is hygroscopic. It is deliquescence with the atmospheric moisture.

Optical rotation <*2.49*> $[\alpha]_D^{20}$: +159 – +170° (50 mg calculated on the anhydrous basis, diluted ammonia solution (28) (1 in 1000), 5 mL, 100 mm).

Purity Related substances—Dissolve 3 mg of manninotriose for thin-layer chromatography in 1 mL of a mixture of water and methanol (1:1), and use this solution as the sample solution. Perform the test with the sample solution as directed under Thin-layer chromatography <*2.03*>. Spot 2 μL of the sample solution on a plate of silica gel for thin-layer chromatography. Develop the plate with a mixture of 2-propanol, water and methanol (3:2:2) to a distance of about 7 cm, and air-dry the plate. Spray evenly 1,3-naphthalenediol TS to the plate, and heat the plate at 105°C for 10 minutes: a spot other than the principle spot with an *Rf* value of about 0.4 is not observed.

D-Mannitol $C_6H_{14}O_6$ [Same as the monograph D-Mannitol]

D-Mannosamine hydrochloride $C_6H_{13}NO_5.HCl$ White powder. Melting point: about 168°C (with decomposition).

Optical rotation <*2.49*> $[\alpha]_D^{20}$: −4.2 – −3.2° (0.4 g, water, 20 mL, 100 mm).

D-Mannose $C_6H_{12}O_6$ White, crystal or crystalline powder. It is very soluble in water. Melting point: about 132°C (with decomposition).

Optical rotation <*2.49*> $[\alpha]_D^{20}$: +13.7 – +14.7° (4 g, diluted ammonia TS (1 in 200), 20 mL, 100 mm).

Marker protein for celmoleukin molecular mass determination Add 10 μL of cytochrome C prepared to a concentration of 2 mg per mL to 10 μL of a commercially available marker protein with a known molecular weight (6 ingredients: phosphorylase b, bovine serum albumin, ovalbumin, carbonic dehydratase, soy trypsin inhibitor, and lysozyme) and then dilute 10-fold with buffer solution for celmoleukin.

Meat extract Concentrated extract of fresh meat of bovine, equine or other animals. A yellow-brown to dark brown, paste-like mass, having a meat-like odor.

Mebendazole $C_{16}H_{13}N_3O_3$ White powder. Practically insoluble in water and in ethanol (95).

Medium for float culture Dissolve 6.000 g of sodium chloride, 0.400 g of potassium chloride, 0.677 g of anhydrous sodium dihydrogen phosphate, 0.100 g of calcium nitrite tetrahydrate, 0.100 g of magnesium sulfate heptahydrate, 2.000 g of glucose, 0.164 g of sodium succinate hexahydrate, 46 mg of succinic acid, 0.240 g of L-arginine hydrochloride, 56.8 mg of L-asparagine monohydrate, 20 mg of L-aspartic acid, 72.9 mg of L-cysteine hydrochloride monohydrate, 20 mg of L-glutamic acid, 1 mg of glutathione, 10 mg of glycine, 20.3 mg of L-histidine hydrochloride monohydrate, 20 mg of L-hydroxyproline, 50 mg of L-isoleucine, 40 mg of L-lysine hydrochloride, 15 mg of methionine, 20 mg of L-threonine, 5 mg of L-tryptophan, 20 mg of L-valine, 50 mg of L-leucine, 15 mg of L-phenylalanine, 20 mg of L-proline, 30 mg of L-serine, 20 mg of L-tyrosine, 0.2 mg of D-biotin (crystals), 0.25 mg of calcium pantothenate, 3 mg of choline chloride, 35 mg of *i*-inositol, 1 mg of 4-aminobenzoic acid, 5 μg of cyanocobalamin, 1 mg of folic acid, 1 mg of nicotinamide, 0.2 mg of riboflavin, 1 mg of thiamine hydrochloride, 1 mg of pyridoxine hydrochloride, and 5 mg of phenol red in a suitable amount of water, add 1 mL of kanamycin sulfate solution (3 in 50), add water to make 1000 mL, and then sterilize by autoclaving at 121°C for 15 minutes. After cooling, add 10 mL of L-glutamine solution (3 in 100) and 20 mL of 7% sodium bicarbonate injection, and then mix. Store at 4°C.

Mefloquin hydrochloride $C_{17}H_{16}F_6N_2O.HCl$ [Same as the namesake monograph]

Mefruside for assay $C_{13}H_{19}ClN_2O_5S_2$ [Same as the monograph Mefruside. When dried, it contains not less than 99.0% of mefruside ($C_{13}H_{19}ClN_2O_5S_2$).]

Meglumine $C_7H_{17}NO_5$ [same as the namesake monograph]

Mentha herb [Same as the namesake monograph]

Mentha oil [Same as the namesake monograph]

Menthol $C_{10}H_{20}O$ [Same as the monograph *dl*-Menthol or *l*-Menthol]

***l*-Menthol for assay** $C_{10}H_{20}O$ [Same as the monograph *l*-Menthol. It contains not less than 99.0% of *l*-menthol ($C_{10}H_{20}O$) and meets the following additional specifications.]

Optical rotation <*2.49*> $[\alpha]_D^{20}$: −48.0 – −51.0° (2.5 g, ethanol (95), 25 mL, 100 mm).

Purity Related substances—Dissolve 0.10 g of *l*-menthol for assay in 10 mL of dichloromethane, and use this solution as the sample solution. Pipet 1 mL of the sample solution, add dichloromethane to make exactly 100 mL, and use this solution as the standard solution (1). Perform the test with exactly 5 μL each of the sample solution and standard solution (1) as directed under Gas Chromatography <*2.02*> according to the following conditions, determine each peak area of these solutions by the automatic integration method: the total area of the peaks other than *l*-menthol obtained from the sample solution is not larger than the peak area of *l*-menthol from the standard solution (1).

Operatin conditions

Proceed the operating conditions in the Assay under Mentha Oil except time span of measurement.

Time span of measurement: About twice as long as the retention time of *l*-menthol, beginning after the solvent peak.
System suitability

Test for required detectability: Pipet 1 mL of the standard solution (1), add dichloromethane to make exactly 20 mL, and use this solution as the standard solution (2). Adjust the detection sensitivity so that the peak area of *l*-menthol obtained with 5 μL of the standard solution (2) can be measured and the peak height of *l*-menthol with 5 μL of the standard solution (1) is about 20% of the full scale.

Mepivacaine hydrochloride for assay $C_{15}H_{22}N_2O.HCl$ [Same as the monograph Mepivacaine Hydrochloride. When dried, it contains not less than 99.0% of mepivacaine hydrochloride ($C_{15}H_{22}N_2O.HCl$).]

Mequitazine for assay $C_{20}H_{22}N_2S$ [Same as the monograph Mequitazine. When dried, it contains not less than 99.5% of mequitazine ($C_{20}H_{22}N_2S$).]

Mercapto acetic acid $HSCH_2COOH$ [K 8630, Special class] Place in an ampule, and preserve in a dark, cold place. Do not use after storing for a long period.

Mercaptoethanesulfonic acid $C_2H_6O_3S_2$ Prepared for amino acid analysis or biochemistry.

2-Mercaptoethanol $HSCH_2CH_2OH$ Clear and colorless liquid.

Specific gravity <2.56> d_4^{20}: 1.112 – 1.117

Content: not less than 97.0%. Assay—Perform the test with 0.6 μL of the substance to be examined as directed under Gas Chromatography <2.02> according to the following conditions, and determine the peak areas of each component by the automatic integration method.

Content (%) = (the peak area of 2-mercaptoethanol/the total of the peak areas of each component) × 100

Operating conditions

Detector: A hydrogen flame-ionization detector.

Column: A glass column 3 mm in inside diameter and 2 m in length, packed with siliceous earth for gas chromatography (177–250 μm in particle diameter) coated in 20% with 50% phenyl-methyl silicone polymer for gas chromatography.

Column temperature: A constant temperature of about 120°C.

Carrier gas: Helium.

Flow rate: about 50 mL per minute (the retention time of 2-mercaptoethanol is 3 to 4 minutes.)

Time span of measurement: About 7 times as long as the retention time of 2-mercaptoethanol.

2-Mercaptoethanol for epoetin beta $HSCH_2CH_2OH$ Prepared for study of sulfoprotein.

Mercaptopurine See mercaptopurine hydrate.

Mercaptopurine hydrate $C_5H_4N_4S.H_2O$ [Same as the namesake monograph]

Mercuric acetate See mercury (II) acetate.

Mercuric acetate TS for nonaqueous titration See mercury (II) acetate TS for nonaqueous titration.

Mercuric chloride See mercury (II) chloride.

Mercury Hg [K 8572, Special class]

Mercury (II) acetate $Hg(CH_3COO)_2$ White, crystals or crystalline powder.

Identification—(1) Dissolve 1 g of mercury (II) chloride in 1 mL of diluted nitric acid (1 in 7), add 20 mL of water, and use this solution as the sample solution. To 10 mL of the sample solution add 0.8 mL of iron (III) chloride TS: a red-brown color is developed.

(2) To 10 mL of the sample solution obtained in (1) add 2 mL of potassium iodate TS: a red precipitate is produced.

Storage—Preserve in a light-resistant tight container.

Mercury (II) acetate TS for nonaqueous titration Dissolve 5 g of mercury (II) acetate in acetic acid (100) for nonaqueous titration to make 100 mL.

Mercury (II) chloride $HgCl_2$ [K 8139, Special class]

Mesaconitine for purity $C_{33}H_{45}NO_{11}$ White, crystals or crystalline powder. Slightly soluble in acetonitrile and in ethanol (99.5), very slightly soluble in diethyl ether, and practically insoluble in water. Melting point: about 190°C (with decomposition).

Identification—Determine the infrared absorption spectrum of mesaconitine for purity as directed in the potassium bromide disk method under Infrared Spectrophotometry <2.25>: it exhibits absorption at the wave numbers of about 3510 cm^{-1}, 1713 cm^{-1}, 1277 cm^{-1}, 1116 cm^{-1}, 1098 cm^{-1} and 717 cm^{-1}.

Absorbance <2.24> $E_{1\,cm}^{1\%}$ (230 nm): 211 – 247 (5 mg, ethanol (99.5), 200 mL).

Purity Related substances—(1) Dissolve 5.0 mg of mesaconitine for purity in 2 mL of acetonitrile, and use this solution as the sample solution. Pipet 1 mL of the sample solution, add acetonitrile to make exactly 50 mL, and use this solution as the standard solution. Perform the test with these solutions as directed under Thin-layer Chromatography <2.03>. Spot 20 μL each of the sample solution and standard solution on a plate of silica gel for thin-layer chromatography, and proceed the test as directed in the Identification under Processed Aconite Root: the spot other than the principal spot obtained from the sample solution is not more intense than the spot from the standard solution.

(2) Dissolve 5.0 mg of mesaconitine for purity in 5 mL of acetonitrile, and use this solution as the sample solution. Pipet 1 mL of the sample solution, add acetonitrile to make exactly 50 mL, and use this solution as the standard solution. Perform the test with exactly 10 μL each of the sample solution and standard solution as directed under Liquid Chromatography <2.01> according to the following conditions, and determine each peak area by the automatic integration method: the total area of the peaks other than mesaconitine obtained from the sample solution is not larger than the peak area of mesaconitine from the standard solution.

Operating conditions

Detector, column, and column temperature: Proceed as directed in the operating conditions in the Purity (3) under Processed Aconite Root.

Mobile phase: A mixture of phosphate buffer solution for processed aconite root and tetrahydrofuran (9:1).

Flow rate: Adjust so that the retention time of mesaconitine is about 19 minutes.

Time span of measurement: About 3 times as long as the retention time of mesaconitine, beginning after the solvent peak.

System suitability

Test for required detectability: Pipet 1 mL of the standard solution, and add acetonitrile to make exactly 20 mL. Confirm that the peak area of mesaconitine with 10 μL of this solution is equivalent to 3.5 to 6.5% of that with 10 μL of the standard solution.

System performance: Dissolve 1 mg each of mesaconitine

for purity, aconitine for purity and hypaconitine for purity, and 8 mg of jesaconitine for purity in 200 mL of acetonitrile. When the procedure is run with 10 μL of this solution under the above operating conditions, mesaconitine, hypaconitine, aconitine and jesaconitine are eluted in this order, and each resolution between these peaks is not less than 1.5, respectively.

System repeatability: When the test is repeated 6 times with 10 μL of the standard solution under the above operating conditions, the relative standard deviation of the peak area of mesaconitine is not more than 1.5%.

Water <2.48>: not more than 1.0% (5 mg, coulometric titration).

Mesalazine for assay $C_7H_7NO_3$ [Same as the monograph Mesalazine. When dried, it contains not less than 99.0% of mesalazine ($C_7H_7NO_3$).]

Mesityl oxide $CH_3COCH = C(CH_3)_2$ A colorless or pale yellow, clear liquid, having a characteristic odor.

Specific gravity <2.56> d_{20}^{20}: 0.850 – 0.860

Metacresol purple $C_{21}H_{18}O_5S$ [K 8889, Special class]

Metacresol purple TS Dissolve 0.10 g of metacresol purple in 13 mL of 0.01 mol/L sodium hydroxide TS, and add water to make 100 mL. Filter if necessary.

Metacycline hydrochloride $C_{22}H_{22}N_2O_8.HCl$ Yellow to dark yellow, crystals or crystalline powder.

Purity Related substances—Dissolve 20 mg of metacycline hydrochloride in 25 mL of 0.01 mol/L hydrochloric acid TS, and use this solution as the sample solution. Proceed the test with 20 μL of the sample solution as directed in the Purity (2) under Doxycycline Hydrochloride Hydrate, determine each peak area by the automatic integration method, and calculate the amounts of them by the area percentage method: the total area of peaks other than metacycline is not more than 10%.

Metallic sodium See sodium.

Metanil yellow $C_{18}H_{14}N_3NaO_3S$ Yellow-brown powder. Sparingly soluble in water, and very slightly soluble in ethanol (95) and in *N,N*-dimethylformamide.

Metanil yellow TS Dissolve 0.1 g of metanil yellow in 200 mL of *N,N*-dimethylformamide.

Metaphosphoric acid HPO_3 A colorless, deliquescent, stick or masses.

Identification—(1) Dissolve 1 g of metaphosphoric acid in 50 mL of water, and use this solution as the sample solution. To 10 mL of the sample solution add 0.2 mL of ammonia TS and 1 mL of silver nitrate TS: a yellowish white precipitate is produced.

(2) To 10 mL of the sample solution obtained in (1) add 10 mL of albumin TS: a white precipitate is produced.

Metaphosphoric acid-acetic acid TS Dissolve 15 g of metaphosphoric acid and 40 mL of acetic acid (100) in water to make 500 mL. Preserve in a cold place, and use within 2 days.

Metenolone enanthate $C_{27}H_{42}O_3$ [Same as the namesake monograph]

Metenolone enanthate for assay $C_{27}H_{42}O_3$ To 1 g of metenolone enanthate add 30 mL of water, and add slowly 70 mL of methanol with warming to dissolve. Filter while hot, and allow the filtrate to stand on a water bath for 30 minutes. Allow to stand overnight in a cold place, collect the crystals thus formed, and wash with a small amount of diluted methanol (1 in 3). Recrystallize in the same manner, and dry the crystals in a desiccator (in vacuum, phosphorus (V) oxide) for 4 hours. It is white, odorless crystals.

Absorbance <2.24> $E_{1\,cm}^{1\%}$ (242 nm): 321 – 328 (1 mg, methanol, 100 mL).

Optical rotation <2.49> $[\alpha]_D^{20}$: +40 – +42° (0.2 g, chloroform, 10 mL, 100 mm).

Melting point <2.60>: 69 – 72°C

Purity Related substances—Dissolve 50 mg of metenolone enanthate for assay in chloroform to make exactly 10 mL, and perform the test with 10 μL of this solution as directed in the Purity (3) under Metenolone Enanthate: any spot other than the principal spot does not appear.

Metformin hydrochloride for assay $C_4H_{11}N_5.HCl$ [Same as the monograph Metformin Hydrochloride. When dried, it contains not less than 99.0% of metformin hydrochloride ($C_4H_{11}N_5.HCl$).]

Methanesulfonic acid CH_3SO_3H Clear, colorless liquid or colorless or white, crystalline mass, having a characteristic odor. Miscible with water, with ethanol (95) and with diethyl ether.

Congealing point <2.42>: 15 – 20°C

Specific gravity <2.56> d_{20}^{20}: 1.483 – 1.488

Content: not less than 99.0%. Assay—Weigh accurately about 2 g of methanesulfonic acid, dissolve in 40 mL of water, and titrate <2.50> with 1 mol/L sodium hydroxide VS (indicator: 2 drops of bromothymol blue TS).

Each mL of 1 mol/L sodium hydroxide VS
= 96.11 mg of CH_3SO_3H

Methanesulfonic acid TS To 35 mL of methanesulfonic acid add 20 mL of acetic acid (100) and water to make 500 mL.

0.1 mol/L Methanesulfonic acid TS To 4.8 g of methanesulfonic acid add water to make 500 mL.

Methanol CH_3OH [K 8891, Special class]

Methanol, anhydrous CH_4O To 1000 mL of methanol add 5 g of magnesium powder. After the evolving of a gas is stopped, distillate the solution, and preserve the distillate protecting from moisture. Water content per mL is not more than 0.3 mg.

Methanol for liquid chromatography CH_3OH A clear, colorless liquid. Miscible with water.

Purity Ultraviolet-absorbing substances—Perform the test as directed in Ultraviolet-visible Spectrophotometry <2.24> using water as the blank: the absorbances at 210 nm, at 220 nm, at 230 nm, at 240 nm and at 254 nm are not more than 0.70, 0.30, 0.15, 0.07 and 0.02, respectively.

Methanol for water determination To 1000 mL of methanol add 30 g of synthetic zeolite for drying, stopper tightly, allow to stand for about 8 hours with occasional gentle shaking, then allow to stand for about 16 hours, and collect the clear layer of methanol. Preserve the methanol, protecting it from moisture. The water content of this methanol should not be more than 0.1 mg per mL.

Methanol-free ethanol See ethanol (95), methanol-free.

Methanol-free ethanol (95) See ethanol (95), methanol-free.

Methanol, purified Distil methanol before use.

Methionin See L-methionine.

L-Methionine $C_5H_{11}NO_2S$ [Same as the namesake

monograph]

Methotrexate $C_{20}H_{22}N_8O_5$ [Same as the namesake monograph]

4′-Methoxyacetophenone $C_9H_{10}O_2$ White to light brown, crystals or crystalline powder.

Melting point <*2.60*>: 34 – 39°C

4-Methoxybenzaldehyde $C_8H_8O_2$ Clear, colorless to light yellow liquid. Miscible with ethanol (95) and with diethyl ether, and practically insoluble in water.

Specific gravity <*2.56*> d_4^{20}: 1.123 – 1.129

Content: not less than 97.0%. Assay—Weigh accurately about 0.8 g of 4-methoxybenzaldehyde, add exactly 75 mL of hydroxylamine TS, shake well, allow to stand for 30 minutes, and titrate <*2.50*> with 0.5 mol/L hydrochloric acid VS (indicator: 3 drops of bromophenol blue TS) until the color of the solution changes from blue through green to yellow-green. Perform a blank determination in the same manner.

Each mL of 0.5 mol/L hydrochloric acid VS
= 68.08 mg of $C_8H_8O_2$

4-Methoxybenzaldehyde-acetic acid TS To 0.5 mL of 4-methoxybenzaldehyde add acetic acid (100) to make 100 mL.

4-Methoxybenzaldehyde-sulfuric acid TS To 9 mL of ethanol (95) add 0.5 mL of 4-methoxybenzaldehyde and 0.5 mL of sulfuric acid, and mix thoroughly.

4-Methoxybenzaldehyde-sulfuric acid-acetic acid-ethanol TS for spraying To 9 mL of ethanol (95) add 0.5 mL of 4-methoxybenzaldehyde, mix gently, add gently 0.5 mL of sulfuric acid and 0.1 mL of acetic acid (100) in this order, and mix well.

4-Methoxybenzaldehyde-sulfuric acid-acetic acid TS To 50 mL of acetic acid (100) add 1 mL of sulfuric acid and 0.5 mL of 4-methoxybenzaldehyde, and stir well. Prepare before use.

(*E*)-2-Methoxycinnamaldehyde for thin-layer chromatography $C_{10}H_{10}O_2$ White to yellow, crystalline powder or powder. Freely soluble in methanol and in ethanol (99.5), and practically insoluble in water. Melting point: 44 – 50°C.

Identification—(1) Determine the absorption spectrum of a solution of (*E*)-2-methoxycinnamaldehyde for thin-layer chromatography in methanol (1 in 200,000) as directed under Ultraviolet-visible Spectrophotometry <*2.24*>: it exhibits maxima between 282 nm and 286 nm, and between 331 nm and 335 nm.

(2) Determine the infrared absorption spectrum of (*E*)-2-methoxycinnamaldehyde for thin-layer chromatography as directed in the potassium bromide disk method under Infrared Spectrophotometry <*2.25*>: it exhibits absorption at the wave numbers of about 1675 cm^{-1}, 1620 cm^{-1}, 1490 cm^{-1}, 1470 cm^{-1}, 1295 cm^{-1}, 1165 cm^{-1}, 1130 cm^{-1}, 1025 cm^{-1} and 600 cm^{-1}.

Purity Related substances—Dissolve 10 mg of (*E*)-2-methoxycinnamaldehyde for thin-layer chromatography in 5 mL of methanol, and use this solution as the sample solution. Pipet 1 mL of the sample solution, add methanol to make exactly 50 mL, and use this as the standard solution. Perform the test with 5 μL each of the sample solution and standard solution as directed in the Identification (5) (ii) under Goshajinkigan Extract: the spots other than the principal spot appeared at *Rf* value of about 0.4 obtained from the sample solution are not more intense than the spot from the standard solution.

2-Methoxyethanol $CH_3OCH_2CH_2OH$ [K 8895, Special class]

2-Methoxy-4-methylphenol $C_8H_{10}O_2$ Colorless to pale yellow liquid. Miscible with methanol and with ethanol (99.5), and slightly soluble in water. Congealing point: 3 – 8°C.

Identification—Determine the infrared absorption spectrum of 2-methoxy-4-methylphenol as directed in the ATR method under Infrared Spectrophotometry <*2.25*>: it exhibits absorption at the wave numbers of about 1511 cm^{-1}, 1423 cm^{-1}, 1361 cm^{-1}, 1268 cm^{-1}, 1231 cm^{-1}, 1202 cm^{-1}, 1148 cm^{-1}, 1120 cm^{-1}, 1031 cm^{-1}, 919 cm^{-1}, 807 cm^{-1} and 788 cm^{-1}.

Purity Related substances—Perform the test with 0.2 μL of 2-methoxy-4-methylphenol as directed under Gas Chromatography <*2.02*> according to the following conditions. Determine each peak area by the automatic integration method: the total area of the peaks other than 2-methoxy-4-methylphenol is not more than 3.0%.

Operating conditions

Detector: A hydrogen flame-ionization detector.

Column: A fused silica column 0.25 mm in inside diameter and 60 m in length, coated inside with polymethylsiloxane for gas chromatography in 0.25 to 0.5 μm in thickness.

Column temperature: Inject at a constant temperature of about 100°C, raise the temperature to 130°C at a rate of 5°C per minute, raise to 140°C at a rate of 2°C per minute, raise to 200°C at a rate of 15°C per minute, and maintain at 200°C for 2 minutes.

Injection port temperature: 200°C.

Detector temperature: 250°C.

Carrier gas: Helium.

Flow rate: Adjust so that the retention time of 2-methoxy-4-methylphenol is about 10 minutes.

Split ratio: 1:50.

System suitability

System performance: Dissolve 60 mg of 2-methoxy-4-methylphenol in methanol to make 100 mL, and use this solution as the solution for system suitability test. Proceed with 1 μL of the solution for system suitability test under the above operating conditions, the symmetry factor of the peak of 2-methoxy-4-methylphenol is not more than 1.5.

System repeatability: When the test is repeated 6 times with 1 μL of the solution for system suitability test under the above operating conditions, the relative standard deviation of the peak area of 2-methoxy-4-methylphenol is not more than 2.0%.

1-Methoxy-2-propanol $C_4H_{10}O_2$ A colorless, clear liquid.

Refractive index <*2.45*> n_D^{20}: 1.402 – 1.405

Specific gravity <*2.56*> d_4^{20}: 0.920 – 0.925

Purity Clarity of solution—To 5 mL of 1-methoxy-2-propanol add 20 mL of water, and mix: the solution is clear.

Water <*2.48*>: not more than 0.5% (5 g).

Content: not less than 98.0%. Assay—Proceed as directed under Gas Chromatography <*2.02*> using the area percentage method according to the following conditions:

Operating conditions

Detector: Thermal conductivity detector.

Column: A glass column about 3 mm in inside diameter and about 2 m in length, packed with siliceous earth for gas chromatography (150 to 180 μm) coated with polyethylene glycol 20 M for gas chromatography in 20%.

Column temperature: A constant temperature of about 90°C.

Carrier gas: Helium.

Flow rate: A constant flow rate of 20 mL per minute.

Methyl acetate CH_3COOCH_3 [K 8382, Special class]

Methyl 4-aminobenzoate $H_2NC_6H_4COOCH_3$ Pale yellow, crystals or crystalline powder.
Melting point <2.60>: 111 - 114°C

***p*-Methyl aminophenol sulfate** See 4-methyl aminophenol sulfate.

4-Methyl aminophenol sulfate $(HOC_6H_4NHCH_3)_2.H_2SO_4$ White to pale yellow or very pale gray, crystals or crystalline powder. Melting point: about 260°C (with decomposition).

***p*-Methyl aminophenol sulfate TS** See 4-methyl aminophenol sulfate TS.

4-Methyl aminophenol sulfate TS Dissolve 0.35 g of 4-methyl aminophenol sulfate and 20 g of sodium hydrogen sulfite in water to make 100 mL. Prepare before use.

2-Methylaminopyridine $C_6H_8N_2$ A light yellow liquid.
Specific gravity <2.56> d_{20}^{20}: 1.050 - 1.065
Boiling point <2.57>: 200 - 202°C
Water <2.48>: less than 0.1%.

2-Methylamino pyridine for water determination Distill and preserve 2-methylaminopyridine, protecting it from moisture. The water content of this 2-methylaminopyridine should not be more than 1 mg per mL.

Methyl arachidate for gas chromatography $C_{21}H_{42}O_2$ White to light yellow, crystals or crystalline masses.
Melting point <2.60>: 45 - 50°C

Methyl behenate $C_{23}H_{46}O_2$ White, odorless and tasteless, scaly crystals or powder. Dissolves in acetone, in diethyl ether and in chloroform.
Melting point <2.60>: 54°C
Saponification value <1.13>: 155.5 - 158.5

Methyl benzoate $C_6H_5COOCH_3$ Clear, colorless liquid.
Refractive index <2.45> n_D^{20}: 1.515 - 1.520
Specific gravity <2.56> d_{20}^{20}: 1.087 - 1.095
Purity—Dissolve 0.1 mL of methyl benzoate in the mobile phase in Assay under Thiamine Chloride Hydrochloride to make 50 mL. Perform the test as directed under Liquid Chromatography <2.01> with 10 μL of this solution according to the operating conditions in the Assay under Thiamine Chloride Hydrochloride. Determine each peak area by the automatic integration method in a range about twice the retention time of methyl benzoate, and calculate the amount of methyl benzoate by the area percentage method: it shows the purity of not less than 99.0%.

Methyl benzoate for estriol test $C_6H_5COOCH_3$ Clear, colorless liquid, having a characteristic odor.
Refractive index <2.45> n_D^{20}: 1.515 - 1.520
Specific gravity <2.56> d_{20}^{20}: 1.087 - 1.095
Acid value <1.13>: not more than 0.5.

4-Methylbenzophenone $C_{14}H_{12}O$ White crystals.

3-Methyl-2-benzothiazolonehydrazone hydrochloride monohydrate $C_8H_{10}ClN_3S.H_2O$ A white to light yellow-white crystalline powder. Melting point: about 270°C (with decomposition).

D-(+)-α-Methylbenzylamine $C_6H_5CH(CH_3)NH_2$ Colorless or pale yellow, clear liquid, having an amine like odor. Very soluble in ethanol (95) and in acetone, and slightly soluble in water.
Refractive index <2.45> n_D^{20}: 1.524–1.529
Optical rotation <2.49> $[\alpha]_D^{20}$: + 37 - + 41° (50 mm).
Purity—Perform the test with 0.6 μL of D-(+)-α-methylbenzylamine as directed under Gas Chromatography <2.02> according to the following conditions. Determine each peak area by the automatic integration method, and calculate the amount of D-(+)-α-methylbenzylamine by the area percentage method: not less than 98.0%.
Operating conditions
Detector: A hydrogen flame-ionization detector.
Column: A glass column about 3 mm in inside diameter and about 2 m in length, packed with siliceous earth for gas chromatography (180 to 250 μm in particle diameter) coated with polyethylene glycol 20 M for gas chromatography and potassium hydroxide at the ratio of 10% and 5%, respectively.
Column temperature: A constant temperature of about 140°C.
Carrier gas: Helium.
Flow rate: Adjust so that the retention time of D-(+)-α-methylbenzylamine is about 5 minutes.
Selection of column: To 5 mL of D-(+)-α-methylbenzylamine add 1 mL of pyridine. Proceed with 0.6 μL of this solution under the above operating conditions, and calculate the resolution. Use a column giving elution of pyridine and D-(+)-α-methylbenzylamine in this order with the resolution between these peaks being not less than 3.
Detection sensitivity: Adjust the detection sensitivity so that the peak height of D-(+)-α-methylbenzylamine obtained with 0.6 μL of the D-(+)-α-methylbenzylamine is not less than about 90% of the full scale.
Time span of measurement: About 3 times as long as the retention time of D-(+)-α-methylbenzylamine.

3-Methyl-1-butanol $C_5H_{12}O$ [K 8051, Special class]

3-Methylbutyl acetate $CH_3COOCH_2CH_2CH(CH_3)_2$ A clear and colorless liquid. Boiling point: about 140°C.
Specific gravity <2.56> d_{20}^{20}: 0.868 - 0.879
Storage—Preserve in a light-resistant tight container.

Methyl cellosolve See 2-methoxyethanol.

Methylcyclohexane C_7H_{14} A clear and colorless liquid.
Refractive index <2.45> n_D^{20}: 1.420 - 1.425
Density <2.56> (20°C): 0.766 - 0.772 g/mL

Methyl docosanate $C_{23}H_{46}O_2$ White, tabular crystals or crystalline powder.
Melting point <2.60>: 51.0 - 56.0°C

Methyldopa See methyldopa hydrate.

Methyldopa for assay See methyldopa hydrate for assay.

Methyldopa hydrate $C_{10}H_{13}NO_4.1\frac{1}{2}H_2O$ [Same as the namesake monograph]

Methyldopa hydrate for assay $C_{10}H_{13}NO_4.1\frac{1}{2}H_2O$ [Same as the monograph Methyldopa Hydrate. It contains not less than 99.0% of methyldopa ($C_{10}H_{13}NO_4$), calculated on the anhydrous basis.]

***N,N′*-Methylenebisacrylamide** $CH_2(NHCOCHCH_2)_2$ White crystalline powder.
Content: not less than 97.0%.

Methyl eicosenoate for gas chromatography $C_{21}H_{40}O_2$ A clear and colorless, liquid.

Methylene blue See methylene blue trihydrate.

Methylene blue-sulfuric acid-sodium dihydrogenphosphate TS To 30 mL of a solution of methylene blue (1 in

1000) add 500 mL of water, 6.8 mL of sulfuric acid and 50 g of sodium dihydrogenphosphate dihydrate, dissolve, and add water to make 1000 mL.

Methylene blue trihydrate $C_{16}H_{18}ClN_3S.3H_2O$ [K 8897, Special class]

Methylene blue TS Dissolve 0.1 g of methylene blue trihydrate in water to make 100 mL. Filter if necessary.

***dl*-Methylephedrine hydrochloride** $C_{11}H_{17}NO.HCl$ [Same as the namesake monograph]

***dl*-Methylephedrine hydrochloride for assay** [Same as the monograph *dl*-Methylephedrine Hydrochloride]

Methylergometrine maleate for assay $C_{20}H_{25}N_3O_2.C_4H_4O_4$ [Same as the monograph Methylergometrine Maleate. When dried, it contains not less than 99.0% of methylergometrine maleate ($C_{20}H_{25}N_3O_2.C_4H_4O_4$).]

Methyl ethyl ketone See 2-butanone.

Methyl iodide See iodomethane.

Methyl iodide for assay See iodomethane for assay.

Methyl isobutyl ketone See 4-methyl-2-pentanone.

Methyl laurate for gas chromatography $C_{13}H_{26}O_2$ A colorless to yellow, liquid.

Refractive index <2.45> n_D^{20}: 1.431 – 1.433

Specific gravity <2.56> d_{20}^{20}: 0.870 – 0.872

Methyl lignocerate for gas chromatography $C_{25}H_{50}O_2$ A white crystalline powder.

Melting point <2.60>: 58 – 61°C

Methyl linoleate for gas chromatography $C_{19}H_{34}O_2$ A colorless to light yellow, liquid.

Specific gravity <2.56> d_{20}^{20}: 0.880 – 0.889

Methyl linolenate for gas chromatography $C_{19}H_{32}O_2$ A colorless to light yellow, liquid.

Specific gravity <2.56> d_{20}^{20}: 0.890 – 0.901

3-O-Methylmethyldopa for thin-layer chromatography $C_{11}H_{15}NO_4$

Purity Related substances—Dissolve 5 mg of 3-O-methylmethyldopa for thin-layer chromatography in methanol to make exactly 100 mL. Perform the test with 20 μL of this solution as directed in the Purity (5) under Methyldopa Hydrate: any spot other than the principal spot at the *R*f value of about 0.7 does not appear.

Methyl myristate for gas chromatography $C_{15}H_{30}O_2$ A colorless to light yellow, liquid.

Specific gravity <2.56> d_{20}^{20}: about 0.866 – 0.874

2-Methyl-5-nitroimidazole for thin-layer chromatography $C_4H_5N_3O_2$ White crystalline powder. Slightly soluble in water and in acetone. Melting point: about 253°C (with decomposition).

Purity Related substances—Dissolve 40 mg of 2-methyl-5-nitroimidazole for thin-layer chromatography in 8 mL of acetone, and use this solution as the sample solution. Pipet 2.5 mL of the sample solution, add acetone to make exactly 100 mL, and use this solution as the standard solution. Perform the test as directed in the Purity (2) under Metronidazole: the spots other than the principal spot obtained from the sample solution are not more intense than the spot from the standard solution.

Methyl oleate for gas chromatography $C_{19}H_{36}O_2$ A clear, colorless to light yellow, liquid.

Specific gravity <2.56> d_{20}^{20}: 0.866 – 0.882

Methyl orange $C_{14}H_{14}N_3NaO_3S$ [K 8893, Special class]

Methyl orange-boric acid TS Add 0.5 g of methyl orange and 5.2 g of boric acid in 500 mL of water, and dissolve by warming on a water bath. After cooling, wash this solution with three 50-mL portions of chloroform.

Methyl orange TS Dissolve 0.1 g of methyl orange in 100 mL of water, and filter if necessary.

Methyl orange-xylenecyanol FF TS Dissolve 1 g of methyl orange and 1.4 g of xylene cyanol FF in 500 mL of dilute ethanol.

Methyl palmitate for gas chromatography $C_{17}H_{34}O_2$ White, crystals or waxy masses.

Congealing point <2.42>: 25 – 31°C

Methyl palmitoleate for gas chromatography $C_{17}H_{32}O_2$

Specific gravity <2.56> d_{20}^{20}: 0.876 – 0.881

Methyl parahydroxybenzoate $HOC_6H_4COOCH_3$ [Same as the namesake monograph]

Methyl parahydroxybenzoate for resolution check $C_8H_8O_3$ Colorless crystals or a white crystalline powder. Freely soluble in methanol, in ethanol (95) and in acetone, and very slightly soluble in water. Melting point: 125 – 128°C.

Identification—Determine the infrared absorption spectrum of methyl parahydroxybenzoate for resolution check as directed in the potassium bromide disk method under Infrared Spectrophotometry <2.25>, and compare the spectrum with the Reference Spectrum of Methyl Parahydroxybenzoate or the spectrum of Methyl Parahydroxybenzoate RS: both spectra exhibit similar intensities of absorption at the same wave numbers.

Purity Related substances—Dissolve 50 mg of methyl parahydroxybenzoate for resolution check in 2.5 mL of methanol, and add the mobile phase to make 50 mL. To 10 mL of this solution add the mobile phase to make 100 mL, and use this solution as the sample solution. Pipet 1 mL of the sample solution, add the mobile phase to make exactly 10 mL, and use this solution as the standard solution. Perform the test with exactly 10 μL each of the sample solution and standard solution as directed under Liquid Chromatography <2.01> according to the following conditions. Determine each peak area by the automatic integration method: total area of the peaks other than methyl parahydroxybenzoate obtained from the sample solution is not larger than the peak area of methyl parahydroxybenzoate from the standard solution.

Operating conditions

Detector, column, column temperature, mobile phase, and flow rate: Proceed as directed in the operating conditions in the Assay under Methyl Parahydroxybenzoate.

Time span of measurement: About 5 times as long as the retention time of methyl parahydroxybenzoate.

System suitability

Test for required detectability: Pipet 1 mL of the standard solution, and add methanol to make exactly 20 mL. Confirm that the peak area of methyl parahydroxybenzoate obtained with 10 μL of this solution is equivalent to 3.5 to 6.5% of that with 10 μL of the standard solution.

System performance: When the procedure is run with 10 μL of the standard solution under the above operating conditions, the number of theoretical plates and the symmetry factor of the peak of methyl parahydroxybenzoate are not less than 2500 and not more than 2.0, respectively.

System repeatability: When the test is repeated 6 times

with 10 μL of the standard solution under the above operating conditions, the relative standard deviation of the peak area of methyl parahydroxybenzoate is not more than 5.0%.

4-Methylpentan-2-ol $C_6H_{14}O$ A clear and colorless, volatile liquid.

Refractive index ‹2.45› n_D^{20}: about 1.411

Specific gravity ‹2.56› d_{20}^{20}: about 0.802

Boiling point ‹2.57›: about 132°C

4-Methyl-2-pentanone $CH_3COCH_2CH(CH_3)_2$ [K 8903, Special class]

3-Methyl-1-phenyl-5-pyrazolone $C_{10}H_{10}N_{20}O$ [K 9548, Special class]

Methyl prednisolone $C_{22}H_{30}O_3$ [Same as the namesake monograph]

2-Methyl-1-propanol $(CH_3)_2CHCH_2OH$ [K 8811, Special class]

***N*-Methylpyrrolidine** $C_5H_{11}N$ Colorless, clear liquid, having a characteristic order.

Identification—Determine the spectrum of *N*-methylpyrrolidine in a solution of deuterated chloroform for nuclear magnetic resonance spectroscopy (2 in 25) as directed under Nuclear Magnetic Resonance Spectroscopy ‹2.21› (^{1}H): it exhibits a big signal, at around δ 2.3 ppm.

Content: not less than 95%. Assay—Put 30 mL of water in a beaker, weigh accurately the beaker, add dropwise about 0.15 g of *N*-methylpyrrolidine, weigh accurately the beaker again, and titrate ‹2.50› with 0.05 mol/L sulfuric acid VS (potentiometric titration). Perform a blank determination in the same manner, and make any necessary correction.

Each mL of 0.05 mol/L sulfuric acid VS
= 8.515 mg of $C_5H_{11}N$

Methyl red $C_{15}H_{15}N_3O_2$ [K 8896, Special class]

Methyl red-methylene blue TS Dissolve 0.1 g of methyl red and 0.1 g of methylene blue in ethanol (95) to make 100 mL, and filter if necessary.

Storage—Preserve in light-resistant containers.

Methyl red-sodium hydroxide TS Dissolve 50 mg of methyl red in a mixture of 1.86 mL of 0.1 mol/L sodium hydroxide VS and 50 mL of ethanol (95), and add water to make 100 mL.

Methyl red TS Dissolve 0.1 g of methyl red in 100 mL of ethanol (95), and filter if necessary.

Methyl red TS, dilute Dissolve 25 mg of methyl red in 100 mL of ethanol (99.5), and filter if necessary. Prepare before use.

Methyl red TS for acidity or alkalinity test To 0.1 g of methyl red add 7.4 mL of 0.05 mol/L sodium hydroxide VS or 3.7 mL of 0.1 mol/L sodium hydroxide VS, triturate to dissolve in a mortar, and add freshly boiled and cooled water to make 200 mL.

Storage—Preserve in light-resistant, glass-stoppered bottles.

Methylrosaniline chloride See crystal violet.

Methylrosaniline chloride TS See crystal violet TS.

Methyl salicylate $C_8H_8O_3$ [Same as the namesake monograph]

Methylsilicone polymer for gas chromatography Prepared for gas chromatography.

Methyl stearate for gas chromatography $C_{19}H_{38}O_2$ White, crystals or crystalline masses.

Melting point ‹2.60›: 36 – 42°C

Methyltestosterone $C_{20}H_{30}O_2$ [Same as the namesake monograph]

1-Methyl-1*H*-tetrazole-5-thiol $C_2H_4N_4S$ White, crystals or crystalline powder.

Identification (1) Determine the ultraviolet-visible absorption spectrum of a solution of 1-methyl-1*H*-tetrazole-5-thiol (1 in 200,000) as directed under Ultraviolet-visible Spectrophotometry ‹2.24›: it exhibits a maximum between 222 nm and 226 nm.

(2) Determine the infrared absorption spectrum of 1-methyl-1*H*-tetrazole-5-thiol according to the potassium bromide disk method under Infrared Spectrophotometry ‹2.25›: it exhibits absorption at the wave numbers of about 3060 cm^{-1}, 2920 cm^{-1}, 2780 cm^{-1}, 1500 cm^{-1}, 1430 cm^{-1} and 1410 cm^{-1}.

Melting point ‹2.60›: 125 – 129°C

Purity Related substances—Dissolve 0.10 g of 1-methyl-1*H*-tetrazole-5-thiol in exactly 100 mL of water. Perform the test with 1 μL of this solution as directed in the Purity (4) under Cefmetazole Sodium: any spot other than the principal spot at the *Rf* value of about 0.77 does not appear.

1-Methyl-1*H*-tetrazole-5-thiol for liquid chromatography $C_2H_4N_4S$ White, crystals or crystalline powder. Very soluble in methanol, and freely soluble in water.

Melting point ‹2.60›: 123 – 127°C

Loss on drying ‹2.41›: not more than 1.0% (1 g, in vacuum, phosphorous (V) oxide, 2 hours).

Content: not less than 99.0%. Assay—Weigh accurately about 0.2 g of 1-methyl-1*H*-tetrazole-5-thiol, previously dried, dissolve in 80 mL of *N*,*N*-dimethylformamide, and titrate ‹2.50› with 0.1 mol/L sodium methoxide VS (indicator: 3 drops of thymol blue-*N*,*N*-dimethylformamide TS). Perform a blank determination in the same manner, and make any necessary correction.

Each mL of 0.1 mol/L sodium methoxide VS
= 11.61 mg of $C_2H_4N_4S$

Methylthymol blue $C_{37}H_{43}N_2NaO_{13}S$ [K 9552, Special class]

Methylthymol blue-potassium nitrate indicator Mix 0.1 g of methylthymol blue with 9.9 g of potassium nitrate, and triturate until the mixture becomes homogeneous.

Sensitivity—When 20 mg of methylthymol blue-potassium nitrate indicator is dissolved in 100 mL of 0.02 mol/L sodium hydroxide VS, the solution is slightly blue in color. On adding 0.05 mL of 0.01 mol/L barium chloride VS to this solution, the solution shows a blue color, then on the subsequent addition of 0.1 mL of 0.01 mol/L disodium dihydrogen ethylenediamine tetraacetate VS, it becomes colorless.

Methylthymol blue-sodium chloride indicator Mix 0.25 g of methylthymol blue and 10 g of sodium chloride, and grind to homogenize.

Methyl yellow $C_{14}H_{15}N_3$ [K 8494, Special class]

Methyl yellow TS Dissolve 0.1 g of methyl yellow in 200 mL of ethanol (95).

Metoclopramide for assay $C_{14}H_{22}ClN_3O_2$ [Same as the monograph]

Metoprolol tartrate for assay $(C_{15}H_{25}NO_3)_2.C_4H_6O_6$

[Same as the monograph Metoprolol Tartrate. When dried, it contains not less than 99.5% of metoprolol tartrate $((C_{15}H_{25}NO_3)_2.C_4H_6O_6)$.]

Metronidazole $C_6H_9N_3O_3$ [Same as the namesake monograph]

Metronidazole for assay $C_6H_9N_3O_3$ [Same as the monograph Metronidazole. It meets the following additional requirement.]

Purity Related substances—Dissolive about 25 mg of metronidazole for assay in 100 mL of a mixture of water and methanol (4:1), and use this solution as the sample solution. Pipet 2 mL of the sample solution, and add the mixture of water and methanol (4:1) to make exactly 50 mL. Pipet 2.5 mL of this solution, add the mixture of water and methanol (4:1) to make exactly 20 mL, and use this solution as the standard solution. Perform the test with exactly 10 μL each of the sample solution and standard solution as directed under Liquid Chromatography *<2.01>* according to the following conditions, and determine each peak area by the automatic integration method: the total area of the peaks other than metronidazole obtained from the sample solution is not more than the peak area of metronidazole from the standard solution.

Operating conditions

Detector, column, column temperature, mobile phase, and flow rate: Proceed as directed in the operating conditions in the Assay under Metronidazole Tablets.

Time span of measurement: About 4 times as long as the retention time of metronidazole.

System suitability

Test for required detectability: Measure exactly 2 mL of the standard solution, add a mixture of water and methanol (4:1) to make exactly 20 mL. Confirm that the peak area of metronidazole obtained with 10 μL of this solution is equivalent to 7 to 13% of that with the standard solution.

System performance: When the procedure is run with 10 μL of the standard solution under the above operating conditions, the number of theoretical plates and the symmetry factor of the peak of metronidazole are not less than 3000 and not more than 1.5, respectively.

System repeatability: When the test is repeated 6 times with 10 μL of the standard solution under the above operating conditions, the relative standard deviation of the peak area of metronidazole is not more than 2.0%.

Miconazole nitrate $C_{18}H_{14}Cl_4N_2O.HNO_3$ [Same as the namesake monograph]

Microplate A plate having multiple wells. It ordinarily has 96 or more wells and is about 128 mm × about 85 mm × about 14 mm in size. Select the material, surface treatment, and other conditions of the microplate suitable to tests for use.

Miglitol $C_8H_{17}NO_5$ [Same as the namesake monograph]

Milk casein See casein, milk.

Milk of lime Place 10 g of calcium oxide in a mortar, and add gradually 40 mL of water under grinding.

Minocycline hydrochloride $C_{23}H_{27}N_3O_7.HCl$ [Same as the namesake monograph]

Mitiglinide calcium hydrate $C_{38}H_{48}CaN_2O_6.2H_2O$ [Same as the namesake monograph]

Mixture of petroleum hexamethyl tetracosane branching hydrocarbons (L) for gas chromatography Prepared for gas chromatography.

Molecular mass marker for epoetin alfa A solution containing about 0.4 mg each of egg albumin, carbonic anhydrase, soybean trypsin inhibitor and lysozyme in 200 μL.

Molecular mass marker for interferon alfa Molecular mass known marker proteins, which are adjusted for molecular mass determination [4 components: egg albumin, carbonic anhydrase, soybean trypsin inhibitor, and α-lactalbumin].

Identification Use a solution of the molecular mass marker for interferon alfa as the sample solution. Separately, add water to an amount of egg albumin so that each mL contains 100 μg as protein content of egg albumin, and use this solution as the standard solution. Perform SDS-polyacrylamide gel electrophoresis with the sample solution and standard solution under the test conditions for molecular mass of Interferon Alfa (NAMALWA). The sample solution indicates 4 main electrophoretic bands. In addition, the mobility of egg albumin obtained from the sample solution corresponds with that of the band from the standard solution.

Molecular mass marker for nartograstim test A solution containing the following proteins. Egg albumin, carbonic anhydrase, soybean trypsin inhibitor and lysozyme.

Molecular mass standard stock solution Dissolve 1.2 g of 2-amino-2-hydroxymethyl-1,3-propanediol and 3.2 g of sodium lauryl sulfate in a suitable amount of water, adjust to pH 6.8 with 6 mol/L hydrochloric acid TS, 1 mol/L hydrochloric acid TS or 0.1 mol/L hydrochloric acid TS, add 32 mg of bromophenol blue and 16 mL of glycerin, and add water to make 40 mL. To 500 μL of this solution add 100 μL of molecular mass marker for epoetin alfa and 1400 μL of water, and heat at 100°C for 5 minutes. It meets the following requirement.

Identification—Dissolve 0.1 mg each of egg albumin, carbonic anhydrase, soybean trypsin inhibitor and lysozyme in 250 μL of buffer solution for epoetin alfa sample, add water to them to make 1 mL and heat at 100°C for 5 minutes, and use these solutions as each standard solution. When perform the test with the solution to be examined and each standard solution by the SDS-polyacrylamide gel electrophoresis as directed in the Molecular mass under Epoetin Alfa (Genetical recombination), the each band in the chromatogram obtained from the solution to be examined shows the same mobility as the band corresponding to egg albumin, carbonic anhydrase, soybean trypsin inhibitor or lysozyme obtained from each standard solution.

Molecular mass markers for teceleukin Dissolve 0.4 mg each of lysozyme, soybean trypsin inhibitor, carbonic anhydrase, egg albumin, bovine serum albumin, and phosphorylase b in 200 μL of diluted glycerin (1 in 2).

Molybdenum (VI) oxide MoO_3 A white to yellowish green powder.

Identification—Dissolve 0.5 g of molybdenum (VI) oxide in 5 mL of ammonia solution (28), acidify 1 mL of this solution with a suitable amount of nitric acid, add 5 mL of sodium phosphate TS, and warm: yellow precipitates appear.

Molybdenum (VI) oxide-citric acid TS To 54 g of molybdenum (VI) oxide and 11 g of sodium hydroxide add 200 mL of water, and dissolve by heating while stirring. Separately, dissolve 60 g of citric acid monohydrate in 250 mL of water, and add 140 mL of hydrochloric acid. Mix these solutions, filter if necessary, add water to make 1000 mL, and add a solution of potassium bromate (1 in 100) until a yellow-green color appears.

Storage—Preserve in tightly stoppered containers, protected from light.

Molybdenium-sulfuric acid TS Dissolve 2.5 g of hexaammonium heptamolybdate tetrahydrate in 20 mL of water by heating. To this solution add a solution, prepared by careful adding 28 mL of sulfuric acid to 50 mL of water, mixing and cooling, and add water to make 100 mL. Reserve in a polyethylene container.

Molybdenum trioxide See molybdenum (VI) oxide.

Molybdenum trioxide-citric acid TS See molybdenum (VI) oxide-citric acid TS.

Monoammonium glycyrrhizinate for resolution check $C_{42}H_{61}O_{16}NH_4$ Mainly composed with monoammonium glycyrrhizinate and its isomers. It is white, crystals or crystalline powder.

Identification—Dissolve 1 mg of monoammonium glycyrrhizinate for resolution check in 2 mL of diluted ethanol (2 in 5). Perform the test with 2 μL of this solution as directed under Liquid Chromatography <*2.01*> according to the following conditions: a peak having a relative retention time of about 0.9 to glycyrrhizic acid is observed, and when performed the test with these two peaks by liquid chromatography-mass spectrometry (ESI method, positive mode) their mass charge ratios (*m/z* values) are observed at 823 or 840 or at the both of them, respectively.

Operating conditions

Detector: An ultraviolet absorption photometer (wavelength: 254 nm) and mass spectrometer.

Column: A stainless steel column 2 mm in inside diameter and 15 cm in length, packed with octadecylsilanized silica gel for liquid chromatography (3 μm in particle diameter).

Column temperature: A constant temperature of about 40°C.

Mobile phase: Dissolve 0.63 g of ammonium formate in water to make 1000 mL. To 800 mL of this solution add 200 mL of acetonitrile.

Flow rate: About 0.5 mL per minute.

Monobasic ammonium phosphate See ammonium dihydrogenphosphate.

0.02 mol/L Monobasic ammonium phosphate TS See 0.02 mol/L ammonium dihydrogenphosphate TS.

Monobasic potassium phosphate See potassium dihydrogenphosphate.

Monobasic potassium phosphate for pH determination See potassium dihydrogenphosphate for pH determination.

0.05 mol/L Monobasic potassium phosphate (pH 3.0) See 0.05 mol/L potassium dihydrogenphosphate (pH 3.0).

0.05 mol/L Monobasic potassium phosphate TS (pH 4.7) See 0.05 mol/L potassium dihydrogenphosphate TS (pH 4.7).

0.02 mol/L Monobasic potassium phosphate TS See 0.02 mol/L potassium dihydrogenphosphate TS.

0.05 mol/L Monobasic potassium phosphate TS See 0.05 mol/L potassium dihydrogenphosphate TS.

0.2 mol/L Monobasic potassium phosphate TS See 0.2 mol/L potassium dihydrogenphosphate TS.

0.2 mol/L Monobasic potassium phosphate TS for buffer solution See 0.2 mol/L potassium dihydrogenphosphate TS for buffer solution.

Monobasic sodium phosphate See sodium dihydrogenphosphate dihydrate.

0.05 mol/L Monobasic sodium phosphate TS (pH 2.6) See 0.05 mol/L sodium dihydrogenphosphate TS (pH 2.6).

0.05 mol/L Monobasic sodium phosphate TS (pH 3.0) See 0.05 mol/L sodium dihydrogenphosphate TS (pH 3.0).

0.1 mol/L Monobasic sodium phosphate TS (pH 3.0) See 0.1 mol/L sodium dihydrogenphosphate TS (pH 3.0).

0.05 mol/L Monobasic sodium phosphate TS See 0.05 mol/L sodium dihydrogenphosphate TS.

0.1 mol/L Monobasic sodium phosphate TS See 0.1 mol/L sodium dihydrogenphosphate TS.

2 mol/L Monobasic sodium phosphate TS See 2 mol/L sodium dihydrogenphosphate TS.

Monoethanolamine See 2-Aminoethanol.

Morphine hydrochloride See morphine hydrochloride hydrate.

Morphine hydrochloride for assay See morphine hydrochloride hydrate for assay.

Morphine hydrochloride hydrate $C_{17}H_{19}NO_3.HCl.3H_2O$ [Same as the namesake monograph]

Morphine hydrochloride hydrate for assay $C_{17}H_{19}NO_3.HCl.3H_2O$ [Same as the monograph Morphine Hydrochloride Hydrate. It contains not less than 99.0% of morphine hydrochloride ($C_{17}H_{19}NO_3.HCl$), calculated on the anhydrous basis.]

3-(*N*-Morpholino)propanesulfonic acid $C_7H_{15}NO_4S$ White crystalline powder, freely soluble in water, and practically insoluble in ethanol (99.5).

Melting point <*2.60*>: 275 – 280°C

0.02 mol/L 3-(*N*-Morpholino)propanesulfonic acid buffer solution (pH 7.0) Dissolve 4.2 g of 3-(*N*-morpholino)propanesulfonic acid in 900 mL of water, adjust the pH to 7.0 with dilute sodium hydroxide TS, and add water to make 1000 mL.

0.1 mol/L 3-(*N*-Morpholino)propanesulfonic acid buffer solution (pH 7.0) Dissolve 20.92 g of 3-(*N*-morpholino) propanesulfonic acid in 900 mL of water, adjust the pH to 7.0 with sodium hydroxide TS, and add water to make 1000 mL.

0.02 mol/L 3-(*N*-Morpholino)propanesulfonic acid buffer solution (pH 8.0) Dissolve 4.2 g of 3-(*N*-morpholino)propanesulfonic acid in 700 mL of water, adjust the pH to 8.0 with dilute sodium hydroxide TS, and add water to make 1000 mL.

Mosapride citrate for assay See mosapride citrate hydrate for assay.

Mosapride citrate hydrate for assay $C_{21}H_{25}ClFN_3O_3.C_6H_8O_7.2H_2O$ [Same as the monograph Mosapride Citrate Hydrate. It contains not less than 99.0% of mosapride citrate ($C_{21}H_{25}ClFN_3O_3.C_6H_8O_7$) calculated on the anhydrous basis.]

Mouse anti-epoetin alfa monoclonal antibody A solution of the monoclonal antibody in phosphate-buffered sodium chloride TS, which is obtained from mouse immunized with a synthetic peptide having the amino acid sequence corresponding to N-terminal 20 residues of epoetin alfa (genetical recombination). When perform the Western blotting against Epoetin Alfa RS, it is reactable.

MTT TS Dissolve 8 g of sodium chloride, 0.2 g of potassium chloride, 1.15 g of anhydrous disodium hydrogen phosphate and 0.2 g of potassium dihydrogen phosphate in water to make 1000 mL, and sterilize in an autoclave for 15 minutes at 121°C to make the PBS(−) solution. Dissolve 0.3 g of 3-(4,5-dimethylthiazole-2-yl)-2,5-diphenyl-2*H*-tetrazolium bromide in this PBS(−) solution to make 100 mL. Sterilize by membrane filtration (pore size, 0.45 μm), and store in a cool place shielded from light.

Murexide $C_8H_8N_6O_6$ Red-purple powder. Practically insoluble in water, in ethanol (95) and in diethyl ether.

Purity Clarity of solution—Dissolve 10 mg of murexide in 100 mL of water: the solution is clear.

Residue on ignition <2.44>: not more than 0.1% (1 g).

Sensitivity—Dissolve 10 mg of murexide in 2 mL of ammonia-ammonium chloride buffer solution (pH 10.0), and add water to make 100 mL, and use this solution as the sample solution. Separately, add 2 mL of ammonia-ammonium chloride buffer solution (pH 10.0) to 5 mL of diluted Standard Calcium Solution (1 in 10), add water to make 25 mL, and render the solution to pH 11.3 with sodium hydroxide TS. Add 2 mL of the sample solution and water to this solution to make 50 mL: a red-purple color develops.

Murexide-sodium chloride indicator Prepared by mixing 0.1 g of murexide and 10 g of sodium chloride and grinding to get homogeneous.

Storage—Preserve in light-resistant containers.

Myoglobin A hemoprotein obtained from horse heart muscle. White crystalline powder. It contains not less than 95% of myoglobin in the total protein.

Myoinositol $C_6H_6(OH)_6$ White, crystals or crystalline powder.

Myristicin for thin-layer chromatography $C_{11}H_{12}O_3$ Colorless, clear liquid, having a characteristic odor. Miscible with ethanol (95), and practically insoluble in water.

Identification—Determine the infrared absorption spectrum of myristicin for thin-layer chromatography as directed in the liquid film method under Infrared Spectrophotometry <2.25>: it exhibits absorption at the wave numbers of about 3080 cm^{-1}, 2890 cm^{-1}, 1633 cm^{-1}, 1508 cm^{-1}, 1357 cm^{-1}, 1318 cm^{-1}, 1239 cm^{-1}, 1194 cm^{-1}, 1044 cm^{-1}, 994 cm^{-1}, 918 cm^{-1}, 828 cm^{-1} and 806 cm^{-1}.

Purity Related substances—Dissolve 20 mg of myristicin for thin-layer chromatography in 1 mL of ethanol (95), and use this solution as the sample solution. Pipet 0.5 mL of the sample solution, add ethanol (95) to make exactly 25 mL, and use this solution as the standard solution. Perform the test with 5 μL each of the sample solution and standard solution as directed in the Identification under Nutmeg: the spots other than the principle spot at the *R*f value of about 0.4 obtained from the sample solution are not more intense than the spot from the standard solution.

NADH peroxidase One unit indicates an amount of the enzyme which consumes 1 μmol of β-NADH in 1 minute at 25°C and pH 8.0 using β-nicotinamide adenine dinucleotide (β-NADH) and hydrogen peroxide as the substrate.

NADH peroxidase TS Suspend NADH peroxidase in ammonium sulfate TS so that each mL contains 10 units of the activity.

Storage—Between 0 and 8°C.

Naftopidil for assay $C_{24}H_{28}N_2O_3$ [Same as the monograph Naftopidil. When dried, it contains not less than 99.5% of naftopidil ($C_{24}H_{28}N_2O_3$).]

Nalidixic acid $C_{12}H_{12}N_2O_3$ [Same as the namesake monograph]

Namalwa cell Human cell line derived from B lymphoblasts, taken from patients with Burkitt's lymphoma.

Naphazoline hydrochloride $C_{14}H_{14}N_2.HCl$ [Same as the namesake monograph]

Naphazoline nitrate $C_{14}H_{14}N_2.HNO_3$ [Same as the namesake monograph]

Naphazoline nitrate for assay $C_{14}H_{14}N_2.HNO_3$ [Same as the monograph Naphazoline Nitrate. When dried, it contains not less than 99.0% of naphazoline nitrate ($C_{14}H_{14}N_2.NHO_3$).]

Naphthalene $C_{10}H_8$ Colorless flake-like or lustrous stick-like crystals, having a characteristic odor.

Melting point <2.60>: 78 – 82°C

1,3-Naphthalenediol $C_{10}H_8O_2$ Red-brown crystals or gray-brown powder. Freely soluble in water, in methanol and in ethanol (99.5). Melting point: about 124°C.

1,3-Naphthalenediol TS Dissolve 50 mg of 1,3-naphthalenediol in 25 mL of ethanol (99.5), and add 2.5 mL of phosphoric acid.

2-Naphthalenesulfonic acid See 2-naphthalenesulfonic acid monohydrate.

2-Naphthalenesulfonic acid monohydrate $C_{10}H_8O_3S.H_2O$ White to pale yellow-white powder. Very soluble in water, in methanol and in ethanol (95), and sparingly soluble in diethyl ether and in chloroform.

Water <2.48>: 7.0 – 11.5% (0.5 g, volumetric titration, direct titration).

Content: not less than 95.0%, calculated on the anhydrous basis. Assay—Weigh accurately about 0.5 g of 2-naphthalenesulfonic acid monohydrate, dissolve in 30 mL of water, and titrate <2.50> with 0.1 mol/L sodium hydroxide VS (indicator: 3 drops of bromothymol blue TS). Perform a blank determination in the same manner, and make any necessary correction.

Each mL of 0.1 mol/L sodim hydroxide VS
= 20.82 mg of $C_{10}H_8O_3S$

1-Naphthol $C_{10}H_7OH$ [K 8698, Special class] Preserve in light-resistant containers.

2-Naphthol $C_{10}H_7OH$ [K 8699, Special class] Preserve in light-resistant containers.

α-Naphthol See 1-naphthol.

β-Naphthol See 2-naphthol.

***p*-Naphtholbenzein** $C_{27}H_{18}O_2$ [K 8693, Special class]

α-Naphtholbenzein See *p*-naphtholbenzein.

***p*-Naphtholbenzein TS** Dissolve 0.2 g of *p*-naphtholbenzein in acetic acid (100) to make 100 mL.

Purity Clarity and color of solution—Dissolve 0.10 g of *p*-naphtholbenzein in 100 mL of ethanol (95): the solution is red in color and clear.

Sensitivity—Add 100 mL of freshly boiled and cooled water to 0.2 mL of a solution of *p*-naphtholbenzein in ethanol (95) (1 in 1000), and add 0.1 mL of 0.1 mol/L sodium hydroxide VS: a green color develops. Add subsequently 0.2 mL of 0.1 mol/L hydrochloric acid VS: the color of the solution changes to yellow-red.

α-Naphtholbenzein TS See *p*-naphtholbenzein TS.

1-Naphthol-sulfuric acid TS Dissolve 1.5 g of 1-naphthol in 50 mL of ethanol (95), add 3 mL of water and 7 mL of sulfuric acid, and mix well. Prepare before use.

1-Naphthol TS Dissolve 6 g of sodium hydroxide and 16 g of anhydrous sodium carbonate in water to make 100 mL. In this solution dissolve 1 g of 1-naphthol. Prepare before use.

2-Naphthol TS Dissolve 1 g of 2-naphthol in sodium carbonate TS to make 100 mL. Prepare before use.

α-Naphthol TS See 1-naphthol TS.

β-Naphthol TS See 2-naphthol TS.

Naphthoresorcin-phosphoric acid TS Dissolve 0.2 g of 1,3-dihydroxynaphthalene in ethanol (99.5) to make 100 mL. To this solution add 10 mL of phosphoric acid.

1-Naphthylamine $C_{10}H_7NH_2$ [K 8692, Special class] Preserve in light-resistant containers.

α-Naphthylamine See 1-naphthylamine.

***N*-(1-Naphthyl)-*N′*-diethylethylenediamine oxalate** See *N,N*-diethyl-*N′*-1-naphthylethylenediamine oxalate.

***N*-(1-Naphthyl)-*N′*-diethylethylenediamine oxalate-acetone TS** See *N,N*-diethyl-*N′*-1-naphthylethylenediamine oxalate-acetone TS.

***N*-(1-Naphthyl)-*N′*-diethylethylenediamine oxalate TS** See *N,N*-diethyl-*N′*-1-naphthylethylenediamine oxalate TS.

***N*-1-Naphthylethylenediamine dihydrochloride** $C_{10}H_7NHCH_2CH_2NH_2.2HCl$ [K 8197, Special class]

Naphthylethylenediamine TS Dissolve 0.1 g of *N*-1-naphthylethylenediamine dihydrochloride in water to make 100 mL. Prepare before use.

Naringin for thin-layer chromatography $C_{27}H_{32}O_{14}$ White to light yellow crystalline powder. Freely soluble in ethanol (95) and in acetone, and slightly soluble in water. Melting point: about 170°C (with decomposition).

Optical rotation <2.49> $[\alpha]_D^{20}$: −87 – −93° (0.1 g, ethanol (95), 10 mL, 100 mm).

Purity Related substances—Proceed with 10 μL of a solution, prepared by dissolving 10 mg of naringin for thin-layer chromatography in 10 mL of ethanol (95), as directed in the Identification under Bitter Orange Peel: any spot other than the principal spot with an *Rf* value of about 0.4 does not appear.

Neocarzinostatin $C_{511}H_{768}N_{132}O_{179}S_4$ A white or pale yellow-white powder.

Identification—Determine the absorption spectrum of a solution of the substance to be examined (1 in 3000) as directed under Ultraviolet-visible Spectrophotometry <2.24>: it exhibits a maximum between 270 nm and 275 nm, and shoulders between 288 nm and 292 nm and between 330 nm and 360 nm.

Purity—Dissolve 10 mg of the substance to be examined in the mobile phase to make 50 mL, and use this solution as the sample solution. Perform the test with 0.25 mL of the sample solution as directed under Liquid Chromatography <2.01>, determine each peak area by the automatic integration method, and calculate the amount of neocarzinostatin by the area percentage method: not less than 90.0%.

Operating conditions

Detector: An ultraviolet absorption photometer (wavelength: 254 nm).

Column: Pre-column is a stainless steel column 7.5 mm in inside diameter and 75 mm in length, packed with silica gel for liquid chromatography (10 μm in particle size). Separation column is a stainless steel column 7.5 mm in inside diameter and 60 cm in length, packed with silica gel for liquid chromatography (10 μm in particle size), which is coupled to the pre-column.

Column temperature: A constant temperature of about 25°C.

Mobile phase: Dissolve 3.78 g of potassium dihydrogen phosphate and 5.52 g of anhydrous disodium hydrogen phosphate in water to make 1000 mL.

Flow rate: Adjust so that the retention time of neocarzinostatin is about 21 minutes.

Time span of measurement: About 2 times as long as the retention time of neocarzinostatin.

System suitability

System performance: When the procedure is run with 0.25 mL of the sample solution under the above operating conditions, the number of theoretical plates and the symmetry factor of the peak of neocarzinostatin are not less than 2000 and not more than 2.5, respectively.

System repeatability: When the test is repeated 6 times with 0.25 mL of the sample solution under the above operating conditions, the relative standard deviation of the peak area of neocarzinostatin is not more than 2.0%.

Water <2.48> Not more than 10.0% (10 mg, coulometric titration).

Neocarzinostatin-styrene-maleic acid alternating copolymer partial butyl ester condensate (2:3) Condensate of neocarzinostatin and styrene-maleic acid alternating copolymer partial butyl ester in a rate of 2:3 by amide bond. Average molecular mass: about 28,400. A pale yellow powder.

Identification—Dissolve 4 mg of the substance to be examined in 0.05 mol/L phosphate buffer solution (pH 7.0) to make 10 mL. Determine the absorption spectrum of this solution as directed under Ultraviolet-visible Spectrophotometry <2.24>: it exhibits a maximum between 266 nm and 270 nm, and shoulders between 257 nm and 262 nm, between 286 nm and 291 nm and between 318 nm and 348 nm.

Absorbance <2.24> $E^{1\%}_{1\,cm}$ (268 nm): 13.0 – 17.5 [4 mg calculated on the anhydrous basis, 0.05 mol/L phosphate buffer solution (pH 7.0), 10 mL].

Purity (i) Test solutions

Solution A: Dissolve 36.6 g of 2-amino-2-hydroxymethyl-1,3-propanediol in 48 mL of 1 mol/L hydrochloric acid TS, 0.23 mL of *N,N,N′,N′*-tetramethylethylenediamine and water to make 100 mL.

Solution B: Dissolve 33.3 g of acrylamide and 0.89 g of *N,N′*-methylenebisacrylamide in water to make 100 mL. Preserve in a cold place, avoiding exposure to light.

Solution C: Dissolve 5.98 g of 2-amino-2-hydroxymethyl-1,3-propanediol in 48 mL of 1 mol/L hydrochloric acid TS, 0.46 mL of *N,N,N′,N′*-tetramethylethylenediamine and water to make 100 mL.

Solution D: Dissolve 10.0 g of acrylamide and 2.5 g of *N,N′*-methylenebisacrylamide in water to make 100 mL. Preserve in a cold place, avoiding exposure to light.

Solution E: Dissolve 4 mg of riboflavin in water to make 100 mL. Preserve in a cold place, avoiding exposure to light.

Solution F: Dissolve 3.0 g of 2-amino-2-hydroxymethyl-1,3-propanediol and 14.4 g of glycine in water to make 500 mL.

Buffer solution for sample: To 50 mL of Solution C add 20 mL of water and 10 mL of glycerin solution (3 in 5).

(ii) Gels

Resolving gel: Mix 2.5 mL of Solution A and 7.5 mL of Solution B. Mix the mixture with 10 mL of freshly prepared ammonium peroxodisulfate solution (7 in 5000) after degassing under reduced pressure. Pour this mixture into a glass tube, 5 mm in inside diameter and 10 cm in length, to make 7 cm height, put water gently on the upper surface of the mixture, and allow to polymerize for 60 minutes. After polymerization, remove the water from the upper surface of the gel.

Stacking gel: Mix 1 mL of Solution C, 2 mL of Solution D, 1 mL of Solution E and 4 mL of water, pour 0.2 mL of the mixture on the resolving gel, put water gently on the upper surface of the mixture, and allow to polymerize under a fluorescent light for 60 minutes. After polymerization, remove the water from the upper surface of the gel.

iii) Sample solution Dissolve 3.0 mg of the substance to be examined in the buffer solution for sample to make 10 mL.

(iv) Procedure Mount the gel in electrophoresis apparatus. Add a mixture of 200 mL of Solution F and 2 mL of bromophenol blue solution (1 in 100,000) to the upper reservoir (cathode) and 300 mL of Solution F to the lower reservoir (anode). Introduce carefully exactly 100 μL of the sample solution onto the surface of the gel, and allow electrophoresis at room temperature to take place with a current of 2 mA per tube as a bromophenol blue band is passing in the stacking gel and then increase the current to 4 mA per tube as the bromophenol blue band is passing in the resolving gel, and stop the current when the band reached 5 cm from the upper end of the gel.

(v) Staining and decolorization Dissolve 0.1 g of Coomassie brilliant blue G-250 in 100 mL of trichloroacetic acid solution (1 in 2), and mix 1 volume of this solution and 2 volumes of water before using. Immerse the gels for 15 hours in this mixture, and transfer into about 20 mL of acetic acid (100) solution (7 in 100) to remove the excess of dye. Replace the acetic acid (100) solution (7 in 100) until the back ground of the gel becomes colorless.

(vi) Determination Determine the peak area, A_T, of neocarzinostatin-styrene-maleic acid alternating copolymer partial butyl ester condensate (2:3) and the total area, A, of the peaks other than neocarzinostatin-styrene-maleic acid alternating copolymer partial butyl ester condensate (2:3), based on the absorbance at 600 nm of the gel determined by using a densitometer. Calculate the amount of neocarzinostatin-styrene-maleic acid alternating copolymer partial butyl ester condensate (2:3) by the following formula: not less than 90.0%.

Amount (%) of neocarzinostatin-styrene-maleic acid alternating copolymer partial butyl ester condensate (2:3)
$= A_T/(A_T + A) \times 100$

Water <2.48> Not more than 12.0% (10 mg, coulometric titration).

Neutral alumina containing 4% of water Take 50 g of neutral alumina for column chromatography, previously dried at 105°C for 2 hours, in a tight container, add 2.0 mL of water, shake well to make homogeneous, and allow to stand for more than 2 hours.

Neutral detergent Synthetic detergent containing anionic or non-ionic surfactant, and pH of its 0.25% solution is between 6.0 and 8.0. Dilute to a suitable concentration before use.

Neutralized ethanol See ethanol, neutralized.

Neutral red $C_{15}H_{17}N_4Cl$ Slightly metallic, dark green powder or masses.

Identification—Determine the infrared absorption spectrum as directed in the potassium bromide disk method under Infrared Spectrophotometry <2.25>: it exhibits absorption at the wave numbers of about 3310 cm^{-1}, 3160 cm^{-1}, 1621 cm^{-1}, 1503 cm^{-1}, 1323 cm^{-1}, 1199 cm^{-1} and 732 cm^{-1}.

Neutral red TS Dissolve 0.1 g of neutral red in acetic acid (100) to make 100 mL.

Neutral red-Eagle's minimum essential medium containing bovine serum To Eagle's minimum essential medium containing bovine serum, which contains *N*-2-hydroxyethylpiperazine-*N*′-2-ethanesulfonic acid but not sodium hydrogen carbonate, add a solution of neutral red (1 in 100), and adjust to pH 6.7 – 6.8 with sodium hydroxide TS.

NFS-60 cell Prepared from leukemia mouse, infected with retrovirus (Cas-Br-M). After conditioning with a suitable medium, preserve the strain established by J. N. Ihle, *et al.* (*Proc. Natl. Acad. Sci. USA*, 1985, 82, 6687) at not exceeding −150°C in conveniently sized packets.

Nicardipine hydrochloride for assay $C_{26}H_{29}N_3O_6.HCl$ [Same as the monograph Nicardipine Hydrochloride. When dried, it contains not less than 99.0% of nicardipine hydrochloride ($C_{26}H_{29}N_3O_6.HCl$).]

Nicergoline for assay $C_{24}H_{26}BrN_3O_3$ [Same as the monograph Nicergoline, or Nicergoline purified according to the method below. When dried, it contains not less than 99.0% of nicergoline ($C_{24}H_{26}BrN_3O_3$), and when perform the test of the Purity (2) under Nicergoline, the total area of the peaks other than nicergoline obtained from the sample solution is not more than 2.5 times the peak area of nicergoline from the standard solution.

Method of purification: Dissolve 1 g of Nicergoline in 20 mL of acetonitrile, allow to stand in a dark place for about 36 hours, filter, and dry the crystals so obtained at 60°C for 2 hours in vacuum.]

Nickel (II) sulfate hexahydrate $NiSO_4.6H_2O$ [K 8989, Special class]

Nicomol for assay $C_{34}H_{32}N_4O_9$ [Same as the monograph Nicomol. When dried, it contains not less than 99.0% of nicomol ($C_{34}H_{32}N_4O_9$).]

Nicotinamide $C_6H_6N_2O$ [Same as the namesake monograph]

***β*-Nicotinamide-adenine dinucleotide (*β*-NAD)** $C_{21}H_{27}N_7O_{14}P_2$ [K 9802 *β*-NAD$^+$, and meets the following requirement.]

Content: not less than 94.5%. Assay—Weigh accurately about 25 mg of *β*-nicotinamide-adenine dinucleotide, and dissolve in water to make exactly 25 mL. Pipet 0.2 mL of this solution, add 0.1 mol/L phosphate buffer solution (pH 7.0) to make exactly 10 mL, and use this solution as the sample solution. Determine the absorbances, A_T and A_B, of the sample solution and 0.1 mol/L phosphate buffer solution (pH 7.0) at 260 nm as directed under Ultraviolet-visible Spectrophotometry <2.24>, using water as the blank.

Amount (mg) of *β*-nicotinamide-adenine dinucleotide ($C_{21}H_{27}N_7O_{14}P_2$)

$$= \frac{0.6634 \times 10}{17.6 \times 0.20} \times (A_T - A_B) \times 25$$

β-Nicotinamide adenine dinucleotide TS Dissolve 40 mg of β-nicotinamide adenine dinucleotide (β-NAD) in 10 mL of water. Prepare before use.

β-Nicotinamide adenine dinucleotide reduced form (β-NADH) $C_{21}H_{27}N_7O_{14}P_2.Na_2$ A white to light yellow-white powder.

Absorbance ratio: Determine the absorbances at 260 nm and at 340 nm, A_{260} and A_{340}, of a solution of β-nicotinamide adenine dinucleotide reduced form (β-NADH) in diluted phosphate buffer solution (pH 7.4) (1 in 50,000) as directed under Ultraviolet-visible Spectrophotometry <*2.24*>: the result of A_{260}/A_{340} is between 2.2 and 2.4.

Water <*2.48*>: not more than 8.0% (0.3 g, volumetric titration, direct titration).

β-Nicotinamide adenine dinucleotide reduced form TS Dissolve 0.4 mg of β-nicotinamide adenine dinucleotide reduced form (β-NADH) in 1 mL of 0.6 mol/L 2,2′,2″-nitrilotriethanol hydrochloride buffer solution (pH 8.0). Prepare before use.

Nicotinic acid $C_6H_5NO_2$ White, crystals or crystalline powder.

Identification—Determine the infrared absorption spectrum of nicotinic acid as directed in the potassium bromide disk method under Infrared Spectrophotometry <*2.25*>: it exhibits absorption at the wave numbers of about 2440 cm^{-1}, 1707 cm^{-1}, 1418 cm^{-1}, 811 cm^{-1}, 747 cm^{-1} and 641 cm^{-1}.

Nifedipine $C_{17}H_{18}N_2O_6$ [Same as the namesake monograph]

Nifedipine for assay $C_{17}H_{18}N_2O_6$ [Same as the monograph Nifedipine. When dried, it contains not less than 99.0% of nifedipine ($C_{17}H_{18}N_2O_6$) and meets the following requirement.]

Purity Related substances—Conduct this procedure without exposure to light, using light-resistant vessels. Dissolve 25 mg of nifedipine for assay in 25 mL of the mobile phase, and use this solution as the sample solution. Pipet 1 mL of the sample solution, add the mobile phase to make exactly 10 mL. Pipet 2 mL of this solution, add the mobile phase to make exactly 25 mL, and use this solution as the standard solution. Perform the test with exactly 10 μL each of the sample solution and standard solution as directed under Liquid Chromatography <*2.01*> according to the following conditions, and determine the peak area by the automatic integration method: the total area of the peaks other than nifedipine obtained from the sample solution is not larger than the peak area of nifedipine from the standard solution.

Operating conditions

Detector: An ultraviolet absorption photometer (wavelength: 230 nm).

Column: A stainless steel column 4.6 mm in inside diameter and 15 cm in length, packed with octadecylsilanized silica gel for liquid chromatography (5 μm in particle diameter).

Column temperature: A constant temperature of about 40°C.

Mobile phase: Adjust to pH 6.1 of a mixture of methanol and diluted 0.05 mol/L disodium hydrogen phosphate TS (1 in 5) (11:9) with phosphoric acid.

Flow rate: Adjust so that the retention time of nifedipine is about 6 minutes.

Time span of measurement: About 2 times as long as the retention time of nifedipine, beginning after the solvent peak.

System suitability

Test for required detectability: To exactly 5 mL of the standard solution add the mobile phase to make exactly 20 mL. Confirm that the peak area of nifedipine obtained with 10 μL of this solution is equivalent to 18 to 32% of that with 10 μL of the standard solution.

System performance: When the procedure is run with 10 μL of the standard solution under the above operating conditions, the number of theoretical plates and the symmetry factor of the peak of nifedipine are not less than 4000 and not more than 1.2, respectively.

System repeatability: When the test is repeated 6 times with 10 μL of the standard solution under the above operating conditions, the relative standard deviation of the peak area of nifedipine is not more than 2.0%.

Nile blue $C_{20}H_{20}ClN_3O$ Blue-green powder.

Ninhydrin $C_9H_6O_4$ [K 8870, Special class]

Ninhydrin TS Dissolve 0.2 g of ninhydrin in water to make 10 mL. Prepare before use.

Ninhydrin-acetic acid TS Dissolve 1.0 g of ninhydrin in 50 mL of ethanol (95), and add 10 mL of acetic acid (100).

Ninhydrin-L-ascorbic acid TS Dissolve 0.25 g of ninhydrin and 10 mg of L-ascorbic acid in water to make 50 mL. Prepare before use.

Ninhydrin-butanol TS Dissolve 0.3 g of ninhydrin in 100 mL of 1-butanol, and add 3 mL of acetic acid (100).

Ninhydrin-citric acid-acetic acid TS Dissolve 70 g of citric acid monohydrate in 500 mL of water, add 58 mL of acetic acid (100), 70 mL of a solution of sodium hydroxide (21 in 50) and water to make 1000 mL. In 100 mL of this solution dissolve 0.2 g of ninhydrin.

Ninhydrin-ethanol TS for spraying Dissolve 1 g of ninhydrin in 50 mL of ethanol (95).

Ninhydrin-stannous chloride TS See ninhydrin-tin (II) chloride TS.

Ninhydrin-sulfuric acid TS Dissolve 0.1 g of ninhydrin in 100 mL of sulfuric acid. Prepare before use.

Ninhydrin-tin (II) chloride TS Dissolve 21.0 g of citric acid monohydrate in water to make 200 mL, adjust the pH to 5.6 ± 0.2 with sodium hydroxide TS, add water to make 500 mL, and dissolve 1.3 g of tin (II) chloride dihydrate. To 50 mL of the solution, add 50 mL of a 2-methoxyethanol solution of ninhydrin (1 in 25). Prepare before use.

0.2% Ninhydrin-water saturated 1-butanol TS Dissolve 2 g of ninhydrin in 1-butanol saturated with water to make 1000 mL.

Nitrendipine for assay $C_{18}H_{20}N_2O_6$ [Same as the monograph Nitrendipine. It, when dried, contains not less than 99.0% of nitrendipine ($C_{18}H_{20}N_2O_6$), and meets the following requirement. When perform the test as directed in the Purity (2) under Nitrendipine, the area of the peak of dimethyl ester, having the relative retention time of about 0.8 to nitrendipine obtained from the sample solution is not larger than 1/2 times the peak area of nitrendipine from the standard solution, the area of the peak other than nitrendipine and the dimethyl ester is not larger than 1/5 times the peak area of nitrendipine from the standard solution, and the total area of the peak other than nitrendipine is not larger than 1/2 times the peak area of nitrendipine from the standard solution.]

Nitric acid HNO_3 [K 8541, Special class, Concentration: 69 – 70%, Density: about 1.42 g/mL]

Nitric acid, dilute Dilute 10.5 mL of nitric acid with water to make 100 mL.

Nitric acid, fuming [K 8739, Special class, Concentration: not less than 97%, Density: about 1.52 g/mL]

Nitric acid TS, 2 mol/L Dilute 12.9 mL of nitric acid with water to make 100 mL.

Nitrilotriacetic acid $C_6H_9NO_6$ A white crystalline powder. Melting point: about 240°C (with decomposition).

Identification—Determine the infrared absorption spectrum of nitrilotriacetic acid as directed in the paste method under Infrared Spectrophotometry <*2.25*>: it exhibits absorption at the wave numbers of about 1718 cm^{-1}, 1243 cm^{-1}, 1205 cm^{-1}, 968 cm^{-1}, 903 cm^{-1}, 746 cm^{-1} and 484 cm^{-1}.

Loss on drying <*2.41*>: not more than 0.5% (1 g, 105°C, 3 hours).

Content: not less than 97.0%. Assay—Weigh accurately about 0.2 g of nitrilotriacetic acid, dissolve in 50 mL of water by heating, and titrate <*2.50*> after cooling with 0.1 mol/L sodium hydroxide VS (potentiometric titration). Perform a blank determination in the same manner, and make any necessary correction.

Each mL of 0.1 mol/L sodium hydroxide VS
= 9.557 mg of $C_6H_9NO_6$

2,2′,2″-Nitrilotriethanol $(CH_2CH_2OH)_3N$ [K 8663, Special class]

2,2′,2″-Nitrilotriethanol buffer solution (pH 7.8) Dissolve 149.2 g of 2,2′,2″-nitrilotriethanol in about 4500 mL of water, adjust to pH 7.8 with diluted 6 mol/L hydrochloric acid TS (2 in 3), and add water to make 5000 mL.

2,2′,2″-Nitrilotriethanol hydrochloride $(CH_2CH_2OH)_3N.HCl$ White, crystals or powder.

Purity Clarity of solution—A solution (1 in 20) is clear.

Content: not less than 98%. Assay—Dissolve 0.3 g of 2,2′,2″-nitrilotriethanol hydrochloride, accurately weighed, in 50 mL of water, add 5 mL of diluted nitric acid (1 in 3), and titrate <*2.50*> with 0.1 mol/L silver nitrate VS (potentiometric titration).

Each mL of 0.1 mol/L silver nitrate VS
= 18.57 mg of $(CH_2CH_2OH)_3N.HCl$

0.6 mol/L 2,2′,2″-Nitrilotriethanol hydrochloride buffer solution (pH 8.0) Dissolve 5.57 g of 2,2′,2″-nitrilotriethanol hydrochloride in 40 mL of water, adjust to pH 8.0 with 5 mol/L sodium hydroxide TS, and add water to make 50 mL.

3-Nitroaniline $C_6H_6N_2O_2$ Yellow, crystals or crystalline powder.

Melting point <*2.60*>: 112 – 116°C

4-Nitroaniline $C_6H_4NO_2NH_2$ Yellow to yellowish-red, crystals or crystalline powder.

Melting point <*2.60*>: 147 – 150°C.

Storage—Preserve in a light-resistant tight container.

***p*-Nitroaniline** See 4-nitroaniline.

***p*-Nitroaniline-sodium nitrite TS** See 4-nitroaniline-sodium nitrite TS.

4-Nitroaniline-sodium nitrite TS To 90 mL of a solution of 0.3 g of 4-nitroaniline in 100 mL of 10 mol/L hydrochloric acid TS add 10 mL of a solution of sodium nitrite (1 in 20), and mix well. Prepare before use.

***o*-Nitrobenzaldehyde** See 2-nitrobenzaldehyde.

2-Nitrobenzaldehyde $O_2NC_6H_4CHO$ Pale yellow, crystals or crystalline powder.

Melting point <*2.60*>: 42 – 44°C

Nitrobenzene $C_6H_5NO_2$ [K 8723, Special class]

***p*-Nitrobenzenediazonium chloride TS** See 4-nitrobenzenediazonium chloride TS.

4-Nitrobenzenediazonium chloride TS Dissolve 1.1 g of 4-nitroaniline in 1.5 mL of hydrochloric acid, add 1.5 mL of water, and then add a solution prepared by dissolving 0.5 g of sodium nitrite in 5 mL of water, while cooling in an ice bath. Prepare before use.

***p*-Nitrobenzenediazonium chloride TS for spraying** See 4-nitrobenzenediazonium chloride TS for spraying.

4-Nitrobenzenediazonium chloride TS for spraying Dissolve 0.4 g of 4-nitroaniline in 60 mL of 1 mol/L hydrochloric acid TS, and add, while cooling in an ice bath, sodium nitrite TS until the mixture turns potassium iodide-starch paper to blue in color. Prepare before use.

***p*-Nitrobenzenediazonium fluoroborate** See 4-nitrobenzenediazonium fluoroborate.

4-Nitrobenzenediazonium fluoroborate $O_2NC_6H_4N_2BF_4$ Light yellow-white, almost odorless powder. Freely soluble in dilute hydrochloric acid, slightly soluble in water, and very slightly solute in ethanol (95) and in chloroform. Melting point: about 148°C (with decomposition).

Identification—Add 1 mL each of a solution of phenol (1 in 1000) and sodium hydroxide TS to 10 mL of a solution of 4-nitrobenzenediazonium fluoroborate (1 in 1000): a red color develops.

Loss on drying <*2.41*>: not more than 1.0% (1 g, silica gel, 2 hours).

***p*-Nitrobenzoyl chloride** See 4-nitrobenzoyl chloride.

4-Nitrobenzoyl chloride $O_2NC_6H_4COCl$ Light yellow crystals.

Melting point <*2.60*>: 70 – 74°C

Content: not less than 98.0%. Assay—Weigh accurately about 0.5 g of 4-nitrobenzoyl chloride, add an excess of silver nitrate-ethanol TS, and boil under a reflux condenser for 1 hour. After cooling, filter the precipitate, wash with water, dry at 105°C to constant mass, and weigh. The mass of 4-nitrobenzoyl chloride, multiplied by 1.107, represents the mass of 4-nitrobenzoyl chloride ($C_7H_4ClNO_3$).

***p*-Nitrobenzyl chloride** See 4-nitrobenzyl chloride.

4-Nitrobenzyl chloride $O_2NC_6H_4CH_2Cl$ Light yellow, crystals or crystalline powder. Soluble in ethanol (95).

Melting point <*2.60*>: 71 – 73°C

Content: not less than 98.0%. Assay—Weigh accurately about 0.5 g of 4-nitrobenzyl chloride, add 15 mL of a solution prepared by dissolving 4 g of silver nitrate in 10 mL of water and adding ethanol (95) to make 100 mL, and heat on a water bath under a reflux condenser for 1 hour. After cooling, filter the precipitate with a glass filter, wash with water, dry at 105°C to constant mass, and weigh. The mass of the precipitate represents the amount of silver chloride (AgCl: 143.32).

Amount (mg) of 4-nitrobenzyl chloride ($C_7H_6ClNO_2$)
= amount (mg) of silver chloride (AgCl) × 1.1972

4-(4-Nitrobenzyl)pyridine $C_{12}H_{10}N_2O_2$ Pale yellow, crystalline powder. Freely soluble in acetone, and soluble in ethanol (95).

Melting point <*2.60*>: 69 – 71°C

Nitroethane $C_2H_5NO_2$

Density <*2.56*>: 1.048 – 1.053 g/cm³ (20°C)

Water <*2.48*>: not more than 0.1%.

Nitrogen N_2 [Same as the namesake monograph]

Nitrogen monoxide NO A colorless gas. Prepare by adding sodium nitrite TS to a solution of iron (II) sulfate heptahydrate in dilute sulfuric acid. Nitrogen monoxide from a metal cylinder may be used.

Nitromethane CH_3NO_2 [K 9523, Special class]

2-Nitrophenol $C_6H_5NO_3$ A yellow crystalline powder.

Melting points <*2.60*>: 44.5 – 49.0°C

3-Nitrophenol $C_6H_5NO_3$ A light yellow crystalline powder.

Melting point <*2.60*>: 96 – 99°C

4-Nitrophenol $C_6H_5NO_3$ [K 8721, *p*-nitrophenol, Special class]

***o*-Nitrophenyl-*β*-D-galactopyranoside** See 2-nitrophenyl-*β*-D-galactopyranoside.

2-Nitrophenyl-*β*-D-galactopyranoside $C_{12}H_{15}NO_8$ White crystalline powder. Odorless. It is sparingly soluble in water, slightly soluble in ethanol (95), and practically insoluble in diethyl ether.

Melting point <*2.60*>: 193 – 194°C

Purity Clarity and color of solution—A solution of 2-nitrophenyl-*β*-D-galactopyranoside (1 in 100) is clear and colorless.

Loss on drying <*2.41*>: not more than 0.1% (0.5 g, 105°C, 2 hours).

Content: not less than 98.0%. Assay—Weigh accurately about 50 mg of 2-nitrophenyl-*β*-D-galactopyranoside, previously dried, dissolve in water to make exactly 100 mL. Pipet 20 mL of this solution, and add water to make exactly 50 mL. Determine the absorbance, A, of this solution at 262 nm as directed under Ultraviolet-visible Spectrophotometry <*2.24*>.

Amount (mg) of 2-nitrophenyl-*β*-D-galactopyranoside

$$= \frac{A}{133} \times 25{,}000$$

1-Nitroso-2-naphthol $C_{10}H_7NO_2$ A yellow-brawn to red-brown crystalline powder.

Melting point <*2.60*>: 106 – 110°C

Storage—Preserve in a light-resistant tight container.

1-Nitroso-2-naphthol TS Dissolve 60 mg of 1-nitroso-2-naphthol in 80 mL of acetic acid (100), and add water to make 100 mL.

***α*-Nitroso-*β*-naphthol** See 1-nitroso-2-naphthol.

***α*-Nitroso-*β*-naphthol TS** See 1-nitroso-2-naphthol TS.

Nitrous oxide N_2O Colorless and odorless gas. Use nitrous oxide from a metal cylinder.

NK-7 cells Cells derived from mouse NK cells.

NN Indicator Mix 0.5 g of 2-hydroxy-1-(2-hydroxy-4-sulfo-1-naphthylazo)-3-naphthoic acid with 50 g of anhydrous sodium sulfate, and triturate until the mixture becomes homogeneous.

Nodakenin for thin-layer chromatography $C_{20}H_{24}O_9$ White powder. Slightly soluble in water and in methanol, and very slightly soluble in ethanol (99.5). Melting point: about 220°C (with decomposition).

Identification—Determine the absorption spectrum of a solution of nodakenin for thin-layer chromatography in methanol (1 in 100,000) as directed under Ultraviolet-visible Spectrophotometry <*2.24*>: it exhibits a maximum between 333 nm and 337 nm.

Optical rotation <*2.49*> $[\alpha]_D^{20}$: +50 – +68° (5 mg, methanol, 10 mL, 100 mm).

Purity Related substances—Dissolve 1 mg of nodakenin for thin-layer chromatography in 3 mL of methanol, and use this solution as the sample solution. Pipet 1 mL of the sample solution, add methanol to make exactly 100 mL, and use this solution as the standard solution. Proceed with 5 μL each of these solutions as directed in the Identification (2) under Peucedanum Root: the spot other than the principal spot of around *Rf* value of 0.3 obtained from the sample solution is not more intense than the spot from the standard solution.

Nonessential amino acid TS Dissolve 89 mg of L-alanine, 150 mg of L-asparagine monohydrate, 133 mg of L-aspartic acid, 147 mg of L-glutamic acid, 75 mg of glycine, 115 mg of L-proline and 105 mg of L-serine in 100 mL of water, and sterilize by filtration through a membrane filter with a pore size not exceeding 0.22 μm.

Nonylphenoxypoly(ethyleneoxy)ethanol for gas chromatography Prepared for gas chromatography.

L-Norleucine $C_6H_{13}NO_2$ White, crystals or powder. Dissolves in water.

Normal agar media for teceleukin Dissolve 5.0 g of meat extract, 10.0 g of peptone, 5.0 g of sodium chloride, and 15.0 to 20.0 g of agar in water to make 1000 mL, and sterilize. Adjust the pH to 6.9 to 7.1.

Nortriptyline hydrochloride $C_{19}H_{21}N.HCl$ [Same as the namesake monograph]

Nortriptyline hydrochloride for assay $C_{19}H_{21}N.HCl$ [Same as the monograph Nortriptyline Hydrochloride. When dried, it contains not less than 99.0% of nortriptyline hydrochloride ($C_{19}H_{21}N.HCl$).]

Nuclease-free water See water, nuclease-free.

***n*-Octadecane** $C_{18}H_{38}$ Colorless or white solid at ordinary temperature.

Purity Clarity of solution—A solution of *n*-octadecane in chloroform (1 in 25) is clear.

Octadecylsilanized silica gel for pretreatment Prepared for pretreatment.

***n*-Octane** C_8H_{18}

Specific gravity <*2.56*> d_4^{20}: 0.700 – 0.705

Purity—Perform the test with 2 μL of *n*-octane as directed under Gas Chromatography <*2.02*> according to the operating conditions in the Assay under Hypromellose. Determine each peak area by the automatic integration method, and calculate the amount of *n*-octane by the area percentage method: not less than 99.0%.

Octane, iso A colorless liquid. Practically insoluble in water. Miscible with diethyl ether and with chloroform.

Purity—Determine the absorbances of isooctane at 230 nm, 250 nm and 280 nm as directed under Ultraviolet-visible Spectrophotometry <*2.24*>, using water as the blank solution:

these values are not more than 0.050, 0.010 and 0.005, respectively.

1-Octanol $CH_3(CH_2)_6CH_2OH$ [K 8213, Special class]

Octyl alcohol See 1-octanol.

***n*-Octylbenzene** $C_{14}H_{22}$ Clear and colorless liquid, having a characteristic odor.
Specific gravity <2.56> d_4^{20}: 0.854 – 0.863
Distillation test <2.57>: 263 – 265°C, not less than 95 vol%.

Ofloxacin $C_{18}H_{20}FN_3O_4$ [Same as the namesake monograph]

Ofloxacin demethyl substance (±)-9-Fluoro-2,3-dihydro-3-methyl-7-oxo-7*H*-10-(1-piperazinyl)-pyrido[1,2,3-*de*] [1,4] benzoxazine-6-carboxylic acid $C_{17}H_{18}FN_3O_4$ White to light green-yellow-white, crystals or crystalline powder.
Identification—Determine the infrared absorption spectrum of ofloxacin demethyl substance as directed in the potassium bromide disk method under Infrared Spectrophotometry <2.25>: it exhibits absorption at the wave numbers of about 3050 cm^{-1}, 2840 cm^{-1}, 1619 cm^{-1}, 1581 cm^{-1}, 1466 cm^{-1}, 1267 cm^{-1}, 1090 cm^{-1}, 1051 cm^{-1} and 816 cm^{-1}.

Oleic acid $C_{18}H_{34}O_2$ Occurs as a colorless or pale yellow transparent liquid and has a slightly distinct odor. It is miscible with ethanol (95) and with diethyl ether, and practically insoluble in water.
Specific gravity <2.56> d_{20}^{20}: about 0.9.
Content: not less than 99.0%. Assay—To 40 μL of oleic acid add 1 mL of a solution of boron trifluoride in methanol (3 in 20), mix, and heat on a water bath for 3 minutes. After cooling, add 10 mL of petroleum ether and 10 mL of water, shake, collect the ether layer after allowing to stand, and use this solution as the sample solution. Perform the test with 0.2 μL of the sample solution as directed under Gas Chromatography <2.02> according to the following conditions, determine each peak area by the automatic integration method, and calculate the amount of methyl oleate by the area percentage method.
Operating conditions
Detector: A hydrogen flame-ionization detector
Column: A glass column 3 mm in inside diameter and 2 m in length, packed with siliceous earth for gas chromatography (149 – 177 μm) coated with methyl polyacrylate in a rate of 5 – 10%.
Column temperature: A constant temperature of about 220°C.
Carrier gas: Helium.
Flow rate: Adjust so that the retention time of methyl oleate is about 10 minutes.
Time span of measurement: About 2 times as long as the retention time of methyl oleate, beginning after the solvent peak.

Olive oil [Same as the namesake monograph]

Olopatadine hydrochloride for assay $C_{21}H_{23}NO_3.HCl$ [Same as the monograph Olopatadine Hydrochloride. When dried, it contains not less than 99.5% of olopatadine hydrochloride ($C_{21}H_{23}NO_3.HCl$).]

Omeprazole for assay $C_{17}H_{19}N_3O_3S$ [Same as the monograph Omeprazole]

Ophiopogon root [Same as the namesake monograph]

Orcine $C_7H_3O_2$ White to light red-brown, crystals or crystalline powder, having an unpleasant sweet taste. It turns to red in color when oxidized in air. Soluble in water, in ethanol (95), and in diethyl ether.
Meting point <2.60>: 107 – 111°C

Orcine-ferric chloride TS See orcine-iron (III) chloride TS.

Orcine-iron (III) chloride TS Dissolve 10 mg of orcine in 1 mL of a solution of iron (III) chloride hexahydrate in hydrochloric acid (1 in 1000). Prepare before use.

Ordinary agar medium Dissolve 25 to 30 g of agar in 1000 mL of ordinary broth with the aid of heat, add water to make up for the loss, adjust the pH to between 6.4 and 7.0, and filter. Dispense the filtrate, and sterilize by autoclaving. When powdered agar is used, 15 to 20 g of it is dissolved.

Ordinary broth Dissolve 5 g of beef extract and 10 g of peptone in 1000 mL of water by gentle heating. Adjust the pH of the mixture between 6.4 and 7.0 after sterilization, cool, add water to make up for the loss, and filter. Sterilize the filtrate by autoclaving for 30 minutes at 121°C.

Osthole for thin-layer chromatography $C_{15}H_{16}O_3$ A white crystalline powder, having no odor. Freely soluble in methanol and in ethyl acetate, soluble in ethanol (99.5), and practically insoluble in water. Melting point: 83 – 84°C.
Purity Related substances—Dissolve 1.0 mg of osthole for thin-layer chromatography in 1 mL of methanol. Perform the test with 10 μL of this solution as directed in the Identification under Cnidium Monnieri Fruit: on spot appears other than the principal spot at around *Rf* value of 0.3.

Oxalate pH standard solution See pH Determination <2.54>.

Oxalic acid See oxalic acid dihydrate.

Oxalic acid dihydrate $H_2C_2O_4.2H_2O$ [K 8519, Special class]

Oxalic acid TS Dissolve 6.3 g of oxalic acid dihydrate in water to make 100 mL (0.5 mol/L).

Oxycodone hydrochloride for assay See oxycodone hydrochloride hydrate for assay.

Oxycodone hydrochloride hydrate for assay $C_{18}H_{21}NO_4.HCl.3H_2O$ [Same as the monograph Oxycodone Hydrochloride Hydrate. It contains not less than 99.0% of oxycodone hydrochloride ($C_{18}H_{21}NO_4.HCl$), calculated on the anhydrous basis.]

Oxygen O_2 [K 1101]

Oxygen reference gas for assay Containing not less than 99.99 vol% of oxygen in a sealed pressure-resistant container.

Oxygen span gas for assay Containing not less than 99.7 vol% of oxygen in a sealed pressure-resistant container.

Oxygen zero gas for assay Containing not less than 99.99 vol% of nitrogen or argon in a sealed pressure-resistant container. Or, containing oxygen of 98 to 99 vol% of a minimum scale within the measuring range, and nitrogen or argon is employed as a diluent gas.

2-Oxy-1-(2′-oxy-4′-sulfo-1′-naphthylazo)-3-naphthoic acid See 2-hydroxy-1-(2-hydroxy-4-sulfo-1-naphthylazo)-3-naphthoic acid.

8-Oxyquinoline See 8-quinolinol.

Oxytocin $C_{43}H_{66}N_{12}O_{12}S_2$ [Same as the namesake

monograph]

Paeoniflorin for thin-layer chromatography $C_{23}H_{28}O_{11}$ A white powder. Freely soluble in water, in methanol and in ethanol (99.5).

Identification Determine the infrared absorption spectrum of paeoniflorin to be examined as directed in the potassium bromide disk method under Infrared Spectrophotometry <2.25>: it exhibits absorption at the wave numbers of about 3410 cm^{-1}, 1711 cm^{-1}, 1279 cm^{-1}, 823 cm^{-1} and 714 cm^{-1}.

Purity Related substances—Dissolve 1 mg of paeoniflorin to be examined in exactly 1 mL of methanol. Perform the test with 20 μL of this solution as directed in the Identification (2) under Peony Root: any spot other than the principal spot with an *Rf* value of about 0.3 does not appear.

Paeonol for assay $C_9H_{10}O_3$ Use paeonol for thin-layer chromatography meeting the following additional specifications. Correct the content based on the amount (%) obtained in the Assay.

Unity of peak—Dissolve 5 mg of paeonol for assay in 50 mL of the mobile phase. To 1 mL of this solution add the mobile phase to make 50 mL, and use this solution as the sample solution. Perform the test with 10 μL of the sample solution as directed under Liquid Chromatography <2.01> according to the following conditions, and compare the absorption spectra of at least 3 points including the top of paeonol peak and around the two middle peak heights of before and after the top: no difference in form is observed between their spectra.

Operating conditions

Column, column temperature, mobile phase, and flow rate: Proceed as directed in the operating conditions in the Assay under Moutan Bark.

Detector: A photodiode array detector (wavelength: 274 nm, spectrum range of measurement: 220 – 400 nm).

System suitability

System performance: Proceed as directed in the system suitability in the Assay under Moutan Bark.

Assay—Weigh accurately 5 mg of paeonol for assay and 1 mg of 1,4-BTMSB-d_4 for nuclear magnetic resonance spectroscopy using an ultramicrobalance, dissolve in 1 mL of deuterated methanol for nuclear magnetic resonance spectroscopy, and use this solution as the sample solution. Transfer the sample solution into an NMR tube 5 mm in outer diameter, measure ^{1}H-NMR as directed under Nuclear Magnetic Resonance Spectroscopy <2.21> and Crude Drugs Test <5.01> according to the following conditions, using 1,4-BTMSB-d_4 for nuclear magnetic resonance spectroscopy as the reference standard for qNMR. Calculate the resonance intensities, A_1 (equivalent to 2 hydrogen) and A_2 (equivalent to 1 hydrogen), of the signals around δ 6.17 – 6.25 ppm and δ 7.54 ppm assuming the signal of the reference standard for qNMR as δ 0 ppm.

$$\text{Amount (\%) of paeonol } (C_9H_{10}O_3) = M_S \times I \times P/(M \times N) \times 0.7336$$

M: Amount (mg) of paeonol for assay taken

M_S: Amount (mg) of 1,4-BTMSB-d_4 for nuclear magnetic resonance spectroscopy taken

I: Sum of the signal resonance intensities, A_1 and A_2, based on the signal resonance intensity of 1,4-BTMSB-d_4 for nuclear magnetic resonance spectroscopy as 18.000

N: Sum of numbers of the hydrogen derived from A_1 and A_2

P: Purity (%) of 1,4-BTMSB-d_4 for nuclear magnetic resonance spectroscopy

Operating conditions

Apparatus: An apparatus of nuclear magnetic resonance spectrum measurement having ^{1}H resonance frequency of not less than 400 MHz.

Target nucleus: ^{1}H.

Digital resolution: 0.25 Hz or lower.

Measuring spectrum range: 20 ppm or upper, including between −5 ppm and 15 ppm.

Spinning: off.

Pulse angle: 90°.

^{13}C decoupling: on.

Delay time: Repeating pulse waiting time not less than 60 seconds.

Integrating times: 8 or more times.

Dummy scanning: 2 or more times.

Measuring temperature: A constant temperature between 20°C and 30°C.

System suitability

Test for required detectability: When the procedure is run with the sample solution under the above operating conditions, SN ratio of the two signals of around δ 6.17 – δ 6.25 ppm and δ 7.54 ppm is not less than 100.

System performance: When the procedure is run with the sample solution under the above operating conditions, the two signals of around δ 6.17 – δ 6.25 ppm and δ 7.54 ppm are not overlapped with any signal of obvious foreign substance, and the ratios of the resonance intensities, $(A_1/2)/A_2$, of each signal around δ 6.17 – δ 6.25 ppm and δ 7.54 ppm are between 0.99 and 1.01, respectively.

System repeatability: When the test is repeated 6 times with the sample solution under the above operating conditions, the relative standard deviation of the ratio of the resonance intensity, A_1 or A_2, to that of the reference standard for qNMR is not more than 1.0%.

Paeonol for component determination See paeonol for assay.

Paeonol for thin-layer chromatography $C_9H_{10}O_3$ White, crystals or crystalline powder, having a specific odor. Freely soluble in methanol and in diethyl ether, and slightly soluble in water. Melting point: about 50°C.

Purity Related substances—Dissolve 1.0 mg of paeonol for thin-layer chromatography in exactly 1 mL of methanol, and perform the test with 10 μL of this solution as directed in the Identification under Moutan Bark: any spot other than the principal spot at the *Rf* value of near 0.5 does not appear.

Palladium chloride See palladium (II) chloride.

Palladium chloride TS See palladium (II) chloride TS.

Palladium (II) chloride $PdCl_2$ [K 8154, Special class]

Palladium (II) chloride TS Dissolve 0.2 g of palladium (II) chloride in 500 mL of 0.25 mol/L sulfuric acid TS, by heating if necessary, cool, and add 0.25 mol/L sulfuric acid TS to make 1000 mL.

Palmatin chloride $C_{21}H_{22}ClNO_4$ A yellow-brown crystalline powder.

Purity Related substances—Dissolve 1 mg of palmatin chloride in 10 mL of methanol, and use this solution as the sample solution. Proceed with 20 μL of the sample solution as directed in the Assay under Phellodendron Bark: when measure the peak areas for 2 times the retention time of berberine, the total area of the peaks other than palmatin is not larger than 1/10 times the total area except the area of solvent peak.

Palmitic acid for gas chromatography $C_{16}H_{32}O_2$ [K 8756, Special class]

Pancreatic digest of casein See Peptone, casein.

Pancreatic digest of gelatin See Peptone, gelatin.

Papaic digest of soya bean See Peptone, soybean.

Papaverine hydrochloride $C_{20}H_{21}NO_4.HCl$ [Same as the namesake monograph]

Papaverine hydrochloride for assay $C_{20}H_{21}NO_4.HCl$ [Same as the monograph Papaverine Hydrochloride. When dried, it contains not less than 99.0% of papaverine hydrochloride ($C_{20}H_{21}NO_4.HCl$).]

Paraffin [Same as the namesake monograph]

Paraffin, light liquid [Same as the namesake monograph]

Parahydroxybenzoic acid $C_7H_6O_3$ White crystals.
Melting point <2.60>: 212 – 216°C
Content: not less than 98.0 %. Assay—Weigh accurately about 0.7 g of parahydroxybenzoic acid, dissolve in 50 mL of acetone, add 100 mL of water, and titrate <2.50> with 0.5 mol/L sodium hydroxide VS (potentiometric titration). Perform a blank determination in the same manner, and make any necessary correction.

Each mL of 0.5 mol/L sodium hydroxide VS
= 69.06 mg of $C_7H_6O_3$

Particle counter apparatus An apparatus that is able to count the fine particles derived from reticulocyte similar cells.

Patent blue $C_{27}H_{31}N_2NaO_6S_2$ Red-purple-brown to dark red-brown, crystalline powder to powder, or masses.
Identification—(1) To 5 mg of patent blue add 20 mL of ethanol (99.5): a dark blue color develops.
(2) Determine the infrared absorption spectrum of patent blue as directed in the potassium bromide disk method under Infrared Spectrophotometry <2.25>: it exhibits absorption at the wave numbers of about 1580 cm^{-1}, 1420 cm^{-1}, 1340 cm^{-1}, 1180 cm^{-1}, 1150 cm^{-1}, 1070 cm^{-1}, 1030 cm^{-1}, 910 cm^{-1}, 790 cm^{-1}, 700 cm^{-1} and 620 cm^{-1}.

2-fold PCR reaction solution containing SYBR Green 2-Fold reaction solution for real-time PCR, containing SYBR Green.

Peanut oil [Same as the namesake monograph]

Pemirolast potassium $C_{10}H_7KN_6O$ [Same as the namesake monograph]

Pentane $CH_3(CH_2)_3CH_3$ Clear and colorless liquid.
Specific gravity <2.56> d_{20}^{20}: 0.620 – 0.650
Distilling range <2.57>: 35.5 – 37°C, not less than 98 vol%.

Peptic digest of animal tissue See Peptone, animal tissue.

Peptone Prepared for microbial test.

Peptone, animal tissue Prepared for microbial test.

Peptone, casein Grayish yellow powder, having a characteristic but not putrescent odor. It dissolves in water, but not in ethanol (95) and in diethyl ether.
Loss on drying <2.41>: not more than 7% (0.5 g, 105°C, constant mass).
Residue on ignition <2.44>: not more than 15% (0.5 g).
Degree of digestion—Dissolve 1 g of casein peptone in 10 mL of water, and perform the following test using this solution as the sample solution:
(1) Overlay 1 mL of the sample solution with 0.5 mL of a mixture of 1 mL of acetic acid (100) and 10 mL of dilute ethanol: no ring or precipitate forms at the junction of the two liquids, and on shaking, no turbidity results.
(2) Mix 1 mL of the sample solution with 4 mL of a saturated solution of zinc sulfate heptahydrate: a small quantity of precipitate is produced (proteoses).
(3) Filter the mixture of (2), and to 1 mL of the filtrate add 3 mL of water and 4 drops of bromine TS: a red-purple color is produced.
Nitrogen content <1.08>: not less than 10% (105°C, constant mass, after drying).

Peptone, gelatin Prepared for microbial test.

Peptone, soybean Prepared for microbial test.

Perchloric acid $HClO_4$ [K 8223, Special class, Density: about 1.67 g/mL. Concentration: 70.0 – 72.0%]

Perchloric acid-dehydrated ethanol TS See perchloric acid-ethanol TS.

Perchloric acid-ethanol TS Add cautiously 25.5 mL of perchloric acid to 50 mL of ethanol (99.5), cool, and add ethanol (99.5) to make 100 mL (3 mol/L).

Performic acid Mix 9 volumes of formic acid and 1 volume of hydrogen peroxide (30), and leave at room temperature for 2 hours.
Storage—Store in a cool place.

Perillaldehyde for assay $C_{10}H_{14}O$ Perillaldehyde for thin-layer chromatography meeting the following specifications.
Absorbance <2.24> $E_{1cm}^{1\%}$ (230 nm): 850 – 950 (10 mg, methanol, 2000 mL).
Purity Related substances—Dissolve 10 mg of perillaldehyde for assay in 250 mL of methanol, and use this solution as the sample solution. Pipet 1 mL of this solution, add methanol to make exactly 50 mL, and use this solution as the standard solution. Perform the test with exactly 10 μL each of the sample solution and standard solution as directed under Liquid Chromatography <2.01> according to the following conditions. Determine each peak area from both solutions by the automatic integration method: the total area of the peaks other than perillaldehyde obtained from the sample solution is not larger than perillaldehyde from the standard solution.
Operating conditions
Detector: An ultraviolet absorption photometer (wavelength: 230 nm).
Column: A stainless steel column 4.6 mm in inside diameter and 15 cm in length, packed with octadecylsilanized silica gel for liquid chromatography (5 μm in particle diameter).
Column temperature: A constant temperature of about 40°C.
Mobile phase: A mixture of water and acetonitrile (13:7).
Flow rate: 1.0 mL per minute.
Time span of measurement: About 3 times as long as the retention time of perillaldehyde, beginning after the solvent peak.
System suitability
Test for required detectability: Pipet 1 mL of the standard solution, and add methanol to make exactly 20 mL. Confirm

that the peak area of perillaldehyde obtained with 10 μL of this solution is equivalent to 3.5 to 6.5% of that with 10 μL of the standard solution.

System performance: Dissolve 1 mg of (*E*)-asarone in 50 mL of the standard solution. When the procedure is run with 10 μL of this solution under the above operating conditions, perillaldehyde and (*E*)-asarone are eluted in this order with the resolution between these peaks being not less than 1.5.

System repeatability: When the test is repeated 6 times with 10 μL of the standard solution under the above operating conditions, the relative standard deviation of the peak area of perillaldehyde is not more than 1.5%.

Perillaldehyde for component determination See perillaldehyde for assay.

Perillaldehyde for thin-layer chromatography $C_{10}H_{14}O$ Colorless to light brown transparent liquid, having a characteristic odor. Miscible with methanol and with ethanol (99.5), and very slightly soluble in water.

Identification—Determine the infrared absorption spectrum of perillaldehyde for thin-layer chromatography as directed in the liquid film method under Infrared Spectrophotometry <2.25>: it exhibits absorption at the wave numbers of about 3080 cm^{-1}, 2930 cm^{-1}, 1685 cm^{-1}, 1644 cm^{-1}, 1435 cm^{-1} and 890 cm^{-1}.

Purity Related substances—Dissolve 1.0 mg of perillaldehyde for thin-layer chromatography in 10 mL of methanol, and perform the test with 10 μL of this solution as directed in the Identification under Perilla Herb: no spot other than the principal spot at around *R*f value of 0.5 appears.

Peroxidase Obtained from horse-radish. A red-brown powder. It is freely soluble in water. It contains about 250 units per mg. One unit indicates an amount of the enzyme which produces 1 mg of purpurogallin in 20 seconds at 20°C and pH 6.0, from pyrogallol and hydrogen peroxide (30) used as the substrate.

Peroxidase labeled anti-rabbit antibody It is prepared as follows: Immunize small animals with rabbit immunoglobulin G to obtain the antiserum. From the obtained antiserum the specific antibody is separated by the affinity chromatography using a column coupled with rabbit immunoglobulin G, and the specific antibody is labeled with peroxidase by the periodic acid method.

Peroxidase labeled anti-rabbit antibody TS Dissolve 0.10 g of bovine serum albumin in phosphate-buffered sodium chloride TS to make 100 mL. To 15 mL of this solution add 5 μL of peroxidase labeled anti-rabbit antibody. Prepare before use.

Peroxidase-labeled avidin A solution of avidin conjugated with horseradish peroxidase in an appropriate buffer solution.

Peroxidase-labeled avidin TS Dilute peroxidase-labeled avidin with 0.01 mol/L tris buffer solution-sodium chloride TS (pH 7.4) so that the concentration of peroxidase-labeled avidin is 0.3 μg/mL. Prepare before use.

Peroxidase-labeled bradykinin A solution of horseradish origin peroxidase-binding bradykinin in gelatin-phosphate buffer solution (pH 7.0). A colorless to light brown clear solution.

Peroxidase-labeled bradykinin TS To 0.08 mL of peroxidase-labeled bradykinin, 8 mg of sodium tetraborate decahydrate, 8 mg of bovine serum albumin and 0.8 mL of gelatin-phosphate buffer solution (pH 7.0) add water to make 8 mL, and lyophilize. Dissolve this in 8 mL of water. Prepare before use.

Perphenazine maleate for assay $C_{21}H_{26}ClN_3OS.2C_4H_4O_4$ [Same as the monograph Perphenazine Maleate. When dried, it contains not less than 99.0% of perphenazine maleate ($C_{21}H_{26}ClN_3OS.2C_4H_4O_4$).]

Pethidine hydrochloride for assay $C_{15}H_{21}NO_2.HCl$ [Same as the monograph Pethidine Hydrochloride. When dried, it contains not less than 99.0% of pethidine hydrochloride $C_{15}H_{21}NO_2.HCl$.]

Petrolatum [Same as the monograph Yellow Petrolatum or White Petrolatum]

Petroleum benzine [K 8594, Special class]

Petroleum ether [K 8593, Special class]

Peucedanum·ledebourielloides for purity Powder of the root and rhizome of *Peucedanum ledebourielloides* K. T. Fu (*Umbelliferae*).

Identification—Place 1.0 g of peucedanum·ledebourielloides for purity in a glass-stoppered centrifuge tube, add 5 mL of hexane, shake for 10 minutes, centrifuge, and use the supernatant liquid as the sample solution. Perform the test with the sample solution as directed under Thin-layer Chromatography <2.03>. Spot 5 μL of the sample solution on a plate of silica gel for thin-layer chromatography. Develop the plate with a mixture of hexane, ethyl acetate and acetic acid (100) (20:10:1) to a distance of about 7 cm, and air-dry the plate. Examine under ultraviolet light (main wavelength: 365 nm): blue fluorescent spots at *R*f values of about 0.35 (agasyllin) and about 0.4 [xanthalin ($C_{24}H_{26}O_7$)] are observed.

Phenacetin $C_{10}H_{13}NO_2$ White, crystals or crystalline powder. Soluble in ethanol (95), and very slightly soluble in water.

Melting point <2.60>: 134 – 137°C

Loss on drying <2.41>: not more than 0.5% (1 g, 105°C, 2 hours).

***o*-Phenanthroline** See 1,10-phenanthroline monohydrate.

***o*-Phenanthroline hydrochloride** See 1,10-phenanthrolinium chloride monohydrate.

1,10-Phenanthroline monohydrate $C_{12}H_8N_2.H_2O$ [K 8789, Special class]

***o*-Phenanthroline TS** See 1,10-phenanthroline TS.

1,10-Phenanthroline TS Dissolve 0.15 g of 1,10-phenanthroline monohydrate in 10 mL of a freshly prepared iron (II) sulfate heptahydrate solution (37 in 2500) and 1 mL of dilute sulfuric acid. Preserve in tightly stoppered containers.

1,10-Phenanthrolinium chloride monohydrate $C_{12}H_8N_2.HCl.H_2O$ [K 8202, Special class]

Phenethylamine hydrochloride $C_6H_5CH_2CH_2NH_2.HCl$ White, crystals or crystalline powder.

Melting point: <2.60> 220 – 225°C

Phenobarbital for assay $C_{12}H_{12}N_2O_3$ [Same as the monograph Phenobarbital]

Phenol C_6H_5OH [K 8798, Special class]

Phenol for assay C_6H_5OH [K 8798, Phenol, Special class]

Phenol-hydrochloric acid TS Dissolve 0.2 g of phenol in 10 mL of 6 mol/L hydrochloric acid TS.

Phenolphthalein $C_{20}H_{14}O_4$ [K 8799, Special class]

Phenolphthalein-thymol blue TS Solution A: Dissolve 0.1 g of phenolphthalein in 100 mL of diluted ethanol (4 in 5). Solution B: Dissolve 0.1 g of thymol blue in 50 mL of a mixture of ethanol (95) and dilute sodium hydroxide TS (250:11), add water to make 100 mL. Mix 2 volumes of solution A and 3 volumes of solution B before use.

Phenolphthalein TS Dissolve 1 g of phenolphthalein in 100 mL of ethanol (95).

Phenolphthalein TS, alkaline See Alcohol Number Determination *<1.01>*.

Phenolphthalein TS, dilute Dissolve 0.1 g of phenolphthalein in 80 mL of ethanol (95), and add water to make 100 mL.

Phenol red $C_{19}H_{14}O_5S$ [K 8800, Special class]

Phenol red TS Dissolve 0.1 g of phenol red in 100 mL of ethanol (95), and filter if necessary.

Phenol red TS, dilute To 235 mL of a solution of ammonium nitrate (1 in 9400) add 105 mL of 2 mol/L sodium hydroxide TS and 135 mL of a solution prepared by dissolving 24 g of acetic acid (100) in water to make 200 mL. To this solution add 25 mL of a solution prepared by dissolving 33 mg of phenol red in 1.5 mL of 2 mol/L sodium hydroxide TS and adding water to make 100 mL. If necessary, adjust the pH to 4.7.

Phenol-sodium nitroprusside TS See phenol-sodium pentacyanonitrosylferrate (III) TS.

Phenol-sodium pentacyanonitrosylferrate (III) TS Dissolve 5 g of phenol and 25 mg of sodium pentacyanonitrosylferrate (III) dihydrate in sufficient water to make 500 mL. Preserve in a dark, cold place.

Phenolsulfonphthalein for assay $C_{19}H_{14}O_5S$ [Same as the monograph Phenolsulfonphthalein. When dried, it contains not less than 99.0% of phenolsulfonphthalein ($C_{19}H_{14}O_5S$).]

Phenylalanine See L-phenylalanine.

L-Phenylalanine $C_9H_{11}NO_2$ [Same as the namesake monograph]

***H*-D-phenylalanyl-L-pipecolyl-L-arginyl-*p*-nitroanilide dihydrochloride** A white powder. Slightly soluble in water.

Absorbance *<2.24>* $E^{1\%}_{1\,cm}$ (316 nm): 192 – 214 (10 mg, water, 300 mL).

Phenyl benzoate $C_6H_5COOC_6H_5$ White, crystals or crystalline powder, having a slight, characteristic odor.

Melting point *<2.60>*: 68 – 70°C

Purity Clarity of solution—Dissolve 1.0 g of phenyl benzoate in 20 mL of methanol: the solution is clear.

25% Phenyl-25% cyanopropyl-methylsilicone polymer for gas chromatography Prepared for gas chromatography.

***o*-Phenylenediamine** $H_2NC_6H_4NH_2$ White to dark brown, crystals or crystalline powder. Freely soluble in ethanol (95) and in acetone, and soluble in water.

Content: not less than 95.0%. Assay—Accurately weigh about 0.15 g of *o*-phenylenediamine, add 50 mL of acetic acid for nonaqueous titration to dissolve, and then titrate *<2.50>* with 0.1 mol/L of perchloric acid VS (potentiometric titration). Perform a blank determination in the same manner, and make any necessary correction.

Each mL of 0.1 mol/L perchloric acid VS
= 10.81 mg of $H_2NC_6H_4NH_2$

***o*-Phenylenediamine dihydrochloride** $H_2NC_6H_4NH_2.2HCl$ White to pale yellow or pale red, crystals or crystalline powder.

Purity Clarity—a solution (1 in 20) is clear.

Content: not less than 98.0%. Assay—Weigh accurately about 0.15 g of *o*-phenylenediamine dihydrochloride, dissolve in 50 mL of water, and titrate *<2.50>* with 0.1 mol/L sodium hydroxide VS (potentiometric titration).

Each mL of 0.1 mol/L sodium hydroxide VS
= 9.053 mg of $H_2NC_6H_4NH_2.2HCl$

1,3-Phenylenediamine hydrochloride $C_6H_8N_2.2HCl$ A white or faintly reddish crystalline powder. It is colored to red or brown by light.

Identification—To 3 mL of a solution of 1,3-phenylenediamine hydrochloride (1 in 6000) add 0.5 mL of a solution of sodium nitrite (3 in 20,000), then add 2 to 3 drops of hydrochloric acid: a yellow color is produced.

(*S*)-1-Phenylethyl isocyanate $C_6H_5CH(CH_3)NCO$ Colorless to light yellow, clear liquid, having a characteristic odor.

Optical rotation *<2.49>* α_D^{20}: −8.5 – −11.5° (100 mm).

Specific gravity *<2.56>* d_4^{20}: 1.040 – 1.050

Phenylfluorone $C_{19}H_{12}O_5$ [K 9547, Special class]

Phenylfluorone-ethanol TS Dissolve 50 mg of phenylfluorone in ethanol (95) and in 10 mL of diluted hydrochloric acid (1 in 3), and add ethanol (95) to make exactly 500 mL.

D-Phenylglycine $C_8H_9NO_2$ White, crystals or crystalline powder. Slightly soluble in water.

Loss on drying *<2.41>*: not more than 0.5% (1 g, 105°C, 3 hours).

Content: not less than 98.5%. Assay—Weigh accurately about 0.3 g of D-phenylglycine, previously dried, dissolve in 3 mL of formic acid, add 50 mL of acetic acid (100), and titrate *<2.50>* with 0.1 mol/L perchloric acid VS (potentiometric titration). Perform a blank determination in the same manner, and make any necessary correction.

Each mL of 0.1 mol/L perchloric acid VS
= 15.12 mg of $C_8H_9NO_2$

Phenylhydrazine $C_6H_5NHNH_2$ Colorless or light yellow, clear liquid, having a faint aromatic odor.

Content: not less than 99.0%. Assay—Weigh accurately about 1 g of phenylhydrazine, add 30 mL of diluted hydrochloric acid (1 in 100) and water to make exactly 100 mL. Put exactly 20 mL of this solution in a glass-stoppered conical flask, and add 40 mL of diluted hydrochloric acid (3 in 4). After cooling, add 5 mL of chloroform, and titrate *<2.50>* with 0.05 mol/L potassium iodate VS while shaking vigorously until the red color of the chloroform layer disappears. Perform a blank determination in the same manner, and make any necessary correction.

Each mL of 0.05 mol/L potassium iodate VS
= 5.407 mg of $C_6H_5NHNH_2$

Phenylhydrazine hydrochloride See phenylhydrazinium chloride.

Phenylhydrazine hydrochloride TS See phenylhydrazinium chloride TS.

Phenylhydrazinium chloride $C_6H_5NHNH_2.HCl$

[K 8203, Special class]

Phenylhydrazinium chloride TS Dissolve 65 mg of phenylhydrazinium chloride recrystallized from dilute ethanol, in 100 mL of a solution previously prepared by adding cautiously 170 mL of sulfuric acid to 80 mL of water.

Phenyl isothiocyanate C_7H_5NS Prepared for amino acid analysis or biochemistry.

1-phenyl-3-methyl-5-pyrazolone See 3-methyl-1-phenyl-5-pyrazolone.

50% Phenyl-50% methylpolysiloxane for gas chromatography Prepared for gas chromatography.

5% Phenyl-methyl silicone polymer for gas chromatography Prepared for gas chromatography.

35% Phenyl-methyl silicone polymer for gas chromatography Prepared for gas chromatography.

50% Phenyl-methyl silicone polymer for gas chromatography Prepared for gas chromatography.

65% Phenyl-methyl silicone polymer for gas chromatography Prepared for gas chromatography.

Phenylpiperazine hydrochloride See 1-phenylpiperazine monohydrochloride.

1-Phenylpiperazine monohydrochloride $C_{10}H_{14}N_2.HCl$ A white powder. Melting point: about 247°C (with decomposition).

Phenytoin for assay $C_{15}H_{12}N_2O_2$ [Same as the monograph Phenytoin. It meets the following requirements.]

Purity Related substances—Dissolve 25 mg of phenytoin for assay in 50 mL of the mobile phase, and use this solution as the sample solution. To exactly 1 mL of the sample solution add the mobile phase to make exactly 200 mL, and use this solution as the standard solution. Perform the test with exactly 10 μL each of the sample solution and standard solution as directed under Liquid Chromatography *<2.01>* according to the following conditions, and determine each peak area by the automatic integration method: the total area of the peaks other than phenytoin obtained from the sample solution is not larger than the peak area of phenytoin from the standard solution.

Operating conditions

Column, column temperature, and flow rate: Proceed as directed in the operating conditions in the Assay under Phenytoin Tablets.

Detector: An ultraviolet absorption photometer (wavelength: 220 nm).

Mobile phase: A mixture of 0.02 mol/L phosphate buffer solution (pH 3.5) and acetonitrile for liquid chromatography (11:9).

Time span of measurement: About 5 times as long as the retention time of phenytoin, beginning after the solvent peak.

System suitability

Test for required detectability: To exactly 2 mL of the standard solution add the mobile phase to make exactly 20 mL. Confirm that the peak area of phenytoin obtained with 10 μL of this solution is equivalent to 8 to 12% of that with 10 μL of the standard solution.

System performance: When the procedure is run with 10 μL of the standard solution under the above operating conditions, the number of theoretical plates and the symmetry factor of the peak of phenytoin are not less than 6000 and not more than 2.0, respectively.

System repeatability: When the test is repeated 6 times with 10 μL of the standard solution under the above operating conditions, the relative standard deviation of the peak area of phenytoin is not more than 2.0%.

Phloroglucin See phloroglucinol dihydrate.

Phloroglucin dihydrate See phloroglucinol dihydrate.

Phloroglucinol dihydrate $C_6H_3(OH)_3.2H_2O$ White to pale yellow, crystals or crystalline powder.

Melting point <2.60>: 215 – 219°C (after drying).

Loss on drying <2.41>: 18.0 – 24.0% (1 g, 105°C, 1 hour).

Phosphatase, alkaline Obtained from bovine small intestine. A white to grayish white or yellow-brown, lyophilized powder.

It contains not less than 1 unit per mg, not containing any saline. One unit indicates an amount of the enzyme which produces 1 μmol of 4-nitrophenol at 37°C and pH 9.8 in 1 minute from 4-nitrophenyl phosphate used as the substrate.

Phosphatase TS, alkaline Dissolve 0.1 g of alkaline phosphatase in 10 mL of boric acid-magnesium chloride buffer solution (pH 9.0). Prepare before use.

Phosphate-buffered sodium chloride TS Dissolve 8.0 g of sodium chloride, 0.2 g of potassium chloride, 2.9 g of disodium hydrogen phosphate dodecahydrate, and 0.2 g of potassium dihydrogen phosphate in water to make 1000 mL.

0.01 mol/L Phosphate buffer-sodium chloride TS (pH 7.4) Dissolve 2.93 g of disodium hydrogen phosphate dodecahydrate, 0.25 g of potassium dihydrogen phosphate, and 9 g of sodium chloride in water to make 1000 mL.

Phosphate buffer solution for assay of bupleurum root To 100 mL of 0.2 mol/L potassium dihydrogen phosphate TS add 59 mL of 0.2 mol/L sodium hydroxide TS.

Phosphate buffer solution for component determination of bupleurum root See phosphate buffer solution for assay of bupleurum root.

Phosphate buffer solution for cytotoxicity test Dissolve 0.20 g of potassium chloride, 0.20 g of potassium dihydrogen phosphate, 8.00 g of sodium chloride and 1.15 g of anhydrous disodium hydrogen phosphate in water to make 1000 mL, and sterilize in an autoclave at 121°C for 15 minutes.

Phosphate buffer solution for epoetin alfa Dissolve 0.247 g of sodium dihydrogen phosphate dihydrate, 0.151 g of disodium hydrogen phosphate dodecahydrate and 8.77 g of sodium chloride in water to make 1000 mL.

Phosphate buffer solution for microplate washing Dissolve 0.62 g of sodium dihydrogen phosphate dihydrate, 9.48 g of disodium hydrogen phosphate dodecahydrate, 52.6 g of sodium chloride, 3.0 g of polysorbate 80 and 1.8 g of polyoxyethylene (40) octylphenyl ether in water to make 600 mL. Dilute this solution 10 times with water before use.

Phosphate buffer solution for pancreatin Dissolve 3.3 g of anhydrous disodium hydrogen phosphate, 1.4 g of potassium dihydrogen phosphate and 0.33 g of sodium chloride in water to make 100 mL.

Phosphate buffer solution for processed aconite root Dissolve 19.3 g of disodium hydrogen phosphate dodecahydrate in 3660 mL of water, and add 12.7 g of phosphoric acid.

Phosphate buffer solution (pH 3.0) Dissolve 136 g of potassium dihydrogen phosphate in water to make 1000 mL, and adjust to pH 3.0 with phosphoric acid.

0.02 mol/L Phosphate buffer solution (pH 3.0) Dissolve 3.1 g of sodium dihydrogen phosphate dihydrate in 1000 mL of water, and adjust the pH to 3.0 with diluted phosphoric acid (1 in 10).

Phosphate buffer solution (pH 3.1) Dissolve 136.1 g of potassium dihydrogen phosphate in 500 mL of water, and add 6.3 mL of phosphoric acid and water to make 1000 mL.

0.02 mol/L Phosphate buffer solution (pH 3.5) Dissolve 3.1 g of sodium dihydrogen phosphate dihydrate in 1000 mL of water, and adjust the pH to 3.5 with diluted phosphoric acid (1 in 10).

0.05 mol/L Phosphate buffer solution (pH 3.5) To 1000 mL of 0.05 mol/L potassium dihydrogen phosphate TS add a suitable amount of a solution of diluted phosphoric acid (49 in 10,000) to make a solution having (pH 3.5).

Phosphate buffer solution (pH 4.0) Adjust the pH of 0.05 mol/L potassium dihydrogen phosphate TS to 4.0 with diluted phosphoric acid (1 in 10).

0.1 mol/L Phosphate buffer solution (pH 4.5) Dissolve 13.61 g of potassium dihydrogen phosphate in 750 mL of water, adjust to pH 4.5 with potassium hydroxide TS, and add water to make 1000 mL.

0.1 mol/L Phosphate buffer solution (pH 5.3) Dissolve 0.44 g of disodium hydrogen phosphate dodecahydrate and 13.32 g of potassium dihydrogen phosphate in 750 mL of water, adjust the pH to 5.3 with sodium hydroxide TS or phosphoric acid, and add water to make 1000 mL.

0.1 mol/L Phosphate buffer solution (pH 7) Dissolve 13.6 g of potassium dihydrogen phosphate in 800 mL of water, adjust the pH to 7 ± 0.4 with sodium hydroxide TS, and add water to make 1000 mL.

1/15 mol/L Phosphate buffer solution (pH 5.6) Dissolve 9.07 g of potassium dihydrogen phosphate in about 750 mL of water, adjust the pH to 5.6 with potassium hydroxide TS, and add water to make 1000 mL.

Phosphate buffer solution (pH 5.9) Dissolve 6.8 g of potassium dihydrogen phosphate in 800 mL of water, adjust the pH to 5.9 with diluted potassium hydroxide TS (1 in 10), and add water to make 1000 mL.

Phosphate buffer solution (pH 6.0) Dissolve 8.63 g of potassium dihydrogen phosphate and 1.37 g of anhydrous disodium hydrogen phosphate in 750 mL of water, adjust the pH to 6.0 with sodium hydroxide TS or diluted phosphoric acid (1 in 15), and add water to make 1000 mL.

0.05 mol/L Phosphate buffer solution (pH 6.0) To 50 mL of 0.2 mol/L potassium dihydrogen phosphate TS for buffer solution add 5.70 mL of 0.2 mol/L sodium hydroxide TS and water to make 200 mL.

Phosphate buffer solution (pH 6.2) Dissolve 9.08 g of potassium dihydrogen phosphate in 1000 mL of water (solution A). Dissolve 9.46 g of anhydrous disodium hydrogen phosphate in 1000 mL of water (solution B). Mix 800 mL of the solution A and 200 mL of the solution B, and adjust the pH to 6.2 with the solution A or the solution B if necessary.

Phosphate buffer solution (pH 6.5) Mix 50 mL of 0.2 mol/L potassium dihydrogen phosphate TS for buffer solution and 15.20 mL of 0.2 mol/L sodium hydroxide TS, and add water to make 200 mL.

Phosphate buffer solution for antibiotics (pH 6.5) Dissolve 10.5 g of disodium hydrogen phosphate dodecahydrate and 5.8 g of potassium dihydrogen phosphate in 750 mL of water, adjust the pH to 6.5 with sodium hydroxide TS, and add water to make 1000 mL.

Phosphate buffer solution (pH 6.8) Dissolve 3.40 g of potassium dihydrogen phosphate and 3.55 g of anhydrous disodium hydrogen phosphate in water to make 1000 mL.

0.01 mol/L Phosphate buffer solution (pH 6.8) Dissolve 1.36 g of potassium dihydrogen phosphate in 900 mL of water, adjust the pH to 6.8 with 0.2 mol/L sodium hydroxide TS, and add water to make 1000 mL.

0.1 mol/L Phosphate buffer solution (pH 6.8) Dissolve 6.4 g of potassium dihydrogen phosphate and 18.9 g of disodium hydrogen phosphate dodecahydrate in 750 mL of water, adjust the pH to 6.8 with sodium hydroxide TS and add water to make 1000 mL.

Phosphate buffer solution (pH 7.0) Mix 50 mL of 0.2 mol/L potassium dihydrogen phosphate TS for buffer solution and 29.54 mL of 0.2 mol/L sodium hydroxide TS, and add water to make 200 mL.

0.05 mol/L Phosphate buffer solution (pH 7.0) Dissolve 4.83 g of dipotassium hydrogen phosphate and 3.02 g of potassium dihydrogen phosphate in 1000 mL of water, and adjust to (pH 7.0) with phosphoric acid or potassium hydroxide TS.

0.1 mol/L Phosphate buffer solution (pH 7) Dissolve 13.6 g of potassium dihydrogen phosphate in 800 mL of water, adjust the pH to 7 ± 0.4 with sodium hydroxide TS, and add water to make 1000 mL.

0.1 mol/L Phosphate buffer solution (pH 7.0) Dissolve 17.9 g of disodium hydrogen phosphate dodecahydrate in water to make 500 mL (solution A). Dissolve 6.8 g of potassium dihydrogen phosphate in water to make 500 mL (solution B). To a volume of solution A add solution B until the mixture is adjusted to pH 7.0 (about 2:1 by volume of solutions A and B).

Phosphate buffer solution (pH 7.2) Mix 50 mL of 0.2 mol/L potassium dihydrogen phosphate TS for buffer solution and 34.7 mL of 0.2 mol/L sodium hydroxide TS, and add water to make 200 mL.

Phosphate buffer solution (pH 7.4) Mix 50 mL of 0.2 mol/L potassium dihydrogen phosphate TS for buffer solution and 39.50 mL of 0.2 mol/L sodium hydroxide TS, and add water to make 200 mL.

0.02 mol/L Phosphate buffer solution (pH 7.5) Dissolve 2.72 g of potassium dihydrogen phosphate in 900 mL of water, adjust to pH 7.5 with 0.2 mol/L sodium hydroxide TS, and add water to make 1000 mL.

0.03 mol/L Phosphate buffer solution (pH 7.5) Dissolve 4.083 g of potassium dihydrogen phosphate in 800 mL of water, adjust the pH to 7.5 with 0.2 mol/L sodium hydroxide TS, and add water to make 1000 mL.

Phosphate buffer solution (pH 8.0) Mix 50 mL of 0.2 mol/L potassium dihydrogen phosphate TS for buffer solution and 46.1 mL of 0.2 mol/L sodium hydroxide TS, and add water to make 200 mL.

0.02 mol/L Phosphate buffer solution (pH 8.0) To 50 mL of 0.2 mol/L potassium dihydrogen phosphate TS add 300 mL of water, adjust the pH to 8.0 with sodium hydroxide TS, and add water to make 500 mL.

0.1 mol/L Phosphate buffer solution (pH 8.0) Dissolve 13.2 g of anhydrous disodium hydrogen phosphate and 0.91 g of potassium dihydrogen phosphate in about 750 mL of water, adjust to pH 8.0 with phosphoric acid, and add water to make 1000 mL.

0.1 mol/L Phosphate buffer solution for antibiotics (pH 8.0) Dissolve 16.73 g of dipotassium hydrogen phosphate and 0.523 g of potassium dihydrogen phosphate in 750 mL of water, adjust the pH to 8.0 with phosphoric acid, and add water to make 1000 mL.

0.2 mol/L Phosphate buffer solution (pH 10.5) Dissolve 34.8 g of dipotassium hydrogen phosphate in 750 mL of water, adjust to pH 10.5 with 8 mol/L sodium hydroxide TS, and add water to make 1000 mL.

Phosphate buffer solution (pH 12) To 5.44 g of anhydrous disodium hydrogen phosphate add 36.5 mL of sodium hydroxide TS and about 40 mL of water, dissolve by shaking well, and add water to make 100 mL.

0.01 mol/L Phosphate buffer solution Dissolve 1.15 g of anhydrous disodium hydrogen phosphate, 0.2 g of potassium dihydrogen phosphate, 8.0 g of sodium chloride and 0.2 g of potassium chloride in water to make 1000 mL.

Phosphinic acid H_3PO_2 Colorless or pale yellow viscous liquid.

Identification—(1) To 0.5 mL of phosphinic acid add 0.5 mL of hydrogen peroxide (30) and 0.5 mL of diluted sulfuric acid (1 in 6), and evaporate to nearly dryness on a water bath. After cooling, add 10 mL of water and 5 mL of ammonia TS, and add 5 mL of magnesia TS: a white precipitate is produced.

(2) To 1 mL of phosphinic acid add the mixture of iodine TS (1 mL) and water (20 mL): the iodine color disappears.

Content: 30.0 – 32.0%. Assay—Weigh accurately about 1.5 g of phosphinic acid, and dissolve in water to make exactly 250 mL. Pipet 25 mL of this solution into an iodine bottle, add exactly 50 mL of 0.05 mol/L bromine VS, 100 mL of water and 10 mL of diluted sulfuric acid (1 in 6), immediately stoppered, gently shake, and allow to stand for 3 hours. Then add 20 mL of potassium iodide TS, stopper immediately, shake vigorously, and titrate *<2.50>* liberated iodine with 0.1 mol/L sodium thiosulfate VS (indicator: 1 mL of starch TS). Perform a blank determination in the same manner.

Each mL of 0.05 mol/L bromine VS
= 1.650 mg of H_3PO_2

Phosphate TS Dissolve 2.0 g of dipotassium hydrogen phosphate and 8.0 g of potassium dihydrogen phosphate in water to make 1000 mL.

Phosphomolybdic acid See phosphomolybdic acid *n*-hydrate.

Phosphomolybdic acid *n*-hydrate $P_2O_5.24MoO_3.xH_2O$ Yellow, crystals or crystalline powder.

Identification (1) To 10 mL of a solution (1 in 10) add 0.5 mL of ammonia TS: yellow precipitates appear, which disappear by the addition of 2 mL of ammonia TS, and yellow precipitates appear by further addition of 5 mL of diluted nitric acid (1 in 2).

(2) To 5 mL of a solution (1 in 10) add 1 mL of ammonia TS and 1 mL of magnesia TS: white precipitates appear.

Phosphoric acid H_3PO_4 [K 9005, Special class]

Phosphoric acid-acetic acid-boric acid buffer solution (pH 2.0) Dissolve 6.77 mL of phosphoric acid, 5.72 mL of acetic acid (100) and 6.18 g of boric acid in water to make 1000 mL. Adjust the pH of this solution to 2.0 with 0.5 mol/L sodium hydroxide VS.

Phosphoric acid-sodium sulfate buffer solution (pH 2.3) Dissolve 28.4 g of anhydrous sodium sulfate in 1000 mL of water, and add 2.7 mL of phosphoric acid. If necessary, adjust to pH 2.3 with 2-aminoethanol.

Phosphorus pentoxide See phosphorus (V) oxide.

Phosphorus, red P An odorless dark red powder. Practically insoluble in carbon disulfide and in water.

Purity Free phosphoric acid: Not more than 0.5%.

To 5 g add 10 mL of a solution of sodium chloride (1 in 5), mix, then add 50 mL of the solution of sodium chloride (1 in 5), allow to stand for 1 hour, and filter. Wash the residue with three 10-mL portions of the solution of sodium chloride (1 in 5), combine the filtrate and the washings, and titrate *<2.50>* with 0.1 mol/L sodium hydroxide VS (indicator: 3 drops of thymol blue TS). Perform a blank determination in the same manner, and make any necessary correction.

Each mL of 0.1 mol/L sodium hydroxide VS
= 4.90 mg of H_3PO_4

Phosphorus (V) oxide P_2O_5 [K 8342, Special class]

Phosphotungstic acid See phosphotungstic acid *n*-hydrate.

Phosphotungstic acid *n*-hydrate $P_2O_5.24WO_3.xH_2O$ White to yellowish green, crystals or crystalline powder.

Identification—To 5 mL of a solution (1 in 10) add 1 mL of acidic tin (II) chloride TS, and heat: blue precipitates appear.

Phosphotungstic acid TS Dissolve 1 g of phosphotungstic acid *n*-hydrate in water to make 100 mL.

***o*-Phthalaldehyde** $C_6H_4(CHO)_2$ Light yellow to yellow crystals.

Content: not less than 99%. Assay—Dissolve 1 g of *o*-phthalaldehyde in 10 mL of ethanol (95). Perform the test with 2 μL of this solution as directed in Gas Chromatography *<2.02>* according to the following conditions, and determine each peak area by the automatic integration method.

Content (%) = peak area of *o*-phthalaldehyde/total area of all peaks × 100

Operating conditions

Detector: A thermal conductivity detector.

Column: A glass column 3 mm in inside diameter and 2 m in length, packed with siliceous earth for gas chromatography treated with acid and silane (177 – 250 μm), coated with methyl silicon polymer for gas chromatography in 10%.

Column temperature: A constant temperature of about 180°C.

Carrier gas: Helium.

Flow rate: Adjust so that the retention time of *o*-phthalaldehyde is 3 – 4 minutes.

Time span of measurement: About 7 times as long as the retention time of *o*-phthalaldehyde, beginning after the solvent peak.

Phthalate buffer solution (pH 5.8) Dissolve 100.0 g of potassium hydrogen phthalate in about 800 mL of water, adjust to pH 5.8 with a solution of sodium hydroxide (1 in 2), and add water to make 1000 mL.

Phthalein purple $C_{32}H_{32}N_2O_{12}.xH_2O$ Yellow-white to brown power. Soluble in ethanol (95), and practically insoluble in water.

Sensitivity test—Dissolve 10 mg of phthalein purple in 1 mL of ammonia solution (28), and add water to make 100 mL. To 5 mL of this solution add 95 mL of water, 4 mL of ammonia solution (28), 50 mL of ethanol (95) and 0.1 mL of diluted barium chloride TS (1 in 5): the solution shows a blue-purple color which disappears on the addition of 0.15 mL of 0.1 mol/L disodium dihydrogen ethylenediamine tetraacetate TS.

Phthalic acid $C_8H_6O_4$ Colorless or white crystalline powder. Soluble in methanol and in ethanol (95), sparingly soluble in water, and practically insoluble in chloroform. Melting point: about 200°C (with decomposition).

Content: not less than 98%. Assay—Weigh accurately about 2.8 g of phthalic acid, add exactly 50 mL of 1 mol/L sodium hydroxide VS and 25 mL of water, and dissolve by heating on a hot plate. After cooling, add 5 drops of phenolphthalein TS, and titrate the excess sodium hydroxide with 0.5 mol/L sulfuric acid VS. Perform a blank determination in the same manner, and make any necessary correction.

Each mL of 1 mol/L sodium hydroxide VS
= 83.07 mg of $C_8H_6O_4$

Phthalic anhydride $C_8H_4O_3$ White, crystals or crystalline powder.

Melting point <2.60>: 131 – 134°C

Phthalimide $C_8H_5NO_2$ White to pale brown, crystals or powder.

Melting point <2.60>: 232 – 237°C

Purity Clarity—1.0 g of phthalimide dissolves in 20 mL of sodium hydroxide TS as a slight turbid solution.

Content: not less than 98.0%. Assay—Weigh accurately about 0.3 g of the substance to be tested, dissolve in 40 mL of *N,N*-dimethylformamide, and titrate <2.50> with 0.1 mol/L sodium methoxide VS (potentiometric titration). Perform a blank determination in the same manner, and make any necessary correction.

Each mL of 0.1 mol/L sodium methoxide VS
= 14.71 mg of $C_8H_5NO_2$

Phytonadione $C_{31}H_{46}O_2$ [Same as the namesake monograph]

Picric acid See 2,4,6-trinitrophenol.

Picric acid-ethanol TS See 2,4,6-trinitrophenol-ethanol TS.

Picric acid TS See 2,4,6-trinitrophenol TS.

Picric acid TS, alkaline See 2,4,6-trinitrophenol TS, alkaline.

Pig bile powder for thin-layer chromatography A yellow-gray to yellow-brown powder, having a characteristic odor and a bitter taste. It is practically insoluble in water, in methanol and in ethanol (99.5).

Identification—To 0.1 g of pig bile powder for thin-layer chromatography in a screw-capped test tube, add 1 mL of sodium hydroxide solution (3 in 25), and shake. Heat the tube in an oil bath at 120°C for 4 hours, allow to cool to a lukewarm temperature, add 2 mL of 3 mol/L hydrochloric acid TS and 2 mL of ethyl acetate, shake at 50°C for 30 minutes, and separate ethyl acetate layer as the sample solution. Separately, dissolve 10 mg of hyodeoxycholic acid for thin-layer chromatography in 5 mL of methanol, and use this solution as the standard solution. Perform the test with these solutions as directed under Thin-layer Chromatography <2.03>. Spot 2 μL each of the sample solution and standard solution on a plate of silica gel for thin-layer chromatography. Develop the plate with a mixture of chloroform, acetone and acetic acid (100) (7:2:1) to a distance of about 10 cm, and air-dry the plate. Spray evenly dilute sulfuric acid on the plate, and heat the plate at 105°C for 10 minutes: one of the several spots obtained from the sample solution shows the same color tone and the same *Rf* value as the spot from the standard solution.

Pilocarpine hydrochloride for assay $C_{11}H_{16}N_2O_2.HCl$ [Same as the monograph Pilocarpine Hydrochloride. It meets the following additional requirements.]

Purity Related substances—Dissolve 40 mg of pilocarpine hydrochloride for assay in 100 mL of phosphate buffer solution (pH 4.0) and use this solution as the sample solution. Pipet 1 mL of the sample solution, add phosphate buffer solution (pH 4.0) to make exactly 100 mL, and use this solution as the standard solution. Perform the test with exactly 10 μL each of the sample solution and standard solution as directed under Liquid Chromatography <2.01> according to the following conditions, and determine each peak area by the automatic integration method: the area of the peaks, having the relative retention time of about 0.78 and about 0.92 to pilocarpine obtained from the sample solution, is not larger than 1/2 times the peak area of pilocarpine from the standard solution, the area of the peak, other than pilocarpine and the peaks mentioned above from the sample solution, is not larger than 1/5 times the peak area of pilocarpine from the standard solution, and the total area of the peaks other than pilocarpine from the sample solution is not larger than the peak area of pilocarpine from the standard solution.

Operating conditions

Detector, column, column temperature, mobile phase, and flow rate: Proceed as directed in the operating conditions in the Assay under Pilocarpine Hydrochloride Tablets.

Time span of measurement: About 1.3 times as long as the retention time of pilocarpine, beginning after the solvent peak.

System suitability

Proceed as directed in the system suitability in the Purity under Pilocarpine Hydrochloride Tablets.

Pilsicainide hydrochloride hydrate for assay $C_{17}H_{24}N_2O.HCl.½H_2O$ [Same as the monograph Pilsicainide Hydrochloride Hydrate. It contains not less than 99.3% of pilsicainide hydrochloride hydrate ($C_{17}H_{24}N_2O.HCl.½H_2O$).]

Piperacillin hydrate $C_{23}H_{27}N_5O_7S.H_2O$ [Same as the namesake monograph]

Piperidine hydrochloride $C_5H_{11}N.HCl$ A white crystalline powder. Dissolves in water and in methanol. The pH of a solution of 1.0 g of piperidine hydrochloride in 20 mL of water is between 3.0 and 5.0.

Melting point <2.60>: 247 – 252°C

Purity Clarity and color of solution—Dissolve 1.0 g of piperidine hydrochloride in 20 mL of water: the solution is clear and colorless.

Residue on ignition <2.44>: not more than 0.1% (1 g).

Content: not less than 99.0%. Assay—Dissolve about 0.25 g of piperidine hydrochloride, accurately weighed, in 50 mL of water, add 5 mL of diluted nitric acid (1 in 3), and titrate <2.50> with 0.1 mol/L silver nitrate VS (potentiometric titration). Perform a blank determination in the same manner, and make any necessary correction.

Each mL of 0.1 mol/L silver nitrate VS
= 12.16 mg of $C_5H_{11}N.HCl$

Plantago seed for thin-layer chromatography [Same as the monograph Plantago Seed meeting the following additional specifications.]

Identification (1) To 1 g of pulverized plantago seed for thin-layer chromatography add 3 mL of methanol, and warm on a water bath for 3 minutes. After cooling, centrifuge, and use the supernatant liquid as the sample solution. Perform the test with the sample solution as directed under Thin-layer Chromatography *<2.03>*. Spot 10 μL of the sample solution on a plate of silica gel for thin-layer chromatography. Develop the plate with a mixture of acetone, ethyl acetate, water and acetic acid (100) (10:10:3:1) to a distance of about 10 cm, and air-dry the plate. Spray evenly 4-methoxybenzaldehyde-sulfuric acid TS on the plate, heat the plate at 105°C for 10 minutes: spots equivalent to those described below appear.

Rf value	Color and shape of the spot
Around 0	A strong spot, very dark blue
Around 0.08	A very dark blue spot
Around 0.1 - 0.2	A leading spot, very dark blue
Around 0.25	A strong spot, deep blue (corresponding to plantagoguanidinic acid)
Around 0.35	A strong spot, dark grayish blue (corresponding to geniposidic acid)
Around 0.45	A weak spot, grayish yellowish green
Around 0.50	A strong spot, deep yellow-green (corresponding to verbascoside)
Around 0.6	A weak spot, light blue
Around 0.85	A deep blue spot
Around 0.9 - 0.95	A tailing spot, grayish blue

(2) Proceed with the sample solution and the standard solution obtained under (1) as directed in the method under (1), except using a mixture of ethyl acetate, water and formic acid (6:1:1) as developing solvent: spots equivalent to those described below appear.

Rf value	Color and shape of the spot
Around 0	A yellow-greenish dark gray spot
Around 0.05	A weak spot, dark grayish yellow-green
Around 0.2	A weak spot, dark green
Around 0.25	A strong spot, dark reddish purple (corresponding to geniposidic acid)
Around 0.35	A weak spot, bright blue
Around 0.4 - 0.45	A weak tailing spot, dull greenish blue
Around 0.45	A strong spot, deep yellow-green (corresponding to verbascoside)
Around 0.5	A strong spot, deep blue (corresponding to plantagoguanidinic acid)
Around 0.95	A strong spot, dark grayish blue-green
Around 0.97	A dark grayish blue-green spot

Platycodin D for thin-layer chromatography $C_{57}H_{92}O_{28}$ A white powder. Freely soluble in methanol.

Identification Determine the infrared absorption spectrum of platycodin D for thin-layer chromatography as directed in the potassium bromide disk method under Infrared Spectrophotometry *<2.25>*: it exhibits absorption at the wave numbers of about 1734 cm^{-1}, 1637 cm^{-1}, 1385 cm^{-1}, 825 cm^{-1} and 783 cm^{-1}.

Purity Related substances—Dissolve 2 mg of platycodin D for thin-layer chromatography in 2 mL of methanol, and use this solution as the sample solution. Pipet 1 mL of the sample solution, add methanol to make exactly 50 mL, and use this solution as the standard solution. Perform the test with these solutions as directed under Thin-layer Chromatography *<2.03>*. Spot 5 μL each of the sample solution and standard solution on a plate of silica gel for thin-layer chromatography. Develop the plate with a mixture of 1-propanol, ethyl acetate, water and acetic acid (100) (5:3:2:1) to a distance of about 10 cm, and air-dry the plate. Spray dilute sulfuric acid on the plate, and heat the plate at 105°C for 10 minutes: the spots other than the principal spot with an *Rf* value of about 0.5 obtained from the sample solution are not more intense than the spot from the standard solution.

Platycodon Root [Same as the namesake monograph.]

Polyacrylamide gel for epoetin alfa A polyacrylamide gel composed with the resolving gel 12.5% in acrylamide concentration.

Polyacrylamide gel for filgrastim A polyacrylamide gel composed with the resolving gel 15% in acrylamide concentration.

Polyacrylamide gel for nartograstim A polyacrylamide gel composed with the resolving gel 14% in acrylamide concentration.

Polyalkylene glycol for gas chromatography Prepared for gas chromatography.

Polyalkylene glycol monoether for gas chromatography Prepared for gas chromatography.

Polyethylene glycol 15000-diepoxide for gas chromatography Prepared for gas chromatography.

Polyethylene glycol ester for gas chromatography Prepared for gas chromatography.

Polyethylene glycol 20 M for gas chromatography Prepared for gas chromatography.

Polyethylene glycol 400 for gas chromatography Prepared for gas chromatography.

Polyethylene glycol 600 for gas chromatography Prepared for gas chromatography.

Polyethylene glycol 1500 for gas chromatography Prepared for gas chromatography.

Polyethylene glycol 6000 for gas chromatography Prepared for gas chromatography.

Polyethylene glycol 2-nitroterephthalate for gas chromatography Prepared for gas chromatography.

Polygala root [Same as the namesake monograph]

Polymethyl acrylate for gas chromatography Prepared for gas chromatography.

Polymethylsiloxane for gas chromatography Prepared for gas chromatography.

Polyoxyethylene hydrogenated castor oil 60 A nonionic surfactant prepared by addition polymerization of ethylene oxide with hydrogenated castor oil. Average molar number of ethylene oxide added is about 60. A white or pale yellow petrolatum-like or waxy substance, having a faint, characteristic odor and a slight bitter taste. Very soluble in ethyl acetate and in chloroform, freely soluble in ethanol (95), slightly soluble in water, and practically insoluble in diethyl ether.

Identification (1) To 0.5 g of polyoxyethylene hydrogenated castor oil 60 add 10 mL of water and 5 mL of ammonium thiocyanate-cobalt (II) nitrate TS, and shake thoroughly. Add 5 mL of chloroform, shake, and allow to stand: a blue color develops in the chloroform layer.

(2) To 0.2 g of polyoxyethylene hydrogenated castor oil 60 add 0.5 g of potassium bisulfate, and heat: an acrolein-like, irritating odor is perceptible.

(3) To 0.5 g of polyoxyethylene hydrogenated castor oil 60 add 10 mL of water, shake, and add 5 drops of bromine TS: the color of the test solution does not disappear.

Congealing point <*2.42*>: 30 – 34°C

pH <*2.54*>—To 1.0 g of polyoxyethylene hydrogenated castor oil 60 add 20 mL of water, and dissolve by heating: the pH of the solution is between 3.6 and 6.0.

Acid value <*1.13*>: not more than 1.0.

Saponification value <*1.13*>: 41 – 51

Hydroxyl value <*1.13*>: 39 – 49

Purity (1) Clarity and color of solution—Dissolve 1.0 g of polyoxyethylene hydrogenated castor oil 60 in 20 mL of ethanol (95): the solution is clear and colorless.

(2) Heavy metals <*1.07*>—Proceed with 1.0 g of polyoxyethylene hydrogenated castor oil 60 according to Method 2, and perform the test. Prepare the control solution with 2.0 mL of Standard Lead Solution (not more than 20 ppm).

(3) Arsenic <*1.11*>—Prepare the test solution with 1.0 g of polyoxyethylene hydrogenated castor oil 60 according to Method 3, and perform the test (not more than 2 ppm).

Water <*2.48*>: not more than 2.0% (1 g).

Residue on ignition <*2.44*>: not more than 0.1% (1 g).

Storage—Preserve in tight containers.

Polyoxyethylene (23) lauryl ether $C_{12}H_{25}(OCH_2CH_2)_nOH$ White masses. Melting point: about 40°C.

Polyoxyethylene (40) octylphenyl ether Obtained by the addition polymerization with ethylene oxide to octylphenol. A colorless or white to pale yellow, liquid, vaseline-like or waxy, having slightly a characteristic odor.

pH <*2.54*>: 7.0 – 9.5 (5 w/v%, 25°C).

Specific gravity <*2.56*> d_4^{25}: 1.10 – 1.11

Purity Clarity of solution—Dissolve 1.0 g of polyoxyethylene (40) octylphenyl ether in 20 mL of water: the solution is clear.

Polysorbate 20 Chiefly consists of addition polymer of sorbitan monolaurate and ethylene oxide. Pale yellow to yellow liquid, having a faint, characteristic odor.

Identification (1) To 0.5 g of polysorbate 20 add 10 mL of water and 10 mL of sodium hydroxide TS, boil for 5 minutes, and acidify with dilute hydrochloric acid: an oily fraction is separated.

(2) To 0.5 g of polysorbate 20 add 10 mL of water, shake, and add 5 drops of bromine TS: the red color of the test solution does not disappear.

(3) Place 0.1 g of polysorbate 20 in a flask, dissolve in 2 mL of a solution of sodium hydroxide in methanol (1 in 50), and heat under a reflux condenser for 30 minutes. Add 2 mL of boron trifluoride-methanol TS through the condenser, and heat for 30 minutes. Then, add 4 mL of heptane through the condenser, and heat for 5 minutes. After cooling, add 10 mL of saturated sodium chloride solution, shake for about 15 seconds, then add sufficient saturated sodium chloride solution such that the upper layer of the content reaches the neck of the flask. Take 2 mL of the upper layer, wash 3 times with each 2-mL portion of water, dry with anhydrous sodium sulfate, and use this solution as the sample solution. Separately, dissolve 50 mg of methyl laurate for gas chromatography, 50 mg of methyl palmitate for gas chromatography, 80 mg of methyl stearate for gas chromatography and 100 mg of methyl oleate for gas chromatography in heptane to make 50 mL, and use this solution as the standard solution. Perform the test with 1 μL each of the sample solution and standard solution as directed under Gas Chromatography <*2.02*> according to the following conditions: the retention time of the principal peak obtained from the sample solution is the same with that of the peak of methyl laurate from the standard solution.

Operating conditions

Detector: A hydrogen flame-ionization detector.

Column: A fused silica column 0.25 mm in inside diameter and 30 m in length, coated the inside surface with polyethylene glycol 20 M for gas chromatography 0.5 μm in thickness.

Column temperature: Inject at a constant temperature of 80°C, raise the temperature at the rate of 10°C per minute to 220°C, and maintain the temperature at 220°C for 40 minutes.

Injection port temperature: A constant temperature of about 250°C.

Detector temperature: A constant temperature of about 250°C.

Carrier gas: Helium.

Flow rate: Adjust so that the retention time of the peak of methyl laurate is about 10 minutes.

Split ratio: 1:50.

System suitability

System performance: When the procedure is run with 1 μL of the standard solution under the above operating conditions, methyl laurate, methyl palmitate, methyl stearate and methyl oleate are eluted in this order, and the resolution between the peaks of methyl stearate and methyl oleate is not less than 2.0.

Acid value <*1.13*>: not more than 4.0.

Saponification value <*1.13*>: 43 – 55

Loss on drying <*2.41*>: not more than 3.0% (5 g, 105°C, 1 hour).

Residue on ignition—Weigh accurately about 3 g of polysorbate 20, heat gently at first, and ignite gradually (800 – 1200°C) until the residue is completely incinerated. If any carbonized substance remains, extract with hot water, filter through a filter paper for quantitative analysis (5C), and ignite the residue with the filter paper. Add the filtrate to it, evaporate to dryness, and ignite carefully until the carbonized substance does not remain. If any carbonized substance still remains, add 15 mL of ethanol (95), crush the carbonized substance with a glass rod, burn the ethanol, and ignite carefully. Cool in a desiccator (silica gel), and weigh the residue accurately: not more than 1.0%.

Polysorbate 20 for epoetin beta A clear to slightly turbid, yellow-brown liquid.

Viscosity <*2.53*>: 300 – 500 mPa·s

Acid value <*1.13*>: not more than 3.

Saponification value <*1.13*>: 40 – 50

Hydroxyl value <*1.13*>: 95 – 110

Water <*2.48*>: not more than 5.0%.

Polysorbate 80 [Same as the namesake monograph].

Polyvinyl alcohol $(-CH_2CHOH-)_n$ [K 9550, Special class]

Polyvinyl alcohol I Colorless to white or pale yellow, granules or powder. It is odorless, or has a faint odor of acetic acid. It is tasteless. Practically insoluble in ethanol (95) and in diethyl ether. To polyvinyl alcohol I add water, and heat: a clear, viscous solution is obtained. Polyvinyl alcohol I is hygroscopic.

Viscosity 〈*2.53*〉 25.0 - 31.0 mm^2/s. Weigh 4.000 g of polyvinyl alcohol I, previously dried, add 95 mL of water, allow to stand for 30 minutes, and heat to dissolve on a water bath under a reflux condenser for 2 hours while stirring. After cooling, add water to make 100.0 g, and mix. Allow to stand still to remove bubbles, and perform the test at 20 ± 0.1°C as directed in Method 1.

pH 〈*2.54*〉—The pH of a solution of 1.0 g of polyvinyl alcohol I in 25 mL of water is between 5.0 and 8.0.

Purity Clarity and color of solution—To 20 mL of water add 1.0 g of polyvinyl alcohol I, disperse by thorough stirring, warm between 60°C and 80°C for 2 hours, and cool: the solution is clear and colorless.

Saponification value 98.0 - 99.0 mol%. Weigh accurately about 3.0 g of polyvinyl alcohol I, previously dried, transfer to a glass-stoppered conical flask, add 100 mL of water, and dissolve by heating on a water bath. After cooling, add exactly 25 mL of 0.1 mol/L sodium hydroxide VS, stopper tightly, and allow to stand for 2 hours. Then add exactly 30 mL of 0.05 mol/L sulfuric acid VS, shake thoroughly, and titrate 〈*2.50*〉 with 0.1 mol/L sodium hydroxide VS (indicator: 3 drops of phenolphthalein TS). Perform a blank determination in the same manner, and make any necessary correction. However, when the volume of 0.1 mol/L sodium hydroxide VS consumed in the test is 25 mL or more, use about 2.0 g of the sample.

$$\text{Saponification value (mol\%)} = 100 - \frac{44.05A}{60.05 - 0.42A}$$

$$A = \frac{0.6005 \times (a - b)}{\text{amount (g) of polyvinyl alcohol I taken}}$$

a: Volume (mL) of 0.1 mol/L sodium hydroxide VS consumed in the test

b: Volume (mL) of 0.1 mol/L sodium hydroxide VS consumed in the blank test

Polyvinyl alcohol II Colorless to white or pale yellow, granules or powder. It is odorless, or has a faint odor of acetic acid. It is tasteless. Practically insoluble in ethanol (95) and in diethyl ether. To polyvinyl alcohol II add water, and heat: a clear, viscous solution is obtained. Polyvinyl alcohol II is hygroscopic.

Viscosity 〈*2.53*〉 4.6 - 5.4 mm^2/s. Weigh 4.000 g of polyvinyl alcohol II, previously dried, add 95 mL of water, allow to stand for 30 minutes, and dissolve by stirring on a water bath between 60°C and 80°C for 2 hours. After cooling, add water to make 100.0 g, and mix. Allow to stand still to remove bubbles, and perform the test at 20 ± 0.1°C as directed in Method 1.

pH 〈*2.54*〉—The pH of a solution of 1.0 g of polyvinyl alcohol II in 25 mL of water is between 5.0 and 8.0.

Purity Clarity and color of solution—To 20 mL of water add 1.0 g of polyvinyl alcohol II, disperse by thorough stirring, heat on a water bath for 2 hours, and cool: the solution is clear and colorless.

Saponification value 86.5 - 89.5 mol%. Weigh accurately about 2 g of polyvinyl alcohol II, previously dried, transfer to a glass-stoppered conical flask, add 100 mL of water, and warm while stirring for 2 hours. After cooling, add exactly 25 mL of 0.5 mol/L sodium hydroxide VS, stopper tightly, and allow to stand for 2 hours. Then add exactly 30 mL of 0.25 mol/L sulfuric acid VS, shake thoroughly, and titrate 〈*2.50*〉 with 0.5 mol/L sodium hydroxide VS (indicator: 3 drops of phenolphthalein TS). Perform a blank determination in the same manner, and make any necessary correction.

$$\text{Saponification value (mol\%)} = 100 - \frac{44.05A}{60.05 - 0.42A}$$

$$A = \frac{3.0025 \times (a - b)}{\text{amount (g) of polyvinyl alcohol II taken}}$$

a: Volume (mL) of 0.5 mol/L sodium hydroxide VS consumed in the test

b: Volume (mL) of 0.5 mol/L sodium hydroxide VS consumed in the blank test

Polyvinyl alcohol TS Weigh exactly 0.50 g of polyvinyl alcohol, and add water to make exactly 100 mL.

Polyvinylidene fluoride membrane For Western blotting.

Potassium acetate CH_3COOK [K 8363, Special class]

Potassium acetate TS Dissolve 10 g of potassium acetate in water to make 100 mL (1 mol/L).

Potassium aluminum sulfate See aluminum potassium sulfate dodecahydrate.

Potassium bicarbonate See potassium hydrogen carbonate.

Potassium biphthalate See potassium hydrogen phthalate.

Potassium biphthalate buffer solution (pH 3.5) See potassium hydrogen phthalate buffer solution (pH 3.5).

Potassium biphthalate buffer solution (pH 4.6) See potassium hydrogen phthalate buffer solution (pH 4.6).

Potassium biphthalate buffer solution (pH 5.6) See potassium hydrogen phthalate buffer solution (pH 5.6).

Potassium biphthalate for pH determination See potassium hydrogen phthalate for pH determination.

Potassium biphthalate (standard reagent) See potassium hydrogen phthalate (standard reagent).

0.2 mol/L Potassium biphthalate TS for buffer solution See 0.2 mol/L potassium hydrogen phthalate TS for buffer solution.

Potassium bisulfate See potassium hydrogen sulfate.

Potassium bromate $KBrO_3$ [K 8530, Special class]

Potassium bromide KBr [K 8506, Special class]

Potassium bromide for infrared spectrophotometry Crush homocrystals of potassium bromide or potassium bromide, collect a powder passed through a No. 200 (75 μm) sieve, and dry at 120°C for 10 hours or at 500°C for 5 hours. Prepare tablets with this powder, and determine the infrared absorption spectrum 〈*2.25*〉: any abnormal absorption does not appear.

Potassium carbonate K_2CO_3 [K 8615, Special class]

Potassium carbonate, anhydrous See potassium carbonate.

Potassium carbonate-sodium carbonate TS Dissolve

1.7 g of potassium carbonate and 1.3 g of anhydrous sodium carbonate in water to make 100 mL.

Potassium chlorate $KClO_3$ [K 8207, Special class]

Potassium chloride KCl [K 8121, Special class]

Potassium chloride for assay KCl [Same as the monograph, Potassium Chloride]

Potassium chloride for conductivity measurement [K 8121, Potassium chloride for conductivity measurement]

Potassium chloride for infrared spectrophotometry Crush homocrystals of potassium chloride or potassium chloride, collect the powder passed through a No. 200 (75 μm) sieve, and dry at 120°C for 10 hours or at 500°C for 5 hours. Prepare tablets with this powder, and determine the infrared absorption spectrum <2.25>: any abnormal absorption does not appear.

Potassium chloride-hydrochloric acid buffer solution To 250 mL of a solution of potassium chloride (3 in 20) add 53 mL of 2 mol/L hydrochloric acid TS and water to make 1000 mL.

Potassium chloride TS, acidic Dissolve 250 g of potassium chloride in water to make 1000 mL, and add 8.5 mL of hydrochloric acid.

0.2 mol/L Potassium chloride TS Dissolve 14.9 g of potassium chloride in water to make 1000 mL. Prepare before use.

Potassium chromate K_2CrO_4 [K 8312, Special class]

Potassium chromate TS Dissolve 10 g of potassium chromate in water to make 100 mL.

Potassium cyanide KCN [K 8443, Special class]

Potassium cyanide TS Dissolve 1 g of potassium cyanide in water to make 10 mL. Prepare before use.

Potassium dichromate $K_2Cr_2O_7$ [K 8517, Special class]

Potassium dichromate (standard reagent) $K_2Cr_2O_7$ In addition to JIS K 8005 standard reagent for volumetric analysis, certified reference material which can be used for volumetric analysis may be used.

Potassium dichromate-sulfuric acid TS Dissolve 0.5 g of potassium dichromate in diluted sulfuric acid (1 in 5) to make 100 mL.

Potassium dichromate TS Dissolve 7.5 g of potassium dichromate in water to make 100 mL.

Potassium dihydrogen phosphate KH_2PO_4 [K 9007, Special class]

Potassium dihydrogen phosphate for pH determination KH_2PO_4 [K 9007, for pH determination]

0.1 mol/L Potassium dihydrogen phosphate TS (pH 2.0) Dissolve 13.6 g of potassium dihydrogen phosphate in water to make 1000 mL. Adjust the pH to 2.0 with phosphoric acid.

0.05 mol/L Potassium dihydrogen phosphate (pH 3.0) Adjust the pH of 0.05 mol/L potassium dihydrogen phosphate TS to 3.0 with phosphoric acid.

0.25 mol/L Potassium dihydrogen phosphate TS (pH 3.5) Dissolve 34 g of potassium dihydrogen phosphate in 900 mL of water, adjust the pH to 3.5 with phosphoric acid, and add water to make 1000 mL.

0.01 mol/L Potassium dihydrogen phosphate TS (pH 4.0) Dissolve 1.4 g of potassium dihydrogen phosphate in 1000 mL of water, and adjust the pH to 4.0 with phosphoric acid.

0.05 mol/L Potassium dihydrogen phosphate TS (pH 4.7) Dissolve 6.80 g of potassium dihydrogen phosphate in 900 mL of water, adjust the pH to exactly 4.7 with dilute sodium hydrochloride TS, and add water to make 1000 mL.

0.02 mol/L Potassium dihydrogen phosphate TS Dissolve 2.72 g of potassium dihydrogen phosphate in water to make 1000 mL.

0.05 mol/L Potassium dihydrogen phosphate TS Dissolve 6.80 g of potassium dihydrogen phosphate in water to make 1000 mL.

0.33 mol/L Potassium dihydrogen phosphate TS Dissolve 4.491 g of potassium dihydrogen phosphate in water to make 100 mL.

0.1 mol/L Potassium dihydrogen phosphate TS Dissolve 13.61 g of potassium dihydrogen phosphate in water to make 1000 mL.

0.2 mol/L Potassium dihydrogen phosphate TS Dissolve 27.22 g of potassium dihydrogen phosphate in water to make 1000 mL.

0.2 mol/L Potassium dihydrogen phosphate TS for buffer solution Dissolve 27.218 g of potassium dihydrogen phosphate for pH determination in water to make 1000 mL.

Potassium disulfate $K_2S_2O_7$ [K 8783, Special class]

Potassium ferricyanide See potassium hexacyanoferrate (III).

Potassium ferricyanide TS See potassium hexacyanoferrate (III) TS.

Potassium ferricyanide TS, alkaline See potassium hexacyanoferrate (III) TS, alkaline.

Potassium ferrocyanide See potassium hexacyanoferrate (II) trihydrate.

Potassium ferrocyanide TS See potassium hexacyanoferrate (II) TS.

Potassium guaiacolsulfonate $C_7H_7KO_5S$ [Same as the namesake monograph]

Potassium hexacyanoferrate (II) trihydrate $K_4Fe(CN)_6.3H_2O$ [K 8802, Special class]

Potassium hexacyanoferrate (II) TS Dissolve 1 g of potassium hexacyanoferrate (II) trihydrate in water to make 10 mL (0.25 mol/L). Prepare before use.

Potassium hexacyanoferrate (III) $K_3Fe(CN)_6$ [K 8801, Special class]

Potassium hexacyanoferrate (III) TS Dissolve 1 g of potassium hexacyanoferrate (III) in water to make 10 mL (0.3 mol/L). Prepare before use.

Potassium hexacyanoferrate (III) TS, alkaline Dissolve 1.65 g of potassium hexacyanoferrate (III) and 10.6 g of anhydrous sodium carbonate in water to make 1000 mL. Preserve in light-resistant containers.

Potassium hexahydroxoantimonate (V) $K[Sb(OH)_6]$ White, granules or crystalline powder.

Identification—To 1 g add 100 mL of water, and dissolve by warming. To 20 mL of this solution add 0.2 mL of sodium chloride TS: white precipitates appear. Rubbing the inside wall of the vessel with a glass rod accelerates the forming of the precipitates.

Potassium hexahydroxoantimonate (V) TS To 2 g of potassium hexahydroxoantimonate (V) add 100 mL of water. Boil the solution for about 5 minutes, cool quickly, add 10 mL of a solution of potassium hydroxide (3 in 20), allow to stand for 1 day, and filter.

Potassium hydrogen carbonate $KHCO_3$ [K 8621, Special class]

Potassium hydrogen phthalate $C_6H_4(COOK)(COOH)$ [K 8809, Special class]

Potassium hydrogen phthalate (standard reagent) $C_6H_4(COOK)(COOH)$ In addition to JIS K 8005 standard reagent for volumetric analysis, certified reference material which can be used for volumetric analysis may be used.

Potassium hydrogen phthalate buffer solution (pH 3.5) Dilute 50 mL of 0.2 mol/L potassium hydrogen phthalate TS for buffer solution and 7.97 mL of 0.2 mol/L hydrochloric acid VS with water to make 200 mL.

Potassium hydrogen phthalate buffer solution (pH 4.6) Dilute 50 mL of 0.2 mol/L potassium hydrogen phthalate TS for buffer solution and 12.0 mL of 0.2 mol/L sodium hydroxide VS with water to make 200 mL.

0.3 mol/L Potassium hydrogen phthalate buffer solution (pH 4.6) Dissolve 61.26 g of potassium hydrogen phthalate in about 800 mL of water, adjust the pH to 4.6 with sodium hydroxide TS, and add water to make 1000 mL.

Potassium hydrogen phthalate buffer solution (pH 5.6) Dilute 50 mL of 0.2 mol/L potassium hydrogen phthalate TS for buffer solution and 39.7 mL of 0.2 mol/L sodium hydroxide VS with water to make 200 mL.

Potassium hydrogen phthalate for pH determination $C_6H_4(COOK)(COOH)$ [K 8809, For pH determination]

0.2 mol/L Potassium hydrogen phthalate TS for buffer solution Dissolve 40.843 g of potassium hydrogen phthalate for pH determination in water to make 1000 mL.

Potassium hydrogen sulfate $KHSO_4$ [K 8972, Special class]

Potassium hydroxide KOH [K 8574, Special class]

Potassium hydroxide-ethanol TS Dissolve 10 g of potassium hydroxide in ethanol (95) to make 100 mL. Prepare before use.

0.1 mol/L Potassium hydroxide-ethanol TS To 1 mL of dilute potassium hydroxide-ethanol TS add ethanol (95) to make 5 mL. Prepare before use.

Potassium hydroxide-ethanol TS, dilute Dissolve 35 g of potassium hydroxide in 20 mL of water, and add ethanol (95) to make 1000 mL (0.5 mol/L). Preserve in tightly stoppered bottles.

Potassium hydroxide TS Dissolve 6.5 g of potassium hydroxide in water to make 100 mL (1 mol/L). Preserve in polyethylene bottles.

0.02 mol/L Potassium hydroxide TS Dilute 2 mL of potassium hydroxide TS with water to make 100 mL. Prepare before use.

0.05 mol/L Potassium hydroxide TS Dilute 5 mL of potassium hydroxide TS with water to make 100 mL. Prepare before use.

8 mol/L Potassium hydroxide TS Dissolve 52 g of potassium hydroxide in water to make 100 mL. Preserve in polyethylene bottles.

Potassium iodate KIO_3 [K 8922, Special class]

Potassium iodate (standard reagent) KIO_3 In addition to JIS K 8005 standard reagent for volumetric analysis, certified reference material which can be used for volumetric analysis may be used.

Potassium iodide KI [K 8913, Special class]

Potassium iodide for assay [Same as the monograph Potassium Iodide]

Potassium iodide-starch TS Dissolve 0.5 g of potassium iodide in 100 mL of freshly prepared starch TS. Prepare before use.

Potassium iodide TS Dissolve 16.5 g of potassium iodide in water to make 100 mL. Preserve in light-resistant containers. Prepare before use (1 mol/L).

Potassium iodide TS, concentrated Dissolve 30 g of potassium iodide in 70 mL of water. Prepare before use.
Storage—Preserve in light-resistant containers.

Potassium iodide TS, saturated Saturate 20 g of potassium iodide in 10 mL of fleshly boiled and cooled water. Prepare before use.

Potassium iodide-zinc sulfate TS Dissolve 5 g of potassium iodide, 10 g of zinc sulfate heptahydrate, and 50 g of sodium chloride in water to make 200 mL.

Potassium methanesulfonate CH_3SO_3K White, crystals or crystalline powder.
Purity Clarity and color of solution—Dissolve 1.0 g of potassium methanesulfonate in 20 mL of water: the solution is transparent and colorless.
Content: not less than 98.0%. Assay—Dissolve about 0.1 g of potassium methanesulfonate, accurately weighed, in 10 mL of acetic acid (100), add 20 mL of acetic anhydride, and titrate *<2.50>* with 0.1 mol/L perchloric acid VS (potentiometric titration). Perform a blank determination in the same manner, and make any necessary correction.

Each mL of 0.1 mol/L perchloric acid VS
= 13.42 mg of CH_3SO_3K

Potassium naphthoquinone sulfonate See potassium 1,2-naphthoquinone-4-sulfonate.

Potassium 1,2-naphthoquinone-4-sulfonate $C_{10}H_5O_2SO_3K$ [K 8696, Special class]

Potassium 1,2-naphthoquinone-4-sulfonate TS Dissolve 0.5 g of potassium 1,2-naphthoquinone-4-sulfonate in water to make 100 mL. Prepare before use.

Potassium nitrate KNO_3 [K 8548, Special class]

Potassium nitrite KNO_2 A white to pale yellow crystalline powder. It is deliquescent.
Identification—(1) Dissolve 1 g of potassium nitrite in 20 mL of water, and use this solution as the sample solution. To 5 mL of the sample solution add 1 mL of sulfuric acid: a yellow-brown gas is evolved.
(2) The sample solution obtained in (1) responds to Qualitative Tests *<1.09>* (1) for potassium salt.
Storage—Preserve in a light-resistant tight container.

Potassium periodate KIO_4 [K 8249, Special class]

Potassium periodate TS To 2.8 g of potassium periodate

add 200 mL of water, dissolve by adding dropwise 20 mL of sulfuric acid under shaking, cool, and add water to make 1000 mL.

1.6% Potassium periodate-0.2% potassium permanganate TS, alkaline Dissolve 1 g of potassium permanganate, 8 g of potassium periodate and 10 g of potassium carbonate in 500 mL of water. After allowing to stand for 16 hours, filter through a filter paper.

Potassium permanganate $KMnO_4$ [K 8247, Special class]

Potassium permanganate TS Dissolve 3.3 g of potassium permanganate in water to make 1000 mL (0.02 mol/L).

Potassium permanganate TS, acidic To 100 mL of potassium permanganate TS add 0.3 mL of sulfuric acid.

Potassium peroxodisulfate $K_2S_2O_8$ [K 8253, Special class]

Potassium persulfate See potassium peroxodisulfate.

Potassium pyroantimonate See potassium hexahydroxoantimonate (V).

Potassium pyroantimonate TS See potassium hexahydroxoantimonate (V) TS.

Potassium pyrophosphate $K_4O_7P_2$ White crystalline powder, very soluble in water. Melting point: 1109°C.

Potassium pyrosulfate See potassium disulfate.

Potassium sodium tartarate See potassium sodium tartarate tetrahydrate.

Potassium sodium tartarate tetrahydrate $KNaC_4H_4O_6.4H_2O$ [K 8536, (+)-Potassium sodium tartrate tetrahydrate, Special class]

Potassium sulfate K_2SO_4 [K 8962, Special class]

Potassium sulfate TS Dissolve 1 g of potassium sulfate in water to make 100 mL.

Potassium tartrate $2C_4H_4K_2O_6.H_2O$ [K 8535, (+)-Potassium Tartrate-Water (2/1), Special class]

Potassium tellurite K_2TeO_3 White, powder or small masses obtained by melting an equimolar mixture of tellurium dioxide and potassium carbonate in a stream of carbon dioxide. Soluble in water.

Content: not less than 90.0%. Assay—Dissolve about 1.0 g of potassium tellurite, accurately weighed, in 100 mL of water, add 5 mL of diluted acetic acid (31) (1 in 3), and boil. After cooling, filter by suction through a crucible glass filter (1G4) [previously dried at 105 ± 2°C for 1 hour to constant mass (*b* (g)]. Wash the filtrate with water, dry the glass filter at 110°C for 3 hours, and measure the mass *a* (g).

Content (%) of potassium tellurite (K_2TeO_3)

$$= \frac{(a - b) \times 1.5902}{S} \times 100$$

S: Amount (g) of potassium tellurite taken

Potassium tetraoxalate for pH determination See potassium trihydrogen dioxalate dihydrate for pH determination.

Potassium tetraphenylborate TS Add 1 mL of acetic acid (31) to 50 mL of a solution of potassium biphthalate (1 in 500), then to this solution add 20 mL of a solution of sodium tetraphenylborate (7 in 1000), shake well, and allow to stand for 1 hour. Collect the produced precipitate on filter paper, and wash it with water. To 1/3 quantity of the precipitate add 100 mL of water, warm, with shaking, at about 50°C for 5 minutes, cool quickly, allow to stand for 2 hours with occasional shaking, and filter, discarding the first 30 mL of the filtrate.

Potassium thiocyanate KSCN [K 9001, Special class]

Potassium thiocyanate TS Dissolve 1 g of potassium thiocyanate in water to make 10 mL.

Potassium trihydrogen dioxalate dihydrate for pH determination $KH_3(C_2O_4)_2.2H_2O$ [K 8474, for pH determination]

Potato extract Prepared for microbial test.

Potato starch [Same as the namesake monograph]

Potato starch TS Prepare as directed under starch TS with 1 g of potato starch.

Potato starch TS for amylolytic activity test Dry about 1 g of potato starch, accurately weighed, at 105°C for 2 hours, and measure the loss. Weigh accurately an amount of potato starch, equivalent to 1.000 g on the dried basis, place into a conical flask, add 20 mL of water, and make it pasty by gradually adding 5 mL of a solution of sodium hydroxide (2 in 25) while shaking well. Heat in a water bath for 3 minutes while shaking, add 25 mL of water, and cool. Neutralize exactly with 2 mol/L hydrochloric acid TS, add 10 mL of 1 mol/L acetic acid-sodium acetate buffer solution (pH 5.0) and add water to make exactly 100 mL. Prepare before use.

Potency measuring medium for nartograstim test Dissolve 10.4 g of RPMI-1640 medium in a suitable amount of water, add 16 mL of sodium hydrogen carbonate solution (3 in 40), then add water to make 1000 mL, adjust to pH 7.0 by passing carbon dioxide through the solution, and sterilize by filtration. To 90 mL of this solution add 10 mL of fetal bovine serum, previously heat at 56°C for 30 minutes, 1 mL of a solution dissolved 1.0×10^5 units of potassium benzylpenicillin and 0.1 g (potency) of streptomycin sulfate in 10 mL of isotonic sodium chloride solution, and add 5 μL of 2-mercaptoethanol solution (9 in 125). Sterilize this solution by filtration.

Potency measuring medium for teceleukin Add 100 mL of fetal calf serum to 1000 mL of medium for float culture. Store at 4°C.

Powdered tragacanth [Same as the namesake monograph]

(±)-Praeruptorin A for thin-layer chromatography $C_{21}H_{22}O_7$ White, crystals or crystalline powder. Soluble in methanol, sparingly slightly soluble in ethanol (99.5), and practically insoluble in water.

Identification—Determine the absorption spectrum of a solution of (±)-praeruptorin A for thin-layer chromatography in methanol (1 in 100,000) as directed under Ultraviolet-visible Spectrophotometry <2.24>: it exhibits a maximum between 320 nm and 324 nm.

Melting point <2.60>: 152 – 156°C

Purity Related substances—Dissolve 2 mg of (±)-praeruptorin A for thin-layer chromatography in 2 mL of methanol, and use this solution as the sample solution. Pipet 1 mL of the sample solution, add methanol to make exactly 100 mL, and use this solution as the standard solution. Proceed with 5 μL each of the sample solution and standard solution as directed in the Identification (1) under Peucedanum

Root: the spot other than the principal spot of around *Rf* value of 0.3 obtained from the sample solution is not more intense than the spot from the standard solution.

Pravastatin sodium $C_{23}H_{35}NaO_7$ [Same as the namesake monograph]

Prazepam for assay $C_{19}H_{17}ClN_2O$ [Same as the monograph Prazepam. When dried, it contains not less than 99.0% of prazepam ($C_{19}H_{17}ClN_2O$).]

Prednisolone $C_{21}H_{28}O_5$ [Same as the namesake monograph]

Prednisolone acetate $C_{23}H_{30}O_6$ [Same as the namesake monograph]

Prednisone $C_{21}H_{26}O_5$ White crystalline powder. Slightly soluble in methanol, in ethanol (95) and in chloroform, and very slightly soluble in water.

Optical rotation <2.49> $[\alpha]_D^{20}$: +167 – +175° (after drying, 0.1 g, 1,4-dioxane, 10 mL, 100 mm).

Loss on drying <2.41>: not more than 1.0% (1 g, 105°C, 3 hours).

Content: 96.0 – 104.0%. Assay—Weigh accurately about 20 mg of prednisone, previously dried, and dissolve in methanol to make exactly 100 mL. Pipet 5 mL of this solution, dilute with methanol to make exactly 100 mL. Perform the test with this solution as directed under Ultraviolet-visible Spectrophotometry <2.24>, and read the absorbance *A* at the wavelength of maximum absorption at about 238 nm.

$$\text{Amount (mg) of prednisone } (C_{21}H_{26}O_5) = \frac{A}{440} \times 20{,}000$$

Primary antibody TS To a mixture of 1.5 mL of blocking TS for epoetin alfa and 13.5 mL of sodium azide-phosphate-buffered sodium chloride TS add a volume of mouse anti-epoetin alfa monoclonal antibody corresponding to 100 μg of protein, 50 μL of a solution of aprotinin containing 1×10^5 units in 5 mL of water and 100 μL of phenylmethylsulfonyl fluoride solution containing 1.74 mg in 100 mL of methanol.

Primer F A primer corresponding to the Alu sequence. Synthesize an oligonucleotide which nucleotide sequence is represented by "5′-CATCCTGGCYAACAYGGTGAAAC-3′", and use.

Primer F TS To primer F add TE buffer solution so that primer F is 100 μmol/L. Then add tris-glycine buffer solution (pH 6.8) so that primer F is 25 μmol/L.

Primer R A primer corresponding to the Alu sequence. Synthesize an oligonucleotide which nucleotide sequence is represented by "5′-ATTCTCCTGCCTCAGCCTCC-3′", and use.

Primer R TS To primer R add TE buffer solution so that primer R is 100 μmol/L. Then, add tris-glycine buffer solution (pH 6.8) so that primer R is 25 μmol/L.

Probenecid $C_{13}H_{19}NO_4S$ [Same as the namesake monograph]

Procainamide hydrochloride $C_{13}H_{21}N_3O.HCl$ [Same as the namesake monograph]

Procainamide hydrochloride for assay $C_{13}H_{21}N_3O.HCl$ [Same as the monograph Procainamide Hydrochloride. When dried, it contains not less than 99.0% of procainamide hydrochloride ($C_{13}H_{21}N_3O.HCl$).]

Procaine hydrochloride $C_{13}H_{20}N_2O_2.HCl$ [Same as the namesake monograph]

Procaine hydrochloride for assay See procaine hydrochloride.

Procaterol hydrochloride See procaterol hydrochloride hydrate.

Procaterol hydrochloride hydrate $C_{16}H_{22}N_2O_3.HCl.\frac{1}{2}H_2O$ [Same as the namesake monograph]

Progesterone $C_{21}H_{30}O_2$ [Same as the namesake monograph]

L-Proline $C_5H_9NO_2$ [K 9107, L(−)-proline, Special class]

Propafenone hydrochloride for assay $C_{21}H_{27}NO_3.HCl$ [Same as the monograph Propafenone Hydrochloride. When dried, it contains not less than 99.0% of propafenone hydrochloride ($C_{21}H_{27}NO_3.HCl$). When perform the test as directed in the Purity (2), the total area of the peaks other than propafenone is not larger than 3 times the peak area of propafenone from the standard solution.]

***n*-Propanol** See 1-propanol.

1-Propanol $CH_3CH_2CH_2OH$ [K 8838, Special class]

2-Propanol $(CH_3)_2CHOH$ [K 8839, Special class]

2-Propanol for vitamin A assay $(CH_3)_2CHOH$ [K 8839, Special class] When the absorbances at 300 nm and between 320 nm and 350 nm are determined as directed under Ultraviolet-visible Spectrophotometry <2.24>, using water as the control, they are not more than 0.05 and not more than 0.01, respectively. If necessary, purify by distillation.

2-Propanol for liquid chromatography $(CH_3)_2CHOH$ Clear, colorless and volatile liquid, having a characteristic odor. Miscible with water, with ethanol (95) and with diethyl ether. Boiling point: about 82°C.

Refractive index <2.45> n_D^{20}: 1.376 – 1.378

Specific gravity <2.56> d_{20}^{20}: 0.785 – 0.788

Purity (1) Ultraviolet absorbing substances—Perform the test with 2-propanol for liquid chromatography as directed under Ultraviolet-visible Spectrophotometry <2.24>, using water as the blank: the absorbance at 230 nm is not more than 0.2; at 250 nm, not more than 0.03; and between 280 nm and 400 nm, not more than 0.01.

(2) Peroxide—Mix 100 mL of water and 25 mL of dilute sulfuric acid, and add 25 mL of a solution of potassium iodide (1 in 10). Add this solution to 20 g of 2-propanol for liquid chromatography. Stopper tightly, shake, allow to stand for 15 minutes in a dark place, and titrate <2.50> with 0.01 mol/L sodium thiosulfate VS (indicator: 1 mL of starch TS). Perform a blank determination in the same manner, and make any necessary correction (not more than 0.0005%).

Propanol, iso See 2-propanol.

Propranolol hydrochloride for assay $C_{16}H_{21}NO_2.HCl$ [Same as the monograph Propranolol Hydrochloride. When dried, it contains not less than 99.5% of propranolol hydrochloride ($C_{16}H_{21}NO_2.HCl$).]

Propantheline bromide $C_{23}H_{30}BrNO_3$ [Same as the namesake monograph]

Propionic acid CH_3CH_2COOH Colorless liquid.

Purity—Clarity and color of solution—Dissolve 1.0 g of

propionic acid in 20 mL of ethanol (95): the solution is clear and colorless.

Specific gravity <2.56> d_{20}^{20}: 0.998 – 1.004

Distilling range <2.57>: 139 – 143°C, not less than 95 vol%.

Propylamine, iso $(CH_3)_2CHNH_2$ Colorless liquid, having a characteristic, amine-like odor. Miscible with water, with ethanol (95) and with diethyl ether.

Refractive index <2.45> n_D^{20}: 1.374 – 1.376

Specific gravity <2.56> d_{20}^{20}: 0.685 – 0.690

Distilling range <2.57>: 31 – 33°C, not less than 95 vol%.

Propyl benzoate $C_6H_5COOC_3H_7$ Clear, colorless liquid, having a characteristic odor.

Refractive index <2.45> n_D^{20}: 1.498 – 1.503

Specific gravity <2.56> d_{20}^{20}: 1.022 – 1.027

Propylene carbonate $C_4H_6O_3$ Colorless liquid.

Boiling point <2.57>: 240 – 242°C

Water <2.48>: less than 0.1%.

Propylene carbonate for water determination To 1000 mL of propylene carbonate add 30 g of synthetic zeolite for drying, stopper tightly, allow to stand for about 8 hours with occasional gentle shaking, then allow to stand for about 16 hours, and collect the clear propylene carbonate layer. Preserve this protecting from moisture. The water content should not be more than 0.3 mg per mL.

Propylene glycol $CH_3CH(OH)CH_2OH$ [K 8837, Special class]

Propylene glycol cefatrizine $C_{18}H_{18}N_6O_5S_2.C_3H_8O_2$ [Same as the namesake monograph]

Propylene glycol for gas chromatography $C_3H_8O_2$ [K 8837, Special class] When perform the test as directed in the Purity (7) under Propylene Glycol, it does not show any peak at the retention times corresponding to ethylene glycol and diethylene glycol.

Propylether, iso $(CH_3)_2CHOCH(CH_3)_2$ Clear, colorless liquid, having a characteristic odor. Not miscible with water.

Refractive index <2.45> n_D^{20}: 1.368 – 1.369

Specific gravity <2.56> d_4^{20}: 0.723 – 0.725

Propyl parahydroxybenzoate $HOC_6H_4COOCH_2CH_2CH_3$ [Same as the namesake monograph]

Propyl parahydroxybenzoate for resolution check $C_{10}H_{12}O_3$ Colorless crystals or a white crystalline powder. Freely soluble in methanol, in ethanol (95) and in acetone, and very slightly soluble in water. Melting point: 96 – 99°C.

Identification—Determine the infrared absorption spectrum of propyl parahydroxybenzoate for resolution check as directed in the potassium bromide disk method under Infrared Spectrophotometry <2.25>, and compare the spectrum with the Reference Spectrum of Propyl Parahydroxybenzoate or the spectrum of Propyl Parahydroxybenzoate RS: both spectra exhibit similar intensities of absorption at the same wave numbers.

Purity Related substances—Dissolve 50 mg of propyl parahydroxybenzoate for resolution check in 2.5 mL of methanol, and add the mobile phase to make 50 mL. To 10 mL of this solution add the mobile phase to make 100 mL, and use this solution as the sample solution. Pipet 1 mL of the sample solution, add the mobile phase to make exactly 10 mL, and use this solution as the standard solution. Perform the test with exactly 10 μL each of the sample solution and standard solution as directed under Liquid Chromatography <2.01> according to the following conditions. Determine each peak area by the automatic integration method: total area of the peaks other than propyl parahydroxybenzoate obtained from the sample solution is not larger than the peak area of propyl parahydroxybenzoate from the standard solution.

Operating conditions

Detector, column, column temperature, mobile phase, and flow rate: Proceed as directed in the operating conditions in the Assay under Propyl Parahydroxybenzoate.

Time span of measurement: About 2.5 times as long as the retention time of propyl parahydroxybenzoate.

System suitability

Test for required detectability: Pipet 1 mL of the standard solution, and add methanol to make exactly 20 mL. Confirm that the peak area of propyl parahydroxybenzoate obtained with 10 μL of this solution is equivalent to 3.5 to 6.5% of that with 10 μL of the standard solution.

System performance: When the procedure is run with 10 μL of the standard solution under the above operating conditions, the number of theoretical plates and the symmetry factor of the peak of propyl parahydroxybenzoate are not less than 2500 and not more than 2.0, respectively.

System repeatability: When the test is repeated 6 times with 10 μL of the standard solution under the above operating conditions, the relative standard deviation of the peak area of propyl parahydroxybenzoate is not more than 5.0%.

Propylthiouracil for assay $C_7H_{10}N_2OS$ [Same as the monograph Propylthiouracil. When dried, it contains not less than 99.0% of propylthiouracil ($C_7H_{10}N_2OS$).]

Prostaglandin A₁ $C_{20}H_{32}O_4$ White, crystals or crystalline powder. Very soluble in ethanol (95) and in ethyl acetate, and very slightly soluble in water.

Purity Related substances—Dissolve 5 mg of prostaglandin A_1 in 10 mL of ethanol (95), and use this solution as the sample solution. Pipet 3 mL of the sample solution, add ethanol (95) to make exactly 100 mL, and use this solution as the standard solution. Perform the test with exactly 10 μL each of the sample solution and standard solution as directed under Liquid Chromatography <2.01> according to the following conditions. Determine areas of all peaks of both solutions by the automatic integration method: the total area of the peaks other than prostaglandin A_1 obtained from the sample solution is not larger than the peak area of prostaglandin A_1 from the standard solution.

Operating conditions

Detector, column, column temperature, mobile phase, flow rate, and selection of column: Proceed the operating conditions in the Assay under Alprostadil Alfadex.

Detection sensitivity: Adjust the detection sensitivity so that the peak height of prostaglandin A_1 obtained with 10 μL of the standard solution is 5 to 10% of the full scale.

Time span of measurement: About twice as long as the retention time of prostaglandin A_1, beginning after the solvent peak.

Protein digestive enzyme TS A solution of lysyl endopeptidase in 0.05 mol/L tris buffer solution (pH 8.6) (1 in 50,000).

Pseudoephedrine hydrochloride $C_{10}H_{15}NO.HCl$ White, crystals or crystalline powder. Freely soluble in water, in methanol and in acetic acid (100), soluble in ethanol (99.5), and practically insoluble in acetic anhydride. Melting point: 182 – 186°C.

Purity Related substances—Dissolve 1 mg of pseudoephedrine hydrochloride in 10 mL of diluted methanol (1 in 2), and use this solution as the sample solution. Perform the test with 10 μL of the sample solution for twice as long as the retention time of ephedrine as directed in the Assay (1) under Kakkonto Extract: the total area of the peaks other than pseudoephedrine and the solvent is not larger than 1/10 times the total area of the peaks other than the solvent.

Puerarin for thin-layer chromatography $C_{21}H_{20}O_9$ White, crystals or crystalline powder. Freely soluble in methanol, soluble in ethanol (99.5), and practically insoluble in water.

Identification Determine the infrared absorption spectrum of puerarin to be examined as directed in the potassium bromide disk method under Infrared Spectrophotometry <*2.25*>: it exhibits absorption at the wave numbers of about 3370 cm^{-1}, 1632 cm^{-1}, 1447 cm^{-1}, 1060 cm^{-1} and 836 cm^{-1}.

Purity Related substances—Dissolve 1 mg of puerarin to be examined in methanol to make exactly 1 mL. Perform the test with 2 μL of this solution as directed in the Identification under Pueraria Root: any spot other than the principal spot with an *Rf* value of about 0.4 does not appear.

Pullulanase An enzyme obtained from *Klebsiella pneumoniae*. White crystals. It contains not less than 30 units per mg. One unit is an enzymatic activity to produce 1 μmol of maltotriose from pullulan per minute at pH 5.0 and 30°C.

Pullulanase TS A solution of pullulanase containing 10 units per mL.

Purified hydrochloric acid See hydrochloric acid, purified.

Purified sodium hyaluronate See sodium hyaluronate, purified.

Purified methanol See methanol, purified.

Purified sulfuric acid See sulfuric acid, purified.

Purified water [Use the water prescribed by the monographs of Purified Water or Purified Water in Containers. It is not necessary to check the conformity to all the specification items of the monograph, if it is confirmed that the water to be used is suitable for the purpose of the relevant test.]

Pyrazole $C_3H_4N_2$ White to pale yellow, crystals or crystalline powder.

Melting point <*2.60*>: 67 – 71°C

Pyridine C_5H_5N [K 8777, Special class]

Pyridine-acetic acid TS Dilute 20 mL of pyridine with sufficient diluted acetic acid (100) (1 in 25) to make 100 mL. Prepare before use.

Pyridine, dehydrated C_5H_5N To 100 mL of pyridine add 10 g of sodium hydroxide, and allow to stand for 24 hours. Decant the supernatant liquid, and distill.

Pyridine for water determination Add potassium hydroxide or barium oxide to pyridine, stopper tightly, and allow to stand for several days. Distill and preserve the purified and dried pyridine, protecting it from moisture. The water content of this pyridine for water determination should not be more than 1 mg per mL.

0.2 mol/L Pyridine-formic acid buffer solution (pH 3.0) To 15.82 g of pyridine add 900 mL of water, mix well, adjust the pH to 3.0 with diluted formic acid (1 in 2), and add water to make 1000 mL.

Pyridine-pyrazolone TS Dissolve, with thorough shaking, 0.1 g of 3-methyl-1-phenyl-5-pyrazolone in 100 mL of water by heating between 65°C and 70°C, and cool below 30°C. Mix this solution with a solution prepared by dissolving 20 mg of bis-(1-phenyl-3-methyl-5-pyrazolone) in 20 mL of pyridine. Prepare before use.

Pyridoxine hydrochloride $C_8H_{11}NO_3.HCl$ [Same as the namesake monograph]

1-(2-Pyridylazo)-2-naphthol $C_{15}H_{11}N_3O$ Orange-yellow or orange-red powder.

Absorbance—Dissolve 25 mg of 1-(2-pyridylazo)-2-naphthol in methanol to make exactly 100 mL. Pipet 2.0 mL of this solution, and add methanol to make exactly 50 mL. Perform the test with this solution as directed under Ultraviolet-visible Spectrophotometry <*2.24*>: absorbance at the wavelength of 470 nm is not less than 0.55.

Melting point <*2.60*>: 137 – 140°C

Purity Clarity and color of solution—Dissolve 25 mg of 1-(2-pyridylazo)-2-naphthol in 100 mL of methanol: the solution is clear and orange-yellow.

Residue on ignition <*2.44*>: not more than 1.0%.

Sensitivity—On adding 50 mL of water, 30 mL of methanol and 10 mL of acetic acid-sodium acetate buffer solution (pH 5.5) to 0.2 mL of a solution of 1-(2-pyridylazo)-2-naphthol in methanol (1 in 4000), the solution is yellow in color. Add 1 drop of a solution of copper (II) chloride dihydrate (1 in 600) to this solution: the solution is red-purple in color. Add a subsequent 1 drop of diluted 0.1 mol/L disodium dihydrogen ethylenediamine tetraacetate TS (1 in 10): the color of the solution changes to yellow again.

1-(4-Pyridyl)pyridinium chloride hydrochloride $C_{10}H_9ClN_2.HCl$ White to yellow-white crystalline powder. Very soluble in water, very slightly soluble in ethanol (95), and practically insoluble in diethyl ether.

Melting point <*2.60*>: 154 – 156°C

Pyrogallol $C_6H_3(OH)_3$ [K 8780, Special class]

L-Pyroglutamylglycyl-L-arginine-*p*-nitroaniline hydrochloride $C_{19}H_{26}N_8O_6.HCl$ White to light yellow powder. Freely soluble in water, in methanol and in acetic acid (100).

Absorbance <*2.24*> $E^{1\%}_{1\,cm}$ (316 nm): 242 – 268 (2 mg, water, 100 mL).

Optical rotation <*2.49*> $[\alpha]^{25}_{D}$: −51 – −56° [0.1 g, diluted acetic acid (100) (1 in 2), 10 mL, 100 mm].

Purity Related substances—Dissolve 50 mg of L-pyroglutamylglycyl-L-arginine-*p*-nitroaniline hydrochloride in 10 mL of methanol, and use this solution as the sample solution. Pipet 1 mL of the sample solution, add methanol to make exactly 50 mL, and use this solution as the standard solution. Perform the test with these solutions as directed under Thin-layer Chromatography <*2.03*>. Spot 20 μL each of the sample solution and standard solution on a plate of silica gel with fluorescent indicator for thin-layer chromatography. Develop the plate with a mixture of 1-butanol, water, pyridine and acetic acid (100) (15:12:10:3) to a distance of about 10 cm, and air-dry the plate. Examine under ultraviolet light (main wavelength: 254 nm): the spots other than the principal spot obtained from the sample solution are not more intense than the spot from the standard solution.

L-Pyroglutamylglycyl-L-arginine-*p*-nitroaniline hydrochloride TS Dissolve 25 mg of L-pyroglutamylglycyl-L-arginine-*p*-nitroaniline hydrochloride and 40 mg of D-mannitol in 2 to 3 mL of water, lyophilize, and add 16.7 mL of water to dissolve. To 1 volume of this solution add 9 volumes of water before use.

Pyrrole C_4H_5N Clear, colorless liquid, having a characteristic odor. Soluble in ethanol (95) and in diethyl ether, and practically insoluble in water.

Specific gravity <2.56> d^{20}_{20}: 0.965 – 0.975

Pyrophosphate buffer solution (pH 9.0) Dissolve 3.3 g of potassium pyrophosphate, 15 mg of dithiothreitol and 40 mg of disodium dihydrogen ethylenediamine tetraacetate dihydrate in 70 mL of water, adjust the pH with a solution of citric acid monohydrate (21 in 100) to exactly 9.0, and add water to make 100 mL.

2-Pyrrolidone C_4H_7NO Clear, colorless to pale yellow liquid, or white to pale yellow, masses or powder. Odorless.

Congealing point <2.42>: 22 – 26°C

Purity Dissolve about 1 g of 2-pyrrolidone in 10 mL of methanol, and use this solution as the sample solution. Perform the test with 1 μL of the sample solution as directed under Gas Chromatography <2.02> according to the following conditions. Determine each peak area by the automatic integration method, and calculate the amount of 2-pyrrolidone by the area percentage method: not less than 98.0%.

Operating conditions

Detector: Hydrogen flame-ionization detector.

Column: A capillary glass column 0.53 mm in inside diameter and 30 m in length, coated with a 1.0-μm layer of polyethylene glycol 20 M for gas chromatography on the inner surface.

Column temperature: Maintain the temperature at 80°C for 1 minute, then raise at the rate of 10°C per minute to 190°C, and maintain at this temperature for 20 minutes.

Temperature of sample vaporization chamber: A constant temperature of about 200°C.

Carrier gas: Helium.

Flow rate: Adjust so that the retention time of 2-pyrrolidone is about 10 minutes.

Split ratio: 1:20.

Time span of measurement: About 2 times as long as the retention time of 2-pyrrolidone.

Water <2.48> Not more than 0.2% (5 g, volumetric titration, direct titration).

0.05 mol/L Pyrophosphate buffer solution (pH 9.0) Dissolve 0.83 g of potassium pyrophosphate in 40 mL of water, adjust the pH with 1 mol/L hydrochloric acid TS to 9.0, and add water to make 50 mL. Adjust the temperature to 22 ± 2°C before use.

Quinapril hydrochloride for assay $C_{25}H_{30}N_2O_5.HCl$ [Same as the monograph Quinapril Hydrochloride. When perform the test as directed in the Purity (2) of Quinapril Hydrochloride, the area of the peaks, having the relative retention time of about 0.5 and about 2.0 to quinapril obtained from the sample solution, is not larger than the peak area of quinapril from the standard solution, the area of peak other than quinapril and the peak mentioned above from the sample solution is not larger than 2/5 times the peak area of quinapril from the standard solution, and the total area of the peaks other than quinapril from the sample solution is not larger than 2 times the peak area of quinapril from the standard solution.]

Quinhydrone $C_6H_4(OH)_2.C_6H_4O_2$ Green, crystals or crystalline powder.

Melting point <2.60>: 169 – 172°C

Quinidine sulfate See quinidine sulfate hydrate.

Quinidine sulfate hydrate $(C_{20}H_{24}N_2O_2)_2.H_2SO_4.2H_2O$ [Same as the namesake monograph]

Quinine sulfate See quinine sulfate hydrate.

Quinine sulfate hydrate $(C_{20}H_{24}N_2O_2)_2.H_2SO_4.2H_2O$ [Same as the namesake monograph]

Quinoline C_9H_7N [K 8279, Special class]

Quinoline TS Mix 50 mL of quinoline with 360 mL of diluted hydrochloric acid (1 in 6), previously heated, cool, and filter if necessary.

8-Quinolinol C_9H_7NO [K 8775, Special class]

Rabbit anti-nartograstim antibody Dissolve the antibody obtained from rabbit antiserum, prepared by immunizing with Nartograstim (Genetical Recombination), in tris-acetic acid buffer solution (pH 8.0) so that each mL contains 1 mg of rabbit anti-nartograstim antibody. Storage at −80°C.

Performance test: When perform the test by Ouchterlony method, a precipitation line is appeared against Nartograstim (Genetical Recombination).

Protein concentration: Determine the absorbance at 280 nm as directed under Ultraviolet-visible Spectrophotometry <2.24>, and calculate the protein concentration using the specific absorbance $E^{1\%}_{1\,\mathrm{cm}}$ 15.

Rabbit anti-nartograstim antibody TS To rabbit anti-nartograstim antibody add bovine serum albumin TS for nartograstim test so that each mL contains 0.2 μg of rabbit anti-nartograstim antibody. Prepare before use.

Raney nickel catalyst Grayish black powder. An alloy containing 40 to 50% of nickel and 50 to 60% of aluminum.

Ranitidinediamine $(C_{10}H_{18}N_2OS)_2.C_4H_4O_4$ White to pale yellow crystalline powder.

Identification—Determine the infrared absorption spectrum of ranitidinediamine as directed in the paste method under Infrared Spectrophotometry <2.25>: it exhibits absorption at the wave numbers of about 2780 cm^{-1}, 1637 cm^{-1}, 1015 cm^{-1} and 788 cm^{-1}.

Content: not less than 95%. Assay—Weigh accurately about 0.1 g of ranitidinediamine, dissolve in 50 mL of acetic acid (100), and titrate <2.50> with 0.1 mol/L perchloric acid VS until the color of the solution changes from purple to green through blue (indicator: crystal violet TS). Perform the blank determination in the same manner, and make any necessary correction.

Each mL of 0.1 mol/L perchloric acid VS
= 13.62 mg of $(C_{10}H_{18}N_2OS)_2.C_4H_4O_4$

Rebamipide for assay $C_{19}H_{15}ClN_2O_4$ [Same as the monograph Rebamipide. When dried, it contains not less than 99.5% of rebamipide ($C_{19}H_{15}ClN_2O_4$).]

Reduced iron See iron powder.

Reduction buffer solution for nartograstim sample Mix 0.8 mL of sodium lauryl sulfate solution (1 in 10), 0.5 mL of 0.5 mol/L tris buffer solution (pH 6.8), 0.4 mL of glycerin, 0.3 mL of 2-mercaptoethanol and 0.1 mL of bromophenol blue solution (1 in 200). Prepare before use.

Reduction liquid for molecular mass determination Dissolve 10.6 g of sodium lauryl sulfate and 3.9 g of 2-amino-2-hydroxymethyl-1,3-propanediol in 60 mL of water, adjust to pH 6.8 with hydrochloric acid, dissolve 31 g of sucrose, and add water to make 100 mL. To 97 mL of this solution add 3 mL of bromophenol blue solution (11 in 2500). To 0.4 mL of this solution add 0.1 mL of 2-mercaptoethanol. Prepare before use.

Reference anti-interleukin-2 antibody for teceleukin Monoclonal antibody obtained from a fusion cell strain from mouse spleen cells sensitized to teceleukin and mouse melanoma cells, or alternately, rabbit antiserum towards human interleukin-2, that is purified using affinity chromatography. When determining the neutralizing activity, taking 1 neutralizing unit as the titer that neutralizes one unit of activity of teceleukin, contains at least 2000 neutralizing units per mL.

Reference anti-interleukin-2 antiserum TS Anti-interleukin-2 antiserum is diluted with culture media for celmoleukin, so that the diluted antiserum solution neutralizes the same volume of about 800 unit per mL solution of Celmoleukin (Genetical Recombination).

Reference suspension 1 To 5.0 mL of formazin opalescence standard solution add 95.0 mL of water. Mix and shake before use.

Reinecke salt See reinecke salt monohydrate.

Reinecke salt monohydrate $NH_4[Cr(NH_3)_2(SCN)_4].H_2O$ Dark red, crystals or crystalline powder.

Identification—Determine the infrared absorption spectrum of Reinecke salt monohydrate as directed in the potassium bromide disk method as directed under Infrared Spectrophotometry <*2.25*>: it exhibits absorption at the wave numbers of about 3310 cm^{-1}, 2130 cm^{-1}, 1633 cm^{-1}, 1400 cm^{-1}, 1261 cm^{-1} and 711 cm^{-1}.

Reinecke salt TS To 20 mL of water add 0.5 g of Reinecke salt monohydrate, shake frequently for 1 hour, then filter. Use within 48 hours.

Resazurin $C_{12}H_6NNaO_4$ Brownish purple powder. It dissolves in water and the solution is purple in color.

Residue on ignition <*2.44*>: not less than 28.5% (1 g).

Resazurin solution Prepared for the test for measurement of living cell.

Resibufogenin for assay $C_{24}H_{32}O_4$ Odorless white crystalline powder.

Absorbance <*2.24*> $E^{1\%}_{1\,cm}$ (300 nm): 131 – 145 (10 mg, methanol, 250 mL), dried in a desiccator (silica gel) for 24 hours.

Purity Related substances—Weigh accurately 40 mg of resibufogenin for assay and proceed as directed in the Purity under bufalin for assay.

Content: not less than 98.0%. Assay—Weigh accurately about 10 mg of resibufogenin for assay, previously dried in a desiccator (silica gel) for 24 hours, add methanol to make exactly 10 mL, and use this solution as the sample solution. Perform the test with 20 µL of the sample solution as directed under Liquid Chromatography <*2.01*> according to the following conditions. Determine each peak area by the automatic integration method, and calculate the amount of resibufogenin by the area percentage method.

Operating conditions

Detector: An ultraviolet absorption photometer (wavelength: 300 nm).

Column: A stainless steel column about 4 to 6 mm in inside diameter and 15 to 30 cm in length, packed with octadecylsilanized silica gel for liquid chromatography (5 to 10 mm in particle diameter).

Column temperature: A constant temperature of about 40°C.

Mobile phase: A mixture of water and acetonitrile (1:1).

Flow rate: Adjust so that the retention time of resibufogenin is about 9 minutes.

Time span of measurement: About twice as long as the retention time of resibufogenin, beginning after the peak of solvent.

System suitability

Test for required detectability: Pipet 1 mL of the sample solution, add methanol to make exactly 100 mL, and use this solution as the standard solution (1). Pipet 1 mL of the standard solution (1), add methanol to make exactly 20 mL, and use this solution as the standard solution (2). Adjust the detection sensitivity so that the peak area of resibufogenin obtained with 20 µL of standard solution (2) can be measured by the automatic integration method and the peak height of resibufogenin with 20 µL of the standard solution (1) is about 20% of the full scale.

System performance: Dissolve 10 mg each of resibufogenin for assay, bufalin for assay and cinobufagin for assay in methanol to make 200 mL. When the procedure is run with 20 µL of this solution according to the above operating conditions, bufalin, cinobufagin and resibufogenin are eluted in this order, and each resolution between these peaks is not less than 1.5, respectively.

Resibufogenin for component determination See resibufogenin for assay.

Resibufogenin for thin-layer chromatography $C_{24}H_{32}O_4$ White crystalline powder having no odor. It is freely soluble in acetone and in methanol.

Purity Related substances—Dissolve 5.0 mg of resibufogenin for thin-layer chromatography in exactly 5 mL of acetone. Perform the test with 5 µL of this solution as directed in the Identification under Toad Cake: no spot other than the principal spot with an *R*f value of about 0.4 appear.

Resolving gel for celmoleukin Prepare the resolving gel in tris buffer solution (pH 8.8) using ammonium persulfate and *N*,*N*,*N′*,*N′*-tetramethylethylenediamine so the concentrations of acrylamide and sodium lauryl sulfate are 13.5% and 0.1%, respectively.

Resorcin See resorcinol.

Resorcinol $C_6H_4(OH)_2$ [K 9032, Special class]

Resorcinol sulfuric acid TS Dissolve 0.1 g of resorcinol in 10 mL of diluted sulfuric acid (1 in 10).

Resorcinol TS Dissolve 0.1 g of resorcinol in 10 mL of hydrochloric acid. Prepare before use.

Resorcinol-copper (II) sulfate TS Dissolve 0.1 g of resorcinol in 5 mL of water, add 125 µL of 0.1 mol/L copper (II) sulfate solution, 24 mL of hydrochloric acid, and add water to make 50 mL. Prepare this TS at least 4 hours before the time of use.

Resorcin sulfuric acid TS See resorcinol sulfuric acid TS.

Resorcin TS See resorcinol TS.

L-Rhamnose monohydrate $C_6H_{12}O.H_2O$ White crystalline powder having sweet taste. Freely soluble in water, and sparingly soluble in ethanol (95).

Optical rotation <*2.49*> $[\alpha]^{20}_{D}$: +7.8 – +8.3° (1 g, 20 mL of water, 2 drops of ammonia TS, 100 mm).

Melting point <*2.60*>: 87 – 91°C

Purity Related substances—Dissolve 1.0 mg of L-rhamnose monohydrate in 1 mL of water, and add methanol to make exactly 10 mL. Proceed with 20 µL of this solution as directed in the Identification under Acacia: any spot other than the principal spot at the *R*f value of about 0.5 does not appear.

Rhaponticin for purity $C_{21}H_{24}O_9$ A white to pale yellow-brown crystalline powder, having no odor. Slightly soluble in methanol, and practically insoluble in water and in ethanol (99.5).

Identification—Determine the infrared absorption spectrum of rhaponticin for purity as directed in the potassium bromide disk method under Infrared Spectrophotometry <*2.25*>: it exhibits absorption at the wave numbers of about 1612 cm^{-1}, 1577 cm^{-1}, 1513 cm^{-1}, 948 cm^{-1}, 831 cm^{-1} and 798 cm^{-1}.

Purity Related substances—Dissolve 4 mg of rhaponticin for purity in 2 mL of methanol, and use this solution as the sample solution. Pipet 1 mL of the sample solution, add methanol to make exactly 50 mL, and use this solution as the standard solution. Perform the test with 10 μL each of the sample solution and standard solution as directed in the Purity (3) under Rhubarb: the spot other than the principal spot that appears at an *R*f value of about 0.3 obtained with the sample solution is not more intense than the spot with the standard solution.

Rhein for assay $C_{15}H_8O_6$ Use rhein for thin-layer chromatography meeting the following additional specifications. Its content is corrected based on the amount (%) of rhein obtained in the Assay.

Absorbance <*2.24*> $E^{1\%}_{1\,cm}$ (257 nm): 678 – 720 (3 mg, methanol, 500 mL).

Unity of peak—Dissolve 1 mg of rhein for assay in 100 mL of acetone, and use this solution as the sample solution. Perform the test with 10 μL of the sample solution as directed under Liquid Chromatography <*2.01*> according to the following conditions, and compare the absorption spectra of at least 3 points including the top of rhein peak and around the two middle peak heights of before and after the top: no difference in form is observed between their spectra.

Operating conditions

Detector: An ultraviolet absorption photometer (wavelength: 257 nm).

Column: A stainless steel column 4.6 mm in inside diameter and 15 cm in length, packed with octadecylsilanized silica gel for liquid chromatography (5 μm in particle diameter).

Column temperature: A constant temperature of about 50°C.

Mobile phase: A mixture of water, acetonitrile, and phosphoric acid (650:350:1).

Flow rate: Adjust so that the retention time of rhein is about 14 minutes.

System suitability

System performance: Proceed as directed in the system suitability in the Assay (5) under Otsujito Extract.

Assay—Weigh accurately 5 mg of rhein for assay and 1 mg of DSS-d_6 for nuclear magnetic resonance spectroscopy using an ultramicrobalance, dissolve in 1 mL of deuterated dimethyl sulfoxide for nuclear magnetic resonance spectroscopy, and use this solution as the sample solution. Transfer the sample solution into an NMR tube 5 mm in outer diameter, measure ^{1}H-NMR as directed under Nuclear Magnetic Resonance Spectroscopy <*2.21*> and Crude Drugs Test <*5.01*> according to the following conditions, using DSS-d_6 for nuclear magnetic resonance spectroscopy as the reference standard for qNMR. Calculate the resonance intensity *A* (equivalent to 1 hydrogen) of the signal around δ 8.16 ppm assuming the signal of the reference standard for qNMR as δ 0 ppm.

$$\text{Amount (\%) of rhein } (C_{15}H_8O_6) = M_S \times I \times P/(M \times N) \times 1.2668$$

M: Amount (mg) of rhein for assay taken

M_S: Amount (mg) of DSS-d_6 for nuclear magnetic resonance spectroscopy taken

I: Signal resonance intensity based on the signal resonance intensity of DSS-d_6 for nuclear magnetic resonance spectroscopy as 9.000

N: Number of the hydrogen derived from *A*

P: Purity (%) of DSS-d_6 for nuclear magnetic resonance spectroscopy

Operating conditions

Apparatus: A nuclear magnetic resonance spectrometer having ^{1}H resonance frequency of not less than 400 MHz.

Target nucleus: ^{1}H.

Digital resolution: 0.25 Hz or lower.

Measuring spectrum range: 20 ppm or upper, including between − 5 ppm and 15 ppm.

Spinning: off.

Pulse angle: 90°.

^{13}C decoupling: on.

Delay time: Repeating pulse waiting time is not less than 60 seconds.

Integrating times: 8 or more times.

Dummy scanning: 2 or more times.

Measuring temperature: A constant temperature between 20°C and 30°C.

System suitability

Test for required detectability: When the procedure is run with the sample solution under the above operating conditions, the SN ratio of the signal of around δ 8.16 ppm is not less than 100.

System performance: When the procedure is run with the sample solution under the above operating conditions, the signal of around δ 8.16 ppm is not overlapped with any signal of obvious foreign substance.

System repeatability: When the test is repeated 6 times with the sample solution under the above operating conditions, the relative standard deviation of the resonance intensity *A* to that of the reference standard for qNMR is not more than 1.0%.

Rhein for thin-layer chromatography $C_{15}H_8O_6$ A yellow to reddish yellow powder. Very slightly soluble in acetone, and practically insoluble in water, in methanol, and in ethanol (99.5).

Identification—Determine the absorption spectrum of a solution in methanol (3 in 500,000) as directed under Ultraviolet-visible Spectrophotometry <*2.24*>: it exhibits maxima between 228 nm and 232 nm, between 255 nm and 259 nm, and between 429 nm and 433 nm.

Purity Related substances—Dissolve 1 mg of rhein for thin-layer chromatography in 10 mL of acetone, and perform the test with 2 μL of this solution as directed in the Identification (1) under Daiokanzoto Extract: no spot other than the principal spot at an *R*f value of about 0.3 appears.

Rhyncophylline for assay $C_{22}H_{28}N_2O_4$ Rhyncophylline for thin-layer chromatography. It meets the following requirements.

Absorbance <*2.24*>: $E^{1\%}_{1\,cm}$ (245 nm): 473 – 502 (5 mg of the dried substance in a desiccator (silica gel) for 24 hours, a mixture of methanol and dilute acetic acid (7:3), 500 mL).

Purity Related substances—Dissolve 5 mg of rhyncophylline for assay in 100 mL of a mixture of methanol and dilute acetic acid (7:3), and use this solution as the sample solution. Pipet 1 mL of the sample solution, add a mixture of methanol and dilute acetic acid (7:3) to make exactly 100 mL, and use this solution as the standard solution. Perform the test with exactly 20 μL each of the sample solution and standard solution as directed under Liquid-chromatography

<*2.01*> according to the following conditions. Determine the peak area of each solution by the automatic integration method: the total area of the peaks other than rhyncophylline obtained from the sample solution is not larger than the peak area of rhyncophylline from the standard solution.
Operating conditions

Detector, column, column temperature, mobile phase, and flow rate: Proceed as directed in the operating conditions in the Assay under Uncaria Hook.

Time span of measurement: About 4 times as long as the retention time of rhyncophylline, beginning after the solvent peak.
System suitability

System performance and system repeatability: Proceed as directed in the system suitability in the Assay under Uncaria Hook.

Test for required detectability: Pipet 1 mL of the standard solution, add a mixture of methanol and dilute acetic acid (7:3) to make exactly 20 mL. Confirm that the peak area of rhyncophylline obtained with 20 μL of this solution is equivalent to 3.5 to 6.5% of that with 20 μL of the standard solution.

Rhynchophylline for component determination See rhynchophylline for assay.

Rhyncophylline for thin-layer chromatography $C_{22}H_{28}N_2O_4$ White, crystals or crystalline powder. Slightly soluble in ethanol (99.5) and in acetone, and practically insoluble in water. Melting point: 205 - 209°C.

Identification—Determine the absorption spectrum of a solution of rhyncophylline for thin-layer chromatography in a mixture of methanol and dilute acetic acid (7:3) (1 in 100,000) as directed under Ultraviolet-visible Spectrophotometry <*2.24*>: it exhibits a maximum between 242 nm and 246 nm.

Purity Related substances—Dissolve 1.0 mg of rhyncophylline for thin-layer chromatography in 1 mL of acetone, and use this solution as the sample solution. Perform the test with the sample solution as directed under Thin-layer Chromatography <*2.03*>. Spot 10 μL of the sample solution on a plate of silica gel with fluorescent indicator for thin-layer chromatography. Develop the plate with a mixture of 1-butanol, water and acetic acid (100) (7:2:1) to a distance of about 10 cm, and air-dry the plate. Examine under ultraviolet light (main wavelength: 254 nm): no spot other than the principal spot at around *R*f value of 0.5 appears.

Ribavirin $C_8H_{12}N_4O_5$ [Same as the namesake monograph]

Riboflavin $C_{17}H_{20}N_4O_6$ [Same as the namesake monograph]

Riboflavin sodium phosphate $C_{17}H_{20}N_4NaO_9P$ [Same as the namesake monograph]

Ribonuclease A for gel filtration molecular mass marker Obtained from bovine pancreas, for gel filtration chromatography.

Rilmazafone hydrochloride hydrate $C_{21}H_{20}Cl_2N_6O_3.HCl.2H_2O$ [Same as the namesake monograph]

Risperidone for assay $C_{23}H_{27}FN_4O_2$ [Same as the monograph Risperidone. It contains not less than 99.5% of risperidone ($C_{23}H_{27}FN_4O_2$), calculated on the dried basis.]

Ritodrine hydrochloride $C_{17}H_{21}NO_3.HCl$ [Same as the namesake monograph]

Rose Bengal $C_{20}H_2Cl_4I_4Na_2O_5$ [Special class] A red-brown powder, and shows a purple red when dissolved in water.

Rosmarinic acid for assay $C_{18}H_{16}O_8$ Use rosmarinic acid for thin-layer chromatography meeting the following additional specifications. Its content is corrected based on the amount (%) of rosmarinic acid obtained in the Assay.

Unity of peak—Conduct this procedure without exposure to light, using light-resistant vessels. Dissolve 1 mg of rosmarinic acid for assay in 50 mL of ethanol, and use this solution as the sample solution. Perform the test with 10 μL of the sample solution as directed under Liquid Chromatography <*2.01*> according to the following conditions, and compare the absorption spectra of at least 3 points including the top of rosmarinic acid peak and around the two middle peak heights of before and after the top: no difference in form is observed between their spectra.
Operating conditions

Detector: A photodiode array detector (wavelength: 330 nm, spectrum range of measurement: 220 - 400 nm).

Column: A stainless steel column 4.6 mm in inside diameter and 15 cm in length, packed with octadecylsilanized silica gel for liquid chromatography (5 μm in particle diameter).

Column temperature: A constant temperature of about 40°C.

Mobile phase: A mixture of diluted acetic acid (1 in 100) and methanol (13:7).

Flow rate: Adjust so that the retention time of rosmarinic acid is about 10 minutes.
System suitability

System performance: When the procedure is run with 10 μL of the sample solution, previously irradiated ultraviolet light (main wavelength: 365 nm) for 30 minutes, under the above operating conditions, an obvious peak is observed just before the peak of rosmarinic acid, and the resolution between these peaks is not less than 1.5.

Assay—Weigh accurately 5 mg of rosmarinic acid for assay and 1 mg of DSS-d_6 for nuclear magnetic resonance spectroscopy using an ultramicrobalance, dissolve in 1 mL of deuterated dimethylsulfoxide for nuclear magnetic resonance spectroscopy, and use this solution as the sample solution. Transfer the sample solution into an NMR tube 5 mm in outer diameter, measure ^{1}H-NMR as directed under Nuclear Magnetic Resonance Spectroscopy <*2.21*> and Crude Drugs Test <*5.01*> according to the following conditions, using DSS-d_6 for nuclear magnetic resonance spectroscopy as the reference standard for qNMR. Calculate the resonance intensity *A* (equivalent to 1 hydrogen) of the signal around δ 6.27 ppm assuming the signal of the reference standard for qNMR as δ 0 ppm.

$$\text{Amount (\%) of rosmarinic acid } (C_{18}H_{16}O_8) = M_S \times I \times P/(M \times N) \times 1.6059$$

M: Amount (mg) of rosmarinic acid for assay 2 taken
M_S: Amount (mg) of DSS-d_6 for nuclear magnetic resonance spectroscopy taken
I: Signal resonance intensity *A* based on the signal resonance intensity of DSS-d_6 for nuclear magnetic resonance spectroscopy as 9.000
N: Number of the hydrogen derived from *A*
P: Purity (%) of DSS-d_6 for nuclear magnetic resonance spectroscopy

Operating conditions

Apparatus: A nuclear magnetic resonance spectrometer having ^{1}H resonance frequency of not less than 400 MHz.

Target nucleus: ^{1}H.

Digital resolution: 0.25 Hz or lower.

Measuring spectrum range: 20 ppm or upper, including between −5 ppm and 15 ppm.

Spinning: off.

Pulse angle: 90°.

^{13}C decoupling: on.

Delay time: Repeating pulse waiting time not less than 60 seconds.

Integrating times: 8 or more times.

Dummy scanning: 2 or more times.

Measuring temperature: A constant temperature between 20°C and 30°C.

System suitability

Test for required detectability: When the procedure is run with the sample solution under the above operating conditions, the SN ratio of the signal of around δ 6.27 ppm is not less than 100.

System performance: When the procedure is run with the sample solution under the above operating conditions, the signal of around δ 6.27 ppm is not overlapped with any obvious signal of foreign substance.

System repeatability: When the test is repeated 6 times with the sample solution under the above operating conditions, the relative standard deviation of the ratio of the resonance intensity A to that of the reference standard for qNMR is not more than 1.0%.

Rosmarinic acid for component determination See rosmarinic acid for assay.

Rosmarinic acid for thin-layer chromatography $C_{18}H_{16}O_8$ White to pale yellow, crystals or crystalline powder. Freely soluble in ethanol (99.5), and slightly soluble in water. Melting point: about 170°C (with decomposition).

Identification—Determine the absorption spectrum of a solution of rosmarinic acid for thin-layer chromatography (1 in 100,000) as directed under Ultraviolet-visible Spectrophotometry <2.24>: it exhibits maxima between 215 nm and 219 nm and between 322 nm and 326 nm.

Purity Related substances—Conduct this procedure using light-resistance vessels. Dissolve 10 mg of rosmarinic acid for thin-layer chromatography in 2 mL of ethanol (99.5), and use this solution as the sample solution. Pipet 1 mL of the sample solution, add ethanol (99.5) to make exactly 50 mL, and use this solution as the standard solution. Proceed with 10 μL each of the sample solution and standard solution as directed in the Identification (2) under Hangekobokuto Extract: the spot other than the principal spot of around Rf value of 0.5 obtained from the sample solution is not more intense than the spot from the standard solution.

Rosuvastatin calcium $(C_{22}H_{27}FN_3O_6S)_2Ca$ [Same as the namesake monograph]

Rosuvastatin calcium enantiomer $(C_{22}H_{27}FN_3O_6S)_2Ca$ White powder.

Identification—(1) Proceed the test as directed in the system performance of the system suitability in the Purity (4) under Rosuvastatin Calcium: the relative retention time of rosuvastatin enantiomer to rosuvastatin peak is about 0.92.

(2) Determine the ^{1}H spectrum of a solution of Rosuvastatin calcium enantiomer in deuterated dimethyl sulfoxide for nuclear magnetic resonance spectroscopy (3 in 100) as directed under Nuclear Magnetic Resonance Spectroscopy <2.21>, using tetramethylsilane for nuclear magnetic resonance spectroscopy as an internal reference compound: it exhibits a double triplet signal A at around δ 1.5 ppm, a multiplet signal B at around δ 4.2 ppm, a double doublet signal C at around δ 5.5 ppm, a double doublet signal D at around δ 6.5 ppm, a multiplet signal E at around δ 7.3 ppm, and a multiplet signal F at around δ 7.7 ppm. The ratio of integrated intensity of each signal, A:B:C:D:E:F, is about 1:1:1:1:2:2.

Roxatidine acetate hydrochloride $C_{19}H_{28}N_2O_4.HCl$ [Same as the namesake monograph]

RPMI-1640 powdered medium Powdered medium for cell culture containing 6 g of sodium chloride, 400 mg of potassium chloride, 800 mg of anhydrous sodium dihydrogen phosphate, 100 mg of anhydrous calcium nitrate, 49 mg of anhydrous magnesium sulfate, 2 g of dextrose, 200 mg of L-arginine, 1 mg of glutathione, 50 mg of L-isoleucine, 15 mg of L-phenylalanine, 5 mg of L-tryptophan, 0.2 mg of biotin, 1 mg of nicotinamide, 1 mg thiamine hydrochloride, 300 mg of L-glutamine, 56.8 mg of L-asparagine, 10 mg of glycine, 50 mg of L-leucine, 20 mg of L-proline, 20 mg of L-tyrosine, 0.25 mg of D-calcium pantothenate, 5 μg of cyanocobalamin, 1 mg of aminobenzoic acid, 20 mg of L-aspartic acid, 15 mg of L-histidine, 40 mg of L-lysine hydrochloride, 30 mg of L-serine, 20 mg of L-valine, 1 mg of folic acid, 1 mg of pyridoxine hydrochloride, 20 mg of L-glutamic acid, 20 mg of L-hydroxyproline, 15 mg of L-methionine, 20 mg of L-threonine, 3 mg of choline chloride, 35 mg of *i*-inositol, 0.2 mg of riboflavin, 59 mg of L-cystine, and 5 mg of phenol red per 1 L.

Rubidium chloride RbCl White, crystals or crystalline powder.

Content: Not less than 99.0%. Assay—Weigh accurately about 0.2 g of rubidium chloride, dissolve in 100 mL of water, add 5 mL of diluted nitric acid (1 in 2), and titrate <2.50> with 0.1 mol/L silver nitrate VS (potentiometric titration).

Each mL of 0.1 mol/L silver nitrate VS
= 12.09 mg of RbCl

Rutin for thin-layer chromatography $C_{27}H_{30}O_{16}$ Pale yellow to yellow-green, crystals or crystalline powder, having no odor. Soluble in methanol, slightly soluble in ethanol (99.5), and practically insoluble in water.

Identification (1) Determine the absorption spectrum of a solution of rutin for thin-layer chromatography in methanol (1 in 100,000) as directed under Ultraviolet-visible Spectrophotometry <2.24>: it exhibits maxima between 255 nm and 259 nm, and between 356 nm and 360 nm.

(2) Determine the infrared absorption spectrum of rutin for thin-layer chromatography as directed in the potassium bromide disk method under Infrared Spectrophotometry <2.25>: it exhibits absorption at the wave numbers of about 1655 cm^{-1}, 1600 cm^{-1}, 1507 cm^{-1} and 1363 cm^{-1}.

Purity Related substances—Dissolve 10 mg of rutin for thin-layer chromatography in 2 mL of methanol, and use this solution as the sample solution. Pipet 1 mL of the sample solution, add methanol to make exactly 20 mL, and use this solution as the standard solution. Perform the test with 2 μL each of the sample solution and standard solution as directed in Identification (1) under Crataegus Fruit: the spot other than the principal spot appeared at an Rf value of about 0.3 obtained from the sample solution is not more intense than the spot from the standard solution.

Saccharated pepsin [Same as the namesake monograph]

Saikosaponin a for assay $C_{42}H_{68}O_{13}$ Use saikosaponin a for thin-layer chromatography meeting the following additional specifications, 1) Saikosaponin a for assay 1 or 2) Saikosaponin a for assay 2 (Purity value by quantitative NMR).

The former is used after drying in a desiccator (silica gel) for 24 hour, and the latter is corrected based on the amount (%) obtained in the Assay.

1) Saikosaponin a for assay 1

Absorbance ⟨*2.24*⟩ $E^{1\%}_{1\,\mathrm{cm}}$ (206 nm): 65 – 73 (15 mg, methanol, 200 mL). Previously dried in a desiccator (in vacuum, silica gel) for 24 hours.

Purity Related substances—Dissolve 10 mg of saikosaponin a for assay 1 in 20 mL of methanol, and use this solution as the sample solution. Pipet 1 mL of the sample solution, add methanol to make exactly 100 mL, and use this solution as the standard solution. Perform the test with exactly 20 μL each of the sample solution and standard solution as directed under Liquid Chromatography ⟨*2.01*⟩ according to the following conditions, and determine each peak area by the automatic integration method: the total area of the peaks other than saikosaponin a obtained from the sample solution is not more than the peak area of saikosaponin a from the standard solution.

Operating conditions

Detector, and column: Proceed as directed in the operating conditions in the Assay under Bupleurum Root.

Column temperature: A constant temperature of about 40°C.

Mobile phase: A mixture of water and acetonitrile (13:7).

Flow rate: Adjust so that the retention time of saikosaponin a is about 16 minutes.

Time span of measurement: About 6 times as long as the retention time of saikosaponin a, beginning after the solvent peak.

System suitability

Test for required detectability: Measure exactly 1 mL of the standard solution, and add methanol to make exactly 20 mL. Confirm that the peak area of saikosaponin a obtained with 20 μL of this solution is equivalent to 3.5 to 6.5% of that with 20 μL of the standard solution.

System performance: Dissolve 6 mg each of saikosaponin a for assay and saikosaponin b_2 for assay in methanol to make 100 mL. When the procedure is run with 20 μL of this solution under the above operating conditions, saikosaponin a and saikosaponin b_2 are eluted in this order with the resolution between these peaks being not less than 1.5.

System repeatability: When the test is repeated 6 times with 20 μL of the standard solution under the above operating conditions, the relative standard deviation of the peak area of saikosaponin a is not more than 1.0%.

2) Saikosaponin a for assay 2 (Purity value by quantitative NMR)

Unity of peak—Dissolve 1 mg of saikosaponin a for assay 2 in 2 mL of methanol, and use this solution as the sample solution. Perform the test with 20 μL of the sample solution as directed under Liquid Chromatography ⟨*2.01*⟩ according to the following conditions, and compare the absorption spectra of at least 3 points including the top of saikosaponin a peak and around the two middle peak heights of before and after the top: no difference in form is observed between their spectra.

Operating conditions

Column, column temperature, mobile phase, and flow rate: Proceed as directed in the operating conditions in the Assay under Bupleurum Root.

Detector: A photodiode array detector (wavelength: 206 nm, spectrum range of measurement: 200 – 400 nm).

System suitability

System performance: Dissolve 1 mL of the sample solution and 1 mg of saikosaponin d for assay 2 in 2 mL of methanol. To 1 mL of this solution add methanol to make 10 mL. When the procedure is run with 20 μL of this solution under the above operating conditions, saikosaponin a and saikosaponin d are eluted in this order, and the numbers of theoretical plates and the symmetry factors of these peaks are not less than 4000 and not more than 1.4, respectively.

Assay—Weigh accurately 5 mg of saikosaponin a for assay 2 and 1 mg of 1,4-BTMSB-d_4 for nuclear magnetic resonance spectroscopy using an ultramicrobalance, dissolve in 1 mL of deuterated methanol for nuclear magnetic resonance spectroscopy, and use this solution as the sample solution. Transfer the sample solution into an NMR tube 5 mm in outer diameter, measure ^{1}H-NMR as directed under Nuclear Magnetic Resonance Spectroscopy ⟨*2.21*⟩ and Crude Drugs Test ⟨*5.01*⟩ according to the following conditions, using 1,4-BTMSB-d_4 for nuclear magnetic resonance spectroscopy as the reference standard for qNMR. Calculate the resonance intensity *A* (equivalent to 1 hydrogen atom) of the signal around δ 5.70 ppm assuming the signal of the reference standard for qNMR as δ 0 ppm.

$$\text{Amount (\%) of saikosaponin a } (C_{42}H_{68}O_{13}) = M_S \times I \times P/(M \times N) \times 3.4480$$

M: Amount (mg) of saikosaponin a for assay 2 taken

M_S: Amount (mg) of 1,4-BTMSB-d_4 for nuclear magnetic resonance spectroscopy taken

I: Signal resonance intensity *A* based on the signal resonance intensity of 1,4-BTMSB-d_4 for nuclear magnetic resonance spectroscopy as 18.000

N: Number of the hydrogen derived from *A*

P: Purity (%) of 1,4-BTMSB-d_4 for nuclear magnetic resonance spectroscopy

Operating conditions

Apparatus: A nuclear magnetic resonance spectrometer having ^{1}H resonance frequency of not less than 400 MHz.

Target nucleus: ^{1}H.

Digital resolution: 0.25 Hz or lower.

Measuring spectrum range: 20 ppm or upper, including between −5 ppm and 15 ppm.

Spinning: off.

Pulse angle: 90°

^{13}C Decoupling: on.

Delay time: Repeating pulse waiting time not less than 60 seconds.

Integrating times: 8 or more times.

Dummy scanning: 2 or more times.

Measuring temperature: A constant temperature between 20°C and 30°C.

System suitability

Test for required detectability: When the procedure is run with the sample solution under the above operating conditions, the SN ratio of the signal around δ 5.70 ppm is not less than 100.

System performance: When the procedure is run with the sample solution under the above operating conditions, the signal of around δ 5.70 ppm is not overlapped with any obvious signal of foreign substance.

System repeatability: When the test is repeated 6 times with the sample solution under the above operating conditions, the relative standard deviation of the ratio of the resonance intensity *A* to that of the reference standard for qNMR is not more than 1.0%.

Saikosaponin a for component determination See saikosaponin a for assay.

Saikosaponin a for thin-layer chromatography $C_{42}H_{68}O_{13}$ A white, crystalline powder or powder. Freely soluble in methanol and in ethanol (99.5), and practically insoluble in water. Melting point: 225 – 232°C (with decomposition).

Purity Related substances—Dissolve 1.0 mg of saikosaponin a for thin-layer chromatography in exactly 1 mL of methanol, and perform the test with 10 μL of this solution as directed in the Identification (2) under Bupleurum Root: any spot other than the principal spot at the *R*f value of about 0.4 does not appear.

Saikosaponins a and d standard TS for assay Prepare as described in the following 1), 2)-1 or 2)-2.

1) Weigh accurately about 10 mg each of saikosaponin a for assay (for assay 1) and saikosaponin d for assay (for assay 1), previously dried in a desiccator (silica gel) for 24 hours, dissolve in methanol to make exactly 200 mL, and use this solution as the saikosaponins a and d standard TS for assay.

2)-1 Weigh accurately about 10 mg each of saikosaponin a (for assay 2) and saikosaponin d (for assay 2), and dissolve in methanol to make exactly 100 mL. Pipet 500 μL of this solution, and evaporate the solvent under low pressure (in vacuo). Before using, add exactly 1 mL of methanol, and use this solution as the saikosaponins a and d TS for assay. It contains 10 mg each of saikosaponin a for assay and saikosaponin d for assay in 200 mL of methanol. This standard TS is corrected by the content obtained in the Assay for saikosaponin a for assay (for assay 2) and saikosaponin d for assay(for assay 2).

2)-2 Weigh accurately about 10 mg each of saikosaponin a (for assay 2) and saikosaponin d (for assay 2), dissolve in methanol to make exactly 200 mL, and use this solution as the saikosaponins a and d TS for assay. This standard TS is corrected by the content obtained in the Assay for saikosaponin a for assay (for assay 2) and saikosaponin d for assay (for assay 2).

Saikosaponin b_2 for assay $C_{42}H_{68}O_{13}$ Saikosaponin b_2 for thin-layer chromatography. It meets the the following requirements. It is used with correction for its amount based on the result obtained in the Assay.

Unity of peak—Dissolve 1 mg of saikosaponin b_2 for assay in 50 mL of the mobile phase, and use this solution as the sample solution. Perform the test with 10 μL of the sample solution as directed under Liquid Chromatography <*2.01*> according to the following conditions, and compare the absorption spectra of at least 3 points including the top of saikosaponin b_2 peak and around the two middle peak heights of before and after the top: no difference in form is observed between their spectra.

Operating conditions

Column, column temperature, mobile phase, and flow rate: Proceed as directed in the operating conditions in the Assay (1) under Saireito Extract.

Detector: A photodiode array detector (wavelength: 252 nm, spectrum range of measurment: 220 – 400 nm).

System suitability

System performance: Proceed as directed in the system suitability in the Assay (1) under Saireito Extract.

Assay—Weigh accurately 5 mg of saikosaponin b_2 for assay and 1 mg of 1,4-BTMSB-d_4 for nuclear magnetic resonance spectroscopy using an ultramicrobalance, dissolve in 1 mL of deuterated methanol for nuclear magnetic resonance spectroscopy, and use this solution as the sample solution. Transfer the sample solution into an NMR tube 5 mm in outer diameter, measure ^{1}H-NMR as directed under Nuclear Magnetic Resonance Spectroscopy <*2.21*> and Crude Drugs Test <*5.01*> according to the following conditions, using 1,4-BTMSB-d_4 for nuclear magnetic resonance spectroscopy as the reference standard for qNMR. Calculate the resonance intensity *A* (equivalent to 1 hydrogen) of the signal around δ 6.20 ppm assuming the signal of the reference standard for qNMR as δ 0 ppm.

$$\text{Amount (\%) of saikosaponin } b_2\ (C_{42}H_{68}O_{13}) = M_S \times I \times P/(M \times N) \times 3.4480$$

M: Amount (mg) of saikosaponin b_2 for assay taken
M_S: Amount (mg) of 1,4-BTMSB-d_4 for nuclear magnetic resonance spectroscopy taken
I: Signal resonance intensity *A* based on the signal resonance intensity of 1,4-BTMSB-d_4 for nuclear magnetic resonance spectroscopy as 18.000
N: Number of the hydrogen derived from *A*
P: Purity (%) of 1,4-BTMSB-d_4 for nuclear magnetic resonance spectroscopy

Operating conditions

Apparatus: A nuclear magnetic resonance spectrometer having ^{1}H resonance frequency of not less than 400 MHz.

Target nucleus: ^{1}H.

Digital resolution: 0.25 Hz or lower.

Measuring spectrum range: 20 ppm or upper, including between −5 ppm and 15 ppm.

Spinning: off.

Pulse angle: 90°

^{13}C Decoupling: on.

Delay time: Repeating pulse waiting time not less than 60 seconds.

Integrating times: 8 or more times.

Dummy scanning: 2 or more times.

Measuring temperature: A constant temperature between 20°C and 30°C.

System suitability

Test for required detectability: When the procedure is run with the sample solution under the above operating conditions, the SN ratio of the signal of around δ 6.20 ppm is not less than 100.

System performance: When the procedure is run with the sample solution under the above operating conditions, the signal of around δ 6.20 ppm is no overlapped with any obvious signal of foreign substance.

System repeatability: When the test is repeated 6 times with the sample solution under the above operating conditions, the relative standard deviation of the ratio of the resonance intensity *A* to that of the reference standard for qNMR is not more than 1.0%.

Saikosaponin b_2 for component determination See saikosaponin b_2 for assay.

Saikosaponin b_2 standard TS for assay Prepare as described in the following 1) or 2).

1) Weigh accurately about 10 mg of saikosaponin b_2 for assay, and dissolve in methanol to make exactly 250 mL. Pipet 500 μL of this solution, and evaporate the solvent under reduced pressure. Before using, add exactly 2 mL of a mixture of water and methanol (1:1), and use this solution as the saikosaponin b_2 standard TS for assay. It contains 10 mg of saikosaponin b_2 for assay in 1000 mL of a mixture of water and methanol (1:1). This standard TS is corrected by the content obtained in the Assay for saikosaponin b_2 for assay.

2) Weigh accurately about 10 mg of saikosaponin b_2 for assay, dissolve in 50 mL of methanol, and add water to make exactly 100 mL. Pipet 10 mL of this solution, add a mixture of water and methanol (1:1) to make exactly 100

mL, and use this solution as saikosaponin b_2 standard TS for assay. This standard TS is corrected by the content obtained in the Assay for saikosaponin b_2 for assay.

Saikosaponin b_2 for thin-layer chromatography $C_{42}H_{68}O_{13}$ White, crystals or crystalline powder. Freely soluble in ethanol (99.5), soluble in methanol, and practically insoluble in water. Melting point: about 240°C.

Identification—Determine the absorption spectrum of a solution of saikosaponin b_2 for thin-layer chromatography in methanol (1 in 50,000) as directed under Ultraviolet-visible Spectrophotometry *<2.24>*: it exhibits maxima between 241 nm and 245 nm, between 250 nm and 254 nm, and between 259 nm and 263 nm.

Purity Related substances—Dissolve 2 mg of saikosaponin b_2 for thin-layer chromatography in 2 mL of methanol, and use this solution as the sample solution. Pipet 1 mL of the sample solution, add methanol to make exactly 50 mL, and use this solution as the standard solution. Proceed the test with 10 μL each of the sample solution and standard solution as directed in the Identification (1) under Saireito Extract: the spot other than the principle spot, having *Rf* value of about 0.3, obtained from the sample solution is not more intense than the spot from the standard solution.

Saikosaponin d for assay $C_{42}H_{68}O_{13}$ A white, crystalline powder or powder. Freely soluble in methanol and in ethanol (99.5), and practically insoluble in water. Melting point: about 240°C. It meets the requirements of the following Saikosaponin d for assay 1 and Saikosaponin d for assay 2 (Purity value by quantitative NMR). The former is used after drying in a desiccator (silica gel) for 24 hour in the Assay 1, and the latter is corrected the content based on the amount (%) obtained in the Assay 2.

1) Saikosaponin d for assay 1

Absorbance *<2.24>* $E^{1\%}_{1\,\mathrm{cm}}$ (206 nm): 66 – 74 (15 mg, methanol, 200 mL). Previously dried in a desiccator (in vacuum, silica gel) for 24 hours.

Purity Related substances—

(1) Dissolve 2.0 mg of saikosaponin d for assay in 2 mL of methanol, and use this solution as the sample solution. Pipet 1 mL of the sample solution, add methanol to make exactly 100 mL, and use this as the standard solution. Proceed the test with 10 μL each of the sample solution and standard solution as directed in the Identification (2) under Bupleurum Root: the spot other than the principal spot around *Rf* value of 0.4 obtained from the sample solution is not larger and not more intense than the spot from the standard solution.

(2) Dissolve 10 mg of saikosaponin d for assay in 20 mL of methanol, and use this solution as the sample solution. Pipet 1 mL of the sample solution, add methanol to make exactly 100 mL, and use this solution as the standard solution. Perform the test with exactly 20 μL each of the sample solution and standard solution as directed under Liquid Chromatography *<2.01>* according to the following conditions, and determine each peak area by the automatic integration method: the total area of the peaks other than saikosaponin d obtained from the sample solution is not more than the peak area of saikosaponin d from the standard solution.

Operating conditions

Detector, and column: Proceed as directed in the operating conditions in the Assay under Bupleurum Root.

Column temperature: A constant temperature of about 40°C.

Mobile phase: A mixture of water and acetonitrile (11:9).

Flow rate: Adjust so that the retention time of saikosaponin d is about 13 minutes.

Time span of measurement: About 4 times as long as the retention time of saikosaponin d, beginning after the solvent peak.

System suitability

Test for required detectability: Measure exactly 1 mL of the standard solution, and add methanol to make exactly 20 mL. Confirm that the peak area of saikosaponin d obtained with 20 μL of this solution is equivalent to 3.5 to 6.5% of that with 20 μL of the standard solution.

System performance: Dissolve 6 mg each of saikosaponin d for assay and saikosaponin a for assay in methanol to make 100 mL. When the procedure is run with 20 μL of this solution under the above operating conditions, saikosaponin a and saikosaponin d are eluted in this order with the resolution between these peaks being not less than 1.5.

System repeatability: When the test is repeated 6 times with 20 μL of the standard solution under the above operating conditions, the relative standard deviation of the peak area of saikosaponin d is not more than 1.0%.

2) Saikosaponin d for assay 2 (Purity value by quantitative NMR)

Unity of peak—Dissolve 1 mg of saikosaponin d for assay in 2 mL of methanol, and use this solution as the sample solution. Perform the test with 20 μL of the sample solution as directed under Liquid Chromatography *<2.01>* according to the following conditions, and compare the absorption spectra of at least 3 points including the top of saikosaponin d peak and around the two middle peak heights of before and after the top: no difference in form is observed between their spectra.

Operating conditions

Column, column temperature, mobile phase, and flow rate: Proceed as directed in the operating conditions in the Assay under Bupleurum Root.

Detector: A photodiode array detector (wavelength: 206 nm, spectrum range of measurement: 200 – 400 nm).

System suitability

System performance: Dissolve 1 mL of the sample solution and 1 mg of saikosaponin a for assay 2 in 2 mL of methanol. To 1 mL of this solution add methanol to make 10 mL. When the procedure is run with 20 μL of this solution under the above operating conditions, saikosaponin a and saikosaponin d are eluted in this order, and the numbers of theoretical plates and the symmetry factors of these peaks are not less than 4000 and not more than 1.4, respectively.

Assay—Weigh accurately 5 mg of saikosaponin d for assay 2 and 1 mg of 1,4-BTMSB-d_4 for nuclear magnetic resonance spectroscopy using an ultramicrobalance, dissolve in 1 mL of deuterated methanol for nuclear magnetic resonance spectroscopy, and use this solution as the sample solution. Transfer the sample solution into an NMR tube 5 mm in outer diameter, measure ^{1}H-NMR as directed under Nuclear Magnetic Resonance Spectroscopy *<2.21>* and Crude Drugs Test *<5.01>* according to the following conditions, using 1,4-BTMSB-d_4 for nuclear magnetic resonance spectroscopy as the reference standard for qNMR. Calculate the resonance intensity *A* (equivalent to 1 hydrogen atom) of the signal around δ 5.70 ppm assuming the signal of the reference standard for qNMR as δ 0 ppm.

Amount (%) of saikosaponin d ($C_{42}H_{68}O_{13}$)
$$= M_S \times I \times P/(M \times N) \times 3.4480$$

M: Amount (mg) of saikosaponin a for assay 2 taken

M_S: Amount (mg) of 1,4-BTMSB-d_4 for nuclear magnetic resonance spectroscopy taken

I: Signal resonance intensity *A* based on the signal

resonance intensity of 1,4-BTMSB-d_4 for nuclear magnetic resonance spectroscopy as 18.000

N: Number of the hydrogen derived from A

P: Purity (%) of 1,4-BTMSB-d_4 for nuclear magnetic resonance spectroscopy

Operating conditions

Apparatus: A nuclear magnetic resonance spectrometer having ^1H resonance frequency of not less than 400 MHz.

Target nucleus: ^1H.

Digital resolution: 0.25 Hz or lower.

Measuring spectrum range: 20 ppm or upper, including between −5 ppm and 15 ppm.

Spinning: off.

Pulse angle: 90°

^{13}C Decoupling: on.

Delay time: Repeating pulse waiting time not less than 60 seconds.

Integrating times: 8 or more times.

Dummy scanning: 2 or more times.

Measuring temperature: A constant temperature between 20°C and 30°C.

System suitability

Test for required detectability: When the procedure is run with the sample solution under the above operating conditions, the SN ratio of the signal of around δ 5.70 ppm is not less than 100.

System performance: When the procedure is run with the sample solution under the above operating conditions, the signal of around δ 5.70 ppm is no overlapped with any obvious signal of foreign substance.

System repeatability: When the test is repeated 6 times with the sample solution under the above operating conditions, the relative standard deviation of the ratio of the resonance intensity A to that of the reference standard for qNMR is not more than 1.0%.

Saikosaponin d for component determination See saikosaponin d for assay.

Salicylaldazine $C_{14}H_{12}N_2O_2$ Dissolve 0.30 g of hydrazinium sulfate in 5 mL of water. To this solution add 1 mL of acetic acid (100) and 2 mL of a freshly prepared solution of salicylaldehyde in 2-propanol (1 in 5), shake well, and allow to stand until a yellow precipitate is produced. Extract with two 15 mL portions of dichloromethane, to the combined dichloromethane extracts add 5 g of anhydrous sodium sulfate, shake, decant or filter, and evaporate the dichloromethane in the supernatant liquid or filtrate. Dissolve the residue in a warmed mixture of toluene and methanol (3:2), and cool. Filter the crystals produced, and dry in a desiccator (in vacuum, silica gel) for 24 hours. It is a yellow, crystalline powder.

Melting point <2.60>: 213 – 219°C

Purity Related substances—Dissolve 90 mg of salicylaldazine in toluene to make exactly 100 mL. Pipet 1 mL of this solution, add toluene to make exactly 100 mL, and perform the test with this solution as directed in the Purity (6) under Povidone: any spot other than the principal spot does not appear.

Salicylaldehyde HOC_6H_4CHO [K 8390, Special class]

Salicylamide $C_7H_7NO_2$ White, crystals or crystalline powder, and it is odorless and tasteless. Very soluble in N,N-dimethylformamide, freely soluble in ethanol (95), soluble in propylene glycol, sparingly soluble in diethyl ether, and slightly soluble in water and in chloroform. It dissolves in sodium hydroxide TS.

Melting point <2.60>: 139 – 143°C

Purity Ammonium <1.02>—Shake 1.0 g of salicylamide with 40 mL of water, and filter through filter paper previously washed well with water. Discard the first 10 mL of the filtrate, transfer the subsequent 20 mL to a Nessler tube, and add water to make 30 mL. Perform the test using this solution as the test solution. Prepare the control solution as follows: transfer 2.5 mL of Standard Ammonium Solution to a Nessler tube, and add water to make 30 mL.

Loss on drying <2.41>: not more than 0.5% (1 g, silica gel, 4 hours).

Residue on ignition <2.44>: not more than 0.1% (1 g).

Content: not less than 98.5%. Assay—Weigh accurately about 0.2 g of salicylamide, previously dried, dissolve in 70 mL of N,N-dimethylformamide, and titrate <2.50> with 0.1 mol/L tetramethylammonium hydroxide VS (potentiometric titration). Separately, perform a blank determination in the same manner with a solution of 70 mL of N,N-dimethylformamide in 15 mL of water, and make any necessary correction.

Each mL of 0.1 mol/L tetramethylammonium hydroxide VS
= 13.71 mg of $C_7H_7NO_2$

Salicylic acid HOC_6H_4COOH [K 8392, Special class]

Salicylic acid for assay HOC_6H_4COOH [K 8392, Special class]

Salicylic acid TS Dissolve 0.1 g of salicylic acid in 10 mL of sulfuric acid. Prepare before use.

Salmon sperm DNA Salmon sperm or nuclear fraction extracted from salmon sperm, which is sonicated and dried.

Santonin $C_{15}H_{18}O_3$ [Same as the namesake monograph]

Santonin for assay $C_{15}H_{18}O_3$ [Same as the monograph Santonin. It contains not less than 99.0% of santonin ($C_{15}H_{18}O_3$).]

Sarpogrelate hydrochloride $C_{24}H_{31}NO_6.HCl$ [Same as the namesake monograph]

Sarsasapogenin for thin-layer chromatography $C_{27}H_{44}O_3$ It is a white or slightly greyish white, crystalline powder or powder. Slightly soluble in methanol and in ethanol (99.5), and practically insoluble in water.

Identification Determine the infrared absorption spectrum of the substance to be examined as directed in the potassium bromide disk method under Infrared Spectrophotometry <2.25>: it exhibits absorption at the wave numbers of about 2930 cm^{-1}, 1448 cm^{-1}, 1173 cm^{-1}, 985 cm^{-1} and 850 cm^{-1}.

Purity Related substances—Dissolve 1 mg of sarsasapogenin for thin-layer chromatography in 1 mL of methanol, and use this solution as the sample solution. Pipet 0.5 mL of the sample solution, add methanol to make exactly 25 mL, and use this solution as the standard solution. Perform the test with these solutions as directed under Thin-layer Chromatography <2.03>. Perform the test with 5 μL each of the sample solution and standard solution as directed in the Identification (2) under Anemarrhena Rhizome: any spot other than the principal spot with an Rf value of about 0.4 obtained from the sample solution is not more intense than the spot from the standard solution.

Saussurea root [Same as the namesake monograph]

Schisandrin for thin-layer chromatography $C_{24}H_{32}O_7$ White, crystals or crystalline powder. Freely soluble in methanol and in diethyl ether, and practically insoluble in water.

Melting point <*2.60*>: 130 – 135°C

Purity Related substances—Dissolve 1.0 mg of schisandrin for thin-layer chromatography in exactly 1 mL of methanol. Perform the test with 5 μL of this solution as directed in the Identification under Schisandra Fruit: any spot other than the principal spot at the *Rf* value of about 0.4 does not appear.

Scopolamine hydrobromide See scopolamine hydrobromide hydrate.

Scopolamine hydrobromide for thin-layer chromatography See scopolamine hydrobromide hydrate for thin-layer chromatography.

Scopolamine hydrobromide hydrate
$C_{17}H_{21}NO_4.HBr.3H_2O$ [Same as the namesake monograph]

Scopolamine hydrobromide hydrate for thin-layer chromatography $C_{17}H_{21}NO_4.HBr.3H_2O$ [Same as the monograph Scopolamine Hydrobromide Hydrate], or scopolamine hydrobromide hydrate meeting the following requirements. Colorless or white crystals, or white, grains or powder. Freely soluble in water, sparingly soluble in ethanol (95) and in acetic acid (100), and practically insoluble in diethyl ether.

Identification Determine the infrared absorption spectrum of scopolamine hydrobromide hydrate for thin-layer chromatography as directed in the potassium bromide disk method under Infrared Spectrophotometry <*2.25*>: it exhibits absorption at the wave numbers of about 1731 cm^{-1}, 1204 cm^{-1}, 1070 cm^{-1} and 735 cm^{-1}.

Purity Related substances—Dissolve 5 mg of scopolamine hydrobromide hydrate for thin-layer chromatography in 1 mL of ethanol (95), and use this solution as the sample solution. Pipet 0.5 mL of the sample solution, add ethanol (95) to make exactly 25 mL, and use this solution as the standard solution. Perform the test with these solutions as directed under Thin-layer Chromatography <*2.03*>. Spot 20 μL each of the sample solution and standard solution on a plate of silica gel for thin-layer chromatography. Develop the plate with a mixture of acetone, water and ammonia solution (28) (90:7:3) to a distance of about 10 cm, and dry the plate at 80°C for 10 minutes. After cooling, spray evenly Dragendorff's TS for spraying on the plate: any spot other than the principal spot with an *Rf* value of about 0.6 obtained from the sample solution is not more intense than the spot from the standard solution.

Scopoletin for thin-layer chromatography $C_{10}H_8O_4$ White or light brown, crystalline powder or powder. Sparingly soluble in methanol and in ethanol (99.5), and practically insoluble in water. Melting point: about 206°C.

Identification—(1) Determine the absorption spectrum of a solution of scopoletin for thin-layer chromatography in methanol (1 in 250,000) as directed under Ultraviolet-visible Spectrophotometry <*2.24*>: it exhibits maxima between 226 nm and 230 nm, between 295 nm and 299 nm and between 343 nm and 347 nm.

(2) Determine the infrared absorption spectrum of scopoletin for thin-layer chromatography as directed in the potassium bromide disk method under Infrared Spectrophotometry <*2.25*>: it exhibits absorption at the wave numbers of about 3340 cm^{-1}, 1702 cm^{-1}, 1566 cm^{-1}, 1436 cm^{-1} and 923 cm^{-1}.

Purity Related substances – Dissolve 1.0 mg of scopoletin for thin-layer chromatography in 10 mL of methanol, and use this solution as the sample solution. Pipet 1 mL of the sample solution, add methanol to make exactly 50 mL, and use this solution as the standard solution. Perform the test with 5 μL each of the sample solution and standard solution as directed in the Identification under Artemisia Leaf: the spot other than the principal spot, having an *Rf* value of about 0.4, obtained from the sample solution is not more intense than the spot from the standard solution.

Sea sand A mixture of white, grey, brown or black grains, 0.3 to 1.0 mm in particle size.

Secondary antibody TS To a mixture of 1.5 mL of blocking TS for epoetin alfa and 13.5 mL of sodium azide-phosphate-buffered sodium chloride TS, add 1 drop of biotinylated equine anti-mouse IgG antibody.

2nd Fluid for disintegration test To 250 mL of 0.2 mol/L potassium dihydrogen phosphate TS add 118 mL of 0.2 mol/L sodium hydroxide TS and water to make 1000 mL. It is clear and colorless, and has a pH about 6.8.

2nd Fluid for dissolution test A mixture of phosphate buffer solution (pH 6.8) and water (1:1).

Selenious acid H_2SeO_3 Colorless or white crystals. It is hygroscopic.

Identification—(1) Dissolve 0.2 g of selenious acid in 20 mL of water, and use this solution as the sample solution. To 10 mL of the sample solution add 2 mL of tin (II) chloride TS: a red precipitate is produced.

(2) To 10 mL of the sample solution obtained in (1) add 1 mL of diluted hydrochloric acid (2 in 3) and 1 mL of potassium iodide TS: a brown color is produced.

Storage—Preserve in a light-resistant tight container.

Selenious acid-sulfuric acid TS Dissolve 50 mg of selenious acid in 10 mL of sulfuric acid.

Selenium Se [K 8598, Special class]

Selenium dioxide SeO_2 White, crystals or crystalline powder.

Identification—(1) To 10 mL of a solution of selenium dioxide (1 in 100) add 2 mL of tin (II) chloride TS: a red precipitate is produced.

(2) To 10 mL of a solution of selenium dioxide (1 in 100) add 1 mL of diluted hydrochloric acid (2 in 3) and 1 mL of potassium iodide TS: a brown color is produced.

Content: not less than 97.0%. Assay—Weigh accurately about 0.6 g of selenium dioxide, and dissolve in water to make exactly 200 mL. Pipet 20 mL of this solution into an iodine bottle, add 80 mL of water, 3 g of potassium iodide and 5 mL of diluted hydrochloric acid (2 in 3), allow to stand at a dark place for 5 minutes, and titrate <*2.50*> with 0.1 mol/L sodium thiosulfate VS (indicator: starch TS). Perform a blank determination in the same manner, and make any necessary correction.

Each mL of 0.1 mol/L sodium thiosulfate VS
= 2.774 mg of SeO_2

Semicarbazide acetate TS Place 2.5 g of semicarbazide hydrochloride, 2.5 g of anhydrous sodium acetate and 30 mL of methanol in a flask, heat on a water bath for 2 hours, cool to 20°C, and filter. To the filtrate add methanol to make 100 mL. Preserve in a cold place. Do not use the solution showing a yellow color.

Semicarbazide hydrochloride $H_2NNHCONH_2.HCl$ White to light yellow crystals.

Identification (1) To 10 mL of a solution of semicarbazide hydrochloride (1 in 100) add 1 mL of silver nitrate

TS: white precipitates appear.

(2) Determine the infrared absorption spectrum as directed in the potassium bromide disk method under Infrared Spectrophotometry <2.25>: it exhibits absorption at the wave numbers of about 3420 cm^{-1}, 3260 cm^{-1}, 2670 cm^{-1}, 1684 cm^{-1}, 1582 cm^{-1}, 1474 cm^{-1}, 1386 cm^{-1}, 1210 cm^{-1}, 1181 cm^{-1}, 770 cm^{-1} and 719 cm^{-1}.

Sendai virus RNA virus of *Paramyxoviridae*, which is grown in the allantoic cavity of embryonated chicken eggs. Measure hemagglutination titer (HA titer) with chicken red blood cells, and use it with 800 to 3200 HA titer/mL.

Sennoside A for thin-layer chromatography $C_{42}H_{38}O_{20}$ A yellow powder. Practically insoluble in water and in ethanol (99.5).

Identification Determine the infrared absorption spectrum of sennoside A to be examined as directed in the potassium bromide disk method under Infrared Spectrophotometry <2.25>: it exhibits absorption at the wave numbers of about 3420 cm^{-1}, 1712 cm^{-1}, 1637 cm^{-1}, 1597 cm^{-1} and 1074 cm^{-1}.

Purity Related substances—Conduct this procedure without exposure to light, using light-resistant vessels. Dissolve 1 mg of sennoside A to be examined in 1 mL of a mixture of tetrahydrofuran and water (7:3), and use this solution as the sample solution. Pipet 0.5 mL of the sample solution, add a mixture of tetrahydrofuran and water (7:3) to make exactly 25 mL, and use this solution as the standard solution. Then, perform the test with 5 μL each of the sample solution and standard solution as directed in the Identification (2) under Senna Leaf: any spot other than the principal spot with an *R*f value of about 0.3 obtained from the sample solution is not more intense than the spot from the standard solution.

L-Serine $C_3H_7NO_3$ [K 9105, Special class]

Sesame oil [Same as the namesake monograph]

Sesamin for thin-layer chromatography $C_{20}H_{18}O_6$ White, crystals or crystalline powder. Slightly soluble in methanol and in ethanol (99.5), and practically insoluble in water.

Identification Determine the absorption spectrum of a solution of sesame for thin-layer chromatography in methanol (3 in 200,000) as directed under Ultraviolet-visible Spectrophotometry <2.24>: it exhibits maxima between 235 nm and 239 nm and between 285 nm and 289 nm.

Melting point <2.60>: 122 – 124°C

Purity Related substances—Dissolve 2.0 mg of sesamin for thin-layer chromatography in 2 mL of methanol, and use this solution as the sample solution. Pipet 1 mL of the sample solution, add methanol to make exactly 50 mL, and use this solution as the standard solution. Perform the test with 5 μL each of the sample solution and standard solution as directed in the Identification under Sesame: the spot other than the principal spot obtained from the sample solution is not more intense than the spot from the standard solution.

[6]-Shogaol for assay $C_{17}H_{24}O_3$ [6]-Shogaol for thin-layer chromatography. It meets the following 1) [6]-Shogaol for assay 1 or 2) [6]-Shogaol for assay 2 (Purity value by quantitative NMR). The latter is used with correction for its amount based on the result obtained in the Assay.

1) [6]-Shogaol for assay 1

Absorbance <2.24>: $E^{1\%}_{1\,cm}$ (225 nm): 727 – 781 (5 mg, ethanol (99.5), 500 mL).

Purity Related substances—Dissolve 5 mg of [6]-shogaol for assay in 10 mL of a mixture of acetonitrile and water (2:1), and use this solution as the sample solution. Pipet 1 mL of the sample solution, add a mixture of acetonitrile and water (2:1) to make exactly 100 mL, and use this solution as the standard solution. Perform the test with exactly 10 μL each of the sample solution and standard solution as directed under Liquid Chromatography <2.01> according to the following conditions, and determine each peak area by the automatic integration method: the total area of the peaks other than [6]-shogaol obtained from the sample solution is not larger than the peak area of [6]-shogaol from the standard solution.

Operating conditions

Detector, column, column temperature, mobile phase, and flow rate: Proceed as directed in the operating conditions under Assay (2) of Mukoi-Daikenchuto Extract.

Time span of measurement: 3 times as long as the retention time of [6]-shogaol, beginning after the solvent peak.

System suitability

Test for required detectability: Pipet 1 mL of the standard solution, and add a mixture of acetonitrile and water (2:1) to make exactly 20 mL. Confirm that the peak area of [6]-shogaol obtained with 10 μL of this solution is equivalent to 3.5 to 6.5% of that with 10 μL of the standard solution.

System performance: When the procedure is run with 10 μL of the standard solution under the above operating conditions, the number of theoretical plates and the symmetry factor of the peak of [6]-shogaol are not less than 5000 and not more than 1.5%, respectively.

System repeatability: When the test is repeated 6 times with 10 μL of the standard solution under the above operating conditions, the relative standard deviation of the peak area of [6]-shogaol is not more than 1.5%.

2) [6]-Shogaol for assay 2 (Purity value by quantitative NMR)

Unity of peak—Dissolve 5 mg of [6]-shogaol for assay 2 in 10 mL of a mixture of acetonitrile and water (2:1), and use this solution as the sample solution. Perform the test with 10 μL of the sample solution as directed under Liquid Chromatography <2.01> according to the following conditions, and compare the absorption spectra of at least 3 points including the top of [6]-shogaol peak and around the two middle peak heights of before and after the top: no difference in form is observed among their spectra.

Operating conditions

Column, column temperature, mobile phase, and flow rate: Proceed as directed in the operating conditions in the Assay (2) under Mukoi-Daikenchuto Extract.

Detector: A photodiode array detector (wavelength: 225 nm, spectrum range of measurement: 220 – 400 nm).

System suitability

System performance: Proceed as directed in the system suitability in the Assay (2) under Mukoi-Daikenchuto Extract.

Assay—Weigh accurately 5 mg of [6]-shogaol for assay 2 and 1 mg of 1,4-BTMSB-d_4 for nuclear magnetic resonance spectroscopy using an ultramicrobalance, dissolve in 1 mL of deuterated methanol for nuclear magnetic resonance spectroscopy, and use this solution as the sample solution. Transfer the sample solution into an NMR tube 5 mm in outer diameter, and measure ^{1}H-NMR as directed under Nuclear Magnetic Resonance Spectroscopy <2.21> and Crude Drugs Test <5.01> according to the following conditions, using 1,4-BTMSB-d_4 for nuclear magnetic resonance spectroscopy as the reference standard for qNMR. Calculate the resonance intensity *A* (equivalent to 3 hydrogens) of the signal around δ 3.57 ppm assuming the signal of the reference standard for qNMR as δ 0 ppm.

Amount (%) of [6]-shogaol ($C_{17}H_{24}O_3$)
$= M_S \times I \times P/(M \times N) \times 1.2202$

M: Amount (mg) of [6]-shogaol for assay 2 taken
M_S: Amount (mg) of 1,4-BTMSB-d_4 for nuclear magnetic resonance spectroscopy taken
I: Signal resonance intensity *A* based on the signal resonance intensity of 1,4-BTMSB-d_4 for nuclear magnetic resonance spectroscopy as 18.000
N: Number of the hydrogen derived from *A*
P: Purity (%) of 1,4-BTMSB-d_4 for nuclear magnetic resonance spectroscopy

Operating conditions
Apparatus: A nuclear magnetic resonance spectrometer having ^1H resonance frequency of not less than 400 MHz.
Target nucleus: ^1H.
Digital resolution: 0.25 Hz or lower.
Measuring spectrum range: 20 ppm or upper, including between − 5 ppm and 15 ppm.
Spinning: off.
Pulse angle: 90°.
^{13}C decoupling: on.
Delay time: Repeating pulse waiting time not less than 60 seconds.
Integrating times: 8 or more times.
Dummy scanning: 2 or more times.
Measuring temperature: A constant temperature between 20°C and 30°C.
System suitability
Test for required detectability: When the procedure is run with the sample solution under the above operating conditions, the SN ratio of each signal around δ 3.57 ppm and δ 6.37 – 6.43 ppm is not less than 100.
System performance: When the procedure is run with the sample solution under the above operating conditions, the two signals around δ 3.57 ppm and δ 6.37 – 6.43 ppm are not overlapped with any signal of obvious foreign substance. Furthermore, when determined the resonance intensities, *A* (equivalent to 3 hydrogens) and A_1 (equivalent to 2 hydrogens) of each signal around δ 3.57 ppm and δ 6.37 – 6.43 ppm, the ratio of the resonance intensities, $(A_1/2)/(A/3)$, of each signal around δ 3.57 ppm and δ 6.37 – 6.43 ppm is between 0.99 and 1.01.
System repeatability: When the test is repeated 6 times with the sample solution under the above operating conditions, the relative standard deviation of the ratio of the resonance intensity *A* to that of the reference standard for qNMR is not more than 1.0%.

[6]-Shogaol for thin-layer chromatography $C_{17}H_{24}O_3$ A pale yellow, clear liquid. Miscible with methanol and with ethanol (99.5), and practically insoluble in water.
Purity Related substances—Dissolve 1.0 mg of [6]-shogaol for thin-layer chromatography in 2 mL of methanol, and use this solution as the sample solution. Perform the test with the sample solution as directed under Thin-layer Chromatography <2.03>. Spot 10 μL of the sample solution on a plate of silica gel for thin-layer chromatography. Develop the plate with a mixture of ethyl acetate and hexane (1:1) to a distance of about 10 cm, and air-dry the plate. Spray evenly 4-dimethylaminobenzaldehyde TS for spraying on the plate, heat the plate at 105°C for 5 minutes, and allow to cool: any spot other than the principal spot at an *Rf* value of about 0.5 does not appear.

Silica gel An amorphous, partly hydrated silicic acid occurring in glassy granules of various sizes. When used as a desiccant, it is frequently coated with a substance that changes color when the capacity to absorb water is exhausted. Such colored products may be regenerated by being heated at 110°C until the gel assumes the original color.
Loss on ignition <2.43>: not more than 6% (2 g, 950 ± 50°C).
Water absorption: not less than 31%. Weigh accurately about 10 g of silica gel, and allow to stand for 24 hours in a closed container in which the atmosphere is maintained at 80% relative humidity with sulfuric acid having a specific gravity of 1.19. Weigh again, and calculate the increase in mass.

Siliceous earth [K 8330, Diatomaceous earth, First class]

Silicone oil Colorless clear liquid, having no odor.
Viscosity <2.53>: 50 – 100 mm²/s.

Silicone resin Light gray, half-clear, viscous liquid or a pasty material. It is almost odorless.
Viscosity and refractive index—Place 15 g of silicone resin in a Soxhlet extractor, then extract with 150 mL of carbon tetrachloride for 3 hours. The kinematic viscosity of the residual liquid, obtained by evaporating carbon tetrachloride from the extract on a water bath, is 100 to 1100 mm²/s (25°C). Its refractive index is 1.400 to 1.410 (25°C).
Specific gravity <2.56> *d*: 0.98 – 1.02
Loss on drying <2.41>: 0.45 – 2.25 g with the extracted residue obtained in the Viscosity and refractive index (100°C, 1 hour).

Silicotungstic acid 26-water $SiO_2.12WO_3.26H_2O$ White to slightly yellowish, crystals. Deliquescent. Very soluble in water and in ethanol (95).
Purity Clarity and color of solution—a solution (1 in 20) is clear and colorless.
Loss on ignition <2.43>: 14 – 15% (2 g, dry at 110°C for 2 hours then 700 – 750°C, constant mass).

Silodosin $C_{25}H_{32}F_3N_3O_4$ [Same as the namesake monograph]

Silver chromate-saturated potassium chromate TS Dissolve 5 g of potassium chromate in 50 mL of water, add silver nitrate TS until a pale red precipitate is produced, and filter. To the filtrate add water to make 100 mL.

Silver diethyldithiocarbamate See silver *N,N*-diethyldithiocarbamate.

Silver nitrate $AgNO_3$ [K 8550, Special class]

Silver nitrate-ammonia TS Dissolve 1 g of silver nitrate in 20 mL of water, and add ammonia TS dropwise with stirring until the precipitate is almost entirely dissolved.
Storage—Preserve in tight, light-resistant containers.

Silver nitrate TS Dissolve 17.5 g of silver nitrate in water to make 1000 mL (0.1 mol/L).
Storage—Preserve in light-resistant containers.

Silver *N,N*-diethyldithiocarbamate $C_5H_{10}AgNS_2$ [K 9512, Special class]

Sindbis virus RNA virus of *Togaviridae*, proliferated by chick embryo cell primary culture. Determine the number of plaques on the cell culture, and use the virus with not less than 1 × 10⁸ PFU/mL.

Sinomenine for assay $C_{19}H_{23}NO_4$ Sinomenine for thin-layer chromatography. It meets the requirements of the following 1) sinomenine for assay 1 or 2) sinomenine for assay 2 (Purity value by quantitative NMR). The former is used after drying in a desiccator (silica gel) for 24 hours, and latter is used with correction for its amount based on the result obtained in the Assay.

1) Sinomenine for assay 1

Identification Determine the absorption spectrum of a solution of sinomenine for assay in methanol (1 in 25,000) as directed under Ultraviolet-visible Spectrophotometry <*2.24*>: it exhibits the maximum between 259 nm and 263 nm.

Purity Related substances—Dissolve 5 mg of sinomenine for assay 1 in 10 mL of a mixture of water and acetonitrile (7:3), and use this solution as the sample solution. Pipet 1 mL of the sample solution, add the mixture of water and acetonitrile (7:3) to make exactly 100 mL, and use this solution as the standard solution. Perform the test with exactly 10 μL each of the sample solution and standard solution as directed under Liquid Chromatography <*2.01*> according to the following conditions, and determine each peak area by the automatic integration method: the total area of the peaks other than sinomenine obtained from the sample solution is not larger than the peak area of sinomenine from the standard solution.

Operating conditions

Column, column temperature, mobile phase and flow rate: Proceed as directed in the operating conditions in the Assay (1) under Boiogito Extract.

Detector: An ultraviolet absorption photometer (wavelength: 261 nm).

Time span of measurement: About 3 times as long as the retention time of sinomenine, beginning after the solvent peak.

System suitability

Test for required detectability: Pipet 1 mL of the standard solution, and add a mixture of water and acetonitrile (7:3) to make exactly 20 mL. Confirm that the peak area of sinomenine obtained with 10 μL of this solution is equivalent to 3.5 to 6.5% of that with 10 μL of the standard solution.

System performance: When the procedure is run with 10 μL of the standard solution under the above operating conditions, the number of theoretical plates and the symmetry factor of the peak of sinomenine are not less than 5000 and not more than 1.5, respectively.

System repeatability: When the test is repeated 6 times with 10 μL of the standard solution under the above operating conditions, the relative standard deviation of the peak area of sinomenine is not more than 1.5%.

2) Sinomenine for assay 2 (Purity value by quantitative NMR)

Unity of peak—Dissolve 5 mg of sinomenine for assay 2 in 10 mL of a mixture of water and acetonitrile (7:3), and use this solution as the sample solution. Perform the test with 10 μL of the sample solution as directed under Liquid Chromatography <*2.01*> according to the following conditions, and compare the absorption spectra of at least 3 points including the top of sinomenine peak and around the two middle peak heights of before and after the top: no difference in form is observed among their spectra.

Operating conditions

Column, column temperature, mobile phase and flow rate: Proceed as directed in the operating conditions in the Assay (1) under Boiogito Extract.

Detector: A photodiode array detector (wavelength: 261 nm, spectrum range of measurement: 220 – 400 nm).

System suitability

System performance: When the procedure is run with 10 μL of the sample solution under the above operating conditions, the number of theoretical plates and the symmetry factor of the peak of sinomenine are not less than 5000 and not more than 1.5, respectively.

Assay—Weigh accurately 5 mg of sinomenine for assay 2 and 1 mg of 1,4-BTMSB-d_4 for nuclear magnetic resonance spectroscopy using an ultramicrobalance, dissolve in 1 mL of deuterated acetone for nuclear magnetic resonance spectroscopy, and use this solution as the sample solution. Transfer the sample solution into an NMR tube 5 mm in outer diameter, and measure ^{1}H-NMR as directed under Nuclear Magnetic Resonance Spectroscopy <*2.21*> and Crude Drugs Test <*5.01*> according to the following conditions, using 1,4-BTMSB-d_4 for nuclear magnetic resonance spectroscopy as the reference standard for qNMR. Calculate the resonance intensity A (equivalent to 1 hydrogen) of the signal around δ 5.42 ppm assuming the signal of the reference standard for qNMR as δ 0 ppm.

$$\text{Amount (\%) of sinomenine } (C_{19}H_{23}NO_4) = M_S \times I \times P/(M \times N) \times 1.4543$$

M: Amount (mg) of sinomenine for assay 2 taken

M_S: Amount (mg) of 1,4-BTMSB-d_4 for nuclear magnetic resonance spectroscopy taken

I: Signal resonance intensity A based on the signal resonance intensity of 1,4-BTMSB-d_4 for nuclear magnetic resonance spectroscopy as 18.000

N: Number of hydrogen derived from A

P: Purity (%) of 1,4-BTMSB-d_4 for nuclear magnetic resonance spectroscopy

Operating conditions

Apparatus: A nuclear magnetic resonance spectrometer having ^{1}H resonance frequency of not less than 400 MHz.

Target nucleus: ^{1}H.

Digital resolution: 0.25 Hz or lower.

Measuring spectrum range: 20 ppm or upper, including between −5 ppm and 15 ppm.

Spinning: off.

Pulse angle: 90°.

^{13}C decoupling: on.

Delay time: Repeating pulse waiting time not less than 60 seconds.

Integrating times: 8 or more times.

Dummy scanning: 2 or more times.

Measuring temperature: A constant temperature between 20°C and 30°C.

System suitability

Test for required detectability: When the procedure is run with the sample solution under the above operating conditions, the SN ratio of the signal around δ 5.42 ppm is not less than 100.

System performance: When the procedure is run with the sample solution under the above operating conditions, the signal around δ 5.42 ppm is not overlapped with any signal of obvious foreign substances.

System repeatability: When the test is repeated 6 times with the sample solution under the above operating conditions, the relative standard deviation of the ratio of the resonance intensity A to that of the reference standard for qNMR is not more than 1.0%.

Sinomenine for thin-layer chromatography $C_{19}H_{23}NO_4$ A white or pale brown crystalline powder. Freely soluble in methanol, soluble in ethanol (99.5), and very slightly soluble in water.

Identification Determine the infrared absorption spectrum of sinomenine for thin-layer chromatography as directed in the potassium bromide disk method under Infrared Spectrophotometry <*2.25*>: it exhibits absorption at the wave numbers of about 2830 cm^{-1}, 1687 cm^{-1}, 1630 cm^{-1}, 1441 cm^{-1} and 1279 cm^{-1}.

Purity Related substances—Dissolve 5 mg of sinomenine for thin-layer chromatography in 2 mL of methanol, and use this solution as the sample solution. Pipet 1 mL of the sample solution, add methanol to make exactly 100 mL, and use this solution as the standard solution. Perform the test with 10 μL each of the sample solution and standard solution as directed in the Identification (1) under Boiogito Extract: the spot other than the principal spot at an *R*f value of about 0.2 obtained from the sample solution is not more colored than the spot from the standard solution.

Sivelestat sodium hydrate $C_{20}H_{21}N_2NaO_7S.4H_2O$ [Same as the namesake monograph]

Soda lime [K 8603, For carbon dioxide absorption]

Sodium Na [K 8687, special class]

Sodium acetate See sodium acetate trihydrate.

Sodium acetate-acetone TS Dissolve 8.15 g of sodium acetate trihydrate and 42 g of sodium chloride in 100 mL of water, and add 68 mL of 0.1 mol/L hydrochloric acid VS, 150 mL of acetone and water to make 500 mL.

Sodium acetate, anhydrous CH_3COONa [K 8372, Special class]

Sodium acetate trihydrate $CH_3COONa.3H_2O$ [K 8371, Special class]

Sodium acetate TS Dissolve 13.6 g of sodium acetate trihydrate in water to make 100 mL (1 mol/L).

Sodium azide NaN_3 [K 9501, Special class]

Sodium azide-phosphate-buffered sodium chloride TS Dissolve 8.0 g of sodium chloride, 0.2 g of potassium chloride, 2.9 g of disodium hydrogen phosphate dodecahydrate and 0.2 g of potassium dihydrogen phosphate in water to make 1000 mL. Dissolve 0.25 g of sodium azide in this solution.

Sodium benzoate $C_7H_5NaO_2$ [Same as the namesake monograph]

Sodium bicarbonate See sodium hydrogen carbonate.

Sodium bicarbonate for pH determination See sodium hydrogen carbonate for pH determination.

Sodium bicarbonate TS See sodium hydrogen carbonate TS.

7% **Sodium bicarbonate injection** [Same as the monograph Sodium Bicarbonate Injection. However, labeled amount should be 7 w/v%.]

Sodium bismuthate See bismuth sodium trioxide.

Sodium bisulfite See sodium hydrogen sulfite.

Sodium bisulfite TS See sodium hydrogen sulfite TS.

Sodium bitartrate See sodium hydrogen tartrate monohydrate.

Sodium bitartrate TS See sodium hydrogen tartrate TS.

Sodium borate See sodium tetraborate decahydrate.

Sodium borate for pH determination See sodium tetraborate decahydrate for pH determination.

Sodium borohydride $NaBH_4$ White to grayish white, crystals, powder or masses. Freely soluble in water.

Content: not less than 95%. Assay—Weigh accurately 0.25 g of sodium borohydride, dissolve in 20 mL of diluted sodium hydroxide TS (3 in 10), and add water to make exactly 500 mL. Pipet 20 mL of this solution, put in a glassstoppered iodine flask, and cool in ice. Add exactly 40 mL of iodine TS, allow to stand at a dark place for 10 minutes, add exactly 10 mL of diluted sulfuric acid (1 in 6), and titrate <*2.50*> with 0.1 mol/L sodium thiosulfate VS (back titration) (indicator: starch solution). Perform a blank determination in the same manner, and make any necessary correction.

Each mL of 0.1 mol/L sodium thiosulfate VS
= 0.4729 mg of $NaBH_4$

Sodium bromide NaBr [K 8514, Special class]

Sodium carbonate See sodium carbonate decahydrate.

Sodium carbonate, anhydrous Na_2CO_3 [K 8625, Sodium carbonate, Special class]

Sodium carbonate decahydrate $Na_2CO_3.10H_2O$ [K 8624, Special class]

Sodium carbonate for pH determination Na_2CO_3 [K 8625, for pH determination]

Sodium carbonate (standard reagent) Na_2CO_3 In addition to JIS K 8005 standard reagent for volumetric analysis, certified reference material which can be used for volumetric analysis may be used.

Sodium carbonate TS Dissolve 10.5 g of anhydrous sodium carbonate in water to make 100 mL (1 mol/L).

0.55 mol/L Sodium carbonate TS Dissolve 5.83 g of anhydrous sodium carbonate in water to make 100 mL.

Sodium chloride NaCl [K 8150, Special class]

Sodium chloride (standard reagent) NaCl In addition to JIS K 8005 standard reagent for volumetric analysis, certified reference material which can be used for volumetric analysis may be used.

Sodium chloride for assay NaCl [Same as the monograph, Sodium Chloride]

Sodium chloride TS Dissolve 10 g of sodium chloride in water to make 100 mL.

0.1 mol/L Sodium chloride TS Dissolve 6 g of sodium chloride in water to make 1000 mL.

0.2 mol/L Sodium chloride TS Dissolve 11.7 g of sodium chloride in water to make 1000 mL.

1 mol/L Sodium chloride TS Dissolve 29.22 g of sodium chloride in water to make 500 mL.

Sodium cholate hydrate $C_{24}H_{39}O_5Na.H_2O$ A white powder.

Identification—Determine the infrared absorption spectrum of sodium cholate hydrate as directed in the potassium bromide disk method under Infrared Spectrophotometry <*2.25*>: it exhibits absorption at the wave numbers of about 3400 cm^{-1}, 2940 cm^{-1}, 1579 cm^{-1}, 1408 cm^{-1} and 1082 cm^{-1}.

Water <*2.48*>: 3.5 – 5.0% (40 mg, coulometric titration).

Content: not less than 99.0% of sodium cholate ($C_{24}H_{39}O_5Na$), calculated on the anhydrous basis. Assay—Weigh accurately about 0.35 g of sodium cholate hydrate, dissolve in 60 mL of acetic acid (100), and titrate <*2.50*> with 0.1 mol/L perchloric acid VS (potentiometric titration). Perform a blank determination in the same manner, and make any necessary correction.

Each mL of 0.1 mol/L perchloric acid VS
= 43.06 mg of $C_{24}H_{39}O_5Na$

Sodium citrate See sodium citrate hydrate.

Sodium citrate hydrate $C_6H_5Na_3O_7.2H_2O$ [K 8288, Trisodium citrate dihydrate, or same as the namesake monograph]

0.1 mol/L Sodium citrate TS Dissolve 29.4 g of trisodium citrate dihydrate in water to make 1000 mL

Sodium cobaltinitrite See sodium hexanitrocobaltate (III).

Sodium cobaltinitrite TS See sodium hexanitrocobaltate (III) TS.

Sodium 1-decanesulfonate $C_{10}H_{21}NaO_3S$ A white powder.

Purity Clarity and color of solution—Dissolve 1.0 g of sodium decanesulfonate in 20 mL of water: the solution is clear and colorless.

Loss on drying <*2.41*>: not more than 3.0% (1 g, 105°C, 3 hours).

Content: not less than 98.0%. Assay—Weigh accurately about 0.45 g of sodium 1-decanesulfonate, dissolve in 50 mL of water, and pass through a column, about 1.2 cm in inside diameter and about 25 cm in length, packed with about 20 mL of strongly acidic ion-exchange resin (0.3 to 1.0 mm, H type) for column chromatography at a flow rate of about 4 mL per minute. Wash with 150 mL of water at a flow rate of about 4 mL per minute. Combine the washing and the elute, and titrate <*2.50*> with 0.1 mol/L sodium hydroxide VS (potentiometric titration). Perform a blank determination in the same manner, and make any necessary correction.

Each mL of 0.1 mol/L sodium hydroxide VS
= 24.43 mg of $C_{10}H_{21}NaO_3S$

0.0375 mol/L Sodium 1-decanesulfonate TS Dissolve 3.665 g of sodium 1-decanesulfonate in 400 mL of water.

Sodium desoxycholate $C_{24}H_{39}NaO_4$ White, odorless, crystalline powder.

Identification—Determine the infrared absorption spectrum of sodium desoxycholate, previously dried, according to the potassium bromide disk method under Infrared Spectrophotometry <*2.25*>: it exhibits absorption at the wave numbers of about 3400 cm^{-1}, 2940 cm^{-1}, 1562 cm^{-1} and 1408 cm^{-1}.

Purity Related substances—Dissolve 0.10 g of sodium desoxycholate in 10 mL of methanol, and use this solution as the sample solution. Pipet 1 mL of this solution, add methanol to make exactly 100 mL, and use this solution as the standard solution. Perform the test with these solutions as directed under Thin-layer Chromatography <*2.03*>. Spot 10 μL each of the sample solution and standard solution on a plate of silica gel for thin-layer chromatography. Develop the plate with a mixture of 1-butanol, methanol and acetic acid (100) (80:40:1) to a distance of about 10 cm, and air-dry the plate. Spray evenly concentrated sulfuric acid on the plate, and heat the plate at 105°C for 10 minutes: the spots other than the principal spot obtained from the sample solution are not more intense than the spot from the standard solution.

Sodium 2,6-dichloroindophenol-sodium acetate TS Mix before use an equal volume of sodium 2,6-dichloroindophenol dihydrate solution (1 in 20) and acetic acid-sodium acetate TS (pH 7.0).

Sodium diethyldithiocarbamate See sodium *N,N*-diethyldithiocarbamate trihydrate.

Sodium *N,N*-diethyldithiocarbamate trihydrate $(C_2H_5)_2NCS_2Na.3H_2O$ [K 8454, Special class]

Sodium di-2-ethylhexyl sulfosuccinate $C_8H_{17}COOCH_2(C_8H_{17}COO)CHSO_3Na$ White or translucent white mucilaginous soft masses. Sparingly soluble in water.

Purity Clarity and color of solution—A solution prepared by dissolving 1.0 g of sodium di-2-ethylhexyl sulfosuccinate in 100 mL of water is clear and colorless.

Loss on drying <*2.41*>: not more than 5.0% (1 g, 105°C, 2 hours).

Sodium dihydrogen phosphate See sodium dihydrogen phosphate dihydrate.

Sodium dihydrogen phosphate anhydrous NaH_2PO_4 A white, powder or crystalline powder. Freely soluble in water, and very slightly soluble in ethanol (99.5). It has a hygroscopic property.

A solution is acidic.

Sodium dihydrogen phosphate dihydrate $NaH_2PO_4.2H_2O$ [K 9009, Special class]

Sodium dihydrogen phosphate-ethanol TS To 500 mL of sodium dihydrogen phosphate solution (39 in 2500) add 200 mL of water, and add 300 mL of ethanol (99.5).

Sodium dihydrogen phosphate monohydrate $NaH_2PO_4.H_2O$ White, crystals or crystalline powder. It slightly deliquesces in moist air. It is freely soluble in water, and practically insoluble in ethanol (99.5).

pH <*2.54*>—The pH of a solution of 1.0 g of sodium dihydrogen phosphate monohydrate in 20 mL of water is between 4.1 and 4.5.

Sodium dihydrogen phosphate TS (pH 2.2) Dissolve 1.56 g of sodium dihydrogen phosphate dihydrate in 800 mL of water, adjust the pH to 2.2 with phosphoric acid, and add water to make 1000 mL.

Sodium dihydrogen phosphate TS (pH 2.5) Dissolve 2.7 g of sodium dihydrogen phosphate dihydrate in 1000 mL of water, and adjust the pH to 2.5 with phosphoric acid.

0.05 mol/L Sodium dihydrogen phosphate TS (pH 2.6) Dissolve 7.80 g of sodium dihydrogen phosphate dihydrate in 900 mL of water, adjust the pH to 2.6 with phosphoric acid and add water to make 1000 mL.

0.05 mol/L Sodium dihydrogen phosphate TS (pH 3.0) Dissolve 3.45 g of sodium dihydrogen phosphate dihydrate in 500 mL of water (solution A). Dilute 2.45 g of phosphoric acid with water to make 500 mL (solution B). To a volume of solution A add solution B until the mixture is adjusted to (pH 3.0).

0.1 mol/L Sodium dihydrogen phosphate TS (pH 3.0) Dissolve 15.60 g of sodium dihydrogen phosphate dihydrate in 900 mL of water, adjust the pH to 3.0 with phosphoric acid, and add water to make 1000 mL.

0.05 mol/L Sodium dihydrogen phosphate TS (pH 5.5) Dissolve 7.80 g of sodium dihydrogen phosphate dihydrate in 900 mL of water, adjust to pH 5.5 with sodium hydroxide TS, and add water to make 1000 mL.

0.01 mol/L sodium dihydrogen phosphate TS (pH 7.5) Dissolve 1.56 g of sodium dihydrogen phosphate dihydrate in 900 mL of water, adjust to pH 7.5 with sodium hydroxide

TS, and add water to make 1000 mL.

0.05 mol/L Sodium dihydrogen phosphate TS Dissolve 7.80 g of sodium dihydrogen phosphate dihydrate in water to make 1000 mL.

0.1 mol/L Sodium dihydrogen phosphate TS Dissolve 7.80 g of sodium dihydrogen phosphate dihydrate in 450 mL of water, adjust to a pH of 5.8 exactly with sodium hydroxide TS, and add water to make 500 mL.

2 mol/L Sodium dihydrogen phosphate TS Dissolve 312.02 g of sodium dihydrogen phosphate dihydrate in water to make 1000 mL.

Sodium disulfite $Na_2S_2O_5$ [K 8501, First class]

Sodium disulfite TS Dissolve 0.10 g of sodium disulfite in 10 mL of 1 mol/L hydrochloric acid TS, and add acetone to make 100 mL.

Sodium dithionite $Na_2S_2O_4$ A white to grayish white crystalline powder, having a strong irritating odor. It is decomposed with moisture or atmospheric oxygen.

Identification—(1) Dissolve 0.5 g of sodium dithionite in 50 mL of water, and use this solution as the sample solution. To 10 mL of the sample solution add 1 mL of copper (II) sulfate TS: a grayish brown color is produced.

(2) The sample solution obtained in (1) responds to Qualitative Tests *<1.09>* (1) for sodium salt.

Storage—Preserve in a light-resistant tight container.

Sodium dodecylbenzene sulfonate $C_{18}H_{29}SO_3Na$ White, crystalline powder or mass.

pH <2.54>—The pH of a solution of 0.5 g of sodium dodecylbenzene sulfonate in 50 mL of freshly boiled and cooled water is between 5.0 and 7.0. Measure the pH at 25°C passing nitrogen with stirring.

Loss on drying <2.41>: not more than 0.5% (1 g, 105°C, 2 hours).

Content: not less than 99.0%. Assay—Weigh accurately about 40 mg of sodium dodecylbenzene sulfonate, previously dried, and perform the test as directed in (4) Sulfur in the Procedure of determination under Oxygen Flask Combustion Method *<1.06>*, using a mixture of 20 mL of water and 2 mL of strong hydrogen peroxide water as absorbing solution.

Each mL of 0.005 mol/L barium perchlorate VS
= 1.742 mg of $C_{18}H_{29}SO_3Na$

Sodium fluoride NaF [K 8821, Special class]

Sodium fluoride (standard reagent) NaF In addition to JIS K 8005 standard reagent for volumetric analysis, certified reference material which can be used for volumetric analysis may be used.

Sodium fluoride-hydrochloric acid TS Dissolve 0.5 g of sodium fluoride in 100 mL of 0.5 mol/L hydrochloric acid TS. Prepare before use.

Sodium fluoride TS Dissolve 0.5 g of sodium fluoride in 100 mL of 0.1 mol/L hydrochloric acid TS. Prepare before use.

Sodium gluconate $C_6H_{11}NaO_7$ A white or pale yellow-brown crystalline powder.

Purity Clarity and color of solution—A solution obtained by dissolving 1.0 g of sodium gluconate in 10 mL of water is clear and colorless or pale yellow.

Sodium glycocholate for thin-layer chromatography $C_{26}H_{42}NNaO_6$ White to pale brown, crystalline powder or powder. Freely soluble in water and in methanol, and slightly soluble in ethanol (99.5).

Identification—(1) Determine the infrared absorption spectrum of sodium glycocholate for thin-layer chromatography as directed in the potassium bromide disk method under Infrared Spectrophotometry *<2.25>*: it exhibits absorption at the wave numbers of about 2940 cm^{-1}, 1599 cm^{-1}, 1398 cm^{-1}, 1309 cm^{-1}, 1078 cm^{-1}, 1040 cm^{-1}, 982 cm^{-1} and 915 cm^{-1}.

(2) Sodium glycocholate for thin-layer chromatography responds to Qualitative Tests *<1.09>* (1) for sodium salt.

Optical rotation <2.49> $[\alpha]_D^{20}$: +25 – +35° (60 mg, methanol, 20 mL, 100 mm).

Purity Related substances—Dissolve 5 mg of sodium glycocholate for thin-layer chromatography in 1 mL of methanol, and use this solution as the sample solution. Pipet 0.2 mL of the sample solution, add methanol to make exactly 10 mL, and use this solution as the standard solution. Perform the test with these solutions as directed under Thin-layer Chromatography *<2.03>*. Proceed with 5 μL each of the sample solution and standard solution as directed in the Identification under Bear Bile: the spots other than the principal spot with an *Rf* value of about 0.2 obtained from the sample solution are not more intense than the spot from the standard solution.

Sodium 1-heptane sulfonate $C_7H_{15}NaO_3S$ White, crystals or crystalline powder.

Purity Clarity and color of solution—Dissolve 1.0 g of sodium 1-heptane sulfonate in 10 mL of water: the solution is clear and colorless.

Loss on drying <2.41>: not more than 3.0% (1 g, 105°C, 3 hours).

Content: not less than 98.0%. Assay—Dissolve about 0.4 g of sodium 1-heptane sulfonate, previously dried and weighed accurately, in 50 mL of water, transfer to a chromatographic column, prepared by packing a chromatographic tube 9 mm in inside diameter and 160 mm in height with 10 mL of strongly acidic ion exchange resin for column chromatography (425 to 600 μm in particle diameter, H type), and flow at a flow rate of about 4 mL per minute. Wash the column at the same flow rate with 150 mL of water, combine the washings with the effluent solution, and titrate *<2.50>* with 0.1 mol/L sodium hydroxide VS (indicator: 10 drops of bromothymol blue TS) until the color of the solution changes from yellow to blue.

Each mL of 0.1 mol/L sodium hydroxide VS
= 20.23 mg of $C_7H_{15}NaO_3S$

Sodium 1-hexane sulfonate $C_6H_{13}NaO_3S$ White, crystals or crystalline powder.

Loss on drying <2.41>: not more than 3.0% (1 g, 105°C, 2 hours).

Content: not less than 98.0%. Assay—Weigh accurately about 0.4 g of sodium 1-hexane sulfonate, previously dried, and dissolve in 25 mL of water. Transfer 15–20 mL of this solution into a chromatographic column about 11 mm in diameter and about 500 mm in height of strongly acidic ion exchange resin for column chromatography (246 μm to 833 μm in particle diameter, type H), and elute at the rate of 5 – 10 mL per minute, then wash the column with five 50-mL portions of water at the rate of 5 – 10 mL per minute. Combine the washings to the eluate, and titrate *<2.50>* with 0.1 mol/L sodium hydroxide VS (indicator: 3 drops of phenolphthalein TS).

Each mL of 0.1 mol/L sodium hydroxide VS
= 18.82 mg of $C_6H_{13}NaO_3S$

Sodium hexanitrocobaltate (III) $Na_3Co(NO_2)_6$ [K 8347, Special class]

Sodium hexanitrocobaltate (III) TS Dissolve 10 g of sodium hexanitrocobaltate (III) in water to make 50 mL, and filter if necessary. Prepare before use.

Sodium hyaluronate, purified $(C_{14}H_{20}NNaO_{11})_n$ [Same as the namesake monograph]

Sodium hyaluronate for assay $(C_{14}H_{20}NNaO_{11})_n$ [Same as the monograph Purified Sodium Hyaluronate. It contains not less than 99.0% of sodium hyaluronate $[(C_{14}H_{20}NNaO_{11})_n]$, calculated on the dried basis.]

Sodium hydrogen carbonate $NaHCO_3$ [K 8622, Special class]

Sodium hydrogen carbonate for pH determination $NaHCO_3$ [K 8622, for pH determination]

Sodium hydrogen carbonate TS Dissolve 5.0 g of sodium hydrogen carbonate in water to make 100 mL.

10% Sodium hydrogen carbonate TS Dissolve 10 g of sodium hydrogen carbonate in water to make 100 mL, and sterilize in a tight container in an autoclave at 121°C for 15 minutes or by filtration through a membrane filter with a pore size not exceeding 0.22 μm.

7% Sodium hydrogen carbonate injection See 7% sodium bicarbonate injection.

Sodium hydrogen sulfite [K 8059, Special class]

Sodium hydrogen sulfite TS Dissolve 10 g of sodium hydrogen sulfite in water to make 30 mL. Prepare before use.

Sodium hydrogen tartrate monohydrate $NaHC_4H_4O_6.H_2O$ [K 8538, (+)-Sodium hydrogen tartrate monohydrate, Special class]

Sodium hydrogen tartrate TS Dissolve 1 g of sodium hydrogen tartrate monohydrate in water to make 10 mL (0.5 mol/L). Prepare before use.

Sodium hydroxide NaOH [K 8576, Special class]

Sodium hydroxide-dioxane TS Dissolve 0.80 g of sodium hydroxide in a mixture of 1,4-dioxane and water (3:1) to make 100 mL.

Sodium hydroxide-methanol TS Dissolve by thorough shaking 4 g of sodium hydroxide in methanol to make 100 mL. To the supernatant liquid obtained by centrifugation add methanol to make 500 mL. Prepare before use.

Sodium hydroxide TS Dissolve 4.3 g of sodium hydroxide in water to make 100 mL (1 mol/L). Preserve in polyethylene bottles.

Sodium hydroxide TS, dilute Dissolve 4.3 g of sodium hydroxide in freshly boiled and cooled water to make 1000 mL. Prepare before use (0.1 mol/L).

0.01 mol/L Sodium hydroxide TS Dilute 10 mL of sodium hydroxide TS with water to make 1000 mL. Prepare before use.

0.05 mol/L Sodium hydroxide TS To 10 mL of 0.5 mol/L sodium hydroxide TS add water to make 100 mL.

0.2 mol/L Sodium hydroxide TS Dissolve 8.0 g of sodium hydroxide in freshly boiled and cooled water to make 1000 mL. Prepare before use.

0.5 mol/L Sodium hydroxide TS Dissolve 22 g of sodium hydroxide in water to make 1000 mL. Preserve in polyethylene bottles.

2 mol/L Sodium hydroxide TS Dissolve 86 g of sodium hydroxide in water to make 1000 mL. Preserve in polyethylene bottles.

4 mol/L Sodium hydroxide TS Dissolve 168 g of sodium hydroxide in water to make 1000 mL. Preserve in polyethylene bottles.

5 mol/L Sodium hydroxide TS Dissolve 210 g of sodium hydroxide in water to make 1000 mL. Preserve in a polyethylene bottle.

6 mol/L Sodium hydroxide TS Dissolve 252 g of sodium hydroxide in water to make 1000 mL. Preserve in a polyethylene bottle.

8 mol/L Sodium hydroxide TS Dissolve 336 g of sodium hydroxide in water to make 1000 mL. Preserve in polyethylene bottles.

Sodium hypobromite TS To 8 mL of bromine TS add 25 mL of water and 25 mL of sodium carbonate TS. Prepare before use.

Sodium hypochlorite-sodium hydroxide TS To a volume of sodium hypochlorite TS for ammonium limit test, equivalent to 1.05 g of sodium hypochlorite (NaClO: 74.44), add 15 g of sodium hydroxide and water to make 1000 mL. Prepare before use.

Sodium hypochlorite TS Prepare the solution by passing chlorine into sodium hydroxide TS while cooling with ice, so as to contain 5% of sodium hypochlorite (NaClO: 74.44). Prepare before use.

10% Sodium hypochlorite TS Prepare by introducing chlorine into an aqueous solution of sodium hydroxide while ice-cooling so that the content of sodium hypochlorite (NaClO: 74.44) is 10%. Prepare before use.

Sodium hypochlorite TS for ammonium limit test Clear, colorless or light green-yellow solution prepared by passing chlorine into sodium hydroxide or sodium carbonate decahydrate solution, having the odor of chlorine.

Content: not less than 4.2 g/d L as sodium hypochlorite (NaClO: 74.44). Assay—Pipet 10 mL of sodium hypochlorite TS for ammonium limit test, and add water to make exactly 100 mL. Transfer exactly 10 mL of this solution to a glass-stoppered flask, add 90 mL of water, then add 2 g of potassium iodide and 6 mL of diluted acetic acid (31) (1 in 2), stopper tightly, shake well, and allow to stand for 5 minutes in a dark place. Titrate <*2.50*> the liberated iodine with 0.1 mol/L sodium thiosulfate VS (indicator: 3 mL of starch TS). Perform a blank determination in the same manner, and make any necessary correction.

Each mL of 0.1 mol/L sodium thiosulfate VS
= 3.722 mg of NaClO.

Sodium L-lactate solution for assay $C_3H_5NaO_3$ [Same as the monograph, Sodium L-Lactate Solution]

Sodium lauryl sulfate [Same as the namesake monograph]

Sodium lauryl sulfate TS Dissolve 100 g of sodium lauryl sulfate in 900 mL of water, add 10 mL of 1 mol/L hydrochloric acid TS, and add water to make 1000 mL.

0.2% Sodium lauryl sulfate TS Dissolve 0.1 g of sodium

lauryl sulfate in 0.1 mol/L sodium phosphate buffer (pH 7.0) to make 50 mL.

Sodium metabisulfite See sodium disulfite.

Sodium metabisulfite TS See sodium disulfite TS.

Sodium, metallic See sodium

Sodium 1-methyl-1*H*-tetrazole-5-thiolate See sodium 1-methyl-1*H*-tetrazole-5-thiolate dihydrate.

Sodium 1-methyl-1*H*-tetrazole-5-thiolate dihydrate $C_2H_3N_4NaS.2H_2O$ White, crystals or crystalline powder.

Melting point <2.60>: 90 – 94°C

Purity Related substances—Dissolve 10 mg of sodium 1-methyl-1*H*-tetrazole-5-thiolate dihydrate in 10 mL of water, and use this solution as the sample solution. Perform the test with the sample solution as directed under Thin-layer Chromatography <2.03>. Spot 5 μL of the sample solution on a plate of silica gel with fluorescent indicator for thin-layer chromatography. Develop the plate with a mixture of ethyl acetate, acetone, water and acetic acid (100) (10:2:1:1) to a distance of about 10 cm, and air-dry the plate. Examine under ultraviolet light (main wavelength: 254 nm): any spot other than the principal spot does not appear.

Sodium molybdate See sodium molybdate (VI) dihydrate.

Sodium molybdate (VI) dihydrate $Na_2MoO_4.2H_2O$ [K 8906, disodium molybdate (VI) dihydrate, Special class]

Sodium 2-naphthalenesulfonate $C_{10}H_7NaO_3S$ Pale brown, crystals or powder.

Content: not less than 98.0%.

Sodium β-naphthoquinone sulfonate $C_{10}H_5NaO_5S$ Yellow to orange-yellow, crystals or crystalline powder. Soluble in water, and practically insoluble in ethanol (95).

Loss on drying <2.41>: Not more than 2.0% (1 g, in vacuum, 50°C).

Residue on ignition <2.44>: 26.5 – 28.0% (1 g, after drying).

Sodium naphthoquinone sulfonate TS Dissolve 0.25 g of sodium β-naphthoquinone sulfonate in methanol to make 100 mL.

Sodium nitrate $NaNO_3$ [K 8562, Special class]

Sodium nitrite $NaNO_2$ [K 8019, Special class]

Sodium nitrite TS Dissolve 10 g of sodium nitrite in water to make 100 mL. Prepare before use.

Sodium nitroprusside See sodium pentacyanonitrosylferrate (III) dihydrate.

Sodium nitroprusside TS See sodium pentacyanonitrosylferrate (III) TS.

Sodium 1-nonanesulfonate $CH_3(CH_2)_8SO_3Na$ White crystalline powder. Freely soluble in water.

Loss on drying <2.41>: Not more than 1.0% (1 g, 105°C, 3 hours).

Residue on ignition <2.44>: 30 – 32% (0.5 g).

Sodium 1-octane sulfonate $CH_3(CH_2)_7SO_3Na$ White, crystals or powder.

Residue on ignition <2.44>: 32.2 – 33.0% (1.0 g).

Sodium oxalate (standard reagent) $C_2Na_2O_4$ In addition to JIS K 8005 standard reagent for volumetric analysis, certified reference material which can be used for volumetric analysis may be used.

Sodium pentacyanoammine ferroate (II) *n*-hydrate $Na_3[Fe(CN)_5NH_3].xH_2O$ A light yellow to light green-yellow crystalline powder.

Identification—(1) Dissolve 0.2 g of sodium pentacyanoammine ferroate (II) *x*-hydrate in 5 mL of water, add 2 mL of sodium hydroxide solution (1 in 10), and heat: ammonia gas is evolved and a brown precipitate is produced.

(2) Dissolve 0.25 g of sodium pentacyanoammine ferroate (II) *n*-hydrate in 20 mL of water. To 1 mL of this solution add 0.2 mL of iron (II) sulfate TS: a green-blue color develops, which changes to a dark blue color on the addition of 2 drops of diluted sodium hypochlorite TS (2 in 5) and 0.2 mL of acetic acid (100).

Sodium pentacyanonitrosylferrate (III) dihydrate $Na_2[Fe(CN)_5(NO)].2H_2O$ [K 8722, Special class]

Sodium pentacyanonitrosylferrate (III)-potassium hexacyanoferrate (III) TS Mix an equal volume of a solution of sodium pentacyanonitrosylferrate (III) dihydrate (1 in 10), a solution of potassium hexacyanoferrate (III) (1 in 10) and a solution of sodium hydroxide (1 in 10), and allow to stand for 30 minutes. Use after the color of the solution is changed from a dark red to yellow. Prepare before use.

Sodium pentacyanonitrosylferrate (III)-potassium hexacyanoferrate (III) TS, dilute To 5 mL of a solution of pentacyanonitrosylferrate (III) dihydrate (3 in 50) add 5 mL of a solution of potassium hexacyanoferrate (III) (13 in 200) and 2.5 mL of a solution of sodium hydroxide (1 in 10), add water to make 25 mL, mix, and use after changing the color of the solution from a dark red to light yellow. Prepare before use.

Sodium pentacyanonitrosylferrate (III) TS Dissolve 1 g of sodium pentacyanonitrosylferrate (III) dihydrate in water to make 20 mL. Prepare before use.

Sodium 1-pentane sulfonate $C_5H_{11}NaO_3S$ White, crystals or crystalline powder. Freely soluble in water, and practically insoluble in acetonitrile.

Purity Clarity and color of solution—Dissolve 1.0 g of sodium 1-pentane sulfonate in 10 mL of water: the solution is colorless and clear.

Water <2.48>: not more than 3.0% (0.2 g).

Content: not less than 99.0%, calculated on the anhydrous basis. Assay—Dissolve about 0.3 g of sodium 1-pentane sulfonate, accurately weighed, in 50 mL of water. Transfer this solution to a chromatographic column, prepared by pouring 10 mL of strongly acidic ion-exchange resin (H type) (425 – 600 μm in particle diameter) into a chromatographic tube, 9 mm in inside diameter and 160 mm in height, and elute at the rate of about 4 mL per minute. Wash the chromatographic column with 50 mL of water at the rate of about 4 mL per minute, and wash again with 100 mL of water in the same manner. Combine the washings with the eluate, and titrate <2.50> with 0.1 mol/L sodium hydroxide VS (indicator: 10 drops of bromothymol blue TS) until the yellow color of the solution changes to blue.

Each mL of 0.1 mol/L sodium hydroxide VS
= 17.42 mg of $C_5H_{11}NaO_3S$

Sodium perchlorate See sodium perchlorate monohydrate.

Sodium perchlorate monohydrate $NaClO_4.H_2O$ [K 8227, Special class]

Sodium periodate $NaIO_4$ [K 8256, Special class]

Sodium periodate TS Dissolve 60.0 g of sodium periodate in 120 mL of 0.05 mol/L sulfuric acid TS, and add water to make 1000 mL. Keep in a light-resistant vessel.

Sodium peroxide Na_2O_2 [K 8231, Special class]

Sodium *p*-phenol sulfonate See sodium *p*-phenol sulfonate dihydrate.

Sodium *p*-phenol sulfonate dihydrate $C_6H_5O_4NaS.2H_2O$ White to light yellow, crystals or crystalline powder, having a specific odor.

Identification (1) To 10 mL of a solution of sodium *p*-phenol sulfonate dihydrate (1 in 10) add 1 drop of iron (III) chloride TS: a purple color develops.

(2) Determine the absorption spectrum of a solution of sodium *p*-phenol sulfonate dihydrate (1 in 5000) as directed under Ultraviolet-visible Spectrophotometry <*2.24*>: it exhibits maxima between 269 nm and 273 nm and between 276 nm and 280 nm.

Purity Clarity and color of solution—Dissolve 1.0 g of sodium *p*-phenol sulfonate dihydrate in 25 mL of water: the solution is clear and colorless.

Content: not less than 90.0%. Assay—Dissolve about 0.5 g of sodium *p*-phenol sulfonate dihydrate, accurately weighed, in 50 mL of water. Transfer the solution to a chromatographic column, prepared by pouring 20 mL of strongly acidic ion exchange resin (H type) for column chromatography (150 to 300 μm in particle diameter) into a chromatographic tube about 1 cm in inside diameter and about 30 cm in height, and allow to flow. Wash the chromatographic column with water until the washing is no longer acidic, combine the washings with the above effluent solution, and titrate <*2.50*> with 0.1 mol/L sodium hydroxide VS (indicator: 5 drops of bromocresol green-methyl red TS). Separately, dissolve 0.5 g of sodium *p*-phenol sulfonate dihydrate, weighed accurately, in 50 mL of water and titrate with 0.1 mol/L sodium hydroxide VS, and make any necessary correction.

Each mL of 0.1 mol/L sodium hydroxide VS
= 23.22 mg of $C_6H_5O_4NaS.2H_2O$

Sodium phosphate See trisodium phosphate dodecahydrate.

Sodium phosphate TS Dissolve 5.68 g of anhydrous disodium hydrogen phosphate and 6.24 g of sodium dihydrogen phosphate dihydrate in water to make 1000 mL.

0.1 mol/L Sodium phosphate buffer solution (pH 7.0) Dissolve 17.9 g of disodium hydrogen phosphate dodecahydrate in water to make 500 mL. Add to this solution to a 500 mL solution prepared by dissolving 7.8 g of sodium dihydrogen phosphate dihydrate in water until the pH becomes 7.0.

Sodium pyruvate $CH_3COCOONa$ A white to pale yellow crystalline powder. Freely soluble in water, and slightly soluble in ethanol (99.5) and in acetone.

Identification (1) Determine the infrared absorption spectrum of sodium pyruvate as directed in the potassium bromide disk method under Infrared Spectrophotometry <*2.25*>: it exhibits absorption at the wave numbers of about 1710 cm^{-1}, 1630 cm^{-1}, 1410 cm^{-1}, 1360 cm^{-1}, 1190 cm^{-1}, 1020 cm^{-1}, 980 cm^{-1}, 830 cm^{-1},750 cm^{-1}, 630 cm^{-1} and 430 cm^{-1}.

(2) A solution of sodium pyruvate (1 in 20) responds to Qualitative Tests <*1.09*> (1) for sodium salt.

Content: Not less than 97.0%. Assay—Weigh accurately about 0.4 g of sodium pyruvate, and dissolve in water to make exactly 200 mL. Pipet 20 mL of this solution into an iodine bottle, cool to 10°C or lower, add exactly 40 mL of 0.05 mol/L iodine VS, then add 20 mL of a solution of sodium hydroxide (17 in 100), and allow to stand at a dark place for 2 hours. Then add 15 mL of diluted sulfuric acid (1 in 6), and titrate <*2.50*> with 0.1 mol/L sodium thiosulfate VS (indicator: starch TS). Perform a blank determination in the same manner, and make any necessary correction.

Each mL of 0.05 mol/L iodine VS
= 1.834 mg of $C_3H_3NaO_3$

100 mmol/L Sodium pyruvate TS Dissolve 1.1 g of sodium pyruvate in water to make 100 mL, and sterilize by filtration through a membrane filter with a pore size not exceeding 0.22 μm.

Sodium salicylate HOC_6H_4COONa [K 8397, Special class]

Sodium salicylate-sodium hydroxide TS Dissolve 1 g of sodium salicylate in 0.01 mol/L sodium hydroxide VS to make 100 mL.

Sodium selenite Na_2SeO_3 A white crystalline powder.

Identification—(1) Dissolve 1 g of sodium selenite in 100 mL of water, and use this solution as the sample solution. To 10 mL of the sample solution add 2 mL of tin (II) chloride TS: a red precipitate is produced.

(2) The sample solution obtained in (1) responds to Qualitative Tests <*1.09*> (1) for sodium salt.

Storage—Preserve in a light-resistant tight container.

Sodium stearyl fumarate $C_{22}H_{39}NaO_4$ A white crystalline powder.

Identification (1) Determine the infrared absorption spectrum of sodium stearyl fumarate as directed in the potassium bromide disk method under Infrared Spectrophotometry <*2.25*>: it exhibits absorption at the wave numbers of about 2950 cm^{-1}, 2920 cm^{-1}, 2850 cm^{-1}, 1720 cm^{-1}, 1610 cm^{-1}, 1313 cm^{-1}, 1186 cm^{-1}, 980 cm^{-1}, and 665 cm^{-1}.

(2) Sodium stearyl fumarate responds to Qualitative Tests <*1.09*> (1) for sodium salt.

Sodium *p*-styrenesulfonate $C_8H_7NaO_3S$ White, crystals or crystalline powder. Freely soluble in water, slightly soluble in ethanol (99.5), and practically insoluble in diethyl ether.

Recrystalize from diluted ethanol (1 in 2), and dry in vacuum.

Identification—Determine the infrared absorption spectrum of sodium *p*-styrenesulfonate according to the potassium bromide disk method under Infrared Spectrophotometry <*2.25*>: it exhibits absorption at the wave numbers of about 1236 cm^{-1}, 1192 cm^{-1}, 1136 cm^{-1}, 1052 cm^{-1}, 844 cm^{-1} and 688 cm^{-1}.

Purity—Perform the test with 10 μL of a solution of sodium *p*-styrenesulfonate (1 in 1000) as directed in the Assay under Panipenem: Any obstructive peaks for determination of panipenem are not observed.

Sodium sulfate See sodium sulfate decahydrate.

Sodium sulfate, anhydrous Na_2SO_4 [K 8987, Special class]

Sodium sulfate decahydrate $Na_2SO_4.10H_2O$ [K 8986, Special class]

Sodium sulfide See sodium sulfide enneahydrate.

Sodium sulfide enneahydrate $Na_2S.9H_2O$ [K 8949, Special class]

Sodium sulfide TS Dissolve 5 g of sodium sulfide enneahydrate in a mixture of 10 mL of water and 30 mL of glycerin. Or dissolve 5 g of sodium hydroxide in a mixture of 30 mL of water and 90 mL of glycerin, saturate a half volume of this solution with hydrogen sulfide, while cooling, and mix with the remaining half. Preserve in well-filled, light-resistant bottles. Use within 3 months.

Sodium sulfite See sodium sulfite heptahydrate.

Sodium sulfite, anhydrous Na_2SO_3 [K 8061, Sodium sulfite, Special class]

Sodium sulfite heptahydrate $Na_2SO_3.7H_2O$ [K 8060, Special class]

1 mol/L Sodium sulfite TS Dissolve 1.26 g of anhydrous sodium sulfite in water to make 10 mL.

Sodium sulfite-sodium dihydrogen phosphate TS Mix 1.5 mL of a solution dissolved 1.26 g of anhydrous sodium sulfite in 100 mL of water and 98.5 mL of a solution dissolved 1.56 g of sodium dihydrogen phosphate dihydrate in 100 mL of water. Prepare before use.

Sodium tartrate See sodium tartrate dihydrate.

Sodium tartrate dihydrate $C_4H_4Na_2O_6.2H_2O$ [K 8540, sodium (+)-tartrate dihydrate, Special class]

Sodium tauroursodeoxycholate for thin-layer chromatography $C_{26}H_{44}NNaO_6S$ White to pale brown, crystalline powder or powder. Freely soluble in methanol, soluble in water, and sparingly soluble in ethanol (99.5).

Identification—(1) Determine the infrared absorption spectrum of sodium tauroursodeoxycholate for thin-layer chromatography as directed in the potassium bromide disk method under Infrared Spectrophotometry <*2.25*>: it exhibits absorption at the wave numbers of about 2930 cm^{-1}, 1645 cm^{-1}, 1556 cm^{-1}, 1453 cm^{-1}, 1215 cm^{-1} and 1049 cm^{-1}.

(2) Sodium tauroursodeoxycholate for thin-layer chromatography responds to Qualitative Tests <*1.09*> (1) for sodium salt.

Optical rotation <*2.49*> $[\alpha]_D^{20}$: +40 – +50° (40 mg, methanol, 20 mL, 100 mm).

Purity Related substances—Dissolve 10 mg of sodium tauroursodeoxycholate for thin-layer chromatography in 1 mL of methanol, and use this solution as the sample solution. Pipet 0.2 mL of the sample solution, add methanol to make exactly 10 mL, and use this solution as the standard solution. Perform the test with these solutions as directed under Thin-layer Chromatography <*2.03*>. Perform the test with 5 μL each of the sample solution and standard solution as directed in the Identification under Bear Bile: the spots other than the principal spot with an *Rf* value of about 0.2 obtained from the sample solution are not more intense than the spot from the standard solution.

Sodium tetraborate-calcium chloride buffer solution (pH 8.0) Dissolve 0.572 g of sodium tetraborate decahydrate and 2.94 g of calcium chloride dihydrate in 800 mL of freshly boiled and cooled water, adjust the pH to 8.0 with 1 mol/L hydrochloric acid TS, and add water to make 1000 mL.

Sodium tetraborate decahydrate $Na_2B_4O_7.10H_2O$ [K 8866, Special class]

Sodium tetraborate decahydrate for pH determination [K 8866, for pH standard solution]

Sodium tetraborate-sulfuric acid TS To 9.5 g of sodium tetraborate decahydrate add 1000 mL of sulfuric acid, and dissolve by shaking for a night.

Purity: To 5 mL of sodium tetraborate-sulfuric acid TS, previously cooled in ice water, add gently 1 mL of water, stir while cooling, then heat in a water bath for 10 minutes, and cool in ice water. Add exactly 0.2 mL of carbazole TS, stir thoroughly, then heat in a water bath for 15 minutes, and cool in ice water to room temperature: a green color does not appear.

Sodium tetraphenylborate $(C_6H_5)_4BNa$ [K 9521, Special class]

Sodium thioglycolate $HSCH_2COONa$ A white powder, having a characteristic odor.

Identification (1) To a solution (1 in 10) add 0.1 mL of ammonia solution (28) and 1 drop of iron (III) chloride TS: a dark red-purple color appears.

(2) Perform the test as directed under Flame Coloration Test <*1.04*> (1): a yellow color appears.

Purity Clarity and color of solution—Dissolve 1 g in 10 mL of water: the solution is clear and colorless.

Sodium thiosulfate See sodium thiosulfate pentahydrate.

Sodium thiosulfate pentahydrate $Na_2S_2O_3.5H_2O$ [K 8637, Special class]

Sodium thiosulfate TS Dissolve 26 g of sodium thiosulfate pentahydrate and 0.2 g of anhydrous sodium carbonate in freshly boiled and cooled water to make 1000 mL (0.1 mol/L).

Sodium toluenesulfonchloramide trihydrate $C_7H_7ClNNaO_2S.3H_2O$ [K 8318, Sodium *p*-toluenesulfonchloramide trihydrate, Special class]

Sodium toluenesulfonchloramide TS Dissolve 1 g of sodium toluenesulfonchloramide trihydrate in water to make 100 mL. Prepare before use.

Sodium tridecanesulfonate $C_{13}H_{27}SO_3Na$ White, crystals or powder.

Purity Absorbance—Dissolve 1.43 g of sodium tridecanesulfonate in 1000 mL of water, and perform the test with this solution as directed under Ultraviolet-visible Spectrophotometry <*2.24*>: the absorbances at 230 nm and 254 nm are not more than 0.05 and 0.01, respectively.

Sodium 3-trimethylsilylpropanesulfonate for nuclear magnetic resonance spectroscopy $(CH_3)_3SiCH_2CH_2CH_2SO_3Na$ Prepared for nuclear magnetic resonance spectroscopy.

Sodium 3-trimethylsilylpropionate-d_4 for nuclear magnetic resonance spectroscopy $(CH_3)_3SiCD_2CD_2COONa$ Prepared for nuclear magnetic resonance spectroscopy.

Sodium 2,4,6-trinitrobenzenesulfonate dihydrate $C_6H_2N_3NaO_9S.2H_2O$ White or pale yellowish, crystals or powder.

Sodium tungstate See sodium tungstate (VI) dihydrate.

Sodium tungstate (VI) dihydrate $Na_2WO_4.2H_2O$ [K 8612, Special class]

Sodium valproate for assay $C_8H_{15}NaO_2$ [Same as the monograph Sodium Valproate. When dried, it contains not less than 99.0% of sodium valproate ($C_8H_{15}NaO_2$).]

Soluble starch See starch, soluble.

Soluble starch TS Triturate 1 g of soluble starch in 10 mL of cooled water, pour gradually into 90 mL of boiled water while constantly stirring, boil gently for 3 minutes, and cool. Prepare before use.

Sorbitan sesquioleate [Same as the namesake monograph]

D-Sorbitol $C_6H_{14}O_6$ [Same as the namesake monograph]

D-Sorbitol for gas chromatography Prepared for gas chromatography.

Soybean-casein digest medium See Sterility Test <4.06>.

Soybean oil [Same as the namesake monograph]

Soybean peptone See peptone, soybean.

Stachyose for thin-layer chromatography $C_{24}H_{42}O_{21}$ A white powder. Very soluble in water, and practically insoluble in ethanol (99.5). It is deliquescence with the atmospheric moisture.

Optical rotation <2.49> $[\alpha]_D^{20}$: +144 – +154° (50 mg calculated on the anhydrous basis, diluted ammonia solution (28) (1 in 1000), 5 mL, 100 mm).

Purity Related substances—Dissolve 2 mg of stachyose for thin-layer chromatography in 1 mL of a mixture of water and methanol (1:1), and use this solution as the sample solution. Perform the test with the sample solution as directed under Thin-layer chromatography <2.03>. Spot 2 μL of the sample solution on a plate of silica gel for thin-layer chromatography. Develop the plate with a mixture of 2-propanol, water and methanol (3:2:2) to a distance of about 7 cm, and air-dry the plate. Spray evenly 1,3-naphthalenediol TS to the plate, and heat at 105°C for 10 minutes: a spot other than the principle spot with an *R*f value of about 0.5 is not observed.

Stacking gel for celmoleukin In 0.5 mol/L Tris buffer solution (pH 6.8), prepare stacking the gel using ammonium persulfate and *N*,*N*,*N'*,*N'*-tetramethylenediamine so the acrylamide concentration is 5.2% and the sodium lauryl sulfate concentration is 0.1%.

Stannous chloride See tin (II) chloride dihydrate.

Stannous chloride-sulfuric acid TS See tin (II) chloride-sulfuric acid TS.

Stannous chloride TS See tin (II) chloride TS.

Stannous chloride TS, acidic See tin (II) chloride TS, acidic.

Starch [K 8658, Special class]

Starch-sodium chloride TS Saturate starch TS with sodium chloride. Use within 5 to 6 days.

Starch, soluble [K 8659, Starch, soluble, First class]

Starch TS Triturate 1 g of starch with 10 mL of cold water, and pour the mixture slowly, with constant stirring, into 200 mL of boiling water. Boil the mixture until a thin, translucent fluid is obtained. Allow to settle, and use the supernatant liquid. Prepare before use.

Stearic acid for gas chromatography $C_{18}H_{36}O_2$ [K 8585, Special class]

Stearyl alcohol [Same as the namesake monograph]

Sterile purified water [Same as the monograph Sterile Purified Water in Containers. It is not necessary to confirm if they meet all of the requirement, provided that they are confirmed to be suitable for the purpose of the relevant test.]

Strong ammonia water See ammonia solution (28).

Strong cupric acetate TS See copper (II) acetate TS, strong.

Strong hydrogen peroxide water See hydrogen peroxide (30).

Strongly acidic ion exchange resin Contains strong acid ion exchange residues. Particle diameter is about 100 μm.

Strongly basic ion exchange resin Contains strong basic ion exchange residues. Particle diameter is about 100 μm.

Strontium TS Dissolve 76.5 g of strontium chloride in water to make exactly 500 mL. Pipet 20 mL of this solution, and add water to make exactly 1000 mL (1000 ppm).

Strontium chloride See strontium chloride hexahydrate.

Strontium chloride hexahydrate $SrCl_2.6H_2O$ [K 8132, Special class]

Strychnine nitrate for assay $C_{21}H_{22}N_2O_2.HNO_3$ To 1 g of strychnine nitrate add 14 mL of water and about 10 mg of active carbon, heat in a water bath for 10 minutes, filter while hot, cool the filtrate quickly to form crystals, and filter the crystals. Add 8 mL of water to the crystals, dissolve by heating in a water bath, filter while hot, cool quickly, and filter the crystals formed. Repeat this procedure with 8 mL of water, and dry the crystals in a desiccator (in vacuum, silica gel) for 24 hours. Colorless or white, crystals or crystalline powder. Sparingly soluble in water and in glycerin, slightly soluble in ethanol (95), and practically insoluble in diethyl ether.

Purity Related substances—Dissolve 35 mg of strychnine nitrate for assay in 100 mL of the mobile phase and use this solution as the sample solution. Pipet 2 mL of the sample solution, add the mobile phase to make exactly 100 mL, and use this solution as the standard solution (1). Perform the test with exactly 20 μL each of the sample solution and standard solution (1) as directed under Liquid Chromatography <2.01> according to the following conditions. Determine each peak area of these solutions by the automatic integration method: the total area of the peaks other than strychnine obtained from the sample solution is not larger than the peak area of strychnine from the standard solution (1).

Operating conditions

Proceed the operating conditions in the Assay under Nux Vomica except time span of measurement.

Time span of measurement: About 3 times as long as the retention time of strychnine, beginning after the solvent peak.

System suitability

Test for required detectability: Pipet 1 mL of the standard solution (1), add the mobile phase to make exactly 40 mL, and use this solution as the standard solution (2). Adjust the detection sensitivity so that the peak area of strychnine obtained with 20 μL of the standard solution (2) can be measured by the automatic integration method and the peak height of strychnine with 20 μL of the standard solution (1) is about 20% of the full scale.

Loss on drying <2.41>: not more than 0.5% (0.2 g, 105°C, 3 hours).

Content: not less than 99.0% calculated on the dried basis. Assay—Dissolve about 0.5 g of strychnine nitrate for assay, accurately weighed, in 40 mL of a mixture of acetic anhydride and acetic acid (100) (4:1), heat if necessary, cool, and titrate <2.50> with 0.1 mol/L perchloric acid VS (potentiometric titration). Perform a blank determination in the same manner, and make any necessary correction.

Each mL of 0.1 mol/L perchloric acid VS
= 39.74 mg of $C_{21}H_{22}N_2O_2.HNO_3$

Styrene C_8H_8 Colorless, clear liquid.

Specific gravity <2.56> *d*: 0.902 – 0.910

Purity—Perform the test with 1 μL of styrene as directed under Gas Chromatography <2.02> according to the following conditions. Determine each peak area by the automatic integration method and calculate the amount of styrene by the area percentage method: it shows the purity of not less than 99%.

Operating conditions

Detector: Thermal conductivity detector.

Column: A glass column, about 3 mm in inside diameter and about 2 m in length, packed with siliceous earth (180 to 250 μm in particle diameter) coated with polyethylene glycol 20 M at the ratio of 10%.

Column temperature: A constant temperature of about 100°C.

Temperature of sample vaporization chamber: A constant temperature of about 150°C.

Carrier gas: Helium.

Flow rate: Adjust so that the retention time of styrene is about 10 minutes.

Time span of measurement: About twice as long as the retention time of styrene.

Styrene-maleic acid alternating copolymer partial butyl ester Polymerize styrene and maleic anhydride using cumene as solvent, and add 1-butanol or water to the maleic anhydride groups. Average molecular mass: about 1600. A white to pale yellow-white powder.

Identification—Dissolve 5 mg of the substance to be examined in sodium hydrogen carbonate solution (1 in 15) to make 10 mL. Determine the absorption spectrum of this solution as directed under Ultraviolet-visible Spectrophotometry <2.24>: it exhibits a maximum between 256 nm and 260 nm, and a shoulder between 251 nm and 256 nm.

Absorbance <2.24> $E^{1\%}_{1cm}$ (258 nm): 6.3 – 7.3 [5 mg calculated on the anhydrous basis, sodium hydrogen carbonate solution (1 in 15), 10 mL].

Purity (i) Test solutions

Solution A: Dissolve 36.6 g of 2-amino-2-hydroxymethyl-1,3-propanediol in 48 mL of 1 mol/L hydrochloric acid TS, 0.23 mL of *N,N,N′,N′*-tetramethylethylenediamine and water to make 100 mL.

Solution B: Dissolve 33.3 g of acrylamide and 0.89 g of *N,N′*-methylenebisacrylamide in water to make 100 mL. Preserve in a cold place, avoiding exposure to light.

Solution C: Dissolve 5.98 g of 2-amino-2-hydroxymethyl-1,3-propanediol in 48 mL of 1 mol/L hydrochloric acid TS, 0.46 mL of *N,N,N′,N′*-tetramethylethylenediamine and water to make 100 mL.

Solution D: Dissolve 10.0 g of acrylamide and 2.5 g of *N,N′*-methylenebisacrylamide in water to make 100 mL. Preserve in a cold place, avoiding exposure to light.

Solution E: Dissolve 4 mg of riboflavin in water to make 100 mL. Preserve in a cold place, avoiding exposure to light.

Solution F: Dissolve 3.0 g of 2-amino-2-hydroxymethyl-1,3-propanediol and 14.4 g of glycine in water to make 500 mL.

Buffer solution for sample: To 50 mL of Solution C add 20 mL of water and 10 mL of glycerin solution (3 in 5).

(ii) Gels

Resolving gel: Mix 2.5 mL of Solution A and 7.5 mL of Solution B. Mix the mixture with 10 mL of freshly prepared ammonium peroxodisulfate solution (7 in 5000) after degassing under reduced pressure. Pour this mixture into a glass tube, 5 mm in inside diameter and 10 cm in length, to make 7 cm height, put water gently on the upper surface of the mixture, and allow to polymerize for 60 minutes. After polymerization, remove the water from the upper surface of the gel.

Stacking gel: Mix 1 mL of Solution C, 2 mL of Solution D, 1 mL of Solution E and 4 mL of water, pour 0.2 mL of the mixture on the resolving gel, put water gently on the upper surface of the mixture, and allow to polymerize under a fluorescent light for 60 minutes. After polymerization, remove the water from the upper surface of the gel.

(iii) Sample solution Dissolve 3.0 mg of the substance to be examined in the buffer solution for sample to make 20 mL.

(iv) Procedure Mount the gel in an electrophoresis apparatus. Add a mixture of 200 mL of Solution F and 2 mL of bromophenol blue solution (1 in 100,000) to the upper reservoir (cathode) and 300 mL of Solution F to the lower reservoir (anode). Introduce carefully exactly 100 μL of the sample solution onto the surface of the gel, and allow electrophoresis at room temperature to take place with a current of 2 mA per tube as a bromophenol blue band is passing in the stacking gel and then increase the current to 4 mA per tube as the bromophenol blue band is passing in the resolving gel, and stop the current when the band reached 5 cm from the upper end of the gel.

(v) Staining and decolorization Dissolve 0.1 g of Coomassie brilliant blue G-250 in 100 mL of trichloroacetic acid solution (1 in 2), and mix 1 volume of this solution and 2 volumes of water before using. Immerse the gels for 15 hours in this mixture, and transfer into about 20 mL of acetic acid (100) solution (7 in 100) to remove the excess of dye. Replace the acetic acid (100) solution until the back ground of the gel becomes colorless.

(vi) Determination Determine the peak area, A_T, of styrene-maleic acid alternating copolymer partial butyl ester and the total area, A, of the peaks other than styrene-maleic acid alternating copolymer partial butyl ester, based on the absorbance at 600 nm of the gel determined by using a densitometer. Calculate the amount of styrene-maleic acid alternating copolymer partial butyl ester by the following formula: not less than 98.0%.

Amount (%) of styrene-maleic acid alternating copolymer partial butyl ester

$$= A_T/(A_T + A) \times 100$$

Water <2.48>: Not more than 10.0% (10 mg, coulometric titration).

Subculture medium for nartograstim test Dissolve an amount of Nartograstim (Genetical Recombination), equivalent to 0.20 mg in 20 mL of phosphate-buffered sodium chloride TS. To 0.1 mL of this solution add 100 mL of potency measuring medium for nartograstim test.

Substrate buffer for celmoleukin Dissolve 32.4 g of tripotassium citrate monohydrate in water to make 1000 mL, and add 1 mol/L citric acid TS for buffer solution to adjust the pH to 5.5. To 100 mL of this solution add and dissolve 0.44 g of *o*-phenylenediamine and then 60 μL of hydrogen peroxide (30). Prepare at the time of use.

Substrate TS for epoetin alfa Dissolve 30 mg of 4-chloro-1-naphthol in 10 ml of methanol, and use as Solution A. Mix 30 μL of hydrogen peroxide (30) and 50 mL of 0.02 mol/L tris buffer solution (pH 7.5) and use as Solution B. Mix Solutions A and B before use.

Substrate TS for interferon alfa confirmation Dissolve 9 mg of 3,3′-diaminobenzidine tetrahydrochloride in phosphate-buffered sodium chloride TS to make 30 mL. Add 5

μL of hydrogen peroxide (30) to this solution. Prepare before use.

Substrate TS for peroxidase determination Dissolve 0.195 mL of hydrogen peroxidase (30), 8.38 g of disodium hydrogen phosphate dodecahydrate and 1.41 g of citric acid monohydrate in water to make 300 mL. To 15 mL of this solution add 13 mg of *o*-phenylenediamine dihydrochloride before use.

Substrate TS for kallidinogenase assay (1) Dissolve an appropriate amount of *H*-D-valyl-L-leucyl-L-arginine-4-nitroanilide dihydrochloride in 0.1 mol/L tris buffer solution (pH 8.0) to prepare a solution containing 1 mg of *H*-D-valyl-L-leucyl-L-arginine-4-nitroanilide dihydrochloride in 5 mL.

Substrate TS for kallidinogenase assay (2) Dissolve 17.7 mg of *N*-α-benzoyl-L-arginine ethyl ester hydrochloride in 0.1 mol/L tris buffer solution (pH 8.0) to make 100 mL.

Substrate TS for kallidinogenase assay (3) Suspend 0.6 g of milk casein purified by the Hammerstein's method in 80 mL of 0.05 mol/L sodium hydrogen phosphate TS, and dissolve by warming at 65°C for 20 minutes. After cooling, adjust to pH 8.0 with 1 mol/L hydrochloric acid TS or sodium hydroxide TS, and add water to make exactly 100 mL. Prepare before use.

Substrate TS for kallidinogenase assay (4) Dissolve 25 mg of *H*-D-valyl-L-leucyl-L-arginine-4-nitroanilide dihydrochloride in 28.8 mL of water.

Substrate TS for lysozyme hydrochloride To a suitable amount of dried cells of *Micrococcus luteus* add a suitable amount of phosphate buffer solution (pH 6.2) gently shake to make a suspension, and add the substrate cells or the same buffer solution so that the absorbance of the suspension at 640 nm is about 0.65. Prepare before use.

***N*-Succinimidyl 4-(*N*-maleidomethyl)cyclohexane-1-carboxylate** See 4-(*N*-Maleidomethyl cyclohexane-1-carboxylic acid *N*-succinimidyl ester.

Succinic acid $C_4H_6O_4$ Colorless or white crystalline powder. Very soluble in hot water, soluble in water and in ethanol (99.5), and sparingly soluble in diethyl ether.

Melting point <*2.60*>: About 185°C.

Residue on ignition <*2.44*>: not more than 0.02% (1 g).

Content: not less than 99.5%. Assay—Weigh accurately about 1 g of succinic acid, dissolve in 50 mL of water, add 5 drops of phenolphthalein TS, and titrate <*2.50*> with 1 mol/L sodium hydroxide VS. Perform a blank titration in the same manner, and make any necessary correction.

Each mL of 1 mol/L sodium hydroxide VS
= 59.05 mg of $C_4H_6O_4$

Succinic acid, anhydrous $C_4H_4O_3$ White or pale yellow-white, crystals or flakes. It is odorless. Soluble in water, freely soluble in hot water, and sparingly soluble in ethanol (95).

Purity (1) Chloride <*1.03*>: not more than 0.005%.

(2) Iron <*1.10*>: not more than 0.001%.

Residue on ignition <*2.44*>: not more than 0.1% (1 g).

Content: not less than 98.0%. Assay—Dissolve about 1 g of anhydrous succinic acid, accurately weighed, in 50 mL of water by warming, cool, and titrate <*2.50*> with 1 mol/L sodium hydroxide VS (indicator: 2 drops of phenolphthalein TS).

Each mL of 1 mol/L sodium hydroxide VS
= 50.04 mg of $C_4H_4O_3$.

Sucrose $C_{12}H_{22}O_{11}$ [K 8383, Special class]

Sucrose for optical rotation $C_{12}H_{22}O_{11}$ [K 8383, Sucrose, Special class]

Sudan III $C_{22}H_{16}N_4O$ Red-brown powder. It dissolves in acetic acid (100) and in chloroform, and insoluble in water, in ethanol (95), in acetone and in diethyl ether.

Melting point <*2.60*>: 170 - 190°C

Sudan III TS Dissolve 10 mg of sudan III in 5 mL of ethanol (95), filter, and add 5 mL of glycerin to the filtrate. Prepare before use.

Sulbactam sodium for sulbactam penicillamine $C_8H_{10}NNaO_5S$ White to yellowish white crystalline powder. Freely soluble in water, and slightly soluble in ethanol (95).

Identification—Determine the infrared absorption spectrum of sulbactam sodium for sulbactam penicillamine according to the potassium bromide disk method under Infrared Spectrophotometry <*2.25*>: it exhibits the absorption at the wave numbers of about 1780 cm^{-1}, 1600 cm^{-1}, 1410 cm^{-1}, 1400 cm^{-1}, 1320 cm^{-1}, 1300 cm^{-1}, 1200 cm^{-1} and 1130 cm^{-1}.

Water <*2.48*>: not more than 1.0% (0.5 g).

Content: not less than 875 μg (potency) per mg, calculated on the anhydrous basis. Assay—Weigh accurately an amount of sulbactam sodium for sulbactam penicillamine and Sulbactam RS, equivalent to about 0.10 g (potency), dissolve each in a suitable volume of the mobile phase, add exactly 10 mL of the internal standard solution and the mobile phase to make 100 mL, and use these solutions as the sample solution and the standard solution, respectively. Perform the test with 10 μL each of these solutions as directed under Liquid Chromatography <*2.01*> according to the following conditions, and calculate the ratios, Q_T and Q_S, of the peak area of sulbactam to that of the internal standard.

Amount [μg (potency)] of sulbactam ($C_8H_{11}NO_5S$)
$= M_S \times Q_T/Q_S \times 1000$

M_S: amount [mg (potency)] of Sulbactam RS taken

Internal standard solution—A solution of ethyl parahydroxybenzoate in the mobile phase (7 in 1000).

Operating conditions

Detector: An ultraviolet absorption photometer (wavelength: 220 nm).

Column: A stainless steel column 3.9 mm in inside diameter and 30 cm in length, packed with octadecylsilanized silica gel for liquid chromatography (10 μm in particle diameter).

Column temperature: A constant temperature of about 35°C.

Mobile phase: To 750 mL of 0.005 mol/L tetrabutylammonium hydroxide TS add 250 mL of acetonitrile for liquid chromatography.

Flow rate: Adjust so that the retention time of sulbactam is about 6 minutes.

System suitability

System performance: When the procedure is run with 10 μL of the standard solution according to the above operating conditions, sulbactam and the internal standard are eluted in this order with the resolution between these peaks being not less than 1.5.

System repeatability: When the test is repeated 6 times with 10 μL of the standard solution according to the above operating conditions, the relative standard deviation of the peak areas of sulbactam is not more than 2.0%.

Sulfamic acid (standard reagent) See amido sulfuric acid (standard reagent).

Sulfanilamide $H_2NC_6H_4SO_2NH_2$ [K 9066, Special class]

Sulfanilamide for titration of diazotization $H_2NC_6H_4SO_2NH_2$ [K 9066, For titration of diazotization]

Sulfanilic acid $H_2NC_6H_4SO_3H$ [K 8586, Special class]

Sulfathiazole $C_9H_9N_3O_2S_2$ White crystalline powder.
Melting point <*2.60*>: 200 - 204°C

Sulfite oxidase One unit indicates an amount of the enzyme which consumes 1 μmol of oxygen in 1 minute at 25°C and pH 8.0 using sulfur dioxide and oxygen as the substrate.

Sulfite oxidase TS Suspend sulfite oxidase in ammonium sulfate TS so that each mL contains 2.5 units of the activity.
Storage—Between 0 and 8°C.

Sulfosalicylic acid See 5-sulfosalicylic acid dihydrate.

5-Sulfosalicylic acid dihydrate $C_7H_6O_6S.2H_2O$ [K 8589, Special class]

Sulfosalicylic acid TS Dissolve 5 g of 5-sulfosalicylic acid dihydrate in water to make 100 mL.

Sulfur S [K 8088, Special class]

Sulfur dioxide SO_2 Prepare by adding sulfuric acid dropwise to a concentrated solution of sodium bisulfite. Colorless gas, having a characteristic odor.

Sulfuric acid H_2SO_4 [K 8951, Special class]

Sulfuric acid, dilute Cautiously add 5.7 mL of sulfuric acid to 10 mL of water, cool, and dilute with water to make 100 mL (10%).

Sulfuric acid-ethanol TS With stirring, add slowly 3 mL of sulfuric acid to 1000 mL of ethanol (99.5), and cool.

Sulfuric acid for readily carbonizable substances To sulfuric acid, the content of which has previously been determined by the following method, add water cautiously, and adjust the final concentration to 94.5% to 95.5% of sulfuric acid (H_2SO_4). When the concentration is changed owing to absorption of water during storage, prepare freshly.
Assay—Weigh accurately about 2 g of sulfuric acid in a glass-stoppered flask rapidly, add 30 mL of water, cool, and titrate <*2.50*> the solution with 1 mol/L sodium hydroxide VS (indicator: 2 to 3 drops of bromothymol blue TS).

Each mL of 1 mol/L sodium hydroxide VS
= 49.04 mg of H_2SO_4

Sulfuric acid, fuming $H_2SO_4.nSO_3$ [K 8741, Special class]

Sulfuric acid-hexane-methanol TS To 230 mL of a mixture of methanol and hexane (3:1) add cautiously 2 mL of sulfuric acid.

Sulfuric acid-methanol TS Prepare carefully by adding 60 mL of sulfuric acid to 40 mL of methanol.

0.05 mol/L Sulfuric acid-methanol TS Add gradually 3 mL of sulfuric acid to 1000 mL of methanol, while stirring, and allow to cool.

Sulfuric acid-monobasic sodium phosphate TS See sulfuric acid-sodium dihydrogenphosphate TS.

Sulfuric acid, purified Place sulfuric acid in a beaker, heat until white fumes are evolved, then heat for 3 minutes cautiously and gently. Use after cooling.

Sulfuric acid-sodium dihydrogenphosphate TS Add 6.8 mL of sulfuric acid to 500 mL of water, then dissolve 50 g of sodium dihydrogenphosphate dihydrate in this solution, and add water to make 1000 mL.

Sulfuric acid-sodium hydroxide TS With stirring add slowly 120 mL of sulfuric acid to 1000 mL of water, and cool (solution A). Dissolve 88.0 g of sodium hydroxide in 1000 mL of freshly boiled and cooled water (solution B). Mix equal volumes of solution A and solution B.

Sulfuric acid TS Cautiously add 1 volume of sulfuric acid to 2 volumes of water, and while warming on a water bath add dropwise potassium permanganate TS until a pale red color of the solution remains.

0.05 mol/L Sulfuric acid TS Dilute 100 mL of 0.5 mol/L sulfuric acid TS with water to make 1000 mL.

0.25 mol/L Sulfuric acid TS With stirring, add slowly 15 mL of sulfuric acid to 1000 mL of water, then cool.

0.5 mol/L Sulfuric acid TS With stirring, add slowly 30 mL of sulfuric acid to 1000 mL of water, then cool.

1 mol/L Sulfuric acid TS Add 60 mL of sulfuric acid in 1000 mL of water slowly with stirring, then allow to cool.

2 mol/L Sulfuric acid TS To 1000 mL of water add gradually 120 mL of sulfuric acid with stirring, and cool.

5 mol/L Sulfuric acid TS Add 300 mL of sulfuric acid in 1000 mL of water slowly with stirring, then allow to cool.

Sulfurous acid solution A clear and colorless liquid containing more than 5% of SO_2, having a pungent odor. Specific gravity: about 1.03 g/mL.
Identification—To 1 mL of iodine TS add 20 mL of water, and add 1 mL of sulfurous acid solution: the color of the solution disappears, and this solution forms a white precipitate upon addition of 1 mL of barium chloride TS.
Storage—Preserve at a cold place.

Sulpiride for assay $C_{15}H_{23}N_3O_4S$ [Same as the monograph Sulpiride. When dried, it contains not less than 99.0% of sulpiride ($C_{15}H_{23}N_3O_4S$).]

Sulpyrine See sulpyrine hydrate.

Sulpyrine for assay See sulpyrine hydrate for assay.

Sulpyrine hydrate $C_{13}H_{16}N_3NaO_4S.H_2O$ [Same as the namesake monograph]

Sulpyrine hydrate for assay $C_{13}H_{16}N_3NaO_4S.H_2O$ [Same as the monograph Sulpyrine Hydrate. Calculated on the dried basis, it contains not less than 99.0% of sulpyrine ($C_{13}H_{16}N_3NaO_4S$).]

Suxamethonium chloride for thin-layer chromatography See suxamethonium chloride hydrate for thin-layer chromatography.

Suxamethonium chloride hydrate for thin-layer chromatography $C_{14}H_{30}Cl_2N_2O_4.2H_2O$ [Same as the monograph Suxamethonium Chloride Hydrate]

Sweet hydrangea leaf dihydroisocoumarin for thin-layer chromatography White to light yellow-brown crystalline powder of mainly two components, generally obtained from activated charcoal treated fraction of acetone or methanol extracts of crumping upped leaves or tip branches of

Hydrangea macrophylla Seringe var. *thunbergii* Makino (*Saxifragaceae*).

Identification Dissolve 2 mg of the substance to be examined in 1 mL of methanol, and perform the test with 5 μL of this solution as directed in the Identification under Sweet Hydrangea Leaf: two consecutive spots are observed at *R*f values of about 0.3.

Swertia herb [Same as the namesake monograph]

Swertiamarin for thin-layer chromatography $C_{16}H_{22}O_{10}$ A white to light yellow powder. Freely soluble in water and in ethanol (95).

Identification Determine the infrared absorption spectrum of swertiamarin for thin-layer chromatography as directed in the potassium bromide disk method under Infrared Spectrophotometry <2.25>: it exhibits absorption at the wave numbers of about 3380 cm^{-1}, 1693 cm^{-1}, 1618 cm^{-1} and 1068 cm^{-1}.

Purity Related substances—Dissolve 2 mg of swertiamarin for thin-layer chromatography in 1 mL of ethanol (95), and use this solution as the sample solution. Pipet 0.5 mL of the sample solution, add ethanol (95) to make exactly 25 mL, and use this solution as the standard solution. Perform the test with these solutions as directed under Thin-layer Chromatography <2.03>. Spot 20 μL each of the sample solution and standard solution on a plate of silica gel with fluorescent indicator for thin-layer chromatography. Develop the plate with a mixture of ethyl acetate, 1-propanol and water (6:4:3) to a distance of about 10 cm and air-dry the plate. Examine under ultraviolet light (main wavelength: 254 nm): any spot other than the principal spot with an *R*f value of about 0.5 obtained from the sample solution is not more intense than the spot from the standard solution.

Synthetic zeolite for drying A mixture of $6(Na_2O).6(Al_2O_3).12(SiO_2)$ and $6(K_2O).6(Al_2O_3).12(SiO_2)$ prepared for drying. Usually, use the spherically molded form, 2 mm in diameter, prepared by adding a binder. White to grayish white, or color transition by adsorbing water. Average fine pore diameter is about 0.3 nm, and the surface area is 500 to 700 m^2 per g.

Loss on ignition <2.43>: not more than 2.0% [2 g, 550 – 600°C, 4 hours, allow to stand in a desiccator (phosphorus (V) oxide).]

System suitability test solution for filgrastim Filgrastim (Genetical Recombination) containing about 2% charge isomer.

Talc [Same as the namesake monograph]

Taltirelin hydrate for assay $C_{17}H_{23}N_7O_5.4H_2O$ [Same as the monograph Taltirelin Hydrate. It contains not less than 99.0% of taltirelin ($C_{17}H_{23}N_7O_5$), calculated on the anhydrous basis.]

Tamsulosin hydrochloride $C_{20}H_{28}N_2O_5S.HCl$ [Same as the namesake monograph]

Tamsulosin hydrochloride for assay $C_{20}H_{28}N_2O_5S.HCl$ [Same as the monograph Tamsulosin Hydrochloride. When dried, it contains not less than 99.0% of tamsulosin hydrochloride ($C_{20}H_{28}N_2O_5S.HCl$).]

Tannic acid [Same as the namesake monograph]

Tannic acid TS Dissolve 1 g of tannic acid in 1 mL of ethanol (95), and add water to make 10 mL. Prepare before use.

Tartaric acid See L-tartaric acid.

L-Tartaric acid $C_4H_6O_6$ [K 8532, L(+)-Tartaric acid, Special class].

Tartrate buffer solution (pH 3.0) Dissolve 1.5 g of L-tartaric acid and 2.3 g of sodium tartarate dihydrate in water to make 1000 mL.

Taurine $H_2NCH_2CH_2SO_3H$ White, crystals or crystalline powder.

Contents: not less than 95.0%. Assay—Weigh accurately about 0.2 g, dissolve in 50 mL of water, add 5 mL of formaldehyde solution, and titrate <2.50> with 0.1 mol/L sodium hydroxide VS (indicator: 3 drops of phenolphthalein TS). Perform a blank determination in the same manner, and make any necessary correction.

Each mL of 0.1 mol/L sodium hydroxide VS
= 12.52 mg of $C_2H_7NO_3S$

Telmisartan for assay $C_{33}H_{30}N_4O_2$ [Same as the monograph Telmisartan]

Temocapril hydrochloride for assay $C_{23}H_{28}N_2O_5S_2.HCl$ [Same as the monograph Temocapril Hydrochloride. It contains not less than 99.5% of temocapril hydrochloride ($C_{23}H_{28}N_2O_5S_2.HCl$: 513.07), calculated on the anhydrous basis.]

Terbinafine hydrochloride for assay $C_{21}H_{25}N.HCl$ [Same as the monograph Terbinafine Hydrochloride]

Terephthalic acid $C_6H_4(COOH)_2$ White, crystals or crystalline powder. Slightly soluble in ethanol (95), and practically insoluble in water and in diethyl ether.

Residue on ignition <2.44>: not more than 0.3% (1 g).

Content: not less than 95.0%. Assay—Weigh accurately about 2 g of terephthalic acid, dissolve in exactly 50 mL of 1 mol/L sodium hydroxide VS, and titrate <2.50> with 1 mol/L hydrochloric acid VS (indicator: 3 drops of phenolphthalein TS). Perform a blank determination in the same manner.

Each mL of 1 mol/L sodium hydroxide VS
= 83.07 mg of $C_8H_6O_4$

Terphenyl $C_{18}H_{14}$ White crystalline powder.

Identification—Determine the absorption spectrum of a solution of terphenyl in methanol (1 in 250,000) as directed under Ultraviolet-visible Spectrophotometry <2.24>: it exhibits a maximum between 276 nm and 280 nm.

Melting point <2.60>: 208 – 213°C

***p*-Terphenyl** See terphenyl.

Test bacteria inoculation medium for teceleukin Dissolve 6.0 g of peptone, 3.0 g of yeast extract, 1.5 g of meat extract, 1.0 g of glucose, and 13.0 to 20.0 g of agar in water to make 1000 mL and sterilize. The pH is 6.5 to 6.6.

Test bacteria inoculation medium slant for teceleukin Sterilized slant culture obtained by adding approximately 9 mL of test bacteria inoculation medium for teceleukin to a test tube with an inside diameter of 16 mm.

Testosterone $C_{19}H_{28}O_2$ White, crystals or crystalline powder.

Identification—Determine the infrared absorption spectrum of testosterone as directed in the potassium bromide disk method under Infrared Spectrophotometry <2.25>: it exhibits the absorption at the wave numbers of about 3530 cm^{-1}, 3380 cm^{-1}, 1612 cm^{-1}, 1233 cm^{-1}, 1067 cm^{-1} and 1056 cm^{-1}.

Testosterone propionate $C_{22}H_{32}O_3$ [Same as the namesake monograph]

Tetrabromophenolphthalein ethyl ester potassium salt $C_{22}H_{13}Br_4KO_4$ [K 9042, Special class]

Tetrabromophenolphthalein ethyl ester TS Dissolve 0.1 g of tetrabromophenolphthalein ethyl ester potassium salt in acetic acid (100) to make 100 mL. Prepare before use.

Tetra-*n*-butylammonium bromide $[CH_3(CH_2)_3]_4NBr$ White, crystals or crystalline powder, having a slight, characteristic odor.

Melting point <2.60>: 101 – 105°C

Purity Clarity and color of solution—Dissolve 1.0 g of tetra-*n*-butylammonium bromide in 20 mL of water: the solution is clear and colorless.

Content: not less than 98.0%. Assay—Dissolve about 0.5 g of tetra-*n*-butylammonium bromide, accurately weighed, in 50 mL of water, add 5 mL of dilute nitric acid, and titrate <2.50> with 0.1 mol/L silver nitrate VS while strongly shaking (potentiometric titration). Perform a blank determination in the same manner, and make any necessary correction.

Each mL of 0.1 mol/L silver nitrate VS
= 32.24 mg of $C_{16}H_{36}NBr$

Tetra-*n*-butylammonium chloride $C_{16}H_{36}ClN$ White crystals, and it is deliquescent.

Water <2.48>: not more than 6.0% (0.1 g).

Content: not less than 95.0%, calculated on the anhydrous basis. Assay—Weigh accurately about 0.25 g of tetra-*n*-butylammonium chloride, dissolve in 50 mL of water, and titrate <2.50> with 0.1 mol/L silver nitrate VS (potentiometric titration).

Each mL of 0.1 mol/L silver nitrate VS
= 27.79 mg of $C_{16}H_{36}ClN$

Tetrabutylammonium dihydrogen phosphate $(C_4H_9)_4NH_2PO_4$ White powder. It is soluble in water. For Eribulin Mesilate, when perform the test as directed in the system suitability in the Purity (2) under Eribulin Mesilate, the height of a peak appeared in the gradient mode is not more than 6 times the peak height of eribulin obtained from the standard solution.

Content: not less than 97.0%. Assay—Weigh accurately 1.5 g of tetrabutylammonium dihydrogen phosphate, dissolve in 80 mL of water, and titrate <2.50> with 0.5 mol/L sodium hydroxide VS (potentiometric titration). Perform a blank determination in the same manner, and make any necessary correction.

Each mL of 0.5 mol/L sodium hydroxide VS
= 169.7 mg of $(C_4H_9)_4NH_2PO_4$

Tetrabutylammonium hydrogensulfate $C_{16}H_{37}NO_4S$ White crystalline powder.

Content: not less than 98.0%. Assay—Weigh accurately about 0.7 g of tetrabutylammonium hydrogensulfate, dissolve in 100 mL of freshly boiled and cooled water, and titrate <2.50> with 0.1 mol/L sodium hydroxide VS (indicator: 3 drops of bromocresol green-methyl red TS).

Each mL of 0.1 mol/L sodium hydroxide VS
= 33.95 mg of $C_{16}H_{37}NO_4S$

40% Tetrabutylammonium hydroxide TS A solution containing 40 g/dL of tetrabutylammonium hydroxide $[(C_4H_9)_4NOH: 259.47]$.

Content: 36 – 44 g/dL. Assay—Pipet 10 mL of 40% tetrabutylammonium hydroxide TS, and titrate <2.50> with 1 mol/L hydrochloric acid VS (indicator: 3 drops of methyl red TS).

Each mL of 1 mol/L hydrochloric acid VS
= 259.5 mg of $C_{16}H_{37}NO$

0.005 mol/L Tetrabutylammonium hydroxide TS To 10 mL of tetrabutylammonium hydroxide TS add 700 mL of water, adjust to pH 4.0 with diluted phosphoric acid (1 in 10), and add water to make 1000 mL.

Tetrabutylammonium hydroxide-methanol TS Methanol solution containing 25 g/dL of tetrabutylammonium hydroxide $[(C_4H_9)_4NOH: 259.47]$. Colorless to pale yellow solution, having an ammonium-like odor.

Content: 22.5 – 27.5 g/dL. Assay—Pipet 15 mL of tetrabutylammonium hydroxide-methanol TS and titrate <2.50> with 1 mol/L hydrochloric acid VS (indicator: 3 drops of methyl red TS).

Each mL of 1 mol/L hydrochloric acid VS
= 259.5 mg of $C_{16}H_{37}NO$

10% Tetrabutylammonium hydroxide-methanol TS A methanol solution containing 10 g/dL of tetrabutylammonium hydroxide $[(C_4H_9)_4NOH: 259.47]$.

Content: 9.0 – 11.0 g/dL. Assay—Pipet 2 mL of 10% tetrabutylammonium hydroxide-methanol TS, transfer to a glass-stoppered flask containing 20 mL of water, and titrate <2.50> with 0.1 mol/L hydrochloric acid VS (indicator: 3 drops of methyl red TS).

Each mL of 0.1 mol/L hydrochloric acid VS
= 25.95 mg of $C_{16}H_{37}NO$

Tetrabutylammonium hydroxide TS A solution containing 13 g/dL of tetrabutylammonium hydroxide $[(C_4H_9)_4NOH: 259.47]$.

Content: 11.7 – 14.3 g/dL. Assay—Pipet a quantity, equivalent to about 0.3 g of tetrabutylammonium hydroxide $[(C_4H_9)_4NOH]$, transfer to a glass-stoppered flask containing 15 mL of water, accurately weighed, and titrate <2.50> with 0.1 mol/L hydrochloric acid VS (indicator: 3 drops of methyl red TS).

Each mL of 0.1 mol/L hydrochloric acid VS
= 25.95 mg of $C_{16}H_{37}NO$

Tetrabutylammonium phosphate See tetrabuthylammonium dihydrogen phosphate.

Tetracycline $C_{22}H_{24}N_2O_8$ Yellow to dark yellow, crystals or crystalline powder. Sparingly soluble in ethanol, and very slightly soluble in water.

Content: it contains not less than 870 μg (potency) per mg. Assay—Proceed as directed in the Assay under Tetracycline Hydrochloride. However, use the following formula.

Amount [μg (potency)] of tetracycline ($C_{22}H_{24}N_2O_8$)
$= M_S \times (A_T/A_S) \times 1000$

M_S: Amount [mg (potency)] of Tetracycline Hydrochloride RS taken

Tetracycline Hydrochloride $C_{22}H_{24}N_2O_8.HCl$ Yellow, crystals or crystalline powder.

Purity Related substances—Dissolve 20 mg of tetracycline hydrochloride in 0.01 mol/L hydrochloric acid TS to make 25 mL, and use this solution as the sample solution. Proceed the test with 20 μL of the sample solution as directed in the Purity (2) under Oxytetracycline Hydrochloride, determine each peak area by the automatic integration method, and calculate the amounts of them by the area percentage method: the total amount of the peaks other than tetracycline is not more than 10%.

Tetradecyl trimethylammonium bromide $CH_3(CH_2)_{13}N(CH_3)_3Br$ A white powder.

Purity Clarity and color of solution—Dissolve 1.0 g of tetradecyl trimethylammonium bromide in 20 mL of water: the solution is clear and colorless.

Content: not less than 98.0%. Assay—Weigh accurately about 0.5 g of tetradecyl trimethylammonium bromide, dissolve in 100 mL of water, add 5 mL of a mixture of water and nitric acid (2:1), and titrate <*2.50*> with 0.1 mol/L silver nitrate VS (potentiometric titration). Perform a blank test in the same manner, and make any necessary correction.

Each mL of 0.1 mol/L silver nitrate VS
= 33.64 mg of $C_{17}H_{38}NBr$

Tetraethylammonium hydroxide TS A solution containing 10% of tetraethylammonium hydroxide [$(C_2H_5)_4NOH$: 147.26]. A clear, colorless liquid, having a strong ammonia odor. It is a strong basic and easily absorbs carbon dioxide from the air.

Content: 10.0 – 11.0% Assay—Weigh accurately about 3 g of tetraethylammonium hydroxide in a glass-stoppered flask containing 15 mL of water, and titrate <*2.50*> with 0.1 mol/L hydrochloric acid VS (indicator: 3 drops of methyl red TS). Perform a blank determination in the same manner, and make any necessary correction.

Each mL of 0.1 mol/L hydrochloric acid VS
= 14.73 mg of $C_8H_{21}NO$

Tetra-*n*-heptylammonium bromide $[CH_3(CH_2)_6]_4NBr$ White, crystals or crystalline powder, having a slight, characteristic odor.

Melting point <*2.60*>: 89 – 93°C

Content: not less than 98.0%. Assay—Dissolve about 0.5 g of tetra-*n*-heptylammonium bromide, accurately weighed, in 50 mL of diluted acetonitrile (3 in 5), and 5 mL of dilute nitric acid, and titrate <*2.50*> with 0.1 mol/L silver nitrate VS while strongly shaking (potentiometric titration). Perform a blank determination in the same manner, and make any necessary correction.

Each mL of 0.1 mol/L silver nitrate VS
= 49.07 mg $C_{28}H_{60}NBr$

Tetrahydrofuran $CH_2(CH_2)_2CH_2O$ [K 9705, Special class]

Tetrahydrofuran for gas chromatography Use tetrahydrofuran prepared by distilling with iron (II) sulfate heptahydrate.

Storage—Preserve in containers, in which the air has been displaced by nitrogen, in a dark, cold place.

Tetrahydrofuran for liquid chromatography C_4H_8O Clear and colorless liquid.

Refractive index <*2.45*> n_D^{20}: 1.406 – 1.409

Density <*2.56*> 0.884 – 0.889 g/mL (20°C)

Purity Ultraviolet absorbing substances—Determine the absorption spectrum of tetrahydrofuran for liquid chromatography as directed under Ultraviolet-visible Spectrophotometry <*2.24*>, using water as the blank: the absorbances at 240 nm, 254 nm, 280 nm, 290 nm, and between 300 nm and 400 nm are not more than 0.35, 0.20, 0.05, 0.02 and 0.01, respectively.

Peroxide—Perform the test according to the method described in JIS K 9705: not more than 0.01%.

Tetrahydroxyquinone $C_6H_4O_6$ Dark blue crystals. Its color changes to yellow on exposure to light. Soluble in ethanol (95) and sparingly soluble in water.

Tetrahydroxyquinone indicator Mix 1 g of tetrahydroxyquinone with 100 g of sucrose homogeneously.

Tetrakishydroxypropylethylenediamine for gas chromatography Prepared for gas chromatography.

Tetramethylammonium hydroxide $(CH_3)_4NOH$ Ordinarily, available as an approximately 10% aqueous solution, which is clear and colorless, and has a strong ammonia-like odor. Tetramethylammonium hydroxide is a stronger base than ammonia, and rapidly absorbs carbon dioxide from the air. Use a 10% aqueous solution.

Purity Ammonia and other amines—Weigh accurately a quantity of the solution, corresponding to about 0.3 g of tetramethylammonium hydroxide [$(CH_3)_4NOH$], in a weighing bottle already containing 5 mL of water. Add a slight excess of 1 mol/L hydrochloric acid TS (about 4 mL), and evaporate on a water bath to dryness. The mass of the residue (tetramethylammonium chloride), dried at 105°C for 2 hours and multiplied by 0.8317, represents the quantity of tetramethylammonium hydroxide [$(CH_3)_4NOH$], and corresponds to ±0.2% of that found in the Assay.

Residue on evaporation: not more than 0.02% (5 mL, 105°C, 1 hour).

Content: not less than 98% of the labeled amount. Assay—Accurately weigh a glass-stoppered flask containing about 15 mL of water. Add a quantity of the solution, equivalent to about 0.2 g of tetramethylammonium hydroxide [$(CH_3)_4NOH$], weigh again, and titrate <*2.50*> with 0.1 mol/L hydrochloric acid VS (indicator: methyl red TS).

Each mL of 0.1 mol/L hydrochloric acid VS
= 9.115 mg of $C_4H_{13}NO$

Tetramethylammonium hydroxide-methanol TS A methanol solution containing of 10 g/dL of tetramethylammonium hydroxide [$(CH_3)_4NOH$: 91.15]

Content: 9.0 – 11.0 g/dL. Assay—Pipet 2 mL of tetramethylammonium hydroxide-methanol TS, transfer to a glass-stoppered flask containing 20 mL of water, and titrate <*2.50*> with 0.1 mol/L hydrochloric acid VS (indicator: bromocresol green-methyl red TS).

Each mL of 0.1 mol/L hydrochloric acid VS
= 9.115 mg of $C_4H_{13}NO$

Tetramethylammonium hydroxide TS Pipet 15 mL of tetramethylammonium hydroxide, and add ethanol (99.5) to make exactly 100 mL.

Tetramethylammonium hydroxide TS (pH 5.5) To 10 mL of tetramethylammonium hydroxide add 990 mL of water, and adjust the pH to 5.5 with diluted phosphoric acid (1 in 10).

3,3′,5,5′-Tetramethylbenzidine dihydrochloride dihydrate $C_{16}H_{22}Cl_2N_2.2H_2O$ White to pale red-white crystalline powder.

***N,N,N′,N′*-Tetramethylethylenediamine** $(CH_3)_2NCH_2CH_2N(CH_3)_2$ Pale yellow clear liquid.

Specific gravity <*2.56*> d_4^{20}: 0.774 – 0.799

Content: not less than 99.0%.

Tetramethylsilane for nuclear magnetic resonance spectroscopy $(CH_3)_4Si$ Prepared for nuclear magnetic resonance spectroscopy.

Tetra-*n*-pentylammonium bromide $[CH_3(CH_2)_4]_4NBr$ White, crystals or crystalline powder. It is hygroscopic.

Melting point ⟨*2.60*⟩: 100 – 101°C

Tetraphenylboron sodium See sodium tetraphenylborate.

Tetra-*n*-propylammonium bromide $[CH_3CH_2CH_2]_4NBr$ White, crystals or crystalline powder.

Purity Clarity and color of solution—Dissolve 1.0 g of tetra-*n*-propylammonium bromide in 20 mL of water: the solution is clear and colorless.

Content: not less than 98.0%. Assay—Weigh accurately about 0.4 g of tetra-*n*-propylammonium bromide, dissolve in 50 mL of water, add 5 mL of dilute nitric acid, and titrate ⟨*2.50*⟩ with 0.1 mol/L silver nitrate VS while shaking strongly (potentiometric titration). Perform a blank determination in the same manner, and make any necessary correction.

Each mL of 0.1 mol/L silver nitrate VS
= 26.63 mg of $C_{12}H_{28}NBr$

Theophylline $C_7H_8N_4O_2$ White powder. Slightly soluble in water.

Melting point ⟨*2.60*⟩: 269 – 274°C

Purity Caffeine, theobromine or paraxanthine—To 0.20 g of theophylline add 5 mL of potassium hydroxide TS or 5 mL of ammonia TS: each solution is clear.

Loss on drying ⟨*2.41*⟩: not more than 0.5% (1 g, 105°C, 4 hours).

Content: not less than 99.0%. Assay—Weigh accurately about 0.25 g of theophylline, previously dried, dissolve it in 40 mL of *N*,*N*-dimethylformamide, and titrate ⟨*2.50*⟩ with 0.1 mol/L sodium methoxide VS (indicator: 3 drops of thymol blue-*N*,*N*-dimethylformamide TS). Perform a blank determination in the same manner, and make any necessary correction.

Each mL of 0.1 mol/L sodium methoxide VS
= 18.02 mg of $C_7H_8N_4O_2$

Theophylline for assay $C_7H_8N_4O_2$ [Same as the monograph Theophylline meeting the following additional specifications.]

Purity Related substances—Dissolve 50 mg of theophylline for assay in water to make 100 mL, and use this solution as the sample solution. Pipet 1 mL of the sample solution, add water to make exactly 200 mL, and use this solution as the standard solution. Perform the test with exactly 20 μL of the sample solution and standard solution as directed under Liquid Chromatography ⟨*2.01*⟩ according to the following conditions. Determine each peak area from both solutions by the automatic integration method: the total area of peaks other than theophylline obtained from the sample solution is not larger than the peak area of theophylline from the standard solution.

Operating conditions

Detector: An ultraviolet absorption photometer (wavelength: 270 nm).

Column: A stainless steel column 6 mm in inside diameter and 15 cm in length, packed with octadecylsilanized silica gel for liquid chromatography (5 μm in particle diameter).

Column temperature: A constant temperature of about 40°C.

Mobile phase: A mixture of diluted acetic acid (100) (1 in 100) and methanol (4:1).

Flow rate: Adjust so that the retention time of theophylline is about 10 minutes.

Time span of measurement: About 3 times as long as the retention time of theophylline.

System suitability

Test for required detectability: Pipet 5 mL of the standard solution, and add water to make exactly 25 mL. Confirm that the peak area of theophylline obtained with 20 μL of this solution is equivalent to 15 to 25% of that of theophylline with 20 μL of the standard solution.

System performance: When the procedure is run with 20 μL of the standard solution under the above operating conditions, the number of theoretical plates and the symmetry factor of the peak of theophylline are not less than 3000 and not more than 1.5, respectively.

System repeatability: When the test is repeated 6 times with 20 μL of the standard solution under the above operating conditions, the relative standard deviation of the peak area of theophylline is not more than 3.0%.

Thermolysin It has the activity of 50 – 100 units per mg protein. Origin: *Bacillus thermoproteolyticus rokko*.

Thiamine nitrate $C_{12}H_{17}N_5O_4S$ [Same as the namesake monograph]

Thianthol [Same as the monograph Thianthol. Proceed as directed in the Identification (3) under Sulfur, Salicylic Acid and Thianthol Ointment: any spot other than the principal spot does not appear.]

3-Thienylethylpenicillin sodium $C_{14}H_{15}N_2NaO_4S_2$ White to pale yellow-white powder. Very soluble in water, freely soluble in methanol, and sparingly soluble in ethanol (95).

Optical rotation ⟨*2.49*⟩ $[\alpha]_D^{20}$: +265 – +290° (0.5 g calculated on the anhydrous bases, water, 50 mL, 100 mm).

Water ⟨*2.48*⟩: Not more than 10.0% (0.2 g, volumetric titration, direct titration).

Content: not less than 90% calculated on the anhydrous basis. Assay—Weigh accurately about 0.1 g of 3-thienylethylpenicillin sodium, dissolve in 35 mL of water, add 0.75 mL of 0.1 mol/L hydrochloric acid TS, and adjust to pH 8.5 with 0.1 mol/L sodium hydroxide TS. To this solution add 2 mL of a penicillinase solution prepared by dissolving penicillinase, equivalent to 513,000 Levy units, in 25 mL of water and neutralizing with dilute sodium hydroxide TS until a pale red color appears with 1 drop of a solution of phenolphthalein in ethanol (95) (1 in 1000) as indicator, and allow to stand at 25°C for 5 minutes. Titrate ⟨*2.50*⟩ this solution with 0.1 mol/L sodium hydroxide VS until the solution reaches pH 8.5 (potentiometric titration). Use the water freshly boiled and cooled.

Each mL of 0.1 mol/L sodium hydroxide VS
= 36.24 mg of $C_{14}H_{15}N_2NaO_4S_2$

Thioacetamide C_2H_5NS A white crystalline powder or colorless crystals, having a characteristic odor. Freely soluble in water and in ethanol (99.5). Melting point: 112 – 116°C.

Thioacetamide-alkaline glycerin TS To 0.2 mL of a solution of thioacetamide (1 in 25) add 1 mL of alkaline glycerin TS, and heat for 20 seconds in a water bath. Prepare before use.

Thioacetamide TS To 0.2 mL of a solution of thioacetamide (1 in 25) add 1 mL of a mixture of 15 mL of sodium hydroxide TS, 5 mL of water and 20 mL of 85% glycerin, and heat in a water bath for 20 seconds. Prepare before use.

Thiodiglycol $S(CH_2CH_2OH)_2$ [*β*-Thiodiglycol for amino acid autoanalysis] Colorless or pale yellow, clear liquid.

Specific gravity <2.56> d_{20}^{20}: 1.180 – 1.190

Water <2.48>: not more than 0.7%.

Thioglycolate medium I for sterility test See fluid thioglycolate medium.

Thioglycolate medium II for sterility test See alternative thioglycolate medium.

Thioglycolic acid See mercapto acetic acid.

Thionyl chloride $SOCl_2$ A colorless or light yellow, clear liquid, having a pungent odor.

Specific gravity <2.56> d_{20}^{20}: about 1.65 (Method 3).

Content: not less than 95.0%. Assay—Weigh accurately 0.1 g of thionyl chloride in a weighing bottle, put the bottle in a glass-stoppered conical flask containing 50 mL of water cooled to about 5°C, stopper immediately, dissolve the sample thoroughly, and transfer the solution to a 200-mL beaker. Wash the conical flask and the weighing bottle in it with 30 mL of water, and combine the washings and the solution in the beaker. Add 1 drop of an aqueous solution of polyvinyl alcohol (1 in 10), and titrate <2.50> with 0.1 mol/L silver nitrate VS (potentiometric titration). Perform a blank determination in the same manner, and make any necessary correction.

Each mL of 0.1 mol/L silver nitrate VS
= 5.949 mg of $SOCl_2$

Thiopental for assay $C_{11}H_{18}N_2O_2S$ Dissolve 10 g of thiopental sodium in 300 mL of water. To this solution add slowly 50 mL of dilute hydrochloric acid with stirring. Take the produced crystals by filtration, wash with water until the filtrate indicates no reaction to chloride, and air-dry. Add diluted ethanol (3 in 5), dissolve by heating in a water bath, allow to stand, and take the produced crystals by filtration. Air-dry the crystals, and dry again at 105°C for 4 hours. White, odorless crystals.

Melting point <2.60>: 159 – 162°C

Purity (1) Clarity and color of solution—Dissolve 1.0 g of thiopental for assay in 10 mL of ethanol (99.5): the solution is clear and light yellow.

(2) Related substances—Dissolve 50 mg of thiopental for assay in 15 mL of acetonitrile, add water to make 50 mL, and use this solution as the sample solution. Pipet 1 mL of the sample solution, add the mobile phase in the Purity (4) under Thiopental Sodium to make exactly 200 mL, and use this solution as the standard solution. Proceed as directed in Purity (4) under Thiopental Sodium.

Loss on drying <2.41>: not more than 0.20% (1 g, 105°C, 3 hours).

Content: not less than 99.0%. Assay—Weigh accurately about 0.35 g of thiopental for assay, previously dried, dissolve in 5 mL of ethanol (99.5) and 50 mL of chloroform, and titrate <2.50> with 0.1 mol/L potassium hydroxide-ethanol VS (potentiometric titration). Perform a blank determination in the same manner, and make any necessary correction.

Each mL of 0.1 mol/L potassium hydroxide-ethanol VS
= 24.23 mg of $C_{11}H_{18}N_2O_2S$

Thiopental sodium $C_{11}H_{17}N_2NaO_2S$ [Same as the namesake monograph]

Thiosemicarbazide $H_2NCSNHNH_2$ White, crystals or crystalline powder.

Identification—Determine the infrared absorption spectrum as directed in the potassium bromide disk method under Infrared Spectrophotometry <2.25>: it exhibits absorption at the wave numbers of about 3370 cm^{-1}, 3180 cm^{-1}, 1648 cm^{-1}, 1622 cm^{-1}, 1535 cm^{-1}, 1288 cm^{-1}, 1167 cm^{-1}, 1003 cm^{-1} and 803 cm^{-1}.

Thiourea H_2NCSNH_2 [K 8635, Special class]

Thiourea TS Dissolve 10 g of thiourea in water to make 100 mL.

L-Threonine $C_4H_9NO_3$ [Same as the namesake monograph]

Threoprocaterol hydrochloride $C_{16}H_{22}N_2O_3.HCl$ To procaterol hydrochloride add 10 volumes of 3 mol/L hydrochloric acid TS, heat, and reflux for 3 hours. After cooling, neutralize (pH 8.5) with sodium hydroxide TS, and collect the crystals produced. Suspend the crystals in water, dissolve by acidifying the solution at pH 1 to 2 with addition of hydrochloric acid, neutralize (pH 8.5) by adding sodium hydroxide TS, and separate the crystals produced. Suspend the crystals in 2-propanol, and acidify the solution at pH 1 to 2 by adding hydrochloric acid. The crystals are dissolved and reproduced. Collect the crystals, dry at about 60°C while passing air. White to pale yellow-white, odorless, crystals or crystalline powder. Melting point: about 207°C (with decomposition).

Purity—Dissolve 0.10 g of threoprocaterol hydrochloride in 100 mL of diluted methanol (1 in 2), and use this solution as the sample solution. Perform the test with 2 μL of the sample solution as directed under Liquid Chromatography <2.01> according to the operating conditions in the Purity (3) under Procaterol Hydrochloride Hydrate. Measure each peak area by the automatic integration method, and calculate the amount of threoprocaterol by the area percentage method: it shows the purity of not less than 95.0%. Adjust the detection sensitivity so that the peak height of threoprocaterol obtained with 2 μL of the solution prepared by diluting 5.0 mL of the sample solution with diluted methanol (1 in 2) to make 100 mL, is 5 to 10% of the full scale, and the time span of measurement is about twice as long as the retention time of threoprocaterol, beginning after the solvent peak.

Thrombin [Same as the namesake monograph]

Thymine for liquid chromatography $C_5H_6N_2O_2$ Occurs as a white powder.

Purity—Dissolve 10 mg of the substance to be examined in 100 mL of methanol, add the mobile phase to make 250 mL, and use this solution as the sample solution. Pipet 5 mL of the sample solution, add the mobile phase to make exactly 100 mL, and use this solution as the standard solution. Perform the test with 10 μL each of these solutions as directed in the Purity (3) under Zidovudine. Determine each peak area by the automatic integration method: the total area of peaks other than thymine obtained from the sample solution is not larger than that from the standard solution. However, the time span of measurement is about 10 times the retention time of thymine, beginning after the solvent peak.

Thymol $CH_3C_6H_3(OH)CH(CH_3)_2$ [Same as the namesake monograph]

Thymol blue $C_{27}H_{30}O_5S$ [K 8643, Special class]

Thymol blue-*N*,*N*-dimethylformamide TS Dissolve 0.1 g of thymol blue in 100 mL of *N*,*N*-dimethylformamide.

Thymol blue-1,4-dioxane TS Dissolve 50 mg of thymol blue in 100 mL of 1,4-dioxane, and filter if necessary. Prepare before use.

Thymol blue TS Dissolve 0.1 g of thymol blue in 100 mL of ethanol (95), and filter if necessary.

Thymol blue TS, dilute Dissolve 50 mg of thymol blue in 100 mL of ethanol (99.5), and filter if necessary. Prepare before use.

Thymol for assay $C_{10}H_{14}O$ [Same as the monograph Thymol. It contains not less than 99.0% of thymol ($C_{10}H_{14}O$).]

Thymol for spraying test solution $C_{10}H_{14}O$ White, crystals or crystalline powder, having an aromatic odor. Very soluble in methanol and in ethanol (99.5), and practically insoluble in water.

Identification—Determine the infrared absorption spectrum as directed in the potassium bromide disk method under Infrared Spectrophotometry <*2.25*>: it exhibits absorption at the wave numbers of about 2960 cm^{-1}, 1420 cm^{-1}, 1290 cm^{-1}, 1090 cm^{-1} and 810 cm^{-1}.

Melting point <*2.60*>: 49 – 52°C

Purity Other phenols—Shake vigorously 1.0 g of the substance to be examined with 20 mL of warm water for 1 minute, and filter. To 5 mL of the filtrate add 1 drop of a solution of iron (III) chloride hexahydrate (27 in 100): the solution reveals a green but not a blue to purple color.

Thymolphthalein $C_{28}H_{30}O_4$ [K 8642, Special class]

Thymolphthalein TS Dissolve 0.1 g of thymolphthalein in 100 mL of ethanol (95), and filter if necessary.

Thymol-sulfuric acid-methanol TS for spraying Dissolve 1.5 g of thymol for spraying test solution in 100 mL of methanol, and add 5.7 mL of sulfuric acid.

Tiaramide hydrochloride for assay $C_{15}H_{18}ClN_3O_3S.HCl$ [Same as the monograph Tiaramide Hydrochloride. When dried, it contains not less than 99.0% of tiaramide hydrochloride ($C_{15}H_{18}ClN_3O_3S.HCl$).]

Tiapride hydrochloride for assay $C_{15}H_{24}N_2O_4S.HCl$ [Same as the monograph Tiapride Hydrochloride]

Ticlopidine hydrochloride for assay $C_{14}H_{14}ClNS.HCl$ [Same as the monograph Ticlopidine Hydrochloride. It meets the following additional requirements.]

Purity Related substances—Dissolve 0.2 g of ticlopidine hydrochloride for assay in 100 mL of a mixture of water and methanol (1:1), and use this solution as the sample solution. Pipet 1 mL of the sample solution, add a mixture of water and methanol (1:1) to make exactly 100 mL. Pipet 1 mL of this solution, add a mixture of water and methanol (1:1) to make exactly 10 mL, and use this solution as the standard solution. Perform the test with exactly 10 μL each of the sample solution and standard solution as directed under Liquid Chromatography <*2.01*> according to the following conditions, and determine each peak area by the automatic integration method: the area of the peak other than ticlopidine obtained from the sample solution is not larger than the peak area of ticlopidine from the standard solution, and the total area of the peaks other than ticlopidine from the sample solution is not larger than 2 times the peak area of ticlopidine from the standard solution.

Operating conditions

Detector: An ultraviolet absorption photometer (wavelength: 220 nm).

Column: A stainless steel column 4.6 mm in inside diameter and 15 cm in length, packed with octadecylsilanized silica gel for liquid chromatography (5 μm in particle diameter).

Column temperature: A constant temperature of about 40°C.

Mobile phase: A mixture of 0.05 mol/L phosphate buffer solution (pH 3.5) and methanol (1:1).

Flow rate: Adjust so that the retention time of ticlopidine is about 8 minutes.

Time span of measurement: About 7 times as long as the retention time of ticlopidine, beginning after the solvent peak.

System suitability

Test for required detectability: Pipet 2 mL of the standard solution, and add a mixture of water and methanol (1:1) to make exactly 10 mL. Confirm that the peak area of ticlopidine obtained with 10 μL of this solution is equivalent to 14 to 26% of that with 10 μL of the standard solution.

System performance: When the procedure is run with 10 μL of the standard solution under the above operating conditions, the number of theoretical plates and the symmetry factor of the peak of ticlopidine are not less than 5000 and not more than 1.5, respectively.

System repeatability: When the test is repeated 6 times with 10 μL of the standard solution under the above operating conditions, the relative standard deviation of the peak area of ticlopidine is not more than 2.0%.

Tin Sn [K 8580, Special class]

Tin (II) chloride dihydrate $SnCl_2.2H_2O$ [K 8136, Special class]

Tin (II) chloride-hydrochloric acid TS To 20 g of tin add 85 mL of hydrochloric acid, heat until hydrogen gas no longer are evolved, and allow to cool. Mix 1 volume of this solution and 10 volume of dilute hydrochloric acid. Prepare before use.

Tin (II) chloride-sulfuric acid TS Dissolve 10 g of tin (II) chloride dihydrate in diluted sulfuric acid (3 in 200) to make 100 mL.

Tin (II) chloride TS Dissolve 1.5 g of Tin (II) chloride dihydrate in 10 mL of water containing a small amount of hydrochloric acid. Preserve in glass-stoppered bottles in which a fragment of tin has been placed. Use within 1 month.

Tin (II) chloride TS, acidic Dissolve 8 g of Tin (II) chloride dihydrate in 500 mL of hydrochloric acid. Preserve in glass-stoppered bottles. Use within 3 months.

Tipepidine hibenzate for assay $C_{15}H_{17}NS_2.C_{14}H_{10}O_4$ [Same as the monograph Tipepidine Hibenzate. When dried, it contains not less than 99.0% of tipepidine hibenzate ($C_{15}H_{17}NS_2.C_{14}H_{10}O_4$).]

Titanium dioxide See titanium (IV) oxide.

Titanium dioxide TS See titanium (IV) oxide TS.

Titanium (III) chloride (20) $TiCl_3$ [K 8401, Titanium (III) chloride solution, Special class] Store in light-resistant, glass-stoppered containers.

Titanium (III) chloride-sulfuric acid TS Mix carefully 20 mL of titanium (III) chloride TS and 13 mL of sulfuric acid, add carefully hydrogen peroxide (30) in small portions until a yellow color develops, and heat until white fumes evolve. After cooling, add water, heat again in the same manner, repeat this procedure until the solution is colorless, and add water to make 100 mL.

Titanium (III) chloride TS To titanium (III) chloride (20) add dilute hydrochloric acid to obtain a solution containing 15 g/dL of titanium (III) chloride ($TiCl_3$). Prepare before use.

Content: 14.0 - 16.0 g/dL. Assay—To exactly 2 mL of titanium (III) chloride TS add 200 mL of water and 5 mL of a hydrochloric acid solution (2 in 3), and titrate <*2.50*> with 0.1 mol/L ammonium iron (III) sulfate VS under carbon dioxide until a slight red color develops in the solution (indicator: 5 mL of ammonium thiocyanate TS).

Each mL of 0.1 mol/L ferric ammonium sulfate VS
= 15.42 mg of $TiCl_3$

Titanium (IV) oxide TiO_2 [K 8703, Special class]

Titanium (IV) oxide TS To 100 mL of sulfuric acid add 0.1 g of titanium (IV) oxide, and dissolve by gradually heating on a flame with occasional gentle shaking.

Titanium trichloride See titanium (III) chloride (20).

Titanium trichloride-sulfuric acid TS See titanium (III) chloride-sulfuric acid TS.

Titanium trichloride TS See titanium (III) chloride TS.

Titanium yellow $C_{28}H_{19}N_5Na_2O_6S_4$ A dark yellow to dark yellow-brown, powder or masses.

Identification—Determine the infrared absorption spectrum of titanium yellow, previously dried at 105°C for 4 hours, as directed in the potassium bromide disk method under Infrared Spectrophotometry <*2.25*>: it exhibits absorption at the wave numbers of about 1603 cm^{-1}, 1467 cm^{-1}, 1394 cm^{-1}, 1306 cm^{-1}, 1040 cm^{-1}, 988 cm^{-1}, 820 cm^{-1} and 644 cm^{-1}.

Storage—Preserve in a light-resistant tight container.

Tocopherol $C_{29}H_{50}O_2$ [Same as the namesake monograph]

Tocopherol acetate $C_{31}H_{52}O_3$ [Same as the namesake monograph]

Tocopherol calcium succinate $C_{66}H_{106}CaO_{10}$ [Same as the namesake monograph]

Tocopherol succinate $C_{33}H_{54}O_5$ Wet 0.5 g of tocopherol calcium succinate with 5 mL of acetic acid (100), add 10 mL of toluene, and warm at 70°C for 30 minutes with occasional shaking. After cooling, add 30 mL of water, shake thoroughly, and allow to stand. Remove the water layer, wash the toluene layer with several 30-mL portions of water until the washings become neutral, and allow to stand. Shake the toluene extract with 3 g of anhydrous sodium sulfate, decant the toluene layer, distil the toluene under reduced pressure, and obtain a light yellow, viscous liquid. When preserved at room temperature for a long time, it becomes a pale yellowish solid.

Absorbance <*2.24*> $E^{1\%}_{1\,cm}$ (286 nm): 38.0 - 42.0 (10 mg, chloroform, 100 mL).

Tolbutamide $C_{12}H_{18}N_2O_3S$ [Same as the namesake monograph]

Toluene $C_6H_5CH_3$ [K 8680, Special class]

***o*-Toluene sulfonamide** $C_7H_9NO_2S$ Colorless crystals or white crystalline powder. Soluble in ethanol (95), and sparingly soluble in water.

Melting point <*2.60*>: 157 - 160°C

Purity *p*-Toluene sulfonamide—Use a solution of *o*-toluene sulfonamide in ethyl acetate (1 in 5000) as the sample solution. Perform the test with 10 μL of the sample solution as directed under Gas Chromatography <*2.02*> according to the operating conditions in the Purity (5) under Saccharin Sodium Hydrate: any peak other than the peak of *o*-toluene sulfonamide does not appear. Adjust the flow rate so that the retention time of *o*-toluene sulfonamide is about 10 minutes, and adjust the detection sensitivity so that the peak height of *o*-toluene sulfonamide obtained from 10 μL of the sample solution is about 50% of the full scale. Time span of measurement is about twice as long as the retention time of *o*-toluene sulfonamide, beginning after the solvent peak.

Water <*2.48*>: not more than 0.5% (4 g, use 25 mL of methanol for water determination and 5 mL of pyridine for water determination).

Content: not less than 98.5%, calculated on the anhydrous basis. Assay—Weigh accurately about 25 mg of *o*-toluene sulfonamide, and perform the test as directed under Nitrogen Determination <*1.08*>.

Each mL of 0.005 mol/L sulfuric acid VS
= 1.712 mg of $C_7H_9NO_2S$

***p*-Toluenesulfonamide** $CH_3C_6H_4SO_2NH_2$ White, crystals or crystalline powder. Melting point: about 137°C.

Purity Related substances—Dissolve 30 mg of *p*-toluenesulfonamide in acetone to make exactly 200 mL. Spot 10 μL of this solution on a plate of silica gel for thin-layer chromatography. Develop the plate with a mixture of chloroform, methanol, cyclohexane and diluted ammonia solution (28) (10 in 11) (200:100:60:23) to a distance of about 12 cm, and air-dry the plate. Heat the plate at 110°C for 10 minutes, and immediately expose to chlorine for 2 minutes. Expose the plate to cold wind until a very pale blue color develops when 1 drop of potassium iodide-starch TS is placed on a site below the starting line on the plate. Spray evenly potassium iodide-starch TS on the plate: no spot other than the principal spot at an *R*f value of about 0.6 appears.

***p*-Toluene sulfonic acid** See *p*-toluenesulfonic acid monohydrate.

***p*-Toluenesulfonic acid monohydrate**
$CH_3C_6H_4SO_3H.H_2O$ [K 8681, Special class]

***o*-Toluic acid** $C_8H_8O_2$ White, crystals or crystalline powder.

Melting point <*2.60*>: 102 - 105°C

Content: not less than 98.0%.

Toluidine blue See toluidine blue O

Toluidine blue O $C_{15}H_{16}ClN_3S$ Dark green powder, soluble in water, and slightly soluble in ethanol (95).

Identification—

(1) A solution (1 in 100) shows a blue to purple color.

(2) A solution in ethanol (95) (1 in 200) shows a blue color.

(3) A solution shows a maximum absorption at around 630 nm.

Tranilast for assay $C_{18}H_{17}NO_5$ [Same as the monograph Tranilast. When dried, it contains not less than 99.5% of tranilast ($C_{18}H_{17}NO_5$).]

Triamcinolone acetonide $C_{24}H_{31}FO_6$ [Same as the namesake monograph]

Trichloroacetic acid CCl_3COOH [K 8667, Special class]

Trichloroacetic acid-gelatin-tris buffer solution To 1 volume of a solution of trichloroacetic acid (1 in 5) add 6 volume of gelatin-tris buffer solution (pH 8.0) and 5 volume of water.

Trichloroacetic acid TS Dissolve 1.80 g of trichloroacetic acid, 2.99 g of sodium acetate trihydrate and 1.98 g of acetic acid (31) in water to make 100 mL.

Trichloroethylene C_2HCl_3 [K 8666, Special class]

Trichlorofluoromethane CCl_3F A colorless liquid or gas.

Specific gravity <*2.56*> $d_4^{17.2}$: 1.494

Boiling point <*2.57*>: 23.7°C

1,1,2-Trichloro-1,2,2-trifluoroethane $CFCl_2CF_2Cl$ Colorless volatile liquid. Miscible with acetone and with diethyl ether, and not with water.

Purity Related substances—Perform the test with 0.1 μL of 1,1,2-trichloro-1,2,2-trifluroethane as directed under Gas Chromatography <*2.02*> according to the operating conditions in the Purity (5) under Halothane: any peak other than the peak of 1,1,2-trichloro-1,2,2-trifluoroethane does not appear.

Tricine $C_6H_{13}NO_5$ White crystalline powder. Melting point: 182 to 184°C (with decomposition).

Trientine hydrochloride for assay $C_6H_{18}N_4.2HCl$ [Same as the monograph Trientine Hydrochloride or purified Trientine Hydrochloride according to the method of purification shown below. It contains not less than 98.0% of trientine hydrochloride ($C_6H_{18}N_4.2HCl$), calculated on the dried basis, and meets the following requirements.]

Purity Related substances—Dissolve 0.10 g of trientine hydrochloride for assay in 10 mL of methanol, and use this solution as the sample solution. Pipet 5 mL of the sample solution, and add methanol to make exactly 50 mL. Pipet 3 mL of this solution, add methanol to make exactly 100 mL, and use this solution as the standard solution. Perform the test with these solutions as directed under Thin-layer Chromatography <*2.03*>. Spot 3 μL each of the sample solution and standard solution on two plates of silica gel for thin-layer chromatography. Develop one of the plates with a mixture of 2-propanol and ammonia solution (28) (3:2) to a distance of about 6 cm, and air-dry the plate. Spray evenly ninhydrin-butanol TS on the plate, and heat the plate at 130°C for 5 minutes: the spot other than the principal spot and the spot nearby the original point obtained from the sample solution is not more intense than the spot from the standard solution. Develop the other plate with a mixture of ammonia solution (28), diethyl ether, acetonitrile and ethanol (99.5) (10:4:3:3), and perform the test in the same manner as above: the spot nearby the original point from the sample solution is not more intense than the spot from the standard solution.

Method of purification: Dissolve Trientine Hydrochloride in water while warming, and recrystallize by addition of ethanol (99.5). Or dissolve Trientine Hydrochloride in water while warming, allow to stand after addition of activated charcoal in a cool and dark place for one night, and filter. To the filtrate add ethanol (99.5), allow to stand in a cool and dark place, and recrystallize. Dry the crystals under reduced pressure not exceeding 0.67 kPa at 40°C until ethanol odor disappears.

Triethanolamine See 2,2′,2″-nitrilotriethanol.

Triethylamine $(C_2H_5)_3N$ Clear colorless liquid, having a strong amines odor. Miscible with methanol, with ethanol (95) and with diethyl ether.

Specific gravity <*2.56*> d_4^{25}: 0.722 - 0.730

Boiling point <*2.57*>: 89 - 90°C

Triethylamine buffer solution (pH 3.2) To 4 mL of triethylamine add 2000 mL of water, and adjust the pH to 3.2 with phosphoric acid.

Triethylamine for epoetin beta $(C_2H_5)_3N$ A clear and colorless liquid.

Specific gravity <*2.56*> d_4^{20}: 0.724 - 0.730

Water <*2.48*>: not more than 0.2%.

1% Triethylamine-phosphate buffer solution (pH 3.0) Dissolve 10 g of triethylamine in 950 mL of water, adjust the pH to 3.0 with phosphoric acid, and make exactly 1000 mL.

Triethylamine-phosphate buffer solution (pH 5.0) To 1.0 mL of triethylamine add 900 mL of water, adjust the pH to 5.0 with diluted phosphoric acid (1 in 10), and add water to make 1000 mL.

Trifluoroacetic acid CF_3COOH Colorless, clear liquid, having a pungent odor. Miscible well with water.

Specific gravity <*2.56*> d_{20}^{20}: 1.535

Boiling point <*2.57*>: 72 - 73°C

Trifluoroacetic acid for epoetin beta CF_3COOH A clear and colorless liquid.

Purity: When determine the absorbance of 50 vol% solution of trifluoroacetic acid for epoetin beta as directed under Ultraviolet-visible Spectrophotometry <*2.24*>: not more than 0.10 at 270 nm, not more than 0.02 at 280 nm, and not more than 0.01 between 300 nm and 400 nm.

Trifluoroacetic acid for nuclear magnetic resonance spectroscopy CF_3COOH Prepared for nuclear magnetic resonance spectroscopy.

Trifluoroacetic acid TS To 1 mL of trifluoroacetic acid add water to make 1000 mL.

Trifluoroacetic anhydride for gas chromatography $(CF_3CO)_2O$ Colorless, clear liquid, having a pungent odor.

Boiling point <*2.57*>: 40 - 45°C

Trimetazidine hydrochloride for assay $C_{14}H_{22}N_2O_3.2HCl$ [Same as the monograph Trimetazidine Hydrochloride. It contains not less than 99.0% of trimetazidine hydrochloride ($C_{14}H_{22}N_2O_3.2HCl$), calculated on the anhydrous basis.]

Trimethylsilyl imidazole $C_6H_{12}N_2Si$ Clear, colorless to pale yellow liquid.

Refractive index <*2.45*> n_D^{20}: 1.4744 - 1.4764

2,4,6-trinitrobenzenesulfonic acid See 2,4,6-trinitrobenzenesulfonic acid dihydrate.

2,4,6-Trinitrobenzenesulfonic acid dihydrate $C_6H_2(NO_2)_3SO_3H.2H_2O$ Pale yellow to light yellow powder.

Water <*2.48*>: 11 - 15% (0.1 g, volumetric titration, direct titration).

Content: not less than 98%, calculated on the anhydrous basis. Assay—Weigh accurately about 0.3 g of 2,4,6-trinitrobenzenesulfonic acid, dissolve in 50 mL of a mixture of water and ethanol (99.5) (1:1), and titrate <*2.50*> with 0.1 mol/L sodium hydroxide VS (potentiometric titration). Perform a blank determination in the same manner, and make any necessary correction.

Each mL of 0.1 mol/L sodium hydroxide VS
= 29.32 mg of $C_6H_2(NO_2)_3SO_3H$

2,4,6-Trinitrophenol $HOC_6H_2(NO_2)_3$ Light yellow to yellow, moist crystals. It is added 15 to 25% of water for the sake of safety, because it might explode by heating, mechanical shocking and friction when it is dried.

Identification—To 0.1 g add 10 mL of water, dissolve by warming, and add 12 mL of a mixture of 1% copper (II) sulfate solution and ammonia TS (5:1): green precipitates appear.

Content: not less than 99.5%. Assay—Weigh accurately about 0.25 g, previously dried in a desiccator (silica gel) for 24 hours, dissolve in 50 mL of water by warming, and titrate *<2.50>* with 0.1 mL sodium hydroxide VS (indicator: 3 drops of phenolphthalein TS). Perform a blank determination in the same manner, and make any necessary correction.

Each mL of 0.1 mol/L sodium hydroxide VS
= 22.91 mg of $HOC_6H_2(NO_2)_3$

2,4,6-Trinitrophenol-ethanol TS Dissolve 1.8 g of 2,4,6-trinitrophenol in 50 mL of diluted ethanol (99.5) (9 in 10) and 30 mL of water, and add water to make 100 mL.

2,4,6-Trinitrophenol TS Dissolve 1 g of 2,4,6-trinitrophenol in 100 mL of hot water, cool, and filter if necessary.

2,4,6-Trinitrophenol TS, alkaline Mix 20 mL of 2,4,6-trinitrophenol TS with 10 mL of a solution of sodium hydroxide (1 in 20), and add water to make 100 mL. Use within 2 days.

Triphenylantimony $Sb(C_6H_5)_3$ White to pale yellow-brown, crystals or crystalline powder or masses.

Content: not less than 95.0%. Assay—Weigh accurately about 0.3 g of triphenylantimony, dissolve in 100 mL of ethanol (95), add 1 g of sodium hydrogen carbonate, and titrate *<2.50>* with 0.05 mol/L iodine VS. Perform a blank determination in the same manner.

Each mL of 0.05 mol/L iodine VS
= 17.65 mg of $Sb(C_6H_5)_3$

Triphenylchloromethane $(C_6H_5)_3CCl$ White to grayish or yellowish white, crystals or crystalline powder.

Melting point <2.60>: 107 – 115°C

Triphenylmethane $C_{19}H_{16}$ A white to pale yellow, crystalline powder.

Melting point <2.60>: 93 – 95°C

Triphenylmethanol for thin-layer chromatography $C_{19}H_{15}OH$ Occurs as a white powder.

Purity—Dissolve 0.1 g of triphenylmethanol for thin-layer chromatography in 100 mL of methanol and perform the test as directed in the Purity (2) under Zidovudine: spots other than the principal spot with an *R*f value of about 0.73 are not observed.

Triphenyltetrazolium chloride See 2,3,5-triphenyl-2*H*-tetrazolium chloride.

Triphenyltetrazolium chloride TS See 2,3,5-triphenyl-2*H*-tetrazolium chloride TS.

2,3,5-Triphenyl-2*H*-tetrazolium chloride $C_{19}H_{15}ClN_4$ [K 8214, Special class]

2,3,5-Triphenyl-2*H*-tetrazolium chloride TS Dissolve 0.25 g of 2,3,5-triphenyl-2*H*-tetrazolium chloride in ethanol (99.5) to make 100 mL. Prepare before use.

2,3,5-Triphenyl-2*H*-tetrazolium chloride-methanol TS for spraying Solution A: A solution of 2,3,5-triphenyl-2*H*-tetrazolium chloride in methanol (1 in 25). Solution B: A solution of sodium hydroxide in methanol (1 in 125). Mix an equal volume of the solution A and solution B just before use.

Tripotassium citrate monohydrate $C_6H_5K_3O_7.H_2O$ White, crystals or crystalline powder. Very soluble in water, and practically insoluble in ethanol (95).

Content: 99.0% or more Assay—Accurately weigh about 0.2 g of tripotassium citrate monohydrate, add 50 mL of acetic acid for nonaqueous titration, dissolve by warming on a water bath, cool, and then titrate *<2.50>* with 0.1 mol/L of perchloric acid VS (potentiometric titration). Perform a blank determination in the same manner, and make any necessary correction.

Each mL of 0.1 mol/L perchloric acid VS
= 32.44 mg of $C_6H_5K_3O_7.H_2O$

Tris-acetic acid buffer solution (pH 6.5) Dissolve 13.57 g of 2-amino-2-hydroxymethyl-1,3-propanediol and 6.73 g of acetic acid (100) in water to make 1000 mL.

Tris-acetic acid buffer solution (pH 8.0) Dissolve 1.2 g of 2-amino-2-hydroxymethyl-1,3-propanediol in 800 mL of water, adjust to pH 8.0 with acetic acid (100), and add water to make 1000 mL.

Tris buffer solution for bacterial endotoxins test Dissolve 18.2 g of 2-amino-2-hydroxymethyl-1,3-propanediol in 800 mL of water for bacterial endotoxins test, add 100 mL of 0.1 mol/L hydrochloric acid TS and water for bacterial endotoxins test to make 1000 mL, and sterilize by heating in an autoclave at 121°C for 90 minutes.

Tris buffer solution (pH 6.8) Dissolve 30.3 g of 2-amino-2-hydroxymethyl-1,3-propanediol and 2.0 g of sodium lauryl sulfate in 800 mL of water, adjust to pH 6.8 with 5 mol/L hydrochloric acid TS, and add water to make 1000 mL.

0.5 mol/L Tris buffer solution (pH 6.8) Dissolve 6 g of 2-amino-2-hydroxymethyl-1,3-propanediol in 50 mL of water, add 2 mol/L hydrochloric acid TS to adjust the pH to 6.8, and then add water to make 100 mL. Filter if necessary.

0.05 mol/L Tris buffer solution (pH 7.0) Dissolve 6.06 g of 2-amino-2-hydroxymethyl-1,3-propanediol in about 750 mL of water, adjust to pH 7.0 with 1 mol/L hydrochloric acid TS, and add water to make 1000 mL.

Tris buffer solution (pH 7.0) Dissolve 24.3 g of 2-amino-2-hydroxymethyl-1,3-propanediol in 1000 mL of water, and adjust the pH to 7.0 with 0.1 mol/L hydrochloric acid TS.

0.1 mol/L Tris buffer solution (pH 7.3) Dissolve 2.42 g of 2-amino-2-hydroxymethyl-1,3-propanediol in a suitable amount of water, adjust to pH 7.3 with hydrochloric acid or 6 mol/L hydrochloric acid TS, and add water to make 200 mL.

0.02 mol/L Tris buffer solution (pH 7.4) Dissolve 2.4 g of 2-amino-2-hydroxymethyl-1,3-propanediol in 800 mL of water, adjust to pH 7.4 with 1 mol/L hydrochloric acid TS, and add water to make 1000 mL.

0.02 mol/L Tris buffer solution (pH 7.5) Dissolve 2.4 g of 2-amino-2-hydroxymethyl-1,3-propanediol and 29.2 g of sodium chloride in a suitable amount of water, adjust to pH 7.5 with hydrochloric acid, and add water to make 1000 mL.

1 mol/L Tris buffer solution (pH 7.5) Dissolve 12.11 g of 2-amino-2-hydroxymethyl-1,3-propanediol in 90 mL of water, adjust to pH 7.5 with hydrochloric acid, and add water to make 100 mL.

0.1 mol/L Tris buffer solution (pH 8.0) Dissolve 2.42 g of 2-amino-2-hydroxymethyl-1,3-propanediol in 100 mL of water, adjust the pH to 8.0 with 0.2 mol/L hydrochloric acid TS, and add water to make 200 mL.

1 mol/L Tris buffer solution (pH 8.0) Dissolve 121 g of 2-amino-2-hydroxymethyl-1,3-propanediol in 800 mL of water, adjust to pH 8.0 with hydrochloric acid, add water to make 1000 mL, and sterilize in an autoclave.

0.2 mol/L Tris buffer solution (pH 8.1) Dissolve 24.2 g of 2-amino-2-hydroxymethyl-1,3-propanediol in water to make 1000 mL, and adjust to pH 8.1 with hydrochloric acid.

0.5 mol/L Tris buffer solution (pH 8.1) Dissolve 12.1 g of 2-amino-2-hydroxymethyl-1,3-propanediol in 100 mL of water, adjust to pH 8.1 with 1 mol/L hydrochloric acid TS, and add water to make 200 mL.

Tris buffer solution (pH 8.2) Dissolve 24.2 g of 2-amino-2-hydroxymethyl-1,3-propanediol and 0.5 g of polysorbate 20 in 800 mL of water, adjust to pH 8.2 with 1 mol/L hydrochloric acid TS, and add water to make 1000 mL.

Tris buffer solution (pH 8.3) Dissolve 3.03 g of 2-amino-2-hydroxymethyl-1,3-propanediol, 1.0 g of sodium lauryl sulfate, and 14.4 g of glycine in 900 mL of water, adjust to pH 8.3 with 5 mol/L hydrochloric acid TS, and add water to make 1000 mL.

Tris buffer solution (pH 8.4) Dissolve 6.1 g of 2-amino-2-hydroxymethyl-1,3-propanediol and 10.2 g of sodium chloride in 800 mL of water, adjust to pH 8.4 with 1 mol/L hydrochloride TS, and add water to make 1000 mL.

0.05 mol/L Tris buffer solution (pH 8.6) Dissolve 6.1 g of 2-amino-2-hydroxymethyl-1,3-propanediol in 950 mL of water, add 2 mol/L hydrochloric acid TS to adjust the pH to 8.6, and then add water to make 1000 mL.

Tris buffer solution (pH 8.8) Dissolve 22.7 g of 2-amino-2-hydroxymethyl-1,3-propanediol and 1.5 g of sodium lauryl sulfate in 140 mL of water, adjust to pH 8.8 with 5 mol/L hydrochloric acid TS, and add water to make 200 mL.

1.5 mol/L Tris buffer solution (pH 8.8) Dissolve 18.2 g of 2-amino-2-hydroxymethyl-1,3-propanediol in 75 mL of water, add 5 mol/L hydrochloric acid TS to adjust the pH to 8.8, and then add water to make 100 mL. Filter if necessary.

Tris buffer solution (pH 9.5) Dissolve 36.3 g of 2-amino-2-hydroxymethyl-1,3-propanediol in 1000 mL of water, and adjust the pH to 9.5 by adding 1 mol/L hydrochloric acid TS.

0.01 mol/L tris buffer solution - sodium chloride TS (pH 7.4) Dissolve 1.2 g of 2-amino-2-hydroxymethyl-1,3-propanediol, 29.2 g of sodium chloride and 0.5 g of polysorbate 20 in 800 mL of water, adjust to pH 7.4 with 1 mol/L hydrochloric acid TS, and add water to make 1000 mL.

Tris(4-*t*-butylphenyl)phosphate $[(CH_3)_3CC_6H_4O]_3PO$ White, crystals or crystalline powder.

Melting point <2.60>: 100 - 104°C

Tris-calcium chloride buffer solution (pH 6.5) Dissolve 6.1 g of 2-amino-2-hydroxymethyl-1,3-propanediol and 15 mg of calcium chloride dihydrate in 800 mL of water, adjust to pH 6.5 with dilute hydrochloric acid, and add water to make 1000 mL.

Tris-glycine buffer solution (pH 6.8) Dissolve 1.22 g of 2-amino-2-hydroxymethyl-1,3-propanediol, 0.76 g of glycine, 8.8 g of sodium chloride and 0.1 g of polysorbate 80 in 800 mL of water, adjust to pH 6.8 with 1 mol/L hydrochloric acid TS, and add water to make 1000 mL.

0.2 mol/L Tris-hydrochloride buffer solution (pH 7.4) Dissolve 6.61 g of 2-amino-2-hydroxymethyl-1,3-propanediol hydrochloride and 0.97 g of 2-amino-2-hydroxymethyl-1,3-propanediol in water to make 250 mL.

0.05 mol/L Tris-hydrochloride buffer solution (pH 7.5) Dissolve 6.35 g of 2-amino-2-hydroxymethyl-1,3-propanediol hydrochloride and 1.18 g of 2-amino-2-hydroxymethyl-1,3-propanediol in water to make 1000 mL.

Tris-sodium chloride buffer solution (pH 8.0) Dissolve 2.42 g of 2-amino-2-hydroxymethyl-1,3-propanediol and 1.64 g of sodium chloride in 900 mL of water, adjust to pH 8.0 with dilute hydrochloric acid, and add water to make 1000 mL.

Trishydroxymethylaminomethane See 2-amino-2-hydroxymethyl-1,3-propanediol.

Trisodium citrate dihydrate See sodium citrate hydrate.

0.1 mol/L Trisodium citrate TS Dissolve 29.4 g of trisodium citrate dihydrate in water to make 1000 mL.

Trisodium ferrous pentacyanoamine TS See iron (II) trisodium pentacyanoamine TS.

Trisodium phosphate dodecahydrate $Na_3PO_4.12H_2O$ [K 9012, Special class]

Trypsin Obtained from bovine or hog pancreas, and prepared for biochemistry or to meet the following requirements. White to light yellow, crystals or powder.

Loss on drying: Not more than 5.0% (60°C, in vacuum, 4 hours).

Content: Not less than 220 trypsin units per mg. Assay (i) Sample solution—Weigh accurately about 20 mg of the substance to be assayed, and dissolve in 0.001 mol/L hydrochloric acid TS so that each mL contains about 3000 trypsin units. To a suitable amount of this solution add 0.001 mol/L hydrochloric acid TS so that each mL contains about 40 trypsin units, and use this solution as the sample solution.

(ii) Diluting solution—Dissolve 4.54 g of potassium dihydrogen phosphate in water to make exactly 500 mL (Solution I). Dissolve 4.73 g of anhydrous disodium hydrogen phosphate in water to make exactly 500 mL (Solution II). To 80 mL of Solution II add a suitable amount of Solution I to adjust to pH 7.6.

(iii) Substrate solution—Dissolve 85.7 mg of *N*-α-benzoyl-L-ethylarginine hydrochloride in water to make exactly 100 mL, and use this solution as the substrate stock solution. Pipet 10 mL of the substrate stock solution add the diluting solution to make exactly 100 mL, and use this solution as the substrate solution. The substrate solution gives an absorbance of between 0.575 and 0.585 at 253 nm when determined as directed under Ultraviolet-visible spectrophotometry <2.24> using water as the blank. If necessary adjust the absorbance by addition of the diluting solution or substrate stock solution.

(iv) Procedure—Transfer exactly 3 mL of the substrate solution, previously warmed to 25 ± 0.1°C, into a 1-cm quartz cell, add exactly 0.2 mL of the sample solution, immediately start the timer, and determine the change of the absorbance at 253 nm at 25 ± 0.1°C for 5 minutes, using the control prepared by adding exactly 0.2 mL of 0.001 mol/L hydrochloric acid TS to exact 3 mL of the substrate solution. Obtain the variation per minute of the absorbance, A, from the part where the changing rate of the absorbance is constant for at least 3 minutes.

(v) Calculation—Calculate trypsin unit per mg using the following equation. Where, one trypsin unit is the quantity of enzyme that gives the variation of the absorbance 0.003 per minute.

$$\text{Trypsin unit per mg} = A/0.003 \times 1/M$$

M: Amount (mg) of the substance to be assayed in 0.2 mL of the sample solution

Storage—At a cold place.

Trypsin for epoetin alfa liquid chromatography Bovine pancreas origin. It has not less than 180 units per mg, as 1 unit is equivalent to the amount of enzyme necessary to hydrolysis 1 μmol of *p*-toluenesulfonyl-L-arginine methyl ester per minute at 25°C, pH 8.2.

Trypsin for liquid chromatography An enzyme obtained from the bovine pancreas. This one part digests 250 parts of casein in the following reaction system.

Casein solution—To 0.1 g of milk casein add 30 mL of water, disperse the casein well, add 1.0 mL of diluted sodium hydroxide TS (1 in 10) to dissolve, and add water to make 50 mL. Prepare before use.

Sample solution—Dissolve 10 mg of trypsin for liquid chromatography in 500 mL of water.

Procedure—To 5 mL of the casein solution add 2 mL of the sample solution and 3 mL of water, mix, then allow to stand at 40°C for 1 hour, and add 3 drops of a mixture of ethanol (95), water and acetic acid (100) (10:9:1): no precipitate appears.

Trypsin inhibitor Produced by purifying soybean. Each mg of trypsin inhibitor inhibits 10,000 to 30,000 BAEE Units of trypsin. One BAEE Unit means a trypsin activity to indicate an absorbance difference of 0.001 at 253 nm per minute when 3.2 mL of the solution is reacted at 25°C and pH 7.6, using *N*-α-benzoyl-L-arginine ethyl ester as substrate.

Trypsin inhibitor TS Dissolve 5 mg of trypsin inhibitor in 0.05 mol/L phosphate buffer solution (pH 7.0) to make 10 mL.

Trypsin TS Dissolve 0.5 g of trypsin and 0.2 g of disodium dihydrogen ethylenediamine tetraacetate dihydrate in phosphate buffer solution for cytotoxicity test to make 1000 mL, and sterilize by filtration through a membrane filter with a pore size not exceeding 0.22 μm.

Trypsin TS for epoetin alfa Dissolve 0.5 mg of trypsin for epoetin alfa liquid chromatography in 2.5 mL of water.

Trypsin TS for test of elcatonin Dissolve 5 mg of trypsin for liquid chromatography in 20 mL of a solution of ammonium hydrogen carbonate (1 in 100). Prepare before use.

Trypsin TS for test of ulinastatin Dissolve crystalline trypsin for ulinastatin assay in ice-cooled 1 mmol/L hydrochloric acid TS containing 1 mmol/L calcium chloride dihydrate so that each mL of the solution contains 180 μg of trypsin. Prepare before use, and preserve in an ice-cooled water bath.

L-Tryptophan $C_{11}H_{12}N_2O_2$ [Same as the namesake monograph]

Tulobuterol for assay $C_{12}H_{18}ClNO$ [Same as the monograph Tulobuterol. It contains not less than 99.0% of tulobuterol ($C_{12}H_{18}ClNO$), calculated on the anhydrous basis.]

Turpentine oil [Same as the namesake monograph]

L-Tyrosine $C_9H_{11}NO_3$ White, crystals or crystalline powder. Odorless and tasteless. Freely soluble in formic acid, very slightly soluble in water, and practically insoluble in ethanol (95) and in diethyl ether. It dissolves in dilute hydrochloric acid and in dilute nitric acid.

Optical rotation <2.49> $[\alpha]_D^{20}$: −10.5 – −12.5° (after drying, 2.5 g, 1 mol/L hydrochloric acid TS, 50 mL, 100 mm).

Loss on drying <2.41>: not more than 0.30% (1 g, 105°C, 3 hours).

Content: not less than 99.0%. Assay—Weigh accurately about 0.3 g of L-tyrosine, previously dried, dissolve in 6 mL of formic acid, add 50 mL of acetic acid (100), and titrate <2.50> with 0.1 mol/L perchloric acid VS (potentiometric titration). Perform a blank determination in the same manner, and make any necessary correction.

Each mL of 0.1 mol/L perchloric acid VS
= 18.12 mg of $C_9H_{11}NO_3$

Ubenimex for assay $C_{16}H_{24}N_2O_4$ [Same as the monograph Ubenimex. When dried, it contains not less than 99.0% of ubenimex ($C_{16}H_{24}N_2O_4$).]

Ubiquinone-9 Yellow to orange crystalline powder. Odorless and no taste.

Absorbance <2.24> $E_{1\,cm}^{1\%}$ (275 nm): 163 – 190 (ethanol (99.5))

Melting point <2.60>: about 44°C

Umbelliferone for thin-layer chromatography $C_9H_6O_3$ White or light brown powder. Sparingly soluble in methanol and in ethanol (99.5), and practically insoluble in water. Melting point: about 232°C.

Identification—(1) Determine the absorption spectrum of a solution of umbelliferone for thin-layer chromatography in methanol (1 in 300,000) as directed under Ultraviolet-visible Spectrophotometry <2.24>: it exhibits maxima between 214 nm and 218 nm, and between 322 nm and 326 nm.

(2) Determine the infrared absorption spectrum of umbelliferone for thin-layer chromatography as directed in the potassium bromide disk method under Infrared Spectrophotometry <2.25>: it exhibits absorption at the wave numbers of about 3160 cm^{-1}, 1681 cm^{-1}, 1604 cm^{-1}, 1323 cm^{-1}, 990 cm^{-1} and 903 cm^{-1}.

Purity Related substances – Dissolve 1.0 mg of umbelliferone for thin-layer chromatography in 10 mL of methanol, and use this solution as the sample solution. Pipet 1 mL of the sample solution, add methanol to make exactly 50 mL, and use this solution as the standard solution. Perform the test with 5 μL each of the sample solution and standard solution as directed in the Identification under Artemisia Leaf: the spot other than the principal spot having an *R*f value of about 0.5 obtained from the sample solution is not more intense than the spot from the standard solution.

Uracil $C_4H_4N_2O_2$ Needle crystals. Freely soluble in hot water, and slightly soluble in cold water.

Melting point <2.60>: 335°C

Urea H_2NCONH_2 [K 8731, Special class]

Urea-EDTA TS Dissolve 48.0 g of urea and 0.2 g of disodium ethylenediamine tetraacetate dihydrate in 0.5 mol/L tris buffer solution (pH 8.1) to make 100 mL.

Urethane See ethyl carbamate.

Ursodeoxycholic acid $C_{24}H_{40}O_4$ [Same as the namesake monograph]

Ursodeoxycholic acid for assay $C_{24}H_{40}O_4$ [Same as the monograph Ursodeoxycholic Acid. However, when dried, it contains not less than 99.0% of ursodeoxycholic acid ($C_{24}H_{40}O_4$) meeting the following additional specifications.]

Purity Related substances—Dissolve 0.15 g of ursodeoxycholic acid for assay in 5 mL of methanol for liquid chromatography, and use this solution as the sample solution. Pipet 2 mL of the sample solution and add methanol for liquid chromatography to make exactly 50 mL. Pipet 2.5 mL of this solution, add methanol for liquid chromatography to make exactly 20 mL, and use this solution as the standard solution. Perform the test with exactly 5 μL each of the sample solution and standard solution as directed under Liquid Chromatography <*2.01*> according to the following conditions. Determine each peak area of both solutions by the automatic integration method: the area of the peak, having the relative retention time of about 2.5 to ursodeoxycholic acid, obtained from the sample solution is not larger than the peak area of ursodeoxycholic acid from the standard solution, and the area of the peak, having the relative retention time of about 5.5, from the sample solution is not larger than 1/5 times the peak area of ursodeoxycholic acid from the standard solution. Furthermore, the total area of the peaks other than ursodeoxycholic acid and the peaks mentioned above from the sample solution is not larger than 1/5 times the peak area of ursodeoxycholic acid from the standard solution.

Operating conditions

Detector: An ultraviolet absorption photometer (wavelength: 210 nm).

Column: A stainless steel column 3 mm in inside diameter and 7.5 cm in length, packed with octylsilanized silica gel for liquid chromatography (5 μm in particle diameter).

Column temperature: A constant temperature of about 40°C.

Mobile phase: A mixture of methanol for liquid chromatography, diluted phosphoric acid (1 in 1000) and acetonitrile for liquid chromatography (96:69:35).

Flow rate: Adjust so that the retention time of ursodeoxycholic acid is about 2.3 minutes.

Time span of measurement: About 7 times as long as the retention time of ursodeoxycholic acid, beginning after the solvent peak.

System suitability

Test for required detectability: Pipet 2 mL of the standard solution, and add methanol for liquid chromatography to make exactly 20 mL. Confirm that the peak area of ursodeoxycholic acid obtained with 5 μL of this solution is equivalent to 8 to 12% of that with 5 μL of the standard solution.

System performance: To 30 mg of chenodeoxycholic acid for thin-layer chromatography and 30 mg of lithocholic acid for thin-layer chromatography, add 1 mL of the sample solution, dissolve in methanol for liquid chromatography to make 50 mL. When the procedure is run with 5 μL of this solution under the above operating conditions, ursodeoxycholic acid, chenodeoxycholic acid, and lithocholic acid are eluted in this order with the resolution between these peaks being not less than 7, respectively.

System repeatability: When the test is repeated 6 times with 5 μL of the standard solution under the above conditions, the relative standard deviation of the peak area of ursodeoxycholic acid is not more than 2.0%.

***n*-Valerianic acid** $CH_3(CH_2)_3COOH$ Clear, colorless to pale yellow liquid, having a characteristic odor. Miscible with ethanol (95) and with diethyl ether, and soluble in water.

Specific gravity <*2.56*> d_4^{20}: 0.936 – 0.942

Distilling range <*2.57*>: 186 – 188°C, not less than 98 vol%.

L-Valine $C_5H_{11}NO_2$ [Same as the namesake monograph]

L-Valine for assay $C_5H_{11}NO_2$ [Same as the monograph L-Valine. When dried, it contains not less than 99.0% of L-valine ($C_5H_{11}NO_2$).]

Valsartan $C_{24}H_{29}N_5O_3$ [Same as the namesake monograph]

***H*-D-Valyl-L-leucyl-L-arginine-4-nitroanilide dihydrochloride** $C_{23}H_{38}N_8O_5.2HCl$ White to pale yellow, powder or masses. Sparingly soluble in water.

Absorbance <*2.24*> $E^{1\%}_{1\,cm}$ (316 nm): 214 – 236 (10 mg, water, 500 mL).

Vanadium pentoxide See vanadium (V) oxide.

Vanadium pentoxide TS See vanadium (V) oxide TS.

Vanadium pentoxide TS, dilute See vanadium (V) oxide TS, dilute.

Vanadium (V) oxide V_2O_5 Orangish yellow to yellow-brown powder.

Identification—Dissolve 0.3 g in 10 mL of ammonia TS and 15 mL of water. To 2 mL of this solution add 20 mL of water, mix, and add gently 1 mL of copper (II) sulfate TS: yellow precipitates appear.

Vanadium (V) oxide TS Add vanadium (V) oxide to phosphoric acid, saturate with vanadium (V) oxide by shaking vigorously for 2 hours, and filter through a glass filter.

Vanadium (V) oxide TS, dilute Dilute 10 mL of vanadium (V) oxide TS with water to make 100 mL. Prepare before use.

Vanillin $C_6H_3CHO(OCH_3)(OH)$ A white to light yellow crystalline powder, having a characteristic odor.

Melting point <*2.60*>: 80.5 – 83.5°C

Storage—Preserve in a light-resistant tight container.

Vanillin-hydrochloric acid TS Dissolve 5 mg of vanillin in 0.5 mL of ethanol (95), and to this solution add 0.5 mL of water and 3 mL of hydrochloric acid. Prepare before use.

Vanillin-sulfuric acid-ethanol TS Dissolve 3 g of vanillin in ethanol (99.5) to make 100 mL, and add 0.5 mL of sulfuric acid.

Vanillin-sulfuric acid-ethanol TS for spraying Dissolve 3 g of vanillin in 30 mL of ethanol (99.5), and add 100 mL of dilute sulfuric acid.

Vanillin-sulfuric acid TS Add cautiously 75 mL of sulfuric acid to 25 mL of ice-cold ethanol (95). After cooling, add 1 g of vanillin to dissolve. Prepare before use.

Vasopressin $C_{46}H_{65}N_{15}O_{12}S_2$ A white powder.

Constituent amino acids—Perform the test as directed in the Constituent amino acids under Oxytocin, and calculate the respective molar ratios with respect to glycine: 0.9 – 1.1 for aspartic acid, 0.9 – 1.1 for glutamic acid, 0.9 – 1.1 for proline, 0.8 – 1.1 for tyrosine, 0.9 – 1.1 for phenylalanine, 0.9 – 1.1 for arginine and 0.8 – 1.1 for cystine, and not more than 0.03 for other amino acids.

Verapamil hydrochloride for assay $C_{27}H_{38}N_2O_4.HCl$ [Same as the monograph Verapamil Hydrochloride. When dried, it contains not less than 99.0% of verapamil hydrochloride ($C_{27}H_{38}N_2O_4.HCl$).]

Verbascoside for thin-layer chromatography $C_{29}H_{36}O_{15}$ A white to very pale yellow, odorless, crystalline powder or powder. Soluble in methanol, sparingly soluble in ethanol (99.5), and slightly soluble in water.

Identification Determine the infrared absorption spectrum of verbascoside for thin-layer chromatography as directed in the potassium bromide disk method under Infrared Spectrophotometry <2.25>: it exhibits absorption at the wave numbers of about 1604 cm^{-1}, 1446 cm^{-1}, 1272 cm^{-1} and 815 cm^{-1}.

Purity Related substances—Dissolve 10 mg of verbascoside for thin-layer chromatography in 2 mL of methanol, and use this solution as the sample solution. Pipet 1 mL of the sample solution, add methanol to make exactly 50 mL, and use this solution as the standard solution. Perform the test with 20 μL each of the sample solution and standard solution as directed in the Identification under Cistanche Herb: the spot other than the principal spot at an *Rf* value of about 0.35 obtained from the sample solution is not more intense than the spot from the standard solution.

Vinblastine sulfate $C_{46}H_{58}N_4O_9.H_2SO_4$ [Same as the namesake monograph]

Vincristine sulfate $C_{46}H_{56}N_4O_{10}.H_2SO_4$ [Same as the namesake monograph]

Vinyl acetate $C_4H_6O_2$ Clear, colorless liquid.
Specific gravity <2.56>: 0.932 – 0.936
Water <2.48>: not more than 0.2%

Vinyl chloride C_2H_3Cl Colorless gas.
Boiling point <2.57>: −14°C
Melting point <2.60>: −160°C

2-Vinylpyridine C_7H_7N A clear, colorless or dark brown liquid.
Refractive index <2.45> n_D^{20}: 1.546 – 1.552
Specific gravity <2.56> d_{20}^{20}: 0.975 – 0.982

4-Vinylpyridine C_7H_7N A pale yellow to black-brown liquid.
Refractive index <2.45> n_D^{20}: 1.5500 – 1.5530
Specific gravity <2.56> d_{20}^{20}: 0.9850 – 0.9880

1-Vinyl-2-pyrrolidone C_6H_9NO Clear liquid.

Purity—Perform the test with 0.5 μL of 1-vinyl-2-pyrrolidone as directed under Gas Chromatography <2.02> according to the following conditions. Determine each peak area of the solutions by the automatic integration method, and calculate the amount of 1-vinyl-2-pyrrolidone by the area percentage method: it is not less than 99.0%.

Operating conditions

Detector: A hydrogen flame-ionization detector.

Column: A hollow, capillary glass column about 0.53 mm in inside diameter and about 30 m in length, having an about 1.0 μm layer of polyethylene glycol 20 M for gas chromatography on the inner side.

Column temperature: Maintain the temperature at 80°C for 1 minute, then raise at the rate of 10°C per minute to 190°C, and hold constant to the temperature for 20 minutes.

Temperature of sample vaporization chamber: A constant temperature of about 190°C.

Carrier gas: Helium.

Flow rate: Adjust so that the retention time of 1-vinyl-2-pyrrolidone is about 15 minutes.

Detection sensitivity: Adjust the detection sensitivity so that the peak height of 1-vinyl-2-pyrrolidone with 0.5 μL of 1-vinyl-2-pyrrolidone is about 70% of the full scale.

Time span of measurement: About twice as long as the retention time of 1-vinyl-2-pyrrolidone.

Water <2.48>—Take 50 mL of methanol for water determination and 10 mL of butyrolactone in a dry titration flask, and titrate with Karl Fischer TS for water determination until end point. Weigh accurately about 2.5 g of 1-vinyl-2-pyrrolidone, transfer immediately to a titration flask, and perform the test: water is not more than 0.1%.

V8 protease A protease obtained from *Staphylococcus aureus* strain. When an amount of the enzyme hydrolyzes 1 μmol of *N-t*-butoxycarbonyl-L-glutamic acid-α-phenyl ester in 1 minute at pH 7.8 and 37°C is defined as 1 unit, it contains 500 – 1000 units per mg.

V8 protease for insulin glargine A protease obtained from *Staphylococcus aureus* strain. When an amount of the enzyme which hydrolyzes 1 μmol of carbobenzoxy-phenylalanyl-leucyl-glutamyl-4-nitroanilide in 1 minute at pH 7.8 and 25°C is defined as 1 unit, it contains not less than 20 units per mg.

V8 protease TS Dissolve V8 protease in water to make a solution of 1 mg per mL. Keep at a cold place and use within 6 days after preparation.

Voglibose for assay $C_{10}H_{21}NO_7$ [Same as the monograph Voglibose]

Voriconazole $C_{16}H_{14}F_3N_5O$ [Same as the namesake monograph]

Warfarin potassium for assay $C_{19}H_{15}KO_4$ [Same as the monograph Warfarin Potassium. When dried, it contains not less than 99.0% of warfarin potassium ($C_{19}H_{15}KO_4$).]

Washing fluid for nartograstim test Dissolve 1 mL of polysorbate 20 in phosphate-buffered sodium chloride TS to make 1000 mL.

25% Water containing benzoyl peroxide See Benzoyl peroxide, 25% water containing.

Water for ammonium limit test To 1500 mL of water add cautiously 4.5 mL of sulfuric acid, distil using a hard glass distiller, discard the sufficient volume of first distillate, and use the remaining distillate (ammonium-free water) as the water for ammonium limit test.

Purity—Mix 40 mL of water for ammonium limit test with 6.0 mL of phenol-sodium pentacyanonitrosylferrate (III) TS. Add 4.0 mL of sodium hypochlorite-sodium hydroxide TS, mix, and allow to stand for 60 minutes. Perform the test with this solution as directed under Ultraviolet-visible Spectrophotometry <2.24>, using water as the blank: the absorbance at 640 nm is not more than 0.010.

Water for bacterial endotoxins test Use the water prescribed by the monographs of Water for Injection or Sterile Water for Injection in Containers, or the water produced by other procedures that shows no reaction with the lysate reagent employed, at the detection limit of the reagent, and is suitable for bacterial endotoxins test.

Water for ICP analysis See Inductively Coupled Plasma-Atomic Emission Spectrometry and Inductively Coupled Plasma-Mass Spectrometry <2.63>.

Water for injection [Use the water prescribed by the monographs of Water for Injection or Sterile Water for Injection in Containers. It is not necessary to check the conformity to all the specification items of the monograph, if it is confirmed that the water to be used is suitable for the purpose of relevant test.]

Water, nuclease-free Water in which nuclease is not included.

Water, sterile purified [Use the water prescribed by the monograph of Sterile Purified Water in Containers. It is not necessary to check the conformity to all the specification items of the monograph, if it is confirmed that the water to be used is suitable for the purpose of relevant test.]

Wijs' TS Transfer 7.9 g of iodine trichloride and 8.9 g of iodine to separate flasks, dissolve each with acetic acid (100), mix both solutions, and add acetic acid (100) to make 1000 mL. Preserve in light-resistant, glass containers.

Wogonin for thin-layer chromatography $C_{16}H_{12}O_5$ Yellow, crystals or crystalline powder. Slightly soluble in methanol and in ethanol (99.5), and practically insoluble in water. Melting point: 204 – 208°C.

Identification—Determine the absorption spectrum of a solution in methanol (1 in 200,000) as directed under Ultraviolet-visible Spectrophotometry <2.24>: it exhibits maxima between 207 nm and 211 nm, and between 273 nm and 277 nm.

Purity Related substances—Dissolve 1 mg of wogonin for thin-layer chromatography in 1 mL of methanol, and perform the test with 10 μL of this solution as directed in the Identification (3) under Saireito Extract: no spot other than the principal spot at an *R*f value of about 0.4 appears.

Xanthene $C_{13}H_{10}O$ White to light yellow, crystals or crystalline powder, having a slight, characteristic odor.

Melting point <2.60>: 98 – 102°C

Water <2.48>: not more than 0.5% (0.15 g).

Xanthene-9-carboxylic acid $C_{14}H_{10}O_3$ Dissolve 0.25 g of propantheline bromide in 5 mL of water and 10 mL of sodium hydroxide TS, heat the mixture to boiling, then continue to heat for 2 minutes. Cool to 60°C, add 5 mL of dilute sulfuric acid, cool, filter the precipitate, and wash thoroughly with water. Recrystallize the residue from dilute ethanol, and dry for 3 hours in a desiccator (in vacuum, silica gel).

Melting point <2.60>: 217 – 222°C

Xanthone $C_{13}H_8O_2$ Light yellow powder. Freely soluble in chloroform, and slightly soluble in hot water and in diethyl ether.

Melting point <2.60>: 174 – 176°C

Purity Related substances—Dissolve 50 mg of xanthone in chloroform to make exactly 10 mL. Perform the test with 5 μL of this solution as directed in the Purity under Propantheline Bromide: any spot other than the principal spot at the *R*f value of about 0.7 does not appear.

Xanthydrol $C_{13}H_{10}O_2$ White to pale yellow powder. Dissolves in ethanol (95), in acetic acid (100), in chloroform, and in diethyl ether, and is practically insoluble in water.

Melting point <2.60>: 121 – 124°C

Residue on ignition <2.44>: not more than 2.0% (0.5 g).

Xylene $C_6H_4(CH_3)_2$ [K 8271, First class]

***o*-Xylene** $C_6H_4(CH_3)_2$ Colorless, clear liquid.

Refractive index <2.45> n_D^{20}: 1.501 – 1.506

Specific gravity <2.56> d_4^{20}: 0.875 – 0.885

Distilling range <2.57>: 143 – 146°C, not less than 95 vol%.

Xylene cyanol FF $C_{25}H_{27}N_2NaO_6S_2$ [K 8272, Special class]

Xylenol orange $C_{31}H_{30}N_2Na_2O_{13}S$ [K 9563, Special class]

Xylenol orange TS Dissolve 0.1 g of xylenol orange in water to make 100 mL.

Xylitol $C_5H_{12}O_5$ [Same as the namesake monograph]

Xylose See D-xylose.

D-Xylose $C_5H_{10}O_5$ [Same as the monograph D-Xylose of the Japanese Standards of Food Additives]

Yeast extract A peptone-like substance which represents all the soluble product of yeast cells (*Saccharomyces*) prepared under optimum conditions, clarified, and dried by evaporating to a powder. Yeast extract (1 g) represents not less than 7.5 g of yeast. A reddish yellow to brown powder, having a characteristic but not putrescent odor. Soluble in water, forming a yellow to brown solution, having a slight acidic reaction. It contains no added carbohydrate.

Purity (1) Chloride <1.03> (calculated as NaCl): not more than 5%.

(2) Coagulable protein—On heating a solution of yeast extract (1 in 20) to boiling, no precipitate is produced.

Loss on drying <2.41>: not more than 5% (105°C, constant mass).

Residue on ignition <2.44>: not more than 15% (0.5 g).

Nitrogen content <1.08>: 7.2 – 9.5% (after drying).

Yellow beeswax [Same as the namesake monograph]

Zaltoprofen $C_{17}H_{14}O_3S$ [Same as the namesake monograph]

Zaltoprofen for assay $C_{17}H_{14}O_3S$ [Same as the monograph Zaltoprofen. When dried, it contains not less than 99.5% of zaltoprofen ($C_{17}H_{14}O_3S$)].

Zero oxygen gas for assay Nitrogen or argon, not less than 99.99 vol%, packed in a pressure-resistant sealed container. Or nitrogen or argon, 98 to 99 vol%, packed in a pressure-resistant sealed container containing oxygen within a minimum scale in the range of measurement.

Zinc Zn [K 8012, Special class]

Zinc (standard reagent) Zn In addition to JIS K 8005 standard reagent for volumetric analysis, certified reference material which can be used for volumetric analysis may be used.

Zinc acetate See zinc acetate dihydrate.

0.25 mol/L Zinc acetate buffer solution (pH 6.4) Dissolve 54.9 g of zinc acetate dihydrate in 150 mL of acetic acid (100) and 600 mL of water, add 150 mL of ammonia water (28), gently mix, and allow to cool to a room temperature. Adjust to pH 6.4 with ammonia water (28), and add water to make 1000 mL.

Zinc acetate dihydrate $Zn(CH_3COO)_2.2H_2O$ [K 8356, Special class]

Zinc, arsenic-free See zinc for arsenic analysis.

Zinc chloride $ZnCl_2$ [K 8111, Special class]

Zinc chloride TS Dissolve 10 g of zinc chloride and 10 g of potassium hydrogen phthalate in 900 mL of water, adjust the pH to 4.0 with sodium hydroxide TS, and add water to make 1000 mL.

0.04 mol/L Zinc chloride TS Dissolve 5.452 g of zinc chloride in water to make 1000 mL.

Zinc dibutyldithiocarbamate $[(C_4H_9)_2NCSS]_2Zn$ A white powder. Melting point: 106 – 110°C.

Content: Not less than 95.0%. Assay—Weigh accurately 1.0 g of zinc dibutyldithiocarbamate, add 10 mL of water and 5 mL of hydrochloric acid, and evaporate to dryness on a hot plate. To the residue add 15 mL of diluted hydrochloric acid (1 in 3), dissolve by warming, then add 50 mL of water and 40 mL of ammonia-ammonium chloride buffer solution (pH 10.7) and titrate <2.50> with 0.1 mol/L disodium dihydrogen ethylenediamine tetraacetate VS until the color of the solution changes from red to blue (indicator: 0.1 mL of eriochrome black T TS).

Each mL of 0.1 mol/L disodium dihydrogen ethylenediamine tetraacetate VS
= 47.41 mg of $[(C_4H_9)_2NCSS]_2Zn$

Zinc diethyldithiocarbamate $[(C_2H_5)_2NCSS]_2Zn$ A white to pale yellow powder. Melting point: 177 – 182°C.

Content: 94.0 – 108.0%. Assay—Weigh accurately about 0.8 g of zinc diethyldithiocarbamate, add 50 mL of water and 15 mL of diluted hydrochloric acid (1 in 3), and boil to dissolve. After cooling, add 40 mL of ammonia-ammonium chloride buffer solution (pH 10.7) and titrate <*2.50*> with 0.1 mol/L disodium dihydrogen ethylenediamine tetraacetate VS until the color of the solution changes from red to blue (indicator: 0.1 mL of eriochrome black T TS).

Each mL of 0.1 mol/L disodium dihydrogen ethylenediamine tetraacetate VS
= 36.19 mg of $[(C_2H_5)_2NCSS]_2Zn$

Zinc disodium ethylenediamine tetraacetate See zinc disodium ethylenediamine tetraacetate tetrahydrate.

Zinc disodium ethylenediamine tetraacetate tetrahydrate $C_{10}H_{12}N_2Na_2O_8Zn.4H_2O$ White powder. The pH of a solution of zinc disodium ethylenediamine tetraacetate tetrahydrate (1 in 100) is between 6.0 and 9.0.

Purity Clarity and color of solution—Dissolve 0.10 g of zinc disodium ethylenediamine tetraacetate tetrahydrate in 10 mL of freshly boiled and cooled water: the solution is clear and colorless.

Content: not less than 98.0%. Assay—Dissolve about 0.5 g of zinc disodium ethylenediamine tetraacetate tetrahydrate, accurately weighed, in water to make exactly 100 mL. Pipet 10 mL of this solution, adjust the pH to about 2 with 80 mL of water and dilute nitric acid, and titrate <*2.50*> with 0.01 mol/L bismuth nitrate VS until the color of the solution changes from yellow to red (indicator: 2 drops of xylenol orange TS).

Each mL of 0.01 mol/L bismuth nitrate VS
= 4.716 mg of $C_{10}H_{12}N_2Na_2O_8Zn.4H_2O$

Zinc dust See zinc powder.

Zinc for arsenic analysis Zn [K 8012] Use granules of about 800 μm.

Zinc iodide-starch TS To 100 mL of boiling water add a solution of 0.75 g of potassium iodide in 5 mL of water, a solution of 2 g of zinc chloride in 10 mL of water and a smooth suspension of 5 g of starch in 30 mL of water, with stirring. Continue to boil for 2 minutes, then cool.

Sensitivity—Dip a glass rod into a mixture of 1 mL of 0.1 mol/L sodium nitrite VS, 500 mL of water and 10 mL of hydrochloric acid, and touch on zinc iodide-starch TS: an apparently blue color appears.

Storage—Preserve in tightly stoppered bottles, in a cold place.

Zincon $C_{20}H_{15}N_4NaO_6S$ A dark red to purple powder.

Identification—Determine the infrared absorption spectrum of zincon, previously dried at 105°C for 4 hours, as directed in the potassium bromide disk method as directed under Infrared Spectrophotometry <*2.25*>: it exhibits absorption at the wave numbers of about 1604 cm^{-1}, 1494 cm^{-1}, 1294 cm^{-1}, 1194 cm^{-1}, 1110 cm^{-1}, 1046 cm^{-1} and 764 cm^{-1}.

Storage—Preserve in a light-resistant tight container.

Zincon TS Dissolve 0.1 g of zincon in 2 mL of 1 mol/L sodium hydroxide VS, and add water to make 100 mL.

Zinc powder Zn [K 8013, for nitrogen oxides analysis or arsenic analysis]

Zinc sulfate See zinc sulfate heptahydrate.

Zinc sulfate for volumetric analysis See zinc sulfate heptahydrate.

Zinc sulfate heptahydrate $ZnSO_4.7H_2O$ [K 8953, Special class]

Zinc sulfate TS Dissolve 10 g of zinc sulfate heptahydrate in water to make 100 mL.

Zirconyl-alizarin red S TS Dissolve 0.2 g of zirconyl nitrate dihydrate in 5 mL of dilute hydrochloric acid, add 10 mL of alizarin red S TS, and then add water to make 30 mL.

Zirconyl-alizarin S TS See zirconyl-alizarin red S TS.

Zirconyl nitrate See zirconyl nitrate dihydrate.

Zirconyl nitrate dihydrate $ZrO(NO_3)_2.2H_2O$ A white crystalline powder. Freely soluble in water.

Identification—(1) To 5 mL of a solution (1 in 20) add 5 mL of sodium hydroxide TS: a white, milky precipitate is formed.

(2) To 10 mL of a solution (1 in 20) add 10 mL of sulfuric acid, cool, and superimpose 2 mL of iron (II) sulfate TS: a brown ring is produced at the zone of contact.

Zolpidem tartrate for assay $(C_{19}H_{21}N_3O)_2.C_4H_6O_6$ [Same as the monograph Zolpidem Tartrate. It contains not less than 99.5% of zolpidem tartrate $[(C_{19}H_{21}N_3O)_2.C_4H_6O_6]$, calculated on the anhydrous basis.]

Zopiclone for assay $C_{17}H_{17}ClN_6O_3$ [Same as the monograph Zopiclone. It contains not less than 99.5% of zopiclone ($C_{17}H_{17}ClN_6O_3$), calculated on the dried basis.]

9.42 Solid Supports/Column Packings for Chromatography

α_1-Acid glycoprotein binding silica gel for liquid chromatography Silica gel bond α_1-acid glycoprotein, prepared for liquid chromatography.

Aminopropylsilanized silica gel for liquid chromatography Prepared for liquid chromatography.

Amylose tris-(3,5-dimethylphenylcarbamate)-coated silica gel for liquid chromatography Prepared for liquid chromatography.

Butylsilanized silica gel for liquid chromatography Prepared for liquid chromatography.

Carbamoyl group bound silica gel for liquid chromatography Prepared for liquid chromatography.

Cellulose derivative-coated silica gel for liquid chromatography Prepared for liquid chromatography.

Cellulose for thin-layer chromatography Prepared for thin-layer chromatography.

Cellulose with fluorescent indicator for thin-layer chromatography Use cellulose for thin-layer chromatography containing a suitable fluorescent substance.

Cellulose tris (4-methyl benzoate)-coated silica gel for liq-

uid chromatography Prepared for liquid chromatography.

18-Crown ether-immobilized silica gel for liquid chromatography Prepared for liquid chromatography.

14% Cyanopropylphenyl-86% dimethyl silicone polymer for gas chromatography Prepared for gas chromatography.

Cyanopropylsilanized silica gel for liquid chromatography Prepared for liquid chromatography.

β-Cyclodextrin binding silica gel for liquid chromatography A silica gel bound with β-cyclodextrin, prepared for liquid chromatography.

Dextran-highly cross-linked agarose gel filtration carrier for liquid chromatography Prepared for liquid chromatography.

DEAE-cross-linking dextran anion exchanger (Cl type), slightly alkaline Slightly alkaline anion exchanger prepared by introducing diethylaminoethyl group into cross-linking dextran of gel filtration carrier.

Diethylaminoethyl cellulose for column chromatography Prepared for column chromatography.

Diethylaminoethyl group bound to synthetic polymer for liquid chromatography Produced by binding diethylaminoethyl group to a hydrophilic synthetic polymer, for liquid chromatography. Exchange volume is about 0.1 mg equivalents/cm^3.

Dimethylaminopropylsilanized silica gel for liquid chromatography Prepared for liquid chromatography.

Dimethylsilanized silica gel with fluorescent indicator for thin-layer chromatography Dimethylsilanized silica gel for thin-layer chromatography to which a fluorescent indicator is added.

Diol silica gel for liquid chromatography Prepared for liquid chromatography.

Divinylbenzene-methacrylate co-polymer for liquid chromatography Prepared for liquid chromatography.

Divinylbenzene-*N*-vinyl pyrrolidone copolymer for column chromatography Prepared for column chromatography.

Ethylsilanized silica gel for column chromatography Prepared for column chromatography.

Fluorosilanized silica gel for liquid chromatography Prepared for liquid chromatography.

Gel-type strong acid cation-exchange resin for liquid chromatography (degree of cross-linkage: 8 %) Prepared for liquid chromatography.

Gel type strong acid ion-exchange resin for liquid chromatography (degree of cross-linkage: 6 %) Prepared for liquid chromatography.

Gel type strong basic ion-exchange resin for liquid chromatography Prepared for liquid chromatography.

Glycol etherifized silica gel for liquid chromatography Glycol group is bound to silica gel for liquid chromatography.

Graphite carbon for gas chromatography Prepared for gas chromatography.

Graphite carbon for liquid chromatography Prepared for liquid chromatography.

Hexasilanized silica gel for liquid chromatography Prepared for liquid chromatography.

Human albumin chemically bonded silica gel for liquid chromatography Prepared for liquid chromatography.

Hydrophilic silica gel for liquid chromatography Diolized porous silica gel prepared for liquid chromatography (5–10 μm in particle diameter).

2-Hydroxypropyl-β-cyclodextrin onto silica gel for liquid chromatography Prepared for liquid chromatography.

Hydroxypropylsilanized silica gel for liquid chromatography Prepared for liquid chromatography.

Neutral alumina for chromatography Prepared for chromatography (75 – 180 μm in particle diameter).

Neutral alumina for column chromatography Prepared for column chromatography.

Octadecylsilanized monolithic silica for liquid chromatography Prepared for liquid chromatography.

Octadecylsilanized polyvinyl alcohol gel polymer for liquid chromatography Prepared for liquid chromatography.

Octadecylsilanized porous glass for liquid chromatography Prepared for liquid chromatography.

Octadecylsilanized silica gel for liquid chromatography Prepared for liquid chromatography.

Octadecylsilanized silica gel for thin-layer chromatography Octadecylsilanized silica gel prepared for thin-layer chromatography.

Octadecylsilanized silica gel with fluorescent indicator for thin-layer chromatography Octadecylsilanized silica gel for thin-layer chromatography containing fluorescent indicator.

Octadecylsilanized silicone polymer coated silica gel for liquid chromatography Prepared for liquid chromatography.

Octadecyl-strong anion exchange-silanized silica gel for liquid chromatography Prepared for liquid chromatography.

Octylsilanized silica gel for liquid chromatography Prepared for liquid chromatography.

Ovomucoid-chemically bonded amino silica gel for liquid chromatography Prepared for liquid chromatography.

Palmitamide propylsilanized silica gel for liquid chromatography Prepared for liquid chromatography.

Pentaethylenehexaaminated polyvinyl alcohol polymer beads for liquid chromatography Prepared for liquid chromatography.

Perfluorohexylpropylsilanized silica gel for liquid chromatography Prepared for liquid chromatography.

Phenylated silica gel for liquid chromatography Prepared for liquid chromatography.

Phenylhexylsilanized silica gel for liquid chromatography Prepared for liquid chromatography.

Phenylsilanized silica gel for liquid chromatography Prepared for liquid chromatography.

Polyamide for column chromatography Prepared for column chromatography.

Polyamide for thin-layer chromatography Prepared for thin-layer chromatography.

Polyamide with fluorescent indicator for thin-layer chromatography Add a fluorescent indicator to polyamide for thin-layer chromatography.

Poly tetrafluoroethylene for gas chromatography Prepared for gas chromatography.

Porous acrylonitrile-divinylbenzene copolymer for gas chromatography (pore diameter: 0.06 – 0.08 μm, 100 – 200 m²/g) Prepared for gas chromatography.

Porous ethyl vinylbenzene-divinylbenzene copolymer for gas chromatography Prepared for gas chromatography.

Porous ethylvinylbenzene-divinylbenzene copolymer for gas chromatography (average pore diameter: 0.0075 μm, 500 – 600 m²/g) A porous ethylvinylbenzene-divinylbenzene copolymer prepared for gas chromatography. The average pore diameter is 0.0075 μm, and surface area is 500 to 600 m²/g.

Porous polymer beads for gas chromatography Prepared for gas chromatography.

Porous polymethacrylate for liquid chromatography Prepared for liquid chromatography.

Porous silica gel for gas chromatography Prepared for gas chromatography.

Porous silica gel for liquid chromatography Prepared for liquid chromatography.

Porous styrene-divinylbenzene copolymer for gas chromatography (average pore diameter: 0.0085 μm, 300 – 400 m²/g) Prepared for gas chromatography. The average pore diameter is 0.0085 μm, and surface area is 300 to 400 m²/g.

Porous styrene-divinylbenzene copolymer for gas chromatography (0.3 – 0.4 μm in mean pore size, not exceeding 50 m²/g) Prepared for gas chromatography.

Porous styrene-divinylbenzene copolymer for liquid chromatography Prepared for liquid chromatography.

Quaternary alkylaminated styrene-divinylbenzene copolymer for liquid chromatography Prepared for liquid chromatography.

Quaternary ammonium group bound to hydrophilic vinyl polymer gel for liquid chromatography Prepared for liquid chromatography.

Silica gel coated with cellulose tris(4-methylbenzoate) for liquid chromatography Prepared for liquid chromatography.

Silica gel for gas chromatography Prepared for gas chromatography.

Silica gel for liquid chromatography Prepared for liquid chromatography.

Silica gel with attached carbamoyl groups for liquid chromatography Prepared for liquid chromatography.

Silica gel for thin-layer chromatography Prepared for thin-layer chromatography.

Silica gel for thin-layer chromatography (particle size 5 – 7 μm, with fluorescent indication) Prepared for high-performance thin-layer chromatography.

Silica gel with complex fluorescent indicator for thin-layer chromatography A silica gel for thin-layer chromatography containing suitable complex fluorescent indicators.

Silica gel with fluorescent indicator for thin-layer chromatography A silica gel for thin-layer chromatography containing a suitable fluorescent indicator.

Siliceous earth for chromatography A siliceous earth prepared for chromatography.

Siliceous earth for gas chromatography A siliceous earth prepared for gas chromatography.

Slightly acidic ion-exchange silica gel for liquid chromatography Prepared for liquid chromatography.

Spherical porous ethylvinylbenzene-divinylbenzene copolymer for gas chromatography Prepared for gas chromatography.

Strongly acidic ion-exchange non-porous resin for liquid chromatography Prepared for liquid chromatography.

Strongly acidic ion-exchange resin for column chromatography Prepared for column chromatography.

Strongly acidic ion-exchange resin for liquid chromatography Prepared for liquid chromatography.

Strongly acidic ion-exchange silica gel for liquid chromatography Prepared for liquid chromatography.

Strongly basic ion-exchange resin for column chromatography Prepared for column chromatography.

Strongly basic ion-exchange resin for liquid chromatography Prepared for liquid chromatography.

Styrene-divinylbenzene copolymer for liquid chromatography Prepared for liquid chromatography.

Sulfonamide group bound to hexadecylsilanized silica gel for liquid chromatography Prepared for column chromatography.

Synthetic magnesium silicate for column chromatography Prepared for column chromatography (150 – 250 μm in particle diameter).

Terephthalic acid for gas chromatography $C_6H_4(COOH)_2$ Prepared for gas chromatography.

Tetrafluoroethylene polymer for gas chromatography Prepared for gas chromatography.

Triacontylsilanized silica gel for liquid chromatography Prepared for liquid chromatography.

Trimethylsilanized silica gel for liquid chromatography Prepared for liquid chromatography.

Weakly acidic CM-bridged cellulose cation exchanger (H type) Weakly acidic cation exchanger, intensified by crosslinking porous spherical cellulose, into which carboxymethyl groups have been introduced.

Weakly acidic ion exchange resin for liquid chromatography Prepared for liquid chromatography.

Weakly acidic ion exchange silica gel for liquid chromatography Prepared for liquid chromatography.

Zeolite for gas chromatography (0.5 nm in pore diameter) Prepared for gas chromatography.

9.43 Filter Papers, Filters for filtration, Test Papers, Crucibles, etc.

Filter paper [P 3801, Filter paper (for chemical analysis), Filter paper for qualitative analysis]
No.1: For bulky gelatinous precipitate
No.2: For moderate-sized precipitate
No.3: For fine precipitate
No.4: Hardened filter paper for fine precipitate

Filter paper for quantitative analysis [P 3801, Filter paper (for chemical analysis), Filter paper for quantitative analysis]
No. 5A: For bulky gelatinous precipitate
No. 5B: For moderate-sized precipitate
No. 5C: For fine precipitate
No. 6: Thin filter paper for fine precipitate

Porcelain crucible [R 1301, Porcelain crucible for chemical analysis]

Sintered glass filter [R 3503, Glass appliance for chemical analysis, Buchner funnel glass filter]
G3: 20–30 μm in pore size
G4: 5–10 μm in pore size

Sintered glass filter for cupric oxide filtration A glass filter with a pore size of 10 – 16 μm.

Blue litmus paper See litmus paper, blue.

Congo red paper Immerse filter paper in congo red TS, and air-dry.

Glass fiber See glass wool.

Glass wool [K 8251, Special class]

Lead acetate paper See lead (II) acetate paper.

Lead (II) acetate paper Usually, immerse strips of filter paper, 6 cm × 8 cm in size, in lead (II) acetate TS, drain off the excess liquid, and dry the paper at 100°C, avoiding contact with metals.

Litmus paper, blue [K 9071, Litmus paper, Blue litmus paper]

Litmus paper, red [K 9071, Litmus paper, Red litmus paper]

Peroxide test strip A strip that is prepared to be able to assay the concentration of hydrogen peroxide in the range of 0 to 25 ppm. The test strips have the suitable color scale covering the range from 0 to 25 ppm hydrogen peroxide.

Phosgene test paper Dissolve 5 g of 4-dimethylaminobenzaldehyde and 5 g of diphenylamine in 100 mL of ethanol (99.5). Immerse a filter paper 5 cm in width in this solution, and allow to dry spontaneously while the paper is suspended in a dark place under clear air. Then cut off the 5-cm portions from the upper side and lower side of the paper, and cut the remaining paper to a length of 7.5 cm.

Storage—Preserve in tight, light-resistant containers. Do not use the paper, which has changed to a yellow color.

Potassium iodate-starch paper Impregnate filter paper with a mixture of equivalent volumes of a solution of potassium iodate (1 in 20) and freshly prepared starch TS, and dry in a clean room.

Storage—Preserve in a glass-stoppered bottle, protected from light and moisture.

Potassium iodide-starch paper Impregnate filter paper with freshly prepared potassium iodide-starch TS, and dry in a clean room.

Storage—Store in a glass-stoppered bottle, protected from light and moisture.

Red litmus paper See litmus paper, red.

Turmeric paper Macerate 20 g of powdered dried rhizome of *Curcuma longa* Linné with four 100 mL-portions of cold water, decant the supernatant liquid each time, and discard it. Dry the residue at a temperature not over 100°C. Macerate the dried residue with 100 mL of ethanol (95) for several days, and filter. Immerse filter paper in this ethanol decoction, and allow the ethanol (95) to evaporate spontaneously in clean air.

Sensitivity—Dip a strip of turmeric paper, about 1.5 cm length, in a solution of 1 mg of boric acid in a mixture of 1 mL of hydrochloric acid and 4 mL of water, after 1 minute remove the paper from the liquid, and allow it to dry spontaneously: the yellow color changes to brown. When the strip is moistened with ammonia TS, the color of the strip changes to greenish black.

Zinc iodide-starch paper Impregnate the filter paper for quantitative analysis with freshly prepared zinc iodide-starch TS, and dry in the clean room.

Storage—Preserve in a glass-stoppered bottle, protected from light and moisture.

9.44 Standard Particles, etc.

α-Alumina for specific surface area determination α-Al_2O_3 Prepared for specific surface area determination.

Calibration ball for particle density measurement Calibration ball with a known volume prepared for measurement of particle density. The volume of the calibration ball must be accurately determined to the nearest 0.001 cm^3.

Indium for thermal analysis Prepared for thermal analysis.

Content: not less than 99.99%.

Standard particles for calibrating light-shielded automatic fine particle counter Use plastic spherical particles of known size and number.

Tin for thermal analysis Sn [K 8580 (Tin). Content: not less than 99.99%]

Measuring Instruments and Appliances, Thermometers, etc.

9.61 Optical Filters for Wavelength and Transmission Rate Calibration

Use optical filters for wavelength calibration and those for transmission rate calibration shown in Table 9.61-1 and Table 9.61-2, respectively. The optical filters for transmission rate calibration are also used for the calibration of absorbances.

Table 9.61-1 Optical Filters for Wavelength Calibration

Type of filter	Range of wavelength calibration (nm)	Product name
Neodymium optical filter for wavelength calibration	400 – 750	JCRM 001
Holmium optical filter for wavelength calibration	250 – 600	JCRM 002

Table 9.61-2 Optical Filters for Transmission Rate Calibration

Type of filter	Transmission rate for calibration (%)	Product name
Optical filter for calibration within the visible wavelength range	1	JCRM 101
	10	JCRM 110
	20	JCRM 120
	30	JCRM 130
	40	JCRM 140
	50	JCRM 150
Optical filter for calibration within the ultraviolet wavelength range	10	JCRM 210 A
	50	JCRM 250 A
Optical filter for calibration within the near-ultraviolet wavelength range	10	JCRM 310
	30	JCRM 330
	50	JCRM 350

9.62 Measuring Instruments, Appliances

Measuring Instruments are the instruments or machines used for measuring mass or volume in the JP tests, and Appliances are the instruments specified in order to make test conditions as consistent as possible in those tests.

Balances and weights **(1)** Chemical balances—Use balances readable to the extent of 0.1 mg.

(2) Semimicrobalances—Use balances readable to the extent of 10 μg.

(3) Microbalances—Use balances readable to the extent of 1 μg.

(4) Ultramicrobalances—Use balances readable to the extent of 0.1 μg.

(5) Weights—Use calibrated weights.

Carbon dioxide measuring detector tube [Gas detector tube measurement system K 0804] Packed with measurement packing for carbon dioxide.

Carbon monoxide measuring detector tube [Gas detector tube measurement system K 0804] Packed with measurement packing for carbon monoxide.

Cassia flask Use glass-stoppered flasks, shown in Fig. 9.62-1, made of hard glass and having graduation lines of volume on the neck.

Gas mixer Use the apparatus, shown in Fig. 9.62-3, made of hard glass.

Nessler tube Use colorless, glass-stoppered cylinders 1.0 to 1.5 mm in thickness, shown in Fig. 9.62-2, made of hard glass. The difference of the height of the graduation line of 50 mL from the bottom among cylinders does not exceed 2 mm.

Sieves Sieves conform to the specifications in Table 9.62-1. Use the sieve number of nominal size as the designation.

Volumetric measures Use volumetric flasks, transfer pipets, piston pipets, burets and measuring cylinders conforming to the Japanese Industrial Standards. For volumetric glassware with Class A error limits specified in the

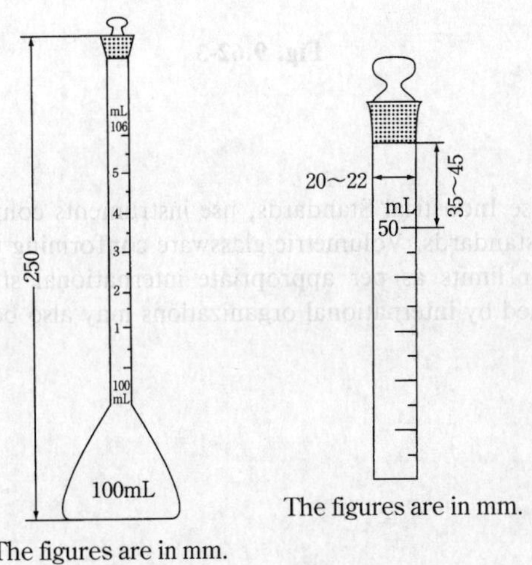

The figures are in mm.

The figures are in mm.

Fig. 9.62-1 **Fig. 9.62-2**

The JP Drugs are to be tested according to the provisions given in the pertinent monographs, General Notices, General Rules for Crude Drugs, General Rules for Preparations, and General Tests for their conformity to the Japanese Pharmacopoeia. (See the General Notices 5.)

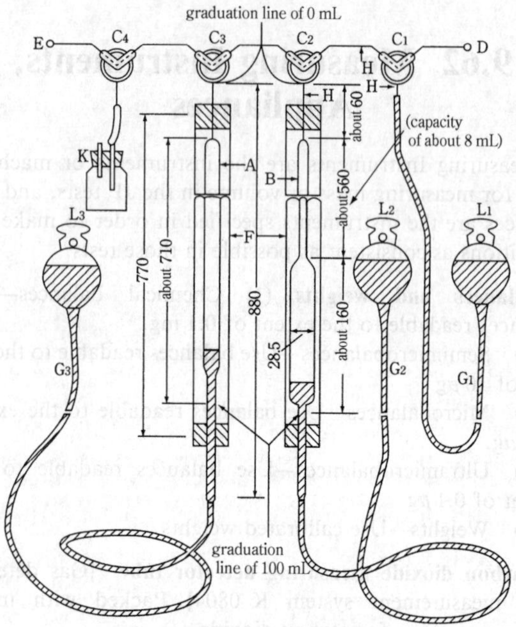

The figures are in mm.

A: Gas buret (capacity of 100 mL, about 13.7 mm in inside diameter, graduated in 0.2 mL divisions, and graduated in 0.1 mL divisions at the lower, narrow part).
B: Gas buret (capacity of 100 mL, about 4.2 mm in inside diameter at the upper stem with graduation in 0.02-mL division, about 28.5 mm in inside diameter at the lower stem with graduation in 1-mL divisions).
C: (C_1, C_2, C_3 and C_4): Three-way stopcock.
D: Inlet of sample (bent forward at 20 mm in length).
E: Outlet of mixed gas (bent forward at 20 mm in-length).
F: Jacket (about 770 mm in length, about 40 mm in outside diameter, almost completely filled with water at room temperature).
G: Rubber pressure tubing, about 4 mm in inside diameter (G_1: about 80 cm in length; G_2 and G_3: about 120 cm in length).
H: Heavy-wall capillary tube (about 1 mm in inside diameter).
K: Receiver.
L: Leveling bulb (L_1: filled with about 50 mL of mercury; L_2 and L_3: filled with about 150 mL of mercury).

Fig. 9.62-3

Japanese Industrial Standards, use instruments conforming to the standards. Volumetric glassware conforming to Class A error limits as per appropriate international standards published by international organizations may also be used.

9.63 Thermometers

Thermometers Ordinarily, use calibrated thermometers with an immersion line (rod) or calibrated total immersion mercury-filled thermometers according to the Japanese Industrial Standards. Use the thermometers with the immersion line (rod), shown in Table 9.63-1, for the tests in Congealing Point, Melting Point (Method 1), Boiling Point and Distilling Range.

Table 9.62-1 Specification of Sieves

Sieve number	Nominal size (μm)	Nominal opening (mm)	Permissible variation of opening (mm)		Diameter of wire (mm)		
			Average	Maximum	Recommended	Maximum	Minimum
3.5	5600	5.60	±0.18	0.47	1.60	1.90	1.30
4	4750	4.75	±0.15	0.41	1.60	1.90	1.30
4.7	4000	4.00	±0.13	0.37	1.40	1.70	1.20
5.5	3350	3.35	±0.11	0.32	1.25	1.50	1.06
6.5	2800	2.80	±0.09	0.29	1.12	1.30	0.95
7.5	2360	2.36	±0.08	0.25	1.00	1.15	0.85
8.6	2000	2.00	±0.07	0.23	0.90	1.04	0.77
10	1700	1.70	±0.06	0.20	0.80	0.92	0.68
12	1400	1.40	±0.05	0.18	0.71	0.82	0.60
14	1180	1.18	±0.04	0.16	0.63	0.72	0.54
16	1000	1.00	±0.03	0.14	0.56	0.64	0.48
18	850	0.850	±0.029	0.127	0.500	0.580	0.430
22	710	0.710	±0.025	0.112	0.450	0.520	0.380
26	600	0.600	±0.021	0.101	0.400	0.460	0.340
30	500	0.500	±0.018	0.089	0.315	0.360	0.270
36	425	0.425	±0.016	0.081	0.280	0.320	0.240
42	355	0.355	±0.013	0.072	0.224	0.260	0.190
50	300	0.300	±0.012	0.065	0.200	0.230	0.170
60	250	0.250	±0.0099	0.058	0.160	0.190	0.130
70	212	0.212	±0.0087	0.052	0.140	0.170	0.120
83	180	0.180	±0.0076	0.047	0.125	0.150	0.106
100	150	0.150	±0.0066	0.043	0.100	0.115	0.085
119	125	0.125	±0.0058	0.038	0.090	0.104	0.077
140	106	0.106	±0.0052	0.035	0.071	0.082	0.060
166	90	0.090	±0.0046	0.032	0.063	0.072	0.054
200	75	0.075	±0.0041	0.029	0.050	0.058	0.043
235	63	0.063	±0.0037	0.026	0.045	0.052	0.038
282	53	0.053	±0.0034	0.024	0.036	0.041	0.031
330	45	0.045	±0.0031	0.022	0.032	0.037	0.027
391	38	0.038	±0.0029	0.020	0.030	0.035	0.024

Table 9.63-1 Thermometers with Immersion Line

	No. 1	No. 2	No. 3	No. 4	No. 5	No. 6
Liquid	Mercury	Mercury	Mercury	Mercury	Mercury	Mercury
Gas filled above liquid	Nitrogen or Argon	Nitrogen or Argon	Nitrogen or Argon	Nitrogen or Argon	Nitrogen or Argon	Nitrogen or Argon
Temperature range	− 17 – 50°C	40 – 100°C	90 – 150°C	140 – 200°C	190 – 250°C	240 – 320°C
Minimum graduation	0.2°C	0.2°C	0.2°C	0.2°C	0.2°C	0.2°C
Longer graduation lines at	each 1°C	each 1°C	each 1°C	each 1°C	each 1°C	each 1°C
Graduation numbered at	each 2°C	each 2°C	each 2°C	each 2°C	each 2°C	each 2°C
Total length (mm)	280 – 300	280 – 300	280 – 300	280 – 300	280 – 300	280 – 300
Stem diameter (mm)	6.0 ± 0.3	6.0 ± 0.3	6.0 ± 0.3	6.0 ± 0.3	6.0 ± 0.3	6.0 ± 0.3
Bulb length (mm)	12 – 18	12 – 18	12 – 18	12 – 18	12 – 18	12 – 18
Distance from bottom of bulb to graduation at the lowest temperature (mm)	75 – 90	75 – 90	75 – 90	75 – 90	75 – 90	75 – 90
Distance from top of thermometer to graduation at the highest temperature (mm)	35 – 65	35 – 65	35 – 65	35 – 65	35 – 65	35 – 65
Distance from bottom of bulb to immersion line(mm)	58 – 62	58 – 62	58 – 62	58 – 62	58 – 62	58 – 62
Shape of top of thermometer	loop	loop	loop	loop	loop	loop
Test temperature	− 15°C, 15°C, 45°C	45°C, 70°C, 95°C	95°C, 120°C, 145°C	145°C, 170°C, 195°C	195°C, 220°C, 245°C	245°C, 280°C, 315°C
Maximum scale error at any point	0.2°C	0.2°C	0.2°C	0.2°C	195°C : 0.2°C 220°C : 0.3°C 245°C : 0.3°C	245°C : 0.3°C 280°C : 0.4°C 315°C : 0.5°C

Official Monographs

Acebutolol Hydrochloride

アセブトロール塩酸塩

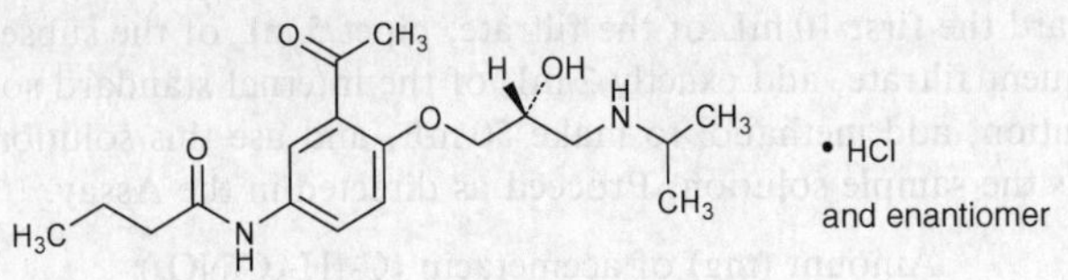

$C_{18}H_{28}N_2O_4.HCl$: 372.89
N-{3-Acetyl-4-[(2*RS*)-2-hydroxy-3-(1-methylethyl)aminopropyloxy]phenyl}butanamide monohydrochloride
[*34381-68-5*]

Acebutolol Hydrochloride, when dried, contains not less than 98.0% and not more than 102.0% of acebutolol hydrochloride ($C_{18}H_{28}N_2O_4.HCl$).

Description Acebutolol Hydrochloride occurs as white to pale yellow-white, crystals or crystalline powder.

It is freely soluble in water, in methanol, in ethanol (95) and in acetic acid (100), and practically insoluble in diethyl ether.

A solution of Acebutolol Hydrochloride (1 in 20) shows no optical rotation.

Identification (1) Determine the absorption spectrum of a solution of Acebutolol Hydrochloride in 0.01 mol/L hydrochloric acid TS (1 in 100,000) as directed under Ultraviolet-visible Spectrophotometry ⟨*2.24*⟩, and compare the spectrum with the Reference Spectrum: both spectra exhibit similar intensities of absorption at the same wavelengths.

(2) Determine the infrared absorption spectrum of Acebutolol Hydrochloride, previously dried, as directed in the potassium bromide disk method under Infrared Spectrophotometry ⟨*2.25*⟩, and compare the spectrum with the Reference Spectrum: both spectra exhibit similar intensities of absorption at the same wave numbers.

(3) A solution of Acebutolol Hydrochloride (1 in 100) responds to Qualitative Tests ⟨*1.09*⟩ for chloride.

Melting point ⟨*2.60*⟩ 141 – 145°C

Purity (1) Heavy metals ⟨*1.07*⟩—Proceed with 1.0 g of Acebutolol Hydrochloride according to Method 2, and perform the test. Prepare the control solution with 1.0 mL of Standard Lead Solution (not more than 10 ppm).

(2) Arsenic ⟨*1.11*⟩—Prepare the test solution with 1.0 g of Acebutolol Hydrochloride according to Method 3, and perform the test (not more than 2 ppm).

(3) Related substances—Dissolve 40 mg of Acebutolol Hydrochloride in 2 mL of methanol, and use this solution as the sample solution. Pipet 1 mL of the sample solution, add methanol to make exactly 25 mL, and pipet 1 mL of this solution, add methanol to make exactly 20 mL, and use this solution as the standard solution. Perform the test with these solutions as directed under Thin-layer Chromatography ⟨*2.03*⟩. Spot 5 μL each of the sample solution and standard solution on a plate of silica gel for thin-layer chromatography. Develop the plate with the upper layer of a mixture of water, 1-butanol and acetic acid (100) (5:4:1) to a distance of about 10 cm, and air-dry the plate. Examine under ultraviolet light (main wavelength: 365 nm): the spots other than the principal spot obtained from the sample solution are not more intense than the spot from the standard solution.

Loss on drying ⟨*2.41*⟩ Not more than 1.0% (0.5 g, 105°C, 3 hours).

Residue on ignition ⟨*2.44*⟩ Not more than 0.2% (1 g).

Assay Weigh accurately about 0.25 g of Acebutolol Hydrochloride, previously dried, dissolve in 20 mL of acetic acid (100), add 80 mL of acetic anhydride, and titrate ⟨*2.50*⟩ with 0.1 mol/L perchloric acid VS (potentiometric titration). Perform a blank determination in the same manner, and make any necessary correction.

Each mL of 0.1 mol/L perchloric acid VS
= 37.29 mg of $C_{18}H_{28}N_2O_4.HCl$

Containers and storage Containers—Well-closed containers.

Acemetacin

アセメタシン

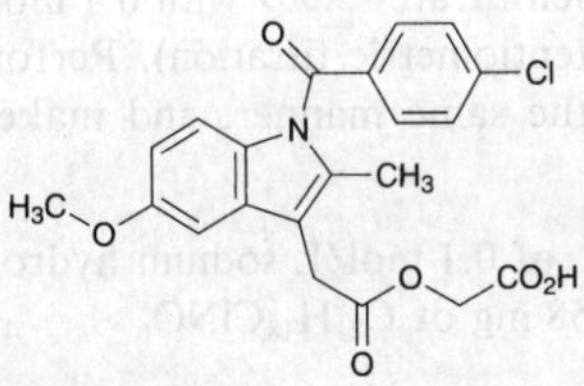

$C_{21}H_{18}ClNO_6$: 415.82
2-{2-[1-(4-Chlorobenzoyl)-5-methoxy-2-methyl-1*H*-indol-3-yl]acetyloxy}acetic acid
[*53164-05-9*]

Acemetacin, when dried, contains not less than 99.0% and not more than 101.0% of acemetacin ($C_{21}H_{18}ClNO_6$).

Description Acemetacin occurs as a light yellow crystalline powder.

It is soluble in acetone, sparingly soluble in methanol, slightly soluble in ethanol (99.5), and practically insoluble in water.

Identification (1) To 1 mg of Acemetacin add 1 mL of concentrated chromotropic acid TS, and heat in a water bath for 5 minutes: a red-purple color develops.

(2) Determine the absorption spectrum of a solution of Acemetacin in methanol (1 in 50,000) as directed under Ultraviolet-visible Spectrophotometry ⟨*2.24*⟩, and compare the spectrum with the Reference Spectrum: both spectra exhibit similar intensities of absorption at the same wavelengths.

(3) Determine the infrared absorption spectrum of Acemetacin as directed in the potassium bromide disk method under Infrared Spectrometry ⟨*2.25*⟩, and compare the spectrum with the Reference Spectrum: both spectra exhibit similar intensities of absorption at the same wave

numbers.

(4) Perform the test with Acemetacin as directed under Flame Coloration Test <1.04> (2): a green color appears.

Melting point <2.60> 151 - 154°C

Purity **(1)** Heavy metals <1.07>—Proceed with 1.0 g of Acemetacin according to Method 4, and perform the test. Prepare the control solution with 2.0 mL of Standard Lead Solution (not more than 20 ppm).

(2) Related substances—Dissolve 0.40 g of Acemetacin in 10 mL of acetone, and use this solution as the sample solution. Pipet 1 mL of the sample solution, and add acetone to make exactly 50 mL. Pipet 1 mL of this solution, add acetone to make exactly 10 mL, and use this solution as the standard solution. Perform the test with these solutions as directed under Thin Layer Chromatography <2.03>. Spot 5 μL each of the sample solution and standard solution on a plate of silica gel with fluorescent indicator for thin layer chromatography. Develop the plate with a mixture of hexane, 4-methyl-2-pentanone and acetic acid (100) (3:2:1) to a distance of about 10 cm, and air-dry the plate. Examine under ultraviolet light (main wavelength: 254 nm): the number of spots other than the principal spot obtained from the sample solution is not more than 2, and these spots are not more intense than the spot from the standard solution.

Loss on drying <2.41> Not more than 0.5% (1 g, 105°C, 2 hours).

Residue on ignition <2.44> Not more than 0.1% (1 g).

Assay Weigh accurately about 0.35 g of Acemetacin, previously dried, dissolve in 20 mL of acetone, add 10 mL of water, and then titrate <2.50> with 0.1 mol/L sodium hydroxide VS (potentiometric titration). Perform a blank determination in the same manner, and make any necessary correction.

Each mL of 0.1 mol/L sodium hydroxide VS
= 41.58 mg of $C_{21}H_{18}ClNO_6$

Containers and storage Containers—Tight containers.

Acemetacin Capsules

アセメタシンカプセル

Acemetacin Capsules contain not less than 93.0% and not more than 107.0% of the labeled amount of acemetacin ($C_{21}H_{18}ClNO_6$: 415.82).

Method of preparation Prepare as directed under Capsules, with Acemetacin.

Identification To an amount of powdered contents of Acemetacin Capsules, equivalent to 0.1 g of Acemetacin, add 100 mL of methanol, shake well, and filter. Take 10 mL of the filtrate, and distil the methanol under reduced pressure. To the residue add 1 mL of methanol, shake well, centrifuge, and use the supernatant liquid as the sample solution. Separately, dissolve 10 mg of acemetacin in 1 mL of methanol, and use this solution as the standard solution. Perform the test with these solutions as directed under Thin-layer Chromatography <2.03>. Spot 2 μL each of the sample solution and standard solution on a plate of silica gel with fluorescent indicator for thin-layer chromatography. Develop the plate with a mixture of hexane, 4-methyl-2-pentanone and acetic acid (100) (3:2:1) to a distance of about 10 cm, and air-dry the plate. Examine under ultraviolet light (main wavelength: 254 nm): the spots obtained from the sample solution and standard solution show the same *Rf* value.

Uniformity of dosage units <6.02> Perform the test according to the following method: it meets the requirement of the Content uniformity test.

Take out the contents of 1 capsule of Acemetacin Capsules, add 40 mL of methanol, shake well, and add methanol to make exactly *V* mL so that each mL contains about 0.6 mg of acemetacin ($C_{21}H_{18}ClNO_6$). Filter this solution, discard the first 10 mL of the filtrate, pipet 5 mL of the subsequent filtrate, add exactly 2 mL of the internal standard solution, add methanol to make 50 mL, and use this solution as the sample solution. Proceed as directed in the Assay.

Amount (mg) of acemetacin ($C_{21}H_{18}ClNO_6$)
$= M_S \times Q_T/Q_S \times V/50$

M_S: Amount (mg) of acemetacin for assay taken

Internal standard solution—A solution of hexyl parahydroxybenzoate in methanol (1 in 1000).

Dissolution <6.10> When the test is performed at 50 revolutions per minute according to the Paddle method using the sinker, using 900 mL of 2nd fluid for dissolution test as the dissolution medium, the dissolution rate in 30 minutes of Acemetacin Capsules is not less than 70%.

Start the test with 1 capsule of Acemetacin Capsules, withdraw not less than 20 mL of the medium at the specified minute after starting the test, and filter through a membrane filter with a pore size not exceeding 0.45 μm. Discard not less than 10 mL of the first filtrate, pipet *V* mL of the subsequent filtrate, add the dissolution medium to make exactly *V′* mL so that each mL contains about 33 μg of acemetacin ($C_{21}H_{18}ClNO_6$), and use this solution as the sample solution. Separately, weigh accurately about 17 mg of acemetacin for assay, previously dried at 105°C for 2 hours, dissolve in the dissolution medium to make exactly 100 mL. Pipet 4 mL of this solution, add the dissolution medium to make exactly 20 mL, and use this solution as the standard solution. Determine the absorbances, A_T and A_S, of the sample solution and standard solution at 319 nm as directed under Ultraviolet-visible Spectrophotometry <2.24>.

Dissolution rate (%) with respect to the labeled amount of acemetacin ($C_{21}H_{18}ClNO_6$)
$= M_S \times A_T/A_S \times V'/V \times 1/C \times 180$

M_S: Amount (mg) of acemetacin for assay taken
C: Labeled amount (mg) of acemetacin ($C_{21}H_{18}ClNO_6$) in 1 capsule

Assay Take out the contents of not less than 20 Acemetacin Capsules, weigh accurately the mass of the contents, and powder. Weigh accurately a portion of the powder, equivalent to about 30 mg of acemetacin ($C_{21}H_{18}ClNO_6$), add 40 mL of methanol, shake well, and add methanol to make exactly 50 mL. Filter this solution, discard the first 10 mL of the filtrate, pipet 5 mL of the subsequent filtrate, add exactly 2 mL of the internal standard solution, add methanol to make 50 mL, and use this solution as the sample solution. Separately, weigh accurately about 30 mg of acemetacin for assay, previously dried at 105°C for 2 hours, and dissolve in methanol to make exactly 50 mL. Pipet 5 mL of this solution, add exactly 2 mL of the internal standard solution, add methanol to make 50 mL, and use this solution as the standard solution. Perform the test with 20 μL each of the sample solution and standard solution as directed under Liquid Chromatography <2.01> according to the following conditions, and calculate the ratios, Q_T and Q_S, of the peak area of acemetacin to that of the internal standard.

$$\text{Amount (mg) of acemetacin } (C_{21}H_{18}ClNO_6) = M_S \times Q_T/Q_S$$

M_S: Amount (mg) of acemetacin for assay taken

Internal standard solution—A solution of hexyl parahydroxybenzoate in methanol (1 in 1000).

Operating conditions—

Detector: An ultraviolet absorption photometer (wavelength 254 nm).

Column: A stainless steel column 4.6 mm in inside diameter and 25 cm in length, packed with octadecylsilanized silica gel for liquid chromatography (5 μm in particle diameter).

Column temperature: A constant temperature of about 40°C.

Mobile phase: To 6 g of acetic acid (100) add water to make 1000 mL, and adjust the pH to 3.2 with a solution of 1.36 g of sodium acetate trihydrate in 100 mL of water. To 200 mL of this solution add 300 mL of acetonitrile.

Flow rate: Adjust so that the retention time of acemetacin is about 7 minutes.

System suitability—

System performance: Dissolve 75 mg of acemetacin and 75 mg of indometacin in 50 mL of methanol. To 2 mL of this solution add 2 mL of the internal standard solution, and add methanol to make 50 mL. When the procedure is run with 20 μL of this solution under the above operating conditions, acemetacin, indometacin and the internal standard are eluted in this order with the resolutions between the peaks of acemetacin and indometacin and between the peaks of indometacin and the internal standard being not less than 3, respectively.

System repeatability: When the test is repeated 6 times with 20 μL of the standard solution under the above operating conditions, the relative standard deviation of the ratio of the peak area of acemetacin to that of the internal standard is not more than 1.0%.

Containers and storage Containers—Tight containers.

Acemetacin Tablets

アセメタシン錠

Acemetacin Tablets contain not less than 93.0% and not more than 107.0% of the labeled amount of acemetacin ($C_{21}H_{18}ClNO_6$: 415.82).

Method of preparation Prepare as directed under Tablets, with Acemetacin.

Identification To a quantity of powdered Acemetacin Tablets, equivalent to 0.1 g of Acemetacin, add 100 mL of methanol, shake well, and filter. Take 10 mL of the filtrate, and distil the methanol under reduced pressure. Dissolve the residue in 1 mL of methanol, centrifuge, and use the supernatant liquid as the sample solution. Separately, dissolve 10 mg of acemetacin in 1 mL of methanol, and use this solution as the standard solution. Perform the test with these solutions as directed under Thin-layer Chromatography <*2.03*>. Spot 2 μL each of the sample solution and standard solution on a plate of silica gel with fluorescent indicator for thin-layer chromatography. Develop the plate with a mixture of hexane, 4-methyl-2-pentanone and acetic acid (100) (3:2:1) to a distance of about 10 cm, and air-dry the plate. Examine under ultraviolet light (main wavelength: 254 nm): the spots obtained from the sample solution and standard solution show the same *R*f value.

Uniformity of dosage units <*6.02*> Perform the test according to the following method: it meets the requirement of the Content uniformity test.

To 1 tablet of Acemetacin Tablets add 3 mL of water, and shake until the tablet is disintegrated. Add 15 mL of methanol, shake for 20 minutes, and add methanol to make exactly *V* mL so that each mL contains about 1.2 mg of acemetacin ($C_{21}H_{18}ClNO_6$). Centrifuge this solution, filter the supernatant liquid, discard the first 10 mL of the filtrate, pipet 5 mL of the subsequent filtrate, add exactly 1 mL of the internal standard solution, add methanol to make 50 mL, and use this solution as the sample solution. Proceed as directed in the Assay.

$$\text{Amount (mg) of acemetacin } (C_{21}H_{18}ClNO_6) = M_S \times Q_T/Q_S \times V/25$$

M_S: Amount (mg) of acemetacin for assay taken

Internal standard solution—A solution of hexyl parahydroxybenzoate in methanol (1 in 250).

Dissolution <*6.10*> When the test is performed at 50 revolutions per minute according to the Paddle method, using 900 mL of 2nd fluid for dissolution test as the dissolution medium, the dissolution rate in 45 minutes of Acemetacin Tablets is not less than 80%.

Start the test with 1 tablet of Acemetacin Tablets, withdraw not less than 20 mL of the medium at the specified minute after starting the test, and filter through a membrane filter with a pore size not exceeding 0.45 μm. Discard not less than 10 mL of the first filtrate, pipet *V* mL of the subsequent filtrate, add the dissolution medium to make exactly *V′* mL so that each mL contains about 33 μg of acemetacin ($C_{21}H_{18}ClNO_6$), and use this solution as the sample solution. Separately, weigh accurately about 17 mg of acemetacin for assay, previously dried at 105°C for 2 hours, dissolve in the dissolution medium to make exactly 100 mL. Pipet 4 mL of this solution, add the dissolution medium to make exactly 20 mL, and use this solution as the standard solution. Determine the absorbances, A_T and A_S, of the sample solution and standard solution at 319 nm as directed under Ultraviolet-visible Spectrophotometry <*2.24*>.

$$\text{Dissolution rate (\%) with respect to the labeled amount of acemetacin } (C_{21}H_{18}ClNO_6) = M_S \times A_T/A_S \times V'/V \times 1/C \times 180$$

M_S: Amount (mg) of acemetacin for assay taken

C: Labeled amount (mg) of acemetacin ($C_{21}H_{18}ClNO_6$) in 1 tablet

Assay Weigh accurately the mass of not less than 20 Acemetacin Tablets, and powder. Weigh accurately a portion of the powder, equivalent to about 0.6 g of acemetacin ($C_{21}H_{18}ClNO_6$), add 120 mL of methanol, shake for 20 minutes, and add methanol to make exactly 200 mL. Centrifuge this solution, filter the supernatant liquid, discard the first 10 mL of the filtrate, pipet 2 mL of the subsequent filtrate, add exactly 1 mL of the internal standard solution, add methanol to make 50 mL, and use this solution as the sample solution. Separately, weigh accurately about 30 mg of acemetacin for assay, previously dried at 105°C for 2 hours, and dissolve in methanol to make exactly 25 mL. Pipet 5 mL of this solution, add exactly 1 mL of the internal standard solution, add methanol to make 50 mL, and use this solution as the standard solution. Perform the test with

10 μL each of the sample solution and standard solution as directed under Liquid Chromatography <*2.01*> according to the following conditions, and calculate the ratios, Q_T and Q_S, of the peak area of acemetacin to that of the internal standard.

Amount (mg) of acemetacin ($C_{21}H_{18}ClNO_6$)
$= M_S \times Q_T/Q_S \times 20$

M_S: Amount (mg) of acemetacin for assay taken

Internal standard solution—A solution of hexyl parahydroxybenzoate in methanol (1 in 250).

Operating conditions—

Detector: An ultraviolet absorption photometer (wavelength 254 nm).

Column: A stainless steel column 4.6 mm in inside diameter and 25 cm in length, packed with octadecylsilanized silica gel for liquid chromatography (5 μm in particle diameter).

Column temperature: A constant temperature of about 40°C.

Mobile phase: To 6 g of acetic acid (100) add water to make 1000 mL, and adjust the pH to 3.2 with a solution of 1.36 g of sodium acetate trihydrate in 100 mL of water. To 200 mL of this solution add 300 mL of acetonitrile.

Flow rate: Adjust so that the retention time of acemetacin is about 7 minutes.

System suitability—

System performance: Dissolve 75 mg of acemetacin and 75 mg of indometacin in 50 mL of methanol. To 4 mL of this solution add 1 mL of the internal standard solution, and add methanol to make 50 mL. When the procedure is run with 10 μL of this solution under the above operating conditions, acemetacin, indometacin and the internal standard are eluted in this order with the resolutions between the peaks of acemetacin and indometacin and between the peaks of indometacin and the internal standard being not less than 3, respectively.

System repeatability: When the test is repeated 6 times with 10 μL of the standard solution under the above operating conditions, the relative standard deviation of the ratio of the peak area of acemetacin to that of the internal standard is not more than 1.0%.

Containers and storage Containers—Tight containers.

Acetaminophen

Paracetamol

アセトアミノフェン

$C_8H_9NO_2$: 151.16
N-(4-Hydroxyphenyl)acetamide
[*103-90-2*]

Acetaminophen, when dried, contains not less than 98.0% of acetaminophen ($C_8H_9NO_2$).

Description Acetaminophen occurs as white, crystals or crystalline powder.

It is freely soluble in methanol and in ethanol (95), sparingly soluble in water, and very slightly, soluble in diethyl ether.

It dissolves in sodium hydroxide TS.

Identification Determine the infrared absorption spectra of Acetaminophen, previously dried, as directed in the potassium bromide disk method under Infrared Spectrophotometry <*2.25*>, and compare the spectrum with the Reference Spectrum or the spectrum of dried Acetaminophen RS: both spectra exhibit similar intensities of absorption at the same wave numbers.

Melting point <*2.60*> 169 – 172°C

Purity **(1)** Chloride <*1.03*>—Dissolve 4.0 g of Acetaminophen in 100 mL of water by heating, cool with shaking in ice water, allow to stand until ordinary temperature is attained, add water to make 100 mL, and filter. To 25 mL of the filtrate add 6 mL of dilute nitric acid and water to make 50 mL, and perform the test using this solution as the test solution. Prepare the control solution with 0.40 mL of 0.01 mol/L hydrochloric acid VS (not more than 0.014%).

(2) Sulfate <*1.14*>—To 25 mL of the filtrate obtained in (1) add 1 mL of dilute hydrochloric acid and water to make 50 mL, and perform the test using this solution as the test solution. Prepare the control solution with 0.40 mL of 0.005 mol/L sulfuric acid VS (not more than 0.019%).

(3) Heavy metals <*1.07*>—Proceed with 2.0 g of Acetaminophen according to Method 4, and perform the test. Prepare the control solution with 2.0 mL of Standard Lead Solution (not more than 10 ppm).

(4) Arsenic <*1.11*>—Prepare the test solution with 1.0 g of Acetaminophen according to Method 3, and perform the test (not more than 2 ppm).

(5) Related substances—Dissolve 50 mg of Acetaminophen in 1 mL of methanol, add the mobile phase to make 50 mL, and use this solution as the sample solution. Pipet 1 mL of the sample solution, add the mobile phase to make exactly 200 mL, and use this solution as the standard solution. Perform the test with exactly 10 μL each of the sample solution and standard solution as directed under Liquid Chromatography <*2.01*> according to the following conditions. Determine each peak area of both solutions by the automatic integration method: the total area of all peaks other than acetaminophen obtained from the sample solution is not larger than the peak area of acetaminophen from the standard solution.

Operating conditions—

Detector: An ultraviolet absorption photometer (wavelength: 225 nm).

Column: A stainless steel column about 4 mm in inside diameter and about 15 cm in length, packed with octadecylsilanized silica gel for liquid chromatography (5 μm in particle diameter).

Column temperature: A constant temperature of about 40°C.

Mobile phase: A mixture of 0.05 mol/L potassium dihydrogenphosphate (pH 4.7) and methanol (4:1).

Flow rate: Adjust so that the retention time of acetaminophen is about 5 minutes.

Selection of column: Dissolve 0.01 g each of Acetaminophen and 4-aminophenol hydrochloride in 1 mL of methanol, add the mobile phase to make 50 mL, to 1 mL of this solution add the mobile phase to make 10 mL. Proceed with 10 μL of this solution under the above operating conditions, and calculate the resolution. Use a column giving elution of 4-aminophenol and acetaminophen in this order with the resolution between these peaks being not less than 7.

Detection sensitivity: Adjust the detection sensitivity so that the peak height of acetaminophen obtained from 10 μL of the standard solution is about 15% of the full scale.

Time span of measurement: About 6 times as long as the retention time of acetaminophen, beginning after the solvent peak.

Loss on drying *<2.41>* Not more than 0.3% (0.5 g, 105°C, 2 hours).

Residue on ignition *<2.44>* Not more than 0.1% (1 g).

Assay Weigh accurately about 20 mg each of Acetaminophen and Acetaminophen RS, previously dried, dissolve in 2 mL of methanol, and add water to make exactly 100 mL. Pipet 3 mL each of these solutions, add water to make exactly 100 mL, and use these solutions as the sample solution and the standard solution, respectively. Determine the absorbances, A_T and A_S, of the sample solution and standard solution at the wavelength of maximum absorption at about 244 nm as directed under Ultraviolet-visible Spectrophotometry *<2.24>*, using water as the blank.

Amount (mg) of acetaminophen ($C_8H_9NO_2$)
$= M_S \times A_T/A_S$

M_S: Amount (mg) of Acetaminophen RS taken

Containers and storage Containers—Tight containers.

Storage—Light-resistant.

Acetazolamide

アセタゾラミド

$C_4H_6N_4O_3S_2$: 222.25
N-(5-Sulfamoyl-1,3,4-thiadiazol-2-yl)acetamide
[59-66-5]

Acetazolamide contains not less than 98.0% and not more than 102.0% of acetazolamide ($C_4H_6N_4O_3S_2$), calculated on the dried basis.

Description Acetazolamide occurs as a white to pale yellow-white crystalline powder. It is odorless, and has a slight bitter taste.

It is slightly soluble in ethanol (95), very slightly soluble in water, and practically insoluble in diethyl ether.

Melting point: about 255°C (with decomposition).

Identification **(1)** To 0.1 g of Acetazolamide add 5 mL of sodium hydroxide TS, then add 5 mL of a solution of 0.1 g of hydroxylammonium chloride and 0.05 g of copper (II) sulfate pentahydrate in 10 mL of water: a light yellow color develops. Then heat this solution for 5 minutes: a deep yellow color is produced gradually.

(2) To 0.02 g of Acetazolamide add 2 mL of dilute hydrochloric acid, boil for 10 minutes, cool, and add 8 mL of water: this solution responds to Qualitative Tests *<1.09>* for primary aromatic amines.

(3) To 0.2 g of Acetazolamide add 0.5 g of granulated zinc and 5 mL of diluted hydrochloric acid (1 in 2): the gas evolved darkens moistened lead (II) acetate paper.

Purity **(1)** Clarity and color of solution—Dissolve 1.0 g of Acetazolamide in 10 mL of sodium hydroxide TS: the solution is clear and colorless to pale yellow.

(2) Chloride *<1.03>*—To 1.5 g of Acetazolamide add 75 mL of water, and warm at 70°C for 20 minutes with occasional shaking. After cooling, filter, and to 25 mL of the filtrate add 6 mL of dilute nitric acid and water to make 50 mL. Perform the test using this solution as the test solution. Prepare the control solution with 0.20 mL of 0.01 mol/L hydrochloric acid VS (not more than 0.014%).

(3) Sulfate *<1.14>*—To 25 mL of the filtrate obtained in (2) add 1 mL of dilute hydrochloric acid and water to make 50 mL. Perform the test using this solution as the test solution. Prepare the control solution with 0.40 mL of 0.005 mol/L sulfuric acid VS (not more than 0.038%).

(4) Heavy metals *<1.07>*—Proceed with 1.0 g of Acetazolamide according to Method 2, and perform the test. Prepare the control solution with 2.0 mL of Standard Lead Solution (not more than 20 ppm).

(5) Silver-reducing substances—Wet 5 g of Acetazolamide with 5 mL of aldehyde-free ethanol, and add 125 mL of water, 10 mL of nitric acid and exactly 5 mL of 0.1 mol/L silver nitrate VS. Stir for 30 minutes by protecting from light, filter through a glass filter (G3), and wash the residue on the glass filter with two 10-mL portions of water. Combine the filtrate with the washings, to the solution add 5 mL of ammonium iron (III) sulfate TS, and titrate *<2.50>* with 0.1 mol/L ammonium thiocyanate VS: not less than 4.8 mL of 0.1 mol/L ammonium thiocyanate VS is consumed.

Loss on drying *<2.41>* Not more than 0.5% (0.5 g, 105°C, 3 hours).

Residue on ignition *<2.44>* Not more than 0.1% (0.5 g).

Assay Weigh accurately about 0.15 g of Acetazolamide, and dissolve in 400 mL of water in a water bath by heating. After cooling, add water to make exactly 1000 mL. Pipet 5 mL of the solution, add 10 mL of 1 mol/L hydrochloric acid TS, and then add water to make exactly 100 mL. Determine the absorbance A of this solution at the wavelength of maximum absorption at about 265 nm as directed under Ultraviolet-visible Spectrophotometry *<2.24>*.

Amount (mg) of acetazolamide ($C_4H_6N_4O_3S_2$)
$= A/474 \times 200{,}000$

Containers and storage Containers—Well-closed containers.

Storage—Light-resistant.

Acetic Acid

酢酸

Acetic Acid contains not less than 30.0 w/v% and not more than 32.0 w/v% of acetic acid ($C_2H_4O_2$: 60.05).

Description Acetic Acid is a clear, colorless liquid. It has a pungent, characteristic odor and an acid taste.

It is miscible with water, with ethanol (95) and with glycerin.

Specific gravity d_{20}^{20}: about 1.04

Identification Acetic Acid changes blue litmus paper to red, and responds to Qualitative Tests *<1.09>* for acetate.

Purity **(1)** Chloride—To 20 mL of Acetic Acid add 40 mL of water, and use this solution as the sample solution. To 10 mL of the sample solution add 5 drops of silver nitrate TS: no opalescence is produced.

(2) Sulfate—To 10 mL of the sample solution obtained in (1) add 1 mL of barium chloride TS: no turbidity is produced.

(3) Heavy metals *<1.07>*—Evaporate 10 mL of Acetic Acid on a water bath to dryness, and to the residue add 2 mL of dilute acetic acid and water to make 50 mL. Perform the test with this solution as the test solution. Prepare the control solution with 3.0 mL of Standard Lead Solution by adding 2 mL of dilute acetic acid and water to make 50 mL (not more than 3 ppm).

(4) Potassium permanganate-reducing substances—To 20 mL of the sample solution obtained in (1) add 0.10 mL of 0.02 mol/L potassium permanganate VS: the red color does not disappear within 30 minutes.

(5) Non-volatile residue—Evaporate 30 mL of Acetic Acid on a water bath to dryness, and dry at 105°C for 1 hour: the mass of the residue is not more than 1.0 mg.

Assay Measure exactly 5 mL of Acetic Acid, add 30 mL of water, and titrate *<2.50>* with 1 mol/L sodium hydroxide VS (indicator: 2 drops of phenolphthalein TS).

Each mL of 1 mol/L sodium hydroxide VS
= 60.05 mg of $C_2H_4O_2$

Containers and storage Containers—Tight containers.

Glacial Acetic Acid

氷酢酸

$H_3C—CO_2H$

$C_2H_4O_2$: 60.05
Acetic acid
[64-19-7]

Glacial Acetic Acid contains not less than 99.0% of acetic acid ($C_2H_4O_2$).

Description Glacial Acetic Acid is a clear, colorless, volatile liquid, or colorless or white, crystalline masses. It has a pungent, characteristic odor.

It is miscible with water, with ethanol (95) and with diethyl ether.

Boiling point: about 118°C
Specific gravity d^{20}_{20}: about 1.049

Identification A solution of Glacial Acetic Acid (1 in 3) changes blue litmus paper to red, and responds to Qualitative Tests *<1.09>* for acetate.

Congealing point *<2.42>* Not less than 14.5°C.

Purity **(1)** Chloride—To 10 mL of Glacial Acetic Acid add water to make 100 mL, and use this solution as the sample solution. To 10 mL of the sample solution add 5 drops of silver nitrate TS: no opalescence is produced.

(2) Sulfate—To 10 mL of the sample solution obtained in (1) add 1 mL of barium chloride TS: no turbidity is produced.

(3) Heavy metals *<1.07>*—Evaporate 2.0 mL of Glacial Acetic Acid on a water bath to dryness. Dissolve the residue in 2 mL of dilute acetic acid and water to make 50 mL, and perform the test using this solution as the test solution. Prepare the control solution with 2.0 mL of Standard Lead Solution by adding 2.0 mL of dilute acetic acid and water to make 50 mL (not more than 10 ppm).

(4) Potassium permanganate-reducing substances—To 20 mL of the sample solution obtained in (1) add 0.10 mL of 0.02 mol/L potassium permanganate VS: the red color does not disappear within 30 minutes.

(5) Non-volatile residue—Evaporate 10 mL of Glacial Acetic Acid on a water bath to dryness, and dry at 105°C for 1 hour: the mass of the residue is not more than 1.0 mg.

Assay Place 10 mL of water in a glass-stoppered flask, and weigh accurately. Add about 1.5 g of Glacial Acetic Acid, weigh accurately again, then add 30 mL of water, and titrate *<2.50>* with 1 mol/L sodium hydroxide VS (indicator: 2 drops of phenolphthalein TS).

Each mL of 1 mol/L sodium hydroxide VS
= 60.05 mg of $C_2H_4O_2$

Containers and storage Containers—Tight containers.

Acetohexamide

アセトヘキサミド

$C_{15}H_{20}N_2O_4S$: 324.40
4-Acetyl-*N*-(cyclohexylcarbamoyl)benzenesulfonamide
[968-81-0]

Acetohexamide, when dried, contains not less than 98.0% and not more than 101.0% of acetohexamide ($C_{15}H_{20}N_2O_4S$).

Description Acetohexamide occurs as a white to yellowish white powder.

It is freely soluble in *N,N*-dimethylformamide, sparingly soluble in acetone, slightly soluble in methanol and in ethanol (99.5), and practically insoluble in water.

Melting point: about 185°C (with decomposition).

Identification **(1)** Dissolve 0.10 g of Acetohexamide in 100 mL of methanol. To 5 mL of the solution add 20 mL of 0.5 mol/L hydrochloric acid TS and 75 mL of methanol, and use the solution as the sample solution (1). Determine the absorption spectrum of the sample solution (1) as directed under Ultraviolet-visible Spectrophotometry *<2.24>*, using methanol as the blank, and compare the spectrum with the Reference Spectrum 1: both spectra exhibit similar intensities of absorption at the same wavelengths. Separately, to exactly 10 mL of the sample solution (1) add methanol to make exactly 50 mL, and use the solution as the sample solution (2). Determine the absorption spectrum of the sample solution (2) as directed under Ultraviolet-visible Spectrophotometry *<2.24>*, using methanol as the blank, and compare the spectrum with the Reference Spectrum 2: both spectra exhibit similar intensities of absorption at the same wavelengths.

(2) Determine the infrared absorption spectrum of Acetohexamide, previously dried, as directed in the potassium bromide disk method under Infrared Spectrophotometry *<2.25>*, and compare the spectrum with the Reference Spectrum: both spectra exhibit similar intensities of absorption at the same wave numbers.

Purity **(1)** Chloride *<1.03>*—Dissolve 1.5 g of Acetohexamide in 40 mL of *N,N*-dimethylformamide, add 6 mL of dilute nitric acid and *N,N*-dimethylformamide to make 50 mL. Perform the test using this solution as the test solution.

Prepare the control solution as follows: to 0.45 mL of 0.01 mol/L hydrochloric acid VS add 6 mL of dilute nitric acid and *N,N*-dimethylformamide to make 50 mL (not more than 0.011%).

(2) Sulfate *<1.14>*—Dissolve 2.0 g of Acetohexamide in 40 mL of *N,N*-dimethylformamide, and add 1 mL of dilute hydrochloric acid and *N,N*-dimethylformamide to make 50 mL. Perform the test using this solution as the test solution. Prepare the control solution as follows: to 0.40 mL of 0.005 mol/L sulfuric acid VS add 1 mL of dilute hydrochloric acid and *N,N*-dimethylformamide to make 50 mL (not more than 0.010%).

(3) Heavy metals *<1.07>*—Proceed with 1.0 g of Acetohexamide according to Method 2, and perform the test. Prepare the control solution with 2.0 mL of Standard Lead Solution (not more than 20 ppm).

(4) Related substances (i) Cyclohexylamine—Dissolve exactly 1.0 g of Acetohexamide in exactly 30 mL of 0.5 mol/L sodium hydroxide TS, add exactly 5 mL of hexane, shake vigorously for 60 minutes, allow to stand for 5 minutes, and use the upper layer as the sample solution. Separately, dissolve exactly 50 mg of cyclohexylamine in 0.5 mol/L sodium hydroxide TS to make exactly 50 mL. Pipet 2 mL of this solution, and add 0.5 mol/L sodium hydroxide TS to make exactly 300 mL. Pipet 30 mL of this solution, add exactly 5 mL of hexane, shake vigorously for 60 minutes, allow to stand for 5 minutes, and use the upper layer as the standard solution. Perform the test with exactly 2 μL each of the sample solution and standard solution as directed under Gas Chromatography *<2.02>* according to the following conditions, and determine the peak area of cyclohexylamine by the automatic integration method: the peak area of cyclohexylamine obtained from the sample solution is not more than that from the standard solution.

Operating conditions—

Detector: A hydrogen flame-ionization detector.

Column: A fused-silica column 0.53 mm in inside diameter and 30 m in length, coated the inner surface with methylsilicone polymer for gas chromatography 1.5 μm in thickness.

Column temperature: A constant temperature of about 90°C.

Injection port temperature: A constant temperature of about 150°C.

Detector temperature: A constant temperature of about 210°C.

Carrier gas: Helium.

Flow rate: Adjust so that the retention time of cyclohexylamine is about 4 minutes.

Split ratio: 1:1.

System suitability—

System performance: When the procedure is run with 2 μL of the standard solution under the above operating conditions, the number of theoretical plates of the peak of cyclohexylamine is not less than 8000.

System repeatability: When the test is repeated 6 times with 2 μL of the standard solution under the above operating conditions, the relative standard deviation of the peak area of cyclohexylamine is not more than 5%.

(ii) Dicyclohexylurea—Dissolve exactly 1.0 g of Acetohexamide in exactly 10 mL of 0.5 mol/L sodium hydroxide TS, add exactly 20 mL of methanol, shake, then add exactly 5 mL of diluted hydrochloric acid (1 in 10), shake vigorously for 15 minutes, and centrifuge. Filter 10 mL or more of the supernatant liquid through a membrane filter with pore size of not larger than 0.5 μm. Discard the first 5 mL of the filtrate, and use the subsequent filtrate as the sample solution. Separately, dissolve exactly 50 mg of dicyclohexylurea in methanol to make exactly 100 mL. Pipet 2 mL of this solution, and add methanol to make exactly 100 mL. Pipet 20 mL of this solution, add exactly 10 mL of 0.5 mol/L sodium hydroxide TS, shake, then add exactly 5 mL of diluted hydrochloric acid (1 in 10), shake, and use this solution as the standard solution. Perform the test with exactly 50 μL each of the sample solution and standard solution as directed under Liquid Chromatography *<2.01>* according to the following conditions, and determine the peak area of dicyclohexylurea by the automatic integration method: the peak area of dicyclohexylurea obtained from the sample solution is not more than that from the standard solution.

Operating conditions—

Detector: An ultraviolet absorption photometer (wavelength: 210 nm).

Column: A stainless steel column 4.6 mm in inside diameter and 25 cm in length, packed with octadecylsilanized silica gel for liquid chromatography (5 μm in particle diameter).

Column temperature: A constant temperature of about 25°C.

Mobile phase: Dissolve 0.5 g of sodium hydroxide in 1000 mL of 0.05 mol/L sodium dihydrogen phosphate TS, and adjust the pH to 6.5 with 0.5 mol/L sodium hydroxide TS. To 500 mL of this solution add 500 mL of acetonitrile.

Flow rate: Adjust so that the retention time of dicyclohexylurea is about 10 minutes.

System suitability—

System performance: When the procedure is run with 50 μL of the standard solution under the above operating conditions, the number of theoretical plates of the peak of dicyclohexylurea is not less than 10,000.

System repeatability: When the test is repeated 6 times with 50 μL of the standard solution under the above operating conditions, the relative standard deviation of the peak area of dicyclohexylurea is not more than 2.0%.

(iii) Other related substances—Dissolve 0.10 g of Acetohexamide in 10 mL of acetone, and use this solution as the sample solution. Pipet 1 mL of the sample solution, and add acetone to make exactly 20 mL. Pipet two 1 mL portions of this solution, add acetone to make exactly 10 mL and 25 mL, respectively, and use these solutions as the standard solution (1) and the standard solution (2). Perform the test with these solutions as directed under Thin-layer Chromatography *<2.03>*. Spot 10 μL each of the sample solution and standard solutions (1) and (2) on a plate of silica gel with fluorescent indicator for thin-layer chromatography. Develop the plate with a mixture of ethyl acetate, methanol, ammonia solution (28) and cyclohexane (6:2:1:1) to a distance of about 10 cm, and air-dry the plate. Examine under ultraviolet light (main wavelength: 254 nm): the spots other than the principal spot obtained from the sample solution are not more intense than the spot from the standard solution (1), and the number of them which are more intense than the spot from the standard solution (2) is not more than 4.

Loss on drying *<2.41>* Not more than 1.0% (1 g, 105°C, 4 hours).

Residue on ignition *<2.44>* Not more than 0.1% (1 g).

Assay Weigh accurately about 0.3 g of Acetohexamide, previously dried, dissolve in 30 mL of *N,N*-dimethylformamide, add 10 mL of water, and titrate *<2.50>* with 0.1 mol/L sodium hydroxide VS (potentiometric titration). Perform a blank determination in the same manner using a solution prepared by adding 19 mL of water to 30 mL of *N,N*-dimethylformamide, and make any necessary correction.

Each mL of 0.1 mol/L sodium hydroxide VS
= 32.44 mg of $C_{15}H_{20}N_2O_4S$

Containers and storage Containers—Well-closed containers.

Acetylcholine Chloride for Injection

注射用アセチルコリン塩化物

$C_7H_{16}ClNO_2$: 181.66
2-Acetoxy-*N*,*N*,*N*-trimethylethylaminium chloride
[60-31-1]

Acetylcholine Chloride for Injection is a preparation for injection which is dissolved before use.

It contains not less than 98.0% and not more than 102.0% of acetylcholine chloride ($C_7H_{16}ClNO_2$), and not less than 19.3% and not more than 19.8% of chlorine (Cl: 35.45), calculated on the dried basis.

It contains not less than 93.0% and not more than 107.0% of the labeled amount of acetylcholine chloride ($C_7H_{16}ClNO_2$).

Method of preparation Prepare as directed under Injections.

Description Acetylcholine Chloride for Injection occurs as white, crystals or crystalline powder.

It is very soluble in water, and freely soluble in ethanol (95).

It is extremely hygroscopic.

Identification **(1)** Determine the infrared absorption spectrum of Acetylcholine Chloride for Injection, previously dried, as directed in the potassium bromide disk method under Infrared Spectrophotometry 〈*2.25*〉, and compare the spectrum with the Reference Spectrum: both spectra exhibit similar intensities of absorption at the same wave numbers.

(2) A solution of Acetylcholine Chloride for Injection (1 in 10) responds to Qualitative Tests 〈*1.09*〉 (2) for chloride.

Melting point 〈*2.60*〉 149 – 152°C. Seal Acetylcholine Chloride for Injection in a capillary tube for melting point immediately after drying both of the sample and the tube at 105°C for 3 hours, and determine the melting point.

Purity **(1)** Clarity and color of solution—Dissolve 1.0 g of Acetylcholine Chloride for Injection in 10 mL of water: the solution is clear and colorless.

(2) Acidity—Dissolve 0.10 g of Acetylcholine Chloride for Injection in 10 mL of freshly boiled and cooled water, and add 1 drop of bromothymol blue TS, and 0.30 mL of 0.01 mol/L sodium hydroxide VS: the solution is blue in color.

(3) Heavy metals 〈*1.07*〉—Proceed with 2.0 g of Acetylcholine Chloride for Injection according to Method 1, and perform the test. Prepare the control solution with 2.0 mL of Standard Lead Solution (not more than 10 ppm).

Loss on drying 〈*2.41*〉 Not more than 1.0% (1 g, 105°C, 3 hours).

Residue on ignition 〈*2.44*〉 Not more than 0.1% (1 g).

Uniformity of dosage units 〈*6.02*〉 It meets the requirement of the Mass variation test.

Foreign insoluble matter 〈*6.06*〉 Perform the test according to Method 2: it meets the requirement.

Insoluble particulate matter 〈*6.07*〉 It meets the requirement.

Sterility 〈*4.06*〉 Perform the test according to the Membrane filtration method: it meets the requirement.

Assay **(1)** Acetylcholine chloride—Weigh accurately the contents of not less than 10 Acetylcholine Chloride for Injections. Weigh accurately about 0.5 g of the contents, dissolve in 15 mL of water, then add exactly 40 mL of 0.1 mol/L sodium hydroxide VS, stopper loosely, and heat on a water bath for 30 minutes. Cool quickly, and titrate 〈*2.50*〉 the excess sodium hydroxide with 0.05 mol/L sulfuric acid VS (indicator: 3 drops of phenolphthalein TS). Perform a blank determination in the same manner.

Each mL of 0.1 mol/L sodium hydroxide VS
= 18.17 mg of $C_7H_{16}ClNO_2$

(2) Chlorine—Titrate 〈*2.50*〉 the solution, which has been titrated in (1), with 0.1 mol/L silver nitrate VS (indicator: 3 drops of fluorescein sodium TS).

Each mL of 0.1 mol/L silver nitrate VS
= 3.545 mg of Cl

Containers and storage Containers—Hermetic containers.

Acetylcysteine

アセチルシステイン

$C_5H_9NO_3S$: 163.19
(2*R*)-2-Acetylamino-3-sulfanylpropanoic acid
[616-91-1]

Acetylcysteine contains not less than 99.0% and not more than 101.0% of acetylcysteine ($C_5H_9NO_3S$), calculated on the dried basis.

Description Acetylcysteine occurs as white, crystals or crystalline powder.

It is freely soluble in water and in ethanol (99.5).

It dissolves in sodium hydroxide TS.

Identification Determine the infrared absorption spectrum of Acetylcysteine as directed in the potassium bromide disk method under Infrared Spectrophotometry 〈*2.25*〉, and compare the spectrum with the Reference Spectrum: both spectra exhibit similar intensities of absorption at the same wave numbers.

Optical rotation 〈*2.49*〉 $[\alpha]_D^{20}$: +21.0 – +27.0° Weigh accurately an amount of Acetylcysteine, equivalent to about 2.5 g calculated on the dried basis, and dissolve with 2 mL of a solution of disodium dihydrogen ethylenediamine tetraacetate dihydrate (1 in 100) and 15 mL of a solution of sodium hydroxide (1 in 25). To this solution add a solution, prepared by adjusting the pH to 7.0 of 500 mL of a solution of potassium dihydrogen phosphate (17 in 125) with sodium hydroxide TS and adding water to make 1000 mL, to make exactly 50 mL. Determine the optical rotation of this solution using a 100-mm cell.

Melting point *<2.60>* 107 - 111°C

Purity **(1)** Chloride *<1.03>*—Dissolve 0.40 g of Acetylcysteine in 25 mL of sodium hydroxide TS, add 4 mL of hydrogen peroxide (30), heat in a water bath for 45 minutes, and cool. Then add 5 mL of nitric acid, add water to make 50 mL, and perform the test using this solution as the test solution. Prepare the control solution with 0.45 mL of 0.01 mol/L hydrochloric acid VS (not more than 0.040%).

(2) Sulfate *<1.14>*—Perform the test with 0.8 g of Acetylcysteine. Prepare the control solution with 0.50 mL of 0.005 mol/L sulfuric acid VS (not more than 0.030%).

(3) Ammonium *<1.02>*—Perform the test with 0.10 g of Acetylcysteine, using the distillation under reduced pressure. Prepare the control solution with 2.0 mL of Standard Ammonium Solution (not more than 0.02%).

(4) Heavy metals *<1.07>*—Dissolve 1.0 g of Acetylcysteine in 40 mL of water, add 3 mL of sodium hydroxide TS, 2 mL of dilute acetic acid and water to make 50 mL, and perform the test using this solution as the test solution. Prepare the control solution as follows: To 1.0 mL of Standard Lead Solution add 2 mL of dilute acetic acid and water to make 50 mL (not more than 10 ppm).

(5) Iron *<1.10>*—Prepare the test solution with 1.0 g of Acetylcysteine according to Method 1, and perform the test according to Method A. Prepare the control solution with 1.0 mL of Standard Iron Solution (not more than 10 ppm).

(6) Related substances—Dissolve 50 mg of Acetylcysteine in 25 mL of the mobile phase, and use this solution as the sample solution. The sample solution is prepared before using. Perform the test with 10 μL of the sample solution as directed under Liquid Chromatography *<2.01>* according to the following conditions, determine each peak area by the automatic integration method, and calculate their amounts by the area percentage method: the area of the peak other than acetylcysteine is not more than 0.3%, and the total area of the peak other than acetylcysteine is not more than 0.6%.

Operating conditions—

Detector: An ultraviolet absorption photometer (wavelength: 220 nm).

Column: A stainless steel column 4.6 mm in inside diameter and 25 cm in length, packed with octadecylsilanized silica gel for liquid chromatography (5 μm in particle diameter).

Column temperature: A constant temperature of about 40°C.

Mobile phase: A mixture of diluted phosphoric acid (1 in 2500) and acetonitrile (19:1).

Flow rate: Adjust so that the retention time of acetylcysteine is about 7 minutes.

Time span of measurement: About 4 times as long as the retention time of acetylcysteine, beginning after the solvent peak.

System suitability—

Test for required detectability: To 1 mL of the sample solution add the mobile phase to make 10 mL. To 1 mL of this solution, add the mobile phase to make 20 mL, and use this solution as the solution for system suitability test. Pipet 5 mL of the solution for system suitability test, and add the mobile phase to make exactly 25 mL. Confirm that the peak area of acetylcysteine obtained with 10 μL of this solution is equivalent to 15 to 25% of that with 10 μL of the solution for system suitability test.

System performance: When the procedure is run with 10 μL of the solution for system suitability test under the above operating conditions, the number of theoretical plates and the symmetry factor of the peak of acetylcysteine are not less than 15,000 and not more than 1.5, respectively.

System repeatability: When the test is repeated 6 times with 10 μL of the solution for system suitability test under the above operating conditions, the relative standard deviation of the peak area of acetylcysteine is not more than 2.0%.

Loss on drying *<2.41>* Not more than 0.5% (1 g, 80°C, 3 hours).

Residue on ignition *<2.44>* Not more than 0.3% (1 g).

Assay Weigh accurately about 0.2 g of Acetylcysteine, place it in a stoppered flask, dissolve in 20 mL of water, add 4 g of potassium iodide and 5 mL of dilute hydrochloric acid, then add exactly 25 mL of 0.05 mol/L iodine VS, stopper tightly, allow to stand for 20 minutes in an ice cold water in the dark, and titrate *<2.50>* the excess of iodine with 0.1 mol/L sodium thiosulfate VS (indicator: 1 mL of starch TS). Perform a blank determination in the same manner.

Each mL of 0.05 mol/L iodine VS
= 16.32 mg of $C_5H_9NO_3S$

Containers and storage Containers—Tight containers.

Aciclovir

アシクロビル

$C_8H_{11}N_5O_3$: 225.20

2-Amino-9-[(2-hydroxyethoxy)methyl]-1,9-dihydro-6*H*-purin-6-one

[59277-89-3]

Aciclovir contains not less than 98.5% and not more than 101.0% of aciclovir ($C_8H_{11}N_5O_3$), calculated on the anhydrous basis.

Description Aciclovir occurs as a white to pale yellow-white crystalline powder.

It is slightly soluble in water and very slightly soluble in ethanol (99.5).

It dissolves in 0.1 mol/L hydrochloric acid TS and in dilute sodium hydroxide TS.

Identification **(1)** Determine the absorption spectrum of a solution of Aciclovir in 0.1 mol/L hydrochloric acid TS (1 in 100,000) as directed under Ultraviolet-visible Spectrophotometry *<2.24>*, and compare the spectrum with the Reference Spectrum or the spectrum of a solution of Aciclovir RS prepared in the same manner as the sample solution: both spectra exhibit similar intensities of absorption at the same wavelengths.

(2) Determine the infrared absorption spectrum of Aciclovir as directed in the potassium bromide disk method under Infrared Spectrophotometry *<2.25>*, and compare the spectrum with the Reference Spectrum or the spectrum of Aciclovir RS: both spectra exhibit similar intensities of absorption at the same wave numbers.

Purity **(1)** Clarity and color of solution—Dissolve 0.5 g of Aciclovir in 20 mL of dilute sodium hydroxide TS: the solution is clear and is not more colored than the following control solution.

Control solution: To 2.5 mL of Matching Fluid F add diluted dilute hydrochloric acid (1 in 10) to make 100 mL.

(2) Heavy metals <*1.07*>—Proceed with 1.0 g of Aciclovir according to Method 2, and perform the test. Prepare the control solution with 1.0 mL of Standard Lead Solution (not more than 10 ppm).

(3) Related substances—Use the sample solution obtained in the Assay as the sample solution. Separately, weigh accurately about 25 mg of guanine, dissolve in 50 mL of dilute sodium hydroxide TS, and add the mobile phase to make exactly 100 mL. Pipet 2 mL of this solution, add the mobile phase to make exactly 100 mL, and use this solution as the standard solution. Perform the test with exactly 10 μL each of the sample solution and standard solution as directed under Liquid Chromatography <*2.01*> according to the following conditions. Determine the peak areas of guanine, A_T and A_S, and calculate the amount of guanine by the following equation: it is not more than 0.7%. Determine each peak area from the sample solution by the automatic integration method, and calculate the amount of each related substance other than aciclovir and guanine by the area percentage method: it is not more than 0.2%. Furthermore, the sum of the amount of guanine calculated above and the amounts of related substances determined by the area percentage method is not more than 1.5%.

$$\text{Amount (\%) of guanine} = M_S/M_T \times A_T/A_S \times 2/5$$

M_S: Amount (mg) of guanine taken

M_T: Amount (mg) of Aciclovir taken

Operating conditions—

Detector, column, column temperature, mobile phase, and flow rate: Proceed as directed in the operating conditions in the Assay.

Time span of measurement: About 8 times as long as the retention time of aciclovir, beginning after the solvent peak.

System suitability—

System performance: Proceed as directed in the system suitability in the Assay.

Test for required detectability: To 1 mL of the sample solution add the mobile phase to make 100 mL, and use this solution as the solution for system suitability test. Pipet 1 mL of the solution for system suitability test, and add the mobile phase to make exactly 10 mL. Confirm that the peak area of aciclovir obtained with 10 μL of this solution is equivalent to 7 to 13% of that with 10 μL of the solution for system suitability test.

System repeatability: When the test is repeated 6 times with 10 μL of the standard solution under the above operating conditions, the relative standard deviation of the peak area of guanine is not more than 2.0%.

Water <*2.48*> Not more than 6.0% (50 mg, coulometric titration).

Residue on ignition <*2.44*> Not more than 0.1% (1 g).

Assay Weigh accurately about 20 mg each of Aciclovir and Aciclovir RS (separately determine the water <*2.48*> in the same manner as Aciclovir), dissolve each in 1 mL of dilute sodium hydroxide TS, add the mobile phase to make exactly 20 mL each, and use these solutions as the sample solution and the standard solution, respectively. Perform the test with exactly 10 μL each of the sample solution and standard solution as directed under Liquid Chromatography <*2.01*> according to the following conditions, and determine the peak areas, A_T and A_S, of aciclovir in each solution.

$$\text{Amount (mg) of aciclovir } (C_8H_{11}N_5O_3) = M_S \times A_T/A_S$$

M_S: Amount (mg) of Aciclovir RS taken, calculated on the anhydrous basis

Operating conditions—

Detector: An ultraviolet absorption photometer (wavelength: 254 nm).

Column: A stainless steel column 4.6 mm in inside diameter and 10 cm in length, packed with octadecylsilanized silica gel for liquid chromatography (3 μm in particle diameter).

Column temperature: A constant temperature of about 20°C.

Mobile phase: Dissolve 1.0 g of sodium 1-decanesulfonate and 6.0 g of sodium dihydrogen phosphate dihydrate in 1000 mL of water, and adjust the pH to 3.0 with phosphoric acid. To this solution add 40 mL of acetonitrile.

Flow rate: Adjust so that the retention time of aciclovir is about 3 minutes.

System suitability—

System performance: Dissolve 0.1 g of Aciclovir in 5 mL of dilute sodium hydroxide TS, add 2 mL of a solution of guanine in dilute sodium hydroxide TS (1 in 4000), and add the mobile phase to make 100 mL. When the procedure is run with 10 μL of this solution under the above operating conditions, aciclovir and guanine are eluted in this order with the resolution between these peaks being not less than 17.

System repeatability: When the test is repeated 6 times with 10 μL of the standard solution under the above operating conditions, the relative standard deviation of the peak area of aciclovir is not more than 1.0%.

Containers and storage Containers—Well-closed containers.

Aciclovir Granules

アシクロビル顆粒

Aciclovir Granules contain not less than 93.0% and not more than 107.0% of the labeled amount of aciclovir ($C_8H_{11}N_5O_3$: 225.20).

Method of preparation Prepare as directed under Granules, with Aciclovir.

Identification Determine the absorption spectrum of the sample solution obtained in the Assay as directed under Ultraviolet-visible Spectrophotometry <*2.24*>: it exhibits a maximum between 254 nm and 258 nm.

Uniformity of dosage units <*6.02*> Perform the test according to the following method: Aciclovir Granules in single-dose packages meet the requirement of the Content uniformity test.

To the total amount of the content of 1 package of Aciclovir Granules, add 100 mL of dilute sodium hydroxide TS, sonicate with occasional shaking, and add dilute sodium hydroxide TS to make exactly 200 mL. Filter this solution, discard the first 20 mL of the filtrate, pipet V mL of the subsequent filtrate, add dilute sodium hydroxide TS to make exactly V' mL so that each mL contains about 1 mg of aciclovir ($C_8H_{11}N_5O_3$). Pipet 15 mL of this solution, add 50 mL of water and 5.8 mL of 2 mol/L hydrochloric acid TS, add water to make exactly 100 mL. Pipet 5 mL of this solution, add 0.1 mol/L hydrochloric acid TS to make exactly 100 mL, and use this solution as the sample solution. Then, proceed as directed in the Assay.

$$\text{Amount (mg) of acyclovir } (C_8H_{11}N_5O_3) = M_S \times A_T/A_S \times V'/V \times 8$$

M_S: Amount (mg) of Aciclovir RS taken, calculated on the anhydrous basis

Dissolution ⟨6.10⟩ When the test is performed at 50 revolutions per minute according to the Paddle method, using 900 mL of water as the dissolution medium, the dissolution rate in 30 minutes of Aciclovir Granules is not less than 85%.

Start the test with an accurately weighed amount of Aciclovir Granules, equivalent to about 0.4 g of aciclovir ($C_8H_{11}N_5O_3$), withdraw not less than 20 mL of the medium at the specified minute after starting the test, and filter through a membrane filter with a pore size not exceeding 0.45 μm. Discard not less than 10 mL of the first filtrate, pipet 2 mL of the subsequent filtrate, add water to make exactly 100 mL, and use this solution as the sample solution. Separately, weigh accurately about 22 mg of Aciclovir RS (separately determine the water ⟨2.48⟩ in the same manner as Aciclovir), and dissolve in water to make exactly 100 mL. Pipet 4 mL of this solution, add water to make exactly 100 mL, and use this solution as the standard solution. Determine the absorbances, A_T and A_S, at 252 nm of the sample solution and standard solution as directed under Ultraviolet-visible Spectrophotometry ⟨2.24⟩.

$$\text{Dissolution rate (\%) with respect to the labeled amount of aciclovir } (C_8H_{11}N_5O_3) = M_S/M_T \times A_T/A_S \times 1/C \times 1800$$

M_S: Amount (mg) of aciclovir RS taken, calculated on the anhydrous basis

M_T: Amount (g) of Aciclovir Granules taken

C: Labeled amount (mg) of aciclovir ($C_8H_{11}N_5O_3$) in 1 g

Assay Powder Aciclovir Granules, and weigh accurately a portion of the powder, equivalent to about 0.1 g of aciclovir ($C_8H_{11}N_5O_3$), add 60 mL of dilute sodium hydroxide TS, sonicate for 15 minutes, then add dilute sodium hydroxide TS to make exactly 100 mL, and filter. Discard the first 20 mL of filtrate, pipet 15 mL of the subsequent filtrate, add 50 mL of water and 5.8 mL of 2 mol/L hydrochloric acid TS, and add water to make exactly 100 mL. Pipet 5 mL of this solution, add 0.1 mol/L hydrochloric acid TS to make exactly 100 mL, and use this solution as the sample solution. Separately, weigh accurately about 25 mg of Aciclovir RS (separately determine the water ⟨2.48⟩ in the same manner as Aciclovir), and dissolve in dilute sodium hydroxide TS to make exactly 25 mL. Pipet 15 mL of this solution, add 50 mL of water and 5.8 mL of 2 mol/L hydrochloric acid TS, add water to make exactly 100 mL. Pipet 5 mL of this solution, add 0.1 mol/L hydrochloric acid TS to make exactly 100 mL, and use this solution as the standard solution. Determine the absorbances, A_T and A_S, at 255 nm of the sample solution and standard solution as directed under Ultraviolet-visible Spectrophotometry ⟨2.24⟩, using 0.1 mol/L hydrochloric acid TS as the blank.

$$\text{Amount (mg) of acyclovir } (C_8H_{11}N_5O_3) = M_S \times A_T/A_S \times 4$$

M_S: Amount (mg) of Aciclovir RS taken, calculated on the anhydrous basis

Containers and storage Containers—Tight containers.

Aciclovir Injection

アシクロビル注射液

Aciclovir Injection is an aqueous injection.

It contains not less than 95.0% and not more than 105.0% of the labeled amount of aciclovir ($C_8H_{11}N_5O_3$: 225.20).

Method of preparation Prepare as directed under Injections, with Aciclovir.

Description Aciclovir Injection occurs as a colorless or pale yellow, clear liquid.

Identification To a volume of Aciclovir Injection, equivalent to 25 mg of Aciclovir, add 0.5 mol/L hydrochloric acid TS to make 100 mL. To 2 mL of this solution add 0.5 mol/L hydrochloric acid TS to make 50 mL. Determine the absorption spectrum of this solution as directed under Ultraviolet-visible Spectrophotometry ⟨2.24⟩: it exhibits a maximum between 254 nm and 258 nm.

Bacterial endotoxins ⟨4.01⟩ Less than 0.5 EU/mg.

Extractable volume ⟨6.05⟩ It meets the requirement.

Foreign insoluble matter ⟨6.06⟩ Perform the test according to Method 1: it meets the requirement.

Insoluble particulate matter ⟨6.07⟩ It meets the requirement.

Sterility ⟨4.06⟩ Perform the test according to the Membrane filtration method: it meets the requirement.

Assay To an exact volume of Aciclovir Injection, equivalent to about 25 mg of aciclovir ($C_8H_{11}N_5O_3$), add 0.1 mol/L hydrochloric acid TS to make exactly 100 mL. Pipet 2 mL of this solution, add exactly 5 mL of the internal standard solution, then add 0.1 mol/L hydrochloric acid TS to make 50 mL, and use this solution as the sample solution. Separately, weigh accurately about 25 mg of Aciclovir RS (separately determine the water ⟨2.48⟩ in the same manner as Aciclovir), and dissolve in 0.1 mol/L hydrochloric acid TS to make exactly 100 mL. Pipet 2 mL of this solution, add exactly 5 mL of the internal standard solution, then add 0.1 mol/L hydrochloric acid TS to make 50 mL, and use this solution as the standard solution. Perform the test with 20 μL each of the sample solution and standard solution as directed under Liquid Chromatography ⟨2.01⟩ according to the following conditions, and calculate the ratios, Q_T and Q_S, of the peak area of aciclovir to that of the internal standard.

$$\text{Amount (mg) of aciclovir } (C_8H_{11}N_5O_3) = M_S \times Q_T/Q_S$$

M_S: Amount (mg) of Aciclovir RS taken, calculated on the anhydrous basis

Internal standard solution—A solution of nicotinic acid in 0.1 mol/L hydrochloric acid TS (3 in 20,000).

Operating conditions—

Detector: An ultraviolet absorption photometer (wavelength: 254 nm).

Column: A stainless steel column 4.6 mm in inside diameter and 15 cm in length, packed with octadecylsilanized silica gel for liquid chromatography (5 μm in particle diameter).

Column temperature: A constant temperature of about 25°C.

Mobile phase: To 1.45 g of phosphoric acid and 25 mL of

dilute acetic acid add water to make 900 mL. Adjust this solution to pH 2.5 with 1 mol/L sodium hydroxide TS, and add water to make 1000 mL. To 950 mL of this solution add 50 mL of methanol.

Flow rate: Adjust so that the retention time of aciclovir is about 7 minutes.

System suitability—

System performance: When the procedure is run with 20 μL of the standard solution under the above operating conditions, the internal standard and aciclovir are eluted in this order with the resolution between these peaks being not less than 3.

System repeatability: When the test is repeated 6 times with 20 μL of the standard solution under the above operating conditions, the relative standard deviation of the ratio of the peak area of aciclovir to that of the internal standard is not more than 1.0%.

Containers and storage Containers—Hermetic containers.

Aciclovir for Injection

注射用アシクロビル

Aciclovir for Injection is a preparation for injection which is dissolved before use.

It contains not less than 95.0% and not more than 105.0% of the labeled amount of aciclovir ($C_8H_{11}N_5O_3$: 225.20).

Method of preparation Prepare as directed under Injections, with Aciclovir.

Description Aciclovir for Injection occurs as white to pale yellow-white, light masses or powder.

Identification Determine the absorption spectrum of the sample solution obtained in the Assay as directed under Ultraviolet-visible Spectrophotometry *<2.24>*: it exhibits a maximum between 254 nm and 258 nm.

pH Being specified separately when the drug is granted approval based on the Law.

Purity Clarity and color of solution—Dissolve an amount of Aciclovir for Injection, equivalent to 0.25 g of Aciclovir, in 10 mL of water: the solution is clear and is not more colored than the following control solution.

Control solution: To 2.5 mL of Matching Fluid F add diluted dilute hydrochloric acid (1 in 10) to make 100 mL.

Water *<2.48>* Not more than 7.5% (0.1 g, volumetric titration, direct titration).

Bacterial endotoxins *<4.01>* Less than 0.25 EU/mg.

Uniformity of dosage units *<6.02>* It meets the requirement of the Mass variation test.

Foreign insoluble matter *<6.06>* Perform the test according to Method 2: it meets the requirement.

Insoluble particulate matter *<6.07>* It meets the requirement.

Sterility *<4.06>* Perform the test according to the Membrane filtration method: it meets the requirement.

Assay Weigh accurately the mass of the contents of not less than 10 Aciclovir for Injection. Weigh accurately an amount of the contents, equivalent to about 0.1 g of aciclovir ($C_8H_{11}N_5O_3$), and dissolve in dilute sodium hydroxide TS to make exactly 100 mL. Pipet 15 mL of this solution, add 70 mL of water and 5 mL of 2 mol/L hydrochloric acid TS, then add water to make exactly 100 mL. Pipet 5 mL of this solution, add 0.1 mol/L hydrochloric acid TS to make exactly 100 mL, and use this solution as the sample solution. Separately, weigh accurately about 20 mg of Aciclovir RS (separately determine the water *<2.48>* in the same manner as Aciclovir), and dissolve in dilute sodium hydroxide TS to make exactly 20 mL. Pipet 15 mL of this solution, add 70 mL of water and 5 mL of 2 mol/L hydrochloric acid TS, then add water to make exactly 100 mL. Pipet 5 mL of this solution, add 0.1 mol/L hydrochloric acid TS to make exactly 100 mL, and use this solution as the standard solution. Determine the absorbances, A_T and A_S, at 255 nm of the sample solution and standard solution as directed under Ultraviolet-visible Spectrophotometry *<2.24>*, using 0.1 mol/L hydrochloric acid TS as the blank.

$$\text{Amount (mg) of aciclovir } (C_8H_{11}N_5O_3) = M_S \times A_T/A_S \times 5$$

M_S: Amount (mg) of Aciclovir RS taken, calculated on the anhydrous basis

Containers and storage Containers—Hermetic containers.

Aciclovir Ointment

アシクロビル軟膏

Aciclovir Ointment contains not less than 95.0% and not more than 105.0% of the labeled amount of aciclovir ($C_8H_{11}N_5O_3$: 225.20).

Method of preparation Prepare as directed under Ointments, with Aciclovir.

Identification Determine the absorption spectrum of the sample solution obtained in the Assay as directed under Ultraviolet-visible Spectrophotometry *<2.24>*: it exhibits a maximum between 254 nm and 258 nm.

Assay Weigh accurately an amount of Aciclovir Ointment, equivalent to about 10 mg of aciclovir ($C_8H_{11}N_5O_3$), add 25 mL of dilute sodium hydroxide TS, warm if necessary, and dissolve by shaking. After cooling, add water to make exactly 100 mL. Pipet 15 mL of this solution, add 0.1 mol/L hydrochloric acid TS to make exactly 200 mL, and use this solution as the sample solution. Separately, weigh accurately about 20 mg of Aciclovir RS (separately, determine the water *<2.48>* in the same manner as Aciclovir), and dissolve in dilute sodium hydroxide TS to make exactly 20 mL. Pipet 10 mL of this solution, and add 15 mL of dilute sodium hydroxide TS and water to make exactly 100 mL. Pipet 15 mL of this solution, add 0.1 mol/L hydrochloric acid TS to make exactly 200 mL, and use this solution as the standard solution. Determine the absorbances, A_T and A_S, at 255 nm of the sample solution and standard solution as directed under Ultraviolet-visible Spectrophotometry *<2.24>*, using 0.1 mol/L hydrochloric acid TS as the blank.

$$\text{Amount (mg) of aciclovir } (C_8H_{11}N_5O_3) = M_S \times A_T/A_S \times 1/2$$

M_S: Amount (mg) of Aciclovir RS taken, calculated on the anhydrous basis

Containers and storage Containers—Tight containers.

Aciclovir Ophthalmic Ointment

アシクロビル眼軟膏

Aciclovir Ophthalmic Ointment contains not less than 90.0% and not more than 110.0% of the labeled amount of aciclovir ($C_8H_{11}N_5O_3$: 225.20).

Method of preparation Prepare as directed under Ophthalmic Ointments, with Aciclovir.

Identification Determine the absorption spectrum of the sample solution obtained in the Assay as directed under Ultraviolet-visible Spectrophotometry <*2.24*>: it exhibits a maximum between 254 nm and 258 nm.

Metal Particles <*6.01*> It meets the requirement.

Sterility <*4.06*> Perform the test according to the Membrane filtration method: it meets the requirement.

Particle diameter Being specified separately when the drug is granted approval based on the Law.

Assay Weigh accurately a portion of Aciclovir Ophthalmic Ointment, equivalent to about 15 mg of aciclovir ($C_8H_{11}N_5O_3$), add exactly 20 mL of hexane and exactly 20 mL of dilute sodium hydroxide TS, and shake vigorously. Centrifuge this mixture, discard the upper layer, pipet 1 mL of the lower layer, add 70 mL of water and 5 mL of 2 mol/L hydrochloric acid TS, then add water to make exactly 100 mL, and use this solution as the sample solution. Separately, weigh accurately about 15 mg of Aciclovir RS (separately determine the water <*2.48*> in the same manner as Aciclovir), and dissolve in dilute sodium hydroxide TS to make exactly 20 mL. Pipet 1 mL of this solution, add 70 mL of water and 5 mL of 2 mol/L hydrochloric acid TS, then add water to make exactly 100 mL, and use this solution as the standard solution. Determine the absorbances, A_T and A_S, at 255 nm of the sample solution and standard solution as directed under Ultraviolet-visible Spectrophotometry <*2.24*>, using water as the blank.

Amount (mg) of acyclovir ($C_8H_{11}N_5O_3$) = $M_S \times A_T/A_S$

M_S: Amount (mg) of Aciclovir RS taken, calculated on the anhydrous basis

Containers and storage Containers—Tight containers.

Aciclovir Syrup

アシクロビルシロップ

Aciclovir Syrup is a suspension syrup.

It contains not less than 93.0% and not more than 107.0% of the labeled amount of aciclovir ($C_8H_{11}N_5O_3$: 225.20).

Method of preparation Prepare as directed under Syrups, with Aciclovir.

Identification To a volume of thoroughly shaken Aciclovir Syrup, equivalent to 80 mg of Aciclovir, add 0.1 mol/L hydrochloric acid TS to make 100 mL. Centrifuge this solution, to 1 mL of the supernatant liquid add 0.1 mol/L hydrochloric acid TS to make 100 mL. Determine the absorption spectrum of this solution as directed under Ultraviolet-visible Spectrophotometry <*2.24*>: it exhibits a maximum between 254 nm and 258 nm.

Dissolution <*6.10*> When the test is performed at 50 revolutions per minute according to the Paddle method, using 900 mL of water as the dissolution medium, the dissolution rate in 15 minutes of Aciclovir Syrup is not less than 85%.

Start the test with an exact volume of thoroughly shaken Aciclovir Syrup, equivalent to about 0.4 g of aciclovir ($C_8H_{11}N_5O_3$), withdraw not less than 20 mL of the medium at the specified minute after starting the test, and centrifuge. Pipet 2 mL of the supernatant liquid, add water to make exactly 100 mL, and use this solution as the sample solution. Separately, weigh accurately about 22 mg of Aciclovir RS (separately determine the water <*2.48*> in the same manner as Aciclovir), and dissolve in water to make exactly 100 mL. Pipet 4 mL of this solution, add water to make exactly 100 mL, and use this solution as the standard solution. Determine the absorbances, A_T and A_S, at 252 nm of the sample solution and standard solution as directed under Ultraviolet-visible Spectrophotometry <*2.24*>.

Dissolution rate (%) with respect to the labeled amount of aciclovir ($C_8H_{11}N_5O_3$)
$= M_S/V_T \times A_T/A_S \times 1/C \times 1800$

M_S: Amount (mg) of Aciclovir RS taken, calculated on the anhydrous basis
V_T: Amount (mL) of Aciclovir Syrup taken
C: Labeled amount (mg) of aciclovir ($C_8H_{11}N_5O_3$) in 1 mL

Assay Shake thoroughly Aciclovir Syrup. To an exact volume of the syrup, equivalent to about 80 mg of aciclovir ($C_8H_{11}N_5O_3$), add 0.1 mol/L hydrochloric acid TS to make exactly 100 mL. Centrifuge this solution, pipet 2 mL of the supernatant liquid, add exactly 5 mL of the internal standard solution, then add 0.1 mol/L hydrochloric acid TS to make 50 mL, and use this solution as the sample solution. Separately, weigh accurately about 40 mg of Aciclovir RS (separately determine the water <*2.48*> in the same manner as Aciclovir), and dissolve in 0.1 mol/L hydrochloric acid TS to make exactly 50 mL. Pipet 2 mL of this solution, add exactly 5 mL of the internal standard solution, then add 0.1 mol/L hydrochloric acid TS to make 50 mL, and use this solution as the standard solution. Perform the test with 20 μL each of the sample solution and standard solution as directed under Liquid Chromatography <*2.01*> according to the following conditions, and calculate the ratios, Q_T and Q_S, of the peak area of aciclovir to that of the internal standard.

Amount (mg) of aciclovir ($C_8H_{11}N_5O_3$)
$= M_S \times Q_T/Q_S \times 2$

M_S: Amount (mg) of Aciclovir RS taken, calculated on the anhydrous basis

Internal standard solution—A solution of nicotinic acid in 0.1 mol/L hydrochloric acid TS (1 in 2000).

Operating conditions—

Detector: An ultraviolet absorption photometer (wavelength: 254 nm).

Column: A stainless steel column 4.6 mm in inside diameter and 15 cm in length, packed with octadecylsilanized silica gel for liquid chromatography (5 μm in particle diameter).

Column temperature: A constant temperature of about 25°C.

Mobile phase: To 1.45 g of phosphoric acid and 25 mL of dilute acetic acid add water to make 900 mL. Adjust this solution to pH 2.5 with 1 mol/L sodium hydroxide TS, and add water to make 1000 mL. To 950 mL of this solution add 50 mL of methanol.

Flow rate: Adjust so that the retention time of aciclovir is about 7 minutes.

System suitability—

System performance: When the procedure is run with 20 μL of the standard solution under the above operating conditions, the internal standard and aciclovir are eluted in this order with the resolution between these peaks being not less than 3.

System repeatability: When the test is repeated 6 times with 20 μL of the standard solution under the above operating conditions, the relative standard deviation of the ratio of the peak area of aciclovir to that of the internal standard is not more than 1.0%.

Containers and storage Containers—Tight containers.

Aciclovir for Syrup

シロップ用アシクロビル

Aciclovir for Syrup is a preparation for syrup, which is suspended before use.

It contains not less than 95.0% and not more than 105.0% of the labeled amount of aciclovir ($C_8H_{11}N_5O_3$: 225.20).

Method of preparation Prepare as directed under Preparations for Syrup, with Aciclovir.

Identification Dissolve an amount of Aciclovir for Syrup, equivalent to 12 mg of Aciclovir, in 0.1 mol/L hydrochloric acid TS to make 50 mL. To 2 mL of this solution add 0.1 mol/L hydrochloric acid TS to make 50 mL, and determine the absorption spectrum of this solution as directed under Ultraviolet-visible Spectrophotometry <*2.24*>: it exhibits a maximum between 254 nm and 258 nm.

Uniformity of dosage units <*6.02*> Perform the test according to the following method: Aciclovir for Syrup in single-dose packages meets the requirement of the Content uniformity test.

To the total content of 1 package of Aciclovir for Syrup add $2V/25$ mL of diluted sodium hydroxide TS (1 in 10), and sonicate to disintegrate, add water to make exactly V mL so that each mL contains about 0.8 mg of aciclovir ($C_8H_{11}N_5O_3$), and filter this solution through a membrane filter with a pore size not exceeding 0.45 μm. Discard the first 2 mL of the filtrate, pipet 5 mL of the subsequent filtrate, add exactly 5 mL of the internal standard solution, then add the mobile phase to make 50 mL, and use this solution as the sample solution. Then, proceed as directed in the Assay.

$$\text{Amount (mg) of aciclovir } (C_8H_{11}N_5O_3) = M_S \times Q_T/Q_S \times V/10$$

M_S: Amount (mg) of Aciclovir RS taken, calculated on the anhydrous basis

Internal standard solution—A solution of parahydroxybenzoic acid in the mobile phase (1 in 1250).

Dissolution <*6.10*> When the test is performed at 50 revolutions per minute according to the Paddle method, using 900 mL of water as the dissolution medium, the dissolution rate in 45 minutes of Aciclovir for Syrup is not less than 85%.

Start the test with an accurately weighed amount of Aciclovir for Syrup, equivalent to about 0.2 g of aciclovir ($C_8H_{11}N_5O_3$), withdraw not less than 5 mL of the medium at the specified minute after starting the test, and filter through a membrane filter with a pore size not exceeding 0.45 μm. Discard not less than 2 mL of the first filtrate, pipet 2 mL of the subsequent filtrate, add water to make exactly 50 mL, and use this solution as the sample solution. Separately, weigh accurately about 11 mg of Aciclovir RS (separately determine the water <*2.48*> in the same manner as Aciclovir), and dissolve in water to make exactly 50 mL. Pipet 2 mL of this solution, add water to make exactly 50 mL, and use this solution as the standard solution. Determine the absorbances, A_T and A_S, at 254 nm of the sample solution and standard solution as directed under Ultraviolet-visible Spectrophotometry <*2.24*>.

$$\text{Dissolution rate (\%) with respect to the labeled amount of aciclovir } (C_8H_{11}N_5O_3) = M_S/M_T \times A_T/A_S \times 1/C \times 1800$$

M_S: Amount (mg) of Aciclovir RS taken, calculated on the anhydrous basis

M_T: Amount (g) of Aciclovir for Syrup taken

C: Labeled amount (mg) of aciclovir ($C_8H_{11}N_5O_3$) in 1 g

Assay Weigh accurately an amount of Aciclovir for Syrup, previously powdered if necessary, equivalent to about 0.2 g of aciclovir ($C_8H_{11}N_5O_3$), add 20 mL of diluted sodium hydroxide TS (1 in 10), sonicate to disintegrate, then add water to make exactly 200 mL, and filter this solution through a membrane filter with a pore size not exceeding 0.45 μm. Discard the first 2 mL of the filtrate, pipet 5 mL of the subsequent filtrate, add exactly 5 mL of the internal standard solution, then add the mobile phase to make 50 mL, and use this solution as the sample solution. Separately, weigh accurately about 10 mg of Aciclovir RS (separately determine the water <*2.48*> in the same manner as Aciclovir), add exactly 10 mL of the internal standard solution, then add the mobile phase to make 100 mL, and use this solution as the standard solution. Perform the test with 20 μL each of the sample solution and standard solution as directed under Liquid Chromatography <*2.01*> according to the following conditions, and calculate the ratios, Q_T and Q_S, of the peak area of aciclovir to that of the internal standard.

$$\text{Amount (mg) of aciclovir } (C_8H_{11}N_5O_3) = M_S \times Q_T/Q_S \times 20$$

M_S: Amount (mg) of Aciclovir RS taken, calculated on the anhydrous basis

Internal standard solution—A solution of parahydroxybenzoic acid in the mobile phase (1 in 1250).

Operating conditions—

Detector: An ultraviolet absorption photometer (wavelength: 254 nm).

Column: A stainless steel column 4.6 mm in inside diameter and 25 cm in length, packed with octadecylsilanized silica gel for liquid chromatography (5 μm in particle diameter).

Column temperature: A constant temperature of about 40°C.

Mobile phase: Dissolve 7.8 g of sodium dihydrogen phosphate dihydrate and 0.85 g of sodium 1-octanesulfonate in 900 mL of water, adjust to pH 3.0 with phosphoric acid, add water to make 950 mL, and add 50 mL of acetonitrile.

Flow rate: Adjust so that the retention time of aciclovir is about 5 minutes.

System suitability—

System performance: When the procedure is run with 20 μL of the standard solution under the above operating conditions, aciclovir and the internal standard are eluted in this order with the resolution between these peaks being not less than 20.

System repeatability: When the test is repeated 6 times with 20 μL of the standard solution under the above operating conditions, the relative standard deviation of the ratio of the peak area of aciclovir to that of the internal standard is not more than 1.0%.

Containers and storage Containers—Tight containers.

Aciclovir Tablets

アシクロビル錠

Aciclovir Tablets contain not less than 95.0% and not more than 105.0% of the labeled amount of aciclovir ($C_8H_{11}N_5O_3$: 225.20).

Method of preparation Prepare as directed under Tablets, with Aciclovir.

Identification Determine the absorption spectrum of the sample solution obtained in the Assay as directed under Ultraviolet-visible Spectrophotometry *<2.24>*: it exhibits a maximum between 254 nm and 258 nm.

Uniformity of dosage units *<6.02>* It meets the requirement of the Mass variation test.

Dissolution *<6.10>* When the test is performed at 50 revolutions per minute according to the Paddle method, using 900 mL of water as the dissolution medium, the dissolution rate in 30 minutes of Aciclovir Tablets is not less than 80%.

Start the test with 1 tablet of Aciclovir Tablets, withdraw not less than 20 mL of the medium at the specified minute after starting the test, and filter through a membrane filter with a pore size not exceeding 0.45 μm. Discard not less than 10 mL of the first filtrate, pipet V mL of the subsequent filtrate, add water to make exactly V' mL so that each mL contains about 8.9 μg of aciclovir ($C_8H_{11}N_5O_3$), and use this solution as the sample solution. Separately, weigh accurately about 22 mg of aciclovir RS (separately determine the water *<2.48>* in the same manner as Aciclovir), and dissolve in water to make exactly 100 mL. Pipet 4 mL of this solution, add water to make exactly 100 mL, and use this solution as the standard solution. Determine the absorbances, A_T and A_S, at 252 nm of the sample solution and standard solution as directed under Ultraviolet-visible Spectrophotometry *<2.24>*.

Dissolution rate (%) with respect to the labeled amount of aciclovir ($C_8H_{11}N_5O_3$)
$= M_S \times A_T/A_S \times V'/V \times 1/C \times 36$

M_S: Amount (mg) of Acyclovir RS taken, calculated on the anhydrous basis

C: Labeled amount (mg) of aciclovir ($C_8H_{11}N_5O_3$) in 1 tablet

Assay Weigh accurately the mass of not less than 20 Aciclovir Tablets, and powder. Weigh accurately a portion of the powder, equivalent to about 0.1 g of aciclovir ($C_8H_{11}N_5O_3$), add 60 mL of dilute sodium hydroxide TS, and sonicate for 15 minutes, then add dilute sodium hydroxide TS to make exactly 100 mL, and filter. Discard the first 20 mL of filtrate, pipet 15 mL of the subsequent filtrate, add 50 mL of water and 5.8 mL of 2 mol/L hydrochloric acid TS, and add water to make exactly 100 mL. Pipet 5 mL of this solution, add 0.1 mol/L hydrochloric acid TS to make exactly 100 mL, and use this solution as the sample solution. Separately, weigh accurately about 25 mg of Aciclovir RS (separately determine the water *<2.48>* in the same manner as Aciclovir), and dissolve in dilute sodium hydroxide TS to make exactly 25 mL. Pipet 15 mL of this solution, add 50 mL of water and 5.8 mL of 2 mol/L hydrochloric acid TS, add water to make exactly 100 mL. Pipet 5 mL of this solution, add 0.1 mol/L hydrochloric acid TS to make exactly 100 mL, and use this solution as the standard solution. Determine the absorbances, A_T and A_S, at 255 nm of the sample solution and standard solution as directed under Ultraviolet-visible Spectrophotometry *<2.24>*, using 0.1 mol/L hydrochloric acid TS as the blank.

Amount (mg) of aciclovir ($C_8H_{11}N_5O_3$)
$= M_S \times A_T/A_S \times 4$

M_S: Amount (mg) of Aciclovir RS taken, calculated on the anhydrous basis

Containers and storage Containers—Well-closed containers.

Aclarubicin Hydrochloride

アクラルビシン塩酸塩

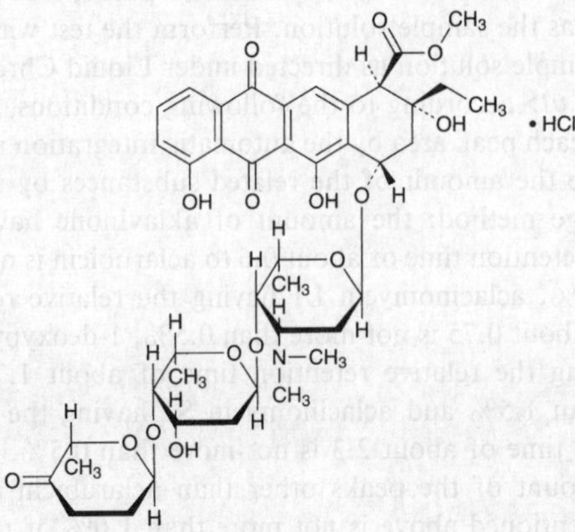

$C_{42}H_{53}NO_{15}$.HCl: 848.33
Methyl (1*R*,2*R*,4*S*)-4-{2,6-dideoxy-4-*O*-[(2*R*,6*S*)-6-methyl-5-oxo-3,4,5,6-tetrahydro-2*H*-pyran-2-yl]-α-L-*lyxo*-hexopyranosyl-(1→4)-2,3,6-trideoxy-3-dimethylamino-α-L-*lyxo*-hexopyranosyloxy}-2-ethyl-2,5,7-trihydroxy-6,11-dioxo-1,2,3,4-tetrahydrotetracene-1-carboxylate monohydrochloride
[75443-99-1]

Aclarubicin Hydrochloride is the hydrochloride of an anthracycline substance having antitumor activity produced by the growth of *Streptomyces galilaeus*.

It contains not less than 920 μg (potency) and not more than 975 μg (potency) per mg, calculated on the anhydrous basis. The potency of Aclarubicin Hydrochloride is expressed as mass (potency) of aclarubicin ($C_{42}H_{53}NO_{15}$: 811.87).

Description Aclarubicin Hydrochloride occurs as a yellow to pale orange-yellow powder.

It is very soluble in chloroform and in methanol, freely soluble in water, and slightly soluble in ethanol (95).

Identification **(1)** Determine the absorption spectrum of a solution of Aclarubicin Hydrochloride in diluted methanol (4 in 5) (3 in 100,000) as directed under Ultraviolet-visible Spectrophotometry *<2.24>*, and compare the spectrum with the Reference Spectrum: both spectra exhibit similar intensities of absorption at the same wavelengths.

(2) Determine the infrared absorption spectrum of Aclarubicin Hydrochloride as directed in the potassium bromide disk method under Infrared Spectrophotometry <*2.25*>, and compare the spectrum with the Reference Spectrum: both spectra exhibit similar intensities of absorption at the same wave numbers.

(3) A solution of Aclarubicin Hydrochloride in methanol (1 in 200) responds to Qualitative Tests <*1.09*> (2) for chloride.

Optical rotation <*2.49*> $[\alpha]_D^{20}$: −146 − −162° (50 mg calculated on the anhydrous basis, water, 10 mL, 100 mm).

pH <*2.54*> The pH of a solution obtained by dissolving 0.05 g of Aclarubicin Hydrochloride in 10 mL of water is between 5.5 and 6.5.

Purity **(1)** Clarity and color of solution—Dissolve 0.10 g of Aclarubicin Hydrochloride in 10 mL of water: the solution is clear and yellow to pale orange-yellow.

(2) Heavy metals <*1.07*>—Proceed with 1.0 g of Aclarubicin Hydrochloride according to Method 2, and perform the test. Prepare the control solution with 2.0 mL of Standard Lead Solution (not more than 20 ppm).

(3) Related substances—Dissolve 10 mg of Aclarubicin Hydrochloride in 10 mL of the mobile phase, and use this solution as the sample solution. Perform the test with 20 μL of the sample solution as directed under Liquid Chromatography <*2.01*> according to the following conditions, and determine each peak area by the automatic integration method. Calculate the amount of the related substances by the area percentage method: the amount of aklavinone having the relative retention time of about 0.6 to aclarubicin is not more than 0.2%, aclacinomycin L1 having the relative retention time of about 0.75 is not more than 0.5%, 1-deoxypyrromycin having the relative retention time of about 1.7 is not more than 1.5% and aclacinomycin S1 having the relative retention time of about 2.3 is not more than 0.5%, and the total amount of the peaks other than aclarubicin and the peaks mentioned above is not more than 1.0% of the peak area of aclarubicin.

Operating conditions—

Detector: A visible absorption photometer (wavelength: 436 nm).

Column: A stainless steel column 3.9 mm in inside diameter and 30 cm in length, packed with silica gel for liquid chromatography (10 μm in particle diameter).

Column temperature: A constant temperature of about 25°C.

Mobile phase: A mixture of chloroform, methanol, acetic acid (100), water and triethylamine (6800:2000:1000:200:1).

Flow rate: Adjust so that the retention time of aclarubicin is about 5 minutes.

Time span of measurement: As long as about 4 times of the retention time of aclarubicin, beginning after the solvent peak.

System suitability—

Test for required detectability: To 1 mL of the sample solution, add the mobile phase to make 100 mL, and use this solution as the solution for system suitability test. Pipet 1 mL of the solution for system suitability test, and add the mobile phase to make exactly 10 mL. Confirm that the peak area of aclarubicin obtained with 20 μL of this solution is equivalent to 7 to 13% of that with 20 μL of the solution for system suitability test.

System performance: Dissolve 5 mg of Aclarubicin Hydrochloride in 10 mL of 0.1 mol/L hydrochloric acid TS, and allow to stand for 60 minutes. To 1.0 mL of this solution add 1.0 mL of 0.2 mol/L sodium hydroxide TS, 1.0 mL of phosphate buffer solution (pH 8.0) and 1.0 mL of chloroform, shake vigorously, and take the chloroform layer. When the procedure is run with 20 μL of the chloroform under the above operating conditions, aclarubicin and 1-deoxypyrromycin are eluted in this order with the resolution between these peaks being not less than 3.0.

System repeatability: When the test is repeated 5 times with 20 μL of the sample solution under the above operating conditions, the relative standard deviation of the peak area of aclarubicin is not more than 2.0%.

Water <*2.48*> Not more than 3.5% (0.1 g, volumetric titration, direct titration).

Residue on ignition <*2.44*> Not more than 0.1% (1 g).

Assay Weigh accurately an amount of Aclarubicin Hydrochloride, equivalent to about 20 mg (potency), and dissolve in diluted methanol (4 in 5) to make exactly 100 mL. Pipet 15 mL of this solution, add diluted methanol (4 in 5) to make exactly 100 mL, and use this solution as the sample solution. Separately, weigh accurately an amount of Aclarubicin RS, equivalent to about 20 mg (potency), add 0.6 mL of diluted hydrochloric acid (1 in 250) and diluted methanol (4 in 5) to make exactly 100 mL. Pipet 15 mL of this solution, add diluted methanol (4 in 5) to make exactly 100 mL, and use this solution as the standard solution. Perform the test with the sample solution and standard solution as directed under Ultraviolet-visible Spectrophotometry <*2.24*>, and determine the absorbances, A_T and A_S, at 433 nm.

Amount [μg (potency)] of aclarubicin ($C_{42}H_{53}NO_{15}$)
$= M_S \times A_T/A_S \times 1000$

M_S: Amount [mg (potency)] of Aclarubicin RS taken

Containers and storage Containers—Tight containers.
Storage—Light-resistant and at 5°C or below.

Acrinol Hydrate

Ethacridine Lactate

アクリノール水和物

$C_{15}H_{15}N_3O.C_3H_6O_3.H_2O$: 361.39
2-Ethoxy-6,9-diaminoacridine monolactate monohydrate
[6402-23-9]

Acrinol Hydrate contains not less than 98.5% and not more than 101.0% of acrinol ($C_{15}H_{15}N_3O.C_3H_6O_3$: 343.38), calculated on the anhydrous basis.

Description Acrinol Hydrate occurs as a yellow crystalline powder.

It is sparingly soluble in water, in methanol and in ethanol (99.5).

Melting point: about 245°C (with decomposition).

The pH of a solution of Acrinol Hydrate (1 in 100) is between 5.5 and 7.0.

Identification **(1)** Determine the absorption spectrum of a solution of Acrinol Hydrate (3 in 250,000) as directed under

Ultraviolet-visible Spectrophotometry <2.24>, and compare the spectrum with the Reference Spectrum: both spectra exhibit similar intensities of absorption at the same wavelengths.

(2) Determine the infrared absorption spectrum of Acrinol Hydrate as directed in the potassium bromide disk method under Infrared Spectrophotometry <2.25>, and compare the spectrum with the Reference Spectrum: both spectra exhibit similar intensities of absorption at the same wave numbers.

(3) To 5 mL of a solution of Acrinol Hydrate (1 in 100) add 5 mL of dilute sulfuric acid, shake well, allow to stand for about 10 minutes at room temperature, and filter: the filtrate responds to Qualitative Tests <1.09> for lactate.

Purity **(1)** Chloride <1.03>—Dissolve 1.0 g of Acrinol Hydrate in 80 mL of water by warming on a water bath, cool, and add 10 mL of sodium hydroxide TS and water to make 100 mL. Shake well, allow to stand for 30 minutes, filter, to 40 mL of the filtrate add 7 mL of dilute nitric acid and water to make 50 mL, and perform the test using this solution as the test solution. Prepare 50 mL of the control solution with 4 mL of sodium hydroxide TS, 7 mL of dilute nitric acid, 0.30 mL of 0.01 mol/L hydrochloric acid VS and sufficient water (not more than 0.026%).

(2) Heavy metals <1.07>—Proceed with 1.0 g of Acrinol Hydrate according to Method 2, and perform the test. Prepare the control solution with 2.0 mL of Standard Lead Solution (not more than 20 ppm).

(3) Volatile fatty acids—Dissolve 0.5 g of Acrinol Hydrate in a mixture of 20 mL of water and 5 mL of dilute sulfuric acid, shake well, filter, and heat the filtrate: no odor of volatile fatty acids is perceptible.

(4) Related substances—Dissolve 10 mg of Acrinol Hydrate in 25 mL of the mobile phase, and use this solution as the sample solution. Pipet 1 mL of the sample solution, add the mobile phase to make exactly 100 mL, and use this solution as the standard solution (1). Pipet 1 mL of the standard solution (1), add the mobile phase to make exactly 10 mL, and use this solution as the standard solution (2). Perform the test with exactly 10 μL each of the sample solution and standard solutions (1) and (2) as directed under Liquid Chromatography <2.01> according to the following conditions, and determine each peak area by the automatic integration method: the area of the peak other than acrinol obtained from the sample solution is not larger than 3 times the peak area of acrinol from the standard solution (2), and the total area of the peaks other than acrinol from the sample solution is not larger than the peak area of acrinol from the standard solution (1).

Operating conditions—

Detector: An ultraviolet absorption photometer (wavelength: 268 nm).

Column: A stainless steel column 4.6 mm in inside diameter and 25 cm in length, packed with octadecylsilanized silica gel for liquid chromatography (5 μm in particle diameter).

Column temperature: A constant temperature of about 25°C.

Mobile phase: Dissolve 7.8 g of sodium dihydrogen phosphate in 900 mL of water, adjust to pH 2.8 with phosphoric acid, and add water to make 1000 mL. To 700 mL of this solution add 300 mL of acetonitrile for liquid chromatography, and add 1.0 g of sodium 1-octanesulfonate to dissolve.

Flow rate: Adjust so that the retention time of acrinol is about 15 minutes.

Time span of measurement: About 3 times as long as the retention time of acrinol, beginning after the solvent peak.

System suitability—

Test for required detectability: Confirm that the peak area of acrinol obtained with 10 μL of the standard solution (2) is equivalent to 7 to 13% of that with 10 μL of the standard solution (1).

System performance: When the procedure is run with 10 μL of the standard solution (1) under the above operating conditions, the number of theoretical plates and the symmetry factor of the peak of acrinol are not less than 5000 and not more than 2.0, respectively.

System repeatability: When the test is repeated 6 times with 10 μL of the standard solution (1) under the above operating conditions, the relative standard deviation of the peak area of acrinol is not more than 1.5%.

Water <2.48> 4.5 – 5.5% (0.2 g, volumetric titration, direct titration)

Residue on ignition <2.44> Not more than 0.1% (1 g).

Assay Weigh accurately about 0.27 g of Acrinol Hydrate, dissolve in 5 mL of formic acid, add 60 mL of a mixture of acetic anhydride and acetic acid (100) (1:1), and titrate <2.50> immediately with 0.1 mol/L perchloric acid VS (potentiometric titration). Perform a blank determination in the same manner, and make any necessary correction.

Each mL of 0.1 mol/L perchloric acid VS
= 34.34 mg of $C_{15}H_{15}N_3O.C_3H_6O_3$

Containers and storage Containers—Tight containers.
Storage—Light-resistant.

Acrinol and Zinc Oxide Oil

アクリノール·チンク油

Acrinol and Zinc Oxide Oil contains not less than 44.6% and not more than 54.4% of zinc oxide (ZnO: 81.38).

Method of preparation

Acrinol Hydrate, very finely powdered	10 g
Zinc Oxide Oil	990 g
To make	1000 g

Prepare by mixing the above ingredients. Acrinol Hydrate may be mixed after being dissolved in a little amount of warmed Purified Water or Purified Water in Containers. Instead of Zinc Oxide Oil adequate amounts of Zinc Oxide and vegetable oil may be used, and an adequate amount of Castor Oil or polysorbate 20 may be substituted for a part of the vegetable oil.

Description Acrinol and Zinc Oxide Oil is a yellow-white, slimy substance. Separation of a part of its ingredients occurs on prolonged standing.

Identification **(1)** Shake well 1 g of Acrinol and Zinc Oxide Oil with 10 mL of diethyl ether, 2 mL of acetic acid (100) and 10 mL of water, and separate the water layer. Shake the layer with 5 mL of hydrochloric acid and 2 to 3 drops of sodium nitrite TS, and allow to stand: a dark red color is produced (acrinol).

(2) Place 1 g of Acrinol and Zinc Oxide Oil in a crucible, melt by warming, heat, gradually raising the temperature until the mass is thoroughly charred, and then ignite strongly: a yellow color is produced, and disappears on cooling. To the residue add 10 mL of water and 5 mL of dilute hydrochloric acid, filter after thorough shaking, and to the filtrate add 2 to 3 drops of potassium hexacyanoferrate (II) TS: a white precipitate is formed (zinc oxide).

(3) Shake well 0.2 g of Acrinol and Zinc Oxide Oil with 20 mL of ethanol (95) and 1 mL of acetic acid (100), centrifuge, filter, and use the filtrate as the sample solution. Separately, dissolve 5 mg of acrinol in 50 mL of ethanol (95) and 2.5 mL of acetic acid (100), and use this solution as the standard solution. Perform the test with these solutions as directed under Thin-layer Chromatography <*2.03*>. Spot 5 μL each of the sample solution and standard solution on a plate of silica gel for thin-layer chromatography. Develop the plate with a mixture of 2-propanol and acetic acid (100) (9:1) to a distance of about 10 cm, and air-dry the plate. Examine under ultraviolet light (main wavelength: 365 nm): the spots from the sample solution and standard solution exhibit a blue fluorescence and show the same *Rf* value.

Assay Transfer about 0.8 g of well-mixed Acrinol and Zinc Oxide Oil, accurately weighed, to a crucible, heat, gradually raising the temperature until the mass is throughly charred, then strongly heat until the residue becomes yellow. After cooling, dissolve the residue by addition of 1 mL of water and 1.5 mL of hydrochloric acid, and add water to make exactly 100 mL. Pipet 20 mL of this solution, add 80 mL of water, then add sodium hydroxide solution (1 in 50) until slightly precipitates appear, and add 5 mL of ammonia-ammonium chloride buffer solution (pH 10.7). Titrate <*2.50*> with 0.05 mol/L disodium dihydrogen ethylenediamine tetraacetate VS (indicator: 40 mg of eriochrome black T-sodium chloride indicator).

Each mL of 0.05 mol/L disodium dihydrogen ethylenediamine tetraacetate VS
= 4.069 mg of ZnO

Containers and storage Containers—Tight containers.
Storage—Light-resistant.

Compound Acrinol and Zinc Oxide Oil

複方アクリノール·チンク油

Method of preparation

Acrinol Hydrate, very finely powdered	10 g
Zinc Oxide Oil	650 g
Ethyl Aminobenzoate, finely powdered	50 g
White Beeswax	20 g
Hydrophilic Petrolatum	270 g
To make	1000 g

Prepare by mixing the above ingredients.

Description Compound Acrinol and Zinc Oxide Oil is light yellow to yellow in color.

Identification **(1)** Shake well 1 g of Compound Acrinol and Zinc Oxide Oil with 10 mL of diethyl ether, 2 mL of acetic acid (100) and 10 mL of water, and separate the water layer. Shake the layer with 5 mL of hydrochloric acid and 2 to 3 drops of sodium nitrite TS, and allow to stand: a dark red color is produced (acrinol).

(2) Place 1 g of Compound Acrinol and Zinc Oxide Oil in a crucible, melt by warming, heat, gradually raising the temperature until the mass is thoroughly charred, and then ignite strongly: a yellow color is produced, and disappears on cooling. To the residue add 10 mL of water and 5 mL of dilute hydrochloric acid, shake well, and filter. To the filtrate add 2 to 3 drops of potassium hexacyanoferrate (II) TS: a white precipitate is produced (zinc oxide).

(3) Shake well 0.2 g of Compound Acrinol and Zinc Oxide Oil with 20 mL of ethanol (95) and 1 mL of acetic acid (100), centrifuge, filter, and use the filtrate as the sample solution. Separately, dissolve 5 mg of acrinol and 25 mg of ethyl aminobenzoate in 50 mL of ethanol (95) and in 2.5 mL of acetic acid (100), respectively, and use both solutions as the standard solutions (1) and (2). Perform the test with these solutions as directed under Thin-layer Chromatography <*2.03*>. Spot 5 μL each of the sample solution and standard solutions on a plate of silica gel with fluorescent indicator for thin-layer chromatography. Develop the plate with a mixture of 2-propanol and acetic acid (100) (9:1) to a distance of about 10 cm, and air-dry the plate. Examine under ultraviolet light (main wavelength: 365 nm): the spots from the sample solution and standard solution (1) exhibit a blue fluorescence, and show the same *Rf* value. Also examine under ultraviolet light (main wavelength: 254 nm): the spots from the sample solution and standard solution (2) exhibit a purple color, and show the same *Rf* value.

Containers and storage Containers—Tight containers.
Storage—Light-resistant.

Acrinol and Zinc Oxide Ointment

アクリノール·亜鉛華軟膏

Method of preparation

Acrinol Hydrate, very finely powdered	10 g
Zinc Oxide Ointment	990 g
To make	1000 g

Prepare as directed under Ointments, with the above ingredients.

Description Acrinol and Zinc oxide Ointment is yellow in color.

Identification **(1)** Shake 0.5 g of Acrinol and Zinc Oxide Ointment with 5 mL of diethyl ether, 5 mL of dilute hydrochloric acid and 2 to 3 drops of sodium nitrite TS, and allow to stand: a dark red color develops in the water layer (acrinol).

(2) Ignite 0.5 g of Acrinol and Zinc Oxide Ointment to char, and dissolve the residue in 5 mL of dilute hydrochloric acid: the solution responds to Qualitative Tests <*1.09*> for zinc salt.

(3) Shake 0.5 g of Acrinol and Zinc Oxide Ointment with 5 mL of diethyl ether, 1 mL of acetic acid (100) and 5 mL of water, separate the water layer, and use the water layer as the sample solution. Dissolve 5 mg of acrinol in 1 mL of acetic acid (100) and 5 mL of water, and use this solution as the standard solution. Perform the test with these solutions as directed under Thin-layer Chromatography <*2.03*>. Spot 5 μL each of the sample solution and standard solution on a plate of silica gel for thin-layer chromatography. Develop the plate with a mixture of diethyl ether, ethanol (95) and acetic acid (100) (40:10:1) to a distance of about 10 cm, and air-dry the plate. Examine under ultraviolet light (main wavelength: 365 nm): the spots from the sample solution and the standard solution exhibit a blue fluorescence and show the same *Rf* value.

Containers and storage Containers—Tight containers.
Storage—Light-resistant.

Actinomycin D

Dactinomycin

アクチノマイシンD

MeGly = *N*-Methylglycine
MeVal = *N*-Methylvaline

$C_{62}H_{86}N_{12}O_{16}$: 1255.42
[50-76-0]

Actinomycin D is a peptide substance having antitumor activity produced by the growth of *Streptomyces parvulus*.

It, when dried, contains not less than 950 μg (potency) and not more than 1030 μg (potency) per mg. The potency of Actinomycin D is expressed as mass (potency) of actinomycin D ($C_{62}H_{86}N_{12}O_{16}$).

Description Actinomycin D occurs as an orange-red to red crystalline powder.

It is freely soluble in acetone, sparingly soluble in acetonitrile and in methanol, slightly soluble in ethanol (99.5), and very slightly soluble in water.

Identification **(1)** Determine the absorption spectrum of a solution of Actinomycin D in methanol (3 in 100,000) as directed under Ultraviolet-visible Spectrophotometry <*2.24*>, and compare the spectrum with the Reference Spectrum or the spectrum of a solution of Actinomycin D RS prepared in the same manner as the sample solution: both spectra exhibit similar intensities of absorption at the same wavelengths.

(2) Dissolve 0.1 g each of Actinomycin D and Actinomycin D RS in 10 mL of acetone, and use these solutions as the sample solution and standard solution. Perform the test with these solutions as directed under Thin-layer Chromatography <*2.03*>. Spot 10 μL each of the sample solution and standard solution on a plate of silica gel with fluorescent indicator for thin-layer chromatography. Develop the plate with a mixture of 1-butanol, water and methanol (4:2:1) to a distance of about 10 cm, and air-dry the plate. Examine under ultraviolet light (main wavelength: 254 nm): the *R*f value of the principal spot from the sample solution is the same as that from the standard solution.

Optical rotation <*2.49*> $[\alpha]_D^{20}$: $-293 - -329°$ (after drying, 10 mg, methanol, 10 mL, 100 mm).

Loss on drying <*2.41*> Not more than 5.0% (1 g, in vacuum, 60°C, 3 hours).

Assay Weigh accurately an amount of Actinomycin D and Actinomycin D RS, previously dried, equivalent to about 60 mg (potency), dissolve each in the mobile phase to make exactly 50 mL, and use these solutions as the sample solution and standard solution. Perform the test with exactly 25 μL each of the sample solution and standard solution as directed under Liquid Chromatography <*2.01*> according to the following conditions, and determine the peak area of actinomycin D, A_T and A_S, in each solution.

Amount [μg (potency)] of actinomycin D ($C_{62}H_{86}N_{12}O_{16}$)
$= M_S \times A_T/A_S \times 1000$

M_S: Amount [mg (potency)] of Actinomycin D RS taken

Operating conditions—

Detector: An ultraviolet absorption photometer (wavelength: 254 nm).

Column: A stainless steel column 3.9 mm in inside diameter and 30 cm in length, packed with octadecylsilanized silica gel for liquid chromatography (10 μm in particle diameter).

Column temperature: A constant temperature of about 25°C.

Mobile phase: A mixture of 0.02 mol/L acetic acid-sodium acetate TS and acetonitrile (25:23).

Flow rate: Adjust so that the retention time of actinomycin D is about 23 minutes.

System suitability—

System performance: When the procedure is run with 25 μL of the standard solution under the above operating conditions, the number of theoretical plates and the symmetry factor of the peak of actinomycin D are not less than 2000 and not more than 1.5, respectively.

System repeatability: When the test is repeated 5 times with 25 μL of the standard solution under the above operating conditions, the relative standard deviation of the peak area of actinomycin D is not more than 2.0%.

Containers and storage Containers—Tight containers.
Storage—Light-resistant.

Adrenaline

Epinephrine

アドレナリン

$C_9H_{13}NO_3$: 183.20
4-[(1*R*)-1-Hydroxy-2-(methylamino)ethyl]benzene-1,2-diol
[51-43-4]

Adrenaline, when dried, contains not less than 98.0% and not more than 101.0% of adrenaline ($C_9H_{13}NO_3$).

Description Adrenaline occurs as a white to grayish white crystalline powder.

It is freely soluble in formic acid and in acetic acid (100), very slightly soluble in water, and practically insoluble in methanol and in ethanol (99.5).

It dissolves in dilute hydrochloric acid.

It gradually changes to brown in color by air and by light.

Identification **(1)** Determine the absorption spectrum of a solution of Adrenaline in 0.01 mol/L hydrochloric acid TS (1 in 25,000) as directed under Ultraviolet-visible Spectrophotometry <*2.24*>, and compare the spectrum with the Reference Spectrum: both spectra exhibit similar intensities of absorption at the same wavelengths.

(2) Determine the infrared absorption spectrum of Adrenaline as directed in the potassium bromide disk method under Infrared Spectrophotometry <*2.25*>, and compare the spectrum with the Reference Spectrum: both spectra exhibit similar intensities of absorption at the same wave numbers.

Optical rotation <*2.49*> $[\alpha]_D^{20}$: −50.0 − −53.5° (after drying, 1 g, 1 mol/L hydrochloric acid TS, 25 mL, 100 mm).

Purity **(1)** Clarity and color of solution—Dissolve 0.10 g of Adrenaline in 10 mL of dilute hydrochloric acid: the solution is clear, and is not more colored than Matching Fluid A.

(2) Heavy metals <*1.07*>—Proceed with 1.0 g of Adrenaline according to Method 4, and perform the test. Prepare the control solution with 2.0 mL of Standard Lead Solution (not more than 20 ppm).

(3) Adrenalone—Dissolve 50 mg of Adrenaline in 0.05 mol/L hydrochloric acid TS to make exactly 25 mL, and determine the absorbance of this solution at 310 nm as directed under Ultraviolet-visible Spectrophotometry <*2.24*>: it is not more than 0.2.

(4) Noradrenaline—Dissolve 0.20 g of Adrenaline in 1 mL of formic acid, add methanol to make exactly 10 mL, and use this solution as the sample solution. Separately, dissolve 8.0 mg of Noradrenaline Bitartrate RS in methanol to make exactly 10 mL, and use this solution as the standard solution. Perform the test with these solutions as directed under Thin-layer Chromatography <*2.03*>. Spot 5 μL each of the sample solution and standard solution on a plate of silica gel with fluorescent indicator for thin-layer chromatography. Develop the plate with a mixture of 1-butanol, water and formic acid (7:2:1) to a distance of about 10 cm, and air-dry the plate. Spray evenly Folin's TS on the plate: the spot obtained from the sample solution, corresponding to the spot from the standard solution, is not more intense than the spot from the standard solution.

Loss on drying <*2.41*> Not more than 1.0% (1 g, in vacuum, silica gel, 18 hours).

Residue on ignition <*2.44*> Not more than 0.1% (1 g).

Assay Weigh accurately about 0.3 g of Adrenaline, previously dried, dissolve in 50 mL of acetic acid (100), and titrate <*2.50*> with 0.1 mol/L perchloric acid VS (potentiometric titration). Perform a blank determination in the same manner, and make any necessary correction.

Each mL of 0.1 mol/L perchloric acid VS
= 18.32 mg of $C_9H_{13}NO_3$

Containers and storage Containers—Tight containers.

Storage—Light-resistant, and under Nitrogen atmosphere.

Adrenaline Injection

Epinephrine Injection

アドレナリン注射液

Adrenaline Injection is an aqueous injection.

It contains not less than 0.085 w/v% and not more than 0.115 w/v% of adrenaline ($C_9H_{13}NO_3$: 183.20).

Method of preparation Dissolve Adrenaline in diluted Hydrochloric Acid (9 in 10,000), and prepare as directed under Injections.

Description Adrenaline Injection is a colorless, clear liquid.

It changes gradually to pale red and then to brown on exposure to air and light.

pH: 2.3 − 5.0

Identification **(1)** To 1 mL of Adrenaline Injection add 4 mL of water and 1 drop of iron (III) chloride TS: a deep green color is produced, and it gradually changes to red.

(2) Place 1 mL each of Adrenaline Injection in test tubes A and B, and proceed as directed in the Identification (2) under Adrenaline.

Extractable volume <*6.05*> It meets the requirement.

Assay Pipet 30 mL of Adrenaline Injection into a separator, add 25 mL of carbon tetrachloride, shake vigorously for 1 minute, allow the liquids to separate, and discard the carbon tetrachloride. Repeat this procedure three times. Rinse the stopper and mouth of the separator with a small amount of water. Add 0.2 mL of starch TS, then while swirling the separator add iodine TS dropwise until a persistent blue color develops, and immediately add sodium thiosulfate TS to discharge the blue color. Add 2.1 g of sodium hydrogen carbonate to the liquid in the separator, preventing it from coming in contact with the mouth of the separator, and shake until most of the sodium hydrogen carbonate dissolves. Rapidly inject 1.0 mL of acetic anhydride into the contents of the separator. Immediately stopper the separator loosely, and allow to stand until the evolution of gas ceases. Shake vigorously, allow to stand for 5 minutes, extract with six 25-mL portions of chloroform, and filter each chloroform extract through a pledget of absorbent cotton. Evaporate the combined chloroform extracts on a water bath in a current of air to 3 mL, completely transfer this residue by means of small portions of chloroform to a tared beaker, and heat again to evaporate to dryness. Dry the residue at 105°C for 30 minutes, cool in a desiccator (silica gel), and accurately measure the mass M (mg) of the dried residue. Dissolve in chloroform to make exactly 5 mL, and determine the optical rotation <*2.49*> $[\alpha]_D^{20}$ using a 100-mm cell.

Amount (mg) of adrenaline ($C_9H_{13}NO_3$)
$= M \times \{0.5 + (0.5 \times |[\alpha]_D^{20}|)/93\} \times 0.592$

Containers and storage Containers—Hermetic containers, and colored containers may be used.

Storage—Light-resistant.

Adrenaline Solution

Epinephrine Solution

アドレナリン液

Adrenaline Solution contains not less than 0.085 w/v% and not more than 0.115 w/v% of adrenaline ($C_9H_{13}NO_3$: 183.20).

Method of preparation

Adrenaline	1 g
Sodium Chloride	8.5 g
Diluted Hydrochloric Acid (9 in 100)	10 mL
Stabilizer	a suitable quantity
Preservative	a suitable quantity
Purified Water or Purified Water in Containers	a sufficient quantity
To make	1000 mL

Prepare by mixing the above ingredients.

Description Adrenaline Solution is clear, colorless or

slightly reddish liquid.

It changes gradually to pale red and then to brown on exposure to air and light.

pH: 2.3 – 5.0

Identification Proceed as directed in the Identification under Adrenaline Injection.

Assay Proceed as directed in the Assay under Adrenaline Injection.

$$\text{Amount (mg) of adrenaline } (C_9H_{13}NO_3) = M \times \{0.5 + (0.5 \times |[\alpha]_D^{20}|)/93\} \times 0.592$$

Containers and storage Containers—Tight containers.

Storage—Light-resistant.

Afloqualone

アフロクアロン

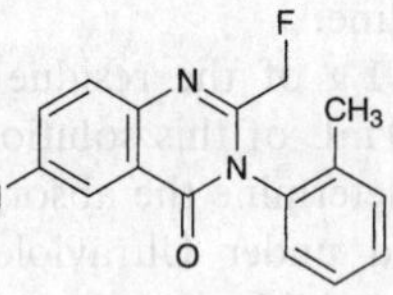

$C_{16}H_{14}FN_3O$: 283.30

6-Amino-2-fluoromethyl-3-(2-tolyl)-3*H*-quinazolin-4-one

[56287-74-2]

Afloqualone, when dried, contains not less than 98.5% of afloqualone ($C_{16}H_{14}FN_3O$).

Description Afloqualone occurs as white to light yellow, crystals or crystalline powder.

It is soluble in acetonitrile, sparingly soluble in ethanol (99.5), and practically insoluble in water.

It is gradually colored by light.

Melting point: about 197°C (with decomposition).

Identification **(1)** Conduct this procedure without exposure to light, using light-resistant containers. Determine the absorption spectrum of a solution of Afloqualone in ethanol (99.5) (1 in 150,000) as directed under Ultraviolet-visible Spectrophotometry <*2.24*>, and compare the spectrum with the Reference Spectrum: both spectra exhibit similar intensities of absorption at the same wavelengths.

(2) Determine the infrared absorption spectrum of Afloqualone, previously dried, as directed in the potassium bromide disk method under Infrared Spectrophotometry <*2.25*>, and compare the spectrum with the Reference Spectrum: both spectra exhibit similar intensities of absorption at the same wave numbers.

Purity **(1)** Acidity or alkalinity—Take 1.0 g of Afloqualone in a light-resistant vessel, add 20 mL of freshly boiled and cooled water, shake well, and filter. To 10 mL of the filtrate add 2 drops of bromothymol blue TS: a yellow color develops. The color changes to blue by adding 0.20 mL of 0.01 mol/L sodium hydroxide TS.

(2) Heavy metals <*1.07*>—Proceed with 2.0 g of Afloqualone in a platinum crucible according to Method 2, and perform the test. Prepare the control solution with 2.0 mL of Standard Lead Solution (not more than 10 ppm).

(3) Related substances—Conduct this procedure without exposure to light, using light-resistant vessels. Dissolve 10 mg of Afloqualone in 25 mL of the mobile phase, and use this solution as the sample solution. Pipet 3 mL of the sample solution, add the mobile phase to make exactly 100 mL. Pipet 2 mL of this solution, add the mobile phase to make exactly 20 mL, and use this solution as the standard solution. Perform the test with exactly 20 μL each of the sample solution and standard solution as directed under Liquid Chromatography <*2.01*> according to the following conditions. Determine each peak area by the automatic integration method: the total area of the peaks other than afloqualone from the sample solution is not larger than the peak area of afloqualone from the standard solution.

Operating conditions—

Detector: An ultraviolet absorption photometer (wavelength: 254 nm).

Column: A stainless steel column 4.6 mm in inside diameter and 15 cm in length, packed with octylsilanized silica gel for liquid chromatography (5 μm in particle diameter).

Column temperature: A constant temperature of about 40°C.

Mobile phase: Dissolve 7.2 g of disodium hydrogen phosphate dodecahydrate in 1000 mL of water, adjust to pH 5.5 with diluted phosphoric acid (1 in 10). To 600 mL of this solution add 400 mL of acetonitrile.

Flow rate: Adjust so that the retention time of afloqualone is about 5.5 minutes.

Time span of measurement: About 4 times as long as the retention time of afloqualone, beginning after the solvent peak.

System suitability—

Test for required detectability: Pipet 5 mL of the standard solution, add the mobile phase to make exactly 25 mL, and confirm that the peak area of afloqualone obtained with 20 μL of this solution is equivalent to 15 to 25% of that with 20 μL of the standard solution.

System performance: Dissolve 0.01 g of Afloqualone in a suitable amount of the mobile phase, add 5 mL of a solution of propyl parahydroxybenzoate in the mobile phase (1 in 2000) and the mobile phase to make 100 mL. When the procedure is run with 20 μL of this solution under the above operating conditions, afloqualone and propyl parahydroxybenzoate are eluted in this order with the resolution between these peaks being not less than 4.

System repeatability: When the test is repeated 6 times with 20 μL of the standard solution under the above operating conditions, the relative standard deviation of the peak areas of afloqualone is not more than 5%.

Loss on drying <*2.41*> Not more than 0.5% (1 g, in vacuum, 60°C, 2 hours).

Residue on ignition <*2.44*> Not more than 0.1% (1.0 g, platinum crucible).

Assay Weigh accurately about 0.4 g of Afloqualone, previously dried, dissolve in 10 mL of hydrochloric acid and 40 mL of water, and add 10 mL of a solution of potassium bromide (3 in 10). After cooling at 15°C or below, titrate <*2.50*> with 0.1 mol/L sodium nitrite VS according to the potentiometric titration or amperometric titration under the Electrometric Titration method.

$$\text{Each mL of 0.1 mol/L sodium nitrite} = 28.33 \text{ mg of } C_{16}H_{14}FN_3O$$

Containers and storage Containers—Tight containers.

Storage—Light-resistant.

Ajmaline

アジマリン

$C_{20}H_{26}N_2O_2$: 326.43
(17*R*,21*R*)-Ajmalan-17,21-diol
[*4360-12-7*]

Ajmaline, when dried, contains not less than 96.0% of ajmaline ($C_{20}H_{26}N_2O_2$).

Description Ajmaline occurs as a white to pale yellow crystalline powder. It is odorless, and has a bitter taste.

It is freely soluble in acetic anhydride and in chloroform, sparingly soluble in methanol, in ethanol (95), in acetone and in diethyl ether, and very slightly soluble in water.

It dissolves in dilute hydrochloric acid.

Melting point: about 195°C (with decomposition).

Identification **(1)** Dissolve 0.05 g of Ajmaline in 5 mL of methanol, and use this solution as the sample solution. Add 3 mL of nitric acid to 1 mL of the sample solution: a deep red color develops.

(2) Spot the sample solution of (1) on filter paper, and spray Dragendorff's TS: an orange color develops.

Absorbance <*2.24*> $E^{1\%}_{1\,cm}$ (249 nm): 257 – 271 (after drying, 2 mg, ethanol (95), 100 mL).

$E^{1\%}_{1\,cm}$ (292 nm): 85 – 95 (after drying, 2 mg, ethanol (95), 100 mL).

Optical rotation <*2.49*> $[\alpha]^{20}_{D}$: +136 – +151° (after drying, 0.5 g, chloroform, 50 mL, 100 mm).

Purity Related substances—Dissolve 0.10 g of Ajmaline in 10 mL of chloroform, and use this solution as the sample solution. Pipet 1 mL of the sample solution, add chloroform to make exactly 100 mL, and use this solution as the standard solution. Perform the test with these solutions as directed under Thin-layer Chromatography <*2.03*>. Spot 10 μL each of the sample solution and standard solution on a plate of silica gel with fluorescent indicator for thin-layer chromatography. Develop the plate with a mixture of chloroform, acetone and diethylamine (5:4:1) to a distance of about 10 cm, and air-dry the plate. Examine under ultraviolet light (main wavelength: 254 nm): the spots other than the principal spot obtained from the sample solution are not more intense than the spot from the standard solution.

Loss on drying <*2.41*> Not more than 1.0% (0.6 g, in vacuum, 80°C, 3 hours).

Residue on ignition <*2.44*> Not more than 0.2% (0.5 g).

Assay Weigh accurately about 0.3 g of Ajmaline, previously dried, dissolve in 50 mL of acetic anhydride and 50 mL of acetone for nonaqueous titration, and titrate <*2.50*> with 0.05 mol/L perchloric acid VS (potentiometric titration). Perform a blank determination in the same manner, and make any necessary correction.

Each mL of 0.05 mol/L perchloric acid VS
= 16.32 mg of $C_{20}H_{26}N_2O_2$

Containers and storage Containers—Well-closed containers.

Storage—Light-resistant.

Ajmaline Tablets

アジマリン錠

Ajmaline Tablets contain not less than 90.0% and not more than 110.0% of the labeled amount of ajmaline ($C_{20}H_{26}N_2O_2$: 326.43).

Method of preparation Prepare as directed under Tablets, with Ajmaline.

Identification **(1)** Shake a quantity of powdered Ajmaline Tablets, equivalent to 0.1 g of Ajmaline, with 30 mL of chloroform, and filter. Evaporate the filtrate on a water bath to dryness. With the residue, proceed as directed in the Identification under Ajmaline.

(2) Dissolve 0.01 g of the residue of (1) in 100 mL of ethanol (95). To 10 mL of this solution add ethanol (95) to make 50 mL, and determine the absorption spectrum of the solution as directed under Ultraviolet-visible Spectrophotometry <*2.24*>: it exhibits maxima between 247 nm and 251 nm and between 291 nm and 294 nm, and a minimum between 269 nm and 273 nm.

Uniformity of dosage units <*6.02*> Perform the test according to the following method: it meets the requirement of the Content uniformity test.

To 1 tablet of Ajmaline Tablets add 150 mL of 2nd fluid for dissolution test, shake to disintegrate the tablet, then add 2nd fluid for dissolution test to make exactly 200 mL, and filter this solution through a membrane filter with a pore size not exceeding 0.8 μm. Discard the first 10 mL of the filtrate, pipet *V* mL of the subsequent filtrate equivalent to about 0.5 mg of ajmaline ($C_{20}H_{26}N_2O_2$), add 2nd fluid for dissolution test to make exactly 10 mL, and use this solution as the sample solution. Separately, weigh accurately about 25 mg of ajmaline for assay, previously dried in vacuum at 80°C for 3 hours, dissolve in 2nd fluid for dissolution test to make exactly 500 mL, and use this solution as the standard solution. Determine the absorbances at 288 nm, A_T and A_S, of the sample solution and standard solution as directed under Ultraviolet-visible Spectrophotometry <*2.24*>.

$$\text{Amount (mg) of ajmaline } (C_{20}H_{26}N_2O_2) = M_S \times A_T/A_S \times 1/V \times 4$$

M_S: Amount (mg) of ajmaline for assay taken

Dissolution <*6.10*> When the test is performed at 100 revolutions per minute according to the Paddle method, using 900 mL of 2nd fluid for dissolution test as the dissolution medium, the dissolution rate in 60 minutes of Ajmaline Tablets is not less than 75%.

Start the test with 1 tablet of Ajmaline Tablets, withdraw not less than 20 mL of the medium at the specified minute after starting the test, and filter through a membrane filter with a pore size not exceeding 0.8 μm. Discard not less than 10 mL of the first filtrate, pipet *V* mL of the subsequent filtrate, add the dissolution medium to make exactly *V′* mL so that each mL contains about 56 μg of ajmaline ($C_{20}H_{26}N_2O_2$), and use this solution as the sample solution. Separately, weigh accurately about 28 mg of ajmaline for assay, previously dried in vacuum at 80°C for 3 hours, dissolve in the dissolution medium to make exactly 500 mL, and use this solution as the standard solution. Determine the absorbances, A_T and A_S, of the sample solution and standard solution at 288 nm as directed under Ultraviolet-visible Spectrophotometry ⟨*2.24*⟩.

Dissolution rate (%) with respect to the labeled amount of ajmaline ($C_{20}H_{26}N_2O_2$)

$$= M_S \times A_T/A_S \times V'/V \times 1/C \times 180$$

M_S: Amount (mg) of ajmaline for assay taken

C: Labeled amount (mg) of ajmaline ($C_{20}H_{26}N_2O_2$) in 1 tablet

Assay Weigh accurately and powder not less than 20 Ajmaline Tablets. Weigh accurately a portion of the powder, equivalent to about 0.3 g of ajmaline ($C_{20}H_{26}N_2O_2$), add 15 mL of ammonia solution (28), and extract with four 25-mL portions of chloroform. Combine the chloroform extracts, wash with 10 mL of water, add 5 g of anhydrous sodium sulfate, shake well, and filter. Wash the container and the residue with two 10-mL portions of chloroform, and filter. Evaporate the combined filtrate on a water bath to dryness, dissolve the residue in 50 mL of acetic anhydride and 50 mL of acetone for nonaqueous titration, and titrate ⟨*2.50*⟩ with 0.05 mol/L perchloric acid VS (potentiometric titration). Perform a blank determination in the same manner, and make any necessary correction.

Each mL of 0.05 mol/L perchloric acid VS
$= 16.32$ mg of $C_{20}H_{26}N_2O_2$

Containers and storage Containers—Well-closed containers.

Storage—Light-resistant.

Alacepril

アラセプリル

$C_{20}H_{26}N_2O_5S$: 406.50

(2*S*)-2-{(2*S*)-1-[(2*S*)-3-(Acetylsulfanyl)-2-methylpropanoyl]pyrrolidine-2-carbonyl}amino-3-phenylpropanoic acid

[*74258-86-9*]

Alacepril, when dried, contains not less than 98.5% and not more than 101.0% of alacepril ($C_{20}H_{26}N_2O_5S$).

Description Alacepril occurs as white, crystals or crystalline powder.

It is freely soluble in methanol, soluble in ethanol (95), and slightly soluble in water.

It dissolves in sodium hydroxide TS.

Identification **(1)** To 20 mg of Alacepril add 0.1 g of sodium hydroxide, and heat gradually to melt: the gas evolved changes the color of a moisten red litmus paper to blue. After cooling, to the melted substance add 2 mL of water, shake, and add 1 mL of lead (II) acetate TS: a brown to black precipitate is formed.

(2) Determine the infrared absorption spectrum of Alacepril, previously dried, as directed in the potassium bromide disk method under Infrared Spectrophotometry ⟨*2.25*⟩, and compare the spectrum with the Reference Spectrum: both spectra exhibit similar intensities of absorption at the same wave numbers.

Optical rotation ⟨*2.49*⟩ $[\alpha]_D^{20}$: −81 – −85° (after drying, 0.25 g, ethanol (95), 25 mL, 100 mm).

Melting point ⟨*2.60*⟩ 153 – 157°C

Purity **(1)** Chloride ⟨*1.03*⟩—Dissolve 0.5 g of Alacepril in 30 mL of methanol, add 6 mL of dilute nitric acid and water to make 50 mL, and perform the test with this solution as the test solution. Prepare the control solution as follows: to 0.30 mL of 0.01 mol/L hydrochloric acid VS add 30 mL of methanol, 6 mL of dilute nitric acid and water to make 50 mL (not more than 0.021%).

(2) Sulfate ⟨*1.14*⟩—Dissolve 0.5 g of Alacepril in 30 mL of methanol, add 1 mL of dilute hydrochloric acid and water to make 50 mL, and perform the test using this solution as the test solution. Prepare the control solution as follows: to 0.50 mL of 0.005 mol/L sulfuric acid VS add 30 mL of methanol, 1 mL of dilute hydrochloric acid and water to make 50 mL (not more than 0.048%).

(3) Heavy metals ⟨*1.07*⟩—Proceed with 1.0 g of Alacepril according to Method 2, and perform the test. Prepare the control solution with 2.0 mL of Standard Lead Solution (not more than 20 ppm).

(4) Related substances—Dissolve 50 mg of Alacepril in 5 mL of ethanol (95), and use this solution as the sample solution. Pipet 1 mL of the sample solution, add ethanol (95) to make exactly 200 mL, and use this solution as the standard solution. Perform the test with exactly 10 μL each of the sample solution and standard solution as directed under Liquid Chromatography ⟨*2.01*⟩ according to the following conditions, and determine each peak area by the automatic integration method: the area of the peak other than alacepril from the sample solution is not larger than 2/5 times the peak area of alacepril from the standard solution, and the total area of the peaks other than alacepril from the sample solution is not larger than the peak area of alacepril from the standard solution. For the areas of the peaks, having the relative retention times of about 2.3 and about 2.6 to alacepril, multiply their correction factors, 1.5 and 1.9, respectively.

Operating conditions—

Detector: An ultraviolet absorption photometer (wavelength: 254 nm).

Column: A stainless steel column 4.6 mm in inside diameter and 15 cm in length, packed with octadecylsilanized silica gel for liquid chromatography (5 μm in particle diameter).

Column temperature: A constant temperature of about 40°C.

Mobile phase: A mixture of diluted acetic acid (100) (1 in 100), acetonitrile, methanol and tetrahydrofuran (6:2:1:1).

Flow rate: Adjust so that the retention time of alacepril is about 5 minutes.

Time span of measurement: About 3 times as long as the retention time of alacepril, beginning after the solvent peak.

System suitability—

Test for required detectability: To exactly 4 mL of the standard solution add ethanol (95) to make exactly 10 mL. Confirm that the peak area of alacepril obtained with 10 μL of this solution is equivalent to 30 to 50% of that obtained with 10 μL of the standard solution.

System performance: Dissolve 20 mg of Alacepril in 50 mL of a solution of propyl parahydroxybenzoate in ethanol (95) (1 in 80,000). When the procedure is run with 10 μL of this solution under the above operating conditions, alacepril and propyl parahydroxybenzoate are eluted in this order with the resolution between these peaks being not less than 7.

System repeatability: When the test is repeated 6 times with 10 μL of the standard solution under the above operating conditions, the relative standard deviation of the peak area of alacepril is not more than 2.0%.

Loss on drying *<2.41>* Not more than 1.0% (1 g, 105°C, 3 hours).

Residue on ignition *<2.44>* Not more than 0.1% (1 g).

Assay Weigh accurately about 0.6 g of Alacepril, previously dried, dissolve in 75 mL of a mixture of methanol and water (2:1), and titrate *<2.50>* with 0.1 mol/L sodium hydroxide VS (potentiometric titration). Perform a blank determination in the same manner, and make any necessary correction.

Each mL of 0.1 mol/L sodium hydroxide VS
= 40.65 mg of $C_{20}H_{26}N_2O_5S$

Containers and storage Containers—Tight containers.

Alacepril Tablets

アラセプリル錠

Alacepril Tablets contain not less than 95.0% and not more than 105.0% of the labeled amount of alacepril ($C_{20}H_{26}N_2O_5S$: 406.50).

Method of preparation Prepare as directed under Tablets, with Alacepril.

Identification Shake well a quantity of powdered Alacepril Tablets, equivalent to 0.1 g of Alacepril, with 10 mL of ethanol (95), filter, and use the filtrate as the sample solution. Separately, dissolve 10 mg of alacepril in 1 mL of ethanol (95), and use this solution as the standard solution. Perform the test with these solutions as directed under Thin-layer Chromatography *<2.03>*. Spot 5 μL each of the sample solution and standard solution on a plate of silica gel with fluorescent indicator for thin-layer chromatography, develop the plate with a mixture of ethanol (99.5) and hexane (2:1) to a distance of about 10 cm, and air-dry the plate. Examine under ultraviolet light (main wavelength: 254 nm): the principal spot from the sample solution and the spot from the standard solution show the same color tone and *R*f value.

Uniformity of dosage units *<6.02>* Perform the Mass variation test, or the Content uniformity test according to the following method: it meets the requirement.

To 1 tablet of Alacepril Tablets add 2 mL of water, sonicate to disperse the particle, and add exactly 2 mL of the internal standard solution for every 10 mg of alacepril ($C_{20}H_{26}N_2O_5S$). To this solution add a suitable amount of methanol, extract for 15 minutes with the aid of ultrasonic wave while occasional shaking, and shake more 15 minutes. Add methanol to make *V* mL so that each mL of the solution contains about 0.5 mg of alacepril ($C_{20}H_{26}N_2O_5S$), centrifuge, and use the supernatant liquid as the sample solution. Separately, weigh accurately about 25 mg of alacepril for assay, previously dried at 105°C for 3 hours, add exactly 5 mL of the internal standard solution and methanol to make 50 mL, and use this solution as the standard solution. Perform the test with 10 μL each of the sample solution and standard solution as directed under Liquid Chromatography *<2.01>* according to the following conditions, and calculate the ratios, Q_T and Q_S, of the peak area of alacepril to that of the internal standard.

$$\text{Amount (mg) of alacepril } (C_{20}H_{26}N_2O_5S) = M_S \times Q_T/Q_S \times V/50$$

M_S: Amount (mg) of alacepril for assay taken

Internal standard solution—A solution of propyl parahydroxybenzoate in methanol (3 in 20,000).

Operating conditions—

Proceed as directed in the operating conditions in the Assay.

System suitability—

Proceed as directed in the system suitability in the Assay.

Dissolution *<6.10>* When the test is performed at 50 revolutions per minute according to the Paddle method, using 900 mL of water as the dissolution medium, the dissolution rate of a 12.5-mg tablet and a 25-mg tablet in 30 minutes is not less than 75%, and that of a 50-mg tablet in 30 minutes is not less than 70%.

Start the test with 1 tablet of Alacepril Tablets, withdraw not less than 20 mL of the medium at the specified minute after starting the test, and filter through a membrane filter with a pore size not exceeding 0.45 μm. Discard not less than 10 mL of the first filtrate, pipet *V* mL of the subsequent filtrate, add water to make exactly *V′* mL so that each mL contains about 14 μg of alacepril ($C_{20}H_{26}N_2O_5S$), and use this solution as the sample solution. Separately, weigh accurately about 14 mg of alacepril for assay, previously dried at 105°C for 3 hours, dissolve in 2 mL of methanol, and add water to make exactly 100 mL. Pipet 5 mL of this solution, add water to make exactly 50 mL, and use this solution as the standard solution. Determine the absorbances, A_{T1} and A_{S1}, at 230 nm, and A_{T2} and A_{S2}, at 300 nm, of the sample solution and standard solution as directed under Ultraviolet-visible Spectrophotometry *<2.24>*, using water as the blank.

Dissolution rate (%) with respect to the labeled amount of alacepril ($C_{20}H_{26}N_2O_5S$)

$$= M_S \times (A_{T1} - A_{T2})/(A_{S1} - A_{S2}) \times V'/V \times 1/C \times 90$$

M_S: Amount (mg) of alacepril for assay taken
C: Labeled amount (mg) of alacepril ($C_{20}H_{26}N_2O_5S$) in 1 tablet

Assay Weigh accurately, and powder not less than 20 Alacepril Tablets. Weigh accurately a portion of the powder, equivalent to about 50 mg of alacepril ($C_{20}H_{26}N_2O_5S$), moisten with 2 mL of water, add exactly 3 mL of the internal standard solution and 40 mL of methanol, sonicate for 15 minutes, cool, and add methanol to make 50 mL. Centrifuge this solution, and use the supernatant liquid as the sample solution. Separately, weigh accurately about 50 mg of alacepril for assay, previously dried at 105°C for 3 hours, add exactly 3 mL of the internal standard solution, dissolve with methanol to make 50 mL, and use this solution as the standard solution. Perform the test with 10 μL each of the sample solution and standard solution as directed under Liquid Chromatography *<2.01>* according to the following conditions, and calculate the ratios, Q_T and Q_S, of the peak area of alacepril to that of the internal standard.

$$\text{Amount (mg) of alacepril } (C_{20}H_{26}N_2O_5S) = M_S \times Q_T/Q_S$$

M_S: Amount (mg) of alacepril for assay taken

Internal standard solution—A solution of propyl parahydroxybenzoate in methanol (1 in 2000).

Operating conditions—

Detector: An ultraviolet absorption photometer (wavelength: 254 nm).

Column: A stainless steel column 4.6 mm in inside diameter and 15 cm in length, packed with octadecylsilanized silica gel for liquid chromatography (5 μm in particle diameter).

Column temperature: A constant temperature of about 40°C.

Mobile phase: A mixture of diluted acetic acid (100) (1 in 100), acetonitrile, methanol and tetrahydrofuran (13:5:1:1).

Flow rate: Adjust so that the retention time of alacepril is about 6 minutes.

System suitability—

System performance: When the procedure is run with 10 μL of the standard solution under the above operating conditions, alacepril and the internal standard are eluted in this order with the resolution between these peaks being not less than 7.

System repeatability: When the test is repeated 6 times with 10 μL of the standard solution under the above operating conditions, the relative standard deviation of the ratio of the peak area of alacepril to that of the internal standard is not more than 1.0%.

Containers and storage Containers—Tight containers.

L-Alanine

L-アラニン

$C_3H_7NO_2$: 89.09
(2*S*)-2-Aminopropanoic acid
[*56-41-7*]

L-Alanine, when dried, contains not less than 98.5% and not more than 101.0% of L-alanine ($C_3H_7NO_2$).

Description L-Alanine occurs as white, crystals or crystalline powder. It has a slightly sweet taste.

It is freely soluble in water and in formic acid, and practically insoluble in ethanol (99.5).

It dissolves in 6 mol/L hydrochloric acid TS.

Identification Determine the infrared absorption spectrum of L-Alanine as directed in the potassium bromide disk method under Infrared Spectrophotometry <*2.25*>, and compare the spectrum with the Reference Spectrum: both spectra exhibit similar intensities of absorption at the same wave numbers.

Optical rotation <*2.49*> $[\alpha]_D^{20}$: +13.5 – +15.5° (after drying, 2.5 g, 6 mol/L hydrochloric acid TS, 25 mL, 100 mm).

pH <*2.54*> Dissolve 1.0 g of L-Alanine in 20 mL of water: the pH of the solution is between 5.7 and 6.7.

Purity **(1)** Clarity and color of solution—Dissolve 1.0 g of L-Alanine in 10 mL of water: the solution is clear and colorless.

(2) Chloride <*1.03*>—Perform the test with 0.5 g of L-Alanine. Prepare the control solution with 0.30 mL of 0.01 mol/L hydrochloric acid VS (not more than 0.021%).

(3) Sulfate <*1.14*>—Perform the test with 0.6 g of L-Alanine. Prepare the control solution with 0.35 mL of 0.005 mol/L sulfuric acid VS (not more than 0.028%).

(4) Ammonium <*1.02*>—Perform the test with 0.25 g of L-Alanine. Prepare the control solution with 5.0 mL of Standard Ammonium Solution (not more than 0.02%).

(5) Heavy metals <*1.07*>—Proceed with 1.0 g of L-Alanine according to Method 1, and perform the test. Prepare the control solution with 1.0 mL of Standard Lead Solution (not more than 10 ppm).

(6) Iron <*1.10*>—Prepare the test solution with 1.0 g of L-Alanine according to Method 1, and perform the test according to Method A. Prepare the control solution with 1.0 mL of Standard Iron Solution (not more than 10 ppm).

(7) Related substances—Weigh accurately about 0.5 g of L-Alanine, dissolve in 0.5 mL of hydrochloric acid and water to make exactly 100 mL. Pipet 10 mL of this solution, add 0.02 mol/L hydrochloric acid TS to make exactly 50 mL, and use this solution as the sample solution. Separately, accurately measure 2.5 mmol amounts of L-aspartic acid, L-threonine, L-serine, L-glutamic acid, glycine, L-alanine, L-cystine, L-valine, L-methionine, L-isoleucine, L-leucine, L-tyrosine, L-phenylalanine, L-lysine hydrochloride, ammonium chloride, L-histidine and L-arginine, dissolve in 0.1 mol/L hydrochloric acid TS to make exactly 1000 mL, and use this solution as the standard stock solution. Pipet 5 mL of the standard stock solution, add 0.02 mol/L hydrochloric acid TS to make exactly 100 mL. Pipet 4 mL of this solution, add 0.02 mol/L hydrochloric acid TS to make exactly 50 mL, and use this solution as the standard solution. Perform the test with exactly 20 μL each of the sample solution and standard solution as directed under Liquid Chromatography <*2.01*> according to the following conditions. Based on the peak heights obtained from the sample solution and standard solution, determine the mass of the amino acids other than alanine contained in 1 mL of the sample solution, and calculate the mass percent: the amount of each amino acid other than alanine is not more than 0.1%.

Operating conditions—

Detector: A visible spectrophotometer (wavelength: 570 nm).

Column: A stainless steel column 4.6 mm in inside diameter and 8 cm in length, packed with strongly acidic ion-exchange resin for liquid chromatography (Na type) composed with a sulfonated polystyrene copolymer (3 μm in particle diameter).

Column temperature: A constant temperature of about 57°C.

Chemical reaction bath temperature: A constant temperature of about 130°C.

Reaction time: About 1 minute.

Mobile phase: Prepare mobile phases A, B, C, D and E according to the following table, and add 0.1 mL of capric acid to each mobile phase.

	Mobile phase A	Mobile phase B	Mobile phase C	Mobile phase D	Mobile phase E
Citric acid monohydrate	19.80 g	22.00 g	12.80 g	6.10 g	—
Trisodium citrate dihydrate	6.19 g	7.74 g	13.31 g	26.67 g	—
Sodium chloride	5.66 g	7.07 g	3.74 g	54.35 g	—
Sodium hydroxide	—	—	—	—	8.00 g
Ethanol (99.5)	130 mL	20 mL	4 mL	—	100 mL
Thiodiglycol	5 mL	5 mL	5 mL	—	—
Benzyl alcohol	—	—	—	5 mL	—
Lauromacrogol solution (1 in 4)	4 mL	4 mL	4 mL	4 mL	4 mL
Water	Appropriate amount	Appropriate amount	Appropriate amount	Appropriate amount	Appropriate amount
Total volume	1000 mL	1000 mL	1000 mL	1000 mL	1000 mL

Changing mobile phases: When the procedure is run with 20 μL of the standard solution under the above operating conditions, switchover in sequence to mobile phases A, B, C, D and E so that aspartic acid, threonine, serine, glutamic acid, glycine, alanine, cystine, valine, methionine, isoleucine, leucine, tyrosine, phenylalanine, lysine, ammonia, histidine, and arginine are eluted in this order with the resolution between the peaks of isoleucine and leucine being not less than 1.2.

Reaction reagents: Dissolve 204 g of lithium acetate dihydrate in water, add 123 mL of acetic acid (100) and 401 mL of 1-methoxy-2-propanol, and water to make 1000 mL, introduce nitrogen for 10 minutes, and use this solution as solution (I). Separately, add 39 g of ninhydrin to 979 mL of 1-methoxy-2-propanol, introduce nitrogen for 5 minutes, add 81 mg of sodium borohydride, introduce nitrogen for 30 minutes, and use this solution as solution (II). To 1 volume of solution (I) add 1 volume of solution (II). Prepare before use.

Flow rate of mobile phase: 0.20 mL per minute.

Flow rate of reaction reagent: 0.24 mL per minute.

System suitability—

System performance: When the procedure is run with 20 μL of the standard solution under the above operating conditions, the resolution between the peaks of glycine and alanine is not less than 1.2.

System repeatability: When the test is repeated 6 times with 20 μL of the standard solution under the above operating conditions, the relative standard deviations of the peak height and retention time of each amino acid obtained from the standard solution are not more than 5.0% and not more than 1.0%, respectively.

Loss on drying *<2.41>* Not more than 0.3% (1 g, 105°C, 3 hours).

Residue on ignition *<2.44>* Not more than 0.1% (1 g).

Assay Weigh accurately about 90 mg of L-Alanine, previously dried, dissolve in 3 mL of formic acid, add 50 mL of acetic acid (100), and titrate *<2.50>* with 0.1 mol/L perchloric acid VS (potentiometric titration). Perform a blank determination in the same manner, and make any necessary correction.

Each mL of 0.1 mol/L perchloric acid VS
= 8.909 mg of $C_3H_7NO_2$

Containers and storage Containers—Tight containers.

Albumin Tannate

タンニン酸アルブミン

Albumin Tannate is a compound of tannic acid and a protein.

The label states the origin of the protein of Albumin Tannate.

Description Albumin Tannate occurs as a light brown powder. It is odorless, or has a faint, characteristic odor.

It is practically insoluble in water and in ethanol (95).

It dissolves in sodium hydroxide TS with turbidity.

Identification **(1)** To 0.1 g of Albumin Tannate add 10 mL of ethanol (95), and heat in a water bath for 3 minutes with shaking. After cooling, filter, and to 5 mL of the filtrate add 1 drop of iron (III) chloride TS: a blue-purple to bluish black color is produced. On standing, a bluish black precipitate is produced.

(2) To 0.1 g of Albumin Tannate add 5 mL of nitric acid: an orange-yellow color develops.

Purity **(1)** Acidity—Shake 1.0 g of Albumin Tannate with 50 mL of water for 5 minutes, and filter. To 25 mL of the filtrate add 1.0 mL of 0.1 mol/L sodium hydroxide VS and 2 drops of phenolphthalein TS: a red color develops.

(2) Fats—To 2.0 g of Albumin Tannate add 20 mL of petroleum benzine, shake vigorously for 15 minutes, and filter. Evaporate 10 mL of the filtrate on a water bath: the mass of the residue is not more than 50 mg.

Loss on drying *<2.41>* Not more than 6.0% (1 g, 105°C, 3 hours).

Residue on ignition *<2.44>* Not more than 1.0% (0.5 g).

Digestion test To 1.00 g of Albumin Tannate add 0.25 g of saccharated pepsin and 100 mL of water, shake well, and allow to stand for 20 minutes at 40 ± 1°C in a water bath. Add 1.0 mL of dilute hydrochloric acid, shake, and allow to stand for 3 hours at 40 ± 1°C. Cool rapidly to ordinary temperature, and filter. Wash the residue with three 10-mL portions of water, dry in a desiccator (silica gel) for 18 hours, and dry at 105°C for 5 hours: the mass of the residue is 0.50 to 0.58 g.

Containers and storage Containers—Tight containers.

Storage—Light-resistant.

Aldioxa

アルジオキサ

$C_4H_7AlN_4O_5$: 218.10

Dihydroxo[(4*RS*)-5-oxo-4-ureido-4,5-dihydro-1*H*-imidazol-2-yl]oxoaluminium

[*5579-81-7*]

Aldioxa is a condensation product of allantoin and aluminum hydroxide.

When dried, it contains not less than 65.3% and not

more than 74.3% of allantoin ($C_4H_6N_4O_3$: 158.12), and not less than 11.1% and not more than 13.0% of aluminum (Al: 26.98).

Description Aldioxa occurs as a white powder.

It is practically insoluble in water and in ethanol (99.5).

It dissolves in dilute hydrochloric acid.

A solution of Aldioxa in sodium fluoride-hydrochloric acid TS (1 in 100) shows no optical rotation.

Melting point: about 230°C (with decomposition).

Identification **(1)** Determine the infrared absorption spectrum of Aldioxa, previously dried, as directed in the potassium bromide disk method under Infrared Spectrophotometry *<2.25>*, and compare the spectrum with the Reference Spectrum: both spectra exhibit similar intensities of absorption at the same wave numbers.

(2) To 0.2 g of Aldioxa add 10 mL of dilute hydrochloric acid, dissolve by warming, and cool: the solution responds to Qualitative Tests *<1.09>* for aluminum salt.

Purity **(1)** Chloride *<1.03>*—To 0.10 g of Aldioxa add 6 mL of dilute nitric acid, boil to dissolve with shaking for 5 minutes, cool, and add water to make 50 mL. Perform the test using this solution as the test solution. Prepare the control solution with 0.40 mL of 0.01 mol/L hydrochloric acid VS (not more than 0.142%).

(2) Heavy metals *<1.07>*—To 1.0 g of Aldioxa add 3 mL of hydrochloric acid and 3 mL of water, heat gently to boil with shaking, and evaporate on a water bath to dryness. To the residue add 30 mL of water, shake under warming, cool, filter, and to the filtrate add 2 mL of dilute acetic acid and water to make 50 mL. Perform the test using this solution as the test solution. Prepare the control solution as follows: evaporate 3 mL of hydrochloric acid on a water bath to dryness, and add 2.0 mL of Standard Lead Solution, 2 mL of dilute acetic acid and water to make 50 mL (not more than 20 ppm).

Loss on drying *<2.41>* Not more than 4.0% (1 g, 105°C, 2 hours).

Assay **(1)** Allantoin—Weigh accurately about 0.1 g of Aldioxa, previously dried, dissolve in 50 mL of dilute sulfuric acid by heating, cool, and add water to make exactly 100 mL. Pipet 10 mL of this solution, and perform the test as directed under Nitrogen Determination *<1.08>*.

Each mL of 0.005 mol/L sulfuric acid VS
= 0.3953 mg of $C_4H_6N_4O_3$

(2) Aluminum—Weigh accurately about 0.2 g of Aldioxa, previously dried, dissolve carefully in 50 mL of dilute hydrochloric acid by heating, cool, and add dilute hydrochloric acid to make exactly 100 mL. Pipet 4 mL of this solution, add water to make exactly 25 mL, and use this solution as the sample solution. Separately, pipet a suitable quantity of Standard Aluminum Stock Solution, dilute with water so that each mL of the solution contains not less than 16.0 μg and not more than 64.0 μg of aluminum (Al: 26.98), and use this solution as the standard solution. Perform the test with the sample solution and standard solution as directed under Atomic Absorption Spectrophotometry *<2.23>* according to the following conditions, and calculate the aluminum content of the sample solution from the calibration curve obtained from the absorbance of the standard solution.

Gas: Combustible gas—Acetylene.
Supporting gas—Nitrous oxide.
Lamp: An aluminum hollow cathode lamp.
Wavelength: 309.2 nm.

Containers and storage Containers—Well-closed containers.

Aldioxa Granules

アルジオキサ顆粒

Aldioxa Granules contain not less than 95.0% and not more than 105.0% of the labeled amount of aldioxa ($C_4H_7AlN_4O_5$: 218.10).

Method of preparation Prepare as directed under Granules, with Aldioxa.

Identification **(1)** Determine the absorption spectrum of the sample solution obtained in the Assay as directed under Ultraviolet-visible Spectrophotometry *<2.24>*: it exhibits a maximum between 221 nm and 225 nm.

(2) To a quantity of powdered Aldioxa Granules, equivalent to 0.2 g of Aldioxa, add 10 mL of dilute hydrochloric acid, boil for 5 minutes, and filter: the cooled filtrate responds to Qualitative Tests *<1.09>* for aluminum salt.

Uniformity of dosage units *<6.02>* Perform the test according to the following method: Aldioxa Granules in single-dose packages meet the requirement of the Content uniformity test.

To the total content of 1 package of Aldioxa Granules add 80 mL of sodium fluoride-hydrochloric acid TS, shake for 20 minutes, add sodium fluoride-hydrochloric acid TS to make exactly 100 mL, and filter. Pipet V mL of the filtrate, add diluted ammonia-ammonium chloride buffer solution (pH 10.0) (1 in 10) to make exactly V' mL so that each mL contains about 20 μg of aldioxa ($C_4H_7AlN_4O_5$), and use this solution as the sample solution. Then, proceed as directed in the Assay.

$$\text{Amount (mg) of aldioxa } (C_4H_7AlN_4O_5) = M_S \times A_T/A_S \times V'/V \times 1/25$$

M_S: Amount (mg) of aldioxa for assay taken

Dissolution *<6.10>* When the test is performed at 50 revolutions per minute according to the Paddle method, using 900 mL of water as the dissolution medium, the dissolution rate in 15 minutes of Aldioxa Granules is not less than 85%.

Start the test with an accurately weighed amount of Aldioxa Granules, equivalent to about 0.1 g of aldioxa ($C_4H_7AlN_4O_5$), withdraw not less than 20 mL of the medium at the specified minute after starting the test, and filter through a membrane filter with a pore size not exceeding 0.45 μm. Discard not less than 10 mL of the first filtrate, pipet 10 mL of the subsequent filtrate, add diluted ammonia-ammonium chloride buffer solution (pH 10.0) (1 in 10) to make exactly 50 mL, and use this solution as the sample solution. Separately, weigh accurately about 28 mg of aldioxa for assay, previously dried at 105°C for 2 hours, and dissolve in sodium fluoride-hydrochloric acid TS to make exactly 25 mL. Pipet 1 mL of this solution, add diluted ammonia-ammonium chloride buffer solution (pH 10.0) (1 in 10) to make exactly 50 mL, and use this solution as the standard solution. Determine the absorbances, A_T and A_S, at 223 nm of the sample solution and standard solution as directed under Ultraviolet-visible Spectrophotometry *<2.24>*.

Dissolution rate (%) with respect to the labeled amount of aldioxa ($C_4H_7AlN_4O_5$)

$$= M_S/M_T \times A_T/A_S \times 1/C \times 360$$

M_S: Amount (mg) of aldioxa for assay taken
M_T: Amount (g) of Aldioxa Granules taken
C: Labeled amount (mg) of aldioxa ($C_4H_7AlN_4O_5$) in 1 g

Assay Weigh accurately an amount of powdered Aldioxa Granules, equivalent to about 0.1 g of aldioxa ($C_4H_7AlN_4O_5$), add 80 mL of sodium fluoride-hydrochloric acid TS, shake for 20 minutes, add sodium fluoride-hydrochloric acid TS to make exactly 100 mL, and filter. Pipet 2 mL of the filtrate, add diluted ammonia-ammonium chloride buffer solution (pH 10.0) (1 in 10) to make exactly 100 mL, and use this solution as the sample solution. Separately, weigh accurately about 50 mg of aldioxa for assay, previously dried at 105°C for 2 hours, and dissolve in sodium fluoride-hydrochloric acid TS to make exactly 100 mL. Pipet 4 mL of this solution, add diluted ammonia-ammonium chloride buffer solution (pH 10.0) (1 in 10) to make exactly 100 mL, and use this solution as the standard solution. Determine the absorbances, A_T and A_S, at 223 nm of the sample solution and standard solution as directed under Ultraviolet-visible Spectrophotometry <*2.24*>.

Amount (mg) of aldioxa ($C_4H_7AlN_4O_5$)

$$= M_S \times A_T/A_S \times 2$$

M_S: Amount (mg) of aldioxa for assay taken

Containers and storage Containers—Tight containers.

Aldioxa Tablets

アルジオキサ錠

Aldioxa Tablets contain not less than 95.0% and not more than 105.0% of the labeled amount of aldioxa ($C_4H_7AlN_4O_5$: 218.10).

Method of preparation Prepare as directed under Tablets, with Aldioxa.

Identification Determine the absorption spectrum of the sample solution obtained in the Assay as directed under Ultraviolet-visible Spectrophotometry <*2.24*>: it exhibits a maximum between 221 nm and 225 nm.

Uniformity of dosage units <*6.02*> Perform the Mass variation test, or the Content uniformity test according to the following method: it meets the requirement.

To 1 tablet of Aldioxa Tablets add 80 mL of sodium fluoride-hydrochloric acid TS, shake for 20 minutes, add sodium fluoride-hydrochloric acid TS to make exactly 100 mL, and filter. Pipet V mL of the filtrate, add diluted ammonia-ammonium chloride buffer solution (pH 10.0) (1 in 10) to make exactly V' mL so that each mL contains about 20 μg of aldioxa ($C_4H_7AlN_4O_5$), and use this solution as the sample solution. Then, proceed as directed in the Assay.

Amount (mg) of aldioxa ($C_4H_7AlN_4O_5$)

$$= M_S \times A_T/A_S \times V'/V \times 1/25$$

M_S: Amount (mg) of aldioxa for assay taken

Dissolution <*6.10*> When the test is performed at 50 revolutions per minute according to the Paddle method, using 900 mL of water as the dissolution medium, the dissolution rates in 15 minutes of 50-mg tablet and in 30 minutes of 100-mg tablet are not less than 80% and not less than 70%, respectively.

Start the test with 1 tablet of Aldioxa Tablets, withdraw not less than 20 mL of the medium at the specified minute after starting the test, and filter through a membrane filter with a pore size not exceeding 0.45 μm. Discard not less than 10 mL of the first filtrate, pipet V mL of the subsequent filtrate, add diluted ammonia-ammonium chloride buffer solution (pH 10.0) (1 in 10) to make exactly V' mL so that each mL contains about 22 μg of aldioxa ($C_4H_7AlN_4O_5$), and use this solution as the sample solution. Separately, weigh accurately about 28 mg of aldioxa for assay, previously dried at 105°C for 2 hours, and dissolve in sodium fluoride-hydrochloric acid TS to make exactly 25 mL. Pipet 1 mL of this solution, add diluted ammonia-ammonium chloride buffer solution (pH 10.0) (1 in 10) to make exactly 50 mL, and use this solution as the standard solution. Determine the absorbances, A_T and A_S, at 223 nm of the sample solution and standard solution as directed under Ultraviolet-visible Spectrophotometry <*2.24*>.

Dissolution rate (%) with respect to the labeled amount of aldioxa ($C_4H_7AlN_4O_5$)

$$= M_S \times A_T/A_S \times V'/V \times 1/C \times 72$$

M_S: Amount (mg) of aldioxa for assay taken
C: Labeled amount (mg) of aldioxa ($C_4H_7AlN_4O_5$) in 1 tablet

Assay Weigh accurately, and powder not less than 20 Aldioxa Tablets. Weigh accurately a portion of the powder, equivalent to about 0.1 g of aldioxa ($C_4H_7AlN_4O_5$), add 80 mL of sodium fluoride-hydrochloric acid TS, shake for 20 minutes, add sodium fluoride-hydrochloric acid TS to make exactly 100 mL, and filter. Pipet 2 mL of the filtrate, add diluted ammonia-ammonium chloride buffer solution (pH 10.0) (1 in 10) to make exactly 100 mL, and use this solution as the sample solution. Separately, weigh accurately about 50 mg of aldioxa for assay, previously dried at 105°C for 2 hours, and dissolve in sodium fluoride-hydrochloric acid TS to make exactly 100 mL. Pipet 4 mL of this solution, add diluted ammonia-ammonium chloride buffer solution (pH 10.0) (1 in 10) to make exactly 100 mL, and use this solution as the standard solution. Determine the absorbances, A_T and A_S, at 223 nm of the sample solution and standard solution as directed under Ultraviolet-visible Spectrophotometry <*2.24*>.

Amount (mg) of aldioxa ($C_4H_7AlN_4O_5$)

$$= M_S \times A_T/A_S \times 2$$

M_S: Amount (mg) of aldioxa for assay taken

Containers and storage Containers—Tight containers.

Alendronate Sodium Hydrate

アレンドロン酸ナトリウム水和物

$C_4H_{12}NNaO_7P_2.3H_2O$: 325.12
Monosodium trihydrogen 4-amino-1-hydroxybutane-1,1-diyldiphosphonate trihydrate
[121268-17-5]

Alendronate Sodium Hydrate contains not less than 99.0% and not more than 101.0% of alendronate sodium ($C_4H_{12}NNaO_7P_2$: 271.08), calculated on the dried basis.

Description Alendronate Sodium Hydrate occurs as a white crystalline powder.

It is sparingly soluble in water, and practically insoluble in ethanol (99.5).

It dissolves in 0.1 mol/L trisodium citrate TS.

Melting point: about 252°C (with decomposition, after drying).

Identification **(1)** To 5 mL of a solution of Alendronate Sodium Hydrate (1 in 50) add 1 mL of ninhydrin TS, and heat: a blue-purple color develops.

(2) Determine the infrared absorption spectrum of Alendronate Sodium Hydrate as directed in the potassium bromide disk method under Infrared Spectrophotometry *<2.25>*, and compare the spectrum with the Reference Spectrum or the spectrum of Alendronate Sodium RS: both spectra exhibit similar intensities of absorption at the same wave numbers.

(3) To 0.1 g of Alendronate Sodium Hydrate add 10 mL of a mixture of nitric acid and perchloric acid (1:1). Heat to concentrate to about 1 mL, add about 10 mL of water while hot, and neutralize with a solution of sodium hydroxide (2 in 5): the solution responds to Qualitative Tests *<1.09>* for phosphate.

(4) A solution of Alendronate Sodium Hydrate (1 in 100) responds to Qualitative Tests *<1.09>* for sodium salt.

pH *<2.54>* The pH of a solution of 1.0 g of Alendronate Sodium Hydrate in 100 mL of freshly boiled and cooled water is between 4.0 and 5.0.

Purity **(1)** Heavy metals *<1.07>*—Put 1.0 g of Alendronate Sodium Hydrate in a Kjeldahl flask, add 9 mL of a mixture of nitric acid and sulfuric acid (5:4), and heat until the solution becomes brown. After cooling, add 9 mL of a mixture of nitric acid and sulfuric acid (5:4), and heat again until the color changes from colorless to brown. After cooling, add 2 mL of nitric acid, strongly heat until brown fumes are no longer evolved, and heat until large amounts of white fumes are evolved. After cooling, add carefully 5 mL of water and 1 mL of hydrogen peroxide (30), heat until white fumes are no longer evolved, and continue heating for more 5 minutes. After cooling, if any yellow color remains, add 2 mL of nitric acid, and repeat the same procedure. After cooling, transfer the solution in the Kjeldahl flask to a beaker, wash out the inside of the flask with 5 mL of water, and add the washing to the beaker. Adjust to pH 3 – 5 with ammonia solution (28), transfer to a Nessler tube, add water to make 50 mL, and perform the test with this solution as the test solution. Prepare the control solution in the same procedure using the same amount of the reagents used for the preparation of the sample solution, add 1.0 mL of Standard Lead Solution and add water to make 50 mL (not more than 10 ppm).

(2) Related substances—Dissolve 15 mg of Alendronate Sodium Hydrate in 25 mL of 0.1 mol/L trisodium citrate TS, and use this solution as the sample stock solution. Pipet 5 mL of the sample stock solution, and add 0.1 mol/L trisodium citrate TS to make exactly 50 mL. Pipet 1 mL of this solution, add 0.1 mol/L trisodium citrate TS to make exactly 100 mL, and use this solution as the standard stock solution. To exactly 5 mL each of the sample stock solution and standard stock solution, add exactly 5 mL each of a solution of sodium tetraborate decahydrate (19 in 1000), acetonitrile and a solution of 9-fluorenylmethyl chloroformate in acetonitrile (1 in 250), shake for 45 seconds, and allow to stand for 30 minutes at room temperature. Then, add 20 mL of dichloromethane to them, shake for 60 seconds, centrifuge, and use the supernatant liquids so obtained as the sample solution and the standard solution, respectively. Perform the test with exactly 20 μL each of the sample solution and standard solution as directed under Liquid Chromatography *<2.01>* according to the following conditions. Determine each peak area of these solutions by the automatic integration method: each peak area other than alendronic acid obtained from the sample solution is not larger than the peak area of alendronic acid from the standard solution.

Operating conditions—

Detector: An ultraviolet absorption photometer (wavelength: 266 nm).

Column: A stainless steel column 4.1 mm in inside diameter and 25 cm in length, packed with styrene-divinylbenzene copolymer for liquid chromatography (10 μm in particle diameter).

Column temperature: A constant temperature of about 45°C.

Mobile phase A: Dissolve 2.94 g of trisodium citrate dihydrate and 1.42 g of anhydrous disodium hydrogen phosphate in 900 mL of water, adjust to pH 8.0 with phosphoric acid, and add water to make 1000 mL. To 850 mL of this solution add 150 mL of acetonitrile for liquid chromatography.

Mobile phase B: Dissolve 2.94 g of trisodium citrate dihydrate and 1.42 g of anhydrous disodium hydrogen phosphate in 900 mL of water, adjust to pH 8.0 with phosphoric acid, and add water to make 1000 mL. To 300 mL of this solution add 700 mL of acetonitrile for liquid chromatography.

Flowing of mobile phase: Control the gradient by mixing the mobile phases A and B as directed in the following table.

Time after injection of sample (min)	Mobile phase A (vol%)	Mobile phase B (vol%)
0 – 15	100 → 50	0 → 50
15 – 25	50 → 0	50 → 100

Flow rate: About 1.8 mL per minute.

Time span of measurement: About 5 times as long as the retention time of alendronic acid, beginning after the solvent peak.

System suitability—

System performance: Dissolve 15 mg of Alendronate Sodium Hydrate and 2 mg of 4-aminobutylic acid in 100 mL of 0.1 mol/L trisodium citrate TS. To 5 mL of this solution add 5 mL each of a solution of sodium tetraborate decahydrate (19 in 1000), acetonitrile and a solution of 9-fluorenylmethyl chloroformate in acetonitrile (1 in 250), then, proceed in the same manner as the sample solution. When the procedure is run with 20 μL of this solution under the above operating conditions, alendronic acid and 4-aminobutylic acid are eluted in this order with the resolution between these peaks being not less than 6.

System repeatability: When the test is repeated 6 times with 20 μL of the standard solution under the above operating conditions, the relative standard deviation of the peak area of alendronic acid is not more than 2.0%.

Loss on drying *<2.41>* 16.1 – 17.1% (1 g, 140°C, 3 hours).

Assay Weigh accurately about 10 mg each of Alendronate Sodium Hydrate and Alendronate Sodium RS (separately determine the loss on drying *<2.41>* in the same conditions as Alendronate Sodium Hydrate), dissolve in 0.1 mol/L trisodium citrate TS to make exactly 100 mL, and use these solutions as the sample stock solution and the standard stock solution, respectively. To exactly 5 mL each of these solutions add exactly 5 mL each of a solution of sodium tetraborate decahydrate (19 in 1000) and a solution of 9-fluorenylmethyl chloroformate in acetonitrile (1 in 2000), shake for 30 seconds, and allow to stand for 25 minutes. Then, add 25 mL of dichloromethane, shake for 60 seconds, centrifuge, and use the supernatant liquids so obtained as the sample solution and the standard solution, respectively. Perform the test with exactly 10 μL each of the sample solution and standard solution as directed under Liquid Chromatography <2.01> according to the following conditions, and determine the peak areas, A_T and A_S, of alendronic acid in each solution.

Amount (mg) of alendronate sodium ($C_4H_{12}NNaO_7P_2$)
$= M_S \times A_T/A_S$

M_S: Amount (mg) of Alendronate Sodium RS taken, calculated on the dried basis

Operating conditions—

Detector: An ultraviolet absorption photometer (wavelength: 266 nm).

Column: A stainless steel column 4.1 mm in inside diameter and 25 cm in length, packed with styrene-divinylbenzene copolymer for liquid chromatography (10 μm in particle diameter).

Column temperature: A constant temperature of about 35°C.

Mobile phase: Dissolve 14.7 g of trisodium citrate dihydrate and 7.1 g of anhydrous disodium hydrogen phosphate in 900 mL of water, adjust to pH 8.0 with phosphoric acid, and add water to make 1000 mL. To 700 mL of this solution add 250 mL of acetonitrile for liquid chromatography and 50 mL of methanol.

Flow rate: Adjust so that the retention time of alendronic acid is about 3 minutes.

System suitability—

System performance: When the procedure is run with 10 μL of the standard solution under the above operating conditions, the number of theoretical plates and the symmetry factor of the peak of alendronic acid are not less than 1500 and not more than 1.5, respectively.

System repeatability: When the test is repeated 6 times with 10 μL of the standard solution under the above operating conditions, the relative standard deviation of the peak area of alendronic acid is not more than 1.0%.

Containers and storage Containers—Tight containers.

Alendronate Sodium Injection

アレンドロン酸ナトリウム注射液

Alendronate Sodium Injection is an aqueous injection.

It contains not less than 95.0% and not more than 105.0% of the labeled amount of alendronic acid ($C_4H_{13}NO_7P_2$: 249.10).

Method of preparation Prepare as directed under Injections, with Alendronate Sodium Hydrate.

Description Alendronate Sodium Injection is a clear, colorless liquid.

Identification Use Alendronate Sodium Injection as the sample solution. Separately, dissolve 33 mg of alendronate sodium hydrate in 10 mL of water, and use this solution as the standard solution. Perform the test with these solutions as directed under Thin-layer Chromatography <2.03>. Spot 5 μL each of the sample solution and standard solution on a plate of cellulose for thin-layer chromatography. Develop the plate with a mixture of water, pyridine, acetic acid (100) and ethyl acetate (1:1:1:1) to a distance of about 10 cm, and air-dry the plate. Spray evenly a solution of ninhydrin in acetone (1 in 50) on the plate, and heat at 100°C for 10 minutes: the principal spots from the sample solution and standard solution show a blue-purple color and the same *R*f value.

pH Being specified separately when the drug is granted approval based on the Law.

Bacterial endotoxins <4.01> Less than 119 EU/mg.

Extractable volume <6.05> It meets the requirement.

Foreign insoluble matter <6.06> Perform the test according to Method 1: it meets the requirement.

Insoluble particulate matter <6.07> It meets the requirement.

Sterility <4.06> Perform the test according to Membrane-filter method: it meets the requirement.

Assay To an exactly measured volume of Alendronate Sodium Injection, equivalent to about 5 mg of alendronic acid ($C_4H_{13}NO_7P_2$), add a solution of disodium dihydrogen ethylenediamine tetraacetate dihydrate (1 in 500) to make exactly 100 mL, and use this solution as the sample stock solution. Separately, weigh accurately about 33 mg of Alendronate Sodium RS (separately determine the loss on drying <2.41> under the same conditions as Alendronate Sodium Hydrate), and dissolve in a solution of disodium dihydrogen ethylenediamine tetraacetate dihydrate (1 in 500) to make exactly 100 mL. Pipet 10 mL of this solution, add a solution of disodium dihydrogen ethylenediamine tetraacetate dihydrate (1 in 500) to make exactly 50 mL, and use this solution as the standard stock solution. Pipet 5 mL each of the sample stock solution and standard stock solution, add exactly 5 mL of a solution of sodium tetraborate decahydrate (19 in 500) and exactly 4 mL of a solution of 9-fluorenylmethyl chloroformate in acetonitrile (1 in 1000), shake for 30 seconds, and allow to stand at room temperature for 25 minutes. Then, add 25 mL of dichloromethane to them, shake for 45 seconds, centrifuge, and use the supernatant liquid so obtained as the sample solution and the standard solution, respectively. Perform the test with 50 μL each of the sample solution and standard solution as directed under Liquid Chromatography <2.01> according to the following conditions, and determine the peak areas, A_T and A_S, of alendronic acid in each solution.

Amount (mg) of alendronic acid ($C_4H_{13}NO_7P_2$)
$= M_S \times A_T/A_S \times 1/5 \times 0.919$

M_S: Amount (mg) of Alendronate Sodium RS taken, calculated on the dried basis

Operating conditions—

Detector: An ultraviolet absorption photometer (wavelength: 265 nm).

Column: A stainless steel column 4.1 mm in inside diameter and 25 cm in length, packed with styrene-divinylbenzene copolymer for liquid chromatography (10 μm in particle diameter).

Column temperature: A constant temperature of about 40°C.

Mobile phase: Dissolve 14.7 g of trisodium citrate dihydrate and 8.7 g of dipotassium hydrogen phosphate in 900 mL of water, adjust to pH 8.0 with phosphoric acid, and add water to make 1000 mL. To 750 mL of this solution add 200 mL of acetonitrile for liquid chromatography and 50 mL of methanol.

Flow rate: Adjust so that the retention time of alendronic acid is about 7 minutes.

System suitability—

System performance: When the procedure is run with 50 μL of the standard solution under the above operating conditions, the number of theoretical plates and the symmetry factor of the peak of alendronic acid are not less than 1500 and not more than 1.5, respectively.

System repeatability: When the test is repeated 6 times with 50 μL of the standard solution under the above operations conditions, the relative standard deviation of the peak of alendronic acid is not more than 1.0%.

Containers and storage Containers—Hermetic containers.

Alendronate Sodium Tablets

アレンドロン酸ナトリウム錠

Alendronate Sodium Tablets contain not less than 95.0% and not more than 105.0% of the labeled amount of alendronic acid ($C_4H_{13}NO_7P_2$: 249.10).

Method of preparation Prepare as directed under Tablets, with Alendronate Sodium Hydrate.

Identification To a quantity of powdered Alendronate Sodium Tablets, equivalent to 25 mg of alendronic acid ($C_4H_{13}NO_7P_2$), add 25 mL of water, shake, centrifuge, and use the supernatant liquid as the sample solution. Separately, weigh 33 mg of alendronate sodium hydrate, and dissolve in 25 mL of water, and use this solution as the standard solution. Perform the test with these solutions as directed under Thin-layer Chromatography <*2.03*>. Spot 5 μL each of the sample solution and standard solution on a plate of cellulose for thin-layer chromatography. Develop the plate with a mixture of water, pyridine, acetic acid (100) and ethyl acetate (1:1:1:1) to a distance of about 10 cm, and air-dry the plate. Spray evenly a solution of ninhydrin in acetone (1 in 50) on the plate, and heat the plate at 100°C for 10 minutes: the principal spots from the sample solution and standard solution show a blue-purple color and the same *R*f value.

Uniformity of dosage units <*6.02*> Perform the Mass variation test, or the Content uniformity test according to the following method: it meets the requirement.

To 1 tablet of Alendronate Sodium Tablets add 0.1 mol/L trisodium citrate TS to make exactly 100 mL, and stir until the tablet is completely disintegrated. Centrifuge this solution, pipet *V* mL of the supernatant liquid, and add 0.1 mol/L trisodium citrate TS to make exactly *V′* mL so that each mL contains about 25 μg of alendronic acid ($C_4H_{13}NO_7P_2$), and use this solution as the sample stock solution. Then, proceed as directed in the Assay.

$$\text{Amount (mg) of alendronic acid } (C_4H_{13}NO_7P_2) = M_S \times A_T/A_S \times V'/V \times 2/25 \times 0.919$$

M_S: Amount (mg) of Alendronate Sodium RS taken, calculated on the dried basis

Dissolution <*6.10*> When the test is performed at 50 revolutions per minute according to the Paddle method, using 900 mL of water as the dissolution medium, the dissolution rate in 15 minutes of Alendronate Sodium Tablets is not less than 85%.

Start the test with 1 tablet of Alendronate Sodium Tablets, withdraw not less than 10 mL of the medium at the specified minute after starting the test, and centrifuge. Pipet *V* mL of the supernatant liquid, add water to make exactly *V′* mL so that each mL contains about 6 μg of alendronic acid ($C_4H_{13}NO_7P_2$), and use this solution as the sample stock solution. Separately, weigh accurately about 29 mg of Alendronate Sodium RS (separately determine the loss on drying <*2.41*> under the same conditions as Alendronate Sodium Hydrate), and dissolve in water to make exactly 250 mL. Pipet 3 mL of this solution, add water to make exactly 50 mL, and use this solution as the standard stock solution. Pipet 5 mL each of the sample stock solution and standard stock solution, add exactly 1 mL of trisodium citrate dihydrate solution (22 in 125), exactly 5 mL of a solution obtained by dissolving 6.2 g of boric acid in 950 mL of water, adjusting to pH 9.0 with sodium hydrate TS, and adding water to make 1000 mL, and add exactly 4 mL of a solution of 9-fluorenylmethyl chloroformate in acetonitrile (1 in 2000), shake for 30 seconds, and allow to stand at room temperature for 25 minutes. Add 25 mL of dichloromethane, shake for 45 seconds, then centrifuge, and use the supernatant liquid as the sample solution and the standard solution, respectively. Then, proceed as directed in the Assay.

$$\text{Dissolution rate (\%) with respect to the labeled amount of alendronic acid } (C_4H_{13}NO_7P_2) = M_S \times A_T/A_S \times V'/V \times 1/C \times 108/5 \times 0.919$$

M_S: Amount (mg) of Alendronate Sodium RS taken, calculated on the dried basis

C: Labeled amount (mg) of alendronic acid ($C_4H_{13}NO_7P_2$) in 1 tablet

Assay Weigh accurately and powder not less than 20 Alendronate Sodium Tablets. Weigh accurately a portion of the powder, equivalent to about 50 mg of alendronic acid ($C_4H_{13}NO_7P_2$), add 0.1 mol/L trisodium citrate TS to make exactly 1000 mL, stir for 30 minutes, and centrifuge. Pipet 5 mL of the supernatant liquid, add 0.1 mol/L trisodium citrate TS to make exactly 10 mL, and use this solution as the sample stock solution. Separately, weigh accurately about 39 mg of Alendronate Sodium RS (separately determine the loss on drying <*2.41*> under the same conditions as Alendronate Sodium Hydrate), dissolve in 0.1 mol/L trisodium citrate TS to make exactly 50 mL. Pipet 2 mL of this solution, add 0.1 mol/L trisodium citrate TS to make exactly 50 mL, and use this solution as the standard stock solution. Pipet 5 mL each of the sample stock solution and standard stock solution, add exactly 5 mL of a solution of sodium tetraborate decahydrate (19 in 500) and exactly 4 mL of a solution of 9-fluprenylmethyl chloroformate in acetonitrile (1 in 1000), shake for 30 seconds, and allow to stand at room temperature for 25 minutes. Then, add 25 mL of dichloromethane to them, shake for 45 seconds, centrifuge, and use the supernatant liquid so obtained as the sample solution and the standard solution, respectively. Perform the test with exactly 50 μL each of the sample solution and standard solution as directed under Liquid Chromatography <*2.01*> according to the following conditions, and determine the peak areas, A_T and A_S, of alendronic acid in each solution.

$$\text{Amount (mg) of alendronic acid } (C_4H_{13}NO_7P_2) = M_S \times A_T/A_S \times 8/5 \times 0.919$$

M_S: Amount (mg) of Alendronate Sodium RS taken, calculated on the dried basis

The JP Drugs are to be tested according to the provisions given in the pertinent monographs, General Notices, General Rules for Crude Drugs, General Rules for Preparations, and General Tests for their conformity to the Japanese Pharmacopoeia. (See the General Notices 5.)

Operating conditions—

Detector: An ultraviolet absorption photometer (wavelength: 266 nm).

Column: A stainless steel column 4.1 mm in inside diameter and 25 cm in length, packed with styrene-divinylbenzene copolymer for liquid chromatography (10 μm in particle diameter).

Column temperature: A constant temperature of about 35°C.

Mobile phase: Dissolve 14.7 g of trisodium citrate dihydrate and 7.1 g of anhydrous disodium hydrogen phosphate in 900 mL of water, adjust to pH 8.0 with phosphoric acid, and add water to make 1000 mL. To 750 mL of this solution add 200 mL of acetonitrile for liquid chromatography and 50 mL of methanol.

Flow rate: Adjust so that the retention time of alendronic acid is about 7 minutes.

System suitability—

System performance: When the procedure is run with 50 μL of the standard solution under the above operating conditions, the number of theoretical plates and the symmetry factor of the peak of alendronic acid are not less than 1500 and not more than 1.5, respectively.

System repeatability: When the test is repeated 6 times with 50 μL of the standard solution under the above operations conditions, the relative standard deviation of the peak of alendronic acid is not more than 1.0%.

Containers and storage Containers—Well-closed containers.

Alimemazine Tartrate

アリメマジン酒石酸塩

$(C_{18}H_{22}N_2S)_2.C_4H_6O_6$: 746.98
N,*N*,2-Trimethyl-3-(10*H*-phenothiazin-10-yl)propylamine hemitartrate
[*41375-66-0*]

Alimemazine Tartrate, when dried, contains not less than 98.0% of alimemazine tartrate [$(C_{18}H_{22}N_2S)_2.C_4H_6O_6$].

Description Alimemazine Tartrate occurs as a white powder. It is odorless, and has a bitter taste.

It is freely soluble in water and in acetic acid (100), sparingly soluble in ethanol (95), and practically insoluble in diethyl ether.

The pH of a solution of 1.0 g of Alimemazine Tartrate in 50 mL of water is between 5.0 and 6.5.

It is gradually colored by light.

Identification **(1)** To 2 mL of a solution of Alimemazine Tartrate (1 in 100) add 1 drop of iron (III) chloride TS: a red-brown color is produced, and immediately a yellow precipitate is formed.

(2) Dissolve 1 g of Alimemazine Tartrate in 5 mL of water, add 3 mL of sodium hydroxide TS, extract with two 10-mL portions of diethyl ether [use the aqueous layer obtained in the Identification (4)]. Shake the combined diethyl ether extracts with 3 g of anhydrous sodium sulfate, filter, and evaporate the diethyl ether with the aid of a current of air. Dry the residue in a desiccator (in vacuum, phosphorus (V) oxide) for 16 hours: it melts *<2.60>* between 66°C and 70°C.

(3) Determine the absorption spectrum of a solution of Alimemazine Tartrate (1 in 100,000) as directed under Ultraviolet-visible Spectrophotometry *<2.24>*, and compare the spectrum with the Reference Spectrum: both spectra exhibit similar intensities of absorption at the same wavelengths.

(4) The aqueous layer, obtained in the identification (2), when neutralized with dilute acetic acid, responds to Qualitative Tests *<1.09>* (1) and (2) for tartrate.

Melting point *<2.60>* 159 – 163°C

Purity **(1)** Clarity and color of solution—Dissolve 1.0 g of Alimemazine Tartrate in 20 mL of water: the solution is clear and colorless.

(2) Heavy metals *<1.07>*—Proceed with 1.0 g of Alimemazine Tartrate according to Method 2, and perform the test. Prepare the control solution with 2.0 mL of Standard Lead Solution (not more than 20 ppm).

(3) Arsenic *<1.11>*—Prepare the test solution with 1.0 g of Alimemazine Tartrate according to Method 3, and perform the test. Use a solution of magnesium nitrate hexahydrate in ethanol (95) (1 in 5) (not more than 2 ppm).

Loss on drying *<2.41>* Not more than 0.5% (1 g, 105°C, 3 hours).

Residue on ignition *<2.44>* Not more than 0.1% (1 g).

Assay Weigh accurately about 0.8 g of Alimemazine Tartrate, previously dried, dissolve in 50 mL of acetic acid (100), and titrate *<2.50>* with 0.1 mol/L perchloric acid VS until the color of the solution changes from red through brown to green-brown (indicator: 2 mL of *p*-naphtholbenzein TS). Perform a blank determination in the same manner, and make any necessary correction.

Each mL of 0.1 mol/L perchloric acid VS
= 37.35 mg of $(C_{18}H_{22}N_2S)_2.C_4H_6O_6$

Containers and storage Containers—Tight containers.
Storage—Light-resistant.

Allopurinol

アロプリノール

$C_5H_4N_4O$: 136.11
1*H*-Pyrazolo[3,4-*d*]pyrimidin-4-ol
[*315-30-0*]

Allopurinol, when dried, contains not less than 98.0% and not more than 101.0% of allopurinol ($C_5H_4N_4O$).

Description Allopurinol occurs as white to pale yellow-white, crystals or crystalline powder.

It is slightly soluble in *N*,*N*-dimethylformamide, and very slightly soluble in water and in ethanol (99.5).

It dissolves in ammonia TS.

Identification **(1)** Determine the absorption spectrum of a solution of Allopurinol (1 in 200,000) as directed under Ultraviolet-visible Spectrophotometry <*2.24*>, and compare the spectrum with the Reference Spectrum: both spectra exhibit similar intensities of absorption at the same wavelengths.

(2) Determine the infrared absorption spectrum of Allopurinol, previously dried, as directed in the potassium bromide disk method under Infrared Spectrophotometry <*2.25*>, and compare the spectrum with the Reference Spectrum: both spectra exhibit similar intensities of absorption at the same wave numbers.

Purity **(1)** Heavy metals <*1.07*>—Proceed with 1.0 g of Allopurinol according to Method 2, and perform the test. Prepare the control solution with 2.0 mL of Standard Lead Solution (not more than 20 ppm).

(2) Arsenic <*1.11*>—Prepare the test solution with 1.0 g of Allopurinol according to Method 3, and perform the test (not more than 2 ppm).

(3) Related substances—Dissolve 50 mg of Allopurinol in 10 mL of ammonia TS, and use this solution as the sample solution. Pipet 1 mL of the sample solution, add ammonia TS to make exactly 500 mL, and use this solution as the standard solution. Perform the test with these solutions as directed under Thin-layer Chromatography <*2.03*>. Spot 5 μL each of the sample solution and standard solution on a plate of cellulose with fluorescent indicator for thin-layer chromatography. Develop the plate with ammonia TS-saturated 1-butanol to a distance of about 10 cm, and air-dry the plate. Examine under ultraviolet light (main wavelength: 254 nm): the spots other than the principal spot obtained from the sample solution are not more intense than the spot from the standard solution.

Loss on drying <*2.41*> Not more than 0.5% (1 g, 105°C, 4 hours).

Residue on ignition <*2.44*> Not more than 0.1% (1 g).

Assay Weigh accurately about 0.16 g of Allopurinol, previously dried, dissolve in 70 mL of *N,N*-dimethylformamide by warming. Cool, and titrate <*2.50*> with 0.1 mol/L tetramethylammonium hydroxide VS (potentiometric titration). To 70 mL of *N,N*-dimethylformamide add 12 mL of water, perform a blank determination in the same manner, and make any necessary correction.

Each mL of 0.1 mol/L tetramethylammonium hydroxide VS
= 13.61 mg of $C_5H_4N_4O$

Containers and storage Containers—Tight containers.

Allopurinol Tablets

アロプリノール錠

Allopurinol Tablets contain not less than 93.0% and not more than 107.0% of the labeled amount of allopurinol ($C_5H_4N_4O$: 136.11).

Method of preparation Prepare as directed under Tablets, with Allopurinol.

Identification **(1)** Determine the absorption spectrum of the sample solution obtained in the Assay as directed under Ultraviolet-visible Spectrophotometry <*2.24*>: it exhibits a maximum between 248 nm and 252 nm.

(2) To a quantity of powdered Allopurinol Tablets, equivalent to 0.1 g of Allopurinol, add 5 mL of a solution of diethylamine (1 in 10), shake well, add 5 mL of methanol, centrifuge, and use the supernatant liquid as the sample solution. Separately, dissolve 0.1 g of allopurinol in 5 mL of a solution of diethylamine (1 in 10), add 5 mL of methanol, and use this solution as the standard solution. Perform the test with these solutions as directed under Thin-layer Chromatography <*2.03*>. Spot 2.5 μL each of the sample solution and standard solution on a plate of silica gel with fluorescent indicator for thin-layer chromatography. Develop the plate with a mixture of 2-butanone, ammonia solution (28) and 2-methoxyethanol (3:1:1) to a distance of about 10 cm, and air-dry the plate. Examine under ultraviolet light (main wavelength: 254 nm): the principal spots obtained from the sample solution and standard solution show the same *R*f value.

Uniformity of dosage units <*6.02*> Perform the Mass variation test, or the Content uniformity test according to the following method: it meets the requirement.

To 1 tablet of Allopurinol Tablets add *V*/10 mL of 0.05 mol/L sodium hydroxide TS, shake well, and sonicate for 10 minutes. After cooling, add 0.1 mol/L hydrochloric acid TS to make exactly *V* mL so that each mL contains about 0.5 mg of allopurinol ($C_5H_4N_4O$), and filter through a membrane filter with a pore size not exceeding 0.8 μm. Discard the first 10 mL of the filtrate, pipet 2 mL of the subsequent filtrate, add 0.1 mol/L of hydrochloric acid TS to make exactly 100 mL, and use this solution as the sample solution. Separately, weigh accurately about 50 mg of allopurinol for assay, previously dried at 105°C for 4 hours, dissolve in 10 mL of 0.05 mol/L sodium hydroxide TS, and add 0.1 mol/L hydrochloric acid TS to make exactly 100 mL. Pipet 2 mL of this solution, add 0.1 mol/L hydrochloric acid TS to make exactly 100 mL, and use this solution as the standard solution. Determine the absorbances, A_T and A_S, of the sample solution and standard solution at 250 nm as directed under Ultraviolet-visible Spectrophotometry <*2.24*>.

Amount (mg) of allopurinol ($C_5H_4N_4O$)
$= M_S \times A_T/A_S \times V/100$

M_S: Amount (mg) of allopurinol for assay taken

Dissolution <*6.10*> When the test is performed at 50 revolutions per minute according to the Paddle method, using 900 mL of water as the dissolution medium, the dissolution rate in 30 minutes of Allopurinol Tablets is not less than 80%.

Start the test with 1 tablet of Allopurinol Tablets, withdraw not less than 20 mL of the medium at the specified minute after starting the test, and filter through a membrane filter with a pore size not exceeding 0.8 μm. Discard not less than 10 mL of the first filtrate, pipet *V* mL of the subsequent filtrate, add water to make exactly *V′* mL so that each mL contains about 11 μg of allopurinol ($C_5H_4N_4O$), and use this solution as the sample solution. Separately, weigh accurately about 11 mg of allopurinol for assay, previously dried at 105 °C for 4 hours, and dissolve in water to make exactly 100 mL. Pipet 5 mL of this solution, add water to make exactly 50 mL, and use this solution as the standard solution. Determine the absorbances, A_T and A_S, of the sample solution and standard solution at 250 nm as directed under Ultraviolet-visible Spectrophotometry <*2.24*>.

Dissolution rate (%) with respect to the labeled amount of allopurinol ($C_5H_4N_4O$)
$= M_S \times A_T/A_S \times V'/V \times 1/C \times 90$

M_S: Amount (mg) of allopurinol for assay taken
C: Labeled amount (mg) of allopurinol ($C_5H_4N_4O$) in 1 tablet

Assay Weigh accurately the mass of not less than 20 Allopurinol Tablets, and powder. Weigh accurately a portion of the powder, equivalent to about 0.1 g of allopurinol ($C_5H_4N_4O$), add 20 mL of 0.05 mol/L sodium hydroxide TS, shake well, and treat with ultrasonic waves for 10 minutes. After cooling, add 0.1 mol/L hydrochloric acid TS to make exactly 200 mL, and filter through a membrane filter with a pore size not exceeding 0.8 μm. Discard the first 10 mL of the filtrate, pipet 2 mL of the subsequent filtrate, add 0.1 mol/L hydrochloric acid TS to make exactly 100 mL, and use this solution as the sample solution. Separately, weigh accurately about 0.1 g of allopurinol for assay, previously dried at 105°C for 4 hours, dissolve in 20 mL of 0.05 mol/L sodium hydroxide TS, and add 0.1 mol/L hydrochloric acid TS to make exactly 200 mL. Pipet 2 mL of this solution, add 0.1 mol/L hydrochloric acid TS to make exactly 100 mL, and use this solution as the standard solution. Determine the absorbances, A_T and A_S, of the sample solution and standard solution at 250 nm as directed under Ultraviolet-visible Spectrophotometry *<2.24>*.

Amount (mg) of allopurinol ($C_5H_4N_4O$) = $M_S \times A_T/A_S$

M_S: Amount (mg) of allopurinol for assay taken

Containers and storage Containers—Well-closed containers.

Alminoprofen

アルミノプロフェン

and enantiomer

$C_{13}H_{17}NO_2$: 219.28
(2*RS*)-2-{[4-(2-Methylprop-2-en-1-yl)amino]phenyl}propanoic acid
[39718-89-3]

Alminoprofen, when dried, contains not less than 99.0% and not more than 101.0% of alminoprofen ($C_{13}H_{17}NO_2$).

Description Alminoprofen occurs as white to pale yellow, crystals or crystalline powder.

It is freely soluble in ethanol (99.5) and in acetic acid (100), and very slightly soluble in water.

It gradually turns brown on exposure to light.

A solution of Alminoprofen in ethanol (99.5) (1 in 10) shows no optical rotation.

Identification (1) Determine the absorption spectrum of a solution of Alminoprofen in ethanol (99.5) (3 in 500,000) as directed under Ultraviolet-visible Spectrophotometry *<2.24>*, and compare the spectrum with the Reference Spectrum: both spectra exhibit similar intensities of absorption at the same wavelengths.

(2) Determine the infrared absorption spectrum of Alminoprofen as directed in the potassium bromide disk method under Infrared Spectrophotometry *<2.25>*, and compare the spectrum with the Reference Spectrum: both spectra exhibit similar intensities of absorption at the same wave numbers.

Melting point *<2.60>* 106 - 108°C

Purity (1) Heavy metals *<1.07>*—Proceed with 2.0 g of Alminoprofen according to Method 2, and perform the test. Prepare the control solution with 2.0 mL of Standard Lead Solution (not more than 10 ppm).

(2) Arsenic *<1.11>*—Prepare the test solution with 1.0 g of Alminoprofen according to Method 3, and perform the test (not more than 2 ppm).

(3) Related substances—Conduct this procedure using light-resistant vessels. Dissolve 50 mg of Alminoprofen in 100 mL of the mobile phase, and use this solution as the sample solution. Pipet 2 mL of the sample solution, add the mobile phase to make exactly 200 mL, and use this solution as the standard solution. Perform the test with exactly 5 μL each of the sample solution and standard solution as directed under Liquid Chromatography *<2.01>* according to the following conditions. Determine each peak area of these solutions by the automatic integration method: the area of the peak other than alminoprofen obtained from the sample solution is not larger than 1/5 times the peak area of alminoprofen from the standard solution. Furthermore, the total area of the peaks other than alminoprofen from the sample solution is not larger than the peak area of alminoprofen from the standard solution.

Operating conditions—

Detector: An ultraviolet absorption photometer (wavelength: 254 nm).

Column: A stainless steel column 6.0 mm in inside diameter and 15 cm in length, packed with octadecylsilanized silica gel for liquid chromatography (5 μm in particle diameter).

Column temperature: A constant temperature of about 25°C.

Mobile phase: A mixture of methanol and diluted acetic acid (100) (1 in 1000) (4:1).

Flow rate: Adjust so that the retention time of alminoprofen is about 5 minutes.

Time span of measurement: About 5 times as long as the retention time of alminoprofen, beginning after the solvent peak.

System suitability—

Test for required detectability: Pipet 1 mL of the standard solution, and add the mobile phase to make exactly 10 mL. Confirm that the peak area of alminoprofen obtained with 5 μL of this solution is equivalent to 7 to 13% of that with 5 μL of the standard solution.

System performance: Dissolve 10 mg each of Alminoprofen and butyl parahydroxybenzoate in 100 mL of methanol. Pipet 10 mL of this solution, and add methanol to make exactly 50 mL. When the procedure is run with 5 μL of this solution under the above operating conditions, alminoprofen and butyl parahydroxybenzoate are eluted in this order with the resolution between these peaks being not less than 2.0.

System repeatability: When the test is repeated 6 times with 5 μL of the standard solution under the above operating conditions, the relative standard deviation of the peak area of alminoprofen is not more than 2.0%.

Loss on drying *<2.41>* Not more than 0.5% (1 g, in vacuum, phosphorus (V) oxide, 1 hour).

Residue on ignition *<2.44>* Not more than 0.1% (1 g).

Assay Weigh accurately about 0.3 g of Alminoprofen, previously dried, dissolve in 50 mL of acetic acid (100), and titrate *<2.50>* with 0.1 mol/L perchloric acid VS (potentiometric titration). Perform a blank determination in the same manner, and make any necessary correction.

Each mL of 0.1 mol/L perchloric acid VS
= 21.93 mg of $C_{13}H_{17}NO_2$

Containers and storage Containers—Well-closed containers.

Storage—Light-resistant.

Alminoprofen Tablets

アルミノプロフェン錠

Alminoprofen Tablets contain not less than 93.0% and not more than 107.0% of the labeled amount of alminoprofen ($C_{13}H_{17}NO_2$: 219.28).

Method of preparation Prepare as directed under Tablets, with Alminoprofen.

Identification Take an amount of powdered Alminoprofen Tablets, equivalent to 30 mg of Alminoprofen, add ethanol (99.5) to make 100 mL, shake thoroughly, and centrifuge. To 2 mL of the supernatant liquid add ethanol (99.5) to make 100 mL, and determine the absorption spectrum of this solution as directed under Ultraviolet-visible Spectrophotometry *<2.24>*: it exhibits maxima between 253 nm and 257 nm, and between 298 nm and 302 nm.

Purity Related substances—Conduct this procedure using light-resistant vessels. Powder 10 tablets of Alminoprofen Tablets, weigh a portion of the powder equivalent to 50 mg of Alminoprofen, add 50 mL of the mobile phase, shake for 15 minutes, add the mobile phase to make exactly 100 mL, centrifuge, and use the supernatant liquid as the sample solution. Pipet 2 mL of the sample solution, add the mobile phase to make exactly 200 mL, and use this solution as the standard solution. Perform the test with exactly 5 μL each of the sample solution and standard solution as directed under Liquid Chromatography *<2.01>* according to the following conditions. Determine each peak area of each solution by the automatic integration method: the area of the peak other than alminoprofen obtained from the sample solution is not larger than 1/2 times the peak area of alminoprofen from the standard solution. Furthermore, the total area of the peaks other than alminoprofen from the sample solution is not larger than 2 times the peak area of alminoprofen from the standard solution.

Operating conditions—

Proceed as directed in the operating conditions in the Purity (3) under Alminoprofen.

System suitability—

Proceed as directed in the system suitability in the Purity (3) in Assay under Alminoprofen.

Uniformity of dosage units *<6.02>* Perform the test according to the following method: it meets the requirement of the Content uniformity test.

To 1 tablet of Alminoprofen Tablets add 5 mL of water, shake until the tablet is disintegrated, add 50 mL of ethanol (99.5), shake for 20 minutes, then add ethanol (99.5) to make exactly 100 mL, and centrifuge. Pipet 3 mL of the supernatant liquid, add ethanol (99.5) to make exactly 50 mL. Pipet V mL of this solution, add ethanol (99.5) to make exactly V' mL so that each mL contains about 6 μg of alminoprofen ($C_{13}H_{17}NO_2$), and use this solution as the sample solution. Then, proceed as directed in the Assay.

Amount (mg) of alminoprofen ($C_{13}H_{17}NO_2$)
$$= M_S \times A_T/A_S \times V'/V \times 1/3$$

M_S: Amount (mg) of alminoprofen for assay taken

Dissolution *<6.10>* When the test is performed at 50 revolutions per minute according to the Paddle method, using 900 mL of 2nd fluid for dissolution test as the dissolution medium, the dissolution rate in 45 minutes of Alminoprofen Tablets is not less than 80%.

Start the test with 1 tablet of Alminoprofen Tablets, withdraw not less than 20 mL of the medium at specified minute after starting the test, and filter through a membrane filter with a pore size not exceeding 0.45 μm. Discard not less than 10 mL of the first filtrate, pipet V mL of the subsequent filtrate, add 0.05 mol/L sodium hydroxide TS to make exactly V' mL so that each mL contains about 8.9 μg of alminoprofen ($C_{13}H_{17}NO_2$), and use this solution as the sample solution. Separately, weigh accurately about 30 mg of alminoprofen for assay, previously dried in vacuum for 1 hour using phosphorus (V) oxide as the dessicant, and dissolve in 0.05 mol/L sodium hydroxide TS to make exactly 100 mL. Pipet 3 mL of this solution, add 0.05 mol/L sodium hydroxide TS to make exactly 100 mL, and use this solution as the standard solution. Determine the absorbances, A_T and A_S, at 245 nm of the sample solution and standard solution as directed under Ultraviolet-visible Spectrophotometry *<2.24>*.

Dissolution rate (%) with respect to the labeled amount of alminoprofen ($C_{13}H_{17}NO_2$)
$$= M_S \times A_T/A_S \times V'/V \times 1/C \times 27$$

M_S: Amount (mg) of alminoprofen for assay taken
C: Labeled amount (mg) of alminoprofen ($C_{13}H_{17}NO_2$) in 1 tablet

Assay Weigh accurately the mass of not less than 20 tablets of Alminoprofen Tablets, and powder. Weigh accurately an amount equivalent to about 60 mg of alminoprofen ($C_{13}H_{17}NO_2$), add ethanol (99.5) and shake well, add ethanol (99.5) to make exactly 200 mL, and centrifuge. Pipet 2 mL of the supernatant liquid, add ethanol (99.5) to make exactly 100 mL, and use this solution as the sample solution. Separately, weigh accurately about 30 mg of alminoprofen for assay, previously dried in vacuum for 1 hour using phosphorus (V) oxide as the dessicant, dissolve in ethanol (99.5) to make exactly 100 mL. Pipet 2 mL of this solution, add ethanol (99.5) to make exactly 100 mL, and use this solution as the standard solution. Determine the absorbances, A_T and A_S, at the wavelength of maximum absorption at about 255 nm of the sample solution and standard solution as directed under Ultraviolet-visible Spectrophotometry *<2.24>*.

Amount (mg) of alminoprofen ($C_{13}H_{17}NO_2$)
$$= M_S \times A_T/A_S \times 2$$

M_S: Amount (mg) of alminoprofen for assay taken

Containers and storage Containers—Well-closed containers.

Alprazolam

アルプラゾラム

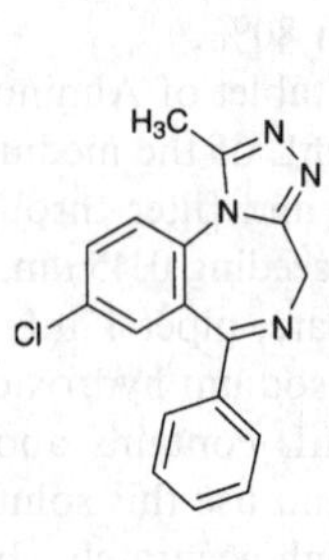

$C_{17}H_{13}ClN_4$: 308.76
8-Chloro-1-methyl-6-phenyl-4*H*-[1,2,4]triazolo[4,3-*a*][1,4]benzodiazepine
[28981-97-7]

Alprazolam, when dried, contains not less than 98.5% of alprazolam ($C_{17}H_{13}ClN_4$).

Description Alprazolam occurs as white, crystals or crystalline powder.

It is freely soluble in chloroform, soluble in methanol and in ethanol (95), sparingly soluble in acetic anhydride, and practically insoluble in water.

It dissolves in dilute nitric acid.

Identification **(1)** Determine the absorption spectrum of a solution of Alprazolam in ethanol (95) (1 in 200,000) as directed under Ultraviolet-visible Spectrophotometry <*2.24*>, and compare the spectrum with the Reference Spectrum: both spectra exhibit similar intensities of absorption at the same wavelengths.

(2) Dissolve 0.05 g of Alprazolam in 0.7 mL of deuterochloroform for nuclear magnetic resonance spectroscopy, and determine the spectrum of this solution using tetramethylsilane for nuclear magnetic resonance spectroscopy as an internal reference compound, as directed under Nuclear Magnetic Resonance Spectroscopy <*2.21*> (^{1}H): it exhibits a single signal A at around δ 2.6 ppm, doublet signals B and C at around δ 4.0 ppm and δ 5.4 ppm, and a broad signal D between δ 7.1 ppm and 7.9 ppm. The ratio of integrated intensity of each signal, A:B:C:D, is about 3:1:1:8.

(3) Perform the test with Alprazolam as directed under Flame Coloration Test <*1.04*> (2): a green color appears.

Melting point <*2.60*> 228 – 232°C

Purity **(1)** Chloride <*1.03*>—Dissolve 0.5 g of Alprazolam in 10 mL of dilute nitric acid, and add water to make 50 mL. Perform the test using this solution as the test solution. Prepare the control solution with 0.20 mL of 0.01 mol/L hydrochloric acid VS (not more than 0.014%).

(2) Heavy metals <*1.07*>—Proceed with 2.0 g of Alprazolam according to Method 4, and perform the test. Prepare the control solution with 2.0 mL of Standard Lead Solution (not more than 10 ppm).

(3) Related substances—Dissolve 50 mg of Alprazolam in 10 mL of methanol, and use this solution as the sample solution. Pipet 1 mL of the sample solution, add methanol to make exactly 100 mL, then pipet 1 mL of this solution, add methanol to make exactly 10 mL, and use this solution as the standard solution. Perform the test with these solutions as directed under Thin-layer Chromatography <*2.03*>. Spot 20 μL each of the sample solution and standard solution on a plate of silica gel with fluorescent indicator for thin-layer chromatography. Develop with a mixture of acetone, hexane, ethyl acetate and ethanol (95) (4:2:2:1) to a distance of about 10 cm, and air-dry the plate. Examine under ultraviolet light (main wavelength: 254 nm): the spots other than the principal spot obtained from the sample solution are not more intense than the spot from the standard solution.

Loss on drying <*2.41*> Not more than 0.5% (1 g, reduced pressure not exceeding 0.67 kPa, 60°C, 4 hours).

Residue on ignition <*2.44*> Not more than 0.1% (1 g).

Assay Weigh accurately about 0.25 g of Alprazolam, previously dried, dissolve in 100 mL of acetic anhydride, and titrate <*2.50*> with 0.1 mol/L perchloric acid VS (potentiometric titration). Perform a blank determination in the same manner, and make any necessary correction.

Each mL of 0.1 mol/L perchloric acid VS
= 15.44 mg of $C_{17}H_{13}ClN_4$

Containers and storage Containers—Well-closed containers.

Alprenolol Hydrochloride

アルプレノロール塩酸塩

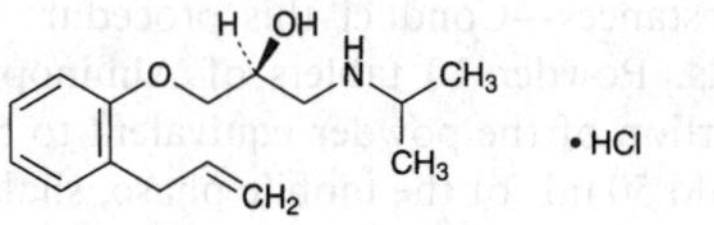

and enantiomer

$C_{15}H_{23}NO_2.HCl$: 285.81
(2*RS*)-1-(2-Allylphenoxy)-3-[(1-methylethyl)amino]propan-2-ol monohydrochloride
[13707-88-5]

Alprenolol Hydrochloride, when dried, contains not less than 99.0% of alprenolol hydrochloride ($C_{15}H_{23}NO_2.HCl$).

Description Alprenolol Hydrochloride occurs as white, crystals or crystalline powder.

It is freely soluble in water, in ethanol (95) and in acetic acid (100), slightly soluble in acetic anhydride, and practically insoluble in diethyl ether.

Identification **(1)** To 2 mL of a solution of Alprenolol Hydrochloride (1 in 100) add 0.05 mL of copper (II) sulfate TS and 2 mL of sodium hydroxide TS: a blue-purple color develops. To this solution add 1 mL of diethyl ether, shake well, and allow to stand: a red-purple color develops in the diethyl ether layer.

(2) Dissolve 0.05 g of Alprenolol Hydrochloride in 5 mL of water, add 1 to 2 drops of bromine TS, and shake: the color of the test solution disappears.

(3) Determine the absorption spectrum of a solution of Alprenolol Hydrochloride in ethanol (95) (1 in 10,000) as directed under Ultraviolet-visible Spectrophotometry <*2.24*>, and compare the spectrum with the Reference Spectrum: both spectra exhibit similar intensities of absorption at the same wavelengths.

(4) Determine the infrared absorption spectrum of Alprenolol Hydrochloride, previously dried, as directed in the potassium chloride disk method under Infrared Spectrophotometry <*2.25*>, and compare the spectrum with the Reference Spectrum: both spectra exhibit similar intensities of absorption at the same wave numbers.

(5) A solution of Alprenolol Hydrochloride (1 in 50) responds to Qualitative Tests <*1.09*> for chloride.

pH <*2.54*> Dissolve 1.0 g of Alprenolol Hydrochloride in 10 mL of water: the pH of this solution is between 4.5 and 6.0.

Melting point <*2.60*> 108 - 112°C

Purity **(1)** Clarity and color of solution—Dissolve 1.0 g of Alprenolol Hydrochloride in 10 mL of water: the solution is clear and colorless.

(2) Heavy metals <*1.07*>—Proceed with 2.0 g of Alprenolol Hydrochloride according to Method 2, and perform the test. Prepare the control solution with 2.0 mL of Standard Lead Solution (not more than 10 ppm).

(3) Arsenic <*1.11*>—Prepare the test solution with 1.0 g of Alprenolol Hydrochloride according to Method 3, and perform the test (not more than 2 ppm).

(4) Related substances—Dissolve 0.10 g of Alprenolol Hydrochloride in 10 mL of ethanol (95), and use this solution as the sample solution. Pipet 1 mL of the sample solution, and add ethanol (95) to make exactly 100 mL. Pipet 2.5 mL of this solution, add ethanol (95) to make exactly 10 mL, and use this solution as the standard solution. Perform the test with these solutions as directed under Thin-layer Chromatography <*2.03*>. Spot 10 μL each of the sample solution and standard solution on a plate of silica gel for thin-layer chromatography. Develop the plate with a mixture of dichloromethane, acetone, acetic acid (100) and water (60:42:5:3) to a distance of about 10 cm, air-dry the plate, and then dry at 80°C for 30 minutes. After cooling, allow the plate to stand in iodine vapor for 30 minutes: the spots other than the principal spot and the spot on the starting point obtained from the sample solution are not more intense than the spot from the standard solution.

Loss on drying <*2.41*> Not more than 0.5% (1 g, in vacuum, silica gel, 4 hours).

Residue on ignition <*2.44*> Not more than 0.1% (1 g).

Assay Weigh accurately about 0.5 g of Alprenolol Hydrochloride, previously dried, dissolve in 50 mL of a mixture of acetic anhydride and acetic acid (100) (7:3), and titrate <*2.50*> with 0.1 mol/L perchloric acid VS (potentiometric titration). Perform a blank determination in the same manner, and make any necessary correction.

Each mL of 0.1 mol/L perchloric acid VS
= 28.58 mg of $C_{15}H_{23}NO_2.HCl$

Containers and storage Containers—Well-closed containers.

Alprostadil

アルプロスタジル

$C_{20}H_{34}O_5$: 354.48
7-{(1*R*,2*R*,3*R*)-3-Hydroxy-2-[(1*E*,3*S*)-3-hydroxyoct-1-en-1-yl]-5-oxocyclopentyl}heptanoic acid
[*745-65-3*]

Alprostadil, when dried, contains not less than 97.0% and not more than 103.0% of alprostadil ($C_{20}H_{34}O_5$).

Description Alprostadil occurs as white, crystals or crystalline powder.

It is freely soluble in ethanol (99.5) and in tetrahydrofuran, slightly soluble in acetonitrile, and practically insoluble in water.

Identification **(1)** The absorption spectrum of a solution of Alprostadil in ethanol (99.5) (1 in 100,000) determined as directed under Ultraviolet-visible Spectrophotometry <*2.24*> shows no absorption between 210 nm and 350 nm. Separately, to 10 mL of this solution add 1 mL of potassium hydroxide-ethanol TS, allow to stand for 15 minutes, and determine the absorption spectrum in the same way. Compare the spectrum so obtained with the Reference Spectrum or the spectrum of a solution of Alprostadil RS prepared in the same manner as the sample solution: both spectra exhibit similar intensities of absorption at the same wavelengths.

(2) Determine the infrared absorption spectrum of Alprostadil, previously dried, as directed in the potassium bromide disk method under Infrared Spectrophotometry <*2.25*>, and compare the spectrum with the Reference Spectrum or the spectrum of previously dried Alprostadil RS: both spectra exhibit similar intensities of absorption at the same wave numbers.

Optical rotation <*2.49*> $[\alpha]_D^{20}$: −53 - −61° (after drying, 25 mg, tetrahydrofuran, 5 mL, 100 mm).

Melting point <*2.60*> 114 - 118°C

Purity Related substances—Dissolve 4 mg of Alprostadil in 2 mL of a mixture of acetonitrile for liquid chromatography and water (9:1), and use this solution as the sample solution. Pipet 0.5 mL of the sample solution, and add the mixture of acetonitrile for liquid chromatography and water (9:1) to make exactly 10 mL. Pipet 2 mL of this solution, add the mixture of acetonitrile for liquid chromatography and water (9:1) to make exactly 10 mL, and use this solution as the standard solution. Perform the test with exactly 5 μL each of the sample solution and standard solution as directed under Liquid Chromatography <*2.01*> according to the following conditions, and determine each peak area by the automatic integration method: the area of the peaks, having the relative retention time of about 0.70 and 1.26 to alprostadil, obtained from the sample solution is not larger than 1/2 times the peak area of alprostadil from the standard solution, the area of the peaks, having the relative retention time of about 0.88 and 1.18 to alprostadil, is not larger than the peak area of alprostadil from the standard solution, the area of the peaks other than alprostadil and the peaks mentioned above is not larger than 1/10 times the peak area of alprostadil from the standard solution and the total area of the peaks other than alprostadil is not larger than 2 times the peak area of alprostadil from the standard solution.

Operating conditions—

Detector, column, column temperature, mobile phase, and flow rate: Proceed as directed in the operating conditions in the Assay.

Time span of measurement: About 5 times as long as the retention time of alprostadil, beginning after the solvent peak.

System suitability—

System performance: Proceed as directed in the system suitability in the Assay.

Test for required detectability: Measure exactly 2 mL of the standard solution, add the mixture of acetonitrile for liquid chromatography and water (9:1) to make exactly 20 mL. Confirm that the peak area of alprostadil obtained with 5 μL of this solution is equivalent to 7 to 13% of that with 5 μL of the standard solution.

System repeatability: When the test is repeated 6 times with 5 μL of the standard solution under the above operating conditions, the relative standard deviation of the peak area of alprostadil is not more than 1.5%.

Loss on drying <*2.41*> Not more than 1.0% (0.1 g, in vacuum, phosphorus (V) oxide, 4 hours).

Assay Weigh accurately about 5 mg each of Alprostadil and Alprostadil RS, previously dried, dissolve in exactly 5 mL of the internal standard solution, add a mixture of acetonitrile for liquid chromatography and water (9:1) to make 50 mL, and use these solutions as the sample solution and standard solution, respectively. Perform the test with 5 μL each of the sample solution and standard solution as directed under Liquid Chromatography <*2.01*> according to the following conditions, and calculate the ratios, Q_T and Q_S, of the peak area of alprostadil to that of the internal standard.

Amount (mg) of alprostadil ($C_{20}H_{34}O_5$) = $M_S \times Q_T/Q_S$

M_S: Amount (mg) of Alprostadil RS taken

Internal standard solution—A solution of dimethyl phthalate in the mixture of acetonitrile for liquid chromatography and water (9:1) (1 in 10,000).

Operating conditions—

Detector: An ultraviolet absorption photometer (wavelength: 196 nm).

Column: A stainless steel column 4.6 mm in inside diameter and 15 cm in length, packed with octadecylsilanized silica gel for liquid chromatography (5 μm in particle diameter).

Column temperature: A constant temperature of about 40°C.

Mobile phase: Dissolve 9.07 g of potassium dihydrogen phosphate in water to make 1000 mL. Adjust the pH to 6.3 with a solution prepared by dissolving 9.46 g of disodium hydrogen phosphate in water to make 1000 mL, and dilute to 10 times its volume with water. To 360 mL of this solution add 110 mL of acetonitrile for liquid chromatography and 30 mL of methanol for liquid chromatography.

Flow rate: Adjust so that the retention time of alprostadil is about 10 minutes.

System suitability—

System performance: When the procedure is run with 5 μL of the standard solution under the above operating conditions, alprostadil and the internal standard are eluted in this order with the resolution between these peaks being not less than 9.

System repeatability: When the test is repeated 6 times with 5 μL of the standard solution under the above operating conditions, the relative standard deviation of the ratio of the peak area of alprostadil to that of the internal standard is not more than 1.0%.

Containers and storage Containers—Tight containers.

Storage—Light-resistant, and at a temperature not exceeding 5°C.

Alprostadil Injection

アルプロスタジル注射液

Alprostadil Injection is an emulsion-type injection.

It contains not less than 80.0% and not more than 125.0% of the labeled amount of alprostadil ($C_{20}H_{34}O_5$: 354.48).

Method of preparation Prepare as directed under Injections, with Alprostadil.

Description Alprostadil Injection occurs as a white emulsion and is slightly viscous. It has a distinctive odor.

Identification To a quantity of Alprostadil Injection, corresponding to 10 μg of Alprostadil, add 2 mL of acetonitrile, shake well, and centrifuge. To 3.5 mL of the supernatant liquid add 7 mL of diluted phosphoric acid (1 in 1000), and then run this solution on a column (prepared by filling a 10 mm inside diameter, 9 mm long chromatography tube with 0.4 g of 70 μm octadecylsilanized silica gel for pretreatment) prewashed with 10 mL of methanol and then 10 mL of water. Wash the column with 10 mL of water and then 20 mL of petroleum ether, followed by elution with 2.5 mL of a mixture of methanol and water (4:1). Remove the solvent from the effluent under reduced pressure, dissolve the residue in 100 μL of ethyl acetate, and use this solution as the sample solution. Separately, dissolve 1 mg of Alprostadil RS in 10 mL of ethyl acetate, and use this solution as the standard solution. Perform the test with these solutions as directed under Thin-layer Chromatography <*2.03*>. Spot the entire volume of the sample solution and 100 μL of the standard solution on a plate of silica gel for thin-layer chromatography. Then, develop the plate with a mixture of ethyl acetate, ethanol (99.5) and acetic acid (100) (100:5:1) to a distance of about 10 cm, and air-dry the plate. Spray evenly a solution of phosphomolybdic acid *n*-hydrate in ethanol (99.5) (1 in 10) on the plate, and heat at 100°C for 5 minutes: the color of the spot obtained from the standard solution and the spot corresponding to that location obtained from the sample solution is dark blue.

pH Being specified separately when the drug is granted approval based on the Law.

Purity **(1)** Heavy metals <*1.07*>—Proceed with 4.0 mL of Alprostadil Injection according to Method 2, and perform the test. Prepare the control solution with 2.0 mL of Standard Lead Solution (not more than 5 ppm).

(2) Prostaglandin A_1—Use the sample solution obtained in the Assay as the sample solution. Separately, weigh accurately about 10 mg of prostaglandin A_1, previously dried for 4 hours in a desiccator (in vacuum, phosphorus (V) oxide), and dissolve in ethanol (99.5) to make exactly 100 mL. Pipet 2.5 mL of this solution, and add the mobile phase to make exactly 50 mL. Pipet 1 mL of this solution, add exactly 1 mL of the internal standard solution, and use this solution as the standard solution. Perform the test with 40 μL each of the sample solution and standard solution as directed under Liquid Chromatography <*2.01*> according to the following conditions, calculate the ratios, Q_T and Q_S, of the peak area of prostaglandin A_1 to that of the internal standard, and calculate the amount of prostaglandin A_1 converted to alprostadil using the following equation: not more than 3.0 μg per a volume, equivalent to 5 μg of alprostadil ($C_{20}H_{34}O_5$).

Amount (μg) of prostaglandin A_1 ($C_{20}H_{32}O_4$), converted to alprostadil
$= M_S \times Q_T/Q_S \times 1/2 \times 1.054$

M_S: Amount (mg) of prostaglandin A_1 taken

Internal standard solution—Dissolve 50 mg of 1-naphthol in 20 mL of ethanol (99.5). To 3 mL of this solution add the mobile phase to make 100 mL.
Operating conditions—

Proceed as directed in the operating conditions in the Assay.
System suitability—

System performance, and system repeatability: Proceed as directed in the system suitability in the Assay.

Test for required detectability: To exactly 1 mL of the standard solution add the mobile phase to make exactly 5 mL. Confirm that the peak area of prostaglandin A_1 obtained with 40 μL of this solution is equivalent to 14 to 26% of that with 40 μL of the standard solution.

(3) Peroxide—Pipet 4 mL of Alprostadil Injection, place in a glass-stoppered flask, add 15 mL of a mixture of acetic acid (100) and isooctane (3:2), previously having undergone a 30 minute nitrogen substitution, and dissolve with gentle shaking. To this solution add 0.5 mL of saturated potassium iodide TS, replace the inside of the vessel with nitrogen, and shake for exactly 5 minutes. Then, add 0.5 mL of starch TS, shake vigorously, add 15 mL of water, and shake vigorously. Under a stream of nitrogen, titrate *<2.50>* with 0.01 mol/L sodium thiosulfate VS until the color of the solution disappears. Separately, perform a blank determination using 4 mL of water, and make any necessary correction. Calculate the amount of peroxides using the following equation: not more than 0.5 meq/L.

Amount (meq/L) of peroxides $= V \times 2.5$

V: Amount (mL) of 0.01 mol/L sodium thiosulfate VS consumed

(4) Free fatty acids—Pipet 3 mL of Alprostadil Injection, add exactly 15 mL of a mixture of 2-propanol, heptane and 0.5 mol/L sulfuric acid TS (40:10:1), and shake for 1 minute. After leaving for 10 minutes, add exactly 9 mL of heptane and exactly 9 mL of water, shake the test tube by inverting 10 times, leave for 15 minutes, and pipet 9 mL of the supernatant liquid. To this solution, add 3 mL of a solution prepared by combining 1 volume of Nile blue solution (1 in 5000) washed 5 times with heptane and 9 volumes of ethanol (99.5), and use this solution as the sample solution. Titrate *<2.50>* this solution with 0.02 mol/L sodium hydroxide VS under a stream of nitrogen. Separately, dissolve 5.65 g of oleic acid in heptane to make exactly 200 mL, and use this solution as the standard solution. Pipet 25 mL of the standard solution, add 2 drops of phenolphthalein TS, titrate *<2.50>* with 0.1 mol/L potassium hydroxide-ethanol VS until a light red color develops, and determine the correction factor f. Pipet 30 mL of the standard solution and add heptane to make exactly 200 mL. Pipet 3 mL of this solution, add exactly 15 mL of a mixture of 2-propanol, heptane and 0.5 mol/L sulfuric acid TS (40:10:1), and shake for 1 minute. After leaving for 10 minutes, add exactly 6 mL of heptane and exactly 12 mL of water, shake the test tube by inverting 10 times, and then titrate *<2.50>* in the same manner as for the sample solution. Determine the volume (mL), V_T and V_S, of 0.02 mol/L sodium hydroxide VS consumed by the sample and standard solutions: the amount of free fatty acid is not more than 12.0 meq/L.

Amount (meq/L) of free fatty acids $= V_T/V_S \times f \times 15$

Bacterial endotoxins *<4.01>* Less than 10 EU/mL.

Extractable volume *<6.05>* It meets the requirement.

Foreign insoluble matter *<6.06>* Perform the test according to Method 1: it meets the requirement.

Sterility *<4.06>* Perform the test according to the Membrane filter method: it meets the requirement. However, use the sample solution consisting of equal volume of Alprostadil Injection and a solution prepared by adding water to 0.1 g of polysorbate 80 to make 100 mL.

Particle diameter Being specified separately when the drug is granted approval based on the Law.

Assay Measure exactly a volume of Alprostadil Injection corresponding to 5 μg of alprostadil ($C_{20}H_{34}O_5$), add exactly 1 mL of the internal standard solution, shake, and use this solution as the sample solution. Separately, weigh accurately about 5 mg of Alprostadil RS, previously dried in a desiccator (in vacuum, phosphorus (V) oxide) for 4 hours, dissolve in ethanol (99.5) to make exactly 50 mL, and use this solution as standard stock solution. Pipet 2.5 mL of the standard stock solution, add the mobile phase to make exactly 50 mL, pipet 1 mL, add exactly 1 mL of the internal standard solution, and use this solution as the standard solution. Perform the test with 40 μL each of the sample solution and standard solution as directed under Liquid Chromatography *<2.01>* according to the following conditions using an apparatus equipped with an automatic pretreatment device (using a postcolumn reaction), and calculate the ratios, Q_T and Q_S, of the peak area of alprostadil to that of the internal standard.

Amount (μg) of alprostadil ($C_{20}H_{34}O_5$) $= M_S \times Q_T/Q_S$

M_S: Amount (mg) of Alprostadil RS taken

Internal standard solution—Dissolve 50 mg of 1-naphthol in 20 mL of ethanol (99.5). To 3 mL of this solution add the mobile phase to make 100 mL.
Operating conditions—

Equipment: Liquid chromatograph consisting of 2 pumps for pumping the mobile phase and the reaction reagent, an automatic pretreatment device, column, reaction coil, detector, and recording apparatus. Use a reaction coil that is maintained at a constant temperature.

Detector: An ultraviolet absorption photometer (wavelength: 278 nm).

Column: A stainless steel column 4.6 mm in inside diameter and 15 cm in length, packed with octadecylsilanized silica gel for liquid chromatography (5 μm in particle diameter).

Column temperature: A constant temperature of about 60°C.

Reaction coil: Polytetrafluoroethylene tube 0.5 mm in inside diameter and 10 m in length.

Mobile phase: Dissolve 9.07 g of potassium dihydrogen phosphate in water to make 1000 mL and adjust the pH to 6.3 by adding a solution prepared by dissolving 9.46 g of disodium hydrogen phosphate in water to make 1000 mL. To 1 volume of this solution add 9 volumes of water. To 3 volumes of this solution add 1 volume of acetonitrile for liquid chromatography.

Reaction reagent: Potassium hydroxide TS.

Reaction temperature: A constant temperature of about 60°C.

Mobile phase flow rate: Adjust so that the retention time of alprostadil is about 7 minutes.

Reaction reagent flow rate: 0.5 mL per minute.

Automatic pretreatment device: Composed of a pretreatment column, pump for pumping pretreatment column wash solution, and routing valve for 2 high pressure flow paths.

Pretreatment column: A stainless steel column 4 mm in inside diameter and 2.5 cm in length, packed with octadecylsilanized silica gel for liquid chromatography (5 μm in particle diameter).

Pretreatment column wash solution: Ethanol (99.5).

Flow rate of wash solution: A constant flow rate of about 2.0 mL per minute.

Flow path operating conditions: Change the flow path operating conditions at the times shown in the table below using the valves shown in the figure.

	Time of switchover (minutes)				
Valve	0	9.0	9.1	*1)	*2)
RVA	0	0	1	0	0
RVB	0	1	1	1	0

*1) After the internal standard has completely eluted
*2) 0.1 minutes after *1)

System suitability—

System performance: Dissolve 10 mg of prostaglandin A_1, previously dried in a desiccator (in vacuum, phosphorus (V) oxide) for 4 hours, in ethanol (99.5) to make 100 mL. To 2.5 mL of this solution add 2.5 mL of the standard stock solution, and add the mobile phase to make 50 mL. To 1 mL of this solution add 1 mL of the internal standard solution, shake, and perform the test under the above conditions with 40 μL of the solution. Alprostadil, prostaglandin A_1 and the internal standard are eluted in this order, and the resolution between the peaks of alprostadil and prostaglandin A_1 is not less than 10, and that between prostaglandin A_1 and the internal standard is not less than 2.0.

System repeatability: When the test is repeated 6 times with 40 μL of the standard solution under the above conditions, the relative standard deviation of the ratio of the peak area of alprostadil to that of the internal standard is not more than 2.0%.

Containers and storage Containers—Hermetic containers.

Storage—Light-resistant, not exceeding 5°C, avoiding freezing.

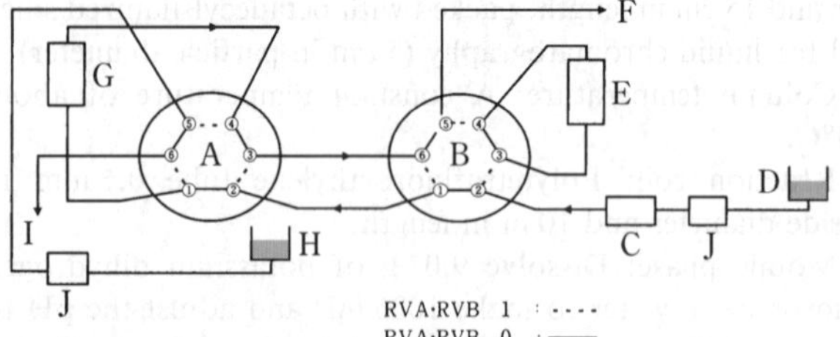

A: RVA valve
B: RVB valve
C: Sample injector
D: Mobile phase
E: Column for pressure correction
F: Column
G: Pretreatment column
H: Wash solution
I: Drain
J: Pump

Figure Components of automatic pretreatment system

Alprostadil Alfadex

アルプロスタジル　アルファデクス

$C_{20}H_{34}O_5 \cdot \chi C_{36}H_{60}O_{30}$
7-{(1*R*,2*R*,3*R*)-3-Hydroxy-2-[(1*E*,3*S*)-3-hydroxyoct-1-en-1-yl]-5-oxocyclopentyl}heptanoic acid—α-cyclodextrin
[*55648-20-9*]

Alprostadil Alfadex is a α-cyclodextrin clathrate compound of alprostadil.

It contains not less than 2.8% and not more than 3.2% of alprostadil ($C_{20}H_{34}O_5$: 354.48), calculated on the anhydrous basis.

Description Alprostadil Alfadex occurs as a white powder.

It is freely soluble in water, and practically insoluble in ethanol (95), in ethyl acetate and in diethyl ether.

It is hygroscopic.

Identification **(1)** Dissolve 0.02 g of Alprostadil Alfadex in 5 mL of water, add 5 mL of ethyl acetate, shake, and centrifuge. Use the supernatant liquid as the sample solution (1). Separately, to 0.02 g of Alprostadil Alfadex add 5 mL of ethyl acetate, shake, and centrifuge. Use the supernatant liquid as the sample solution (2). Evaporate the solvent from these solutions under reduced pressure, add 2 mL of sulfuric acid to the residue, and shake for 5 minutes: the liquid obtained from the sample solution (1) shows an orange-yellow color, while the liquid obtained from the sample solution (2) does not show that color.

(2) Dissolve 0.02 g of Alprostadil Alfadex in 5 mL of water, add 5 mL of ethyl acetate, shake, centrifuge, and evaporate the solvent from the supernatant liquid under reduced pressure. Dissolve the residue in 2 mL of ethanol (95), add 5 mL of 1,3-dinitrobenzene TS, then add 5 mL of a solution of potassium hydroxide in ethanol (95) (17 in 100) under ice-cooling, and allow to stand for 20 minutes in a dark place under ice-cooling: a purple color develops.

(3) Dissolve 0.05 g of Alprostadil Alfadex in 1 mL of iodine TS, by heating on a water bath, and allow to stand: a dark blue precipitate is formed.

(4) Determine the absorption spectrum of a solution of Alprostadil Alfadex in dilute ethanol (3 in 10,000) as directed under Ultraviolet-visible Spectrophotometry <*2.24*>: it exhibits no absorption between 220 nm and 400 nm. Separately, to 10 mL of the solution add 1 mL of potassium hydroxide-ethanol TS, allow to stand for 15 minutes, and determine the absorption spectrum as directed under Ultraviolet-visible Spectrophotometry <*2.24*>, and compare the spectrum with the Reference Spectrum: both spectra exhibit similar intensities of absorption at the same wavelengths.

Optical rotation <*2.49*> $[\alpha]_D^{20}$: +126 – +138° (0.1 g calculated on the anhydrous basis, dilute ethanol, 20 mL, 100 mm).

pH <*2.54*> Dissolve 0.10 g of Alprostadil Alfadex in 20 mL of water: the pH of this solution is between 4.0 and 5.0.

Purity **(1)** Clarity and color of solution—Dissolve 1.0 g of Alprostadil Alfadex in 10 mL of water: the solution is colorless. Perform the test with this solution as directed under Ultraviolet-visible Spectrophotometry within 30 minutes after preparation of the solution: the absorbance at 450 nm is not larger than 0.10.

(2) Prostaglandin A_1—Dissolve 0.10 g of Alprostadil Alfadex in 5 mL of water, add exactly 5 mL of the internal standard solution and ethanol (95) to make 15 mL, and use this solution as the sample solution. Separately, dissolve 1.5 mg of prostaglandin A_1 in ethanol (95) to make exactly 100 mL. Pipet 3 mL of this solution, add exactly 5 mL of the internal standard solution, 2 mL of ethanol (95) and water to make 15 mL, and use this solution as the standard solution. Perform the test with 10 μL each of the sample solution and standard solution as directed under Liquid Chromatography <*2.01*> according to the operating conditions described in the Assay, and calculate the ratios, Q_T and Q_S, of the peak area of prostaglandin A_1 to that of the internal standard: Q_T is not larger than Q_S.

Internal standard solution—A solution of propyl parahydroxybenzoate in dilute ethanol (1 in 15,000).

(3) Related substances—Dissolve 0.10 g of Alprostadil Alfadex in 3 mL of water, add exactly 3 mL of ethyl acetate, shake, centrifuge, and use the supernatant liquid obtained as the sample solution. Separately, dissolve 1.0 mg of prostaglandin A_1 in ethyl acetate to make exactly 100 mL, and use this solution as the standard solution. Perform the test with these solutions as directed under Thin-layer Chromatography <*2.03*>. Spot 10 μL each of the sample solution and standard solution on a plate of silica gel for thin-layer chromatography. Develop the plate with a mixture of ethyl acetate, hexane and acetic acid (100) (10:2:1) to a distance of about 10 cm, and air-dry the plate. Spray evenly a solution of phosphomolybdic acid *n*-hydrate in ethanol (95) (1 in 4) on the plate, and heat the plate at 100°C for 5 minutes: the spots other than the principal spot obtained from the sample solution, and the spots other than the spot corresponding to the spot from the standard solution are all not more intense than the spot from the standard solution.

Water <*2.48*> Not more than 6.0% (0.2 g, direct titration).

Assay Weigh accurately about 0.1 g of Alprostadil Alfadex, dissolve in 5 mL of water, add exactly 5 mL of the internal standard solution and water to make 15 mL, and use this solution as the sample solution. Separately, weigh accurately about 3 mg of Alprostadil RS, dissolve in 5 mL of ethanol (95), add exactly 5 mL of the internal standard solution and water to make 15 mL, and use this solution as the standard solution. Perform the test with 10 μL each of the sample solution and standard solution as directed under Liquid Chromatography <*2.01*> according to the following conditions, and calculate the ratios, Q_T and Q_S, of the peak area of alprostadil to that of the internal standard.

Amount (mg) of alprostadil ($C_{20}H_{34}O_5$)
$= M_S \times Q_T/Q_S$

M_S: Amount (mg) of Alprostadil RS taken

Internal standard solution—A solution of propyl parahydroxybenzoate in dilute ethanol (1 in 15,000).

Operating conditions—

Detector: An ultraviolet absorption photometer (wavelength: 205 nm).

Column: A stainless steel column about 5 mm in inside diameter and about 15 cm in length, packed with octadecylsilanized silica gel for liquid chromatography (5 μm in particle diameter).

Column temperature: A constant temperature of about 25°C.

Mobile phase: A mixture of 0.02 mol/L potassium dihydrogenphosphate and acetonitrile (3:2).

Flow rate: Adjust so that the retention time of alprostadil is about 6 minutes.

Selection of column: Dissolve about 0.1 g of Alprostadil Alfadex in 5 mL of water, add 5 mL of a solution of prostaglandin A_1 in ethanol (95) (3 in 200,000) and 5 mL of the internal standard solution. Proceed with 10 μL of this solution under the above operating conditions, and calculate the resolution. Use a column giving elution of alprostadil, the internal standard and prostaglandin A_1 in this order and complete separation of these peaks.

Containers and storage Containers—Tight containers.

Storage—Light-resistant, at a temperature not exceeding 5°C.

Alum Solution

ミョウバン水

Alum Solution contains not less than 0.27 w/v% and not more than 0.33 w/v% of aluminum potassium sulfate Hydrate [$AlK(SO_4)_2.12H_2O$: 474.39].

Method of preparation

Aluminum Potassium Sulfate Hydrate	3 g
Mentha Water	50 mL
Water, Purified Water or Purified Water in Containers	a sufficient quantity
To make	1000 mL

Dissolve and mix the above ingredients.

Description Alum Solution is a clear, colorless liquid. It has the odor of the mentha oil and an astringent taste.

Identification **(1)** To 5 mL of Alum Solution add 3 mL of ammonium chloride TS and 1 mL of ammonia TS: a white, gelatinous precipitate is produced, which changes to red upon the addition of 5 drops of alizarin red S TS (aluminum sulfate).

(2) Place 100 mL of Alum Solution in an evaporating dish, evaporate on a water bath to dryness, and dissolve the residue in 5 mL of water: the solution responds to Qualitative Tests <*1.09*> for potassium salt.

(3) Alum Solution responds to the Qualitative Tests <*1.09*> (1) and (2) for sulfate.

Assay Pipet 50 mL of Alum Solution, add exactly 30 mL of 0.02 mol/L disodium dihydrogen ethylenediamine tetraacetate VS, and further add 20 mL of acetic acid-ammonium acetate buffer solution (pH 4.8). Boil for 5 minutes, cool, add 55 mL of ethanol (95), and titrate <*2.50*> with 0.02 mol/L zinc acetate VS (indicator: 2 mL of dithizone TS), until the color of the solution changes from light dark green to light red. Perform a blank determination in the same manner.

Each mL of 0.02 mol/L disodium dihydrogen ethylenediamine tetraacetate VS
$= 9.488$ mg of $AlK(SO_4)_2.12H_2O$

Containers and storage Containers—Tight containers.

Dried Aluminum Hydroxide Gel

乾燥水酸化アルミニウムゲル

Dried Aluminum Hydroxide Gel contains not less than 50.0% of aluminum oxide (Al_2O_3: 101.96).

Description Dried Aluminum Hydroxide Gel occurs as a white, amorphous powder. It is odorless and tasteless.

It is practically insoluble in water, in ethanol (95) and in diethyl ether.

Most of it dissolves in dilute hydrochloric acid and in sodium hydroxide TS.

Identification To 0.2 g of Dried Aluminum Hydroxide Gel add 20 mL of dilute hydrochloric acid, warm, and centrifuge: the supernatant liquid responds to Qualitative Tests <*1.09*> for aluminum salt.

Purity **(1)** Acidity or alkalinity—To 1.0 g of Dried Aluminum Hydroxide Gel add 25 mL of water, shake well, and centrifuge: the supernatant liquid is neutral.

(2) Chloride <*1.03*>—To 1.0 g of Dried Aluminum Hydroxide Gel add 30 mL of dilute nitric acid, heat gently to boil while shaking, cool, add water to make 100 mL, and centrifuge. To 5 mL of the supernatant liquid add 6 mL of dilute nitric acid and water to make 50 mL. Perform the test using this solution as the test solution. Prepare the control solution with 0.40 mL of 0.01 mol/L hydrochloric acid VS (not more than 0.284%).

(3) Sulfate <*1.14*>—To 1.0 g of Dried Aluminum Hydroxide Gel add 15 mL of dilute hydrochloric acid, heat gently to boil while shaking, cool, add water to make 250 mL, and centrifuge. To 25 mL of the supernatant liquid add 1 mL of dilute hydrochloric acid and water to make 50 mL. Perform the test using this solution as the test solution. Prepare the control solution with 1.0 mL of 0.005 mol/L sulfuric acid VS (not more than 0.480%).

(4) Nitrate—To 0.10 g of Dried Aluminum Hydroxide Gel add 5 mL of water, then carefully add 5 mL of sulfuric acid, shake well to dissolve, and cool. Superimpose the solution on 2 mL of iron (II) sulfate TS: no brown-colored ring is produced at the zone of contact.

(5) Heavy metals <*1.07*>—Dissolve 2.0 g of Dried Aluminum Hydroxide Gel in 10 mL of dilute hydrochloric acid by heating, filter if necessary, and add water to make 50 mL. Perform the test with this solution as the test solution. Prepare the control solution as follows: evaporate 10 mL of dilute hydrochloric acid to dryness, and add 2.0 mL of Standard Lead Solution, 2 mL of dilute acetic acid and water to make 50 mL (not more than 10 ppm).

(6) Arsenic <*1.11*>—To 0.8 g of Dried Aluminum Hydroxide Gel add 10 mL of dilute sulfuric acid, heat gently to boil while shaking, cool, and filter. Take 5 mL of the filtrate, use this solution as the test solution, and perform the test (not more than 5 ppm).

Acid-consuming capacity Weigh accurately about 0.2 g of Dried Aluminum Hydroxide Gel, and transfer to a glass-stoppered flask. Add exactly 100 mL of 0.1 mol/L hydrochloric acid VS, stopper the flask, shake at 37 ± 2°C for 1 hour, and filter. Measure exactly 50 mL of the filtrate, and titrate <*2.50*> while thoroughly stirring, the excess hydrochloric acid with 0.1 mol/L sodium hydroxide VS until the pH of the solution becomes to 3.5. The volume of 0.1 mol/L hydrochloric acid VS consumed is not less than 250 mL per g of Dried Aluminum Hydroxide Gel.

Assay Weigh accurately about 2 g of Dried Aluminum Hydroxide Gel, add 15 mL of hydrochloric acid, heat on a water bath with shaking for 30 minutes, cool, and add water to make exactly 500 mL. Pipet 20 mL of this solution, add exactly 30 mL of 0.05 mol/L disodium dihydrogen ethylenediamine tetraacetate VS and 20 mL of acetic acid (31)-ammonium acetate buffer solution (pH 4.8), boil for 5 minutes, and cool. Add 55 mL of ethanol (95), and titrate <*2.50*> with 0.05 mol/L zinc acetate VS until the color of the solution changes from light dark green to light red. (indicator: 2 mL of dithizone TS). Perform a blank determination in the same manner, and make any necessary correction.

Each mL of 0.05 mol/L disodium dihydrogen ethylenediamine tetraacetate VS
= 2.549 mg of Al_2O_3

Containers and storage Containers—Tight containers.

Dried Aluminum Hydroxide Gel Fine Granules

乾燥水酸化アルミニウムゲル細粒

Dried Aluminum Hydroxide Gel Fine Granules contain not less than 47.0% of aluminum oxide (Al_2O_3: 101.96).

Method of preparation Prepare as directed under Granules, with Dried Aluminum Hydroxide Gel.

Identification To 0.2 g of Dried Aluminum Hydroxide Gel Fine Granules add 20 mL of dilute hydrochloric acid, warm and centrifuge: the supernatant liquid responds to Qualitative Tests <*1.09*> for aluminum salt.

Acid-consuming capacity Proceed as directed for Acid-consuming capacity under Dried Aluminum Hydroxide Gel: the volume of 0.1 mol/L hydrochloric acid VS consumed is not less than 235 mL per g of Dried Aluminum Hydroxide Gel Fine Granules.

Assay Proceed as directed in the Assay under Dried Aluminum Hydroxide Gel.

Each mL of 0.05 mol/L disodium dihydrogen ethylenediamine tetraacetate VS
= 2.549 mg of Al_2O_3

Containers and storage Containers—Tight containers.

Aluminum Monostearate

モノステアリン酸アルミニウム

Aluminum Monostearate is mainly aluminum compounds of stearic acid ($C_{18}H_{36}O_2$: 284.48) and palmitic acid ($C_{16}H_{32}O_2$: 256.42).

Aluminum Monostearate, when dried, contains not less than 7.2% and not more than 8.9% of aluminum (Al: 26.98).

Description Aluminum Monostearate occurs as a white to yellow-white powder. It is odorless or has a faint, characteristic odor.

It is practically insoluble in water, in ethanol (95) and in diethyl ether.

Identification **(1)** Heat 3 g of Aluminum Monostearate with 30 mL of hydrochloric acid in a water bath with occasional shaking for 10 minutes. After cooling, shake the mixture vigorously with 50 mL of water and 30 mL of diethyl ether for 3 minutes, and allow to stand. To the separated aqueous layer add sodium hydroxide TS until the solution becomes slightly turbid, and filter: the filtrate responds to Qualitative Tests <*1.09*> for aluminum salt.

(2) Wash the diethyl ether layer separated in (1) with two 20-mL portions of water, and evaporate the diethyl ether layer on a water bath: the residue melts <*1.13*> at above 54°C.

Acid value for fatty acid <*1.13*> 193 – 210. Weigh accurately about 1 g of fatty acid obtained in the Identification (2), transfer a 250-mL glass-stoppered flask, add 100 mL of a mixture of diethyl ether and ethanol (95) (2:1), warm to dissolve, add several drops of phenolphthalein TS, and proceed as directed under Acid Value.

Purity **(1)** Free fatty acid—Mix 1.0 g of Aluminum Monostearate with about 50 mL of a mixture of neutralized ethanol and diethyl ether (1:1), filter through dry filter paper, wash the vessel and the filter paper with a small amount of a mixture of neutralized ethanol and diethyl ether (1:1), combine the filtrate and the washings, and add 2.1 mL of 0.1 mol/L potassium hydroxide VS: a red color develops.

(2) Water-soluble salts—Heat 2.0 g of Aluminum Monostearate with 80 mL of water in a loosely stoppered conical flask on a water bath for 30 minutes with occasional shaking. After cooling, filter through dry filter paper, wash the residue with a small amount of water, combine the washings with the filtrate, add water to make 100 mL, evaporate 50 mL of this solution on a water bath, and heat strongly at 600°C: the mass of the residue is not more than 10.0 mg.

(3) Heavy metals <*1.07*>—Heat 1.0 g of Aluminum Monostearate over a small flame with caution at the beginning, and continue the heating, gradually raising the temperature, to ash. After cooling, add 10 mL of diluted hydrochloric acid (1 in 2), evaporate on a water bath, and boil the residue with 20 mL of water for 1 minute. Cool, filter, wash the residue with water, combine the filtrate and the washings, and add 2 mL of dilute acetic acid and water to make 50 mL. Perform the test using this solution as the test solution. Evaporate 10 mL of diluted hydrochloric acid (1 in 2) on a water bath to dryness, add 2 mL of dilute acetic acid and 5.0 mL of Standard Lead Solution, dilute with water to make 50 mL, and use this solution as the control solution (not more than 50 ppm).

(4) Arsenic <*1.11*>—Mix 1.0 g of Aluminum Monostearate with 2 g of magnesium nitrate hexahydrate, ignite over a small flame, moisten the residue after cooling with 0.5 mL of nitric acid, and heat. Heat again the residue with 10 mL of dilute sulfuric acid until white fumes evolve, add water to make 5 mL, and perform the test with this solution as the test solution (not more than 2 ppm).

Loss on drying <*2.41*> Not more than 3.0% (1 g, 105°C, 3 hours).

Assay Weigh accurately about 1 g of Aluminum Monostearate, previously dried, ignite gently to ash, and cool. Add dropwise 0.5 mL of nitric acid, evaporate on a water bath by heating, and then heat strongly between 900°C and 1100°C to a constant mass. After cooling, weigh rapidly the ignited residue, and designate the mass as aluminum oxide (Al_2O_3: 101.96).

Amount (mg) of aluminum (Al)
= amount (mg) of aluminum oxide (Al_2O_3) × 0.529

Containers and storage Containers—Well-closed containers.

Dried Aluminum Potassium Sulfate

Burnt Alum

乾燥硫酸アルミニウムカリウム

$AlK(SO_4)_2$: 258.21

Dried Aluminum Potassium Sulfate, when dried, contains not less than 98.0% of aluminum potassium sulfate [$AlK(SO_4)_2$].

Description Dried Aluminum Potassium Sulfate occurs as white masses or white powder. It is odorless. It has a slightly sweet, astringent taste.

It is freely soluble in hot water and practically insoluble in ethanol (95).

It dissolves slowly in water.

Identification A solution of Dried Aluminum Potassium Sulfate (1 in 20) responds to Qualitative Tests <*1.09*> for aluminum salt, to Qualitative Tests <*1.09*> (1), (3) and (4) for potassium salt, and to Qualitative Tests <*1.09*> (1) and (3) for sulfate.

Purity **(1)** Water-insoluble substances—To 2.0 g of Dried Aluminum Potassium Sulfate add 40 mL of water, shake frequently, and allow to stand for 48 hours. Collect the insoluble residue on a glass filter (G4), wash with 50 mL of water, and dry at 105°C for 2 hours: the mass of the residue is not more than 50 mg.

(2) Heavy metals <*1.07*>—Dissolve 0.5 g of Dried Aluminum Potassium Sulfate in 45 mL of water, and filter, if necessary. Add 2 mL of dilute acetic acid and water to make 50 mL, and perform the test using this solution as the test solution. Prepare the control solution with 2.0 mL of Standard Lead Solution, 2 mL of dilute acetic acid and water to make 50 mL (not more than 40 ppm).

(3) Iron <*1.10*>—Prepare the test solution with 0.54 g of Dried Aluminum Potassium Sulfate according to Method 1, and perform the test according to Method A. Prepare the control solution with 2.0 mL of Standard Iron Solution (not more than 37 ppm).

(4) Arsenic <*1.11*>—Prepare the test solution with 0.40 g of Dried Aluminum Potassium Sulfate, according to Method 1, and perform the test (not more than 5 ppm).

Loss on drying <*2.41*> Not more than 15.0% (2 g, 200°C, 4 hours).

Assay Weigh accurately about 1.2 g of Dried Aluminum Potassium Sulfate, previously dried, add 80 mL of water, and heat on a water bath with occasional shaking for 20 minutes. Cool, add water to make exactly 100 mL, and filter, if necessary. Discard the first 30 mL of the filtrate, take exactly the subsequent 20 mL of the filtrate, and add exactly 30 mL of 0.05 mol/L disodium dihydrogen ethylenediamine tetraacetate VS and 20 mL of acetic acid-ammonium acetate buffer solution (pH 4.8), boil for 5 minutes, and cool. Add 55 mL of ethanol (95), and titrate <*2.50*> with 0.05 mol/L zinc acetate VS (indicator: 2 mL of dithizone TS), until the color of the solution changes from light dark green to light red. Perform a blank determination in the same manner.

Each mL of 0.05 mol/L disodium dihydrogen ethylenediamine tetraacetate VS
= 12.91 mg of $AlK(SO_4)_2$

Containers and storage Containers—Tight containers.

Aluminum Potassium Sulfate Hydrate

Alum

硫酸アルミニウムカリウム水和物

$AlK(SO_4)_2.12H_2O$: 474.39

Aluminum Potassium Sulfate Hydrate contains not less than 99.5% of aluminum potassium sulfate hydrate [$AlK(SO_4)_2.12H_2O$].

Description Aluminum Potassium Sulfate Hydrate occurs as colorless or white, crystals or powder. It is odorless. It has a slightly sweet, strongly astringent taste.

It is freely soluble in water, and practically insoluble in ethanol (95) and in diethyl ether.

A solution of Aluminum Potassium Sulfate Hydrate (1 in 20) is acid.

Identification A solution of Aluminum Potassium Sulfate Hydrate (1 in 10) responds to Qualitative Tests <*1.09*> for aluminum salt, to Qualitative Tests <*1.09*> (1), (3) and (4) for potassium salt, and to the Qualitative Tests <*1.09*> (1) and (3) for sulfate.

Purity (1) Heavy metals <*1.07*>—Proceed with 1.0 g of Aluminum Potassium Sulfate Hydrate according to Method 1, and perform the test. Prepare the control solution with 2.0 mL of Standard Lead Solution (not more than 20 ppm).

(2) Iron <*1.10*>—Prepare the test solution with 1.0 g of Aluminum Potassium Sulfate Hydrate according to Method 1, and perform the test according to Method A. Prepare the control solution with 2.0 mL of Standard Iron Solution (not more than 20 ppm).

(3) Arsenic <*1.11*>—Prepare the test solution with 0.6 g of Aluminum Potassium Sulfate Hydrate, according to Method 1, and perform the test (not more than 3.3 ppm).

Assay Weigh accurately about 4.5 g of Aluminum Potassium Sulfate Hydrate, and dissolve in water to make exactly 200 mL. Take exactly 20 mL of this solution, and add exactly 30 mL of 0.05 mol/L disodium dihydrogen ethylenediamine tetraacetate VS and 20 mL of acetic acid-ammonium acetate buffer solution (pH 4.8), boil for 5 minutes, and cool. Add 55 mL of ethanol (95), and titrate <*2.50*> with 0.05 mol/L zinc acetate VS (indicator: 2 mL of dithizone TS), until the color of the solution changes from light dark green to light red. Perform a blank determination in the same manner.

Each mL of 0.05 mol/L disodium dihydorogen ethylenediamine tetraacetate VS
= 23.72 mg of $AlK(SO_4)_2.12H_2O$

Containers and storage Containers—Tight containers.

Natural Aluminum Silicate

天然ケイ酸アルミニウム

Description Natural Aluminum Silicate occurs as a white or slightly colored powder. It is odorless and tasteless.

It is practically insoluble in water, in ethanol (95) and in diethyl ether.

Natural Aluminum Silicate (1 g) dissolves when heated in 20 mL of a solution of sodium hydroxide (1 in 5), with some decomposition, leaving a large amount of insoluble substance.

Identification (1) To 0.5 g of Natural Aluminum Silicate add 3 mL of diluted sulfuric acid (1 in 3), heat until white fumes evolve, cool, add 20 mL of water, and filter. Render the filtrate slightly acid with ammonia TS: the solution responds to Qualitative Tests <*1.09*> for aluminum salt.

(2) Prepare a bead by fusing ammonium sodium hydrogenphosphate tetrahydrate on a platinum loop. Place the bead in contact with Natural Aluminum Silicate, and fuse again: an infusible material appears in the bead, producing, upon cooling, an opaque bead with a web-like structure.

Purity (1) Acidity or alkalinity—Shake 5.0 g of Natural Aluminum Silicate with 100 mL of water, and centrifuge: the supernatant liquid so obtained is neutral.

(2) Chloride <*1.03*>—To 5.0 g of Natural Aluminum Silicate add 100 mL of water, boil gently for 15 minutes while shaking, then cool, add water to restore the original volume, and centrifuge. To 10 mL of the supernatant liquid add 6 mL of dilute nitric acid, dilute to 50 mL with water, and perform the test using this solution as the test solution. Prepare the control solution with 0.30 mL of 0.01 mol/L hydrochloric acid VS (not more than 0.021%).

(3) Sulfate <*1.14*>—To the residue obtained in (6) add 3 mL of dilute hydrochloric acid, heat on a water bath for 10 minutes, dilute to 50 mL with water, and filter. To 2.0 mL of the filtrate add 1 mL of dilute hydrochloric acid and water to make 50 mL. Perform the test using this solution as the test solution. Prepare the control solution with 1.0 mL of 0.005 mol/L sulfuric acid VS (not more than 0.480%).

(4) Heavy metals <*1.07*>—To 1.5 g of Natural Aluminum Silicate add 50 mL of water and 5 mL of hydrochloric acid, boil gently for 20 minutes while shaking, then cool, centrifuge, remove the supernatant liquid, wash the residue with two 10-mL portions of water, centrifuging each time, combine these washings with the filtrate, and add ammonia solution (28) dropwise, until a precipitate just appears. Add dropwise dilute hydrochloric acid with vigorous shaking and redissolve the precipitate. Heat the mixture with 0.45 g of hydroxylammonium chloride, cool, and add 0.45 g of sodium acetate trihydrate, 6 mL of dilute acetic acid and water to make 150 mL. Perform the test, using 50 mL of this solution as the test solution. Prepare the control solution with 2.0 mL of Standard Lead Solution, 0.15 g of hydroxylammonium chloride, 0.15 g of sodium acetate trihydrate, 2 mL of dilute acetic acid and water to make 50 mL (not more than 40 ppm).

(5) Arsenic <*1.11*>—To 1.0 g of Natural Aluminum Silicate, add 5 mL of dilute hydrochloric acid, heat gently to boil while shaking well, cool rapidly, and centrifuge. Mix the residue with 5 mL of dilute hydrochloric acid with shaking, centrifuge, then add 10 mL of water to the residue, and repeat the extraction in the same manner. Concentrate the

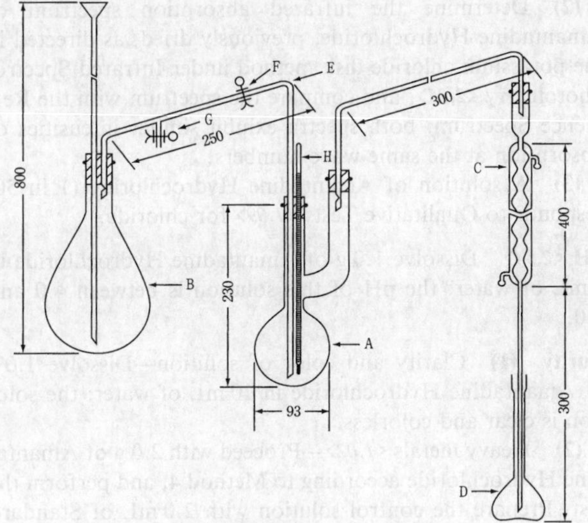

The figures are in mm.

A: Distilling flask of about 300-mL capacity.
B: Steam generator of about 1000-mL capacity, containing a few boiling tips to prevent bumping
C: Condenser
D: Receiver: 200-mL volumetric flask
E: Steam-introducing tube having an internal diameter of about 8 mm
F, G: Rubber tube with a clamp
H: Thermometer

combined extracts on a water bath to 5 mL. Use this solution as the test solution, and perform the test (not more than 2 ppm).

(6) Soluble salts—Evaporate 50 mL of the supernatant liquid obtained in (1) on a water bath to dryness, and ignite the residue at 700°C for 2 hours: the mass of the ignited residue is not more than 40 mg.

(7) Fluoride—(i) Apparatus: Use a hard glass apparatus as illustrated in the figure. Ground-glass joints may be used.

(ii) Procedure: Transfer 5.0 g of Natural Aluminum Silicate to the distilling flask A with the aid of 20 mL of water, add about 1 g of glass wool and 50 mL of diluted purified sulfuric acid (1 in 2), and connect A to the distillation apparatus, previously washed with steam streamed through the steam introducing tube E. Connect the condenser C with the receiver D containing 10 mL of 0.01 mol/L sodium hydroxide VS and 10 mL of water so that the lower end of C is immersed in the solution. Heat A gradually until the temperature of the solution in A reaches 130°C, then open the rubber tube F, close the rubber tube G, boil water in the steam generator B vigorously, and introduce the generated steam into F. Simultaneously, heat A, and maintain the temperature of the solution in A between 135°C and 145°C. Adjust the distilling rate to about 10 mL per minute. Collect about 170 mL of the distillate, then stop the distillation, wash C with a small quantity of water, combine the washings with the distillate, add water to make exactly 200 mL, and use this solution as the test solution. Perform the test with the test solution as directed in the procedure of determination for fluoride under Oxygen Flask Combustion Method <*1.06*>. No corrective solution is used in this procedure. The content of fluoride (F) is not more than 0.01%.

Amount (mg) of fluoride (F: 19.00) in the test solution
= amount (mg) of fluoride in 5 mL of the standard solution $\times A_T/A_S \times 200/V$

Loss on drying <*2.41*> Not more than 20.0% (1 g, 105°C, 3 hours).

Adsorptive power To 0.10 g of Natural Aluminum Silicate add 20 mL of a solution of methylene blue trihydrate (3 in 2000), shake for 15 minutes, allow to stand for 5 hours at 37 ± 2°C, and centrifuge. Dilute 1.0 mL of the supernatant liquid with water to 200 mL. Place 50 mL of the solution in a Nessler tube and observe horizontally or vertically against a white background: the color of the solution is not deeper than that of the following control solution.

Control solution: Dilute 1.0 mL of a solution of methylene blue trihydrate (3 in 2000) with water to 400 mL, and use 50 mL of this solution.

Containers and storage Containers—Well-closed containers.

Synthetic Aluminum Silicate

合成ケイ酸アルミニウム

Description Synthetic Aluminum Silicate occurs as a white powder. It is odorless and tasteless.

It is practically insoluble in water, in ethanol (95) and in diethyl ether.

Synthetic Aluminum Silicate (1 g) dissolves when heated in 20 mL of a solution of sodium hydroxide (1 in 5), leaving a small amount of insoluble substance .

Identification **(1)** To 0.5 g of Synthetic Aluminum Silicate add 3 mL of diluted sulfuric acid (1 in 3), heat until white fumes evolve, cool, add 20 mL of water, and filter. Render the filtrate slightly acid with ammonia TS: the solution responds to Qualitative Tests <*1.09*> for aluminum salt.

(2) Prepare a bead by fusing ammonium sodium hydrogenphosphate tetrahydrate on a platinum loop. Place the bead in contact with Synthetic Aluminum Silicate, and fuse again: an infusible material appears in the bead, producing, upon cooling, an opaque bead with a web-like structure.

Purity **(1)** Acidity or alkalinity—Shake 1.0 g of Synthetic Aluminum Silicate with 20 mL of water, and centrifuge: the supernatant liquid so obtained is neutral.

(2) Chloride <*1.03*>—To 5.0 g of Synthetic Aluminum Silicate add 100 mL of water, boil gently for 15 minutes while shaking, then cool, add water to restore the original volume, and centrifuge. To 10 mL of the supernatant liquid add 6 mL of dilute nitric acid and water to make 50 mL, and perform the test using this solution as the test solution. Prepare the control solution with 0.30 mL of 0.01 mol/L hydrochloric acid VS (not more than 0.021%).

(3) Sulfate <*1.14*>—To 2.0 mL of the supernatant liquid obtained in (2) add 1 mL of dilute hydrochloric acid and water to make 50 mL. Perform the test using this solution as the test solution. Prepare the control solution with 1.0 mL of 0.005 mol/L sulfuric acid VS (not more than 0.480%).

(4) Heavy metals <*1.07*>—To 3.0 g of Synthetic Aluminum Silicate add 50 mL of water and 5 mL of hydrochloric acid, boil gently for 20 minutes while shaking, then after cooling, centrifuge, remove the supernatant liquid, wash the precipitate with two 10-mL portions of water, centrifuging each time, combine these washings with the filtrate, and add ammonia solution (28) dropwise until a precipitate just appears. Add dropwise dilute hydrochloric acid with vigorous shaking to redissolve the precipitate. Heat the solution with 0.45 g of hydroxylammonium chloride, and after cooling, add 0.45 g of sodium acetate trihydrate, 6 mL of dilute acetic acid and water to make 150 mL. Perform the test with 50 mL of this solution as the test solution. Prepare the control solution with 3.0 mL of Standard Lead Solution, 0.15 g of hydroxylammonium chloride, 0.15 g of sodium acetate trihydrate, 2 mL of dilute acetic acid and water to make 50 mL (not more than 30 ppm).

(5) Arsenic *<1.11>*—To 1.0 g of Synthetic Aluminum Silicate add 10 mL of dilute hydrochloric acid, heat gently to boiling while shaking well, cool rapidly, and centrifuge. Mix the residue with 5 mL of dilute hydrochloric acid with shaking, centrifuge, then add 10 mL of water to the residue, and repeat the extraction in the same manner. Concentrate the combined extracts on a water bath to 5 mL. Use this solution as the test solution, and perform the test (not more than 2 ppm).

Loss on drying *<2.41>* Not more than 20.0% (1 g, 105°C, 3 hours).

Acid-consuming capacity *<6.04>* Weigh accurately about 1 g of Synthetic Aluminum Silicate, transfer to a glass-stoppered flask, add 200 mL of 0.1 mol/L hydrochloric acid VS, exactly measured, stopper the flask, and shake at 37 ± 2°C for 1 hour. Filter, pipet 50 mL of the filtrate, and titrate *<2.50>* by stirring well the excess hydrochloric acid with 0.1 mol/L sodium hydroxide VS until the pH of the solution changes to 3.5. The volume of 0.1 mol/L hydrochloric acid VS consumed is not less than 50.0 mL per g of Synthetic Aluminum Silicate.

Containers and storage Containers—Well-closed containers.

Amantadine Hydrochloride

アマンタジン塩酸塩

$C_{10}H_{17}N.HCl$: 187.71
Tricyclo[3.3.1.1^{3,7}]dec-1-ylamine monohydrochloride
[665-66-7]

Amantadine Hydrochloride, when dried, contains not less than 99.0% of amantadine hydrochloride ($C_{10}H_{17}N.HCl$).

Description Amantadine Hydrochloride occurs as a white crystalline powder. It is odorless, and has a bitter taste.

It is very soluble in formic acid, freely soluble in water, in methanol and in ethanol (95), and practically insoluble in diethyl ether.

Identification **(1)** To 0.1 g of Amantadine Hydrochloride add 1 mL of pyridine and 0.1 mL of acetic anhydride, dissolve by boiling for 1 minute, add 10 mL of dilute hydrochloric acid, and cool in ice water. Filter the crystals separated, wash with water, and dry at 105°C for 1 hour: the residue melts *<2.60>* between 147°C and 151°C.

(2) Determine the infrared absorption spectrum of Amantadine Hydrochloride, previously dried, as directed in the potassium chloride disk method under Infrared Spectrophotometry *<2.25>*, and compare the spectrum with the Reference Spectrum: both spectra exhibit similar intensities of absorption at the same wave numbers.

(3) A solution of Amantadine Hydrochloride (1 in 50) responds to Qualitative Tests *<1.09>* for chloride.

pH *<2.54>* Dissolve 1.0 g of Amantadine Hydrochloride in 5 mL of water: the pH of this solution is between 4.0 and 6.0.

Purity **(1)** Clarity and color of solution—Dissolve 1.0 g of Amantadine Hydrochloride in 10 mL of water: the solution is clear and colorless.

(2) Heavy metals *<1.07>*—Proceed with 2.0 g of Amantadine Hydrochloride according to Method 4, and perform the test. Prepare the control solution with 2.0 mL of Standard Lead Solution (not more than 10 ppm).

(3) Arsenic *<1.11>*—Prepare the test solution with 1.0 g of Amantadine Hydrochloride according to Method 3, and perform the test (not more than 2 ppm).

(4) Related substances—Dissolve 0.50 g of Amantadine Hydrochloride in 10 mL of water, add 10 mL of sodium hydroxide TS and 10 mL of chloroform, and shake. Filter the chloroform layer through absorbent cotton with 3 g of anhydrous sodium sulfate on a funnel, and use the filtrate as the sample solution. Pipet 1 mL of the sample solution, add chloroform to make exactly 100 mL, and use this solution as the standard solution. Perform the test with exactly 2 μL each of the sample solution and standard solution as directed under Gas Chromatography *<2.02>* according to the following conditions. Determine each peak area of these solutions by the automatic integration method: each peak area other than amantadine obtained from the sample solution is not larger than 1/3 times the peak area of amantadine from the standard solution, and the total area of each peak is not larger than the peak area of amantadine from the standard solution.

Operating conditions—

Detector: A hydrogen flame-ionization detector.

Column: A glass column about 3 mm in inside diameter and about 2 m in length, packed with siliceous earth for gas chromatography (150 to 180 μm in particle diameter) coated with a mixture (L) of branched hydrocarbon of petroleum hexamethyltetracosane group for gas chromatography and potassium hydroxide at the ratios of 2% and 1%, respectively.

Column temperature: Inject at a constant temperature of about 125°C, maintain the temperature for 5 minutes, raise at the rate of 5°C per minute to 150°C, and maintain at a constant temperature of about 150°C for 15 minutes.

Carrier gas: Nitrogen.

Flow rate: Adjust so that the retention time of amantadine is about 11 minutes.

Selection of column: Dissolve 0.15 g of naphthalene in 5 mL of the sample solution, and add chloroform to make 100 mL. Proceed with 2 μL of this solution under the above operating conditions, and calculate the resolution. Use a column giving elution of naphthalene and amantadine in this order with the resolution between these peaks being not less than 2.5.

Detection sensitivity: Adjust the detection sensitivity so that the peak height of amantadine obtained from 2 μL of the standard solution composes about 10% of the full scale.

Time span of measurement: About twice as long as the retention time of amantadine, beginning after the solvent peak.

Loss on drying <2.41> Not more than 0.5% (1 g, 105°C, 3 hours).

Residue on ignition <2.44> Not more than 0.2% (1 g).

Assay Weigh accurately about 0.2 g of Amantadine Hydrochloride, previously dried, dissolve in 2 mL of formic acid, add exactly 15 mL of 0.1 mol/L perchloric acid VS, and heat on a water bath for 30 minutes. After cooling, add acetic acid (100) to make 70 mL, and titrate <2.50> the excess perchloric acid with 0.1 mol/L sodium acetate VS (potentiometric titration). Perform a blank determination in the same manner, and make any necessary correction.

Each mL of 0.1 mol/L perchloric acid VS
= 18.77 mg of $C_{10}H_{17}N.HCl$

Containers and storage Containers—Well-closed containers.

Ambenonium Chloride

アンベノニウム塩化物

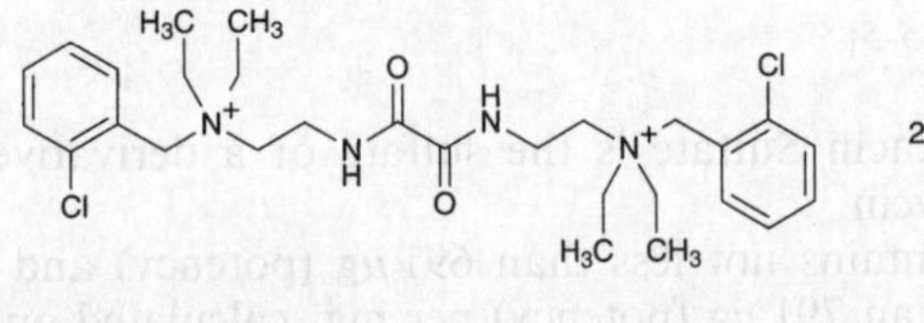

$C_{28}H_{42}Cl_4N_4O_2$: 608.47
2,2′-[(1,2-Dioxoethane-1,2-diyl)diimino]bis[*N*-(2-chlorobenzyl)-*N*,*N*-diethylethylaminium] dichloride
[*115-79-7*]

Ambenonium Chloride contains not less than 98.5% of ambenonium chloride ($C_{28}H_{42}Cl_4N_4O_2$), calculated on the dried basis.

Description Ambenonium Chloride occurs as a white powder.

It is freely soluble in water, in methanol and in acetic acid (100), soluble in ethanol (95), and slightly soluble in acetic anhydride.

It is hygroscopic.

Melting point: about 205°C (with decomposition).

Identification (1) Determine the absorption spectrum of a solution of Ambenonium Chloride in methanol (1 in 5000) as directed under Ultraviolet-visible Spectrophotometry <2.24>, and compare the spectrum with the Reference Spectrum: both spectra exhibit similar intensities of absorption at the same wavelengths.

(2) Determine the infrared absorption spectrum of Ambenonium Chloride, previously dried, as directed in the potassium chloride disk method under Infrared Spectrophotometry <2.25>, and compare the spectrum with the Reference Spectrum: both spectra exhibit similar intensities of absorption at the same wave numbers.

(3) A solution of Ambenonium Chloride (1 in 100) responds to Qualitative Tests <1.09> for chloride.

Purity (1) Clarity and color of solution—Dissolve 1.0 g of Ambenonium Chloride in 10 mL of water: the solution is clear and colorless.

(2) Heavy metals <1.07>—Proceed with 1.0 g of Ambenonium Chloride according to Method 4, and perform the test. Use a solution of magnesium nitrate in ethanol (95) (1 in 5). Prepare the control solution with 2.0 mL of Standard Lead Solution (not more than 20 ppm).

(3) Related substances—Dissolve 0.10 g of Ambenonium Chloride in 10 mL of methanol, and use this solution as the sample solution. Pipet 1 mL of the sample solution, and add methanol to make exactly 20 mL. Pipet 1 mL of this solution, add methanol to make exactly 10 mL, and use this solution as the standard solution. Perform the test with these solutions as directed under Thin-layer Chromatography <2.03>. Spot 5 μL each of the sample solution and standard solution on a plate of silica gel for thin-layer chromatography. Develop the plate with a mixture of 1-butanol, formic acid and water (12:6:5) to a distance of about 10 cm, and air-dry the plate. Allow the plate to stand in iodine vapor: the spots other than the principal spot obtained from the sample solution are not more intense than the spot from the standard solution.

Loss on drying <2.41> Not more than 11.5% (1 g, 105°C, 4 hours).

Residue on ignition <2.44> Not more than 0.2% (1 g).

Assay Weigh accurately about 0.3 g of Ambenonium Chloride, and dissolve in 50 mL of a mixture of acetic anhydride and acetic acid (100) (7:3). Titrate <2.50> with 0.1 mol/L perchloric acid VS (potentiometric titration). Perform a blank determination in the same manner, and make any necessary correction.

Each mL of 0.1 mol/L perchloric acid VS
= 30.42 mg of $C_{28}H_{42}Cl_4N_4O_2$

Containers and storage Containers—Tight containers.

Amidotrizoic Acid

アミドトリゾ酸

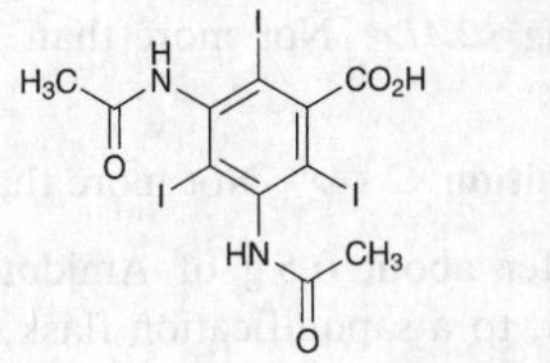

$C_{11}H_9I_3N_2O_4$: 613.91
3,5-Bis(acetylamino)-2,4,6-triiodobenzoic acid
[*117-96-4*]

Amidotrizoic Acid, calculated on the dried basis, contains not less than 98.0% of amidotrizoic acid ($C_{11}H_9I_3N_2O_4$).

Description Amidotrizoic Acid occurs as a white crystalline powder. It is odorless.

It is slightly soluble in ethanol (95), very slightly soluble in water, and practically insoluble in diethyl ether.

It dissolves in sodium hydroxide TS.

Identification (1) Heat 0.1 g of Amidotrizoic Acid over a flame: a purple gas is evolved.

(2) Determine the infrared absorption spectrum of Amidotrizoic Acid as directed in the potassium bromide disk method under Infrared Spectrophotometry <2.25>, and compare the spectrum with the Reference Spectrum: both spectra exhibit similar intensities of absorption at the same wave numbers.

Purity (1) Clarity and color of solution—Dissolve 1.0 g

of Amidotrizoic Acid in 10 mL of 0.2 mol/L sodium hydroxide TS: the solution is clear and colorless.

(2) Primary aromatic amines—Dissolve 0.20 g of Amidotrizoic Acid in 5 mL of water and 1 mL of sodium hydroxide TS, add 4 mL of a solution of sodium nitrite (1 in 100) and 10 mL of 1 mol/L hydrochloric acid TS, shake, and allow to stand for 2 minutes. Add 5 mL of ammonium amidosulfate TS, shake well, allow to stand for 1 minute, and add 0.4 mL of a solution of 1-naphthol in ethanol (95) (1 in 10), 15 mL of sodium hydroxide TS and water to make exactly 50 mL. Determine the absorbance of this solution at 485 nm as directed under Ultraviolet-visible Spectrophotometry *<2.24>* using a solution, prepared in the same manner, as the blank: the absorbance is not more than 0.15.

(3) Soluble halides—Dissolve 2.5 g of Amidotrizoic Acid in 20 mL of water and 2.5 mL of ammonia TS, add 20 mL of dilute nitric acid and water to make 100 mL, allow to stand for 15 minutes with occasional shaking, and filter. Discard the first 10 mL of the filtrate, transfer the subsequent 25 mL of the filtrate to a Nessler tube, and add ethanol (95) to make 50 mL. Proceed as directed under Chloride Limit Test *<1.03>* using this solution as the test solution. Prepare the control solution as follows: to 0.10 mL of 0.01 mol/L hydrochloric acid VS, add 6 mL of dilute nitric acid and water to make 25 mL, then ethanol (95) to make 50 mL.

(4) Iodine—Dissolve 0.20 g of Amidotrizoic Acid in 2.0 mL of sodium hydroxide TS, add 2.5 mL of 0.5 mol/L sulfuric acid TS, allow to stand for 10 minutes with occasional shaking, add 5 mL of chloroform, shake well, and allow to stand: the solution is colorless in the chloroform layer.

(5) Heavy metals *<1.07>*—Proceed with 2.0 g of Amidotrizoic Acid according to Method 2, and perform the test. Prepare the control solution with 2.0 mL of Standard Lead Solution (not more than 10 ppm).

(6) Arsenic *<1.11>*—Prepare the test solution with 0.6 g of Amidotrizoic Acid according to Method 3, and perform the test (not more than 3.3 ppm).

Loss on drying *<2.41>* Not more than 7.0% (1 g, 105°C, 4 hours).

Residue on ignition *<2.44>* Not more than 0.1% (1 g).

Assay Transfer about 0.5 g of Amidotrizoic Acid, accurately weighed, to a saponification flask, dissolve in 40 mL of sodium hydroxide TS, add 1 g of zinc powder, connect to a reflux condenser, boil for 30 minutes, cool, and filter. Wash the flask and the filter paper with 50 mL of water, and combine the washings and the filtrate. Add 5 mL of acetic acid (100) to this solution, and titrate *<2.50>* with 0.1 mol/L silver nitrate VS until the color of the precipitate changes from yellow to green (indicator: 1 mL of tetrabromophenolphthalein ethyl ester TS).

Each mL of 0.1 mol/L silver nitrate VS
= 20.46 mg of $C_{11}H_9I_3N_2O_4$

Containers and storage Containers—Tight containers.
Storage—Light-resistant.

Amikacin Sulfate

アミカシン硫酸塩

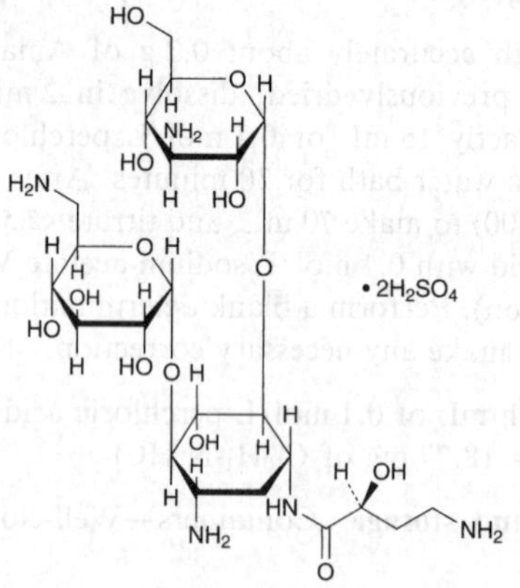

$C_{22}H_{43}N_5O_{13}.2H_2SO_4$: 781.76
3-Amino-3-deoxy-α-D-glucopyranosyl-(1→6)-[6-amino-6-deoxy-α-D-glucopyranosyl-(1→4)]-1-*N*-[(2*S*)-4-amino-2-hydroxybutanoyl]-2-deoxy-D-streptamine disulfate
[39831-55-5]

Amikacin Sulfate is the sulfate of a derivative of kanamycin.

It contains not less than 691 μg (potency) and not more than 791 μg (potency) per mg, calculated on the dried basis. The potency of Amikacin Sulfate is expressed as mass (potency) of amikacin ($C_{22}H_{43}N_5O_{13}$: 585.60).

Description Amikacin Sulfate occurs as a white to yellow-white powder.

It is very soluble in water, and practically insoluble in ethanol (95).

Identification **(1)** Determine the infrared absorption spectrum of Amikacin Sulfate, previously dried, as directed in the potassium bromide disk method under Infrared Spectrophotometry *<2.25>*, and compare the spectrum with the Reference Spectrum or the spectrum of Amikacin Sulfate RS previously dried: both spectra exhibit similar intensities of absorption at the same wave numbers.

(2) Dissolve 0.1 g each of Amikacin Sulfate and Amikacin Sulfate RS in 4 mL of water, and use these solutions as the sample solution and standard solution. Perform the test with these solutions as directed under Thin-layer chromatography *<2.03>*. Spot 2 μL each of the sample solution and standard solution on a plate of silica gel for thin-layer chromatography. Develop the plate with a mixture of water, ammonia water (28), methanol and tetrahydrofuran (1:1:1:1) to a distance of about 10 cm, and air-dry the plate. Spray evenly ninhydrin-citric acid-acetic acid TS on the plate, and heat at 100°C for 10 minutes: the principal spot obtained from the sample solution and the spot from the standard solution show a red-purple color and the same *Rf* value.

(3) A solution of Amikacin Sulfate (1 in 100) responds to Qualitative Tests *<1.09>* (1) for sulfate.

Optical rotation *<2.49>* $[\alpha]_D^{20}$: +76 – +84° (1 g, water, 100 mL, 100 mm).

pH *<2.54>* Dissolve 1.0 g of Amikacin Sulfate in 100 mL of water: the pH of the solution is between 6.0 and 7.5.

Purity **(1)** Heavy metals *<1.07>*—Proceed with 1.0 g of

Amikacin Sulfate according to Method 2, and perform the test. Prepare the control solution with 2.0 mL Standard Lead Solution (not more than 20 ppm).

(2) Related substances—Dissolve 0.10 g of Amikacin Sulfate in 4 mL of a water, and use this solution as the sample solution. Pipet 1 mL of the sample solution, add water to make exactly 100 mL, and use this solution as the standard solution. Perform the test with these solutions as directed under Thin-layer chromatography *<2.03>*. Spot 2 μL each of the sample solution and standard solution on a plate of silica gel for thin-layer chromatography. Develop the plate with a mixture of water, ammonia water (28), methanol and tetrahydrofuran (1:1:1:1) to a distance of about 10 cm, and air-dry the plate. Spray evenly ninhydrin-citric acid-acetic acid TS on the plate, and heat the plate at 100°C for 10 minutes: the spots other than the principal spot obtained from the sample solution are not more intense than the spot from the standard solution.

Loss on drying *<2.41>* Not more than 4.0% (1 g, in vacuum, 60°C, 3 hours).

Assay Weigh accurately an amount of Amikacin Sulfate and Amikacin Sulfate RS, equivalent to about 50 mg (potency), dissolve each in water to make exactly 50 mL. Pipet 200 μL each of these solutions in the test tube with glass stopper, add exactly 3 mL of pyridine and exactly 2 mL of a solution of 2,4,6-trinitrobenzenesulfonic acid (1 in 100), stopper tightly, and heat in a water bath at 70°C for 30 minutes. After cooling, add exactly 2 mL each of acetic aid (100), and use these solutions as the sample solution and standard solution, respectively. Perform the test with exactly 20 μL each of these solutions as directed under Liquid Chromatography *<2.01>* according to the following conditions, and determine the heights, H_T and H_S, of the peak of amikacin derivative in each solution.

Amount [μg (potency)] of amikacin ($C_{22}H_{43}N_5O_{13}$)
$= M_S \times H_T/H_S \times 1000$

M_S: Amount [mg (potency)] of Amikacin Sulfate RS taken

Operating conditions—

Detector: An ultraviolet absorption photometer (wavelength: 340 nm).

Column: A stainless steel column 4.6 mm in inside diameter and 25 cm in length, packed with octadecylsilanized silica gel for liquid chromatography (5 μm in particle diameter).

Column temperature: A constant temperature of about 35°C.

Mobile phase: Dissolve 2.72 g of potassium dihydrogenphosphate in 800 mL of water, adjust to pH 6.5 with a solution of potassium hydroxide (1 in 40), and add water to make 1000 mL. To 280 mL of this solution add 720 mL of methanol, and mix.

Flow rate: Adjust so that the retention time of amikacin derivative is about 9 minutes.

System suitability—

System performance: Dissolve about 5 mg (potency) of Amikacin Sulfate and about 5 mg (potency) of Kanamycin Sulfate in 5 mL of water. Transfer 200 μL of this solution in a glass-stoppered test tube, add 3 mL of pyridine and 2 mL of a solution of 2,4,6-trinitrobenzenesulfonic acid (1 in 100), stopper tightly, heat in a water bath at 70°C for 30 minutes. After cooling, add 2 mL of acetic acid (100). When the procedure is run with 20 μL of this solution under the above operating conditions, amikacin derivative and kanamycin derivative are eluted in this order with the resolution between these peaks being not less than 5.

System repeatability: When the test is repeated 6 times with 20 μL of the standard solution under the above operating conditions, the relative standard deviation of the ratios of the peak height of amikacin derivative is not more than 2.0%.

Containers and storage Containers—Hermetic containers.

Amikacin Sulfate Injection

アミカシン硫酸塩注射液

Amikacin Sulfate Injection is an aqueous injection.

It contains not less than 90.0% and not more than 115.0% of the labeled potency of amikacin ($C_{22}H_{43}N_5O_{13}$: 585.60).

Method of preparation Prepare as directed under Injections, with Amikacin Sulfate.

Description Amikacin Sulfate Injection occurs as a colorless or pale yellow clear liquid.

Identification To a volume of Amikacin Sulfate Injection, equivalent to 0.1 g (potency) of Amikacin Sulfate, add water to make 4 mL, and use this solution as the sample solution. Separately, dissolve 25 mg (potency) of Amikacin Sulfate RS in 1 mL of water, and use this solution as the standard solution. Then, proceed as directed in the Identifiction (2) under Amikacin Sulfate.

Osmotic pressure ratio Being specified separately when the drug is granted approval based on the Law.

pH *<2.54>* 6.0 – 7.5

Bacterial endotoxins *<4.01>* Less than 0.50 EU/mg (potency).

Extractable volume *<6.05>* It meets the requirement.

Foreign insoluble matter *<6.06>* Perform the test according to Method 1: it meets the requirement.

Insoluble particulate matter *<6.07>* It meets the requirement.

Sterility *<4.06>* Perform the test according to the Membrane filtration method: it meets the requirement.

Assay Take exactly a volume of Amikacin Sulfate Injection, equivalent to about 0.1 g (potency) of Amikacin Sulfate, and add water to make exactly 100 mL. Separately, weigh accurately an amount of Amikacin Sulfate RS, equivalent to about 50 mg (potency), and add water to make exactly 50 mL. Take exactly 200 μL each of these solutions into stoppered test tubes, then proceed as directed in the Assay under Amikacin Sulfate.

Amount [mg (potency)] of amikacin ($C_{22}H_{43}N_5O_{13}$)
$= M_S \times H_T/H_S \times 2$

M_S: Amount [mg (potency)] of Amikacin Sulfate RS taken

Containers and storage Containers—Hermetic containers.

Amikacin Sulfate for Injection

注射用アミカシン硫酸塩

Amikacin Sulfate for Injection is a preparation for injection, which is dissolved before use.

It contains not less than 90.0% and not more than 115.0% of the labeled potency of amikacin ($C_{22}H_{43}N_5O_{13}$: 585.60).

Method of preparation Prepare as directed under Injections, with Amikacin Sulfate.

Description Amikacin Sulfate for Injection occurs as white to yellow-white masses or powder.

Identification Dissolve an amount of Amikacin Sulfate for Injection, equivalent to 25 mg (potency) of Amikacin Sulfate, in 1 mL of water, and use this solution as the sample solution. Separately, dissolve 25 mg (potency) of Amikacin Sulfate RS in 1 mL of water, and use this solution as the standard solution. Then, proceed as directed in the Identification (2) under Amikacin Sulfate.

Osmotic pressure ratio Being specified separately when the drug is granted approval based on the Law.

pH 〈*2.54*〉 Dissolve an amount of Amikacin Sulfate for Injection, equivalent to 0.1 g (potency) of Amikacin Sulfate, in 10 mL of water: the pH of this solution is 6.0 to 7.5.

Purity Clarity and color of solution—Dissolve an amount of Amikacin Sulfate for Injection, equivalent to 0.5 g (potency) of Amikacin Sulfate, in 5 mL of water: the solution is clear, and the absorbance at 405 nm of the solution determined as directed under Ultraviolet-visible Spectrophotometry 〈*2.24*〉 is not more than 0.15.

Loss on drying 〈*2.41*〉 Not more than 4.0% (1 g, in vacuum, 60°C, 3 hours).

Bacterial endotoxins 〈*4.01*〉 Less than 0.50 EU/mg (potency).

Uniformity of dosage units 〈*6.02*〉 It meets the requirement of the Mass variation test.

Foreign insoluble matter 〈*6.06*〉 Perform the test according to Method 2: it meets the requirement.

Insoluble particulate matter 〈*6.07*〉 It meets the requirement.

Sterility 〈*4.06*〉 Perform the test according to the Membrane filtration method: it meets the requirement.

Assay Weigh accurately the mass of the content of not less than 10 Amikacin Sulfate for Injection. Weigh accurately a portion of the content, equivalent to about 50 mg (potency) of Amikacin Sulfate, dissolve in water to make exactly 50 mL. Separately, weigh accurately an amount of Amikacin Sulfate RS, equivalent to about 50 mg (potency), and dissolve in water to make exactly 50 mL. Transfer exactly 200 μL each of these solutions to separate glass stoppered tubes, and proceed as directed in the Assay under Amikacin Sulfate.

Amount [mg (potency)] of amikacin ($C_{22}H_{43}N_5O_{13}$)
$= M_S \times H_T/H_S$

M_S: Amount [mg (potency)] of Amikacin Sulfate RS taken

Containers and storage Containers—Hermetic containers.

Aminophylline Hydrate

アミノフィリン水和物

$C_{14}H_{16}N_8O_4.C_2H_8N_2.xH_2O$
1,3-Dimethyl-1*H*-purine-2,6(3*H*,7*H*)-dione hemi(ethane-1,2-diamine) hydrate
[*76970-41-7*, monohydrate]

Aminophylline Hydrate contains not less than 84.0% and not more than 86.0% of theophylline ($C_7H_8N_4O_2$: 180.16), and not less than 14.0% and not more than 15.0% of ethylenediamine ($C_2H_8N_2$: 60.10), calculated on the anhydrous basis.

Description Aminophylline Hydrate occurs as white to pale yellow, granules or powder. It is odorless or slightly ammonia-like odor, and has a bitter taste.

It is soluble in water, slightly soluble in methanol, and practically insoluble in ethanol (95) and in diethyl ether.

To 1 g of Aminophylline Hydrate add 5 mL of water, and shake: it dissolves almost completely. Separation of crystals begins in 2 to 3 minutes, and these crystals dissolve on the addition of a small amount of ethylenediamine.

It is gradually affected by light, and gradually loses ethylenediamine in air.

Identification **(1)** Dissolve 0.75 g of Aminophylline Hydrate in 30 mL of water, and use this solution as the sample solution. To 20 mL of the sample solution add 1 mL of dilute hydrochloric acid: a precipitate is gradually formed. Filter the precipitate, recrystallize from water, and dry at 105°C for 1 hour: the crystals so obtained melt 〈*2.60*〉 between 271°C and 275°C.

(2) Dissolve 0.1 g of the crystals obtained in (1) in 50 mL of water, and to 2 mL of this solution add tannic acid TS dropwise: a white precipitate is produced, and this precipitate dissolves upon dropwise addition of tannic acid TS.

(3) To 0.01 g of the crystals obtained in (1) add 10 drops of hydrogen peroxide TS and 1 drop of hydrochloric acid, and evaporate on a water bath to dryness: the residue shows a yellow-red color. Invert the dish containing the residue over a vessel containing 2 to 3 drops of ammonia TS: the color of the residue changes to red-purple, which is destroyed on the addition of 2 to 3 drops of sodium hydroxide TS.

(4) Dissolve 0.01 g of the crystals obtained in (1) in 5 mL of water, add 3 mL of ammonia-ammonium chloride buffer solution (pH 8.0) and 1 mL of copper (II) sulfate-pyridine TS, and mix. Add 5 mL of chloroform to the mixture, and shake: the chloroform layer develops a green color.

(5) To 5 mL of the sample solution obtained in (1) add 2 drops of copper (II) sulfate TS: a purple color develops. Add 1 mL of copper (II) sulfate TS: the color changes to blue, and green precipitates are formed on standing.

pH 〈*2.54*〉 Dissolve 1.0 g of Aminophylline Hydrate in 25 mL of water: the pH of the solution is between 8.0 and 9.5.

Purity **(1)** Clarity and color of solution—Dissolve 1.0 g of Aminophylline Hydrate in 10 mL of hot water: the solution is clear and colorless to pale yellow.

(2) Heavy metals *<1.07>*—Proceed with 1.0 g of Aminophylline Hydrate according to Method 2, and perform the test. Prepare the control solution with 2.0 mL of Standard Lead Solution (not more than 20 ppm).

Water *<2.48>* Not more than 7.9% (0.3 g, direct titration).

Residue on ignition *<2.44>* Not more than 0.1% (1 g).

Assay (1) Theophylline—Weigh accurately about 0.25 g of Aminophylline Hydrate, and dissolve in 50 mL of water and 8 mL of ammonia TS by gentle warming on a water bath. Add exactly 20 mL of 0.1 mol/L silver nitrate VS, warm on a water bath for 15 minutes, allow to stand between 5°C and 10°C for 20 minutes, collect the precipitate by suction, and wash with three 10-mL portions of water. Combine the filtrate and washings, and add dilute nitric acid to make neutral. Add 3 mL of dilute nitric acid, and titrate *<2.50>* the excess silver nitrate with 0.1 mol/L ammonium thiocyanate VS (indicator: 2 mL of ammonium iron (III) sulfate TS). Perform a blank determination in the same manner.

Each mL of 0.1 mol/L silver nitrate VS
= 18.02 mg of $C_7H_8N_4O_2$

(2) Ethylenediamine—Weigh accurately about 0.5 g of Aminophylline Hydrate, dissolve in 30 mL of water, and titrate *<2.50>* with 0.1 mol/L hydrochloric acid VS (indicator: 3 drops of bromophenol blue TS).

Each mL of 0.1 mol/L hydrochloric acid VS
= 3.005 mg of $C_2H_8N_2$

Containers and storage Containers—Tight containers.
Storage—Light-resistant.

Aminophylline Injection

アミノフィリン注射液

Aminophylline Injection is an aqueous injection.

It contains not less than 75.0% and not more than 86.0% of the labeled amount of theophylline ($C_7H_8N_4O_2$: 180.16), and not less than 13.0% and not more than 20.0% of ethylenediamine ($C_2H_8N_2$: 60.10).

The concentration of Aminophylline Injection is expressed as the quantity of aminophylline dihydrate ($C_{16}H_{24}N_{10}O_4.2H_2O$: 456.46).

Method of preparation Prepare as directed under Injections, with Aminophylline Hydrate. It may be prepared with Theophylline and its equivalent Ethylenediamine, instead of Aminophylline Hydrate.

It may contain not more than 60 mg of Ethylenediamine as a stabilizer for each g of Aminophylline Hydrate.

Description Aminophylline Injection is a clear and colorless liquid. It has a slightly bitter taste.

It gradually changes in color by light.

pH: 8.0 - 10.0

Identification To a volume of Aminophylline Injection, equivalent to 0.75 g of Aminophylline Hydrate, add water to make 30 mL. Proceed with this solution as directed in the Identification under Aminophylline Hydrate.

Bacterial endotoxins *<4.01>* Less than 0.6 EU/mg.

Extractable volume *<6.05>* It meets the requirement.

Foreign insoluble matter *<6.06>* Perform the test according to Method 1: it meets the requirement.

Insoluble particulate matter *<6.07>* It meets the requirement.

Sterility *<4.06>* Perform the test according to the Membrane filtration method: it meets the requirement.

Assay (1) Theophylline—Pipet a volume of Aminophylline Injection, equivalent to about 39.4 mg of theophylline ($C_7H_8N_4O_2$) (about 50 mg of Aminophylline Hydrate), add water to make exactly 50 mL, and use this solution as the sample solution. Separately, weigh accurately about 40 mg of theophylline for assay, previously dried at 105°C for 4 hours, dissolve in water to make exactly 50 mL, and use this solution as the standard solution. Perform the test with exactly 5 μL each of the sample solution and standard solution as directed under Liquid Chromatography *<2.01>* according to the following conditions, and determine the peak areas, A_T and A_S, of theophylline in each solution.

Amount (mg) of theophylline ($C_7H_8N_4O_2$)
$= M_S \times A_T/A_S$

M_S: Amount (mg) of theophylline for assay taken

Operating conditions—

Detector: An ultraviolet absorption photometer (wavelength: 270 nm).

Column: A stainless steel column 6 mm in inside diameter and 15 cm in length, packed with octadecylsilanized silica gel for liquid chromatography (5 μm in particle diameter).

Column temperature: A constant temperature of about 40°C.

Mobile phase: A mixture of diluted acetic acid (100) (1 in 100) and methanol (4:1).

Flow rate: Adjust so that the retention time of theophylline is about 5 minutes.

System suitability—

System performance: When the procedure is run with 5 μL of the standard solution under the above operating conditions, the number of theoretical plates and the symmetry factor of the peak of theophylline are not less than 3000 and not more than 1.5, respectively.

System repeatability: When the test is repeated 6 times with 5 μL of the standard solution under the above operating conditions, the relative standard deviation of the peak area of theophylline is not more than 1.0%.

(2) Ethylenediamine—To an accurately measured volume of Aminophylline Injection, equivalent to about 30 mg of ethylenediamine ($C_2H_8N_2$) (about 0.2 g of Aminophylline Hydrate), add water to make 30 mL, and titrate *<2.50>* with 0.1 mol/L hydrochloric acid VS (indicator: 2 to 3 drops of bromophenol blue TS).

Each mL of 0.1 mol/L hydrochloric acid VS
= 3.005 mg of $C_2H_8N_2$

Containers and storage Containers—Hermetic containers. Plastic containers for aqueous injections may be used.
Storage—Light-resistant.

Amiodarone Hydrochloride

アミオダロン塩酸塩

$C_{25}H_{29}I_2NO_3.HCl$: 681.77
(2-Butylbenzofuran-3-yl){4-[2-(diethylamino)ethoxy]-3,5-diiodophenyl}methanone monohydrochloride
[*19774-82-4*]

Amiodarone Hydrochloride, when dried, contains not less than 98.5% and not more than 101.0% of amiodarone hydrochloride ($C_{25}H_{29}I_2NO_3.HCl$).

Description Amiodarone Hydrochloride occurs as a white to pale yellow-white crystalline powder.

It is very soluble in water at 80°C, freely soluble in dichloromethane, soluble in methanol, sparingly soluble in ethanol (95), and very slightly soluble in water.

Melting point: about 161°C (with decomposition).

Identification **(1)** Determine the absorption spectrum of a solution of Amiodarone Hydrochloride in ethanol (95) (1 in 100,000) as directed under Ultraviolet-visible Spectrophotometry <*2.24*>, and compare the spectrum with the Reference Spectrum: both spectra exhibit similar intensities of absorption at the same wavelengths.

(2) Determine the infrared absorption spectrum of Amiodarone Hydrochloride as directed in the potassium bromide disk method under Infrared Spectrophotometry <*2.25*>, and compare the spectrum with the Reference Spectrum: both spectra exhibit similar intensities of absorption at the same wave numbers.

(3) To 0.1 g of Amiodarone Hydrochloride add 10 mL of water, dissolve by warming at 80°C, and cool: the solution responds to Qualitative Tests <*1.09*> (2) for chloride.

pH <*2.54*> To 1.0 g of Amiodarone Hydrochloride add 20 mL of freshly boiled and cooled water, dissolve by warming at 80°C, and cool: the pH of this solution is between 3.2 and 3.8.

Purity **(1)** Clarity and color of solution—Dissolve 0.5 g of Amiodarone Hydrochloride in 10 mL of methanol: the solution is clear, and is not more colored than the following control solutions (1) and (2).

Control solution (1): To a mixture of 1.0 mL of Cobalt (II) Chloride CS, 2.4 mL of Iron (III) Chloride CS and 0.4 mL of Copper (II) Sulfate CS, add diluted hydrochloric acid (1 in 40) to make 10.0 mL. To 2.5 mL of this solution add diluted hydrochloric acid (1 in 40) to make 20 mL.

Control solution (2): To 3.0 mL of a mixture of 0.2 mL of Cobalt (II) Chloride CS, 9.6 mL of Iron (III) Chloride CS and 0.2 mL of Copper (II) Sulfate CS, add diluted hydrochloric acid (1 in 40) to make 100 mL.

(2) Iodine—To 1.50 g of Amiodarone Hydrochloride add 40 mL of water, dissolve by warming at 80°C, cool, add water to make exactly 50 mL, and use this solution as the sample stock solution. Pipet 15 mL of this solution, add exactly 1 mL of 0.1 mol/L hydrochloric acid TS and exactly 1 mL of a solution of potassium iodate (107 in 10,000), add water to make exactly 20 mL, and use this solution as the sample solution. Separately, pipet 15 mL of the sample stock solution, add exactly 1 mL of 0.1 mol/L hydrochloric acid TS, exactly 1 mL of a solution of potassium iodide (441 in 5,000,000) and exactly 1 mL of a solution of potassium iodate (107 in 10,000), add water to make exactly 20 mL, and use this solution as the standard solution. Separately, pipet 15 mL of the sample stock solution, add exactly 1 mL of 0.1 mol/L hydrochloric acid TS, add water to make exactly 20 mL, and use this solution as the control solution. Allow the sample solution, standard solution and control solution to stand in a dark place for 4 hours. Perform the test with the sample solution and standard solution as directed under Ultraviolet-visible Spectrophotometry <*2.24*>, using the control solution as the blank: the absorbance of the sample solution at 420 nm is not larger than 1/2 times the absorbance of the standard solution.

(3) Heavy metals <*1.07*>—Proceed with 1.0 g of Amiodarone Hydrochloride according to Method 4, and perform the test. Prepare the control solution with 2.0 mL of Standard Lead Solution (not more than 20 ppm).

(4) Related substance 1—Dissolve 0.5 g of Amiodarone Hydrochloride in 5 mL of dichloromethane, and use this solution as the sample solution. Separately, dissolve 10 mg of 2-chloroethyl diethylamine hydrochloride in 50 mL of dichloromethane, and use this solution as the standard solution. Perform the test with these solutions as directed under Thin-layer Chromatography <*2.03*>. Spot 5 μL each of the sample solution and standard solution on a plate of silica gel with fluorescent indicator for thin-layer chromatography. Develop the plate with a mixture of dichloromethane, methanol and formic acid (17:2:1) to a distance of about 15 cm, and air-dry the plate. Spray evenly bismuth subnitrate TS and then hydrogen peroxide TS: the spot obtained from the sample solution corresponding to the spot from the standard solution is not more intense than the spot from the standard solution.

(5) Related substance 2—Dissolve 0.125 g of Amiodarone Hydrochloride in 25 mL of a mixture of water and acetonitrile for liquid chromatography (1:1), and use this solution as the sample solution. Pipet 2 mL of the sample solution, and add a mixture of water and acetonitrile for liquid chromatography (1:1) to make exactly 50 mL. Pipet 1 mL of this solution, add a mixture of water and acetonitrile for liquid chromatography (1:1) to make exactly 20 mL, and use this solution as the standard solution. Perform the test with exactly 10 μL each of the sample solution and standard solution as directed under Liquid Chromatography <*2.01*> according to the following conditions. Determine each peak area by the automatic integration method: the area of the peak other than amiodarone obtained from the sample solution is not larger than the peak area of amiodarone from the standard solution, and the total area of the peaks other than amiodarone from the sample solution is not larger than 2.5 times the peak area of amiodarone from the standard solution.

Operating conditions—

Detector: An ultraviolet absorption photometer (wavelength: 240 nm).

Column: A stainless steel column 4.6 mm in inside diameter and 15 cm in length, packed with octadecylsilanized silica gel for liquid chromatography (5 μm in particle diameter).

Column temperature: A constant temperature of about 30°C.

Mobile phase: To 800 mL of water add 3.0 mL of acetic acid (100), adjust the pH to 4.95 with ammonia solution (28), and add water to make 1000 mL. To 300 mL of this solution add 400 mL of acetonitrile for liquid chromatography and 300 mL of methanol for liquid chromatography.

Flow rate: Adjust so that the retention time of amiodarone is about 24 minutes.

Time span of measurement: About 2 times as long as the retention time of amiodarone.

System suitability—

Test for required detectability: Pipet 5 mL of the standard solution, and add a mixture of water and acetonitrile for liquid chromatography (1:1) to make exactly 25 mL. Confirm that the peak area of amiodarone obtained with 10 μL of this solution is equivalent to 14 to 26% of that with 10 μL of the standard solution.

System performance: When the procedure is run with 10 μL of the standard solution under the above operating conditions, the number of theoretical plates and the symmetry factor of the peak of amiodarone are not less than 5000 and not more than 1.5, respectively.

System repeatability: When the test is repeated 6 times with 10 μL of the standard solution under the above operating conditions, the relative standard deviation of the peak area of amiodarone is not more than 1.0%.

Loss on drying <*2.41*> Not more than 0.5% (1 g, reduced pressure not exceeding 0.3 kPa, 50°C, 4 hours).

Residue on ignition <*2.44*> Not more than 0.1% (1 g).

Assay Weigh accurately about 0.6 g of Amiodarone Hydrochloride, previously dried, dissolve in 40 mL of a mixture of acetic anhydride and acetic acid (100) (3:1), and titrate <*2.50*> with 0.1 mol/L perchloric acid VS (potentiometric titration). Perform a blank determination in the same manner, and make any necessary correction.

Each mL of 0.1 mol/L perchloric acid VS
= 68.18 mg of $C_{25}H_{29}I_2NO_3.HCl$

Containers and storage Containers—Tight containers.
Storage—Light-resistant.

Amiodarone Hydrochloride Tablets

アミオダロン塩酸塩錠

Amiodarone Hydrochloride Tablets contain not less than 93.0% and not more than 107.0% of the labeled amount of amiodarone hydrochloride ($C_{25}H_{29}I_2NO_3.HCl$: 681.77).

Method of preparation Prepare as directed under Tablets, with Amiodarone Hydrochloride.

Identification To 1 mL of the sample stock solution obtained in the Assay add the mobile phase to make 50 mL. Determine the absorption spectrum of this solution as directed under Ultraviolet-visible Spectrophotometry <*2.24*>: it exhibits a maximum between 239 nm and 243 nm.

Uniformity of dosage units <*6.02*> Perform the Mass variation test, or the Content uniformity test according to the following method: it meets the requirement.

To 1 tablet of Amiodarone Hydrochloride Tablets add 160 mL of the mobile phase, sonicate for 10 minutes, add the mobile phase to make exactly 200 mL, and centrifuge. Pipet *V* mL of the supernatant liquid, equivalent to about 1 mg of amiodarone hydrochloride ($C_{25}H_{29}I_2NO_3.HCl$), add the mobile phase to make exactly 50 mL, and use this solution as the sample solution. Separately, weigh accurately about 25 mg of amiodarone hydrochloride for assay, previously dried at 50°C for 4 hours under reduced pressure not exceeding 0.3 kPa, and dissolve in the mobile phase to make exactly 50 mL. Pipet 2 mL of this solution, add the mobile phase to make exactly 50 mL, and use this solution as the standard solution. Perform the test with exactly 10 μL each of the sample solution and standard solution as directed under Liquid Chromatography <*2.01*> according to the following conditions, and determine the peak areas, A_T and A_S, of amiodarone in each solution.

Amount (mg) of amiodarone hydrochloride
($C_{25}H_{29}I_2NO_3.HCl$)
$= M_S \times A_T/A_S \times 8/V$

M_S: Amount (mg) of amiodarone for assay taken

Operating conditions—

Proceed as directed in the operating conditions in the Assay.

System suitability—

System performance: When the procedure is run with 10 μL of the standard solution under the above operating conditions, the number of theoretical plates and the symmetry factor of the peak of amiodarone are not less than 5000 and not more than 1.5, respectively.

System repeatability: When the test is repeated 6 times with 10 μL of the standard solution under the above operating conditions, the relative standard deviation of the peak area of amiodarone is not more than 1.0%.

Dissolution <*6.10*> When the test is performed at 50 revolutions per minute according to the Paddle method, using 900 mL of acetic acid-sodium acetate buffer solution (pH 4.0) as the dissolution medium, the dissolution rate in 30 minutes of Amiodarone Hydrochloride Tablets is not less than 80%.

Start the test with 1 tablet of Amiodarone Hydrochloride Tablets, withdraw not less than 20 mL of the medium at the specified minute after starting the test, and filter through a membrane filter with a pore size not exceeding 0.45 μm. Discard not less than 10 mL of the first filtrate, pipet *V* mL of the subsequent filtrate, add exactly *V* mL of methanol, then add a mixture of the dissolution medium and methanol (1:1) to make exactly *V′* mL so that each mL contains about 11 μg of amiodarone hydrochloride ($C_{25}H_{29}I_2NO_3.HCl$), and use this solution as the sample solution. Separately, weigh accurately about 28 mg of amiodarone hydrochloride for assay, previously dried at 50°C for 4 hours under reduced pressure not exceeding 0.3 kPa, and dissolve in methanol to make exactly 50 mL. Pipet 2 mL of this solution, add exactly 2 mL of the dissolution medium, then add a mixture of the dissolution medium and methanol (1:1) to make exactly 100 mL, and use this solution as the standard solution. Determine the absorbances, A_T and A_S, of the sample solution and standard solution at 241 nm as directed under Ultraviolet-visible Spectrophotometry <*2.24*>, using a mixture of the dissolution medium and methanol (1:1) as the blank.

Dissolution rate (%) with respect to the labeled amount
of amiodarone hydrochloride ($C_{25}H_{29}I_2NO_3.HCl$)
$= M_S \times A_T/A_S \times V'/V \times 1/C \times 36$

M_S: Amount (mg) of amiodarone hydrochloride for assay taken

C: Labeled amount (mg) of amiodarone hydrochloride ($C_{25}H_{29}I_2NO_3.HCl$) in 1 tablet

Assay Weigh accurately the mass of not less than 20 Amiodarone Hydrochloride Tablets, and powder. Weigh accurately a portion of the powder, equivalent to about 50 mg of amiodarone hydrochloride ($C_{25}H_{29}I_2NO_3.HCl$), add 80 mL of the mobile phase, sonicate for 10 minutes, and add the mobile phase to make exactly 100 mL. Centrifuge this solution, and use the supernatant liquid as the sample stock solution. Pipet 2 mL of the stock solution, add exactly 2 mL of the internal standard solution, add the mobile phase to make 50 mL, and use this solution as the sample solution. Separately, weigh accurately 25 mg of amiodarone hydrochloride for assay, previously dried at 50°C for 4 hours under reduced pressure not exceeding 0.3 kPa, and dissolve in the mobile phase to make exactly 50 mL. Pipet 2 mL of this solution, add exactly 2 mL of the internal standard solution, add the mobile phase to make 50 mL, and use this solution as the standard solution. Perform the test with 10 μL each of the sample solution and standard solution as directed under Liquid Chromatography <2.01> according to the following conditions, and calculate the ratios, Q_T and Q_S, of the peak area of amiodarone to that of the internal standard.

Amount (mg) of amiodarone hydrochloride ($C_{25}H_{29}I_2NO_3.HCl$)
$= M_S \times Q_T/Q_S \times 2$

M_S: Amount (mg) of amiodarone hydrochloride for assay taken

Internal standard solution—A solution of chlorhexidine hydrochloride in the mobile phase (1 in 2500).
Operating conditions—

Detector: An ultraviolet absorption photometer (wavelength: 242 nm).

Column: A stainless steel column 4 mm in inside diameter and 15 cm in length, packed with octadecylsilanized silica gel for liquid chromatography (5 μm in particle diameter).

Column temperature: A constant temperature of about 50°C.

Mobile phase: A mixture of acetonitrile for liquid chromatography, a solution of sodium laurylsulfate (1 in 50) and phosphoric acid (750:250:1).

Flow rate: Adjust so that the retention time of amiodarone is about 7 minutes.
System suitability—

System performance: When the procedure is run with 10 μL of the standard solution under the above operating conditions, the internal standard and amiodarone are eluted in this order with the resolution between these peaks being not less than 5.

System repeatability: When the test is repeated 6 times with 10 μL of the standard solution under the above operating conditions, the relative standard deviation of the ratio of the peak area of amiodarone to that of the internal standard is not more than 1.0%.

Containers and storage Containers—Tight containers.
Storage—Light-resistant.

Amitriptyline Hydrochloride

アミトリプチリン塩酸塩

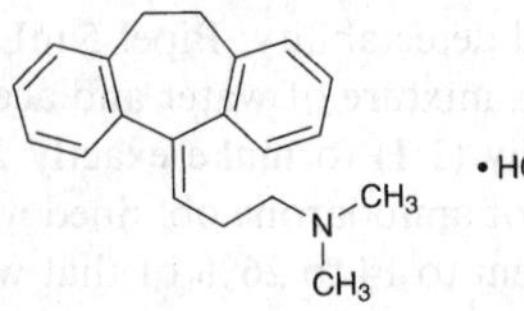

$C_{20}H_{23}N.HCl$: 313.86
3-(10,11-Dihydro-5*H*-dibenzo[*a*,*d*]cyclohepten-5-ylidene)-*N*,*N*-dimethylpropylamine monohydrochloride
[*549-18-8*]

Amitriptyline Hydrochloride, when dried, contains not less than 99.0% of amitriptyline hydrochloride ($C_{20}H_{23}N.HCl$).

Description Amitriptyline Hydrochloride occurs as colorless crystals or a white to pale yellow crystalline powder. It has a bitter taste and a numbing effect.

It is freely soluble in water, in ethanol (95) and in acetic acid (100), soluble in acetic anhydride, and practically insoluble in diethyl ether.

The pH of a solution of 1.0 g of Amitriptyline Hydrochloride in 20 mL of water is between 4.0 and 5.0.

Identification **(1)** Dissolve 5 mg of Amitriptyline Hydrochloride in 3 mL of sulfuric acid: a red color develops. Add 5 drops of potassium dichromate TS to this solution: it turns dark brown.

(2) Acidify 1 mL of a solution of Amitriptyline Hydrochloride (1 in 500) with 0.5 mL of dilute nitric acid, and add 1 drop of silver nitrate TS: a white, opalescent precipitate is produced.

(3) Determine the absorption spectrum of a solution of Amitriptyline Hydrochloride (1 in 100,000) as directed under Ultraviolet-visible Spectrophotometry <2.24>, and compare the spectrum with the Reference Spectrum or the spectrum of a solution of Amitriptyline Hydrochloride RS prepared in the same manner as the sample solution: both spectra exhibit similar intensities of absorption at the same wavelengths.

Melting point <2.60> 195 – 198°C

Purity **(1)** Clarity and color of solution—Dissolve 1.0 g of Amitriptyline Hydrochloride in 20 mL of water: the solution is clear and colorless.

(2) Heavy metals <1.07>—Proceed with 2.0 g of Amitriptyline Hydrochloride according to Method 2, and perform the test. Prepare the control solution with 2.0 mL of Standard Lead Solution (not more than 10 ppm).

Loss on drying <2.41> Not more than 0.5% (1 g, 105°C, 2 hours).

Residue on ignition <2.44> Not more than 0.1% (1 g).

Assay Weigh accurately about 0.5 g of Amitriptyline Hydrochloride, previously dried, dissolve in 50 mL of a mixture of acetic anhydride and acetic acid (100) (7:3), and titrate <2.50> with 0.1 mol/L perchloric acid VS (potentiometric titration). Perform a blank determination in the same manner, and make any necessary correction.

Each mL of 0.1 mol/L perchloric acid VS
$= 31.39$ mg of $C_{20}H_{23}N.HCl$

Containers and storage Containers—Tight containers.

Storage—Light-resistant.

Amitriptyline Hydrochloride Tablets

アミトリプチリン塩酸塩錠

Amitriptyline Hydrochloride Tablets contain not less than 90.0% and not more than 110.0% of the labeled amount of amitriptyline hydrochloride ($C_{20}H_{23}N.HCl$: 313.86).

Method of preparation Prepare as directed under Tablets, with Amitriptyline Hydrochloride.

Identification **(1)** Weigh a quantity of powdered Amitriptyline Hydrochloride Tablets, equivalent to 0.1 g of Amitriptyline Hydrochloride. Add 10 mL of chloroform, shake thoroughly, and filter. Evaporate the filtrate on a water bath to about 2 mL, add diethyl ether until turbidity is produced, and allow to stand. Filter the crystals formed through a glass filter (G4), and proceed as directed in the Identification (1) and (2) under Amitriptyline Hydrochloride.

(2) Determine the absorption spectrum of a solution of the crystals obtained in (1) (1 in 100,000) as directed under Ultraviolet-visible Spectrophotometry *<2.24>*: it exhibits a maximum between 238 nm and 240 nm, and a minimum between 228 nm and 230 nm.

Uniformity of dosage units *<6.02>* Perform the test according to the following method: it meets the requirement of the Content uniformity test.

To 1 tablet of Amitriptyline Hydrochloride Tablets add 50 mL of diluted methanol (1 in 2), shake to disintegrate the tablet, then add diluted methanol (1 in 2) to make exactly 100 mL, and filter. Discard the first 20 mL of the filtrate, pipet V mL of the subsequent filtrate, add methanol to make exactly V' mL so that each mL contains about 10 μg of amitriptyline hydrochloride ($C_{20}H_{23}N.HCl$), and use this solution as the sample solution. Then, proceed as directed in the Assay.

Amount (mg) of amitriptyline hydrochloride ($C_{20}H_{23}N.HCl$)
$= M_S \times A_T/A_S \times V'/V \times 1/20$

M_S: Amount (mg) of Amitriptyline Hydrochloride RS taken

Dissolution *<6.10>* When the test is performed at 50 revolutions per minute according to the Paddle method, using 900 mL of 2nd fluid for dissolution test as the dissolution medium, the dissolution rate in 60 minutes of Amitriptyline Hydrochloride Tablets is not less than 70%.

Start the test with 1 tablet of Amitriptyline Hydrochloride Tablets, withdraw not less than 20 mL of the medium at the specified minute after starting the test, and filter through a membrane filter with a pore size not exceeding 0.8 μm. Discard not less than 10 mL of the first filtrate, pipet the subsequent V mL of the filtrate, add the dissolution medium to make exactly V' mL so that each mL contains about 11 μg of amitriptyline hydrochloride ($C_{20}H_{23}N.HCl$), and use this solution as the sample solution. Separately, weigh accurately about 55 mg of Amitriptyline Hydrochloride RS, previously dried at 105°C for 2 hours, and dissolve in the dissolution medium to make exactly 250 mL. Pipet 5 mL of this solution, add the dissolution medium to make exactly 100 mL, and use this solution as the standard solution. Determine the absorbances, A_T and A_S, of the sample solution and standard solution at 239 nm as directed under Ultraviolet-visible Spectrophotometry *<2.24>*.

Dissolution rate (%) with respect to the labeled amount of amitriptyline hydrochloride ($C_{20}H_{23}N.HCl$)
$= M_S \times A_T/A_S \times V'/V \times 1/C \times 18$

M_S: Amount (mg) of Amitriptyline Hydrochloride RS taken

C: Labeled amount (mg) of amitriptyline hydrochloride ($C_{20}H_{23}N.HCl$) in 1 tablet

Assay Weigh accurately and powder not less than 20 Amitriptyline Hydrochloride Tablets. Weigh accurately a portion of the powder, equivalent to about 20 mg of amitriptyline hydrochloride ($C_{20}H_{23}N.HCl$), and add 75 mL of diluted methanol (1 in 2). After shaking for 30 minutes, add diluted methanol (1 in 2) to make exactly 100 mL, and filter. Discard the first 20-mL portion of the filtrate, measure exactly the subsequent 5-mL portion, add methanol to make exactly 100 mL, and use this solution as the sample solution. Separately, weigh accurately about 20 mg of Amitriptyline Hydrochloride RS, previously dried at 105°C for 2 hours, and dissolve in diluted methanol (1 in 2) to make exactly 100 mL. Measure exactly 5 mL of this solution, add methanol to make exactly 100 mL, and use this solution as the standard solution. Determine the absorbances, A_T and A_S, of the sample solution and standard solution at 239 nm as directed under Ultraviolet-visible Spectrophotometry *<2.24>*, respectively.

Amount (mg) of amitriptyline hydrochloride ($C_{20}H_{23}N.HCl$)
$= M_S \times A_T/A_S$

M_S: Amount (mg) of Amitriptyline Hydrochloride RS taken

Containers and storage Containers—Tight containers.

Amlexanox

アンレキサノクス

$C_{16}H_{14}N_2O_4$: 298.29
2-Amino-7-(1-methylethyl)-5-oxo-
5*H*-[1]benzopyrano[2,3-*b*]pyridine-3-carboxylic acid
[68302-57-8]

Amlexanox, when dried, contains not less than 98.0% and not more than 102.0% of amlexanox ($C_{16}H_{14}N_2O_4$).

Description Amlexanox occurs as white to yellowish white, crystals or crystalline powder.

It is very slightly soluble in ethanol (99.5), and practically insoluble in water.

It dissolves in diluted sodium hydroxide TS (1 in 3).

Identification **(1)** Determine the absorption spectrum of a solution of Amlexanox in ethanol (99.5) (1 in 250,000) as directed under Ultraviolet-visible Spectrophotometry *<2.24>*, and compare the spectrum with the Reference Spectrum or the spectrum of a solution of Amlexanox RS prepared in the same manner as the sample solution: both spectra exhibit similar intensities of absorption at the same wavelengths.

(2) Determine the infrared absorption spectrum of Amlexanox as directed in the potassium bromide disk method under Infrared Spectrophotometry <2.25>, and compare the spectrum with the Reference Spectrum or the spectrum of Amlexanox RS: both spectra exhibit similar intensities of absorption at the same wave numbers.

Purity (1) Chloride <1.03>—Dissolve 1.0 g of Amlexanox in 20 mL of water and 10 mL of sodium hydroxide TS, add 15 mL of dilute nitric acid and water to make 50 mL, centrifuge, and then filter the supernatant liquid. To 25 mL of this filtrate add water to make 50 mL. Perform the test using this solution as the test solution. The control solution consists of 5 mL of sodium hydroxide TS, 7.5 mL of dilute nitric acid, 0.30 mL of 0.01 mol/L hydrochloric acid VS, and water added to make 50 mL (not more than 0.021%).

(2) Heavy metals <1.07>—Proceed with 1.0 g of Amlexanox according to Method 2, and perform the test. Prepare the control solution with 2.0 mL of Standard Lead Solution (not more than 20 ppm).

(3) Related substances—(i) Dissolve 30 mg of Amlexanox in 50 mL of the mobile phase, and use this solution as the sample solution. Pipet 1 mL of the sample solution, and add the mobile phase to make exactly 50 mL. Pipet 1 mL of this solution, add the mobile phase to make exactly 20 mL, and use this solution as the standard solution. Perform the test with exactly 10 μL each of the sample solution and standard solution as directed under Liquid Chromatography <2.01> according to the following conditions. Determine each peak area of these solutions by the automatic integration method: the area of the peak other than amlexanox obtained from the sample solution is not larger than 2 times the peak area of amlexanox from the standard solution.

Operating conditions—

The detector, column, column temperature, mobile phase, and flow rate: Proceed as directed in the operating conditions in the Assay.

Time span of measurement: Until completion of the elution of amlexanox, beginning after the solvent peak.

System suitability—

System performance: Proceed as directed in the system suitability in the Assay.

Test for required detectability: Pipet 10 mL of the standard solution, and add the mobile phase to make exactly 100 mL. Confirm that the peak area of amlexanox obtained with 10 μL of this solution is equivalent to 7 to 13% of that with 10 μL of the standard solution.

System repeatability: When the test is repeated 6 times with 10 μL of the standard solution under the above operating conditions, the relative standard deviation of the peak area of amlexanox is not more than 2.0%.

(ii) Dissolve 30 mg of Amlexanox in 50 mL of the mobile phase, and use this solution as the sample solution. Pipet 1 mL of the sample solution, and add the mobile phase to make exactly 50 mL. Pipet 1 mL of this solution, add the mobile phase to make exactly 20 mL, and use this solution as the standard solution. Perform the test with exactly 10 μL each of the sample solution and standard solution as directed under Liquid Chromatography <2.01> according to the following conditions, and determine each peak area of these solutions by the automatic integration method: the area of the peak other than amlexanox obtained from the sample solution is not larger than 2 times the peak area of amlexanox from the standard solution.

Operating conditions—

Detector, column, and column temperature: Proceed as directed in the operating conditions in the Assay.

Mobile phase: Dissolve 7.2 g of disodium hydrogen phosphate dodecahydrate in water to make 1000 mL. Adjust the pH of this solution to 8.0 by adding a solution prepared by dissolving 3.1 g of sodium dihydrogen phosphate dihydrate in 1000 mL of water. To 400 mL of this solution add 600 mL of acetonitrile.

Flow rate: To 15 mL of a solution of benzophenone in the mobile phase (3 in 1,000,000) add the mobile phase to make 20 mL. Adjust so that the retention time of benzophenone is about 6.5 minutes when perform the test with 10 μL of this solution under the conditions described above.

Time span of measurement: About 3 times as long as the retention time of benzophenone, beginning after the peak of amlexanox.

System suitability—

Test for required detectability: Pipet 5 mL of the standard solution, and add the mobile phase to make exactly 50 mL. Confirm that the peak area of amlexanox obtained with 10 μL of this solution is equivalent to 7 to 13% of that with 10 μL of the standard solution.

System performance: Pipet 1 mL of the sample solution, and add the mobile phase to make 100 mL. To 5 mL of this solution add 15 mL of the solution of benzophenone in the mobile phase (3 in 1,000,000). When perform the test with 10 μL of this solution according to the above conditions, amlexanox and benzophenone are eluted in this order with the resolution between these peaks being not less than 10.

System repeatability: When the test is repeated 6 times with 10 μL of the standard solution under the above operating conditions, the relative standard deviation of the peak area of amlexanox is not more than 2.0%.

(iii) The total amount of related substances, when calculated according to the following formula, is not more than 0.5%.

$$\text{Total amount (\%) of related substances} = \{(A_{T1}/A_{S1}) + (A_{T2}/A_{S2})\} \times 1/10$$

A_{T1}: Total area of the peaks other than amlexanox from the sample solution obtained in (i)

A_{T2}: Total area of the peaks other than amlexanox from the sample solution obtained in (ii)

A_{S1}: Peak area of amlexanox from the standard solution obtained in (i)

A_{S2}: Peak area of amlexanox from the standard solution obtained in (ii)

Loss on drying <2.41> Not more than 0.3% (1 g, 105°C, 2 hours).

Residue on ignition <2.44> Not more than 0.1% (1 g).

Assay Weigh accurately about 30 mg each of Amlexanox and Amlexanox RS, both dried, and dissolve them separately in the mobile phase to make exactly 50 mL. Pipet 5 mL each of these solutions, and add exactly 15 mL of the internal standard solution, and use these solutions as the sample solution and the standard solution, respectively. Perform the test with 10 μL each of the sample solution and standard solution as directed under Liquid Chromatography <2.01> according to the following conditions, and calculate the ratios, Q_T and Q_S, of the peak area of amlexanox to that of the internal standard, respectively.

$$\text{Amount (mg) of amlexanox } (C_{16}H_{14}N_2O_4) = M_S \times Q_T/Q_S$$

M_S: Amount (mg) of Amlexanox RS taken

Internal standard solution—A solution of 3-nitroaniline in the mobile phase (1 in 4000).

Operating conditions—

Detector: An ultraviolet absorption photometer (wavelength: 254 nm).

Column: A stainless steel column 4.0 mm in inside diameter and 15 cm in length, packed with octadecylsilanized silica gel for liquid chromatography (5 μm in particle diameter).

Column temperature: A constant temperature of about 25°C.

Mobile phase: Dissolve 17.9 g of disodium hydrogen phosphate dodecahydrate in water to make 1000 mL. Adjust the pH of this solution to 8.0 by adding a solution prepared by dissolving 7.8 g of sodium dihydrogen phosphate dihydrate in 1000 mL of water. To 760 mL of this solution add 240 mL of acetonitrile.

Flow rate: Adjust so that the retention time of amlexanox is about 10 minutes.

System suitability—

System performance: When the procedure is run with 10 μL of the standard solution according to the above conditions, amlexanox and the internal standard are eluted in this order with the resolution between these peaks being not less than 2.0.

System repeatability: When the test is repeated 6 times with 10 μL of the standard solution under the above conditions, the relative standard deviation of the ratio of the peak area of amlexanox to that of the internal standard is not more than 1.0%.

Containers and storage Containers—Well-closed containers.

Amlexanox Tablets

アンレキサノクス錠

Amlexanox Tablets contain not less than 93.0% and not more than 107.0% of the labeled amount of amlexanox ($C_{16}H_{14}N_2O_4$: 298.29).

Method of preparation Prepare as directed under Tablets, with Amlexanox.

Identification **(1)** Take an amount of powdered Amlexanox Tablets, equivalent to 10 mg of Amlexanox, add 100 mL of ethanol (99.5), shake vigorously, and filter. Pipet 1 mL of the filtrate, add 25 mL of ethanol (99.5), and use this solution as the sample solution. Determine the absorption spectrum of the sample solution as directed under Ultraviolet-visible Spectrophotometry <*2.24*>: it exhibits absorption maxima between 240 nm and 244 nm, between 285 nm and 289 nm, and between 341 nm and 352 nm.

(2) Observe the sample solution obtained in (1) under ultraviolet light (main wavelength: 365 nm): the solution shows a blue-white fluorescence.

Uniformity of dosage units <*6.02*> Perform the Mass variation test, or the Content uniformity test according to the following method: it meets the requirement.

Take 1 tablet of Amlexanox Tablets, add exactly 0.6 mL of the internal standard solution per 1 mg of amlexanox ($C_{16}H_{14}N_2O_4$), add the mobile phase to make exactly V mL so there is about 167 μg of amlexanox ($C_{16}H_{14}N_2O_4$) per mL, disintegrate the tablet, and then shake vigorously for 5 minutes. Centrifuge this solution, and use the supernatant liquid as the sample solution. Separately, weigh accurately about 30 mg of Amlexanox RS, previously dried at 105°C for 2 hours, and dissolve in the mobile phase to make exactly 50 mL. Pipet 25 mL of this solution, add exactly 10 mL of the internal standard solution, add the mobile phase to make 100 mL, and use this solution as the standard solution. Then, proceed as directed in the Assay under Amlexanox.

$$\text{Amount (mg) of amlexanox } (C_{16}H_{14}N_2O_4) = M_S \times Q_T/Q_S \times V/200$$

M_S: Amount (mg) of Amlexanox RS taken

Internal standard solution—A solution of 3-nitroaniline in the mobile phase (1 in 500).

Dissolution <*6.10*> When the test is performed at 50 revolutions per minute according to the Paddle method, using 900 mL of 2nd fluid for dissolution test as the dissolution medium, the dissolution rate in 45 minutes of Amlexanox Tablets is not less than 80%.

Start the test with 1 tablet of Amlexanox Tablets, withdraw not less than 20 mL of the medium at the specified minute after starting the test, and filter through a membrane filter with a pore size not exceeding 0.45 μm. Discard not less than 10 mL of the first filtrate, pipet V mL of the subsequent filtrate, add the dissolution medium to make exactly V' mL so that each mL contains about 5.6 μg of amlexanox ($C_{16}H_{14}N_2O_4$), and use this solution as the sample solution. Separately, weigh accurately about 28 mg of Amlexanox RS, previously dried at 105°C for 2 hours, and dissolve in 2 mL of dilute sodium hydroxide TS, add the dissolution medium to make exactly 50 mL. Pipet 1 mL of this solution, add the dissolution medium to make exactly 100 mL, and use this solution as the standard solution. Determine the absorbances, A_T and A_S, at 350 nm of the sample solution and standard solution as directed under Ultraviolet-visible Spectrophotometry <*2.24*>.

$$\text{Dissolution rate (\%) with respect to the labeled amount of amlexanox } (C_{16}H_{14}N_2O_4) = M_S \times A_T/A_S \times V'/V \times 1/C \times 18$$

M_S: Amount (mg) of Amlexanox RS taken

C: Labeled amount (mg) of amlexanox ($C_{16}H_{14}N_2O_4$) in 1 tablet

Assay Weigh accurately not less than 20 Amlexanox Tablets, and powder. Weigh accurately a portion of the powder, equivalent to about 15 mg of amlexanox ($C_{16}H_{14}N_2O_4$), add exactly 10 mL of the internal standard solution, add 80 mL of the mobile phase, shake vigorously for 5 minutes, and then add the mobile phase to make 100 mL. Centrifuge this solution, and use the supernatant liquid as the sample solution. Separately, weigh accurately about 30 mg of Amlexanox RS, previously dried at 105°C for 2 hours, and dissolve in the mobile phase to make exactly 50 mL. Pipet 25 mL of this solution, add exactly 10 mL of the internal standard solution, add the mobile phase to make 100 mL, and use this solution as the standard solution. Then, proceed as directed in the Assay under Amlexanox.

$$\text{Amount (mg) of amlexanox } (C_{16}H_{14}N_2O_4) = M_S \times Q_T/Q_S \times 1/2$$

M_S: Amount (mg) of Amlexanox RS taken

Internal standard solution—A solution of 3-nitroaniline in the mobile phase (1 in 500).

Containers and storage Containers—Tight containers.

Amlodipine Besilate

アムロジピンベシル酸塩

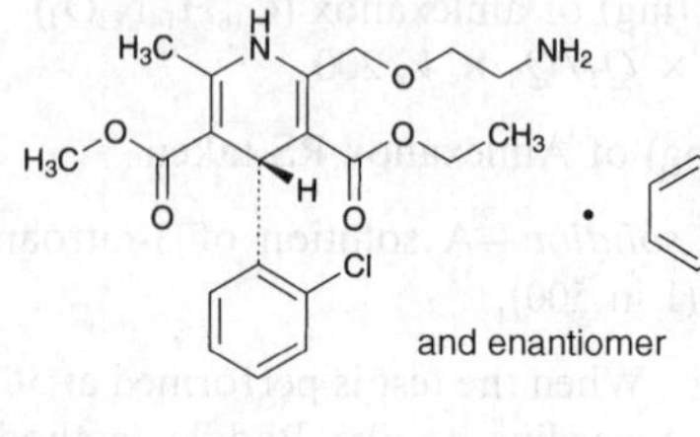

$C_{20}H_{25}ClN_2O_5.C_6H_6O_3S$: 567.05
3-Ethyl 5-methyl (4*RS*)-2-[(2-aminoethoxy)methyl]-4-(2-chlorophenyl)-6-methyl-1,4-dihydropyridine-3,5-dicarboxylate monobenzenesulfonate
[*111470-99-6*]

Amlodipine Besilate contains not less than 98.0% and not more than 102.0% of amlodipine besilate ($C_{20}H_{25}ClN_2O_5.C_6H_6O_3S$), calculated on the anhydrous basis.

Description Amlodipine Besilate occurs as a white to yellowish white crystalline powder.

It is freely soluble in methanol, sparingly soluble in ethanol (99.5), and slightly soluble in water.

A solution of Amlodipine Besilate in methanol (1 in 100) shows no optical rotation.

Melting point: about 198°C (with decomposition).

Identification **(1)** Determine the absorption spectrum of a solution of Amlodipine Besilate in 0.01 mol/L hydrochloric acid-methanol TS (1 in 40,000) as directed under Ultraviolet-visible Spectrophotometry <*2.24*>, and compare the spectrum with the Reference Spectrum or the spectrum of a solution of Amlodipine Besilate RS prepared in the same manner as the sample solution: both spectra exhibit similar intensities of absorption at the same wavelengths.

(2) Determine the infrared absorption spectrum of Amlodipine Besilate as directed in the potassium bromide disk method under Infrared Spectrophotometry <*2.25*>, and compare the spectrum with the Reference Spectrum or the spectrum of Amlodipine Besilate RS: both spectra exhibit similar intensities of absorption at the same wave numbers.

(3) To 30 mg of Amlodipine Besilate add 0.1 g of sodium nitrate and 0.1 g of anhydrous sodium carbonate, mix, and gradually ignite. After cooling, dissolve the residue in 2 mL of dilute hydrochloric acid and 10 mL of water, filter if necessary, and add barium chloride TS: a white precipitate is formed.

Purity **(1)** Heavy metals <*1.07*>—Proceed with 1.0 g of Amlodipine Besilate according to Method 4, and perform the test. Prepare the control solution with 2.5 mL of Standard Lead Solution (not more than 25 ppm).

(2) Related substances—Dissolve 0.10 g of Amlodipine Besilate in 50 mL of a mixture of water and acetonitrile (1:1), and use this solution as the sample solution. Pipet 1 mL of the sample solution, and add the mixture of water and acetonitrile (1:1) to make exactly 100 mL. Pipet 3 mL of this solution, add the mixture of water and acetonitrile (1:1) to make exactly 10 mL, and use this solution as the standard solution. Perform the test with exactly 10 μL each of the sample solution and standard solution as directed under Liquid Chromatography <*2.01*> according to the following conditions, and determine each peak area by the automatic integration method: the area of the peak having the relative retention time of 0.90 to amlodipine, obtained from the sample solution is not larger than the peak area of amlodipine from the standard solution, and the area of the peak other than amlodipine, benzenesulfonic acid having the relative retention time of about 0.15, and the peak mentioned above from the sample solution is not larger than 1/3 times the peak area of amlodipine from the standard solution. Furthermore, the total area of the peaks other than amlodipine and benzenesulfonic acid from the sample solution is not larger than 2.7 times the peak area of amlodipine from the standard solution.

Operating conditions—

Detector: An ultraviolet absorption photometer (wavelength: 237 nm).

Column: A stainless steel column 4.6 mm in inside diameter and 15 cm in length, packed with octadecylsilanized silica gel for liquid chromatography (3 μm in particle diameter).

Column temperature: A constant temperature of about 35°C.

Mobile phase A: A mixture of water and trifluoroacetic acid (5000:1).

Mobile phase B: A mixture of acetonitrile and trifluoroacetic acid (5000:1).

Flowing of mobile phase: Control the gradient by mixing the mobile phases A and B as directed in the following table.

Time after injection of sample (min)	Mobile phase A (vol%)	Mobile phase B (vol%)
0 – 30	80 → 20	20 → 80
30 – 45	20	80

Flow rate: 1.0 mL per minute.

Time span of measurement: About 3 times as long as the retention time of amlodipine, beginning after the solvent peak.

System suitability—

Test for required detectability: Pipet 1 mL of the standard solution, and add a mixture of water and acetonitrile (1:1) to make exactly 10 mL. Confirm that the peak area of amlodipine obtained with 10 μL of this solution is equivalent to 7 to 13% of that with 10 μL of the standard solution.

System performance: When the procedure is run with 10 μL of the standard solution under the above operating conditions, the number of theoretical plates and the symmetry factor of the peak of amlodipine are not less than 70,000 and not more than 1.5, respectively.

System repeatability: When the test is repeated 6 times with 10 μL of the standard solution under the above operating conditions, the relative standard deviation of the peak area of amlodipine is not more than 2.0%.

Water <*2.48*> Not more than 0.5% (1 g, volumetric titration, direct titration).

Residue on ignition <*2.44*> Not more than 0.2% (1 g).

Assay Weigh accurately about 35 mg each of Amlodipine Besilate and Amlodipine Besilate RS (separately determine the water <*2.48*> using the same manner as Amlodipine Besilate), dissolve them separately in the mobile phase to make exactly 250 mL. Pipet 5 mL each of these solutions, add exactly 5 mL each of the internal standard solution, add the mobile phase to make 25 mL, and use these solutions as the sample solution and standard solution. Perform the test with 20 μL of the sample solution and standard solution as directed under Liquid Chromatography <*2.01*> according to the following conditions, and calculate the ratios, Q_T and

Q_S, of the peak area of amlodipine to that of the internal standard.

Amount (mg) of amlodipine besilate ($C_{20}H_{25}ClN_2O_5.C_6H_6O_3S$)
$= M_S \times Q_T/Q_S$

M_S: Amount (mg) of Amlodipine Besilate RS taken, calculated on the anhydrous basis

Internal standard solution—A solution of isobutyl parahydroxybenzoate in the mobile phase (3 in 20,000).

Operating conditions—

Detector: An ultraviolet absorption photometer (wavelength: 237 nm).

Column: A stainless steel column 4.6 mm in inside diameter and 15 cm in length, packed with octadecylsilanized silica gel for liquid chromatography (5 μm in particle diameter).

Column temperature: A constant temperature of about 25°C.

Mobile phase: A mixture of methanol and a solution of potassium dihydrogen phosphate (41 in 10,000) (13:7).

Flow rate: Adjust so that the retention time of amlodipine is about 8 minutes.

System suitability—

System performance: When the procedure is run with 20 μL of the standard solution under the above operating conditions, amlodipine and the internal standard are eluted in this order with the resolution between these peaks being not less than 3.

System repeatability: When the test is repeated 6 times with 20 μL of the standard solution under the above operating conditions, the relative standard deviation of the ratio of the peak area of amlodipine to that of the internal standard is not more than 1.0%.

Containers and storage Containers—Well-closed containers.

Storage—Light-resistant.

Amlodipine Besilate Orally Disintegrating Tablets

アムロジピンベシル酸塩口腔内崩壊錠

Amlodipine Besilate Orally Disintegrating Tablets contain not less than 95.0% and not more than 105.0% of the labeled amount of amlodipine besilate ($C_{20}H_{25}ClN_2O_5.C_6H_6O_3S$: 567.05).

Method of preparation Prepare as directed under Tablets, with Amlodipine Besilate.

Identification To an amount of powdered Amlodipine Besilate Orally Disintegrating Tablets, equivalent to 7 mg of Amlodipine Besilate, add 200 mL of 0.01 mol/L hydrochloric acid-methanol TS, treat with ultrasonic waves, and filter. Determine the absorption spectrum of the filtrate as directed under Ultraviolet-visible Spectrophotometry *<2.24>*: it exhibits a maximum between 358 nm and 362 nm.

Purity Related substances—Use the sample solution obtained in the Assay as the sample solution. Pipet 1 mL of the sample solution, add a mixture of methanol and the mobile phase A (3:2) to make exactly 200 mL, and use this solution as the standard solution. Perform the test with exactly 30 μL each of the sample solution and standard solution as directed under Liquid Chromatography *<2.01>* according to the following conditions, and determine each peak area by the automatic integration method: the area of the peak having the relative retention time of about 0.45 to amlodipine obtained from the sample solution is not larger than the peak area of amlodipine from the standard solution, the area of the peak having the relative retention time of about 4.5 to amlodipine from the sample solution is not larger than 1.8 times the peak area of amlodipine from the standard solution, and the area of the peak having the relative retention time of about 0.16 to amlodipine and the peaks other than mentioned above from the sample solution is not larger than 2/5 times the peak area of amlodipine from the standard solution. Furthermore, the total area of the peaks other than amlodipine and the peak having the relative retention time of about 0.16 to amlodipine from the sample solution is not larger than 2.8 times the peak area of amlodipine from the standard solution. For the areas of the peaks, having the relative retention time of about 0.45 and about 4.5 to amlodipine, multiply their correction factors, 2.0 and 1.9, respectively.

Operating conditions—

Detector: An ultraviolet absorption photometer (wavelength: 237 nm).

Column: A stainless steel column 4.6 mm in inside diameter and 15 cm in length, packed with octadecylsilanized silica gel for liquid chromatography (5 μm in particle diameter).

Column temperature: A constant temperature of about 25°C.

Mobile phase A: Dissolve 4.1 g of potassium dihydrogen phosphate in 1000 mL of water, adjust to pH 6.0 with a solution of 5.4 g of disodium hydrogen phosphate dodecahydrate in 500 mL of water. To 500 mL of this solution add 500 mL of methanol.

Mobile phase B: Dissolve 4.1 g of potassium dihydrogen phosphate in 1000 mL of water, adjust to pH 6.0 with a solution of 5.4 g of disodium hydrogen phosphate dodecahydrate in 500 mL of water. To 50 mL of this solution add 950 mL of methanol.

Flowing of mobile phase: Control the gradient by mixing the mobile phases A and B as directed in the following table.

Time after injection of sample (min)	Mobile phase A (vol%)	Mobile phase B (vol%)
0 – 10	80	20
10 – 35	80 → 0	20 → 100
35 – 50	0	100

Flow rate: Adjust so that the retention time of amlodipine is about 10 minutes.

Time span of measurement: About 5 times as long as the retention time of amlodipine.

System suitability—

Test for required detectability: Pipet 10 mL of the standard solution, and add a mixture of methanol and the mobile phase A (3:2) to make exactly 50 mL. Confirm that the peak area of amlodipine obtained with 30 μL of this solution is equivalent to 14 to 26% of that with 30 μL of the standard solution.

System performance: When the procedure is run with 30 μL of the standard solution under the above operating conditions, the number of theoretical plates and the symmetry factor of the peak of amlodipine are not less than 3000 and not more than 1.5, respectively.

System repeatability: When the test is repeated 6 times with 30 μL of the standard solution under the above operating conditions, the relative standard deviation of the peak area of amlodipine is not more than 2.0%.

Uniformity of dosage units <*6.02*> Perform the test according to the following method: it meets the requirement of the Content uniformity test.

To 1 tablet of Amlodipine Besilate Orally Disintegrating Tablets add $4V/5$ mL of a mixture of the mobile phase and methanol (1:1), disperse the particles by sonicating, add a mixture of the mobile phase and methanol (1:1) to make exactly V mL so that each mL of the solution contains about 0.14 mg of amlodipine besilate ($C_{20}H_{25}ClN_2O_5.C_6H_6O_3S$). Centrifuge this solution, and use the supernatant liquid as the sample solution. Then, proceed as directed in the Assay.

Amount (mg) of amlodipine besilate
($C_{20}H_{25}ClN_2O_5.C_6H_6O_3S$)
$= M_S \times A_T/A_S \times V \times 1/250$

M_S: Amount (mg) of Amlodipine Besilate RS taken, calculated on the anhydrous basis

Disintegration Being specified separately when the drug is granted approval based on the Law.

Dissolution Being specified separately when the drug is granted approval based on the Law.

Assay Weigh accurately the mass of not less than 20 Amlodipine Besilate Orally Disintegrating Tablets, and powder them. Weigh accurately a portion of this powder, equivalent to about 7 mg of amlodipine besilate ($C_{20}H_{25}ClN_2O_5.C_6H_6O_3S$), add 40 mL of a mixture of the mobile phase and methanol (1:1), disperse the particles with the aid of ultrasonic waves, and add a mixture of the mobile phase and methanol (1:1) to make exactly 50 mL. Centrifuge this solution, and use the supernatant liquid as the sample solution. Separately, weigh accurately about 35 mg of Amlodipine Besilate RS (separately, determine the water <*2.48*> in the same manner as Amlodipine Besilate), add 150 mL of a mixture of the mobile phase and methanol (1:1), dissolve with the aid of ultrasonic waves, then add a mixture of the mobile phase and methanol (1:1) to make exactly 250 mL, and use this solution as the standard solution. Perform the test with exactly 30 μL each of the sample solution and standard solution as directed under Liquid Chromatography <*2.01*>, and determine the peak areas, A_T and A_S, of amlodipine in each solution.

Amount (mg) of amlodipine besilate
($C_{20}H_{25}ClN_2O_5.C_6H_6O_3S$)
$= M_S \times A_T/A_S \times 1/5$

M_S: Amount (mg) of Amlodipine Besilate RS taken, calculated on the anhydrous basis

Operating conditions—

Detector: An ultraviolet absorption photometer (wavelength: 237 nm).

Column: A stainless steel column 4.6 mm in inside diameter and 15 cm in length, packed with octadecylsilanized silica gel for liquid chromatography (5 μm in particle diameter).

Column temperature: A constant temperature of about 25°C.

Mobile phase: Dissolve 4.1 g of potassium dihydrogen phosphate in 1000 mL of water, adjust to pH 6.0 with a solution of 5.4 g of disodium hydrogen phosphate dodecahydrate in 500 mL of water. To 400 mL of this solution add 600 mL of methanol.

Flow rate: Adjust so that the retention time of amlodipine is about 10 minutes.

System suitability—

System performance: When the procedure is run with 30 μL of the standard solution under the above operating conditions, the number of theoretical plates and the symmetry factor of the peak of amlodipine are not less than 3000 and not more than 2.0, respectively.

System repeatability: When the test is repeated 6 times with 30 μL of the standard solution under the above operating conditions, the relative standard deviation of the peak area of amlodipine is not more than 1.0%.

Containers and storage Containers—Tight containers.

Amlodipine Besilate Tablets

アムロジピンベシル酸塩錠

Amlodipine Besilate Tablets contain not less than 95.0% and not more than 105.0% of the labeled amount of amlodipine besilate ($C_{20}H_{25}ClN_2O_5.C_6H_6O_3S$: 567.05).

Method of preparation Prepare as directed under Tablets, with Amlodipine Besilate.

Identification To a quantity of powdered Amlodipine Besilate Tablets, equivalent to 2.5 mg of Amlodipine Besilate, add 100 mL of 0.01 mol/L hydrochloric acid-methanol TS, shake vigorously, and filter. Determine the absorption spectrum of the filtrate as directed under Ultraviolet-visible Spectrophotometry <*2.24*>: it exhibits maxima between 235 nm and 239 nm, and between 358 nm and 362 nm.

Uniformity of dosage units <*6.02*> Perform the test according to the following method: it meets the requirement of the Content uniformity test.

To 1 tablet of Amlodipine Besilate Tablets add 10 mL of water to disintegrate, disperse by sonicating with occasional shaking, add the mobile phase to make exactly V mL so that each mL contains about 69 μg of amlodipine besilate ($C_{20}H_{25}ClN_2O_5.C_6H_6O_3S$), and shake for 60 minutes. Centrifuge this solution, pipet 10 mL of the supernatant liquid, add exactly 5 mL of the internal standard solution, add the mobile phase to make 25 mL, and use this solution as the sample solution. Proceed as directed in the Assay.

Amount (mg) of amlodipine besilate
($C_{20}H_{25}ClN_2O_5.C_6H_6O_3S$)
$= M_S \times Q_T/Q_S \times V/500$

M_S: Amount (mg) of Amlodipine Besilate RS taken, calculated on the anhydrous basis

Internal standard solution—A solution of isobutyl parahydroxybenzoate in the mobile phase (3 in 20,000).

Dissolution Being specified separately when the drug is granted approval based on the Law.

Assay To 20 Amlodipine Besilate Tablets add 100 mL of water to disintegrate, disperse with the aid of ultrasonic waves with occasional shaking, add the mobile phase to make exactly 1000 mL, and shake for 60 minutes. Centrifuge this solution, pipet a volume of the supernatant liquid, equivalent to about 0.7 mg of amlodipine besilate ($C_{20}H_{25}ClN_2O_5.C_6H_6O_3S$), add exactly 5 mL of the internal standard solution, add the mobile phase to make 25 mL, and use this solution as the sample solution. Separately, weigh accurately about 35 mg of Amlodipine Besilate RS (separately, determine the water <*2.48*> in the same manner as Amlodipine Besilate), and dissolve in the mobile phase to make exactly 250 mL. Pipet 5 mL of this solution, add exactly 5 mL of the internal standard solution, add the mobile phase to make 25 mL, and use this solution as the standard solution. Perform the test with 20 μL each of the sample solution and standard solution as directed under Liquid Chromatography <*2.01*> according to the following conditions, and calculate the ratios, Q_T and Q_S, of the peak area of amlodipine to that of the internal standard.

Amount (mg) of amlodipine besilate ($C_{20}H_{25}ClN_2O_5.C_6H_6O_3S$)
$= M_S \times Q_T/Q_S \times 1/50$

M_S: Amount (mg) of Amlodipine Besilate RS taken, calculated on the anhydrous basis

Internal standard solution—A solution of isobutyl parahydroxybenzoate in the mobile phase (3 in 20,000).

Operating conditions—

Detector: An ultraviolet absorption photometer (wavelength: 237 nm).

Column: A stainless steel column 4.6 mm in inside diameter and 15 cm in length, packed with octadecylsilanized silica gel for liquid chromatography (5 μm in particle diameter).

Column temperature: A constant temperature of about 25°C.

Mobile phase: A mixture of methanol and potassium dihydrogen phosphate (41 in 10,000) (13:7).

Flow rate: Adjust so that the retention time of amlodipine is about 8 minutes.

System suitability—

System performance: When the procedure is run with 20 μL of the standard solution under the above operating conditions, amlodipine and the internal standard are eluted in this order with the resolution between these peaks being not less than 5.

System repeatability: When the test is repeated 6 times with 20 μL of the standard solution under the above operating conditions, the relative standard deviation of the ratios of the peak area of amlodipine to that of the internal standard is not more than 1.0%.

Containers and storage Containers—Well-closed containers.

Ammonia Water

アンモニア水

Ammonia Water contains not less than 9.5 w/v% and not more than 10.5 w/v% of ammonia (NH_3: 17.03).

Description Ammonia Water occurs as a clear, colorless liquid, having a very pungent, characteristic odor.

It is alkaline.

Specific gravity d^{20}_{20}: 0.95 – 0.96

Identification **(1)** Hold a glass rod moistened with hydrochloric acid near the surface of Ammonia Water: dense white fumes are produced.

(2) Hold moistened red litmus paper near the surface of Ammonia Water: it turns blue.

Purity **(1)** Residue on evaporation—Evaporate 10.0 mL of Ammonia Water to dryness, and dry the residue at 105°C for 1 hour: the mass of the residue is not more than 2.0 mg.

(2) Heavy metals <*1.07*>—Evaporate 5.0 mL of Ammonia Water to dryness on a water bath, add 1 mL of dilute hydrochloric acid to the residue, and evaporate to dryness. Dissolve the residue in 2 mL of dilute acetic acid, add water to make 50 mL, and perform the test using this solution as the test solution. Prepare the control solution with 2.5 mL of Standard Lead Solution, 2 mL of dilute acetic acid and water to make 50 mL (not more than 5 ppm).

(3) Potassium permanganate-reducing substances—To 10.0 mL of Ammonia Water add 40 mL of dilute sulfuric acid while cooling, and add 0.10 mL of 0.02 mol/L potassium permanganate VS: the red color of the potassium permanganate does not disappear within 10 minutes.

Assay Pipet 5 mL of Ammonia Water, add 25 mL of water, and titrate <*2.50*> with 0.5 mol/L sulfuric acid VS (indicator: 2 drops of methyl red TS).

Each mL of 0.5 mol/L sulfuric acid VS
= 17.03 mg of NH_3

Containers and storage Containers—Tight containers.

Storage—Not exceeding 30°C.

Amobarbital

アモバルビタール

$C_{11}H_{18}N_2O_3$: 226.27
5-Ethyl-5-(3-methylbutyl)pyrimidine-2,4,6(1*H*,3*H*,5*H*)-trione
[*57-43-2*]

Amobarbital, when dried, contains not less than 99.0% of amobarbital ($C_{11}H_{18}N_2O_3$).

Description Amobarbital occurs as white, crystals or crystalline powder. It is odorless, and has a slightly bitter taste.

It is freely soluble in ethanol (95), in acetone and in diethyl ether, sparingly soluble in chloroform, and practically insoluble in water.

It dissolves in sodium hydroxide TS and in sodium carbonate TS.

The pH of a saturated solution of Amobarbital is between 5.0 and 5.6.

Identification **(1)** Boil 0.2 g of Amobarbital with 10 mL of sodium hydroxide TS: the gas evolved changes moistened red litmus paper to blue.

(2) Dissolve 0.05 g of Amobarbital in 2 to 3 drops of ammonia-ammonium chloride buffer solution (pH 10.7) and 5 mL of diluted pyridine (1 in 10). Add 5 mL of chloroform and 0.3 mL of copper (II) sulfate TS to the solution: a red-purple precipitate is produced in the aqueous layer. Shake the mixture: a red-purple color is produced in the chloroform layer.

(3) To 0.4 g of Amobarbital add 0.1 g of anhydrous sodium carbonate and 4 mL of water, shake, and add a solution of 0.3 g of 4-nitrobenzyl chloride in 7 mL of ethanol (95). Heat the mixture on a water bath for 30 minutes under a reflux condenser, and allow to stand for 1 hour. Filter the crystals produced, wash with 7 mL of sodium hydroxide TS and a small portion of water, recrystallize from ethanol, and dry at 105°C for 30 minutes: the crystals so obtained melt <*2.60*> between 168°C and 173°C or between 150°C and 154°C.

Melting point <*2.60*> 157 – 160°C

Purity (1) Clarity and color of solution—Dissolve 0.5 g of Amobarbital in 5 mL of sodium hydroxide TS: the solution is clear and colorless.

(2) Chloride <*1.03*>—Dissolve 0.30 g of Amobarbital in 20 mL of acetone, and add 6 mL of dilute nitric acid and water to make 50 mL. Perform the test using this solution as the test solution. Prepare the control solution as follows: take 0.30 mL of 0.01 mol/L hydrochloric acid VS, 20 mL of acetone and 6 mL of dilute nitric acid, and add water to make 50 mL (not more than 0.035%).

(3) Sulfate <*1.14*>—Dissolve 0.40 g of Amobarbital in 20 mL of acetone, and add 1 mL of dilute hydrochloric acid and water to make 50 mL. Perform the test using this solution as the test solution. Prepare the control solution as follows: take 0.40 mL of 0.005 mol/L sulfuric acid VS, 20 mL of acetone, and 1 mL of dilute hydrochloric acid, and add water to make 50 mL (not more than 0.048%).

(4) Heavy metals <*1.07*>—Proceed with 1.0 g of Amobarbital according to Method 2, and perform the test. Prepare the control solution with 2.0 mL of Standard Lead Solution (not more than 20 ppm).

(5) Readily carbonizable substances <*1.15*>—Perform the test with 0.5 g of Amobarbital. The solution is not more colored than Matching Fluid A.

Loss on drying <*2.41*> Not more than 1.0% (1 g, 105°C, 4 hours).

Residue on ignition <*2.44*> Not more than 0.1% (1 g).

Assay Weigh accurately about 0.5 g of Amobarbital, previously dried, and dissolve in 5 mL of ethanol (95) and 50 mL of chloroform. Titrate <*2.50*> with 0.1 mol/L potassium hydroxide-ethanol VS until the color of the solution changes from yellow through light blue to purple (indicator: 1 mL of alizarin yellow GG-thymolphthalein TS). Perform a blank determination in the same manner, and make any necessary correction.

Each mL of 0.1 mol/L potassium hydroxide-ethanol VS
= 22.63 mg of $C_{11}H_{18}N_2O_3$

Containers and storage Containers—Well-closed containers.

Amosulalol Hydrochloride

アモスラロール塩酸塩

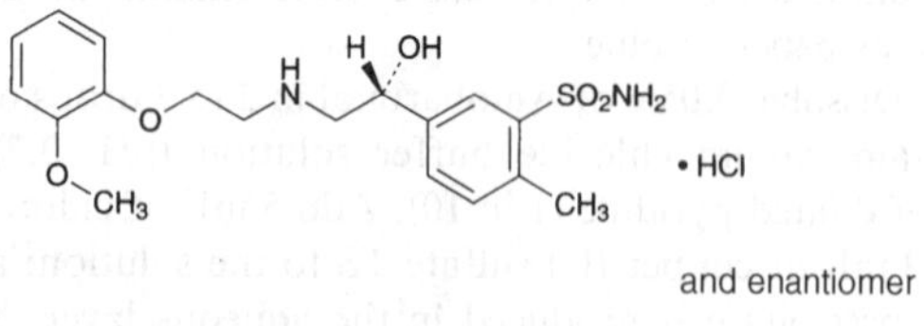

and enantiomer

$C_{18}H_{24}N_2O_5S.HCl$: 416.92
5-((1*RS*)-1-Hydroxy-2-{[2-(2-methoxyphenoxy)ethyl]amino}ethyl)-2-methylbenzenesulfonamide monohydrochloride
[*70958-86-0*]

Amosulalol Hydrochloride contains not less than 98.5% and not more than 101.0% of amosulalol hydrochloride ($C_{18}H_{24}N_2O_5S.HCl$), calculated on the anhydrous basis.

Description Amosulalol Hydrochloride occurs as white crystals or a white crystalline powder. It has a bitter taste.

It is very soluble in formic acid, freely soluble in methanol, and sparingly soluble in water and in ethanol (99.5).

It is hygroscopic.

A solution of Amosulalol Hydrochloride in methanol (1 in 100) shows no optical rotation.

Identification (1) Determine the absorption spectrum of a solution of Amosulalol Hydrochloride (1 in 20,000) as directed under Ultraviolet-visible Spectrophotometry <*2.24*>, and compare the spectrum with the Reference Spectrum: both spectra exhibit similar intensities of absorption at the same wavelengths.

(2) Determine the infrared absorption spectrum of Amosulalol Hydrochloride as directed in the potassium chloride disk method under Infrared Spectrophotometry <*2.25*>, and compare the spectrum with the Reference Spectrum: both spectra exhibit similar intensities of absorption at the same wave numbers.

(3) A solution of Amosulalol Hydrochloride (1 in 100) responds to Qualitative Tests <*1.09*> for chloride.

Melting point <*2.60*> 158 – 162°C

Purity (1) Heavy metals <*1.07*>—Place 1.0 g of Amosulalol Hydrochloride in a porcelain crucible, add 1.5 mL of sulfuric acid, cover loosely, and heat gently to carbonize. After cooling, add 2 mL of nitric acid, heat carefully until white fumes no longer are evolved, and then heat intensely to 500 – 600°C to incinerate. After cooling, add 2 mL of hydrochloric acid, proceed according to Method 2, and perform the test. The control solution, processed in the same manner as the test solution using the same amounts of reagents, is prepared by combining 2.0 mL of Standard Lead Solution and water to make 50 mL (not more than 20 ppm).

(2) Related substances—Dissolve 0.10 g of Amosulalol Hydrochloride in 20 mL of the mobile phase, and use this solution as the sample solution. Pipet 1 mL of the sample solution, add the mobile phase to make exactly 200 mL, and use this solution as the standard solution. Perform the test with exactly 10 μL each of the sample solution and standard solution as directed under Liquid Chromatography <*2.01*> according to the following conditions, and determine each peak area of both solutions by the automatic integration method: the total area of the peaks other than amosulalol obtained from the sample solution is not larger than 2/5 times the peak area of amosulalol from the standard solution.

Operating conditions—

Detector: An ultraviolet absorption photometer (wavelength: 272 nm).

Column: A stainless steel column 4.6 mm in inside diameter and 15 cm in length, packed with octadecylsilanized silica gel for liquid chromatography (5 μm in particle diameter).

Column temperature: A constant temperature of about 30°C.

Mobile phase: Dissolve 1.36 g of potassium dihydrogen phosphate in water to make 1000 mL, and adjust to pH 5.7 by adding a solution prepared by dissolving 3.58 g of disodium hydrogen phosphate dodecahydrate in water to make 1000 mL. To 670 mL of this solution add 330 mL of acetonitrile.

Flow rate: Adjust so that the retention time of amosulalol is about 7 minutes.

Time span of measurement: About 2 times as long as the retention time of amosulalol, beginning after the solvent peak.

System suitability—

Test for required detectability: Pipet 1 mL of the standard solution, and add the mobile phase to make exactly 10 mL.

Confirm that the peak area of amosulalol obtained with 10 μL of this solution is equivalent to 7 to 13% of that with 10 μL of the standard solution.

System performance: When the procedure is run with 10 μL of the standard solution under the above operating conditions, the number of theoretical plates and the symmetry factor of the peak of amosulalol are not less than 4000 and not more than 1.7, respectively.

System repeatability: When the test is repeated 6 times with 10 μL of the standard solution under the above operating conditions, the relative standard deviation of the peak area of amosulalol is not more than 1.0%.

Water <*2.48*> Not more than 4.0% (1 g, volumetric titration, direct titration).

Residue on ignition <*2.44*> Not more than 0.1% (1 g).

Assay Weigh accurately about 0.6 g of Amosulalol Hydrochloride, dissolve in 3 mL of formic acid, add 80 mL of a mixture of acetic acid (100) and acetic anhydride (3:2), and titrate <*2.50*> within 5 minutes with 0.1 mol/L perchloric acid VS (potentiometric titration). Perform a blank determination in the same manner, and make any necessary correction.

Each mL of 0.1 mol/L perchloric acid VS
= 41.69 mg of $C_{18}H_{24}N_2O_5S.HCl$

Containers and storage Containers—Tight containers.

Amosulalol Hydrochloride Tablets

アモスラロール塩酸塩錠

Amosulalol Hydrochloride Tablets contain not less than 95.0% and not more than 105.0% of the labeled amount of amosulalol hydrochloride ($C_{18}H_{24}N_2O_5S.HCl$: 416.92).

Method of preparation Prepare as directed under Tablets, with Amosulalol Hydrochloride.

Identification To a quantity of powdered Amosulalol Hydrochloride Tablets, equivalent to 50 mg of Amosulalol Hydrochloride, add 25 mL of 0.1 mol/L hydrochloric acid TS, shake well, and then centrifuge. To 2.5 mL of the supernatant liquid add water to make 100 mL. Determine the absorption spectrum of this solution as directed under Ultraviolet-visible Spectrophotometry <*2.24*>: it exhibits a maximum between 270 nm and 274 nm, and a shoulder between 275 nm and 281 nm.

Uniformity of dosage units <*6.02*> Perform the test according to the following method: it meets the requirement of the Content uniformity test.

Take 1 tablet of Amosulalol Hydrochloride Tablets, disintegrate by adding 2 mL of 0.1 mol/L hydrochloric acid TS, add 15 mL of methanol, and shake well. Add methanol to make exactly V mL so that each mL contains about 0.4 mg of amosulalol hydrochloride ($C_{18}H_{24}N_2O_5S.HCl$), and centrifuge. Pipet 5 mL of the supernatant liquid, add exactly 2 mL of the internal standard solution and the mobile phase to make 20 mL, and use this solution as the sample solution. Separately, weigh accurately about 20 mg of amosulalol hydrochloride for assay (separately determine the water <*2.48*> in the same manner as Amosulalol Hydrochloride), and dissolve in methanol to make exactly 50 mL. Pipet 5 mL of this solution, add exactly 2 mL of the internal standard solution, add the mobile phase to make 20 mL, and use this solution as the standard solution. Then, proceed as directed in the Assay.

Amount (mg) of amosulalol hydrochloride ($C_{18}H_{24}N_2O_5S.HCl$)
$= M_S \times Q_T/Q_S \times V/50$

M_S: Amount (mg) of amosulalol hydrochloride for assay taken, calculated on the anhydrous basis

Internal standard solution—A solution of ethyl parahydroxybenzoate in methanol (1 in 6250).

Dissolution <*6.10*> When the test is performed at 50 revolutions per minute according to the Paddle method, using 900 mL of water as the dissolution medium, the dissolution rate in 30 minutes of Amosulalol Hydrochloride Tablets is not less than 75%.

Start the test with 1 tablet of Amosulalol Hydrochloride Tablets, withdraw not less than 20 mL of the medium at the specified minute after starting the test, and filter through a membrane filter with a pore size not exceeding 0.5 μm. Discard not less than 10 mL of the first filtrate, pipet V mL of the subsequent filtrate, add water to make exactly V' mL so that each mL contains about 5.5 μg of amosulalol hydrochloride ($C_{18}H_{24}N_2O_5S.HCl$), and use this solution as the sample solution. Separately, weigh accurately about 22 mg of amosulalol hydrochloride for assay (separately determine the water <*2.48*> in the same manner as Amosulalol Hydrochloride), and dissolve in water to make exactly 200 mL. Pipet 5 mL of this solution, add water to make exactly 100 mL, and use this solution as the standard solution. Perform the test with exactly 50 μL each of the sample solution and standard solution as directed under Liquid Chromatography <*2.01*> according to the following conditions, and determine the amosulalol peak areas, A_T and A_S, in each solution.

Dissolution rate (%) with respect to the labeled amount of amosulalol hydrochloride ($C_{18}H_{24}N_2O_5S.HCl$)
$= M_S \times A_T/A_S \times V'/V \times 1/C \times 45/2$

M_S: Amount (mg) of amosulalol hydrochloride for assay taken, calculated on the anhydrous basis
C: Labeled amount (mg) of amosulalol hydrochloride ($C_{18}H_{24}N_2O_5S.HCl$) in 1 tablet

Operating conditions—

Detector: An ultraviolet absorption photometer (wavelength: 272 nm).

Column: A stainless steel column 4.6 mm in inside diameter and 15 cm in length, packed with octadecylsilanized silica gel for liquid chromatography (5 μm in particle diameter).

Column temperature: A constant temperature of about 30°C.

Mobile phase: Dissolve 1.36 g of potassium dihydrogen phosphate in water to make 1000 mL, and adjust to pH 5.7 by adding a soluion prepared by dissolving 3.58 g of disodium hydrogen phosphate dodecahydrate in water to make 1000 mL. To 670 mL of this solution add 330 mL of acetonitrile.

Flow rate: Adjust so that the retention time of amosulalol is about 5 minutes.

System suitability—

System performance: When the procedure is run with 50 μL of the standard solution under the above operating conditions, the number of theoretical plates and the symmetry factor of the peak of amosulalol are not less than 4000 and not more than 1.7, respectively.

System repeatability: When the test is repeated 6 times

with 50 μL of the standard solution under the above operating conditions, the relative standard deviation of the peak area of amosulalol is not more than 1.0%.

Assay Take 10 Amosulalol Hydrochloride Tablets, add 20 mL of 0.1 mol/L hydrochloric acid TS, and shake well to disintegrate. Add 120 mL of methanol, again shake well, add methanol to make exactly 200 mL, and then centrifuge. Pipet a volume of supernatant liquid corresponding to about 5 mg of amosulalol hydrochloride ($C_{18}H_{24}N_2O_5S.HCl$), add exactly 5 mL of the internal standard solution, add the mobile phase to make 50 mL, and use this solution as the sample solution. Separately, weigh accurately about 25 mg of amosulalol hydrochloride for assay (separately determine the water *<2.48>* in the same manner as Amosulalol Hydrochloride), and dissolve in methanol to make exactly 25 mL. Pipet 5 mL of this solution, add exactly 5 mL of the internal standard solution, add the mobile phase to make 50 mL, and use this solution as the standard solution. Perform the test with 10 μL each of the sample solution and standard solution as directed under Liquid Chromatography *<2.01>* according to the following conditions, and calculate the ratios, Q_T and Q_S, of the peak area of amosulalol to that of the internal standard.

$$\text{Amount (mg) of amosulalol hydrochloride } (C_{18}H_{24}N_2O_5S.HCl) = M_S \times Q_T/Q_S \times 1/5$$

M_S: Amount (mg) of amosulalol hydrochloride for assay taken, calculated on the anhydrous basis

Internal standard solution—A solution of ethyl parahydroxybenzoate in methanol (1 in 6250).

Operating conditions—

Detector: An ultraviolet absorption photometer (wavelength: 272 nm).

Column: A stainless steel column 4.6 mm in inside diameter and 15 cm in length, packed with octadecylsilanized silica gel for liquid chromatography (5 μm in particle diameter).

Column temperature: A constant temperature of about 25°C.

Mobile phase: A mixture of diluted acetic acid (100) (1 in 25), acetonitrile and a solution of ammonium acetate (1 in 250) (5:3:2).

Flow rate: Adjust so that the retention time of amosulalol is about 4 minutes.

System suitability—

System performance: When the procedure is run with 10 μL of the standard solution under the above operating conditions, amosulalol and the internal standard are eluted in this order with the resolution between these peaks being not less than 7.

System repeatability: When the test is repeated 6 times with 10 μL of the standard solution under the above operating conditions, the relative standard deviation of the ratio of the peak area of amosulalol to that of the internal standard is not more than 1.0%.

Containers and storage Containers—Tight containers.

Amoxapine

アモキサピン

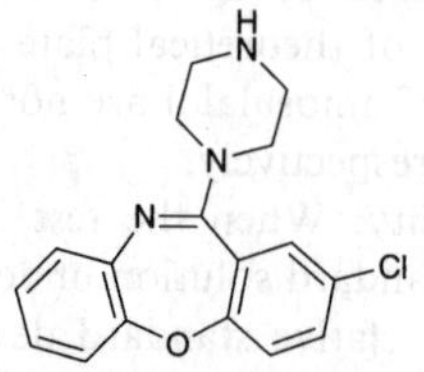

$C_{17}H_{16}ClN_3O$: 313.78

2-Chloro-11-(piperazin-1-yl)dibenzo[*b,f*][1,4]oxazepine

[*14028-44-5*]

Amoxapine, when dried, contains not less than 98.5% of amoxapine ($C_{17}H_{16}ClN_3O$).

Description Amoxapine occurs as white to light yellow-white, crystals or crystalline powder.

It is freely soluble in acetic acid (100), slightly soluble in ethanol (95) and in diethyl ether, and practically insoluble in water.

Identification **(1)** Determine the absorption spectrum of a solution of Amoxapine in 0.1 mol/L hydrochloric acid TS (1 in 50,000) as directed under Ultraviolet-visible Spectrophotometry *<2.24>*, and compare the spectrum with the Reference Spectrum: both spectra exhibit similar intensities of absorption as the same wavelengths.

(2) Determine the infrared absorption spectrum of Amoxapine, previously dried, as directed in the potassium bromide disk method under Infrared Spectrophotometry *<2.25>*, and compare the spectrum with the Reference Spectrum: both spectra exhibit similar intensities of absorption at the same wave numbers.

(3) Perform the test with Amoxapine as directed under Flame Coloration Test *<1.04>* (2): a green color appears.

Melting point *<2.60>* 178 – 182°C

Purity **(1)** Heavy metals *<1.07>*—Proceed with 2.0 g of Amoxapine according to Method 2, and perform the test. Prepare the control solution with 3.0 mL of Standard Lead Solution (not more than 15 ppm).

(2) Related substances—Dissolve 0.5 g of Amoxapine in 10 mL of a mixture of ethanol (95) and acetic acid (100) (9:1), and use this solution as the sample solution. Pipet 1 mL of the sample solution, and add a mixture of ethanol (95) and acetic acid (100) (9:1) to make exactly 10 mL. Pipet 1 mL of this solution, add a mixture of ethanol (95) and acetic acid (100) (9:1) to make exactly 20 mL, and use this solution as the standard solution. Perform the test with these solutions as directed under Thin-layer Chromatography *<2.03>*. Spot 5 μL each of the sample solution and standard solution on a plate of silica gel with fluorescent indicator for thin-layer chromatography. Develop the plate with a mixture of ethanol (95) and acetic acid (100) (9:1) to a distance of about 10 cm, and air-dry the plate. Examine under ultraviolet light (main wavelength: 254 nm): the spots other than the principal spot obtained from the sample solution are not more intense than the spot from the standard solution.

Loss on drying *<2.41>* Not more than 0.4% (1 g, in vacuum, 60°C, 3 hours).

Residue on ignition *<2.44>* Not more than 0.1% (1 g).

Assay Weigh accurately about 0.3 g of Amoxapine, previously dried, dissolve in 50 mL of acetic acid (100), and titrate <*2.50*> with 0.1 mol/L perchloric acid VS until the color of the solution changes from purple through blue to greenish blue (indicator: 2 drops of crystal violet TS). Perform a blank determination in the same manner, and make any necessary correction.

Each mL of 0.1 mol/L perchloric acid VS
= 15.69 mg of $C_{17}H_{16}ClN_3O$

Containers and storage Containers—Tight containers.

Amoxicillin Hydrate

アモキシシリン水和物

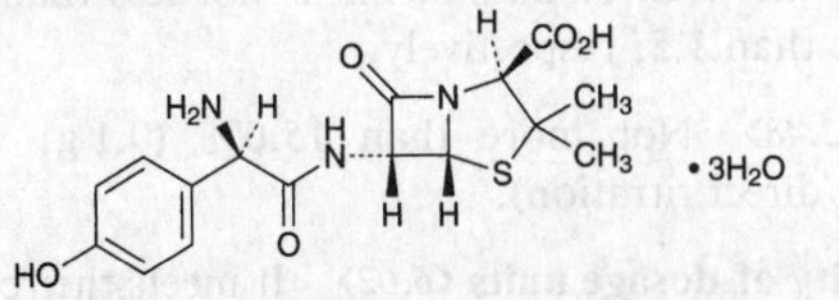

$C_{16}H_{19}N_3O_5S.3H_2O$: 419.45
(2*S*,5*R*,6*R*)-6-[(2*R*)-2-Amino-2-(4-hydroxyphenyl)-acetylamino]-3,3-dimethyl-7-oxo-4-thia-1-azabicyclo[3.2.0]heptane-2-carboxylic acid trihydrate
[*61336-70-7*]

Amoxicillin Hydrate contains not less than 950 μg (potency) and not more than 1010 μg (potency) per mg, calculated on the anhydrous basis. The potency of Amoxicillin Hydrate is expressed as mass (potency) of amoxicillin ($C_{16}H_{19}N_3O_5S$: 365.40).

Description Amoxicillin Hydrate occurs as white to light yellow-white, crystals or crystalline powder.

It is slightly soluble in water and in methanol, and very slightly soluble in ethanol (95).

Identification Determine the infrared absorption spectrum of Amoxicillin Hydrate as directed in the potassium bromide disk method under Infrared Spectrophotometry <*2.25*>, and compare the spectrum with the Reference Spectrum or the spectrum of Amoxicillin RS: both spectra exhibit similar intensities of absorption at the same wave numbers.

Optical rotation <*2.49*> $[\alpha]_D^{20}$: +290 – +315° (0.1 g calculated on the anhydrous basis, water, 100 mL, 100 mm).

Purity **(1)** Heavy metals <*1.07*>—To 1.0 g of Amoxicillin Hydrate add 2 mL of a solution of magnesium sulfate heptahydrate (1 in 4), mix, and heat on a water bath to dryness. Carbonize the residue by gently heating. After cooling, add 1 mL of sulfuric acid, heat carefully, then heat at 500 – 600°C to incinerate. After cooling, add 1 mL of hydrochloric acid to the residue, and heat on a water bath to dryness. Then add 10 mL of water to the residue, and heat on a water bath to dissolve. After cooling, add ammonia TS to adjust the pH to 3 – 4, and add 2 mL of dilute acetic acid. If necessary, filter, wash the residue on the filter with 10 mL of water, transfer the filtrate and washings into a Nessler tube, add water to make 50 mL, and use this solution as the test solution. Prepare the control solution as follows: To 2.0 mL of Standard Lead Solution add 2 mL of a solution of magnesium sulfate heptahydrate (1 in 4), then proceed in the same manner as for preparation of the test solution (not more than 20 ppm).

(2) Arsenic <*1.11*>—Prepare the test solution with 1.0 g of Amoxicillin Hydrate according to Method 4, and perform the test (not more than 2 ppm).

(3) Related substances—Dissolve 0.10 g of Amoxicillin Hydrate in 50 mL of a solution of boric acid (1 in 200), and use this solution as the sample solution. Pipet 1 mL of the sample solution, add a solution of boric acid (1 in 200) to make exactly 100 mL, and use this solution as the standard solution. Perform the test with exactly 10 μL each of the sample solution and standard solution as directed under Liquid Chromatography <*2.01*> according to the following conditions. Determine each peak area of both solutions by the automatic integration method: the area of the peak other than amoxicillin obtained from the sample solution is not larger than the peak area of amoxicillin from the standard solution. Furthermore, the total area of the peaks other than amoxicillin from the sample solution is not larger than 3 times the peak area of amoxicillin from the standard solution.

Operating conditions—

Detector: An ultraviolet absorption photometer (wavelength: 254 nm).

Column: A stainless steel column 4 mm in inside diameter and 30 cm in length, packed with octadecylsilanized silica gel for liquid chromatography (10 μm in particle diameter).

Column temperature: A constant temperature of about 25°C.

Mobile phase: Dissolve 1.36 g of sodium acetate trihydrate in 750 mL of water, adjust to pH 4.5 with acetic acid (31), and add water to make 1000 mL. To 950 mL of this solution add 50 mL of methanol.

Flow rate: Adjust so that the retention time of amoxicillin is about 8 minutes.

Time span of measurement: About 4 times as long as the retention time of amoxicillin, beginning after the solvent peak.

System suitability—

Test for required detectability: To exactly 1 mL of the standard solution add a solution of boric acid (1 in 200) to make exactly 10 mL. Confirm that the peak area of amoxicillin obtained with 10 μL of this solution is equivalent to 7 to 13% of that with 10 μL of the standard solution.

System performance: When the procedure is run with 10 μL of the standard solution under the above operating conditions, the number of theoretical plates and the symmetry factor of the peak of amoxicillin are not less than 2500 and not more than 1.5, respectively.

System repeatability: When the test is repeated 6 times with 10 μL of the standard solution under the above operating conditions, the relative standard deviation of the peak area of amoxicillin is not more than 1.0%.

Water <*2.48*> Not less than 11.0% and not more than 15.0% (0.1 g, volumetric titration, direct titration).

Assay Weigh accurately an amount of Amoxicillin Hydrate and Amoxicillin RS, equivalent to about 30 mg (potency), dissolve each in a solution of boric acid (1 in 200) to make exactly 100 mL, and use these solutions as the sample solution and standard solution. Perform the test with exactly 10 μL each of the sample solution and standard solution as directed under Liquid Chromatography <*2.01*> according to the following conditions, and calculate the peak areas, A_T and A_S, of amoxicillin in each solution.

Amount [μg (potency)] of amoxicillin ($C_{16}H_{19}N_3O_5S$)
$= M_S \times A_T/A_S \times 1000$

M_S: Amount [mg (potency)] of Amoxicillin RS taken

Operating conditions—

Detector: An ultraviolet absorption photometer (wavelength: 230 nm).

Column: A stainless steel column 4.6 mm in inside diameter and 15 cm in length, packed with octadecylsilanized silica gel for liquid chromatography (5 μm in particle diameter).

Column temperature: A constant temperature of about 25°C.

Mobile phase: Dissolve 1.361 g of sodium acetate trihydrate in 750 mL of water, adjust to pH 4.5 with acetic acid (31), and add water to make 1000 mL. To 950 mL of this solution add 50 mL of methanol.

Flow rate: Adjust so that the retention time of amoxicillin is about 8 minutes.

System suitability—

System performance: When the procedure is run with 10 μL of the standard solution under the above operating conditions, the number of theoretical plates of the peak of amoxicillin is not less than 2500.

System repeatability: When the test is repeated 6 times with 10 μL of the standard solution under the above operating conditions, the relative standard deviation of the peak area of amoxicillin is not more than 1.0%.

Containers and storage Containers—Tight containers.

Amoxicillin Capsules

アモキシシリンカプセル

Amoxicillin Capsules contain not less than 92.0% and not more than 105.0% of the labeled potency of Amoxicillin ($C_{16}H_{19}N_3O_5S$: 365.40).

Method of preparation Prepare as directed under Capsules, with Amoxicillin Hydrate.

Identification Take out the contents of Amoxicillin Capsules, to a quantity of the contents, equivalent to 8 mg (potency) of Amoxicillin Hydrate, add 2 mL of 0.01 mol/L hydrochloric acid TS, shake for 30 minutes, filter, and use the filtrate as the sample solution. Separately, dissolve an amount equivalent to 8 mg (potency) of Amoxicillin RS in 2 mL of 0.01 mol/L hydrochloric acid TS, and use this solution as the standard solution. Perform the test with these solutions as directed under Thin-layer Chromatography <*2.03*>. Spot 5 μL each of the sample solution and standard solution on a plate of silica gel for thin-layer chromatography. Develop the plate with a mixture of tetrahydrofuran, water and formic acid (50:5:2) to a distance of about 10 cm, and air-dry the plate. Spray evenly a solution of ninhydrin in ethanol (95) (1 in 20) on the plate, and heat the plate at 110°C for 15 minutes: the principal spot obtained from the sample solution and the spot from the standard solution show a red-purple color and the same *R*f value.

Purity Related substances—Take out the contents of Amoxicillin Capsules, to a quantity of the contents, equivalent to 0.1 g (potency) of Amoxicillin Hydrate, add 30 mL of a solution of boric acid (1 in 200), shake for 15 minutes, and add a solution of boric acid (1 in 200) to make 50 mL. Centrifuge this solution, and use the supernatant liquid as the sample solution. Pipet 1 mL of the sample solution, add a solution of boric acid (1 in 200) to make exactly 100 mL, and use this solution as the standard solution. Perform the test with exactly 10 μL each of the sample solution and standard solution as directed under Liquid Chromatography <*2.01*> according to the following conditions. Determine each peak area of both solutions by the automatic integration method: the area of each peak other than amoxicillin obtained from the sample solution is not larger than the peak area of amoxicillin from the standard solution.

Operating conditions—

Proceed as directed in the operating conditions in the Purity (3) under Amoxicillin Hydrate.

System suitability—

Test for required detectability and system repeatability: Proceed as directed in the system suitability in the Purity (3) under Amoxicillin Hydrate.

System performance: When the procedure is run with 10 μL of the standard solution under the above operating conditions, the number of theoretical plates and the symmetry factor of the peak of amoxicillin is not less than 2500 and not more than 1.5, respectively.

Water <*2.48*> Not more than 15.0% (0.1 g, volumetric titration, direct titration).

Uniformity of dosage units <*6.02*> It meets the requirement of the Mass variation test.

Dissolution <*6.10*> When the test is performed at 100 revolutions per minute according to the Paddle method using the sinker, using 900 mL of water as the dissolution medium, the dissolution rate in 60 minutes of Amoxicillin Capsules is not less than 75%.

Start the test with 1 capsule of Amoxicillin Capsules, withdraw not less than 20 mL of the medium at the specified minute after starting the test, and filter through a membrane filter with a pore size not exceeding 0.45 μm. Discard not less than 10 mL of the first filtrate, pipet *V* mL of the subsequent filtrate, add water to make exactly *V′* mL so that each mL contains about 56 μg (potency) of Amoxicillin Hydrate, and use this solution as the sample solution. Separately, weigh accurately an amount equivalent to about 28 mg (potency) of Amoxicillin RS, dissolve in water to make exactly 100 mL. Pipet 5 mL of this solution, add water to make exactly 25 mL, and use this solution as the standard solution. Perform the test with exactly 50 μL each of the sample solution and standard solution as directed under Liquid Chromatography <*2.01*> according to the following conditions, and determine the peak areas, A_T and A_S, of amoxicillin in each solution.

Dissolution rate (%) with respect to the labeled amount of amoxicillin ($C_{16}H_{19}N_3O_5S$)

$$= M_S \times A_T/A_S \times V'/V \times 1/C \times 180$$

M_S: Amount [mg (potency)] of Amoxicillin RS taken

C: Labeled amount [mg (potency)] of amoxicillin ($C_{16}H_{19}N_3O_5S$) in 1 capsule

Operating conditions—

Proceed as directed in the operating conditions in the Assay under Amoxicillin Hydrate.

System suitability—

System performance: When the procedure is run with 50 μL of the standard solution under the above operating conditions, the number of theoretical plates and the symmetry factor of the peak of amoxicillin are not less than 2500 and not more than 2.0, respectively.

System repeatability: When the test is repeated 6 times with 50 μL of the standard solution under the above operating conditions, the relative standard deviation of the peak area of amoxicillin is not more than 1.5%.

Assay Weigh accurately the mass of not less than 10 Amoxicillin Capsules, take out the contents, and weigh accurately the mass of the emptied shells. Weigh accurately an amount equivalent to about 0.1 g (potency) of Amoxicillin Hydrate, add 70 mL of water, shake for 15 minutes, and add water to make exactly 100 mL. Centrifuge this solution, and use the supernatant liquid as the sample solution. Separately, weigh accurately an amount equivalent to about 20 mg (potency) of Amoxicillin RS, dissolve in water to make exactly 20 mL, and use this solution as the standard solution. Perform the test with exactly 10 μL each of the sample solution and standard solution as directed under Liquid Chromatography *<2.01>* according to the following conditions, and determine the peak areas, A_T and A_S, of amoxicillin in each solution.

$$\text{Amount [mg (potency)] of amoxicillin } (C_{16}H_{19}N_3O_5S) = M_S \times A_T/A_S \times 5$$

M_S: Amount [mg (potency)] of Amoxicillin RS taken

Operating conditions—

Column temperature, mobile phase, and flow rate: Proceed as directed in the operating conditions in the Assay under Amoxicillin Hydrate.

Detector: An ultraviolet absorption photometer (wavelength: 254 nm).

Column: A stainless steel column 4 mm in inside diameter and 30 cm in length, packed with octadecylsilanized silica gel for liquid chromatography (10 μm in particle diameter).

System suitability—

System performance: When the procedure is run with 10 μL of the standard solution under the above operating conditions, the number of theoretical plates and the symmetry factor of the peak of amoxicillin are not less than 2500 and not more than 1.5, respectively.

System repeatability: When the test is repeated 6 times with 10 μL of the standard solution under the above operating conditions, the relative standard deviation of peak areas of amoxicillin is not more than 1.0%.

Containers and storage Containers—Tight containers.

Amphotericin B

アムホテリシンB

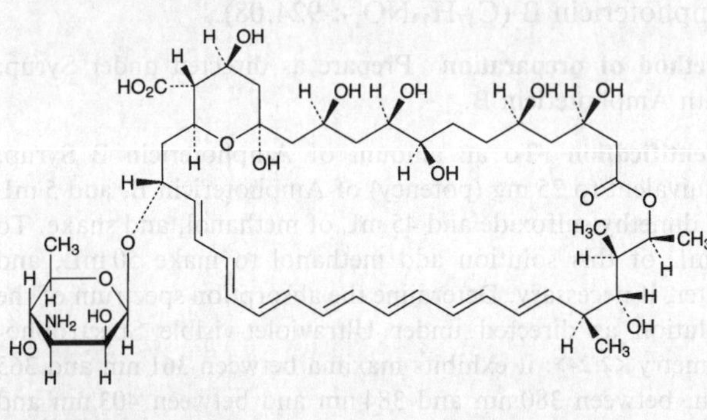

$C_{47}H_{73}NO_{17}$: 924.08

(1*R*,3*S*,5*R*,6*R*,9*R*,11*R*,15*S*,16*R*,17*R*,18*S*,19*E*,21*E*,23*E*,25*E*,27*E*,29*E*,31*E*,33*R*,35*S*,36*R*,37*S*)-33-(3-Amino-3,6-dideoxy-β-D-mannopyranosyloxy)-1,3,5,6,9,11,17,37-octahydroxy-15,16,18-trimethyl-13-oxo-14,39-dioxabicyclo[33.3.1]nonatriaconta-19,21,23,25,27,29,31-heptaene-36-carboxylic acid

[1397-89-3]

Amphotericin B is a polyene macrolide substance having antifungal activity produced by the growth of *Streptomyces nodosus*.

It contains not less than 840 μg (potency) per mg, calculated on the dried basis. The potency of Amphotericin B is expressed as mass (potency) of amphotericin B ($C_{47}H_{73}NO_{17}$).

Description Amphotericin B occurs as a yellow to orange powder.

It is freely soluble in dimethylsulfoxide and practically insoluble in water and in ethanol (95).

Identification (1) Dissolve 5 mg of Amphotericin B in 10 mL of dimethylsulfoxide. To 1 mL of this solution add 5 mL of phosphoric acid: a blue color develops between the two layers, and the solution becomes blue by shaking. After addition of 15 mL of water it becomes yellow to light yellow-brown by shaking.

(2) Dissolve 25 mg of Amphotericin B in 5 mL of dimethylsulfoxide, and add methanol to make 50 mL. To 1 mL of this solution add methanol to make 50 mL. Determine the absorption spectrum of this solution as directed under Ultraviolet-visible Spectrophotometry *<2.24>*, and compare the spectrum with the Reference Spectrum or the spectrum of a solution of Amphotericin B RS prepared in the same manner as the sample solution: both spectra exhibit similar intensities of absorption at the same wavelengths.

Purity Amphotericin A—Weigh accurately about 50 mg each of Amphotericin B and Amphotericin B RS, add exactly 10 mL each of dimethylsulfoxide to dissolve, and add methanol to make exactly 50 mL. Pipet 4 mL each of these solutions, add methanol to make exactly 50 mL, and use these solutions as the sample solution and standard solution (1), respectively. Separately, weigh accurately about 20 mg of Nystatin RS, add exactly 40 mL of dimethylsulfoxide to dissolve, then add methanol to make exactly 200 mL. Pipet 4 mL of this solution, add methanol to make exactly 50 mL, and use this solution as the standard solution (2). Perform the test with these solutions as directed under Ultraviolet-visible Spectrophotometry *<2.24>* using a solution obtained in the same manner as the sample solution as the blank, and determine the absorbances at 282 nm and at 304 nm. Calculate the amount of amphotericin A by the following equation: not more than 5% for Amphotericin B used for injections, and not more than 15% for Amphotericin B not used for injections.

$$\text{Amount (\%) of amphotericin A} = \frac{M_S \times \{(A_{Sa1} \times A_{T2}) - (A_{Sa2} \times A_{T1})\} \times 25}{M_T \times \{(A_{Sa1} \times A_{Sb2}) - (A_{Sa2} \times A_{Sb1})\}}$$

M_S: Amount (mg) of Nystatin RS taken
M_T: Amount (mg) of Amphotericin B taken
A_{Sa1}: Absorbance at 282 nm of the standard solution (1)
A_{Sb1}: Absorbance at 282 nm of the standard solution (2)
A_{Sa2}: Absorbance at 304 nm of the standard solution (1)
A_{Sb2}: Absorbance at 304 nm of the standard solution (2)
A_{T1}: Absorbance at 282 nm of the sample solution
A_{T2}: Absorbance at 304 nm of the sample solution

Loss on drying *<2.41>* Not more than 5.0% (0.1 g, in vacuum, 60°C, 3 hours).

Assay Perform the test according to the Cylinder-plate method as directed under Microbial Assay for Antibiotics *<4.02>* according to the following conditions.

(i) Test organism—*Saccharomyces cerevisiae* ATCC 9763

(ii) Culture medium—Use the medium 2) under (1) Agar media for seed and base layer.

(iii) Preparation of cylinder-agar plate—Proceed as directed in 1.5 Preparation of agar base layer plates under the Cylinder plate method, using Petri dish plates not dispensing the agar medium for base layer and dispensing 8.0 mL of the seeded agar medium.

(iv) Standard solution—Use light-resistant vessels. Weigh accurately an amount of Amphotericin B RS equivalent to about 20 mg (potency), dissolve in dimethylsulfoxide to make exactly 20 mL, and use this solution as the standard stock solution. Keep the standard stock solution at 5°C or below and use within 24 hours. Take exactly a suitable amount of the standard stock solution before use, and add dimethylsulfoxide to make solutions so that each mL contains 200 μg (potency) and 50 μg (potency). Pipet 1 mL each of these solutions, add 0.2 mol/L phosphate buffer solution (pH 10.5) to make exactly 20 mL, and use these solutions as the high concentration standard solution and low concentration standard solution, respectively.

(v) Sample solution—Use light-resistant vessels. Weigh accurately an amount of Amphotericin B equivalent to about 20 mg (potency), dissolve in dimethylsulfoxide to make exactly 20 mL, and use this solution as the sample stock solution. Take exactly a suitable amount of the sample stock solution, add dimethylsulfoxide to make solutions so that each mL contains 200 μg (potency) and 50 μg (potency). Pipet 1 mL each of these solutions, add 0.2 mol/L phosphate buffer solution (pH 10.5) to make exactly 20 mL, and use these solutions as the high concentration sample solution and low concentration sample solution, respectively.

Containers and storage Containers—Tight containers.

Storage—Light-resistant, and in a cold place.

Amphotericin B for Injection

注射用アムホテリシンB

Amphotericin B for Injection is a preparation for injection which is dissolved before use.

It contains not less than 90.0% and not more than 120.0% of the labeled potency of amphotericin B ($C_{47}H_{73}NO_{17}$: 924.08).

Method of preparation Prepare as directed under Injections, with Amphotericin B.

Description Amphotericin B for Injection occurs as yellow to orange, powder or masses.

Identification To an amount of Amphotericin B for Injection, equivalent to 25 mg (potency) of Amphotericin B, add 5 mL of dimethylsulfoxide and 45 mL of methanol, and shake. To 1 mL of this solution add methanol to make 50 mL, and filter if necessary. Determine the absorption spectrum of the solution as directed under Ultraviolet-visible Spectrophotometry ⟨*2.24*⟩: it exhibits maxima between 361 nm and 365 nm, between 380 nm and 384 nm and between 403 nm and 407 nm.

pH ⟨*2.54*⟩ Dissolve an amount of Amphotericin B for Injection, equivalent to 50 mg (potency) of Amphotericin B, in 10 mL of water. To 1 mL of this solution add water to make 50 mL: 7.2 – 8.0.

Purity Clarity and color of solution—Dissolve an amount of Amphotericin B for Injection, equivalent to 50 mg (potency) of Amphotericin B, in 10 mL of water: the solution is clear and yellow to orange.

Loss on drying ⟨*2.41*⟩ Not more than 8.0% (0.3 g, in vacuum, 60°C, 3 hours).

Bacterial endotoxins ⟨*4.01*⟩ Less than 3.0 EU/mg (potency).

Uniformity of dosage units ⟨*6.02*⟩ It meets the requirement of the Mass variation test (*T*: 105.0%).

Foreign insoluble matter ⟨*6.06*⟩ Perform the test according to Method 2: it meets the requirement.

Insoluble particulate matter ⟨*6.07*⟩ It meets the requirement.

Sterility ⟨*4.06*⟩ Perform the test according to the Membrane filtration method: it meets the requirement.

Assay Perform the test according to the Cylinder-plate method as directed under Microbial Assay for Antibiotics ⟨*4.02*⟩ according to the following conditions.

(i) Test organism, culture medium, preparation of cylinder-agar plate and standard solutions—Proceed as directed in the Assay under Amphotericin B.

(ii) Sample solutions—Prepare using light-resistant containers. Weigh accurately an amount of Amphotericin B for Injection, equivalent to about 50 mg (potency), dissolve in dimethylsulfoxide to make exactly 50 mL, and use this solution as the sample stock solution. Measure exactly a suitable quantity of the sample stock solution, add dimethylsulfoxide to make solutions so that each mL contains about 200 μg (potency) and 50 μg (potency). Pipet 1 mL each of these solutions, add 0.2 mol/L phosphate buffer solution (pH 10.5) to make exactly 20 mL, and use these solutions as the high concentration sample solution and low concentration sample solution, respectively.

Containers and storage Containers—Hermetic containers.

Storage—Light-resistant, at a cold place.

Amphotericin B Syrup

アムホテリシンBシロップ

Amphotericin B Syrup contain not less than 90.0% and not more than 115.0% of the labeled potency of amphotericin B ($C_{47}H_{73}NO_{17}$: 924.08).

Method of preparation Prepare as directed under Syrup, with Amphotericin B.

Identification To an amount of Amphotericin B Syrup, equivalent to 25 mg (potency) of Amphotericin B, add 5 mL of dimethylsulfoxide and 45 mL of methanol, and shake. To 1 mL of this solution add methanol to make 50 mL, and filter, if necessary. Determine the absorption spectrum of the solution as directed under Ultraviolet-visible Spectrophotometry ⟨*2.24*⟩: it exhibits maxima between 361 nm and 365 nm, between 380 nm and 384 nm and between 403 nm and 407 nm.

pH ⟨*2.54*⟩ 5.0 – 7.0

Microbial limit ⟨*4.05*⟩ The acceptance criteria of TAMC and TYMC are 10^2 CFU/mL and 5×10^1 CFU/mL, respectively.

Assay Perform the test according to the Cylinder-plate method as directed under Microbial Assay for Antibiotics ⟨*4.02*⟩ according to the following conditions.

(i) Test organism, culture medium, preparation of cylinder-agar plate and standard solutions—Proceed as directed in the Assay under Amphotericin B.

(ii) Sample solutions—Prepare using light-resistant containers. Weigh accurately an amount of Amphotericin B Syrup, equivalent to about 0.1 g (potency), add about 70 mL of dimethylsulfoxide, shake, then add dimethylsulfoxide to make exactly 100 mL, and use this solution as the sample stock solution. Measure exactly a suitable amount of the sample stock solution, add dimethylsulfoxide to make solutions so that each mL contains about 200 μg (potency) and 50 μg (potency). Pipet 1 mL each of these solutions, add 0.2 mol/L phosphate buffer solution (pH 10.5) to make exactly 20 mL, and use these solutions as the high concentration sample solution and low concentration sample solution, respectively.

Containers and storage Containers—Tight containers.

Storage—Light-resistant.

Amphotericin B Tablets

アムホテリシンB錠

Amphotericin B Tablets contain not less than 90.0% and not more than 120.0% of the labeled potency of amphotericin B ($C_{47}H_{73}NO_{17}$: 924.08).

Method of preparation Prepare as directed under Tablets, with Amphotericin B.

Identification To an amount of pulverized Amphotericin B Tablets, equivalent to 25 mg (potency) of Amphotericin B, add 5 mL of dimethylsulfoxide and 45 mL of methanol, and shake. To 1 mL of this solution add methanol to make 50 mL, and filter, if necessary. Determine the absorption spectrum of the solution as directed under Ultraviolet-visible Spectrophotometry ⟨*2.24*⟩: it exhibits maxima between 361 nm and 365 nm, between 380 nm and 384 nm and between 403 nm and 407 nm.

Loss on drying ⟨*2.41*⟩ Not more than 5.0% (0.3 g, in vacuum, 60°C, 3 hours).

Uniformity of dosage units ⟨*6.02*⟩ It meets the requirement of the Mass variation test (*T*: 105.0%).

Disintegration ⟨*6.09*⟩ Perform the test using the disk: it meets the requirement.

Assay Perform the test according to the Cylinder-plate method as directed under Microbial Assay for Antibiotics ⟨*4.02*⟩ according to the following conditions.

(i) Test organism, culture medium, preparation of cylinder-agar plate and standard solutions—Proceed as directed in the Assay under Amphotericin B.

(ii) Sample solutions—Prepare using light-resistant containers. Weigh accurately and powder not less than 20 tablets of Amphotericin B Tablets. Weigh accurately a part of the powder, equivalent to about 0.1 g (potency), add about 70 mL of dimethylsulfoxide, shake, then add dimethylsulfoxide to make exactly 100 mL, centrifuge, and use the supernatant liquid as the sample stock solution. Measure exactly a suitable amount of the sample stock solution, add dimethylsulfoxide to make solutions so that each mL contains 200 μg (potency) and 50 μg (potency). Pipet 1 mL each of these solutions, add 0.2 mol/L phosphate buffer solution (pH 10.5) to make exactly 20 mL, and use these solutions as the high concentration sample solution and low concentration sample solution, respectively.

Containers and storage Containers—Well-closed containers.

Anhydrous Ampicillin

無水アンピシリン

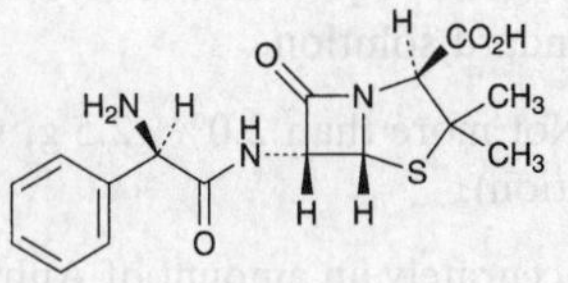

$C_{16}H_{19}N_3O_4S$: 349.40

(2*S*,5*R*,6*R*)-6-[(2*R*)-2-Amino-2-phenylacetylamino]-3,3-dimethyl-7-oxo-4-thia-1-azabicyclo[3.2.0]heptane-2-carboxylic acid

[69-53-4]

Anhydrous Ampicillin contains not less than 960 μg (potency) and not more than 1005 μg (potency) per mg, calculated on the anhydrous basis. The potency of Anhydrous Ampicillin is expressed as mass (potency) of ampicillin ($C_{16}H_{19}N_3O_4S$).

Description Anhydrous Ampicillin occurs as white to light yellow-white, crystals or crystalline powder.

It is sparingly soluble in water, slightly soluble in methanol, very slightly soluble in ethanol (95), and practically insoluble in acetonitrile.

Identification Determine the infrared absorption spectrum of Anhydrous Ampicillin as directed in the potassium bromide disk method under Infrared Spectrophotometry ⟨*2.25*⟩, and compare the spectrum with the Reference Spectrum: both spectra exhibit similar intensities of absorption at the same wave numbers.

Optical rotation ⟨*2.49*⟩ $[\alpha]_D^{20}$: +280 – +305° (0.5 g calculated on the anhydrous basis, water, 100 mL, 100 mm).

pH ⟨*2.54*⟩ The pH of a solution obtained by dissolving 1.0 g of Anhydrous Ampicillin in 100 mL of water is between 4.0 and 5.5.

Purity **(1)** Heavy metals ⟨*1.07*⟩—Proceed with 1.0 g of Anhydrous Ampicillin according to Method 2, and perform the test. Prepare the control solution with 2.0 mL of Standard Lead Solution (not more than 20 ppm).

(2) Arsenic ⟨*1.11*⟩—Prepare the test solution with 1.0 g of Anhydrous Ampicillin according to Method 3, and perform the test (not more than 2 ppm).

(3) Related substances—Dissolve 0.05 g of Anhydrous Ampicillin in the mobile phase to make 50 mL, and use this solution as the sample solution. Pipet 1 mL of the sample solution, add the mobile phase to make exactly 100 mL, and use this solution as the standard solution. Perform the test with exactly 10 μL each of the sample solution and standard solution as directed under Liquid Chromatography ⟨*2.01*⟩ according to the following conditions, and determine each peak area by the automatic integration method: the area of each peak other than ampicillin obtained from the sample solution is not larger than the peak area of ampicillin from the standard solution.

Operating conditions—

Detector, column, column temperature, mobile phase, and flow rate: Proceed as directed in the operating conditions in the Assay.

Time span of measurement: As long as about 10 times of

the retention time of ampicillin.

System suitability—

System performance, and system repeatability: Proceed as directed in the system suitability in the Assay.

Test for required detectability: To exactly 1 mL of the standard solution add the mobile phase to make exactly 10 mL. Confirm that the peak area of ampicillin obtained with 10 μL of this solution is equivalent to 7 to 13% of that with 10 μL of the standard solution.

Water <2.48> Not more than 2.0% (2.5 g, volumetric titration, direct titration).

Assay Weigh accurately an amount of Anhydrous Ampicillin and Ampicillin RS, equivalent to about 50 mg (potency), add exactly 5 mL each of the internal standard solution and the mobile phase to make 50 mL, and use these solutions as the sample solution and standard solution. Perform the test with 10 μL each of the sample solution and standard solution as directed under Liquid Chromatography <2.01> according to the following conditions, and calculate the ratios, Q_T and Q_S, of the peak area of ampicillin to that of the internal standard.

Amount [μg (potency)] of ampicillin ($C_{16}H_{19}N_3O_4S$)
$= M_S \times Q_T/Q_S \times 1000$

M_S: Amount [mg (potency)] of Ampicillin RS taken

Internal standard solution—A solution of guaifenesin in the mobile phase (1 in 200).

Operating conditions—

Detector: An ultraviolet absorption photometer (wavelength: 230 nm).

Column: A stainless steel column 4.6 mm in inside diameter and 15 cm in length, packed with octadecylsilanized silica gel for liquid chromatography (5 μm in particle diameter).

Column temperature: A constant temperature of about 25°C.

Mobile phase: Dissolve 5.94 g of diammonium hydrogen phosphate in 850 mL of water, add 100 mL of acetonitrile, adjust the pH to 5.0 with phosphoric acid, and add water to make exactly 1000 mL.

Flow rate: Adjust so that the retention time of ampicillin is about 6 minutes.

System suitability—

System performance: When the procedure is run with 10 μL of the standard solution under the above operating conditions, ampicillin and the internal standard are eluted in this order with the resolution between these peaks being not less than 40.

System repeatability: When the test is repeated 6 times with 10 μL of the standard solution under the above operating conditions, the relative standard deviation of the ratios of the peak area of ampicillin to that of the internal standard is not more than 1.0%.

Containers and storage Containers—Tight containers.

Ampicillin Hydrate

アンピシリン水和物

$C_{16}H_{19}N_3O_4S.3H_2O$: 403.45
(2*S*,5*R*,6*R*)-6-[(2*R*)-2-Amino-2-phenylacetylamino]-3,3-dimethyl-7-oxo-4-thia-1-azabicyclo[3.2.0]heptane-2-carboxylic acid trihydrate
[*7177-48-2*]

Ampicillin Hydrate contains not less than 960 μg (potency) and not more than 1005 μg (potency) per mg, calculated on the anhydrous basis. The potency of Ampicillin Hydrate is expressed as mass (potency) of ampicillin ($C_{16}H_{19}N_3O_4S$: 349.40).

Description Ampicillin Hydrate occurs as a white to light yellow-white, crystals or crystalline powder.

It is sparingly soluble in water, slightly soluble in methanol, very slightly soluble in ethanol (95), and practically insoluble in acetonitrile.

Identification Determine the infrared absorption spectrum of Ampicillin Hydrate as directed in the potassium bromide disk method under Infrared Spectrophotometry <2.25>, and compare the spectrum with the Reference Spectrum or the spectrum of Ampicillin RS: both spectra exhibit similar intensities of absorption at the same wave numbers.

Optical rotation <2.49> $[\alpha]_D^{20}$: +280 – +305° (0.5 g calculated on the anhydrous basis, water, 100 mL, 100 mm).

pH <2.54> The pH of a solution obtained by dissolving 1.0 g of Ampicillin Hydrate in 400 mL of water is between 3.5 and 5.5.

Purity (1) Heavy metals <1.07>—Proceed with 1.0 g of Ampicillin Hydrate according to Method 2, and perform the test. Prepare the control solution with 2.0 mL of Standard Lead Solution (not more than 20 ppm).

(2) Arsenic <1.11>—Prepare the test solution with 1.0 g of Ampicillin hydrate according to Method 3, and perform the test (not more than 2 ppm).

(3) Related substances—Dissolve 50 mg of Ampicillin Hydrate in 50 mL of the mobile phase, and use this solution as the sample solution. Pipet 1 mL of the sample solution, add the mobile phase to make exactly 100 mL, and use this solution as the standard solution. Perform the test with exactly 10 μL each of the sample solution and standard solution as directed under Liquid Chromatography <2.01> according to the following conditions, and determine each peak area by the automatic integration method: the area of the peak other than ampicillin obtained from the sample solution is not larger than the peak area of ampicillin from the standard solution, and the total area of the peaks other than ampicillin from the sample solution is not larger than 2 times the peak area of ampicillin from the standard solution.

Operating conditions—

Detector, column, column temperature, mobile phase, and flow rate: Proceed as directed in the operating conditions in the Assay.

Time span of measurement: About 10 times as long as the retention time of ampicillin.

System suitability—

Test for required detectability: Pipet 1 mL of the standard solution, and add the mobile phase to make exactly 10 mL. Confirm that the peak area of ampicillin obtained with 10 μL of this solution is equivalent to 7 to 13% of that with 10 μL of the standard solution.

System performance: When the procedure is run with 10 μL of the standard solution under the above operating conditions, the number of theoretical plates and the symmetry factor of the peak of ampicillin are not less than 5000 and not more than 1.5, respectively.

System repeatability: When the test is repeated 6 times with 10 μL of the standard solution under the above operating conditions, the relative standard deviation of the peak area of ampicillin is not more than 1.0%.

(4) *N,N*-Dimethylaniline—Weigh accurately about 1 g of Ampicillin Hydrate, dissolve in 5 mL of sodium hydroxide TS, add exactly 1 mL of the internal standard solution, shake vigorously for 1 minute, and use the upper layer liquid obtained after allowing it to stand as the sample solution. Separately, weigh accurately about 50 mg of *N,N*-dimethylaniline, dissolve in 2 mL of hydrochloric acid and 20 mL of water, add water to make exactly 50 mL, and use this solution as the standard stock solution. Pipet 5 mL of the standard stock solution, and add water to make exactly 250 mL. Pipet 1 mL of this solution, add 5 mL of sodium hydroxide TS and exactly 1 mL of the internal standard solution, shake vigorously for 1 minute, and use the upper layer liquid obtained after allowing it to stand as the standard solution. Perform the test with 1 μL each of the sample solution and standard solution as directed under Gas Chromatography <*2.02*> according to the following conditions, calculate the ratios, Q_T and Q_S, of the peak area of *N,N*-dimethylaniline to that of the internal standard, and calculate the amount of *N,N*-dimethylaniline by the following equation: not more than 20 ppm.

$$\text{Amount (ppm) of } N,N\text{-dimethylaniline} = M_S/M_T \times Q_T/Q_S \times 400$$

M_S: Amount (g) of *N,N*-dimethylaniline taken
M_T: Amount (g) of Ampicillin Hydrate taken

*Internal standard solution—*A solution of naphthalene in cyclohexane (1 in 20,000).

Operating conditions—

Detector: A hydrogen flame-ionization detector.

Column: A glass column 2.6 mm in inside diameter and 2 m in length, packed with siliceous earth for gas chromatography (180 – 250 μm in particle diameter) coated with 50% phenyl-50% methyl polysiloxane for gas chromatography at the ratio of 3%.

Column temperature: A constant temperature of about 120°C.

Carrier gas: Helium.

Flow rate: Adjust so that the retention time of *N,N*-dimethylaniline is about 5 minutes.

System suitability—

Test for required detectability: Measure exactly 1 mL of the standard stock solution, and add water to make exactly 250 mL. Pipet 1 mL of this solution, add 5 mL of sodium hydroxide TS and exactly 1 mL of the internal standard solution, shake vigorously for 1 minute, and use the upper layer liquid obtained after allowing it to stand for the test. Confirm that when the procedure is run with 1 μL of the upper layer liquid under the above operating conditions, the ratio of the peak area of *N,N*-dimethylaniline to that of the internal standard is equivalent to 15 to 25% of the ratio of the peak area of *N,N*-dimethylaniline to that of the internal standard with the standard solution.

System performance: Dissolve 50 mg of *N,N*-dimethylaniline in cyclohexane to make 50 mL. To 1 mL of this solution add the internal standard solution to make 50 mL, and use this solution as the solution for system suitability test. When the procedure is run with 1 μL of the solution for system suitability test under the above operating conditions, *N,N*-dimethylaniline and the internal standard are eluted in this order with the resolution between these peaks being not less than 3.

System repeatability: When the test is repeated 6 times with 1 μL of the solution for system suitability test under the above operating conditions, the relative standard deviation of the ratios of the peak area of *N,N*-dimethylaniline to that of the internal standard is not more than 2.0%.

Water <*2.48*> 12.0 – 15.0% (0.1 g, volumetric titration, direct titration).

Assay Weigh accurately an amount of Ampicillin Hydrate and Ampicillin RS, equivalent to about 50 mg (potency), dissolve in a suitable volume of the mobile phase, add exactly 5 mL each of the internal standard solution and the mobile phase to make 50 mL, and use these solutions as the sample solution and standard solution. Perform the test with 10 μL each of the sample solution and standard solution as directed under Liquid Chromatography <*2.01*> according to the following conditions, and calculate the ratios, Q_T and Q_S, of the peak area of ampicillin to that of the internal standard.

$$\text{Amount [}\mu\text{g (potency)] of ampicillin } (C_{16}H_{19}N_3O_4S) = M_S \times Q_T/Q_S \times 1000$$

M_S: Amount [mg (potency)] of Ampicillin RS taken

*Internal standard solution—*A solution of guaifenesin in the mobile phase (1 in 200).

Operating conditions—

Detector: An ultraviolet absorption photometer (wavelength: 230 nm).

Column: A stainless steel column 4.6 mm in inside diameter and 15 cm in length, packed with octadecylsilanized silica gel for liquid chromatography (5 μm in particle diameter).

Column temperature: A constant temperature of about 25°C.

Mobile phase: Dissolve 5.94 g of diammonium hydrogenphosphate in 850 mL of water, add 100 mL of acetonitrile, adjust the pH to 5.0 with phosphoric acid, and add water to make exactly 1000 mL.

Flow rate: Adjust so that the retention time of ampicillin is about 6 minutes.

System suitability—

System performance: When the procedure is run with 10 μL of the standard solution under the above operating conditions, ampicillin and the internal standard are eluted in this order with the resolution between these peaks being not less than 40.

System repeatability: When the test is repeated 6 times with 10 μL of the standard solution under the above operating conditions, the relative standard deviation of the ratios of the peak area of ampicillin to that of the internal standard is not more than 1.0%.

Containers and storage Containers—Tight containers.

Ampicillin Sodium

アンピシリンナトリウム

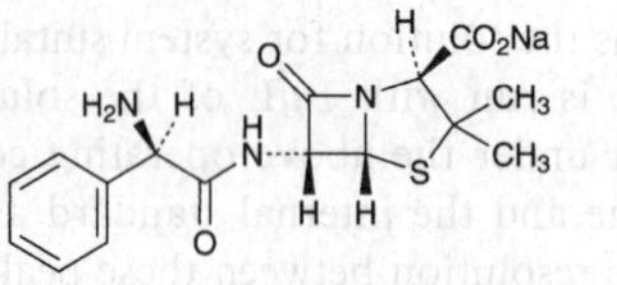

$C_{16}H_{18}N_3NaO_4S$: 371.39
Monosodium (2*S*,5*R*,6*R*)-6-[(2*R*)-2-amino-2-phenylacetylamino]-3,3-dimethyl-7-oxo-4-thia-1-azabicyclo[3.2.0]heptane-2-carboxylate
[*69-52-3*]

Ampicillin Sodium contains not less than 850 μg (potency) and not more than 950 μg (potency) per mg, calculated on the anhydrous basis. The potency of Ampicillin Sodium is expressed as mass (potency) of ampicillin ($C_{16}H_{19}N_3O_4S$: 349.40).

Description Ampicillin Sodium occurs as white to light yellow-white, crystals or crystalline powder.

It is very soluble in water, and sparingly soluble in ethanol (99.5).

Identification **(1)** Determine the infrared absorption spectrum of Ampicillin Sodium, previously dried in a desiccator (reduced pressure not exceeding 0.67 kPa, 60°C) for 3 hours, as directed in the potassium bromide disk method under Infrared Spectrophotometry <*2.25*>, and compare the spectrum with the Reference Spectrum: both spectra exhibit similar intensities of absorption at the same wave numbers.

(2) Ampicillin Sodium responds to Qualitative Tests <*1.09*> (1) for sodium salt.

Optical rotation <*2.49*> $[\alpha]_D^{20}$: +246 – +272° (1 g calculated on the anhydrous basis, water, 100 mL, 100 mm).

pH <*2.54*> The pH of a solution obtained by dissolving 1.0 g of Ampicillin Sodium in 10 mL of water is between 8.0 and 10.0.

Purity **(1)** Clarity and color of solution—Dissolve 0.25 g (potency) of Ampicillin Sodium in 0.75 mL of water: the solution is clear, and its absorbance at 400 nm, determined as directed under Ultraviolet-visible Spectrophotometry <*2.24*>, is not more than 0.40.

(2) Heavy metals <*1.07*>—Proceed with 1.0 g of Ampicillin Sodium according to Method 1, and perform the test. Prepare the control solution with 2.0 mL of Standard Lead Solution (not more than 20 ppm).

(3) Arsenic <*1.11*>—Prepare the test solution with 1.0 g of Ampicillin Sodium according to Method 1, and perform the test (not more than 2 ppm).

(4) Related substances—Dissolve 50 mg of Ampicillin Sodium in 50 mL of the mobile phase, and use this solution as the sample solution. Pipet 1 mL of the sample solution, add the mobile phase to make exactly 100 mL, and use this solution as the standard solution. Perform the test with exactly 10 μL each of the sample solution and standard solution as directed under Liquid Chromatography <*2.01*> according to the following conditions, and determine each peak area by the automatic integration method: the area of the peaks other than ampicillin obtained from the sample solution is not larger than the peak area of ampicillin from the standard solution.

Operating conditions—

Detector, column, column temperature, mobile phase, and flow rate: Proceed as directed in the operating conditions in the Assay.

Time span of measurement: About 10 times as long as the retention time of ampicillin.

System suitability—

Test for required detectability: Measure exactly 1 mL of the standard solution, and add the mobile phase to make exactly 10 mL. Confirm that the peak area of ampicillin obtained with 10 μL of this solution is equivalent to 7 to 13% of that with 10 μL of the standard solution.

System performance: Dissolve 50 mg of Ampicillin RS in a suitable amount of the mobile phase, add 5 mL of a solution of guaifenesin in the mobile phase (1 in 200) and the mobile phase to make 50 mL, and use this solution as the solution for system suitability test. When the procedure is run with 10 μL of the solution for system suitability test under the above operating conditions, ampicillin and guaifenesin are eluted in this order with the resolution between these peaks being not less than 35.

System repeatability: When the test is repeated 6 times with 10 μL of the solution for system suitability test under the above operating conditions, the relative standard deviation of the peak area of ampicillin is not more than 1.0%.

Water <*2.48*> Not more than 2.0% (0.2 g, volumetric titration, direct titration).

Assay Weigh accurately an amount of Ampicillin Sodium and Ampicillin RS, equivalent to about 50 mg (potency), dissolve them in a suitable amount of the mobile phase, add exactly 5 mL of the internal standard solution, then add the mobile phase to make 50 mL, and use these solutions as the sample solution and the standard solution, respectively. Perform the test with 10 μL each of the sample solution and standard solution as directed under Liquid Chromatography <*2.01*> according to the following conditions, and calculate the ratios, Q_T and Q_S, of the peak area of ampicillin to that of the internal standard.

$$\text{Amount [}\mu\text{g (potency)] of ampicillin } (C_{16}H_{19}N_3O_4S) = M_S \times Q_T/Q_S \times 1000$$

M_S: Amount [mg (potency)] of Ampicillin RS taken

Internal standard solution—A solution of guaifenesin in the mobile phase (1 in 200).

Operating conditions—

Detector: An ultraviolet absorption photometer (wavelength: 230 nm).

Column: A stainless steel column 4.6 mm in inside diameter and 15 cm in length, packed with octadecylsilanized silica gel for liquid chromatography (5 μm in particle diameter).

Column temperature: A constant temperature of about 25°C.

Mobile phase: Dissolve 5.94 g of diammonium hydrogen phosphate in 850 mL of water, add 100 mL of acetonitrile, adjust to pH 5.0 with phosphoric acid, and add water to make 1000 mL.

Flow rate: Adjust so that the retention time of ampicillin is about 6 minutes.

System suitability—

System performance: When the procedure is run with 10 μL of the standard solution under the above operating conditions, ampicillin and guaifenesin are eluted in this order with the resolution between these peaks being not less than 35.

System repeatability: When the test is repeated 6 times

with 10 μL of the standard solution under the above operating conditions, the relative standard deviation of the ratio of the peak area of ampicillin to that of the internal standard is not more than 1.0%.

Containers and storage Containers—Tight containers.

Ampicillin Sodium for Injection

注射用アンピシリンナトリウム

Ampicillin Sodium for Injection is a preparation for injection which is dissolved before use.

It contains not less than 90.0% and not more than 110.0% of the labeled potency of ampicillin ($C_{16}H_{19}N_3O_4S$: 349.40).

Method of preparation Prepare as directed under Injections, with Ampicillin Sodium.

Description Ampicillin Sodium for Injection occurs as white to light yellow-white, crystals or crystalline powder.

Identification Proceed as directed in the Identification (1) under Ampicillin Sodium.

Osmotic pressure ratio Being specified separately when the drug is granted approval based on the Law.

pH <*2.54*> The pH of a solution prepared by dissolving an amount of Ampicillin Sodium for Injection, equivalent to 1.0 g (potency) of Ampicillin Sodium, in 10 mL of water is 8.0 to 10.0.

Purity Clarity and color of solution—Dissolve an amount of Ampicillin Sodium for Injection, equivalent to 0.25 g (potency) of Ampicillin Sodium, in 0.75 mL of water: the solution is clear. Perform the test with the solution as directed under Ultraviolet-visible Spectrophotometry <*2.24*>: the absorbance at 400 nm is not more than 0.40.

Water <*2.48*> Not more than 3.0% (0.2 g, volumetric titration, direct titration).

Bacterial endotoxins <*4.01*> Less than 0.075 EU/mg (potency).

Uniformity of dosage units <*6.02*> It meets the requirement of the Mass variation test.

Foreign insoluble matter <*6.06*> Perform the test according to Method 2: it meets the requirement.

Insoluble particulate matter <*6.07*> It meets the requirement.

Sterility <*4.06*> Perform the test according to the Membrane filtration method: it meets the requirement.

Assay Weigh accurately the mass of the contents of not less than 10 containers of Ampicillin Sodium for Injection. Weigh accurately an amount of a portion of the contents, equivalent to about 50 mg (potency) of Ampicillin Sodium, add exactly 5 mL of the internal standard solution and dissolve. Then add the mobile phase to make 50 mL, and use this solution as the sample solution. Separately, weigh accurately an amount of Ampicillin RS, equivalent to about 50 mg (potency), add exactly 5 mL of the internal standard solution and dissolve. Then add the mobile phase to make 50 mL, and use this solution as the standard solution. Perform the test with 10 μL each of the sample solution and standard solution as directed under Liquid Chromatography <*2.01*> according to the following conditions, and calculate the ratios, Q_T and Q_S, of the peak area of ampicillin to that of the internal standard.

Amount [mg (potency)] of ampicillin ($C_{16}H_{19}N_3O_4S$)
$= M_S \times Q_T/Q_S$

M_S: Amount [mg (potency)] of Ampicillin RS taken

Internal standard solution—A solution of guaifenesin in the mobile phase (1 in 200).

Operating conditions—

Detector: An ultraviolet absorption photometer (wavelength: 230 nm).

Column: A stainless steel column 4.6 mm in inside diameter and 15 cm in length, packed with octadecylsilanized silica gel for liquid chromatography (5 μm in particle diameter).

Column temperature: A constant temperature of about 25°C.

Mobile phase: Dissolve 5.94 mg of diammonium hydrogen phosphate in 850 mL of water, add 100 mL of acetonitrile, add phosphoric acid to adjust the pH to 5.0, then add water to make exactly 1000 mL.

Flow rate: Adjust so that the retention time of ampicillin is about 6 minutes.

System suitability—

System performance: When the procedure is run with 10 μL of the standard solution under the above operating conditions, ampicillin and the internal standard are eluted in this order with the resolution between these peaks being not less than 26.

System repeatability: When the test is repeated 6 times with 10 μL of the standard solution under the above operating conditions, the relative standard deviation of the ratio of the peak area of ampicillin to that of the internal standard is not more than1.0%.

Containers and storage Containers—Hermetic containers.

Ampicillin Sodium and Sulbactam Sodium for Injection

注射用アンピシリンナトリウム·スルバクタムナトリウム

Ampicillin Sodium and Sulbactam Sodium for Injection is a preparation for injection which is dissolved before use.

It contains not less than 95.0% and not more than 112.0% of the labeled potency of ampicillin ($C_{16}H_{19}N_3O_4S$: 349.40) and sulbactam ($C_8H_{11}NO_5S$: 233.24).

Method of preparation Prepare as directed under Injections, with Ampicillin Sodium and Sulbactam Sodium.

Description Ampicillin Sodium and Sulbactam Sodium for Injection occurs as a white to yellowish white powder.

Identification **(1)** The retention times of ampicillin obtained from the sample solution and the standard solution observed in the Assay are the same, and the peak area of ampicillin observed in the Assay obtained from the sample solution is 2.8 to 3.6 times the peak area of ampicillin observed in the test performed with 10 μL of the sample solution obtained in the Assay as directed under Liquid Chromatography <*2.01*> according to the following conditions.

Operating conditions—

Column, column temperature, mobile phase, and flow

rate: Proceed as directed in the operating conditions in the Assay.

Detector: An ultraviolet absorption photometer (wavelength: 230 nm).

System suitability—

System performance: Proceed as directed in the system suitability in the Assay.

(2) The retention times of sulbactam obtained from the sample solution and the standard solution observed in the Assay are the same, and the peak area of sulbactam observed in the Assay obtained from the sample solution is 2.0 to 2.6 times the peak area of sulbactam observed in the test performed with 10 μL of the sample solution obtained in the Assay as directed under Liquid Chromatography <*2.01*> according to the following conditions.

Operating conditions—

Column, column temperature, mobile phase, and flow rate: Proceed as directed in the operating conditions in the Assay.

Detector: An ultraviolet absorption photometer (wavelength: 230 nm).

System suitability—

System performance: Proceed as directed in the system suitability in the Assay.

pH <*2.54*> The pH of a solution prepared by dissolving an amount of Ampicillin Sodium and Sulbactam Sodium for Injection, equivalent to 1.0 g (potency) of ampicillin ($C_{16}H_{19}N_3O_4S$), in 10 mL of water is between 8.0 and 10.0.

Purity **(1)** Clarity and color of solution—Dissolve an amount of Ampicillin Sodium and Sulbactam Sodium for Injection, equivalent to 1.0 g (potency) of ampicillin ($C_{16}H_{19}N_3O_4S$), in 10 mL of water: the solution is clear. Determine the absorption of this solution as directed under Ultraviolet-visible Spectrophotometry <*2.24*>: the absorbance at 425 nm is not more than 0.10.

(2) Total penicilloic acid—Weigh accurately about 25 mg of Ampicillin Sodium and Sulbactam Sodium for Injection, place in a glass-stoppered flask, dissolve in 25 mL of 0.02 mol/L phosphate buffer solution (pH 3.0), add exactly 5 mL of 0.005 mol/L iodine VS, stopper the flask, allow to stand for 5 minutes, and titrate <*2.50*> with 0.005 mol/L sodium thiosulfate VS (indicator: 1.0 mL of starch TS). Perform a blank determination in the same manner, and make any necessary correction: the amount of total penicilloic acid (as $C_{16}H_{21}N_3O_5S$: 367.42) is not more than 3.0%.

Each mL of 0.005 mol/L sodium thiosulfate VS
= 0.2064 mg of $C_{16}H_{21}N_3O_5S$

Water <*2.48*> Not more than 2.0% (0.5 g, volumetric titration, direct titration).

Bacterial endotoxins <*4.01*> Less than 0.10 EU/mg (potency).

Uniformity of dosage units <*6.02*> Perform the test according to the following method: it meets the requirement of the Content uniformity test (*T*: 105.0%).

Dissolve 1 Ampicillin Sodium and Sulbactam Sodium for Injection in the mobile phase to make exactly *V* mL so that each mL contains 5 mg (potency) of ampicillin ($C_{16}H_{19}N_3O_4S$). Pipet 5 mL of this solution, add exactly 5 mL of the internal standard solution, then add the mobile phase to make 50 mL, and use this solution as the sample solution. Then, proceed as directed in the Assay.

Amount [mg (potency)] of ampicillin ($C_{16}H_{19}N_3O_4S$)
$= M_{S1} \times Q_{Ta}/Q_{Sa} \times V/10$

Amount [mg (potency)] of sulbactam ($C_8H_{11}NO_5S$)
$= M_{S2} \times Q_{Tb}/Q_{Sb} \times V/10$

M_{S1}: Amount [mg (potency)] of Ampicillin RS taken
M_{S2}: Amount [mg (potency)] of Sulbactam RS taken

Internal standard solution—A solution of parahydroxybenzoic acid in the mobile phase (1 in 1000).

Foreign insoluble matter <*6.06*> Perform the test according to Method 2: it meets the requirement.

Insoluble particulate matter <*6.07*> It meets the requirement.

Sterility <*4.06*> Perform the test according to the Membrane filtration method: it meets the requirement.

Assay Weigh accurately the mass of the contents of not less than 10 containers of Ampicillin Sodium and Sulbactam Sodium for Injection. Weigh accurately an amount of a portion of the contents, equivalent to about 0.25 g (potency) of ampicillin ($C_{16}H_{19}N_3O_4S$), and dissolve in the mobile phase to make exactly 50 mL. Pipet 5 mL of this solution, add exactly 5 mL of the internal standard solution, add the mobile phase to make 50 mL, and use this solution as the sample solution. Separately, weigh accurately an amount of Ampicillin RS, equivalent to about 50 mg (potency), and an amount of Sulbactam RS, equivalent to about 25 mg (potency), dissolve in the mobile phase, add exactly 10 mL of the internal standard solution, add the mobile phase to make 100 mL, and use this solution as the standard solution. Perform the test with 10 μL each of the sample solution and standard solution as directed under Liquid Chromatography <*2.01*> according to the following conditions, and calculate the ratios, Q_{Ta} and Q_{Tb}, of the peak areas of ampicillin and sulbactam to that of the internal standard obtained from the sample solution, and the ratios, Q_{Sa} and Q_{Sb}, of the peak areas of ampicillin and sulbactam to that of the internal standard from the standard solution.

Amount [mg (potency)] of ampicillin ($C_{16}H_{19}N_3O_4S$)
$= M_{S1} \times Q_{Ta}/Q_{Sa} \times 5$

Amount [mg (potency)] of sulbactam ($C_8H_{11}NO_5S$)
$= M_{S2} \times Q_{Tb}/Q_{Sb} \times 5$

M_{S1}: Amount [mg (potency)] of Ampicillin RS taken
M_{S2}: Amount [mg (potency)] of Sulbactam RS taken

Internal standard solution—A solution of parahydroxybenzoic acid in the mobile phase (1 in 1000).

Operating conditions—

Detector: An ultraviolet absorption photometer (wavelength: 215 nm).

Column: A stainless steel column 4.6 mm in inside diameter and 15 cm in length, packed with octadecylsilanized silica gel for liquid chromatography (10 μm in particle diameter).

Column temperature: A constant temperature of about 35°C.

Mobile phase: A mixture of 0.02 mol/L phosphate buffer (pH 3.0) and acetonitrile for liquid chromatography (23:2).

Flow rate: Adjust so that the retention time of the internal standard is about 9 minutes.

System suitability—

System performance: When the procedure is run with 10 μL of the standard solution under the above operating conditions, sulbactam, the internal standard and ampicillin are eluted in this order, and either resolution between these peaks is not less than 2.0.

System repeatability: When the test is repeated 6 times with 10 μL of the standard solution under the above operat-

ing conditions, the relative standard deviation of the peak area of sulbactam is not more than 1.0%.

Containers and storage—Hermetic containers. Plastic containers for aqueous injections may be used.

Ampiroxicam

アンピロキシカム

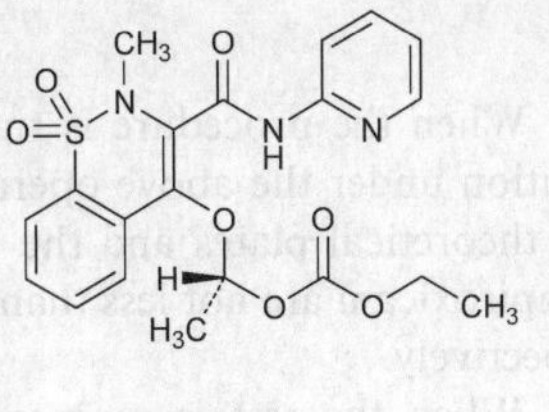

$C_{20}H_{21}N_3O_7S$: 447.46

Ethyl (1*RS*)-1-({2-methyl-1,1-dioxido-3-[(pyridin-2-ylamino)carbonyl]-2*H*-1,2-benzothiazin-4-yl}oxy)ethyl carbonate

[*99464-64-9*]

Ampiroxicam, when dried, contains not less than 99.0% and not more than 101.0% of ampiroxicam ($C_{20}H_{21}N_3O_7S$).

Description Ampiroxicam occurs as a white to yellowish white crystalline powder.

It is freely soluble in acetic acid (100), soluble in acetonitrile, very slightly soluble in ethanol (99.5), and practically insoluble in water.

A solution of Ampiroxicam in acetonitrile (1 in 20) shows no optical rotation.

It shows crystal polymorphism.

Identification **(1)** Determine the absorption spectrum of a solution of Ampiroxicam in 0.01 mol/L hydrochloric acid-methanol TS (1 in 100,000) as directed under Ultraviolet-visible Spectrophotometry *<2.24>*, and compare the spectrum with the Reference Spectrum: both spectra exhibit similar intensities of absorption at the same wavelengths.

(2) Determine the infrared absorption spectrum of Ampiroxicam as directed in the potassium bromide disk method under Infrared Spectrophotometry *<2.25>*, and compare the spectrum with the Reference Spectrum: both spectra exhibit similar intensities of absorption at the same wave numbers.

Purity **(1)** Heavy metals *<1.07>*—Proceed with 1.0 g of Ampiroxicam according to Method 2, and perform the test. Prepare the control solution with 2.0 mL of Standard Lead solution (not more than 20 ppm).

(2) Related substances—Dissolve 20 mg of Ampiroxicam in 50 mL of acetonitrile, and use this solution as the sample solution. Pipet 1 mL of the sample solution, add acetonitrile to make exactly 200 mL, and use this solution as the standard solution. Perform the test with exactly 10 μL each of the sample solution and standard solution as directed under Liquid Chromatography *<2.01>* according to the following conditions, and determine each peak area by the automatic integration method: the area of the peak, having a relative retention time of about 0.17 to ampiroxicam, obtained from the sample solution is not larger than 1/2 times the peak area of ampiroxicam from the standard solution, the area of the peak other than ampiroxicam and the peak mentioned above from the sample solution is not larger than 2/5 times the peak area of ampiroxicam from the standard solution, and the total area of the peaks other than ampiroxicam from the sample solution is not larger than the peak area of ampiroxicam from the standard solution. For the area of the peaks, having the relative retention time of about 0.17 and about 0.46 to ampiroxicam, multiply the correction factor, 0.37 and 0.60, respectively.

Operating conditions—

Detector: An ultraviolet absorption photometer (wavelength: 254 nm).

Column: A stainless steel column 3.9 mm in inside diameter and 15 cm in length, packed with octadecylsilanized silica gel for liquid chromatography (4 μm in particle diameter).

Column temperature: A constant temperature of about 25°C.

Mobile phase: A mixture of diluted acetic acid (100) (3 in 500), methanol and acetonitrile (5:3:2).

Flow rate: Adjust so that the retention time of ampiroxicam is about 9 minutes.

Time span of measurement: About 2 times as long as the retention time of ampiroxicam, beginning after the solvent peak.

System suitability—

Test for required detectability: Pipet 5 mL of the standard solution, add acetonitrile to make exactly 50 mL. Confirm that the peak area of ampiroxicam obtained with 10 μL of this solution is equivalent to 7 to 13% of that with 10 μL of the standard solution.

System performance: When the procedure is run with 10 μL of the standard solution under the above operating conditions, the number of theoretical plates and the symmetry factor of the peak of ampiroxicam are not less than 3000 and not more than 2.0, respectively.

System repeatability: When the test is repeated 6 times with 10 μL of the standard solution under the above operating conditions, the relative standard deviation of the peak area of ampiroxicam is not more than 5%.

Loss on drying *<2.41>* Not more than 0.5% (1 g, 105°C, 3 hours).

Residue on ignition *<2.44>* Not more than 0.2% (1 g).

Assay Weigh accurately about 0.22 g of Ampiroxicam, previously dried, dissolve in 50 mL of acetic acid (100), and titrate *<2.50>* with 0.1 mol/L perchloric acid VS (potentiometric titration). Perform a blank determination in the same manner, and make any necessary correction.

Each mL of 0.1 mol/L perchloric acid VS
= 44.75 mg of $C_{20}H_{21}N_3O_7S$

Containers and storage Containers—Tight containers.

Storage—Light-resistant.

Ampiroxicam Capsules

アンピロキシカムカプセル

Ampiroxicam Capsules contain not less than 95.0% and not more than 105.0% of the labeled amount of ampiroxicam ($C_{20}H_{21}N_3O_7S$: 447.46).

Method of Preparation Prepare as directed under Capsules, with Ampiroxicam.

Identification Take out the contents of Ampiroxicam Capsules, to a quantity of the contents, equivalent to 10 mg of Ampiroxicam, add 100 mL of 0.01 mol/L hydrochloric acid-methanol TS, shake well, and centrifuge. To 5 mL of the supernatant liquid add 0.01 mol/L hydrochloric acid-methanol TS to make 50 mL. Determine the absorption spectrum of this solution as directed under Ultraviolet-visible Spectrophotometry <2.24>: it exhibits a maximum between 318 nm and 322 nm.

Uniformity of dosage units <*6.02*> Perform the test according to the following method: it meets the requirement of the Content uniformity test.

Take out the contents of 1 capsule of Ampiroxicam Capsules, add acetonitrile to make exactly *V* mL so that each mL contains about 0.27 mg of ampiroxicam ($C_{20}H_{21}N_3O_7S$). Stir for 30 minutes, then centrifuge, and use the supernatant liquid as the sample solution. Then, proceed as directed in the Assay.

$$\text{Amount (mg) of ampiroxicam } (C_{20}H_{21}N_3O_7S) = M_S \times A_T/A_S \times V/100$$

M_S: Amount (mg) of ampiroxicam for assay taken

Dissolution <*6.10*> When the test is performed at 50 revolutions per minute according to the Paddle method using the sinker, using 900 mL of 1st fluid for dissolution test as the dissolution medium, the dissolution rate in 30 minutes of Ampiroxicam Capsules is not less than 70%.

Start the test with 1 capsule of Ampiroxicam Capsules, withdraw not less than 20 mL of the medium at the specified minute after starting the test, and filter through a membrane filter with a pore size not exceeding 0.45 µm. Discard not less than 10 mL of the first filtrate, pipet *V* mL of the subsequent filtrate, add the dissolution medium to make exactly *V′* mL so that each mL contains about 15 µg of ampiroxicam ($C_{20}H_{21}N_3O_7S$), and use this solution as the sample solution. Separately, weigh accurately about 30 mg of ampiroxicam for assay, previously dried at 105°C for 3 hours, dissolve in 5 mL of acetonitrile, and add the dissolution medium to make exactly 100 mL. Pipet 5 mL of this solution, add the dissolution medium to make exactly 100 mL, and use this solution as the standard solution. Determine the absorbances, A_T and A_S, at 320 nm of the sample solution and standard solution as directed under Ultraviolet-visible Spectrophotometry <*2.24*>, using the dissolution medium as the blank.

$$\text{Dissolution rate (\%) with respect to the labeled amount of ampiroxicam } (C_{20}H_{21}N_3O_7S) = M_S \times A_T/A_S \times V'/V \times 1/C \times 45$$

M_S: Amount (mg) of ampiroxicam for assay taken
C: Labeled amount (mg) of ampiroxicam ($C_{20}H_{21}N_3O_7S$) in 1 capsule

Assay Take out the contents of not less than 20 Ampiroxicam Capsules, weigh accurately the mass of the contents, and powder if necessary. Weigh accurately a portion of the powder, equivalent to about 13.5 mg of ampiroxicam ($C_{20}H_{21}N_3O_7S$), and add acetonitrile to make exactly 50 mL. Stir for 30 minutes, centrifuge, and use the supernatant liquid as the sample solution. Separately, weigh accurately about 27 mg of ampiroxicam for assay, previously dried at 105°C for 3 hours, dissolve in acetonitrile to make exactly 100 mL, and use this solution as the standard solution. Perform the test with exactly 10 µL each of the sample solution and standard solution as directed under Liquid Chromatography <*2.01*> according to the following condition, and determine the peak areas, A_T and A_S, of ampiroxicam in each solution.

$$\text{Amount (mg) of ampiroxicam } (C_{20}H_{21}N_3O_7S) = M_S \times A_T/A_S \times 1/2$$

M_S: Amount (mg) of ampiroxicam for assay taken

Operating conditions—

Detector: An ultraviolet absorption photometer (wavelength: 254 nm).

Column: A stainless steel column 3.9 mm in inside diameter and 15 cm in length, packed with octadecylsilanized silica gel for liquid chromatography (4 µm in particle diameter).

Column temperature: A constant temperature of about 25°C.

Mobile phase: A mixture of diluted acetic acid (100) (3 in 500), methanol, and acetonitrile (5:3:2).

Flow rate: Adjust so that the retention time of ampiroxicam is about 9 minutes.

System suitability—

System performance: When the procedure is run with 10 µL of the standard solution under the above operating conditions, the number of theoretical plates and the symmetry factor of the peak of ampiroxicam are not less than 4000 and not more than 2.0, respectively.

System repeatability: When the test is repeated 6 times with 10 µL of the standard solution under the above operating conditions, the relative standard deviation of the peak area of ampiroxicam is not more than 1.0%.

Containers and storage Containers—Well-closed containers.

Amyl Nitrite

亜硝酸アミル

$C_5H_{11}NO_2$: 117.15

Amyl Nitrite is the nitrous acid ester of 3-methylbutanol-1 and contains a small quantity of 2-methylbutanol-1 and the nitrous acid esters of other homologues.

It contains not less than 90.0% of amyl nitrite ($C_5H_{11}NO_2$).

Description Amyl Nitrite is a clear, light yellow-liquid, and has a characteristic, fruity odor.

It is miscible with ethanol (95), and with diethyl ether.

It is practically insoluble in water.

It is affected by light and by heat.

It is volatile at ordinary temperature and flammable even at a low temperature.

Boiling point: about 97°C

Identification Determine the infrared spectrum of Amyl Nitrite as directed in the liquid film method under Infrared Spectrophotometry <*2.25*>, and compare the spectrum with the Reference Spectrum: both spectra exhibit similar intensities of absorption at the same wave numbers.

Specific gravity <*2.56*> d^{20}_{20}: 0.871 – 0.880

Purity (1) Acidity—To 5 mL of Amyl Nitrite add a mixture of 1.0 mL of 1 mol/L sodium hydroxide VS, 10 mL of water and 1 drop of phenolphthalein TS, shake, and allow to stand for 1 minute: the light red color of the water layer does not disappear.

(2) Water—Allow 2.0 mL of Amyl Nitrite to stand in ice water: no turbidity is produced.

(3) Aldehyde—To 3 mL of a mixture of equal volumes of silver nitrate TS and aldehyde free-ethanol add ammonia TS dropwise until the precipitate first formed is redissolved. Add 1.0 mL of Amyl Nitrite, and warm between 60°C and 70°C for 1 minute: a brown to black color is not produced.

(4) Residue on evaporation—Evaporate 10.0 mL of

Amyl Nitrite on a water bath in a draft chamber, carefully protecting from flame, and dry the residue at 105°C for 1 hour: the mass of the residue is not more than 1.0 mg.

Assay Weigh accurately a volumetric flask containing 10 mL of ethanol (95), add about 0.5 g of Amyl Nitrite, and weigh accurately again. Add exactly 25 mL of 0.1 mol/L silver nitrate VS, then add 15 mL of potassium chlorate solution (1 in 20) and 10 mL of dilute nitric acid, stopper the flask immediately, and shake it vigorously for 5 minutes. Dilute with water to make exactly 100 mL, shake, and filter through dry filter paper. Discard the first 20 mL of the filtrate, measure exactly 50 mL of the subsequent filtrate, and titrate *<2.50>* the excess silver nitrate with 0.1 mol/L ammonium thiocyanate VS (indicator: 2 mL of ammonium iron (III) sulfate TS). Perform a blank determination in the same manner.

Each mL of 0.1 mol/L silver nitrate VS
= 35.15 mg of $C_5H_{11}NO_2$

Containers and storage Containers—Hermetic containers not exceeding 10-ml capacity.

Storage—Light-resistant, in a cold place, and remote from fire.

Dental Antiformin

Dental Sodium Hypochlorite Solution

歯科用アンチホルミン

Dental Antiformin contains not less than 3.0 w/v% and not more than 6.0 w/v% of sodium hypochlorite (NaClO: 74.44).

Description Dental Antiformin is a slightly light yellow-green, clear liquid. It has a slight odor of chlorine.

It gradually changes by light.

Identification **(1)** Dental Antiformin changes red litmus paper to blue, and then decolorizes it.

(2) To Dental Antiformin add dilute hydrochloric acid: it evolves the odor of chlorine, and the gas changes potassium iodide starch paper moistened with water to blue.

(3) Dental Antiformin responds to Qualitative Tests *<1.09>* (1) for sodium salt.

Assay Measure exactly 3 mL of Dental Antiformin in a glass-stoppered flask, add 50 mL of water, 2 g of potassium iodide and 10 mL of acetic acid (31), and titrate *<2.50>* the liberated iodine with 0.1 mol/L sodium thiosulfate VS (indicator: 3 mL of starch TS).

Each mL of 0.1 mol/L sodium thiosulfate VS
= 3.722 mg of NaClO

Containers and storage Containers—Tight containers.

Storage—Light-resistant, and not exceeding 10°C.

Antipyrine

Phenazone

アンチピリン

$C_{11}H_{12}N_2O$: 188.23
1,5-Dimethyl-2-phenyl-1,2-dihydro-3*H*-pyrazol-3-one
[60-80-0]

Antipyrine, when dried, contains not less than 99.0% of antipyrine ($C_{11}H_{12}N_2O$).

Description Antipyrine occurs as colorless or white crystals, or a white, crystalline powder. It is odorless, and has a slightly bitter taste.

It is very soluble in water, freely soluble in ethanol (95), and sparingly soluble in diethyl ether.

A solution of Antipyrine (1 in 10) is neutral.

Identification **(1)** To 5 mL of a solution of Antipyrine (1 in 100) add 2 drops of sodium nitrite TS and 1 mL of dilute sulfuric acid: a deep green color develops.

(2) To 2 mL of a solution of Antipyrine (1 in 100) add 4 drops of dilute iron (III) chloride TS: a yellow-red color develops. Then add 10 drops of dilute sulfuric acid: the color changes to light yellow.

(3) To 5 mL of a solution of Antipyrine (1 in 100) add 2 to 3 drops of tannic acid TS: a white precipitate is produced.

(4) To 0.1 g of Antipyrine add 0.1 g of vanillin, 5 mL of water and 2 mL of sulfuric acid, boil the mixture, and cool: a yellow-red precipitate is produced.

Melting point *<2.60>* 111 - 113°C

Purity **(1)** Chloride *<1.03>*—Perform the test with 1.0 g of Antipyrine. Prepare the control solution with 0.40 mL of 0.01 mol/L hydrochloric acid VS (not more than 0.014%).

(2) Heavy metals *<1.07>*—Proceed with 1.0 g of Antipyrine according to Method 1, and perform the test. Prepare the control solution with 2.0 mL of Standard Lead Solution (not more than 20 ppm).

(3) Readily carbonizable substances*<1.15>*—Perform the test with 0.5 g of Antipyrine: the solution remains colorless.

Loss on drying *<2.41>* Not more than 0.5% (1 g, silica gel, 4 hours).

Residue on ignition *<2.44>* Not more than 0.1% (1 g).

Assay Dissolve about 0.2 g of Antipyrine, previously dried and accurately weighed, in 20 mL of sodium acetate TS, add exactly 30 mL of 0.05 mol/L iodine VS, and allow to stand for 20 minutes with occasional shaking. Dissolve the precipitate in 10 mL of chloroform, and titrate *<2.50>* the excess iodine with 0.1 mol/L sodium thiosulfate VS (indicator: 3 mL of starch TS). Perform a blank determination in the same manner.

Each mL of 0.05 mol/L iodine VS
= 9.412 mg of $C_{11}H_{12}N_2O$

Containers and storage Containers—Well-closed containers.

Aprindine Hydrochloride

アプリンジン塩酸塩

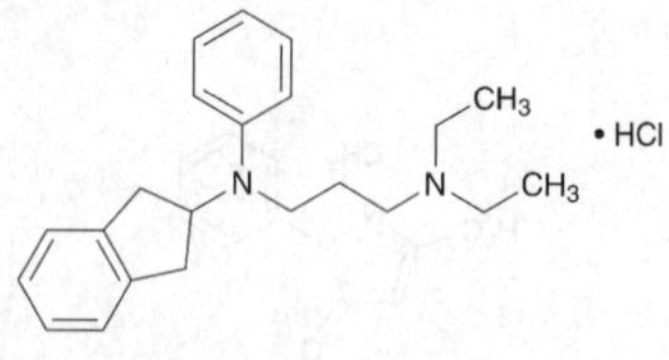

$C_{22}H_{30}N_2.HCl$: 358.95
N-(2,3-Dihydro-1*H*-inden-2-yl)-*N'*,*N'*-diethyl-*N*-phenylpropane-1,3-diamine monohydrochloride
[33237-74-0]

Aprindine Hydrochloride, when dried, contains not less than 98.5% and not more than 101.0% of aprindine hydrochloride ($C_{22}H_{30}N_2.HCl$).

Description Aprindine Hydrochloride occurs as a white to pale yellow-white crystalline powder. It has a bitter taste, numbing the tongue.

It is very soluble in water, in methanol and in acetic acid (100), and freely soluble in ethanol (99.5).

It gradually turns brown on exposure to light.

Identification **(1)** Dissolve 10 mg of Aprindine Hydrochloride in a solution of hydrochloric acid in diluted ethanol (1 in 2) (1 in 125) to make 50 mL. Determine the absorption spectrum of this solution as directed under Ultraviolet-visible Spectrophotometry ⟨*2.24*⟩, and compare the spectrum with the Reference Spectrum: both spectra exhibit similar intensities of absorption at the same wavelengths.

(2) Determine the infrared absorption spectrum of Aprindine Hydrochloride as directed in the potassium chloride disk method under Infrared Spectrophotometry ⟨*2.25*⟩, and compare the spectrum with the Reference Spectrum: both spectra exhibit similar intensities of absorption at the same wave numbers.

(3) To 5 mL of a solution of Aprindine Hydrochloride (1 in 50) add 1 mL of dilute nitric acid: this solution responds to Qualitative Tests ⟨*1.09*⟩ for chloride.

pH ⟨*2.54*⟩ Dissolve 1.0 g of Aprindine Hydrochloride in 50 mL of water: the pH of the solution is between 6.4 and 7.0.

Melting point ⟨*2.60*⟩ 127 – 131°C

Purity **(1)** Clarity and color of solution—Dissolve 1.0 g of Aprindine Hydrochloride in 10 mL of methanol: the solution is clear, and its absorbance at 420 nm determined as directed under Ultraviolet-visible Spectrophotometry ⟨*2.24*⟩ is not more than 0.10.

(2) Heavy metals ⟨*1.07*⟩—Proceed with 1.0 g of Aprindine Hydrochloride according to Method 2, and perform the test. Prepare the control solution with 1.0 mL of Standard Lead Solution (not more than 10 ppm).

(3) Related substances—Dissolve 25 mg of Aprindine Hydrochloride in 10 mL of the mobile phase, and use this solution as the sample solution. Pipet 1 mL of the sample solution, add the mobile phase to make exactly 100 mL, and use this solution as the standard solution. Perform the test with exactly 10 μL each of the sample solution and standard solution as directed under Liquid Chromatography ⟨*2.01*⟩ according to the following conditions. Determine each peak area of both solutions by the automatic integration method: the area of the peak other than aprindine obtained from the sample solution is not larger than 1/10 times the peak area of aprindine from the standard solution.

Operating conditions—

Detector: An ultraviolet absorption photometer (wavelength: 254 nm).

Column: A stainless steel column 4.6 mm in inside diameter and 15 cm in length, packed with octadecylsilanized silica gel for liquid chromatography (5 μm in particle diameter).

Column temperature: A constant temperature of about 40°C.

Mobile phase: Dissolve 3.40 g of potassium dihydrogen phosphate in 500 mL of water, and adjust the pH to 3.0 with hydrochloric acid. To 500 mL of this solution add 500 mL of acetonitrile.

Flow rate: Adjust so that the retention time of aprindine is about 6 minutes.

Time span of measurement: About 4 times as long as the retention time of aprindine.

System suitability—

Test for required detectability: Pipet 1 mL of the standard solution, and add the mobile phase to make exactly 10 mL. Confirm that the peak area of aprindine obtained with 10 μL of this solution is equivalent to 7 to 13% of that with 10 μL of the standard solution.

System performance: When the procedure is run with 10 μL of the standard solution under the above operating conditions, the number of theoretical plates and the symmetry factor of the peak of aprindine are not less than 3000 and not more than 2.0, respectively.

System repeatability: When the test is repeated 6 times with 10 μL of the standard solution under the above operating conditions, the relative standard deviation of the peak area of aprindine is not more than 1.5%.

Loss on drying ⟨*2.41*⟩ Not more than 0.5% (1 g, in vacuum, 60°C, 4 hours).

Residue on ignition ⟨*2.44*⟩ Not more than 0.1% (1 g).

Assay Weigh accurately about 0.5 g of Aprindine Hydrochloride, previously dried, dissolve in 80 mL of acetic acid (100), and titrate ⟨*2.50*⟩ with 0.1 mol/L perchloric acid VS (potentiometric titration). Perform a blank determination in the same manner, and make any necessary correction.

Each mL of 0.1 mol/L perchloric acid VS
= 35.90 mg of $C_{22}H_{30}N_2.HCl$

Containers and storage Containers—Well-closed containers.

Storage—Light-resistant.

Aprindine Hydrochloride Capsules

アプリンジン塩酸塩カプセル

Aprindine Hydrochloride Capsules contain not less than 95.0% and not more than 105.0% of the labeled amount of aprindine hydrochloride ($C_{22}H_{30}N_2.HCl$: 358.95).

Method of preparation Prepare as directed under Capsules, with Aprindine Hydrochloride.

Identification Determine the absorption spectrum of the sample solution obtained in the Assay as directed under Ultraviolet-visible Spectrophotometry ⟨*2.24*⟩, it exhibits maxima between 264 nm and 268 nm, and between 271 nm and 275 nm.

Uniformity of dosage units <*6.02*> Perform the test according to the following method: it meets the requirement of the Content uniformity test.

Take out the contents of 1 capsule of Aprindine Hydrochloride Capsules, add 30 mL of a solution of hydrochloric acid in diluted ethanol (1 in 2) (1 in 125), shake vigorously for 20 minutes, add a solution of hydrochloric acid in diluted ethanol (1 in 2) (1 in 125) to make exactly *V* mL so that each mL contains about 0.2 mg of aprindine hydrochloride ($C_{22}H_{30}N_2.HCl$), and filter. Discard the first 5 mL of the filtrate, and use the subsequent filtrate as the sample solution. Proceed as directed in the Assay.

Amount (mg) of aprindine hydrochloride ($C_{22}H_{30}N_2.HCl$)
$= M_S \times A_T/A_S \times V/250$

M_S: Amount (mg) of aprindine hydrochloride for assay taken

Dissolution <*6.10*> When the test is performed at 50 revolutions per minute according to the Paddle method using the sinker, using 900 mL of water as the dissolution medium, the dissolution rate in 15 minutes of Aprindine Hydrochloride Capsules is not less than 80%.

Start the test with 1 capsule of Aprindine Hydrochloride Capsules, withdraw not less than 20 mL of the medium at the specified minute after starting the test, and filter through a membrane filter with a pore size not exceeding 0.45 μm. Discard not less than 10 mL of the first filtrate, pipet *V* mL of the subsequent filtrate, add water to make exactly *V′* mL so that each mL contains about 11 μg of aprindine hydrochloride ($C_{22}H_{30}N_2.HCl$), and use this solution as the sample solution. Separately, weigh accurately about 28 mg of aprindine hydrochloride for assay, previously dried in vacuum at 60°C for 4 hours, and dissolve in water to make exactly 100 mL. Pipet 2 mL of this solution, add water to make exactly 50 mL, and use this solution as the standard solution. Perform the test with exactly 20 μL each of the sample solution and standard solution as directed under Liquid Chromatography <*2.01*> according to the following conditions, and determine the peak areas, A_T and A_S, of aprindine in each solution.

Dissolution rate (%) with respect to the labeled amount of aprindine hydrochloride ($C_{22}H_{30}N_2.HCl$)
$= M_S \times A_T/A_S \times V'/V \times 1/C \times 36$

M_S: Amount (mg) of aprindine hydrochloride for assay taken
C: Labeled amount (mg) of aprindine hydrochloride ($C_{22}H_{30}N_2.HCl$) in 1 capsule

Operating conditions—

Detector: An ultraviolet absorption photometer (wavelength: 254 nm).

Column: A stainless steel column 4.6 mm in inside diameter and 15 cm in length, packed with octadecylsilanized silica gel for liquid chromatography (5 μm in particle diameter).

Column temperature: A constant temperature of about 40°C.

Mobile phase: Dissolve 3.40 g of potassium dihydrogen phosphate in 500 mL of water, and adjust the pH to 3.0 with hydrochloric acid. To 500 mL of this solution add 500 mL of acetonitrile.

Flow rate: Adjust so that the retention time of aprindine is about 6 minutes.

System suitability—

System performance: When the procedure is run with 20 μL of the standard solution under the above operating conditions, the number of theoretical plates and the symmetry factor of the peak of aprindine are not less than 3000 and not more than 2.0, respectively.

System repeatability: When the test is repeated 6 times with 20 μL of the standard solution under the above operating conditions, the relative standard deviation of the peak area of aprindine is not more than 1.5%.

Assay Take out the contents of not less than 20 Aprindine Hydrochloride Capsules, weigh accurately the mass of the contents, and powder. Weigh accurately a portion of the powder, equivalent to about 0.1 g of aprindine hydrochloride ($C_{22}H_{30}N_2.HCl$), add 60 mL of a solution of hydrochloric acid in diluted ethanol (1 in 2) (1 in 125), shake vigorously for 20 minutes, and add a solution of hydrochloric acid in diluted ethanol (1 in 2) (1 in 125) to make exactly 100 mL. Pipet 10 mL of this solution, add a solution of hydrochloric acid in diluted ethanol (1 in 2) (1 in 125) to make exactly 50 mL, and filter, Discard the first 5 mL of the filtrate, and use the subsequent filtrate as the sample solution. Separately, weigh accurately about 50 mg of aprindine hydrochloride for assay, previously dried in vacuum at 60°C for 4 hours, and dissolve in a solution of hydrochloric acid in diluted ethanol (1 in 2) (1 in 125) to make exactly 50 mL. Pipet 10 mL of this solution, add a solution of hydrochloric acid in diluted ethanol (1 in 2) (1 in 125) to make exactly 50 mL, and use this solution as the standard solution. Determine the absorbances, A_T and A_S, of the sample solution and standard solution at 265 nm as directed under Ultraviolet-visible Spectrophotometry <*2.24*>.

Amount (mg) of aprindine hydrochloride ($C_{22}H_{30}N_2.HCl$)
$= M_S \times A_T/A_S \times 2$

M_S: Amount (mg) of aprindine hydrochloride for assay taken

Containers and storage Containers—Tight containers.
Storage—Light-resistant.

Arbekacin Sulfate

アルベカシン硫酸塩

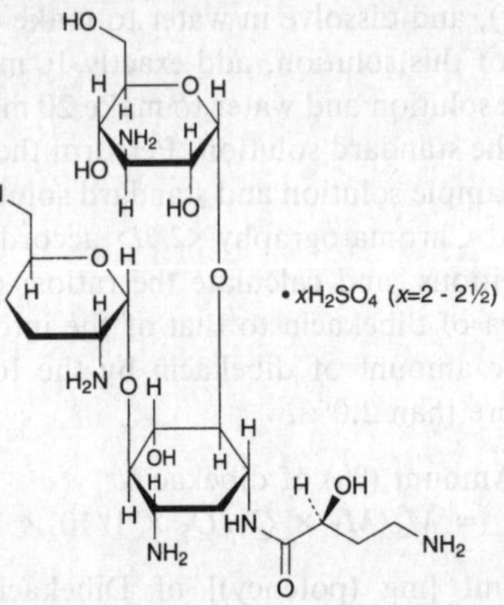

$C_{22}H_{44}N_6O_{10}.xH_2SO_4$ ($x = 2 - 2½$)
3-Amino-3-deoxy-*α*-D-glucopyranosyl-(1→6)-[2,6-diamino-2,3,4,6-tetradeoxy-*α*-D-*erythro*-hexopyranosyl-(1→4)]-1-*N*-[(2*S*)-4-amino-2-hydroxybutanoyl]-2-deoxy-D-streptamine sulfate
[*51025-85-5*, Arbekacin]

Arbekacin Sulfate is the sulfate of a derivative of dibekacin.

It contains not less than 670 μg (potency) and not more than 750 μg (potency) per mg, calculated on the dried basis. The potency of Arbekacin Sulfate is expressed as mass (potency) of arbekacin ($C_{22}H_{44}N_6O_{10}$: 552.62).

Description Arbekacin Sulfate occurs as a white powder.

It is very soluble in water, and practically insoluble in ethanol (99.5).

Identification (1) Dissolve 10 mg each of Arbekacin Sulfate and Arbekacin Sulfate RS in 1 mL of water, and use these solutions as the sample solution and standard solution. Perform the test with these solutions as directed under Thin-layer Chromatography <*2.03*>. Spot 2 μL each of the sample solution and standard solution on a plate of silica gel for thin-layer chromatography. Develop the plate with a mixture of ammonia solution (28), methanol, chloroform and ethanol (95) (7:6:4:1) to a distance of about 10 cm, and air-dry the plate. Spray evenly 0.2% ninhydrin-water saturated 1-butanol TS on the plate, and heat the plate at 100°C for 10 minutes: the principal spot obtained from the sample solution and the spot from the standard solution are purple-brown in color and their *Rf* values are the same.

(2) A solution of Arbekacin Sulfate (1 in 50) responds to Qualitative Tests <*1.09*> (1) for sulfate.

Optical rotation <*2.49*> $[\alpha]_D^{20}$: +69 – +79° (0.25 g after drying, water, 25 mL, 100 mm).

pH <*2.54*> The pH of a solution obtained by dissolving 0.75 g of Arbekacin Sulfate in 10 mL of water is between 6.0 and 8.0.

Purity (1) Clarity and color of solution—A solution obtained by dissolving 1.0 g of Arbekacin Sulfate in 5 mL of water is clear and colorless.

(2) Heavy metals <*1.07*>—Proceed with 2.0 g of Arbekacin Sulfate according to Method 1, and perform the test. Prepare the control solution with 2.0 mL of Standard Lead Solution (not more than 10 ppm).

(3) Dibekacin—Weigh accurately about 20 mg of Arbekacin Sulfate, add exactly 10 mL of the internal standard solution to dissolve, add water to make 20 mL, and use this solution as the sample solution. Separately, weigh accurately an amount of Dibekacin Sulfate RS, equivalent to about 10 mg (potency), and dissolve in water to make exactly 50 mL. Pipet 5 mL of this solution, add exactly 10 mL of the internal standard solution and water to make 20 mL, and use this solution as the standard solution. Perform the test with 5 μL each of the sample solution and standard solution as directed under Liquid Chromatography <*2.01*> according to the following conditions, and calculate the ratios, Q_T and Q_S, of the peak area of dibekacin to that of the internal standard. Calculate the amount of dibekacin by the following equation: not more than 2.0%.

$$\text{Amount (\%) of dibekacin} = M_S/M_T \times Q_T/Q_S \times 1/10 \times 100$$

M_S: Amount [mg (potency)] of Dibekacin Sulfate RS taken

M_T: Amount (mg) of Arbekacin Sulfate taken

Internal standard solution—A solution of bekanamycin sulfate (1 in 2000).

Operating conditions—

Detector: Fluorometric detector (excitation wavelength: 340 nm, detection wavelength: 460 nm).

Column: A stainless steel column 4.6 mm in inside diameter and 15 cm in length, packed with octadecylsilanized silica gel for liquid chromatography (5 μm in particle diameter).

Column temperature: A constant temperature of about 40°C.

Reaction coil: A column about 0.3 mm in inside diameter and about 3 m in length.

Reaction coil temperature: A constant temperature of about 50°C.

Mobile phase: Dissolve 8.70 g of sodium 1-pentane sulfonate and 8.52 g of anhydrous sodium sulfate in 980 mL of water, adjust the pH to 4.0 with acetic acid (100), and add water to make 1000 mL. To 230 mL of this solution add 20 mL of methanol.

Reagent: Dissolve 12.36 g of boric acid in 960 mL of water, add 10 mL of a solution of *o*-phthalaldehyde in ethanol (99.5) (1 in 25), adjust the pH to 10.5 with 8 mol/L potassium hydroxide TS, and add water to make 1000 mL. To this solution add 1 mL of 2-mercaptoethanol.

Reaction temperature: A constant temperature of about 50°C.

Flow rate of mobile phase: 0.5 mL per minute.

Flow rate of reagent: 1 mL per minute.

System suitability—

System performance: Dissolve 20 mg each of Arbekacin Sulfate, becanamycin sulfate and dibekacin sulfate in 200 mL of water. When the procedure is run with 5 μL of this solution under the above operating conditions, becanamycin, arbekacin and dibekacin are eluted in this order, and the resolution between the peaks, becanamycin and arbekacin is not less than 5 and arbekacin and dibekacin is not less than 1.5, respectively.

System repeatability: When the test is repeated 6 times with 5 μL of the standard solution under the above operating conditions, the relative standard deviation of the ratio of the peak area of dibekacin to that of the internal standard is not more than 2.0%.

(4) Related substances—Dissolve 20 mg of Arbekacin Sulfate in 20 mL of water, and use this solution as the sample solution. Pipet 3 mL of the sample solution, add water to make exactly 250 mL, and use this solution as the standard solution. Perform the test with exactly 5 μL each of the sample solution and standard solution as directed under Liquid Chromatography <*2.01*> according to the following conditions, and determine the area of each peak by the automatic integration method: the total area of the peaks other than arbekacin and dibekacin obtained from the sample solution is not larger than the peak area of arbekacin from the standard solution.

Operating conditions—

Detector, column, column temperature, reaction coil, reaction coil temperature, mobile phase, reagent, reaction temperature, flow rate of mobile phase, and flow rate of reagent: Proceed as directed in the operating conditions in the Purity (3).

Time span of measurement: About 1.5 times as long as the retention time of arbekacin.

System suitability—

System performance: Dissolve 10 mg each of Arbekacin Sulfate and dibekacin sulfate in 200 mL of water. When the procedure is run with 5 μL of this solution under the above operating conditions, arbekacin and dibekacin are eluted in this order with the resolution between these peaks being not less than 1.5.

System repeatability: When the test is repeated 6 times with 5 μL of the standard solution under the above operating conditions, the relative standard deviation of the peak area of arbekacin is not more than 5.0%.

Loss on drying <*2.41*> Not more than 5.0% (0.5 g, reduced pressure not exceeding 0.67 kPa, 60°C, 3 hours).

Assay Perform the test according to the Cylinder-plate method as directed under Microbial Assay for Antibiotics <4.02> according to the following conditions.

(i) Test organism—*Bacillus subtilis* ATCC 6633

(ii) Culture medium—Use the medium i in 1) under (1) Agar media for seed and base layer, having pH 7.8 – 8.0 after sterilization.

(iii) Standard solutions—Weigh accurately an amount of Arbekacin Sulfate RS, previously dried, equivalent to about 20 mg (potency), dissolve in diluted phosphate buffer solution (pH 6.0) (1 in 2) to make exactly 50 mL, and use this solution as the standard stock solution. Keep the standard stock solution at 5 to 15°C and use within 30 days. Take exactly a suitable amount of the standard stock solution before use, add 0.1 mol/L phosphate buffer solution (pH 8.0) to make solutions so that each mL contains 20 μg (potency) and 5 μg (potency), and use these solutions as the high concentration standard solution and low concentration standard solution, respectively.

(iv) Sample solutions—Weigh accurately an amount of Arbekacin Sulfate, equivalent to about 20 mg (potency), and dissolve in water to make exactly 50 mL. Take exactly a suitable amount of this solution, add 0.1 mol/L phosphate buffer solution (pH 8.0) to make solutions so that each mL contains 20 μg (potency) and 5 μg (potency), and use these solutions as the high concentration sample solution and low concentration sample solution, respectively.

Containers and storage Containers—Tight containers.

Arbekacin Sulfate Injection

アルベカシン硫酸塩注射液

Arbekacin Sulfate Injection is an aqueous injection. It contains not less than 90.0% and not more than 110.0% of the labeled potency of arbekacin sulfate ($C_{22}H_{44}N_6O_{10}$: 552.62).

Method of preparation Prepare as directed under Injections, with Arbekacin Sulfate.

Description Arbekacin Sulfate Injection occurs as a clear and colorless liquid.

Identification To 0.2 mL of Arbekacin Sulfate Injection add 1 mL of water, and use this solution as the sample solution. Separately, dissolve 10 mg of Arbekacin Sulfate RS in 1 mL of water, and use this solution as the standard solution. Perform the test with these solutions as directed under Thin-layer Chromatography <2.03>. Spot 2 μL each of the sample solution and standard solution on a plate of silica gel for thin-layer chromatography. Develop with a mixture of ammonia solution (28), methanol, chloroform and ethanol (95) (7:6:4:1) to a distance of about 12 cm, and air-dry the plate. Spray evenly 0.2% ninhydrin-water saturated 1-butanol TS on the plate, and heat the plate at 80°C for 10 minutes: the principal spot obtained from the sample solution and the spot from the standard solution show a purple-brown color and the same *Rf* value.

Osmotic pressure ratio <2.47> 0.8 – 1.2 (for the preparation intended for intramuscular use).

pH <2.54> 6.0 – 8.0

Bacterial endotoxins <4.01> Less than 0.50 EU/mg (potency).

Extractable volume <6.05> It meets the requirement.

Foreign insoluble matter <6.06> Perform the test according to Method 1: it meets the requirement.

Insoluble particulate matter <6.07> It meets the requirement.

Sterility <4.06> Perform the test according to the Membrane filtration method: it meets the requirement.

Assay Perform the test according to the Cylinder-plate method as directed under Microbial Assay for Antibiotics <4.02> according to the following conditions.

(i) Test organism, Culture medium and Standard solutions: Proceed as directed in the Assay under Arbekacin Sulfate.

(ii) Sample solutions—Take exactly a volume of Arbekacin Sulfate Injection, equivalent to about 20 mg (potency), and add water to make exactly 50 mL. Take exactly a suitable amount of this solution, add 0.1 mol/L phosphate buffer solution (pH 8.0) to make solutions so that each mL contains 20 μg (potency) and 5 μg (potency), and use these solutions as the high concentration sample solution and low concentration sample solution, respectively.

Containers and storage Containers—Hermetic containers.

Argatroban Hydrate

アルガトロバン水和物

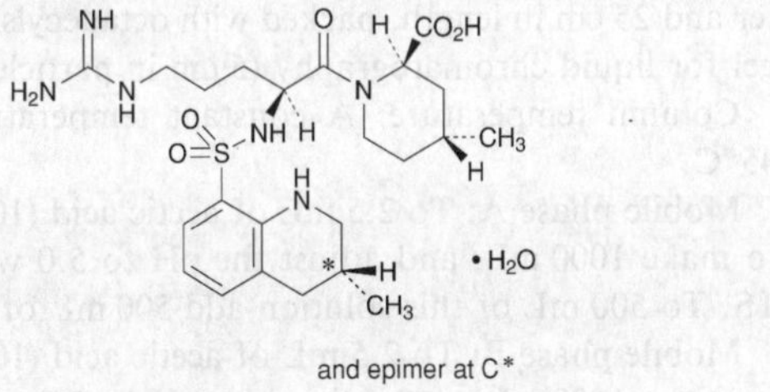

and epimer at C*

$C_{23}H_{36}N_6O_5S.H_2O$: 526.65

(2*R*,4*R*)-4-Methyl-1-((2*S*)-2-{[(3*RS*)-3-methyl-1,2,3,4-tetrahydroquinolin-8-yl]sulfonyl}amino-5-guanidinopentanoyl)piperidine-2-carboxylic acid monohydrate

[*141396-28-3*]

Argatroban Hydrate contains not less than 98.5% and not more than 101.0% of argatroban ($C_{23}H_{36}N_6O_5S$: 508.63), calculated on the anhydrous basis.

Description Argatroban Hydrate occurs as white, crystals or crystalline powder. It has a bitter taste.

It is freely soluble in acetic acid (100), sparingly soluble in methanol, slightly soluble in ethanol (99.5), and very slightly soluble in water.

It is gradually decomposed on exposure to light.

Identification **(1)** Determine the absorption spectrum of a solution of Argatroban Hydrate in ethanol (99.5) (1 in 20,000) as directed under Ultraviolet-visible Spectrophotometry <2.24>, and compare the spectrum with the Reference Spectrum: both spectra exhibit similar intensities of absorption at the same wavelengths.

(2) Determine the infrared absorption spectrum of Argatroban Hydrate as directed in the potassium bromide disk method under Infrared Spectrophotometry <2.25>, and compare the spectrum with the Reference Spectrum: both spectra exhibit similar intensities of absorption at the same wave numbers.

Optical rotation <2.49> $[\alpha]_D^{20}$: +175 – +185° (0.2 g calculated on the anhydrous basis, methanol, 25 mL, 100 mm).

Purity (1) Heavy metals <1.07>—Proceed with 2.0 g of Argatroban Hydrate according to Method 2, and perform the test. Prepare the control solution with 2.0 mL of Standard Lead Solution (not more than 10 ppm).

(2) Arsenic <1.11>—Incinerate 2.0 g of Argatroban Hydrate according to Method 4. After cooling, add 10 mL of dilute hydrochloric acid to the residue, dissolve by warming on a water bath, and perform the test using this solution as the test solution. Add 10 mL of a solution of magnesium nitrate hexahydrate in ethanol (95) (1 in 10), then add 1.5 mL of hydrogen peroxide (30), and fire to burn (not more than 1 ppm).

(3) Related substance 1—Dissolve 50 mg of Argatroban Hydrate in 40 mL of methanol, add water to make 100 mL, and use this solution as the sample solution. Perform the test with 10 μL of the sample solution as directed under Liquid Chromatography <2.01> according to the following conditions. Determine each peak area from the sample solution by the automatic integration method, and calculate the amount of them by the area percentage method: the amount of each peak other than argatroban is not more than 0.1%.

Operating conditions—

Detector: An ultraviolet absorption photometer (wavelength: 254 nm).

Column: A stainless steel column 4.6 mm in inside diameter and 25 cm in length, packed with octadecylsilanized silica gel for liquid chromatography (5 μm in particle diameter).

Column temperature: A constant temperature of about 45°C.

Mobile phase A: To 2.5 mL of acetic acid (100) add water to make 1000 mL, and adjust the pH to 5.0 with ammonia TS. To 500 mL of this solution add 500 mL of methanol.

Mobile phase B: To 2.5 mL of acetic acid (100) add water to make 1000 mL, and adjust the pH to 5.0 with ammonia TS. To 200 mL of this solution add 800 mL of methanol.

Flowing of mobile phase: Control the gradient by mixing the mobile phases A and B as directed in the following table.

Time after injection of sample (min)	Mobile phase A (vol%)	Mobile phase B (vol%)
0 – 5	100	0
5 – 35	100 → 5	0 → 95

Flow rate: About 1.0 mL per minute.

Time span of measurement: About 1.5 times as long as the retention time of argatroban, beginning after the solvent peak.

System suitability—

Test for required detectability: To 1 mL of the sample solution add the mobile phase A to make 100 mL, and use this solution as the solution for system suitability test. Pipet 1 mL of the solution for system suitability test, and add the mobile phase A to make exactly 10 mL. Confirm that the peak area of argatroban obtained with 10 μL of this solution is equivalent to 7 to 13% of that with 10 μL of the solution for system suitability test.

System performance: Dissolve 5 mg of Argatroban Hydrate and 5 μL of methyl benzoate in 40 mL of methanol, and add water to make 100 mL. To 5 mL of this solution add 40 mL of methanol and water to make 100 mL. When the procedure is run with 10 μL of this solution under the above operating conditions, methyl benzoate and argatroban are eluted in this order with the resolution between these peaks being not less than 3.

System repeatability: When the test is repeated 6 times with 10 μL of the solution for system suitability test under the above operating conditions, the relative standard deviation of the peak area of argatroban is not more than 2.0%.

(4) Related substance 2—Dissolve 0.10 g of Argatroban Hydrate in 10 mL of methanol, and use this solution as the sample solution. Pipet 3 mL of the sample solution, and add methanol to make exactly 100 mL. Pipet 5 mL of this solution, add methanol to make exactly 50 mL, and use this solution as the standard solution. Perform the test with these solutions as directed under Thin-layer Chromatography <2.03>. Spot 10 μL each of the sample solution and standard solution on a plate of silica gel with fluorescent indicator for thin-layer chromatography. Develop the plate with a mixture of methanol, ethyl acetate and water (10:10:1) to a distance of about 10 cm, and air-dry the plate. Examine under ultraviolet light (main wavelength: 254 nm): the number of spots other than the principal spot obtained from the sample solution is not more than 2, and they are not more intense than the spot from the standard solution.

Water <2.48> 2.5 – 4.5% (0.2 g, volumetric titration, direct titration).

Residue on ignition <2.44> Not more than 0.1% (1 g).

Isomer ratio Dissolve 50 mg of Argatroban Hydrate in 50 mL of methanol, add water to make 100 mL, and use this solution as the sample solution. Perform the test with 10 μL of the sample solution as directed under Liquid Chromatography <2.01> according to the following conditions. Determine the areas of two adjacent peaks, A_a and A_b, having the retention times of about 40 minutes, where A_a is the peak area of shorter retention time and A_b is the peak area of longer retention time: $A_b/(A_a + A_b)$ is between 0.30 and 0.40.

Operating conditions—

Detector: An ultraviolet absorption photometer (wavelength: 254 nm).

Column: A stainless steel column 6.0 mm in inside diameter and 15 cm in length, packed with octadecylsilanized silica gel for liquid chromatography (5 μm in particle diameter).

Column temperature: A constant temperature of about 40°C.

Mobile phase: To 500 mL of water add 500 mL of methanol, 13 mL of diluted 40% tetrabutylammonium hydroxide TS (1 in 4) and 0.68 mL of phosphoric acid, and adjust the pH to 6.8 with ammonia TS and diluted ammonia solution (28) (1 in 20).

Flow rate: Adjust so that the retention time of the peak having the shorter retention time of the two peaks of argatroban is about 40 minutes.

System suitability—

System performance: When the procedure is run with 10 μL of the sample solution under the above operating conditions, the resolution between the two peaks is not less than 1.2.

System repeatability: When the test is repeated 6 times with 10 μL of the sample solution under the above operating conditions, the relative standard deviation of the total area of the two separate peaks of argatroban is not more than 2.0%.

Assay Weigh accurately about 0.5 g of Argatroban Hydrate, dissolve in 20 mL of acetic acid for nonaqueous titration, add 40 mL of acetone for nonaqueous titration, and titrate *<2.50>* with 0.1 mol/L perchloric acid VS (potentiometric titration). Perform a blank determination in the same manner, and make any necessary correction.

Each mL of 0.1 mol/L perchloric acid VS
= 50.86 mg of $C_{23}H_{36}N_6O_5S$

Containers and storage Containers—Tight containers.
Storage—Light-resistant.

L-Arginine

L-アルギニン

$C_6H_{14}N_4O_2$: 174.20
(2*S*)-2-Amino-5-guanidinopentanoic acid
[*74-79-3*]

L-Arginine, when dried, contains not less than 98.5% and not more than 101.0% of L-arginine ($C_6H_{14}N_4O_2$).

Description L-Arginine occurs as white, crystals or crystalline powder. It has a characteristic odor.

It is freely soluble in water and in formic acid, and practically insoluble in ethanol (99.5).

It dissolves in dilute hydrochloric acid.

It is hygroscopic.

Identification Determine the infrared absorption spectrum of previously dried L-Arginine as directed in the potassium bromide disk method under Infrared Spectrophotometry *<2.25>*, and compare the spectrum with the Reference Spectrum: both spectra exhibit similar intensities of absorption at the same wave numbers.

Optical rotation *<2.49>* $[\alpha]_D^{20}$: +26.9 – +27.9° (after drying, 2 g, 6 mol/L hydrochloric acid TS, 25 mL, 100 mm).

pH *<2.54>* The pH of a solution prepared by dissolving 1.0 g of L-Arginine in 10 mL of water is between 10.5 and 12.0.

Purity **(1)** Clarity and color of solution—A solution obtained by dissolving 1.0 g of L-Arginine in 10 mL of water is clear and colorless.

(2) Chloride *<1.03>*—Perform the test with 0.5 g of L-Arginine. Prepare the control solution with 0.30 mL of 0.01 mol/L hydrochloric acid VS (not more than 0.021%).

(3) Sulfate *<1.14>*—Perform the test with 0.6 g of L-Arginine. Prepare the control solution with 0.35 mL of 0.005 mol/L sulfuric acid VS (not more than 0.028%).

(4) Ammonium *<1.02>*—Perform the test with 0.25 g of L-Arginine, using the distillation under reduced pressure. Prepare the control solution with 5.0 mL of Standard Ammonium Solution (not more than 0.02%).

(5) Heavy metals *<1.07>*—Dissolve 2.0 g of L-Arginine in 30 mL of water, add 1 drop of phenolphthalein TS, neutralize with dilute hydrochloric acid, add 2 mL of dilute acetic acid and water to make 50 mL, and perform the test. Prepare the control solution with 2.0 mL of Standard Lead Solution (not more than 10 ppm).

(6) Iron *<1.10>*—Prepare the test solution with 1.0 g of L-Arginine according to Method 1, and perform the test according to Method A. Prepare the control solution with 1.0 mL of Standard Iron Solution (not more than 10 ppm).

(7) Related substances—Dissolve 0.10 g of L-Arginine in 10 mL of water, and use this solution as the sample solution. Pipet 1 mL of the sample solution, and add water to make exactly 50 mL. Pipet 2 mL of this solution, add water to make exactly 20 mL, and use this solution as the standard solution. Perform the test with these solutions as directed under Thin-layer Chromatography *<2.03>*. Spot 5 μL each of the sample solution and standard solution on a plate of silica gel for thin-layer chromatography. Develop the plate with a mixture of 2-propanol and ammonia solution (28) (7:3) to a distance of about 10 cm, and dry the plate at 80°C for 30 minutes. Spray evenly ninhydrin-butanol TS on the plate, and heat the plate at 80°C for 10 minutes: the spot other than the principal spot obtained from the sample solution is not more intense than the spot from the standard solution.

Loss on drying *<2.41>* Not more than 0.30% (1 g, 105°C, 3 hours).

Residue on ignition *<2.44>* Not more than 0.1% (1 g).

Assay Weigh accurately about 80 mg of L-Arginine, previously dried, dissolve in 3 mL of formic acid, add 50 mL of acetic acid (100), and titrate *<2.50>* with 0.1 mol/L perchloric acid VS (potentiometric titration). Perform a blank determination in the same manner, and make any necessary correction.

Each mL of 0.1 mol/L perchloric acid VS
= 8.710 mg of $C_6H_{14}N_4O_2$

Containers and storage Containers—Tight containers.

L-Arginine Hydrochloride

L-アルギニン塩酸塩

$C_6H_{14}N_4O_2.HCl$: 210.66
(2*S*)-2-Amino-5-guanidinopentanoic acid
monohydrochloride
[*1119-34-2*]

L-Arginine Hydrochloride, when dried, contains not less than 98.5% of L-arginine hydrochloride ($C_6H_{14}N_4O_2.HCl$).

Description L-Arginine Hydrochloride occurs as white, crystals or crystalline powder. It is odorless, and has a slight, characteristic taste.

It is freely soluble in water and in formic acid, and very slightly soluble in ethanol (95).

Identification **(1)** Determine the infrared absorption spectrum of L-Arginine Hydrochloride, previously dried, as directed in the potassium bromide disk method under Infrared Spectrophotometry *<2.25>*, and compare the spectrum with the Reference Spectrum: both spectra exhibit similar intensities of absorption at the same wave numbers.

(2) A solution of L-Arginine Hydrochloride (1 in 50) responds to the Qualitative Tests *<1.09>* for chloride.

Optical rotation *<2.49>* $[\alpha]_D^{20}$: +21.5 – +23.5° (after drying, 2 g, 6 mol/L hydrochloric acid TS, 25 mL, 100 mm).

pH *<2.54>* Dissolve 1.0 g of L-Arginine Hydrochloride in 10 mL of water: the pH of this solution is between 4.7 and 6.2.

Purity (1) Clarity and color of solution—Dissolve 1.0 g of L-Arginine Hydrochloride in 10 mL of water: the solution is clear and colorless.

(2) Sulfate *<1.14>*—Perform the test with 0.6 g of L-Arginine Hydrochloride. Prepare the control solution with 0.35 mL of 0.005 mol/L sulfuric acid VS (not more than 0.028%).

(3) Ammonium *<1.02>*—Perform the test with 0.25 g of L-Arginine Hydrochloride, using the distillation under reduced pressure. Prepare the control solution with 5.0 mL of Standard Ammonium Solution (not more than 0.02%).

(4) Heavy metals *<1.07>*—Proceed with 1.0 g of L-Arginine Hydrochloride according to Method 1, and perform the test. Prepare the control solution with 2.0 mL of Standard Lead Solution (not more than 20 ppm).

(5) Arsenic *<1.11>*—Prepare the test solution with 1.0 g of L-Arginine Hydrochloride according to Method 1, and perform the test (not more than 2 ppm).

(6) Related substances—Dissolve 0.20 g of L-Arginine Hydrochloride in 10 mL of water, and use this solution as the sample solution. Pipet 1 mL of the sample solution, and add water to make exactly 10 mL. Pipet 1 mL of this solution, add water to make exactly 25 mL, and use this solution as the standard solution. Perform the test with these solutions as directed under Thin-layer Chromatography *<2.03>*. Spot 5 μL each of the sample solution and standard solution on a plate of silica gel for thin-layer chromatography. Develop the plate with a mixture of ethanol (99.5), water, 1-butanol and ammonia water (28) (2:1:1:1) to a distance of about 10 cm, and dry the plate at 100°C for 30 minutes. Spray evenly a solution of ninhydrin in acetone (1 in 50) on the plate, and heat the plate at 80°C for 5 minutes: the spots other than the principal spot obtained from the sample solution are not more intense than the spot from the standard solution.

Loss on drying *<2.41>* Not more than 0.20% (1 g, 105°C, 3 hours).

Residue on ignition *<2.44>* Not more than 0.1% (1 g).

Assay Weigh accurately about 0.1 g of L-Arginine Hydrochloride, previously dried, dissolve in 2 mL of formic acid, add exactly 15 mL of 0.1 mol/L perchloric acid VS, and heat on a water bath for 30 minutes. After cooling, add 45 mL of acetic acid (100), and titrate *<2.50>* the excess perchloric acid with 0.1 mol/L sodium acetate VS (potentiometric titration). Perform a blank determination in the same manner.

Each mL of 0.1 mol/L perchloric acid VS
= 10.53 mg of $C_6H_{14}N_4O_2.HCl$

Containers and storage Containers—Tight containers.

L-Arginine Hydrochloride Injection

L-アルギニン塩酸塩注射液

L-Arginine Hydrochloride Injection is an aqueous injection.

It contains not less than 9.5 w/v% and not more than 10.5 w/v% of L-arginine hydrochloride ($C_6H_{14}N_4O_2.HCl$: 210.66).

Method of preparation

L-Arginine Hydrochloride	100 g
Water for Injection or Sterile Water for Injection in Containers	a sufficient quantity
To make	1000 mL

Prepare as directed under Injections, with the above ingredients.

No preservative is added.

Description L-Arginine Hydrochloride Injection is a clear, colorless liquid.

Identification (1) To 5 mL of a solution of L-Arginine Hydrochloride Injection (1 in 100) add 1 mL of ninhydrin TS, and heat for 3 minutes: a blue-purple color develops.

(2) To 5 mL of a solution of L-Arginine Hydrochloride Injection (1 in 10) add 2 mL of sodium hydroxide TS and 1 to 2 drops of a solution of 1-naphthol in ethanol (95) (1 in 1000), allow to stand for 5 minutes, and add 1 to 2 drops of sodium hypochlorite TS: a red-orange color develops.

pH *<2.54>* 5.0 – 6.0

Bacterial endotoxins *<4.01>* Less than 0.50 EU/mL.

Extractable volume *<6.05>* It meets the requirement.

Foreign insoluble matter *<6.06>* Perform the test according to Method 1: it meets the requirement.

Insoluble particulate matter *<6.07>* It meets the requirement.

Sterility *<4.06>* Perform the test according to the Membrane filtration method: it meets the requirement.

Assay Pipet 20 mL of L-Arginine Hydrochloride Injection, add 7.5 mol/L hydrochloric acid TS to make exactly 100 mL, and determine the optical rotation α_D as directed under Optical Rotation Determination *<2.49>* at 20 ± 1°C in a 100-mm cell.

Amount (mg) of L-arginine hydrochloride ($C_6H_{14}N_4O_2.HCl$)
= $\alpha_D \times 4444$

Containers and storage Containers—Hermetic containers.

Arotinolol Hydrochloride

アロチノロール塩酸塩

and enantiomer

$C_{15}H_{21}N_3O_2S_3.HCl$: 408.00
5-{2-[(2*RS*)-3-(1,1-Dimethylethyl)amino-2-hydroxypropylsulfanyl]-1,3-thiazol-4-yl}thiophene-2-carboxamide monohydrochloride
[68377-91-3]

Arotinolol Hydrochloride, when dried, contains not less than 99.0% of arotinolol hydrochloride ($C_{15}H_{21}N_3O_2S_3.HCl$).

Description Arotinolol Hydrochloride occurs as a white to light yellow crystalline powder.

It is freely soluble in dimethylsulfoxide, slightly soluble in methanol and in water, very slightly soluble in ethanol (99.5), and practically insoluble in diethyl ether.

A solution of Arotinolol Hydrochloride in methanol (1 in 125) does not show optical rotation.

Identification **(1)** Determine the absorption spectrum of a solution of Arotinolol Hydrochloride in methanol (1 in 75,000) as directed under Ultraviolet-visible Spectrophotometry <*2.24*>, and compare the spectrum with the Reference Spectrum: both spectra exhibit similar intensities of absorption at the same wavelengths.

(2) Determine the infrared absorption spectrum of Arotinolol Hydrochloride, previously dried, as directed in the potassium bromide disk method under Infrared Spectrophotometry <*2.25*>, and compare the spectrum with the Reference Spectrum: both spectra exhibit similar intensities of absorption at the same wave numbers.

(3) A solution of Arotinolol Hydrochloride (1 in 200) responds to Qualitative Tests <*1.09*> (2) for chloride.

Purity **(1)** Heavy metals <*1.07*>—Proceed with 1.0 g of Arotinolol Hydrochloride according to Method 2, and perform the test. Prepare the control solution with 1.0 mL of Standard Lead Solution (not more than 10 ppm).

(2) Related substances—Dissolve 0.05 g of Arotinolol Hydrochloride in 10 mL of methanol, and use this solution as the sample solution. Pipet 1 mL of the sample solution, add methanol to make exactly 100 mL. Pipet 1 mL of this solution, add methanol to make exactly 10 mL, and use this solution as the standard solution. Perform the test with these solutions as directed under Thin-layer Chromatography <*2.03*>. Spot 40 μL each of the sample solution and standard solution on a plate of silica gel with fluorescent indicator for thin-layer chromatography. Develop the plate with a mixture of chloroform, methanol, acetone and ammonia solution (28) (30:10:10:1) to a distance of about 12 cm, and air-dry the plate. Examine under ultraviolet light (main wavelength: 254 nm): the spots other than the principal spot obtained from the sample solution are not more intense than the spot from the standard solution.

Loss on drying <*2.41*> Not more than 0.20% (1 g, in vacuum, 105°C, 4 hours).

Residue on ignition <*2.44*> Not more than 0.1% (1 g).

Assay Weigh accurately about 1.5 g of Arotinolol Hydrochloride, previously dried, dissolve in dimethylsulfoxide to make exactly 25 mL. Pipet 5 mL of this solution, add 100 mL of water and 5 mL of sodium hydroxide TS, and extract with three 50-mL portions of dichloromethane. Filter each dichloromethane extract through a pledget of absorbent cotton with anhydrous sodium sulfate on it. Evaporate combined filtrate to dryness in vacuum. Dissolve the residue in 70 mL of acetic acid (100), and titrate <*2.50*> with 0.05 mol/L perchloric acid VS (potentiometric titration). Perform a blank determination in the same manner, and make any necessary correction.

Each mL of 0.05 mol/L perchloric acid VS
= 20.40 mg of $C_{15}H_{21}N_3O_2S_3.HCl$

Containers and storage Containers—Tight containers.
Storage—Light-resistant.

Arsenical Paste

亜ヒ酸パスタ

Arsenical Paste contains not less than 36.0% and not more than 44.0% of arsenic trioxide (As_2O_3: 197.84).

Method of preparation

Arsenic Trioxide, finely powdered	40 g
Procaine Hydrochloride, finely powdered	10 g
Hydrophilic Cream	30 g
Clove Oil	a suitable quantity
Medicinal Carbon	a suitable quantity
To make	100 g

Mix Arsenic Trioxide and Procaine Hydrochloride with Hydrophilic Cream, and add Clove Oil to make a suitably viscous liquid, followed by Medicinal Carbon for coloring.

Description Arsenical Paste is grayish black and has the odor of clove oil.

Identification **(1)** Place 0.1 g of Arsenical Paste in a small flask, add 5 mL of fuming nitric acid and 5 mL of sulfuric acid, and heat over a flame until the reacting liquid becomes colorless and white fumes begin to evolve. After cooling, add the reacting liquid to 20 mL of water cautiously, and add 10 mL of hydrogen sulfide TS while warming: a yellow precipitate is produced (arsenic trioxide).

(2) Shake thoroughly 0.5 g of Arsenical Paste with 25 mL of diethyl ether, 5 mL of dilute hydrochloric acid and 20 mL of water, separate the water layer, and filter: 5 mL of the filtrate responds to Qualitative Tests <*1.09*> for primary aromatic amines (procaine hydrochloride).

(3) Shake thoroughly 0.5 g of Arsenical Paste with 25 mL of diethyl ether and 25 mL of water, separate the water layer, filter, and use the filtrate as the sample solution. Dissolve 0.01 g of procaine hydrochloride in 5 mL of water, and use this solution as the standard solution. Perform the test with these solutions as directed under Thin-layer Chromatography <*2.03*>. Spot 5 μL each of the sample solution and standard solution on a plate of silica gel with fluorescent indicator for thin-layer chromatography. Develop the plate with a mixture of ethyl acetate, ethanol (99.5) and ammonia solution (28) (50:5:1) to a distance of about 10 cm, and air-dry the plate. Examine under ultraviolet light (main wavelength: 254 mm): the spots obtained from the sample solution and standard solution exhibit the same *R*f value.

Assay Weigh accurately about 0.3 g of Arsenical Paste into a 150-mL Kjeldahl flask, add 5 mL of fuming nitric acid and 10 mL of sulfuric acid, and shake thoroughly. Heat cautiously the mixture, gently at first, and then continue strong heating, until red fumes of nitrogen oxide are sparingly evolved. After cooling, add 5 mL of fuming nitric acid, heat again until red fumes of nitrogen oxide are no longer evolved and the reacting liquid becomes clear, and cool. Add 30 mL of a saturated solution of ammonium oxalate monohydrate, heat again until white fumes of sulfuric acid are evolved, and continue the heating for 10 minutes. Decompose completely oxalic acid, cool, transfer cautiously the colorless reacting liquid to a glass-stoppered flask, containing 40 mL of water. Wash thoroughly the Kjeldahl flask with 60 mL of water, add the washings to the content of the glass-stoppered flask, and cool. Dissolve 3 g of potassium iodide in this solution, allow to stand in a dark place at room temperature for 45 minutes, and titrate 〈*2.50*〉 the liberated iodine with 0.1 mol/L sodium thiosulfate VS (indicator: 5 mL of starch TS). Perform a blank determination in the same manner, and make any necessary correction.

Each mL of 0.1 mol/L sodium thiosulfate VS
= 4.946 mg of As_2O_3

Containers and storage Containers—Tight containers.

Arsenic Trioxide

三酸化二ヒ素

As_2O_3: 197.84

Arsenic Trioxide, when dried, contains not less than 99.5% of arsenic trioxide (As_2O_3).

Description Arsenic Trioxide occurs as a white powder.

It is odorless. It is practically insoluble in water, in ethanol (95) and in diethyl ether.

It dissolves in sodium hydroxide TS.

Identification Dissolve 0.2 g of Arsenic Trioxide in 40 mL of water by heating on a water bath: the solution responds to Qualitative Tests 〈*1.09*〉 for arsenite.

Purity Clarity of solution—To 1.0 g of Arsenic Trioxide add 10 mL of ammonia TS, and heat gently: the solution is clear.

Loss on drying 〈*2.41*〉 Not more than 0.5% (1 g, 105°C, 3 hours).

Assay Weigh accurately about 0.15 g of Arsenic Trioxide, previously dried, dissolve in 20 mL of a solution of sodium hydroxide (1 in 25), by warming, if necessary. Add 40 mL of water and 2 drops of methyl orange TS, then add dilute hydrochloric acid until the color of the solution becomes light red. Add 2 g of sodium hydrogen carbonate and 50 mL of water to this solution, and titrate 〈*2.50*〉 with 0.05 mol/L iodine VS (indicator: 3 mL of starch TS).

Each mL of 0.05 mol/L iodine VS = 4.946 mg of As_2O_3

Containers and storage Containers—Tight containers.

Ascorbic Acid

Vitamin C

アスコルビン酸

$C_6H_8O_6$: 176.12
L-*threo*-Hex-2-enono-1,4-lactone
[*50-81-7*]

Ascorbic Acid, when dried, contains not less than 99.0% of L-ascorbic acid ($C_6H_8O_6$).

Description Ascorbic Acid occurs as white crystals or a white crystalline powder. It is odorless, and has an acid taste.

It is freely soluble in water, sparingly soluble in ethanol (95), and practically insoluble in diethyl ether.

Melting point: about 190°C (with decomposition).

Identification **(1)** To 5 mL each of a solution of Ascorbic Acid (1 in 50) add 1 drop of potassium permanganate TS or 1 to 2 drops of 2,6-dichloroindophenol sodium TS: the color of the solution is discharged immediately in each case.

(2) Dissolve 0.1 g of Ascorbic Acid in 100 mL of a solution of metaphosphoric acid (1 in 50). To 5 mL of the solution add iodine TS until the color of the solution becomes light yellow. Then add 1 drop of a solution of copper (II) sulfate pentahydrate (1 in 1000) and 1 drop of pyrrole, and warm the mixture at 50°C for 5 minutes: a blue color develops.

Optical rotation 〈*2.49*〉 $[\alpha]_D^{20}$: +20.5 – +21.5° (2.5 g, water, 25 mL, 100 mm).

pH 〈*2.54*〉 Dissolve 1.0 g of Ascorbic Acid in 20 mL of water: the pH of this solution is between 2.2 and 2.5.

Purity **(1)** Clarity and color of solution—Dissolve 1.0 g of Ascorbic Acid in 20 mL of water: the solution is clear and colorless.

(2) Heavy metals 〈*1.07*〉—Perform the test with 1.0 g of Ascorbic Acid according to Method 1. Prepare the control solution with 2.0 mL of Standard Lead Solution (not more than 20 ppm).

Loss on drying 〈*2.41*〉 Not more than 0.20% (1 g, silica gel, 24 hours).

Residue on ignition 〈*2.44*〉 Not more than 0.1% (1 g).

Assay Weigh accurately about 0.2 g of Ascorbic Acid, previously dried, dissolve in 50 mL of a solution of metaphosphoric acid (1 in 50), and titrate 〈*2.50*〉 with 0.05 mol/L iodine VS (indicator: 1 mL of starch TS).

Each mL of 0.05 mol/L iodine VS
= 8.806 mg of $C_6H_8O_6$

Containers and storage Containers—Tight containers.
Storage—Light-resistant.

Ascorbic Acid Injection

Vitamin C Injection

アスコルビン酸注射液

Ascorbic Acid Injection is an aqueous injection.
It contains not less than 95.0% and not more than 115.0% of the labeled amount of L-ascorbic acid ($C_6H_8O_6$: 176.12).

Method of preparation Prepare as directed under Injections, with the sodium salt of Ascorbic Acid.

Description Ascorbic Acid Injection occurs as a clear, colorless liquid.

Identification **(1)** Measure a volume of Ascorbic Acid Injection, equivalent to 0.5 g of Ascorbic Acid, and add water to make 25 mL. Proceed with 5 mL each of the solution as directed in the Identification (1) under Ascorbic Acid.

(2) Measure a volume of Ascorbic Acid Injection, equivalent to 5 mg of Ascorbic Acid. Add a solution of metaphosphoric acid (1 in 50) to make 5 mL, and proceed with this solution as directed in the Identification (2) under Ascorbic Acid.

(3) Ascorbic Acid Injection responds to Qualitative Tests (1) for sodium salt.

pH <2.54> 5.6 – 7.4

Bacterial endotoxins <4.01> Less than 0.15 EU/mg.

Extractable volume <6.05> It meets requirement.

Foreign insoluble matter <6.06> Perform the test according to Method 1: it meets the requirement.

Insoluble particulate matter <6.07> It meets the requirement.

Sterility <4.06> Perform the test according to the Membrane filtration method: it meets the requirement.

Assay Measure exactly a volume of Ascorbic Acid Injection, equivalent to about 0.1 g of L-ascorbic acid ($C_6H_8O_6$), previously diluted with metaphosphoric acid-acetic acid TS, if necessary, and add metaphosphoric acid-acetic acid TS to make exactly 200 mL. Measure exactly 2 mL of the solution, and shake with 8 mL of metaphosphoric acid-acetic acid TS and 2 mL of hydrogen peroxide TS. Titrate <2.50> with 2,6-dichloroindophenol sodium TS for titration until a light red color persists for 5 seconds. Perform a blank determination in the same manner, and make any necessary correction.

Each mL of 2, 6-dichlorophenol-indophenol sodium TS for titration
= *A* mg of $C_6H_8O_6$

A is decided by the following standardization of 2,6-dichloroindophenol sodium TS for titration.

2,6-Dichlorophenol-indophenol sodium TS for titration: *Preparation*—Dissolve 42 mg of sodium hydrogen carbonate in 50 mL of water, add 0.5 g of 2,6-dichloroindophenol sodium dihydrate and water to make 200 mL, and filter. Prepare before use.

Standardization—Weigh accurately about 50 mg of Ascorbic Acid RS, previously dried in a desiccator (silica gel) for 24 hours, and dissolve in metaphosphoric acid-acetic acid TS to make exactly 100 mL. Pipet 2 mL of this solution, shake with 8 mL of metaphosphoric acid-acetic acid TS and 2 mL of hydrogen peroxide TS, and titrate <2.50> with 2,6-dichloroindophenol sodium TS for titration until a light red color persists for 5 seconds. Perform a blank determination in the same manner, and make any necessary correction. Calculate the quantity (A mg) of L-ascorbic acid ($C_6H_8O_6$) equivalent to 1 mL of this test solution.

Containers and storage Containers—Hermetic containers.
Storage—Under nitrogen atmosphere.

Ascorbic Acid Powder

Vitamin C Powder

アスコルビン酸散

Ascorbic Acid Powder contains not less than 95.0% and not more than 120.0% of the labeled amount of L-ascorbic acid ($C_6H_8O_6$: 176.12).

Method of preparation Prepare as directed under Granules or Powders, with Ascorbic Acid.

Identification (1) Weigh a portion of Ascorbic Acid Powder, equivalent to 0.5 g of Ascorbic Acid, add 30 mL of water, shake for 1 minute, and filter. Proceed with 5 mL each of the filtrate as directed in the Identification (1) under Ascorbic Acid.

(2) Weigh a portion of Ascorbic Acid Powder, equivalent to about 0.01 g of Ascorbic Acid, add 10 mL of a solution of metaphosphoric acid (1 in 50), shake for 1 minute, and filter. Proceed with 5 mL of the filtrate as directed in the Identification (2) under Ascorbic Acid.

Purity Rancidity—Ascorbic Acid Powder is free from any unpleasant or rancid odor and taste.

Assay Weigh accurately a portion of Ascorbic Acid Powder, equivalent to about 0.1 g of L-ascorbic acid ($C_6H_8O_6$), extract with several successive portions of metaphosphoric acid-acetic acid TS, combine the extracts, and filter. Wash the residue with metaphosphoric acid-acetic acid TS. Combine the filtrates and washings, and add metaphosphoric acid-acetic acid to make exactly 200 mL. Pipet 2 mL of the solution, and shake with 8 mL of metaphosphoric acid-acetic acid TS and 2 mL of hydrogen peroxide TS. Titrate <2.50> with 2,6-dichloroindophenol sodium TS for titration until a light red color persists for 5 seconds. Perform a blank determination in the same manner, and make any necessary correction.

Each mL of 2,6-dichlorophenol-indophenol sodium TS for titration
= *A* mg of $C_6H_8O_6$

A is decided by the following standardization of 2,6-dichloroindophenol sodium TS for titration.

2,6-Dichlorophenol-indophenol sodium TS for titration: *Preparation*—Dissolve 42 mg of sodium hydrogen carbonate in 50 mL of water, add 0.05 g of 2,6-dichloroindophenol sodium dihydrate and water to make 200 mL, and filter. Prepare before use.

Standardization—Weigh accurately about 50 mg of Ascorbic Acid RS, previously dried in a desiccator (silica gel) for 24 hours, and dissolve in metaphosphoric acid-acetic acid TS to make exactly 100 mL. Pipet 2 mL of this solution, shake with 8 mL of metaphosphoric acid-acetic acid TS and 2 mL of hydrogen peroxide TS, and titrate <2.50> with 2,6-dichloroindophenol sodium TS for titration until a light red color persists for 5 seconds. Perform a blank determination in the same manner, and make any necessary correction. Calculate the quantity (*A* mg) of L-ascorbic acid ($C_6H_8O_6$) equivalent to 1 mL of this test solution.

Containers and storage Containers—Tight containers.

Ascorbic Acid and Calcium Pantothenate Tablets

アスコルビン酸・パントテン酸カルシウム錠

Ascorbic Acid and Calcium Pantothenate Tablets contain not less than 95.0% and not more than 105.0% of the labeled amount of L-ascorbic acid ($C_6H_8O_6$: 176.12) and not less than 93.0% and not more than 107.0% of the labeled amount of calcium pantothenate ($C_{18}H_{32}CaN_2O_{10}$: 476.53).

Method of preparation Prepare as directed under Tablets, with Ascorbic Acid and Calcium Pantothenate.

Identification (1) To a quantity of powdered Ascorbic

Acid and Calcium Pantothenate Tablets, equivalent to 0.5 g of Ascorbic Acid, add 30 mL of water, shake for 1 minute, and filter. Proceed as directed in the Identification (1) under Ascorbic Acid using 5 mL each of the filtrate.

(2) To a quantity of powdered Ascorbic Acid and Calcium Pantothenate Tablets, equivalent to 3 mg of Calcium Pantothenate, add 20 mL of ethanol (95), shake vigorously for 10 minutes, centrifuge, and use the supernatant liquid as the sample solution. Separately, dissolve 3 mg of calcium pantothenate in 20 mL of ethanol (95), and use this solution as the standard solution. Perform the test with these solutions as directed under Thin-layer Chromatography <*2.03*>. Spot 10 μL each of the sample solution and standard solution on a plate of silica gel for thin-layer chromatography. Develop the plate with a mixture of ethyl acetate, methanol and dilute acetic acid (5:3:2) to a distance of about 10 cm, and air-dry the plate. Spray evenly a solution of ninhydrin in ethanol (95) (1 in 200) on the plate, and heat the plate at 120°C for 20 minutes: one of the spots obtained from the sample solution and the spot from the standard solution are purple in color and their *Rf* value are the same.

Uniformity of dosage units <*6.02*> **(1)** L-Ascorbic acid—Perform the Mass variation test, or the Content uniformity test according to the following method: it meets the requirement.

To 1 tablet of Ascorbic Acid and Calcium Pantothenate Tablets add 100 mL of a solution of metaphosphoric acid (1 in 50), stir thoroughly, and titrate <*2.50*> with 0.05 mol/L iodine VS (indicator: 1 mL of starch TS).

Each mL of 0.05 mol/L iodine VS = 8.806 mg of $C_6H_8O_6$

(2) Calcium pantothenate—Perform the test according to the following method: it meets the requirement of the Content uniformity test.

To 1 tablet of Ascorbic Acid and Calcium Pantothenate Tablets add exactly *V* mL of the internal standard solution so that each mL contains about 0.15 mg of calcium pantothenate ($C_{18}H_{32}CaN_2O_{10}$), shake vigorously for 15 minutes, filter through a membrane filter with a pore size not exceeding 0.45 μm, and use the filtrate as the sample solution. Then, proceed as directed in the Assay (2).

Amount (mg) of calcium pantothenate ($C_{18}H_{32}CaN_2O_{10}$)
$= M_S \times Q_T/Q_S \times V/200$

M_S: Amount (mg) of Calcium Pantothenate RS taken, calculated on the dried basis

Internal Standard Solution—A solution of acetaminophen (1 in 50,000).

Dissolution <*6.10*> **(1)** L-Ascorbic acid—When the test is performed at 50 revolutions per minute according to the Paddle method, using 900 mL of water as the dissolution medium, the dissolution rate in 60 minutes of Ascorbic Acid and Calcium Pantothenate Tablets is not less than 85%.

Start the test with 1 tablet of Ascorbic Acid and Calcium Pantothenate Tablets, withdraw 20 mL of the medium at the specified minute after starting the test, and filter through a membrane filter with a pore size not exceeding 0.45 μm. Discard not less than 10 mL of the first filtrate, pipet *V* mL of the subsequent filtrate, add 1st fluid for dissolution test to make exactly *V′* mL so that each mL contains about 11 μg of L-ascorbic acid ($C_6H_8O_6$), and use this solution as the sample solution. Separately, weigh accurately about 22 mg of Ascorbic Acid RS, previously dried in a desiccator (silica gel) for 24 hours, dissolve in water to make exactly 100 mL, and warm at 37°C for 1 hour. Pipet 5 mL of this solution, add 1st fluid for dissolution test to make exactly 100 mL, and use this solution as the standard solution. Determine the absorbances, A_T and A_S, at 243 nm of the sample solution and standard solution as directed under Ultraviolet-visible Spectrophotometry <*2.24*> within 1 hour after withdrawing the medium, using 1st fluid for dissolution test as the blank.

Dissolution rate (%) with respect to the labeled amount of L-ascorbic acid ($C_6H_8O_6$)
$= M_S \times A_T/A_S \times V'/V \times 1/C \times 45$

M_S: Amount (mg) of Ascorbic Acid RS taken
C: Labeled amount (mg) of L-ascorbic acid ($C_6H_8O_6$) in 1 tablet

(2) Calcium pantothenate—When the test is performed at 50 revolutions per minute according to the Paddle method, using 900 mL of water as the dissolution medium, the dissolution rate in 90 minutes of Ascorbic Acid and Calcium Pantothenate Tablets is not less than 75%.

Start the test with 1 tablet of Ascorbic Acid and Calcium Pantothenate Tablets, withdraw 20 mL of the medium at the specified minute after starting the test, and filter through a membrane filter with a pore size not exceeding 0.45 μm. Discard not less than 10 mL of the first filtrate, pipet *V* mL of the subsequent filtrate, add 1st fluid for dissolution test to make exactly *V′* mL so that each mL contains about 3.3 μg of calcium pantothenate ($C_{18}H_{32}CaN_2O_{10}$), and use this solution as the sample solution. Separately, weigh accurately about 16.5 mg of Calcium Pantothenate RS (separately determine the loss on drying <*2.41*> under the same conditions as Calcium Pantothenate), and dissolve in water to make exactly 100 mL. Pipet 2 mL of this solution, add water to make exactly 100 mL, and use this solution as the standard solution. Perform the test with exactly 100 μL each of the sample solution and standard solution as directed under Liquid Chromatography <*2.01*> according to the following conditions, and determine the peak areas, A_T and A_S, of pantothenic acid in each solution.

Dissolution rate (%) with respect to the labeled amount of calcium pantothenate ($C_{18}H_{32}CaN_2O_{10}$)
$= M_S \times A_T/A_S \times V'/V \times 1/C \times 18$

M_S: Amount (mg) of Calcium Pantothenate RS taken, calculated on the dried basis
C: Labeled amount (mg) of calcium pantothenate ($C_{18}H_{32}CaN_2O_{10}$) in 1 tablet

Operating conditions—

Detector: An ultraviolet absorption photometer (wavelength: 210 nm).

Column: A stainless steel column 4.6 mm in inside diameter and 15 cm in length, packed with octadecylsilanized silicone polymer coated silica gel for liquid chromatography (5 μm in particle diameter).

Column temperature: A constant temperature of about 35°C.

Mobile phase: Dissolve 7.80 g of sodium dihydrogen phosphate dihydrate in 900 mL of water, adjust to pH 2.6 with phosphoric acid, and add water to make 1000 mL. To 970 mL of this solution add 30 mL of acetonitrile for liquid chromatography.

Flow rate: Adjust so that the retention time of pantothenic acid is about 10 minutes.

System suitability—

System performance: When the procedure is run with 100 μL of the standard solution under the above operating conditions, the number of theoretical plates and the symmetry factor of the peak of pantothenic acid are not less than 5000

and not more than 2.0, respectively.

System repeatability: When the test is repeated 6 times with 100 μL of the standard solution under the above operating conditions, the relative standard deviation of the peak area of pantothenic acid is not more than 2.0%.

Assay **(1)** L-Ascorbic acid—Weigh accurately the mass of not less than 20 tablets of Ascorbic Acid and Calcium Pantothenate Tablets, and powder. Weigh accurately a portion of the powder, equivalent to about 0.1 g of L-ascorbic acid ($C_6H_8O_6$), add 50 mL of a solution of metaphosphoric acid (1 in 50), stir thoroughly, and titrate <*2.50*> with 0.05 mol/L iodine VS (indicator: 1 mL of starch TS).

Each mL of 0.05 mol/L iodine VS = 8.806 mg of $C_6H_8O_6$

(2) Calcium pantothenate—Weigh accurately the mass of not less than 20 tablets of Ascorbic Acid and Calcium Pantothenate Tablets, and powder. Weigh accurately a portion of the powder, equivalent to about 3 mg of calcium pantothenate ($C_{18}H_{32}CaN_2O_{10}$), add exactly 20 mL of the internal standard solution, shake for 15 minutes, filter through a membrane filter with a pore size not exceeding 0.45 μm, and use the filtrate as the sample solution. Separately, weigh accurately about 30 mg of Calcium Pantothenate RS (separately determine the loss on drying <*2.41*> under the same conditions as Calcium Pantothenate), and dissolve in water to make exactly 50 mL. Pipet 5 mL of this solution, add exactly 20 mL of the internal standard solution, and use this solution as the standard solution. Perform the test with 5 μL each of the sample solution and standard solution as directed under Liquid Chromatography <*2.01*> according to the following conditions, and calculate the ratios, Q_T and Q_S, of the peak area of pantothenic acid to that of the internal standard.

Amount (mg) of calcium pantothenate ($C_{18}H_{32}CaN_2O_{10}$)
$= M_S \times Q_T/Q_S \times 1/10$

M_S: Amount (mg) of Calcium Pantothenate RS taken, calculated on the dried basis

Internal standard solution—A solution of acetaminophen (1 in 50,000).

Operating conditions—

Detector: An ultraviolet absorption photometer (wavelength: 200 nm).

Column: A stainless steel column 4.6 mm in inside diameter and 5 cm in length, packed with octadecylsilanized silica gel for liquid chromatography (3 μm in particle diameter).

Column temperature: A constant temperature of about 25°C.

Mobile phase: A mixture of 0.05 mol/L sodium dihydrogen phosphate TS and acetonitrile for liquid chromatography (97:3).

Flow rate: Adjust so that the retention time of pantothenic acid is about 3 minutes.

System suitability—

System performance: When the procedure is run with 5 μL of the standard solution under the above operating conditions, pantothenic acid and the internal standard are eluted in this order with the resolution between these peaks being not less than 4.

System repeatability: When the test is repeated 6 times with 5 μL of the standard solution under the above operating conditions, the relative standard deviation of the ratio of the peak area of pantothenic acid to that of the internal standard is not more than 1.0%.

Containers and storage Containers—Tight containers.

L-Aspartic Acid

L-アスパラギン酸

HO2C–CH2–C(H)(NH2)–CO2H

$C_4H_7NO_4$: 133.10
(2*S*)-2-Aminobutanedioic acid
[*56-84-8*]

L-Aspartic Acid, when dried, contains not less than 98.5% and not more than 101.0% of L-aspartic acid ($C_4H_7NO_4$).

Description L-Aspartic Acid occurs as white, crystals or crystalline powder.

It is sparingly soluble in water, and practically insoluble in ethanol (99.5).

It dissolves in dilute hydrochloric acid and in 0.2 mol/L sodium hydroxide TS.

Identification Determine the infrared absorption spectrum of L-Aspartic Acid as directed in the potassium bromide disk method under Infrared Spectrophotometry <*2.25*>, and compare the spectrum with the Reference Spectrum: both spectra exhibit similar intensities of absorption at the same wave numbers.

Optical rotation <*2.49*> $[\alpha]_D^{20}$: +24.0 – +26.0° (2 g, after drying, 6 mol/L hydrochloric acid TS, 25 mL, 100 mm).

pH <*2.54*> Dissolve 0.4 g of L-Aspartic Acid in 100 mL of water by warming, and allow to cool: between 2.5 and 3.5.

Purity **(1)** Clarity and color of solution—Dissolve 1.0 g of L-Aspartic Acid in 20 mL of 1 mol/L hydrochloric acid TS: the solution is clear and colorless.

(2) Chloride <*1.03*>—Dissolve 0.5 g of L-Aspartic Acid in 6 mL of dilute nitric acid and 20 mL of water, add water to make 50 mL, and perform the test with this solution as the test solution. Prepare the control solution with 0.30 mL of 0.01 mol/L hydrochloric acid VS (not more than 0.021%).

(3) Sulfate <*1.14*>—Dissolve 0.6 g of L-Aspartic Acid in 5 mL of dilute hydrochloric acid and 30 mL of water, add water to make 45 mL, and add 5 mL of barium chloride TS. Perform the test with this solution as the test solution. Prepare the control solution with 0.35 mL of 0.005 mol/L sulfuric acid VS, add 5 mL of dilute hydrochloric acid and water to make 45 mL, and add 5 mL of barium chloride (not more than 0.028%).

(4) Ammonium <*1.02*>—Perform the test with 0.25 g of L-Aspartic Acid. Prepare the control solution with 5.0 mL of Standard Ammonium Solution (not more than 0.02%).

(5) Heavy metals <*1.07*>—Proceed with 1.0 g of L-Aspartic Acid according to Method 4, and perform the test. Prepare the control solution with 1.0 mL of Standard Lead Solution (not more than 10 ppm).

(6) Iron <*1.10*>—Prepare the test solution with 1.0 g of L-Aspartic Acid according to Method 1, and perform the test according to Method A. Prepare the control solution with 1.0 mL of Standard Iron Solution (not more than 10 ppm).

(7) Related substances—Dissolve 0.20 g of L-Aspartic Acid in 10 mL of 0.2 mol/L sodium hydroxide TS, and use this solution as the sample solution. Pipet 1 mL of the sample solution, add water to make exactly 10 mL. Pipet 1 mL of this solution, add water to make exactly 50 mL, and use this solution as the standard solution. Perform the test with these solutions as directed under Thin-layer Chromatography <*2.03*>. Spot 5 μL each of the sample solution and standard solution on a plate of silica gel for thin-layer chromatography, develop with a mixture of 1-butanol, water and acetic acid (100) (3:1:1) to a distance of about 10 cm, and dry the plate at 80°C for 30 minutes. Spray evenly a solution of ninhydrin in a mixture of methanol and acetic acid (100) (97:3) (1 in 100), and heat the plate at 80°C for 10 minutes: the spot other than the principal spot obtained from the sample solution is not more intense than the spot from the standard solution.

Loss on drying <*2.41*> Not more than 0.30% (1 g, 105°C, 3 hours).

Residue on ignition <*2.44*> Not more than 0.1% (1 g).

Assay Weigh accurately about 0.15 g of L-Aspartic Acid, previously dried, dissolve in 50 mL of water by warming. After cooling, titrate <*2.50*> with 0.1 mol/L sodium hydroxide VS (potentiometric titration). Perform a blank determination in the same manner, and make any necessary correction.

Each mL of 0.1 mol/L sodium hydroxide VS
= 13.31 mg of $C_4H_7NO_4$

Containers and storage Containers—Tight containers.

Aspirin

Acetylsalicylic Acid

アスピリン

$C_9H_8O_4$: 180.16
2-Acetoxybenzoic acid
[50-78-2]

Aspirin, when dried, contains not less than 99.5% of aspirin ($C_9H_8O_4$).

Description Aspirin occurs as white, crystals, granules or powder. It is odorless, and has a slight acid taste.

It is freely soluble in ethanol (95) and in acetone, soluble in diethyl ether, and slightly soluble in water.

It dissolves in sodium hydroxide TS and in sodium carbonate TS.

In moist air, it gradually hydrolyzes to salicylic acid and acetic acid.

Melting point: about 136°C (bath fluid is heated at 130°C previously).

Identification **(1)** Boil 0.1 g of Aspirin in 5 mL of water for 5 to 6 minutes, cool, and add 1 to 2 drops of iron (III) chloride TS: a red-purple color is produced.

(2) Boil 0.5 g of Aspirin in 10 mL of sodium carbonate TS for 5 minutes, and add 10 mL of dilute sulfuric acid: the odor of acetic acid is perceptible, and a white precipitate is produced. Filter the precipitate, add 3 mL of ethanol (95) and 3 mL of sulfuric acid to the filtrate, and heat: the odor of ethyl acetate is perceptible.

Purity **(1)** Clarity of solution—Dissolve 0.5 g of Aspirin in 10 mL of warm sodium carbonate TS: the solution is clear.

(2) Salicylic acid—Dissolve 2.5 g of Aspirin in 25 mL of ethanol (95), and add 1.0 mL of this solution to a solution which is prepared by transferring 1 mL of a freshly prepared dilute ammonium iron (III) sulfate TS to a Nessler tube and diluting with water to 50 mL. Allow to stand for 30 seconds: the solution has no more color than the following control solution.

Control solution: Dissolve 0.100 g of salicylic acid in water, and add 1 mL of acetic acid (100) and water to make 1000 mL. Add 1.0 mL of this solution to a solution which is prepared by transferring 1 mL of freshly prepared dilute ammonium iron (III) sulfate TS and 1 mL of ethanol (95) to a Nessler tube and diluting with water to 50 mL. Allow to stand for 30 seconds.

(3) Chloride <*1.03*>—Boil 1.8 g of Aspirin in 75 mL of water for 5 minutes, cool, add water to make 75 mL, and filter. To 25 mL of the filtrate add 6 mL of dilute nitric acid and water to make 50 mL, and perform the test using this solution as the test solution. Prepare the control solution with 0.25 mL of 0.01 mol/L hydrochloric acid VS (not more than 0.015%).

(4) Sulfate <*1.14*>—To 25 mL of the filtrate obtained in (3) add 1 mL of dilute hydrochloric acid and water to make 50 mL. Perform the test using this solution as the test solution. Prepare the control solution with 0.50 mL of 0.005 mol/L sulfuric acid VS (not more than 0.040%).

(5) Heavy metals <*1.07*>—Dissolve 2.5 g of Aspirin in 30 mL of acetone, add 2 mL of dilute acetic acid and water to make 50 mL, and perform the test using this solution as the test solution. Prepare the control solution with 2.5 mL of Standard Lead Solution, 30 mL of acetone, 2 mL of dilute acetic acid and water to make 50 mL (not more than 10 ppm).

(6) Readily carbonizable substances <*1.15*>—Weigh 0.5 g of Aspirin, and perform the test. The solution has no more color than Matching Fluid Q.

Loss on drying <*2.41*> Not more than 0.5% (3 g, silica gel, 5 hours).

Residue on ignition <*2.44*> Not more than 0.1% (1 g).

Assay Weigh accurately about 1.5 g of Aspirin, previously dried, add exactly 50 mL of 0.5 mol/L sodium hydroxide VS, and boil gently for 10 minutes under a reflux condenser with a carbon dioxide-absorbing tube (soda lime). Cool, and titrate <*2.50*> immediately the excess sodium hydroxide with 0.25 mol/L sulfuric acid VS (indicator: 3 drops of phenolphthalein TS). Perform a blank determination in the same manner.

Each mL of 0.5 mol/L sodium hydroxide VS
= 45.04 mg of $C_9H_8O_4$

Containers and storage Containers—Well-closed containers.

Aspirin Tablets

Acetylsalicylic Acid Tablets

アスピリン錠

Aspirin Tablets contain not less than 95.0% and not more than 105.0% of the labeled amount of aspirin ($C_9H_8O_4$: 180.16).

Method of preparation Prepare as directed under Tablets, with Aspirin.

Identification **(1)** Weigh a quantity of powdered Aspirin Tablets, equivalent to 0.1 g of Aspirin, add 10 mL of water, and boil for 5 to 6 minutes. After cooling, filter, and add 1 to 2 drops of iron (III) chloride TS to the filtrate: a red-violet color develops.

(2) Weigh a portion of powdered Aspirin Tablets, equivalent to 0.5 g of Aspirin, extract with two 10-mL portions of warm ethanol (95), and filter the combined extracts. Evaporate the filtrate to dryness, and boil the residue with 10 mL of sodium carbonate TS for 5 minutes. Proceed as directed in the Identification (2) under Aspirin.

Purity Salicylic acid—Take a portion of the powdered Aspirin Tablets, equivalent to 1.0 g of Aspirin, shake with 15 mL of ethanol (95) for 5 minutes, filter, discard the first 5 mL of the filtrate, and add 1.0 mL of the subsequent filtrate to a solution which is prepared by transferring 1 mL of freshly prepared dilute ammonium iron (III) sulfate TS to a Nessler tube and diluting with water to make 50 mL. Proceed as directed in the Purity (2) under Aspirin.

Assay Weigh accurately and powder not less than 20 Aspirin Tablets. Weigh accurately a portion of the powder, equivalent to about 1.5 g of aspirin ($C_9H_8O_4$), add exactly 50 mL of 0.5 mol/L sodium hydroxide VS, and proceed as directed in the Assay under Aspirin.

Each mL of 0.5 mol/L sodium hydroxide VS
= 45.04 mg of $C_9H_8O_4$

Containers and storage Containers—Well-closed containers.

Aspirin Aluminum

Aluminum Acetylsalicylate

アスピリンアルミニウム

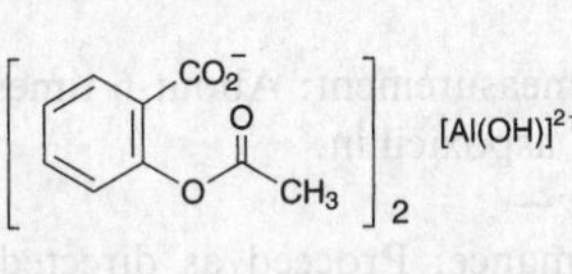

$C_{18}H_{15}AlO_9$: 402.29
Bis(2-acetoxybenzoato)hydroxoaluminium
[23413-80-1]

Aspirin Aluminum contains not less than 83.0% and not more than 90.0% of aspirin ($C_9H_8O_4$: 180.16), and not less than 6.0% and not more than 7.0% of aluminum (Al: 26.98), calculated on the anhydrous basis.

Description Aspirin Aluminum occurs as a white crystalline powder. It is odorless or has a slight, acetic odor.

It is practically insoluble in water, in methanol, in ethanol (95) and in diethyl ether.

It dissolves, with decomposition, in sodium hydroxide TS and in sodium carbonate TS.

Identification **(1)** Dissolve 0.1 g of Aspirin Aluminum in 10 mL of sodium hydroxide TS by heating, if necessary. Neutralize 2 mL of the solution with hydrochloric acid, and add 1 to 2 drops of iron (III) chloride TS: a red-purple color develops.

(2) Determine the absorption spectrum of the sample solution obtained in the Assay (1) as directed under Ultraviolet-visible Spectrophotometry <*2.24*>: it exhibits a maximum between 277 nm and 279 nm.

(3) Place 2 g of Aspirin Aluminum in a platinum crucible, and ignite until charred. To the residue add 1 g of anhydrous sodium carbonate, and ignite for 20 minutes. After cooling, to the residue add 15 mL of dilute hydrochloric acid, shake, and filter: the filtrate responds to Qualitative Tests <*1.09*> for aluminum salt.

Purity **(1)** Salicylate—Using A_{T2} and A_{S2} obtained in the Assay (1), calculate the amount of salicylate [as salicylic acid ($C_7H_6O_3$: 138.12)] by the following equation: salicylate content is not more than 7.5%, calculated on the anhydrous basis.

Amount (mg) of salicylic acid ($C_7H_6O_3$)
$= M_S \times A_{T2}/A_{S2} \times 1/4$

M_S: Amount (mg) of salicylic acid for assay taken

(2) Heavy metals <*1.07*>—Place 2.0 g of Aspirin Aluminum in a porcelain crucible, cover the crucible loosely, and ignite at a low temperature until charred. After cooling, add 2 mL of nitric acid and 1 mL of sulfuric acid to the content of the crucible, heat gently the crucible until white fumes are evolved, and continue the heating until white fumes are no longer evolved, then ignite between 500°C and 600°C until the carbon is incinerated. When the incineration is not completed, add 2 mL of nitric acid and 1 mL of sulfuric acid, and heat gently in the same manner, then ignite between 500°C and 600°C to incinerate completely. After cooling, add 2 mL of hydrochloric acid, and proceed as directed in Method 2, and perform the test. Prepare the control solution by using the same quantities of the same reagents as directed for the preparation of the test solution, and add 2.0 mL of Standard Lead Solution and water to make 50 mL (not more than 10 ppm).

(3) Arsenic <*1.11*>—Dissolve 1.0 g of Aspirin Aluminum in 15 mL of sodium hydroxide TS. To this solution add 1 drop of phenolphthalein TS, and with stirring, add dropwise hydrochloric acid until the red color of the solution disappears. Then add 2 mL of hydrochloric acid, cool with occasional shaking for 10 minutes, and filter with a glass filter (G3). Wash the residue with two 5 mL portions of 1 mol/L hydrochloric acid TS, and combine the filtrate and the washings. Use this solution as the test solution, and perform the test (not more than 2 ppm).

Water <*2.48*> Not more than 4.0% (0.15 g, direct titration).

Assay **(1)** Aspirin—Weigh accurately about 0.1 g of Aspirin Aluminum, add 40 mL of sodium fluoride TS, and shake for 5 minutes. Allow the solution to stand for 10 minutes with frequent shaking. Extract the solution with six 20-mL portions of chloroform. Combine all chloroform extracts, and add chloroform to make exactly 200 mL. Measure exactly 10 mL of this solution, add chloroform to make exactly 100 mL, and use this solution as the sample solution. Separately, weigh accurately about 90 mg of salicylic acid for assay, previously dried in a desiccator (silica gel) for 3 hours, and dissolve in chloroform to make exactly 200 mL. Measure exactly 5 mL of this solution, add chloroform to make exactly 200 mL, and use this solution as the standard solution (1). Then weigh accurately about 90 mg of Aspirin RS, previously dried in a desiccator (silica gel) for 5 hours, and dissolve in chloroform to make exactly 200 mL. Measure exactly 10 mL of this solution, add chloroform to make exactly 100 mL, and use this solution as the standard solution (2). Perform the test with these solutions as directed under Ultraviolet-visible Spectrophotometry <*2.24*>. Determine the absorbances, A_{T1} and A_{S1}, of the sample solution and standard solution (1) at 278 nm, and absorbances, A_{T2} and A_{S2}, of these solution, at 308 nm, respectively. Then determine the absorbance A_{S3} of the standard solution (2) at 278 nm.

$$\text{Amount (mg) of aspirin } (C_9H_8O_4) = M_S \times \left(\frac{A_{T1} - \dfrac{A_{T2} \times A_{S1}}{A_{S2}}}{A_{S3}} \right)$$

M_S: Amount (mg) of Aspirin RS taken

(2) Aluminum—Weigh accurately about 0.4 g of Aspirin Aluminum, and dissolve in 10 mL of sodium hydroxide TS. Add dropwise 1 mol/L hydrochloric acid TS to adjust the solution to a pH of about 1, add 20 mL of acetic acid-ammonium acetate buffer solution (pH 3.0) and 0.5 mL of Cu-PAN TS, and heat. While boiling, titrate ⟨2.50⟩ with 0.05 mol/L disodium dihydrogen ethylenediamine tetraacetate VS until the color of the solution changes from red to yellow and persists for 1 minute. Perform a blank determination in the same manner, and make any necessary correction.

Each mL of 0.05 mol/L disodium dihydrogen ethylenediamine tetraacetate VS
= 1.349 mg of Al

Containers and storage Containers—Well-closed containers.

Aspoxicillin Hydrate

アスポキシシリン水和物

$C_{21}H_{27}N_5O_7S.3H_2O$: 547.58
(2*S*,5*R*,6*R*)-6-[(2*R*)-2-[(2*R*)-2-Amino-3-methylcarbamoylpropanoylamino]-2-(4-hydroxyphenyl)acetylamino]-3,3-dimethyl-7-oxo-4-thia-1-azabicyclo[3.2.0]heptane-2-carboxylic acid trihydrate
[*63358-49-6*, anhydride]

Aspoxicillin Hydrate contains not less than 950 μg (potency) and not more than 1020 μg (potency) per mg, calculated on the anhydrous basis. The potency of Aspoxicillin Hydrate is expressed as mass (potency) of aspoxicillin ($C_{21}H_{27}N_5O_7S$: 493.53).

Description Aspoxicillin Hydrate occurs as a white, crystals or crystalline powder.

It is freely soluble in *N,N*-dimethylformamide, sparingly soluble in water, and practically insoluble in acetonitrile, in methanol and in ethanol (95).

Identification **(1)** Determine the absorption spectrum of a solution of Aspoxicillin Hydrate (1 in 4000) as directed under Ultraviolet-visible Spectrophotometry ⟨2.24⟩, and compare the spectrum with the Reference Spectrum or the spectrum of a solution of Aspoxicillin RS prepared in the same manner as the sample solution: both spectra exhibit similar intensities of absorption at the same wavelengths.

(2) Determine the infrared absorption spectrum of Aspoxicillin Hydrate as directed in the potassium bromide disk method under Infrared Spectrophotometry ⟨2.25⟩, and compare the spectrum with the Reference Spectrum or spectrum of Aspoxicillin RS: both spectra exhibit similar intensities of absorption at the same wave numbers.

Optical rotation ⟨2.49⟩ $[\alpha]_D^{20}$: +170 – +185° (0.2 g calculated on the anhydrous bases, water, 20 mL, 100 mm).

pH ⟨2.54⟩ Dissolve 1.0 g of Aspoxicillin Hydrate in 50 mL of water: the pH of the solution is between 4.2 and 5.2.

Purity **(1)** Clarity and color of solution—Dissolve 1.0 g of Aspoxicillin Hydrate in 50 mL of water: the solution is clear and colorless.

(2) Heavy metals ⟨1.07⟩—Proceed with 2.0 g of Aspoxicillin Hydrate according to Method 2, and perform the test. Prepare the control solution with 2.0 mL of Standard Lead Solution (not more than 10 ppm).

(3) Arsenic ⟨1.11⟩—Prepare the test solution with 2.0 g of Aspoxicillin Hydrate according to Method 5, and perform the test (not more than 1 ppm).

(4) Related substances—Dissolve 0.05 g of Aspoxicillin Hydrate in 10 mL of the mobile phase, and use this solution as the sample solution. Pipet 1 mL of the sample solution, add the mobile phase to make exactly 100 mL, and use this solution as the standard solution. Perform the test with exactly 10 μL each of these solutions as directed under Liquid Chromatography ⟨2.01⟩ according to the following conditions, and determine the areas of each peak by the automatic integration method: the area of each peak other than aspoxicillin obtained from the sample solution is not larger than 3/10 times the peak area of aspoxicillin from the standard solution, and the total of peak areas other than aspoxicillin from the sample solution is not larger than the peak area of aspoxicillin from the standard solution.

Operating conditions—

Detector, column, column temperature, mobile phase, and flow rate: Proceed as directed in the operating conditions in the Assay.

Time span of measurement: About 6 times as long as the retention time of aspoxicillin.

System suitability—

System performance: Proceed as directed in the system suitability in the Assay.

Test for required detectability: Pipet 2 mL of the standard solution, add the mobile phase to make exactly 10 mL. Confirm that the peak area of aspoxicillin obtained with 10 μL of this solution is equivalent to 15 to 25% of that with 10 μL of the standard solution.

System repeatability: When the test is repeated 6 times with 10 μL of the standard solution under the above operating conditions, the relative standard deviation of the peak areas of aspoxicillin is not more than 5%.

Water ⟨2.48⟩ Not less than 9.5% and not more than 13.0% (0.2 g, volumetric titration, direct titration).

Assay Weigh accurately an amount of Aspoxicillin Hydrate and Aspoxicillin RS, equivalent to about 0.1 g (potency), dissolve each in a suitable amount of water, add exactly 10 mL of the internal standard solution, 6.5 mL of acetonitrile and water to make 50 mL, and use these solutions as the sample solution and the standard solution, respectively. Perform the test with 10 μL each of these solutions as directed under Liquid Chromatography ⟨2.01⟩ according to the following conditions, and calculate the ratios, Q_T and Q_S, of the peak area of aspoxicillin to that of the internal standard.

$$\text{Amount [}\mu\text{g (potency)] of aspoxicillin } (C_{21}H_{27}N_5O_7S) = M_S \times Q_T/Q_S \times 1000$$

M_S: Amount [mg (potency)] of Aspoxicillin RS taken

Internal standard solution—A solution of *N*-(3-hydroxyphenyl)acetamide (1 in 1000).

Operating conditions—

Detector: An ultraviolet absorption photometer (wavelength: 280 nm).

Column: A stainless steel column 4.6 mm in inside diameter and 15 cm in length, packed with octadecylsilanized silica gel for liquid chromatography (5 μm in particle diameter).

Column temperature: A constant temperature of about 40°C.

Mobile phase: To 130 mL of acetonitrile add potassium dihydrogenphosphate TS (pH 3.0) to make 1000 mL.

Flow rate: Adjust so that the retention time of aspoxicillin is about 3 minutes.

System suitability—

System performance: When the procedure is run with 10 μL of the standard solution under the above operating conditions, aspoxicillin and the internal standard are eluted in this order with the resolution between these peaks being not less than 8.

System repeatability: When the test is repeated 6 times with 10 μL of the standard solution under the above operating conditions, the relative standard deviation of the ratios of the peak area of aspoxicillin to that of the internal standard is not more than 0.8%.

Containers and storage Containers—Tight containers.

Atenolol

アテノロール

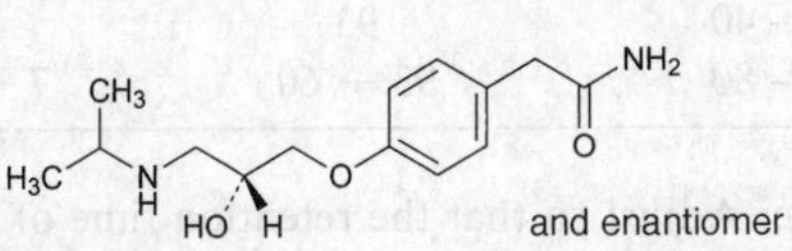

and enantiomer

$C_{14}H_{22}N_2O_3$: 266.34
2-(4-{(2*RS*)-2-Hydroxy-3-[(1-methylethyl)amino]propyloxy}phenyl)acetamide
[*29122-68-7*]

Atenolol, when dried, contains not less than 99.0% and not more than 101.0% of atenolol ($C_{14}H_{22}N_2O_3$).

Description Atenolol occurs as a white to pale yellow crystalline powder.

It is freely soluble in methanol and in acetic acid (100), soluble in ethanol (99.5), and slightly soluble in water.

A solution of Atenolol in methanol (1 in 25) shows no optical rotation.

Identification **(1)** Determine the absorption spectrum of a solution of Atenolol in methanol (1 in 50,000) as directed under Ultraviolet-visible Spectrophotometry *<2.24>*, and compare the spectrum with the Reference Spectrum: both spectra exhibit similar intensities of absorption at the same wavelengths.

(2) Determine the infrared absorption spectrum of Atenolol as directed in the potassium bromide disk method under Infrared Spectrophotometry *<2.25>*, and compare the spectrum with the Reference Spectrum: both spectra exhibit similar intensities of absorption at the same wave numbers.

Melting Pint *<2.60>* 152 – 156°C

Purity **(1)** Heavy metals *<1.07>*—Proceed with 1.0 g of Atenolol according to Method 2, and perform the test. Prepare the control solution with 2.0 mL of Standard Lead Solution (not more than 20 ppm).

(2) Related substances—Dissolve 50 mg of Atenolol in 25 mL of the mobile phase, and use this solution as the sample solution. Pipet 1 mL of the sample solution, add the mobile phase to make exactly 200 mL, and use this solution as the standard solution. Perform the test with exactly 10 μL each of the sample solution and standard solution as directed under Liquid Chromatography *<2.01>* according to the following conditions, and determine each peak area by the automatic integration method: the area of the peak other than atenolol obtained from the sample solution is not larger than 1/2 times the peak area of atenolol from the standard solution, and the total area of the peaks other than atenolol from the sample solution is not larger than the peak area of atenolol from the standard solution.

Operating conditions—

Detector: An ultraviolet absorption photometer (wavelength: 226 nm).

Column: A stainless steel column 4.6 mm in inside diameter and 15 cm in length, packed with octadecylsilanized silica gel for liquid chromatography (5 μm in particle diameter).

Column temperature: A constant temperature of about 25°C.

Mobile phase: Dissolve 3.4 g of potassium dihydrogen phosphate in 1000 mL of water, and adjust to pH 3.0 with phosphoric acid. To 40 volume of this solution add 9 volume of methanol and 1 volume of tetrahydrofuran. Dissolve 1 g of sodium 1-octanesulfonate and 0.4 g of tetrabutylammonium hydrogensulfate in 1000 mL of this solution.

Flow rate: Adjust so that the retention time of atenolol is about 8 minutes.

Time span of measurement: About 4 times as long as the retention time of atenolol.

System suitability—

Test for required detectability: To exactly 10 mL of the standard solution add the mobile phase to make exactly 50 mL. Confirm that the peak area of atenolol obtained with 10 μL of this solution is equivalent to 14 to 26% of that with 10 μL of the standard solution.

System performance: When the procedure is run with 10 μL of the standard solution under the above operating conditions, the number of theoretical plates and the symmetry factor of the peak of atenolol are not less than 5000 and not more than 1.5, respectively.

System repeatability: When the test is repeated 6 times with 10 μL of the standard solution under the above operating conditions, the relative standard deviation of the peak area of atenolol is not more than 1.0%.

Loss on drying *<2.41>* Not more than 0.5% (1 g, 105°C, 3 hours).

Residue on ignition *<2.44>* Not more than 0.2% (1 g).

Assay Weigh accurately about 0.3 g of Atenolol, previously dried, dissolve in 100 mL of acetic acid (100), and titrate *<2.50>* with 0.1 mol/L perchloric acid VS (potentiometric titration). Perform a blank determination in the same manner, and make any necessary correction.

$$\text{Each mL of 0.1 mol/L perchloric acid VS} = 26.63 \text{ mg of } C_{14}H_{22}N_2O_3$$

Containers and storage Containers—Tight containers.

Atorvastatin Calcium Hydrate

アトルバスタチンカルシウム水和物

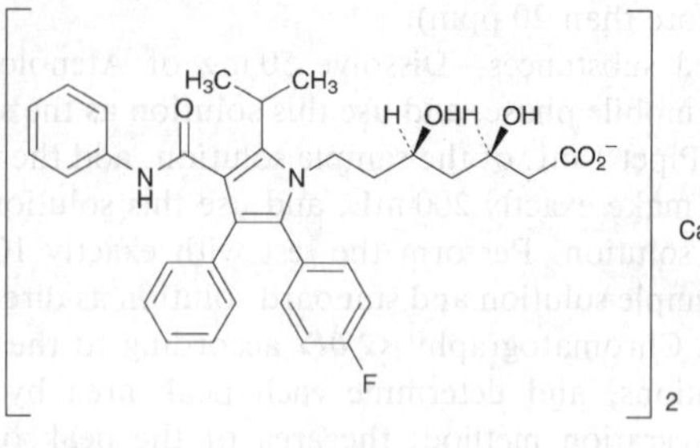

$C_{66}H_{68}CaF_2N_4O_{10}.3H_2O$: 1209.39
Monocalcium bis{(3*R*,5*R*)-7-[2-(4-fluorophenyl)-5-(1-methylethyl)-3-phenyl-4-(phenylcarbamoyl)-1*H*-pyrrol-1-yl]-3,5-dihydroxyheptanoate} trihydrate
[*344423-98-9*]

Atorvastatin Calcium Hydrate contains not less than 98.0% and not more than 102.0% of atorvastatin calcium ($C_{66}H_{68}CaF_2N_4O_{10}$: 1155.34), calculated on the anhydrous basis.

Description Atorvastatin Calcium Hydrate occurs as a white to pale yellow-white crystalline powder.

It is very soluble in methanol, freely soluble in dimethylsulfoxide, and very slightly soluble in water and in ethanol (99.5).

It gradually turns yellowish white on exposure to light.

It shows crystal polymorphism.

Identification **(1)** Determine the absorption spectrum of a solution of Atorvastatin Calcium Hydrate in methanol (1 in 62,500) as directed under Ultraviolet-visible Spectrophotometry <*2.24*>, and compare the spectrum with the Reference Spectrum or the spectrum of a solution of Atorvastatin Calcium RS prepared in the same manner as the sample solution: both spectra exhibit similar intensities of absorption at the same wavelengths.

(2) Determine the infrared absorption spectrum of Atorvastatin Calcium Hydrate as directed in the potassium bromide disk method under Infrared Spectrophotometry <*2.25*>, and compare the spectrum with the Reference Spectrum or the spectrum of Atorvastatin Calcium RS: both spectra exhibit similar intensities of absorption at the same wave numbers. If any difference appears between the spectra, recrystallize the sample and the reference standard according to the method otherwise specified, filter and dry the crystals, and perform the test with the crystals.

(3) A gruel-like liquid of Atorvastatin Calcium Hydrate prepared by adding a small amount of dilute hydrochloric acid responds to the Qualitative Tests <*1.09*> (1) for calcium salt. A solution of Atorvastatin Calcium Hydrate in a mixture of methanol and water (7:3) (1 in 250) is also responds to Qualitative Tests <*1.09*> (3) for calcium salt.

Optical rotation <*2.49*> $[\alpha]_D^{25}$: −7 – −10° (0.2 g, calculated on the anhydrous basis, dimethylsulfoxide, 20 mL, 100 mm).

Purity **(1)** Heavy metals <*1.07*>—Proceed with 1.0 g of Atorvastatin Calcium Hydrate according to Method 4, and perform the test. Prepare the control solution with 1.0 mL of Standard Lead Solution (not more than 10 ppm).

(2) Related substances—Dissolve 20 mg of Atorvastatin Calcium Hydrate in 20 mL of a mixture of water and acetonitrile (1:1), and use this solution as the sample solution. Pipet 1 mL of the sample solution, add a mixture of water and acetonitrile (1:1) to make exactly 100 mL, and use this solution as the standard solution. Perform the test with exactly 20 μL each of the sample solution and standard solution as directed under Liquid Chromatography <*2.01*> according to the following conditions, and determine each peak area by the automatic integration method: the area of the peak, having the relative retention time of about 0.8 to atorvastatin, obtained from the sample solution is not larger than 3/10 times the peak area of atorvastatin from the standard solution, the area of the peak other than atorvastatin and the peak mentioned above from the sample solution is not larger than 1/10 times the peak area of atorvastatin from the standard solution, and the total area of the peaks other than atorvastatin from the sample solution is not larger than the peak area of atorvastatin from the standard solution.

Operating conditions—

Detector: An ultraviolet absorption photometer (wavelength: 254 nm).

Column: A stainless steel column 4.6 mm in inside diameter and 25 cm in length, packed with octadecylsilanized silica gel for liquid chromatography (5 μm in particle diameter).

Column temperature: A constant temperature of about 40°C.

Mobile phase A: Dissolve 10.5 g of citric acid monohydrate in 900 mL of water, adjust to pH 5.0 with ammonia solution (28), and add water to make 1000 mL. To 400 mL of this solution add 100 mL of acetonitrile and 100 mL of tetrahydrofuran.

Mobile phase B: A mixture of acetonitrile and tetrahydrofuran (1:1).

Flowing of mobile phase: Control the gradient by mixing the mobile phases A and B as directed in the following table.

Time after injection of sample (min)	Mobile phase A (vol%)	Mobile phase B (vol%)
0 – 40	93	7
40 – 80	93 → 60	7 → 40

Flow rate: Adjust so that the retention time of atorvastatin is about 16 minutes.

Time span of measurement: About 5 times as long as the retention time of atorvastatin, beginning after the solvent peak.

System suitability—

Test for required detectability: Pipet 5 mL of the standard solution, and add a mixture of water and acetonitrile (1:1) to make exactly 100 mL. Confirm that the peak area of atorvastatin obtained with 20 μL of this solution is equivalent to 3.5 to 6.5% of that with 20 μL of the standard solution.

System performance: When the procedure is run with 20 μL of the standard solution under the above operating conditions, the number of theoretical plates and the symmetry factor of the peak of atorvastatin are not less than 8000 and not more than 1.5, respectively.

System repeatability: When the test is repeated 6 times with 20 μL of the standard solution under the above operating conditions, the relative standard deviation of the peak area of atorvastatin is not more than 2.0%.

Water <*2.48*> 3.5 – 5.5% (50 mg, coulometric titration).

Assay Weigh accurately about 20 mg each of Atorvastatin Calcium Hydrate and Atorvastatin Calcium RS (separately determine the water <*2.48*> in the same manner as Atorvastatin Calcium Hydrate), dissolve each in an adequate amount of a mixture of water and acetonitrile (1:1), add exactly 10 mL of the internal standard solution, then add a mixture of water and acetonitrile (1:1) to make 50 mL, and use these solutions as the sample solution and the standard solution, respectively. Perform the test with 10 μL each of the sample solution and standard solution as directed under Liquid Chromatography ⟨*2.01*⟩ according to the following conditions, and calculate the ratios, Q_T and Q_S, of the peak area of atorvastatin to that of the internal standard.

Amount (mg) of atorvastatin calcium ($C_{66}H_{68}CaF_2N_4O_{10}$)
$= M_S \times Q_T/Q_S$

M_S: Amount (mg) of Atorvastatin Calcium RS taken, calculated on the anhydrous basis

Internal standard solution—A solution of butyl parahydroxybenzoate in a mixture of water and acetonitrile (1:1) (1 in 1500).

Operating conditions—

Detector: An ultraviolet absorption photometer (wavelength: 254 nm).

Column: A stainless steel column 4.6 mm in inside diameter and 25 cm in length, packed with octadecylsilanized silica gel for liquid chromatography (5 μm in particle diameter).

Column temperature: A constant temperature of about 40°C.

Mobile phase: Dissolve 10.5 g of citric acid monohydrate in 900 mL of water, adjust to pH 4.0 with ammonia solution (28), and add water to make 1000 mL. To 530 mL of this solution add 270 mL of acetonitrile and 200 mL of tetrahydrofuran.

Flow rate: Adjust so that the retention time of atorvastatin is about 10 minutes.

System suitability—

System performance: When the procedure is run with 10 μL of the standard solution under the above operating conditions, the internal standard and atorvastatin are eluted in this order with the resolution between these peaks being not less than 5.

System repeatability: When the test is repeated 6 times with 10 μL of the standard solution under the above operating conditions, the relative standard deviation of the ratio of the peak area of atorvastatin to that of the internal standard is not more than 1.0%.

Containers and storage Containers—Well-closed containers.

Storage—Light-resistant.

Atorvastatin Calcium Tablets

アトルバスタチンカルシウム錠

Atorvastatin Calcium Tablets contain not less than 95.0% and not more than 105.0% of the labeled amount of atorvastatin calcium hydrate ($C_{66}H_{68}CaF_2N_4O_{10}.3H_2O$: 1209.39).

Method of preparation Prepare as directed under Tablets, with Atorvastatin Calcium Hydrate.

Identification To a quantity of powdered Atorvastatin Calcium Tablets, equivalent to 10 mg of Atorvastatin Calcium Hydrate, add 50 mL of methanol, shake thoroughly, and centrifuge. To 2.5 mL of the supernatant liquid add methanol to make 50 mL, and determine the absorption spectrum of this solution as directed under Ultraviolet-visible Spectrophotometry ⟨*2.24*⟩: it exhibits a maximum between 244 nm and 248 nm.

Uniformity of dosage units ⟨*6.02*⟩ Perform the test according to the following method: it meets the requirement of the Content uniformity test.

To 1 tablet of Atorvastatin Calcium Tablets add 3*V*/5 mL of a mixture of water and methanol (1:1), and disintegrate the tablet by shaking. Add exactly *V*/10 mL of the internal standard solution, and add a mixture of water and methanol (1:1) to make *V* mL so that each mL contains about 0.1 mg of atorvastatin calcium hydrate ($C_{66}H_{68}CaF_2N_4O_{10}.3H_2O$). Centrifuge this solution, and use the supernatant liquid as the sample solution. Separately, weigh accurately about 22 mg of Atorvastatin Calcium RS (separately determine the water ⟨*2.48*⟩ in the same manner as Atorvastatin Calcium Hydrate), and dissolve in a mixture of water and methanol (1:1) to make exactly 20 mL. Pipet 5 mL of this solution, add exactly 5 mL of the internal standard solution, then add a mixture of water and methanol (1:1) to make 50 mL, and use this solution as the standard solution. Perform the test with 10 μL each of the sample solution and standard solution as directed under Liquid Chromatography ⟨*2.01*⟩ according to the following conditions, and calculate the ratios, Q_T and Q_S, of the peak area of atorvastatin to that of the internal standard.

Amount (mg) of atorvastatin calcium hydrate
($C_{66}H_{68}CaF_2N_4O_{10}.3H_2O$)
$= M_S \times Q_T/Q_S \times V/200 \times 1.047$

M_S: Amount (mg) of Atorvastatin Calcium RS taken, calculated on the anhydrous basis

Internal standard solution—A solution of 1,3-dinitrobenzene in methanol (1 in 2500).

Operating conditions—

Proceed as directed in the operating conditions in the Assay.

System suitability—

System performance: When the procedure is run with 10 μL of the standard solution under the above operating conditions, the internal standard and atorvastatin are eluted in this order with the resolution between these peaks being not less than 10.

System repeatability: When the test is repeated 6 times with 10 μL of the standard solution under the above operating conditions, the relative standard deviation of the ratio of the peak area of atorvastatin to that of the internal standard is not more than 1.0%.

Dissolution ⟨*6.10*⟩ When the test is performed at 75 revolutions per minute according to the Paddle method, using 900 mL of water as the dissolution medium, the dissolution rate in 15 minutes of Atorvastatin Calcium Tablets is not less than 80%.

Start the test with 1 tablet of Atorvastatin Calcium Tablets, withdraw not less than 20 mL of the medium at the specified minute after starting the test, and filter through a membrane filter with a pore size not exceeding 0.45 μm. Discard not less than 10 mL of the first filtrate, pipet *V* mL of the subsequent filtrate, add water to make exactly *V′* mL so that each mL contains about 6 μg of atorvastatin calcium hydrate ($C_{66}H_{68}CaF_2N_4O_{10}.3H_2O$), and use this solution as the sample solution. Separately, weigh accurately about 60 mg of Atorvastatin Calcium RS (separately determine the water ⟨*2.48*⟩ in the same manner as Atorvastatin Calcium Hydrate), and dissolve in a mixture of water and methanol (1:1) to make exactly 100 mL. Pipet 5 mL of this solution, add water to make exactly 50 mL. Pipet 5 mL of this solution, add water to make exactly 50 mL, and use this solution as the standard solution. Perform the test with exactly 50 μL each of the sample solution and standard solution as directed under Liquid Chromatography <*2.01*>, and determine the peak areas, A_T and A_S, of atorvastatin in each solution.

Dissolution rate (%) with respect to the labeled amount of atorvastatin calcium hydrate ($C_{66}H_{68}CaF_2N_4O_{10}.3H_2O$)
$= M_S \times A_T/A_S \times V'/V \times 1/C \times 9 \times 1.047$

M_S: Amount (mg) of Atorvastatin Calcium RS taken, calculated on the anhydrous basis
C: Labeled amount (mg) of atorvastatin calcium hydrate ($C_{66}H_{68}CaF_2N_4O_{10}.3H_2O$) in 1 tablet

Operating conditions—
Proceed as directed in the operating conditions in the Assay.

System suitability—
System performance: When the procedure is run with 50 μL of the standard solution under the above operating conditions, the number of theoretical plates and the symmetry factor of the peak of atorvastatin are not less than 6000 and not more than 2.0, respectively.

System repeatability: When the test is repeated 6 times with 50 μL of the standard solution under the above operating conditions, the relative standard deviation of the peak area of atorvastatin is not more than 2.0%.

Assay To 20 Atorvastatin Calcium Tablets add 3V/5 mL of a mixture of water and methanol (1:1), and disintegrate the tablet by shaking. Add exactly V/10 mL of the internal standard solution, add a mixture of water and methanol (1:1) to make V mL so that each mL contains about 2 mg of atorvastatin calcium hydrate ($C_{66}H_{68}CaF_2N_4O_{10}.3H_2O$), and centrifuge. To 2.5 mL of the supernatant liquid add a mixture of water and methanol (1:1) to make 50 mL, and use this solution as the sample solution. Separately, weigh accurately about 44 mg of Atorvastatin Calcium RS (separately determine the water <*2.48*> in the same manner as Atorvastatin Calcium Hydrate), add exactly 2 mL of the internal standard solution, and add a mixture of water and methanol (1:1) to make 20 mL. Pipet 2.5 mL of this solution, add a mixture of water and methanol (1:1) to make 50 mL, and use this solution as the standard solution. Perform the test with 10 μL each of the sample solution and standard solution as directed under Liquid Chromatography <*2.01*> according to the following conditions, and calculate the ratios, Q_T and Q_S, of the peak area of atorvastatin to that of the internal standard.

Amount (mg) of atorvastatin calcium hydrate ($C_{66}H_{68}CaF_2N_4O_{10}.3H_2O$)
in 1 tablet of Atorvastatin Calcium Tablets
$= M_S \times Q_T/Q_S \times V/400 \times 1.047$

M_S: Amount (mg) of Atorvastatin Calcium RS taken, calculated on the anhydrous basis

Internal standard solution—A solution of 1,3-dinitrobenzene in methanol (1 in 125).

Operating conditions—
Detector: An ultraviolet absorption photometer (wavelength: 244 nm).

Column: A stainless steel column 4.6 mm in inside diameter and 25 cm in length, packed with octadecylsilanized silica gel for liquid chromatography (5 μm in particle diameter).

Column temperature: A constant temperature of about 30°C.

Mobile phase: Dissolve 10.5 g of citric acid monohydrate in 900 mL of water, adjust to pH 4.0 with ammonia solution (28), and add water to make 1000 mL. To 530 mL of this solution add 270 mL of acetonitrile and 200 mL of tetrahydrofuran.

Flow rate: Adjust so that the retention time of atorvastatin is about 9 minutes.

System suitability—
System performance: When the procedure is run with 10 μL of the standard solution under the above operating conditions, the internal standard and atorvastatin are eluted in this order with the resolution between these peaks being not less than 10.

System repeatability: When the test is repeated 6 times with 10 μL of the standard solution under the above operating conditions, the relative standard deviation of the ratio of the peak area of atorvastatin to that of the internal standard is not more than 1.0%.

Containers and storage Containers—Tight containers.

Atropine Sulfate Hydrate

アトロピン硫酸塩水和物

$(C_{17}H_{23}NO_3)_2.H_2SO_4.H_2O$: 694.83
(1*R*,3*r*,5*S*)-8-Methyl-8-azabicyclo[3.2.1]oct-3-yl [(2*RS*)-3-hydroxy-2-phenyl]propanoate hemisulfate hemihydrate
[*5908-99-6*]

Atropine Sulfate Hydrate, when dried, contains not less than 98.0% of atropine sulfate [$(C_{17}H_{23}NO_3)_2.H_2SO_4$: 676.82].

Description Atropine Sulfate Hydrate occurs as colorless crystals or a white crystalline powder. It is odorless.

It is very soluble in water and in acetic acid (100), freely soluble in ethanol (95), and practically insoluble in diethyl ether.

Melting point: 188 – 194°C (with decomposition). Introduce a capillary tube charged with dried sample into a bath previously heated to 180°C, and continue to heat at a rate of rise of about 3°C per minute.

It is affected by light.

Identification **(1)** To 1 mg of Atropine Sulfate Hydrate add 3 drops of fuming nitric acid, and evaporate the mixture on a water bath to dryness. Dissolve the residue in 1 mL of *N*,*N*-dimethylformamide, and add 5 to 6 drops of tetraethylammonium hydroxide TS: a red-purple color develops.

(2) To 2 mL of a solution of Atropine Sulfate Hydrate (1 in 50) add 4 to 5 drops of hydrogen tetrachloroaurate (III) TS: a lusterless, yellow-white precipitate is formed.

(3) To 5 mL of a solution of Atropine Sulfate Hydrate (1 in 25) add 2 mL of ammonia TS, and allow to stand for 2 to 3 minutes. Collect the precipitate, wash with water, and dry in a desiccator (in vacuum, silica gel) for 4 hours: it melts <*2.60*> between 115°C and 118°C.

(4) A solution of Atropine Sulfate Hydrate (1 in 20) responds to Qualitative Tests <*1.09*> for sulfate.

Purity **(1)** Clarity and color of solution —Dissolve 0.5 g of Atropine Sulfate Hydrate in 10 mL of water: the solution is clear and colorless.

(2) Acidity—Dissolve 1.0 g of Atropine Sulfate Hydrate in 20 mL of water, and add 0.30 mL of 0.02 mol/L sodium hydroxide VS and 1 drop of methyl red-methylene blue TS: a green color develops.

(3) Related substances—Dissolve 0.25 g of Atropine Sulfate Hydrate in 1 mL of diluted hydrochloric acid (1 in 10), add water to make 15 mL, and use this solution as the sample solution.

(i) To 5 mL of the sample solution add 2 to 3 drops of hydrogen hexachloroplatinate (IV) TS: no precipitate is formed.

(ii) To 5 mL of the sample solution add 2 mL of ammonia TS, and shake vigorously: the turbidity of the solution is not greater than that of the following control solution.

Control solution: To 0.30 mL of 0.01 mol/L hydrochloric acid VS add 6 mL of dilute nitric acid and water to make 50 mL. To this solution add 1 mL of silver nitrate TS, and allow 7 mL of the mixture to stand for 5 minutes.

(4) Hyoscyamine—Weigh accurately about 1 g of Atropine Sulfate Hydrate, previously dried, and dissolve in water to make exactly 10 mL: the specific optical rotation $[\alpha]_D^{20}$ <*2.49*> of this solution in a 100-mm cell is between −0.60° and +0.10°.

(5) Readily carbonizable substances <*1.15*>—Take 0.20 g of Atropine Sulfate Hydrate, and perform the test: the solution has no more color than Matching Fluid A.

Loss on drying <*2.41*> Not more than 4.0% (0.5 g, in vacuum, phosphorus (V) oxide, 110°C, 4 hours).

Residue on ignition <*2.44*> Not more than 0.1% (0.5 g).

Assay Dissolve about 0.25 g of Atropine Sulfate Hydrate, previously dried and accurately weighed, in 30 mL of acetic acid (100). If necessary, dissolve it by warming, and cool. Titrate <*2.50*> with 0.05 mol/L perchloric acid VS until the color of the solution changes from purple through blue to blue-green (indicator: 3 drops of crystal violet TS). Perform a blank determination in the same manner, and make any necessary correction.

Each mL of 0.05 mol/L perchloric acid VS
= 33.84 mg of $(C_{17}H_{23}NO_3)_2.H_2SO_4$

Containers and storage Containers—Tight containers.
Storage—Light-resistant.

Atropine Sulfate Injection

アトロピン硫酸塩注射液

Atropine Sulfate Injection is an aqueous injection.

It contains not less than 93.0% and not more than 107.0% of the labeled amount of atropine sulfate hydrate [$(C_{17}H_{23}NO_3)_2.H_2SO_4.H_2O$: 694.83].

Method of preparation Prepare as directed under Injections, with Atropine Sulfate Hydrate.

Description Atropine Sulfate Injection is a clear, colorless liquid.

pH: 4.0 – 6.0

Identification **(1)** Evaporate a volume of Atropine Sulfate Injection, equivalent to 1 mg of Atropine Sulfate Hydrate, on a water bath to dryness. Proceed with the residue as directed in the Identification (1) under Atropine Sulfate Hydrate.

(2) Evaporate an exactly measured volume of Atropine Sulfate Injection, equivalent to 5 mg of Atropine Sulfate Hydrate, on a water bath to dryness. After cooling, dissolve the residue in 1 mL of ethanol (95), and use this solution as the sample solution. If insoluble substance remains, crush it, allow to stand, and use the supernatant liquid as the sample solution. Separately, dissolve 10 mg of Atropine Sulfate RS in 2 mL of ethanol (95), and use this solution as the standard solution. Perform the test with these solutions as directed under Thin-layer Chromatography <*2.03*>. Spot 5 μL each of the sample solution and standard solution on a plate of silica gel for thin-layer chromatography. Develop the plate with a mixture of acetone, water and ammonia water (28) (90:7:3) to a distance of about 10 cm, and dry the plate at 80°C for 10 minutes. After cooling, spray evenly Dragendorff's TS for spraying on the plate: the spots obtained from the sample solution and the standard solution show an orange color and the same *R*f value.

(3) Atropine Sulfate Injection responds to Qualitative Tests <*1.09*> for sulfate.

Bacterial endotoxins <*4.01*> Less than 75 EU/mg.

Extractable volume <*6.05*> It meets the requirements.

Foreign insoluble matter <*6.06*> Perform the test according to Method 1: it meets the requirement.

Insoluble particulate matter <*6.07*> It meets the requirement.

Sterility <*4.06*> Perform the test: it meets the requirement.

Assay To an exactly measured volume of Atropine Sulfate Injection, equivalent to about 5 mg of atropine sulfate hydrate [$(C_{17}H_{23}NO_3)_2.H_2SO_4.H_2O$], add exactly 3 mL of the internal standard solution and water to make 50 mL, and use this solution as the sample solution. Separately, weigh accurately about 25 mg of Atropine Sulfate RS (separately determine the loss on drying <*2.41*> under the same conditions as Atropine Sulfate Hydrate), and dissolve in water to make exactly 50 mL. Pipet 10 mL of this solution, add exactly 3 mL of the internal standard solution and water to make 50 mL, and use this solution as the standard solution. Perform the test with 20 μL each of the sample solution and standard solution as directed under Liquid Chromatography <*2.01*> according to the following conditions, and calculate the ratios, Q_T and Q_S, of the peak area of atropine to that of the internal standard.

Amount (mg) of atropine sulfate hydrate
[$(C_{17}H_{23}NO_3)_2.H_2SO_4.H_2O$]
$= M_S \times Q_T/Q_S \times 1/5 \times 1.027$

M_S: Amount (mg) of Atropine Sulfate RS taken, calculated based on the dried basis

Internal standard solution—A solution of etilefrine hydrochloride (1 in 1000).

Operating conditions—

Detector: An ultraviolet absorption photometer (wavelength: 210 nm).

Column: A stainless steel column 4.6 mm in inside diameter and 15 cm in length, packed with octadecylsilanized silica gel for liquid chromatography (5 μm in particle diameter).

Column temperature: A constant temperature of about 40°C.

Mobile phase: To 0.4 g of sodium lauryl sulfate add 500 mL of diluted phosphoric acid (1 in 1000) to dissolve, and adjust the pH to 3.0 with sodium hydroxide TS. To 240 mL of this solution add 70 mL of tetrahydrofuran, and mix.

Flow rate: Adjust so that the retention time of atropine is about 16 minutes.

System suitability—

System performance: When the procedure is run with 20 μL of the standard solution under the above operating conditions, the internal standard and atropine are eluted in this order with the resolution between these peaks being not less than 3.

System repeatability: When the test is repeated 6 times with 20 μL of the standard solution under the above operating conditions, the relative standard deviation of the ratio of the peak area of atropine to that of the internal standard is not more than 1.5%.

Containers and storage Containers—Hermetic containers.

Storage—Light-resistant.

Auranofin

オーラノフィン

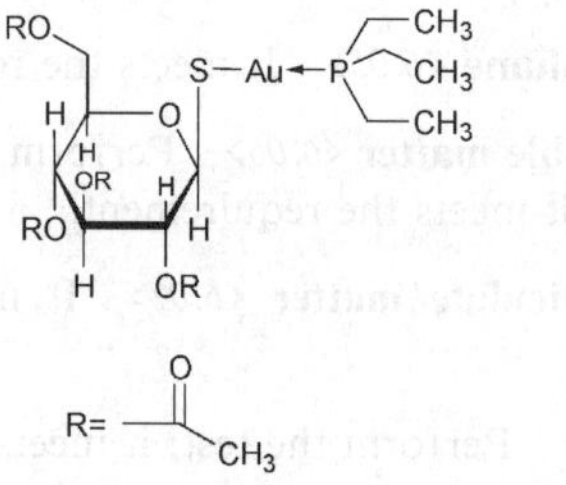

$C_{20}H_{34}AuO_9PS$: 678.48
(2,3,4,6-Tetra-*O*-acetyl-1-thio-
β-D-glucopyranosato)(triethylphosphine)gold
[*34031-32-8*]

Auranofin, when dried, contains not less than 98.0% and not more than 102.0% of auranofin ($C_{20}H_{34}AuO_9PS$).

Description Auranofin occurs as a white crystalline powder.

It is very soluble in chloroform, freely soluble in methanol, sparingly soluble in ethanol (99.5), and practically insoluble in water.

It shows crystal polymorphism.

Identification **(1)** To 50 mg of Auranofin add 3 mL of water, 3 mL of nitric acid and 3 mL of sulfuric acid, shake, and allow to stand: golden colored suspended matters are produced.

(2) Determine the infrared absorption spectrum of Auranofin as directed in the paste method under Infrared Spectrophotometry *<2.25>*, and compare the spectrum with the Reference Spectrum or the spectrum of Auranofin RS: both spectra exhibit similar intensities of absorption at the same wave numbers.

(3) Prepare the test solution with 1 mg of Auranofin as directed under Oxygen Flask Combustion Method *<1.06>*, using 10 mL of water as the absorbing liquid. Wash out the test solution into a Nessler tube with water to make 30 mL. Add 10 mL of dilute sulfuric acid, 3 mL of hexaammonium heptamolybdate-sulfuric acid TS and 0.1 mL of tin (II) chloride TS, shake, and allow to stand for 10 to 15 minutes: a blue color is developed.

Optical rotation *<2.49>* $[\alpha]_D^{20}$: $-54.0 - -62.0°$ (after drying, 0.2 g, methanol, 20 mL, 100 mm).

Melting point *<2.60>* 113 - 116°C

Purity **(1)** Chloride *<1.03>*—Put 0.5 g of Auranofin in a porcelain crucible, add 0.25 g of anhydrous sodium carbonate, mix well, and ignite until the carbonized substance is disappeared. After cooling, add 20 mL of water, heat, and filter after cooling. Wash the residue with 20 mL of water, combine the filtrate and the washings, neutralize with dilute nitric acid, then add 6 mL of dilute nitric acid and water to make 50 mL. Perform the test using this solution as the test solution. Prepare the control solution as follows: Dissolve 0.25 g of anhydrous sodium carbonate in 20 mL of water, neutralize with dilute nitric acid, add 0.50 mL of 0.01 mol/L hydrochloric acid, 6 mL of dilute nitric acid, and water to make 50 mL (not more than 0.036%).

(2) Heavy metals *<1.07>*—Proceed with 1.0 g of Auranofin according to Method 2, and perform the test. Prepare the control solution with 2.0 mL of Standard Lead Solution (not more than 20 ppm).

(3) Arsenic *<1.11>*—Put 0.5 g of Auranofin in a Kjeldahl flask, add cautiously 2 mL of sulfuric acid and 5 mL of nitric acid, and heat until the solution becomes almost colorless. After cooling, add 15 mL of a saturated solution of ammonium oxalate monohydrate, heat until white fumes are evolved, and concentrate to 1 to 2 mL. Then, add 3 mL of water and 1 drop of methyl orange TS, neutralize with ammonia solution (28), filter, and perform the test using the filtrate as the test solution: the color is not darker than that of the following control solution.

Control solution: Heat a mixture of 2 mL of sulfuric acid and 5 mL of nitric acid until white fumes are no longer evolved. After cooling, add 15 mL of a saturated solution of ammonium oxalate monohydrate, heat until white fumes are evolved, and concentrate to 1 to 2 mL. Add 3 mL of water and 1 drop of methyl orange TS, neutralize with ammonia solution (28), and filter. To the filtrate add 2.0 mL of Standard Arsenic Solution, then proceed in the same manner as for the test solution (not more than 4 ppm).

(4) Related substances—Dissolve 50 mg of Auranofin in 5 mL of chloroform, and use this solution as the sample solution. Pipet 1 mL of the sample solution, and add chloroform to make exactly 100 mL. To exactly 3 mL of this solution add chloroform to make exactly 10 mL, and use this solution as the standard solution. Perform the test with these solutions as directed under Thin-layer Chromatography *<2.03>*. Spot 10 μL each of the sample solution and standard solution on a plate of silica gel for thin-layer chromatography. Develop the plate with a mixture of chloroform and acetone (4:1) to a distance of about 10 cm, and air-dry the plate. Dry the plate, furthermore, at 80°C for 30 minutes. After cooling, allow the plate to stand in a iodine vapor for 30 minutes: the spots other than the principal spot obtained from the sample solution are not more intense than the spot from the standard solution.

Loss on drying *<2.41>* Not more than 0.5% (1 g, 105°C, 3 hours).

Assay Weigh accurately about 20 mg each of Auranofin and Auranofin RS, both previously dried, dissolve each in 10 mL of a mixture of water and acetonitrile (1:1), and add exactly 5 mL each of the internal standard solution. Then add a mixture of water and acetonitrile (1:1) to make 100 mL, and use these solutions as the sample solution and the standard solution, respectively. Perform the test with 10 μL each of the sample solution and standard solution as directed under Liquid Chromatography *<2.01>* according to the following conditions, and calculate the ratios, Q_T and Q_S, of the peak area of auranofin to that of the internal standard.

Amount (mg) of auranofin ($C_{20}H_{34}AuO_9PS$)
$= M_S \times Q_T/Q_S$

M_S: Amount (mg) of Auranofin RS taken

Internal standard solution—A solution of butyl parahydroxybenzoate in a mixture of water and acetonitrile (1:1) (3 in 1250).

Operating conditions—

Detector: An ultraviolet absorption photometer (wavelength: 230 nm).

Column: A stainless steel column 4 mm in inside diameter and 15 cm in length, packed with octadecylsilanized silica gel for liquid chromatography (5 μm in particle diameter).

Column temperature: A constant temperature of about 25°C.

Mobile phase: A mixture of sodium dihydrogen phosphate dihydrate solution (1 in 100), tetrahydrofuran and acetonitrile (12:5:3).

Flow rate: Adjust so that the retention time of auranofin is about 6 minutes.

System suitability—

System performance: When the procedure is run with 10 μL of the standard solution under the above operating conditions, auranofin and the internal standard are eluted in this order with the resolution between these peaks being not less than 9.

System repeatability: When the test is repeated 6 times with 10 μL of the standard solution under the above operating conditions, the relative standard deviation of the ratio of the peak area of auranofin to that of the internal standard is not more than 1.0%.

Containers and storage Containers—Tight containers.

Auranofin Tablets

オーラノフィン錠

Auranofin Tablets contain not less than 93.0% and not more than 107.0% of the labeled amount of auranofin ($C_{20}H_{34}AuO_9PS$: 678.48).

Method of preparation Prepare as directed under Tablets, with Auranofin.

Identification Put an amount of powdered Auranofin Tablets, equivalent to 11 mg of Auranofin, in a porcelain crucible, and heat weakly to carbonize. After cooling, add 2 mL of nitric acid and 5 drops of sulfuric acid, heat cautiously at first then incinerate by ignition. After cooling, add 4 mL of aqua regia to the residue, dissolve by warming, and add 16 mL of water. To 5 mL of this solution add 0.5 mL of tin (II) chloride TS: a purple to red-brown color is developed.

Uniformity of dosage units <*6.02*> Perform the test according to the following method: it meets the requirement of the Content uniformity test.

To 1 tablet of Auranofin Tablets add 2 mL of water, disintegrate the tablet by sonicating, add exactly 2 mL of the internal standard solution for every 3 mg of auranofin ($C_{20}H_{34}AuO_9PS$), and add 2 mL of a mixture of water and acetonitrile (1:1). Shake for 15 minutes, then add a mixture of water and acetonitrile (1:1) to make V mL so that each mL contains 0.3 mg of auranofin ($C_{20}H_{34}AuO_9PS$), centrifuge, and use the supernatant liquid as the sample solution. Then, proceed as directed in the Assay.

Amount (mg) of auranofin ($C_{20}H_{34}AuO_9PS$)
$= M_S \times Q_T/Q_S \times V/100$

M_S: Amount (mg) of Auranofin RS taken

Internal standard solution—A solution of butyl parahydroxybenzoate in acetonitrile (9 in 10,000).

Dissolution <*6.10*> When the test is performed at 50 revolutions per minute according to the Paddle method, using 900 mL of water as the dissolution medium, the dissolution rate in 15 minutes of Auranofin Tablets is not less than 85%.

Start the test with 1 tablet of Auranofin Tablets, withdraw not less than 20 mL of the medium at the specified minute after starting the test, and filter through a membrane filter with a pore size not exceeding 0.45 μm. Discard not less than 10 mL of the first filtrate, pipet V mL of the subsequent filtrate, add water to make exactly V' mL so that each mL contains about 3.3 μg of auranofin ($C_{20}H_{34}AuO_9PS$), and use this solution as the sample solution. Separately, weigh accurately about 30 mg of Auranofin RS, previously dried at 105°C for 3 hours, and dissolve in acetonitrile to make exactly 50 mL. Pipet 5 mL of this solution, and add water to make exactly 100 mL. Pipet 10 mL of this solution, add water to make exactly 100 mL, and use this solution as the standard solution. Perform the test with exactly 50 μL each of the sample solution and standard solution as directed under Liquid Chromatography <*2.01*> under the following conditions, and determine the peak areas, A_T and A_S, of auranofin in each solution.

Dissolution rate (%) with respect to the labeled amount of auranofin ($C_{20}H_{34}AuO_9PS$)
$= M_S \times A_T/A_S \times V'/V \times 1/C \times 9$

M_S: Amount (mg) of Auranofin RS taken
C: Labeled amount (mg) of auranofin ($C_{20}H_{34}AuO_9PS$) in 1 tablet

Operating conditions—

Proceed as directed in the operating conditions in the Assay under Auranofin.

System suitability—

System performance: When the procedure is run with 50 μL of the standard solution under the above operating conditions, the number of theoretical plates and the symmetry factor of the peak of auranofin are not less than 5000 and not more than 2.0, respectively.

System repeatability: When the test is repeated 6 times with 50 μL of the standard solution under the above operating conditions, the relative standard deviation of the peak area of auranofin is not more than 1.0%.

Assay Accurately weigh the mass of not less than 20 Auranofin Tablets, and powder them. Weigh accurately a portion of the powder, equivalent to about 60 mg of auranofin ($C_{20}H_{34}AuO_9PS$), add 40 mL of water, disperse the particles with the aid of ultrasonic waves, then add exactly 40 mL of the internal standard solution, add 40 mL of a mixture of water and acetonitrile (1:1), and shake for 15 minutes. To this solution add a mixture of water and acetonitrile (1:1) to make 200 mL, centrifuge, and use the supernatant liquid as the sample solution. Separately, weigh accurately about 30 mg of Auranofin RS, previously dried at 105°C for 3 hours, dissolve in 60 mL of a mixture of water and acetonitrile (1:1), add exactly 20 mL of the internal standard solution, then add water to make 100 mL, and use this solution as the standard solution. Perform the test with 10 μL each of the sample solution and standard solution as directed under Liquid Chromatography *<2.01>* according to the following conditions, and calculate the ratios, Q_T and Q_S, of the peak area of auranofin to that of the internal standard.

Amount (mg) of auranofin ($C_{20}H_{34}AuO_9PS$)
$= M_S \times Q_T/Q_S \times 2$

M_S: Amount (mg) of Auranofin RS taken

Internal standard solution—A solution of butyl parahydroxybenzoate in acetonitrile (9 in 10,000).

Operating conditions—

Proceed as directed in the operating conditions in the Assay under Auranofin.

System suitability—

System performance: When the procedure is run with 10 μL of the standard solution under the above operating conditions, auranofin and the internal standard are eluted in this order with the resolution between these peaks being not less than 9.

System repeatability: When the test is repeated 6 times with 10 μL of the standard solution under the above operating conditions, the relative standard deviation of the ratio of the peak area of auranofin to that of the internal standard is not more than 1.0%.

Containers and storage Containers—Tight containers.

Azathioprine

アザチオプリン

$C_9H_7N_7O_2S$: 277.26
6-(1-Methyl-4-nitro-1*H*-imidazol-5-ylthio)purine
[446-86-6]

Azathioprine, when dried, contains not less than 98.5% of azathioprine ($C_9H_7N_7O_2S$).

Description Azathioprine is light yellow, crystals or crystalline powder. It is odorless.

It is sparingly soluble in *N,N*-dimethylformamide and in pyridine, very slightly soluble in water and in ethanol (99.5), and practically insoluble in chloroform and in diethyl ether.

It dissolves in sodium hydroxide TS and in ammonia TS.

It is gradually colored by light.

Melting point: about 240°C (with decomposition).

Identification **(1)** Dissolve 0.01 g of Azathioprine in 50 mL of water by warming. To 5 mL of this solution add 1 mL of dilute hydrochloric acid and 0.01 g of zinc powder, and allow to stand for 5 minutes: a yellow color is produced. Filter this solution: the filtrate responds to Qualitative Tests *<1.09>* for primary aromatic amines, and a red color is produced.

(2) Dissolve 0.01 g of Azathioprine in 50 mL of water by warming. To 1 mL of this solution add 0.5 mL of phosphotungstic acid TS and 0.5 mL of dilute hydrochloric acid: a white precipitate is formed.

(3) Prepare the test solution by proceeding with 0.03 g of Azathioprine according to Oxygen Flask Combustion Method *<1.06>*, using 20 mL of water as the absorbing liquid: the test solution responds to Qualitative Tests *<1.09>* (1) for sulfate.

(4) Dissolve 0.01 g of Azathioprine in 2 mol/L hydrochloric acid TS to make 100 mL. Dilute 5 mL of the solution with water to make 50 mL. Determine the absorption spectrum of the solution as directed under Ultraviolet-visible Spectrophotometry *<2.24>*, and compare the spectrum with the Reference Spectrum or the spectrum of a solution of Azathioprine RS prepared in the same manner as the sample solution: both spectra exhibit similar intensities of absorption at the same wavelengths.

Purity **(1)** Clarity and color of solution—Dissolve 0.5 g of Azathioprine in 50 mL of *N,N*-dimethylformamide: the solution is clear and shows a light yellow color.

(2) Acidity or alkalinity—Add 100 mL of water to 2.0 g of Azathioprine, shake well for 15 minutes, centrifuge for 5 minutes at 10,000 revolutions per minute, and filter. Discard the first 20 mL of the filtrate, add 2 drops of methyl red TS to 40 mL of the subsequent filtrate, and use this solution as the sample solution.

(i) Add 0.10 mL of 0.02 mol/L hydrochloric acid VS to 20 mL of the sample solution: a red color develops.

(ii) Add 0.10 mL of 0.02 mol/L sodium hydroxide VS to 20 mL of the sample solution: a yellow color develops.

(3) Sulfate *<1.14>*—To 25 mL of the filtrate obtained in (2) add 1 mL of dilute hydrochloric acid and water to make 50 mL, and perform the test using this solution as the test solution. Prepare the control solution with 0.40 mL of 0.005 mol/L sulfuric acid VS (not more than 0.038%).

(4) Heavy metals *<1.07>*—Proceed with 2.0 g of Azathioprine according to Method 2, and perform the test. Prepare the control solution with 2.0 mL of Standard Lead Solution (not more than 10 ppm).

(5) Arsenic *<1.11>*—Prepare the test solution with 1.0 g of Azathioprine, according to Method 3, and perform the test (not more than 2 ppm).

(6) Related substances—Dissolve 10 mg of Azathioprine in 80 mL of the mobile phase by warming, cool, add the mobile phase to make 100 mL, and use this solution as the sample solution. Pipet 1 mL of the sample solution, add water to make exactly 100 mL, and use this solution as the standard solution. Perform the test with exactly 20 μL each of the sample solution and standard solution as directed under Liquid Chromatography *<2.01>* according to the following conditions. Determine each peak area by the automatic integration method: the total area of the peaks other than azathioprine obtained from the sample solution is not larger than 1/2 times the peak area of azathioprine from the standard solution.

Operating conditions—

Detector: An ultraviolet absorption photometer (wavelength: 296 nm).

Column: A stainless steel column 4.6 mm in inside diameter and 15 cm in length, packed with octadecylsilanized silica gel for liquid chromatography (5 μm in particle diameter).

Column temperature: A constant temperature of about 40°C.

Mobile phase: Adjust to pH 2.5 of a solution of 0.05 mol/L potassium dihydrogenphosphate TS (1 in 2) with diluted phosphoric acid (3 in 2000). To 800 mL of this solution add 200 mL of methanol.

Flow rate: Adjust so that the retention time of azathioprine is about 8 minutes.

Time span of measurement: About three times as long as the retention time of azathioprine, beginning after the solvent peak.

System suitability—

Test for required detectability: To exactly 5 mL of the standard solution add water to make exactly 50 mL. Confirm that the peak area of azathioprine obtained with 20 μL of this solution is equivalent to 8 to 12% of that with 20 μL of the standard solution.

System performance: Dissolve 10 mg of Azathioprine in 80 mL of water by warming, cool, and add water to make 100 mL. To 2 mL of this solution add 2 mL of a solution, separately prepared by dissolving 0.06 g of benzoic acid in 3 mL of methanol and diluting with water to make 10 mL, and add the mobile phase to make 25 mL. When the procedure is run with 20 μL of this solution under the above operating conditions, azathioprine and benzoic acid are eluted in this order with the resolution between these peaks being not less than 9.

System repeatability: When the test is repeated 6 times with 20 μL of the standard solution under the above operating conditions, the relative standard deviation of the peak areas of azathioprine is not more than 2.0%.

Loss on drying ⟨*2.41*⟩ Not more than 0.5% (1 g, 105°C, 5 hours).

Residue on ignition ⟨*2.44*⟩ Not more than 0.1% (1 g).

Assay Weigh accurately about 0.5 g of Azathioprine, previously dried, add 80 mL of *N*,*N*-dimethylformamide, and warm to dissolve. After cooling, titrate ⟨*2.50*⟩ with 0.1 mol/L tetramethylammonium hydroxide VS until the color of the solution changes from yellow through yellow-green to blue-green (indicator: 1 mL of thymol blue-dimethylformamide TS). Perform a blank determination in the same manner, and make any necessary correction.

Each mL of 0.1 mol/L tetramethylammonium hydroxide VS
= 27.73 mg of $C_9H_7O_7O_2S$

Containers and storage Containers—Well-closed containers.

Storage—Light-resistant.

Azathioprine Tablets

アザチオプリン錠

Azathioprine Tablets contain not less than 95.0% and not more than 105.0% of the labeled amount of azathioprine ($C_9H_7N_7O_2S$: 277.26).

Method of preparation Prepare as directed under Tablets, with Azathioprine.

Identification **(1)** Weigh a quantity of powdered Azathioprine Tablets, equivalent to 0.01 g of Azathioprine. Add 50 mL of water, shake well while warming, and filter. Proceed with 5 mL of the filtrate as directed in the Identification (1) under Azathioprine.

(2) Proceed with 1 mL of the filtrate obtained in (1) as directed in the Identification (2) under Azathioprine.

(3) Determine the absorption spectrum of the sample solution in the Assay as directed under Ultraviolet-visible Spectrophotometry ⟨*2.24*⟩: it exhibits a maximum between 278 nm and 282 nm.

(4) Weigh a quantity of powdered Azathioprine Tablets, equivalent to 0.1 g of Azathioprine to the labeled amount. Add 10 mL of a solution of ammonia solution (28) in ethanol (95) (1 in 10), shake well, filter, and use the filtrate as the sample solution. Separately, dissolve 0.1 g of Azathioprine RS in 10 mL of a solution of ammonia solution (28) in ethanol (95) (1 in 10), and use this solution as the standard solution. Perform the test with these solutions as directed under Thin-layer Chromatography ⟨*2.03*⟩. Spot 5 μL each of the sample solution and standard solution on a plate of silica gel with fluorescent indicator for thin-layer chromatography. Develop the plate with a mixture of ethanol (95), ethyl acetate, and ammonia solution (28) (5:5:1) to a distance of about 7 cm, and air-dry the plate. Examine under ultraviolet light (main wavelength: 254 nm): the spots obtained from the sample solution and the standard solution show the same *R*f value.

Uniformity of dosage units ⟨*6.02*⟩ Perform the Mass variation test, or the Content uniformity test according to the following method: it meets the requirement.

To 1 tablet of Azathioprine Tablets add 1 mL of dimethylsulfoxide for ultraviolet-visible spectrophotometry per 5 mg of azathioprine ($C_9H_7N_7O_2S$), shake well, add 0.1 mol/L hydrochloric acid TS to make exactly *V* mL so that each mL contains about 0.2 mg of azathioprine ($C_9H_7N_7O_2S$), and filter. Discard the first 20 mL of the filtrate, pipet 3 mL of the subsequent filtrate, add 0.1 mol/L hydrochloric acid TS to make exactly 100 mL, and use this solution as the sample solution. Then, proceed as directed in the Assay.

$$\text{Amount (mg) of azathioprine } (C_9H_7N_7O_2S) = M_S \times A_T/A_S \times V/500$$

M_S: Amount (mg) of Azathioprine RS taken

Dissolution ⟨*6.10*⟩ When the test is performed at 50 revolutions per minute according to the Paddle method, using 900 mL of water as the dissolution medium, the dissolution rate in 45 minutes of Azathioprine Tablets is not less than 80%.

Start the test with 1 tablet of Azathioprine Tablets, withdraw not less than 20 mL of the medium at the specified minute after starting the test, and filter through a membrane filter with a pore size not exceeding 0.8 μm. Discard not less than 10 mL of the first filtrate, pipet *V* mL of the subsequent filtrate, add water to make exactly *V′* mL so that each mL contains about 11 μg of azathioprine ($C_9H_7N_7O_2S$), and use this solution as the sample solution. Separately, weigh accurately about 10 mg of Azathioprine RS, previously dried at 105°C for 5 hours, and dissolve in water to make exactly 100 mL. Pipet 6 mL of this solution, add water to make exactly 50 mL, and use this solution as the standard solution. Determine the absorbances, A_T and A_S, at 280 nm of the sample solution and standard solution as directed under Ultraviolet-visible Spectrophotometry ⟨*2.24*⟩.

$$\text{Dissolution rate (\%) with respect to the labeled amount of azathioprine } (C_9H_7N_7O_2S) = M_S \times A_T/A_S \times V'/V \times 1/C \times 108$$

M_S: Amount (mg) of Azathioprine RS taken

C: Labeled amount (mg) of azathioprine ($C_9H_7N_7O_2S$) in 1 tablet

Assay Weigh accurately and powder not less than 20 Azathioprine Tablets. Weigh accurately a portion of the powder, equivalent to about 0.1 g of azathioprine ($C_9H_7N_7O_2S$), add 20 mL of dimethylsulfoxide for ultraviolet-visible spectrophotometry, shake well, add 0.1 mol/L hydrochloric acid TS to make exactly 500 mL, and filter. Discard the first 20 mL of the filtrate, measure exactly 3 mL of the subsequent filtrate, add 0.1 mol/L hydrochloric acid TS to make exactly 100 mL, and use this solution as the sample solution. Separately, weigh accurately about 0.1 g of

Azathioprine RS, previously dried at 105°C for 5 hours, dissolve in 20 mL of dimethylsulfoxide for ultraviolet-visible spectrophotometry, and add 0.1 mol/L hydrochloric acid TS to make exactly 500 mL. Measure exactly 3 mL of this solution, add 0.1 mol/L hydrochloric acid TS to make exactly 100 mL, and use this solution as the standard solution. Determine the absorbances, A_T and A_S, of the sample solution and standard solution at 280 nm as directed under Ultraviolet-visible Spectrophotometry <2.24>.

Amount (mg) of azathioprine ($C_9H_7N_7O_2S$)
$= M_S \times A_T/A_S$

M_S: Amount (mg) of Azathioprine RS taken

Containers and storage Containers—Tight containers.
Storage—Light-resistant.

Azelastine Hydrochloride

アゼラスチン塩酸塩

• HCl

and enantiomer

$C_{22}H_{24}ClN_3O.HCl$: 418.36
4-[(4-Chlorophenyl)methyl]-2-[(4*RS*)-(1-methylazepan-4-yl)]phthalazin-1(2*H*)-one monohydrochloride
[*79307-93-0*]

Azelastine Hydrochloride, when dried, contains not less than 99.0% and not more than 101.0% of azelastine hydrochloride ($C_{22}H_{24}ClN_3O.HCl$).

Description Azelastine Hydrochloride occurs as a white crystalline powder.

It is freely soluble in formic acid, and slightly soluble in water and in ethanol (99.5).

Melting point: about 225°C (with decomposition).

A solution of Azelastine Hydrochloride (1 in 200) shows no optical rotation.

Identification (1) Determine the absorption spectrum of a solution of Azelastine Hydrochloride (3 in 100,000) as directed under Ultraviolet-visible Spectrophotometry <2.24>, and compare the spectrum with the Reference Spectrum: both spectra exhibit similar intensities of absorption at the same wavelengths.

(2) Determine the infrared absorption spectrum of Azelastine Hydrochloride as directed in the potassium chloride disk method under Infrared Spectrophotometry <2.25>: both spectra exhibit similar intensities of absorption at the same wave numbers.

(3) To 10 mL of a saturated solution of Azelastine Hydrochloride add 1 mL of dilute nitric acid, and filter to separate formed crystals: the filtrate responds to Qualitative Tests <1.09> (2) for chloride.

Purity (1) Heavy metals <1.07>—Proceed with 1.0 g of Azelastine Hydrochloride according to Method 2, and perform the test. Prepare the control solution with 2.0 mL of Standard Lead Solution (not more than 20 ppm).

(2) Arsenic <1.11>—Prepare the test solution with 1.0 g of Azelastine Hydrochloride according to Method 3, and perform the test (not more than 2 ppm).

(3) Related substances—Dissolve 50 mg of Azelastine Hydrochloride in 100 mL of the mobile phase, and use this solution as the sample solution. Pipet 1 mL of the sample solution, add the mobile phase to make exactly 100 mL, and use this solution as the standard solution. Perform the test with exactly 20 μL each of the sample solution and standard solution as directed under Liquid Chromatography <2.01> according to the following conditions. Determine each peak area of these solutions by the automatic integration method: each peak area other than azelastine obtained from the sample solution is not larger than 1/10 times the peak area of azelastine from the standard solution, and the total area of the peaks other than the peak of azelastine from the sample solution is not larger than 1/2 times the peak area of azelastine from the standard solution.

Operating conditions—

Detector: An ultraviolet absorption photometer (wavelength: 240 nm).

Column: A stainless steel column 4.6 mm in inside diameter and 15 cm in length, packed with octadecylsilanized silica gel for liquid chromatography (5 μm in particle diameter).

Column temperature: A constant temperature of about 35°C.

Mobile phase: A mixture of water, acetonitrile and perchloric acid (660:340:1).

Flow rate: Adjust so that the retention time of azelastine is about 10 minutes.

Time span of measurement: About 2 times as long as the retention time of azelastine, beginning after the solvent peak.

System suitability—

Test for required detectability: Pipet 5 mL of the standard solution, and add the mobile phase to make exactly 50 mL. Confirm that the peak area of azelastine obtained with 20 μL of this solution is equivalent to 7 to 13% of that with 20 μL of the standard solution.

System performance: When the procedure is run with 20 μL of the standard solution under the above operating conditions, the number of theoretical plates and the symmetry factor of the peak of azelastine is not less than 5000 and not more than 1.5, respectively.

System repeatability: When the test is repeated 6 times with 20 μL of the standard solution under the above operating conditions, the relative standard deviation of the peak area of azelastine is not more than 1.0%.

Loss on drying <2.41> Not more than 1.0% (1 g, 105°C, 2 hours).

Residue on ignition <2.44> Not more than 0.1% (1 g).

Assay Weigh accurately about 0.6 g of previously dried Azelastine Hydrochloride, dissolve in 5 mL of formic acid, add 70 mL of acetic anhydride, and titrate <2.50> with 0.1 mol/L perchloric acid VS (potentiometric titration). Perform a blank determination in the same manner, and make any necessary correction.

Each mL of 0.1 mol/L perchloric acid VS
$= 41.84$ mg of $C_{22}H_{24}ClN_3O.HCl$

Containers and storage Containers—Tight containers.
Storage—Light-resistant.

Azelastine Hydrochloride Granules

アゼラスチン塩酸塩顆粒

Azelastine Hydrochloride Granules contain not less than 93.0% and not more than 107.0% of the labeled amount of azelastine hydrochloride ($C_{22}H_{24}ClN_3O.HCl$: 418.36).

Method of preparation Prepare as directed under Granules, with Azelastine Hydrochloride.

Identification To a quantity of Azelastine Hydrochloride Granules, equivalent to 2 mg of Azelastine Hydrochloride, add 30 mL of 0.1 mol/L hydrochloric acid TS, and sonicate for 30 minutes. After cooling, add 0.1 mol/L hydrochloric acid TS to make 50 mL, and centrifuge. Determine the absorption spectrum of the supernatant liquid as directed under Ultraviolet-visible Spectrophotometry <2.24>: it exhibits a maximum between 283 nm and 287 nm.

Dissolution <6.10> When the test is performed at 50 revolutions per minute according to the Paddle method, using 900 mL of 0.05 mol/L acetic acid-sodium acetate buffer solution (pH 4.0) as the dissolution medium, the dissolution rate in 45 minutes of Azelastine Hydrochloride Granules is not less than 80%.

Start the test with accurately weighed amount of Azelastine Hydrochloride Granules, equivalent to about 1 mg of azelastine hydrochloride ($C_{22}H_{24}ClN_3O.HCl$), withdraw not less than 20 mL of the medium at the specified minute after starting the test, and filter through a membrane filter with a pore size not exceeding 0.5 μm. Discard not less than 10 mL of the first filtrate, and use the subsequent filtrate as the sample solution. Separately, weigh accurately about 50 mg of azelastine hydrochloride for assay, previously dried at 105°C for 2 hours, and dissolve in the dissolution medium to make exactly 250 mL. Pipet 1 mL of this solution, add the dissolution medium to make exactly 200 mL, and use this solution as the standard solution. Perform the test with exactly 50 μL each of the sample solution and standard solution as directed under Liquid Chromatography <2.01> according to the following conditions, and determine the peak areas, A_T and A_S, of azelastine in each solution.

Dissolution rate (%) with respect to the labeled amount of azelastine hydrochloride ($C_{22}H_{24}ClN_3O.HCl$)
$= M_S/M_T \times A_T/A_S \times 1/C \times 9/5$

M_S: Amount (mg) of azelastine hydrochloride for assay taken
M_T: Amount (g) of Azelastine Hydrochloride Granules taken
C: Labeled amount (mg) of azelastine hydrochloride ($C_{22}H_{24}ClN_3O.HCl$) in 1 g

Operating conditions—

Proceed as directed in the operating conditions in the Assay.

System suitability—

System performance: When the procedure is run with 50 μL of the standard solution under the above operating conditions, the number of theoretical plates and the symmetry factor of the peak of azelastine are not less than 2000 and not more than 1.5, respectively.

System repeatability: When the test is repeated 6 times with 50 μL of the standard solution under the above operating conditions, the relative standard deviation of the peak area of azelastine is not more than 2.0%.

Assay Weigh accurately an amount of Azelastine Hydrochloride Granules, equivalent to about 2 mg of azelastine hydrochloride ($C_{22}H_{24}ClN_3O.HCl$), add 50 mL of 0.1 mol/L hydrochloric acid TS, sonicate for 20 minutes, add 40 mL of ethanol (99.5), add exactly 5 mL of the internal standard solution, and add ethanol (99.5) to make 100 mL. Centrifuge this solution, and use the supernatant liquid as the sample solution. Separately, weigh accurately about 50 mg of azelastine hydrochloride for assay, previously dried at 105°C for 2 hours, and dissolve in water to make exactly 50 mL. Pipet 10 mL of this solution, and add 0.1 mol/L hydrochloric acid TS to make exactly 50 mL. Pipet 10 mL of this solution, add 40 mL of 0.1 mol/L hydrochloric acid TS and 40 mL of ethanol (99.5), add exactly 5 mL of the internal standard solution, add ethanol (99.5) to make 100 mL, and use this solution as the standard solution. Perform the test with 20 μL each of the sample solution and standard solution as directed under Liquid Chromatography <2.01> according to the following conditions, and calculate the ratios, Q_T and Q_S, of the peak area of azelastine to that of the internal standard.

Amount (mg) of azelastine hydrochloride ($C_{22}H_{24}ClN_3O.HCl$)
$= M_S \times Q_T/Q_S \times 1/25$

M_S: Amount (mg) of azelastine hydrochloride for assay taken

*Internal standard solution—*Dissolve 0.2 g of 2-ethylhexyl parahydroxybenzoate in ethanol (99.5) to make 100 mL.

Operating conditions—

Detector: An ultraviolet absorption photometer (wavelength: 285 nm).

Column: A stainless steel column 4.6 mm in inside diameter and 15 cm in length, packed with octadecylsilanized silica gel for liquid chromatography (5 μm in particle diameter).

Column temperature: A constant temperature of about 40°C.

Mobile phase: A mixture of acetonitrile and a solution of sodium lauryl sulfate in diluted acetic acid (100) (1 in 250) (1 in 500) (11:9).

Flow rate: Adjust so that the retention time of azelastine is about 6 minutes.

System suitability—

System performance: When the procedure is run with 20 μL of the standard solution under the above operating conditions, azelastine and the internal standard are eluted in this order with the resolution between these peaks being not less than 2.0.

System repeatability: When the test is repeated 6 times with 20 μL of the standard solution under the above operating conditions, the relative standard deviation of the ratio of the peak area of azelastine to that of the internal standard is not more than 1.0%.

Containers and storage Containers—Tight containers.

Azelnidipine

アゼルニジピン

and enantiomer

$C_{33}H_{34}N_4O_6$: 582.65
3-[1-(Diphenylmethyl)azetidin-3-yl] 5-(1-methylethyl) (4*RS*)-2-amino-6-methyl-4-(3-nitrophenyl)-1,4-dihydropyridine-3,5-dicarboxylate
[*123524-52-7*]

Azelnidipine contains not less than 99.0% and not more than 101.0% of azelnidipine ($C_{33}H_{34}N_4O_6$), calculated on the dried basis.

Description Azelnidipine occurs as a light yellow to yellow, crystalline powder or powder containing masses.

It is freely soluble in ethanol (99.5) and in acetic acid (100), and practically insoluble in water.

A solution of Azelnidipine in ethanol (99.5) (1 in 100) shows no optical rotation.

Azelnidipine shows crystal polymorphism.

Identification **(1)** Determine the absorption spectrum of a solution of Azelnidipine in ethanol (99.5) (1 in 50,000) as directed under Ultraviolet-visible Spectrophotometry *<2.24>*, and compare the spectrum with the Reference Spectrum: both spectra exhibit similar intensities of absorption at the same wavelengths.

(2) Determine the infrared absorption spectrum of Azelnidipine as directed in the paste method under Infrared Spectrophotometry *<2.25>*, and compare the spectrum with the Reference Spectrum: both spectra exhibit similar intensities of absorption at the same wave numbers.

Purity **(1)** Heavy metals *<1.07>*—Proceed with 1.0 g of Azelnidipine according to Method 2, and perform the test. Prepare the control solution with 1.0 mL of Standard Lead Solution (not more than 10 ppm).

(2) Related substances—Dissolve 0.10 g of Azelnidipine in a mixture of acetonitrile and water (4:1) to make 100 mL, and use this solution as the sample solution. Pipet 2 mL of the sample solution, add a mixture of acetonitrile and water (4:1) to make exactly 200 mL, and use this solution as the standard solution. Perform the test with exactly 10 μL each of the sample solution and standard solution as directed under Liquid Chromatography *<2.01>* according to the following conditions. Determine each peak area by the automatic integration method: the areas of the peak, having the relative retention time of about 0.50 and about 1.42 to azelnidipine, obtained from the sample solution are not larger than 1/5 times and 3/10 times the peak area of azelnidipine from the standard solution, respectively, the area of the peak other than azelnidipine and the peaks mentioned above from the sample solution is not larger than 1/10 times the peak area of azelnidipine from the standard solution, and the total area of the peaks other than azelnidipine from the sample solution is not larger than 7/10 times the peak area of azelnidipine from the standard solution.

Operating conditions—

Detector: An ultraviolet absorption photometer (wavelength: 220 nm).

Column: A stainless steel column 4.6 mm in inside diameter and 25 cm in length, packed with octadecylsilanized silica gel for liquid chromatography (5 μm in particle diameter).

Column temperature: A constant temperature of about 40°C.

Mobile phase: Dissolve 1.05 g of potassium dihydrogen phosphate in 350 mL of water, add 650 mL of a mixture of acetonitrile and methanol (7:3), and adjust to pH 5.5 with diluted phosphoric acid (1 in 10).

Flow rate: Adjust so that the retention time of azelnidipine is about 36 minutes.

Time span of measurement: About 2 times as long as the retention time of azelnidipine, beginning after the solvent peak.

System suitability—

Test for required detectability: To exactly 1 mL of the standard solution add a mixture of acetonitrile and water (4:1) to make exactly 20 mL. Confirm that the peak area of azelnidipine obtained with 10 μL of this solution is equivalent to 3.5 to 6.5% of that with 10 μL of the standard solution.

System performance: When the procedure is run with 10 μL of the standard solution under the above operating conditions, the number of theoretical plates and the symmetry factor of the peak of azelnidipine are not less than 15,000 and 0.8 to 1.5, respectively.

System repeatability: When the test is repeated 6 times with 10 μL of the standard solution under the above operating conditions, the relative standard deviation of the peak area of azelnidipine is not more than 1.0%.

Loss on drying *<2.41>* Not more than 0.5% (1 g, in vacuum, 70°C, 5 hours).

Residue on ignition *<2.44>* Not more than 0.1% (1 g).

Assay Weigh accurately about 0.4 g of Azelnidipine, dissolve in 50 mL of acetic acid (100), and titrate *<2.50>* with 0.1 mol/L perchloric acid VS (potentiometric titration). Perform a blank determination in the same manner, and make any necessary correction.

Each mL of 0.1 mol/L perchloric acid VS
= 29.13 mg of $C_{33}H_{34}N_4O_6$

Containers and storage Containers—Tight containers.

Azelnidipine Tablets

アゼルニジピン錠

Azelnidipine Tablets contain not less than 95.0% and not more than 105.0% of the labeled amount of azelnidipine ($C_{33}H_{34}N_4O_6$: 582.65).

Method of preparation Prepare as directed under Tablets, with Azelnidipine.

Identification Powder Azelnidipine Tablets. Weigh a portion of the powder, equivalent to 4 mg of Azelnidipine, add 150 mL of ethanol (99.5), sonicate for 15 minutes, then add ethanol (99.5) to make 200 mL. Centrifuge this solution, filter the supernatant liquid through a glass wool filter with a pore size not exceeding 0.7 μm. Discard the first 10 mL of the filtrate, and use the subsequent filtrate as the sample solution. Determine the absorption spectrum of the sample solution as directed under Ultraviolet-visible Spectrophotometry *<2.24>*: it exhibits maxima between 253 nm and 257

The JP Drugs are to be tested according to the provisions given in the pertinent monographs, General Notices, General Rules for Crude Drugs, General Rules for Preparations, and General Tests for their conformity to the Japanese Pharmacopoeia. (See the General Notices 5.)

nm and between 339 nm and 346 nm.

Purity Related substances—Conduct this procedure using light-resistant vessels. Powder Azelnidipine Tablets. Weigh a portion of the powder, equivalent to 10 mg of Azelnidipine, add 10 mL of a mixture of acetonitrile and water (4:1), agitate gently, then disperse to fine particles by sonicating for 15 minutes. Centrifuge this solution, and use the supernatant liquid as the sample solution. Pipet 2 mL of the sample solution, add a mixture of acetonitrile and water (4:1) to make exactly 100 mL, and use this solution as the standard solution. Perform the test with exactly 10 μL each of the sample solution and standard solution as directed under Liquid Chromatography <*2.01*> according to the following conditions, and determine each peak area by the automatic integration method: the areas of the peaks, having the relative retention times of about 0.10, about 0.13, about 0.50, and about 1.42 to azelnidipine, obtained from the sample solution, are not larger than 9/20 times, 1/5 times, 2/5 times, and 2/5 times the peak area of azelnidipine obtained from the standard solution, respectively, the area of the peak, other than azelnidipine and the peaks mentioned above, is not larger than 1/10 times the peak area of azelnidipine from the standard solution. Furthermore, the total area of these peaks other than azelnidipine is not larger than 1.75 times the peak area of azelnidipine from the standard solution.

Operating conditions—

Detector, column, column temperature, mobile phase, and flow rate: Proceed as directed in the operating conditions in the Purity (2) under Azelnidipine.

Time span of measurement: About 2 times as long as the retention time of azelnidipine.

System suitability—

Test for required detectability: To exactly 1 mL of the standard solution add a mixture of acetonitrile and water (4:1) to make exactly 20 mL. Confirm that the peak area of azelnidipine obtained with 10 μL of this solution is equivalent to 3.5 to 6.5% of that with 10 μL of the standard solution.

System performance: When the procedure is run with 10 μL of the standard solution under the above operating conditions, the number of theoretical plates and the symmetry factor of the peak of azelnidipine are not less than 15,000 and not more than 1.5, respectively.

System repeatability: When the test is repeated 6 times with 10 μL of the standard solution under the above operating conditions, the relative standard deviation of the peak area of azelnidipine is not more than 1.0%.

Uniformity of dosage units <*6.02*> Perform the test according to the following method: it meets the requirement of the Content uniformity test.

To 1 tablet of Azelnidipine Tablets add exactly 1 mL of the internal standard solution per 2 mg of azelnidipine ($C_{33}H_{34}N_4O_6$), and add a mixture of acetonitrile and water (4:1) to make 32 mL. Disintegrate the tablet with occasional shaking, and sonicate for 10 minutes. Centrifuge this solution, pipet V mL of the supernatant liquid, equivalent to 2.5 mg of azelnidipine ($C_{33}H_{34}N_4O_6$), add a mixture of acetonitrile and water (4:1) to make 50 mL, and use this solution as the sample solution. Then, proceed as directed in the Assay.

Amount (mg) of azelnidipine ($C_{33}H_{34}N_4O_6$)
$= M_S \times Q_T/Q_S \times 8/5V$

M_S: Amount (mg) of azelnidipine for assay taken

Internal standard solution—A solution of 2,2′-dinaphthylether in a mixture of acetonitrile and water (4:1) (1 in 1000).

Dissolution <*6.10*> When the test is performed at 50 revolutions per minute according to the Paddle method, using 900 mL of 1st fluid for dissolution test as the dissolution medium, the dissolution rate in 45 minutes of Azelnidipine Tablets is not less than 75%.

Start the test with 1 tablet of Azelnidipine Tablets, withdraw not less than 20 mL of the medium at the specified minute after starting the test, and filter through a membrane filter with a pore size not exceeding 0.45 μm. Discard not less than 10 mL of the first filtrate, pipet V mL of the subsequent filtrate, add the dissolution medium to make exactly V' mL so that each mL contains about 8.9 μg of azelnidipine ($C_{33}H_{34}N_4O_6$), and use this solution as the sample solution. Separately, weigh accurately about 45 mg of azelnidipine for assay, previously dried in vacuum at 70°C for 5 hours, dissolve in ethanol (99.5) to make exactly 25 mL. Pipet 1 mL of this solution, add the dissolution medium to make exactly 200 mL, and use this solution as the standard solution. Determine the absorbances, A_T and A_S, at 270 nm of the sample solution and standard solution as directed under Ultraviolet-visible Spectrophotometry <*2.24*>, using the dissolution medium as the blank.

Dissolution rate (%) with respect to the labeled amount of azelnidipine ($C_{33}H_{34}N_4O_6$)
$= M_S \times A_T/A_S \times V'/V \times 1/C \times 18$

M_S: Amount (mg) of azelnidipine for assay taken
C: Labeled amount (mg) of azelnidipine ($C_{33}H_{34}N_4O_6$) in 1 tablet

Assay Weigh accurately the mass of not less than 20 Azelnidipine Tablets, and powder. Weigh accurately a portion of the powder, equivalent to about 50 mg of azelnidipine ($C_{33}H_{34}N_4O_6$), add exactly 25 mL of the internal standard solution, add 50 mL of a mixture of acetonitrile and water (4:1). After sonicating for 10 minutes, add a mixture of acetonitrile and water (4:1) to make 100 mL. Centrifuge this solution, to 5 mL of the supernatant liquid add a mixture of acetonitrile and water (4:1) to make 50 mL, and use this solution as the sample solution. Separately, weigh accurately about 50 mg of azelnidipine for assay, previously dried in vacuum at 70°C for 5 hours, dissolve in exactly 25 mL of the internal standard solution, and add a mixture of acetonitrile and water (4:1) to make 100 mL. To 5 mL of this solution add a mixture of acetonitrile and water (4:1) to make 50 mL, and use this solution as the standard solution. Perform the test with 10 μL each of the sample solution and standard solution as directed under Liquid Chromatography <*2.01*> according to the following conditions, and calculate the ratios, Q_T and Q_S, of the peak area of azelnidipine to that of the internal standard.

Amount (mg) of azelnidipine ($C_{33}H_{34}N_4O_6$) $= M_S \times Q_T/Q_S$

M_S: Amount (mg) of azelnidipine for assay taken

Internal standard solution—2,2′-dinaphthylether in a mixture of acetonitrile and water (4:1) (1 in 1000).

Operating conditions—

Detector: An ultraviolet absorption photometer (wavelength: 254 nm).

Column: A stainless steel column 4.6 mm in inside diameter and 25 cm in length, packed with octadecylsilanized silica gel for liquid chromatography (5 μm in particle diameter).

Column temperature: A constant temperature of about 40°C.

Mobile phase: Dissolve 0.9 g of potassium dihydrogen

phosphate in 300 mL of water, add 700 mL of acetonitrile, then adjust to pH 6.0 with dilute sodium hydroxide TS.

Flow rate: Adjust so that the retention time of azelnidipine is about 13 minutes.

System suitability—

System performance: When the procedure is run with 10 μL of the standard solution under the above operating conditions, azelnidipine and the internal standard are eluted in this order with the resolution between these peaks being not less than 12.

System repeatability: When the test is repeated 6 times with 10 μL of the standard solution under the above operating conditions, the relative standard deviation of the ratio of the peak area of azelnidipine to that of the internal standard is not more than 1.0%.

Containers and storage Containers—Tight containers.

Storage—Light-resistant.

Azithromycin Hydrate

アジスロマイシン水和物

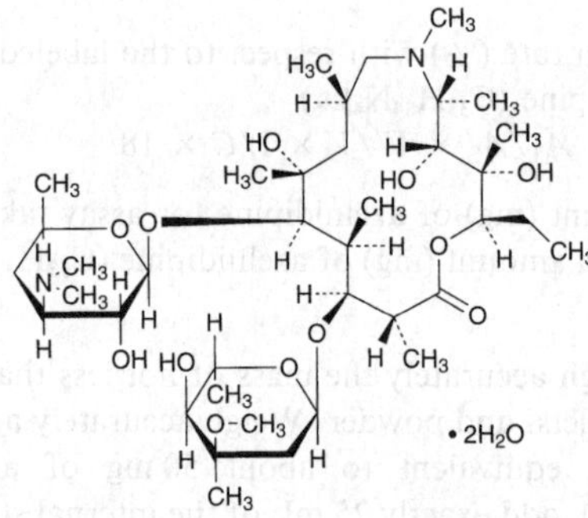

$C_{38}H_{72}N_2O_{12}.2H_2O$: 785.02

(2*R*,3*S*,4*S*,5*R*,6*R*,8*R*,11*R*,12*R*,13*S*,14*R*)-5-(3,4,6-Trideoxy-3-dimethylamino-*β*-D-*xylo*-hexopyranosyloxy)-3-(2,6-dideoxy-3-*C*-methyl-3-*O*-methyl-*α*-L-ribo-hexopyranosyloxy)-10-aza-6,12,13-trihydroxy-2,4,6,8,10,11,13-heptamethylhexadecan-14-olide dihydrate

[*117772-70-0*]

Azithromycin Hydrate is the derivative of erythromycin.

It contains not less than 945 μg (potency) and not more than 1030 μg (potency) per mg, calculated on the anhydrous basis. The potency of Azithromycin Hydrate is expressed as mass (potency) of azithromycin ($C_{38}H_{72}N_2O_{12}$: 748.98).

Description Azithromycin Hydrate occurs as a white crystalline powder.

It is freely soluble in methanol and in ethanol (99.5), and practically insoluble in water.

Identification Determine the infrared absorption spectrum of Azithromycin Hydrate as directed in the potassium bromide disk method under the Infrared Spectrophotometry <*2.25*>, and compare the spectrum with the Reference Spectrum or the spectrum of Azithromycin RS: both spectra exhibit similar intensities of absorption at the same wave numbers.

Optical rotation <*2.49*> $[\alpha]_D^{20}$: −45 – −49° (0.4 g calculated on the anhydrous basis, ethanol (99.5), 20 mL, 100 mm).

Purity (1) Heavy metals <*1.07*>—Proceed with 1.0 g of Azithromycin Hydrate according to Method 2, and perform the test. Prepare the control solution with 1.0 mL of Standard Lead Solution (not more than 10 ppm).

(2) Related substances—Being specified separately when the drug is granted approval based on the Law.

Water <*2.48*> Not less than 4.0% and not more than 5.0% (0.4 g, volumetric titration, direct titration).

Residue on ignition <*2.44*> Not more than 0.1% (1 g).

Assay Weigh accurately an amount of Azithromycin Hydrate and Azithromycin RS, equivalent to about 50 mg (potency), dissolve each in an adequate amount of a mixture of acetonitrile and water (3:2), add exactly 2 mL of the internal standard solution and the mixture of acetonitrile and water (3:2) to make 50 mL, and use these solutions as the sample solution and standard solution. Perform the test with 5 μL each of the sample solution and standard solution as directed under Liquid Chromatography <*2.01*> according to the following conditions, and calculate the ratios, Q_T and Q_S, of the peak area of azithromycin to that of the internal standard.

Amount [μg (potency)] of azithromycin ($C_{38}H_{72}N_2O_{12}$)
$= M_S \times Q_T/Q_S \times 1000$

M_S: Amount [mg (potency)] of Azithromycin RS taken

Internal standard solution—A solution of 4,4′-bis(diethylamino)benzophenone in acetonitrile (3 in 4000).

Operating conditions—

Detector: An ultraviolet absorption photometer (wavelength: 215 nm).

Column: A stainless steel column 4.6 mm in inside diameter and 25 cm in length, packed with octadecylsilanized polyvinyl alcohol gel polymer for liquid chromatography (5 μm in particle diameter).

Column temperature: A constant temperature of about 40°C.

Mobile phase: Dissolve 6.97 g of dipotassium hydrogen phosphate in about 750 mL of water, adjust the pH to 11.0 with potassium hydroxide TS, and add water to make 1000 mL. To 400 mL of this solution add 600 mL of acetonitrile for liquid chromatography.

Flow rate: Adjust so that the retention time of azithromycin is about 10 minutes.

System suitability—

System performance: When the procedure is run with 5 μL of the standard solution under the above operating conditions, azithromycin and the internal standard are eluted in this order with the resolution between these peaks being not less than 2.0.

System repeatability: When the test is repeated 6 times with 5 μL of the standard solution under the above operating conditions, the relative standard deviation of the ratios of the peak area of azithromycin to that of the internal standard is not more than 1.0%.

Containers and storage Containers—Tight containers.

Azosemide

アゾセミド

$C_{12}H_{11}ClN_6O_2S_2$: 370.84
2-Chloro-5-(1*H*-tetrazol-5-yl)-4-[(thien-2-ylmethyl)amino]
benzenesulfonamide
[*27589-33-9*]

Azosemide, when dried, contains not less than 99.0% and not more than 101.0% of azosemide ($C_{12}H_{11}ClN_6O_2S_2$).

Description Azosemide occurs as a white to yellow-white crystalline powder.

It is freely soluble in *N*,*N*-dimethylformamide, slightly soluble in methanol and in ethanol (99.5), and practically insoluble in water.

It dissolves in dilute sodium hydroxide TS.

It is gradually colored to yellow by light.

Melting point: about 226°C (with decomposition).

Identification **(1)** Determine the absorption spectrum of a solution of Azosemide in dilute sodium hydroxide TS (3 in 500,000) as directed under Ultraviolet-visible Spectrophotometry 〈*2.24*〉, and compare the spectrum with the Reference Spectrum: both spectra exhibit similar intensities of absorption at the same wavelengths.

(2) Determine the infrared absorption spectrum of Azosemide, previously dried, as directed in the potassium bromide disk method under Infrared Spectrophotometry 〈*2.25*〉, and compare the spectrum with the Reference Spectrum: both spectra exhibit similar intensities of absorption at the same wave numbers.

Purity **(1)** Chloride 〈*1.03*〉—To 1.0 g of Azosemide add 60 mL of dilute sodium hydroxide TS, dissolve by warming. After cooling, add 0.5 mL of nitric acid and filter. To 30 mL of the filtrate add 6 mL of dilute nitric acid and water to make 50 mL. Perform the test using this solution as the test solution. Prepare the control solution with 0.45 mL of 0.01 mol/L hydrochloric acid VS (not more than 0.032%).

(2) Heavy metal 〈*1.07*〉—Proceed with 1.0 g of Azosemide according to Method 2, and perform the test. Prepare the control solution with 2.0 mL of Standard Lead Solution (not more than 20 ppm).

(3) Primary aromatic amines—Dissolve 20 mg of Azosemide in 5 mL of *N*,*N*-dimethylformamide, add 12 mL of water, 1.0 mL of a solution of sodium nitrite (1 in 200) and 2.0 mL of diluted hydrochloric acid (1 in 10) under ice-cooling, shake, and allow to stand for 3 minutes. Add 1.0 mL of ammonium amidosulfate TS, shake thoroughly, allow to stand for 3 minutes, and add 1.0 mL of a solution of *N*-1-naphthylethylenediamine dihydrochloride (1 in 200). Shake this solution, and add *N*,*N*-dimethylformamide to make exactly 50 mL. Determine the absorbance of this solution at 540 nm as directed under Ultraviolet-visible Spectrophotometry 〈*2.24*〉, using a solution prepared in the same manner with 5 mL of *N*,*N*-dimethylformamide as the blank: the absorbance is not more than 0.15.

Loss on drying 〈*2.41*〉 Not more than 0.5% (1 g, 105°C, 3 hours).

Residue on ignition 〈*2.44*〉 Not more than 0.1% (1 g).

Assay Weigh accurately about 0.6 g of Azosemide, previously dried, dissolve in 50 mL of *N*,*N*-dimethylformamide, and titrate 〈*2.50*〉 with 0.1 mol/L potassium hydroxide-ethanol VS until the color of the solution changes from yellow to yellow-green (indicator: 10 drops of thymol blue-*N*,*N*-dimethylformamide TS). Perform a blank determination in the same manner with a solution prepared by adding 15 mL of ethanol (95) to 50 mL of *N*,*N*-dimethylformamide, and make any necessary correction.

Each mL of 0.1 mol/L potassium hydroxide-ethanol VS
= 37.08 mg of $C_{12}H_{11}ClN_6O_2S_2$

Containers and storage Containers—Tight containers.
Storage—Light-resistant.

Azosemide Tablets

アゾセミド錠

Azosemide Tablets contain not less than 95.0% and not more than 105.0% of the labeled amount of azosemide ($C_{12}H_{11}ClN_6O_2S_2$: 370.84).

Method of preparation Prepare as directed under Tablets, with Azosemide.

Identification To a quantity of powdered Azosemide Tablets, equivalent to 60 mg of Azosemide, add dilute sodium hydroxide TS to make 100 mL, shake, and filter. To 1 mL of the filtrate add dilute sodium hydroxide TS to make 100 mL. Determine the absorption spectrum of this solution as directed under Ultraviolet-visible Spectrophotometry 〈*2.24*〉: it exhibits maxima between 234 nm and 238 nm, between 272 nm and 276 nm and between 324 nm and 330 nm.

Purity Primary aromatic amines—To a quantity of powdered Azosemide Tablets, equivalent to 20 mg of Azosemide, add 5 mL of *N*,*N*-dimethylformamide, and allow to stand with occasional shaking. Add 12 mL of water, 1.0 mL of a solution of sodium nitrite (1 in 200) and 2.0 mL of diluted hydrochloric acid (1 in 10) under ice-cooling, shake, and allow to stand for 3 minutes. Add 1.0 mL of ammonium amidosulfate TS, shake thoroughly, and allow to stand for 3 minutes. Add 1.0 mL of a solution of *N*-1-naphthylethylenediamine dihydrochloride (1 in 200), and shake. Add *N*,*N*-dimethylformamide to make exactly 50 mL, centrifuge, and use the supernatant liquid as the sample solution. Determine the absorbance of the sample solution at 540 nm as directed under Ultraviolet-visible Spectrophotometry 〈*2.24*〉, using a solution prepared in the same manner with 5 mL of *N*,*N*-dimethylformamide as the blank: the absorbance is not more than 0.15.

Uniformity of dosage unit 〈*6.02*〉 Perform the Mass variation test, or the Content uniformity test according to the following method: it meets the requirement.

To 1 tablet of Azosemide Tablets add dilute sodium hydroxide TS to make exactly *V* mL so that each mL contains about 0.6 mg of azosemide ($C_{12}H_{11}ClN_6O_2S_2$), shake thoroughly, and centrifuge. Pipet 10 mL of the supernatant liquid, and add dilute sodium hydroxide TS to make exactly 100 mL. Pipet 10 mL of this solution, add dilute sodium hydroxide TS to make exactly 50 mL, and use this solution as the sample solution. Separately, weigh accurately about 60 mg of azosemide for assay, previously dried at 105°C for 3 hours, and dissolve in dilute sodium hydroxide TS to make exactly 100 mL. Pipet 10 mL of this solution, and add dilute sodium hydroxide TS to make exactly 100 mL. Pipet 10 mL of this solution, add dilute sodium hydroxide TS to make exactly 50 mL, and use this solution as the standard solution. Determine the absorbances, A_T and A_S, of the sample solution and standard solution at 274 nm as directed under Ultraviolet-visible Spectrophotometry <2.24>.

$$\text{Amount (mg) of azosemide } (C_{12}H_{11}ClN_6O_2S_2) = M_S \times A_T/A_S \times V/100$$

M_S: Amount (mg) of azosemide for assay taken

Dissolution *<6.10>* When the test is performed at 50 revolutions per minute according to the Paddle method, using 900 mL of 2nd fluid for dissolution test as the dissolution medium, the dissolution rate in 60 minutes of a 30-mg tablet and in 90 minutes of a 60-mg tablet are not less than 70%, respectively.

Start the test with 1 tablet of Azosemide Tablets, withdraw not less than 20 mL of the medium at the specified minute after starting the test, and filter through a membrane filter with a pore size not exceeding 0.5 μm. Discard not less than 10 mL of the first filtrate, pipet V mL of the subsequent filtrate, and add the dissolution medium to make exactly V' mL so that each mL contains about 33 μg of azosemide ($C_{12}H_{11}ClN_6O_2S_2$). Pipet 8 mL of this solution, add 0.2 mol/L sodium hydroxide TS to make exactly 20 mL, and use this solution as the sample solution. Separately, weigh accurately about 22 mg of azosemide for assay, previously dried at 105°C for 3 hours, and dissolve in 0.2 mol/L sodium hydroxide TS to make exactly 100 mL. Pipet 5 mL of this solution, and add 0.2 mol/L sodium hydroxide TS to make exactly 50 mL. Pipet 15 mL of this solution, add the dissolution medium to make exactly 25 mL, and use this solution as the standard solution. Determine the absorbances, A_T and A_S, of the sample solution and standard solution at 274 nm as directed under Ultraviolet-visible Spectrophotometry <2.24>, using a solution prepared by adding 0.2 mol/L sodium hydroxide TS to 8 mL of the dissolution medium to make 20 mL as the blank.

$$\text{Dissolution rate (\%) with respect to the labeled amount of azosemide } (C_{12}H_{11}ClN_6O_2S_2) = M_S \times A_T/A_S \times V'/V \times 1/C \times 135$$

M_S: Amount (mg) of azosemide for assay taken
C: Labeled amount (mg) of azosemide ($C_{12}H_{11}ClN_6O_2S_2$) in 1 tablet

Assay Weigh accurately the mass of not less than 20 tablets of Azosemide Tablets, and powder. Weigh accurately a portion of the powder, equivalent to about 60 mg of azosemide ($C_{12}H_{11}ClN_6O_2S_2$), add dilute sodium hydroxide TS to make exactly 100 mL, shake thoroughly, and filter. Discard the first 5 mL of the filtrate, pipet 5 mL of the subsequent filtrate, add exactly 10 mL of the internal standard solution, add the mobile phase to make 100 mL, and use this solution as the sample solution. Separately, weigh accurately about 60 mg of azosemide for assay, previously dried at 105°C for 3 hours, and dissolve in dilute sodium hydroxide TS to make exactly 100 mL. Pipet 5 mL of this solution, add exactly 10 mL of the internal standard solution, add the mobile phase to make 100 mL, and use this solution as the standard solution. Perform the test with 10 μL each of the sample solution and standard solution as directed under Liquid Chromatography <2.01> according to the following conditions, and calculate the ratios, Q_T and Q_S, of the peak area of azosemide to that of the internal standard.

$$\text{Amount (mg) of azosemide } (C_{12}H_{11}ClN_6O_2S_2) = M_S \times Q_T/Q_S$$

M_S: Amount (mg) of azosemide for assay taken

Internal standard solution—A solution of propyl parahydroxybenzoate in the mobile phase (3 in 5000).
Operating conditions—

Detector: An ultraviolet absorption photometer (wavelength: 280 nm).

Column: A stainless steel column 4.6 mm in inside diameter and 15 cm in length, packed with octadecylsilanized silica gel for liquid chromatography (5 μm in particle diameter).

Column temperature: A constant temperature of about 25°C.

Mobile phase: A mixture of 0.03 mol/L potassium dihydrogen phosphate solution, acetonitrile and methanol (55:27:18).

Flow rate: Adjust so that the retention time of azosemide is about 5 minutes.

System suitability—

System performance: When the procedure is run with 10 μL of the standard solution under the above operating conditions, azosemide and the internal standard are eluted in this order with the resolution between these peaks being not less than 8.

System repeatability: When the test is repeated 6 times with 10 μL of the standard solution under the above operating conditions, the relative standard deviation of the ratio of the peak area of azosemide to that of the internal standard is not more than 1.0%.

Containers and storage Containers—Tight containers.

Aztreonam

アズトレオナム

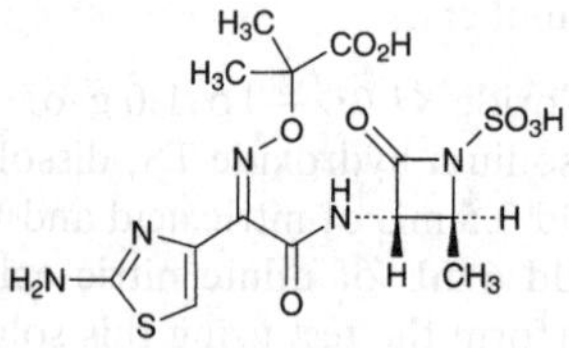

$C_{13}H_{17}N_5O_8S_2$: 435.43
2-{(*Z*)-(2-Aminothiazol-4-yl)-[(2*S*,3*S*)-2-methyl-4-oxo-1-sulfoazetidin-3-ylcarbamoyl]methyleneaminooxy}-2-methyl-1-propanoic acid
[*78110-38-0*]

Aztreonam contains not less than 920 μg (potency) and not more than 1030 μg (potency) per mg, calculated on the anhydrous basis. The potency of Aztreonam is expressed as mass (potency) of aztreonam ($C_{13}H_{17}N_5O_8S_2$).

Description Aztreonam occurs as a white to yellowish white crystalline powder.

It is freely soluble in dimethylsulfoxide, slightly soluble in water and in methanol, and very slightly soluble in ethanol (95).

Identification (1) Determine the absorption spectrum of a solution of Aztreonam (3 in 100,000) as directed under Ultraviolet-visible Spectrophotometry <2.24>, and compare the spectrum with the Reference Spectrum or the spectrum of a solution of Aztreonam RS prepared in the same manner as the sample solution: both spectra exhibit similar intensities of absorption at the same wavelengths.

(2) Determine the spectrum of a solution of Aztreonam in deuterated dimethylsulfoxide for nuclear magnetic resonance spectroscopy (1 in 10), using a light hydrogen substance existing in deuterated dimethylsulfoxide for nuclear magnetic resonance spectroscopy as an internal reference compound and 2.50 ppm for its chemical shift, as directed under Nuclear Magnetic Resonance Spectroscopy *<2.21>* (^{1}H): it exhibits a multiple signal at around δ 1.5 ppm, and a single signal at around δ 7.0 ppm. The ratio of integrated intensity of each signal is 9:1.

Optical rotation *<2.49>* $[\alpha]_D^{20}$: −26 – −32° (0.25 g calculated on the anhydrous bases, water, 50 mL, 100 mm).

pH *<2.54>* Dissolve 0.05 g of Aztreonam in 10 mL of water: the pH of this solution is between 2.2 and 2.8.

Purity **(1)** Clarity and color of solution—Dissolve 1.0 g of Aztreonam in 20 mL of dimethylsulfoxide: the solution is clear, and its absorbance at 420 nm, determined as directed under Ultraviolet-visible Spectrophotometry *<2.24>*, is not more than 0.06.

(2) Heavy metals *<1.07>*—Proceed with 2.0 g of Aztreonam according to Method 2, and perform the test. Prepare the control solution with 2.0 mL of Standard Lead Solution (not more than 10 ppm).

(3) Related substances—Dissolve 40 mg of Aztreonam in 100 mL of water, and use this solution as the sample solution. Pipet 2 mL of the sample solution, add water to make exactly 100 mL, and use this solution as the standard solution. Perform the test with exactly 25 μL each of the sample solution and standard solution as directed under Liquid Chromatography *<2.01>* according to the following conditions, and determine each peak area of both solutions by the automatic integration method: the area of the peak other than aztreonam obtained from the sample solution is not larger than the peak area of aztreonam from the standard solution, and the total area of peaks other than aztreonam from the sample solution is not larger than 2.5 times the peak area of aztreonam from the standard solution.

Operating conditions—

Column, column temperature, mobile phase, and flow rate: Proceed as directed in the operating conditions in the Assay.

Detector: An ultraviolet absorption photometer (wavelength: 254 nm).

Time span of measurement: About 4 times as long as the retention time of aztreonam, beginning after the solvent peak.

System suitability—

Test for required detectability: To 5 mL of the standard solution add water to make 10 mL, and use this solution as the solution for system suitability test. Pipet 1 mL of the solution for system suitability test, and add water to make exactly 10 mL. Confirm that the peak area of aztreonam obtained with 25 μL of this solution is equivalent to 7 to 13% of that with 25 μL of the solution for system suitability test.

System performance: When the procedure is run under the above operating conditions with 25 μL of the standard solution obtained in the Assay, the internal standard and aztreonam are eluted in this order with the resolution between these peaks being not less than 4.

System repeatability: When the test is repeated 6 times with 25 μL of the standard solution under the above operating conditions, the relative standard deviation of the peak areas of aztreonam is not more than 2.0%.

Water *<2.48>* Not more than 2.0% (0.5 g, volumetric titration, direct titration).

Residue on ignition *<2.44>* Not more than 0.1% (1 g).

Assay Weigh accurately an amount of Aztreonam and Aztreonam RS, equivalent to about 20 mg (potency), dissolve each in 70 mL of water, add exactly 10 mL of the internal standard solution and water to make 100 mL, and use these solutions as the sample solution and standard solution, respectively. Perform the test with 25 μL each of these solutions as directed under Liquid Chromatography *<2.01>* according to the following conditions, and calculate the ratios, Q_T and Q_S, of the peak area of aztreonam to that of the internal standard.

Amount [μg (potency)] of aztreonam ($C_{13}H_{17}N_5O_8S_2$)
$= M_S \times Q_T/Q_S \times 1000$

M_S: Amount [mg (potency)] of Aztreonam RS taken

Internal standard solution—A solution of 4-aminobenzoic acid (1 in 6250).

Operating conditions—

Detector: An ultraviolet absorption photometer (wavelength: 280 nm).

Column: A stainless steel column 4.6 mm in inside diameter and 25 cm in length, packed with octadecylsilanized silica gel for liquid chromatography (10 μm in particle diameter).

Column temperature: A constant temperature of about 40°C.

Mobile phase: Dissolve 1.7 g of tetrabutylammonium hydrogensulfate in 300 mL of water, adjust to pH 3.0 with 0.5 mol/L disodium hydrogenphosphate TS, and add water to make 1000 mL. To 650 mL of this solution add 350 mL of methanol.

Flow rate: Adjust so that the retention time of aztreonam is about 8 minutes.

System suitability—

System performance: When the procedure is run with 25 μL of the standard solution under the above operating conditions, the internal standard and aztreonam are eluted in this order with the resolution between these peaks being not less than 4.

System repeatability: When the test is repeated 6 times with 25 μL of the standard solution under the above operating conditions, the relative standard deviation of the ratios of the peak area of aztreonam to that of the internal standard is not more than 1.5%.

Containers and storage Containers—Tight containers.
Storage—Light-resistant.

Aztreonam for Injection

注射用アズトレオナム

Aztreonam for Injection is a preparation for injection which is dissolved before use.

It contains not less than 93.0% and not more than 107.0% of the labeled potency of aztreonam ($C_{13}H_{17}N_5O_8S_2$: 435.43).

Method of preparation Prepare as directed under Injections, with Aztreonam.

Description Aztreonam for Injection is white to yellow-white masses or powder.

Identification **(1)** Dissolve an amount of Aztreonam for Injection, equivalent to 6 mg (potency) of Aztreonam, in 1 mL of hydroxylammonium chloride-ethanol TS, allow to stand for 3 minutes, add 1 mL of acidic ammonium iron (III) sulfate TS, and mix: a red-brown color develops.

(2) Dissolve an amount of Aztreonam for Injection, equivalent to 3 mg (potency) of Aztreonam, in 100 mL of water, and determine the absorption spectrum of the solution as directed under Ultraviolet-visible Spectrophotometry *<2.24>*: it exhibits a maximum between 289 nm and 293 nm.

pH *<2.54>* The pH of a solution prepared by dissolving an amount of Aztreonam for Injection, equivalent to 1.0 g (potency) of Aztreonam, in 10 mL of water is 4.5 to 7.0.

Purity Clarity and color of solution—Dissolve an amount of Aztreonam for Injection, equivalent to 1.0 g (potency) of Aztreonam, in 10 mL of water: the solution is clear, and its absorbance *<2.24>* at 450 nm is not more than 0.06.

Water *<2.48>* Not more than 2.0% (0.5 g, volumetric titration, direct titration).

Bacterial endotoxins *<4.01>* Less than 0.10 EU/mg (potency).

Uniformity of dosage units *<6.02>* It meets the requirement of the Mass variation test.

Foreign insoluble matter *<6.06>* Perform the test according to Method 2: it meets the requirement.

Insoluble particulate matter *<6.07>* It meets the requirement.

Sterility *<4.06>* Perform the test according to the Membrane filtration method: it meets the requirement.

Assay Take an amount of Aztreonam for Injection, equivalent to about 5 g (potency) of Aztreonam, dissolve the contents with a suitable amount of water, and transfer to a 100-mL volumetric flask. Wash each container with water, combine the washings and the solution, and add water to make exactly 100 mL. Pipet 10 mL of this solution, and add water to make exactly 50 mL. Pipet 2 mL of this solution, add exactly 10 mL of the internal standard solution and water to make 100 mL, and use this solution as the sample solution. Separately, weigh accurately an amount of Aztreonam RS, equivalent to about 20 mg (potency), dissolve in a suitable amount of water, add exactly 10 mL of the internal standard solution and water to make 100 mL, and use this solution as the standard solution. Then, proceed as directed in the Assay under Aztreonam.

Amount [mg (potency)] of aztreonam ($C_{13}H_{17}N_5O_8S_2$)
$= M_S \times Q_T/Q_S \times 250$

M_S: Amount [mg (potency)] of Aztreonam RS taken

Internal standard solution—A solution of 4-aminobenzoic acid (1 in 6250).

Containers and storage Containers—Hermetic containers.
Storage—Light-resistant.

Bacampicillin Hydrochloride

バカンピシリン塩酸塩

$C_{21}H_{27}N_3O_7S.HCl$: 501.98

1-Ethoxycarbonyloxyethyl (2*S*,5*R*,6*R*)-6-[(2*R*)-2-amino-2-phenylacetylamino]-3,3-dimethyl-7-oxo-4-thia-1-azabicyclo[3.2.0]heptane-2-carboxylate monohydrochloride
[37661-08-8]

Bacampicillin Hydrochloride is a hydrochloride of ampicillin ethoxycarbonyloxyethyl ester.

It contains not less than 626 μg (potency) and not more than 710 μg (potency) per mg, calculated on the anhydrous basis. The potency of Bacampicillin Hydrochloride is expressed as mass (potency) of ampicillin ($C_{16}H_{19}N_3O_4S$: 349.40).

Description Bacampicillin Hydrochloride occurs as a white to pale yellow crystalline powder.

It is freely soluble in methanol and in ethanol (95), and soluble in water.

Identification **(1)** Determine the absorption spectrum of a solution of Bacampicillin Hydrochloride in methanol (1 in 1000) as directed under Ultraviolet-visible Spectrophotometry *<2.24>*, and compare the spectrum with the Reference Spectrum or the spectrum of a solution of Bacampicillin Hydrochloride RS prepared in the same manner as the sample solution: both spectra exhibit similar intensities of absorption at the same wavelengths.

(2) Determine the infrared absorption spectrum of Bacampicillin Hydrochloride as directed in the potassium chloride disk method under Infrared Spectrophotometry *<2.25>*, and compare the spectrum with the Reference Spectrum or the spectrum of Bacampicillin Hydrochloride RS: both spectra exhibit similar intensities of absorption at the same wave numbers.

(3) A solution of Bacampicillin Hydrochloride (1 in 50) responds to Qualitative Tests *<1.09>* for chloride.

Optical rotation *<2.49>* $[\alpha]_D^{20}$: +140 – +170° (0.1 g calculated on the anhydrous basis, ethanol (95), 25 mL, 100 mm).

Purity **(1)** Heavy metals *<1.07>*—Proceed with 1.0 g of Bacampicillin Hydrochloride according to Method 2, and perform the test. Prepare the control solution with 2.0 mL of Standard Lead Solution (not more than 20 ppm).

(2) Arsenic *<1.11>*—Prepare the test solution with 1.0 g of Bacampicillin Hydrochloride according to Method 3, and perform the test (not more than 2 ppm).

(3) Free ampicillin—Carry out the determination immediately after preparing the sample solution. Weigh accurately about 0.1 g of Bacampicillin Hydrochloride, dissolve in exactly 10 mL of the internal standard solution, add the mobile phase to make 20 mL, and use this solution as the sample solution. Separately, weigh accurately an amount of Ampicillin RS, equivalent to about 25 mg (potency), and dissolve in water to make exactly 100 mL. Pipet 4 mL of this solution, add exactly 10 mL of the internal standard solution, add the mobile phase to make 20 mL, and use this solution as the standard solution. Perform the test with 10 μL each of the sample solution and standard solution as directed under Liquid Chromatography <*2.01*> according to the following conditions, and calculate the ratios, Q_T and Q_S, of the peak area of ampicillin to that of the internal standard in each solution. The amount of ampicillin, calculated by the following equation, is not more than 1.0%.

$$\text{Amount (\%) of ampicillin } (C_{16}H_{19}N_3O_4S) = M_S/M_T \times Q_T/Q_S \times 4$$

M_S: Amount [mg (potency)] of Ampicillin RS taken
M_T: Amount (mg) of Bacampicillin Hydrochloride taken

Internal standard solution—A solution of anhydrous caffeine in the mobile phase (1 in 25,000).
Operating conditions—

Detector: An ultraviolet absorption photometer (wavelength: 230 nm).

Column: A stainless steel column 4.6 mm in inside diameter and 15 cm in length, packed with octadecylsilanized silica gel for liquid chromatography (5 μm in particle diameter).

Column temperature: A constant temperature of about 25°C.

Mobile phase: Dissolve 1.22 g of potassium dihydrogen phosphate in water to make 900 mL, and add 100 mL of acetonitrile.

Flow rate: Adjust so that the retention time of ampicillin is about 7 minutes.
System suitability—

System performance: When the procedure is run with 10 μL of the standard solution under the above operating conditions, ampicillin and the internal standard are eluted in this order with the resolution between these peaks being not less than 5.

System repeatability: When the test is repeated 6 times with 10 μL of the standard solution under the above operating conditions, the relative standard deviation of the ratio of the peak area of ampicillin to that of the internal standard is not more than 2.0%.

Water <*2.48*> Not more than 1.0% (0.5 g, volumetric titration, direct titration).

Residue on ignition <*2.44*> Not more than 1.5% (1 g).

Assay Weigh accurately an amount of Bacampicillin Hydrochloride and Bacampicillin Hydrochloride RS, equivalent to about 40 mg (potency), dissolve each in water to make exactly 100 mL, and use these solutions as the sample solution and standard solution. Perform the test with exactly 20 μL each of the sample solution and standard solution as directed under Liquid Chromatography <*2.01*> according to the following conditions, and determine the peak areas, A_T and A_S, of bacampicillin in each solution.

$$\text{Amount [}\mu\text{g (potency)] of ampicillin } (C_{16}H_{19}N_3O_4S) = M_S \times A_T/A_S \times 1000$$

M_S: Amount [mg (potency)] of Bacampicillin Hydrochloride RS taken

Operating conditions—

Detector: An ultraviolet absorption photometer (wavelength: 254 nm).

Column: A stainless steel column 4.6 mm in inside diameter and 15 cm in length, packed with octadecylsilanized silica gel for liquid chromatography (5 μm in particle diameter).

Column temperature: A constant temperature of about 25°C.

Mobile phase: To 500 mL of diluted 2 mol/L sodium dihydrogen phosphate TS (1 in 100), add diluted 0.05 mol/L disodium hydrogen phosphate TS (2 in 5) to adjust the pH to 6.8. To 500 mL of this solution add 500 mL of acetonitrile.

Flow rate: Adjust so that the retention time of bacampicillin is about 6.5 minutes.
System suitability—

System performance: When the procedure is run with 20 μL of the standard solution under the above operating conditions, the number of theoretical plates and the symmetry factor of the peak of bacampicillin are not less than 10,000 and not more than 2, respectively.

System repeatability: When the test is repeated 6 times with 20 μL of the standard solution under the above operating conditions, the relative standard deviation of peak areas of bacampicillin is not more than 2.0%.

Containers and storage Containers—Tight containers.

Bacitracin

バシトラシン

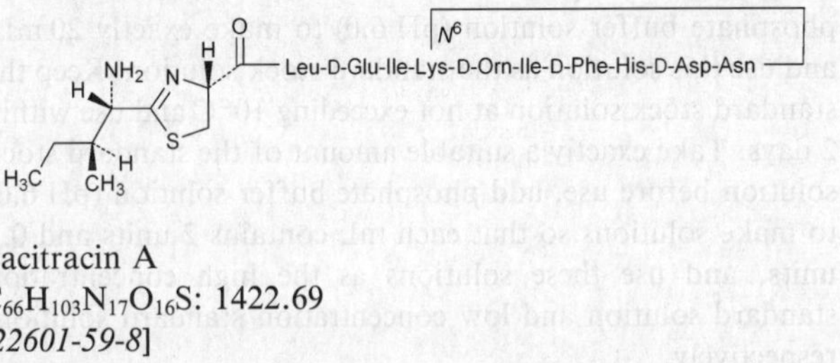

Leu-D-Glu-Ile-Lys-D-Orn-Ile-D-Phe-His-D-Asp-Asn

Bacitracin A
$C_{66}H_{103}N_{17}O_{16}S$: 1422.69
[*22601-59-8*]
[*1405-87-4*, Bacitracin]

Bacitracin is a mixture of peptide substances having antibacterial activity including bacitracin A as the main component produced by the growth of *Bacillus subtilis* or *Bacillus licheniformis*.

It contains not less than 60 Units per mg, calculated on the dried basis. The potency of Bacitracin is expressed as unit calculated from the amount of bacitracin A ($C_{66}H_{103}N_{17}O_{16}S$: 1422.69). One unit of Bacitracin is equivalent to 23.8 μg of bacitracin A ($C_{66}H_{103}N_{17}O_{16}S$).

Description Bacitracin occurs as a white to light brown powder.

It is freely soluble in water, and slightly soluble in ethanol (99.5).

Identification **(1)** To 3 mL of a solution of Bacitracin (1 in 100) add 3 mL of 4-dimethylaminobenzaldehyde TS, shake until red-rosy to red-purple color appears, then add several drops of a solution of sodium nitrite (1 in 100), and shake: a green to dark green color is produced.

(2) Dissolve 60 mg each of Bacitracin and Bacitracin RS in 10 mL of water, and use these solutions as the sample solution and standard solution. Perform the test with these solutions as directed under Thin-layer Chromatography <*2.03*>. Spot 1 μL each of the sample solution and standard solution on a plate of silica gel for thin-layer chromatography. Develop the plate with a mixture of 1-butanol, acetic acid (100), water, pyridine and ethanol (99.5) (30:15:10:6:5) to a distance of about 10 cm, and air-dry the plate. Spray evenly ninhydrin TS on the plate, and heat the plate at 110°C for 5 minutes: the spots obtained from the sample solution and standard solution show the same *Rf* value.

Purity **(1)** Heavy metals <*1.07*>—Proceed with 1.0 g of Bacitracin according to Method 2, and perform the test.

Prepare the control solution with 2.0 mL of Standard Lead Solution (not more than 20 ppm).

(2) Related substances—Dissolve 0.15 g of Bacitracin in 0.05 mol/L sulfuric acid TS to make 100 mL. To 2 mL of this solution add 0.05 mol/L sulfuric acid TS to make 10 mL, and determine the absorbances of this solution, A_1 and A_2, at 252 nm and 290 nm as directed under Ultraviolet-visible Spectrophotometry <*2.24*>: A_2/A_1 is not more than 0.20.

Loss on drying <*2.41*> Not more than 5.0% (1 g, in vacuum, 60°C, 3 hours).

Residue on ignition <*2.44*> Not more than 1.0% (1 g).

Assay Perform the test according to the Cylinder-plate method as directed under Microbial Assay for Antibiotics <*4.02*> according to the following conditions.

(i) Test organism—*Micrococcus luteus* ATCC 10240.

(ii) Culture medium—Use the medium iii in 3) under (1) Agar media for seed and base layer.

(iii) Standard solutions—Weigh accurately an amount of Bacitracin RS, equivalent to about 400 units, dissolve in phosphate buffer solution (pH 6.0) to make exactly 20 mL, and use this solution as the standard stock solution. Keep the standard stock solution at not exceeding 10°C and use within 2 days. Take exactly a suitable amount of the standard stock solution before use, add phosphate buffer solution (pH 6.0) to make solutions so that each mL contains 2 units and 0.5 units, and use these solutions as the high concentration standard solution and low concentration standard solution, respectively.

(iv) Sample solutions—Weigh accurately an amount of Bacitracin, equivalent about 400 units, dissolve in phosphate buffer solution (pH 6.0) to make exactly 20 mL. Take exactly a suitable amount of this solution, add phosphate buffer solution (pH 6.0) to make solutions so that each mL contains 2 units and 0.5 units, and use these solutions as the high concentration sample solution and low concentration sample solution, respectively.

Containers and storage Containers—Tight containers.

Storage—In a cold place.

Baclofen

バクロフェン

and enantiomer

$C_{10}H_{12}ClNO_2$: 213.66

(3*RS*)-4-Amino-3-(4-chlorophenyl)butanoic acid

[*1134-47-0*]

Baclofen contains not less than 98.5% of baclofen ($C_{10}H_{12}ClNO_2$), calculated on the anhydrous basis.

Description Baclofen occurs as a white to pale yellow-white crystalline powder.

It is freely soluble in acetic acid (100), slightly soluble in water, very slightly soluble in methanol and in ethanol (95), and practically insoluble in diethyl ether.

It dissolves in dilute hydrochloric acid.

Identification **(1)** To 5 mL of a solution of Baclofen (1 in 1000) add 1 mL of ninhydrin TS, and heat on a water bath for 3 minutes: a blue-purple color develops.

(2) Determine the absorption spectrum of a solution of Baclofen in 0.1 mol/L hydrochloric acid TS (1 in 2000) as directed under Ultraviolet-visible Spectrophotometry <*2.24*>, and compare the spectrum with the Reference Spectrum or the spectrum of a solution of Baclofen RS prepared in the same manner as the sample solution: both spectra exhibit similar intensities of absorption at the same wavelengths.

(3) Perform the test with Baclofen as directed under Flame Coloration Test <*1.04*> (2): a green color appears.

Purity **(1)** Chloride <*1.03*>—Dissolve 0.5 g of Baclofen in 50 mL of acetic acid (100), and add water to make 100 mL. To 10 mL of this solution add 6 mL of dilute nitric acid and water to make 50 mL. Perform the test using this solution as the test solution. Prepare the control solution as follows: to 0.30 mL of 0.01 mol/L hydrochloric acid VS add 5 mL of acetic acid (100), 6 mL of dilute nitric acid and water to make 50 mL (not more than 0.21%).

(2) Heavy metals <*1.07*>—Proceed with 2.0 g of Baclofen according to Method 2, and perform the test. Prepare the control solution with 2.0 mL of Standard Lead Solution (not more than 10 ppm).

(3) Arsenic <*1.11*>—Prepare the test solution with 1.0 g of Baclofen according to Method 3, and perform the test (not more than 2 ppm).

(4) Related substances—Dissolve 50 mg of Baclofen in 50 mL of the mobile phase, and use this solution as the sample solution. Pipet 1.0 mL and 1.5 mL of the sample solution, to each add the mobile phase to make exactly 100 mL, and use these solutions as the standard solutions (1) and (2), respectively. Perform the test with exactly 25 μL each of the sample solution and standard solutions (1) and (2) as directed under Liquid Chromatography <*2.01*> according to the following conditions. Determine each peak height of these solutions: each height of the peaks other than the peak of baclofen obtained from the sample solution is not larger than the peak height of baclofen from the standard solution (1), and the total height of these peaks is not larger than the peak height of baclofen from the standard solution (2).

Operating conditions—

Detector: An ultraviolet absorption photometer (wavelength: 268 nm).

Column: A stainless steel column 4 mm in inside diameter and 25 cm in length, packed with octadecylsilanized silica gel for liquid chromatography (10 μm in particle diameter).

Column temperature: A constant temperature of about 25°C.

Mobile phase: A mixture of methanol and diluted acetic acid (100) (1 in 900) (3:2).

Flow rate: Adjust so that the retention time of baclofen is about 4 minutes.

Time span of measurement: About 3 times as long as the retention time of baclofen, beginning after the solvent peak.

System suitability—

Test for required detectability: Adjust the sensitivity so that the peak height of baclofen obtained with 25 μL of the standard solution (1) is between 5 and 10 mm.

System performance: Dissolve 0.40 g of Baclofen and 5 mg of methyl parahydroxybenzoate in 200 mL of the mobile phase. To 10 mL of this solution add the mobile phase to make 100 mL. When the procedure is run with 25 μL of this solution under the above operating conditions, baclofen and methyl parahydroxybenzoate are eluted in this order with the resolution between these peaks being not less than 5.

System repeatability: When the test is repeated 6 times with 25 μL of the standard solution (1) under the above operating conditions, the relative standard deviation of the peak heights of baclofen is not more than 3.0%.

Water <2.48> Not more than 1.0% (1 g, direct titration).

Residue on ignition <2.44> Not more than 0.3% (1 g).

Assay Weigh accurately about 0.5 g of Baclofen, dissolve in 80 mL of acetic acid (100), and titrate <2.50> with 0.1 mol/L perchloric acid VS until the color of the solution changes from purple through blue to greenish blue (indicator: 2 drops of crystal violet TS). Perform a blank determination in the same manner, and make any necessary correction.

Each mL of 0.1 mol/L perchloric acid VS
= 21.37 mg of $C_{10}H_{12}ClNO_2$

Containers and storage Containers—Well-closed containers.

Baclofen Tablets

バクロフェン錠

Baclofen Tablets contain not less than 93.0% and not more than 107.0% of the labeled amount of baclofen ($C_{10}H_{12}ClNO_2$: 213.66).

Method of preparation Prepare as directed under Tablets, with Baclofen.

Identification **(1)** To a portion of powdered Baclofen Tablets, equivalent to 0.01 g of Baclofen, add 10 mL of water, shake well, and filter. To 5 mL of the filtrate add 1 mL of ninhydrin TS, and proceed as directed in the Identification (1) under Baclofen.

(2) To a portion of powdered Baclofen Tablets, equivalent to 25 mg of Baclofen, add 50 mL of 0.1 mol/L hydrochloric acid TS, shake for 15 minutes, and filter. Determine the absorption spectrum of the filtrate as directed under Ultraviolet-visible Spectrophotometry <2.24>: it exhibits maxima between 257 nm and 261 nm, between 264 nm and 268 nm, and between 272 nm and 276 nm.

(3) To a portion of powdered Baclofen Tablets, equivalent to 0.01 g of Baclofen, add 2 mL of a mixture of methanol and acetic acid (100) (4:1), shake well, centrifuge, and use the supernatant liquid as the sample solution. Separately, dissolve 0.01 g of Baclofen RS in 2 mL of a mixture of methanol and acetic acid (100) (4:1), and use this solution as the standard solution. Perform the test with these solutions as directed under Thin-layer Chromatography <2.03>. Spot 20 μL each of the sample solution and standard solution on a plate of silica gel with fluorescent indicator for thin-layer chromatography. Develop the plate with a mixture of 1-butanol, water and acetic acid (100) (4:1:1) to a distance of about 10 cm, and air-dry the plate. Examine under ultraviolet light (main wavelength: 254 nm): the spot from the sample solution and that from the standard solution show the same *R*f value.

Uniformity of dosage units <6.02> Perform the test according to the following method: it meets the requirement of the Content uniformity test.

To 1 tablet of Baclofen Tablets add 5 mL of 0.1 mol/L hydrochloric acid TS, disperse the tablet into small particles by sonicating, then shake for 10 minutes, and add 0.1 mol/L hydrochloric acid TS to make exactly V mL so that each mL contains about 0.5 mg of baclofen ($C_{10}H_{12}ClNO_2$). Centrifuge, pipet 5 mL of the supernatant liquid, add 2 drops of phenolphthalein TS, neutralize with dilute sodium hydroxide TS, then add water to make exactly 50 mL, and use this solution as the sample solution. Separately, weigh accurately about 25 mg of Baclofen RS (separately determine the water <2.48> in the same manner as Baclofen), and dissolve in 0.1 mol/L hydrochloric acid TS to make exactly 50 mL. Pipet 5 mL of this solution, add 2 drops of phenolphthalein TS, neutralize with dilute sodium hydroxide TS, then add water to make exactly 50 mL, and use this solution as the standard solution. To exactly 2 mL each of the sample solution and standard solution add 4 mL of ninhydrin-tin (II) chloride TS, mix, heat on a water bath for 20 minutes, then immediately shake vigorously for 2 minutes. After cooling, add a mixture of water and 1-propanol (1:1) to make them exactly 25 mL, and determine the absorbances, A_T and A_S, of them at 570 nm as directed under Ultraviolet-visible Spectrophotometry <2.24>, using a solution obtained with 2 mL of water by the same procedure as above as the blank.

$$\text{Amount (mg) of baclofen } (C_{10}H_{12}ClNO_2) = M_S \times A_T/A_S \times V/50$$

M_S: Amount (mg) of Baclofen RS taken, calculated on the anhydrous basis

Dissolution <6.10> When the test is performed at 50 revolutions per minute according to the Paddle method, using 500 mL of water as the dissolution medium, the dissolution rate in 45 minutes of Baclofen Tablets is not less than 70%.

Start the test with 1 tablet of Baclofen Tablets, withdraw not less than 20 mL of the medium at the specified minute after starting the test, and filter through a membrane filter with a pore size not exceeding 0.8 μm. Discard not less than 10 mL of the first filtrate, pipet V mL of the subsequent, add water to make exactly V' mL so that each mL contains about 10 μg of baclofen ($C_{10}H_{12}ClNO_2$), and use this solution as the sample solution. Separately, weigh accurately about 10 mg of Baclofen RS (separately determine the water <2.48> in the same manner as Baclofen), dissolve in water to make exactly 100 mL, then pipet 10 mL of this solution, add water to make exactly 100 mL, and use this solution as the standard solution. Determine the absorbances, A_T and A_S, of the sample solution and the standard solution at 220 nm as directed under Ultraviolet-visible Spectrophotometry <2.24>.

$$\text{Dissolution rate (\%) with respect to the labeled amount of baclofen } (C_{10}H_{12}ClNO_2) = M_S \times A_T/A_S \times V'/V \times 1/C \times 50$$

M_S: Amount (mg) of Baclofen RS taken, calculated on the anhydrous basis

C: Labeled amount (mg) of baclofen ($C_{10}H_{12}ClNO_2$) in 1 tablet

Assay Weigh accurately and powder not less than 20 Baclofen Tablets. Weigh accurately a portion of the powder, equivalent to about 50 mg of baclofen ($C_{10}H_{12}ClNO_2$), add 130 mL of 0.1 mol/L hydrochloric acid TS, shake for 10 minutes, add 0.1 mol/L hydrochloric acid TS to make exactly 200 mL, and centrifuge. Pipet 10 mL of the supernatant liquid, add 2 drops of phenolphthalein TS, neutralize with dilute sodium hydroxide TS, add water to make exactly 50 mL, and use this solution as the sample solution. Separately, weigh accurately about 0.25 g of Baclofen RS (separately determine the water content <2.48> in the same manner as Baclofen), and dissolve in 0.1 mol/L hydrochloric acid TS to make exactly 100 mL. Pipet 10 mL of this solution, and add 0.1 mol/L hydrochloric acid TS to make exactly 100 mL. Pipet 10 mL of this solution, add 2 drops of phenolphthalein TS, neutralize with dilute sodium hydroxide TS, add water to make exactly 50 mL, and use this solution as the standard solution. Pipet 2 mL each of the sample solution and the standard solution, to each add 4 mL of ninhydrin-stannous chloride TS, shake, heat on a water bath for 20 minutes, and shake at once vigorously for 2 minutes. After cooling, to each solution add a mixture of water and 1-propanol (1:1) to make exactly 25 mL. Determine the absorbances, A_T and A_S, of these solutions at 570 nm as directed under Ultraviolet-visible Spectrophotometry <2.24>, using a blank prepared with 2 mL of water in the same manner.

$$\text{Amount (mg) of baclofen } (C_{10}H_{12}ClNO_2) = M_S \times A_T/A_S \times 1/5$$

M_S: Amount (mg) of Baclofen RS taken, calculated on the anhydrous basis

Containers and storage Containers—Well-closed containers.

Bamethan Sulfate

バメタン硫酸塩

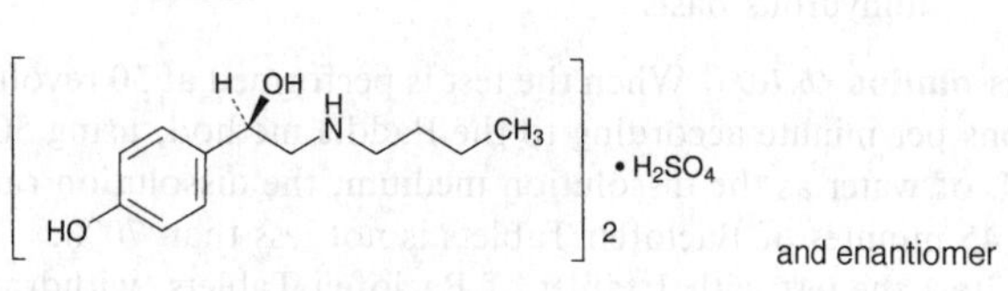

$(C_{12}H_{19}NO_2)_2.H_2SO_4$: 516.65
(1*RS*)-2-Butylamino-1-(4-hydroxyphenyl)ethanol hemisulfate
[*5716-20-1*]

Bamethan Sulfate, when dried, contains not less than 99.0% of bamethan sulfate $[(C_{12}H_{19}NO_2)_2.H_2SO_4]$.

Description Bamethan Sulfate occurs as white, crystals or crystalline powder. It is odorless, and has a bitter taste.

It is freely soluble in water and in acetic acid (100), soluble in methanol, slightly soluble in ethanol (95), and practically insoluble in diethyl ether.

Melting point: about 169°C (with decomposition).

Identification (1) To 1 mL of a solution of Bamethan Sulfate (1 in 1000) add 5 mL of a solution of 4-nitrobenzenediazonium fluoroborate (1 in 2000) and 10 mL of boric acid-potassium chloride-sodium hydroxide buffer solution (pH 9.2): an orange-red color develops.

(2) Determine the absorption spectrum of a solution of Bamethan Sulfate in 0.01 mol/L hydrochloric acid TS (1 in 10,000) as directed under Ultraviolet-visible Spectrophotometry <2.24>, and compare the spectrum with the Reference Spectrum: both spectra exhibit similar intensities of absorption at the same wavelengths.

(3) Determine the infrared absorption spectrum of Bamethan Sulfate, previously dried, as directed in the potassium bromide disk method under Infrared Spectrophotometry <2.25>: it exhibits absorption at the wave numbers of about 1618, 1597, 1518, 1118 and 833 cm^{-1}.

(4) A solution of Bamethan Sulfate (1 in 100) responds to Qualitative Tests <1.09> for sulfate.

pH <2.54> Dissolve 1.0 g of Bamethan Sulfate in 10 mL of water: the pH of this solution is between 4.0 and 5.5.

Purity (1) Clarity and color of solution—Dissolve 1.0 g of Bamethan Sulfate in 20 mL of water: the solution is clear, and has no more color than the following control solution.

Control solution: To 1.5 mL of Matching Fluid O add diluted hydrochloric acid (1 in 40) to make 200 mL.

(2) Chloride <1.03>—Perform the test with 3.5 g of Bamethan Sulfate. Prepare the control solution with 0.25 mL of 0.01 mol/L hydrochloric acid VS (not more than 0.002%).

(3) Heavy metals <1.07>—Proceed with 2.0 g of Bamethan Sulfate according to Method 1, and perform the test. Prepare the control solution with 2.0 mL of Standard Lead Solution (not more than 10 ppm).

(4) Arsenic <1.11>—Prepare the test solution with 1.0 g of Bamethan Sulfate according to Method 3, and perform the test (not more than 2 ppm).

(5) Related substances—Dissolve 0.10 g of Bamethan Sulfate in 2 mL of methanol, and use this solution as the sample solution. Pipet 1 mL of the sample solution, add methanol to make exactly 100 mL, and use this solution as the standard solution. Perform the test with these solutions as directed under Thin-layer Chromatography <2.03>. Spot 2 μL each of the sample solution and standard solution on a plate of silica gel for thin-layer chromatography. Develop the plate with a mixture of chloroform and methanol (7:2) in a developing vessel saturated with ammonia vapor to a distance of about 12 cm, and air-dry the plate. Spray evenly Dragendorff's TS for spraying on the plate, air-dry for 15 minutes, spray Dragendorff's TS for spraying again, then, after 1 minute, spray evenly a solution of sodium nitrite (1 in 20), and immediately put a glass plate on the plate. Examine the plate after 30 minutes: the spots other than the principal spot obtained from the sample solution are not more intense than the spot from the standard solution.

Loss on drying <2.41> Not more than 0.5% (1 g, 105°C, 4 hours).

Residue on ignition <2.44> Not more than 0.1% (1 g).

Assay Weigh accurately about 0.75 g of Bamethan Sulfate, previously dried, dissolve in 80 mL of acetic acid (100), and titrate with 0.1 mol/L perchloric acid VS (potentiometric titration). Perform a blank determination in the same manner, and make any necessary correction.

$$\text{Each mL of 0.1 mol/L perchloric acid VS} = 51.67 \text{ mg of } (C_{12}H_{19}NO_2)_2.H_2SO_4$$

Containers and storage Containers—Tight containers.

Barbital

バルビタール

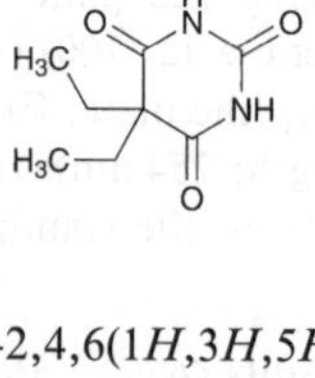

$C_8H_{12}N_2O_3$: 184.19
5,5-Diethylpyrimidine-2,4,6(1*H*,3*H*,5*H*)-trione
[*57-44-3*]

Barbital, when dried, contains not less than 99.0% of barbital ($C_8H_{12}N_2O_3$).

Description Barbital occurs as colorless or white crystals or a white crystalline powder. It is odorless, and has a slightly bitter taste.

It is freely soluble in acetone and in pyridine, soluble in ethanol (95), sparingly soluble in diethyl ether, and slightly soluble in water and in chloroform.

It dissolves in sodium hydroxide TS and in ammonia TS.

The pH of its saturated solution is between 5.0 and 6.0.

Identification **(1)** Boil 0.2 g of Barbital with 10 mL of sodium hydroxide TS: the gas evolved changes moistened red litmus paper to blue.

(2) Dissolve 0.05 g of Barbital in 5 mL of diluted pyridine (1 in 10), add 0.3 mL of copper (II) sulfate TS, shake, and allow to stand for 5 minutes: a red-purple precipitate is formed. Shake the mixture with 5 mL of chloroform: a red-purple color develops in the chloroform layer. Separately, dissolve 0.05 g of Barbital in 2 to 3 drops of ammonia-ammonium chloride buffer solution (pH 10.7) and 5 mL of diluted pyridine (1 in 10). Add 5 mL of chloroform and 0.3 mL of copper (II) sulfate TS to the solution: a red-purple precipitate is produced in the aqueous layer. The red-purple precipitate is not dissolved in the chloroform by shaking.

(3) To 0.4 g of Barbital add 0.1 g of anhydrous sodium carbonate and 4 mL of water, shake, and add a solution of 0.3 g of 4-nitrobenzyl chloride in 7 mL of ethanol (95). Heat the mixture on a water bath under a reflux condenser for 30 minutes, and allow to stand for 1 hour. Collect the separated crystals, wash with 7 mL of sodium hydroxide TS and a small amount of water, recrystallize from a mixture of ethanol (95) and chloroform (1:1), and dry at 105°C for 30 minutes: the crystals melt *<2.60>* between 192°C and 196°C.

Melting point *<2.60>* 189 - 192°C

Purity **(1)** Clarity and color of solution—Dissolve 0.5 g of Barbital in 5 mL of sodium hydroxide TS: the solution is clear and colorless.

(2) Chloride *<1.03>*—Dissolve 0.30 g of Barbital in 20 mL of acetone, and add 6 mL of dilute nitric acid and water to make 50 mL. Perform the test using this solution as the test solution. Prepare the control solution as follows: take 0.30 mL of 0.01 mol/L hydrochloric acid VS, 20 mL of acetone and 6 mL of dilute nitric acid, and add water to make 50 mL (not more than 0.035%).

(3) Sulfate *<1.14>*—Dissolve 0.40 g of Barbital in 20 mL of acetone, and add 1 mL of dilute hydrochloric acid and water to make 50 mL. Perform the test using this solution as the test solution. Prepare the control solution as follows: take 0.40 mL of 0.005 mol/L sulfuric acid VS, 20 mL of acetone, and 1 mL of dilute hydrochloric acid, and add water to make 50 mL (not more than 0.048%).

(4) Heavy metals *<1.07>*—Proceed with 1.0 g of Barbital according to Method 2, and perform the test. Prepare the control solution with 2.0 mL of Standard Lead solution (not more than 20 ppm).

(5) Readily carbonizable substances *<1.15>*—Perform the test with 0.5 g of Barbital. The solution is not more colored than Matching Fluid A.

Loss on drying *<2.41>* Not more than 1.0% (1 g, 105°C, 2 hours).

Residue on ignition *<2.44>* Not more than 0.1% (1 g).

Assay Weigh accurately about 0.4 g of Barbital, previously dried, and dissolve in 5 mL of ethanol (95) and 50 mL of chloroform. Titrate *<2.50>* with 0.1 mol/L potassium hydroxide-ethanol VS until the color of the solution changes from yellow through light blue to purple (indicator: 1 mL of alizarin yellow GG-thymolphthalein TS). Perform a blank determination in the same manner, and make any necessary correction.

Each mL of 0.1 mol/L potassium hydroxide-ethanol VS
= 18.42 mg of $C_8H_{12}N_2O_3$

Containers and storage Containers—Well-closed containers.

Barium Sulfate

硫酸バリウム

$BaSO_4$: 233.39

Description Barium Sulfate occurs as a white powder. It is odorless and tasteless.

It is practically insoluble in water, in ethanol (95) and in diethyl ether.

It does not dissolve in hydrochloric acid, in nitric acid and in sodium hydroxide TS.

Identification **(1)** Mix 0.5 g of Barium Sulfate with 2 g each of anhydrous sodium carbonate and potassium carbonate in a crucible, heat the mixture until fusion is complete, treat the cooled mass with hot water, and filter. The filtrate, acidified with hydrochloric acid, responds to Qualitative Tests *<1.09>* for sulfate.

(2) Wash the hot water-insoluble residue obtained in (1) with water, dissolve in 2 mL of acetic acid (31), and filter, if necessary: the solution responds to Qualitative Tests *<1.09>* for barium salt.

Purity **(1)** Acidity or alkalinity—Agitate 1.0 g of Barium Sulfate with 20 mL of water for 5 minutes: the solution is neutral.

(2) Phosphate—Boil 1.0 g of Barium Sulfate with 3 mL of nitric acid and 5 mL of water for 5 minutes, cool, and add water to restore the original volume. Filter through a filter paper, previously washed with dilute nitric acid, to the filtrate add an equal volume of hexaammonium heptamolybdate TS, and allow to stand between 50°C and 60°C for 1 hour: no yellow precipitate is produced.

(3) Sulfide—Place 10 g of Barium Sulfate in a 250-mL conical flask, add 10 mL of dilute hydrochloric acid and water to make 100 mL, and boil for 10 minutes: the gas evolved does not darken moistened lead (II) acetate paper.

(4) Heavy metals *<1.07>*—Boil 5.0 g of Barium Sulfate with 2.5 mL of acetic acid (100) and 50 mL of water for 10 minutes, cool, add 0.5 mL of ammonia TS and water to make 100 mL, and filter. Perform the test with a 50-mL portion of this filtrate. Prepare the control solution with 2.5 mL of Standard Lead Solution, 1.25 mL of acetic acid (100), 0.25 mL of ammonia TS and water to make 50 mL (not more than 10 ppm).

(5) Arsenic *<1.11>*—Prepare the test solution with 2.0 g of Barium Sulfate according to Method 1, and perform the test (not more than 1 ppm).

(6) Hydrochloric acid-soluble substances and soluble barium salts—Cool the solution obtained in (3), add water to make 100 mL, and filter. Evaporate 50 mL of the filtrate on a water bath to dryness, add 2 drops of hydrochloric acid and 10 mL of warm water, filter through a filter paper for quantitative analysis, and wash with 10 mL of warm water. Evaporate the combined filtrate and washings on a water bath to dryness, and dry the residue at 105°C for 1 hour: the residue weighs not more than 15 mg. Shake the residue, if any, with 10 mL of water, and filter. To the filtrate add 0.5 mL of dilute sulfuric acid, and allow to stand for 30 minutes: no turbidity is produced.

Containers and storage Containers—Well-closed containers.

Freeze-dried BCG Vaccine (for Percutaneous Use)

乾燥 **BCG** ワクチン

Freeze-dried BCG Vaccine (for Percutaneous Use) is a preparation for injection which is dissolved before use.

It contains live bacteria derived from a culture of the bacillus of Calmette and Guérin.

It conforms to the requirements of Freeze-dried BCG Vaccine (for Percutaneous Use) in the Minimum Requirements for Biological Products.

Description Freeze-dried BCG Vaccine (for Percutaneous Use) becomes a white to light yellow, turbid liquid on addition of solvent.

Beclometasone Dipropionate

ベクロメタゾンプロピオン酸エステル

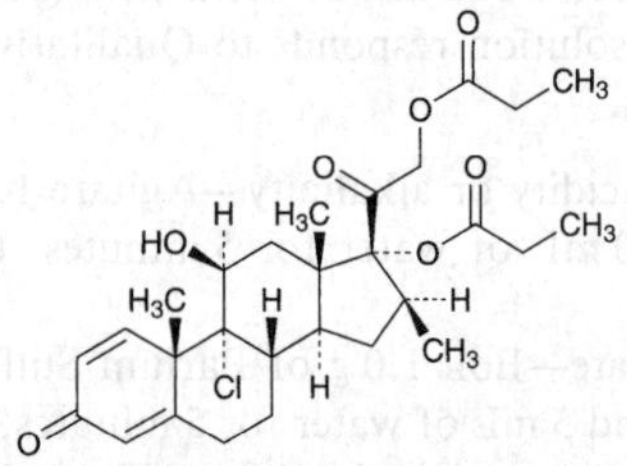

$C_{28}H_{37}ClO_7$: 521.04
9-Chloro-11β,17,21-trihydroxy-16β-methylpregna-1,4-diene-3,20-dione 17,21-dipropanoate
[*5534-09-8*]

Beclometasone Dipropionate, when dried, contains not less than 97.0% and not more than 103.0% of beclometasone dipropionate ($C_{28}H_{37}ClO_7$).

Description Beclometasone Dipropionate occurs as a white to pale yellow powder.

It is soluble in methanol, sparingly soluble in ethanol (99.5), and practically insoluble in water.

Melting point: about 208°C (with decomposition).

It shows crystal polymorphism.

Identification **(1)** Dissolve 2 mg of Beclometasone Dipropionate in 2 mL of sulfuric acid: initially a yellowish color develops, and gradually changes through orange to dark red-brown. To this solution add carefully 10 mL of water: the color changes to bluish green, and a flocculent precipitate is formed.

(2) Dissolve 0.01 g of Beclometasone Dipropionate in 1 mL of methanol, add 1 mL of Fehling's TS, and heat: a red to red-brown precipitate is formed.

(3) Perform the test with 0.02 g of Beclometasone Dipropionate as directed under Oxygen Flask Combustion Method <*1.06*>, using a mixture of 1 mL of sodium hydroxide TS and 20 mL of water as an absorbing liquid: the test solution responds to Qualitative Tests <*1.09*> for chloride.

(4) Determine the infrared absorption spectrum of Beclometasone Dipropionate, previously dried, as directed in the potassium bromide disk method under Infrared Spectrophotometry <*2.25*>, and compare the spectrum with the Reference Spectrum or the spectrum of previously dried Beclometasone Dipropionate RS: both spectra exhibit similar intensities of absorption at the same wave numbers. If any difference appears between the spectra, dissolve Beclometasone Dipropionate and Beclometasone Dipropionate RS in ethanol (95), respectively, then evaporate the ethanol to dryness, and repeat the test on the residues.

Optical rotation <*2.49*> $[\alpha]_D^{25}$: +106 – +114° (after drying, 0.1 g, ethanol (99.5), 10 mL, 100 mm).

Purity **(1)** Heavy metals <*1.07*>—Proceed with 0.5 g of Beclometasone Dipropionate according to Method 2, and perform the test. Prepare the control solution with 1.5 mL of Standard Lead Solution (not more than 30 ppm).

(2) Related substances—Dissolve 20 mg of Beclometasone Dipropionate in 5 mL of a mixture of chloroform and methanol (9:1), and use this solution as the sample solution. Pipet 1 mL of the sample solution, add a mixture of chloroform and methanol (9:1) to make exactly 50 mL, and use this solution as the standard solution. Perform the test with these solutions as directed under Thin-layer Chromatography <*2.03*>. Spot 5 μL each of the sample solution and standard solution on a plate of silica gel for thin-layer chromatography. Develop the plate with a mixture of 1,2-dichloroethane, methanol and water (475:25:1) to a distance of about 15 cm, and air-dry the plate. Spray evenly alkaline blue tetrazolium TS on the plate: the spots other than the principal spot obtained from the sample solution are not more intense than the spot from the standard solution.

Loss on drying <*2.41*> Not more than 0.5% (0.5 g, 105°C, 3 hours).

Residue on ignition <*2.44*> Not more than 0.1% (0.5 g).

Assay Weigh accurately about 20 mg each of Beclometasone Dipropionate and Beclometasone Dipropionate RS, previously dried, and dissolve each in methanol to make exactly 50 mL. Pipet 10 mL each of these solutions, add exactly 10 mL of the internal standard solution and methanol to make 50 mL, and use these solutions as the sample solution and the standard solution, respectively. Perform the test with 20 μL each of the sample solution and standard solution as directed under Liquid Chromatography <*2.01*> according to the following conditions, and calculate the ratios, Q_T and Q_S, of the peak area of beclometasone dipropionate to that of the internal standard, respectively.

Amount (mg) of beclometasone dipropionate ($C_{28}H_{37}ClO_7$)
$= M_S \times Q_T/Q_S$

M_S: Amount (mg) of Beclometasone Dipropionate RS taken

Internal standard solution—A solution of testosterone propionate in methanol (1 in 4000).

Operating conditions—

Detector: An ultraviolet absorption photometer (wavelength: 254 nm).

Column: A stainless steel column 4.6 mm in inside diameter and 20 cm in length, packed with octadecylsilanized silica gel for liquid chromatography (5 μm in particle diameter).

Column temperature: A constant temperature of about 25°C.

Mobile phase: A mixture of acetonitrile and water (3:2).

Flow rate: Adjust so that the retention time of beclometasone dipropionate is about 6 minutes.

System suitability—

System performance: When the procedure is run with 20 μL of the standard solution under the above operating conditions, beclometasone dipropionate and the internal standard are eluted in this order with the resolution between these peaks being not less than 8.

System repeatability: When the test is repeated 6 times with 20 μL of the standard solution under the above operating conditions, the relative standard deviation of the ratios of the peak area of beclometasone dipropionate to that of the internal standard is not more than 1.0%.

Containers and storage Containers—Tight containers.

Bekanamycin Sulfate

ベカナマイシン硫酸塩

$C_{18}H_{37}N_5O_{10}.xH_2SO_4$
3-Amino-3-deoxy-α-D-glucopyranosyl-(1→6)-[2,6-diamino-2,6-dideoxy-α-D-glucopyranosyl-(1→4)]-2-deoxy-D-streptamine sulfate
[*70550-99-1*]

Bekanamycin Sulfate is the sulfate of an aminoglycoside substance having antibacterial activity produced by the growth of the mutant of *Streptomyces kanamyceticus*.

It contains not less than 680 μg (potency) and not more than 770 μg (potency) per mg, calculated on the dried basis. The potency of Bekanamycin Sulfate is expressed as mass (potency) of bekanamycin ($C_{18}H_{37}N_5O_{10}$: 483.51).

Description Bekanamycin Sulfate occurs as a white powder.

It is freely soluble in water, and practically insoluble in ethanol (99.5).

Identification **(1)** Dissolve 20 mg of Bekanamycin Sulfate in 2 mL of 1/15 mol/L phosphate buffer solution (pH 5.6), add 1 mL of ninhydrin TS, and boil: a blue-purple color develops.

(2) Dissolve 30 mg each of Bekanamycin Sulfate and Bekanamycin Sulfate RS in 5 mL of water, and use these solutions as the sample solution and standard solution. Perform the test with these solutions as directed under Thin-layer Chromatography ⟨*2.03*⟩. Spot 5 μL each of the sample solution and standard solution on a plate of silica gel for thin-layer chromatography. Develop the plate with a solution of potassium dihydrogen phosphate (3 in 40) to a distance of about 10 cm, and air-dry the plate. Spray evenly 0.2% ninhydrin-water saturated 1-butanol TS on the plate, and heat the plate at 100°C for 10 minutes: the principal spots obtained from the sample solution and the standard solution show a purple-brown color and the same *R*f value.

(3) To a solution of Bekanamycin Sulfate (1 in 5) add 1 drop of barium chloride TS: a white turbidity is produced.

Optical rotation ⟨*2.49*⟩ $[\alpha]_D^{20}$: +102 – +116° (after drying, 0.25 g, water, 25 mL, 100 mm).

pH ⟨*2.54*⟩ The pH of a solution obtained by dissolving 0.50 g of Bekanamycin Sulfate in 10 mL of water is between 6.0 and 8.5.

Purity **(1)** Clarity and color of solution—Dissolve 0.5 g of Bekanamycin Sulfate in 5 mL of water: the solution is clear and colorless.

(2) Heavy metals ⟨*1.07*⟩—Proceed with 1.0 g of Bekanamycin Sulfate according to Method 4, and perform the test. Prepare the control solution with 3.0 mL of Standard Lead Solution (not more than 30 ppm).

(3) Arsenic ⟨*1.11*⟩—Prepare the test solution with 2.0 g of Bekanamycin Sulfate according to Method 1, and perform the test (not more than 1 ppm).

(4) Related substances—Dissolve 60 mg of Bekanamycin Sulfate in 10 mL of water, and use this solution as the sample solution. Pipet 3 mL of the sample solution, add water to make exactly 100 mL, and use this solution as the standard solution. Perform the test with these solutions as directed under Thin-layer Chromatography ⟨*2.03*⟩. Spot 5 μL each of the sample solution and standard solution on a plate of silica gel for thin-layer chromatography. Develop the plate with a solution of potassium dihydrogen phosphate (3 in 40) to a distance of about 10 cm, and air-dry the plate. Spray evenly 0.2% ninhydrin-water saturated 1-butanol TS on the plate, and heat the plate at 100°C for 10 minutes: the spot other than the principal spot obtained from the sample solution is not more intense than the spot from the standard solution.

Loss on drying ⟨*2.41*⟩ Not more than 5.0% (0.5 g, reduced pressure not exceeding 0.67 kPa, 60°C, 3 hours).

Residue on ignition ⟨*2.44*⟩ Not more than 0.5% (1 g).

Assay Perform the test according to the Cylinder-plate method as directed under Microbial Assay for Antibiotics ⟨*4.02*⟩ according to the following conditions.

(i) Test organism—*Bacillus subtilis* ATCC 6633

(ii) Culture medium—Use the medium i in 1) under (1) Agar media for seed and base layer having pH ⟨*2.54*⟩ 7.8 to 8.0 after sterilization.

(iii) Standard solutions—Weigh accurately an amount of Bekanamycin Sulfate RS, previously dried, equivalent to about 20 mg (potency), dissolve in diluted phosphate buffer solution (pH 6.0) (1 in 2) to make exactly 50 mL, and use this solution as the standard stock solution. Keep the standard stock solution at 5 to 15°C and use within 30 days. Take exactly a suitable amount of the standard stock solution before use, add 0.1 mol/L phosphate buffer solution (pH 8.0) to make solutions so that each mL contains 10 μg (potency) and 2.5 μg (potency), and use these solutions as the high concentration standard solution and low concentration standard solution, respectively.

(iv) Sample solutions—Weigh accurately an amount of Bekanamycin Sulfate, equivalent to about 20 mg (potency), and dissolve in water to make exactly 50 mL. Take exactly a suitable amount of this solution, add 0.1 mol/L phosphate buffer solution (pH 8.0) to make solutions so that each mL contains 10 μg (potency) and 2.5 μg (potency), and use these solutions as the high concentration sample solution and low concentration sample solution, respectively.

Containers and storage Containers—Tight containers.

Benidipine Hydrochloride

ベニジピン塩酸塩

$C_{28}H_{31}N_3O_6.HCl$: 542.02
3-[(3*RS*)-1-Benzylpiperidin-3-yl] 5-methyl (4*RS*)-2,6-dimethyl-4-(3-nitrophenyl)-1,4-dihydropyridine-3,5-dicarboxylate monohydrochloride
[*91599-74-5*]

Benidipine Hydrochloride, when dried, contains not less than 99.0% and not more than 101.0% of benidipine hydrochloride ($C_{28}H_{31}N_3O_6.HCl$).

Description Benidipine Hydrochloride occurs as a yellow crystalline powder.

It is very soluble in formic acid, soluble in methanol, sparingly soluble in ethanol (99.5), and practically insoluble in water.

A solution of Benidipine Hydrochloride in methanol (1 in 100) shows no optical rotation.

Melting point: about 200°C (with decomposition).

Identification (1) Determine the absorption spectrum of a solution of Benidipine Hydrochloride in methanol (1 in 100,000) as directed under Ultraviolet-visible Spectrophotometry 〈*2.24*〉, and compare the spectrum with the Reference Spectrum: both spectra exhibit similar intensities of absorption at the same wavelengths.

(2) Determine the infrared absorption spectrum of Benidipine Hydrochloride, previously dried, as directed in the potassium chloride disk method under Infrared Spectrophotometry 〈*2.25*〉, and compare the spectrum with the Reference Spectrum: both spectra exhibit similar intensities of absorption at the same wave numbers.

(3) To 5 mL of a solution of Benidipine Hydrochloride (1 in 10) add 5 mL of ammonia TS, heat on a water bath for 5 minutes, cool, and filter. The filtrate, which is acidified with dilute nitric acid, responds to Qualitative Tests 〈*1.09*〉 (2) for chloride.

Purity (1) Heavy metals 〈*1.07*〉—Proceed with 1.0 g of Benidipine Hydrochloride according to Method 2, and perform the test. Prepare the control solution with 2.0 mL of Standard Lead Solution (not more than 20 ppm).

(2) Related substances—Dissolve 20 mg of Benidipine Hydrochloride in 100 mL of a mixture of water and methanol (1:1), and use this solution as the sample solution. Pipet 1 mL of the sample solution, add the mixture of water and methanol (1:1) to make exactly 500 mL, and use this solution as the standard solution. Perform the test with exactly 10 μL each of the sample solution and standard solution as directed under Liquid Chromatography 〈*2.01*〉 according to the following conditions, and determine each peak area by the automatic integration method: the peak areas of bisbenzylpiperidyl ester having the relative retention time of about 0.35 to benidipine, dehydro derivative having the relative retention time of about 0.75 and other related substances obtained from the sample solution are not larger than 1/2 times the peak area of benidipine from the standard solution, and the total area of the peaks other than benidipine from the sample solution is not larger than the peak area of benidipine from the standard solution. For the areas of the peaks of bisbenzylpiperidyl ester and dehydro derivative, multiply their correction factor 1.6, respectively.

Operating conditions—

Detector: An ultraviolet absorption photometer (wavelength: 237 nm).

Column: A stainless steel column 4.6 mm in inside diameter and 10 cm in length, packed with octadecylsilanized silica gel for liquid chromatography (3 μm in particle diameter).

Column temperature: A constant temperature of about 25°C.

Mobile phase: A mixture of 0.05 mol/L potassium dihydrogen phosphate TS (pH 3.0), methanol and tetrahydrofuran (65:27:8).

Flow rate: Adjust so that the retention time of benidipine is about 20 minutes.

Time span of measurement: About 2 times as long as the retention time of benidipine, beginning after the solvent peak.

System suitability—

Test for required detectability: Measure exactly 5 mL of the standard solution, and add the mixture of water and methanol (1:1) to make exactly 20 mL. Confirm that the peak area of benidipine obtained with 10 μL of this solution is equivalent to 18 to 32% of that obtained with 10 μL of the standard solution.

System performance: Dissolve 6 mg of Benidipine Hydrochloride and 5 mg of benzoin in 200 mL of the mixture of water and methanol (1:1). When the procedure is run with 10 μL of this solution under the above operating conditions, benzoin and benidipine are eluted in this order with the resolution between these peaks being not less than 8.

System repeatability: When the test is repeated 6 times with 10 μL of the standard solution under the above operating conditions, the relative standard deviation of the peak area of benidipine is not more than 3.5%.

Loss on drying 〈*2.41*〉 Not more than 0.5% (0.5 g, 105°C, 2 hours).

Residue on ignition 〈*2.44*〉 Not more than 0.1% (1 g).

Assay Weigh accurately about 0.7 g of Benidipine Hydrochloride, previously dried, dissolve in 10 mL of formic acid, add 70 mL of acetic anhydride, and titrate 〈*2.50*〉 with 0.1 mol/L perchloric acid VS (potentiometric titration). Perform a blank determination in the same manner, and make any necessary correction.

Each mL of 0.1 mol/L perchloric acid VS
= 54.20 mg of $C_{28}H_{31}N_3O_6.HCl$

Containers and storage Containers—Tight containers.

Benidipine Hydrochloride Tablets

ベニジピン塩酸塩錠

Benidipine Hydrochloride Tablets contain not less than 95.0% and not more than 105.0% of the labeled amount of benidipine hydrochloride ($C_{28}H_{31}N_3O_6.HCl$: 542.02).

Method of preparation Prepare as directed under Tablets, with Benidipine Hydrochloride.

Identification Shake well a quantity of powdered Benidipine Hydrochloride Tablets, equivalent to 10 mg of Benidipine Hydrochloride, with 100 mL of methanol, and centrifuge. To 10 mL of the supernatant liquid add methanol to make 100 mL, and use this solution as the sample solution. Determine the absorption spectrum of the sample solution as directed under Ultraviolet-visible Spectrophotometry <*2.24*>: it exhibits maxima between 235 nm and 239 nm, and between 350 nm and 360 nm.

Purity Dehydro derivative—Powder Benidipine Hydrochloride Tablets in an agate mortar. To an amount of the powder, equivalent to 20 mg of Benidipine Hydrochloride, add about 80 mL of a mixture of diluted phosphoric acid (1 in 500) and methanol (1:1), shake well, and add the mixture of diluted phosphoric acid (1 in 500) and methanol (1:1) to make exactly 100 mL. Filter through a membrane filter with pore size of 0.45 μm, and use the filtrate as the sample solution. Separately, dissolve 20 mg of benidipine hydrochloride for assay in the mixture of diluted phosphoric acid (1 in 500) and methanol (1:1) to make exactly 100 mL. Pipet 1 mL of this solution, add the mixture of diluted phosphoric acid (1 in 500) and methanol (1:1) to make exactly 100 mL, and use this solution as the standard solution. Perform the test with exactly 10 μL each of the sample solution and standard solution as directed under Liquid Chromatography <*2.01*> according to the following conditions, and determine each peak area by the automatic integration method: the peak area of dehydro derivative having the relative retention time of about 0.75 to benidipine obtained from the sample solution is not larger than 1/2 times the peak area of benidipine from the standard solution. For the area of the peak of dehydro derivative, multiply the correction factor 1.6.

Operating conditions—

Perform as directed in the operating conditions in the Assay.

System suitability—

Test for required detectability: Measure exactly 2 mL of the standard solution, and add the mixture of diluted phosphoric acid (1 in 500) and methanol (1:1) to make exactly 20 mL. Confirm that the peak area of benidipine obtained with 10 μL of this solution is equivalent to 7 to 13% of that with 10 μL of the standard solution.

System performance: Dissolve 6 mg of benidipine hydrochloride and 5 mg of benzoin in 200 mL of a mixture of water and methanol (1:1). When the procedure is run with 10 μL of this solution under the above operating conditions, benzoin and benidipine are eluted in this order with the resolution between these peaks being not less than 8.

System repeatability: When the test is repeated 6 times with 10 μL of the standard solution under the above operating conditions, the relative standard deviation of the peak area of benidipine is not more than 2.0%.

Uniformity of dosage units <*6.02*> Perform the test according to the following method: it meets the requirement of the Content uniformity test.

To 1 tablet of Benidipine Hydrochloride Tablets add 40 mL of a mixture of diluted phosphoric acid (1 in 500) and methanol (1:1), shake to disintegrate, and add a suitable amount of the mixture of diluted phosphoric acid (1 in 500) and methanol (1:1) to make exactly V mL of a solution, containing 40 μg of benidipine hydrochloride ($C_{28}H_{31}N_3O_6.HCl$) per mL. Centrifuge the solution, pipet 20 mL of the supernatant liquid, add exactly 10 mL of the internal standard solution and the mixture of diluted phosphoric acid (1 in 500) and methanol (1:1) to make 50 mL, and use this solution as the sample solution. Then, proceed as directed in the Assay.

$$\text{Amount (mg) of benidipine hydrochloride } (C_{28}H_{31}N_3O_6.HCl) = M_S \times Q_T/Q_S \times V/1000$$

M_S: Amount (mg) of benidipine hydrochloride for assay taken

Internal standard solution—A solution of benzoin in a mixture of water and methanol (1:1) (13 in 200,000).

Dissolution <*6.10*> When the test is performed at 50 revolutions per minute according to the Paddle method using the sinker, using 900 mL of 1st fluid for dissolution test as the dissolution medium, the dissolution rate of a 2-mg tablet and a 4-mg tablet in 30 minutes is not less than 80%, and that of a 8-mg tablet in 45 minutes is not less than 85%.

Start the test with 1 tablet of Benidipine Hydrochloride Tablets, withdraw not less than 20 mL of the medium at the specified minute after starting the test, and filter through a membrane filter with a pore size not exceeding 0.45 μm. Discard not less than 10 mL of the first filtrate, pipet the subsequent V mL, and add the dissolution medium to make exactly V' mL so that each mL contains about 2.2 μg of benidipine hydrochloride ($C_{28}H_{31}N_3O_6.HCl$). Pipet 5 mL of this solution, add exactly 5 mL of the mobile phase, and use this solution as the sample solution. Separately, weigh accurately about 22 mg of benidipine hydrochloride for assay, previously dried at 105°C for 2 hours, and dissolve in the mobile phase to make exactly 100 mL. Pipet 2 mL of this solution, and add the mobile phase to make exactly 50 mL. Pipet 5 mL of this solution, and add the mobile phase to make exactly 20 mL. Pipet 5 mL of this solution, add exactly 5 mL of the dissolution medium, and use this solution as the standard solution. Perform the test with exactly 50 μL each of the sample solution and standard solution as directed under Liquid Chromatography <*2.01*> according to the following conditions, and determine the peak areas, A_T and A_S, of benidipine in each solution.

$$\text{Dissolution rate (\%) of benidipine hydrochloride } (C_{28}H_{31}N_3O_6.HCl) \text{ with respect to the labeled amount} = M_S \times A_T/A_S \times V'/V \times 1/C \times 9$$

M_S: Amount (mg) of benidipine hydrochloride for assay taken

C: Labeled amount (mg) of benidipine hydrochloride ($C_{28}H_{31}N_3O_6.HCl$) in 1 tablet.

Operating conditions—

Detector: An ultraviolet absorption photometer (wavelength: 237 nm).

Column: A stainless steel column 4.6 mm in inside diameter and 15 cm in length, packed with octadecylsilanized silica gel for liquid chromatography (5 μm in particle diameter).

Column temperature: A constant temperature of about 25°C.

Mobile phase: A mixture of 0.05 mol/L potassium dihydrogen phosphate TS (pH 3.0) and acetonitrile (11:9).

Flow rate: Adjust so that the retention time of benidipine is about 5 minutes.

System suitability—

System performance: When the procedure is run with 50 μL of the standard solution under the above operating conditions, the number of theoretical plates and the symmetry factor of the peak of benidipine are not less than 3000 and not more than 2.0, respectively.

System repeatability: When the test is repeated 6 times with 50 μL of the standard solution under the above operating conditions, the relative standard deviation of the peak area of benidipine is not more than 1.5%.

Assay Weigh accurately the mass of not less than 20 Benidipine Hydrochloride Tablets, and powder using an agate mortar. Weigh accurately a part of the powder, equivalent to about 8 mg of benidipine hydrochloride ($C_{28}H_{31}N_3O_6.HCl$), add about 150 mL of a mixture of diluted phosphoric acid (1 in 500) and methanol (1:1), shake, then add the mixture of diluted phosphoric acid (1 in 500) and methanol (1:1) to make exactly 200 mL, and centrifuge. Pipet 20 mL of the supernatant liquid, add exactly 10 mL of the internal standard solution and the mixture of diluted phosphoric acid (1 in 500) and methanol (1:1) to make 50 mL, and use this solution as the sample solution. Separately, weigh accurately about 40 mg of benidipine hydrochloride for assay, previously dried at 105°C for 2 hours, and dissolve in the mixture of diluted phosphoric acid (1 in 500) and methanol (1:1) to make exactly 100 mL. Pipet 2 mL of this solution, add exactly 10 mL of the internal standard solution and the mixture of diluted phosphoric acid (1 in 500) and methanol (1:1) to make 50 mL, and use this solution as the standard solution. Perform the test with 10 μL each of the sample solution and standard solution as directed under Liquid Chromatography <*2.01*> according to the following conditions, and calculate the ratios, Q_T and Q_S, of the peak area of benidipine to that of the internal standard.

Amount (mg) of benidipine hydrochloride ($C_{28}H_{31}N_3O_6.HCl$)
$= M_S \times Q_T/Q_S \times 1/5$

M_S: Amount (mg) of benidipine hydrochloride for assay taken

Internal standard solution—A solution of benzoin in a mixture of water and methanol (1:1) (13 in 200,000).

Operating conditions—

Detector: An ultraviolet absorption photometer (wavelength: 237 nm).

Column: A stainless steel column 4.6 mm in inside diameter and 10 cm in length, packed with octadecylsilanized silica gel for liquid chromatography (3 μm in particle diameter).

Column temperature: A constant temperature of about 25°C.

Mobile phase: A mixture of 0.05 mol/L potassium dihydrogen phosphate TS (pH 3.0), methanol and tetrahydrofuran (65:27:8).

Flow rate: Adjust so that the retention time of benidipine is about 20 minutes.

System suitability—

System performance: When the procedure is run with 10 μL of the standard solution under the above operating conditions, the internal standard and benidipine are eluted in this order with the resolution between these peaks being not less than 8.

System repeatability: When the test is repeated 6 times with 10 μL of the standard solution under the above operating conditions, the relative standard deviation of the ratio of the peak area of benidipine to that of the internal standard is not more than 1.0%.

Containers and storage Containers—Well-closed containers.

Benserazide Hydrochloride

ベンセラジド塩酸塩

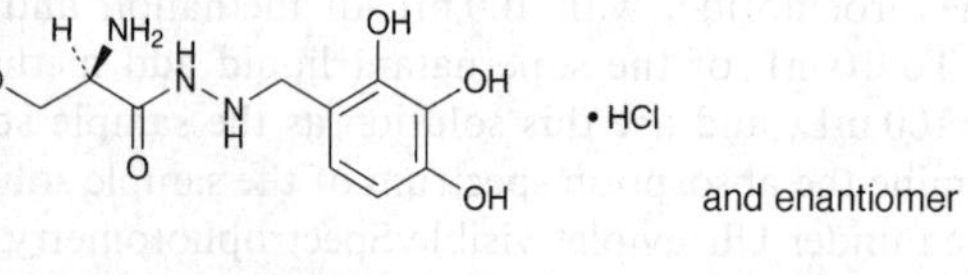

$C_{10}H_{15}N_3O_5.HCl$: 293.70
(2*RS*)-2-Amino-3-hydroxy-
N′-(2,3,4-trihydroxybenzyl)propanoylhydrazide
monohydrochloride
[*14919-77-8*]

Benserazide Hydrochloride contains not less than 98.0% and not more than 101.0% of benserazide hydrochloride ($C_{10}H_{15}N_3O_5.HCl$), calculated on the anhydrous basis.

Description Benserazide Hydrochloride occurs as a white to grayish white crystalline powder.

It is freely soluble in water and in formic acid, soluble in methanol, very slightly soluble in ethanol (95).

It dissolves in 0.1 mol/L hydrochloric acid TS.

The pH of a solution of 1.0 g of Benserazide Hydrochloride in 100 mL of water is between 4.0 and 5.0.

It is hygroscopic.

It is gradually colored by light.

A solution of Benserazide Hydrochloride (1 in 100) shows no optical rotation.

Identification (1) Determine the absorption spectrum of a solution of Benserazide Hydrochloride in 0.1 mol/L hydrochloric acid TS (1 in 10,000) as directed under Ultraviolet-visible Spectrophotometry <*2.24*>, and compare the spectrum with the Reference Spectrum: both spectra exhibit similar intensities of absorption at the same wavelengths.

(2) Determine the infrared absorption spectrum of Benserazide Hydrochloride as directed in the potassium chloride disk method under Infrared Spectrophotometry <*2.25*>, and compare the spectrum with the Reference Spectrum: both spectra exhibit similar intensities of absorption at the same wave numbers.

(3) To 10 mL of a solution of Benserazide Hydrochloride (1 in 30) add silver nitrate TS: a white precipitate is formed. To a portion of this precipitate add dilute nitric acid: the precipitation does not dissolve.

Purity (1) Clarity and color of solution—Dissolve 0.5 g of Benserazide Hydrochloride in 10 mL of water, and perform the test with this solution as directed under Ultraviolet-visible Spectrophotometry <*2.24*>: the absorbance of this solution at 430 nm is not more than 0.10.

(2) Heavy metals <*1.07*>—Proceed with 1.0 g of Benserazide Hydrochloride according to Method 2, and perform the test. Prepare the control solution with 2.0 mL of Standard Lead Solution (not more than 20 ppm).

(3) Related substances—Conduct this procedure without exposure to light, using light-resistant vessels. Dissolve 0.25 g of Benserazide Hydrochloride in 10 mL of methanol, and use this solution as the sample solution. Pipet 1 mL and 3 mL of the sample solution, add methanol to make exactly 200 mL, and use these solutions as the standard solution (1) and (2), respectively. Perform the test with these solutions as directed under Thin-layer Chromatography <*2.03*>. Spot 2 μL each of the sample solution and standard solutions (1) and (2) on a plate of cellulose for thin-layer chromatogra-

phy. Develop the plate with a solution of formic acid in sodium chloride TS (1 in 1000) to a distance of about 10 cm, and air-dry the plate. Spray evenly sodium carbonate TS, air-dry, and then spray evenly Folin's TS on the plate: the spots other than the principal spot obtained from the sample solution are not more intense than the spot from the standard solution (2), and the number of the spots which intense more than the spot from the standard solution (1) are not more than 2.

Water *<2.48>* Not more than 2.5% (0.5 g, volumetric titration, direct titration). Use a solution of salicylic acid in methanol for water determination (3 in 20) instead of methanol for water determination.

Residue on ignition *<2.44>* Not more than 0.1% (1 g).

Assay Weigh accurately about 0.3 g of Benserazide Hydrochloride, dissolve in 5 mL of formic acid, add 50 mL of acetic acid (100), and titrate *<2.50>* immediately with 0.1 mol/L perchloric acid VS (potentiometric titration). Perform a blank determination in the same manner, and make any necessary correction.

Each mL of 0.1 mol/L perchloric acid VS
= 29.37 mg of $C_{10}H_{15}N_3O_5.HCl$

Containers and storage Containers—Tight containers.
Storage—Light-resistant.

Bentonite

ベントナイト

Bentonite is a natural, colloidal, hydrated aluminum silicate.

Description Bentonite occurs as a very fine, white to light yellow-brown powder. It is odorless. It has a slightly earthy taste.

It is practically insoluble in water, in ethanol (95) and in diethyl ether.

It swells in water.

Identification **(1)** Add 0.5 g of Bentonite to 3 mL of diluted sulfuric acid (1 in 3), and heat until white fumes are evolved. Cool, add 20 mL of water, and filter. To 5 mL of the filtrate add 3 mL of ammonia TS: a white, gelatinous precipitate is produced, which turns red on the addition of 5 drops of alizarin red S TS.

(2) Wash the residue obtained in (1) with water, add 2 mL of a solution of methylene blue trihydrate (1 in 10,000), and wash again with water: the residue is blue in color.

pH *<2.54>* To 1.0 g of Bentonite add 50 mL of water, and shake: the pH of the suspension is between 9.0 and 10.5.

Purity **(1)** Heavy metals *<1.07>*—To 1.5 g of Bentonite add 80 mL of water and 5 mL of hydrochloric acid, and boil gently for 20 minutes with thorough stirring. Cool, centrifuge, collect the supernatant liquid, wash the residue with two 10-mL portions of water, and centrifuge each. Combine the supernatant liquid and the washings, and add dropwise ammonia solution (28). When a precipitate is produced, add dropwise dilute hydrochloric acid with vigorous stirring, and dissolve. To the solution add 0.45 g of hydroxylammonium chloride, and heat. Cool, and add 0.45 g of sodium acetate trihydrate, 6 mL of dilute acetic acid and water to make 150 mL. Pipet 50 mL of the solution, and perform the test using this solution as the test solution. Prepare the control solution as follows: mix 2.5 mL of Standard Lead Solution, 0.15 g of hydroxylammonium chloride, 0.15 g of sodium acetate trihydrate, and 2 mL of dilute acetic acid, and add water to make 50 mL (not more than 50 ppm).

(2) Arsenic *<1.11>*—To 1.0 g of Bentonite add 5 mL of dilute hydrochloric acid, and gently heat to boil while stirring well. Cool immediately, and centrifuge. To the residue add 5 mL of dilute hydrochloric acid, shake well, and centrifuge. To the residue add 10 mL of water, and perform the same operations. Combine all the extracts, and heat on a water bath to concentrate to 5 mL. Perform the test with this solution as the test solution (not more than 2 ppm).

(3) Foreign matter—Place 2.0 g of Bentonite in a mortar, add 20 mL of water to swell, disperse evenly with a pestle, and dilute with water to 100 mL. Pour the suspension through a No. 200 (74 μm) sieve, and wash the sieve thoroughly with water. No grit is felt when the fingers are rubbed over the wire mesh of the sieve.

Loss on drying *<2.41>* 5.0 – 10.0% (2 g, 105°C, 2 hours).

Gel formation Mix 6.0 g of Bentonite with 0.30 g of magnesium oxide. Add the mixture, in several portions, to 200 mL of water contained in a glass-stoppered 500-mL cylinder. Agitate for 1 hour, transfer 100 mL of the suspension to a 100-mL graduated cylinder, and allow to stand for 24 hours: not more than 2 mL of supernatant appears on the surface.

Swelling power To 100 mL of water in a glass-stoppered 100-mL cylinder add 2.0 g of Bentonite in ten portions, allowing each portion to settle before adding the next, and allow to stand for 24 hours: the apparent volume of the sediment at the bottom is not less than 20 mL.

Containers and storage Containers—Well-closed containers.

Benzalkonium Chloride

ベンザルコニウム塩化物

Benzalkonium Chloride is represented by the formula $[C_6H_5CH_2N(CH_3)_2R]Cl$, in which R extends from C_8H_{17} to $C_{18}H_{37}$, with $C_{12}H_{25}$ and $C_{14}H_{29}$ comprising the major portion.

It contains not less than 95.0% and not more than 105.0% of benzalkonium chloride (as $C_{22}H_{40}ClN$: 354.01), calculated on the anhydrous basis.

Description Benzalkonium Chloride occurs as a white to yellow-white powder, colorless to light yellow, gelatinous pieces, or jelly-like fluid or mass. It has a characteristic odor.

It is very soluble in water and in ethanol (95), and practically insoluble in diethyl ether.

A solution of Benzalkonium Chloride foams strongly when shaken.

Identification **(1)** Dissolve 0.2 g of Benzalkonium Chloride in 1 mL of sulfuric acid, add 0.1 g of sodium nitrate, and heat for 5 minutes on a water bath. After cooling, add 10 mL of water and 0.5 g of zinc powder, heat for 5 minutes, cool, and filter: the filtrate responds to Qualitative Tests *<1.09>* for primary aromatic amines. The color of the solution is red.

(2) To 2 mL of a solution of Benzalkonium Chloride (1 in 1000) add a mixture of 0.2 mL of a solution of bromophenol blue (1 in 2000) and 0.5 mL of sodium hydroxide TS: a blue color develops. Add 4 mL of chloroform to this solution, and shake vigorously: the blue color shifts to the chloroform layer. Collect the chloroform layer, and add dropwise, with stirring, a solution of sodium lauryl sulfate (1 in 1000): the chloroform layer turns colorless.

(3) Determine the absorption spectrum of a solution of Benzalkonium Chloride in 0.1 mol/L hydrochloric acid TS (1 in 2000) as directed under Ultraviolet-visible Spectrophotometry *<2.24>*, and compare the spectrum with the Reference Spectrum: both spectra exhibit similar intensities of absorption at the same wavelengths.

(4) To 1 mL of a solution of Benzalkonium Chloride (1 in 100) add 2 mL of ethanol (95), 0.5 mL of dilute nitric acid and 1 mL of silver nitrate TS: a white precipitate is produced. This precipitate does not dissolve on the addition of dilute nitric acid, but dissolves on the addition of ammonia TS.

Purity **(1)** Clarity and color of solution—Dissolve 1.0 g of Benzalkonium Chloride in 10 mL of water: the solution is clear and colorless to light yellow.

(2) Petroleum ether-soluble substances—To 3.0 g of Benzalkonium Chloride add water to make 50 mL, then add 50 mL of ethanol (99.5) and 5 mL of 0.5 mol/L sodium hydroxide TS, and extract with three 50-mL portions of petroleum ether. Combine the petroleum ether extracts, and wash with three 50-mL portions of dilute ethanol. After shaking well with 10 g of anhydrous sodium sulfate, filter through a dry filter paper, and wash the filter paper with two 10-mL portions of petroleum ether. Evaporate the petroleum ether on a water bath by heating, and dry the residue at 105°C for 1 hour: the residue is not more than 1.0%.

Water *<2.48>* Not more than 15.0% (volumetric titration, direct titration).

Residue on ignition *<2.44>* Not more than 0.2% (1 g).

Assay Weigh accurately about 0.15 g of Benzalkonium Chloride, and dissolve in 75 mL of water. Adjust the pH between 2.6 and 3.4 by adding dropwise diluted dilute hydrochloric acid (1 in 2), add 1 drop of methyl orange TS, and titrate *<2.50>* with 0.02 mol/L sodium tetraphenylboron VS until the color of the solution becomes red.

Each mL of 0.02 mol/L sodium tetraphenylboron VS
= 7.080 mg of $C_{22}H_{40}ClN$

Containers and storage Containers—Tight containers.

Benzalkonium Chloride Solution

ベンザルコニウム塩化物液

Benzalkonium Chloride Solution is an aqueous solution containing not more than 50.0 w/v% of benzalkonium chloride.

It contains not less than 93.0% and not more than 107.0% of the labeled amount of benzalkonium chloride ($C_{22}H_{40}ClN$: 354.01).

Method of preparation Dissolve Benzalkonium Chloride in Water, Purified Water or Purified Water in Containers. It is also prepared by diluting Concentrated Benzalkonium Chloride Solution 50 with Water, Purified Water or Purified Water in Containers.

Description Benzalkonium Chloride Solution is a clear, colorless to light yellow liquid, having a characteristic odor.

It foams strongly on shaking.

Identification **(1)** Evaporate a volume of Benzalkonium Chloride Solution, equivalent to 0.2 g of Benzalkonium Chloride, on a water bath to dryness, and proceed with the residue as directed in the Identification (1) under Benzalkonium Chloride.

(2) To a volume of Benzalkonium Chloride Solution, equivalent to 0.01 g of Benzalkonium Chloride, add water to make 10 mL. Proceed with 2 mL of this solution as directed in the Identification (2) under Benzalkonium Chloride.

(3) To a volume of Benzalkonium Chloride Solution, equivalent to 1 g of Benzalkonium Chloride, add water or concentrate on a water bath, if necessary, to make 10 mL. To 1 mL of this solution add 0.1 mol/L hydrochloric acid VS to make 200 mL, and proceed as directed in the Identification (3) under Benzalkonium Chloride.

(4) To a volume of Benzalkonium Chloride Solution, equivalent to 0.1 g of Benzalkonium Chloride, add water or concentrate on a water bath, if necessary, to make 10 mL. Proceed with 1 mL of this solution as directed in the Identification (4) under Benzalkonium Chloride.

Assay Pipet a volume of Benzalkonium Chloride Solution, equivalent to about 0.15 g of benzalkonium chloride ($C_{22}H_{40}ClN$), dilute with water to make 75 mL, if necessary, and proceed as directed in the Assay under Benzalkonium Chloride.

Each mL of 0.02 mol/L sodium tetraphenylboron VS
= 7.080 mg of $C_{22}H_{40}ClN$

Containers and storage Containers—Tight containers.

Benzalkonium Chloride Concentrated Solution 50

濃ベンザルコニウム塩化物液 50

Benzalkonium Chloride Concentrated Solution 50 is an aqueous solution, presented as $[C_6H_5CH_2N(CH_3)_2R]Cl$, where R ranges from C_8H_{17} to $C_{18}H_{37}$, and mainly consisting of $C_{12}H_{25}$ and $C_{14}H_{29}$.

It contains more than 50.0% and not more than 55.0% of benzalkonium chloride ($C_{22}H_{40}ClN$: 354.01).

Description Benzalkonium Chloride Concentrated Solution 50 is a colorless to light yellow liquid or jelly-like fluid, and has a characteristic odor.

It is very soluble in water and in ethanol (95), and practically insoluble in diethyl ether.

A solution prepared by adding water to it vigorously foams when shaken.

Identification **(1)** Dissolve 0.4 g of Benzalkonium Chloride Concentrated Solution 50 in 1 mL of sulfuric acid, add 0.1 g of sodium nitrate, and heat for 5 minutes on a water bath. After cooling, add 10 mL of water and 0.5 g of zinc powder, heat for 5 minutes, cool, and filter: the filtrate responds to Qualitative Tests *<1.09>* for primary aromatic amines. The color of the solution is red.

(2) To 2 mL of a solution of Benzalkonium Chloride Concentrated Solution 50 (1 in 500) add a mixture of 0.2 mL of a solution of bromophenol blue (1 in 2000) and 0.5 mL of sodium hydroxide TS: a blue color develops. Add 4 mL of chloroform to this solution, and shake vigorously: the blue color shifts to the chloroform layer. Collect the chloroform layer, and add dropwise, with stirring, a solution of sodium lauryl sulfate (1 in 1000): the chloroform layer turns colorless.

(3) Determine the absorption spectrum of a solution of Benzalkonium Chloride Concentrated Solution 50 in 0.1 mol/L hydrochloric acid TS (1 in 1000) as directed under Ultraviolet-visible Spectrophotometry *<2.24>*, and compare the spectrum with the Reference Spectrum of Benzalkonium Chloride: both spectra exhibit similar intensities of absorption at the same wavelengths.

(4) To 1 mL of a solution of Benzalkonium Chloride Concentrated Solution 50 (1 in 50) add 2 mL of ethanol (95), 0.5 mL of dilute nitric acid and 1 mL of silver nitrate TS: a white precipitate is produced. This precipitate does not dissolve on the addition of dilute nitric acid, but dissolves on the addition of ammonia TS.

Purity **(1)** Clarity and color of solution—Dissolve 2.0 g of Benzalkonium Chloride Concentrated Solution 50 in 10 mL of water: the solution is clear and colorless to light yellow.

(2) Petroleum ether-soluble substances—To 6.0 g of Benzalkonium Chloride Concentrated Solution 50 add water to make 50 mL, then add 50 mL of ethanol (99.5) and 5 mL of 0.5 mol/L sodium hydroxide TS, and extract with three 50-mL portions of petroleum ether. Combine the petroleum ether extracts, and wash with three 50-mL portions of dilute ethanol. After shaking well with 10 g of anhydrous sodium sulfate, filter through a dry filter paper, and wash the filter paper with two 10-mL portions of petroleum ether. Evaporate the petroleum ether on a water bath by heating, and dry the residue at 105°C for 1 hour: the residue is not more than 1.0%.

Residue on ignition *<2.44>* Not more than 0.2% (1 g).

Assay Weigh accurately about 0.3 g of Benzalkonium Chloride Concentrated Solution 50, and dissolve in 75 mL of water. Adjust the pH to between 2.6 and 3.4 by adding dropwise diluted dilute hydrochloric acid (1 in 2), add 1 drop of methyl orange TS, and titrate *<2.50>* with 0.02 mol/L sodium tetraphenylboron VS until the color of the solution becomes red.

Each mL of 0.02 mol/L sodium tetraphenylborate VS
= 7.080 mg of $C_{22}H_{40}ClN$

Containers and storage Containers—Tight containers.

Benzbromarone

ベンズブロマロン

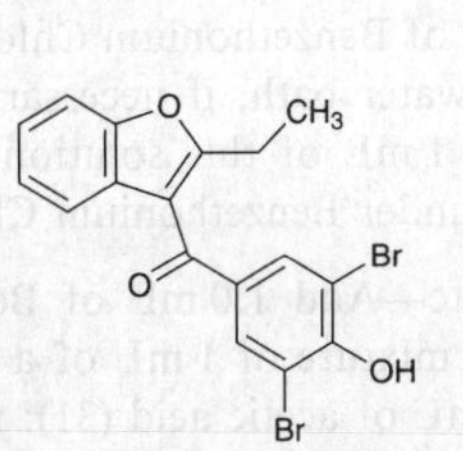

$C_{17}H_{12}Br_2O_3$: 424.08
3,5-Dibromo-4-hydroxyphenyl 2-ethylbenzo[*b*]furan-3-yl ketone
[3562-84-3]

Benzbromarone, when dried, contains not less than 98.5% and not more than 101.0% of benzbromarone ($C_{17}H_{12}Br_2O_3$).

Description Benzbromarone occurs as a white to light yellow crystalline powder.

It is very soluble in *N,N*-dimethylformamide, freely soluble in acetone, sparingly soluble in ethanol (99.5), and practically insoluble in water.

It dissolves in dilute sodium hydroxide TS.

Identification **(1)** Determine the absorption spectrum of a solution of Benzbromarone in 0.01 mol/L sodium hydroxide TS (1 in 100,000) as directed under Ultraviolet-visible Spectrophotometry *<2.24>*, and compare the spectrum with the Reference Spectrum: both spectra exhibit similar intensities of absorption at the same wavelengths.

(2) Determine the infrared absorption spectrum of Benzbromarone, previously dried, as directed in the potassium bromide disk method under Infrared Spectrophotometry *<2.25>*, and compare the spectrum with the Reference Spectrum: both spectra exhibit similar intensities of absorption at the same wave numbers.

Melting point *<2.60>* 149 – 153°C

Purity **(1)** Sulfate *<1.14>*—Dissolve 1.0 g of Benzbromarone in 40 mL of acetone, and add 1 mL of dilute hydrochloric acid and water to make 50 mL. Perform the test using this solution as the test solution. Prepare the control solution as follows: to 0.40 mL of 0.005 mol/L sulfuric acid VS add 40 mL of acetone, 1 mL of dilute hydrochloric acid and water to make 50 mL (not more than 0.019%).

(2) Soluble halides—Dissolve 0.5 g of Benzbromarone in 40 mL of acetone, and add 6 mL of dilute nitric acid and water to make 50 mL. Proceed with this solution as directed under Chloride Limit Test *<1.03>*. Prepare the control solution as follows: to 0.25 mL of 0.01 mol/L hydrochloric acid VS add 40 mL of acetone, 6 mL of dilute nitric acid and water to make 50 mL.

(3) Heavy metals *<1.07>*—Proceed with 2.0 g of Benzbromarone according to Method 2, and perform the test. Prepare the control solution with 2.0 mL of Standard Lead Solution (not more than 10 ppm).

(4) Iron *<1.10>*—Prepare the test solution with 1.0 g of Benzbromarone according to Method 3, and perform the test according to Method A. Prepare the control solution with 2.0 mL of Standard Iron Solution (not more than 20 ppm).

(5) Related substances—Dissolve 0.10 g of Benzbromarone in 10 mL of acetone, and use this solution as the sample solution. Pipet 1 mL of the sample solution, add acetone to make exactly 100 mL, and use this solution as the standard solution. Perform the test with these solutions as directed under Thin-layer Chromatography *<2.03>*. Spot 10 μL each of the sample solution and standard solution on a plate of silica gel with fluorescent indicator for thin-layer chromatography. Develop the plate with a mixture of cyclohexane, 4-methyl-2-pentanone, ethanol (99.5) and acetic acid (100) (100:20:2:1) to a distance of about 15 cm, and air-dry the plate. Examine under ultraviolet light (main wavelength: 254 nm): the spots other than the principal spot obtained from the sample solution are not more intense than the spot from the standard solution.

Loss on drying *<2.41>* Not more than 0.5% (1 g, in vacuum at a pressure not exceeding 0.67 kPa, phosphorus (V) oxide, 50°C, 4 hours).

Residue on ignition *<2.44>* Not more than 0.1% (1 g).

Assay Weigh accurately about 0.6 g of Benzbromarone, previously dried, dissolve in 30 mL of *N,N*-dimethylformamide, and titrate *<2.50>* with 0.1 mol/L tetramethylammonium hydroxide VS (indicator: 5 drops of thymol blue dimethylformamide TS). Perform a blank determination in the same manner, and make any necessary correction.

Each mL of 0.1 mol/L tetramethylammonium hydroxide VS
= 42.41 mg of $C_{17}H_{12}Br_2O_3$

Containers and storage Containers—Tight containers.
Storage—Light-resistant.

Benzethonium Chloride

ベンゼトニウム塩化物

$C_{27}H_{42}ClNO_2$: 448.08
N-Benzyl-*N*,*N*-dimethyl-2-{2-[4-(1,1,3,3-tetramethylbutyl)phenoxy]ethoxy}ethylaminium chloride
[*121-54-0*]

Benzethonium Chloride, when dried, contains not less than 97.0% of benzethonium chloride ($C_{27}H_{42}ClNO_2$).

Description Benzethonium Chloride occurs as colorless or white crystals. It is odorless.

It is very soluble in ethanol (95), freely soluble in water, and practically insoluble in diethyl ether.

A solution of Benzethonium Chloride foams strongly when shaken.

Identification **(1)** Dissolve 0.2 g of Benzethonium Chloride in 1 mL of sulfuric acid, add 0.1 g of sodium nitrate, and heat for 5 minutes on a water bath. After cooling, add 10 mL of water and 0.5 g of zinc powder, heat for 5 minutes, cool, and filter: the filtrate responds to Qualitative Tests 〈*1.09*〉 for primary aromatic amines, developing a red color.

(2) To 2 mL of a solution of Benzethonium Chloride (1 in 1000) add a mixture of 0.2 mL of a solution of bromophenol blue (1 in 2000) and 0.5 mL of sodium hydroxide TS: a blue color develops. Add 4 mL of chloroform to this solution, and shake vigorously: the blue color shifts to the chloroform layer. Collect the chloroform layer, and add dropwise a solution of sodium lauryl sulfate (1 in 1000) with stirring: the chloroform layer turns colorless.

(3) Determine the absorption spectrum of a solution of Benzethonium Chloride in 0.1 mol/L hydrochloric acid TS (1 in 5000) as directed under Ultraviolet-visible Spectrophotometry 〈*2.24*〉, and compare the spectrum with the Reference Spectrum: both spectra exhibit similar intensities of absorption at the same wavelengths.

(4) To 1 mL of a solution of Benzethonium Chloride (1 in 100) add 2 mL of ethanol (95), 0.5 mL of dilute nitric acid and 1 mL of silver nitrate TS: a white precipitate is produced. This precipitate does not dissolve on addition of dilute nitric acid, but dissolves on addition of ammonia TS.

Melting point 〈*2.60*〉 158 - 164°C (after drying).

Purity Ammonium—Dissolve 0.10 g of Benzethonium Chloride in 5 mL of water, and boil with 3 mL of sodium hydroxide TS: the evolving gas dose not change moistened red litmus paper to blue.

Loss on drying 〈*2.41*〉 Not more than 5.0% (1 g, 105°C, 4 hours).

Residue on ignition 〈*2.44*〉 Not more than 0.1% (1 g).

Assay Weigh accurately about 0.2 g of Benzethonium Chloride, previously dried, dissolve in 75 mL of water, add diluted dilute hydrochloric acid (1 in 2) dropwise to adjust the pH to 2.6–3.4, then add 1 drop of methyl orange TS, and titrate 〈*2.50*〉 with 0.02 mol/L tetraphenylboron VS until the solution develops a red.

Each mL of 0.02 mol/L sodium tetraphenylboron VS
= 8.962 mg of $C_{27}H_{42}ClNO_2$

Containers and storage Containers—Tight containers.
Storage—Light-resistant.

Benzethonium Chloride Solution

ベンゼトニウム塩化物液

Benzethonium Chloride Solution contains not less than 93.0% and not more than 107.0% of the labeled amount of benzethonium chloride ($C_{27}H_{42}ClNO_2$: 448.08).

Method of preparation Dissolve Benzethonium Chloride in Water, Purified Water or Purified Water in Containers.

Description Benzethonium Chloride Solution is a clear, colorless liquid. It is odorless.

It foams strongly when shaken.

Identification **(1)** Evaporate a volume of Benzethonium Chloride Solution, equivalent to 0.2 g of Benzethonium Chloride, on a water bath to dryness, and proceed with the residue as directed in the Identification (1) under Benzethonium Chloride.

(2) To a volume of Benzethonium Chloride Solution, equivalent to 0.01 g of Benzethonium Chloride, add water to make 10 mL, proceed with 2 mL of this solution as directed in the Identification (2) under Benzethonium Chloride.

(3) To a volume of Benzethonium Chloride Solution, equivalent to 1 g of Benzethonium Chloride, and add water or concentrate on a water bath to make 10 mL. To 1 mL of this solution add 0.1 mol/L hydrochloric acid TS to make 500 mL, and determine the abosorption spectrum as directed under Ultraviolet-visible Spectrophotometry 〈*2.24*〉: it exhibits maxima between 262 nm and 264 nm, between 268 nm and 270 nm, and between 274 nm and 276 nm.

(4) To a volume of Benzethonium Chloride Solution, equivalent to 0.1 g of Benzethonium Chloride, add water, or concentrate on a water bath, if necessary, to make 10 mL, and proceed with 1 mL of this solution as directed in the Identification (4) under Benzethonium Chloride.

Purity **(1)** Nitrite—Add 1.0 mL of Benzethonium Chloride Solution to a mixture of 1 mL of a solution of glycine (1 in 10) and 0.5 mL of acetic acid (31): no gas is evolved.

(2) Oxidizing substances—To 5 mL of Benzethonium Chloride Solution add 0.5 mL of potassium iodide TS and 2 to 3 drops of dilute hydrochloric acid: no yellow color is produced.

Assay Pipet a volume of Benzethonium Chloride Solution, equivalent to about 0.2 g of benzethonium chloride ($C_{27}H_{42}ClNO_2$), dilute with water to make 75 mL, if necessary, and proceed as directed in the Assay under Benzethonium Chloride.

Each mL of 0.02 mol/L sodium tetraphenylboron VS
= 8.962 mg of $C_{27}H_{42}ClNO_2$

Containers and storage Containers—Tight containers.
Storage—Light-resistant.

Benzoic Acid

安息香酸

$C_7H_6O_2$: 122.12
Benzoic acid
[65-85-0]

Benzoic Acid, when dried, contains not less than 99.5% of benzoic acid ($C_7H_6O_2$).

Description Benzoic Acid occurs as white, crystals or crystalline powder. It is odorless, or has a faint, benzaldehyde-like odor.

It is freely soluble in ethanol (95), in acetone and in diethyl ether, soluble in hot water, and slightly soluble in water.

Identification Dissolve 1 g of Benzoic Acid in 8 mL of sodium hydroxide TS, and add water to make 100 mL. This solution responds to Qualitative Tests <*1.09*> (2) for benzoate.

Melting point <*2.60*> 121 – 124°C

Purity **(1)** Heavy metals <*1.07*>—Dissolve 1.0 g of Benzoic Acid in 25 mL of acetone, add 2 mL of dilute acetic acid and water to make 50 mL, and perform the test using this solution as the test solution. Prepare the control solution as follows: to 2.0 mL of Standard Lead Solution add 2 mL of dilute acetic acid, 25 mL of acetone and water to make 50 mL (not more than 20 ppm).

(2) Chlorinated compounds—Take 0.5 g of Benzoic Acid and 0.7 g of calcium carbonate in a crucible, mix with a small amount of water, and dry. Ignite it at about 600°C, dissolve in 20 mL of dilute nitric acid, and filter. Wash the residue with 15 mL of water, combine the filtrate and the washing, add water to make 50 mL, and add 0.5 mL of silver nitrate TS: this solution has not more turbid than the following control solution.

Control solution: Dissolve 0.7 g of calcium carbonate in 20 mL of dilute nitric acid, and filter. Wash the residue with 15 mL of water, combine the filtrate and the washings, add 1.2 mL of 0.01 mol/L hydrochloric acid VS and water to make 50 mL, and add 0.5 mL of silver nitrate TS.

(3) Potassium permanganate-reducing substances—Add 0.02 mol/L potassium permanganate VS dropwise to a boiling mixture of 100 mL of water and 1.5 mL of sulfuric acid, until a red color persists for 30 seconds. Dissolve 1.0 g of Benzoic Acid in this boiling solution, and add 0.50 mL of 0.02 mol/L potassium permanganate VS: a red color persists for at least 15 seconds.

(4) Phthalic acid—To 0.10 g of Benzoic Acid add 1 mL of water and 1 mL of resorcinol-sulfuric acid TS, and heat the mixture in an oil bath heated at a temperature between 120°C and 125°C. After evaporating the water, heat the residue for 90 minutes, cool, and dissolve in 5 mL of water. To 1 mL of the solution add 10 mL of a solution of sodium hydroxide (43 in 500), shake, then examine under light at a wavelength between 470 nm and 490 nm: the green fluorescence of the solution is not more intense than that of the following control solution.

Control solution: Dissolve 61 mg of potassium hydrogen phthalate in water to make exactly 1000 mL. Measure exactly 1 mL of the solution, add 1 mL of resorcinol-sulfuric acid TS, and proceed as directed above.

(5) Readily carbonizable substances <*1.15*>—Perform the test with 0.5 g of Benzoic Acid. The solution is not more colored than Matching Fluid Q.

Loss on drying <*2.41*> Not more than 0.5% (1 g, silica gel, 3 hours).

Residue on ignition <*2.44*> Not more than 0.05% (1 g).

Assay Weigh accurately about 0.5 g of Benzoic Acid, previously dried, dissolve in 25 mL of neutralized ethanol and 25 mL of water, and titrate <*2.50*> with 0.1 mol/L sodium hydroxide VS (indicator: 3 drops of phenolphthalein TS).

Each mL of 0.1 mol/L sodium hydroxide VS
= 12.21 mg of $C_7H_6O_2$

Containers and storage Containers—Well-closed containers.

Benzyl Alcohol

ベンジルアルコール

C_7H_8O: 108.14
Benzyl alcohol
[100-51-6]

This monograph is harmonized with the European Pharmacopoeia and the U.S. Pharmacopeia.

The parts of the text that are not harmonized are marked with symbols (◆ ◆).

Information on the harmonization with the European Pharmacopoeia and the U.S. Pharmacopeia is available on the website of the Pharmaceuticals and Medical Devices Agency.

Benzyl Alcohol contains not less than 98.0% and not more than 100.5% of benzyl alcohol (C_7H_8O).

◆The label states, where applicable, that it is suitable for use in the manufacture of injection forms.◆

◆**Description** Benzyl Alcohol is a clear, colorless oily liquid.

It is miscible with ethanol (95), with fatty oils and with essential oils.

It is soluble in water.

Specific gravity d^{20}_{20}: 1.043 – 1.049◆

◆**Identification** Determine the infrared absorption spectrum of Benzyl Alcohol as directed in the liquid film method under Infrared Spectrophotometry <*2.25*>, and compare the spectrum with the Reference Spectrum: both spectra exhibit similar intensities of absorption at the same wave numbers.◆

Refractive index <*2.45*> n^{20}_{D}: 1.538 – 1.541

Purity ◆**(1)** Clarity and color of solution—Dissolve 2.0 mL of Benzyl Alcohol in 60 mL of water: the solution is clear and colorless.◆

(2) Acidity—To 10 mL of Benzyl Alcohol add 10 mL of ethanol (95) and 2 drops of phenolphthalein TS, and add dropwise 0.1 mol/L sodium hydroxide VS until the solution acquires a light red color: the amount of 0.1 mol/L sodium hydroxide VS used is not more than 1.0 mL.

(3) Benzaldehyde and other related substances—Use Benzyl Alcohol as the sample solution. Separately, dissolve exactly 0.100 g of ethylbenzene in Benzyl Alcohol to make exactly 10 mL. Pipet 2 mL of this solution, add Benzyl Alcohol to make exactly 20 mL, and use this solution as the ethylbenzene stock solution. Separately, dissolve exactly 2.000 g of dicyclohexyl in Benzyl Alcohol to make exactly 10 mL. Pipet 2 mL of this solution, add Benzyl Alcohol to make exactly 20 mL, and use this solution as the dicyclohexyl stock solution. Separately, weigh exactly 0.750 g of benzaldehyde and 0.500 g of cyclohexylmethanol, and add Benzyl Alcohol to make exactly 25 mL. Pipet 1 mL of this solution, add exactly 2 mL of ethylbenzene stock solution and exactly 3 mL of dicyclohexyl stock solution, then add Benzyl Alcohol to make exactly 20 mL, and use this solution as the standard solution (1). Perform the test with exactly 0.1 μL each of the sample solution and standard solution (1) as directed under Gas Chromatography <*2.02*> according to the following conditions, and when the peak having the retention time corresponding to ethylbenzene and dicyclohexyl appears on the chromatogram obtained from the sample solution, correct the peak areas of ethylbenzene and dicyclohexyl from the standard solution (1) by deducting the relevant peak area from the sample solution, the peak area of benzaldehyde from the sample solution is not more than the difference between the peak areas of benzaldehyde of the sample solution and the standard solution (1) (0.15%), and the peak area of cyclohexylmethanol from the sample solution is not more than the difference between the peak areas of cyclohexylmethanol of the sample solution and the standard solution (1) (0.10%). The total area of the peaks having smaller retention time than benzyl alcohol and other than benzaldehyde and cyclohexylmethanol from the sample solution is not more than 4 times the peak area or the corrected peak area of ethylbenzene from the standard solution (1) (0.04%). The total area of the peaks having larger retention time than benzyl alcohol from the sample solution is not more than the peak area or the corrected peak area of dicyclohexyl from the standard solution (1) (0.3%). For these calculations the peak areas less than 1/100 times the peak area or the corrected peak area of ethylbenzene with the standard solution (1) are excluded.

Benzyl Alcohol labeled that it is suitable for use in the manufacture of injection forms meets the following requirements.

Use Benzyl Alcohol as the sample solution. Separately, weigh exactly 0.250 g of benzaldehyde and 0.500 g of cyclohexylmethanol, and add Benzyl Alcohol to make exactly 25 mL. Pipet 1 mL of this solution, add exactly 2 mL of the ethylbenzene stock solution and exactly 2 mL of the dicyclohexyl stock solution, then add Benzyl Alcohol to make exactly 20 mL, and use this solution as the standard solution (2). Perform the test with exactly 0.1 μL each of the sample solution and standard solution (2) as directed under Gas Chromatography <*2.02*> according to the following conditions, and when the peak having the retention time corresponding to ethylbenzene and dicyclohexyl appears on the chromatogram obtained from the sample solution, correct the peak areas of ethylbenzene and dicyclohexyl from the standard solution (2) by deducting the relevant peak area from the sample solution, the peak area of benzaldehyde from the sample solution is not more than the difference between the peak areas of benzaldehyde of the sample solution and the standard solution (2) (0.05%), and the peak area of cyclohexylmethanol from the sample solution is not more than the difference between the peak areas of cyclohexylmethanol of the sample solution and the standard solution (2) (0.10%). The total area of the peaks having smaller retention time than benzyl alcohol and other than benzaldehyde and cyclohexylmethanol from the sample solution is not more than 2 times the peak area or the corrected peak area of ethylbenzene from the standard solution (2) (0.02%). The total area of the peaks having larger retention time than benzyl alcohol from the sample solution is not more than the peak area of or the corrected peak area dicyclohexyl from the standard solution (2) (0.2%). For these calculation the peak areas less than 1/100 times the peak area or the corrected peak area of ethylbenzene from the standard solution (2) are excluded.

Operating conditions—

Detector: A hydrogen flame-ionization detector.

Column: A fused silica column 0.32 mm in inside diameter and 30 m in length, coated inside with polyethylene glycol 20 M for gas chromatography in 0.5 μm thickness.

Column temperature: Inject at a constant temperature of about 50°C, raise the temperature at a rate of 5°C per minute to 220°C, and maintain at 220°C for 35 minutes.

Temperature of injection port: A constant temperature of about 200°C.

Temperature of detector: A constant temperature of about 310°C.

Carrier gas: Helium.

Flow rate: 25 cm/second.

Splitless.

Detection sensitivity: When 0.1 μL of the standard solution (1) is injected, adjust the sensitivity of the detector so that the height of the peak of ethylbenzene is not less than 30% of the full scale of the recorder. For Benzyl Alcohol labeled to use for injection, use the standard solution (2) instead of the standard solution (1).

System suitability—

System performance: When the procedure is run with the standard solution (1) under the above operating conditions, the retention time of benzyl alcohol is about 26 minutes, the relative retention times of ethylbenzene, dicyclohexyl, benzaldehyde and cyclohexylmethanol to benzyl alcohol are about 0.28, about 0.59, about 0.68 and about 0.71, respectively, and the resolution between the peaks of benzaldehyde and cyclohexylmethanol is not less than 3.0. In the case of Benzyl Alcohol labeled to use for injection, proceed with the standard solution (2) instead of the standard solution (1).

(4) Peroxide value—Weigh accurately about 5 g of Benzyl Alcohol, and dissolve in 30 mL of a mixture of acetic acid (100) and chloroform (3:2) in a 250-mL glass-stoppered conical flask. Add 0.5 mL of saturated potassium iodide solution, shake for exactly 1 minute, add 30 mL of water, and titrate <*2.50*> with 0.01 mol/L sodium thiosulfate VS, adding the titrant slowly with continuous vigorous shaking, until the blue color of the solution disappears after addition of 5 mL of starch TS near the end point where the solution is a pale yellow color. Perform a blank determination in the same manner. Calculate the amount of peroxide by the following formula: not more than 5. In the blank determination, the required amount of 0.01 mol/L sodium thiosulfate VS must not exceed 0.1 mL.

$$\text{Amount (mEq/kg) of peroxide} = 10 \times (V_1 - V_0)/M$$

V_1: Volume (mL) of 0.01 mol/L sodium thiosulfate VS consumed in the test

V_0: Volume (mL) of 0.01 mol/L sodium thiosulfate VS consumed in the blank determination

M: Amount (g) of Benzyl Alcohol taken

(5) Residue on evaporation—Perform the test after conformation that the sample meets the requirement of the peroxide value. Transfer 10.0 g of Benzyl Alcohol to a porcelain or quartz crucible or platinum dish, previously weighed accurately, and heat on a hot-plate at not exceeding 200°C, taking care to avoid boiling, to evaporate to dryness. Dry the residue on the hot-plate for 1 hour, and allow to cool in a desiccator: not more than 5 mg.

Assay Weigh accurately about 0.9 g of Benzyl Alcohol, add exactly 15 mL of a freshly prepared mixture of dehydrated pyridine and acetic anhydride (7:1), and heat on a water bath under a reflux condenser for 30 minutes. Cool, add 25 mL of water, and titrate *<2.50>* the excess acetic acid with 1 mol/L sodium hydroxide VS (indicator: 2 drops of phenolphthalein TS). Perform a blank determination in the same manner.

Each mL of 1 mol/L sodium hydroxide VS
= 108.1 mg of C_7H_8O

◆**Containers and storage** Containers—Tight containers.
Storage—Light-resistant.◆

Benzyl Benzoate

安息香酸ベンジル

$C_{14}H_{12}O_2$: 212.24
Benzyl benzoate
[120-51-4]

Benzyl Benzoate contains not less than 99.0% of benzyl benzoate ($C_{14}H_{12}O_2$).

Description Benzyl Benzoate is a colorless, clear, viscous liquid. It has a faint, aromatic odor and a pungent, burning taste.

It is miscible with ethanol (95) and with diethyl ether.

It is practically insoluble in water.

Congealing point: about 17°C

Specific gravity d_{20}^{20}: about 1.123

Boiling point: about 323°C

Identification **(1)** Heat gently 1 mL of Benzyl Benzoate with 5 mL of sodium carbonate TS and 2 mL of potassium permanganate TS: the odor of benzaldehyde is perceptible.

(2) Warm the titrated mixture obtained in the Assay on a water bath to remove ethanol, and add 0.5 mL of iron (III) chloride TS: a light yellow-red precipitate is produced, which turns white on the addition of dilute hydrochloric acid.

Refractive index *<2.45>* n_D^{20}: 1.568 – 1.570

Purity Acidity—Dissolve 5.0 mL of Benzyl Benzoate in 25 mL of neutralized ethanol, and add 0.50 mL of 0.1 mol/L sodium hydroxide VS: a red color develops.

Residue on ignition *<2.44>* Not more than 0.05% (2 g).

Assay Weigh accurately about 2 g of Benzyl Benzoate, add exactly 50 mL of 0.5 mol/L potassium hydroxide-ethanol VS, and boil gently for 1 hour under a reflux condenser with a carbon dioxide-absorbing tube (soda lime). Cool, and titrate *<2.50>* the excess potassium hydroxide with 0.5 mol/L hydrochloric acid VS (indicator: 2 drops of phenolphthalein TS). Perform a blank determination in the same manner.

Each mL of 0.5 mol/L potassium hydroxide-ethanol VS
= 106.1 mg of $C_{14}H_{12}O_2$

Containers and storage Containers—Tight containers.
Storage—Light-resistant.

Benzylpenicillin Benzathine Hydrate

ベンジルペニシリンベンザチン水和物

$(C_{16}H_{18}N_2O_4S)_2.C_{16}H_{20}N_2.4H_2O$: 981.18
(2*S*,5*R*,6*R*)-3,3-Dimethyl-7-oxo-6-[(phenylacetyl)amino]-4-thia-1-azabicyclo[3.2.0]heptane-2-carboxylic acid hemi(*N*,*N′*-dibenzylethane-1,2-diamine)dihydrate
[41372-02-5]

Benzylpenicillin Benzathine Hydrate is the *N*,*N′*-dibenzylethylenediamine salt of a penicillin compound having antibacterial activity produced by the growth of *Penicillium* species.

It contains not less than 1213 Units and not more than 1333 Units per mg, calculated on the anhydrous basis. The potency of Benzylpenicillin Benzathine Hydrate is expressed as unit calculated from the amount of benzylpenicillin sodium ($C_{16}H_{17}N_2NaO_4S$: 356.37). 1 Unit of Benzylpenicillin Benzathine Hydrate is equivalent to 0.6 μg of benzylpenicillin sodium ($C_{16}H_{17}N_2NaO_4S$). It contains not less than 24.0% and not more than 27.0% of *N*,*N′*-dibenzylethylenediamine ($C_{16}H_{20}N_2$: 240.34), calculated on the anhydrous basis.

Description Benzylpenicillin Benzathine Hydrate occurs as a white crystalline powder.

It is slightly soluble in methanol and in ethanol (99.5), and practically insoluble in water.

Identification **(1)** Determine the absorption spectrum of a solution of Benzylpenicillin Benzathine Hydrate in methanol (1 in 2000) as directed under Ultraviolet-visible Spectrophotometry *<2.24>*, and compare the spectrum with the Reference Spectrum: both spectra exhibit similar intensities of absorption at the same wavelengths.

(2) Determine the infrared absorption spectrum of Benzylpenicillin Benzathine Hydrate as directed in the potassium bromide disk method under Infrared Spectrophotometry *<2.25>*, and compare the spectrum with the Reference Spectrum: both spectra exhibit similar intensities of absorption at the same wave numbers.

Optical rotation *<2.49>* $[\alpha]_D^{20}$: +217 – +233° (0.1 g calculated on the anhydrous basis, methanol, 20 mL, 100 mm).

Purity **(1)** Heavy metals *<1.07>*—Proceed with 1.0 g of Benzylpenicillin Benzathine Hydrate according to Method 2, and perform the test. Prepare the control solution with 2.0 mL of Standard Lead Solution (not more than 20 ppm).

(2) Arsenic *<1.11>*—Prepare the test solution with 1.0 g of Benzylpenicillin Benzathine Hydrate according to Method 3, and perform the test (not more than 2 ppm).

(3) Related substances—Dissolve 70 mg of Benzylpenicillin Benzathine Hydrate in 25 mL of methanol, add a solution prepared by dissolving 1.02 g of disodium hydrogen phosphate and 6.80 g of potassium dihydrogen phosphate in water to make 1000 mL to make 50 mL, and use this solution as the sample solution. Pipet 1 mL of the sample solution, add the mobile phase A to make exactly 100 mL, and use this solution as the standard solution. Perform the test with exactly 20 μL each of the sample solution and standard solution as directed under Liquid Chromatography <*2.01*> according to the following conditions, and determine each peak area by the automatic integration method: the area of the peak having the relative retention time of about 2.4 to benzylpenicillin obtained from the sample solution is not larger than 2 times the total area of the peaks of benzylpenicillin and *N,N′*-dibenzylethylenediamine from the standard solution, and the area of the peak other than benzylpenicillin, *N,N′*-dibenzylethylenediamine and the peak having the relative retention time of about 2.4 to benzylpenicillin from the sample solution is not larger than the total area of the peaks of benzylpenicillin and *N,N′*-dibenzylethylenediamine from the standard solution.

Operating conditions—

Detector: An ultraviolet absorption photometer (wavelength: 220 nm).

Column: A stainless steel column 4.0 mm in inside diameter and 25 cm in length, packed with octadecylsilanized silica gel for liquid chromatography (5 μm in particle diameter).

Column temperature: A constant temperature of about 40°C.

Mobile phase A: A mixture of water, methanol and 0.25 mol/L potassium dihydrogen phosphate TS (pH 3.5) (6:3:1).

Mobile phase B: A mixture of methanol, water and 0.25 mol/L potassium dihydrogen phosphate TS (pH 3.5) (6:3:1).

Flowing of mobile phase: Control the gradient by mixing the mobile phases A and B as directed in the following table.

Time after injection of sample (min)	Mobile phase A (vol%)	Mobile phase B (vol%)
0 – 10	75	25
10 – 20	75 → 0	25 → 100
20 – 55	0	100

Flow rate: 1.0 mL per minute.

Time span of measurement: About 3 times as long as the retention time of benzylpenicillin, beginning after the solvent peak.

System suitability—

Test for required detectability: To exactly 1 mL of the standard solution add the mobile phase A to make exactly 20 mL. Confirm that the peak area of benzylpenicillin obtained with 20 μL of this solution is equivalent to 3.5 to 6.5% of that with 20 μL of the standard solution.

System performance: When the procedure is run with 20 μL of the standard solution under the above operating conditions, *N,N′*-dibenzylethylenediamine and benzylpenicillin are eluted in this order with the resolution between these peaks being not less than 25.

System repeatability: When the test is repeated 3 times with 20 μL of the standard solution under the above operating conditions, the relative standard deviation of the peak areas of benzylpenicillin is not more than 2.0%.

Water <*2.48*> 5.0 – 8.0% (1 g, volumetric titration, direct titration).

Assay **(1)** Benzylpenicillin—Weigh accurately an amount of Benzylpenicillin Benzathine Hydrate, equivalent to about 85,000 Units, dissolve in 25 mL of methanol, and add a solution containing 1.02 g of disodium hydrogen phosphate and 6.80 g of potassium dihydrogen phosphate in 1000 mL of water to make exactly 50 mL. Pipet 5 mL of this solution, add a mixture of the solution containing 1.02 g of disodium hydrogen phosphate and 6.80 g of potassium dihydrogen phosphate in 1000 mL of water and methanol (1:1) to make exactly 20 mL, and use this solution as the sample solution. Separately, weigh accurately an amount of Benzylpenicillin Potassium RS, equivalent to about 85,000 Units, and about 25 mg of *N,N′*-dibenzylethylenediamine diacetate, dissolve in 25 mL of methanol, and add the solution containing 1.02 g of disodium hydrogen phosphate and 6.80 g of potassium dihydrogen phosphate in 1000 mL of water to make exactly 50 mL. Pipet 5 mL of this solution, add a mixture of the solution containing 1.02 g of disodium hydrogen phosphate and 6.80 g of potassium dihydrogen phosphate in 1000 mL of water and methanol (1:1) to make exactly 20 mL, and use this solution as the standard solution. Perform the test with exactly 20 μL each of the sample solution and standard solution as directed under Liquid Chromatography <*2.01*> according to the following conditions, and determine the peak areas, A_T ands A_S, of benzylpenicillin in each solution.

Amount (unit) of benzylpenicillin sodium ($C_{16}H_{17}N_2NaO_4S$)
$= M_S \times A_T/A_S$

M_S: Amount (unit) of Benzylpenicillin Potassium RS taken

Operating conditions—

Detector: An ultraviolet absorption photometer (wavelength: 220 nm).

Column: A stainless steel column 4.6 mm in inside diameter and 25 cm in length, packed with octadecylsilanized silica gel for liquid chromatography (5 μm in particle diameter).

Column temperature: A constant temperature of about 40°C.

Mobile phase: A mixture of water, methanol and 0.25 mol/L potassium dihydrogen phosphate TS (pH 3.5) (11:7:2).

Flow rate: Adjust so that the retention time of benzylpenicillin is about 18 minutes.

System suitability—

System performance: When the procedure is run with 20 μL of the standard solution under the above operating conditions, *N,N′*-dibenzylethylenediamine and benzylpenicillin are eluted in this order with the resolution between these peaks being not less than 20.

System repeatability: When the test is repeated 6 times with 20 μL of the standard solution under the above operating conditions, the relative standard deviations of the peak areas of *N,N′*-dibenzylethylenediamine and benzylpenicillin are not more than 2.0%, respectively.

(2) *N,N′*-Dibenzylethylenediamine—Determine the areas, A_T and A_S, of the peak corresponding to *N,N′*-dibenzylethylenediamine on the chromatograms obtained in (1) with the sample solution and standard solution.

Amount (%) of *N,N′*-dibenzylethylenediamine ($C_{16}H_{20}N_2$)
$= M_S/M_T \times A_T/A_S \times 100 \times 0.667$

M_S: Amount (mg) of *N,N′*-dibenzylethylenediamine diacetate taken

M_T: Amount (mg) of Benzylpenicillin Benzathine Hydrate taken

0.667: Conversion factor for the molecular mass of *N,N′*-dibenzylethylenediamine diacetate ($C_{16}H_{20}N_2 \cdot 2CH_3COOH$) to that of *N,N′*-dibenzylethylenediamine (benzathine, $C_{16}H_{20}N_2$)

Containers and storage Containers—Tight containers.
Storage—Light-resistant.

Benzylpenicillin Potassium

Penicillin G Potassium

ベンジルペニシリンカリウム

$C_{16}H_{17}KN_2O_4S$: 372.48
Monopotassium (2*S*,5*R*,6*R*)-3,3-dimethyl-7-oxo-6-[(phenylacetyl)amino]-4-thia-1-azabicyclo[3.2.0]heptane-2-carboxylate
[*113-98-4*]

Benzylpenicillin Potassium is the potassium salt of a penicillin substance having antibacterial activity produced by the growth of *Penicillium* species.

It contains not less than 1430 units and not more than 1630 units per mg, calculated on the dried basis. The potency of Benzylpenicillin Potassium is expressed as mass unit of benzylpenicillin potassium ($C_{16}H_{17}KN_2O_4S$). One unit of Benzylpenicillin Potassium is equivalent to 0.63 μg of benzylpenicillin potassium.

Description Benzylpenicillin Potassium occurs as white, crystals or crystalline powder.

It is very soluble in water, and slightly soluble in ethanol (99.5).

Identification **(1)** Determine the absorption spectrum of a solution of Benzylpenicillin Potassium (1 in 1000) as directed under Ultraviolet-visible Spectrophotometry <*2.24*>, and compare the spectrum with the Reference Spectrum or the spectrum of a solution of Benzylpenicillin Potassium RS prepared in the same manner as the sample solution: both spectra exhibit similar intensities of absorption at the same wavelengths.

(2) Determine the infrared absorption spectrum of Benzylpenicillin Potassium as directed in the potassium bromide disk method under Infrared Spectrophotometry <*2.25*>, and compare the spectrum with the Reference Spectrum or the spectrum of Benzylpenicillin Potassium RS: both spectra exhibit similar intensities of absorption at the same wave numbers.

(3) Benzylpenicillin Potassium responds to Qualitative Tests <*1.09*> (1) for potassium salt.

Optical rotation <*2.49*> $[\alpha]_D^{20}$: +270 – +300° (1.0 g calculated on the dried basis, water, 50 mL, 100 mm).

pH <*2.54*> The pH of a solution obtained by dissolving 1.0 g of Benzylpenicillin Potassium in 100 mL of water is between 5.0 and 7.5.

Purity **(1)** Clarity and color of solution—A solution obtained by dissolving 1.0 g of Benzylpenicillin Potassium in 10 mL of water is clear, and its absorbance at 400 nm determined as directed under Ultraviolet-visible Spectrophotometry <*2.24*> is not more than 0.10.

(2) Heavy metals <*1.07*>—Proceed with 2.0 g of Benzylpenicillin Potassium according to Method 4, and perform the test. Prepare the control solution with 2.0 mL of Standard Lead Solution (not more than 10 ppm).

(3) Arsenic <*1.11*>—Prepare the test solution by incinerating 1.0 g of Benzylpenicillin Potassium according to Method 4, and perform the test. In the incineration, use a crucible of porcelain, and after addition of 10 mL of a solution of magnesium nitrate hexahydrate in ethanol (95) (1 in 10) add 1 mL of hydrogen peroxide (30), then burn the ethanol (not more than 2 ppm).

(4) Related substances—Dissolve 40 mg of Benzylpenicillin Potassium in 20 mL of water, and use this solution as the sample solution. Pipet 1 mL of the sample solution, add water to make exactly 100 mL, and use this solution as the standard solution. Perform the test with exactly 20 μL each of the sample solution and standard solution as directed under Liquid Chromatography <*2.01*> according to the following conditions, and determine each peak area by the automatic integration method: the area of the peak other than benzylpenicillin obtained from the sample solution is not larger than the peak area of benzylpenicillin from the standard solution, and the total area of the peaks other than benzylpenicillin from the sample solution is not larger than 3 times the peak area of benzylpenicillin from the standard solution.

Operating conditions—

Detector, column, column temperature, mobile phase, and flow rate: Proceed as directed in the operating conditions in the Assay.

Time span of measurement: About 5 times as long as the retention time of benzylpenicillin, beginning after the solvent peak.

System suitability—

Test for required detectability: Pipet 10 mL of the standard solution, and add water to make exactly 100 mL. Confirm that the peak area of benzylpenicillin obtained with 20 μL of this solution is equivalent to 7 to 13% of that with 20 μL of the standard solution.

System performance: When the procedure is run with 20 μL of the standard solution under the above operating conditions, the number of theoretical plates and the symmetry factor of the peak of benzylpenicillin are not less than 4000 and 0.7 to 1.2, respectively.

System repeatability: When the test is repeated 6 times with 20 μL of the standard solution under the above operating conditions, the relative standard deviation of the peak area of benzylpenicillin is not more than 1.0%.

Loss on drying <*2.41*> Not more than 1.0% (3 g, reduced pressure not exceeding 0.67 kPa, 60°C, 3 hours).

Assay Weigh accurately amounts of Benzylpenicillin Potassium and Benzylpenicillin Potassium RS, equivalent to about 6 × 10^4 Units, dissolve each in water to make exactly 20 mL, and use these solutions as the sample solution and the standard solution, respectively. Perform the test with exactly 20 μL each of the sample solution and standard solution as directed under Liquid Chromatography <*2.01*> according to the following conditions, and determine the peak areas, A_T and A_S, of benzylpenicillin in each solution.

Amount (unit) of benzylpenicillin potassium ($C_{16}H_{17}KN_2O_4S$)
$$= M_S \times A_T/A_S$$

M_S: Amount (unit) of benzylpenicillin potassium RS taken

Operating conditions—

Detector: An ultraviolet absorption photometer (wavelength: 254 nm).

Column: A stainless steel column 4.6 mm in inside diameter and 25 cm in length, packed with octadecylsilanized silica gel for liquid chromatography (7 μm in particle diameter).

Column temperature: A constant temperature of about 25°C.

Mobile phase: A mixture of diammonium hydrogen phosphate solution (33 in 5000) and acetonitrile (19:6), adjusted to pH 8.0 with phosphoric acid.

Flow rate: Adjust so that the retention time of benzylpenicillin is about 7.5 minutes.

System suitability—

System performance: When the procedure is run with 20 μL of the standard solution under the above operating conditions, the number of theoretical plates and the symmetry factor of the peak of benzylpenicillin are not less than 2000 and not more than 3.0, respectively.

System repeatability: When the test is repeated 6 times with 20 μL of the standard solution under the above operating conditions, the relative standard deviation of the peak area of benzylpenicillin is not more than 1.0%.

Containers and storage Containers—Tight containers.

Benzylpenicillin Potassium for Injection

Penicillin G Potassium for Injection

注射用ベンジルペニシリンカリウム

Benzylpenicillin Potassium for Injection is a preparation for injection which is dissolved before use.

It contains not less than 93.0% and not more than 107.0% of the labeled potency of benzylpenicillin potassium ($C_{16}H_{17}KN_2O_4S$: 372.48).

Method of preparation Prepare as directed under Injections, with Benzylpenicillin Potassium.

Description Benzylpenicillin Potassium for Injection occurs as white, crystals or crystalline powder.

Identification Proceed as directed in the Identification (2) under Benzylpenicillin Potassium.

Osmotic pressure ratio Being specified separately when the drug is granted approval based on the Law.

pH <*2.54*> The pH of a solution prepared by dissolving an amount of Benzylpenicillin Potassium for Injection, equivalent to 1.0 × 10^5 Units of Benzylpenicillin Potassium, in 10 mL of water is 5.0 to 7.5.

Purity Clarity and color of solution—A solution prepared by dissolving an amount of Benzylpenicillin Potassium for Injection, equivalent to 1.0 × 10^6 Units of Benzylpenicillin Potassium, in 10 mL of water is clear. Perform the test with this solution as directed under Ultraviolet-visible Spectrophotometry <*2.24*>: the absorbance at 400 nm is not more than 0.10.

Loss on drying <*2.41*> Not more than 1.2% (3 g, in vacuum, below 0.67 kPa, 60°C, 3 hours).

Bacterial endotoxins <*4.01*> Less than 1.25 × 10^{-4} EU/Unit.

Uniformity of dosage units <*6.02*> It meets the requirement of the Mass variation test.

Foreign insoluble matter <*6.06*> Perform the test according to Method 2: it meets the requirement.

Insoluble particulate matter <*6.07*> It meets the requirement.

Sterility <*4.06*> Perform the test according to the Membrane filtration method: it meets the requirement.

Assay Weigh accurately the mass of the contents of not less than 10 containers of Benzylpenicillin Potassium for Injection. Weigh accurately an amount of a portion of the contents, equivalent to about 6 × 10^4 Units of Benzylpenicillin Potassium, dissolve in water to make exactly 20 mL, and use this solution as the sample solution. Separately, weigh accurately an amount of Benzylpenicillin Potassium RS, equivalent to about 6 × 10^4 Units, dissolve in water to make exactly 20 mL, and use this solution as the standard solution. Perform the test with exactly 5 μL each of the sample solution and standard solution as directed under Liquid Chromatography <*2.01*> according to the following conditions. Determine the peak areas, A_T and A_S, of benzylpenicillin in each solution.

$$\text{Amount (unit) of Benzylpenicillin Potassium } (C_{16}H_{17}KN_2O_4S) = M_S \times A_T/A_S$$

M_S: Amount (unit) of Benzylpenicillin Potassium RS taken

Operating conditions—

Detector: An ultraviolet absorption photometer (wavelength: 254 nm).

Column: A stainless steel column 4.6 mm in inside diameter and 25 cm in length, packed with octadecylsilanized silica gel for liquid chromatography (7 μm in particle diameter).

Column temperature: A constant temperature of about 25°C.

Mobile phase: To a mixture of diammonium hydrogen phosphate solution (33 in 5000) and acetonitril (19:6), add phosphoric acid to adjust the pH of this solution to 8.0.

Flow rate: Adjust so that the retention time of benzylpenicillin is about 7.5 minutes.

System suitability—

System performance: When the procedure is run with 5 μL of the standard solution under the above operating conditions, the number of theoretical plates and the symmetry factor of the peak of benzylpenicillin are not less than 6000 and not more than 2.0, respectively.

System repeatability: When the test is repeated 6 times with 5 μL of the standard solution under the above operating conditions, the relative standard deviation of the peak area of benzylpenicillin is not more than 1.0%.

Containers and storage Containers—Hermetic containers.

Bepotastine Besilate

ベポタスチンベシル酸塩

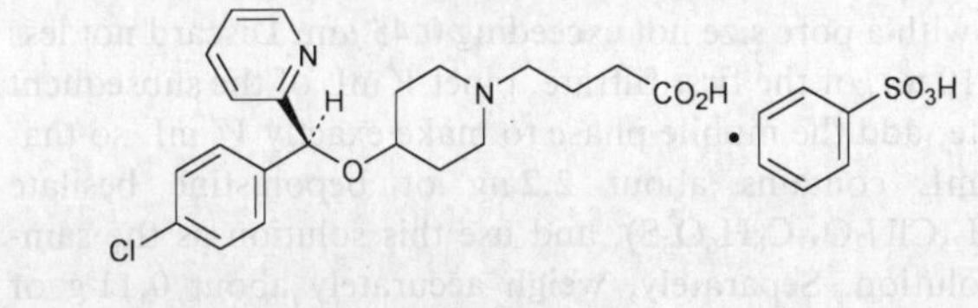

$C_{21}H_{25}ClN_2O_3.C_6H_6O_3S$: 547.06
(*S*)-4-{4-[(4-Chlorophenyl)(pyridin-2-yl)methoxy]piperidin-1-yl}butanoic acid monobenzenesulfonate
[*190786-44-8*]

Bepotastine Besilate contains not less than 99.0% and not more than 101.0% of bepotastine besilate ($C_{21}H_{25}ClN_2O_3.C_6H_6O_3S$), calculated on the anhydrous and residual solvent-free basis.

Description Bepotastine Besilate occurs as white to pale yellow-white, crystals or crystalline powder.

It is very soluble in acetic acid (100), and sparingly soluble in water and in ethanol (99.5).

The pH of a solution of 1 g of Bepotastine Besilate in 100 mL of water is about 3.8.

Identification **(1)** Determine the absorption spectrum of a solution of Bepotastine Besilate (1 in 20,000) as directed under Ultraviolet-visible Spectrophotometry 〈*2.24*〉, and compare the spectrum with the Reference Spectrum: both spectra exhibit similar intensities of absorption at the same wavelengths.

(2) Determine the infrared absorption spectrum of Bepotastine Besilate as directed in the potassium bromide disk method under Infrared Spectrophotometry 〈*2.25*〉, and compare the spectrum with the Reference Spectrum: both spectra exhibit similar intensities of absorption at the same wave numbers.

(3) Perform the test with Bepotastine Besilate as directed under Flame Coloration Test 〈*1.04*〉 (2): a green color appears.

(4) Mix well 30 mg of Bepotastine Besilate with 0.1 g of sodium nitrate and 0.1 g of anhydrous sodium carbonate, and gradually ignite. After cooling, dissolve the residue in 2 mL of dilute hydrochloric acid and 10 mL of water, filter if necessary, and add barium chloride TS: a white precipitate is produced.

Melting point 〈*2.60*〉 159–163°C

Purity **(1)** Heavy metals 〈*1.07*〉—Proceed with 2.0 g of Bepotastine Besilate according to Method 4, and perform the test. Prepare the control solution with 2.0 mL of Standard Lead Solution (not more than 10 ppm).

(2) Related substances—Dissolve 10 mg of Bepotastine Besilate in 25 mL of the mobile phase, and use this solution as the sample solution. Pipet 1 mL of the sample solution, add the mobile phase to make exactly 100 mL, and use this solution as the standard solution. Perform the test with exactly 20 μL each of the sample solution and standard solution as directed under Liquid Chromatography 〈*2.01*〉 according to the following conditions, and determine each peak area by the automatic integration method: the area of the peak, having a relative retention time of about 2.5 to bepotastine, obtained from the sample solution is not larger than the peak area of bepotastine from the standard solution, and the area of the peak other than bepotastine and the peak mentioned above from the sample solution is not larger than 1/10 times the peak area of bepotastine from the standard solution. Furthermore, the total area of the peaks other than bepotastine from the sample solution is not larger than the peak area of bepotastine from the standard solution.

Operating conditions—

Detector: An ultraviolet absorption photometer (wavelength: 220 nm).

Column: A stainless steel column 4.6 mm in inside diameter and 15 cm in length, packed with octylsilanized silica gel for liquid chromatography (5 μm in particle diameter).

Column temperature: A constant temperature of about 40°C.

Mobile phase: Dissolve 1.0 g of sodium 1-pentane sulfonate in a mixture of 0.05 mol/L potassium dihydrogen phosphate TS (pH 3.0) and acetonitrile (7:3) to make 1000 mL.

Flow rate: Adjust so that the retention time of bepotastine is about 6 minutes.

Time span of measurement: About 5 times as long as the retention time of bepotastine, beginning after the peak of benzenesulfonic acid.

System suitability—

Test for required detectability: Pipet 2.5 mL of the standard solution, and add the mobile phase to make exactly 50 mL. Confirm that the peak area of bepotastine obtained with 20 μL of this solution is equivalent to 3.5 to 6.5% of that with 20 μL of the standard solution.

System performance: When the procedure is run with 20 μL of the standard solution under the above operating conditions, the number of theoretical plates and the symmetry factor of the peak of bepotastine are not less than 3000 and 0.8 to 1.5, respectively.

System repeatability: When the test is repeated 6 times with 20 μL of the standard solution under the above operating conditions, the relative standard deviation of the peak area of bepotastine is not more than 2.0%.

(3) Enantiomer—Dissolve 5.0 mg of Bepotastine Besilate in 25 mL of the mobile phase, and use this solution as the sample solution. Pipet 1 mL of the sample solution, add the mobile phase to make exactly 200 mL, and use this solution as the standard solution. Perform the test with exactly 10 μL each of the sample solution and standard solution as directed under Liquid Chromatography 〈*2.01*〉 according to the following conditions, and determine the area of each peak by the automatic integration method: the peak area of the enantiomer having the relative retention time of about 0.9 to bepotastine obtained from the sample solution is not larger than the peak area of bepotastine from the standard solution.

Operating conditions—

Detector: An ultraviolet absorption photometer (wavelength: 225 nm).

Column: A stainless steel column 6.0 mm in inside diameter and 15 cm in length, packed with β-cyclodextrin binding silica gel for liquid chromatography (5 μm in particle diameter).

Column temperature: A constant temperature of about 40°C.

Mobile phase: A mixture of 0.02 mol/L potassium dihydrogen phosphate TS and acetonitrile (3:1).

Flow rate: Adjust so that the retention time of bepotastine is about 17 minutes.

System suitability—

System performance: When the procedure is run with 10 μL of the standard solution under the above operating con-

ditions, the number of theoretical plates and the symmetry factor of the peak of bepotastine are not less than 3000 and 0.8 to 1.5, respectively.

System repeatability: When the test is repeated 6 times with 10 μL of the standard solution under the above operating conditions, the relative standard deviation of the peak area of bepotastine is not more than 5.0%.

Water <*2.48*> Not more than 0.1% (0.3 g, coulometric titration).

Residue on ignition <*2.44*> Not more than 0.1% (1 g).

Assay Weigh accurately about 0.8 g of Bepotastine Besilate, dissolve in 60 mL of acetic acid (100), and titrate <*2.50*> with 0.1 mol/L perchloric acid VS (potentiometric titration). Perform a blank determination in the same manner, and make any necessary correction.

Each mL of 0.1 mol/L perchloric acid VS
= 54.71 mg of $C_{21}H_{25}ClN_2O_3.C_6H_6O_3S$

Containers and storage Containers—Tight containers.

Bepotastine Besilate Tablets

ベポタスチンベシル酸塩錠

Bepotastine Besilate Tablets contain not less than 95.0% and not more than 105.0% of the labeled amount of bepotastine besilate ($C_{21}H_{25}ClN_2O_3.C_6H_6O_3S$: 547.06).

Method of preparation Prepare as directed under Tablets, with Bepotastine Besilate.

Identification To an amount of powdered Bepotastine Besilate Tablets, equivalent to 2 mg of Bepotastine Besilate, add 40 mL of water, shake thoroughly, and filter. Determine the absorption spectrum of the filtrate as directed under Ultraviolet-visible Spectrophotometry <*2.24*>: it exhibits a maximum between 260 nm and 264 nm.

Uniformity of dosage units <*6.02*> Perform the test according to the following method: it meets the requirement of the Content uniformity test.

To 1 tablet of Bepotastine Besilate Tablets add exactly $V/5$ mL of the internal standard solution, then add the mobile phase to make V mL so that each mL contains about 0.4 mg of bepotastine besilate ($C_{21}H_{25}ClN_2O_3.C_6H_6O_3S$), shake vigorously for 10 minutes, and filter through a membrane filter with a pore size not exceeding 0.45 μm. Discard the first 5 mL of the filtrate, to 2 mL of the subsequent filtrate add the mobile phase to make 10 mL, and use this solution as the sample solution. Then, proceed as directed in the Assay.

Amount (mg) of bepotastine besilate
($C_{21}H_{25}ClN_2O_3.C_6H_6O_3S$)
$= M_S \times Q_T/Q_S \times V/50$

M_S: Amount (mg) of bepotastine besilate for assay taken, calculated on the anhydrous and residual solvent-free basis

Internal standard solution—A solution of ethyl parahydroxybenzoate in acetonitrile (1 in 4500).

Dissolution <*6.10*> When the test is performed at 50 revolutions per minute according to the Paddle method, using 900 mL of water as the dissolution medium, the dissolution rate in 30 minutes of Bepotastine Besilate Tablets is not less than 85%.

Start the test with 1 tablet of Bepotastine Besilate Tablets, withdraw not less than 20 mL of the medium at the specified minute after starting the test, and filter through a membrane filter with a pore size not exceeding 0.45 μm. Discard not less than 10 mL of the first filtrate, pipet V mL of the subsequent filtrate, add the mobile phase to make exactly V' mL so that each mL contains about 2.2 μg of bepotastine besilate ($C_{21}H_{25}ClN_2O_3.C_6H_6O_3S$), and use this solution as the sample solution. Separately, weigh accurately about 0.11 g of bepotastine besilate for assay (separately determine the water <*2.48*> and the residual solvent in the same manner as Bepotastine Besilate), and dissolve in water to make exactly 100 mL. Pipet 1 mL of this solution, add water to make exactly 100 mL. Pipet 2 mL of this solution, add the mobile phase to make exactly 10 mL, and use this solution as the standard solution. Perform the test with exactly 50 μL each of the sample solution and standard solution as directed under Liquid Chromatography <*2.01*> according to the following conditions, and determine the peak areas, A_T and A_S, of bepotastine in each solution.

Dissolution rate (%) with respect to the labeled amount of bepotastine besilate ($C_{21}H_{25}ClN_2O_3.C_6H_6O_3S$)
$= M_S \times A_T/A_S \times V'/V \times 1/C \times 9/5$

M_S: Amount (mg) of bepotastine besilate for assay taken, calculated on the anhydrous and residual solvent-free basis

C: Labeled amount (mg) of bepotastine besilate ($C_{21}H_{25}ClN_2O_3.C_6H_6O_3S$) in 1 tablet

Operating conditions—

Proceed as directed in the operating conditions in the Assay.

System suitability—

System performance: When the procedure is run with 50 μL of the standard solution under the above operating conditions, the number of theoretical plates and the symmetry factor of the peak of bepotastine are not less than 5000 and not more than 1.5, respectively.

System repeatability: When the test is repeated 6 times with 50 μL of the standard solution under the above operating conditions, the relative standard deviation of the peak area of bepotastine is not more than 1.5%.

Assay Weigh accurately the mass of not less than 20 tablets of Bepotastine Besilate Tablets, and powder. Weigh accurately a portion of the powder, equivalent to about 10 mg of bepotastine besilate ($C_{21}H_{25}ClN_2O_3.C_6H_6O_3S$), add exactly 5 mL of the internal standard solution, then add 20 mL of the mobile phase, shake thoroughly for 10 minutes, and filter through a membrane filter with a pore size not exceeding 0.45 μm. Discard the first 5 mL of the filtrate, to 2 mL of the subsequent filtrate add the mobile phase to make 10 mL, and use this solution as the sample solution. Separately, weigh accurately about 20 mg of bepotastine besilate for assay (separately determine the water <*2.48*> and the residual solvent in the same manner as Bepotastine Besilate), add exactly 10 mL of the internal standard solution, and dissolve in the mobile phase to make 50 mL. To 2 mL of this solution add the mobile phase to make 10 mL, and use this solution as the standard solution. Perform the test with 20 μL each of the sample solution and standard solution as directed under Liquid Chromatography <*2.01*> according to the following conditions, and calculate the ratios, Q_T and Q_S, of the peak area of bepotastine to that of the internal standard.

Amount (mg) of bepotastine besilate ($C_{21}H_{25}ClN_2O_3.C_6H_6O_3S$)
$= M_S \times Q_T/Q_S \times 1/2$

M_S: Amount (mg) of bepotastine besilate for assay taken, calculated on the anhydrous and residual solvent-free basis

Internal standard solution—A solution of ethyl parahydroxybenzoate in acetonitrile (1 in 4500).

Operating conditions—

Detector: An ultraviolet absorption photometer (wavelength: 260 nm).

Column: A stainless steel column 4.6 mm in inside diameter and 15 cm in length, packed with octylsilanized silica gel for liquid chromatography (5 μm in particle diameter).

Column temperature: A constant temperature of about 40°C.

Mobile phase: A solution of sodium 1-pentanesulfonate in a mixture of 0.05 mol/L potassium dihydrogen phosphate TS (pH 3.0) and acetonitrile (7:3) (1 in 1000).

Flow rate: Adjust so that the retention time of bepotastine is about 6 minutes.

System suitability—

System performance: When the procedure is run with 20 μL of the standard solution under the above operating conditions, bepotastine and the internal standard are eluted in this order with the resolution between these peaks being not less than 5.

System repeatability: When the test is repeated 6 times with 20 μL of the standard solution under the above operating conditions, the relative standard deviation of the ratio of the peak area of bepotastine to that of the internal standard is not more than 1.0%.

Containers and storage Containers—Tight containers.

Beraprost Sodium

ベラプロストナトリウム

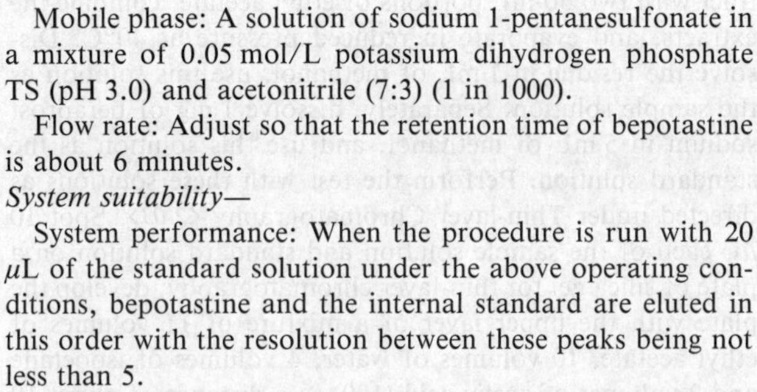

$C_{24}H_{29}NaO_5$: 420.47

Monosodium (1*RS*,2*RS*,3a*SR*,8b*SR*)-2,3,3a,8b-tetrahydro-2-hydroxy-1-[(1*E*,3*SR*,4*RS*)-3-hydroxy-4-methyloct-1-en-6-yn-1-yl]-1*H*-cyclopenta[*b*]benzofuran-5-butanoate

Monosodium (1*RS*,2*RS*,3a*SR*,8b*SR*)-2,3,3a,8b-tetrahydro-2-hydroxy-1-[(1*E*,3*SR*,4*SR*)-3-hydroxy-4-methyloct-1-en-6-yn-1-yl]-1*H*-cyclopenta[*b*]benzofuran-5-butanoate

[88475-69-8]

Beraprost Sodium, when dried, contains not less than 98.5% and not more than 101.0% of beraprost sodium ($C_{24}H_{29}NaO_5$).

Description Beraprost Sodium occurs as a white powder.

It is very soluble in methanol, and freely soluble in water and in ethanol (99.5).

It is hygroscopic.

A solution of Beraprost Sodium (1 in 200) shows no optical rotation.

Identification (1) Determine the absorption spectrum of a solution of Beraprost Sodium in methanol (3 in 50,000) as directed under Ultraviolet-visible Spectrophotometry <*2.24*>, and compare the spectrum with the Reference Spectrum: both spectra exhibit similar intensities of absorption at the same wavelengths.

(2) Determine the infrared absorption spectrum of previously dried Beraprost Sodium as directed in the potassium bromide disk method under Infrared Spectrophotometry <*2.25*>, and compare the spectrum with the Reference Spectrum: both spectra exhibit similar intensities of absorption at the same wave numbers.

(3) A solution of Beraprost Sodium in methanol (1 in 1000) responds to Qualitative Tests <*1.09*> (1) for sodium salt.

Purity Related substances—Dissolve 20 mg of Beraprost Sodium in 2 mL of methanol, and use this solution as the sample solution. Perform the test with 15 μL of the sample solution as directed under Liquid Chromatography <*2.01*> according to the following conditions. Determine each peak area by the automatic integration method, and calculate their amounts by the area percentage method: the amount of the peak having the relative retention time of about 0.5 to the second eluting principal peak of beraprost and the two adjacent peaks at the relative retention time of about 1.7 and another two adjacent peaks at the relative retention time of about 2.0 are not more than 0.2%, respectively, the amount of the peak at the relative retention time of about 1.2 is not more than 0.3%, the amount of the peak, other than the two peaks of beraprost and the peaks mentioned above, is less than 0.1%, and the total amount of the peaks, other than the two peaks of beraprost, is not more than 1.5%.

Operating conditions—

Detector: An ultraviolet absorption photometer (wavelength: 285 nm).

Column: A stainless steel column 4 mm in inside diameter and 25 cm in length, packed with octadecylsilanized silica gel for liquid chromatography (4 μm in particle diameter).

Column temperature: A constant temperature of about 35°C.

Mobile phase A: A mixture of water, acetonitrile, methanol and acetic acid (100) (640:330:30:1).

Mobile phase B: A mixture of acetonitrile, water and acetic acid (100) (900:100:1).

Flowing of mobile phase: Control the gradient by mixing the mobile phases A and B as directed in the following table.

Time after injection of sample (min)	Mobile phase A (vol%)	Mobile phase B (vol%)
0 – 30	100	0
30 – 45	100 → 56	0 → 44
45 – 60	56	44
60 – 70	56 → 0	44 → 100
70 – 80	0	100

Flow rate: Adjust so that the retention time of the second peak of beraprost is about 23 minutes.

Time span of measurement: For 80 minutes after injection, beginning after the solvent peak.

System suitability—

Test for required detectability: To 1 mL of the sample solution add methanol to make 20 mL. To 1 mL of this solution add methanol to make 20 mL, and use this solution as the solution for system suitability test. Pipet 2 mL of the solution for system suitability test, and add methanol to make exactly 10 mL. Confirm that the total area of the two peaks of beraprost obtained with 15 μL of this solution is equivalent to 14 to 26% of that with 15 μL of the solution for system suitability test.

System performance: When the procedure is run with 15 μL of the solution for system suitability test under the above operating conditions, the resolution between the two peaks of beraprost is not less than 1.5.

System repeatability: When the test is repeated 6 times with 15 μL of the solution for system suitability test under the above operating conditions, the relative standard deviation of the total area of the two peaks of beraprost is not more than 2.0%.

Loss on drying ⟨*2.41*⟩ Not more than 3.0% (0.5 g, reduced pressure not exceeding 0.67 kPa, silica gel, 60°C, 5 hours).

Isomer ratio Dissolve 10 mg of Beraprost Sodium in 5 mL of methanol, and use this solution as the sample solution. Perform the test with 15 μL of the sample solution as directed under Liquid Chromatography ⟨*2.01*⟩ according to the following conditions, and determine the areas, A_a of the peak which appears at the retention time about 25 minutes, and A_b of the peak which appears at about 27 minutes: A_b/A_a is between 0.90 and 1.10.

Operating conditions—

Detector: An ultraviolet absorption photometer (wavelength: 285 nm).

Column: A stainless steel column 6 mm in inside diameter and 15 cm in length, packed with octadecylsilanized silica gel for liquid chromatography (5 μm in particle diameter).

Column temperature: A constant temperature of about 40°C.

Mobile phase: A mixture of methanol, water and acetic acid (100) (600:400:1).

Flow rate: Adjust so that the retention time of the second eluting peak of beraprost is about 27 minutes.

System suitability—

System performance: When the procedure is run with 15 μL of the sample solution under the above operating conditions, the resolution between the two peaks of beraprost is not less than 1.2.

System repeatability: When the test is repeated 6 times with 15 μL of the sample solution under the above operating conditions, the relative standard deviation of the total area of the two peak of beraprost is not more than 2.0%.

Assay Weigh accurately about 0.1 g of Beraprost Sodium, previously dried, dissolve in 30 mL of diluted ethanol with freshly boiled and cooled water (7 in 10), add exactly 2 mL of 0.2 mol/L hydrochloric acid TS, and titrate ⟨*2.50*⟩ with 0.025 mol/L sodium hydroxide-ethanol VS from the first equivalence point to the second equivalence point (potentiometric titration).

Each mL of 0.025 mol/L sodium hydroxide-ethanol VS
= 10.51 mg of $C_{24}H_{29}NaO_5$

Containers and storage Containers—Tight containers.
Storage—Light-resistant.

Beraprost Sodium Tablets

ベラプロストナトリウム錠

Beraprost Sodium Tablets contain not less than 95.0% and not more than 105.0% of the labeled amount of beraprost sodium ($C_{24}H_{29}NaO_5$: 420.47).

Method of preparation Prepare as directed under Tablets, with Beraprost Sodium.

Identification Powder Beraprost Sodium Tablets. To a portion of the powder, equivalent to 0.2 mg of Beraprost Sodium, add 10 mL of water, shake, and filter through a membrane filter with a pore size not exceeding 0.45 μm. To the filtrate add 1 mL of 0.1 mol/L hydrochloric acid TS, extract with two 50-mL portions of ethyl acetate, combine the extracts, and evaporate in reduced pressure at 40°C. Dissolve the residue in 1 mL of methanol, use this solution as the sample solution. Separately, dissolve 1 mg of beraprost sodium in 5 mL of methanol, and use this solution as the standard solution. Perform the test with these solutions as directed under Thin-layer Chromatography ⟨*2.03*⟩. Spot 10 μL each of the sample solution and standard solution on a plate of silica gel for thin-layer chromatography, develop the plate with the upper layer of a mixture of 11 volumes of ethyl acetate, 10 volumes of water, 4 volumes of isooctane and 2 volumes of acetic acid (100) to a distance of about 10 cm, air-dry the plate, and heat at 120°C for 30 minutes. After cooling, spray evenly a mixture of ethanol (99.5), water, sulfuric acid and 4-methoxybenzaldehide (17:2:1:1) on the plate, and heat the plate at 120°C for 3 minutes: the principal spot obtained from the sample solution and the spot from the standard solution show the same *R*f value.

Uniformity of dosage units ⟨*6.02*⟩ Perform the test according to the following method: it meets the requirement of the Content uniformity test.

To 1 tablet of Beraprost Sodium Tablets add exactly *V* mL of the internal standard solution so that each mL contains about 2 μg of beraprost sodium ($C_{24}H_{29}NaO_5$), shake at 30°C for 30 minutes, filter through a membrane filter with a pore size not exceeding 0.45 μm, and use the filtrate as the sample solution. Then, proceed as directed in the Assay.

Amount (mg) of beraprost sodium ($C_{24}H_{29}NaO_5$)
$= M_S \times Q_T/Q_S \times V/10,000$

M_S: Amount (mg) of beraprost sodium for assay taken

Internal standard solution—A mixture of water and a solution of 4-isopropylphenol in methanol (1 in 250,000) (1:1).

Dissolution ⟨*6.10*⟩ When the test is performed at 50 revolutions per minute according to the Paddle method, using 900 mL of water as the dissolution medium, the dissolution rate in 30 minutes of Beraprost Sodium Tablets is not less than 85%.

Start the test with 1 tablet of Beraprost Sodium Tablets, withdraw not less than 20 mL of the medium at the specified minute after starting the test, and filter through a membrane filter with a pore size not exceeding 0.45 μm. Discard not less than 10 mL of the first filtrate, pipet *V* mL of the subsequent filtrate, add water to make exactly *V′* mL so that each mL contains about 22 ng of beraprost sodium ($C_{24}H_{29}NaO_5$), and use this solution as the sample solution. Separately, weigh accurately about 20 mg of beraprost sodium for assay, previously dried in reduced pressure not exceeding 0.67 kPa at 60°C for 5 hours using silica gel as a desiccant, and dissolve in methanol to make exactly 100 mL. Pipet 2 mL of this solution, and add water to make exactly 200 mL. Pipet 2 mL of this solution, add water to make exactly 200 mL, and use this solution as the standard solution. Perform the test with exactly 200 μL each of the sample solution and standard solution as directed under Liquid Chromatography <*2.01*> according to the following conditions, and determine the total areas, A_T and A_S, of the two peaks of beraprost in each solution.

Dissolution rate (%) with respect to the labeled amount of beraprost sodium ($C_{24}H_{29}NaO_5$)
$= M_S \times A_T/A_S \times V'/V \times 1/C \times 9/100$

M_S: Amount (mg) of beraprost sodium for assay taken
C: Labeled amount (mg) of beraprost sodium ($C_{24}H_{29}NaO_5$) in 1 tablet

Operating conditions—

Detector, column temperature, and mobile phase: Proceed as directed in the operating conditions in the Assay.

Column: A stainless steel column 4.6 mm in inside diameter and 15 cm in length, packed with octadecylsilanized silica gel for liquid chromatography (5 μm in particle diameter).

Flow rate: Adjust so that the retention time of the first eluting peak of beraprost is about 10 minutes.

System suitability—

System performance: When the procedure is run with 200 μL of the standard solution under the above operating conditions, the resolution between the two peaks of beraprost is not less than 1.2.

System repeatability: When the test is repeated 6 times with 200 μL of the standard solution under the above operating conditions, the relative standard deviation of the total area of the two peaks of beraprost is not more than 2.0%.

Assay Weigh accurately the mass of not less than 20 Beraprost Sodium Tablets, and powder. Weigh accurately a portion of the powder, equivalent to about 40 μg of beraprost sodium ($C_{24}H_{29}NaO_5$), add exactly 20 mL of the internal standard solution, shake at 30°C for 30 minutes, filter through a membrane filter with a pore size not exceeding 0.45 μm, and use the filtrate as the sample solution. Separately, weigh accurately about 20 mg of beraprost sodium for assay, previously dried in reduced pressure not exceeding 0.67 kPa at 60°C for 5 hours using silica gel as a desiccant, and dissolve in methanol to make exactly 100 mL. Pipet 10 mL of this solution, and add methanol to make exactly 200 mL. Pipet 4 mL of this solution, and evaporate under reduced pressure at 40°C. To the residue add exactly 20 mL of the internal standard solution, and use this solution as the standard solution. Perform the test with 20 μL each of the sample solution and standard solution as directed under Liquid Chromatography <*2.01*> according to the following conditions, and calculate the ratios, Q_T and Q_S, of the total area of the two peaks of beraprost to the peak area of the internal standard.

Amount (mg) of beraprost sodium ($C_{24}H_{29}NaO_5$)
$= M_S \times Q_T/Q_S \times 1/500$

M_S: Amount (mg) of beraprost sodium for assay taken

Internal standard solution—A mixture of water and a solution of 4-isopropylphenol in methanol (1 in 250,000) (1:1).

Operating conditions—

Detector: A fluorophotometer (excitation wavelength: 285 nm, fluorescence wavelength: 614 nm).

Column: A stainless steel column 6 mm in inside diameter and 15 cm in length, packed with octadecylsilanized silica gel for liquid chromatography (5 μm in particle diameter).

Column temperature: A constant temperature of about 40°C.

Mobile phase: A mixture of methanol, water and acetic acid (100) (650:350:1).

Flow rate: Adjust so that the retention time of the first eluting peak of beraprost is about 15 minutes.

System suitability—

System performance: When the procedure is run with 20 μL of the standard solution under the above operating conditions, the internal standard and beraprost are eluted in this order and the resolution between the internal standard peak and the first eluting peak of beraprost is not less than 11, and the resolution between the two peaks of beraprost is not less than 1.5.

System repeatability: When the test is repeated 6 times with 20 μL of the standard solution under the above operating conditions, the relative standard deviation of the ratio of the total area of the two peaks of beraprost to the peak area of the internal standard is not more than 2.0%.

Containers and storage Containers—Well-closed containers.

Berberine Chloride Hydrate

ベルベリン塩化物水和物

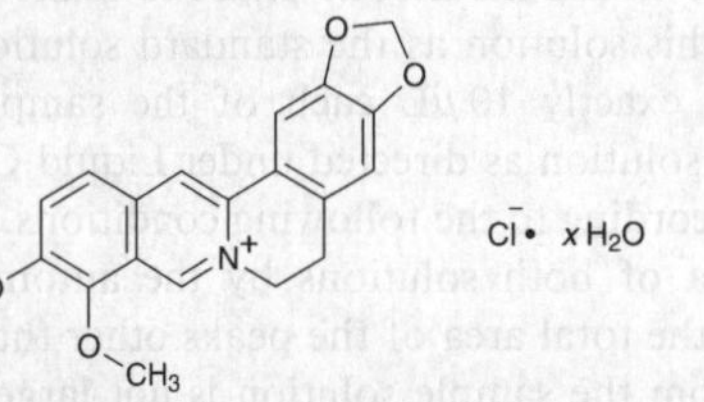

$Cl^- \cdot xH_2O$ H_3C O N^+ CH_3

$C_{20}H_{18}ClNO_4.xH_2O$
9,10-Dimethoxy-5,6-dihydro[1,3]dioxolo[4,5-*g*]isoquino[3,2-*a*]isoquinolin-7-ium chloride hydrate
[*633-65-8*, anhydride]

Berberine Chloride Hydrate contains not less than 95.0% and not more than 102.0% of berberine chloride ($C_{20}H_{18}ClNO_4$: 371.81), calculated on the anhydrous basis.

Description Berberine Chloride Hydrate occurs as yellow, crystals or crystalline powder. It is odorless or has a faint, characteristic odor. It has a very bitter taste.

It is sparingly soluble in methanol, slightly soluble in ethanol (95), and very slightly soluble in water.

Identification **(1)** Determine the absorption spectrum of a solution of Berberine Chloride Hydrate (1 in 100,000) as directed under Ultraviolet-visible Spectrophotometry <*2.24*>, and compare the spectrum with the Reference Spectrum or the spectrum of a solution of Berberine Chloride RS prepared in the same manner as the sample solution: both spectra exhibit similar intensities of absorption at the same wavelengths.

(2) Determine the infrared absorption spectrum of Berberine Chloride Hydrate as directed in the potassium bromide disk method under Infrared Spectrophotometry <*2.25*>, and compare the spectrum with the Reference Spectrum or the spectrum of Berberine Chloride RS: both spectra exhibit similar intensities of absorption at the same wave numbers.

(3) Dissolve 0.1 g of Berberine Chloride Hydrate in 20

mL of water by warming, add 0.5 mL of nitric acid, cool, and filter after allowing to stand for 10 minutes. To 3 mL of the filtrate add 1 mL of silver nitrate TS, and collect the produced precipitate: the precipitate does not dissolve in dilute nitric acid, but it dissolves in an excess amount of ammonia TS.

Purity **(1)** Acidity—Shake thoroughly 0.10 g of Berberine Chloride Hydrate with 30 mL of water, and filter. To the filtrate add 2 drops of phenolphthalein TS and 0.10 mL of 0.1 mol/L sodium hydroxide VS: the yellow color changes to an orange to red color.

(2) Sulfate *<1.14>*—Shake 1.0 g of Berberine Chloride Hydrate with 48 mL of water and 2 mL of dilute hydrochloric acid for 1 minute, and filter. Discard the first 5 mL of the filtrate, take the subsequent 25 mL of the filtrate, add water to make 50 mL, and perform the test using this solution as the test solution. Prepare the control solution with 0.50 mL of 0.005 mol/L sulfuric acid VS, 1 mL of dilute hydrochloric acid, 5 to 10 drops of bromophenol blue TS and water to make 50 mL (not more than 0.048%).

(3) Heavy metals *<1.07>*—Proceed with 1.0 g of Berberine Chloride Hydrate according to Method 2, and perform the test. Prepare the control solution with 3.0 mL of Standard Lead Solution (not more than 30 ppm).

(4) Related substances—Dissolve 10 mg of Berberine Chloride Hydrate in 100 mL of the mobile phase, and use this solution as the sample solution. Pipet 4 mL of the sample solution, add the mobile phase to make exactly 100 mL, and use this solution as the standard solution. Perform the test with exactly 10 μL each of the sample solution and standard solution as directed under Liquid Chromatography *<2.01>* according to the following conditions. Determine each peak area of both solutions by the automatic integration method: the total area of the peaks other than berberine obtained from the sample solution is not larger than the peak area of berberine from the standard solution.

Operating conditions—

Detector, column, column temperature, mobile phase, flow rate, and selection of column: Proceed as directed in the operating conditions in the Assay.

Time span of measurement: About 2 times as long as the retention time of berberine, beginning after the solvent peak.

Detection sensitivity: Adjust so that the peak height of berberine obtained from 10 μL of the standard solution is about 10% of the full scale.

Water *<2.48>* 8 – 12% (0.1 g, volumetric titration, direct titration).

Residue on ignition *<2.44>* Not more than 0.1% (1 g).

Assay Weigh accurately about 10 mg of Berberine Chloride Hydrate, dissolve in the mobile phase to make exactly 100 mL, and use this solution as the sample solution. Separately, weigh accurately about 10 mg of Berberine Chloride RS (separately, determine the water content *<2.48>* in the same manner as Berberine Chloride Hydrate), and dissolve in the mobile phase to make exactly 100 mL, and use this solution as the standard solution. Perform the test with exactly 10 μL each of the sample solution and standard solution as directed under Liquid Chromatography *<2.01>* according to the following conditions. Determine the peak areas, A_T and A_S of berberine in each solution.

Amount (mg) of berberine chloride ($C_{20}H_{18}ClNO_4$)
$= M_S \times A_T/A_S$

M_S: Amount (mg) of Berberine Chloride RS taken, calculated on the anhydrous basis

Operating conditions—

Detector: An ultraviolet absorption photometer (wavelength: 345 nm).

Column: A stainless steel column about 4 mm in inside diameter and about 25 cm in length, packed with octadecylsilanized silica gel for liquid chromatography (5 μm in particle diameter).

Column temperature: A constant temperature of about 40°C.

Mobile phase: Dissolve 3.4 g of monobasic potassium phosphate and 1.7 g of sodium lauryl sulfate in 1000 mL of a mixture of water and acetonitrile (1:1).

Flow rate: Adjust so that the retention time of berberine is about 10 minutes.

Selection of column: Dissolve each 1 mg of berberine chloride and palmatin chloride in the mobile phase to make 10 mL. Proceed with 10 μL of this solution under the above operating conditions, and calculate the resolution. Use a column giving elution of palmatin and berberine in this order with the resolution between these peaks being not less than 1.5.

System repeatability: When the test is repeated 5 times with the standard solution under the above operating conditions, the relative standard deviation of the peak areas of berberine is not more than 1.5%.

Containers and storage Containers—Tight containers.

Storage—Light-resistant.

Berberine Tannate

タンニン酸ベルベリン

Berberine Tannate is a compound of berberine and tannic acid.

It contains not less than 27.0% and not more than 33.0% of berberine ($C_{20}H_{19}NO_5$: 353.37), calculated on the anhydrous basis.

Description Berberine Tannate occurs as a yellow to light yellow-brown powder. It is odorless or has a faint, characteristic odor, and is tasteless.

It is practically insoluble in water, in acetonitrile, in methanol and in ethanol (95).

Identification **(1)** To 0.1 g of Berberine Tannate add 10 mL of ethanol (95), and heat in a water bath for 3 minutes with shaking. Cool, filter, and to 5 mL of the filtrate add 1 drop of iron (III) chloride TS: a blue-green color is produced, and on allowing to stand, a bluish black precipitate is formed.

(2) Dissolve 0.01 g of Berberine Tannate in 10 mL of methanol and 0.4 mL of 1 mol/L hydrochloric acid TS, and add water to make 200 mL. To 8 mL of the solution add water to make 25 mL. Determine the absorption spectrum of the solution as directed under Ultraviolet-visible Spectrophotometry *<2.24>*, and compare the spectrum with the Reference Spectrum: both spectra exhibit similar intensities of absorption at the same wavelengths.

(3) Determine the infrared absorption spectrum of Berberine Tannate as directed in the potassium bromide disk method under Infrared Spectrophotometry *<2.25>*, and compare the spectrum with the Reference Spectrum: both spectra exhibit similar intensities of absorption at the same wave numbers.

Purity **(1)** Acidity—To 0.10 g of Berberine Tannate add

30 mL of water, and filter after shaking well. To the filtrate add 2 drops of phenolphthalein TS and 0.10 mL of 0.1 mol/L sodium hydroxide VS: the color of the solution changes from yellow to orange to red.

(2) Chloride <*1.03*>—Shake 1.0 g of Berberine Tannate with 38 mL of water and 12 mL of dilute nitric acid for 5 minutes, and filter. Discard the first 5 mL of the filtrate, to 25 mL of the subsequent filtrate add water to make 50 mL, and perform the test using this solution as the test solution. Prepare the control solution with 0.50 mL of 0.01 mol/L hydrochloric acid VS by adding 6 mL of dilute nitric acid, 10 to 15 drops of bromophenol blue TS and water to make 50 mL (not more than 0.035%).

(3) Sulfate <*1.14*>—Shake 1.0 g of Berberine Tannate with 48 mL of water and 2 mL of dilute hydrochloric acid for 1 minute, and filter. Discard the first 5 mL of the filtrate, take the subsequent 25 mL of the filtrate, add water to make 50 mL, and perform the test using this solution as the test solution. Prepare the control solution with 0.50 mL of 0.005 mol/L sulfuric acid VS, 1 mL of dilute hydrochloric acid, 5 to 10 drops of bromophenol blue TS and water to make 50 mL (not more than 0.048%).

(4) Heavy metals <*1.07*>—Proceed with 1.0 g of Berberine Tannate according to Method 2, and perform the test. Prepare the control solution with 3.0 mL of Standard Lead Solution (not more than 30 ppm).

(5) Related substances—Dissolve 10 mg of Berberine Tannate in 100 mL of the mobile phase, and use this solution as the sample solution. Pipet 4 mL of the sample solution, add the mobile phase to make exactly 100 mL, and use this solution as the standard solution. Perform the test with exactly 10 μL each of the sample solution and standard solution as directed under Liquid Chromatography <*2.01*> according to the following conditions. Determine each peak area of both solutions by the automatic integration method: the total area of the peaks other than berberine obtained from the sample solution is not larger than the peak area of berberine from the standard solution.

Operating conditions—

Detector, column, column temperature, mobile phase, and flow rate: Proceed as directed in the operating conditions in the Assay.

Time span of measurement: About 2 times as long as the retention time of berberine, beginning after the solvent peak.

System suitability—

System performance: Proceed as directed in the system suitability in the Assay.

Test for required detectability: To exactly 2 mL of the standard solution add the mobile phase to make exactly 20 mL. Confirm that the peak area of berberine obtained with 10 μL of this solution is equivalent to 7 to 13% of that with 10 μL of the standard solution.

System repeatability: When the test is repeated 6 times with 10 μL of the standard solution under the above operating conditions, the relative standard deviation of the peak area of berberine is not more than 3.0%.

Water <*2.48*> Not more than 6.0% (0.7 g, volumetric titration, direct titration).

Residue on ignition <*2.44*> Not more than 1.0% (1 g).

Assay Weigh accurately about 30 mg of Berberine Tannate, dissolve in the mobile phase to make exactly 100 mL, and use this solution as the sample solution. Separately, weigh accurately about 10 mg of Berberine Chloride RS (separately, determine the water <*2.48*> in the same manner as Berberine Chloride Hydrate), dissolve in the mobile phase to make exactly 100 mL, and use this solution as the standard solution. Perform the test with exactly 10 μL each of the sample solution and standard solution as directed under Liquid Chromatography <*2.01*> according to the following conditions. Determine the peak areas, A_T and A_S, of berberine in each solution.

$$\text{Amount (mg) of berberine } (C_{20}H_{19}NO_5) = M_S \times A_T/A_S \times 0.950$$

M_S: Amount (mg) of Berberine Chloride RS taken, calculated on the anhydrous basis

Operating conditions—

Detector: An ultraviolet absorption photometer (wavelength: 345 nm).

Column: A stainless steel column 4.6 mm in inside diameter and 25 cm in length, packed with octadecylsilanized silica gel for liquid chromatography (5 μm in particle diameter).

Column temperature: A constant temperature of about 40°C.

Mobile phase: Dissolve 3.4 g of potassium dihydrogen phosphate and 1.7 g of sodium lauryl sulfate in 1000 mL of a mixture of water and acetonitrile (1:1).

Flow rate: Adjust so that the retention time of berberine is about 10 minutes.

System suitability—

System performance: Dissolve 1 mg each of berberine chloride and palmatin chloride in the mobile phase to make 10 mL. When the procedure is run with 10 μL of this solution under the above operating conditions, palmatin and berberine are eluted in this order with the resolution between these peaks being not less than 1.5.

System repeatability: When the test is repeated 6 times with 10 μL of the standard solution under the above operating conditions, the relative standard deviation of the peak area of berberine is not more than 1.5%.

Containers and storage Containers—Tight containers.

Storage—Light-resistant.

Betahistine Mesilate

ベタヒスチンメシル酸塩

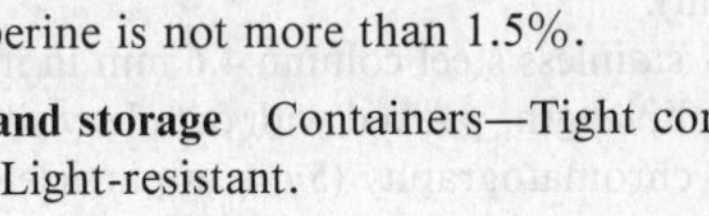

$C_8H_{12}N_2.2CH_4O_3S$: 328.41

N-Methyl-2-pyridin-2-ylethylamine dimethanesulfonate

[*5638-76-6*, Betahistine]

Betahistine Mesilate, when dried, contains not less than 98.0% and not more than 101.0% of betahistine mesilate ($C_8H_{12}N_2.2CH_4O_3S$).

Description Betahistine Mesilate occurs as white, crystals or crystalline powder.

It is very soluble in water, freely soluble in acetic acid (100), and sparingly soluble in ethanol (99.5).

It dissolves in dilute hydrochloric acid.

It is hygroscopic.

Identification **(1)** Determine the absorption spectrum of a solution of Betahistine Mesilate in 0.1 mol/L hydrochloric acid (1 in 50,000) as directed under Ultraviolet-visible Spectrophotometry <*2.24*>, and compare the spectrum with the

Reference Spectrum: both spectra exhibit similar intensities of absorption at the same wavelengths.

(2) Determine the infrared absorption spectrum of Betahistine Mesilate, previously dried, as directed in the potassium bromide disk method under Infrared Spectrophotometry *<2.25>*, and compare the spectrum with the Reference Spectrum: both spectra exhibit similar intensities of absorption at the same wave numbers.

(3) A 30 mg portion of Betahistine Mesilate responds to Qualitative Tests *<1.09>* (2) for mesilate.

Melting point *<2.60>* 110 – 114°C (after drying).

Purity **(1)** Heavy metals *<1.07>*—Proceed with 1.0 g of Betahistine Mesilate according to Method 4, and perform the test. Prepare the control solution with 2.0 mL of Standard Lead Solution (not more than 20 ppm).

(2) Related substances—Dissolve 50 mg of Betahistine Mesilate in 10 mL of a mixture of water and acetonitrile (63:37), and use this solution as the sample solution. Pipet 1 mL of the sample solution, add the mixture of water and acetonitrile (63:37) to make exactly 100 mL, and use this solution as the standard solution. Perform the test with exactly 20 μL each of the sample solution and standard solution as directed under Liquid Chromatography *<2.01>* according to the following conditions, and determine each peak area by the automatic integration method: the area of the peak other than betahistine obtained from the sample solution is not larger than 1/10 times the peak area of betahistine from the standard solution, and the total area of the peaks other than the peak of betahistine from the sample solution is not larger than 1/2 times the peak area of betahistine from the standard solution.

Operating conditions—

Detector: An ultraviolet absorption photometer (wavelength: 261 nm).

Column: A stainless steel column 4.6 mm in inside diameter and 15 cm in length, packed with octadecylsilanized silica gel for liquid chromatography (5 μm in particle diameter).

Column temperature: A constant temperature of about 35°C.

Mobile phase: To 5 mL of diethylamine and 20 mL of acetic acid (100) add water to make 1000 mL. Dissolve 2.3 g of sodium lauryl sulfate in 630 mL of this solution, and add 370 mL of acetonitrile.

Flow rate: Adjust so that the retention time of betahistine is about 5 minutes.

Time span of measurement: About 3 times as long as the retention time of betahistine, beginning after the solvent peak.

System suitability—

Test for required detectability: To exactly 5 mL of the standard solution add the mixture of water and acetonitrile (63:37) to make exactly 50 mL. Confirm that the peak area of betahistine obtained with 20 μL of this solution is equivalent to 7 to 13% of that with 20 μL of the standard solution.

System performance: Dissolve 10 mg of betahistine mesilate and 10 mg of 2-vinylpyridine in 50 mL of the mixture of water and acetonitrile (63:37). To 2 mL of this solution add the mixture of water and acetonitrile (63:37) to make 50 mL. When the procedure is run with 20 μL of this solution under the above operating conditions, 2-vinylpyridine and betahistine are eluted in this order with the resolution between these peaks being not less than 5.

System repeatability: When the test is repeated 6 times with 20 μL of the standard solution under the above operating conditions, the relative standard deviation of the peak area of betahistine is not more than 1.0%

Loss on drying *<2.41>* Not more than 1.0% (1 g, in vacuum, phosphorus (V) oxide, 70°C, 24 hours).

Residue on ignition *<2.44>* Not more than 0.1% (1 g).

Assay Weigh accurately about 0.2 g of Betahistine Mesilate, previously dried, dissolve in 1 mL of acetic acid (100), add 50 mL of acetic anhydride, and titrate *<2.50>* with 0.1 mol/L perchloric acid VS (potentiometric titration). Perform a blank determination in the same manner, and make any necessary correction.

Each mL of 0.1 mol/L perchloric acid VS
= 16.42 mg of $C_8H_{12}N_2.2CH_4O_3S$

Containers and storage Containers—Tight containers.

Betahistine Mesilate Tablets

ベタヒスチンメシル酸塩錠

Betahistine Mesilate Tablets contain not less than 93.0% and not more than 107.0% of the labeled amount of betahistine mesilate ($C_8H_{12}N_2.2CH_4O_3S$: 328.41).

Method of preparation Prepare as directed under Tablets, with Betahistine Mesilate.

Identification To 5 mL of the sample solution obtained in the Assay add 0.1 mol/L hydrochloric acid TS to make 100 mL, and determine the absorption spectrum of this solution as directed under Ultraviolet-visible Spectrophotometry *<2.24>*: it exhibits a maximum between 259 nm and 263 nm.

Purity Related substances—Powder not less than 20 Betahistine Mesilate Tablets. To a portion of the powder, equivalent to about 50 mg of Betahistine Mesilate, add 10 mL of a mixture of water and acetonitrile (63:37), agitate for 10 minutes by sonicating, centrifuge, and use the supernatant liquid as the sample solution. Pipet 1 mL of the sample solution, add the mixture of water and acetonitrile (63:37) to make exactly 100 mL, and use this solution as the standard solution. Perform the test with exactly 20 μL each of the sample solution and standard solution as directed under Liquid Chromatography *<2.01>* according to the following conditions, and determine each peak area by the automatic integration method: the area of the peak, having the relative retention time of about 1.9 to betahistine obtained from the sample solution, is not larger than 3/5 times the peak area of betahistine from the standard solution, and the total area of the peaks other than betahistine from the sample solution is not larger than the peak area of betahistine from the standard solution.

Operating conditions—

Detector, column, column temperature, mobile phase, and flow rate: Proceed as directed in the operating conditions in the Assay.

Time span of measurement: About 8 times as long as the retention time of betahistine, beginning after the solvent peak.

System suitability—

Test for required detectability: To exactly 5 mL of the standard solution add the mixture of water and acetonitrile (63:37) to make exactly 50 mL. Confirm that the peak area of betahistine obtained with 20 μL of this solution is equivalent to 7 to 13% of that with 20 μL of the standard solution.

System performance: Dissolve 10 mg of betahistine mesilate and 10 mg of 2-vinylpyridine in 50 mL of the mixture of water and acetonitrile (63:37). To 2 mL of this solution add the mixture of water and acetonitrile (63:37) to make 50 mL. When the procedure is run with 20 μL of this solution under the above operating conditions, 2-vinylpyridine and betahistine are eluted in this order with the resolution between these peaks being not less than 5.

System repeatability: When the test is repeated 6 times with 20 μL of the standard solution under the above operating conditions, the relative standard deviation of the peak area of betahistine is not more than 1.0%.

Uniformity of dosage units <*6.02*> Perform the test according to the following method: it meets the requirement of the Content uniformity test.

To 1 tablet of Betahistine Mesilate Tablets add exactly *V* mL of 0.1 mol/L hydrochloric acid TS so that each mL contains about 0.4 mg of betahistine mesilate ($C_8H_{12}N_2.2CH_4O_3S$), agitate for about 10 minutes by sonicating to disintegrate the tablet, then centrifuge, and use the supernatant liquid as the sample solution. Proceed as directed in the Assay.

$$\text{Amount (mg) of betahistine mesilate } (C_8H_{12}N_2.2CH_4O_3S) = M_S \times A_T/A_S \times V/250$$

M_S: Amount (mg) of betahistine mesilate for assay taken

Dissolution <*6.10*> When the test is performed at 50 revolutions per minute according to the Paddle method, using 900 mL of water as the dissolution medium, the dissolution rate in 15 minutes of Betahistine Mesilate Tablets is not less than 85%.

Start the test with 1 tablet of Betahistine Mesilate Tablets, withdraw not less than 20 mL of the medium at the specified minute after starting the test, and filter through a membrane filter with a pore size not exceeding 0.45 μm. Discard not less than 10 mL of the first filtrate, pipet *V* mL of the subsequent filtrate, add water to make exactly *V′* mL so that each mL contains about 6.7 μg of betahistine mesilate ($C_8H_{12}N_2.2CH_4O_3S$), and use this solution as the sample solution. Separately, weigh accurately about 17 mg of betahistine mesilate for assay, previously dried under reduced pressure with phosphorous (V) oxide at 70°C for 24 hours, and dissolve in water to make exactly 100 mL. Pipet 4 mL of this solution, add water to make exactly 100 mL, and use this solution as the standard solution. Perform the test with exactly 20 μL each of the sample solution and standard solution as directed under Liquid Chromatography <*2.01*> according to the following conditions, and determine the peak areas, A_T and A_S, of betahistine in each solution.

$$\text{Dissolution rate (\%) with respect to the labeled amount of betahistine mesilate } (C_8H_{12}N_2.2CH_4O_3S) = M_S \times A_T/A_S \times V'/V \times 1/C \times 36$$

M_S: Amount (mg) of betahistine mesilate for assay taken
C: Labeled amount (mg) of betahistine mesilate ($C_8H_{12}N_2.2CH_4O_3S$) in 1 tablet

Operating conditions—

Proceed as directed in the operating conditions in the Assay.

System suitability—

System performance: When the procedure is run with 20 μL of the standard solution under the above operating conditions, the number of theoretical plates and the symmetry factor of the peak of betahistine are not less than 2000 and not more than 1.5, respectively.

System repeatability: When the test is repeated 6 times with 20 μL of the standard solution under the above operating conditions, the relative standard deviation of the peak area of betahistine is not more than 2.0%.

Assay Weigh accurately the mass of not less than 20 Betahistine Mesilate Tablets, and powder. Weigh accurately a portion of the powder, equivalent to about 20 mg of betahistine mesilate ($C_8H_{12}N_2.2CH_4O_3S$), add 40 mL of 0.1 mol/L hydrochloric acid TS, agitate for 10 minutes by sonicating, and add 0.1 mol/L hydrochloric acid TS to make exactly 50 mL. Centrifuge, and use the supernatant liquid as the sample solution. Separately, weigh accurately about 0.1 g of betahistine mesilate for assay, previously dried under reduced pressure with phosphorous (V) oxide at 70°C for 24 hours, and dissolve in 0.1 mol/L hydrochloric acid TS to make exactly 50 mL. Pipet 10 mL of this solution, add 0.1 mol/L hydrochloric acid TS to make exactly 50 mL, and use this solution as the standard solution. Perform the test with exactly 5 μL each of the sample solution and standard solution as directed under Liquid Chromatography <*2.01*>, according to the following conditions, and determine the peak areas, A_T and A_S, of betahistine in each solution.

$$\text{Amount (mg) of betahistine mesilate } (C_8H_{12}N_2.2CH_4O_3S) = M_S \times A_T/A_S \times 1/5$$

M_S: Amount (mg) of betahistine mesilate for assay taken

Operating conditions—

Detector: An ultraviolet absorption photometer (wavelength: 261 nm).

Column: A stainless steel column 4.6 mm in inside diameter and 15 cm in length, packed with octadecylsilanized silica gel for liquid chromatography (5 μm in particle diameter).

Column temperature: A constant temperature of about 35°C.

Mobile phase: To 5 mL of diethylamine and 20 mL of acetic acid (100) add water to make 1000 mL. In 630 mL of this solution dissolve 2.3 g of sodium lauryl sulfate, and add 370 mL of acetonitrile.

Flow rate: Adjust so that the retention time of betahistine is about 5 minutes.

System suitability—

System performance: When the procedure is run with 5 μL of the standard solution under the above operating conditions, the number of theoretical plates and the symmetry factor of the peak of betahistine are not less than 2000 and not more than 1.5, respectively.

System repeatability: When the test is repeated 6 times with 5 μL of the standard solution under the above operating conditions, the relative standard deviation of the peak area of betahistine is not more than 1.0%.

Containers and storage Containers—Tight containers.

Betamethasone

ベタメタゾン

$C_{22}H_{29}FO_5$: 392.46
9-Fluoro-11β,17,21-trihydroxy-16β-methylpregna-1,4-diene-3,20-dione
[378-44-9]

Betamethasone, when dried, contains not less than 96.0% and not more than 103.0% of betamethasone ($C_{22}H_{29}FO_5$).

Description Betamethasone occurs as a white to pale yellow-white crystalline powder.

It is sparingly soluble in methanol, in ethanol (95) and in acetone, and practically insoluble in water.

Melting point: about 240°C (with decomposition).

It shows crystal polymorphism.

Identification **(1)** Proceed with 10 mg of Betamethasone as directed under Oxygen Flask Combustion Method *<1.06>*, using a mixture of 0.5 mL of 0.01 mol/L sodium hydroxide TS and 20 mL of water as the absorbing liquid: the test solution so obtained responds to Qualitative Tests *<1.09>* for fluoride.

(2) Dissolve 1.0 mg of Betamethasone in 10 mL of ethanol (95). Mix 2.0 mL of the solution with 10 mL of phenylhydrazinium hydrochloride TS, heat in a water bath at 60°C for 20 minutes, and cool the solution. Determine the absorption spectrum of the solution as directed under Ultraviolet-visible Spectrophotometry *<2.24>*, using as the blank the solution prepared with 2.0 mL of ethanol (95) in the same manner as the former solution, and compare the spectrum with the Reference Spectrum or the spectrum of a solution of Betamethasone RS prepared in the same manner as the sample solution: both spectra exhibit similar intensities of absorption at the same wavelengths.

(3) Determine the infrared absorption spectrum of Betamethasone, previously dried, as directed in the potassium bromide disk method under Infrared Spectrophotometry *<2.25>*, and compare the spectrum with the Reference Spectrum or the spectrum of previously dried Betamethasone RS: both spectra exhibit similar intensities of absorption at the same wave numbers. If any difference appears between the spectra, dissolve Betamethasone and Betamethasone RS in acetone, respectively, then evaporate the acetone to dryness, and repeat the test on the residues.

Optical rotation *<2.49>* $[\alpha]_D^{20}$: +118 – +126° (after drying, 0.1 g, methanol, 20 mL, 100 mm).

Purity **(1)** Heavy metals *<1.07>*—Proceed with 0.5 g of Betamethasone according to Method 2, and perform the test. Prepare the control solution with 1.5 mL of Standard Lead Solution (not more than 30 ppm).

(2) Related substances—Dissolve 10 mg of Betamethasone in 5 mL of a mixture of chloroform and methanol (9:1), and use this solution as the sample solution. Pipet 1 mL of the sample solution, add a mixture of chloroform and methanol (9:1) to make exactly 100 mL, and use this solution as the standard solution. Perform the test with these solutions as directed under Thin-layer Chromatography *<2.03>*. Spot 5 μL each of the sample solution and standard solution on a plate of silica gel with fluorescent indicator for thin-layer chromatography. Develop the plate with a mixture of dichloromethane, diethyl ether, methanol and water (385:75:40:6) to a distance of about 12 cm, and air-dry the plate. Examine under ultraviolet light (main wavelength: 254 nm): the spots other than the principal spot obtained from the sample solution are not more intense than the spot from the standard solution.

Loss on drying *<2.41>* Not more than 0.5% (0.5 g, in vacuum, phosphorus (V) oxide, 4 hours).

Residue on ignition *<2.44>* Not more than 0.5% (0.1 g, platinum crucible).

Assay Dissolve about 20 mg each of Betamethasone and Betamethasone RS, previously dried and accurately weighed, in methanol to make exactly 50 mL. Pipet 5 mL each of these solutions, add exactly 5 mL each of the internal standard solution, then add methanol to make 50 mL, and use these solutions as the sample solution and standard solution, respectively. Perform the test with 10 μL each of these solutions as directed under Liquid Chromatography *<2.01>* according to the following conditions, and calculate the ratios, Q_T and Q_S, of the peak area of betamethasone to that of the internal standard.

$$\text{Amount (mg) of betamethasone } (C_{22}H_{29}FO_5) = M_S \times Q_T/Q_S$$

M_S: Amount (mg) of Betamethasone RS taken

Internal standard solution—A solution of butyl parahydroxybenzoate in methanol (1 in 1750).

Operating conditions—

Detector: An ultraviolet absorption photometer (wavelength: 240 nm).

Column: A stainless steel column about 4.0 mm in inside diameter and 15 cm in length, packed with octadecylsilanized silica gel for liquid chromatography (5 μm in particle diameter).

Column temperature: A constant temperature of about 25°C.

Mobile phase: A mixture of water and acetonitrile (3:2).

Flow rate: Adjust so that the retention time of betamethasone is about 4 minutes.

System suitability—

System performance: When proceed the test with 10 μL of the standard solution under the above operating conditions, betamethasone and the internal standard are eluted in this order with the resolution between these peaks being not less than 10.

System repeatability: When the test is repeated 6 times with 10 μL of the standard solution under the above operating conditions, the relative standard deviation of the ratio of the peak area of betamethasone to that of the internal standard is not more than 1.0%.

Containers and storage Containers—Tight containers.

Storage—Light-resistant.

Betamethasone Tablets

ベタメタゾン錠

Betamethasone Tablets contain not less than 90.0% and not more than 107.0% of the labeled amount of betamethasone ($C_{22}H_{29}FO_5$: 392.46).

Method of preparation Prepare as directed under Tablets, with Betamethasone.

Identification Pulverize Betamethasone Tablets. To a portion of the powder, equivalent to 2 mg of Betamethasone, add 20 mL of methanol, shake for 5 minutes, and filter. Evaporate the filtrate on a water bath to dryness, dissolve the residue after cooling in 2 mL of methanol, filter if necessary, and use this as the sample solution. Separately, dissolve 2 mg of Betamethasone RS in 2 mL of methanol, and use this solution as the standard solution. Perform the test with these solutions as directed under Thin-layer Chromatography <*2.03*>. Spot 5 μL each of the sample solution and standard solution on a plate of silica gel with fluorescent indicator for thin-layer chromatography, develop with a mixture of 1-butanol, water and acetic anhydride (3:1:1) to a distance of about 10 cm, and air-dry the plate. Examine under ultraviolet light (main wavelength: 254 nm): the principal spot obtained from the sample solution and the spot from the standard solution show the same *R*f value.

Uniformity of dosage units <*6.02*> Perform the test according to the following method: it meets the requirement of the Content uniformity test.

To 1 tablet of Betamethasone Tablets add *V* mL of water so that each mL contains about 50 μg of betamethasone ($C_{22}H_{29}FO_5$). Add exactly 2*V* mL of the internal standard solution, shake vigorously for 10 minutes, centrifuge, and use the supernatant liquid as the sample solution. Separately, weigh accurately about 20 mg of Betamethasone RS, previously dried for 4 hours in a desiccator (in vacuum, phosphorus (V) oxide), dissolve in acetonitrile to make exactly 200 mL. Pipet 5 mL of this solution, add exactly 20 mL of the internal standard solution, add 5 mL of water, and use this solution as the standard solution. Perform the test with 20 μL each of the sample solution and standard solution as directed under Liquid Chromatography <*2.01*> according to the following conditions, and calculate the ratios, Q_T and Q_S, of the peak area of betamethasone to that of the internal standard.

Amount (mg) of betamethasone ($C_{22}H_{29}FO_5$)
$= M_S \times Q_T/Q_S \times V/400$

M_S: Amount (mg) of Betamethasone RS taken

Internal standard solution—A solution of butyl parahydroxybenzoate in acetonitrile (1 in 40,000).

Operating conditions—

Proceed as directed in the operating conditions in the Assay.

System suitability—

System performance: When the procedure is run with 20 μL of the standard solution under the above operating conditions, betamethasone and the internal standard are eluted in this order with the resolution between these peaks being not less than 10.

System repeatability: When the test is repeated 6 times with 20 μL of the standard solution under the above operating conditions, the relative standard deviation of the ratio of the peak area of betamethasone to that of the internal standard is not more than 1.0%.

Dissolution <*6.10*> When the test is performed at 50 revolutions per minute according to the Paddle method, using 900 mL of water as the dissolution medium, the dissolution rate in 30 minutes of Betamethasone Tablets is not less than 85%.

Start the test with 1 tablet of Betamethasone Tablets, withdraw not less than 20 mL of the medium at the specified minute after starting the test, and filter through a membrane filter with a pore size not exceeding 0.45 μm. Discard not less than 10 mL of the first filtrate, pipet the subsequent *V* mL of the filtrate, add water to make exactly *V′* mL so that each mL contains about 0.56 μg of betamethasone ($C_{22}H_{29}FO_5$), and use this solution as the sample solution. Separately, weigh accurately about 28 mg of Betamethasone RS, previously dried in a desiccator (in vacuum, phosphorus (V) oxide) for 4 hours, dissolve in methanol to make exactly 100 mL. Pipet 5 mL of this solution, and add water to make exactly 100 mL. Pipet 4 mL of this solution, add water to make exactly 100 mL, and use this solution as the standard solution. Perform the test with exactly 100 μL each of the sample solution and standard solution as directed under Liquid Chromatography <*2.01*> according to the following conditions, and determine the peak areas, A_T and A_S, of betamethasone in each solution.

Dissolution rate (%) with respect to the labeled amount of betamethasone ($C_{22}H_{29}FO_5$)
$= M_S \times A_T/A_S \times V'/V \times 1/C \times 9/5$

M_S: Amount (mg) of Betamethasone RS taken
C: Labeled amount (mg) of betamethasone ($C_{22}H_{29}FO_5$) in 1 tablet

Operating conditions—

Detector: An ultraviolet absorption photometer (wavelength: 241 nm).

Column: A stainless steel column 4.6 mm in inside diameter and 15 cm in length, packed with octadecylsilanized silica gel for liquid chromatography (5 μm in particle diameter).

Column temperature: A constant temperature of about 25°C.

Mobile phase: A mixture of methanol and water (3:2).

Flow rate: Adjust so that the retention time of betamethasone is about 7 minutes.

System suitability—

System performance: When the procedure is run with 100 μL of the standard solution under the above operating conditions, the number of theoretical plates and the symmetry factor of the peak of betamethasone are not less than 3000 and not more than 2.0, respectively.

System repeatability: When the test is repeated 6 times with 100 μL of the standard solution under the above operating conditions, the relative standard deviation of the peak area of betamethasone is not more than 2.0%.

Assay Weigh accurately the mass of not less than 20 Betamethasone Tablets, and powder. Weigh accurately a portion of the powder, equivalent to about 5 mg of betamethasone ($C_{22}H_{29}FO_5$), add 25 mL of water, then add exactly 50 mL of the internal standard solution, and shake vigorously for 10 minutes. Filter through a membrane filter with pore size not exceeding 0.5 μm, discard the first 5 mL of the filtrate, and use the subsequent filtrate as the sample solution. Separately, weigh accurately about 20 mg of Betamethasone RS, previously dried in a desiccator (in vacuum, phosphorus (V) oxide) for 4 hours, and dissolve in acetonitrile to make exactly 50 mL. Pipet 5 mL of this solution, add exactly 20 mL of the internal standard solution and 5 mL of water, and use this solution as the standard solution. Perform the test with 20 μL each of the sample solution and standard solution as directed under Liquid Chromatography *<2.01>* according to the following conditions, and calculate the ratios, Q_T and Q_S, of the peak area of betamethasone to that of the internal standard.

$$\text{Amount (mg) of betamethasone } (C_{22}H_{29}FO_5) = M_S \times Q_T/Q_S \times 1/4$$

M_S: Amount (mg) of Betamethasone RS taken

Internal standard solution—A solution of butyl parahydroxybenzoate in acetonitrile (1 in 10,000).

Operating conditions—

Detector: An ultraviolet absorption photometer (wavelength: 240 nm).

Column: A stainless steel column 4 mm in inside diameter and 15 cm in length, packed with octadecylsilanized silica gel for liquid chromatography (5 μm in particle diameter).

Column temperature: A constant temperature of about 25°C.

Mobile phase: A mixture of water and acetonitrile (3:2).

Flow rate: Adjust so that the retention time of betamethasone is about 4 minutes.

System suitability—

System performance: When the procedure is run with 20 μL of the standard solution under the above operating conditions, betamethasone and the internal standard are eluted in this order with the resolution between these peaks being not less than 10.

System repeatability: When the test is repeated 6 times with 20 μL of the standard solution under the above operating conditions, the relative standard deviation of the ratio of the peak area of betamethasone to that of the internal standard is not more than 1.0%.

Containers and storage Containers—Tight containers.

Storage—Light-resistant.

Betamethasone Dipropionate

ベタメタゾンジプロピオン酸エステル

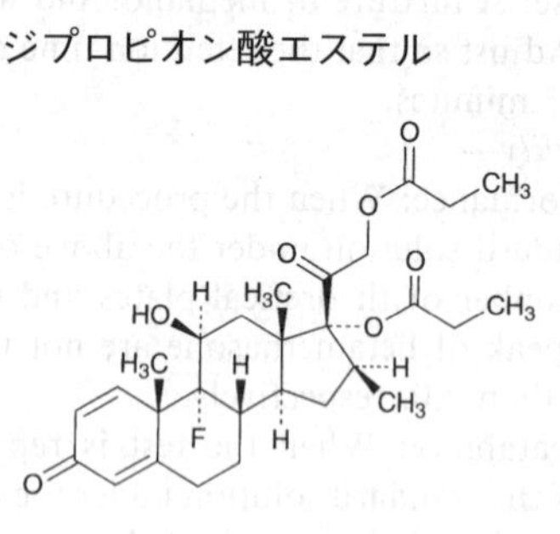

$C_{28}H_{37}FO_7$: 504.59

9-Fluoro-11β,17,21-trihydroxy-16β-methylpregna-1,4-diene-3,20-dione 17,21-dipropanoate

[5593-20-4]

Betamethasone Dipropionate, when dried, contains not less than 97.0% and not more than 103.0% of betamethasone dipropionate ($C_{28}H_{37}FO_7$), and not less than 3.4% and not more than 4.1% of fluorine (F:19.00).

Description Betamethasone Dipropionate occurs as a white to pale yellow-white crystalline powder. It is odorless.

It is freely soluble in acetone and in chloroform, soluble in methanol and in ethanol (99.5), and practically insoluble in water.

It is gradually affected by light.

Identification **(1)** To 1 mL of a solution of Betamethasone Dipropionate in methanol (1 in 10,000) add 4 mL of isoniazid TS, and heat on a water bath for 2 minutes: a yellow color develops.

(2) Proceed with 0.01 g of Betamethasone Dipropionate as directed under Oxygen Flask Combustion Method *<1.06>*, using a mixture of 0.5 mL of 0.01 mol/L sodium hydroxide TS and 20 mL of water as the absorbing liquid: the test solution so obtained responds to the Qualitative Tests *<1.09>* for fluoride.

(3) Determine the absorption spectrum of a solution of Betamethasone Dipropionate in methanol (3 in 200,000) as directed under Ultraviolet-visible Spectrophotometry *<2.24>*, and compare the spectrum with the Reference Spectrum: both spectra exhibit similar intensities of absorption at the same wavelengths.

(4) Determine the infrared absorption spectrum of Betamethasone Dipropionate, previously dried, as directed in the potassium bromide disk method under Infrared Spectrophotometry *<2.25>*, and compare the spectrum with the Reference Spectrum: both spectra exhibit similar intensities of absorption at the same wave numbers.

Optical rotation *<2.49>* $[\alpha]_D^{25}$: +84 – +89° (after drying, 50 mg, ethanol (99.5), 10 mL, 100 mm).

Melting point *<2.60>* 176 – 180°C

Purity **(1)** Fluoride—To 0.10 g of Betamethasone Dipropionate add 10.0 mL of diluted 0.01 mol/L sodium hydroxide TS (1 in 20), shake for 10 minutes, and filter through a membrane filter (0.4-μm pore size). Place 5.0 mL of the filtrate in a 20-mL volumetric flask, and add 10 mL of a mixture of alizarin complexone TS, acetic acid-potassium acetate buffer solution (pH 4.3) and cerium (III) nitrate TS (1:1:1), add water to make 20 mL, allow to stand for 1 hour, and use this solution as the sample solution. Separately, place 1.0 mL of Standard Fluorine Solution in a 20-mL volumetric flask, add 5.0 mL of diluted 0.01 mol/L sodium hydroxide TS (1 in 20), then 10 mL of a mixture of alizarin complexone TS, acetic acid-potassium acetate buffer solution (pH 4.3) and cerium (III) nitrate TS (1:1:1), proceed in the same manner as the preparation of the sample solution, and use this solution as the standard solution. Place 5.0 mL of diluted 0.01 mol/L sodium hydroxide TS (1 in 20) in a 20-mL volumetric flask, and proceed in the same manner as the preparation of the sample solution. Using this solution as the blank, determine the absorbances of the sample solution and standard solution at 600 nm as directed under Ultraviolet-visible Spectrophotometry *<2.24>*: the absorbance of the sample solution is not more than that of the standard solution (not more than 0.012%).

(2) Heavy metals *<1.07>*—Proceed with 1.0 g of Betamethasone Dipropionate according to Method 2, and perform the test. Prepare the control solution with 2.0 mL of Standard Lead Solution (not more than 20 ppm).

(3) Related substances—Conduct this procedure without exposure to light, using light-resistant vessels. Dissolve 10 mg of Betamethasone Dipropionate in 10 mL of chloroform, and use this solution as the sample solution. Pipet 3 mL of the sample solution, add chloroform to make exactly 100 mL, and use this solution as the standard solution. Perform the test as directed under Thin-layer Chromatography *<2.03>* with these solutions. Spot 20 μL each of the sample solution and standard solution on a plate of silica gel with fluorescent indicator for thin-layer chromatography. Develop the plate with a mixture of chloroform and acetone (7:1) to a distance of about 10 cm, and air-dry the plate. Examine under ultraviolet light (main wavelength: 254 nm): the spots other than the principal spot obtained from the sample solution are not more intense than the spot from the standard solution.

Loss on drying <*2.41*> Not more than 1.0% (0.5 g, 105°C, 3 hours).

Residue on ignition <*2.44*> Not more than 0.2% (0.5 g, platinum crucible).

Assay **(1)** Betamethasone dipropionate—Weigh accurately about 15 mg of Betamethasone Dipropionate, previously dried, and dissolve in methanol to make exactly 100 mL. Pipet 5 mL of this solution, and dilute with methanol to exactly 50 mL. Determine the absorbance A of this solution at the wavelength of maximum absorption at about 239 nm as directed under Ultraviolet-visible Spectrophotometry <*2.24*>.

Amount (mg) of betamethasone dipropionate ($C_{28}H_{37}FO_7$)
$= A/312 \times 10{,}000$

(2) Fluorine—Weigh accurately about 10 mg of Betamethasone Dipropionate, previously dried, and proceed as directed in the procedure of determination for fluorine under Oxygen Flask Combustion Method <*1.06*>, using a mixture of 0.5 mL of 0.01 mol/L sodium hydroxide TS and 20 mL of water as the absorbing liquid.

Containers and storage Containers—Tight containers.
Storage—Light-resistant.

Betamethasone Sodium Phosphate

ベタメタゾンリン酸エステルナトリウム

$C_{22}H_{28}FNa_2O_8P$: 516.40
9-Fluoro-11β,17,21-trihydroxy-16β-methylpregna-1,4-diene-3,20-dione 21-(disodium phosphate)
[*151-73-5*]

Betamethasone Sodium Phosphate contains not less than 97.0% and not more than 103.0% of betamethasone sodium phosphate ($C_{22}H_{28}FNa_2O_8P$), calculated on the anhydrous basis.

Description Betamethasone Sodium Phosphate occurs as white to pale yellow-white, crystalline powder or masses. It is odorless.

It is freely soluble in water, sparingly soluble in methanol, slightly soluble in ethanol (95), and practically insoluble in diethyl ether.

It is hygroscopic.

Melting point: about 213°C (with decomposition).

Identification **(1)** Dissolve 2 mg of Betamethasone Sodium Phosphate in 2 mL of sulfuric acid: a brown color develops, and gradually changes to blackish brown.

(2) Prepare the test solution with 0.01 g of Betamethasone Sodium Phosphate as directed under Oxygen Flask Combustion Method <*1.06*>, using a mixture of 0.5 mL of 0.01 mol/L sodium hydroxide TS and 20 mL of water as an absorbing liquid: the test solution responds to Qualitative Tests <*1.09*> (2) for fluoride.

(3) Take 40 mg of Betamethasone Sodium Phosphate in a platinum crucible, and carbonize by heating. After cooling, add 5 drops of nitric acid, and incinerate by heating. To the residue add 10 mL of diluted nitric acid (1 in 50), and boil for several minutes. After cooling, filter if necessary, and use this solution as the sample solution. The sample solution responds to Qualitative Tests <*1.09*> (2) for phosphate. The sample solution neutralized with ammonia TS responds to Qualitative Tests <*1.09*> for sodium salt, and to Qualitative Tests <*1.09*> (1) and (3) for phosphate.

(4) Determine the infrared absorption spectrum of Betamethasone Sodium Phosphate, as directed in the potassium bromide disk method under Infrared Spectrophotometry <*2.25*>, and compare the spectrum with the Reference Spectrum or the spectrum of Betamethasone Sodium Phosphate RS: both spectra exhibit similar intensities of absorption at the same wave numbers.

Optical rotation <*2.49*> $[\alpha]_D^{20}$: +99 – +105° (0.1 g calculated on the anhydrous basis, water, 10 mL, 100 mm).

pH <*2.54*> Dissolve 0.10 g of Betamethasone Sodium Phosphate in 20 mL of water: the pH of this solution is between 7.5 and 9.0.

Purity **(1)** Clarity and color of solution—Dissolve 0.25 g of Betamethasone Sodium Phosphate in 10 mL of water: the solution is clear and colorless.

(2) Free phosphoric acid—Weigh accurately about 20 mg of Betamethasone Sodium Phosphate, dissolve in 20 mL of water, and use this solution as the sample solution. Separately, pipet 4 mL of Standard Phosphoric Acid Solution, add 20 mL of water, and use this solution as the standard solution. To each of the sample solution and the standard solution add exactly 7 mL of dilute sulfuric acid, exactly 2 mL of hexaammonium heptamolybdate-sulfuric acid TS and exactly 2 mL of *p*-methylaminophenol sulfate TS, shake well, and allow to stand at 20 ± 1°C for 15 minutes. To each add water to make exactly 50 mL, and allow to stand at 20 ± 1°C for 15 minutes. Perform the test with these solutions as directed under Ultraviolet-visible Spectrophotometry <*2.24*>, using a solution prepared with 20 mL of water in the same manner as the blank. Determine the absorbances, A_T and A_S, of each solution from the sample solution and standard solution at 730 nm: the amount of free phosphoric acid is not more than 0.5%.

Amount (%) of free phosphoric acid (H_3PO_4)
$= A_T/A_S \times 1/M \times 10.32$

M: Amount (mg) of Betamethasone Sodium Phosphate taken, calculated on the anhydrous basis

(3) Betamethasone—Dissolve 20 mg of Betamethasone Sodium Phosphate in exactly 2 mL of methanol, and use this solution as the sample solution. Separately, dissolve 20 mg of Betamethasone RS in exactly 10 mL of methanol. Pipet 1 mL of this solution, add methanol to make exactly 20 mL, and use this solution as the standard solution. Perform the test with these solutions as directed under Thin-layer Chromatography <*2.03*>. Spot 5 μL each of the sample solution and standard solution on a plate of silica gel with fluorescent indicator for thin-layer chromatography. Develop the plate with a freshly prepared mixture of 1-butanol, water and acetic anhydride (3:1:1) to a distance of about 10 cm, and air-dry the plate. Examine under ultraviolet light (main wavelength: 254 nm): the spot from the sample solution corresponding to the spot obtained from the standard solution is not more intense than the spot from the standard solution.

Water <*2.48*> Not more than 10.0% (0.2 g, volumetric titration, back titration).

Assay Weigh accurately about 20 mg each of Betamethasone Sodium Phosphate and Betamethasone Sodium Phosphate RS (separately, determine the water <*2.48*> in the same manner as Betamethasone Sodium Phosphate), and dissolve each in methanol to make exactly 20 mL. Pipet 5 mL each of these solutions, and exactly 5 mL of the internal standard solution, then add methanol to make 50 mL, and use these solutions as the sample solution and standard solution, respectively. Perform the test with 10 μL each of the sample solution and standard solution as directed under Liquid Chromatography <*2.01*> according to the following conditions, and calculate the ratios, Q_T and Q_S, of the peak area of betamethasone phosphate to that of the internal standard.

Amount (mg) of betamethasone sodium phosphate ($C_{22}H_{28}FNa_2O_8P$) $= M_S \times Q_T/Q_S$

M_S: Amount (mg) of Betamethasone Sodium Phosphate RS taken, calculated on the anhydrous basis

Internal standard solution—A solution of butyl parahydroxybenzoate in methanol (1 in 5000).

Operating conditions—

Detector: An ultraviolet absorption photometer (wavelength: 254 nm).

Column: A stainless steel column 4.0 mm in inside diameter and 25 cm in length, packed with octadecylsilanized silica gel for liquid chromatography (7 μm in particle diameter).

Column temperature: A constant temperature of about 25°C.

Mobile phase: Dissolve 1.6 g of tetra-*n*-butylammonium bromide, 3.2 g of disodium hydrogen phosphate dodecahydrate and 6.9 g of potassium dihydrogen phosphate in 1000 mL of water, and add 1500 mL of methanol.

Flow rate: Adjust so that the retention time of betamethasone phosphate is about 5 minutes.

System suitability—

System performance: When the procedure is run with 10 μL of the standard solution under the above operating conditions, betamethasone phosphate and the internal standard are eluted in this order with the resolution between these peaks being not less than 10.

System repeatability: When the test is repeated 6 times with 10 μL of the standard solution under the above operating conditions, the relative standard deviation of the ratios of the peak area of betamethasone phosphate to that of the internal standard is not more than 1.0%.

Containers and storage Containers—Tight containers.

Betamethasone Valerate

ベタメタゾン吉草酸エステル

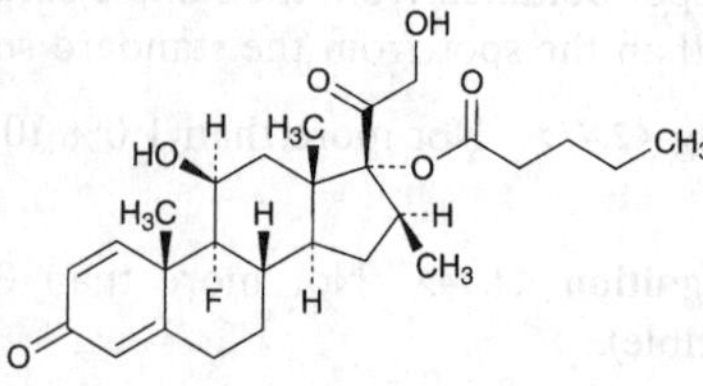

$C_{27}H_{37}FO_6$: 476.58
9-Fluoro-11β,17,21-trihydroxy-16β-methylpregna-1,4-diene-3,20-dione 17-pentanoate
[*2152-44-5*]

Betamethasone Valerate, when dried, contains not less than 97.0% and not more than 103.0% of betamethasone valerate ($C_{27}H_{37}FO_6$).

Description Betamethasone Valerate occurs as a white crystalline powder. It is odorless.

It is freely soluble in chloroform, soluble in ethanol (95), sparingly soluble in methanol, slightly soluble in diethyl ether, and practically insoluble in water.

Melting point: about 190°C (with decomposition).

Identification **(1)** Proceed with 0.01 g of Betamethasone Valerate as directed under Oxygen Flask Combustion Method <*1.06*>, using a mixture of 0.5 mL of 0.01 mol/L sodium hydroxide TS and 20 mL of water as the absorbing liquid: the test solution so obtained responds to Qualitative Tests <*1.09*> for fluoride.

(2) Determine the infrared absorption spectrum of Betamethasone Valerate, previously dried, as directed in the potassium bromide disk method under Infrared Spectrophotometry <*2.25*>, and compare the spectrum with the Reference Spectrum or the spectrum of dried Betamethasone Valerate RS: both spectra exhibit similar intensities of absorption at the same wave numbers.

Optical rotation <*2.49*> $[\alpha]_D^{20}$: +77 – +83° (after drying, 0.1 g, methanol, 20 mL, 100 mm).

Purity Related substances—Conduct this procedure without exposure to daylight. Dissolve 0.02 g of Betamethasone Valerate in 5 mL of a mixture of chloroform and methanol (9:1), and use this solution as the sample solution. Pipet 1 mL of the sample solution, add a mixture of chloroform and methanol (9:1) to make exactly 50 mL, and use this solution as the standard solution. Perform the test with these solutions as directed under Thin-layer Chromatography <*2.03*>. Spot 5 μL each of the sample solution and standard solution on a plate of silica gel for thin-layer chromatography. Develop the plate with a mixture of chloroform and methanol (9:1) to a distance of about 12 cm, and air-dry the plate. Spray evenly alkaline blue tetrazolium TS on the plate: the spots other than the principal spot obtained from the sample solution are not more intense than the spot from the standard solution.

Loss on drying <*2.41*> Not more than 0.5% (1 g, 105°C, 3 hours).

Residue on ignition <*2.44*> Not more than 0.2% (0.5 g, platinum crucible).

Assay Dissolve about 10 mg each of Betamethasone Valerate and Betamethasone Valerate RS, previously dried and accurately weighed, in methanol to make exactly 100 mL. Pipet 10 mL each of these solutions, add 10 mL each of the internal standard solution, and use these solutions as the sample solution and the standard solution, respectively. Perform the test with 10 μL each of the sample solution and standard solution as directed under Liquid Chromatography *<2.01>* according to the following conditions, and calculate the ratios, Q_T and Q_S, of the peak area of betamethasone valerate to that of the internal standard.

Amount (mg) of betamethasone valerate ($C_{27}H_{37}FO_6$)
$= M_S \times Q_T/Q_S$

M_S: Amount (mg) of Betamethasone Valerate RS taken

Internal standard solution—A solution of isoamyl benzoate in methanol (1 in 1000).

Operating conditions—

Detector: An ultraviolet absorption photometer (wavelength: 254 nm).

Column: A stainless steel column 4.0 mm in inside diameter and 20 cm in length, packed with octadecylsilanized silica gel for liquid chromatography (7 μm in particle diameter).

Column temperature: A constant temperature of about 25°C.

Mobile phase: A mixture of methanol and water (7:3).

Flow rate: Adjust so that the retention time of betamethasone valerate is about 10 minutes.

System suitability—

System performance: When the procedure is run with 10 μL of the standard solution under the above operating conditions, betamethasone valerate and the internal standard are eluted in this order with the resolution between these peaks being not less than 5.

System repeatability: When the test is repeated 6 times with 10 μL of the standard solution under the above operating conditions, the relative standard deviation of the ratio of the peak area of betamethasone valerate to that of the internal standard is not more than 1.0%.

Containers and storage Containers—Tight containers.

Betamethasone Valerate and Gentamicin Sulfate Cream

ベタメタゾン吉草酸エステル·ゲンタマイシン硫酸塩クリーム

Betamethasone Valerate and Gentamicin Sulfate Cream contains not less than 90.0% and not more than 110.0% of the labeled amount of betamethasone valerate ($C_{27}H_{37}FO_6$: 476.58) and not less than 90.0% and not more than 115.0% of the labeled amount of gentamicin C_1 ($C_{21}H_{43}N_5O_7$: 477.60).

Method of preparation Prepare as directed under Creams, with Betamethasone Valerate and Gentamicin Sulfate.

Identification **(1)** To a quantity of Betamethasone Valerate and Gentamicin Sulfate Cream, equivalent to about 1.2 mg of Betamethasone Valerate, add 20 mL of methanol and 20 mL of hexane, shake vigorously for 10 minutes, and allow to stand. Take 15 mL of the lower layer, evaporate the layer to dryness on a water bath under a current of nitrogen. To the residue add 1 mL of ethyl acetate, mix, and use as the sample solution. Separately, dissolve about 18 mg of Betamethasone Valerate RS in 20 mL of ethyl acetate, and use this solution as the standard solution. Perform the test with these solutions as directed under Thin-layer Chromatography *<2.03>*. Spot 5 μL each of the sample solution and standard solution on a plate of silica gel for thin-layer chromatography, develop the plate with ethyl acetate to a distance of about 10 cm, and air-dry the plate. Spray evenly alkaline blue tetrazolium TS on the plate, and heat the plate at 100°C: the principal spot obtained from the sample solution and the spot from the standard solution are purple in color, and their *R*f values are the same.

(2) To a quantity of Betamethasone Valerate and Gentamicin Sulfate Cream, equivalent to about 2 mg (potency) of Gentamicin Sulfate, add 20 mL of ethyl acetate and 10 mL of water, shake vigorously for 10 minutes, and centrifuge. To 3 mL of the lower layer add 1 mL of dilute sodium hydroxide TS and 2 mL of ninhydrin TS, and heat in a water bath at 90 – 95°C for 10 minutes: a purple to dark purple color develops.

pH *<2.54>* To a quantity of Betamethasone Valerate and Gentamicin Sulfate Cream, equivalent to 6 mg of Betamethasone Valerate, add 15 mL of water, and mix while warming on a water bath to make a milky liquid: the pH of the cooled liquid is between 4.0 and 6.0.

Purity Related substances—Weigh accurately an amount of Betamethasone Valerate and Gentamicin Sulfate Cream, equivalent to about 1 mg of Betamethasone Valerate, and add 10 mL of a mixture of methanol and water (7:3). Warm in a water bath at 60°C for 5 minutes, and shake vigorously for 20 minutes. Repeat this procedure 2 times. After cooling for 15 minutes with ice, centrifuge for 5 minutes, take away the bubbles from the upper surface, and filter the remaining liquid. Discard first 2 mL of the filtrate, and use the subsequent filtrate as the sample solution. Perform the test with 150 μL of the sample solution as directed under Liquid Chromatography *<2.01>* according to the following conditions, determine each peak area by the automatic integration method, and calculate these amounts by the area percentage method: the amount of the substance other than betamethasone valerate is not more than 3.5%, and the total amount of them is not more than 7.0%.

Operating conditions—

Detector: An ultraviolet absorption photometer (wavelength: 240 nm).

Column: A stainless steel column 4.6 mm in inside diameter and 15 cm in length, packed with octadecylsilanized silica gel for liquid chromatography (5 μm in particle diameter).

Column temperature: A constant temperature of about 45°C.

Mobile phase: A mixture of water, acetonitrile and methanol (12:7:1).

Flow rate: Adjust so that the retention time of betamethasone valerate is about 16 minutes.

Time span of measurement: About 2.5 times as long as the retention time of betamethasone valerate beginning after the solvent peak. The peaks of the compounding ingredients are not determined.

System suitability—

Test for required detectability: Dissolve 20 mg of Betamethasone Valerate in 100 mL of a mixture of methanol and water (7:3). To exactly 1 mL of this solution add the mixture of methanol and water (7:3) to make exactly 100 mL, and use this solution as the solution for system suitability test. To exactly 2.5 mL of the solution for system suitability test add the mixture of methanol and water (7:3) to make exactly 50 mL. Confirm that the peak area of betamethasone valerate obtained with 150 μL of this solution is equivalent to 3.5 to 6.5% of that with 150 μL of the solution for system suitability test.

System performance: When the procedure is run with 150 μL of the solution for system suitability test under the above operating conditions, the number of theoretical plates and the symmetry factor of the peak of betamethasone valerate are not less than 4000 and 0.8 to 1.3, respectively.

System repeatability: When the test is repeated 6 times with 150 μL of the solution for system suitability test under the above operating conditions, the relative standard deviation of the peak area of betamethasone valerate is not more than 2.0%.

Assay **(1)** Betamethasone valerate—Weigh accurately an amount of Betamethasone Valerate and Gentamicin Sulfate Cream, equivalent to about 1 mg of betamethasone valerate ($C_{27}H_{37}FO_6$), add 10 mL of a mixture of methanol and water (7:3), and add exactly 10 mL of the internal standard solution. After warming in a water bath at 60°C for 5 minutes, shake vigorously for 20 minutes. Repeat this procedure twice, cool with ice for 15 minutes, centrifuge for 5 minutes, then filter the supernatant liquid, discard the first 5 mL of filtrate, and use the subsequent filtrate as the sample solution. Separately, weigh accurately about 25 mg of Betamethasone Valerate RS, previously dried at 105°C for 3 hours, and dissolve in methanol to make exactly 25 mL. Pipet 5 mL of this solution, and add the mixture of methanol and water (7:3) to make exactly 50 mL. Pipet 10 mL of this solution, add exactly 10 mL of the internal standard solution, mix, and use this solution as the standard solution. Perform the test with 3 μL each of the sample solution and standard solution as directed under Liquid Chromatography <*2.01*> according to the following conditions, and calculate the ratios, Q_T and Q_S, of the peak area of betamethasone valerate to that of the internal standard.

Amount (mg) of betamethasone valerate ($C_{27}H_{37}FO_6$)
$= M_S \times Q_T/Q_S \times 1/25$

M_S: Amount (mg) of Betamethasone Valerate RS taken

Internal standard solution—Dissolve 20 mg of beclometasone dipropionate in 10 mL of methanol, and add the mixture of methanol and water (7:3) to make 200 mL.

Operating conditions—

Detector: An ultraviolet absorption photometer (wavelength: 254 nm).

Column: A stainless steel column 2.1 mm in inside diameter and 10 cm in length, packed with octadecylsilanized silica gel for liquid chromatography (3.5 μm in particle diameter).

Column temperature: A constant temperature of about 25°C.

Mobile phase: A mixture of methanol and water (13:7).

Flow rate: Adjust so that the retention time of betamethasone valerate is about 16 minutes.

System suitability—

System performance: When the procedure is run with 3 μL of the standard solution under the above operating conditions, betamethasone valerate and the internal standard are eluted in this order with the resolution between these peaks being not less than 4.

System repeatability: When the test is repeated 6 times with 3 μL of the standard solution under the above operating conditions, the relative standard deviation of the ratio of the peak area of betamethasone valerate to that of the internal standard is not more than 1.0%.

(2) Gentamicin sulfate—Perform the test according to the Cylinder-plate method as directed under Microbial Assay for Antibiotics <*4.02*> according to the following conditions.

(i) Test organism, agar media for base layer and seed layer, agar medium for transferring test organisms, and standard solutions—Proceed as directed in the Assay under Gentamicin Sulfate.

(ii) Sample solutions—Weigh accurately an amount of Betamethasone Valerate and Gentamicin Sulfate Cream, equivalent to about 1 mg (potency) of Gentamicin Sulfate, add 100 mL of 0.1 mol/L phosphate buffer solution (pH 8.0) previously warmed to about 85°C, and shake well to dissolve. After cooling, add 0.1 mol/L phosphate buffer solution (pH 8.0) to make exactly 250 mL to make the high concentration sample solution, which contains 4 μg (potency) per mL. Pipet a suitable amount of the high concentration sample solution, add 0.1 mol/L phosphate buffer solution (pH 8.0) so that each mL contains 1 μg (potency), and use this solution as the low concentration sample solution.

Containers and storage Containers—Tight containers.

Storage—Light-resistant.

Betamethasone Valerate and Gentamicin Sulfate Ointment

ベタメタゾン吉草酸エステル·ゲンタマイシン硫酸塩軟膏

Betamethasone Valerate and Gentamicin Sulfate Ointment contains not less than 95.0% and not more than 110.0% of the labeled amount of betamethasone valerate ($C_{27}H_{37}FO_6$: 476.58) and not less than 90.0% and not more than 115.0% of the labeled potency of gentamicin C_1 ($C_{21}H_{43}N_5O_7$: 477.60).

Method of preparation Prepare as directed under Ointment, with Betamethasone Valerate and Gentamicin Sulfate.

Identification **(1)** To a quantity of Betamethasone Valerate and Gentamicin Sulfate Ointment, equivalent to 1.2 mg of Betamethasone Valerate, add 20 mL of methanol and 20 mL of hexane, and disperse the ointment by sonicating. Shake vigorously for 5 minutes, centrifuge for 5 minutes, cool for 15 minutes with ice, and take 15 mL of the lower layer. Evaporate the layer to dryness on a water bath under a current of nitrogen. To the residue add 1 mL of ethyl acetate, sonicate, filter, if necessary, and use the filtrate as the sample solution. Separately, dissolve 18 mg of Betamethasone Valerate RS in 20 mL of ethyl acetate, and use this solution as the standard solution. Perform the test with these solutions as directed under Thin-layer Chromatography <*2.03*>. Spot 5 μL each of the sample solution and standard solution on a plate of silica gel for thin-layer chromatography, develop the plate with ethyl acetate to a distance of about 10 cm, and air-dry the plate. Spray evenly alkaline blue tetrazolium TS on the plate, and heat the plate at 100°C: the principal spot obtained from the sample solution and the spot from the standard solution are purple in color, and their *Rf* values are the same.

(2) To a quantity of Betamethasone Valerate and Gentamicin Sulfate Ointment, equivalent to 2 mg (potency) of Gentamicin Sulfate, add 20 mL of hexane and 10 mL of water, shake vigorously for 10 minutes, and centrifuge. To 3 mL of the lower layer add 1 mL of dilute sodium hydroxide TS and 2 mL of ninhydrin TS, and heat in a water bath at 90 – 95°C for 10 minutes: a red-brown color develops.

pH <*2.54*> To a quantity of Betamethasone Valerate and Gentamicin Sulfate Ointment, equivalent to 6 mg of Betamethasone Valerate, add 15 mL of water, and warm on a water bath to dissolve. After cooling, separate the water layer: the pH of the layer is between 4.0 and 7.0.

Assay (1) Betamethasone valerate—Weigh accurately an amount of Betamethasone Valerate and Gentamicin Sulfate Ointment, equivalent to about 1 mg of betamethasone valerate ($C_{27}H_{37}FO_6$), add 10 mL of a mixture of methanol and water (7:3), and add exactly 10 mL of the internal standard solution. After warming in a water bath at 75°C for 5 minutes, shake vigorously for 10 minutes. Repeat this procedure once more, cool with ice for 15 minutes, filter, discard the first 5 mL of filtrate, and use the subsequent filtrate as the sample solution. Separately, weigh accurately about 25 mg of Betamethasone Valerate RS, previously dried at 105°C for 3 hours, and dissolve in methanol to make exactly 25 mL. Pipet 5 mL of this solution, and add the mixture of methanol and water (7:3) to make exactly 50 mL. Pipet 10 mL of this solution, add exactly 10 mL of the internal standard solution, mix, and use this solution as the standard solution. Perform the test with 3 μL each of the sample solution and standard solution as directed under Liquid Chromatography <*2.01*> according to the following conditions, and calculate the ratios, Q_T and Q_S, of the peak area of betamethasone valerate to that of the internal standard.

Amount (mg) of betamethasone valerate ($C_{27}H_{37}FO_6$)
$= M_S \times Q_T/Q_S \times 1/25$

M_S: Amount (mg) of Betamethasone Valerate RS taken

Internal standard solution—Dissolve 20 mg of beclometasone dipropionate in 10 mL of methanol, and add the mixture of methanol and water (7:3) to make 200 mL.

Operating conditions—

Detector: An ultraviolet absorption photometer (wavelength: 254 nm).

Column: A stainless steel column 2.1 mm in inside diameter and 10 cm in length, packed with octadecylsilanized silica gel for liquid chromatography (3.5 μm in particle diameter).

Column temperature: A constant temperature of about 25°C.

Mobile phase: A mixture of methanol and water (13:7).

Flow rate: Adjust so that the retention time of betamethasone valerate is about 16 minutes.

System suitability—

System performance: When the procedure is run with 3 μL of the standard solution under the above operating conditions, betamethasone valerate and the internal standard are eluted in this order with the resolution between these peaks being not less than 4.

System repeatability: When the test is repeated 6 times with 3 μL of the standard solution under the above operating conditions, the relative standard deviation of the ratio of the peak area of betamethasone valerate to that of the internal standard is not more than 1.0%.

(2) Gentamicin sulfate—Perform the test according to the Cylinder-plate method as directed under Microbial Assay for Antibiotics <*4.02*> according to the following conditions.

(i) Test organism, agar media for base layer and seed layer, agar medium for transferring test organisms, and standard solutions—Proceed as directed in the Assay under Gentamicin Sulfate.

(ii) Sample solutions—Weigh accurately an amount of Betamethasone Valerate and Gentamicin Sulfate Ointment, equivalent to about 1 mg (potency) of Gentamicin Sulfate, transfer to a separator, add 50 mL of petroleum ether and exactly 100 mL of 0.1 mol/L phosphate buffer solution (pH 8.0), shake for 10 minutes, and allow to stand. Pipet a suitable amount of the water layer, add 0.1 mol/L phosphate buffer solution (pH 8.0) to make solutions so that each mL contains 4 μg (potency) and 1 μg (potency), and use these solutions as the high concentration sample solution and low concentration sample solution, respectively.

Containers and storage Containers—Tight containers.

Storage—Light-resistant.

Betamipron

ベタミプロン

$C_{10}H_{11}NO_3$: 193.20
3-Benzoylaminopropanoic acid
[*3440-28-6*]

Betamipron contains not less than 99.0% and not more than 101.0% of betamipron ($C_{10}H_{11}NO_3$), calculated on the anhydrous basis.

Description Betamipron occurs as white, crystals or crystalline powder.

It is freely soluble in methanol, soluble in ethanol (99.5), and slightly soluble in water.

It dissolves in sodium hydroxide TS.

Identification (1) Determine the absorption spectrum of a solution of Betamipron in ethanol (99.5) (1 in 100,000) as directed under Ultraviolet-visible Spectrophotometry <*2.24*>, and compare the spectrum with the Reference Spectrum: both spectra exhibit similar intensities of absorption at the same wavelengths.

(2) Determine the infrared absorption spectrum of Betamipron as directed in the potassium bromide disk method under Infrared Spectrophotometry <*2.25*>, and compare the spectrum with the Reference Spectrum: both spectra exhibit similar intensities of absorption at the same wave numbers.

pH <*2.54*> Dissolve 0.25 g of Betamipron in 100 mL of water by warming, and cool: the pH of this solution is between 3.0 and 3.4.

Melting point <*2.60*> 132 – 135°C

Purity (1) Clarity and color of solution—Dissolve 1.0 g of Betamipron in 10 mL of sodium hydroxide TS: the solution is clear and colorless.

(2) Heavy metals <*1.07*>—Proceed with 1.0 g of Betamipron according to Method 4, and perform the test. Prepare the control solution with 1.0 mL of Standard Lead Solution (not more than 10 ppm).

(3) β-Alanine—Dissolve 0.25 g of Betamipron in 10 mL of methanol, and use this solution as the sample solution. Separately, dissolve 50 mg of β-alanine in methanol to make exactly 100 mL. Pipet 1 mL of this solution, add methanol to make exactly 10 mL, and use this solution as the standard solution. Perform the test with these solutions as directed under Thin-layer Chromatography <*2.03*>. Spot 5 μL each of the sample solution and standard solution on a plate of silica gel for thin-layer chromatography, develop the plate with a mixture of methanol, ethyl acetate, ammonia solution (28) and water (200:200:63:37) to a distance of about 10 cm, and air-dry the plate. Spray evenly ninhydrin-butanol TS on the plate, and heat the plate at 105°C for 5 minutes: the spot obtained from the sample solution corresponding to the spot

from the standard solution is not more intense than the spot from the standard solution.

(4) Related substances—Dissolve 20 mg of Betamipron in 100 mL of the mobile phase, and use this solution as the sample solution. Pipet 1 mL of the sample solution, add the mobile phase to make exactly 200 mL, and use this solution as the standard solution. Perform the test with exactly 10 μL each of the sample solution and standard solution as directed under Liquid Chromatography *<2.01>* according to the following conditions, and determine each peak area by the automatic integration method: the area of the peak other than betamipron from the sample solution is not larger than 2/5 times the peak area of betamipron from the standard solution, and the total area of the peaks other than betamipron from the sample solution is not larger than the peak area of betamipron from the standard solution.

Operating conditions—

Detector: An ultraviolet absorption photometer (wavelength: 225 nm).

Column: A stainless steel column 6 mm in inside diameter and 15 cm in length, packed with octadecylsilanized silica gel for liquid chromatography (5 μm in particle diameter).

Column temperature: A constant temperature of about 40°C.

Mobile phase: Dissolve 3.12 g of sodium dihydrogen phosphate dihydrate in 800 mL of water, adjust to pH 7.0 with dilute sodium hydroxide TS, and add water to make 1000 mL. To 900 mL of this solution add 100 mL of acetonitrile.

Flow rate: Adjust so that the retention time of betamipron is about 6 minutes.

Time span of measurement: About 2 times as long as the retention time of betamipron, beginning after the solvent peak.

System suitability—

Test for required detectability: To exactly 1 mL of the standard solution add the mobile phase to make exactly 10 mL. Confirm that the peak area of betamipron obtained with 10 μL of this solution is equivalent to 7 to 13% of that with 10 μL of the standard solution.

System performance: Dissolve 5 mg of Betamipron and 5 mg of benzoic acid in 200 mL of the mobile phase. When the procedure is run with 10 μL of this solution under the above operating conditions, benzoic acid and betamipron are eluted in this order with the resolution between these peaks being not less than 5.

System repeatability: When the test is repeated 6 times with 10 μL of the standard solution under the above operating conditions, the relative standard deviation of the peak area of betamipron is not more than 2.0%.

Water *<2.48>* Not more than 0.5% (1 g, volumetric titration, direct titration).

Residue on ignition *<2.44>* Not more than 0.1% (1 g).

Assay Weigh accurately about 0.25 g of Betamipron, dissolve in 25 mL of ethanol (99.5), add 25 mL of water, and titrate *<2.50>* with 0.1 mol/L sodium hydroxide VS (potentiometric titration). Perform the blank determination in the same manner, and make any necessary correction.

Each mL of 0.1 mol/L sodium hydroxide VS
= 19.32 mg of $C_{10}H_{11}NO_3$

Containers and storage Containers—Tight containers.

Betaxolol Hydrochloride

ベタキソロール塩酸塩

and enantiomer

$C_{18}H_{29}NO_3.HCl$: 343.89
(2*RS*)-1-{4-[2-(Cyclopropylmethoxy)ethyl]phenoxy}-3-[(1-methylethyl)amino]propan-2-ol monohydrochloride
[*63659-19-8*]

Betaxolol Hydrochloride, when dried, contains not less than 99.0% and not more than 101.0% of betaxolol hydrochloride ($C_{18}H_{29}NO_3.HCl$).

Description Betaxolol Hydrochloride occurs as white, crystals or crystalline powder.

It is very soluble in water, and freely soluble in methanol, in ethanol (99.5) and in acetic acid (100).

Dissolve 1.0 g of Betaxolol Hydrochloride in 50 mL of water: the pH of the solution is between 4.5 and 6.5.

A solution of Betaxolol Hydrochloride (1 in 100) shows no optical rotation.

Identification **(1)** Determine the absorption spectrum of a solution of Betaxolol Hydrochloride in ethanol (99.5) (1 in 10,000) as directed under Ultraviolet-visible Spectrophotometry *<2.24>*, and compare the spectrum with the Reference Spectrum: both spectra exhibit similar intensities of absorption at the same wavelengths.

(2) Determine the infrared absorption spectrum of Betaxolol Hydrochloride as directed in the potassium chloride disk method under Infrared Spectrophotometry *<2.25>*, and compare the spectrum with the Reference Spectrum: both spectra exhibit similar intensities of absorption at the same wave numbers.

(3) A solution of Betaxolol Hydrochloride (1 in 10) responds to Qualitative Tests *<1.09>* (2) for chloride.

Melting point *<2.60>* 114 – 117°C

Purity **(1)** Clarity and color of solution—Dissolve 1.0 g of Betaxolol Hydrochloride in 10 mL of water: the solution is clear and colorless.

(2) Heavy metals *<1.07>*—Proceed with 2.0 g of Betaxolol Hydrochloride according to Method 4, and perform the test. Prepare the control solution with 2.0 mL of Standard Lead Solution (not more than 10 ppm).

(3) Arsenic *<1.11>*—Prepare the test solution with 2.0 g of Betaxolol Hydrochloride according to Method 3, and perform the test (not more than 1 ppm).

(4) Related substance I—Dissolve 0.10 g of Betaxolol Hydrochloride in 10 mL of methanol, and use this solution as the sample solution. Pipet 3 mL of the sample solution, and add methanol to make exactly 50 mL. Pipet 1 mL of this solution, add methanol to make exactly 20 mL, and use this solution as the standard solution. Perform the test with these solutions as directed under Thin-layer Chromatography *<2.03>*. Spot 10 μL each of the sample solution and standard solution on a plate of silica gel for thin-layer chromatography. Develop the plate with a mixture of ethyl acetate, water and acetic acid (100) (10:3:3) to a distance of about 10 cm, and air-dry the plate. Allow the plate to stand in iodine vapor for 1 hour: the number of the spots other than the principal spot obtained from the sample solution is not more than 3, and they are not more intense than the spot from the standard solution.

(5) Related substance II—Dissolve 0.10 g of Betaxolol Hydrochloride in 50 mL of the mobile phase, and use this solution as the sample solution. Pipet 1 mL of the sample solution, add the mobile phase to make exactly 200 mL, and use this solution as the standard solution. Perform the test with exactly 10 μL each of the sample solution and standard solution as directed under Liquid Chromatography <*2.01*> according to the following conditions. Determine each peak area of both solutions by the automatic integration method: the area of the peak other than betaxolol obtained from the sample solution is not larger than the peak area of betaxolol from the standard solution, and the total area of the peaks other than the peak of betaxolol from the sample solution is not larger than 2 times the peak area of betaxolol from the standard solution.

Operating conditions—

Detector: An ultraviolet absorption photometer (wavelength: 273 nm).

Column: A stainless steel column 4.6 mm in inside diameter and 15 cm in length, packed with octylsilanized silica gel for liquid chromatography (5 μm in particle diameter).

Column temperature: A constant temperature of about 25°C.

Mobile phase: A mixture of diluted 0.05 mol/L potassium dihydrogen phosphate TS (1 in 2) with the pH adjusted to 3.0 with 1 mol/L hydrochloric acid TS, acetonitrile and methanol (26:7:7).

Flow rate: Adjust so that the retention time of betaxolol is about 9 minutes.

Time span of measurement: About 2 times as long as the retention time of betaxolol, beginning after the solvent peak.

System suitability—

Test for required detectability: Pipet 4 mL of the standard solution, and add the mobile phase to make exactly 20 mL. Confirm that the peak area of betaxolol obtained with 10 μL of this solution is equivalent to 14 to 26% of that with 10 μL of the standard solution.

System performance: Dissolve 50 mg of Betaxolol Hydrochloride and 5 mg of 2-naphthol in 200 mL of the mobile phase. When the procedure is run with 10 μL of this solution under the above operating conditions, betaxolol and 2-naphthol are eluted in this order with the resolution between these peaks being not less than 10.

System repeatability: When the test is repeated 6 times with 10 μL of the standard solution under the above operating conditions, the relative standard deviation of the peak area of betaxolol is not more than 2.0%.

Loss on drying <*2.41*> Not more than 0.5% (1 g, 105°C, 4 hours).

Residue on ignition <*2.44*> Not more than 0.1% (1 g).

Assay Weigh accurately about 0.3 g of Betaxolol Hydrochloride, previously dried, dissolve in 30 mL of acetic acid (100), add 30 mL of acetic anhydride, and titrate <*2.50*> with 0.1 mol/L perchloric acid VS (potentiometric titration). Perform a blank determination in the same manner, and make any necessary correction.

Each mL of 0.1 mol/L perchloric acid VS
= 34.39 mg of $C_{18}H_{29}NO_3.HCl$

Containers and storage Containers—Tight containers.

Bethanechol Chloride

ベタネコール塩化物

and enantiomer

$C_7H_{17}ClN_2O_2$: 196.68
(2*RS*)-2-Carbamoyloxy-*N*,*N*,*N*-trimethylpropylaminium chloride
[*590-63-6*]

Bethanechol Chloride, when dried, contains not less than 98.0% and not more than 101.0% of bethanechol chloride ($C_7H_{17}ClN_2O_2$).

Description Bethanechol Chloride occurs as colorless or white crystals or a white, crystalline powder.

It is very soluble in water, freely soluble in acetic acid (100), and sparingly soluble in ethanol (99.5).

It is hygroscopic.

A solution of Bethanechol Chloride (1 in 10) shows no optical rotation.

Identification **(1)** To 2 mL of a solution of Bethanechol Chloride (1 in 40) add 0.1 mL of a solution of cobalt (II) chloride hexahydrate (1 in 100), then add 0.1 mL of potassium hexacyanoferrate (II) TS: A green color is produced, and almost entirely fades within 10 minutes.

(2) To 1 mL of a solution of Bethanechol Chloride (1 in 100) add 0.1 mL of iodine TS: a brown precipitate is produced, and the solution shows a greenish brown color.

(3) Determine the infrared absorption spectrum of Bethanechol Chloride as directed in the paste method under Infrared Spectrophotometry <*2.25*>, and compare the spectrum with the Reference Spectrum: both spectra exhibit similar intensities of absorption at the same wave numbers.

(4) A solution of Bethanechol Chloride (1 in 100) responds to Qualitative Tests <*1.09*> for chloride.

Melting point <*2.60*> 217 – 221°C (after drying).

Purity **(1)** Heavy metals <*1.07*>—Proceed with 1.0 g of Bethanechol Chloride according to Method 1, and perform the test. Prepare the control solution with 2.0 mL of Standard Lead Solution (not more than 20 ppm).

(2) Related substances—Dissolve 1.0 g of Bethanechol Chloride in 2.5 mL of water, and use this solution as the sample solution. Pipet 1 mL of the sample solution, add water to make exactly 100 mL, and use this solution as the standard solution. Perform the test with these solutions as directed under Thin-layer Chromatography <*2.03*>. Spot 1 μL each of the sample solution and standard solution on a plate of cellulose for thin-layer chromatography. Develop the plate with a mixture of a solution of ammonium acetate (1 in 100), acetone, 1-butanol and formic acid (20:20:20:1) to a distance of about 10 cm, and dry the plate at 105°C for 15 minutes. Spray evenly hydrogen hexachloroplatinate (IV)-potassium iodide TS on the plate, and allow to stand for 30 minutes: the spot other than the principal spot obtained from the sample solution is not more intense than the spot from the standard solution.

Loss on drying <*2.41*> Not more than 1.0% (1 g, 105°C, 2 hours).

Residue on ignition <*2.44*> Not more than 0.1% (1 g).

Assay Weigh accurately about 0.4 g of Bethanechol Chloride, previously dried, dissolve in 2 mL of acetic acid (100), add 40 mL of acetic anhydride, and titrate ⟨*2.50*⟩ with 0.1 mol/L perchloric acid VS (potentiometric titration). Perform a blank determination in the same manner, and make any necessary correction.

Each mL of 0.1 mol/L perchloric acid VS
= 19.67 mg of $C_7H_{17}ClN_2O_2$

Containers and storage Containers—Tight containers.

Bezafibrate

ベザフィブラート

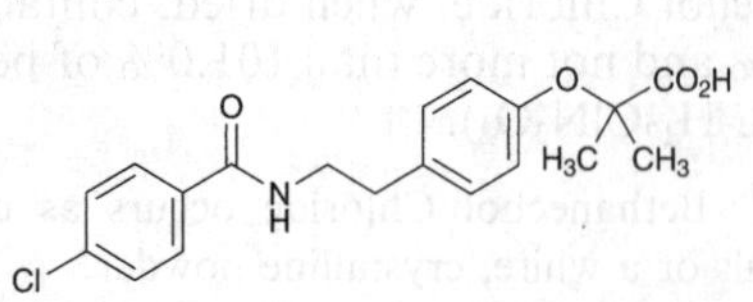

$C_{19}H_{20}ClNO_4$: 361.82
2-(4-{2-[(4-Chlorobenzoyl)amino]ethyl}phenoxy)-2-methylpropanoic acid
[41859-67-0]

Bezafibrate, when dried, contains not less than 98.5% and not more than 101.0% of bezafibrate ($C_{19}H_{20}ClNO_4$).

Description Bezafibrate occurs as a white crystalline powder.

It is freely soluble in *N*,*N*-dimethylformamide, soluble in methanol, slightly soluble in ethanol (99.5), and practically insoluble in water.

Identification (1) Determine the absorption spectrum of a solution of Bezafibrate in methanol (1 in 100,000) as directed under Ultraviolet-visible Spectrophotometry ⟨*2.24*⟩, and compare the spectrum with the Reference Spectrum: both spectra exhibit similar intensities of absorption at the same wavelengths.

(2) Determine the infrared absorption spectrum of Bezafibrate, previously dried, as directed in the potassium bromide disk method under Infrared Spectrophotometry ⟨*2.25*⟩, and compare the spectrum with the Reference Spectrum: both spectra exhibit similar intensities of absorption at the same wave numbers.

(3) Perform the test with Bezafibrate as directed under Flame Coloration Test ⟨*1.04*⟩ (2): a green color appears.

Melting point ⟨*2.60*⟩ 181 – 186°C

Purity (1) Chloride ⟨*1.03*⟩—Dissolve 3.0 g of Bezafibrate in 15 mL of *N*,*N*-dimethylformamide, add water to make 60 mL, shake well, allow to stand for more than 12 hours, and filter. To 40 mL of the filtrate add 6 mL of dilute nitric acid and water to make 50 mL, and perform the test using this solution as the test solution. Prepare the control solution as follows: To 0.70 mL of 0.01 mol/L hydrochloric acid VS add 10 mL of *N*,*N*-dimethylformamide, 6 mL of dilute nitric acid and water to make 50 mL (not more than 0.012%).

(2) Heavy metals ⟨*1.07*⟩—Proceed with 2.0 g of Bezafibrate according to Method 4, and perform the test. Prepare the control solution with 2.0 mL of Standard Lead Solution (not more than 10 ppm).

(3) Related substances—Dissolve 0.10 g of Bezafibrate in 35 mL of methanol, add diluted 0.5 mol/L ammonium acetate TS (1 in 50) to make 50 mL, and use this solution as the sample solution. Pipet 1 mL of the sample solution, add 70 mL of methanol and diluted 0.5 mol/L ammonium acetate TS (1 in 50) to make exactly 100 mL, and use this solution as the standard solution. Perform the test with exactly 5 μL each of the sample solution and standard solution as directed under Liquid Chromatography ⟨*2.01*⟩ according to the following conditions, and determine each peak area by the automatic integration method: the areas of the peaks having the relative retention times of about 0.65 and 1.86 to bezafibrate obtained from the sample solution are not larger than 1/2 times the peak area of bezafibrate from the standard solution, the area of the peaks other bezafibrate and the peaks mentioned above from the sample solution is not larger than 1/5 times the peak area of bezafibrate from the standard solution, and the total area of the peaks other than the peak of bezafibrate from the sample solution is not larger than 3/4 times the peak area of bezafibrate from the standard solution.

Operating conditions—

Detector: An ultraviolet absorption photometer (wavelength: 230 nm).

Column: A stainless steel column 4.6 mm in inside diameter and 15 cm in length, packed with octadecylsilanized silica gel for liquid chromatography (5 μm in particle diameter).

Column temperature: A constant temperature of about 25°C.

Mobile phase: A mixture of methanol and diluted acetic acid (100) (1 in 100) (9:4).

Flow rate: Adjust so that the retention time of bezafibrate is about 6 minutes.

Time span of measurement: About 2.5 times as long as the retention time of bezafibrate, beginning after the solvent peak.

System suitability—

Test for required detectability: Measure exactly 5 mL of the standard solution, and add a mixture of methanol and diluted 0.5 mol/L ammonium acetate TS (1 in 50) (7:3) to make exactly 50 mL. Confirm that the peak area of bezafibrate obtained with 5 μL of this solution is equivalent to 7 to 13% of that with 5 μL of the standard solution.

System performance: Dissolve 20 mg of Bezafibrate and 10 mg of 4-chlorobenzoate in 70 mL of methanol, and add diluted 0.5 mol/L ammonium acetate TS (1 in 50) to make 100 mL. When the procedure is run with 5 μL of this solution under the above operating conditions, 4-chlorobenzoate and bezafibrate are eluted in this order with the resolution between these peaks being not less than 3.

System repeatability: When the test is repeated 6 times with 5 μL of the standard solution under the above operating conditions, the relative standard deviation of the peak area of bezafibrate is not more than 2.0%.

Loss on drying ⟨*2.41*⟩ Not more than 0.5% (1 g, 105°C, 3 hours).

Residue on ignition ⟨*2.44*⟩ Not more than 0.1% (1 g).

Assay Weigh accurately about 0.7 g of Bezafibrate, previously dried, dissolve in 50 mL of ethanol (99.5), and titrate ⟨*2.50*⟩ with 0.1 mol/L sodium hydroxide VS (indicator: 3 drops of phenolphthalein TS). Perform a blank determination in the same manner, and make any necessary correction.

Each mL of 0.1 mol/L sodium hydroxide VS
= 36.18 mg of $C_{19}H_{20}ClNO_4$

Containers and storage Containers—Tight containers.

Bezafibrate Extended-release Tablets

ベザフィブラート徐放錠

Bezafibrate Extended-release Tablets contain not less than 95.0% and not more than 105.0% of the labeled amount of bezafibrate ($C_{19}H_{20}ClNO_4$: 361.82).

Method of preparation Prepare as directed under Tablets, with Bezafibrate.

Identification Mix well an amount of powdered Bezafibrate Extended-release Tablets, equivalent to 0.1 g of Bezafibrate, with 100 mL of methanol, and filter. To 1 mL of the filtrate add methanol to make 100 mL. Determine the absorption spectrum of this solution as directed under Ultraviolet-visible Spectrophotometry *<2.24>*: it exhibits a maximum between 227 nm and 231 nm.

Uniformity of dosage units *<6.02>* It meets the requirement of the Mass variation test.

Dissolution *<6.10>* When the test is performed at 50 revolutions per minute according to the Paddle method, using 900 mL of disodium hydrogen phosphate-citric acid buffer solution (pH 7.2) as the dissolution medium, the dissolution rates of a 100-mg tablet in 1.5 hours, in 2.5 hours and in 8 hours are 15 – 45%, 35 – 65% and not less than 80%, respectively, and those of a 200-mg tablet in 1.5 hours, in 2.5 hours and in 8 hours are 15 – 45%, 30 – 60% and not less than 75%, respectively.

Start the test with 1 tablet of Bezafibrate Extended-release Tablets, withdraw exactly 20 mL of the medium at the specified minutes after starting the test, and immediately fill up the dissolution medium each time with exactly 20 mL of fresh dissolution medium, previously warmed to 37 ± 0.5°C. Filter these media through a membrane filter with a pore size not exceeding 0.45 µm. Discard not less than 10 mL of the first filtrate, pipet the subsequent V mL, add the dissolution medium to make exactly V' mL so that each mL contains about 13 µg of bezafibrate ($C_{19}H_{20}ClNO_4$), and use these solutions as the sample solutions. Separately, weigh accurately about 66 mg of bezafibrate for assay, previously dried at 105°C for 3 hours, and dissolve in methanol to make exactly 50 mL. Pipet 2 mL of this solution, add the dissolution medium to make exactly 200 mL, and use this solution as the standard solution. Determine the absorbances, $A_{T(n)}$ (n = 1,2,3) and A_S, of the sample solutions and standard solution at 228 nm as directed under Ultraviolet-visible Spectrophotometry *<2.24>*, using the dissolution medium as the blank.

Dissolution rate (%) in each case of n with respect to the labeled amount of bezafibrate ($C_{19}H_{20}ClNO_4$)

$$= M_S \times \left\{\frac{A_{T(n)}}{A_S} + \sum_{i=1}^{n-1}\left(\frac{A_{T(i)}}{A_S} \times \frac{1}{45}\right)\right\} \times \frac{V'}{V} \times \frac{1}{C} \times 18$$

M_S: Amount (mg) of bezafibrate for assay taken
C: Labeled amount (mg) of bezafibrate ($C_{19}H_{20}ClNO_4$) in 1 tablet

Assay Weigh accurately, and powder not less than 20 Bezafibrate Extended-release Tablets. Weigh accurately a portion of the powder, equivalent to about 20 mg of bezafibrate ($C_{19}H_{20}ClNO_4$), add 60 mL of methanol and exactly 10 mL of the internal standard solution, and shake for 20 minutes. Add diluted 0.5 mol/L ammonium acetate TS (1 in 50) to make 100 mL, filter, and use the filtrate as the sample solution. Separately, weigh accurately about 20 mg of bezafibrate for assay, previously dried at 105°C for 3 hours, dissolve in 60 mL of methanol, add exactly 10 mL of the internal standard solution and diluted 0.5 mol/L ammonium acetate TS (1 in 50) to make 100 mL, and use this solution as the standard solution. Perform the test with 2 µL each of the sample solution and standard solution as directed under Liquid Chromatography *<2.01>* according to the following conditions, and calculate the ratios, Q_T and Q_S, of the peak area of bezafibrate to that of the internal standard.

Amount (mg) of bezafibrate ($C_{19}H_{20}ClNO_4$) = $M_S \times Q_T/Q_S$

M_S: Amount (mg) of bezafibrate for assay taken

Internal standard solution—A solution of 4-nitrophenol in methanol (1 in 500).
Operating conditions—

Detector: An ultraviolet absorption photometer (wavelength: 230 nm).

Column: A stainless steel column 4.6 mm in inside diameter and 15 cm in length, packed with octadecylsilanized silica gel for liquid chromatography (5 µm in particle diameter).

Column temperature: A constant temperature of about 25°C.

Mobile phase: A mixture of methanol and diluted acetic acid (100) (1 in 100) (9:4).

Flow rate: Adjust so that the retention time of bezafibrate is about 6 minutes.
System suitability—

System performance: When the procedure is run with 2 µL of the standard solution under the above operating conditions, the internal standard and bezafibrate are eluted in this order with the resolution between these peaks being not less than 4.

System repeatability: When the test is repeated 6 times with 2 µL of the standard solution under the above operating conditions, the relative standard deviation of the ratio of the peak area of bezafibrate to that of the internal standard is not more than 1.0%.

Containers and storage Containers—Tight containers.

Bicalutamide

ビカルタミド

and enantiomer

$C_{18}H_{14}F_4N_2O_4S$: 430.37
(2*RS*)-*N*-[4-Cyano-3-(trifluoromethyl)phenyl]-3-[(4-fluorophenyl)sulfonyl]-2-hydroxy-2-methylpropanamide
[90357-06-5]

Bicalutamide contains not less than 98.0% and not more than 102.0% of bicalutamide ($C_{18}H_{14}F_4N_2O_4S$), calculated on the dried basis.

Description Bicalutamide occurs as a white, powder or crystalline powder.

It is freely soluble in acetone, sparingly soluble in methanol, slightly soluble in ethanol (99.5), and practically insoluble in water.

A solution of Bicalutamide in acetone (1 in 100) shows no optical rotation.

Melting point <*2.60*> 192 – 197°C

Bicalutamide shows crystal polymorphism.

Identification (1) Determine the absorption spectrum of a solution of Bicalutamide in methanol (1 in 100,000) as directed under Ultraviolet-visible Spectrophotometry <*2.24*>, and compare the spectrum with the Reference Spectrum or the spectrum of a solution of Bicalutamide RS prepared in the same manner as the sample solution: both spectra exhibit similar intensities of absorption at the same wavelengths.

(2) Determine the infrared absorption spectrum of Bicalutamide as directed in the potassium bromide disk method under Infrared Spectrophotometry <*2.25*>, and compare the spectrum with the Reference Spectrum or the spectrum of Bicalutamide RS: both spectra exhibit similar intensities of absorption at the same wave numbers. Alternatively, perform the test by the ATR method, and compare the spectrum with the spectrum of Bicalutamide RS: both spectra exhibit similar intensities of absorption at the same wave numbers. If any difference appears between the spectra, recrystallize Bicalutamide and Bicalutamide RS with acetone, respectively, filter and dry the crystals, and perform the test by the potassium bromide disk method or the ATR method in the same manner.

Purity (1) Heavy metals <*1.07*>—Proceed with 2.0 g of Bicalutamide according to Method 2, and perform the test. Prepare the control solution with 2.0 mL of Standard Lead Solution (not more than 10 ppm).

(2) Related substances—Dissolve 25 mg of Bicalutamide in 25 mL of a mixture of water, acetonitrile and phosphoric acid (1000:1000:1), and use this solution as the sample solution. Pipet 1 mL of the sample solution, and add a mixture of water, acetonitrile and phosphoric acid (1000:1000:1) to make exactly 100 mL. Pipet 10 mL of this solution, add a mixture of water, acetonitrile and phosphoric acid (1000:1000:1) to make exactly 100 mL, and use this solution as the standard solution. Perform the test with exactly 10 μL each of the sample solution and standard solution as directed under Liquid Chromatography <*2.01*> according to the following conditions. Determine each peak area by the automatic integration method: the peak areas of related substance M, having the relative retention time of about 0.26 to bicalutamide, related substance N, having the relative retention time of about 0.34, related substance L, having the relative retention time of about 1.03 and related substance K, having the relative retention time of about 1.13, obtained from the sample solution, are not larger than the peak area of bicalutamide from the standard solution, and the area of the peak other than bicalutamide and the peaks mentioned above from the sample solution is not larger than the peak area of bicalutamide from the standard solution. Furthermore, the total area of the peaks other than bicalutamide from the sample solution is not larger than 5 times the peak area of bicalutamide from the standard solution. For the areas of the peaks, related substance G, having the relative retention times of about 0.21 and about 0.25, related substance I, having the relative retention time of about 0.23, related substance M, related substance N, related substance O, having the relative retention time of about 0.55, related substance A, having the relative retention time of about 0.95, and related substance L, and related substance P, having the relative retention time of about 1.09 from the sample solution, multiply their correction factors, 0.5, 0.5, 0.5, 0.4, 0.7, 0.5, 1.1, 0.9 and 0.7, respectively.

Operating conditions—

Detector, column, column temperature, mobile phase and flow rate: Proceed as directed in the operating conditions in the Assay.

Time span of measurement: For 47 minutes after injection, beginning after the solvent peak.

System suitability—

Test for required detectability: Pipet 5 mL of the standard solution, and add a mixture of water, acetonitrile and phosphoric acid (1000:1000:1) to make exactly 10 mL. When the procedure is run with 10 μL of this solution under the above operating conditions, the SN ratio of the peak of bicalutamide is not less than 10.

System performance: When the procedure is run with 10 μL of the standard solution under the above operating conditions, the number of theoretical plates and the symmetry factor of the peak of bicalutamide are not less than 10,000 and not more than 1.5, respectively.

System repeatability: When the test is repeated 6 times with 10 μL of the standard solution under the above operating conditions, the relative standard deviation of the peak area of bicalutamide is not more than 5.0%.

Loss on drying <*2.41*> Not more than 0.5% (1 g, 105°C, 4 hours).

Residue on ignition <*2.44*> Not more than 0.1% (1 g, platinum crucible).

Assay Weigh accurately about 25 mg each of Bicalutamide and Bicalutamide RS (separately determine the loss on drying <*2.41*> in the same conditions as Bicalutamide), and dissolve each in a mixture of water, acetonitrile and phosphoric acid (1000:1000 1) to make exactly 25 mL. Pipet 5 mL each of these solutions, add a mixture of water, acetonitrile and phosphoric acid (1000:1000:1) to make exactly 25 mL, and use these solutions as the sample solution and the standard solution, respectively. Perform the test with exactly 10 μL each of the sample solution and standard solution as directed under Liquid Chromatography <*2.01*> according to the following conditions, and determine the peak areas, A_T and A_S, of bicalutamide in each solution.

Amount (mg) of bicalutamide ($C_{18}H_{14}F_4N_2O_4S$)
$= M_S \times A_T/A_S$

M_S: Amount (mg) of Bicalutamide RS taken, calculated on the dried basis

Operating conditions—

Detector: An ultraviolet absorption photometer (wavelength: 210 nm).

Column: A stainless steel column 4 mm in inside diameter and 25 cm in length, packed with octadecylsilanized silica gel for liquid chromatography (5 μm in particle diameter).

Column temperature: A constant temperature of about 50°C.

Mobile phase A: A mixture of diluted phosphoric acid (1 in 1000) and acetonitrile for liquid chromatography (19:1).

Mobile phase B: A mixture of acetonitrile for liquid chromatography and diluted phosphoric acid (1 in 1000) (19:1).

Flowing of mobile phase: Control the gradient by mixing the mobile phases A and B as directed in the following table.

Time after injection of sample (min)	Mobile phase A (vol%)	Mobile phase B (vol%)
0 – 20	92 → 67	8 → 33
20 – 40	67 → 50	33 → 50
40 – 47	50	50

Flow rate: 1.0 mL per minute.

System suitability—

System performance: When the procedure is run with 10 μL of the standard solution under the above operating conditions, the number of theoretical plates and the symmetry factor of the peak of bicalutamide are not less than 10,000 and not more than 1.5, respectively.

System repeatability: When the test is repeated 6 times with 10 μL of the standard solution under the above operating conditions, the relative standard deviation of the peak area of bicalutamide is not more than 1.0%.

Containers and storage Containers—Well-closed containers.

Others

Related substance G:
(2*RS*)-3-[(*RS*)-(4-Fluorophenyl)sulfinyl]-2-hydroxy-2-methylpropanoic acid

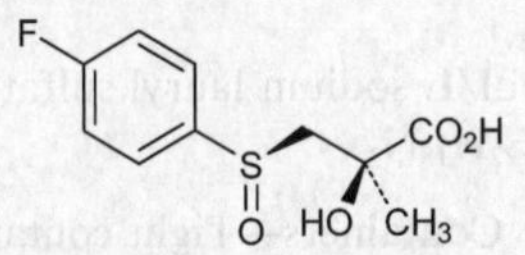

and enantiomer

(2*RS*)-3-[(*SR*)-(4-Fluorophenyl)sulfinyl]-2-hydroxy-2-methylpropanoic acid

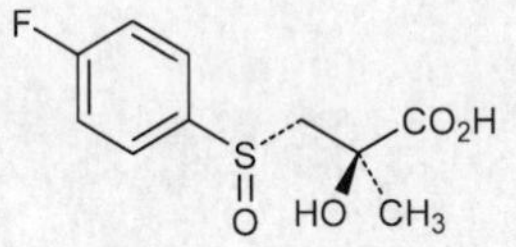

and enantiomer

Related substance I:
(2*RS*)-3-[(2-Fluorophenyl)sulfonyl]-2-hydroxy-2-methylpropanoic acid

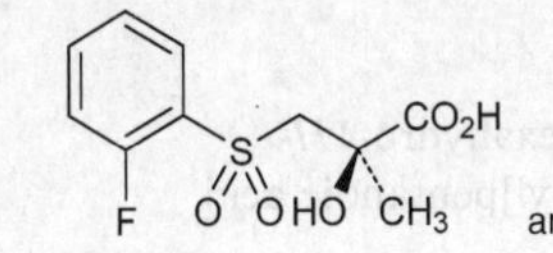

and enantiomer

Related substance M:
(2*RS*)-3-[(4-Fluorophenyl)sulfonyl]-2-hydroxy-2-methylpropanoic acid

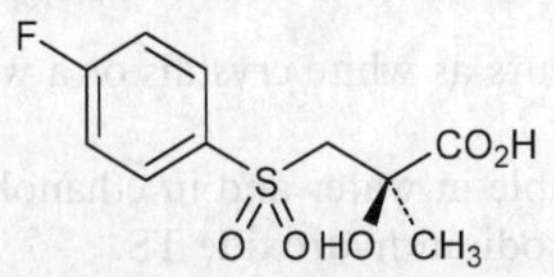

and enantiomer

Related substance N:
1-Fluoro-4-(methylsulfonyl)benzene

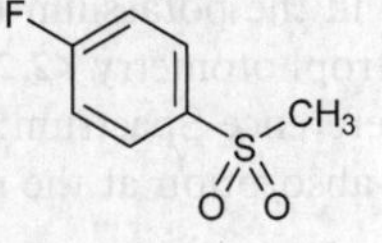

Related substance O:
(2*RS*)-3-[(4-Fluorophenyl)sulfanyl]-2-hydroxy-2-methylpropanoic acid

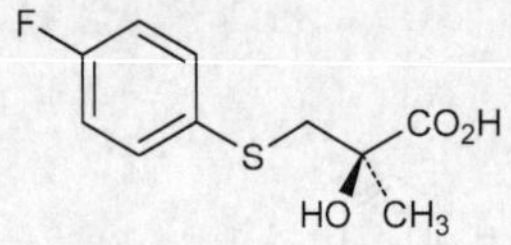

and enantiomer

Related substance A:
(2*RS*)-*N*-[4-Cyano-3-(trifluoromethyl)phenyl]-2-hydroxy-2-methyl-3-(phenylsulfonyl)propanamide

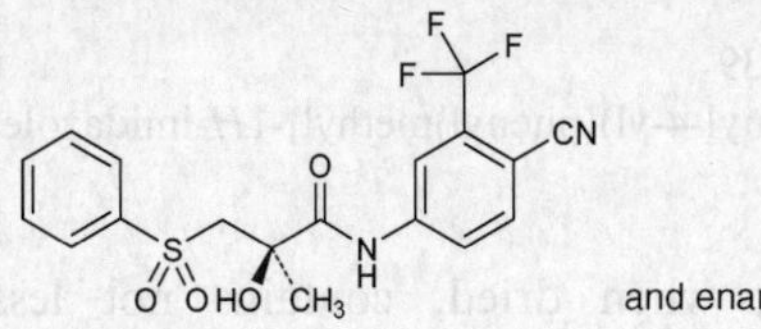

and enantiomer

Related substance L:
(2*RS*,2′*RS*)-3,3′-Sulfonylbis{*N*-[4-cyano-3-(trifluoromethyl)phenyl]-2-hydroxy-2-methylpropanamide}

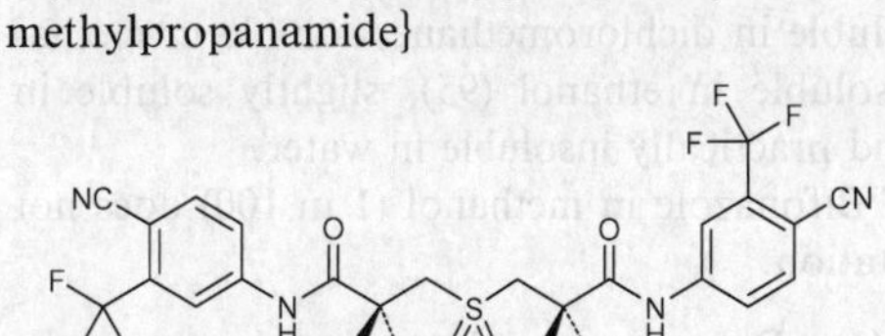

and enantiomer

Related substance P:
(2*RS*)-3-[(4-Fluorophenyl)sulfonyl]-2-hydroxy-2-methyl-*N*-[4-nitro-3-(trifluoromethyl)phenyl]propanamide

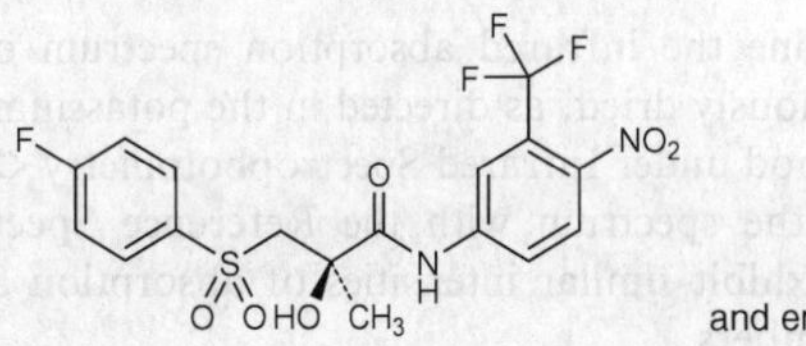

and enantiomer

Related substance K:
(2*R*,2′*S*)-3,3′-Sulfonylbis{*N*-[4-cyano-3-(trifluoromethyl)phenyl]-2-hydroxy-2-methylpropanamide}

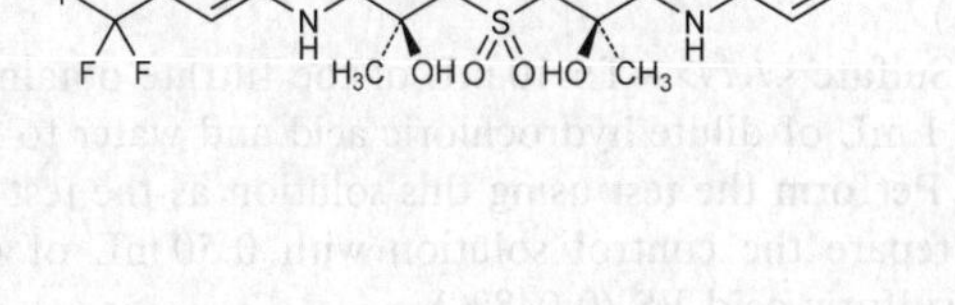

Bifonazole

ビホナゾール

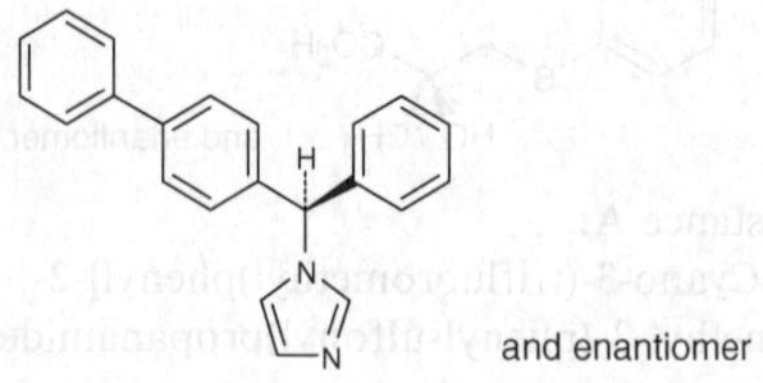

$C_{22}H_{18}N_2$: 310.39
1-[(*RS*)-(Biphenyl-4-yl)(phenyl)methyl]-1*H*-imidazole
[*60628-96-8*]

Bifonazole, when dried, contains not less than 98.5% of bifonazole ($C_{22}H_{18}N_2$).

Description Bifonazole occurs as a white to pale yellow powder. It is odorless and tasteless.

It is freely soluble in dichloromethane, soluble in methanol, sparingly soluble in ethanol (95), slightly soluble in diethyl ether, and practically insoluble in water.

A solution of Bifonazole in methanol (1 in 100) does not show optical rotation.

Identification **(1)** Determine the absorption spectrum of a solution of Bifonazole in methanol (1 in 100,000) as directed under Ultraviolet-visible Spectrophotometry 〈*2.24*〉, and compare the spectrum with the Reference Spectrum: both spectra exhibit similar intensities of absorption at the same wavelengths.

(2) Determine the infrared absorption spectrum of Bifonazole, previously dried, as directed in the potassium bromide disk method under Infrared Spectrophotometry 〈*2.25*〉, and compare the spectrum with the Reference Spectrum: both spectra exhibit similar intensities of absorption at the same wave numbers.

Melting point 〈*2.60*〉 147 – 151°C

Purity **(1)** Chloride 〈*1.03*〉—To 2.0 g of Bifonazole add 40 mL of water, warm for 5 minutes, and after cooling, filter. To 10 mL of the filtrate add 6 mL of dilute nitric acid and water to make 50 mL. Perform the test using this solution as the test solution. Prepare the control solution with 0.30 mL of 0.01 mol/L hydrochloric acid VS (not more than 0.021%).

(2) Sulfate 〈*1.14*〉—To 10 mL of the filtrate obtained in (1) add 1 mL of dilute hydrochloric acid and water to make 50 mL. Perform the test using this solution as the test solution. Prepare the control solution with 0.50 mL of 0.005 mol/L sulfuric acid VS (0.048%).

(3) Heavy metals 〈*1.07*〉—Proceed with 2.0 g of Bifonazole according to Method 2, and perform the test. Prepare the control solution with 2.0 mL of Standard Lead Solution (not more than 10 ppm).

(4) Related substances—Conduct this procedure without exposure to light, using light-resistant vessels. Dissolve 0.10 g of Bifonazole in 10 mL of methanol, and use this solution as the sample solution. Pipet 3 mL of the sample solution, and add methanol to make exactly 100 mL. Pipet 25 mL and 5 mL of this solution, add methanol to make exactly 50 mL each, and use these solutions as the standard solutions (1) and (2), respectively. Perform the test with these solutions as directed under Thin-layer Chromatography 〈*2.03*〉. Spot 10 μL each of the sample solution and standard solutions (1) and (2) on a plate of silica gel with fluorescent indicator for thin-layer chromatography. Develop the plate with a mixture of ethyl acetate and ammonia solution (28) (49:1) to a distance of about 10 cm, and air-dry the plate. Examine under ultraviolet light (main wavelength: 254 nm): the spot with *R*f value of about 0.20 obtained from the sample solution is not more intense than the spot from the standard solution (1). And the spots other than the spot mentioned above and the principal spot from the sample solution are not more intense than the spot from the standard solution (2).

Loss on drying 〈*2.41*〉 Not more than 0.5% (0.5 g, in vacuum, phosphorus (V) oxide, 2 hours).

Residue on ignition 〈*2.44*〉 Not more than 0.1% (1 g).

Assay Weigh accurately about 0.15 g of Bifonazole, previously dried, and dissolve in dichloromethane to make exactly 50 mL. Pipet 5 mL of this solution in a glass-stoppered conical flask, add 10 mL of water, 5 mL of dilute sulfuric acid and 25 mL of dichloromethane, and add 2 to 3 drops of a solution of methyl yellow in dichloromethane (1 in 500) as indicator, and titrate 〈*2.50*〉, while shaking vigorously, with 0.01 mol/L sodium lauryl sulfate VS by a buret with 0.02-mL minimum graduation. The end point is reached when the color of the dichloromethane layer changes from yellow to orange-red after dropwise addition of 0.01 mol/L sodium lauryl sulfate VS, strong shaking, and standing for a while.

Each mL of 0.01 mol/L sodium lauryl sulfate VS
= 3.104 mg of $C_{22}H_{18}N_2$

Containers and storage Containers—Tight containers.
Storage—Light-resistant.

Biotin

ビオチン

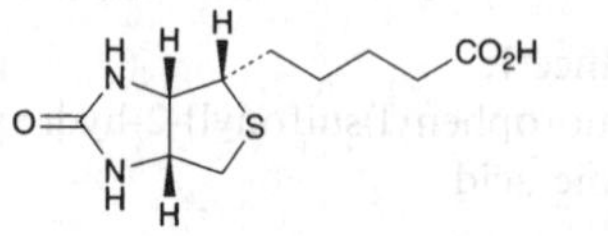

$C_{10}H_{16}N_2O_3S$: 244.31
5-[(3a*S*,4*S*,6a*R*)-2-Oxohexahydro-1*H*-thieno[3,4-*d*]imidazol-4-yl]pentanoic acid
[*58-85-5*]

Biotin, when dried, contains not less than 98.5% and not more than 101.0% of biotin ($C_{10}H_{16}N_2O_3S$).

Description Biotin occurs as white crystals or a white crystalline powder.

It is very slightly soluble in water and in ethanol (99.5).

It dissolves in dilute sodium hydroxide TS.

Melting point: about 231°C (with decomposition).

Identification Determine the infrared absorption spectrum of Biotin as directed in the potassium bromide disc method under Infrared Spectrophotometry 〈*2.25*〉, and compare the spectrum with the Reference Spectrum: both spectra exhibit similar intensities of absorption at the same wave numbers.

Optical rotation 〈*2.49*〉 $[\alpha]_D^{20}$: +89 – +93° (after drying, 0.4 g, dilute sodium hydroxide TS, 20 mL, 100 mm).

Purity **(1)** Clarity and color of solution—Dissolve 1.0 g of Biotin in 10 mL of 0.5 mol/L sodium hydroxide TS: the solution is clear and colorless.

(2) Heavy metals 〈*1.07*〉—Proceed with 2.0 g of Biotin

according to Method 2, and perform the test. Prepare the control solution with 2.0 mL of Standard Lead Solution (not more than 10 ppm).

(3) Arsenic *⟨1.11⟩*—Place 0.7 g of Biotin in a Kjeldahl flask, add 5 mL of nitric acid and 2 mL of sulfuric acid, place a small funnel on the mouth of the flask, and carefully heat until white fumes are evolved. After cooling, add 2 mL of nitric acid twice, heat, add 2 mL of hydrogen peroxide (30) several times, and heat until the color of the solution becomes colorless or pale yellow. After cooling, add 2 mL of saturated ammonium oxalate solution, and heat to concentrate until white fumes are evolved again. After cooling, add water to make 5 mL, and perform the test using this solution as the test solution (not more than 2.8 ppm).

(4) Related substances—Dissolve 0.10 g of Biotin in 10 mL of diluted ammonia solution (28) (7 in 100), and use this solution as the sample solution. Pipet 1 mL of the sample solution, and add diluted ammonia solution (28) (7 in 100) to make exactly 100 mL. Pipet 10 mL of this solution, add diluted ammonia solution (28) (7 in 100) to make exactly 50 mL, and use this solution as the standard solution. Perform the test with these solutions as directed under Thin-layer Chromatography *⟨2.03⟩*. Spot 5 μL each of the sample solution and standard solution on a plate of silica gel for thin-layer chromatography. Develop the plate with a mixture of 1-butanol, water, and acetic acid (100) (5:2:1) to a distance of about 10 cm, air-dry the plate, and then dry for 30 minutes at 105°C. Spray the plate evenly with a mixture of a solution of 4-dimethylaminocinnamaldehyde in ethanol (99.5) (1 in 500) and a solution of sulfuric acid in ethanol (99.5) (1 in 50) (1:1): the spots other than the principal spot obtained from the sample solution are not more intense than the spot from the standard solution.

Loss on drying *⟨2.41⟩* Not more than 0.5% (0.5 g, 105°C, 4 hours).

Residue on ignition *⟨2.44⟩* Not more than 0.1% (1 g).

Assay Weigh accurately about 0.25 g of Biotin, previously dried, dissolve by adding exactly 20 mL of 0.1 mol/L sodium hydroxide VS, and titrate *⟨2.50⟩* the excess sodium hydroxide with 0.1 mol/L hydrochloric acid VS (indicator: 2 drops of phenolphthalein TS). Perform a blank determination in the same manner.

Each mL of 0.1 mol/L sodium hydroxide VS
= 24.43 mg of $C_{10}H_{16}N_2O_3S$

Containers and storage Containers—Tight containers.

Biperiden Hydrochloride

ビペリデン塩酸塩

$C_{21}H_{29}NO.HCl$: 347.92
1-(Bicyclo[2.2.1]hept-5-en-2-yl)-1-phenyl-3-(piperidin-1-yl)propan-1-ol monohydrochloride
[1235-82-1]

Biperiden Hydrochloride, when dried, contains not less than 99.0% of biperiden hydrochloride ($C_{21}H_{29}NO.HCl$).

Description Biperiden Hydrochloride occurs as a white to brownish yellow-white crystalline powder.

It is freely soluble in formic acid, slightly soluble in water, in methanol and in ethanol (95), and practically insoluble in diethyl ether.

Melting point: about 270°C (with decomposition).

Identification **(1)** Dissolve 0.02 g of Biperiden Hydrochloride in 5 mL of phosphoric acid: a green color develops.

(2) Dissolve 0.01 g of Biperiden Hydrochloride in 5 mL of water by heating, cool, and add 5 to 6 drops of bromine TS: a yellow precipitate is formed.

(3) Determine the absorption spectrum of a solution of Biperiden Hydrochloride (1 in 2000) as directed under Ultraviolet-visible Spectrophotometry *⟨2.24⟩*, and compare the spectrum with the Reference Spectrum: both spectra exhibit similar intensities of absorption at the same wavelengths.

(4) Determine the infrared absorption spectrum of Biperiden Hydrochloride, previously dried, as directed in the potassium chloride disk method under Infrared Spectrophotometry *⟨2.25⟩*, and compare the spectrum with the Reference Spectrum: both spectra exhibit similar intensities of absorption at the same wave numbers.

(5) Dissolve 0.02 g of Biperiden Hydrochloride in 10 mL of water by heating, and cool: the solution responds to Qualitative Tests *⟨1.09⟩* for chloride.

Purity **(1)** Acidity or alkalinity—To 1.0 g of Biperiden Hydrochloride add 50 mL of water, shake vigorously, filter, and to 20 mL of the filtrate add 1 drop of methyl red TS: no red to yellow color develops.

(2) Heavy metals *⟨1.07⟩*—Proceed with 1.0 g of Biperiden Hydrochloride according to Method 2, and perform the test. Prepare the control solution with 2.0 mL of Standard Lead Solution (not more than 20 ppm).

(3) Arsenic *⟨1.11⟩*—Prepare the test solution with 1.0 g of Biperiden Hydrochloride according to Method 3, and perform the test (not more than 2 ppm).

(4) Related substances—Dissolve 0.10 g of Biperiden Hydrochloride in 20 mL of methanol, and use this solution as the sample solution. Pipet 1 mL of the sample solution, add methanol to make exactly 200 mL, and use this solution as the standard solution. Perform the test with these solutions as directed under Thin-layer Chromatography *⟨2.03⟩*. Spot 50 μL each of the sample solution and standard solution on a plate of silica gel for thin-layer chromatography. Develop the plate with a mixture of chloroform, methanol and ammonia solution (28) (80:15:2) to a distance of about 15 cm, and air-dry the plate. Spray evenly Dragendorff's TS for spraying on the plate: the spots other than the principal spot obtained from the sample solution are not more intense than the spot from the standard solution.

Loss on drying *⟨2.41⟩* Not more than 0.5% (1 g, 105°C, 3 hours).

Residue on ignition *⟨2.44⟩* Not more than 0.1% (1 g).

Assay Weigh accurately about 0.4 g of Biperiden Hydrochloride, previously dried, dissolve in 5 mL of formic acid, add 60 mL of acetic anhydride, and titrate *⟨2.50⟩* with 0.1 mol/L perchloric acid VS (potentiometric titration). Perform a blank determination in the same manner, and make any necessary correction.

Each mL of 0.1 mol/L perchloric acid VS
= 34.79 mg of $C_{21}H_{29}NO.HCl$

Containers and storage Containers—Well-closed contain-

ers.

Storage—Light-resistant.

Bisacodyl

ビサコジル

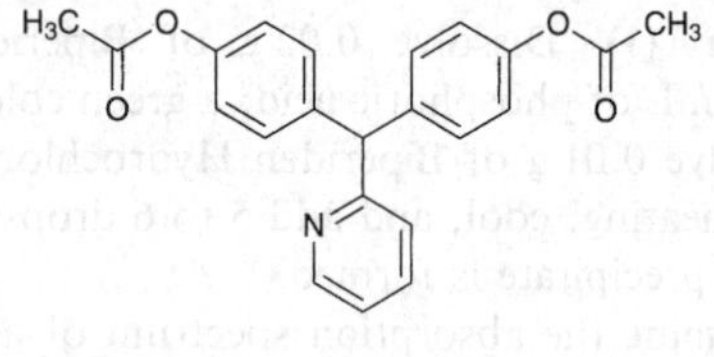

$C_{22}H_{19}NO_4$: 361.39
4,4′-(Pyridin-2-ylmethylene)bis(phenyl acetate)
[603-50-9]

Bisacodyl, when dried, contains not less than 98.5% of bisacodyl ($C_{22}H_{19}NO_4$).

Description Bisacodyl occurs as a white crystalline powder.

It is freely soluble in acetic acid (100), soluble in acetone, slightly soluble in ethanol (95) and in diethyl ether, and practically insoluble in water.

It dissolves in dilute hydrochloric acid.

Identification **(1)** Determine the absorption spectrum of a solution of Bisacodyl in ethanol (95) (3 in 100,000) as directed under Ultraviolet-visible Spectrophotometry *<2.24>*, and compare the spectrum with the Reference Spectrum or the spectrum of a solution of Bisacodyl RS prepared in the same manner as the sample solution: both spectra exhibit similar intensities of absorption at the same wavelengths.

(2) Determine the infrared absorption spectrum of Bisacodyl, previously dried, as directed in the potassium bromide disk method under Infrared Spectrophotometry *<2.25>*, and compare the spectrum with the Reference Spectrum or the spectrum of dried Bisacodyl RS: both spectra exhibit similar intensities of absorption at the same wave numbers.

Melting point *<2.60>* 132 – 136°C

Purity **(1)** Chloride *<1.03>*—Dissolve 1.0 g of Bisacodyl in 30 mL of acetone, and add 6 mL of dilute nitric acid and water to make 50 mL. Perform the test using this solution as the test solution. Prepare the control solution as follows: to 0.35 mL of 0.01 mol/L hydrochloric acid VS add 30 mL of acetone, 6 mL of dilute nitric acid and water to make 50 mL (not more than 0.012%).

(2) Sulfate *<1.14>*—Dissolve 1.0 g of Bisacodyl in 2 mL of dilute hydrochloric acid, and add water to make 50 mL. Perform the test using this solution as the test solution. Prepare the control solution as follows: to 0.35 mL of 0.005 mol/L sulfuric acid VS add 2 mL of dilute hydrochloric acid and water to make 50 mL (not more than 0.017%).

(3) Heavy metals *<1.07>*—Proceed with 2.0 g of Bisacodyl according to Method 4, and perform the test. Prepare the control solution with 2.0 mL of Standard Lead Solution (not more than 10 ppm).

(4) Related substances—Dissolve 0.20 g of Bisacodyl in 10 mL of acetone, and use this solution as the sample solution. Pipet 1 mL of the sample solution, add acetone to make exactly 200 mL, and use this solution as the standard solution. Perform the test with these solutions as directed under Thin-layer Chromatography *<2.03>*. Spot 10 μL each of the sample solution and standard solution on a plate of silica gel with fluorescent indicator for thin-layer chromatography. Develop the plate with a mixture of 2-butanone, chloroform and xylene (1:1:1) to a distance of about 10 cm, and air-dry the plate. Examine under ultraviolet light (main wavelength: 254 nm): the spots other than the principal spot obtained from the sample solution are not more intense than the spot from the standard solution.

Loss on drying *<2.41>* Not more than 0.5% (1 g, 105°C, 2 hours).

Residue on ignition *<2.44>* Not more than 0.1% (1 g).

Assay Weigh accurately about 0.5 g of Bisacodyl, previously dried, dissolve in 50 mL of acetic acid (100), and titrate *<2.50>* with 0.1 mol/L perchloric acid VS until the color of the solution changes from orange-yellow to green (indicator: 0.5 mL of *p*-naphtholbenzein TS). Perform a blank determination in the same manner, and make any necessary correction.

Each mL of 0.1 mol/L perchloric acid VS
= 36.14 mg of $C_{22}H_{19}NO_4$

Containers and storage Containers—Well-closed containers.

Bisacodyl Suppositories

ビサコジル坐剤

Bisacodyl Suppositories contain not less than 90.0% and not more than 110.0% of the labeled amount of bisacodyl ($C_{22}H_{19}NO_4$: 361.39).

Method of preparation Prepare as directed under Suppositories, with Bisacodyl.

Identification **(1)** To a quantity of Bisacodyl Suppositories, equivalent to 6 mg of Bisacodyl, add 20 mL of ethanol (95), warm on a water bath for 10 minutes, shake vigorously for 10 minutes, and allow to stand in ice water for 1 hour. Centrifuge the solution, filter the supernatant liquid, and to 2 mL of the filtrate add ethanol (95) to make 20 mL. Determine the absorption spectrum of the solution as directed under Ultraviolet-visible Spectrophotometry *<2.24>*: it exhibits a maximum between 261 nm and 265 nm.

(2) Use the filtrate obtained in (1) as the sample solution. Separately, dissolve 6 mg of Bisacodyl RS in 20 mL of ethanol (95), and use this solution as the standard solution. Perform the test with these solutions as directed under Thin-layer Chromatography *<2.03>*. Spot 20 μL each of the sample solution and standard solution on a plate of silica gel with fluorescent indicator for thin-layer chromatography. Develop the plate with a mixture of 2-butanone, chloroform and xylene (1:1:1) to a distance of about 10 cm, and air-dry the plate. Examine under ultraviolet light (main wavelength: 254 nm): the spot obtained from the sample solution and that from the standard solution show the same *Rf* value.

Uniformity of dosage units *<6.02>* Perform the test according to the following method: it meets the requirement of the Content uniformity test.

To 1 suppository of Bisacodyl Suppositories add a suitable amount of tetrahydrofuran, warm to 40°C, and shake to dissolve. After cooling, add tetrahydrofuran to make exactly V mL so that each mL contains about 0.2 mg of bisacodyl ($C_{22}H_{19}NO_4$). Pipet 5 mL of this solution, and proceed as directed in the Assay.

Amount (mg) of bisacodyl ($C_{22}H_{19}NO_4$)
$= M_S \times Q_T/Q_S \times V/50$

M_S: Amount (mg) of Bisacodyl RS taken

Internal standard solution—A solution of ethyl parahydroxybenzoate in acetonitrile (3 in 100,000).

Assay Weigh accurately not less than 20 Bisacodyl Suppositories, make them fine fragments carefully, and mix uniformly. Weigh accurately a portion of the fragments, equivalent to about 10 mg of bisacodyl ($C_{22}H_{19}NO_4$), add 40 mL of tetrahydrofuran, warm to 40°C, dissolve by shaking, cool, and add tetrahydrofuran to make exactly 50 mL. Pipet 5 mL of this solution, add exactly 5 mL of the internal standard solution, and add the mobile phase to make 100 mL. Cool this solution in ice for 30 minutes, centrifuge, filter the supernatant liquid through a membrane filter with pore size of 0.5 μm, discard the first 10 mL of the filtrate, and use the subsequent filtrate as the sample solution. Separately, weigh accurately about 10 mg of Bisacodyl RS, previously dried at 105°C for 2 hours, and dissolve in tetrahydrofuran to make exactly 50 mL. Pipet 5 mL of this solution, proceed in the same manner as the sample solution, and use this solution as the standard solution. Perform the test with 20 μL each of the sample solution and standard solution as directed under Liquid Chromatography *<2.01>* according to the following conditions, and calculate the ratios, Q_T and Q_S, of the peak area of bisacodyl to that of the internal standard.

$$\text{Amount (mg) of bisacodyl } (C_{22}H_{19}NO_4) = M_S \times Q_T/Q_S$$

M_S: Amount (mg) of Bisacodyl RS taken

Internal standard solution—A solution of ethyl parahydroxybenzoate in acetonitrile (3 in 100,000).

Operating conditions—

Detector: An ultraviolet absorption photometer (wavelength: 254 nm).

Column: A stainless steel column 4 mm in inside diameter and 30 cm in length, packed with octadecylsilanized silica gel for liquid chromatography (10 μm in particle diameter).

Column temperature: A constant temperature of about 25°C.

Mobile phase: A mixture of 0.01 mol/L citric acid TS, acetonitrile and methanol (2:1:1).

Flow rate: Adjust so that the retention time of bisacodyl is about 8 minutes.

System suitability—

System performance: When the procedure is run with 20 μL of the standard solution under the above operating conditions, the internal standard and bisacodyl are eluted in this order with the resolution between these peaks being not less than 2.0.

System repeatability: When the test is repeated 6 times with 20 μL of the standard solution under the above operating conditions, the relative standard deviation of the ratios of the peak area of bisacodyl to that of the internal standard is not more than 1.0%.

Containers and storage Containers—Tight containers.

Bismuth Subgallate

次没食子酸ビスマス

Bismuth Subgallate, when dried, contains not less than 47.0% and not more than 51.0% of bismuth (Bi: 208.98).

Description Bismuth Subgallate occurs as a yellow powder. It is odorless and tasteless.

It is practically insoluble in water, in ethanol (95) and in diethyl ether.

It dissolves in dilute hydrochloric acid, in dilute nitric acid and in dilute sulfuric acid on warming. It dissolves in sodium hydroxide TS, forming a clear, yellow solution, which turns red immediately.

It is affected by light.

Identification **(1)** Ignite 0.5 g of Bismuth Subgallate: it chars at first, and leaves finally a yellow residue. The residue responds to Qualitative Tests *<1.09>* for bismuth salt.

(2) To 0.5 g of Bismuth Subgallate add 25 mL of water and 20 mL of hydrogen sulfide TS, and shake well. Filter off the blackish brown precipitate, and add 1 drop of iron (III) chloride TS to the filtrate: a blue-black color is produced.

Purity **(1)** Clarity of solution—Dissolve 1.0 g of Bismuth Subgallate in 40 mL of diluted sodium hydroxide TS (1 in 8): the solution is clear.

(2) Sulfate—Ignite 3.0 g of Bismuth Subgallate in a porcelain crucible, and cautiously dissolve the residue in 2.5 mL of nitric acid by warming. Pour the solution into 100 mL of water, shake, and filter. Evaporate 50 mL of the filtrate on a water bath to 15 mL. Add water to make 20 mL, filter again, and use the filtrate as the sample solution. To 5 mL of the sample solution add 2 to 3 drops of barium nitrate TS: no turbidity is produced.

(3) Nitrate—To 0.5 g of Bismuth Subgallate add 5 mL of dilute sulfuric acid and 25 mL of iron (II) sulfate TS, shake well, and filter. Superimpose carefully 5 mL of the filtrate on sulfuric acid: no red-brown color develops at the zone of contact.

(4) Ammonium—Dissolve 1.0 g of Bismuth Subgallate in 5 mL of sodium hydroxide TS, and heat: the gas evolved does not change moistened red litmus paper to blue.

(5) Copper—To 5 mL of the sample solution obtained in (2) add 1 mL of ammonia TS, and filter: no blue color develops in the filtrate.

(6) Lead—Ignite 1.0 g of Bismuth Subgallate at about 500°C in a porcelain crucible, dissolve the residue in a smallest possible amount of nitric acid added dropwise, evaporate over a low flame to dryness , and cool. Add 5 mL of a solution of potassium hydroxide (1 in 6) to the residue, boil carefully for 2 minutes, cool, and centrifuge. Take the supernatant liquid in a test tube, add 10 drops of potassium chromate TS, and acidify the solution by adding acetic acid (100) dropwise: neither turbidity nor a yellow precipitate is produced.

(7) Silver—To 5 mL of the sample solution obtained in (2) add 0.5 mL of nitric acid and 2 to 3 drops of dilute hydrochloric acid: no turbidity is produced.

(8) Alkaline earth metals and alkali metals—Boil 1.0 g of Bismuth Subgallate with 40 mL of diluted acetic acid (31) (1 in 2) for 2 minutes, cool, add water to make 40 mL, and filter. To 20 mL of the filtrate add 2 mL of dilute hydrochloric acid, boil, immediately pass hydrogen sulfide thoroughly through the solution, filter the precipitate produced, and wash with water. Combine the filtrate and the washings, add 5 drops of sulfuric acid, and evaporate to dryness. Ignite as directed under Residue on Ignition *<2.44>*: the mass of the residue is not more than 5.0 mg.

(9) Arsenic *<1.11>*—Mix well 0.20 g of Bismuth Subgallate with 0.20 g of calcium hydroxide, and ignite the mixture. Dissolve the residue in 5 mL of dilute hydrochloric acid, use this solution as the test solution, and perform the test (not more than 10 ppm).

(10) Gallic acid—To 1.0 g of Bismuth Subgallate add 20 mL of ethanol (95), shake for 1 minute, and filter.

Evaporate the filtrate on a water bath to dryness: the mass of the residue is not more than 5.0 mg.

Loss on drying *<2.41>* Not more than 6.0% (1 g, 105°C, 3 hours).

Assay Weigh accurately about 0.5 g of Bismuth Subgallate, previously dried, ignite at about 500°C for 30 minutes, and cool. Dissolve the residue in 5 mL of diluted nitric acid (2 in 5) by warming, and add water to make exactly 100 mL. Measure exactly 30 mL of this solution, add 200 mL of water, and titrate *<2.50>* with 0.02 mol/L disodium dihydrogen ethylenediamine tetraacetate VS until the color of the solution changes from red-purple to yellow (indicator: 2 to 3 drops of xylenol orange TS).

Each mL of 0.02 mol/L disodium dihydrogen ethylenediamine tetraacetate VS
= 4.180 mg of Bi

Containers and storage Containers—Well-closed containers.

Storage—Light-resistant.

Bismuth Subnitrate

次硝酸ビスマス

Bismuth Subnitrate, when dried, contains not less than 71.5% and not more than 74.5% of bismuth (Bi: 208.98).

Description Bismuth Subnitrate occurs as a white powder.

It is practically insoluble in water, in ethanol (95) and in diethyl ether.

It readily dissolves in hydrochloric acid and in nitric acid without effervescence.

It is slightly hygroscopic, and changes moistened blue litmus paper to red.

Identification Bismuth Subnitrate responds to Qualitative Tests *<1.09>* for bismuth salt and nitrate.

Purity **(1)** Chloride *<1.03>*—Dissolve 0.7 g of Bismuth Subnitrate in 2 mL of water and 2 mL of nitric acid, and add 6 mL of dilute nitric acid and water to make 50 mL. Perform the test using this solution as the test solution. Prepare the control solution as follows: evaporate 2 mL of nitric acid on a water bath to dryness, add 0.70 mL of 0.01 mol/L hydrochloric acid VS, 6 mL of dilute nitric acid and water to make 50 mL (not more than 0.035%).

(2) Sulfate—Dissolve 3.0 g of Bismuth Subnitrate in 3.0 mL of warmed nitric acid, pour this solution into 100 mL of water, shake, and filter. Concentrate the filtrate on a water bath to 30 mL, filter, and use this filtrate as the sample solution. To 5 mL of the sample solution add 2 to 3 drops of barium nitrate TS: no turbidity is produced.

(3) Ammonium—Boil 0.10 g of bismuth Subnitrate with 5 mL of sodium hydroxide TS: the gas evolved does not change moistened red litmus paper to blue.

(4) Copper—To 5 mL of the sample solution obtained in (2) add 2 mL of ammonia TS, and filter: no blue color develops.

(5) Lead—To 1.0 g of Bismuth Subnitrate add 5 mL of a solution of sodium hydroxide (1 in 6), boil carefully for 2 minutes, cool and centrifuge. Transfer the supernatant liquid to a test tube, add 10 drops of potassium chromate TS, and add dropwise acetic acid (31) to render the solution acid: no turbidity or yellow precipitate is produced.

(6) Silver—To 5 mL of the sample solution obtained in (2) add 0.5 mL of nitric acid and 2 to 3 drops of dilute hydrochloric acid: no turbidity is produced.

(7) Alkaline earth metals and alkali metals—Boil 2.0 g of Bismuth Subnitrate with 40 mL of diluted acetic acid (31) (1 in 2) for 2 minutes, cool, add water to make 40 mL, and filter. To 20 mL of the filtrate add 2 mL of dilute hydrochloric acid, boil, immediately pass hydrogen sulfide thoroughly through the solution, filter, and wash the residue with water. Combine the filtrate and the washings, add 5 drops of sulfuric acid, evaporate to dryness, and ignite as directed under Residue on Ignition *<2.44>*: the residue is not exceed 5.0 mg

(8) Arsenic *<1.11>*—To 0.20 g of Bismuth Subnitrate add 2 mL of sulfuric acid, heat until white fumes evolve, dilute cautiously with water to 5 mL, use this solution as the test solution, and perform the test (not more than 10 ppm).

Loss on drying *<2.41>* Not more than 3.0% (2 g, 105°C, 2 hours).

Assay Weigh accurately about 0.4 g of Bismuth Subnitrate, previously dried, dissolve in 5 mL of diluted nitric acid (2 in 5) by warming, and add water to make exactly 100 mL. Pipet 25 mL of the solution, add 200 mL of water and titrate *<2.50>* with 0.02 mol/L disodium dihydrogen ethylenediamine tetraacetate VS until the color of the solution changes from red-purple to yellow (indicator: 5 drops of xylenol orange TS)

Each mL of 0.02 mol/L disodium dihydrogen ethylenediamine tetraacetate VS
= 4.180 mg of Bi

Containers and storage Containers—Well-closed containers.

Bisoprolol Fumarate

ビソプロロールフマル酸塩

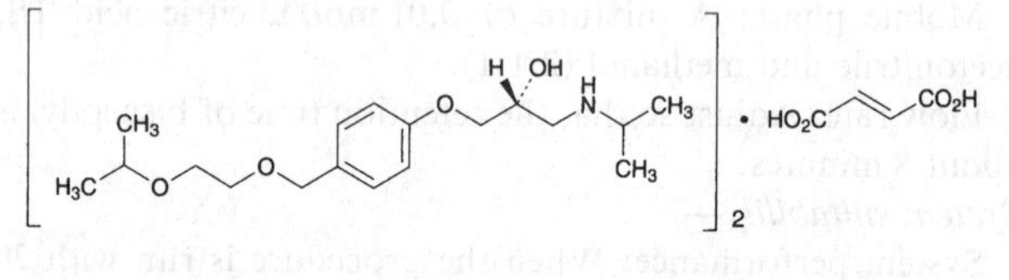

and enantiomer

$(C_{18}H_{31}NO_4)_2.C_4H_4O_4$: 766.96
(2*RS*)-1-(4-{[2-(1-Methylethoxy)ethoxy]methyl}phenoxy)-3-[(1-methylethyl)amino]propan-2-ol hemifumarate
[*104344-23-2*]

Bisoprolol Fumarate, when dried, contains not less than 98.5% and not more than 101.0% of bisoprolol fumarate $[(C_{18}H_{31}NO_4)_2.C_4H_4O_4]$.

Description Bisoprolol Fumarate occurs as white crystals or a white crystalline powder.

It is very soluble in water and in methanol, and freely soluble in ethanol (99.5) and in acetic acid (100).

A solution of Bisoprolol Fumarate (1 in 10) shows no optical rotation.

Identification **(1)** Determine the absorption spectrum of a solution of Bisoprolol Fumarate in methanol (1 in 10,000) as directed under Ultraviolet-visible Spectrophotometry *<2.24>*, and compare the spectrum with the Reference Spectrum: both spectra exhibit similar intensities of absorption at the same wavelengths.

(2) Determine the infrared absorption spectrum of Bisoprolol Fumarate as directed in the potassium bromide disc method under Infrared Spectrophotometry <*2.25*>, and compare the spectrum with the Reference Spectrum: both spectra exhibit similar intensities of absorption at the same wave numbers.

Melting point <*2.60*> 101 – 105°C

Purity **(1)** Heavy metals <*1.07*>—Proceed with 2.0 g of Bisoprolol Fumarate according to Method 2, and perform the test. Prepare the control solution with 2.0 mL of Standard Lead Solution (not more than 10 ppm).

(2) Related substances—Dissolve 50 mg of Bisoprolol Fumarate in 100 mL of a mixture of water and acetonitrile (4:1), and use this solution as the sample solution. Pipet 1 mL of the sample solution, add the mixture of water and acetonitrile (4:1) to make exactly 100 mL, and use this solution as the standard solution. Perform the test with exactly 20 μL each of the sample solution and standard solution as directed under Liquid Chromatography <*2.01*> according to the following conditions. Determine each peak area of both solutions by the automatic integration method: the area of the peaks other than bisoprolol obtained from the sample solution is not larger than 1/2 times the peak area of bisoprolol from the standard solution. Furthermore, the total of the areas of peaks other than bisoprolol from the sample solution is not larger than the peak area of bisoprolol from the standard solution.

Operating conditions—

Detector: An ultraviolet absorption photometer (wavelength: 225 nm).

Column: A stainless steel column 4.6 mm in inside diameter and 15 cm in length, packed with octylsilanized silica gel for liquid chromatography (5 μm in particle diameter).

Column temperature: A constant temperature of about 40°C.

Mobile phase: Dissolve 4.08 g of potassium dihydrogen phosphate in 1000 mL of water, and adjust to pH 2.5 with phosphoric acid. To 800 mL of this solution add 200 mL of acetonitrile.

Flow rate: Adjust so that the retention time of bisoprolol is about 8 minutes.

Time span of measurement: About 2 times as long as the retention time of bisoprolol, beginning after the fumaric acid peak.

System suitability—

Test for required detectability: Pipet 2 mL of the standard solution, and add a mixture of water and acetonitrile (4:1) to make exactly 20 mL. Confirm that the peak area of bisoprolol obtained with 20 μL of this solution is equivalent to 7 to 13% of that with 20 μL of the standard solution.

System performance: When the procedure is run with 20 μL of the standard solution under the above operating conditions, the number of theoretical plates and the symmetry factor of the peak of bisoprolol are not less than 5000 and not more than 1.5, respectively.

System repeatability: When the test is repeated 6 times with 20 μL of the standard solution under the above operating conditions, the relative standard deviation of the peak area of bisoprolol is not more than 1.5%.

Loss on drying <*2.41*> Not more than 0.5% (1 g, in vacuum, phosphorus (V) oxide, 80°C, 5 hours).

Residue on ignition <*2.44*> Not more than 0.1% (1 g).

Assay Weigh accurately about 0.6 g of Bisoprolol Fumarate, previously dried, dissolve in 70 mL of acetic acid (100), and titrate <*2.50*> with 0.1 mol/L perchloric acid VS (indicator: 2 drops of crystal violet TS). The endpoint of titration is when the purple color of the solution turns blue and then blue-green. Perform a blank determination in the same manner, and make any necessary correction.

Each mL of 0.1 mol/L perchloric acid VS
= 38.35 mg of $(C_{18}H_{31}NO_4)_2.C_4H_4O_4$

Containers and storage Containers—Tight containers.

Bisoprolol Fumarate Tablets

ビソプロロールフマル酸塩錠

Bisoprolol Fumarate Tablets contain not less than 95.0% and not more than 105.0% of the labeled amount of bisoprolol fumarate $[(C_{18}H_{31}NO_4)_2.C_4H_4O_4$: 766.96].

Method of preparation Prepare as directed under Tablets, with Bisoprolol Fumarate.

Identification To a quantity of powdered Bisoprolol Fumarate Tablets, equivalent to 10 mg of Bisoprolol Fumarate, add 60 mL of methanol, shake vigorously for 10 minutes, add methanol to make 100 mL, and filter through a membrane filter with a pore size not exceeding 0.45 μm. Determine the absorption spectrum of the filtrate as directed under Ultraviolet-visible Spectrophotometry <*2.24*>: it exhibits a maximum between 271 nm and 275 nm.

Purity Related substances—This is applied to 0.625-mg tablets. Shake vigorously for 10 minutes a portion of powdered Bisoprolol Fumarate Tablets, equivalent to 5 mg of Bisoprolol Fumarate, with exactly 20 mL of a mixture of water and acetonitrile (3:1), filter through a membrane filter with a pore size not exceeding 0.45 μm. Discard the first 3 mL of the filtrate, and use the subsequent filtrate as the sample solution. Perform the test with 20 μL of the sample solution as directed under Liquid Chromatography <*2.01*> according to the following conditions. Determine each peak area by the automatic integration method, and calculate the amount of the peak other than bisoprolol and the peak having the relative retention time of about 0.8 to bisoprolol by the area percentage method: the amount of the two peaks, having relative retention time of about 1.2 and about 3.8 to bisoprolol, are not more than 1.0%, respectively, the amount of the peak other than the peaks mentioned above is not more than 0.2%, and the total amount of the peaks other than bisoprolol is not more than 2.5%. For the area of the peak, having the relative retention time of about 1.2 to bisoprolol, multiply the correction factor 5.

Operating conditions—

Detector, column, column temperature, and flow rate: Proceed as directed in the operating conditions in the Assay.

Mobile phase: Dissolve 4.08 g of potassium dihydrogen phosphate in water to make 1000 mL, and adjust to pH 2.5 with phosphoric acid. To 750 mL of this solution add 250 mL of acetonitrile.

Time span of measurement: About 5 times as long as the retention time of bisoprolol, beginning after the peak of fumaric acid.

System suitability—

Test for required detectability: To 1 mL of the sample solution add a mixture of water and acetonitrile (3:1) to make 100 mL, and use this solution as the solution for system suitability test. Pipet 2 mL of the solution for system suitability test, and add a mixture of water and acetonitrile (3:1) to make exactly 20 mL. Confirm that the peak area of bisoprolol obtained with 20 μL of this solution is equivalent to 7 to 13% of that with 20 μL of the solution for system suitability test.

System performance: When the procedure is run with 20 μL of the solution for system suitability test under the above operating conditions, the number of theoretical plates and the symmetry factor of the peak of bisoprolol are not less than 5000 and not more than 2.0, respectively.

System repeatability: When the test is repeated 6 times with 20 μL of the solution for system suitability test under the above operating conditions, the relative standard deviation of the peak area of bisoprolol is not more than 1.5%.

Uniformity of dosage units <*6.02*> Perform the test according to the following method: it meets the requirement of the Content uniformity test.

Take 1 tablet of Bisoprolol Fumarate Tablets, disintegrate by adding 8 mL of water, and add water to make exactly 10 mL, and then filter through a membrane filter with a pore size not exceeding 0.45 μm. Discard the first 3 mL of the filtrate, pipet V mL of the subsequent filtrate, add water to make exactly V' mL so that each mL contains about 62.5 μg of bisoprolol fumarate [$(C_{18}H_{31}NO_4)_2.C_4H_4O_4$], and use this solution as the sample solution. Separately, weigh accurately about 20 mg of bisoprolol fumarate for assay, previously dried under reduced pressure at 80°C for 5 hours, using phosphorus (V) oxide as a dessicant, and dissolve in water to make exactly 200 mL. Pipet 15 mL of this solution, add water to make exactly 25 mL, and use this solution as the standard solution. Determine the absorbances, A_T and A_S, at 271.5 nm of the sample solution and standard solution as directed under Ultraviolet-visible Spectrophotometry <*2.24*>.

Amount (mg) of bisoprolol fumarate [$(C_{18}H_{31}NO_4)_2.C_4H_4O_4$]
$$= M_S \times A_T/A_S \times V'/V \times 3/100$$

M_S: Amount (mg) of bisoprolol fumarate for assay taken

Dissolution <*6.10*> When the test is performed at 50 revolutions per minute according to the Paddle method, using 900 mL of 2nd fluid for dissolution test as the dissolution medium, the dissolution rate in 30 minutes of Bisoprolol Fumarate Tablets is not less than 85%.

Start the test with 1 tablet of Bisoprolol Fumarate Tablets, withdraw not less than 20 mL of the medium at the specified minute after starting the test, and filter through a membrane filter with a pore size not exceeding 0.45 μm. Discard not less than 10 mL of the first filtrate, pipet V mL of the subsequent filtrate, add the dissolution medium to make exactly V' mL so that each mL contains about 0.7 μg of bisoprolol fumarate [$(C_{18}H_{31}NO_4)_2.C_4H_4O_4$], and use this solution as the sample solution. Separately, weigh accurately about 14 mg of bisoprolol fumarate for assay, previously dried in vacuum at 80°C for 5 hours, using phosphorus (V) oxide as a dessicant, and dissolve in the dissolution medium to make exactly 100 mL. Pipet 1 mL of this solution, add the dissolution medium to make exactly 200 mL, and use this solution as the standard solution. Perform the test with exactly 50 μL each of the sample solution and standard solution as directed under Liquid Chromatography <*2.01*>, and determine the peak areas, A_T and A_S, of bisoprolol in each solution.

Dissolution rate (%) with respect to the labeled amount of bisoprolol fumarate [$(C_{18}H_{31}NO_4)_2.C_4H_4O_4$]
$$= M_S \times A_T/A_S \times V'/V \times 1/C \times 9/2$$

M_S: Amount (mg) of bisoprolol fumarate for assay taken
C: Labeled amount (mg) of bisoprolol fumarate [$(C_{18}H_{31}NO_4)_2.C_4H_4O_4$] in 1 tablet

Operating conditions—

Detector, column, column temperature, and flow rate: Proceed as directed in the operating conditions in the Assay.

Mobile phase: Dissolve 4.08 g of potassium dihydrogen phosphate in 1000 mL of water, and adjust to pH 2.5 with phosphoric acid. To 750 mL of this solution add 250 mL of acetonitrile.

System suitability—

System performance: When the procedure is run with 50 μL of the standard solution under the above operating conditions, the number of theoretical plates and the symmetry factor of the peak of bisoprolol are not less than 3000 and not more than 2.0, respectively.

System repeatability: When the test is repeated 6 times with 50 μL of the standard solution under the above operating conditions, the relative standard deviation of the peak area of bisoprolol is not more than 2.0%.

Assay Weigh accurately not less than 20 Bisoprolol Fumarate Tablets and powder. Weigh accurately a portion of the powder, equivalent to about 20 mg of bisoprolol fumarate [$(C_{18}H_{31}NO_4)_2.C_4H_4O_4$], add 70 mL of a mixture of water and acetonitrile (3:1) and exactly 10 mL of the internal standard solution, shake vigorously for 10 minutes, and add the mixture of water and acetonitrile (3:1) to make 100 mL. Filter this solution through a membrane filter with a pore size not exceeding 0.45 μm, discard the first 3 mL of the filtrate, and use the subsequent filtrate as the sample solution. Separately, weigh accurately about 20 mg of bisoprolol fumarate for assay, previously dried in vacuum at 80°C for 5 hours using phosphorus (V) oxide as the dessicant, add exactly 10 mL of the internal standard solution, dissolve in the mixture of water and acetonitrile (3:1) to make 100 mL, and use this solution as the standard solution. Perform the test with 20 μL each of the sample solution and standard solution as directed under Liquid Chromatography <*2.01*> according to the following conditions, and calculate the ratios, Q_T and Q_S, of the peak area of bisoprolol to that of the internal standard.

Amount (mg) of bisoprolol fumarate [$(C_{18}H_{31}NO_4)_2.C_4H_4O_4$]
$$= M_S \times Q_T/Q_S$$

M_S: Amount (mg) of bisoprolol fumarate for assay taken

*Internal standard solution—*A solution of isopropyl parahydroxybenzoate in the mixture of water and acetonitrile (3:1) (1 in 250).

Operating conditions—

Detector: An ultraviolet absorption photometer (wavelength: 225 nm).

Column: A stainless steel column 4.6 mm in inside diameter and 15 cm in length, packed with octylsilanized silica gel for liquid chromatography (5 μm in particle diameter).

Column temperature: A constant temperature of about 40°C.

Mobile phase: Dissolve 4.08 g of potassium dihydrogen phosphate in 1000 mL of water, and adjust to pH 2.5 with phosphoric acid. To 800 mL of this solution add 200 mL of acetonitrile.

Flow rate: Adjust so that the retention time of bisoprolol is about 8 minutes.

System suitability—

System performance: When the procedure is run with 20 μL of the standard solution under the above operating con-

ditions, fumaric acid, bisoprolol and the internal standard are eluted in this order with the resolution between the peaks of bisoprolol and the internal standard being not less than 12.

System repeatability: When the test is repeated 6 times with 20 μL of the standard solution under the above operating conditions, the relative standard deviation of the ratio of the peak area of bisoprolol to that of the internal standard is not more than 1.0%.

Containers and storage Containers—Tight containers.

Bleomycin Hydrochloride

ブレオマイシン塩酸塩

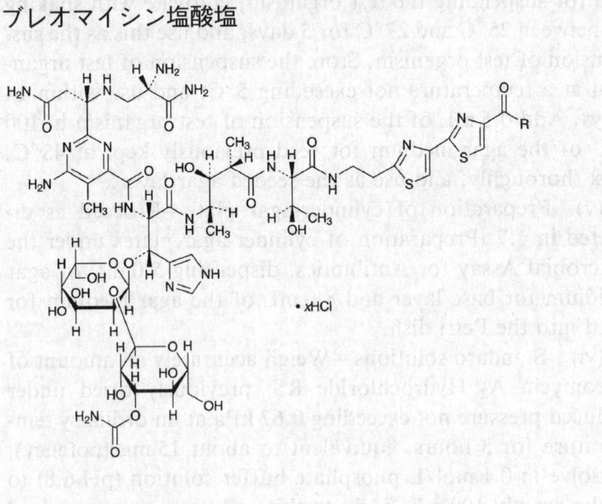

Bleomycinoic Acid hydrochloride
1-Bleomycinoic acid hydrochloride

Bleomycin A_1 hydrochloride
N^1-[3-(Methylsulfinyl)propyl]bleomycinamide hydrochloride

Bleomycin Demethyl-A_2 hydrochloride
N^1-[3-(Methylsulfanyl)propyl]bleomycinamide hydrochloride

Bleomycin A_2 hydrochloride
N^1-[3-(Dimethylsulfonio)propyl]bleomycinamide hydrochloride

Bleomycin $A_{2'\text{-a}}$ hydrochloride
N^1-(4-Aminobutyl)bleomycinamide hydrochloride

Bleomycin $A_{2'\text{-b}}$ hydrochloride
N^1-(3-Aminopropyl)bleomycinamide hydrochloride

Bleomycin A_5 hydrochloride
N^1-{3-[(4-Aminobutyl)amino]propyl}bleomycinamide hydrochloride

Bleomycin $B_{1'}$ hydrochloride
Bleomycinamide hydrochloride

Bleomycin B_2 hydrochloride
N^1-(4-Guanidinobutyl)bleomycinamide hydrochloride

Bleomycin B_4 hydrochloride
N^1-{4-[3-(4-Guanidinobutyl)guanidino]butyl}-bleomycinamide hydrochloride
[*11056-06-7*, Bleomycin]

Bleomycin Hydrochloride is the hydrochloride of a mixture of substances having antitumor activity produced by the growth of *Streptomyces verticillus*.

It contains not less than 1400 μg (potency) and not more than 2000 μg (potency) per mg, calculated on the dried basis. The potency of Bleomycin Hydrochloride is expressed as mass (potency) of bleomycin A_2 ($C_{55}H_{84}ClN_{17}O_{21}S_3$: 1451.00).

Description Bleomycin Hydrochloride occurs as a white to yellow-white powder.

It is freely soluble in water, and slightly soluble in ethanol (95).

It is hygroscopic.

Identification (1) To 4 mg of Bleomycin Hydrochloride add 5 μL of copper (II) sulfate TS, and dissolve in water to make 100 mL. Determine the absorption spectrum of this solution as directed under Ultraviolet-visible Spectrophotometry <*2.24*>, and compare the spectrum with the Reference Spectrum: both spectra exhibit similar intensities of absorption at the same wavelengths.

(2) Determine the infrared absorption spectrum of Bleomycin Hydrochloride as directed in the potassium bromide disk method under Infrared Spectrophotometry <*2.25*>, and compare the spectrum with the Reference Spectrum: both spectra exhibit similar intensities of absorption at the same wave numbers.

(3) A solution of Bleomycin Hydrochloride (1 in 100) responds to Qualitative Tests <*1.09*> (2) for chloride.

pH <*2.54*> The pH of a solution obtained by dissolving 0.10 g of Bleomycin Hydrochloride in 20 mL of water is between 4.5 and 6.0.

Content ratio of the active principle Dissolve 10 mg of Bleomycin Hydrochloride in 20 mL of water, and use this solution as the sample solution. Perform the test with 20 μL of the sample solution as directed under Liquid Chromatography <*2.01*> according to the following conditions, and determine each peak area by the automatic integration method, and calculate their amounts by the area percentage method: the amount of the peak of bleomycin A_2 (the first principal peak) is between 55% and 70%, that of bleomycin B_2 (the second principal peak) is between 25% and 32%, the total amount of the peak of bleomycin A_2 and bleomycin B_2 is not less than 85%, the amount of the peak of demethylbleomycin A_2 (a peak having the relative retention time of 1.5 – 2.5 to bleomycin A_2) is not more than 5.5%, and the total amount of the rest peaks is not more than 9.5%.

Operating conditions—

Detector: An ultraviolet absorption photometer (wavelength: 254 nm).

Column: A stainless steel column 4.6 mm in inside diameter and 25 cm in length, packed with octadecylsilanized silica gel for liquid chromatography (7 μm in particle diameter).

Column temperature: A constant temperature of about 40°C.

Mobile phase stock solution: Dissolve 0.96 g of sodium 1-pentanesulfonate and 1.86 g of disodium dihydrogen ethylenediamine tetraacetate dihydrate in 1000 mL of water and 5 mL of acetic acid (100), and adjust the pH to 4.3 with ammonia TS.

Mobile phase A: A mixture of the mobile phase stock solution and methanol (9:1).

Mobile phase B: A mixture of the mobile phase stock solution and methanol (3:2).

Flowing of mobile phase: Control the gradient by mixing the mobile phases A and B as directed in the following table.

Time after injection of sample (min)	Mobile phase A (vol%)	Mobile phase B (vol%)
0 – 60	100 → 0	0 → 100
60 – 75	0	100

Flow rate: About 1.2 mL per minute.

Time span of measurement: 20 minutes after elution of the peak of demethylbreomycin A_2, beginning after the solvent peak.

System suitability—

System performance: When the procedure is run with 20 μL of the sample solution under the above operating conditions, bleomycin A_2 and bleomycin B_2 are eluted in this order with the resolution between these peaks being not less than 5.

System repeatability: When the test is repeated 6 times with 20 μL of the sample solution under the above operating conditions, the relative standard deviation of the peak area of bleomycin A_2 is not more than 2.0%.

Purity **(1)** Clarity and color of solution—A solution obtained by dissolving 80 mg of Bleomycin Hydrochloride in 4 mL of water is clear and colorless.

(2) Copper—Dissolve exactly 75 mg of Bleomycin Hydrochloride in exactly 10 mL of diluted nitric acid (1 in 100), and use this solution as the sample solution. Separately, to exactly 15 mL of Standard Copper Solution add diluted nitric acid (1 in 100) to make exactly 100 mL, and use this solution as the standard solution. Perform the test with the sample solution and standard solution as directed under Atomic Absorption Spectrophotometry <2.23> according to the following conditions: the absorbance of the sample solution is not more than that of the standard solution (not more than 200 ppm).

Gas: Combustible gas—Acetylene.

Supporting gas—Air.

Lamp: Copper hollow-cathode lamp.

Wavelength: 324.8 nm.

Loss on drying <*2.41*> Not more than 5.0% (60 mg, in vacuum, phosphorus (V) oxide, 60°C, 3 hours. Take the sample to be tested while avoiding moisture absorption).

Assay Perform the test according to the Cylinder-plate method as directed under Microbial Assay for Antibiotics <*4.02*> according to the following conditions.

(i) Test organism—*Mycobacterium smegmatis* ATCC 607

(ii) Agar medium for seed, base layer and transferring the test organism

Glycerin	10.0 g
Peptone	10.0 g
Meat extract	10.0 g
Sodium chloride	3.0 g
Agar	15.0 g
Water	1000 mL

Mix all the components, and sterilize. Adjust the pH after sterilization to 6.9 – 7.1 with sodium hydroxide TS.

(iii) Liquid media for suspending the test organism

Glycerin	10.0 g
Peptone	10.0 g
Meat extract	10.0 g
Sodium chloride	3.0 g
Water	1000 mL

Mix all the components, and sterilize. Adjust the pH after sterilization to 6.9 – 7.1 with sodium hydroxide TS.

(iv) Preparation of seeded agar layer—Cultivate the test organism on the slant of the agar medium for transferring the test organism at 27°C for 40 to 48 hours, then inoculate the test organism thus obtained in 100 mL of the liquid media for suspending the test organism, cultivate with shaking at between 25°C and 27°C for 5 days, and use this as the suspension of test organism. Store the suspension of test organism at a temperature not exceeding 5°C, and use within 14 days. Add 0.5 mL of the suspension of test organism in 100 mL of the agar medium for seed previously kept at 48°C, mix thoroughly, and use as the seeded agar layer.

(v) Preparation of cylinder-agar plate—Proceed as directed in 1.7. Preparation of cylinder-agar plates under the Microbial Assay for Antibiotics, dispensing 5.0 mL of agar medium for base layer and 8.0 mL of the agar medium for seed into the Petri dish.

(vi) Standard solutions—Weigh accurately an amount of Bleomycin A_2 Hydrochloride RS, previously dried under reduced pressure not exceeding 0.67 kPa at an ordinary temperature for 3 hours, equivalent to about 15 mg (potency), dissolve in 0.1 mol/L phosphate buffer solution (pH 6.8) to make exactly 100 mL, and use this solution as the standard stock solution. Keep the standard stock solution at 5°C or below, and use within 30 days. Take exactly a suitable amount of the standard stock solution before use, add 0.1 mol/L phosphate buffer solution (pH 6.8) to make solutions so that each mL contains 30 μg (potency) and 15 μg (potency), and use these solutions as the high concentration standard solution and low concentration standard solution, respectively.

(vii) Sample solutions—Weigh accurately an amount of Bleomycin Hydrochloride, equivalent to about 15 mg (potency), and dissolve in 0.1 mol/L phosphate buffer solution (pH 6.8) to make exactly 100 mL. Take exactly a suitable amount of this solution, add 0.1 mol/L phosphate buffer solution (pH 6.8) to make solutions so that each mL contains 30 μg (potency) and 15 μg (potency), and use these solutions as the high concentration sample solution and low concentration sample solution, respectively.

Containers and storage Containers—Tight containers.

Bleomycin Sulfate

ブレオマイシン硫酸塩

Bleomycinoic Acid sulfate
1-Bleomycinoic acid sulfate

Bleomycin A_1 sulfate
N^1-[3-(Methylsulfinyl)propyl]bleomycinamide sulfate

Bleomycin Demethyl-A_2 sulfate
N^1-[3-(Methylsulfanyl)propyl]bleomycinamide sulfate

Bleomycin A_2 sulfate
N^1-[3-(Dimethylsulfonium)propyl]bleomycinamide sulfate

Bleomycin $A_{2'\text{-a}}$ sulfate
N^1-(4-Aminobutyl)bleomycinamide sulfate

Bleomycin $A_{2'\text{-b}}$ sulfate
N^1-(3-Aminopropyl)bleomycinamide sulfate

Bleomycin A_5 sulfate
N^1-{3-[(4-Aminobutyl)amino]propyl}bleomycinamide sulfate

Bleomycin $B_1{}'$ sulfate
Bleomycinamide sulfate

Bleomycin B_2 sulfate
N^1-(4-Guanidinobutyl)bleomycinamide sulfate

Bleomycin B_4 sulfate
N^1-{4-[3-(4-Guanidinobutyl)guanidino]butyl}-bleomycinamide sulfate
[*9041-93-4*, Bleomycin Sulfate]

Bleomycin Sulfate is the sulfate of a mixture of substances having antitumor activity produced by the growth of *Streptomyces verticillus*.

It contains not less than 1400 μg (potency) and not more than 2000 μg (potency) per mg, calculated on the dried basis. The potency of Bleomycin Sulfate is expressed as mass (potency) of bleomycin A_2 ($C_{55}H_{84}ClN_{17}O_{21}S_3$: 1451.00).

Description Bleomycin Sulfate occurs as a white to yellow-white powder.

It is freely soluble in water, and slightly soluble in ethanol (95).

It is hygroscopic.

Identification **(1)** To 4 mg of Bleomycin Sulfate add 5 μL of copper (II) sulfate TS, and dissolve in water to make 100 mL. Determine the absorption spectrum of this solution as directed under Ultraviolet-visible Spectrophotometry <*2.24*>, and compare the spectrum with the Reference Spectrum: both spectra exhibit similar intensities of absorption at the same wavelengths.

(2) Determine the infrared absorption spectrum of Bleomycin Sulfate as directed in the potassium bromide disk method under Infrared Spectrophotometry <*2.25*>, and compare the spectrum with the Reference Spectrum: both spectra exhibit similar intensities of absorption at the same wave numbers.

(3) A solution of Bleomycin Sulfate (1 in 200) responds to Qualitative Tests <*1.09*> (1) and (2) for sulfate.

pH <*2.54*> The pH of a solution obtained by dissolving 10 mg of Bleomycin Sulfate in 20 mL of water is between 4.5 and 6.0.

Content ratio of the active principle Dissolve 10 mg of Bleomycin Sulfate in 20 mL of water, and use this solution as the sample solution. Perform the test with 20 μL of the sample solution as directed under Liquid Chromatography <*2.01*> according to the following conditions, and determine each peak area by the automatic integration method, and calculate their amounts by the area percentage method: the amount of the peak of bleomycin A_2 (the first principal peak) is between 55% and 70%, that of bleomycin B_2 (the second principal peak) is between 25% and 32%, the total amount of the peak of bleomycin A_2 and bleomycin B_2 is not less than 85%, the amount of the peak of demethylbleomycin A_2 (a peak having the relative retention time of 1.5 – 2.5 to bleomycin A_2) is not more than 5.5%, and the total amount of the rest peaks is not more than 9.5%.

Operating conditions—

Detector: An ultraviolet absorption photometer (wavelength: 254 nm).

Column: A stainless steel column 4.6 mm in inside diameter and 25 cm in length, packed with octadecylsilanized silica gel for liquid chromatography (7 μm in particle diameter).

Column temperature: A constant temperature of about 40°C.

Mobile phase stock solution: Dissolve 0.96 g of sodium 1-pentanesulfonate and 1.86 g of disodium dihydrogen ethylenediamine tetraacetate dihydrate in 1000 mL of water and 5 mL of acetic acid (100), and adjust the pH to 4.3 with ammonia TS.

Mobile phase A: A mixture of the mobile phase stock solution and methanol (9:1).

Mobile phase B: A mixture of the mobile phase stock solution and methanol (3:2).

Flowing of mobile phase: Control the gradient by mixing the mobile phases A and B as directed in the following table.

Time after injection of sample (min)	Mobile phase A (vol%)	Mobile phase B (vol%)
0 - 60	100 → 0	0 → 100
60 - 75	0	100

Flow rate: About 1.2 mL per minute.

Time span of measurement: Twenty minutes after elution of the peak of demethylbleomycin A_2, beginning after the solvent peak.

System suitability—

System performance: When the procedure is run with 20 μL of the sample solution under the above operating conditions, bleomycin A_2 and bleomycin B_2 are eluted in this order with the resolution between these peaks being not less than 5.

System repeatability: When the test is repeated 6 times with 20 μL of the sample solution under the above operating conditions, the relative standard deviation of the peak area of bleomycin A_2 is not more than 2.0%.

Purity (1) Clarity and color of solution—A solution obtained by dissolving 80 mg of Bleomycin Sulfate in 4 mL of water is clear and colorless.

(2) Copper—Dissolve exactly 75 mg of Bleomycin Sulfate in 10 mL of diluted nitric acid (1 in 100), and use this solution as the sample solution. Separately, to exactly 15 mL of Standard Copper Solution add diluted nitric acid (1 in 100) to make exactly 100 mL, and use this solution as the standard solution. Perform the test with the sample solution and standard solution as directed under Atomic Absorption Spectrophotometry <*2.23*> according to the following conditions: the absorbance of the sample solution is not more than that of the standard solution (not more than 200 ppm).

Gas: Combustible gas—Acetylene.

Supporting gas—Air.

Lamp: Copper hollow-cathode lamp.

Wavelength: 324.8 nm.

Loss on drying <*2.41*> Not more than 3.0% (60 mg, in vacuum, phosphorus (V) oxide, 60°C, 3 hours. Take the sample to be tested while avoiding moisture absorption).

Assay Perform the test according to the Cylinder-plate method as directed under Microbial Assay for Antibiotics <*4.02*> according to the following conditions.

(i) Test organism—*Mycrobacterium smegmatis* ATCC 607

(ii) Agar medium for seed, base layer and transferring the test organism

Glycerin	10.0 g
Peptone	10.0 g
Meat extract	10.0 g
Sodium chloride	3.0 g
Agar	15.0 g
Water	1000 mL

Mix all the components and sterilize. Adjust the pH after sterilization to 6.9 - 7.1 with sodium hydroxide TS.

(iii) Liquid media for suspending the test organism

Glycerin	10.0 g
Peptone	10.0 g
Meat extract	10.0 g
Sodium chloride	3.0 g
Water	1000 mL

Mix all the components and sterilize. Adjust the pH after sterilization to 6.9 - 7.1 with sodium hydroxide TS.

(iv) Preparation of seeded agar layer—Cultivate the test organism on the slant of the agar medium for transferring the test organism at 27°C for 40 to 48 hours, then inoculate the test organism thus obtained in 100 mL of the liquid media for suspending the test organism, cultivate with shaking at between 25°C and 27°C for 5 days, and use this as the suspension of test organism. Store the suspension of test organism at a temperature not exceeding 5°C, and use within 14 days. Add 0.5 mL of the suspension of test organism in 100 mL of the agar medium for seed previously kept at 48°C, mix thoroughly, and use as the seeded agar layer.

(v) Preparation of cylinder-agar plate—Proceed as directed in 1.7. Preparation of cylinder-agar plates under the Microbial Assay for Antibiotics, dispensing 5.0 mL of agar medium for base layer and 8.0 mL of the agar medium for seed into the Petri dish.

(vi) Standard solutions—Weigh accurately an amount of Bleomycin A_2 Hydrochloride RS, previously dried under reduced pressure not exceeding 0.67 kPa at an ordinary temperature for 3 hours, equivalent to about 15 mg (potency), dissolve in 0.1 mol/L phosphate buffer solution (pH 6.8) to make exactly 100 mL, and use this solution as the standard stock solution. Keep the standard stock solution at 5°C or below, and use within 30 days. Take exactly a suitable amount of the standard stock solution before use, add 0.1 mol/L phosphate buffer solution (pH 6.8) to make solutions so that each mL contains 30 μg (potency) and 15 μg (potency), and use these solutions as the high concentration standard solution and low concentration standard solution, respectively.

(vii) Sample solutions—Weigh accurately an amount of Bleomycin Sulfate, equivalent to about 15 mg (potency), dissolve in 0.1 mol/L phosphate buffer solution (pH 6.8) to make exactly 100 mL. Take exactly a suitable amount of this solution, add 0.1 mol/L phosphate buffer solution (pH 6.8) to make solutions so that each mL contains 30 μg (potency) and 15 μg (potency), and use these solutions as the high concentration sample solution and low concentration sample solution, respectively.

Containers and storage Containers—Tight containers.

Boric Acid

ホウ酸

H_3BO_3: 61.83

Boric Acid, when dried, contains not less than 99.5% of boric acid (H_3BO_3).

Description Boric Acid occurs as colorless or white, crystals or crystalline powder. It is odorless, and has a slight, characteristic taste.

It is freely soluble in warm water, in hot ethanol (95) and in glycerin, soluble in water and in ethanol (95), and practically insoluble in diethyl ether.

The pH of a solution of 1.0 g of Boric Acid in 20 mL of water is between 3.5 and 4.1.

Identification A solution of Boric Acid (1 in 20) responds to Qualitative Tests <*1.09*> for borate.

Purity (1) Clarity and color of solution—Dissolve 1.0 g of Boric Acid in 25 mL of water or in 10 mL of hot ethanol (95): the solution is clear and colorless.

(2) Heavy metals <*1.07*>—Proceed with 2.0 g of Boric Acid according to Method 1, and perform the test. Prepare the control solution with 2.0 mL of Standard Lead Solution (not more than 10 ppm).

(3) Arsenic <*1.11*>—Prepare the test solution with 0.40 g of Boric Acid according to Method 1, and perform the test (not more than 5 ppm).

Loss on drying <*2.41*> Not more than 0.5% (2 g, silica gel, 5 hours).

Assay Weigh accurately about 1.5 g of Boric Acid, previously dried, add 15 g of D-sorbitol and 50 mL of water, and dissolve by warming. After cooling, titrate <*2.50*> with 1 mol/L sodium hydroxide VS (indicator: 2 drops of phenolphthalein TS).

Each mL of 1 mol/L sodium hydroxide VS
= 61.83 mg of H_3BO_3

Containers and storage Containers—Well-closed containers.

Freeze-dried Botulism Antitoxin, Equine

乾燥ボツリヌスウマ抗毒素

Freeze-dried Botulism Antitoxin, Equine, is a preparation for injection which is dissolved before use.

It contains botulism antitoxin type A, botulism antitoxin type B, botulism antitoxin type E and botulism antitoxin type F in immunoglobulin of horse origin. It may contain one, two or three of these four antitoxins.

It conforms to the requirements of Freeze-dried Botulism Antitoxin, Equine, in the Minimum Requirements for Biological Products.

Description Freeze-dried Botulism Antitoxin, Equine, becomes a colorless or yellow-brown, clear liquid or a slightly white-turbid liquid on the addition of solvent.

Bromazepam

ブロマゼパム

$C_{14}H_{10}BrN_3O$: 316.15
7-Bromo-5-(pyridin-2-yl)-1,3-dihydro-2*H*-1,4-benzodiazepin-2-one
[*1812-30-2*]

Bromazepam, when dried, contains not less than 99.0% and not more than 101.0% of bromazepam ($C_{14}H_{10}BrN_3O$).

Description Bromazepam occurs as white to light yellow-white, crystals or crystalline powder.

It is freely soluble in acetic acid (100), slightly soluble in methanol, in ethanol (99.5) and in acetone, and practically insoluble in water.

Melting point: about 245°C (with decomposition).

Identification **(1)** Determine the absorption spectrum of a solution of Bromazepam in ethanol (99.5) (1 in 200,000) as directed under Ultraviolet-visible Spectrophotometry <*2.24*>, and compare the spectrum with the Reference Spectrum: both spectra exhibit similar intensities of absorption at the same wavelengths.

(2) Determine the infrared absorption spectrum of Bromazepam, previously dried, as directed in the potassium bromide disk method under Infrared Spectrophotometry <*2.25*>, and compare the spectrum with the Reference Spectrum: both spectra exhibit similar intensities of absorption at the same wave numbers.

Purity **(1)** Heavy metals <*1.07*>—Proceed with 1.0 g of Bromazepam in a platinum crucible according to Method 4, and perform the test. Prepare the control solution with 2.0 mL of Standard Lead Solution (not more than 20 ppm).

(2) Related substances—Dissolve 50 mg of Bromazepam in 5 mL of a mixture of acetone and methanol (3:2), and use this solution as the sample solution. Pipet 1 mL of the sample solution, and add the mixture of acetone and methanol (3:2) to make exactly 50 mL. Pipet 5 mL of this solution, add the mixture of acetone and methanol (3:2) to make exactly 50 mL, and use this solution as the standard solution. Perform the test with these solutions as directed under Thin-layer Chromatography <*2.03*>. Spot 20 μL each of the sample solution and standard solution on a plate of silica gel with fluorescent indicator for thin-layer chromatography. Develop the plate with a mixture of ethyl acetate, ammonia solution (28) and ethanol (99.5) (38:1:1) to a distance of about 12 cm, and air-dry the plate. Examine under ultraviolet light (main wavelength: 254 nm): the spots other than the principal spot obtained from the sample solution and the spot of the starting point are not more than 2, and not more intense than the spot from the standard solution.

Loss on drying <*2.41*> Not more than 0.20% (1 g, 105°C, 4 hours).

Residue on ignition <*2.44*> Not more than 0.1% (1 g).

Assay Weigh accurately about 0.4 g of Bromazepam, previously dried, dissolve in 80 mL of acetic acid (100), and titrate <*2.50*> with 0.1 mol/L perchloric acid VS (potentiometric titration). Perform a blank determination in the same manner, and make any necessary correction.

Each mL of 0.1 mol/L perchloric acid VS
= 31.62 mg of $C_{14}H_{10}BrN_3O$

Containers and storage Containers—Well-closed containers.

Bromfenac Sodium Hydrate

ブロムフェナクナトリウム水和物

$C_{15}H_{11}BrNNaO_3 \cdot 1\frac{1}{2}H_2O$: 383.17
Sodium 2-[2-amino-3-(4-bromobenzoyl)phenyl]acetate sesquihydrate
[*120638-55-3*]

Bromfenac Sodium Hydrate contains not less than 97.5% and not more than 101.5% of bromfenac sodium ($C_{15}H_{11}BrNNaO_3$: 356.15), calculated on the anhydrous basis.

Description Bromfenac Sodium Hydrate occurs as a yellow to orange crystalline powder.

It is freely soluble in water, soluble in methanol, and slightly soluble in ethanol (99.5).

It dissolves in a solution of sodium hydrogen carbonate (21 in 2500).

Identification (1) Dissolve 10 mg of Bromfenac Sodium Hydrate in 500 mL of a solution of sodium hydrogen carbonate (21 in 2500). Determine the absorption spectrum of this solution as directed under Ultraviolet-visible Spectrophotometry *<2.24>*, and compare the spectrum with the Reference Spectrum or the spectrum of a solution of Bromfenac Sodium RS prepared in the same manner as the sample solution: both spectra exhibit similar intensities of absorption at the same wavelengths.

(2) Determine the infrared absorption spectrum of Bromfenac Sodium Hydrate as directed in the potassium bromide disk method under Infrared Spectrophotometry *<2.25>*, and compare the spectrum with the Reference Spectrum or the spectrum of Bromfenac Sodium RS: both spectra exhibit similar intensities of absorption at the same wave numbers.

(3) A solution of Bromfenac Sodium Hydrate (1 in 20) responds to Qualitative Tests *<1.09>* (1) for sodium salt.

pH *<2.54>* Dissolve 1.0 g of Bromfenac Sodium Hydrate in 20 mL of water: the pH of the solution is between 8.4 and 10.2.

Purity (1) Heavy metals *<1.07>*—Proceed with 1.0 g of Bromfenac Sodium Hydrate according to Method 2, and perform the test. Prepare the control solution with 2.0 mL of Standard Lead Solution (not more than 20 ppm).

(2) Related substances—Dissolve 50 mg of Bromfenac Sodium Hydrate in 100 mL of methanol, and use this solution as the sample solution. Pipet 1 mL of the sample solution, add methanol to make exactly 100 mL, and use this solution as the standard solution. Perform the test with exactly 20 μL each of the sample solution and standard solution as directed under Liquid Chromatography *<2.01>* according to the following conditions, and determine each peak area by the automatic integration method: the area of the peak other than bromfenac obtained from the sample solution is not larger than 1/10 times the peak area of bromfenac from the standard solution, and the total area of the peaks other than bromfenac from the sample solution is not larger than the peak area of bromfenac from the standard solution.

Operating conditions—

Detector, column and column temperature: Proceed as directed in the operating conditions in the Assay.

Mobile phase: Dissolve 3.85 g of ammonium acetate in 1000 mL of water, and adjust to pH 4.0 with acetic acid (100). To 570 mL of this solution add 430 mL of acetonitrile.

Flow rate: Adjust so that the retention time of bromfenac is about 8 minutes.

Time span of measurement: About 3 times as long as the retention time of bromfenac, beginning after the solvent peak.

System suitability—

Test for required detectability: Pipet 2 mL of the standard solution, and add methanol to make exactly 20 mL. Confirm that the peak area of bromfenac obtained with 20 μL of this solution is equivalent to 7 to 13% of that with 20 μL of the standard solution.

System performance: When the procedure is run with 20 μL of the standard solution under the above operating conditions, the number of theoretical plates and the symmetry factor of the peak of bromfenac are not less than 5000 and not more than 1.5, respectively.

System repeatability: When the test is repeated 6 times with 20 μL of the standard solution under the above operating conditions, the relative standard deviation of the peak area of bromfenac is not more than 2.0%.

Water *<2.48>* 6.9 – 8.5% (0.15 g, volumetric titration, direct titration. Use a solution of imidazole for water determination in methanol for water determination (1 in 80) instead of methanol for water determination).

Assay Weigh accurately about 30 mg each of Bromfenac Sodium Hydrate and Bromfenac Sodium RS (separately determine the water *<2.48>* in the same manner as Bromfenac Sodium Hydrate), dissolve each in methanol to make exactly 50 mL. Pipet 5 mL each of these solutions, add the mobile phase to make them exactly 100 mL, and use these solutions as the sample solution and the standard solution, respectively. Perform the test with exactly 20 μL each of the sample solution and standard solution as directed under Liquid Chromatography *<2.01>* according to the following conditions, and determine the peak areas, A_T and A_S, of bromfenac in each solution.

Amount (mg) of bromfenac sodium ($C_{15}H_{11}BrNNaO_3$)
$= M_S \times A_T/A_S$

M_S: Amount (mg) of Bromfenac Sodium RS taken, calculated on the anhydrous basis

Operating conditions—

Detector: An ultraviolet absorption photometer (wavelength: 266 nm).

Column: A stainless steel column 4.6 mm in inside diameter and 15 cm in length, packed with octadecylsilanized silica gel for liquid chromatography (5 μm in particle diameter).

Column temperature: A constant temperature of about 35°C.

Mobile phase: Dissolve 3.85 g of ammonium acetate in 1000 mL of water. To 600 mL of this solution add 250 mL of methanol and 150 mL of tetrahydrofuran.

Flow rate: Adjust so that the retention time of bromfenac is about 9 minutes.

System suitability—

System performance: When the procedure is run with 20 μL of the standard solution under the above operating conditions, the number of theoretical plates and the symmetry factor of the peak of bromfenac are not less than 5000 and not more than 1.5, respectively.

System repeatability: When the test is repeated 6 times with 20 μL of the standard solution under the above operating conditions, the relative standard deviation of the peak area of bromfenac is not more than 1.0%.

Containers and storage Containers—Tight containers.

Storage—Light-resistant.

Bromfenac Sodium Ophthalmic Solution

ブロムフェナクナトリウム点眼液

Bromfenac Sodium Ophthalmic Solution is an aqueous ophthalmic preparation.

It contains not less than 90.0% and not more than 110.0% of the labeled amount of Bromfenac Sodium Hydrate ($C_{15}H_{11}BrNNaO_3.1\frac{1}{2}H_2O$: 383.17).

Method of preparation Prepare as directed under Ophthalmic Liquids and Solutions, with Bromfenac Sodium Hydrate.

Description Bromfenac Sodium Ophthalmic Solution occurs as a clear and yellow liquid.

Identification To a volume of Bromfenac Sodium Ophthalmic Solution, equivalent to 1 mg of Bromfenac Sodium Hydrate, add a solution of sodium hydrogen carbonate (21 in 2500) to make 50 mL, and determine the absorption spectrum of this solution as directed under Ultraviolet-visible Spectrophotometry *<2.24>*: it exhibits maxima between 266 nm and 270 nm, and between 377 nm and 381 nm.

pH Being specified separately when the drug is granted approval based on the Law.

Purity Related substances—Being specified separately when the drug is granted approval based on the Law.

Foreign insoluble matter *<6.11>* It meets the requirement.

Insoluble particulate matter *<6.08>* It meets the requirement.

Sterility *<4.06>* Perform the test according to the Membrane filtration method: it meets the requirement.

Assay Pipet a volume of Bromfenac Sodium Ophthalmic Solution, equivalent to about 2 mg of bromfenac sodium hydrate ($C_{15}H_{11}BrNNaO_3.1\frac{1}{2}H_2O$), add the mobile phase to make exactly 20 mL, and use this solution as the sample solution. Separately, weigh accurately about 20 mg of Bromfenac Sodium RS (separately determine the water *<2.48>* in the same manner as Bromfenac Sodium Hydrate), and dissolve in the mobile phase to make exactly 20 mL. Pipet 2 mL of this solution, add the mobile phase to make exactly 20 mL, and use this solution as the standard solution. Perform the test with exactly 10 μL each of the sample solution and standard solution as directed under Liquid Chromatography *<2.01>* according to the following conditions, and determine the peak areas, A_T and A_S, of bromfenac in each solution.

Amount (mg) of bromfenac sodium hydrate ($C_{15}H_{11}BrNNaO_3.1\frac{1}{2}H_2O$)
$= M_S \times A_T/A_S \times 1/10 \times 1.076$

M_S: Amount (mg) of Bromfenac Sodium RS taken, calculated on the anhydrous basis

Operating conditions—

Detector: An ultraviolet absorption photometer (wavelength: 266 nm).

Column: A stainless steel column 4.6 mm in inside diameter and 25 cm in length, packed with octadecylsilanized silica gel for liquid chromatography (5 μm in particle diameter).

Column temperature: A constant temperature of about 40°C.

Mobile phase: Dissolve 1.98 g of diammonium hydrogen phosphate in 750 mL of water, adjust to pH 7.3 with phosphoric acid, and add 250 mL of acetonitrile.

Flow rate: Adjust so that the retention time of bromfenac is about 18 minutes.

System suitability—

System performance: When the procedure is run with 10 μL of the standard solution under the above operating conditions, the number of theoretical plates and the symmetry factor of the peak of bromfenac are not less than 13,000 and not more than 2.0, respectively.

System repeatability: When the test is repeated 6 times with 10 μL of the standard solution under the above operating conditions, the relative standard deviation of the peak area of bromfenac is not more than 1.0%.

Containers and storage Containers—Tight containers.

Bromhexine Hydrochloride

ブロムヘキシン塩酸塩

$C_{14}H_{20}Br_2N_2.HCl$: 412.59
2-Amino-3,5-dibromo-*N*-cyclohexyl-*N*-methylbenzylamine monohydrochloride
[611-75-6]

Bromhexine Hydrochloride, when dried, contains not less than 98.5% of bromhexine hydrochloride ($C_{14}H_{20}Br_2N_2.HCl$).

Description Bromhexine Hydrochloride occurs as white, crystals or crystalline powder.

It is freely soluble in formic acid, sparingly soluble in methanol, and slightly soluble in water and in ethanol (95).

The pH of its saturated solution is between 3.0 and 5.0.

Melting point: about 239°C (with decomposition).

Identification **(1)** Dissolve 3 mg of Bromhexine Hydrochloride in 0.01 mol/L hydrochloric acid TS to make 100 mL. Determine the absorption spectrum of the solution as directed under Ultraviolet-visible Spectrophotometry *<2.24>*, and compare the spectrum with the Reference Spectrum: both spectra exhibit similar intensities of absorption at the same wavelengths.

(2) Determine the infrared absorption spectrum of Bromhexine Hydrochloride, previously dried, as directed in the potassium bromide disk method under Spectrophotometry *<2.25>*, and compare the spectrum with the Reference Spectrum: both spectra exhibit similar intensities of absorption at the same wave numbers.

(3) Add 20 mL of water to 1 g of Bromhexine Hydrochloride. After thorough shaking, add 3 mL of sodium hydroxide TS, and extract with four 20-mL portions of diethyl ether. Neutralize the water layer with dilute nitric acid: the solution responds to Qualitative Tests *<1.09>* (2) for chloride.

Purity **(1)** Heavy metals *<1.07>*—Proceed with 2.0 g of Bromhexine Hydrochloride according to Method 2, and perform the test. Prepare the control solution with 2.0 mL of Standard Lead Solution (not more than 10 ppm).

(2) Related substances—Conduct this procedure without exposure to light, using light-resistant vessels. Dissolve 50

mg of Bromhexine Hydrochloride in 10 mL of methanol, and use this solution as the sample solution. Pipet 1 mL of the sample solution, and add the mobile phase to make exactly 20 mL. Pipet 1 mL of this solution, add the mobile phase to make exactly 25 mL, and use this solution as the standard solution. Perform the test with exactly 5 μL each of the sample solution and standard solution as directed under Liquid Chromatography *<2.01>* according to the following conditions, and determine each peak area by the automatic integration method: each peak area other than bromhexine obtained from the sample solution is not larger than the peak area of bromhexine from the standard solution.

Operating conditions—

Detector: An ultraviolet absorption photometer (wavelength: 245 nm).

Column: A stainless steel column about 5 mm in inside diameter and about 15 cm in length, packed with octadecylsilanized silica gel for liquid chromatography (5 μm in particle diameter).

Column temperature: A constant temperature of about 40°C.

Mobile phase: Dissolve 1.0 g of potassium dihydrogen phosphate in 900 mL of water, adjust the pH to 7.0 with 0.5 mol/L sodium hydroxide TS, and add water to make 1000 mL. To 200 mL of this solution add 800 mL of acetonitrile.

Flow rate: Adjust so that the retention time of bromhexine is about 6 minutes.

Selection of column: To 0.05 g of bamethan sulfate add 0.5 mL of the sample solution, and add the mobile phase to make 10 mL. Proceed with 5 μL of this solution under the above operating conditions, and calculate the resolution. Use a column giving elution of bamethan and bromhexine in this order with the resolution between these peaks being not less than 7.

Detection sensitivity: Adjust the detection sensitivity so that the peak height of bromhexine from 5 μL of the standard solution is between 5 mm and 15 mm.

Time span of measurement: About 2 times as long as the retention time of bromhexine, beginning after the solvent peak.

Loss on drying *<2.41>* Not more than 0.5% (1 g, 105°C, 4 hours).

Residue on ignition *<2.44>* Not more than 0.1% (1 g).

Assay Weigh accurately about 0.5 g of Bromhexine Hydrochloride, previously dried, dissolve in 2 mL of formic acid, add 60 mL of acetic anhydride, and warm in a water bath at 50°C for 15 minutes. After cooling, titrate *<2.50>* with 0.1 mol/L perchloric acid VS until the color of the solution changes from purple through blue-green to yellow-green (indicator: 2 drops of crystal violet TS). Perform a blank determination in the same manner, and make any necessary correction.

Each mL of 0.1 mol/L perchloric acid VS
= 41.26 mg of $C_{14}H_{20}Br_2N_2.HCl$

Containers and storage Containers—Well-closed containers.

Storage—Light-resistant.

Bromocriptine Mesilate

ブロモクリプチンメシル酸塩

$C_{32}H_{40}BrN_5O_5.CH_4O_3S$: 750.70
(5′*S*)-2-Bromo-12′-hydroxy-2′-(1-methylethyl)-5′-(2-methylpropyl)ergotaman-3′,6′,18-trione monomethanesulfonate
[22260-51-1]

Bromocriptine Mesilate contains not less than 98.0% of bromocriptine mesilate ($C_{32}H_{40}BrN_5O_5$.CH_4O_3S), calculated on the dried basis.

Description Bromocriptine Mesilate occurs as a white to pale yellowish white or pale brownish white crystalline powder. It is odorless, or has a faint characteristic odor.

It is very soluble in acetic acid (100), freely soluble in methanol, sparingly soluble in ethanol (95), very slightly soluble in acetic anhydride, in dichloromethane and in chloroform, and practically insoluble in water and in diethyl ether.

It is gradually colored by light.

Identification **(1)** Dissolve 2 mg of Bromocriptine Mesilate in 1 mL of methanol, add 2 mL of 4-dimethylaminobenzaldehyde-ferric chloride TS, and shake: a purplish blue color develops.

(2) Determine the absorption spectrum of a solution of Bromocriptine Mesilate in methanol (3 in 100,000) as directed under Ultraviolet-visible Spectrophotometry *<2.24>*, and compare the spectrum with the Reference Spectrum: both spectra exhibit similar intensities of absorption at the same wavelengths.

(3) Determine the infrared absorption spectrum of Bromocriptine Mesilate as directed in the paste method under Infrared Spectrophotometry *<2.25>*, and compare the spectrum with the Reference Spectrum: both spectra exhibit similar intensities of absorption at the same wave numbers.

(4) Perform the test with Bromocriptine Mesilate as directed under Flame Coloration Test *<1.04>* (2): a green color appears.

Optical rotation *<2.49>* $[\alpha]_D^{20}$: +95 – +105° [0.1 g, calculated on the dried basis, a mixture of methanol and dichloromethane (1:1), 10 mL, 100 mm].

Purity **(1)** Clarity and color of solution—Dissolve 0.10 g of Bromocriptine Mesilate in 10 mL of methanol: the solution is clear, and has no more color than the following control solution.

Control solution: To 2.5 mL of Cobalt (II) Chloride CS, 6.0 mL of Iron (III) Chloride CS and 1.0 mL of Copper (II) Sulfate CS add diluted hydrochloric acid (1 in 40) to make exactly 100 mL.

(2) Heavy metals *<1.07>*—Proceed with 1.0 g of Bromocriptine Mesilate according to Method 2, and perform the test. Prepare the control solution with 2.0 mL of Standard Lead Solution (not more than 20 ppm).

(3) Related substances—Conduct this procedure without exposure to light, using light-resistant vessels. Dissolve 0.10 g of Bromocriptine Mesilate in 10 mL of a mixture of methanol and chloroform (1:1), and use this solution as the sample solution. Pipet 1 mL of the sample solution, add a mixture of methanol and chloroform (1:1) to make exactly 200 mL, and use this solution as the standard solution (1). Pipet 10 mL of the standard solution (1), add a mixture of methanol and chloroform (1:1) to make exactly 20 mL, and use this solution as the standard solution (2). Perform the test with these solutions as directed under Thin-layer Chromatography ⟨*2.03*⟩. Spot 10 μL each of the sample solution and standard solutions (1) and (2), as a band with 1 cm in width, on a plate of silica gel for thin-layer chromatography. Develop the plate immediately with a mixture of dichloromethane, 1,4-dioxane, ethanol (95) and ammonia solution (28) (1800:150:50:1) to a distance of about 10 cm, and dry the plate under reduced pressure for 30 minutes. Spray evenly Dragendorff's TS for spraying on the plate, then spray evenly hydrogen peroxide TS, cover the plate with a glass plate, and examine: the spots other than the principal spot obtained from the sample solution are not more intense than the spot from the standard solution (1), and the spot other than the principal spot, which is more intense than the spot from the standard solution (2), is not more than one.

Loss on drying ⟨*2.41*⟩ Not more than 3.0% (1 g, in vacuum at a pressure not exceeding 0.67 kPa, 80°C, 5 hours).

Residue on ignition ⟨*2.44*⟩ Not more than 0.1% (1 g).

Assay Weigh accurately about 0.6 g of Bromocriptine Mesilate, dissolve in 80 mL of a mixture of acetic anhydride and acetic acid (100) (7:1), and titrate ⟨*2.50*⟩ with 0.1 mol/L perchloric acid VS (potentiometric titration). Perform a blank determination in the same manner, and make any necessary correction.

Each mL of 0.1 mol/L perchloric acid VS
= 75.07 mg of $C_{32}H_{40}BrN_5O_5.CH_4O_3S$

Containers and storage Containers—Tight containers.
Storage—Light-resistant, and not exceeding −18°C.

Bromovalerylurea

ブロモバレリル尿素

and enantiomer

$C_6H_{11}BrN_2O_2$: 223.07
(2*RS*)-(2-Bromo-3-methylbutanoyl)urea
[*496-67-3*]

Bromovalerylurea, when dried, contains not less than 98.0% of bromovalerylurea ($C_6H_{11}BrN_2O_2$).

Description Bromovalerylurea occurs as colorless or white, crystals or crystalline powder. It is odorless, and has a slightly bitter taste.

It is soluble in ethanol (95), sparingly soluble in diethyl ether, and very slightly soluble in water.

It dissolves in sulfuric acid, in nitric acid and in hydrochloric acid, and precipitates are produced on the addition of water.

It dissolves in sodium hydroxide TS.

Identification **(1)** Boil 0.2 g of Bromovalerylurea with 5 mL of a solution of sodium hydroxide (1 in 10): the gas evolved changes moistened red litmus paper to blue. Boil this solution with an excess of dilute sulfuric acid: the odor of valeric acid is perceptible.

(2) To 0.1 g of Bromovalerylurea add 0.5 g of anhydrous sodium carbonate, and decompose thoroughly by gentle heating. Dissolve the residue in 5 mL of hot water, cool, acidify with acetic acid (31), and filter: the filtrate responds to Qualitative Tests ⟨*1.09*⟩ (2) for bromide.

Melting point ⟨*2.60*⟩ 151 – 155°C

Purity **(1)** Acidity or alkalinity—To 1.5 g of Bromovalerylurea add 30 mL of water, shake for 5 minutes, and filter: the filtrate is neutral.

(2) Chloride ⟨*1.03*⟩—Perform the test with a 10-mL portion of the filtrate obtained in (1). Prepare the control solution with 0.40 mL of 0.01 mol/L hydrochloric acid VS (not more than 0.028%).

(3) Sulfate ⟨*1.14*⟩—Perform the test with 10 mL of the filtrate obtained in (1). Prepare the control solution with 0.40 mL of 0.005 mol/L sulfuric acid VS (not more than 0.038%).

(4) Heavy metals ⟨*1.07*⟩—Proceed with 2.0 g of Bromovalerylurea according to Method 2, and perform the test. Prepare the control solution with 2.0 mL of Standard Lead Solution (not more than 10 ppm).

(5) Arsenic ⟨*1.11*⟩—Dissolve 0.5 g of Bromovalerylurea in 5 mL of sodium hydroxide TS, use this solution as the test solution, and perform the test (not more than 4 ppm).

(6) Readily carbonizable substances ⟨*1.15*⟩—Perform the test with 0.5 g of Bromovalerylurea: the solution is not more colored than Matching Fluid A.

Loss on drying ⟨*2.41*⟩ Not more than 0.5% (1 g, 80°C, 2 hours).

Residue on ignition ⟨*2.44*⟩ Not more than 0.1% (1 g).

Assay Weigh accurately about 0.4 g of Bromovalerylurea, previously dried, in a 300-mL conical flask, add 40 mL of sodium hydroxide TS, and boil gently for 20 minutes under a reflux condenser. Cool, wash the lower part of the reflux condenser and the mouth of the flask with 30 mL of water, and combine the washings with the solution in the conical flask. Add 5 mL of nitric acid and exactly 30 mL of 0.1 mol/L silver nitrate VS, and titrate ⟨*2.50*⟩ the excess silver nitrate with 0.1 mol/L ammonium thiocyanate VS (indicator: 2 mL of ammonium iron (III) sulfate TS). Perform a blank determination in the same manner.

Each mL of 0.1 mol/L silver nitrate VS
= 22.31 mg of $C_6H_{11}BrN_2O_2$

Containers and storage Containers—Well-closed containers.

Brotizolam

ブロチゾラム

$C_{15}H_{10}BrClN_4S$: 393.69
2-Bromo-4-(2-chlorophenyl)-9-methyl-
6*H*-thieno[3,2-*f*][1,2,4]triazolo[4,3-*a*][1,4]diazepine
[*57801-81-7*]

Brotizolam, when dried, contains not less than 98.5% and not more than 101.0% of brotizolam ($C_{15}H_{10}BrClN_4S$).

Description Brotizolam occurs as a white or pale yellow crystalline powder.

It is sparingly soluble in methanol, slightly soluble in acetonitrile and in ethanol (99.5), and practically insoluble in water.

Identification (1) Determine the absorption spectrum of a solution of Brotizolam in methanol (1 in 100,000) as directed under Ultraviolet-visible Spectrophotometry <*2.24*>, and compare the spectrum with the Reference Spectrum: both spectra exhibit similar intensities of absorption at the same wavelengths.

(2) Determine the infrared absorption spectrum of Brotizolam as directed in the potassium bromide disk method under Infrared Spectrophotometry <*2.25*>, and compare the spectrum with the Reference Spectrum: both spectra exhibit similar intensities of absorption at the same wave numbers.

Melting point <*2.60*> 208 – 212°C

Purity (1) Heavy metals <*1.07*>—Proceed with 2.0 g of Brotizolam according to Method 2, and perform the test. Prepare the control solution with 2.0 mL of Standard Lead Solution (not more than 10 ppm).

(2) Related substances—Dissolve 50 mg of Brotizolam in 50 mL of acetonitrile, and use this solution as the sample solution. Pipet 2 mL of the sample solution, and add acetonitrile to make exactly 100 mL. Pipet 1 mL of this solution, add acetonitrile to make exactly 10 mL, and use this solution as the standard solution. Perform the test with exactly 5 μL each of the sample solution and standard solution as directed under Liquid Chromatography <*2.01*> according to the following conditions. Determine each peak area by the automatic integration method: each peak area other than brotizolam obtained from the sample solution is not larger than 1/2 times the peak area of brotizolam from the standard solution, and the total area of the peaks other than brotizolam from the sample solution is not larger than the peak area of brotizolam from the standard solution.

Operating conditions—

Detector: An ultraviolet absorption photometer (wavelength: 242 nm).

Column: A stainless steel column 3.9 mm in inside diameter and 15 cm in length, packed with octylsilanized silica gel for liquid chromatography (5 μm in particle diameter).

Column temperature: A constant temperature of about 40°C.

Mobile phase A: Dissolve 1.84 g of sodium 1-heptanesulfonate in 1000 mL of water.

Mobile phase B: Dissolve 0.46 g of sodium 1-heptanesulfonate in 250 mL of water and 750 mL of acetonitrile.

Flowing of mobile phase: Control the gradient by mixing the mobile phases A and B as directed in the following table.

Time after injection of sample (min)	Mobile phase A (vol%)	Mobile phase B (vol%)
0 – 4	63	37
4 – 15	63 → 12	37 → 88

Flow rate: About 2 mL per minute.

Time span of measurement: About 2 times as long as the retention time of brotizolam, beginning after the solvent peak.

System suitability—

Test for required detectability: Pipet 5 mL of the standard solution, and add acetonitrile to make exactly 20 mL. Confirm that the peak area of brotizolam obtained with 5 μL of this solution is equivalent to 18 to 32% of that with 5 μL of the standard solution.

System performance: When the procedure is run with 5 μL of the standard solution under the above operating conditions, the number of theoretical plates and the symmetry factor of the peak of brotizolam are not less than 5000 and not more than 2.0, respectively.

System repeatability: When the test is repeated 6 times with 5 μL of the standard solution under the above operating conditions, the relative standard deviation of the peak area of brotizolam is not more than 2.0%.

Loss on drying <*2.41*> Not more than 0.5% (1 g, 105°C, 3 hours).

Residue on ignition <*2.44*> Not more than 0.1% (1 g).

Assay Weigh accurately about 0.15 g of Brotizolam, previously dried, dissolve in 75 mL of a mixture of acetic anhydride and acetic acid (100) (2:1), and titrate <*2.50*> with 0.1 mol/L perchloric acid VS (potentiometric titration). Perform a blank determination in the same manner, and make any necessary correction.

Each mL of 0.1 mol/L perchloric acid VS
= 19.68 mg of $C_{15}H_{10}BrClN_4S$

Containers and storage Containers—Tight containers.
Storage—Light-resistant.

Brotizolam Tablets

ブロチゾラム錠

Brotizolam Tablets contain not less than 95.0% and not more than 105.0% of the labeled amount of brotizolam ($C_{15}H_{10}BrClN_4S$: 393.69).

Method of preparation Prepare as directed under Tablets, with Brotizolam.

Identification Shake a quantity of powdered Brotizolam Tablets, equivalent to 0.1 mg of Brotizolam, with 10 mL of methanol, and centrifuge. Determine the absorption spectrum of the supernatant liquid as directed under Ultraviolet-visible Spectrophotometry <*2.24*>: it exhibits a maximum between 239 nm and 243 nm.

Purity Related substances—Use the sample solution obtained in the Assay as the sample solution. Pipet 1 mL of the sample solution, add the mobile phase to make exactly 100 mL, and use this solution as the standard solution. Perform the test with exactly 40 μL each of the sample solution and standard solution as directed under Liquid Chromatography <*2.01*> according to the following conditions, and determine each peak area by the automatic integration method: the total area of the peaks other than brotizolam obtained from the sample solution is not larger than 1.5 times the peak area of brotizolam from the standard solution.

Operating conditions—

Detector, column, column temperature, mobile phase, and flow rate: Proceed as directed in the operating conditions in the Assay.

Time span of measurement: About 3 times as long as the retention time of brotizolam, beginning after the solvent peak.

System suitability—

Test for required detectability: To exactly 10 mL of the standard solution add the mobile phase to make exactly 100 mL. Confirm that the peak area of brotizolam obtained with 40 μL of this solution is equivalent to 7 to 13% of that obtained with 40 μL of the standard solution.

System performance: When the procedure is run with 40 μL of the standard solution under the above operating conditions, the number of theoretical plates and the symmetry factor of the peak of brotizolam are not less than 3000 and not more than 2.0, respectively.

System repeatability: When the test is repeated 6 times with 40 μL of the standard solution under the above operating conditions, the relative standard deviation of the peak area of brotizolam is not more than 2.0%.

Uniformity of dosage units <*6.02*> Perform the test according to the following method: it meets the requirement of the Content uniformity test.

To 1 tablet of Brotizolam Tablets add exactly *V* mL of the mobile phase so that each mL contains about 25 μg of brotizolam ($C_{15}H_{10}BrClN_4S$), shake for 15 minutes, centrifuge, and use the supernatant liquid as the sample solution. Then, proceed as directed in the Assay.

$$\text{Amount (mg) of brotizolam } (C_{15}H_{10}BrClN_4S) = M_S \times A_T/A_S \times V/1000$$

M_S: Amount (mg) of brotizolam for assay taken

Dissolution <*6.10*> When the test is performed at 50 revolutions per minute according to the Paddle method, using 900 mL of water as the dissolution medium, the dissolution rate in 15 minutes of Brotizolam Tablets is not less than 85%.

Start the test with 1 tablet of Brotizolam Tablets, withdraw not less than 20 mL of the medium at the specified minute after starting the test, and filter through a membrane filter with a pore size not exceeding 0.5 μm. Discard not less than 10 mL of the first filtrate, pipet *V* mL of the subsequent filtrate, add water to make exactly *V'* mL so that each mL contains about 0.14 μg of brotizolam ($C_{15}H_{10}BrClN_4S$), and use this solution as the sample solution. Separately, weigh accurately about 28 mg of brotizolam for assay, previously dried at 105°C for 3 hours, dissolve in 10 mL of methanol, and add water to make exactly 100 mL. Pipet 5 mL of this solution, add water to make exactly 200 mL. Pipet 2 mL of this solution, add water to make exactly 100 mL, and use this solution as the standard solution. Perform the test with exactly 200 μL each of the sample solution and standard solution as directed under Liquid Chromatography <*2.01*> according to the following conditions, and determine the peak areas, A_T and A_S, of brotizolam in each solution.

$$\text{Dissolution rate (\%) with respect to the labeled amount of brotizolam } (C_{15}H_{10}BrClN_4S) = M_S \times A_T/A_S \times V'/V \times 1/C \times 9/20$$

M_S: Amount (mg) of brotizolam for assay taken

C: Labeled amount (mg) of brotizolam ($C_{15}H_{10}BrClN_4S$) in 1 tablet

Operating conditions—

Detector, column, and column temperature: Proceed as directed in the operating conditions in the Assay.

Mobile phase: A mixture of water and acetonitrile (63:37).

Flow rate: Adjust so that the retention time of brotizolam is about 7 minutes.

System suitability—

System performance: When the procedure is run with 200 μL of the standard solution under the above operating conditions, the number of theoretical plates and the symmetry factor of the peak of brotizolam are not less than 2000 and not more than 2.0, respectively.

System repeatability: When the test is repeated 6 times with 200 μL of the standard solution under the above operating conditions, the relative standard deviation of the peak area of brotizolam is not more than 2.0%.

Assay Weigh accurately the mass of not less than 20 Brotizolam Tablets, and powder. Weigh accurately a portion of the powder, equivalent to about 0.25 mg of brotizolam ($C_{15}H_{10}BrClN_4S$), add exactly 10 mL of the mobile phase, and shake for 15 minutes. Centrifuge this solution, and use the supernatant liquid as the sample solution. Separately, weigh accurately about 25 mg of brotizolam for assay, previously dried at 105°C for 3 hours, and dissolve in the mobile phase to make exactly 50 mL. Pipet 5 mL of this solution, add the mobile phase to make exactly 100 mL, and use this solution as the standard solution. Perform the test with exactly 40 μL each of the sample solution and standard solution as directed under Liquid Chromatography <*2.01*> according to the following conditions, and determine the peak areas, A_T and A_S, of brotizolam in each solution.

$$\text{Amount (mg) of brotizolam } (C_{15}H_{10}BrClN_4S) = M_S \times A_T/A_S \times 1/100$$

M_S: Amount (mg) of brotizolam for assay taken

Operating conditions—

Detector: An ultraviolet absorption photometer (wavelength: 240 nm).

Column: A stainless steel column 4.6 mm in inside diameter and 15 cm in length, packed with octadecylsilanized silica gel for liquid chromatography (5 μm in particle diameter).

Column temperature: A constant temperature of about 30°C.

Mobile phase: Dissolve 1.1 g of ammonium carbonate in 1000 mL of water. To 600 mL of this solution add 500 mL of acetonitrile.

Flow rate: Adjust so that the retention time of brotizolam is about 3 minutes.

System suitability—

System performance: When the procedure is run with 40 μL of the standard solution under the above operating conditions, the number of theoretical plates and the symmetry factor of the peak of brotizolam are not less than 3000 and not more than 2.0, respectively.

System repeatability: When the test is repeated 6 times with 40 μL of the standard solution under the above operating conditions, the relative standard deviation of the peak

area of brotizolam is not more than 1.0%.

Containers and storage Containers—Tight containers.
Storage—Light-resistant.

Bucillamine

ブシラミン

$C_7H_{13}NO_3S_2$: 223.31
(2*R*)-2-(2-Methyl-2-sulfanylpropanoylamino)-3-sulfanylpropanoic acid
[65002-17-7]

Bucillamine, when dried, contains not less than 98.5% and not more than 101.0% of bucillamine ($C_7H_{13}NO_3S_2$).

Description Bucillamine occurs as white, crystals or crystalline powder.

It is freely soluble in methanol and in ethanol (95), and slightly soluble in water.

Identification **(1)** To 5 mL of a solution of Bucillamine (1 in 250) add 2 mL of sodium hydroxide TS and 2 drops of sodium pentacyanonitrosylferrate (III) TS: the solution reveals a red-purple color.

(2) Determine the infrared absorption spectrum of Bucillamine as directed in the potassium bromide disk method under Infrared Spectrophotometry *〈2.25〉*, and compare the spectrum with the Reference Spectrum: both spectra exhibit similar intensities of absorption at the same wave numbers.

Optical rotation *〈2.49〉* $[\alpha]_D^{20}$: +33.0 – +36.5° (after drying, 2 g, ethanol (95), 50 mL, 100 mm).

Melting point *〈2.60〉* 136 – 140°C

Purity **(1)** Heavy metals *〈1.07〉*—Proceed with 1.0 g of Bucillamine according to Method 2, and perform the test. Prepare the control solution with 2.0 mL of Standard Lead Solution (not more than 20 ppm).

(2) Arsenic *〈1.11〉*—Prepare the test solution with 1.0 g of Bucillamine according to Method 3, and perform the test (not more than 2 ppm).

(3) Related substances—Dissolve 60 mg of Bucillamine in 20 mL of a mixture of water and methanol (1:1), and use this solution as the sample solution. Pipet 3 mL of the sample solution, add the mixture of water and methanol (1:1) to make exactly 200 mL, and use this solution as the standard solution. Immediately perform the test with exactly 20 μL each of the sample solution and standard solution as directed under Liquid Chromatography *〈2.01〉* according to the following conditions, and determine each peak area by the automatic integration method: the peak areas of related substances, having the relative retention time of about 2.3 and about 3.1 to bucillamine, obtained from the sample solution are not larger than 8/15 times and 2/5 times the peak area of bucillamine from the standard solution, respectively, and the area of the peak other than the bucillamine and the peaks mentioned above from the sample solution is not larger than 1/5 times the peak area of bucillamine from the standard solution. The total area of the peaks other than bucillamine from the sample solution is not larger than the peak area of bucillamine from the standard solution.

Operating conditions—

Detector: An ultraviolet absorption photometer (wavelength: 254 nm).

Column: A stainless steel column 6.0 mm in inside diameter and 15 cm in length, packed with octadecylsilanized silica gel for liquid chromatography (5 μm in particle diameter).

Column temperature: A constant temperature of about 40°C.

Mobile phase: A mixture of 0.01 mol/L citric acid TS and methanol (1:1).

Flow rate: Adjust so that the retention time of bucillamine is about 5 minutes.

Time span of measurement: About 7 times as long as the retention time of bucillamine, beginning after the solvent peak.

System suitability—

Test for required detectability: To exactly 1 mL of the standard solution add the mixture of water and methanol (1:1) to make exactly 10 mL. Confirm that the peak area of bucillamine obtained with 20 μL of this solution is equivalent to 7 to 13% of that with 20 μL of the standard solution.

System performance: Dissolve 0.10 g of bucillamine and 10 mg of 4-fluorobenzoic acid in 100 mL of methanol. To 10 mL of this solution add water to make exactly 50 mL. When the procedure is run with 20 μL of this solution under the above operating conditions, bucillamine and 4-fluorobenzoic acid are eluted in this order with the resolution between these peaks being not less than 3.

System repeatability: When the test is repeated 6 times with 20 μL of the standard solution under the above operating conditions, the relative standard deviation of the peak area of bucillamine is not more than 2.0%.

Loss on drying *〈2.41〉* Not more than 0.5% (1 g, in vacuum, phosphorus (V) oxide, 60°C, 6 hours).

Residue on ignition *〈2.44〉* Not more than 0.1% (1 g).

Assay Weigh accurately about 0.25 g of Bucillamine, dissolve in 35 mL of methanol, add 15 mL of water, and titrate *〈2.50〉* with 0.05 mol/L iodine VS (potentiometric titration). Perform a blank determination in the same manner, and make any necessary correction.

Each mL of 0.05 mol/L iodine VS
= 11.17 mg of $C_7H_{13}NO_3S_2$

Containers and storage Containers—Tight containers.

Bucillamine Tablets

ブシラミン錠

Bucillamine Tablets contain not less than 95.0% and not more than 105.0% of the labeled amount of bucillamine ($C_7H_{13}NO_3S_2$: 223.31).

Method of preparation Prepare as directed under Tablets, with Bucillamine.

Identification **(1)** To a quantity of powdered Bucillamine Tablets, equivalent to 0.1 g of Bucillamine, add 0.1 g of sodium hydrogen carbonate and 10 mL of water, shake well, filter, and add 1 or 2 drops of ninhydrin TS to the filtrate: it exhibits a red-brown color.

(2) To a quantity of powdered Bucillamine Tablets, equivalent to 0.1 g of Bucillamine, add 25 mL of water, shake well, and filter. To 5 mL of the filtrate, add 2 mL of dilute sodium hydroxide TS and 1 or 2 drops of sodium pentacyanonitrosylferrate (III) TS: it exhibits a red-purple color.

Uniformity of dosage units <*6.02*>—Perform the Mass variation test, or the Content uniformity test according to the following method: it meets the requirement.

Store the sample solution and standard solution in a cold place until performing the measurements. Take 1 tablet of Bucillamine Tablets, add exactly 1 mL of the internal standard solution per 0.1 g of bucillamine ($C_7H_{13}NO_3S_2$), then add 3 mL of water and 6 mL of methanol per 0.1 g of bucillamine ($C_7H_{13}NO_3S_2$), and stir well until the tablet completely disintegrated. To 1 mL of this solution add the mobile phase to make 25 mL, filter through a membrane filter with a pore size not exceeding 0.45 μm, and use the filtrate as the sample solution. Then, proceed as directed in the Assay.

Amount (mg) of bucillamine ($C_7H_{13}NO_3S_2$)
$= M_S \times Q_T/Q_S \times C \times 1/200$

M_S: Amount (mg) of bucillamine for assay taken
C: Labeled amount (mg) of bucillamine ($C_7H_{13}NO_3S_2$) in 1 tablet

Internal standard solution—A solution of 4-fluorobenzoic acid in methanol (1 in 100).

Dissolution <*6.10*>—When the test is performed at 50 revolutions per minute according to the Paddle method, using 900 mL of water as the dissolution medium, the dissolution rate in 30 minutes of Bucillamine Tablets is not less than 80%.

Store the sample solution and standard solution in a cold place until performing the measurements. Start the test with 1 tablet of Bucillamine Tablets, withdraw not less than 20 mL of the medium at the specified minute after starting the test, and filter through a membrane filter with a pore size not exceeding 0.45 μm. Discard not less than 10 mL of the first filtrate, and use the subsequent filtrate as the sample solution. Separately, weigh accurately an amount of bucillamine for assay equivalent to the labeled amount of the tablet, previously dried in vacuum at 60°C for 6 hours using phosphorus (V) oxide as a dessicant, and dissolve in methanol to make exactly 10 mL. Pipet 1 mL of this solution, add water to make exactly 100 mL, and use this solution as the standard solution. Perform the test with exactly 20 μL each of the sample solution and standard solution as directed under Liquid Chromatography <*2.01*> according to the following conditions, and determine the peak areas, A_T and A_S, of bucillamine in each solution.

Dissolution rate (%) with respect to the labeled amount of bucillamine ($C_7H_{13}NO_3S_2$)
$= M_S \times A_T/A_S \times 1/C \times 90$

M_S: Amount (mg) of bucillamine for assay taken
C: Labeled amount (mg) of bucillamine ($C_7H_{13}NO_3S_2$) in 1 tablet

Operating conditions—

Detector, column, and column temperature: Proceed as directed in the operating conditions in the Assay.

Mobile phase: A mixture of diluted phosphoric acid (1 in 1000) and methanol (11:9).

Flow rate: Adjust so that the retention time of bucillamine is about 4 minutes.

System suitability—

System performance: When the procedure is run with 20 μL of the standard solution under the above operating conditions, the number of theoretical plates and the symmetry factor of the peak of bucillamine are not less than 3000 and not more than 1.5, respectively.

System repeatability: When the test is repeated 6 times with 20 μL of the standard solution under the above operating conditions, the relative standard deviation of the peak area of bucillamine is not more than 2.0%.

Assay Store the sample solution and standard solution in a cold place until performing the measurements. Take 10 tablets of Bucillamine Tablets, add exactly 1 mL of the internal standard solution per 0.1 g of bucillamine ($C_7H_{13}NO_3S_2$), add 3 mL of water and 6 mL of methanol, and stir well until the tablets completely disintegrated. To 1 mL of this solution add the mobile phase to make 25 mL, filter through a membrane filter with a pore size not exceeding 0.45 μm, and use this solution as the sample solution. Separately, weigh accurately about 0.2 g of bucillamine for assay, previously dried in vacuum at 60°C for 6 hours using phosphorus (V) oxide as a dessicant, add exactly 2 mL of the internal standard solution, and add 6 mL of water and 12 mL of methanol. To 1 mL of this solution add the mobile phase to make 25 mL, filter through a membrane filter with a pore size not exceeding 0.45 μm, and use this solution as the standard solution. Perform the test with 10 μL each of the sample solution and standard solution as directed under Liquid Chromatography <*2.01*> according to the following conditions, and calculate the ratios, Q_T and Q_S, of the peak area of bucillamine to that of the internal standard.

Amount (mg) of bucillamine ($C_7H_{13}NO_3S_2$)
$= M_S \times Q_T/Q_S \times C \times 1/200$

M_S: Amount (mg) of bucillamine for assay taken
C: Labeled amount (mg) of bucillamine ($C_7H_{13}NO_3S_2$) in 1 tablet

Internal standard solution—A solution of 4-fluorobenzoic acid in methanol (1 in 100).

Operating conditions—

Detector: An ultraviolet absorption photometer (wavelength: 254 nm).

Column: A stainless steel column 4.6 mm in inside diameter and 15 cm in length, packed with octadecylsilanized silica gel for liquid chromatography (5 μm in particle diameter).

Column temperature: A constant temperature of about 40°C.

Mobile phase: A mixture of diluted phosphoric acid (1 in 1000) and methanol (3:2).

Flow rate: Adjust so that the retention time of bucillamine is about 5 minutes.

System suitability—

System performance: When the procedure is run with 10 μL of the standard solution under the above operating conditions, bucillamine and the internal standard are eluted in this order with the resolution between these peaks being not less than 3.

System repeatability: When the test is repeated 6 times with 10 μL of the standard solution under the above operating conditions, the relative standard deviation of the ratio of the peak area of bucillamine to that of the internal standard is not more than 1.0%.

Containers and storage Containers—Tight containers.

Bucumolol Hydrochloride

ブクモロール塩酸塩

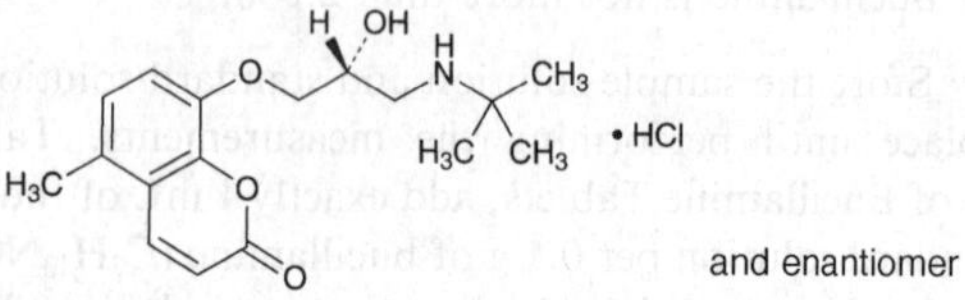

and enantiomer

$C_{17}H_{23}NO_4.HCl$: 341.83

8-{(2*RS*)-3-[(1,1-Dimethylethyl)amino]-2-hydroxypropyloxy}-5-methylchromen-2-one monohydrochloride

[*36556-75-9*]

Bucumolol Hydrochloride, when dried, contains not less than 99.0% of bucumolol hydrochloride ($C_{17}H_{23}NO_4.HCl$).

Description Bucumolol Hydrochloride occurs as white, crystals or crystalline powder.

It is freely soluble in water, sparingly soluble in methanol and in ethanol (95), slightly soluble in acetic acid (100), and practically insoluble in diethyl ether.

Melting point: about 228°C (with decomposition).

Identification **(1)** Dissolve 0.01 g of Bucumolol Hydrochloride in 10 mL of diluted ethanol (95) (1 in 2), and observe under ultraviolet light (main wavelength: 365 nm): the solution shows a yellow-green fluorescence. Render this solution alkaline by adding sodium hydroxide TS: the fluorescence disappears. Acidify the solution by adding dilute hydrochloric acid: the fluorescence reappears.

(2) Dissolve 0.1 g of Bucumolol Hydrochloride in 5 mL of water, and add 5 drops of Reinecke salt TS: a light red precipitate is formed.

(3) Determine the absorption spectrum of a solution of Bucumolol Hydrochloride (1 in 60,000) as directed under Ultraviolet-visible Spectrophotometry <*2.24*>, and compare the spectrum with the Reference Spectrum: both spectra exhibit similar intensities of absorption at the same wavelengths.

(4) Determine the infrared absorption spectrum of Bucumolol Hydrochloride, previously dried, as directed in the potassium chloride disk method under Infrared Spectrophotometry <*2.25*>, and compare the spectrum with the Reference Spectrum: both spectra exhibit similar intensities of absorption at the same wave numbers.

(5) A solution of Bucumolol Hydrochloride (1 in 50) responds to Qualitative Tests <*1.09*> for chloride.

Absorbance <*2.24*> $E^{1\%}_{1\,cm}$ (296 nm): 330 – 360 (after drying, 40 mg, water, 2500 mL).

Purity **(1)** Clarity and color of solution—Dissolve 1.0 g of Bucumolol Hydrochloride in 20 mL of water: the solution is clear and colorless to pale yellow.

(2) Heavy metals <*1.07*>—Proceed with 1.0 g of Bucumolol Hydrochloride according to Method 2, and perform the test. Prepare the control solution with 2.0 mL of Standard Lead Solution (not more than 20 ppm).

(3) Arsenic <*1.11*>—Prepare the test solution with 1.0 g of Bucumolol Hydrochloride according to Method 3, and perform the test (not more than 2 ppm).

(4) Related substances—Dissolve 0.10 g of Bucumolol Hydrochloride in 10 mL of methanol, and use this solution as the sample solution. Pipet 1 mL of the sample solution, and add methanol to make exactly 50 mL. Pipet 5 mL of this solution, add methanol to make exactly 25 mL, and use this solution as the standard solution. Perform the test with these solutions as directed under Thin-layer Chromatography <*2.03*>. Spot 5 μL each of the sample solution and standard solution on a plate of silica gel with fluorescent indicator for thin-layer chromatography. Develop the plate with a mixture of methanol and ammonia-ammonium chloride buffer solution (pH 10.7) (30:1) to a distance of about 12 cm, and air-dry the plate. Examine under ultraviolet light (main wavelength: 254 nm): the spots other than the principal spot obtained from the sample solution are not more intense than the spot from the standard solution.

Loss on drying <*2.41*> Not more than 0.5% (1 g, 105°C, 5 hours).

Residue on ignition <*2.44*> Not more than 0.1% (1 g).

Assay Weigh accurately about 0.4 g of Bucumolol Hydrochloride, previously dried, add 45 mL of acetic acid (100), dissolve by warming at 60°C, and cool. Add 105 mL of acetic anhydride, and titrate <*2.50*> with 0.1 mol/L perchloric acid VS (potentiometric titration). Perform a blank determination in the same manner, and make any necessary correction.

Each mL of 0.1 mol/L perchloric acid VS
= 34.18 mg of $C_{17}H_{23}NO_4.HCl$

Containers and storage Containers—Well-closed containers.

Bufetolol Hydrochloride

ブフェトロール塩酸塩

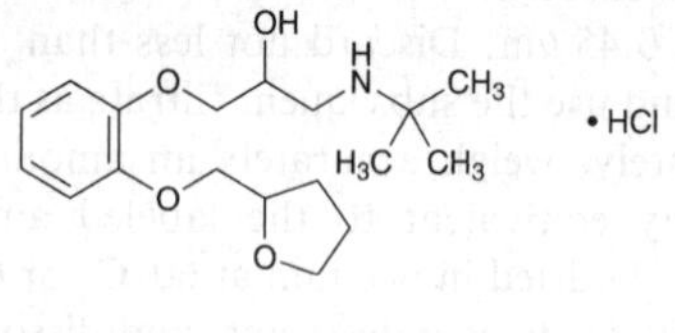

$C_{18}H_{29}NO_4.HCl$: 359.89

1-(1,1-Dimethylethyl)amino-3-[2-(tetrahydrofuran-2-ylmethoxy)phenoxy]propan-2-ol monohydrochloride

[*35108-88-4*]

Bufetolol Hydrochloride, when dried, contains not less than 98.5% of bufetolol hydrochloride ($C_{18}H_{29}NO_4.HCl$).

Description Bufetolol Hydrochloride occurs as white, crystals or crystalline powder.

It is freely soluble in water and in methanol, soluble in ethanol (95) and in acetic acid (100), and practically insoluble in diethyl ether.

A solution of Bufetolol Hydrochloride (1 in 10) shows no optical rotation.

Identification **(1)** To 5 mL of a solution of Bufetolol Hydrochloride (1 in 100) add 5 drops of Reinecke salt TS: a light red precipitate is formed.

(2) Determine the absorption spectrum of a solution of Bufetolol Hydrochloride (1 in 20,000) as directed under Ultraviolet-visible Spectrophotometry <*2.24*>, and compare the spectrum with the Reference Spectrum: both spectra exhibit similar intensities of absorption at the same wavelengths.

(3) Determine the infrared absorption spectrum of Bufetolol Hydrochloride, previously dried, as directed in the potassium chloride disk method under Infrared Spectrophotometry ⟨*2.25*⟩, and compare the spectrum with the Reference Spectrum: both spectra exhibit similar intensities of absorption at the same wave numbers.

(4) A solution of Bufetolol Hydrochloride (1 in 50) responds to Qualitative Tests ⟨*1.09*⟩ for chloride.

Melting point ⟨*2.60*⟩ 153 – 157°C

Purity **(1)** Clarity and color of solution—Dissolve 1.0 g of Bufetolol Hydrochloride in 10 mL of water: the solution is clear and colorless.

(2) Sulfate ⟨*1.14*⟩—Perform the test with 0.5 g of Bufetolol Hydrochloride. Prepare the control solution with 0.40 mL of 0.005 mol/L sulfuric acid VS (not more than 0.038%).

(3) Heavy metals ⟨*1.07*⟩—Proceed with 2.0 g of Bufetolol Hydrochloride according to Method 2, and perform the test. Prepare the control solution with 2.0 mL of Standard Lead Solution (not more than 10 ppm).

(4) Related substances—Dissolve 0.20 g of Bufetolol Hydrochloride in 5 mL of methanol, and use this solution as the sample solution. Pipet 1 mL of the sample solution, add methanol to make exactly 200 mL, and use this solution as the standard solution. Perform the test with these solutions as directed under Thin-layer Chromatography ⟨*2.03*⟩. Spot 10 μL each of the sample solution and standard solution on a plate of silica gel with fluorescent indicator for thin-layer chromatography. Develop the plate with a mixture of chloroform, acetone, ethanol (95) and ammonia solution (28) (40:20:5:1) to a distance of about 10 cm, and air-dry the plate. Examine under ultraviolet light (main wavelength: 254 nm): the spots other than the principal spot obtained from the sample solution are not more intense than the spot from the standard solution.

Loss on drying ⟨*2.41*⟩ Not more than 0.5% (1 g, 105°C, 4 hours).

Residue on ignition ⟨*2.44*⟩ Not more than 0.1% (1 g).

Assay Weigh accurately about 0.4 g of Bufetolol Hydrochloride, previously dried, dissolve in 10 mL of acetic acid (100), add 50 mL of acetic anhydride, and titrate ⟨*2.50*⟩ with 0.1 mol/L perchloric acid VS (potentiometric titration). Perform a blank determination in the same manner, and make any necessary correction.

Each mL of 0.1 mol/L perchloric acid VS
= 35.99 mg of $C_{18}H_{29}NO_4.HCl$

Containers and storage Containers—Tight containers.

Buformin Hydrochloride

ブホルミン塩酸塩

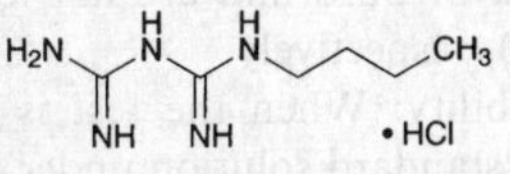

$C_6H_{15}N_5.HCl$: 193.68
1-Butylbiguanide hydrochloride
[*1190-53-0*]

Buformin Hydrochloride, when dried, contains not less than 98.5% and not more than 101.0% of buformin hydrochloride ($C_6H_{15}N_5.HCl$).

Description Buformin Hydrochloride occurs as a white crystalline powder.

It is freely soluble in water and in ethanol (99.5).

Identification **(1)** To 5 mL of a solution of Buformin Hydrochloride (1 in 2000) add 1 mL of dilute sodium pentacyanonitrosylferrate (III)-potassium hexacyanoferrate (III) TS: a red-brown color develops.

(2) Determine the absorption spectrum of a solution of Buformin Hydrochloride (1 in 125,000) as directed under Ultraviolet-visible Spectrophotometry ⟨*2.24*⟩, and compare the spectrum with the Reference Spectrum: both spectra exhibit similar intensities of absorption at the same wavelengths.

(3) Determine the infrared absorption spectrum of Buformin Hydrochloride as directed in the potassium chloride disk method under Infrared Spectrophotometry ⟨*2.25*⟩, and compare the spectrum with the Reference Spectrum: both spectra exhibit similar intensities of absorption at the same wave numbers.

(4) A solution of Buformin Hydrochloride (1 in 20) responds to the Qualitative Tests ⟨*1.09*⟩ for chlorides.

Melting point ⟨*2.60*⟩ 175 – 180°C

Purity **(1)** Heavy metals ⟨*1.07*⟩—Proceed with 1.0 g of Buformin Hydrochloride according to Method 1, and perform the test. Prepare the control solution with 2.0 mL of Standard Lead Solution (not more than 20 ppm).

(2) Arsenic ⟨*1.11*⟩—Prepare the test solution with 1.0 g of Buformin Hydrochloride according to Method 1, and perform the test (not more than 2 ppm).

(3) Related substances—Dissolve 0.10 g of Buformin Hydrochloride in 200 mL of the mobile phase, and use this solution as the sample solution. Pipet 1 mL of the sample solution, add the mobile phase to make exactly 100 mL, and use this solution as the standard solution. Perform the test with exactly 10 μL each of the sample solution and standard solution as directed under Liquid Chromatography ⟨*2.01*⟩ according to the following conditions, and determine each peak area of both solutions by the automatic integration method: the area of the peak other than buformin obtained from the sample solution is not larger than 1/5 times the peak area of buformin from the standard solution. Furthermore, the total areas of all peaks other than the buformin peak from the sample solution is not larger than 1/2 times the peak area of buformin from the standard solution.

Operating conditions—

Detector: An ultraviolet absorption photometer (wavelength: 230 nm).

Column: A stainless steel column 4.6 mm in inside diameter and 15 cm in length, packed with octadecylsilanized silica gel for liquid chromatography (5 μm in particle diameter).

Column temperature: A constant temperature of about 35°C.

Mobile phase: A mixture of a solution of sodium perchlorate monohydrate in diluted phosphoric acid (1 in 1000) (7 in 250) and acetonitrile (7:1).

Flow rate: Adjust so that the retention time of buformin is about 6 minutes.

Time span of measurement: About 2 times as long as the retention time of buformin, beginning after the solvent peak.

System suitability—

Test for required detectability: Pipet 1 mL of the standard solution, and add the mobile phase to make exactly 10 mL. Confirm that the peak area of buformin obtained with 10 μL of this solution is equivalent to 7 to 13% of that with 10 μL of the standard solution.

System performance: When the procedure is run with 10 μL of the standard solution under the above operating conditions, the number of theoretical plates and the symmetry factor of the peak of buformin are not less than 5000 and

not more than 2.0, respectively.

System repeatability: When the test is repeated 6 times with 10 μL of the standard solution under the above operating conditions, the relative standard deviation of the peak area of buformin is not more than 1.0%.

Loss on drying <2.41> Not more than 0.5% (1 g, 105°C, 3 hours).

Residue on ignition <2.44> Not more than 0.1% (1 g).

Assay Weigh accurately about 0.15 g of Buformin Hydrochloride, previously dried, dissolve in 50 mL of a mixture of acetic anhydride and acetic acid (100) (7:3), and immediately titrate <2.50> with 0.1 mol/L perchloric acid VS (potentiometric titration). Perform a blank determination in the same manner, and make any necessary correction.

Each mL of 0.1 mol/L perchloric acid VS
= 9.684 mg of $C_6H_{15}N_5.HCl$

Containers and storage Containers—Tight containers.

Buformin Hydrochloride Delayed-release Tablets

ブホルミン塩酸塩腸溶錠

Buformin Hydrochloride Delayed-release Tablets contain not less than 93.0% and not more than 107.0% of the labeled amount of buformin hydrochloride ($C_6H_{15}N_5.HCl$: 193.68).

Method of preparation Prepare as directed under Tablets, with Buformin Hydrochloride.

Identification To a quantity of powdered Buformin Hydrochloride Delayed-release Tablets, equivalent to 0.1 g of Buformin Hydrochloride, add 10 mL of water, shake well, and then filter. To 4 mL of the filtrate add 1 mL of a mixture of hydrogen peroxide TS, sodium pentacyanonitrosylferrate (III) TS and a solution of sodium hydroxide (1 in 10) (2:1:1): the solution exhibits a red to red-purple color.

Uniformity of dosage units <6.02> Perform the test according to the following method: it meets the requirement of the Content uniformity test.

To 1 tablet of Buformin Hydrochloride Delayed-release Tablets add 5 mL of a mixture of ethanol (99.5) and acetone (1:1), disperse the pellicle to smaller using ultrasonic waves, add exactly 10 mL of the internal standard solution per 50 mg of buformin hydrochloride ($C_6H_{15}N_5.HCl$), and then add diluted acetonitrile (1 in 2) to make 13*V*/20 mL. Disintegrate the tablet using ultrasonic waves, then shake for 20 minutes, and add diluted acetonitrile (1 in 2) to make *V* mL so that each mL contains about 0.5 mg of buformin hydrochloride ($C_6H_{15}N_5.HCl$) per mL. Centrifuge this solution, to 1 mL of the supernatant liquid, add the mobile phase to make 50 mL. If necessary, filter this solution through a membrane filter with a pore size not exceeding 0.5 μm, and use the filtrate as the sample solution. Then, proceed as directed in the Assay.

Amount (mg) of buformin hydrochloride ($C_6H_{15}N_5.HCl$)
$= M_S \times Q_T/Q_S \times V/50$

M_S: Amount (mg) of buformin hydrochloride for assay taken

Internal standard solution—A solution of *p*-acetanisidide in diluted acetonitrile (1 in 2) (1 in 150).

Dissolution <6.10> When the tests are performed at 50 revolutions per minute according to the Paddle method, using 900 mL each of 1st fluid for dissolution test and 2nd fluid for dissolution test as the dissolution medium, the dissolution rate in 120 minutes of Buformin Hydrochloride Delayed-release Tablets using 1st fluid is not more than 5%, and that in 90 minutes of Buformin Hydrochloride Delayed-release Tablets using 2nd fluid is not less than 80%.

Start the test with 1 tablet of Buformin Hydrochloride Delayed-release Tablets, withdraw not less than 20 mL of the medium at the specified minute after starting the test, and filter through a membrane filter with a pore size not exceeding 0.5 μm. Discard not less than 10 mL of the first filtrate, pipet *V* mL of the subsequent filtrate, add the relevant dissolution medium to make exactly *V′* mL so that each mL contains about 56 μg of buformin hydrochloride ($C_6H_{15}N_5.HCl$), and use this solution as the sample solution. Separately, weigh accurately about 28 mg of buformin hydrochloride for assay, previously dried at 105°C for 3 hours, and dissolve in the relevant dissolution medium to make exactly 100 mL. Pipet 4 mL of this solution, add the relevant dissolution medium to make exactly 20 mL, and use this solution as the standard solution. Perform the test with exactly 20 μL each of the sample solution and standard solution as directed under Liquid Chromatography <2.01> according to the following conditions, and determine the peak areas, A_T and A_S, of buformin in each solution.

Dissolution rate (%) with respect to the labeled amount of buformin hydrochloride ($C_6H_{15}N_5.HCl$)
$= M_S \times A_T/A_S \times V'/V \times 1/C \times 180$

M_S: Amount (mg) of buformin hydrochloride for assay taken

C: Labeled amount (mg) of buformin hydrochloride ($C_6H_{15}N_5.HCl$) in 1 tablet

Operating conditions—

Detector: An ultraviolet absorption photometer (wavelength: 230 nm).

Column: A stainless steel column 4.6 mm in inside diameter and 15 cm in length, packed with octadecylsilanized silica gel for liquid chromatography (5 μm in particle diameter).

Column temperature: A constant temperature of about 35°C.

Mobile phase: A mixture of a solution of sodium perchlorate in diluted phosphoric acid (1 in 1000) (7 in 500) and acetonitrile (7:1).

Flow rate: Adjust so that the retention time of buformin is about 6 minutes.

System suitability—

System performance: When the procedure is run with 20 μL of the standard solution under the above operating conditions, the number of theoretical plates and the symmetry factor of the peak of buformin are not less than 3000 and not more than 2.0, respectively.

System repeatability: When the test is repeated 6 times with 20 μL of the standard solution under the above operating conditions, the relative standard deviation of the peak area of buformin is not more than 2.0%.

Assay Add 20 mL of a mixture of ethanol (99.5) and acetone (1:1) to an amount of Buformin Hydrochloride Delayed-release Tablets equivalent to 0.5 g of buformin hydrochloride ($C_6H_{15}N_5.HCl$), disperse the pellicles to smaller using ultrasonic waves, and then add 100 mL of diluted acetonitrile (1 in 2). Disintegrate the tablets with the aid of ultrasonic waves, shake for 20 minutes, and then add diluted acetonitrile (1 in 2) to make exactly 200 mL. Centrifuge this solution, pipet 10 mL of the supernatant liquid, add exactly 5 mL of the internal standard solution, and then add diluted acetonitrile (1 in 2) to make 50 mL. Pipet 1 mL of this solution, and add the mobile phase to make 50 mL. If necessary, filter this solution through a membrane filter with a pore size not exceeding 0.5 μm, and use the filtrate as the sample solution. Separately, weigh accurately about 25 mg of buformin hydrochloride for assay, previously dried at 105°C for 3 hours, dissolve in an adequate amount of diluted acetonitrile (1 in 2), add exactly 5 mL of the internal standard solution, and then add diluted acetonitrile (1 in 2) to make 50 mL. To 1 mL of this solution add the mobile phase to make 50 mL, and use this solution as the standard solution. Perform the test with 10 μL each of the sample solution and standard solution as directed under Liquid Chromatography <*2.01*> according to the following conditions, and calculate the ratios, Q_T and Q_S, of the peak area of buformin to that of the internal standard.

Amount (mg) of buformin hydrochloride ($C_6H_{15}N_5.HCl$)
$= M_S \times Q_T/Q_S \times 20$

M_S: Amount (mg) of buformin hydrochloride for assay taken

Internal standard solution—A solution of *p*-acetanisidide in diluted acetonitrile (1 in 2) (1 in 150).
Operating conditions—

Detector: An ultraviolet absorption photometer (wavelength: 233 nm).

Column: A stainless steel column 4.6 mm in inside diameter and 15 cm in length, packed with octadecylsilanized silica gel for liquid chromatography (5 μm in particle diameter).

Column temperature: A constant temperature of about 35°C.

Mobile phase: A mixture of a solution of sodium perchlorate (7 in 250) and acetonitrile (7:1).

Flow rate: Adjust so that the retention time of buformin is about 7 minutes.
System suitability—

System performance: When the procedure is run with 10 μL of the standard solution under the above operating conditions, buformin and the internal standard are eluted in this order with the resolution between these peaks being not less than 5.

System repeatability: When the test is repeated 6 times with 10 μL of the standard solution under the above operating conditions, the relative standard deviation of the ratio of the peak area of buformin to that of the internal standard is not more than 1.0%.

Containers and storage Containers—Well-closed containers.

Buformin Hydrochloride Tablets

ブホルミン塩酸塩錠

Buformin Hydrochloride Tablets contain not less than 95.0% and not more than 105.0% of the labeled amount of buformin hydrochloride ($C_6H_{15}N_5.HCl$: 193.68).

Method of preparation Prepare as directed under Tablets, with Buformin Hydrochloride.

Identification To a quantity of powdered Buformin Hydrochloride Tablets, equivalent to 1 g of Buformin Hydrochloride, add 100 mL of water, shake well, and then filter. To 4 mL of the filtrate add 1 mL of dilute sodium pentacyanonitrosylferrate (III)-potassium hexacyanoferrate (III) TS: the solution exhibits a red-brown color.

Uniformity of dosage units <*6.02*> Perform the Mass variation test, or the Content uniformity test according to the following method: it meets the requirement.

Take 1 tablet of Buformin Hydrochloride Tablets, add water to make exactly 200 mL, and then treat with ultrasonic waves for 5 minutes. Take 40 mL of this solution and centrifuge. Pipet V mL of the supernatant liquid equivalent to about 0.5 mg of buformin hydrochloride ($C_6H_{15}N_5.HCl$), add water to make exactly 100 mL, and use this solution as the sample solution. Separately, weigh accurately about 50 mg of buformin hydrochloride for assay, previously dried at 105°C for 3 hours, and dissolve in water to make exactly 200 mL. Pipet 2 mL of this solution, add water to make exactly 100 mL, and use this solution as the standard solution. Determine the absorbances, A_T and A_S, of the sample solution and standard solution at 233 nm as directed under Ultraviolet-visible Spectrophotometry <*2.24*>.

Amount (mg) of buformin hydrochloride ($C_6H_{15}N_5.HCl$)
$= M_S \times A_T/A_S \times 2/V$

M_S: Amount (mg) of buformin hydrochloride for assay taken

Dissolution <*6.10*> When the test is performed at 50 revolutions per minute according to the Paddle method, using 900 mL of water as the dissolution medium, the dissolution rate in 15 minutes of Buformin Hydrochloride Tablets is not less than 80%.

Start the test with 1 tablet of Buformin Hydrochloride Tablets, withdraw not less than 20 mL of the medium at the specified minute after starting the test, and filter through a membrane filter with a pore size not exceeding 0.5 μm. Discard not less than 10 mL of the first filtrate, pipet V mL of the subsequent filtrate, and add water to make exactly V' mL so that each mL contains about 5.6 μg of buformin hydrochloride ($C_6H_{15}N_5.HCl$), and use this solution as the sample solution. Separately, weigh accurately about 28 mg of buformin hydrochloride for assay, previously dried at 105°C for 3 hours, and dissolve in water to make exactly 100 mL. Pipet 2 mL of this solution, add water to make exactly 100 mL, and use this solution as the standard solution. Perform the test with the sample solution and standard solution as directed under Ultraviolet-visible Spectrophotometry <*2.24*>, and determine the absorbances, A_T and A_S, at 233 nm.

Dissolution rate (%) with respect to the labeled amount of buformin hydrochloride ($C_6H_{15}N_5.HCl$)
$= M_S \times A_T/A_S \times V'/V \times 1/C \times 18$

M_S: Amount (mg) of buformin hydrochloride for assay taken
C: Labeled amount (mg) of buformin hydrochloride ($C_6H_{15}N_5.HCl$) in 1 tablet

Assay Weigh accurately not less than 20 Buformin Hydrochloride Tablets, and powder. Weigh accurately a portion of the powder, equivalent to about 60 mg of buformin hydrochloride ($C_6H_{15}N_5.HCl$), add water to make exactly 200 mL, and treat with ultrasonic waves for 5 minutes. Take 40 mL of this solution, centrifuge, pipet 2 mL of the supernatant liquid, add water to make exactly 100 mL, and use this solution as the sample solution. Separately, weigh accurately about 60 mg of buformin hydrochloride for assay, previously dried at 105°C for 3 hours, and dissolve in water to make exactly 200 mL. Pipet 2 mL of this solution, add water to make exactly 100 mL, and use this solution as the standard solution. Perform the test with the sample solution and standard solution as directed under Ultraviolet-visible Spectrophotometry 〈*2.24*〉, and determine the absorbances, A_T and A_S, at 233 nm.

Amount (mg) of buformin hydrochloride ($C_6H_{15}N_5.HCl$)
$= M_S \times A_T/A_S$

M_S: Amount (mg) of buformin hydrochloride for assay taken

Containers and storage Containers—Well-closed containers.

Bumetanide

ブメタニド

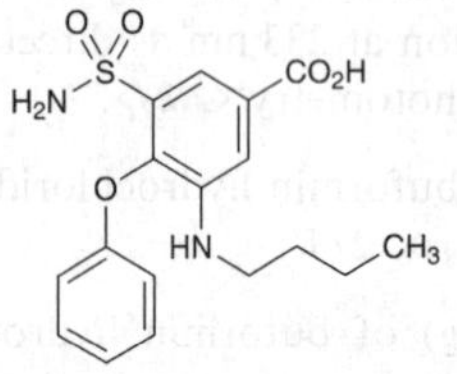

$C_{17}H_{20}N_2O_5S$: 364.42
3-Butylamino-4-phenoxy-5-sulfamoylbenzoic acid
[*28395-03-1*]

Bumetanide, when dried, contains not less than 98.5% of bumetanide ($C_{17}H_{20}N_2O_5S$).

Description Bumetanide occurs as white, crystals or crystalline powder.

It is freely soluble in pyridine, soluble in methanol and in ethanol (95), slightly soluble in diethyl ether, and practically insoluble in water.

It dissolves in potassium hydroxide TS.

It is gradually colored by light.

Identification **(1)** Dissolve 0.01 g of Bumetanide in 1 mL of pyridine, add 2 drops of copper (II) sulfate TS, shake, add 3 mL of water and 5 mL of chloroform, shake, and allow to stand: a light blue color develops in the chloroform layer.

(2) Dissolve 0.04 g of Bumetanide in 100 mL of phosphate buffer solution (pH 7.0) and dilute 10 mL of the solution with water to make 100 mL. Determine the absorption spectrum of the solution as directed under Ultraviolet-visible Spectrophotometry 〈*2.24*〉, and compare the spectrum with the Reference Spectrum: both spectra exhibit similar intensities of absorption at the same wavelengths.

(3) Determine the infrared absorption spectrum of Bumetanide, previously dried, as directed in the potassium bromide disk method under Infrared Spectrophotometry 〈*2.25*〉, and compare the spectrum with the Reference Spectrum: both spectra exhibit similar intensities of absorption at the same wave numbers.

Melting point 〈*2.60*〉 232 – 237°C

Purity **(1)** Clarity and color of solution—Dissolve 50 mg of Bumetanide in 2 mL of a solution of potassium hydroxide (1 in 30) and 8 mL of water: the solution is clear, and is not more colored than the following control solution.

Control solution: Pipet 0.5 mL each of Cobalt (II) Chloride CS, Iron (III) Chloride CS and Copper (II) Sulfate CS, mix them, and add diluted hydrochloric acid (1 in 40) to make exactly 100 mL.

(2) Chloride 〈*1.03*〉—Mix well 0.5 g of Bumetanide with 0.7 g of potassium nitrate and 1.2 g of anhydrous sodium carbonate, transfer, in small portions, to a red-hot platinum crucible, and heat to red-hot until the reaction is complete. After cooling, to the residue add 14 mL of dilute sulfuric acid and 6 mL of water, boil for 5 minutes, filter, wash the residue with 10 mL of water, combine the filtrate and the washing, and add 6 mL of dilute nitric acid and water to make 50 mL. Perform the test using this solution as the test solution. Prepare the control solution with 0.30 mL of 0.01 mol/L hydrochloric acid VS (not more than 0.021%).

(3) Heavy metals 〈*1.07*〉—Proceed with 2.0 g of Bumetanide according to Method 2, and perform the test. Prepare the control solution with 2.0 mL of Standard Lead Solution (not more than 10 ppm).

(4) Arsenic 〈*1.11*〉—Prepare the test solution with 1.0 g of Bumetanide according to Method 3, and perform the test (not more than 2 ppm).

(5) Related substances—Conduct this procedure without exposure to light, using light-resistant vessels. Dissolve 0.10 g of Bumetanide in 10 mL of methanol, and use this solution as the sample solution. Pipet 1 mL of the sample solution, and add methanol to make exactly 100 mL. Pipet 2 mL of this solution, add methanol to make exactly 10 mL, and use this solution as the standard solution. Perform the test with these solutions as directed under Thin-layer Chromatography 〈*2.03*〉. Spot 10 μL each of the sample solution and standard solution on a plate of silica gel with fluorescent indicator for thin-layer chromatography. Develop the plate with a mixture of chloroform, acetic acid (100), cyclohexane and methanol (32:4:4:1) to a distance of about 12 cm, and air-dry the plate. Examine under ultraviolet light (main wavelength: 254 nm): the spots other than the principal spot obtained from the sample solution are not more intense than the spot from the standard solution.

Loss on drying 〈*2.41*〉 Not more than 0.5% (1 g, 105°C, 2 hours).

Residue on ignition 〈*2.44*〉 Not more than 0.1% (1 g).

Assay Weigh accurately about 0.5 g of Bumetanide, previously dried, dissolve in 50 mL of ethanol (95), and titrate 〈*2.50*〉 with 0.1 mol/L sodium hydroxide VS (potentiometric titration). Perform a blank determination in the same manner, and make any necessary correction.

Each mL of 0.1 mol/L sodium hydroxide VS
$= 36.44$ mg of $C_{17}H_{20}N_2O_5S$

Containers and storage Containers—Tight containers.
Storage—Light-resistant.

Bunazosin Hydrochloride

ブナゾシン塩酸塩

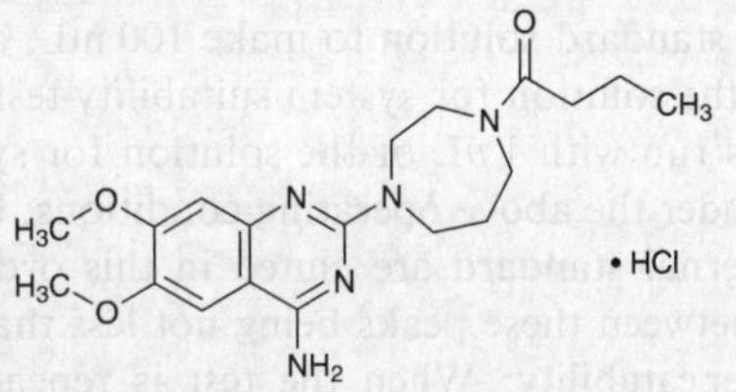

$C_{19}H_{27}N_5O_3.HCl$: 409.91
4-Amino-2-(4-butanoyl-1,4-diazepan-1-yl)-6,7-dimethoxyquinazoline monohydrochloride
[*52712-76-2*]

Bunazosin Hydrochloride, when dried, contains not less than 98.0% of bunazosin hydrochloride ($C_{19}H_{27}N_5O_3.HCl$).

Description Bunazosin Hydrochloride occurs as a white crystalline powder.

It is very soluble in formic acid, slightly soluble in water and in methanol, very slightly soluble in ethanol (99.5), and practically insoluble in diethyl ether.

Melting point: about 273°C (with decomposition).

Identification **(1)** Dissolve 0.1 g of Bunazosin Hydrochloride in 10 mL of 0.2 mol/L hydrochloric acid TS, and boil for 3 minutes over a flame: butylic acid like odor is perceptible.

(2) Determine the infrared absorption spectrum of Bunazosin Hydrochloride, previously dried, as directed in the potassium bromide disk method under Infrared Spectrophotometry *<2.25>*, and compare the spectrum with the Reference Spectrum: both spectra exhibit similar intensities of absorption at the same wave numbers.

(3) A solution of Bunazosin Hydrochloride (1 in 100) responds to Qualitative Tests *<1.09>* for chloride.

Purity **(1)** Heavy metals *<1.07>*—Proceed with 1.0 g of Bunazosin Hydrochloride according to Method 4, and perform the test. Prepare the control solution with 2.0 mL of Standard Lead Solution (not more than 20 ppm).

(2) Related substances—Dissolve 0.05 g of Bunazosin Hydrochloride in 50 mL of the mobile phase, and use this solution as the sample solution. To exactly 1 mL of the sample solution add the mobile phase to make exactly 200 mL, and use this solution as the standard solution. Perform the test with exactly 10 μL each of the sample solution and standard solution as directed under Liquid Chromatography *<2.01>* according to the following conditions. Determine each peak area of both solutions by the automatic integration method: the total area of the peaks other than bunazosin obtained from the sample solution is not larger than the peak area of bunazosin from the standard solution.

Operating conditions—

Detector: An ultraviolet absorption photometer (wavelength: 254 nm).

Column: A stainless steel column about 4 mm in inside diameter and about 15 cm in length, packed with octadecylsilanized silica gel for liquid chromatography (5 μm in particle diameter).

Column temperature: A constant temperature of about 30°C.

Mobile phase: Dissolve 1.44 g of sodium lauryl sulfate in a suitable amount of water, add 10 mL of acetic acid (100), 500 mL of acetonitrile and water to make 1000 mL.

Flow rate: Adjust so that the retention time of bunazosin is about 5 minutes.

Selection of column: Proceed with 20 μL of a mixture of the standard solution and a solution of procaine hydrochloride in the mobile phase (1 in 20,000) (1:1) under the above operating conditions, and calculate the resolution. Use a column giving elution of procaine and bunazosin in this order with the resolution between these peaks being not less than 3.0.

Detection sensitivity: Adjust the detection sensitivity so that the peak height of bunazosin obtained from 20 μL of the standard solution is 20 to 60% of the full-scale.

Time span of measurement: About 6 times of the retention time of bunazosin.

Loss on drying *<2.41>* Not more than 0.5% (1 g, 105°C, 2 hours).

Residue on ignition *<2.44>* Not more than 0.1% (1 g).

Assay Weigh accurately about 0.3 g of Bunazosin Hydrochloride, previously dried, dissolve in 6 mL of formic acid, add exactly 15 mL of 0.1 mol/L perchloric acid, and heat for 20 minutes on a water bath. After cooling, add 20 mL of acetic acid (100), and titrate *<2.50>* the excess perchloric acid with 0.1 mol/L sodium acetate VS (potentiometric titration). Perform a blank determination in the same manner.

Each mL of 0.1 mol/L perchloric acid VS
= 40.99 mg of $C_{19}H_{27}N_5O_3.HCl$

Containers and storage Containers—Well-closed containers.

Storage—Light-resistant.

Bupivacaine Hydrochloride Hydrate

ブピバカイン塩酸塩水和物

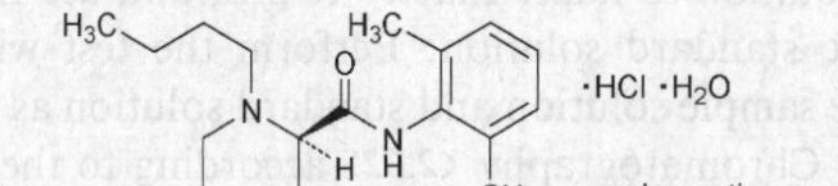

and enantiomer

$C_{18}H_{28}N_2O.HCl.H_2O$: 342.90
(2*RS*)-1-Butyl-*N*-(2,6-dimethylphenyl)piperidine-2-carboxamide monohydrochloride monohydrate
[*14252-80-3*]

Bupivacaine Hydrochloride Hydrate contains not less than 98.5% and not more than 101.0% of bupivacaine hydrochloride ($C_{18}H_{28}N_2O.HCl$: 324.89), calculated on the anhydrous basis.

Description Bupivacaine Hydrochloride Hydrate occurs as a white crystalline powder.

It is freely soluble in acetic acid (100), and soluble in water, in methanol and in ethanol (99.5).

It dissolves in 0.01 mol/L hydrochloric acid TS.

A solution of 0.5 g of Bupivacaine Hydrochloride Hydrate in 50 mL of a mixture of ethanol (99.5), water and 5 mol/L sodium hydroxide TS (34:15:1) shows no optical rotation.

Melting point: about 252°C (with decomposition).

Identification **(1)** Determine the absorption spectrum of a solution of Bupivacaine Hydrochloride Hydrate in 0.01 mol/L hydrochloric acid TS (1 in 2000) as directed under Ultraviolet-visible Spectrophotometry <*2.24*>, and compare the spectrum with the Reference Spectrum: both spectra exhibit similar intensities of absorption at the same wavelengths.

(2) Determine the infrared absorption spectrum of Bupivacaine Hydrochloride Hydrate as directed in the potassium chloride disk method under Infrared Spectrophotometry <*2.25*>, and compare the spectrum with the Reference Spectrum: both spectra exhibit similar intensities of absorption at the same wave numbers.

(3) A solution of Bupivacaine Hydrochloride Hydrate (1 in 50) responds to Qualitative Tests <*1.09*> for chloride.

pH <*2.54*> The pH of a solution obtained by dissolving 1.0 g of Bupivacaine Hydrochloride Hydrate in 100 mL of freshly boiled and cooled water is between 4.5 to 6.0.

Purity **(1)** Clarity and color of solution—Dissolve 1.0 g of Bupivacaine Hydrochloride Hydrate in 50 mL of water: the solution is clear and colorless.

(2) Heavy metals <*1.07*>—Proceed with 1.0 g of Bupivacaine Hydrochloride Hydrate according to Method 1, and perform the test. Prepare the control solution with 2.0 mL of Standard Lead Solution (not more than 20 ppm).

(3) 2,6-Dimethylaniline—Dissolve exactly 0.50 g of Bupivacaine Hydrochloride Hydrate in 10 mL of methanol. To 2 mL of this solution add 1 mL of a freshly prepared solution of 4-dimethylaminobenzaldehyde in methanol (1 in 100) and 2 mL of acetic acid (100), and allow to stand for 10 minutes: the color of the solution is not more colored than the following control solution.

Control solution: Prepare by proceeding in the same manner as above, using 2 mL of a solution of 2,6-dimethylaniline in methanol (1 in 200,000).

(4) Related substances—Dissolve 50 mg of Bupivacaine Hydrochloride Hydrate in 2.5 mL of water, add 2.5 mL of 2 mol/L sodium hydroxide TS and 5 mL of the internal standard solution, shake, collect the lower layer, filter, and use the filtrate as the sample solution. Pipet 1 mL of the sample solution, and add the internal standard solution to make exactly 100 mL. Pipet 1 mL of this solution, add the internal standard solution to make exactly 10 mL, and use this solution as the standard solution. Perform the test with 1 μL each of the sample solution and standard solution as directed under Gas Chromatography <*2.02*> according to the following conditions, and determine each peak area by the automatic integration method: the ratio of the area of the peak other than bupivacaine to the peak area of the internal standard obtained from the sample solution is not larger than the ratio of the peak area of bupivacaine to that of the internal standard from the standard solution.

Internal standard solution—A solution of methyl behenate in dichloromethane (1 in 20,000).

Operating conditions—

Detector: A hydrogen flame-ionization detector.

Column: A quartz tube 0.32 mm in inside diameter and 30 m in length, coated the inside surface with 5% diphenyl-95% dimethylpolysiloxane for gas chromatography 0.25 μm in thickness.

Column temperature: Rise the temperature from 180°C to 230°C at the rate of 5°C per minute, and maintain at 230°C for 5 minutes.

Injection port temperature: A constant temperature of about 250°C.

Detector temperature: A constant temperature of about 250°C.

Carrier gas: Helium.

Flow rate: Adjust so that the retention time of bupivacaine is about 10 minutes.

Split ratio: 1:12.

Time span of measurement: About 1.5 times as long as the retention time of bupivacaine.

System suitability—

System performance: To 1 mL of the sample solution add the internal standard solution to make 100 mL, and use this solution as the solution for system suitability test. When the procedure is run with 1 μL of the solution for system suitability test under the above operating conditions, bupivacaine and the internal standard are eluted in this order with the resolution between these peaks being not less than 20.

System repeatability: When the test is repeated 6 times with 1 μL of the solution for system suitability test under the above operating conditions, the relative standard deviation of the ratio of the peak area of bupivacaine to that of the internal standard is not more than 2.0%.

Water <*2.48*> 4.0 – 6.0% (0.25 g, volumetric titration, direct titration).

Residue on ignition <*2.44*> Not more than 0.1% (1 g).

Assay Weigh accurately about 0.5 g of Bupivacaine Hydrochloride Hydrate, dissolve in 20 mL of acetic acid (100), add 50 mL of acetic anhydride, and titrate <*2.50*> with 0.1 mol/L perchloric acid VS (potentiometric titration). Perform a blank determination in the same manner, and make any necessary correction.

Each mL of 0.1 mol/L perchloric acid VS
= 32.49 mg of $C_{18}H_{28}N_2O.HCl$

Containers and storage Containers—Tight containers.

Bupranolol Hydrochloride

ブプラノロール塩酸塩

and enantiomer

$C_{14}H_{22}ClNO_2.HCl$: 308.24

(2*RS*)-3-(2-Chloro-5-methylphenoxy)-1-(1,1-dimethylethyl)aminopropan-2-ol monohydrochloride

[*15148-80-8*]

Bupranolol Hydrochloride, when dried, contains not less than 98.0% of bupranolol hydrochloride ($C_{14}H_{22}ClNO_2.HCl$).

Description Bupranolol Hydrochloride occurs as a white crystalline powder.

It is sparingly soluble in methanol, slightly soluble in water, in ethanol (95) and in acetic acid (100), very slightly soluble in acetic anhydride, and practically insoluble in diethyl ether.

The pH of a solution of 1.0 g of Bupranolol Hydrochloride in 1000 mL of water is between 5.2 and 6.2.

Identification **(1)** Take 0.01 g of Bupranolol Hydrochloride in a test tube, mix with 25 mg of potassium iodide and 25 mg of oxalic acid dihydrate, cover the mouth of the test tube with filter paper moistened with a solution of 2,6-dibromo-*N*-chloro-1,4-benzoquinone monoimine in ethanol (95) (1 in 100), and heat gently for several minutes. Expose the filter paper to ammonia gas: the filter paper acquires a blue color.

(2) Determine the absorption spectrum of a solution of

Bupranolol Hydrochloride in 0.1 mol/L hydrochloric acid TS (1 in 10,000) as directed under Ultraviolet-visible Spectrophotometry <*2.24*>, and compare the spectrum with the Reference Spectrum: both spectra exhibit similar intensities of absorption at the same wavelengths.

(3) Determine the infrared absorption spectrum of Bupranolol Hydrochloride, previously dried, as directed in the potassium chloride disk method under Infrared Spectrophotometry <*2.25*>, and compare the spectrum with the Reference Spectrum: both spectra exhibit similar intensities of absorption at the same wave numbers.

(4) A solution of Bupranolol Hydrochloride (1 in 200) responds to Qualitative Tests <*1.09*> for chloride.

Absorbance <*2.24*> $E^{1\%}_{1\,cm}$ (275 nm): 57 – 60 (after drying, 50 mg, 0.1 mol/L hydrochloric acid TS, 500 mL).

Melting point <*2.60*> 223 – 226°C

Purity **(1)** Clarity and color of solution—Dissolve 0.10 g of Bupranolol Hydrochloride in 15 mL of water: the solution is clear and colorless.

(2) Acidity—Dissolve 0.10 g of Bupranolol Hydrochloride in 15 mL of freshly boiled and cooled water, and add 1 drop of methyl red TS: a light red color develops. To this solution add 0.05 mL of 0.01 mol/L sodium hydroxide VS: the color changes to yellow.

(3) Sulfate <*1.14*>—Perform the test with 0.10 g of Bupranolol Hydrochloride. Prepare the control solution with 0.35 mL of 0.005 mol/L sulfuric acid VS (not more than 0.168%).

(4) Heavy metals <*1.07*>—Proceed with 1.0 g of Bupranolol Hydrochloride according to Method 4, and perform the test. Prepare the control solution with 2.0 mL of Standard Lead Solution (not more than 20 ppm).

(5) Arsenic <*1.11*>—Prepare the test solution with 1.0 g of Bupranolol Hydrochloride according to Method 3, and perform the test (not more than 2 ppm).

(6) Related substances—Dissolve 0.30 g of Bupranolol Hydrochloride in 10 mL of methanol, and use this solution as the sample solution. Pipet 1 mL of the sample solution, add methanol to make exactly 100 mL, and use this solution as the standard solution. Perform the test with these solutions as directed under Thin-layer Chromatography <*2.03*>. Spot 10 μL each of the sample solution and standard solution on a plate of polyamide with fluorescent indicator for thin-layer chromatography. Develop the plate with a mixture of methanol, ammonia solution (28) and water (16:4:1) to a distance of about 10 cm, and air-dry the plate. Examine under ultraviolet light (main wavelength: 254 nm): the spots other than the principal spot obtained from the sample solution are not more intense than the spot from the standard solution.

Loss on drying <*2.41*> Not more than 0.5% (0.5 g, 105°C, 4 hours).

Residue on ignition <*2.44*> Not more than 0.1% (1 g).

Assay Weigh accurately about 0.18 g of Bupranolol Hydrochloride, previously dried, dissolve in 60 mL of a mixture of acetic anhydride and acetic acid (100) (2:1) by warming, cool, and titrate <*2.50*> with 0.1 mol/L perchloric acid VS (potentiometric titration). Perform a blank determination in the same manner, and make any necessary correction.

Each mL of 0.1 mol/L perchloric acid VS
= 30.82 mg of $C_{14}H_{22}ClNO_2.HCl$

Containers and storage Containers—Well-closed containers.

Buprenorphine Hydrochloride

ブプレノルフィン塩酸塩

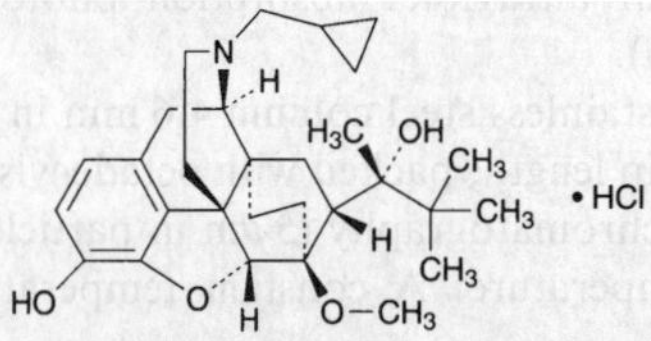

$C_{29}H_{41}NO_4.HCl$: 504.10
(2*S*)-2-[(5*R*,6*R*,7*R*,14*S*)-17-(Cyclopropylmethyl)-4,5-epoxy-3-hydroxy-6-methoxy-6,14-ethanomorphinan-7-yl]-3,3-dimethylbutan-2-ol monohydrochloride
[*53152-21-9*]

Buprenorphine Hydrochloride, when dried, contains not less than 98.5% and not more than 101.0% of buprenorphine hydrochloride ($C_{29}H_{41}NO_4.HCl$).

Description Buprenorphine Hydrochloride occurs as white to yellowish white, crystals or a crystalline powder.

It is freely soluble in methanol and in acetic acid (100), and sparingly soluble in water and in ethanol (99.5).

Melting point: about 268°C (with decomposition).

Identification **(1)** Determine the absorption spectrum of a solution of Buprenorphine Hydrochloride (1 in 5000) as directed under Ultraviolet-visible Spectrophotometry <*2.24*>, and compare the spectrum with the Reference Spectrum: both spectra exhibit similar intensities of absorption at the same wavelengths.

(2) Determine the infrared absorption spectrum of Buprenorphine Hydrochloride as directed in the potassium chloride disk method under Infrared Spectrophotometry <*2.25*>, and compare the spectrum with the Reference Spectrum: both spectra exhibit similar intensities of absorption at the same wave numbers.

(3) A solution of Buprenorphine Hydrochloride (1 in 100) responds to Qualitative Tests <*1.09*> for chloride.

Optical rotation <*2.49*> $[\alpha]_D^{20}$: −92 – −98° (after drying, 0.4 g, methanol, 20 mL, 100 mm).

pH <*2.54*> The pH of a solution prepared by dissolving 1.0 g of Buprenorphine Hydrochloride in 200 mL of water is between 4.0 and 6.0.

Purity **(1)** Clarity and color of solution—A solution obtained by dissolving 0.1 g of Buprenorphine Hydrochloride in 10 mL of water is clear and colorless.

(2) Heavy metals <*1.07*>—Proceed with 1.0 g of Buprenorphine Hydrochloride according to Method 4, and perform the test. Prepare the control solution with 1.0 mL of Standard Lead Solution (not more than 10 ppm).

(3) Related substances—Dissolve 0.10 g of Buprenorphine Hydrochloride in 20 mL of the mobile phase, and use this solution as the sample solution. Pipet 1 mL of the sample solution, add the mobile phase to make exactly 100 mL, and use this solution as the standard solution. Perform the test with exactly 20 μL each of the sample solution and standard solution as directed under Liquid Chromatography <*2.01*> according to the following conditions. Determine each peak area of both solutions by the automatic integration method: the area of each peak other than buprenorphine obtained from the sample solution is not larger than 1/4 times the peak area of buprenorphine obtained from the standard solution. Furthermore, the total area of the peaks other than buprenorphine from the sample solution is not larger than 13/20 times the peak area of buprenorphine from the standard solution.

Operating conditions—

Detector: An ultraviolet absorption photometer (wavelength: 288 nm).

Column: A stainless steel column 4.6 mm in inside diameter and 25 cm in length, packed with octadecylsilanized silica gel for liquid chromatography (5 μm in particle diameter).

Column temperature: A constant temperature of about 40°C.

Mobile phase: A mixture of methanol, ammonium acetate solution (1 in 100), and acetic acid (100) (6000:1000:1).

Flow rate: Adjust so that the retention time of buprenorphine is about 17 minutes.

Time span of measurement: About 2.5 times as long as the retention time of buprenorphine, beginning after the solvent peak.

System suitability—

Test for required detectability: Pipet 5 mL of the standard solution, and add the mobile phase to make exactly 50 mL. Confirm that the peak area of buprenorphine obtained with 20 μL of this solution is equivalent to 7 to 13% of that with 20 μL of the standard solution.

System performance: When the procedure is run with 20 μL of the standard solution under the above operating conditions, the number of theoretical plates and the symmetry factor of the peak of buprenorphine are not less than 6500 and not more than 1.2, respectively.

System repeatability: When the test is repeated 6 times with 20 μL of the standard solution under the above operating conditions, the relative standard deviation of the peak area of buprenorphine is not more than 2.0%.

Loss on drying 〈*2.41*〉 Not more than 1.0% (1 g, 115°C, 3 hours).

Residue on ignition 〈*2.44*〉 Not more than 0.1% (1 g).

Assay Weigh accurately about 0.5 g of Buprenorphine Hydrochloride, previously dried, dissolve in 5 mL of acetic acid (100), add 50 mL of acetic anhydride, and titrate 〈*2.50*〉 with 0.1 mol/L perchloric acid VS (potentiometric titration). Perform a blank determination in the same manner, and make any necessary correction.

Each mL of 0.1 mol/L perchloric acid VS
= 50.41 mg of $C_{29}H_{41}NO_4$.HCl

Containers and storage Containers—Well-closed containers.

Busulfan

ブスルファン

$C_6H_{14}O_6S_2$: 246.30
Tetramethylenedimethanesulfonate
[55-98-1]

Busulfan contains not less than 98.5% of busulfan ($C_6H_{14}O_6S_2$), calculated on the dried basis.

Description Busulfan occurs as a white crystalline powder.

It is slightly soluble in diethyl ether, very slightly soluble in ethanol (95), and practically insoluble in water.

Identification **(1)** To 0.1 g of Busulfan add 10 mL of water and 5 mL of sodium hydroxide TS, dissolve by heating, and use this solution as the sample solution.

(i) To 7 mL of the sample solution add 1 drop of potassium permanganate TS: the red-purple color of potassium permanganate TS changes from blue-purple through blue to green.

(ii) Acidify 7 mL of the sample solution with dilute sulfuric acid, and add 1 drop of potassium permanganate TS: the color of potassium permanganate TS remains.

(2) Determine the infrared absorption spectrum of Busulfan, previously dried, as directed in the potassium bromide disk method under Infrared Spectrophotometry 〈*2.25*〉, and compare the spectrum with the Reference Spectrum: both spectra exhibit similar intensities of absorption at the same wave numbers.

Melting point 〈*2.60*〉 115 – 118°C

Purity **(1)** Sulfate 〈*1.14*〉—To 1.0 g of Busulfan add 40 mL of water, and dissolve by heating. Cool in ice for 15 minutes, and filter. Wash the residue with 5 mL of water, combine the washings with the filtrate, and add 1 mL of dilute hydrochloric acid and water to make 50 mL. Perform the test using this solution as the test solution. Prepare the control solution with 0.40 mL of 0.005 mol/L sulfuric acid VS (not more than 0.019%).

(2) Heavy metals 〈*1.07*〉—Proceed with 1.0 g of Busulfan according to Method 2, and perform the test. Prepare the control solution with 2.0 mL of Standard Lead Solution (not more than 20 ppm).

Loss on drying 〈*2.41*〉 Not more than 2.0% (1 g, in vacuum, phosphorus (V) oxide, 60°C, 4 hours).

Residue on ignition 〈*2.44*〉 Not more than 0.1% (1 g).

Assay Weigh accurately about 0.2 g of Busulfan, add 40 mL of water, and boil gently under a reflux condenser for 30 minutes. Cool, and titrate 〈*2.50*〉 with 0.1 mol/L sodium hydroxide VS (indicator: 3 drops of phenolphthalein TS).

Each mL of 0.1 mol/L sodium hydroxide VS
= 12.32 mg of $C_6H_{14}O_6S_2$

Containers and storage Containers—Well-closed containers.

Storage—Light-resistant.

Butenafine Hydrochloride

ブテナフィン塩酸塩

$C_{23}H_{27}N.HCl$: 353.93
N-[4-(1,1-Dimethylethyl)benzyl]-*N*-methyl-1-(naphthalen-1-yl)methylamine monohydrochloride
[101827-46-7]

Butenafine Hydrochloride, when dried, contains not less than 99.0% and not more than 101.0% of butenafine hydrochloride ($C_{23}H_{27}N.HCl$).

Description Butenafine Hydrochloride occurs as white, crystals or crystalline powder.

It is very soluble in formic acid, freely soluble in methanol and in ethanol (99.5), and slightly soluble in water.

The pH of a solution dissolved 0.20 g of Butenafine Hydrochloride in 100 mL of water by warming and cooled is 3.0 to 4.0.

Melting point: about 214°C (with decomposition).

Identification (1) Determine the absorption spectrum of a solution of Butenafine Hydrochloride in methanol (1 in 40,000) as directed under Ultraviolet-visible Spectrophotometry <*2.24*>, and compare the spectrum with the Reference Spectrum: both spectra exhibit similar intensities of absorption at the same wavelengths.

(2) Determine the infrared absorption spectrum of Butenafine Hydrochloride, previously dried, as directed in the potassium chloride disk method under Infrared Spectrophotometry <*2.25*>, and compare the spectrum with the Reference Spectrum: both spectra exhibit similar intensities of absorption at the same wave numbers.

(3) A solution of Butenafine Hydrochloride in dilute ethanol (1 in 200) responds to Qualitative Tests <*1.09*> (1) for chloride.

Purity (1) Heavy metals <*1.07*>—Dissolve 2.0 g of Butenafine Hydrochloride in 20 mL of ethanol (99.5), add 2 mL of dilute acetic acid and ethanol (99.5) to make 50 mL, and perform the test using this solution as the test solution. The control solution: To 2.0 mL of Standard Lead Solution add 2 mL of dilute acetic acid, and add ethanol (99.5) to make 50 mL (not more than 10 ppm).

(2) Related substances—Dissolve 30 mg of Butenafine Hydrochloride in 50 mL of a mixture of water and acetonitrile for liquid chromatography (3:2), and use this solution as the sample solution. Pipet 1 mL of the sample solution, add a mixture of water and acetonitrile for liquid chromatography (3:2) to make exactly 50 mL. Pipet 1 mL of this solution, add a mixture of water and acetonitrile for liquid chromatography (3:2) to make exactly 20 mL, and use this solution as the standard solution. Perform the test with exactly 10 μL each of the sample solution and standard solution as directed under Liquid Chromatography <*2.01*> according to the following conditions, and determine each peak area of both solutions by the automatic integration method: the area of the peak, having the relative retention time of about 0.16 to butenafine, obtained from the sample solution is not larger than 3/10 times the peak area of butenafine from the standard solution, and the area of the peak other than butenafine and the peak mentioned above from the sample solution is not larger than the peak area of butenafine from the standard solution.

Operating conditions—

Detector: An ultraviolet absorption photometer (wavelength: 217 nm).

Column: A stainless steel column 3.0 mm in inside diameter and 15 cm in length, packed with octadecylsilanized silica gel for liquid chromatography (3 μm in particle diameter).

Column temperature: A constant temperature of about 40°C.

Mobile phase A: Diluted 0.5 mol/L ammonium acetate TS (1 in 1000).

Mobile phase B: Acetonitrile for liquid chromatography.

Flowing of mobile phase: Control the gradient by mixing the mobile phases A and B as directed in the following table.

Time after injection of sample (min)	Mobile phase A (vol%)	Mobile phase B (vol%)
0 – 10	60 → 20	40 → 80
10 – 60	20	80

Flow rate: 0.4 mL per minute.

Time span of measurement: For 60 minutes after injection, beginning after the solvent peak.

System suitability—

Test for required detectability: Pipet 2 mL of the standard solution, and add a mixture of water and acetonitrile for liquid chromatography (3:2) to make exactly 10 mL. Confirm that the peak area of butenafine obtained with 10 μL of this solution is equivalent to 14 to 26% of that with 10 μL of the standard solution.

System performance: When the procedure is run with 10 μL of the standard solution under the above operating conditions, the number of theoretical plates and the symmetry factor of the peak of butenafine are not less than 20,000 and 0.9 to 1.2, respectively.

System repeatability: When the test is repeated 6 times with 10 μL of the standard solution under the above operating conditions, the relative standard deviation of the peak area of butenafine is not more than 2.0%.

Loss on drying <*2.41*> Not more than 0.1% (1 g, in vacuum, phosphorus (V) oxide, 60°C, 3 hours).

Residue on ignition <*2.44*> Not more than 0.1% (1 g).

Assay Weigh accurately about 0.3 g of Butenafine Hydrochloride, previously dried, dissolve in 5 mL of formic acid, add 80 mL of acetic anhydride, and titrate <*2.50*> with 0.1 mol/L perchloric acid VS (potentiometric titration). Perform a blank determination in the same manner, and make any necessary correction.

Each mL of 0.1 mol/L perchloric acid VS
= 35.39 mg of $C_{23}H_{27}N.HCl$

Containers and storage Containers—Tight containers.

Butenafine Hydrochloride Cream

ブテナフィン塩酸塩クリーム

Butenafine Hydrochloride Cream contains not less than 95.0% and not more than 105.0% of the labeled amount of butenafine hydrochloride ($C_{23}H_{27}N.HCl$: 353.93).

Method of preparation Prepare as directed under Creams, with Butenafine Hydrochloride.

Identification To an amount of Butenafine Hydrochloride Cream, equivalent to 20 mg of Butenafine Hydrochloride, add 20 mL of acetonitrile, and warm on a water bath to melt the bases. Shake thoroughly, add an appropriate amount of sodium chloride, and allow to stand for 30 minutes in an ice cold water keeping not exceeding 0°C to separate out the bases. Centrifuge, collect the supernatant liquid, add an appropriate amount of sodium chloride to the liquid, allow to stand for 1 hour in an ice cold water keeping not exceeding 0°C, and filter while cooling. To 1 mL of the filtrate add methanol to make 20 mL, and determine the absorption spectrum of this solution as directed under Ultraviolet-visible Spectrophotometry <*2.24*>: it exhibits maxima between 272 nm and 276 nm, between 281 nm and 285 nm, between 311 nm and 315 nm, and between 316 nm and 320 nm, and a shoulder between 289 nm and 299 nm.

Assay Weigh accurately a quantity of Butenafine Hydrochloride Cream, equivalent to about 5 mg of butenafine hydrochloride ($C_{23}H_{27}N.HCl$), add 20 mL of methanol, and add exactly 10 mL of the internal standard solution. Warm this in a water bath for 5 minutes, and shake vigorously for 20 minutes. Then, cool in an ice bath for 15 minutes, centrifuge, and filter the supernatant liquid with a membrane filter with a pore size not exceeding 0.45 μm. Discard the first 5 mL of the filtrate, and use the subsequent filtrate as the sample solution. Separately, weigh accurately about 25 mg of butenafine hydrochloride for assay, previously dried in vacuum at 60°C for 3 hours using phosphorus (V) oxide as desiccant, and dissolve in methanol to make exactly 100 mL. Pipet 20 mL of this solution, add exactly 10 mL of the internal standard solution, and use this solution as the standard solution. Perform the test with 5 μL each of the sample solution and standard solution as directed under Liquid Chromatography <2.01> according to the following conditions, and calculate the ratios, Q_T and Q_S, of the peak area of butenafine to that of the internal standard.

Amount (mg) of butenafine hydrochloride ($C_{23}H_{27}N.HCl$)
$= M_S \times Q_T/Q_S \times 1/5$

M_S: Amount (mg) of butenafine hydrochloride for assay taken

Internal standard solution—A solution of diphenyl in methanol (3 in 2000).
Operating conditions—

Detector: An ultraviolet absorption photometer (wavelength: 282 nm).

Column: A stainless steel column 3.0 mm in inside diameter and 5 cm in length, packed with octylsilanized silica gel for liquid chromatography (3 μm in particle diameter).

Column temperature: A constant temperature of about 40°C.

Mobile phase: A mixture of acetonitrile and diluted 0.5 mol/L ammonium acetate TS (1 in 500) (4:1).

Flow rate: Adjust so that the retention time of butenafine is about 2.5 minutes.

System suitability—

System performance: When the procedure is run with 5 μL of the standard solution under the above operating conditions, the internal standard and butenafine are eluted in this order with the resolution between these peaks being not less than 6.

System repeatability: When the test is repeated 6 times with 5 μL of the standard solution under the above operating conditions, the relative standard deviation of the ratio of the peak area of butenafine to that of the internal standard is not more than 1.0%.

Containers and storage Containers—Tight containers.
Storage—Light-resistant.

Butenafine Hydrochloride Solution

ブテナフィン塩酸塩液

Butenafine Hydrochloride Solution is a liquid for external use.

It contains not less than 95.0% and not more than 105.0% of the labeled amount of butenafine hydrochloride ($C_{23}H_{27}N.HCl$: 353.93).

Method of preparation Prepare as directed under Liquids and Solutions for Cutaneous Application, with Butenafine Hydrochloride.

Identification To an amount of Butenafine Hydrochloride Solution, equivalent to 10 mg of Butenafine Hydrochloride, add methanol to make 200 mL, and determine the absorption spectrum of this solution as directed under Ultraviolet-visible Spectrophotometry <2.24>: it exhibits maxima between 272 nm and 276 nm, between 281 nm and 285 nm, between 311 nm and 315 nm, and between 316 nm and 320 nm, and a shoulder between 289 nm and 299 nm.

Assay To an exact volume of Butenafine Hydrochloride Solution, equivalent to about 20 mg of butenafine hydrochloride ($C_{23}H_{27}N.HCl$), add methanol to make exactly 50 mL. Pipet 5 mL of this solution, add exactly 4 mL of the internal standard solution, then add methanol to make 25 mL, and use this solution as the sample solution. Separately, weigh accurately about 20 mg of butenafine hydrochloride for assay, previously dried in vacuum at 60°C for 3 hours using phosphorus (V) oxide as desiccant, and dissolve in methanol to make exactly 50 mL. Pipet 5 mL of this solution, add exactly 4 mL of the internal standard solution, then add methanol to make 25 mL, and use this solution as the standard solution. Perform the test with 5 μL each of the sample solution and standard solution as directed under Liquid Chromatography <2.01> according to the following conditions, and calculate the ratios, Q_T and Q_S, of the peak area of butenafine to that of the internal standard.

Amount (mg) of butenafine hydrochloride ($C_{23}H_{27}N.HCl$)
$= M_S \times Q_T/Q_S$

M_S: Amount (mg) of butenafine hydrochloride for assay taken

Internal standard solution—A solution of diphenyl in methanol (3 in 2000).
Operating conditions—

Detector: An ultraviolet absorption photometer (wavelength: 282 nm).

Column: A stainless steel column 3.0 mm in inside diameter and 5 cm in length, packed with octylsilanized silica gel for liquid chromatography (3 μm in particle diameter).

Column temperature: A constant temperature of about 40°C.

Mobile phase: A mixture of acetonitrile and diluted 0.5 mol/L ammonium acetate TS (1 in 500) (4:1).

Flow rate: Adjust so that the retention time of butenafine is about 2.5 minutes.

System suitability—

System performance: When the procedure is run with 5 μL of the standard solution under the above operating conditions, the internal standard and butenafine are eluted in this order with the resolution between these peaks being not less than 6.

System repeatability: When the test is repeated 6 times

with 5 μL of the standard solution under the above operating conditions, the relative standard deviation of the ratio of the peak area of butenafine to that of the internal standard is not more than 1.0%.

Containers and storage Containers—Tight containers.
Storage—Light-resistant.

Butenafine Hydrochloride Spray

ブテナフィン塩酸塩スプレー

Butenafine Hydrochloride Spray contains not less than 95.0% and not more than 105.0% of the labeled amount of butenafine hydrochloride ($C_{23}H_{27}N.HCl$: 353.93).

Method of preparation Prepare as directed under Pump Sprays for Cutaneous Application, with Butenafine Hydrochloride.

Identification To an amount of Butenafine Hydrochloride Spray, equivalent to 10 mg of Butenafine Hydrochloride, add methanol to make 200 mL, and determine the absorption spectrum of this solution as directed under Ultraviolet-visible Spectrophotometry <*2.24*>: it exhibits maxima between 272 nm and 276 nm, between 281 nm and 285 nm, between 311 nm and 315 nm, and between 316 nm and 320 nm, and a shoulder between 289 nm and 299 nm.

Assay To an exact volume of Butenafine Hydrochloride Spray, equivalent to about 20 mg of butenafine hydrochloride ($C_{23}H_{27}N.HCl$), add methanol to make exactly 50 mL. Pipet 5 mL of this solution, add exactly 4 mL of the internal standard solution, then add methanol to make 25 mL, and use this solution as the sample solution. Separately, weigh accurately about 20 mg of butenafine hydrochloride for assay, previously dried in vacuum at 60°C for 3 hours using phosphorus (V) oxide as desiccant, and dissolve in methanol to make exactly 50 mL. Pipet 5 mL of this solution, add exactly 4 mL of the internal standard solution, then add methanol to make 25 mL, and use this solution as the standard solution. Perform the test with 5 μL each of the sample solution and standard solution as directed under Liquid Chromatography <*2.01*> according to the following conditions, and calculate the ratios, Q_T and Q_S, of the peak area of butenafine to that of the internal standard.

Amount (mg) of butenafine hydrochloride ($C_{23}H_{27}N.HCl$)
$= M_S \times Q_T/Q_S$

M_S: Amount (mg) of butenafine hydrochloride for assay taken

Internal standard solution—A solution of diphenyl in methanol (3 in 2000).

Operating conditions—

Detector: An ultraviolet absorption photometer (wavelength: 282 nm).

Column: A stainless steel column 3.0 mm in inside diameter and 5 cm in length, packed with octylsilanized silica gel for liquid chromatography (3 μm in particle diameter).

Column temperature: A constant temperature of about 40°C.

Mobile phase: A mixture of acetonitrile and diluted 0.5 mol/L ammonium acetate TS (1 in 500) (4:1).

Flow rate: Adjust so that the retention time of butenafine is about 2.5 minutes.

System suitability—

System performance: When the procedure is run with 5 μL of the standard solution under the above operating conditions, the internal standard and butenafine are eluted in this order with the resolution between these peaks being not less than 6.

System repeatability: When the test is repeated 6 times with 5 μL of the standard solution under the above operating conditions, the relative standard deviation of the ratio of the peak area of butenafine to that of the internal standard is not more than 1.0%.

Containers and storage Containers—Tight containers.
Storage—Light-resistant.

Butropium Bromide

ブトロピウム臭化物

$C_{28}H_{38}BrNO_4$: 532.51
(1*R*,3*r*,5*S*)-8-(4-Butoxybenzyl)-3-[(2*S*)-hydroxy-2-phenylpropanoyloxy]-8-methyl-8-azoniabicyclo[3.2.1]octane bromide
[*29025-14-7*]

Butropium Bromide, when dried, contains not less than 98.0% of butropium bromide ($C_{28}H_{38}BrNO_4$).

Description Butropium Bromide occurs as white, crystals or crystalline powder.

It is very soluble in formic acid, freely soluble in methanol, soluble in ethanol (95), slightly soluble in water, and practically insoluble in diethyl ether and in acetic anhydride.

Identification **(1)** To 1 mg of Butropium Bromide add 3 drops of fuming nitric acid, and evaporate on a water bath to dryness. Dissolve the residue in 1 mL of *N*,*N*-dimethylformamide, and add 5 to 6 drops of tetraethylammonium hydroxide TS: a red-purple color develops.

(2) Determine the absorption spectrum of a solution of Butropium Bromide in methanol (1 in 100,000) as directed under Ultraviolet-visible Spectrophotometry <*2.24*>, and compare the spectrum with the Reference Spectrum 1: both spectra exhibit similar intensities of absorption at the same wavelengths. Separately, determine the absorption spectrum of a solution of Butropium Bromide in methanol (1 in 5000) as directed under Ultraviolet-visible Spectrophotometry <*2.24*>, and compare the spectrum with the Reference Spectrum 2: both spectra exhibit similar intensities of absorption at the same wavelengths.

(3) A solution of Butropium Bromide in methanol (1 in 20) responds to Qualitative Tests <*1.09*> (1) for bromide.

Optical rotation <*2.49*> $[\alpha]_D^{20}$: −14.0 – −17.0° (after drying, 0.5 g, methanol, 20 mL, 100 mm).

Purity **(1)** Heavy metals <*1.07*>—Dissolve 1.0 g of Butropium Bromide in 40 mL of ethanol (95), add 2 mL of dilute acetic acid and water to make 50 mL. Perform the test, using this solution as the test solution. Prepare the control solution with 2.0 mL of Standard Lead Solution (not more than 20 ppm).

(2) Related substances—Dissolve 50 mg of Butropium

Bromide in 10 mL of the mobile phase, and use this solution as the sample solution. Pipet 1 mL of the sample solution, add the mobile phase to make exactly 100 mL, and use this solution as the standard solution. Perform the test with exactly 5 μL each of the sample solution and standard solution as directed under Liquid Chromatography <*2.01*> according to the following conditions. Determine each peak area of both solutions by the automatic integration method: the peak area, having the relative retention time about 0.5 to butropium obtained from the sample solution is not larger than 1/4 times the peak area from the standard solution, and the total area of all peaks other than the peak eluted first, the peak, having the relative retention time to butropium about 0.5 and butropium peak from the sample solution is not larger than the peak area from the standard solution.

Operating conditions—

Detector: An ultraviolet absorption photometer (wavelength: 220 nm).

Column: A stainless steel column about 5 mm in inside diameter and about 15 cm in length, packed with octadecylsilanized silica gel for liquid chromatography (5 μm in particle diameter).

Column temperature: A constant temperature of about 40°C.

Mobile phase: Dissolve 1.15 g of sodium lauryl sulfate in 1000 mL of a mixture of acetonitrile and 0.005 mol/L sulfuric acid (3:2).

Flow rate: Adjust so that the retention time of butropium is about 5 minutes.

Selection of column: Dissolve 0.50 g of Butropium Bromide in 9 mL of ethanol (99.5) and 1 mL of 0.1 mol/L potassium hydroxide-ethanol TS, and heat at 70°C for 15 minutes. After cooling, to 1 mL of this solution add the mobile phase to make 100 mL. Proceed with 5 μL of this solution under the above operating conditions, and calculate the resolution. Use a column giving elution of the peak of butropium and the peak having a ratio of the retention time about 0.7 to butropium with the resolution between these peaks being not less than 2.5.

Detection sensitivity: Adjust the detection sensitivity so that the peak height of the butropium obtained from 5 μL of the standard solution is between 10 mm and 30 mm.

Time span of measurement: About twice as long as the retention time of butropium.

Loss on drying <*2.41*> Not more than 1.0% (1 g, 105°C, 3 hours).

Residue on ignition <*2.44*> Not more than 0.2% (1 g).

Assay Weigh accurately about 0.8 g of Butropium Bromide, previously dried, dissolve in 5 mL of formic acid, add 100 mL of acetic anhydride, and titrate <*2.50*> with 0.1 mol/L perchloric acid-dioxane VS (potentiometric titration). Perform a blank determination in the same manner, and make any necessary correction.

Each mL of 0.1 mol/L perchloric acid-dioxane VS
= 53.25 mg of $C_{28}H_{38}BrNO_4$

Containers and storage Containers—Well-closed containers.

Storage—Light-resistant.

Butyl Parahydroxybenzoate

パラオキシ安息香酸ブチル

$C_{11}H_{14}O_3$: 194.23
Butyl 4-hydroxybenzoate
[*94-26-8*]

This monograph is harmonized with the European Pharmacopoeia and the U.S. Pharmacopeia.

The parts of the text that are not harmonized are marked with symbols (◆ ◆)

Information on the harmonization with the European Pharmacopoeia and the U.S. Pharmacopeia is available on the website of the Pharmaceuticals and Medical Devices Agency.

Butyl Parahydroxybenzoate contains not less than 98.0% and not more than 102.0% of butyl parahydroxybenzoate ($C_{11}H_{14}O_3$).

◆**Description** Butyl Parahydroxybenzoate occurs as colorless crystals or white crystalline powder.

It is very soluble in methanol, freely soluble in ethanol (95) and in acetone, and practically insoluble in water.◆

Identification Determine the infrared absorption spectrum of Butyl Parahydroxybenzoate as directed in the potassium bromide disk method under Infrared Spectrophotometry <*2.25*>, and compare the spectrum with the Reference Spectrum or the spectrum of Butyl Parahydroxybenzoate RS: both spectra exhibit similar intensities of absorption at the same wave numbers.

Melting point <*2.60*> 68 - 71°C

Purity **(1)** Clarity and color of solution—Dissolve 1.0 g of Butyl Parahydroxybenzoate in ethanol (95) to make 10 mL: the solution is clear and not more intensely colored than the following control solution.

Control solution: To 5.0 mL of Cobalt (II) Chloride CS, 12.0 mL of Iron (III) Chloride CS and 2.0 mL of Copper (II) Sulfate CS add diluted dilute hydrochloric acid (1 in 10) to make 1000 mL.

(2) Acidity—To 2 mL of the solution of Butyl Parahydroxybenzoate obtained in (1) add 3 mL of ethanol (95), add 5 mL of freshly boiled and cooled water and 0.1 mL of bromocresol green-sodium hydroxide-ethanol TS, then add 0.1 mol/L sodium hydroxide VS until the solution shows a blue color: the volume of 0.1 mol/L sodium hydroxide VS used does not exceed 0.1 mL.

◆**(3)** Heavy metals <*1.07*>—Dissolve 1.0 g of Butyl Parahydroxybenzoate in 25 mL of acetone, add 2 mL of dilute acetic acid and water to make 50 mL, and perform the test using this solution as the test solution. Prepare the control solution as follows: to 2.0 mL of Standard Lead Solution add 25 mL of acetone, 2 mL of dilute acetic acid, and water to make 50 mL (not more than 20 ppm).◆

(4) Related substances—Dissolve 50.0 mg of Butyl Parahydroxybenzoate in 2.5 mL of methanol, and add the mobile phase to make exactly 50 mL. Pipet 10 mL of this solution, add the mobile phase to make exactly 100 mL, and use this solution as the sample solution. Pipet 1 mL of the sample solution, and add the mobile phase to make exactly

20 mL. Pipet 1 mL of this solution, add the mobile phase to make exactly 10 mL, and use this solution as the standard solution. Perform the test with exactly 10 μL each of the sample solution and standard solution as directed under Liquid Chromatography <*2.01*> according to the following conditions, and determine each peak area by the automatic integration method: the peak area of parahydroxybenzoic acid having a relative retention time of about 0.1 to butyl parahydroxybenzoate obtained from the sample solution is not larger than the peak area of butyl parahydroxybenzoate from the standard solution (0.5%). For the area of the peak of parahydroxybenzoic acid multiply the correction factor, 1.4. Furthermore, the area of the peak other than butyl parahydroxybenzoate and parahydroxybenzoic acid from the sample solution is not larger than the peak area of butyl parahydroxybenzoate from the standard solution (0.5%), and the total area of the peaks other than butyl parahydroxybenzoate is not larger than 2 times the peak area of butyl parahydroxybenzoate from the standard solution (1.0%). For this calculation the peak area not larger than 1/5 times the peak area of butyl parahydroxybenzoate from the standard solution is excluded (0.1%).

Operating conditions—

Detector, column, column temperature, mobile phase, and flow rate: Proceed as directed in the operating conditions in the Assay.

Time span of measurement: About 1.5 times as long as the retention time of butyl parahydroxybenzoate.

System suitability—

System performance: Proceed as directed in the system suitability in the Assay.

◆Test for required detectability: To exactly 2 mL of the standard solution add the mobile phase to make exactly 10 mL. Confirm that the peak area of butyl parahydroxybenzoate obtained with 10 μL of this solution is equivalent to 14 to 26% of that with 10 μL of the standard solution.◆

◆System repeatability: When the test is repeated 6 times with 10 μL of the standard solution under the above operating conditions, the relative standard deviation of the peak area of butyl parahydroxybenzoate is not more than 2.0%.◆

Residue on ignition <*2.44*> Not more than 0.1% (1 g).

Assay Weigh accurately about 50.0 mg each of Butyl Parahydroxybenzoate and Butyl Parahydroxybenzoate RS, dissolve separately in 2.5 mL each of methanol, and add the mobile phase to make exactly 50 mL. Pipet 10 mL each of these solutions, add the mobile phase to make exactly 100 mL, and use these solutions as the sample solution and the standard solution, respectively. Perform the test with exactly 10 μL each of the sample solution and standard solution as directed under Liquid Chromatography <*2.01*> according to the following conditions, and determine the peak areas, A_T and A_S, of butyl parahydroxybenzoate in each solution.

Amount (mg) of butyl parahydroxybenzoate ($C_{11}H_{14}O_3$)
$= M_S \times A_T/A_S$

M_S: Amount (mg) of Butyl Parahydroxybenzoate RS taken

Operating conditions—

Detector: An ultraviolet absorption photometer (wavelength: 272 nm).

Column: A stainless steel column 4.6 mm in inside diameter and 15 cm in length, packed with octadecylsilanized silica gel for liquid chromatography (5 μm in particle diameter).

Column temperature: A constant temperature of about 35°C.

Mobile phase: A mixture of methanol and potassium dihydrogen phosphate solution (17 in 2500) (1:1).

Flow rate: 1.3 mL per minute.

System suitability—

System performance: Dissolve 5 mg each of Butyl Parahydroxybenzoate, propyl parahydroxybenzoate and parahydroxybenzoic acid in the mobile phase to make exactly 100 mL. Pipet 1 mL of this solution, add the mobile phase to make exactly 10 mL, and use this solution as the solution for system suitability test (1). Separately, dissolve 5 mg of isobutyl parahydroxybenzoate in the mobile phase to make exactly 100 mL. Pipet 0.5 mL of this solution, add the standard solution to make exactly 50 mL, and use this solution as the solution for system suitability test (2). When the procedure is run with 10 μL each of the solution for system suitability test (1) and (2) under the above operating conditions, parahydroxybenzoic acid, propyl parahydroxybenzoate, isobutyl parahydroxybenzoate and butyl parahydroxybenzoate are eluted in this order, the relative retention times of parahydroxybenzoic acid, propyl parahydroxybenzoate and isobutyl parahydoxybenzoate to butyl parahydroxybenzoate are about 0.1, about 0.5 and about 0.9, respectively, the resolution between the peaks of propyl parahydroxybenzoate and butyl parahydroxybenzoate is not less than 5.0, and the resolution between the peaks of isobutyl parahydroxybenzoate and butyl parahydroxybenzoate is not less than 1.5.

System repeatability: When the test is repeated 6 times with 10 μL of the standard solution under the above operating conditions, the relative standard deviation of the peak area of butyl parahydroxybenzoate is not more than 0.85%.

◆**Containers and storage** Containers—Well-closed containers.◆

Cabergoline

カベルゴリン

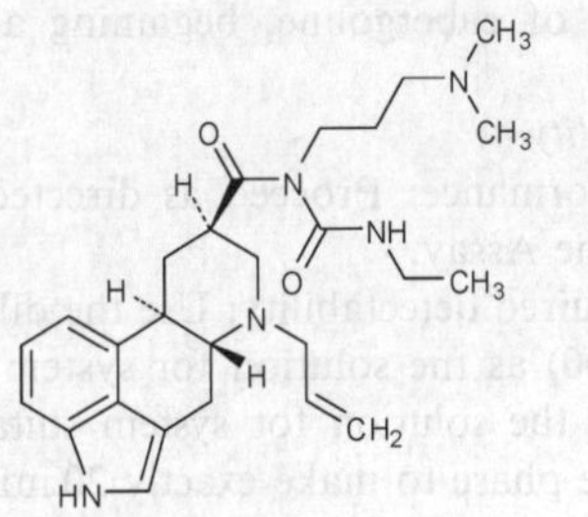

$C_{26}H_{37}N_5O_2$: 451.60
(8*R*)-6-Allyl-*N*-[3-(dimethylamino)propyl]-*N*-(ethylcarbamoyl)ergoline-8-carboxamide
[81409-90-7]

Cabergoline contains not less than 98.0% and not more than 102.0% of cabergoline ($C_{26}H_{37}N_5O_2$), calculated on the anhydrous basis.

Description Cabergoline occurs as a white crystalline powder.

It is very soluble in methanol, freely soluble in ethanol (95), and very slightly soluble in water.

It is gradually colored to yellow by light.

It shows crystal polymorphism.

Identification **(1)** Determine the absorption spectrum of a solution of Cabergoline in ethanol (95) (1 in 30,000) as directed under Ultraviolet-visible Spectrophotometry <*2.24*>, and compare the spectrum with the Reference Spectrum or the spectrum of a solution of Cabergoline RS prepared in the same manner as the sample solution: both spectra exhibit similar intensities of absorption at the same wavelengths.

(2) Determine the infrared absorption spectrum of Cabergoline as directed in the potassium bromide disk method under Infrared Spectrophotometry <*2.25*>, and compare the spectrum with the Reference Spectrum or the spectrum of Cabergoline RS: both spectra exhibit similar intensities of absorption at the same wave numbers. If any difference appears between the spectra, dissolve Cabergoline and Cabergoline RS in ethanol (95), respectively, then evaporate the ethanol, dry the residues, and repeat the test on the residues.

Optical rotation <*2.49*> $[\alpha]_D^{20}$: −77 – −83° (0.1 g calculated on the anhydrous basis, ethanol (95), 50 mL, 100 mm).

Purity **(1)** Heavy metals <*1.07*>—Proceed with 1.0 g of Cabergoline according to Method 4, and perform the test. Prepare the control solution with 2.0 mL of Standard Lead Solution (not more than 20 ppm).

(2) Related substances—Conduct this procedure using light-resistant vessels. Perform the test with 20 μL of the sample solution obtained in the Assay as directed under Liquid Chromatography <*2.01*> according to the following conditions. Determine each peak area by the automatic integration method, and calculate the amounts of them by the area percentage method: the amount of related substances A and B, having the relative retention times of about 0.8 and about 2.8 to cabergoline are not more than 0.5%, respectively, and the amount of the peak other than cabergoline and the peaks mentioned above is not more than 0.1%. Furthermore, the total amount of the peaks other than cabergoline is not more than 1.5%.

Operating conditions—

Detector, column, column temperature, mobile phase, and flow rate: Proceed as directed in the operating conditions in the Assay.

Time span of measurement: About 4 times as long as the retention time of cabergoline, beginning after the solvent peak.

System suitability—

System performance: Proceed as directed in the system suitability in the Assay.

Test for required detectability: Use the diluted sample solution (1 in 500) as the solution for system suitability test. Pipet 5 mL of the solution for system suitability test, and add the mobile phase to make exactly 20 mL. Confirm that the peak area of cabergoline obtained with 20 μL of this solution is equivalent to 18 to 32% of that with 20 μL of the solution for system suitability test.

System repeatability: When the test is repeated 6 times with 20 μL of the solution for system suitability test under the above operating conditions, the relative standard deviation of the peak area of cabergoline is not more than 2.0%.

Water <*2.48*> Not more than 0.5% (1 g, volumetric titration, direct titration).

Assay Conduct this procedure using light-resistant vessels. Weigh accurately about 30 mg each of Cabergoline and Cabergoline RS (separately determine the water <*2.48*> in the same manner as Cabergoline), dissolve each in the mobile phase to make exactly 25 mL, and use these solutions as the sample solution and the standard solution, respectively. Perform the test with exactly 20 μL each of the sample solution and standard solution as directed under Liquid Chromatography <*2.01*> according to the following conditions, and determine the peak areas, A_T and A_S, of cabergoline in each solution.

Amount (mg) of cabergoline ($C_{26}H_{37}N_5O_2$) = $M_S \times A_T/A_S$

M_S: Amount (mg) of Cabergoline RS taken, calculated on the anhydrous basis

Operating conditions—

Detector: An ultraviolet absorption photometer (wavelength: 280 nm).

Column: A stainless steel column 4.0 mm in inside diameter and 25 cm in length, packed with octadecylsilanized silica gel for liquid chromatography (10 μm in particle diameter).

Column temperature: A constant temperature of about 25°C.

Mobile phase: Dissolve 6.8 g of potassium dihydrogen phosphate in 900 mL of water, adjust to pH 2.0 with phosphoric acid, and add water to make 1000 mL. To this solution add 0.2 mL of triethylamine. To 840 mL of this solution add 160 mL of acetonitrile.

Flow rate: Adjust so that the retention time of cabergoline is about 12 minutes.

System suitability—

System performance: Suspend 50 mg of Cabergoline in 10 mL of 0.1 mol/L sodium hydroxide TS, and stir for 15 minutes. To 1 mL of this solution add 1 mL of 0.1 mol/L hydrochloric acid TS, and add the mobile phase to make 10 mL. When the procedure is run with 20 μL of this solution under the above operating conditions, the resolution between the peaks of related substance A having the relative retention time of about 0.8 to cabergoline and cabergoline is not less than 3.

System repeatability: When the test is repeated 6 times with 20 μL of the standard solution under the above operating conditions, the relative standard deviation of the peak area of cabergoline is not more than 1.0%.

Containers and storage Containers—Tight containers.

Storage—Light-resistant.

Others

Related substance A:

(8*R*)-6-Allylergoline-8-carboxylic acid

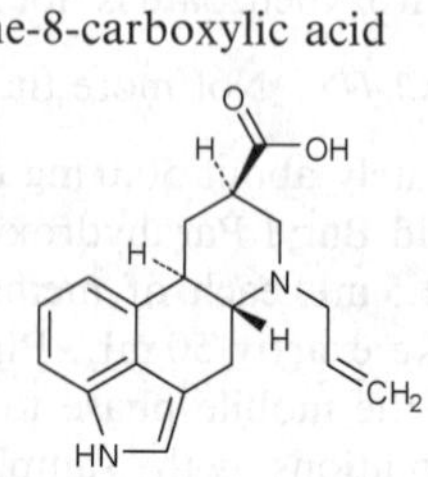

Related substance B:

(8*R*)-6-Allyl-*N*-[3-(dimethylamino)propyl]-*N*,1-bis(ethylcarbamoyl)ergoline-8-carboxamide

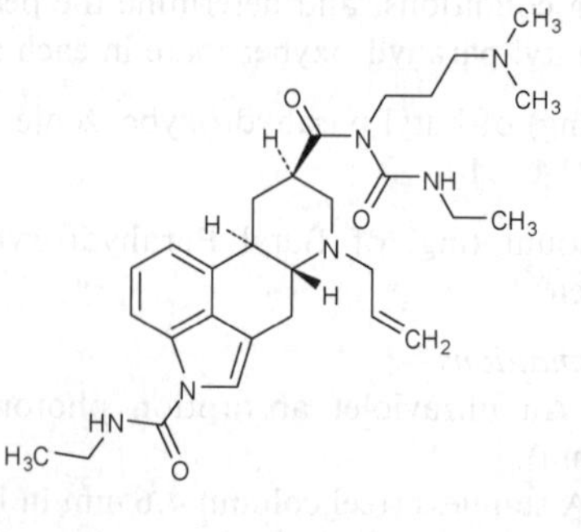

Cadralazine

カドララジン

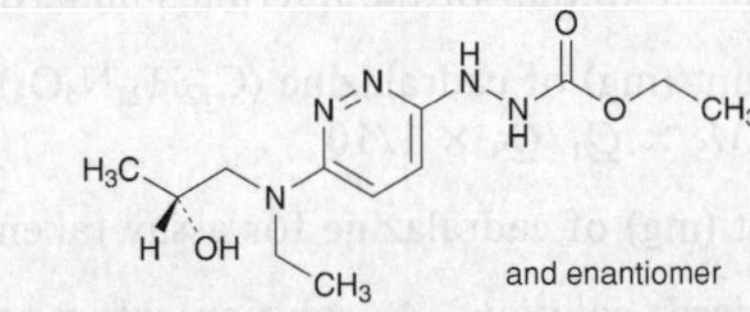

$C_{12}H_{21}N_5O_3$: 283.33
Ethyl 3-(6-{ethyl[(2*RS*)-2-hydroxypropyl]amino}pyridazin-3-yl)carbazate
[*64241-34-5*]

Cadralazine, when dried, contains not less than 98.5% and not more than 101.0% of cadralazine ($C_{12}H_{21}N_5O_3$).

Description Cadralazine occurs as a pale yellow to light yellow crystalline powder.

It is freely soluble in acetic acid (100), soluble in methanol, sparingly soluble in ethanol (99.5), and slightly soluble in water.

It dissolves in 0.05 mol/L sulfuric acid TS.

A solution of Cadralazine in methanol (1 in 40) shows no optical rotation.

Melting point: about 165°C (with decomposition).

Identification **(1)** Determine the absorption spectrum of a solution of Cadralazine in 0.05 mol/L sulfuric acid TS (1 in 125,000) as directed under Ultraviolet-visible Spectrophotometry *<2.24>*, and compare the spectrum with the Reference Spectrum: both spectra exhibit similar intensities of absorption at the same wavelengths.

(2) Determine the infrared absorption spectrum of Cadralazine, previously dried, as directed in the potassium bromide disk method under Infrared Spectrophotometry *<2.25>*, and compare the spectrum with the Reference Spectrum: both spectra exhibit similar intensities of absorption at the same wave numbers.

Purity **(1)** Chloride *<1.03>*—Dissolve 0.40 g of Cadralazine in 15 mL of methanol, add 6 mL of dilute nitric acid and water to make 50 mL. Perform the test using this solution as the test solution. Prepare the control solution with 0.40 mL of 0.01 mol/L hydrochloric acid VS by adding 15 mL of methanol, 6 mL of dilute nitric acid, and water to make 50 mL (not more than 0.036%).

(2) Heavy metals *<1.07>*—Proceed with 1.0 g of Cadralazine according to Method 4, and perform the test. Prepare the control solution with 2.0 mL of Standard Lead Solution (not more than 20 ppm).

(3) Related substances—Dissolve 50 mg of Cadralazine in 20 mL of 0.05 mol/L sulfuric acid TS, add water to 100 mL, and use this solution as the sample solution. Pipet 1 mL of the sample solution, add water to make exactly 200 mL, and use this solution as the standard solution. Perform the test with exactly 10 μL each of the sample solution and standard solution as directed under Liquid Chromatography *<2.01>* according to the following conditions. Determine each peak area of both solutions by the automatic integration method: the area of the peak, having the relative retention time of about 2.1 to cadralazine, obtained from the sample solution is not larger than the peak area of cadralazine from the standard solution, and the area of the peak other than cadralazine and the peak mentioned above is not larger than 2/5 times the peak area of cadralazine from the standard solution. Furthermore, the total area of the peaks other than cadralazine from the sample solution is not larger than 2 times the peak area of cadralazine from the standard solution. For the areas of the peaks, having the relative retention time of about 0.49 and about 2.1 to cadralazine, multiply their correction factors, 0.65 and 1.25, respectively.

Operating conditions—

Detector: An ultraviolet absorption photometer (wavelength: 250 nm).

Column: A stainless steel column 4.6 mm in inside diameter and 15 cm in length, packed with octadecylsilanized silica gel for liquid chromatography (5 μm in particle diameter).

Column temperature: A constant temperature of about 40°C.

Mobile phase: Dissolve 13.6 g of sodium acetate trihydrate in 800 mL of water, adjust the pH to 5.8 with dilute acetic acid, and add water to make 1000 mL. To 860 mL of this solution add 140 mL of acetonitrile.

Flow rate: Adjust so that the retention time of cadralazine is about 10 minutes.

Time span of measurement: About 3 times as long as the retention time of cadralazine.

System suitability—

Test for required detectability: Pipet 5 mL of the standard solution, and add water to make exactly 25 mL. Confirm that the peak area of cadralazine obtained with 10 μL of this solution is equivalent to 15 to 25% of that with 10 μL of the standard solution.

System performance: When the procedure is run with 10 μL of the standard solution under the above operating conditions, the number of theoretical plates and the symmetry factor of the peak of cadralazine are not less than 4000 and not more than 1.5, respectively.

System repeatability: When the test is repeated 6 times with 10 μL of the standard solution under the above operating conditions, the relative standard deviation of the peak area of cadralazine is not more than 4.0%.

Loss on drying *<2.41>* Not more than 1.0% (1 g, 105°C, 3 hours).

Residue on ignition *<2.44>* Not more than 0.1% (1 g).

Assay Weigh accurately about 0.5 g of Cadralazine, previously dried, dissolve in 50 mL of acetic acid (100), and titrate *<2.50>* with 0.1 mol/L perchloric acid VS (potentiometric titration). Perform a blank determination in the same manner, and make any necessary correction.

Each mL of 0.1 mol/L perchloric acid VS
= 28.33 mg of $C_{12}H_{21}N_5O_3$

Containers and storage Containers—Well-closed containers.

Cadralazine Tablets

カドララジン錠

Cadralazine Tablets contain not less than 95.0% and not more than 105.0% of the labeled amount of cadralazine ($C_{12}H_{21}N_5O_3$: 283.33).

Method of preparation Prepare as directed under Tablets, with Cadralazine.

Identification To a quantity of powdered Cadralazine Tablets, equivalent to 20 mg of Cadralazine, add 50 mL of 0.05 mol/L sulfuric acid TS, shake well, and centrifuge. To

1 mL of the supernatant liquid add 0.05 mol/L sulfuric acid TS to make 50 mL. Determine the absorption spectrum of this solution as directed under Ultraviolet-visible Spectrophotometry *<2.24>*: it exhibits a maximum between 247 nm and 251 nm.

Uniformity of dosage units *<6.02>* Perform the test according to the following method: it meets the requirement of the Content uniformity test.

To 1 tablet of Cadralazine Tablets add 30 mL of 0.05 mol/L sulfuric acid TS, shake well to disintegrate, and add 0.05 mol/L sulfuric acid TS to make exactly 50 mL. Centrifuge this solution, pipet 3 mL of the supernatant liquid, add 0.05 mol/L sulfuric acid TS to make exactly V mL so that each mL contains about 6 μg of cadralazine ($C_{12}H_{21}N_5O_3$), and use this solution as the sample solution. Separately, weigh accurately about 20 mg of cadralazine for assay, previously dried at 105°C for 3 hours, and dissolve in 0.05 mol/L sulfuric acid TS to make exactly 100 mL. Pipet 3 mL of this solution, add 0.05 mol/L sulfuric acid TS to make exactly 100 mL, and use this solution as the standard solution. Determine the absorbances, A_T and A_S, of the sample solution and standard solution at 249 nm as directed under Ultraviolet-visible Spectrophotometry *<2.24>*.

Amount (mg) of cadralazine ($C_{12}H_{21}N_5O_3$)
$$= M_S \times A_T/A_S \times V/200$$

M_S: Amount (mg) of cadralazine for assay taken

Dissolution *<6.10>* When the test is performed at 50 revolutions per minute according to the Paddle method, using 900 mL of water as the dissolution medium, the dissolution rate in 30 minutes of Cadralazine Tablets is not less than 80%.

Start the test with 1 tablet of Cadralazine Tablets, withdraw not less than 20 mL of the medium at the specified minute after starting the test, and filter through a membrane filter with a pore size not exceeding 0.5 μm. Discard not less than 10 mL of the first filtrate, pipet V mL of the subsequent filtrate, add water to make exactly V' mL so that each mL contains about 5.6 μg of cadralazine ($C_{12}H_{21}N_5O_3$), and use this solution as the sample solution. Separately, weigh accurately about 30 mg of cadralazine for assay, previously dried at 105°C for 3 hours, and dissolve in water to make exactly 200 mL. Pipet 4 mL of this solution, add water to make exactly 100 mL, and use this solution as the standard solution. Determine the absorbances, A_T and A_S, of the sample solution and standard solution at 254 nm as directed under Ultraviolet-visible Spectrophotometry *<2.24>*.

Dissolution rate (%) with respect to the labeled amount of cadralazine ($C_{12}H_{21}N_5O_3$)
$$= M_S \times A_T/A_S \times V'/V \times 1/C \times 18$$

M_S: Amount (mg) of cadralazine for assay taken
C: Labeled amount (mg) of cadralazine ($C_{12}H_{21}N_5O_3$) in 1 tablet

Assay To 10 Cadralazine Tablets add 70 mL of 0.05 mol/L sulfuric acid TS, shake well to disintegrate, add 0.05 mol/L sulfuric acid TS to make exactly 200 mL. Centrifuge this solution, pipet a volume of the supernatant liquid, equivalent to about 2.5 mg of cadralazine ($C_{12}H_{21}N_5O_3$), add exactly 5 mL of the internal standard solution, add water to make 25 mL, and use this solution as the sample solution. Separately, weigh accurately about 25 mg of cadralazine for assay, previously dried at 105°C for 3 hours, and dissolve in 0.05 mol/L of sulfuric acid TS to make exactly 50 mL. Pipet 5 mL of this solution, add exactly 5 mL of the internal standard solution, add water to make 25 mL, and use this solution as the standard solution. Perform the test with 5 μL each of the sample solution and standard solution as directed under Liquid Chromatography *<2.01>* according to the following conditions, and calculate the ratios, Q_T and Q_S, of the peak area of cadralazine to that of the internal standard.

Amount (mg) of cadralazine ($C_{12}H_{21}N_5O_3$)
$$= M_S \times Q_T/Q_S \times 1/10$$

M_S: Amount (mg) of cadralazine for assay taken

Internal standard solution—A solution of *p*-toluenesulfonamide in acetonitrile (1 in 50).
Operating conditions—

Detector: An ultraviolet absorption photometer (wavelength: 250 nm).

Column: A stainless steel column 4.6 mm in inside diameter and 15 cm in length, packed with octadecylsilanized silica gel for liquid chromatography (5 μm in particle diameter).

Column temperature: A constant temperature of about 40°C.

Mobile phase: Dissolve 13.6 g of sodium acetate trihydrate in 800 mL of water, adjust the pH to 5.8 with dilute acetic acid, and add water to make 1000 mL. To 860 mL of this solution add 140 mL of acetonitrile.

Flow rate: Adjust so that the retention time of cadralazine is about 10 minutes.
System suitability—

System performance: When the procedure is run with 5 μL of the standard solution under the above operating conditions, cadralazine and the internal standard are eluted in this order with the resolution between these peaks being not less than 3.

System repeatability: When the test is repeated 6 times with 5 μL of the standard solution under the above operating conditions, the relative standard deviation of the ratio of the peak area of cadralazine to that of the internal standard is not more than 1.0%.

Containers and storage Containers—Well-closed containers.

Anhydrous Caffeine

無水カフェイン

$C_8H_{10}N_4O_2$: 194.19
1,3,7-Trimethyl-1*H*-purine-2,6(3*H*,7*H*)-dione
[58-08-2]

Anhydrous Caffeine, when dried, contains not less than 98.5% of caffeine ($C_8H_{10}N_4O_2$).

Description Anhydrous Caffeine occurs as white, crystals or powder. It is odorless, and has a bitter taste.

It is freely soluble in chloroform, sparingly soluble in water, in acetic acid (100) and in acetic anhydride, and slightly soluble in ethanol (95) and in diethyl ether.

The pH of a solution of 1.0 g of Anhydrous Caffeine in 100 mL of water is between 5.5 and 6.5.

Identification (1) To 2 mL of a solution of Anhydrous Caffeine (1 in 500) add tannic acid TS dropwise: a white precipitate, which dissolves upon the dropwise addition of tannic acid TS, is produced.

(2) To 0.01 g of Anhydrous Caffeine add 10 drops of hydrogen peroxide TS and 1 drop of hydrochloric acid, and evaporate on a water bath to dryness: the residue acquires a yellow-red color. Invert the residue over a vessel containing 2 to 3 drops of ammonia TS: the color turns red-purple, and disappears upon the addition of 2 to 3 drops of sodium hydroxide TS.

(3) Dissolve 0.01 g of Anhydrous Caffeine in water to make 50 mL. To 5 mL of this solution add 3 mL of diluted acetic acid (31) (3 in 100) and 5 mL of pyridine (1 in 10), mix, add 2 mL of diluted sodium hypochlorite TS (1 in 5), and allow to stand for 1 minute. Add 2 mL of sodium thiosulfate TS and 5 mL of sodium hydroxide TS to the solution: a yellow color develops.

Melting point 〈*2.60*〉 235 – 238°C

Purity **(1)** Chloride 〈*1.03*〉—Dissolve 2.0 g of Anhydrous Caffeine in 80 mL of hot water, cool rapidly to 20°C, add water to make 100 mL, and use this solution as the sample solution. To 40 mL of the sample solution add 6 mL of dilute nitric acid and water to make 50 mL. Perform the test using this solution as the test solution. Prepare the control solution with 0.25 mL of 0.01 mol/L hydrochloric acid VS (not more than 0.011%).

(2) Sulfate 〈*1.14*〉—To 40 mL of the sample solution obtained in (1) add 1 mL of dilute hydrochloric acid and water to make 50 mL. Perform the test using this solution as the test solution. Prepare the control solution with 0.40 mL of 0.005 mol/L sulfuric acid VS (not more than 0.024%).

(3) Heavy metals 〈*1.07*〉—Proceed with 2.0 g of Anhydrous Caffeine according to Method 2, and perform the test. Prepare the control solution with 2.0 mL of Standard Lead Solution (not more than 10 ppm).

(4) Related substances—Dissolve 0.10 g of Anhydrous Caffeine in 10 mL of chloroform, and use this solution as the sample solution. Pipet 1 mL of the sample solution, and add chloroform to make exactly 100 mL. Pipet 1 mL of this solution, add chloroform to make exactly 10 mL, and use this solution as the standard solution. Perform the test with these solutions as directed under Thin-layer Chromatography 〈*2.03*〉. Spot 10 μL each of the sample solution and standard solution on a plate of silica gel with fluorescent indicator for thin-layer chromatography. Develop the plate with a mixture of chloroform and ethanol (95) (9:1) to a distance of about 10 cm, and air-dry the plate. Examine under ultraviolet light (main wavelength: 254 nm): the spots other than the principal spot obtained from the sample solution are not more intense than the spot from the standard solution.

(5) Readily carbonizable substances 〈*1.15*〉—Perform the test using 0.5 g of Anhydrous Caffeine: the solution is not more colored than Matching Fluid D.

Loss on drying 〈*2.41*〉 Not more than 0.5% (1 g, 80°C, 4 hours).

Residue on ignition 〈*2.44*〉 Not more than 0.1% (0.5 g).

Assay Weigh accurately about 0.4 g of Anhydrous Caffeine, previously dried, dissolve in 70 mL of a mixture of acetic anhydride and acetic acid (100) (6:1), and titrate 〈*2.50*〉 with 0.1 mol/L perchloric acid VS until the solution changes from purple through green to yellow (indicator: 3 drops of crystal violet TS). Perform a blank determination in the same manner, and make any necessary correction.

Each mL of 0.1 mol/L perchloric acid VS
= 19.42 mg of $C_8H_{10}N_4O_2$

Containers and storage Containers—Tight containers.

Caffeine Hydrate

カフェイン水和物

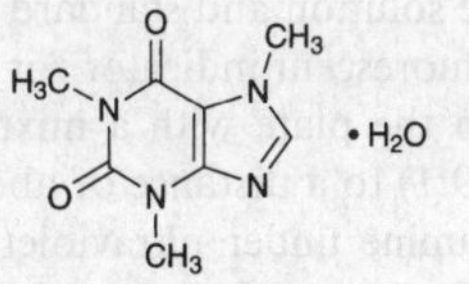

$C_8H_{10}N_4O_2.H_2O$: 212.21
1,3,7-Trimethyl-1*H*-purine-2,6(3*H*,7*H*)-dione monohydrate
[*5743-12-4*]

Caffeine Hydrate, when dried, contains not less than 98.5% of caffeine ($C_8H_{10}N_4O_2$: 194.19).

Description Caffeine Hydrate occurs as white, soft crystals or powder. It is odorless, and has a slightly bitter taste.

It is freely soluble in chloroform, sparingly soluble in water, in acetic acid (100) and in acetic anhydride, slightly soluble in ethanol (95), and very slightly soluble in diethyl ether.

The pH of a solution of 1.0 g of Caffeine Hydrate in 100 mL of water is between 5.5 and 6.5.

It effloresces in dry air.

Identification **(1)** To 2 mL of a solution of Caffeine Hydrate (1 in 500) add tannic acid TS dropwise: a white precipitate, which dissolves upon the dropwise addition of tannic acid TS, is produced.

(2) To 0.01 g of Caffeine Hydrate add 10 drops of hydrogen peroxide TS and 1 drop of hydrochloric acid, and evaporate to dryness on a water bath: the residue acquires a yellow-red color. Invert the residue over a vessel containing 2 to 3 drops of ammonia TS: the color turns red-purple, and disappears upon the addition of 2 to 3 drops of sodium hydroxide TS.

(3) Dissolve 0.01 g of Caffeine Hydrate in water to make 50 mL. To 5 mL of this solution add 3 mL of diluted acetic acid (31) (3 in 100) and 5 mL of a solution of pyridine (1 in 10), mix, add 2 mL of diluted sodium hypochlorite TS (1 in 5), and allow to stand for 1 minute. Add 2 mL of sodium thiosulfate TS and 5 mL of sodium hydroxide TS to the solution: a yellow color develops.

Melting point 〈*2.60*〉 235 – 238°C (after drying).

Purity **(1)** Chloride 〈*1.03*〉—Dissolve 2.0 g of Caffeine Hydrate in 80 mL of hot water, cool rapidly to 20°C, add water to make 100 mL, and use this solution as the sample solution. To 40 mL of the sample solution add 6 mL of dilute nitric acid and water to make 50 mL. Perform the test using this solution as the test solution. Prepare the control solution with 0.25 mL of 0.01 mol/L hydrochloric acid VS (not more than 0.011%).

(2) Sulfate 〈*1.14*〉—To 40 mL of the sample solution obtained in (1) add 1 mL of dilute hydrochloric acid and water to make 50 mL. Perform the test using this solution as the test solution. Prepare the control solution with 0.40 mL of 0.005 mol/L sulfuric acid VS (not more than 0.024%).

(3) Heavy metals 〈*1.07*〉—Proceed with 2.0 g of Caffeine Hydrate according to Method 2, and perform the test. Prepare the control solution with 2.0 mL of Standard Lead Solution (not more than 10 ppm).

(4) Related substances—Dissolve 0.10 g of Caffeine Hydrate in 10 mL of chloroform, and use this solution as the sample solution. Pipet 1 mL of the sample solution, and add chloroform to make exactly 100 mL. Pipet 1 mL of this solution, add chloroform to make exactly 10 mL, and use this solution as the standard solution. Perform the test as directed under Thin-layer Chromatography <*2.03*>. Spot 10 μL each of the sample solution and standard solution on a plate of silica gel with fluorescent indicator for thin-layer chromatography. Develop the plate with a mixture of chloroform and ethanol (95) (9:1) to a distance of about 10 cm, and air-dry the plate. Examine under ultraviolet light (main wavelength: 254 nm): the spots other than the principal spot obtained from the sample solution are not more intense than the spot from the standard solution.

(5) Readily carbonizable substances <*1.15*>—Perform the test using 0.5 g of Caffeine Hydrate: the solution is not more colored than Matching Fluid D.

Loss on drying <*2.41*> 0.5 - 8.5% (1 g, 80°C, 4 hours).

Residue on ignition <*2.44*> Not more than 0.1% (0.5 g).

Assay Weigh accurately about 0.4 g of Caffeine Hydrate, previously dried, dissolve in 70 mL of a mixture of acetic anhydride and acetic acid (100) (6:1), and titrate <*2.50*> with 0.1 mol/L perchloric acid VS until the solution changes from purple through green to yellow (indicator: 3 drops of crystal violet TS). Perform a blank determination in the same manner, and make any necessary correction.

Each mL of 0.1 mol/L perchloric acid VS
= 19.42 mg of $C_8H_{10}N_4O_2$

Containers and storage Containers—Tight containers.

Caffeine and Sodium Benzoate

安息香酸ナトリウムカフェイン

Caffeine and Sodium Benzoate, when dried, contains not less than 48.0% and not more than 50.0% of caffeine ($C_8H_{10}N_4O_2$: 194.19), and not less than 50.0% and not more than 52.0% of sodium benzoate ($C_7H_5NaO_2$: 144.10).

Description Caffeine and Sodium Benzoate occurs as a white powder. It is odorless, and has a slightly bitter taste.

It is freely soluble in water, soluble in acetic acid (100) and in acetic anhydride, sparingly soluble in ethanol (95), and practically insoluble in diethyl ether.

Identification **(1)** Dissolve 1 g of Caffeine and Sodium Benzoate in 10 mL of water in a separator, add 1 drop of phenolphthalein TS, and add carefully 0.01 mol/L sodium hydroxide VS dropwise until a faint red color develops. Extract with three 20-mL portions of chloroform by thorough shaking, and separate the chloroform layer from the water layer. [Use the water layer for test (2).] Filter the combined chloroform extracts, evaporate the filtrate to dryness on a water bath, and proceed the following tests with the residue:

(i) To 2 mL of a solution of the residue (1 in 500) add tannic acid TS dropwise: a white precipitate, which dissolves upon the dropwise addition of tannic acid TS, is produced.

(ii) To 0.01 g of the residue add 10 drops of hydrogen peroxide TS and 1 drop of hydrochloric acid, evaporate to dryness on a water bath: the residue acquires a yellow-red color. Invert the residue over a vessel containing 2 to 3 drops of ammonia TS: the color turns red-purple, and disappears upon the addition of 2 to 3 drops of sodium hydroxide TS.

(iii) Dissolve 0.01 g of the residue in water to make 50 mL. To 5 mL of this solution add 3 mL of diluted acetic acid (31) (3 in 100) and 5 mL of a solution of pyridine (1 in 10), mix, add 2 mL of diluted sodium hypochlorite TS (1 in 5), and allow to stand for 1 minute. Add 2 mL of sodium thiosulfate TS and 5 mL of sodium hydroxide TS to the solution: a yellow color develops.

(2) To 5 mL of the water layer obtained in (1) add 5 mL of water: the solution responds to the Qualitative Tests <*1.09*> (2) for benzoate.

(3) Heat Caffeine and Sodium Benzoate: white fumes are evolved. Ignite furthermore, and to the residue add hydrochloric acid: bubbles are produced, and the solution responds to Qualitative Tests <*1.09*> (1) for sodium salt.

Purity **(1)** Clarity and color of solution—Dissolve 1.0 g of Caffeine and Sodium Benzoate in 5 mL of water: the solution is clear and colorless.

(2) Alkalinity—Dissolve 1.0 g of Caffeine and Sodium Benzoate in 20 mL of water, and add 1 or 2 drops of phenolphthalein TS: no red color develops.

(3) Chloride <*1.03*>—Dissolve 0.5 g of Caffeine and Sodium Benzoate in 10 mL of water, and add 30 mL of ethanol (95), 6 mL of dilute nitric acid and water to make 50 mL. Perform the test using this solution as the test solution. Prepare the control solution with 0.70 mL of 0.01 mol/L hydrochloric acid VS, 30 mL of ethanol (95) and water to make 50 mL (not more than 0.050%).

(4) Chlorinated compounds—Dissolve 1.0 g of Caffeine and Sodium Benzoate in 40 mL of water, add 10 mL of dilute sulfuric acid, and extract with two 20-mL portions of diethyl ether. Allow the combined diethyl ether extracts to evaporate at room temperature to dryness. Place this residue and 0.7 g of calcium carbonate in a crucible, mix with a small amount of water, and dry. Ignite at about 600°C, dissolve the residue in 20 mL of dilute nitric acid, and filter. Wash the residue with 15 mL of water, combine the filtrate and the washings, and add water to make 50 mL. To this solution add 0.5 mL of silver nitrate TS: the solution is not more turbid than the following control solution to which 0.5 mL of silver nitrate TS has been added.

Control solution: Dissolve 0.7 g of calcium carbonate in 20 mL of dilute nitric acid, and filter. Wash the residue with 15 mL of water, combine the filtrate and the washings, and add 1.2 mL of 0.01 mol/L hydrochloric acid VS and water to make 50 mL.

(5) Heavy metals <*1.07*>—Dissolve 2.0 g of Caffeine and Sodium Benzoate in 47 mL of water, add slowly, with vigorous stirring, 3 mL of dilute hydrochloric acid, and filter. Discard the first 5 mL of the filtrate, neutralize the subsequent 25 mL of the filtrate with ammonia TS, and add 2 mL of dilute acetic acid and water to make 50 mL. Perform the test using this solution as the test solution. Prepare the control solution with 2.0 mL of Standard Lead Solution by adding 2 mL of dilute acetic acid and water to make 50 mL (not more than 20 ppm).

(6) Arsenic <*1.11*>—Prepare the test solution with 1.0 g of Caffeine and Sodium Benzoate according to Method 1, and perform the test (not more than 2 ppm).

(7) Phthalic acid—To 0.10 g of Caffeine and Sodium Benzoate add 1 mL of water and 1 mL of resorcinol-sulfuric acid TS, and heat the mixture in an oil bath heated at a temperature between 120°C and 125°C to evaporate the water, then heat the residue for further 90 minutes, cool, and dissolve in 5 mL of water. To 1 mL of the solution add 10 mL of a solution of sodium hydroxide (43 in 500), shake, then examine under light at a wavelength between 470 nm and 490 nm: the green fluorescence of the solution is not more intense than that of the following control solution.

Control solution: Dissolve 61 mg of potassium hydrogen phthalate in water to make exactly 1000 mL. Pipet exactly 1 mL of the solution, add 1 mL of resorcinol-sulfuric acid TS, and proceed as directed above.

(8) Readily carbonizable substances *<1.15>*—Proceed with 0.5 g of Caffeine and Sodium Benzoate, and perform the test: the solution is not more colored than Matching Fluid A.

Loss on drying *<2.41>* Not more than 3.0% (2 g, 80°C, 4 hours).

Assay **(1)** Sodium benzoate—Weigh accurately about 0.2 g of Caffeine and Sodium Benzoate, previously dried, dissolve by warming in 50 mL of a mixture of acetic anhydride and acetic acid (100) (6:1), cool, and titrate *<2.50>* with 0.1 mol/L perchloric acid-dioxane VS to the first equivalence point (potentiometric titration). Perform a blank determination in the same manner, and make any ncessary correction.

Each mL of 0.1 mol/L perchloric acid-dioxane VS
= 14.41 mg of $C_7H_5NaO_2$

(2) Caffeine—Continue the titration *<2.50>* in (1) with 0.1 mol/L perchloric acid-dioxane VS from the first equivalence point to the second equivalence point (potentiometric titration).

Each mL of 0.1 mol/L perchloric acid-dioxane VS
= 19.42 mg of $C_8H_{10}N_4O_2$

Containers and storage Containers—Well-closed containers.

Calcitonin Salmon

カルシトニン サケ

CSNLSTCVLG KLSQELHKLQ TYPRTNTGSG TP-NH_2

$C_{145}H_{240}N_{44}O_{48}S_2$: 3431.85
[47931-85-1]

Calcitonin Salmon is synthetic salmon calcitonin, and is a peptide consisting of 32 amino acid residues.

It contains not less than 4000 Units of calcitonin salmon per 1 mg of peptide.

Description Calcitonin Salmon occurs as a white powder.

It is freely soluble in water.

It dissolves in dilute acetic acid.

Dissolve 20 mg of Calcitonin Salmon in 2 mL of water: the pH of the solution is between 5.0 and 7.0.

It is hygroscopic.

Identification Dissolve 1 mg of Calcitonin Salmon in 1 mL of dilute acetic acid. Determine the absorption spectrum of this solution as directed under Ultraviolet-visible Spectrophotometry *<2.24>*, and compare the spectrum with the Reference Spectrum: both spectra exhibit similar intensities of absorption at the same wavelengths.

Absorbance *<2.24>* $E^{1\%}_{1\,cm}$ (275 nm): 3.3 – 4.0 (1 mg, dilute acetic acid, 1 mL).

Optical rotation *<2.49>* $[\alpha]^{20}_D$: −24 – −32° (25 mg, diluted acetic acid (100) (1 in 2), 10 mL, 100 mm).

Constituent amino acids Weigh accurately about 1 mg of Calcitonin Salmon, put in a test tube for hydrolysis, dissolve in 0.5 mL of diluted hydrochloric acid (1 in 2), freeze in a dry ice-acetone bath, seal the tube under reduced pressure, and heat at 110 ± 2°C for 24 hours. After cooling, open the tube, evaporate the hydrolyzate to dryness under reduced pressure, dissolve the residue in exactly 5 mL of 0.02 mol/L hydrochloric acid TS, and use this solution as the sample solution. Separately, weigh accurately about 27 mg of L-aspartic acid, about 24 mg of L-threonine, about 21 mg of L-serine, about 29 mg of L-glutamic acid, about 23 mg of L-proline, about 15 mg of glycine, about 18 mg of L-alanine, about 23 mg of L-valine, about 48 mg of L-cystine, about 30 mg of methionine, about 26 mg of L-isoleucine, about 26 mg of L-leucine, about 36 mg of L-tyrosine, about 33 mg of phenylalanine, about 37 mg of L-lysine hydrochloride, about 42 mg of L-histidine hydrochloride monohydrate and about 42 mg of L-arginine hydrochloride, dissolve them in 10 mL of 1 mol/L hydrochloric acid TS, and add water to make exactly 100 mL. Pipet 5 mL of this solution, add 0.02 mol/L hydrochloric acid TS to make exactly 50 mL, and use this solution as the standard solution. Perform the test with exactly 10 μL each of the sample solution and standard solution as directed under Liquid Chromatography *<2.01>* according to the following conditions: 13 peaks of amino acids appear on the chromatogram obtained from the sample solution, and their respective molar ratios with respect to leucine (=5) are 1.9 – 2.3 for lysine, 0.8 – 1.1 for histidine, 0.9 – 1.1 for arginine, 1.9 – 2.1 for aspartic acid, 4.5 – 4.9 for threonine, 3.2 – 3.8 for serine, 2.8 – 3.1 for glutamic acid, 1.9 – 2.4 for proline, 2.7 – 3.3 for glycine, 1.5 – 2.5 for 1/2 cystine, 0.9 – 1.0 for valine, and 0.8 – 1.0 for tyrosine.

Operating conditions—

Detector: A visible spectrophotometer (wavelength: 440 nm and 570 nm).

Column: A stainless steel column 4.6 mm in inside diameter and 6 cm in length, packed with strongly acidic ion-exchange resin for liquid chromatography (Na type) composed with a sulfonated polystyrene copolymer (3 μm in particle diameter).

Column temperature: A constant temperature of about 57°C.

Chemical reaction bath temperature: A constant temperature of about 130°C.

Color developing time: About 1 minute.

Mobile phase: Prepare mobile phases A, B, C, D and E according to the following table.

	Mobile phase A	Mobile phase B	Mobile phase C	Mobile phase D	Mobile phase E
Citric acid monohydrate	19.80 g	22.00 g	12.80 g	6.10 g	—
Trisodium citrate dihydrate	6.19 g	7.74 g	13.31 g	26.67 g	—
Sodium hydroxide	—	—	—	—	8.00 g
Sodium chloride	5.66 g	7.07 g	3.74 g	54.35 g	—
Ethanol (99.5)	130.0 mL	20.0 mL	4.0 mL	—	100.0 mL
Benzyl alcohol	—	—	—	5.0 mL	—
Thiodiglycol	5.0 mL	5.0 mL	5.0 mL	—	—
Lauromacrogol solution (1 in 4)	4.0 mL	4.0 mL	4.0 mL	4.0 mL	4.0 mL
Caprylic acid	0.1 mL	0.1 mL	0.1 mL	0.1 mL	0.1 mL
Water	a sufficient amount	a sufficient amount	a sufficient amount	a sufficient amount	a sufficient amount
Total volume	1000 mL	1000 mL	1000 mL	1000 mL	1000 mL

Flowing of mobile phase: Control the gradient by mixing the mobile phases A, B, C, D and E as directed in the following table.

Time after injection of sample (min)	Mobile phase A (vol%)	Mobile phase B (vol%)	Mobile phase C (vol%)	Mobile phase D (vol%)	Mobile phase E (vol%)
0 – 1.5	100	0	0	0	0
1.5 – 4	0	100	0	0	0
4 – 12	0	0	100	0	0
12 – 26	0	0	0	100	0
26 – 30	0	0	0	0	100

Reaction reagent: Mix 407 g of lithium acetate dihydrate, 245 mL of acetic acid (100) and 801 mL of 1-methoxy-2-propanol, add water to make 2000 mL, stir for 10 minutes while passing nitrogen, and use this solution as solution A. Separately, to 1957 mL of 1-methoxy-2-propanol add 77 g of ninhydrin and 0.134 g of sodium borohydride, stir for 30 minutes while passing nitrogen, and use this solution as solution B. Mix solution A and solution B before use.

Flow rate of mobile phase: About 0.4 mL per minute.

Flow rate of reaction reagent: About 0.35 mL per minute.

System suitability—

System performance: When the procedure is run with 10 μL of the standard solution under the above operating conditions, aspartic acid, threonine, serine, glutamic acid, proline, glycine, alanine, cystine, valine, methionine, isoleucine, leucine, tyrosine, phenylalanine, lysine, histidine and arginine are eluted in this order with the resolutions between the peaks of threonine and serine, glycine and alanine, and isoleucine and leucine being not less than 1.2, 1.0 and 1.2, respectively.

System repeatability: When the test is repeated 3 times with 10 μL of the standard solution under the above operating conditions, the relative standard deviations of the peak areas of aspartic acid, proline, valine and arginine are not more than 2.0%, respectively.

Peptide content Calculate the peptide content in Calcitonin Salmon by the following equation using amino acid analysis values (μmol/mL) obtained in the Constituent amino acids: it is not less than 80.0%.

$$\text{Peptide content (\%)} = 3431.85 \times 5/M \times A/11 \times 100$$

A: Total (μmol/mL) of the amino acid analysis values of valine, leucine, glycine and proline

M: Amount (μg) of Calcitonin Salmon taken

11: Total of the theoretical residue numbers of valine, leucine, glycine and proline per one mole of calcitonin salmon

Purity **(1)** Acetic acid—Weigh accurately about 10 mg of Calcitonin Salmon, dissolve in water to make exactly 10 mL, and use this solution as the sample solution. Separately, weigh accurately about 1 g of acetic acid (100), and dissolve in water to make exactly 100 mL. Pipet 2 mL of this solution, add water to make exactly 200 mL, and use this solution as the standard solution. Perform the test with exactly 100 μL each of the sample solution and standard solution as directed under Liquid Chromatography <*2.01*> according to the following conditions. Determine the peak areas, A_T and A_S, of acetic acid in each solution, and calculate the amount of acetic acid by the following equation: the amount of acetic acid is not more than 7.0%.

$$\text{Amount (\%) of acetic acid } (CH_3COOH) = M_S/M_T \times A_T/A_S \times 1/10$$

M_S: Amount (mg) of acetic acid (100) taken

M_T: Amount (mg) of Calcitonin Salmon taken

Operating conditions—

Detector: An ultraviolet absorption photometer (wavelength: 210 nm).

Column: A stainless steel column 4.6 mm in inside diameter and 25 cm in length, packed with octadecylsilanized silica gel for liquid chromatography (5 μm in particle diameter).

Column temperature: A constant temperature of about 40°C.

Mobile phase A: To 0.7 mL of phosphoric acid add 900 mL of water, adjust the pH to 3.0 with 8 mol/L sodium hydroxide TS, and add water to make 1000 mL.

Mobile phase B: Methanol.

Flowing of mobile phase: Control the gradient by mixing the mobile phases A and B as directed in the following table.

Time after injection of sample (min)	Mobile phase A (vol%)	Mobile phase B (vol%)
0 – 5	95	5
5 – 10	95 → 50	5 → 50
10 – 20	50	50
20 – 22	50 → 95	50 → 5
22 – 30	95	5

Flow rate: Adjust so that the retention time of acetic acid is about 4 minutes.

System suitability—

System performance: When the procedure is run with 100 μL of the standard solution under the above operating conditions, the number of theoretical plates and the symmetry factor of the peak of acetic acid are not less than 3000 and not more than 2.0, respectively.

System repeatability: When the test is repeated 6 times with 100 μL of the standard solution under the above operating conditions, the relative standard deviation of the peak areas of acetic acid is not more than 2.0%.

(2) Related substances—Dissolve 2 mg of Calcitonin Salmon in 2 mL of dilute acetic acid, and use this solution as the sample solution. Perform the test with 20 μL of the sample solution as directed under Liquid Chromatography

<2.01> according to the following conditions. Determine each peak area from the sample solution by the automatic integration method, and calculate the amount of them by the area percentage method: the total amount of the peaks other than calcitonin salmon is not more than 3%.

Operating conditions—

Detector: An ultraviolet absorption photometer (wavelength: 210 nm).

Column: A stainless steel column 3.9 mm in inside diameter and 30 cm in length, packed with octadecylsilanized silica gel for liquid chromatography (10 μm in particle diameter).

Column temperature: A constant temperature of about 25°C.

Mobile phase: A mixture of 1% trimethylamine-phosphate buffer solution (pH 3.0) and acetonitrile (27:13).

Flow rate: Adjust so that the retention time of calcitonin salmon is about 9 minutes.

Time span of measurement: About 2 times as long as the retention time of calcitonin salmon, beginning after the solvent peak.

System suitability—

Test for required detectability: To 1 mL of the sample solution add the mobile phase to make 100 mL, and use this solution as the solution for system suitability test. Pipet 1 mL of the solution for system suitability test, and add the mobile phase to make exactly 10 mL. Confirm that the peak area of calcitonin salmon obtained with 20 μL of this solution is equivalent to 5 to 15% of that with 20 μL of the solution for system suitability test.

System performance: Dissolve 5 mg of methyl parahydroxybenzoate and 7 mg of ethyl parahydroxybenzoate in 100 mL of acetonitrile. When the procedure is run with 20 μL of this solution under the above operating conditions methyl parahydroxybenzoate and ethyl parahydroxybenzoate are eluted in this order with the resolution between these peaks being not less than 5.

System repeatability: When the test is repeated 6 times with 20 μL of the solution for system suitability test under the above operating conditions, the relative standard deviation of the peak areas of calcitonin salmon is not more than 2.0%.

Water <2.48> Not more than 10.0% (5 mg, coulometric titration).

Assay (i) Test animals: Select healthy albino rats weighing between 55 and 180 g, fasted for 24 hours before the test but allowed to drink water ad libitum.

(ii) Standard solutions: Dissolve a quantity of Calcitonin Salmon RS in acetic acid buffer solution containing 0.1% bovine serum albumin, and prepare a high-dose standard solution S_H and a low-dose standard solution S_L containing exactly 0.050 and 0.025 Units per mL, respectively.

(iii) Sample solutions: According to the labeled units, weigh accurately a suitable amount of Calcitonin Salmon, and dissolve in acetic acid buffer solution containing 0.1% bovine serum albumin, and prepare a high-dose sample solution T_H and the low-dose sample solution T_L having Units equal to the standard solutions in equal volumes, respectively.

(iv) Dose for injection: Inject 0.3 mL per animal.

(v) Procedure: Divide the test animals at random into 4 groups, A, B, C and D, with not less than 8 animals and equal numbers in each group. Inject S_H, S_L, T_H and T_L into the tail vein or subcutaneously into the neck of each animal of the respective groups. At 1 hour after the injection, collect blood from the abdominal aorta in a way that minimizes the suffering of the animals, allow the blood samples to stand at room temperature for about 30 minutes, and centrifuge at 3000 revolutions per minute for 10 minutes to separate serum.

(vi) Serum calcium determination: Pipet 0.1 mL of the serum, add exactly 6.9 mL of strontium TS, mix well, and use this solution as the sample solution for calcium determination. Separately, pipet a suitable volume of Standard Calcium Solution for Atomic Absorption Spectrophotometry, dissolve in strontium TS to make a solution so that each mL contains 0.2 to 3 μg of calcium (Ca: 40.08), and use this solution as the standard solution for calcium determination. Perform the test as directed under Atomic Absorption Spectrometry <2.23> according to the following conditions, and calculate the calcium content of the sample solution for calcium determination from the calibration curve obtained from the absorbance of the standard solution for calcium determination.

Amount (mg) of Calcium (Ca) in 100 mL of the serum
= Calcium content (ppm) in the sample solution for calcium determination × 7

Gas: Combustible gas—Acetylene.
Supporting gas—Air.
Lamp: Calcium hollow-cathode lamp.
Wavelength: 422.7 nm.

(vii) Calculation: Amounts of calcium in the serum obtained with S_H, S_L, T_H and T_L are symbolized as y_1, y_2, y_3 and y_4, respectively. Sum up y_1, y_2, y_3 and y_4 on each set to obtain Y_1, Y_2, Y_3 and Y_4, respectively.

Units per mg of peptide = antilog $M \times b/a \times 1/c \times 5$

$M = 0.3010 \times (Y_a/Y_b)$
$Y_a = -Y_1 - Y_2 + Y_3 + Y_4$
$Y_b = Y_1 - Y_2 + Y_3 - Y_4$

a: Amount (mg) of Calcitonin Salmon taken
b: Total volume (mL) of the high-dose sample solution prepared by dissolving Calcitonin Salmon in acetic acid buffer solution containing 0.1% bovine serum albumin.
c: Peptide content (%)

F' computed by the following equation should be smaller than F_1 shown in the table against n with which s^2 is calculated. Calculate L (P = 0.95) by use of the following equation: L should be not more than 0.20. If F' exceeds F_1, or if L exceeds 0.20, repeat the test, increasing the number of animals or arranging the assay conditions so that F' is not more than F_1 and L is not more than 0.20.

$F' = (-Y_1 + Y_2 + Y_3 - Y_4)^2/4fs^2$
f: Number of the test animals of each group.
$s^2 = \{\Sigma y^2 - (Y/f)\}/n$
Σy^2: The sum of squares of y_1, y_2, y_3 and y_4 in each group.
$Y = Y_1^2 + Y_2^2 + Y_3^2 + Y_4^2$
$n = 4(f - 1)$
$L = 2\sqrt{(C - 1)(CM^2 + 0.09062)}$
$C = Y_b^2/(Y_b^2 - 4fs^2t^2)$
t^2: Value shown in the following table against n used to calculate s^2.

n	$t^2 = F_1$	n	$t^2 = F_1$	n	$t^2 = F_1$
1	161.45	13	4.667	25	4.242
2	18.51	14	4.600	26	4.225
3	10.129	15	4.543	27	4.210
4	7.709	16	4.494	28	4.196
5	6.608	17	4.451	29	4.183
6	5.987	18	4.414	30	4.171
7	5.591	19	4.381	40	4.085
8	5.318	20	4.351	60	4.001
9	5.117	21	4.325	120	3.920
10	4.965	22	4.301	∞	3.841
11	4.844	23	4.279		
12	4.747	24	4.260		

Containers and storage Containers—Hermetic containers.

Storage—Light-resistant, not exceeding 10°C.

Precipitated Calcium Carbonate

沈降炭酸カルシウム

$CaCO_3$: 100.09

Precipitated Calcium Carbonate, when dried, contains not less than 98.5% of calcium carbonate ($CaCO_3$).

Description Precipitated Calcium Carbonate occurs as a white, fine crystalline powder. It is odorless and tasteless.

It is practically insoluble in water, but its solubility in water is increased in the presence of carbon dioxide.

It is practically insoluble in ethanol (95) and in diethyl ether.

It dissolves with effervescence in dilute acetic acid, in dilute hydrochloric acid and in dilute nitric acid.

Identification (1) Dissolve 0.5 g of Precipitated Calcium Carbonate in 10 mL of dilute hydrochloric acid, boil, then cool, and neutralize with ammonia TS: the solution responds to Qualitative Tests <*1.09*> for calcium salt.

(2) Precipitated Calcium Carbonate responds to Qualitative Tests <*1.09*> (1) for carbonate.

Purity (1) Acid-insoluble substances—To 5.0 g of Precipitated Calcium Carbonate add 50 mL of water, then add 20 mL of hydrochloric acid dropwise with stirring, boil for 5 minutes, cool, add water to make 200 mL, and filter through filter paper for quantitative analysis. Wash the residue until the last washing shows no turbidity with silver nitrate TS, and ignite the residue together with the filter paper: the mass of the residue is not more than 10.0 mg.

(2) Heavy metals <*1.07*>—Mix 2.0 g of Precipitated Calcium Carbonate with 5 mL of water, add slowly 6 mL of dilute hydrochloric acid, and evaporate on a water bath to dryness. Dissolve the residue in 50 mL of water, and filter. To 25 mL of the filtrate add 2 mL of dilute acetic acid, 1 drop of ammonia TS and water to make 50 mL, and perform the test using this solution as the test solution. Prepare the control solution as follows: evaporate 3 mL of hydrochloric acid on a water bath to dryness, and add 2.0 mL of Standard Lead Solution, 2 mL of dilute acetic acid and water to make 50 mL (not more than 20 ppm).

(3) Barium—Mix 1.0 g of Precipitated Calcium Carbonate with 10 mL of water, add dropwise 4 mL of hydrochloric acid with stirring, boil for 5 minutes, cool, add water to make 40 mL, and filter. With the filtrate, perform the test as directed under Flame Coloration Test <*1.04*> (1): no green color appears.

(4) Magnesium and alkali metals—Dissolve 1.0 g of Precipitated Calcium Carbonate in a mixture of 20 mL of water and 10 mL of dilute hydrochloric acid, boil, neutralize with ammonia TS, and add ammonium oxalate TS until precipitation of calcium oxalate is completed. Heat the mixture on a water bath for 1 hour, cool, dilute with water to 100 mL, shake well, and filter. To 50 mL of the filtrate add 0.5 mL of sulfuric acid, evaporate to dryness, and ignite at 600°C to constant mass: the mass of the residue is not more than 5.0 mg.

(5) Arsenic <*1.11*>—Moisten 0.40 g of Precipitated Calcium Carbonate with 1 mL of water, then dissolve in 4 mL of dilute hydrochloric acid, use this solution as the test solution, and perform the test (not more than 5 ppm).

Loss on drying <*2.41*> Not more than 1.0% (1 g, 180°C, 4 hours).

Assay Weigh accurately about 0.12 g of Precipitated Calcium Carbonate, previously dried, and dissolve in 20 mL of water and 3 mL of dilute hydrochloric acid. Add 80 mL of water, 15 mL of a solution of potassium hydroxide (1 in 10) and 0.05 g of NN indicator, and titrate <*2.50*> immediately with 0.05 mol/L disodium dihydrogen ethylenediamine tetraacetate VS until the color of the solution changes from red-purple to blue.

Each mL of 0.05 mol/L disodium dihydrogen
ethylenediamine tetraacetate VS
= 5.005 mg of $CaCO_3$

Containers and storage Containers—Tight containers.

Precipitated Calcium Carbonate Fine Granules

沈降炭酸カルシウム細粒

Precipitated Calcium Carbonate Fine Granules contain not less than 95.0% and not more than 105.0% of the labeled amount of calcium carbonate ($CaCO_3$: 100.09).

Method of preparation Prepare as directed under Granules, with Precipitated Calcium Carbonate.

Identification (1) To a quantity of powdered Precipitated Calcium Carbonate Fine Granules, equivalent to 0.5 g of Precipitated Calcium Carbonate, add 10 mL of dilute hydrochloric acid, shake thoroughly, and filter. Boil the filtrate, then cool, and neutralize with ammonia TS: the solution responds to Qualitative Tests <*1.09*> (1), (2) and (3) for calcium salt.

(2) Powdered Precipitated Calcium Carbonate Fine Granules responds to Qualitative Tests <*1.09*> (1) for carbonate.

Uniformity of dosage units <*6.02*> The granules in single-dose packages meet the requirement of the Mass variation test.

Dissolution <*6.10*> When the test is performed at 50 revolutions per minute according to the Paddle method, using 900 mL of 1st fluid for dissolution test as the dissolution medium, the dissolution rate in 10 minutes of Precipitated Calcium Carbonate Fine Granules is not less than 80%.

Start the test with an accurately weighed amount of

Precipitated Calcium Carbonate Fine Granules, equivalent to about 0.5 g of calcium carbonate ($CaCO_3$), withdraw not less than 20 mL of the medium at the specified minute after starting the test, and filter through a membrane filter with a pore size not exceeding 0.45 μm. Discard not less than 10 mL of the first filtrate, pipet 2 mL of the subsequent filtrate, add the mobile phase to make exactly 20 mL, and use this solution as the sample solution. Separately, weigh accurately about 28 mg of calcium carbonate for assay, previously dried at 180°C for 4 hours, and dissolve in the dissolution medium to make exactly 100 mL. Pipet 10 mL of this solution, add the mobile phase to make exactly 50 mL, and use this solution as the standard solution. Perform the test with exactly 20 μL each of the sample solution and standard solution as directed under Liquid Chromatography ⟨*2.01*⟩ according to the following conditions, and determine the peak areas, A_T and A_S, of calcium in each solution.

Dissolution rate (%) with respect to the labeled amount of calcium carbonate ($CaCO_3$)

$$= M_S/M_T \times A_T/A_S \times 1/C \times 1800$$

M_S: Amount (mg) of calcium carbonate for assay taken
M_T: Amount (mg) of Precipitated Calcium Carbonate Fine Granules taken
C: Labeled amount (mg) of calcium carbonate ($CaCO_3$) in 1 g

Operating conditions—

Detector: An electric conductivity detector.

Column: A polyether ether ketone tube 4.6 mm in inside diameter and 10 cm in length, packed with slightly acidic ion-exchange silica gel for liquid chromatography (7 μm in particle diameter).

Column temperature: A constant temperature of about 40°C.

Mobile phase: A mixture of a solution of tartaric acid (3 in 2000) and a solution of dipicolinic acid (1 in 3000) (1:1).

Flow rate: Adjust so that the retention time of calcium is about 8 minutes.

System suitability—

System performance: When the procedure is run with 20 μL of the standard solution under the above operating conditions, sodium and calcium are eluted in this order with the resolution between these peaks being not less than 4.5.

System repeatability: When the test is repeated 5 times with 20 μL of the standard solution under the above operating conditions, the relative standard deviation of the peak area of calcium is not more than 2.0%.

Assay Weigh accurately a quantity of powdered Precipitated Calcium Carbonate Fine Granules, equivalent to about 0.12 g of calcium carbonate ($CaCO_3$), add 20 mL of water and 3 mL of dilute hydrochloric acid, and agitate for 15 minutes with the aid of ultrasonic waves. Then, add 80 mL of water, 15 mL of a solution of potassium hydroxide (1 in 10) and 50 mg of NN indicator, and titrate ⟨*2.50*⟩ immediately with 0.05 mol/L disodium dihydrogen ethylenediamine tetraacetate VS until the color of the solution changes from red-purple to blue.

Each mL of 0.05 mol/L disodium dihydrogen ethylenediamine tetraacetate VS
= 5.005 mg of $CaCO_3$

Containers and storage Containers—Well-closed containers.

Precipitated Calcium Carbonate Tablets

沈降炭酸カルシウム錠

Precipitated Calcium Carbonate Tablets contain not less than 95.0% and not more than 105.0% of the labeled amount of calcium carbonate ($CaCO_3$: 100.09).

Method of preparation Prepare as directed under Tablets, with Precipitated Calcium Carbonate.

Identification **(1)** To a quantity of powdered Precipitated Calcium Carbonate Tablets, equivalent to 0.5 g of Precipitated Calcium Carbonate, add 10 mL of dilute hydrochloric acid, shake throughly, and filter, if necessary. Boil, then cool, and neutralize with ammonia TS: the solution responds to Qualitative Tests ⟨*1.09*⟩ (1), (2) and (3) for calcium salt.

(2) Powdered Precipitated Calcium Carbonate Tablets responds to Qualitative Tests ⟨*1.09*⟩ (1) for carbonate.

Uniformity of dosage units ⟨*6.02*⟩ It meets the requirement of the Mass variation test.

Disintegration ⟨*6.09*⟩ Apply to the preparation intended to be used as antacid.

Perform the test using the disk: it meets the requirement.

Dissolution ⟨*6.10*⟩ Apply to the preparation intended to be used as hyperphosphatemia.

When the test is performed at 50 revolutions per minute according to the Paddle method, using 900 mL of 1st fluid for dissolution test as the dissolution medium, the dissolution rate in 10 minutes of Precipitated Calcium Carbonate Tablets is not less than 80%.

Start the test with 1 tablet of Precipitated Calcium Carbonate Tablets, withdraw not less than 20 mL of the medium at the specified minute after starting the test, and filter through a membrane filter with a pore size not exceeding 0.45 μm. Discard not less than 10 mL of the first filtrate, pipet V mL of the subsequent filtrate, add the mobile phase to make exactly V' mL so that each mL contains about 56 μg of calcium carbonate ($CaCo_3$), and use this solution as the sample solution. Separately, weigh accurately about 28 mg of calcium carbonate for assay, previously dried at 180°C for 4 hours, and dissolve in the dissolution medium to make exactly 100 mL. Pipet 10 mL of this solution, add the mobile phase to make exactly 50 mL, and use this solution as the standard solution. Perform the test with exactly 20 μL each of the sample solution and standard solution as directed under Liquid Chromatography ⟨*2.01*⟩ according to the following conditions, and determine the peak areas, A_T and A_S, of calcium in each solution.

Dissolution rate (%) with respect to the labeled amount of calcium carbonate ($CaCO_3$)

$$= M_S \times A_T/A_S \times V'/V \times 1/C \times 180$$

M_S: Amount (mg) of calcium carbonate for assay taken
C: Labeled amount (mg) of calcium carbonate ($CaCO_3$) in 1 tablet

Operating conditions—

Detector: An electric conductivity detector.

Column: A polyether ether ketone tube 4.6 mm in inside diameter and 10 cm in length, packed with slightly acidic ion-exchange silica gel for liquid chromatography (7 μm in particle diameter).

Column temperature: A constant temperature of about 40°C.

Mobile phase: A mixture of a solution of tartaric acid (3 in 2000) and a solution of dipicolinic acid (1 in 3000) (1:1).

Flow rate: Adjust so that the retention time of calcium is about 8 minutes.

System suitability—

System performance: When the procedure is run with 20 μL of the standard solution under the above operating conditions, sodium and calcium are eluted in this order with the resolution between these peaks being not less than 4.5.

System repeatability: When the test is repeated 5 times with 20 μL of the standard solution under the above operating conditions, the relative standard deviation of the peak area of calcium is not more than 2.0%.

Acid-neutralizing capacity <*6.04*> Apply to the preparation intended to be used as antacid.

Weigh accurately and powder not less than 40 Precipitated Calcium Carbonate Tablets. Perform the test with an accurately weighed amount of the powder, equivalent to about 0.25 g of Calcium Carbonate: the amount of 0.1 mol/L hydrochloric acid VS consumed per 1 g of Precipitated Calcium Carbonate is not less than 190 mL.

Assay Weigh accurately and powder not less than 20 Precipitated Calcium Carbonate Tablets. To an accurately weighed portion of the powder, equivalent to about 0.12 g of calcium carbonate ($CaCO_3$), add 20 mL of water, 3 mL of dilute hydrochloric acid, and agitate, if necessary, for 15 minutes with the aid of ultrasonic waves. Then, add 80 mL of water, 15 mL of a solution of potassium hydroxide (1 in 10) and 50 mg of NN indicator, and titrate <*2.50*> immediately with 0.05 mol/L disodium dihydrogen ethylenediamine tetraacetate VS until the color of the solution changes from red-purple to blue.

Each mL of 0.05 mol/L disodium dihydrogen ethylenediamine tetraacetate VS
= 5.005 mg of $CaCO_3$

Containers and storage Containers—Tight containers.

Calcium Chloride Hydrate

塩化カルシウム水和物

$CaCl_2.2H_2O$: 147.01

Calcium Chloride Hydrate contains not less than 96.7% and not more than 103.3% of calcium chloride hydrate ($CaCl_2.2H_2O$).

Description Calcium Chloride Hydrate occurs as white, granules or masses. It is odorless.

It is very soluble in water, and soluble in ethanol (95), and practically insoluble in diethyl ether.

It is deliquescent.

Identification A solution of Calcium Chloride Hydrate (1 in 10) responds to Qualitative Tests <*1.09*> for calcium salt and for chloride.

pH <*2.54*> The pH of a solution of 1.0 g of Calcium Chloride Hydrate in 20 mL of freshly boiled and cooled water is between 4.5 and 9.2.

Purity (1) Clarity and color of solution—A solution of 1.0 g of Calcium Chloride Hydrate in 20 mL of water is clear and colorless.

(2) Sulfate <*1.14*>—Take 1.0 g of Calcium Chloride Hydrate, and perform the test. Prepare the control solution with 0.50 mL of 0.005 mol/L sulfuric acid VS (not more than 0.024%).

(3) Hypochlorite—Dissolve 0.5 g of Calcium Chloride Hydrate in 5 mL of water, add 2 to 3 drops of dilute hydrochloric acid and 2 to 3 drops of zinc iodide-starch TS: no blue color develops immediately.

(4) Heavy metals <*1.07*>—Proceed with 2.0 g of Calcium Chloride Hydrate according to Method 1, and perform the test. Prepare the control solution with 2.0 mL of Standard Lead Solution (not more than 10 ppm).

(5) Iron, aluminum or phosphate—Dissolve, in a Nessler tube, 1.0 g of Calcium Chloride Hydrate in 20 mL of water and 1 drop of dilute hydrochloric acid, boil, then cool, add 3 drops of ammonia TS, and heat the solution to boil: no turbidity or precipitate is produced.

(6) Barium—Dissolve 0.5 g of Calcium Chloride Hydrate in 5 mL of water, add 2 drops of dilute hydrochloric acid and 2 mL of potassium sulfate TS, and allow to stand for 10 minutes: no turbidity is produced.

(7) Arsenic <*1.11*>—Prepare the test solution with 1.0 g of Calcium Chloride Hydrate according to Method 1, and perform the test (not more than 2 ppm).

Assay Weigh accurately about 0.4 g of Calcium Chloride Hydrate, and dissolve in water to make exactly 200 mL. Measure exactly 20 mL of this solution, add 40 mL of water, 2 mL of 8 mol/L potassium hydroxide TS and 0.1 g of NN indicator, and titrate <*2.50*> immediately with 0.02 mol/L disodium dihydrogen ethylenediamine tetraacetate VS until the color of the solution changes from red-purple to blue.

Each mL of 0.02 mol/L disodium dihydrogen ethylenediamine tetraacetate VS
= 2.940 mg of $CaCl_2.2H_2O$

Containers and storage Containers—Tight containers.

Calcium Chloride Injection

塩化カルシウム注射液

Calcium Chloride Injection is an aqueous injection. It contains not less than 95.0% and not more than 105.0% of the labeled amount of calcium chloride ($CaCl_2$: 110.98).

The concentration of Calcium Chloride Injection is expressed as the quantity of calcium chloride ($CaCl_2$).

Method of preparation Prepare as directed under Injection, with Calcium Chloride Hydrate.

Description Calcium Chloride Injection is a clear, colorless liquid.

Identification Calcium Chloride Injection responds to Qualitative Tests <*1.09*> for calcium salt and for chloride.

pH <*2.54*> 4.5 – 7.5

Bacterial endotoxins <*4.01*> Less than 0.30 EU/mg.

Extractable volume <*6.05*> It meets the requirement.

Foreign insoluble matter <*6.06*> Perform the test according to Method 1: it meets the requirement.

Insoluble particulate matter <*6.07*> It meets the requirement.

Sterility 〈*4.06*〉 Perform the test according to the Membrane filtration method: it meets the requirement.

Assay Measure exactly a volume of Calcium Chloride Injection, equivalent to about 0.4 g of calcium chloride ($CaCl_2$), and proceed as directed in the Assay under Calcium Chloride Hydrate.

Each mL of 0.02 mol/L disodium dihydrogen ethylenediamine tetraacetate VS
= 2.220 mg of $CaCl_2$

Containers and storage Containers—Hermetic containers. Plastic containers for aqueous injections may be used.

Calcium Folinate Hydrate

Calcium Folinate

Calcium Leucovorin

ホリナートカルシウム水和物

$C_{20}H_{21}CaN_7O_7.xH_2O$
Monocalcium *N*-(4-{[(2-amino-5-formyl-4-oxo-1,4,5,6,7,8-hexahydropteridin-6-yl)methyl]amino}benzoyl)-L-glutamate hydrate
[*1492-18-8*, anhydride]

Calcium Folinate Hydrate contains not less than 95.0% and not more than 102.0% of calcium folinate ($C_{20}H_{21}CaN_7O_7$), calculated on the anhydrous basis.

Description Calcium Folinate Hydrate occurs as a white to light yellow crystalline powder.

It is sparingly soluble in water, and practically insoluble in methanol and in ethanol (99.5).

Identification **(1)** Determine the absorption spectrum of a solution of Calcium Folinate Hydrate (1 in 100,000) as directed under Ultraviolet-visible Spectrophotometry 〈*2.24*〉, and compare the spectrum with the Reference Spectrum or the spectrum of a solution of Calcium Folinate Hydrate RS prepared in the same manner as the sample solution: both spectra exhibit similar intensities of absorption at the same wavelengths.

(2) Determine the infrared absorption spectrum of Calcium Folinate Hydrate as directed in the potassium bromide disk method under Infrared Spectrophotometry 〈*2.25*〉, and compare the spectrum with the Reference Spectrum: both spectra exhibit similar intensities of absorption at the same wave numbers.

(3) A solution of Calcium Folinate Hydrate (1 in 100) responds to Qualitative Tests 〈*1.09*〉 (2) and (3) for calcium salt.

Optical rotation 〈*2.49*〉 $[\alpha]_D^{20}$: +14 – +19° (0.1 g calculated on the anhydrous basis, water, 10 mL, 100 mm).

pH 〈*2.54*〉 To 1.25 g of Calcium Folinate Hydrate add 50 mL of freshly boiled and cooled water, and warm to 40°C, if necessary, to dissolve: the pH of this solution is between 6.8 and 8.0.

Purity **(1)** Clarity and color of solution—To 1.25 g of Calcium Folinate Hydrate add 50 mL of freshly boiled and cooled water, and warm to 40°C, if necessary, to dissolve: the solution is clear, and the absorbance at 420 nm of it, determined as directed under Ultraviolet-visible Spectrophotometry 〈*2.24*〉, is not more than 0.25.

(2) Heavy metals 〈*1.07*〉—Proceed with 0.40 g of Calcium Folinate Hydrate according to Method 2, and perform the test. Prepare the control solution with 2.0 mL of Standard Lead Solution (not more than 50 ppm).

(3) Related substances—Dissolve 10 mg of Calcium Folinate Hydrate in 25 mL of water, and use this solution as the sample solution. Pipet 2 mL of the sample solution, add water to make exactly 200 mL, and use this solution as the standard solution. Perform the test with exactly 20 μL each of the sample solution and standard solution as directed under Liquid Chromatography 〈*2.01*〉 according to the following conditions, and determine each peak area by the automatic integration method: the area of the peak other than folinate obtained from the sample solution is not larger than the peak area of folinate from the standard solution, and the total area of the peaks other than folinate from the sample solution is not larger than 5 times the peak area of folinate from the standard solution.

Operating conditions—

Detector, column, column temperature, mobile phase, and flow rate: Proceed as directed in the operating conditions in the Assay.

Time span of measurement: About 2.5 times as long as the retention time of folinate, beginning after the solvent peak.

System suitability—

System performance: Proceed as directed in the system suitability in the Assay.

Test for required detectability: Pipet 5 mL of the standard solution, and add water to make exactly 50 mL. Confirm that the peak area of folinate obtained with 20 μL of this solution is equivalent to 7 to 13% of that with 20 μL of the standard solution.

System repeatability: When the test is repeated 6 times with 20 μL of the standard solution under the above operating conditions, the relative standard deviation of the peak area of folinate is not more than 2.0%.

Water 〈*2.48*〉 Not less than 7.0% and not more than 17.0% (0.2 g, volumetric titration, direct titration).

Assay Weigh accurately about 10 mg each of Calcium Folinate Hydrate and Calcium Folinate Hydrate RS (separately determine the water 〈*2.48*〉 in the same manner as Calcium Folinate Hydrate), dissolve in water to make them exactly 25 mL. Pipet 5 mL each of these solutions, add the mobile phase to make exactly 25 mL, and use these solutions as the sample solution and the standard solution, respectively. Perform the test with exactly 20 μL each of the sample solution and standard solution as directed under Liquid Chromatography 〈*2.01*〉 according to the following conditions, and determine the peak areas, A_T and A_S, of folinate in each solution.

Amount (mg) of calcium folinate ($C_{20}H_{21}CaN_7O_7$)
$= M_S \times A_T/A_S$

M_S: Amount (mg) of Calcium Folinate Hydrate RS taken, calculated on the anhydrous basis

Operating conditions—

Detector: An ultraviolet absorption photometer (wavelength: 254 nm).

Column: A stainless steel column 4.6 mm in inside diame-

ter and 15 cm in length, packed with octadecylsilanized silica gel for liquid chromatography (5 μm in particle diameter).

Column temperature: A constant temperature of about 45°C.

Mobile phase: A mixture of disodium hydrogen phosphate dodecahydrate solution (287 in 100,000), methanol and tetrabutylammonium hydroxide TS (385:110:4), adjusted to pH7.5 with phosphoric acid.

Flow rate: Adjust so that the retention time of folinate is about 10 minutes.

System suitability—

System performance: Dissolve 10 mg each of Calcium Folinate Hydrate and folic acid in 100 mL of the mobile phase. When the procedure is run with 20 μL of this solution under the above operating conditions, folinate and folic acid are eluted in this order with the resolution between these peaks being not less than 10.

System repeatability: When the test is repeated 6 times with 20 μL of the standard solution under the above operating conditions, the relative standard deviation of the peak area of folinate is not more than 1.0%.

Containers and storage Containers—Tight containers.

Storage—Light-resistant.

Calcium Gluconate Hydrate

グルコン酸カルシウム水和物

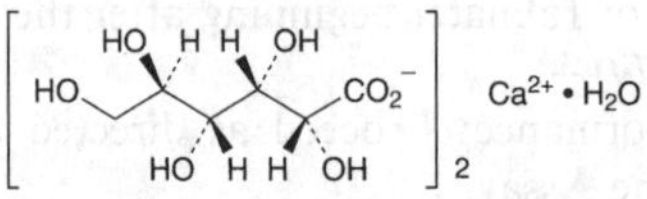

$C_{12}H_{22}CaO_{14}.H_2O$: 448.39

Monocalcium di-D-gluconate monohydrate

[299-28-5]

Calcium Gluconate Hydrate, when dried, contains not less than 99.0% and not more than 104.0% of calcium gluconate hydrate ($C_{12}H_{22}CaO_{14}.H_2O$).

Description Calcium Gluconate Hydrate occurs as a white, crystalline powder or granules.

It is soluble in water, and practically insoluble in ethanol (99.5).

Identification **(1)** To separately 10 mg each of Calcium Gluconate Hydrate and calcium gluconate for thin-layer chromatography add 1 mL of water, dissolve by warming, and use these solutions as the sample solution and the standard solution, respectively. Perform the test with these solutions as directed under Thin-layer Chromatography <*2.03*>. Spot 5 μL each of the sample solution and standard solution on a plate of silica gel for thin-layer chromatography. Develop the plate with a mixture of ethanol (95), water, ammonia solution (28) and ethyl acetate (5:3:1:1) to a distance of about 10 cm, air-dry the plate, and heat the plate at 110°C for 20 minutes. After cooling, spray evenly hexaammonium heptamolybdate-cerium (IV) sulfate TS on the plate, air-dry, and heat at 110°C for 10 minutes: the spots with the sample solution and the standard solution are the same in the *R*f value and color tone.

(2) A solution of Calcium Gluconate Hydrate (1 in 40) responds to Qualitative Tests <*1.09*> (1), (2) and (3) for calcium salt.

Optical rotation <*2.49*> $[\alpha]_D^{20}$: +6 – +11° (after drying, 0.5 g, water, warming, after cooling, 25 mL, 100 mm).

pH <*2.54*> Dissolve 1.0 g of Calcium Gluconate Hydrate in 20 mL of water by warming: the pH of the solution is between 6.0 and 8.0.

Purity **(1)** Clarity and color of solution—Dissolve 1.0 g of Calcium Gluconate Hydrate in 50 mL of water by warming: the solution is clear and colorless.

(2) Chloride <*1.03*>—Take 0.40 g of Calcium Gluconate Hydrate, and perform the test. Prepare the control solution with 0.80 mL of 0.01 mol/L hydrochloric acid VS (not more than 0.071%).

(3) Sulfate <*1.14*>—Take 1.0 g of Calcium Gluconate Hydrate, and perform the test. Prepare the control solution with 1.0 mL of 0.005 mol/L sulfuric acid VS (not more than 0.048%).

(4) Heavy metals <*1.07*>—Dissolve 1.0 g of Calcium Gluconate Hydrate in 30 mL of water and 2 mL of dilute acetic acid by warming, cool, and add water to make 50 mL. Perform the test using this solution as the test solution. Prepare the control solution with 2.0 mL of Standard Lead Solution, 2 mL of dilute acetic acid, and water to make 50 mL (not more than 20 ppm).

(5) Arsenic <*1.11*>—Dissolve 0.6 g of Calcium Gluconate Hydrate in 5 mL of water by warming, add 5 mL of dilute sulfuric acid and 1 mL of bromine TS, and concentrate on a water bath to 5 mL. Perform the test with this solution as the test solution (not more than 3.3 ppm).

(6) Sucrose and reducing sugars—To 0.5 g of Calcium Gluconate Hydrate add 10 mL of water and 2 mL of dilute hydrochloric acid, and boil the solution for 2 minutes. After cooling, add 5 mL of sodium carbonate TS, allow to stand for 5 minutes, add water to make 20 mL, and filter. To 5 mL of the filtrate add 2 mL of Fehling's TS, and boil for 1 minute: no orange-yellow to red precipitate is formed immediately.

Loss on drying <*2.41*> Not more than 1.0% (1 g, 80°C, 2 hours).

Assay Weigh accurately about 0.4 g of Calcium Gluconate Hydrate, previously dried, dissolve in 100 mL of water, add 2 mL of 8 mol/L potassium hydroxide TS and 0.1 g of NN indicator, and titrate <*2.50*> immediately with 0.05 mol/L disodium dihydrogen ethylenediamine tetraacetate VS until the color of the solution changes from red-purple to blue.

Each mL of 0.05 mol/L disodium dihydrogen ethylenediamine tetraacetate VS
= 22.42 mg of $C_{12}H_{22}CaO_{14}.H_2O$

Containers and storage Containers—Well-closed containers.

Calcium Hydroxide

水酸化カルシウム

$Ca(OH)_2$: 74.09

Calcium Hydroxide contains not less than 90.0% of calcium hydrate [$Ca(OH)_2$].

Description Calcium Hydroxide occurs as a white powder. It has a slightly bitter taste.

It is slightly soluble in water, very slightly soluble in boiling water, and practically insoluble in ethanol (95) and in diethyl ether.

It dissolves in dilute acetic acid, in dilute hydrochloric acid and in dilute nitric acid.

It absorbs carbon dioxide from air.

Identification **(1)** Mix Calcium Hydroxide with 3 to 4 times its mass of water: the mixture is slushy and is alkaline.

(2) Dissolve 1 g of Calcium Hydroxide in 30 mL of dilute acetic acid, and boil. After cooling, neutralize with ammonia TS: the solution responds to Qualitative tests *<1.09>* (2) and (3) for calcium salt.

Purity **(1)** Acid-insoluble substances—To 5 g of Calcium Hydroxide add 100 mL of water, add hydrochloric acid dropwise with strring until the solution becomes acidic, and further add 1 mL of hydrochloric acid. Boil this solution for 5 minutes, cool, and filter through a tared glass filter (G4). Wash the residue with boiling water until the last washing exhibits no turbidity upon addition of silver nitrate TS, and dry at 105°C to constant mass: the mass is not more than 25 mg.

(2) Heavy metals *<1.07>*—Dissolve 1.0 g of Calcium Hydroxide in 10 mL of dilute hydrochloric acid, evaporate on a water bath to dryness, dissolve the residue in 40 mL of water, and filter. To 20 mL of the filtrate add 2 mL of dilute acetic acid and water to make 50 mL, and perform the test using this solution as the test solution. Prepare the control solution as follows: evaporate 5 mL of dilute hydrochloric acid on a water bath to dryness, and add 2 mL of dilute acetic acid, 2.0 mL of Standard Lead Solution and water to make 50 mL (not more than 40 ppm).

(3) Magnesium and alkali metals—Dissolve 1.0 g of Calcium Hydroxide in a mixture of 20 mL of water and 10 mL of dilute hydrochloric acid, boil, neutralize with ammonia TS, and precipitate calcium oxalate completely by adding dropwise ammonium oxalate TS. Heat the mixture on a water bath for 1 hour, cool, dilute with water to 100 mL, shake, and filter. To 50 mL of the filtrate add 0.5 mL of sulfuric acid, evaporate to dryness, and ignite at 600°C to constant mass: the mass of the residue does not exceed 24 mg.

(4) Arsenic *<1.11>*—Dissolve 0.5 g of Calcium Hydroxide in 5 mL of dilute hydrochloric acid, and perform the test with this solution as the test solution (not more than 4 ppm).

Assay Weigh accurately about 1 g of Calcium Hydroxide, dissolve by adding 10 mL of dilute hydrochloric acid, and add water to make exactly 100 mL. Measure exactly 10 mL of this solution, add 90 mL of water and 1.5 mL of 8 mol/L potassium hydroxide TS, shake, allow to stand for 3 to 5 minutes, and then add 0.1 g of NN indicator. Titrate *<2.50>* immediately with 0.05 mol/L disodium dihydrogen ethylenediamine tetraacetate VS, until the red-purple color of the solution changes to blue.

Each mL of 0.05 mol/L disodium dihydrogen ethylenediamine tetraacetate VS
= 3.705 mg of $Ca(OH)_2$

Containers and storage Containers—Tight containers.

Calcium Lactate Hydrate

乳酸カルシウム水和物

$$\left[H_3C-CH(OH)-CO_2^- \right]_2 \; Ca^{2+} \cdot 5H_2O$$

and enantiomer

$C_6H_{10}CaO_6.5H_2O$: 308.29
Monocalcium bis[(2*RS*)-2-hydroxypropanonate] pentahydrate
[63690-56-2]

Calcium Lactate Hydrate, when dried, contains not less than 97.0% of calcium lactate ($C_6H_{10}CaO_6$: 218.22).

Description Calcium Lactate Hydrate occurs as white, powder or granules. It is odorless, and has a slightly acid taste.

A 1 g portion of it dissolves gradually in 20 mL of water, and it is slightly soluble in ethanol (95), and practically insoluble in diethyl ether.

It is partly efflorescent at ordinary temperature, and yields the anhydride at 120°C.

Identification A solution of Calcium Lactate Hydrate (1 in 20) responds to Qualitative Tests *<1.09>* for calcium salt and for lactate.

Purity **(1)** Clarity of solution—Dissolve 1.0 g of Calcium Lactate Hydrate in 20 mL of water by warming: the solution is clear.

(2) Acidity or alkalinity—To the solution obtained in (1) add 2 drops of phenolphthalein TS: no red color is produced. Then add 0.50 mL of 0.1 mol/L sodium hydroxide VS: a red color develops.

(3) Heavy metals *<1.07>*—Dissolve 1.0 g of Calcium Lactate Hydrate in 30 mL of water and 5 mL of dilute acetic acid by warming, cool, add water to make 50 mL, and perform the test using this solution as the test solution. Prepare the control solution from 2.0 mL of Standard Lead Solution and 2 mL of dilute acetic acid, and dilute with water to 50 mL (not more than 20 ppm).

(4) Magnesium or alkali metals—Dissolve 1.0 g of Calcium Lactate Hydrate in 40 mL of water, add 0.5 g of ammonium chloride, boil, then add 20 mL of ammonium oxalate TS. Heat the mixture on a water bath for 1 hour, cool, dilute with water to 100 mL, and filter. To 50 mL of the filtrate add 0.5 mL of sulfuric acid, evaporate to dryness, and ignite between 450°C and 550°C to constant mass: the mass of the residue is not more than 5 mg.

(5) Arsenic *<1.11>*—Dissolve 0.5 g of Calcium Lactate Hydrate in 2 mL of water and 3 mL of hydrochloric acid, and perform the test with this solution as the test solution (not more than 4 ppm).

(6) Volatile fatty acid—Warm 1.0 g of Calcium Lactate Hydrate with 2 mL of sulfuric acid: an odor of acetic acid or butyric acid is not perceptible.

Loss on drying *<2.41>* 25.0 – 30.0% (1 g, 80°C, 1 hour at first, then 120°C, 4 hours).

Assay Weigh accurately about 0.5 g of Calcium Lactate Hydrate, previously dried, add water, dissolve by heating on a water bath, cool, and add water to make exactly 100 mL. Pipet 20 mL of this solution, then 80 mL of water and 1.5 mL of 8 mol/L potassium hydroxide TS, and allow to stand for 3 to 5 minutes. Add 0.1 g of NN indicator, and titrate

<*2.50*> immediately with 0.02 mol/L disodium dihydrogen ethylenediamine tetraacetate VS until the color of the solution changes from red to blue.

Each mL of 0.02 mol/L disodium dihydrogen ethylenediamine tetraacetate VS
= 4.364 mg of $C_6H_{10}CaO_6$

Containers and storage Containers—Tight containers.

Calcium Levofolinate Hydrate

レボホリナートカルシウム水和物

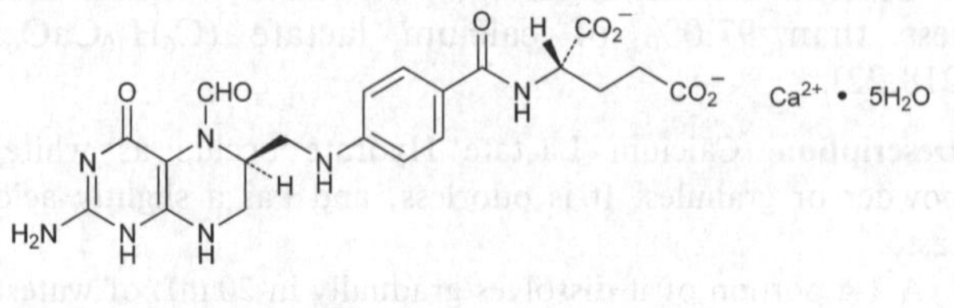

$C_{20}H_{21}CaN_7O_7.5H_2O$: 601.58
Monocalcium *N*-[4-({[(6*S*)-2-amino-5-formyl-4-oxo-1,4,5,6,7,8-hexahydropteridin-6-yl]methyl}amino)benzoyl]-L-glutamate pentahydrate
[*419573-16-3*]

Calcium Levofolinate Hydrate contains not less than 97.0% and not more than 102.0% of calcium levofolinate ($C_{20}H_{21}CaN_7O_7$: 511.50), calculated on the anhydrous and residual solvent-free basis.

Description Calcium Levofolinate Hydrate occurs as a white to light yellow crystalline powder.

It is sparingly soluble in water, and practically insoluble in methanol and in ethanol (99.5).

It is hygroscopic.

Optical rotation $[\alpha]_D^{25}$: −10 – −15° (0.25 g calculated on the anhydrous and residual solvent-free basis, 0.2 mol/L tris buffer solution (pH 8.1), 25 mL, 100 mm).

Identification **(1)** Determine the absorption spectrum of a solution of Calcium Levofolinate Hydrate (1 in 100,000) as directed under Ultraviolet-visible Spectrophotometry <*2.24*>, and compare the spectrum with the Reference Spectrum: both spectra exhibit similar intensities of absorption at the same wavelengths.

(2) Determine the infrared absorption spectrum of Calcium Levofolinate Hydrate as directed in the potassium bromide disk method under Infrared Spectrophotometry <*2.25*>, and compare the spectrum with the Reference Spectrum: both spectra exhibit similar intensities of absorption at the same wave numbers.

(3) A solution of Calcium Levofolinate Hydrate (1 in 200) responds to Qualitative Tests <*1.09*> (2) and (3) for calcium salt.

pH <*2.54*> To 0.4 g of Calcium Levofolinate Hydrate add 50 mL of freshly boiled and cooled water, and warm to 40°C, if necessary, to dissolve: the pH of the solution is between 7.0 and 8.5.

Purity **(1)** Clarity and color of solution—To 0.4 g of Calcium Levofolinate Hydrate add 50 mL of water, and warm to 40°C, if necessary, to dissolve: the solution is clear, and its absorbance at 420 nm determined as directed under Ultraviolet-visible Spectrophotometry <*2.24*> is not more than 0.25.

(2) Chloride—To 0.300 g of Calcium Levofolinate Hydrate add 50 mL of water, warm to 40°C, if necessary, to dissolve, add 10 mL of 2 mol/L nitric acid TS, and titrate <*2.50*> with 0.005 mol/L silver nitrate VS (potentiometric titration) (not more than 0.5%).

Each mL of 0.005 mol/L silver nitrate VS
= 0.177 mg of Cl

(3) Heavy metals <*1.07*>—Proceed with 1.0 g of Calcium Levofolinate Hydrate according to Method 2, and perform the test. Prepare the control solution with 2.0 mL of Standard Lead Solution (not more than 20 ppm).

(4) Platinum—Being specified separately when the drug is granted approval based on the Law (not more than 5 ppm).

(5) Related substances—Dissolve 20 mg of Calcium Levofolinate Hydrate in 25 mL of water, and use this solution as the sample solution. Pipet 1 mL of the sample solution, add water to make exactly 200 mL, and use this solution as the standard solution. Perform the test with exactly 20 μL each of the sample solution and standard solution as directed under Liquid Chromatography <*2.01*> according to the following conditions. Determine each peak area by the automatic integration method: the area of the peak other than levofolinate obtained from the sample solution is not larger than the peak area of levofolinate from the standard solution, and the total area of the peaks other than levofolinate from the sample solution is not larger than 5 times the peak area of levofolinate from the standard solution.

Operating conditions—

Detector, column, column temperature, mobile phase, and flow rate: Proceed as directed in the operating conditions in the Assay.

Time span of measurement: About 3 times as long as the retention time of levofolinate, beginning after the solvent peak.

System suitability—

Test for required detectability: To exactly 5 mL of the standard solution add water to make exactly 25 mL. Confirm that the peak area of levofolinate obtained with 20 μL of this solution is equivalent to 14 to 26% of that with 20 μL of the standard solution.

System performance: When the procedure is run with 20 μL of the standard solution under the above operating conditions, the number of theoretical plates and the symmetry factor of the peak of levofolinate are not less than 1500 and not more than 1.5, respectively.

System repeatability: When the test is repeated 6 times with 20 μL of the standard solution under the above operating conditions, the relative standard deviation of the peak area of levofolinate is not more than 2.0%.

(6) Diastereomer—Dissolve 50 mg of Calcium Levofolinate Hydrate in 100 mL of water, and use this solution as the sample solution. Perform the test with 10 μL of the sample solution as directed under Liquid Chromatography <*2.01*> according to the following conditions. Determine each peak area by the automatic integration method, and calculate their amounts by the area percentage method: the amount of the peak of the diastereomer, having the relative retention time of about 2.0 to levofolinate, is not more than 0.3%.

Operating conditions—

Detector: An ultraviolet absorption photometer (wavelength: 286 nm).

Column: A stainless steel column 4 mm in inside diameter and 15 cm in length, packed with human albumin chemically bonded silica gel for liquid chromatography (5 μm in particle diameter).

Column temperature: A constant temperature of about 40°C.

Mobile phase: Dissolve 3.4 g of sodium dihydrogen phosphate dihydrate in 870 mL of water, adjust to pH 4.9 with sodium hydroxide TS or phosphoric acid, and add 110 mL of 2-propanol and 20 mL of acetonitrile.

Flow rate: Adjust so that the retention time of levofolinate is about 16 minutes.

System suitability—

Test for required detectability: Dissolve 10 mg of Calcium Folinate RS in water to make 50 mL. To 1 mL of this solution add the sample solution to make 20 mL, and use this solution as the solution for system suitability test. Pipet 1 mL of the solution for system suitability test, and add water to make exactly 10 mL. Confirm that the peak area of the diastereomer obtained with 10 μL of this solution is equivalent to 7 to 13% of that with 10 μL of the solution for system suitability test.

System performance: When the procedure is run with 10 μL of the solution for system suitability test under the above operating conditions, levofolinate and the diastereomer are eluted in this order with the resolution between these peaks being not less than 5.

System repeatability: When the test is repeated 6 times with 10 μL of the solution for system suitability test under the above operating conditions, the relative standard deviation of the peak area of the diastereomer is not more than 2.0%.

Water *<2.48>* 12.0 – 17.0% (0.2 g, volumetric titration, direct titration).

Assay Weigh accurately about 10 mg each of Calcium Levofolinate Hydrate and Calcium Folinate RS (separately determine the water *<2.48>* in the same manner as Calcium Folinate Hydrate), and dissolve each in water to make exactly 25 mL, and use these solutions as the sample solution and the standard solution, respectively. Perform the test with exactly 20 μL each of the sample solution and standard solution as directed under Liquid Chromatography *<2.01>* according to the following conditions, and determine the peak area, A_T, of levofolinate with the sample solution, and the peak area, A_S, of folinate with the standard solution.

Amount (mg) of calcium levofolinate ($C_{20}H_{21}CaN_7O_7$)
$= M_S \times A_T/A_S$

M_S: Amount (mg) of Calcium Folinate RS taken, calculated on the anhydrous basis

Operating conditions—

Detector: An ultraviolet absorption photometer (wavelength: 254 nm).

Column: A stainless steel column 4.6 mm in inside diameter and 15 cm in length, packed with octadecylsilanized silica gel for liquid chromatography (5 μm in particle diameter).

Column temperature: A constant temperature of about 45°C.

Mobile phase: Adjust the pH of a mixture of diluted 0.05 mol/L disodium hydrogen phosphate TS (4 in 25), methanol and tetrabutylammonium hydroxide TS (385:110:4) to 7.5 with phosphoric acid.

Flow rate: Adjust so that the retention time of folinate is about 10 minutes.

System suitability—

System performance: Dissolve 10 mg of folic acid in 50 mL of the mobile phase. To 5 mL of this solution add 5 mL of the standard solution. When the procedure is run with 20 μL of this solution under the above operating conditions, folinate and folic acid are eluted in this order with the resolution between these peaks being not less than 10.

System repeatability: When the test is repeated 6 times with 20 μL of the standard solution under the above operating conditions, the relative standard deviation of the peak area of folinate is not more than 1.0%.

Containers and storage Containers—Tight containers.
Storage—Light-resistant.

Calcium Oxide

酸化カルシウム

CaO: 56.08

Calcium Oxide, when incinerated, contains not less than 98.0% of calcium oxide (CaO).

Description Calcium Oxide occurs as hard, white masses, containing a powder. It is odorless.

It is very slightly soluble in boiling water, and practically insoluble in ethanol (95).

One gram of Calcium Oxide dissolves almost completely in 2500 mL of water.

It slowly absorbs moisture and carbon dioxide from air.

Identification **(1)** Moisten Calcium Oxide with water: heat is generated and a white powder is obtained. Mix the powder with about 5 times its mass of water: the mixture is alkaline.

(2) Dissolve 1 g of Calcium Oxide in 20 mL of water by adding a few drops of acetic acid (31): the solution responds to Qualitative Tests *<1.09>* for calcium salt.

Purity **(1)** Acid-insoluble substances—Disintegrate 5.0 g of Calcium Oxide with a small amount of water, add 100 mL of water, add dropwise hydrochloric acid with stirring until the solution becomes acidic, and further add 1 mL of hydrochloric acid. Boil the solution for 5 minutes, cool, filter through a glass filter (G4), wash the residue with boiling water until no turbidity is produced when silver nitrate TS is added to the last washing, and dry at 105°C to constant mass: the mass of the residue is not more than 10.0 mg.

(2) Carbonate—Disintegrate 1.0 g of Calcium Oxide with a small amount of water, mix thoroughly with 50 mL of water, allow to stand for a while, remove most of the supernatant milky liquid by decantation, and add an excess of dilute hydrochloric acid to the residue: no vigorous effervescence is produced.

(3) Magnesium and alkali metals—Dissolve 1.0 g of Calcium Oxide in 75 mL of water by adding dropwise hydrochloric acid, and further add 1 mL of hydrochloric acid. Boil for 1 to 2 minutes, neutralize with ammonia TS, add dropwise an excess of hot ammonium oxalate TS, heat the mixture on a water bath for 2 hours, cool, add water to make 200 mL, mix thoroughly, and filter. Evaporate 50 mL of the filtrate with 0.5 mL of sulfuric acid to dryness, and heat the residue strongly at 600°C to constant mass: the mass of the residue is not more than 15 mg.

Loss on ignition *<2.43>* Not more than 10.0% (1 g, 900°C, constant mass).

Assay Weigh accurately about 0.7 g of Calcium Oxide, previously incinerated at 900°C to constant mass and cooled in a desiccator (silica gel), and dissolve in 50 mL of water and 8

mL of diluted hydrochloric acid (1 in 3) by heating. Cool, and add water to make exactly 250 mL. Pipet 10 mL of the solution, add 50 mL of water, 2 mL of 8 mol/L potassium hydroxide TS and 0.1 g of NN indicator, and titrate <*2.50*> with 0.02 mol/L disodium dihydrogen ethylenediamine tetraacetate VS, until the red-purple color of the solution changes to blue.

Each mL of 0.02 mol/L disodium dihydrogen ethylenediamine tetraacetate VS
= 1.122 mg of CaO

Containers and storage Containers—Tight containers.

Calcium Pantothenate

パントテン酸カルシウム

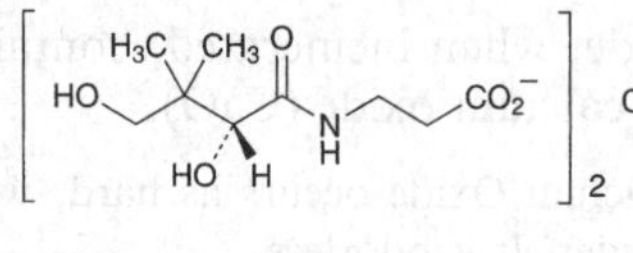

$C_{18}H_{32}CaN_2O_{10}$: 476.53
Monocalcium bis{3-[(2*R*)-2,4-dihydroxy-3,3-dimethylbutanoylamino]propanoate}
[*137-08-6*]

Calcium Pantothenate contains not less than 98.0% and not more than 102.0% of calcium pantothenate ($C_{18}H_{32}CaN_2O_{10}$), calculated on the dried basis.

Description Calcium Pantothenate occurs as a white powder.

It is freely soluble in water, and practically insoluble in ethanol (99.5).

The pH of a solution prepared by dissolving 1.0 g of Calcium Pantothenate in 20 mL of water is between 7.0 and 9.0.

It is hygroscopic.

It shows crystal polymorphism.

Identification **(1)** Determine the infrared absorption spectrum of previously dried Calcium Pantothenate as directed in the potassium bromide disk method under Infrared Spectrophotometry <*2.25*>, and compare the spectrum with the Reference Spectrum or the spectrum of dried Calcium Pantothenate RS: both spectra exhibit similar intensities of absorption at the same wave numbers. If any difference appears between the spectra, dissolve the sample and the Reference Standard separately in water, evaporate water, dry the residues in vacuum for 24 hours using silica gel as a desiccant, and perform the test using these residues.

(2) A solution of Calcium Pantothenate (1 in 10) responds to Qualitative Tests <*1.09*> (1), (2) and (3) for calcium salt.

Optical rotation <*2.49*> $[\alpha]_D^{20}$: +25.0 – +28.5° (1 g calculated on the dried basis, water, 20 mL, 100 mm).

Purity **(1)** Heavy metals <*1.07*>—Proceed with 1.0 g of Calcium Pantothenate according to Method 1, and perform the test. Prepare the control solution with 2.0 mL of Standard Lead Solution (not more than 20 ppm).

(2) Related substances—Dissolve 0.30 g of Calcium Pantothenate in 20 mL of water, and use this solution as the sample solution. Pipet 1 mL of the sample solution, add water to make exactly 200 mL, and use this solution as the standard solution. Perform the test with exactly 10 μL each of the sample solution and standard solution as directed under Liquid Chromatography <*2.01*> according to the following conditions, and determine each peak area by the automatic integration method: the area of the peak, having the relative retention time of about 0.6 to pantothenic acid obtained from the sample solution is not larger than 1.2 times the peak area of pantothenic acid from the standard solution, the area of the peak, having the relative retention time of about 0.8 is not larger than the peak area of pantothenic acid from the standard solution, the area of the peak, having the relative retention time of about 1.5 is not larger than 3/5 times the peak area of pantothenic acid from the standard solution, and the area of the peak other than pantothenic acid and the peaks mentioned above is not larger than 3/10 times the peak area of pantothenic acid from the standard solution. Additionally, the total area of the peaks other than pantothenic acid from the sample solution is not larger than 2.4 times the peak area of pantothenic acid from the standard solution. For the areas of the peaks, having the relative retention time of about 0.6 and about 0.8 to pantothenic acid, multiply their correction factors, 19 and 13, respectively.

Operating conditions—

Detector, column, column temperature, mobile phase, and flow rate: Proceed as directed in the operating conditions in the Assay.

Time span of measurement: About 2 times as long as the retention time of pantothenic acid, beginning after the solvent peak.

System suitability—

Test for required detectability: To exactly 2 mL of the standard solution add water to make exactly 10 mL. Confirm that the peak area of pantothenic acid obtained with 10 μL of this solution is equivalent to 14 to 26% of that with 10 μL of the standard solution.

System performance: When the procedure is run with 10 μL of the standard solution under the above operating conditions, the number of theoretical plates and the symmetry factor of the peak of pantothenic acid are not less than 10,000 and not more than 1.5, respectively.

System repeatability: When the test is repeated 6 times with 10 μL of the standard solution under the above operating conditions, the relative standard deviation of the peak area of pantothenic acid is not more than 2.0%.

(3) Alkaloids—Dissolve 50 mg of Calcium Pantothenate in 5 mL of water, add 0.5 mL of hexaammonium heptamolybdate TS and 0.5 mL of a solution of phosphoric acid (1 in 10): no white turbidity is produced.

Loss on drying <*2.41*> Not more than 5.0% (1 g, 105°C, 4 hours).

Assay Weigh accurately about 20 mg each of Calcium Pantothenate and Calcium Pantothenate RS (separately determine the loss on drying <*2.41*> in the same conditions as Calcium Pantothenate), dissolve each in water to make exactly 100 mL, and use these solutions as the sample solution and the standard solution, respectively. Perform the test with exactly 10 μL each of the sample solution and standard solution as directed under Liquid Chromatography <*2.01*> according to the following conditions, and determine the peak areas, A_T and A_S, of pantothenic acid in each solution.

Amount (mg) of calcium pantothenate ($C_{18}H_{32}CaN_2O_{10}$)
$= M_S \times A_T/A_S$

M_S: Amount (mg) of Calcium Pantothenate RS taken, calculated on the dried basis

Operating conditions—

Detector: An ultraviolet absorption photometer (wave-

length: 210 nm).

Column: A stainless steel column 4.6 mm in inside diameter and 25 cm in length, packed with octadecylsilanized silica gel for liquid chromatography (5 μm in particle diameter).

Column temperature: A constant temperature of about 40°C.

Mobile phase: Dissolve 0.81 g of sodium 1-heptanesulfonate and 1.36 g of potassium dihydrogen phosphate in water to make 1000 mL, and adjust to pH 2.1 with phosphoric acid. To 980 mL of this solution add 10 mL of acetonitrile and 10 mL of methanol.

Flow rate: Adjust so that the retention time of pantothenic acid is about 17 minutes.

System suitability—

System performance: When the procedure is run with 10 μL of the standard solution under the above operating conditions, the number of theoretical plates and the symmetry factor of the peak of pantothenic acid are not less than 10,000 and not more than 1.5, respectively.

System repeatability: When the test is repeated 6 times with 10 μL of the standard solution under the above operating conditions, the relative standard deviation of the peak area of pantothenic acid is not more than 1.0%.

Containers and storage Containers—Tight containers.

Calcium Paraaminosalicylate Hydrate

Pas-calcium Hydrate

パラアミノサリチル酸カルシウム水和物

$C_7H_5CaNO_3 \cdot 3\frac{1}{2}H_2O$: 254.25

Monocalcium 4-amino-2-oxidobenzoate hemiheptahydrate

[*137422-1-08-5*, anhydride]

Calcium Paraaminosalicylate Hydrate contains not less than 97.0% and not more than 103.0% of calcium paraaminosalicylic acid ($C_7H_5CaNO_3$: 191.20), calculated on the anhydrous basis.

Description Calcium Paraaminosalicylate Hydrate occurs as a white to slightly colored powder. It has a slightly bitter taste.

It is very slightly soluble in water, and practically insoluble in methanol and in ethanol (99.5).

It is gradually colored to brown by light.

Identification **(1)** To 50 mg of Calcium Paraaminosalicylate Hydrate add 100 mL of water, shake well, and filter. To 10 mL of the filtrate add 1 mL of 1 mol/L hydrochloric acid TS, shake, and add 1 drop of iron (III) chloride TS: a red-purple color develops.

(2) Determine the infrared absorption spectrum of Calcium Paraaminosalicylate Hydrate as directed in the potassium bromide disk method under Infrared Spectrophotometry *<2.25>*, and compare the spectrum with the Reference Spectrum: both spectra exhibit similar intensities of absorption at the same wave numbers.

(3) To 3 g of Calcium Paraaminosalicylate Hydrate add 15 mL of ammonium chloride TS and 15 mL of water, heat on a water bath until almost dissolved, and filter after cooling: the filtrate responds to Qualitative Tests *<1.09>* (1), (2) and (3) for calcium salt.

Purity **(1)** Chloride *<1.03>*—Dissolve 1.0 g of Calcium Paraaminosalicylate Hydrate in 15 mL of dilute nitric acid, and add water to make 50 mL. Perform the test using this solution as the test solution. Prepare the control solution with 0.70 mL of 0.01 mol/L hydrochloric acid VS (not more than 0.025%).

(2) Heavy metals *<1.07>*—Proceed with 1.0 g of Calcium Paraaminosalicylate Hydrate according to method 3, and perform the test. Prepare the control solution with 2.0 mL of Standard Lead Solution (not more than 20 ppm).

(3) Arsenic *<1.11>*—Dissolve 0.40 g of Calcium Paraaminosalicylate Hydrate in 20 mL of 0.1 mol/L hydrochloric acid TS by warming on a water bath, use this solution as the test solution, and perform the test (not more than 5 ppm).

(4) 3-Aminophenol—To 0.10 g of Calcium Paraaminosalicylate Hydrate add 5 mL of 0.1 mol/L disodium dihydrogen ethylenediamine tetraacetate TS, previously cooled in ice-water, and dissolve by shaking vigorously. Add immediately 3 mL of ammonia-ammonium chloride buffer solution (pH 11.0) previously cooled in ice water, and shake. Add 2 mL of 4-amino-*N,N*-diethylaniline sulfate TS, shake, add 10.0 mL of cyclohexane and 4 mL of diluted potassium hexacyanoferrate (III) TS (1 in 10), and shake immediately for 20 seconds. Centrifuge this solution, wash the separated cyclohexane layer with two 5-mL portions of diluted ammonia TS (1 in 14), add 1 g of anhydrous sodium sulfate, shake, and allow to stand for 5 minutes: the clear cyclohexane layer is not more colored than the following control solution.

Control solution: Dissolve 50 mg of 3-aminophenol in water, and dilute with water to exactly 500 mL. Measure exactly 20 mL of this solution, and add water to make exactly 100 mL. Take 5.0 mL of this solution, add 3 mL of ammonia-ammonium chloride buffer solution (pH 11.0) previously cooled in ice-water, and treat this solution in the same manner as the sample.

Water *<2.48>* 23.3 – 26.3% (0.1 g, volumetric titration, direct titration).

Assay Weigh accurately about 0.2 g of Calcium Paraaminosalicylate Hydrate, dissolve in 60 mL of water and 0.75 mL of dilute hydrochloric acid by warming on a water bath. After cooling, add water to make exactly 100 mL, and use this solution as the sample solution. Measure exactly 30 mL of the sample solution, transfer to an iodine flask, and add exactly 25 mL of 0.05 mol/L bromine VS and 20 mL of a solution of potassium bromide (1 in 4). Add immediately 14 mL of a mixture of acetic acid (100) and hydrochloric acid (5:2), stopper the flask immediately, and allow to stand for 10 minutes with occasional shaking. Add cautiously 6 mL of potassium iodide TS, and shake gently. After 5 minutes, titrate *<2.50>* the produced iodine with 0.1 mol/L sodium thiosulfate VS (indicator: 1 mL of starch TS). Perform a blank determination in the same manner.

Each mL of 0.05 mol/L bromine VS
= 3.187 mg of $C_7H_5CaNO_3$

Containers and storage Containers—Tight containers.

Storage—Light-resistant.

Calcium Paraaminosalicylate Granules

Pas-calcium Granules

パラアミノサリチル酸カルシウム顆粒

Calcium Paraaminosalicylate Granules contain not less than 95.0% and not more than 105.0% of the labeled amount of calcium paraaminosalicylate hydrate ($C_7H_5CaNO_3.3\frac{1}{2}H_2O$: 254.25).

Method of preparation Prepare as directed under Granules, with Calcium Paraaminosalicylate Hydrate.

Identification Powder Calcium Paraaminosalicylate Granules, weigh a portion of the powder, equivalent to 50 mg of Calcium Paraaminosalicylate Hydrate, add 100 mL of water, shake, and filter. To 10 mL of the filtrate add 1 mL of 1 mol/L hydrochloric acid TS, shake, and add 1 drop of iron (III) chloride TS: a red-purple color develops.

Dissolution <*6.10*> When the test is performed at 75 revolutions per minute according to the Paddle method, using 900 mL of water as the dissolution medium, the dissolution rate in 60 minutes of Calcium Paraaminosalicylate Granules is not less than 75%.

Start the test with an accurately weighed amount of Calcium Paraaminosalicylate Granules, equivalent to about 0.25 g of calcium paraaminosalicylate hydrate ($C_7H_5CaNO_3.3\frac{1}{2}H_2O$), withdraw not less than 20 mL of the medium at the specified minute after starting the test, and filter through a membrane filter with a pore size not exceeding 0.5 μm. Discard not less than 10 mL of the first filtrate, pipet 5 mL of the subsequent filtrate, add water to make exactly 100 mL, and use this solution as the sample solution. Separately, weigh accurately about 28 mg of calcium paraaminosalicylate hydrate for assay (separately determine the water <*2.48*> in the same manner as Calcium Paraaminosalicylate Hydrate), and dissolve in water to make exactly 100 mL. Pipet 5 mL of this solution, add water to make exactly 100 mL, and use this solution as the standard solution. Determine the absorbances, A_T and A_S, at 300 nm of the sample solution and standard solution as directed under Ultraviolet-visible Spectrophotometry <*2.24*>.

Dissolution rate (%) with respect to the labeled amount of calcium paraaminosalicylate hydrate ($C_7H_5CaNO_3.3\frac{1}{2}H_2O$)
$= M_S/M_T \times A_T/A_S \times 1/C \times 900 \times 1.330$

M_S: Amount (mg) of calcium paraaminosalicylate hydrate for assay taken, calculated on the anhydrous basis
M_T: Amount (g) of Calcium Paraaminosalicylate Granules taken
C: Labeled amount (mg) of calcium paraaminosalicylate hydrate ($C_7H_5CaNO_3.3\frac{1}{2}H_2O$) in 1 g

Assay Powder Calcium Paraaminosalicylate Granules, weigh accurately a portion of the powder, equivalent to about 0.2 g of calcium paraaminosalicylate hydrate ($C_7H_5CaNO_3.3\frac{1}{2}H_2O$), add 60 mL of water and 0.75 mL of dilute hydrochloric acid, and dissolve by heating on a water bath. After cooling, add water to make exactly 100 mL, and filter. Pipet 30 mL of the filtrate, transfer to an iodine flask, and proceed as directed in the Assay under Calcium Paraaminosalicylate Hydrate.

Each mL of 0.05 mol/L bromine VS
$= 4.238$ mg of $C_7H_5CaNO_3.3\frac{1}{2}H_2O$

Containers and storage Containers—Tight containers.
Storage—Light-resistant.

Anhydrous Dibasic Calcium Phosphate

無水リン酸水素カルシウム

$CaHPO_4$: 136.06
[*7757-93-9*]

This monograph is harmonized with the European Pharmacopoeia and the U.S. Pharmacopeia.

The corresponding part of the attributes/provisions which are agreed as non-harmonized within the scope of the harmonization is marked with symbols (◆ ◆), and the corresponding parts which are agreed as the JP local requirement other than the scope of the harmonization are marked with symbols (◇ ◇).

Information on the harmonization with the European Pharmacopoeia and the U.S. Pharmacopeia is available on the website of the Pharmaceuticals and Medical Devices Agency.

Anhydrous Dibasic Calcium Phosphate contains not less than 97.5% and not more than 102.5% of dibasic calcium phosphate ($CaHPO_4$).

◆**Description** Anhydrous Dibasic Calcium Phosphate occurs as white, crystalline powder or granules.

It is practically insoluble in water and in ethanol (99.5).

It dissolves in dilute hydrochloric acid and in dilute nitric acid.◆

Identification **(1)** Dissolve 0.1 g of Anhydrous Dibasic Calcium Phosphate in 10 mL of 2 mol/L hydrochloric acid TS by warming, add 2.5 mL of ammonia TS dropwise with shaking, and add 5 mL of ammonium oxalate TS: a white precipitate is produced.

(2) Dissolve 0.1 g of Anhydrous Dibasic Calcium Phosphate in 5 mL of dilute nitric acid, and add 2 mL of hexaammonium heptamolybdate TS after warming at 70°C for 1 to 2 minutes: a yellow precipitate is produced.

Purity **(1)** Acid-insoluble substances—Dissolve 5.0 g of Anhydrous Dibasic Calcium Phosphate in 40 mL of water and 10 mL of hydrochloric acid, and boil gently for 5 minutes. After cooling, collect the insoluble substance using a filter paper for quantitative analysis. Wash with water until no more turbidity of the washings is produced when silver nitrate TS is added. Ignite to incinerate the residue and the filter paper at 600 ± 50°C: the mass is not more than 10 mg (not more than 0.2%).

(2) Chloride—To 0.20 g of Anhydrous Dibasic Calcium Phosphate add 20 mL of water and 13 mL of dilute nitric acid, dissolve by warming, if necessary, add water to make 100 mL, and filter, if necessary. Put 50 mL of this solution in a Nessler tube, and use this as the sample solution. Separately, transfer 0.70 mL of 0.01 mol/L hydrochloric acid VS to another Nessler tube, add 6 mL of dilute nitric acid and water to make 50 mL, and use this solution as the control solution. Add 1 mL of silver nitrate TS to the sample solution and control solution, mix well, and allow to stand for 5 minutes protecting from light. Compare the opalescence developed in both solutions against a black background by viewing downward or transversely. The opalescence developed in the sample solution is not more than that of the control solution (not more than 0.25%).

(3) Sulfate—Dissolve 0.50 g of Anhydrous Dibasic Calcium Phosphate in 5 mL of water and 5 mL of dilute hydrochloric acid, add water to make 100 mL, and filter, if necessary. Put 20 mL of this solution in a Nessler tube, add 1 mL of dilute hydrochloric acid, and add water to make 50 mL, and use this as the sample solution. Transfer 1.0 mL of 0.005 mol/L sulfuric acid VS to another Nessler tube, add 1 mL of dilute hydrochloride acid and water to make 50 mL, and use this solution as the control solution. Add 2 mL of barium chloride TS to the sample solution and control solution, mix well, and allow to stand for 10 minutes. Compare the white turbidity produced in both solutions against a black background by viewing downward or transversely. The turbidity produced in the sample solution is not thicker than that of the control solution (not more than 0.48%).

(4) Carbonate—Shake 1.0 g of Anhydrous Dibasic Calcium Phosphate with 5 mL of freshly boiled and cooled water, and add immediately 2 mL of hydrochloric acid: no effervescence occurs.

◇**(5)** Heavy metals <*1.07*>—Dissolve 0.65 g of Anhydrous Dibasic Calcium Phosphate in a mixture of 5 mL of water and 5 mL of dilute hydrochloric acid by warming, cool, and add ammonia TS until precipitates begin to form in the solution. Dissolve the precipitates by adding a small amount of dilute hydrochloric acid dropwise, add 10 mL of hydrochloric acid-ammonium acetate buffer solution (pH 3.5) and water to make 50 mL, and perform the test using this solution as the sample solution. Prepare the control solution as follows: to 10 mL of hydrochloric acid-ammonium acetate buffer solution (pH 3.5) add 2.0 mL of Standard Lead Solution and water to make 50 mL (not more than 31 ppm).◇

(6) Barium—Heat 0.5 g of Anhydrous Dibasic Calcium Phosphate with 10 mL of water, add 1 mL of hydrochloric acid dropwise with stirring, and filter after cooling, if necessary. Add 2 mL of potassium sulfate TS to this solution, and allow to stand for 10 minutes: no turbidity forms.

◆**(7)** Arsenic <*1.11*>—Dissolve 1.0 g of Anhydrous Dibasic Calcium Phosphate in 5 mL of dilute hydrochloric acid, and perform the test with this solution as the test solution (not more than 2 ppm).◆

Loss on ignition <*2.43*> Not less than 6.6% and not more than 8.7% (1 g, 800 - 825°C, constant mass).

Assay Weigh accurately about 0.4 g of Anhydrous Dibasic Calcium Phosphate, dissolve in 12 mL of dilute hydrochloric acid by heating on a water bath, if necessary, and add water to make exactly 200 mL. Pipet 20 mL of this solution, add exactly 25 mL of 0.02 mol/L disodium dihydrogen ethylenediamine tetraacetate VS, 50 mL of water and 5 mL of ammonia-ammonium chloride buffer solution (pH 10.7), and titrate <*2.50*> the excess disodium dihydrogen ethylenediamine tetraacetate with 0.02 mol/L zinc sulfate VS (indicator: 25 mg of eriochrome black T-sodium chloride indicator). Perform a blank determination in the same manner.

Each mL of 0.02 mol/L disodium dihydrogen ethylenediamine tetraacetate VS
= 2.721 mg of $CaHPO_4$

◆**Containers and storage** Containers—Well-closed containers.◆

Dibasic Calcium Phosphate Hydrate

リン酸水素カルシウム水和物

$CaHPO_4.2H_2O$: 172.09
[*7789-77-7*]

This monograph is harmonized with the European Pharmacopoeia and the U.S. Pharmacopeia.

The parts of the text that are not harmonized are marked with symbols (◆ ◆).

Information on the harmonization with the European Pharmacopoeia and the U.S. Pharmacopeia is available on the website of the Pharmaceuticals and Medical Devices Agency.

Dibasic Calcium Phosphate Hydrate contains not less than 98.0% and not more than 105.0% of dibasic calcium phosphate hydrate ($CaHPO_4.2H_2O$).

◆**Description** Dibasic Calcium Phosphate Hydrate occurs as a white crystalline powder.

It is practically insoluble in water and in ethanol (99.5).

It dissolves in dilute hydrochloric acid and in dilute nitric acid.◆

Identification **(1)** Dissolve 0.1 g of Dibasic Calcium Phosphate Hydrate in 10 mL of 2 mol/L hydrochloric acid TS by warming, add 2.5 mL of ammonia TS dropwise with shaking, and add 5 mL of ammonium oxalate TS: a white precipitate is produced.

(2) Dissolve 0.1 g of Dibasic Calcium Phosphate Hydrate in 5 mL of dilute nitric acid, and add 2 mL of hexaammonium heptamolybdate TS after warming at 70°C for 1 to 2 minutes: a yellow precipitate is produced.

Purity **(1)** Acid-insoluble substance—Dissolve 5.0 g of Dibasic Calcium Phosphate Hydrate in 40 mL of water and 10 mL of hydrochloric acid, and boil gently for 5 minutes. After cooling, collect the insoluble substance using a filter paper for quantitative analysis. Wash with water until no more turbidity of the washing is produced when silver nitrate TS is added. Ignite to incinerate the residue and filter paper at 600 ± 50°C: the mass is not more than 10 mg (not more than 0.2%).

(2) Chloride—To 0.20 g of Dibasic Calcium Phosphate Hydrate add 20 mL of water and 13 mL of dilute nitric acid, dissolve by warming, if necessary, add water to make 100 mL, and filter, if necessary. Put 50 mL of this solution in a Nessler tube, and use this as the test solution. Transfer 0.70 mL of 0.01 mol/L hydrochloric acid VS to another Nessler tube, add 6 mL of dilute nitric acid and water to make 50 mL, and use this solution as the control solution. Add 1 mL of silver nitrate TS to the test solution and the control solution, mix well, and allow to stand for 5 minutes protecting from light. Compare the opalescence developed in both solutions against a black background by viewing downward or transversely. The opalescence developed in the test solution is not more than that of the control solution. (not more than 0.25%)

(3) Sulfate—Dissolve 0.50 g of Dibasic Calcium Phosphate Hydrate in 5 mL of water and 5 mL of dilute hydrochloric acid, add water to make 100 mL, and filter, if necessary. Put 20 mL of this solution in a Nessler tube, add 1 mL of dilute hydrochloric acid, and add water to make 50 mL, and use this as the test solution. Transfer 1.0 mL of 0.005 mol/L sulfuric acid VS to another Nessler tube, add 1 mL of dilute hydrochloride acid and water to make 50 mL, and use this solution as the control solution. Add 2 mL of barium chloride TS to the test solution and the control solution, mix well, and allow to stand for 10 minutes. Compare the white turbidity produced in both solutions against a black background by viewing downward or transversely. The turbidity produced in the test solution is not thicker than that of the control solution. (not more than 0.48%)

(4) Carbonate—Mix 1.0 g of Dibasic Calcium Phosphate Hydrate with 5 mL of freshly boiled and cooled water, and add immediately 2 mL of hydrochloric acid: no effervescence occurs.

◆**(5)** Heavy metals <*1.07*>—Dissolve 0.65 g of Dibasic Calcium Phosphate Hydrate in a mixture of 5 mL of water and 5 mL of dilute hydrochloric acid by warming, cool, and add ammonia TS until precipitates begin to form in the solution. Dissolve the precipitates by adding a small amount of dilute hydrochloric acid dropwise, add 10 mL of hydrochloric acid-ammonium acetate buffer solution (pH 3.5) and water to make 50 mL, and perform the test using this solution as the test solution. Prepare the control solution as follows: to 10 mL of hydrochloric acid-ammonium acetate buffer solution (pH 3.5) add 2.0 mL of Standard Lead Solution and water to make 50 mL (not more than 31 ppm).◆

(6) Barium—Heat 0.5 g of Dibasic Calcium Phosphate Hydrate with 10 mL of water, add 1 mL of hydrochloric acid dropwise with stirring, and filter after cooling, if necessary. Add 2 mL of potassium sulfate TS to this solution, and allow to stand for 10 minutes: no turbidity forms.

◆**(7)** Arsenic <*1.11*>—Dissolve 1.0 g of Dibasic Calcium Phosphate Hydrate in 5 mL of dilute hydrochloric acid, and perform the test with this solution as the test solution (not more than 2 ppm).◆

Loss on ignition <*2.43*> Not less than 24.5% and not more than 26.5% (1 g, 800 - 825°C, constant mass).

Assay Weigh accurately about 0.4 g of Dibasic Calcium Phosphate Hydrate, dissolve in 12 mL of dilute hydrochloric acid by warming on a water bath, if necessary, and add water to make exactly 200 mL. Pipet 20 mL of this solution, add exactly 25 mL of 0.02 mol/L disodium dihydrogen ethylenediamine tetraacetate VS, 50 mL of water and 5 mL of ammonia-ammonium chloride buffer solution (pH 10.7), and titrate <*2.50*> the excess disodium dihydrogen ethylenediamine tetraacetate with 0.02 mol/L zinc sulfate VS (indicator: 25 mg of eriochrome black T-sodium chloride indicator). Perform a blank determination in the same manner.

Each mL of 0.02 mol/L disodium dihydrogen ethylenediamine tetraacetate VS
= 3.442 mg of $CaHPO_4.2H_2O$

◆**Containers and storage** Containers—Well-closed containers.◆

Monobasic Calcium Phosphate Hydrate

リン酸二水素カルシウム水和物

$Ca(H_2PO_4)_2.H_2O$: 252.07

Monobasic Calcium Phosphate Hydrate, when dried, contains not less than 90.0% of monobasic calcium phosphate hydrate [$Ca(H_2PO_4)_2.H_2O$].

Description Monobasic Calcium Phosphate Hydrate occurs as white, crystals or crystalline powder. It is odorless and has an acid taste.

It is sparingly soluble in water, and practically insoluble in ethanol (95) and in diethyl ether.

It dissolves in dilute hydrochloric acid and in dilute nitric acid.

It is slightly deliquescent.

Identification **(1)** Dissolve 0.1 g of Monobasic Calcium Phosphate Hydrate in 10 mL of diluted hydrochloric acid (1 in 6) by warming, add 2.5 mL of ammonia TS dropwise with shaking, and add 5 mL of ammonium oxalate TS: a white precipitate is produced.

(2) Dissolve 0.1 g of Monobasic Calcium Phosphate Hydrate in 5 mL of dilute nitric acid, and add 2 mL of hexaammonium heptamolybdate TS after warming for 1 to 2 minutes at 70°C: a yellow precipitate is produced.

Purity **(1)** Clarity and color of solution—Dissolve 1.0 g of Monobasic Calcium Phosphate Hydrate in 19 mL of water and 2 mL of diluted hydrochloric acid (3 in 4), and heat on a water bath for 5 minutes with occasional shaking: the solution is clear and colorless.

(2) Dibasic phosphate and acid—Triturate 1.0 g of Monobasic Calcium Phosphate Hydrate with 3 mL of water, and add 100 mL of water and 1 drop of methyl orange TS: a red color develops. Then add 1.0 mL of 1 mol/L sodium hydroxide VS: the color changes to yellow.

(3) Chloride <*1.03*>—Dissolve 1.0 g of Monobasic Calcium Phosphate Hydrate in 20 mL of water and 12 mL of dilute nitric acid, add water to make 100 mL, and filter, if necessary. Perform the test using 50 mL of this solution as the test solution. Prepare the control solution with 0.25 mL of 0.01 mol/L hydrochloric acid VS (not more than 0.018%).

(4) Sulfate <*1.14*>—Dissolve 1.0 g of Monobasic Calcium Phosphate Hydrate in 20 mL of water and 1 mL of hydrochloric acid, add water to make 100 mL, and filter, if necessary. Perform the test using 50 mL of this solution as the test solution. Prepare the control solution with 0.50 mL of 0.005 mol/L sulfuric acid VS (not more than 0.048%).

(5) Heavy metals <*1.07*>—Dissolve 0.65 g of Monobasic Calcium Phosphate Hydrate in a mixture of 5 mL of water and 5 mL of dilute hydrochloric acid by warming, cool, and add ammonia TS until precipitates begin to form in the solution. Dissolve the precipitates by adding a small amount of dilute hydrochloric acid dropwise, add 10 mL of hydrochloric acid-ammonium acetate buffer solution (pH 3.5) and water to make 50 mL, and perform the test using this solution as the test solution. Prepare the control solution as follows: to 10 mL of hydrochloric acid-ammonium acetate buffer solution (pH 3.5) add 2.0 mL of Standard Lead Solution and water to make 50 mL (not more than 31 ppm).

(6) Arsenic <*1.11*>—Dissolve 1.0 g of Monobasic Calcium Phosphate Hydrate in 5 mL of dilute hydrochloric acid, and perform the test with this solution as the test solution (not more than 2 ppm).

Loss on drying <*2.41*> Not more than 3.0% (1 g, silica gel, 24 hours).

Assay Weigh accurately about 0.4 g of Monobasic Calcium Phosphate Hydrate, previously dried, dissolve in 3 mL of dilute hydrochloric acid, and add water to make exactly 100 mL. Pipet 20 mL of this solution, add exactly 25 mL of 0.02 mol/L disodium dihydrogen ethylenediamine tetraacetate VS, 50 mL of water and 5 mL of ammonia-ammonium chloride buffer solution (pH 10.7), and titrate <*2.50*> the excess disodium dihydrogen ethylenediamine tetraacetate with 0.02 mol/L zinc acetate VS (indicator: 25 mg of eriochrome black T-sodium chloride indicator). Perform a blank determination in the same manner.

Each mL of 0.02 mol/L disodium dihydrogen ethylenediamine tetraacetate VS
= 5.041 mg of $Ca(H_2PO_4)_2.H_2O$

Containers and storage Containers—Tight containers.

Calcium Polystyrene Sulfonate

ポリスチレンスルホン酸カルシウム

Calcium Polystyrene Sulfonate is a cation exchange resin prepared as the calcium form of the sulfonated styrene divinylbenzene copolymer.

When dried, it contains not less than 7.0% and not more than 9.0% of calcium (Ca: 40.08).

Each g of Calcium Polystyrene Sulfonate, when dried, exchanges with 53 to 71 mg of potassium (K: 39.10).

Description Calcium Polystyrene Sulfonate occurs as a pale yellow-white to light yellow powder. It is odorless and tasteless.

It is practically insoluble in water, in ethanol (95) and in diethyl ether.

Identification **(1)** Determine the infrared absorption spectrum of Calcium Polystyrene Sulfonate, previously dried, as directed in the potassium bromide disk method under Infrared Spectrophotometry <*2.25*>, and compare the spectrum with the Reference Spectrum: both spectra exhibit similar intensities of absorption at the same wave numbers.

(2) Mix 0.5 g of Calcium Polystyrene Sulfonate with 10 mL of dilute hydrochloric acid, filter, and neutralize the filtrate with ammonia TS: the solution responds to Qualitative Tests <*1.09*> for calcium salt.

Purity **(1)** Ammonium—Place 1.0 g of Calcium Polystyrene Sulfonate in a flask, add 5 mL of sodium hydroxide TS, cover the flask with a watch glass having a moistened strip of red litmus paper on the underside, and boil for 15 minutes: the gas evolved does not change the red litmus paper to blue (not more than 5 ppm).

(2) Heavy metals <*1.07*>—Proceed with 2.0 g of Calcium Polystyrene Sulfonate according to Method 2, and perform the test. Prepare the control solution with 2.0 mL of Standard Lead Solution (not more than 10 ppm).

(3) Arsenic <*1.11*>—Prepare the test solution with 1.0 g of Calcium Polystyrene Sulfonate according to Method 3, and perform the test (not more than 2 ppm).

(4) Styrene—To 10.0 g of Calcium Polystyrene Sulfonate add 10 mL of acetone, shake for 30 minutes, centrifuge, and use the supernatant liquid as the sample solution. Separately, dissolve 10 mg of styrene in acetone to make exactly 100 mL. Pipet 1 mL of this solution, dilute with acetone to make exactly 100 mL, and use this solution as the standard solution. Perform the test with exactly 5 μL each of the sample solution and standard solution as directed under Gas Chromatography <*2.02*> according to the following conditions. Determine the peak heights, H_T and H_S, of styrene in each solution: H_T is not larger than H_S.

Operating conditions—

Detector: A hydrogen flame-ionization detector.

Column: A stainless steel column 3 mm in inside diameter and 2 m in length, having polyethylene glycol 20 M coated at the ratio of 15% on siliceous earth for gas chromatography (150 to 180 μm in particle diameter).

Column temperature: A constant temperature of about 90°C.

Carrier gas: Nitrogen.

Flow rate: Adjust so that the retention time of styrene is about 9 minutes.

System suitability—

System performance: Mix 10 mg of styrene with 1000 mL of acetone. When the procedure is run with 5 μL of this solution under the above operating conditions, the number of theoretical plates and the symmetry factor of the peak of styrene are not less than 800 and 0.8 to 1.2, respectively.

System repeatability: When the test is repeated 6 times with 5 μL of the standard solution under the above operating conditions, the relative standard deviation of the peak heights of styrene is not more than 5%.

(5) Sodium—Pipet 2 mL of the 50-mL solution obtained in the Assay (1), add 0.02 mol/L hydrochloric acid TS to make exactly 500 mL, and use this solution as the sample solution. Separately, weigh accurately 0.2542 g of sodium chloride, previously dried at 130°C for 2 hours, and dissolve in 0.02 mol/L hydrochloric acid TS to make exactly 1000 mL. Pipet a suitable volume of this solution, and dilute with 0.02 mol/L hydrochloric acid TS to make a solution containing 1 to 3 μg of sodium (Na: 22.99) per mL, and use these solutions as the standard solutions. Perform the test with the sample solution and standard solutions according to Atomic Absorption Spectrophotometry <*2.23*> under the following conditions, and determine the amount of sodium in the sample solution using the calibration curve obtained from the standard solutions: the amount of sodium is not more than 1%.

Gas: Combustible gas—Acetylene.
Supporting gas—Air.

Lamp: A sodium hollow-cathode lamp.

Wavelength: 589.0 nm.

Loss on drying <*2.41*> Not more than 10.0% (1 g, in vacuum, 80°C, 5 hours).

Microparticles (i) Apparatus: Use an apparatus as shown in the illustration.

(ii) Procedure: Weigh accurately about 5.5 g of Calcium Polystyrene Sulfonate, previously dried, add 300 mL of water of 25°C, and mix for 5 minutes. Transfer this turbid solution to the sedimentation tube J, keeping a temperature at 25°C, add water of 25°C to 2 mm below the mark F of 20 cm of the sedimentation tube J, and then insert the pipet. Open the two-way stopcock C, exhaust air, add exactly water from the vent-hole D to the mark F of 20 cm, and close the two-way stopcock C. Shake the apparatus well vertically and horizontally, disperse Calcium Polystyrene Sulfonate in water, and then open the two-way stopcock, and allow to stand at 25 ± 1°C for 5 hours and 15 minutes.

Then, draw exactly the meniscus of the turbid solution in sedimentation tube J up to the mark of pipet bulb A by suction, open the two-way stopcock C to the outlet of pipet H, and transfer exactly measured 20 mL of the turbid solution to a weighing bottle. Repeat the procedure, and combine exactly measured 20 mL of the turbid solution. Evaporate 20 mL of this turbid solution on a water bath to dryness, dry to constant mass at 105°C, and weigh the residue as M_S (g). Pipet 20 mL of used water, and weigh the residue in the same manner as M_B (g). Calculate the difference *mi* (g) between M_S and M_B, and calculate the amount of microparticles (*S*) by the following equation: the amount of microparticles is

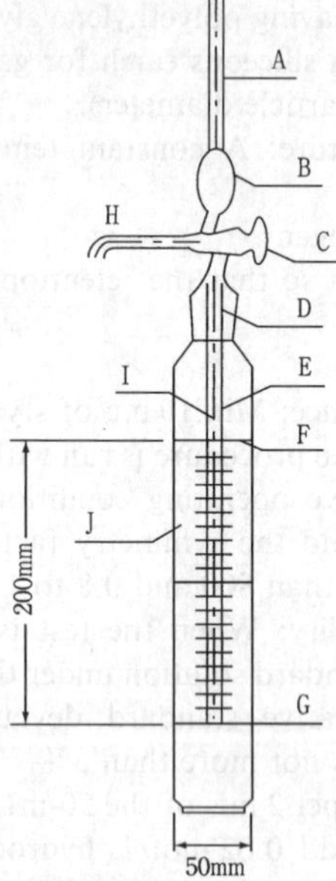

Actual volume to the mark of 20 cm at which the sedimentation tube is inserted: 550 mL
Single suction volume: 10 mL

A: Mark of pipet bulb
B: Pipet bulb for suction
C: Two-way stopcock
D: Vent-hole
E: Suction part of pipet
F: Mark of 20 cm
G: Base line of 0 cm
H: Outlet of pipet
I: Capillary tube of pipet
J: Sedimentation tube

Fig. Andreasen pipet

not more than 0.1%.

$$S\ (\%) = (mi \times V)/(20 \times M_T) \times 100$$

M_T: Amount (g) of Calcium Polystyrene Sulfonate taken
V: Actual volume (mL) to the mark of 20 cm at which the suction part of pipet is inserted

Assay **(1)** Calcium—Weigh accurately about 1 g of Calcium Polystyrene Sulfonate, previously dried, and disperse in 5 mL of 3 mol/L hydrochloric acid TS. Transfer this mixture, and wash out completely with the aid of a small quantity of 3 mol/L hydrochloric acid TS to a column 12 mm in inside diameter and 70 mm in length, packed with a pledged of fine glass wool in the bottom of it, placing a 50-mL volumetric flask as a receiver under the column. Then collect about 45 mL of eluate, adding 3 mol/L hydrochloric acid TS to the column, and add water to make exactly 50 mL. Pipet 20 mL of this solution, adjust with ammonia TS to a pH of exactly 10. Titrate *<2.50>* immediately with 0.05 mol/L disodium dihydrogen ethylenediamine tetraacetate VS until the red-purple color of the solution disappears, and a blue color develops (indicator: 0.04 g eriochrome black T-sodium chloride indicator). Perform a blank determination in the same manner, and make any necessary correction.

Each mL of 0.05 mol/L disodium dihydrogen ethylenediamine tetraacetate VS
= 2.004 mg of Ca

(2) Potassium exchange capacity—Pipet 50 mL of Standard Potassium Stock Solution into a glass-stoppered flask containing about 1 g of dried Calcium Polystyrene Sulfonate, accurately weighed, stir for 120 minutes, filter, and discard the first 20 mL of the filtrate. Pipet 5 mL of the subsequent filtrate, and add 0.02 mol/L hydrochloric acid TS to make exactly 100 mL. Pipet 10 mL of this solution, add 0.02 mol/L hydrochloric acid TS to make exactly 1000 mL, and use this solution as the sample solution. Separately, measure exactly a suitable volume of Standard Potassium Stock Solution, dilute with 0.02 mol/L hydrochloric acid TS to make solutions containing 0.5 to 2.5 μg of potassium (K: 39.10) per mL, and use these solutions as the standard solutions. Perform the test with the sample solution and standard solutions as directed under Atomic Absorption Spectrophotometry *<2.23>* according to the following conditions, and determine the amount, Y (mg), of potassium in 1000 mL of the sample solution, using the calibration curve obtained from the standard solutions. The exchange quantity for potassium per g of dried Calcium Polystyrene Sulfonate is 53 to 71 mg, calculating by the following equation.

Exchange quantity (mg) for potassium (K) per g of dried Calcium Polystyrene Sulfonate
$= (X - 100\ Y)/M$

X: The amount (mg) of potassium in 50 mL of Standard Potassium Stock Solution before exchange
M: The amount (g) of dried Calcium Polystyrene Sulfonate taken

Gas: Combustible gas—Acetylene.
Supporting gas—Air.
Lamp: A potassium hollow-cathode lamp.
Wavelength: 766.5 nm.

Containers and storage Containers—Tight containers.

Calcium Sodium Edetate Hydrate

エデト酸カルシウムナトリウム水和物

$C_{10}H_{12}CaN_2Na_2O_8.xH_2O$
Disodium [{*N*,*N'*-ethane-1,2-diylbis[*N*-(carboxymethyl)glycinato]}(4-)-*N*,*N'*,*O*,*O'*,*O*^{N},*O*$^{N'}$]calciate(2-) hydrate
[*23411-34-9*]

This monograph is harmonized with the European Pharmacopoeia and the U.S. Pharmacopeia.

The parts of the text that are not harmonized are marked with symbols (◆ ◆).

Information on the harmonization with the European Pharmacopoeia and the U.S. Pharmacopeia is available on the website of the Pharmaceuticals and Medical Devices Agency.

Calcium Sodium Edetate Hydrate contains not less than 98.0% and not more than 102.0% of calcium disodium edetate ($C_{10}H_{12}CaN_2Na_2O_8$: 374.27), calculated on the anhydrous basis.

◆**Description** Calcium Sodium Edetate Hydrate occurs as

white, powder or particles.

It is freely soluble in water, sparingly soluble in methanol, and practically insoluble in ethanol (99.5).

It is hygroscopic.◆

Identification (1) Dissolve 2 g of Calcium Sodium Edetate Hydrate in 10 mL of water, add 6 mL of a solution of lead (II) nitrate (33 in 1000), shake, and add 3 mL of potassium iodide TS: no yellow precipitate is formed. Make this solution alkaline by the addition of diluted ammonia solution (28) (7 in 50), and add 3 mL of ammonium oxalate TS: a white precipitate is formed.

◆(2) Determine the infrared absorption spectrum of Calcium Sodium Edetate Hydrate as directed in the potassium bromide disk method under Infrared Spectrophotometry <2.25>, and compare the spectrum with the Reference Spectrum: both spectra exhibit similar intensities of absorption at the same wave numbers.◆

(3) A solution of Calcium Sodium Edetate Hydrate (1 in 20) responds to Qualitative Tests <1.09> (2) for sodium salt.

pH <2.54> The pH of a solution of 2.0 g of Calcium Sodium Edetate Hydrate in 10 mL of water is 6.5 to 8.0.

Purity ◆(1) Clarity and color of solution—Dissolve 0.25 g of Calcium Sodium Edetate Hydrate in 10 mL of water: the solution is clear and colorless.◆

(2) Chloride <1.03>—Dissolve 0.70 g of Calcium Sodium Edetate Hydrate in water to make 20 mL. To this solution add 30 mL of dilute nitric acid, allow to stand for 30 minutes, and filter. To 10 mL of the filtrate add water to make 50 mL, and perform the test using this solution as the test solution. Prepare the control solution with 0.40 mL of 0.01 mol/L hydrochloric acid VS (not more than 0.10%).

◆(3) Heavy metals <1.07>—Proceed with 1.0 g of Calcium Sodium Edetate Hydrate according to Method 2, and perform the test. Prepare the control solution with 2.0 mL of Standard Lead Solution (not more than 20 ppm).◆

(4) Disodium edetate—Dissolve 1.00 g of Calcium Sodium Edetate Hydrate in 50 mL of water, add 5 mL of ammonia-ammonium chloride buffer solution (pH 10.7), and titrate <2.50> with 0.01 mol/L magnesium chloride VS until the color of the solution changes from blue to red-purple (indicator: 40 mg of eriochrome black T-sodium chloride indicator): the amount of 0.01 mol/L magnesium chloride VS consumed is not more than 3.0 mL (not more than 1.0%).

◆(5) Nitrilotriacetic acid—Conduct this procedure using light-resistant vessels. Dissolve 0.100 g of Calcium Sodium Edetate Hydrate in diluting solution to make exactly 25 mL, and use this solution as the sample solution. Separately, dissolve 40.0 mg of nitrilotriacetic acid in diluting solution to make exactly 100 mL. Pipet 1 mL of this solution, add 0.1 mL of the sample solution, then add diluting solution to make exactly 100 mL, and use this solution as the standard solution. Perform the test with exactly 20 μL each of the sample solution and standard solution as directed under Liquid Chromatography <2.01> according to the following conditions, and determine the peak areas, A_T and A_S, of nitrilotriacetic acid in each solution: A_T is not larger than A_S (not more than 0.1%).

Diluting solution: Dissolve 10.0 g of iron (III) sulfate *n*-hydrate in 20 mL of 0.5 mol/L sulfuric acid TS and 780 mL of water, adjust to pH 2.0 with sodium hydroxide TS, and add water to make 1000 mL.

Operating conditions—

Detector: An ultraviolet absorption photometer (wavelength: 273 nm).

Column: A stainless steel column 4.6 mm in inside diameter and 10 cm in length, packed with graphite carbon for liquid chromatography (mean pore size: 25 nm, specific surface: 120 m^2/g, 5 μm in particle diameter).

Column temperature: A constant temperature of about 40°C.

Mobile phase: Dissolve 50.0 mg of iron (III) sulfate *n*-hydrate in 50 mL of 0.5 mol/L sulfuric acid TS, add 750 mL of water, adjust to pH 1.5 with 0.5 mol/L sulfuric acid TS or sodium hydroxide TS, and add 20 mL of ethylene glycol and water to make 1000 mL.

Flow rate: 1.0 mL per minute (the retention time of nitrilotriacetic acid is about 5 minutes).

System suitability—

Test for required detectability: When perform the test with 20 μL of the standard solution under the above operating conditions, the SN ratio of the peak of nitrilotriacetic acid is not less than 50.

System performance: When the procedure is run with 20 μL of the standard solution under the above operating conditions, nitrilotriacetic acid and edetic acid are eluted in this order with the resolution between these peaks being not less than 7.

System repeatability: When the test is repeated 6 times with 20 μL of the standard solution under the above operating conditions, the relative standard deviation of the peak area of nitrilotriacetic acid is not more than 1.0%.◆

Water <2.48> 5.0 – 13.0% (0.2 g, volumetric titration, direct titration).

Assay Weigh accurately about 0.5 g of Calcium Sodium Edetate Hydrate, and dissolve in water to make exactly 200 mL. Pipet 20 mL of this solution, add 80 mL of water, adjust to pH 2 – 3 with dilute nitric acid, and titrate <2.50> with 0.01 mol/L bismuth nitrate VS until the color of the solution changes from yellow to red (indicator: 2 drops of xylenol orange TS).

Each mL of 0.01 mol/L bismuth nitrate VS
= 3.743 mg of $C_{10}H_{12}CaN_2Na_2O_8$

◆**Containers and storage** Containers—Tight containers.◆

Calcium Stearate

ステアリン酸カルシウム

Calcium Stearate mainly consists of calcium salts of stearic acid ($C_{18}H_{36}O_2$: 284.48) and palmitic acid ($C_{16}H_{32}O_2$: 256.42).

Calcium Stearate, when dried, contains not less than 6.4% and not more than 7.1% of calcium (Ca: 40.08).

Description Calcium Stearate occurs as a white, light, bulky powder. It feels smooth when touched, and is adhesive to the skin. It is odorless or has a faint, characteristic odor.

It is practically insoluble in water, in ethanol (95) and in diethyl ether.

Identification (1) Shake vigorously 3 g of Calcium Stearate with 20 mL of diluted hydrochloric acid (1 in 2) and 30 mL of diethyl ether for 3 minutes, and allow to stand: the separated aqueous layer responds to Qualitative Tests <1.09> (1), (2) and (4) for calcium salt.

(2) Wash the diethyl ether layer obtained in (1) with 20 mL and 10 mL of dilute hydrochloric acid and 20 mL of water successively, and evaporate the diethyl ether on a water bath: the residue melts <1.13> at a temperature not

below 54°C.

Purity (1) Heavy metals <*1.07*>—Heat gently 1.0 g of Calcium Stearate with caution at the beginning, and heat further, gradually raising the temperature, to incineration. After cooling, add 2 mL of hydrochloric acid, evaporate on a water bath to dryness, warm the residue with 20 mL of water and 2 mL of dilute acetic acid for 2 minutes, cool, filter, and wash the residue with 15 mL of water. Combine the filtrate and the washings, add water to make 50 mL, and perform the test using this solution as the test solution. Prepare the control solution by evaporating 2 mL of hydrochloric acid on a water bath to dryness and by adding 2 mL of dilute acetic acid, 2.0 mL of Standard Lead Solution and water to make 50 mL (not more than 20 ppm).

(2) Arsenic <*1.11*>—To 1.0 g of Calcium Stearate add 5 mL of diluted hydrochloric acid (1 in 2) and 20 mL of chloroform, shake vigorously for 3 minutes, allow to stand, and separate the water layer. Perform the test with the water layer as the test solution (not more than 2 ppm).

Loss on drying <*2.41*> Not more than 4.0% (1 g, 105°C, 3 hours).

Assay Weigh accurately about 0.5 g of Calcium Stearate, previously dried, heat gently with caution at first, and then ignite gradually to ash. Cool, add 10 mL of dilute hydrochloric acid to the residue, warm for 10 minutes on a water bath, and transfer the contents to a flask with the aid of 10-mL, 10-mL, and 5-mL portions of hot water. Add sodium hydroxide TS until the solution becomes slightly turbid, and then add 25 mL of 0.05 mol/L disodium dihydrogen ethylenediamine tetraacetate VS, 10 mL of ammonia-ammonium chloride buffer solution (pH 10.7), 4 drops of eriochrome black T TS and 5 drops of methyl yellow TS, and titrate <*2.50*> rapidly the excess disodium dihydrogen ethylenediamine tetraacetate with 0.05 mol/L magnesium chloride VS, until the green color of the solution disappears and a red color develops. Perform a blank determination in the same manner.

Each mL of 0.05 mol/L disodium dihydrogen ethylenediamine tetraacetate VS
= 2.004 mg of Ca

Containers and storage Containers—Well-closed containers.

Camostat Mesilate

カモスタットメシル酸塩

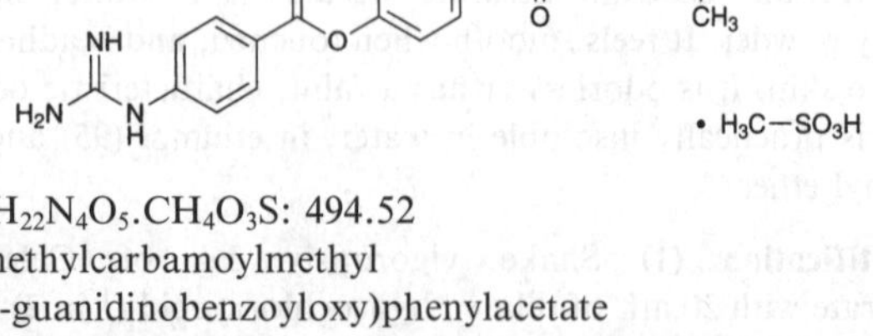

$C_{20}H_{22}N_4O_5.CH_4O_3S$: 494.52
Dimethylcarbamoylmethyl
4-(4-guanidinobenzoyloxy)phenylacetate
monomethanesulfonate
[*59721-29-8*]

Camostat Mesilate, when dried, contains not less than 98.5% of camostat mesilate ($C_{20}H_{22}N_4O_5.CH_4O_3S$).

Description Camostat Mesilate occurs as white, crystals or crystalline powder.

It is sparingly soluble in water, slightly soluble in ethanol (95), and practically insoluble in diethyl ether.

Identification (1) To 4 mL of a solution of Camostat Mesilate (1 in 2000) add 2 mL of 1-naphthol TS and 1 mL of diacetyl TS, and allow to stand for 10 minutes: a red color develops.

(2) Determine the absorption spectrum of a solution of Camostat Mesilate (1 in 100,000) as directed under Ultraviolet-visible Spectrophotometry <*2.24*>, and compare the spectrum with the Reference Spectrum or the spectrum of a solution of Camostat Mesilate RS prepared in the same manner as the sample solution: both spectra exhibit similar intensities of absorption at the same wavelengths.

(3) A 0.1 g portion of Camostat Mesilate responds to Qualitative Tests <*1.09*> (1) for mesilate.

Melting point <*2.60*> 194 – 198°C

Purity (1) Heavy metals <*1.07*>—Dissolve 1.0 g of Camostat Mesilate in 40 mL of water by warming, and add 2 mL of dilute acetic acid and water to make 50 mL. Perform the test using this solution as the test solution. Prepare the control solution with 2.0 mL of Standard Lead Solution and 2 mL of dilute acetic acid (not more than 20 ppm).

(2) Arsenic <*1.11*>—Dissolve 2.0 g of Camostat Mesilate in 20 mL of 2 mol/L hydrochloric acid TS by heating in a water bath, and continue to heat for 20 minutes. After cooling, centrifuge, take 10 mL of the supernatant liquid, and use this solution as the test solution. Perform the test (not more than 2 ppm).

(3) Related substances—Dissolve 30 mg of Camostat Mesilate in 10 mL of ethanol (95), and use this solution as the sample solution. Pipet 1 mL of the sample solution, add ethanol (95) to make exactly 200 mL, and use this solution as the standard solution. Perform the test with these solutions as directed under Thin-layer Chromatography <*2.03*>. Spot 10 μL each of the sample solution and standard solution on a plate of silica gel for thin-layer chromatography. Develop the plate with a mixture of ethyl acetate, water and acetic acid (100) (3:1:1) to a distance of about 10 cm, and air-dry the plate. Allow the plate to stand overnight in iodine vapor: the spots other than the principal spot obtained from the sample solution are not more intense than the spot from the standard solution.

Loss on drying <*2.41*> Not more than 1.0% (1 g, silica gel, 105°C, 3 hours).

Residue on ignition <*2.44*> Not more than 0.2% (1 g).

Assay Weigh accurately about 50 mg each of Camostat Mesilate and Camostat Mesilate RS, previously dried, and dissolve each in water to make exactly 50 mL. Pipet 5 mL each of these solutions, add exactly 5 mL of the internal standard solution, and use these solutions as the sample solution and the standard solution, respectively. Perform the test with 2 μL each of the sample solution and standard solution as directed under Liquid Chromatography <*2.01*> according to the following conditions, and calculate the ratios, Q_T and Q_S, of the peak area of camostat to that of the internal standard.

$$\text{Amount (mg) of camostat mesilate } (C_{20}H_{22}N_4O_5.CH_4O_3S) = M_S \times Q_T/Q_S$$

M_S: Amount (mg) of Camostat Mesilate RS taken

Internal standard solution—A solution of butyl parahydroxybenzoate in ethanol (95) (1 in 1500).

Operating conditions—

Detector: An ultraviolet absorption photometer (wavelength: 265 nm).

Column: A stainless steel column 4.6 mm in inside diameter and 15 cm in length, packed with octadecylsilanized silica gel for liquid chromatography (5 μm in particle diameter).

Column temperature: A constant temperature of about 25°C.

Mobile phase: A mixture of methanol, a solution of sodium 1-heptane sulfonate (1 in 500), a solution of sodium lauryl sulfate (1 in 1000) and acetic acid (100) (200:100:50:1).

Flow rate: Adjust so that the retention time of camostat is about 10 minutes.

System suitability—

System performance: When the procedure is run with 2 μL of the standard solution under the above operating conditions, camostat and the internal standard are eluted in this order with the resolution between these peaks being not less than 5.

System repeatability: When the test is repeated 6 times with 2 μL of the standard solution under the above operating conditions, the relative standard deviation of the ratio of the peak area of camostat to that of the internal standard is not more than 1.0%.

Containers and storage Containers—Tight containers.

d-Camphor

d-カンフル

$C_{10}H_{16}O$: 152.23
(1*R*,4*R*)-1,7,7-Trimethylbicyclo[2.2.1]heptan-2-one
[*464-49-3*]

d-Camphor contains not less than 96.0% of *d*-camphor ($C_{10}H_{16}O$).

Description *d*-Camphor occurs as colorless or white, translucent crystals, crystalline powder or masses. It has a characteristic, agreeable odor, and a slightly bitter taste, followed by a pleasant, cooling sensation.

It is freely soluble in ethanol (95), in diethyl ether and in carbon disulfide, and slightly soluble in water.

It slowly volatilizes at room temperature.

Identification Dissolve 0.1 g of *d*-Camphor in 2 mL of methanol, add 1 mL of 2,4-dinitrophenylhydradine TS, and heat for 5 minutes on a water bath: an orange-red precipitate is formed.

Optical rotation <*2.49*> $[\alpha]_D^{20}$: +41.0 – +43.0° (5 g, ethanol (95), 50 mL, 100 mm).

Melting point <*2.60*> 177 – 182°C

Purity **(1)** Water—Shake 1.0 g of *d*-Camphor with 10 mL of carbon disulfide: the solution is clear.

(2) Chlorinated compounds—Mix 0.20 g of finely powdered *d*-Camphor with 0.4 g of sodium peroxide in a dried porcelain crucible. Heat the crucible gently by the open flame until the incineration is complete. Dissolve the residue in 20 mL of warm water, acidify with 12 mL of dilute nitric acid, and filter the solution into a Nessler tube. Wash the filter paper with three 5-mL portions of hot water, adding the washings to the filtrate. After cooling, add water to make 50 mL, then add 1 mL of silver nitrate TS, mix well, and allow to stand for 5 minutes: the turbidity of the solution does not exceed that of the following control solution.

Control solution: Prepare in the same manner as described above, using 0.20 mL of 0.01 mol/L hydrochloric acid VS.

(3) Non-volatile residue—Heat 2.0 g of *d*-Camphor on a water bath until sublimation is complete, then dry the residue at 105°C for 3 hours: the mass of the residue does not exceed 1.0 mg.

Assay Weigh accurately about 0.1 g each of *d*-Camphor and *d*-Camphor RS, add exactly 5 mL each of the internal standard solution, dissolve in ethanol (99.5) to make 100 mL, and use these solutions as the sample solution and the standard solution. Perform the test with 2 μL each of the sample solution and standard solution as directed under Gas Chromatography <*2.02*> according to the following conditions, and calculate the ratios, Q_T and Q_S, of the peak area of *d*-camphor to that of the internal standard.

Amount (mg) of *d*-camphor ($C_{10}H_{16}O$) = $M_S \times Q_T/Q_S$

M_S: Amount (mg) of *d*-Camphor RS taken

*Internal standard solution—*A solution of methyl salicylate in ethanol (99.5) (1 in 25).

Operating conditions—

Detector: A hydrogen flame-ionization detector.

Column: A glass column 3 mm in inside diameter and 3 m in length, which is packed with 10% of polyethylene glycol 20 M for gas chromatography supported on 180 to 250 μm mesh silanized siliceous earth for gas chromatography.

Column temperature: A constant temperature of about 160°C.

Carrier gas: Nitrogen.

Flow rate: Adjust so that the retention time of *d*-camphor is about 6 minutes.

System suitability—

System performance: When the procedure is run with 2 μL of the standard solution under the above operating conditions, *d*-camphor and the internal standard are eluted in this order with the resolution between these peaks being not less than 7.

System repeatability: When the test is repeated 6 times with 2 μL of the standard solution under the above operating conditions, the relative standard deviation of the ratios of the peak area of *d*-camphor to that of the internal standard is not more than 1.0%.

Containers and storage Containers—Tight containers.

dl-Camphor

dl-カンフル

and enantiomer

$C_{10}H_{16}O$: 152.23
(1*RS*,4*RS*)-1,7,7-Trimethylbicyclo[2.2.1]heptan-2-one
[*76-22-2*]

dl-Camphor contains not less than 96.0% of *dl*-camphor ($C_{10}H_{16}O$).

Description *dl*-Camphor occurs as colorless or white, translucent crystals, crystalline powder or masses. It has a characteristic, agreeable odor, and has a slightly bitter taste followed by a pleasant, cooling sensation.

It is freely soluble in ethanol (95), in diethyl ether and in carbon disulfide, and slightly soluble in water.

It slowly volatilizes at room temperature.

Identification Dissolve 0.1 g of *dl*-Camphor in 2 mL of methanol, add 1 mL of 2,4-dinitrophenylhydradine TS, and heat for 5 minutes on a water bath: an orange-red precipitate is formed.

Optical rotation <*2.49*> $[\alpha]_D^{20}$: −1.5 – +1.5° (5 g, ethanol (95), 50 mL, 100 mm).

Melting point <*2.60*> 175 – 180°C

Purity **(1)** Water—Shake 1.0 g of *dl*-Camphor with 10 mL of carbon disulfide: the solution is clear.

(2) Chlorinated compounds—Mix 0.20 g of finely powdered *dl*-Camphor with 0.4 g of sodium peroxide in a dried porcelain crucible. Heat the crucible gently by the open flame until the incineration is complete. Dissolve the residue in 20 mL of warm water, acidify with 12 mL of dilute nitric acid, and filter the solution into a Nessler tube. Wash the filter paper with three 5-mL portions of hot water, adding the washings to the filtrate. After cooling, add water to make 50 mL, then add 1 mL of silver nitrate TS, mix well, and allow to stand for 5 minutes: the turbidity of the solution does not exceed that of the following control solution.

Control solution: Prepare in the same manner as described above, using 0.20 mL of 0.01 mol/L hydrochloric acid VS.

(3) Non-volatile residue—Heat 2.0 g of *dl*-Camphor on a water bath until sublimation is complete, then dry the residue at 105°C for 3 hours: the mass of the residue does not exceed 1.0 mg.

Assay Weigh accurately about 0.1 g each of *dl*-Camphor and *dl*-Camphor RS, add exactly 5 mL each of the internal standard solution, dissolve in ethanol (99.5) to make 100 mL, and use these solutions as the sample solution and standard solution, respectively. Perform the test with 2 μL each of the sample solution and standard solution as directed under Gas Chromatography <*2.02*> according to the following conditions, and calculate the ratios, Q_T and Q_S, of the peak area of *dl*-camphor to that of the internal standard.

Amount (mg) of *dl*-camphor ($C_{10}H_{16}O$) = $M_S \times Q_T/Q_S$

M_S: Amount (mg) of *dl*-Camphor RS taken

Internal standard solution—A solution of methyl salicylate in ethanol (99.5) (1 in 25).

Operating conditions—

Detector: A hydrogen flame-ionization detector.

Column: A glass column 3 mm in inside diameter and 3 m in length, which is packed with 10% of polyethylene glycol 20 M for gas chromatography supported on 180 to 250 μm mesh silanized siliceous earth for gas chromatography.

Column temperature: A constant temperature of about 160°C.

Carrier gas: Nitrogen.

Flow rate: Adjust so that the retention time of *dl*-camphor is about 6 minutes.

System suitability—

System performance: When the procedure is run with 2 μL of the standard solution under the above operating conditions, *dl*-camphor and the internal standard are eluted in this order with the resolution between these peaks being not less than 7.

System repeatability: When the test is repeated 6 times with 2 μL of the standard solution under the above operating conditions, the relative standard deviation of the ratios of the peak area of *dl*-camphor to that of the internal standard is not more than 1.0%.

Containers and storage Containers—Tight containers.

Candesartan Cilexetil

カンデサルタン シレキセチル

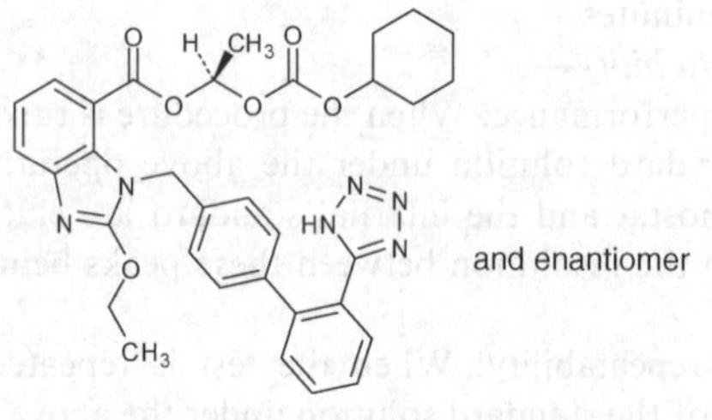

and enantiomer

$C_{33}H_{34}N_6O_6$: 610.66

(1*RS*)-1-(Cyclohexyloxycarbonyloxy)ethyl-2-ethoxy-1-{[2′-(1*H*-tetrazol-5-yl)biphenyl-4-yl]methyl}-1*H*-benzimidazole-7-carboxylate

[*145040-37-5*]

Candesartan Cilexetil contains not less than 99.0% and not more than 101.0% of candesartan cilexetil ($C_{33}H_{34}N_6O_6$), calculated on the anhydrous basis.

Description Candesartan Cilexetil occurs as white, crystals or crystalline powder.

It is soluble in acetic acid (100), sparingly soluble in methanol, slightly soluble in ethanol (99.5), and practically insoluble in water.

A solution of Candesartan Cilexetil in methanol (1 in 100) shows no optical rotation.

Candesartan Cilexetil shows crystal polymorphism.

Identification **(1)** Determine the absorption spectrum of a solution of Candesartan Cilexetil in methanol (1 in 50,000) as directed under Ultraviolet-visible Spectrophotometry <*2.24*>, and compare the spectrum with the Reference Spectrum: both spectra exhibit similar intensities of absorption at the same wavelengths.

(2) Determine the infrared absorption spectrum of Candesartan Cilexetil as directed in the potassium bromide disk method under Infrared Spectrophotometry <*2.25*>, and compare the spectrum with the Reference Spectrum: both spectra exhibit similar intensities of absorption at the same wave numbers. If any difference appears between the spectra, recrystallize the sample and the RS according to the method otherwise specified, filter and dry the crystals, and perform the test with the crystals.

Purity **(1)** Heavy metals <*1.07*>—Proceed with 1.0 g of Candesartan Cilexetil according to Method 4, and perform the test. Prepare the control solution with 2.0 mL of Standard Lead Solution (not more than 20 ppm).

(2) Related substances—Dissolve 20 mg of Candesartan Cilexetil in 50 mL of a mixture of acetonitrile and water (3:2), and use this solution as the sample solution. Pipet 1 mL of the sample solution, add a mixture of acetonitrile and water (3:2) to make exactly 100 mL, and use this solution as the standard solution. Perform the test with exactly 10 μL each of the sample solution and standard solution as directed under Liquid Chromatography <*2.01*> according to the following conditions, and determine each peak area by the automatic integration method: the area of the peaks, having the relative retention time of about 0.4 and about 2.0 to candesartan cilexetil, obtained from the sample solution is not larger than 1/5 times the peak area of candesartan cilexetil from the standard solution, the area of the peak, having the relative retention time of about 0.5 to candesartan cilexetil, from the sample solution is not larger than 3/10 times the peak area of candesartan cilexetil from the standard solution, the area of the peak other than candesartan cilexetil and the peaks mentioned above from the sample solution is smaller than 1/10 times the peak area of candesartan cilexetil from the standard solution, and the total area of the peaks other than candesartan cilexetil from the sample solution is not larger than 3/5 times the peak area of candesartan cilexetil from the standard solution.

Operating conditions—

Detector: An ultraviolet absorption photometer (wavelength: 254 nm).

Column: A stainless steel column 4 mm in inside diameter and 15 cm in length, packed with octadecylsilanized silica gel for liquid chromatography (4 μm in particle diameter).

Column temperature: A constant temperature of about 25°C.

Mobile phase A: A mixture of acetonitrile, water and acetic acid (100) (57:43:1).

Mobile phase B: A mixture of acetonitrile, water and acetic acid (100) (90:10:1).

Flowing of mobile phase: Control the gradient by mixing the mobile phases A and B as directed in the following table.

Time after injection of sample (min)	Mobile phase A (vol%)	Mobile phase B (vol%)
0 – 30	100 → 0	0 → 100

Flow rate: 0.8 mL per minute.

Time span of measurement: For 30 minutes after injection, beginning after the solvent peak.

System suitability—

Test for required detectability: Pipet 2 mL of the standard solution, and add a mixture of acetonitrile and water (3:2) to make exactly 20 mL. Confirm that the peak area of candesartan cilexetil obtained with 10 μL of this solution is equivalent to 7 to 13% of that with 10 μL of the standard solution.

System performance: When the procedure is run with 10 μL of the standard solution under the above operating conditions, the number of theoretical plates and the symmetry factor of the peak of candesartan cilexetil are not less than 12,000 and not more than 1.5, respectively.

System repeatability: When the test is repeated 6 times with 10 μL of the standard solution under the above operating conditions, the relative standard deviation of the peak area of candesartan cilexetil is not more than 2.0%.

Water <2.48> Not more than 0.3% (0.5 g, coulometric titration).

Residue on ignition <2.44> Not more than 0.1% (1 g).

Assay Weigh accurately about 0.5 g of Candesartan Cilexetil, dissolve in 60 mL of acetic acid (100), and titrate <2.50> with 0.1 mol/L perchloric acid VS (potentiometric titration). Perform a blank determination in the same manner, and make any necessary correction.

Each mL of 0.1 mol/L perchloric acid VS
= 61.07 mg of $C_{33}H_{34}N_6O_6$

Containers and storage Containers—Well-closed containers.

Candesartan Cilexetil Tablets

カンデサルタン　シレキセチル錠

Candesartan Cilexetil Tablets contain not less than 95.0% and not more than 105.0% of the labeled amount of candesartan cilexetil ($C_{33}H_{34}N_6O_6$: 610.66).

Method of preparation Prepare as directed under Tablets, with Candesartan Cilexetil.

Identification Powder Candesartan Cilexetil Tablets. To a portion of the powder, equivalent to 1 mg of Candesartan Cilexetil, add 50 mL of methanol, shake vigorously for 10 minutes, and filter. Determine the absorption spectrum of the filtrate as directed under Ultraviolet-visible Spectrophotometry <2.24>: it exhibits absorption maxima between 252 nm and 256 nm and between 302 nm and 307 nm.

Purity Related substances—Powder not less than 10 Candesartan Cilexetil Tablets. To a portion of the powder, equivalent to 6 mg of Candesartan Cilexetil, add 15 mL of a mixture of acetonitrile and water (3:2), shake vigorously for 10 minutes, and centrifuge. Filter the supernatant liquid through a membrane filter with a pore size not exceeding 0.45 μm. Discard the first 3 mL of the filtrate, and use the subsequent filtrate as the sample solution. Pipet 1 mL of the sample solution, add a mixture of acetonitrile and water (3:2) to make exactly 100 mL, and use this solution as the standard solution. Perform the test with exactly 10 μL each of the sample solution and standard solution as directed under Liquid Chromatography <2.01> according to the following conditions, and determine each peak area by the automatic integration method: the area of the peak having the relative retention time of about 0.5 to candesartan cilexetil obtained from the sample solution is not larger than 1.5 times the peak area of candesartan cilexetil from the standard solution, the area of the peak having the relative retention time of about 0.8, about 1.1 and about 1.5 to candesartan cilexetil from the sample solution is not larger than 1/2 times the peak area of candesartan cilexetil from the standard solution, the area of the peak having the relative retention time of about 2.0 to candesartan cilexetil from the sample solution is not larger than the peak area of candesartan cilexetil from the standard solution, the area of the peak other than candesartan cilexetil, the peak having the relative retention time of about 0.4 to candesartan cilexetil and the peaks mentioned above from the sample solution is smaller than 1/10 times the peak area of candesartan cilexetil from the standard solution, and the total area of the peaks other than candesartan cilexetil from the sample solution is not larger than 4 times the peak area of candesartan cilexetil from the standard solution.

Operating conditions—

Detector: An ultraviolet absorption photometer (wavelength: 254 nm).

Column: A stainless steel column 3.9 mm in inside diameter and 15 cm in length, packed with octadecylsilanized silica gel for liquid chromatography (4 μm in particle diameter).

Column temperature: A constant temperature of about 25°C.

Mobile phase A: A mixture of acetonitrile, water and acetic acid (100) (57:43:1).

Mobile phase B: A mixture of acetonitrile, water and acetic acid (100) (90:10:1).

Flowing of mobile phase: Control the gradient by mixing the mobile phases A and B as directed in the following table.

Time after injection of sample (min)	Mobile phase A (vol%)	Mobile phase B (vol%)
0 - 30	100 → 0	0 → 100

Flow rate: 0.8 mL per minute.

Time span of measurement: For 30 minutes after injection, beginning after the solvent peak.

System suitability—

Test for required detectability: Pipet 2 mL of the standard solution, and add a mixture of acetonitrile and water (3:2) to make exactly 20 mL. Confirm that the peak area of candesartan cilexetil obtained with 10 μL of this solution is equivalent to 7 to 13% of that with 10 μL of the standard solution.

System performance: When the procedure is run with 10 μL of the standard solution under the above operating conditions, the number of theoretical plates and the symmetry factor of the peak of candesartan cilexetil are not less than 12,000 and not more than 1.5, respectively.

System repeatability: When the test is repeated 6 times with 10 μL of the standard solution under the above operating conditions, the relative standard deviation of the peak area of candesartan cilexetil is not more than 2.0%.

Uniformity of dosage units <*6.02*> Perform the test according to the following method: it meets the requirement of the Content uniformity test.

To 1 tablet of Candesartan Cilexetil Tablets add 30 mL of a mixture of acetonitrile and water (3:2), shake vigorously for 20 minutes, then add a mixture of acetonitrile and water (3:2) to make exactly *V* mL so that each mL contains about 40 μg of candesartan cilexetil ($C_{33}H_{34}N_6O_6$), centrifuge, and use the supernatant liquid as the sample solution. Separately, weigh accurately about 50 mg of candesartan cilexetil for assay (separately determine the water <*2.48*> in the same manner as Candesartan Cilexetil), and dissolve in acetonitrile to make exactly 50 mL. Pipet 4 mL of this solution, add a mixture of acetonitrile and water (3:2) to make exactly 100 mL, and use this solution as the standard solution. Determine the absorbances, A_T and A_S, of the sample solution and standard solution at 305 nm as directed under Ultraviolet-visible Spectrophotometry <*2.24*>.

Amount (mg) of candesartan cilexetil ($C_{33}H_{34}N_6O_6$)
$= M_S \times A_T/A_S \times V/1250$

M_S: Amount (mg) of candesartan cilexetil for assay taken, calculated on the anhydrous basis

Dissolution <*6.10*> When the test is performed at 50 revolutions per minute according to the Paddle method, using 900 mL of a solution of polysorbate 20 (1 in 100) as the dissolution medium, the dissolution rate in 45 minutes of Candesartan Cilexetil Tablets is not less than 75%.

Start the test with 1 tablet of Candesartan Cilexetil Tablets, withdraw not less than 20 mL of the medium at the specified minute after starting the test, and filter through a membrane filter with a pore size not exceeding 0.45 μm. Discard not less than 5 mL of the first filtrate, pipet *V* mL of the subsequent filtrate, add the dissolution medium to make exactly *V′* mL so that each mL contains about 2.2 μg of candesartan cilexetil ($C_{33}H_{34}N_6O_6$), and use this solution as the sample solution. Separately, weigh accurately about 50 mg of candesartan cilexetil for assay (separately determine the water <*2.48*> in the same manner as Candesartan Cilexetil), and dissolve in acetonitrile to make exactly 50 mL. Pipet 5 mL of this solution, add acetonitrile to make exactly 50 mL. Pipet 1 mL of this solution, add the dissolution medium to make exactly 50 mL, and use this solution as the standard solution. Perform the test with exactly 50 μL each of the sample solution and standard solution as directed under Liquid Chromatography <*2.01*>, and determine the peak areas, A_T and A_S, of candesartan cilexetil in each solution.

Dissolution rate (%) with respect to the labeled amount of candesartan cilexetil ($C_{33}H_{34}N_6O_6$)
$= M_S \times A_T/A_S \times V'/V \times 1/C \times 18/5$

M_S: Amount (mg) of candesartan cilexetil for assay taken, calculated on the anhydrous basis

C: Labeled amount (mg) of candesartan cilexetil ($C_{33}H_{34}N_6O_6$) in 1 tablet

Operating conditions—

Proceed as directed in the operating conditions in the Assay.

System suitability—

System performance: When the procedure is run with 50 μL of the standard solution under the above operating conditions, the number of theoretical plates and the symmetry factor of the peak of candesartan cilexetil are not less than 7000 and not more than 1.5, respectively.

System repeatability: When the test is repeated 6 times with 50 μL of the standard solution under the above operating conditions, the relative standard deviation of the peak area of candesartan cilexetil is not more than 2.0%.

Assay Weigh accurately the mass of not less than 20 Candesartan Cilexetil Tablets, and powder. Weigh accurately a portion of the powder, equivalent to about 6 mg of candesartan cilexetil ($C_{33}H_{34}N_6O_6$), add exactly 15 mL of the internal standard solution, then add a mixture of acetonitrile and water (3:2) to make 150 mL, shake vigorously for 10 minutes, and allow to stand. Filter the supernatant liquid through a membrane filter with a pore size not exceeding 0.45 μm. Discard the first 5 mL of the filtrate, and use the subsequent filtrate as the sample solution. Separately, weigh accurately about 50 mg of candesartan cilexetil for assay (separately determine the water <*2.48*> in the same manner as Candesartan Cilexetil), dissolve in acetonitrile to make exactly 50 mL. Pipet 4 mL of this solution, add exactly 10 mL of the internal standard solution, then add a mixture of acetonitrile and water (3:2) to make 100 mL, and use this solution as the standard solution. Perform the test with 10 μL each of the sample solution and standard solution as directed under Liquid Chromatography <*2.01*> according to the following conditions, and calculate the ratios, Q_T and Q_S, of the peak area of candesartan cilexetil to that of the internal standard.

Amount (mg) of candesartan cilexetil ($C_{33}H_{34}N_6O_6$)
$= M_S \times Q_T/Q_S \times 3/25$

M_S: Amount (mg) of candesartan cilexetil for assay taken, calculated on the anhydrous basis

*Internal standard solution—*A solution of acenaphthene in acetonitrile (1 in 800).

Operating conditions—

Detector: An ultraviolet absorption photometer (wave-

length: 254 nm).

Column: A stainless steel column 3.9 mm in inside diameter and 15 cm in length, packed with octadecylsilanized silica gel for liquid chromatography (4 μm in particle diameter).

Column temperature: A constant temperature of about 25°C.

Mobile phase: A mixture of acetonitrile, water and acetic acid (100) (57:43:1).

Flow rate: Adjust so that the retention time of candesartan cilexetil is about 13 minutes.

System suitability—

System performance: When the procedure is run with 10 μL of the standard solution under the above operating conditions, the internal standard and candesartan cilexetil are eluted in this order with the resolution between these peaks being not less than 5.

System repeatability: When the test is repeated 6 times with 10 μL of the standard solution under the above operating conditions, the relative standard deviation of the ratio of the peak area of candesartan cilexetil to that of the internal standard is not more than 1.0%.

Containers and storage Containers—Tight containers.

Candesartan Cilexetil and Amlodipine Besylate Tablets

カンデサルタン　シレキセチル･アムロジピンベシル酸塩錠

Candesartan Cilexetil and Amlodipine Besylate Tablets contain not less than 95.0% and not more than 105.0% of the labeled amount of candesartan cilexetil ($C_{33}H_{34}N_6O_6$: 610.66) and amlodipine besylate ($C_{20}H_{25}ClN_2O_5.C_6H_6O_3S$: 567.05).

Method of preparation Prepare as directed under Tablets, with Candesartan Cilexetil and Amlodipine Besylate.

Identification **(1)** Shake thoroughly a quantity of powdered Candesartan Cilexetil and Amlodipine Besylate Tablets, equivalent to 8 mg of Candesartan Cilexetil, with 20 mL of 0.01 mol/L hydrochloric acid TS, and centrifuge. Remove the supernatant liquid, to the residue add 20 mL of 0.01 mol/L hydrochloric acid TS, shake thoroughly, and centrifuge. Remove the supernatant liquid, to the residue add 40 mL of methanol, shake thoroughly, and filter through a membrane filter with a pore size not exceeding 0.45 μm. To 5 mL of the filtrate add methanol to make 50 mL, and determine the absorption spectrum of this solution as directed under Ultraviolet-visible Spectrophotometry <2.24>: it exhibits maxima between 252 nm and 256 nm, and between 302 nm and 307 nm.

(2) Shake thoroughly a quantity of powdered Candesartan Cilexetil and Amlodipine Besylate Tablets, equivalent to 2.5 mg of Amlodipine Besylate, with 20 mL of 0.01 mol/L hydrochloric acid TS, and centrifuge. Filter the supernatant liquid through a membrane filter with a pore size not exceeding 0.45 μm. To 5 mL of the filtrate add methanol to make 25 mL, and determine the absorption spectrum of this solution as directed under Ultraviolet-visible Spectrophotometry <2.24>: it exhibits maxima between 236 nm and 240 nm, and between 360 nm and 364 nm.

Purity Related substances—Shake vigorously for 20 minutes a quantity of powdered Candesartan Cilexetil and Amlodipine Besylate Tablets, equivalent to 8 mg of Candesartan Cilexetil, with 20 mL of diluting solution, and filter this solution through a membrane filter with a pore size not exceeding 0.45 μm. Discard the first 5 mL of the filtrate, and use the subsequent filtrate as the sample solution. Pipet 1 mL of the sample solution, add diluting solution to make exactly 100 mL, and use this solution as the standard solution. Perform the test with exactly 20 μL each of the sample solution and standard solution as directed under Liquid Chromatography <2.01> according to the following conditions. Determine each peak area by the automatic integration method: the area of the peak, having the relative retention time of about 0.8 to candesartan cilexetil, obtained from the sample solution is not larger than 1.5 times the peak area of candesartan cilexetil from the standard solution, the area of the peaks, having a relative retention time of about 0.9, about 1.1 and about 1.2 from the sample solution is not larger than 1/2 times the peak area of candesartan cilexetil from the standard solution, the area of the peak, having a relative retention time of about 1.4 from the sample solution, is not larger than the peak area of candesartan cilexetil from the standard solution, and the area of the peak other than candesartan cilexetil and the peaks mentioned above from the sample solution is smaller than 1/10 times the peak area of candesartan cilexetil from the standard solution. Furthermore, the total area of the peaks other than candesartan cilexetil from the sample solution is not larger than 4 times the peak area of candesartan cilexetil from the standard solution.

Diluting solution: To 3.5 mL of triethylamine add water to make 500 mL, and adjust to pH 3.0 with phosphoric acid. To 400 mL of this solution add 600 mL of acetonitrile.

Operating conditions—

Detector: An ultraviolet absorption photometer (wavelength: 253 nm).

Column: A stainless steel column 4.6 mm in inside diameter and 15 cm in length, packed with octadecylsilanized silica gel for liquid chromatography (5 μm in particle diameter).

Column temperature: A constant temperature of about 25°C.

Mobile phase A: A mixture of water, acetonitrile and trifluoroacetic acid (4000:1000:1).

Mobile phase B: A mixture of acetonitrile, water and trifluoroacetic acid (4000:1000:1).

Flowing of mobile phase: Control the gradient by mixing the mobile phases A and B as directed in the following table.

Time after injection of sample (min)	Mobile phase A (vol%)	Mobile phase B (vol%)
0 – 15	100 → 50	0 → 50
15 – 50	50 → 0	50 → 100
50 – 60	0	100

Flow rate: 1.0 mL per minute.

Time span of measurement: For 60 minutes after injection, beginning after the solvent peak.

System suitability—

Test for required detectability: To exactly 1 mL of the standard solution add diluting solution to make exactly 50 mL. Confirm that the peak area of candesartan cilexetil obtained with 20 μL of this solution is equivalent to 1.4 to 2.6% of that obtained with 20 μL of the standard solution.

System performance: When the procedure is run with 20 μL of the standard solution under the above operating conditions, the number of theoretical plates and the symmetry factor of the peak of candesartan cilexetil are not less than 100,000 and not more than 1.5, respectively.

System repeatability: When the test is repeated 6 times with 20 μL of the standard solution under the above operating conditions, the relative standard deviation of the peak area of candesartan cilexetil is not more than 2.0%.

Uniformity of dosage units *<6.02>* Perform the test according to the following methods: it meets the requirements of the Content uniformity test.

(1) Candesartan cilexetil—To 1 tablet of Candesartan Cilexetil and Amlodipine Besylate Tablets add exactly 20 mL of diluting solution, shake for 20 minutes to disintegrate the tablet, and filter through a membrane filter with a pore size not exceeding 0.45 μm. Discard the first 5 mL of the filtrate, pipet V mL of the subsequent filtrate, add exactly $V'/5$ mL of the internal standard solution, then add diluting solution to make V' mL so that each mL contains about 0.16 mg of candesartan cilexetil ($C_{33}H_{34}N_6O_6$), and use this solution as the sample solution. Then, proceed as directed in the Assay (1).

Amount (mg) of candesartan cilexetil ($C_{33}H_{34}N_6O_6$)
$= M_S \times Q_T/Q_S \times V'/V \times 2/25$

M_S: Amount (mg) of candesartan cilexetil for assay taken, calculated on the anhydrous basis

Internal standard solution—A solution of butyl parahydroxybenzoate in diluting solution (1 in 2500).

Diluting solution: To 3.5 mL of triethylamine add water to make 500 mL, and adjust to pH 3.0 with phosphoric acid. To 400 mL of this solution add 600 mL of acetonitrile.

(2) Amlodipine besylate—To 1 tablet of Candesartan Cilexetil and Amlodipine Besylate Tablets add exactly 20 mL of diluting solution, shake for 20 minutes to disintegrate the tablet, and filter through a membrane filter with a pore size not exceeding 0.45 μm. Discard the first 5 mL of the filtrate, pipet V mL of the subsequent filtrate, add exactly $V'/5$ mL of the internal standard solution, then add diluting solution to make V' mL so that each mL contains about 70 μg of amlodipine besylate ($C_{20}H_{25}ClN_2O_5.C_6H_6O_3S$), and use this solution as the sample solution. Then, proceed as directed in the Assay (2).

Amount (mg) of amlodipine besylate
($C_{20}H_{25}ClN_2O_5.C_6H_6O_3S$)
$= M_S \times Q_T/Q_S \times V'/V \times 1/25$

M_S: Amount (mg) of Amlodipine Besylate RS taken, calculated on the anhydrous basis

Internal standard solution—A solution of butyl parahydroxybenzoate in diluting solution (1 in 2500).

Diluting solution: To 3.5 mL of triethylamine add water to make 500 mL, and adjust to pH 3.0 with phosphoric acid. To 400 mL of this solution add 600 mL of acetonitrile.

Dissolution *<6.10>* **(1)** Candesartan cilexetil—When the test is performed at 75 revolutions per minute according to the Paddle method, using 900 mL of a solution, prepared by dissolving 1 g of polysorbate 80 in 2nd fluid for dissolution test to make 1000 mL, as the dissolution medium, the dissolution rate in 45 minutes of Candesartan Cilexetil and Amlodipine Besylate Tablets is not less than 80%.

Start the test with 1 tablet of Candesartan Cilexetil and Amlodipine Besylate Tablets, withdraw not less than 10 mL of the medium at the specified minute after starting the test, and filter through a membrane filter with a pore size not exceeding 0.45 μm. Discard not less than 5 mL of the first filtrate, pipet V mL of the subsequent filtrate, add the dissolution medium to make exactly V' mL so that each mL contains about 8.9 μg of candesartan cilexetil ($C_{33}H_{34}N_6O_6$), and use this solution as the sample solution. Separately, weigh accurately about 45 mg of candesartan cilexetil for assay (separately, determine the water *<2.48>* in the same manner as Candesartan Cilexetil), and dissolve in acetonitrile to make exactly 50 mL. Pipet 1 mL of this solution, add the dissolution medium to make exactly 100 mL, and use this solution as the standard solution. Perform the test with exactly 20 μL each of the sample solution and standard solution as directed under Liquid Chromatography *<2.01>* according to the following conditions, and determine the peak areas, A_T and A_S, of candesartan cilexetil in each solution.

Dissolution rate (%) with respect to the labeled amount of candesartan cilexetil ($C_{33}H_{34}N_6O_6$)
$= M_S \times A_T/A_S \times V'/V \times 1/C \times 18$

M_S: Amount (mg) of candesartan cilexetil for assay taken, calculated on the anhydrous basis

C: Labeled amount (mg) of candesartan cilexetil ($C_{33}H_{34}N_6O_6$) in 1 tablet

Operating conditions—

Detector: An ultraviolet absorption photometer (wavelength: 254 nm).

Column: A stainless steel column 4.6 mm in inside diameter and 5 cm in length, packed with octadecylsilanized silica gel for liquid chromatography (5 μm in particle diameter).

Column temperature: A constant temperature of about 25°C.

Mobile phase: A mixture of acetonitrile, water and acetic acid (100) (57:43:1).

Flow rate: Adjust so that the retention time of candesartan cilexetil is about 6.5 minutes.

System suitability—

System performance: When the procedure is run with 20 μL of the standard solution under the above operating conditions, the number of theoretical plates and the symmetry factor of the peak of candesartan cilexetil are not less than 2000 and not more than 1.5, respectively.

System repeatability: When the test is repeated 6 times with 20 μL of the standard solution under the above operating conditions, the relative standard deviation of the peak area of candesartan cilexetil is not more than 1.0%.

(2) Amlodipine besylate—When the test is performed at 50 revolutions per minute according to the Paddle method, using 900 mL of 0.05 mol/L acetic acid-sodium acetate buffer solution (pH 4.0) as the dissolution medium, the dissolution rate in 30 minutes of Candesartan Cilexetil and Amlodipine Besylate Tablets is not less than 80%.

Start the test with 1 tablet of Candesartan Cilexetil and Amlodipine Besylate Tablets, withdraw not less than 10 mL of the medium at the specified minute after starting the test, and filter through a membrane filter with a pore size not exceeding 0.45 μm. Discard not less than 5 mL of the first filtrate, pipet V mL of the subsequent filtrate, add the dissolution medium to make exactly V' mL so that each mL contains about 3.9 μg of amlodipine besylate ($C_{20}H_{25}ClN_2O_5.C_6H_6O_3S$), and use this solution as the sample solution. Separately, weigh accurately about 39 mg of Amlodipine Besylate RS (separately, determine the water *<2.48>* in the same manner as Amlodipine Besylate), and dissolve in acetonitrile to make exactly 50 mL. Pipet 5 mL of this solution, add acetonitrile to make exactly 50 mL. Pipet 5 mL of this solution, add the dissolution medium to make exactly 100 mL, and use this solution as the standard solution. Perform the test with exactly 50 μL each of the sample solution and standard solution as directed under Liquid Chromatography *<2.01>* according to the following conditions, and determine the peak areas, A_T and A_S, of amlodipine in each solution.

Dissolution rate (%) with respect to the labeled amount of amlodipine besylate ($C_{20}H_{25}ClN_2O_5.C_6H_6O_3S$)

$$= M_S \times A_T/A_S \times V'/V \times 1/C \times 9$$

M_S: Amount (mg) of Amlodipine Besylate RS taken, calculated on the anhydrous basis

C: Labeled amount (mg) of amlodipine besylate ($C_{20}H_{25}ClN_2O_5.C_6H_6O_3S$) in 1 tablet

Operating conditions—

Detector, column, column temperature, and mobile phase: Proceed as directed in the operating conditions in the Assay (1).

Flow rate: Adjust so that the retention time of amlodipine is about 4 minutes.

System suitability—

System performance: When the procedure is run with 50 μL of the standard solution under the above operating conditions, the number of theoretical plates and the symmetry factor of the peak of amlodipine are not less than 3000 and not more than 2.0, respectively.

System repeatability: When the test is repeated 6 times with 50 μL of the standard solution under the above operating conditions, the relative standard deviation of the peak area of amlodipine is not more than 1.0%.

Assay (1) Candesartan cilexetil—Weigh accurately the mass of not less than 20 Candesartan Cilexetil and Amlodipine Besylate Tablets, and powder. Weigh accurately a portion of the powder, equivalent to about 8 mg of candesartan cilexetil ($C_{33}H_{34}N_6O_6$), add exactly 20 mL of diluting solution, shake vigorously for 20 minutes, and filter through a membrane filter with a pore size not exceeding 0.45 μm. Discard the first 5 mL of the filtrate, pipet 10 mL of the subsequent filtrate, add exactly 5 mL of the internal standard solution, then add diluting solution to make 25 mL, and use this solution as the sample solution. Separately, weigh accurately about 40 mg of candesartan cilexetil for assay (separately, determine the water <2.48> in the same manner as Candesartan Cilexetil), dissolve in diluting solution to make exactly 100 mL, and use this solution as the candesartan cilexetil standard stock solution. Pipet 10 mL of the candesartan cilexetil standard stock solution, add exactly 5 mL of the internal standard solution, then add diluting solution to make 25 mL, and use this solution as the standard solution. Perform the test with 10 μL each of the sample solution and standard solution as directed under Liquid Chromatography <2.01> according to the following conditions, and calculate the ratios, Q_T and Q_S, of the peak area of candesartan cilexetil to that of the internal standard.

Amount (mg) of candesartan cilexetil ($C_{33}H_{34}N_6O_6$)

$$= M_S \times Q_T/Q_S \times 1/5$$

M_S: Amount (mg) of candesartan cilexetil for assay taken, calculated on the anhydrous basis

Internal standard solution—A solution of butyl parahydroxybenzoate in diluting solution (1 in 2500).

Diluting solution: To 3.5 mL of triethylamine add water to make 500 mL, and adjust to pH 3.0 with phosphoric acid. To 400 mL of this solution add 600 mL of acetonitrile.

Operating conditions—

Detector: An ultraviolet absorption photometer (wavelength: 238 nm).

Column: A stainless steel column 3.9 mm in inside diameter and 15 cm in length, packed with octadecylsilanized silica gel for liquid chromatography (5 μm in particle diameter).

Column temperature: A constant temperature of about 25°C.

Mobile phase: To 7 mL of triethylamine add water to make 1000 mL, and adjust to pH 6.5 with phosphoric acid. To 800 mL of this solution add 500 mL of acetonitrile.

Flow rate: Adjust so that the retention time of candesartan cilexetil is about 31 minutes.

System suitability—

System performance: Mix 10 mL of the candesartan cilexetil standard stock solution and 5 mL of the amlodipine besylate standard stock solution prepared in the Assay (2), add 5 mL of the internal standard solution, then add diluting solution to make 25 mL. When the procedure is run with 10 μL of this solution under the above operating conditions, amlodipine, the internal standard and candesartan cilexetil are eluted in this order and the resolution between the peaks of the internal standard and candesartan cilexetil is not less than 15.

System repeatability: When the test is repeated 6 times with 10 μL of the standard solution under the above operating conditions, the relative standard deviation of the ratio of the peak area of candesartan cilexetil to that of the internal standard is not more than 1.0%.

(2) Amlodipine besylate—Weigh accurately the mass of not less than 20 Candesartan Cilexetil and Amlodipine Besylate Tablets, and powder. Weigh accurately a portion of the powder, equivalent to about 3.5 mg of amlodipine besylate ($C_{20}H_{25}ClN_2O_5.C_6H_6O_3S$), add exactly 20 mL of diluting solution, shake vigorously for 20 minutes, and filter through a membrane filter with a pore size not exceeding 0.45 μm. Discard the first 5 mL of the filtrate, pipet 10 mL of the subsequent filtrate, add exactly 5 mL of the internal standard solution, then add diluting solution to make 25 mL, and use this solution as the sample solution. Separately, weigh accurately about 35 mg of Amlodipine Besylate RS (separately, determine the water <2.48> in the same manner as Amlodipine Besylate), dissolve in diluting solution to make exactly 100 mL, and use this solution as the amlodipine besylate standard stock solution. Pipet 5 mL of the amlodipine besylate standard stock solution, add exactly 5 mL of the internal standard solution, then add diluting solution to make 25 mL, and use this solution as the standard solution. Perform the test with 10 μL each of the sample solution and standard solution as directed under Liquid Chromatography <2.01> according to the following conditions, and calculate the ratios, Q_T and Q_S, of the peak area of amlodipine to that of the internal standard.

Amount (mg) of amlodipine besylate ($C_{20}H_{25}ClN_2O_5.C_6H_6O_3S$)

$$= M_S \times Q_T/Q_S \times 1/10$$

M_S: Amount (mg) of Amlodipine Besylate RS taken, calculated on the anhydrous basis

Internal standard solution—A solution of butyl parahydroxybenzoate in diluting solution (1 in 2500).

Diluting solution: To 3.5 mL of triethylamine add water to make 500 mL, and adjust to pH 3.0 with phosphoric acid. To 400 mL of this solution add 600 mL of acetonitrile.

Operating conditions—

Detector, column, column temperature, and mobile phase: Proceed as directed in the operating conditions in the Assay (1).

Flow rate: Adjust so that the retention time of amlodipine is about 2.5 minutes.

System suitability—

System performance: Mix 10 mL of the candesartan cilexetil standard stock solution prepared in the Assay (1) and 5 mL of the amlodipine besylate standard stock solution, add 5 mL of the internal standard solution, then add diluting solution to make 25 mL. When the procedure is run with 10 μL of this solution under the above operating conditions, amlodipine, the internal standard and candesartan cilexetil are eluted in this order and the resolution between the peaks of amlodipine and the internal standard is not less than 15.

System repeatability: When the test is repeated 6 times with 10 μL of the standard solution under the above operating conditions, the relative standard deviation of the ratio of the peak area of amlodipine to that of the internal standard is not more than 1.0%.

Containers and storage Containers—Tight containers.

Candesartan Cilexetil and Hydrochlorothiazide Tablets

カンデサルタン シレキセチル・ヒドロクロロチアジド錠

Candesartan Cilexetil and Hydrochlorothiazide Tablets contain not less than 95.0% and not more than 105.0% of the labeled amount of candesartan cilexetil ($C_{33}H_{34}N_6O_6$: 610.66) and hydrochlorothiazide ($C_7H_8ClN_3O_4S_2$: 297.74).

Method of preparation Prepare as directed under Tablets, with Candesartan Cilexetil and Hydrochlorothiazide.

Identification **(1)** To an amount of powdered Candesartan Cilexetil and Hydrochlorothiazide Tablets, equivalent to 4 mg of Candesartan Cilexetil, add 5 mL of acetone, shake thoroughly, centrifuge, and filter the supernatant liquid through a membrane filter with a pore size not exceeding 0.45 μm. Evaporate the filtrate to dryness with the aid of a current of nitrogen. Dissolve the residue in 0.5 mL of acetone, and use this solution as the sample solution. Separately, dissolve 40 mg of candesartan cilexetil in 5 mL of acetone, and use this solution as the standard solution. Perform the test with these solutions as directed under Thin-layer Chromatography *<2.03>*. Spot 2 μL each of the sample solution and standard solution on a plate of silica gel with fluorescent indicator for thin-layer chromatography. Develop the plate with a mixture of ethyl acetate and acetic acid (100) (10:1) to a distance of about 10 cm, and air-dry the plate. Examine under ultraviolet light (main wavelength: 254 nm): the *R*f value of the spot having a larger *R*f value among the spots obtained from the sample solution is the same with that of the spot from the standard solution.

(2) To an amount of powdered Candesartan Cilexetil and Hydrochlorothiazide Tablets, equivalent to 6.25 mg of Hydrochlorothiazide, add 5 mL of acetone, shake thoroughly, centrifuge, and filter the supernatant liquid through a membrane filter with a pore size not exceeding 0.45 μm. Evaporate the filtrate to dryness with the aid of a current of nitrogen. Dissolve the residue in 0.5 mL of acetone, and use this solution as the sample solution. Separately, dissolve 50 mg of hydrochlorothiazide in 4 mL of acetone, and use this solution as the standard solution. Perform the test with these solutions as directed under Thin-layer Chromatography *<2.03>*. Spot 2 μL each of the sample solution and standard solution on a plate of silica gel with fluorescent indicator for thin-layer chromatography. Develop the plate with a mixture of ethyl acetate and acetic acid (100) (10:1) to a distance of about 10 cm, and air-dry the plate. Examine under ultraviolet light (main wavelength: 254 nm): the *R*f value of the spot having a smaller *R*f value among the spots obtained from the sample solution is the same with that of the spot from the standard solution.

Purity Related substances—(i) To an amount of powdered Candesartan Cilexetil and Hydrochlorothiazide Tablets, equivalent to 4 mg of Candesartan Cilexetil, add 10 mL of a mixture of acetonitrile and water (3:2), shake vigorously for 10 minutes, centrifuge, and filter the supernatant liquid through a membrane filter with a pore size not exceeding 0.45 μm. Discard the first 5 mL of the filtrate, and use the subsequent filtrate as the sample solution. Pipet 1 mL of the sample solution, add a mixture of acetonitrile and water (3:2) to make exactly 100 mL, and use this solution as the standard solution. Perform the test with exactly 10 μL each of the sample solution and standard solution as directed under Liquid Chromatography *<2.01>* according to the following conditions, and determine each peak area by the automatic integration method: the area of the peak, having a relative retention time of about 0.5 to candesartan cilexetil, obtained from the sample solution is not larger than 1.5 times the peak area of candesartan cilexetil from the standard solution, the area of the peak, having a relative retention time of about 0.8, about 1.1 and about 1.5, from the sample solution is not larger than 1/2 times the peak area of candesartan cilexetil from the standard solution, the area of the peak, having a relative retention time of about 2.0, from the sample solution is not larger than the peak area of candesartan cilexetil from the standard solution, and the area of the peak, other than candesartan cilexetil and the peaks mentioned above, from the sample solution is smaller than 1/10 times the peak area of candesartan cilexetil from the standard solution. Furthermore, the total area of the peaks other than candesartan cilexetil from the sample solution is not larger than 4 times the peak area of candesartan cilexetil from the standard solution.

Operating conditions—

Detector, column, column temperature, mobile phases A and B, flowing of mobile phase, and time span of measurement: Proceed as directed in the operating conditions in the Purity (2) under Candesartan Cilexetil.

Flow rate: 0.6 mL per minute.

System suitability—

Test for required detectability: To exactly 1 mL of the standard solution add a mixture of acetonitrile and water (3:2) to make exactly 50 mL. Confirm that the peak area of candesartan cilexetil obtained with 10 μL of this solution is equivalent to 1.4% to 2.6% of that with 10 μL of the standard solution.

System performance: When the procedure is run with 10 μL of the standard solution under the above operating conditions, the number of theoretical plates and the symmetry factor of the peak of candesartan cilexetil are not less than 12,000 and not more than 1.5, respectively.

System repeatability: When the test is repeated 6 times with 10 μL of the standard solution under the above operating conditions, the relative standard deviation of the peak area of candesartan cilexetil is not more than 2.0%.

(ii) To an amount of powdered Candesartan Cilexetil and Hydrochlorothiazide Tablets, equivalent to 6.25 mg of Hydrochlorothiazide, add 10 mL of a mixture of 0.05 mol/L sodium dihydrogen phosphate TS (pH 3.0) and acetonitrile (3:1), shake vigorously for 10 minutes, centrifuge, and filter the supernatant liquid through a membrane filter with a pore size not exceeding 0.45 μm. Discard the first 5 mL of the filtrate, and use the subsequent filtrate as the sample solution.

Pipet 1 mL of the sample solution, add a mixture of 0.05 mol/L sodium dihydrogen phosphate TS (pH 3.0) and acetonitrile (3:1) to make exactly 100 mL, and use this solution as the standard solution. Perform the test with exactly 10 μL each of the sample solution and standard solution as directed under Liquid Chromatography <*2.01*> according to the following conditions, and determine each peak area by the automatic integration method: the area of the peak, having a relative retention time of about 0.9 and about 3.2 to hydrochlorothiazide, obtained from the sample solution is not larger than the peak area of hydrochlorothiazide from the standard solution, and the area of the peak, other than hydrochlorothiazide and the peaks mentioned above, from the sample solution is not larger than 1/5 times the peak area of hydrochlorothiazide from the standard solution. Furthermore, the total area of the peaks other than hydrochlorothiazide from the sample solution is not larger than 2 times the peak area of hydrochlorothiazide from the standard solution. For the area of the peak, having a relative retention time of about 0.8 and about 0.9 to hydrochlorothiazide, multiply their correction factors, 1.4 and 0.5, respectively.

Operating conditions—

Detector, column, column temperature, mobile phase, and flow rate: Proceed as directed in the operating conditions in the Assay (2).

Time span of measurement: For 30 minutes after injection, beginning after the solvent peak.

System suitability—

Test for required detectability: To exactly 1 mL of the standard solution add a mixture of 0.05 mol/L sodium dihydrogen phosphate TS (pH 3.0) and acetonitrile (3:1) to make exactly 50 mL. Confirm that the peak area of hydrochlorothiazide obtained with 10 μL of this solution is equivalent to 1.4% to 2.6% of that obtained with 10 μL of the standard solution.

System performance: When the procedure is run with 10 μL of the standard solution under the above operating conditions, the number of theoretical plates and the symmetry factor of the peak of hydrochlorothiazide are not less than 5000 and not more than 1.5, respectively.

System repeatability: When the test is repeated 6 times with 10 μL of the standard solution under the above operating conditions, the relative standard deviation of the peak area of hydrochlorothiazide is not more than 2.0%.

Uniformity of dosage units <*6.02*> Perform the test according to the following methods: it meets the requirements of the Content uniformity test.

(1) Candesartan cilexetil—To 1 tablet of Candesartan Cilexetil and Hydrochlorothiazide Tablets add exactly *V*/10 mL of the internal standard solution, add a mixture of acetonitrile and 0.05 mol/L sodium dihydrogen phosphate TS (pH 3.0) (3:2) to make *V* mL so that each mL contains about 40 μg of candesartan cilexetil ($C_{33}H_{34}N_6O_6$). Shake for 20 minutes to disintegrate the tablet, centrifuge, and use the supernatant liquid as the sample solution. Separately, weigh accurately about 50 mg of candesartan cilexetil for assay (separately determine the water <*2.48*> in the same manner as Candesartan Cilexetil), dissolve in acetonitrile to make exactly 50 mL, and use this solution as the candesartan cilexetil standard stock solution. Pipet 4 mL of the candesartan cilexetil standard stock solution, add exactly 10 mL of the internal standard solution, add a mixture of acetonitrile and 0.05 mol/L sodium dihydrogen phosphate TS (pH 3.0) (3:2) to make 100 mL, and use this solution as the standard solution. Perform the test with 10 μL each of the sample solution and standard solution as directed under Liquid Chromatography <*2.01*> according to the following conditions, and calculate the ratios, Q_T and Q_S, of the peak area of candesartan cilexetil to that of the internal standard.

$$\text{Amount (mg) of candesartan cilexetil } (C_{33}H_{34}N_6O_6) = M_S \times Q_T/Q_S \times V \times 1/1250$$

M_S: Amount (mg) of candesartan cilexetil for assay taken, calculated on the anhydrous basis.

*Internal standard solution—*A solution of benzophenone in acetonitrile (1 in 10,000).

Operating conditions—

Detector: An ultraviolet absorption photometer (wavelength: 254 nm).

Column: A stainless steel column 4.6 mm in inside diameter and 15 cm in length, packed with octadecylsilanized silica gel for liquid chromatography (4 μm in particle diameter).

Column temperature: A constant temperature of about 25°C.

Mobile phase: A mixture of acetonitrile and 0.05 mol/L sodium dihydrogen phosphate TS (pH 5.5) (11:9).

Flow rate: Adjust so that the retention time of candesartan cilexetil is about 7 minutes.

System suitability—

System performance: Mix 4 mL of the candesartan cilexetil standard stock solution and 10 mL of the hydrochlorothiazide standard stock solution obtained in (2), add 10 mL of the internal standard solution, and add a mixture of acetonitrile and 0.05 mol/L sodium dihydrogen phosphate TS (pH 3.0) (3:2) to make 100 mL. When the procedure is run with 10 μL of this solution under the above operating conditions, hydrochlorothiazide, candesartan cilexetil and the internal standard are eluted in this order, and the resolution between the peaks of hydrochlorothiazide and candesartan cilexetil is not less than 7, and the resolution between the peaks of candesartan cilexetil and the internal standard is not less than 6.

System repeatability: When the test is repeated 6 times with 10 μL of the standard solution under the above operating conditions, the relative standard deviation of the ratio of the peak area of candesartan cilexetil to that of the internal standard is not more than 1.0%.

(2) Hydrochlorothiazide—To 1 tablet of Candesartan Cilexetil and Hydrochlorothiazide Tablets add exactly *V*/10 mL of the internal standard solution, add a mixture of acetonitrile and 0.05 mol/L sodium dihydrogen phosphate TS (pH 3.0) (3:2) to make *V* mL so that each mL contains about 63 μg of hydrochlorothiazide ($C_7H_8ClN_3O_4S_2$). Shake for 20 minutes, centrifuge, and use the supernatant liquid as the sample solution. Separately, weigh accurately about 31 mg of Hydrochlorothiazide RS (separately determine the loss on drying <*2.41*> under the same conditions as Hydrochlorothiazide), dissolve in acetonitrile to make exactly 50 mL, and use this solution as the hydrochlorothiazide standard stock solution. Pipet 10 mL of the hydrochlorothiazide standard stock solution, add exactly 10 mL of the internal standard solution, add a mixture of acetonitrile and 0.05 mol/L sodium dihydrogen phosphate TS (pH 3.0) (3:2) to make 100 mL, and use this solution as the standard solution. Perform the test with 10 μL each of the sample solution and standard solution as directed under Liquid Chromatography <*2.01*> according to the following conditions, and calculate the ratios, Q_T and Q_S, of the peak area of hydrochlorothiazide to that of the internal standard.

$$\text{Amount (mg) of hydrochlorothiazide } (C_7H_8ClN_3O_4S_2) = M_S \times Q_T/Q_S \times V \times 1/500$$

M_S: Amount (mg) of Hydrochlorothiazide RS taken, calculated on the dried basis.

Internal standard solution—A solution of benzophenone in acetonitrile (1 in 10,000).

Operating conditions—

Detector, column, and column temperature: Proceed as directed in the operating conditions in the Assay (2).

Mobile phase: A mixture of acetonitrile and 0.05 mol/L sodium dihydrogen phosphate TS (pH 5.5) (11:9).

Flow rate: Adjust so that the retention time of hydrochlorothiazide is about 3.5 minutes.

System suitability—

System performance: Mix 4 mL of the candesartan cilexetil standard stock solution obtained in (1) and 10 mL of the hydrochlorothiazide standard stock solution, add 10 mL of the internal standard solution, and add a mixture of acetonitrile and 0.05 mol/L sodium dihydrogen phosphate TS (pH 3.0) (3:2) to make 100 mL. When the procedure is run with 10 μL of this solution under the above operating conditions, hydrochlorothiazide, candesartan cilexetil and the internal standard are eluted in this order, and the resolution between the peaks of hydrochlorothiazide and candesartan cilexetil is not less than 7, and the resolution between the peaks of candesartan cilexetil and the internal standard is not less than 6.

System repeatability: When the test is repeated 6 times with 10 μL of the standard solution under the above operating conditions, the relative standard deviation of the ratio of the peak area of hydrochlorothiazide to that of the internal standard is not more than 1.0%.

Dissolution *<6.10>* **(1)** Candesartan cilexetil—When the test is performed at 50 revolutions per minute according to the Paddle method, using 900 mL of a solution, prepared by dissolving 1 g of polysorbate 80 in 2nd fluid for dissolution test to make 1000 mL, as the dissolution medium, the dissolution rate in 45 minutes of Candesartan Cilexetil and Hydrochlorothiazide Tablets is not less than 75%.

Start the test with 1 tablet of Candesartan Cilexetil and Hydrochlorothiazide Tablets, withdraw not less than 10 mL of the medium at the specified minute after starting the test, and filter through a membrane filter with a pore size not exceeding 0.45 μm. Discard not less than 5 mL of the first filtrate, pipet *V* mL of the subsequent filtrate, add 0.05 mol/L sodium dihydrogen phosphate TS (pH 3.0) to make exactly *V′* mL so that each mL contains about 2.2 μg of candesartan cilexetil ($C_{33}H_{34}N_6O_6$), and use this solution as the sample solution. Separately, weigh accurately about 25 mg of candesartan cilexetil for assay (separately determine the water *<2.48>* in the same manner as Candesartan Cilexetil), dissolve in acetonitrile to make exactly 100 mL, and use this solution as the candesartan cilexetil standard stock solution. Pipet 2 mL of the candesartan cilexetil standard stock solution, add dissolution medium to make exactly 100 mL. Pipet 10 mL of this solution, add 0.05 mol/L sodium dihydrogen phosphate TS (pH 3.0) to make exactly 20 mL, and use this solution as the standard solution. Perform the test with exactly 40 μL each of the sample solution and standard solution as directed under Liquid Chromatography *<2.01>* according to the following conditions, and determine the peak areas, A_T and A_S, of candesartan cilexetil in each solution.

Dissolution rate (%) with respect to the labeled amount of candesartan cilexetil ($C_{33}H_{34}N_6O_6$)

$$= M_S \times A_T/A_S \times V'/V \times 1/C \times 9$$

M_S: Amount (mg) of candesartan cilexetil for assay taken, calculated on the anhydrous basis

C: Labeled amount (mg) of candesartan cilexetil ($C_{33}H_{34}N_6O_6$) in 1 tablet

Operating conditions—

Proceed as directed in the operating conditions in the Uniformity of dosage units (1).

System suitability—

System performance: Mix 2 mL each of the candesartan cilexetil standard stock solution and the hydrochlorothiazide standard stock solution obtained in (2), and add the dissolution medium to make 100 mL. To 10 mL of this solution add 10 mL of 0.05 mol/L sodium dihydrogen phosphate TS (pH 3.0). When the procedure is run with 40 μL of this solution under the above operating conditions, hydrochlorothiazide and candesartan cilexetil are eluted in this order with the resolution between these peaks being not less than 6.

System repeatability: When the test is repeated 6 times with 40 μL of the standard solution under the above operating conditions, the relative standard deviation of the peak area of candesartan cilexetil is not more than 1.0%.

(2) Hydrochlorothiazide—When the test is performed at 50 revolutions per minute according to the Paddle method, using 900 mL of a solution, prepared by dissolving 1 g of polysorbate 80 in 2nd fluid for dissolution test to make 1000 mL, as the dissolution medium, the dissolution rate in 45 minutes of Candesartan Cilexetil and Hydrochlorothiazide Tablets is not less than 80%.

Start the test with 1 tablet of Candesartan Cilexetil and Hydrochlorothiazide Tablets, withdraw not less than 10 mL of the medium at the specified minute after starting the test, and filter through a membrane filter with a pore size not exceeding 0.45 μm. Discard not less than 5 mL of the first filtrate, pipet *V* mL of the subsequent filtrate, add 0.05 mol/L sodium dihydrogen phosphate TS (pH 3.0) to make exactly *V′* mL so that each mL contains about 3.5 μg of hydrochlorothiazide ($C_7H_8ClN_3O_4S_2$), and use this solution as the sample solution. Separately, weigh accurately about 38 mg of Hydrochlorothiazide RS (separately determine the loss on drying *<2.41>* under the same conditions as Hydrochlorothiazide), dissolve in acetonitrile to make exactly 100 mL, and use this solution as the hydrochlorothiazide standard stock solution. Pipet 2 mL of the hydrochlorothiazide standard stock solution, add dissolution medium to make exactly 100 mL. Pipet 10 mL of this solution, add 0.05 mol/L sodium dihydrogen phosphate TS (pH 3.0) to make exactly 20 mL, and use this solution as the standard solution. Perform the test with exactly 40 μL each of the sample solution and standard solution as directed under Liquid Chromatography *<2.01>* according to the following conditions, and determine the peak areas, A_T and A_S, of hydrochlorothiazide in each solution.

Dissolution rate (%) with respect to the labeled amount of hydrochlorothiazide ($C_7H_8ClN_3O_4S_2$)

$$= M_S \times A_T/A_S \times V'/V \times 1/C \times 9$$

M_S: Amount (mg) of Hydrochlorothiazide RS taken, calculated on the dried basis

C: Labeled amount (mg) of hydrochlorothiazide ($C_7H_8ClN_3O_4S_2$) in 1 tablet

Operating conditions—

Detector, column, and column temperature: Proceed as directed in the operating conditions in the Assay (2).

Mobile phase: A mixture of acetonitrile and 0.05 mol/L sodium dihydrogen phosphate TS (pH 5.5) (11:9).

Flow rate: Adjust so that the retention time of hydrochlorothiazide is about 3.5 minutes.

System suitability—

System performance: Mix 2 mL each of the candesartan cilexetil standard stock solution obtained in (1) and the hydrochlorothiazide standard stock solution, and add the dissolution medium to make 100 mL. To 10 mL of this solution add 10 mL of 0.05 mol/L sodium dihydrogen phosphate TS (pH 3.0). When the procedure is run with 40 μL of this solution under the above operating conditions, hydrochlorothiazide and candesartan cilexetil are eluted in this order with the resolution between these peaks being not less than 6.

System repeatability: When the test is repeated 6 times with 40 μL of the standard solution under the above operating conditions, the relative standard deviation of the peak area of hydrochlorothiazide is not more than 1.0%.

Assay **(1)** Candesartan cilexetil—Weigh accurately the mass of not less than 20 Candesartan Cilexetil and Hydrochlorothiazide Tablets, and powder. Weigh accurately a portion of the powder, equivalent to about 4 mg of candesartan cilexetil ($C_{33}H_{34}N_6O_6$), add exactly 10 mL of the internal standard solution, add a mixture of acetonitrile and water (3:2) to make 100 mL, and shake vigorously for 10 minutes. Allow to stand for 5 minutes, and filter the supernatant liquid through a membrane filter with a pore size not exceeding 0.45 μm. Discard the first 5 mL of the filtrate, and use the subsequent filtrate as the sample solution. Separately, weigh accurately about 50 mg of candesartan cilexetil for assay (separately determine the water *<2.48>* in the same manner as Candesartan Cilexetil), dissolve in acetonitrile to make exactly 50 mL. Pipet 4 mL of this solution, add exactly 10 mL of the internal standard solution, add a mixture of acetonitrile and water (3:2) to make 100 mL, and use this solution as the standard solution. Perform the test with 10 μL each of the sample solution and standard solution as directed under Liquid Chromatography *<2.01>* according to the following conditions, and calculate the ratios, Q_T and Q_S, of the peak area of candesartan cilexetil to that of the internal standard.

Amount (mg) of candesartan cilexetil ($C_{33}H_{34}N_6O_6$)
$= M_S \times Q_T/Q_S \times 2/25$

M_S: Amount (mg) of candesartan cilexetil for assay taken, calculated on the anhydrous basis

*Internal standard solution—*A solution of acenaphthene in acetonitrile (1 in 800).

Operating conditions—

Detector: An ultraviolet absorption photometer (wavelength: 254 nm).

Column: A stainless steel column 4 mm in inside diameter and 15 cm in length, packed with octadecylsilanized silica gel for liquid chromatography (4 μm in particle diameter).

Column temperature: A constant temperature of about 25°C.

Mobile phase: A mixture of acetonitrile, water and acetic acid (100) (57:43:1).

Flow rate: Adjust so that the retention time of candesartan cilexetil is about 13 minutes.

System suitability—

System performance: When the procedure is run with 10 μL of the standard solution under the above operating conditions, the internal standard and candesartan cilexetil are eluted in this order with the resolution between these peaks being not less than 5.

System repeatability: When the test is repeated 6 times with 10 μL of the standard solution under the above operating conditions, the relative standard deviation of the ratio of the peak area of candesartan cilexetil to that of the internal standard is not more than 1.0%.

(2) Hydrochlorothiazide—Weigh accurately the mass of not less than 20 Candesartan Cilexetil and Hydrochlorothiazide Tablets, and powder. Weigh accurately a portion of the powder, equivalent to about 6.25 mg of hydrochlorothiazide ($C_7H_8ClN_3O_4S_2$), add exactly 10 mL of the internal standard solution, add a mixture of 0.05 mol/L sodium dihydrogen phosphate TS (pH 3.0) and acetonitrile (3:1) to make 100 mL, and shake vigorously for 10 minutes. Allow to stand for 5 minutes, and filter the supernatant liquid through a membrane filter with a pore size not exceeding 0.45 μm. Discard the first 5 mL of the filtrate, and use the subsequent filtrate as the sample solution. Separately, weigh accurately about 31 mg of Hydrochlorothiazide RS (separately determine the loss on drying *<2.41>* under the same conditions as Hydrochlorothiazide), dissolve in acetonitrile to make exactly 50 mL. Pipet 10 mL of this solution, add exactly 10 mL of the internal standard solution, add a mixture of 0.05 mol/L sodium dihydrogen phosphate TS (pH 3.0) and acetonitrile (3:1) to make 100 mL, and use this solution as the standard solution. Perform the test with 10 μL each of the sample solution and standard solution as directed under Liquid Chromatography *<2.01>* according to the following conditions, and calculate the ratios, Q_T and Q_S, of the peak area of hydrochlorothiazide to that of the internal standard.

Amount (mg) of hydrochlorothiazide ($C_7H_8ClN_3O_4S_2$)
$= M_S \times Q_T/Q_S \times 1/5$

M_S: Amount (mg) of Hydrochlorothiazide RS taken, calculated on the dried basis

*Internal standard solution—*A solution of *m*-hydroxyacetophenone in acetonitrile (1 in 6500).

Operating conditions—

Detector: An ultraviolet absorption photometer (wavelength: 254 nm).

Column: A stainless steel column 4.6 mm in inside diameter and 15 cm in length, packed with octadecylsilanized silica gel for liquid chromatography (4 μm in particle diameter).

Column temperature: A constant temperature of about 25°C.

Mobile phase: A mixture of 0.05 mol/L sodium dihydrogen phosphate TS (pH 5.5) and acetonitrile (3:1).

Flow rate: Adjust so that the retention time of hydrochlorothiazide is about 6 minutes.

System suitability—

System performance: When the procedure is run with 10 μL of the standard solution under the above operating conditions, hydrochlorothiazide and the internal standard are eluted in this order with the resolution between these peaks being not less than 5.

System repeatability: When the test is repeated 6 times with 10 μL of the standard solution under the above operating conditions, the relative standard deviation of the ratio of the peak area of hydrochlorothiazide to that of the internal standard is not more than 1.0%.

Containers and storage Containers—Tight containers.

Capsules

カプセル

Capsules are made of Gelatin, and their shape is a pair of cylinders with one end closed which can be overlapped on each other.

Method of preparation Dissolve Gelatin in water by warming, add Glycerin or D-Sorbitol, Macrogol 4000, emulsifier, dispersing agent, preservatives, coloring substances and so forth, if necessary, to make a viscous liquid, and form into capsules while warm.

Capsules may be coated with a lubricant, if necessary.

Solubility and acidity or alkalinity Place, without overlapping of the parts, 1 piece (1 pair) of Capsules in a 100-mL conical flask, add 50 mL of water, and shake often, keeping the temperature at 37 ± 2°C. Perform this test 5 times: they all dissolve within 10 minutes. All these solutions are odorless, and neutral or slightly acidic.

Loss on drying <*2.41*> 13 - 16% (1 g, 105°C, 2 hours).

Microbial limit <*4.05*> The acceptance criteria of TAMC and TYMC are 10^3 CFU/g and 10^2 CFU/g, respectively.

Containers and storage Containers—Well-closed containers.

Hypromellose Capsules

ヒプロメロースカプセル

Hypromellose Capsules are made of Hypromellose as the base material, and their shape is a pair of cylinders with one end closed which can be overlapped on each other.

The label states the use or nonuse of the gelling agent and its name.

Method of preparation Dissolve Hypromellose in water by warming, add, if necessary, Glycerin or D-Sorbitol, emulsifiers, dispersing agents, preservatives, coloring agents, gelling agents, and gelling aid, etc. to make a viscous liquid, and form into a certain shape while warming.

They may be coated with a lubricant as necessary.

Solubility and acidity or alkalinity Place one pair of Hypromellose Capsules without snapping in a 100-mL conical flask, add 50 mL of water, and shake occasionally at 37 ± 2°C. When perform this test 5 times, either capsule dissolves within 15 minutes and their solutions are neutral or slightly acidic.

Loss on drying <*2.41*> 2 - 7% (1 g, 105°C, 2 hours).

Microbial limit <*4.05*> The acceptance criteria of TAMC and TYMC are 10^3 CFU/g and 10^2 CFU/g, respectively.

Containers and storage Containers—Well-closed containers.

Pullulan Capsules

プルランカプセル

Pullulan Capsules are made of Pullulan as the base material, and their shape is a pair of cylinders with one end closed which can be overlapped on each other.

The label states the use or nonuse of the gelling agent and its name.

Method of preparation Dissolve Pullulan in water by warming, add, if necessary, emulsifiers, dispersing agents, preservatives, coloring agents, gelling agents, and gelling aid, etc. to make a viscous liquid, and form into a certain shape while warming.

They may be coated with a lubricant as necessary.

Solubility and acidity or alkalinity Place one pair of Pullulan Capsules without snapping in a 100-mL conical flask, add 50 mL of water, and shake occasionally at 37 ± 2°C. When perform this test 5 times, either capsule dissolves within 10 minutes and these solutions are neutral or slightly acidic.

Loss on drying <*2.41*> 10 - 14% (1 g, 105°C, 6 hours).

Microbial limit <*4.05*> The acceptance criteria of TAMC and TYMC are 10^3 CFU/g and 10^2 CFU/g, respectively.

Containers and storage Containers—Well-closed containers.

Captopril

カプトプリル

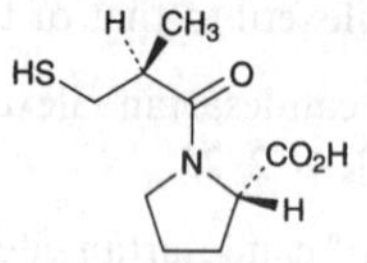

$C_9H_{15}NO_3S$: 217.29

(2*S*)-1-[(2*S*)-2-Methyl-3-sulfanylpropanoyl]pyrrolidine-2-carboxylic acid

[*62571-86-2*]

Captopril contains not less than 98.0% of captopril ($C_9H_{15}NO_3S$), calculated on the dried basis.

Description Captopril occurs as white, crystals or crystalline powder.

It is very soluble in methanol, freely soluble in ethanol (99.5), and soluble in water.

Identification Determine the infrared absorption spectrum of Captopril as directed in the potassium bromide disk method under Infrared Spectrophotometry <*2.25*>, and compare the spectrum with the Reference Spectrum: both spectra exhibit similar intensities of absorption at the same wave numbers.

Optical rotation <*2.49*> $[\alpha]_D^{25}$: −125 − −134° (after drying, 0.1 g, ethanol (99.5), 10 mL, 100 mm).

Melting point <*2.60*> 105 - 110°C

Purity (1) Heavy metals <*1.07*>—Proceed with 1.0 g of Captopril according to Method 2, and perform the test. Prepare the control solution with 2.0 mL of Standard Lead So-

lution (not more than 20 ppm).

(2) Arsenic 〈*1.11*〉—Prepare the test solution with 1.0 g of Captopril according to Method 1, and perform the test (not more than 2 ppm).

(3) Related substances—Dissolve 0.20 g of Captopril in methanol to make exactly 10 mL, and use this solution as the sample solution. Separately, dissolve 15 mg of 1,1′-[3,3′-dithiobis(2-methyl-1-oxopropyl)]-L-diproline in methanol to make exactly 250 mL, and use this solution as the standard solution. Perform the test with these solutions as directed under Thin-layer Chromatography 〈*2.03*〉. Spot 10 μL each of the sample solution and standard solution on a plate of silica gel for thin-layer chromatography. Develop with a mixture of toluene and acetic acid (100) (13:7) to a distance of about 15 cm, and air-dry the plate. Place the plate in a chamber filled with iodine vapor, and allow to stand for 30 minutes: the number of the spots other than the spot corresponding to that obtained from the standard solution and the principal spot from the sample solution is not more than two, and they are not more intense than the spot from the standard solution.

(4) 1,1′-[3,3′-Dithiobis(2-methyl-1-oxopropyl)]-L-diproline—Dissolve 0.10 g of Captopril in methanol to make exactly 20 mL, and use this solution as the sample solution. Separately, dissolve 25 mg of 1,1′-[3,3′-dithiobis(2-methyl-1-oxopropyl)]-L-diproline in methanol to make exactly 250 mL, and use this solution as the standard solution. Perform the test with exactly 20 μL each of the sample solution and standard solution as directed under Liquid Chromatography 〈*2.01*〉 according to the following conditions, and determine the peak areas, A_T and A_S, of 1,1′-[3,3′-dithiobis(2-methyl-1-oxopropyl)]-L-diproline in each solution: A_T is not larger than A_S.

Operating conditions—

Detector: An ultraviolet absorption photometer (wavelength: 220 nm).

Column: A stainless steel column 3.9 mm in inside diameter and 30 cm in length, packed with octadecylsilanized silica gel for liquid chromatography (10 μm in particle diameter).

Column temperature: A constant temperature of about 25°C.

Mobile phase: A mixture of water, methanol and phosphoric acid (1000:1000:1).

Flow rate: Adjust so that the retention time of 1,1′-[3,3′-dithiobis(2-methyl-1-oxopropyl)]-L-diproline is about 10 minutes.

System suitability—

System performance: Dissolve 25 mg each of Captopril and 1,1′-[3,3′-dithiobis(2-methyl-1-oxopropyl)]-L-diproline in 200 mL of methanol. When the procedure is run with 20 μL of this solution under the above operating conditions, captopril and 1,1′-[3,3′-dithiobis(2-methyl-1-oxopropyl)]-L-diproline are eluted in this order with the resolution between these peaks being not less than 3.

System repeatability: When the test is repeated 5 times with 20 μL of the standard solution under the above operating conditions, the relative standard deviation of the peak areas of 1,1′-[3,3′-dithiobis(2-methyl-1-oxopropyl)]-L-diproline is not more than 2.0%.

Loss on drying 〈*2.41*〉 Not more than 1.0% (1 g, in vacuum, 80°C, 3 hours).

Residue on ignition 〈*2.44*〉 Not more than 0.2% (1 g).

Assay Weigh accurately about 0.3 g of Captopril, dissolve in 100 mL of water, add 20 mL of dilute sulfuric acid and 1 g of potassium iodide, and shake. Titrate 〈*2.50*〉 with 1/60 mol/L potassium iodate VS (indicator: 2 mL of starch TS). Perform a blank determination in the same manner, and make any necessary correction.

Each mL of 1/60 mol/L potassium iodate VS
= 21.73 mg of $C_9H_{15}NO_3S$

Containers and storage Containers—Tight containers.

Carbamazepine

カルバマゼピン

$C_{15}H_{12}N_2O$: 236.27
5*H*-Dibenz[*b*,*f*]azepine-5-carboxamide
[*298-46-4*]

Carbamazepine, when dried, contains not less than 97.0% and not more than 103.0% of carbamazepine ($C_{15}H_{12}N_2O$).

Description Carbamazepine occurs as a white to slightly yellow-white powder. It is odorless and tasteless at first, and leaves a slightly bitter aftertaste.

It is freely soluble in chloroform, sparingly soluble in ethanol (95) and in acetone, and very slightly soluble in water and in diethyl ether.

Identification **(1)** To 0.1 g of Carbamazepine add 2 mL of nitric acid, and heat on a water bath for 3 minutes: an orange-red color is produced.

(2) To 0.1 g of Carbamazepine add 2 mL of sulfuric acid, and heat on a water bath for 3 minutes: a yellow color is produced with a green fluorescence.

(3) Examine Carbamazepine under ultraviolet light: the solution shows an intense blue fluorescence.

(4) Determine the absorption spectrum of the solution obtained in the Assay as directed under Ultraviolet-visible Spectrophotometry 〈*2.24*〉, and compare the spectrum with the Reference Spectrum: both spectra exhibit similar intensities of absorption at the same wavelengths.

Melting point 〈*2.60*〉 189 – 193°C

Purity **(1)** Clarity and color of solution—Dissolve 1.0 g of Carbamazepine in 10 mL of chloroform: the solution is clear and colorless to pale yellow.

(2) Acidity—To 2.0 g of Carbamazepine add exactly 40 mL of water, stir well for 15 minutes, and filter through a glass filter (G3). To 10 mL of this filtrate add 1 drop of phenolphthalein TS and 0.50 mL of 0.01 mol/L sodium hydroxide VS: a red color is produced.

(3) Alkalinity—To 10 mL of the filtrate obtained in (2) add 1 drop of methyl red TS and 0.50 mL of 0.01 mol/L hydrochloric acid VS: a red color is produced.

(4) Chloride 〈*1.03*〉—Dissolve 0.25 g of Carbamazepine in 30 mL of acetone, add 6 mL of dilute nitric acid and water to make 50 mL, and perform the test using this solution as the test solution. Prepare the control solution as follows: to 0.20 mL of 0.01 mol/L hydrochloric acid VS add 30 mL of acetone, 6 mL of dilute nitric acid and water to make 50 mL (not more than 0.028%).

(5) Heavy metals 〈*1.07*〉—Proceed with 2.0 g of Carbamazepine according to Method 2, and perform the test.

Prepare the control solution with 2.0 mL of Standard Lead Solution (not more than 10 ppm).

(6) Related substances—Dissolve 0.25 g of Carbamazepine in 10 mL of chloroform, and use this solution as the sample solution. Separately, dissolve 5.0 mg of iminodibenzyl in chloroform to make exactly 100 mL, and use this solution as the standard solution. Perform the test with these solutions as directed under Thin-layer Chromatography *<2.03>*. Spot 10 μL each of the sample solution and standard solution on a plate of silica gel for thin-layer chromatography. Develop the plate with a mixture of toluene and methanol (19:1) to a distance of about 10 cm, and air-dry the plate. Spray evenly potassium dichromate-sulfuric acid TS on the plate: the spots other than the principal spot obtained from the sample solution is not more intense than the spot from the standard solution.

Loss on drying *<2.41>* Not more than 0.5% (1 g, 105°C, 2 hours).

Residue on ignition *<2.44>* Not more than 0.1% (1 g).

Assay Dissolve about 50 mg of Carbamazepine, previously dried and accurately weighed, in ethanol (95) to make exactly 250 mL. Pipet 5 mL of this solution and add ethanol (95) to make exactly 100 mL. Perform the test as directed under Ultraviolet-visible Spectrophotometry *<2.24>*, and determine the absorbance *A* of this solution at the wavelength of maximum absorption at about 285 nm.

$$\text{Amount (mg) of carbamazepine } (C_{15}H_{12}N_2O) = A/490 \times 50{,}000$$

Containers and storage Containers—Tight containers.

Carbazochrome Sodium Sulfonate Hydrate

カルバゾクロムスルホン酸ナトリウム水和物

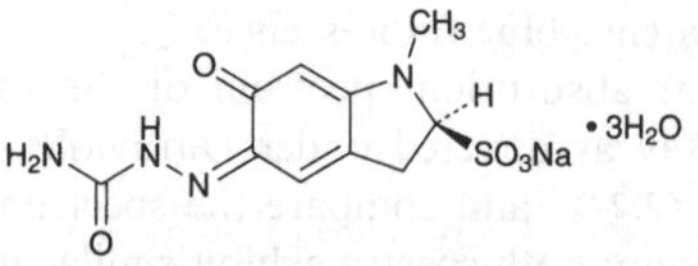

and enantiomer

$C_{10}H_{11}N_4NaO_5S.3H_2O$: 376.32
Monosodium (2*RS*)-1-methyl-6-oxo-5-semicarbazono-2,3,5,6-tetrahydroindole-2-sulfonate trihydrate
[*51460-26-5*, anhydride]

Carbazochrome Sodium Sulfonate Hydrate contains not less than 98.0% and not more than 102.0% of carbazochrome sodium sulfonate ($C_{10}H_{11}N_4NaO_5S$: 322.27), calculated on the anhydrous basis.

Description Carbazochrome Sodium Sulfonate Hydrate occurs as orange-yellow, crystals or crystalline powder.

It is sparingly soluble in water, very slightly soluble in methanol and in ethanol (95), and practically insoluble in diethyl ether.

A solution of Carbazochrome Sodium Sulfonate Hydrate (1 in 100) shows no optical rotation.

Melting point: about 210°C (with decomposition).

Identification **(1)** Determine the absorption spectrum of a solution of Carbazochrome Sodium Sulfonate Hydrate (1 in 100,000) as directed under Ultraviolet-visible Spectrophotometry *<2.24>*, and compare the spectrum with the Reference Spectrum: both spectra exhibit similar intensities of absorption at the same wavelengths.

(2) Determine the infrared absorption spectrum of Carbazochrome Sodium Sulfonate Hydrate as directed in the potassium bromide disk method under Infrared Spectrophotometry *<2.25>*, and compare the spectrum with the Reference Spectrum: both spectra exhibit similar intensities of absorption at the same wave numbers.

(3) A solution of Carbazochrome Sodium Sulfonate Hydrate (1 in 100) responds to Qualitative Tests *<1.09>* (1) for sodium salt.

pH *<2.54>* Dissolve 0.8 g of Carbazochrome Sodium Sulfonate Hydrate in 50 mL of water by warming, and cool: the pH of this solution is between 5.0 and 6.0.

Purity **(1)** Clarity and color of solution—Dissolve 1.0 g of Carbazochrome Sodium Sulfonate Hydrate in 50 mL of water by warming, and allow to cool: the solution is clear. Perform the test with this solution as directed under Ultraviolet-visible Spectrophotometry *<2.24>*: the absorbance at 590 nm is not more than 0.070.

(2) Heavy metals *<1.07>*—Proceed with 1.0 g of Carbazochrome Sodium Sulfonate Hydrate according to Method 2, and perform the test. Prepare the control solution with 2.0 mL of Standard Lead Solution (not more than 20 ppm).

(3) Related substances—Dissolve 50 mg of Carbazochrome Sodium Sulfonate Hydrate in 100 mL of water, and use this solution as the sample solution. Pipet 2 mL of the sample solution, add water to make exactly 200 mL, and use this solution as the standard solution. Perform the test with exactly 10 μL each of the sample solution and standard solution as directed under Liquid Chromatography *<2.01>* according to the following conditions. Determine each peak area of these solutions by the automatic integration method: the total area of the peaks other than carbazochrome sulfonate obtained from the sample solution is not larger than the peak area of carbazochrome sulfonate from the standard solution.

Operating conditions—

Detector: An ultraviolet absorption photometer (wavelength: 360 nm).

Column: A stainless steel column 4.6 mm in inside diameter and 25 cm in length, packed with octadecylsilanized silica gel for liquid chromatography (7 μm in particle diameter).

Column temperature: A constant temperature of about 40°C.

Mobile phase: Dissolve 1.2 g of ammonium dihydrogen phosphate in 1000 mL of water, and filter through a membrane filter (0.4 μm in pore size) if necessary. To 925 mL of this solution add 75 mL of ethanol (95), shake, and adjust the pH to 3 with phosphoric acid.

Flow rate: Adjust so that the retention time of carbazochrome sulfonate is about 7 minutes.

Time span of measurement: About 3 times as long as the retention time of carbazochrome sulfonate, beginning after the solvent peak.

System suitability—

Test for required detectability: To exactly 2 mL of the standard solution add the mobile phase to make exactly 20 mL. Confirm that the peak area of carbazochrome sulfonate obtained with 10 μL of this solution is equivalent to 7 to 13% of that with 10 μL of the standard solution.

System performance: Dissolve 10 mg each of Carbazochrome Sodium Sulfonate Hydrate and carbazochrome in 100 mL of water by warming. When the procedure is run with 10 μL of this solution under the above operating conditions, carbazochrome sulfonate and carbazochrome are eluted in this order with the resolution between these peaks being not less than 3.

System repeatability: When the test is repeated 6 times with 10 μL of the standard solution under the above operating conditions, the relative standard deviation of the peak area of carbazochrome sulfonate is not more than 2.0%.

Water ⟨*2.48*⟩ 13.0 - 16.0% (0.3 g, volumetric titration, direct titration).

Assay Weigh accurately about 0.25 g of Carbazochrome Sodium Sulfonate Hydrate, dissolve in 50 mL of water, apply to a chromatographic column, 10 mm in diameter, previously prepared with 20 mL of strongly acidic ion exchange resin for column chromatography (type H), and allow to flow at a rate of 4 mL per minute. Wash the column with 150 mL of water, combine the washing and the former effluent solution, and titrate ⟨*2.50*⟩ with 0.05 mol/L sodium hydroxide VS (potentiometric titration). Perform a blank determination in the same manner, and make any necessary correction.

Each mL of 0.05 mol/L sodium hydroxide VS
= 16.11 mg of $C_{10}H_{11}N_4NaO_5S$

Containers and storage Containers—Well-closed containers.

Carbidopa Hydrate

カルビドパ水和物

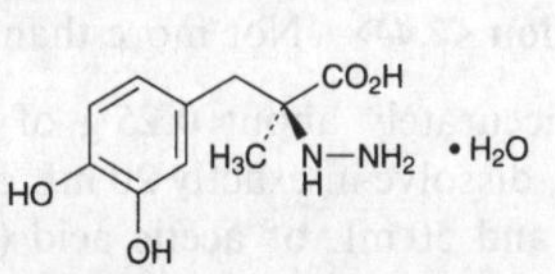

$C_{10}H_{14}N_2O_4.H_2O$: 244.24
(2*S*)-2-(3,4-Dihydroxybenzyl)-2-hydrazinopropanoic acid monohydrate
[*38821-49-7*]

Carbidopa Hydrate contains not less than 98.0% of carbidopa hydrate ($C_{10}H_{14}N_2O_4.H_2O$).

Description Carbidopa Hydrate occurs as a white to yellowish white powder.

It is sparingly soluble in methanol, slightly soluble in water, very slightly soluble in ethanol (95), and practically insoluble in diethyl ether.

Melting point: about 197°C (with decomposition).

Identification **(1)** Dissolve 0.01 g of Carbidopa Hydrate in 250 mL of a solution of hydrochloric acid in methanol (9 in 1000). Determine the absorption spectrum of this solution as directed under Ultraviolet-visible Spectrophotometry ⟨*2.24*⟩, and compare the spectrum with the Reference Spectrum or the spectrum of a solution of Carbidopa RS prepared in the same manner as the sample solution: both spectra exhibit similar intensities of absorption at the same wavelengths.

(2) Determine the infrared absorption spectrum of Carbidopa Hydrate as directed in the potassium bromide disk method under Infrared Spectrophotometry ⟨*2.25*⟩, and compare the spectrum with the Reference Spectrum or the spectrum of Carbidopa RS: both spectra exhibit similar intensities of absorption at the same wave numbers.

Optical rotation ⟨*2.49*⟩ $[\alpha]_D^{20}$: −21.0 − −23.5° (1 g, aluminum (III) chloride TS, 100 mL, 100 mm).

Purity **(1)** Heavy metals ⟨*1.07*⟩—Proceed with 2.0 g of Carbidopa Hydrate according to Method 2, and perform the test. Prepare the control solution with 2.0 mL of Standard Lead Solution (not more than 10 ppm).

(2) Related substances—Dissolve 50 mg of Carbidopa Hydrate in 70 mL of the mobile phase, by warming and using ultrasonication, if necessary. After cooling, add the mobile phase to make 100 mL, and use this solution as the sample solution. Pipet 1 mL of the sample solution, add the mobile phase to make exactly 100 mL, and use this solution as the standard solution. Perform the test with exactly 20 μL each of the sample solution and standard solution as directed under Liquid Chromatography ⟨*2.01*⟩ according to the following conditions. Determine each peak area from both solutions by the automatic integration method: the total area of the peaks other than carbidopa obtained from the sample solution is not larger than the peak area of carbidopa from the standard solution.

Operating conditions—

Detector, column, column temperature, mobile phase, and flow rate: Proceed as directed in the operating conditions in the Assay.

Time span of measurement: About 3 times as long as the retention time of carbidopa.

System suitability—

System performance, and system repeatability: Proceed as directed in the system suitability in the Assay.

Test for required detectability: To exactly 2 mL of the standard solution add the mobile phase to make exactly 20 mL. Confirm that the peak area of carbidopa obtained with 20 μL of this solution is equivalent to 7 to 13% of that with 20 μL of the standard solution.

Loss on drying ⟨*2.41*⟩ 6.9 - 7.9% (1 g, in vacuum not exceeding 0.67 kPa, 100°C, 6 hours).

Residue on ignition ⟨*2.44*⟩ Not more than 0.1% (1 g).

Assay Weigh accurately about 50 mg each of Carbidopa Hydrate and Carbidopa RS (separately determine the loss on drying ⟨*2.41*⟩ under the same conditions as Carbidopa Hydrate), and dissolve each in 70 mL of the mobile phase, by warming and using ultrasonication if necessary. After cooling, add the mobile phase to make exactly 100 mL, and use these solutions as the sample solution and the standard solution, respectively. Perform the test with exactly 20 μL each of the sample solution and standard solution as directed under Liquid Chromatography ⟨*2.01*⟩ according to the following conditions, and determine the peak areas, A_T and A_S, of carbidopa in each solution.

Amount (mg) of carbidopa hydrate ($C_{10}H_{14}N_2O_4.H_2O$)
$= M_S \times A_T/A_S \times 1.080$

M_S: Amount (mg) of Carbidopa RS taken, calculated on the dried basis

Operating conditions—

Detector: An ultraviolet absorption photometer (wavelength: 280 nm).

Column: A stainless steel column 4 mm in inside diameter and 25 cm in length, packed with octadecylsilanized silica gel for liquid chromatography (7 μm in particle diameter).

Column temperature: A constant temperature of about 25°C.

Mobile phase: To 950 mL of 0.05 mol/L sodium dihydrogen phosphate TS add 50 mL of ethanol (95), and adjust the pH to 2.7 with phosphoric acid.

Flow rate: Adjust so that the retention time of carbidopa is about 6 minutes.

System suitability—

System performance: Dissolve 50 mg each of Carbidopa Hydrate and methyldopa in 100 mL of the mobile phase. When the procedure is run with 20 µL of this solution under the above operating conditions, methyldopa and carbidopa are eluted in this order with the resolution between these peaks being not less than 0.9.

System repeatability: When the test is repeated 6 times with 20 µL of the standard solution under the above operating conditions, the relative standard deviation of the peak area of carbidopa is not more than 1.0%.

Containers and storage Containers—Tight containers.

Storage—Light-resistant.

L-Carbocisteine

L-カルボシステイン

HO2C S CO2H H NH2

$C_5H_9NO_4S$: 179.19

(2*R*)-2-Amino-3-carboxymethylsulfanylpropanoic acid

[*638-23-3*]

L-Carbocisteine, when dried, contains not less than 98.5% of L-carbocisteine ($C_5H_9NO_4S$).

Description L-Carbocisteine occurs as a white crystalline powder. It is odorless, and has a slightly acid taste.

It is very slightly soluble in water, and practically insoluble in ethanol (95).

It dissolves in dilute hydrochloric acid or in sodium hydroxide TS.

Melting point: about 186°C (with decomposition).

Identification **(1)** To 0.2 g of L-Carbocisteine add 1 mL of lead acetate TS and 3 mL of water, shake, add 0.2 g of sodium hydroxide, and heat over a flame for 1 minute: a dark brown to black precipitate is formed.

(2) Determine the infrared absorption spectrum of L-Carbocisteine as directed in the potassium bromide disk method under Infrared Spectrophotometry <*2.25*>, and compare the spectrum with the Reference Spectrum: both spectra exhibit similar intensities of absorption at the same wave numbers.

Optical rotation <*2.49*> $[\alpha]_D^{20}$: −33.5 – −36.5° Weigh accurately about 5 g of L-Carbocisteine, previously dried, dissolve in 20 mL of water and a suitable amount of a solution of sodium hydroxide (13 in 100), and adjust the pH with 1 mol/L hydrochloric acid TS or 0.1 mol/L hydrochloric acid TS to 6.0, and add water to make exactly 50 mL. Determine the optical rotation of this solution in a 100-mm cell.

Purity **(1)** Clarity and color of solution—Dissolve 1.0 g of L-Carbocisteine in 10 mL of sodium hydroxide TS: the solution is clear and colorless.

(2) Chloride <*1.03*>—Dissolve 0.20 g of L-Carbocisteine in 10 mL of water and 20 mL of nitric acid, and add water to make 50 mL. Perform the test using this solution as the test solution. Prepare the control solution as follows. To 0.40 mL of 0.01 mol/L hydrochloric acid VS add 20 mL of nitric acid and water to make 50 mL (not more than 0.071%).

(3) Ammonium <*1.02*>—Perform the test with 0.25 g of L-Carbocisteine using the distillation under reduced pressure. Prepare the control solution with 5.0 mL of Standard Ammonium Solution (not more than 0.02%).

(4) Heavy metals <*1.07*>—Proceed with 1.0 g of L-Carbocisteine according to Method 2, and perform the test. Prepare the control solution with 2.0 mL of Standard Lead Solution (not more than 20 ppm).

(5) Arsenic <*1.11*>—Prepare the test solution with 1.0 g of L-Carbocisteine according to Method 3, and perform the test (not more than 2 ppm).

(6) Related substances—Dissolve 0.30 g of L-Carbocisteine in 10 mL of 0.2 mol/L sodium hydroxide TS, and use this solution as the sample solution. Pipet 2 mL of the sample solution, and add 0.2 mol/L sodium hydroxide TS to make exactly 100 mL. Pipet 1 mL of this solution, and add 0.2 mol/L sodium hydroxide TS to make exactly 10 mL, and use this solution as the standard solution. Perform the test with these solutions as directed under Thin-layer Chromatography <*2.03*>. Spot 5 µL each of the sample solution and standard solution, in 15 mm length along the starting line on a plate of silica gel for thin-layer chromatography. Develop the plate with a mixture of 1-butanol, water and acetic acid (100) (3:1:1) to a distance of about 10 cm, and dry the plate at 80°C for 30 minutes. Spray evenly a solution of ninhydrin in acetone (1 in 50) on the plate, and heat the plate at 80°C for 5 minutes: the spots other than the principal spot obtained from the sample solution are not more intense than the spot from the standard solution.

Loss on drying <*2.41*> Not more than 0.30% (1 g, 105°C, 2 hours).

Residue on ignition <*2.44*> Not more than 0.1% (1 g).

Assay Weigh accurately about 0.25 g of L-Carbocisteine, previously dried, dissolve in exactly 20 mL of 0.1 mol/L perchloric acid VS and 50 mL of acetic acid (100), and titrate <*2.50*> the excess perchloric acid with 0.1 mol/L sodium acetate VS (potentiometric titration). Perform a blank determination in the same manner.

Each mL of 0.1 mol/L perchloric acid VS
= 17.92 mg of $C_5H_9NO_4S$

Containers and storage Containers—Tight containers.

L-Carbocisteine Tablets

L-カルボシステイン錠

L-Carbocisteine Tablets contain not less than 95.0% and not more than 105.0% of the labeled amount of L-carbocisteine ($C_5H_9NO_4S$: 179.19).

Method of Preparation Prepare as directed under Tablets, with L-Carbocisteine.

Identification Powder L-Carbocisteine Tablets. To a portion of the powder, equivalent to 0.18 g of L-Carbocisteine, add 50 mL of water, stir for 10 minutes, and filter. To 5 mL of the filtrate add 1 mL of ninhydrin TS, and heat in a water bath for 3 minutes: a purple color develops.

Uniformity of dosage units <*6.02*> It meets the requirement of the Mass variation test.

Dissolution <*6.10*> When the test is performed at 75 revolutions per minute according to the Paddle method, using 900 mL of water as the dissolution medium, the dissolution rates in 15 minutes of 250-mg tablet and in 30 minutes of 500-mg tablet are not less than 80% and not less than 85%, respectively.

Start the test with 1 tablet of L-Carbocisteine Tablets, withdraw not less than 20 mL of the medium at the specified minute after starting the test, and filter through a membrane filter with a pore size not exceeding 0.45 μm. Discard not less than 10 mL of the first filtrate, pipet V mL of the subsequent filtrate, add the mobile phase to make exactly V' mL so that each mL contains about 0.14 mg of L-carbocisteine ($C_5H_9NO_4S$), and use this solution as the sample solution. Separately, weigh accurately about 28 mg of L-carbocisteine for assay, previously dried at 105°C for 2 hours, and dissolve in the mobile phase to make exactly 200 mL, and use this solution as the standard solution. Perform the test with exactly 20 μL each of the sample solution and standard solution as directed under Liquid Chromatography *<2.01>* according to the following condition, and determine the peak areas, A_T and A_S, of L-carbocisteine in each solution.

Dissolution rate (%) with respect to the labeled amount of L-carbocisteine ($C_5H_9NO_4S$)

$$= M_S \times A_T/A_S \times V'/V \times 1/C \times 450$$

M_S: Amount (mg) of L-carbocisteine for assay taken
C: Labeled amount (mg) of L-carbocisteine ($C_5H_9NO_4S$) in 1 tablet

Operating conditions—
Proceed as directed in the operating conditions in the Assay.

System suitability—
System performance: When the procedure is run with 20 μL of the standard solution under the above operating conditions, the number of theoretical plates and the symmetry factor of the peak of L-carbocisteine are not less than 1500 and not more than 2.0, respectively.

System repeatability: When the test is repeated 6 times with 20 μL of the standard solution under the above operating conditions, the relative standard deviation of the peak area of L-carbocisteine is not more than 1.0%.

Assay To 10 L-Carbocisteine Tablets add 220 mL of 0.5 mol/L hydrochloric acid TS, stir for 30 minutes, add 0.5 mol/L hydrochloric acid TS to make exactly 250 mL, and stir additionally for 30 minutes. Filter this solution, discard the first 20 mL of the filtrate, pipet 2 mL of the subsequent filtrate, add (V—50)/25 mL of 0.5 mol/L hydrochloric acid TS, then add exactly V/25 mL of the internal standard solution, add water to make V mL so that each mL contains about 0.4 mg of L-carbocisteine ($C_5H_9NO_4S$), and use this solution as the sample solution. Separately, weigh accurately about 20 mg of L-carbocisteine for assay, previously dried at 105°C for 2 hours, add 2 mL of 0.5 mol/L hydrochloric acid TS, and exactly 2 mL of the internal standard solution. Then add water to dissolve to make 50 mL, and use this solution as the standard solution. Perform the test with 5 μL each of the sample solution and standard solution as directed under Liquid Chromatography *<2.01>* according to the following conditions, and calculate the ratios, Q_T and Q_S, of the peak area of L-carbocisteine to that of the internal standard.

Amount (mg) of L-carbocisteine ($C_5H_9NO_4S$) in 1 tablet
$$= M_S \times Q_T/Q_S \times V/4$$

M_S: Amount of L-carbocisteine for assay taken

Internal standard solution—A solution of nicotinic acid (9 in 10,000).

Operating conditions—
Detector: An ultraviolet absorption photometer (wavelength: 240 nm).

Column: A stainless steel column 4.6 mm in inside diameter and 15 cm in length, packed with octadecylsilanized silica gel for liquid chromatography (5 μm in particle diameter).

Column temperature: A constant temperature of about 20°C.

Mobile phase: Diluted trifluoroacetic acid (1 in 1000).

Flow rate: Adjust so that the retention time of L-carbocisteine is about 2 minutes.

System suitability—
System performance: When the procedure is run with 5 μL of the standard solution under the above operating conditions, L-carbocisteine and the internal standard are eluted in this order with the resolution between these peaks being not less than 4.

System repeatability: When the test is repeated 6 times with 5 μL of the standard solution under the above operating conditions, the relative standard deviation of the ratio of the peak area of L-carbocisteine to that of the internal standard is not more than 1.0%.

Containers and storage Containers—Tight containers.

Carbon Dioxide

二酸化炭素

CO_2: 44.01
[124-38-9]

Carbon Dioxide contains not less than 99.5 vol% of carbon dioxide (CO_2).

Description Carbon Dioxide is a colorless gas at room temperature and under atmospheric pressure. It is odorless.

A 1 mL volume of Carbon Dioxide dissolves in 1 mL of water, and the solution is slightly acid.

1000 mL of Carbon Dioxide at 0°C and under a pressure of 101.3 kPa weighs 1.978 g.

Identification **(1)** Pass 100 mL of Carbon Dioxide through a carbon dioxide measuring detector tube: the detector tube is changed to a stipulated color tone by each detector tube, provided that the detector tube with a upper limit of measurement of not less than 10% is used.

(2) Pass Carbon Dioxide into calcium hydroxide TS: a white precipitate is produced. Collect the precipitate, and add acetic acid (31): it dissolves with effervescence.

Purity **(1)** Acidity—Place 50 mL of freshly boiled and cooled water in a Nessler tube, and pass 1000 mL of Carbon Dioxide into it for 15 minutes through an introducing tube about 1 mm in diameter extending to 2 mm from the bottom of the Nessler tube, then add 0.10 mL of methyl orange TS: the solution is not more colored than the following control solution.

Control solution: To 50 mL of freshly boiled and cooled water in a Nessler tube add 0.10 mL of methyl orange TS and 1.0 mL of 0.01 mol/L hydrochloric acid VS.

(2) Hydrogen phosphide, hydrogen sulfide or reducing organic substances—Place 25 mL of silver nitrate-ammonia TS and 3 mL of ammonia TS in each of two Nessler tubes A and B, and designate the solution in each tube as solution A and solution B, respectively. Pass 1000 mL of Carbon Dioxide into solution A in the same manner as directed in (1): the turbidity and color of this solution are the same as that of solution B.

(3) Carbon monoxide—Pass a specified amount of Carbon Dioxide through a carbon monoxide measuring detector tube: the concentration of carbon monoxide is less than 15 ppm, provided that the passing amount (mL) of Carbon Dioxide is stipulated according to each detector tube.

Assay Place 125 mL of a solution of potassium hydroxide (1 in 2) in a gas pipet of suitable capacity. Measure exactly about 100 mL of Carbon Dioxide in a 100-mL gas buret filled with water. Force the entire volume of gas into the gas pipet, and shake for 5 minutes. Draw some of the unabsorbed gas into the gas buret, measure the volume, force the residual back upon the surface of the liquid in the gas pipet, and repeat this procedure until a constant volume of the residual reading is obtained. Determine the volume V (mL) of the residual gas. Calculate the volume of the sample and V on the basis of the gas volume at 20°C and at 101.3 kPa.

Volume (mL) of carbon dioxide (CO_2)
= volume (mL) of the sample − V (mL)

Containers and storage Containers—Cylinders.
Storage—Not exceeding 40°C.

Carboplatin

カルボプラチン

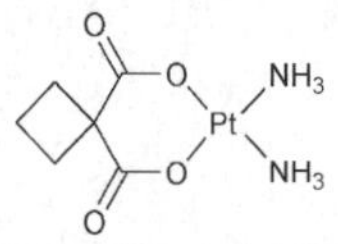

$C_6H_{12}N_2O_4Pt$: 371.25
(*SP*-4-2)-Diammine[cyclobutan-1,1-dicarboxylato(2-)-*O*,*O'*]platinum
[*41575-94-4*]

Carboplatin contains not less than 98.5% and not more than 101.0% of carboplatin ($C_6H_{12}N_2O_4Pt$), calculated on the dried basis.

Description Carboplatin occurs as white, crystals or crystalline powder.

It is sparingly soluble in water, and very slightly soluble in ethanol (99.5).

Melting point: about 200°C (with decomposition).

Identification **(1)** To 2 mL of a solution of Carboplatin (1 in 100) add 2 to 3 drops of diluted tin (II) chloride TS (1 in 15), and allow to stand for 30 minutes: a yellowish brown precipitate is formed.

(2) Determine the infrared absorption spectrum of Carboplatin as directed in the potassium bromide disk method under Infrared Spectrophotometry *<2.25>*, and compare the spectrum with the Reference Spectrum or the spectrum of Carboplatin RS: both spectra exhibit similar intensities of absorption at the same wave numbers.

pH *<2.54>* Dissolve 0.10 g of Carboplatin in 10 mL of water: the pH of this solution is 5.0 to 7.0.

Purity **(1)** 1,1-Cyclobutanedicarboxylic acid—Weigh accurately about 40 mg of Carboplatin, dissolve in the mobile phase to make exactly 20 mL, and use this solution as the sample solution. Separately, weigh accurately about 25 mg of 1,1-cyclobutanedicarboxylic acid, and dissolve in the mobile phase to make exactly 100 mL. Pipet 4 mL of this solution, add the mobile phase to make exactly 50 mL, and use this solution as the standard solution. Perform the test with exactly 25 μL each of the sample solution and standard solution as directed under Liquid Chromatography *<2.01>* according to the following conditions. Determine the peak areas, A_T and A_S, of 1,1-cyclobutanedicarboxylic acid in each solution, and calculate the amount of 1,1-cyclobutanedicarboxylic acid by the following formula: it is not more than 0.2%.

Amount (%) of 1,1-cyclobutanedicarboxylic acid
$= M_S/M_T \times A_T/A_S \times 8/5$

M_S: Amount (mg) of 1,1-cyclobutanedicarboxylic acid taken
M_T: Amount (mg) of Carboplatin taken

Operating conditions—

Detector: An ultraviolet absorption photometer (wavelength: 220 nm).

Column: A stainless steel column 4.0 mm in inside diameter and 30 cm in length, packed with octadecylsilanized silica gel for liquid chromatography (7 μm in particle diameter).

Column temperature: A constant temperature of about 35°C.

Mobile phase: Dissolve 8.5 g of tetrabutylammonium hydrogensulfate in 80 mL of water, add 3.4 mL of phosphoric acid, and adjust to pH 7.5 with a solution of sodium hydroxide (43 in 100). To 10 mL of this solution add 430 mL of water and 60 mL of acetonitrile.

Flow rate: Adjust so that the retention time of 1,1-cyclobutanedicarboxylic acid is about 5 minutes.

System suitability—

Test for required detectability: To exactly 2 mL of the standard solution add the mobile phase to make exactly 10 mL. Confirm that the peak area of 1,1-cyclobutanedicarboxylic acid obtained with 25 μL of this solution is equivalent to 14 to 26% of that with 25 μL of the standard solution.

System performance: Dissolve 25 mg each of 1,1-cyclobutanedicarboxylic acid and cyclobutanecarboxylic acid in 100 mL of water. To 10 mL of this solution add the mobile phase to make 25 mL. When the procedure is run with 25 μL of this solution under the above operating conditions, cyclobutanecarboxylic acid and 1,1-cyclobutanedicarboxylic acid are eluded in this order with the resolution between these peaks being not less than 3.

System repeatability: When the test is repeated 6 times with 25 μL of the standard solution under the above operating conditions, the relative standard deviation of the peak area of 1,1-cyclobutanedicarboxylic acid is not more than 2.0%.

(2) Related substances—Dissolve 25 mg of Carboplatin in 25 mL of water, and use this solution as the sample solution. Perform the test with 10 μL of the sample solution as directed under Liquid Chromatography *<2.01>* according to the following conditions, and determine each peak area by the automatic integration method. Calculate the amount of the peaks by the area percentage method: the amount of the peak, having the relative retention time of about 0.8 to carboplatin, is not more than 0.25%, the amount of the peak other than carboplatin and the peak mentioned above is not more than 0.1%, and the total amount of the peaks other than carboplatin is not more than 0.5%.

Operating conditions—

Detector, column, column temperature, mobile phases A and B, and flow rate: Proceed as directed in the operating conditions in the Assay.

Flowing of mobile phase: Control the gradient by mixing the mobile phases A and B as directed in the following table.

Time after injection of sample (min)	Mobile phase A (vol%)	Mobile phase B (vol%)
0 – 15	100	0
15 – 35	100 → 0	0 → 100
35 – 50	0	100

Time span of measurement: About 2.5 times as long as the retention time of carboplatin, beginning after the solvent peak.

System suitability—

System performance: Proceed as directed in the system suitability in the Assay.

Test for required detectability: To 1 mL of the sample solution add water to make 100 mL, and use this solution as the solution for system suitability test. Pipet 1 mL of the solution for system suitability test, and add water to make exactly 20 mL. Confirm that the peak area of carboplatin obtained with 10 μL of this solution is equivalent to 3.5 to 6.5% of that with 10 μL of the solution for system suitability test.

System repeatability: When the test is repeated 6 times with 10 μL of the solution for system suitability test under the above operating conditions, the relative standard deviation of the peak area of carboplatin is not more than 2.0%.

Loss on drying <*2.41*> Not more than 0.1% (0.5 g, 105°C, 4 hours).

Assay Weigh accurately about 25 mg each of Carboplatin and Carboplatin RS (separately determine the loss on drying <*2.41*> under the same conditions as Carboplatin), dissolve separately in water to make exactly 25 mL, and use these solutions as the sample solution and the standard solution, respectively. Perform the test with exactly 10 μL each of the sample solution and standard solution as directed under Liquid Chromatography <*2.01*> according to the following conditions, and determine the peak areas, A_T and A_S, of carboplatin in each solution.

$$\text{Amount (mg) of carboplatin } (C_6H_{12}N_2O_4Pt) = M_S \times A_T/A_S$$

M_S: Amount (mg) of Carboplatin RS taken, calculated on the dried basis

Operating conditions—

Detector: An ultraviolet absorption photometer (wavelength: 220 nm).

Column: A stainless steel column 4.6 mm in inside diameter and 25 cm in length, packed with phenylhexylsilanized silica gel for liquid chromatography (5 μm in particle diameter).

Column temperature: A constant temperature of about 27°C.

Mobile phase A: Dissolve 8.5 g of tetrabutylammonium hydrogensulfate in 80 mL of water, add 3.4 mL of phosphoric acid, and adjust to pH 7.5 with a solution of sodium hydroxide (43 in 100). To 20 mL of this solution add water to make 1000 mL.

Mobile phase B: Dissolve 8.5 g of tetrabutylammonium hydrogensulfate in 80 mL of water, add 3.4 mL of phosphoric acid, and adjust to pH 7.5 with a solution of sodium hydroxide (43 in 100). To 20 mL of this solution add water to make 800 mL, and add 200 mL of acetonitrile.

Flowing of mobile phase: Control the gradient by mixing the mobile phases A and B as directed in the following table.

Time after injection of sample (min)	Mobile phase A (vol%)	Mobile phase B (vol%)
0 – 15	100	0
15 – 35	100 → 0	0 → 100

Flow rate: 0.5 mL per minute.

System suitability—

System performance: To 9 mL of the standard solution add 1 mL of diluted hydrogen peroxide TS (1 in 60), and allow to stand at room temperature for not less than 1 hour. When the procedure is run with 10 μL of this solution under the above operating conditions, the resolution between the peak of carboplatin and the peak having the relative retention time about 0.93 to carboplatin is not less than 1.2.

System repeatability: When the test is repeated 6 times with 10 μL of the standard solution under the above operating conditions, the relative standard deviation of the peak area of carboplatin is not more than 1.0%.

Containers and storage Containers—Tight containers.

Storage—Light-resistant.

Carboplatin Injection

カルボプラチン注射液

Carboplatin Injection is an aqueous injection.

It contains not less than 95.0% and not more than 105.0% of the labeled amount of carboplatin ($C_6H_{12}N_2O_4Pt$: 371.25).

Method of preparation Prepare as directed under Injections, with Carboplatin.

Description Carboplatin Injection is a clear, colorless to pale yellow liquid.

Identification **(1)** To an amount of Carboplatin Injection, equivalent to 20 mg of Carboplatin, add 2 to 3 drops of diluted tin (II) chloride TS (1 in 15), and allow to stand for 30 minutes: a yellowish brown precipitate is formed.

(2) Evaporate to dryness a volume of Carboplatin Injection, equivalent to 10 mg of Carboplatin, in a water bath at not exceeding 30°C under vacuum. Determine the infrared absorption spectrum of the residue as directed in the potassium bromide disk method under Infrared Spectrophotometry <*2.25*>: it exhibits absorption at the wave numbers of about 3270 cm^{-1}, 2990 cm^{-1}, 2960 cm^{-1}, 1645 cm^{-1}, 1610 cm^{-1}, 1381 cm^{-1} and 1348 cm^{-1}.

pH Being specified separately when the drug is granted approval based on the Law.

Purity **(1)** 1,1-Cyclobutanedicarboxylic acid—To an exact volume of Carboplatin Injection, equivalent to 20 mg of Carboplatin, add the mobile phase to make exactly 10 mL, and use this solution as the sample solution. Separately, weigh accurately about 25 mg of 1,1-cyclobutanedicarboxylic acid, and dissolve in the mobile phase to make exactly 100 mL. Pipet 4 mL of this solution, add the mobile phase to make exactly 50 mL, and use this solution as the standard solution. Perform the test with exactly 25 μL each of the sample solution and standard solution as directed under Liquid Chromatography <*2.01*> according to the following conditions. Determine the peak areas, A_T and A_S, of 1,1-cyclobutanedicarboxylic acid in each solution, and calculate the amount of 1,1-cyclobutanedicarboxylic acid by the following formula: it is not more than 0.7%.

Amount (%) of 1,1-cyclobutanedicarboxylic acid
$= M_S \times A_T/A_S \times 1/25$

M_S: Amount (mg) of 1,1-cyclobutanedicarboxylic acid taken

Operating conditions—

Proceed as directed in the operating conditions in the Purity (1) under Carboplatin.

System suitability—

Proceed as directed in the system suitability in the Purity (1) under Carboplatin.

(2) Related substances—To a volume of Carboplatin Injection, equivalent to 10 mg of Carboplatin, add water to make 10 mL, and use this solution as the sample solution. Perform the test with 10 μL of the sample solution as directed under Liquid Chromatography <*2.01*> according to the following conditions, and determine each peak area by the automatic integration method. Calculate the amount of these peaks by the area percentage method: the total amount of the peaks other than carboplatin is not more than 2.0%.

Operating conditions—

Detector, column, column temperature, mobile phases A and B, and flow rate: Proceed as directed in the operating conditions in the Assay under Carboplatin.

Flowing of mobile phase, and time span of measurement: Proceed as directed in the operating conditions in the Purity (2) under Carboplatin.

System suitability—

System performance: Proceed as directed in the system suitability in the Assay under Carboplatin.

Test for required detectability, and system repeatability: Proceed as directed in the system suitability in the Purity (2) under Carboplatin.

Bacterial endotoxins <*4.01*> Less than 0.2 EU/mg.

Extractable volume <*6.05*> It meets the requirement.

Foreign insoluble matter <*6.06*> Perform the test according to Method 1: it meets the requirement.

Insoluble particulate matter <*6.07*> It meets the requirement.

Sterility <*4.06*> Perform the test according to the Membrane filtration method: it meets the requirement.

Assay To an exact volume of Carboplatin Injection, equivalent to about 20 mg of carboplatin ($C_6H_{12}N_2O_4Pt$), add water to make exactly 20 mL, and use this solution as the sample solution. Separately, weigh accurately about 25 mg of Carboplatin RS (separately determine the loss on drying <*2.41*> under the same conditions as Carboplatin), dissolve in water to make exactly 25 mL, and use this solution as the standard solution. Perform the test with exactly 10 μL each of the sample solution and standard solution as directed under Liquid Chromatography <*2.01*> according to the following conditions, and determine the peak areas, A_T and A_S, of carboplatin in each solution.

Amount (mg) of carboplatin ($C_6H_{12}N_2O_4Pt$)
$= M_S \times A_T/A_S \times 4/5$

M_S: Amount (mg) of Carboplatin RS taken, calculated on the dried basis

Operating conditions—

Detector: An ultraviolet absorption photometer (wavelength: 230 nm).

Column: A stainless steel column 4.0 mm in inside diameter and 25 cm in length, packed with octadecylsilanized silica gel for liquid chromatography (10 μm in particle diameter).

Column temperature: A constant temperature of about 35°C.

Mobile phase: Dissolve 8.5 g of tetrabutylammonium hydrogensulfate in 80 mL of water, add 3.4 mL of phosphoric acid, and adjust to pH 7.5 with a solution of sodium hydroxide (43 in 100). To 10 mL of this solution add 880 mL of water and 10 mL of acetonitrile.

Flow rate: Adjust so that the retention time of carboplatin is about 4 minutes.

System suitability—

System performance: To a solution of 25 mg of carboplatin in 20 mL of water add 2.5 mL of a solution of 65 mg of 1,3-phenylenediamine hydrochloride in 50 mL of water, and add water to make 25 mL. When the procedure is run with 10 μL of this solution under the above operating conditions, carboplatin and 1,3-phenylenediamine are eluted in this order with the resolution between these peaks being not less than 2.0.

System repeatability: When the test is repeated 6 times with 10 μL of the standard solution under the above operating conditions, the relative standard deviation of the peak area of carboplatin is not more than 1.0%.

Containers and storage Containers—Hermetic containers.
Storage—Light-resistant.

Shelf life 24 months after preparation.

Carmellose

Carboxymethylcellulose

カルメロース

[*9000-11-7*]

This monograph is harmonized with the European Pharmacopoeia and the U.S. Pharmacopeia.

The parts of the text that are not harmonized are marked with symbols (◆ ◆).

Information on the harmonization with the European Pharmacopoeia and the U.S. Pharmacopeia is available on the website of the Pharmaceuticals and Medical Devices Agency.

Carmellose is partly *O*-carboxymethylated cellulose.

◆**Description** Carmellose occurs as a white powder.
It is practically insoluble in ethanol (95).
It swells with water to form suspension.
It becomes viscid in sodium hydroxide TS.
It is hygroscopic.◆

Identification **(1)** Determine the infrared absorption spectrum of Carmellose as directed in the potassium bromide disk method under Infrared Spectrophotometry <*2.25*>, and compare the spectrum with the Reference Spectrum: both spectra exhibit similar intensities of absorption at the same wave numbers.

(2) The pH <*2.54*> of a suspension, obtained by shaking 1 g of Carmellose with 100 mL of water, is between 3.5 and 5.0.

Purity **(1)** Chloride—Shake well 0.8 g of Carmellose with 50 mL of water, add 10 mL of sodium hydroxide TS to dissolve, and add water to make 100 mL. Heat 20 mL of this solution with 10 mL of dilute nitric acid in a water bath until a flocculent precipitate is produced, cool, centrifuge, and take out the supernatant liquid. Wash the precipitate with three 10-mL portions of water by centrifuge each time, combine the supernatant liquid and the washings, and add water to make 100 mL. Take 25 mL of this solution in a Nessler tube, add 6 mL of dilute nitric acid and water to make 50 mL, and use this solution as the test solution. Separately, to 0.40 mL of 0.01 mol/L hydrochloric acid VS add 6 mL of dilute nitric acid and water to make 50 mL, and use this solution as the control solution. To the test solution and the control solution add 1 mL each of silver nitrate TS, ◆mix,◆ and allow to stand protected from light for 5 minutes. Compare the opalescence developed in both solutions ◆against a black background by viewing downward or transversely◆. The opalescence in the test solution is not more intense than that in the control solution (not more than 0.36%).

(2) Sulfate—Shake well 0.40 g of Carmellose with 25 mL of water, add 5 mL of sodium hydroxide TS to dissolve, and add 20 mL of water. Heat this solution with 2.5 mL of hydrochloric acid in a water bath until a flocculent precipitate is produced, cool, centrifuge, and take out the supernatant liquid. Wash the precipitate with three 10-mL portions of water by centrifuge each time, combine the supernatant liquid and the washings, and add water to make 100 mL. Filter this solution, discard the first 5 mL of the filtrate, take 25 mL of the subsequent filtrate in a Nessler tube, add 1 mL of dilute hydrochloric acid and water to make 50 mL, and use this solution as the test solution. Separately, to 1.5 mL of 0.005 mol/L sulfuric acid VS add 1 mL of dilute hydrochloric acid and water to make 50 mL, and use this solution as the control solution. To the test solution and the control solution add 2 mL each of barium chloride TS, mix, and allow to stand for 10 minutes. Compare the opalescence developed in both solutions ◆against a black background by viewing downward or transversely◆. The opalescence in the test solution is not more intense than that in the control solution (not more than 0.72%).

◆**(3)** Heavy metals *<1.07>*—Proceed with 1.0 g of Carmellose according to Method 2, and perform the test. Prepare the control solution with 2.0 mL of Standard Lead Solution (not more than 20 ppm).◆

Loss on drying *<2.41>* Not more than 8.0% (1 g, 105°C, 4 hours).

Residue on ignition *<2.44>* Not more than 1.5% (after drying, 1 g).

◆**Containers and storage** Containers—Tight containers.◆

Carmellose Calcium

Carboxymethylcellulose Calcium

カルメロースカルシウム

[9050-04-8]

This monograph is harmonized with the European Pharmacopoeia and the U.S. Pharmacopeia.

The parts of the text that are not harmonized are marked with symbols (◆ ◆).

Information on the harmonization with the European Pharmacopoeia and the U.S. Pharmacopeia is available on the website of the Pharmaceuticals and Medical Devices Agency.

Carmellose Calcium is the calcium salt of partly *O*-carboxymethylated cellulose.

◆**Description** Carmellose Calcium occurs as a white to yellowish white powder.

It is practically insoluble in ethanol (95) and in diethyl ether.

It swells with water to form a suspension.

The pH of a suspension, obtained by shaking 1.0 g of Carmellose Calcium with 100 mL of water, is between 4.5 and 6.0.

It is hygroscopic.◆

Identification **(1)** Shake thoroughly 0.1 g of Carmellose Calcium with 10 mL of water, followed by 2 mL of sodium hydroxide TS, allow to stand for 10 minutes, and use this solution as the sample solution. To 1 mL of the sample solution add water to make 5 mL. To 1 drop of this solution add 0.5 mL of chromotropic acid TS, and heat in a water bath for 10 minutes: a red-purple color develops.

(2) Shake 5 mL of the sample solution obtained in (1) with 10 mL of acetone: a white, flocculent precipitate is produced.

(3) Shake 5 mL of the sample solution obtained in (1) with 1 mL of iron (III) chloride TS: a brown, flocculent precipitate is produced.

(4) Ignite 1 g of Carmellose Calcium to ash, dissolve the residue in 10 mL of water and 6 mL of acetic acid (31), and filter, if necessary. Boil the filtrate, cool, and neutralize with ammonia TS: the solution responds to Qualitative Tests *<1.09>* (1) and (3) for calcium salt.

Purity **(1)** Alkalinity—Shake thoroughly 1.0 g of Carmellose Calcium with 50 mL of freshly boiled and cooled water, and add 2 drops of phenolphthalein TS: no red color develops.

(2) Chloride *<1.03>*—Shake thoroughly 0.80 g of Carmellose Calcium with 50 mL of water, add 10 mL of sodium hydroxide TS to dissolved, add water to make 100 mL, and use this solution as the sample solution. Heat 20 mL of the sample solution with 10 mL of 2 mol/L nitric acid TS on a water bath until a flocculent precipitate is produced. After cooling, centrifuge, and take out the supernatant liquid. Wash the precipitate with three 10-mL portions of water by centrifuging each time, combine the supernatant and the washings, and add water to make 100 mL. Take 25 mL of this solution, and add 1 mL of nitric acid and water to make 50 mL. Perform the test using this solution as the test solution. Prepare the control solution with 0.40 mL of 0.01 mol/L hydrochloric acid VS (not more than 0.36%).

(3) Sulfate *<1.14>*—Heat 10 mL of the sample solution obtained in (2) with 1 mL of hydrochloric acid in a water bath until a flocculent precipitate is produced. Cool, centrifuge, and take out the supernatant liquid. Wash the precipitate with three 10-mL portions of water by centrifuging each time, combine the supernatant and the washings, and add water to make 100 mL. Perform the test with 25 mL this solution as the test solution. Prepare the control solution with 0.42 mL of 0.005 mol/L sulfuric acid VS. To the test solution and the control solution add 1 mL of 3 mol/L hydrochloric acid TS and 3 mL of barium chloride TS, then add water to make 50 mL, and mix. Allow to stand for 10 minutes, and compare the turbidity of these solutions: the turbidity obtained with the test solution is not more than that obtained with the control solution (not more than 1.0%).

◆**(4)** Heavy metals <*1.07*>—Proceed with 1.0 g of Carmellose Calcium according to Method 2, and perform the test. Prepare the control solution with 2.0 mL of Standard Lead Solution (not more than 20 ppm).◆

Loss on drying <*2.41*> Not more than 10.0% (1 g, 105°C, 4 hours).

Residue on ignition <*2.44*> 10 - 20% (after drying 1 g).

◆**Containers and storage** Containers—Tight containers.◆

Carmellose Sodium

Carboxymethylcellulose Sodium

カルメロースナトリウム

[*9004-32-4*]

Carmellose Sodium is the sodium salt of partly *O*-carboxymethylated cellulose.

It, when dried, contains not less than 6.5% and not more than 8.5% of sodium (Na: 22.99).

Description Carmellose Sodium occurs as a white to yellowish white, powder or granules. It has no taste.

It is practically insoluble in methanol, in ethanol (95), in acetic acid (100) and in diethyl ether.

It forms a viscid solution in water and in warm water.

It is hygroscopic.

Identification **(1)** Dissolve 0.2 g of Carmellose Sodium in 20 mL of warm water with stirring, cool, and use this solution as the sample solution. To 1 mL of the sample solution add water to make 5 mL. To 1 drop of this solution add 0.5 mL of concentrated chromotropic acid TS, and heat in a water bath for 10 minutes: a red-purple color develops.

(2) To 10 mL of the sample solution obtained in test (1) add 1 mL of copper (II) sulfate TS: a blue flocculent precipitate is produced.

(3) To 3 g of Carmellose Sodium add 20 mL of methanol and 2 mL of dilute hydrochloric acid, boil gently on a water bath for 5 minutes, and filter. Evaporate the filtrate to dryness, and add 20 mL of water to the residue: the solution responds to Qualitative Tests <*1.09*> for sodium salt.

pH <*2.54*> Add 1.0 g of Carmellose Sodium in small portions to 100 mL of warm water with stirring, dissolve, and cool: the pH of this solution is between 6.0 and 8.0.

Purity **(1)** Clarity and color of solution—Firmly attach a glass plate of good quality 2 mm in thickness, to the bottom of a glass column 250 mm in height, 25 mm in inner diameter and 2 mm in thickness. This is used as an outer tube. Similarly prepare an inner tube by attaching a glass plate of good quality 2 mm in thickness to the bottom of a glass column 300 mm in height, 15 mm in inner diameter and 2 mm in thickness. Dissolve 1.0 g of Carmellose Sodium in 100 mL of water, pour this solution into the outer tube, and place on a piece of white paper on which 15 parallel black lines 1 mm in width and 1 mm in interval are drawn. Moving the inner tube up and down and observing from the upper part, determine the height of the solution up to the lower edge of the inner tube when the distinction of the lines becomes impossible. Repeat the operation 3 times, and calculate the mean value: it is larger than that calculated from the similar operation, using the following control solution.

Control solution: To 5.50 mL of 0.005 mol/L sulfuric acid VS add 1 mL of dilute hydrochloric acid, 5 mL of ethanol (95) and water to make 50 mL. Add 2 mL of barium chloride TS, mix well, and allow to stand for 10 minutes. Shake well this solution before use.

(2) Chloride <*1.03*>—Dissolve 0.5 g of Carmellose Sodium in 50 mL of water, and use this solution as the sample solution. Shake 10 mL of the sample solution with 10 mL of dilute nitric acid, heat to produce a flocculent precipitate in a water bath, cool, and centrifuge. Separate the supernatant liquid, wash the precipitate with three 10-mL portions of water, centrifuging each time, combine the supernatant liquid with the washings, and dilute with water to 200 mL. Perform the test using 50 mL of this solution as the test solution. Prepare the control solution with 0.45 mL of 0.01 mol/L hydrochloric acid VS (not more than 0.640%).

(3) Sulfate <*1.14*>—Add 1 mL of hydrochloric acid to 10 mL of the sample solution obtained in (2), shake well, heat to produce a flocculent precipitate in a water bath, cool, and centrifuge. Separate the supernatant liquid, wash the precipitate with three 10-mL portions of water, centrifuging each time, combine the washings with the supernatant liquid mentioned above, and dilute to 50 mL with water. Take 10 mL of this solution, dilute with water to 50 mL, and perform the test using this solution as the test solution. Prepare the control solution with 0.40 mL of 0.005 mol/L sulfuric acid VS (not more than 0.960%).

(4) Silicate—Weigh accurately about 1 g of Carmellose Sodium, ignite in a platinum dish, add 20 mL of dilute hydrochloric acid, cover with a watch glass, and boil gently for 30 minutes. Remove the watch glass, and evaporate on a water bath to dryness with the aid of a current of air. Continue heating for further 1 hour, add 10 mL of hot water, stir well, and filter through a filter paper for quantitative analysis. Wash the residue with hot water, dry together with the filter paper after no turbidity is produced on the addition of silver nitrate TS to the last washing, and then ignite to constant mass: the mass of the residue is not more than 0.5%.

(5) Heavy metals <*1.07*>—Proceed with 1.0 g of Carmellose Sodium according to Method 2, and perform the test. Prepare the control solution with 2.0 mL of Standard Lead Solution (not more than 20 ppm).

(6) Arsenic <*1.11*>—To 1.0 g of Carmellose Sodium add 20 mL of nitric acid, heat gently until it becomes fluid, cool, add 5 mL of sulfuric acid, and heat until white fumes are evolved. Add, if necessary, 5 mL of nitric acid after cooling, and heat again. Repeat this operation until the solution becomes colorless or slightly yellow. After cooling, add 15 mL of a saturated solution of ammonium oxalate monohydrate, and heat until white fumes are evolved again, cool, and dilute with water to 25 mL. Take 5 mL of this solution as the test solution, and perform the test. The solution has no more color than the following color standard.

Color standard: Without using Carmellose Sodium, proceed in the same manner, then transfer 5 mL of this solution to a generator bottle, add exactly 2 mL of Standard Arsenic Solution, and proceed as directed for the test with the test solution (not more than 10 ppm).

(7) Starch—Add 2 drops of iodine TS to 10 mL of the sample solution obtained in (2): no blue color develops.

Loss on drying <*2.41*> Not more than 10.0% (1 g, 105°C, 4 hours).

Assay Weigh accurately about 0.5 g of Carmellose Sodium, previously dried, add 80 mL of acetic acid (100), connect with a reflux condenser, and heat in an oil bath maintained at 130°C for 2 hours. Cool, and titrate <*2.50*> with 0.1 mol/L perchloric acid VS (potentiometric titration). Perform a blank determination in the same manner, and make any necessary correction.

Each mL of 0.1 mol/L perchloric acid VS
= 2.299 mg of Na

Containers and storage Containers—Tight containers.

Croscarmellose Sodium

クロスカルメロースナトリウム

[74811-65-7]

This monograph is harmonized with the European Pharmacopoeia and the U.S. Pharmacopeia.

The parts of the text that are not harmonized are marked with symbol (◆ ◆).

Information on the harmonization with the European Pharmacopoeia and the U.S. Pharmacopeia is available on the website of the Pharmaceuticals and Medical Devices Agency.

Croscarmellose Sodium is the sodium salt of cross-linked, partly *O*-carboxymethylated cellulose.

◆**Description** Croscarmellose Sodium occurs as a white to yellowish white powder.

It is practically insoluble in ethanol (99.5) and in diethyl ether.

It swells with water and becomes a suspension.

It is hygroscopic.◆

Identification **(1)** To 1 g of Croscarmellose Sodium add 100 mL of a solution of methylene blue (1 in 250,000), stir well, and allow to stand: blue cotton-like precipitates appear.

(2) To 1 g of Croscarmellose Sodium add 50 mL of water, and stir well to make a suspension. To 1 mL of this suspension add 1 mL of water and 5 drops of fleshly prepared solution of 1-naphtol in methanol (1 in 25), and gently add 2 mL of sulfuric acid along a wall of the vessel: a red-purple color appears at the zone of contact.

(3) The suspension obtained in (2) responds to Qualitative Tests *<1.09>* (1) for sodium salt.

pH *<2.54>* To 1.0 g of Croscarmellose Sodium add 100 mL of water, and stir for 5 minutes: the pH of the supernatant liquid is between 5.0 and 7.0.

Purity ◆**(1)** Heavy metals *<1.07>*—Proceed with 2.0 g of Croscarmellose Sodium according to Method 2, and perform the test. Prepare the control solution with 2.0 mL of Standard Lead Solution (not more than 10 ppm).◆

◆**(2)** Sodium chloride and sodium glycolate—The total amount of sodium chloride and sodium glycolate is not more than 0.5%, calculated on the dried basis.

(i) Sodium chloride: Weigh accurately about 5 g of Croscarmellose Sodium, add 50 mL of water and 5 mL of hydrogen peroxide (30), and heat on a water bath for 20 minutes with occasional stirring. After cooling, add 100 mL of water and 10 mL of nitric acid, and titrate *<2.50>* with 0.1 mol/L silver nitrate VS (potentiometric titration). Perform a blank determination in the same manner, and make any necessary correction.

Each mL of 0.1 mol/L silver nitrate VS
= 5.844 mg of NaCl

(ii) Sodium glycolate: Weigh accurately about 0.5 g of Croscarmellose Sodium, add 2 mL of acetic acid (100) and 5 mL of water, and stir for 15 minutes. Add gradually 50 mL of acetone with stirring, then add 1 g of sodium chloride, stir for 3 minutes, and filter through a filter paper moistened with acetone. Wash the residue thoroughly with 30 mL of acetone, combine the filtrate and washings, add acetone to make exactly 100 mL, and use this solution as the sample stock solution. Separately, dissolve 0.100 g of glycolic acid in water to make 200 mL. Pipet 0.5 mL, 1 mL, 2 mL, 3 mL and 4 mL of this solution, add water to make them exactly 5 mL, then add 5 mL of acetic acid (100) and acetone to make exactly 100 mL, and designate them standard stock solution (1), standard stock solution (2), standard stock solution (3), standard stock solution (4) and standard stock solution (5), respectively. Pipet 2 mL each of the sample stock solution and the standard stock solutions (1), (2), (3), (4) and (5), and heat them in a water bath for 20 minutes to evaporate acetone. After cooling, add exactly 5 mL of 2,7-dihydroxynaphthalene TS, mix, then add 15 mL of 2,7-dihydroxynaphthalene TS, mix, cover the mouth of the vessels with aluminum foil, and heat in a water bath for 20 minutes. After cooling, add sulfuric acid to make exactly 25 mL, mix, and designate them sample solution, standard solution (1), standard solution (2), standard solution (3), standard solution (4) and standard solution (5), respectively. Separately, to 10 mL of a mixture of water and acetic acid (100) (1:1) add acetone to make exactly 100 mL, and proceed with exactly 2 mL of this solution in the same manner for preparation of the sample solution, and use the solution so obtained as the blank solution. Determine the absorbances, A_T, A_{S1}, A_{S2}, A_{S3}, A_{S4} and A_{S5}, of the sample solution and the standard solutions (1), (2), (3), (4) and (5), respectively, at 540 nm as directed under Ultraviolet-visible Spectrophotometry *<2.24>*, using the blank solution as the control. Determine the amount (g) of glycolic acid, X, in 100 mL of the sample stock solution from the calibration curve obtained with the standard solutions, and calculate the amount of sodium glycolate by the following formula.

$$\text{Amount (\%) of sodium glycolate} = X/M \times 100 \times 1.289$$

M: Amount (g) of sample taken, calculated on the dried basis◆

◆**(3)** Water-soluble substance—Weigh accurately about 10 g of Croscarmellose Sodium, disperse in 800 mL of water by stirring for 1 minute every 10 minutes during 30 minutes, and allow to stand for at most 1 hour to precipitate. Filter by suction or centrifuge the clear upper portion, and weigh accurately the mass of about 150 mL of the filtrate or supernatant liquid. Heat to concentrate this liquid avoiding to dryness, then dry at 105°C for 4 hours, and weigh the mass of the residue accurately. Calculate the amount of the water-soluble substance by the following formula: not less than 1.0% and not more than 10.0%.

$$\text{Amount (\%) of water-soluble substance} = 100\, M_3\, (800 + M_1)/M_1M_2$$

M_1: Amount (g) of sample taken, calculated on the dried basis

M_2: Amount (g) of the filtrate or supernatant liquid of about 150 mL

M_3: Amount (g) of the residue◆

Precipitation test Put 75 mL of water in a 100-mL glass-stoppered graduated cylinder, and add portion by portion with 1.5 g of Croscarmellose Sodium divided into three portions while shaking vigorously at each time. Then, add water to make 100 mL, shake until to get a homogenous dispersion, and allow to stand for 4 hours: the volume of the settled layer is not less than 10.0 mL and not more than 30.0 mL.

Degree of substitution Weigh accurately about 1 g of Croscarmellose Sodium, put in a 500-mL glass-stoppered conical flask, add 300 mL of sodium chloride TS, then add 25.0 mL of 0.1 mol/L sodium hydroxide VS, stopper, and allow to stand for 5 minutes with occasional shaking. Add 5 drops of *m*-cresol purple TS, then add exactly 15 mL of 0.1 mol/L hydrochloric acid VS using a buret, stopper the flask, and shake. If the color of the solution is purple, add exactly 1-mL portions of 0.1 mol/L hydrochloric acid VS using the buret, with shaking each time, until the color of the solution changes to yellow, then titrate <2.50> with 0.1 mol/L sodium hydroxide VS until the color changes from yellow to purple. Perform a blank determination in the same manner. Calculate the degrees of substitution of acid-carboxymethyl group and sodium-carboxymethyl group, A and S: $A + S$ is not less than 0.60 and not more than 0.85.

$$A = 1150M/(7102 - 412M - 80C)$$
$$S = (162 + 58A)C/(7102 - 80C)$$

M: Amount (mmol) of sodium hydroxide needed to neutralize 1 g of sample taken, calculated on the dried basis

C: The value (%) obtained in Residue on ignition

Loss on drying <2.41> Not more than 10.0% (1 g, 105°C, 6 hours).

Residue on ignition <2.44> 14.0 - 28.0% (after drying, 1 g).

Containers and storage Containers—Tight containers.

Carmofur

カルモフール

$C_{11}H_{16}FN_3O_3$: 257.26
5-Fluoro-1-(hexylaminocarbonyl)uracil
[61422-45-5]

Carmofur, when dried, contains not less than 98.0% of carmofur ($C_{11}H_{16}FN_3O_3$).

Description Carmofur occurs as a white crystalline powder.

It is very soluble in *N,N*-dimethylformamide, freely soluble in acetic acid (100), soluble in diethyl ether, sparingly soluble in methanol and in ethanol (99.5), and practically insoluble in water.

Melting point: about 111°C (with decomposition).

Identification **(1)** Proceed with 5 mg of Carmofur as directed under Oxygen Flask Combustion Method <1.06>, using a mixture of 0.5 mL of 0.01 mol/L sodium hydroxide TS and 20 mL of water as the absorbing liquid, and prepare the test solution: the test solution responds to Qualitative Tests <1.09> (2) for fluoride.

(2) Determine the absorption spectrum of a solution of Carmofur in a mixture of methanol and phosphoric acid-acetic acid-boric acid buffer solution (pH 2.0) (9:1) (1 in 100,000) as directed under Ultraviolet-visible Spectrophotometry <2.24>, and compare the spectrum with the Reference Spectrum: both spectra exhibit similar intensities of absorption at the same wavelengths.

(3) Determine the infrared absorption spectrum of Carmofur, previously dried, as directed in the potassium bromide disk method under Infrared Spectrophotometry <2.25>, and compare the spectrum with the Reference Spectrum: both spectra exhibit similar intensities of absorption at the same wave numbers.

Purity **(1)** Heavy metals <1.07>—Proceed with 2.0 g of Carmofur according to Method 2, and perform the test. Prepare the control solution with 2.0 mL of Standard Lead Solution (not more than 10 ppm).

(2) Related substances—Dissolve 0.20 g of Carmofur in 10 mL of a mixture of methanol and acetic acid (100) (99:1), and use this solution as the sample solution. Pipet 1 mL of the sample solution, add a mixture of methanol and acetic acid (100) (99:1) to make exactly 500 mL, and use this solution as the standard solution. Perform the test with these solutions as directed under Thin-layer Chromatography <2.03>. Spot 15 μL each of the sample solution and standard solution on a plate of silica gel with fluorescent indicator for thin-layer chromatography. Develop the plate with a mixture of toluene and acetone (5:3) to a distance of about 12 cm, and air-dry the plate. Examine under ultraviolet light (main wavelength: 254 nm): the spots other than the principal spot from the sample solution are not more intense than the spot from the standard solution. After exposure of the plate to bromine vapor for 30 second, spray evenly a solution of fluorescein in ethanol (95) (1 in 2500): the spots other than the principal spot obtained from the sample solution are not more intense than the spot from the standard solution.

Loss on drying <2.41> Not more than 0.5% (1 g, in vacuum, 50°C, 3 hours).

Residue on ignition <2.44> Not more than 0.1% (1 g).

Assay Weigh accurately about 0.5 g of Carmofur, previously dried, dissolve in 20 mL of *N,N*-dimethylformamide, and titrate <2.50> with 0.1 mol/L tetramethylammonium hydroxide-methanol VS until the color of the solution changes from yellow through blue-green to blue (indicator: 3 drops of thymol blue-dimethylformamide TS).

Each mL of 0.1 mol/L tetramethylammonium hydroxide-methanol VS
= 25.73 mg of $C_{11}H_{16}FN_3O_3$

Containers and storage Containers—Tight containers.

Carteolol Hydrochloride

カルテオロール塩酸塩

and enantiomer

$C_{16}H_{24}N_2O_3.HCl$: 328.83
5-[(2*RS*)-3-(1,1-Dimethylethyl)amino-2-hydroxypropyloxy]-3,4-dihydroquinolin-2(1*H*)-one monohydrochloride
[*51781-21-6*]

Carteolol Hydrochloride, when dried, contains not less than 99.0% of carteolol hydrochloride ($C_{16}H_{24}N_2O_3.HCl$).

Description Carteolol Hydrochloride occurs as white, crystals or crystalline powder.

It is soluble in water, sparingly soluble in methanol, very slightly soluble in ethanol (95) and in acetic acid (100), and practically insoluble in diethyl ether.

The pH of a solution of 1.0 g of Carteolol Hydrochloride in 100 mL of water is between 5.0 and 6.0.

The solution of Carteolol Hydrochloride (1 in 20) shows no optical rotation.

Melting point: about 277°C (with decomposition).

Identification **(1)** Dissolve 0.1 g of Carteolol Hydrochloride in 5 mL of water, and add 5 drops of Reinecke salt TS: a light red precipitate is formed.

(2) Determine the absorption spectrum of a solution of Carteolol Hydrochloride (1 in 100,000) as directed under Ultraviolet-visible Spectrophotometry <*2.24*>, and compare the spectrum with the Reference Spectrum: both spectra exhibit similar intensities of absorption at the same wavelengths.

(3) Determine the infrared absorption spectrum of Carteolol Hydrochloride as directed in the potassium chloride disk method under Infrared Spectrophotometry <*2.25*>, and compare the spectrum with the Reference Spectrum: both spectra exhibit similar intensities of absorption at the same wave numbers.

(4) A solution of Carteolol Hydrochloride (1 in 50) responds to Qualitative Tests <*1.09*> for chloride.

Purity **(1)** Clarity and color of solution—Dissolve 1.0 g of Carteolol Hydrochloride in 30 mL of water: the solution is clear and colorless.

(2) Heavy metals <*1.07*>—Proceed with 2.0 g of Carteolol Hydrochloride according to Method 2, and perform the test. Prepare the control solution with 2.0 mL of Standard Lead Solution (not more than 10 ppm).

(3) Arsenic <*1.11*>—Prepare the test solution with 1.0 g of Carteolol Hydrochloride according to Method 3, and perform the test (not more than 2 ppm).

(4) Related substances—Dissolve 0.20 g of Carteolol Hydrochloride in 10 mL of methanol, and use this solution as the sample solution. Pipet 2 mL of the sample solution, and add methanol to make exactly 100 mL. Pipet 1 mL of this solution, add methanol to make exactly 10 mL, and use this solution as the standard solution. Perform the test with these solutions as directed under Thin-layer Chromatography <*2.03*>. Spot 10 μL each of the sample solution and standard solution on a plate of silica gel with fluorescent indicator for thin-layer chromatography. Develop the plate with a mixture of chloroform, methanol and ammonia solution (28) (50:20:1) to a distance of about 12 cm, and air-dry the plate. Examine under ultraviolet light (main wavelength: 254 nm): the spots other than the principal spot obtained from the sample solution are not more intense than the spot from the standard solution.

Loss on drying <*2.41*> Not more than 0.5% (1 g, 105°C, 3 hours).

Residue on ignition <*2.44*> Not more than 0.1% (1 g).

Assay Weigh accurately about 0.5 g of Carteolol Hydrochloride, previously dried, add 30 mL of acetic acid (100), dissolve by heating on a water bath, and cool. After adding 70 mL of acetic anhydride, titrate <*2.50*> with 0.1 mol/L perchloric acid VS (potentiometric titration). Perform a blank determination in the same manner, and make any necessary correction.

Each mL of 0.1 mol/L perchloric acid VS
= 32.88 mg of $C_{16}H_{24}N_2O_3.HCl$

Containers and storage Containers—Well-closed containers.

Carumonam Sodium

カルモナムナトリウム

$C_{12}H_{12}N_6Na_2O_{10}S_2$: 510.37
Disodium (*Z*)-{(2-aminothiazol-4-yl)[(2*S*,3*S*)-2-carbamoyloxymethyl-4-oxo-1-sulfonatoazetidin-3-ylcarbamoyl]methyleneaminooxy}acetate
[*86832-68-0*]

Carumonam Sodium contains not less than 850 μg (potency) and not more than 920 μg (potency) per mg, calculated on the anhydrous basis. The potency of Carumonam Sodium is expressed as mass (potency) of carumonam ($C_{12}H_{14}N_6O_{10}S_2$: 466.40).

Description Carumonam Sodium occurs as a white to yellowish white, crystals or crystalline powder.

It is freely soluble in water, soluble in formamide, very slightly soluble in methanol, and practically insoluble in ethanol (99.5) and in acetic acid (100).

Identification **(1)** Determine the absorption spectrum of a solution of Carumonam Sodium (3 in 100,000) as directed under Ultraviolet-visible Spectrophotometry <*2.24*>, and compare the spectrum with the Reference Spectrum or the spectrum of a solution of Carumonam Sodium RS prepared in the same manner as the sample solution: both spectra exhibit similar intensities of absorption at the same wavelengths.

(2) Determine the infrared absorption spectrum of Carumonam Sodium as directed in the potassium bromide disk method under Infrared Spectrophotometry <*2.25*>, and compare the spectrum with the Reference Spectrum or the spectrum of Carumonam Sodium RS: both spectra exhibit similar intensities of absorption at the same wave numbers.

(3) Determine the ^1H spectrum of a solution of

Carumonam Sodium in heavy water for nuclear magnetic resonance spectroscopy (1 in 10) as directed under Nuclear Magnetic Resonance Spectroscopy <*2.21*>, using sodium 3-trimethylsilylpropionate-d_4 for nuclear magnetic resonance spectroscopy as an internal reference compound: it exhibits a doublet signal A at around δ 5.5 ppm, and a singlet signal B at around δ 7.0 ppm. The ratio of the integrated intensity of these signals, A:B, is about 1:1.

(4) Carumonam Sodium responds to Qualitative Tests <*1.09*> (1) for sodium salt.

Optical rotation <*2.49*> $[\alpha]_D^{20}$: +18.5 – +21.0° (0.1 g calculated on the anhydrous basis, water, 10 mL, 100 mm).

pH <*2.54*> The pH of a solution obtained by dissolving 1.0 g of Carumonam Sodium in 10 mL of water is between 5.0 and 6.5.

Purity **(1)** Clarity and color of solution—Dissolve 0.5 g of Carumonam Sodium in 5 mL of water: the solution is clear and colorless to pale yellow.

(2) Heavy metals <*1.07*>—Proceed with 2.0 g of Carumonam Sodium according to Method 2, and perform the test. Prepare the control solution with 3.0 mL of Standard Lead Solution (not more than 15 ppm).

(3) Arsenic <*1.11*>—Prepare the test solution with 2.0 g of Carumonam Sodium according to Method 4, and perform the test (not more than 1 ppm).

(4) Related substance 1—Weigh accurately about 0.1 g of Carumonam Sodium, and dissolve in the mobile phase to make exactly 50 mL. Pipet 5 mL of this solution, add the mobile phase to make exactly 25 mL, and use this solution as the sample solution. Separately, weigh accurately about 0.1 g of Carumonam Sodium RS, and dissolve in the mobile phase to make exactly 50 mL. Pipet 5 mL of this solution, and add the mobile phase to make exactly 25 mL. Pipet 1 mL of this solution, add the mobile phase to make exactly 100 mL, and use this solution as the standard solution. Perform the test with exactly 10 μL each of the sample solution and standard solution as directed under Liquid Chromatography <*2.01*> according to the following conditions, and determine each peak area by the automatic integration method. Calculate the amount of the related substances by the following equation: the amount of the related substance having the relative retention time of about 0.7 to carumonam is not more than 4.0%, and each amount of the related substances other than the related substance having the relative retention time of about 0.7 is not more than 1.0%.

$$\text{Amount (\%) of related substance} = M_S/M_T \times A_T/A_S$$

M_S: Amount (g) of Carumonam Sodium RS taken
M_T: Amount (g) of Carumonam Sodium taken
A_S: Peak area of carumonam from the standard solution
A_T: Each peak area other than carumonam from the sample solution

Operating conditions—

Detector, column, column temperature, mobile phase, and flow rate: Proceed as directed in the operating conditions in the Assay.

Time span of measurement: About 3 times as long as the retention time of carumonam.

System suitability—

Test for required detectability: Measure exactly 5 mL of the standard solution, and add the mobile phase to make exactly 50 mL. Confirm that the peak area of carumonam obtained with 10 μL of this solution is equivalent to 7 to 13% of that with 10 μL of the standard solution.

System performance: Dissolve 40 mg of Carumonam Sodium in 20 mL of the mobile phase. To 5 mL of this solution add 5 mL of a solution of resorcinol in the mobile phase (9 in 1000) and the mobile phase to make 25 mL. When the procedure is run with 10 μL of this solution under the above operating conditions, resorcinol and carumonam are eluted in this order with the resolution between these peaks being not less than 2.5.

System repeatability: When the test is repeated 3 times with 10 μL of the standard solution under the above operating conditions, the relative standard deviation of the peak area of carumonam is not more than 2.0%.

(5) Related substance 2—Weigh accurately about 0.1 g of Carumonam Sodium, and dissolve in the mobile phase to make exactly 50 mL. Pipet 5 mL of this solution, add the mobile phase to make exactly 25 mL, and use this solution as the sample solution. Separately, weigh accurately about 0.1 g of Carumonam Sodium RS, and dissolve in the mobile phase to make exactly 50 mL. Pipet 5 mL of this solution, and add the mobile phase to make exactly 25 mL. Pipet 1 mL of this solution, add the mobile phase to make exactly 100 mL, and use this solution as the standard solution. Perform the test with exactly 10 μL each of the sample solution and standard solution as directed under Liquid Chromatography <*2.01*> according to the following conditions, and determine each peak area by the automatic integration method. Calculate the amount of the related substances by the following equation: the amount of each related substance is not more than 1.0%.

$$\text{Amount (\%) of related substance} = M_S/M_T \times A_T/A_S$$

M_S: Amount (g) of Carumonam Sodium RS taken
M_T: Amount (g) of Carumonam Sodium taken
A_S: Peak area of carumonam from the standard solution
A_T: Each area of the peaks appeared after the peak of carumonam from the sample solution

Operating conditions—

Detector, column, and column temperature: Proceed as directed in the operating conditions in the Assay.

Mobile phase: A mixture of a solution of ammonium sulfate (1 in 10,000), methanol and acetic acid (100) (74:25:1).

Flow rate: Dissolve 0.01 g of phthalic acid in the mobile phase to make 100 mL. Adjust so that the retention time of phthalic acid is about 6.5 minutes when the procedure is run with 10 μL of this solution.

Time span of measurement: About 10 times as long as the retention time of carumonam.

System suitability—

Test for required detectability: Measure exactly 5 mL of the standard solution, and add the mobile phase to make exactly 50 mL. Confirm that the peak area of carumonam obtained with 10 μL of this solution is equivalent to 7 to 13% of that with 10 μL of the standard solution.

System performance: Dissolve 40 mg of Carumonam Sodium in 20 mL of the mobile phase. To 5 mL of this solution add 5 mL of a solution of resorcinol in the mobile phase (9 in 1000) and the mobile phase to make 25 mL. When the procedure is run with 10 μL of this solution under the above operating conditions, resorcinol and carumonam are eluted in this order with the resolution between these peaks being not less than 7.

System repeatability: When the test is repeated 3 times with 10 μL of the standard solution under the above operating conditions, the relative standard deviation of the peak area of carumonam is not more than 2.0%.

(6) Total amount of related substances—The total of the amounts of the related substances obtained in the Related substance 1 and the Related substance 2 is not more than 6.0%.

Water <*2.48*> Not more than 2.0% (0.2 g, volumetric titration, direct titration; Use a mixture of formamide for water determination and methanol for water determination (3:1) instead of methanol for water determination).

Assay Weigh accurately an amount of Carumonam Sodium and Carumonam Sodium RS, equivalent to about 40 mg (potency), and dissolve each in the mobile phase to make exactly 20 mL. Measure exactly 5 mL each of these solutions, add exactly 5 mL of the internal standard solution and the mobile phase to make 25 mL, and use these solutions as the sample solution and standard solution. Perform the test with 10 μL each of the sample solution and standard solution as directed under Liquid Chromatography <*2.01*> according to the following conditions, and calculate the ratios, Q_T and Q_S, of the peak area of carumonam to that of the internal standard.

Amount [μg (potency)] of carumonam ($C_{12}H_{14}N_6O_{10}S_2$)
$= M_S \times Q_T/Q_S \times 1000$

M_S: Amount [mg (potency)] of Carumonam Sodium RS taken

Internal standard solution—A solution of resorcinol in the mobile phase (9 in 1000).

Operating conditions—

Detector: An ultraviolet absorption photometer (wavelength: 254 nm).

Column: A stainless steel column 4 mm in inside diameter and 15 cm in length, packed with octadecylsilanized silica gel for liquid chromatography (5 μm in particle diameter).

Column temperature: A constant temperature of about 25°C.

Mobile phase: A mixture of a solution of ammonium sulfate (1 in 10,000), methanol and acetic acid (100) (97:2:1).

Flow rate: Adjust so that the retention time of carumonam is about 10 minutes.

System suitability—

System performance: When the procedure is run with 10 μL of the standard solution under the above operating conditions, the internal standard and carumonam are eluted in this order with the resolution between these peaks being not less than 2.5.

System repeatability: When the test is repeated 6 times with 10 μL of the standard solution under the above operating conditions, the relative standard deviation of the ratios of the peak area of carumonam to that of the internal standard is not more than 1.0%.

Containers and storage Containers—Hermetic containers.

Storage—Light-resistant.

Carvedilol

カルベジロール

and enantiomer

$C_{24}H_{26}N_2O_4$: 406.47
(2*RS*)-1-(9*H*-Carbazol-4-yloxy)-
3-{[2-(2-methoxyphenoxy)ethyl]amino}propan-2-ol
[*72956-09-3*]

Carvedilol, when dried, contains not less than 99.0% and not more than 101.0% of carvedilol ($C_{24}H_{26}N_2O_4$).

Description Carvedilol occurs as white to pale yellowish-white, crystals or crystalline powder.

It is freely soluble in acetic acid (100), sparingly soluble in methanol, slightly soluble in ethanol (99.5), and practically insoluble in water.

A solution of Carvedilol in methanol (1 in 100) shows no optical rotation.

Identification **(1)** Determine the absorption spectrum of a solution of Carvedilol in methanol (1 in 200,000) as directed under Ultraviolet-visible Spectrophotometry <*2.24*>, and compare the spectrum with the Reference Spectrum: both spectra exhibit similar intensities of absorption at the same wavelengths.

(2) Determine the infrared absorption spectrum of Carvedilol as directed in the potassium bromide disk method under Infrared Spectrophotometry <*2.25*>, and compare the spectrum with the Reference Spectrum: both spectra exhibit similar intensities of absorption at the same wave numbers.

Melting point <*2.60*> 114 – 119°C

Purity **(1)** Heavy metals <*1.07*>—Wrap 2.0 g of Carvedilol with a filter paper for quantitative analysis, then proceed according to Method 4, and perform the test. Prepare the control solution as follows: Put a filter paper for quantitative analysis in a crucible, add 10 mL of a solution of magnesium nitrate hexahydrate in ethanol (95) (1 in 10), then proceed as directed for the test solution, and add 2.0 mL of Standard Lead Solution and water to make 50 mL (not more than 10 ppm).

(2) Related substances—Dissolve 65 mg of Carvedilol in 100 mL of the mobile phase. To 1 mL of this solution add the mobile phase to make 10 mL, and use this solution as the sample solution. Pipet 1 mL of the sample solution, add the mobile phase to make exactly 100 mL, and use this solution as the standard solution. Perform the test with exactly 20 μL each of the sample solution and standard solution as directed under Liquid Chromatography <*2.01*> according to the following conditions. Determine each peak area by the automatic integration method: the area of the peak other than carvedilol obtained from the sample solution is not larger than 3/20 times the peak area of carvedilol from the standard solution, and the total area of the peaks other than carvedilol from the sample solution is not larger than 1/2 times the peak area of carvedilol from the standard solution.

Operating conditions—

Detector: An ultraviolet absorption photometer (wavelength: 240 nm).

Column: A stainless steel column 4.6 mm in inside diameter and 15 cm in length, packed with octylsilanized silica gel for liquid chromatography (5 μm in particle diameter).

Column temperature: A constant temperature of about 55°C.

Mobile phase: Dissolve 2.72 g of potassium dihydrogen phosphate in 900 mL of water, adjust to pH 2.0 with phosphoric acid, and add water to make 1000 mL. To 650 mL of this solution add 350 mL of acetonitrile.

Flow rate: Adjust so that the retention time of carvedilol is about 4 minutes.

Time span of measurement: About 9 times as long as the retention time of carvedilol, beginning after the solvent peak.

System suitability—

Test for required detectability: Pipet 2 mL of the standard solution, add the mobile phase to make exactly 20 mL. Confirm that the peak area of carvedilol obtained with 20 μL of this solution is equivalent to 7 to 13% of that with 20 μL of the standard solution.

System performance: When the procedure is run with 20 μL of the standard solution under the above operating conditions, the number of theoretical plates and the symmetry factor of the peak of carvedilol are not less than 6000 and not more than 1.5, respectively.

System repeatability: When the test is repeated 6 times with 20 μL of the standard solution under the above operating conditions, the relative standard deviation of the peak area of carvedilol is not more than 2.0%.

Loss on drying <*2.41*> Not more than 0.5% (1 g, 105°C, 2 hours).

Residue on ignition <*2.44*> Not more than 0.1% (1 g).

Assay Weigh accurately about 0.5 g of Carvedilol, previously dried, dissolve in 60 mL of acetic acid (100), and titrate <*2.50*> with 0.1 mol/L perchloric acid VS (potentiometric titration). Perform the blank determination in the same manner, and make any necessary correction.

Each mL of 0.1 mol/L perchloric acid VS
= 40.65 mg of $C_{24}H_{26}N_2O_4$

Containers and storage Containers—Tight containers.

Carvedilol Tablets

カルベジロール錠

Carvedilol Tablets contain not less than 95.0% and not more than 105.0% of the labeled amount of carvedilol ($C_{24}H_{26}N_2O_4$: 406.47).

Method of preparation Prepare as directed under Tablets, with Carvedilol.

Identification Powder Carvedilol Tablets. To a portion of the powder, equivalent to 20 mg of Carvedilol, add 10 mL of methanol, shake well, and filter. To 0.5 mL of the filtrate add methanol to make 200 mL, and determine the absorption spectrum of this solution as directed under Ultraviolet-visible Spectrophotometry <*2.24*>: it exhibits maxima between 222 nm and 226 nm, between 241 nm and 245 nm, between 284 nm and 288 nm, between 317 nm and 321 nm and between 330 nm and 334 nm.

Purity Related substances—In this procedure the sample solution should be stored not exceeding 5°C and used within 24 hours after preparation. Powder Carvedilol Tablets. Dissolve a portion of the powder, equivalent to 12.5 mg of Carvedilol, add an adequate amount of the mobile phase and disperse the particles with the aid of ultrasonic waves, if necessary, add the mobile phase to make 100 mL, and shake for 30 minutes. Filter through a membrane filter with a pore size not exceeding 0.22 μm, discard the first 5 mL of the filtrate, and use the subsequent filtrate as the sample solution. Pipet 1 mL of the sample solution, add the mobile phase to make exactly 100 mL, and use this solution as the standard solution. Perform the test with exactly 50 μL each of the sample solution and standard solution as directed under Liquid Chromatography <*2.01*> according to the following conditions, and determine each peak area by the automatic integration method: the area of the two peaks, having the relative retention time between 1.7 and 1.9 and between 2.0 and 3.1 to carvedilol, obtained from the sample solution of 1.25-mg or 2.5-mg tablet is not larger than 3/10 times and 1.6 times the peak area of carvedilol from the standard solution, respectively, the area of the peak other than carvedilol and the peaks mentioned above from the sample solution is not larger than 1/5 times the peak area of carvedilol from the standard solution, and the total area of the peaks other than carvedilol from the sample solution is not larger than 2.2 times the peak area of carvedilol from the standard solution. The area of the two peaks, having the relative retention time between 1.7 and 1.9 and between 2.0 and 3.1, from the sample solution of 10-mg or 20-mg tablet is not larger than 1/10 times and 2/5 times the peak area of carvedilol from the standard solution, respectively, the area of the peak other than carvedilol and the peak mentioned above from the sample solution is not larger than 1/10 times the peak area of carvedilol from the standard solution, and the total area of the peaks other than carvedilol from the sample solution is not larger than 3/5 times the peak area of carvedilol from the standard solution. For the area of the peak, having the relative retention time between 1.7 and 1.9 to carvedilol, multiply the correction factor 1.25.

Operating conditions—

Detector, column, column temperature, mobile phase, and flow rate: Proceed as directed in the operating conditions in the Assay.

Time span of measurement: About 10 times as long as the retention time of carvedilol, beginning after the solvent peak.

System suitability—

Test for required detectability: To exactly 5 mL of the standard solution add the mobile phase to make exactly 100 mL. Confirm that the peak area of carvedilol obtained with 50 μL of this solution is equivalent to 3.5 to 6.5% of that with 50 μL of the standard solution.

System performance: When the procedure is run with 50 μL of the standard solution under the above operating conditions, the number of theoretical plates and the symmetry factor of the peak of carvedilol are not less than 3000 and not more than 2.0, respectively.

System repeatability: When the test is repeated 6 times with 50 μL of the standard solution under the above operating conditions, the relative standard deviation of the peak area of carvedilol is not more than 1.0%.

Uniformity of dosage units <*6.02*> Perform the test according to the following method: it meets the requirement of the Content uniformity test.

To 1 tablet of Carvedilol Tablets add 70 mL of a mixture of 0.1 mol/L hydrochloric acid TS and methanol (1:1), shake until the tablet is completely disintegrated, then add a mixture of 0.1 mol/L hydrochloric acid TS and methanol (1:1) to make exactly 100 mL, and filter through a membrane filter with a pore size not exceeding 0.45 μm. Discard the first 10 mL of the filtrate, pipet V mL of the subsequent filtrate, add a mixture of 0.1 mol/L hydrochloric acid TS and methanol (1:1) to make exactly V' mL so that each mL contains about 5 μg of carvedilol ($C_{24}H_{26}N_2O_4$), and use this solution as the sample solution. Separately, weigh accurately about 25 mg of carvedilol for assay, previously dried at 105°C for 2 hours, and dissolve in a mixture of 0.1 mol/L hydrochloric acid TS and methanol (1:1) to make exactly 100 mL. Pipet 2 mL of this solution, add a mixture of 0.1 mol/L hydrochloric acid TS and methanol (1:1) to make exactly 100 mL, and use this solution as the standard solution. Determine the absorbances, A_T and A_S, of the sample solution and standard solution at 240 nm as directed under Ultraviolet-visible Spectrophotometry <2.24>.

Amount (mg) of carvedilol ($C_{24}H_{26}N_2O_4$)
$= M_S \times A_T/A_S \times V'/V \times 1/50$

M_S: Amount (mg) of carvedilol for assay taken

Dissolution <*6.10*> **(1)** 10-mg tablet and 20-mg tablet When the test is performed at 75 revolutions per minute according to the Paddle method, using 900 mL of 0.05 mol/L acetic acid-sodium acetate buffer solution (pH 4.0) as the dissolution medium, the dissolution rate in 30 minutes of Carvedilol Tablets is not less than 80%.

Start the test with 1 tablet of Carvedilol Tablets, withdraw not less than 20 mL of the medium at the specified minute after starting the test, and filter through a membrane filter with a pore size not exceeding 0.45 μm. Discard not less than 10 mL of the first filtrate, pipet V mL of the subsequent filtrate, add the dissolution medium to make exactly V' mL so that each mL contains about 11 μg of carvedilol ($C_{24}H_{26}N_2O_4$), and use this solution as the sample solution. Separately, weigh accurately about 28 mg of carvedilol for assay, previously dried at 105°C for 2 hours, and dissolve in methanol to make exactly 50 mL. Pipet 2 mL of this solution, add the dissolution medium to make exactly 100 mL, and use this solution as the standard solution. Determine the absorbances, A_T and A_S, at 285 nm of the sample solution and standard solution as directed under Ultraviolet-visible Spectrophotometry <*2.24*>, using the dissolution medium as the blank.

Dissolution rate (%) with respect to the labeled amount of carvedilol ($C_{24}H_{26}N_2O_4$)
$= M_S \times A_T/A_S \times V'/V \times 1/C \times 36$

M_S: Amount (mg) of carvedilol for assay taken
C: Labeled amount (mg) of carvedilol ($C_{24}H_{26}N_2O_4$) in 1 tablet

(2) 1.25-mg tablet and 2.5-mg tablet When the test is performed at 50 revolutions per minute according to the Paddle method, using 900 mL of 0.05 mol/L acetic acid-sodium acetate buffer solution (pH 4.0) as the dissolution medium, the dissolution rate in 20 minutes is not less than 75%.

Start the test with 1 tablet of Carvedilol Tablets, withdraw not less than 20 mL of the medium at the specified minute after starting the test, and filter through a membrane filter with a pore size not exceeding 0.45 μm. Discard not less than 10 mL of the first filtrate, pipet V mL of the subsequent filtrate, add the dissolution medium to make exactly V' mL so that each mL contains about 1.4 μg of carvedilol ($C_{24}H_{26}N_2O_4$), and use this solution as the sample solution. Separately, weigh accurately about 28 mg of carvedilol for assay, previously dried at 105°C for 2 hours, and dissolve in methanol to make exactly 200 mL. Pipet 2 mL of this solution, add the dissolution medium to make exactly 200 mL, and use this solution as the standard solution. Determine the absorbances, A_T and A_S, at 240 nm of the sample solution and standard solution as directed under Ultraviolet-visible Spectrophotometry <*2.24*>, using the dissolution medium as the blank.

Dissolution rate (%) with respect to the labeled amount of carvedilol ($C_{24}H_{26}N_2O_4$)
$= M_S \times A_T/A_S \times V'/V \times 1/C \times 9/2$

M_S: Amount (mg) of carvedilol for assay taken
C: Labeled amount (mg) of carvedilol ($C_{24}H_{26}N_2O_4$) in 1 tablet

Assay Weigh accurately the mass of not less than 20 Carvedilol Tablets, and powder. Weigh accurately a portion of the powder, equivalent to about 25 mg of carvedilol ($C_{24}H_{26}N_2O_4$), add exactly 5 mL of the internal standard solution, add a mixture of 0.1 mol/L hydrochloric acid TS and methanol (1:1) to make 250 mL, and shake for 30 minutes. To 2 mL of this solution, add the mobile phase to make 20 mL, and filter through a membrane filter with a pore size not exceeding 0.45 μm. Discard the first 10 mL of the filtrate, and use the subsequent filtrate as the sample solution. Separately, weigh accurately about 25 mg of carvedilol for assay, previously dried at 105°C for 2 hours, add exactly 5 mL of the internal standard solution, and add a mixture of 0.1 mol/L hydrochloric acid TS and methanol (1:1) to make 250 mL. To 2 mL of this solution add the mobile phase to make 20 mL, and use this solution as the standard solution. Perform the test with 10 μL each of the sample solution and standard solution as directed under Liquid Chromatography <*2.01*> under the following conditions, and calculate the ratios, Q_T and Q_S, of the peak area of carvedilol to that of the internal standard.

Amount (mg) of carvedilol ($C_{24}H_{26}N_2O_4$)
$= M_S \times Q_T/Q_S$

M_S: Amount (mg) of carvedilol for assay taken

Internal standard solution—A solution of isoamyl parahydroxybenzoate in the mobile phase (1 in 70).

Operating conditions—

Detector: An ultraviolet absorption photometer (wavelength: 240 nm).

Column: A stainless steel column 4.6 mm in inside diameter and 15 cm in length, packed with octadecylsilanized silica gel for liquid chromatography (5 μm in particle diameter).

Column temperature: A constant temperature of about 40°C.

Mobile phase: Dissolve 2.7 g of potassium dihydrogen phosphate in water to make 1000 mL, and adjust to pH 5.0 with a solution prepared by dissolving 0.7 g of dipotassium hydrogen phosphate in water to make 200 mL. To 450 mL of this solution add 550 mL of methanol.

Flow rate: Adjust so that the retention time of carvedilol is about 5 minutes.

System suitability—

System performance: When the procedure is run with 10 μL of the standard solution under the above operating conditions, carvedilol and the internal standard are eluted in this order with the resolution between these peaks being not less than 20.

System repeatability: When the test is repeated 6 times with 10 μL of the standard solution under the above operating conditions, the relative standard deviation of the ratio of the peak area of carvedilol to that of the internal standard is not more than 1.0%.

Containers and storage Containers—Tight containers.

Cefaclor

セファクロル

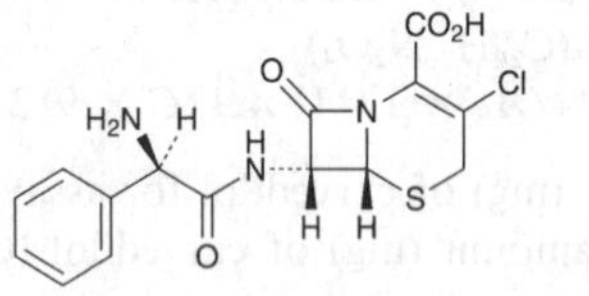

$C_{15}H_{14}ClN_3O_4S$: 367.81
(6*R*,7*R*)-7-[(2*R*)-2-Amino-2-phenylacetylamino]-3-chloro-8-oxo-5-thia-1-azabicyclo[4.2.0]oct-2-ene-2-carboxylic acid
[*53994-73-3*]

Cefaclor contains not less than 950 μg (potency) and not more than 1020 μg (potency) per mg, calculated on the anhydrous basis. The potency of Cefaclor is expressed as mass (potency) of cefaclor ($C_{15}H_{14}ClN_3O_4S$).

Description Cefaclor occurs as a white to yellow-white crystalline powder.

It is slightly soluble in water and in methanol, and practically insoluble in *N*,*N*-dimethylformamide and in ethanol (99.5).

Identification **(1)** Determine the absorption spectrum of a solution of Cefaclor (1 in 50,000) as directed under Ultraviolet-visible Spectrophotometry <*2.24*>, and compare the spectrum with the Reference Spectrum: both spectra exhibit similar intensities of absorption at the same wavelengths.

(2) Determine the infrared absorption spectrum of Cefaclor as directed in the potassium bromide disk method under Infrared Spectrophotometry <*2.25*>, and compare the spectrum with the Reference Spectrum: both spectra exhibit similar intensities of absorption at the same wave numbers.

(3) Dissolve 40 mg of Cefaclor in 0.5 mL of heavy water for nuclear magnetic resonance spectroscopy and 1 drop of deuterated hydrochloric acid for nuclear magnetic resonance spectroscopy, and determine the ^1H spectrum of this solution as directed under Nuclear Magnetic Resonance Spectroscopy <*2.21*>, using sodium 3-trimethylsilylpropanesulfonate for nuclear magnetic resonance spectroscopy as an internal reference compound: it exhibits an AB type quartet signal A at around δ 3.7 ppm, and a singlet signal or a sharp multiplet signal B at around δ 7.6 ppm. The ratio of the integrated intensity of each signal, A:B, is about 2:5.

(4) Perform the test with Cefaclor as directed under Flame Coloration Test <*1.04*> (2): a green color appears.

Optical rotation <*2.49*> $[\alpha]_D^{20}$: +105 – +120° (0.1 g calculated on the anhydrous basis, water, 25 mL, 100 mm).

Purity **(1)** Heavy metals <*1.07*>—Proceed with 1.0 g of Cefaclor according to Method 2, and perform the test. Prepare the control solution with 2.0 mL of Standard Lead Solution (not more than 20 ppm).

(2) Arsenic <*1.11*>—Prepare the test solution by suspending 1.0 g of Cefaclor in 10 mL of *N*,*N*-dimethylformamide, and perform the test (not more than 2 ppm).

(3) Related substances—Dissolve 50 mg of Cefaclor in 10 mL of sodium dihydrogen phosphate TS (pH 2.5), and use this solution as the sample solution. Pipet 1 mL of the sample solution, add sodium dihydrogen phosphate TS (pH 2.5) to make exactly 100 mL, and use this solution as the standard solution. Perform the test with exactly 20 μL each of the sample solution and standard solution as directed under Liquid Chromatography <*2.01*> according to the following conditions, and determine each peak area by the automatic integration method: the area of the peaks other than cefaclor obtained from the sample solution are not larger than 1/2 times the peak area of cefaclor from the standard solution, and the total area of the peaks other than cefaclor from the sample solution is not larger than 2 times of the peak area of cefaclor from the standard solution. If necessary, proceed with 20 μL of sodium dihydrogen phosphate TS (pH 2.5) in the same manner as above to compensate the base line.

Operating conditions—

Detector: An ultraviolet absorption photometer (wavelength: 220 nm).

Column: A stainless steel column 4.6 mm in inside diameter and 25 cm in length, packed with octadecylsilanized silica gel for liquid chromatography (5 μm in particle diameter).

Column temperature: A constant temperature of about 25°C.

Mobile phase A: Dissolve 7.8 g of sodium dihydrogen phosphate dihydrate in 1000 mL of water, and adjust the pH to 4.0 with phosphoric acid.

Mobile phase B: To 550 mL of the mobile phase A add 450 mL of acetonitrile for liquid chromatography.

Flowing of mobile phase: Control the gradient by mixing the mobile phases A and B as directed in the following table.

Time after injection of sample (min)	Mobile phase A (vol%)	Mobile phase B (vol%)
0 – 30	95 → 75	5 → 25
30 – 45	75 → 0	25 → 100
45 – 55	0	100

Flow rate: 1.0 mL per minute.

Time span of measurement: About 2.5 times as long as the retention time of cefaclor, beginning after the solvent peak.

System suitability—

Test for required detectability: Measure exactly 1 mL of the standard solution, and add sodium dihydrogen phosphate TS, pH 2.5 to make exactly 20 mL. Confirm that the peak area of cefaclor obtained with 20 μL of this solution is equivalent to 4 to 6% of that with 20 μL of the standard solution.

System performance: When the procedure is run with 20 μL of the standard solution under the above operating conditions, the number of theoretical plates and the symmetry factor of the peak of cefaclor are not less than 40,000 and 0.8 to 1.3, respectively.

System repeatability: When the test is repeated 3 times with 20 μL of the standard solution under the above operating conditions, the relative standard deviations of the peak areas and the retention times of cefaclor are not more than 2.0%, respectively.

Water <*2.48*> Not more than 6.5% (0.2 g, volumetric titration, back titration).

Assay Weigh accurately an amount of Cefaclor and Cefaclor RS, equivalent to about 50 mg (potency), and dissolve each in 0.1 mol/L phosphate buffer solution (pH 4.5) to make exactly 50 mL. Pipet 10 mL each of these solutions, add exactly 10 mL of the internal standard solution, add 0.1

mol/L phosphate buffer solution (pH 4.5) to make 50 mL, and use these solutions as the sample solution and the standard solution, respectively. Perform the test with 10 μL each of the sample solution and standard solution as directed under Liquid Chromatography <2.01> according to the following conditions, and calculate the ratios, Q_T and Q_S, of the peak area of cefaclor to that of the internal standard.

Amount [μg (potency)] of cefaclor ($C_{15}H_{14}ClN_3O_4S$)
$= M_S \times Q_T/Q_S \times 1000$

M_S: Amount [mg (potency)] of Cefaclor RS taken

Internal standard solution—A solution of 4-aminoacetophenone in 0.1 mol/L phosphate buffer solution (pH 4.5) (1 in 700).

Operating conditions—

Detector: An ultraviolet absorption photometer (wavelength: 254 nm).

Column: A stainless steel column 4.6 mm in inside diameter and 15 cm in length, packed with octadecylsilanized silica gel for liquid chromatography (5 μm in particle diameter).

Column temperature: A constant temperature of about 25°C.

Mobile phase: Dissolve 6.8 g of potassium dihydrogen phosphate in 1000 mL of water, and adjust the pH to 3.4 with diluted phosphoric acid (3 in 500). To 940 mL of this solution add 60 mL of acetonitrile.

Flow rate: Adjust so that the retention time of cefaclor is about 7 minutes.

System suitability—

System performance: When the procedure is run with 10 μL of the standard solution under the above operating conditions, cefaclor and the internal standard are eluted in this order with the resolution between these peaks being not less than 5.

System repeatability: When the test is repeated 6 times with 10 μL of the standard solution under the above operating conditions, the relative standard deviation of the ratios of the peak area of cefaclor to that of the internal standard is not more than 1.0%.

Containers and storage Containers—Tight containers.

Storage—Light-resistant.

Cefaclor Capsules

セファクロルカプセル

Cefaclor Capsules contain not less than 90.0% and not more than 110.0% of the labeled potency of cefaclor ($C_{15}H_{14}ClN_3O_4S$: 367.81).

Method of preparation Prepare as directed under Capsules, with Cefaclor.

Identification Shake vigorously a quantity of the contents of Cefaclor Capsules, equivalent to 20 mg (potency) of Cefaclor, with 10 mL of water, centrifuge, and use the supernatant liquid as the sample solution. Separately, dissolve 20 mg of Cefaclor RS in 10 mL of water, and use this solution as the standard solution. Perform the test with these solutions as directed under Thin-layer Chromatography <2.03>. Spot 2 μL each of the sample solution and standard solution on a plate of silica gel with fluorescent indicator for thin-layer chromatography, develop the plate with a mixture of acetonitrile, water, ethyl acetate and formic acid (30:10:10:1) to a distance of about 10 cm, and air-dry the plate. Examine under ultraviolet light (main wavelength: 254 nm): the principal spot obtained from the sample solution and the spot from the standard solution show the same *R*f value.

Purity Related substances—Weigh accurately not less than 5 Cefaclor Capsules, open the capsules and carefully take out the contents, mix well, and powder, if necessary. Wash the empty capsules with a little amount of diethyl ether, if necessary, allow the capsules to stand at room temperature to vaporize adhering diethyl ether, and weigh accurately the capsules to calculate the mass of the contents. Weigh accurately a quantity of the contents, equivalent to about 0.25 g (potency) of Cefaclor, shake with 40 mL of 0.1 mol/L phosphate buffer solution (pH 4.5) for 10 minutes, add the same buffer solution to make exactly 50 mL, and filter through a 0.45-μm pore-size membrane filter. Discard the first 1 mL of the filtrate, and use the subsequent filtrate as the sample solution. Separately, weigh accurately an amount of Cefaclor RS, equivalent to about 20 mg (potency), and dissolve in 0.1 mol/L phosphate buffer solution (pH 4.5) to make exactly 20 mL. Pipet 2.5 mL of this solution, add the same buffer solution to make exactly 50 mL, and use this solution as the standard solution. Perform the test with exactly 20 μL each of the sample solution and standard solution as directed under Liquid Chromatography <2.01> according to the following conditions, and determine the peak areas by the automatic integration method. Calculate the amount of each related substance by the following equation: the amount of each related substance is not more than 0.5%, and the total amount of the related substances is not more than 2.5%. If necessary, correct the fluctuation of the base line by performing the test in the same manner with 20 μL of 0.1 mol/L phosphate buffer solution (pH 4.5).

Amount (%) of each related substance
$= M_S/M_T \times A_T/A_S \times M_M/C \times 25/2$

Total amount (%) of the related substances
$= M_S/M_T \times \Sigma A_T/A_S \times M_M/C \times 25/2$

M_S: Amount [mg (potency)] of Cefaclor RS taken
M_T: Amount (mg) of the contents of Cefaclor Capsules taken
M_M: Average mass (mg) of the contents in 1 capsule
A_T: Area of each peak other than cefaclor and solvent from the sample solution
A_S: Peak area of cefaclor from the standard solution
C: Labeled potency [mg (potency)] of Cefaclor in 1 capsule

Operating conditions—

Proceed as directed in the operating conditions in the Purity (3) under Cefaclor.

System suitability—

Test for required detectability: Pipet 1 mL of the standard solution, and add 0.1 mol/L phosphate buffer solution (pH 4.5) to make exactly 20 mL. Confirm that the peak area of cefaclor obtained with 20 μL of this solution is equivalent to 3.5 to 6.5% of that with 20 μL of the standard solution.

System performance: When the procedure is run with 20 μL of the standard solution under the above operating conditions, the number of theoretical plates and the symmetry factor of the peak of cefaclor are not less than 40,000 and 0.8 to 1.3, respectively.

System repeatability: When the test is repeated 3 times with 20 μL of the standard solution under the above operating conditions, the relative standard deviation of the peak area of cefaclor is not more than 2.0%.

Water <2.48> Not more than 8.0% (0.2 g, volumetric titration, back titration).

Uniformity of dosage units <*6.02*> It meets the requirement of the Mass variation test.

Dissolution <*6.10*> When the test is performed at 50 revolutions per minute according to the Paddle method, using 900 mL of water as the dissolution medium, the dissolution rate in 15 minutes of Cefaclor Capsules is not less than 80%.

Start the test with 1 capsule of Cefaclor Capsules, withdraw not less than 20 mL of the medium at the specified minute after starting the test, and filter through a membrane filter with a pore size not exceeding 0.5 μm. Discard not less than 10 mL of the first filtrate, pipet V mL of the subsequent filtrate, add water to make exactly V' mL so that each mL contains about 20 μg (potency) of Cefaclor, and use this solution as the sample solution. Separately, weigh accurately about 20 mg (potency) of Cefaclor RS, and dissolve in water to make exactly 20 mL. Pipet 1 mL of this solution, add water to make exactly 50 mL, and use this solution as the standard solution. Determine the absorbances, A_T and A_S, at 265 nm of the sample solution and standard solution as directed under Ultraviolet-visible Spectrophotometry <*2.24*>.

Dissolution rate (%) with respect to the labeled amount of cefaclor ($C_{15}H_{14}ClN_3O_4S$)
$= M_S \times A_T/A_S \times V'/V \times 1/C \times 90$

M_S: Amount [mg (potency)] of Cefaclor RS taken
C: Labeled amount [mg (potency)] of Cefaclor in 1 capsule

Assay Weigh accurately not less than 5 Cefaclor Capsules, open the capsules and carefully take out the contents, mix well, and powder, if necessary. Wash the empty capsules with a little amount of diethyl ether, if necessary, allow the capsules to stand at room temperature to vaporize adhering diethyl ether, and weigh accurately the capsules to calculate the mass of the contents. Weigh accurately a quantity of the contents, equivalent to about 0.1 g (potency) of Cefaclor, shake vigorously with 60 mL of 0.1 mol/L phosphate buffer solution (pH 4.5) for 10 minutes, add the same buffer solution to make exactly 100 mL, and centrifuge. Pipet 10 mL of the supernatant liquid, add exactly 10 mL of the internal standard solution and the same buffer solution to make 50 mL, and use this solution as the sample solution. Separately, weigh accurately an amount of Cefaclor RS, equivalent to about 50 mg (potency), and dissolve in 0.1 mol/L phosphate buffer solution (pH 4.5) to make exactly 50 mL. Pipet 10 mL of this solution, add exactly 10 mL of the internal standard solution and the same buffer solution to make 50 mL, and use this solution as the standard solution. Proceed as directed in the Assay under Cefaclor.

Amount [mg (potency)] of cefaclor ($C_{15}H_{14}ClN_3O_4S$)
$= M_S \times Q_T/Q_S \times 2$

M_S: Amount [mg (potency)] of Cefaclor RS taken

Internal standard solution—A solution of 4-aminoacetophenone in 0.1 mol/L phosphate buffer solution (pH 4.5) (1 in 700).

Containers and storage Containers—Tight containers.
Storage—Light-resistant.

Cefaclor Combination Granules

セファクロル複合顆粒

Cefaclor Combination Granules contain gastric-soluble granules and enteric-soluble granules in one package.

It contains cefaclor ($C_{15}H_{14}ClN_3O_4S$: 367.81) equivalent to not less than 90.0% and not more than 110.0% of the labeled total potency and the labeled potency of gastric-soluble granule, respectively.

Method of preparation Prepare as directed under Granules, with Cefaclor, and divide into single-dose packages.

Identification Shake vigorously a quantity of Cefaclor Combination Granules, equivalent to 20 mg (potency) of Cefaclor according to the labeled total potency, with 10 mL of water, centrifuge, and use the supernatant liquid as the sample solution. Separately, dissolve 20 mg of Cefaclor RS in 10 mL of water, and use this solution as the standard solution. Perform the test with these solutions as directed under Thin-layer Chromatography <*2.03*>. Spot 2 μL each of the sample solution and standard solution on a plate of silica gel with fluorescent indicator for thin-layer chromatography, develop the plate with a mixture of acetonitrile, water, ethyl acetate and formic acid (30:10:10:1) to a distance of about 10 cm, and air-dry the plate. Examine under ultraviolet light (main wavelength: 254 nm): the principal spot obtained from the sample solution and the spot from the standard solution show the same Rf value.

Purity Related substances—Take out the total content of not less than 5 packages of Cefaclor Combination Granules, add a small amount of 0.1 mol/L phosphate buffer solution (pH 4.5), grind, add 0.1 mol/L phosphate buffer solution (pH 4.5), shake vigorously for 10 minutes, and add 0.1 mol/L phosphate buffer solution (pH 4.5) to make exactly V mL so that each mL contains about 5 mg (potency) of Cefaclor according to the labeled total potency. Pipet 10 mL of this solution, add 0.1 mol/L phosphate buffer solution (pH 4.5) to make exactly 25 mL, and filter through a membrane filter with a pore size not exceeding 0.45 μm. Discard the first 1 mL of the filtrate, and use the subsequent filtrate as the sample solution. Separately, weigh accurately an amount of Cefaclor RS, equivalent to about 20 mg (potency), and dissolve in 0.1 mol/L phosphate buffer solution (pH 4.5) to make exactly 20 mL. Pipet 2 mL of this solution, add 0.1 mol/L phosphate buffer solution (pH 4.5) to make exactly 100 mL, and use this solution as the standard solution. Perform the test with exactly 50 μL each of the sample solution and standard solution as directed under Liquid Chromatography <*2.01*> according to the following conditions, and determine each peak area in each solution by the automatic integration method. Calculate the amount of each related substance by the following equation: the amount of each related substance is not more than 0.6%, and the total amount of the related substances is not more than 2.8%. If necessary, correct the fluctuation of the base line by performing the test in the same manner with 50 μL of 0.1 mol/L phosphate buffer solution (pH 4.5).

Amount (%) of each related substance
$= M_S \times A_T/A_S \times V/4 \times \{1/(C \times T)\}$

Total amount (%) of the related substances
$= M_S \times \Sigma A_T/A_S \times V/4 \times \{1/(C \times T)\}$

M_S: Amount [mg (potency)] of Cefaclor RS taken
A_T: Area of each peak other than cefaclor, solvent and excipient from the sample solution
ΣA_T: Total area of the peaks other than cefaclor, solvent and excipient from the sample solution
A_S: Peak area of cefaclor from the standard solution
C: Labeled total potency [mg (potency)] of Cefaclor in 1 package
T: Number (pack) of Cefaclor Combination Granules

Operating conditions—

Proceed as directed in the operating conditions in the Purity (3) under Cefaclor.

System suitability—

Test for required detectability: Pipet 1 mL of standard solution, and add 0.1 mol/L phosphate buffer solution (pH 4.5) to make exactly 20 mL. Confirm that the peak area of cefaclor obtained from 50 μL of this solution is equivalent to 3.5 to 6.5% of that obtained from 50 μL of the standard solution.

System performance: When the procedure is run with 50 μL of the standard solution under the above operating conditions, the number of theoretical plates and the symmetry factor of the peak of cefaclor are not less than 40,000 and between 0.8 and 1.3, respectively.

System repeatability: When the test is repeated 3 times with 50 μL of the standard solution under the above operating conditions, the relative standard deviation of the peak area of cefaclor is not more than 2.0%.

Water <*2.48*> Not more than 5.5% (0.3 g, volumetric titration, back titration).

Uniformity of dosage units <*6.02*> Perform the test according to the following method: it meets the requirement of the Content uniformity test.

(1) Total potency—Take out the total content of 1 package of Cefaclor Combination Granules, add a little amount of 0.1 mol/L phosphate buffer solution (pH 4.5), grind well, add the same buffer solutions to make exactly V mL so that each mL contains about 3.8 mg (potency) of Cefaclor according to the labeled total potency after shaking vigorously for 10 minutes, and centrifuge. Pipet 3 mL of the supernatant liquid, add exactly 10 mL of the internal standard solution and the same buffer solution to make 50 mL, and use this solution as the sample solution. Separately, weigh accurately an amount of Cefaclor RS, equivalent to about 50 mg (potency), and dissolve in 0.1 mol/L phosphate buffer solution (pH 4.5) to make exactly 50 mL. Pipet 10 mL of this solution, add exactly 10 mL of the internal standard solution and the same buffer solution to make 50 mL, and use this solution as the standard solution. Then, proceed as directed in the Assay under Cefaclor.

Amount [mg (potency)] of cefaclor ($C_{15}H_{14}ClN_3O_4S$)
$= M_S \times Q_T/Q_S \times V/15$

M_S: Amount [mg (potency)] of Cefaclor RS taken

Internal standard solution—A solution of 4-aminoacetophenone in 0.1 mol/L phosphate buffer solution (pH 4.5) (1 in 700).

(2) Potency of gastric-soluble granule—Take out the total content of 1 package of Cefaclor Combination Granules stir gently with 60 mL of 0.1 mol/L phosphate buffer solution (pH 4.5) for 5 minutes, add the same buffer solution to make exactly V mL so that each mL contains about 1.5 mg (potency) of Cefaclor according to the labeled potency of gastric-soluble granule, and centrifuge. Pipet 7 mL of the supernatant liquid, add exactly 10 mL of the internal standard solution and the same buffer solution to make 50 mL, and use this solution as the sample solution. Separately, weigh accurately an amount of Cefaclor RS, equivalent to about 50 mg (potency), and dissolve in 0.1 mol/L phosphate buffer solution (pH 4.5) to make exactly 50 mL. Pipet 10 mL of this solution, add exactly 10 mL of the internal standard solution and the same buffer solution to make 50 mL, and use this solution as the standard solution. Then, proceed as directed in the Assay under Cefaclor.

Amount [mg (potency)] of cefaclor ($C_{15}H_{14}ClN_3O_4S$)
$= M_S \times Q_T/Q_S \times V/35$

M_S: Amount [mg (potency)] of Cefaclor RS taken

Internal standard solution—A solution of 4-aminoacetophenone in 0.1 mol/L phosphate buffer solution (pH 4.5) (1 in 700).

Dissolution <*6.10*> When the test is performed at 50 revolutions per minute according to the Paddle method, using 900 mL of 1st fluid for dissolution test as the dissolution medium, the dissolution rate in 60 minutes of Cefaclor Combination Granules is between 35% and 45%.

Start the test with the total content of 1 package of Cefaclor Combination Granules, withdraw not less than 20 mL of the medium at the specified minute after starting the test, and filter through a membrane filter with a pore size not exceeding 0.5 μm. Discard not less than 10 mL of the first filtrate, pipet V mL of the subsequent filtrate, add the dissolution medium to make exactly V' mL so that each mL contains about 20 μg (potency) of Cefaclor according to the labeled potency of gastric-soluble granule, and use this solution as the sample solution. Separately, weigh accurately an amount of Cefaclor RS, equivalent to about 20 mg (potency), and dissolve in the dissolution medium to make exactly 20 mL. Pipet 2 mL of this solution, add the dissolution medium to make exactly 100 mL, and use this solution as the standard solution. Determine the absorbances, A_T and A_S, at 265 nm of the sample solution and standard solution as directed under Ultraviolet-visible Spectrophotometry <*2.24*>.

Dissolution rate (%) of cefaclor ($C_{15}H_{14}ClN_3O_4S$) with respect to the labeled potency
$= M_S \times A_T/A_S \times V'/V \times 1/C \times 90$

M_S: Amount [mg (potency)] of Cefaclor RS taken
C: Labeled total potency [mg (potency)] of Cefaclor in 1 pack

Separately, when the test is performed at 50 revolutions per minute according to the Paddle method, using 900 mL of 2nd fluid for dissolution test as the dissolution medium, the dissolution rate in 60 minutes of Cefaclor Combination Granules is not less than 70%.

Start the test with the total content of 1 package of Cefaclor Combination Granules, withdraw not less than 20 mL of the medium at the specified minute after starting the test, and filter through a membrane filter with a pore size not exceeding 0.5 μm. Discard not less than 10 mL of the first filtrate, pipet V mL of the subsequent filtrate, add 0.01 mol/L hydrochloric acid TS to make exactly V' mL so that each mL contains about 20 μg (potency) of Cefaclor according to the labeled total potency, and use this solution as the sample solution. Separately, weigh accurately an amount of Cefaclor RS, equivalent to about 20 mg (potency), dissolve in the dissolution medium to make exactly 100 mL, and warm at 37°C for 60 minutes. Pipet 2 mL of this solution, add 0.01 mol/L hydrochloric acid TS to make exactly 20 mL, and use this solution as the standard solution. Determine the absorbances, A_T and A_S, at 265 nm of the sample solution and standard solution as directed under Ultraviolet-visible Spectrophotometry <*2.24*>, using 0.01 mol/L hydrochloric acid TS as the blank.

Dissolution rate (%) of cefaclor ($C_{15}H_{14}ClN_3O_4S$) with respect to the labeled potency
$= M_S \times A_T/A_S \times V'/V \times 1/C \times 90$

M_S: Amount [mg (potency)] of Cefaclor RS taken
C: Labeled total potency [mg (potency)] of Cefaclor in 1 package

Assay **(1)** Total potency—Take out the total content of not less than 5 Cefaclor Combination Granules, add a small amount of 0.1 mol/L phosphate buffer solution (pH 4.5), grind well, add the same buffer solution so that each mL containing about 5 mg (potency) of Cefaclor according to the labeled total potency after shaking vigorously for 10 minutes, and centrifuge. Pipet 2 mL of the supernatant liquid, add exactly 10 mL of the internal standard solution and the same buffer solution to make 50 mL, and use this solution as the sample solution. Separately, weigh accurately an amount of Cefaclor RS, equivalent to about 50 mg (potency), and dissolve in 0.1 mol/L phosphate buffer solution (pH 4.5) to make exactly 50 mL. Pipet 10 mL of this solution, add exactly 10 mL of the internal standard solution and the same buffer solution to make 50 mL, and use this solution as the standard solution. Then, proceed as directed in the Assay under Cefaclor.

Amount [mg (potency)] of cefaclor ($C_{15}H_{14}ClN_3O_4S$)
$= M_S \times Q_T/Q_S \times 1/5$

M_S: Amount [mg (potency)] of Cefaclor RS taken

Internal standard solution—A solution of 4-aminoacetophenone in 0.1 mol/L phosphate buffer solution (pH 4.5) (1 in 700).

(2) Potency of gastric-soluble granule—Stir gentry the total content of not less than 5 Cefaclor Combination Granules with about 100 mL of 0.1 mol/L phosphate buffer solution (pH 4.5) for 5 minutes, add the same buffer solution so that each mL containing about 2 mg (potency) of Cefaclor according to the labeled potency of gastric-soluble granule, and centrifuge. Pipet 5 mL of the supernatant liquid, add exactly 10 mL of the internal standard solution and the same buffer solution to make 50 mL, and use this solution as the sample solution. Separately, weigh accurately an amount of Cefaclor RS, equivalent to about 50 mg (potency), and dissolve in 0.1 mol/L phosphate buffer solution (pH 4.5) to make exactly 50 mL. Pipet 10 mL of this solution, add exactly 10 mL of the internal standard solution and the same buffer solution to make 50 mL, and use this solution as the standard solution. Then, proceed as directed in the Assay under Cefaclor.

Amount [mg (potency)] of cefaclor ($C_{15}H_{14}ClN_3O_4S$)
$= M_S \times Q_T/Q_S \times 1/5$

M_S: Amount [mg (potency)] of Cefaclor RS taken

Internal standard solution—A solution of 4-aminoacetophenone in 0.1 mol/L phosphate buffer solution (pH 4.5) (1 in 700).

Containers and storage Containers—Tight containers.
Storage—Light-resistant.

Cefaclor Fine Granules

セファクロル細粒

Cefaclor Fine Granules contain not less than 90.0% and not more than 110.0% of the labeled potency of cefaclor ($C_{15}H_{14}ClN_3O_4S$: 367.81).

Method of preparation Prepare as directed under Granules, with Cefaclor.

Identification Shake vigorously a quantity of Cefaclor Fine Granules, equivalent to 20 mg (potency) of Cefaclor, with 10 mL of water, centrifuge, and use the supernatant liquid as the sample solution. Separately, dissolve 20 mg (potency) of Cefaclor RS in 10 mL of water, and use this solution as the standard solution. Perform the test with these solutions as directed under Thin-layer Chromatography <*2.03*>. Spot 2 μL each of the sample solution and standard solution on a plate of silica gel with fluorescent indicator for thin-layer chromatography, develop the plate with a mixture of acetonitrile, water, ethyl acetate and formic acid (30:10:10:1) to a distance of about 10 cm, and air-dry the plate. Examine under ultraviolet light (main wavelength: 254 nm): the principal spot from the sample solution and the spot from the standard solution show the same *Rf* value.

Purity Related substances—Weigh accurately a quantity of Cefaclor Fine Granules after powdered if necessary, equivalent to about 0.1 g (potency) of Cefaclor, shake with 40 mL of 0.1 mol/L phosphate buffer solution (pH 4.5) for 10 minutes, add the same buffer solution to make exactly 50 mL, and filter through a 0.45-μm pore-size membrane filter. Discard the first 1 mL of the filtrate, and use the subsequent filtrate as the sample solution. Separately, weigh accurately an amount of Cefaclor RS, equivalent to about 20 mg (potency), and dissolve in 0.1 mol/L phosphate buffer solution (pH 4.5) to make exactly 20 mL. Pipet 2 mL of this solution, add the same buffer solution to make exactly 100 mL, and use this solution as the standard solution. Perform the test with exactly 50 μL each of the sample solution and standard solution as directed under Liquid Chromatography <*2.01*> according to the following conditions, and determine the peak areas by the automatic integration method. Calculate the amount of each related substance by the following equation: the amount of each related substance is not more than 0.5%, and the total amount of the related substances is not more than 3.0%. If necessary, correct the fluctuation of the base line by performing the test in the same manner with 50 μL of 0.1 mol/L phosphate buffer solution (pH 4.5).

Amount (%) of each related substance
$= M_S/M_T \times A_T/A_S \times 1/C \times 5$

Total amount (%) of the related substances
$= M_S/M_T \times \Sigma A_T/A_S \times 1/C \times 5$

M_S: Amount [mg (potency)] of Cefaclor RS taken
M_T: Amount (g) of Cefaclor Fine Granules taken
A_T: Area of the peak other than cefaclor and the solvent from the sample solution
A_S: Peak area of cefaclor from the standard solution
C: Labeled potency [mg (potency)] of cefaclor ($C_{15}H_{14}ClN_3O_4S$) in 1 g

Operating conditions—
Proceed as directed in the operating conditions in the Purity (3) under Cefaclor.

System suitability—

Test for required detectability: Pipet 1 mL of the standard solution, and add 0.1 mol/L phosphate buffer solution (pH 4.5) to make exactly 20 mL. Confirm that the peak area of cefaclor obtained with 50 μL of this solution is equivalent to 3.5 to 6.5% of that with 50 μL of the standard solution.

System performance: When the procedure is run with 50 μL of the standard solution under the above operating conditions, the number of theoretical plates and the symmetry factor of the peak of cefaclor are not less than 40,000 and between 0.8 and 1.3, respectively.

System repeatability: When the test is repeated 3 times with 50 μL of the standard solution under the above operating conditions, the relative standard deviation of the peak area of cefaclor is not more than 2.0%.

Water ⟨*2.48*⟩ Not more than 1.5% (1 g, volumetric titration, back titration).

Uniformity of dosage units ⟨*6.02*⟩ The granules in single-dose packages meet the requirement of the Mass variation test.

Dissolution ⟨*6.10*⟩ When the test is performed at 50 revolutions per minute according to the Paddle method, using 900 mL of water as the dissolution medium, the dissolution rate in 15 minutes of Cefaclor Fine Granules is not less than 85%.

Start the test with an accurately weighed amount of Cefaclor Fine Granules, equivalent to about 0.25 g (potency) of Cefaclor, withdraw not less than about 20 mL of the medium at the specified minute after starting the test, and filter through a membrane filter with a pore size not exceeding 0.5 μm. Discard not less than 10 mL of the first filtrate, pipet V mL of the subsequent filtrate, add water to make exactly V' mL so that each mL contains about 20 μg (potency) of Cefaclor, and use this solution as the sample solution. Separately, weigh accurately about 20 mg (potency) of Cefaclor RS, and dissolve in water to make exactly 20 mL. Pipet 1 mL of this solution, add water to make exactly 50 mL, and use this solution as the standard solution. Determine the absorbances, A_T and A_S, at 265 nm of the sample solution and standard solution as directed under Ultraviolet-visible Spectrophotometry ⟨*2.24*⟩.

Dissolution rate (%) with respect to the labeled amount of cefaclor ($C_{15}H_{14}ClN_3O_4S$)

$$= M_S/M_T \times A_T/A_S \times V'/V \times 1/C \times 90$$

M_S: Amount [mg (potency)] of Cefaclor RS taken

M_T: Amount [mg (potency)] of Cefaclor Fine Granules taken

C: Labeled amount [mg (potency)] of cefaclor ($C_{15}H_{14}ClN_3O_4S$) in 1 g

Assay Weigh accurately a quantity of Cefaclor Fine Granules after powdered if necessary, equivalent to about 0.1 g (potency) of Cefaclor, shake vigorously with 60 mL of 0.1 mol/L phosphate buffer solution (pH 4.5) for 10 minutes, add the same buffer solution to make exactly 100 mL, and centrifuge. Pipet 10 mL of the supernatant liquid, add exactly 10 mL of the internal standard solution and the same buffer solution to make 50 mL, and use this solution as the sample solution. Separately, weigh accurately about 50 mg (potency) of Cefaclor RS, and dissolve in 0.1 mol/L phosphate buffer solution (pH 4.5) to make exactly 50 mL. Pipet 10 mL of this solution, add exactly 10 mL of the internal standard solution and the same buffer solution to make 50 mL, and use this solution as standard solution. Proceed as directed in the Assay under Cefaclor.

Amount [mg (potency)] of cefaclor ($C_{15}H_{14}ClN_3O_4S$)

$$= M_S \times Q_T/Q_S \times 2$$

M_S: Amount [mg (potency)] of Cefaclor RS taken

Internal standard solution—A solution of 4-aminoacetophenone in 0.1 mol/L phosphate buffer solution (pH 4.5) (1 in 700).

Containers and storage Containers—Tight containers.
Storage—Light-resistant.

Cefadroxil

セファドロキシル

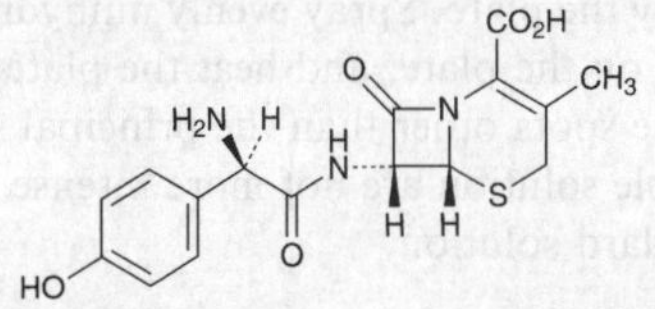

$C_{16}H_{17}N_3O_5S$: 363.39
(6*R*,7*R*)-7-[(2*R*)-2-Amino-2-(4-hydroxyphenyl)acetylamino]-3-methyl-8-oxo-5-thia-1-azabicyclo[4.2.0]oct-2-ene-2-carboxylic acid
[*50370-12-2*]

Cefadroxil contains not less than 950 μg (potency) and not more than 1020 μg (potency) per mg, calculated on the anhydrous basis. The potency of Cefadroxil is expressed as mass (potency) of cefadroxil ($C_{16}H_{17}N_3O_5S$).

Description Cefadroxil occurs as a white to light yellowish white powder.

It is sparingly soluble in water, slightly soluble in methanol, and very slightly soluble in ethanol (95).

Identification **(1)** Determine the absorption spectrum of a solution of Cefadroxil (1 in 50,000) as directed under Ultraviolet-visible Spectrophotometry ⟨*2.24*⟩, and compare the spectrum with the Reference Spectrum or the spectrum of a solution of Cefadroxil RS prepared in the same manner as the sample solution: both spectra exhibit similar intensities of absorption at the same wavelengths.

(2) Determine the infrared absorption spectrum of Cefadroxil as directed in the potassium bromide disk method under Infrared Spectrophotometry ⟨*2.25*⟩, and compare the spectrum with the Reference Spectrum or the spectrum of Cefadroxil RS: both spectra exhibit similar intensities of absorption at the same wave numbers.

(3) Determine the ^{1}H spectrum of a solution of Cefadroxil in a mixture of heavy water for nuclear magnetic resonance spectroscopy and deuterated hydrochloric acid (3:1) (1 in 10), using sodium 3-(trimethylsilyl)propionate-d_4 for nuclear magnetic resonance spectroscopy as an internal reference compound, as directed under Nuclear Magnetic Resonance Spectroscopy ⟨*2.21*⟩: it exhibits a singlet signal A at around δ 2.1 ppm, a doublet signal B at around δ 7.0 ppm, and a doublet signal C at around δ 7.5 ppm. The ratio of integrated intensity of each signal, A:B:C, is about 3:2:2.

Optical rotation ⟨*2.49*⟩ $[\alpha]_D^{25}$: +164 – +182° (0.6 g calculated on the anhydrous basis, water, 100 mL, 100 mm).

pH ⟨*2.54*⟩ Dissolve 1.0 g of Cefadroxil in 200 mL of water: pH of the solution is between 4.0 and 6.0.

Purity **(1)** Heavy metals ⟨*1.07*⟩—Proceed with 1.0 g of

Cefadroxil according to Method 2, and perform the test. Prepare the control solution with 2.0 mL of Standard Lead Solution (not more than 20 ppm).

(2) Related substances—Dissolve 0.1 g of Cefadroxil in 4 mL of a mixture of ethanol (99.5), water and diluted hydrochloric acid (1 in 5) (75:22:3), and use this solution as the sample solution. Pipet 1 mL of the sample solution, add a mixture of ethanol (99.5), water and diluted hydrochloric acid (1 in 5) (75:22:3) to make exactly 100 mL, and use this solution as the standard solution. Perform the test with these solutions as directed under Thin-layer Chromatography <*2.03*>. Spot 2 μL each of the sample solution and standard solution on a plate of silica gel for thin-layer chromatography. Develop with a mixture of ethyl acetate, water, ethanol (99.5) and formic acid (14:5:5:1) to a distance of about 12 cm, and air-dry the plate. Spray evenly ninhydrin-citric acid-acetic acid TS on the plate, and heat the plate at 100°C for 10 minutes: the spots other than the principal spot obtained from the sample solution are not more intense than the spot from the standard solution.

Water <*2.48*> Not less than 4.2% and not more than 6.0% (0.5 g, volumetric titration, direct titration).

Assay Weigh accurately an amount of Cefadroxil and Cefadroxil RS, equivalent to about 50 mg (potency), dissolve each in water to make exactly 500 mL, and use these solutions as the sample solution and the standard solution, respectively. Perform the test with exactly 10 μL each of the sample solution and standard solution as directed under Liquid Chromatography <*2.01*> according to the following conditions, and determine the peak areas, A_T and A_S, of cefadroxil in each solution.

Amount [μg (potency)] of cefadroxil ($C_{16}H_{17}N_3O_5S$)
$= M_S \times A_T/A_S \times 1000$

M_S: amount [mg (potency)] of Cefadroxil RS taken

Operating conditions—

Detector: An ultraviolet absorption photometer (wavelength: 262 nm).

Column: A stainless steel column 4.6 mm in inside diameter and 25 cm in length, packed with octadecylsilanized silica gel for liquid chromatography (5 μm in particle diameter).

Column temperature: A constant temperature of about 40°C.

Mobile phase: A mixture of a solution of potassium dihydrogenphosphate (17 in 12,500) and methanol (17:3).

Flow rate: Adjust so that the retention time of cefadroxil is about 5 minutes.

System suitability—

System performance: Dissolve about 5 mg (potency) of Cefadroxil and about 10 mg (potency) of propylene glycol cefatrizine in 50 mL of water. When the procedure is run with 10 μL of this solution under the above operating conditions, cefadroxil and cefatrizine are eluted in this order with the resolution between these peaks being not less than 4.

System repeatability: When the test is repeated 6 times with 10 μL of the standard solution under the above operating conditions, the relative standard deviation of the peak areas of cefadroxil is not more than 1.0%.

Containers and storage Containers—Tight containers.

Cefadroxil Capsules

セファドロキシルカプセル

Cefadroxil Capsules contain not less than 95.0% and not more than 105.0% of the labeled potency of cefadroxil ($C_{16}H_{17}N_3O_5S$: 363.39).

Method of preparation Prepare as directed under Capsules, with Cefadroxil.

Identification Dissolve the contents of Cefadroxil Capsules, equivalent to 10 mg (potency) of Cefadroxil, in 500 mL of water, and filter. Determine the absorption spectrum of the filtrate as directed under Ultraviolet-visible Spectrophotometry <*2.24*>: it exhibits maxima between 228 nm and 232 nm, and between 261 nm and 265 nm.

Water <*2.48*> Not more than 7.0% (0.15 g, volumetric titration, direct titration).

Uniformity of dosage units <*6.02*> Perform the test according to the following method: it meets the requirement of the Content uniformity test.

Place 1 capsule of Cefadroxil Capsules in 300 mL of water, disperse with the aid of ultrasonic waves, shake for 30 minutes, and add water to make exactly 500 mL. Pipet 5 mL of this solution, and add water to make exactly V mL so that each mL contains about 0.1 mg (potency) of Cefadroxil. Filter the solution, discard the first 10 mL of the filtrate, and use the subsequent filtrate as the sample solution. Separately, weigh accurately about 20 mg (potency) of Cefadroxil RS, dissolve in water to make exactly 200 mL, and use this solution as the standard solution. Then, proceed as directed in the Assay under Cefadroxil.

Amount [mg (potency)] of cefadroxil ($C_{16}H_{17}N_3O_5S$)
$= M_S \times A_T/A_S \times V/2$

M_S: Amount [mg (potency)] of Cefadroxil RS taken

Dissolution <*6.10*> When the test is performed at 50 revolutions per minute according to the Paddle method, using 900 mL of 0.05 mol/L acetic acid-sodium acetate buffer solution (pH 4.0) as the dissolution medium, the dissolution rate in 90 minutes of Cefadroxil Capsules is not less than 80%.

Start the test with 1 capsule of Cefadroxil Capsules, withdraw not less than 20 mL of the medium at the specified minute after starting the test, and filter through a membrane filter with a pore size not exceeding 0.45 μm. Discard not less than 10 mL of the first filtrate, pipet V mL of the subsequent filtrate, add water to make exactly V' mL so that each mL contains about 22 μg (potency) of Cefadroxil, and use this solution as the sample solution. Separately, weigh accurately about 22 mg (potency) of Cefadroxil RS, and add water to make exactly 100 mL. Pipet 5 mL of this solution, add water to make exactly 50 mL, and use this solution as the standard solution. Determine the absorbances, A_T and A_S, at 263 nm of the sample solution and standard solution as directed under Ultraviolet-visible Spectrophotometry <*2.24*>, using water as the blank.

Dissolution rate (%) with respect to the labeled amount of cefadroxil ($C_{16}H_{17}N_3O_5S$)
$= M_S \times A_T/A_S \times V'/V \times 1/C \times 90$

M_S: Amount [mg (potency)] of Cefadroxil RS taken
C: Labeled amount [mg (potency)] of cefadroxil in 1 capsule

Assay Take out the contents of 20 Cefadroxil Capsules, and combine. Weigh accurately the mass of the combined contents, and powder. Weigh accurately a portion of the powder, equivalent to about 50 mg (potency) of Cefadroxil, add 300 mL of water, shake for 30 minutes, then add water to make exactly 500 mL, and filter. Discard the first 10 mL of the filtrate, and use the subsequent filtrate as the sample solution. Separately, weigh accurately an amount of Cefadroxil RS, equivalent to about 20 mg (potency), dissolve in water to make exactly 200 mL, and use this solution as the standard solution. Then, proceed as directed in the Assay under Cefadroxil.

Amount [mg (potency)] of cefadroxil ($C_{16}H_{17}N_3O_5S$)
$= M_S \times A_T/A_S \times 5/2$

M_S: Amount [mg (potency)] of Cefadroxil RS taken

Containers and storage Containers—Tight containers.

Cefadroxil for Syrup

シロップ用セファドロキシル

Cefadroxil for Syrup is a preparation for syrup, which is suspended before use.

It contains not less than 95.0% and not more than 110.0% of the labeled potency of cefadroxil ($C_{16}H_{17}N_3O_5S$: 363.39).

Method of preparation Prepare as directed under Preparations for Syrups, with Cefadroxil.

Identification Dissolve an amount of Cefadroxil for Syrup, equivalent to 10 mg (potency) of Cefadroxil, in 500 mL of water, and determine the absorption spectrum of this solution as directed under Ultraviolet-visible Spectrophotometry <*2.24*>: it exhibits maxima between 228 nm and 232 nm, and between 261 nm and 265 nm.

Water <*2.48*> Not more than 3.0% (0.5 g, volumetric titration, direct titration).

Uniformity of dosage units <*6.02*> The syrup in single-dose packages meets the requirement of the Mass variation test.

Dissolution <*6.10*> When the test is performed at 50 revolutions per minute according to the Paddle method (put the sample in the dissolution medium so that it disperses), using 900 mL of water as the dissolution medium, the dissolution rate in 15 minutes of Cefadroxil for Syrup is not less than 85%.

Start the test with accurately weighed amount of Cefadroxil for Syrup, equivalent to about 0.1 g (potency) of Cefadroxil, withdraw not less than 20 mL of the medium at the specified minute after starting the test, and filter through a membrane filter with a pore size not exceeding 0.45 μm. Discard not less than 10 mL of the first filtrate, pipet 4 mL of the subsequent filtrate, add water to make exactly 20 mL, and use this solution as the sample solution. Separately, weigh accurately about 22 mg (potency) of Cefadroxil RS, and dissolve in water to make exactly 100 mL. Pipet 5 mL of this solution, add water to make exactly 50 mL, and use this solution as the standard solution. Determine the absorbances, A_T and A_S, at 263 nm of the sample solution and standard solution as directed under Ultraviolet-visible Spectrophotometry <*2.24*>.

Dissolution rate (%) with respect to the labeled amount of cefadroxil ($C_{16}H_{17}N_3O_5S$)
$= M_S/M_T \times A_T/A_S \times 1/C \times 450$

M_S: Amount [mg (potency)] of Cefadroxil RS taken
M_T: Amount (g) of Cefadroxil for Syrup taken
C: Labeled amount [mg (potency)] of cefadroxil in 1 g

Assay Weigh accurately an amount of powdered Cefadroxil for Syrup, equivalent to about 50 mg (potency) of Cefadroxil, dissolve in water to make exactly 500 mL, and use this solution as the sample solution. Separately, weigh accurately an amount of Cefadroxil RS, equivalent to about 20 mg (potency), dissolve in water to make exactly 200 mL, and use this solution as the standard solution. Then, proceed as directed in the Assay under Cefadroxil.

Amount [mg (potency)] of cefadroxil ($C_{16}H_{17}N_3O_5S$)
$= M_S \times A_T/A_S \times 5/2$

M_S: Amount [mg (potency)] of Cefadroxil RS taken

Containers and storage Containers—Tight containers.

Cefalexin

セファレキシン

$C_{16}H_{17}N_3O_4S$: 347.39
(6*R*,7*R*)-7-[(2*R*)-2-Amino-2-phenylacetylamino]-3-methyl-8-oxo-5-thia-1-azabicyclo[4.2.0]oct-2-ene-2-carboxylic acid
[*15686-71-2*]

Cefalexin contains not less than 950 μg (potency) and not more than 1030 μg (potency) per mg, calculated on the anhydrous basis. The potency of Cefalexin is expressed as mass (potency) of cefalexin ($C_{16}H_{17}N_3O_4S$).

Description Cefalexin occurs as a white to light yellowwhite, crystals or crystalline powder.

It is sparingly soluble in water, slightly soluble in methanol, and practically insoluble in ethanol (95) and in *N,N*-dimethylformamide.

It is hygroscopic.

Identification **(1)** Determine the absorption spectrum of a solution of Cefalexin (3 in 100,000) as directed under Ultraviolet-visible Spectrophotometry <*2.24*>, and compare the spectrum with the Reference Spectrum: both spectra exhibit similar intensities of absorption at the same wavelengths.

(2) Determine the infrared absorption spectrum of Cefalexin as directed in the potassium bromide disk method under Infrared Spectrophotometry <*2.25*>, and compare the spectrum with the Reference Spectrum: both spectra exhibit similar intensities of absorption at the same wave numbers.

(3) Determine the ^1H spectrum of a solution of Cefalexin in heavy water for nuclear magnetic resonance spectroscopy (1 in 200) as directed under Nuclear Magnetic Resonance Spectroscopy <*2.21*>, using sodium 3-trimethylsilylpropanesulfonate for nuclear magnetic resonance spectroscopy as an internal reference compound: it exhibits a singlet signal A at around δ 1.8 ppm, and a singlet or a sharp multiplet signal B at around δ 7.5 ppm. The ratio of integrated intensity of these signals, A:B, is about 3:5.

Optical rotation <*2.49*> $[\alpha]_D^{20}$: +144 – +158° (0.125 g calculated on the anhydrous basis, water, 25 mL, 100 mm).

Purity **(1)** Heavy metals <*1.07*>—Proceed with 2.0 g of Cefalexin according to Method 4, and perform the test. Prepare the control solution with 2.0 mL of Standard Lead Solution (not more than 10 ppm).

(2) Arsenic <*1.11*>—Prepare the test solution with 1.0 g of Cefalexin by suspending in 10 mL of *N,N*-dimethylformamide, and perform the test (not more than 2 ppm).

(3) Related substances—Dissolve about 25 mg of Cefalexin in a solution of potassium dihydrogenphosphate (9 in 500) to make 5 mL, and use this solution as the sample solution. Pipet 1 mL of the sample solution, add a solution of potassium dihydrogenphosphate (9 in 500) to make exactly 100 mL, and use this solution as the standard solution. Perform the test with exactly 20 μL each of the sample solution and standard solution as directed under Liquid Chromatography <*2.01*> according to the following conditions, and determine the areas of each peak by the automatic integration method. If necessary, correct the change of the base-line due to the potassium dihydrogenphosphate solution by proceeding in the same manner with 20 μL of a solution of potassium dihydrogenphosphate (9 in 500): each peak area other than cefalexin from the sample solution is not larger than the peak area of cefalexin from the standard solution, and the total area of the peaks other than cefalexin from the sample solution which are larger than 1/50 times the peak area of cefalexin from the standard solution is not larger than 5 times of the peak area of cefalexin from the standard solution.

Operating conditions—

Detector: An ultraviolet absorption photometer (wavelength: 254 nm).

Column: A stainless steel column 4.6 mm in inside diameter and 25 cm in length, packed with octadecylsilanized silica gel for liquid chromatography (5 μm in particle diameter).

Column temperature: A constant temperature of about 25°C.

Mobile phase A: Dissolve 1.0 g of sodium 1-pentanesulfonate in 1000 mL of water, add 15 mL of triethylamine, and adjust to pH 2.5 with phosphoric acid.

Mobile phase B: Dissolve 1.0 g of sodium 1-pentanesulfonate in 300 mL of water, add 15 mL of triethylamine, and adjust to pH 2.5 with phosphoric acid. To this solution add 350 mL of acetonitrile and 350 mL of methanol.

Flowing of mobile phase: Control the gradient by mixing the mobile phases A and B as directed in the following table.

Time after injection of sample (min)	Mobile phase A (vol%)	Mobile phase B (vol%)
0 – 1	100	0
1 – 34.5	100 → 0	0 → 100
34.5 – 35.5	0	100

Flow rate: 1.0 mL per minute.

Time span of measurement: About 2 times as long as the retention time of cefalexin, beginning after the solvent peak.

System suitability—

Test for required detectability: Pipet 2 mL of the standard solution, add a solution of potassium dihydrogenphosphate (9 in 500) to make exactly 100 mL. Confirm that the peak area of cefalexin obtained with 20 μL of this solution is equivalent to 1.8 to 2.2% of that with 20 μL of the standard solution.

System performance: When the procedure is run with 20 μL of the standard solution under the above operating conditions, the number of theoretical plates and the symmetry factor of the peak of cefalexin are not less than 150,000 and between 0.8 and 1.3, respectively.

System repeatability: When the test is repeated 3 times with 20 μL of the standard solution under the above operating conditions, the relative standard deviation of the retention time and the peak areas of cefalexin are not more than 2.0%, respectively.

Water <*2.48*> Not more than 8.0% (0.2 g, volumetric titration, back titration).

Assay Weigh accurately an amount of Cefalexin and Cefalexin RS, equivalent to about 25 mg (potency), dissolve each in 0.1 mol/L phosphate buffer solution (pH 4.5) to make exactly 25 mL. Pipet 10 mL of these solutions, add exactly 5 mL of the internal standard solution, then add 0.1 mol/L phosphate buffer solution (pH 4.5) to make 50 mL, and use these solutions as the sample solution and standard solution. Perform the test with 10 μL each of the sample solution and standard solution as directed under Liquid Chromatography <*2.01*> according to the following conditions, and calculate the ratios, Q_T and Q_S, of the peak area of cefalexin to that of the internal standard.

Amount [μg (potency)] of cefalexin ($C_{16}H_{17}N_3O_4S$)
$= M_S \times Q_T/Q_S \times 1000$

M_S: amount [mg (potency)] of Cefalexin RS taken

Internal standard solution—A solution of *m*-hydroxyacetophenone in 0.1 mol/L phosphate buffer solution (pH 4.5) (1 in 1500).

Operating conditions—

Detector: An ultraviolet absorption photometer (wavelength: 254 nm).

Column: A stainless steel column 4.6 mm in inside diameter and 15 cm in length, packed with octadecylsilanized silica gel for liquid chromatography (5 μm in particle diameter).

Column temperature: A constant temperature of about 25°C.

Mobile phase: Dissolve 6.8 g of potassium dihydrogenphosphate in 1000 mL of water, adjust to pH 3.0 with diluted phosphoric acid (3 in 500). To 800 mL of this solution add 200 mL of methanol.

Flow rate: Adjust so that the retention time of cefalexin is about 7 minutes.

System suitability—

System performance: When the procedure is run with 10 μL of the standard solution under the above operating conditions, cefalexin and the internal standard are eluted in this order with the resolution between these peaks being not less than 6.

System repeatability: When the test is repeated 5 times with 10 μL of the standard solution under the above operating conditions, the relative standard deviation of the ratios of the peak area of cefalexin to that of the internal standard is not more than 1.0%.

Containers and storage Containers—Tight containers.

Cefalexin Capsules

セファレキシンカプセル

Cefalexin Capsules contain not less than 93.0% and not more than 107.0% of the labeled potency of cefalexin ($C_{16}H_{17}N_3O_4S$: 347.39).

Method of preparation Prepare as directed under Capsules, with Cefalexin.

Identification Take out the contents of Cefalexin Capsules, to a quantity of the contents, equivalent to 70 mg (potency) of Cefalexin, add 25 mL of water, shake vigorously for 5 minutes, and filter. To 1 mL of the filtrate add water to make 100 mL. Determine the absorption spectrum of this solution as directed under Ultraviolet-visible Spectrophotometry <2.24>: it exhibits a maximum between 260 nm and 264 nm.

Water <2.48> Not more than 10.0% (0.2 g, volumetric titration, back titration).

Uniformity of dosage units <6.02> Perform the Mass variation test, or the Content uniformity test according to the following method: it meets the requirement.

Open 1 capsule of Cefalexin Capsules, add 3*V*/5 mL of 0.1 mol/L phosphate buffer solution (pH 4.5), shake vigorously for 10 minutes, add 0.1 mol/L phosphate buffer solution (pH 4.5) to make exactly *V* mL so that each mL contains about 1.25 mg (potency) of Cefalexin. Centrifuge this solution, pipet 2 mL of the supernatant liquid, add exactly 10 mL of the internal standard solution, add 0.1 mol/L phosphate buffer solution (pH 4.5) to make 100 mL, and use this solution as the sample solution. Separately, weigh accurately an amount of Cefalexin RS, equivalent to about 25 mg (potency), dissolve in 0.1 mol/L phosphate buffer solution (pH 4.5) to make exactly 100 mL. Pipet 10 mL of this solution, add exactly 10 mL of the internal standard solution, add 0.1 mol/L phosphate buffer solution (pH 4.5) to make 100 mL, and use this solution as the standard solution. Perform the test with 10 μL each of the sample solution and standard solution as directed under Liquid Chromatography <2.01> according to the following conditions, and calculate the ratios, Q_T and Q_S, of the peak area of cefalexin to that of the internal standard.

Amount [mg (potency)] of cefalexin ($C_{16}H_{17}N_3O_4S$)
$= M_S \times Q_T/Q_S \times V/20$

M_S: Amount [mg (potency)] of Cefalexin RS taken

Internal standard solution—A solution of *m*-hydroxyacetophenone in 0.1 mol/L phosphate buffer solution (pH 4.5) (1 in 15,000).

Operating conditions—

Proceed as directed in the operating conditions in the Assay.

System suitability—

System performance: When the procedure is run with 10 μL of the standard solution under the above operating conditions, cefalexin and the internal standard are eluted in this order with the resolution between these peaks being not less than 8.

System repeatability: When the test is repeated 6 times with 10 μL of the standard solution under the above operating conditions, the relative standard deviation of the ratio of the peak area of cefalexin to that of the internal standard substance is not more than 1.0%.

Dissolution <6.10> When the test is performed at 50 revolutions per minute according to the Paddle method, using 900 mL of water as the dissolution medium, the dissolution rates in 30 minutes of 125-mg (potency) capsule and in 60 minutes of 250-mg (potency) capsule are not less than 75% and 80%, respectively.

Start the test with 1 capsule of Cefalexin Capsules, withdraw not less than 20 mL of the medium at the specified minute after starting the test, and filter through a membrane filter with a pore size not exceeding 0.5 μm. Discard not less than 10 mL of the first filtrate, pipet *V* mL of the subsequent filtrate, add water to make exactly *V′* mL so that each mL contains about 22 μg (potency) of Cefalexin, and use this solution as the sample solution. Separately, weigh accurately an amount of Cefalexin RS, equivalent to about 22 mg (potency), and dissolve in water to make exactly 50 mL. Pipet 5 mL of this solution, add water to make exactly 100 mL, and use this solution as the standard solution. Perform the test with the sample solution and standard solution as directed under Ultraviolet-visible Spectrophotometry <2.24>, and determine the absorbances, A_T and A_S, at 262 nm.

Dissolution rate (%) with respect to the labeled amount of cefalexin ($C_{16}H_{17}N_3O_4S$)
$= M_S \times A_T/A_S \times V'/V \times 1/C \times 90$

M_S: Amount [mg (potency)] of Cefalexin RS taken
C: Labeled amount [mg (potency)] of cefalexin ($C_{16}H_{17}N_3O_4S$) in 1 capsule

Assay Take out the contents of not less than 20 capsules of Cefalexin Capsules, weigh accurately the mass of the contents, and powder. Weigh accurately a portion of the powder, equivalent to about 0.1 g (potency) of Cefalexin, add 60 mL of 0.1 mol/L phosphate buffer solution (pH 4.5), shake vigorously for 10 minutes, add 0.1 mol/L phosphate buffer solution (pH 4.5) to make exactly 100 mL, and centrifuge. Pipet 2 mL of the supernatant liquid, add exactly 10 mL of the internal standard solution, add 0.1 mol/L phosphate buffer solution (pH 4.5) to make 100 mL, and use this solution as the sample solution. Separately, weigh accurately an amount of Cefalexin RS, equivalent to about 20 mg (potency), dissolve in 0.1 mol/L phosphate buffer solution (pH 4.5) to make exactly 100 mL. Pipet 10 mL of this solution, add exactly 10 mL of the internal standard solution, add 0.1 mol/L phosphate buffer solution (pH 4.5) to make 100 mL, and use this solution as the standard solution. Perform the test with 10 μL each of the sample solution and standard solution as directed under Liquid Chromatography <2.01> according to the following conditions, and calculate the ratios, Q_T and Q_S, of the peak area of cefalexin to that of the internal standard.

Amount [mg (potency)] of cefalexin ($C_{16}H_{17}N_3O_4S$)
$= M_S \times Q_T/Q_S \times 5$

M_S: Amount [mg (potency)] of Cefalexin RS taken

Internal standard solution—A solution of *m*-hydroxyacetophenone in 0.1 mol/L phosphate buffer solution (pH 4.5) (1 in 15,000).

Operating conditions—

Detector: An ultraviolet absorption photometer (wavelength: 254 nm).

Column: A stainless steel column 3.0 mm in inside diameter and 7.5 cm in length, packed with octadecylsilanized silica gel for liquid chromatography (3 μm in particle diameter).

Column temperature: A constant temperature of about 25°C.

Mobile phase: Dissolve 2.72 g of potassium dihydrogen phosphate in 1000 mL of water, and adjust the pH to 3.0 with diluted phosphoric acid (3 in 500). To 800 mL of this solution add 200 mL of methanol.

Flow rate: Adjust so that the retention time of cefalexin is about 6 minutes.

System suitability—

System performance: When the procedure is run with 10 μL of the standard solution under the above operating conditions, cefalexin and the internal standard are eluted in this order with the resolution between these peaks being not less than 8.

System repeatability: When the test is repeated 6 times with 10 μL of the standard solution under the above operating conditions, the relative standard deviation of the ratio of the peak area of cefalexin to that of the internal standard is not more than 1.0%.

Containers and storage Containers—Tight containers.

Cefalexin Combination Granules

セファレキシン複合顆粒

Cefalexin Combination Granules contain gastric-soluble granules and enteric-soluble granules in one package.

It contains not less than 90.0% and not more than 110.0% of cefalexin ($C_{16}H_{17}N_3O_4S$: 347.39) for the labeled total potency and the labeled potency of gastric-soluble granules, respectively.

Method of preparation Prepare as directed under Granules, with Cefalexin, and pack into single-dose packages.

Identification Powder Cefalexin Combination Granules, weigh a portion of the powder, equivalent to 30 mg (potency) of Cefalexin according to the labeled total potency, shake vigorously for 5 minutes with 100 mL of water, and centrifuge. To 2 mL of the supernatant liquid add water to make 20 mL. Determine the absorption spectrum of this solution as directed under Ultraviolet-visible Spectrophotometry <*2.24*>: it exhibits a maximum between 260 nm and 264 nm.

Water <*2.48*> Not more than 5.0% (0.5 g, volumetric titration, direct titration).

Uniformity of dosage units <*6.02*> Perform the test according to the following method: it meets the requirement of the Content uniformity test.

(1) Total potency—To the total content of 1 package of Cefalexin Combination Granules add a small amount of 0.1 mol/L phosphate buffer solution (pH 4.5), grind, add 3 V/5 mL of 0.1 mol/L phosphate buffer solution (pH 4.5), shake vigorously for 10 minutes, add 0.1 mol/L phosphate buffer solution (pH 4.5) to make exactly V mL so that each mL contains about 2 mg (potency) of Cefalexin according to the labeled total potency, and centrifuge. Pipet 2 mL of the supernatant liquid, add exactly 20 mL of the internal standard solution, add 0.1 mol/L phosphate buffer solution (pH 4.5) to make 200 mL, and use this solution as the sample solution. Then, proceed as directed in the Assay (1) Total potency.

Amount [mg (potency)] of cefalexin ($C_{16}H_{17}N_3O_4S$)
$= M_S \times Q_T/Q_S \times V/10$

M_S: Amount [mg (potency)] of Cefalexin RS taken

Internal standard solution—A solution of *m*-hydroxyacetophenone in 0.1 mol/L phosphate buffer solution (pH 4.5) (1 in 15,000).

(2) Potency of gastric-soluble granules—To the total content of 1 package of Cefalexin Combination Granules, add 3 V/5 mL of 0.1 mol/L phosphate buffer solution (pH 4.5), shake gently for 5 minutes, add 0.1 mol/L phosphate buffer solution (pH 4.5) to make exactly V mL so that each mL contains about 0.6 mg (potency) of Cefalexin according to the labeled potency of gastric-soluble granules, and centrifuge. Pipet 7 mL of the supernatant liquid, add exactly 20 mL of the internal standard solution, add 0.1 mol/L phosphate buffer solution (pH 4.5) to make 200 mL, and use this solution as the sample solution. Then, proceed as directed in the Assay (1) Total potency.

Amount [mg (potency)] of cefalexin ($C_{16}H_{17}N_3O_4S$)
$= M_S \times Q_T/Q_S \times V/35$

M_S: Amount [mg (potency)] of Cefalexin RS taken

Internal standard solution—A solution of *m*-hydroxyacetophenone in 0.1 mol/L phosphate buffer solution (pH 4.5) (1 in 15,000).

Dissolution <*6.10*> When the test is performed at 50 revolutions per minute according to the Paddle method, using 900 mL of 1st fluid for dissolution test as the dissolution medium, the dissolution rate in 30 minutes of Cefalexin Combination Granules is between 25% and 35%.

Start the test with the total content of 1 package of Cefalexin Combination Granules, withdraw not less than 20 mL of the medium at the specified minute after starting the test, and filter through a membrane filter with a pore size not exceeding 0.5 μm. Discard not less than 10 mL of the first filtrate, pipet V mL of the subsequent filtrate, add the dissolution medium to make exactly V' mL so that each mL contains about 22 μg (potency) of Cefalexin according to the labeled potency of gastric-soluble granules, and use this solution as the sample solution. Separately, weigh accurately an amount of Cefalexin RS, equivalent to about 22 mg (potency), and dissolve in the dissolution medium to make exactly 50 mL. Pipet 5 mL of this solution, add the dissolution medium to make exactly 100 mL, and use this solution as the standard solution. Determine the absorbances, A_T and A_S, at 262 nm of the sample solution and standard solution as directed under Ultraviolet-visible Spectrophotometry <*2.24*>.

Dissolution rate (%) of cefalexin ($C_{16}H_{17}N_3O_4S$) with respect to the labeled potency
$= M_S \times A_T/A_S \times V'/V \times 1/C \times 90$

M_S: Amount [mg (potency)] of Cefalexin RS taken
C: Labeled total potency [mg (potency)] of Cefalexin in 1 package

When the test is performed at 50 revolutions per minute according to the Paddle method, using 900 mL of 2nd fluid for dissolution test as the dissolution medium, the dissolution rate in 60 minutes of 200 mg (potency) preparation is not less than 80%, and the dissolution rate in 45 minutes of 500 mg (potency) preparation is not less than 75%.

Start the test with the total content of 1 package of Cefalexin Combination Granules, withdraw not less than 20 mL of the medium at the specified minute after starting the test, and filter through a membrane filter with a pore size not exceeding 0.5 μm. Discard not less than 10 mL of the first filtrate, pipet V mL of the subsequent filtrate, add the dissolution medium to make exactly V' mL so that each mL contains about 22 μg (potency) of Cefalexin according to the labeled total potency, and use this solution as the sample solution. Separately, weigh accurately an amount of Cefalexin RS, equivalent to about 22 mg (potency), dissolve in the dissolution medium to make exactly 50 mL. Pipet 5 mL of this solution, add the dissolution medium to make exactly 100 mL, and use this solution as the standard solution. Determine the absorbances, A_T and A_S, at 262 nm of the sample solution and standard solution as directed under Ultraviolet-visible Spectrophotometry <*2.24*>.

Dissolution rate (%) of cefalexin ($C_{16}H_{17}N_3O_4S$) with respect to the labeled potency

$$= M_S \times A_T/A_S \times V'/V \times 1/C \times 90$$

M_S: Amount [mg (potency)] of Cefalexin RS taken

C: Labeled total potency [mg (potency)] of Cefalexin in 1 package

Assay **(1)** Total potency—Powder the total content obtained from not less than 20 packages of Cefalexin Combination Granules, weigh accurately a portion of the powder, equivalent to about 0.5 g (potency) of Cefalexin, shake vigorously for 10 minutes with 150 mL of 0.1 mol/L phosphate buffer solution (pH 4.5), add 0.1 mol/L phosphate buffer solution (pH 4.5) to make exactly 250 mL, and centrifuge. Pipet 2 mL of this solution, add exactly 20 mL of the internal standard solution, and add 0.1 mol/L phosphate buffer solution (pH 4.5) to make 200 mL, and use this solution as the sample solution. Separately, weigh accurately an amount of Cefalexin RS, equivalent to about 20 mg (potency), and dissolve in 0.1 mol/L phosphate buffer solution (pH 4.5) to make exactly 100 mL. Pipet 10 mL of this solution, add exactly 10 mL of the internal standard solution, and add 0.1 mol/L phosphate buffer solution (pH 4.5) to make 100 mL, and use this solution as the standard solution. Perform the test with 10 μL each of the sample solution and standard solution as directed under Liquid Chromatography <*2.01*> according to the following conditions, and calculate the ratios, Q_T and Q_S, of the peak area of cefalexin to that of the internal standard.

Amount [mg (potency)] of cefalexin ($C_{16}H_{17}N_3O_4S$)

$$= M_S \times Q_T/Q_S \times 25$$

M_S: Amount [mg (potency)] of Cefalexin RS taken

Internal standard solution—A solution of *m*-hydroxyacetophenone in 0.1 mol/L phosphate buffer solution (pH 4.5) (1 in 15,000).

Operating conditions—

Detector: An ultraviolet absorption photometer (wavelength: 254 nm).

Column: A stainless steel column 3.0 mm in inside diameter and 7.5 cm in length, packed with octadecylsilanized silica gel for liquid chromatography (3 μm in particle diameter).

Column temperature: A constant temperature of about 25°C.

Mobile phase: Dissolve 2.72 g of potassium dihydrogen phosphate in 1000 mL of water, and adjust to pH 3.0 with diluted phosphoric acid (3 in 500). To 800 mL of this solution add 200 mL of methanol.

Flow rate: Adjust so that the retention time of cefalexin is about 6 minutes.

System suitability—

System performance: When the procedure is run with 10 μL of the standard solution under the above operating conditions, cefalexin and the internal standard are eluted in this order with the resolution between these peaks being not less than 8.

System repeatability: When the test is repeated 6 times with 10 μL of the standard solution under the above operating conditions, the relative standard deviation of the ratio of the peak area of cefalexin to that of the internal standard is not more than 1.0%.

(2) Potency of gastric-soluble granules—Take out the content from not less than 20 packages of Cefalexin Combination Granules, weigh accurately a quantity, equivalent to about 0.3 g (potency) of Cefalexin according to the labeled potency of gastric-soluble granules, shake gently for 5 minutes with 200 mL of 0.1 mol/L phosphate buffer solution (pH 4.5), add 0.1 mol/L phosphate buffer solution (pH 4.5) to make exactly 300 mL, and centrifuge. Pipet 2 mL of the supernatant liquid, add exactly 10 mL of the internal standard solution, and add 0.1 mol/L phosphate buffer solution (pH 4.5) to make 100 mL, and use this solution as the sample solution. Then, proceed as directed in the Assay (1) Total potency.

Amount [mg (potency)] of cefalexin ($C_{16}H_{17}N_3O_4S$)

$$= M_S \times Q_T/Q_S \times 15$$

M_S: Amount [mg (potency)] of Cefalexin RS taken

Internal standard solution—A solution of *m*-hydroxyacetophenone in 0.1 mol/L phosphate buffer solution (pH 4.5) (1 in 15,000).

Containers and storage Containers—Tight containers.

Cefalexin for Syrup

シロップ用セファレキシン

Cefalexin for Syrup is a preparation for syrup, which is dissolved or suspended before use.

It contains not less than 90.0% and not more than 110.0% of the labeled potency of cefalexin ($C_{16}H_{17}N_3O_4S$: 347.39).

Method of preparation Prepare as directed under Preparations for Syrups, with Cefalexin.

Identification Dissolve a quantity of Cefalexin for Syrup, equivalent to 3 mg (potency) of Cefalexin, in water to make 100 mL. Determine the absorption spectrum of this solution as directed under Ultraviolet-visible Spectrophotometry <*2.24*>: it exhibits a maximum between 260 nm and 264 nm.

Water <*2.48*> Not more than 5.0% (0.4 g, volumetric titration, back titration).

Uniformity of dosage units <*6.02*> Perform the test according to the following method: Cefalexin for Syrup in single-dose packages meets the requirement of the Content uniformity test.

Take out the total content of 1 package of Cefalexin for Syrup, add $3V/5$ mL of 0.1 mol/L phosphate buffer solution (pH 4.5), shake vigorously for 10 minutes, add 0.1 mol/L phosphate buffer solution (pH 4.5) to make exactly V mL so that each mL contains about 1 mg (potency) of Cefalexin, and centrifuge. Pipet 2 mL of the supernatant liquid, add exactly 10 mL of the internal standard solution, add 0.1 mol/L phosphate buffer solution (pH 4.5) to make 100 mL, and use this solution as the sample solution. Then, proceed as directed in the Assay.

Amount [mg (potency)] of cefalexin ($C_{16}H_{17}N_3O_4S$)

$$= M_S \times Q_T/Q_S \times V/20$$

M_S: Amount [mg (potency)] of Cefalexin RS taken

Internal standard solution—A solution of *m*-hydroxyacetophenone in 0.1 mol/L phosphate buffer solution (pH 4.5) (1 in 15,000).

Dissolution <*6.10*> When the test is performed at 50 revolutions per minute according to the Paddle method, using 900 mL of water as the dissolution medium, the dissolution rate in 15 minutes of Cefalexin for Syrup is not less than 80%.

Start the test with an accurately weighed amount of Cefalexin, equivalent to about 0.25 g (potency) of Cefalexin for Syrup, withdraw not less than 20 mL of the medium at the specified minute after starting the test, and filter through a membrane filter with a pore size not exceeding 0.5 μm. Discard not less than 10 mL of the first filtrate, pipet 2 mL of the subsequent filtrate, add water to make exactly 25 mL, and use this solution as the sample solution. Separately, weigh accurately an amount of Cefalexin RS, equivalent to about 22 mg (potency), and dissolve in water to make exactly 50 mL. Pipet 5 mL of this solution, add water to make exactly 100 mL, and use this solution as the standard solution. Perform the test with the sample solution and standard solution as directed under Ultraviolet-visible Spectrophotometry <*2.24*>, and determine the absorbances, A_T and A_S, at 262 nm.

Dissolution rate (%) with respect to the labeled amount of cefalexin ($C_{16}H_{17}N_3O_4S$)
$= M_S/M_T \times A_T/A_S \times 1/C \times 1125$

M_S: Amount [mg (potency)] of Cefalexin RS taken
M_T: Amount (g) of Cefalexin for Syrup taken
C: Labeled amount [mg (potency)] of cefalexin ($C_{16}H_{17}N_3O_4S$) in 1 g

Assay Powder Cefalexin for Syrup, if necessary, and weigh accurately a portion of the powder, equivalent to about 0.1 g (potency) of Cefalexin, add 60 mL of 0.1 mol/L phosphate buffer solution (pH 4.5), shake vigorously for 10 minutes, add 0.1 mol/L phosphate buffer solution (pH 4.5) to make exactly 100 mL, and centrifuge. Pipet 2 mL of the supernatant liquid, add exactly 10 mL of the internal standard solution, add 0.1 mol/L phosphate buffer solution (pH 4.5) to make 100 mL, and use this solution as the sample solution. Separately, weigh accurately an amount of Cefalexin RS, equivalent to about 20 mg (potency), dissolve in 0.1 mol/L phosphate buffer solution (pH 4.5) to make exactly 100 mL. Pipet 10 mL of this solution, add exactly 10 mL of the internal standard solution, add 0.1 mol/L phosphate buffer solution (pH 4.5) to make 100 mL, and use this solution as the standard solution. Perform the test with 10 μL each of the sample solution and standard solution as directed under Liquid Chromatography <*2.01*> according to the following conditions, and calculate the ratios, Q_T and Q_S, of the peak area of cefalexin to that of the internal standard.

Amount [mg (potency)] of cefalexin ($C_{16}H_{17}N_3O_4S$)
$= M_S \times Q_T/Q_S \times 5$

M_S: Amount [mg (potency)] of Cefalexin RS taken

Internal standard solution—A solution of *m*-hydroxyacetophenone in 0.1 mol/L phosphate buffer solution (pH 4.5) (1 in 15,000).

Operating conditions—

Detector: An ultraviolet absorption photometer (wavelength: 254 nm).

Column: A stainless steel column 3.0 mm in inside diameter and 7.5 cm in length, packed with octadecylsilanized silica gel for liquid chromatography (3 μm in particle diameter).

Column temperature: A constant temperature of about 25°C.

Mobile phase: Dissolve 2.72 g of potassium dihydrogen phosphate in 1000 mL of water, and adjust the pH to 3.0 with diluted phosphoric acid (3 in 500). To 800 mL of this solution add 200 mL of methanol.

Flow rate: Adjust so that the retention time of cefalexin is about 6 minutes.

System suitability—

System performance: When the procedure is run with 10 μL of the standard solution under the above operating conditions, cefalexin and the internal standard are eluted in this order with the resolution between these peaks being not less than 8.

System repeatability: When the test is repeated 6 times with 10 μL of the standard solution under the above operating conditions, the relative standard deviation of the ratio of the peak area of cefalexin to that of the internal standard is not more than 1.0%.

Containers and storage Containers—Tight containers.
Storage—Light-resistant.

Cefalotin Sodium

セファロチンナトリウム

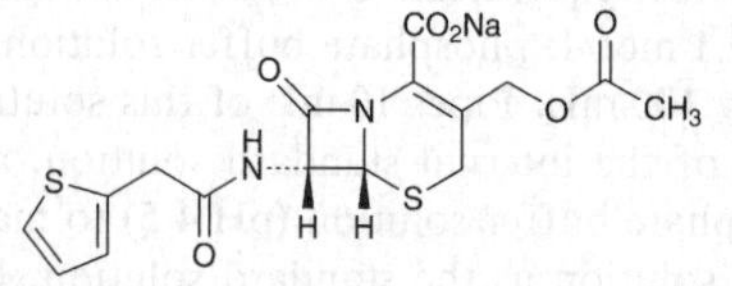

$C_{16}H_{15}N_2NaO_6S_2$: 418.42
Monosodium (6*R*,7*R*)-3-acetoxymethyl-8-oxo-7-[2-(thiophen-2-yl)acetylamino]-5-thia-1-azabicyclo[4.2.0]oct-2-ene-2-carboxylate
[*58-71-9*]

Cefalotin Sodium contains not less than 920 μg (potency) and not more than 980 μg (potency) per mg, calculated on the anhydrous basis. The potency of Cefalotin Sodium is expressed as mass (potency) of cefalotin ($C_{16}H_{16}N_2O_6S_2$: 396.44).

Description Cefalotin Sodium occurs as white to light yellow-white, crystals or crystalline powder.

It is freely soluble in water, slightly soluble in methanol, very slightly soluble in ethanol (95), and practically insoluble in acetonitrile.

Identification **(1)** Determine the absorption spectrum of a solution of Cefalotin Sodium (1 in 50,000) as directed under Ultraviolet-visible Spectrophotometry <*2.24*>, and compare the spectrum with the Reference Spectrum or the spectrum of a solution of Cefalotin Sodium RS prepared in the same manner as the sample solution: both spectra exhibit similar intensities of absorption at the same wavelengths.

(2) Determine the infrared absorption spectrum of Cefalotin Sodium as directed in the potassium bromide disk method under Infrared Spectrophotometry <*2.25*>, and compare the spectrum with the Reference Spectrum or the spectrum of Cefalotin Sodium RS: both spectra exhibit similar intensities of absorption at the same wave numbers.

(3) Determine the ^{1}H spectrum of a solution of Cefalotin Sodium in heavy water for nuclear magnetic resonance spectroscopy (1 in 10) as directed under Nuclear Magnetic

Resonance Spectroscopy 〈*2.21*〉, using sodium 3-trimethylsilylpropanesulfonate for nuclear magnetic resonance spectroscopy as an internal reference compound: it exhibits a singlet signal A at around δ 2.1 ppm, a singlet or sharp multiplet signal B at around δ 3.9 ppm, and a multiplet signal C at around δ 7.0 ppm. The ratio of the integrated intensity of these signals, A:B:C, is about 3:2:2.

(4) Cefalotin Sodium responds to Qualitative Tests 〈*1.09*〉 (1) for sodium salt.

Optical rotation 〈*2.49*〉 $[\alpha]_D^{25}$: +124 – +134° (5 g, water, 100 mL, 100 mm).

pH 〈*2.54*〉 The pH of a solution obtained by dissolving 1.0 g of Cefalotin Sodium in 10 mL of water is between 4.5 and 7.0.

Purity **(1)** Clarity and color of solution—Dissolve 1.0 g of Cefalotin Sodium in 10 mL of water: the solution is clear. The absorbance of this solution at 450 nm, determined as directed under Ultraviolet-visible Spectrophotometry 〈*2.24*〉, is not more than 0.20.

(2) Heavy metals 〈*1.07*〉—Proceed with 1.0 g of Cefalotin Sodium according to Method 2, and perform the test. Prepare the control solution with 2.0 mL of Standard Lead Solution (not more than 20 ppm).

(3) Arsenic 〈*1.11*〉—Prepare the test solution with 1.0 g of Cefalotin Sodium according to Method 3, and perform the test (not more than 2 ppm).

(4) Related substances—Pipet 1 mL of the standard solution obtained in the Assay, add the mobile phase to make exactly 100 mL, and use this solution as the standard solution. Perform the test with exactly 10 μL each of the sample solution obtained in the Assay and the standard solution prepared here as directed under Liquid Chromatography 〈*2.01*〉 according to the following conditions, and determine each peak area by the automatic integration method: the area of the peaks other than cefalotin from the sample solution is not larger than the peak area of cefalotin from the standard solution, and the total area of the peaks other than cefalotin obtained from the sample solution is not larger than 3 times the peak area of cefalotin from the standard solution.

Operating conditions—

Detector, column, column temperature, mobile phase, and flow rate: Proceed as directed in the operating conditions in the Assay.

Time span of measurement: About 4 times as long as the retention time of cefalotin.

System suitability—

Test for required detectability: Measure exactly 1 mL of the standard solution, and add the mobile phase to make exactly 10 mL. Confirm that the peak area of cefalotin obtained with 10 μL of this solution is equivalent to 7 to 13% of that with 10 μL of the standard solution.

System performance: Heat the standard solution in a water bath of 90°C for 10 minutes, and cool. Measure exactly 2.5 mL of this solution, and add the mobile phase to make exactly 100 mL. When the procedure is run with 10 μL of this solution under the above operating conditions, the resolution between the peak of cefalotin and the peak, having the relative retention time of about 0.5 to cefalotin, is not less than 9, and the symmetry factor of the peak of cefalotin is not more than 1.8.

System repeatability: When the test is repeated 3 times with 10 μL of the standard solution under the above operating conditions, the relative standard deviation of the peak area of cefalotin is not more than 2.0%.

Water 〈*2.48*〉 Not more than 1.0% (0.5 g, volumetric titration, back titration).

Assay Weigh accurately an amount of Cefalotin Sodium and Cefalotin Sodium RS, equivalent to about 25 mg (potency), and dissolve each in the mobile phase to make exactly 25 mL, and use these solutions as the sample solution and standard solution. Perform the test with exactly 10 μL each of the sample solution and standard solution as directed under Liquid Chromatography 〈*2.01*〉 according to the following conditions, and determine the peak areas, A_T and A_S, of cefalotin in each solution.

$$\text{Amount [}\mu\text{g (potency)] of cefalotin } (C_{16}H_{16}N_2O_6S_2) = M_S \times A_T/A_S \times 1000$$

M_S: Amount [mg (potency)] of Cefalotin Sodium RS taken

Operating conditions—

Detector: An ultraviolet absorption photometer (wavelength: 254 nm).

Column: A stainless steel column 4.6 mm in inside diameter and 25 cm in length, packed with octadecylsilanized silica gel for liquid chromatography (5 μm in particle diameter).

Column temperature: A constant temperature of about 40°C.

Mobile phase: Dissolve 17 g of sodium acetate trihydrate in 790 mL of water, and add 0.6 mL of acetic acid (100). If necessary adjust the pH to 5.9 ± 0.1 with diluted sodium hydroxide TS (1 in 10) or acetic acid (100). To this solution add 150 mL of acetonitrile and 70 mL of ethanol (95).

Flow rate: Adjust so that the retention time of cefalotin is about 12 minutes.

System suitability—

System performance: Heat the standard solution in a water bath of 90°C for 10 minutes, and cool. Measure exactly 2.5 mL of this solution, and add the mobile phase to make exactly 100 mL. When the procedure is run with 10 μL of this solution under the above operating conditions, the resolution between the peak of cefalotin and the peak, having the relative retention time of about 0.5 to cefalotin is not less than 9, and the symmetry factor of the peak of cefalotin is not more than 1.8.

System repeatability: When the test is repeated 6 times with 10 μL of the standard solution under the above operating conditions, the relative standard deviation of the peak area of cefalotin is not more than 1.0%.

Containers and storage Containers—Tight containers.

Cefalotin Sodium for Injection

注射用セファロチンナトリウム

Cefalotin Sodium for Injection is a preparation for injection, which is dissolved before use.

It contains not less than 90.0% and not more than 110.0% of the labeled potency of cefalotin ($C_{16}H_{16}N_2O_6S_2$: 396.44).

Method of preparation Prepare as directed under Injections, with Cefalotin Sodium.

Description Cefalotin Sodium for Injection occurs as white to light yellow-white, crystals or crystalline powder.

Identification Determine the infrared absorption spectrum of Cefalotin Sodium for Injection as directed in the potassium bromide disk method under Infrared Spectrophotometry <*2.25*>, and compare the spectrum with the Reference Spectrum of Cefalotin Sodium or the spectrum of Cefalotin Sodium RS: both spectra exhibit similar intensities of absorption at the same wave numbers.

pH <*2.54*> Dissolve an amount of Cefalotin Sodium for Injection, equivalent to 0.5 g (potency) of Cefalotin Sodium, in 5 mL of water: the pH of the solution is between 4.5 and 7.0.

Purity **(1)** Clarity and color of solution—Dissolve 1.0 g of Cefalotin Sodium for Injection in 10 mL of water: the solution is clear. Perform the test with this solution as directed under Ultraviolet-visible Spectrophotometry <*2.24*>: the absorbance at 450 nm is not more than 0.20.

(2) Related substances—Dissolve an amount of Cefalotin Sodium for Injection, equivalent to 25 mg (potency), in the mobile phase to make 25 mL, and use this solution as the sample solution. Pipet 1 mL of the sample solution, and add the mobile phase to make exactly 100 mL, and use this solution as the standard solution. Perform the test with exactly 10 μL each of the sample solution and standard solution as directed under Liquid Chromatography <*2.01*> according to the following conditions, and determine each peak area by the automatic integration method: the area of the peak other than cefalotin obtained from the sample solution is not larger than the peak area of cefalotin from the standard solution, and the total area of the peaks other than cefalotin from the sample solution is not larger than 3 times the peak area of cefalotin from the standard solution.

Operating conditions—

Detector, column, column temperature, mobile phase and flow rate: Proceed as directed in the operating conditions in the Assay under Cefalotin Sodium.

Time span of measurement: About 4 times as long as the retention time of cefalotin.

System suitability—

Proceed as directed in the system suitability in the Purity (4) under Cefalotin Sodium.

Water <*2.48*> Not more than 1.0% (0.5 g, volumetric titration, back titration).

Bacterial endotoxins <*4.01*> Less than 0.2 EU/mg (potency).

Uniformity of dosage units <*6.02*> It meets the requirement of the Mass variation test.

Foreign insoluble matter <*6.06*> Perform the test according to Method 2: it meets the requirement.

Insoluble particulate matter <*6.07*> It meets the requirement.

Sterility <*4.06*> Perform the test according to the Membrane filtration method: it meets the requirement.

Assay Weigh accurately the mass of the contents of not less than 10 containers of Cefalotin Sodium for Injection. Weigh accurately an amount of the contents, equivalent to about 25 mg (potency) of Cefalotin Sodium, dissolve in the mobile phase to make exactly 25 mL, and use this solution as the sample solution. Separately, weigh accurately about 25 mg (potency) of Cefalotin Sodium RS, and dissolve in the mobile phase to make exactly 25 mL, and use this solution as the standard solution. Then, proceed as directed in the Assay under Cefalotin Sodium.

Amount [μg(potency)] of cefalotin ($C_{16}H_{16}N_2O_6S_2$)
$= M_S \times A_T/A_S \times 1000$

M_S: Amount [mg(potency)] of Cefalotin Sodium RS taken

Containers and storage Containers—Hermetic containers.

Cefatrizine Propylene Glycolate

セファトリジンプロピレングリコール

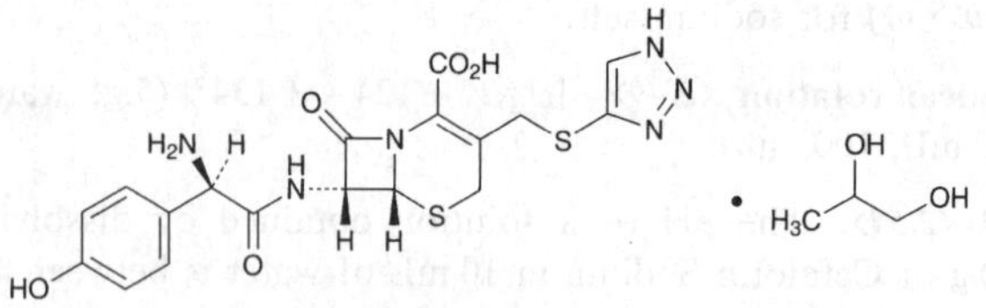

$C_{18}H_{18}N_6O_5S_2.C_3H_8O_2$: 538.60
(6*R*,7*R*)-7-[(2*R*)-2-Amino-2-(4-hydroxyphenyl)acetylamino]-8-oxo-3-[2-(1*H*-1,2,3-triazol-4-yl)sulfanylmethyl]-5-thia-1-azabicyclo[4.2.0]oct-2-ene-2-carboxylic acid monopropane-1,2-diolate (1/1)
[*51627-14-6*, Cefatrizine]

Cefatrizine Propylene Glycolate contains not less than 816 μg (potency) and not more than 876 μg (potency) per mg, calculated on the anhydrous basis. The potency of Cefatrizine Propylene Glycolate is expressed as mass (potency) of cefatrizine ($C_{18}H_{18}N_6O_5S_2$: 462.50).

Description Cefatrizine Propylene Glycolate occurs as a white to yellowish white powder.

It is sparingly soluble in water, and practically insoluble in methanol and in ethanol (95).

Identification **(1)** Determine the absorption spectrum of a solution of Cefatrizine Propylene Glycolate (1 in 50,000) as directed under Ultraviolet-visible Spectrophotometry <*2.24*>, and compare the spectrum with the Reference Spectrum or the spectrum of a solution of Cefatrizine Propylene Glycolate RS prepared in the same manner as the sample solution: both spectra exhibit similar intensities of absorption at the same wavelengths.

(2) Determine the infrared absorption spectrum of Cefatrizine Propylene Glycolate as directed in the potassium bromide disk method under Infrared Spectrophotometry <*2.25*>, and compare the spectrum with the Reference Spectrum or the spectrum of Cefatrizine Propylene Glycolate RS: both spectra exhibit similar intensities of absorption at the same wave numbers.

(3) Determine the ^{1}H spectrum of a solution of Cefatrizine Propylene Glycolate in a mixture of heavy water for nuclear magnetic resonance spectroscopy and deuterated hydrochloric acid for nuclear magnetic resonance spectroscopy (3:1) (1 in 10), using sodium 3-(trimethylsilyl)propionate-d_4 for nuclear magnetic resonance spectroscopy as an internal reference compound, as directed under Nuclear Magnetic Resonance Spectroscopy <*2.21*>: it exhibits a doublet signal A at around δ 1.2 ppm, a doublet signal B at around δ 7.0 ppm, a doublet signal C at around δ 7.5 ppm and a singlet signal D at around δ 8.3 ppm. The ratio of integrated intensity of these signals, A:B:C:D, is about 3:2:2:1.

Optical rotation <*2.49*> $[\alpha]_D^{20}$: +52 – +58° (2.5 g calculated on the anhydrous bases, 1 mol/L hydrochloric acid TS, 50 mL, 100 mm).

Purity **(1)** Heavy metals <*1.07*>—Proceed with 1.0 g of Cefatrizine Propylene Glycolate according to Method 2, and

perform the test. Prepare the control solution with 2.0 mL of Standard Lead Solution (not more than 20 ppm).

(2) Arsenic <*1.11*>—Prepare the test solution with 1.0 g of Cefatrizine Propylene Glycolate according to Method 3, and perform the test (not more than 2 ppm). Use a solution of magnesium nitrate hexahydrate in ethanol (1 in 25).

(3) Related substances—Dissolve 25 mg of Cefatrizine Propylene Glycolate in 5 mL of water, and use this solution as the sample solution. Pipet 1 mL of the sample solution, add water to make exactly 20 mL, and use this solution as the standard solution. Perform the test with these solutions as directed under Thin-layer Chromatography <*2.03*>. Spot 5 μL each of the sample solution and standard solution on a plate of silica gel for thin-layer chromatography. Develop with a mixture of 1-butanol, water and acetic acid (100) (3:1:1) to a distance of about 12 cm, and air-dry the plate. Spray evenly ninhydrin-citric acid-acetic acid TS on the plate, and heat the plate at 100°C for 10 minutes: the spots other than the principal spot obtained from the sample solution are not more intense than the spot from the standard solution.

Water <*2.48*> Not more than 2.0% (0.5 g, volumetric titration, direct titration).

Assay Weigh accurately an amount of Cefatrizine Propylene Glycolate and Cefatrizine Propylene Glycolate RS, equivalent to about 0.1 g (potency), dissolve each in water to make exactly 500 mL, and use these solutions as the sample solution and the standard solution, respectively. Perform the test with exactly 10 μL each of the sample solution and standard solution as directed under Liquid Chromatography <*2.01*> according to the following conditions, and determine the peak areas, A_T and A_S, of cefatrizine in each solution.

$$\text{Amount [}\mu\text{g (potency)] of cefatrizine } (C_{18}H_{18}N_6O_5S_2) = M_S \times A_T/A_S \times 1000$$

M_S: Amount [mg (potency)] of Cefatrizine Propylene Glycolate RS taken

Operating conditions—

Detector: An ultraviolet absorption photometer (wavelength: 270 nm).

Column: A stainless steel column 4.6 mm in inside diameter and 25 cm in length, packed with octadecylsilanized silica gel for liquid chromatography (5 μm in particle diameter).

Column temperature: A constant temperature of about 40°C.

Mobile phase: A mixture of a solution of potassium dihydrogenphosphate (17 in 12,500) and methanol (17:3).

Flow rate: Adjust so that the retention time of cefatrizine is about 11 minutes.

System suitability—

System performance: Dissolve about 10 mg (potency) of Cefatrizine Propylene Glycolate and about 5 mg (potency) of Cefadroxil in 50 mL of water. When the procedure is run with 10 μL of this solution under the above operating conditions, cefadroxil and cefatrizine are eluted in this order with the resolution between these peaks being not less than 4.

System repeatability: When the test is repeated 6 times with 10 μL of the standard solution under the above operating conditions, the relative standard deviation of peak areas of cefatrizine is not more than 1.0%.

Containers and storage Containers—Tight containers.

Cefatrizine Propylene Glycolate for Syrup

シロップ用セファトリジンプロピレングリコール

Cefatrizine Propylene Glycolate for Syrup is a preparation for syrup, which is dissolved before use.

It contains not less than 90.0% and not more than 105.0% of the labeled potency of Cefatrizine ($C_{18}H_{18}N_6O_5S_2$: 462.50).

Method of preparation Prepare as directed under Preparations for Syrup, with Cefatrizine Propylene Glycolate.

Identification Powder Cefatrizine Propylene Glycolate for Syrup, weigh a portion of the powder, equivalent to 10 mg (potency) of Cefatrizine Propylene Glycolate, and dissolve in 10 mL of water. To 2 mL of this solution add water to make 100 mL. Determine the absorption spectrum of this solution as directed under Ultraviolet-visible Spectrophotometry <*2.24*>: it exhibits maxima between 225 nm and 229 nm, and between 266 nm and 271 nm.

pH <*2.54*> Take an amount of Cefatrizine Propylene Glycolate for Syrup, equivalent to 0.4 g (potency) of Cefatrizine Propylene Glycolate, and suspend in 10 mL of water: the pH of this suspension is between 4.0 and 6.0.

Purity Related substances—Use the sample solution obtained in the Assay as the sample solution. Pipet 1 mL of the sample solution, add water to make exactly 100 mL, and use this solution as the standard solution. Perform the test with exactly 10 μL each of the sample solution and standard solution as directed under Liquid Chromatography <*2.01*> according to the following conditions. Determine each peak area in each solution by the automatic integration method: the area of each peak other than cefatrizine obtained from the sample solution is not larger than the peak area of cefatrizine from the standard solution, and the total area of the peaks other than cefatrizine from the sample solution is not larger than 2 times the peak area of cefatrizine from the standard solution.

Operating conditions—

Detector, column, column temperature, mobile phase and flow rate: Proceed as directed in the operating conditions in the Assay under Cefatrizine Propylene Glycolate.

Time span of measurement: About 2.5 times as long as the retention time of cefatrizine, beginning after the solvent peak.

System suitability—

System performance: Proceed as directed in the system suitability in the Assay under Cefatrizine Propylene Glycolate.

Test for required detectability: Pipet 2 mL of the standard solution, and add water to make exactly 10 mL. Confirm that the peak area of cefatrizine obtained with 10 μL of this solution is equivalent to 15 to 25% of that with 10 μL of the standard solution.

System repeatability: When the test is repeated 6 times with 10 μL of the standard solution under the above operating conditions, the relative standard deviation of the peak area of cefatrizine is not more than 2.0%.

Uniformity of dosage units <*6.02*> Cefatrizine Propylene Glycolate for Syrup in single-dose packages meets the requirement of the Mass variation test.

Assay Powder Cefatrizine Propylene Glycolate for Syrup,

weigh accurately a portion of the powder, equivalent to about 0.1 g (potency) of Cefatrizine Propylene Glycolate, dissolve in water to make exactly 500 mL, and use this solution as the sample solution. Separately, weigh accurately an amount of Cefatrizine Propylene Glycolate RS, equivalent to about 20 mg (potency), dissolve in water to make exactly 100 mL, and use this solution as the standard solution. Then, proceed as directed in the Assay under Cefatrizine Propylene Glycolate.

Amount [mg (potency)] of cefatrizine ($C_{18}H_{18}N_6O_5S_2$)
$= M_S \times A_T/A_S \times 5$

M_S: Amount [mg (potency)] of Cefatrizine Propylene Glycolate RS taken

Containers and storage Containers—Tight containers.

Cefazolin Sodium

セファゾリンナトリウム

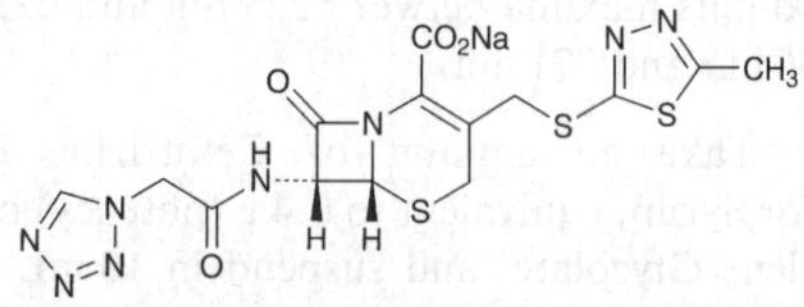

$C_{14}H_{13}N_8NaO_4S_3$: 476.49
Monosodium (6*R*,7*R*)-3-(5-methyl-1,3,4-thiadiazol-2-ylsulfanylmethyl)-8-oxo-7-[2-(1*H*-tetrazol-1-yl)acetylamino]-5-thia-1-azabicyclo[4.2.0]oct-2-ene-2-carboxylate
[*27164-46-1*]

Cefazolin Sodium contains not less than 900 μg (potency) and not more than 975 μg (potency) per mg, calculated on the anhydrous basis. The potency of Cefazolin Sodium is expressed as mass (potency) of cefazolin ($C_{14}H_{14}N_8O_4S_3$: 454.51).

Description Cefazolin Sodium occurs as a white to light yellow-white, crystals or crystalline powder.

It is freely soluble in water and in formamide, slightly soluble in methanol, and practically insoluble in ethanol (95).

Identification (1) Determine the absorption spectrum of a solution of Cefazolin Sodium (1 in 50,000) as directed under Ultraviolet-visible Spectrophotometry <*2.24*>, and compare the spectrum with the Reference Spectrum: both spectra exhibit similar intensities of absorption at the same wavelengths.

(2) Determine the infrared absorption spectrum of Cefazolin Sodium as directed in the potassium bromide disk method under Infrared Spectrophotometry <*2.25*>, and compare the spectrum with the Reference Spectrum: both spectra exhibit similar intensities of absorption at the same wave numbers.

(3) Determine the ^1H spectrum of a solution of Cefazolin Sodium in heavy water for nuclear magnetic resonance spectroscopy (1 in 10), using sodium 3-trimethylsilylpropionate-d_4 for nuclear magnetic resonance spectroscopy as an internal reference compound, as directed under Nuclear Magnetic Resonance Spectroscopy <*2.21*>: it exhibits singlet signals, A and B, at around δ 2.7 ppm and at around δ 9.3 ppm, respectively. The ratio of integrated intensity of these signals, A:B, is about 3:1.

(4) Cefazolin Sodium responds to Qualitative Tests <*1.09*> (1) for sodium salt.

Optical rotation <*2.49*> $[\alpha]_D^{20}$: −19 – −23° (2.5 g calculated as the anhydrous basis, water, 25 mL, 100 mm).

pH <*2.54*> Dissolve 1.0 g of Cefazolin Sodium in 10 mL of water: pH of the solution is between 4.8 and 6.3.

Purity (1) Clarity and color of solution—Dissolve 1.0 g of Cefazolin Sodium in 10 mL of water: the solution is clear and colorless to pale yellow, and its absorbance at 400 nm determined as directed under Ultraviolet-visible Spectrophotometry <*2.24*> is not more than 0.35. The test should be performed within 10 minutes after preparing of the solution.

(2) Heavy metals <*1.07*>—Proceed with 2.0 g of Cefazolin Sodium according to Method 2, and perform the test. Prepare the control solution with 2.0 mL of Standard Lead Solution (not more than 10 ppm).

(3) Arsenic <*1.11*>—Prepare the test solution with 2.0 g of Cefazolin Sodium according to Method 3, and perform the test. When prepare the test solution, add 1.5 mL of hydrogen peroxide (30) after addition of 10 mL of a solution of magnesium nitrate hexahydrate in ethanol (95) (1 in 50), and then ignite (not more than 1 ppm).

(4) Related substances—Dissolve 0.10 g of Cefazolin Sodium in 20 mL of 0.1 mol/L phosphate buffer solution (pH 7.0) and use this solution as the sample solution. Prepare the sample solution before use. Perform the test with 5 μL of the sample solution as directed under Liquid Chromatography <*2.01*> according to the following conditions. Determine each peak area by the automatic integration method, and calculate the amount of the peaks by the area percentage method: the amount of the peak, having the relative retention time of about 0.2 to cefazolin and the amount of the peak other than cefazolin and the peak mentioned above are not more than 1.5%, respectively. The total amount of the peaks other than cefazolin is not more than 2.5%. For the area of the peak, having the relative retention time of about 0.2 to the cefazolin, multiply the correction factor, 1.43.

Operating conditions—

Detector, column, column temperature, mobile phase, and flow rate: Proceed as directed in the operating conditions in the Assay.

Time span of measurement: About 3 times as long as the retention time of cefazolin, beginning after the solvent peak.

System suitability—

System performance: Proceed as directed in the system suitability in the Assay.

Test for required detectability: Dissolve about 80 mg of Cefazolin RS in 0.1 mol/L phosphate buffer solution (pH 7.0) to make 100 mL, and use this solution as the solution for system suitability test. Pipet 1 mL of the solution for system suitability test, and add 0.1 mol/L phosphate buffer solution (pH 7.0) to make exactly 20 mL. Confirm that the peak area of cefazolin obtained with 5 μL of this solution is equivalent to 3 to 7% of that with 5 μL of the solution for system suitability test.

System repeatability: When the test is repeated 6 times with 5 μL of the solution for system suitability test under the above operating conditions, the relative standard deviation of the peak areas of cefazolin is not more than 1.0%.

Water <*2.48*> Not more than 2.5% (1.0 g, volumetric titration, direct titration. Use a mixture of formamide for water determination and methanol for water determination (2:1) instead of methanol for water determination).

Assay Weigh accurately an amount of Cefazolin Sodium

and Cefazolin RS, equivalent to about 20 mg (potency), dissolve each in the internal standard solution to make exactly 20 mL, and use these solutions as the sample solution and the standard solution, respectively. Perform the test with 5 μL each of the sample solution and standard solution as directed under Liquid Chromatography <2.01> according to the following conditions, and calculate the ratios, Q_T and Q_S, of the peak area of cefazolin to that of the internal standard.

Amount [μg (potency)] of cefazolin ($C_{14}H_{14}N_8O_4S_3$)
$= M_S \times Q_T/Q_S \times 1000$

M_S: Amount [mg (potency)] of Cefazolin RS taken

Internal standard solution—A solution of *p*-acetanisidide in 0.1 mol/L phosphate buffer solution (pH 7.0) (11 in 20,000).
Operating conditions—

Detector: An ultraviolet absorption photometer (wavelength: 254 nm).

Column: A stainless steel column 4 mm in inside diameter and 15 cm in length, packed with octadecylsilanized silica gel for liquid chromatography (10 μm in particle diameter).

Column temperature: A constant temperature of about 25°C.

Mobile phase: Dissolve 2.27 g of disodium hydrogen phosphate dodecahydrate and 0.47 g of citric acid monohydrate in water to make 935 mL, and add 65 mL of acetonitrile.

Flow rate: Adjust so that the retention time of cefazolin is about 8 minutes.
System suitability—

System performance: When the procedure is run with 5 μL of the standard solution under the above operating conditions, cefazolin and the internal standard are eluted in this order with the resolution between these peaks being not less than 4.

System repeatability: When the test is repeated 6 times with 5 μL of the standard solution under the above operating conditions, the relative standard deviation of the ratios of the peak area of cefazolin to that of the internal standard is not more than 1.0%.

Containers and storage Containers—Tight containers.

Cefazolin Sodium for Injection

注射用セファゾリンナトリウム

Cefazolin Sodium for Injection is a preparation for injection which is dissolved before use.

It contains not less than 90.0% and not more than 110.0% of the labeled potency of cefazolin ($C_{14}H_{14}N_8O_4S_3$: 454.51).

Method of preparation Prepare as directed under Injections, with Cefazolin Sodium.

Description Cefazolin Sodium for Injection occurs as white to light yellow-white, crystals or crystalline powder or masses.

Identification (1) Determine the absorption spectrum of a solution of Cefazolin Sodium for Injection (1 in 50,000) as directed under Ultraviolet-visible Spectrophotometry <2.24>: it exhibits a maximum between 270 nm and 274 nm.

(2) Cefazolin Sodium for Injection responds to Qualitative Tests <1.09> (1) for chloride.

Osmotic pressure ratio Being specified separately when the drug is granted approval based on the Law.

pH <2.54> The pH of a solution prepared by dissolving an amount of Cefazolin Sodium for Injection, equivalent to 1.0 g (potency) of Cefazolin Sodium, in 10 mL of water is 4.5 to 6.5.

Purity (1) Clarity and color of solution—Conduct this procedure within 10 minutes after the preparation of the solutions. A solution prepared by dissolving an amount of Cefazolin Sodium for Injection, equivalent to 1.0 g (potency) of Cefazolin Sodium, in 10 mL of water is clear, and the absorbance of this solution at 400 nm, determined as directed under Ultraviolet-visible Spectrophotometry <2.24>, is not more than 0.35.

(2) Related substances—Dissolve an amount of Cefazolin Sodium for Injection, equivalent to 0.10 g (potency) of Cefazolin Sodium, in 20 mL of 0.1 mol/L phosphate buffer solution (pH 7.0) and use this solution as the sample solution. Prepare the sample solution before use. Perform the test with 5 μL of the sample solution as directed under Liquid Chromatography <2.01> according to the following conditions, and determine each peak area by the automatic integration method. Calculate the amount of each peak by the area percentage method: the amount of the peaks other than cefazolin is not more than 1.5%. Furthermore the total amount of the peaks other than cefazolin is not more than 2.5%. For the area of the peak, having the relative retention time of about 0.2 to cefazolin, multiply the correction factor, 1.43.
Operating conditions—

Detector, column, column temperature, mobile phase, and flow rate: Proceed as directed in the operating conditions in the Assay under Cefazolin Sodium.

Time span of measurement: About 3 times as long as the retention time of cefazolin, beginning after the solvent peak.
System suitability—

System performance: Proceed as directed in the system suitability in the Assay under Cefazolin Sodium.

Test for required detectability: To 8 mL of the sample solution, add 0.1 mol/L phosphate buffer solution (pH 7.0) to make 50 mL, and use this solution as the solution for system suitability test. Pipet 1 mL of the solution for system suitability test, add 0.1 mol/L phosphate buffer solution (pH 7.0) to make exactly 20 mL. Confirm that the peak area of cefazolin obtained with 5 μL of this solution is equivalent to 3 to 7% of that with 5 μL of the solution for system suitability test.

System repeatability: When the test is repeated 6 times with 5 μL of the solution for system suitability test under the above operating conditions, the relative standard deviation of the peak area of cefazolin is not more than 1.0%.

Water <2.48> Not more than 3.0% (0.5 g, volumetric titration, direct titration). Use a mixture of formamide for water determination and methanol for water determination (2:1) instead of methanol for water determination.

Bacterial endotoxins <4.01> Less than 0.05 EU/mg (potency).

Uniformity of dosage units <6.02> It meets the requirement of the Mass variation test.

Foreign insoluble matter <6.06> Perform the test according to Method 2: it meets the requirement.

Insoluble particulate matter <6.07> It meets the requirement.

Sterility <4.06> Perform the test according to the Mem-

brane filtration method: it meets the requirement.

Assay Weigh accurately the mass of the contents of not less than 10 containers of Cefazolin Sodium for Injection. Weigh accurately an amount of the contents, equivalent to about 50 mg (potency) of Cefazolin Sodium, dissolve in the internal standard solution to make exactly 50 mL, and use this solution as the sample solution. Separately, weigh accurately an amount of Cefazolin RS, equivalent to about 50 mg (potency), dissolve in the internal standard solution to make exactly 50 mL, and use this solution as the standard solution. Then, proceed as directed in the Assay under Cefazolin Sodium.

Amount [mg (potency)] of cefazolin ($C_{14}H_{14}N_8O_4S_3$)
$= M_S \times Q_T/Q_S$

M_S: Amount [mg (potency)] of Cefazolin RS taken

Internal standard solution—A solution of *p*-acetanisidide in 0.1 mol/L phosphate buffer solution (pH 7.0) (11 in 20,000).

Containers and storage Containers—Hermetic containers. Plastic containers for aqueous injections may be used.

Cefazolin Sodium Hydrate

セファゾリンナトリウム水和物

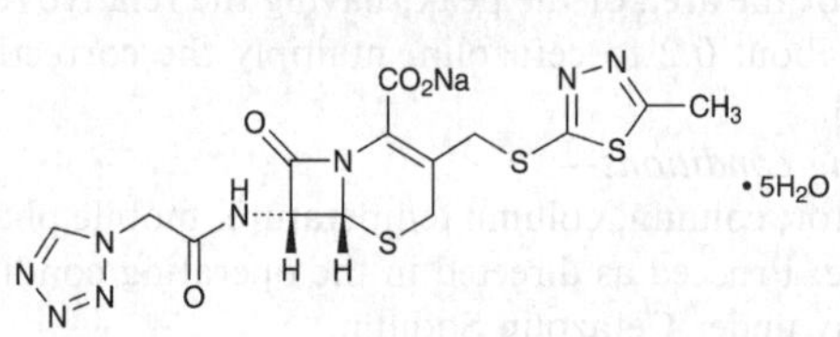

$C_{14}H_{13}N_8NaO_4S_3.5H_2O$: 566.57
Monosodium (6*R*,7*R*)-3-(5-methyl-1,3,4-thiadiazol-2-ylsulfanylmethyl)-8-oxo-7-[2-(1*H*-tetrazol-1-yl)acetylamino]-5-thia-1-azabicyclo[4.2.0]oct-2-ene-2-carboxylate pentahydrate
[*115850-11-8*]

Cefazolin Sodium Hydrate contains not less than 920 μg (potency) and not more than 975 μg (potency) per mg, calculated on the anhydrous basis. The potency of Cefazolin Sodium Hydrate is expressed as mass (potency) of cefazolin ($C_{14}H_{14}N_8O_4S_3$: 454.51).

Description Cefazolin Sodium Hydrate occurs as white to pale yellowish white crystals.

It is freely soluble in water, sparingly soluble in methanol, slightly soluble in ethanol (95), and practically insoluble in diethyl ether.

Identification **(1)** Determine the absorption spectrum of a solution of Cefazolin Sodium Hydrate (1 in 50,000) as directed under Ultraviolet-visible Spectrophotometry *<2.24>*, and compare the spectrum with the Reference Spectrum: both spectra exhibit similar intensities of absorption at the same wavelengths.

(2) Determine the infrared absorption spectrum of Cefazolin Sodium Hydrate as directed in the potassium bromide disk method under Infrared Spectrophotometry *<2.25>*, and compare the spectrum with the Reference Spectrum: both spectra exhibit similar intensities of absorption at the same wave numbers.

(3) Determine the ^1H spectrum of a solution of Cefazolin Sodium Hydrate in heavy water for nuclear magnetic resonance spectroscopy (1 in 10), using sodium 3-trimethylsilylpropionate-d_4 for nuclear magnetic resonance spectroscopy as an internal reference compound, as directed under Nuclear Magnetic Resonance Spectroscopy *<2.21>*: it exhibits singlet signals, A and B, at around δ 2.7 ppm and at around δ 9.3 ppm. The ratio of integrated intensity of each signal, A:B, is about 3:1.

(4) Cefazolin Sodium Hydrate responds to Qualitative Tests *<1.09>* (1) for sodium salt.

Absorbance *<2.24>* $E^{1\%}_{1\,cm}$ (272 nm): 272 – 292 (80 mg calculated on the anhydrous basis, water, 5000 mL).

Optical rotation *<2.49>* $[\alpha]^{20}_D$: -20 – $-25°$ (2.5 g calculated on the anhydrous basis, water, 25 mL, 100 mm).

pH *<2.54>* Dissolve 1.0 g of Cefazolin Sodium Hydrate in 10 mL of water: the pH of the solution is between 4.8 and 6.3.

Purity **(1)** Clarity and color of solution—Dissolve 1.0 g of Cefazolin Sodium Hydrate in 10 mL of water: the solution is clear, and when determine the absorbance at 400 nm of this solution as directed under Ultraviolet-visible Spectrophotometry *<2.24>*, it is not more than 0.15.

(2) Heavy metals *<1.07>*—Proceed with 2.0 g of Cefazolin Sodium Hydrate according to Method 2, and perform the test. Prepare the control solution with 2.0 mL of Standard Lead Solution (not more than 10 ppm).

(3) Related substances—Dissolve 0.10 of Cefazolin Sodium Hydrate in 20 mL of 0.1 mol/L phosphate buffer solution (pH 7.0) and use this solution as the sample solution. Perform the test with 5 μL of the sample solution as directed under Liquid Chromatography *<2.01>* according to the following conditions. Determine each peak area by the automatic integration method, and calculate the amount of them by the area percentage method: the amount of the peak having the relative retention time of about 0.2 to cefazolin is not more than 1.0%, the amount of the peak other than cefazolin and the peak mentioned above is not more than 0.5%, and the total amount of the peaks other than cefazolin is not more than 2.0%. For the area of the peak, having the relative retention time of about 0.2 to cefazolin, multiply the correction factor 1.43.

Operating conditions—

Detector, column, column temperature, mobile phase, and flow rate: Proceed as directed in the operating conditions in the Assay.

Time span of measurement: About 3 times as long as the retention time of cefazolin, beginning after the solvent peak.

System suitability—

Test for required detectability: To 1 mL of the sample solution add 0.1 mol/L phosphate buffer solution (pH 7.0) to make 100 mL, and use this solution as the solution for system suitability test. Pipet 1 mL of the solution for system suitability test, add 0.1 mol/L phosphate buffer solution (pH 7.0) to make exactly 10 mL. Confirm that the peak area of cefazolin obtained with 5 μL of this solution is equivalent to 7 to 13% of that with 5 μL of the solution for system suitability test.

System performance: Dissolve 20 mg of Cefazolin Sodium Hydrate in 20 mL of a solution of *p*-acetanisidide in 0.1 mol/L phosphate buffer solution (pH 7.0) (11 in 20,000). When the procedure is run with 5 μL of this solution under the above operating conditions, cefazolin and *p*-acetanisidide are eluted in this order with the resolution between these peaks being not less than 4.

System repeatability: When the test is repeated 6 times with 5 μL of the solution for system suitability test under the above operating conditions, the relative standard deviation of the peak area of cefazolin is not more than 2.0%.

Water <2.48> Not less than 13.7% and not more than 16.0% (0.1 g, volumetric titration, direct titration. Use a mixture of formamide for water determination and methanol for water determination (2:1) instead of methanol for water determination).

Bacterial endotoxins <4.01> Less than 0.10 EU/mg (potency).

Assay Weigh accurately an amount of Cefazolin Sodium Hydrate and Cefazolin RS, equivalent to about 20 mg (potency), dissolve in exactly 20 mL of the internal standard solution, and use these solutions as the sample solution and standard solution. Perform the test with 5 μL each of the sample solution and standard solution as directed under Liquid Chromatography <2.01> according to the following conditions, and calculate the ratios, Q_T and Q_S, of the peak area of cefazolin to that of the internal standard.

Amount [μg (potency)] of cefazolin ($C_{14}H_{14}N_8O_4S_3$)
$= M_S \times Q_T/Q_S \times 1000$

M_S: Amount [mg (potency)] of Cefazolin RS taken

Internal standard solution—A solution of *p*-acetanisidide in 0.1 mol/L phosphate buffer solution (pH 7.0) (11 in 20,000).
Operating conditions—

Detector: An ultraviolet absorption photometer (wavelength: 254 nm).

Column: A stainless steel column 4 mm in inside diameter and 15 cm in length, packed with octadecylsilanized silica gel for liquid chromatography (10 μm in particle diameter).

Column temperature: A constant temperature of about 25°C.

Mobile phase: Dissolve 2.27 g of disodium hydrogen phosphate dodecahydrate and 0.47 g of citric acid monohydrate in water to make 935 mL. To this solution, add 65 mL of acetonitrile.

Flow rate: Adjust so that the retention time of cefazolin is about 8 minutes.
System suitability—

System performance: When the procedure is run with 5 μL of the standard solution under the above operating conditions, cefazolin and the internal standard are eluted in this order with the resolution between these peaks being not less than 4.

System repeatability: When the test is repeated 6 times with 5 μL of the standard solution under the above operating conditions, the relative standard deviation of the peak area of cefazolin is not more than 1.0%.

Containers and storage Containers—Hermetic containers.
Storage—Light-resistant.

Cefbuperazone Sodium

セフブペラゾンナトリウム

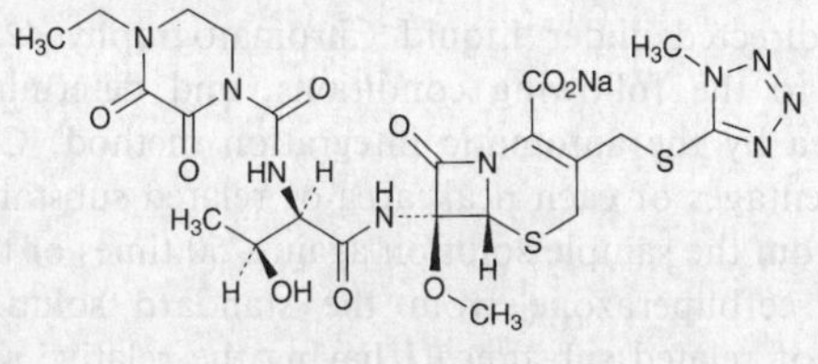

$C_{22}H_{28}N_9NaO_9S_2$: 649.63
Monosodium (6*R*,7*S*)-7-{(2*R*,3*S*)-2-[(4-ethyl-2,3-dioxopiperazine-1-carbonyl)amino]-3-hydroxybutanoylamino}-7-methoxy-3-(1-methyl-1*H*-tetrazol-5-ylsulfanylmethyl)-8-oxo-5-thia-1-azabicyclo[4.2.0]oct-2-ene-2-carboxylate
[*76648-01-6*]

Cefbuperazone Sodium contains not less than 870 μg (potency) per mg, calculated on the anhydrous basis. The potency of Cefbuperazone Sodium is expressed as mass (potency) of cefbuperazone ($C_{22}H_{29}N_9O_9S_2$: 627.65).

Description Cefbuperazone Sodium occurs as white to light yellow-white, powder or masses.

It is very soluble in water, freely soluble in methanol and in pyridine, sparingly soluble in ethanol (95), and very slightly soluble in acetonitrile.

Identification **(1)** Determine the absorption spectrum of a solution of Cefbuperazone Sodium (1 in 50,000) as directed under Ultraviolet-visible Spectrophotometry <2.24>, and compare the spectrum with the Reference Spectrum: both spectra exhibit similar intensities of absorption at the same wavelengths.

(2) Dissolve 0.1 g of Cefbuperazone Sodium in 0.5 mL of deuterated pyridine for nuclear magnetic resonance spectroscopy and 1 drop of heavy water for nuclear magnetic resonance spectroscopy, and determine the ^{1}H spectrum of this solution as directed under Nuclear Magnetic Resonance Spectroscopy <2.21>, using tetramethylsilane for nuclear magnetic resonance spectroscopy as an internal reference compound: it exhibits a triplet signal A at around δ 1.1 ppm, and two doublet signals, B and C, at around δ 1.6 ppm and at around δ 5.1 ppm, respectively. The ratio of the integrated intensity of each signal, A:B:C, is about 3:3:1.

(3) Cefbuperazone Sodium responds to Qualitative Tests <1.09> (1) for sodium salt.

Optical rotation <2.49> $[\alpha]_D^{20}$: +48 – +56° (0.4 g calculated on the anhydrous basis, water, 20 mL, 100 mm).

pH <2.54> Dissolve 1.0 g of Cefbuperazone Sodium in 4 mL of water: the pH of the solution is between 4.0 and 6.0.

Purity **(1)** Clarity and color of solution—Dissolve 1.0 g of Cefbuperazone Sodium in 4 mL of water: the solution is clear and light yellow.

(2) Heavy metals <1.07>—Proceed with 2.0 g of Cefbuperazone Sodium according to Method 4, and perform the test. Prepare the control solution with 2.0 mL of Standard Lead Solution (not more than 10 ppm).

(3) Arsenic <1.11>—Prepare the test solution with 1.0 g of Cefbuperazone Sodium according to Method 4, and perform the test (not more than 2 ppm).

(4) Related substances—Dissolve 0.10 g of Cefbuperazone Sodium in 100 mL of the mobile phase, and use this solution as the sample solution. Pipet 1 mL of the sample solution, add the mobile phase to make exactly 50 mL, and use this solution as the standard solution. Perform the test with exactly 25 μL each of the sample solution and standard solution as directed under Liquid Chromatography <2.01> according to the following conditions, and determine each peak area by the automatic integration method. Calculate the percentages of each peak area of related substances obtained from the sample solution against 50 times of the peak area of cefbuperazone from the standard solution; the amount of related substance I having the relative retention time of about 0.2 to cefbuperazone is not more than 2.0%, the amount of related substance II having the relative retention time of about 0.6 is not more than 4.5% and the amount of related substance III having the relative retention time of about 1.6 is not more than 1.0%, and the total amount of these related substances is not more than 6.0%. For the peak areas of the related substances I and III, multiply their correction factors, 0.72 and 0.69, respectively.

Operating conditions—

Detector, column, column temperature, mobile phase, and flow rate: Proceed as directed in the operating conditions in the Assay.

Time span of measurement: About 2 times as long as the retention time of cefbuperazone.

System suitability—

Test for required detectability: Measure exactly 1 mL of the standard solution, and add the mobile phase to make exactly 10 mL. Confirm that the peak area of cefbuperazone obtained with 25 μL of this solution is equivalent to 7 to 13% of that with 25 μL of the standard solution.

System performance: When the procedure is run with 25 μL of the standard solution under the above operating conditions, the number of theoretical plates and the symmetry factor of the peak of cefbuperazone are not less than 5000 and not more than 1.5, respectively.

System repeatability: When the test is repeated 6 times with 25 μL of the standard solution under the above operating conditions, the relative standard deviation of the peak area of cefbuperazone is not more than 2.0%.

Water <2.48> Not more than 1.0% (3 g, volumetric titration, direct titration).

Assay Weigh accurately an amount of Cefbuperazone Sodium and Cefbuperazone RS, equivalent to about 0.1 g (potency), and dissolve each in the mobile phase to make exactly 100 mL. Measure exactly 10 mL each of these solutions, add exactly 10 mL of the internal standard solution and the mobile phase to make 50 mL, and use these solutions as the sample solution and standard solution. Perform the test with 10 μL each of the sample solution and standard solution as directed under Liquid Chromatography <2.01> according to the following conditions, and calculate the ratios, Q_T and Q_S, of the peak area of cefbuperazone to that of the internal standard.

Amount [μg (potency)] of cefbuperazone ($C_{22}H_{29}N_9O_9S_2$)
$= M_S \times Q_T/Q_S \times 1000$

M_S: Amount [mg (potency)] of Cefbuperazone RS taken

*Internal standard solution—*A solution of acetanilide in the mobile phase (1 in 4000).

Operating conditions—

Detector: An ultraviolet absorption photometer (wavelength: 254 nm).

Column: A stainless steel column 4.6 mm in inside diameter and 15 cm in length, packed with octadecylsilanized silica gel for liquid chromatography (5 μm in particle diameter).

Column temperature: A constant temperature of about 25°C.

Mobile phase: Dissolve 2.0 g of tetra-*n*-propylammonium bromide in 1000 mL of a mixture of water, acetonitrile and acetic acid-sodium acetate buffer solution (pH 5.0) (83:13:4).

Flow rate: Adjust so that the retention time of cefbuperazone is about 16 minutes.

System suitability—

System performance: When the procedure is run with 10 μL of the standard solution under the above operating conditions, the internal standard and cefbuperazone are eluted in this order with the resolution between these peaks being not less than 3.

System repeatability: When the test is repeated 6 times with 10 μL of the standard solution under the above operating conditions, the relative standard deviation of the ratios of the peak area of cefbuperazone to that of the internal standard is not more than 1.0%.

Containers and storage Containers—Hermetic containers. Storage—In a cold place.

Cefcapene Pivoxil Hydrochloride Hydrate

セフカペン　ピボキシル塩酸塩水和物

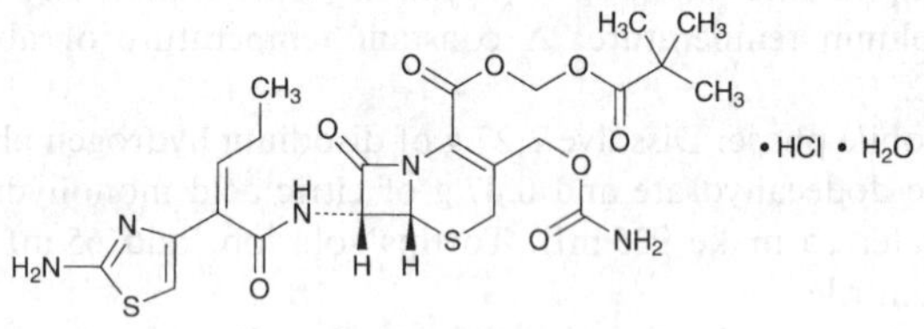

$C_{23}H_{29}N_5O_8S_2.HCl.H_2O$: 622.11
2,2-Dimethylpropanoyloxymethyl (6*R*,7*R*)-7-[(2*Z*)-2-(2-aminothiazol-4-yl)pent-2-enoylamino]-3-carbamoyloxymethyl-8-oxo-5-thia-1-azabicyclo[4.2.0]oct-2-ene-2-caboxylate monohydrochloride monohydrate
[*147816-24-8*]

Cefcapene Pivoxil Hydrochloride Hydrate contains not less than 722 μg (potency) and not more than 764 μg (potency) per mg, calculated on the anhydrous basis. The potency of Cefcapene Pivoxil Hydrochloride Hydrate is expressed as mass (potency) of cefcapene ($C_{17}H_{19}N_5O_6S_2$: 453.49).

Description Cefcapene Pivoxil Hydrochloride Hydrate occurs as a white to pale yellow-white, crystalline powder or mass. It has slightly a characteristic odor.

It is freely soluble in *N*,*N*-dimethylformamide and in methanol, soluble in ethanol (99.5), slightly soluble in water, and practically insoluble in diethyl ether.

Identification **(1)** Determine the absorption spectrum of a solution of Cefcapene Pivoxil Hydrochloride Hydrate in methanol (1 in 50,000) as directed under Ultraviolet-visible Spectrophotometry <2.24>, and compare the spectrum with the Reference Spectrum or the spectrum of a solution of Cefcapene Pivoxil Hydrochloride RS prepared in the same manner as the sample solution: both spectra exhibit similar intensities of absorption at the same wavelengths.

(2) Determine the infrared absorption spectra of Cefcapene Pivoxil Hydrochloride Hydrate and Cefcapene Pivoxil Hydrochloride RS as directed in the paste method under Infrared Spectrophotometry *<2.25>*, and compare these spectra: both spectra exhibit similar intensities of absorption at the same wave numbers.

(3) Determine the ^{1}H spectrum of a solution of Cefcapene Pivoxil Hydrochloride Hydrate in deuterated methanol for nuclear magnetic resonance spectroscopy (1 in 50) as directed under Nuclear Magnetic Resonance Spectroscopy *<2.21>*, using tetramethylsilane for nuclear magnetic resonance spectroscopy as an internal reference compound: it exhibits a triplet signal A at around δ 6.3 ppm, and a single signal B at around δ 6.7 ppm, and the ratio of integrated intensity of each signal, A:B, is about 1:1.

(4) Dissolve 10 mg of Cefcapene Pivoxil Hydrochloride Hydrate in 2 mL of a mixture of water and methanol (1:1), and add 1 drop of silver nitrate TS: a white precipitate is formed.

Optical rotation *<2.49>* $[\alpha]_D^{20}$: +51 – +54° (0.1 g calculated on the anhydrous basis, methanol, 10 mL, 100 mm).

Purity (1) Heavy metals *<1.07>*—Proceed with 2.0 g of Cefcapene Pivoxil Hydrochloride Hydrate according to Method 4, and perform the test. Prepare the control solution with 2.0 mL of Standard Lead Solution (not more than 10 ppm).

(2) Related substance I—Dissolve an amount of Cefcapene Pivoxil Hydrochloride Hydrate, equivalent to about 10 mg (potency), in 2 mL of methanol, add a mixture of water and methanol (1:1) to make 50 mL, and use this solution as the sample solution. Perform the test with 30 μL of the sample solution as directed under Liquid Chromatography *<2.01>* according to the following conditions, and determine each peak area by the automatic integration method. If necessary, compensate the base-line by performing in the same manner as the test with 30 μL of a mixture of water and methanol (1:1). Measure the amount of the peak other than cefcapene pivoxil by the area percentage method: the amounts of the peaks, having the relative retention times of about 1.5 and about 1.7 to cefcapene pivoxil, are not more than 0.2%, respectively. The amount of the peaks other than the peaks mentioned above is not more than 0.1%, and the total of them is not more than 1.5%.

Operating conditions—

Detector: An ultraviolet absorption photometer (wavelength: 265 nm).

Column: A stainless steel column 4.6 mm in inside diameter and 15 cm in length, packed with octadecylsilanized silica gel for liquid chromatography (5 μm in particle diameter).

Column temperature: A constant temperature of about 20°C.

Mobile phase A: Dissolve 5.99 g of potassium dihydrogen phosphate in water to make 1100 mL. To this solution add a solution prepared by dissolving 1.89 g of tetra-*n*-pentylammonium bromide in methanol to make 1000 mL.

Mobile phase B: A mixture of methanol and water (22:3).

Flowing of mobile phase: Control the gradient by mixing the mobile phases A and B as directed in the following table.

Time after injection of sample (min)	Mobile phase A (vol%)	Mobile phase B (vol%)
0 – 20	98	2
20 – 40	98 → 50	2 → 50
40 – 50	50	50

Flow rate: 0.8 mL per minute.

Time span of measurement: About 2.5 times as long as the retention time of cefcapene pivoxil.

System suitability—

Test for required detectability: To exactly 1 mL of the sample solution add a mixture of water and methanol (1:1) to make 100 mL, and use this solution as the solution for system suitability test. Pipet 1 mL of the solution for system suitability test, and add the mixture of water and methanol (1:1) to make exactly 10 mL. Confirm that the peak area of cefcapene pivoxil obtained with 30 μL of this solution is equivalent to 7 to 13% of that with 30 μL of the solution for system suitability test.

System performance: Dissolve 10 mg of Cefcapene Pivoxil Hydrochloride Hydrate and 10 mg of propyl parahydroxybenzoate in 25 mL of methanol, and add water to make 50 mL. To 5 mL of this solution add the mixture of water and methanol (1:1) to make 50 mL. When the procedure is run with 30 μL of this solution under the above operating conditions, cefcapene pivoxil and propyl parahydroxybenzoate are eluted in this order with the resolution between these peaks being not less than 7.

System repeatability: When the test is repeated 3 times with 30 μL of the solution for system suitability test under the above operating conditions, the relative standard deviation of the peak area of cefcapene pivoxil is not more than 4.0%.

(3) Related substance II—Dissolve an amount of Cefcapene Pivoxil Hydrochloride Hydrate, equivalent to about 2 mg (potency), in *N*,*N*-dimethylformamide for liquid chromatography to make 20 mL, and use this solution as the sample solution. Perform the test with 20 μL of the sample solution as directed under Liquid Chromatography *<2.01>* according to the following conditions, and determine each peak area by the automatic integration method: the total area of the peaks which appear earlier than cefcapene pivoxil is not more than 1.7% of the total area of the peaks other than the solvent.

Operating conditions—

Detector: An ultraviolet absorption photometer (wavelength: 280 nm).

Column: A stainless steel column 7.8 mm in inside diameter and 30 cm in length, packed with styrene-divinylbenzene copolymer for liquid chromatography.

Column temperature: A constant temperature of about 25°C.

Mobile phase: A solution of lithium bromide in *N*,*N*-dimethylformamide for liquid chromatography (13 in 5000).

Flow rate: Adjust so that the retention time of cefcapene pivoxil is about 22 minutes.

Time span of measurement: About 1.8 times as long as the retention time of cefcapene pivoxil.

System suitability—

Test for required detectability: To exactly 1 mL of the sample solution add *N*,*N*-dimethylformamide for liquid chromatography to make 100 mL, and use this solution as the solution for system suitability test. Pipet 3 mL of the solution for system suitability test, and add *N*,*N*-dimethylformamide for liquid chromatography to make exactly 10 mL. Conform that the peak area of cefcapene pivoxil obtained with 20 μL of this solution is equivalent to 20 to 40% of that with 20 μL of the solution for system suitability test.

System performance: When the procedure is run with 20 μL of the sample solution under the above operating conditions, the number of theoretical plates of the peak of cefcapene pivoxil is not less than 12,000.

System repeatability: When the test is repeated 6 times

with 20 μL of the solution for system suitability test under the above operating conditions, the relative standard deviation of the peak areas of cefcapene pivoxil is not more than 4.0%.

Water <*2.48*> Not less than 2.8% and not more than 3.7% (0.5 g, volumetric titration, back titration).

Assay Weigh accurately an amount of Cefcapene Pivoxil Hydrochloride Hydrate and Cefcapene Pivoxil Hydrochloride RS, equivalent to about 20 mg (potency), and dissolve each in a mixture of water and methanol (1:1) to make exactly 50 mL. Pipet 10 mL each of these solutions, add exactly 10 mL of the internal standard solution and the mixture of water and methanol (1:1) to them to make 50 mL, and use these solutions as the sample solution and the standard solution, respectively. Perform the test with 10 μL each of the sample solution and standard solution as directed under Liquid Chromatography <*2.01*> according to the following conditions, and calculate the ratios, Q_T and Q_S, of the peak area of cefcapene pivoxil to that of the internal standard.

Amount [μg (potency)] of cefcapene ($C_{17}H_{19}N_5O_6S_2$)
$= M_S \times Q_T/Q_S \times 1000$

M_S: Amount [mg (potency)] of Cefcapene Pivoxil Hydrochloride RS taken

Internal standard solution—A solution of *p*-benzylphenol in a mixture of water and methanol (1:1) (7 in 4000).
Operating conditions—

Detector: An ultraviolet absorption photometer (wavelength: 265 nm).

Column: A stainless steel column 3.0 mm in inside diameter and 7.5 cm in length, packed with octadecylsilanized silica gel for liquid chromatography (3 μm in particle diameter).

Column temperature: A constant temperature of about 40°C.

Mobile phase: Dissolve 1.56 g of sodium dihydrogenphosphate dihydrate and 1.22 g of sodium 1-decanesulfonate in water to make 1000 mL. To 700 mL of this solution add 300 mL of acetonitrile and 100 mL of methanol.

Flow rate: Adjust so that the retention time of cefcapene pivoxil is about 5 minutes.
System suitability—

System performance: Dissolve 0.2 g of Cefcapene Pivoxil Hydrochloride Hydrate in 10 mL of methanol, and warm in a water bath at 60°C for 20 minutes. After cooling, pipet 1 mL of this solution, and add exactly 10 mL of the internal standard solution and the mixture of water and methanol (1:1) to make 50 mL. When the procedure is run with 10 μL of this solution under the above operating conditions, cefcapene pivoxil, *trans*-cefcapene pivoxil and the internal standard are eluted in this order, the relative retention time of trans-cefcapene pivoxil and the internal standard to that of cefcapene pivoxil are about 1.7 and about 2.0, respectively, and the resolution between the peaks of *trans*-cefcapene pivoxil and the internal standard is not less than 1.5.

System repeatability: When the test is repeated 5 times with 10 μL of the standard solution under the above operating conditions, the relative standard deviation of the ratio of the peak area of cefcapene pivoxil to that of the internal standard is not more than 1.0%.

Containers and storage Containers—Tight containers.

Storage—Light-resistant, at a temperature not exceeding 5°C.

Cefcapene Pivoxil Hydrochloride Fine Granules

セフカペン　ピボキシル塩酸塩細粒

Cefcapene Pivoxil Hydrochloride Fine Granules contain not less than 90.0% and not more than 110.0% of the labeled potency of cefcapene ($C_{17}H_{19}N_5O_6S_2$: 453.49).

Method of preparation Prepare as directed under Granules, with Cefcapene Pivoxil Hydrochloride Hydrate.

Identification Powder Cefcapene Pivoxil Hydrochloride Fine Granules. To a portion of the powder, equivalent to 10 mg (potency) of Cefcapene Pivoxil Hydrochloride Hydrate, add 40 mL of methanol, shake vigorously, and add methanol to make 50 mL. To 4 mL of this solution add methanol to make 50 mL, and filter through a membrane filter with a pore size of 0.45 μm. Determine the absorption spectrum of the filtrate as directed under Ultraviolet-visible Spectrophotometry <*2.24*>: it exhibits a maximum between 264 nm and 268 nm.

Purity **(1)** Related substances I—Powder Cefcapene Pivoxil Hydrochloride Fine Granules. To a portion of the powder, equivalent to 5 mg (potency) of Cefcapene Pivoxil Hydrochloride Hydrate, add 1 mL of methanol, and shake. Add 25 mL of a mixture of water and methanol (1:1), shake vigorously for 5 minutes, and filter through a membrane filter with a pore size of 0.45 μm. Discard the first 3 mL of the filtrate, and use the subsequent filtrate as the sample solution. Perform the test with 30 μL of the sample solution as directed under Liquid Chromatography <*2.01*> according to the following conditions. Determine each peak area by the automatic integration method. If necessary, compensate the base-line by performing in the same manner as the test with 30 μL of a mixture of water and methanol (1:1). Calculate the amount of the peaks other than the peak of cefcapene pivoxil by the area percentage method: the amount of the substance, having the relative retention time of about 1.3 to cefcapene pivoxil, is not more than 0.4%, the amount of the trans-isomer of cefcapene pivoxil, having the relative retention time of about 1.5, is not more than 1.1%, the amount of the substance other than that mentioned above is not more than 0.3%, and the total amount of these substances is not more than 2.8%.
Operating conditions—

Proceed as directed in the operating conditions in the Purity (2) under Cefcapene Pivoxil Hydrochloride Hydrate.
System suitability—

Proceed as directed in the system suitability in the Purity (2) under Cefcapene Pivoxil Hydrochloride Hydrate.

(2) Related substances II—Powder Cefcapene Pivoxil Hydrochloride Fine Granules. To a portion of the powder, equivalent to 2 mg (potency) of Cefcapene Pivoxil Hydrochloride Hydrate, add 20 mL of *N,N*-dimethylformamide for liquid chromatography, shake vigorously for 10 minutes, and filter through a membrane filter with a pore size of 0.45 μm. Discard the first 3 mL of the filtrate, and use the subsequent filtrate as the sample solution. Perform the test with 20 μL of the sample solution as directed under Liquid Chromatography <*2.01*> according to the following conditions, and determine each peak area by the automatic integration method: the total area of the peaks eluted before that of cefcapene pivoxil is not more than 4.0% of the total area of all peaks other than the solvent peak.

Operating conditions—

Proceed as directed in the operating conditions in the Purity (3) under Cefcapene Pivoxil Hydrochloride Hydrate.

System suitability—

Proceed as directed in the system suitability in the Purity (3) under Cefcapene Pivoxil Hydrochloride Hydrate.

Water <*2.48*> Not more than 1.4% (0.5 g, volumetric titration, back titration). Perform the test without pulverizing the sample, and handling the sample under a relative humidity of less than 30%.

Uniformity of dosage units <*6.02*> The granules in single-dose packages meet the requirement of the Mass variation test.

Dissolution Being specified separately when the drug is granted approval based on the Law.

Assay Weigh accurately an amount of Cefcapene Pivoxil Hydrochloride Fine Granules, equivalent to about 0.2 g (potency) of and Cefcapene Pivoxil Hydrochloride Hydrate, add 100 mL of the mixture of water and methanol (1:1), shake vigorously for 10 minutes, add the mixture of water and methanol (1:1) to make exactly 200 mL, and centrifuge at 3000 rpm for 5 minutes. Filter the supernatant liquid through a membrane filter with a pore size of 0.45 μm, discard the first 1 mL of the filtrate, pipet 2 mL of the subsequent filtrate, add exactly 5 mL of the internal standard solution and the mixture of water and methanol (1:1) to make 25 mL, and use this solution as the sample solution. Separately, weigh accurately about 20 mg (potency) of Cefcapene Pivoxil Hydrochloride RS, and dissolve in the mixture of water and methanol (1:1) to make exactly 50 mL. Pipet 10 mL of this solution, add exactly 10 mL of the internal standard solution and the mixture of water and methanol (1:1) to make 50 mL, and use this solution as the standard solution. Proceed as directed in the Assay under Cefcapene Pivoxil Hydrochloride Hydrate.

Amount [mg (potency)] of cefcapene ($C_{17}H_{19}N_5O_6S_2$)
$= M_S \times Q_T/Q_S \times 10$

M_S: Amount [mg (potency)] of Cefcapene Pivoxil Hydrochloride RS taken

Internal standard solution—A solution of *p*-benzylphenol in the mixture of water and methanol (1:1) (7 in 4000).

Containers and storage Containers—Tight containers.

Storage—Light-resistant.

Cefcapene Pivoxil Hydrochloride Tablets

セフカペン　ピボキシル塩酸塩錠

Cefcapene Pivoxil Hydrochloride Tablets contain not less than 90.0% and not more than 105.0% of the labeled potency of cefcapene ($C_{17}H_{19}N_5O_6S_2$: 453.49).

Method of preparation Prepare as directed under Tablets, with Cefcapene Pivoxil Hydrochloride Hydrate.

Identification To an amount of powdered Cefcapene Pivoxil Hydrochloride Tablets, equivalent to about 10 mg (potency) of Cefcapene Pivoxil Hydrochloride Hydrate, add 40 mL of methanol, shake vigorously, and add methanol to make 50 mL. To 4 mL of this solution add methanol to make 50 mL, filter through a membrane filter with pore size of 0.45 μm, and use the filtrate as the sample solution. Determine the absorption spectrum of the sample solution as directed under Ultraviolet-visible Spectrophotometry <*2.24*>: it exhibits a maximum between 263 nm and 267 nm.

Purity **(1)** Related substances I—To an amount of powdered Cefcapene Pivoxil Hydrochloride Tables, equivalent to about 5 mg (potency) of Cefcapene Pivoxil Hydrochloride Hydrate, add 1 mL of methanol, and shake. Add 25 mL of a mixture of water and methanol (1:1), shake vigorously for 5 minutes, and filter through a membrane filter with pore size of 0.45 μm. Discard the first 3 mL of the filtrate, and use the subsequent filtrate as the sample solution. Perform the test with 30 μL of the sample solution as directed under Liquid Chromatography <*2.01*> according to the following conditions, and determine each peak area by the automatic integration method. If necessary, proceed with 30 μL of the mixture of water and methanol (1:1) in the same manner as the sample solution to compensate the base line. Calculate the amounts of the peaks other than cefcapene pivoxil by the area percentage method: the amount of the peak, having the relative retention time of about 1.3 to cefcapene pivoxil, is not more than 0.4%, the amount of the peak of cefcapene pivoxil trans-isomer, having the relative retention time of about 1.5, is not more than 0.5%, the amount of the peaks other than the peaks mentioned above are not more than 0.3%, respectively, and the total amount of these peaks is not more than 2.0%.

Operating conditions—

Proceed as directed in the operating conditions in the Purity (2) under Cefcapene Pivoxil Hydrochloride Hydrate.

System suitability—

Proceed as directed in the system suitability in the Purity (2) under Cefcapene Pivoxil Hydrochloride Hydrate.

(2) Related substances II—To an amount of powdered Cefcapene Pivoxil Hydrochloride Tablets, equivalent to 2 mg (potency) of Cefcapene Pivoxil Hydrochloride Hydrate, add 20 mL of *N*,*N*-dimethylformamide for liquid chromatography, shake vigorously for 10 minutes, and filter through a membrane filter with pore size of 0.45 μm. Discard the first 3 mL of the filtrate, and use the subsequent filtrate as the sample solution. Perform the test with 20 μL of the sample solution as directed under Liquid Chromatography <*2.01*> according to the following conditions, and determine each peak area by the automatic integration method: the total area of the peaks which are eluted before cefcapene pivoxil is not more than 3.3% of the total area of the peaks other than the solvent peak.

Operating conditions—

Proceed as directed in the operating conditions in the Purity (3) under Cefcapene Pivoxil Hydrochloride Hydrate.

System suitability—

Proceed as directed in the system suitability in the Purity (3) under Cefcapene Pivoxil Hydrochloride Hydrate.

Water <*2.48*> Not more than 3.9% (0.5 g, volumetric titration, back titration). Powdering of the sample tablets and handling of the powder are performed under the relative humidity of not exceeding 30%.

Uniformity of dosage units <*6.02*> Perform the Mass variation test, or the Content uniformity test according to the following method: it meets the requirement.

To 1 tablet of Cefcapene Pivoxil Hydrochloride Tablets add 5 mL of water, and shake vigorously for 5 minutes to disintegrate. Add 20 mL of methanol, shake vigorously for 5 minutes, add a mixture of methanol and water (4:1) to make exactly 50 mL, and centrifuge at 3000 rpm for 5 minutes. Filter the supernatant liquid through a membrane filter with pore size of 0.45 μm, and discard the first 1 mL of the filtrate. Pipet *V* mL of the subsequent filtrate, equivalent to about 6 mg (potency) of Cefcapene Pivoxil Hydrochloride Hydrate, add exactly 15 mL of the internal standard solution, add a mixture of water and methanol (1:1) to make 75 mL, and use this solution as the sample solution. Then, proceed as directed in the Assay.

Amount [mg (potency)] of cefcapene ($C_{17}H_{19}N_5O_6S_2$)
$= M_S \times Q_T/Q_S \times 15/V$

M_S: Amount [mg (potency)] of Cefcapene Pivoxil Hydrochloride RS taken

Internal standard solution—A solution of *p*-benzylphenol in a mixture of water and methanol (1:1) (7 in 4000).

Dissolution Being specified separately when the drug is granted approval based on the Law.

Assay To an amount of Cefcapene Pivoxil Hydrochloride Tablets, equivalent to about 0.6 g (potency) of Cefcapene Pivoxil Hydrochloride Hydrate, add 20 mL of water, and shake for 5 minutes to disintegrate. Add 80 mL of methanol, shake vigorously for 5 minutes, add a mixture of methanol and water (4:1) to make exactly 200 mL, and centrifuge at 3000 rpm for 5 minutes. Filter the supernatant liquid through a membrane filter with pore size of 0.45 μm, and discard the first 1 mL of the filtrate. Pipet 2 mL of the subsequent filtrate, add exactly 15 mL of the internal standard solution, add the mixture of water and methanol (1:1) to make 75 mL, and use this solution as the sample solution. Separately, weigh accurately an amount of Cefcapene Pivoxil Hydrochloride RS, equivalent to about 20 mg (potency), and dissolve in the mixture of water and methanol (1:1) to make exactly 50 mL. Pipet 10 mL of this solution, add exactly 10 mL of the internal standard solution, add the mixture of water and methanol (1:1) to make 50 mL, and use this solution as the standard solution. Proceed as directed in the Assay under Cefcapene Pivoxil Hydrochloride Hydrate.

Amount [mg (potency)] of cefcapene ($C_{17}H_{19}N_5O_6S_2$)
$= M_S \times Q_T/Q_S \times 30$

M_S: Amount [mg (potency)] of Cefcapene Pivoxil Hydrochloride RS taken

Internal standard solution—A solution of *p*-benzylphenol in the mixture of water and methanol (1:1) (7 in 4000).

Containers and storage Containers—Tight containers.

Cefdinir

セフジニル

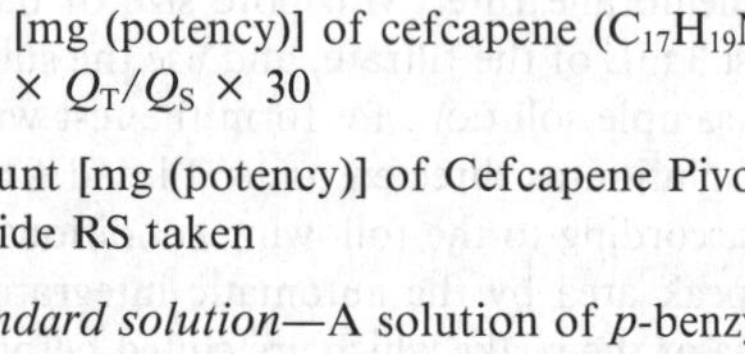

$C_{14}H_{13}N_5O_5S_2$: 395.41
(6*R*,7*R*)-7-[(*Z*)-2-(2-Aminothiazol-4-yl)-2-(hydroxyimino)acetylamino]-8-oxo-3-vinyl-5-thia-1-azabicyclo[4.2.0]oct-2-ene-2-carboxylic acid
[*91832-40-5*]

Cefdinir contains not less than 930 μg (potency) and not more than 1020 μg (potency) per mg. The potency of Cefdinir is expressed as mass (potency) of cefdinir ($C_{14}H_{13}N_5O_5S_2$).

Description Cefdinir occurs as a white to light yellow crystalline powder.

It is practically insoluble in water, in ethanol (95) and in diethyl ether.

It dissolves in 0.1 mol/L phosphate buffer solution (pH 7.0).

Identification **(1)** Determine the absorption spectra of solutions of Cefdinir and Cefdinir RS in 0.1 mol/L phosphate buffer solution (pH 7.0) (1 in 100,000) as directed under Ultraviolet-visible Spectrophotometry *<2.24>*, and compare these spectra: both spectra exhibit similar intensities of absorption at the same wavelengths.

(2) Determine the infrared absorption spectra of Cefdinir and Cefdinir RS as directed in the paste method under Infrared Spectrophotometry *<2.25>*, and compare these spectra: both spectra exhibit similar intensities of absorption at the same wave numbers.

(3) Determine the ^1H spectrum of a solution of Cefdinir in a mixture of deuterated dimethyl sulfoxide for nuclear magnetic resonance spectroscopy and heavy water for nuclear magnetic resonance spectroscopy (4:1) (1 in 10), using tetramethylsilane for nuclear magnetic resonance spectroscopy as an internal reference compound, as directed under Nuclear Magnetic Resonance Spectroscopy *<2.21>*: it exhibits multiplet signals, A at around δ 5.0 – 6.1 ppm and B at around δ 6.4 – 7.5 ppm. The ratio of integrated intensity of each signal, A:B is about 2:1.

Optical rotation *<2.49>* $[\alpha]_D^{20}$: −58 – −66° (0.25 g, 0.1 mol/L phosphate buffer solution (pH 7.0), 25 mL, 100 mm).

Purity **(1)** Heavy metals *<1.07>*—Proceed with 2.0 g of Cefdinir according to Method 2, and perform the test. Prepare the control solution with 2.0 mL of Standard Lead Solution (not more than 10 ppm).

(2) Related substances—Dissolve about 0.1 g of Cefdinir in 10 mL of 0.1 mol/L phosphate buffer solution (pH 7.0). To 3 mL of this solution add tetramethylammonium hydroxide TS (pH 5.5) to make 20 mL, and use this solution as the sample solution. Perform the test with 10 μL of the sample solution as directed under Liquid Chromatography *<2.01>* according to the following conditions. Determine each peak area by the automatic integration method, and calculate the amounts of their peaks by the area percentage method: the amount of the peaks, having the relative retention time of about 0.7, about 1.2 and about 1.5 to cefdinir, are not more than 0.7%, not more than 0.3% and not more than 0.8%, respectively, the total amount of the peaks, having the relative retention time of about 0.85, about 0.93, about 1.11 and about 1.14, is not more than 0.4%, and the amount of the peak other than cefdinir and the peaks mentioned above is not more than 0.2%. And the total amount of the peaks other than cefdinir is not more than 3.0%.

Operating conditions—

Detector: An ultraviolet absorption photometer (wavelength: 254 nm).

Column: A stainless steel column 4.6 mm in inside diameter and 15 cm in length, packed with octadecylsilanized silica gel for liquid chromatography (5 μm in particle diameter).

Column temperature: A constant temperature of about 40°C.

Mobile phase A: To 1000 mL of tetramethylammonium hydroxide TS (pH 5.5) add 0.4 mL of 0.1 mol/L disodium dihydrogen ethylenediamine tetraacetate TS.

Mobile phase B: To 500 mL of tetramethylammonium hydroxide TS (pH 5.5) add 300 mL of acetonitrile for liquid chromatography and 200 mL of methanol, and add 0.4 mL of 0.1 mol/L disodium dihydrogen ethylenediamine tetraacetate TS.

Flowing of mobile phase: Control the gradient by mixing the mobile phases A and B as directed in the following table.

Time after injection of sample (min)	Mobile phase A (vol%)	Mobile phase B (vol%)
0 - 2	95	5
2 - 22	95 → 75	5 → 25
22 - 32	75 → 50	25 → 50
32 - 37	50	50

Flow rate: 1.0 mL per minute (the retention time of cefdinir is about 22 minutes).

Time span of measurement: For 37 minutes after injection, beginning after the solvent peak.

System suitability—

Test for required detectability: To 1 mL of the sample solution add tetramethylammonium hydroxide TS (pH 5.5) to make 100 mL, and use this solution as the solution for system suitability test. Pipet 1 mL of the solution for system suitability test, add tetramethylammonium hydroxide TS (pH 5.5) to make exactly 10 mL. Confirm that the peak area of cefdinir obtained with 10 μL of this solution is equivalent to 7 to 13% of that with 10 μL of the solution for system suitability test.

System performance: Dissolve 30 mg of Cefdinir RS and 2 mg of cefdinir lactam ring-cleavage lactones in 3 mL of 0.1 mol/L phosphate buffer solution (pH 7.0), add tetramethylammonium hydroxide TS (pH 5.5) to make 20 mL. When the procedure is run with 10 μL of this solution under the above operating conditions, peak 1 and peak 2 of cefdinir lactam ring-cleavage lactones separated into 4 peaks, cefdinir, peak 3 and peak 4 of remaining cefdinir lactam ring-cleavage lactones are eluted in this order. Relative retention time of peak 3 of cefdinir lactam ring-cleavage lactone to cefdinir is about 1.11. The number of theoretical plates and the symmetry factor of the peak of cefdinir are not less than 7000 and not more than 3.0, respectively.

System repeatability: When the test is repeated 3 times with 10 μL of the solution for system suitability test under the above operating conditions, the relative standard deviation of the peak areas of cefdinir is not more than 2.0%.

Water *<2.48>* Not more than 2.0% (1 g, volumetric titration, direct titration. Use a mixture of formamide for water determination and methanol for water determination (2:1) instead of methanol for water determination).

Assay Weigh accurately an amount of Cefdinir and Cefdinir RS equivalent to about 20 mg (potency), dissolve each in 0.1 mol/L phosphate buffer solution (pH 7.0) to make exactly 100 mL, and use these solutions as the sample solution and standard solution. Perform the test with exactly 5 μL of the sample solution and standard solution as directed under Liquid Chromatography *<2.01>* according to the following conditions, and determine the peak areas, A_T and A_S, of cefdinir in each solution.

$$\text{Amount [}\mu\text{g (potency)] of cefdinir } (C_{14}H_{13}N_5O_5S_2) = M_S \times A_T/A_S \times 1000$$

M_S: Amount [mg (potency)] of Cefdinir RS taken

Operating conditions—

Detector: An ultraviolet absorption photometer (wavelength: 254 nm).

Column: A stainless steel column 4.6 mm in inside diameter and 15 cm in length, packed with octadecylsilanized silica gel for liquid chromatography (5 μm in particle diameter).

Column temperature: A constant temperature of about 40°C.

Mobile phase: To 1000 mL of tetramethylammonium hydroxide TS (pH 5.5) add 0.4 mL of 0.1 mol/L disodium dihydrogen ethylenediamine tetraacetate TS. To 900 mL of this solution add 60 mL of acetonitrile for liquid chromatography and 40 mL of methanol.

Flow rate: Adjust so that the retention time of cefdinir is about 8 minutes.

System suitability—

System performance: Dissolve 2 mg of Cefdinir RS and 5 mg of cefdinir lactam ring-cleavage lactones in 10 mL of 0.1 mol/L phosphate buffer solution, pH 7.0. When the procedure is run with 5 μL of this solution under the above operating conditions, peak 1 and peak 2 of cefdinir lactam ring-cleavage lactones separated into 4 peaks, cefdinir, peak 3 and peak 4 of remaining cefdinir lactam ring-cleavage lactones are eluted in this order. The resolution between the peak 2 of cefdinir lactam ring-cleavage lactone and that of cefdinir is not less than 1.2. The number of theoretical plates and the symmetry factor of the peak of cefdinir are not less than 2000 and not more than 1.5, respectively.

System repeatability: When the test is repeated 6 times with 5 μL of the standard solution under the above operating conditions, the relative standard deviation of the peak areas of cefdinir is not more than 1.0%.

Containers and storage Containers—Tight containers.
Storage—Light-resistant.

Cefdinir Capsules

セフジニルカプセル

Cefdinir Capsules contain not less than 90.0% and not more than 110.0% of the labeled potency of cefdinir ($C_{14}H_{13}N_5O_5S_2$: 395.41).

Method of preparation Prepare as directed under Capsules, with Cefdinir.

Identification To an amount of the contents of Cefdinir Capsules, equivalent to 10 mg (potency) of Cefdinir, add 100 mL of 0.1 mol/L phosphate buffer solution (pH 7.0), exposure to ultrasonic waves for 1 minute, and filter. To 2 mL of the filtrate add 0.1 mol/L phosphate buffer solution (pH 7.0) to make 20 mL, and determine the absorption spectrum of this solution as directed under Ultraviolet-visible Spectrophotometry *<2.24>*: it exhibits maxima between 221 nm and 225 nm and between 285 nm and 289 nm.

Uniformity of dosage units *<6.02>* It meets the requirement of the Mass variation test.

Dissolution *<6.10>* When the test is performed at 50 revolutions per minute according to the Paddle method using the sinker, using 900 mL of 2nd fluid for dissolution test as the dissolution medium, the dissolution rate of a 50-mg capsule in 30 minutes is not less than 80%, and that of a 100-mg capsule in 45 minutes is not less than 75%.

Start the test with 1 capsule of Cefdinir Capsules, withdraw not less than 20 mL of the medium at the specified minute after starting the test, and filter through a membrane filter with a pore size not exceeding 0.5 μm. Discard not less than 10 mL of the first filtrate, pipet V mL of the subsequent filtrate, add the dissolution medium to make exactly V' mL so that each mL contains about 56 μg (potency) of Cefdinir, and use this solution as the sample solution. Separately, weigh accurately about 28 mg (potency) of Cefdinir RS, and dissolve in the dissolution medium to make exactly 100 mL. Pipet 4 mL of this solution, add the dissolution medium to make exactly 20 mL, and use this solution as the standard solution. Perform the test with exactly 20 μL each of the sample solution and standard solution as directed under Liquid Chromatography <*2.01*>, and determine the peak areas, A_T and A_S, of cefdinir in each solution.

Dissolution rate (%) with respect to the labeled amount of cefdinir ($C_{14}H_{13}N_5O_5S_2$)
$= M_S \times A_T/A_S \times V'/V \times 1/C \times 180$

M_S: Amount [mg (potency)] of Cefdinir RS taken
C: Labeled amount [mg (potency)] of cefdinir ($C_{14}H_{13}N_5O_5S_2$) in 1 capsule

Operating conditions—

Proceed as directed in the operating conditions in the Assay under Cefdinir.

System suitability—

System performance: When the procedure is run with 20 μL of the standard solution under the above operating conditions, the number of theoretical plates and the symmetry factor of the peak of cefdinir are not less than 2000 and not more than 2.0, respectively.

System repeatability: When the test is repeated 6 times with 20 μL of the standard solution under the above operating conditions, the relative standard deviation of the peak area of cefdinir is not more than 1.0%.

Assay Weigh accurately not less than 5 Cefdinir Capsules, take out the contents, and powder. Wash the empty capsules with a little amount of diethyl ether, if necessary, allow to stand at a room temperature to vaporize the adhering diethyl ether, and weigh accurately the mass of the capsules to calculate the mass of the contents. Weigh accurately an amount of the contents, equivalent to about 0.1 g (potency) of Cefdinir, add 70 mL of 0.1 mol/L phosphate buffer solution (pH 7.0), shake for 30 minutes, and add 0.1 mol/L phosphate buffer solution (pH 7.0) to make exactly 100 mL. Centrifuge this solution at 3000 revolutions per minute for 10 minutes, pipet 4 mL of the supernatant liquid, add 0.1 mol/L phosphate buffer solution (pH 7.0) to make exactly 20 mL, and use this solution as the sample solution. Separately, weigh accurately an amount of Cefdinir RS, equivalent to about 20 mg (potency), dissolve in 0.1 mol/L phosphate buffer solution (pH 7.0) to make exactly 100 mL, and use this solution as the standard solution. Proceed as directed in the Assay under Cefdinir.

Amount [mg (potency)] of cefdinir ($C_{14}H_{13}N_5O_5S_2$)
$= M_S \times A_T/A_S \times 5$

M_S: Amount [mg (potency)] of Cefdinir RS taken

Containers and storage Containers—Tight containers.

Cefdinir Fine Granules

セフジニル細粒

Cefdinir Fine Granules contain not less than 93.0% and not more than 107.0% of the labeled potency of cefdinir ($C_{14}H_{13}N_5O_5S_2$: 395.41).

Method of preparation Prepare as directed under Granules, with Cefdinir.

Identification To an amount of Cefdinir Fine Granules, equivalent to 10 mg (potency) of Cefdinir, add 100 mL of 0.1 mol/L phosphate buffer solution (pH 7.0), exposure to ultrasonic waves for 1 minute, and filter. To 2 mL of the filtrate add 0.1 mol/L phosphate buffer solution (pH 7.0) to make 20 mL, and determine the absorption spectrum of this solution as directed under Ultraviolet-visible Spectrophotometry <*2.24*>: it exhibits maxima between 221 nm and 225 nm and between 285 nm and 289 nm.

Uniformity of dosage units <*6.02*> The granules in single-dose packages meet the requirement of the Mass variation test.

Dissolution <*6.10*> When the test is performed at 50 revolutions per minute according to the Paddle method, using 900 mL of 2nd fluid for dissolution test as the dissolution medium, the dissolution rate in 30 minutes of Cefdinir Fine Granules is not less than 75%.

Start the test with an accurate amount of Cefdinir Fine Granules, equivalent to about 0.1 g (potency) of Cefdinir, withdraw not less than about 20 mL of the medium at the specified minute after starting the test, and filter through a membrane filter with a pore size not exceeding 0.5 μm. Discard not less than 10 mL of the first filtrate, and use the subsequent filtrate as the sample solution. Separately, weigh accurately about 28 mg (potency) of Cefdinir RS, and dissolve in the dissolution medium to make exactly 50 mL. Pipet 4 mL of this solution, add the dissolution medium to make exactly 20 mL, and use this solution as the standard solution. Perform the test with exactly 20 μL each of the sample solution and standard solution as directed under Liquid Chromatography <*2.01*>, and determine the peak areas, A_T and A_S, of cefdinir in each solution.

Dissolution rate (%) with respect to the labeled amount of cefdinir ($C_{14}H_{13}N_5O_5S_2$)
$= M_S/M_T \times A_T/A_S \times 1/C \times 360$

M_S: Amount [mg (potency)] of Cefdinir RS taken
M_T: Amount (g) of Cefdinir Fine Granules taken
C: Labeled amount [mg (potency)] of cefdinir ($C_{14}H_{13}N_5O_5S_2$) in 1 g

Operating conditions—

Proceed as directed in the operating conditions in the Assay under Cefdinir.

System suitability—

System performance: When the procedure is run with 20 μL of the standard solution under the above operating conditions, the number of theoretical plates and the symmetry factor of the peak of cefdinir are not less than 2000 and not more than 2.0, respectively.

System repeatability: When the test is repeated 6 times with 20 μL of the standard solution under the above operating conditions, the relative standard deviation of the peak area of cefdinir is not more than 1.0%.

Assay Powder, if necessary, and weigh accurately an amount of Cefdinir Fine Granules, equivalent to about 0.1 g (potency) of Cefdinir, add 70 mL of 0.1 mol/L phosphate buffer solution (pH 7.0), shake for 30 minutes, and add 0.1 mol/L phosphate buffer solution (pH 7.0) to make exactly 100 mL. Centrifuge at 3000 revolutions per minute for 10 minutes, pipet 4 mL of the supernatant liquid, add 0.1 mol/L phosphate buffer solution (pH 7.0) to make 20 mL, and use this solution as the sample solution. Separately, weigh accurately an amount of Cefdinir RS, equivalent to about 20 mg (potency), dissolve in 0.1 mol/L phosphate buffer solution (pH 7.0) to make exactly 100 mL, and use this solution as the standard solution. Proceed as directed in the Assay under Cefdinir.

Amount [mg (potency)] of cefdinir ($C_{14}H_{13}N_5O_5S_2$)
$= M_S \times A_T/A_S \times 5$

M_S: Amount [mg (potency)] of Cefdinir RS taken

Containers and storage Containers—Tight containers.
Storage—Light-resistant.

Cefditoren Pivoxil

セフジトレン ピボキシル

$C_{25}H_{28}N_6O_7S_3$: 620.72
2,2-Dimethylpropanoyloxymethyl (6*R*,7*R*)-7-[(*Z*)-2-(2-aminothiazol-4-yl)-2-(methoxyimino)acetylamino]-3-[(1*Z*)-2-(4-methylthiazol-5-yl)ethenyl]-8-oxo-5-thia-1-azabicyclo[4.2.0]oct-2-ene-2-carboxylate
[*117467-28-4*]

Cefditoren Pivoxil contains not less than 770 μg (potency) and not more than 820 μg (potency) per mg, calculated on the anhydrous basis. The potency of Cefditoren Pivoxil is expressed as mass (potency) of cefditoren ($C_{19}H_{18}N_6O_5S_3$: 506.58).

Description Cefditoren Pivoxil occurs as a light yellow-white to light yellow crystalline powder.

It is sparingly soluble in methanol, slightly soluble in acetonitrile and in ethanol (95), very slightly soluble in diethyleter and practically insoluble in water.

It dissolves in dilute hydrochloric acid.

Identification **(1)** Dissolve 5 mg of Cefditoren Pivoxil in 3 mL of hydroxylammonium chloride-ethanol TS, allow to stand for 5 minutes, add 1 mL of acidic ammonium iron (III) sulfate TS and shake: a red-brown color develops.

(2) Dissolve 1 mg of Cefditoren Pivoxil in 1 mL of dilute hydrochloric acid and 4 mL of water, add 3 drops of sodium nitrite TS under ice-cooling, shake, and allow to stand for 2 minutes. Then add 1 mL of ammonium amidosulfate TS, shake well, and allow to stand for 1 minute, and add 1 mL of *N*,*N*-diethyl-*N*′-1-naphthylethylenediamine oxalate TS: a purple color develops.

(3) Determine the absorption spectrum of a solution of Cefditoren Pivoxil in methanol (1 in 50,000) as directed under Ultraviolet-visible Spectrophotometry ⟨*2.24*⟩, and compare the spectrum with the Reference Spectrum or the spectrum of a solution of Cefditoren Pivoxil RS prepared in the same manner as the sample solution: both spectra exhibit similar intensities of absorption at the same wavelengths.

(4) Determine the ^{1}H spectrum of a solution of Cefditoren Pivoxil in deuterated chloroform for nuclear magnetic resonance spectroscopy (1 in 50), using tetramethylsilane for nuclear magnetic resonance spectroscopy as an internal reference compound, as directed under Nuclear Magnetic Resonance Spectroscopy ⟨*2.21*⟩: it exhibits singlet signals A, B and C, at around δ 1.1 ppm, at around δ 2.4 ppm and at around δ 4.0 ppm, doublet signals D and E, at around δ 6.4 ppm and at around δ 6.7 ppm, and a singlet signal F at around δ 8.6 ppm. The ratio of integrated intensity of each signal A:B:C:D:E:F, is about 9:3:3:1:1:1.

Absorbance ⟨*2.24*⟩ $E^{1\%}_{1\,cm}$ (231 nm): 340 – 360 (50 mg, methanol, 2500 mL).

Optical rotation ⟨*2.49*⟩ $[\alpha]^{20}_D$: −45 – −52° (50 mg, methanol, 10 mL, 100 mm).

Purity **(1)** Heavy metals ⟨*1.07*⟩—Proceed with 2.0 g of Cefditoren Pivoxil according to Method 2, and perform the test. Prepare the control solution with 2.0 mL of Standard Lead Solution (not more than 10 ppm).

(2) Related substances—Being specified separately when the drug is granted approval based on the Law.

Water ⟨*2.48*⟩ Not more than 1.5% (0.5 g, volumetric titration, direct titration).

Residue on ignition Being specified separately when the drug is granted approval based on the Law.

Assay Conduct this procedure using light-resistant vessels. Weigh accurately an amount of Cefditoren Pivoxil and Cefditoren Pivoxil RS, equivalent to about 40 mg (potency), dissolve in 40 mL of acetonitrile, add exactly 10 mL each of the internal standard solution, and add acetonitrile to make 100 mL, and use these solutions as the sample solution and standard solution. Perform the test with 10 μL each of the sample solution and standard solution as directed under Liquid Chromatography ⟨*2.01*⟩ according to the following conditions, and calculate the ratios, Q_T and Q_S, of the peak area of cefditoren pivoxil to that of the internal standard.

Amount [μg (potency)] of cefditoren ($C_{19}H_{18}N_6O_5S_3$)
$= M_S \times Q_T/Q_S \times 1000$

M_S: Amount [mg (potency)] of Cefditoren Pivoxil RS taken

Internal standard solution—A solution of propyl *p*-hydroxybenzoate in acetonitrile (1 in 200).
Operating conditions—

Detector: An ultraviolet absorption photometer (wavelength: 230 nm).

Column: A stainless steel column 4.6 mm in inside diameter and 25 cm in length, packed with octadecylsilanized silica gel for liquid chromatography (5 μm in particle diameter).

Column temperature: A constant temperature of about 25°C.

Mobile phase: Dissolve 1.58 g of ammonium formate in 900 mL of water, adjust to pH 6.0 with diluted formic acid (1 in 250), and add water to make 1000 mL. To 450 mL of this solution add 275 mL of acetonitrile and 275 mL of methanol.

Flow rate: Adjust so that the retention time of cefditoren pivoxil is about 15 minutes.

System suitability—

System performance: When the procedure is run with 10 μL of the standard solution under the above operating conditions, the internal standard and cefditoren pivoxil are eluted in this order with the resolution between these peaks being not less than 5.

System repeatability: When the test is repeated 5 times with 10 μL of the standard solution under the above operating conditions, the relative standard deviation of the ratios of the peak area of cefditoren pivoxil to that of the internal standard is not more than 1.0%.

Containers and storage Containers—Tight containers.
Storage—Light-resistant.

Cefditoren Pivoxil Fine Granules

セフジトレン　ピボキシル細粒

Cefditoren Pivoxil Fine Granules contain not less than 90.0% and not more than 110.0% of the labeled potency of cefditoren ($C_{19}H_{18}N_6O_5S_3$: 506.58).

Method of preparation Prepare as directed under Granules, with Cefditoren Pivoxil.

Identification To an amount of powdered Cefditoren Pivoxil Fine Granules, equivalent to 0.1 g (potency) of Cefditoren Pivoxil, add 10 mL of acetonitrile, shake vigorously, and filter. To 1 mL of the filtrate add acetonitrile to make 50 mL. To 1 mL of this solution add acetonitrile to make 20 mL, and determine the absorption spectrum of this solution as directed under Ultraviolet-visible Spectrophotometry <*2.24*>: it exhibits a maximum between 230 nm and 234 nm.

Purity Related substances—Being specified separately when the drug is granted approval based on the Law.

Loss on drying <*2.41*> Not more than 4.5% (0.5 g, reduced pressure not exceeding 0.67 kPa, 60°C, 3 hours).

Uniformity of dosage units <*6.02*> The granules in single-dose packages meet the requirement of the Mass variation test.

Dissolution <*6.10*> When the test is performed at 50 revolutions per minute according to the Paddle method, using 900 mL of 1st fluid for dissolution test as the dissolution medium, the dissolution rate in 15 minutes of Cefditoren Pivoxil Fine Granules is not less than 80%.

Start the test with an accurately weighed amount of Cefditoren Pivoxil Fine Granules, equivalent to about 0.1 g (potency) of Cefditoren Pivoxil, withdraw not less than 20 mL of the medium at the specified minute after starting the test, and filter through a membrane filter with a pore size not exceeding 0.45 μm. Discard not less than 10 mL of the first filtrate, pipet 2 mL of the subsequent filtrate, add water to make exactly 20 mL, and use this solution as the sample solution. Separately, weigh accurately an amount of Cefditoren Pivoxil RS, equivalent to about 22 mg (potency), dissolve in 20 mL of diluted acetonitrile (3 in 4), and add the dissolution medium to make exactly 200 mL. Pipet 2 mL of this solution, add water to make exactly 20 mL, and use this solution as the standard solution. Determine the absorbances, A_T and A_S, at 272 nm of the sample solution and standard solution as directed under Ultraviolet-visible Spectrophotometry <*2.24*>, using water as the control.

Dissolution rate (%) with respect to the labeled amount of cefditoren pivoxil ($C_{25}H_{28}N_6O_7S_3$)
$= M_S/M_T \times A_T/A_S \times 1/C \times 450$

M_S: Amount [mg(potency)] of Cefditoren Pivoxil RS taken
M_T: Amount (g) of Cefditoren Pivoxil Fine Granules taken
C: Labeled amount [mg(potency)] of cefditoren pivoxil ($C_{25}H_{28}N_6O_7S_3$) in 1 g

Assay Conduct this procedure using light-resistant vessels. Weigh accurately an amount of powdered Cefditoren Pivoxil Fine Granules, equivalent to about 40 mg (potency) of Cefditoren Pivoxil, add 70 mL of diluted acetonitrile (3 in 4), and shake vigorously. To this solution add exactly 10 mL of the internal standard solution, then add acetonitrile to make 100 mL, filter, and use the filtrate as the sample solution. Separately, weigh accurately an amount of Cefditoren Pivoxil RS, equivalent to about 20 mg (potency), dissolve in 20 mL of acetonitrile, add exactly 5 mL of the internal standard solution, then add acetonitrile to make 50 mL, and use this solution as the standard solution. Proceed as directed in the Assay under Cefditoren Pivoxil.

Amount [mg (potency)] of cefditoren ($C_{19}H_{18}N_6O_5S_3$)
$= M_S \times Q_T/Q_S \times 2$

M_S: Amount [mg (potency)] of Cefditoren Pivoxil RS taken

Internal standard solution—A solution of propyl parahydroxybenzoate in acetonitrile (1 in 200).

Containers and storage Containers—Tight containers.
Storage—Light-resistant.

Cefditoren Pivoxil Tablets

セフジトレン　ピボキシル錠

Cefditoren Pivoxil Tablets contain not less than 90.0% and not more than 110.0% of the labeled potency of cefditoren ($C_{19}H_{18}N_6O_5S_3$: 506.58).

Method of preparation Prepare as directed under Tablets, with Cefditoren Pivoxil.

Identification To an amount of powdered Cefditoren Pivoxil Tablets, equivalent to 35 mg (potency) of Cefditoren Pivoxil, add 100 mL of methanol, shake, and filter. To 5 mL of the filtrate add methanol to make 100 mL, and determine the absorption spectrum of this solution as directed under Ultraviolet-visible Spectrophotometry <*2.24*>: it exhibits a maximum between 229 nm and 233 nm.

Purity Related substances—Being specified separately when the drug is granted approval based on the Law.

Loss on drying <*2.41*> Not more than 4.0% (0.5 g, reduced pressure not exceeding 0.67 kPa, 60°C, 3 hours).

Uniformity of dosage units <*6.02*> Perform the Mass variation test, or the Content uniformity test according to the following method: it meets the requirement.

Conduct this procedure using light-resistant vessels. To 1 tablet of Cefditoren Pivoxil Tablets add 12.5 mL of the 1st fluid for disintegration test, shake vigorously, add about 25 mL of acetonitrile, shake again, and add acetonitrile to make exactly 50 mL. Pipet V mL of this solution, equivalent to about 20 mg (potency) of Cefditoren Pivoxil, add exactly

5 mL of the internal standard solution, then add diluted acetonitrile (3 in 4) to make 50 mL, filter, and use the filtrate as the sample solution. Separately, weigh accurately an amount of Cefditoren Pivoxil RS, equivalent to about 20 mg (potency), dissolve in 20 mL of acetonitrile, add exactly 5 mL of the internal standard solution, then add acetonitrile to make 50 mL, and use this solution as the standard solution. Proceed as directed in the Assay under Cefditoren Pivoxil.

Amount [mg (potency)] of cefditoren ($C_{19}H_{18}N_6O_5S_3$)
$= M_S \times Q_T/Q_S \times 50/V$

M_S: Amount [mg (potency)] of Cefditoren Pivoxil RS taken

Internal standard solution—A solution of propyl parahydroxybezoate in acetonitrile (1 in 200).

Dissolution ⟨*6.10*⟩ When the test is performed at 50 revolutions per minute according to the Paddle method, using 900 mL of 1st fluid for dissolution test as the dissolution medium, the dissolution rate in 20 minutes of Cefditoren Pivoxil Tablets is not less than 85%.

Start the test with 1 tablet of Cefditoren Pivoxil Tablets, withdraw not less than 20 mL of the medium at the specified minute after starting the test, and filter through a membrane filter with a pore size not exceeding 0.45 μm. Discard not less than 10 mL of the first filtrate, pipet V mL of the subsequent filtrate, add water to make exactly V' mL so that each mL contains about 11 μg (potency) of Cefditoren Pivoxil, and use this solution as the sample solution. Separately, weigh accurately an amount of Cefditoren Pivoxil RS, equivalent to about 22 mg (potency), dissolve in 20 mL of diluted acetonitrile (3 in 4), then add the dissolution medium to make exactly 200 mL. Pipet 2 mL of this solution, add water to make exactly 20 mL, and use this solution as the standard solution. Determine the absorbances, A_T and A_S, at 272 nm of the sample solution and standard solution as directed under Ultraviolet-visible Spectrophotometry ⟨*2.24*⟩ using water as the control.

Dissolution rate (%) with respect to the labeled amount of cefditoren pivoxil ($C_{25}H_{28}N_6O_7S_3$)
$= M_S \times A_T/A_S \times V'/V \times 1/C \times 45$

M_S: Amount [mg (potency)] of Cefditoren Pivoxil RS taken
C: Labeled amount [mg (potency)] of cefditoren pivoxil ($C_{25}H_{28}N_6O_7S_3$) in 1 tablet

Assay Conduct this procedure using light-resistant vessels. To an amount of Cefditoren Pivoxil Tablets, equivalent to 0.5 g (potency) of Cefditoren Pivoxil, add 63 mL of the 1st fluid for disintegration test, shake vigorously, add about 125 mL of acetonitrile, shake again, and add acetonitrile to make exactly 250 mL. Pipet 10 mL of this solution, add exactly 5 mL of the internal standard solution, then add diluted acetonitrile (3 in 4) to make 50 mL, filter, and use the filtrate as the sample solution. Separately, weigh accurately an amount of Cefditoren Pivoxil RS, equivalent to about 20 mg (potency), dissolve in 20 mL of acetonitrile, add exactly 5 mL of the internal standard solution, then add acetonitrile to make 50 mL, and use this solution as the standard solution. Proceed as directed in the Assay under Cefditoren Pivoxil.

Amount [mg (potency)] of cefditoren ($C_{19}H_{18}N_6O_5S_3$)
$= M_S \times Q_T/Q_S \times 25$

M_S: Amount [mg (potency)] of Cefditoren Pivoxil RS taken

Internal standard solution—A solution of propyl parahydroxybenzoate in acetonitrile (1 in 200).

Containers and storage Containers—Tight containers.

Cefepime Dihydrochloride Hydrate

セフェピム塩酸塩水和物

$C_{19}H_{24}N_6O_5S_2.2HCl.H_2O$: 571.50
(6*R*,7*R*)-7-[(*Z*)-2-(2-Aminothiazol-4-yl)-2-(methoxyimino)acetylamino]-3-(1-methylpyrrolidinium-1-ylmethyl)-8-oxo-5-thia-1-azabicyclo[4.2.0]oct-2-ene-2-carboxylate dihydrochloride monohydrate
[*123171-59-5*]

Cefepime Dihydrochloride Hydrate contains not less than 835 μg (potency) and not more than 886 μg (potency) per mg, calculated on the anhydrous basis. The potency of Cefepime Dihydrochloride Hydrate is expressed as mass (potency) of cefepime ($C_{19}H_{24}N_6O_5S_2$: 480.56).

Description Cefepime Dihydrochloride Hydrate occurs as a white to yellowish white, crystals or crystalline powder.

It is freely soluble in water and in methanol, and slightly soluble in ethanol (95), and practically in soluble in diethyl ether.

Identification **(1)** Dissolve 0.02 g of Cefepime Dihydrochloride Hydrate in 2 mL of water, add 1 mL of a solution of hydroxylammonium chloride (1 in 10) and 2 mL of sodium hydroxide TS, allow to stand for 5 minutes, then add 3 mL of 1 mol/L hydrochloric acid TS and 3 drops of iron (III) chloride TS: a red-brown color develops.

(2) Determine the absorption spectra of solutions (1 in 20,000) of Cefepime Dihydrochloride Hydrate and Cefepime Dihydrochloride RS as directed under Ultraviolet-visible Spectrophotometry ⟨*2.24*⟩, and compare these spectra: both spectra exhibit similar intensities of absorption at the same wavelengths.

(3) Determine the infrared absorption spectra of Cefepime Dihydrochloride Hydrate and Cefepime Dihydrochloride RS as directed in the potassium bromide disk method under Infrared Spectrophotometry ⟨*2.25*⟩, and compare these spectra: both spectra exhibit similar intensities of absorption at the same wave numbers.

(4) Determine the ^1H spectrum of a solution of Cefepime Dihydrochloride Hydrate in heavy water for nuclear magnetic resonance spectroscopy (1 in 10) as directed under Nuclear Magnetic Resonance Spectroscopy ⟨*2.21*⟩, using sodium 3-trimethylsilylpropionate-d_4 for nuclear magnetic resonance spectroscopy as an internal reference compound: it exhibits single signals, A and B, at around δ 3.1 ppm and at around δ 7.2 ppm, respectively, and the ratio of integrated intensity of each signal, A:B, is about 3:1.

(5) Dissolve 15 mg of Cefepime Dihydrochloride Hydrate in 5 mL of water, and add 2 drops of silver nitrate TS: a white turbidity is produced.

Absorbance ⟨*2.24*⟩ $E^{1\%}_{1\,cm}$ (259 nm): 310 – 340 (50 mg calculated on the anhydrous basis, water, 1000 mL).

Optical rotation ⟨*2.49*⟩ $[\alpha]_D^{20}$: +39 - +47° (60 mg calculated on the anhydrous basis, water, 20 mL, 100 mm).

pH ⟨*2.54*⟩ Dissolve 0.1 g of Cefepime Dihydrochloride Hydrate in 10 mL of water: the pH of this solution is between 1.6 and 2.1.

Purity **(1)** Clarity and color of solution—Dissolve 0.5 g of Cefepime Dihydrochloride Hydrate in 5 mL of a solution of L-arginine (3 in 50): the solution is clear and has no more color than Matching Fluid H.

(2) Heavy metals ⟨*1.07*⟩—Proceed with 1.0 g of Cefepime Dihydrochloride Hydrate according to Method 2, and perform the test. Prepare the control solution with 2.0 mL of Standard Lead Solution (not more than 20 ppm).

(3) *N*-Methylpyrrolidine—Weigh accurately an amount of Cefepime Dihydrochloride Hydrate equivalent to about 80 mg (potency), dissolve in diluted nitric acid (2 in 3125) to make exactly 10 mL, and use this solution as the sample solution. Separately, put 30 mL of water in a 100-mL volumetric flask, weigh accurately the mass of flask, then add about 0.125 g of *N*-methylpyrrolidine, weigh accurately the mass of the flask again, and add water to make exactly 100 mL. Pipet 4 mL of this solution, add diluted nitric acid (2 in 3125) to make exactly 100 mL, and use this solution as the standard solution. Perform the test with exactly 100 μL each of the sample solution and standard solution as directed under Liquid Chromatography ⟨*2.01*⟩ according to the following conditions, and determine the peak areas, A_T and A_S, of *N*-methylpyrrolidine by the automatic integration method. Calculate the amount of *N*-methylpyrrolidine per 1 mg (potency) of Cefepime Dihydrochloride Hydrate by the following equation: not more than 0.5%. The sample solution must be tested within 20 minutes after preparation.

$$\text{Amount (\%) of } N\text{-methylpyrrolidine} = (M_S \times f)/M_T \times A_T/A_S \times 1/250$$

M_S: Amount (mg) of *N*-methylpyrrolidine taken
M_T: Amount [mg (potency)] of Cefepime Dihydrochloride Hydrate taken
f: Purity (%) of *N*-methylpyrrolidine

Operating conditions—

Detector: An electric conductivity detector.

Column: A plastic tube 4.6 mm in inside diameter and 5 cm in length, packed with hydrophilic silica gel for liquid chromatography carrying sulfonic acid groups having the exchange capacity of about 0.3 meq per g (5 μm in particle diameter).

Column temperature: A constant temperature of about 35°C.

Mobile phase: To 990 mL of diluted nitric acid (2 in 3125) add 10 mL of acetonitrile.

Flow rate: 1.0 mL per minute.

System suitability—

System performance: To 20 mL of a solution of sodium chloride (3 in 1000) add 0.125 g of *N*-methylpyrrolidine, and add water to make 100 mL. To 4 mL of this solution add diluted nitric acid (2 in 3125) to make 100 mL. When the procedure is run with 100 μL of this solution under the above operating conditions, sodium and *N*-methylpyrrolidine are eluted in this order with the resolution between these peaks being not less than 2.0.

System repeatability: When the test is repeated 5 times with 100 μL of the standard solution under the above operating conditions, the relative standard deviation of the peak areas of *N*-methylpyrrolidine is not more than 4.0%.

(4) Related substances—Dissolve about 0.1 g of Cefepime Dihydrochloride Hydrate in the mobile phase A to make 50 mL, and use this solution as the sample solution. Perform the test with 5 μL of the sample solution as directed under Liquid Chromatography ⟨*2.01*⟩ according to the following conditions, and determine the area of each peak by the automatic integration method. Calculate the total amount of the peaks other than cefepime by the area percentage method: not more than 0.5%.

Operating conditions—

Detector: An ultraviolet absorption photometer (wavelength: 254 nm).

Column: A stainless steel column 4.6 mm in inside diameter and 25 cm in length, packed with octadecylsilanized silica gel for liquid chromatography (10 μm in particle diameter).

Column temperature: A constant temperature of about 25°C.

Mobile phase A: Dissolve 0.57 g of ammonium dihydrogenphosphate in 1000 mL of water.

Mobile phase B: Acetonitrile.

Flowing of mobile phase: Control the gradient by mixing the mobile phases A and B as directed in the following table.

Time after injection of the sample (min)	Mobile phase A (vol%)	Mobile phase B (vol%)
0 - 25	100 → 75	0 → 25

Flow rate: Adjust so that the retention time of cefepime is about 9.5 minutes.

Time span of measurement: About 2.5 times as long as the retention time of cefepime.

System suitability—

Test for required detectability: To 1 mL of the sample solution add the mobile phase A to make 10 mL, and use this solution as the solution for system suitability test. To 1 mL of the solution for system suitability test add the mobile phase A to make 10 mL, and use this solution as the solution for test for required detectability. Pipet 1 mL of the solution for test for required detectability, add the mobile phase A to make exactly 10 mL. Conform that the peak area of cefepime obtained with 5 μL of this solution is equivalent to 7 to 13% of that with 5 μL of the solution for test for required detectability.

System performance: When the procedure is run with 5 μL of the solution for system suitability test under the above operating conditions, the number of theoretical plates of the peak of cefepime is not less than 6000.

System repeatability: When the test is repeated 3 times with 5 μL of the solution for system suitability test under the above operating conditions, the relative standard deviation of the peak areas of cefepime is not more than 2.0%.

Water ⟨*2.48*⟩ Not less than 3.0% and not more than 4.5% (Weigh accurately about 50 mg of Cefepime Dihydrochloride Hydrate, dissolve in exactly 2 mL of methanol for water determination and perform the test with exactly 0.5 mL of this solution; coulometric titration).

Residue on ignition ⟨*2.44*⟩ Not more than 0.1% (1 g).

Bacterial endotoxins ⟨*4.01*⟩ Less than 0.04 EU/mg (potency).

Assay Weigh accurately an amount of Cefepime Dihydrochloride Hydrate and Cefepime Dihydrochloride RS, equivalent to about 60 mg (potency), dissolve in the mobile phase to make exactly 50 mL, and use these solutions as the sample solution and the standard solution, respectively. Perform the test with exactly 10 μL each of the sample solution and standard solution as directed under Liquid Chromatography <*2.01*> according to the following conditions, and determine the peak areas, A_T and A_S, of cefepime in each solution.

Amount [μg (potency)] of cefepime ($C_{19}H_{24}N_6O_5S_2$)
$= M_S \times A_T/A_S \times 1000$

M_S: Amount [mg (potency)] of Cefepime Dihydrochloride RS taken

Operating conditions—

Detector: An ultraviolet absorption photometer (wavelength: 254 nm).

Column: A stainless steel column 3.9 mm in inside diameter and 30 cm in length, packed with octadecylsilanized silica gel for liquid chromatography (10 μm in particle diameter).

Column temperature: A constant temperature of about 40°C.

Mobile phase: Adjust a solution of sodium 1-pentanesulfonate (261 in 100,000) to pH 3.4 with acetic acid (100), then adjust this solution to pH 4.0 with a solution of potassium hydroxide (13 in 20). To 950 mL of this solution add 50 mL of acetonitrile.

Flow rate: Adjust so that the retention time of cefepime is about 8 minutes.

System suitability—

System performance: When the procedure is run with 10 μL of the standard solution under the above operating conditions, the number of theoretical plates of the peak of cefepime is not less than 1500.

System repeatability: When the test is repeated 5 times with 10 μL of the standard solution under the above operating conditions, the relative standard deviation of the peak areas of cefepime is not more than 2.0%.

Containers and storage Containers—Hermetic containers. Storage—Light-resistant.

Cefepime Dihydrochloride for Injection

注射用セフェピム塩酸塩

Cefepime Dihydrochloride for Injection is a preparation for injection, which is dissolved before use.

It contains not less than 95.0% and not more than 110.0% of the labeled potency of cefepime ($C_{19}H_{24}N_6O_5S_2$: 480.56).

Method of preparation Prepare as directed under Injections, with Cefepime Dihydrochloride Hydrate.

Description Cefepime Dihydrochloride for Injection occurs as a white to pale yellow powder.

Identification **(1)** Dissolve 40 mg of Cefepime Dihydrochloride in 2 mL of water, add 1 mL of a solution of hydroxylammonium chloride (1 in 10) and 2 mL of sodium hydroxide TS, allow to stand for 5 minutes, then add 3 mL of 1 mol/L hydrochloric acid TS and 3 drops of iron (III) chloride TS: a red-brown color develops.

(2) Determine the absorption spectrum of a solution of Cefepime Dihydrochloride for Injection (1 in 12,500) as directed under Ultraviolet-visible Spectrophotometry <*2.24*>: it exhibits maxima between 233 nm and 237 nm and between 255 nm and 259 nm.

pH <*2.54*> The pH of a solution obtained by dissolving an amount of Cefepime Dihydrochloride for Injection, equivalent to 0.5 g (potency) of Cefepime Dihydrochloride Hydrate, in 5 mL of water is between 4.0 and 6.0.

Purity **(1)** Clarity and color of solution—Dissolve an amount of Cefepime Dihydrochloride for Injection, equivalent to 0.5 g (potency) of Cefepime Dihydrochloride Hydrate, in 5 mL of water: the solution is clear and colorless or light yellow. The color is not darker than Matching Fluid I.

(2) *N*-Methylpyrrolidine—Weigh accurately an amount of Cefepime Dihydrochloride for Injection, equivalent to about 0.2 g (potency) of Cefepime Dihydrochloride Hydrate, dissolve in diluted nitric acid (2 in 625) to make exactly 20 mL, and use this solution as the sample solution. Separately, transfer 30 mL of water into a 100-mL volumetric flask, weigh accurately the mass of the flask, add about 0.125 g of *N*-methylpyrrolidine, then weigh accurately the mass, and add water to make exactly 100 mL. Pipet 4 mL of this solution, add diluted nitric acid (2 in 3125) to make exactly 100 mL, and use this solution as the standard solution. Perform the test with exactly 100 μL each of the sample solution and standard solution as directed under Liquid Chromatography <*2.01*> according to the following conditions, and determine the peak areas of *N*-methylpyrrolidine, A_T and A_S, by the automatic integration method within 20 minutes after the sample solution is prepared. Calculate the amount of *N*-methylpyrrolidine per mg (potency) of Cefepime Dihydrochloride for Injection by the following formula: not more than 1.0%.

Amount (%) of *N*-methylpyrrolidine
$= (M_S \times f)/M_T \times A_T/A_S \times 1/125$

M_S: Amount (mg) of *N*-methylpyrrolidine taken
M_T: Amount [mg (potency)] of Cefepime Dihydrochloride for Injection taken
f: Purity (%) of *N*-methylpyrrolidine

Operating conditions—

Proceed as directed in the operating conditions in the Purity (3) under Cefepime Dihydrochloride Hydrate.

System suitability—

Proceed as directed in the system suitability in the Purity (3) under Cefepime Dihydrochloride Hydrate.

Water <*2.48*> Not more than 4.0% (Weigh accurately about 50 mg of Cefepime Dihydrochloride for Injection, dissolve in exactly 2 mL of methanol for water determination, and perform the test with exactly 0.5 mL of this solution: coulometric titration).

Bacterial endotoxins <*4.01*> Less than 0.06 EU/mg (potency).

Uniformity of dosage units <*6.02*> It meets the requirement of the Mass variation test.

Foreign insoluble matter <*6.06*> Perform the test according to Method 2: it meets the requirement.

Insoluble particulate matter <*6.07*> It meets the requirement.

Sterility <*4.06*> Perform the test according to the Membrane filtration method: it meets the requirement.

Assay Weigh accurately the mass of the contents of not less than 10 Cefepime Dihydrochloride for Injection. Weigh accurately an amount of the content, equivalent to about 60 mg (potency) of Cefepime Dihydrochloride Hydrate, dissolve in the mobile phase to make exactly 50 mL, and use this solution as the sample solution. Separately, weigh accurately an amount of Cefepime Dihydrochloride RS, equivalent to about 60 mg (potency), dissolve in the mobile phase to make exactly 50 mL, and use this solution as the standard solution. Proceed as directed in the Assay under Cefepime Dihydrochloride Hydrate.

Amount [μg (potency)] of cefepime ($C_{19}H_{24}N_6O_5S_2$)
$= M_S \times A_T/A_S \times 1000$

M_S: Amount [mg (potency)] of Cefepime Dihydrochloride RS taken

Containers and storage Containers—Hermetic containers. Storage—Light-resistant.

Cefixime Hydrate

セフィキシム水和物

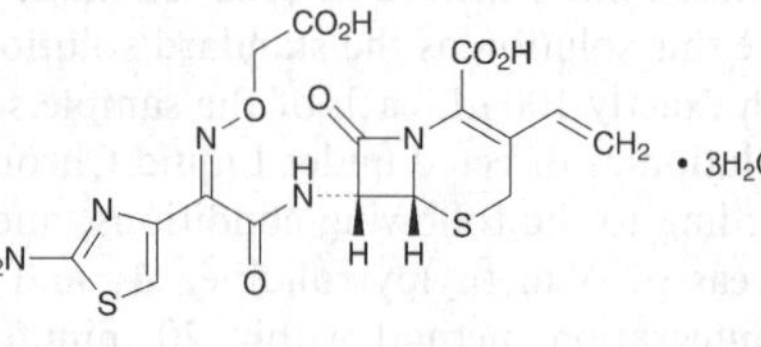

$C_{16}H_{15}N_5O_7S_2.3H_2O$: 507.50
(6*R*,7*R*)-7-[(*Z*)-2-(2-Aminothiazol-4-yl)-2-(carboxymethoxyimino)acetylamino]-8-oxo-3-vinyl-5-thia-1-azabicyclo[4.2.0]oct-2-ene-2-carboxylic acid trihydrate
[*125110-14-7*]

Cefixime Hydrate contains not less than 930 μg (potency) and not more than 1020 μg (potency) per mg, calculated on the anhydrous basis. The potency of Cefixime Hydrate is expressed as mass (potency) of cefixime ($C_{16}H_{15}N_5O_7S_2$: 453.45).

Description Cefixime Hydrate occurs as a white to light yellow crystalline powder.

It is freely soluble in methanol and in dimethylsulfoxide, sparingly soluble in ethanol (99.5), and practically insoluble in water.

Identification **(1)** Determine the absorption spectrum of a solution of Cefixime Hydrate in 0.1 mol/L phosphate buffer solution (pH 7.0) (1 in 62,500) as directed under Ultraviolet-visible Spectrophotometry *<2.24>*, and compare the spectrum with the Reference Spectrum or the spectrum of a solution of Cefixime RS prepared in the same manner as the sample solution: both spectra exhibit similar intensities of absorption at the same wavelengths.

(2) Determine the infrared absorption spectrum of Cefixime Hydrate as directed in the potassium bromide disk method under Infrared Spectrophotometry *<2.25>*, and compare the spectrum with the Reference Spectrum or the spectrum of Cefixime RS: both spectra exhibit similar intensities of absorption at the same wave numbers.

(3) Dissolve 50 mg of Cefixime Hydrate in 0.5 mL of a mixture of deuterated dimethylsulfoxide for nuclear magnetic resonance spectroscopy and heavy water for nuclear magnetic resonance spectroscopy (4:1). Determine the ^{1}H spectrum of this solution, as directed under Nuclear Magnetic Resonance Spectroscopy *<2.21>*, using tetramethylsilane for nuclear magnetic resonance spectroscopy as an internal reference compound: it exhibits a singlet signal A at around δ 4.7 ppm, and a multiplet signal B between δ 6.5 ppm and δ 7.4 ppm. The ratio of integrated intensity of these signals, A:B, is about 1:1.

Optical rotation *<2.49>* $[\alpha]_D^{20}$: $-75 - -88°$ (0.45 g calculated on the anhydrous bases, a solution of sodium hydrogen carbonate (1 in 50), 50 mL, 100 mm).

Purity Dissolve 0.1 g of Cefixime Hydrate in 100 mL of 0.1 mol/L phosphate buffer solution (pH 7.0), and use this solution as the sample solution. Perform the test with 10 μL of the sample solution as directed under Liquid Chromatography *<2.01>* according to the following conditions. Determine each peak area by the automatic integration method, and calculate their amounts by the area percentage method: the amount of the peak other than cefixime is not more than 1.0%, and the total amount of the peaks other than cefixime is not more than 2.5%.

Operating conditions—

Detector, column, column temperature, mobile phase, and flow rate: Proceed as directed in the operating conditions in the Assay.

Time span of measurement: About 3 times as long as the retention time of cefixime, beginning after the solvent peak.

System suitability—

Test for required detectability: To 1 mL of the sample solution add 0.1 mol/L phosphate buffer solution (pH 7.0) to make 100 mL, and use this solution as the solution for system suitability test. Pipet 1 mL of the solution for system suitability test, add 0.1 mol/L phosphate buffer solution (pH 7.0) to make exactly 10 mL. Confirm that the peak area of cefixime obtained with 10 μL of this solution is equivalent to 7 to 13% of that with 10 μL of the solution for system suitability test.

System performance: When the procedure is run with 10 μL of the solution for system suitability test under the above operating conditions, the number of theoretical plates and the symmetry factor of the peak of cefixime are not less than 4000 and not more than 2.0, respectively.

System repeatability: When the test is repeated 6 times with 10 μL of the solution for system suitability test under the above operating conditions, the relative standard deviation of the peak areas of cefixime is not more than 2.0%.

Water *<2.48>* Not less than 9.0 and not more than 12.0% (0.1 g, volumetric titration, direct titration).

Residue on ignition *<2.44>* Not more than 0.1% (1 g).

Assay Weigh accurately an amount of Cefixime Hydrate, equivalent to about 0.1 g (potency), and dissolve in 0.1 mol/L phosphate buffer solution (pH 7.0) to make exactly 100 mL. Pipet 10 mL of this solution, add 0.1 mol/L phosphate buffer solution (pH 7.0) to make exactly 50 mL, and use this solution as the sample solution. Separately, weigh accurately an amount of Cefixime RS, equivalent to about 20 mg (potency), and dissolve in 0.1 mol/L phosphate buffer solution (pH 7.0) to make exactly 20 mL. Pipet 10 mL of this solution, add 0.1 mol/L phosphate buffer solution (pH 7.0) to make exactly 50 mL, and use this solution as the standard solution. Perform the test with exactly 10 μL each of the sample solution and standard solution as directed under Liquid Chromatography *<2.01>* according to the following conditions, and determine the peak areas, A_T and A_S, of cefixime in each solution.

Amount [μg (potency)] of cefixime ($C_{16}H_{15}N_5O_7S_2$)
$= M_S \times A_T/A_S \times 5000$

M_S: Amount [mg (potency)] of Cefixime RS taken

Operating conditions—

Detector: An ultraviolet absorption photometer (wavelength: 254 nm).

Column: A stainless steel column 4 mm in inside diameter and 125 mm in length, packed with octadecylsilanized silica gel for liquid chromatography (4 μm in particle diameter).

Column temperature: A constant temperature of about 40°C.

Mobile phase: To 25 mL of a solution of tetrabutylammonium hydroxide TS (10 in 13) add water to make 1000 mL, and adjust to pH 6.5 with diluted phosphoric acid (1 in 10). To 300 mL of this solution add 100 mL of acetonitrile.

Flow rate: Adjust so that the retention time of cefixime is about 10 minutes.

System suitability—

System performance: When the procedure is run with 10 μL of the standard solution under the above operating conditions, the number of theoretical plates and the symmetry factor of the peak of cefixime are not less than 4000 and not more than 2.0, respectively.

System repeatability: When the test is repeated 6 times with 10 μL of the standard solution under the above operating conditions, the relative standard deviation of peak area of cefixime is not more than 2.0%.

Containers and storage Containers—Hermetic containers.

Storage—Light-resistant.

Cefixime Capsules

セフィキシムカプセル

Cefixime Capsules contain not less than 90.0% and not more than 105.0% of the labeled potency of cefixime ($C_{16}H_{15}N_5O_7S_2$: 453.45).

Method of preparation Prepare as directed under Capsules, with Cefixime Hydrate.

Identification Take out the contents of Cefixime Capsules, to a quantity of the contents of Cefixime Capsules, equivalent to 70 mg (potency) of Cefixime Hydrate, add 100 mL of 0.1 mol/L phosphate buffer solution (pH 7.0), shake for 30 minutes, and filter. To 1 mL of the filtrate add 0.1 mol/L phosphate buffer solution (pH 7.0) to make 50 mL. Determine the absorption spectrum of this solution as directed under Ultraviolet-visible Spectrophotometry *<2.24>*: it exhibits a maximum between 286 nm and 290 nm.

Purity Related substances—Take out the contents of Cefixime Capsules, to a quantity of the contents of Cefixime Capsules, equivalent to 0.1 g (potency) of Cefixime Hydrate, add 100 mL of 0.1 mol/L phosphate buffer solution (pH 7.0), shake for 30 minutes, filter, and use the filtrate as the sample solution. Perform the test with 10 μL of the sample solution as directed under Liquid Chromatography *<2.01>* according to the following conditions. Determine each peak area from the sample solution by the automatic integration method, and calculate the amount of them by the area percentage method: the amount of each peak other than cefixime is not more than 1.0%, and the total amount of the peaks other than cefixime is not more than 2.5%.

Operating conditions—

Detector, column, column temperature, mobile phase and flow rate: Proceed as directed in the operating conditions in the Assay under Cefixime Hydrate.

Time span for measurement: Proceed as directed in the operating conditions in the Purity under Cefixime Hydrate.

System suitability—

Test for required detectability: Pipet 1 mL of the sample solution, and add 0.1 mol/L phosphate buffer solution (pH 7.0) to make exactly 100 mL, and use this solution as the solution for system suitability test. Pipet 1 mL of the solution for system suitability test, and add 0.1 mol/L phosphate buffer solution (pH 7.0) to make exactly 10 mL. Confirm that the peak area of cefixime obtained with 10 μL of this solution is equivalent to 7 to 13% of that with 10 μL of the solution for system suitability test.

System performance: When the procedure is run with 10 μL of the solution for system suitability test under the above operating conditions, the number of theoretical plates and the symmetry factor of the peak of cefixime are not less than 4000 and not more than 2.0, respectively.

System repeatability: When the test is repeated 6 times with 10 μL of the solution for system suitability test under the above operating conditions, the relative standard deviation of the peak area of cefixime is not more than 2.0%.

Water *<2.48>* Not more than 12.0% (0.1 g of the contents, volumetric titration, direct titration).

Uniformity of dosage units *<6.02>* Perform the Mass variation test, or the Content uniformity test according to the following method: it meets the requirement.

Take out the contents of 1 capsule of Cefixime Capsules, and to the contents and the capsule shells add $7V/10$ mL of 0.1 mol/L phosphate buffer solution (pH 7.0), shake for 30 minutes, and add 0.1 mol/L phosphate buffer solution (pH 7.0) to make exactly V mL so that each mL contains about 1 mg (potency) of Cefixime Hydrate. Centrifuge this solution, pipet 10 mL of the supernatant liquid, add 0.1 mol/L phosphate buffer solution (pH 7.0) to make exactly 50 mL, and use this solution as the sample solution. Separately, weigh accurately an amount of Cefixime RS, equivalent to about 20 mg (potency), dissolve in 0.1 mol/L phosphate buffer solution (pH 7.0) to make exactly 100 mL, and use this solution as the standard solution. Then, proceed as directed in the Assay under Cefixime Hydrate.

$$\text{Amount [mg (potency)] of cefixime } (C_{16}H_{15}N_5O_7S_2) = M_S \times A_T/A_S \times V/20$$

M_S: Amount [mg (potency)] of Cefixime RS taken

Dissolution *<6.10>* When the test is performed at 50 revolutions per minute according to the Paddle method using the sinker, using 900 mL of disodium hydrogen phosphate-citric acid buffer solution (pH 7.5) as the dissolution medium, the dissolution rates in 60 minutes of 50-mg (potency) capsule and in 90 minutes of 100-mg (potency) capsule are not less than 80%, respectively.

Start the test with 1 capsule of Cefixime Capsules, withdraw not less than 20 mL of the medium at the specified minute after starting the test, and filter through a membrane filter with a pore size not exceeding 0.5 μm. Discard not less than 10 mL of the first filtrate, pipet V mL of the subsequent filtrate, add the dissolution medium to make exactly V' mL so that each mL contains about 56 μg (potency) of Cefixime Hydrate, and use this solution as the sample solution. Separately, weigh accurately an amount of Cefixime RS, equivalent to about 28 mg (potency), and dissolve in the dissolution medium to make exactly 100 mL. Pipet 4 mL of this solution, add the dissolution medium to make exactly 20 mL, and use this solution as the standard solution. Perform the test with exactly 20 μL each of the sample solution and standard solution as directed under Liquid Chromatography *<2.01>* according to the following conditions, and determine the peak areas, A_T and A_S, of cefixime in each solution.

Dissolution rate (%) with respect to the labeled amount of cefixime ($C_{16}H_{15}N_5O_7S_2$)
$= M_S \times A_T/A_S \times V'/V \times 1/C \times 180$

M_S: Amount [mg (potency)] of Cefixime RS taken
C: Labeled amount [mg (potency)] of Cefixime Hydrate in 1 capsule

Operating conditions—

Proceed as directed in the operating conditions in the Assay under Cefixime Hydrate.

System suitability—

System performance: When the procedure is run with 20 μL of the standard solution under the above operating conditions, the number of theoretical plates and the symmetry factor of the peak of cefixime are not less than 4000 and not more than 2.0, respectively.

System repeatability: When the test is repeated 6 times with 20 μL of the standard solution under the above operating conditions, the relative standard deviation of the peak area of cefixime is not more than 2.0%.

Assay Take out the contents of not less than 20 Cefixime Capsules, weigh accurately the mass of the contents, and powder. Weigh accurately a portion of the powder, equivalent to about 0.1 g (potency) of Cefixime Hydrate, add 70 mL of 0.1 mol/L phosphate buffer solution (pH 7.0) and shake for 30 minutes, add 0.1 mol/L phosphate buffer solution (pH 7.0) to make exactly 100 mL. Centrifuge this solution, pipet 10 mL of the supernatant liquid, add 0.1 mol/L phosphate buffer solution (pH 7.0) to make exactly 50 mL, and use this solution as the sample solution. Separately, weigh accurately an amount of Cefixime RS, equivalent to about 20 mg (potency), dissolve in 0.1 mol/L phosphate buffer solution (pH 7.0) to make exactly 100 mL, and use this solution as the standard solution. Then, proceed as directed in the Assay under Cefixime Hydrate.

Amount [mg (potency)] of cefixime ($C_{16}H_{15}N_5O_7S_2$)
$= M_S \times A_T/A_S \times 5$

M_S: Amount [mg (potency)] of Cefixime RS taken

Containers and storage Containers—Tight containers.

Cefixime Fine Granules

セフィキシム細粒

Cefixime Fine Granules contain not less than 90.0% and not more than 105.0% of the labeled potency of cefixime ($C_{16}H_{15}N_5O_7S_2$: 453.45).

Method of preparation Prepare as directed under Granules, with Cefixime Hydrate.

Identification To a quantity of powdered Cefixime Fine Granules, equivalent to 2 mg (potency) of Cefixime Hydrate, add 150 mL of 0.1 mol/L phosphate buffer solution (pH 7.0), and shake. If necessary, filter or centrifuge. Determine the absorption spectrum of this solution as directed under Ultraviolet-visible Spectrophotometry *<2.24>*: it exhibits maximum between 286 nm and 290 nm.

Purity Related substances—To a quantity of powdered Cefixime Fine Granules, equivalent to 0.1 g (potency) of Cefixime Hydrate, add 100 mL of 0.1 mol/L phosphate buffer solution (pH 7.0), shake, filter through a membrane filter with a pore size not exceeding 0.45 μm, and use the filtrate as the sample solution. Perform the test with 10 μL of the sample solution as directed under Liquid Chromatography *<2.01>* according to the following conditions. Determine each peak area by the automatic integration method, and calculate their amounts by the area percentage method: the amount of the peak other than cefixime is not more than 1.0%, and the total amount of the peaks other than cefixime is not more than 2.5%.

Operating conditions—

Detector, column, column temperature, mobile phase and flow rate: Proceed as directed in the operating conditions in the Assay under Cefixime Hydrate.

Time span of measurement: Proceed as directed in the operating conditions in the Purity under Cefixime Hydrate.

System suitability—

Test for required detectability: To 1 mL of the sample solution add 0.1 mol/L phosphate buffer solution (pH 7.0) to make 100 mL, and use this solution as the solution for system suitability test. Pipet 1 mL of the solution for system suitability test, and add 0.1 mol/L phosphate buffer solution (pH 7.0) to make exactly 10 mL. Confirm that the peak area of cefixime obtained with 10 μL of this solution is equivalent to 7 to 13% of that with 10 μL of the solution for system suitability test.

System performance: When the procedure is run with 10 μL of the solution for system suitability test under the above operating conditions, the number of theoretical plates and the symmetry factor of the peak of cefixime are not less than 4000 and not more than 2.0, respectively.

System repeatability: When the test is repeated 6 times with 10 μL of the solution for system suitability test under the above operating conditions, the relative standard deviation of the peak area of cefixime is not more than 2.0%.

Water *<2.48>* Not more than 3.0% (1 g, volumetric titration, direct titration. Use a mixture of formamide for water determination and methanol for water determination (2:1) instead of methanol for water determination).

Uniformity of dosage units *<6.02>* Perform the test according to the following method: Cefixime Fine Granules in single-dose packages meet the requirement of the Content uniformity test.

To the total content of 1 package of Cefixime Fine Granules add 7 V/10 mL of 0.1 mol/L phosphate buffer solution (pH 7.0), shake, add 0.1 mol/L phosphate buffer solution (pH 7.0) to make exactly V mL so that each mL contains about 1 mg (potency) of Cefixime Hydrate. Centrifuge this solution, pipet 10 mL of the supernatant liquid, add 0.1 mol/L phosphate buffer solution (pH 7.0) to make exactly 50 mL, and use this solution as the sample solution. Separately, weigh accurately an amount of Cefixime RS, equivalent to about 20 mg (potency), dissolve in 0.1 mol/L phosphate buffer solution (pH 7.0) to make exactly 100 mL, and use this solution as the standard solution. Then, proceed as directed in the Assay under Cefixime Hydrate.

Amount [mg (potency)] of cefixime ($C_{16}H_{15}N_5O_7S_2$)
$= M_S \times A_T/A_S \times V/20$

M_S: Amount [mg (potency)] of Cefixime RS taken

Dissolution *<6.10>* When the test is performed at 50 revolutions per minute according to the Paddle method, using 900 mL of 2nd fluid for dissolution test as the dissolution medium, the dissolution rates in 30 minutes of Cefixime Fine Granules is not less than 75%.

Start the test with an accurately weighed amount of Cefixime Fine Granules, equivalent to about 0.1 g (potency) of Cefixime Hydrate, withdraw not less than 20 mL of the medium at the specified minute after starting the test, and filter through a membrane filter with a pore size not exceeding 0.45 μm. Discard not less than 10 mL of the first filtrate, and use the subsequent filtrate as the sample solution. Separately, weigh accurately an amount of Cefixime RS, equivalent to about 28 mg (potency), and dissolve in the dissolution medium to make exactly 50 mL. Pipet 4 mL of this solution, add the dissolution medium to make exactly 20 mL, and use this solution as the standard solution. Perform the test with exactly 20 μL each of the sample solution and standard solution as directed under Liquid Chromatography *<2.01>* according to the following conditions, and determine the peak areas, A_T and A_S, of cefixime in each solution.

Dissolution rate (%) with respect to the labeled amount of cefixime ($C_{16}H_{15}N_5O_7S_2$)
$= M_S/M_T \times A_T/A_S \times 1/C \times 360$

M_S: Amount [mg (potency)] of Cefixime RS taken
M_T: Amount (g) of Cefixime Fine Granules taken
C: Labeled amount [mg (potency)] of cefixime ($C_{16}H_{15}N_5O_7S_2$) in 1 g

Operating conditions—

Proceed as directed in the operating conditions in the Assay under Cefixime Hydrate.

System suitability—

System performance: When the procedure is run with 20 μL of the standard solution under the above operating conditions, the number of theoretical plates and the symmetry factor of the peak of cefixime are not less than 4000 and not more than 2.0, respectively.

System repeatability: When the test is repeated 6 times with 20 μL of the standard solution under the above operating conditions, the relative standard deviation of the peak area of cefixime is not more than 2.0%.

Assay Weigh accurately an amount of powdered Cefixime Fine Granules, equivalent to about 0.1 g (potency) of Cefixime Hydrate, add 70 mL of 0.1 mol/L phosphate buffer solution (pH 7.0), shake, and add 0.1 mol/L phosphate buffer solution (pH 7.0) to make exactly 100 mL. Centrifuge this solution, pipet 10 mL of the supernatant liquid, add 0.1 mol/L phosphate buffer solution (pH 7.0) to make exactly 50 mL, and use this solution as the sample solution. Separately, weigh accurately an amount of Cefixime RS, equivalent to about 20 mg (potency), dissolve in 0.1 mol/L phosphate buffer solution (pH 7.0) to make exactly 100 mL, and use this solution as the standard solution. Then, proceed as directed in the Assay under Cefixime Hydrate.

Amount [mg (potency)] of cefixime ($C_{16}H_{15}N_5O_7S_2$)
$= M_S \times A_T/A_S \times 5$

M_S: Amount [mg (potency)] of Cefixime RS taken

Containers and storage Containers—Tight containers.

Cefmenoxime Hydrochloride

セフメノキシム塩酸塩

$(C_{16}H_{17}N_9O_5S_3.)_2.HCl$: 1059.58
(6*R*,7*R*)-7-[(*Z*)-2-(2-Aminothiazol-4-yl)-2-(methoxyimino)acetylamino]-3-(1-methyl-1*H*-tetrazol-5-ylsulfanylmethyl)-8-oxo-5-thia-1-azabicyclo[4.2.0]oct-2-ene-2-carboxylic acid hemihydrochloride
[75738-58-8]

Cefmenoxime Hydrochloride contains not less than 890 μg (potency) and not more than 975 μg (potency) per mg, calculated on the anhydrous basis. The potency of Cefmenoxime Hydrochloride is expressed as mass (potency) of cefmenoxime ($C_{16}H_{17}N_9O_5S_3$: 511.56).

Description Cefmenoxime Hydrochloride occurs as white to light orange-yellow, crystals or crystalline powder.

It is freely soluble in formamide and in dimethylsulfoxide, slightly soluble in methanol, very slightly soluble in water, and practically insoluble in ethanol (95).

Identification **(1)** Determine the absorption spectrum of a solution of Cefmenoxime Hydrochloride in 0.1 mol/L phosphate buffer solution (pH 6.8) (3 in 200,000) as directed under Ultraviolet-visible Spectrophotometry *<2.24>*, and compare the spectrum with the Reference Spectrum or the spectrum of a solution of Cefmenoxime Hydrochloride RS prepared in the same manner as the sample solution: both spectra exhibit similar intensities of absorption at the same wavelengths.

(2) Determine the infrared absorption spectrum of Cefmenoxime Hydrochloride as directed in the potassium bromide disk method under Infrared Spectrophotometry *<2.25>*, and compare the spectrum with the Reference Spectrum or the spectrum of Cefmenoxime Hydrochloride RS: both spectra exhibit similar intensities of absorption at the same wave numbers.

(3) Determine the ^1H spectrum of a solution of Cefmenoxime Hydrochloride in deuterated dimethylsulfoxide for nuclear magnetic resonance spectroscopy (1 in 10) as directed under Nuclear Magnetic Resonance Spectroscopy *<2.21>*, using tetramethylsilane for nuclear magnetic resonance spectroscopy as an internal reference compound: it exhibits two singlet signals, A and B, at around δ 3.9 ppm, and a singlet signal C at around δ 6.8 ppm. The ratio of the integrated intensity of each signal, A:B:C, is about 3:3:1.

(4) Dissolve 10 mg of Cefmenoxime Hydrochloride in 1 mL of diluted sodium carbonate TS (1 in 20), add 5 mL of acetic acid (100) and 2 drops of silver nitrate TS: a white precipitate is formed.

Optical rotation *<2.49>* $[\alpha]_D^{20}$: $-27 - -35°$ (1 g, 0.1 mol/L phosphate buffer solution (pH 6.8), 100 mL, 100 mm).

pH *<2.54>* The pH of a solution obtained by dissolving 0.10 g of Cefmenoxime Hydrochloride in 150 mL of water is between 2.8 and 3.3.

Purity **(1)** Clarity and color of solution—A solution obtained by dissolving 1.0 g of Cefmenoxime Hydrochloride in 10 mL of diluted sodium carbonate TS (1 in 4) is clear and colorless to light yellow.

(2) Heavy metals *<1.07>*—Proceed with 1.0 g of Cefmenoxime Hydrochloride according to Method 4, and perform the test. Prepare the control solution with 2.0 mL of Standard Lead Solution (not more than 20 ppm).

(3) Arsenic *<1.11>*—Prepare the test solution with 1.0 g of Cefmenoxime Hydrochloride according to Method 4 and adding 10 mL of dilute hydrochloric acid to the residue after cooling, and perform the test (not more than 2 ppm).

(4) Related substances—Weigh accurately about 0.1 g of Cefmenoxime Hydrochloride, dissolve in 20 mL of 0.1 mol/L phosphate buffer solution (pH 6.8) and add the mobile phase to make exactly 100 mL. Pipet 4 mL of this solution, add the mobile phase to make exactly 50 mL, and use this solution as the sample solution. Separately, weigh accurately about 10 mg of 1-methyl-1*H*-tetrazol-5-thiol, and dissolve in the mobile phase to make exactly 100 mL. Pipet 4 mL of this solution, add the mobile phase to make exactly 250 mL, and use this solution as the standard solution (1). Weigh accurately about 0.1 g of Cefmenoxime Hydrochloride RS, dissolve in 20 mL of 0.1 mol/L phosphate buffer solution (pH 6.8) and add the mobile phase to make exactly 100 mL. Pipet 1 mL of this solution, add the mobile phase to make exactly 250 mL, and use this solution as the standard solution (2). Perform the test immediately after preparation of these solutions with exactly 10 μL each of the sample solution and standard solutions (1) and (2) as directed under Liquid Chromatography *<2.01>* according to the following conditions. Determine each peak area of these solutions by the automatic integration method, and calculate the amounts of 1-methyl-1*H*-tetrazol-5-thiol and the total related substance by the following formula: the amount of 1-methyl-1*H*-tetrazol-5-thiol is not more than 1.0%, and the total related substance is not more than 3.0%.

Amount (%) of 1-methyl-1*H*-tetrazol-5-thiol
$$= M_{Sa}/M_T \times A_{Ta}/A_{Sa} \times 20$$

Amount (%) of total related substances
$$= M_{Sa}/M_T \times A_{Ta}/A_{Sa} \times 20 + M_{Sb}/M_T \times S_T/A_{Sb} \times 5$$

M_{Sa}: Amount (g) of 1-methyl-1*H*-tetrazol-5-thiol taken
M_{Sb}: Amount (g) of Cefmenoxime Hydrochloride RS taken
M_T: Amount (g) of Cefmenoxime Hydrochloride taken
A_{Sa}: Peak area of 1-methyl-1*H*-tetrazol-5-thiol from the standard solution (1)
A_{Sb}: Peak area of cefmenoxime from the standard solution (2)
A_{Ta}: Peak area of 1-methyl-1*H*-tetrazol-5-thiol from the sample solution
S_T: Total area of the peaks other than 1-methyl-1*H*-tetrazol-5-thiol and other than cefmenoxime from the sample solution

Operating conditions—

Detector, column, column temperature, mobile phase, and flow rate: Proceed as directed in the operating conditions in the Assay.

Time span of measurement: About 2.5 times as long as the retention time of cefmenoxime.

System suitability—

System performance: Proceed as directed in the system suitability in the Assay.

Test for required detectability: Measure exactly 5 mL of the standard solution (1), add the mobile phase to make exactly 100 mL. Confirm that the peak area of 1-methyl-1*H*-tetrazol-5-thiol obtained with 10 μL of this solution is equivalent to 4.5 to 5.5% of that with 10 μL of the standard solution (1). Then, measure exactly 2 mL of the standard solution (2), add the mobile phase to make exactly 100 mL. Confirm that the peak area of cefmenoxime obtained with 10 μL of this solution is equivalent to 1.5 to 2.5% of that with 10 μL of the standard solution (2).

System repeatability: When the test is repeated 6 times with 10 μL of the standard solution (1) under the above operating conditions, the relative standard deviation of the peak area of 1-methyl-1*H*-tetrazol-5-thiol is not more than 1.0%.

Water *<2.48>* Not more than 1.5% (1 g, volumetric titration, direct titration. Use a mixture of formamide for water determination and methanol for water determination (2:1)).

Assay Weigh accurately an amount of Cefmenoxime Hydrochloride and Cefmenoxime Hydrochloride RS, equivalent to about 50 mg (potency), dissolve each in 10 mL of 0.1 mol/L phosphate buffer solution (pH 6.8) and add the mobile phase to make exactly 50 mL. Pipet 4 mL each of these solutions, add exactly 20 mL of the internal standard solution and the mobile phase to make 50 mL, and use these solutions as the sample solution and the standard solution, respectively. Perform the test with 10 μL each of the sample solution and standard solution as directed under Liquid Chromatography *<2.01>* according to the following conditions, and calculate the ratios, Q_T and Q_S, of the peak area of cefmenoxime to that of the internal standard.

Amount [μg (potency)] of cefmenoxime ($C_{16}H_{17}N_9O_5S_3$)
$$= M_S \times Q_T/Q_S \times 1000$$

M_S: Amount [mg (potency)] of Cefmenoxime Hydrochloride RS taken

Internal standard solution—A solution of phthalimide in methanol (3 in 2000).

Operating conditions—

Detector: An ultraviolet absorption photometer (wavelength: 254 nm).

Column: A stainless steel column 4 mm in inside diameter and 15 cm in length, packed with octadecylsilanized silica gel for liquid chromatography (5 μm in particle diameter).

Column temperature: A constant temperature of about 25°C.

Mobile phase: A mixture of water, acetonitrile and acetic acid (100) (50:10:1).

Flow rate: Adjust so that the retention time of cefmenoxime is about 8 minutes.

System suitability—

System performance: When the procedure is run with 10 μL of the standard solution under the above operating conditions, cefmenoxime and the internal standard are eluted in this order with the resolution between these peaks being not less than 2.3.

System repeatability: When the test is repeated 6 times with 10 μL of the standard solution under the above operating conditions, the relative standard deviation of the ratios of the peak areas of cefmenoxime to that of the internal standard is not more than 1.0%.

Containers and storage Containers—Hermetic containers.

Cefmetazole Sodium

セフメタゾールナトリウム

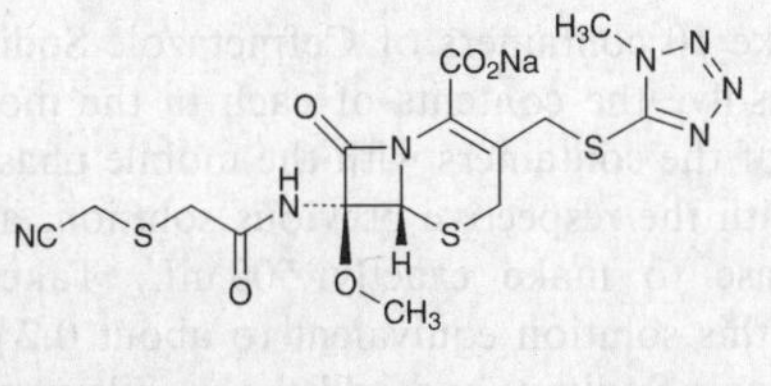

$C_{15}H_{16}N_7NaO_5S_3$: 493.52
Monosodium (6*R*,7*R*)-7-{[(cyanomethylsulfanyl)acetyl]amino}-7-methoxy-3-(1-methyl-1*H*-tetrazol-5-ylsulfanylmethyl)-8-oxo-5-thia-1-azabicyclo[4.2.0]oct-2-ene-2-carboxylate
[56796-20-4]

Cefmetazole Sodium contains not less than 860 μg (potency) and not more than 965 μg (potency) per mg, calculated on the anhydrous basis. The potency of Cefmetazole Sodium is expressed as mass (potency) of cefmetazole ($C_{15}H_{17}N_7O_5S_3$: 471.53).

Description Cefmetazole Sodium occurs as a white to light yellow-white, powder or mass.

It is very soluble in water, freely soluble in methanol, slightly soluble in ethanol (95), and very slightly soluble in tetrahydrofuran.

It is hygroscopic.

Identification (1) Determine the absorption spectrum of a solution of Cefmetazole Sodium (1 in 40,000) as directed under Ultraviolet-visible Spectrophotometry ⟨*2.24*⟩, and compare the spectrum with the Reference Spectrum: both spectra exhibit similar intensities of absorption at the same wavelengths.

(2) Determine the infrared absorption spectrum of Cefmetazole Sodium as directed in the potassium bromide disk method under Infrared Spectrophotometry ⟨*2.25*⟩, and compare the spectrum with the Reference Spectrum: both spectra exhibit similar intensities of absorption at the same wave numbers.

(3) Determine the ^{1}H spectrum of a solution of Cefmetazole Sodium in heavy water for nuclear magnetic resonance spectroscopy (1 in 10) as directed under Nuclear Magnetic Resonance Spectroscopy ⟨*2.21*⟩, using sodium 3-trimethylsilylpropanesulfonate for nuclear magnetic resonance spectroscopy as an internal reference compound: it exhibits singlet signals, A, B and C, at around δ 3.6 ppm, at around δ 4.1 ppm and at around δ 5.2 ppm, respectively. The ratio of integrated intensity of each signal, A:B:C, is about 3:3:1.

(4) Cefmetazole Sodium responds to Qualitative Tests ⟨*1.09*⟩ (1) for sodium salt.

Optical rotation ⟨*2.49*⟩ $[\alpha]_D^{20}$: +73 – +85° (0.25 g, water, 25 mL, 100 mm).

pH ⟨*2.54*⟩ Dissolve 1.0 g of Cefmetazole Sodium in 10 mL of water: the pH of the solution is between 4.2 and 6.2.

Purity (1) Clarity and color of solution—Dissolve 1.0 g of Cefmetazole Sodium in 10 mL of water: the solution is clear, and has no more color than the following control solution.

Control solution: To a mixture of exactly 0.5 mL of Cobalt (II) Chloride CS and exactly 5 mL of Iron (III) Chloride CS add water to make exactly 50 mL. To exactly 15 mL of this solution add water to make exactly 20 mL.

(2) Heavy metals ⟨*1.07*⟩—Proceed with 1.0 g of Cefmetazole Sodium according to Method 2, and perform the test. Prepare the control solution with 2.0 mL of Standard Lead Solution (not more than 20 ppm).

(3) Arsenic ⟨*1.11*⟩—Prepare the test solution with 1.0 g of Cefmetazole Sodium according to Method 3, and perform the test (not more than 2 ppm).

(4) Related substances—Dissolve 0.50 g of Cefmetazole Sodium in 10 mL of water, and use this solution as the sample solution. Pipet 4 mL, 2 mL, 1 mL, 0.5 mL and 0.25 mL of the sample solution, add water to them to make exactly 100 mL, and use these solutions as the standard solutions (1), (2), (3), (4) and (5), respectively. Separately, dissolve 0.10 g of 1-methyl-1*H*-tetrazole-5-thiol in water to make exactly 100 mL, and use this solution as the standard solution (6). Perform the test with these solutions as directed under Thin-layer Chromatography ⟨*2.03*⟩. Spot 1 μL each of the sample solution and standard solutions (1) to (6) on a plate of silica gel for thin-layer chromatography. Develop with a mixture of 1-butanol, water and acetic acid (100) (4:1:1) to a distance of about 12 cm, and air-dry the plate. Allow the plate to stand in iodine vapor: the spot obtained from the sample solution corresponding to the spot from the standard solution (6) is not more intense than the spot from the standard solution (6), and the spots other than this spot and other than the principal spot are not more intense than the spot from the standard solution (1). Furthermore, the total amount of the spots other than the principal spot from the sample solution, calculated by the comparison with the spots from the standard solutions (1), (2), (3), (4) and (5), is not more than 8.0%.

Water ⟨*2.48*⟩ Not more than 1.0% (1 g, volumetric titration, direct titration).

Assay Weigh accurately an amount of Cefmetazole Sodium and Cefmetazole RS, equivalent to about 50 mg (potency), and dissolve each in the mobile phase to make exactly 25 mL. Pipet 1 mL each of these solutions, add exactly 10 mL of the internal standard solution, and use these solutions as the sample solution and the standard solution, respectively. Perform the test with 10 μL each of the sample solution and standard solution as directed under Liquid Chromatography ⟨*2.01*⟩ according to the following conditions, and calculate the ratios, Q_T and Q_S, of the peak area of cefmetazole to that of the internal standard.

Amount [μg (potency)] of cefmetazole ($C_{15}H_{17}N_7O_5S_3$)
$= M_S \times Q_T/Q_S \times 1000$

M_S: Amount [mg (potency)] of Cefmetazole RS taken

Internal standard solution—A solution of methyl parahydroxybenzoate in the mobile phase (1 in 10,000).
Operating conditions—

Detector: An ultraviolet absorption photometer (wavelength: 214 nm).

Column: A stainless steel column 4.6 mm in inside diameter and 25 cm in length, packed with octadecylsilanized silica gel for liquid chromatography (5 μm in particle diameter).

Column temperature: A constant temperature of about 25°C.

Mobile phase: Dissolve 5.75 g of ammonium dihydrogenphosphate in 700 mL of water, add 280 mL of methanol, 20 mL of tetrahydrofuran and 3.2 mL of 40% tetrabutylammonium hydroxide TS, and adjust to pH 4.5 with phosphoric acid.

Flow rate: Adjust so that the retention time of cefmetazole is about 8 minutes.

System suitability—

System performance: When the procedure is run with 10 μL of the standard solution under the above operating conditions, cefmetazole and the internal standard are eluted in this order with the resolution between these peaks being not less than 10.

System repeatability: When the test is repeated 5 times with 10 μL of the standard solution under the above operating conditions, the relative standard deviation of the ratios of the peak area of cefmetazole to that of the internal standard is not more than 1.0%.

Containers and storage Containers—Hermetic containers.

Cefmetazole Sodium for Injection

注射用セフメタゾールナトリウム

Cefmetazole Sodium for Injection is a preparation for injection which is dissolved before use.

It contains not less than 90.0% and not more than 110.0% of the labeled potency of cefmetazole ($C_{15}H_{17}N_7O_5S_3$: 471.53).

Method of preparation Prepare as directed under Injections, with Cefmetazole Sodium.

Description Cefmetazole Sodium for Injection is a white to light yellow powder or masses.

It is hygroscopic.

Identification **(1)** Determine the absorption spectrum of a solution of Cefmetazole Sodium for Injection (1 in 40,000) as directed under Ultraviolet-visible Spectrophotometry *<2.24>*, and compare the spectrum with the Reference Spectrum: both spectra exhibit similar intensities of absorption at the same wavelengths.

(2) Determine the infrared absorption spectrum of Cefmetazole Sodium for Injection as directed in the potassium bromide disk method under Infrared Spectrophotometry *<2.25>*, and compare the spectrum with the Reference Spectrum: both spectra exhibit similar intensities of absorption at the same wave numbers.

pH *<2.54>* Take an amount of Cefmetazole Sodium for Injection equivalent to 1.0 g (potency) of Cefmetazole Sodium, and dissolve in 10 mL of water: the pH of the solution is 4.2 to 6.2.

Purity **(1)** Clarity and color of solution—Dissolve an amount of Cefmetazole Sodium for Injection, equivalent to 1.0 g (potency) of Cefmetazole Sodium, in 10 mL of water: the solution is clear and the color is not darker than the following control solution.

Control solution: Pipet 5 mL of Iron (III) Chloride CS and 0.5 mL of Cobalt (II) Chloride CS, and add water to make exactly 50 mL. Pipet 15 mL of this solution, and add water to make exactly 20 mL.

(2) Related substances—Proceed as directed in the Purity (4) under Cefmetazole Sodium.

Bacterial endotoxins *<4.01>* Less than 0.06 EU/mg (potency).

Uniformity of dosage units *<6.02>* It meets the requirement of the Mass variation test.

Foreign particulate matter *<6.06>* Perform the test according to Method 2: it meets the requirement.

Insoluble particulate matter *<6.07>* It meets the requirement.

Sterility *<4.06>* Perform the test according to the Membrane filtration method: it meets the requirement.

Assay Take 10 containers of Cefmetazole Sodium for Injection, dissolve the contents of each in the mobile phase, rinse each of the containers with the mobile phase, combine the rinse with the respective previous solution, and add the mobile phase to make exactly 500 mL. Take exactly a volume of this solution equivalent to about 0.2 g (potency) of Cefmetazole Sodium, and add the mobile phase to make exactly 100 mL. Pipet 1 mL of this solution, add exactly 10 mL of the internal standard solution, and use this solution as the sample solution. Separately, weigh accurately an amount of Cefmetazole RS, equivalent to about 50 mg (potency), and dissolve in the mobile phase to make exactly 25 mL. Pipet 1 mL of this solution, add exactly 10 mL of the internal standard solution, and use this solution as the standard solution. Then, proceed as directed in the Assay under Cefmetazole Sodium.

Amount [mg (potency)] of cefmetazole ($C_{15}H_{17}N_7O_5S_3$)
$= M_S \times Q_T/Q_S \times 4$

M_S: Amount [mg (potency)] of Cefmetazole RS taken

Internal standard solution—A solution of methyl parahydroxybenzoate in the mobile phase (1 in 10,000).

Containers and storage Containers—Hermetic containers. Plastic containers for aqueous injections may be used.

Cefminox Sodium Hydrate

セフミノクスナトリウム水和物

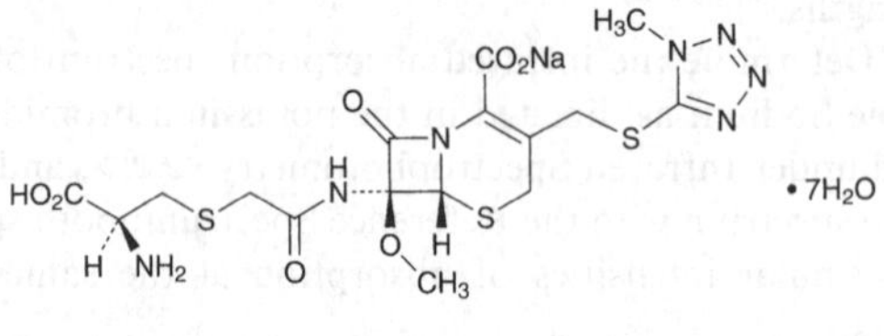

$C_{16}H_{20}N_7NaO_7S_3.7H_2O$: 667.66

Monosodium (6*R*,7*S*)-7-{2-[(2*S*)-2-amino-2-carboxyethylsulfanyl]acetylamino}-7-methoxy-3-(1-methyl-1*H*-tetrazol-5-ylsulfanylmethyl)-8-oxo-5-thia-1-azabicyclo[4.2.0]oct-2-ene-2-carboxylate heptahydrate [*75498-96-3*]

Cefminox Sodium Hydrate contains not less than 900 μg (potency) and not more than 970 μg (potency) per mg, calculated on the anhydrous basis. The potency of Cefminox Sodium Hydrate is expressed as mass (potency) of cefminox ($C_{16}H_{21}N_7O_7S_3$: 519.58).

Description Cefminox Sodium Hydrate occurs as a white to light yellow-white crystalline powder.

It is freely soluble in water, sparingly soluble in methanol, and practically insoluble in ethanol (99.5).

Identification **(1)** Determine the absorption spectrum of a solution of Cefminox Sodium Hydrate (1 in 50,000) as directed under Ultraviolet-visible Spectrophotometry *<2.24>*, and compare the spectrum with the Reference Spectrum or the spectrum of a solution of Cefminox Sodium RS prepared in the same manner as the sample solution: both spectra exhibit similar intensities of absorption at the same wavelengths.

(2) Determine the infrared absorption spectrum of Cefminox Sodium Hydrate as directed in the potassium bromide disk method under Infrared Spectrophotometry <*2.25*>, and compare the spectrum with the Reference Spectrum or the spectrum of Cefminox Sodium RS: both spectra exhibit similar intensities of absorption at the same wave numbers.

(3) Determine the ^1H spectrum of a solution of Cefminox Sodium Hydrate in heavy water for nuclear magnetic resonance spectroscopy (1 in 30) as directed under Nuclear Magnetic Resonance Spectroscopy <*2.21*>, using sodium 3-trimethylsilylpropanesulfonate for nuclear magnetic resonance spectroscopy as an internal reference compound: it exhibits a multiplet signal, A, at around δ 3.2 ppm, a singlet signal, B, at around δ 3.5 ppm, a singlet signal, C, at around δ 4.0 ppm, and a singlet signal, D, at around δ 5.1 ppm. The ratio of integrated intensity of each signal, A:B:C:D, is about 2:3:3:1.

(4) Cefminox Sodium Hydrate responds to Qualitative Tests <*1.09*> (1) for sodium salt.

Optical rotation <*2.49*> $[\alpha]_D^{20}$: +62 – +72° (50 mg, water, 10 mL, 100 mm).

pH <*2.54*> Dissolve 0.70 g of Cefminox Sodium Hydrate in 10 mL of water: the pH of the solution is between 4.5 and 6.0.

Purity **(1)** Heavy metals <*1.07*>—Proceed with 2.0 g of Cefminox Sodium Hydrate according to Method 2, and perform the test. Prepare the control solution with 2.0 mL of Standard Lead Solution (not more than 10 ppm).

(2) Arsenic <*1.11*>—Prepare the test solution with 2.0 g of Cefminox Sodium Hydrate according to Method 3, and perform the test (not more than 1 ppm).

Water <*2.48*> Not less than 18.0% and not more than 20.0% (0.1 g, volumetric titration, direct titration).

Assay Perform the test according to the Cylinder-plate method as directed under Microbial Assay for Antibiotics <*4.02*> according to the following conditions.

(i) Test organism—*Escherichia coli* NIHJ

(ii) Culture medium—Use the medium iii in 3) under (1) Agar media for seed and base layer. Adjust the pH of the medium so that it will be 6.5 to 6.6 after sterilization.

(iii) Standard solution—Weigh accurately an amount of Cefminox Sodium RS, equivalent to about 40 mg (potency), dissolve in 0.05 mol/L phosphate buffer solution (pH 7.0) to make exactly 50 mL, and use this solution as the standard stock solution. Keep the standard stock solution at 5°C or below and use within 7 days. Take exactly a suitable amount of the standard stock solution before use, add 0.05 mol/L phosphate buffer solution (pH 7.0) to make solutions so that each mL contains 40 μg (potency) and 20 μg (potency), and use these solutions as the high concentration standard solution and the low concentration standard solution, respectively.

(iv) Sample solution—Weigh accurately an amount of Cefminox Sodium Hydrate equivalent to about 40 mg (potency), dissolve in 0.05 mol/L phosphate buffer solution (pH 7.0) to make exactly 50 mL. Take exactly a suitable amount of this solution, add 0.05 mol/L phosphate buffer solution (pH 7.0) to make solutions so that each mL contains 40 μg (potency) and 20 μg (potency), and use these solutions as the high concentration sample solution and the low concentration sample solution, respectively.

(v) Procedure—Incubate between 32°C and 35°C.

Containers and storage Containers—Hermetic containers.

Cefodizime Sodium

セフォジジムナトリウム

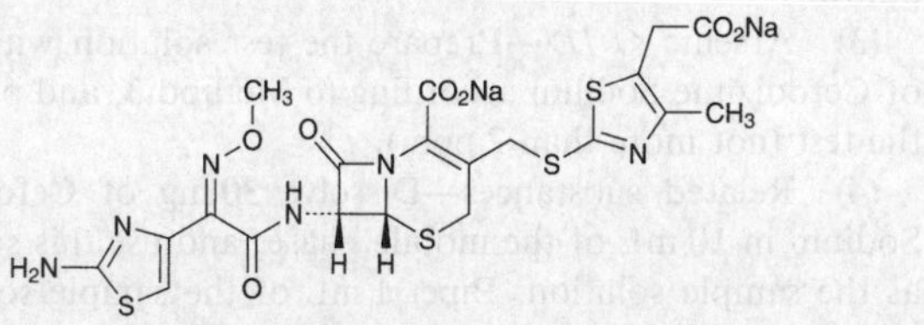

$C_{20}H_{18}N_6Na_2O_7S_4$: 628.63

Disodium (6*R*,7*R*)-7-[(*Z*)-2-(2-aminothiazol-4-yl)-2-(methoxyimino)acetylamino]-3-[(5-carboxylatomethyl-4-methylthiazol-2-yl)sulfanylmethyl]-8-oxo-5-thia-1-azabicyclo[4.2.0]oct-2-ene-2-carboxylate

[*86329-79-5*]

Cefodizime Sodium contains not less than 890 μg (potency) per mg, calculated on the anhydrous and ethanol-free basis. The potency of Cefodizime Sodium is expressed as mass (potency) of cefodizime ($C_{20}H_{20}N_6O_7S_4$: 584.67).

Description Cefodizime Sodium occurs as a white to light yellow-white crystalline powder.

It is very soluble in water, and practically insoluble in acetonitrile and in ethanol (99.5).

Identification **(1)** Determine the absorption spectrum of a solution of Cefodizime Sodium (1 in 50,000) as directed under Ultraviolet-visible Spectrophotometry <*2.24*>, and compare the spectrum with the Reference Spectrum or the spectrum of a solution of Cefodizime Sodium RS prepared in the same manner as the sample solution: both spectra exhibit similar intensities of absorption at the same wavelengths.

(2) Determine the infrared absorption spectrum of Cefodizime Sodium as directed in the potassium bromide disk method under Infrared Spectrophotometry <*2.25*>, and compare the spectrum with the Reference Spectrum or the spectrum of Cefodizime Sodium RS: both spectra exhibit similar intensities of absorption at the same wave numbers.

(3) Determine the ^1H spectrum of a solution of Cefodizime Sodium in heavy water for nuclear magnetic resonance spectroscopy (1 in 10) as directed under Nuclear Magnetic Resonance Spectroscopy <*2.21*>, using sodium 3-trimethylsilylpropanesulfonate for nuclear magnetic resonance spectroscopy as an internal reference compound: it exhibits singlet signals, A, B and C, at around δ 2.3 ppm, at around δ 4.0 ppm, and at around δ 7.0 ppm. The ratio of the integrated intensity of these signals, A:B:C, is about 3:3:1.

(4) Cefodizime Sodium responds to Qualitative Tests <*1.09*> (1) for sodium salt.

Optical rotation <*2.49*> $[\alpha]_D^{20}$: −56 – −62° (0.2 g calculated on the anhydrous and ethanol-free basis, water, 20 mL, 100 mm).

pH <*2.54*> Dissolve 1.0 g of Cefodizime Sodium in 10 mL of water: the pH of the solution is between 5.5 and 7.5.

Purity **(1)** Clarity and color of solution—Dissolve 1.0 g of Cefodizime Sodium in 10 mL of water: the solution is clear and pale yellow to light yellow.

(2) Heavy metals <*1.07*>—Weigh 1.0 g of Cefodizime Sodium in a crucible, cover loosely, and carbonize by gentle heating. After cooling, add 2 mL of sulfuric acid, heat gradually until the white fumes are no longer evolved, and ignite between 500°C and 600°C. Proceed according to Method 2, and perform the test. Prepare the control solution with 2.0 mL of Standard Lead Solution (not more than 20 ppm).

(3) Arsenic <*1.11*>—Prepare the test solution with 1.0 g of Cefodizime Sodium according to Method 3, and perform the test (not more than 2 ppm).

(4) Related substances—Dissolve 30 mg of Cefodizime Sodium in 10 mL of the mobile phase, and use this solution as the sample solution. Pipet 1 mL of the sample solution, add the mobile phase to make exactly 100 mL, and use this solution as the standard solution. Perform the test with exactly 5 μL each of the sample solution and standard solution as directed under Liquid Chromatography <*2.01*> according to the following conditions, and determine each peak area by the automatic integration method: the area of the peaks other than cefodizime obtained from the sample solution is not larger than the peak area of cefodizime from the standard solution, and the total area of the peaks other than cefodizime from the sample solution is not larger than 3 times the peak area of cefodizime from the standard solution.

Operating conditions—

Detector, column, column temperature, mobile phase, and flow rate: Proceed as directed in the operating conditions in the Assay.

Time span of measurement: About 4 times as long as the retention time of cefodizime, beginning after the solvent peak.

System suitability—

System performance, and system repeatability: Proceed as directed in the system suitability in the Assay.

Test for required detectability: Measure exactly 2 mL of the standard solution, and add the mobile phase to make exactly 20 mL. Confirm that the peak area of cefodizime obtained with 5 μL of this solution is equivalent to 7 to 13% of that with 5 μL of the standard solution.

(5) Ethanol—Weigh accurately about 1 g of Cefodizime Sodium, and dissolve in water to make exactly 10 mL. Pipet 2 mL of this solution, add exactly 2 mL of the internal standard solution, and use this solution as the sample solution. Separately, weigh accurately about 2 g of ethanol for gas chromatography, and add water to make exactly 1000 mL. Pipet 2 mL of this solution, add exactly 2 mL of the internal standard solution, and use this solution as the standard solution. Perform the test with 10 μL each of the sample solution and standard solution as directed under Gas Chromatography <*2.02*> according to the following conditions, and calculate the ratios, Q_T and Q_S, of the peak area of ethanol to that of the internal standard: the amount of ethanol is not more than 2.0%.

$$\text{Amount (\%) of ethanol} = M_S/M_T \times Q_T/Q_S$$

M_S: Amount (g) of ethanol for gas chromatography taken
M_T: Amount (g) of Cefodizime Sodium taken

Internal standard solution—A solution of 1-propanol (1 in 400).

Operating conditions—

Detector: A hydrogen flame-ionization detector.

Column: A glass column 3.2 mm in inside diameter and 3 m in length, packed with tetrafluoroethylene polymer for gas chromatography (180 – 250 μm in particle diameter) coated in 15% with polyethylene glycol 20 M.

Column temperature: A constant temperature of about 100°C.

Carrier gas: Nitrogen.

Flow rate: Adjust so that the retention time of ethanol is about 3 minutes.

System suitability—

System performance: When the procedure is run with 10 μL of the standard solution under the above operating conditions, ethanol and the internal standard are eluted in this order with the resolution between these peaks being not less than 2.5.

System repeatability: When the test is repeated 6 times with 10 μL of the standard solution under the above operating conditions, the relative standard deviation of the ratios of the peak area of ethanol to that of the internal standard is not more than 2.0%.

Water <*2.48*> Not more than 4.0% (0.5 g, volumetric titration, direct titration).

Assay Weigh accurately an amount of Cefodizime Sodium and Cefodizime Sodium RS, equivalent to about 50 mg (potency), add exactly 10 mL of the internal standard solution to dissolve, add water to make 100 mL, and use these solutions as the sample solution and standard solution. Perform the test with 10 μL each of the sample solution and standard solution as directed under Liquid Chromatography <*2.01*> according to the following conditions, and calculate the ratios, Q_T and Q_S, of the peak area of cefodizime to that of the internal standard.

$$\text{Amount [μg (potency)] of cefodizime } (C_{20}H_{20}N_6O_7S_4) = M_S \times Q_T/Q_S \times 1000$$

M_S: Amount [mg (potency)] of Cefodizime Sodium RS taken

Internal standard solution—A solution of anhydrous caffeine (3 in 400).

Operating conditions—

Detector: An ultraviolet absorption photometer (wavelength: 254 nm).

Column: A stainless steel column 4.6 mm in inside diameter and 25 cm in length, packed with octadecylsilanized silica gel for liquid chromatography (10 μm in particle diameter).

Column temperature: A constant temperature of about 25°C.

Mobile phase: Dissolve 0.80 g of potassium dihydrogen phosphate and 0.20 g of anhydrous disodium hydrogen phosphate in a suitable amount of water, and add 80 mL of acetonitrile and water to make 1000 mL.

Flow rate: Adjust so that the retention time of cefodizime is about 5 minutes.

System suitability—

System performance: When the procedure is run with 10 μL of the standard solution under the above operating conditions, cefodizime and the internal standard are eluted in this order with the resolution between these peaks being not less than 6.

System repeatability: When the test is repeated 6 times with 10 μL of the standard solution under the above operating conditions, the relative standard deviation of the ratios of the peak area of cefodizime to that of the internal standard is not more than 2.0%.

Containers and storage Containers—Tight containers.

Cefoperazone Sodium

セフォペラゾンナトリウム

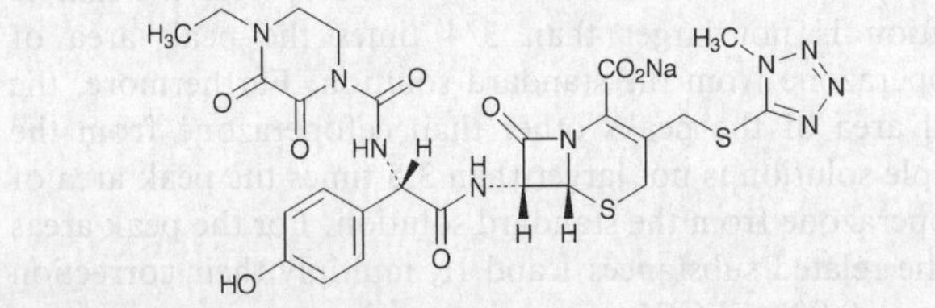

$C_{25}H_{26}N_9NaO_8S_2$: 667.65
Monosodium (6*R*,7*R*)-7-{(2*R*)-2-[(4-ethyl-2,3-dioxopiperazine-1-carbonyl)amino]-2-(4-hydroxyphenyl)acetylamino}-3-(1-methyl-1*H*-tetrazol-5-ylsulfanylmethyl)-8-oxo-5-thia-1-azabicyclo[4.2.0]oct-2-ene-2-carboxylate
[*62893-20-3*]

Cefoperazone Sodium contains not less than 871 μg (potency) and not more than 986 μg (potency) per mg, calculated on the anhydrous basis. The potency of Cefoperazone Sodium is expressed as mass (potency) of cefoperazone ($C_{25}H_{27}N_9O_8S_2$: 645.67).

Description Cefoperazone Sodium occurs as a white to yellowish white crystalline powder.

It is very soluble in water, soluble in methanol, and slightly soluble in ethanol (99.5).

Identification **(1)** Determine the absorption spectrum of a solution of Cefoperazone Sodium (1 in 50,000) as directed under Ultraviolet-visible Spectrophotometry <*2.24*>, and compare the spectrum with the Reference Spectrum: both spectra exhibit similar intensities of absorption at the same wavelengths.

(2) Determine the ^{1}H spectrum of a solution of Cefoperazone Sodium in heavy water for nuclear magnetic resonance spectroscopy (1 in 10) as directed under Nuclear Magnetic Resonance Spectroscopy <*2.21*>, using sodium 3-trimethylsilylpropanesulfonate for nuclear magnetic resonance spectroscopy as an internal reference compound: it exhibits a triplet signal A at around δ 1.2 ppm, a doublet signal B at around δ 6.8 ppm, and a doublet signal C at around δ 7.3 ppm. The ratio of integrated intensity of these signals, A:B:C, is about 3:2:2.

(3) Cefoperazone Sodium responds to the Qualitative Tests <*1.09*> (1) for sodium salt.

Optical rotation <*2.49*> $[\alpha]_D^{20}$: $-15 - -25°$ (1 g, water, 100 mL, 100 mm).

pH <*2.54*> Dissolve 1.0 g of Cefoperazone Sodium in 4 mL of water: the pH of the solution is between 4.5 and 6.5.

Purity **(1)** Clarity and color of solution—Dissolve 1.0 g of Cefoperazone Sodium in 10 mL of water: the solution is clear, and its absorbance at 400 nm, determined as directed under Ultraviolet-visible Spectrophotometry <*2.24*>, is not more than 0.18.

(2) Heavy metals <*1.07*>—Proceed with 1.0 g of Cefoperazone Sodium according to Method 4, and perform the test. Prepare the control solution with 2.0 mL of Standard Lead Solution (not more than 20 ppm).

(3) Arsenic <*1.11*>—Prepare the test solution with 1.0 g of Cefoperazone Sodium according to Method 4, and perform the test (not more than 2 ppm).

(4) Related substances—Dissolve 0.1 g of Cefoperazone Sodium in 100 mL of water, and use this solution as the sample solution. Pipet 1 mL of the sample solution, add water to make exactly 50 mL, and use this solution as the standard solution. Perform the test with exactly 25 μL each of the sample solution and standard solution as directed under Liquid Chromatography <*2.01*> according to the following conditions, and determine each peak area by the automatic integration method. Calculate the percentages of each peak area obtained from the sample solution against 50 times of the peak area of cefoperazone from the standard solution: the related substance I with the retention time of about 8 minutes is not more than 5.0%, the related substance II with that of about 17 minutes is not more than 1.5%, and the total amount of all related substances is not more than 7.0 %. For the peak areas of the related substances I and II, multiply their correction factors, 0.90 and 0.75, respectively.

Operating conditions—

Detector, column, column temperature, mobile phase, and flow rate: Proceed as directed in the operating conditions in the Assay.

Time span of measurement: About 3 times as long as the retention time of cefoperazone, beginning after the solvent peak.

System suitability—

Test for required detectability: Pipet 1 mL of the standard solution, and add the mobile phase to make exactly 20 mL. Confirm that the peak area of cefoperazone obtained with 25 μL of this solution is equivalent to 3.5 to 6.5% of that with 25 μL of the standard solution.

System performance: When the procedure is run with 25 μL of the standard solution under the above operating conditions, the number of theoretical plates and the symmetry factor of the peak of cefoperazone are not less than 5000 and not more than 1.5, respectively.

System repeatability: When the test is repeated 6 times with 25 μL of the standard solution under the above operating conditions, the relative standard deviation of the peak areas of cefoperazone is not more than 2.0%.

Water <*2.48*> Not more than 1.0% (3 g, volumetric titration, direct titration).

Assay Weigh accurately an amount of Cefoperazone Sodium equivalent to about 0.1 g (potency), and dissolve in water to make exactly 100 mL. Pipet 5 mL of this solution, add exactly 5 mL of the internal standard solution, and use this solution as the sample solution. Separately, weigh accurately an amount of Cefoperazone RS equivalent to about 20 mg (potency), dissolve in 1 mL of 0.1 mol/L phosphate buffer solution (pH 7.0) and add water to make exactly 20 mL. Pipet 5 mL of this solution, add exactly 5 mL of the internal standard solution, and use this solution as the standard solution. Perform the test with 10 μL each of the sample solution and standard solution as directed under Liquid Chromatography <*2.01*> according to the following conditions, and calculate the ratios, Q_T and Q_S, of the peak area of cefoperazone to that of the internal standard.

$$\text{Amount [}\mu\text{g (potency)] of cefoperazone } (C_{25}H_{27}N_9O_8S_2) = M_S \times Q_T/Q_S \times 5000$$

M_S: Amount [mg (potency)] of Cefoperazone RS taken

Internal standard solution—A solution of acetanilide in a mixture of water and acetonitrile (43:7) (3 in 8000).

Operating conditions—

Detector: An ultraviolet absorption photometer (wavelength: 254 nm).

Column: A stainless steel column 4.6 mm in inside diame-

ter and 15 cm in length, packed with octadecylsilanized silica gel for liquid chromatography (5 μm in particle diameter).

Column temperature: A constant temperature of about 35°C.

Mobile phase: To 57 mL of acetic acid (100) add 139 mL of triethylamine and water to make 1000 mL. To 20 mL of this solution add 835 mL of water, 140 mL of acetonitrile and 5 mL of dilute acetic acid.

Flow rate: Adjust so that the retention time of cefoperazone is about 10 minutes.

System suitability—

System performance: When the procedure is run with 10 μL of the standard solution under the above operating conditions, the internal standard and cefoperazone are eluted in this order with the resolution between these peaks being not less than 5.

System repeatability: When the test is repeated 6 times with 10 μL of the standard solution under the above operating conditions, the relative standard deviation of the ratios of the peak area of cefoperazone to that of the internal standard is not more than 1.0%.

Containers and storage Containers—Hermetic containers.
Storage—In a cold place.

Cefoperazone Sodium for Injection

注射用セフォペラゾンナトリウム

Cefoperazone Sodium for Injection is a preparation for injection which is dissolved before use.

It contains not less than 93.0% and not more than 107.0% of the labeled potency of cefoperazone ($C_{25}H_{27}N_9O_8S_2$: 645.67).

Method of preparation Prepare as directed under Injections, with Cefoperazone Sodium.

Description Cefoperazone Sodium for Injection occurs as a white to yellowish white, crystalline powder or masses.

Identification Determine the absorption spectrum of a solution of Cefoperazone Sodium for Injection (1 in 50,000) as directed under Ultraviolet-visible Spectrophotometry <2.24>: it exhibits maxima between 226 nm and 230 nm, and between 263 nm and 267 nm.

pH <2.54> The pH of a solution prepared by dissolving an amount of Cefoperazone Sodium for Injection, equivalent to 1.0 g (potency) of Cefoperazone Sodium, in 4 mL of water is between 4.5 and 6.5.

Purity **(1)** Clarity and color of solution—Dissolve an amount of Cefoperazone Sodium for Injection, equivalent to 1.0 g (potency) of Cefoperazone Sodium, in 10 mL of water: the solution is clear, and its absorbance at 400 nm, determined as directed under Ultraviolet-visible Spectrophotometry <2.24>, is not more than 0.22.

(2) Related substances—Dissolve an amount of Cefoperazone Sodium for Injection, equivalent to 0.1 g (potency) of Cefoperazone Sodium, in 100 mL of water, and use this solution as the sample solution. Pipet 1 mL of the sample solution, add water to make exactly 50 mL, and use this solution as the standard solution. Perform the test with exactly 25 μL each of the sample solution and standard solution as directed under Liquid Chromatography <2.01> according to the following conditions, and determine each peak area by the automatic integration method: the peak area of related substance I, having the relative retention time of about 0.8 to cefoperazone, obtained from the sample solution is not larger than 2.5 times the peak area of cefoperazone from the standard solution, the peak area of related substance II, having the relative retention time of about 1.7, from the sample solution is not larger than 3/4 times the peak area of cefoperazone from the standard solution. Furthermore, the total area of the peaks other than cefoperazone from the sample solution is not larger than 3.5 times the peak area of cefoperazone from the standard solution. For the peak areas of the related substances I and II, multiply their correction factors, 0.90 and 0.75, respectively.

Operating conditions—

Detector, column, column temperature, mobile phase and flow rate: Proceed as directed in the operating conditions in the Assay under Cefoperazone Sodium.

Time span of measurement: About 3 times as long as the retention time of cefoperazone, beginning after the solvent peak.

System suitability—

Proceed as directed in the system suitability in the Purity (4) under Cefoperazone Sodium.

Water <2.48> Not more than 1.0% (3 g, volumetric titration, direct titration).

Bacterial endotoxins <4.01> Less than 0.05 EU/mg (potency).

Uniformity of dosage units <6.02> It meets the requirement of the Mass variation test.

Foreign insoluble matter <6.06> Perform the test according to Method 2: it meets the requirement.

Insoluble particulate matter <6.07> It meets the requirement.

Sterility <4.06> Perform the test according to the Membrane filtration method: it meets the requirement.

Assay Weigh accurately the mass of the contents of not less than 10 Cefoperazone Sodium for Injection. Weigh accurately a portion of the content, equivalent to about 0.1 g (potency) of Cefoperazone Sodium, and dissolve in water to make exactly 100 mL. Pipet 5 mL of this solution, add exactly 5 mL of the internal standard solution, and use this solution as the sample solution. Then, proceed as directed in the Assay under Cefoperazone Sodium.

$$\text{Amount [mg (potency)] of cefoperazone } (C_{25}H_{27}N_9O_8S_2) = M_S \times Q_T/Q_S \times 5$$

M_S: Amount [mg (potency)] of Cefoperazone RS taken

Internal standard solution—A solution of acetanilide in a mixture of water and acetonitrile (43:7) (3 in 8000).

Containers and storage Containers—Hermetic containers.
Storage—In a cold place.

Shelf life 24 months after preparation.

Cefoperazone Sodium and Sulbactam Sodium for Injection

注射用セフォペラゾンナトリウム・スルバクタムナトリウム

Cefoperazone Sodium and Sulbactam Sodium for Injection is a preparation for injection which is dissolved before use.

It contains not less than 90.0% and not more than 110.0% of the labeled potency of cefoperazone ($C_{25}H_{27}N_9O_8S_2$: 645.67), and not less than 95.0% and not more than 110.0% of the labeled potency of sulbactam ($C_8H_{11}NO_5S$: 233.24).

Method of Preparation Prepare as directed under Injections, with Cefoperazone Sodium and Sulbactam Sodium.

Description Cefoperazone Sodium and Sulbactam Sodium for Injection occurs as white to pale yellowish white, masses or powder.

Identification **(1)** The retention times of cefoperazone in the chromatogram obtained from the sample solution and the standard solution in the Assay are the same, and the peak area of cefoperazone obtained from the sample solution in the Assay is 0.8 to 1.1 times the peak area of cefoperazone obtained by the test performed with 10 μL of the sample solution obtained in the Assay as directed under Liquid Chromatography <*2.01*> according to the following conditions.

Operating conditions—

Column, column temperature, mobile phase, and flow rate: Proceed as directed in the operating conditions in the Assay.

Detector: An ultraviolet absorption photometer (wavelength: 230 nm).

System suitability—

System performance: Proceed as directed in the system suitability in the Assay.

(2) The retention times of sulbactam in the chromatogram obtained from the sample solution and the standard solution in the Assay are the same, and the peak area of sulbactam obtained from the sample solution in the Assay is 1.4 to 1.9 times the peak area of sulbactam obtained by the test performed with 10 μL of the sample solution obtained in the Assay as directed under Liquid Chromatography <*2.01*> according to the following conditions.

Operating conditions—

Column, column temperature, mobile phase, and flow rate: Proceed as directed in the operating conditions in the Assay.

Detector: An ultraviolet absorption photometer (wavelength: 230 nm).

System suitability—

System performance: Proceed as directed in the system suitability in the Assay.

pH <*2.54*> The pH of a solution prepared by dissolving an amount of Cefoperazone Sodium and Sulbactam Sodium for Injection, equivalent to 1.0 g (potency) of Cefoperazone Sodium, in 20 mL of water is 4.5 to 6.5.

Purity **(1)** Clarity and color of solution—A solution of an amount of Cefoperazone Sodium and Sulbactam Sodium for Injection, equivalent to 0.5 g (potency) of Cefoperazone Sodium, in 10 mL of water is clear. Perform the test with this solution as directed under Ultraviolet Spectrophotometry <*2.24*>: the absorbance at 425 nm is not more than 0.10.

(2) Related substances—Weigh accurately an amount of Cefoperazone Sodium and Sulbactam Sodium for Injection, equivalent to 0.1 g (potency) of Cefoperazone Sodium, dissolve in the mobile phase to make exactly 50 mL, and use this solution as the sample solution. Pipet 2 mL of the sample solution, add the mobile phase to make exactly 50 mL, and use this solution as the standard solution (1). Weigh accurately about 40 mg of sulbactam sodium for sulbactam penicillamine, dissolve in 2 mL of water, add 0.5 mL of sodium hydroxide TS, allow to stand at room temperature for 10 minutes, then add 0.5 mL of 1 mol/L hydrochloric acid TS, and add the mobile phase to make exactly 100 mL. Pipet 5 mL of this solution, add the mobile phase to make exactly 50 mL, and use this solution as the standard solution (2). Perform the test with exactly 10 μL each of the sample solution and the standard solutions (1) and (2) as directed under Liquid Chromatography <*2.01*> according to the following conditions, and determine each peak area by the automatic integration method: the area of the peak, having a relative retention time of about 0.3 (related substance I) to cefoperazone, obtained from the sample solution is not larger than 1.75 times the peak area of cefoperazone from the standard solution (1), the area of the peak, having a relative retention time of about 0.4 (related substance III) and about 1.3 (related substance II), obtained from the sample solution is not larger than 1/2 times the peak area of cefoperazone from the standard solution (1). When determine the peak areas, A_T and A_S, of sulbactam penicillamine with the sample solution and the standard solution (2), and calculate the amount of sulbactam penicillamine by the following equation, it is not more than 1.0%. For the area of the peak of related substance III, multiply the correction factor 0.4.

$$\text{Amount of sulbactam penicillamine (\%)} = M_S/M_T \times A_T/A_S \times 5$$

M_S: Amount (mg) of sulbactam sodium for sulbactam penicillamine taken

M_T: Amount (mg) of Cefoperazone Sodium and Sulbactam Sodium for Injection taken

Operating conditions—

Column, column temperature, mobile phase, and flow rate: Proceed as directed in the operating conditions in the Assay.

Detector: An ultraviolet absorption photometer (wavelength: 230 nm).

System suitability—

System performance: To 1 mL of the standard solution (1) add 1 mL of the standard solution (2). When the procedure is run with 10 μL of this solution under the above operating conditions, sulbactam penicillamine, sulbactam and cefoperazone are eluted in this order with the resolutions between the peaks, sulbactam penicillamine and sulbactam, and sulbactam and cefoperazone, being not less than 4 and not less than 5, respectively.

System repeatability: When the test is repeated 6 times with 10 μL of the standard solution (2) under the above operating conditions, the relative standard deviation of the peak area of sulbactam penicillamine is not more than 2.0%.

Water <*2.48*> Not more than 1.0% (1 g, volumetric titration, direct titration).

Bacterial endotoxins <*4.01*> Less than 0.060 EU/mg (potency).

Uniformity of dosage units <*6.02*> It meets the requirement of the Mass variation test (T: 105.0%).

Foreign insoluble matter ⟨*6.06*⟩ Perform the test according to Method 2: it meets the requirement.

Insoluble particulate matter ⟨*6.07*⟩ It meets the requirement.

Sterility ⟨*4.06*⟩ Perform the test according to the Membrane filtration method: it meets the requirement.

Assay Weigh accurately the mass of the content of not less than 5 Cefoperazone Sodium and Sulbactam Sodium for Injection. Weigh accurately a portion of the content, equivalent to about 50 mg (potency) of Cefoperazone Sodium, dissolve in suitable amount of the mobile phase, add exactly 5 mL of the internal standard solution, add the mobile phase to make 50 mL, and use this solution as the sample solution. Separately, weigh accurately about 50 mg (potency) each of Sulbactam RS and Cefoperazone RS, dissolve in suitable amount of the mobile phase, add exactly 5 mL of the internal standard solution, add the mobile phase to make 50 mL, and use this solution as the standard solution. Perform the test with 10 μL each of the sample solution and standard solution as directed under Liquid Chromatography ⟨*2.01*⟩ according to the following conditions, and calculate the ratios, Q_{Ta} and Q_{Tb} of the peak areas of sulbactam and cefoperazone to that of the internal standard obtained from the sample solution, and the ratios, Q_{Sa} and Q_{Sb} of the peak areas of sulbactam and cefoperazone to that of the internal standard obtained from the standard solution.

Amount [mg (potency)] of sulbactam ($C_8H_{11}NO_5S$)
$= M_{S1} \times Q_{Ta}/Q_{Sa}$

Amount [mg (potency)] of cefoperazone ($C_{25}H_{27}N_9O_8S_2$)
$= M_{S2} \times Q_{Tb}/Q_{Sb}$

M_{S1}: Amount [mg (potency)] of Sulbactam RS taken
M_{S2}: Amount [mg (potency)] of Cefoperazone RS taken

Internal standard solution—A solution of ethyl parahydroxybenzoate (7 in 1000).

Operating conditions—

Detector: An ultraviolet absorption photometer (wavelength: 220 nm).

Column: A stainless steel column 3.9 mm in inside diameter and 30 cm in length, packed with octadecylsilanized silica gel for liquid chromatography (10 μm in particle diameter).

Column temperature: A constant temperature of about 35°C.

Mobile phase: A mixture of 0.005 mol/L tetrabutylammonium hydroxide TS and acetonitrile for liquid chromatography (3:1).

Flow rate: Adjust so that the retention time of sulbactam is about 7 minutes.

System suitability—

System performance: When the procedure is run with 10 μL of the standard solution under the above operating conditions, sulbactam, the internal standard, and cefoperazone are eluted in this order with the resolution between these peaks being not less than 1.5.

System repeatability: When the test is repeated 6 times with 10 μL of the standard solution under the above operating conditions, the relative standard deviation of the peak of sulbactam is not more than 1.0%.

Containers and storage Containers—Hermetic containers. Plastic containers for aqueous injections may be used.

Cefotaxime Sodium

セフォタキシムナトリウム

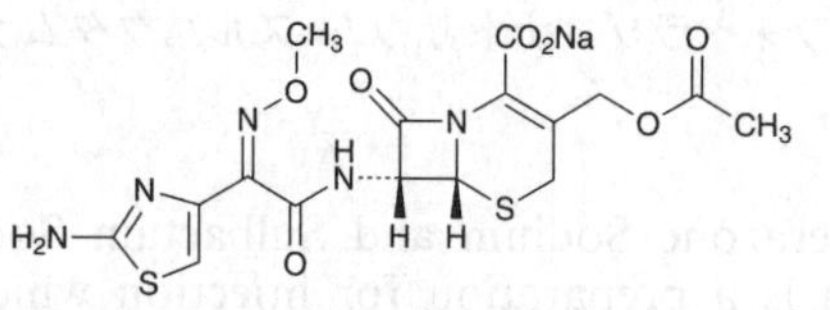

$C_{16}H_{16}N_5NaO_7S_2$: 477.45
Monosodium (6*R*,7*R*)-3-acetoxymethyl-7-[(*Z*)-2-(2-aminothiazol-4-yl)-2-(methoxyimino)acetylamino]-8-oxo-5-thia-1-azabicyclo[4.2.0]oct-2-ene-2-carboxylate
[64485-93-4]

Cefotaxime Sodium contains not less than 916 μg (potency) and not more than 978 μg (potency) per mg, calculated on the dried basis. The potency of Cefotaxime Sodium is expressed as mass (potency) of cefotaxime ($C_{16}H_{17}N_5O_7S_2$: 455.47).

Description Cefotaxime Sodium occurs as white to light yellow-white crystalline powder.

It is freely soluble in water, sparingly soluble in methanol, and very slightly soluble in ethanol (95).

Identification **(1)** Dissolve 2 mg of Cefotaxime Sodium in 0.01 mol/L hydrochloric acid TS to make 100 mL. Determine the absorption spectrum of this solution as directed under Ultraviolet-visible Spectrophotometry ⟨*2.24*⟩, and compare the spectrum with the Reference Spectrum: both spectra exhibit similar intensities of absorption at the same wavelengths.

(2) Determine the infrared absorption spectrum of Cefotaxime Sodium as directed in the potassium bromide disk method under Infrared Spectrophotometry ⟨*2.25*⟩, and compare the spectrum with the Reference Spectrum: both spectra exhibit similar intensities of absorption at the same wave numbers.

(3) Determine the ^1H spectrum of a solution of Cefotaxime Sodium in heavy water for nuclear magnetic resonance spectroscopy (1 in 125) as directed under Nuclear Magnetic Resonance Spectroscopy ⟨*2.21*⟩, using sodium 3-trimethylsilylpropanesulfonate for nuclear magnetic resonance spectroscopy as an internal reference compound: it exhibits three single signals, A, B and C, at around δ 2.1 ppm, at around δ 4.0 ppm and at around δ 7.0 ppm. The ratio of the integrated intensity of each signal, A:B:C, is about 3:3:1.

(4) Cefotaxime Sodium responds to Qualitative Tests ⟨*1.09*⟩ (1) for sodium salt.

Optical rotation ⟨*2.49*⟩ $[\alpha]_D^{20}$: +58 – +64° (0.25 g calculated on the dried basis, water, 25 mL, 100 mm).

pH ⟨*2.54*⟩ The pH of a solution obtained by dissolving 1.0 g of Cefotaxime Sodium in 10 mL of water is between 4.5 and 6.5.

Purity **(1)** Clarity and color of solution—Dissolve 1.0 g of Cefotaxime Sodium in 10 mL of water: the solution is clear, and its absorbance at 430 nm, determined as directed under Ultraviolet-visible Spectrophotometry ⟨*2.24*⟩, is not more than 0.40.

(2) Sulfate ⟨*1.14*⟩—Dissolve 2.0 g of Cefotaxime Sodium in 40 mL of water, add 2 mL of dilute hydrochloric acid and water to make 50 mL, shake well, and filter. Discard first 10 mL of the filtrate, and to the subsequent 25 mL of the filtrate add water to make 50 mL. Perform the test with this solution as the test solution. Prepare the control solution as follows: To 1.0 mL of 0.005 mol/L sulfuric acid VS add 1 mL of dilute hydrochloric acid and water to make 50 mL (not more than 0.048%).

(3) Heavy metals <*1.07*>—Proceed with 1.0 g of Cefotaxime Sodium according to Method 2, and perform the test. Prepare the control solution with 2.0 mL of Standard Lead Solution (not more than 20 ppm).

(4) Arsenic <*1.11*>—Prepare the test solution with 1.0 g of Cefotaxime Sodium according to Method 3, and perform the test (not more than 2 ppm).

(5) Related substances—Perform the test with 10 μL of the sample solution obtained in the Assay as directed under Liquid Chromatography <*2.01*> according to the following conditions, and determine each peak area obtained from the chromatogram by the automatic integration method, and calculated the amounts of them by the area percentage method: the amount of the peak other than cefotaxime is not more than 1.0% and the total amount of these peaks is not more than 3.0%.

Operating conditions—

Detector, column, column temperature, mobile phase A, mobile phase B, flowing of mobile phase, and flow rate: Proceed as directed in the operating conditions in the Assay.

Time span of measurement: About 3.5 times as long as the retention time of cefotaxime, beginning after the solvent peak.

System suitability—

System performance, and system repeatability: Proceed as directed in the system suitability in the Assay.

Test for required detectability: Measure exactly 2 mL of the standard solution, and add the mobile phase A to make exactly 100 mL. Pipet 2 mL of this solution, and add the mobile phase A to make exactly 20 mL. Confirm that the peak area of cefotaxime obtained with 10 μL of this solution is equivalent to 0.15 to 0.25% of that with 10 μL of the standard solution.

Loss on drying <*2.41*> Not more than 3.0% (1 g, 105°C, 3 hours).

Assay Weigh accurately an amount of Cefotaxime Sodium and Cefotaxime RS, equivalent to about 40 mg (potency), dissolve each in the mobile phase A to make exactly 50 mL, and use these solutions as the sample solution and standard solution. Perform the test with exactly 10 μL each of the sample solution and standard solution as directed under Liquid Chromatography <*2.01*> according to the following conditions, and determine the peak areas, A_T and A_S, of cefotaxime in each solution.

Amount [μg (potency)] of cefotaxime ($C_{16}H_{17}N_5O_7S_2$)
$= M_S \times A_T/A_S \times 1000$

M_S: Amount [mg (potency)] of Cefotaxime RS taken

Operating conditions—

Detector: An ultraviolet absorption photometer (wavelength: 235 nm).

Column: A stainless steel column 4.6 mm in inside diameter and 15 cm in length, packed with octadecylsilanized silica gel for liquid chromatography (5 μm in particle diameter).

Column temperature: A constant temperature of about 30°C.

Mobile phase A: To 0.05 mol/L disodium hydrogen phosphate TS add phosphoric acid to adjust the pH to 6.25. To 860 mL of this solution add 140 mL of methanol.

Mobile phase B: To 0.05 mol/L disodium hydrogen phosphate TS add phosphoric acid to adjust the pH to 6.25. To 600 mL of this solution add 400 mL of methanol.

Flowing of mobile phase: Control the gradient by mixing the mobile phases A and B as directed in the following table.

Time after injection of sample (min)	Mobile phase A (vol%)	Mobile phase B (vol%)
0 – 7	100	0
7 – 9	100 → 80	0 → 20
9 – 16	80	20
16 – 45	80 → 0	20 → 100
45 – 50	0	100

Flow rate: 1.3 mL per minute (the retention time of cefotaxime is about 14 minutes).

System suitability—

System performance: To 1 mL of the standard solution add 7.0 mL of water and 2.0 mL of methanol, mix, then add 25 mg of sodium carbonate decahydrate, and shake. After allowing to stand for 10 minutes, add 3 drops of acetic acid (100) and 1 mL of the standard solution, and mix. When the procedure is run with 10 μL of this solution under the above operating conditions, desacetyl cefotaxime with the relative retention time being about 0.3 to cefotaxime and cefotaxime are eluted in this order with the resolution between these peaks being not less than 20, and the symmetry factor of the peak of cefotaxime is not more than 2.

System repeatability: When the test is repeated 6 times with 10 μL of the standard solution under the above operating conditions, the relative standard deviation of the peak area of cefotaxime is not more than 2.0%.

Containers and storage Containers—Tight containers.

Cefotetan

セフォテタン

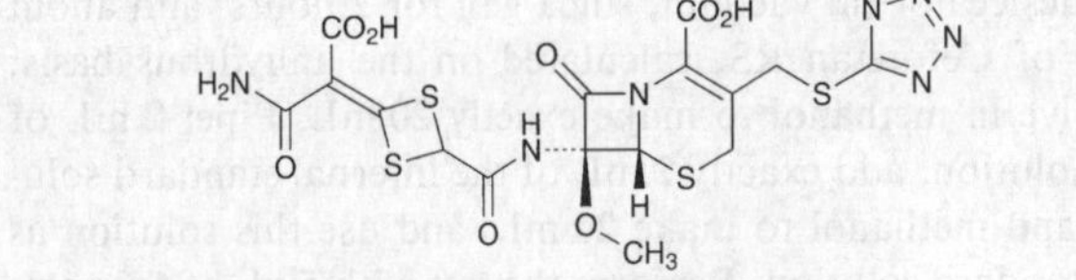

$C_{17}H_{17}N_7O_8S_4$: 575.62
(6*R*,7*R*)-7-{[4-(Carbamoylcarboxymethylidene)-1,3-dithietane-2-carbonyl]amino}-7-methoxy-3-(1-methyl-1*H*-tetrazol-5-ylsulfanylmethyl)-8-oxo-5-thia-1-azabicyclo[4.2.0]oct-2-ene-2-carboxylic acid
[*69712-56-7*]

Cefotetan contains not less than 960 μg (potency) and not more than 1010 μg (potency) per mg, calculated on the anhydrous basis. The potency of Cefotetan is expressed as mass (potency) of cefotetan ($C_{17}H_{17}N_7O_8S_4$).

Description Cefotetan occurs as white to light yellow-white powder.

It is sparingly soluble in methanol, and slightly soluble in water and in ethanol (99.5).

Identification **(1)** Determine the absorption spectrum of a solution of Cefotetan in phosphate buffer solution for antibiotics, pH 6.5 (1 in 100,000) as directed under Ultraviolet-visible Spectrophotometry <*2.24*>, and compare the spectrum with the Reference Spectrum or the spectrum of a solution of Cefotetan RS prepared in the same manner as the sample solution: both spectra exhibit similar intensities of absorption at the same wavelengths.

(2) Determine the infrared absorption spectrum of Cefotetan as directed in the potassium bromide disk method under Infrared Spectrophotometry <*2.25*>, and compare the spectrum with the Reference Spectrum or the spectrum of Cefotetan RS: both spectra exhibit similar intensities of absorption at the same wave numbers.

(3) Dissolve 50 mg of Cefotetan in 0.5 mL of a solution of sodium hydrogen carbonate in heavy water for nuclear magnetic resonance spectroscopy (1 in 25). Determine the ^{1}H spectrum of this solution as directed under Nuclear Magnetic Resonance Spectroscopy <*2.21*>, using sodium 3-trimethylsilylpropanesulfonate for nuclear magnetic resonance spectroscopy as an internal reference compound: it exhibits singlet signals, A, B, C and D, at around δ 3.6 ppm, at around δ 4.0 ppm, at around δ 5.1 ppm and at around δ 5.2 ppm, respectively. The ratio of the integrated intensity of each signal, A:B:C:D, is about 3:3:1:1.

Optical rotation <*2.49*> $[\alpha]_D^{20}$: +112 – +124° (0.5 g calculated on the anhydrous basis, a solution of sodium hydrogen carbonate (1 in 200), 50 mL, 100 mm).

Purity (1) Clarity and color of solution—Dissolve 1.0 g of Cefotetan in 10 mL of a solution of sodium hydrogen carbonate (1 in 30): the solution is clear, and colorless or light yellow.

(2) Heavy metals <*1.07*>—Proceed with 1.0 g of Cefotetan according to Method 2, and perform the test. Prepare the control solution with 2.0 mL of Standard Lead Solution (not more than 20 ppm).

(3) Related substances—Weigh accurately about 0.1 g of Cefotetan, dissolve in a suitable amount of methanol, add exactly 2 mL of the internal standard solution and methanol to make 20 mL, and use this solution as the sample solution. Separately, weigh accurately about 3 mg of 1-methyl-1*H*-tetrazole-5-thiol for liquid chromatography, previously dried in a desiccator (in vacuum, silica gel) for 2 hours, and about 2 mg of Cefotetan RS, calculated on the anhydrous basis, dissolve in methanol to make exactly 20 mL. Pipet 2 mL of this solution, add exactly 2 mL of the internal standard solution and methanol to make 20 mL, and use this solution as the standard solution. Perform the test with 5 μL of the sample solution and standard solution as directed under Liquid Chromatography <*2.01*> according to the following conditions, and calculate the ratios, Q_{Ta}, Q_{Tb}, Q_{Tc}, Q_{Td}, Q_{Te} and Q_{Tf}, of the peak areas of 1-methyl-1*H*-tetrazole-5-thiol, cefotetan lactone having the relative retention time of about 0.5 to cefotetan, Δ_2-cefotetan having the relative retention time of about 1.2, isothiazole substance having the relative retention time of about 1.3, each of other related substances and the total of other related substances, to the peak area of the internal standard, respectively, obtained from the sample solution, and the ratios, Q_{Sa} and Q_{Sb}, of the peak areas of 1-methyl-1*H*-tetrazole-5-thiol and cefotetan, to the peak area of the internal standard, respectively, from the standard solution. Calculate the amount of 1-methyl-1*H*-tetrazole-5-thiol, cefotetan lactone, Δ_2-cefotetan, isothiazole substance, each of other related substances and the total of other related substances from the following equations: the amount of 1-methyl-1*H*-tetrazole-5-thiol is not more than 0.3%, cefotetan lactone is not more than 0.3%, Δ_2-cefotetan is not more than 0.5%, isothiazole substance is not more than 0.5%, each of other related substances is not more than 0.2% and the total of other related substances is not more than 0.4%.

1-Methyl-1*H*-tetrazole-5-thiol (%)
$= M_{Sa}/M_T \times Q_{Ta}/Q_{Sa} \times 1/100$

Cefotetan lactone (%)
$= M_{Sb}/M_T \times Q_{Tb}/Q_{Sb} \times 1/100$

Δ_2-Cefotetan (%)
$= M_{Sb}/M_T \times Q_{Tc}/Q_{Sb} \times 1/100$

Isothiazole substance (%)
$= M_{Sb}/M_T \times Q_{Td}/Q_{Sb} \times 1/100$

Each of other related substances (%)
$= M_{Sb}/M_T \times Q_{Te}/Q_{Sb} \times 1/100$

Total of other related substances (%)
$= M_{Sb}/M_T \times Q_{Tf}/Q_{Sb} \times 1/100$

M_{Sa}: Amount (mg) of 1-methyl-1*H*-tetrazole-5-thiol taken
M_{Sb}: Amount (mg) of Cefotetan RS, calculated on the anhydrous basis taken
M_T: Amount (g) of Cefotetan taken

Internal standard solution—A solution of anhydrous caffeine in methanol (3 in 10,000).

Operating conditions—

Detector, column, column temperature, mobile phase, and flow rate: Proceed as directed in the operating conditions in the Assay.

Time span of measurement: About 3.5 times as long as the retention time of cefotetan.

System suitability—

System performance: Proceed as directed in the system suitability in the Assay.

Test for required detectability: Measure exactly 15 mL of the standard solution, and add methanol to make exactly 100 mL. Confirm that the peak area of cefotetan obtained with 5 μL of this solution is equivalent to 12 to 18% of that with 5 μL of the standard solution.

System repeatability: When the test is repeated 6 times with 5 μL of the standard solution under the above operating conditions, the relative standard deviation of the ratio of the peak area of cefotetan to that of the internal standard is not more than 2.0%.

Water <*2.48*> Not more than 2.5% (1 g, volumetric titration, direct titration).

Residue on ignition <*2.44*> Not more than 0.1% (1 g).

Isomer ratio Dissolve 10 mg of Cefotetan in 20 mL of methanol, and use this solution as the sample solution. Perform the test with 5 μL of the sample solution as directed under Liquid Chromatography <*2.01*> according to the following conditions, and determine each peak area by the automatic integration method. Calculate the amount of the adjacent two peaks appeared at around the retention time of 40 minutes, one having shorter retention time is *l*-substance and another having longer retention time is *d*-substance, by the area percentage method: the amount of *l*-substance is not less than 35% and not more than 45%.

Operating conditions—

Detector: An ultraviolet absorption photometer (wavelength: 254 nm).

Column: A stainless steel column 4 mm in inside diameter and 15 cm in length, packed with octadecylsilanized silica gel for liquid chromatography (5 μm in particle diameter).

Column temperature: A constant temperature of about 40°C.

Mobile phase: A mixture of 0.1 mol/L phosphate buffer

solution (pH 7.0), water and a solution of tetrabutylammonium hydrogensulfate in acetonitrile (1 in 150) (9:9:2).

Flow rate: Adjust so that the retention time of *l*-substance is about 40 minutes.

System suitability—

System performance: When the procedure is run with 5 μL of the sample solution under the above operating conditions, *l*-substance and *d*-substance are eluted in this order with the resolution between these peaks being not less than 1.5.

System repeatability: To exactly 1 mL of the sample solution add methanol to make exactly 10 mL. When the test is repeated 6 times with 5 μL of this solution under the above operating conditions, the relative standard deviation of the peak area of *l*-substance is not more than 5.0%.

Assay Weigh accurately an amount of Cefotetan and Cefotetan RS, equivalent to about 50 mg (potency), and dissolve each in phosphate buffer solution for antibiotics, pH 6.5 to make exactly 50 mL. Pipet 15 mL each of these solutions, add exactly 10 mL of the internal standard solution and phosphate buffer solution for antibiotics, pH 6.5 to make 50 mL, and use these solutions as the sample solution and standard solution. Perform the test with 5 μL each of the sample solution and standard solution as directed under Liquid Chromatography <2.01> according to the following conditions, and calculate the ratios, Q_T and Q_S, of the peak area of cefotetan to that of the internal standard.

Amount [μg (potency)] of cefotetan ($C_{17}H_{17}N_7O_8S_4$)
$= M_S \times Q_T/Q_S \times 1000$

M_S: Amount [mg (potency)] of Cefotetan RS taken

*Internal standard solution—*A solution of anhydrous caffeine (1 in 1000).

Operating conditions—

Detector: An ultraviolet absorption photometer (wavelength: 254 nm).

Column: A stainless steel column 4.6 mm in inside diameter and 15 cm in length, packed with octadecylsilanized silica gel for liquid chromatography (5 μm in particle diameter).

Column temperature: A constant temperature of about 40°C.

Mobile phase: Dissolve 11.53 g of phosphoric acid in 1000 mL of water. To 850 mL of this solution add 50 mL of acetonitrile, 50 mL of acetic acid (100) and 50 mL of methanol.

Flow rate: Adjust so that the retention time of cefotetan is about 17 minutes.

System suitability—

System performance: When the procedure is run with 5 μL of the standard solution under the above operating conditions, the internal standard and cefotetan are eluted in this order with the resolution between these peaks being not less than 8.

System repeatability: When the test is repeated 5 times with 5 μL of the standard solution under the above operating conditions, the relative standard deviation of the ratio of the peak area of cefotetan to that of the internal standard is not more than 1.0%.

Containers and storage Containers—Tight containers.

Storage—Light-resistant, and at a temperature not exceeding 5°C.

Cefotiam Hexetil Hydrochloride

セフォチアム　ヘキセチル塩酸塩

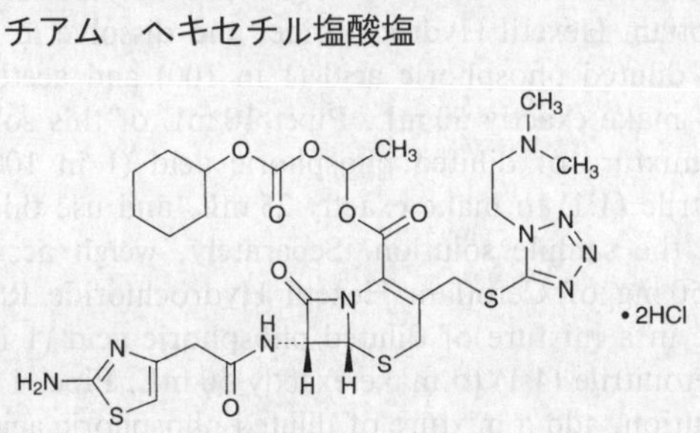

$C_{27}H_{37}N_9O_7S_3.2HCl$: 768.76
(1*RS*)-1-Cyclohexyloxycarbonyloxyethyl (6*R*,7*R*)-7-[2-(2-aminothiazol-4-yl)acetylamino]-3-[1-(2-dimethylaminoethyl)-1*H*-tetrazol-5-ylsulfanylmethyl]-8-oxo-5-thia-1-azabicyclo[4.2.0]oct-2-ene-2-carboxylate dihydrochloride
[*95789-30-3*]

Cefotiam Hexetil Hydrochloride contains not less than 615 μg (potency) and not more than 690 μg (potency) per mg, calculated on the anhydrous basis. The potency of Cefotiam Hexetil Hydrochloride is expressed as mass (potency) of cefotiam ($C_{18}H_{23}N_9O_4S_3$: 525.63).

Description Cefotiam Hexetil Hydrochloride occurs as a white to light yellow powder.

It is very soluble in water, in methanol and in ethanol (95), freely soluble in dimethylsulfoxide, and slightly soluble in acetonitrile.

It dissolves in 0.1 mol/L hydrochloric acid TS.

It is hygroscopic.

Identification **(1)** Determine the absorption spectrum of a solution of Cefotiam Hexetil Hydrochloride in 0.1 mol/L hydrochloric acid TS (3 in 125,000) as directed under Ultraviolet-visible Spectrophotometry <2.24>, and compare the spectrum with the Reference Spectrum or the spectrum of a solution of Cefotiam Hexetil Hydrochloride RS prepared in the same manner as the sample solution: both spectra exhibit similar intensities of absorption at the same wavelengths.

(2) Determine the ^1H spectrum of a solution of Cefotiam Hexetil Hydrochloride in deuterated dimethylsulfoxide for nuclear magnetic resonance spectroscopy (1 in 20) as directed under Nuclear Magnetic Resonance Spectroscopy <2.21>, using tetramethylsilane for nuclear magnetic resonance spectroscopy as an internal reference compound: it exhibits two singlet signals, A and B, at around δ 2.8 ppm and at around δ 6.6 ppm, and a multiplet signal, C, at around δ 6.9 ppm. The ratio of the integrated intensity of each signal, A:B:C, is about 6:1:1.

(3) To a solution of Cefotiam Hexetil Hydrochloride (1 in 200) add 2 mL of dilute nitric acid and 1 mL of silver nitrate TS, and mix: a white precipitate is formed.

Optical rotation <2.49> $[\alpha]_D^{20}$: +52 – +60° (0.1 g calculated on the anhydrous basis, 0.1 mol/L hydrochloric acid TS, 10 mL, 100 mm).

Purity **(1)** Heavy metals <1.07>—Proceed with 2.0 g of Cefotiam Hexetil Hydrochloride according to Method 2, and perform the test. Prepare the control solution with 2.0 mL of Standard Lead Solution (not more than 10 ppm).

(2) Arsenic <1.11>—Prepare the test solution with 2.0 g of Cefotiam Hexetil Hydrochloride according to Method 3, and perform the test, using a solution of magnesium nitrate hexahydrate in ethanol (95) (1 in 5) (not more than 1 ppm).

(3) Related substance 1—Weigh accurately about 50 mg of Cefotiam Hexetil Hydrochloride, and dissolve in a mixture of diluted phosphoric acid (1 in 100) and acetonitrile (4:1) to make exactly 50 mL. Pipet 10 mL of this solution, add a mixture of diluted phosphoric acid (1 in 100) and acetonitrile (4:1) to make exactly 25 mL, and use this solution as the sample solution. Separately, weigh accurately about 50 mg of Cefotiam Hexetil Hydrochloride RS, and dissolve in a mixture of diluted phosphoric acid (1 in 100) and acetonitrile (4:1) to make exactly 50 mL. Pipet 1 mL of this solution, add a mixture of diluted phosphoric acid (1 in 100) and acetonitrile (4:1) to make exactly 50 mL, and use this solution as the standard solution. Perform the test with exactly 10 μL each of the sample solution and standard solution as directed under Liquid Chromatography <*2.01*> according to the following conditions, and determine each peak area by the automatic integration method. Calculate the amount of the related substances by the following equation: the amount of the related substance having the relative retention time of about 1.2 to one of the peaks of cefotiam hexetil, which has the larger retention time, is not more than 2.0%, and each amount of the other related substances is not more than 0.5%. For the peak area, having the relative retention time of about 1.2 to one of the peaks of cefotiam hexetil, which has the larger retention time, multiply the correction factor, 0.78.

$$\text{Amount (\%) of related substance} = M_S/M_T \times A_T/A_S \times 5$$

M_S: Amount (g) of Cefotiam Hexetil Hydrochloride RS taken
M_T: Amount (g) of Cefotiam Hexetil Hydrochloride taken
A_S: Total of two peak areas of cefotiam hexetil from the standard solution
A_T: Each peak area of related substance from the sample solution

Operating conditions—

Detector: An ultraviolet absorption photometer (wavelength: 254 nm).

Column: A stainless steel column 4 mm in inside diameter and 15 cm in length, packed with octadecylsilanized silica gel for liquid chromatography (5 μm in particle diameter).

Column temperature: A constant temperature of about 25°C.

Mobile phase A: A mixture of diluted 0.2 mol/L potassium dihydrogen phosphate TS (1 in 2), acetonitrile and acetic acid (100) (72:28:1).

Mobile phase B: A mixture of acetonitrile, diluted 0.2 mol/L potassium dihydrogen phosphate TS (1 in 2) and acetic acid (100) (60:40:1).

Flowing of mobile phase: Adjust so that the mixing rate of the mobile phase A and the mobile phase B is changed lineally from 1:0 to 0:1 for 30 minutes.

Flow rate: 0.7 mL per minute.

Time span of measurement: As long as about 3 times of the retention time of one of the cefotiam hexetil peaks, which appears first, beginning after the solvent peak.

System suitability—

Test for required detectability: Measure exactly 1 mL of the standard solution, and add a mixture of diluted phosphoric acid (1 in 100) and acetonitrile (4:1) to make exactly 50 mL. Confirm that each area of the two peaks of cefotiam hexetil obtained with 10 μL of this solution is equivalent to 1.6 to 2.4% of that with 10 μL of the standard solution.

System performance: When the procedure is run with 10 μL of the standard solution under the above operating conditions, the resolution between the two peaks of cefotiam hexetil is not less than 2.0.

System repeatability: When the test is repeated 6 times with 10 μL of the standard solution under the above operating conditions, the relative standard deviation of the total of the two peak areas of cefotiam hexetil is not more than 2.0%.

(4) Related substance 2—Weigh accurately about 20 mg of Cefotiam Hexetil Hydrochloride, dissolve in 2 mL of methanol, add a mixture of a solution of diammonium hydrogen phosphate (79 in 20,000) and acetic acid (100) (200:3) to make exactly 50 mL, and use this solution as the sample solution. Separately, weigh accurately about 25 mg of Cefotiam Hydrochloride RS, and dissolve in the mobile phase to make exactly 50 mL. Pipet 2 mL of this solution, add the mobile phase to make exactly 50 mL, and use this solution as the standard solution. Perform the test with exactly 10 μL each of the sample solution and standard solution as directed under Liquid Chromatography <*2.01*> according to the following conditions, and determine each peak area by the automatic integration method. Calculate the amount of the related substances by the following equation: the amounts of the related substances having the relative retention time of about 0.1 and about 0.9 are not more than 1.0%, respectively, and each amount of the related substances other than the related substances having the relative retention time of about 0.1 and about 0.9 is not more than 0.5%. For the peak area, having the relative retention time of about 0.9 to cefotiam, multiply the correction factor, 0.76.

$$\text{Amount (\%) of related substance} = M_S/M_T \times A_T/A_S \times 4$$

M_S: Amount (g) of Cefotiam Hydrochloride RS taken
M_T: Amount (g) of Cefotiam Hexetil Hydrochloride taken
A_S: Peak area of cefotiam from the standard solution
A_T: Each peak area from the sample solution

Operating conditions—

Detector: An ultraviolet absorption photometer (wavelength: 254 nm).

Column: A stainless steel column 4 mm in inside diameter and 15 cm in length, packed with octadecylsilanized silica gel for liquid chromatography (5 μm in particle diameter).

Column temperature: A constant temperature of about 25°C.

Mobile phase: A mixture of a solution of diammonium hydrogen phosphate (79 in 20,000), methanol and acetic acid (100) (200:10:3).

Flow rate: Adjust so that the retention time of cefotiam is about 15 minutes.

Time span of measurement: As long as about 2 times of the retention time of cefotiam, beginning after the solvent peak.

System suitability—

Test for required detectability: Measure exactly 1 mL of the standard solution, and add the mobile phase to make exactly 50 mL. Confirm that the peak area of cefotiam obtained with 10 μL of this solution is equivalent to 1.6 to 2.4% of that with 10 μL of the standard solution.

System performance: To 1 mL of a solution of acetaminophen in the mobile phase (1 in 50,000) add 3 mL of the standard solution, and mix well. When the procedure is run with 10 μL of this solution under the above operating conditions, acetaminophen and cefotiam are eluted in this order with the resolution between these peaks being not less than 4.

System repeatability: When the test is repeated 6 times with 10 μL of the standard solution under the above operating conditions, the relative standard deviation of the peak area of cefotiam is not more than 2.0%.

(5) Total amount of related substances—The total of the amount of related substances obtained in the Related substance 1 and the Related substance 2 is not more than 6.5%.

Water <*2.48*> Not more than 3.5% (0.1 g, volumetric titration, direct titration).

Residue on ignition <*2.44*> Not more than 0.1% (1 g).

Isomer ratio Proceed the test with 20 μL of the sample solution obtained in the Assay as directed under Liquid Chromatography <*2.01*> according to the conditions directed in the Assay, and determine the areas of the two peaks, A_a for the faster peak and A_b for the later peak, closely appeared each other at the retention time of around 10 minutes: $A_a/(A_a + A_b)$ is not less than 0.45 and not more than 0.55.

Assay Weigh accurately an amount of Cefotiam Hexetil Hydrochloride and Cefotiam Hexetil Hydrochloride RS, equivalent to about 30 mg (potency), and dissolve each in a mixture of diluted phosphoric acid (1 in 100) and acetonitrile (4:1) to make exactly 50 mL. Measure exactly 5 mL each of these solutions, add exactly 5 mL of the internal standard solution and a mixture of diluted phosphoric acid (1 in 100) and acetonitrile (4:1) to make 50 mL, and use these solutions as the sample solution and standard solution. Perform the test with 20 μL each of the sample solution and standard solution as directed under Liquid Chromatography <*2.01*> according to the following conditions, and calculate the ratios, Q_T and Q_S, of the peak area of cefotiam hexetil to that of the internal standard. For this calculation, the total of the areas of the two peaks appeared closely each other at the retention time of around 10 minutes is used as the peak area of cefotiam hexetil.

Amount [μg (potency)] of cefotiam ($C_{18}H_{23}N_9O_4S_3$)
$= M_S \times Q_T/Q_S \times 1000$

M_S: Amount [mg (potency)] of Cefotiam Hexetil Hydrochloride RS taken

Internal standard solution—A solution of benzoic acid in a mixture of diluted phosphoric acid (1 in 100) and acetonitrile (4:1) (7 in 10,000).

Operating conditions—

Detector: An ultraviolet absorption photometer (wavelength: 254 nm).

Column: A stainless steel column 4 mm in inside diameter and 15 cm in length, packed with octadecylsilanized silica gel for liquid chromatography (5 μm in particle diameter).

Column temperature: A constant temperature of about 25°C.

Mobile phase: A mixture of diluted 0.2 mol/L potassium dihydrogen phosphate TS (1 in 2), acetonitrile and acetic acid (100) (72:28:1).

Flow rate: Adjust so that the retention time of the faster peak of cefotiam hexetil is about 9 minutes.

System suitability—

System performance: When the procedure is run with 20 μL of the standard solution under the above operating conditions, the internal standard and cefotiam hexetil are eluted in this order with the resolution between the two peaks of cefotiam hexetil being not less than 2.0.

System repeatability: When the test is repeated 6 times with 20 μL of the standard solution under the above operating conditions, the relative standard deviation of the ratios of the peak area of cefotiam hexetil to that of the internal standard is not more than 1.0%.

Containers and storage Containers—Tight containers.

Cefotiam Hydrochloride

セフォチアム塩酸塩

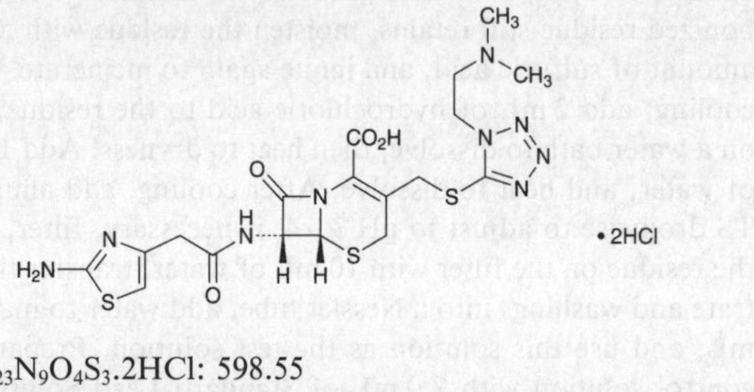

$C_{18}H_{23}N_9O_4S_3.2HCl$: 598.55
(6*R*,7*R*)-7-[2-(2-Aminothiazol-4-yl)acetylamino]-3-[1-(2-dimethylaminoethyl)-1*H*-tetrazol-5-ylsulfanylmethyl]-8-oxo-5-thia-1-azabicyclo[4.2.0]oct-2-ene-2-carboxylic acid dihydrochloride
[*66309-69-1*]

Cefotiam Hydrochloride contains not less than 810 μg (potency) and not more than 890 μg (potency) per mg, calculated on the anhydrous basis. The potency of Cefotiam Hydrochloride is expressed as mass (potency) of cefotiam ($C_{18}H_{23}N_9O_4S_3$: 525.63).

Description Cefotiam Hydrochloride occurs as white to light yellow, crystals or crystalline powder.

It is freely soluble in water, in methanol and in formamide, slightly soluble in ethanol (95), and practically insoluble in acetonitrile.

Identification **(1)** Determine the absorption spectrum of a solution of Cefotiam Hydrochloride (1 in 50,000) as directed under Ultraviolet-visible Spectrophotometry <*2.24*>, and compare the spectrum with the Reference Spectrum or the spectrum of a solution of Cefotiam Hydrochloride RS prepared in the same manner as the sample solution: both spectra exhibit similar intensities of absorption at the same wavelengths.

(2) Determine the infrared absorption spectrum of Cefotiam Hydrochloride as directed in the potassium chloride disk method under Infrared Spectrophotometry <*2.25*>, and compare the spectrum with the Reference Spectrum or the spectrum of Cefotiam Hydrochloride RS: both spectra exhibit similar intensities of absorption at the same wave numbers.

(3) Determine the ^{1}H spectrum of a solution of Cefotiam Hydrochloride in heavy water for nuclear magnetic resonance spectroscopy (1 in 10) as directed under Nuclear Magnetic Resonance Spectroscopy <*2.21*>, using sodium 3-trimethylsilylpropanesulfonate for nuclear magnetic resonance spectroscopy as an internal reference compound: it exhibits singlet signals, A and B, at around δ 3.1 ppm and at around δ 6.7 ppm, respectively. The ratio of integrated intensity of each signal, A:B, is about 6:1.

(4) Dissolve 0.1 g of Cefotiam Hydrochloride in 5 mL of dilute nitric acid, and immediately add 1 mL of silver nitrate TS: a white precipitate is formed.

Optical rotation <*2.49*> $[\alpha]_D^{20}$: +60 – +72° (1 g calculated on the anhydrous bases, water, 100 mL, 100 mm).

pH <2.54> Dissolve 1.0 g of Cefotiam Hydrochloride in 10 mL of water: the pH of the solution is between 1.2 and 1.7.

Purity **(1)** Clarity and color of solution—Dissolve 1.0 g of Cefotiam Hydrochloride in 10 mL of water: the solution is clear, and colorless to yellow.

(2) Heavy metals <1.07>—To 1.0 g of Cefotiam Hydrochloride add 1 mL of sulfuric acid, and heat gently to carbonize. After cooling, add 10 mL of a solution of magnesium nitrate hexahydrate in ethanol (95) (1 in 10), fire the ethanol to burn, then heat gradually to incinerate. If a carbonized residue still retains, moisten the residue with a little amount of sulfuric acid, and ignite again to incinerate. After cooling, add 2 mL of hydrochloric acid to the residue, heat on a water bath to dissolve, then heat to dryness. Add 10 mL of water, and heat to dissolve. After cooling, add ammonia TS dropwise to adjust to pH 3 - 4, if necessary, filter, wash the residue on the filter with 10 mL of water, transfer the filtrate and washings into a Nessler tube, add water to make 50 mL, and use this solution as the test solution. Prepare the control solution with 2.0 mL of Standard Lead Solution in the same manner as for preparation of the test solution (not more than 20 ppm).

(3) Arsenic <1.11>—Incinerate 1.0 g of Cefotiam Hydrochloride according to Method 4. After cooling, add 10 mL of dilute hydrochloric acid to the residue, heat to dissolve on the water bath, and use this solution as the test solution. Perform the test (not more than 2 ppm).

Water <2.48> Not more than 7.0% (0.25 g, volumetric titration, direct titration. Use a mixture of formamide for water determination and methanol for water determination (2:1) instead of methanol for water determination).

Assay Weigh accurately an amount of Cefotiam Hydrochloride and Cefotiam Hydrochloride RS, equivalent to about 0.1 g (potency), and dissolve each in the mobile phase to make exactly 100 mL, and use these solutions as the sample solution and the standard solution, respectively. Perform the test with exactly 10 μL each of the sample solution and standard solution as directed under Liquid Chromatography <2.01> according to the following conditions, and determine the peak areas, A_T and A_S, of cefotiam in each solution.

$$\text{Amount } [\mu\text{g (potency)}] \text{ of cefotiam } (C_{18}H_{23}N_9O_4S_3) = M_S \times A_T/A_S \times 1000$$

M_S: Amount [mg (potency)] of Cefotiam Hydrochloride RS taken

Operating conditions—

Detector: An ultraviolet absorption photometer (wavelength: 254 nm).

Column: A stainless steel column 4.0 mm in inside diameter and 125 mm in length, packed with octadecylsilanized silica gel for liquid chromatography (5 μm in particle diameter).

Column temperature: A constant temperature of about 25°C.

Mobile phase: To 800 mL of 0.05 mol/L disodium hydrogenphosphate TS add 0.05 mol/L potassium dihydrogenphosphate TS to adjust the pH to 7.7. To 440 mL of this solution add 60 mL of acetonitrile.

Flow rate: Adjust so that the retention time of cefotiam is about 14 minutes.

System suitability—

System performance: Dissolve 0.04 g of orcine in 10 mL of the standard solution. When the procedure is run with 10 μL of the standard solution under the above operating conditions, orcine and cefotiam are eluted in this order with the resolution between these peaks being not less than 5.

System repeatability: When the test is repeated 6 times with 10 μL of the standard solution under the above operating conditions, the relative standard deviation of the peak areas of cefotiam is not more than 1.0%.

Containers and storage Containers—Hermetic containers.

Cefotiam Hydrochloride for Injection

注射用セフォチアム塩酸塩

Cefotiam Hydrochloride for Injection is a preparation for injection which is dissolved before use.

It contains not less than 90.0% and not more than 110.0% of the labeled potency of cefotiam ($C_{18}H_{23}N_9O_4S_3$: 525.63).

Method of Preparation Prepare as directed under Injection, with Cefotiam Hydrochloride.

Description Cefotiam Hydrochloride for Injection occurs as a white to light yellow powder.

Identification **(1)** Determine the absorption spectrum of a solution of Cefotiam Hydrochloride for Injection (1 in 50,000) as directed under Ultraviolet-visible Spectrophotometry <2.24>: it exhibits a maximum between 257 nm and 261 nm.

(2) Determine the ^{1}H spectrum of a solution of Cefotiam Hydrochloride for Injection in heavy water for nuclear magnetic resonance spectroscopy (1 in 10) as directed under Nuclear Magnetic Resonance Spectroscopy <2.21>, using sodium 3-trimethylsilylpropanesulfonate for nuclear magnetic resonance spectroscopy as an internal reference compound: it exhibits a singlet signal A between δ 2.7 ppm and δ 3.0 ppm, and a singlet signal B at around δ 6.5 ppm. The ratio of the integrated intensity of each signal, A:B, is about 6:1.

pH <2.54> The pH of a solution prepared by dissolving an amount of Cefotiam Hydrochloride for Injection, equivalent to 0.5 g (potency), in 5 mL of water is between 5.7 and 7.2.

Purity Clarity and color of solution—Dissolve an amount of Cefotiam Hydrochloride for Injection, equivalent to 1.0 g (potency) of Cefotiam Hydrochloride, in 10 mL of water: the solution is clear, and the absorbance of this solution, determined at 450 nm 10 minutes after dissolving as directed under Ultraviolet-visible Spectrophotometry <2.24>, is not more than 0.20.

Loss on drying <2.41> Not more than 6.0% (0.5 g, in vacuum, 60°C, 3 hours).

Bacterial endotoxins <4.01> Less than 0.125 EU/mg (potency).

Uniformity of dosage units <6.02> It meets the requirement of the Mass variation test.

Foreign insoluble matter <6.06> Perform the test according to Method 2: it meets the requirement.

Insoluble particulate matter <6.07> It meets the requirement.

Sterility <4.06> Perform the test according to the Membrane filtration method: it meets the requirement.

Assay Weigh accurately the contents of not less than 10

Cefotiam Hydrochloride for Injection. Weigh accurately an amount of the content, equivalent to about 50 mg (potency) of Cefotiam Hydrochloride, dissolve in the mobile phase to make exactly 50 mL, and use this solution as the sample solution. Separately, weigh accurately about 50 mg (potency) of Cefotiam Hydrochloride RS, dissolve in the mobile phase to make exactly 50 mL, and use this solution as the standard solution. Proceed as directed in the Assay under Cefotiam Hydrochloride.

Amount [μg (potency)] of cefotiam ($C_{18}H_{23}N_9O_4S_3$)
$= M_S \times A_T/A_S \times 1000$

M_S: Amount [mg (potency)] of Cefotiam Hydrochloride RS taken

Containers and storage Containers—Hermetic containers. Plastic containers for aqueous injections may be used.

Cefozopran Hydrochloride

セフォゾプラン塩酸塩

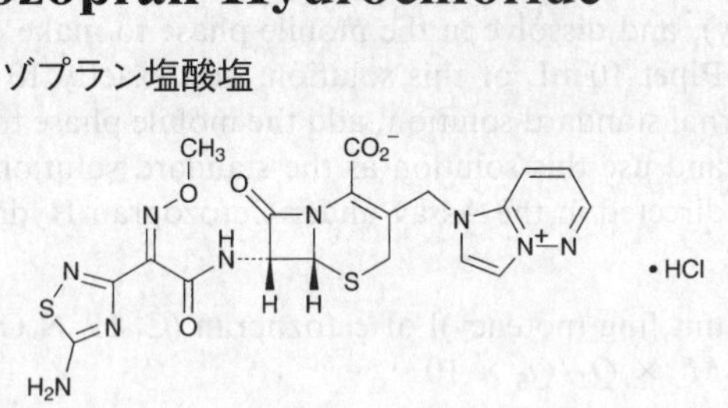

$C_{19}H_{17}N_9O_5S_2$.HCl: 551.99
(6*R*,7*R*)-7-[(*Z*)-2-(5-Amino-1,2,4-thiadiazol-3-yl)-2-(methoxyimino)acetylamino]-3-(1*H*-imidazo[1,2-*b*]pyridazin-4-ium-1-ylmethyl)-8-oxo-5-thia-1-azabicyclo[4.2.0]oct-2-ene-2-carboxylate monohydrochloride
[*113359-04-9*, Cefozopran]

Cefozopran Hydrochloride contains not less than 860 μg (potency) and not more than 960 μg (potency) per mg, calculated on the anhydrous basis. The potency of Cefozopran Hydrochloride is expressed as mass (potency) of cefozopran ($C_{19}H_{17}N_9O_5S_2$: 515.53).

Description Cefozopran Hydrochloride occurs as white to pale yellow, crystals or crystalline powder.

It is freely soluble in dimethylsulfoxide and in formamide, slightly soluble in water, in methanol and in ethanol (95), and practically insoluble in acetonitrile and diethylether.

Identification **(1)** Dissolve 0.02 g of Cefozopran Hydrochloride in 10 mL of water, add 1 mL of a solution of hydroxylammonium chloride (1 in 10) and 2 mL of sodium hydroxide TS, allow to stand for 5 minutes, then add 3 mL of 1 mol/L hydrochloric acid TS and 3 drops of iron (III) chloride TS, and mix: a red-purple color develops.

(2) Determine the absorption spectra of solutions of Cefozopran Hydrochloride and Cefozopran Hydrochloride RS in a mixture of sodium chloride TS and methanol (3:2) (1 in 100,000) as directed under Ultraviolet-visible Spectrophotometry 〈*2.24*〉, and compare these spectra: both spectra exhibit similar intensities of absorption at the same wavelengths.

(3) Determine the ^{1}H spectrum of a solution of Cefozopran Hydrochloride in deuterated dimethylsulfoxide for nuclear magnetic resonance spectroscopy (1 in 20) as directed under Nuclear Magnetic Resonance Spectroscopy 〈*2.21*〉, using tetramethylsilane for nuclear magnetic resonance spectroscopy as an internal reference compound: it exhibits a singlet signal A at around δ 3.9 ppm, a doublet signal B at around δ 5.2 ppm, and a quartet signal C at around δ 8.0 ppm, and the ratio of integrated intensity of each signal, A:B:C, is about 3:1:1.

(4) Dissolve 0.01 g of Cefozopran Hydrochloride in 1 mL of water and 2 mL of acetic acid (100), add 2 drops of silver nitrate TS, and mix: a white turbidity is formed.

Absorbance 〈*2.24*〉 $E^{1\%}_{1\,cm}$ (238 nm): 455 – 485 (50 mg calculated on the anhydrous basis, a mixture of sodium chloride TS and methanol (3:2), 5000 mL).

Optical rotation 〈*2.49*〉 $[\alpha]^{20}_D$: −73 – −78° (0.1 g calculated on the anhydrous basis, a mixture of sodium chloride TS and methanol (3:2), 10 mL, 100 mm).

Purity **(1)** Clarity and color of solution—Being specified separately when the drug is granted approval based on the Law.

(2) Heavy metals 〈*1.07*〉—Proceed with 2.0 g of Cefozopran Hydrochloride according to Method 2, and perform the test. Prepare the control solution with 2.0 mL of Standard Lead Solution (not more than 10 ppm).

(3) Arsenic—Being specified separately when the drug is granted approval based on the Law.

(4) Related substances—Being specified separately when the drug is granted approval based on the Law.

Water 〈*2.48*〉 Not more than 2.5% (0.5 g, volumetric titration, direct titration. Use a mixture of formamide for water determination and methanol for water determination (2:1) instead of methanol for water determination).

Residue on ignition Being specified separately when the drug is granted approval based on the Law.

Bacterial endotoxins 〈*4.01*〉 Less than 0.05 EU/mg (potency).

Assay Weigh accurately an amount of Cefozopran Hydrochloride and Cefozopran Hydrochloride RS, equivalent to about 50 mg (potency), and dissolve each in the mobile phase to make exactly 50 mL. Pipet 10 mL each of these solutions, add exactly 10 mL of the internal standard solution and the mobile phase to make 25 mL, and use these solutions as the sample solution and the standard solution, respectively. Perform the test with 10 μL each of the sample solution and standard solution as directed under Liquid Chromatography 〈*2.01*〉 according to the following conditions, and calculate the ratios, Q_T and Q_S, of the peak area of cefozopran to that of the internal standard.

Amount [μg (potency)] of cefozopran ($C_{19}H_{17}N_9O_5S_2$)
$= M_S \times Q_T/Q_S \times 1000$

M_S: Amount [mg (potency)] of Cefozopran Hydrochloride RS taken

Internal standard solution—A solution of 2,4-dihydroxybenzoic acid in the mobile phase (1 in 1250).

Operating conditions—

Detector: An ultraviolet absorption photometer (wavelength: 254 nm).

Column: A stainless steel column 4.6 mm in inside diameter and 15 cm in length, packed with octadecylsilanized silica gel for liquid chromatography (5 μm in particle diameter).

Column temperature: A constant temperature of about 25°C.

Mobile phase: Mix 0.366 g of diethylamine with water to make 1000 mL, and add 60 mL of acetonitrile and 5 mL of acetic acid (100).

Flow rate: Adjust so that the retention time of cefozopran

is about 9 minutes.

System suitability—

System performance: When the procedure is run with 10 μL of the standard solution under the above operating conditions, cefozopran and the internal standard are eluted in this order with the resolution between these peaks being not less than 10.

System repeatability: When the test is repeated 6 times with 10 μL of the standard solution under the above operating conditions, the relative standard deviation of the ratios of the peak area of cefozopran to that of the internal standard is not more than 1.0%.

Containers and storage Containers—Hermetic containers.

Storage—Light-resistant.

Cefozopran Hydrochloride for Injection

注射用セフォゾプラン塩酸塩

Cefozopran Hydrochloride for Injection is a preparation for injection which is dissolved before use.

It contains not less than 90.0% and not more than 115.0% of the labeled potency of cefozopran ($C_{19}H_{17}N_9O_5S_2$: 515.53).

Method of Preparation Prepare as directed under the Injections, with Cefozopran Hydrochloride.

Description Cefozopran Hydrochloride for Injection occurs as a white to light yellow, powder or masses.

Identification **(1)** Determine the absorption spectrum of a solution of Cefozopran Hydrochloride for Injection (1 in 100,000) as directed under Ultraviolet-visible Spectrophotometry <*2.24*>: it exhibits a maximum between 236 nm and 241 nm.

(2) To 50 mg of Cefozopran Hydrochloride for Injection add 0.8 mL of deuterated dimethylsulfoxide for nuclear magnetic resonance spectroscopy, and filter after shaking, and determine the ^{1}H spectrum of the filtrate as directed under Nuclear Magnetic Resonance Spectroscopy <*2.21*>, using tetramethylsilane for nuclear magnetic resonance spectroscopy as an internal reference compound: it exhibits a singlet signal A at around δ 3.9 ppm, a doublet signal B at around δ 5.0 ppm, and a quartet signal C at around δ 8.0 ppm. The ratio of the integrated intensity of each signal, A:B:C, is about 3:1:1.

pH <*2.54*> Dissolve an amount of Cefozopran Hydrochloride for Injection, equivalent to 0.5 g (potency) of Cefozopran Hydrochloride, in 5 mL of water: the pH of this solution is between 7.5 and 9.0.

Purity **(1)** Clarity and color of solution—Dissolve an amount of Cefozopran Hydrochloride for Injection, equivalent to 1 g (potency) of Cefozopran Hydrochloride, in 10 mL of water: the solution is clear and has no more color than Matching Fluid N.

(2) Related substances—Being specified separately when the drug is granted approval based on the Law.

Water <*2.48*> Not more than 2.5% (0.5 g, volumetric titration, direct titration. Use a mixture of formamide for water determination and methanol for water determination (2:1) instead of methanol for water determination).

Bacterial endotoxins <*4.01*> Less than 0.05 EU/mg (potency).

Uniformity of dosage units <*6.02*> It meets the requirement of the Mass variation test.

Foreign insoluble matter <*6.06*> It meets the requirement.

Insoluble particulate matter <*6.07*> It meets the requirement.

Sterility <*4.06*> Perform the test according to the Membrane filtration method: it meets the requirement.

Assay Weigh accurately the mass of the contents of not less than 10 Cefozopran Hydrochloride for Injection. Weigh accurately an amount of the contents, equivalent to about 0.5 g (potency) of Cefozopran Hydrochloride, and add water to make exactly 100 mL. Pipet 2 mL of this solution, add exactly 10 mL of the internal standard solution, add the mobile phase to make 25 mL, and use this solution as the sample solution. Separately, weigh accurately an amount of Cefozopran Hydrochloride RS, equivalent to about 50 mg (potency), and dissolve in the mobile phase to make exactly 50 mL. Pipet 10 mL of this solution, add exactly 10 mL of the internal standard solution, add the mobile phase to make 25 mL, and use this solution as the standard solution. Proceed as directed in the Assay under Cefozopran Hydrochloride.

Amount [mg (potency)] of cefozopran ($C_{19}H_{17}N_9O_5S_2$)
$= M_S \times Q_T/Q_S \times 10$

M_S: Amount [mg (potency)] of Cefozopran Hydrochloride RS taken

Internal standard solution—A solution 2,4-dihydroxybenzoic acid in the mobile phase (1 in 1250).

Containers and storage Containers—Hermetic containers. Plastic containers for aqueous injections may be used.

Storage—Light-resistant.

Cefpiramide Sodium

セフピラミドナトリウム

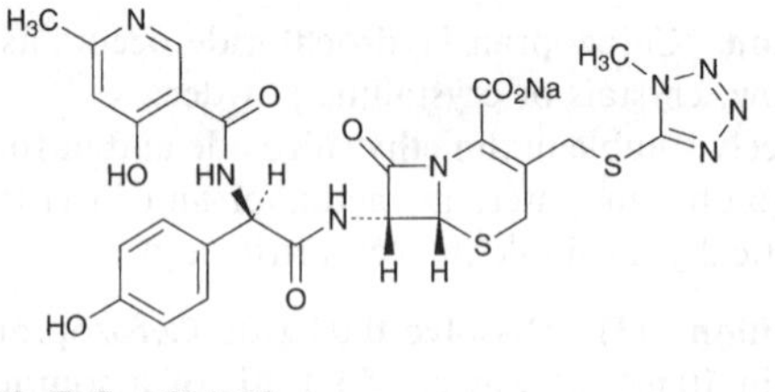

$C_{25}H_{23}N_8NaO_7S_2$: 634.62

Monosodium (6*R*,7*R*)-7-{(2*R*)-2-[(4-hydroxy-6-methylpyridine-3-carbonyl)amino]-2-(4-hydroxyphenyl)acetylamino}-3-(1-methyl-1*H*-tetrazol-5-ylsulfanylmethyl)-8-oxo-5-thia-1-azabicyclo[4.2.0]oct-2-ene-2-carboxylate

[*74849-93-7*]

Cefpiramide Sodium contains not less than 900 μg (potency) and not more than 990 μg (potency) per mg, calculated on the anhydrous basis. The potency of Cefpiramide Sodium is expressed as mass (potency) of cefpiramide ($C_{25}H_{24}N_8O_7S_2$: 612.64).

Description Cefpiramide Sodium occurs as white to yellowish white powder.

It is very soluble in dimethylsulfoxide, freely soluble in water, sparingly soluble in methanol, and slightly soluble in ethanol (95).

Identification (1) Determine the absorption spectrum of a solution of Cefpiramide Sodium in 0.05 mol/L phosphate buffer solution (pH 7.0) (1 in 50,000) as directed under Ultraviolet-visible Spectrophotometry <*2.24*>, and compare the spectrum with the Reference Spectrum: both spectra exhibit similar intensities of absorption at the same wavelengths.

(2) Determine the ^{1}H spectrum of a solution of Cefpiramide Sodium in deuterated dimethylsulfoxide for nuclear magnetic resonance spectroscopy (1 in 10) as directed under Nuclear Magnetic Resonance Spectroscopy <*2.21*>, using tetramethylsilane for nuclear magnetic resonance spectroscopy as an internal reference compound: it exhibits singlet signals, A, B and C, at around δ 2.3 ppm, at around δ 3.9 ppm and at around δ 8.2 ppm, respectively. The ratio of the integrated intensity of each signal, A:B:C, is about 3:3:1.

(3) Cefpiramide Sodium responds to the Qualitative Tests <*1.09*> (1) for sodium salt.

Optical rotation <*2.49*> $[\alpha]_D^{20}$: −33 − −40° (0.2 g calculated on the anhydrous basis, 0.05 mol/L phosphate buffer solution (pH 7.0), 10 mL, 100 mm).

pH <*2.54*> The pH of a solution obtained by dissolving 2.0 g of Cefpiramide Sodium in 20 mL of water is between 5.5 and 8.0.

Purity (1) Clarity and color of solution—Dissolve 1.0 g of Cefpiramide Sodium in 10 mL of 0.05 mol/L phosphate buffer solution (pH 7.0): the solution is clear, and colorless or light yellow.

(2) Heavy metals <*1.07*>—Proceed with 1.0 g of Cefpiramide Sodium according to Method 2, and perform the test. Prepare the control solution with 2.0 mL of Standard Lead Solution (not more than 20 ppm).

(3) Related substances—Weigh accurately about 25 mg of Cefpiramide Sodium, dissolve in 0.03 mol/L phosphate buffer solution (pH 7.5) to make exactly 50 mL, and use this solution as the sample solution. Separately, weigh accurately about 25 mg of 1-methyl-1*H*-tetrazole-5-thiol for liquid chromatography, previously dried in a desiccator (in vacuum, silica gel) for 2 hours, and an amount of Cefpiramide RS, equivalent to about 75 mg (potency), dissolve them in 0.03 mol/L phosphate buffer solution (pH 7.5) to make exactly 100 mL. Pipet 2 mL of this solution, add 0.03 mol/L phosphate buffer solution (pH 7.5) to make exactly 100 mL, and use this solution as the standard solution. Perform the test with exactly 5 μL of the sample solution and standard solution as directed under Liquid Chromatography <*2.01*> according to the following conditions, and determine each peak area by the automatic integration method. Calculate the amount of 1-methyl-1*H*-tetrazole-5-thiol, each of the other related substances and the total of the other related substances by the following equations: the amount of 1-methyl-1*H*-tetrazole-5-thiol, each of the other related substances and the total of the other related substances are not more than 1.0%, not more than 1.5% and not more than 4.0%, respectively.

Amount (%) of 1-methyl-1*H*-tetrazole-5-thiol ($C_2H_4N_4S$)
$= M_{Sa}/M_T \times A_{Ta}/A_{Sa}$

Amount (%) of each of other related substances
$= M_{Sb}/M_T \times A_{Tc}/A_{Sb}$

M_{Sa}: Amount (mg) of 1-methyl-1*H*-tetrazole-5-thiol taken
M_{Sb}: Amount [mg (potency)] of Cefpiramide RS taken
M_T: Amount (mg) of Cefpiramide Sodium taken
A_{Sa}: Peak area of 1-methyl-1*H*-tetrazole-5-thiol from the standard solution
A_{Sb}: Peak area of cefpiramide from the standard solution
A_{Ta}: Peak area of 1-methyl-1*H*-tetrazole-5-thiol from the sample solution
A_{Tc}: Area of each peak other than 1-methyl-1*H*-tetrazole-5-thiol and cefpiramide from the sample solution

Operating conditions—

Detector: An ultraviolet absorption photometer (wavelength: 254 nm).

Column: A stainless steel column 4 mm in inside diameter and 30 cm in length, packed with octylsilanized silica gel for liquid chromatography (10 μm in particle diameter).

Column temperature: A constant temperature of about 25°C.

Mobile phase: A mixture of 0.03 mol/L phosphate buffer solution (pH 7.5) and methanol (3:1).

Flow rate: Adjust so that the retention time of cefpiramide is about 11 minutes.

Time span of measurement: About 2 times as long as the retention time of cefpiramide.

System suitability—

Test for required detectability: Measure exactly 5 mL of the standard solution, and add 0.03 mol/L phosphate buffer solution (pH 7.5) to make exactly 50 mL. Confirm that the peak area of 1-methyl-1*H*-tetrazole-5-thiol obtained with 5 μL of this solution is equivalent to 8 to 12% of that with 5 μL of the standard solution.

System performance: Dissolve 25 mg of Cefpiramide RS and 7 mg of cinnamic acid in the mobile phase to make 50 mL. When the procedure is run with 5 μL of this solution under the above operating conditions, cinnamic acid and cefpiramide are eluted in this order with the resolution between these peaks being not less than 3.

System repeatability: When the test is repeated 6 times with 5 μL of the standard solution under the above operating conditions, the relative standard deviation of the peak area of 1-methyl-1*H*-tetrazole-5-thiol is not more than 2.0%.

Water <*2.48*> Not more than 7.0% (0.35 g, volumetric titration, direct titration).

Assay Weigh accurately an amount of Cefpiramide Sodium and Cefpiramide RS, equivalent to about 50 mg (potency), add exactly 5 mL of the internal standard solution to dissolve, then add the mobile phase to make 100 mL, and use these solutions as the sample solution and standard solution. Perform the test with 5 μL each of the sample solution and standard solution as directed under Liquid Chromatography <*2.01*> according to the following conditions, and calculate the ratios, Q_T and Q_S, of the peak area of cefpiramide to that of the internal standard.

Amount [μg (potency)] of cefpiramide ($C_{25}H_{24}N_8O_7S_2$)
$= M_S \times Q_T/Q_S \times 1000$

M_S: Amount [mg (potency)] of Cefpiramide RS taken

Internal standard solution—A solution of 4-dimethylaminoantipyrine (1 in 100).

Operating conditions—

Detector: An ultraviolet absorption photometer (wavelength: 254 nm).

Column: A stainless steel column 4 mm in inside diameter and 30 cm in length, packed with octylsilanized silica gel for liquid chromatography (10 μm in particle diameter).

Column temperature: A constant temperature of about 25°C.

Mobile phase: A mixture of 0.01 mol/L phosphate buffer

solution (pH 6.8), acetonitrile, methanol and tetrahydrofuran (22:1:1:1).

Flow rate: Adjust so that the retention time of cefpiramide is about 7 minutes.

System suitability—

System performance: When the procedure is run with 5 μL of the standard solution under the above operating conditions, cefpiramide and the internal standard are eluted in this order with the resolution between these peaks being not less than 7.

System repeatability: When the test is repeated 6 times with 5 μL of the standard solution under the above operating conditions, the relative standard deviation of the ratio of the peak area of cefpiramide to that of the internal standard is not more than 2.0%.

Containers and storage Containers—Tight containers.

Storage—Light-resistant, and at a temperature not exceeding 5°C.

Cefpirome Sulfate

セフピロム硫酸塩

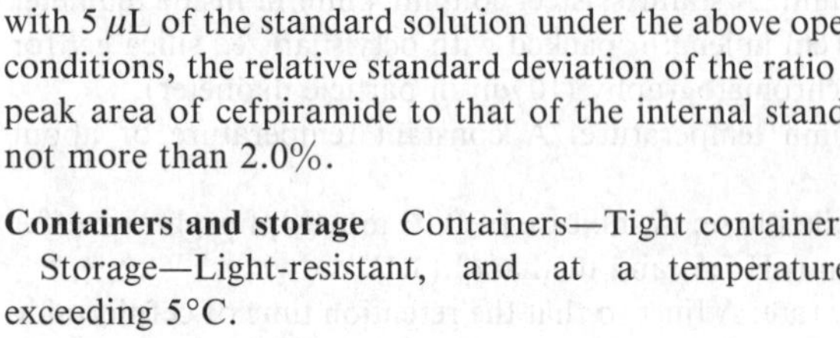

$C_{22}H_{22}N_6O_5S_2.H_2SO_4$: 612.66
(6*R*,7*R*)-7-[(*Z*)-2-(2-Aminothiazol-4-yl)-2-(methoxyimino)acetylamino]-3-(6,7-dihydro-5*H*-cyclopenta[*b*]pyridinium-1-ylmethyl)-8-oxo-5-thia-1-azabicyclo[4.2.0]oct-2-ene-2-carboxylate monosulfate
[*98753-19-6*]

Cefpirome Sulfate contains not less than 760 μg (potency) per mg, calculated on the anhydrous basis. The potency of Cefpirome Sulfate is expressed as mass (potency) of cefpirome ($C_{22}H_{22}N_6O_5S_2$: 514.58).

Description Cefpirome Sulfate occurs as a white to pale yellow-white crystalline powder, and has a slight, characteristic odor.

It is soluble in water, and practically insoluble in ethanol (95) and in diethyl ether.

It is hygroscopic.

Identification **(1)** Dissolve 10 mg of Cefpirome Sulfate in 2 mL of water, add 3 mL of hydroxylammonium hydrochloride-ethanol TS, allow to stand for 5 minutes, add 1 mL of acidic ammonium iron (III) sulfate TS, and shake: a red-brown color develops.

(2) Dissolve 1 mg of Cefpirome Sulfate in 4 mL of water, add 1 mL of dilute hydrochloric acid while cooling in ice, add 1 mL of a freshly prepared solution of sodium nitrite (1 in 100), and allow to stand for 2 minutes. Add 1 mL of ammonium amidosulfuric acid TS while cooling in ice bath, allow to stand for 1 minute, and add 1 mL of a solution of *N*-1-naphthylethylene dihydrochloride (1 in 1000): a purple color develops.

(3) Take 5 mg of Cefpirome Sulfate, dissolve in 1 mL of ethanol (95) and 1 mL of water, add 100 mg of 1-chloro-2,4-dinitrobenzene, and heat on a water bath for 5 minutes. After cooling, add 2 or 3 drops of a solution of sodium hydroxide (1 in 10) and 3 mL of ethanol (95): a red-brown color develops.

(4) Determine the absorption spectra of solutions of Cefpirome Sulfate and Cefpirome Sulfate RS in 0.01 mol/L hydrochloric acid TS (1 in 50,000) as directed under Ultraviolet-visible Spectrophotometry 〈*2.24*〉, and compare the spectra: both spectra exhibit similar intensities of absorption at the same wavelengths.

(5) Determine the ^{1}H spectrum of a solution of Cefpirome Sulfate in heavy water for nuclear magnetic resonance spectroscopy (1 in 25) as directed under Nuclear Magnetic Resonance Spectroscopy 〈*2.21*〉, using sodium 3-trimethylsilylpropanesulfonate for nuclear magnetic resonance spectroscopy as an internal reference compound: it exhibits a singlet signal A at around δ 4.1 ppm, a doublet signal B at around δ 5.9 ppm, a singlet signal C at around δ 7.1 ppm, and a multiplet signal D at around δ 7.8 ppm. The ratio of integrated intensity of each signal, A:B:C:D, is about 3:1:1:1.

(6) A solution of Cefpirome Sulfate (1 in 250) responds to Qualitative Tests 〈*1.09*〉 (1) for sulfate salt.

Absorbance 〈*2.24*〉 $E^{1\%}_{1\,cm}$ (270 nm): 405 – 435 (50 mg calculated on the anhydrous basis, 0.01 mol/L hydrochloric acid TS, 2500 mL).

Optical rotation 〈*2.49*〉 $[\alpha]^{20}_D$: −27 – −33° (50 mg calculated on the anhydrous basis, a solution prepared by addition of water to 25 mL of acetonitrile to make 50 mL, 20 mL, 100 mm).

pH 〈*2.54*〉 Dissolve 0.1 g of Cefpirome Sulfate in 10 mL of water: the pH of the solution is between 1.6 and 2.6.

Purity **(1)** Clarity and color of solution—Being specified separately when the drug is granted approval based on the Law.

(2) Heavy metals 〈*1.07*〉—Proceed with 1.0 g of Cefpirome Sulfate according to Method 2, and perform the test. Prepare the control solution with 2.0 mL of Standard Lead Solution (not more than 20 ppm).

(3) Arsenic—Being specified separately when the drug is granted approval based on the Law.

(4) Related substances—Being specified separately when the drug is granted approval based on the Law.

Water 〈*2.48*〉 Not more than 2.5% (0.5 g, volumetric titration, direct titration).

Residue on ignition Being specified separately when the drug is granted approval based on the Law.

Bacterial endotoxins 〈*4.01*〉 Less than 0.10 EU/mg (potency).

Assay Weigh accurately an amount of Cefpirome Sulfate and Cefpirome Sulfate RS, equivalent to about 50 mg (potency), dissolve each in water to make exactly 100 mL. Pipet 5 mL of these solutions, add each in water to make exactly 20 mL, and use these solutions as the sample solution and standard solution. Perform the test with exactly 20 μL of the sample solution and standard solution as directed under Liquid Chromatography 〈*2.01*〉 according to the following conditions, and determine the peak areas, A_T and A_S, of cefpirome in each solution.

Amount [μg (potency)] of cefpirome ($C_{22}H_{22}N_6O_5S_2$)
$= M_S \times A_T/A_S \times 1000$

M_S: Amount [mg (potency)] of Cefpirome Sulfate RS taken

Operating conditions—

Detector: An ultraviolet absorption photometer (wavelength: 270 nm).

Column: A stainless steel column 4.6 mm in inside diameter and 25 cm in length, packed with octadecylsilanized silica gel for liquid chromatography (5 μm in particle diameter).

Column temperature: A constant temperature of about 25°C.

Mobile phase: Dissolve 3.45 g of ammonium dihydrogenphosphate in 1000 mL of water, and adjust the pH to 3.3 with phosphoric acid. To 800 mL of this solution add 100 mL of acetonitrile.

Flow rate: Adjust so that the retention time of cefpirome is about 7.5 minutes.

System suitability—

System performance: When the procedure is run with 20 μL of the standard solution under the above operating conditions, the number of theoretical plates of the peak of cefpirome is not less than 3600.

System repeatability: When the test is repeated 5 times with 20 μL of the standard solution under the above operating conditions, the relative standard deviation of the peak areas of cefpirome is not more than 1.0%.

Containers and storage Containers—Hermetic containers.

Storage—At a temperature between 2°C and 8°C.

Cefpodoxime Proxetil

セフポドキシム　プロキセチル

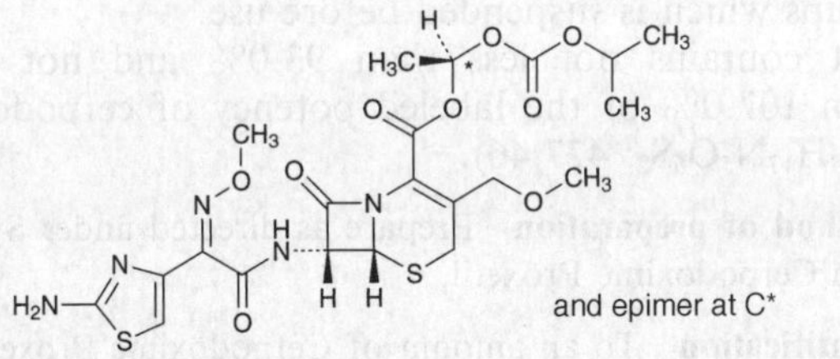

and epimer at C*

$C_{21}H_{27}N_5O_9S_2$: 557.60
(1*RS*)-1-[(1-Methylethoxy)carbonyloxy]ethyl
(6*R*,7*R*)-7-[(*Z*)-2-(2-aminothiazol-4-yl)-2-(methoxyimino)acetylamino]-3-methoxymethyl-8-oxo-5-thia-1-azabicyclo[4.2.0]oct-2-ene-2-carboxylate
[*87239-81-4*]

Cefpodoxime Proxetil contains not less than 706 μg (potency) and not more than 774 μg (potency) per mg, calculated on the anhydrous basis. The potency of Cefpodoxime Proxetil is expressed as mass (potency) of cefpodoxime ($C_{15}H_{17}N_5O_6S_2$: 427.46).

Description Cefpodoxime Proxetil occurs as a white to light brown-white powder.

It is very soluble in acetonitrile, in methanol and in chloroform, freely soluble in ethanol (99.5), and very slightly soluble in water.

Identification (1) Determine the absorption spectrum of a solution of Cefpodoxime Proxetil in acetonitrile (3 in 200,000) as directed under Ultraviolet-visible Spectrophotometry <*2.24*>, and compare the spectrum with the Reference Spectrum or the spectrum of a solution of Cefpodoxime Proxetil RS prepared in the same manner as the sample solution: both spectra exhibit similar intensities of absorption at the same wavelengths.

(2) Determine the infrared absorption spectrum of Cefpodoxime Proxetil as directed in the potassium bromide disk method under Infrared Spectrophotometry <*2.25*>, and compare the spectrum with the Reference Spectrum or the spectrum of Cefpodoxime Proxetil RS: both spectra exhibit similar intensities of absorption at the same wave numbers.

(3) Determine the ^{1}H spectrum of a solution of Cefpodoxime Proxetil in deuterochloroform for nuclear magnetic resonance spectroscopy (1 in 10) as directed under Nuclear Magnetic Resonance Spectroscopy <*2.21*>, using tetramethylsilane for nuclear magnetic resonance spectroscopy as an internal reference compound: it exhibits doublet signals, A and B, at around δ 1.3 ppm and at around δ 1.6 ppm, and singlet signals, C and D, at around δ 3.3 ppm and at around δ 4.0 ppm. The ratio of the integrated intensity of these signals, A:B:C:D, is about 2:1:1:1.

Optical rotation <*2.49*> $[\alpha]_D^{20}$: +24.0 – +31.4° (0.1 g calculated on the anhydrous basis, acetonitrile, 20 mL, 100 mm).

Purity (1) Heavy metals <*1.07*>—Proceed with 1.0 g of Cefpodoxime Proxetil according to Method 2, and perform the test. Prepare the control solution with 2.0 mL of Standard Lead Solution (not more than 20 ppm).

(2) Related substances—Dissolve 50 mg of Cefpodoxime Proxetil in 50 mL of a mixture of water, acetonitrile and acetic acid (100) (99:99:2), and use this solution as the sample solution. Perform the test with 20 μL of the sample solution as directed under Liquid Chromatography <*2.01*> according to the following conditions. Determine each peak area by the automatic integration method, and calculate the amounts of them by the area percentage method: the amount of the peak, having the relative retention time of about 0.8 to the isomer B of cefpodoxime proxetil, is not more than 2.0%, the amount of the peak other than cefpodoxime proxetil is not more than 1.0%, and the total amount of the peaks other than cefpodoxime proxetil is not more than 6.0%.

Operating conditions—

Detector: An ultraviolet absorption photometer (wavelength: 254 nm).

Column: A stainless steel column 4.6 mm in inside diameter and 15 cm in length, packed with octadecylsilanized silica gel for liquid chromatography (5 μm in particle diameter).

Column temperature: A constant temperature of about 22°C.

Mobile phase A: A mixture of water, methanol and a solution of formic acid (1 in 50) (11:8:1).

Mobile phase B: A mixture of methanol and a solution of formic acid (1 in 50) (19:1).

Flowing of mobile phase: Control the gradient by mixing the mobile phases A and B as directed in the following table.

Time after injection of sample (min)	Mobile phase A (vol%)	Mobile phase B (vol%)
0 – 65	95	5
65 – 145	95 → 15	5 → 85
145 – 155	15	85

Flow rate: 0.7 mL per minute (the retention time of the isomer B of cefpodoxime proxetil is about 60 minutes).

Time span of measurement: For 155 minutes after injection, beginning after the solvent peak.

System suitability—

Test for required detectability: To 5 mL of the sample solution add a mixture of water, acetonitrile and acetic acid (100) (99:99:2) to make 200 mL, and use this solution as the solution for system suitability test. Pipet 2 mL of the solution for system suitability test, and add the mixture of water, acetonitrile and acetic acid (100) (99:99:2) to make exactly 100 mL. Confirm that the peak areas of the isomer A and the isomer B of cefpodoxime proxetil obtained with 20 μL of this solution are equivalent to 1.4 to 2.6% of them with 20 μL of the solution for system suitability test, respectively.

System performance: When the procedure is run with 20 μL of the solution for system suitability test under the above operating conditions, the isomer A and the isomer B of cefpodoxime proxetil are eluted in this order with the resolution between these peaks being not less than 6.

System repeatability: When the test is repeated 5 times with 20 μL of the solution for system suitability test under the above operating conditions, the relative standard deviation of the peak area of the isomer A and the isomer B of cefpodoxime proxetil is not more than 2.0%.

Water <*2.48*> Not more than 2.5% (0.5 g, volumetric titration, direct titration).

Residue on ignition <*2.44*> Not more than 0.2% (1 g).

Isomer ratio Perform the test with 5 μL of the sample solution obtained in the Assay as directed under Liquid Chromatography <*2.01*> according to the following conditions, and determine the peak areas of the two isomers of cefpodoxime proxetil, A_a, for the isomer having the smaller retention time, and A_b, for the isomer having the larger retention time, by the automatic integration method: $A_b/(A_a + A_b)$ is between 0.50 and 0.60.

Operating conditions—

Proceed as directed in the operating conditions in the Assay.

System suitability—

System performance: When the procedure is run with 5 μL of the standard solution obtained in the Assay under the above operating conditions, the internal standard, the isomer A and the isomer B of cefpodoxime proxetil are eluted in this order with the resolution between the peaks of the isomers being not less than 4.

System repeatability: When the test is repeated 5 times with 5 μL of the standard solution obtained in the Assay under the above operating conditions, the relative standard deviation of the ratio of the peak area of the isomer B of cefpodoxime proxetil to that of the internal standard is not more than 1.0%.

Assay Weigh accurately an amount of Cefpodoxime Proxetil and Cefpodoxime Proxetil RS, equivalent to about 60 mg (potency), dissolve in 80 mL of acetonitrile, add exactly 4 mL of the internal standard solution, add acetonitrile to make 100 mL, and use these solutions as the sample solution and standard solution. Perform the test with 5 μL each of the sample solution and standard solution as directed under Liquid Chromatography <*2.01*> according to the following conditions, and calculate the ratios, Q_{T1}, Q_{S1}, Q_{T2} and Q_{S2}, of the areas of the two peaks of the isomers of cefpodoxime proxetil to the peak area of the internal standard.

Amount [μg (potency)] of cefpodoxime ($C_{15}H_{17}N_5O_6S_2$)
$= M_S \times (Q_{T1} + Q_{T2})/(Q_{S1} + Q_{S2}) \times 1000$

M_S: Amount [mg (potency)] of Cefpodoxime Proxetil RS taken

*Internal standard solution—*Dissolve 0.3 g of ethyl parahydroxybenzoate in a solution of citric acid in acetonitrile (1 in 2000) to make 100 mL.

Operating conditions—

Detector: An ultraviolet absorption photometer (wavelength: 240 nm).

Column: A stainless steel column 4.6 mm in inside diameter and 15 cm in length, packed with octadecylsilanized silica gel for liquid chromatography (5 μm in particle diameter).

Column temperature: A constant temperature of about 40°C.

Mobile phase: A mixture of water and methanol (11:9).

Flow rate: Adjust so that the retention time of the internal standard is about 11 minutes.

System suitability—

System performance: When the procedure is run with 5 μL of the standard solution under the above operating conditions, the internal standard, the isomer A and the isomer B are eluted in this order with the resolution between these peaks being not less than 4.

System repeatability: When the test is repeated 5 times with 5 μL of the standard solution under the above operating conditions, the relative standard deviation of the ratios of the peak area of the isomer B of cefpodoxime proxetil to that of the internal standard is not more than 1.0%.

Containers and storage Containers—Tight containers.

Cefpodoxime Proxetil for Syrup

シロップ用セフポドキシム　プロキセチル

Cefpodoxime Proxetil for Syrup is a preparation for syrups which is suspended before use.

It contains not less than 93.0% and not more than 107.0% of the labeled potency of cefpodoxime ($C_{15}H_{17}N_5O_6S_2$: 427.46).

Method of preparation Prepare as directed under Syrups, with Cefpodoxime Proxetil.

Identification To an amount of Cefpodoxime Proxetil for Syrup, equivalent to 15 mg (potency) of Cefpodoxime Proxetil, add 10 mL of 0.1 mol/L phosphate buffer solution (pH 8.0), treat with ultrasonic waves for 5 minutes while occasional shaking. Then, add 20 mL of ethyl acetate, shake for 5 minutes, and centrifuge. Take 3 mL of the supernatant liquid, evaporate the ethyl acetate by warming at 40°C under reduced pressure. Dissolve the residue in acetonitrile to make 200 mL, and determine the absorption spectrum of this solution as directed under Ultraviolet-visible Spectrophotometry <*2.24*>: it exhibits a maximum between 232 nm and 236 nm.

Uniformity of dosage units <*6.02*> Perform the test according to the following method: Cefpodoxime Proxetil for Syrup in single-dose packages meet the requirement of the Content uniformity test.

To the total content of 1 package of Cefpodoxime Proxetil for Syrup add exactly 30 mL of the internal standard solution, treat with ultrasonic waves for 10 minutes while occasional shaking, and centrifuge. Take 3 mL of the supernatant liquid, add a mixture of water, acetonitrile and acetic acid (100) (99:99:2) to make 20 mL, and use this solution as the sample solution. Separately, weigh accurately an amount of Cefpodoxime Proxetil RS, equivalent to about 50 mg (potency), dissolve in a suitable amount of a mixture of water, acetonitrile and acetic acid (100) (99:99:2), add exactly 15 mL of the internal standard solution, then add a mixture of water, acetonitrile and acetic acid (100) (99:99:2) to make 100 mL, and use this solution as the standard solution.

Then, proceed as directed in the Assay under Cefpodoxime Proxetil.

Amount [mg (potency)] of cefpodoxime ($C_{15}H_{17}N_5O_6S_2$)
$= M_S \times (Q_{T1} + Q_{T2})/(Q_{S1} + Q_{S2}) \times 2$

M_S: Amount [mg (potency)] of Cefpodoxime Proxetil RS taken

Internal standard solution—Dissolve 0.2 g of ethyl parahydroxybenzoate in a mixture of water, acetonitrile and acetic acid (100) (99:99:2) to make 300 mL.

Dissolution <*6.10*> When the test is performed at 50 revolutions per minute according to the Paddle method, using 900 mL of water as the dissolution medium, the dissolution rates in 15 minutes of Cefpodoxime Proxetil for Syrup is not less than 85%.

Start the test with an accurately weighed amount of Cefpodoxime Proxetil for Syrup, equivalent to about 50 mg (potency) of Cefpodoxime Proxetil, withdraw not less than 20 mL of the medium at the specified minute after starting the test, and filter through a membrane filter with a pore size not exceeding 0.5 μm. Discard not less than 10 mL of the first filtrate, pipet 5 mL of the subsequent filtrate, add a solution of citric acid monohydrate in the mobile phase (1 in 2000) to make exactly 25 mL, and use this solution as the sample solution. Separately, weigh accurately an amount of Cefpodoxime Proxetil RS, equivalent to about 22 mg (potency), dissolve in a solution of citric acid monohydrate in the mobile phase (1 in 2000) to make exactly 100 mL. Pipet 5 mL of this solution, add a solution of citric acid monohydrate in the mobile phase (1 in 2000) to make exactly 100 mL, and use this solution as the standard solution. Perform the test with exactly 10 μL each of the sample solution and standard solution as directed under Liquid Chromatography <*2.01*> according to the following conditions, and determine the areas, A_{Ta} and A_{Sa}, of the one peak which appears at the retention time of about 24 minutes among the two peaks obtainable from cefpodoxime proxetil, and the areas, A_{Tb} and A_{Sb}, of the peak which appears at the retention time of about 30 minutes, in each solution.

Dissolution rate (%) with respect to the labeled amount of cefpodoxime proxetil ($C_{21}H_{27}N_5O_9S_2$)
$= M_S/M_T \times (A_{Ta} + A_{Tb})/(A_{Sa} + A_{Sb}) \times 1/C \times 225$

M_S: Amount [mg (potency)] of Cefpodoxime Proxetil RS taken
M_T: Amount (g) of Cefpodoxime Proxetil for Syrup taken
C: Labeled amount [mg (potency)] of cefpodoxime proxetil ($C_{21}H_{27}N_5O_9S_2$) in 1 g

Operating conditions—

Detector, column, column temperature, and mobile phase: Proceed as directed in the operating conditions in the Assay under Cefpodoxime Proxetil.

Flow rate: Adjust so that the retention time of the peak, which elutes faster among the two peaks obtained from cefpodoxime proxetil, is about 24 minutes.

System suitability—

System performance: When the procedure is run with 10 μL of the standard solution under the above operating conditions, the resolution between the two peaks obtained from cefpodoxime proxetil is not less than 4.

System repeatability: When the test is repeated 6 times with 10 μL of the standard solution under the above operating conditions, the relative standard deviation of the sum of the areas of the two peaks obtained from cefpodoxime proxetil is not more than 2.0%.

Assay Weigh accurately an amount of powdered Cefpodoxime Proxetil for Syrup, equivalent to about 0.1 g (potency) of Cefpodoxime Proxetil, add exactly 30 mL of the internal standard solution, treat with ultrasonic waves for 10 minutes while occasional shaking, and centrifuge. Take 3 mL of the supernatant liquid, add a mixture of water, acetonitrile and acetic acid (100) (99:99:2) to make 20 mL, and use this solution as the sample solution. Separately, weigh accurately an amount of Cefpodoxime Proxetil RS, equivalent to about 50 mg (potency), dissolve in a suitable amount of a mixture of water, acetonitrile and acetic acid (100) (99:99:2), add exactly 15 mL of the internal standard solution, then add a mixture of water, acetonitrile and acetic acid (100) (99:99:2) to make 100 mL, and use this solution as the standard solution. Then, proceed as directed in the Assay under Cefpodoxime Proxetil.

Amount [mg (potency)] of cefpodoxime ($C_{15}H_{17}N_5O_6S_2$)
$= M_S \times (Q_{T1} + Q_{T2})/(Q_{S1} + Q_{S2}) \times 2$

M_S: Amount [mg (potency)] of Cefpodoxime Proxetil RS taken

Internal standard solution—Dissolve 0.2 g of ethyl parahydroxybenzoate in a mixture of water, acetonitrile and acetic acid (100) (99:99:2) to make 300 mL.

Containers and storage Containers—Tight containers.

Cefpodoxime Proxetil Tablets

セフポドキシム　プロキセチル錠

Cefpodoxime Proxetil Tablets contain not less than 93.0% and not more than 107.0% of the labeled potency of cefpodoxime ($C_{15}H_{17}N_5O_6S_2$: 427.46).

Method of preparation Prepare as directed under Tablets, with Cefpodoxime Proxetil.

Identification Powder Cefpodoxime Proxetil Tablets. To a portion of the powder, equivalent to 65 mg (potency) of Cefpodoxime Proxetil, add 25 mL of acetonitrile, shake thoroughly, and centrifuge. To 2 mL of the supernatant liquid add acetonitrile to make 50 mL. To 5 mL of this solution add acetonitrile to make 50 mL. Determine the absorption spectrum of this solution as directed under Ultraviolet-visible Spectrophotometry <*2.24*>: it exhibits a maximum between 232 nm and 236 nm.

Uniformity of dosage units <*6.02*> Perform the Mass variation test, or the Content uniformity test according to the following method: it meets the requirement.

To 1 tablet of Cefpodoxime Proxetil Tablets, add exactly 20 mL of a mixture of water, acetonitrile and acetic acid (100) (99:99:2), agitate with the aid of ultrasonic waves for 10 minutes, and filter through a membrane filter with a pore size not exceeding 0.45 μm. Discard the first 10 mL of the filtrate, pipet V mL of the subsequent filtrate, equivalent to 30 mg (potency) of Cefpodoxime Proxetil, add exactly 6 mL of the internal standard solution, then add a mixture of water, acetonitrile and acetic acid (100) (99:99:2) to make 50 mL, and use this solution as the sample solution. Separately, weigh accurately an amount of Cefpodoxime Proxetil RS, equivalent to about 60 mg (potency), dissolve in 60 mL of a mixture of water, acetonitrile and acetic acid (100) (99:99:2), add exactly 12 mL of the internal standard solution, then add a mixture of water, acetonitrile and acetic acid (100) (99:99:2) to make 100 mL, and use this solution as the standard solution. Then, proceed as directed in the Assay under Cefpodoxime Proxetil.

Amount [mg (potency)] of cefpodoxime ($C_{15}H_{17}N_5O_6S_2$)
$= M_S \times (Q_{T1} + Q_{T2})/(Q_{S1} + Q_{S2}) \times 10/V$

M_S: Amount [mg (potency)] of Cefpodoxime Proxetil RS taken

Internal standard solution—Dissolve 0.1 g of ethyl parahydroxybenzoate in a mixture of water, acetonitrile and acetic acid (100) (99:99:2) to make 100 mL.

Dissolution <6.10> When the test is performed at 50 revolutions per minute according to the Paddle method, using 900 mL of water as the dissolution medium, the dissolution rate in 45 minutes of Cefpodoxime Proxetil Tablets is not less than 70%.

Start the test with 1 tablet of Cefpodoxime Proxetil Tablets, withdraw not less than 20 mL of the medium at the specified minute after starting the test, and filter through a membrane filter with a pore size not exceeding 0.5 μm. Discard not less than 10 mL of the first filtrate, pipet V mL of the subsequent filtrate, add a solution of citric acid monohydrate in the mobile phase (1 in 2000) to make exactly V' mL so that each mL contains about 11 μg (potency) of Cefpodoxime Proxetil, and use this solution as the sample solution. Separately, weigh accurately an amount of Cefpodoxime Proxetil RS, equivalent to about 22 mg (potency), and dissolve in a solution of citric acid monohydrate in the mobile phase (1 in 2000) to make exactly 100 mL. Pipet 5 mL of this solution, add a solution of citric acid monohydrate in the mobile phase (1 in 2000) to make exactly 100 mL, and use this solution as the standard solution. Perform the test with exactly 10 μL each of the sample solution and standard solution as directed under Liquid Chromatography <2.01> according to the following conditions, and determine the areas of separated two peaks, one has the retention time of about 24 minutes, A_{Ta} and A_{Sa}, and another one has the retention time of about 30 minutes, A_{Tb} and A_{Sb}, in each solution.

Dissolution rate (%) with respect to the labeled amount of cefpodoxime proxetil ($C_{21}H_{27}N_5O_9S_2$)
$= M_S \times (A_{Ta} + A_{Tb})/(A_{Sa} + A_{Sb}) \times V'/V \times 1/C \times 45$

M_S: Amount [mg (potency)] of Cefpodoxime Proxetil RS taken
C: Labeled amount [mg (potency)] of cefpodoxime proxetil ($C_{21}H_{27}N_5O_9S_2$) in 1 tablet

Operating conditions—

Detector: An ultraviolet absorption photometer (wavelength: 240 nm).

Column: A stainless steel column 4.6 mm in inside diameter and 15 cm in length, packed with octadecylsilanized silica gel for liquid chromatography (5 μm in particle diameter).

Column temperature: A constant temperature of about 40°C.

Mobile phase: A mixture of water and methanol (11:9).

Flow rate: Adjust so that the retention time of one of the two peaks that elutes firster is about 24 minutes.

System suitability—

System performance: When the procedure is run with 10 μL of the standard solution under the above operating conditions, the resolution between the two peaks of cefpodoxime proxetil is not less than 4.

System repeatability: When the test is repeated 6 times with 10 μL of the standard solution under the above operating conditions, the relative standard deviation of the total area of the two peaks of cefpodoxime proxetil is not more than 2.0%.

Assay Weigh accurately the mass of not less than 20 Cefpodoxime Proxetil Tablets, and powder. Weigh accurately a portion of the powder, equivalent to about 0.3 g (potency) of Cefpodoxime Proxetil, add 80 mL of a mixture of water, acetonitrile and acetic acid (100) (99:99:2), agitate for 10 minutes with the aid of ultrasonic waves, and add a mixture of water, acetonitrile and acetic acid (100) (99:99:2) to make exactly 100 mL. Filter this solution through a membrane filter with a pore size not exceeding 0.45 μm. Discard the first 10 mL of the filtrate, pipet 10 mL of the subsequent filtrate, add exactly 6 mL of the internal standard solution, then, add a mixture of water, acetonitrile and acetic acid (100) (99:99:2) to make 50 mL, and use this solution as the sample solution. Separately, weigh accurately an amount of Cefpodoxime Proxetil RS, equivalent to about 60 mg (potency), dissolve in 60 mL of a mixture of water, acetonitrile and acetic acid (100) (99:99:2), add exactly 12 mL of the internal standard solution, then add a mixture of water, acetonitrile and acetic acid (100) (99:99:2) to make 100 mL, and use this solution as the standard solution. Then, proceed as directed in the Assay under Cefpodoxime Proxetil.

Amount [mg (potency)] of cefpodoxime ($C_{15}H_{17}N_5O_6S_2$)
$= M_S \times (Q_{T1} + Q_{T2})/(Q_{S1} + Q_{S2}) \times 5$

M_S: Amount [mg (potency)] of Cefpodoxime Proxetil RS taken

Internal standard solution—Dissolve 0.1 g of ethyl parahydroxybenzoate in a mixture of water, acetonitrile and acetic acid (100) (99:99:2) to make 100 mL.

Containers and storage Containers—Tight containers.

Cefroxadine Hydrate

セフロキサジン水和物

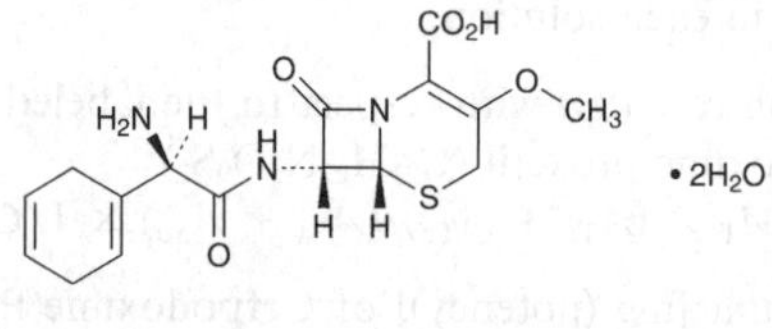

$C_{16}H_{19}N_3O_5S.2H_2O$: 401.43
(6*R*,7*R*)-7-[(2*R*)-2-Amino-2-cyclohexa-1,4-dienylacetylamino]-3-methoxy-8-oxo-5-thia-1-azabicyclo[4.2.0]oct-2-ene-2-carboxylic acid dihydrate
[*51762-05-1*, anhydride]

Cefroxadine Hydrate contains not less than 930 μg (potency) and not more than 1020 μg (potency) per mg, calculated on the anhydrous basis. The potency of Cefroxadine Hydrate is expressed as mass (potency) of cefroxadine ($C_{16}H_{19}N_3O_5S$: 365.40).

Description Cefroxadine Hydrate occurs as pale yellow-white to light yellow, crystalline particles or powder.

It is very soluble in formic acid, slightly soluble in water and in methanol, and very slightly soluble in acetonitrile and in ethanol (95).

It dissolves in 0.001 mol/L hydrochloric acid TS and in dilute acetic acid.

Identification (1) Determine the absorption spectrum of a solution of Cefroxadine Hydrate in 0.001 mol/L hydrochloric acid TS (1 in 50,000) as directed under Ultraviolet-visible

Spectrophotometry <2.24>, and compare the spectrum with the Reference Spectrum or the spectrum of a solution of Cefroxadine RS prepared in the same manner as the sample solution: both spectra exhibit similar intensities of absorption at the same wavelengths.

(2) Determine the infrared absorption spectrum of Cefroxadine Hydrate as directed in the potassium bromide disk method under Infrared Spectrophotometry <2.25>, and compare the spectrum with the Reference Spectrum or the spectrum of Cefroxadine RS: both spectra exhibit similar intensities of absorption at the same wave numbers.

(3) Determine the ^{1}H spectrum of a solution of Cefroxadine Hydrate in deuterated formic acid for nuclear magnetic resonance spectroscopy (1 in 10) as directed under Nuclear Magnetic Resonance Spectroscopy <2.21>, using tetramethylsilane for nuclear magnetic resonance spectroscopy as an internal reference compound: it exhibits three sharp singlet signals, A, B and C, at around δ 2.8 ppm, at around δ 4.1 ppm and at around δ 6.3 ppm. The ratio of the integrated intensity of each signal, A:B:C, is about 4:3:1.

Optical rotation <2.49> $[\alpha]_D^{20}$: +95 – +108° (0.1 g calculated on the anhydrous basis, diluted acetic acid (100) (3 in 25), 100 mL, 100 mm).

Purity (1) Heavy metals <1.07>—Weigh 1.0 g of Cefroxadine Hydrate in a porcelain crucible, add 10 mL of a solution of magnesium nitrate hexahydrate in ethanol (95) (1 in 10), mix, burn the ethanol, and carbonize by gently heating. After cooling, add 2 mL of nitric acid, heat carefully, and incinerate by ignition at 500 – 600°C. If a carbonized substance still remains, moisten it with a small amount of nitric acid, and incinerate again by ignition. After cooling, add 6 mL of hydrochloric acid, and evaporate on a water bath to dryness. Moisten the residue with 3 drops of hydrochloric acid, and add 10 mL of hot water to dissolve the residue by heating on a water bath. After cooling, adjust the pH between 3 and 4 with ammonia TS, add 2 mL of dilute acetic acid, filter if necessary, transfer to a Nessler tube, wash the crucible with 10 mL of water, and add the washing and water to the tube to make 50 mL. Perform the test with this solution. Prepare the control solution as follows: Put 2.0 mL of Standard Lead Solution and 10 mL of a solution of magnesium nitrate hexahydrate in ethanol (95) (1 in 10) in a porcelain crucible, and proceed as directed for the preparation of the test solution (not more than 20 ppm).

(2) Related substances—Dissolve 10 mg of Cefroxadine Hydrate in 100 mL of the mobile phase, and use this solution as the sample solution. Pipet 1 mL of the sample solution, add the mobile phase to make exactly 100 mL, and use this solution as the standard solution. Perform the test with exactly 40 μL each of the sample solution and standard solution as directed under Liquid Chromatography <2.01> according to the following conditions, and determine each peak area by the automatic integration method: the areas of the peaks, having the relative retention times of about 0.07, about 0.6 and about 0.8 to cefroxadine obtained from the sample solution are not larger than 2 times, 4 times and 1 time the peak area of cefroxadine from the standard solution, respectively, and any peak area other than cefroxadine and other than the peaks mentioned above is not larger than 1/2 times the peak area of cefroxadine from the standard solution, and the total area of the peaks other than cefroxadine is not larger than 6 times the peak area of cefroxadine from the standard solution.

Operating conditions—

Detector: An ultraviolet absorption photometer (wavelength: 254 nm).

Column: A stainless steel column 4.6 mm in inside diameter and 10 cm in length, packed with octadecylsilanized silica gel for liquid chromatography (5 μm in particle diameter).

Column temperature: A constant temperature of about 25°C.

Mobile phase: Dissolve 1.4 g of sodium perchlorate in 1000 mL of a mixture of water and acetonitrile (489:11).

Flow rate: Adjust so that the retention time of cefroxadine is about 20 minutes.

Time span of measurement: About 2 times as long as the retention time of cefroxadine.

System suitability—

Test for required detectability: Measure exactly 2 mL of the standard solution, and add the mobile phase to make exactly 20 mL. Confirm that the peak area of cefroxadine obtained with 40 μL of this solution is equivalent to 7 to 13% of that with 40 μL of the standard solution.

System performance: Dissolve 3 mg of Cefroxadine Hydrate and 15 mg of orcin in 100 mL of the mobile phase. When the procedure is run with 40 μL of this solution under the above operating conditions, orcin and cefroxadine are eluted in this order with the resolution between these peaks being not less than 3.

System repeatability: When the test is repeated 6 times with 40 μL of the standard solution under the above operating conditions, the relative standard deviation of the peak area of cefroxadine is not more than 2.0%.

Water <2.48> Not less than 8.5% and not more than 12.0% (0.1 g, volumetric titration, direct titration).

Assay Weigh accurately an amount of Cefroxadine Hydrate and Cefroxadine RS, equivalent to about 50 mg (potency), dissolve each in a suitable amount of a mixture of dilute acetic acid and phosphoric acid (500:1), add exactly 5 mL of the internal standard solution and a mixture of dilute acetic acid and phosphoric acid (500:1) to make 200 mL, and use these solutions as the sample solution and standard solution. Perform the test with 10 μL each of the sample solution and standard solution as directed under Liquid Chromatography <2.01> according to the following conditions, and calculate the ratios, Q_T and Q_S, of the peak area of cefroxadine to that of the internal standard.

$$\text{Amount } [\mu\text{g (potency)}] \text{ of cefroxadine } (C_{16}H_{19}N_3O_5S) = M_S \times Q_T/Q_S \times 1000$$

M_S: Amount [mg (potency)] of Cefroxadine RS taken

*Internal standard solution—*Dissolve 1.6 g of vanillin in 5 mL of methanol, and add a mixture of dilute acetic acid and phosphoric acid (500:1) to make 100 mL.

Operating conditions—

Detector: An ultraviolet absorption photometer (wavelength: 254 nm).

Column: A stainless steel column 4.6 mm in inside diameter and 10 cm in length, packed with octadecylsilanized silica gel for liquid chromatography (5 μm in particle diameter).

Column temperature: A constant temperature of about 25°C.

Mobile phase: A mixture of a solution of ammonium sulfate (1 in 50) and acetonitrile (97:3).

Flow rate: Adjust so that the retention time of cefroxadine is about 10 minutes.

System suitability—

System performance: When the procedure is run with 10 μL of the standard solution under the above operating conditions, cefroxadine and the internal standard are eluted in this order with the resolution between these peaks being not less than 1.5.

System repeatability: When the test is repeated 6 times with 10 μL of the standard solution under the above operating conditions, the relative standard deviation of the ratios of the peak areas of cefroxadine to that of the internal standard is not more than 1.0%.

Containers and storage Containers—Tight containers.

Cefroxadine for Syrup

シロップ用セフロキサジン

Cefroxadine for Syrup is a preparation for syrup, which is suspended before use.

It contains not less than 93.0% and not more than 107.0% of the labeled potency of cefroxadine ($C_{16}H_{19}N_3O_5S$: 365.40).

Method of preparation Prepare as directed under Preparations for Syrups, with Cefroxadine Hydrate.

Identification Powder Cefroxadine for Syrup, if necessary. To a portion of the powder, equivalent to 2 mg (potency) of Cefroxadine Hydrate, add 100 mL of 0.001 mol/L hydrochloric acid TS, shake well, and filter. Determine the absorption spectrum of this filtrate as directed under Ultraviolet-visible Spectrophotometry <*2.24*>: it exhibits a maximum between 267 nm and 271 nm.

Water <*2.48*> Not more than 4.5% (0.1 g, volumetric titration, direct titration).

Uniformity of dosage units <*6.02*> Perform the test according to the following method: Cefroxadine for Syrup in single-dose packages meet the requirement of the Content uniformity test.

Take out the total contents of 1 package of Cefroxadine for Syrup, add $4V/5$ mL of a mixture of dilute acetic acid and phosphoric acid (500:1), shake well for 15 minutes, add exactly 5 mL of the internal standard solution per 50 mg (potency) of Cefroxadine Hydrate, and add a mixture of dilute acetic acid and phosphoric acid (500:1) to make V mL so that each mL contains about 0.25 mg (potency) of Cefroxadine Hydrate. Filter this solution through a membrane filter with pore size of not exceeding 0.45 μm, and use the filtrate as the sample solution. Separately, weigh accurately an amount of Cefroxadine RS, equivalent to about 50 mg (potency), dissolve in a mixture of dilute acetic acid and phosphoric acid (500:1), add exactly 5 mL of the internal standard solution, add a mixture of dilute acetic acid and phosphoric acid (500:1) to make 200 mL, and use this solution as the standard solution. Then, proceed as directed in the Assay under Cefroxadine Hydrate.

Amount [mg (potency)] of cefroxadine ($C_{16}H_{19}N_3O_5S$)
$= M_S \times Q_T/Q_S \times V/200$

M_S: Amount [mg (potency)] of Cefroxadine RS taken

Internal standard solution—Dissolve 1.6 g of vanillin in 5 mL of methanol, and add a mixture of dilute acetic acid and phosphoric acid (500:1) to make 100 mL.

Dissolution <*6.10*> When the test is performed at 50 revolutions per minute according to the Paddle method, using 900 mL of water as the dissolution medium, the dissolution rate in 15 minutes of Cefroxadine for Syrup is not less than 85%.

Start the test with an accurately weighed amount of Cefroxadine for Syrup, equivalent to about 0.1 g (potency) of Cefroxadine Hydrate, withdraw not less than 10 mL of the medium at the specified minute after starting the test, and filter through a membrane filter with a pore size not exceeding 0.8 μm. Discard not less than 5 mL of the first filtrate, pipet 4 mL of the subsequent filtrate, add 0.1 mol/L hydrochloric acid TS to make exactly 20 mL, and use this solution as the sample solution. Separately, weigh accurately an amount of Cefroxadine RS, equivalent to about 22 mg (potency), and dissolve in 0.1 mol/L hydrochloric acid TS to make exactly 100 mL. Pipet 5 mL of this solution, add 10 mL of water, add 0.1 mol/L hydrochloric acid TS to make exactly 50 mL, and use this solution as the standard solution. Perform the test with the sample solution and standard solution as directed under Ultraviolet-visible Spectrophotometry <*2.24*>, and determine the absorbances, A_T and A_S, at 267 nm.

Dissolution rate (%) with respect to the labeled amount of cefroxadine ($C_{16}H_{19}N_3O_5S$)
$= M_S/M_T \times A_T/A_S \times 1/C \times 450$

M_S: Amount [mg (potency)] of Cefroxadine RS taken
M_T: Amount (g) of Cefroxadine for Syrup taken
C: Labeled amount [mg (potency)] of cefroxadine ($C_{16}H_{19}N_3O_5S$) in 1 g

Assay Powder Cefroxadine for Syrup, if necessary, weigh accurately a portion of the powder, equivalent to about 50 mg (potency) of Cefroxadine Hydrate, add 160 mL of a mixture of dilute acetic acid and phosphoric acid (500:1), shake well for 15 minutes, add exactly 5 mL of the internal standard solution, and add a mixture of dilute acetic acid and phosphoric acid (500:1) to make 200 mL. Filter this solution through a membrane filter with a pore size not exceeding 0.45 μm, and use the filtrate as the sample solution. Separately, weigh accurately an amount of Cefroxadine RS, equivalent to about 50 mg (potency), dissolve in a mixture of dilute acetic acid and phosphoric acid (500:1), add exactly 5 mL of the internal standard solution, add a mixture of dilute acetic acid and phosphoric acid (500:1) to make 200 mL, and use this solution as the standard solution. Proceed as directed in the Assay under Cefroxadine Hydrate.

Amount [mg (potency)] of cefroxadine ($C_{16}H_{19}N_3O_5S$)
$= M_S \times Q_T/Q_S$

M_S: Amount [mg (potency)] of Cefroxadine RS taken

Internal standard solution—Dissolve 1.6 g of vanillin in 5 mL of methanol, and add a mixture of dilute acetic acid and phosphoric acid (500:1) to make 100 mL.

Containers and storage Containers—Tight containers.

Cefsulodin Sodium

セフスロジンナトリウム

$C_{22}H_{19}N_4NaO_8S_2$: 554.53
Monosodium (6*R*,7*R*)-3-(4-carbamoylpyridinium-1-ylmethyl)-8-oxo-7-[(2*R*)-2-phenyl-2-sulfonatoacetylamino]-5-thia-1-azabicyclo[4.2.0]oct-2-ene-2-carboxylate
[52152-93-9]

Cefsulodin Sodium contains not less than 900 μg (potency) and not more than 970 μg (potency) per mg, calculated on the anhydrous basis. The potency of Cefsulodin Sodium is expressed as mass (potency) of cefsulodin ($C_{22}H_{20}N_4O_8S_2$: 532.55).

Description Cefsulodin Sodium occurs as white to light yellow, crystals or crystalline powder.

It is freely soluble in water and in formamide, slightly soluble in methanol, and very slightly soluble in ethanol (95).

It is hygroscopic.

Identification **(1)** Determine the absorption spectrum of a solution of Cefsulodin Sodium (1 in 50,000) as directed under Ultraviolet-visible Spectrophotometry ⟨*2.24*⟩, and compare the spectrum with the Reference Spectrum or the spectrum of a solution of Cefsulodin Sodium RS prepared in the same manner as sample solution: both spectra exhibit similar intensities of absorption at the same wavelengths.

(2) Determine the infrared absorption spectrum of Cefsulodin Sodium as directed in the potassium bromide disk method under Infrared Spectrophotometry ⟨*2.25*⟩, and compare the spectrum with the Reference Spectrum or the spectrum of Cefsulodin Sodium RS: both spectra exhibit similar intensities of absorption at the same wave numbers.

(3) Determine the ^1H spectrum of a solution of Cefsulodin Sodium in heavy water for nuclear magnetic resonance spectroscopy (1 in 10) as directed under Nuclear Magnetic Resonance Spectroscopy ⟨*2.21*⟩, using sodium 3-trimethylsilylpropanesulfonate for nuclear magnetic resonance spectroscopy as an internal reference compound: it exhibits a multiplet signal A between δ 7.3 ppm and δ 7.7 ppm, and doublet signals, B and C, at around δ 8.4 ppm and at around δ 9.1 ppm, respectively. The ratio of integrated intensity of these signals, A:B:C, is about 5:2:2.

(4) Cefsulodin Sodium responds to Qualitative Tests ⟨*1.09*⟩ (1) for sodium salt.

Optical rotation ⟨*2.49*⟩ $[\alpha]_D^{20}$: +16.5 – +20.0° (0.1 g calculated on the anhydrous basis, water, 10 mL, 100 mm).

pH ⟨*2.54*⟩ Dissolve 1.0 g of Cefsulodin Sodium in 10 mL of water: the pH of the solution is not less than 3.3 and not more than 4.8.

Purity **(1)** Clarity of solution—Dissolve 1.0 g of Cefsulodin Sodium in 10 mL of water: the solution is clear.

(2) Heavy metals ⟨*1.07*⟩—To 1.0 g of Cefsulodin Sodium add 10 mL of a solution of magnesium nitrate hexahydrate in ethanol (95) (1 in 5), mix, fire the ethanol to burn, then heat gradually to carbonize. After cooling, add 2 mL of nitric acid, heat carefully, then heat at 500 – 600°C to incinerate. If a carbonized residue still retains, add a little amount of nitric acid, and heat again to incinerate. After cooling, add 6 mL of hydrochloric acid to the residue, heat to dryness on a water bath, then moisten the residue with 3 drops of hydrochloric acid, add 10 mL of hot water, and heat on a water bath to dissolve. Add ammonia TS dropwise to adjust to pH 3 – 4, and add 2 mL of dilute acetic acid. If necessary, filter, wash the crucible and residue on the filter with 10 mL of water, transfer the filtrate and washings into a Nessler tube, add water to make 50 mL, and use this solution as the test solution. Prepare the control solution as follows: To 2.0 mL of Standard Lead Solution add 10 mL of a solution of magnesium nitrate hexahydrate in ethanol (95) (1 in 5), fire the ethanol to burn. After cooling, add 2 mL of nitric acid, heat carefully, then heat at 500 – 600°C. After cooling, add 6 mL of hydrochloric acid, then proceed in the same manner as for the preparation of the test solution (not more than 20 ppm).

(3) Arsenic ⟨*1.11*⟩—Prepare the test solution with 1.0 g of Cefsulodin Sodium according to Method 3, using a solution of magnesium nitrate hexahydrate in ethanol (95) (1 in 5) and 15 mL of dilute hydrochloric acid instead of a solution of magnesium nitrate hexahydrate in ethanol (95) (1 in 50) and 3 mL of hydrochloric acid, and perform the test (not more than 2 ppm).

(4) Related substances—Weigh accurately 0.10 g of Cefsulodin Sodium, dissolve in water to make exactly 50 mL, and use this solution as the sample solution. Separately, weigh accurately about 20 mg of isonicotinic acid amide and about 20 mg of Cefsulodin Sodium RS (separately determine the water ⟨*2.48*⟩ in the same manner as Cefsulodin Sodium), and dissolve in water to make exactly 100 mL. Pipet 10 mL of this solution, add water to make exactly 100 mL, and use this solution as the standard solution. Perform the test with exactly 10 μL each of the sample solution and standard solution as directed under Liquid Chromatography ⟨*2.01*⟩ according to the following conditions, and determine the areas of each peak by the automatic integration method. Calculate the amount of the related substances by the following formula: the amount of isonicotinic acid amide is not more than 1.0%, and the total amount of other related substances is not more than 1.2%.

Amount (%) of isonicotinic acid amide
$$= A/B_I \times M_I/M_T \times 5$$

Total amount (%) of the other related substances
$$= B/B_S \times M_S/M_T \times 5$$

A: Peak area of isonicotinic acid amide from the sample solution
B: Total peak area other than cefsulodin and other than isonicotinic acid amide from the sample solution
B_I: Peak area of isonicotinic acid amide from the standard solution
B_S: Peak area of cefsulodin from the standard solution
M_T: Amount (g) of Cefsulodin Sodium taken
M_S: Amount (g) of Cefsulodin Sodium RS taken
M_I: Amount (g) of isonicotinic acid amide taken

Operating conditions—

Detector: An ultraviolet absorption photometer (wavelength: 254 nm).

Column: A stainless steel column 4 mm in inside diameter and 15 cm in length, packed with octadecylsilanized silica gel for liquid chromatography (5 μm in particle diameter).

Column temperature: A constant temperature of about 25°C.

Mobile phase A: A mixture of a solution of ammonium sulfate (1 in 100) and acetonitrile (97:3).

Mobile phase B: A mixture of a solution of ammonium

sulfate (1 in 100) and acetonitrile (23:2).

Flowing of mobile phase: Change the mobile phase A to B at 14 minutes after the injection of sample.

Flow rate: Adjust so that the retention time of cefsulodin is about 9 minutes.

Time span of measurement: About 4 times as long as the retention time of cefsulodin.

System suitability—

Test for required detectability: Pipet 1 mL of the standard solution, add water to make exactly 10 mL. Confirm that the peak areas of isonicotinic acid amide and cefsulodin obtained with 10 μL of this solution are equivalent to 7 to 13% of those with 10 μL of the standard solution.

System performance: When the procedure is run with 10 μL of the standard solution under the above operating conditions, isonicotinic acid amide and cefsulodin are eluted in this order with the resolution between these peaks being not less than 5.

System repeatability: When the test is repeated 5 times with 10 μL of the standard solution under the above operating conditions, the relative standard deviation of the peak areas of cefsulodin is not more than 1.0%.

Water <2.48> Not more than 5.0% (1 g, volumetric titration, direct titration, avoiding moisture absorption of the sample, using a mixture of formamide for water determination and methanol for water determination (2:1) instead of methanol for water determination).

Assay Weigh accurately an amount of Cefsulodin Sodium and Cefsulodin Sodium RS, equivalent to about 0.1 g (potency), dissolve each in water to make exactly 50 mL, and use these solutions as the sample solution and standard solution. Perform the test with exactly 10 μL each of the sample solution and standard solution as directed under Liquid Chromatography <2.01> according to the following conditions, and determine the peak areas, A_T and A_S, of cefsulodin in each solution.

Amount [μg (potency)] of cefsulodin ($C_{22}H_{20}N_4O_8S_2$)
$= M_S \times A_T/A_S \times 1000$

M_S: Amount [mg (potency)] of Cefsulodin Sodium RS taken

Operating conditions—

Detector: An ultraviolet absorption photometer (wavelength: 254 nm).

Column: A stainless steel column 4 mm in inside diameter and 15 cm in length, packed with octadecylsilanized silica gel for liquid chromatography (5 μm in particle diameter).

Column temperature: A constant temperature of about 25°C.

Mobile phase: A mixture of a solution of ammonium sulfate (1 in 100) and acetonitrile (97:3).

Flow rate: Adjust so that the retention time of cefsulodin is about 9 minutes.

System suitability—

System performance: Dissolve 40 mg of isonicotinic acid amide in 25 mL of the standard solution. When the procedure is run with 10 μL of this solution under the above operating conditions, isonicotinic acid amide and cefsulodin are eluted in this order with the resolution between these peaks being not less than 5.

System repeatability: When the test is repeated 5 times with 10 μL of the standard solution under the above operating conditions, the relative standard deviation of the peak areas of cefsulodin is not more than 1.0%.

Containers and storage Containers—Hermetic containers.

Ceftazidime Hydrate

セフタジジム水和物

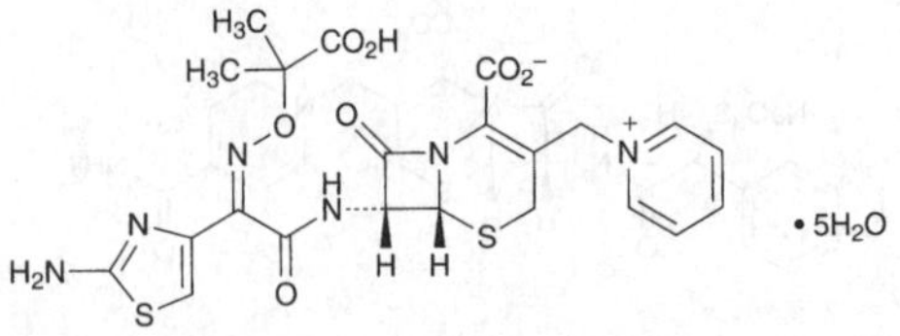

$C_{22}H_{22}N_6O_7S_2.5H_2O$: 636.65
(6*R*,7*R*)-7-[(*Z*)-2-(2-Aminothiazol-4-yl)-2-(1-carboxy-1-methylethoxyimino)acetylamino]-3-(pyridinium-1-ylmethyl)-8-oxo-5-thia-1-azabicyclo[4.2.0]oct-2-ene-2-carboxylate pentahydrate
[*78439-06-2*]

Ceftazidime Hydrate contains not less than 950 μg (potency) and not more than 1020 μg (potency) per mg, calculated on the anhydrous basis. The potency of Ceftazidime Hydrate is expressed as mass (potency) of ceftazidime ($C_{22}H_{22}N_6O_7S_2$: 546.58).

Description Ceftazidime Hydrate occurs as a white to light yellow-white crystalline powder.

It is slightly soluble in water, and very slightly soluble in acetonitrile and in ethanol (95).

Identification **(1)** Determine the absorption spectrum of a solution of Ceftazidime Hydrate in phosphate buffer solution (pH 6.0) (1 in 100,000) as directed under Ultraviolet-visible Spectrophotometry <2.24>, and compare the spectrum with the Reference Spectrum or the spectrum of a solution of Ceftazidime RS prepared in the same manner as the sample solution: both spectra exhibit similar intensities of absorption at the same wavelengths.

(2) Determine the infrared absorption spectrum of Ceftazidime Hydrate as directed in the potassium bromide disk method under Infrared Spectrophotometry <2.25>, and compare the spectrum with the Reference Spectrum or the spectrum of Ceftazidime RS: both spectra exhibit similar intensities of absorption at the same wave numbers.

(3) To 0.05 g of Ceftazidime Hydrate add 5 mg of dried sodium carbonate, and add 0.5 mL of heavy water for nuclear magnetic resonance spectroscopy to dissolve. Determine the ^1H spectrum of this solution as directed under Nuclear Magnetic Resonance Spectroscopy <2.21>, using sodium 3-trimethylsilylpropanesulfonate for nuclear magnetic resonance spectroscopy as an internal reference compound: it exhibits singlet signals, A and B, at around δ 1.5 ppm and at around δ 6.9 ppm, and a multiplet signal C between δ 7.9 ppm and δ 9.2 ppm. The ratio of integrated intensity of each signal, A:B:C, is about 6:1:5.

Optical rotation <2.49> $[\alpha]_D^{20}$: $-28 - -34°$ (0.5 g calculated on the anhydrous basis, phosphate buffer solution (pH 6.0), 100 mL, 100 mm).

pH <2.54> Dissolve 0.5 g of Ceftazidime Hydrate in 100 mL of water: the pH of the solution is between 3.0 and 4.0.

Purity **(1)** Clarity and color of solution—Dissolve 1.0 g of Ceftazidime Hydrate in 10 mL of a solution obtained by dissolving 5 g of anhydrous disodium hydrogen phosphate and 1 g of potassium dihydrogen phosphate in water to make 100 mL: the solution is clear, and its absorbance at 420 nm, determined as directed under Ultraviolet-visible Spectrophotometry <2.24>, is not more than 0.20.

(2) Heavy metals <*1.07*>—Proceed with 1.0 g of Ceftazidime Hydrate according to Method 2, and perform the test. Prepare the control solution with 2.0 mL of Standard Lead Solution (not more than 20 ppm).

(3) Related substances (i) Trityl-*t*-butyl substance and *t*-butyl substance—Dissolve 0.10 g of Ceftazidime Hydrate in 2 mL of diluted disodium hydrogen phosphate TS (1 in 3), and use this solution as the sample solution. Pipet 1 mL of the sample solution, add diluted disodium hydrogenphosphate TS (1 in 3) to make exactly 100 mL, and use this solution as the standard solution. Perform the test with these solutions as directed under Thin-layer Chromatography <*2.03*>. Spot 2 µL each of the sample solution and standard solution on a plate of silica gel with fluorescent indicator for thin-layer chromatography. Develop with a mixture of acetic acid (100), *n*-butyl acetate, acetate buffer solution (pH 4.5) and 1-butanol (16:16:13:3) to a distance of about 12 cm, and air-dry the plate. Examine under ultraviolet light (main wavelength: 254 nm): the spots which appear upper in position than the principal spot obtained from the sample solution are not more intense than the spot from the standard solution.

(ii) Other related substances—Dissolve 20 mg of Ceftazidime Hydrate in 10 mL of the mobile phase, and use this solution as the sample solution. Pipet 1 mL of the sample solution, add the mobile phase to make exactly 200 mL, and use this solution as the standard solution. Perform the test with exactly 5 µL each of the sample solution and standard solution as directed under Liquid Chromatography <*2.01*> according to the following conditions, and determine each peak area by the automatic integration method: the area of the peak other than ceftazidime obtained from the sample solution is not larger than that of ceftazidime from the standard solution, and the total of peak areas other than ceftazidime from the sample solution is not larger than 5 times the peak area of ceftazidime from the standard solution.

Operating conditions—

Detector: An ultraviolet absorption photometer (wavelength: 254 nm).

Column: A stainless steel column 4.6 mm in inside diameter and 20 cm in length, packed with octadecylsilanized silica gel for liquid chromatography (5 µm in particle diameter).

Column temperature: A constant temperature of about 25°C.

Mobile phase: Dissolve 5.0 g of ammonium dihydrogenphosphate in 750 mL of water, adjust to pH 3.5 with phosphoric acid, and add water to make 870 mL. To this solution add 130 mL of acetonitrile.

Flow rate: Adjust so that the retention time of ceftazidime is about 4 minutes.

Time span of measurement: About 3 times as long as the retention time of ceftazidime, beginning after the solvent peak.

System suitability—

Test for required detectability: Pipet 1 mL of the standard solution, add the mobile phase to make exactly 5 mL, and confirm that the peak area of ceftazidime obtained with 5 µL of this solution is equivalent to 15 to 25% of that with 5 µL of the standard solution.

System performance: Dissolve about 10 mg each of Ceftazidime Hydrate and acetanilide in 20 mL of the mobile phase. When the procedure is run with 5 µL of this solution under the above operating conditions, ceftazidime and acetanilide are eluted in this order with the resolution between these peaks being not less than 10.

System repeatability: When the test is repeated 6 times with 5 µL of the standard solution under the above operating conditions, the relative standard deviation of the peak area of ceftazidime is not more than 2.0%.

(4) Free pyridine—Weigh accurately about 50 mg of Ceftazidime Hydrate, dissolve in the mobile phase to make exactly 10 mL, and use this solution as the sample solution. Separately, weigh accurately about 0.1 g of pyridine, and add the mobile phase to make exactly 100 mL. Pipet 1 mL of this solution, add the mobile phase to make exactly 100 mL, and use this solution as the standard solution. Perform the test with exactly 10 µL each of the sample solution and standard solution as directed under Liquid Chromatography <*2.01*> according to the following conditions, and determine the peak heights, H_T and H_S, of pyridine in each solution: the amount of free pyridine is not more than 0.3%.

$$\text{Amount (mg) of free pyridine} = M_S \times H_T/H_S \times 1/1000$$

M_S: Amount (mg) of pyridine taken

Operating conditions—

Detector: An ultraviolet absorption photometer (wavelength: 254 nm).

Column: A stainless steel column 4.6 mm in inside diameter and 20 cm in length, packed with octadecylsilanized silica gel for liquid chromatography (5 µm in particle diameter).

Column temperature: A constant temperature of about 40°C.

Mobile phase: Dissolve 2.88 g of ammonium dihydrogenphosphate in 500 mL of water, add 300 mL of acetonitrile and water to make 1000 mL, and adjust to pH 7.0 with ammonia solution (28).

Flow rate: Adjust so that the retention time of pyridine is about 4 minutes.

System suitability—

System performance: Dissolve 5 mg of Ceftazidime Hydrate in 100 mL of a solution of pyridine in the mobile phase (1 in 20,000). When the procedure is run with 10 µL of this solution under the above operating conditions, ceftazidime and pyridine are eluted in this order with the resolution between these peaks being not less than 9.

System repeatability: When the test is repeated 6 times with 10 µL of the standard solution under the above operating conditions, the relative standard deviation of the peak height of pyridine is not more than 5.0%.

Water <*2.48*> 13.0 – 15.0% (0.1 g, volumetric titration, direct titration).

Assay Weigh accurately an amount of Ceftazidime Hydrate, equivalent to about 0.1 g (potency), and dissolve in 0.05 mol/L phosphate buffer solution (pH 7.0) to make exactly 100 mL. Pipet 10 mL of this solution, add exactly 5 mL of the internal standard solution, then add 0.05 mol/L phosphate buffer solution (pH 7.0) to make 50 mL, and use this solution as the sample solution. Separately, weigh accurately an amount of Ceftazidime RS, equivalent to about 20 mg (potency), dissolve in 0.05 mol/L phosphate buffer solution (pH 7.0) to make exactly 20 mL. Pipet 10 mL of this solution, add exactly 5 mL of the internal standard solution, then add 0.05 mol/L phosphate buffer solution (pH 7.0) to make 50 mL, and use this solution as the standard solution. Perform the test with 5 µL each of the sample solution and standard solution as directed under Liquid Chromatography <*2.01*> according to the following conditions, and calculate the ratios, Q_T and Q_S, of the peak area of ceftazidime to that of the internal standard.

Amount [μg (potency)] of ceftazidime ($C_{22}H_{22}N_6O_7S_2$)
$= M_S \times Q_T/Q_S \times 5000$

M_S: Amount [mg (potency)] of Ceftazidime RS taken

Internal standard solution—A solution of dimedon in 0.05 mol/L phosphate buffer solution (pH 7.0) (11 in 10,000).
Operating conditions—

Detector: An ultraviolet absorption photometer (wavelength: 254 nm).

Column: A stainless steel column 4.6 mm in inside diameter and 10 cm in length, packed with hexasilanized silica gel for liquid chromatography (5 μm in particle diameter).

Column temperature: A constant temperature of about 25°C.

Mobile phase: Dissolve 4.26 g of anhydrous disodium hydrogen phosphate and 2.72 g of potassium dihydrogen phosphate in 980 mL of water, and add 20 mL of acetonitrile.

Flow rate: Adjust so that the retention time of ceftazidime is about 4 minutes.
System suitability—

System performance: When the procedure is run with 5 μL of the standard solution under the above operating conditions, the internal standard and ceftazidime are eluted in this order with the resolution between these peaks being not less than 3.

System repeatability: When the test is repeated 6 times with 5 μL of the standard solution under the above operating conditions, the relative standard deviation of the ratios of the peak area of ceftazidime to that of the internal standard is not more than 1.0%.

Containers and storage Containers—Tight containers.
Storage—Light-resistant.

Ceftazidime for Injection

注射用セフタジジム

Ceftazidime for Injection is a preparation for injection which is dissolved before use.

It contains not less than 93.0% and not more than 107.0% of the labeled potency of ceftazidime ($C_{22}H_{22}N_6O_7S_2$: 546.58).

Method of preparation Prepare as directed under Injections, with Ceftazidime Hydrate.

Description Ceftazidime for Injection is a white to pale yellow-white powder.

Identification Determine the absorption spectrum of a solution of Ceftazidime for Injection (1 in 100,000) in phosphate buffer solution (pH 6.0) as directed under Ultraviolet-visible Spectrophotometry 〈*2.24*〉: it exhibits a maximum between 255 nm and 259 nm.

pH 〈*2.54*〉 Dissolve an amount of Ceftazidime for Injection, equivalent to 1.0 g (potency) of Ceftazidime Hydrate, in 10 mL of water: the pH of this solution is 5.8 to 7.8.

Purity Clarity and color of solution—Dissolve 5 g of disodium hydrogen phosphate and 1 g of potassium dihydrogen phosphate in water to make 100 mL. In 10 mL of this solution dissolve an amount of Ceftazidime for Injection, equivalent to 1.0 g (potency) of Ceftazidime Hydrate: the solution is clear. Also, determine the absorption spectra of this solution as directed under Ultraviolet-visible Spectrophotometry 〈*2.24*〉: the absorbance at 420 nm is not more than 0.3.

Loss on drying 〈*2.41*〉 Not more than 14.0% (0.1 g, in vacuum not exceeding 0.67 kPa, 60°C, 3 hours).

Bacterial endotoxins 〈*4.01*〉 Less than 0.067 EU/mg (potency).

Uniformity of dosage units 〈*6.02*〉 It meets the requirement of the Mass variation test.

Foreign insoluble matter 〈*6.06*〉 Perform the test according to Method 2: it meets the requirement.

Insoluble particulate matter 〈*6.07*〉 It meets the requirement.

Sterility 〈*4.06*〉 Perform the test according to the Membrane filter method: it meets the requirement.

Assay Weigh accurately the mass of the contents of not less than 10 containers of Ceftazidime for Injection. Weigh accurately an amount of Ceftazidime Hydrate, equivalent to about 0.25 g (potency), and dissolve in 0.05 mol/L phosphate buffer solution (pH 7.0) to make exactly 250 mL. Pipet 10 mL of this solution, add exactly 5 mL of the internal standard solution, add more 0.05 mol/L phosphate buffer solution (pH 7.0) to make 50 mL, and use this solution as the sample solution. Separately, weigh accurately an amount of Ceftazidime RS, equivalent to about 25 mg (potency), and dissolve in 0.05 mol/L phosphate buffer solution (pH 7.0) to make exactly 25 mL. Pipet 10 mL of this solution, add exactly 5 mL of the internal standard solution, then add 0.05 mol/L phosphate buffer solution (pH 7.0) to make 50 mL, and use this solution as the standard solution. Then, proceed as directed in the Assay under Ceftazidime Hydrate.

Amount [mg (potency)] of ceftazidime ($C_{22}H_{22}N_6O_7S_2$)
$= M_S \times Q_T/Q_S \times 10$

M_S: Amount [mg(potency)] of Ceftazidime RS taken

Internal standard solution—A solution of dimedon in 0.05 mol/L phosphate buffer solution (pH 7.0) (11 in 10,000).

Containers and storage Containers—Hermetic containers.
Storage—Light-resistant.

Cefteram Pivoxil

セフテラム　ピボキシル

$C_{22}H_{27}N_9O_7S_2$: 593.64
2,2-Dimethylpropanoyloxymethyl (6*R*,7*R*)-7-[(*Z*)-2-(2-aminothiazol-4-yl)-2-(methoxyimino)acetylamino]-3-(5-methyl-2*H*-tetrazol-2-ylmethyl)-8-oxo-5-thia-1-azabicyclo[4.2.0]oct-2-ene-2-carboxylate
[*82547-58-8*, Cefteram]

Cefteram Pivoxil contains not less than 743 μg (potency) and not more than 824 μg (potency) per mg, calculated on the anhydrous basis. The potency of Cefteram Pivoxil is expressed as mass (potency) of cefteram ($C_{16}H_{17}N_9O_5S_2$: 479.49).

Description Cefteram Pivoxil occurs as a white to pale yellow-white powder.

It is very soluble in acetonitrile, freely soluble in methanol, in ethanol (95) and in chloroform, and practically insoluble in water.

Identification **(1)** Determine the absorption spectrum of a solution of Cefteram Pivoxil in 0.05 mol/L hydrochloric acid-methanol TS (1 in 100,000) as directed under Ultraviolet-visible Spectrophotometry <2.24>, and compare the spectrum with the Reference Spectrum: both spectra exhibit similar intensities of absorption at the same wavelengths.

(2) Determine the infrared absorption spectrum of Cefteram Pivoxil as directed in the potassium bromide disk method under Infrared Spectrophotometry <2.25>, and compare the spectrum with the Reference Spectrum: both spectra exhibit similar intensities of absorption at the same wave numbers.

(3) Determine the ^{1}H spectrum of a solution of Cefteram Pivoxil in deuterated chloroform for nuclear magnetic resonance spectroscopy (1 in 10) as directed under Nuclear Magnetic Resonance Spectroscopy <2.21>, using tetramethylsilane for nuclear magnetic resonance spectroscopy as an internal reference compound: it exhibits singlet signals A, B and C, at around δ 1.2 ppm, at around δ 2.5 ppm and at around δ 4.0 ppm, respectively. The ratio of the integrated intensity of these signals, A:B:C, is about 3:1:1.

Optical rotation <2.49> $[\alpha]_D^{20}$: +35 – +43° (0.4 g calculated on the anhydrous basis, methanol, 20 mL, 100 mm).

Purity **(1)** Heavy metals <1.07>—Proceed with 1.0 g of Cefteram Pivoxil according to Method 2, and perform the test. Prepare the control solution with 2.0 mL of Standard Lead Solution (not more than 20 ppm).

(2) Related substances—Dissolve 50 mg of Cefteram Pivoxil in 50 mL of the mobile phase, and use this solution as the sample solution. Pipet 1 mL of the sample solution, add the mobile phase to make exactly 50 mL, and use this solution as the standard solution. Perform the test with exactly 10 μL each of the sample solution and standard solution as directed under Liquid Chromatography <2.01> according to the following conditions, and determine each peak area by the automatic integration method: the each area of the peaks, having the relative retention time of about 0.2 and about 0.9 to cefteram pivoxil, obtained from the sample solution is not larger than 1/2 times and 1.25 times the peak area of cefteram pivoxil from the standard solution, respectively, the area of the peak other than cefteram pivoxil and the peaks mentioned above is not larger than 1/4 times the peak area of cefteram pivoxil from the standard solution, and the total area of the peaks other than cefteram pivoxil is not larger than 2.75 times the peak area of cefteram pivoxil from the standard solution. For the area of the peak, having the relative retention time of about 0.1 to cefteram pivoxil, multiply the correction factor, 0.74.

Operating conditions—

Detector, column, column temperature, mobile phase, and flow rate: Proceed as directed in the operating conditions in the Assay.

Time span of measurement: About 2 times as long as the retention time of cefteram pivoxil.

System suitability—

Test for required detectability: To exactly 1 mL of the standard solution add the mobile phase to make exactly 10 mL. Confirm that the peak area of cefteram pivoxil obtained with 10 μL of this solution is equivalent to 7 to 13% of that with 10 μL of the standard solution.

System performance: When the procedure is run with 10 μL of the standard solution under the above operating conditions, the number of theoretical plates and the symmetry factor of the peak of cefteram pivoxil are not less than 5000 and not more than 1.5, respectively.

System repeatability: When the test is repeated 6 times with 10 μL of the standard solution under the above operating conditions, the relative standard deviation of the peak area of cefteram pivoxil is not more than 3.0%.

Water <2.48> Not more than 3.0% (0.3 g, coulometric titration).

Assay Weigh accurately an amount of Cefteram Pivoxil and Cefteram Pivoxil Mesitylene Sulfonate RS, equivalent to about 40 mg (potency), dissolve each in 20 mL of diluted acetonitrile (1 in 2), add exactly 5 mL of the internal standard solution and diluted acetonitrile (1 in 2) to make 50 mL, and use these solutions as the sample solution and standard solution. Perform the test with 10 μL each of the sample solution and standard solution as directed under Liquid Chromatography <2.01> according to the following conditions, and calculate the ratios, Q_T and Q_S, of the peak area of cefteram pivoxil to that of the internal standard.

Amount [μg (potency)] of cefteram ($C_{16}H_{17}N_9O_5S_2$)
$= M_S \times Q_T/Q_S \times 1000$

M_S: Amount [mg (potency)] of Cefteram Pivoxil Mesitylene Sulfonate RS taken

Internal standard solution—A solution of methyl parahydroxybenzoate in diluted acetonitrile (1 in 2) (1 in 1000).

Operating conditions—

Detector: An ultraviolet absorption photometer (wavelength: 254 nm).

Column: A stainless steel column 4.6 mm in inside diameter and 15 cm in length, packed with octadecylsilanized silica gel for liquid chromatography (5 μm in particle diameter).

Column temperature: A constant temperature of about 25°C.

Mobile phase: To 100 mL of acetic acid-sodium acetate buffer solution (pH 5.0) add 375 mL of acetonitrile and water to make 1000 mL.

Flow rate: Adjust so that the retention time of cefteram pivoxil is about 14 minutes.

System suitability—

System performance: When the procedure is run with 10 μL of the standard solution under the above operating conditions, the internal standard and cefteram pivoxil are eluted in this order with the resolution between these peaks being not less than 3.

System repeatability: When the test is repeated 6 times with 10 μL of the standard solution under the above operating conditions, the relative standard deviation of the ratios of the peak area of cefteram pivoxil to that of the internal standard is not more than 1.0%.

Containers and storage Containers—Tight containers.

Storage—In a cold place.

Cefteram Pivoxil Fine Granules

セフテラム ピボキシル細粒

Cefteram Pivoxil Fine Granules contain not less than 90.0% and not more than 110.0% of the labeled potency of cefteram ($C_{16}H_{17}N_9O_5S_2$: 479.49).

Method of preparation Prepare as directed under Granules, with Cefteram Pivoxil.

Identification Powder Cefteram Pivoxil Fine Granules. To a portion of the powder, equivalent to 0.1 g (potency) of Cefteram Pivoxil, add 20 mL of methanol, shake well, and filter. To 1 mL of the filtrate add 0.05 mol/L hydrochloric acid-methanol TS to make 500 mL, and determine the absorption spectrum as directed under Ultraviolet-visible Spectrophotometry 〈*2.24*〉: it exhibits a maximum between 262 nm and 266 nm.

Purity Related substances—Powder Cefteram Pivoxil Fine Granules, if necessary. To a portion, equivalent to 0.1 g (potency) of Cefteram Pivoxil, add diluted acetonitrile (1 in 2) to make 100 mL, disperse the particle by sonicating, then filter, and use the filtrate as the sample solution. Pipet 1 mL of the sample solution, add the mobile phase to make exactly 50 mL, and use this solution as the standard solution. Perform the test with exactly 10 μL each of the sample solution and standard solution as directed under Liquid Chromatography 〈*2.01*〉 according to the following conditions, and determine each peak area by the automatic integration method: the area of the peak, having the relative retention time of about 0.9 to cefteram pivoxil obtained from the sample solution, is not larger than 1.75 times the peak area of cefteram pivoxil obtained from the standard solution, the area of the peak, having the relative retention time of about 0.1 from the sample solution, is not larger than 17/25 times the peak area of cefteram pivoxil from the standard solution, and the total area of the peaks other than cefteram pivoxil from the sample solution is not larger than 3.7 times the peak area of cefteram pivoxil from the standard solution. For the area of the peak, having the relative retention time of about 0.1 to cefteram pivoxil, multiply the correction factor, 0.74.

Operating conditions—

Proceed as directed in the operating conditions in the Purity (2) under Cefteram Pivoxil.

System suitability—

Proceed as directed in the system suitability in the Purity (2) under Cefteram Pivoxil.

Water 〈*2.48*〉 Not more than 0.3% (0.1 g (potency), coulometric titration).

Uniformity of dosage units 〈*6.02*〉 The Granules in single-dose packages meet the requirement of the Mass variation test.

Dissolution Being specified separately when the drug is granted approval based on the Law.

Assay Powder Cefteram Pivoxil Fine Granules, if necessary. Weigh accurately an amount of the powder, equivalent to about 0.3 g (potency) of Cefteram Pivoxil, add exactly 30 mL of the internal standard solution and diluted acetonitrile (1 in 2) to make 300 mL. Disperse the particle by sonicating, then filter, and use the filtrate as the sample solution. Separately, weigh accurately an amount of Cefteram Pivoxil Mesitylene Sulfonate RS, equivalent to about 50 mg (potency), dissolve in 20 mL of diluted acetonitrile (1 in 2), add exactly 5 mL of the internal standard solution and diluted acetonitrile (1 in 2) to make 50 mL, and use this solution as the standard solution. Perform the test with 10 μL each of the sample solution and standard solution as directed under Liquid Chromatography 〈*2.01*〉 according to the following conditions, and calculate the ratios, Q_T and Q_S, of the peak area of cefteram pivoxil to that of the internal standard.

$$\text{Amount [mg (potency)] of cefteram } (C_{16}H_{17}N_9O_5S_2) = M_S \times Q_T/Q_S \times 6$$

M_S: Amount [mg (potency)] of Cefteram Pivoxil Mesitylene Sulfonate RS taken

Internal standard solution—A solution of methyl parahydroxybenzoate in diluted acetonitrile (1:2) (1 in 1000).

Operating conditions—

Proceed as directed in the operating conditions in the Assay under Cefteram Pivoxil.

System suitability—

Proceed as directed in the system suitability in the Assay under Cefteram Pivoxil.

Containers and storage Containers—Tight containers.

Cefteram Pivoxil Tablets

セフテラム ピボキシル錠

Cefteram Pivoxil Tablets contain not less than 90.0% and not more than 110.0% of the labeled potency of cefteram ($C_{16}H_{17}N_9O_5S_2$: 479.49).

Method of preparation Prepare as directed under Tablets, with Cefteram Pivoxil.

Identification To a quantity of powdered Cefteram Pivoxil Tablets, equivalent to 0.1 g (potency) of Cefteram Pivoxil, add 20 mL of methanol, shake well, and filter. To 1 mL of the filtrate add 0.05 mol/L hydrochloric acid-methanol TS to make 500 mL. Determine the absorption spectrum of this solution as directed under Ultraviolet-visible Spectrophotometry 〈*2.24*〉: it exhibits a maximum between 262 nm and 266 nm.

Purity Related substances—To a quantity of powdered Cefteram Pivoxil Tablets, equivalent to 0.1 g (potency) of Cefteram Pivoxil, add diluted acetonitrile (1 in 2) to make 100 mL. Disperse this solution by sonicating, filter, and use the filtrate as the sample solution. Pipet 1 mL of the sample solution, add the mobile phase to make exactly 50 mL and use this solution as the standard solution. Perform the test with exactly 10 μL each of the sample solution and standard solution as directed under Liquid Chromatography 〈*2.01*〉 according to the following conditions. Determine each peak area of both solutions by the automatic integration method: the area of the peak, having the relative retention time of about 0.9 to cefteram pivoxil, obtained from the sample solution is not larger than 1.75 times the peak area of cefteram pivoxil from the standard solution, and the area of the peak, having the relative retention time of about 0.1 from the sample solution is not larger than 17/25 times the peak area of cefteram pivoxil from the standard solution. Furthermore, the total area of the peaks other than cefteram pivoxil from the sample solution is not larger than 3.7 times the peak area of cefteram pivoxil from the standard solution. For the area of the peak, having the relative retention time of about 0.1 to cefteram pivoxil, multiply the correction factor, 0.74.

Operating conditions—

Proceed as directed in the operating conditions in the Purity (2) under Cefteram Pivoxil.

System suitability—

Proceed as directed in the system suitability in the Purity (2) under Cefteram Pivoxil.

Water <*2.48*> Not more than 4.0% (a quantity equivalent to 0.2 g (potency) of powdered Cefteram Pivoxil Tablets, volumetric titration, direct titration).

Uniformity of dosage units <*6.02*> Perform the Mass variation test, or the Content uniformity test according to the following method: it meets the requirement.

To 1 tablet of Cefteram Pivoxil Tablets add exactly 5 mL of the internal standard solution per 50 mg (potency) of Cefteram Pivoxil, and add diluted acetonitrile (1 in 2) to make V mL so that each mL contains about 1 mg (potency) of Cefteram Pivoxil. Disperse this solution by sonicating, filter through a membrane filter with pore size of not exceeding 0.45 μm, discard the first 10 mL of the filtrate, and use the subsequent filtrate as the sample solution. Separately, weigh accurately an amount of Cefteram Pivoxil Mesitylene Sulfonate RS, equivalent to about 50 mg (potency), dissolve in 20 mL of diluted acetonitrile (1 in 2), add exactly 5 mL of the internal standard solution, add diluted acetonitrile (1 in 2) to make 50 mL, and use this solution as the standard solution. Then, proceed as directed in the Assay under Cefteram Pivoxil.

Amount [mg (potency)] of cefteram ($C_{16}H_{17}N_9O_5S_2$)
$= M_S \times Q_T/Q_S \times V/50$

M_S: Amount [mg (potency)] of Cefteram Pivoxil Mesitylene Sulfonate RS taken

Internal standard solution—A solution of methyl parahydroxybenzoate in diluted acetonitrile (1 in 2) (1 in 1000).

Dissolution <*6.10*> When the test is performed at 75 revolutions per minute according to the Paddle method, using 900 mL of water as the dissolution medium, the dissolution rate in 30 minutes of Cefteram Pivoxil Tablets is not less than 75%.

Start the test with 1 tablet of Cefteram Pivoxil Tablets, withdraw not less than 20 mL of the medium at the specified minute after starting the test, and filter through a membrane filter with a pore size not exceeding 0.45 μm. Discard not less than 10 mL of the first filtrate, pipet V mL of the subsequent filtrate, add water to make exactly V' mL so that each mL contains about 22 μg (potency) of Cefteram Pivoxil, and use this solution as the sample solution. Separately, weigh accurately an amount of Cefteram Pivoxil Mesitylene Sulfonate RS, equivalent to about 22 mg (potency), and dissolve in 20 mL of methanol, and add water to make exactly 50 mL. Pipet 5 mL of this solution, add water to make exactly 100 mL, and use this solution as the standard solution. Perform the test with the sample solution and standard solution as directed under Ultraviolet-visible Spectrophotometry <*2.24*>, using water as the blank, and determine the absorbances, A_T and A_S, at 300 nm.

Dissolution rate (%) with respect to the labeled amount of cefteram ($C_{16}H_{17}N_9O_5S_2$)
$= M_S \times A_T/A_S \times V'/V \times 1/C \times 90$

M_S: Amount [mg (potency)] of Cefteram Pivoxil Mesitylene Sulfonate RS taken

C: Labeled amount [mg (potency)] of cefteram ($C_{16}H_{17}N_9O_5S_2$) in 1 tablet

Assay To a number of tablet of Cefteram Pivoxil Tablets, equivalent to about 1.0 g (potency) of Cefteram Pivoxil, add 120 mL of diluted acetonitrile (1 in 2), disperse by sonicating, and add diluted acetonitrile (1 in 2) to make exactly 200 mL. Centrifuge this solution, pipet 10 mL of the supernatant liquid, add exactly 5 mL of the internal standard solution, add diluted acetonitrile (1 in 2) to make 50 mL, filter through a membrane filter with pore size not exceeding 0.45 μm, discard the first 3 mL of the filtrate, and use the subsequent filtrate as the sample solution. Separately, weigh accurately an amount of Cefteram Pivoxil Mesitylene Sulfonate RS, equivalent to about 50 mg (potency), dissolve in 20 mL of diluted acetonitrile (1 in 2), add exactly 5 mL of the internal standard solution, add diluted acetonitrile (1 in 2) to make 50 mL, and use this solution as the standard solution. Then, proceed as directed in the Assay under Cefteram Pivoxil.

Amount [mg (potency)] of cefteram ($C_{16}H_{17}N_9O_5S_2$)
$= M_S \times Q_T/Q_S \times 20$

M_S: Amount [mg (potency)] of Cefteram Pivoxil Mesitylene Sulfonate RS taken

Internal standard solution—A solution of methyl parahydroxybenzoate in diluted acetonitrile (1 in 2) (1 in 1000).

Containers and storage Containers—Tight containers.

Storage—Light-resistant.

Ceftibuten Hydrate

セフチブテン水和物

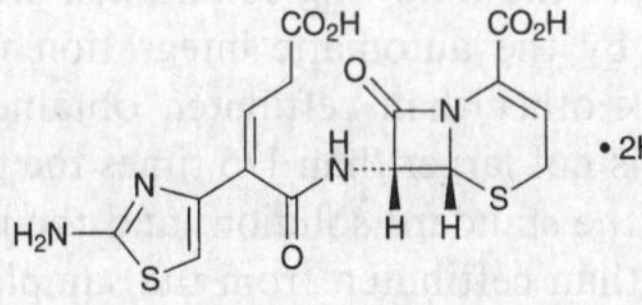

$C_{15}H_{14}N_4O_6S_2.2H_2O$: 446.46

(6*R*,7*R*)-7-[(2*Z*)-2-(2-Aminothiazol-4-yl)-4-carboxybut-2-enoylamino]-8-oxo-5-thia-1-azabicyclo[4.2.0]oct-2-ene-2-carboxylic acid dihydrate

[*118081-34-8*]

Ceftibuten Hydrate contains not less than 900 μg (potency) and not more than 1020 μg (potency) per mg, calculated on the anhydrous basis. The potency of Ceftibuten Hydrate is expressed as mass (potency) of ceftibuten ($C_{15}H_{14}N_4O_6S_2$: 410.42).

Description Ceftibuten Hydrate occurs as a white to pale yellow-white crystalline powder.

It is freely soluble in *N*,*N*-dimethylformamide and in dimethyl sulfoxide, and practically insoluble in water, in ethanol (95) and in diethyl ether.

Identification **(1)** Determine the absorption spectrum of a solution of Ceftibuten Hydrate in 0.1 mol/L phosphate buffer solution for antibiotics (pH 8.0) (1 in 50,000) as directed under Ultraviolet-visible Spectrophotometry <*2.24*>, and compare the spectrum with the Reference Spectrum: both spectra exhibit similar intensities of absorption at the same wavelengths.

(2) Determine the infrared absorption spectrum of Ceftibuten Hydrate as directed in the paste method under the Infrared Spectrophotometry <*2.25*>, and compare the spectrum with the Reference Spectrum: both spectra exhibit similar intensities of absorption at the same wave numbers.

(3) Determine the ^{1}H spectrum of a solution of Ceftibuten Hydrate in deuterated dimethyl sulfoxide for nuclear magnetic resonance spectroscopy (1 in 30), using tetramethylsilane for nuclear magnetic resonance spectroscopy as an internal reference compound, as directed under Nuclear Magnetic Resonance Spectroscopy *<2.21>*: it exhibits doublet signals A and B, at around δ 3.2 ppm and at around δ 5.1 ppm, a quartet signal C, at around δ 5.8 ppm, and a singlet signal D, at around δ 6.3 ppm. The ratio of integrated intensity of each signal except the signal at around δ 3.2 ppm, B:C:D is about 1:1:1.

Optical rotation *<2.49>* $[\alpha]_D^{20}$: +135 – +155° (0.3 g calculated on the anhydrous basis, 0.1 mol/L phosphate buffer solution for antibiotics, pH 8.0, 50 mL, 100 mm).

Purity (1) Heavy metals *<1.07>*—Proceed with 2.0 g of Ceftibuten Hydrate according to Method 2, and perform the test. Prepare the control solution with 2.0 mL of Standard Lead Solution (not more than 10 ppm).

(2) Related substances—(i) Keep the sample solution and the standard solution at not exceeding 5°C and use within 2 hours after preparation. Dissolve 25 mg of Ceftibuten Hydrate in 20 mL of 0.1 mol/L phosphate buffer solution for antibiotics (pH 8.0). To 4 mL of this solution add 0.1 mol/L phosphate buffer solution for antibiotics (pH 8.0) to make 20 mL, and use this solution as the sample solution. Pipet 5 mL of the sample solution, add 0.1 mol/L phosphate buffer solution for antibiotics (pH 8.0) to make exactly 100 mL, and use this solution as the standard solution. Perform the test with exactly 5 μL each of the sample solution and standard solution as directed under Liquid Chromatography *<2.01>* according to the following conditions, and determine each peak area by the automatic integration method: the area of the peak other than ceftibuten obtained from the sample solution is not larger than 1/5 times the peak area of ceftibuten from the standard solution, and the total area of the peaks other than ceftibuten from the sample solution is not larger than the peak area of ceftibuten from the standard solution.

Operating conditions—

Detector, column, column temperature, mobile phase, and flow rate: Proceed as directed in the operating conditions in the Assay.

Time span of measurement: About 1.7 times as long as the retention time of ceftibuten, beginning after the solvent peak.

System suitability—

Test for required detectability: Pipet 2 mL of the standard solution, and add 0.1 mol/L phosphate buffer solution for antibiotics (pH 8.0) to make exactly 20 mL. Confirm that the peak area of ceftibuten obtained with 5 μL of this solution is equivalent to 7 to 13% of that with 5 μL of the standard solution.

System performance: Dissolve 5 mg of Ceftibuten Hydrate in 20 mL of 0.1 mol/L hydrochloric acid TS, and allow to stand at 40°C for 1 hour. To 4 mL of this solution add 0.1 mol/L phosphate buffer solution for antibiotics (pH 8.0) to make 25 mL. When the procedure is run with 5 μL of this solution under the above operating conditions, trans-isomer of ceftibuten and ceftibuten are eluted in this order with the resolution between these peaks being not less than 2.0.

System repeatability: When the test is repeated 5 times with 5 μL of the standard solution under the above operating conditions, the relative standard deviation of the peak area of ceftibuten is not more than 2.0%.

(ii) Keep the sample solution at not exceeding 5°C, and use within 24 hours after preparation. To 5 mg of Ceftibuten Hydrate add 20 mL of the mobile phase, sonicate, if necessary, then shake to dissolve, filter through a membrane filter with a pore size not exceeding 0.45 μm, and use the filtrate as the sample solution. Perform the test with 10 μL of the sample solution as directed under Liquid Chromatography *<2.01>* according to the following conditions. Determine each peak area by the automatic integration method, and calculate their amounts by the area percentage method: the total amount of the peaks that are eluted faster than ceftibuten is not more than 5.0%. For the areas of these peaks, multiply the correction factor, 1.63, respectively.

Operating conditions—

Detector: An ultraviolet absorption photometer (wavelength: 263 nm).

Column: A stainless steel column 7.5 mm in inside diameter and 60 cm in length, packed with glycol etherified silica gel for liquid chromatography (10 μm in particle diameter).

Column temperature: A constant temperature of about 25°C.

Mobile phase: Dissolve 1.05 g of disodium hydrogen phosphate dodecahydrate and 0.58 g of potassium dihydrogen phosphate in water to make 1000 mL.

Flow rate: Adjust so that the retention time of ceftibuten is about 20 minutes.

Time span of measurement: About 1.6 times as long as the retention time of ceftibuten.

System suitability—

Test for required detectability: To 1 mL of the sample solution add the mobile phase to make 20 mL, and use this solution as the solution for system suitability test. Pipet 2 mL of the solution for system suitability test, and add the mobile phase to make exactly 20 mL. Confirm that the peak area of ceftibuten obtained with 10 μL of this solution is equivalent to 7 to 13% of that with 10 μL of the solution for system suitability test.

System performance: When the procedure is run with 10 μL of the solution for system suitability test under the above operating conditions, the number of theoretical plates and the symmetry factor of the peak of ceftibuten are not less than 10,000 and 0.8 – 1.2, respectively.

System repeatability: When the test is repeated 5 times with 10 μL of the solution for system suitability test under the above operating conditions, the relative standard deviation of the peak area of ceftibuten is not more than 1.7%.

Water *<2.48>* Not less than 8.0% and not more than 13.0% (0.2 g, volumetric titration, direct titration. Use a mixture of pyridine for water determination and ethylene glycol for water determination (5:1) instead of methanol for water determination).

Residue on ignition *<2.44>* Not more than 0.1% (1 g).

Assay Keep the sample solution and the standard solution at not exceeding 5°C and use within 2 hours after preparation. Weigh accurately an amount of Ceftibuten Hydrate and Ceftibuten Hydrochloride RS, equivalent to about 10 mg (potency), dissolve each in about 36 mL of 0.1 mol/L phosphate buffer solution for antibiotics (pH 8.0), add exactly 4 mL each of the internal standard solution, shake, and use these solutions as the sample solution and the standard solution, respectively. Perform the test with 5 μL each of the sample solution and standard solution as directed under Liquid Chromatography *<2.01>* according to the following conditions, and calculate the ratios, Q_T and Q_S, of the peak area of ceftibuten to that of the internal standard.

Amount [μg (potency)] of ceftibuten ($C_{15}H_{14}N_4O_6S_2$)
$= M_S \times Q_T/Q_S \times 1000$

M_S: Amount [mg (potency)] of Ceftibuten Hydrochloride RS taken

Internal standard solution—A solution of methyl parahydroxybenzoate in acetonitrile (3 in 4000).

Operating conditions—

Detector: An ultraviolet absorption photometer (wavelength: 263 nm).

Column: A stainless steel column 4 mm in inside diameter and 20 cm in length, packed with octadecylsilanized silica gel for liquid chromatography (7 μm in particle diameter).

Column temperature: A constant temperature of about 25°C.

Mobile phase: A mixture of 0.005 mol/L *n*-decyl trimethylammonium bromide TS and acetonitrile (4:1).

Flow rate: Adjust so that the retention time of ceftibuten is about 10 minutes.

System suitability—

System performance: Dissolve 5 mg of Ceftibuten Hydrate in 20 mL of 0.1 mol/L hydrochloric acid TS, and allow to stand at 40°C for 1 hour. To 4 mL of this solution add 0.1 mol/L phosphate buffer solution for antibiotics (pH 8.0) to make 25 mL. When the procedure is run with 5 μL of this solution under the above operating conditions, trans-isomer of ceftibuten and ceftibuten are eluted in this order with the resolution between these peaks being not less than 1.5.

System repeatability: When the test is repeated 6 times with 5 μL of the standard solution under the above operating conditions, the relative standard deviation of the ratio of the peak area of ceftibuten to that of the internal standard is not more than 1.0%.

Containers and storage Containers—Tight containers.

Storage—Light-resistant, and not exceeding 5°C.

Ceftizoxime Sodium

セフチゾキシムナトリウム

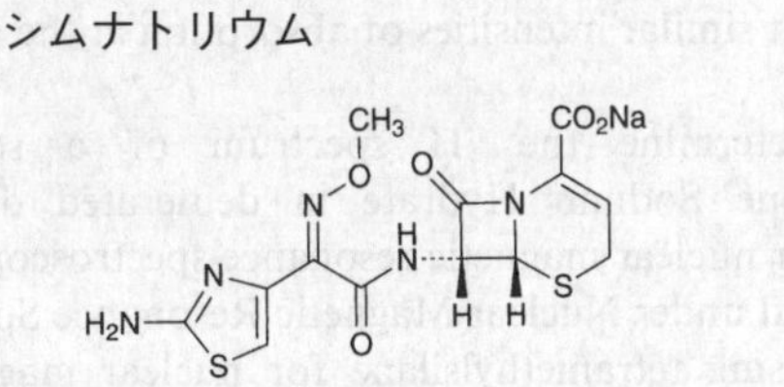

$C_{13}H_{12}N_5NaO_5S_2$: 405.38

Monosodium (6*R*,7*R*)-7-[(*Z*)-2-(2-aminothiazol-4-yl)-2-(methoxyimino)acetylamino]-8-oxo-5-thia-1-azabicyclo[4.2.0]oct-2-ene-2-carboxylate

[*68401-82-1*]

Ceftizoxime Sodium contains not less than 925 μg (potency) and not more than 965 μg (potency) per mg, calculated on the anhydrous basis. The potency of Ceftizoxime Sodium is expressed as mass (potency) of ceftizoxime ($C_{13}H_{13}N_5O_5S_2$: 383.40).

Description Ceftizoxime Sodium occurs as a white to light yellow, crystals or crystalline powder.

It is very soluble in water, sparingly soluble in methanol, and practically insoluble in ethanol (95).

Identification **(1)** Determine the absorption spectrum of a solution of Ceftizoxime Sodium (1 in 63,000) as directed under Ultraviolet-visible Spectrophotometry <*2.24*>, and compare the spectrum with the Reference Spectrum: both spectra exhibit similar intensities of absorption at the same wavelengths.

(2) Determine the infrared absorption spectrum of Ceftizoxime Sodium as directed in the potassium bromide disk method under Infrared Spectrophotometry <*2.25*>, and compare the spectrum with the Reference Spectrum: both spectra exhibit similar intensities of absorption at the same wave numbers.

(3) Determine the ^1H spectrum of a solution of Ceftizoxime Sodium in heavy water for nuclear magnetic resonance spectroscopy (1 in 10) as directed under Nuclear Magnetic Resonance Spectroscopy <*2.21*>, using sodium 3-trimethylsilylpropionate-d_4 for nuclear magnetic resonance spectroscopy as an internal reference compound: it exhibits a singlet signal A at around δ 4.0 ppm, a multiplet signal B around δ 6.3 ppm, and a singlet signal C at around δ 7.0 ppm. The ratio of integrated intensity of each signal, A:B:C, is about 3:1:1.

(4) Ceftizoxime Sodium responds to Qualitative Tests <*1.09*> (1) for sodium salt.

Optical rotation <*2.49*> $[\alpha]_D^{20}$: +125 – +145° (0.25 g calculated on the anhydrous bases, water, 25 mL, 100 mm).

pH <*2.54*> Dissolve 1.0 g of Ceftizoxime Sodium in 10 mL of water: the pH of the solution is between 6.0 and 8.0.

Purity **(1)** Clarity and color of solution—Dissolve 1.0 g of Ceftizoxime Sodium in 10 mL of water: the solution is clear. Perform the test with this solution as directed under Method for Color Matching <*2.65*>: the color is not more colored than Matching Fluid M.

(2) Heavy metals <*1.07*>—Proceed with 2.0 g of Ceftizoxime Sodium according to Method 2, and perform the test. Prepare the control solution with 2.0 mL of Standard Lead Solution (not more than 10 ppm).

(3) Arsenic <*1.11*>—Prepare the test solution with 2.0 g of Ceftizoxime Sodium according to Method 3, and perform the test (not more than 1 ppm).

(4) Related substances—Dissolve 0.11 g of Ceftizoxime Sodium in 100 mL of 0.1 mol/L phosphate buffer solution (pH 7.0) and use this solution as the sample solution. Perform the test with 5 μL of the sample solution as directed under Liquid Chromatography <*2.01*> according to the following conditions, and determine the areas of each peak by the automatic integration method: each peak area other than ceftizoxime is not more than 0.5% of the peak area of ceftizoxime, and the total area of peaks other than ceftizoxime is not more than 1.0% of that of ceftizoxime.

Operating conditions—

Detector, column, and column temperature: Proceed as directed in the operating conditions in the Assay.

Mobile phase: Dissolve 2.31 g of disodium hydrogenphosphate dodecahydrate and 1.42 g of citric acid monohydrate in 1000 mL of water, adjust to pH 3.6 with diluted phosphoric acid (1 in 10) or dilute sodium hydroxide TS. To 200 mL of this solution add 10 mL of acetonitrile.

Flow rate: Adjust so that the retention time of ceftizoxime is about 12 minutes.

Time span of measurement: About 5 times as long as the retention time of ceftizoxime, beginning after the solvent peak.

System suitability—

Test for required detectability: Pipet 1 mL of the sample solution, add 0.1 mol/L phosphate buffer solution (pH 7.0) to make exactly 100 mL, and use this solution as the solution for test for required detectability. Pipet 1 mL of the solution, add 0.1 mol/L phosphate buffer solution (pH 7.0) to make exactly 10 mL, and confirm that the peak area of ceftizoxime obtained with 5 μL of this solution is equivalent to 7 to 13% of that with 5 μL of the solution for test for required detectability.

System performance: Dissolve about 10 mg of Ceftizoxime RS in 100 mL of 0.1 mol/L phosphate buffer solution (pH 7.0) and use this solution as the solution for system suitability test. When the procedure is run with 5 μL of this solution under the above operating conditions, the number of theoretical plates and the symmetry factor of the peak of ceftizoxime are not less than 4000 and not more than 2.0, respectively.

System repeatability: When the test is repeated 6 times with 5 μL of the solution for system suitability test under the above operating conditions, the relative standard deviation of the peak areas of ceftizoxime is not more than 2.0%.

Water <*2.48*> Not more than 8.5% (0.4 g, volumetric titration, direct titration).

Assay Weigh accurately an amount of Ceftizoxime Sodium and Ceftizoxime RS, equivalent to about 25 mg (potency), dissolve each in 0.1 mol/L phosphate buffer solution (pH 7.0), add exactly 20 mL of the internal standard solution, then add 0.1 mol/L phosphate buffer solution (pH 7.0) to make 50 mL, and use these solutions as the sample solution and the standard solution, respectively. Perform the test with 5 μL each of the sample solution and standard solution as directed under Liquid Chromatography <*2.01*> according to the following conditions, and calculate the ratios, Q_T and Q_S, of the peak area of ceftizoxime to that of the internal standard.

Amount [μg (potency)] of ceftizoxime ($C_{13}H_{13}N_5O_5S_2$)
$= M_S \times Q_T/Q_S \times 1000$

M_S: Amount [mg (potency)] of Ceftizoxime RS taken

Internal standard solution—A solution of 3-hydroxybenzoic acid in 0.1 mol/L phosphate buffer solution (pH 7.0) (3 in 400).

Operating conditions—

Detector: An ultraviolet absorption photometer (wavelength: 254 nm).

Column: A stainless steel column 4.6 mm in inside diameter and 25 cm in length, packed with octadecylsilanized silica gel for liquid chromatography (10 μm in particle diameter).

Column temperature: A constant temperature of about 35°C.

Mobile phase: Dissolve 2.31 g of disodium hydrogen phosphate dodecahydrate and 1.42 g of citric acid monohydrate in 1000 mL of water, and adjust to pH 3.6 with diluted phosphoric acid (1 in 10) or dilute sodium hydroxide TS. To 450 mL of this solution add 50 mL of acetonitrile.

Flow rate: Adjust so that the retention time of ceftizoxime is about 4 minutes.

System suitability—

System performance: When the procedure is run with 5 μL of the standard solution under the above operating conditions, ceftizoxime and the internal standard are eluted in this order with the resolution between these peaks being not less than 7.0 and the symmetry factor of each peak is not more than 1.5.

System repeatability: When the test is repeated 6 times with 5 μL of the standard solution under the above operating conditions, the relative standard deviation of the ratio of the peak area of ceftizoxime to that of the internal standard is not more than 1.0%.

Containers and storage Containers—Tight containers.

Storage—Light-resistant.

Ceftriaxone Sodium Hydrate

セフトリアキソンナトリウム水和物

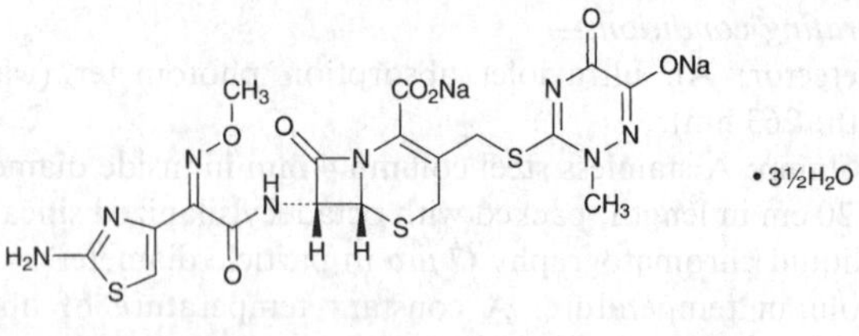

$C_{18}H_{16}N_8Na_2O_7S_3.3\frac{1}{2}H_2O$: 661.60

Disodium (6*R*,7*R*)-7-[(*Z*)-2-(2-aminothiazol-4-yl)-2-(methoxyimino)acetylamino]-3-(6-hydroxy-2-methyl-5-oxo-2,5-dihydro-1,2,4-triazin-3-ylsulfanylmethyl)-8-oxo-5-thia-1-azabicyclo[4.2.0]oct-2-ene-2-carboxylate hemiheptahydrate

[*104376-79-6*]

Ceftriaxone Sodium Hydrate contains not less than 905 μg (potency) and not more than 935 μg (potency) per mg, calculated on the anhydrous basis. The potency of Ceftriaxone Sodium Hydrate is expressed as mass (potency) of ceftriaxone ($C_{18}H_{18}N_8O_7S_3$: 554.58).

Description Ceftriaxone Sodium Hydrate occurs as a white to yellow-white crystalline powder.

It is freely soluble in water and in dimethylsulfoxide, sparingly soluble in methanol, very slightly soluble in ethanol (99.5), and practically insoluble in acetonitrile.

Identification **(1)** Determine the absorption spectrum of a solution of Ceftriaxone Sodium Hydrate (1 in 100,000) as directed under Ultraviolet-visible Spectrophotometry <*2.24*>, and compare the spectrum with the Reference Spectrum or the spectrum of a solution of Ceftriaxone Sodium RS prepared in the same manner as the sample solution: both spectra exhibit similar intensities of absorption at the same wavelengths.

(2) Determine the ^{1}H spectrum of a solution of Ceftriaxone Sodium Hydrate in deuterated dimethylsulfoxide for nuclear magnetic resonance spectroscopy (1 in 10) as directed under Nuclear Magnetic Resonance Spectroscopy <*2.21*>, using tetramethylsilane for nuclear magnetic resonance spectroscopy as an internal reference compound: it exhibits singlet signals, A, B, C and D, at around δ 3.5 ppm, at around δ 3.8 ppm, at around δ 6.7 ppm and at around δ 7.2 ppm, respectively. The ratio of integrated intensity of each signal, A: B: C: D, is about 3:3:1:2. When the signal at around δ 3.5 ppm overlaps with the signal of water, perform the measurement in the probe kept at about 50°C.

(3) Ceftriaxone Sodium Hydrate responds to Qualitative Tests <*1.09*> (1) for sodium salt.

Optical rotation <*2.49*> $[\alpha]_D^{20}$: $-153 - -170°$ (50 mg calculated on the anhydrous basis, water, 2.5 mL, 20 mm).

pH <*2.54*> Dissolve 0.6 g of Ceftriaxone Sodium Hydrate in 5 mL of water: the pH of the solution is between 6.0 and 8.0.

Purity **(1)** Clarity and color of solution—Dissolve 0.6 g of Ceftriaxone Sodium Hydrate in 5 mL of water: the solution is clear and light yellow.

(2) Heavy metals <*1.07*>—Proceed with 1.0 g of Ceftriaxone Sodium Hydrate according to Method 2, and

perform the test. Prepare the control solution with 2.0 mL of Standard Lead Solution (not more than 20 ppm).

(3) Arsenic <*1.11*>—Prepare the test solution with 1.0 g of Ceftriaxone Sodium Hydrate according to Method 3, and perform the test (not more than 2 ppm).

(4) Related substances 1—Dissolve 20 mg of Ceftriaxone Sodium Hydrate in 10 mL of the mobile phase, and use this solution as the sample solution. Pipet 1 mL of the sample solution, add a mixture of water and acetonitrile for liquid chromatography (11:9) to make exactly 100 mL, and use this solution as the standard solution. Perform the test with exactly 10 μL each of the sample solution and standard solution as directed under Liquid Chromatography <*2.01*> according to the following conditions, and determine each peak area by the automatic integration method: the peak areas of the impurity 1 having the relative retention time of about 0.5 and the impurity 2 having the relative retention time of about 1.3 to ceftriaxone obtained from the sample solution are not larger than the peak area of ceftriaxone from the standard solution. For the areas of the peaks, the impurity 1 and the impurity 2, multiply their correction factors 0.9 and 1.2, respectively.

Operating conditions—

Detector: An ultraviolet absorption photometer (wavelength: 254 nm).

Column: A stainless steel column 4.6 mm in inside diameter and 25 cm in length, packed with octadecylsilanized silica gel for liquid chromatography (10 μm in particle diameter).

Column temperature: A constant temperature of about 25°C.

Mobile phase: Dissolve 5.796 g of anhydrous disodium hydrogen phosphate and 3.522 g of potassium dihydrogen phosphate in water to make exactly 1000 mL, and use this solution as the solution A. Separately, dissolve 20.256 g of citric acid monohydrate and 7.840 g of sodium hydroxide in water to make exactly 1000 mL, and use this solution as the solution B. Dissolve 4.00 g of tetra-*n*-heptylammonium bromide in 450 mL of acetonitrile for liquid chromatography, add 55 mL of the solution A, 5 mL of the solution B and 490 mL of water.

Flow rate: Adjust so that the retention time of ceftriaxone is about 7 minutes.

Time span of measurement: About 2 times as long as the retention time of ceftriaxone.

System suitability—

Test for required detectability: To 5 mL of the sample solution, add a mixture of water and acetonitrile for liquid chromatography (11:9) to make 200 mL, and use this solution as the solution for system suitability test. Pipet 1 mL of the solution for system suitability test, and add a mixture of water and acetonitrile for liquid chromatography (11:9) to make exactly 100 mL. Confirm that the peak area of ceftriaxone obtained with 10 μL of this solution is equivalent to 0.9 to 1.1% of that with 10 μL of the solution for system suitability test.

System performance: Dissolve 10 mg of Ceftriaxone Sodium Hydrate in a mixture of water and acetonitrile for liquid chromatography (11:9) to make 5 mL, add 5 mL of a solution of diethyl terephthalate in a mixture of water and acetonitrile for liquid chromatography (11:9) (9 in 5000), and add a mixture of water and acetonitrile for liquid chromatography (11:9) to make 200 mL. When the procedure is run with 10 μL of this solution under the above operating conditions, ceftriaxone and diethyl terephthalate are eluted in this order, with the resolution between these peaks being not less than 6.

System repeatability: When the test is repeated 6 times with 10 μL of the solution for system suitability test under the above operating conditions, the relative standard deviation of the peak area of ceftriaxone is not more than 1.0%.

(5) Related substances 2—Dissolve 10 mg of Ceftriaxone Sodium Hydrate in 10 mL of the mobile phase, and use this solution as the sample solution. Pipet 1 mL of the sample solution, add a mixture of acetonitrile for liquid chromatography and water (23:11) to make exactly 100 mL, and use this solution as standard solution. Perform the test with exactly 10 μL each of the sample solution and standard solution as directed under Liquid Chromatography <*2.01*> according to the following conditions, and determine each peak area by the automatic integration method: the each peak area of the impurities which appear after the peak of ceftriaxone obtained from the sample solution is not larger than the peak area of ceftriaxone from the standard solution, and the total peak area of these impurities is not larger than 2.5 times of the peak area from the standard solution.

Operating conditions—

Detector: An ultraviolet absorption photometer (wavelength: 254 nm).

Column: A stainless steel column 4.6 mm in inside diameter and 25 cm in length, packed with octadecylsilanized silica gel for liquid chromatography (10 μm in particle diameter).

Column temperature: A constant temperature of about 25°C.

Mobile phase: Dissolve 5.796 g of anhydrous disodium hydrogen phosphate and 3.522 g of potassium dihydrogen phosphate in water to make exactly 1000 mL, and use this solution as the solution A. Separately, dissolve 20.256 g of citric acid monohydrate and 7.840 g of sodium hydroxide in water to make exactly 1000 mL, and use this solution as the solution B. Dissolve 4.00 g of tetra-*n*-heptylammonium bromide in 450 mL of acetonitrile for liquid chromatography, and add 55 mL of the solution A, 5 mL of the solution B, 490 mL of water and 700 mL of acetonitrile for liquid chromatography.

Flow rate: Adjust so that the retention time of ceftriaxone is about 3 minutes.

Time span of measurement: About 10 times as long as the retention time of ceftriaxone.

System suitability—

Test for required detectability: Measure 5 mL of the sample solution, add a mixture of acetonitrile for liquid chromatography and water (23:11) to make 100 mL, and use this solution as the solution for system suitability test. Measure exactly 1 mL of the solution for system suitability test, and add a mixture of acetonitrile for liquid chromatography and water (23:11) to make exactly 100 mL. Confirm that the peak area of ceftriaxone obtained with 10 μL of this solution is equivalent to 0.9 to 1.1% of that with 10 μL of the solution for system suitability test.

System performance: Dissolve 10 mg of Ceftriaxone Sodium Hydrate in a mixture of acetonitrile for liquid chromatography and water (23:11) to make 5 mL, add 5 mL of a solution of diethyl terephthalate in a mixture of water and acetonitrile for liquid chromatography (11:9) (9 in 5000), and add a mixture of acetonitrile for liquid chromatography and water (23:11) to make 200 mL. When the procedure is run with 10 μL of this solution under the above operating conditions, ceftriaxone and diethyl terephthalate are eluted in this order with the resolution between these peaks being not less than 3.

System repeatability: When the test is repeated 6 times with 10 μL of the solution for system suitability test under the above operating conditions, the relative standard deviation of the peak area of ceftriaxone is not more than 1.0%.

Water <2.48> Not less than 8.0% and not more than 11.0% (0.15 g, volumetric titration, direct titration).

Assay Weigh accurately an amount of Ceftriaxone Sodium Hydrate and Ceftriaxone Sodium RS, equivalent to about 0.1 g (potency), dissolve each in a mixture of water and acetonitrile for liquid chromatography (11:9) to make exactly 50 mL. Pipet 5 mL of each solution, add exactly 5 mL of the internal standard solution and a mixture of water and acetonitrile for liquid chromatography (11:9) to make 200 mL, and use these solutions as the sample solution and the standard solution, respectively. Perform the test with 10 μL each of the sample solution and standard solution as directed under Liquid Chromatography <2.01> according to the following conditions, and calculate the ratios, Q_T and Q_S, of the peak area of ceftriaxone to that of the internal standard.

$$\text{Amount [}\mu\text{g (potency)] of ceftriaxone } (C_{18}H_{18}N_8O_7S_3) = M_S \times Q_T/Q_S \times 1000$$

M_S: Amount [mg (potency)] of Ceftriaxone Sodium RS taken

Internal standard solution—A solution of diethyl terephthalate in a mixture of water and acetonitrile for liquid chromatography (11:9) (9 in 5000).

Operating conditions—

Detector: An ultraviolet absorption photometer (wavelength: 254 nm).

Column: A stainless steel column 4.6 mm in inside diameter and 25 cm in length, packed with octadecylsilanized silica gel for liquid chromatography (10 μm in particle diameter).

Column temperature: A constant temperature of about 25°C.

Mobile phase: Dissolve 5.796 g of anhydrous disodium hydrogen phosphate and 3.522 g of potassium dihydrogen phosphate in water to make exactly 1000 mL, and use this solution as solution A. Dissolve 20.256 g of citric acid monohydrate and 7.840 g of sodium hydroxide in water to make exactly 1000 mL, and use this solution as solution B. Dissolve 4.00 g of tetra-*n*-heptylammonium bromide in 450 mL of acetonitrile for liquid chromatography, and add 490 mL of water, 55 mL of solution A, and 5 mL of solution B.

Flow rate: Adjust so that the retention time of ceftriaxone is about 7 minutes.

System suitability—

System performance: When the procedure is run with 10 μL of the standard solution under the above operating conditions, ceftriaxone and the internal standard are eluted in this order with the resolution between these peaks being not less than 6.

System repeatability: When the test is repeated 6 times with 10 μL of the standard solution under the above operating conditions, the relative standard deviation of the ratios of the peak area of ceftriaxone to that of the internal standard is not more than 1.0%.

Containers and storage Containers—Tight containers.

Storage—Light-resistant.

Cefuroxime Axetil

セフロキシム アキセチル

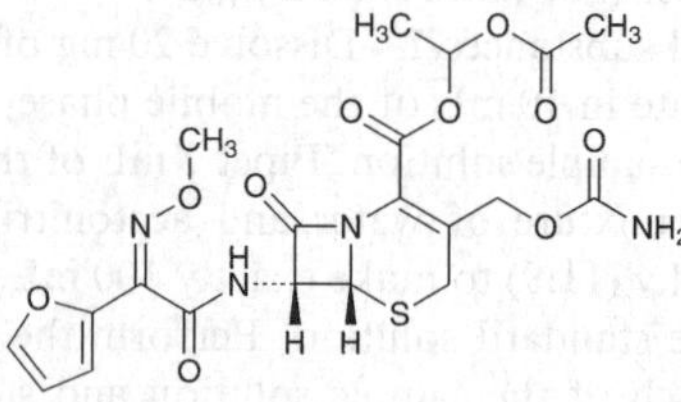

$C_{20}H_{22}N_4O_{10}S$: 510.47

(1*RS*)-1-Acetoxyethyl (6*R*,7*R*)-3-carbamoyloxymethyl-7-[(*Z*)-2-furan-2-yl-2-(methoxyimino)acetylamino]-8-oxo-5-thia-1-azabicyclo[4.2.0]oct-2-ene-2-carboxylate

[64544-07-6]

Cefuroxime Axetil contains not less than 800 μg (potency) and not more than 850 μg (potency) per mg, calculated on the anhydrous and acetone-free basis. The potency of Cefuroxime Axetil is expressed as mass (potency) of cefuroxime ($C_{16}H_{16}N_4O_8S$: 424.39).

Description Cefuroxime Axetil occurs as white to yellow-white non-crystalline powder.

It is freely soluble in dimethylsulfoxide, soluble in methanol, sparingly soluble in ethanol (95), and very slightly soluble in water.

Identification (1) Determine the absorption spectrum of a solution of Cefuroxime Axetil in methanol (3 in 200,000) as directed under Ultraviolet-visible Spectrophotometry <2.24>, and compare the spectrum with the Reference Spectrum or the spectrum of a solution of Cefuroxime Axetil RS prepared in the same manner as the sample solution: both spectra exhibit similar intensities of absorption at the same wavelengths.

(2) Determine the infrared absorption spectrum of Cefuroxime Axetil as directed in the potassium bromide disk method under Infrared Spectrophotometry <2.25>, and compare the spectrum with the Reference Spectrum or the spectrum of Cefuroxime Axetil RS: both spectra exhibit similar intensities of absorption at the same wave numbers.

(3) Determine the ^{1}H spectrum of a solution of Cefuroxime Axetil in deuterated dimethylsulfoxide for nuclear magnetic resonance spectroscopy (1 in 20) as directed under Nuclear Magnetic Resonance Spectroscopy <2.21>, using tetramethylsilane for nuclear magnetic resonance spectroscopy as an internal reference compound: it exhibits a doublet signal or a pair of doublet signals A at around δ 1.5 ppm, a pair of singlet signals B at around δ 2.1 ppm, and a singlet signal C at around δ 3.9 ppm. The ratio of the integrated intensity of each signal, A:B:C, is about 1:1:1.

Optical rotation <2.49> $[\alpha]_D^{20}$: +41 – +47° (0.5 g, methanol, 50 mL, 100 mm).

Purity (1) Heavy metals <1.07>—Proceed with 2.0 g of Cefuroxime Axetil according to Method 2, and perform the test. Prepare the control solution with 2.0 mL of Standard Lead Solution (not more than 10 ppm).

(2) Related substances—Dissolve 25 mg of Cefuroxime Axetil in 4 mL of methanol, add a solution of ammonium dihydrogenphosphate (23 in 1000) to make 10 mL, and use this solution as the sample solution. Pipet 1 mL of the sample solution, add 40 mL of methanol and a solution of ammonium dihydrogenphosphate (23 in 1000) to make exactly

100 mL, and use this solution as the standard solution. Perform the test with exactly 2 μL each of the sample solution and standard solution as directed under Liquid Chromatography <*2.01*> according to the following conditions, and determine each peak area by the automatic integration method: the area of the peak other than cefuroxime axetil obtained from the sample solution is not larger than 1.5 times the total area of the two peaks of cefuroxime axetil from the standard solution, and the total area of the peaks other than cefuroxime axetil from the sample solution is not larger than 4 times the total area of the two peaks of cefuroxime axetil from the standard solution.

Operating conditions—

Detector, column, column temperature, mobile phase, and flow rate: Proceed as directed in the operating conditions in the Assay.

Time span of measurement: About 3 times as long as the retention time of the peak having the larger retention time of the two peaks of cefuroxime axetil, beginning after the solvent peak.

System suitability—

Test for required detectability: Pipet 1 mL of the standard solution, and add 4 mL of methanol and a solution of ammonium dihydrogenphosphate (23 in 1000) to make exactly 10 mL. Confirm that the total area of the two peaks of cefuroxime axetil obtained with 2 μL of this solution is equivalent to 7 to 13% of that with 2 μL of the standard solution.

System performance: When the procedure is run with 2 μL of the standard solution under the above operating conditions, the resolution between the two peaks of cefuroxime axetil is not less than 1.5.

System repeatability: When the test is repeated 6 times with 2 μL of the standard solution under the above operating conditions, the relative standard deviation of the total area of the two peaks of cefuroxime axetil is not more than 2.0%.

(3) Acetone—Weigh accurately about 1 g of Cefuroxime Axetil, add exactly 0.2 mL of the internal standard solution and dimethylsulfoxide to make 10 mL, and use this solution as the sample solution. Separately, weigh accurately about 0.5 g of acetone, and add dimethylsulfoxide to make exactly 100 mL. Pipet 0.2 mL of this solution, add exactly 0.2 mL of the internal standard solution and dimethylsulfoxide to make 10 mL, and use this solution as the standard solution. Perform the test with 1 μL each of the sample solution and standard solution as directed under Gas Chromatography <*2.02*> according to the following conditions, and calculate the ratios, Q_T and Q_S, of the peak area of acetone to that of the internal standard: the amount of acetone is not more than 1.3%.

$$\text{Amount (\%) of acetone} = M_S/M_T \times Q_T/Q_S \times 1/5$$

M_S: Amount (g) of acetone taken

M_T: Amount (g) of Cefuroxime Axetil taken

Internal standard solution—A solution of 1-propanol in dimethylsulfoxide (1 in 200).

Operating conditions—

Detector: A hydrogen flame-ionization detector.

Column: A glass column 3 mm in inside diameter and 2 m in length, packed with siliceous earth for gas chromatography coated with a mixture of polyethylene glycol 600 for gas chromatography and polyethylene glycol 1500 for gas chromatography (1:1) in the ratio of 20% (125 - 150 μm in particle diameter).

Column temperature: A constant temperature of about 90°C.

Temperature of injection port: A constant temperature of about 115°C.

Carrier gas: Nitrogen.

Flow rate: Adjust so that the retention time of the internal standard is about 4 minutes.

System suitability—

System performance: When the procedure is run with 1 μL of the standard solution under the above operating conditions, acetone and the internal standard are eluted in this order with the resolution between these peaks being not less than 5.

System repeatability: When the test is repeated 6 times with 1 μL of the standard solution under the above operating conditions, the relative standard deviation of the ratio of the peak area of acetone to that of the internal standard is not more than 5.0%.

Water <*2.48*> Not more than 2.0% (0.4 g, volumetric titration, direct titration).

Residue on ignition <*2.44*> Not more than 0.2% (0.5 g).

Isomer ratio Perform the test with 10 μL of the sample solution obtained in the Assay as directed under Liquid Chromatography <*2.01*> according to the following conditions, and determine the area, A_a, of the peak having the smaller retention time and the area, A_b, of the peak having the bigger retention time of the two peaks of cefuroxime axetil: $A_b/(A_a + A_b)$ is between 0.48 and 0.55.

Operating conditions—

Detector, column, column temperature, mobile phase, and flow rate: Proceed as directed in the operating conditions in the Assay.

System suitability—

System performance, and system repeatability: Proceed as directed in the system suitability in the Assay.

Assay Weigh accurately an amount of Cefuroxime Axetil and Cefuroxime Axetil RS, equivalent to about 50 mg (potency), and dissolve each in methanol to make exactly 50 mL. Pipet 10 mL each of these solutions, add exactly 5 mL of the internal standard solution, 5 mL of methanol and a solution of ammonium dihydrogen phosphate (23 in 1000) to make 50 mL, and use these solutions as the sample solution and standard solution. Perform the test with 10 μL each of the sample solution and standard solution as directed under Liquid Chromatography <*2.01*> according to the following conditions, and calculate the ratios, Q_T and Q_S, of the sum area of the two peaks of cefuroxime axetil to the peak area of the internal standard.

$$\text{Amount [}\mu\text{g (potency)] of cefuroxime } (C_{16}H_{16}N_4O_8S) = M_S \times Q_T/Q_S \times 1000$$

M_S: Amount [mg (potency)] of Cefuroxime Axetil RS taken

Internal standard solution—A solution of acetanilide in methanol (27 in 5000).

Operating conditions—

Detector: An ultraviolet absorption photometer (wavelength: 278 nm).

Column: A stainless steel column 4.6 mm in inside diameter and 20 cm in length, packed with trimethylsilanized silica gel for liquid chromatography (5 μm in particle diameter).

Column temperature: A constant temperature of about 25°C.

Mobile phase: A mixture of a solution of ammonium dihydrogen phosphate (23 in 1000) and methanol (5:3).

Flow rate: Adjust so that the retention time of the peak

having the smaller retention time of the two peaks of cefuroxime axetil is about 8 minutes.

System suitability—

System performance: When the procedure is run with 10 μL of the standard solution under the above operating conditions, the internal standard and cefuroxime axetil are eluted in this order with the resolution between the two peaks of cefuroxime axetil being not less than 1.5.

System repeatability: When the test is repeated 6 times with 10 μL of the standard solution under the above operating conditions, the relative standard deviation of the ratios of the sum area of the two peaks of cefuroxime axetil to the peak area of the internal standard is not more than 1.0%.

Containers and storage Containers—Tight containers.

Storage—Light-resistant.

Celecoxib

セレコキシブ

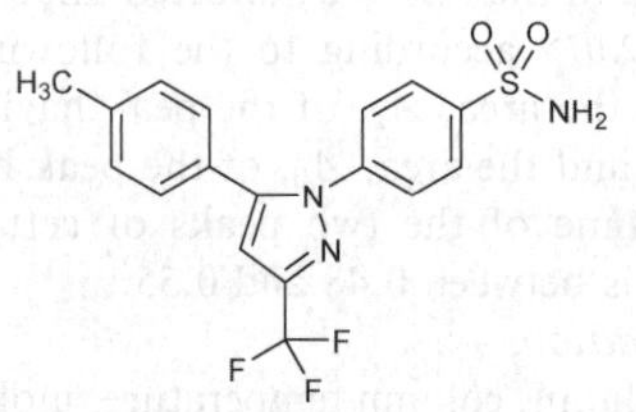

$C_{17}H_{14}F_3N_3O_2S$: 381.37

4-[5-(4-Methylphenyl)-3-(trifluoromethyl)-1*H*-pyrazol-1-yl]benzenesulfonamide

[169590-42-5]

Celecoxib contains not less than 98.0% and not more than 102.0% of celecoxib ($C_{17}H_{14}F_3N_3O_2S$), calculated on the anhydrous basis.

Description Celecoxib occurs as a white, powder or crystalline powder.

It is freely soluble in methanol, soluble in ethanol (99.5), and practically insoluble in water.

Melting point: 161 – 164°C

Celecoxib shows crystal polymorphism.

Identification **(1)** Determine the absorption spectrum of a solution of Celecoxib in methanol (1 in 100,000) as directed under Ultraviolet-visible Spectrophotometry <*2.24*>, and compare the spectrum with the Reference Spectrum or the spectrum of a solution of Celecoxib RS prepared in the same manner as the sample solution: both spectra exhibit similar intensities of absorption at the same wavelengths.

(2) Determine the infrared absorption spectrum of Celecoxib, as directed in the potassium bromide disk method under Infrared Spectrophotometry <*2.25*>, and compare the spectrum with the Reference Spectrum or the spectrum of Celecoxib RS: both spectra exhibit similar intensities of absorption at the same wave numbers.

Purity **(1)** Heavy metals <*1.07*>—Proceed with 1.0 g of Celecoxib according to Method 4, and perform the test. Prepare the control solution with 2.0 mL of Standard Lead Solution (not more than 20 ppm).

(2) Related substances—Use the sample solution obtained in the Assay as the sample solution. Separately, weigh accurately about 50 mg of Celecoxib RS, dissolve in a mixture of methanol and water (3:1) to make exactly 100 mL. Pipet 1 mL of this solution, add a mixture of methanol and water (3:1) to make exactly 100 mL, and use this solution as the standard solution. Perform the test with exactly 25 μL each of the sample solution and standard solution as directed under Liquid Chromatography <*2.01*> according to the following conditions. Determine each peak area, A_T, in the sample solution and the peak area of celecoxib, A_S, in the standard solution by the automatic integration method, and calculate the amount of the related substances by the following equation: the amount of related substance A having the relative retention time of about 0.94 to celecoxib is not more than 0.4%, and each amount of the related substances other than related substance A is not more than 0.10%. Furthermore, the total amount of the related substances is not more than 0.5%.

$$\text{Amount (\%) of related substance} = M_S/M_T \times A_T/A_S$$

M_S: Amount (mg) of Celecoxib RS taken
M_T: Amount (mg) of Celecoxib taken

Operating conditions—

Detector, column, column temperature, mobile phase, and flow rate: Proceed as directed in the operating conditions in the Assay.

Time span of measurement: About 1.5 times as long as the retention time of celecoxib, beginning after the solvent peak.

System suitability—

System performance and system repeatability: Proceed as directed in the system suitability in the Assay.

Test for required detectability: Pipet 5 mL of the standard solution, and add a mixture of methanol and water (3:1) to make exactly 100 mL. Confirm that the peak area of celecoxib obtained with 25 μL of this solution is equivalent to 3.5 to 6.5% of that with 25 μL of the standard solution.

Water <*2.48*> Not more than 0.5% (0.3 g, volumetric titration, direct titration).

Residue on ignition <*2.44*> Not more than 0.2% (1.0 g, platinum crucible).

Assay Weigh accurately about 50 mg each of Celecoxib and Celecoxib RS, and dissolve each in a mixture of methanol and water (3:1) to make exactly 100 mL, and use these solutions as the sample solution and the standard solution, respectively. Perform the test with exactly 25 μL each of the sample solution and standard solution as directed under Liquid Chromatography <*2.01*> according to the following conditions, and determine the peak areas, A_T and A_S, of celecoxib in each solution.

$$\text{Amount (mg) of celecoxib } (C_{17}H_{14}F_3N_3O_2S) = M_S \times A_T/A_S$$

M_S: Amount (mg) of Celecoxib RS taken

Operating conditions—

Detector: An ultraviolet absorption photometer (wavelength: 215 nm).

Column: A stainless steel column 4.6 mm in inside diameter and 25 cm in length, packed with phenylated silica gel for liquid chromatography (5 μm in particle diameter).

Column temperature: A constant temperature of about 60°C.

Mobile phase: Adjust 0.02 mol/L potassium dihydrogen phosphate TS to pH 3.0 with phosphoric acid. To 600 mL of this solution add 300 mL of methanol for liquid chromatography and 100 mL of acetonitrile for liquid chromatography.

Flow rate: Adjust so that the retention time of celecoxib is about 22 minutes.

System suitability—

System performance: When the procedure is run with 25 μL of the standard solution under the above operating conditions, the number of theoretical plates and the symmetry factor of the peak of celecoxib are not less than 6000 and not more than 2.0, respectively.

System repeatability: When the test is repeated 6 times with 25 μL of the standard solution under the above operating conditions, the relative standard deviation of the peak area of celecoxib is not more than 1.0%.

Containers and storage Containers—Well-closed containers.

Others
Related substance A:
4-[5-(3-Methylphenyl)-3-(trifluoromethyl)-1*H*-pyrazol-1-yl]benzenesulfonamide

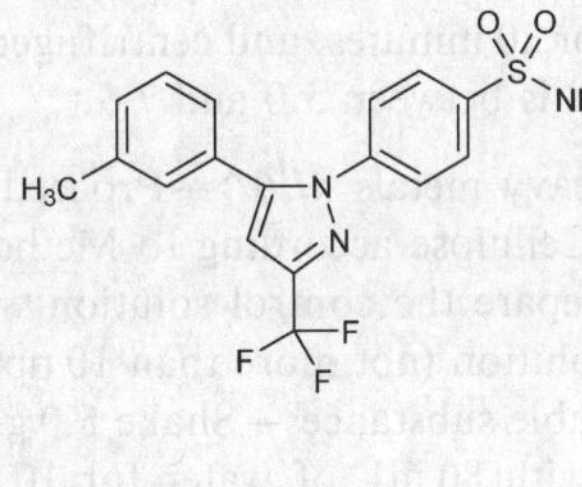

Cellacefate

Cellulose Acetate Phthalate

セラセフェート

[9004-38-0]

This monograph is harmonized with the European Pharmacopoeia and the U.S. Pharmacopeia.

The parts of the text that are not harmonized are marked with symbols (◆ ◆).

Information on the harmonization with the European Pharmacopoeia and the U.S. Pharmacopeia is available on the website of the Pharmaceuticals and Medical Devices Agency.

Cellacefate is a reaction product of phthalic anhydride and partially acetylated cellulose.

It contains not less than 21.5% and not more than 26.0% of acetyl group (-$COCH_3$: 43.04), and not less than 30.0% and not more than 36.0% of carboxybenzoyl group (-COC_6H_4COOH: 149.12), calculated on the anhydrous and free acid-free basis.

◆**Description** Cellacefate occurs as a white, powder or grain.

It is freely soluble in acetone, and practically insoluble in water and in ethanol (99.5).◆

Identification Determine the infrared absorption spectrum of Cellacefate as directed in the potassium bromide disk method under Infrared Spectrophotometry <*2.25*>, and compare the spectrum with the Reference Spectrum or the spectrum of Cellacefate for Identification RS: both spectra exhibit similar intensities of absorption at the same wave numbers.

Viscosity <*2.53*> Weigh accurately a quantity of Cellacefate, equivalent to 15 g calculated on the anhydrous basis, dissolve in 85 g of a mixture of acetone and water (249: 1 in mass), and use this solution as the sample solution. Perform the test with the sample solution at 25 ± 0.2°C as directed in Method 1 to obtain the kinematic viscosity ν. Separately, determine the density, ρ, of the sample solution as directed under Determination of Specific Gravity and Density <*2.56*>, and calculate the viscosity of the sample solution, η, as $\eta = \rho\nu$: not less than 45 mPa·s and not more than 90 mPa·s.

Purity (1) ◆Heavy metals <*1.07*>—Proceed with 2.0 g of Cellacefate according to Method 2, and perform the test. Prepare the control solution with 2.0 mL of Standard Lead Solution (not more than 10 ppm).◆

(2) Free acids—Weigh accurately about 3 g of Cellacefate, put in a glass-stoppered conical flask, add 100 mL of diluted methanol (1 in 2), stopper tightly, and filter after shaking for 2 hours. Wash both the flask and residue with two 10-mL portions each of diluted methanol (1 in 2), combine the washes to the filtrate, and titrate <*2.50*> with 0.1 mol/L sodium hydroxide VS (indicator: 2-3 drops of phenolphthalein TS). Perform the blank determination with 120 mL of diluted methanol (1 in 2), and make any necessary correction.

$$\text{Amount (\%) of free acids} = 0.8306A/M$$

A: Amount (mL) of 0.1 mol/L sodium hydroxide VS consumed

M: Amount (g) of Cellacefate taken, calculated on the anhydrous basis

The amount of free acids is not more than 3.0%, calculated as phthalic acid ($C_8H_6O_4$: 166.13).

Water <*2.48*> Not more than 5.0% (0.5 g, volumetric titration, direct titration, using a mixture of ethanol (99.5) and dichloromethane (3:2) instead of methanol for water determination).

Residue on ignition <*2.44*> Not more than 0.1% (1 g).

Assay (1) Carboxybenzoyl group—Weigh accurately about 1 g of Cellacefate, dissolve in 50 mL of a mixture of ethanol (95) and acetone (3:2), and titrate <*2.50*> with 0.1 mol/L sodium hydroxide VS (indicator: 2 – 3 drops of phenolphthalein TS). Perform a blank determination in the same manner, and make any necessary correction.

$$\text{Content (\%) of carboxybenzoyl group } (C_8H_5O_3) = \frac{\dfrac{1.491 \times A}{M} - (1.795 \times B)}{100 - B} \times 100$$

A: Amount (mL) of 0.1 mol/L sodium hydroxide VS consumed

B: Amount (%) of free acids obtained in the Purity (2)

M: Amount (g) of Cellacefate taken, calculated on the anhydrous basis

(2) Acetyl group—Weigh accurately about 0.1 g of Cellacefate, put in a glass-stoppered conical flask, add exactly 25 mL of 0.1 mol/L sodium hydroxide VS, and boil for 30 minutes under a reflux condenser. After cooling, add 2 – 3 drops of phenolphthalein TS, and titrate <*2.50*> the excess of sodium hydroxide with 0.1 mol/L hydrochloric acid VS. Perform a blank determination in the same manner.

$$\text{Content (\%) of free acids and bound acetyl group } (C_2H_3O) = 0.4305A/M$$

A: Amount (mL) of 0.1 mol/L sodium hydroxide VS consumed, corrected by the blank determination

M: Amount (g) of Cellacefate taken, calculated on the anhydrous basis

Content (%) of acetyl group (C_2H_3O)
$= 100 \times (P - 0.5182B)/(100 - B) - 0.5772C$

B: Amount (%) of free acids obtained in the Purity (2)
C: Content (%) of carboxybenzoyl group
P: Content (%) of free acids and bound acetyl group (C_2H_3O)

◆**Containers and storage** Containers—Tight containers.◆

Microcrystalline Cellulose

結晶セルロース

[*9004-34-6*, cellulose]

This monograph is harmonized with the European Pharmacopoeia and the U.S. Pharmacopeia.

The corresponding part of the attributes/provisions which are agreed as non-harmonized within the scope of the harmonization is marked with symbols (◆ ◆), and the corresponding parts which are agreed as the JP local requirement other than the scope of the harmonization are marked with symbols (◇ ◇).

Information on the harmonization with the European Pharmacopoeia and the U.S. Pharmacopeia is available on the website of the Pharmaceuticals and Medical Devices Agency.

Microcrystalline Cellulose is purified, partially depolymerized α-cellulose, obtained as a pulp from fibrous plant material, with mineral acids.

The label indicates the ◇mean degree of polymerization, loss on drying,◇ and bulk density values with a range.

◆**Description** Microcrystalline Cellulose occurs as a white crystalline powder having fluidity.

It is practically insoluble in water, in ethanol (95) and in diethyl ether.

It swells with sodium hydroxide TS on heating.◆

Identification (1) Dissolve 20 g of zinc chloride and 6.5 g of potassium iodide in 10.5 mL of water, add 0.5 g of iodine, and shake for 15 minutes. Place about 10 mg of Microcrystalline Cellulose on a watch glass, and disperse in 2 mL of this solution: the substance develops a blue-violet color.

(2) Determine the infrared absorption spectrum of Microcrystalline Cellulose as directed in the ATR method under Infrared Spectrophotometry <*2.25*>, and compare the spectrum with the spectrum of Microcrystalline Cellulose for Identification RS: both spectra exhibit similar intensities of absorption at the same wave numbers. If there are absorptions between 800 cm^{-1} and 825 cm^{-1}, and between 950 cm^{-1} and 1000 cm^{-1}, disregard the absorptions.

(3) Transfer about 1.3 g of Microcrystalline Cellulose, accurately weighed, to a 125-mL conical flask, and add exactly 25 mL each of water and 1 mol/L cupriethylenediamine TS. Immediately purge the solution with nitrogen, insert the stopper, and shake on a suitable mechanical shaker to dissolve. Perform the test with a suitable amount of this solution, taken exactly, according to Method 1 under Viscosity Determination <*2.53*> using a capillary viscometer having the viscosity constant (*K*) of approximately 0.03, at 25 ± 0.1°C, and determine the kinematic viscosity, ν. Separately, perform the test with a mixture of exactly 25 mL each of water and 1 mol/L cupriethylenediamine TS in the same manner as above, using a capillary viscometer having *K* of approximately 0.01, and determine the kinematic viscosity, ν_0.

Calculate the relative viscosity, η_{rel}, of Microcrystalline Cellulose by the following formula:

$$\eta_{rel} = \nu/\nu_0$$

Obtain the product, $[\eta]C$, of intrinsic viscosity $[\eta]$(mL/g) and concentration *C* (g/100 mL) from the value η_{rel} of the table. When calculate the degree of polymerization, *P*, by the following formula, *P* is not more than 350 ◇and within the labeled range.◇

$$P = 95[\eta]C/M_T$$

M_T: Amount (g) of the Microcrystalline Cellulose taken, calculated on the dried basis

pH <*2.54*> Shake 5.0 g of Microcrystalline Cellulose with 40 mL of water for 20 minutes, and centrifuge: the pH of the supernatant liquid is between 5.0 and 7.5.

Purity ◇(1) Heavy metals <*1.07*>—Proceed with 2.0 g of Microcrystalline Cellulose according to Method 2, and perform the test. Prepare the control solution with 2.0 mL of Standard Lead Solution (not more than 10 ppm).◇

(2) Water-soluble substances—Shake 5.0 g of Microcrystalline Cellulose with 80 mL of water for 10 minutes, filter with the aid of vacuum through a filter paper for quantitative analysis (5C) into a vacuum flask. Evaporate the filtrate in a tared evaporating dish to dryness without charring, dry at 105°C for 1 hour, cool in a desiccator, and weigh: the difference between the mass of the residue and the mass obtained from a blank determination does not exceed 12.5 mg.

(3) Diethyl ether-soluble substances—Place 10.0 g of Microcrystalline Cellulose in a column having an internal diameter of about 20 mm, and pass 50 mL of peroxide-free diethyl ether through the column. Evaporate the eluate to dryness in a previously dried and tared evaporation dish. Dry the residue at 105°C for 30 minutes, allow to cool in a desiccator, and weigh: the difference between the mass of the residue and the mass obtained from a blank determination does not exceed 5.0 mg.

Conductivity <*2.51*> Perform the test as directed in the Conductivity Measurement with the supernatant liquid obtained in the pH as the sample solution, and determine the conductivity at 25 ± 0.1°C. Determine in the same manner the conductivity of water used for the preparation of the sample solution: the difference between these conductivities is not more than 75 $\mu S \cdot cm^{-1}$.

Loss on drying <*2.41*> Not more than 7.0% ◇and within a range as specified on the label◇ (1 g, 105°C. 3 hours).

Residue on ignition <*2.44*> Not more than 0.1% (2 g).

Bulk density (i) Apparatus—Use a volumeter shown in the figure. Put a No.8.6 sieve (2000 μm) on the top of the volumeter. A funnel is mounted over a baffle box, having four glass baffle plates inside which the sample powder slides as it passes. At the bottom of the baffle box is a funnel that collect the powder, and allows it to pour into a sample receiving cup mounted directly below it.

Table for Conversion of Relative Viscosity (η_{rel}) into the Product of Limiting Viscosity and Concentration ($[\eta]C$)

	$[\eta]C$									
η_{rel}	0.00	0.01	0.02	0.03	0.04	0.05	0.06	0.07	0.08	0.09
1.1	0.098	0.106	0.115	0.125	0.134	0.143	0.152	0.161	0.170	0.180
1.2	0.189	0.198	0.207	0.216	0.225	0.233	0.242	0.250	0.259	0.268
1.3	0.276	0.285	0.293	0.302	0.310	0.318	0.326	0.334	0.342	0.350
1.4	0.358	0.367	0.375	0.383	0.391	0.399	0.407	0.414	0.422	0.430
1.5	0.437	0.445	0.453	0.460	0.468	0.476	0.484	0.491	0.499	0.507
1.6	0.515	0.522	0.529	0.536	0.544	0.551	0.558	0.566	0.573	0.580
1.7	0.587	0.595	0.602	0.608	0.615	0.622	0.629	0.636	0.642	0.649
1.8	0.656	0.663	0.670	0.677	0.683	0.690	0.697	0.704	0.710	0.717
1.9	0.723	0.730	0.736	0.743	0.749	0.756	0.762	0.769	0.775	0.782
2.0	0.788	0.795	0.802	0.809	0.815	0.821	0.827	0.833	0.840	0.846
2.1	0.852	0.858	0.864	0.870	0.876	0.882	0.888	0.894	0.900	0.906
2.2	0.912	0.918	0.924	0.929	0.935	0.941	0.948	0.953	0.959	0.965
2.3	0.971	0.976	0.983	0.988	0.994	1.000	1.006	1.011	1.017	1.022
2.4	1.028	1.033	1.039	1.044	1.050	1.056	1.061	1.067	1.072	1.078
2.5	1.083	1.089	1.094	1.100	1.105	1.111	1.116	1.121	1.126	1.131
2.6	1.137	1.142	1.147	1.153	1.158	1.163	1.169	1.174	1.179	1.184
2.7	1.190	1.195	1.200	1.205	1.210	1.215	1.220	1.225	1.230	1.235
2.8	1.240	1.245	1.250	1.255	1.260	1.265	1.270	1.275	1.280	1.285
2.9	1.290	1.295	1.300	1.305	1.310	1.314	1.319	1.324	1.329	1.333
3.0	1.338	1.343	1.348	1.352	1.357	1.362	1.367	1.371	1.376	1.381
3.1	1.386	1.390	1.395	1.400	1.405	1.409	1.414	1.418	1.423	1.427
3.2	1.432	1.436	1.441	1.446	1.450	1.455	1.459	1.464	1.468	1.473
3.3	1.477	1.482	1.486	1.491	1.496	1.500	1.504	1.508	1.513	1.517
3.4	1.521	1.525	1.529	1.533	1.537	1.542	1.546	1.550	1.554	1.558
3.5	1.562	1.566	1.570	1.575	1.579	1.583	1.587	1.591	1.595	1.600
3.6	1.604	1.608	1.612	1.617	1.621	1.625	1.629	1.633	1.637	1.642
3.7	1.646	1.650	1.654	1.658	1.662	1.666	1.671	1.675	1.679	1.683
3.8	1.687	1.691	1.695	1.700	1.704	1.708	1.712	1.715	1.719	1.723
3.9	1.727	1.731	1.735	1.739	1.742	1.746	1.750	1.754	1.758	1.762
4.0	1.765	1.769	1.773	1.777	1.781	1.785	1.789	1.792	1.796	1.800
4.1	1.804	1.808	1.811	1.815	1.819	1.822	1.826	1.830	1.833	1.837
4.2	1.841	1.845	1.848	1.852	1.856	1.859	1.863	1.867	1.870	1.874
4.3	1.878	1.882	1.885	1.889	1.893	1.896	1.900	1.904	1.907	1.911
4.4	1.914	1.918	1.921	1.925	1.929	1.932	1.936	1.939	1.943	1.946
4.5	1.950	1.954	1.957	1.961	1.964	1.968	1.971	1.975	1.979	1.982
4.6	1.986	1.989	1.993	1.996	2.000	2.003	2.007	2.010	2.013	2.017
4.7	2.020	2.023	2.027	2.030	2.033	2.037	2.040	2.043	2.047	2.050
4.8	2.053	2.057	2.060	2.063	2.067	2.070	2.073	2.077	2.080	2.083
4.9	2.087	2.090	2.093	2.097	2.100	2.103	2.107	2.110	2.113	2.116
5.0	2.119	2.122	2.125	2.129	2.132	2.135	2.139	2.142	2.145	2.148
5.1	2.151	2.154	2.158	2.160	2.164	2.167	2.170	2.173	2.176	2.180
5.2	2.183	2.186	2.190	2.192	2.195	2.197	2.200	2.203	2.206	2.209
5.3	2.212	2.215	2.218	2.221	2.224	2.227	2.230	2.233	2.236	2.240
5.4	2.243	2.246	2.249	2.252	2.255	2.258	2.261	2.264	2.267	2.270
5.5	2.273	2.276	2.279	2.282	2.285	2.288	2.291	2.294	2.297	2.300
5.6	2.303	2.306	2.309	2.312	2.315	2.318	2.320	2.324	2.326	2.329
5.7	2.332	2.335	2.338	2.341	2.344	2.347	2.350	2.353	2.355	2.358
5.8	2.361	2.364	2.367	2.370	2.373	2.376	2.379	2.382	2.384	2.387
5.9	2.390	2.393	2.396	2.400	2.403	2.405	2.408	2.411	2.414	2.417
6.0	2.419	2.422	2.425	2.428	2.431	2.433	2.436	2.439	2.442	2.444
6.1	2.447	2.450	2.453	2.456	2.458	2.461	2.464	2.467	2.470	2.472
6.2	2.475	2.478	2.481	2.483	2.486	2.489	2.492	2.494	2.497	2.500
6.3	2.503	2.505	2.508	2.511	2.513	2.516	2.518	2.521	2.524	2.526
6.4	2.529	2.532	2.534	2.537	2.540	2.542	2.545	2.547	2.550	2.553
6.5	2.555	2.558	2.561	2.563	2.566	2.568	2.571	2.574	2.576	2.579
6.6	2.581	2.584	2.587	2.590	2.592	2.595	2.597	2.600	2.603	2.605
6.7	2.608	2.610	2.613	2.615	2.618	2.620	2.623	2.625	2.627	2.630
6.8	2.633	2.635	2.637	2.640	2.643	2.645	2.648	2.650	2.653	2.655
6.9	2.658	2.660	2.663	2.665	2.668	2.670	2.673	2.675	2.678	2.680

	$[\eta]C$									
η_{rel}	0.00	0.01	0.02	0.03	0.04	0.05	0.06	0.07	0.08	0.09
7.0	2.683	2.685	2.687	2.690	2.693	2.695	2.698	2.700	2.702	2.705
7.1	2.707	2.710	2.712	2.714	2.717	2.719	2.721	2.724	2.726	2.729
7.2	2.731	2.733	2.736	2.738	2.740	2.743	2.745	2.748	2.750	2.752
7.3	2.755	2.757	2.760	2.762	2.764	2.767	2.769	2.771	2.774	2.776
7.4	2.779	2.781	2.783	2.786	2.788	2.790	2.793	2.795	2.798	2.800
7.5	2.802	2.805	2.807	2.809	2.812	2.814	2.816	2.819	2.821	2.823
7.6	2.826	2.828	2.830	2.833	2.835	2.837	2.840	2.842	2.844	2.847
7.7	2.849	2.851	2.854	2.856	2.858	2.860	2.863	2.865	2.868	2.870
7.8	2.873	2.875	2.877	2.879	2.881	2.884	2.887	2.889	2.891	2.893
7.9	2.895	2.898	2.900	2.902	2.905	2.907	2.909	2.911	2.913	2.915
8.0	2.918	2.920	2.922	2.924	2.926	2.928	2.931	2.933	2.935	2.937
8.1	2.939	2.942	2.944	2.946	2.948	2.950	2.952	2.955	2.957	2.959
8.2	2.961	2.963	2.966	2.968	2.970	2.972	2.974	2.976	2.979	2.981
8.3	2.983	2.985	2.987	2.990	2.992	2.994	2.996	2.998	3.000	3.002
8.4	3.004	3.006	3.008	3.010	3.012	3.015	3.017	3.019	3.021	3.023
8.5	3.025	3.027	3.029	3.031	3.033	3.035	3.037	3.040	3.042	3.044
8.6	3.046	3.048	3.050	3.052	3.054	3.056	3.058	3.060	3.062	3.064
8.7	3.067	3.069	3.071	3.073	3.075	3.077	3.079	3.081	3.083	3.085
8.8	3.087	3.089	3.092	3.094	3.096	3.098	3.100	3.102	3.104	3.106
8.9	3.108	3.110	3.112	3.114	3.116	3.118	3.120	3.122	3.124	3.126
9.0	3.128	3.130	3.132	3.134	3.136	3.138	3.140	3.142	3.144	3.146
9.1	3.148	3.150	3.152	3.154	3.156	3.158	3.160	3.162	3.164	3.166
9.2	3.168	3.170	3.172	3.174	3.176	3.178	3.180	3.182	3.184	3.186
9.3	3.188	3.190	3.192	3.194	3.196	3.198	3.200	3.202	3.204	3.206
9.4	3.208	3.210	3.212	3.214	3.215	3.217	3.219	3.221	3.223	3.225
9.5	3.227	3.229	3.231	3.233	3.235	3.237	3.239	3.241	3.242	3.244
9.6	3.246	3.248	3.250	3.252	3.254	3.256	3.258	3.260	3.262	3.264
9.7	3.266	3.268	3.269	3.271	3.273	3.275	3.277	3.279	3.281	3.283
9.8	3.285	3.287	3.289	3.291	3.293	3.295	3.297	3.298	3.300	3.302
9.9	3.304	3.305	3.307	3.309	3.311	3.313	3.316	3.318	3.320	3.321
	0.0	0.1	0.2	0.3	0.4	0.5	0.6	0.7	0.8	0.9
10	3.32	3.34	3.36	3.37	3.39	3.41	3.43	3.45	3.46	3.48
11	3.50	3.52	3.53	3.55	3.56	3.58	3.60	3.61	3.63	3.64
12	3.66	3.68	3.69	3.71	3.72	3.74	3.76	3.77	3.79	3.80
13	3.80	3.83	3.85	3.86	3.88	3.89	3.90	3.92	3.93	3.95
14	3.96	3.97	3.99	4.00	4.02	4.03	4.04	4.06	4.07	4.09
15	4.10	4.11	4.13	4.14	4.15	4.17	4.18	4.19	4.20	4.22
16	4.23	4.24	4.25	4.27	4.28	4.29	4.30	4.31	4.33	4.34
17	4.35	4.36	4.37	4.38	4.39	4.41	4.42	4.43	4.44	4.45
18	4.46	4.47	4.48	4.49	4.50	4.52	4.53	4.54	4.55	4.56
19	4.57	4.58	4.59	4.60	4.61	4.62	4.63	4.64	4.65	4.66

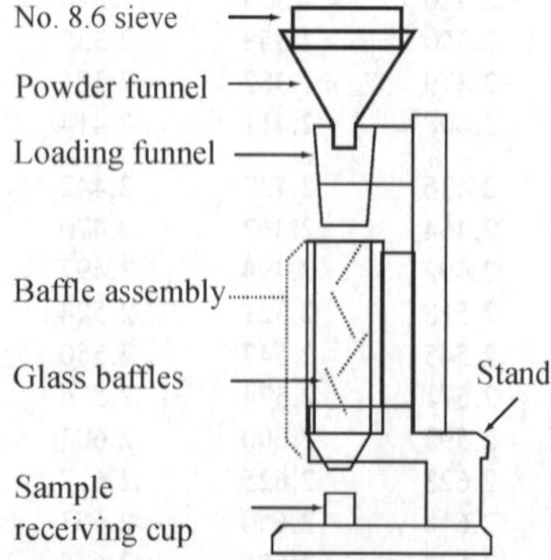

(ii) Procedure—Weigh accurately the mass of a brass or stainless steel cup, which has a capacity of 25.0 ± 0.05 mL and an inside diameter of 30.0 ± 2.0 mm, and put the cup directly below the funnel of the volumeter. Slowly pour Microcrystalline Cellulose 5.1 cm height from the upper part of the powder funnel through the sieve, at a rate suitable to prevent clogging, until the cup overflows. If the clogging occurs, take out the sieve. Level the excess powder with the aid of a slide glass, weigh the filled cup, and weigh accurately the content of the cup, and then calculate the bulk density by the following expression: the bulk density is within the labeled specification.

$$\text{Bulk density (g/cm}^3\text{)} = A/25$$

A: Measured mass (g) of the content of the cup

Microbial limit <*4.05*> The acceptance criteria of TAMC and TYMC are 10^3 CFU/g and 10^2 CFU/g, respectively. *Escherichia coli*, *Salmonella*, *Pseudomonas aeruginosa* and *Staphylococcus aureus* are not observed.

◆**Containers and storage** Containers—Tight containers.◆

Powdered Cellulose

粉末セルロース

[*9004-34-6*, Cellulose]

This monograph is harmonized with the European Pharmacopoeia and the U.S. Pharmacopeia.

The parts of the text that are not harmonized are marked with symbols (◆ ◆).

Information on the harmonization with the European Pharmacopoeia and the U.S. Pharmacopeia is available on the website of the Pharmaceuticals and Medical Devices Agency.

Powdered Cellulose is a purified, mechanically disintegrated alpha cellulose obtained as a pulp, ◆after partial hydrolysis as occasion demands◆, from fibrous plant materials.

The label indicates the mean degree of polymerization value with a range.

◆**Description** Powdered Cellulose occurs as a white powder.

It is practically insoluble in water, in ethanol (95) and in diethyl ether.◆

Identification **(1)** Dissolve 20 g of zinc chloride and 6.5 g of potassium iodide in 10.5 mL of water, add 0.5 g of iodine, and shake for 15 minutes. Place about 10 mg of Powdered Cellulose on a watch glass, and disperse in 2 mL of this solution: the substance develops a blue-violet color.

◆**(2)** Mix 30 g of Powdered Cellulose with 270 mL of water in a high-speed (18,000 revolutions per minute or more) blender for 5 minutes, transfer 100 mL of the dispersion to a 100-mL graduated cylinder, and allow to stand for 1 hour: a supernatant liquid appears above the layer of the cellulose.◆

(3) Transfer 0.25 g of Powdered Cellulose, accurately weighed, to a 125-mL conical flask, add exactly 25 mL each of water and 1 mol/L cupriethylenediamine TS, and proceed as directed in the Identification (3) under Microcrystalline Cellulose. The mean degree of polymerization, P, is not less than 440 and is within the labeled specification.

pH *<2.54>* Mix 10 g of Powdered Cellulose with 90 mL of water, and allow to stand for 1 hour with occasional stirring: the pH of the supernatant liquid is between 5.0 and 7.5.

Purity ◆**(1)** Heavy metals *<1.07>*—Proceed with 2.0 g of Powdered Cellulose according to Method 2, and perform the test. Prepare the control solution with 2.0 mL of Standard Lead Solution (not more than 10 ppm).◆

(2) Water-soluble substances—Shake 6.0 g of Powdered Cellulose with 90 mL of recently boiled and cooled water, and allow to stand for 10 minutes with occasional shaking. Filter, with the aid of vacuum through a filter paper, discard the first 10 mL of the filtrate, and pass the subsequent filtrate through the same filter, if necessary, to obtain a clear filtrate. Evaporate a 15.0-mL portion of the filtrate in a tared evaporating dish to dryness without charring, dry at 105°C for 1 hour, and weigh after allowing to cool in a desiccator: the difference between the mass of the residue and the mass obtained from a blank determination does not exceed 15.0 mg (1.5%).

(3) Diethyl ether-soluble substances—Place 10.0 g of Powdered Cellulose in a column having an internal diameter of about 20 mm, and pass 50 mL of peroxide-free diethyl ether through the column. Evaporate the eluate to dryness in a previously dried and tared evaporation dish. Dry the residue at 105°C for 30 minutes, and weigh after allowing to cool in a desiccator: the difference between the mass of the residue and the mass obtained from a blank determination does not exceed 15.0 mg (0.15%).

Loss on drying *<2.41>* Not more than 6.5% (1 g, 105°C, 3 hours).

Residue on ignition *<2.44>* Not more than 0.3% (1 g calculated on the dried basis).

◆**Microbial limit** *<4.05>* The acceptance criteria of TAMC and TYMC are 10^3 CFU/g and 10^2 CFU/g, respectively. *Escherichia coli*, *Salmonella*, *Pseudomonas aeruginosa* and *Staphylococcus aureus* are not observed.◆

◆**Containers and storage** Containers—Tight containers.◆

Celmoleukin (Genetical Recombination)

セルモロイキン(遺伝子組換え)

```
APTSSSTKKT QLQLEHLLLD LQMILNGINN YKNPKLTRML TFKFYMPKKA
TELKHLQCLE EELKPLEEVL NLAQSKNFHL RPRDLISNIN VIVLELKGSE
TTFMCEYADE TATIVEFLNR WITFCQSIIS TLT
```

$C_{693}H_{1118}N_{178}O_{203}S_7$: 15415.82
[*94218-72-1*]

Celmoleukin (Genetical Recombination) is a recombinant human interleukin-2, and is a protein consisting of 133 amino acid residues. It is a solution.

It contains not less than 0.5 and not more than 1.5 mg of protein per mL, and 1 mg of this protein contains potency not less than 8.0×10^6 units.

Description Celmoleukin (Genetical Recombination) occurs as a clear and colorless liquid.

Identification **(1)** Add 100 μL of protein digestive enzyme TS to 100 μL of Celmoleukin (Genetical Recombination), shake, leave standing at 37°C for 18 to 24 hours, and then add 2 μL of 2-mercaptoethanol. Leave at 37°C for a further 30 minutes, and add 5 μL of trifluoroacetic acid solution (1 in 10). Use this solution as the sample solution. Separately, process with celmoleukin for liquid chromatography by using the same method. Use this solution as the standard solution. Perform the test with 50 μL each of the sample solution and standard solution as directed under Liquid Chromatography *<2.01>* according to the following conditions, and compare the chromatograms obtained from the sample solution and standard solution: the similar peaks are observed at the same retention time.

Operating conditions—

Detector: An ultraviolet absorption photometer (wavelength: 215 nm).

Column: A stainless steel column 4 mm in inside diameter and 30 cm in length, packed with octadecylsilanized silica gel for liquid chromatography (particle size: 5 μm).

Column temperature: A constant temperature of about 25°C.

Mobile phase A: A solution of trifluoroacetic acid (1 in 1000).

Mobile phase B: A solution of trifluoroacetic acid in a

mixture of acetonitrile and water (17:3) (1 in 1000).

Flowing of mobile phase: Control the gradient by mixing the mobile phases A and B as directed in the following table.

Time after injection of sample (min)	Mobile phase A (vol%)	Mobile phase B (vol%)
0 - 5	100	0
5 - 45	100 → 60	0 → 40
45 - 75	60 → 0	40 → 100
75 - 85	0	100

Flow rate: Adjust so that the retention time of celmoleukin is about 70 minutes.

System suitability—

System performance: Add 2 μL of 2-mercaptoethanol to 100 μL of celmoleukin for liquid chromatography, leave at 37°C for 2 hours, and then run this solution under the above operating conditions. Celmoleukin and its reduced form are eluted in this order with the resolution between these peaks being not less than 1.5.

(2) Accurately measure an appropriate amount of Celmoleukin (Genetical Recombination), dilute by adding culture medium for celmoleukin, and prepare a sample solution containing 800 units per mL. Add 25 μL of the sample solution to 2 wells (A and B) of a flat-bottomed microtest plate for tissue culture, and then add 25 μL of reference anti-interleukin-2 antiserum solution diluted with culture medium for celmoleukin to well A and 25 μL of culture medium for celmoleukin to well B. Add 50 μL of culture medium for celmoleukin to another well (well C). After shaking the microtest plate, warm in air containing 5% carbon dioxide at 37°C for 30 minutes to 2 hours. Next, add to each well 50 μL of culture medium for celmoleukin containing the interleukin-2 dependent mouse natural killer cells NKC3 and culture at 37°C for 16 to 24 hours. Add 3-(4,5-dimethylthiazole-2-yl)-2,5-diphenyl-2*H*-tetrazolium bromide TS, culture at 37°C for 4 to 6 hours, and add sodium lauryl sulfate TS and leave for 24 to 48 hours. When the absorbance at 590 nm of the solution in each well is measured, the difference in absorbance between the solutions from wells A and C is not more than 3% of the difference in absorbance between the solutions from wells B and C.

Constituent amino acid When hydrolyze Celmoleukin (Genetical Recombination) according to Method 1 and Method 4 described in "1. Hydrolysis of Protein and Peptide", and perform the test according to Method 1 described in "2. Methodologies of Amino Acid Analysis" under Amino Acid Analysis of Proteins <*2.04*>, the molar ratios of the respective amino acids are as follows: glutamic acid (or glutamine) is 17 or 18, threonine is 11 to 13, aspartic acid (or asparagine) is 11 or 12, lysine is 11, isoleucine is 7 or 8, serine is 6 to 9, phenylalanine is 6, alanine is 5, proline is 5 or 6, arginine is 4, methionine is 4, cysteine is 3 or 4, valine is 3 or 4, tyrosine is 3, histidine is 3, glycine is 2, and tryptophan is 1.

Procedure

(i) Hydrolysis Based on the results of the Assay (1), place an amount of Celmoleukin (Genetical Recombination), equivalent to about 50 μg as the total protein in two hydrolysis tubes, and evaporate to dryness under vacuum. To one of the hydrolysis tubes add 100 μL of a mixture of diluted hydrochloric acid (59 in 125), mercapto acetic acid and phenol (100:10:1), and shake. Place this hydrolysis tube in a vial and humidify the inside of the vial with 200 μL of the mixture of diluted hydrochloric acid (59 in 125), mercapto acetic acid and phenol (100:10:1). Replace the vial interior with inert gas or reduce the pressure, and heat at about 115°C for 24 hours. After drying under vacuum, dissolve in 0.5 mL of 0.02 mol/L hydrochloric acid TS, and use this solution as the sample solution (1). To the other hydrolysis tube, add 100 μL of ice cold performic acid, oxidize for 1.5 hours on ice, add 50 μL of hydrobromic acid, and dry under vacuum. Add 200 μL of water, repeat the dry under vacuum procedure two more times, place the hydrolysis tube in a vial, and humidify the inside of the vial with 200 μL of diluted hydrochloric acid (59 in 125). Replace the vial interior with inert gas or reduce the pressure, and heat at about 115°C for 24 hours. After drying under vacuum, dissolve in 0.5 mL of 0.02 mol/L hydrochloric acid TS, and use this solution as the sample solution (2). Separately, weigh exactly 60 mg of L-aspartic acid, 100 mg of L-glutamic acid, 17 mg of L-alanine, 23 mg of L-methionine, 21 mg of L-tyrosine, 24 mg of L-histidine hydrochloride monohydrate, 58 mg of L-threonine, 22 mg of L-proline, 14 mg of L-cystine, 45 mg of L-isoleucine, 37 mg of L-phenylalanine, 32 mg of L-arginine hydrochloride, 32 mg of L-serine, 6 mg of glycine, 18 mg of L-valine, 109 mg of L-leucine, 76 mg of L-lysine hydrochloride, and 8 mg of L-tryptophan, dissolve with 0.1 mol/L hydrochloric acid TS to make exactly 500 mL, and use this solution as the standard solution. Transfer 40 μL each of the standard solution to two hydrolysis tubes, evaporate to dryness under vacuum, and proceed in the same way for each respective sample solution to make the standard solutions (1) and (2).

(ii) Amino acid analysis Perform the test with exactly 250 μL each of the sample solutions (1) and (2) and standard solutions (1) and (2) as directed under Liquid Chromatography <*2.01*> according to the following conditions, and from the peak areas for each amino acid obtained from the sample solutions (1) and (2) and standard solutions (1) and (2) calculate the molar number of the amino acids contained in 1 mL of the sample solutions (1) and (2). Furthermore, calculate the number of amino acids assuming there are 22 leucine residues in one mole of celmoleukin.

Operating conditions—

Detector: A visible absorption photometer [wavelength: 440 nm (proline) and 570 nm (amino acids other than proline)].

Column: A stainless steel column 4 mm in inside diameter and 25 cm in length, packed with strongly acidic ion-exchange resin for liquid chromatography (Na type) (sulfonic acid group bound divinylbenzenepolystyrene) (5 μm in particle diameter).

Column temperature: Maintaining a constant temperature of about 48°C for 28 minutes after sample injection, then a constant temperature of about 62°C until 121 minutes after the injection.

Reaction temperature: A constant temperature of about 135°C.

Color developing time: About 1 minute.

Mobile phases A, B, C and D: Prepare according to the following table.

Mobile phase	A	B	C	D
Citric acid monohydrate	17.70 g	10.50 g	6.10 g	—
Trisodium citrate dihydrate	7.74 g	15.70 g	26.67 g	—
Sodium chloride	7.07 g	2.92 g	54.35 g	—
Sodium hydroxide	—	—	2.30 g	8.00 g
Methanol (99.5)	40 mL	—	—	—
Benzyl alcohol	—	10 mL	5 mL	—
Thiodiglycol	5 mL	5 mL	5 mL	—
Lauromacrogol solution (1 in 4)	4 mL	4 mL	4 mL	4 mL
Caprylic acid	0.1 mL	0.1 mL	0.1 mL	0.1 mL
Water	a sufficient quantity	a sufficient quantity	a sufficient quantity	a sufficient quantity
Total	1000 mL	1000 mL	1000 mL	1000 mL

Flowing of mobile phase: Control the gradient by mixing the mobile phases A, B, C and D as directed in the following table.

Time after injection of sample (min)	Mobile phase A (vol%)	Mobile phase B (vol%)	Mobile phase C (vol%)	Mobile phase D (vol%)
0 – 35	100	0	0	0
35 – 60	0	100	0	0
60 – 111	0	0	100	0
111 – 121	0	0	0	100

Reaction reagent: Mix 407 g of lithium acetate dihydrate, 245 mL of acetic acid (100) and 801 mL of 1-methoxy-2-propanol, add water to make 2000 mL, stir for 10 minutes while passing a current of nitrogen, and assign as solution A. Separately, to 1957 mL of 1-methoxy-2-propanol add 77 g of ninhydrin and 0.134 g of sodium borohydride, stir for 30 minutes while passing a current of nitrogen, and assign as solution B. Mix solutions A and B before use.

Flow rate of mobile phase: Adjust so that the retention times of serine and leucine are about 30 minutes and about 73 minutes, respectively (about 0.21 mL per minute).

Flow rate of reaction reagent: About 0.25 mL per minute.

System suitability—

System performance: To 2 mL of the standard solution add 0.02 mol/L hydrochloric acid TS to make 25 mL. When the procedure is run with 250 μL of this solution under the above operating conditions, the resolution between the peaks of threonine and serine is not less than 1.2.

System repeatability: To 2 mL of the standard solution add 0.02 mol/L hydrochloric acid TS to make 25 mL. When the test is repeated 3 times with 250 μL of this solution under the above operating conditions, the relative standard deviation of the peak area of aspartic acid, serine, arginine and proline is not more than 2.4%.

Molecular mass Based on the results of the Assay (1), add buffer for celmoleukin and dilute to prepare a sample solution so that there is about 0.5 mg of protein per mL. To vertical uncontinuous buffer SDS-polyacrylamide gel prepared from resolving gel for celmoleukin and stacking gel for celmoleukin add 20 μL of the sample solution or 20 μL of marker protein for celmoleukin molecular mass determination to each stacking gel well, and perform the electrophoresis. The molecular mass of the main electrophoretic band is between 12,500 and 13,800 when the band is stained by immersion in Coomassie staining TS.

pH <*2.54*> 4.5 – 5.5

Purity (1) Related substances—Perform the test with 10 μL each of Celmoleukin (Genetical Recombination) and 0.01 mol/L acetic acid buffer solution (pH 5.0) as directed under Liquid Chromatography <*2.01*> under the following conditions, and measure the area of each peak by an automatic integration method. When the amounts of related substances other than celmoleukin are calculated by the area percentage method, the total amount is not more than 5%.

Operating conditions—

Detector: An ultraviolet absorption photometer (wavelength: 215 nm).

Column: Stainless steel tube with an inside diameter of 4 mm and a length of 30 cm packed with octadecylsilanized silica gel for liquid chromatography (particle size: 5 μm).

Column temperature: A constant temperature of about 25°C.

Mobile phase A: A solution of trifluoroacetic acid in a mixture of acetic acid and water (3:2) (1 in 1000).

Mobile phase B: A solution of trifluoroacetic acid in a mixture of acetic acid and water (13:7) (1 in 1000).

Flowing of mobile phase: Control the gradient by mixing the mobile phases A and B as directed in the following table.

Time after injection of sample (min)	Mobile phase A (vol%)	Mobile phase B (vol%)
0 – 60	70 → 10	30 → 90

Flow rate: Adjust so that the retention time of celmoleukin is about 50 minutes.

Time span of measurement: About 1.3 times as long as the retention time of celmoleukin, beginning after the solvent peak.

System suitability—

Test for required detectability: Measure exactly 0.5 mL of Celmoleukin (Genetical Recombination), and add 0.01 mol/L acetic acid buffer solution (pH 5.0) to make exactly 50 mL. Confirm that the peak area of celmoleukin obtained with 10 μL of this solution is equivalent to 0.9 to 1.1% of the peak area with 10 μL of Celmoleukin (Genetical Recombination).

System performance: Add 2 μL of 2-mercaptoethanol to 100 μL of Celmoleukin (Genetical Recombination), leave at 37°C for 2 hours, and then run this solution under the above conditions. Celmoleukin and its reduced form are eluted in this order with the resolution between these peaks being not less than 3.0.

(2) Multimers—Dilute (at least 4 steps) the sample solution prepared in the Molecular mass with buffer solution for celmoleukin so that the protein content is within the range of 2 to 32 μg per mL to prepare a series of standard solutions. Pipet 20 μL each of the sample solution and the standard solutions into the stacking gel well, and perform vertical uncoupled buffer SDS-polyacrylamide gel electrophoresis followed by immersion in Coomassie staining TS. Each electrophoretic band is stained blue. Next, determine the peak area of the electrophoretic bands obtained from each standard solution using a densitometer and calculate the protein content using the calibration curve mentioned above. When determining the polymer proteins derived from celmoleukin, other than celmoleukin monomer, the amount is not more than 2% in relation to the total protein.

(3) Host cell proteins—Being specified separately when the drug is granted approval based on the Law.

(4) Host cell DNA—Being specified separately when the drug is granted approval based on the Law.

Bacterial endotoxins <*4.01*> Less than 100 EU/mL.

Ammonium acetate Measure exactly 0.1 mL of Celmoleukin (Genetical Recombination), add water to make exactly 10 mL, and use this solution as the sample solution. Separately, weigh accurately about 0.1 g of ammonium chloride, and add water to make exactly 100 mL. Measure exactly 5 mL of this solution, add water to make exactly 100 mL, and use this solution as the standard stock solution. Measure exactly 3 mL of the standard stock solution, add water to make exactly 50 mL, and use this solution as the standard solution. Perform the test with exactly 25 μL each of the sample solution and standard solution as directed under Liquid Chromatography <*2.01*> according to the following conditions. When determining the area of the ammonium ion peak A_T and A_S, Celmoleukin (Genetical Recombination) contains not less than 0.28 mg and not more than 0.49 mg of ammonium acetate per mL.

Amount (mg) of ammonium acetate (CH_3COONH_4) per mL
$= A_T/A_S \times M_S \times 0.003 \times 1.441$

M_S: Amount (mg) of ammonium chloride taken
0.003: Dilution correction factor
1.441: Molecular mass conversion coefficient for converting ammonium chloride to ammonium acetate

Operating conditions—

Detector: An electric conductivity detector.

Column: Resin column 5 mm in inside diameter and 25 cm in length, packed with weakly acidic ion exchange resin for liquid chromatography (particle size: 5.5 μm).

Column temperature: A constant temperature of about 40°C.

Mobile phase: Diluted 0.1 mol/L methanesulfonic acid TS (3 in 10).

Flow rate: Adjust so that the retention time of ammonium is about 8 minutes.

System suitability—

System performance: Measure exactly 1 mL of Standard Sodium Stock Solution and 0.2 mL of Standard Potassium Stock Solution, and then add water to make exactly 100 mL. Measure exactly 5 mL of this solution and 3 mL of Standard Ammonium Solution, and then add water to make exactly 50 mL. When 25 μL of this solution is run under the above conditions, sodium, ammonium and potassium are eluted in this order with the resolution between the peaks of sodium and ammonium being not less than 3.0.

System repeatability: When the test is repeated 5 times with 25 μL of the standard solution under the above conditions, the relative standard deviation of the ammonium peak area is not more than 10%.

Assay (1) Total protein content—Measure accurately 1 mL of Celmoleukin (Genetical Recombination) and add water to make exactly 10 mL. Use this solution as the sample solution. Separately, weigh accurately about 50 mg of bovine serum albumin for assay in water to prepare standard dilution solutions of 50, 100, and 150 μg/mL. Measure exactly 1 mL of the sample solution and each standard dilution solution, add exactly 2.5 mL of alkaline copper TS for protein content determination, shake, and leave for 15 minutes. Next, add exactly 2.5 mL of water and 0.5 mL of dilute Folin's TS, and leave at 37°C for 30 minutes. Measure the absorbances of these solutions at 750 nm as directed under Ultraviolet-visible Spectrophotometry <*2.24*>, using 1 mL of water processed in the same way as control. Using the calibration curve prepared from the absorbance of the standard dilution solution, calculate the protein content of Celmoleukin (Genetical Recombination).

(2) Specific activity—Measure exactly 0.1 mL of Celmoleukin (Genetical Recombination) and add exactly 0.9 mL of culture medium for celmoleukin to make the sample solution. Separately, take one Interleukin-2 RS and add exactly 1 mL of water to dissolve. This is the standard solution. Dilute exactly the sample and standard solutions in serially two-fold steps with culture medium for celmoleukin, and add equal volumes of interleukin-2 dependent mouse natural killer NKC3 cells to the serially diluted solutions. The control solution is a mixture of equal volumes of interleukin-2 dependent mouse natural killer NKC3 and culture medium for celmoleukin. Incubate these solutions at 37°C for 16 to 24 hours. Following this, add a volume of 3-(4,5-dimethylthiazole-2-yl)-2,5-diphenyl-2*H*-tetrazolium bromide TS that is 1/5 that of the volume of culture medium for celmoleukin, incubate at 37°C for 4 to 6 hours, add a volume of sodium lauryl sulfate TS equivalent to the volume of the culture medium for celmoleukin, and leave for 24 to 48 hours. After eluting the blue-colored pigment generated, perform the test on these solutions as directed under Ultraviolet-visible Spectrophotometry <*2.24*>, and measure the absorbance at 590 nm. Taking the absorbance obtained when 1000 to 2000 units of celmoleukin per mL are added as 100% and the absorbance of the control solution as 0%, determine the dilution factor (A) of the Interleukin-2 RS that shows an absorbance of 50% and dilution factor of Celmoleukin (Genetical Recombination) (B). Multiply the B/A value by the unit number of the Interleukin-2 RS to calculate the biological activity of 1 mL of Celmoleukin (Genetical Recombination). Calculate the ratio of biological activity in relation to protein content determined in the total protein content test.

Containers and storage Containers—Tight containers.
Storage—At −20°C or lower.

Cetanol

セタノール

Cetanol is a mixture of solid alcohols, and consists chiefly of cetanol ($C_{16}H_{34}O$: 242.44).

Description Cetanol occurs as unctuous, white, flakes, granules, or masses. It has a faint, characteristic odor. It is tasteless.

It is very soluble in pyridine, freely soluble in ethanol (95), in ethanol (99.5) and in diethyl ether, very slightly soluble in acetic anhydride, and practically insoluble in water.

Melting point <*1.13*> 47 – 53°C Prepare the sample according to Method 2, then attach tightly a capillary tube to the bottom of the thermometer by means of a rubber band or by any suitable means, and make the bottom of the capillary tube equal in position to the lower end of the thermometer. Insert this thermometer into a test tube 17 mm in inside diameter and about 170 mm in height, fasten the thermometer with cork stopper so that the lower end of the thermometer is about 25 mm distant from the bottom of the test tube. Suspend the test tube in a beaker containing water, and heat the beaker with constant stirring until the temperature rises to 5°C below the expected melting point. Then regulate the rate of increase to 1°C per minute. The temperature at which the sample is transparent and no turbidity is produced is taken as the melting point.

Acid value ⟨*1.13*⟩ Not more than 1.0.

Ester value ⟨*1.13*⟩ Not more than 2.0.

Hydroxyl value ⟨*1.13*⟩ 210 – 232

Iodine value ⟨*1.13*⟩ Not more than 2.0.

Purity (1) Clarity of solution—Dissolve 3.0 g of Cetanol in 25 mL of ethanol (99.5) by warming: the solution is clear.

(2) Alkalinity—To the solution obtained in (1) add 2 drops of phenolphthalein TS: no red color develops.

Residue on ignition ⟨*2.44*⟩ Not more than 0.05% (2 g).

Containers and storage Containers—Well-closed containers.

Cetirizine Hydrochloride

セチリジン塩酸塩

2HCl and enantiomer

$C_{21}H_{25}ClN_2O_3.2HCl$: 461.81

2-(2-{4-[(*RS*)-(4-Chlorophenyl)(phenyl)methyl]piperazin-1-yl}ethoxy)acetic acid dihydrochloride

[83881-52-1]

Cetirizine Hydrochloride, when dried, contains not less than 99.0% and not more than 101.0% of cetirizine hydrochloride ($C_{21}H_{25}ClN_2O_3.2HCl$).

Description Cetirizine Hydrochloride occurs as a white crystalline powder.

It is very soluble in water, and slightly soluble in ethanol (99.5).

It dissolves in 0.1 mol/L hydrochloric acid TS.

A solution of Cetirizine Hydrochloride (1 in 10) shows no optical rotation.

Identification (1) Determine the absorption spectrum of a solution of Cetirizine Hydrochloride in 0.1 mol/L hydrochloric acid TS (1 in 50,000) as directed under Ultraviolet-visible Spectrophotometry ⟨*2.24*⟩, and compare the spectrum with the Reference Spectrum: both spectra exhibit similar intensities of absorption at the same wavelengths.

(2) Determine the infrared absorption spectrum of Cetirizine Hydrochloride as directed in the potassium chloride disk method under Infrared Spectrophotometry ⟨*2.25*⟩, and compare the spectrum with the Reference Spectrum: both spectra exhibit similar intensities of absorption at the same wave numbers.

(3) A solution of Cetirizine Hydrochloride (1 in 100) responds to Qualitative Tests ⟨*1.09*⟩ for chloride.

Purity (1) Heavy metals ⟨*1.07*⟩—Proceed with 2.0 g of Cetirizine Hydrochloride according to Method 2, and perform the test. Prepare the control solution with 2.0 mL of Standard Lead Solution (not more than 10 ppm).

(2) Related substances—Dissolve 0.10 g of Cetirizine Hydrochloride in 50 mL of the mobile phase, and use this solution as the sample solution. Pipet 2 mL of the sample solution, add the mobile phase to make exactly 50 mL. Pipet 5 mL of this solution, add the mobile phase to make exactly 100 mL, and use this solution as the standard solution. Perform the test with exactly 10 μL each of the sample solution and standard solution as directed under Liquid Chromatography ⟨*2.01*⟩ according to the following conditions, and determine each peak area of each solution by the automatic integration method: the area of each peak other than cetirizine obtained from the sample solution is not larger than the peak area of cetirizine from the standard solution. And the total area of the peaks other than cetirizine from the sample solution is not larger than 2.5 times the peak area of cetirizine from the standard solution.

Operating conditions—

Detector: An ultraviolet absorption photometer (wavelength: 230 nm).

Column: A stainless steel column 4.0 mm in inside diameter and 25 cm in length, packed with silica gel for liquid chromatography (5 μm in particle diameter).

Column temperature: A constant temperature of about 25°C.

Mobile phase: A mixture of acetonitrile and diluted 0.5 mol/L sulfuric acid TS (2 in 25) (47:3).

Flow rate: Adjust so that the retention time of cetirizine is about 9 minutes.

Time span of measurement: About 3 times as long as the retention time of cetirizine, beginning after the solvent peak.

System suitability—

Test for required detectability: Pipet 5 mL of the standard solution, and add the mobile phase to make exactly 10 mL. Confirm that the peak area of cetirizine obtained with 10 μL of this solution is equivalent to 35 to 65% of that with 10 μL of the standard solution.

System performance: Dissolve 20 mg of Cetirizine Hydrochloride in the mobile phase to make 100 mL. To 5 mL of this solution, add 3 mL of a solution of aminopyrine in the mobile phase (1 in 2500), and add the mobile phase to make 20 mL. When the procedure is run with 10 μL of this solution under the above operating conditions, cetirizine and aminopyrine are eluted in this order with the resolution between these peaks being not less than 7.

System repeatability: When the test is repeated 6 times with 10 μL of the standard solution under the above operating conditions, the relative standard deviation of the peak area of cetirizine is not more than 2.0%.

Loss on drying ⟨*2.41*⟩ Not more than 0.5% (1 g, in vacuum, 60°C, 3 hours).

Residue on ignition ⟨*2.44*⟩ Not more than 0.2% (1 g).

Assay Weigh accurately about 0.1 g of Cetirizine Hydrochloride, previously dried, dissolve in 70 mL of a mixture of acetone and water (7:3), and titrate ⟨*2.50*⟩ to the second equivalence point with 0.1 mol/L sodium hydroxide VS (potentiometric titration). Perform a blank determination in the same manner, and make any necessary correction.

Each mL of 0.1 mol/L sodium hydroxide VS
= 15.39 mg of $C_{21}H_{25}ClN_2O_3.2HCl$

Containers and storage Containers—Well-closed containers.

Cetirizine Hydrochloride Tablets

セチリジン塩酸塩錠

Cetirizine Hydrochloride Tablets contain not less than 95.0% and not more than 105.0% of the labeled amount of cetirizine hydrochloride ($C_{21}H_{25}ClN_2O_3.2HCl$: 461.81).

Method of preparation Prepare as directed under Tablets, with Cetirizine Hydrochloride.

Identification To a quantity of powdered Cetirizine Hydrochloride Tablets, equivalent to 10 mg of Cetirizine Hydrochloride, add about 70 mL of 0.1 mol/L hydrochloric acid TS, shake, add 0.1 mol/L hydrochloric acid TS to make 100 mL, and filter. To 4 mL of the filtrate add 0.1 mol/L hydrochloric acid TS to make 25 mL, and determine the absorption spectrum of this solution as directed under Ultraviolet-visible Spectrophotometry <*2.24*>: it exhibits a maximum between 230 nm and 234 nm.

Uniformity of dosage units <*6.02*> Perform the test according to the following method: it meets the requirement of the Content uniformity test.

Take 1 tablet of Cetirizine Hydrochloride Tablets, add $4V/5$ mL of sodium 1-heptanesulfonate solution (1 in 5000) adjusted to pH 3.0 with 0.5 mol/L sulfuric acid TS, sonicate for 20 minutes, add sodium 1-heptanesulfonate solution (1 in 5000) adjusted to pH 3.0 with 0.5 mol/L sulfuric acid TS to exactly V mL so that each mL contains about 0.2 mg of cetirizine hydrochloride ($C_{21}H_{25}ClN_2O_3.2HCl$), and filter through a membrane filter with a pore size not exceeding 0.45 μm. Discard the first 3 mL of the filtrate, pipet 5 mL of the subsequent filtrate, add exactly 2 mL of the internal standard solution, add acetonitrile to make 10 mL, and use this solution as the sample solution. Then, proceed as directed in the Assay.

Amount (mg) of cetirizine hydrochloride ($C_{21}H_{25}ClN_2O_3.2HCl$)
$= M_S \times Q_T/Q_S \times V/100$

M_S: Amount (mg) of cetirizine hydrochloride for assay taken

Internal standard solution—A solution of propyl parahydroxybenzoate in the mobile phase (1 in 1000).

Dissolution <*6.10*> When the test is performed at 50 revolutions per minute according to the Paddle method, using 900 mL of water as the dissolution medium, the dissolution rates in 15 minutes of 5-mg tablet and in 30 minutes of 10-mg tablet are not less than 85% and not less than 80%, respectively.

Start the test with 1 tablet of Cetirizine Hydrochloride Tablets, withdraw not less than 20 mL of the medium at the specified minute after starting the test, and filter through a membrane filter with a pore size not exceeding 0.45 μm. Discard not less than 10 mL of the first filtrate, pipet V mL of the subsequent filtrate, add water to make exactly V' mL so that each mL contains about 5.6 μg of cetirizine hydrochloride ($C_{21}H_{25}ClN_2O_3.2HCl$), and use this solution as the sample solution. Separately, weigh accurately about 28 mg of cetirizine hydrochloride for assay, previously dried in vacuum at 60°C for 3 hours, and dissolve in water to make exactly 100 mL. Pipet 2 mL of this solution, add water to make exactly 100 mL, and use this solution as the standard solution. Determine the absorbances, A_T and A_S, at 230 nm of the sample solution and the standard solution as directed under Ultraviolet-visible Spectrophotometry <*2.24*>.

Dissolution rate (%) with respect to the labeled amount of cetirizine hydrochloride ($C_{21}H_{25}ClN_2O_3.2HCl$)
$= M_S \times A_T/A_S \times V'/V \times 1/C \times 18$

M_S: Amount (mg) of cetirizine hydrochloride for assay taken

C: Labeled amount (mg) of cetirizine hydrochloride ($C_{21}H_{25}ClN_2O_3.2HCl$) in 1 tablet

Assay Weigh accurately not less than 20 Cetirizine Hydrochloride Tablets, and powder. Weigh accurately a portion of the powder, equivalent to about 10 mg of cetirizine hydrochloride ($C_{21}H_{25}ClN_2O_3.2HCl$), add 40 mL of sodium 1-heptanesulfonate solution (1 in 5000) adjusted to pH 3.0 with 0.5 mol/L sulfuric acid TS, treat with ultrasonic waves for 20 minutes, add sodium 1-heptanesulfonate solution (1 in 5000) adjusted to pH 3.0 with 0.5 mol/L sulfuric acid TS, to make exactly 50 mL, and filter this solution through a membrane filter with a pore size not exceeding 0.45 μm. Discard the first 3 mL of the filtrate, pipet 5 mL of the subsequent filtrate, add exactly 2 mL of the internal standard solution, add acetonitrile to make exactly 10 mL, and use this solution as the sample solution. Separately, weigh accurately about 20 mg of cetirizine hydrochloride for assay, previously dried in vacuum at 60°C for 3 hours, and add sodium 1-heptanesulfonate solution (1 in 5000) adjusted to pH 3.0 with 0.5 mol/L sulfuric acid TS, to make exactly 100 mL. Pipet 5 mL of this solution, add exactly 2 mL of the internal standard solution, add acetonitrile to make 10 mL, and use this solution as the standard solution. Perform the test with 20 μL each of the sample solution and standard solution as directed under Liquid Chromatography <*2.01*> according to the following conditions, and calculate the ratios, Q_T and Q_S, of the peak area of cetirizine to that of the internal standard.

Amount (mg) of cetirizine hydrochloride ($C_{21}H_{25}ClN_2O_3.2HCl$)
$= M_S \times Q_T/Q_S \times 1/2$

M_S: Amount (mg) of cetirizine hydrochloride for assay taken

Internal standard solution—A solution of propyl parahydroxybenzoate in the mobile phase (1 in 1000).

Operating conditions—

Detector: An ultraviolet absorption photometer (wavelength: 230 nm).

Column: A stainless steel column 4.0 mm in inside diameter and 25 cm in length, packed with octylsilanized silica gel for liquid chromatography (5 μm in particle diameter).

Column temperature: A constant temperature of about 25°C.

Mobile phase: A mixture of a solution of sodium 1-heptansulfonate (1 in 2900) and acetonitrile (29:21), adjusted to pH 3.0 with 0.5 mol/L sulfuric acid TS.

Flow rate: Adjust so that the retention time of cetirizine is about 5 minutes.

System suitability—

System performance: When the procedure is run with 20 μL of the standard solution under the above operating conditions, cetirizine and the internal standard are eluted in this order with the resolution between these peaks being not less than 7.

System repeatability: When the test is repeated 6 times with 20 μL of the standard solution under the above operating conditions, the relative standard deviation of the ratio of the peak area of cetirizine to that of the internal standard is not more than 1.0%.

Containers and storage Containers—Well-closed containers.

Cetotiamine Hydrochloride Hydrate

セトチアミン塩酸塩水和物

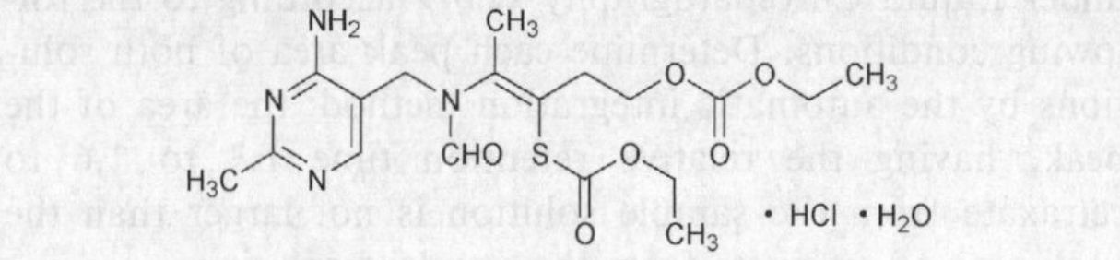

$C_{18}H_{26}N_4O_6S.HCl.H_2O$: 480.96
(3*Z*)-4-{*N*-[(4-Amino-2-methylpyrimidin-5-yl)methyl]-*N*-formylamino}-3-(ethoxycarbonylsulfanyl)pent-3-enyl ethyl carbonate monohydrochloride monohydrate
[*616-96-6*, anhydride]

Cetotiamine Hydrochloride Hydrate contains not less than 98.0% and not more than 102.0% of cetotiamine hydrochloride ($C_{18}H_{26}N_4O_6S.HCl$: 462.95), calculated on the anhydrous basis.

Description Cetotiamine Hydrochloride Hydrate occurs as white, crystals or crystalline powder. It is odorless or has a faint characteristic odor.

It is freely soluble in water and in ethanol (99.5).

It dissolves in 0.01 mol/L hydrochloric acid TS.

Melting point: about 132°C (with decomposition).

Identification **(1)** Determine the absorption spectrum of a solution of Cetotiamine Hydrochloride Hydrate in 0.01 mol/L hydrochloric acid TS (1 in 50,000) as directed under Ultraviolet-visible Spectrophotometry *<2.24>*, and compare the spectrum with the Reference Spectrum or the spectrum of a solution of Cetotiamine Hydrochloride RS prepared in the same manner as the sample solution: both spectra exhibit similar intensities of absorption at the same wavelengths.

(2) Determine the infrared absorption spectrum of Cetotiamine Hydrochloride Hydrate as directed in the potassium bromide disk method under Infrared Spectrophotometry *<2.25>*, and compare the spectrum with the Reference Spectrum or the spectrum of Cetotiamine Hydrochloride RS: both spectra exhibit similar intensities of absorption at the same wave numbers.

(3) A solution of Cetotiamine Hydrochloride Hydrate (1 in 50) responds to Qualitative Tests *<1.09>* for chloride.

Purity **(1)** Clarity and color of solution—A solution obtained by dissolving 1.0 g of Cetotiamine Hydrochloride Hydrate in 10 mL of water is clear and has no more color than the following control solution.

Control solution: Mix exactly 1.5 mL of Cobalt (II) Chloride CS, exactly 36 mL of Iron (III) Chloride CS and exactly 12.5 mL of diluted dilute hydrochloric acid (1 in 10). Pipet 1 mL of this mixture, and add diluted dilute hydrochloric acid (1 in 10) to make exactly 100 mL.

(2) Heavy metals *<1.07>*—Proceed with 1.0 g of Cetotiamine Hydrochloride Hydrate according to Method 1, and perform the test. Prepare the control solution with 2.0 mL of Standard Lead Solution (not more than 20 ppm).

(3) Related substances—Dissolve 50 mg of Cetotiamine Hydrochloride Hydrate in 50 mL of the mobile phase, and use this solution as the sample solution. Pipet 1 mL of the sample solution, add the mobile phase to make exactly 200 mL, and use this solution as the standard solution. Perform the test with exactly 10 μL each of the sample solution and standard solution as directed under Liquid Chromatography *<2.01>* according to the following conditions, and determine each peak area by the automatic integration method: the area of the peak other than cetotiamine obtained from the sample solution is not larger than the peak area of cetotiamine from the standard solution, and the total area of the peaks other than cetotiamine from the sample solution is not larger than 2 times the peak area of cetotiamine from the standard solution.

Operating conditions—

Detector, column, column temperature, mobile phase, and flow rate: Proceed as directed in the operating conditions in the Assay.

Time span of measurement: About 3 times as long as the retention time of cetotiamine, beginning after the solvent peak.

System suitability—

Test for required detectability: To exactly 2 mL of the standard solution add the mobile phase to make exactly 20 mL. Confirm that the peak area of cetotiamine obtained with 10 μL of this solution is equivalent to 7 to 13% of that with 10 μL of the standard solution.

System performance: When the procedure is run with 10 μL of the standard solution under the above operating conditions, the number of theoretical plates and the symmetry factor of the peak of cetotiamine are not less than 3000 and 0.7 – 1.0, respectively.

System repeatability: When the test is repeated 6 times with 10 μL of the standard solution under the above operating conditions, the relative standard deviation of the peak area of cetotiamine is not more than 2.0%.

Water *<2.48>* 3.0 – 5.0% (40 mg, coulometric titration).

Residue on ignition *<2.44>* Not more than 0.2% (1 g).

Assay Weigh accurately about 30 mg each of Cetotiamine Hydrochloride Hydrate and Cetotiamine Hydrochloride RS (separately determine the water *<2.48>* in the same manner as Cetotiamine Hydrochloride Hydrate), add exactly 10 mL each of the internal standard solution, then add a mixture of water and methanol (1:1) to make 50 mL. To 2 mL each of these solutions add a mixture of water and methanol (1:1) to make 10 mL, and use these solutions as the sample solution and the standard solution, respectively. Perform the test with 5 μL each of the sample solution and standard solution as directed under Liquid Chromatography *<2.01>* according to the following conditions, and calculate the ratios, Q_T and Q_S, of the peak area of cetotiamine to that of the internal standard.

Amount (mg) of cetotiamine hydrochloride ($C_{18}H_{26}N_4O_6S.HCl$)
$$= M_S \times Q_T/Q_S$$

M_S: Amount (mg) of Cetotiamine Hydrochloride RS taken, calculated on the anhydrous basis

Internal standard solution—A solution of propyl parahydroxybenzoate in a mixture of water and methanol (1:1) (1 in 800).

Operating conditions—

Detector: An ultraviolet absorption photometer (wavelength: 245 nm).

Column: A stainless steel column 4.6 mm in inside diameter and 15 cm in length, packed with octadecylsilanized silica gel for liquid chromatography (5 μm in particle diameter).

Column temperature: A constant temperature of about 25°C.

Mobile phase: Dissolve 1.0 g of sodium 1-heptanesulfonate in diluted acetic acid (100) (1 in 100) to make 1000 mL. To 1 volume of this solution add 1 volume of methanol.

Flow rate: Adjust so that the retention time of cetotiamine is about 10 minutes.

System suitability—

System performance: When the procedure is run with 5 μL of the standard solution under the above operating conditions, cetotiamine and the internal standard are eluted in this order with the resolution between these peaks being not less than 5.

System repeatability: When the test is repeated 6 times with 5 μL of the standard solution under the above operating conditions, the relative standard deviation of the ratio of the peak area of cetotiamine to that of the internal standard is not more than 1.0%.

Containers and storage Containers—Tight containers.

Cetraxate Hydrochloride

セトラキサート塩酸塩

$C_{17}H_{23}NO_4.HCl$: 341.83
3-{4-[*trans*-4-(Aminomethyl)cyclohexylcarbonyloxy]-phenyl}propanoic acid monohydrochloride
[*27724-96-5*]

Cetraxate Hydrochloride, when dried, contains not less than 98.5% of cetraxate hydrochloride ($C_{17}H_{23}NO_4.HCl$).

Description Cetraxate Hydrochloride occurs as white, crystals or crystalline powder.

It is soluble in methanol, sparingly soluble in water and in ethanol (95), and practically insoluble in diethyl ether.

Melting point: about 236°C (with decomposition).

Identification **(1)** Determine the absorption spectrum of a solution of Cetraxate Hydrochloride in methanol (1 in 2500) as directed under Ultraviolet-visible Spectrophotometry <*2.24*>, and compare the spectrum with the Reference Spectrum: both spectra exhibit similar intensities of absorption at the same wavelengths.

(2) Dissolve 0.5 g of Cetraxate Hydrochloride in 5 mL of a mixture of water and 2-propanol (1:1) by warming, cool to below 25°C. Filter, dry the formed crystals in vacuum for 4 hours, and further dry at 105°C for 1 hour. Determine the infrared absorption spectrum of the dried matter as directed in the potassium chloride disk method under Infrared Spectrophotometry <*2.25*>, and compare the spectrum with the Reference Spectrum: both spectra exhibit similar intensities of absorption at the same wave numbers.

(3) A solution of Cetraxate Hydrochloride (1 in 100) responds to Qualitative Tests <*1.09*> (2) for chloride.

Purity **(1)** Heavy metals <*1.07*>—Proceed with 2.0 g of Cetraxate Hydrochloride according to Method 2, and perform the test. Prepare the control solution with 2.0 mL of Standard Lead Solution (not more than 10 ppm).

(2) Arsenic <*1.11*>—Prepare the test solution with 1.0 g of Cetraxate Hydrochloride according to Method 3, and perform the test with a solution of magnesium nitrate hexahydrate in ethanol (95) (1 in 5) (not more than 2 ppm).

(3) *cis* Isomer—Dissolve 0.10 g of Cetraxate Hydrochloride in 10 mL of water, and use this solution as the sample solution. To exactly 5 mL of the sample solution add water to make exactly 100 mL. To exactly 2 mL of this solution add water to make exactly 50 mL, and use this solution as the standard solution. Perform the test with exactly 10 μL each of the sample solution and standard solution as directed under Liquid Chromatography <*2.01*> according to the following conditions. Determine each peak area of both solutions by the automatic integration method: the area of the peak, having the relative retention time 1.3 to 1.6 to cetraxate from the sample solution is not larger than the peak area of cetraxate from the standard solution.

Operating conditions—

Detector: An ultraviolet absorption photometer (wavelength: 220 nm).

Column: A stainless steel column 6 mm in inside diameter and 15 cm in length, packed with octadecylsilanized silica gel for liquid chromatography (5 μm in particle diameter).

Column temperature: A constant temperature of about 25°C.

Mobile phase: Adjust the pH of a mixture of water, methanol and 0.5 mol/L ammonium acetate TS (15:10:4) to 6.0 with acetic acid (31).

Flow rate: Adjust so that the retention time of cetraxate is about 10 minutes.

System suitability—

System performance: Dissolve 0.02 g of Cetraxate Hydrochloride and 0.01 g of phenol in 100 mL of water. To 2 mL of this solution add water to make 20 mL. When the procedure is run with 10 μL of this solution under the above operating conditions, cetraxate and phenol are eluted in this order with the resolution between these peaks being not less than 5.

System repeatability: When the test is repeated 6 times with 10 μL of the standard solution under the above operating conditions, the relative standard deviation of the peak area of cetraxate is not more than 2.0%.

(4) 3-(*p*-Hydroxyphenyl)propionic acid—To 0.10 g of Cetraxate Hydrochloride add exactly 2 mL of the internal standard solution and methanol to make 10 mL, and use this solution as the sample solution. Separately, dissolve 25 mg of 3-(*p*-hydroxyphenyl)propionic acid in methanol to make exactly 100 mL. To exactly 2 mL of this solution add exactly 2 mL of the internal standard solution and methanol to make 10 mL, and use this solution as the standard solution. Perform the test with 10 μL each of the sample solution and standard solution as directed under Liquid Chromatography <*2.01*> according to the following conditions, and calculate the ratios, Q_T and Q_S, of the peak area of 3-(*p*-hydroxyphenyl)propionic acid to that of the internal standard: Q_T is not larger than Q_S.

Internal standard solution—A solution of caffeine in methanol (1 in 4000).

Operating conditions—

Detector: An ultraviolet absorption photometer (wavelength: 230 nm).

Column: A stainless steel column 6 mm in inside diameter and 15 cm in length, packed with octadecylsilanized silica gel for liquid chromatography (5 μm in particle diameter).

Column temperature: A constant temperature of about 40°C.

Mobile phase: Adjust the pH of a mixture of water, methanol and 0.5 mol/L ammonium acetate TS (15:5:2) to 5.5

with acetic acid (31).

Flow rate: Adjust so that the retention time of 3-(*p*-hydroxyphenyl)propionic acid is about 7 minutes.

System suitability—

System performance: When the procedure is run with 10 μL of the standard solution under the above operating conditions, 3-(*p*-hydroxyphenyl)propionic acid and the internal standard are eluted in this order with the resolution between these peaks being not less than 5.

System repeatability: When the test is repeated 6 times with 10 μL of the standard solution under the above operating conditions, the relative standard deviation of the ratio of the peak area of 3-(*p*-hydroxyphenyl)propionic acid to that of the internal standard is not more than 1.0%.

(5) Related substances—Dissolve 0.10 g of Cetraxate Hydrochloride in 10 mL of methanol, and use this solution as the sample solution. Pipet 1 mL of the sample solution, add methanol to make exactly 100 mL, and use this solution as the standard solution. Perform the test with these solutions as directed under Thin-layer Chromatography *<2.03>*. Spot 5 μL each of the sample solution and standard solution on a plate of silica gel for thin-layer chromatography. Develop the plate with a mixture of chloroform, methanol and acetic acid (100) (20:4:3) to a distance of about 10 cm, and air-dry the plate. Spray evenly ninhydrin TS on the plate, and heat the plate at 90°C for 10 minutes: the spots other than the principal spot obtained from the sample solution are not more intense than the spot from the standard solution.

Loss on drying *<2.41>* Not more than 0.5% (0.5 g, 105°C, 3 hours).

Residue on ignition *<2.44>* Not more than 0.1% (1 g).

Assay Weigh accurately about 0.5 g of Cetraxate Hydrochloride, previously dried, dissolve in 100 mL of water, and adjust the pH of this solution to between 7.0 and 7.5 with dilute sodium hydroxide TS. To this solution add 10 mL of formaldehyde solution, stir for about 5 minutes, and titrate *<2.50>* with 0.1 mol/L sodium hydroxide VS by taking over about 20 minutes (potentiometric titration). Perform a blank determination in the same manner, and make any necessary correction.

Each mL of 0.1 mol/L sodium hydroxide VS
= 34.18 mg of $C_{17}H_{23}NO_4.HCl$

Containers and storage Containers—Tight containers.

Chenodeoxycholic Acid

ケノデオキシコール酸

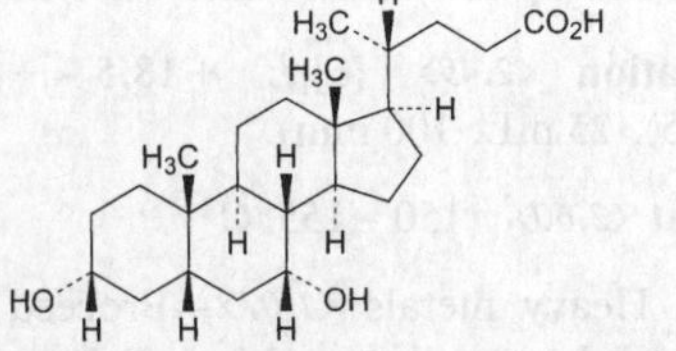

$C_{24}H_{40}O_4$: 392.57

3α,7α-Dihydroxy-5β-cholan-24-oic acid

[*474-25-9*]

Chenodeoxycholic Acid, when dried, contains not less than 98.0% and not more than 101.0% of chenodeoxycholic acid ($C_{24}H_{40}O_4$).

Description Chenodeoxycholic Acid occurs as white, crystals, crystalline powder or powder.

It is freely soluble in methanol and in ethanol (99.5), soluble in acetone, and practically insoluble in water.

Identification Determine the infrared absorption spectrum of Chenodeoxycholic Acid, previously dried, as directed in the potassium bromide disk method under Infrared Spectrophotometry *<2.25>*, and compare the spectrum with the Reference Spectrum: both spectra exhibit similar intensities of absorption at the same wave numbers.

Optical rotation *<2.49>* $[\alpha]_D^{20}$: +11.0 – +13.0° (after drying, 0.4 g, ethanol (99.5), 20 mL, 100 mm).

Melting point *<2.60>* 164 – 169°C

Purity **(1)** Chloride *<1.03>*—Dissolve 0.36 g of Chenodeoxycholic Acid in 30 mL of methanol, add 10 mL of dilute nitric acid and water to make 50 mL, and perform the test with this solution. Prepare the control solution as follows: To 1.0 mL of 0.01 mol/L hydrochloric acid VS add 30 mL of methanol, 10 mL of dilute nitric acid and water to make 50 mL (not more than 0.1%).

(2) Heavy metals *<1.07>*—Proceed with 1.0 g of Chenodeoxycholic Acid according to Method 4, and perform the test. Prepare the control solution with 2.0 mL of Standard Lead Solution (not more than 20 ppm).

(3) Barium—To 2.0 g of Chenodeoxycholic Acid add 100 mL of water, and boil for 2 minutes. To this solution add 2 mL of hydrochloric acid, boil for 2 minutes, filter after cooling, and wash the filter with water until to get 100 mL of the filtrate. To 10 mL of the filtrate add 1 mL of dilute sulfuric acid: no turbidity appears.

(4) Related substances—Dissolve 0.20 g of Chenodeoxycholic Acid in a mixture of acetone and water (9:1) to make exactly 10 mL, and use this solution as the sample solution. Separately, dissolve 10 mg of lithocholic acid for thin-layer chromatography in the mixture of acetone and water (9:1) to make exactly 10 mL. Pipet 2 mL of this solution, add the mixture of acetone and water (9:1) to make exactly 100 mL, and use this solution as the standard solution (1). Separately, dissolve 10 mg of ursodeoxycholic acid in the mixture of acetone and water (9:1) to make exactly 100 mL, and use this solution as the standard solution (2). Separately, dissolve 10 mg of cholic acid for thin-layer chromatography in the mixture of acetone and water (9:1) to make exactly 100 mL, and use this solution as the standard solution (3). Pipet 1 mL of the sample solution, and add the mixture of acetone and water (9:1) to make exactly 20 mL. Pipet 0.5 mL, 1 mL, 2 mL, 3 mL and 5 mL of this solution, add the mixture of acetone and water (9:1) to each of them to make exactly 50 mL, and designate these solutions as standard solution A, standard solution B, standard solution C, standard solution D and standard solution E, respectively. Perform the test with these solutions as directed under Thin-layer Chromatography *<2.03>*. Spot 5 μL each of the sample solution, standard solutions (1), (2), (3) and standard solutions A, B, C, D and E on a plate of silica gel for thin-layer chromatography. Develop the plate with a mixture of 4-methyl-2-pentanone, toluene and formic acid (16:6:1) to a distance of about 15 cm, air-dry the plate, and further dry at 120°C for 30 minutes. Immediately, spray evenly a solution of phosphomolybdic acid *n*-hydrate in ethanol (95) (1 in 5) on the plate, and heat the plate at 120°C for 2 to 3 minutes: the spot corresponding to the spot obtained from the standard solution (1) is not more intense than the spot from the standard solution (1), the spot corresponding to the spot from the standard solution (2) is not more intense than the spot from the standard solution (2), and the spot corresponding to the spot from the standard solution (3) is not more intense than the spot from the standard solution (3). As compared to the spots with the standard solutions A, B, C, D and E, the spots other than the principal spot and the spots mentioned above from the sample solution are not more intense than the spot from the standard solution E, and the total amount of them is not more than 1.5%.

Loss on drying *<2.41>* Not more than 1.5% (1 g, 105°C, 3 hours).

Residue on ignition *<2.44>* Not more than 0.1% (1 g).

Assay Weigh accurately about 0.5 g of Chenodeoxycholic Acid, previously dried, dissolve in 40 mL of ethanol (95) and 20 mL of water, and titrate *<2.50>* with 0.1 mol/L sodium hydroxide VS (potentiometric titration). Perform a blank determination in the same manner, and make any necessary correction.

Each mL of 0.1 mol/L sodium hydroxide VS
= 39.26 mg of $C_{24}H_{40}O_4$

Containers and storage Containers—Tight containers.

Chloral Hydrate

抱水クロラール

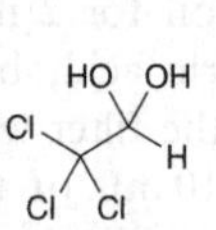

$C_2H_3Cl_3O_2$: 165.40
2,2,2-Trichloroethane-1,1-diol
[302-17-0]

Chloral Hydrate contains not less than 99.5% of chloral hydrate ($C_2H_3Cl_3O_2$).

Description Chloral Hydrate occurs as colorless crystals. It has a pungent odor and an acrid, slightly bitter taste.

It is very soluble in water, and freely soluble in ethanol (95) and in diethyl ether.

It slowly volatilizes in air.

Identification **(1)** Dissolve 0.2 g of Chloral Hydrate in 2 mL of water, and add 2 mL of sodium hydroxide TS: the turbidity is produced, and it separates into two clear layers by warming.

(2) Heat 0.2 g of Chloral Hydrate with 3 drops of aniline and 3 drops of sodium hydroxide TS: the disagreeable odor of phenylisocyanide (poisonous) is perceptible.

Purity **(1)** Clarity and color of solution—Dissolve 1.0 g of Chloral Hydrate in 2 mL of water: the solution is clear and colorless.

(2) Acidity—Dissolve 0.20 g of Chloral Hydrate in 2 mL of water, and add 1 drop of methyl orange TS: a yellow color develops.

(3) Chloride *<1.03>*—Perform the test with 1.0 g of Chloral Hydrate. Prepare the control solution with 0.30 mL of 0.01 mol/L hydrochloric acid VS (not more than 0.011%).

(4) Chloral alcoholate—Warm 1.0 g of Chloral Hydrate with 10 mL of sodium hydroxide TS, filter the upper layer, add iodine TS to the filtrate until a yellow color develops, and allow the solution to stand for 1 hour: no yellow precipitate is produced.

(5) Benzene—Warm the solution obtained in (1) with 3 mL of water: no odor of benzene is perceptible.

Residue on ignition *<2.44>* Not more than 0.1% (1 g).

Assay Weigh accurately about 4 g of Chloral Hydrate in a glass-stoppered flask, add 10 mL of water and exactly 40 mL of 1 mol/L sodium hydroxide VS, and allow the mixture to stand for exactly 2 minutes. Titrate *<2.50>* the excess sodium hydroxide immediately with 0.5 mol/L sulfuric acid VS (indicator: 2 drops of phenolphthalein TS). Perform a blank determination in the same manner, and make any necessary correction.

Each mL of 1 mol/L sodium hydroxide VS
= 165.4 mg of $C_2H_3Cl_3O_2$

Containers and storage Containers—Tight containers.

Chloramphenicol

クロラムフェニコール

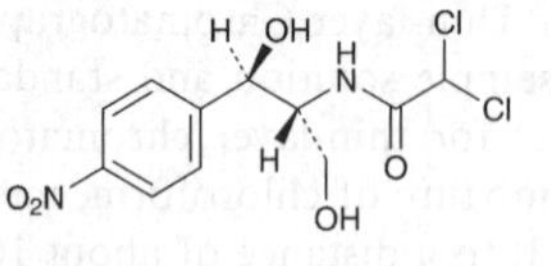

$C_{11}H_{12}Cl_2N_2O_5$: 323.13
2,2-Dichloro-*N*-[(1*R*,2*R*)-1,3-dihydroxy-1-(4-nitrophenyl)propan-2-yl]acetamide
[56-75-7]

Chloramphenicol contains not less than 980 μg (potency) and not more than 1020 μg (potency) per mg, calculated on the dried basis. The potency of Chloramphenicol is expressed as mass (potency) of chloramphenicol ($C_{11}H_{12}Cl_2N_2O_5$).

Description Chloramphenicol occurs as white to yellowwhite, crystals or crystalline powder.

It is freely soluble in methanol and in ethanol (99.5), and slightly soluble in water.

Identification **(1)** Determine the absorption spectrum of the sample solution obtained in the Assay as directed under Ultraviolet-visible Spectrophotometry *<2.24>*, and compare the spectrum with the Reference Spectrum or the spectrum of a solution of Chloramphenicol RS prepared in the same manner as the sample solution: both spectra exhibit similar intensities of absorption at the same wavelengths.

(2) Determine the infrared absorption spectrum of Chloramphenicol as directed in the potassium bromide disk method under Infrared Spectrophotometry *<2.25>*, and compare the spectrum with the Reference Spectrum or the spectrum of Chloramphenicol RS: both spectra exhibit similar intensities of absorption at the same wave numbers.

Optical rotation *<2.49>* $[\alpha]_D^{20}$: +18.5 – +21.5° (1.25 g, ethanol (99.5), 25 mL, 100 mm).

Melting point *<2.60>* 150 – 155°C

Purity **(1)** Heavy metals *<1.07>*—Proceed with 1.0 g of Chloramphenicol according to Method 2, and perform the test. Prepare the control solution with 2.5 mL of Standard Lead Solution (not more than 25 ppm).

(2) Related substances—Dissolve 0.10 g of Chloramphenicol in 10 mL of methanol, and use this solution as the sample solution. Pipet 1 mL of the sample solution, add methanol to make exactly 100 mL, and use this solution as the standard solution (1). Pipet 10 mL of the standard solution (1), add methanol to make exactly 20 mL, and use this solution as the standard solution (2). Perform the test with these solutions as directed under Thin-layer Chromatography *<2.03>*. Spot 20 μL each of the sample solution and standard solutions (1) and (2) on a plate of silica gel with fluorescent indicator for thin-layer chromatography, develop the plate with a mixture of ethyl acetate, methanol and acetic acid (100) (10:1:1) to a distance of about 15 cm, and air-dry the plate. Examine under ultraviolet light (main wavelength: 254 nm): the spots other than the principal spot and the spot of the starting point obtained from the sample solution are not more intense than the spot from the standard solution (1), and the total amount of these spots from the sample solution is not more than 2.0%.

Loss on drying *<2.41>* Not more than 0.5% (1 g, 105°C, 3 hours).

Residue on ignition *<2.44>* Not more than 0.1% (1 g).

Assay Weigh accurately an amount of Chloramphenicol and Chloramphenicol RS, equivalent to about 50 mg (potency), dissolve each in 10 mL of methanol, and add water to make exactly 50 mL. Pipet 20 mL each of these solutions, and add water to make exactly 100 mL. Pipet 10 mL each of these solutions, add water to make exactly 100 mL, and use these solutions as the sample solution and standard solution. Determine the absorbances, A_T and A_S, of the sample solution and standard solution at 278 nm as directed under Ultraviolet-visible Spectrophotometry *<2.24>*.

Amount [μg (potency)] of chloramphenicol ($C_{11}H_{12}Cl_2N_2O_5$)
$= M_S \times A_T/A_S \times 1000$

M_S: Amount [mg (potency)] of Chloramphenicol RS taken

Containers and storage Containers—Tight containers.

Chloramphenicol Palmitate

クロラムフェニコールパルミチン酸エステル

$C_{27}H_{42}Cl_2N_2O_6$: 561.54
(2*R*,3*R*)-2-(Dichloroacetyl)amino-3-hydroxy-3-(4-nitrophenyl)propan-1-yl palmitate
[530-43-8]

Chloramphenicol Palmitate contains not less than 558 μg (potency) and not more than 587 μg (potency) per mg, calculated on the dried basis. The potency of Chloramphenicol Palmitate is expressed as mass (potency) of chloramphenicol ($C_{11}H_{12}Cl_2N_2O_5$: 323.13).

Description Chloramphenicol Palmitate occurs as a white to grayish white, crystalline powder.

It is freely soluble in acetone, sparingly soluble in methanol and in ethanol (99.5), and practically insoluble in water.

Identification (1) Determine the absorption spectrum of a solution of Chloramphenicol Palmitate in ethanol (99.5) (1 in 33,000) as directed under Ultraviolet-visible Spectrophotometry *<2.24>*, and compare the spectrum with the Reference Spectrum or the spectrum of a solution of Chloramphenicol Palmitate RS prepared in the same manner as the sample solution: both spectra exhibit similar intensities of absorption at the same wavelengths.

(2) Dissolve 5 mg each of Chloramphenicol Palmitate and Chloramphenicol Palmitate RS in 1 mL of acetone, and use these solutions as the sample solution and standard solution. Perform the test with these solutions as directed under Thin-layer Chromatography *<2.03>*. Spot 5 μL each of the sample solution and standard solution on a plate of silica gel with fluorescent indicator for thin-layer chromatography. Develop the plate with a mixture of acetone and cyclohexane (1:1) to a distance of about 10 cm, and air-dry the plate. Examine under ultraviolet light (main wavelength: 254 nm): the principal spot obtained from the sample solution has the same *R*f value as the spot from the standard solution.

Optical rotation *<2.49>* $[\alpha]_D^{25}$: +21 – +25° (1 g calculated on the dried basis, ethanol (99.5), 20 mL, 100 mm).

Melting point *<2.60>* 91 - 96°C

Purity (1) Heavy metals *<1.07>*—Proceed with 1.0 g of Chloramphenicol Palmitate according to Method 4, and perform the test. Prepare the control solution with 2.0 mL of Standard Lead Solution (not more than 20 ppm).

(2) Arsenic *<1.11>*—Prepare the test solution with 1.0 g of Chloramphenicol Palmitate according to Method 3, and perform the test (not more than 2 ppm).

(3) Related substances—Dissolve 50 mg of Chloramphenicol Palmitate in 50 mL of methanol, and use this solution as the sample solution. Pipet 1 mL of the sample solution, add methanol to make exactly 100 mL, and use this solution as the standard solution. Perform the test with exactly 20 μL each of the sample solution and standard solution as directed under Liquid Chromatography *<2.01>* according to the following conditions. The test should be performed within 30 minutes after the sample solution and standard solution are prepared. Determine each peak area by the automatic integration method: the total area of the peaks other than the peak of chloramphenicol palmitate obtained from the sample solution is not larger than 3.5 times the peak area of chloramphenicol palmitate from the standard solution. For the peak areas for chloramphenicol, having the relative retention time of about 0.5 to chloramphenicol palmitate, and for chloramphenicol dipalmitate, having the relative retention time of about 5.0, multiply their correction factors, 0.5 and 1.4, respectively.

Operating conditions—

Detector: An ultraviolet absorption photometer (wavelength: 270 nm).

Column: A stainless steel column 6.0 mm in inside diameter and 15 cm in length, packed with octadecylsilanized silica gel for liquid chromatography (5 μm in particle diameter).

Column temperature: A constant temperature of about 20°C.

Mobile phase: Methanol.

Flow rate: Adjust so that the retention time of chloramphenicol palmitate is about 5 minutes.

Time span of measurement: About 6 times as long as the retention time of chloramphenicol palmitate.

System suitability—

Test for required detectability: Dissolve 50 mg of Chloramphenicol Palmitate in 50 mL of methanol. To 1 mL of this solution, add methanol to make 100 mL, and use this solution as the solution for system suitability test. Pipet 5 mL of the solution for system suitability test, and add methanol to make exactly 50 mL. Confirm that the peak area of chloramphenicol palmitate obtained with 20 μL of this solution is equivalent to 7 to 13% of that with 20 μL of the solution for system suitability test.

System performance: When the procedure is run with 20 μL of the solution for system suitability test under the above operating conditions, the number of theoretical plates of the peak of chloramphenicol palmitate is not less than 5000.

System repeatability: When the test is repeated 6 times with 20 μL of the solution for system suitability test under the above operating conditions, the relative standard deviation of the peak area of chloramphenicol palmitate is not more than 1.0%.

Loss on drying *<2.41>* Not more than 1.0% (1 g, reduced pressure not exceeding 0.67 kPa, 60°C, 3 hours).

Assay Weigh accurately an amount of Chloramphenicol Palmitate and Chloramphenicol Palmitate RS, equivalent to about 37 mg (potency), dissolve each in 40 mL of methanol and 1 mL of acetic acid (100), and add methanol to make exactly 50 mL. Pipet 10 mL each of these solutions, add the mobile phase to make exactly 25 mL, and use these solutions as the sample solution and standard solution. Perform the test with exactly 10 μL each of the sample solution and standard solution as directed under Liquid Chromatography *<2.01>* according to the following conditions, and determine the peak areas, A_T and A_S, of chloramphenicol palmitate in each solution.

Amount [μg (potency)] of chloramphenicol ($C_{11}H_{12}Cl_2N_2O_5$)
$= M_S \times A_T/A_S \times 1000$

M_S: Amount [mg (potency)] of Chloramphenicol Palmitate RS taken

Operating conditions—

Detector: An ultraviolet absorption photometer (wavelength: 280 nm).

Column: A stainless steel column 3.9 mm in inside diameter and 30 cm in length, packed with octadecylsilanized silica gel for liquid chromatography (10 μm in particle diameter).

Column temperature: A constant temperature of about 40°C.

Mobile phase: A mixture of methanol, water and acetic acid (100) (172:27:1).

Flow rate: Adjust so that the retention time of chloramphenicol palmitate is about 7 minutes.

System suitability—

System performance: When the procedure is run with 10 μL of the standard solution under the above operating conditions, the number of theoretical plates of the peak of chloramphenicol palmitate is not less than 2400.

System repeatability: When the test is repeated 6 times with 10 μL of the standard solution under the above operating conditions, the relative standard deviation of the peak area of chloramphenicol palmitate is not more than 1.0%.

Containers and storage Containers—Tight containers.

Storage—Light-resistant.

Chloramphenicol Sodium Succinate

クロラムフェニコールコハク酸エステルナトリウム

$C_{15}H_{15}Cl_2N_2NaO_8$: 445.18

Monosodium (2*R*,3*R*)-2-(dichloroacetyl)amino-3-hydroxy-3-(4-nitrophenyl)propan-1-yl succinate

[*982-57-0*]

Chloramphenicol Sodium Succinate contains not less than 711 μg (potency) and not more than 740 μg (potency) per mg, calculated on the anhydrous basis. The potency of Chloramphenicol Sodium Succinate is expressed as mass (potency) of chloramphenicol ($C_{11}H_{12}Cl_2N_2O_5$: 323.13).

Description Chloramphenicol Sodium Succinate occurs as white to yellowish white, crystals or crystalline powder.

It is very soluble in water, and freely soluble in methanol and in ethanol (99.5).

It is hygroscopic.

Identification **(1)** Determine the absorption spectrum of a solution of Chloramphenicol Sodium Succinate (1 in 50,000) as directed under Ultraviolet-visible Spectrophotometry *<2.24>*, and compare the spectrum with the Reference Spectrum: both spectra exhibit similar intensities of absorption at the same wavelengths.

(2) Determine the infrared absorption spectrum of Chloramphenicol Sodium Succinate as directed in the potassium bromide disk method under Infrared Spectrophotometry *<2.25>*, and compare the spectrum with the Reference Spectrum: both spectra exhibit similar intensities of absorption at the same wave numbers.

(3) Chloramphenicol Sodium Succinate responds to Qualitative Tests *<1.09>* (1) for sodium salt.

Optical rotation *<2.49>* $[\alpha]_D^{25}$: +5 – +8° (1.25 g calculated on the anhydrous basis, water, 25 mL, 100 mm).

pH *<2.54>* The pH of a solution obtained by dissolving 1.4 g of Chloramphenicol Sodium Succinate in 5 mL of water is between 6.0 and 7.0.

Purity **(1)** Clarity and color of solution—Dissolve 1.0 g of Chloramphenicol Sodium Succinate in 10 mL of water: the solution is clear, and the absorbance at 420 nm of the solution determined as directed under Ultraviolet-visible Spectrophotometry *<2.24>* is not more than 0.30.

(2) Heavy metals *<1.07>*—Proceed with 1.0 g of Chloramphenicol Sodium Succinate according to Method 2, and perform the test. Prepare the control solution with 2.0 mL of Standard Lead Solution (not more than 20 ppm).

Water *<2.48>* Not more than 2.0% (1.0 g, volumetric titration, direct titration).

Assay Weigh accurately an amount of Chloramphenicol Sodium Succinate, equivalent to about 20 mg (potency), dissolve in water to make exactly 1000 mL, and use this solution as the sample solution. Separately, weigh accurately an amount of Chloramphenicol Succinate RS, equivalent to about 20 mg (potency), add about 50 mL of water to make a suspension, and add gradually about 7 mL of 0.01 mol/L sodium hydroxide TS while stirring to adjust the pH to 7.0. To this solution add water to make exactly 1000 mL, and use this solution as the standard solution. Determine the absorbances, A_T and A_S, at 276 nm of the sample solution and standard solution as directed under Ultraviolet-visible Spectrophotometry <2.24>.

Amount [μg (potency)] of chloramphenicol ($C_{11}H_{12}Cl_2N_2O_5$)
$= M_S \times A_T/A_S \times 1000$

M_S: Amount [mg (potency)] of Chloramphenicol Succinate RS taken

Containers and storage Containers—Hermetic containers.

Chloramphenicol and Colistin Sodium Methanesulfonate Ophthalmic Solution

クロラムフェニコール·コリスチンメタンスルホン酸ナトリウム点眼液

Chloramphenicol and Colistin Sodium Methanesulfonate Ophthalmic Solution is an aqueous ophthalmic preparation.

It contains not less than 90.0% and not more than 120.0% of the labeled potency of chloramphenicol ($C_{11}H_{12}Cl_2N_2O_5$: 323.13) and labeled Units of colistin A ($C_{53}H_{100}N_{16}O_{13}$: 1169.46).

Method of preparation Prepare as directed under Ophthalmic Liquids and Solutions, with Chloramphenicol and Colistin Sodium Methanesulfonate.

Description Chloramphenicol and Colistin Sodium Methanesulfonate Ophthalmic Solution is a clear, colorless to pale yellow liquid.

Identification **(1)** To a volume of Chloramphenicol and Colistin Sodium Methanesulfonate Ophthalmic Solution, equivalent to about 2.5 mg (potency) of Chloramphenicol, and add water to make 100 mL. Determine the absorption spectrum of this solution as directed under Ultraviolet-visible Spectrophotometry <2.24>, using water as a blank: it exhibits a maximum between 276 nm and 280 nm.

(2) To a volume of Chloramphenicol and Colistin Sodium Methanesulfonate Ophthalmic Solution, equivalent to about 5×10^5 Units of Colistin Sodium Methanesulfonate add 0.5 mL of ninhydrin TS, boil for 1 minute, and cool: a blue color develops.

Osmotic pressure ratio Being specified separately when the drug is granted approval based on the Law.

pH <2.54> 6.0 – 8.0

Foreign insoluble matter <6.11> It meets the requirement.

Insoluble particulate matter <6.08> It meets the requirement.

Sterility <4.06> Perform the test according to the Membrane filtration method: it meets the requirement.

Assay Perform the test according to the Cylinder-plate method as directed under Microbial Assay for Antibiotics <4.02> according to the following conditions.

(1) Chloramphenicol

(i) Test organism—*Kocuria rhizophila* ATCC 9341

(ii) Agar media for base layer and seed layer—Use the medium ii in 3) under (1) Agar media for seed and base layer.

(iii) Agar medium for transferring test organisms—Use the medium i in 2) under (2) Agar media for transferring test organisms.

(iv) Liquid medium for suspending test organisms—Use the medium (2) Liquid media for suspending test organisms of 3.2. Culture media.

(v) Standard solutions—Weigh accurately an amount of Chloramphenicol RS, equivalent to about 20 mg (potency), dissolve in 2 mL of ethanol (95), add phosphate buffer solution (pH 6.0) to make exactly 20 mL, and use this solution as the standard stock solution. Keep the standard stock solution at 15°C or below, and use within 30 days. Pipet a suitable amount of the standard stock solution before use, add phosphate buffer solution (pH 6.0) to make solutions so that each mL contains 100 μg (potency) and 25 μg (potency), and use these solutions as the high concentration standard solution and the low concentration standard solution, respectively.

(vi) Sample solutions—Weigh accurately an amount of Chloramphenicol and Colistin Sodium Methanesulfonate Ophthalmic Solution, equivalent to about 10 mg (potency) of Chloramphenicol, add phosphate buffer solution (pH 6.0) to make exactly 100 mL, and filter, if necessary. Pipet a suitable amount of this solution, add phosphate buffer solution (pH 6.0) to make solutions so that each mL contains 100 μg (potency) and 25 μg (potency), and use these solutions as the high concentration sample solution and the low concentration sample solution, respectively.

(2) Colistin Sodium Methanesulfonate

(i) Test organism—*Bordetella bronchiseptica* ATCC 4617

(ii) Agar medium for base layer—

Casein peptone 17.0 g
Sodium chloride 5.0 g
Glucose 2.5 g
Soybean peptone 3.0 g
Dipotassium hydrogen phosphate 2.0 g
Agar 20.0 g
Water 1000 mL

Mix all the ingredients, then add a suitable amount of sodium hydroxide TS so that the pH of the medium will be 7.2 to 7.3 after sterilization, and sterile.

(iii) Agar medium for seed layer—

Casein peptone 17.0 g
Glucose 2.5 g
Soybean peptone 3.0 g
Sodium chloride 5.0 g
Polysorbate 80 10.0 g
Dipotassium hydrogen phosphate 2.5 g
Agar 12.0 g
Water 1000 mL

Mix all the ingredients, then add a suitable amount of sodium hydroxide TS so that the pH of the medium will be 7.2 to 7.3 after sterilization, and sterile.

(iv) Agar medium for transferring test organisms—Use the medium i in 2) under (2) Agar media for transferring test organisms.

(v) Preparation of test organism and seeded agar layer—Cultivate the test organism on the slant of the agar medium for transferring test organism at 32 to 37°C for 16 to 24 hours. Subcultures at least three times. Cultivate the grown organism on the slant of the agar medium for transferring test organism at 32 to 37°C for 16 to 24 hours, add a suitable amount of water to the grown organism, and suspend. Adjust the suspension so that the transmittance at 660 nm is 60% as directed under Ultraviolet-visible Spectrophotometry <*2.24*> using a spectrophotometer or a photoelectric photometer, and use this suspension as the test organism suspension. Keep the test organism suspension at 15°C or below, and use within 3 days. Before use, dissolve 0.13 mL of the test organism suspension, add it to 100 mL of agar medium for seed previously cooled at 48°C, mix thoroughly, and use this as the seeded agar layer.

(vi) Standard solutions—Weigh accurately an amount of Colistin Sodium Methanesulfonate RS, equivalent to about 1×10^6 Units, dissolve in phosphate buffer solution (pH 6.0) to make exactly 100 mL, and use this solution as the standard stock solution. Keep the standard stock solution at 10°C or below, and use within 7 days. Pipet a suitable amount of the standard stock solution before use, add phosphate buffer solution (pH 6.0) to make solutions so that each mL contains 1000 Units and 250 Units, and use these solutions as the high concentration standard solution and the low concentration standard solution, respectively.

(vii) Sample solutions—Weigh accurately an amount of Chloramphenicol and Colistin Sodium Methanesulfonate Ophthalmic Solution, equivalent to about 1×10^5 Units of Colistin Sodium Methanesulfonate, add phosphate buffer solution (pH 6.0) to make a solution so that each mL contains 1000 Units, and use this solution as the high concentration sample solution. Pipet 5 mL of the high concentration sample solution, add phosphate buffer solution (pH 6.0) to make a solution so that each mL contains 250 Units, and use this solution as the low concentration sample solution.

Containers and storage Containers—Tight containers.

Storage—At a temperature between 2°C and 8°C.

Chlordiazepoxide

クロルジアゼポキシド

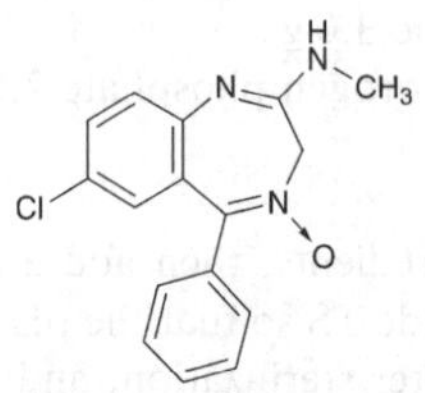

$C_{16}H_{14}ClN_3O$: 299.75

7-Chloro-2-methylamino-5-phenyl-3*H*-1,4-benzodiazepin-4-oxide

[*58-25-3*]

Chlordiazepoxide, when dried, contains not less than 98.5% of chlordiazepoxide ($C_{16}H_{14}ClN_3O$).

Description Chlordiazepoxide occurs as white to light yellow, crystals or crystalline powder.

It is freely soluble in acetic acid (100), sparingly soluble in ethanol (95), very slightly soluble in diethyl ether, and practically insoluble in water.

It dissolves in dilute hydrochloric acid.

It is gradually affected by light.

Melting point: about 240°C (with decomposition).

Identification **(1)** Determine the absorption spectrum of a solution of Chlordiazepoxide in 0.1 mol/L hydrochloric acid TS (1 in 200,000) as directed under Ultraviolet-visible Spectrophotometry <*2.24*>, and compare the spectrum with the Reference Spectrum or the spectrum of a solution of Chlordiazepoxide RS prepared in the same manner as the sample solution: both spectra exhibit similar intensities of absorption at the same wavelengths.

(2) Determine the infrared absorption spectra of Chlordiazepoxide, previously dried, as directed in the potassium bromide disk method under Infrared Spectrophotometry <*2.25*>, and compare the spectrum with the Reference Spectrum or the spectrum of dried Chlordiazepoxide RS: both spectra exhibit similar intensities of absorption at the same wave numbers.

(3) Proceed with Chlordiazepoxide as directed under Flame Coloration Test <*1.04*> (2), and perform the test: a green color develops.

Purity **(1)** Heavy metals <*1.07*>—Proceed with 1.0 g of Chlordiazepoxide according to Method 2, and perform the test. Prepare the control solution with 2.0 mL of Standard Lead Solution (not more than 20 ppm).

(2) Related substances—Conduct this procedure without exposure to light, using light-resistant vessels. Dissolve 0.20 g of Chlordiazepoxide in exactly 10 mL of a mixture of methanol and ammonia TS (97:3), and use this solution as the sample solution. Pipet 1 mL of the sample solution, add a mixture of methanol and ammonia TS (97:3) to make exactly 200 mL, and use this solution as the standard solution (1). Separately, dissolve 10 mg of 2-amino-5-chlorobenzophenone for thin-layer chromatography in methanol to make exactly 200 mL, and use this solution as the standard solution (2). Perform the test with these solutions as directed under Thin-layer Chromatography <*2.03*>. Spot 25 μL of the sample solution and 5 μL each of the standard solutions (1) and (2) on a plate of silica gel with fluorescent indicator for thin-layer chromatography. Develop the plate with a mixture of ethyl acetate and ethanol (99.5) (19:1) to a distance of about 12 cm, and air-dry the plate. Examine under ultraviolet light (main wavelength: 254 nm): the spots other than the principal spot obtained from the sample solution are not more intense than the spot from the standard solution (1). Spray evenly a solution of sodium nitrite in 1 mol/L hydrochloric acid TS (1 in 100) on the plate, allow to stand for 1 minute, and spray evenly *N*-(1-naphthyl)-*N'*-diethylethylenediamine oxalate-acetone TS on the plate: the spots from the sample solution are not more intense than the spots from the standard solution (2).

Loss on drying <*2.41*> Not more than 0.5% (1 g, in vacuum, phosphorus (V) oxide, 60°C, 4 hours).

Residue on ignition <*2.44*> Not more than 0.1% (1 g).

Assay Weigh accurately about 0.6 g of Chlordiazepoxide, previously dried, and dissolve in 50 mL of acetic acid (100). Titrate <*2.50*> with 0.1 mol/L perchloric acid VS until the color of the supernatant liquid changes from purple through blue-purple to blue (indicator: 3 drops of crystal violet TS). Perform a blank determination in the same manner, and make any necessary correction.

Each mL of 0.1 mol/L perchloric acid VS
= 29.98 mg of $C_{16}H_{14}ClN_3O$

Containers and storage Containers—Tight containers.

Storage—Light-resistant.

Chlordiazepoxide Powder

クロルジアゼポキシド散

Chlordiazepoxide Powder contains not less than 93.0% and not more than 107.0% of the labeled amount of chlordiazepoxide ($C_{16}H_{14}ClN_3O$: 299.75).

Method of preparation Prepare as directed under Granules or Powders, with Chlordiazepoxide.

Identification **(1)** Weigh a portion of Chlordiazepoxide Powder, equivalent to 0.01 g of Chlordiazepoxide, add 100 mL of 0.1 mol/L hydrochloric acid TS, shake, and filter. To 5 mL of the filtrate add 0.1 mol/L hydrochloric acid TS to make 100 mL, and determine the absorption spectrum of this solution as directed under Ultraviolet-visible Spectrophotometry *<2.24>*: it exhibits maxima between 244 nm and 248 nm and between 306 nm and 310 nm, and a minimum between 288 nm and 292 nm.

(2) Weigh a portion of Chlordiazepoxide Powder, equivalent to 0.02 g of Chlordiazepoxide, add 10 mL of methanol, shake for 5 minutes, then filter by suction through a glass filter (G4), evaporate the filtrate with the aid of a current of air to dryness, and dry the residue in vacuum at 60°C for 1 hour. Determine the infrared absorption spectrum of the residue as directed in the potassium bromide disk method under Infrared Spectrophotometry *<2.25>*: it exhibits absorption at the wave numbers of about 1625 cm^{-1}, 1465 cm^{-1}, 1265 cm^{-1}, 850 cm^{-1} and 765 cm^{-1}.

Purity Conduct this procedure without exposure to light, using light-resistant vessels. To a portion of Chlordiazepoxide Powder, equivalent to 50 mg of Chlordiazepoxide, add exactly 5 mL of a mixture of methanol and ammonia TS (97:3), shake, centrifuge, and use the supernatant liquid as the sample solution. Separately, dissolve 50 mg of Chlordiazepoxide RS in a mixture of methanol and ammonia TS (97:3) to make exactly 50 mL, and use this solution as the standard solution (1). Dissolve 5.0 mg of 2-amino-5-chlorobenzophenone for thin-layer chromatography in methanol to make exactly 200 mL, and use this solution as the standard solution (2). Perform the test with these solutions as directed under Thin-layer Chromatography *<2.03>*. Spot 25 μL of the sample solution and 10 μL each of the standard solutions (1) and (2) on a plate of silica gel with fluorescent indicator for thin-layer chromatography. Proceed as directed in the Purity (2) under Chlordiazepoxide.

Dissolution *<6.10>* When the test is performed at 100 revolutions per minute according to the Paddle method, using 900 mL of 2nd fluid for dissolution test as the dissolution medium, the dissolution rate in 60 minutes of Chlordiazepoxide Powder is not less than 70%.

Start the test with an accurately weighed amount of Chlordiazepoxide Powder, equivalent to about 3.3 mg of chlordiazepoxide ($C_{16}H_{14}ClN_3O$), withdraw not less than 15 mL of the medium at the specified minute after starting the test, and filter through a membrane filter with a pore size not exceeding 0.45 μm. Discard not less than 10 mL of the first filtrate, and use the subsequent filtrate as the sample solution. Separately, weigh accurately about 12 mg of Chlordiazepoxide RS, previously dried in a desiccator (in vacuum, phosphorus (V) oxide, 60°C) for 4 hours, dissolve in 20 mL of 0.1 mol/L hydrochloric acid TS, and add the dissolution medium to make exactly 200 mL. Pipet 3 mL of this solution, add the dissolution medium to make exactly 50 mL, and use this solution as the standard solution. Determine the absorbances, A_T and A_S, at 260 nm of the sample solution and standard solution as directed under Ultraviolet-visible Spectrophotometry *<2.24>*.

Dissolution rate (%) with respect to the labeled amount of chlordiazepoxide ($C_{16}H_{14}ClN_3O$)
$= M_S/M_T \times A_T/A_S \times 1/C \times 27$

M_S: Amount (mg) of Chlordiazepoxide RS taken
M_T: Amount (g) of Chlordiazepoxide Powder taken
C: Labeled amount (mg) of chlordiazepoxide ($C_{16}H_{14}ClN_3O$) in 1 g

Assay Conduct this procedure without exposure to light, using light-resistant vessels. Weigh accurately a quantity of Chlordiazepoxide Powder, equivalent to about 0.1 g of chlordiazepoxide ($C_{16}H_{14}ClN_3O$), transfer to a glass-stoppered flask, wet with exactly 10 mL of water, add exactly 90 mL of methanol, stopper, shake vigorously for 15 minutes, and centrifuge. Pipet 10 mL of the supernatant liquid, add exactly 5 mL of the internal standard solution, add methanol to make 100 mL, and use this solution as the sample solution. Separately, weigh accurately about 0.1 g of Chlordiazepoxide RS, previously dried in a desiccator (in vacuum, phosphorus (V) oxide, 60°C) for 4 hours, and dissolve in exactly 10 mL of water and exactly 90 mL of methanol. Pipet 10 mL of this solution, add exactly 5 mL of the internal standard solution, add methanol to make 100 mL, and use this solution as the standard solution. Perform the test with 10 μL each of the sample solution and standard solution as directed under Liquid Chromatography *<2.01>* according to the following conditions, and calculate the ratios, Q_T and Q_S, of the peak area of chlordiazepoxide to that of the internal standard.

Amount (mg) of chlordiazepoxide ($C_{16}H_{14}ClN_3O$)
$= M_S \times Q_T/Q_S$

M_S: Amount (mg) of Chlordiazepoxide RS taken

Internal standard solution—A solution of isobutyl salicylate in methanol (1 in 20).
Operating conditions—

Detector: An ultraviolet absorption photometer (wavelength: 254 nm).

Column: A stainless steel column 4 mm in inside diameter and 25 cm in length, packed with octadecylsilanized silica gel for liquid chromatography (10 μm in particle diameter).

Column temperature: A constant temperature of about 25°C.

Mobile phase: A mixture of methanol and 0.02 mol/L ammonium dihydrogenphosphate TS (7:3).

Flow rate: Adjust so that the retention time of chlordiazepoxide is about 5 minutes.

System suitability—

System performance: When the procedure is run with 10 μL of the standard solution under the above operating conditions, chlordiazepoxide and the internal standard are eluted in this order with the resolution between these peaks being not less than 9.

System repeatability: When the test is repeated 6 times with 10 μL of the standard solution under the above operating conditions, the relative standard deviation of the ratios of the peak area of chlordiazepoxide to that of the internal standard is not more than 1.0%.

Containers and storage Containers—Tight containers.
Storage-Light-resistant.

Chlordiazepoxide Tablets

クロルジアゼポキシド錠

Chlordiazepoxide Tablets contain not less than 93.0% and not more than 107.0% of the labeled amount of chlordiazepoxide ($C_{16}H_{14}ClN_3O$: 299.75).

Method of preparation Prepare as directed under Tablets, with Chlordiazepoxide.

Identification **(1)** Weigh a portion of powdered Chlordiazepoxide Tablets, equivalent to 0.01 g of Chlordiazepoxide, add 100 mL of 0.1 mol/L hydrochloric acid TS, shake, and filter. To 5 mL of the filtrate add 0.1 mol/L hydrochloric acid TS to make 100 mL, and determine the absorption spectrum of this solution as directed under Ultraviolet-visible Spectrophotometry *<2.24>*: it exhibits maxima between 244 nm and 248 nm and between 306 nm and 310 nm, and a minimum between 288 nm and 292 nm.

(2) Weigh a portion of powdered Chlordiazepoxide Tablets, equivalent to 0.01 g of Chlordiazepoxide, add 10 mL of diethyl ether, shake vigorously, and centrifuge. Evaporate 5 mL of the supernatant liquid by warming on a water bath to dryness. Determine the infrared absorption spectrum of the residue as directed in the potassium bromide disk method under Infrared Spectrophotometry *<2.25>*: it exhibits absorption at the wave numbers of about 1625 cm^{-1}, 1465 cm^{-1}, 1265 cm^{-1}, 850 cm^{-1} and 765 cm^{-1}.

Purity Related substances—Conduct this procedure without exposure to light, using light-resistant vessels. To a portion of powdered Chlordiazepoxide Tablets, equivalent to 50 mg of Chlordiazepoxide, add exactly 5 mL of a mixture of methanol and ammonia TS (97:3), shake, centrifuge, and use the supernatant liquid as the sample solution. Separately, dissolve 50 mg of Chlordiazepoxide RS in a mixture of methanol and ammonia TS (97:3) to make exactly 50 mL, and use this solution as the standard solution (1). Dissolve 5.0 mg of 2-amino-5-chlorobenzophenone for thin-layer chromatography in methanol to make exactly 200 mL, and use this solution as the standard solution (2). Perform the test with these solutions as directed under Thin-layer Chromatography *<2.03>*. Spot 25 μL of the sample solution and 10 μL each of the standard solutions (1) and (2) on a plate of silica gel with fluorescent indicator for thin-layer chromatography. Proceed as directed in the Purity (2) under Chlordiazepoxide.

Uniformity of dosage units *<6.02>* Perform the test according to the following method: it meets the requirement of the Content uniformity test.

Conduct this procedure without exposure to light, using light-resistant vessels. To 1 tablet of Chlordiazepoxide Tablets add 1 mL of water, shake to disintegrate the tablet, then add 20 mL of methanol, shake, add methanol to make exactly 25 mL, and filter through a membrane filter with a pore size not exceeding 0.5 μm. Discard the first 5 mL of the filtrate, take exactly V mL of the subsequent filtrate equivalent to about 2 mg of chlordiazepoxide ($C_{16}H_{14}ClN_3O$), add exactly 1 mL of the internal standard solution, then add methanol to make 20 mL, and use this solution as the sample solution. Then, proceed as directed in the Assay.

$$\text{Amount (mg) of chlordiazepoxide } (C_{16}H_{14}ClN_3O) = M_S \times Q_T/Q_S \times 5/V$$

M_S: Amount (mg) of Chlordiazepoxide RS taken

Internal standard solution—A solution of isobutyl salicylate in methanol (1 in 20).

Dissolution *<6.10>* When the test is performed at 100 revolutions per minute according to the Paddle method, using 900 mL of 2nd fluid for dissolution test as the dissolution medium, the dissolution rate in 60 minutes of Chlordiazepoxide Tablets is not less than 70%.

Conduct this procedure without exposure to light, using light-resistant vessels. Start the test with 1 tablet of Chlordiazepoxide Tablets, withdraw not less than 30 mL of the medium at the specified minute after starting the test, and filter through a membrane filter with a pore size not exceeding 0.8 μm. Discard not less than 10 mL of the first filtrate, pipet V mL of the subsequent filtrate, add the dissolution medium to make exactly V' mL so that each mL contains about 3.7 μg of chlordiazepoxide ($C_{16}H_{14}ClN_3O$), and use this solution as the sample solution. Separately, weigh accurately about 12 mg of Chlordiazepoxide RS, previously dried under reduced pressure with phosphorus (V) oxide as a dessicant at 60°C for 4 hours, dissolve in 5 mL of 0.1 mol/L hydrochloric acid TS, and add the dissolution medium to make exactly 200 mL. Pipet 3 mL of this solution, add the dissolution medium to make exactly 50 mL, and use this solution as the standard solution. Determine the absorbances, A_T and A_S, at 260 nm of the sample solution and standard solution as directed under Ultraviolet-visible Spectrophotometry *<2.24>*.

$$\text{Dissolution rate (\%) with respect to the labeled amount of chlordiazepoxide } (C_{16}H_{14}ClN_3O) = M_S \times A_T/A_S \times V'/V \times 1/C \times 27$$

M_S: Amount (mg) of Chlordiazepoxide RS taken
C: Labeled amount (mg) of chlordiazepoxide ($C_{16}H_{14}ClN_3O$) in 1 tablet

Assay Conduct this procedure without exposure to light, using light-resistant vessels. Weigh accurately a quantity of Chlordiazepoxide Tablets, equivalent to about 0.1 g of chlordiazepoxide ($C_{16}H_{14}ClN_3O$), add 10 mL of water, and shake well to disintegrate. Add 60 mL of methanol, shake well, add methanol to make exactly 100 mL, and centrifuge. Pipet 10 mL of the supernatant liquid, add exactly 5 mL of the internal standard solution, add methanol to make exactly 100 mL, and use this solution as the sample solution. Separately, weigh accurately about 10 mg of Chlordiazepoxide RS, previously dried in a desiccator (in vacuum, phosphorus (V) oxide, 60°C) for 4 hours, dissolve in 1 mL of water and a suitable amount of methanol, add exactly 5 mL of the internal standard solution, add methanol to make 100 mL, and use this solution as the standard solution. Perform the test with 10 μL each of the sample solution and standard solution as directed under Liquid Chromatography *<2.01>* according to the following conditions, and calculate the ratios, Q_T and Q_S, of the peak area of chlordiazepoxide to that of the internal standard.

$$\text{Amount (mg) of chlordiazepoxide } (C_{16}H_{14}ClN_3O) = M_S \times Q_T/Q_S \times 10$$

M_S: Amount (mg) of Chlordiazepoxide RS taken

Internal standard solution—A solution of isobutyl salicylate in methanol (1 in 20).

Operating conditions—

Detector: An ultraviolet absorption photometer (wavelength: 254 nm).

Column: A stainless steel column 4 mm in inside diameter and 25 cm in length, packed with octadecylsilanized silica gel for liquid chromatography (10 μm in particle diameter).

Column temperature: A constant temperature of about 25°C.

Mobile phase: A mixture of methanol and 0.02 mol/L ammonium dihydrogenphosphate TS (7:3).

Flow rate: Adjust so that the retention time of chlordiazepoxide is about 5 minutes.

System suitability—

System performance: When the procedure is run with 10 μL of the standard solution under the above operating conditions, chlordiazepoxide and the internal standard are eluted in this order with the resolution between these peaks being not less than 9.

System repeatability: When the test is repeated 6 times with 10 μL of the standard solution under the above operating conditions, the relative standard deviation of the ratios of the peak area of chlordiazepoxide to that of the internal standard is not more than 1.0%.

Containers and storage Containers—Tight containers.

Chlorhexidine Gluconate Solution

クロルヘキシジングルコン酸塩液

Chlorhexidine Gluconate Solution is a solution of digluconate of chlorhexidine.

It contains not less than 19.0 w/v% and not more than 21.0 w/v% of chlorhexidine gluconate ($C_{22}H_{30}Cl_2N_{10}.2C_6H_{12}O_7$: 897.76).

Description Chlorhexidine Gluconate Solution is a clear, colorless or pale yellow liquid. It is odorless, and has a bitter taste.

It is miscible with water and with acetic acid (100). 1 mL of Chlorhexidine Gluconate Solution is miscible with not more than 5 mL of ethanol (99.5) and with not more than 3 mL of acetone. By further addition of each of these solvents, a white turbidity is formed.

It is gradually colored by light.

Specific gravity d^{20}_{20}: 1.06 – 1.07

Identification **(1)** To 0.05 mL of Chlorhexidine Gluconate Solution add 5 mL of methanol, 1 mL of bromine TS and 1 mL of 8 mol/L sodium hydroxide TS: a deep red color is produced.

(2) To 0.5 mL of Chlorhexidine Gluconate Solution add 10 mL of water and 0.5 mL of copper (II) sulfate TS: a white precipitate is formed. Heat to boiling: the precipitate changes to light purple.

(3) To 10 mL of Chlorhexidine Gluconate Solution add 5 mL of water, cool on ice, and add 5 mL of sodium hydroxide TS dropwise with stirring: a white precipitate is formed. Collect the precipitate by filtration, wash with water, recrystallize from diluted ethanol (95) (7 in 10), and dry at 105°C for 30 minutes: the crystals thus obtained melt ⟨*2.60*⟩ between 130°C and 134°C.

(4) Neutralize the filtrate obtained in (3) with 5 mol/L hydrochloric acid TS. To 5 mL of this solution add 0.65 mL of acetic acid (100) and 1 mL of freshly distilled phenylhydrazine, and heat on a water bath for 30 minutes. After cooling, scratch the inner wall of the vessel with a glass rod to induce crystallization. Collect the crystals, dissolve in 10 mL of hot water, add a small amount of activated charcoal, and filter. Cool the filtrate, scratch the inner side of the vessel, collect the formed crystals, and dry: the crystals thus obtained melt ⟨*2.60*⟩ at about 195°C (with decomposition).

pH ⟨*2.54*⟩ To 5.0 mL of Chlorhexidine Gluconate Solution add water to make 100 mL: the pH of the solution is between 5.5 and 7.0.

Purity 4-Chloroaniline—To 2.0 mL of Chlorhexidine Gluconate Solution add water to make exactly 100 mL. Pipet 5 mL of the solution, and add 20 mL of water and 5 mL of 1 mol/L hydrochloric acid TS. Add 0.3 mL of sodium nitrite TS, shake, and allow to stand for 2 minutes. Add 4 mL of ammonium amidosulfate TS, and then allow to stand for 1 minute. Add 5 mL of *N*-(1-naphthyl)-*N*′-diethylethylenediamine oxalate-acetone TS, allow to stand for 10 minutes, add 1 mL of ethanol (95), and then add water to make 50 mL: the color of the solution is not more intense than the following control solution.

Control solution: Dissolve 20 mg of 4-chloroaniline in 10 mL of 1 mol/L hydrochloric acid TS, and add water to make exactly 100 mL. Pipet 5 mL of the solution, and add water to make exactly 100 mL. Pipet 5 mL of the solution, add 20 mL of water and 5 mL of 1 mol/L hydrochloric acid TS, and proceed as directed for the preparation of the sample solution.

Residue on ignition ⟨*2.44*⟩ Not more than 0.1% (2 g, after evaporation).

Assay Pipet 2 mL of Chlorhexidine Gluconate Solution, evaporate to dryness on a water bath, dissolve the residue in 60 mL of acetic acid for nonaqueous titration, and titrate ⟨*2.50*⟩ with 0.1 mol/L perchloric acid VS (potentiometric titration). Perform a blank determination in the same manner, and make any necessary correction.

Each mL of 0.1 mol/L perchloric acid VS
= 22.44 mg of $C_{22}H_{30}Cl_2N_{10}.2C_6H_{12}O_7$

Containers and storage Containers—Tight containers.

Storage—Light-resistant.

Chlorhexidine Hydrochloride

クロルヘキシジン塩酸塩

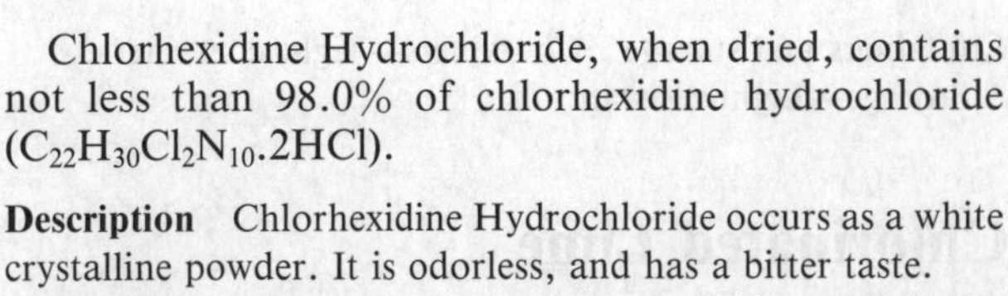

$C_{22}H_{30}Cl_2N_{10}.2HCl$: 578.37

1,1′-Hexamethylenebis[5-(4-chlorophenyl)biguanide] dihydrochloride

[3697-42-5]

Chlorhexidine Hydrochloride, when dried, contains not less than 98.0% of chlorhexidine hydrochloride ($C_{22}H_{30}Cl_2N_{10}.2HCl$).

Description Chlorhexidine Hydrochloride occurs as a white crystalline powder. It is odorless, and has a bitter taste.

It is soluble in formic acid, slightly soluble in methanol and in warm methanol, and practically insoluble in water, in ethanol (95) and in diethyl ether.

It is gradually colored by light.

Identification **(1)** Dissolve 0.01 g of Chlorhexidine Hydrochloride in 5 mL of methanol by warming, and add 1 mL of bromine TS and 1 mL of 8 mol/L sodium hydroxide TS: a deep red color is produced.

(2) Dissolve 0.3 g of Chlorhexidine Hydrochloride in 10

mL of 6 mol/L hydrochloric acid TS, cool in ice, and add 10 mL of 8 mol/L sodium hydroxide TS dropwise with stirring: a white precipitate is produced. Collect the precipitate, wash with water, recrystallize from diluted ethanol (95) (7 in 10), and dry at 105°C for 30 minutes: the crystals so obtained melt <*2.60*> between 130°C and 134°C.

(3) Dissolve 0.1 g of Chlorhexidine Hydrochloride in 50 mL of dilute nitric acid: the solution responds to Qualitative Tests <*1.09*> for chloride.

Purity **(1)** Heavy metals <*1.07*>—Proceed with 2.0 g of Chlorhexidine Hydrochloride according to Method 2, and perform the test. Prepare the control solution with 2.0 mL of Standard Lead Solution (not more than 10 ppm).

(2) Arsenic <*1.11*>—To 1.0 g of Chlorhexidine Hydrochloride in a crucible add 10 mL of a solution of magnesium nitrate hexahydrate in ethanol (95) (1 in 10), fire the ethanol (95) to burn, and heat gradually to incinerate. If a carbonized substance remains, moisten with a small amount of nitric acid, and ignite to incinerate. Cool, add 10 mL of dilute hydrochloric acid to the residue, dissolve by warming on a water bath, use this solution as the test solution, and perform the test (not more than 2 ppm).

(3) *p*-Chloroaniline—Dissolve 0.10 g of Chlorhexidine Hydrochloride in 2 mL of formic acid, and add 15 mL of 1 mol/L hydrochloric acid TS and 20 mL of water immediately. Add 0.3 mL of sodium nitrite TS, shake, and allow to stand for 2 minutes. Add 4 mL of ammonium amidosulfate TS, and then allow to stand for 1 minute. Add 5 mL of *N*-(1-naphthyl)-*N'*-diethylethylenediamine oxalate-acetone TS, allow to stand for 10 minutes, and add 1 mL of ethanol (95) and water to make 50 mL: the solution has no more color than the following control solution.

Control solution: Dissolve 20 mg of 4-chloroaniline in 10 mL of 1 mol/L hydrochloric acid TS, and add water to make exactly 100 mL. Pipet 5 mL of the solution, and add water to make exactly 100 mL. To 2.0 mL of the solution add 2 mL of formic acid, 15 mL of 1 mol/L hydrochloric acid TS and 20 mL of water, and proceed in the same manner.

Loss on drying <*2.41*> Not more than 2.0% (1 g, 130°C, 2 hours).

Residue on ignition <*2.44*> Not more than 0.1% (1 g).

Assay Weigh accurately about 0.2 g of Chlorhexidine Hydrochloride, previously dried, dissolve in 2.0 mL of formic acid, add 60 mL of acetic anhydride, and titrate <*2.50*> with 0.1 mol/L perchloric acid VS (potentiometric titration). Perform a blank determination in the same manner, and make any necessary correction.

Each mL of 0.1 mol/L perchloric acid VS
= 14.46 mg of $C_{22}H_{30}Cl_2N_{10}.2HCl$

Containers and storage Containers—Tight containers.
Storage—Light-resistant.

Chlorinated Lime

サラシ粉

Chlorinated Lime contains not less than 30.0% of available chlorine (Cl: 35.45).

Description Chlorinated Lime occurs as a white powder. It has a chlorine-like odor.

It dissolves partially in water. The solution changes red litmus paper to blue, then gradually decolorizes.

Identification **(1)** To Chlorinated Lime add dilute hydrochloric acid: a gas, which has the odor of chlorine, evolves, and the gas changes moistened starch-potassium iodide paper to blue.

(2) Shake 1 g of Chlorinated Lime with 10 mL of water, and filter: the filtrate responds to Qualitative Tests <*1.09*> (2) and (3) for calcium salt.

Assay Weigh accurately about 5 g of Chlorinated Lime, transfer to a mortar, and triturate thoroughly with 50 mL of water. Transfer to a 500-mL volumetric flask with the aid of water, and add water to make 500 mL. Mix well, immediately take exactly 50 mL of the mixture in an iodine flask, add 10 mL of potassium iodide TS and 10 mL of dilute hydrochloric acid, and titrate <*2.50*> the liberated iodine with 0.1 mol/L sodium thiosulfate VS (indicator: 3 mL of starch TS). Perform a blank determination in the same manner, and make any necessary correction.

Each mL of 0.1 mol/L sodium thiosulfate VS
= 3.545 mg of Cl

Containers and storage Containers—Tight containers.
Storage—Light-resistant, and in a cold place.

Chlormadinone Acetate

クロルマジノン酢酸エステル

$C_{23}H_{29}ClO_4$: 404.93
6-Chloro-3,20-dioxopregna-4,6-dien-17-yl acetate
[*302-22-7*]

Chlormadinone Acetate, when dried, contains not less than 98.0% of chlormadinone acetate ($C_{23}H_{29}ClO_4$).

Description Chlormadinone Acetate occurs as white to light yellow, crystals or crystalline powder. It is odorless.

It is freely soluble in chloroform, soluble in acetonitrile, slightly soluble in ethanol (95) and in diethyl ether, and practically insoluble in water.

Identification **(1)** Dissolve 2 mg of Chlormadinone Acetate in 1 mL of ethanol (95), and add 1 mL of 1,3-dinitrobenzene TS and 1 mL of a solution of potassium hydroxide (1 in 5): a red-purple color develops.

(2) To 0.05 g of Chlormadinone Acetate add 2 mL of potassium hydroxide-ethanol TS, and boil on a water bath for 5 minutes. After cooling, add 2 mL of diluted sulfuric acid (2 in 7), and boil gently for 1 minute: the odor of ethyl acetate is perceptible.

(3) Determine the infrared absorption spectrum of Chlormadinone Acetate, previously dried, as directed in the potassium bromide disk method under Infrared Spectrophotometry <*2.25*>, and compare the spectrum with the Reference Spectrum or the spectrum of previously dried Chlormadinone Acetate RS: both spectra exhibit similar intensities of absorption at the same wave numbers.

(4) Perform the test with Chlormadinone Acetate as directed under Flame Coloration Test <*1.04*> (2): a green color appears.

Optical rotation <*2.49*> $[\alpha]_D^{20}$: −10.0 − −14.0° (after drying, 0.2 g, acetonitrile, 10 mL, 100 mm).

Melting point <*2.60*> 211 − 215°C

Purity (1) Heavy metals <*1.07*>—Proceed with 1.0 g of Chlormadinone Acetate according to Method 2, and perform the test. Prepare the control solution with 2.0 mL of Standard Lead Solution (not more than 20 ppm).

(2) Arsenic <*1.11*>—Prepare the test solution with 1.0 g of Chlormadinone Acetate according to Method 3, and perform the test (not more than 2 ppm).

(3) Related substances—Dissolve 20 mg of Chlormadinone Acetate in 10 mL of acetonitrile, and use this solution as the sample solution. Pipet 1 mL of the sample solution, add acetonitrile to make exactly 100 mL, and use this solution as the standard solution. Perform the test with exactly 10 μL each of the sample solution and standard solution as directed under Liquid Chromatography <*2.01*> according to the following conditions, and determine each peak area by the automatic integration method: the total area of peaks other than the peak of chlormadinone acetate obtained from the sample solution is not larger than the peak area of chlormadinone acetate from the standard solution.

Operating conditions—

Detector: An ultraviolet absorption photometer (wavelength: 236 nm).

Column: A stainless steel column 6 mm in inside diameter and 15 cm in length, packed with octadecylsilanized silica gel for liquid chromatography (5 μm in particle diameter).

Column temperature: A constant temperature of about 30°C.

Mobile phase: A mixture of acetonitrile and water (13:7).

Flow rate: Adjust so that the retention time of chlormadinone acetate is about 10 minutes.

Time span of measurement: About 1.5 times as long as the retention time of chlormadinone acetate, beginning after the solvent peak.

System suitability—

Test for required detectability: To exactly 5 mL of the standard solution add acetonitorile to make exactly 50 mL. Confirm that the peak area of chlormadinone acetate obtained with 10 μL of this solution is equivalent to 7 to 13% of that with 10 μL of the standard solution.

System performance: Dissolve 8 mg of Chlormadinone Acetate and 2 mg of butyl parahydroxybenzoate in 100 mL of acetonitrile. When the procedure is run with 10 μL of this solution under the above operating conditions, butyl parahydroxybenzoate and chlormadinone acetate are eluted in this order with the resolution between these peaks being not less than 8.

System repeatability: When the test is repeated 6 times with 10 μL of the standard solution under the above operating conditions, the relative standard deviation of the peak area of chlormadinone acetate is not more than 1.0%.

Loss on drying <*2.41*> Not more than 0.5% (0.5 g, in vacuum, phosphorus (V) oxide, 4 hours).

Residue on ignition <*2.44*> Not more than 0.1% (0.5 g).

Assay Weigh accurately about 20 mg each of Chlormadinone Acetate and Chlormadinone Acetate RS, previously dried, and dissolve in ethanol (95) to make exactly 100 mL. Pipet 5 mL each of these solutions, to each add ethanol (95) to make exactly 100 mL, and use these solutions as the sample solution and the standard solution, respectively. Perform the test with these solutions as directed under Ultraviolet-visible Spectrophotometry <*2.24*>, and determine the absorbances, A_T and A_S, at 285 nm.

Amount (mg) of chlormadinone acetate ($C_{23}H_{29}ClO_4$)
$= M_S \times A_T/A_S$

M_S: Amount (mg) of Chlormadinone Acetate RS taken

Containers and storage Containers—Tight containers.
Storage—Light-resistant.

Chlorobutanol

クロロブタノール

$C_4H_7Cl_3O$: 177.46
1,1,1-Trichloro-2-methylpropan-2-ol
[*57-15-8*]

Chlorobutanol contains not less than 98.0% of chlorobutanol ($C_4H_7Cl_3O$), calculated on the anhydrous basis.

Description Chlorobutanol occurs as colorless or white crystals. It has a camphoraceous odor.

It is very soluble in methanol, in ethanol (95) and in diethyl ether, and slightly soluble in water.

It slowly volatilizes in air.

Melting point: not lower than about 76°C.

Identification (1) To 5 mL of a solution of Chlorobutanol (1 in 200) add 1 mL of sodium hydroxide TS, then slowly add 3 mL of iodine TS: a yellow precipitate is produced and the odor of iodoform is perceptible.

(2) To 0.1 g of Chlorobutanol add 5 mL of sodium hydroxide TS, shake well the mixture, add 3 to 4 drops of aniline, and warm gently: the disagreeable odor of phenyl isocyanide (poisonous) is perceptible.

Purity (1) Acidity—Shake thoroughly 0.10 g of the powder of Chlorobutanol with 5 mL of water: the solution is neutral.

(2) Chloride <*1.03*>—Dissolve 0.5 g of Chlorobutanol in 25 mL of dilute ethanol, and add 6 mL of dilute nitric acid and water to make 50 mL. Perform the test using this solution as the test solution. Prepare the control solution with 1.0 mL of 0.01 mol/L hydrochloric acid VS by adding 25 mL of dilute ethanol, 6 mL of dilute nitric acid and water to make 50 mL (not more than 0.071%).

Water <*2.48*> Not more than 6.0% (0.2 g, volumetric titration, direct titration).

Residue on ignition <*2.44*> Not more than 0.1% (1 g).

Assay Transfer about 0.1 g of Chlorobutanol, accurately weighed, to a 200-mL conical flask, and dissolve in 10 mL of ethanol (95). Add 10 mL of sodium hydroxide TS, boil under a reflux condenser for 10 minutes, cool, add 40 mL of dilute nitric acid and exactly 25 mL of 0.1 mol/L silver nitrate VS, and shake well. Add 3 mL of nitrobenzene, and shake vigorously until the precipitate is coagulated. Titrate <*2.50*> the excess silver nitrate with 0.1 mol/L ammonium thiocyanate VS (indicator: 2 mL of ammonium iron (III) sulfate TS). Perform a blank determination in the same manner.

Each mL of 0.1 mol/L silver nitrate VS
= 5.915 mg of $C_4H_7Cl_3O$

Containers and storage Containers—Tight containers.

Chlorphenesin Carbamate

クロルフェネシンカルバミン酸エステル

and enantiomer

$C_{10}H_{12}ClNO_4$: 245.66
(2*RS*)-3-(4-Chlorophenoxy)-2-hydroxypropyl carbamate
[*886-74-8*]

Chlorphenesin Carbamate, when dried, contains not less than 98.0% and not more than 102.0% of chlorphenesin carbamate ($C_{10}H_{12}ClNO_4$).

Description Chlorphenesin Carbamate occurs as white, crystals or a crystalline powder.

It is freely soluble in methanol, in ethanol (95) and in pyridine, and slightly soluble in water.

A solution of Chlorphenesin Carbamate in ethanol (95) (1 in 20) shows no optical rotation.

Identification **(1)** Determine the absorption spectrum of a solution of Chlorphenesin Carbamate in ethanol (95) (3 in 200,000) as directed under Ultraviolet-visible Spectrophotometry <*2.24*>, and compare the spectrum with the Reference Spectrum: both spectra exhibit similar intensities of absorption at the same wavelengths.

(2) Determine the infrared absorption spectrum of Chlorphenesin Carbamate, as directed in the potassium bromide disk method under Infrared Spectrophotometry <*2.25*>, and compare the spectrum with the Reference Spectrum: both spectra exhibit similar intensities of absorption at the same wave numbers.

(3) Perform the test with Chlorphenesin Carbamate as directed under Flame Coloration Test <*1.04*> (2): a green color appears.

Melting point <*2.60*> 88 - 91°C

Purity **(1)** Heavy metals <*1.07*>—Dissolve 2.0 g of Chlorphenesin Carbamate in 20 mL of ethanol (95), and add 2 mL of dilute acetic acid and water to make 50 mL. Perform the test using this solution as the test solution. Prepare the control solution as follows: to 2.0 mL of Standard Lead Solution add 20 mL of ethanol (95), 2 mL of dilute acetic acid and water to make 50 mL (not more than 10 ppm).

(2) Arsenic <*1.11*>—Prepare the test solution with 1.0 g of Chlorphenesin Carbamate according to Method 3, and perform the test (not more than 2 ppm).

(3) Chlorphenesin-2-carbamate—Dissolve 0.10 g of Chlorphenesin Carbamate in 20 mL of a mixture of hexane for liquid chromatography and 2-propanol (7:3), and use this solution as the sample solution. Perform the test with 10 μL of the sample solution as directed under Liquid Chromatography <*2.01*> according to the following conditions. Determine the peak area, A_a, of chlorphenesin carbamate and the peak area, A_b, of chlorphenesin-2-carbamate by the automatic integration method: the ratio, $A_b/(A_a + A_b)$, is not more than 0.007.

Operating conditions—

Detector: An ultraviolet absorption photometer (wavelength: 280 nm).

Column: A stainless steel column 4 mm in inside diameter and 30 cm in length, packed with silica gel for liquid chromatography (5 μm in particle diameter).

Column temperature: A constant temperature of about 40°C.

Mobile phase: A mixture of hexane for liquid chromatography, 2-propanol and acetic acid (100) (700:300:1).

Flow rate: Adjust so that the retention time of chlorphenesin carbamate is about 9 minutes.

System suitability—

Test for required detectability: To 1 mL of the sample solution, add a mixture of hexane for liquid chromatography and 2-propanol (7:3) to make 100 mL, and use this solution as the solution for system suitability test. To exactly 5 mL of the solution for system suitability test add the mixture of hexane for liquid chromatography and 2-propanol (7:3) to make exactly 10 mL. Confirm that the peak area of chlorphenesin carbamate obtained with 10 μL of this solution is equivalent to 40 to 60% of that with 10 μL of the solution for system suitability test.

System performance: Dissolve 0.1 g of Chlorphenesin Carbamate in 50 mL of methanol. To 25 mL of this solution add 25 mL of dilute sodium hydroxide TS, and warm at 60°C for 20 minutes. To 20 mL of this solution add 5 mL of 1 mol/L hydrochloric acid TS, shake well with 20 mL of ethyl acetate, and allow to stand to separate the upper layer. When the procedure is run with 10 μL of this layer under the above operating conditions, chlorphenesin, chlorphenesin carbamate and chlorphenesin-2-carbamate are eluted in this order, with the relative retention times of chlorphenesin and chlorphenesin-2-carbamate to chlorphenesin carbamate being about 0.7 and about 1.2, respectively, and with the resolution between the peaks of chlorphenesin and chlorphenesin carbamate being not less than 2.0.

System repeatability: When the test is repeated 6 times with 10 μL of the solution for system suitability test under the above operating conditions, the relative standard deviation of the peak areas of chlorphenesin carbamate is not more than 2.0%.

(4) Related substances—Dissolve 0.10 g of Chlorphenesin Carbamate in 10 mL of ethanol (95), and use this solution as the sample solution. Pipet 1 mL of the sample solution, add ethanol (95) to make exactly 20 mL. Pipet 2 mL of this solution, add ethanol (95) to make exactly 20 mL, and use this solution as the standard solution. Perform the test with these solutions as directed under Thin-layer Chromatography <*2.03*>. Spot 50 μL each of the sample solution and standard solution on a plate of silica gel for thin-layer chromatography. Develop the plate with a mixture of ethyl acetate, methanol and ammonia solution (28) (17:2:1) to a distance of about 10 cm, and air-dry the plate. Allow the plate to stand in iodine vapor for 20 minutes: the spot other than the principal spot obtained from the sample solution is not more than one, and it is not more intense than the spot from the standard solution.

Loss on drying <*2.41*> Not more than 0.20% (1 g, in vacuum, silica gel, 4 hours).

Residue on ignition <*2.44*> Not more than 0.1% (1 g).

Assay Weigh accurately about 0.5 g of Chlorphenesin Carbamate, previously dried, dissolve in 20 mL of pyridine, add exactly 50 mL of 0.1 mol/L potassium hydroxide-ethanol TS, and warm at 70°C for 40 minutes. After cooling, add 100 mL of ethanol (95), and titrate <*2.50*> the excess potassium hydroxide with 0.1 mol/L hydrochloric acid VS until the color of the solution changes from blue through blue-green to yellow (indicator: 1 mL of thymol blue TS). Perform a blank determination in the same manner.

Each mL of 0.1 mol/L potassium hydroxide-ethanol TS
= 24.57 mg of $C_{10}H_{12}ClNO_4$

Containers and storage Containers—Tight containers.

Chlorphenesin Carbamate Tablets

クロルフェネシンカルバミン酸エステル錠

Chlorphenesin Carbamate Tablets contain not less than 93.0% and not more than 107.0% of the labeled amount of chlorphenesin carbamate ($C_{10}H_{12}ClNO_4$: 245.66).

Method of preparation Prepare as directed under Tablets, with Chlorphenesin Carbamate.

Identification To a quantity of powdered Chlorphenesin Carbamate Tablets, equivalent to 0.15 g of Chlorphenesin Carbamate, add 60 mL of ethanol (95), sonicate, and add ethanol (95) to make 100 mL. Centrifuge 20 mL of this solution, add ethanol (95) to 1 mL of the supernatant liquid to make 100 mL, and determine the absorption spectrum of this solution as directed under Ultraviolet-visible Spectrophotometry <*2.24*>: it exhibits maxima between 226 nm and 230 nm, between 279 nm and 283 nm, and between 286 nm and 290 nm.

Uniformity of dosage units <*6.02*> Perform the Mass variation test, or the Content uniformity test according to the following method: it meets the requirement.

To 1 tablet of Chlorphenesin Carbamate Tablets add 10 mL of water to disintegrate the tablet, add 70 mL of a mixture of water and methanol (1:1), sonicate for 15 minutes with occasional stirring, then add the mixture of water and methanol (1:1) to make exactly 100 mL. Centrifuge this solution, pipet V mL of the supernatant liquid equivalent to about 2.5 mg of chlorphenesin carbamate ($C_{10}H_{12}ClNO_4$), add the mixture of water and methanol (1:1) to make exactly 25 mL, and use this solution as the sample solution. Separately, weigh accurately about 50 mg of chlorphenesin carbamate for assay, previously dried in a desiccator (in vacuum, silica gel) for 4 hours, and dissolve in the mixture of water and methanol (1:1) to make exactly 50 mL. Pipet 2 mL of this solution, add the mixture of water and methanol (1:1) to make exactly 20 mL, and use this solution as the standard solution. Determine the absorbances at 280 nm, A_T and A_S, of the sample solution and standard solution as directed under Ultraviolet-visible Spectrophotometry <*2.24*>.

Amount (mg) of chlorphenesin carbamate ($C_{10}H_{12}ClNO_4$)
$= M_S \times A_T/A_S \times 1/V \times 5$

M_S: Amount (mg) of chlorphenesin carbamate for assay taken

Dissolution <*6.10*> When the test is performed at 50 revolutions per minute according to the Paddle method, using 900 mL of water as the dissolution medium, the dissolution rate in 15 minutes of Chlorphenesin Carbamate Tablets is not less than 85%.

Start the test with 1 tablet of Chlorphenesin Carbamate Tablets, withdraw not less than 20 mL of the medium at the specified minute after starting the test, and filter through a membrane filter with a pore size not exceeding 0.45 μm. Discard not less than 10 mL of the first filtrate, pipet V mL of the subsequent filtrate, add water to make exactly V' mL so that each mL contains about 0.14 mg of chlorphenesin carbamate ($C_{10}H_{12}ClNO_4$), and use this solution as the sample solution. Separately, weigh accurately about 28 mg of chlorphenesin carbamate for assay, previously dried in a desiccator (in vacuum, silica gel) for 4 hours, dissolve in 1 mL of methanol, and add water to make exactly 50 mL. Pipet 5 mL of this solution, add water to make exactly 20 mL, and use this solution as the standard solution. Determine the absorbances, A_T and A_S, at 278 nm of the sample solution and standard solution as directed under Ultraviolet-visible Spectrophotometry <*2.24*>.

Dissolution rate (%) with respect to the labeled amount of chlorphenesin carbamate ($C_{10}H_{12}ClNO_4$)
$= M_S \times A_T/A_S \times V'/V \times 1/C \times 450$

M_S: Amount (mg) of chlorphenesin carbamate for assay taken

C: Labeled amount (mg) of chlorphenesin carbamate ($C_{10}H_{12}ClNO_4$) in 1 tablet

Assay Weigh accurately the mass of not less than 20 Chlorphenesin Carbamate Tablets, and powder them in an agate mortar. Weigh accurately a portion of the powder, equivalent to about 0.25 g of chlorphenesin carbamate ($C_{10}H_{12}ClNO_4$), add 30 mL of ethyl acetate, disperse by sonicating, then add ethyl acetate to make exactly 50 mL. Centrifuge 20 mL of this solution, pipet 2 mL of the supernatant liquid, add exactly 2 mL of the internal standard solution, add ethyl acetate to make 20 mL, and use this solution as the sample solution. Separately, weigh accurately about 0.1 g of chlorphenesin carbamate for assay, previously dried in a desiccator (in vacuum, silica gel) for 4 hours, and dissolve in ethyl acetate to make exactly 50 mL. Pipet 5 mL of this solution, add exactly 2 mL of the internal standard solution, then add ethyl acetate to make 20 mL, and use this solution as the standard solution. Perform the test with 10 μL each of the sample solution and standard solution as directed under Liquid Chromatography <*2.01*> according to the following conditions, and calculate the ratios, Q_T and Q_S, of the peak area of chlorphenesin carbamate to that of the internal standard.

Amount (mg) of chlorphenesin carbamate ($C_{10}H_{12}ClNO_4$)
$= M_S \times Q_T/Q_S \times 5/2$

M_S: Amount (mg) of chlorphenesin carbamate for assay taken

Internal standard solution—A solution of ethenzamide in ethyl acetate (1 in 400).

Operating conditions—

Detector: An ultraviolet absorption photometer (wavelength: 280 nm).

Column: A stainless steel column 4 mm in inside diameter and 30 cm in length, packed with silica gel for liquid chromatography (5 μm in particle diameter).

Column temperature: A constant temperature of about 40°C.

Mobile phase: A mixture of hexane for liquid chromatography, 2-propanol and acetic acid (100) (700:300:1).

Flow rate: Adjust so that the retention time of chlorphenesin carbamate is about 9 minutes.

System suitability—

System performance: Proceed as directed in the system suitability in the Purity (3) under Chlorphenesin Carbamate.

System repeatability: When the test is repeated 6 times

with 10 μL of the standard solution under the above operating conditions, the relative standard deviation of the ratio of the peak area of chlorphenesin carbamate to that of the internal standard is not more than 1.5%.

Containers and storage Containers—Well-closed containers.

Chlorpheniramine Maleate

クロルフェニラミンマレイン酸塩

and enantiomer

$C_{16}H_{19}ClN_2.C_4H_4O_4$: 390.86
(3*RS*)-3-(4-Chlorophenyl)-*N*,*N*-dimethyl-3-pyridin-2-ylpropylamine monomaleate
[*113-92-8*]

Chlorpheniramine Maleate, when dried, contains not less than 98.0% and not more than 101.0% of *dl*-chlorpheniramine maleate ($C_{16}H_{19}ClN_2.C_4H_4O_4$).

Description Chlorpheniramine Maleate occurs as white, fine crystals.

It is very soluble in acetic acid (100), freely soluble in water and in methanol, and soluble in ethanol (99.5).

It dissolves in dilute hydrochloric acid.

A solution of Chlorpheniramine Maleate (1 in 20) shows no optical rotation.

Identification (1) Determine the absorption spectrum of a solution of Chlorpheniramine Maleate in 0.1 mol/L hydrochloric acid TS (3 in 100,000) as directed under Ultraviolet-visible Spectrophotometry *<2.24>*, and compare the spectrum with the Reference Spectrum or the spectrum of a solution of Chlorpheniramine Maleate RS prepared in the same manner as the sample solution: both spectra exhibit similar intensities of absorption at the same wavelengths.

(2) Determine the infrared absorption spectrum of Chlorpheniramine Maleate, previously dried, as directed in the paste method under Infrared Spectrophotometry *<2.25>*, and compare the spectrum with the Reference Spectrum or the spectrum of previously dried Chlorpheniramine Maleate RS: both spectra exhibit similar intensities of absorption at the same wave numbers.

(3) Dissolve 0.10 g of Chlorpheniramine Maleate in 5 mL of methanol, and use this solution as the sample solution. Separately, dissolve 56 mg of maleic acid in 10 mL of methanol, and use this solution as the standard solution. Perform the test with these solutions as directed under Thin-layer Chromatography *<2.03>*. Spot 5 μL each of the sample solution and standard solution on a plate of silica gel for thin-layer chromatography. Develop the plate with a mixture of diethyl ether, methanol, acetic acid (100) and water (70:20:7:3) to a distance of about 12 cm, and air-dry the plate. Examine under ultraviolet light (main wavelength: 254 nm): a spot among two of the spots obtained with the sample solution shows the same intense and *Rf* value with the spot obtained with the standard solution.

pH *<2.54>* Dissolve 1.0 g of Chlorpheniramine Maleate in 100 mL of freshly boiled and cooled water: the pH of this solution is between 4.0 and 5.5.

Melting point *<2.60>* 130 – 135°C

Purity (1) Clarity and color of solution—Dissolve 1.0 g of Chlorpheniramine Maleate in 50 mL of water: the solution is clear and colorless.

(2) Heavy metals *<1.07>*—Proceed with 1.0 g of Chlorpheniramine Maleate according to Method 4, and perform the test. Prepare the control solution with 2.0 mL of Standard Lead Solution (not more than 20 ppm).

(3) Related substances—Dissolve 0.10 g of Chlorpheniramine Maleate in 100 mL of the mobile phase, and use this solution as the sample solution. Pipet 3 mL of the sample solution, and add the mobile phase to make exactly 100 mL. Pipet 2 mL of this solution, add the mobile phase to make exactly 20 mL, and use this solution as the standard solution. Perform the test with exactly 20 μL each of the sample solution and standard solution as directed under Liquid Chromatography *<2.01>* according to the following conditions, and determine each peak area by the automatic integration method: the area of the peak other than maleic acid and chlorpheniramine obtained from the sample solution is not larger than 2/3 times the peak area of chlorpheniramine from the standard solution, and the total area of the peaks other than maleic acid and chlorpheniramine from the sample solution is not larger than the peak area of chlorpheniramine from the standard solution.

Operating conditions—

Detector: An ultraviolet absorption photometer (wavelength: 225 nm).

Column: A stainless steel column 3.9 mm in inside diameter and 30 cm in length, packed with octadecylsilanized silica gel for liquid chromatography (10 μm in particle diameter).

Column temperature: A constant temperature of about 25°C.

Mobile phase: Dissolve 8.57 g of ammonium dihydrogenphosphate and 1 mL of phosphoric acid in water to make 1000 mL. To 800 mL of this solution add 200 mL of acetonitrile.

Flow rate: Adjust so that the retention time of chlorpheniramine is about 11 minutes.

Time span of measurement: About 4 times as long as the retention time of chlorpheniramine, beginning after the solvent peak.

System suitability—

Test for required detectability: To exactly 2.5 mL of the standard solution add the mobile phase to make exactly 25 mL. Confirm that the peak area of chlorpheniramine obtained with 20 μL of this solution is equivalent to 7 to 13% of that with 20 μL of the standard solution.

System performance: When the procedure is run with 20 μL of the standard solution under the above operating conditions, the number of theoretical plates and the symmetry factor of the peak of chlorpheniramine are not less than 4000 and not more than 2.0, respectively.

System repeatability: When the test is repeated 6 times with 20 μL of the standard solution under the above operating conditions, the relative standard deviation of the peak area of chlorpheniramine is not more than 4.0%.

Loss on drying *<2.41>* Not more than 0.5% (1 g, 105°C, 3 hours).

Residue on ignition *<2.44>* Not more than 0.1% (1 g).

Assay Dissolve about 0.4 g of Chlorpheniramine Maleate, previously dried and accurately weighed, in 20 mL of acetic acid (100). Titrate *<2.50>* with 0.1 mol/L perchloric acid VS until the color of the solution changes from purple through blue-green to green (indicator: 2 drops of crystal violet TS).

Perform a blank determination in the same manner, and make any necessary correction.

Each mL of 0.1 mol/L perchloric acid VS
= 19.54 mg of $C_{16}H_{19}ClN_2.C_4H_4O_4$

Containers and storage Containers—Tight containers.
Storage—Light-resistant.

Chlorpheniramine Maleate Injection

クロルフェニラミンマレイン酸塩注射液

Chlorpheniramine Maleate Injection is an aqueous injection.

It contains not less than 95.0% and not more than 105.0% of the labeled amount of *dl*-chlorpheniramine maleate ($C_{16}H_{19}ClN_2.C_4H_4O_4$: 390.86).

Method of preparation Prepare as directed under Injections, with Chlorpheniramine Maleate.

Description Chlorpheniramine Maleate Injection is a clear, colorless liquid.

pH: 4.5 – 7.0

Identification Take a volume of Chlorpheniramine Maleate Injection, equivalent to 25 mg of Chlorpheniramine Maleate, add 5 mL of dilute sodium hydroxide TS, and extract with 20 mL of hexane. Wash the hexane layer with 10 mL of water, shake with 0.5 g of anhydrous sodium sulfate for several minutes, and filter. Evaporate the filtrate in a water bath at 50°C under a reduced pressure, and determine the infrared absorption spectrum of the residue as directed in the liquid film method under Infrared Spectrophotometry *<2.25>*: it exhibits absorption at the wave numbers of about 2940 cm^{-1}, 2810 cm^{-1}, 2770 cm^{-1}, 1589 cm^{-1}, 1491 cm^{-1}, 1470 cm^{-1}, 1434 cm^{-1}, 1091 cm^{-1} and 1015 cm^{-1}.

Bacterial endotoxins *<4.01>* Less than 8.8 EU/mg.

Extractable volume *<6.05>* It meets the requirement.

Foreign insoluble matter *<6.06>* Perform the test according to Method 1: it meets the requirement.

Insoluble particulate matter *<6.07>* It meets the requirement.

Sterility *<4.06>* Perform the test according to the Membrane filtration method: it meets the requirement.

Assay Transfer an exactly measured volume of Chlorpheniramine Maleate Injection, equivalent to about 3 mg of chlorpheniramine maleate ($C_{16}H_{19}ClN_2.C_4H_4O_4$), to a 100-mL separator, add 20 mL of water and 2 mL of sodium hydroxide TS, and extract with two 50-mL portions of diethyl ether. Combine the diethyl ether extracts, wash with 20 mL of water, and then extract with 20-mL, 20-mL and 5-mL portions of 0.25 mol/L sulfuric acid TS successively. Combine all acid extracts, and add 0.25 mol/L sulfuric acid TS to make exactly 50 mL. Pipet 10 mL of this solution, add 0.25 mol/L sulfuric acid TS to make exactly 25 mL, and use this solution as the sample solution. Separately, weigh accurately about 30 mg of Chlorpheniramine Maleate RS, previously dried at 105°C for 3 hours, and dissolve in water to make exactly 200 mL. Pipet 20 mL of this solution, transfer to a 100-mL separator, add 2 mL of sodium hydroxide TS, and extract with two 50-mL portions of diethyl ether. Proceed in the same manner as for the preparation of the sample solution, and use the solution so obtained as the standard solution. Determine the absorbances A_T and A_S of the sample solution and standard solution at a wavelength of the maximum absorbance at about 265 nm as directed under Ultraviolet-visible Spectrophotometry *<2.24>*.

Amount (mg) of chlorpheniramine maleate
($C_{16}H_{19}ClN_2.C_4H_4O_4$)
$= M_S \times A_T/A_S \times 1/10$

M_S: Amount (mg) of Chlorpheniramine Maleate RS taken

Containers and storage Containers—Hermetic containers.
Storage—Light-resistant.

Chlorpheniramine Maleate Powder

クロルフェニラミンマレイン酸塩散

Chlorpheniramine Maleate Powder contains not less than 93.0% and not more than 107.0% of the labeled amount of *dl*-chlorpheniramine maleate ($C_{16}H_{19}ClN_2.C_4H_4O_4$: 390.86).

Method of preparation Prepare as directed under Granules or Powders, with Chlorpheniramine Maleate.

Identification Weigh a portion of Chlorpheniramine Maleate Powder, equivalent to 50 mg of Chlorpheniramine Maleate, shake with 40 mL of 0.1 mol/L hydrochloric acid TS, and filter. Transfer the filtrate to a separator, and wash with 40 mL of hexane. Add 10 mL of sodium hydroxide TS, and extract with 20 mL of hexane. Wash the hexane layer with 5 mL of water. Centrifuge, if necessary, shake the hexane extract with 0.5 g of anhydrous sodium sulfate for several minutes, and filter. Evaporate the filtrate in a water bath at about 50°C under reduced pressure, and determine the infrared absorption spectrum of the residue as directed in the liquid film method under Infrared Spectrophotometry *<2.25>*: it exhibits absorption at the wave number of about 2940 cm^{-1}, 2810 cm^{-1}, 2770 cm^{-1}, 1589 cm^{-1}, 1491 cm^{-1}, 1470 cm^{-1}, 1434 cm^{-1}, 1091 cm^{-1} and 1015 cm^{-1}.

Dissolution *<6.10>* When the test is performed at 50 revolutions per minute according to the Paddle method, using 900 mL of water as the dissolution medium, the dissolution rate in 15 minutes of Chlorpheniramine Maleate Powder is not less than 85%.

Start the test with an accurately weighed amount of Chlorpheniramine Maleate Powder, equivalent to about 4 mg of chlorpheniramine maleate ($C_{16}H_{19}ClN_2.C_4H_4O_4$), withdraw not less than 20 mL of the medium at the specified minute after starting the test, and filter through a membrane filter with a pore size not exceeding 0.45 μm. Discard not less than 10 mL of the first filtrate, and use the subsequent filtrate as the sample solution. Separately, weigh accurately about 22 mg of Chlorpheniramine Maleate RS, previously dried at 105°C for 3 hours, and dissolve in water to make exactly 100 mL. Pipet 2 mL of this solution, add water to make exactly 100 mL, and use this solution as the standard solution. Perform the test with exactly 50 μL each of the sample solution and standard solution as directed under Liquid Chromatography *<2.01>* according to the following conditions, and determine the peak areas, A_T and A_S, of chlorpheniramine in each solution.

Dissolution rate (%) with respect to the labeled amount
of chlorpheniramine maleate ($C_{16}H_{19}ClN_2.C_4H_4O_4$)
$= M_S/M_T \times A_T/A_S \times 1/C \times 18$

M_S: Amount (mg) of Chlorpheniramine Maleate RS taken
M_T: Amount (g) of Chlorpheniramine Maleate Powder taken
C: Labeled amount (mg) of chlorpheniramine maleate ($C_{16}H_{19}ClN_2.C_4H_4O_4$) in 1 g

Operating conditions—

Proceed as directed in the operating conditions in the Assay.

System suitability—

System performance: When the procedure is run with 50 μL of the standard solution under the above operating conditions, the number of theoretical plates and the symmetry factor of the peak of chlorpheniramine are not less than 2000 and not more than 2.5, respectively.

System repeatability: When the test is repeated 6 times with 50 μL of the standard solution under the above operating conditions, the relative standard deviation of the peak area of chlorpheniramine is not more than 2.0%.

Assay Weigh accurately an amount of Chlorpheniramine Maleate Powder, equivalent to about 4 mg of chlorpheniramine maleate ($C_{16}H_{19}ClN_2.C_4H_4O_4$), add 70 mL of the internal standard solution, shake for 15 minutes, then add the internal standard solution to make exactly 100 mL, and use this solution as the sample solution. Separately, weigh accurately about 20 mg of Chlorpheniramine Maleate RS, previously dried at 105°C for 3 hours, and add the internal standard to make exactly 100 mL. Pipet 20 mL of this solution, add the internal standard solution to make exactly 100 mL, and use this solution as the standard solution. Perform the test with 30 μL each of the sample solution and standard solution as directed under Liquid Chromatography *<2.01>* according to the following conditions, and calculate the ratios, Q_T and Q_S, of the peak area of chlorpheniramine to that of the internal standard.

Amount (mg) of chlorpheniramine maleate ($C_{16}H_{19}ClN_2.C_4H_4O_4$)
$= M_S \times Q_T/Q_S \times 1/5$

M_S: Amount (mg) of Chlorpheniramine Maleate RS taken

Internal standard solution—To 7 mL of a solultion of methyl parahydroxybenzoate in methanol (1 in 1000) add water to make 1000 mL.

Operating conditions—

Detector: An ultraviolet absorption photometer (wavelength: 265 nm).

Column: A stainless steel column 4.6 mm in inside diameter and 15 cm in length, packed with octadecylsilanized silica gel for liquid chromatography (5 μm in particle diameter).

Column temperature: A constant temperature of about 40°C.

Mobile phase: Dissolve 1 g of sodium 1-heptane sulfonate in 900 mL of water, add 10 mL of acetic acid (100) and water to make 1000 mL. To 650 mL of this solution add 350 mL of acetonitrile.

Flow rate: Adjust so that the retention time of chlorpheniramine is about 8 minutes.

System suitability—

System performance: When the procedure is run with 30 μL of the standard solution under the above operating conditions, the internal standard and chlorpheniramine are eluted in this order with the resolution between these peaks being not less than 2.0.

System repeatability: When the test is repeated 6 times with 30 μL of the standard solution under the above operating conditions, the relative standard deviation of the ratio of the peak area of chlorpheniramine to that of the internal standard is not more than 1.0%.

Containers and storage Containers—Tight containers.

Chlorpheniramine Maleate Tablets

クロルフェニラミンマレイン酸塩錠

Chlorpheniramine Maleate Tablets contain not less than 93.0% and not more than 107.0% of the labeled amount of *dl*-chlorpheniramine maleate ($C_{16}H_{19}ClN_2.C_4H_4O_4$: 390.86).

Method of preparation Prepare as directed under Tablets, with Chlorpheniramine Maleate.

Identification Weigh a portion of powdered Chlorpheniramine Maleate Tablets, equivalent to 50 mg of Chlorpheniramine Maleate, shake with 40 mL of 0.1 mol/L hydrochloric acid TS, and filter. Transfer the filtrate to a separator, and wash with 40 mL of hexane. Add 10 mL of sodium hydroxide TS, and extract with 20 mL of hexane. Wash the hexane layer with 5 mL of water. Centrifuge, if necessary, shake the hexane extract with 0.5 g of anhydrous sodium sulfate for several minutes, and filter. Evaporate the filtrate in a water bath at about 50°C under a reduced pressure, and determine the infrared absorption spectrum of the residue as directed in the liquid film method under Infrared Spectrophotometry *<2.25>*: it exhibits absorption at the wave numbers of about 2940 cm^{-1}, 2810 cm^{-1}, 2770 cm^{-1}, 1589 cm^{-1}, 1491 cm^{-1}, 1470 cm^{-1}, 1434 cm^{-1}, 1091 cm^{-1} and 1015 cm^{-1}.

Uniformity of dosage units *<6.02>* Perform the test according to the following method: it meets the requirement of the Content uniformity test.

To 1 tablet of Chlorpheniramine Maleate Tablets add 10 mL of water, shake to disintegrate the tablet, then add water to make exactly V mL of a solution containing about 80 μg of chlorpheniramine maleate ($C_{16}H_{19}ClN_2.C_4H_4O_4$) per mL, and filter through a membrane filter with a pore size not exceeding 0.5 μm. Pipet 5 mL of the filtrate, add exactly 2.5 mL of the internal standard solution, add water to make 10 mL, and use this solution as the sample solution. Separately, weigh accurately about 20 mg of Chlorpheniramine Maleate RS, previously dried at 105°C for 3 hours, and add water to make exactly 100 mL. Pipet 20 mL of this solution, add exactly 25 mL of the internal standard solution, add water to make 100 mL, and use this solution as the standard solution. Perform the test with 30 μL each of the sample solution and standard solution as directed under Liquid Chromatography *<2.01>* according to the conditions described in the Assay, and calculate the ratios, Q_T and Q_S, of the peak area of chlorpheniramine to that of the internal standard.

Amount (mg) of chlorpheniramine maleate ($C_{16}H_{19}ClN_2.C_4H_4O_4$)
$= M_S \times Q_T/Q_S \times V/250$

M_S: Amount (mg) of Chlorpheniramine Maleate RS taken

Internal standard solution—To 7 mL of a solution of methyl parahydroxybenzoate in methanol (1 in 250) add water to make 1000 mL.

Dissolution *<6.10>* When the test is performed at 50 revolutions per minute according to the Paddle method, using 900 mL of water as the dissolution medium, the dissolution rate in 45 minutes of Chlorpheniramine Maleate Tablets is not less than 75%.

Start the test with 1 tablet of Chlorpheniramine Maleate Tablets, withdraw not less than 20 mL of the medium at the specified minute after starting the test, and filter through a membrane filter with a pore size not exceeding 0.45 μm. Discard not less than 10 mL of the first filtrate, pipet V mL of the subsequent filtrate, add water to make exactly V' mL so that each mL contains about 4.4 μg of chlorpheniramine maleate ($C_{16}H_{19}ClN_2.C_4H_4O_4$), and use this solution as the sample solution. Separately, weigh accurately about 22 mg of Chlorpheniramine Maleate RS, previously dried at 105°C for 3 hours, and dissolve in water to make exactly 100 mL. Pipet 2 mL of this solution, add water to make exactly 100 mL, and use this solution as the standard solution. Perform the test with exactly 50 μL each of the sample solution and standard solution as directed under Liquid Chromatography <2.01>, and determine the peak areas, A_T and A_S, of chlorpheniramine in each solution.

Dissolution rate (%) with respect to the labeled amount of chlorpheniramine maleate ($C_{16}H_{19}ClN_2.C_4H_4O_4$)
$$= M_S \times A_T/A_S \times V'/V \times 1/C \times 18$$

M_S: Amount (mg) of Chlorpheniramine Maleate RS taken
C: Labeled amount (mg) of chlorpheniramine maleate ($C_{16}H_{19}ClN_2.C_4H_4O_4$) in 1 tablet

Operating conditions—

Detector: An ultraviolet absorption photometer (wavelength: 265 nm).

Column: A stainless steel column 4.6 mm in inside diameter and 15 cm in length, packed with octadecylsilanized silica gel for liquid chromatography (5 μm in particle diameter).

Column temperature: A constant temperature of about 40°C.

Mobile phase: Dissolve 1 g of sodium 1-heptane sulfonate in 900 mL of water, add 10 mL of acetic acid (100), and add water to make 1000 mL. To 650 mL of this solution add 350 mL of acetonitrile.

Flow rate: Adjust so that the retention time of chlorpheniramine is about 8 minutes.

System suitability—

System performance: When the procedure is run with 50 μL of the standard solution under the above operating conditions, the number of theoretical plates and the symmetry factor of the peak of chlorpheniramine are not less than 2000 and not more than 2.5, respectively.

System repeatability: When the test is repeated 6 times with 50 μL of the standard solution under the above operating conditions, the relative standard deviation of the peak area of chlorpheniramine is not more than 2.0%.

Assay Weigh accurately the mass of not less than 20 Chlorpheniramine Maleate Tablets, and powder. Weigh accurately a portion of the powder, equivalent to about 4 mg of chlorpheniramine maleate ($C_{16}H_{19}ClN_2.C_4H_4O_4$), add 70 mL of the internal standard solution, shake for 15 minutes, then add the internal standard solution to make exactly 100 mL, filter through a membrane filter with a pore size not exceeding 0.5 μm, and use this solution as the sample solution. Separately, weigh accurately about 20 mg of Chlorpheniramine Maleate RS, previously dried at 105°C for 3 hours, and add the internal standard to make exactly 100 mL. Pipet 20 mL of this solution, add the internal standard solution to make exactly 100 mL, and use this solution as the standard solution. Perform the test with 30 μL each of the sample solution and standard solution as directed under Liquid Chromatography <2.01> according to the following conditions, and calculate the ratios, Q_T and Q_S, of the peak area of chlorpheniramine to that of the internal standard.

Amount (mg) of chlorpheniramine maleate ($C_{16}H_{19}ClN_2.C_4H_4O_4$)
$$= M_S \times Q_T/Q_S \times 1/5$$

M_S: Amount (mg) of Chlorpheniramine Maleate RS taken

*Internal standard solution—*To 7 mL of a solution of methyl parahydroxybenzoate in methanol (1 in 1000) add water to make 1000 mL.

Operating conditions—

Detector: An ultraviolet absorption photometer (wavelength: 265 nm).

Column: A stainless steel column 4.6 mm in inside diameter and 15 cm in length, packed with octadecylsilanized silica gel for liquid chromatography (5 μm in particle diameter).

Column temperature: A constant temperature of about 40°C.

Mobile phase: Dissolve 1 g of sodium 1-heptane sulfonate in 900 mL of water, add 10 mL of acetic acid (100) and water to make 1000 mL. To 650 mL of this solution add 350 mL of acetonitrile.

Flow rate: Adjust so that the retention time of chlorpheniramine is about 8 minutes.

System suitability—

System performance: When the procedure is run with 30 μL of the standard solution under the above operating conditions, the internal standard and chlorpheniramine are eluted in this order with the resolution between these peaks being not less than 2.0.

System repeatability: When the test is repeated 6 times with 30 μL of the standard solution under the above operating conditions, the relative standard deviation of the ratio of the peak area of chlorpheniramine to that of the internal standard is not more than 1.0%.

Containers and storage Containers—Tight containers.

d-Chlorpheniramine Maleate

d-クロルフェニラミンマレイン酸塩

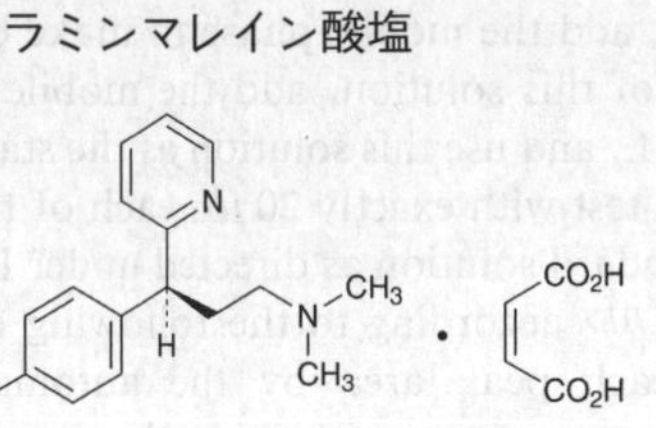

$C_{16}H_{19}ClN_2.C_4H_4O_4$: 390.86
(3*S*)-3-(4-Chlorophenyl)-*N*,*N*-dimethyl-3-pyridin-2-ylpropylamine monomaleate
[*2438-32-6*]

d-Chlorpheniramine Maleate, when dried, contains not less than 99.0% and not more than 101.0% of *d*-chlorpheniramine maleate ($C_{16}H_{19}ClN_2.C_4H_4O_4$).

Description *d*-Chlorpheniramine Maleate occurs as a white crystalline powder.

It is very soluble in water, in methanol and in acetic acid (100), and freely soluble in *N*,*N*-dimethylformamide and in ethanol (99.5).

It dissolves in dilute hydrochloric acid.

Identification **(1)** Determine the absorption spectrum of a solution of *d*-Chlorpheniramine Maleate in 0.1 mol/L hydrochloric acid TS (3 in 100,000) as directed under Ultraviolet-visible Spectrophotometry <2.24>, and compare the spectrum with the Reference Spectrum: both spectra exhibit similar intensities of absorption at the same wavelengths.

(2) Determine the infrared absorption spectrum of *d*-Chlorpheniramine Maleate, previously dried, as directed in the paste method under Infrared Spectrophotometry *<2.25>*, and compare the spectrum with the Reference Spectrum: both spectra exhibit similar intensities of absorption at the same wave numbers.

(3) Dissolve 0.10 g of *d*-Chlorpheniramine Maleate in 5 mL of methanol, and use this solution as the sample solution. Separately, dissolve 56 mg of maleic acid in 10 mL of methanol, and use this solution as the standard solution. Perform the test with these solutions as directed under Thin-layer Chromatography *<2.03>*. Spot 5 μL each of the sample solution and standard solution on a plate of silica gel for thin-layer chromatography. Develop the plate with a mixture of diethyl ether, methanol, acetic acid (100) and water (70:20:7:3) to a distance of about 12 cm, and air-dry the plate. Examine under ultraviolet light (main wavelength: 254 nm): a spot among two of the spots obtained with the sample solution shows the same intense to the spot obtained with the standard solution, and its *R*f value is about 0.4.

Optical rotation *<2.49>* $[\alpha]_D^{20}$: +39.5 – +43.0° (after drying, 0.5 g, *N*,*N*-dimethylformamide, 10 mL, 100 mm).

pH *<2.54>* Dissolve 1.0 g of *d*-Chlorpheniramine Maleate in 100 mL of freshly boiled and cooled water: the pH of this solution is between 4.0 and 5.0.

Melting point *<2.60>* 111 – 115°C

Purity **(1)** Clarity and color of solution—Dissolve 1.0 g of *d*-Chlorpheniramine Maleate in 50 mL of water: the solution is clear and colorless.

(2) Heavy metals *<1.07>*—Proceed with 1.0 g of *d*-Chlorpheniramine Maleate according to Method 4 and perform the test. Prepare the control solution with 2.0 mL of Standard Lead Solution (not more than 20 ppm).

(3) Related substances—Dissolve 0.10 g of *d*-Chlorpheniramine Maleate in 100 mL of the mobile phase, and use this solution as the sample solution. Pipet 3 mL of the sample solution, add the mobile phase to make exactly 100 mL. Pipet 2 mL of this solution, add the mobile phase to make exactly 20 mL, and use this solution as the standard solution. Perform the test with exactly 20 μL each of the sample solution and standard solution as directed under Liquid Chromatography *<2.01>* according to the following conditions, and determine each peak area by the automatic integration method: the area of the peak other than maleic acid and *d*-chlorpheniramine obtained from the sample solution is not larger than 2/3 times the peak area of *d*-chlorpheniramine from the standard solution, and the total area of these peaks is not larger than the peak area of *d*-chlorpheniramine from the standard solution.

Operating conditions—

Detector: An ultraviolet absorption photometer (wavelength: 225 nm).

Column: A stainless steel column 3.9 mm in inside diameter and 30 cm in length, packed with octadecylsilanized silica gel for liquid chromatography (10 μm in particle diameter).

Column temperature: A constant temperature of about 25°C.

Mobile phase: Dissolve 8.57 g of ammonium dihydrogen phosphate and 1 mL of phosphoric acid in water to make 1000 mL. To 800 mL of this solution add 200 mL of acetonitrile.

Flow rate: Adjust so that the retention time of *d*-chlorpheniramine is about 11 minutes.

Time span of measurement: About 4 times as long as the retention time of *d*-chlorpheniramine, beginning after the solvent peak.

System suitability—

Test for required detectability: To exactly 2.5 mL of the standard solution add the mobile phase to make exactly 25 mL. Confirm that the peak area of *d*-chlorpheniramine obtained with 20 μL of this solution is equivalent to 7 to 13% of that with 20 μL of the standard solution.

System performance: When the procedure is run with 20 μL of the standard solution under the above operating conditions, the number of theoretical plates and the symmetry factor of the peak of *d*-chlorpheniramine are not less than 4000 and not more than 2.0, respectively.

System repeatability: When the test is repeated 6 times with 20 μL of the standard solution under the above operating conditions, the relative standard deviation of the peak area of *d*-chlorpheniramine is not more than 4.0%.

Loss on drying *<2.41>* Not more than 0.5% (1 g, 65°C, 4 hours).

Residue on ignition *<2.44>* Not more than 0.1% (1 g).

Assay Weigh accurately about 0.3 g of *d*-Chlorpheniramine Maleate, previously dried, and dissolve in 20 mL of acetic acid (100). Titrate *<2.50>* with 0.1 mol/L perchloric acid VS until the color of the solution changes from purple through blue-green to green (indicator: 2 drops of crystal violet TS). Perform a blank determination in the same manner, and make any necessary correction.

Each mL of 0.1 mol/L perchloric acid VS
= 19.54 mg of $C_{16}H_{19}ClN_2.C_4H_4O_4$

Containers and storage Containers—Tight containers.
Storage—Light-resistant.

Chlorpromazine Hydrochloride

クロルプロマジン塩酸塩

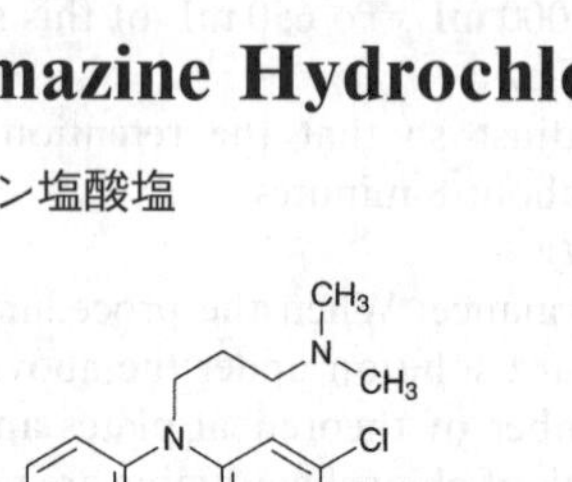

$C_{17}H_{19}ClN_2S.HCl$: 355.33
3-(2-Chloro-10*H*-phenothiazin-10-yl)-*N*,*N*-dimethylpropylamine monohydrochloride
[*69-09-0*]

Chlorpromazine Hydrochloride, when dried, contains not less than 99.0% of chlorpromazine hydrochloride ($C_{17}H_{19}ClN_2S.HCl$).

Description Chlorpromazine Hydrochloride occurs as a white to pale yellow crystalline powder. It is odorless, or has a faint, characteristic odor.

It is very soluble in water, freely soluble in ethanol (95) and in acetic acid (100), sparingly soluble in acetic anhydride, and practically insoluble in diethyl ether.

It is gradually colored by light.

Identification **(1)** To 5 mL of a solution of Chlorpromazine Hydrochloride (1 in 1000) add 1 drop of iron (III) chloride TS: a red color develops.

(2) Dissolve 0.1 g of Chlorpromazine Hydrochloride in

20 mL of water and 3 drops of dilute hydrochloric acid, add 10 mL of 2,4,6-trinitrophenol TS, and allow to stand for 5 hours. Collect the resulting precipitate, wash with water, recrystallize from a small portion of acetone, and dry at 105°C for 1 hour: the crystals so obtained melt <*2.60*> between 175°C and 179°C.

(3) Dissolve 0.5 g of Chlorpromazine Hydrochloride in 5 mL of water, add 2 mL of ammonia TS, and heat on a water bath for 5 minutes. Cool, filter, and render the filtrate acidic with dilute nitric acid: the solution responds to Qualitative Tests <*1.09*> (2) for chloride.

Melting point <*2.60*> 196 – 200°C

pH <*2.54*> Dissolve 1.0 g of Chlorpromazine Hydrochloride in 20 mL of freshly boiled and cooled water, and measure within 10 minutes: the pH of this solution is between 4.0 and 5.0.

Purity **(1)** Clarity and color of solution—A solution of 1.0 g of Chlorpromazine Hydrochloride in 20 mL of water, when observed within 10 minutes, is clear and colorless to pale yellow.

(2) Heavy metals <*1.07*>—Proceed with 1.0 g of Chlorpromazine Hydrochloride according to Method 2, and perform the test. Prepare the control solution with 2.0 mL of Standard Lead Solution (not more than 20 ppm).

Loss on drying <*2.41*> Not more than 0.5% (1 g, 105°C, 2 hours).

Residue on ignition <*2.44*> Not more than 0.1% (1 g).

Assay Weigh accurately about 0.7 g of Chlorpromazine Hydrochloride, previously dried, dissolve in 50 mL of a mixture of acetic anhydride and acetic acid (100) (7:3), and titrate <*2.50*> with 0.1 mol/L perchloric acid VS (potentiometric titration). Perform a blank determination in the same manner, and make any necessary correction.

Each mL of 0.1 mol/L perchloric acid VS
= 35.53 mg of $C_{17}H_{19}ClN_2S.HCl$

Containers and storage Containers—Tight containers.
Storage—Light-resistant.

Chlorpromazine Hydrochloride Injection

クロルプロマジン塩酸塩注射液

Chlorpromazine Hydrochloride Injection is an aqueous injection.

It contains not less than 95.0% and not more than 105.0% of the labeled amount of chlorpromazine hydrochloride ($C_{17}H_{19}ClN_2S.HCl$: 355.33).

Method of preparation Prepare as directed under Injections, with Chlorpromazine Hydrochloride.

Description Chlorpromazine Hydrochloride Injection is a clear, colorless or pale yellow liquid.
pH: 4.0 – 6.5

Identification **(1)** Proceed with a volume of Chlorpromazine Hydrochloride Injection, equivalent to 5 mg of Chlorpromazine Hydrochloride, as directed in the Identification (1) under Chlorpromazine Hydrochloride.

(2) Proceed with a volume of Chlorpromazine Hydrochloride Injection, equivalent to 0.1 g of Chlorpromazine Hydrochloride, as directed in the Identification (2) under Chlorpromazine Hydrochloride.

Extractable volume <*6.05*> It meets the requirement.

Foreign insoluble matter <*6.06*> Perform the test according to Method 1: it meets the requirement.

Insoluble particulate matter <*6.07*> It meets the requirement.

Sterility <*4.06*> Perform the test according to the Membrane filtration method: it meets the requirement.

Assay Transfer an exactly measured volume of Chlorpromazine Hydrochloride Injection, equivalent to about 0.15 g of chlorpromazine hydrochloride ($C_{17}H_{19}ClN_2S.HCl$) to a separator, add 30 mL of water and 10 mL of a solution of sodium hydroxide (1 in 5), and extract with two 30-mL portions and three 20-mL portions of diethyl ether. Wash the combined diethyl ether extracts with successive 10-mL portions of water until the last washing shows no red color upon the addition of phenolphthalein TS. Concentrate the diethyl ether extracts on a water bath to 20 mL, add 5 g of anhydrous sodium sulfate, allow to stand for 20 minutes, and filter through a pledget of absorbent cotton. Wash with diethyl ether, combine the washings with the filtrate, and evaporate the diethyl ether on a water bath. Dissolve the residue in 50 mL of acetone and 5 mL of acetic acid (100), and titrate <*2.50*> with 0.05 mol/L perchloric acid VS until the color of the solution changes from red-purple to blue-purple (indicator: 3 drops of bromocresol green-methylrosaniline chloride TS). Perform a blank determination in the same manner, and make any necessary correction.

Each mL of 0.05 mol/L perchloric acid VS
= 17.77 mg of $C_{17}H_{19}ClN_2S.HCl$

Containers and storage Containers—Hermetic containers, and colored containers may be used.
Storage—Light-resistant.

Chlorpromazine Hydrochloride Tablets

クロルプロマジン塩酸塩錠

Chlorpromazine Hydrochloride Tablets contain not less than 93.0% and not more than 107.0% of the labeled amount of chlorpromazine hydrochloride ($C_{17}H_{19}ClN_2S.HCl$: 355.33).

Method of preparation Prepare as directed under Tablets, with Chlorpromazine Hydrochloride.

Identification **(1)** Shake a quantity of powdered Chlorpromazine Hydrochloride Tablets, equivalent to 0.2 g of Chlorpromazine Hydrochloride, with 40 mL of 0.1 mol/L hydrochloric acid TS, and filter. To 1 mL of the filtrate add 4 mL of water and 1 drop of iron (III) chloride TS: a red color develops.

(2) To 20 mL of the filtrate obtained in (1) add 10 mL of 2,4,6-trinitrophenol TS dropwise, and proceed as directed in the Identification (2) under Chlorpromazine Hydrochloride.

Uniformity of dosage units <*6.02*> Perform the test according to the following method: it meets the requirement of the Content uniformity test.

Conduct this procedures using light-resistant vessels. To 1 tablet of Chlorpromazine Hydrochloride Tablets add an amount of a mixture of diluted phosphoric acid (1 in 500) and ethanol (99.5) (1:1) so that each mL contains about 0.83 mg of chlorpromazine hydrochloride ($C_{17}H_{19}ClN_2S.HCl$), sonicate for 5 minutes, then shake vigorously for 20 minutes, and add the mixture of diluted phosphoric acid (1 in 500) and ethanol (99.5) (1:1) to make exactly V mL so that each mL contains about 0.5 mg of chlorpromazine hydrochloride ($C_{17}H_{19}ClN_2S.HCl$). Filter through a membrane filter with a pore size not exceeding 0.45 μm. Discard the first 3 mL of the filtrate, pipet 2.5 mL of the subsequent filtrate, add exactly 5 mL of the internal standard solution, then add the mixture of diluted phosphoric acid (1 in 500) and ethanol (99.5) (1:1) to make 25 mL, and use this solution as the sample solution. Then, proceed as directed in the Assay.

Amount (mg) of chlorpromazine hydrochloride ($C_{17}H_{19}ClN_2S.HCl$)
$= M_S \times Q_T/Q_S \times V/50$

M_S: Amount (mg) of chlorpromazine hydrochloride for assay taken

Internal standard solution—A solution of ethyl parahydroxybenzoate in the mixture of diluted phosphoric acid (1 in 500) and ethanol (99.5) (1:1) (1 in 4500).

Dissolution <*6.10*> When the test is performed at 75 revolutions per minute according to the Paddle method, using 900 mL of 2nd fluid for dissolution test as the dissolution medium, the dissolution rate in 60 minutes of Chlorpromazine Hydrochloride Tablets is not less than 75%.

Start the test with 1 tablet of Chlorpromazine Hydrochloride Tablets, withdraw not less than 20 mL of the medium at the specified minute after starting the test, and filter through a membrane filter with a pore size not exceeding 0.8 μm. Discard not less than 10 mL of the first filtrate, pipet V mL of the subsequent filtrate, add the dissolution medium to make exactly V' mL so that each mL contains about 5.6 μg of chlorpromazine hydrochloride ($C_{17}H_{19}ClN_2S.HCl$), and use this solution as the sample solution. Separately, weigh accurately about 90 mg of chlorpromazine hydrochloride for assay, previously dried at 105°C for 2 hours, dissolve in the dissolution medium to make exactly 200 mL. Pipet 5 mL of this solution, add the dissolution medium to make exactly 100 mL, further pipet 5 mL of this solution, add the dissolution medium to make exactly 20 mL, and use this solution as the standard solution. Determine the absorbances, A_T and A_S, of the sample solution and standard solution at 254 nm as directed under Ultraviolet-visible Spectrophotometry <*2.24*>.

Dissolution rate (%) with respect to labeled amount of chlorpromazine hydrochloride ($C_{17}H_{19}ClN_2S.HCl$)
$= M_S \times A_T/A_S \times V'/V \times 1/C \times 45/8$

M_S: Amount (mg) of chlorpromazine hydrochloride for assay taken

C: Labeled amount (mg) of chlorpromazine hydrochloride ($C_{17}H_{19}ClN_2S.HCl$) in 1 tablet

Assay Conduct this procedure without exposure to light, using light-resistant vessels. Weigh accurately, and powder not less than 20 Chlorpromazine Hydrochloride Tablets. Weigh accurately a portion of the powder, equivalent to about 50 mg of chlorpromazine hydrochloride ($C_{17}H_{19}ClN_2S.HCl$), add 60 mL of a mixture of diluted phosphoric acid (1 in 500) and ethanol (99.5) (1:1), sonicate for 5 minutes, then shake vigorously for 20 minutes, and add the mixture of diluted phosphoric acid (1 in 500) and ethanol (99.5) (1:1) to make exactly 100 mL. Filter the solution through a membrane filter with a pore size not exceeding 0.45 μm, and discard the first 3 mL of the filtrate. To exactly 2.5 mL of the subsequent filtrate add exactly 5 mL of the internal standard solution, then add the mixture of diluted phosphoric acid (1 in 500) and ethanol (99.5) (1:1) to make 25 mL, and use this solution as the sample solution. Separately, weigh accurately about 25 mg of chlorpromazine hydrochloride for assay, previously dried at 105°C for 2 hours, and dissolve in the mixture of diluted phosphoric acid (1 in 500) and ethanol (99.5) (1:1) to make exactly 100 mL. Pipet 5 mL of this solution, add exactly 5 mL of the internal standard solution and the mixture of diluted phosphoric acid (1 in 500) and ethanol (99.5) (1:1) to make 25 mL, and use this solution as the standard solution. Perform the test with 10 μL each of the sample solution and standard solution as directed under Liquid Chromatography <*2.01*> according to the following conditions, and calculate the ratios, Q_T and Q_S, of the peak area of chlorpromazine to that of the internal standard.

Amount (mg) of chlorpromazine hydrochloride
($C_{17}H_{19}ClN_2S.HCl$) $= M_S \times Q_T/Q_S \times 2$

M_S: Amount (mg) of chlorpromazine hydrochloride for assay taken

Internal standard solution—A solution of ethyl parahydroxybenzoate in a mixture of diluted phosphoric acid (1 in 500) and ethanol (99.5) (1:1) (1 in 4500).

Operating conditions—

Detector: An ultraviolet absorption photometer (wavelength: 256 nm).

Column: A stainless steel column 4.6 mm in inside diameter and 15 cm in length, packed with octadecylsilanized silica gel for liquid chromatography (5 μm in particle diameter).

Column temperature: A constant temperature of about 25°C.

Mobile phase: A mixture of diluted 0.05 mol/L sodium dihydrogen phosphate TS (1 in 2) and acetonitrile (27:13).

Flow rate: Adjust so that the retention time of chlorpromazine is about 15 minutes.

System suitability—

System performance: When the procedure is run with 10 μL of the standard solution under the above operating conditions, the internal standard and chlorpromazine are eluted in this order with the resolution between these peaks being not less than 10.

System repeatability: When the test is repeated 6 times with 10 μL of the standard solution under the above operating conditions, the relative standard deviation of the ratio of the peak area of chlorpromazine to that of the internal standard is not more than 1.0%.

Containers and storage Containers—Tight containers.
Storage—Light-resistant.

Chlorpropamide

クロルプロパミド

$C_{10}H_{13}ClN_2O_3S$: 276.74
4-Chloro-*N*-(propylcarbamoyl)benzenesulfonamide
[94-20-2]

Chlorpropamide, when dried, contains not less than 98.0% of chlorpropamide ($C_{10}H_{13}ClN_2O_3S$).

Description Chlorpropamide occurs as white, crystals or crystalline powder.

It is freely soluble in methanol and in acetone, soluble in ethanol (95), and slightly soluble in diethyl ether, and practically insoluble in water.

Identification **(1)** Dissolve 0.08 g of Chlorpropamide in 50 mL of methanol. To 1 mL of the solution add 0.01 mol/L hydrochloric acid TS to make 200 mL. Determine the absorption spectrum of the solution as directed under Ultraviolet-visible Spectrophotometry 〈*2.24*〉, and compare the spectrum with the Reference Spectrum: both spectra exhibit similar intensities of absorption at the same wavelengths.

(2) Determine the infrared absorption spectrum of Chlorpropamide, previously dried, as directed in the potassium bromide disk method under Infrared Spectrophotometry 〈*2.25*〉, and compare the spectrum with the Reference Spectrum: both spectra exhibit similar intensities of absorption at the same wave numbers.

(3) Perform the test with Chlorpropamide as directed under Flame Coloration Test 〈*1.04*〉 (2): a green color appears.

Melting point 〈*2.60*〉 127 – 131°C

Purity **(1)** Acidity—To 3.0 g Chlorpropamide add 150 mL of water, and warm at 70°C for 5 minutes. Allow to stand in ice water for 1 hour, and filter. To 25 mL of the filtrate add 2 drops of methyl red TS and 0.30 mL of 0.1 mol/L sodium hydroxide VS: a yellow color develops.

(2) Chloride 〈*1.03*〉—To 40 mL of the filtrate obtained in (1) add 6 mL of dilute nitric acid and water to make 50 mL. Perform the test using this solution as the test solution. Prepare the control solution with 0.25 mL of 0.01 mol/L hydrochloric acid VS (not more than 0.011%).

(3) Sulfate 〈*1.14*〉—To 40 mL of the filtrate obtained in (1) add 1 mL of dilute hydrochloric acid and water to make 50 mL. Perform the test using this solution as the test solution. Prepare the control solution with 0.35 mL of 0.005 mol/L sulfuric acid VS (not more than 0.021%).

(4) Heavy metals 〈*1.07*〉—Proceed with 2.0 g of Chlorpropamide according to Method 2, and perform the test. Prepare the control solution with 2.0 mL of Standard Lead Solution (not more than 10 ppm).

(5) Related substances—Dissolve 0.6 g of Chlorpropamide in acetone to make exactly 10 mL, and use this solution as the sample solution. Pipet 1 mL of the sample solution, add acetone to make exactly 300 mL, and use this solution as the standard solution (1). Separately, dissolve 60 mg of 4-chlorobenzene sulfonamide in acetone to make exactly 300 mL, and use this solution as the standard solution (2). Perform the test with these solutions as directed under Thin-layer Chromatography 〈*2.03*〉. Spot 5 μL each of the sample solution and standard solutions (1) and (2) on a plate of silica gel for thin-layer chromatography. Develop the plate with a mixture of cyclohexane, 3-methyl-1-butanol, methanol and ammonia solution (28) (15:10:5:1) to a distance of about 10 cm, and air-dry the plate. After drying the plate at 100°C for 1 hour, spray evenly sodium hypochlorite TS on the plate, and air-dry for 15 minutes. Then spray evenly potassium iodide-starch TS on the plate: the spot obtained from the sample solution equivalent to the spot from the standard solution (2) is not more intense than the spot from the standard solution (2), and the spots other than the spot mentioned above and other than the principal spot is not more intense than the spot from the standard solution (1).

Loss on drying 〈*2.41*〉 Not more than 0.5% (1 g, 105°C, 3 hours).

Residue on ignition 〈*2.44*〉 Not more than 0.2% (1 g).

Assay Weigh accurately about 0.5 g of Chlorpropamide, previously dried, dissolve in 30 mL of neutralized ethanol, and add 20 mL of water. Titrate 〈*2.50*〉 with 0.1 mol/L sodium hydroxide VS (indicator: 3 drops of phenolphthalein TS).

Each mL of 0.1 mol/L sodium hydroxide VS
= 27.67 mg of $C_{10}H_{13}ClN_2O_3S$

Containers and storage Containers—Well-closed containers.

Chlorpropamide Tablets

クロルプロパミド錠

Chlorpropamide Tablets contain not less than 95.0% and not more than 105.0% of the labeled amount of chlorpropamide ($C_{10}H_{13}ClN_2O_3S$: 276.74).

Method of preparation Prepare as directed under Tablets, with Chlorpropamide.

Identification Take a quantity of powdered Chlorpropamide Tablets, equivalent to 0.08 g of Chlorpropamide, add 50 mL of methanol, shake, and filter. To 1 mL of the filtrate add 0.01 mol/L hydrochloric acid TS to make 200 mL, and determine the absorption spectrum of this solution as directed under Ultraviolet-visible Spectrophotometry 〈*2.24*〉: it exhibits a maximum between 231 nm and 235 nm.

Uniformity of dosage units 〈*6.02*〉 Perform the test according to the following method: it meets the requirement of the Content uniformity test.

To 1 tablet of Chlorpropamide Tablets add 75 mL of the mobile phase, sonicate for 20 minutes with occasional strong shaking, then add the mobile phase to make exactly *V* mL so that each mL contains about 2.5 mg of Chlorpropamide. Centrifuge the solution, pipet 2 mL of the supernatant liquid, add the mobile phase to make exactly 100 mL, and use this solution as the sample solution. Then, proceed as directed in the Assay.

$$\text{Amount (mg) of chlorpropamide } (C_{10}H_{13}ClN_2O_3S) = M_S \times A_T/A_S \times V/20$$

M_S: Amount (mg) of chlorpropamide for assay taken

Dissolution 〈*6.10*〉 When the test is performed at 50 revolutions per minute according to the Paddle method, using 900 mL of 2nd fluid for dissolution test as the dissolution medium, the dissolution rate in 45 minutes of Chlorpropamide Tablets is not less than 70%.

Start the test with 1 tablet of Chlorpropamide Tablets, withdraw not less than 20 mL of the medium at the specified minute after starting the test, and filter through a membrane filter with a pore size not exceeding 0.8 μm. Discard not less than 10 mL of the first filtrate, pipet V mL of the subsequent filtrate, add the dissolution medium to make exactly V' mL so that each mL contains about 10 μg of chlorpropamide ($C_{10}H_{13}ClN_2O_3S$), and use this solution as the sample solution. Separately, weigh accurately about 50 mg of chlorpropamide for assay, previously dried at 105°C for 3 hours, dissolve in 10 mL of methanol, and add water to make exactly 50 mL. Pipet 1 mL of this solution, add the dissolution medium to make exactly 100 mL, and use this solution as the standard solution. Determine the absorbances, A_T and A_S, of the sample solution and standard solution at 232 nm as directed under Ultraviolet-visible Spectrophotometry *<2.24>*.

Dissolution rate (%) with respect to the labeled amount of chlorpropamide ($C_{10}H_{13}ClN_2O_3S$)
$= M_S \times A_T/A_S \times V'/V \times 1/C \times 18$

M_S: Amount (mg) of chlorpropamide for assay taken
C: Labeled amount (mg) of chlorpropamide ($C_{10}H_{13}ClN_2O_3S$) in 1 tablet

Assay Weigh accurately and powder not less than 20 Chlorpropamide Tablets. Weigh accurately a quantity of the powder, equivalent to about 50 mg of chlorpropamide ($C_{10}H_{13}ClN_2O_3S$), add 75 mL of the mobile phase, shake for 10 minutes, and add the mobile phase to make exactly 100 mL. Centrifuge this solution, pipet 10 mL of the supernatant liquid, add the mobile phase to make exactly 100 mL, and use this solution as the sample solution. Separately, weigh accurately about 50 mg of chlorpropamide for assay, previously dried at 105°C for 3 hours, dissolve in the mobile phase to make exactly 100 mL. Pipet 10 mL of this solution, add the mobile phase to make exactly 100 mL, and use this solution as the standard solution. Perform the test with exactly 20 μL each of the sample solution and standard solution as directed under Liquid Chromatography *<2.01>* according to the following conditions. Determine the peak areas, A_T and A_S, of chlorpropamide in each solution.

Amount (mg) of chlorpropamide ($C_{10}H_{13}ClN_2O_3S$)
$= M_S \times A_T/A_S$

M_S: Amount (mg) of chlorpropamide for assay taken

Operating conditions—

Detector: An ultraviolet absorption photometer (wavelength: 240 nm).

Column: A stainless steel column 4.6 mm in inside diameter and 25 cm in length, packed with octadecylsilanized silica gel for liquid chromatography (10 μm in particle diameter).

Column temperature: A constant temperature of about 25°C.

Mobile phase: A mixture of diluted acetic acid (100) (1 in 100) and acetonitrile (1:1).

Flow rate: Adjust so that the retention time of chlorpropamide is about 5 minutes.

System suitability—

System performance: When the procedure is run with 20 μL of the standard solution under the above operating conditions, the number of theoretical plates and the symmetry factor of the peak of chlorpropamide are not less than 1500 and not more than 1.5, respectively.

System repeatability: When the test is repeated 6 times with 20 μL of the standard solution under the above operating conditions, the relative standard deviation of the peak area of chlorpropamide is not more than 1.5%.

Containers and storage Containers—Well-closed containers.

Cholecalciferol

Vitamin D_3

コレカルシフェロール

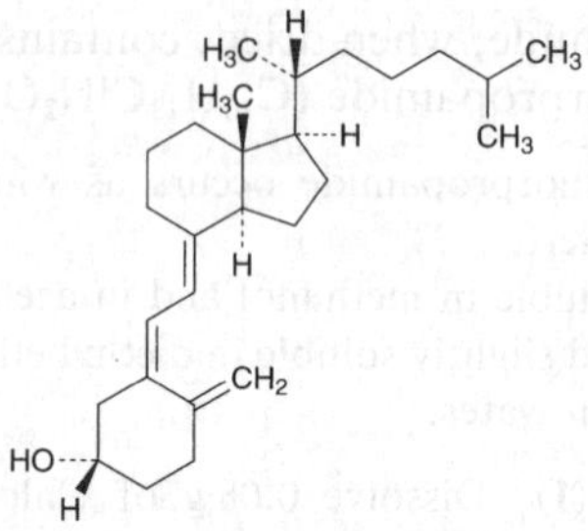

$C_{27}H_{44}O$: 384.64
(3*S*,5*Z*,7*E*)-9,10-Secocholesta-5,7,10(19)-trien-3-ol
[67-97-0]

Cholecalciferol contains not less than 97.0% and not more than 103.0% of cholecalciferol ($C_{27}H_{44}O$).

Description Cholecalciferol occurs as white crystals. It is odorless.

It is freely soluble in ethanol (95), in chloroform, in diethyl ether and in isooctane, and practically insoluble in water.

It is affected by air and by light.

Melting point: 84 – 88°C Transfer Cholecalciferol to a capillary tube, and dry for 3 hours in a desiccator (in vacuum at a pressure not exceeding 2.67 kPa). Immediately fireseal the capillary tube, put it in a bath fluid, previously heated to a temperature about 10°C below the expected melting point, and heat at a rate of rise of about 3°C per minute, and read the melting point.

Identification (1) Dissolve 0.5 mg of Cholecalciferol in 5 mL of chloroform, add 0.3 mL of acetic anhydride and 0.1 mL of sulfuric acid, and shake: a red color is produced, and rapidly changes through purple and blue to green.

(2) Determine the infrared absorption spectrum of Cholecalciferol as directed in the potassium bromide disk method under Infrared Spectrophotometry *<2.25>*, and compare the spectrum with the Reference Spectrum or the spectrum of Cholecalciferol RS: both spectra exhibit similar intensities of absorption at the same wave numbers.

Absorbance *<2.24>* $E^{1\%}_{1\,cm}$ (265 nm): 450 – 490 (10 mg, ethanol (95), 1000 mL).

Optical rotation *<2.49>* $[\alpha]^{20}_D$ + 103 – + 112° (50 mg, ethanol (95), 10 mL, 100 mm). Prepare the solution without delay, using Cholecalciferol from a container opened not longer than 30 minutes, previously, and determine the rotation within 30 minutes after the solution has been prepared.

Purity 7-Dehydrocholesterol—Dissolve 10 mg of Cholecalciferol in 2.0 mL of diluted ethanol (95) (9 in 10), add a solution prepared by dissolving 20 mg of digitonin in 2.0 mL of diluted ethanol (95) (9 in 10), and allow the mixture to stand for 18 hours: no precipitate is formed.

Assay Proceed with the operation avoiding contact with air or other oxidizing agents and using light-resistant containers. Dissolve separately about 30 mg each of Cholecalciferol and Cholecalciferol RS, accurately weighed, in isooctane to make exactly 50 mL. Pipet 10 mL each of these solutions, add 3 mL each of the internal standard solution, then add the mobile phase to make 50 mL, and use these solutions as the sample solution and the standard solution. Perform the test with 10 μL each of the sample solution and standard solution as directed under Liquid Chromatography <*2.01*> according to the following conditions, and calculate the ratios, Q_T and Q_S, of the peak area of cholecalciferol to that of the internal standard.

Amount (mg) of cholecalciferol ($C_{27}H_{44}O$) = $M_S \times Q_T/Q_S$

M_S: Amount (mg) of Cholecalciferol RS taken

Internal standard solution—A solution of dimethyl phthalate in isooctane (1 in 100).

Operating conditions—

Detector: An ultraviolet absorption photometer (wavelength: 254 nm).

Column: A stainless steel column about 4 mm in inside diameter and 10 to 30 cm in length, packed with silica gel for liquid chromatography (5 to 10 μm in particle diameter).

Column temperature: Ordinary temperature.

Mobile phase: A mixture of hexane and *n*-amylalcohol (997:3).

Flow rate: Adjust so that the retention time of cholecalciferol is about 25 minutes.

Selection of column: Dissolve 15 mg of Cholecalciferol RS in 25 mL of isooctane. Transfer this solution to a flask, heat under a reflux condenser in an oil bath for 2 hours, and cool to room temperature rapidly. Transfer this solution to a quartz test tube, and irradiate under a short-wave lamp (main wavelength: 254 nm) and a long-wave lamp (main wavelength: 365 nm) for 3 hours. To this solution add the mobile phase to make 50 mL. Proceed with 10 μL of this solution under the above operating conditions. Use a column with the relative retention time of previtamin D_3, trans-vitamin D_3 and tachysterol D_3 to cholecalciferol being about 0.5, about 0.6 and about 1.1, respectively, and with resolution between previtamin D_3 and trans-vitamin D_3, and that between cholecalciferol and tachysterol D_3 being not less than 1.0.

Containers and storage Containers—Hermetic containers.

Storage—Light-resistant, under nitrogen atmosphere, and in a cold place.

Cholesterol

コレステロール

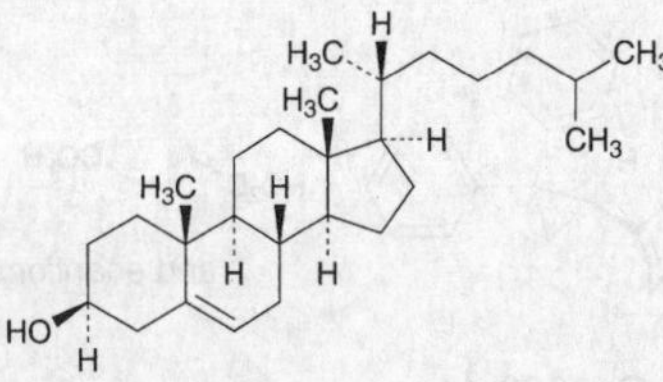

$C_{27}H_{46}O$: 386.65
Cholest-5-en-3β-ol
[*57-88-5*]

Description Cholesterol occurs as white to pale yellow, crystals or grains. It is odorless, or has a slight odor. It is tasteless.

It is freely soluble in chloroform and in diethyl ether, sparingly soluble in ethanol (99.5) and in acetone, and practically insoluble in water.

It gradually changes to a yellow to light yellow-brown color by light.

Identification **(1)** Dissolve 0.01 g of Cholesterol in 1 mL of chloroform, add 1 mL of sulfuric acid, and shake: a red color develops in the chloroform layer, and the sulfuric acid layer shows a green fluorescence.

(2) Dissolve 5 mg of Cholesterol in 2 mL of chloroform, add 1 mL of acetic anhydride and 1 drop of sulfuric acid, and shake: a red color is produced, and it changes to green through blue.

Optical rotation <*2.49*> $[\alpha]_D^{25}$: −29 – −36° (after drying, 0.2 g, acetone, 10 mL, 100 mm).

Melting point <*2.60*> 147 – 150°C

Purity **(1)** Clarity of solution—Place 0.5 g of Cholesterol in a glass-stoppered flask, dissolve in 50 mL of warm ethanol (95), and allow to stand at room temperature for 2 hours: no turbidity or deposit is produced.

(2) Acidity—Place 1.0 g of Cholesterol in a flask, dissolve in 10 mL of diethyl ether, add 10.0 mL of 0.1 mol/L sodium hydroxide VS, and shake for 1 minute. Expel the diethyl ether, and boil for 5 minutes. Cool, add 10 mL of water, and titrate <*2.50*> with 0.05 mol/L sulfuric acid VS (indicator: 2 drops of phenolphthalein TS). Perform a blank determination in the same manner.

The volume of 0.1 mol/L sodium hydroxide VS consumed is not more than 0.30 mL.

Loss on drying <*2.41*> Not more than 0.30% (1 g, in vacuum, 60°C, 4 hours).

Residue on ignition <*2.44*> Not more than 0.1% (1 g).

Containers and storage Containers—Tight containers.

Storage—Light-resistant.

Cibenzoline Succinate

シベンゾリンコハク酸塩

and enantiomer

$C_{18}H_{18}N_2.C_4H_6O_4$: 380.44
2-[(1*RS*)-2,2-Diphenylcyclopropan-1-yl]-4,5-dihydro-1*H*-imidazole monosuccinate
[*100678-32-8*]

Cibenzoline Succinate, when dried, contains not less than 98.5% and not more than 101.0% of cibenzoline succinate ($C_{18}H_{18}N_2.C_4H_6O_4$).

Description Cibenzoline Succinate occurs as a white crystalline powder.

It is freely soluble in methanol and in acetic acid (100), and sparingly soluble in water and in ethanol (99.5).

A solution of Cibenzoline Succinate in methanol (1 in 10) shows no optical rotation.

Identification **(1)** Determine the absorption spectrum of a solution of Cibenzoline Succinate (1 in 50,000) as directed under Ultraviolet-visible Spectrophotometry <*2.24*>, and compare the spectrum with the Reference Spectrum: both spectra exhibit similar intensities of absorption at the same wavelengths.

(2) Determine the infrared absorption spectrum of Cibenzoline Succinate as directed in the paste method under Infrared Spectrophotometry <*2.25*>, and compare the spectrum with the Reference Spectrum: both spectra exhibit similar intensities of absorption at the same wave numbers.

(3) Shake 0.4 g of Cibenzoline Succinate with 2.5 mL of sodium hydroxide TS and 5 mL of ethyl acetate, allow to stand, and to 1 mL of the water layer so obtained add 0.5 mL of 1 mol/L hydrochloric acid TS and 0.5 mL of iron (III) chloride TS: a blown precipitate is formed.

Melting point <*2.60*> 163 - 167°C

pH <*2.54*> Dissolve 0.20 g of Cibenzoline Succinate in 10 mL of water: the pH of this solution is between 4.0 and 6.0.

Purity **(1)** Clarity and color of solution—A solution obtained by dissolving 0.20 g of Cibenzoline Succinate in 10 mL of water is clear and colorless.

(2) Heavy metals <*1.07*>—Proceed with 1.0 g of Cibenzoline Succinate according to Method 2, and perform the test. Prepare the control solution with 2.0 mL of Standard Lead Solution (not more than 20 ppm).

(3) Arsenic <*1.11*>—Prepare the test solution with 1.0 g of Cibenzoline Succinate according to Method 3, using a solution of magnesium nitrate hexahydrate in ethanol (95) (1 in 25), and perform the test (not more than 2 ppm).

(4) Related substances—Dissolve 0.10 g of Cibenzoline Succinate in 10 mL of methanol, and use this solution as the sample solution. Pipet 1 mL of the sample solution, and add methanol to make exactly 100 mL. Pipet 5 mL and 2 mL of this solution, add methanol to make them exactly 10 mL, and use these solutions as the standard solution (1) and the standard solution (2). Perform the test with these solutions as directed under Thin-layer Chromatography <*2.03*>. Spot 10 μL each of the sample solution and standard solutions (1) and (2) on a plate of silica gel with fluorescent indicator for thin-layer chromatography. Develop the plate with a mixture of ethyl acetate, methanol and ammonia solution (28) (20:3:2) to a distance of about 10 cm, air-dry the plate, and dry more at 80°C for 30 minutes. After cooling, examine under ultraviolet light (main wavelength: 254 nm): the spot other than the principal spot obtained from the sample solution is not more intense than the spot from the standard solution (1). Allow the plate to stand for 30 minutes in iodine vapor: the spot other than the principal spot from the sample solution is not more intense than the spot from the standard solution (1), and the spot, which is more intense than the spot from the standard solution (2), is not more than two.

Loss on drying <*2.41*> Not more than 0.3% (1 g, 105°C, 2 hours).

Residue on ignition <*2.44*> Not more than 0.1% (1 g).

Assay Weigh accurately about 0.4 g of Cibenzoline Succinate, previously dried, dissolve in 50 mL of acetic acid (100), and titrate <*2.50*> with 0.1 mol/L perchloric acid VS until the color of the solution changes from violet to blue-green through blue (indicator: 2 drops of crystal violet TS). Perform a blank determination in the same manner, and make any necessary correction.

Each mL of 0.1 mol/L perchloric acid VS
= 38.04 mg of $C_{18}H_{18}N_2.C_4H_6O_4$

Containers and storage Containers—Tight containers.

Cibenzoline Succinate Tablets

シベンゾリンコハク酸塩錠

Cibenzoline Succinate Tablets contain not less than 95.0% and not more than 105.0% of the labeled amount of cibenzoline succinate ($C_{18}H_{18}N_2.C_4H_6O_4$: 380.44).

Method of preparation Prepare as directed under Tablets, with Cibenzoline Succinate.

Identification To a quantity of powdered Cibenzoline Succinate Tablets, equivalent to 50 mg of Cibenzoline Succinate, add 100 mL of water, shake for 10 minutes, and centrifuge. To 2 mL of the supernatant liquid add water to make 50 mL, and determine the absorption spectrum of this solution as directed under Ultraviolet-visible Spectrophotometry <*2.24*>: it exhibits a maximum between 221 nm and 225 nm.

Uniformity of dosage units <*6.02*> Perform the Mass variation test, or the Content uniformity test according to the following method: it meets the requirement.

To 1 tablet of Cibenzoline Succinate Tablets add a suitable amount of water so that each mL contains about 10 mg of cibenzoline succinate ($C_{18}H_{18}N_2.C_4H_6O_4$), and allow standing for 10 minutes while occasional shaking. To this solution add methanol so that each mL contains about 2 mg of cibenzoline succinate ($C_{18}H_{18}N_2.C_4H_6O_4$), add exactly 1 mL of the internal standard solution per 10 mg of cibenzoline succinate ($C_{18}H_{18}N_2.C_4H_6O_4$), then add methanol so that each mL contains about 1 mg of cibenzoline succinate ($C_{18}H_{18}N_2.C_4H_6O_4$). Centrifuge the solution, and use the supernatant liquid as the sample solution. Then, proceed as directed in the Assay.

Amount (mg) of cibenzoline succinate ($C_{18}H_{18}N_2.C_4H_6O_4$)
$= M_S \times Q_T/Q_S \times C/100$

M_S: Amount (mg) of cibenzoline succinate for assay taken
C: Labeled amount (mg) of cibenzoline succinate ($C_{18}H_{18}N_2.C_4H_6O_4$) in 1 tablet

Internal standard solution—Dissolve 0.1 g of 2-ethylhexyl parahydroxybenzoate in methanol to make 100 mL.

Dissolution <6.10> When the test is performed at 50 revolutions per minute according to the Paddle method, using 900 mL of water as the dissolution medium, the dissolution rate in 15 minutes of Cibenzoline Succinate Tablets is not less than 80%.

Start the test with 1 tablet of Cibenzoline Succinate Tablets, withdraw not less than 20 mL of the medium at the specified minute after starting the test, and filter through a membrane filter with a pore size not exceeding 0.45 μm. Discard not less than 10 mL of the first filtrate, pipet V mL of the subsequent filtrate, add water to make exactly V' mL so that each mL contains about 11 μg of cibenzoline succinate ($C_{18}H_{18}N_2.C_4H_6O_4$), and use this solution as the sample solution. Separately, weigh accurately about 28 mg of cibenzoline succinate for assay, previously dried at 105°C for 2 hours, and dissolve in water to make exactly 100 mL. Pipet 2 mL of this solution, add water to make exactly 50 mL, and use this solution as the standard solution. Determine the absorbances, A_T and A_S, of the sample solution and standard solution at 222 nm as directed under Ultraviolet-visible Spectrophotometry <2.24>.

Dissolution rate (%) with respect to the labeled amount of cibenzoline succinate ($C_{18}H_{18}N_2.C_4H_6O_4$)
$= M_S \times A_T/A_S \times V'/V \times 1/C \times 36$

M_S: Amount (mg) of cibenzoline succinate for assay taken
C: Labeled amount (mg) of cibenzoline succinate ($C_{18}H_{18}N_2.C_4H_6O_4$) in 1 tablet

Assay Weigh accurately not less than 20 Cibenzoline Succinate Tablets, and powder. Weigh accurately a portion of the powder, equivalent to about 0.1 g of cibenzoline succinate ($C_{18}H_{18}N_2.C_4H_6O_4$), add 10 mL of water, shake, and add 40 mL of methanol and exactly 10 mL of the internal standard solution. Shake for 20 minutes, add methanol to make 100 mL, centrifuge, and use the supernatant liquid as the sample solution. Separately, weigh accurately about 0.1 g of cibenzoline succinate for assay, previously dried at 105°C for 2 hours, add 10 mL of water and 40 mL of methanol to dissolve, then add exactly 10 mL of the internal standard solution and methanol to make 100 mL, and use this solution as the standard solution. Perform the test with 5 μL each of the sample solution and standard solution as directed under Liquid Chromatography <2.01> according to the following conditions, and calculate the ratios, Q_T and Q_S, of the peak area of cibenzoline to that of the internal standard.

Amount (mg) of cibenzoline succinate ($C_{18}H_{18}N_2.C_4H_6O_4$)
$= M_S \times Q_T/Q_S$

M_S: Amount (mg) of cibenzoline succinate for assay taken

Internal standard solution—Dissolve 0.1 g of 2-ethylhexyl parahydroxybenzoate in methanol to make 100 mL.
Operating conditions—

Detector: An ultraviolet absorption photometer (wavelength: 254 nm).

Column: A stainless steel column 4.6 mm in inside diameter and 5 cm in length, packed with octadecylsilanized silica gel for liquid chromatography (3 μm in particle diameter).

Column temperature: A constant temperature of about 25°C.

Mobile phase: Dissolve 2.67 g of sodium di-2-ethylhexyl sulfosuccinate in 2000 mL of a mixture of water, acetonitrile and diluted phosphoric acid (1 in 10) (1000:1000:1).

Flow rate: Adjust so that the retention time of cibenzoline is about 3 minutes.

System suitability—

System performance: When the procedure is run with 5 μL of the standard solution under the above operating conditions, cibenzoline and the internal standard are eluted in this order with the resolution between these peaks being not less than 6.

System repeatability: When the test is repeated 6 times with 5 μL of the standard solution under the above operating conditions, the relative standard deviation of the ratio of the peak area of cibenzoline to that of the internal standard is not more than 1.0%.

Containers and storage Containers—Tight containers.

Ciclacillin

シクラシリン

$C_{15}H_{23}N_3O_4S$: 341.43
(2*S*,5*R*,6*R*)-6-[(1-Aminocyclohexanecarbonyl)amino]-3,3-dimethyl-7-oxo-4-thia-1-azabicyclo[3.2.0]heptane-2-carboxylic acid
[*3485-14-1*]

Ciclacillin contains not less than 920 μg (potency) and not more than 1010 μg (potency) per mg, calculated on the anhydrous basis. The potency of Ciclacillin is expressed as mass (potency) of ciclacillin ($C_{15}H_{23}N_3O_4S$).

Description Ciclacillin occurs as white to light yellow-white crystalline powder.

It is sparingly soluble in water, slightly soluble in methanol, and practically insoluble in acetonitrile and in ethanol (99.5).

Identification Determine the infrared absorption spectrum of Ciclacillin as directed in the potassium bromide disk method under Infrared Spectrophotometry <2.25>, and compare the spectrum with the Reference Spectrum or the spectrum of Ciclacillin RS: both spectra exhibit similar intensities of absorption at the same wave numbers.

Optical rotation <2.49> $[\alpha]_D^{20}$: +300 – +315° (2 g, water, 100 mL, 100 mm).

Purity (1) Heavy metals <1.07>—Proceed with 1.0 g of Ciclacillin according to Method 2, and perform the test. Prepare the control solution with 2.0 mL of Standard Lead Solution (not more than 20 ppm).

(2) Arsenic <1.11>—Prepare the test solution with 1.0 g of Ciclacillin according to Method 3, and perform the test (not more than 2 ppm).

Water <2.48> Not more than 2.0% (1 g, volumetric titration, direct titration).

Assay Weigh accurately an amount of Ciclacillin and Ciclacillin RS, equivalent to about 50 mg (potency), dissolve each in a suitable amount of the mobile phase, add exactly 5 mL of the internal standard solution and the mobile phase to make 50 mL, and use these solutions as the sample solution and standard solution. Perform the test with 10 μL each of the sample solution and standard solution as directed under Liquid Chromatography <*2.01*> according to the following conditions, and calculate the ratios, Q_T and Q_S, of the peak area of ciclacillin to that of the internal standard.

Amount [μg (potency)] of ciclacillin ($C_{15}H_{23}N_3O_4S$)
$= M_S \times Q_T/Q_S \times 1000$

M_S: Amount [mg (potency)] of Ciclacillin RS taken

Internal standard solution—A solution of orcin in the mobile phase (1 in 500).

Operating conditions—

Detector: An ultraviolet absorption photometer (wavelength: 254 nm).

Column: A stainless steel column 4 mm in inside diameter and 15 cm in length, packed with octadecylsilanized silica gel for liquid chromatography (5 μm in particle diameter).

Column temperature: A constant temperature of about 25°C.

Mobile phase: Dissolve 0.771 g of ammonium acetate in about 900 mL of water, adjust the pH to 4.0 with acetic acid (100), and add water to make 1000 mL. To 850 mL of this solution add 150 mL of acetonitrile.

Flow rate: Adjust so that the retention time of ciclacillin is about 4 minutes.

System suitability—

System performance: When the procedure is run with 10 μL of the standard solution under the above operating conditions, ciclacillin and the internal standard are eluted in this order with the resolution between these peaks being not less than 8.

System repeatability: When the test is repeated 6 times with 10 μL of the standard solution under the above operating conditions, the relative standard deviation of the ratios of the peak areas of ciclacillin to that of the internal standard is not more than 1.0%.

Containers and storage Containers—Tight containers.

Ciclosporin

シクロスポリン

Ala-D-Ala-MeLeu-MeLeu-MeVal—N—Abu-MeGly-MeLeu-Val-MeLeu

Abu = (2*S*)-2-Aminobutyric acid
MeGly = *N*-Methylglycine
MeLeu = *N*-Methylleucine
MeVal = *N*-Methylvaline

$C_{62}H_{111}N_{11}O_{12}$: 1202.61
cyclo{-[(2*S*,3*R*,4*R*,6*E*)-3-Hydroxy-4-methyl-2-methylaminooct-6-enoyl]-L-2-aminobutanoyl-*N*-methylglycyl-*N*-methyl-L-leucyl-L-valyl-*N*-methyl-L-leucyl-L-alanyl-D-alanyl-*N*-methyl-L-leucyl-*N*-methyl-L-leucyl-*N*-methyl-L-valyl-}
[*59865-13-3*]

Ciclosporin contains not less than 98.5% and not more than 101.5% of ciclosporin ($C_{62}H_{111}N_{11}O_{12}$), calculated on the dried basis.

Description Ciclosporin occurs as a white powder.

It is very soluble in acetonitrile, in methanol and in ethanol (95), freely soluble in diethyl ether, and practically insoluble in water.

Identification Determine the infrared absorption spectrum of Ciclosporin as directed in the potassium bromide disk method under Infrared Spectrophotometry <*2.25*>, and compare the spectrum with the Reference Spectrum or the spectrum of Ciclosporin RS: both spectra exhibit similar intensities of absorption at the same wave numbers.

Optical rotation <*2.49*> $[\alpha]_D^{20}$: −185 – −193° (0.1 g calculated on the dried basis, methanol, 20 mL, 100 mm).

Purity (1) Clarity and color of solution—Dissolve 1.0 g of Ciclosporin in 10 mL of ethanol (95): the solution is clear, and has no more color than the following control solutions (1), (2) or (3).

Control solution (1): To exactly 3.0 mL of Iron (III) Chloride CS and exactly 0.8 mL of Cobalt (II) Chloride CS add diluted hydrochloric acid (1 in 40) to make exactly 100 mL.

Control solution (2): To exactly 3.0 mL of Iron (III) Chloride CS, exactly 1.3 mL of Cobalt (II) Chloride CS and exactly 0.5 mL of Copper (II) Sulfate CS add diluted hydrochloric acid (1 in 40) to make exactly 100 mL.

Control solution (3): To exactly 0.5 mL of Iron (III) Chloride CS and exactly 1.0 mL of Cobalt (II) Chloride CS add diluted hydrochloric acid (1 in 40) to make exactly 100 mL.

(2) Heavy metals <*1.07*>—Proceed with 1.0 g of Ciclosporin according to Method 2, and perform the test. Prepare the control solution with 2.0 mL of Standard Lead Solution (not more than 20 ppm).

(3) Related substances—Use the sample solution obtained in the Assay as the sample solution. Pipet 2 mL of the sample solution, add a mixture of water and acetonitrile (1:1) to make exactly 200 mL, and use this solution as the standard solution. Perform the test with exactly 20 μL each of the sample solution and standard soluton as directed under Liquid Chromatography <*2.01*> according to the following conditions. Determine each peak area of both solutions by the automatic integration method: the area of the peak other than the ciclosporin obtained from the sample solution is not larger than 7/10 times the peak area of ciclosporin from the standard solution, and the total area of all peaks other than the ciclosporin from the sample solution is not larger than 1.5 times the peak area of ciclosporin from the standard solution.

Operating conditions—

Detector, column, column temperature, mobile phase, and flow rate: Proceed as directed in the operating conditions in the Assay.

Time span of measurement: About 2 times as long as the retention time of ciclosporin, beginning after the solvent peak.

System suitability—

System performance: Proceed as directed in the system suitability in the Assay.

Test for required detectability: To exactly 2 mL of the standard solution add a mixture of water and acetonitrile (1:1) to make exactly 20 mL. Confirm that the peak area of ciclosporin obtained from 20 μL of this solution is equivalent to 7 to 13% of that of ciclosporin obtained from 20 μL of the standard solution.

System repeatability: When the test is repeated 6 times with 20 μL of the standard solution under the above operating conditions, the relative standard deviation of the peak

area of ciclosporin is not more than 3.0%.

Loss on drying *⟨2.41⟩* Not more than 2.0% (1 g, in vacuum at a pressure not exceeding 0.67 kPa, 60°C, 3 hours).

Residue on ignition *⟨2.44⟩* Not more than 0.1% (0.5 g).

Assay Weigh accurately about 30 mg each of Ciclosporin and Ciclosporin RS (separately determine the loss on drying *⟨2.41⟩* under the same conditions as Ciclosporin), and dissolve each in a mixture of water and acetonitrile (1:1) to make exactly 25 mL, and use these solutions as the sample solution and standard solution. Perform the test with exactly 20 μL each of the sample solution and standard solution as directed under Liquid Chromatography *⟨2.01⟩* according to the following conditions, and determine the peak areas, A_T and A_S, of ciclosporin in each solution.

$$\text{Amount (mg) of ciclosporin } (C_{62}H_{111}N_{11}O_{12}) = M_S \times A_T/A_S$$

M_S: Amount (mg) of Ciclosporin RS taken, calculated on the dried basis

Operating conditions—

Detector: An ultraviolet absorption photometer (wavelength: 210 nm).

Column: A stainless steel column 4 mm in inside diameter and 25 cm in length, packed with octadecylsilanized silica gel for liquid chromatography (5 μm in particle diameter). Connect the sample injection port and the column with a stainless steel tube 0.3 mm in inside diameter and 1 m in length.

Column temperature: A constant temperature of about 80°C (including the sample injection port and the connecting tube).

Mobile phase: A mixture of water, acetonitrile, tert-butyl methyl ether and phosphoric acid (520:430:50:1).

Flow rate: Adjust so that the retention time of ciclosporin is about 27 minutes.

System suitability—

System performance: Dissolve 3 mg of Ciclosporin U in 2.5 mL of a mixture of water and acetonitrile (1:1), and add 2.5 mL of the standard solution. When the procedure is run with 20 μL of this solution under the above operating conditions, ciclosporin U and ciclosporin are eluted in this order with the resolution between these peaks being not less than 1.2.

System repeatability: When the test is repeated 6 times with 20 μL of the standard solution under the above operating conditions, the relative standard deviation of the peak area of ciclosporin is not more than 1.0%.

Containers and storage Containers—Tight containers.

Storage—Light-resistant.

Cilastatin Sodium

シラスタチンナトリウム

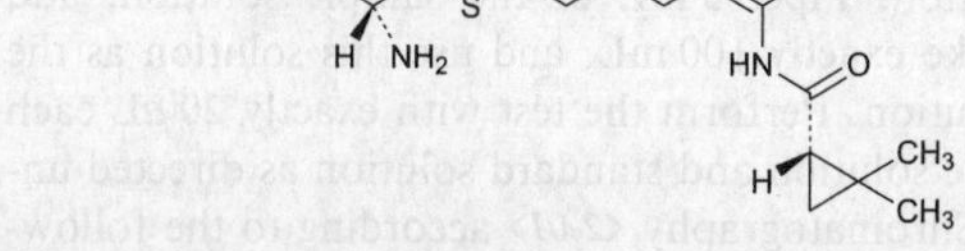

$C_{16}H_{25}N_2NaO_5S$: 380.43

Monosodium (2*Z*)-7-{[(2*R*)-2-amino-2-carboxyethyl]sulfanyl}-2-({[(1*S*)-2,2-dimethylcyclopropyl]carbonyl}amino)hept-2-enoate

[81129-83-1]

Cilastatin Sodium contains not less than 98.0% and not more than 101.0% of cilastatin sodium ($C_{16}H_{25}N_2NaO_5S$), calculated on the anhydrous and residual solvent-free basis.

Description Cilastatin Sodium occurs as a white to pale yellowish white powder.

It is very soluble in water, freely soluble in methanol, and slightly soluble in ethanol (99.5).

It is hygroscopic.

Identification **(1)** Determine the infrared absorption spectrum of Cilastatin Sodium as directed in the potassium bromide disk method under Infrared Spectrophotometry *⟨2.25⟩*, and compare the spectrum with the Reference Spectrum: both spectra exhibit similar intensities of absorption at the same wave numbers.

(2) A solution of Cilastatin Sodium (1 in 10) responds to Qualitative Tests *⟨1.09⟩* for sodium salt.

Optical rotation *⟨2.49⟩* $[\alpha]_D^{20}$: +41.5 – +44.5° (0.1 g calculated on the anhydrous and residual solvent-free basis, a solution of hydrochloric acid in methanol (9 in 1000), 10 mL, 100 mL).

pH *⟨2.54⟩* The pH of a solution prepared by dissolving 1.0 g of Cilastatin Sodium in 100 mL of water is between 6.5 and 7.5.

Purity **(1)** Clarity and color of solution—Dissolve 1.0 g of Cilastatin Sodium in 100 mL of water: the solution is clear and the solution has no more color than the following control solution.

Control solution: To a mixture of 2.4 mL of Iron (III) Chloride CS and 0.6 mL of Cobalt (II) Chloride CS add water to make 10 mL, pipet 5 mL of this solution, and add water to make exactly 100 mL.

(2) Heavy metals *⟨1.07⟩*—Proceed with 1.0 g of Cilastatin Sodium according to Method 2, and perform the test. After carbonization, add 0.5 mL of sulfuric acid instead of nitric acid. Prepare the control solution with 2.0 mL of Standard Lead Solution (not more than 20 ppm).

(3) Arsenic *⟨1.11⟩*—To 2.0 g of Cilastatin Sodium add 5 mL of nitric acid and 1 mL of sulfuric acid, and heat carefully until white fumes are evolved. After cooling, heat with two 2-mL portions of nitric acid, then heat with several 2-mL portions of hydrogen peroxide (30) until a colorless or pale yellow solution is obtained. After cooling, heat again until white fumes are evolved. After cooling, add water to make 5 mL, and perform the test with this solution as the test solution: it shows no more color than the following color standard.

Color standard: Prepare a solution according to the above

procedure without using Cilastatin Sodium, add exactly 2 mL of Standard Arsenic Solution, and perform the test in the same manner as the test solution (not more than 1 ppm).

(4) Related substances—Dissolve about 40 mg of Cilastatin Sodium in 25 mL of water, and use this solution as the sample solution. Pipet 3 mL of the sample solution, add water to make exactly 100 mL, and use this solution as the standard solution. Perform the test with exactly 20 μL each of the sample solution and standard solution as directed under Liquid Chromatography <*2.01*> according to the following conditions, and determine each peak area by the automatic integration method: the area of the peak other than cilastatin obtained from the sample solution is not larger than 1/6 times the peak area of cilastatin from the standard solution, and the total area of the peaks other than the peak of cilastatin from the sample solution is not larger than the peak area of cilastatin from the standard solution.

Operating conditions—

Detector: An ultraviolet absorption photometer (wavelength: 210 nm).

Column: A stainless steel column 4.5 mm in inside diameter and 25 cm in length, packed with octadecylsilanized silica gel for liquid chromatography (5 μm in particle diameter).

Column temperature: A constant temperature of about 50°C.

Mobile phase A: A mixture of diluted phosphoric acid (1 in 1000) and acetonitrile (7:3).

Mobile phase B: Diluted phosphoric acid (1 in 1000).

Flowing of mobile phase: Control the gradient by mixing the mobile phases A and B as directed in the following table.

Time after injection of sample (min)	Mobile phase A (vol%)	Mobile phase B (vol%)
0 – 30	15 → 100	85 → 0
30 – 40	100	0

Flow rate: 2.0 mL per minute.

Time span of measurement: For 40 minutes.

System suitability—

Test for required detectability: Pipet 1 mL of the standard solution, and add water to make exactly 30 mL. Confirm that the peak area of cilastatin obtained with 20 μL of this solution is equivalent to 2.3 to 4.5% of that with 20 μL of the standard solution.

System performance: When the procedure is run with 20 μL of the standard solution under the above operating conditions, the retention time of cilastatin is about 20 minutes, and the number of theoretical plates and the symmetry factor of the peak of cilastatin are not less than 10,000 and not more than 2.5, respectively.

System repeatability: When the test is repeated 3 times with 20 μL of the standard solution under the above operating conditions, the relative standard deviation of the peak area of cilastatin is not more than 2.0%.

(5) Residual solvents <*2.46*>—Weigh accurately about 0.2 g of Cilastatin Sodium, add exactly 2 mL of the internal standard solution, dissolve in water to make 10 mL, and use this solution as the sample solution. Separately, measure exactly 2 mL of acetone, 0.5 mL of methanol and 0.5 mL of mesityl oxide, and add water to make exactly 1000 mL. Pipet 2 mL of this solution, add exactly 2 mL of the internal standard solution, add water to make 10 mL, and use this solution as the standard solution. Perform the test with 2 μL each of the sample solution and standard solution as directed under Gas Chromatography <*2.02*> according to the following conditions. Calculate the ratios of the peak areas of acetone, methanol and mesityl oxide and to the peak area of the internal standard, Q_{Ta} and Q_{Sa}, Q_{Tb} and Q_{Sb}, Q_{Tc} and Q_{Sc}, and calculate the amounts of acetone, methanol and mesityl oxide by the following equation: they are not more than 1.0%, not more 0.5% and not more than 0.4%, respectively.

Amount (%) of acetone (CH_3COCH_3)
$= 1/M_T \times Q_{Ta}/Q_{Sa} \times 400 \times 0.79$

Amount (%) of methanol (CH_3OH)
$= 1/M_T \times Q_{Tb}/Q_{Sb} \times 100 \times 0.79$

Amount (%) of mesityl oxide ($CH_3COCH = C(CH_3)_2$)
$= 1/M_T \times Q_{Tc}/Q_{Sc} \times 100 \times 0.86$

M_T: Amount (mg) of Cilastatin Sodium taken
0.79: Density (g/mL) of acetone and methanol
0.86: Density (g/mL) of mesityl oxide

Internal standard solution—To 0.5 mL of 1-propanol add water to make 1000 mL.

Operating conditions—

Detector: A hydrogen flame-ionization detector.

Column: A glass column 3.2 mm in inside diameter and 2.1 m in length, packed with tetrafluoroethylene polymer for gas chromatography (250 – 420 μm) coated with polyethylene glycol 20 M for gas chromatography at the ratio of 10%.

Column temperature: A constant temperature of about 70°C.

Carrier gas: Helium.

Flow rate: Adjust so that the retention time of the internal standard is about 5 minutes.

Time span of measurement: About 3 times as long as the retention time of the internal standard.

System suitability—

System performance: When the procedure is run with 2 μL of the standard solution under the above operating conditions, acetone, methanol, 1-propanol and mesityl oxide are eluted in this order, and these peaks completely separate each other.

System repeatability: When the test is repeated 6 times with 2 μL of the standard solution under the above operating conditions, the relative standard deviations of the ratio of the peak area of acetone, methanol and mesityl oxide to that of the internal standard are not more than 4.0%, respectively.

Water <*2.48*> Not more than 2.0% (0.5 g, volumetric titration, direct titration).

Assay Weigh accurately about 0.3 g of Cilastatin Sodium, dissolve in 30 mL of methanol, add 5 mL of water, and adjust to pH 3.0 with 0.1 mol/L hydrochloric acid TS. Titrate <*2.50*> with 0.1 mol/L sodium hydroxide VS from the first equivalence point to the third equivalence point (potentiometric titration), and make any necessary correction.

Each mL of 0.1 mol/L sodium hydroxide VS
$= 19.02$ mg of $C_{16}H_{25}N_2NaO_5S$

Containers and storage Containers—Tight containers.
Storage—In a cold place.

Cilazapril Hydrate

シラザプリル水和物

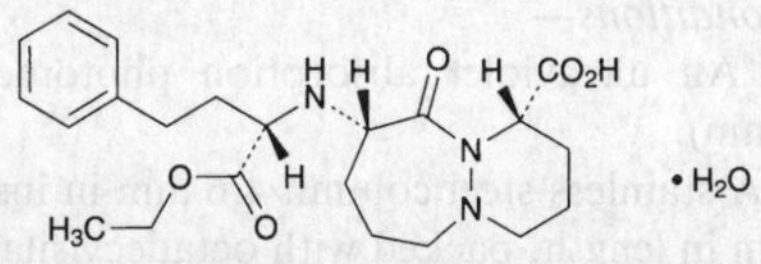

$C_{22}H_{31}N_3O_5.H_2O$: 435.51
(1*S*,9*S*)-9-[(1*S*)-(1-Ethoxycarbonyl-3-phenylpropyl)amino]-10-oxooctahydro-6*H*-pyridazino[1,2-*a*][1,2]diazepine-1-carboxylic acid monohydrate
[*92077-78-6*]

Cilazapril Hydrate contains not less than 98.5% and not more than 101.0% of cilazapril ($C_{22}H_{31}N_3O_5$: 417.50), calculated on the anhydrous basis.

Description Cilazapril Hydrate occurs as white to yellowish white, crystals or crystalline powder.

It is very soluble in methanol, freely soluble in ethanol (99.5) and in acetic acid (100), and slightly soluble in water.

It gradually turns yellow on exposure to light.

Melting point: about 101°C (with decomposition).

Identification **(1)** To 4 mL of a solution of Cilazapril Hydrate (1 in 1000) add 2 mL of Dragendorff's TS: an orange precipitate is produced.

(2) Determine the infrared absorption spectrum of Cilazapril Hydrate as directed in the potassium bromide disk method under Infrared Spectrophotometry *<2.25>*, and compare the spectrum with the Reference Spectrum: both spectra exhibit similar intensities of absorption at the same wave numbers.

Optical rotation *<2.49>* $[\alpha]_D^{20}$: −53 – −58° (0.2 g calculated on the anhydrous basis, methanol, 20 mL, 100 mm).

Purity **(1)** Chloride *<1.03>*—Perform the test using 1.0 g of Cilazapril Hydrate. Prepare the control solution with 0.25 mL of 0.01 mol/L hydrochloric acid VS (not more than 0.009%).

(2) Sulfate *<1.14>*—Dissolve 1.0 g of Cilazapril Hydrate in 40 mL of water and 1.5 mL of dilute hydrochloric acid, and add water to make 50 mL. Perform the test using this solution as the test solution. Prepare the control solution with 0.40 mL of 0.005 mol/L sulfuric acid VS (not more than 0.019%).

(3) Heavy metals *<1.07>*—Proceed with 1.0 g of Cilazapril Hydrate according to Method 4, and perform the test. However, use 10 mL of a solution of magnesium nitrate hexahydrate in ethanol (95) (1 in 8). Prepare the control solution with 2.0 mL of Standard Lead Solution (not more than 20 ppm).

(4) Related substances—Dissolve 0.10 g of Cilazapril Hydrate in 20 mL of methanol, and use this solution as the sample solution. Pipet 1 mL of the sample solution, add methanol to make exactly 100 mL, and use this solution as the standard solution (1). Pipet 3 mL of the standard solution (1), add methanol to make exactly 10 mL, and use this solution as the standard solution (2). Separately, pipet 2 mL of the standard solution (1), add methanol to make exactly 10 mL, and use this solution as the standard solution (3). Perform the test with these solutions as directed under Thin-layer Chromatography *<2.03>*. Spot 20 μL each of the sample solution and three standard solutions on a plate of silica gel with fluorescent indicator for thin-layer chromatography. Develop the plate with a mixture of ethyl acetate, methanol, acetic acid (100), hexane, and water (62:15:10:10:3) to a distance of about 15 cm, and air-dry the plate. Leave the plate in iodine vapor for 2 hours, and examine the plate under ultraviolet light (main wavelength: 254 nm): of the spots other than the principal spot with an *R*f value close to 0.40 obtained from the sample solution, the spot in the vicinity of *R*f value 0.17 is not more intense than the spot from the standard solution (1), and the spot in the vicinity of *R*f value 0.44 is not more intense than the spot from the standard solution (2). The number of all other spot does not exceed 3, and of these spots, no more than one is more intense than the spot from the standard solution (3) and none are more intense than the spot from the standard solution (2).

Water *<2.48>* 3.5 – 5.0% (0.3 g, volumetric titration, direct titration).

Residue on ignition *<2.44>* Not more than 0.1% (0.5 g).

Assay Weigh accurately about 0.2 g of Cilazapril Hydrate, dissolve in 50 mL of acetic acid (100), and titrate *<2.50>* with 0.02 mol/L perchloric acid VS (potentiometric titration). Perform a blank determination in the same manner, and make any necessary correction.

Each mL of 0.02 mol/L perchloric acid VS
= 8.350 mg of $C_{22}H_{31}N_3O_5$

Containers and storage Containers—Tight containers.

Storage—Light-resistant.

Cilazapril Tablets

シラザプリル錠

Cilazapril Tablets contain not less than 93.0% and not more than 107.0% of the labeled amount of cilazapril ($C_{22}H_{31}N_3O_5$: 417.50).

Method of preparation Prepare as directed under Tablets, with Cilazapril Hydrate.

Identification To a quantity of powdered Cilazapril Tablets, equivalent to 2 mg of cilazapril ($C_{22}H_{31}N_3O_5$), add 2 mL of a mixture of acetonitrile and ethyl acetate (3:1), shake, sonicate for 30 seconds, centrifuge, and use the supernatant liquid as the sample solution. Separately, dissolve 5 mg of cilazapril in 5 mL of the mixture of acetonitrile and ethyl acetate (3:1), and use this solution as the standard solution. Perform the test with these solutions as directed under Thin-layer Chromatography *<2.03>*. Spot 20 μL each of the sample solution and standard solution on a plate of silica gel with fluorescent indicator for thin-layer chromatography. Develop the plate with a mixture of ethyl acetate, methanol, acetic acid (100), hexane and water (62:15:10:10:3) to a distance of about 15 cm, and air-dry the plate. Place the plate in iodine vapor for 2 hours, and immediately examine under ultraviolet light (main wavelength: 254 nm): the spots obtained from the sample and standard solutions are dark brown and they show the same *R*f value.

Uniformity of dosage units *<6.02>* Perform the test according to the following method: it meets the requirement of the Content uniformity test.

To 1 tablet of Cilazapril Tablets add 5 mL of a mixture of water and acetonitrile (7:3), shake well until disintegration, add the mixture of water and acetonitrile (7:3) to make exactly V mL so that each mL contains about 25 μg of cilazapril ($C_{22}H_{31}N_3O_5$), and centrifuge. Pipet 4 mL of the supernatant liquid, add exactly 1 mL of the internal standard solution, add the mixture of water and acetonitrile (7:3) to make 10 mL, and use this solution as the sample solution. Separately, weigh accurately about 26 mg of cilazapril for assay (separately determine the water <*2.48*> in the same manner as Cilazapril Hydrate), and dissolve in the mixture of water and acetonitrile (7:3) to make exactly 50 mL. Pipet 2 mL of this solution, add exactly 10 mL of the internal standard solution, add the mixture of water and acetonitrile (7:3) to make 100 mL, and use this solution as the standard solution. Perform the test with 100 μL each of the sample solution and standard solution as directed under Liquid Chromatography <*2.01*> according to the following conditions, and calculate the ratios, Q_T and Q_S, of the peak area of cilazapril to that of the internal standard.

$$\text{Amount (mg) of cilazapril } (C_{22}H_{31}N_3O_5) = M_S \times Q_T/Q_S \times V/1000$$

M_S: Amount (mg) of cilazapril for assay taken, calculated on the anhydrous basis

Internal standard solution—A solution of dimethyl phthalate in a mixture of water and acetonitrile (7:3) (1 in 12,500).

Operating conditions—

Proceed as directed in the operating conditions in the Assay.

System suitability—

System performance: When the procedure is run with 100 μL of the standard solution under the above conditions, cilazapril and the internal standard are eluted in this order with the resolution between these peaks being not less than 6.

System repeatability: When the test is repeated 6 times with 100 μL of the standard solution under the above conditions, the relative standard deviation of the ratio of the peak area of cilazapril to that of the internal standard is not more than 2.0%.

Dissolution <*6.10*> When the test is performed at 50 revolutions per minute according to the Paddle method, using 900 mL of water as the dissolution medium, the dissolution rate in 15 minutes of Cilazapril Tablets is not less than 85%.

Start the test with 1 tablet of Cilazapril Tablets, withdraw not less than 20 mL of the medium at the specified minute after starting the test, and filter through a membrane filter with a pore size not exceeding 0.45 μm. Discard not less than 10 mL of the first filtrate, pipet V mL of the subsequent filtrate, and add water to make exactly V' mL so that each mL contains about 0.28 μg of cilazapril ($C_{22}H_{31}N_3O_5$). Pipet 10 mL of the solution, add exactly 5 mL of acetonitrile, and use this solution as the sample solution. Separately, weigh accurately about 29 mg of cilazapril for assay (separately determine the water <*2.48*> in the same manner as Cilazapril Hydrate), and dissolve in water to make exactly 100 mL. Pipet 5 mL of the solution, add water to make exactly 100 mL. Then, pipet 2 mL of this solution, add water to make exactly 100 mL. Pipet 10 mL of this solution, add exactly 5 mL of acetonitrile, and use this solution as the standard solution. Perform the test with exactly 100 μL each of the sample solution and standard solution as directed under Liquid Chromatography <*2.01*> according to the following conditions, and determine the peak areas, A_T and A_S, of cilazapril in each solution.

$$\text{Dissolution rate (\%) with respect to the labeled amount of cilazapril } (C_{22}H_{31}N_3O_5) = M_S \times A_T/A_S \times V'/V \times 1/C \times 9/10$$

M_S: Amount (mg) of cilazapril for assay taken, calculated on the anhydrous basis

C: Labeled amount (mg) of cilazapril ($C_{22}H_{31}N_3O_5$) in 1 tablet

Operating conditions—

Detector: An ultraviolet absorption photometer (wavelength: 210 nm).

Column: A stainless steel column 4.6 mm in inside diameter and 15 cm in length, packed with octadecylsilanized silica gel for liquid chromatography (5 μm in particle diameter).

Column temperature: A constant temperature of about 25°C.

Mobile phase: To a solution consisting of 180 mL of tetrahydrofuran for liquid chromatography, 120 mL of acetonitrile for liquid chromatography and 3 mL of triethylamine add water to make 1000 mL, and adjust the pH to 2.5 with phosphoric acid.

Flow rate: Adjust so that the retention time of cilazapril is about 10 minutes.

System suitability—

System performance: When the procedure is run with 100 μL of the standard solution under the above operating conditions, the number of theoretical plates and the symmetry factor of the peak of cilazapril are not less than 3000 and not more than 2.0, respectively.

System repeatability: When the test is repeated 6 times with 100 μL of the standard solution under the above operating conditions, the relative standard deviation of the peak area of cilazapril is not more than 2.0%.

Assay Weigh acurately the mass of not less than 20 Cilazapril Tablets, and powder. Weigh accurately a portion of the powder, equivalent to about 1 mg of cilazapril ($C_{22}H_{31}N_3O_5$), add 30 mL of a mixture of water and acetonitrile (7:3), and sonicate for 5 minutes. Next, add exactly 5 mL of the internal standard solution, add the mixture of water and acetonitrile (7:3) to make 50 mL, and centrifuge. Filter the supernatant liquid through a membrane filter with a pore size not exceeding 0.5 μm, and use the filtrate as the sample solution. Separately, weigh accurately about 26 mg of cilazapril for assay (separately determine the water <*2.48*> in the same manner as Cilazapril Hydrate), and dissolve in the mixture of water and acetonitrile (7:3) to make exactly 50 mL. Pipet 2 mL of this solution, add exactly 5 mL of the internal standard solution, add the mixture of water and acetonitrile (7:3) to make 50 mL, and use this solution as the standard solution. Perform the test with 50 μL each of the sample solution and standard solution as directed under Liquid Chromatography <*2.01*> according to the following conditions, and calculate the ratios, Q_T and Q_S, of the peak area of cilazapril to that of the internal standard.

$$\text{Amount (mg) of cilazapril } (C_{22}H_{31}N_3O_5) = M_S \times Q_T/Q_S \times 1/25$$

M_S: Amount (mg) of cilazapril for assay taken, calculated on the anhydrous basis

Internal standard solution—A solution of dimethyl phthalate in a mixture of water and acetonitrile (7:3) (1 in 12,500).

Operating conditions—

Detector: An ultraviolet absorption photometer (wavelength: 210 nm).

Column: A stainless steel column 6 mm in inside diameter and 15 cm in length, packed with octadecylsilanized silica gel for liquid chromatography (5 μm in particle diameter).

Column temperature: A constant temperature of about 23°C.

Mobile phase: To a solution consisting of 180 mL of tetrahydrofuran for liquid chromatography, 120 mL of acetonitrile for liquid chromatography and 3 mL of triethylamine add water to make 1000 mL, and adjust the pH to 2.5 with phosphoric acid.

Flow rate: Adjust so that the retention time of cilazapril is about 10 minutes.

System suitability—

System performance: When the procedure is run with 50 μL of the standard solution under the above operating conditions, cilazapril and the internal standard are eluted in this order with the resolution between these peaks being not less than 6.

System repeatability: When the test is repeated 6 times with 50 μL of the standard solution under the above operating conditions, the relative standard deviation of the ratio of the peak area of cilazapril to that of the internal standard is not more than 1.0%.

Containers and storage Containers—Tight containers.

Cilnidipine

シルニジピン

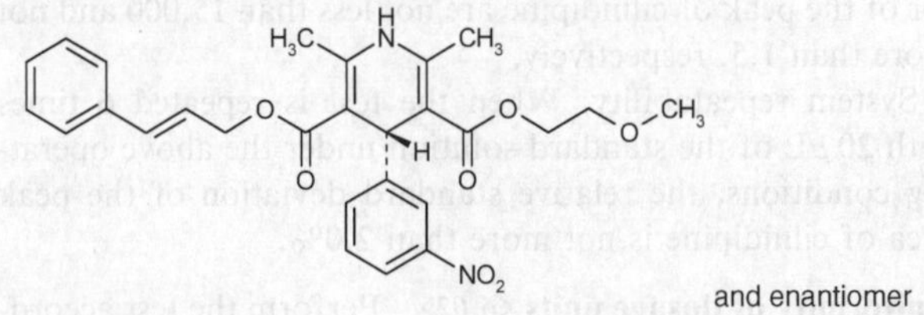

and enantiomer

$C_{27}H_{28}N_2O_7$: 492.52

3-(2-Methoxyethyl) 5-[(2*E*)-3-phenylprop-2-en-1-yl] (4*RS*)-2,6-dimethyl-4-(3-nitrophenyl)-1,4-dihydropyridine-3,5-dicarboxylate

[132203-70-4]

Cilnidipine, when dried, contains not less than 98.0% and not more than 102.0% of cilnidipine ($C_{27}H_{28}N_2O_7$).

Description Cilnidipine occurs as a faint yellow crystalline powder.

It is freely soluble in acetonitrile, sparingly soluble in methanol and in ethanol (99.5), and practically insoluble in water.

A solution of Cilnidipine in acetonitrile (1 in 100) shows no optical rotation.

It is gradually colored to reddish yellow and decomposed by light.

Identification **(1)** Determine the absorption spectrum of a solution of Cilnidipine in methanol (1 in 100,000) as directed under Ultraviolet-visible Spectrophotometry ⟨*2.24*⟩, and compare the spectrum with the Reference Spectrum or the spectrum of a solution of Cilnidipine RS prepared in the same manner as the sample solution: both spectra exhibit similar intensities of absorption at the same wavelengths.

(2) Determine the infrared absorption spectrum of previously dried Cilnidipine as directed in the potassium bromide disk method under Infrared Spectrophotometry ⟨*2.25*⟩, and compare the spectrum with the Reference Spectrum or the spectrum of dried Cilnidipine RS: both spectra exhibit similar intensities of absorption at the same wave numbers.

Melting point ⟨*2.60*⟩ 107 – 112°C

Purity **(1)** Heavy metals ⟨*1.07*⟩—Proceed with 2.0 g of Cilnidipine according to Method 4, and perform the test. Prepare the control solution with 2.0 mL of Standard Lead Solution (not more than 10 ppm).

(2) Related substances—Conduct this procedure using light-resistant vessels. Dissolve 50 mg of Cilnidipine in 20 mL of acetonitrile, add the mobile phase to make 100 mL, and use this solution as the sample solution. Pipet 1 mL of the sample solution, add the mobile phase to make exactly 200 mL, and use this solution as the standard solution. Perform the test with exactly 10 μL each of the sample solution and standard solution as directed under Liquid Chromatography ⟨*2.01*⟩ according to the following conditions, and determine each peak area by the automatic integration method: the area of the peak, having the relative retention time of about 0.5 to cilnidipine, obtained from the sample solution is not larger than 2/5 times the peak area of cilnidipine from the standard solution, the area of the peaks other than cilnidipine and the above mentioned peak from the sample solution is not larger than 1/5 times the peak area of cilnidipine from the standard solution, and the total area of the peaks other than cilnidipine from the sample solution is not larger than the peak area of cilnidipine from the standard solution. For the area of the peak, having the relative retention time of about 1.15, about 1.6, and about 1.7 to cilnidipine, multiply the correction factor, 1.5, 1.4, and 1.6, respectively.

Operating conditions—

Detector, column, column temperature, mobile phase, and flow rate: Proceed as directed in the operating conditions in the Assay.

Time span of measurement: About 3 times as long as the retention time of cilnidipine, beginning after the solvent peak.

System suitability—

System performance: Proceed as directed in the system suitability in the Assay.

Test for required detectability: Pipet 5 mL of the standard solution, add the mobile phase to make exactly 50 mL. Confirm that the peak area of cilnidipine obtained with 10 μL of this solution is equivalent to 7 to 13% of that with 10 μL of the standard solution.

System repeatability: When the test is repeated 6 times with 10 μL of the standard solution under the above operating conditions, the relative standard deviation of the peak area of cilnidipine is not more than 2.0%.

Loss on drying ⟨*2.41*⟩ Not more than 0.5% (1.0 g, in vacuum, 60°C, 3 hours).

Residue on ignition ⟨*2.44*⟩ Not more than 0.1% (1 g).

Assay Conduct this procedure using light-resistant vessels. Weigh accurately about 50 mg each of Cilnidipine and Cilnidipine RS, both previously dried, dissolve in 20 mL of acetonitrile, and add the mobile phase to make exactly 100 mL, respectively. Pipet 5 mL each of these solutions, add exactly 5 mL of the internal standard solution, add the mobile phase to make 25 mL, and use these solutions as the sample solution and the standard solution, respectively. Perform the test with 10 μL each of the sample solution and standard solution as directed under Liquid Chromatography ⟨*2.01*⟩ according to the following conditions, and calculate the ratios, Q_T and Q_S, of the peak area of cilnidipine to that of the internal standard.

Amount (mg) of cilnidipine ($C_{27}H_{28}N_2O_7$) $= M_S \times Q_T/Q_S$

M_S: Amount (mg) of Cilnidipine RS taken

Internal standard solution—A solution of butyl parahydroxybenzoate in acetonitrile (1 in 1000).

Operating conditions—

Detector: An ultraviolet absorption photometer (wavelength: 240 nm).

Column: A stainless steel column 4.6 mm in inside diameter and 25 cm in length, packed with perfluorohexylpropylsilanized silica gel for liquid chromatography (5 μm in particle diameter).

Column temperature: A constant temperature of about 25°C.

Mobile phase: Dissolve 1.36 g of sodium acetate trihydrate in water to make 1000 mL, and adjust to pH 5.5 with diluted acetic acid (100) (1 in 100). To 400 mL of this solution add 600 mL of methanol.

Flow rate: Adjust so that the retention time of cilnidipine is about 20 minutes.

System suitability—

System performance: After exposing Cilnidipine to a fluorescent light (15,000 lx·h), take 10 mg, dissolve in 4 mL of acetonitrile, and add the mobile phase to make 20 mL. When the procedure is run with 10 μL of this solution under the above operating conditions, the resolution between the peak of cilnidipine and the peak having the relative retention time of about 1.07 to cilnidipine is not less than 1.5.

System repeatability: When the test is repeated 6 times with 10 μL of the standard solution under the above operating conditions, the relative standard deviation of the ratio of the peak area of cilnidipine to that of the internal standard is not more than 1.0%.

Containers and storage Containers—Tight containers.
Storage—Light-resistant.

Cilnidipine Tablets

シルニジピン錠

Cilnidipine Tablets contain not less than 95.0% and not more than 105.0% of the labeled amount of cilnidipine ($C_{27}H_{28}N_2O_7$: 492.52).

Method of preparation Prepare as directed under Tablets, with Cilnidipine.

Identification Powder Cilnidipine Tablets. To a portion of the powder, equivalent to 20 mg of Cilnidipine, add 20 mL of methanol, shake well, and centrifuge. To 1 mL of the supernatant liquid add methanol to make 100 mL. Determine the absorption spectrum of this solution as directed under Ultraviolet-visible Spectrophotometry <2.24>: it exhibits maxima between 238 nm and 242 nm and between 350 nm and 360 nm.

Purity Related substances—Conduct this procedure using light-resistant vessels. Powder Cilnidipine Tablets. To a portion of the powder, equivalent to 25 mg of Cilnidipine, add 40 mL of the mobile phase, shake well, and add the mobile phase to make 50 mL. Centrifuge, and use the supernatant liquid as the sample solution. Pipet 3 mL of the sample solution, add the mobile phase to make exactly 200 mL, and use this solution as the standard solution. Perform the test with exactly 20 μL each of the sample solution and standard solution as directed under Liquid Chromatography <2.01> according to the following conditions, and determine each peak area by the automatic integration method: the area of the peak, having the relative retention time of about 1.09 to cilnidipine, obtained from the sample solution is not larger than 1/3 times the peak area of cilnidipine from the standard solution, the area of the peaks other than cilnidipine and the peak mentioned above from the sample solution is not larger than 2/15 times the peak area of cilnidipine from the standard solution, and the total area of the peaks other than cilnidipine from the sample solution is not larger than the peak area of cilnidipine from the standard solution. For the area of the peak, having the relative retention time of about 1.09 to cilnidipine, multiply the correction factor, 1.4.

Operating conditions—

Detector, column, column temperature, mobile phase, and flow rate: Proceed as directed in the operating conditions in the Assay.

Time span of measurement: About 2 times as long as the retention time of cilnidipine, beginning after the solvent peak.

System suitability—

Test for required detectability: Pipet 5 mL of the standard solution, add the mobile phase to make exactly 150 mL. Confirm that the peak area of cilnidipine obtained with 20 μL of this solution is equivalent to 2.4 to 4.3% of that with 20 μL of the standard solution.

System performance: When the procedure is run with 20 μL of standard solution under the above operating conditions, the number of theoretical plates and the symmetry factor of the peak of cilnidipine are not less than 15,000 and not more than 1.5, respectively.

System repeatability: When the test is repeated 6 times with 20 μL of the standard solution under the above operating conditions, the relative standard deviation of the peak area of cilnidipine is not more than 2.0%.

Uniformity of dosage units <6.02> Perform the test according to the following method: it meets the requirement of the Content uniformity test.

Conduct this procedure using light-resistant vessels. To 1 tablet of Cilnidipine Tablets add V/10 mL of water, and shake to completely disintegrate the tablet. Add acetonitrile to make exactly V mL so that each mL contains about 0.2 mg of cilnidipine ($C_{27}H_{28}N_2O_7$), and centrifuge. Pipet 4 mL of the supernatant liquid, add a mixture of acetonitrile and water (9:1) to make exactly 20 mL, filter, if necessary, and use this solution as the sample solution. Separately, weigh accurately about 20 mg of Cilnidipine RS, previously dried in vacuum at 60°C for 3 hours, dissolve in a mixture of acetonitrile and water (9:1) to make exactly 50 mL. Pipet 5 mL of this solution, add a mixture of acetonitrile and water (9:1) to make exactly 50 mL, and use this solution as the standard solution. Determine the absorbances, A_T and A_S, at 355 nm of the sample solution and standard solution as directed under Ultraviolet-visible Spectrophotometry <2.24> using a mixture of acetonitrile and water (9:1) as the control.

$$\text{Amount (mg) of cilnidipine } (C_{27}H_{28}N_2O_7) = M_S \times A_T/A_S \times V/100$$

M_S: Amount (mg) of Cilnidipine RS taken

Dissolution <6.10> When the test is performed at 75 revolutions per minute according to the Paddle method, using 900 mL of a solution of polysorbate 80 (dissolving 1 g of polysorbate 80 in 1000 mL of 2nd fluid for dissolution test) as the dissolution medium, the dissolution rate in 90 minutes of Cilnidipine Tablets is not less than 70%.

Start the test with 1 tablet of Cilnidipine Tablets, withdraw not less than 20 mL of the medium at the specified minute after starting the test, and filter through a membrane filter with a pore size not exceeding 0.45 μm. Discard not less than 10 mL of the first filtrate, pipet V mL of the subsequent filtrate, add the dissolution medium to make exactly V' mL so that each mL contains about 5.6 μg of cilnidipine ($C_{27}H_{28}N_2O_7$), and use this solution as the sample solution. Separately, weigh accurately about 28 mg of Cilnidipine RS, previously dried in vacuum at 60°C for 3 hours, dissolve in acetonitrile to make exactly 100 mL. Pipet 2 mL of this solution, add the dissolution medium to make exactly 100 mL, and use this solution as the standard solution. Perform the test with exactly 20 μL each of the sample solution and standard solution as directed under Liquid Chromatography <*2.01*> according to the following conditions, and determine the peak areas, A_T and A_S, of cilnidipine in each solution.

Dissolution rate (%) with respect to the labeled amount of cilnidipine ($C_{27}H_{28}N_2O_7$)
$= M_S \times A_T/A_S \times V'/V \times 1/C \times 18$

M_S: Amount (mg) of Cilnidipine RS taken
C: Labeled amount (mg) of cilnidipine ($C_{27}H_{28}N_2O_7$) in 1 tablet

Operating conditions—

Detector: An ultraviolet absorption photometer (wavelength: 240 nm).

Column: A stainless steel column 4.6 mm in inside diameter and 15 cm in length, packed with octadecylsilanized silica gel for liquid chromatography (5 μm in particle diameter).

Column temperature: A constant temperature of about 40°C.

Mobile phase: Dissolve 3.58 g of disodium hydrogen phosphate dodecahydrate in 1000 mL of water, and adjust to pH 6.0 with phosphoric acid. To 400 mL of this solution add 600 mL of acetonitrile.

Flow rate: Adjust so that the retention time of cilnidipine is about 8 minutes.

System suitability—

System performance: When the procedure is run with 20 μL of the standard solution under the above operating conditions, the number of theoretical plates and the symmetry factor of the peak of cilnidipine are not less than 2000 and not more than 2.0, respectively.

System repeatability: When the test is repeated 6 times with 20 μL of the standard solution under the above operating conditions, the relative standard deviation of the peak area of cilnidipine is not more than 2.0%.

Assay Conduct this procedure using light-resistant vessels. Weigh accurately the mass of not less than 20 Cilnidipine Tablets, and powder. Weigh accurately a portion of the powder, equivalent to about 25 mg of cilnidipine ($C_{27}H_{28}N_2O_7$), add 40 mL of the mobile phase, shake well, and add the mobile phase to make exactly 50 mL. Centrifuge this solution, pipet 5 mL of the supernatant liquid, add exactly 2.5 mL of the internal standard solution, add the mobile phase to make 25 mL, and use this solution as the sample solution. Separately, weigh accurately about 25 mg of Cilnidipine RS, previously dried in vacuum at 60°C for 3 hours, dissolve in the mobile phase to make exactly 50 mL. Pipet 5 mL of this solution, add exactly 2.5 mL of the internal standard solution, add the mobile phase to make 25 mL, and use this solution as the standard solution. Perform the test with 10 μL each of the sample solution and standard solution as directed under Liquid Chromatography <*2.01*> according to the following conditions, and calculate the ratios, Q_T and Q_S, of the peak area of cilnidipine to that of the internal standard.

Amount (mg) of cilnidipine ($C_{27}H_{28}N_2O_7$) $= M_S \times Q_T/Q_S$

M_S: Amount (mg) of Cilnidipine RS taken

*Internal standard solution—*A solution of 4,4'-difluorobenzophenone in the mobile phase (1 in 500).

Operating conditions—

Detector: An ultraviolet absorption photometer (wavelength: 240 nm).

Column: A stainless steel column 6 mm in inside diameter and 30 cm in length, packed with octadecylsilanized silica gel for liquid chromatography (5 μm in particle diameter).

Column temperature: A constant temperature of about 40°C.

Mobile phase: Dissolve 3.58 g of disodium hydrogen phosphate dodecahydrate in 1000 mL of water, and adjust to pH 6.0 with phosphoric acid. To 400 mL of this solution add 600 mL of acetonitrile.

Flow rate: Adjust so that the retention time of cilnidipine is about 23 minutes.

System suitability—

System performance: When the procedure is run with 10 μL of the standard solution under the above operating conditions, the internal standard and cilnidipine are eluted in this order with the resolution between these peaks being not less than 15.

System repeatability: When the test is repeated 6 times with 10 μL of the standard solution under the above operating conditions, the relative standard deviation of the ratio of the peak area of cilnidipine to that of the internal standard is not more than 1.0%.

Containers and storage Containers—Tight containers. Storage—Light-resistant.

Cilostazol

シロスタゾール

$C_{20}H_{27}N_5O_2$: 369.46
6-[4-(1-Cyclohexyl-1*H*-tetrazol-5-yl)butyloxy]-3,4-dihydroquinolin-2(1*H*)-one
[73963-72-1]

Cilostazol, when dried, contains not less than 98.5% and not more than 101.5% of cilostazol ($C_{20}H_{27}N_5O_2$).

Description Cilostazol occurs as white to pale yellowwhite, crystals or crystalline powder.

It is slightly soluble in methanol, in ethanol (99.5) and in acetonitrile, and practically insoluble in water.

Identification **(1)** Determine the absorption spectrum of a solution of Cilostazol in methanol (1 in 100,000) as directed under Ultraviolet-visible Spectrophotometry <*2.24*>, and compare the spectrum with the Reference Spectrum or the spectrum of a solution of Cilostazol RS prepared in the same manner as the sample solution: both spectra exhibit similar intensities of absorption at the same wavelengths.

(2) Determine the infrared absorption spectrum of Cilostazol as directed in the potassium bromide disk method under Infrared Spectrophotometry <*2.25*>, and compare the spectrum with the Reference Spectrum or the spectrum of Cilostazol RS: both spectra exhibit similar intensities of absorption at the same wave numbers.

Melting point <*2.60*> 158 - 162°C

Purity (1) Heavy metals <*1.07*>—Proceed with 2.0 g of Cilostazol according to Method 2, and perform the test. Prepare the control solution with 2.0 mL of Standard Lead Solution (not more than 10 ppm).

(2) Related substances—Dissolve 25 mg of Cilostazol in 25 mL of acetonitrile, and use this solution as the sample solution. Pipet 1 mL of the sample solution, and add acetonitrile to make exactly 100 mL. Pipet 10 mL of this solution, add acetonitrile to make exactly 50 mL, and use this solution as the standard solution. Perform the test with exactly 10 μL each of the sample solution and standard solution as directed under Liquid Chromatography <*2.01*> according to the following conditions, and determine each peak area by the automatic integration method: the area of the peak other than cilostazol obtained from the sample solution is not larger than 7/10 times the peak area of cilostazol from the standard solution, and the total area of the peaks other than the peak of cilostazol from the sample solution is not larger than 1.2 times the peak area of cilostazol from the standard solution.

Operating conditions—

Detector: An ultraviolet absorption photometer (wavelength: 254 nm).

Column: A stainless steel column 4.6 mm in inside diameter and 15 cm in length, packed with silica gel for liquid chromatography (5 μm in particle diameter).

Column temperature: A constant temperature of about 25°C.

Mobile phase: A mixture of hexane, ethyl acetate and methanol (10:9:1).

Flow rate: Adjust so that the retention time of cilostazol is about 7 minutes.

Time span of measurement: About 3 times as long as the retention time of cilostazol, beginning after the solvent peak.

System suitability—

Test for required detectability: Pipet 1 mL of the standard solution, and add acetonitrile to make exactly 10 mL. Confirm that the peak area of cilostazol obtained with 10 μL of this solution is equivalent to 7 to 13% of that with 10 μL of the standard solution.

System performance: To 1 mL of the sample solution, add 1 mL of a solution prepared by dissolving 5 mg of 3,4-dihydro-6-hydroxy-2(1*H*)-quinolinone in 10 mL of acetonitrile and acetonitrile to make 100 mL. When the procedure is run with 10 μL of this solution under the above operating conditions, 3,4-dihydro-6-hydroxy-2(1*H*)-quinolinone and cilostazol are eluted in this order with the resolution between these peaks being not less than 9.

System repeatability: When the test is repeated 6 times with 10 μL of the standard solution under the above operating conditions, the relative standard deviation of the peak area of cilostazol is not more than 2.0%.

Loss on drying <*2.41*> Not more than 0.1% (1 g, 105°C, 2 hours).

Residue on ignition <*2.44*> Not more than 0.1% (1 g).

Assay Weigh accurately about 50 mg each of Cilostazol and Cilostazol RS, previously dried, dissolve each in a suitable amount of methanol, add exactly 5 mL of the internal standard solution and methanol to make 50 mL. To 1 mL each of these solutions add methanol to make 10 mL, and use these solutions as the sample solution and the standard solution, respectively. Perform the test with 10 μL each of the sample solution and standard solution as directed under Liquid Chromatography <*2.01*> according to the following conditions, and calculate the ratios, Q_T and Q_S, of the peak area of cilostazol to that of the internal standard.

Amount (mg) of cilostazol ($C_{20}H_{27}N_5O_2$) = $M_S \times Q_T/Q_S$

M_S: Amount (mg) of Cilostazol RS taken

Internal standard solution—A solution of benzophenone in methanol (1 in 250).

Operating conditions—

Detector: An ultraviolet absorption photometer (wavelength: 254 nm).

Column: A stainless steel column 4.6 mm in inside diameter and 15 cm in length, packed with octadecylsilanized silica gel for liquid chromatography (5 μm in particle diameter).

Column temperature: A constant temperature of about 25°C.

Mobile phase: A mixture of water, acetonitrile and methanol (10:7:3).

Flow rate: Adjust so that the retention time of cilostazol is about 9 minutes.

System suitability—

System performance: When the procedure is run with 10 μL of the standard solution under the above operating conditions, cilostazol and the internal standard are eluted in this order with the resolution between these peaks being not less than 9.

System repeatability: When the test is repeated 5 times with 10 μL of the standard solution under the above operating conditions, the relative standard deviation of the ratio of the peak area of cilostazol to that of the internal standard is not more than 1.0%.

Containers and storage Containers—Well-closed containers.

Cilostazol Tablets

シロスタゾール錠

Cilostazol Tablets contain not less than 95.0% and not more than 105.0% of the labeled amount of cilostazol ($C_{20}H_{27}N_5O_2$: 369.46).

Method of preparation Prepare as directed under Tablets, with Cilostazol.

Identification Mix well an amount of powdered Cilostazol Tablets, equivalent to 50 mg of Cilostazol, with 10 mL of acetone, centrifuge, and use the supernatant liquid as the sample solution. Separately, dissolve 25 mg of Cilostazol RS in 5 mL of acetone, and use this solution as the standard solution. Perform the test with these solutions as directed under Thin-layer Chromatography <*2.03*>. Spot 6 μL each of the sample solution and standard solution on a plate of silica gel for thin-layer chromatography, develop the plate with a mixture of ethyl acetate, acetonitrile, methanol and formic acid (75:25:5:1) to a distance of about 12 cm, and air-dry the plate. Spray evenly Dragendorff's TS for spraying on the plate: the principal spot obtained from the sample solution and the spot from the standard solution are orange in color and have the same *Rf* value.

Uniformity of dosage units <*6.02*> Perform the Mass variation test, or the Content uniformity test according to the following method: it meets the requirement.

To 1 tablet of Cilostazol Tablets add 2 mL of water to disintegrate the tablet, add the internal standard solution exactly 5 mL for a 50-mg tablet and exactly 10 mL for a 100-mg tablet, and add methanol to make 50 mL. Shake for

10 minutes for the 50-mg tablet and for 20 minutes for the 100-mg tablet. To 1 mL of the solution add methanol to make 10 mL for the 50-mg tablet and 20 mL for the 100-mg tablet, filter through a membrane filter with a pore size not exceeding 0.5 μm, and use the filtrate as the sample solution. Proceed as directed in the Assay.

Amount (mg) of cilostazol ($C_{20}H_{27}N_5O_2$)
$= M_S \times Q_T/Q_S \times C/50$

M_S: Amount (mg) of Cilostazol RS taken
C: Labeled amount (mg) of cilostazol ($C_{20}H_{27}N_5O_2$) in 1 tablet

Internal standard solution—A solution of benzophenone in methanol (1 in 250).

Dissolution 〈*6.10*〉 When the test is performed at 50 revolutions per minute according to the Paddle method, using 900 mL of a solution of sodium lauryl sulfate (3 in 1000) as the dissolution medium, the dissolution rates of a 50-mg tablet in 45 minutes and a 100-mg tablet in 60 minutes are not less than 75% and not less than 70%, respectively.

Start the test with 1 tablet of Cilostazol Tablets, withdraw not less than 20 mL of the medium at the specified minute after starting the test, and filter through a membrane filter with a pore size not exceeding 0.45 μm. Discard not less than 10 mL of the first filtrate, pipet V mL of the subsequent filtrate, add the dissolution medium to make exactly V' mL so that each mL contains about 5.6 μg of cilostazol ($C_{20}H_{27}N_5O_2$), and use this solution as the sample solution. Separately, weigh accurately about 28 mg of Cilostazol RS, previously dried at 105°C for 2 hours, and dissolve in methanol to make exactly 100 mL. Pipet 4 mL of this solution, add the dissolution medium to make exactly 200 mL, and use this solution as the standard solution. Determine the absorbances, A_T and A_S, of the sample solution and standard solution at 257 nm as directed under Ultraviolet-visible Spectrophotometry 〈*2.24*〉 using the dissolution medium as the control.

Dissolution rate (%) with respect to the labeled amount of cilostazol ($C_{20}H_{27}N_5O_2$)
$= M_S \times A_T/A_S \times V'/V \times 1/C \times 18$

M_S: Amount (mg) of Cilostazol RS taken
C: Labeled amount (mg) of cilostazol ($C_{20}H_{27}N_5O_2$) in 1 tablet

Assay Weigh accurately the mass of not less than 20 Cilostazol Tablets, and powder. Weigh accurately a portion of the powder, equivalent to about 50 mg of cilostazol ($C_{20}H_{27}N_5O_2$), add exactly 5 mL of the internal standard solution and methanol to make 50 mL, and shake well for 10 minutes. To 1 mL of this solution add methanol to make 10 mL, filter through a membrane filter with a pore size not exceeding 0.5 μm, and use the filtrate as the sample solution. Separately, weigh accurately about 50 mg of Cilostazol RS, previously dried at 105°C for 2 hours, dissolve in a suitable amount of methanol, and add exactly 5 mL of the internal standard solution, and add methanol to make 50 mL. To 1 mL of this solution add methanol to make 10 mL, and use this solution as the standard solution. Perform the test with 10 μL each of the sample solution and standard solution as directed under Liquid Chromatography 〈*2.01*〉 according to the following conditions, and calculate the ratios, Q_T and Q_S, of the peak area of cilostazol to that of the internal standard.

Amount (mg) of cilostazol ($C_{20}H_{27}N_5O_2$) $= M_S \times Q_T/Q_S$

M_S: Amount (mg) of Cilostazol RS taken

Internal standard solution—A solution of benzophenone in methanol (1 in 250).

Operating conditions—

Proceed as directed in the operating conditions in the Assay under Cilostazol.

System suitability—

System performance: Proceed as directed in the system suitability in the Assay under Cilostazol.

System repeatability: When the test is repeated 6 times with 10 μL of the standard solution under the above operating conditions, the relative standard deviation of the ratio of the peak area of cilostazol to that of the internal standard is not more than 1.5%.

Containers and storage Containers—Well-closed containers.

Cimetidine

シメチジン

$C_{10}H_{16}N_6S$: 252.34
2-Cyano-1-methyl-3-{2-[(5-methyl-1*H*-imidazol-4-yl)methylsulfanyl]ethyl}guanidine
[*51481-61-9*]

Cimetidine, when dried, contains not less than 99.0% of cimetidine ($C_{10}H_{16}N_6S$).

Description Cimetidine occurs as a white crystalline powder. It is odorless, and has a bitter taste.

It is freely soluble in methanol and in acetic acid (100), sparingly soluble in ethanol (95), slightly soluble in water, and practically insoluble in diethyl ether.

It dissolves in dilute hydrochloric acid.

It is gradually colored by light.

Identification **(1)** To 0.1 mL of a solution of Cimetidine in ethanol (95) (1 in 100) add 5 mL of citric acid-acetic anhydride TS, and heat in a water bath for 15 minutes: a red-purple color develops.

(2) Determine the infrared absorption spectrum of Cimetidine, previously dried, as directed in the potassium bromide disk method under the Infrared Spectrophotometry 〈*2.25*〉, and compare the spectrum with the Reference Spectrum: both spectra exhibit similar intensities of absorption at the same wave numbers.

pH 〈*2.54*〉 Dissolve 0.5 g of Cimetidine in 50 mL of freshly boiled and cooled water, shake for 5 minutes and filter: the pH of the filtrate is between 9.0 and 10.5.

Melting point 〈*2.60*〉 140 – 144°C

Purity **(1)** Clarity and color of solution—Dissolve 1.0 g of Cimetidine in 10 mL of methanol: the solution is clear and colorless to pale yellow in color.

(2) Heavy metals 〈*1.07*〉—Proceed with 2.0 g of Cimetidine according to Method 2, and perform the test. Prepare the control solution with 2.0 mL of Standard Lead Solution (not more than 10 ppm).

(3) Arsenic 〈*1.11*〉—Dissolve 1.0 g of Cimetidine in 5 mL of dilute hydrochloric acid, and perform the test with this so-

lution (not more than 2 ppm).

(4) Related substances—Dissolve 0.5 g of Cimetidine in 10 mL of methanol, and use this solution as the sample solution. Pipet 1 mL of the sample solution, add methanol to make exactly 100 mL. Pipet 1 mL of this solution, add methanol to make exactly 10 mL, and use this solution as the standard solution. Perform the test with these solutions as directed under Thin-layer Chromatography 〈*2.03*〉. Spot 4 μL each of the sample solution and standard solution on a plate of silica gel for thin-layer chromatography. Develop the plate with a mixture of ethyl acetate, methanol and ammonia solution (28) (21:2:2) to a distance of about 15 cm, air-dry the plate, and then dry at 80°C for 30 minutes. Allow the plate to stand in iodine vapor for 45 minutes: the spots other than the principal spot obtained from the sample solution are not more intense than the spot from the standard solution.

Loss on drying 〈*2.41*〉 Not more than 0.5% (1 g, 105°C, 3 hours).

Residue on ignition 〈*2.44*〉 Not more than 0.2% (1 g).

Assay Weigh accurately about 0.24 g of Cimetidine, previously dried, dissolve in 75 mL of acetic acid (100), and titrate 〈*2.50*〉 with 0.1 mol/L perchloric acid VS (potentiometric titration). Perform a blank determination in the same manner, and make any necessary correction.

Each mL of 0.1 mol/L perchloric acid VS
= 25.23 mg of $C_{10}H_{16}N_6S$

Containers and storage Containers—Well-closed containers.

Storage—Light-resistant.

Cinoxacin

シノキサシン

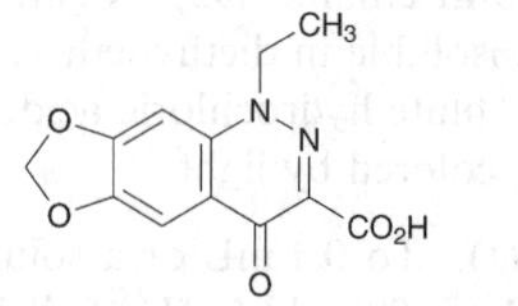

$C_{12}H_{10}N_2O_5$: 262.22
5-Ethyl-8-oxo-5,8-dihydro[1,3]dioxolo[4,5-*g*]cinnoline-7-carboxylic acid
[*28657-80-9*]

Cinoxacin, when dried, contains not less than 98.0% and not more than 101.0% of cinoxacin ($C_{12}H_{10}N_2O_5$).

Description Cinoxacin occurs as a white to pale yellow crystalline powder. It is odorless or has a slight, characteristic odor. It has a bitter taste.

It is slightly soluble in *N,N*-dimethylformamide and in acetone, very slightly soluble in ethanol (99.5), and practically insoluble in water.

It dissolves in sodium hydroxide TS.

Melting point: about 265°C (with decomposition).

Identification (1) Dissolve 30 mg of Cinoxacin in 10 mL of dilute sodium hydroxide TS, and add water to make 100 mL. To 1 mL of this solution add 0.1 mol/L hydrochloric acid TS to make 50 mL. Determine the absorption spectrum of this solution as directed under Ultraviolet-visible Spectrophotometry 〈*2.24*〉, and compare the spectrum with the Reference Spectrum: both spectra exhibit similar intensities of absorption at the same wavelengths.

(2) Determine the infrared absorption spectrum of Cinoxacin as directed in the potassium bromide disk method under Infrared Spectrophotometry 〈*2.25*〉, and compare the spectrum with the Reference Spectrum: both spectra exhibit similar intensities of absorption at the same wave numbers.

Purity (1) Sulfate 〈*1.14*〉—Dissolve 0.20 g of Cinoxacin in 10 mL of dilute sodium hydroxide TS, add 20 mL of 0.1 mol/L hydrochloric acid TS, shake, filter, and add water to the filtrate to make 50 mL. Perform the test using this solution as the test solution. Prepare the control solution with 0.20 mL of 0.005 mol/L sulfuric acid VS by adding 10 mL of dilute sodium hydroxide TS, 20 mL of 0.1 mol/L hydrochloric acid TS, and water to make 50 mL (not more than 0.048%).

(2) Heavy metals 〈*1.07*〉—Proceed with 1.0 g of Cinoxacin according to Method 2, and perform the test. Prepare the control solution with 2.0 mL of Standard Lead Solution (not more than 20 ppm).

(3) Related substances—Dissolve 10 mg of Cinoxacin in 10 mL of acetone, and use this solution as the sample solution. Pipet 1 mL of the sample solution, add acetone to make exactly 200 mL, and use this solution as the standard solution. Perform the test with these solutions as directed under Thin-layer Chromatography 〈*2.03*〉. Spot 10 μL each of the sample solution and standard solution on a plate of silica gel with fluorescent indicator for thin-layer chromatography. Develop the plate with a mixture of acetonitrile, water and ammonia solution (28) (14:4:1) to a distance of about 10 cm, and air-dry the plate. Examine under ultraviolet light (main wavelength: 254 nm): the spots other than the principal spot obtained from the sample solution are not more intense than the spot from the standard solution.

Loss on drying 〈*2.41*〉 Not more than 0.5% (1 g, 105°C, 1 hour).

Residue on ignition 〈*2.44*〉 Not more than 0.2% (1 g).

Assay Weigh accurately about 0.4 g of Cinoxacin, previously dried, add 60 mL of a mixture of acetic anhydride and acetic acid (100) (7:3), and dissolve by warming. After cooling, titrate 〈*2.50*〉 with 0.1 mol/L perchloric acid VS (potentiometric titration). Perform a blank determination in the same manner, and make any necessary correction.

Each mL of 0.1 mol/L perchloric acid VS
= 26.22 mg of $C_{12}H_{10}N_2O_5$

Containers and storage Containers—Tight containers.

Cinoxacin Capsules

シノキサシンカプセル

Cinoxacin Capsules contain not less than 95.0% and not more than 105.0% of the labeled amount of cinoxacin ($C_{12}H_{10}N_2O_5$: 262.22).

Method of preparation Prepare as directed under Capsules, with Cinoxacin.

Identification To a quantity of the contents of Cinoxacin Capsules, equivalent to 10 mg of Cinoxacin, add 20 mL of acetone, shake well, and centrifuge. To 3 mL of the supernatant liquid add acetone to make 10 mL, and use this solution as the sample solution. Separately, dissolve 10 mg of cinoxacin for assay in 20 mL of acetone. To 3 mL of this solution add acetone to make 10 mL, and use this solution as the standard solution. Perform the test with these solutions as directed under Thin-layer Chromatography <*2.03*>. Spot 10 μL each of the sample solution and standard solution on a plate of silica gel with fluorescent indicator for thin-layer chromatography. Develop the plate with a mixture of acetonitrile, water and ammonia solution (28) (14:4:1) to a distance of about 10 cm, and air-dry the plate. Examine under ultraviolet light (main wavelength: 254 nm): the principal spot obtained from the sample solution and the spot from the standard solution show a blue-purple color and the same *Rf* value.

Uniformity of dosage units <*6.02*> Perform the test according to the following method: it meets the requirement of the Content uniformity test.

To 1 capsule of Cinoxacin Capsules add 40 mL of dilute sodium hydroxide TS, and dissolve the capsule in lukewarm water with occasional shaking. After cooling, add water and shake well, add water to make exactly *V* mL so that each mL contains about 1 mg of cinoxacin ($C_{12}H_{10}N_2O_5$), and filter. Discard the first 20 mL of the filtrate, pipet 1 mL of the subsequent filtrate, add 0.1 mol/L hydrochloric acid TS to make exactly 100 mL, and use this solution as the sample solution. Separately, weigh accurately about 0.2 g of cinoxacin for assay, previously dried at 105°C for 1 hour, dissolve in 40 mL of dilute sodium hydroxide TS, and add water to make exactly 200 mL. Pipet 1 mL of this solution, add 0.1 mol/L of hydrochloric acid TS to make exactly 100 mL, and use this solution as the standard solution. Perform the test with the sample solution and standard solution as directed under Ultraviolet-visible Spectrophotometry <*2.24*>, and determine the absorbances, A_T and A_S, at 354 nm.

$$\text{Amount (mg) of cinoxacin } (C_{12}H_{10}N_2O_5) = M_S \times A_T/A_S \times V/200$$

M_S: Amount (mg) of cinoxacin for assay taken

Dissolution <*6.10*> When the test is performed at 50 revolutions per minute according to the Paddle method using the sinker, using 900 mL of 2nd solution for dissolution test as the dissolution medium, the dissolution rate in 90 minutes of Cinoxacin Capsules is not less than 70%.

Start the test with 1 capsule of Cinoxacin Capsules, withdraw not less than 20 mL of the medium at the specified minute after starting the test, and filter through a membrane filter with a pore size not exceeding 0.45 μm. Discard not less than 10 mL of the first filtrate, pipet *V* mL of the subsequent filtrate, add the dissolution medium to make exactly *V′* mL so that each mL contains about 11 μg of cinoxacin ($C_{12}H_{10}N_2O_5$), and use this solution as the sample solution. Separately, weigh accurately about 22 mg of cinoxacin for assay, previously dried at 105°C for 1 hour, and dissolve in the dissolution medium to make exactly 100 mL. Pipet 5 mL of this solution, add the dissolution medium to make exactly 100 mL, and use this solution as the standard solution. Perform the test with the sample solution and standard solution as directed under Ultraviolet-visible Spectrophotometry <*2.24*>, and determine the absorbances, A_T and A_S, at 351 nm.

$$\text{Dissolution rate (\%) with respect to the labeled amount of cinoxacin } (C_{12}H_{10}N_2O_5) = M_S \times A_T/A_S \times V'/V \times 1/C \times 45$$

M_S: Amount (mg) of cinoxacin for assay taken
C: Labeled amount (mg) of cinoxacin ($C_{12}H_{10}N_2O_5$) in 1 capsule

Assay Weigh accurately the mass of not less than 20 Cinoxacin Capsules, take out the contents, and powder. Wash the capsule shells with a small amount of diethyl ether, allow to stand at room temperature to vaporize the diethyl ether, weigh accurately the mass of the capsule shells, and calculate the mass of the contents. Weigh accurately a portion of the powder, equivalent to about 50 mg of cinoxacin ($C_{12}H_{10}N_2O_5$), add 10 mL of dilute sodium hydroxide TS, shake, add water to make exactly 100 mL, and filter. Discard the first 20 mL of the filtrate, pipet 1 mL of the subsequent filtrate, add 0.1 mol/L hydrochloric acid TS to make exactly 50 mL, and use this solution as the sample solution. Separately, weigh accurately about 50 mg of cinoxacin for assay, previously dried at 105°C for 1 hour, dissolve in 10 mL of dilute sodium hydroxide TS, and add water to make exactly 100 mL. Pipet 1 mL of this solution, add 0.1 mol/L hydrochloric acid TS to make exactly 50 mL, and use this solution as the standard solution. Perform the test with the sample solution and standard solution as directed under Ultraviolet-visible Spectrophotometry <*2.24*>, and determine the absorbances, A_T and A_S, at 354 nm.

$$\text{Amount (mg) of cinoxacin } (C_{12}H_{10}N_2O_5) = M_S \times A_T/A_S$$

M_S: Amount (mg) of cinoxacin for assay taken

Containers and storage Containers—Well-closed containers.

Ciprofloxacin

シプロフロキサシン

$C_{17}H_{18}FN_3O_3$: 331.34
1-Cyclopropyl-6-fluoro-4-oxo-7-(piperazin-1-yl)-1,4-dihydroquinoline-3-carboxylic acid
[85721-33-1]

Ciprofloxacin, when dried, contains not less than 98.5% and not more than 101.0% of ciprofloxacin ($C_{17}H_{18}FN_3O_3$).

Description Ciprofloxacin occurs as a white to light yellow-white, crystalline powder.

It is practically insoluble in water and in ethanol (99.5).

It dissolves in ammonia TS.

It is gradually colored to yellow tint by light.

Melting point: about 270°C (with decomposition).

Identification **(1)** Determine the infrared absorption spectrum of Ciprofloxacin, as directed in the potassium bromide disk method under Infrared Spectrophotometry <*2.25*>, and compare the spectrum with the Reference Spectrum or the spectrum of the Ciprofloxacin RS: both spectra exhibit similar intensities of absorption at the same wave numbers.

(2) Conduct this procedure using light-resistant vessels. Dissolve 50 mg each of Ciprofloxacin and Ciprofloxacin RS in 5 mL of ammonia TS, and use these solutions as the sample solution and the standard solution, respectively. Perform the test with these solutions as directed under Thin-layer Chromatography <*2.03*>. Spot 5 μL each of the sample solution and the standard solution on a plate of silica gel with fluorescent indicator for thin-layer chromatography. After allowing to stand this plate in the vapor of ammonia for 15 minutes, develop the plate with a mixture of methanol, dichloromethane, ammonia solution (28) and acetonitrile (4:4:2:1) to a distance of about 10 cm, and air-dry the plate. Examine under ultraviolet light (main wavelength: 254 nm): the principal spot obtained from the sample solution and the spot from the standard solution show the same *Rf* value.

Purity **(1)** Chloride <*1.03*>—To 1.5 g of Ciprofloxacin add 75 mL of water, and boil for 5 minutes. After cooling, add water to make 75 mL, and filter. To 25 mL of the filtrate add 6 mL of dilute nitric acid and water to make 50 mL. Perform the test using this solution as the test solution. Prepare the control solution as follows: to 0.30 mL of 0.01 mol/L hydrochloric acid VS add 6 mL of dilute sulfuric acid and water to make 50 mL (not more than 0.021%).

(2) Heavy metals <*1.07*>—Proceed with 2.0 g of Ciprofloxacin according to Method 4, and perform the test. Prepare the control solution with 2.0 mL of Standard Lead Solution (not more than 10 ppm).

(3) Fluoroquinolonic acid—Conduct this procedure using light-resistant vessels. Dissolve 50 mg of Ciprofloxacin in ammonia TS to make exactly 5 mL, and use this solution as the sample solution. Separately, dissolve 10 mg of fluoroquinolonic acid for thin-layer chromatography in 0.1 mL of ammonia TS and water to make exactly 100 mL. Pipet 2 mL of this solution, add water to make exactly 10 mL, and use this solution as the standard solution. Perform the test with these solutions as directed under Thin-layer Chromatography <*2.03*>. Spot 5 μL each of the sample solution and the standard solution on a plate of silica gel with fluorescent indicator for thin-layer chromatography. After allowing to stand this plate in the vapor of ammonia for 15 minutes, develop the plate with a mixture of methanol, dichloromethane, ammonia solution (28) and acetonitrile (4:4:2:1) to a distance of about 10 cm, and air-dry the plate. Examine under ultraviolet light (main wavelength: 254 nm): the spot obtained from the sample solution, corresponding to the spot obtained from the standard solution, is not more intense than that obtained from the standard solution.

(4) Related substances—Conduct this procedure using light-resistant vessels. To 25 mg of Ciprofloxacin add 2 mL of a mixture of water and phosphoric acid (13:1), then add the mobile phase to make 50 mL, and use this solution as the sample solution. Pipet 2 mL of the sample solution, add the mobile phase to make exactly 20 mL. Pipet 1 mL of this solution, add the mobile phase to make exactly 50 mL, and use this solution as the standard solution. Perform the test with exactly 50 μL each of the sample solution and standard solution as directed under Liquid Chromatography <*2.01*> according to the following conditions. Determine each peak area by the automatic integration method: the area of the peak other than ciprofloxacin obtained from the sample solution is not larger than the peak area of ciprofloxacin from the standard solution, and the total area of the peaks other than ciprofloxacin from the sample solution is not larger than 2.5 times the peak area of ciprofloxacin from the standard solution. For the area of peak, having the relative retention time of about 0.4, about 0.5, and about 1.2 to ciprofloxacin, multiply the correction factor, 6.7, 1.3, and 1.4, respectively.

Operating conditions—

Detector, column, column temperature, mobile phase, and flow rate: Proceed as directed in the operating conditions in the Assay.

Time span of measurement: About 2.3 times as long as the retention time of ciprofloxacin, beginning after the solvent peak.

System suitability—

Test for required detectability: Pipet 5 mL of the standard solution, and add the mobile phase to make exactly 20 mL. Confirm that the peak area of ciprofloxacin obtained with 50 μL of this solution is equivalent to 20 to 30% of that with 50 μL of the standard solution.

System performance: When the procedure is run with 50 μL of the standard solution under the above operating conditions, the number of theoretical plates and the symmetry factor of the peak of ciprofloxacin are not less than 3500 and not more than 1.5, respectively.

System repeatability: When the test is repeated 6 times with 50 μL of the standard solution under the above operating conditions, the relative standard deviation of the peak area of ciprofloxacin is not more than 2.0%.

Loss on drying <*2.41*> Not more than 1.0% (2 g, in vacuum, 120°C, 6 hours).

Residue on ignition <*2.44*> Not more than 0.1% (2 g).

Assay Conduct this procedure using light-resistant vessels. Weigh accurately about 25 mg each of Ciprofloxacin and Ciprofloxacin RS, both dried previously, add 2 mL of a mixture of water and phosphoric acid (13:1), add the mobile phase to make exactly 50 mL, and use these solutions as the sample solution and the standard solution, respectively. Perform the test with exactly 10 μL each of the sample solution and standard solution as directed under Liquid Chromatography <*2.01*> according to the following conditions, and determine the peak areas, A_T and A_S, of ciprofloxacin in each solution.

$$\text{Amount (mg) of ciprofloxacin } (C_{17}H_{18}FN_3O_3) = M_S \times A_T/A_S$$

M_S: Amount (mg) of Ciprofloxacin RS taken

Operating conditions—

Detector: An ultraviolet absorption photometer (wavelength: 278 nm).

Column: A stainless steel column 4 mm in inside diameter and 25 cm in length, packed with octadecylsilanized silica gel for liquid chromatography (5 μm in particle diameter).

Column temperature: A constant temperature of about 40°C.

Mobile phase: To 2.88 g of phosphoric acid add water to make 1000 mL, and adjust to pH 3.0 with triethylamine. To 870 mL of this solution add 130 mL of acetonitrile.

Flow rate: Adjust so that the retention time of ciprofloxacin is about 7 minutes.

System suitability—

System performance: When the procedure is run with 10 μL of the standard solution under the above operating conditions, the number of theoretical plates and the symmetry factor of the peak of ciprofloxacin are not less than 3500 and not more than 2.0, respectively.

System repeatability: When the test is repeated 6 times with 10 μL of the standard solution under the above operating conditions, the relative standard deviation of the peak area of ciprofloxacin is not more than 1.0%.

Containers and storage Containers—Tight containers. Storage—Light-resistant.

Ciprofloxacin Hydrochloride Hydrate

シプロフロキサシン塩酸塩水和物

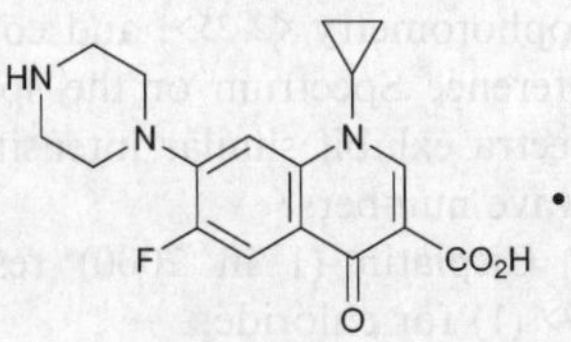

$C_{17}H_{18}FN_3O_3.HCl.xH_2O$
1-Cyclopropyl-6-fluoro-4-oxo-7-(piperazin-1-yl)-1,4-dihydroquinoline-3-carboxylic acid monohydrochloride hydrate
[*86393-32-0*, monohydrochloride monohydrate]

Ciprofloxacin Hydrochloride Hydrate contains not less than 98.0% and not more than 102.0% of ciprofloxacin hydrochloride ($C_{17}H_{18}FN_3O_3.HCl$: 367.80), calculated on the anhydrous basis.

Description Ciprofloxacin Hydrochloride Hydrate occurs as a white to pale yellow crystalline powder.

It is sparingly soluble in water, slightly soluble in methanol, and very slightly soluble in ethanol (99.5).

It is gradually colored to a slightly brownish light yellow by light.

Identification **(1)** Determine the infrared absorption spectrum of Ciprofloxacin Hydrochloride Hydrate, as directed in the potassium chloride disk method under Infrared Spectrophotometry ⟨*2.25*⟩, and compare the spectrum with the Reference Spectrum: both spectra exhibit similar intensities of absorption at the same wave numbers.

(2) Conduct this procedure using light-resistant vessels. Dissolve 50 mg of Ciprofloxacin Hydrochloride Hydrate in 5 mL of water, and use this solution as the sample solution. Separately, dissolve 45 mg of Ciprofloxacin RS in 5 mL of ammonia TS, and use this solution as the standard solution. Perform the test with these solutions, as directed under Thin-layer Chromatography ⟨*2.03*⟩. Spot 5 μL each of the sample solution and standard solution on a plate of silica gel with fluorescent indicator for thin-layer chromatography. After allowing to stand the plate in the vapor of ammonia for 15 minutes, develop the plate with a mixture of methanol, dichloromethane, ammonia solution (28) and acetonitrile (4:4:2:1) to a distance of about 10 cm, and air-dry the plate. Examine under ultraviolet light (main wavelength: 254 nm): the principal spot obtained from the sample solution and the spot obtained from the standard solution show the same *R*f value.

(3) A solution of Ciprofloxacin Hydrochloride Hydrate (1 in 500) responds to Qualitative Tests ⟨*1.09*⟩ for chloride.

Purity **(1)** Sulfate ⟨*1.14*⟩—Perform the test with 0.5 g of Ciprofloxacin Hydrochloride Hydrate. Prepare the control solution with 0.50 mL of 0.005 mol/L sulfuric acid VS (not more than 0.048%).

(2) Heavy metals ⟨*1.07*⟩—Proceed with 1.0 g of Ciprofloxacin Hydrochloride Hydrate according to Method 2, and perform the test. Prepare the control solution with 1.0 ml of Standard Lead Solution (not more than 10 ppm).

(3) Fluoroquinolonic acid—Conduct this procedure using light-resistant vessels. Dissolve 50 mg of Ciprofloxacin Hydrochloride Hydrate in water to make exactly 5 mL, and use this solution as the sample solution. Separately, dissolve 10 mg of fluoroquinolonic acid for thin-layer chromatography in 0.1 mL of ammonia TS and water to make exactly 100 mL. Pipet 2 mL of this solution, add water to make exactly 10 mL, and use this solution as the standard solution. Perform the test with these solutions as directed under Thin-layer Chromatography ⟨*2.03*⟩. Spot 5 μL each of the sample solution and standard solution on a plate of silica gel with fluorescent indicator for thin-layer chromatography. After allowing to stand the plate in the vapor of ammonia for 15 minutes, develop the plate with a mixture of methanol, dichloromethane, ammonia solution (28) and acetonitrile (4:4:2:1) to a distance of about 10 cm, and air-dry the plate. Examine under ultraviolet light (main wavelength: 254 nm): the spot obtained from the sample solution, corresponding to the spot from the standard solution, is not more intense than that from the standard solution.

(4) Related substances—Conduct this procedure using light-resistant vessels. Dissolve 25 mg of Ciprofloxacin Hydrochloride Hydrate in 50 mL of mobile phase, and use this solution as the sample solution. Pipet 2 mL of the sample solution, add the mobile phase to make exactly 20 mL. Pipet 1 mL of this solution, add the mobile phase to make exactly 50 mL, and use this solution as the standard solution. Perform the test with exactly 50 μL each of the sample solution and standard solution as directed under Liquid Chromatography ⟨*2.01*⟩ according to the following conditions. Determine each peak area by the automatic integration method: the area of the peaks other than ciprofloxacin obtained from the sample solution is not larger than the peak area of ciprofloxacin from the standard solution, and the total area of the peaks other than ciprofloxacin from the sample solution is not larger than 2.5 times the peak area of ciprofloxacin from the standard solution. For the area of the peaks, having the relative retention times of about 0.4, about 0.5, and about 1.2 to ciprofloxacin, multiply the correction factors, 6.7, 1.3, and 1.4, respectively.

Operating conditions—

Detector, column, column temperature, mobile phase, and flow rate: Proceed as directed in the operating conditions in the Assay.

Time span of measurement: About 2 times as long as the retention time of ciprofloxacin, beginning after the solvent peak.

System suitability—

Test for required detectability: Pipet 5 mL of the standard solution, and add the mobile phase to make exactly 20 mL. Confirm that the peak area of ciprofloxacin obtained with 50 μL of this solution is equivalent to 20 to 30% of that with 50 μL of the standard solution.

System performance: When the procedure is run with 50 μL of the standard solution under the above operating conditions, the number of theoretical plates and the symmetry factor of the peak of ciprofloxacin are not less than 3500 and not more than 1.5, respectively.

System repeatability: When the test is repeated 6 times with 50 μL of the standard solution under the above operating conditions, the relative standard deviation of the peak area of ciprofloxacin is not more than 2.0%.

Water ⟨*2.48*⟩ 4.7 - 6.7% (0.2 g, volumetric titration, direct titration).

Residue on ignition ⟨*2.44*⟩ Not more than 0.1% (1 g).

Assay Conduct this procedure using light-resistant vessels. Weigh accurately about 25 mg of Ciprofloxacin Hydrochloride Hydrate, dissolve in the mobile phase to make exactly 50 mL, and use this solution as the sample solution. Separately, weigh accurately about 22.5 mg of Ciprofloxacin RS, previously dried at 120°C in vacuum for 6 hours, add 2 mL of a mixture of water and phosphoric acid (13:1), then add the mobile phase to make exactly 50 mL, and use this solution as the standard solution. Perform the test with exactly 10 μL each of the sample solution and standard solution as directed under Liquid Chromatography <*2.01*> according to the following operating conditions, and determine the peak areas, A_T and A_S, of ciprofloxacin in each solution.

Amount (mg) of ciprofloxacin hydrochloride ($C_{17}H_{18}FN_3O_3.HCl$) = $M_S \times A_T/A_S \times 1.110$

M_S: Amount (mg) of Ciprofloxacin RS taken

Operating conditions—

Detector: An ultraviolet absorption photometer (wavelength: 278 nm).

Column: A stainless steel column 4 mm in inside diameter and 25 cm in length, packed with octadecylsilanized silica gel for liquid chromatography (5 μm in particle diameter).

Column temperature: A constant temperature of about 40°C.

Mobile phase: To 2.88 g of phosphoric acid add water to make 1000 mL, and adjust to pH 3.0 with triethylamine. To 870 mL of this solution add 130 mL of acetonitrile for liquid chromatography.

Flow rate: Adjust so that the retention time of ciprofloxacin is about 7 minutes.

System suitability—

System performance: When the procedure is run with 10 μL of the standard solution under the above operating conditions, the number of theoretical plates and the symmetry factor of the peak of ciprofloxacin are not less than 3500 and not more than 2.0, respectively.

System repeatability: When the test is repeated 6 times with 10 μL of the standard solution under the above operating conditions, the relative standard deviation of the peak area of ciprofloxacin is not more than 1.0%.

Containers and storage Containers—Tight containers. Storage—Light-resistant.

Cisplatin

シスプラチン

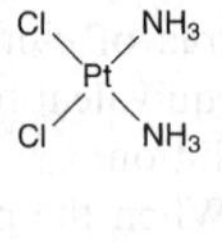

$Cl_2H_6N_2Pt$: 300.05
(*SP*-4-2)-Diamminedichloroplatinum
[*15663-27-1*]

Cisplatin, when dried, contains not less than 98.0% and not more than 102.0% of cisplatin ($Cl_2H_6N_2Pt$).

Description Cisplatin occurs as a yellow crystalline powder.

It is sparingly soluble in *N,N*-dimethylformamide, slightly soluble in water, and practically insoluble in ethanol (99.5).

Identification **(1)** To 5 mL of a solution of Cisplatin (1 in 2000) add 2 to 3 drops of a solution of tin (II) chloride dihydrate (1 in 100): a brown precipitate is formed.

(2) Determine the absorption spectrum of a solution of Cisplatin in a solution of sodium chloride in 0.01 mol/L hydrochloric acid TS (9 in 1000) (1 in 2000) as directed under Ultraviolet-visible Spectrophotometry <*2.24*>, and compare the spectrum with the Reference Spectrum or the spectrum of a solution of Cisplatin RS prepared in the same manner as the sample solution: both spectra exhibit similar intensities of absorption at the same wavelengths.

(3) Determine the infrared absorption spectrum of Cisplatin as directed in the potassium bromide disk method under Infrared Spectrophotometry <*2.25*>, and compare the spectrum with the Reference Spectrum or the spectrum of Cisplatin RS: both spectra exhibit similar intensities of absorption at the same wave numbers.

(4) A solution of Cisplatin (1 in 2000) responds to Qualitative Tests <*1.09*> (1) for chloride.

Purity Ammonium amminetrichloroplatinate—Conduct this procedure using light-resistant vessels. Dissolve 50 mg of Cisplatin in a solution of sodium chloride (9 in 1000) to make exactly 100 mL, and use this solution as the sample solution. Separately, dissolve 10 mg of ammonium amminetrichloroplatinate for liquid chromatography, previously dried at 80°C for 3 hours, in the solution of sodium chloride (9 in 1000) to make exactly 200 mL. Pipet 2 mL of this solution, add the solution of sodium chloride (9 in 1000) to make exactly 20 mL, and use this solution as the standard solution. Perform the test with exactly 40 μL each of the sample solution and standard solution as directed under Liquid Chromatography <*2.01*> according to the following conditions, and determine the peak area of ammonium amminetrichloroplatinate by the automatic integration method: the peak area obtained from the sample solution is not larger than that from the standard solution.

Operating conditions—

Detector: An ultraviolet absorption photometer (wavelength: 209 nm).

Column: A stainless steel column 4.6 mm in inside diameter and 25 cm in length, packed with silica gel for liquid chromatography having quaternary ammonium groups (10 μm in particle diameter).

Column temperature: A constant temperature of about 25°C.

Mobile phase: A solution of ammonium sulfate (1 in 800).

Flow rate: Adjust so that the retention time of ammonium amminetrichloroplatinate is about 8 minutes.

System suitability—

System performance: When the procedure is run with 40 μL of the standard solution under the above operating conditions, the number of theoretical plates and the symmetry factor of the peak of ammonium amminetrichloroplatinate are not less than 1500 and not more than 2.0, respectively.

System repeatability: When the test is repeated 6 times with 40 μL of the standard solution under the above operating conditions, the relative standard deviation of the peak area of ammonium amminetrichloroplatinate is not more than 3.0%.

Loss on drying <*2.41*> Not more than 0.1% (1 g, 105°C, 4 hours).

Assay Conduct this procedure using light-resistant vessels. Weigh accurately about 25 mg each of Cisplatin and Cisplatin RS, previously dried, dissolve in *N,N*-dimethylformamide to make exactly 25 mL, and use these solutions as the sample solution and standard solution. Perform the test with exactly 40 μL each of the sample solution and standard solution as directed under Liquid Chromatography <*2.01*> according to the following conditions, and determine the peak areas, A_T and A_S, of cisplatin in each solution.

Amount (mg) of cisplatin ($Cl_2H_6N_2Pt$) = $M_S \times A_T/A_S$

M_S: Amount (mg) of Cisplatin RS taken

Operating conditions—

Detector: An ultraviolet absorption photometer (wavelength: 310 nm).

Column: A stainless steel column 4.6 mm in inside diameter and 25 cm in length, packed with aminopropylsilanized silica gel for liquid chromatography (5 μm in particle diameter).

Column temperature: A constant temperature of about 25°C.

Mobile phase: A mixture of ethyl acetate, methanol, water and *N,N*-dimethylformamide (25:16:5:5).

Flow rate: Adjust so that the retention time of cisplatin is about 4 minutes.

System suitability—

System performance: When the procedure is run with 40 μL of the standard solution under the above operating conditions, the number of theoretical plates and the symmetry factor of the peak of cisplatin are not less than 3000 and not more than 2.0, respectively.

System repeatability: When the test is repeated 6 times with 40 μL of the standard solution under the above operating conditions, the relative standard deviation of the peak area of cisplatin is not more than 1.0%.

Containers and storage Containers—Tight containers.

Citicoline

シチコリン

$C_{14}H_{26}N_4O_{11}P_2$: 488.32

P'-[2-(Trimethylammonio)ethyl] cytidine 5'-(monohydrogen diphosphate)

[987-78-0]

Citicoline contains not less than 98.0% and not more than 102.0% of citicoline ($C_{14}H_{26}N_4O_{11}P_2$), calculated on the dried basis.

Description Citicoline occurs as a white crystalline powder.

It is very soluble in water, and practically insoluble in ethanol (99.5).

It dissolves in 0.01 mol/L hydrochloric acid TS.

Identification **(1)** Determine the absorption spectrum of a solution of Citicoline in 0.01 mol/L hydrochloric acid TS (3 in 200,000) as directed under Ultraviolet-visible Spectrophotometry <*2.24*>, and compare the spectrum with the Reference Spectrum or the spectrum of a solution of Citicoline RS prepared in the same manner as the sample solution: both spectra exhibit similar intensities of absorption at the same wavelengths.

(2) Determine the infrared absorption spectrum of Citicoline as directed in the potassium bromide disk method under Infrared Spectrophotometry <*2.25*>, and compare the spectrum with the Reference Spectrum or the spectrum of Citicoline RS: both spectra exhibit similar intensities of absorption at the same wave numbers.

pH <*2.54*> The pH of a solution obtained by dissolving 1.0 g of Citicoline in 100 mL of water is between 2.5 and 3.5.

Purity **(1)** Clarity and color of solution—Dissolve 1.0 g of Citicoline in 8 mL of water: the solution is clear and colorless.

(2) Heavy metals <*1.07*>—Proceed with 2.0 g of Citicoline according to Method 1, and perform the test. Prepare the control solution with 2.0 mL of Standard Lead Solution (not more than 10 ppm).

(3) Arsenic <*1.11*>—Prepare the test solution with 1.0 g of Citicoline according to Method 4, and perform the test (not more than 2 ppm).

(4) Free phosphoric acid—Weigh accurately about 0.1 g of Citicoline, dissolve in water to make exactly 10 mL, and use this solution as the sample solution. Separately, pipet 4 mL of Standard Phosphoric Acid Solution, add water to make exactly 10 mL, and use this solution as the standard solution. To each of the sample solution and the standard solution, add exactly 1 mL of hexaammonium heptamolybdate-sulfuric acid TS and exactly 0.5 mL of 1-amino-2-naphthol-4-sulfonic acid TS, and after shaking, allow to stand for 30 minutes at 20 ± 1°C. To exactly 2 mL each of these solutions add water to make exactly 10 mL, and determine the absorbances, A_T and A_S, of the solutions obtained from the sample solution and the standard solution at 730 nm as directed under Ultraviolet-visible Spectrometry <*2.24*>, using the solution, obtained by proceeding with 10 mL of water in the same manner as the sample solution, as the blank. The amount of free phosphoric acid is not more than 0.1%.

$$\text{Amount (\%) of free phosphoric acid } (H_3PO_4) = 1/M \times A_T/A_S \times 10.32$$

M: Amount (mg) of Citicoline taken, calculated on the dried basis

(5) Related substances—Dissolve 0.10 g of Citicoline in water to make 100 mL, and use this solution as the sample solution. Pipet 1 mL of the sample solution, add water to make exactly 200 mL, and use this solution as the standard solution. Perform the test with exactly 10 μL each of the sample solution and standard solution as directed under Liquid Chromatography <*2.01*> according to the following conditions, and determine each peak area by the automatic integration method: the area of the peaks other than citicoline obtained from the sample solution is not larger than 3/5 times the peak area of citicolins from the standard solution, and the total area of the peaks other than citicoline from the sample solution is not larger than the peak area of citicoline from the standard solution. For the area of the peaks, having the relative retention times of about 0.62, about 0.64 and about 1.3 to citicoline, multiply the correction factors, 1.2, 0.7 and 0.5, respectively.

Operating conditions—

Detector, column, column temperature, mobile phase, and flow rate: Proceed as directed in the operating conditions in the Assay.

Time span of measurement: About 2 times as long as the retention time of citicoline.

System suitability—

Test for required detectability: Pipet 4 mL of the standard solution, and add water to make exactly 50 mL. Confirm that the peak area of citicoline obtained with 10 μL of this solution is equivalent to 5.6 to 10.4% of that with 10 μL of the standard solution.

System performance: When the procedure is run with 10 μL of the standard solution under the above operating conditions, the number of theoretical plates and the symmetry factor of the peak of citicoline are not less than 2000 and 0.9 to 1.6, respectively.

System repeatability: When the test is repeated 6 times with 10 μL of the standard solution under the above operating conditions, the relative standard deviation of the peak area of citicoline is not more than 2.0%.

Loss on drying *<2.41>* Not more than 5.0% (1 g, in vacuum, phosphorus (V) oxide, 100°C, 4 hours).

Assay Weigh accurately about 0.1 g of Citicoline, and dissolve in water to make exactly 100 mL. Pipet 1 mL of this solution, add water to make exactly 100 mL, and use this solution as the sample solution. Separately, weigh accurately about 25 mg of Citicoline RS (separately determine the loss on drying *<2.41>* under the same conditions as Citicoline), and dissolve in water to make exactly 25 mL. Pipet 1 mL of this solution, add water to make exactly 100 mL, and use this solution as the standard solution. Perform the test with exactly 10 μL each of the sample solution and standard solution as directed under Liquid Chromatography *<2.01>* according to the following conditions, and determine the peak areas, A_T and A_S, of citicoline in each solution.

$$\text{Amount (mg) of citicoline } (C_{14}H_{26}N_4O_{11}P_2) = M_S \times A_T/A_S \times 4$$

M_S: Amount (mg) of Citicoline RS taken, calculated on the dried basis

Operating conditions—

Detector: An ultraviolet absorption photometer (wavelength: 254 nm).

Column: Combine 2 stainless steel columns (4 mm in inside diameter and 25 cm in length) packed with strongly basic ion exchange resin for liquid chromatography (10 μm in particle diameter) in series.

Column temperature: A constant temperature of about 30°C.

Mobile phase: Dissolve 8.17 g of potassium dihydrogen phosphate in water to make 1000 mL. Adjust the pH of this solution to 3.5 with phosphoric acid.

Flow rate: Adjust so that the retention time of citicoline is about 26 minutes.

System suitability—

System performance: When the procedure is run with 10 μL of the standard solution under the above operating conditions, the number of theoretical plates and the symmetry factor of the peak of citicoline are not less than 2000 and 0.9 to 1.6, respectively.

System repeatability: When the test is repeated 6 times with 10 μL of the standard solution under the above operating conditions, the relative standard deviation of the peak area of citicoline is not more than 1.0%.

Containers and storage Containers—Tight containers.

Anhydrous Citric Acid

無水クエン酸

HO CO₂H / HO₂C CO₂H

$C_6H_8O_7$: 192.12

2-Hydroxypropane-1,2,3-tricarboxylic acid

[77-92-9]

This monograph is harmonized with the European Pharmacopoeia and the U.S. Pharmacopeia.

The parts of the text that are not harmonized are marked with symbol (◆ ◆).

Information on the harmonization with the European Pharmacopoeia and the U.S. Pharmacopeia is available on the website of the Pharmaceuticals and Medical Devices Agency.

Anhydrous Citric Acid contains not less than 99.5% and not more than 100.5% of anhydrous citric acid ($C_6H_8O_7$), calculated on the anhydrous basis.

◆**Description** Anhydrous Citric Acid occurs as colorless crystals, white granules or crystalline powder.

It is very soluble in water, and freely soluble in ethanol (99.5).◆

Identification Determine the infrared absorption spectrum of Anhydrous Citric Acid, previously dried at 105°C for 2 hours, as directed in the potassium bromide disk method under Infrared Spectrophotometry *<2.25>*, and compare the spectrum with the Reference Spectrum: both spectra exhibit similar intensities of absorption at the same wave numbers.

Purity **(1)** Clarity and color of solution—Dissolve 2.0 g of Anhydrous Citric Acid in water to make 10 mL: the solution is clear and colorless or has no more color than the following control solutions (1), (2) or (3).

Control solution (1): To 1.5 mL of Cobalt (II) Chloride CS and 6.0 mL of Iron (III) Chloride CS add diluted dilute hydrochloric acid (1 in 10) to make 1000 mL.

Control solution (2): To 2.5 mL of Cobalt (II) Chloride CS, 6.0 mL of Iron (III) Chloride CS and 1.0 mL of Copper (II) Sulfate CS add diluted dilute hydrochloric acid (1 in 10) to make 1000 mL.

Control solution (3): To 0.15 mL of Cobalt (II) Chloride CS, 7.2 mL of Iron (III) Chloride CS and 0.15 mL of Copper (II) Sulfate CS add diluted dilute hydrochloric acid (1 in 10) to make 1000 mL.

(2) Sulfates—Dissolve 2.0 g of Anhydrous Citric Acid in water to make 30 mL, and use this solution as the sample solution. Separately, dissolve 0.181 g of potassium sulfate in diluted ethanol (3 in 10) to make exactly 500 mL. Pipet 5 mL of this solution, and add diluted ethanol (3 in 10) to make exactly 100 mL. To 4.5 mL of this solution add 3 mL of a solution of barium chloride dihydrate (1 in 4), shake, and allow to stand for 1 minute. To 2.5 mL of this solution add 15 mL of the sample solution and 0.5 mL of acetic acid (31), and allow to stand for 5 minutes: the solution has no more turbidity than the following control solution (not more than 150 ppm).

Control solution: Dissolve 0.181 g of potassium sulfate in water to make exactly 500 mL. Pipet 5 mL of this solution, add water to make exactly 100 mL, and proceed in the same manner as above using this solution instead of the sample solution.

(3) Oxalic acid—Dissolve 0.80 g of Anhydrous Citric Acid in 4 mL of water, add 3 mL of hydrochloric acid and 1 g of zinc, and boil for 1 minute. After allowing to stand for 2 minutes, take the supernatant liquid, add 0.25 mL of a solution of phenylhydrazinium chloride (1 in 100), heat to boil, and then cool quickly. To this solution add the equal volume of hydrochloric acid and 0.25 mL of a solution of potassium hexacyanoferrate (III) (1 in 20), mix, and allow to stand for 30 minutes: the solution has no more color than the following control solution prepared at the same time (not more than 360 ppm expressed as oxalic anhydride).

Control solution: To 4 mL of a solution of oxalic acid dihydrate (1 in 10,000) add 3 mL of hydrochloric acid and 1 g of zinc, and proceed in the same manner as the test solution.

◆**(4)** Heavy metals *<1.07>*—Proceed with 2.0 g of Anhydrous Citric Acid according to Method 2, and perform the test. Prepare the control solution with 2.0 mL of Standard Lead Solution (not more than 10 ppm).◆

(5) Readily carbonizable substances—Place 1.0 g of Anhydrous Citric Acid in a Nessler tube, add 10 mL of sulfuric acid, immediately heat in a 90 ± 1°C water bath for 60 minutes, and cool quickly. Compare the color of 2.0 mL each of this solution and Matching Fluid K, using test tubes 12 mm in outside diameter, from a side against white background: the solution is not more colored than the matching fluid.

Water *<2.48>* Not more than 1.0% (2 g, volumetric titration, direct titration).

Residue on ignition *<2.44>* Not more than 0.1% (1 g).

Assay Weigh accurately about 0.55 g of Anhydrous Citric Acid, dissolve in 50 mL of water, and titrate with 1 mol/L sodium hydroxide VS (indicator: 1 drop of phenolphthalein TS).

Each mL of 1 mol/L sodium hydroxide VS
= 64.04 mg of $C_6H_8O_7$

◆**Containers and storage** Containers—Tight containers.◆

Citric Acid Hydrate

クエン酸水和物

HO CO2H
HO2C CO2H • H2O

$C_6H_8O_7.H_2O$: 210.14
2-Hydroxypropane-1,2,3-tricarboxylic acid monohydrate
[*5949-29-1*]

This monograph is harmonized with the European Pharmacopoeia and the U.S. Pharmacopeia.

The parts of the text that are not harmonized are marked with symbol (◆ ◆).

Information on the harmonization with the European Pharmacopoeia and the U.S. Pharmacopeia is available on the website of the Pharmaceuticals and Medical Devices Agency.

Citric Acid Hydrate contains not less than 99.5% and not more than 100.5% of anhydrous citric acid ($C_6H_8O_7$: 192.12), calculated on the anhydrous basis.

◆**Description** Citric Acid Hydrate occurs as colorless crystals, white granules or crystalline powder.

It is very soluble in water, and freely soluble in ethanol (99.5).

It is efflorescent in dry air.◆

Identification Determine the infrared absorption spectrum of Citric Acid Hydrate, previously dried at 105°C for 2 hours, as directed in the potassium bromide disk method under Infrared Spectrophotometry *<2.25>*, and compare the spectrum with the Reference Spectrum: both spectra exhibit similar intensities of absorption at the same wave numbers.

Purity **(1)** Clarity and color of solution—Dissolve 2.0 g of Citric Acid Hydrate in water to make 10 mL: the solution is clear and colorless or has no more color than the following control solutions (1), (2) or (3).

Control solution (1): To 1.5 mL of Cobalt (II) Chloride CS and 6.0 mL of Iron (III) Chloride CS add diluted dilute hydrochloric acid (1 in 10) to make 1000 mL.

Control solution (2): To 2.5 mL of Cobalt (II) Chloride CS, 6.0 mL of Iron (III) Chloride CS and 1.0 mL of Copper (II) Sulfate CS add diluted dilute hydrochloric acid (1 in 10) to make 1000 mL.

Control solution (3): To 0.15 mL of Cobalt (II) Chloride CS, 7.2 mL of Iron (III) Chloride CS and 0.15 mL of Copper (II) Sulfate CS add diluted dilute hydrochloric acid (1 in 10) to make 1000 mL.

(2) Sulfates—Dissolve 2.0 g of Citric Acid Hydrate in water to make 30 mL, and use this solution as the sample solution. Separately, dissolve 0.181 g of potassium sulfate in diluted ethanol (3 in 10) to make exactly 500 mL. Pipet 5 mL of this solution, and add diluted ethanol (3 in 10) to make exactly 100 mL. To 4.5 mL of this solution add 3 mL of a solution of barium chloride dihydrate (1 in 4), shake, and allow to stand for 1 minute. To 2.5 mL of this solution add 15 mL of the sample solution and 0.5 mL of acetic acid (31), and allow to stand for 5 minutes: the solution has no more turbidity than the following control solution. (not more than 150 ppm).

Control solution: Dissolve 0.181 g of potassium sulfate in water to make exactly 500 mL. Pipet 5 mL of this solution, add water to make exactly 100 mL, and proceed in the same manner as above using this solution instead of the sample solution.

(3) Oxalic acid—Dissolve 0.80 g of Citric Acid Hydrate in 4 mL of water, add 3 mL of hydrochloric acid and 1 g of zinc, and boil for 1 minute. After allowing to stand for 2 minutes, take the supernatant liquid, add 0.25 mL of a solution of phenylhydrazinium chloride (1 in 100), heat to boil, and then cool quickly. To this solution add the equal volume of hydrochloric acid and 0.25 mL of a solution of potassium hexacyanoferrate (III) (1 in 20), mix, and allow to stand for 30 minutes: the solution has no more color than the following control solution prepared at the same time (not more than 360 ppm expressed as oxalic anhydride).

Control solution: To 4 mL of a solution of oxalic acid dihydrate (1 in 10,000) add 3 mL of hydrochloric acid and 1 g of zinc, and proceed in the same manner as the test solution.

◆**(4)** Heavy metals *<1.07>*—Proceed with 2.0 g of Citric Acid Hydrate according to Method 2, and perform the test. Prepare the control solution with 2.0 mL of Standard Lead Solution (not more than 10 ppm).◆

(5) Readily carbonizable substances—Place 1.0 g of Citric Acid Hydrate in a Nessler tube, add 10 mL of sulfuric acid, immediately heat in a 90 ± 1°C water bath for 60 minutes, and cool quickly. Compare the color of 2.0 mL each of this solution and Matching Fluid K, using test tubes 12 mm in outside diameter, from a side against white background: the solution is not more colored than the matching fluid.

Water ⟨*2.48*⟩ Not less than 7.5% and not more than 9.0% (0.5 g, volumetric titration, direct titration).

Residue on ignition ⟨*2.44*⟩ Not more than 0.1% (1 g).

Assay Weigh accurately about 0.55 g of Citric Acid Hydrate, dissolve in 50 mL of water, and titrate ⟨*2.50*⟩ with 1 mol/L sodium hydroxide VS (indicator: 1 drop of phenolphthalein TS).

Each mL of 1 mol/L sodium hydroxide VS
= 64.04 mg of $C_6H_8O_7$

◆**Containers and storage** Containers—Tight containers.◆

Clarithromycin

クラリスロマイシン

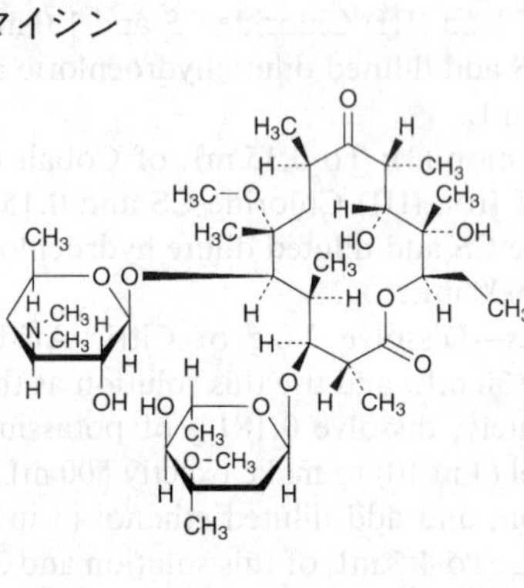

$C_{38}H_{69}NO_{13}$: 747.95
(2*R*,3*S*,4*S*,5*R*,6*R*,8*R*,10*R*,11*R*,12*S*,13*R*)-5-(3,4,6-Trideoxy-3-dimethylamino-*β*-D-*xylo*-hexopyranosyloxy)-3-(2,6-dideoxy-3-*C*-methyl-3-*O*-methyl-*α*-L-*ribo*-hexopyranosyloxy)-11,12-dihydroxy-6-methoxy-2,4,6,8,10,12-hexamethyl-9-oxopentadecan-13-olide
[*81103-11-9*]

Clarithromycin is a derivative of erythromycin.

It contains not less than 950 *μ*g (potency) and not more than 1050 *μ*g (potency) per mg, calculated on the anhydrous basis. The potency of Clarithromycin is expressed as mass (potency) of clarithromycin ($C_{38}H_{69}NO_{13}$).

Description Clarithromycin occurs as a white crystalline powder and has a bitter taste.

It is soluble in acetone and in chloroform, slightly soluble in methanol and in ethanol (95), and practically insoluble in water.

Identification **(1)** To 5 mg of Clarithromycin add 2 mL of sulfuric acid, and shake gently: a red-brown color develops.

(2) Dissolve 3 mg of Clarithromycin in 2 mL of acetone, and add 2 mL of hydrochloric acid: an orange color develops and changes immediately to red to deep purple.

(3) Determine the infrared absorption spectra of Clarithromycin and Clarithromycin RS as directed in the potassium bromide disk method under Infrared Spectrophotometry ⟨*2.25*⟩, and compare these spectra: both spectra exhibit similar intensities of absorption at the same wave numbers.

Optical rotation ⟨*2.49*⟩ $[\alpha]_D^{20}$: −96 – −106° (0.25 g calculated on the anhydrous basis, acetone, 25 mL, 100 mm).

Melting point ⟨*2.60*⟩ 220 – 227°C

Purity **(1)** Heavy metals ⟨*1.07*⟩—Proceed with 2.0 g of Clarithromycin according to Method 4, and perform the test. Prepare the control solution with 2.0 mL of Standard Lead Solution (not more than 10 ppm).

(2) Related substances—Weigh accurately about 0.1 g of Clarithromycin, dissolve in the mobile phase to make exactly 20 mL, and use this solution as the sample solution. Separately, weigh accurately about 10 mg of Clarithromycin RS, dissolve in the mobile phase to make exactly 20 mL, and use this solution as the standard solution. Perform the test with exactly 10 *μ*L each of the sample solution and standard solution as directed under Liquid Chromatography ⟨*2.01*⟩ according to the following conditions, and determine the each peak area by the automatic integration method: the amount of each related substance calculated on the anhydrous basis is not more than 2.0%, and the total amount of them is not more than 5.0%. For these calculations, exclude any peak with an area of less than 0.05%.

Amount (%) of each related substance calculated on the anhydrous basis
$= M_S/M_T \times A_T/A_S \times 100$

Total amount (%) of the related substances calculated on the anhydrous basis
$= M_S/M_T \times \Sigma A_T/A_S \times 100$

M_S: Amount (mg) of Clarithromycin RS taken
M_T: Amount (mg) of Clarithromycin taken, calculated on the anhydrous basis
A_S: Peak area of clarithromycin obtained with the standard solution
A_T: Peak area of each related substance obtained with the sample solution
ΣA_T: Total area of the peaks other than clarithromycin obtained with the sample solution

Operating conditions—

Detector, column, column temperature, mobile phase, and flow rate: Proceed as directed in the operating conditions in the Assay.

Time span of measurement: About 5 times as long as the retention time of the main peak, beginning from 2 minutes after injection of the sample solution.

System suitability—

Test for required detectability: To exactly 2 mL of the standard solution add the mobile phase to make exactly 10 mL, and use this solution as the solution for system suitability test. Pipet 1 mL of the solution for system suitability test, add the mobile phase to make exactly 10 mL. Pipet 2.5 mL of this solution, add the mobile phase to make exactly 10 mL. Confirm that the peak area of clarithromycin obtained with 10 *μ*L of this solution is equivalent to 0.25 – 0.75% of that with 10 *μ*L of the standard solution.

System performance: When the procedure is run with 10 *μ*L of the solution for system suitability test under the above operating conditions, the number of theoretical plates and the symmetry factor of the peak of clarithromycin are not less than 2500 and not more than 2.5, respectively.

System repeatability: When the test is repeated 6 times with 10 *μ*L of the solution for system suitability test under the above operating conditions, the relative standard deviation of the peak area of clarithromycin is not more than 3.0%.

Water ⟨*2.48*⟩ Not more than 2.0% (0.5 g, volumetric titration, direct titration).

Residue on ignition ⟨*2.44*⟩ Not more than 0.1% (2 g).

Assay Weigh accurately an amount of Clarithromycin and Clarithromycin RS, equivalent to about 50 mg (potency), and dissolve each in the mobile phase to make exactly 10 mL. Pipet 2 mL each of these solutions, add exactly 2 mL of the internal standard solution, add the mobile phase to make 20 mL, and use these solutions as the sample solution and the standard solution. Perform the test with 10 μL each of the sample solution and standard solution as directed under Liquid Chromatography <2.01> according to the following conditions, and calculate the ratios, Q_T and Q_S, of the peak area of clarithromycin to that of the internal standard.

Amount [μg (potency)] of clarithromycin ($C_{38}H_{69}NO_{13}$)
$= M_S \times Q_T/Q_S \times 1000$

M_S: Amount [mg (potency)] of Clarithromycin RS taken

Internal standard solution—A solution of butyl parahydroxybenzoate in the mobile phase (1 in 20,000).

Operating conditions—

Detector: An ultraviolet absorption photometer (wavelength: 210 nm).

Column: A stainless steel column 4 mm in inside diameter and 15 cm in length, packed with octadecylsilanized silica gel for liquid chromatography (5 μm in particle diameter).

Column temperature: A constant temperature of about 50°C.

Mobile phase: A mixture of diluted 0.2 mol/L potassium dihydrogen phosphate TS (1 in 3) and acetonitrile (13:7).

Flow rate: Adjust so that the retention time of clarithromycin is about 8 minutes.

System suitability—

System performance: When the procedure is run with 10 μL of the standard solution under the above operating conditions, clarithromycin and the internal standard are eluted in this order with the resolution between these peaks being not less than 3.

System repeatability: When the test is repeated 6 times with 10 μL of the standard solution under the above operating conditions, the relative standard deviation of the ratios of the peak area of clarithromycin to that of the internal standard is not more than 2.0%.

Containers and storage Containers—Well-closed containers.

Clarithromycin for Syrup

シロップ用クラリスロマイシン

Clarithromycin for Syrup is a preparation for syrup, which is suspended before use.

It contains not less than 90.0% and not more than 110.0% of the labeled potency of clarithromycin ($C_{38}H_{69}NO_{13}$: 747.95).

Method of preparation Prepare as directed under Preparations for Syrups, with Clarithromycin.

Identification To an amount of Clarithromycin for Syrup, equivalent to 0.1 g (potency) of Clarithromycin, add 5 mL of acetone, and sonicate. After cooling with ice, centrifuge, take the supernatant liquid, and evaporate the solvent. Dissolve 10 mg of the residue and 2 mg of Clarithromycin RS in separate 2 mL of acetone, and use these solutions as the sample solution and the standard solution, respectively. Perform the test with these solutions as directed under Thin-layer Chromatography <2.03>. Spot 10 μL each of the sample solution and standard solution on a plate of silica gel for thin-layer chromatography. Develop the plate with a mixture of methanol, ethyl acetate and acetic acid (100) (90:10:1) to a distance of about 15 cm, and air-dry the plate. Spray evenly sulfuric acid on the plate, and heat the plate at 105°C for 10 minutes: the principal spot obtained from the sample solution and the spot from the standard solution show a black-purple color and the same *Rf* value.

Water <2.48> Not more than 3.0% (0.5 g, volumetric titration, direct titration).

Uniformity of dosage units <6.02> Perform the test according to the following method: Clarithromycin for Syrup in single-dose packages meet the requirement of the Content uniformity test.

To the total content of 1 package of Clarithromycin for Syrup add 3*V*/5 mL of ethanol (99.5), add exactly *V*/10 mL of the internal standard solution, sonicate with occasional vigorous shaking, and add ethanol (99.5) to make *V* mL so that each mL contains about 0.5 mg (potency) of Clarithromycin. Centrifuge this solution, and filter the supernatant liquid through a membrane filter with a pore size not exceeding 0.45 μm. Discard the first 3 mL of the filtrate, and use the subsequent filtrate as the sample solution. Then, proceed as directed in the Assay.

Amount [mg (potency)] of clarithromycin ($C_{38}H_{69}NO_{13}$)
$= M_S \times Q_T/Q_S \times V/100$

M_S: Amount [mg (potency)] of Clarithromycin RS taken

Internal standard solution—A solution of butyl parahydroxybenzoate in ethanol (99.5) (1 in 12,500).

Dissolution <6.10> When the test is performed at 50 revolutions per minute according to the Paddle method, using 900 mL of disodium hydrogen phosphate-citric acid buffer solution (pH 5.5) as the dissolution medium, the dissolution rate in 90 minutes of Clarithromycin for Syrup is not less than 75%.

Start the test with an accurately weighed amount of Clarithromycin for Syrup, equivalent to about 50 mg (potency) of Clarithromycin, withdraw not less than 20 mL of the medium at the specified minute after starting the test, and filter through a membrane filter with a pore size not exceeding 0.45 μm. Discard not less than 10 mL of the first filtrate, pipet 10 mL of the subsequent filtrate, add the mobile phase to make exactly 20 mL, and use this solution as the sample solution. Separately, weigh accurately an amount of Clarithromycin RS, equivalent to about 28 mg (potency), and dissolve in acetonitrile for liquid chromatography to make exactly 100 mL. Pipet 5 mL of this solution, add the mobile phase to make exactly 50 mL, and use this solution as the standard solution. Perform the test with exactly 100 μL each of the sample solution and standard solution as directed under Liquid Chromatography <2.01> according to the following conditions, and determine the peak areas, A_T and A_S, of clarithromycin in each solution.

Dissolution rate (%) with respect to the labeled amount of clarithromycin ($C_{38}H_{69}NO_{13}$)
$= M_S/M_T \times A_T/A_S \times 1/C \times 180$

M_S: Amount [mg (potency)] of Clarithromycin RS taken
M_T: Amount (g) of Clarithromycin for Syrup taken
C: Labeled amount of [mg (potency)] of clarithromycin ($C_{38}H_{69}NO_{13}$) in 1 g

Operating conditions—

Proceed as directed in the operating conditions in the Assay.

System suitability—

System performance: When the procedure is run with 100 μL of the standard solution under the above operating conditions, the number of theoretical plates and the symmetry factor of the peak of clarithromycin are not less than 3000 and not more than 2.0, respectively.

System repeatability: When the test is repeated 6 times with 100 μL of the standard solution under the above operating conditions, the relative standard deviation of the peak area of clarithromycin is not more than 2.0%.

Assay Weigh accurately an amount of crushed Clarithromycin for Syrup, equivalent to about 50 mg (potency) of Clarithromycin, add 60 mL of ethanol (99.5), add exactly 10 mL of the internal standard solution, sonicate with occasional vigorous shaking, and add ethanol (99.5) to make 100 mL. Centrifuge this solution, and filter the supernatant liquid through a membrane filter with a pore size not exceeding 0.45 μm. Discard the first 3 mL of the filtrate, and use the subsequent filtrate as the sample solution. Separately, weigh accurately an amount of Clarithromycin RS, equivalent about 50 mg (potency), and dissolve in ethanol (99.5) to make exactly 50 mL. Pipet 10 mL of this solution, add exactly 2 mL of the internal standard solution, add ethanol (99.5) to make 20 mL, and use this solution as the standard solution. Perform the test with 10 μL each of the sample solution and standard solution as directed under Liquid Chromatography <2.01> according to the following conditions, and calculate the ratios, Q_T and Q_S, of the peak area of clarithromycin to that of the internal standard.

Amount [mg (potency)] of clarithromycin ($C_{38}H_{69}NO_{13}$)
$= M_S \times Q_T/Q_S$

M_S: Amount [mg (potency)] of Clarithromycin RS taken

*Internal standard solution—*A solution of butyl parahydroxybenzoate in ethanol (99.5) (1 in 12,500).

Operating conditions—

Detector: An ultraviolet absorption photometer (wavelength: 210 nm).

Column: A stainless steel column 4.6 mm in inside diameter and 15 cm in length, packed with octadecylsilanized silica gel for liquid chromatography (5 μm in particle diameter).

Column temperature: A constant temperature of about 50°C.

Mobile phase: A mixture of diluted 0.2 mol/L potassium dihydrogen phosphate TS (1 in 3) and acetonitrile for liquid chromatography (13:7).

Flow rate: Adjust so that the retention time of clarithromycin is about 8 minutes.

System suitability—

System performance: When the procedure is run with 10 μL of the standard solution under the above operating conditions, clarithromycin and the internal standard are eluted in this order with the resolution between these peaks being not less than 3.

System repeatability: When the test is repeated 6 times with 10 μL of the standard solution under the above operating conditions, the relative standard deviation of the ratio of the peak area of clarithromycin to that of the internal standard is not more than 2.0%.

Containers and storage Containers—Tight containers.

Storage—Light-resistant.

Clarithromycin Tablets

クラリスロマイシン錠

Clarithromycin Tablets contain not less than 93.0% and not more than 107.0% of the labeled potency of clarithromycin ($C_{38}H_{69}NO_{13}$: 747.95).

Method of preparation Prepare as directed under Tablets, with Clarithromycin.

Identification Shake a quantity of powdered Clarithromycin Tablets, equivalent to 60 mg (potency) of Clarithromycin, with 40 mL of acetone for 10 minutes, and centrifuge at 4000 rpm for 5 minutes. Evaporate 30 mL of the supernatant liquid, and determine the infrared absorption spectrum of the residue so obtained as directed in the potassium bromide disk method under Infrared Spectrophotometry <2.25>: it exhibits absorption at the wave numbers of about 2980 cm^{-1}, 2940 cm^{-1}, 1734 cm^{-1}, 1693 cm^{-1}, 1459 cm^{-1}, 1379 cm^{-1} and 1171 cm^{-1}.

Uniformity of dosage units <6.02> Perform the Mass variation test, or the Content uniformity test according to the following method: it meets the requirement.

To 1 tablet of Clarithromycin Tablets add exactly $V/20$ mL of the internal standard solution (1), then add the mobile phase so that each mL contains about 5 mg (potency) of clarithromycin ($C_{38}H_{69}NO_{13}$) to make V mL, and disperse to fine particles by sonicating for 20 minutes while occasional vigorous shaking. Centrifuge this solution at 4000 rpm for 15 minutes, and filter the supernatant liquid through a membrane filter with a pore size not exceeding 0.45 μm. Then, proceed as directed in the Assay.

Amount [mg (potency)] of clarithromycin ($C_{38}H_{69}NO_{13}$)
$= M_S \times Q_T/Q_S \times V/10$

M_S: Amount [mg (potency)] of Clarithromycin RS taken

*Internal standard solution (1)—*A solution of butyl parahydroxybenzoate in the mobile phase (1 in 1000).

*Internal standard solution (2)—*To exactly 1 mL of the internal standard solution (1) add the mobile phase to make exactly 20 mL.

Dissolution <6.10> When the test is performed at 50 revolutions per minute according to the Paddle method, using 900 mL of 0.05 mol/L disodium hydrogen phosphate-citric acid buffer solution (pH 6.0) as the dissolution medium, the dissolution rates in 30 minutes of a 50-mg tablet and a 200-mg tablet are not less than 80% and not less than 75%, respectively.

Start the test with 1 tablet of Clarithromycin Tablets, withdraw not less than 20 mL of the medium at the specified minute after starting the test, and filter through a membrane filter with a pore size not exceeding 0.45 μm. Discard not less than 10 mL of the first filtrate, pipet V mL of the subsequent filtrate, add the mobile phase to make exactly V' mL so that each mL contains about 28 μg (potency) of Clarithromycin, and use this solution as the sample solution. Separately, weigh accurately an amount of Clarithromycin RS, equivalent to about 28 mg (potency), and dissolve in acetonitrile for liquid chromatography to make exactly 100 mL. Pipet 5 mL of this solution, add the mobile phase to make exactly 50 mL, and use this solution as the standard solution. Perform the test with exactly 100 μL each of the sample solution and standard solution as directed under Liquid Chromatography <2.01> according to the following conditions, and determine the peak areas, A_T and A_S, of clarithromycin in each solution.

Dissolution rate (%) with respect to the labeled amount of clarithromycin ($C_{38}H_{69}NO_{13}$)
$= M_S \times A_T/A_S \times V'/V \times 1/C \times 90$

M_S: Amount [mg (potency)] of Clarithromycin RS taken
C: Labeled amount [mg (potency)] of clarithromycin ($C_{38}H_{69}NO_{13}$) in 1 tablet

Operating conditions—
Proceed as directed in the operating conditions in the Assay.
System suitability—
System performance: When the procedure is run with 100 μL of the standard solution under the above operating conditions, the number of theoretical plates and the symmetry factor of the peak of clarithromycin are not less than 3000 and not more than 2.0, respectively.
System repeatability: When the test is repeated 6 times with 100 μL of the standard solution under the above operating conditions, the relative standard deviation of the peak area of clarithromycin is not more than 2.0%.

Assay To not less than 5 Clarithromycin Tablets add diluted 0.2 mol/L potassium dihydrogen phosphate TS (1 in 3) so that each mL contains about 8 mg (potency) of clarithromycin ($C_{38}H_{69}NO_{13}$), disperse to fine particles by sonicating, add exactly 1 mL of the internal standard solution (1) per 100 mg (potency) of clarithromycin, then add acetonitrile for liquid chromatography so that each mL contains about 5 mg (potency) of clarithromycin ($C_{38}H_{69}NO_{13}$), and disperse to fine particles by sonicating for 10 minutes while occasional vigorous shaking. Centrifuge of this solution at 4000 rpm for 15 minutes, and filter the supernatant liquid through a membrane filter with a pore size not exceeding 0.45 μm. Discard the first 3 mL of the filtrate, to 2 mL of the subsequent filtrate add the mobile phase to make 20 mL, and use this solution as the sample solution. Separately, weigh accurately an amount of Clarithromycin RS, equivalent to about 50 mg (potency), and dissolve in the mobile phase to make exactly 10 mL. Pipet 2 mL of this solution, add exactly 2 mL of the internal standard solution (2) and the mobile phase to make 20 mL, and use this solution as the standard solution. Perform the test with 10 μL each of the sample solution and standard solution as directed under Liquid Chromatography <*2.01*> according to the following conditions, and calculate the ratios, Q_T and Q_S, of the peak area of clarithromycin to that of the internal standard.

Amount [mg (potency)] of clarithromycin ($C_{38}H_{69}NO_{13}$)
$= M_S \times Q_T/Q_S \times 1/5$

M_S: Amount [mg (potency)] of Clarithromycin RS taken

Internal standard solution (1)—A solution of butyl parahydroxybenzoate in the mobile phase (1 in 1000).
Internal standard solution (2)—To exactly 1 mL of the internal standard solution (1) add the mobile phase to make exactly 20 mL.
Operating conditions—
Detector: An ultraviolet absorption photometer (wavelength: 210 nm).
Column: A stainless steel column 4.6 mm in inside diameter and 15 cm in length, packed with octadecylsilanized silica gel for liquid chromatography (5 μm in particle diameter).
Column temperature: A constant temperature of about 50°C.
Mobile phase: A mixture of diluted 0.2 mol/L potassium dihydrogen phosphate TS (1 in 3) and acetonitrile for liquid chromatography (13:7).
Flow rate: Adjust so that the retention time of clarithromycin is about 8 minutes.
System suitability—
System performance: When the procedure is run with 10 μL of the standard solution under the above operating conditions, clarithromycin and the internal standard are eluted in this order with the resolution between these peaks being not less than 3.
System repeatability: When the test is repeated 6 times with 10 μL of the standard solution under the above operating conditions, the relative standard deviation of the ratio of the peak area of clarithromycin to that of the internal standard is not more than 2.0%.

Containers and storage Containers—Well-closed containers.

Clebopride Malate

クレボプリドリンゴ酸塩

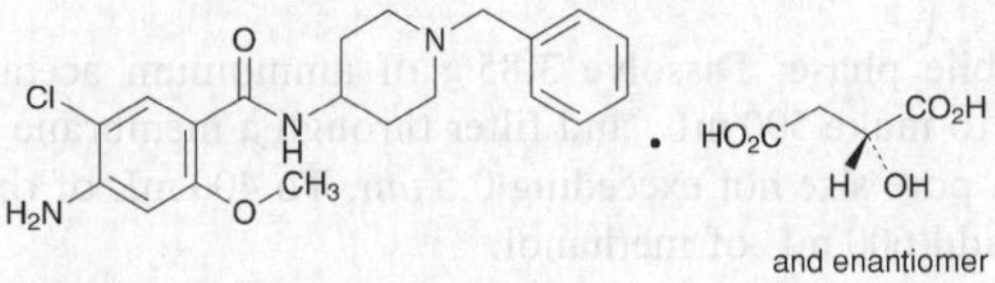

$C_{20}H_{24}ClN_3O_2.C_4H_6O_5$: 507.96
4-Amino-*N*-(1-benzylpiperidin-4-yl)-5-chloro-2-methoxybenzamide mono-(2*RS*)-malate
[*57645-91-7*]

Clebopride Malate, when dried, contains not less than 98.5% and not more than 101.0% of clebopride malate ($C_{20}H_{24}ClN_3O_2.C_4H_6O_5$).

Description Clebopride Malate occurs as a white crystalline powder.
It is freely soluble in acetic acid (100), soluble in methanol, sparingly soluble in water, and slightly soluble in ethanol (99.5).
A solution of Clebopride Malate in methanol (1 in 25) shows no optical rotation.

Identification **(1)** Determine the absorption spectrum of a solution of Clebopride Malate in methanol (1 in 80000) as directed under Ultraviolet-visible Spectrophotometry <*2.24*>, and compare the spectrum with the Reference Spectrum: both spectra exhibit similar intensities of absorption at the same wavelengths.
(2) Determine the infrared absorption spectrum of Clebopride Malate, previously dried, as directed in the potassium bromide disk method under Infrared Spectrophotometry <*2.25*>, and compare the spectrum with the Reference Spectrum: both spectra exhibit similar intensities of absorption at the same wave numbers.
(3) Perform the test with Clebopride Malate under Flame Coloration Test <*1.04*> (2): a green color appears.

Purity **(1)** Chloride <*1.03*>—Dissolve 1.0 g of Clebopride Malate in 20 mL of acetic acid (100), add 6 mL of dilute nitric acid and water to make 50 mL. Perform the test using this solution as the test solution. Prepare the control solution with 0.25 mL of 0.01 mol/L hydrochloric acid VS by adding 20 mL of acetic acid (100), 6 mL of dilute nitric acid and water to make 50 mL (not more than 0.009%).

(2) Heavy metals *<1.07>*—Proceed with 2.0 g of Clebopride Malate according to Method 2, and perform the test. Prepare the control solution with 2.0 mL of Standard Lead Solution (not more than 10 ppm).

(3) Related substances—Dissolve 0.10 g of Clebopride Malate in 10 mL of the mobile phase, and use this solution as the sample solution. Pipet 0.2 mL of the sample solution, add the mobile phase to make exactly 100 mL, and use this solution as the standard solution. Perform the test with exactly 10 μL each of the sample solution and standard solution as directed under Liquid Chromatography *<2.01>* according to the following conditions. Determine each peak area of both solutions by the automatic integration method: the total area of the peaks other than clebopride obtained from the sample solution is not larger than the peak area of clebopride from the standard solution.

Operating conditions—

Detector: An ultraviolet absorption photometer (wavelength: 240 nm).

Column: A stainless steel column 4.6 mm in inside diameter and 25 cm in length, packed with octadecylsilanized silica gel for liquid chromatography (7 μm in particle diameter).

Column temperature: A constant temperature of about 25°C.

Mobile phase: Dissolve 3.85 g of ammonium acetate in water to make 500 mL, and filter through a membrane filter with a pore size not exceeding 0.5 μm. To 400 mL of the filtrate add 600 mL of methanol.

Flow rate: Adjust so that the retention time of clebopride is about 15 minutes.

Time span of measurement: About 2 times as long as the retention time of clebopride.

System suitability—

Test for required detectability: Pipet 10 mL of the standard solution, and add water to make exactly 100 mL. Confirm that the peak area of clebopride obtained with 10 μL of this solution is equivalent to 7 to 13% of that with 10 μL of the standard solution.

System performance: Dissolve 30 mg Clebopride Malate and 5 mg of propyl parahydroxybenzoate in the mobile phase to make 100 mL. When the procedure is run with 10 μL of this solution under the above operating conditions, propyl parahydroxybenzoate and clebopride are eluted in this order with the resolution between these peaks being not less than 3.

System repeatability: When the test is repeated 6 times with 10 μL of the standard solution under the above operating conditions, the relative standard deviation of the peak area of clebopride is not more than 2.5%.

Loss on drying *<2.41>* Not more than 0.5% (1 g, 105°C, 4 hours).

Residue on ignition *<2.44>* Not more than 0.1% (1 g).

Assay Weigh accurately about 0.5 g of Clebopride Malate, previously dried, dissolve in 30 mL of acetic acid (100), and titrate *<2.50>* with 0.1 mol/L perchloric acid VS (potentiometric titration). Perform a blank determination in the same manner, and make any necessary correction.

Each mL of 0.1 mol/L perchloric acid VS
= 50.80 mg of $C_{20}H_{24}ClN_3O_2.C_4H_6O_5$

Containers and storage Containers—Tight containers.

Clemastine Fumarate

クレマスチンフマル酸塩

$C_{21}H_{26}ClNO.C_4H_4O_4$: 459.96

(2*R*)-2-{2-[(1*R*)-1-(4-Chlorophenyl)-1-phenylethoxy]ethyl}-1-methylpyrrolidine monofumarate

[*14976-57-9*]

Clemastine Fumarate, when dried, contains not less than 98.5% of clemastine fumarate ($C_{21}H_{26}ClNO.C_4H_4O_4$).

Description Clemastine Fumarate occurs as a white, crystalline powder. It is odorless.

It is sparingly soluble in methanol and in acetic acid (100), slightly soluble in ethanol (95), very slightly soluble in diethyl ether, and practically insoluble in water.

Identification **(1)** To 5 mg of Clemastine Fumarate add 5 mL of sulfuric acid, and shake to dissolve: a yellow color develops. Slowly drop this solution into 10 mL of water: the yellow color immediately disappears.

(2) To 0.01 g of Clemastine Fumarate add 1 mL of fuming nitric acid, and evaporate on a water bath to dryness. Then add 2 mL of diluted hydrochloric acid (1 in 2) and 0.2 g of zinc powder, heat for 10 minutes on a water bath, cool, and filter. Add 20 mL of water to the filtrate. The solution responds to Qualitative Tests *<1.09>* for primary aromatic amines.

(3) To 5 mL of a solution of Clemastine Fumarate (1 in 50,000), add 5 mL of 4-dimethylaminobenzaldehyde TS, and warm for 10 minutes: a red-purple color develops.

(4) Perform the test with Clemastine Fumarate as directed under Flame Coloration Test *<1.04>* (2): a green color appears.

(5) Dissolve 0.04 g of Clemastine Fumarate and 0.01 g of fumaric acid for thin-layer chromatography in 2 mL each of a mixture of ethanol (95) and water (4:1) by gentle warming, and use these solutions as the sample solution and the standard solution, respectively. Perform the test with these solutions as directed under Thin-layer Chromatography *<2.03>*. Spot 5 μL each of the sample solution and standard solution on a plate of silica gel with fluorescent indicator for thin-layer chromatography. Develop the plate with a mixture of isopropyl ether, formic acid and water (90:7:3) to a distance of about 10 cm, and air-dry the plate. Examine the plate under ultraviolet light (main wavelength: 254 nm): the spot with larger *Rf* value from the sample solution has the same *Rf* value as the spot from the standard solution.

Optical rotation *<2.49>* $[\alpha]_D^{20}$: +16 – +18° (after drying, 0.1 g, methanol, 10 mL, 100 mm).

Melting point *<2.60>* 176 – 180°C (with decomposition).

Purity **(1)** Clarity and color of solution—Dissolve 0.5 g of Clemastine Fumarate in 10 mL of methanol by warming: the solution is clear and colorless.

(2) Heavy metals *<1.07>*—Perform the test with 1.0 g of Clemastine Fumarate according to Method 2. Prepare the control solution with 2.0 mL of Standard Lead Solution (not more than 20 ppm).

(3) Arsenic 〈*1.11*〉—Take 1.0 g of Clemastine Fumarate, prepare the test solution according to Method 3, and perform the test (not more than 2 ppm).

(4) Related Substances—Dissolve 0.10 g of Clemastine Fumarate in 5 mL of methanol, and use this solution as the sample solution. Pipet 1 mL of the sample solution, add methanol to make exactly 250 mL, and use this solution as the standard solution (1). Pipet 5 mL of the standard solution (1), add methanol to make exactly 10 mL, and use this solution as the standard solution (2). Perform the test with these solutions as directed under Thin-layer Chromatography 〈*2.03*〉. Spot 5 μL each of the sample solution and standard solutions (1) and (2) on a plate of silica gel for thin-layer chromatography. Develop the plate with a mixture of chloroform, methanol and ammonia solution (28) (90:10:1) to a distance of about 15 cm, and air-dry the plate. After spraying evenly Dragendorff's TS on the plate, immediately spray evenly hydrogen peroxide TS: the spots other than the principal spot obtained from the sample solution are not more intense than the spot from the standard solution (1), and not more than 2 spots from the sample solution are more intense than the spot from the standard solution (2).

Loss on drying 〈*2.41*〉 Not more than 0.5% (1 g, 105°C, 4 hours).

Residue on ignition 〈*2.44*〉 Not more than 0.2% (1 g).

Assay Weigh accurately about 0.4 g of Clemastine Fumarate, previously dried, dissolved in 50 mL of acetic acid (100), and titrate 〈*2.50*〉 with 0.1 mol/L perchloric acid VS (potentiometric titration). Perform a blank determination in the same manner, and make any necessary correction.

Each mL of 0.1 mol/L perchloric acid VS
= 46.00 mg of $C_{21}H_{26}ClNO.C_4H_4O_4$

Containers and storage Containers—Tight containers.

Clindamycin Hydrochloride

クリンダマイシン塩酸塩

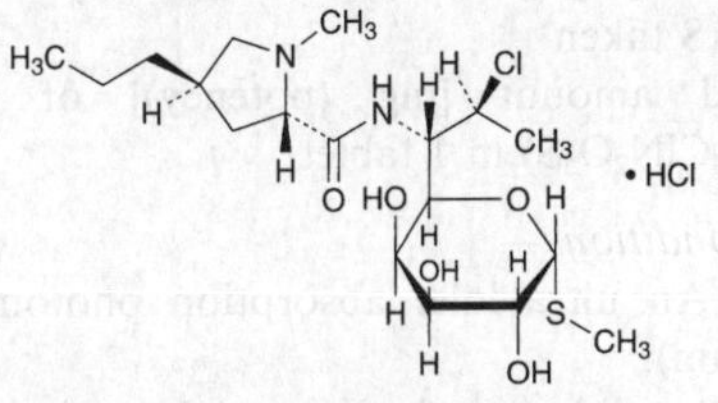

$C_{18}H_{33}ClN_2O_5S.HCl$: 461.44
Methyl 7-chloro-6,7,8-trideoxy-6-[(2*S*,4*R*)-1-methyl-4-propylpyrrolidine-2-carboxamido]-1-thio-L-*threo*-α-D-*galacto*-octopyranoside monohydrochloride
[*21462-39-5*]

Clindamycin Hydrochloride is the hydrochloride of a derivative of lincomycin.

It contains not less than 838 μg (potency) and not more than 940 μg (potency) per mg, calculated on the anhydrous basis. The potency of Clindamycin Hydrochloride is expressed as mass (potency) of clindamycin ($C_{18}H_{33}ClN_2O_5S$: 424.98).

Description Clindamycin Hydrochloride occurs as white to grayish white, crystals or crystalline powder.

It is freely soluble in water and in methanol, and slightly soluble in ethanol (99.5).

Identification **(1)** Determine the infrared absorption spectrum of Clindamycin Hydrochloride as directed in the potassium chloride disk method under Infrared Spectrophotometry 〈*2.25*〉, and compare the spectrum with the Reference Spectrum or the spectrum of Clindamycin Hydrochloride RS: both spectra exhibit similar intensities of absorption at the same wave numbers.

(2) A solution of Clindamycin Hydrochloride (1 in 100) responds to Qualitative Tests 〈*1.09*〉 (2) for chloride.

Optical rotation 〈*2.49*〉 $[\alpha]_D^{25}$: +135 – +150° (0.5 g calculated on the anhydrous basis, water, 25 mL, 100 mm).

Purity **(1)** Heavy metals 〈*1.07*〉—Proceed with 2.0 g of Clindamycin Hydrochloride according to Method 4, and perform the test. Prepare the control solution with 2.0 mL of Standard Lead Solution (not more than 10 ppm).

(2) Related substances—Use the sample solution obtained in the Assay as the sample solution. Pipet 1 mL of the sample solution, add the mobile phase to make exactly 100 mL, and use this solution as the standard solution. Perform the test with exactly 20 μL each of the sample solution and standard solution as directed under Liquid Chromatography 〈*2.01*〉 according to the following conditions, and determine each peak area by the automatic integration method: the peak area of clindamycin B, having the relative retention time of about 0.7 to clindamycin, and that of 7-epiclindamycin, having the relative retention time of about 0.8, obtained from the sample solution are not larger than 2 times the peak area of clindamycin from the standard solution, the area of the peak other than clindamycin and the peaks mentioned above from the sample solution is not larger than the peak area of clindamycin from the standard solution, and the total area of the peaks other than clindamycin from the sample solution is not larger than 4 times the peak area of clindamycin from the standard solution.

Operating conditions—

Detector, column, column temperature, mobile phase, and flow rate: Proceed as directed in the operating conditions in the Assay.

Time span of measurement: About 2 times as long as the retention time of clindamycin, beginning after the solvent peak.

System suitability—

Test for required detectability: Pipet 1 mL of the standard solution, and add the mobile phase to make exactly 10 mL. Confirm that the peak area of clindamycin obtained with 20 μL of this solution is equivalent to 7 to 13% of that with 20 μL of the standard solution.

System performance: When the procedure is run with 20 μL of the standard solution under the above operating conditions, the number of theoretical plates and the symmetry factor of the peak of clindamycin are not less than 6000 and not more than 1.5, respectively.

System repeatability: When the test is repeated 6 times with 20 μL of the standard solution under the above operating conditions, the relative standard deviation of the peak area of clindamycin is not more than 2.0%.

Water 〈*2.48*〉 Not more than 6.0% (0.3 g, volumetric titration, direct titration).

Assay Weigh accurately an amount of Clindamycin Hydrochloride and Clindamycin Hydrochloride RS, equivalent to about 20 mg (potency), dissolve each in the mobile phase to make exactly 20 mL, and use these solutions as the sample solution and the standard solution, respectively. Perform the test with exactly 20 μL each of the sample solution and standard solution as directed under Liquid Chromatography <2.01> according to the following conditions, and determine the peak areas, A_T and A_S, of clindamycin in each solution.

Amount [μg (potency)] of clindamycin ($C_{18}H_{33}ClN_2O_5S$)
$= M_S \times A_T/A_S \times 1000$

M_S: Amount [mg (potency)] of Clindamycin Hydrochloride RS taken

Operating conditions—

Detector: An ultraviolet absorption photometer (wavelength: 210 nm).

Column: A stainless steel column 4.6 mm in inside diameter and 25 cm in length, packed with octadecylsilanized silica gel for liquid chromatography (5 μm in particle diameter).

Column temperature: A constant temperature of about 25°C.

Mobile phase: To 0.05 mol/L potassium dihydrogen phosphate TS add 8 mol/L potassium hydroxide TS to adjust the pH to 7.5. To 550 mL of this solution add 450 mL of acetonitrile for liquid chromatography.

Flow rate: Adjust so that the retention time of clindamycin is about 10 minutes.

System suitability—

System performance: When the procedure is run with 20 μL of the standard solution under the above operating conditions, the number of theoretical plates and the symmetry factor of the peak of clindamycin are not less than 6000 and not more than 1.5, respectively.

System repeatability: When the test is repeated 6 times with 20 μL of the standard solution under the above operating conditions, the relative standard deviation of the peak area of clindamycin is not more than 1.0%.

Containers and storage Containers—Tight containers.

Clindamycin Hydrochloride Capsules

クリンダマイシン塩酸塩カプセル

Clindamycin Hydrochloride Capsules contain not less than 93.0% and not more than 107.0% of the labeled potency of clindamycin ($C_{18}H_{33}ClN_2O_5S$: 424.98).

Method of preparation Prepare as directed under Capsules, with Clindamycin Hydrochloride.

Identification To an amount of the contents of Clindamycin Hydrochloride Capsules, equivalent to 10 mg (potency) of Clindamycin Hydrochloride, add 2 mL of methanol, shake well, centrifuge, and use the supernatant liquid as the sample solution. Separately, dissolve 10 mg of Clindamycin Hydrochloride RS in 2 mL of methanol, and use this solution as the standard solution. Perform the test with these solutions as directed under Thin-layer Chromatography <2.03>. Spot 10 μL each of the sample solution and standard solution on a plate of silica gel for thin-layer chromatography. Develop the plate with a mixture of methanol, toluene and ammonia solution (28) (140:60:3) to a distance of about 12 cm, and air-dry the plate. Spray evenly a mixture of 500 mL of a solution of L-tartaric acid (1 in 5) and 50 mL of bismuth subnitrate TS on the plate: the *Rf* values of the principal spot with the sample solution and the spot with the standard solution are not different each other.

Uniformity of dosage units <6.02> Perform the test according to the following method: it meets the requirement of the Content uniformity test.

To 1 capsule of Clindamycin Hydrochloride Capsules add a suitable amount of the mobile phase, shake for 30 minutes, and add the mobile phase to make exactly *V* mL so that each mL contains 0.75 mg (potency) of Clindamycin Hydrochloride. Centrifuge this solution, and use the supernatant liquid as the sample solution. Then, proceed as directed in the Assay.

Amount [mg (potency)] of clindamycin ($C_{18}H_{33}ClN_2O_5S$)
$= M_S \times A_T/A_S \times V/100$

M_S: Amount [mg (potency)] of Clindamycin Hydrochloride RS taken

Dissolution <6.10> When the test is performed at 50 revolutions per minute according to the Paddle method using the sinker, using 900 mL of water as the dissolution medium, the dissolution rate of a 75-mg capsule in 15 minutes and that of a 150-mg capsule in 30 minutes are not less than 80%, respectively.

Start the test with 1 capsule of Clindamycin Hydrochloride Capsules, withdraw not less than 20 mL of the medium at the specified minute after starting the test, and filter through a membrane filter with a pore size not exceeding 0.45 μm. Discard not less than 10 mL of the first filtrate, pipet *V* mL of the subsequent filtrate, add water to make exactly *V′* so that each mL contains about 83 μg (potency) of Clindamycin Hydrochloride, and use this solution as the sample solution. Separately, weigh accurately an amount of Clindamycin Hydrochloride RS, equivalent to about 17 mg (potency), dissolve in water to make exactly 200 mL, and use this solution as the standard solution. Perform the test with exactly 20 μL each of the sample solution and standard solution as directed under Liquid Chromatography <2.01>, and determine the peak areas, A_T and A_S, of clindamycin in each solution.

Dissolution rate (%) with respect to the labeled amount of clindamycin ($C_{18}H_{33}ClN_2O_5S$)
$= M_S \times A_T/A_S \times V'/V \times 1/C \times 450$

M_S: Amount [mg (potency)] of Clindamycin Hydrochloride RS taken

C: Labeled amount [mg (potency)] of clindamycin ($C_{18}H_{33}ClN_2O_5S$) in 1 tablet

Operating conditions—

Detector: An ultraviolet absorption photometer (wavelength: 210 nm).

Column: A stainless steel column 4.6 mm in inside diameter and 15 cm in length, packed with octadecylsilanized silica gel for liquid chromatography (5 μm in particle diameter).

Column temperature: A constant temperature of about 40°C.

Mobile phase: Adjust the pH of 0.05 mol/L potassium dihydrogen phosphate TS to 7.5 with 8 mol/L potassium hydroxide TS. To 550 mL of this solution add 450 mL of acetonitrile.

Flow rate: Adjust so that the retention time of clindamycin is about 7 minutes.

System suitability—

System performance: When the procedure is run with 20 μL of the standard solution under the above operating conditions, the number of theoretical plates and the symmetry factor of the peak of clindamycin are not less than 3000 and not more than 2.0, respectively.

System repeatability: When the test is repeated 6 times

with 20 μL of the standard solution under the above operating conditions, the relative standard deviation of the peak area of clindamycin is not more than 2.0%.

Assay Take out the contents of not less than 20 Clindamycin Hydrochloride Capsules, weigh accurately the mass of the contents, and powder. Weigh accurately a portion of the powder, equivalent to about 75 mg (potency) of Clindamycin Hydrochloride, add the mobile phase, shake for 30 minutes, and add the mobile phase to make exactly 100 mL. Centrifuge this solution, and use the supernatant liquid as the sample solution. Separately, weigh accurately an amount of Clindamycin Hydrochloride RS, equivalent to about 75 mg (potency), dissolve in the mobile phase to make exactly 100 mL, and use this solution as the standard solution. Perform the test with exactly 20 μL each of the sample solution and standard solution as directed under Liquid Chromatography <2.01> according to the following conditions, and determine the peak areas, A_T and A_S, of clindamycin in each solution.

Amount [mg (potency)] of clindamycin ($C_{18}H_{33}ClN_2O_5S$)
$= M_S \times A_T/A_S$

M_S: Amount [mg (potency)] of Clindamycin Hydrochloride RS taken

Operating conditions—

Detector: An ultraviolet absorption photometer (wavelength: 210 nm).

Column: A stainless steel column 4.6 mm in inside diameter and 15 cm in length, packed with octadecylsilanized silica gel for liquid chromatography (5 μm in particle diameter).

Column temperature: A constant temperature of about 40°C.

Mobile phase: To 0.05 mol/L of potassium dihydrogen phosphate TS add 8 mol/L potassium hydroxide TS to adjust the pH to 7.5. To 550 mL of this solution add 450 mL of acetonitrile for liquid chromatography.

Flow rate: Adjust so that the retention time of clindamycin is about 7 minutes.

System suitability—

System performance: When the procedure is run with 20 μL of the standard solution under the above operating conditions, the number of theoretical plates and the symmetry factor of the peak of clindamycin are not less than 3000 and not more than 2.0, respectively.

System repeatability: When the test is repeated 6 times with 20 μL of the standard solution under the above operating conditions, the relative standard deviation of the peak area of clindamycin is not more than 1.0%.

Containers and storage Containers—Tight containers.

Clindamycin Phosphate

クリンダマイシンリン酸エステル

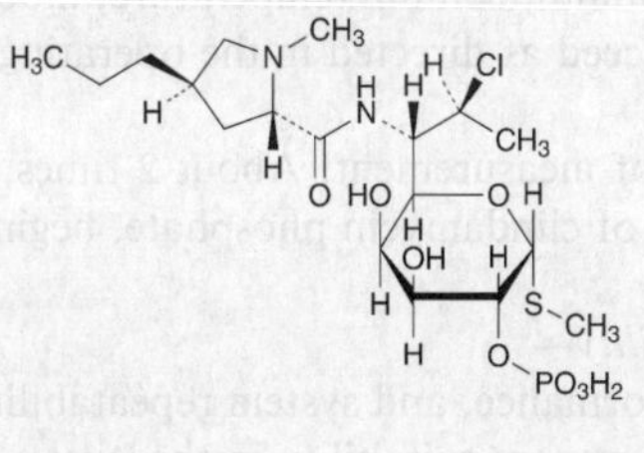

$C_{18}H_{34}ClN_2O_8PS$: 504.96
Methyl 7-chloro-6,7,8-trideoxy-6-[(2*S*,4*R*)-1-methyl-4-propylpyrrolidine-2-carboxamido]-1-thio-L-*threo*-α-D-*galacto*-octopyranoside 2-dihydrogen phosphate
[24729-96-2]

Clindamycin Phosphate is a derivative of clindamycin.

It contains not less than 800 μg (potency) and not more than 846 μg (potency) per mg, calculated on the anhydrous basis. The potency of Clindamycin Phosphate is expressed as mass (potency) of clindamycin ($C_{18}H_{33}ClN_2O_5S$: 424.98).

Description Clindamycin Phosphate occurs as a white to pale yellow-white crystalline powder.

It is freely soluble in water, sparingly soluble in methanol, and practically insoluble in ethanol (95).

Identification Determine the infrared absorption spectrum of Clindamycin Phosphate, previously dried at 100°C for 2 hours, as directed in the paste method under Infrared Spectrophotometry <2.25>, and compare the spectrum with the Reference Spectrum or the spectrum of Clindamycin Phosphate RS previously dried at 100°C for 2 hours: both spectra exhibit similar intensities of absorption at the same wave numbers.

Optical rotation <2.49> $[\alpha]_D^{20}$: +115 – +130° (0.25 g calculated on the anhydrous basis, water, 25 mL, 100 mm).

pH <2.54> Dissolve 0.10 g of Clindamycin Phosphate in 10 mL of water. The pH of the solution is between 3.5 and 4.5.

Purity (1) Clarity and color of solution—Dissolve 1.0 g of Clindamycin Phosphate in 10 mL of freshly boiled and cooled water: the solution is clear and colorless.

(2) Heavy metals <1.07>—Proceed with 2.0 g of Clindamycin Phosphate according to Method 4, and perform the test. Prepare the control solution with 1.0 mL of Standard Lead Solution (not more than 5 ppm).

(3) Arsenic <1.11>—Prepare the test solution with 1.0 g of Clindamycin Phosphate according to Method 4, and perform the test (not more than 2 ppm).

(4) Related substances—Dissolve 0.1 g of Clindamycin Phosphate in 100 mL of the mobile phase, and use this solution as the sample solution. Pipet 1 mL of the sample solution, add the mobile phase to make exactly 100 mL, and use this solution as the standard solution. Perform the test with exactly 20 μL each of the sample solution and standard solution as directed under Liquid Chromatography <2.01> according to the following conditions, and determine each peak area by the automatic integration method: the peak area of clindamycin, having the relative retention time of about 1.8 to clindamycin phosphate, obtained from the sample solution is not larger than 1/2 times the peak area of clindamycin phosphate from the standard solution, and the total

area of the peaks other than clindamycin phosphate from the sample solution is not larger than 4 times the peak area of clindamycin phosphate from the standard solution.

Operating conditions—

Detector, column, column temperature, mobile phase, and flow rate: Proceed as directed in the operating conditions in the Assay.

Time span of measurement: About 2 times as long as the retention time of clindamycin phosphate, beginning after the solvent peak.

System suitability—

System performance, and system repeatability: Proceed as directed in the system suitability in the Assay.

Test for required detectability: Measure exactly 1 mL of the standard solution, and add the mobile phase to make exactly 10 mL. Confirm that the peak area of clindamycin phosphate obtained with 20 μL of this solution is equivalent to 7 to 13% of that with 20 μL of the standard solution.

Water *<2.48>* Not more than 6.0% (0.5 g, volumetric titration, direct titration).

Assay Weigh accurately an amount of Clindamycin Phosphate and Clindamycin Phosphate RS, equivalent to about 20 mg (potency), add exactly 25 mL of the internal standard solution and the mobile phase to make 100 mL, and use these solutions as the sample solution and standard solution. Perform the test with 20 μL each of the sample solution and standard solution as directed under Liquid Chromatography *<2.01>* according to the following conditions, and calculate the ratios, Q_T and Q_S, of the peak area of clindamycin phosphate to that of the internal standard.

Amount [μg (potency)] of clindamycin ($C_{18}H_{33}ClN_2O_5S$)
$= M_S \times Q_T/Q_S \times 1000$

M_S: Amount [mg (potency)] of Clindamycin Phosphate RS taken

Internal standard solution—A solution of methyl parahydroxybenzoate in the mobile phase (3 in 50,000).

Operating conditions—

Detector: An ultraviolet absorption photometer (wavelength: 210 nm).

Column: A stainless steel column 4 mm in inside diameter and 25 cm in length, packed with octylsilanized silica gel for liquid chromatography (5 μm in particle diameter).

Column temperature: A constant temperature of about 25°C.

Mobile phase: Dissolve 10.54 g of potassium dihydrogen phosphate in 775 mL of water, adjust the pH to 2.5 with phosphoric acid, and add 225 mL of acetonitrile.

Flow rate: Adjust so that the retention time of clindamycin phosphate is about 8 minutes.

System suitability—

System performance: When the procedure is run with 20 μL of the standard solution under the above operating conditions, clindamycin phosphate and the internal standard are eluted in this order with the resolution between these peaks being not less than 4.

System repeatability: When the test is repeated 6 times with 20 μL of the standard solution under the above operating conditions, the relative standard deviation of the ratios of the peak area of clindamycin phosphate to that of the internal standard is not more than 2.5%.

Containers and storage Containers—Tight containers.

Clindamycin Phosphate Injection

クリンダマイシンリン酸エステル注射液

Clindamycin Phosphate Injection is an aqueous injection.

It contains not less than 90.0% and not more than 110.0% of the labeled potency of clindamycin phosphate ($C_{18}H_{34}ClN_2O_8PS$: 504.96).

Method of preparation Prepare as directed under Injections, with Clindamycin Phosphate.

Description Clindamycin Phosphate Injection is a clear, colorless or light yellow liquid.

Identification To a volume of Clindamycin Phosphate Injection, equivalent to 0.15 g (potency) of Clindamycin Phosphate, add 4 mL of water, 2 mL of 8 mol/L sodium hydroxide TS and 0.1 mL of sodium pentacyanonitrosylferrate (III) TS, mix, heat in a water bath for 10 minutes, and add 2 mL of hydrochloric acid: a blue-green color develops.

Osmotic pressure ratio Being specified separately when the drug is granted approval based on the Law.

pH *<2.54>* 6.0 – 7.0

Bacterial endotoxins *<4.01>* Less than 0.1 EU/mg (potency).

Extractable volume *<6.05>* It meets the requirement.

Foreign insoluble matter *<6.06>* Perform the test according to Method 1: it meets the requirement.

Insoluble particulate matter *<6.07>* It meets the requirement.

Sterility *<4.06>* Perform the test according to the Membrane filtration method: it meets the requirement.

Assay Measure exactly a volume of Clindamycin Phosphate Injection, equivalent to about 0.3 g (potency) of Clindamycin Phosphate, and add the mobile phase to make exactly 100 mL. Pipet 7 mL of this solution, add exactly 25 mL of the internal standard solution and the mobile phase to make 100 mL, and use this solution as the sample solution. Separately, weigh accurately an amount of Clindamycin Phosphate RS, equivalent to about 20 mg (potency), dissolve in exactly 25 mL of the internal standard solution, add the mobile phase to make 100 mL, and use this solution as the standard solution. Then, proceed as directed in the Assay under Clindamycin Phosphate.

Amount [mg (potency)] of clindamycin phosphate
($C_{18}H_{34}ClN_2O_8PS$)
$= M_S \times Q_T/Q_S \times 100/7$

M_S: Amount [mg (potency)] of Clindamycin Phosphate RS taken

Internal standard solution—A solution of methyl parahydroxybenzoate in the mobile phase (3 in 50,000).

Containers and storage Containers—Hermetic containers.

Clinofibrate

クリノフィブラート

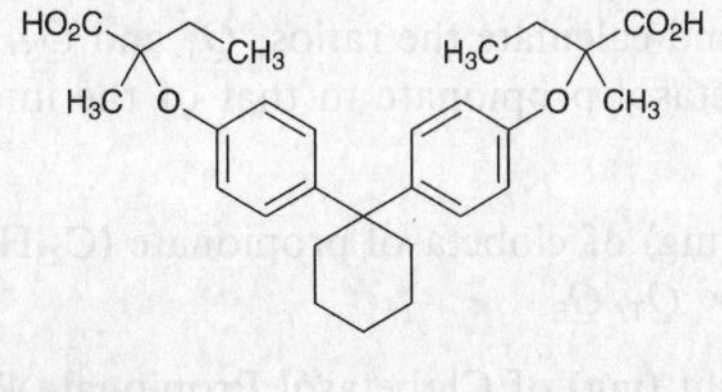

$C_{28}H_{36}O_6$: 468.58
2,2′-[Cyclohexane-1,1-diylbis(4,1-phenyleneoxy)]bis(2-methylbutanoic acid)
[30299-08-2]

Clinofibrate, when dried, contains not less than 98.5% of clinofibrate ($C_{28}H_{36}O_6$).

Description Clinofibrate occurs as a white to yellowish white powder. It is odorless and has no taste.

It is freely soluble in methanol, in ethanol (99.5), in acetone and in diethyl ether, and practically insoluble in water.

A solution of Clinofibrate in methanol (1 in 20) shows no optical rotation.

Melting point: about 146°C (with decomposition).

Identification **(1)** Determine the absorption spectrum of a solution of Clinofibrate in ethanol (99.5) (1 in 50,000) as directed under Ultraviolet-visible Spectrophotometry *<2.24>*, and compare the spectrum with the Reference Spectrum: both spectra exhibit similar intensities of absorption at the same wavelengths.

(2) Determine the infrared absorption spectrum of Clinofibrate, previously dried, as directed in the potassium bromide disk method under Infrared Spectrophotometry *<2.25>*, and compare the spectrum with the Reference Spectrum: both spectra exhibit similar intensities of absorption at the same wave numbers.

Purity **(1)** Heavy metals *<1.07>*—Proceed with 1.0 g of Clinofibrate according to Method 2, and perform the test. Prepare the control solution with 2.0 mL of Standard Lead Solution (not more than 20 ppm).

(2) Arsenic *<1.11>*—Prepare the test solution with 1.0 g of Clinofibrate according to Method 3, and perform the test (not more than 2 ppm).

(3) Related substances—Dissolve 0.10 g of Clinofibrate in 10 mL of acetone, and use this solution as the sample solution. Pipet 1 mL of the sample solution, and add acetone to make exactly 50 mL. Pipet 5 mL of this solution, add acetone to make exactly 20 mL, and use this solution as the standard solution. Perform the test with these solutions as directed under Thin-layer Chromatography *<2.03>*. Spot 50 μL each of the sample solution and standard solution on a plate of silica gel with fluorescent indicator for thin-layer chromatography. Develop the plate with a mixture of chloroform, cyclohexane and acetic acid (100) (12:5:3) to a distance of about 12 cm, and air-dry the plate. Examine under ultraviolet light (main wavelength: 254 nm): the spots other than the principal spot obtained from the sample solution are not more intense than the spot from the standard solution.

Loss on drying *<2.41>* Not more than 1.0% (1 g, in vacuum, 60°C, 3 hours).

Residue on ignition *<2.44>* Not more than 0.2% (1 g).

Isomer ratio To 50 mg of Clinofibrate add 0.4 mL of thionyl chloride, stopper tightly, heat on a water bath of 60°C for 5 minutes with occasional shaking, and evaporate the excess thionyl chloride at a temperature not exceeding 60°C under reduced pressure. Dissolve the residue in 2 mL of toluene previously dried with synthetic zeolite for drying, add 2 mL of a solution of D-(+)-α-methylbenzylamine in toluene previously dried with synthetic zeolite for drying (3 in 100), mix gently, allow to stand for 10 minutes, and evaporate the toluene at a temperature not exceeding 60°C under reduced pressure. Dissolve the residue in 5 mL of chloroform, and use this solution as the sample solution. Perform the test with 5 μL of the sample solution as directed under Liquid Chromatography *<2.01>* according to the following conditions. Determine each peak area, A_a, A_b and A_c, of three peaks appear in order near the retention time of 40 minutes: a value, $A_b/(A_a + A_b + A_c) \times 100$, is between 40 and 70.

Operating conditions—

Detector: An ultraviolet absorption photometer (wavelength: 254 nm).

Column: A stainless steel column about 4 mm in inside diameter and about 30 cm in length, packed with silica gel for liquid chromatography (5 μm in particle diameter).

Column temperature: A constant temperature of about 20°C.

Mobile phase: A mixture of hexane and 2-propanol (500:3).

Flow rate: Adjust so that the retention time of the peak appearing first is about 35 minutes.

Selection of column: Proceed with 5 μL of the sample solution under the above operating conditions. Use a column giving a complete separation of the three peaks.

Assay Weigh accurately about 0.45 g of Clinofibrate, previously dried, dissolve in 40 mL of ethanol (99.5), add 30 mL of water, and titrate *<2.50>* with 0.1 mol/L sodium hydroxide VS (indicator: 3 drops of phenolphthalein TS). Perform a blank determination in the same manner, and make any necessary correction.

Each mL of 0.1 mol/L sodium hydroxide VS
= 23.43 mg of $C_{28}H_{36}O_6$

Containers and storage Containers—Tight containers.

Clobetasol Propionate

クロベタゾールプロピオン酸エステル

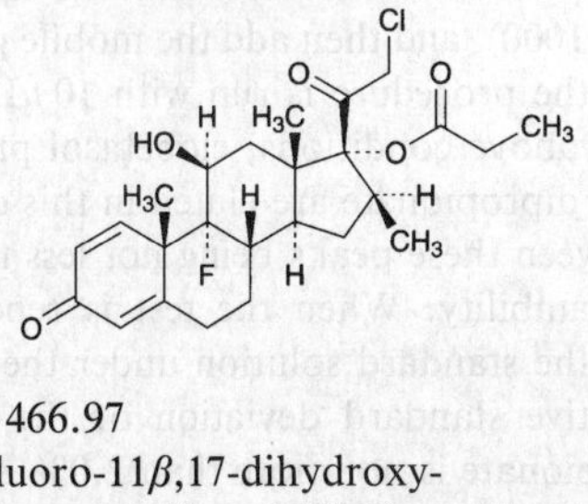

$C_{25}H_{32}ClFO_5$: 466.97
21-Chloro-9-fluoro-11β,17-dihydroxy-16β-methylpregna-1,4-diene-3,20-dione 17-propanoate
[25122-46-7]

Clobetasol Propionate, when dried, contains not less than 97.0% and not more than 102.0% of clobetasol propionate ($C_{25}H_{32}ClFO_5$).

Description Clobetasol Propionate occurs as a white to pale yellow-white crystalline powder.

The JP Drugs are to be tested according to the provisions given in the pertinent monographs, General Notices, General Rules for Crude Drugs, General Rules for Preparations, and General Tests for their conformity to the Japanese Pharmacopoeia. (See the General Notices 5.)

It is soluble in methanol and in ethanol (99.5), and practically insoluble in water.

It gradually turns yellow by light.

Melting point: about 196°C (with decomposition).

Identification Determine the infrared absorption spectra of Clobetasol Propionate as directed in the paste method under Infrared Spectrophotometry 〈*2.25*〉, and compare the spectrum with the Reference Spectrum or the spectrum of Clobetasol Propionate RS: both spectra exhibit similar intensities of absorbance at the same wave numbers.

Optical rotation 〈*2.49*〉 $[\alpha]_D^{20}$: +109 – +115° (after drying, 0.1 g, methanol, 10 mL, 100 mm).

Purity (1) Heavy metals 〈*1.07*〉—Proceed with 1.0 g of Clobetasol Propionate according to Method 2, and perform the test. Prepare the control solution with 2.0 mL of Standard Lead Solution (not more than 20 ppm).

(2) Related substances—Dissolve 10 mg of Clobetasol Propionate in 100 mL of the mobile phase, and use this solution as the sample solution. Pipet 5 mL of the sample solution, add the mobile phase to make exactly 200 mL, and use this solution as the standard solution. Perform the test with exactly 10 μL each of the sample solution and standard solution as directed under Liquid Chromatography 〈*2.01*〉 according to the following conditions, and determine each peak area of these solutions by the automatic integration method: the area of the peak other than clobetasol propionate obtained from the sample solution is not larger than 2/5 times the peak area of clobetasol propionate from the standard solution. Furthermore, the total area of the peaks other than clobetasol propionate from the sample solution is not larger than the peak area of clobetasol propionate from the standard solution.

Operating conditions—

Detector, column, column temperature, mobile phase, and flow rate: Proceed as directed in the operating conditions in the Assay.

Time span of measurement: About 2.5 times as long as the retention time of clobetasol propionate, beginning after the solvent peak.

System suitability—

Test for required detectability: Pipet 2 mL of the standard solution, and add the mobile phase to make exactly 50 mL. Confirm that the peak area of clobetasol propionate obtained with 10 μL of this solution is equivalent to 2.8 to 5.2% of that with 10 μL of the standard solution.

System performance: Dissolve 20 mg of Clobetasol Propionate in 20 mL of methanol. To 5 mL of this solution add 10 mL of a solution of beclometasone dipropionate in methanol (1 in 1000), and then add the mobile phase to make 50 mL. When the procedure is run with 10 μL of this solution under the above conditions, clobetasol propionate and beclometasone dipropionate are eluted in this order with the resolution between these peaks being not less than 8.

System repeatability: When the test is repeated 6 times with 10 μL of the standard solution under the above conditions, the relative standard deviation of the peak area of clobetasol propionate is not more than 2.0%.

Loss on drying 〈*2.41*〉 Not more than 0.5% (1 g, 105°C, 3 hours).

Residue on ignition 〈*2.44*〉 Not more than 0.1% (1 g, platinum crucible).

Assay Weigh accurately about 10 mg each of Clobetasol Propionate and Clobetasol Propionate RS, both previously dried, dissolve each in the mobile phase, add exactly 100 mL of the internal standard solution, add the mobile phase to make 250 mL, and use these solutions as the sample solution and standard solution. Perform the test with 10 μL each of the sample solution and standard solution as directed under Liquid Chromatography 〈*2.01*〉 according to the following conditions, and calculate the ratios, Q_T and Q_S, of the peak area of clobetasol propionate to that of the internal standard.

Amount (mg) of clobetasol propionate ($C_{25}H_{32}ClFO_5$)
$= M_S \times Q_T/Q_S$

M_S: Amount (mg) of Clobetasol Propionate RS taken

Internal standard solution—A solution of beclometasone dipropionate in the mobile phase (1 in 5000).

Operating conditions—

Detector: An ultraviolet absorption photometer (wavelength: 240 nm).

Column: A stainless steel column 4.6 mm in inside diameter and 15 cm in length, packed with octadecylsilanized silica gel for liquid chromatography (5 μm in particle diameter).

Column temperature: A constant temperature of about 25°C.

Mobile phase: Dissolve 7.80 g of sodium dihydrogen phosphate dihydrate in 900 mL of water, adjust the pH to 2.5 with phosphoric acid, and then add water to make 1000 mL. To 425 mL of this solution add 475 mL of acetonitrile and 100 mL of methanol.

Flow rate: Adjust so that the retention time of clobetasol propionate is about 10 minutes.

System suitability—

System performance: When the procedure is run with 10 μL of the standard solution under the above conditions, clobetasol propionate and the internal standard are eluted in this order with the resolution between these peaks being not less than 8.

System repeatability: When the test is repeated 6 times with 10 μL of the standard solution under the above conditions, the relative standard deviation of the ratio of the peak area of clobetasol propionate to that of the internal standard is not more than 1.0%.

Containers and storage Containers—Tight containers.

Storage—Light-resistant.

Clocapramine Hydrochloride Hydrate

クロカプラミン塩酸塩水和物

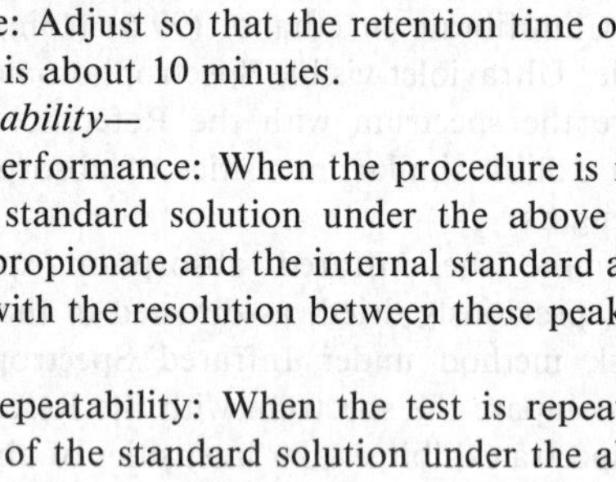

Cl N O NH2 N • 2HCl • H2O

$C_{28}H_{37}ClN_4O.2HCl.H_2O$: 572.01

1′-[3-(3-Chloro-10,11-dihydro-5*H*-dibenz[*b*,*f*]azepin-5-yl)propyl]-1,4′-bipiperidine-4′-carboxamide dihydrochloride monohydrate

[*60789-62-0*]

Clocapramine Hydrochloride Hydrate, when dried, contains not less than 98.0% of clocapramine hydrochloride ($C_{28}H_{37}ClN_4O.2HCl$: 553.99).

Description Clocapramine Hydrochloride Hydrate occurs as white, crystals or crystalline powder. It is odorless, and has a bitter taste.

It is freely soluble in acetic acid (100), sparingly soluble in water and in methanol, slightly soluble in ethanol (95), in chloroform and in isopropylamine, and practically insoluble in acetic anhydride and in diethyl ether.

It is gradually colored by light.

Melting point: about 260°C (with decomposition, after drying).

Identification **(1)** To 5 mL of a solution of Clocapramine Hydrochloride Hydrate (1 in 2500) add 1 mL of nitric acid: a blue color develops at first, and rapidly changes to deep blue, and then changes to green to yellow-green.

(2) Determine the absorption spectrum of a solution of Clocapramine Hydrochloride Hydrate in methanol (1 in 40,000) as directed under Ultraviolet-visible Spectrophotometry ⟨*2.24*⟩, and compare the spectrum with the Reference Spectrum: both spectra exhibit similar intensities of absorption at the same wavelengths.

(3) Determine the infrared absorption spectrum of Clocapramine Hydrochloride Hydrate as directed in the potassium bromide disk method under Infrared Spectrophotometry ⟨*2.25*⟩, and compare the spectrum with the Reference Spectrum: both spectra exhibit similar intensities of absorption at the same wave numbers.

(4) Dissolve 0.1 g of Clocapramine Hydrochloride Hydrate in 10 mL of water by warming, and after cooling, add 2 mL of ammonia TS, and filter. Acidify the filtrate with dilute nitric acid: the solution responds to Qualitative Tests ⟨*1.09*⟩ (2) for chloride.

Purity **(1)** Sulfate ⟨*1.14*⟩—Dissolve 0.5 g of Clocapramine Hydrochloride Hydrate in 40 mL of water by warming, after cooling, and add 1 mL of dilute hydrochloric acid and water to make 50 mL. Perform the test using this solution as the test solution. Prepare the control solution with 0.50 mL of 0.005 mol/L sulfuric acid VS (not more than 0.048%).

(2) Heavy metals ⟨*1.07*⟩—Proceed with 2.0 g of Clocapramine Hydrochloride Hydrate according to Method 2, and perform the test. Prepare the control solution with 2.0 mL of Standard Lead Solution (not more than 10 ppm).

(3) Related substances—Conduct this procedure without exposure to light, using light-resistant vessels. Dissolve 0.10 g of Clocapramine Hydrochloride Hydrate in 10 mL of a mixture of chloroform and isopropylamine (99:1), and use this solution as the sample solution. Pipet 1 mL of the sample solution, add a mixture of chloroform and isopropylamine (99:1) to make exactly 100 mL, and use this solution as the standard solution. Perform the test with these solutions as directed under Thin-layer Chromatography ⟨*2.03*⟩. Spot 10 μL each of the sample solution and standard solution on a plate of silica gel with fluorescent indicator for thin-layer chromatography. Develop the plate with a mixture of diethyl ether, ethyl acetate, methanol and ammonia solution (28) (100:70:40:1) to a distance of about 10 cm, and air-dry the plate. Examine under ultraviolet light (main wavelength: 254 nm): the spots other than the principal spot obtained from the sample solution are not more intense than the spot from the standard solution.

Loss on drying ⟨*2.41*⟩ 2.0 – 3.5% (0.5 g, in vacuum at a pressure not exceeding 0.67 kPa, phosphorus (V) oxide, 105°C, 4 hours).

Residue on ignition ⟨*2.44*⟩ Not more than 0.1% (1 g).

Assay Weigh accurately about 0.5 g of Clocapramine Hydrochloride Hydrate, previously dried, dissolve in 70 mL of a mixture of acetic anhydride and acetic acid (100) (6:1), and titrate ⟨*2.50*⟩ with 0.1 mol/L perchloric acid VS (potentiometric titration). Perform a blank determination in the same manner, and make any necessary correction.

Each mL of 0.1 mol/L perchloric acid VS
= 27.70 mg of $C_{28}H_{37}ClN_4O.2HCl$

Containers and storage Containers—Tight containers.
Storage—Light-resistant.

Clofedanol Hydrochloride

クロフェダノール塩酸塩

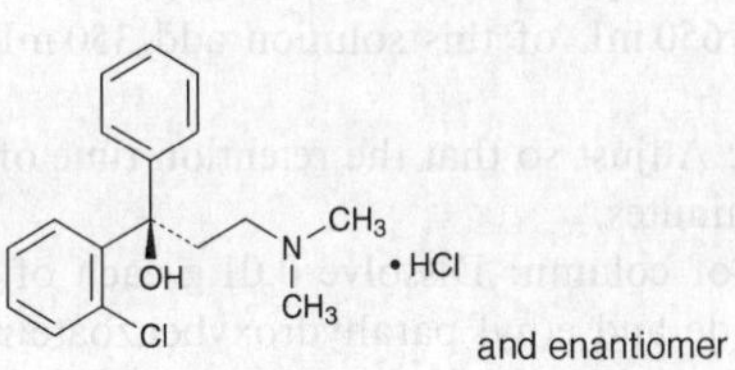

and enantiomer

$C_{17}H_{20}ClNO.HCl$: 326.26
(1*RS*)-1-(2-Chlorophenyl)-3-dimethylamino-1-phenylpropan-1-ol monohydrochloride
[*511-13-7*]

Clofedanol Hydrochloride, when dried, contains not less than 98.5% of clofedanol hydrochloride ($C_{17}H_{20}ClNO.HCl$).

Description Clofedanol Hydrochloride occurs as white, crystals or crystalline powder.

It is freely soluble in methanol, in ethanol (95) and in acetic acid (100), sparingly soluble in water, and practically insoluble in diethyl ether.

A solution of Clofedanol Hydrochloride in methanol (1 in 20) does not show optical rotation.

Melting point: about 190°C (after drying, with decomposition).

Identification **(1)** Determine the absorption spectrum of a solution of Clofedanol Hydrochloride in 0.01 mol/L hydrochloric acid TS (1 in 2500) as directed under Ultraviolet-visible Spectrophotometry ⟨*2.24*⟩, and compare the spectrum with the Reference Spectrum: both spectra exhibit similar intensities of absorption at the same wavelengths.

(2) Determine the infrared absorption spectrum of Clofedanol Hydrochloride, previously dried, as directed in the potassium bromide disk method under Infrared Spectrophotometry ⟨*2.25*⟩, and compare the spectrum with the Reference Spectrum: both spectra exhibit similar intensities of absorption at the same wave numbers.

(3) A solution of Clofedanol Hydrochloride (1 in 100) responds to Qualitative Tests ⟨*1.09*⟩ for chloride.

Purity **(1)** Heavy metals ⟨*1.07*⟩—Proceed with 2.0 g of Clofedanol Hydrochloride according to Method 2, and perform the test. Prepare the control solution with 2.0 mL of Standard Lead Solution (not more than 10 ppm).

(2) Related substances—Dissolve 0.05 g of Clofedanol Hydrochloride in 25 mL of methanol, and use this solution as the sample solution. Pipet 1 mL of the sample solution, add methanol to make exactly 100 mL, and use this solution as the standard solution. Perform the test with exactly 3 μL each of the sample solution and standard solution as directed under Liquid Chromatography <*2.01*> according to the following conditions. Determine each peak area of both solutions by the automatic integration method: the total area of the peaks other than clofedanol obtained from the sample solution is not larger than the peak area of clofedanol from the standard solution.

Operating conditions—

Detector: An ultraviolet absorption photometer (wavelength: 220 nm).

Column: A stainless steel column about 4 mm in inside diameter and about 15 cm in length, packed with octadecylsilanized silica gel for liquid chromatography (5 μm in particle diameter).

Column temperature: A constant temperature of about 40°C.

Mobile phase: Dissolve 1.34 g of potassium methanesulfonate in diluted phosphoric acid (1 in 1000) to make 1000 mL, and to 650 mL of this solution add 350 mL of methanol.

Flow rate: Adjust so that the retention time of clofedanol is about 9 minutes.

Selection of column: Dissolve 0.01 g each of Clofedanol Hydrochloride and ethyl parahydroxybenzoate in methanol to make 100 mL. Proceed with 3 μL of this solution under the above operating conditions, and calculate the resolution. Use a column giving elution of clofedanol and ethyl parahydroxybenzoate in this order with the resolution of these peaks being not less than 4.

Detection sensitivity: Adjust the detection sensitivity so that the peak height of clofedanol obtained from 3 μL of the standard solution composes between 20% and 50% of the full scale.

Time span of measurement: About three times as long as the retention time of clofedanol, beginning after the solvent peak.

Loss on drying <*2.41*> Not more than 2.0% (1 g, in vacuum, silica gel, 80°C, 3 hours).

Residue on ignition <*2.44*> Not more than 0.1% (1 g).

Assay Weigh accurately about 0.5 g of Clofedanol Hydrochloride, previously dried, dissolve in 15 mL of acetic acid (100), add 35 mL of acetic anhydride, and titrate <*2.50*> with 0.1 mol/L perchloric acid VS (potentiometric titration). Perform a blank determination in the same manner, and make any necessary correction.

Each mL of 0.1 mol/L perchloric acid VS
= 32.63 mg of $C_{17}H_{20}ClNO.HCl$

Containers and storage Containers—Tight containers.

Clofibrate

クロフィブラート

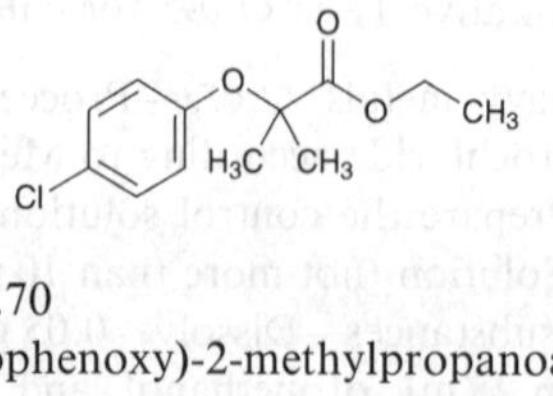

$C_{12}H_{15}ClO_3$: 242.70
Ethyl 2-(4-chlorophenoxy)-2-methylpropanoate
[*637-07-0*]

Clofibrate contains not less than 98.0% of clofibrate ($C_{12}H_{15}ClO_3$), calculated on the anhydrous basis.

Description Clofibrate occurs as a colorless or light yellow, clear, oily liquid. It has a characteristic odor and taste, which is bitter at first, and subsequently sweet.

It is miscible with methanol, with ethanol (95), with ethanol (99.5), with diethyl ether and with hexane, and practically insoluble in water.

It is gradually decomposed by light.

Identification **(1)** Determine the absorption spectrum of a solution of Clofibrate in ethanol (99.5) (1 in 10,000) as directed under Ultraviolet-visible Spectrophotometry <*2.24*>, and compare the spectrum with the Reference Spectrum 1 or the spectrum of a solution of Clofibrate RS prepared in the same manner as the sample solution: both spectra exhibit similar intensities of absorption at the same wavelengths. Separately, determine the absorption spectrum of a solution of Clofibrate in ethanol (99.5) (1 in 100,000) as directed under Ultraviolet-visible Spectrophotometry <*2.24*>, and compare the spectrum with the Reference Spectrum 2 or the spectrum of a solution of Clofibrate RS prepared in the same manner as the sample solution: both spectra exhibit similar intensities of absorption at the same wavelengths.

(2) Determine the infrared absorption spectrum of Clofibrate as directed in the liquid film method under Infrared Spectrophotometry <*2.25*>, and compare the spectrum with the Reference Spectrum or the spectrum of Clofibrate RS: both spectra exhibit similar intensities of absorption at the same wave numbers.

Refractive index <*2.45*> n_D^{20}: 1.500 – 1.505

Specific gravity <*2.56*> d_{20}^{20}: 1.137 – 1.144

Purity **(1)** Acidity—Dissolve 2.0 g of Clofibrate in 100 mL of neutralized ethanol, and add 1 drop of phenolphthalein TS and 0.20 mL of 0.1 mol/L sodium hydroxide VS: the solution is red in color.

(2) Heavy metals <*1.07*>—Proceed with 2.0 g of Clofibrate according to Method 2, and perform the test. Prepare the control solution with 2.0 mL of Standard Lead Solution (not more than 10 ppm).

(3) Arsenic <*1.11*>—To 5.0 g of Clofibrate add 20 mL of nitric acid and 5 mL of sulfuric acid, and heat until white fumes are evolved. After cooling, if necessary, add further 5 mL of nitric acid, heat until white fumes are evolved, and repeat this procedure until the solution is colorless to light yellow. After cooling, add 15 mL of saturated ammonium oxalate solution, and heat again until white fumes are evolved. Cool, add water to make 25 mL, use 5 mL of this solution as the test solution, and perform the test.

Color standard: Prepare a solution according to the above procedure without using Clofibrate as the blank. Transfer 5 mL of the solution to a generator bottle, add 2.0 mL of Standard Arsenic Solution, and then proceed as directed in the test solution (not more than 20 ppm).

(4) *p*-Chlorophenol—To 1.0 g of Clofibrate add exactly 1 mL of the internal standard solution, then add the mobile phase to make 5 mL, and use this solution as the sample solution. Separately, dissolve 10 mg of 4-chlorophenol in a mixture of hexane and 2-propanol (9:1) to make exactly 100 mL. Pipet 10 mL of this solution, and add a mixture of hexane and 2-propanol (9:1) to make exactly 50 mL. Pipet 6 mL of this solution, add exactly 4 mL of the internal standard solution, then add the mobile phase to make 20 mL, and use this solution as the standard solution. Perform the test with 20 μL each of the sample solution and standard solution as directed under Liquid Chromatography <*2.01*> according

to the following conditions, and calculate the ratios, Q_T and Q_S, of the peak area of 4-chlorophenol to that of the internal standard: Q_T is not greater than Q_S.
Internal standard solution—A solution of 4-ethoxyphenol in the mobile phase (1 in 30,000).
Operating conditions—

Detector: An ultraviolet absorption photometer (wavelength: 275 nm).

Column: A stainless steel column about 4 mm in inside diameter and about 30 cm in length, packed with cyanopropylsilanized silica gel for liquid chromatography (5 to 10 μm in particle diameter).

Column temperature: A constant temperature of about 25°C.

Mobile phase: A mixture of hexane, 2-propanol and acetic acid (100) (1970:30:1).

Flow rate: Adjust so that the retention time of clofibrate is about 2 minutes.

Selection of column: Dissolve 10.0 g of Clofibrate, 6 mg of 4-chlorophenol and 6 mg of 4-ethoxyphenol in 1000 mL of hexane. Proceed with 20 μL of this solution under the above operating conditions, and calculate the resolution. Use a column giving elution of clofibrate, 4-chlorophenol and 4-ethoxyphenol in this order, with the resolution between the peaks of clofibrate and 4-chlorophenol is not less than 5, and with the resolution between the peaks of 4-chlorophenol and 4-ethoxyphenol is not less than 2.0.

Water <*2.48*> Not more than 0.2% (5 g, volumetric titration, direct titration).

Residue on ignition <*2.44*> Not more than 0.1% (1 g).

Assay Weigh accurately about 0.5 g of Clofibrate, add exactly 50 mL of 0.1 mol/L potassium hydroxide-ethanol VS, and heat in a water bath under a reflux condenser with a carbon dioxide absorbing tube (soda-lime) for 2 hours with frequent shaking. Cool, and titrate <*2.50*> immediately the excess potassium hydroxide with 0.1 mol/L hydrochloric acid VS (indicator: 3 drops of phenolphthalein TS). Perform a blank determination in the same manner.

Each mL of 0.1 mol/L potassium hydroxide-ethanol VS
= 24.27 mg of $C_{12}H_{15}ClO_3$

Containers and storage Containers—Tight containers.
Storage—Light-resistant.

Clofibrate Capsules

クロフィブラートカプセル

Clofibrate Capsules contain not less than 93.0% and not more than 107.0% of the labeled amount of clofibrate ($C_{12}H_{15}ClO_3$: 242.70).

Method of preparation Prepare as directed under Capsules, with Clofibrate.

Identification Cut and open Clofibrate Capsules, and use the contents as the sample. Determine the absorption spectrum of a solution of the sample in ethanol (99.5) (1 in 10,000) as directed under Ultraviolet-visible Spectrophotometry <*2.24*>: it exhibits a maximum between 278 nm and 282 nm, and it exhibits a maximum between 224 nm and 228 nm after diluting this solution 10 times with ethanol (99.5).

Purity *p*-Chlorophenol—Cut and open not less than 20 Clofibrate Capsules, and proceed with 1.0 g of the well-mixed contents as directed in the Purity (4) under Clofibrate.
Internal standard solution—A solution of 4-ethoxyphenol in the mobile phase (1 in 30,000).

Assay Weigh accurately not less than 20 Clofibrate Capsules, cut and open the capsules, rinse the inside of the capsules with a small amount of diethyl ether after taking out the contents, evaporate the diethyl ether by allowing the capsules to stand at room temperature, and weigh the capsules accurately. Weigh accurately an amount of the contents, equivalent to about 0.1 g of clofibrate ($C_{12}H_{15}ClO_3$), dissolve in acetonitrile to make exactly 100 mL. Pipet 5 mL of this solution, add exactly 5 mL of the internal standard solution, and use this solution as the sample solution. Separately, weigh accurately about 0.1 g of Clofibrate RS, proceed in the same manner as directed for the sample solution, and use the solution so obtained as the standard solution. Perform the test with 10 μL each of the sample solution and standard solution as directed under Liquid Chromatography <*2.01*> according to the following conditions, and calculate the ratios, Q_T and Q_S, of the peak area of clofibrate to that of the internal standard.

Amount (mg) of clofibrate ($C_{12}H_{15}ClO_3$)
$= M_S \times Q_T/Q_S$

M_S: Amount (mg) of Clofibrate RS taken

Internal standard solution—A solution of ibuprofen in the mobile phase (1 in 100).
Operating conditions—

Detector: An ultraviolet absorption photometer (wavelength: 275 nm).

Column: A stainless steel column about 4 mm in inside diameter and about 30 cm in length, packed with octadecylsilanized silica gel for liquid chromatography (5 to 10 μm in particle diameter).

Column temperature: A constant temperature of about 25°C.

Mobile phase: A mixture of acetonitrile and diluted phosphoric acid (1 in 1000) (3:2).

Flow rate: Adjust so that the retention time of clofibrate is about 10 minutes.

Selection of column: Dissolve 0.05 g of clofibrate and 0.3 g of ibuprofen in 50 mL of acetonitrile. Proceed with 10 μL of this solution under the above operating conditions, and calculate the resolution. Use a column giving elution of ibuprofen and clofibrate in this order with the resolution between these peaks being not less than 6.

Containers and storage Containers—Well-closed containers.
Storage—Light-resistant.

Clomifene Citrate

クロミフェンクエン酸塩

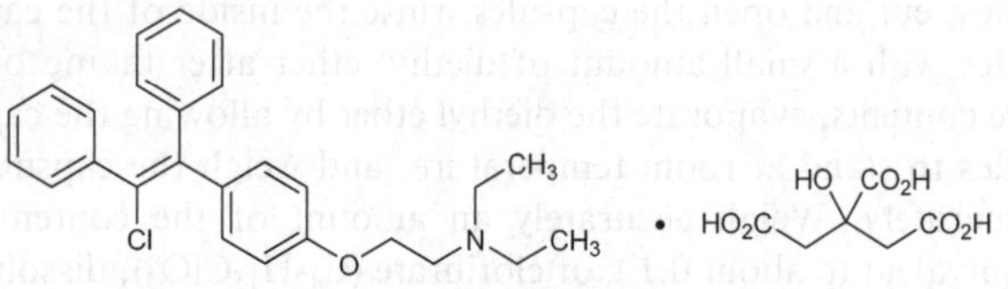

$C_{26}H_{28}ClNO.C_6H_8O_7$: 598.08
2-[4-(2-Chloro-1,2-diphenylvinyl)phenoxy]-*N*,*N*-diethylethylamine monocitrate
[*50-41-9*]

Clomifene Citrate, when dried, contains not less than 98.0% of clomifene citrate ($C_{26}H_{28}ClNO.C_6H_8O_7$).

Description Clomifene Citrate occurs as a white to pale yellow-white powder. It is odorless.

It is freely soluble in methanol and in acetic acid (100), sparingly soluble in ethanol (95), and practically insoluble in diethyl ether.

It gradually changes in color by light.

Melting point: about 115°C

Identification **(1)** To 2 mL of a solution of Clomifene Citrate in methanol (1 in 200) add 2 mL of Reinecke salt TS: a light red precipitate is produced.

(2) Determine the absorption spectrum of a solution of Clomifene Citrate in 0.1 mol/L hydrochloric acid TS (1 in 50,000) as directed under Ultraviolet-visible Spectrophotometry <*2.24*>, and compare the spectrum with the Reference Spectrum or the spectrum of a solution of Clomifene Citrate RS prepared in the same manner as the sample solution: both spectra exhibit similar intensities of absorption at the same wavelengths.

(3) A solution of Clomifene Citrate in methanol (1 in 200) responds to Qualitative Tests <*1.09*> (1) and (2) for citrate salt.

Purity **(1)** Clarity and color of solution—A solution of 1.0 g of Clomifene Citrate in 30 mL of methanol is clear and colorless.

(2) Heavy metals <*1.07*>—Proceed with 2.0 g of Clomifene Citrate according to Method 2, and perform the test. Prepare the control solution with 2.0 mL of Standard Lead Solution (not more than 10 ppm).

Loss on drying <*2.41*> Not more than 1.0% (1 g, in vacuum, phosphorus (V) oxide, 3 hours).

Residue on ignition <*2.44*> Not more than 0.1% (1 g).

Isomer ratio To 10 mg of Clomifene Citrate add 10 mL of water and 1 mL of sodium hydroxide TS, and shake to uniformly disperse. Add 10 mL of ethyl acetate, shake vigorously for 5 minutes, allow to stand for 5 minutes, and use the upper layer as the sample solution. Perform the test with 1 μL of the sample solution as directed under Gas Chromatography <*2.02*> according to the following conditions. Determine the areas of two adjacent peaks, A_a and A_b, having the retention time of about 8 minutes, where A_a is the peak area of shorter retention time and A_b is the peak area of longer retention time: $A_b/(A_a + A_b)$ is between 0.3 and 0.5.

Operating conditions—

Detector: A hydrogen flame-ionization detector.

Column: A fused silica column 0.25 mm in inside diameter and 15 m in length, coated the inside surface with a layer about 0.1 μm thick of dimethylpolysiloxane for gas chromatography.

Column temperature: A constant temperature of about 230°C.

Injection port temperature: A constant temperature of about 270°C.

Detector temperature: A constant temperature of about 300°C.

Carrier gas: Helium.

Flow rate: Adjust so that the retention time of the first peak of clomifene citrate is about 7.5 minutes.

Split ratio: 1:50.

System suitability—

System performance: When the procedure is run with 1 μL of the sample solution under the above operating conditions, the resolution between the two adjacent peaks having the retention time of about 8 minutes is not less than 5.

System repeatability: When the test is repeated 6 times with 1 μL of the sample solution under the above operating conditions, the relative standard deviation of the result of $A_b/(A_a + A_b)$ is not more than 1.0%.

Assay Weigh accurately about 1 g of Clomifene Citrate, previously dried, dissolve in 50 mL of acetic acid (100), and titrate <*2.50*> with 0.1 mol/L perchloric acid VS (indicator: 2 drops of crystal violet TS). Perform a blank determination in the same manner, and make any necessary correction.

Each mL of 0.1 mol/L perchloric acid VS
= 59.81 mg of $C_{26}H_{28}ClNO.C_6H_8O_7$

Containers and storage Containers—Tight containers.
Storage—Light-resistant.

Clomifene Citrate Tablets

クロミフェンクエン酸塩錠

Clomifene Citrate Tablets contain not less than 93.0% and not more than 107.0% of the labeled amount of the clomifene citrate ($C_{26}H_{28}ClNO.C_6H_8O_7$: 598.08).

Method of preparation Prepare as directed under Tablets, with Clomifene Citrate.

Identification Weigh a portion of powdered Clomifene Citrate Tablets, equivalent to 50 mg of Clomifene Citrate, shake vigorously with 50 mL of methanol for 10 minutes, centrifuge, and use the supernatant liquid as the sample solution. Separately, dissolve 10 mg of Clomifene Citrate RS in 10 mL of methanol, and use this solution as the standard solution. Perform the test with these solutions as directed under Thin-layer Chromatography <*2.03*>. Spot 10 μL each of the sample solution and standard solution on a plate of silica gel with fluorescent indicator for thin-layer chromatography. Develop the plate with a mixture of 2-propanol, toluene and diethylamine (10:10:1) to a distance of about 10 cm, and air-dry the plate. Examine under ultraviolet light (main wavelength: 254 nm): the spots from the sample solution and standard solution show the same *Rf* value.

Uniformity of dosage units <*6.02*> Perform the test according to the following method: it meets the requirement of the Content uniformity test.

To 1 tablet of Clomifene Citrate Tablets add 10 mL of water, and shake until the tablets are disintegrated. To this solution add 50 mL of methanol, shake for 10 minutes, and add methanol to make exactly 100 mL. Centrifuge this solution, pipet 4 mL of the supernatant liquid, add methanol to make exactly *V* mL so that each mL contains about 20 μg of clomifene citrate ($C_{26}H_{28}ClNO.C_6H_8O_7$), and use this solution as the sample solution. Proceed as directed in the Assay.

Amount (mg) of clomifene citrate ($C_{26}H_{28}ClNO.C_6H_8O_7$)
$= M_S \times A_T/A_S \times V/100$

M_S: Amount (mg) of Clomifene Citrate RS taken

Dissolution 〈*6.10*〉 When the test is performed at 50 revolutions per minute according to the Paddle method, using 900 mL of 1st fluid for dissolution test as the dissolution medium, the dissolution rate in 30 minutes of Clomifene Citrate Tablets is not less than 80%.

Start the test with 1 tablet of Clomifene Citrate Tablets, withdraw not less than 20 mL of the medium at the specified minute after starting the test, and filter through a membrane filter with a pore size not exceeding 0.45 μm. Discard not less than 10 mL of the first filtrate, pipet *V* mL of the subsequent filtrate, add the dissolution medium to make exactly *V′* mL so that each mL contains about 28 μg of clomifene citrate ($C_{26}H_{28}ClNO.C_6H_8O_7$), and use this solution as the sample solution. Separately, weigh accurately about 28 mg of Clomifene Citrate RS, previously dried in vacuum using phosphorus (V) oxide as a desiccant for 3 hours, and dissolve in methanol to make exactly 50 mL. Pipet 5 mL of this solution, add the dissolution medium to make exactly 100 mL, and use this solution as the standard solution. Determine the absorbances, A_T and A_S, at 291 nm of the sample solution and standard solution as directed under Ultraviolet-visible Spectrophotometry 〈*2.24*〉, using the dissolution medium as the blank.

Dissolution rate (%) with respect to the labeled amount of clomifene citrate ($C_{26}H_{28}ClNO.C_6H_8O_7$)
$= M_S \times A_T/A_S \times V'/V \times 1/C \times 90$

M_S: Amount (mg) of Clomifene Citrate RS taken
C: Labeled amount (mg) of clomifene citrate ($C_{26}H_{28}ClNO.C_6H_8O_7$) in 1 tablet

Assay Weigh accurately, and powder not less than 20 Clomifene Citrate Tablets. Weigh accurately a portion of the powder, equivalent to about 50 mg of clomifene citrate ($C_{26}H_{28}ClNO.C_6H_8O_7$), add 50 mL of methanol, shake for 10 minutes, and add methanol to make exactly 100 mL. Centrifuge a portion of this solution, pipet 4 mL of the supernatant liquid, add methanol to make exactly 100 mL, and use this solution as the sample solution. Separately, weigh accurately about 50 mg of Clomifene Citrate RS, previously dried in a desiccator (in vacuum, phosphorus (V) oxide) for 3 hours, and dissolve in methanol to make exactly 100 mL. Pipet 4 mL of this solution, and dilute with methanol to make exactly 100 mL, and use this solution as the standard solution. Determine the absorbances, A_T and A_S, of the sample solution and the standard solution, respectively, at 295 nm as directed under Ultraviolet-visible Spectrophotometry 〈*2.24*〉.

Amount (mg) of clomifene citrate ($C_{26}H_{28}ClNO.C_6H_8O_7$)
$= M_S \times A_T/A_S$

M_S: Amount (mg) of Clomifene Citrate RS taken

Containers and storage Containers—Tight containers.

Clomipramine Hydrochloride

クロミプラミン塩酸塩

$C_{19}H_{23}ClN_2.HCl$: 351.31
3-(3-Chloro-10,11-dihydro-5*H*-dibenz[*b*,*f*]azepin-5-yl)-*N*,*N*-dimethylpropylamine monohydrochloride
[*17321-77-6*]

Clomipramine Hydrochloride, when dried, contains not less than 98.5% of clomipramine hydrochloride ($C_{19}H_{23}ClN_2.HCl$).

Description Clomipramine Hydrochloride occurs as a white to pale yellow, crystalline powder. It is odorless.

It is very soluble in acetic acid (100), freely soluble in water, in methanol and in chloroform, soluble in ethanol (95), sparingly soluble in acetic anhydride, slightly soluble in acetone, and practically insoluble in ethyl acetate and in diethyl ether.

Identification (1) Dissolve 3 mg of Clomipramine Hydrochloride in 1 mL of nitric acid: a deep blue color develops.

(2) Determine the absorption spectrum of a solution of Clomipramine Hydrochloride in 0.1 mol/L hydrochloric acid TS (3 in 100,000) as directed under Ultraviolet-visible Spectrophotometry 〈*2.24*〉, and compare the spectrum with the Reference Spectrum: both spectra exhibit similar intensities of absorption at the same wavelengths.

(3) Take 1 g of Clomipramine Hydrochloride in a separator, dissolve in 10 mL of water, add 5 mL of sodium hydroxide TS, and extract with two 30-mL portions of diethyl ether [the water layer is used for Identification (4)]. Combine the diethyl ether extracts, add 20 mL of water, and shake. Take diethyl ether layer, dry with a small portion of anhydrous sodium sulfate, and filter. Evaporate the combined extracts by warming on a water bath, and proceed the test with the residue as directed under Flame Coloration Test 〈*1.04*〉 (2): a green color appears.

(4) The solution neutralized by adding dilute nitric acid to the water layer obtained in (3) responds to Qualitative Tests 〈*1.09*〉 for chloride.

pH 〈*2.54*〉 Dissolve 1.0 g of Clomipramine Hydrochloride in 10 mL of water: the pH of this solution is between 3.5 and 5.0.

Melting point 〈*2.60*〉 192 – 196°C

Purity (1) Clarity and color of solution—Dissolve 1.0 g of Clomipramine Hydrochloride in 10 mL of water: the solution is clear and colorless to pale yellow.

(2) Heavy metals 〈*1.07*〉—Proceed with 2.0 g of Clomipramine Hydrochloride according to Method 2, and perform the test. Prepare the control solution with 2.0 mL of Standard Lead Solution (not more than 10 ppm).

(3) Arsenic 〈*1.11*〉—Prepare the test solution with 1.0 g of Clomipramine Hydrochloride according to Method 3, and perform the test (not more than 2 ppm).

(4) Related substances—Dissolve 0.20 g of Clomipramine Hydrochloride in 10 mL of methanol, and use this so-

lution as the sample solution. Separately, weigh 20 mg of Imipramine Hydrochloride, dissolve in methanol to make exactly 100 mL, and use this solution as the standard solution (1). Then pipet 1 mL of the sample solution, and add methanol to make exactly 50 mL. Pipet 5 mL of the solution, add methanol to make exactly 50 mL, and use this solution as the standard solution (2). Perform the test with these solutions as directed under Thin-layer Chromatography <*2.03*>. Spot 5 μL each of the sample solution and standard solutions (1) and (2) on a plate of silica gel for thin-layer chromatography. Develop the plate with a mixture of ethyl acetate, acetone and ammonia solution (28) (15:5:1) to a distance of about 10 cm, and air-dry the plate. Spray evenly potassium dichromate-sulfuric acid TS on the plate: the spot obtained from the sample solution, corresponding to that from the standard solution (1), is not more intense than the spot from the standard solution (1). Each of the spots other than the principal spot and the spot mentioned above from the sample solution is not more intense than the spot from the standard solution (2).

Loss on drying <*2.41*> Not more than 0.5% (1 g, 105°C, 3 hours).

Residue on ignition <*2.44*> Not more than 0.1% (1 g).

Assay Weigh accurately about 0.5 g of Clomipramine Hydrochloride, previously dried, dissolve in 50 mL of a mixture of acetic anhydride and acetic acid (100) (7:3), and titrate <*2.50*> with 0.1 mol/L perchloric acid VS (potentiometric titration). Perform a blank determination in the same manner, and make any necessary correction.

Each mL of 0.1 mol/L perchloric acid VS
= 35.13 mg of $C_{19}H_{23}ClN_2.HCl$

Containers and storage Containers—Well-closed containers.

Storage—Light-resistant.

Clomipramine Hydrochloride Tablets

クロミプラミン塩酸塩錠

Clomipramine Hydrochloride Tablets contain not less than 92.0% and not more than 108.0% of the labeled amount of clomipramine hydrochloride ($C_{19}H_{23}ClN_2.HCl$: 351.31).

Method of preparation Prepare as directed under Tablets, with Clomipramine Hydrochloride.

Identification To a portion of powdered Clomipramine Hydrochloride Tablets, equivalent to 50 mg of Clomipramine Hydrochloride, add a suitable amount of 0.1 mol/L hydrochloric acid TS, shake thoroughly, and add 0.1 mol/L hydrochloric acid TS to make 250 mL. Centrifuge this solution, and to 10 mL of the supernatant liquid add 0.1 mol/L hydrochloric acid TS to make 100 mL. Determine the absorption spectrum of this solution as directed under Ultraviolet-visible Spectrophotometry <*2.24*>: it exhibits a maximum between 250 nm and 254 nm.

Uniformity of dosage unit <*6.02*> Perform the test according to the following method: it meets the requirement of the Content uniformity test.

To 1 tablet of Clomipramine Hydrochloride Tablets add $V/5$ mL of a mixture of methanol and 0.1 mol/L hydrochloric acid TS (3:1), sonicate to disintegrate the tablet, and shake thoroughly for 30 minutes. To this solution add $3V/5$ mL of methanol, shake for 15 minutes, and add methanol to make exactly V mL so that each mL contains about 0.1 mg of clomipramine hydrochloride ($C_{19}H_{23}ClN_2.HCl$). Centrifuge this solution, and use the supernatant liquid as the sample solution. Then, proceed as directed in the Assay.

Amount (mg) of clomipramine hydrochloride ($C_{19}H_{23}ClN_2.HCl$)
$= M_S \times A_T/A_S \times V/250$

M_S: Amount (mg) of clomipramine hydrochloride for assay taken

Dissolution <*6.10*> When the test is performed at 50 revolutions per minute according to the Paddle method, using 900 mL of water as the dissolution medium, the dissolution rates in 45 minutes of 10-mg tablet and in 90 minutes of 25-mg tablet are not less than 80%, respectively.

Start the test with 1 tablet of Clomipramine Hydrochloride Tablets, withdraw not less than 20 mL of the medium at the specified minute after starting the test, and filter through a membrane filter with a pore size not exceeding 0.45 μm. Discard not less than 10 mL of the first filtrate, pipet V mL of the subsequent filtrate, add water to make exactly V' mL so that each mL contains about 11 μg of clomipramine hydrochloride ($C_{19}H_{23}ClN_2.HCl$), and use this solution as the sample solution. Separately, weigh accurately about 28 mg of clomipramine hydrochloride for assay, previously dried at 105°C for 3 hours, and dissolve in water to make exactly 100 mL. Pipet 4 mL of this solution, add water to make exactly 100 mL, and use this solution as the standard solution. Determine the absorbances, A_T and A_S, of the sample solution and standard solution at 252 nm as directed under Ultraviolet-visible Spectrophotometry <*2.24*>.

Dissolution rate (%) with respect to the labeled amount of clomipramine hydrochloride ($C_{19}H_{23}ClN_2.HCl$)
$= M_S \times A_T/A_S \times V'/V \times 1/C \times 36$

M_S: Amount (mg) of clomipramine hydrochloride for assay taken
C: Labeled amount (mg) of clomipramine hydrochloride ($C_{19}H_{23}ClN_2.HCl$) in 1 tablet

Assay Weigh accurately the mass of not less than 20 Clomipramine Hydrochloride Tablets, and powder. Weigh accurately a portion of the powder, equivalent to about 25 mg of clomipramine hydrochloride ($C_{19}H_{23}ClN_2.HCl$), add 50 mL of a mixture of methanol and 0.1 mol/L hydrochloric acid TS (3:1), sonicate, and shake thoroughly for 30 minutes. To this solution add 150 mL of methanol, shake for 15 minutes, and add methanol to make exactly 250 mL. Centrifuge this solution, and use the supernatant liquid as the sample solution. Separately, weigh accurately about 25 mg of clomipramine hydrochloride for assay, previously dried at 105°C for 3 hours, dissolve in 50 mL of a mixture of methanol and 0.1 mol/L hydrochloric acid TS (3:1), add methanol to make exactly 250 mL, and use this solution as the standard solution. Perform the test with exactly 20 μL each of the sample solution and standard solution as directed under Liquid Chromatography <*2.01*> according to the following conditions, and determine the peak areas, A_T and A_S, of clomipramine in each solution.

Amount (mg) of clomipramine hydrochloride ($C_{19}H_{23}ClN_2.HCl$)
$= M_S \times A_T/A_S$

M_S: Amount (mg) of clomipramine hydrochloride for

assay taken

Operating conditions—

Detector: An ultraviolet absorption photometer (wavelength: 254 nm).

Column: A stainless steel column 4.6 mm in inside diameter and 25 cm in length, packed with octadecylsilanized silica gel for liquid chromatography (10 μm in particle diameter).

Column temperature: A constant temperature of about 25°C.

Mobile phase: Dissolve 2 g of sodium 1-octanesulfonate in 300 mL of water, and add 450 mL of methanol, 250 mL of acetonitrile and 1 mL of 0.5 mol/L sulfuric acid TS.

Flow rate: Adjust so that the retention time of clomipramine is about 13 minutes.

System suitability—

System performance: When the procedure is run with 20 μL of the standard solution under the above operating conditions, the number of theoretical plates and the symmetry factor of the peak of clomipramine are not less than 3000 and not more than 1.5, respectively.

System repeatability: When the test is repeated 6 times with 20 μL of the standard solution under the above operating conditions, the relative standard deviation of the peak area of clomipramine is not more than 1.0%.

Containers and storage Containers—Tight containers.

Clonazepam

クロナゼパム

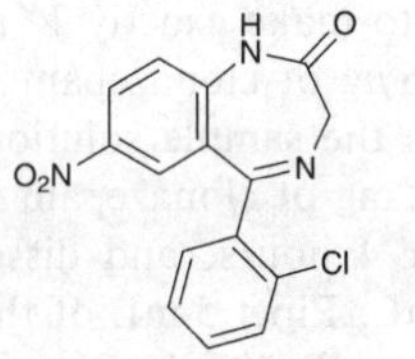

$C_{15}H_{10}ClN_3O_3$: 315.71
5-(2-Chlorophenyl)-7-nitro-1,3-dihydro-2*H*-1,4-benzodiazepin-2-one
[*1622-61-3*]

Clonazepam, when dried, contains not less than 99.0% of clonazepam ($C_{15}H_{10}ClN_3O_3$).

Description Clonazepam occurs as white to light yellow, crystals or crystalline powder.

It is sparingly soluble in acetic anhydride and in acetone, slightly soluble in methanol and in ethanol (95), very slightly soluble in diethyl ether, and practically insoluble in water.

It is gradually colored by light.

Melting point: about 240°C (with decomposition).

Identification (1) Determine the absorption spectrum of a solution of Clonazepam in methanol (1 in 100,000) as directed under Ultraviolet-visible Spectrophotometry <*2.24*>, and compare the spectrum with the Reference Spectrum: both spectra exhibit similar intensities of absorption at the same wavelengths.

(2) Determine the infrared absorption spectrum of Clonazepam, previously dried, as directed in the potassium bromide disk method under Infrared Spectrophotometry <*2.25*>, and compare the spectrum with the Reference Spectrum: both spectra exhibit similar intensities of absorption at the same wave numbers.

(3) Perform the test with Clonazepam as directed under Flame Coloration Test <*1.04*> (2): a green color appears.

Purity (1) Chloride <*1.03*>—To 1.0 g of Clonazepam add 50 mL of water, allow to stand for 1 hour with occasional shaking, and filter. Discard the first 20 mL portion of the filtrate, take the subsequent 20 mL portion of the filtrate, and add 6 mL of dilute nitric acid and water to make 50 mL. Use this solution as the test solution, and perform the test. Prepare the control solution as follows: to 0.25 mL of 0.01 mol/L hydrochloric acid VS add 6 mL of dilute nitric acid and water to make 50 mL (not more than 0.022%).

(2) Heavy metals <*1.07*>—Proceed with 1.0 g of Clonazepam according to Method 4, and perform the test. Prepare the control solution with 2.0 mL of Standard Lead Solution (not more than 20 ppm).

(3) Related substances—Dissolve 0.25 g of Clonazepam in 10 mL of acetone, and use this solution as the sample solution. Pipet 1 mL of the sample solution, add acetone to make exactly 100 mL, then pipet 1 mL of this solution, add acetone to make exactly 10 mL, and use this solution as the standard solution. Perform the test with these solutions as directed under Thin-layer Chromatography <*2.03*>. Spot 10 μL each of the sample solution and standard solution on a plate of silica gel with fluorescent indicator for thin-layer chromatography. Develop the plate with a mixture of nitromethane and acetone (10:1) to a distance of about 12 cm, and air-dry the plate. Examine under ultraviolet light (main wavelength: 254 nm): the spots other than the principal spot obtained from the sample solution are not more intense than the spot from the standard solution.

Loss on drying <*2.41*> Not more than 0.30% (1 g, 105°C, 4 hours).

Residue on ignition <*2.44*> Not more than 0.1% (1 g).

Assay Weigh accurately about 0.5 g of Clonazepam, previously dried, dissolve in 70 mL of acetic anhydride, and titrate <*2.50*> with 0.1 mol/L perchloric acid VS (potentiometric titration). Perform a blank determination in the same manner, and make any necessary correction.

Each mL of 0.1 mol/L perchloric acid VS
= 31.57 mg of $C_{15}H_{10}ClN_3O_3$

Containers and storage Containers—Well-closed containers.

Storage—Light-resistant.

Clonazepam Fine Granules

クロナゼパム細粒

Clonazepam Fine Granules contain not less than 95.0% and not more than 105.0% of the labeled amount of clonazepam ($C_{15}H_{10}ClN_3O_3$: 315.71).

Method of preparation Prepare as directed under Granules, with Clonazepam.

Identification Powder Clonazepam Fine Granules. To a portion of the powder, equivalent to 1 mg of Clonazepam, add an appropriate volume of methanol and shake for 10 minutes, add methanol to make 100 mL, and filter. Determine the absorption spectrum of the filtrate as directed under Ultraviolet-visible Spectrophotometry <*2.24*>: it exhibits a maximum between 307 nm and 311 nm.

Dissolution Being specified separately when the drug is granted approval based on the Law.

Assay Powder Clonazepam Fine Granules. Weigh accurately a portion of the powder, equivalent to about 2.4 mg of clonazepam ($C_{15}H_{10}ClN_3O_3$), add exactly 30 mL of a mixture of methanol and water (7:3), and shake for 15 minutes. Centrifuge this solution, pipet 5 mL of the supernatant liquid, add a mixture of methanol and water (7:3) to make exactly 20 mL, and use this solution as the sample solution. Separately, weigh accurately about 20 mg of clonazepam for assay, previously dried at 105°C for 4 hours, dissolve in methanol to make exactly 50 mL. Pipet 5 mL of this solution, add a mixture of methanol and water (7:3) to make exactly 100 mL, and use this solution as the standard solution. Perform the test with exactly 15 μL each of the sample solution and standard solution as directed under Liquid Chromatography <2.01> according to the following conditions, and determine the peak areas, A_T and A_S, of clonazepam in each solution.

Amount (mg) of clonazepam ($C_{15}H_{10}ClN_3O_3$)
$= M_S \times A_T/A_S \times 3/25$

M_S: Amount (mg) of clonazepam for assay taken

Operating conditions—

Detector: An ultraviolet absorption photometer (wavelength: 310 nm).

Column: A stainless steel column 4.6 mm in inside diameter and 15 cm in length, packed with octadecylsilanized silica gel for liquid chromatography (5 μm in particle diameter).

Column temperature: A constant temperature of about 25°C.

Mobile phase: A mixture of water, acetonitrile and methanol (4:3:3).

Flow rate: Adjust so that the retention time of clonazepam is about 5 minutes.

System suitability—

System performance: When the procedure is run with 15 μL of the standard solution under the above operating conditions, the number of theoretical plates and the symmetry factor of the peak of clonazepam are not less than 3000 and not more than 1.5, respectively.

System repeatability: When the test is repeated 6 times with 15 μL of the standard solution under the above operating conditions, the relative standard deviation of the peak area of clonazepam is not more than 1.0%.

Containers and storage Containers—Tight containers.
Storage—Light-resistant.

Clonazepam Tablets

クロナゼパム錠

Clonazepam Tablets contain not less than 95.0% and not more than 105.0% of the labeled amount of clonazepam ($C_{15}H_{10}ClN_3O_3$: 315.71).

Method of preparation Prepare as directed under Tablets, with Clonazepam.

Identification Powder Clonazepam Tablets. To a portion of the powder, equivalent to 1 mg of Clonazepam, add an appropriate volume of methanol and shake for 10 minutes, then add methanol to make 100 mL, and filter. Determine the absorption spectrum of the filtrate as directed under Ultraviolet-visible Spectrophotometry <2.24>: it exhibits a maximum between 307 nm and 311 nm.

Uniformity of dosage units <6.02> Perform the test according to the following method: it meets the requirement of the Content uniformity test.

To 1 tablet of Clonazepam Tablets, add $V/10$ mL of methanol, shake for 15 minutes, add 2-propanol to make exactly V mL so that each mL contains about 10 μg of clonazepam ($C_{15}H_{10}ClN_3O_3$). Filter this solution through a membrane filter with a pore size not exceeding 0.45 μm. Discard the first 10 mL of the filtrate, and use the subsequent filtrate as the sample solution. Separately, weigh accurately about 20 mg of clonazepam for assay, previously dried at 105°C for 4 hours, dissolve in methanol to make exactly 200 mL. Pipet 10 mL of this solution, add 2-propanol to make exactly 100 mL, and use this solution as the standard solution. Determine the absorbances, A_T and A_S, at 312 nm of the sample solution and standard solution as directed under Ultraviolet-visible Spectrophotometry <2.24>, using a mixture of 2-propanol and methanol (9:1) as the control.

Amount (mg) of clonazepam ($C_{15}H_{10}ClN_3O_3$)
$= M_S \times A_T/A_S \times V/2000$

M_S: Amount (mg) of clonazepam for assay taken

Dissolution <6.10> When the test is performed at 50 revolutions per minute according to the Paddle method, using 900 mL of water as the dissolution medium, the dissolution rate in 30 minutes of 0.5-mg tablet and 1-mg tablet is not less than 80%, and that of 2-mg tablet is not less than 75%.

Start the test with 1 tablet of Clonazepam Tablets, withdraw not less than 20 mL of the medium at the specified minute after starting the test, and filter through a membrane filter with a pore size not exceeding 0.45 μm. Discard not less then 10 mL of the first filtrate, pipet V mL of the subsequent filtrate, add water to make exactly V' mL so that each mL contains about 0.56 μg of clonazepam ($C_{15}H_{10}ClN_3O_3$), and use this solution as the sample solution. Separately, weigh accurately about 22 mg of clonazepam for assay, previously dried at 105°C for 4 hours, and dissolve in methanol to make exactly 100 mL. Pipet 5 mL of this solution, and add methanol to make exactly 50 mL. Pipet 5 mL of this solution and add water to make exactly 200 mL, and use this solution as the standard solution. Perform the test with exactly 100 μL each of the sample solution and standard solution as directed under Liquid Chromatography <2.01> according to the following conditions, and determine the peak areas, A_T and A_S, of clonazepam in each solution.

Dissolution rate (%) with respect to the labeled amount of clonazepam ($C_{15}H_{10}ClN_3O_3$)
$= M_S \times A_T/A_S \times V'/V \times 1/C \times 9/4$

M_S: Amount (mg) of clonazepam for assay taken
C: Labeled amount (mg) of clonazepam ($C_{15}H_{10}ClN_3O_3$) in 1 tablet

Operating conditions—

Proceed as directed in the operating conditions in the Assay.

System suitability—

System performance: When the procedure is run with 100 μL of the standard solution under the above operating conditions, the number of theoretical plates and the symmetry factor of the peak of clonazepam are not less than 2000 and not more than 2.0, respectively.

System repeatability: When the test is repeated 6 times with 100 μL of the standard solution under the above operating conditions, the relative standard deviation of the peak area of clonazepam is not more than 2.0%.

Assay Weigh accurately the mass of not less than 20

Clonazepam Tablets, and powder. Weigh accurately a portion of the powder, equivalent to about 2.5 mg of clonazepam ($C_{15}H_{10}ClN_3O_3$), add exactly 50 mL of a mixture of methanol and water (7:3), and shake for 15 minutes. Centrifuge this solution, and use the supernatant liquid as the sample solution. Separately, weigh accurately about 25 mg of clonazepam for assay, previously dried at 105°C for 4 hours, dissolve in methanol to make exactly 25 mL. Pipet 5 mL of this solution, add a mixture of methanol and water (7:3) to make exactly 100 mL, and use this solution as the standard solution. Perform the test with exactly 10 μL each of the sample solution and standard solution as directed under Liquid Chromatography *<2.01>* according to the following conditions, and determine the peak areas, A_T and A_S, of clonazepam in each solution.

Amount (mg) of clonazepam ($C_{15}H_{10}ClN_3O_3$)
$= M_S \times A_T/A_S \times 1/10$

M_S: Amount (mg) of clonazepam for assay taken

Operating conditions—

Detector: An ultraviolet absorption photometer (wavelength: 310 nm).

Column: A stainless steel column 4.6 mm in inside diameter and 15 cm in length, packed with octadecylsilanized silica gel for liquid chromatography (5 μm in particle diameter).

Column temperature: A constant temperature of about 25°C.

Mobile phase: A mixture of water, acetonitrile and methanol (4:3:3).

Flow rate: Adjust so that the retention time of clonazepam is about 5 minutes.

System suitability—

System performance: When the procedure is run with 10 μL of the standard solution under the above operating conditions, the number of theoretical plates and the symmetry factor of the peak of clonazepam are not less than 3000 and not more than 1.5, respectively.

System repeatability: When the test is repeated 6 times with 10 μL of the standard solution under the above operating conditions, the relative standard deviation of the peak area of clonazepam is not more than 1.0%.

Containers and storage Containers—Tight containers.
Storage—Light-resistant.

Clonidine Hydrochloride

クロニジン塩酸塩

$C_9H_9Cl_2N_3.HCl$: 266.55
2-(2,6-Dichlorophenylimino)imidazolidine monohydrochloride
[*4205-91-8*]

Clonidine Hydrochloride, when dried, contains not less than 99.0% of clonidine hydrochloride ($C_9H_9Cl_2N_3.HCl$).

Description Clonidine Hydrochloride occurs as white, crystals or crystalline powder.

It is freely soluble in methanol, soluble in water and in ethanol (95), slightly soluble in acetic acid (100), and practically insoluble in acetic anhydride and in diethyl ether.

Identification **(1)** To 5 mL of a solution of Clonidine Hydrochloride (1 in 1000) add 6 drops of Dragendorff's TS: an orange precipitate is formed.

(2) Determine the absorption spectrum of a solution of Clonidine Hydrochloride in 0.01 mol/L hydrochloric acid TS (3 in 10,000) as directed under Ultraviolet-visible Spectrophotometry *<2.24>*, and compare the spectrum with the Reference Spectrum: both spectra exhibit similar intensities of absorption at the same wavelengths.

(3) Determine the infrared absorption spectrum of Clonidine Hydrochloride, previously dried, as directed in the potassium chloride disk method under Infrared Spectrophotometry *<2.25>*, and compare the spectrum with the Reference Spectrum: both spectra exhibit similar intensities of absorption at the same wave numbers.

(4) A solution of Clonidine Hydrochloride (1 in 50) responds to Qualitative Tests *<1.09>* for chloride.

pH *<2.54>* Dissolve 1.0 g of Clonidine Hydrochloride in 20 mL of water: the pH of this solution is between 4.0 and 5.5.

Purity **(1)** Clarity and color of solution—Dissolve 1.0 g of Clonidine Hydrochloride in 20 mL of water: the solution is clear and colorless.

(2) Heavy metals *<1.07>*—Proceed with 2.0 g of Clonidine Hydrochloride according to Method 1, and perform the test. Prepare the control solution with 2.0 mL of Standard Lead Solution (not more than 10 ppm).

(3) Arsenic *<1.11>*—Prepare the test solution with 0.5 g of Clonidine Hydrochloride according to Method 3, and perform the test (not more than 4 ppm).

(4) Related substances—Dissolve 0.20 g of Clonidine Hydrochloride in 2 mL of methanol, and use this solution as the sample solution. Pipet 1 mL of the sample solution, and add methanol to make exactly 100 mL. Pipet 1 mL and 2 mL of this solution, to each add methanol to make exactly 20 mL, and use these solutions as the standard solution (1) and the standard solution (2), respectively. Perform the test with these solutions as directed under Thin-layer Chromatography *<2.03>*. Spot 2 μL each of the sample solution and standard solutions (1) and (2) on a plate of silica gel for thin-layer chromatography. Develop the plate with a mixture of toluene, 1,4-dioxane, ethanol (99.5) and ammonia solution (28) (10:8:2:1) to a distance of about 12 cm, air-dry the plate, and then dry at 100°C for 1 hour. Spray evenly sodium hypochlorite TS on the plate, air-dry the plate for 15 minutes, and then spray evenly potassium iodide starch TS on the plate: the spots other than the principal spot and the spot of the starting point obtained from the sample solution are not more intense than the spot from the standard solution (2), and the numbers of spots other than the principal spot and the spot of the starting point, which are more intense than the spot from the standard solution (1), are not more than 3.

Loss on drying *<2.41>* Not more than 0.5% (1 g, 105°C, 4 hours).

Residue on ignition *<2.44>* Not more than 0.1% (1 g).

Assay Weigh accurately about 0.4 g of Clonidine Hydrochloride, previously dried, and dissolve in 30 mL of acetic acid (100) by warming. After cooling, add 70 mL of acetic anhydride, and titrate *<2.50>* with 0.1 mol/L perchloric acid VS (potentiometric titration). Perform a blank determination in the same manner, and make any necessary correction.

Each mL of 0.1 mol/L perchloric acid VS
= 26.66 mg of $C_9H_9Cl_2N_3.HCl$

Containers and storage Containers—Tight containers.

Cloperastine Fendizoate

クロペラスチンフェンジゾ酸塩

and enantiomer

$C_{20}H_{24}ClNO.C_{20}H_{14}O_4$: 648.19
1-{2-[(*RS*)-(4-Chlorophenyl)(phenyl)methoxy]ethyl}piperidine mono{2-[(6-hydroxybiphenyl-3-yl)carbonyl]benzoate}
[85187-37-7]

Cloperastine Fendizoate, when dried, contains not less than 99.0% and not more than 101.0% of cloperastine fendizoate ($C_{20}H_{24}ClNO.\ C_{20}H_{14}O_4$).

Description Cloperastine Fendizoate occurs as white, crystals or crystalline powder.

It is freely soluble in isopropylamine, slightly soluble in methanol, in ethanol (99.5) and in acetic acid (100), and practically insoluble in water.

A solution of Cloperastine Fendizoate in isopropylamine (1 in 20) shows no optical rotation.

Identification **(1)** Determine the absorption spectrum of a solution of Cloperastine Fendizoate in methanol (3 in 200,000) as directed under Ultraviolet-visible Spectrophotometry *<2.24>*, and compare the spectrum with the Reference Spectrum: both spectra exhibit similar intensities of absorption at the same wavelengths.

(2) Determine the infrared absorption spectrum of Cloperastine Fendizoate as directed in the potassium bromide disk method under Infrared Spectrophotometry *<2.25>*, and compare the spectrum with the Reference Spectrum: both spectra exhibit similar intensities of absorption at the same wave numbers.

Melting point *<2.60>* 186 - 190°C

Purity **(1)** Chloride *<1.03>*—To 2.0 g of Cloperastine Fendizoate add 50 mL of water, warm at 70°C for 5 minutes, cool, and filter. To 25 mL of the filtrate add 6 mL of dilute nitric acid and water to make 50 mL. Perform the test using this solution as the test solution. Prepare the control solution with 0.40 mL of 0.01 mol/L hydrochloric acid VS (not more than 0.014%).

(2) Heavy metals *<1.07>*—Proceed with 1.0 g of Cloperastine Fendizoate according to Method 2, and perform the test. Prepare the control solution with 2.0 mL of Standard Lead Solution (not more than 20 ppm).

(3) 4-Chlorobenzophenone—Dissolve exactly 25 mg of Cloperastine Fendizoate in the mobile phase A to make exactly 50 mL, and use this solution as the sample solution. Separately, dissolve exactly 25 mg of 4-chlorobenzophenone in the mobile phase A to make exactly 200 mL. Pipet 1 mL of this solution, add the mobile phase A to make exactly 100 mL, and use this solution as the standard solution. Perform the test with exactly 20 μL each of the sample solution and standard solution as directed under Liquid Chromatography *<2.01>* according to the following conditions, and determine the peak areas of 4-chlorobenzophenone by the automatic integration method: the peak area of 4-chlorobenzophenone obtained from the sample solution is not larger than that from the standard solution.

Operating conditions—

Detector: An ultraviolet absorption photometer (wavelength: 226 nm).

Column: A stainless steel column 4.6 mm in inside diameter and 15 cm in length, packed with octadecylsilanized silica gel for liquid chromatography (5 μm in particle diameter).

Column temperature: A constant temperature of about 25°C.

Mobile phase A: A mixture of 0.1 mol/L potassium dihydrogen phosphate TS, acetonitrile for liquid chromatography and perchloric acid (400:320:1).

Mobile phase B: A mixture of acetonitrile for liquid chromatography, 0.1 mol/L potassium dihydrogen phosphate TS and perchloric acid (1050:450:1).

Flowing of mobile phase: Control the gradient by mixing the mobile phases A and B as directed in the following table.

Time after injection of sample (min)	Mobile phase A (vol%)	Mobile phase B (vol%)
0 - 12	100	0
12 - 22	100 → 0	0 → 100

Flow rate: 1.2 mL per minute.

System suitability—

Test for required detectability: Pipet 2 mL of the standard solution, and add the mobile phase A to make exactly 10 mL. Confirm that the peak area of 4-chlorobenzophenone obtained with 20 μL of this solution is equivalent to 14 to 26% of that with 20 μL of the standard solution.

System performance: When the procedure is run with 20 μL of the standard solution under the above operating conditions, the number of theoretical plates and the symmetry factor of the peak of 4-chlorobenzophenone are not less than 10,000 and not more than 2.0, respectively.

System repeatability: When the test is repeated 6 times with 20 μL of the standard solution under the above operating conditions, the relative standard deviation of the peak area of 4-chlorobenzophenone is not more than 2.0%.

Loss on drying *<2.41>* Not more than 0.5% (1 g, 105°C, 3 hours).

Residue on ignition *<2.44>* Not more than 0.1% (1 g).

Assay Weigh accurately about 1 g of dried Cloperastine Fendizoate, add 100 mL of acetic acid (100), warm to dissolve, cool, and titrate *<2.50>* with 0.1 mol/L perchloric acid VS (potentiometric titration). Perform a blank determination in the same manner, and make any necessary correction.

Each mL of 0.1 mol/L perchloric acid VS
= 64.82 mg of $C_{20}H_{24}ClNO.C_{20}H_{14}O_4$

Containers and storage Containers—Well-closed containers.

Cloperastine Fendizoate Tablets

クロペラスチンフェンジゾ酸塩錠

Cloperastine Fendizoate Tablets contain not less than 95.0% and not more than 105.0% of the labeled amount of cloperastine fendizoate ($C_{20}H_{24}ClNO.C_{20}H_{14}O_4$: 648.19).

Method of preparation Prepare as directed under Tablets, with Cloperastine Fendizoate.

Identification To a quantity of powdered Cloperastine Fendizoate Tablets, equivalent to 1.5 mg of Cloperastine Fendizoate, add methanol, shake thoroughly, add methanol to make 100 mL, and filter. Determine the absorption spectrum of the filtrate as directed under Ultraviolet-visible Spectrophotometry <*2.24*>: it exhibits maxima between 248 nm and 252 nm, and between 282 nm and 286 nm.

Uniformity of dosage units <*6.02*> Perform the test according to the following method: it meets the requirement of the Content uniformity test.

To 1 tablet of Cloperastine Fendizoate Tablets add exactly $V/10$ mL of the internal standard solution, add the mobile phase, shake vigorously until the tablet is disintegrated, add the mobile phase to make V mL so that each mL contains about 88 μg of cloperastine fendizoate ($C_{20}H_{24}ClNO.C_{20}H_{14}O_4$), and filter through a membrane filter with a pore size not exceeding 0.45 μm. Discard the first 10 mL of the filtrate, and use the subsequent filtrate as the sample solution. Then, proceed as directed in the Assay.

Amount (mg) of cloperastine fendizoate ($C_{20}H_{24}ClNO.C_{20}H_{14}O_4$)
$= M_S \times Q_T/Q_S \times V/250$

M_S: Amount (mg) of cloperastine fendizoate for assay taken

Internal standard solution—A solution of ethyl parahydroxybenzoate in the mobile phase (3 in 2000).

Dissolution <*6.10*> When the test is performed at 50 revolutions per minute according to the Paddle method, using 900 mL of 1st fluid for dissolution test as the dissolution medium, the dissolution rate in 90 minutes of Cloperastine Fendizoate Tablets is not less than 75%.

Start the test with 1 tablet of Cloperastine Fendizoate Tablets, withdraw not less than 20 mL of the medium at the specified minute after starting the test, and filter through a membrane filter with a pore size not exceeding 0.45 μm. Discard not less than 10 mL of the first filtrate, pipet V mL of the subsequent filtrate, add the dissolution medium to make exactly V' mL so that each mL contains about 4.9 μg of cloperastine fendizoate ($C_{20}H_{24}ClNO.C_{20}H_{14}O_4$), and use this solution as the sample solution. Separately, weigh accurately about 25 mg of cloperastine fendizoate for assay, previously dried at 105°C for 3 hours, and dissolve in methanol to make exactly 200 mL. Pipet 4 mL of this solution, add the dissolution medium to make exactly 100 mL, and use this solution as the standard solution. Perform the test with exactly 10 μL each of the sample solution and standard solution as directed under Liquid Chromatography <*2.01*> according to the following conditions, and determine the peak areas, A_T and A_S, of cloperastine in each solution.

Dissolution rate (%) with respect to the labeled amount of cloperastine fendizoate ($C_{20}H_{24}ClNO.C_{20}H_{14}O_4$)
$= M_S \times A_T/A_S \times V'/V \times 1/C \times 18$

M_S: Amount (mg) of cloperastine fendizoate for assay taken

C: Labeled amount (mg) of cloperastine fendizoate ($C_{20}H_{24}ClNO.C_{20}H_{14}O_4$) in 1 tablet

Operating conditions—

Proceed as directed in the operating conditions in the Assay.

System suitability—

System performance: When the procedure is run with 10 μL of the standard solution under the above operating conditions, fendizoic acid and cloperastine are eluted in this order with the resolution between these peaks being not less than 6.

System repeatability: When the test is repeated 6 times with 10 μL of the standard solution under the above operating conditions, the relative standard deviation of the peak area of cloperastine is not more than 2.0%.

Assay Weigh accurately the mass of not less than 20 tablets of Cloperastine Fendizoate Tablets, and powder. Weigh accurately a portion of the powder, equivalent to about 4.4 mg of cloperastine fendizoate ($C_{20}H_{24}ClNO.C_{20}H_{14}O_4$), add exactly 5 mL of the internal standard solution, add 20 mL of the mobile phase, shake vigorously for 10 minutes, then add the mobile phase to make 50 mL, and filter through a membrane filter with a pore size not exceeding 0.45 μm. Discard the first 10 mL of the filtrate and use the subsequent filtrate as the sample solution. Separately, weigh accurately about 22 mg of cloperastine fendizoate for assay, previously dried at 105°C for 3 hours, and dissolve in the mobile phase to make exactly 50 mL. Pipet 10 mL of this solution, add exactly 5 mL of the internal standard solution, add the mobile phase to make 50 mL, and use this solution as the standard solution. Perform the test with exactly 20 μL each of the sample solution and standard solution as directed under Liquid Chromatography <*2.01*>, and calculate the ratios, Q_T and Q_S, of the peak area of cloperastine to that of the internal standard.

Amount (mg) of cloperastine fendizoate ($C_{20}H_{24}ClNO.C_{20}H_{14}O_4$)
$= M_S \times Q_T/Q_S \times 1/5$

M_S: Amount (mg) of cloperastine fendizoate for assay taken

Internal standard solution—A solution of ethyl parahydroxybenzoate in the mobile phase (3 in 2000).

Operating conditions—

Detector: An ultraviolet absorption photometer (wavelength: 226 nm).

Column: A stainless steel column 4.6 mm in inside diameter and 15 cm in length, packed with octadecylsilanized silica gel for liquid chromatography (5 μm in particle diameter).

Column temperature: A constant temperature of about 25°C.

Mobile phase: A mixture of 0.1 mol/L potassium dihydrogen phosphate TS, acetonitrile for liquid chromatography and perchloric acid (400:320:1).

Flow rate: Adjust so that the retention time of cloperastine is about 8 minutes.

System suitability—

System performance: When the procedure is run with 20 μL of the standard solution under the above operating conditions, the internal standard, fendizoic acid and cloperastine are eluted in this order, and each resolution between these peaks is not less than 5, respectively.

System repeatability: When the test is repeated 6 times with 20 μL of the standard solution under the above operating conditions, the relative standard deviation of the ratio of the peak area of cloperastine to that of the internal standard is not more than 1.0%.

Containers and storage Containers—Tight containers.

Cloperastine Hydrochloride

クロペラスチン塩酸塩

• HCl

and enantiomer

$C_{20}H_{24}ClNO.HCl$: 366.32
1-{2-[(*RS*)-(4-Chlorophenyl)(phenyl)methoxy]ethyl}piperidine monohydrochloride
[*14984-68-0*]

Cloperastine Hydrochloride, when dried, contains not less than 98.5% of cloperastine hydrochloride ($C_{20}H_{24}ClNO.HCl$).

Description Cloperastine Hydrochloride occurs as white, crystals or crystalline powder.

It is very soluble in water, in methanol, in ethanol (95) and in acetic acid (100), and soluble in acetic anhydride.

A solution of Cloperastine Hydrochloride (1 in 10) shows no optical rotation.

Identification **(1)** Determine the absorption spectrum of a solution of Cloperastine Hydrochloride in 0.1 mol/L hydrochloric acid TS (1 in 2500) as directed under Ultraviolet-visible Spectrophotometry <*2.24*>, and compare the spectrum with the Reference Spectrum 1: both spectra exhibit similar intensities of absorption at the same wavelengths. Separately, determine the absorption spectrum of a solution of Cloperastine Hydrochloride in 0.1 mol/L hydrochloric acid TS (1 in 62,500) as directed under Ultraviolet-visible Spectrophotometry <*2.24*>, and compare the spectrum with the Reference Spectrum 2: both spectra exhibit similar intensities of absorption at the same wavelengths.

(2) Determine the infrared absorption spectrum of Cloperastine Hydrochloride, previously dried, as directed in the potassium chloride disk method under Infrared Spectrophotometry <*2.25*>, and compare the spectrum with the Reference Spectrum: both spectra exhibit similar intensities of absorption at the same wave numbers.

(3) Shake 10 mL of a solution of Cloperastine Hydrochloride (1 in 100) with 2 mL of ammonia TS and 20 mL of diethyl ether, separate the water layer, wash the water layer with 20 mL of diethyl ether, and filter. Acidify the filtrate with dilute nitric acid: the solution responds to Qualitative Tests <*1.09*> for chloride.

Melting point <*2.60*> 149 - 153°C

Purity **(1)** Heavy metals <*1.07*>—Proceed with 1.0 g of Cloperastine Hydrochloride according to Method 2, and perform the test. Prepare the control solution with 2.0 mL of Standard Lead Solution (not more than 20 ppm).

(2) Related substances—Dissolve 40 mg of Cloperastine Hydrochloride in 50 mL of the mobile phase, and use this solution as the sample solution. Pipet 1 mL of the sample solution, add the mobile phase to make exactly 200 mL, and use this solution as the standard solution. Perform the test with exactly 20 μL each of the sample solution and standard solution as directed under Liquid Chromatography <*2.01*> according to the following conditions, and determine each peak area by the automatic integration method: the area of the peaks, having the relative retention times of about 0.8 and about 3.0 to cloperastine obtained from the sample solution are not larger than the peak area of cloperastine from the standard solution, and the area of the peak having the relative retention time about 2.0 from the sample solution is not larger than 5/3 times the peak area of cloperastine from the standard solution. The area of the peak other than cloperastine and the peaks mentioned above from the sample solution are not larger than 3/5 times the peak area of cloperastine from the standard solution, and the total area of these peaks is not larger than 2 times the peak area of cloperastine from the standard solution.

Operating conditions—

Detector: An ultraviolet absorption photometer (wavelength: 222 nm).

Column: A stainless steel column 4.6 mm in inside diameter and 15 cm in length, packed with octadecylsilanized silica gel for liquid chromatography (5 μm in particle diameter).

Column temperature: A constant temperature of about 25°C.

Mobile phase: A mixture of methanol, 0.1 mol/L potassium dihydrogen phosphate TS and perchloric acid (500:250:1).

Flow rate: Adjust so that the retention time of cloperastine is about 7 minutes.

Time span of measurement: About 4 times as long as the retention time of cloperastine, beginning after the solvent peak.

System suitability—

Test for required detectability: Pipet 2 mL of the standard solution, add the mobile phase to make exactly 20 mL. Confirm that the peak area of cloperastine obtained with 20 μL of this solution is equivalent to 7 to 13% of that with 20 μL of the standard solution.

System performance: Dissolve 30 mg of Cloperastine Hydrochloride and 40 mg of benzophenone in 100 mL of the mobile phase. To 2 mL of this solution add the mobile phase to make 50 mL. When the procedure is run with 20 μL of this solution under the above operating conditions, cloperastine and benzophenone are eluted in this order with the resolution between these peaks being not less than 6.

System repeatability: When the test is repeated 6 times with 20 μL of the standard solution under the above operating conditions, the relative standard deviation of the peak area of cloperastine is not more than 2.0%.

Loss on drying <*2.41*> Not more than 0.5% (1 g, 105°C, 3 hours).

Residue on ignition <*2.44*> Not more than 0.1% (1 g).

Assay Weigh accurately about 0.5 g of Cloperastine Hydrochloride, previously dried, dissolve in 70 mL of a mixture of acetic anhydride and acetic acid (100) (7:3), and titrate <*2.50*> with 0.1 mol/L perchloric acid VS (potentiometric titration). Perform a blank determination in the same manner, and make any necessary correction.

Each mL of 0.1 mol/L perchloric acid VS
= 36.63 mg of $C_{20}H_{24}ClNO.HCl$

Containers and storage Containers—Tight containers.
Storage—Light-resistant.

Clopidogrel Sulfate

クロピドグレル硫酸塩

$C_{16}H_{16}ClNO_2S.H_2SO_4$: 419.90
Methyl (2*S*)-2-(2-chlorophenyl)-2-[6,7-dihydrothieno[3,2-*c*]pyridin-5(4*H*)-yl]acetate monosulfate
[*120202-66-6*]

Clopidogrel Sulfate contains not less than 97.0% and not more than 101.5% of clopidogrel sulfate ($C_{16}H_{16}ClNO_2S.H_2SO_4$), calculated on the anhydrous basis.

Description Clopidogrel Sulfate occurs as a white to pale yellow-white, crystalline powder or powder.

It is freely soluble in water and in methanol, and soluble in ethanol (99.5).

It gradually develops a brown color on exposure to light.

Melting point: about 177°C (with decomposition).

It shows crystal polymorphism.

Identification **(1)** Determine the absorption spectrum of a solution of Clopidogrel Sulfate in methanol (3 in 10,000) as directed under Ultraviolet-visible Spectrophotometry *<2.24>*, and compare the spectrum with the Reference Spectrum or the spectrum of a solution of Clopidogrel Sulfate RS prepared in the same manner as the sample solution: both spectra exhibit similar intensities of absorption at the same wavelengths.

(2) Determine the infrared absorption spectrum of Clopidogrel Sulfate as directed in the potassium bromide disk method under Infrared Spectrophotometry *<2.25>*, and compare the spectrum with the Reference Spectrum or the spectrum of Clopidogrel Sulfate RS: both spectra exhibit similar intensities of absorption at the same wave numbers. If any difference appears between the spectra, dissolve Clopidogrel Sulfate, or each of Clopidogrel Sulfate and Clopidogrel Sulfate RS in ethanol (99.5), respectively. Then evaporate the ethanol to dryness, and repeat the test on the residues dried in vacuum.

(3) Perform the test with Clopidogrel Sulfate as directed under Flame Coloration Test *<1.04>* (2): a green color appears.

(4) A solution of Clopidogrel Sulfate in a mixture of water and methanol (1:1) (1 in 100) responds to Qualitative Tests *<1.09>* (1) for sulfate.

Purity **(1)** Heavy metals *<1.07>*—Proceed with 1.0 g of Clopidogrel Sulfate according to Method 4, and perform the test. Prepare the control solution with 2.0 mL of Standard Lead Solution (not more than 20 ppm).

(2) Related substances—Dissolve 65 mg of Clopidogrel Sulfate in 10 mL of a mixture of acetonitrile for liquid chromatography and mobile phase A (3:2), and use this solution as the sample solution. Pipet 2 mL of the sample solution, and add a mixture of acetonitrile for liquid chromatography and the mobile phase A (3:2) to make exactly 100 mL. Pipet 2.5 mL of this solution, add a mixture of acetonitrile for liquid chromatography and the mobile phase A (3:2) to make exactly 50 mL, and use this solution as the standard solution. Perform the test with exactly 10 μL each of the sample solution and standard solution as directed under Liquid Chromatography *<2.01>* according to the following conditions, and determine each peak area by the automatic integration method: the area of the peak, having the relative retention time of about 0.5 and about 1.1 to clopidogrel, obtained from the sample solution is not larger than 2 times the peak area of clopidogrel from the standard solution, the area of the peak other than clopidogrel and the peaks mentioned above from the sample solution is not larger than the peak area of clopidogrel from the standard solution, and the total area of the peaks other than clopidogrel from the sample solution is not larger than 5 times the peak area of clopidogrel from the standard solution.

Operating conditions—

Detector, column and column temperature: Proceed as directed in the operating conditions in the Assay.

Mobile phase A: Dissolve 0.87 g of sodium 1-pentanesufonate in 1000 mL of water, and adjust to pH 2.5 with phosphoric acid. To 950 mL of this solution add 50 mL of methanol.

Mobile phase B: A mixture of acetonitrile for liquid chromatography and methanol (19:1).

Flowing of mobile phase: Control the gradient by mixing the mobile phases A and B as directed in the following table.

Time after injection of sample (min)	Mobile phase A (vol%)	Mobile phase B (vol%)
0 - 3	89.5	10.5
3 - 48	89.5 → 31.5	10.5 → 68.5
48 - 68	31.5	68.5

Flow rate: 1.0 mL per minute.

Time span of measurement: For 68 minutes after injection, beginning after the solvent peak.

System suitability—

Test for required detectability: To exactly 2 mL of the standard solution add a mixture of acetonitrile for liquid chromatography and the mobile phase A (3:2) to make exactly 20 mL. Confirm that the peak area of clopidogrel obtained with 10 μL of this solution is equivalent to 7 to 13% of that with 10 μL of the standard solution.

System performance: When the procedure is run with 10 μL of the standard solution under the above operating conditions, the number of theoretical plates and the symmetry factor of the peak of clopidogrel are not less than 60,000 and not more than 2.0, respectively.

System repeatability: When the test is repeated 6 times with 10 μL of the standard solution under the above operating conditions, the relative standard deviation of the peak area of clopidogrel is not more than 2.0%.

(3) Enantiomer—Dissolve 0.10 g of Clopidogrel Sulfate in 25 mL of ethanol (99.5) for liquid chromatography, add heptane for liquid chromatography to make 50 mL, and use this solution as the sample solution. Pipet 2.5 mL of the sample solution, and add a mixture of ethanol (99.5) for liquid chromatography and heptane for liquid chromatography (1:1) to make exactly 50 mL. Pipet 5 mL of this solution, add a mixture of ethanol (99.5) for liquid chromatography and heptane for liquid chromatography (1:1) to make exactly 50 mL, and use this solution as the standard solution. Perform the test with exactly 10 μL each of the sample solution and standard solution as directed under Liquid Chromatography <2.01> according to the following conditions, and determine each peak area by the automatic integration method: the peak area of the enantiomer, having the relative retention time of about 0.6 to clopidogrel, obtained from the sample solution is not larger than the peak area of clopidogrel from the standard solution.

Operating conditions—

Detector: An ultraviolet absorption photometer (wavelength: 220 nm).

Column: A stainless steel column 4.6 mm in inside diameter and 25 cm in length, packed with cellulose derivative-coated silica gel for liquid chromatography (10 μm in particle diameter).

Column temperature: A constant temperature of about 25°C.

Mobile phase: A mixture of heptane for liquid chromatography and ethanol (99.5) for liquid chromatography (17:3).

Flow rate: Adjust so that the retention time of clopidogrel is about 18 minutes.

System suitability—

System performance: When the procedure is run with 10 μL of the standard solution under the above operating conditions, the number of theoretical plates and the symmetry factor of the peak of clopidogrel are not less than 3500 and not more than 2.0, respectively.

System repeatability: When the test is repeated 6 times with 10 μL of the standard solution under the above operating conditions, the relative standard deviation of the peak area of clopidogrel are not more than 2.0%.

Water <2.48> Not more than 0.5% (1 g, coulometric titration).

Residue on ignition <2.44> Not more than 0.1% (1 g).

Assay Weigh accurately about 45 mg each of Clopidogrel Sulfate and Clopidogrel Sulfate RS (separately, determine the water <2.48> in the same manner as Clopidogrel Sulfate), and dissolve them separately in the mobile phase to make exactly 50 mL. Take exactly 7 mL of each solution, add separately the mobile phase to make exactly 50 mL, and use these solutions as the sample solution and the standard solution, respectively. Perform the test with exactly 10 μL each of the sample solution and standard solution as directed under Liquid Chromatography <2.01> according to the following conditions, and determine the peak areas, A_T and A_S, of clopidogrel in each solution.

Amount (mg) of clopidogrel sulfate ($C_{16}H_{16}ClNO_2S.H_2SO_4$)
$= M_S \times A_T/A_S$

M_S: Amount (mg) of Clopidogrel Sulfate RS taken, calculated on the anhydrous basis

Operating conditions—

Detector: An ultraviolet absorption photometer (wavelength: 220 nm).

Column: A stainless steel column 3.9 mm in inside diameter and 15 cm in length, packed with octadecylsilanized silica gel for liquid chromatography (5 μm in particle diameter).

Column temperature: A constant temperature of about 30°C.

Mobile phase: Dissolve 0.87 g of sodium 1-pentanesufonate in 1000 mL of water, and adjust to pH 2.5 with phosphoric acid. To 950 mL of this solution add 50 mL of methanol. To 600 mL of this solution, add 400 mL of a mixture of acetonitrile for liquid chromatography and methanol (19:1).

Flow rate: Adjust so that the retention time of clopidogrel is about 8 minutes.

System suitability—

System performance: When the procedure is run with 10 μL of the standard solution under the above operating conditions, the number of theoretical plates and the symmetry factor of the peak of clopidogrel are not less than 4500 and not more than 2.0, respectively.

System repeatability: When the test is repeated 6 times with 10 μL of the standard solution under the above operating conditions, the relative standard deviation of the peak area of clopidogrel is not more than 1.0%.

Containers and storage Containers—Tight containers.
Storage—Light-resistant.

Clopidogrel Sulfate Tablets

クロピドグレル硫酸塩錠

Clopidogrel Sulfate Tablets contain not less than 95.0% and not more than 105.0% of the labeled amount of clopidogrel ($C_{16}H_{16}ClNO_2S$: 321.82).

Method of preparation Prepare as directed under Tablets, with Clopidogrel Sulfate.

Identification To a quantity of powdered Clopidogrel Sulfate Tablets, equivalent to 75 mg of clopidogrel ($C_{16}H_{16}ClNO_2S$), add 50 mL of methanol, and after sonicating with ultrasonic waves with occasional shaking, add methanol to make 100 mL. To 10 mL of this solution add methanol to make 30 mL, and filter. Determine the absorption spectrum of the filtrate as directed under Ultraviolet-visible Spectrophotometry <2.24>: it exhibits maxima between 269 nm and 273 nm, and between 276 nm and 280 nm.

Purity Related substances—Keep the sample solution and the standard solution at 5°C or below and use within 24 hours. Take a quantity of Clopidogrel Sulfate Tablets equivalent to 0.15 g of clopidogrel ($C_{16}H_{16}ClNO_2S$), add 120 mL of the mobile phase, sonicate with occasional shaking until the tablets are disintegrated, and add the mobile phase to make 200 mL. Centrifuge this solution, to 10 mL of the supernatant liquid add the mobile phase to make 30 mL, and filter through a membrane filter with a pore size not exceeding 0.45 μm. Discard the first 10 mL of the filtrate, and use the subsequent filtrate as the sample solution. Pipet 2 mL of the sample solution, add the mobile phase to make exactly 200 mL, and use this solution as the standard solution. Perform the test with exactly 10 μL each of the sample solution and standard solution as directed under Liquid Chromatography <2.01> according to the following conditions, and determine each peak area by the automatic integration method: the area of the peaks, having the relative retention times of about 0.3, about 0.5 and about 0.9 to clopidogrel, obtained from the sample solution is not larger than 3/10 times the peak area of clopidogrel from the standard solution. The area of the peak having the relative retention time of about 2.0 from the sample solution is not larger than 1.2 times the peak area of clopidogrel from the standard solution. The area of the peak other than clopidogrel and the peaks mentioned above from the sample solution is not larger than 1/10 times the peak area of clopidogrel from the standard solution. The total area of the peaks other than clopidogrel from the sample solution is not larger than 1.7 times the peak area of clopidogrel from the standard solution.

Operating conditions—

Detector: An ultraviolet absorption photometer (wavelength: 220 nm).

Column: A stainless steel column of 4.6 mm in inside diameter and 15 cm in length, packed with ovomucoid-chemically bonded amino silica gel for liquid chromatography (5 μm in particle diameter).

Column temperature: A constant temperature of about 25°C.

Mobile phase: Dissolve 1.36 g of potassium dihydrogen phosphate in 1000 mL of water, and to 750 mL of this solution add 250 mL of acetonitrile for liquid chromatography.

Flow rate: Adjust so that the retention time of clopidogrel is about 6 minutes.

Time span of measurement: About 2.5 times as long as the retention time of clopidogrel, beginning after the solvent peak.

System suitability—

Test for required detectability: To exactly 5 mL of the standard solution add the mobile phase to make exactly 100 mL. Confirm that the peak area of clopidogrel obtained with 10 μL of this solution is equivalent to 3.5 to 6.5% of that with 10 μL of the standard solution.

System performance: When the procedure is run with 10 μL of the standard solution under the above operating conditions, the number of theoretical plates and the symmetry factor of the peak of clopidogrel are not less than 2500 and not more than 2.0, respectively.

System repeatability: When the test is repeated 6 times with 10 μL of the standard solution under the above operating conditions, the relative standard deviation of the peak area of clopidogrel is not more than 2.0%.

Uniformity of dosage units *<6.02>* Perform the Mass variation test, or the Content uniformity test according to the following method: it meets the requirement.

To 1 tablet of Clopidogrel Sulfate Tablets add a suitable amount of the mobile phase, sonicate with occasional shaking until the tablet is disintegrated, and add the mobile phase to make exactly 50 mL. Filter the solution through a membrane filter with a pore size not exceeding 0.45 μm. Discard the first 10 mL of the filtrate, pipet 2 mL of the subsequent filtrate, add exactly $V/5$ mL of the internal standard solution, and add the mobile phase to make V mL so that each mL contains about 0.1 mg of clopidogrel ($C_{16}H_{16}ClNO_2S$). Use this solution as the sample solution. Then, proceed as directed in the Assay.

$$\text{Amount (mg) of clopidogrel } (C_{16}H_{16}ClNO_2S) = M_S \times Q_T/Q_S \times V/10 \times 0.766$$

M_S: Amount (mg) of Clopidogrel Sulfate RS taken, calculated on the anhydrous basis

*Internal standard solution—*A solution of isopropyl parahydroxybenzoate in the mobile phase (1 in 1500).

Dissolution *<6.10>* When the test is performed at 50 revolutions per minute according to the Paddle method, using 900 mL of water as the dissolution medium, the dissolution rate of 25-mg tablet in 30 minutes is not less than 70%, and that of 75-mg tablet in 45 minutes is not less than 80%.

Start the test with 1 tablet of Clopidogrel Sulfate Tablets, withdraw not less than 20 mL of the medium at the specified minute after starting the test, and filter through a membrane filter with a pore size not exceeding 0.45 μm. Discard not less than 10 mL of the first filtrate, pipet V mL of the subsequent filtrate, add water to make exactly V' mL so that each mL contains about 28 μg of clopidogrel ($C_{16}H_{16}ClNO_2S$), and use this solution as the sample solution. Separately, weigh accurately about 30 mg of Clopidogrel Sulfate RS (separately determine the water *<2.48>* in the same manner as Clopidogrel Sulfate), dissolve in 5 mL of methanol, and add water to make exactly 100 mL. Pipet 6 mL of this solution, add water to make exactly 50 mL, and use this solution as the standard solution. Determine the absorbances, A_T and A_S, at 240 nm of the sample solution and standard solution as directed under Ultraviolet-visible Spectrophotometry *<2.24>*, using water as a blank.

$$\text{Dissolution rate (\%) with respect to the labeled amount of clopidogrel } (C_{16}H_{16}ClNO_2S) = M_S \times A_T/A_S \times V'/V \times 1/C \times 108 \times 0.766$$

M_S: Amount (mg) of Clopidogrel Sulfate RS taken, calculated on the anhydrous basis

C: Labeled amount (mg) of clopidogrel ($C_{16}H_{16}ClNO_2S$) in 1 tablet

Assay To 20 tablets of Clopidogrel Sulfate Tablets add 400 mL of the mobile phase, sonicate with occasional shaking until the tablets are disintegrated, add the mobile phase to make exactly 500 mL, and filter through a membrane filter with a pore size not exceeding 0.45 μm. Discard the first 10 mL of the filtrate, pipet 5 mL of the subsequent filtrate, add the mobile phase to make exactly V mL so that each mL contains about 0.5 mg of clopidogrel ($C_{16}H_{16}ClNO_2S$). Pipet 4 mL of this solution, add exactly 4 mL of the internal standard solution and the mobile phase to make 20 mL, and use this solution as the sample solution. Separately, weigh accurately about 33 mg of Clopidogrel Sulfate RS (separately determine the water *<2.48>* in the same manner as Clopidogrel Sulfate), and dissolve in the mobile phase to make exactly 50 mL. Pipet 4 mL of this solution, add exactly 4 mL of the internal standard solution and the mobile phase to make 20 mL, and use this solution as the standard solution. Perform the test with 10 μL each of the sample solution and standard solution as directed under Liquid Chromatography *<2.01>* according to the following conditions, and calculate the ratios, Q_T and Q_S, of the peak area of clopidogrel to that of the internal standard.

$$\text{Amount (mg) of clopidogrel } (C_{16}H_{16}ClNO_2S) \text{ in 1 tablet of Clopidogrel Sulfate Tablets} = M_S \times Q_T/Q_S \times V/10 \times 0.766$$

M_S: Amount (mg) of Clopidogrel Sulfate RS taken, calculated on the anhydrous basis

*Internal standard solution—*A solution of isopropyl parahydroxybenzoate in the mobile phase (1 in 1500).

Operating conditions—

Detector: An ultraviolet absorption photometer (wavelength: 220 nm).

Column: A stainless steel column of 3.9 mm in inside diameter and 15 cm in length, packed with octadecylsilanized silica gel for liquid chromatography (5 μm in particle diameter).

Column temperature: A constant temperature of about 30°C.

Mobile phase: Dissolve 0.87 g of sodium 1-pentanesulfonate in 1000 mL of water, and adjust to pH 2.5 with phosphoric acid. To 950 mL of this solution add 50 mL of methanol. To 600 mL of this solution add 400 mL of a mixture of acetonitrile for liquid chromatography and methanol (19:1).

Flow rate: Adjust so that the retention time of clopidogrel is about 8 minutes.

System suitability—

System performance: When the procedure is run with 10

μL of the standard solution under the above operating conditions, the internal standard and clopidogrel are eluted in this order with the resolution between these peaks being not less than 4.

System repeatability: When the test is repeated 6 times with 10 μL of the standard solution under the above operating conditions, the relative standard deviation of the ratio of the peak area of clopidogrel to that of the internal standard is not more than 1.0%.

Containers and storage Containers—Tight containers.

Clorazepate Dipotassium

クロラゼプ酸二カリウム

$C_{16}H_{10}ClKN_2O_3.KOH$: 408.92
Monopotassium 7-chloro-2-oxo-5-phenyl-2,3-dihydro-1*H*-1,4-benzodiazepine-3-carboxylate
mono (potassium hydroxide)
[*57109-90-7*]

Clorazepate Dipotassium, when dried, contains not less than 98.5% and not more than 101.0% of clorazepate dipotassium ($C_{16}H_{10}ClKN_2O_3.KOH$).

Description Clorazepate Dipotassium occurs as white to light yellow, crystals or crystalline powder.

It is freely soluble in water, and very slightly soluble in ethanol (99.5).

It dissolves in acetic acid (100).

The pH of a solution obtained by dissolving 1 g of Clorazepate Dipotassium in 100 mL of water is between 11.5 and 12.5.

It gradually turns yellow on exposure to light.

Identification **(1)** Carefully and gradually ignite to redness 30 mg of Clorazepate Dipotassium with 50 mg of sodium. After cooling, add 3 drops of ethanol (99.5) and 5 mL of water, mix well, and filter: the filtrate responds to Qualitative Tests *<1.09>* for chloride.

(2) Determine the absorption spectrum of a solution of Clorazepate Dipotassium (1 in 200,000) as directed under Ultraviolet-visible Spectrophotometry *<2.24>*, and compare the spectrum with the Reference Spectrum: both spectra exhibit similar intensities of absorption at the same wavelengths.

(3) Determine the infrared absorption spectrum of Clorazepate Dipotassium as directed in the potassium bromide disk method under Infrared Spectrophotometry *<2.25>*, and compare the spectrum with the Reference Spectrum: both spectra exhibit similar intensities of absorption at the same wave numbers.

(4) Clorazepate Dipotassium responds to Qualitative Tests *<1.09>* (1) for potassium salt.

Purity **(1)** Chloride *<1.03>*—Dissolve 1.0 g of Clorazepate Dipotassium in 20 mL of water, add 20 mL of acetone, 6 mL of dilute nitric acid and water to make 50 mL. Perform the test with this solution as the test solution. Prepare the control solution as follows: To 0.40 mL of 0.01 mol/L hydrochloric acid VS add 20 mL of acetone, 6 mL of dilute nitric acid and water to make 50 mL (not more than 0.014%).

(2) Heavy metals *<1.07>*—Proceed with 1.0 g of Clorazepate Dipotassium according to Method 2, and perform the test. Prepare the control solution with 2.0 mL of Standard Lead Solution (not more than 20 ppm).

(3) Arsenic *<1.11>*—Prepare the test solution with 1.0 g of Clorazepate Dipotassium according to Method 3, and perform the test (not more than 2 ppm).

(4) Related substances—Dissolve 15 mg of Clorazepate Dipotassium in 25 mL of a mixture of water, potassium carbonate solution (97 in 1000) and acetonitrile (3:1:1), and use this solution as the sample solution. Pipet 1 mL of the sample solution, add the mixture of water, potassium carbonate solution (97 in 1000) and acetonitrile (3:1:1) to make exactly 200 mL, and use this solution as the standard solution. Prepare these solutions quickly and perform the test within 3 minutes. Perform the test with exactly 5 μL each of the sample solution and standard solution as directed under Liquid Chromatography *<2.01>* according to the following conditions, and determine each peak area by the automatic integration method: the peak area of nordiazepam, having the relative retention time of about 3.0 to clorazepic acid, obtained from the sample solution is not larger than the peak area of clorazepic acid from the standard solution, the area of the peak other than clorazepic acid and nordiazepam is not larger than 1/5 times the peak area of clorazepic acid from the standard solution, and the total area of the peaks other than clorazepic acid is not larger than 2 times the peak area of clorazepic acid from the standard solution. For the area of the peak of nordiazepam, multiply the correction factor, 0.64.

Operating conditions—

Detector: An ultraviolet absorption photometer (wavelength: 232 nm).

Column: A stainless steel column 4.6 mm in inside diameter and 15 cm in length, packed with octadecylsilanized silica gel for liquid chromatography (5 μm in particle diameter).

Column temperature: A constant temperature of about 25°C.

Mobile phase: Dissolve 13.8 g of sodium dihydrogen phosphate dihydrate in 500 mL of water, and adjust to pH 8.0 with sodium hydroxide TS. To 100 mL of this solution add 400 mL of acetonitrile and 300 mL of water.

Flow rate: Adjust so that the retention time of clorazepic acid is about 1.3 minutes.

Time span of measurement: About 10 times as long as the retention time of clorazepic acid, beginning after the solvent peak.

System suitability—

Test for required detectability: To exactly 5 mL of the standard solution add the mixture of water, potassium carbonate solution (97 in 1000) and acetonitrile (3:1:1) to make exactly 25 mL. Confirm that the peak area of clorazepic acid obtained with 5 μL of this solution is equivalent to 15 to 25% of that with 5 μL of the standard solution.

System performance: When the procedure is run with 5 μL of the standard solution under the above operating conditions, the number of theoretical plates and the symmetry factor of the peak of clorazepic acid are not less than 3000 and not more than 1.5, respectively.

System repeatability: When the test is repeated 6 times with 5 μL of the standard solution under the above operating conditions, the relative standard deviation of the peak area of clorazepic acid is not more than 1.5%.

Loss on drying *<2.41>* Not more than 0.5% (1 g, in vacuum, phosphorus (V) oxide, 60°C, 5 hours).

Assay Weigh accurately about 0.15 g of Clorazepate Dipotassium, previously dried, dissolve in 100 mL of acetic acid (100), and titrate <*2.50*> with 0.1 mol/L perchloric acid VS until the color of solution changes from violet to blue-green through blue (indicator: 3 drops of crystal violet TS). Perform a blank determination in the same manner, and make any necessary correction.

Each mL of 0.1 mol/L perchloric acid VS
= 13.63 mg of $C_{16}H_{10}ClKN_2O_3.KOH$

Containers and storage Containers—Tight containers.
Storage—Light-resistant.

Clorazepate Dipotassium Capsules

クロラゼプ酸二カリウムカプセル

Clorazepate Dipotassium Capsules contain not less than 93.0% and not more than 107.0% of the labeled amount of clorazepate dipotassium ($C_{16}H_{10}ClKN_2O_3.KOH$: 408.92).

Method of preparation Prepare as directed under Capsules, with Clorazepate Dipotassium.

Identification To 10 mL of the sample solution obtained in the Assay add water to make 20 mL. Determine the absorption spectrum of this solution as directed under Ultraviolet-visible Spectrophotometry <*2.24*>: it exhibits a maximum between 228 nm and 232 nm.

Purity Related substances—Take out the contents of Clorazepate Dipotassium Capsules, and powder. To a portion of the powder, equivalent to 15 mg of Clorazepate Dipotassium, add a mixture of water, potassium carbonate solution (97 in 1000) and acetonitrile (3:1:1) to make 25 mL, and shake for 10 minutes. Filter the solution through a membrane filter with a pore size not exceeding 0.45 μm, discard the first 5 mL of the filtrate, and use the subsequent filtrate as the sample solution. Pipet 1 mL of the sample solution, add a mixture of water, potassium carbonate solution (97 in 1000) and acetonitrile (3:1:1) to make exactly 200 mL, and use this solution as the standard solution. Then, proceed as directed in the Purity (4) under Clorazepate Dipotassium: the peak area of nordiazepam, having the relative retention time of about 3.0 to clorazepic acid, obtained from the sample solution is not larger than 3 times the peak area of clorazepic acid from the standard solution, and the total area of the peaks other than clorazepic acid and nordiazepam is not larger than the peak area of clorazepic acid from the standard solution. For the peak area of nordiazepam, multiply the correction factor, 0.64.

Uniformity of dosage units <*6.02*> Perform the test according to the following method: it meets the requirement of the Content uniformity test.

To 1 capsule of Clorazepate Dipotassium Capsules add 70 mL of water, shake for 15 minutes, and add water to make exactly 100 mL. Centrifuge the solution, pipet V mL of the supernatant liquid, add water to make exactly V' mL so that each mL contains about 12 μg of clorazepate dipotassium ($C_{16}H_{10}ClKN_2O_3.KOH$), and use this solution as the sample solution. Then, proceed as directed in the Assay.

Amount (mg) of clorazepate dipotassium
($C_{16}H_{10}ClKN_2O_3.KOH$)
$= M_S \times A_T/A_S \times V'/V \times 2/25$

M_S: Amount (mg) of clorazepate dipotassium for assay taken

Dissolution <*6.10*> When the test is performed at 50 revolutions per minute according to the Paddle method using the sinker, using 900 mL of water as the dissolution medium, the dissolution rate in 30 minutes of Clorazepate Dipotassium Capsules is not less than 80%.

Start the test with 1 capsule of Clorazepate Dipotassium Capsules, withdraw not less than 20 mL of the medium at the specified minute after starting the test, and filter through a membrane filter with a pore size not exceeding 0.45 μm. Discard not less than 10 mL of the first filtrate, pipet V mL of the subsequent filtrate, add water to make exactly V' mL so that each mL contains about 8.3 μg of clorazepate dipotassium ($C_{16}H_{10}ClKN_2O_3.KOH$), and use this solution as the sample solution. Separately, weigh accurately about 21 mg of clorazepate dipotassium for assay, previously dried in vacuum over phosphorus (V) oxide at 60°C for 5 hours, and dissolve in water to make exactly 100 mL. Pipet 4 mL of this solution, add water to make exactly 100 mL, and use this solution as the standard solution. Determine the absorbances, A_T and A_S, at 252 nm of the sample solution and standard solution as directed under Ultraviolet-visible Spectrophotometry <*2.24*>.

Dissolution rate (%) with respect to the labeled amount of clorazepate dipotassium ($C_{16}H_{10}ClKN_2O_3.KOH$)
$= M_S \times A_T/A_S \times V'/V \times 1/C \times 36$

M_S: Amount (mg) of clorazepate dipotassium for assay taken

C: Labeled amount (mg) of clorazepate dipotassium ($C_{16}H_{10}ClKN_2O_3.KOH$) in 1 capsule

Assay Carefully take out the contents of not less than 20 Clorazepate Dipotassium Capsules, weigh accurately the mass of the contents, and powder. Weigh accurately a portion of the powder, equivalent to about 15 mg of clorazepate dipotassium ($C_{16}H_{10}ClKN_2O_3.KOH$), add 70 mL of water, shake for 15 minutes, and add water to make exactly 100 mL. Centrifuge the solution, pipet 4 mL of the supernatant liquid, add water to make exactly 50 mL, and use this solution as the sample solution. Separately, weigh accurately about 15 mg of clorazepate dipotassium for assay, previously dried in vacuum over phosphorus (V) oxide at 60°C for 5 hours, and dissolve in water to make exactly 100 mL. Pipet 4 mL of this solution, add water to make exactly 50 mL, and use this solution as the standard solution. Perform the test with the sample solution and standard solution as directed under Ultraviolet-visible Spectrophotometry <*2.24*>, and determine the absorbances, A_T and A_S, at 252 nm.

Amount (mg) of clorazepate dipotassium
($C_{16}H_{10}ClKN_2O_3.KOH$)
$= M_S \times A_T/A_S$

M_S: Amount (mg) of clorazepate dipotassium for assay taken

Containers and storage Containers—Tight containers.

Clotiazepam

クロチアゼパム

$C_{16}H_{15}ClN_2OS$: 318.82
5-(2-Chlorophenyl)-7-ethyl-1-methyl-1,3-dihydro-2*H*-thieno[2,3-*e*][1,4]-diazepin-2-one
[*33671-46-4*]

Clotiazepam, when dried, contains not less than 98.5% of clotiazepam ($C_{16}H_{15}ClN_2OS$).

Description Clotiazepam occurs as white to light yellow-white, crystals or crystalline powder. It is odorless, and has a slightly bitter taste.

It is very soluble in chloroform, freely soluble in methanol, in ethanol (95), in acetone, in acetic acid (100) and in ethyl acetate, soluble in diethyl ether, and practically insoluble in water.

It dissolves in 0.1 mol/L hydrochloric acid TS.

It is gradually colored by light.

Identification **(1)** Dissolve 0.01 g of Clotiazepam in 3 mL of sulfuric acid: the solution shows a light yellow fluorescence under ultraviolet light (main wavelength: 365 nm).

(2) Determine the absorption spectrum of a solution of Clotiazepam in 0.1 mol/L hydrochrolic acid TS (1 in 100,000) as directed under Ultraviolet-visible Spectrophotometry <*2.24*>, and compare the spectrum with the Reference Spectrum: both spectra exhibit similar intensities of absorption at the same wavelengths.

(3) Prepare the test solution with 0.01 g of Clotiazepam as directed under Oxygen Flask Combustion Method <*1.06*>, using 10 mL of diluted hydrogen peroxide (30) (1 in 5) as the absorbing liquid. Apply a small amount of water to the upper part of the Apparatus A, pull out C carefully, wash C, B and the inner side of A with 15 mL of methanol, and use the obtained solution as the test solution. Add 0.5 mL of dilute nitric acid to 15 mL of the test solution: this solution responds to Qualitative Tests <*1.09*> (2) for chloride. The remaining test solution responds to Qualitative Tests <*1.09*> (1) for sulfate.

Melting point <*2.60*> 106 - 109°C

Purity **(1)** Clarity and color of solution—Dissolve 1.0 g of Clotiazepam in 10 mL of ethanol (95): the solution is clear and is not more colored than the following control solution.

Control solution: To 5 mL of Matching Fluid C add 0.01 mol/L hydrochloric acid TS to make 10 mL.

(2) Chloride <*1.03*>—To 1.0 g of Clotiazepam add 50 mL of water, shake for 30 minutes, and filter. To 30 mL of the filtrate add 6 mL of dilute nitric acid and water to make 50 mL. Perform the test using this solution as the test solution. Prepare the control solution with 0.25 mL of 0.01 mol/L hydrochloric acid VS (not more than 0.015%).

(3) Heavy metals <*1.07*>—Proceed with 2.0 g of Clotiazepam according to Method 4, and perform the test. Prepare the control solution with 2.0 mL of Standard Lead Solution (not more than 10 ppm).

(4) Arsenic <*1.11*>—Prepare the test solution with 1.0 g of Clotiazepam, according to Method 3, and perform the test (not more than 2 ppm).

(5) Related substances—Dissolve 0.25 g of Clotiazepam in 10 mL of acetone, and use this solution as the sample solution. Pipet 1 mL of the sample solution, add acetone to make exactly 20 mL, pipet 2 mL of this solution, add acetone to make exactly 50 mL, and use this solution as the standard solution. Perform the test with these solutions as directed under Thin-layer Chromatography <*2.03*>. Spot 10 μL each of the sample solution and standard solution on a plate of silica gel with fluorescent indicator for thin-layer chromatography. Develop the plate with a mixture of chloroform and acetone (5:1) to a distance of about 10 cm, and air-dry the plate. Examine under ultraviolet light (main wavelength: 254 nm): the spots other than the principal spot obtained from the sample solution are not more intense than the spot from the standard solution.

Loss on drying <*2.41*> Not more than 0.5% (1 g, 80°C, 3 hours).

Residue on ignition <*2.44*> not more than 0.1% (1 g).

Assay Weigh accurately about 0.5 g of Clotiazepam, previously dried, dissolve in 80 mL of acetic acid (100), and titrate <*2.50*> with 0.1 mol/L perchloric acid (potentiometric titration). Perform a blank determination in the same manner, and make any necessary correction.

Each mL of 0.1 mol/L perchloric acid VS
= 31.88 mg of $C_{16}H_{15}ClN_2OS$

Containers and storage Containers—Tight containers.
Storage—Light-resistant.

Clotiazepam Tablets

クロチアゼパム錠

Clotiazepam Tablets contain not less than 95.0% and not more than 105.0% of the labeled amount of clotiazepam ($C_{16}H_{15}ClN_2OS$: 318.82).

Method of preparation Prepare as directed under Tablets, with Clotiazepam.

Identification Determine the absorption spectrum of the sample solution obtained in the Assay as directed under Ultraviolet-visible Spectrophotometry <*2.24*>: it exhibits a maximum between 260 nm and 264 nm.

Uniformity of dosage unit <*6.02*> Perform the test according to the following method: it meets the requirement of the Content uniformity test.

To 1 tablet of Clotiazepam Tablets add 35 mL of 0.1 mol/L hydrochloric acid TS, stir until the tablet is completely disintegrated, stir for a further 10 minutes, and add 0.1 mol/L hydrochloric acid TS to make exactly 50 mL. Centrifuge this solution, pipet V mL of the supernatant liquid, add 0.1 mol/L hydrochloric acid TS to make exactly V' mL so that each mL contains about 10 μg of clotiazepam ($C_{16}H_{15}ClN_2OS$), and use this solution as the sample solution. Then, proceed as directed in the Assay.

Amount (mg) of clotiazepam ($C_{16}H_{15}ClN_2OS$)
$= M_S \times A_T/A_S \times V'/V \times 1/50$

M_S: Amount (mg) of clotiazepam for assay taken

Dissolution <*6.10*> When the test is performed at 50 revolutions per minute according to the Paddle method, using 900 mL of 1st fluid for dissolution test as the dissolution medium, the dissolution rate in 45 minutes of Clotiazepam Tablets is not less than 80%.

Start the test with 1 tablet of Clotiazepam Tablets, withdraw not less than 20 mL of the medium at the specified minute after starting the test, and filter through a membrane filter with a pore size not exceeding 0.45 μm. Discard not less than 10 mL of the first filtrate, pipet V mL of the subsequent filtrate, add the dissolution medium to make exactly V' mL so that each mL contains about 5.6 μg of clotiazepam ($C_{16}H_{15}ClN_2OS$), and use this solution as the sample solution. Separately, weigh accurately about 28 mg of clotiazepam for assay, previously dried at 80°C for 3 hours, and dissolve in ethanol (95) to make exactly 25 mL. Pipet 5 mL of this solution, and add the dissolution medium to make exactly 100 mL. Pipet 5 mL of this solution, add the dissolution medium to make exactly 50 mL, and use this solution as the standard solution. Determine the absorbances, A_T and A_S, of the sample solution and standard solution at 262 nm as directed under Ultraviolet-visible Spectrophotometry 〈*2.24*〉, using the dissolution medium as the blank.

Dissolution rate (%) with respect to the labeled amount of clotiazepam ($C_{16}H_{15}ClN_2OS$)
$= M_S \times A_T/A_S \times V'/V \times 1/C \times 18$

M_S: Amount (mg) of clotiazepam for assay taken
C: Labeled amount (mg) of clotiazepam ($C_{16}H_{15}ClN_2OS$) in 1 tablet

Assay To 20 Clotiazepam Tablets add 350 mL of 0.1 mol/L hydrochloric acid TS, stir until the tablets are completely disintegrated, stir for a further 10 minutes, and add 0.1 mol/L hydrochloric acid TS to make exactly 500 mL. Centrifuge this solution, pipet V mL of the supernatant liquid, add 0.1 mol/L hydrochloric acid TS to make exactly V' mL so that each mL contains about 10 μg of clotiazepam ($C_{16}H_{15}ClN_2OS$), and use this solution as the sample solution. Separately, weigh accurately about 25 mg of clotiazepam for assay, previously dried at 80°C for 3 hours, and dissolve in 0.1 mol/L hydrochloric acid TS to make exactly 50 mL. Pipet 2 mL of this solution, add 0.1 mol/L hydrochloric acid TS to make exactly 100 mL, and use this solution as the standard solution. Determine the absorbances, A_T and A_S, of the sample solution and standard solution at 261 nm as directed under Ultraviolet-visible Spectrophotometry 〈*2.24*〉.

Amount (mg) of clotiazepam ($C_{16}H_{15}ClN_2OS$) in 1 tablet
$= M_S \times A_T/A_S \times V'/V \times 1/100$

M_S: Amount (mg) of clotiazepam for assay taken

Containers and storage Containers—Tight containers.
Storage—Light-resistant.

Clotrimazole

クロトリマゾール

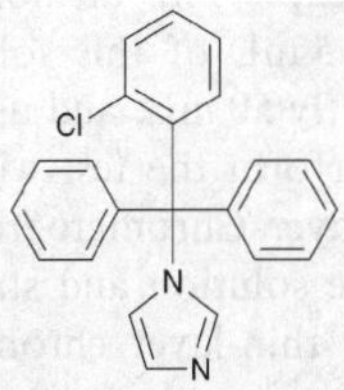

$C_{22}H_{17}ClN_2$: 344.84
1-[(2-Chlorophenyl)(diphenyl)methyl]-1*H*-imidazole
[*23593-75-1*]

Clotrimazole, when dried, contains not less than 98.0% of clotrimazole ($C_{22}H_{17}ClN_2$).

Description Clotrimazole occurs as a white, crystalline powder. It is odorless and tasteless.

It is freely soluble in dichloromethane and in acetic acid (100), soluble in *N,N*-dimethylformamide, in methanol and in ethanol (95), slightly soluble in diethyl ether, and practically insoluble in water.

Identification **(1)** To 0.1 g of Clotrimazole add 10 mL of 5 mol/L hydrochloric acid TS, dissolve by heating, and cool. To this solution add 3 drops of Reinecke salt TS: a light red precipitate is produced.

(2) Determine the absorption spectrum of a solution of Clotrimazole in methanol (1 in 5000) as directed under Ultraviolet-visible Spectrophotometry 〈*2.24*〉, and compare the spectrum with the Reference Spectrum: both spectra exhibit similar intensities of absorption at the same wavelengths.

(3) Determine the infrared absorption spectrum of Clotrimazole, previously dried, as directed in the potassium bromide disk method under Infrared Spectrophotometry 〈*2.25*〉, and compare the spectrum with the Reference Spectrum: both spectra exhibit similar intensities of absorption at the same wave numbers.

(4) Perform the test with Clotrimazole as directed under Flame Coloration Test 〈*1.04*〉 (2): a green color appears.

Melting point 〈*2.60*〉 142 – 145°C

Purity **(1)** Clarity and color of solution—Dissolve 0.5 g of Clotrimazole in 10 mL of dichloromethane: the solution is clear and colorless.

(2) Chloride 〈*1.03*〉—Dissolve 1.0 g of Clotrimazole in 40 mL of *N,N*-dimethylformamide, add 6 mL of dilute nitric acid and water to make 50 mL. Perform the test using this solution as the test solution. Prepare the control solution with 0.60 mL of 0.01 mol/L hydrochloric acid VS, 40 mL of *N,N*-dimethylformamide, 6 mL of dilute nitric acid and water to make 50 mL (not more than 0.021%).

(3) Sulfate 〈*1.14*〉—Dissolve 0.5 g of Clotrimazole in 10 mL of methanol, and add 1 mL of dilute hydrochloric acid and water to make 50 mL. Perform the test using this solution as the test solution. Prepare the control solution with 0.05 mL of 0.005 mol/L sulfuric acid VS, 10 mL of methanol, 1 mL of dilute hydrochloric acid and water to make 50 mL (not more than 0.048%).

(4) Heavy metals 〈*1.07*〉—Proceed with 2.0 g of Clotrimazole according to Method 2, and perform the test. Prepare the control solution with 2.0 mL of Standard Lead Solution (not more than 10 ppm).

(5) Arsenic 〈*1.11*〉—Prepare the test solution with 1.0 g of Clotrimazole according to Method 3, and perform the test (not more than 2 ppm).

(6) Imidazole—Dissolve 0.10 g of Clotrimazole in exactly 10 mL of dichloromethane, and use this solution as the sample solution. Separately, dissolve 25 mg of imidazole for thin-layer chromatography in dichloromethane to make exactly 50 mL. Pipet 5 mL of this solution, add dichloromethane to make exactly 50 mL, and use this solution as the standard solution. Perform the test with these solutions as directed under Thin-layer Chromatography <*2.03*>. Spot 10 μL each of the sample solution and standard solution on a plate of silica gel for thin-layer chromatography. Develop the plate with a mixture of methanol and chloroform (3:2) to a distance of about 10 cm, and air-dry the plate. Spray evenly sodium hypochlorite TS on the plate, and air-dry the plate for 15 minutes, then spray evenly potassium iodide-starch TS on the plate: the spot obtained from the sample solution, corresponding to that from the standard solution, is not more intense than that from the standard solution.

(7) (2-Chlorophenyl)-diphenylmethanol—Dissolve 0.20 g of Clotrimazole in exactly 10 mL of dichloromethane, and use this solution as the sample solution. Separately, dissolve 10 mg of (2-chlorophenyl)-diphenylmethanol for thin-layer chromatography in dichloromethane to make exactly 100 mL, and use this solution as the standard solution. Perform the test with these solutions as directed under Thin-layer Chromatography <*2.03*>. Spot 10 μL each of the sample solution and standard solution on a plate of silica gel with fluorescent indicator for thin-layer chromatography. Develop the plate with a mixture of ethyl acetate and ammonia solution (28) (50:1) to a distance of about 10 cm, and air-dry the plate. Examine under ultraviolet light (main wavelength: 254 nm): the spot obtained from the sample solution, corresponding to that from the standard solution, is not more intense than that from the standard solution.

Loss on drying <*2.41*> Not more than 0.5% (1 g, 105°C, 2 hours).

Residue on ignition <*2.44*> Not more than 0.1% (1 g).

Assay Weigh accurately about 0.35 g of Clotrimazole, previously dried, and dissolve in 80 mL of acetic acid (100), and titrate <*2.50*> with 0.1 mol/L perchloric acid VS (potentiometric titration). Perform a blank determination in the same manner, and make any necessary correction.

Each mL of 0.1 mol/L perchloric acid VS
= 34.48 mg of $C_{22}H_{17}ClN_2$

Containers and storage Containers—Well-closed containers.

Storage—Light-resistant.

Cloxacillin Sodium Hydrate

クロキサシリンナトリウム水和物

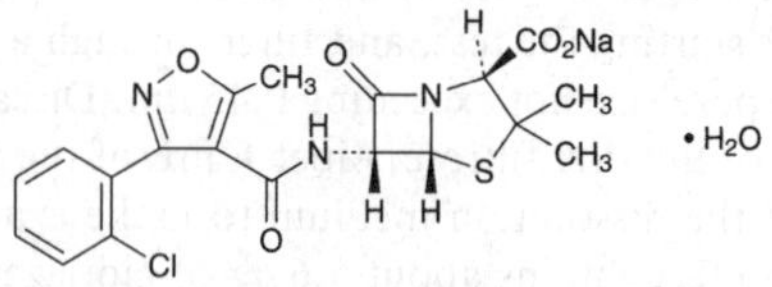

$C_{19}H_{17}ClN_3NaO_5S.H_2O$: 475.88
Monosodium (2*S*,5*R*,6*R*)-6-{[3-(2-chlorophenyl)-5-methylisoxazole-4-carbonyl]amino}-3,3-dimethyl-7-oxo-4-thia-1-azabicyclo[3.2.0]heptane-2-carboxylate monohydrate
[*7081-44-9*]

Cloxacillin Sodium Hydrate contains not less than 900 μg (potency) and not more than 960 μg (potency) per mg, calculated on the anhydrous basis. The potency of Cloxacillin Sodium Hydrate is expressed as mass (potency) of cloxacillin ($C_{19}H_{18}ClN_3O_5S$: 435.88).

Description Cloxacillin Sodium Hydrate occurs as white to light yellow-white, crystals or crystalline powder.

It is freely soluble in water, in *N*,*N*-dimethylformamide and in methanol, and sparingly soluble in ethanol (95).

Identification **(1)** Determine the absorption spectrum of a solution of Cloxacillin Sodium Hydrate in methanol (1 in 2500) as directed under Ultraviolet-visible Spectrophotometry <*2.24*>, and compare the spectrum with the Reference Spectrum or the spectrum of a solution of Cloxacillin Sodium RS prepared in the same manner as the sample solution: both spectra exhibit similar intensities of absorption at the same wavelengths.

(2) Determine the infrared absorption spectrum of Cloxacillin Sodium Hydrate as directed in the potassium bromide disk method under Infrared Spectrophotometry <*2.25*>, and compare the spectrum with the Reference Spectrum or the spectrum of Cloxacillin Sodium RS: both spectra exhibit similar intensities of absorption at the same wave numbers.

(3) Cloxacillin Sodium Hydrate responds to Qualitative Tests <*1.09*> (1) for sodium salt.

Optical rotation <*2.49*> $[\alpha]_D^{20}$: +163 – +171° (1 g calculated on the anhydrous basis, water, 100 mL, 100 mm).

pH <*2.54*> Dissolve 1.0 g of Cloxacillin Sodium Hydrate in 10 mL of water: the pH of the solution is between 5.0 and 7.5.

Purity **(1)** Clarity and color of solution—A solution obtained by dissolving 1.0 g of Cloxacillin Sodium Hydrate in 10 mL of water is clear, and its absorbance at 430 nm, determined as directed under Ultraviolet-visible Spectrophotometry <*2.24*>, is not more than 0.04.

(2) Heavy metals <*1.07*>—Proceed with 1.0 g of Cloxacillin Sodium Hydrate according to Method 2, and perform the test. Prepare the control solution with 2.0 mL of Standard Lead Solution (not more than 20 ppm).

(3) Arsenic <*1.11*>—Prepare the test solution with 1.0 g of Cloxacillin Sodium Hydrate according to Method 5, and perform the test (not more than 2 ppm).

(4) Related substances—Dissolve 50 mg of Cloxacillin Sodium Hydrate in 50 mL of the mobile phase, and use this solution as the sample solution. Pipet 1 mL of the sample solution, add the mobile phase to make exactly 100 mL, and use this solution as the standard solution. Perform the test with exactly 10 μL each of the sample solution and standard solution as directed under Liquid Chromatography <*2.01*> according to the following conditions, and determine each peak area by the automatic integration method: the area of the peak other than cloxacillin obtained from the sample solution is not larger than the peak area of cloxacillin from the standard solution, and the total area of the peaks other than cloxacillin from the sample solution is not larger than 3 times the peak area of cloxacillin from the standard solution.

Operating conditions—

Detector, column, column temperature, mobile phase, and flow rate: Proceed as directed in the operating conditions in the Assay.

Time span of measurement: About 3 times as long as the retention time of cloxacillin.

System suitability—

Test for required detectability: Pipet 1 mL of the standard solution, and add the mobile phase to make exactly 10 mL. Confirm that the peak area of cloxacillin obtained with 10 μL of this solution is equivalent to 7 to 13% of that with 10 μL of the standard solution.

System performance: When the procedure is run with 10 μL of the standard solution under the above operating conditions, the number of theoretical plates and the symmetry factor of the peak of cloxacillin are not less than 5000 and not more than 1.3, respectively.

System repeatability: When the test is repeated 6 times with 10 μL of the standard solution under the above operating conditions, the relative standard deviation of the peak area of cloxacillin is not more than 1.0%.

Water <*2.48*> 3.0 – 4.5% (0.2 g, volumetric titration, direct titration).

Assay Weigh accurately an amount of Cloxacillin Sodium Hydrate and Cloxacillin Sodium RS, equivalent to about 50 mg (potency), dissolve each in a suitable amount of the mobile phase, add exactly 5 mL of the internal standard solution, then add the mobile phase to make 50 mL, and use these solutions as the sample solution and the standard solution, respectively. Perform the test with 10 μL each of the sample solution and standard solution as directed under Liquid Chromatography <*2.01*> according to the following conditions, and calculate the ratios, Q_T and Q_S, of the peak area of cloxacillin to that of the internal standard.

Amount [μg (potency)] of cloxacillin ($C_{19}H_{18}ClN_3O_5S$)
$= M_S \times Q_T/Q_S \times 1000$

M_S: Amount [mg (potency)] of Cloxacillin Sodium RS taken

Internal standard solution—A solution of guaifenesin in the mobile phase (1 in 200).

Operating conditions—

Detector: An ultraviolet absorption photometer (wavelength: 230 nm).

Column: A stainless steel column 6 mm in inside diameter and 15 cm in length, packed with octadecylsilanized silica gel for liquid chromatography (5 μm in particle diameter).

Column temperature: A constant temperature of about 25°C.

Mobile phase: Dissolve 4.95 g of diammonium hydrogen phosphate in 700 mL of water, add 250 mL of acetonitrile, adjust to pH 4.0 with phosphoric acid, and add water to make 1000 mL.

Flow rate: Adjust so that the retention time of cloxacillin is about 24 minutes.

System suitability—

System performance: When the procedure is run with 10 μL of the standard solution under the above operating conditions, guaifenesin and cloxacillin are eluted in this order with the resolution between these peaks being not less than 25.

System repeatability: When the test is repeated 6 times with 10 μL of the standard solution under the above operating conditions, the relative standard deviation of the ratio of the peak area of cloxacillin to that of the internal standard is not more than 1.0%.

Containers and storage Containers—Tight containers.

Cloxazolam

クロキサゾラム

and enantiomer

$C_{17}H_{14}Cl_2N_2O_2$: 349.21
(11b*RS*)-10-Chloro-11b-(2-chlorophenyl)-2,3,7,11b-tetrahydro[1,3]oxazolo[3,2-*d*][1,4]benzodiazepin-6(5*H*)-one
[*24166-13-0*]

Cloxazolam, when dried, contains not less than 99.0% of cloxazolam ($C_{17}H_{14}Cl_2N_2O_2$).

Description Cloxazolam occurs as white, crystals or crystalline powder. It is odorless and tasteless.

It is freely soluble in acetic acid (100), sparingly soluble in dichloromethane, slightly soluble in ethanol (99.5) and in diethyl ether, very slightly soluble in ethanol (95), and practically insoluble in water.

It dissolves in dilute hydrochloric acid.

It is gradually colored by light.

Melting point: about 200°C (with decomposition).

Identification **(1)** Dissolve 0.01 g of Cloxazolam in 10 mL of ethanol (99.5) by heating, and add 1 drop of hydrochloric acid: the solution shows a light yellow color and a yellow-green fluorescence under ultraviolet light (main wavelength: 365 nm). Add 1 mL of sodium hydroxide TS to this solution: the color and fluorescence of this solution disappear immediately.

(2) Dissolve 0.01 g of Cloxazolam in 5 mL of dilute hydrochloric acid by heating in a water bath for 10 minutes. After cooling, 1 mL of this solution responds to Qualitative Tests <*1.09*> for primary aromatic amines.

(3) Place 2 g of Cloxazolam in a 200-mL flask, add 50 mL of ethanol (95) and 25 mL of sodium hydroxide TS, and boil under a reflux condenser for 4 hours. After cooling, neutralize with dilute hydrochloric acid, and extract with 30 mL of dichloromethane. Dehydrate with 3 g of anhydrous sodium sulfate, filter, and evaporate the dichloromethane of the filtrate. Dissolve the residue in 5 mL of methanol by heating on a water bath, and cool immediately in an ice bath. Collect the crystals, and dry the crystals is vacuum at 60°C for 1 hour: it melts <*2.60*> between 87°C and 91°C.

(4) Determine the absorption spectrum of a solution of Cloxazolam in ethanol (99.5) (1 in 100,000) as directed under Ultraviolet-visible Spectrophotometry <*2.24*>, and compare the spectrum with the Reference Spectrum: both spectra exhibit similar intensities of absorption at the same wavelengths.

(5) Proceed with Cloxazolam as directed under Flame Coloration Test <*1.04*> (2), and perform the test: a green color appears.

Absorbance <*2.24*> $E^{1\%}_{1\,\mathrm{cm}}$ (244 nm): 390 – 410 (after drying, 1 mg, ethanol (99.5), 100 mL).

Purity **(1)** Chloride <*1.03*>—To 1.0 g of Cloxazolam add 50 mL of water, allow to stand for 1 hour with occasional shaking, and filter. To 25 mL of this filtrate add 6 mL of dilute nitric acid and water to make 50 mL, and perform the test using this solution as the test solution. Prepare the control solution with 0.20 mL of 0.01 mol/L hydrochloric acid VS (not more than 0.014%).

(2) Heavy metals <*1.07*>—Proceed with 1.0 g of Cloxazolam according to Method 2, and perform the test. Prepare the control solution with 2.0 mL of Standard Lead Solution (not more than 20 ppm).

(3) Arsenic <*1.11*>—Place 1.0 g of Cloxazolam in a Kjeldahl flask, add 5 mL of sulfuric acid and 5 mL of nitric acid, and heat gently. Repeat the addition of 2 to 3 mL of nitric acid at times, and continue heating until a colorless to light yellow solution is obtained. After cooling, add 15 mL of saturated ammonium oxalate solution, and heat the solution until dense white fumes are evolved, and evaporate to a volume of 2 to 3 mL. After cooling, dilute with water to 10 mL, and perform the test with this solution as the test solution (not more than 2 ppm).

(4) Related substances—Dissolve 0.05 g of Cloxazolam in 10 mL of dichloromethane, and use this solution as the sample solution. Pipet 1 mL of the sample solution, add dichloromethane to make exactly 200 mL, and use this solution as the standard solution. Perform the test with these solutions as directed under Thin-layer Chromatography <*2.03*>. Spot 10 μL each of the sample solution and standard solution on a plate of silica gel with fluorescent indicator for thin-layer chromatography. Immediately after air-drying, develop the plate with a mixture of toluene and acetone (5:1) to a distance of about 10 cm, and air-dry the plate. Examine under ultraviolet light (main wavelength: 254 nm): the spots other than the principal spot from the sample solution are not more intense than that from the standard solution.

Loss on drying <*2.41*> Not more than 0.5% (1 g, 105°C, 3 hours).

Residue on ignition <*2.44*> Not more than 0.1% (1 g).

Assay Weigh accurately about 0.5 g of Cloxazolam, previously dried, and dissolve in 50 mL of acetic acid (100). Titrate <*2.50*> with 0.1 mol/L perchloric acid VS until the color of the solution changes from purple through blue to blue-green (indicator: 2 drops of crystal violet TS). Perform a blank determination in the same menner, and make any necessary correction.

Each mL of 0.1 mol/L perchloric acid VS
= 34.92 mg of $C_{17}H_{14}Cl_2N_2O_2$

Containers and storage Containers—Tight containers.

Storage—Light-resistant.

Cocaine Hydrochloride

コカイン塩酸塩

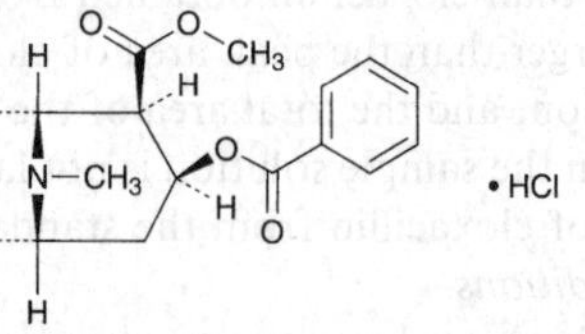

$C_{17}H_{21}NO_4.HCl$: 339.81
(1*R*,2*R*,3*S*,5*S*)-2-Methoxycarbonyl-8-methyl-8-azabicyclo[3.2.1]oct-3-yl benzoate monohydrochloride
[*53-21-4*]

Cocaine Hydrochloride, when dried, contains not less than 98.0% of cocaine hydrochloride ($C_{17}H_{21}NO_4$.HCl).

Description Cocaine Hydrochloride occurs as colorless crystals or a white crystalline powder.

It is very soluble in water, freely soluble in ethanol (95) and in acetic acid (100), slightly soluble in acetic anhydride, and practically insoluble in diethyl ether.

Identification **(1)** Determine the absorption spectrum of a solution of Cocaine Hydrochloride in 0.01 mol/L hydrochloric acid TS (1 in 10,000) as directed under Ultraviolet-visible Spectrophotometry <*2.24*>, and compare the spectrum with the Reference Spectrum 1: both spectra exhibit similar intensities of absorption at the same wavelengths. Separately, determine the absorption spectrum of a solution of Cocaine Hydrochloride in 0.01 mol/L hydrochloric acid TS (1 in 50,000) as directed under Ultraviolet-visible Spectrophotometry <*2.24*>, and compare the spectrum with the Reference Spectrum 2: both spectra exhibit similar intensities of absorption at the same wavelengths.

(2) Determine the infrared absorption spectrum of Cocaine Hydrochloride, previously dried, as directed in the potassium bromide disk method under the Infrared Spectrophotometry <*2.25*>, and compare the spectrum with the Reference Spectrum: both spectra exhibit similar intensities of absorption at the same wave numbers.

(3) A solution of Cocaine Hydrochloride (1 in 50) responds to Qualitative Tests <*1.09*> (2) for chloride.

Optical rotation <*2.49*> $[\alpha]^{20}_{D}$: -70 – $-73°$ (after drying, 0.5 g, water, 20 mL, 100 mm).

Purity **(1)** Acidity—Dissolve 0.5 g of Cocaine Hydrochloride in 10 mL of water, add 1 drop of methyl red TS, and neutralize with 0.01 mol/L sodium hydroxide VS: the consumed volume is not more than 1.0 mL.

(2) Cinnamyl cocaine—Dissolve 0.10 g of Cocaine Hydrochloride in 5 mL of water, and add 0.3 mL of diluted sulfuric acid (1 in 20) and 0.10 mL of 0.02 mol/L potassium permanganate VS: the red color does not disappear within 30 minutes.

(3) Isoatropyl cocaine—Dissolve 0.10 g of Cocaine Hydrochloride in 30 mL of water in a beaker. Transfer 5 mL of this solution to a test tube, add 1 drop of ammonia TS, and mix. After the precipitate is coagulated, add 10 mL of water, and transfer the mixture to the former beaker, to which 30 mL of water has been added previously. Wash the test tube with 10 mL of water, combine the washings with the mixture in the beaker, add 3 drops of ammonia TS to the combined mixture, and mix gently: a crystalline precipitate is produced. Allow to stand for 1 hour: the supernatant liquid is clear.

Loss on drying ⟨*2.41*⟩ Not more than 1.0% (1 g, 105°C, 4 hours).

Residue on ignition ⟨*2.44*⟩ Not more than 0.1% (0.5 g).

Assay Weigh accurately about 0.5 g of Cocaine Hydrochloride, previously dried, dissolve in 50 mL of a mixture of acetic anhydride and acetic acid (100) (7:3), and titrate ⟨*2.50*⟩ with 0.1 mol/L perchloric acid VS (potentiometric titration). Perform a blank determination in the same manner, and make any necessary correction.

Each mL of 0.1 mol/L perchloric acid VS
= 33.98 mg of $C_{17}H_{21}NO_4.HCl$

Containers and storage Containers—Tight containers.
Storage—Light-resistant.

Cod Liver Oil

肝油

Cod Liver Oil is the fatty oils obtained from fresh livers and pyloric appendages of *Gadus macrocephalus* Tilesius or *Theragra chalcogramma* Pallas (*Gadidae*).

Cod Liver Oil contains not less than 2000 Vitamin A Units and not more than 5000 Vitamin A Units per g.

Description Cod Liver Oil is a yellow to orange oily liquid. It has a characteristic, slightly fishy odor and a mild taste.

It is miscible with chloroform.

It is slightly soluble in ethanol (95), and practically insoluble in water.

It is decomposed by air or by light.

Identification Dissolve 0.1 g of Cod Liver Oil in 10 mL of chloroform, and to 1 mL of this solution add 3 mL of antimony (III) chloride TS: a blue color develops immediately, but the color fades rapidly.

Specific gravity ⟨*1.13*⟩ d_{20}^{20}: 0.918 – 0.928

Acid value ⟨*1.13*⟩ Not more than 1.7.

Saponification value ⟨*1.13*⟩ 180 – 192

Unsaponifiable matter ⟨*1.13*⟩ Not more than 3.0%.

Iodine value ⟨*1.13*⟩ 130 – 170

Purity Rancidity—No unpleasant odor of rancid oil is perceptible on warming Cod Liver Oil.

Assay Proceed with about 0.5 g of Cod Liver Oil, accurately weighed, as directed in Method 2 under the Vitamin A Determination ⟨*2.55*⟩, and perform the test.

Containers and storage Containers—Tight containers.

Storage—Light-resistant, and almost well-filled, or under nitrogen atmosphere.

Codeine Phosphate Hydrate

コデインリン酸塩水和物

$\cdot H_3PO_4 \cdot \frac{1}{2}H_2O$

$C_{18}H_{21}NO_3.H_3PO_4.\frac{1}{2}H_2O$: 406.37
(5*R*,6*S*)-4,5-Epoxy-3-methoxy-17-methyl-7,8-didehydromorphinan-6-ol monophosphate hemihydrate
[*41444-62-6*]

Codeine Phosphate Hydrate contains not less than 98.0% of codeine phosphate ($C_{18}H_{21}NO_3.H_3PO_4$: 397.36), calculated on the anhydrous basis.

Description Codeine Phosphate Hydrate occurs as white to yellowish white, crystals or crystalline powder.

It is freely soluble in water and in acetic acid (100), slightly soluble in methanol and in ethanol (95), and practically insoluble in diethyl ether.

The pH of a solution of 1.0 g of Codeine Phosphate Hydrate in 10 mL of water is between 3.0 and 5.0.

It is affected by light.

Identification **(1)** Determine the absorption spectrum of a solution of Codeine Phosphate Hydrate (1 in 10,000) as directed under Ultraviolet-visible Spectrophotometry ⟨*2.24*⟩, and compare the spectrum with the Reference Spectrum: both spectra exhibit similar intensities of absorption at the same wavelengths.

(2) Determine the infrared absorption spectrum of Codeine Phosphate Hydrate, previously dried at 105°C for 4 hours, as directed in the potassium bromide disk method under Infrared Spectrophotometry ⟨*2.25*⟩, and compare the spectrum with the Reference Spectrum: both spectra exhibit similar intensities of absorption at the same wave numbers.

(3) A solution of Codeine Phosphate Hydrate (1 in 20) responds to Qualitative Tests ⟨*1.09*⟩ (1) for phosphate.

Optical rotation ⟨*2.49*⟩ $[\alpha]_D^{20}$: −98 – −102° (0.4 g calculated on the anhydrous basis, water, 20 mL, 100 mm).

Purity **(1)** Chloride ⟨*1.03*⟩—Perform the test with 0.5 g of Codeine Phosphate Hydrate. Prepare the control solution with 0.30 mL of 0.01 mol/L hydrochloric acid VS (not more than 0.021%).

(2) Sulfate ⟨*1.14*⟩—Perform the test with 0.20 g of Codeine Phosphate Hydrate. Prepare the control solution with 1.0 mL of 0.005 mol/L sulfuric acid VS (not more than 0.240%).

(3) Related substances—Dissolve 0.20 g of Codeine Phosphate Hydrate in 10 mL of a mixture of 0.01 mol/L hydrochloric acid TS and ethanol (99.5) (4:1), and use this solution as the sample solution. Pipet 1 mL of the sample solution, add a mixture of 0.01 mol/L hydrochloric acid TS and ethanol (99.5) (4:1) to make exactly 100 mL, and use this solution as the standard solution. Perform the test with these solutions as directed under Thin-layer Chromatography ⟨*2.03*⟩. Spot 10 μL each of the sample solution and standard solution on a plate of silica gel with fluorescent indicator for thin-layer chromatography. Develop the plate with a mixture of ethanol (99.5), toluene, acetone and ammonia solution (28) (14:14:7:1) to a distance of about 10 cm, and air-dry the plate. Examine under ultraviolet light (main wavelength: 254 nm): the spots other than the principal spot obtained from the sample solution are not more intense than the spot from the standard solution.

Water <2.48> 1.5 - 3.0% (0.5 g, volumetric titration, direct titration).

Assay Dissolve about 0.5 g of Codeine Phosphate Hydrate, accurately weighed, in 70 mL of acetic acid (100), and titrate <2.50> with 0.1 mol/L perchloric acid VS until the color of the solution changes from purple through blue to greenish blue (indicator: 3 drops of crystal violet TS). Perform a blank determination in the same manner, and make any necessary correction.

Each mL of 0.1 mol/L perchloric acid VS
= 39.74 mg of $C_{18}H_{21}NO_3.H_3PO_4$

Containers and storage Containers—Tight containers.
Storage—Light-resistant.

1% Codeine Phosphate Powder

コデインリン酸塩散 1%

1% Codeine Phosphate Powder contains not less than 0.90% and not more than 1.10% of codeine phosphate hydrate ($C_{18}H_{21}NO_3.H_3PO_4.{}^1/_2H_2O$: 406.37).

Method of preparation

Codeine Phosphate Hydrate	10 g
Lactose Hydrate	a sufficient quantity
	To make 1000 g

Prepare as directed under Granules or Powders, with the above ingredients.

Identification Determine the absorption spectrum of a solution of 1% Codeine Phosphate Powder (1 in 100) as directed under Ultraviolet-visible Spectrophotometry <2.24>: it exhibits a maximum between 283 nm and 287 nm.

Dissolution <6.10> When the test is performed at 50 revolutions per minute according to the Paddle method, using 900 mL of water as the dissolution medium, the dissolution rate in 15 minutes of 1% Codeine Phosphate Powder is not less than 85%.

Start the test with about 2 g of 1% Codeine Phosphate Powder, accurately weighed, withdraw not less than 20 mL of the medium at the specified minute after starting the test, and filter through a membrane filter with a pore size not exceeding 0.45 μm. Discard not less than 10 mL of the first filtrate, and use the subsequent filtrate as the sample solution. Separately, weigh accurately about 28 mg of codeine phosphate hydrate for assay (separately determine the water <2.48> in the same manner as Codeine Phosphate Hydrate), and dissolve in water to make exactly 100 mL. Pipet 4 mL of this solution, add water to make exactly 50 mL, and use this solution as the standard solution. Perform the test with exactly 50 μL each of the sample solution and standard solution as directed under Liquid Chromatography <2.01> according to the following conditions, and determine the peak areas, A_T and A_S, of codeine in each solution.

Dissolution rate (%) with respect to the labeled amount of codeine phosphate hydrate ($C_{18}H_{21}NO_3.H_3PO_4.{}^1/_2H_2O$)
$= M_S/M_T \times A_T/A_S \times 36/5 \times 1.023$

M_S: Amount (mg) of codeine phosphate hydrate for assay taken, calculated on the anhydrous basis
M_T: Amount (g) of 1% Codeine Phosphate Powder taken

Operating conditions—

Proceed as directed in the operating conditions in the Assay.

System suitability—

System performance: When the procedure is run with 50 μL of the standard solution under the above operating conditions, the number of theoretical plates and the symmetry factor of the peak of codeine are not less than 3000 and not more than 2.0, respectively.

System repeatability: When the test is repeated 6 times with 50 μL of the standard solution under the above operating conditions, the relative standard deviation of the peak area of codeine is not more than 2.0%.

Assay Weigh accurately about 5 g of 1% Codeine Phosphate Powder, dissolve in water to make exactly 100 mL, then pipet 10 mL of this solution, add exactly 10 mL of the internal standard solution, and use this solution as the sample solution. Separately, weigh accurately about 50 mg of codeine phosphate hydrate for assay (previously determine the water <2.48> in the same manner as Codeine Phosphate Hydrate), dissolve in water to make exactly 100 mL, then pipet 10 mL of this solution, add exactly 10 mL of the internal standard solution, and use this solution as the standard solution. Perform the test with 20 μL each of the sample solution and standard solution as directed under Liquid Chromatography <2.01> according to the following conditions, and calculate the ratios, Q_T and Q_S, of the peak area of codeine to that of the internal standard.

Amount (mg) of codeine phosphate hydrate
($C_{18}H_{21}NO_3.H_3PO_4.{}^1/_2H_2O$)
$= M_S \times Q_T/Q_S \times 1.023$

M_S: Amount (mg) of codeine phosphate hydrate for assay taken, calculated on the anhydrous basis

Internal standard solution—A solution of etilefrine hydrochloride (3 in 10,000).

Operating conditions—

Detector: An ultraviolet absorption photometer (wavelength: 280 nm).

Column: A stainless steel column 4.6 mm in inside diameter and 15 cm in length, packed with octadecylsilanized silica gel for liquid chromatography (5 μm in particle diameter).

Column temperature: A constant temperature of about 40°C.

Mobile phase: Dissolve 1.0 g of sodium lauryl sulfate in 500 mL of diluted phosphoric acid (1 in 1000), and adjust the pH to 3.0 with sodium hydroxide TS. To 240 mL of this solution add 70 mL of tetrahydrofuran, and mix.

Flow rate: Adjust so that the retention time of codeine is about 10 minutes.

System suitability—

System performance: When the procedure is run with 20 μL of the standard solution under the above operating conditions, codeine and the internal standard are eluted in this order with the resolution between these peaks being not less than 4.

System repeatability: When the test is repeated 5 times with 20 μL of the standard solution under the above operating conditions, the relative standard deviation of the ratio of the peak area of codeine to that of the internal standard is not more than 1.0%.

Containers and storage Containers—Tight containers.

10% Codeine Phosphate Powder

コデインリン酸塩散 10%

10% Codeine Phosphate Powder contains not less than 9.3% and not more than 10.7% of codeine phosphate hydrate ($C_{18}H_{21}NO_3.H_3PO_4.½H_2O$: 406.37).

Method of preparation

Codeine Phosphate Hydrate	100 g
Lactose Hydrate	a sufficient quantity
To make	1000 g

Prepare as directed under Powders, with the above ingredients.

Identification Determine the absorption spectrum of a solution of 10% Codeine Phosphate Powder (1 in 1000) as directed under Ultraviolet-visible Spectrophotometry <2.24>: it exhibits a maximum between 283 nm and 287 nm.

Dissolution <6.10> When the test is performed at 50 revolutions per minute according to the Paddle method, using 900 mL of water as the dissolution medium, the dissolution rate in 15 minutes of 10% Codeine Phosphate Powder is not less than 85%.

Start the test with about 0.2 g of 10% Codeine Phosphate Powder, accurately weighed, withdraw not less than 20 mL of the medium at the specified minute after starting the test, and filter through a membrane filter with a pore size not exceeding 0.45 µm. Discard not less than 10 mL of the first filtrate, and use the subsequent filtrate as the sample solution. Separately, weigh accurately about 28 mg of codeine phosphate hydrate for assay (separately determine the water <2.48> in the same manner as Codeine Phosphate Hydrate), and dissolve in water to make exactly 100 mL. Pipet 4 mL of this solution, add water to make exactly 50 mL, and use this solution as the standard solution. Perform the test with exactly 50 µL each of the sample solution and standard solution as directed under Liquid Chromatography <2.01> according to the following conditions, and determine the peak areas, A_T and A_S, of codeine in each solution.

Dissolution rate (%) with respect to the labeled amount of codeine phosphate hydrate ($C_{18}H_{21}NO_3.H_3PO_4.½H_2O$)
$= M_S/M_T \times A_T/A_S \times 18/25 \times 1.023$

M_S: Amount (mg) of codeine phosphate hydrate for assay taken, calculated on the anhydrous basis

M_T: Amount (g) of 10% Codeine Phosphate Powder

Operating conditions—

Proceed as directed in the operating conditions in the Assay.

System suitability—

System performance: When the procedure is run with 50 µL of the standard solution under the above operating conditions, the number of theoretical plates and the symmetry factor of the peak of codeine are not less than 3000 and not more than 2.0, respectively.

System repeatability: When the test is repeated 6 times with 50 µL of the standard solution under the above operating conditions, the relative standard deviation of the peak area of codeine is not more than 2.0%.

Assay Weigh accurately about 2.5 g of 10% Codeine Phosphate Powder, dissolve in water to make exactly 100 mL, then pipet 2 mL of this solution, add exactly 10 mL of the internal standard solution and water to make 20 mL, and use this solution as the sample solution. Separately, weigh accurately about 50 mg of codeine phosphate hydrate for assay (previously determine the water <2.48> in the same manner as Codeine Phosphate Hydrate), dissolve in water to make exactly 100 mL, then pipet 10 mL of this solution, add exactly 10 mL of the internal standard solution, and use this solution as the standard solution. Perform the test with 20 µL each of the sample solution and standard solution as directed under Liquid Chromatography <2.01> according to the following conditions, and calculate the ratios, Q_T and Q_S, of the peak area of codeine to that of the internal standard:

Amount (mg) of codeine phosphate hydrate ($C_{18}H_{21}NO_3.H_3PO_4.½H_2O$)
$= M_S \times Q_T/Q_S \times 5 \times 1.023$

M_S: Amount (mg) of codeine phosphate hydrate for assay taken, calculated on the anhydrous basis

Internal standard solution—A solution of etilefrine hydrochloride (3 in 10,000).

Operating conditions—

Detector: An ultraviolet absorption photometer (wavelength: 280 nm).

Column: A stainless steel column 4.6 mm in inside diameter and 15 cm in length, packed with octadecylsilanized silica gel for liquid chromatography (5 µm in particle diameter).

Column temperature: A constant temperature of about 40°C.

Mobile phase: Dissolve 1.0 g of sodium lauryl sulfate in 500 mL of diluted phosphoric acid (1 in 1000), and adjust the pH to 3.0 with sodium hydroxide TS. To 240 mL of this solution add 70 mL of tetrahydrofuran, and mix.

Flow rate: Adjust so that the retention time of codeine is about 10 minutes.

System suitability—

System performance: When the procedure is run with 20 µL of the standard solution under the above operating conditions, codeine and the internal standard are eluted in this order with the resolution between these peaks being not less than 4.

System repeatability: When the test is repeated 5 times with 20 µL of the standard solution under the above operating conditions, the relative standard deviation of the ratios of the peak area of codeine to that of the internal standard is not more than 1.0%.

Containers and storage Containers—Tight containers.

Codeine Phosphate Tablets

コデインリン酸塩錠

Codeine Phosphate Tablets contain not less than 93.0% and not more than 107.0% of the labeled amount of codeine phosphate hydrate ($C_{18}H_{21}NO_3.H_3PO_4.½H_2O$: 406.37)

Method of preparation Prepare as directed under Tablets, with Codeine Phosphate Hydrate.

Identification To a quantity of powdered Codeine Phosphate Tablets, equivalent to 0.1 g of Codeine Phosphate Hydrate, add 20 mL of water, shake, and filter. To 2 mL of the filtrate add water to make 100 mL, and determine the absorption spectrum as directed under Ultraviolet-visible Spectrophotometry <2.24>: it exhibits a maximum between

283 nm and 287 nm.

Uniformity of dosage units <*6.02*> Perform the test according to the following method: it meets the requirement of the Content uniformity test.

To 1 tablet of Codeine Phosphate Tablets add $3V/25$ mL of water to disintegrate, add $2V/25$ mL of diluted dilute sulfuric acid (1 in 20), and sonicate for 10 minutes. To this solution add exactly $2V/25$ mL of the internal standard solution, add water to make V mL so that each mL contains about 0.2 mg of codeine phosphate hydrate ($C_{18}H_{21}NO_3.H_3PO_4.{}^1\!/_2H_2O$), filter, and use the filtrate as the sample solution. Separately, weigh accurately about 50 mg of codeine phosphate hydrate for assay (separately, determine the water <*2.48*> in the same manner as Codeine Phosphate Hydrate), and dissolve in water to make exactly 100 mL. Pipet 10 mL of this solution, add exactly 2 mL of the internal standard solution, add water to make 25 mL, and use this solution as the standard solution. Proceed as directed in the Assay.

Amount (mg) of codeine phosphate hydrate ($C_{18}H_{21}NO_3.H_3PO_4.{}^1\!/_2H_2O$)
$= M_S \times Q_T/Q_S \times V/250 \times 1.023$

M_S: Amount (mg) of codeine phosphate hydrate for assay taken, calculated on the anhydrous basis

Internal standard solution—A solution of ethylefurin hydrochloride (3 in 2000).

Dissolution <*6.10*> When the test is performed at 50 revolutions per minute according to the Paddle method, using 900 mL of water as the dissolution medium, the dissolution rate in 30 minutes of Codeine Phosphate Tablets is not less than 80%.

Start the test with 1 tablet of Codeine Phosphate Tablets, withdraw not less than 20 mL of the medium at the specified minute after starting the test, and filter through a membrane filter with a pore size not exceeding 0.45 μm. Discard not less than 10 mL of the first filtrate, pipet V mL of the subsequent filtrate, add water to make exactly V' mL so that each mL contains about 5.6 μg of codeine phosphate hydrate ($C_{18}H_{21}NO_3.H_3PO_4.{}^1\!/_2H_2O$), and use this solution as the sample solution. Separately, weigh accurately about 28 mg of codeine phosphate hydrate for assay (separately, determine the water <*2.48*> in the same manner as Codeine Phosphate Hydrate), dissolve in water to make exactly 100 mL. Pipet 2 mL of this solution, add water to make exactly 100 mL, and use this solution as the standard solution. Perform the test with exactly 100 μL each of the sample solution and standard solution as directed under Liquid Chromatography <*2.01*> according to the following conditions, and determine the peak areas, A_T and A_S, of codeine in each solution.

Dissolution rate (%) with respect to the labeled amount of codeine phosphate hydrate ($C_{18}H_{21}NO_3.H_3PO_4.{}^1\!/_2H_2O$)
$= M_S \times A_T/A_S \times V'/V \times 1/C \times 18 \times 1.023$

M_S: Amount (mg) of codeine phosphate hydrate for assay taken, calculated on the anhydrous basis

C: Labeled amount (mg) of codeine phosphate hydrate ($C_{18}H_{21}NO_3.H_3PO_4.{}^1\!/_2H_2O$) in 1 tablet

Operating conditions—

Proceed as directed in the operating conditions in the Assay.

System suitability—

System performance: When the procedure is run with 100 μL of the standard solution under the above operating conditions, the number of theoretical plates and the symmetry factor of the peak of codeine are not less than 5000 and not more than 1.5, respectively.

System repeatability: When the test is repeated 6 times with 100 μL of the standard solution under the above operating conditions, the relative standard deviation of the peak area of codeine is not more than 2.0%.

Assay Weigh accurately and powder not less than 20 Codeine Phosphate Tablets. Weigh accurately a portion of the powder, equivalent to about 0.1 g of codeine phosphate hydrate ($C_{18}H_{21}NO_3.H_3PO_4.{}^1\!/_2H_2O$), add 30 mL of water, shake, add 20 mL of diluted dilute sulfuric acid (1 in 20), sonicate the mixture for 10 minutes, and add water to make exactly 100 mL. Filter the solution, then pipet 5 mL of the filtrate, add exactly 10 mL of the internal standard solution and water to make 20 mL, and use this solution as the sample solution. Separately, weigh accurately about 50 mg of codeine phosphate hydrate for assay (previously determine the water <*2.48*> in the same manner as Codeine Phosphate Hydrate), dissolve in water to make exactly 100 mL, then pipet 10 mL of this solution, add exactly 10 mL of the internal standard solution, and use this solution as the standard solution. Perform the test with 20 μL each of the sample solution and standard solution as directed under Liquid Chromatography <*2.01*> according to the following conditions, and calculate the ratios, Q_T and Q_S, of the peak area of codeine to that of the internal standard.

Amount (mg) of codeine phosphate hydrate ($C_{18}H_{21}NO_3.H_3PO_4.{}^1\!/_2H_2O$)
$= M_S \times Q_T/Q_S \times 2 \times 1.023$

M_S: Amount (mg) of codeine phosphate hydrate for assay taken, calculated on the anhydrous basis

Internal standard solution—A solution of etilefrine hydrochloride (3 in 10,000).

Operating conditions—

Detector: An ultraviolet absorption photometer (wavelength: 280 nm).

Column: A stainless steel column 4.6 mm in inside diameter and 15 cm in length, packed with octadecylsilanized silica gel for liquid chromatography (5 μm in particle diameter).

Column temperature: A constant temperature of about 40°C.

Mobile phase: Dissolve 1.0 g of sodium lauryl sulfate in 500 mL of diluted phosphoric acid (1 in 1000), and adjust the pH to 3.0 with sodium hydroxide TS. To 240 mL of this solution add 70 mL of tetrahydrofuran, and mix.

Flow rate: Adjust so that the retention time of codeine is about 10 minutes.

System suitability—

System performance: When the procedure is run with 20 μL of the standard solution under the above operating conditions, codeine and the internal standard are eluted in this order with the resolution between these peaks being not less than 4.

System repeatability: When the test is repeated 5 times with 20 μL of the standard solution under the above operating conditions, the relative standard deviation of the ratios of the peak area of codeine to that of the internal standard is not more than 1.0%.

Containers and storage Containers—Tight containers.

Colchicine

コルヒチン

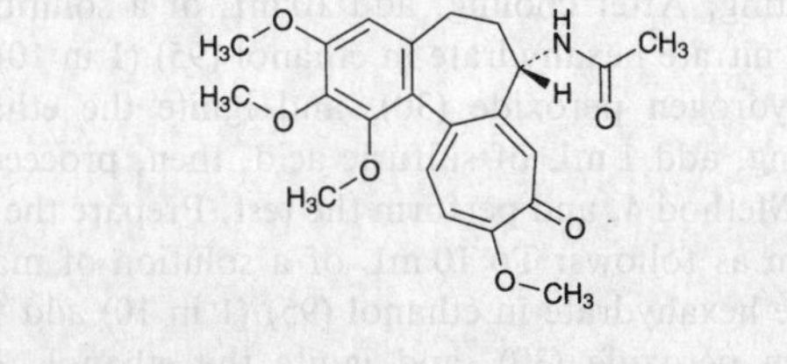

$C_{22}H_{25}NO_6$: 399.44
N-[(7*S*)-(1,2,3,10-Tetramethoxy-9-oxo-5,6,7,9-tetrahydrobenzo[*a*]heptalen-7-yl)]acetamide
[*64-86-8*]

Colchicine contains not less than 97.0% and not more than 102.0% of colchicine ($C_{22}H_{25}NO_6$), calculated on the anhydrous and residual ethyl acetate-free basis.

Description Colchicine occurs as a yellowish white powder.

It is very soluble in methanol, freely soluble in *N*,*N*-dimethylformamide, in ethanol (95) and in acetic anhydride, and sparingly soluble in water.

It is colored by light.

Identification **(1)** Determine the absorption spectrum of a solution of Colchicine in ethanol (95) (1 in 100,000) as directed under Ultraviolet-visible Spectrophotometry *<2.24>*, and compare the spectrum with the Reference Spectrum: both spectra exhibit similar intensities of absorption at the same wavelengths.

(2) To 1 g of potassium bromide for infrared absorption spectrum add 0.5 mL of a solution of Colchicine in methanol (1 in 50), grind thoroughly, and dry in vacuum at 80°C for 1 hour. Determine the infrared absorption spectrum of this powder as directed in the potassium bromide disk method under Infrared Spectrophotometry *<2.25>*, and compare the spectrum with the Reference Spectrum: both spectra exhibit similar intensities of absorption at the same wave numbers.

Optical rotation *<2.49>* $[\alpha]_D^{20}$: −235 – −250° (0.1 g calculated on the anhydrous basis and corrected by the amount of ethyl acetate, ethanol (95), 10 mL, 100 mm).

Purity **(1)** Colchicine—Dissolve 0.10 g of Colchicine in 10 mL of water, and to 5 mL of this solution add 2 drops of iron (III) chloride TS: no definite green color develops.

(2) Chloroform and ethyl acetate—Weigh accurately about 0.6 g of Colchicine, dissolve in exactly 2 mL of the internal standard solution, add *N*,*N*-dimethylformamide to make 10 mL, and use this solution as the sample solution. Separately, weigh 0.30 g of chloroform using a 100-mL volumetric flask containing about 20 mL of *N*,*N*-dimethylformamide, and add *N*,*N*-dimethylformamide to make exactly 100 mL. Pipet 2 mL of this solution, add *N*,*N*-dimethylformamide to make exactly 200 mL, and use this solution as the standard solution (1). Separately, weigh accurately about 1.8 g of ethyl acetate using a 100-mL volumetric flask containing about 20 mL of *N*,*N*-dimethylformamide, and add *N*,*N*-dimethylformamide to make exactly 100 mL. Pipet 2 mL of this solution, add exactly 2 mL of the internal standard solution and *N*,*N*-dimethylformamide to make 10 mL, and use this solution as the standard solution (2). Perform the test with exactly 2 μL each of the sample solution and standard solutions (1) and (2) as directed under Gas Chromatography *<2.02>* according to the following conditions: the peak area of chloroform obtained from sample solution is not larger than that from the standard solution (1). Calculate the ratios of the peak area of ethyl acetate to that of the internal standard, Q_T and Q_S, of the sample solution and standard solution (2), and calculate the amount of ethyl acetate by the following formula: the amount of ethyl acetate is not more than 6.0%.

$$\text{Amount (\%) of ethyl acetate } (C_4H_8O_2) = M_S/M_T \times Q_T/Q_S \times 2$$

M_S: Amount (g) of ethyl acetate taken
M_T: Amount (g) of Colchicine taken

Internal standard solution—A solution of 1-propanol in *N*,*N*-dimethylformamide (3 in 200).

Operating conditions—

Detector: A hydrogen flame-ionization detector.

Column: A fused silica column 0.53 mm in inside diameter and 30 m in length, coated inside surface with polyethylene glycol 20 M for gas chromatography 1.0 μm in thickness.

Column temperature: 60°C for 7 minutes, then up to 100°C at a rate of 40°C per minute if necessary, and hold at 100°C for 10 minutes.

Injection port temperature: A constant temperature of about 130°C.

Detector temperature: A constant temperature of about 200°C.

Carrier gas: Helium.

Flow rate: Adjust so that the retention time of ethyl acetate is about 3 minutes.

Split ratio: 1:20.

System suitability—

Test for required detectability: Pipet 2 mL of the standard solution (2), and add *N*,*N*-dimethylformamide to make exactly 25 mL. Pipet 1 mL of this solution, and add *N*,*N*-dimethylformamide to make exactly 50 mL. Confirm that the peak area of ethyl acetate obtained with 2 μL of this solution is equivalent to 0.11 to 0.21% of that with 2 μL of the standard solution (2).

System performance: To 1 mL of chloroform add *N*,*N*-dimethylformamide to make 10 mL. To 1 mL of this solution add 2 mL of ethyl acetate and *N*,*N*-dimethylformamide to make 100 mL. To 2 mL of this solution add 2 mL of the internal standard solution and *N*,*N*-dimethylformamide to make 10 mL. When the procedure is run with 2 μL of this solution under the above operating conditions, ethyl acetate, chloroform and the internal standard are eluted in this order with the resolution between the peaks of chloroform and the internal standard being not less than 2.0.

System repeatability: When the test is repeated 3 times with 2 μL of the standard solution (2) under the above operating conditions, the relative standard deviation of the ratio of the peak area of ethyl acetate to that of the internal standard is not more than 3.0%.

(3) Related substances—Dissolve 60 mg of Colchicine in 100 mL of diluted methanol (1 in 2). To 1 mL of this solution, add diluted methanol (1 in 2) to make 100 mL, and use this solution as the sample solution. Perform the test with 20 μL of the sample solution as directed under Liquid Chromatography *<2.01>* according to the following conditions, and determine each peak area by the automatic integration method. Calculate the total amount of the peaks other than colchicine by the area percentage method: not more than 5.0%.

Operating conditions—

Detector: An ultraviolet absorption photometer (wavelength: 254 nm).

Column: A stainless steel column 4.6 mm in inside diameter and 25 cm in length, packed with octylsilanized silica gel for liquid chromatography (5 μm in particle diameter).

Column temperature: A constant temperature of about 25°C.

Mobile phase: To 450 mL of 0.05 mol/L potassium dihydrogen phosphate TS add methanol to make 1000 mL. Adjust the pH to 5.5 with diluted phosphoric acid (7 in 200).

Flow rate: Adjust so that the retention time of colchicine is about 7 minutes.

Time span of measurement: About 2 times as long as the retention time of colchicine, beginning after the solvent peak.

System suitability—

Test for required detectability: Pipet 1 mL of the sample solution, and add diluted methanol (1 in 2) to make exactly 50 mL. Confirm that the peak area of colchicine obtained from 20 μL of this solution is equivalent to 1.4 to 2.6% of that obtained from 20 μL of the sample solution.

System performance: When the procedure is run with 20 μL of the sample solution under the above operating conditions, the number of theoretical plates and the symmetry factor of the peak of colchicine are not less than 6000 and not more than 1.5, respectively.

System repeatability: When the test is repeated 6 times with 20 μL of the sample solution under the above operating conditions, the relative standard deviation of the peak area of colchicine is not more than 2.0%.

Water *<2.48>* Not more than 2.0% (0.5 g, volumetric titration, back titration).

Assay Weigh accurately about 0.4 g of Colchicine, dissolve in 25 mL of acetic anhydride, and titrate *<2.50>* with 0.05 mol/L perchloric acid VS (potentiometric titration). Perform a blank determination in the same manner, and make any necessary correction.

Each mL of 0.05 mol/L perchloric acid VS
= 19.97 mg of $C_{22}H_{25}NO_6$

Containers and storage Containers—Tight containers.
Storage—Light-resistant.

Colestimide

コレスチミド

[95522-45-5]

Colestimide is an anion exchange resin, composed of a copolymer of 2-methylimidazole and 1-chloro-2,3-epoxypropane.

It contains not less than 18.0% and not more than 20.0% of chlorine (Cl: 35.45), calculated on the dried basis.

Each g of Colestimide, calculated on the dried basis, exchanges with not less than 2.0 g and not more than 2.4 g of cholic acid ($C_{24}H_{39}O_5$: 407.56).

Description Colestimide occurs as a white to pale yellow-white powder.

It is practically insoluble in water and in ethanol (99.5).

It is hygroscopic.

Identification Determine the infrared absorption spectrum of Colestimide, previously dried, as directed in the potassium chloride disk method under Infrared Spectrophotometry *<2.25>*, and compare the spectrum with the Reference Spectrum: both spectra exhibit similar intensities of absorption at the same wave numbers.

Purity (1) Heavy metals *<1.07>*—Take 2.0 g of Colestimide in a porcelain or platinum crucible, and carbonize by weakly heating. After cooling, add 10 mL of a solution of magnesium nitrate hexahydrate in ethanol (95) (1 in 10) and 5 mL of hydrogen peroxide (30), and ignite the ethanol. After cooling, add 1 mL of sulfuric acid, then, proceed according to Method 4, and perform the test. Prepare the control solution as follows: To 10 mL of a solution of magnesium nitrate hexahydrate in ethanol (95) (1 in 10) add 5 mL of hydrogen peroxide (30), and ignite the ethanol. After cooling, add 1 mL of sulfuric acid, then, proceed in the same manner as for the test solution, and add 2.0 mL of Standard Lead Solution and water to make 50 mL (not more than 10 ppm).

(2) Related substances—To exactly 0.50 g of Colestimide add exactly 20 mL of water, shake for 1 hour, centrifuge, and use the supernatant liquid as the sample solution. Determine the absorbance of the sample solution at 210 nm as directed under Ultraviolet-visible Spectrophotometry *<2.24>*: the absorbance is not more than 0.50.

Loss on drying *<2.41>* Not more than 10.0% (1 g, in vacuum, 105°C, 4 hours).

Residue on ignition *<2.44>* Not more than 0.1% (1 g).

Degree of swelling Weigh accurately about 1 g of Colestimide, put in a 25-mL glass stoppered measuring cylinder (about 11 mm in inside diameter), add 23 mL of water, shake for 2 minutes, and add water to make 25 mL. After standing for 2 hours, measure the volume of the resin layer, and determine the volume per g, calculated on the dried basis: the volume is 12 - 18 mL/g.

Assay (1) Chlorine—Weigh accurately about 0.2 g of Colestimide, add 50 mL of water, and shake. Add 1 mL of nitric acid and 25 mg of potassium nitrate, shake, and titrate *<2.50>* with 0.1 mol/L silver nitrate VS (potentiometric titration). Perform a blank determination in the same manner, and make any necessary correction.

Each mL of 0.1 mol/L silver nitrate VS
= 3.545 mg of Cl

(2) Exchange capacity—Weigh accurately about 0.45 g of sodium cholate hydrate (separately determine the water), dissolve in water to make exactly 100 mL, and use this solution as the sodium cholate standard stock solution. Separately, weigh accurately about 30 mg of Colestimide, add exactly 30 mL of the sodium cholate standard stock solution, shake for 1 hour, and centrifuge or filter through a membrane filter with a pore size not exceeding 0.8 μm. Pipet 5 mL of the supernatant liquid or the filtrate, add exactly 5 mL of the internal standard solution, and use this solution as the sample solution. Separately, pipet 5 mL of the sodium cholate standard stock solution, add exactly 5 mL of the internal standard solution, and use this solution as the standard solution. Perform the test with 10 μL each of the sample solution and standard solution as directed under Liquid Chromatography *<2.01>* according to the following conditions, and calculate the ratios, Q_T and Q_S, of the peak area of cholic acid to that of the internal standard.

Exchanged amount (g) of cholic acid per g of Colestimide, calculated on the dried basis

$$= M_S/M_T \times (Q_S - Q_T)/Q_S \times 3/10 \times 0.947$$

M_S: Amount (mg) of sodium cholate hydrate taken, calculated on the anhydrous basis

M_T: Amount (mg) of Colestimide taken, calculated on the dried basis

Internal standard solution—A solution of butyl parahydroxybenzoate in acetonitrile (1 in 80,000).

Operating conditions—

Detector: An ultraviolet absorption photometer (wavelength: 220 nm).

Column: A stainless steel column 4.6 mm in inside diameter and 25 cm in length, packed with octadecylsilanized silica gel for liquid chromatography (5 μm in particle diameter).

Column temperature: A constant temperature of about 30°C.

Mobile phase: A mixture of diluted phosphoric acid (1 in 1000) and acetonitrile (1:1).

Flow rate: Adjust so that the retention time of cholic acid is about 7 minutes.

System suitability—

System performance: When the procedure is run with 10 μL of the standard solution under the above operating conditions, cholic acid and the internal standard are eluted in this order with the resolution between these peaks being not less than 7.

System repeatability: When the test is repeated 6 times with 10 μL of the standard solution under the above operating conditions, the relative standard deviation of the ratio of the peak area of cholic acid to that of the internal standard is not more than 1.0%.

Containers and storage Containers—Tight containers.

Colestimide Granules

コレスチミド顆粒

Colestimide Granules contain not less than 87.0% and not more than 113.0% of the labeled amount of colestimide.

Method of preparation Prepare as directed under Granules, with Colestimide.

Identification Determine the infrared absorption spectrum of powdered Colestimide Granules as directed in the potassium chloride disk method under Infrared Spectrophotometry <2.25>: it exhibits absorption at the wave numbers of about 1587 cm^{-1}, 1528 cm^{-1} and 1262 cm^{-1}.

Uniformity of dosage units <6.02> Colestimide Granules in single-dose packages meet the requirement of the Mass variation test.

Disintegration <6.09> Carry out the test for 10 minutes with 0.09 - 0.11 g of Colestimide Granules in six glass tubes of the apparatus: it meets the requirement.

Assay Weigh accurately about 4.5 g of sodium cholate hydrate (separately determine the water), dissolve in water to make exactly 1000 mL, and use this solution as the sodium cholate standard stock solution. Take out the contents of not less than 20 single-dose packages of Colestimide Granules, weigh accurately an amount of the contents, equivalent to about 0.2 g of colestimide, add exactly 200 mL of the sodium cholate standard stock solution, shake for 1 hour, and centrifuge. Pipet 5 mL of the supernatant liquid, add exactly 5 mL of the internal standard solution, and use this solution as the sample solution. Then, proceed as directed in the Assay (2) under Colestimide.

Amount (mg) of colestimide
$= M_S \times (Q_S - Q_T)/Q_S \times 1/5 \times 1/2.2 \times 0.947$

M_S: Amount (mg) of sodium cholate hydrate taken, calculated on the anhydrous basis

2.2: Quantity (g) of the cholic acid exchange per mg of colestimide

Internal standard solution—A solution of butyl parahydroxybenzoate in acetonitrile (1 in 80,000).

Containers and storage Containers—Tight containers.

Colestimide Tablets

コレスチミド錠

Colestimide Tablets contain not less than 87.0% and not more than 113.0% of the labeled amount of colestimide.

Method of preparation Prepare as directed under Tablets, with Colestimide.

Identification Powder Colestimide Tablets. Determine the infrared absorption spectrum of a portion of the powder as directed in the potassium chloride disk method under Infrared Spectrophotometry <2.25>: it exhibits absorption at the wave numbers of about 1587 cm^{-1}, 1528 cm^{-1}, 1262 cm^{-1}, 1102 cm^{-1} and 1035 cm^{-1}.

Uniformity of dosage units <6.02> It meets the requirement of the Mass variation test.

Disintegration <6.09> When carry out the test for 10 minutes, it meets the requirement.

Assay Weigh accurately about 0.45 g of sodium cholate hydrate (separately determine the water), dissolve in water to make exactly 100 mL, and use this solution as the sodium cholate standard stock solution. Separately, weigh accurately the mass of not less than 20 Colestimide Tablets, and powder. Weigh accurately a portion of the powder, equivalent to about 30 mg of colestimide, add exactly 30 mL of the sodium cholate standard stock solution, shake for 1 hour, and centrifuge. Pipet 5 mL of the supernatant liquid, add exactly 5 mL of the internal standard solution, and use this solution as the sample solution. Separately, pipet 5 mL of the sodium cholate standard stock solution, add exactly 5 mL of the internal standard solution, and use this solution as the standard solution. Perform the test with 10 μL each of the sample solution and standard solution as directed under Liquid Chromatography <2.01> according to the following conditions, and calculate the ratios, Q_T and Q_S, of the peak area of cholic acid to that of the internal standard.

Amount (mg) of colestimide
$= M_S \times (Q_S - Q_T)/Q_S \times 3/10 \times 1/2.2 \times 0.947$

M_S: Amount (mg) of sodium cholate hydrate taken, calculated on the anhydrous basis

2.2: Exchanged amount (g) of cholic acid per g of colestimide, calculated on the dried basis

Internal standard solution—A solution of butyl parahydroxybenzoate in acetonitrile (1 in 80,000).

Operating conditions—

Detector: An ultraviolet absorption photometer (wavelength: 220 nm).

Column: A stainless steel column 4.6 mm in inside diameter and 25 cm in length, packed with octadecylsilanized silica

gel for liquid chromatography (5 μm in particle diameter).

Column temperature: A constant temperature of about 30°C.

Mobile phase: A mixture of diluted phosphoric acid (1 in 1000) and acetonitrile (1:1).

Flow rate: Adjust so that the retention time of cholic acid is about 7 minutes.

System suitability—

System performance: When the procedure is run with 10 μL of the standard solution under the above operating conditions, cholic acid and the internal standard are eluted in this order with the resolution between these peaks being not less than 7.

System repeatability: When the test is repeated 6 times with 10 μL of the standard solution under the above operating conditions, the relative standard deviation of the ratio of the peak area of cholic acid to that of the internal standard is not more than 1.0%.

Containers and storage Containers—Tight containers.

Colistin Sodium Methanesulfonate

コリスチンメタンスルホン酸ナトリウム

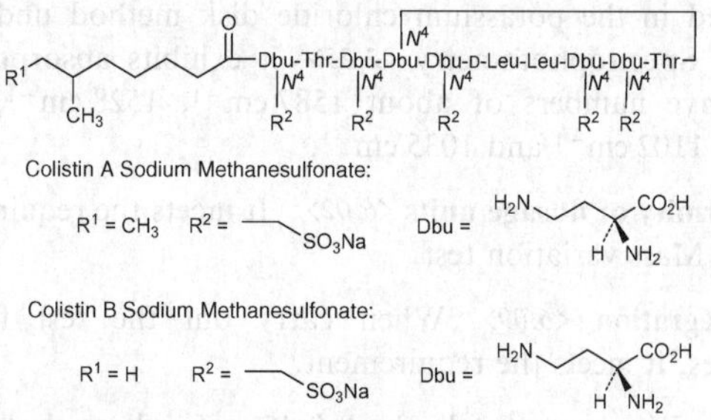

R¹-CH₂-CH(CH₃)-(CH₂)₄-C(=O)-Dbu-Thr-Dbu-Dbu-Dbu-D-Leu-Leu-Dbu-Dbu-Thr (cyclic, N⁴; each Dbu side chain N⁴-R²)

Colistin A Sodium Methanesulfonate:

$R^1 = CH_3$ $R^2 = CH_2SO_3Na$ Dbu = H_2N-CH_2CH_2-C(H)(NH_2)-CO_2H

Colistin B Sodium Methanesulfonate:

$R^1 = H$ $R^2 = CH_2SO_3Na$ Dbu = H_2N-CH_2CH_2-C(H)(NH_2)-CO_2H

Colistin A Sodium Methanesulfonate
$C_{58}H_{105}N_{16}Na_5O_{28}S_5$: 1749.82
Colistin B Sodium Methanesulfonate
$C_{57}H_{103}N_{16}Na_5O_{28}S_5$: 1735.79
[*8068-28-8*, Colistin Sodium Methanesulfonate]

Colistin Sodium Methanesulfonate is the sodium salt of colistin derivatives.

It is a mixture of colistin A sodium methanesulfonate and colistin B sodium methanesulfonate.

It, when dried, contains not less than 11,500 Units and not more than 15,500 Units per mg. The unit of Colistin Sodium Methanesulfonate is expressed as mass of colistin A (R = 6-methyloctanic acid, R′ = H; $C_{53}H_{100}N_{16}O_{13}$: 1169.46).

Description Colistin Sodium Methanesulfonate occurs as a white to light yellow-white powder.

It is freely soluble in water, and practically insoluble in ethanol (95).

Identification **(1)** Dissolve 20 mg of Colistin Sodium Methanesulfonate in 2 mL of water, add 0.5 mL of sodium hydroxide TS, and add 5 drops of copper (II) sulfate TS while shaking: a blue-purple color develops.

(2) Dissolve 40 mg of Colistin Sodium Methanesulfonate in 1 mL of 1 mol/L hydrochloric acid TS, and add 0.5 mL of dilute iodine TS: the color of iodine disappears.

(3) Determine the infrared absorption spectrum of Colistin Sodium Methanesulfonate, previously dried, as directed in the potassium bromide disk method under Infrared Spectrophotometry <*2.25*>, and compare the spectrum with the Reference Spectrum or the spectrum of dried Colistin Sodium Methanesulfonate RS: both spectra exhibit similar intensities of absorption at the same wave numbers.

(4) Colistin Sodium Methanesulfonate responds to Qualitative Tests <*1.09*> (1) for sodium salt.

pH <*2.54*> Dissolve 0.1 g of Colistin Sodium Methanesulfonate in 10 mL of water, and allow to stand for 30 minutes: the pH of the solution is between 6.5 and 8.5.

Purity **(1)** Clarity and color of solution—Dissolve 0.16 g of Colistin Sodium Methanesulfonate in 10 mL of water: the solution is clear and colorless.

(2) Heavy metals <*1.07*>—Proceed with 1.0 g of Colistin Sodium Methanesulfonate according to Method 4, and perform the test. Prepare the control solution with 3.0 mL of Standard Lead Solution (not more than 30 ppm).

(3) Arsenic <*1.11*>—Prepare the test solution with 1.0 g of Colistin Sodium Methanesulfonate according to Method 4, and perform the test (not more than 2 ppm).

(4) Free colistin—Dissolve 80 mg of Colistin Sodium Methanesulfonate in 3 mL of water, add 0.05 mL of a solution of silicotungstic acid 26-water (1 in 10), and immediately compare the solution with the reference suspension described under Test Methods for Plastic Containers <*7.02*>: the turbidity is not greater than that of the reference suspension (not more than 0.25%).

Loss on drying <*2.41*> Not more than 3.0% (0.1 g, reduced pressure, 60°C, 3 hours).

Assay Perform the test according to the Cylinder-plate method as directed under Microbial Assay for Antibiotics <*4.02*> according to the following conditions.

(i) Test organism—*Escherichia coli* NIHJ

(ii) Culture medium—To 10.0 g of peptone, 30.0 g of sodium chloride, 3.0 g of meat extract and 20.0 g of agar add 1000 mL of water, then add a suitable amount of sodium hydroxide TS so that the pH of the medium is being 6.5 to 6.6 after sterilization, sterile, and use this as the seeded agar medium and the agar medium for base layer.

(iii) Standard solutions—Weigh accurately an amount of Colistin Sodium Methanesulfonate RS, previously dried, dissolve in phosphate buffer solution (pH 6.0) to make a solution containing 100,000 Units per mL, and use this solution as the standard stock solution. Keep the standard stock solution at 10°C or below and use within 7 days. Take exactly a suitable amount of the standard stock solution before use, and add phosphate buffer solution (pH 6.0) to make solutions so that each mL contains 10,000 Units and 2500 Units, and use these solutions as the high concentration standard solution and the low concentration standard solution, respectively.

(iv) Sample solutions—Weigh accurately an amount of Colistin Sodium Methanesulfonate, previously dried, dissolve in phosphate buffer solution (pH 6.0) to make a solution containing about 100,000 Units per mL, and use this solution as the sample stock solution. Take exactly a suitable amount of the sample stock solution, add phosphate buffer solution (pH 6.0) to make solutions so that each mL contains 10,000 Units and 2500 Units, and use these solutions as the high concentration sample solution and the low concentration sample solution, respectively.

Containers and storage Containers—Tight containers.

Colistin Sulfate

コリスチン硫酸塩

Dbu-Thr-Dbu-Dbu-Dbu-D-Leu-Leu-Dbu-Dbu-Thr • 2½H_2SO_4

Colistin A Sulfate : R = CH_3

Colistin B Sulfate : R = H

Colistin A Sulfate $C_{53}H_{100}N_{16}O_{13}.2\frac{1}{2}H_2SO_4$: 1414.66
Colistin B Sulfate $C_{52}H_{98}N_{16}O_{13}.2\frac{1}{2}H_2SO_4$: 1400.63
[1264-72-8]

Colistin Sulfate is the sulfate of a mixture of peptide substances having antibacterial activity produced by the growth of *Bacillus polymyxa* var. *colistinus*.

It, when dried, contains not less than 16,000 units per mg. The potency of Colistin Sulfate is expressed as unit calculated from the amount of colistin A ($C_{53}H_{100}N_{16}O_{13}$: 1169.46). One unit of Colistin Sulfate is equivalent to 0.04 μg of colistin A ($C_{53}H_{100}N_{16}O_{13}$).

Description Colistin Sulfate occurs as a white to light yellow-white powder.

It is freely soluble in water, and practically insoluble in ethanol (99.5).

It is hygroscopic.

Identification (1) Dissolve 20 mg of Colistin Sulfate in 2 mL of water, add 0.5 mL of sodium hydroxide TS, then add 5 drops of copper (II) sulfate TS while shaking: a purple color develops.

(2) Dissolve 50 mg of Colistin Sulfate in 10 mL of diluted hydrochloric acid (1 in 2). Transfer 1 mL of this solution in a tube for hydrolysis, seal, and heat at 135°C for 5 hours. After cooling, open the tube, and evaporate the content to dryness until the odor of hydrochloric acid is no more perceptible. Dissolve the residue in 0.5 mL of water, and use this solution as the sample solution. Separately, dissolve 20 mg each of L-leucine, L-threonine, phenylalanine and L-serine in 10 mL of water, and use these solutions as the standard solution (1), (2), (3) and (4). Perform the test with these solutions as directed under Thin-layer Chromatography <*2.03*>. Spot 1 μL each of the sample solution and standard solution (1), (2), (3) and (4) on a plate of cellulose for thin-layer chromatography. Develop the plate with a mixture of 1-butanol, acetic acid (100), water, pyridine and ethanol (99.5) (60:15:10:6:5) to a distance of about 10 cm, and dry the plate at 105°C for 10 minutes. Spray evenly ninhydrin TS on the plate, and heat at 110°C for 5 minutes: three principal spots are obtained from the sample solution, the *R*f values of two spots of them are the same with those of the corresponding spots obtained from the standard solution (1) and the standard solution (2), and the *R*f value of the rest principal spot is about 0.1. No spot is observed at the position corresponding to the spots from the standard solution (3) and the standard solution (4).

(3) A solution of Colistin Sulfate (1 in 20) responds to Qualitative Tests <*1.09*> (1) for sulfate.

Optical rotation <*2.49*> $[\alpha]_D^{20}$: −63 – −73° (1.25 g, after drying, water, 25 mL, 100 mm).

pH <*2.54*> The pH of a solution obtained by dissolving 0.10 g of Colistin Sulfate in 10 mL of water is between 4.0 and 6.0.

Purity (1) Sulfuric acid—Weigh accurately about 0.25 g of previously dried Colistin Sulfate, dissolve in a suitable amount of water, adjust the pH to 11 with ammonia solution (28), and add water to make 100 mL. To this solution add exactly 10 mL of 0.1 mol/L barium chloride VS and 50 mL of ethanol (99.5), and titrate with <*2.50*> 0.1 mol/L disodium dihydrogen ethylenediamine tetraacetate VS until the blue-purple color of the solution disappears (indicator: 0.5 mg of phthalein purple): the amount of sulfuric acid (SO_4) is 16.0 to 18.0%.

Each mL of 0.1 mol/L barium chloride VS
= 9.606 mg of SO_4

(2) Related substances—Dissolve 50 mg of Colistin Sulfate in 10 mL of water, and use this solution as the sample solution. Pipet 1 mL of the sample solution, add water to make exactly 50 mL, and use this solution as the standard solution. Perform the test with these solutions as directed under Thin-layer Chromatography <*2.03*>. Spot 1 μL each of the sample solution and standard solution on a plate of silica gel for thin-layer chromatography. Develop the plate with a mixture of pyridine, 1-butanol, water and acetic acid (100) (6:5:4:1) to a distance of about 10 cm, and dry the plate at 100°C for 30 minutes. Spray evenly ninhydrin-butanol TS on the plate, and heat at 100°C for about 20 minutes: the spot other than the principal spot obtained from the sample solution is not more intense than the spot from the standard solution.

Loss on drying <*2.41*> Not more than 6.0% (1 g, in vacuum, 60°C, 3 hours).

Residue on ignition <*2.44*> Not more than 1.0% (1 g).

Assay Perform the test according to the Cylinder-plate method as directed under Microbial Assay for Antibiotics <*4.02*> according to the following conditions.

(i) Test organism—*Escherichia coli* NIHJ

(ii) Culture medium—Dissolve 10.0 g of peptone, 30.0 g of sodium chloride, 3.0 g of meat extract and 15.0 g of agar in 1000 mL of water, adjust the pH with sodium hydroxide TS so that the solution will be 6.5 to 6.6 after sterilization, and use as the agar media for seed layer and for base layer.

(iii) Standard solutions—Weigh accurately an amount of Colistin Sulfate RS, previously dried, equivalent to about 1,000,000 units, dissolve in phosphate buffer solution (pH 6.0) to make exactly 10 mL, and use this solution as the standard stock solution. Keep the standard stock solution at not exceeding 10°C, and use within 7 days. Take exactly a suitable amount of the standard stock solution before use, add phosphate buffer solution (pH 6.0) to make solutions so that each mL contains 10,000 units and 2500 units, and use these solutions as the high concentration standard solution and the low concentration standard solution, respectively.

(iv) Sample solutions—Weigh accurately an amount of Colistin Sulfate, previously dried, equivalent to about 1,000,000 units, and dissolve in phosphate buffer solution (pH 6.0) to make exactly 10 mL. Take exactly a suitable amount of this solution, add phosphate buffer solution (pH 6.0) to make solutions so that each mL contains 10,000 units and 2500 units, and use these solutions as the high concentration sample solution and the low concentration sample solution, respectively.

Containers and storage Containers—Tight containers.

Copovidone

コポビドン

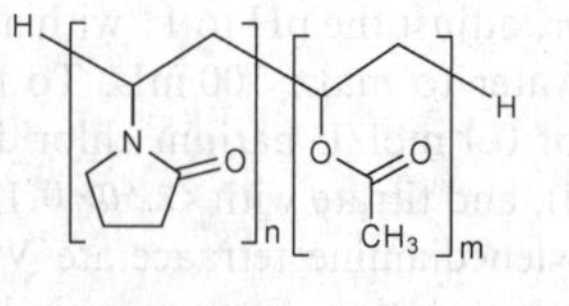

$(C_6H_9NO)_n(C_4H_6O_2)_m$
Poly[(2-oxopyrrolidin-1-yl)ethylene-*co*-(1-acetoxyethylene)]
[*25086-89-9*]

This monograph is harmonized with the European Pharmacopoeia and the U.S. Pharmacopeia.

The corresponding part of the attributes/provisions which are agreed as non-harmonized within the scope of the harmonization is marked with symbols (◆ ◆), and the corresponding parts which are agreed as the JP local requirement other than the scope of the harmonization are marked with symbols (◇ ◇).

Information on the harmonization with the European Pharmacopoeia and the U.S. Pharmacopeia is available on the website of the Pharmaceuticals and Medical Devices Agency.

Copovidone is a copolymer of 1-vinyl-2-pyrrolidone and vinyl acetate at the ratio by mass of 3:2.

It contains not less than 35.3% and not more than 42.0% of vinyl acetate ($C_4H_6O_2$: 86.09), and not less than 7.0% and not more than 8.0% of nitrogen (N: 14.01), calculated on the dried basis.

The nominal K-value is shown on the label.

◆**Description** Copovidone occurs as a white to yellowish white powder. It is odorless or has a faint, characteristic odor.

It is very soluble in methanol and in ethanol (95), and freely soluble in water.

It is hygroscopic.◆

Identification Determine the infrared absorption spectrum of Copovidone, previously dried, as directed in the potassium bromide disk method under Infrared Spectrophotometry *<2.25>*, and compare the spectrum with the Reference Spectrum: both spectra exhibit similar intensities of absorption at the same wave numbers.

pH *<2.54>* Dissolve 1.0 g of Copovidone in 10 mL of water: the pH of this solution is between 3.0 and 7.0.

Purity (1) Clarity and color of solution—Dissolve 1.0 g of Copovidone in 10 mL of water: the solution is clear or slightly opalescent and colorless to pale yellow, or pale red.

◇(2) Heavy metals *<1.07>*—Ignite 2.0 g of Copovidone as directed under Residue on Ignition Test *<2.44>*, add 2 mL of hydrochloric acid to the residue, then proceed according to Method 2, and perform the test. Prepare the control solution with 2.0 mL of Standard Lead Solution (not more than 10 ppm).◇

(3) Aldehydes—Weigh accurately about 1 g of Copovidone, dissolve in 0.05 mol/L pyrophosphate buffer solution (pH 9.0) to make exactly 100 mL. Stopper, heat at 60°C for 60 minutes, allow to cool to room temperature, and use this solution as the sample solution. Separately, dissolve 0.140 g of acetaldehyde ammonia trimer trihydrate in water to make exactly 200 mL. Pipet 1 mL of this solution, add 0.05 mol/L pyrophosphate buffer solution (pH 9.0) to make exactly 100 mL, and use this solution as the standard solution. Measure exactly 0.5 mL each of the sample solution, standard solution and water, transfer to separate 1-cm cells, add 2.5 mL of 0.05 mol/L pyrophosphate buffer solution (pH 9.0) and 0.2 mL of β-nicotinamide adenine dinucleotide TS to each of these cells, mix and stopper tightly. Allow to stand for 2 to 3 minutes at 22 ± 2°C, and perform the test with these solutions as directed under Ultraviolet-visible Spectrophotometry *<2.24>* using water as the control solution. Determine the absorbances, A_{T1}, A_{S1} and A_{B1}, of the subsequent solutions of the sample solution, the standard solution and water (blank) at 340 nm. Then, add 0.05 mL of aldehyde dehydrogenase TS to each of the cells, stir, and stopper tightly. Allow to stand at 22 ± 2°C for 5 minutes. Determine the absorbances, A_{T2}, A_{S2} and A_{B2}, of these solutions in the same manner as above: the content of aldehyde is not more than 500 ppm.

Content (ppm) of aldehydes [as acetaldehyde (CH_3CHO)]
$= C/M \times \{(A_{T2} - A_{T1}) - (A_{B2} - A_{B1})\}/\{(A_{S2} - A_{S1}) - (A_{B2} - A_{B1})\} \times 100{,}000$

M: Amount (g) of Copovidone taken, calculated on the dried basis
C: Concentration (mg/mL) of acetaldehyde in the standard solution, using 0.72 as conversion factor for acetaldehyde ammonia trimer trihydrate to acetaldehyde

(4) 1-Vinyl-2-pyrrolidone and free vinyl acetate—Store the sample solution and the standard solution at 5°C or below, and use within 8 hours. Weigh accurately about 0.25 g of Copovidone, dissolve in a mixture of water and acetonitrile (23:2) to make exactly 10 mL, and use this solution as the sample solution. Separately, dissolve 50 mg each of 1-vinyl-2-pyrrolidone and vinyl acetate in methanol to make exactly 100 mL. Pipet 1 mL of this solution and add methanol to make exactly 100 mL. Pipet 5 mL of this solution, add a mixture of water and acetonitrile (23:2) to make exactly 100 mL, and use this solution as the standard solution. Perform the test with exactly 20 μL each of the sample solution and standard solution as directed under Liquid Chromatography *<2.01>* according to the following conditions, determine the peak areas, A_{Ta}, A_{Tb}, A_{Sa} and A_{Sb}, of 1-vinyl-2-pyrrolidone and free vinyl acetate in each solution, and calculate the content of 1-vinyl-2-pyrrolidone and vinyl acetate by the following equations: they are not more than 10 ppm.

Content (ppm) of 1-vinyl-2-pyrrolidone
$= A_{Ta}/A_{Sa} \times C_{Sa}/C_T \times 1000$

Content (ppm) of free vinyl acetate
$= A_{Tb}/A_{Sb} \times C_{Sb}/C_T \times 1000$

C_{Sa}: Concentration (μg/mL) of 1-vinyl-2-pyrrolidone in the standard solution
C_{Sb}: Concentration (μg/mL) of vinyl acetate in the standard solution
C_T: Concentration (mg/mL) of Copovidone in the sample solution, calculated on the dried basis

Operating conditions—

Detector: An ultraviolet spectrophotometer (wavelength: 235 nm for 1-vinyl-2-pyrrolidone, 205 nm for vinyl acetate).

Column: Two stainless steel columns, one is 4 mm in inside diameter and 33 mm in length and the other is 4 mm in inside diameter and 250 mm in length, packed with octadecylsilanized silica gel for liquid chromatography (5 μm in particle diameter), and use them as the pre-column and the separation column, respectively.

Column temperature: A constant temperature of about

40°C.

Mobile phase: A mixture of water and acetonitrile (23:2).

Flow rate: 1.0 mL per minute (Retention times of 1-vinyl-2-pyrrolidone and vinyl acetate are about 17 and about 22 minutes, respectively).

Time span of measurement: For 40 minutes.

Washing of column: After each test with the sample solution, elute and wash away remaining sample by passing the mobile phase through the separation column or the pre-column backwards at the flow rate mentioned above for about 30 minutes.

System suitability—

System performance: When the procedure is run with 20 μL of the standard solution under the above operating conditions (wavelength: 205 nm), 1-vinyl-2-pyrrolidone and vinyl acetate are eluted in this order with the resolution between these peaks being not less than 2.0.

System repeatability: When the test is repeated 6 times with 20 μL of the standard solution under the above operating conditions, the relative standard deviations of the peak areas of 1-vinyl-2-pyrrolidone and vinyl acetate are not more than 2.0%, respectively.

(5) Peroxides—Weigh exactly an amount of Copovidone, equivalent to 4.0 g calculated on the dried basis, dissolve in water to make exactly 100 mL, and use this solution as the sample solution. To 25 mL of the sample solution add 2 mL of titanium (III) chloride-sulfuric acid TS, and mix. Allow to stand for 30 minutes, and perform the test with this solution as directed under Ultraviolet-visible Spectrophotometry *<2.24>*, using a solution prepared by adding 2 mL of diluted sulfuric acid (13 in 100) to 25 mL of the sample solution as a blank: the absorbance of the sample solution at 405 nm is not more than 0.35 (not more than 400 ppm, as hydrogen peroxide).

(6) Hydrazine—Weigh exactly an amount of Copovidone equivalent to 2.5 g calculated on the dried basis, transfer to a 50-mL centrifuge tube, add 25 mL of water, and stir to dissolve. Add 500 μL of a solution of salicylaldehyde in methanol (1 in 20), stir and warm at 60°C for 15 minutes in a water bath. Allow to cool, add 2.0 mL of toluene, stopper tightly, shake vigorously for 2 minutes, centrifuge, and use the upper layer of the mixture as the sample solution. Separately, dissolve 90 mg of salicylaldazine in toluene to make exactly 100 mL. Pipet 1 mL of this solution, add toluene to make exactly 100 mL, and use this solution as the standard solution. Perform the test with these solutions as directed under Thin-layer Chromatography *<2.03>*. Spot 10 μL each of the sample solution and standard solution on a plate of dimethylsilanized silica gel with fluorescent indicator for thin-layer chromatography. Develop the plate with a mixture of methanol and water (2:1) to a distance of about three-fourths of the length of the plate, and air-dry the plate. Examine under ultraviolet light (main wavelength: 365 nm): the fluorescence of the spot obtained from the sample solution corresponding to the spot having a *R*f value of about 0.3 from the standard solution is not more intense than that of the spot from the standard solution (not more than 1 ppm).

(7) 2-Pyrrolidone—Weigh accurately about 1 g of Copovidone, add 5 mL of methanol for liquid chromatography, and sonicate to dissolve. Add water to make exactly 100 mL, and use this solution as the sample solution. Separately, dissolve 0.150 g of 2-pyrrolidone in a mixture of water and methanol for liquid chromatography (19:1) to make exactly 100 mL. Pipet 3 mL of this solution, add a mixture of water and methanol for liquid chromatography (19:1) to make exactly 100 mL, and use this solution as the standard solution. Perform the test with exactly 20 μL each of the sample solution and standard solution as directed under Liquid Chromatography *<2.01>* according to the following conditions, and determine the peak areas, A_T and A_S, of 2-pyrrolidone in each solution. Calculate the content of 2-pyrrolidone by the following equation: not more than 0.5%.

$$\text{Content (\%) of 2-pyrrolidone} = A_T/A_S \times C_S/C_T \times 100$$

C_S: Concentration (mg/mL) of 2-pyrrolidone in the standard solution

C_T: Concentration (mg/mL) of Copovidone in the sample solution, calculated on the dried basis

Operating conditions—

Detector: An ultraviolet absorption photometer (wavelength: 205 nm).

Column: Two stainless steel columns, one is 4.0 mm in inside diameter and 10 mm in length and the other is 4.6 mm in inside diameter and 150 mm in length, packed with octadecylsilanized silica gel for liquid chromatography (5 μm in particle diameter), and use them as the pre-column and the separation column, respectively.

Column temperature: A constant temperature of about 40°C.

Mobile phase: A mixture of water and methanol for liquid chromatography (19:1).

Flow rate: 0.8 mL per minute (retention time of 2-pyrrolidone is about 7 minutes).

Time span of measurement: For 30 minutes.

Washing of column: After each test with the sample solution, elute and wash away remaining sample by passing the mobile phase through the separation column or the pre-column backwards at the flow rate mentioned above for about 30 minutes.

System suitability—

System performance: When the procedure is run with 20 μL of the standard solution under the above operating conditions, the symmetry factor of the peak of 2-pyrrolidone is not more than 1.5.

System repeatability: When the test is repeated 6 times with 20 μL of the standard solution under the above operating conditions, the relative standard deviation of the peak area of 2-pyrrolidone is not more than 2.0%.

Loss on drying *<2.41>* Not more than 5.0% (0.5 g, 105°C, 3 hours).

Residue on ignition *<2.44>* Not more than 0.1% (1 g).

K-value Weigh accurately an amount of Copovidone, equivalent to 1.00 g, calculated on the dried basis, dissolve in water to make exactly 100 mL, allow to stand for 60 minutes, and use this solution as the sample solution. Perform the test with the sample solution and with water at 25°C as directed in Method 1 under Viscosity Determination *<2.53>*, and calculate the K-value by the following formula: the K-value of Copovidone is not less than 90.0% and not more than 110.0% of the nominal K-value.

$$K = \frac{1.5 \log v_{rel.} - 1}{0.15 + 0.003c} + \frac{\sqrt{300c \log v_{rel.} + (c + 1.5c \log v_{rel.})^2}}{0.15c + 0.003c^2}$$

c: Mass (g) of Copovidone in 100 mL of the solution, calculated on the dried basis

$v_{rel.}$: Kinematic viscosity of the sample solution relative to that of water

Assay **(1)** Vinyl acetate—Weigh accurately about 2 g of

Copovidone, add exactly 25 mL of 0.5 mol/L potassium hydroxide-ethanol VS and a few glass beads, heat under reflux for 30 min. Titrate immediately with 0.5 mol/L hydrochloric acid VS (indicator: 1 mL of phenolphthalein TS). Perform a blank determination in the same manner, and make any necessary correction.

Amount (%) of vinyl acetate

$$= 0.1 \times \frac{86.09}{56.11} \times \frac{28.05\ (n_2 - n_1)}{M}$$

M: Amount (g) of Copovidone taken, calculated on the dried basis

n_1: Volume (mL) of 0.5 mol/L hydrochloric acid VS consumed in the test

n_2: Volume (mL) of 0.5 mol/L hydrochloric acid VS consumed in the blank test

(2) Nitrogen—Weigh accurately about 0.1 g of Copovidone, and place in a Kjeldahl flask. Add 5 g of a decomposition accelerator (a powdered mixture of 33 g of potassium sulfate, 1 g of copper (II) sulfate pentahydrate and 1 g of titanium (IV) oxide), and wash down any adhering sample from the neck of the flask with a small amount of water. Add 7 mL of sulfuric acid allowing to flow down the inside wall of the flask. Heat the flask gradually until the solution has a clear, yellow-green color, and the inside wall of the flask is free from a carbonized material, and then heat for further 45 minutes. After cooling, add cautiously 20 mL of water, and connect the flask to the distillation apparatus previously washed by passing steam through it. To the absorption flask add 30 mL of a solution of boric acid (1 in 25), 3 drops of bromocresol green-methyl red TS and sufficient water to immerse the lower end of the condenser tube. Add 30 mL of a solution of sodium hydroxide (2 in 5) through the funnel, rinse cautiously the funnel with 10 mL of water, immediately close the clamp attached to the rubber tube, then start the distillation with steam to obtain 80 to 100 mL of the distillate. Remove the absorption flask from the lower end of the condenser tube, rinsing the end part with a small quantity of water, and titrate *<2.50>* the distillate with 0.025 mol/L sulfuric acid VS until the color of the solution changes from green through pale grayish blue to pale grayish red-purple. Perform a blank determination in the same manner, and make any necessary correction.

Each mL of 0.025 mol/L sulfuric acid VS = 0.700 mg of N

◆**Containers and storage** Containers—Tight containers.◆

Cortisone Acetate

コルチゾン酢酸エステル

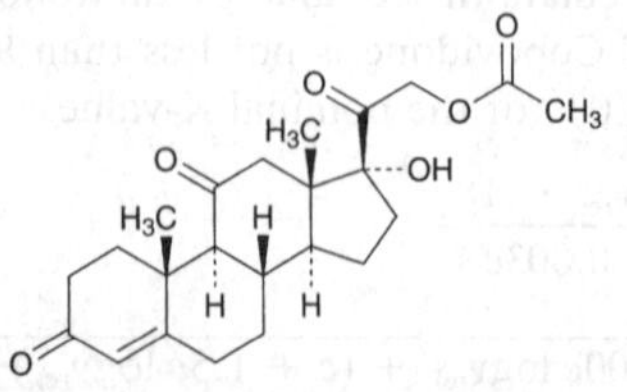

$C_{23}H_{30}O_6$: 402.48
17,21-Dihydroxypregn-4-ene-3,11,20-trione 21-acetate
[50-04-4]

Cortisone Acetate, when dried, contains not less than 97.0% and not more than 102.0% of cortisone acetate ($C_{23}H_{30}O_6$).

Description Cortisone Acetate occurs as white, crystals or crystalline powder.

It is sparingly soluble in methanol, slightly soluble in ethanol (99.5), and practically insoluble in water.

Melting point: about 240°C (with decomposition).

It shows crystal polymorphism.

Identification **(1)** To 2 mg of Cortisone Acetate add 2 mL of sulfuric acid, and allow to stand for a while: a yellowish green color is produced, and it gradually changes to yellow-orange. Examine the solution under ultraviolet light: the solution shows a light green fluorescence. Add carefully 10 mL of water to this solution: the color of the solution is discharged, and the solution remains clear.

(2) Determine the absorption spectrum of a solution of Cortisone Acetate in methanol (1 in 50,000) as directed under Ultraviolet-visible Spectrophotometry *<2.24>*, and compare the spectrum with the Reference Spectrum or the spectrum of a solution of Cortisone Acetate RS prepared in the same manner as the sample solution: both spectra exhibit similar intensities of absorption at the same wavelengths.

(3) Determine the infrared absorption spectrum of Cortisone Acetate, previously dried, as directed in the potassium bromide disk method under Infrared Spectrophotometry *<2.25>*, and compare the spectrum with the Reference Spectrum or the spectrum of previously dried Cortisone Acetate RS: both spectra exhibit similar intensities of absorption at the same wave numbers. If any difference appears between the spectra, dissolve Cortisone Acetate and Cortisone Acetate RS in acetone, respectively, then evaporate the acetone to dryness, and repeat the test on the residues.

Optical rotation *<2.49>* $[\alpha]_D^{20}$: +207 – +216° (after drying, 0.1 g, methanol, 10 mL, 100 mm).

Purity Related substances—Dissolve 25 mg of Cortisone Acetate in 10 mL of a mixture of acetonitrile, water and acetic acid (100) (70:30:1), and use this solution as the sample solution. Pipet 1 mL of the sample solution add the mixture of acetonitrile, water and acetic acid (100) (70:30:1) to make exactly 100 mL, and use this solution as the standard solution. Perform the test with exactly 15 μL each of the sample solution and standard solution as directed under Liquid Chromatography *<2.01>* according to the following conditions, and determine each peak area by the automatic integration method: each peak area other than cortisone acetate obtained from the sample solution is not larger than 1/2 times the peak area of cortisone acetate from the standard solution, and the total area of the peaks other than cortisone acetate is not larger than 1.5 times the peak area of cortisone acetate from the standard solution.

Operating conditions—

Detector: An ultraviolet absorption photometer (wavelength: 254 nm).

Column: A stainless steel column 4.6 mm in inside diameter and 15 cm in length, packed with octadecylsilanized silica gel for liquid chromatography (5 μm in particle diameter).

Column temperature: A constant temperature of about 25°C.

Mobile phase A: A mixture of water and acetonitrile (7:3).

Mobile phase B: A mixture of acetonitrile and water (7:3).

Flowing of mobile phase: Control the gradient by mixing the mobile phases A and B as directed in the following table.

Time after injection of sample (min)	Mobile phase A (vol%)	Mobile phase B (vol%)
0 – 5	90	10
5 – 25	90 → 10	10 → 90
25 – 30	10	90

Flow rate: About 1 mL per minute.

Time span of measurement: About 3 times as long as the retention time of cortisone acetate, beginning after the solvent peak.

System suitability—

Test for required detectability: To exactly 1 mL of the standard solution add a mixture of acetonitrile, water and acetic acid (100) (70:30:1) to make exactly 10 mL. Confirm that the peak area of cortisone acetate obtained with 15 μL of this solution is equivalent to 8 to 12% of that with 15 μL of the standard solution.

System performance: When the procedure is run with 15 μL of the sample solution under the above operating conditions, the number of theoretical plates and the symmetry factor of the peak of cortisone acetate are not less than 10,000 and not more than 1.3, respectively.

System repeatability: When the test is repeated 3 times with 15 μL of the standard solution under the above operating conditions, the relative standard deviation of the peak area of cortisone acetate is not more than 5.0%.

Loss on drying <*2.41*> Not more than 1.0% (0.5 g, 105°C, 3 hours).

Residue on ignition <*2.44*> Not more than 0.1% (0.5 g).

Assay Dissolve about 10 mg each of Cortisone Acetate and Cortisone Acetate RS, previously dried and accurately weighed, in 50 mL of methanol, add exactly 5 mL each of the internal standard solution, then add methanol to make 100 mL, and use these solutions as the sample solution and the standard solution. Perform the test with 10 μL each of the sample solution and standard solution as directed under Liquid Chromatography <*2.01*> according to the following conditions, and calculate the ratios, Q_T and Q_S, of the peak area of cortisone acetate to that of the internal standard.

$$\text{Amount (mg) of cortisone acetate } (C_{23}H_{30}O_6) = M_S \times Q_T/Q_S$$

M_S: Amount (mg) of Cortisone Acetate RS taken

Internal standard solution—A solution of butyl parahydroxybenzoate in methanol (3 in 5000).

Operating conditions—

Detector: An ultraviolet absorption photometer (wavelength: 254 nm).

Column: A stainless steel column 4.6 mm in inside diameter and 30 cm in length, packed with octadecylsilanized silica gel for liquid chromatography (10 μm in particle diameter).

Column temperature: A constant temperature of about 25°C.

Mobile phase: A mixture of water and acetonitrile (13:7).

Flow rate: Adjust so that the retention time of cortisone acetate is about 12 minutes.

System suitability—

System performance: When the procedure is run with 10 μL of the standard solution under the above operating conditions, cortisone acetate and the internal standard are eluted in this order with the resolution between these peaks being not less than 4.

System repeatability: When the test is repeated 6 times with 10 μL of the standard solution under the above operating conditions, the relative standard deviation of the ratios of the peak area of cortisone acetate to that of the internal standard is not more than 1.0%.

Containers and storage Containers—Tight containers.

Absorptive Cream

吸水クリーム

Method of preparation

White Petrolatum	400 g
Cetanol	100 g
White Beeswax	50 g
Sorbitan Sesquioleate	50 g
Lauromacrogol	5 g
Ethyl Parahydroxybenzoate or Methyl Parahydroxybenzoate	1 g
Butyl Parahydroxybenzoate or Propyl Parahydroxybenzoate	1 g
Purified Water or Purified Water in Containers	a sufficient quantity
To make	1000 g

Melt White Petrolatum, Cetanol, White Beeswax, Sorbitan Sesquioleate and Lauromacrogol by heating on a water bath, mix and maintain at about 75°C. Add Methyl Parahydroxybenzoate or Ethyl Parahydroxybenzoate and Propyl Parahydroxybenzoate or Butyl Parahydroxybenzoate to Purified Water or Purified Water in Containers, dissolve by warming at 80°C. Combine both solutions, mix to make emulsion, cool, and stir thoroughly until it congeals.

Description Absorptive Cream is white in color and is lustrous. It has a slightly characteristic odor.

Containers and storage Containers—Tight containers.

Hydrophilic Cream

親水クリーム

Method of preparation

White Petrolatum	250 g
Stearyl Alcohol	200 g
Propylene Glycol	120 g
Polyoxyethylene hydrogenated castor oil 60	40 g
Glycerin Monostearate	10 g
Methyl Parahydroxybenzoate	1 g
Propyl Parahydroxybenzoate	1 g
Purified Water or Purified Water in Containers	a sufficient quantity
To make	1000 g

Melt White Petrolatum, Stearyl Alcohol, polyoxyethylene hydrogenated castor oil 60 and Glycerin Monostearate by heating on a water bath, stir, and keep temperature of the mixture at about 75°C. To Propylene Glycol add Methyl Parahydroxybenzoate and Propyl Parahydroxybenzoate, melt by warming if necessary, dissolve in Purified Water or Purified Water in Containers, and warm to about 75°C. Add this solution to the above mixture, stir to form emulsion, cool, and stir thoroughly until it congeals.

Description Hydrophilic Cream is white in color. It has a slight, characteristic odor.

Containers and storage Containers—Tight containers.

Cresol

クレゾール

C_7H_8O: 108.14

Cresol is a mixture of isomeric cresols.

Description Cresol is a clear, colorless or yellow to yellow-brown liquid. It has a phenol-like odor.

It is miscible with ethanol (95) and with diethyl ether.

It is sparingly soluble in water.

It dissolves in sodium hydroxide TS.

A saturated solution of Cresol is neutral to bromocresol purple TS.

It is a highly refractive liquid.

It becomes dark brown by light or on aging.

Identification To 5 mL of a saturated solution of Cresol add 1 to 2 drops of dilute iron (III) chloride TS: a blue-purple color develops.

Specific gravity <*2.56*> d_{20}^{20}: 1.032 - 1.041

Purity **(1)** Hydrocarbons—Dissolve 1.0 mL of Cresol in 60 mL of water: the solution shows no more turbidity than that produced in the following control solution.

Control solution: To 54 mL of water add 6.0 mL of 0.005 mol/L sulfuric acid VS and 1.0 mL of barium chloride TS, and after thorough shaking, allow to stand for 5 minutes.

(2) Sulfur compounds—Transfer 20 mL of Cresol in a 100-mL conical flask, place a piece of moistened lead (II) acetate paper on the mouth of the flask, and warm for 5 minutes on a water bath: the lead (II) acetate paper may develop a yellow color, but neither a brown nor a dark tint.

Distilling range <*2.57*> 196 - 206°C, not less than 90 vol%.

Containers and storage Containers—Tight containers.

Storage—Light-resistant.

Cresol Solution

クレゾール水

Cresol Solution contains not less than 1.25 vol% and not more than 1.60 vol% of cresol.

Method of preparation

Saponated Cresol Solution	30 mL
Water, Purified Water or Purified Water in Containers	a sufficient quantity
	To make 1000 mL

Prepare by mixing the above ingredients.

Description Cresol Solution is a clear or slightly turbid, yellow solution. It has the odor of cresol.

Identification Shake 0.5 mL of the oily layer obtained in the Assay with 30 mL of water, filter, and perform the following tests using this filtrate as the sample solution:

(1) To 5 mL of the sample solution add 1 to 2 drops of iron (III) chloride TS: a blue-purple color develops.

(2) To 5 mL of the sample solution add 1 to 2 drops of bromine TS: a light yellow, flocculent precipitate is produced.

Assay Transfer 200 mL of Cresol Solution, exactly measured, to a 500-mL distilling flask. Add 40 g of sodium chloride and 3 mL of dilute sulfuric acid, and connect the distilling apparatus with the distilling flask, and distil into a cassia flask which contains 30 g of powdered sodium chloride and 3 mL of kerosene, exactly measured, until the distillate measures 90 mL. Draw off the water from the condenser, and continue the distillation until water vapor begins to come out of the tip of the condenser. Shake often the cassia flask in warm water to dissolve the sodium chloride, and allow to stand for 15 minutes. After cooling to 15°C, add a saturated solution of sodium chloride, and allow to stand for more than 3 hours with occasional shaking. Allow to stand for 1 to 2 minutes with gentle shaking to combine the separated oil drops with the oil layer. The difference between the number of mL of the oil layer measured and 3 mL represents the amount (mL) of cresol.

Containers and storage Containers—Tight containers.

Saponated Cresol Solution

クレゾール石ケン液

Saponated Cresol Solution contains not less than 42 vol% and not more than 52 vol% of cresol.

Method of preparation

Cresol	500 mL
Fixed Oil	300 mL
Potassium Hydroxide	a suitable quantity
Water, Purified Water or Purified Water in Containers	a sufficient quantity
	To make 1000 mL

Dissolve Potassium Hydroxide, in required quantity for saponification, in a sufficient quantity of Water, Purified Water or Purified Water in Containers, add this solution to fixed oil, previously warmed, add a sufficient quantity of Ethanol, if necessary, heat in a water bath by thorough stirring, and continue the saponification. After complete saponification, add Cresol, stir thoroughly until the mixture becomes clear, and add sufficient Water, Purified Water or Purified Water in Containers to make 1000 mL. A corresponding amount of Sodium Hydroxide may be used in place of Potassium Hydroxide.

Description Saponated Cresol Solution is a yellow-brown to red-brown, viscous liquid. It has the odor of cresol.

It is miscible with water, with ethanol (95) and with glycerin.

It is alkaline.

Identification Proceed as directed in the Identification under Cresol, using the distillate in the Purity (3).

Purity **(1)** Alkalinity—Mix well 0.50 mL of Saponated Cresol Solution with 10 mL of neutralized ethanol, add 2 to 3 drops of phenolphthalein TS and 0.10 mL of 1 mol/L hydrochloric acid VS: no red color develops.

(2) Unsaponified matter—To 1.0 mL of Saponated Cresol Solution add 5 mL of water, and shake: the solution is clear.

(3) Cresol fraction—Transfer 180 mL of Saponated Cresol Solution to a 2000-mL distilling flask, add 300 mL of water and 100 mL of dilute sulfuric acid, and distil with steam until the distillate becomes clear. Draw off the water from the condenser, and continue the distillation until water vapor begins to come out of the tip of the condenser. Cool the condenser again, and continue distillation for 5 minutes. Dissolve 20 g of sodium chloride per 100 mL of the distillate, allow to stand, and collect the separated clear oil layer. After adding about 15 g of powdered calcium chloride for drying in small portions with frequent shaking, allow to stand for 4 hours. Filter, and distil exactly 50 mL of the filtrate: the distillate is not less than 43 mL between 196°C and 206°C.

Assay Transfer 5 mL of Saponated Cresol Solution, exactly measured, to a 500-mL distilling flask, holding the pipet vertically for 15 minutes to draw off the solution into the flask. Add 200 mL of water, 40 g of sodium chloride and 3 mL of dilute sulfuric acid, connect the distilling apparatus with the distilling flask, and distil into a cassia flask which contains 30 g of powdered sodium chloride and exactly 3 mL of kerosene, until the distillate reaches 90 mL. Draw off the water from the condenser, and continue the distillation until water vapor begins to come out of the tip of the condenser. Allow the cassia flask to stand in warm water for 15 minutes to dissolve the sodium chloride with frequent shaking. Cool to 15°C, add a saturated solution of sodium chloride, and allow to stand for more than 3 hours with occasional shaking. Allow to stand for 1 to 2 minutes with gentle shaking, and combine the separated oil drops with the oil layer. The volume (mL) subtracted 3 (mL) from the oil layer measured represents the amount (mL) of cresol.

Containers and storage Containers—Tight containers.
Storage—Light-resistant.

Croconazole Hydrochloride

クロコナゾール塩酸塩

$C_{18}H_{15}ClN_2O.HCl$: 347.24
1-{1-[2-(3-Chlorobenzyloxy)phenyl]vinyl}-1*H*-imidazole monohydrochloride
[*77174-66-4*]

Croconazole Hydrochloride, when dried, contains not less than 98.5% of croconazole hydrochloride ($C_{18}H_{15}ClN_2O.HCl$).

Description Croconazole Hydrochloride occurs as white to pale yellow-white, crystals or crystalline powder.

It is very soluble in water, freely soluble in methanol, in ethanol (95) and in acetic acid (100), and practically insoluble in diethyl ether.

Identification (1) Determine the absorption spectrum of a solution of Croconazole Hydrochloride in methanol (1 in 20,000) as directed under Ultraviolet-visible Spectrophotometry <*2.24*>, and compare the spectrum with the Reference Spectrum: both spectra exhibit similar intensities of absorption at the same wavelengths.

(2) Determine the infrared absorption spectrum of Croconazole Hydrochloride, previously dried, as directed in the potassium chloride disk method under Infrared Spectrophotometry <*2.25*>, and compare the spectrum with the Reference Spectrum: both spectra exhibit similar intensities of absorption at the same wave numbers.

(3) Dissolve 0.05 g of Croconazole Hydrochloride in 10 mL of water, add 2 mL of sodium hydroxide TS and 20 mL of diethyl ether, and shake. Wash the separated aqueous layer with two 10-mL portions of diethyl ether, and acidify the solution with 2 mL of dilute nitric acid: the solution responds to Qualitative Tests <*1.09*> for chloride.

Melting point <*2.60*> 148 – 153°C

Purity (1) Heavy metals <*1.07*>—Proceed with 1.0 g of Croconazole Hydrochloride according to Method 4, and perform the test. Prepare the control solution with 1.0 mL of Standard Lead Solution (not more than 10 ppm).

(2) Related substances—Dissolve 50 mg of Croconazole Hydrochloride in 10 mL of methanol, and use this solution as the sample solution. Pipet 1 mL of the sample solution, add methanol to make exactly 100 mL, and use this solution as the standard solution. Perform the test with these solutions as directed under Thin-layer Chromatography <*2.03*>. Spot 10 μL each of the sample solution and standard solution on a plate of silica gel with fluorescent indicator for thin-layer chromatography. Develop the plate with a mixture of ethyl acetate, hexane, methanol and ammonia solution (28) (30:15:5:1) to a distance of about 10 cm, and air-dry the plate. Examine under ultraviolet light (main wavelength: 254 nm): the spots other than the principal spot and the spot of the starting point obtained from the sample solution are not more intense than the spot from the standard solution.

Loss on drying <*2.41*> Not more than 0.5% (1 g, 60°C, 4 hours).

Residue on ignition <*2.44*> Not more than 0.1% (1 g).

Assay Weigh accurately about 0.6 g of Croconazole Hydrochloride, previously dried, dissolve in 10 mL of acetic acid (100), add 40 mL of acetic anhydride, and titrate <*2.50*> with 0.1 mol/L perchloric acid VS [indicator: 1 to 2 drops of a solution of malachite green oxalate in acetic acid (100) (1 in 100)] until the color of the solution changes from blue-green through green to yellow-green. Perform a blank determination in the same manner, and make any necessary correction.

Each mL of 0.1 mol/L perchloric acid VS
= 34.72 mg of $C_{18}H_{15}ClN_2O.HCl$

Containers and storage Containers—Tight containers.
Storage—Light-resistant.

Crospovidone

クロスポビドン

This monograph is harmonized with the European Pharmacopoeia and the U.S. Pharmacopeia.

The parts of the text that are not harmonized are marked with symbols (◆ ◆).

Information on the harmonization with the European Pharmacopoeia and the U.S. Pharmacopeia is available on the website of the Pharmaceuticals and Medical Devices Agency.

Crospovidone is a cross-linked polymer of 1-vinyl-2-pyrrolidone.

It contains not less than 11.0% and not more than 12.8% of nitrogen (N: 14.01), calculated on the dried basis.

Two types of Crospovidone are available, depending on the particle size: type A and type B.

◆The label states the type.◆

◆**Description** Crospovidone occurs as a white to pale yellow-powder.

It is practically insoluble in water, in methanol and in ethanol (99.5).

It is hygroscopic.◆

Identification (1) Suspend 1 g of Crospovidone in 10 mL of water, add 0.1 mL of iodine TS, shake for 30 seconds, then add 1 mL of starch TS, and shake: a blue color is not produced within 30 seconds.

(2) When add 0.1 g of Crospovidone to 10 mL of water, shake to suspend, and allow the suspension to stand, a clear liquid is not produced within 15 minutes.

Particle size Weigh accurately about 20 g of Crospovidone, place in a 1000-mL conical flask, add 500 mL of water, shake for 30 minutes, and pour onto an accurately tared No. 235 (63 μm) sieve, previously washed with hot water and dried at 105°C for a night, and wash the residue with water until the passing water is clear. Dry the residue together with the sieve in a drying machine at 105°C for 5 hours without air-circulation. After cooling down in a desiccator for 30 minutes, weigh the mass of the residue with sieve, and calculate the amount of the residue on the sieve by the following equation: Type A is more than 15%, and type B is not more than 15%.

Amount (%) of the residue of Crospovidone on No. 235 (63 μm) sieve
$= (M_1 - M_3)/M_2 \times 100$

M_1: The mass (g) of the residue with sieve after 5 hours drying

M_2: Amount (g) of Crospovidone taken, calculated on the dried basis

M_3: Mass (g) of the sieve

Purity ◆(1) Heavy metals *<1.07>*—Proceed with 2.0 g of Crospovidone according to Method 2, and perform the test. Prepare the control solution with 2.0 mL of Standard Lead Solution (not more than 10 ppm).◆

(2) Water-soluble substances—Place 25.0 g of Crospovidone in a 400-mL beaker, add 200 mL of water, and stir for 1 hour. Transfer the suspension to a 250-mL volumetric flask, rinsing with water, and dilute to volume with water. Allow the bulk of the solids to settle. Filter about 100 mL of the almost clear supernatant liquid through a 0.45 μm membrane filter, protected by superimposing a 3 μm membrane filter. Transfer exactly 50 mL of the clear filtrate to a tared 100-mL beaker, evaporate to dryness and dry at 105 - 110°C for 3 hours: the mass of the residue is not more than 75 mg.

(3) 1-Vinyl-2-pyrrolidone—To 1.250 g of Crospovidone add exactly 50 mL of methanol, and shake for 60 minutes. Leave bulk to settle, filter through a 0.2 μm membrane filter, and use the filtrate as the sample solution. Separately, dissolve 50 mg of 1-vinyl-2-pyrrolidone in methanol to make exactly 100 mL. Pipet 1 mL of this solution, and add methanol to make exactly 100 mL. To exactly 5 mL of this solution add the mobile phase to make exactly 100 mL, and use this solution as the standard solution. Perform the test with exactly 50 μL each of the sample solution and standard solution as directed under Liquid Chromatography *<2.01>* according to the following conditions: the peak area of 1-vinyl-2-pyrrolidone obtained from the sample solution is not larger than that from the standard solution (not more than 10 ppm).

Operating conditions—

Detector: An ultraviolet absorption photometer (wavelength: 235 nm).

Column: Two stainless steel columns, one is 4 mm in inside diameter and 25 mm in length and the other is 4 mm in inside diameter and 250 mm in length, they are packed with octadecylsilanized silica gel for liquid chromatography (5 μm in particle diameter), and used them as the pre-column and the separation column, respectively.

Column temperature: A constant temperature of about 40°C.

Mobile phase: A mixture of water and acetonitrile (9:1).

Flow rate: 1.0 mL per minute.

Washing of pre-column: After each injection of the sample solution, wash the pre-column by passing the mobile phase backwards, at the same flow rate as applied in the test, for 30 minutes.

System suitability—

System performance: Dissolve 10 mg of 1-vinyl-2-pyrrolidone and 0.50 g of vinyl acetate in methanol to make 100 mL. To 1 mL of this solution add the mobile phase to make 100 mL. When the procedure is run with 50 μL of this solution under the above operating conditions, 1-vinyl-2-pyrrolidone and vinyl acetate are eluted in this order with the resolution between these peaks being not less than 2.0.

System repeatability: When the test is repeated 6 times with 50 μL of the standard solution under the above operating conditions, the relative standard deviation of the peak area of 1-vinyl-2-pyrrolidone is not more than 2.0%.

(4) Peroxides—

Method 1: Apply to the sample labeled as type A. Suspend 4.0 g of Crospovidone in 100 mL of water, and use as the sample suspension. To 25 mL of the sample suspension add 2 mL of titanium (III) chloride-sulfuric acid TS, allow to stand for 30 minutes, and filter. Determine the absorbance of the filtrate at 405 nm as directed under Ultraviolet-visible Spectrophotometry *<2.24>*, using the control, prepared by filtrating the sample suspension and adding 2 mL of diluted sulfuric acid (13 in 100) to 25 mL of this filtrate: not more than 0.35 (not more than 400 ppm expressed as hydrogen peroxide).

Method 2: Apply to the sample labeled as type B. Suspend 2.0 g of Crospovidone in 50 mL of water, and use as the sample suspension. To 10 mL of the sample suspension add water to make 25 mL, add 2 mL of titanium (III) chloride-sulfuric acid TS, allow to stand for 30 minutes, and filter. Determine the absorbance of the filtrate at 405 nm as directed under Ultraviolet-visible Spectrophotometry <*2.24*>, using the control, prepared by filtrating the sample suspension, adding water to 10 mL of this filtrate to make 25 mL and 2 mL of diluted sulfuric acid (13 in 100): not more than 0.35 (not more than 1000 ppm expressed as hydrogen peroxide).

Loss on drying <*2.41*> Not more than 5.0% (0.5 g, 105°C, constant mass).

Residue on ignition <*2.44*> Not more than 0.1% (1 g).

Assay Weigh accurately about 0.1 g of Crospovidone, place in a Kjeldahl flask, add 5 g of a decomposition accelerator (a powdered mixture of 33 g of potassium sulfate, 1 g of copper (II) sulfate pentahydrate and 1 g of titanium (IV) oxide) and 3 glass beads. Wash any adhering particles from the neck into the flask with a small quantity of water. Add 7 mL of sulfuric acid, allowing it to run down the inside wall of the flask. Gradually heat the flask until the solution has a clear, yellowish-green color, and the inside wall of the flask is free from carbonized material, and then heat for a further 45 minutes. After cooling, cautiously add 20 mL of water, and connect the flask to the distillation apparatus previously washed by passing steam through it. To the absorption flask add 30 mL of a solution of boric acid (1 in 25), 3 drops of bromocresol green-methyl red TS and sufficient water to immerse the lower end of the condenser tube. Add 30 mL of a solution of sodium hydroxide (21 in 50) through a funnel, cautiously rinse the funnel with 10 mL of water, immediately close the clamp attached to the rubber tube, then start the distillation with steam to obtain 80 - 100 mL of distillate. Remove the absorption flask from the lower end of the condenser tube, rinsing the end part with a small quantity of water, and titrate <*2.50*> the distillate with 0.025 mol/L sulfuric acid VS until the color of the solution changes from green through pale grayish blue to pale grayish red-purple. Carry out a blank determination in the same manner, and make any necessary correction.

Each mL of 0.025 mol/L sulfuric acid VS
= 0.7003 mg of N

Containers and storage Containers—Tight containers.

Cyanamide

シアナミド

$H_2N—CN$

CH_2N_2: 42.04
Aminonitrile
[*420-04-2*]

Cyanamide contains not less than 97.0% and not more than 101.0% of cyanamide (CH_2N_2), calculated on the anhydrous basis.

Description Cyanamide occurs as white, crystals or crystalline powder.

It is very soluble in water, in methanol, in ethanol (99.5) and in acetone.

The pH of a solution of 1.0 g of Cyanamide in 100 mL of water is between 5.0 and 6.5.

It is hygroscopic.

Melting point: about 46°C

Identification **(1)** To 1 mL of a solution of Cyanamide (1 in 100) add 1 mL of potassium 1,2-naphthoquinone-4-sulfonate TS and 0.2 mL of sodium hydroxide TS: a deep red color develops.

(2) Drop one or two drops of a solution of Cyanamide in acetone (1 in 100) onto a potassium bromide disk prepared as directed in the potassium bromide disk method under Infrared Spectrophotometry <*2.25*>, and air-dry the disk. Determine the infrared absorption spectrum of the disk as directed in the film method under Infrared Spectrophotometry <*2.25*>, and compare the spectrum with the Reference Spectrum: both spectra exhibit similar intensities of absorption at the same wave numbers.

Purity **(1)** Clarity and color of solution—Dissolve 1.0 g of Cyanamide in 10 mL of water: the solution is clear and colorless.

(2) Heavy metals <*1.07*>—Proceed with 2.0 g of Cyanamide according to Method 1, and perform the test. Prepare the control solution with 2.0 mL of Standard Lead Solution (not more than 10 ppm).

Water <*2.48*> Not more than 1.0% (1 g, volumetric titration, direct titration).

Residue on ignition <*2.44*> Not more than 0.1% (1 g).

Assay Weigh accurately about 1 g of Cyanamide, and dissolve in water to make exactly 250 mL. Pipet 15 mL of this solution, add 2 to 3 drops of dilute nitric acid, 10 mL of ammonia TS and exactly 50 mL of 0.1 mol/L silver nitrate VS, and allow to stand for 15 minutes with occasional shaking. Add water to make exactly 100 mL, filter, discard the first 20 mL of the filtrate, and pipet 50 mL of the subsequent filtrate. After neutralizing this solution with dilute nitric acid, add 3 mL of dilute nitric acid, and titrate <*2.50*> the excess silver nitrate with 0.1 mol/L ammonium thiocyanate VS (indicator: 2 mL of ammonium iron (III) sulfate TS). Perform a blank determination in the same manner.

Each mL of 0.1 mol/L silver nitrate VS
= 2.102 mg of CH_2N_2

Containers and storage Containers—Tight containers.
Storage—In a cold place.

Cyanocobalamin

Vitamin B_{12}

シアノコバラミン

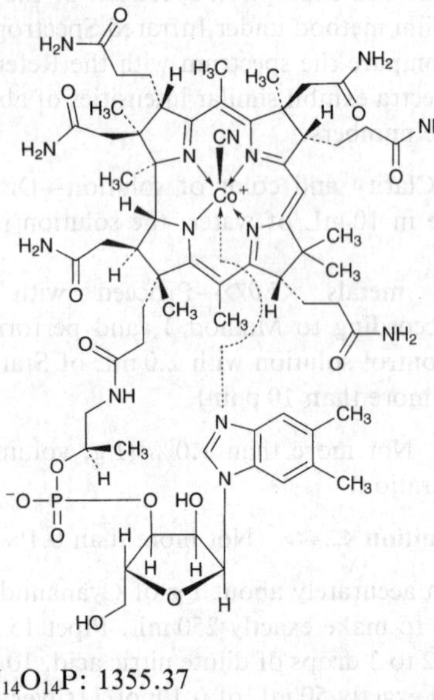

$C_{63}H_{88}CoN_{14}O_{14}P$: 1355.37
Coα-[α-(5,6-Dimethyl-1*H*-benzimidazol-1-yl)]-*Coβ*-cyanocobamide
[68-19-9]

Cyanocobalamin contains not less than 96.0% and not more than 102.0% of cyanocobalamin ($C_{63}H_{88}CoN_{14}O_{14}P$), calculated on the dried basis.

Description Cyanocobalamin occurs as dark red, crystals or powder.

It is sparingly soluble in water, and slightly soluble in ethanol (99.5).

It is hygroscopic.

Identification **(1)** Determine the absorption spectrum of the sample solution obtained in the Assay as directed under Ultraviolet-visible Spectrophotometry *<2.24>*, and compare the spectrum with the Reference Spectrum or the spectrum of a solution of Cyanocobalamin RS prepared in the same manner as the sample solution: both spectra exhibit similar intensities of absorption at the same wavelengths.

(2) Mix 1 mg of Cyanocobalamin with 50 mg of potassium hydrogen sulfate, and fuse by igniting. Cool, break up the mass with a glass rod, add 3 mL of water, and dissolve by boiling. Add 1 drop of phenolphthalein TS, then add dropwise sodium hydroxide TS until a light red color just develops. Add 0.5 g of sodium acetate trihydrate, 0.5 mL of dilute acetic acid and 0.5 mL of a solution of disodium 1-nitroso-2-naphthol-3,6-disulfonate (1 in 500): a red to orange-red color is immediately produced. Then add 0.5 mL of hydrochloric acid, and boil for 1 minute: the red color does not disappear.

(3) Transfer 5 mg of Cyanocobalamin to a 50-mL distilling flask, dissolve in 5 mL of water, and add 2.5 mL of hypophosphorous acid. Connect the flask with a short condenser, and dips its tip into a test tube containing 1 mL of a solution of sodium hydroxide (1 in 50). Heat gently for 10 minutes, then distil 1 mL into a test tube. To the test tube add 4 drops of a saturated solution of ammonium iron (II) sulfate hexahydrate, shake gently, then add about 30 mg of sodium fluoride, and heat the contents to boil. Immediately add dropwise diluted sulfuric acid (1 in 7) until a clear solution results, then add 3 to 5 drops more of diluted sulfuric acid (1 in 7): a blue to blue-green color develops.

pH *<2.54>* Dissolve 0.10 g of Cyanocobalamin in 20 mL of water: the pH of this solution is between 4.2 and 7.0.

Purity **(1)** Clarity and color of solution—Dissolve 20 mg of Cyanocobalamin in 10 mL of water: the solution is clear and red in color.

(2) Related substances—Conduct this procedure using light-resistant vessels. Dissolve 10 mg of Cyanocobalamin in 10 mL of the mobile phase, and use this solution as the sample solution. Pipet 3 mL of the sample solution, add the mobile phase to make exactly 100 mL, and use this solution as the standard solution. Perform the test with exactly 20 μL each of the sample solution and standard solution as directed under Liquid Chromatography *<2.01>* according to the following conditions, and determine each peak area by the automatic integration method: the total area of the peak other than cyanocobalamin obtained from the sample solution is not larger than the peak area of cyanocobalamin from the standard solution.

Operating conditions—

Detector: An ultraviolet absorption photometer (wavelength: 361 nm).

Column: A stainless steel column 4.6 mm in inside diameter and 25 cm in length, packed with octylsilanized silica gel for liquid chromatography (5 μm in particle diameter).

Column temperature: A constant temperature of about 30°C.

Mobile phase: Dissolve 10 g of anhydrous disodium hydrogen phosphate in 1000 mL of water, and adjust to pH 3.5 with phosphoric acid. To 147 mL of this solution add 53 mL of methanol.

Flow rate: Adjust so that the retention time of cyanocobalamin is about 7 minutes.

Time span of measurement: About 4 times as long as the retention time of cyanocobalamin, beginning after the solvent peak.

System suitability—

Test for required detectability: To 1 mL of the sample solution, add the mobile phase to make 100 mL, and use this solution as the solution for system suitability test. Pipet 1 mL of the solution for system suitability test, and add the mobile phase to make exactly 10 mL. Confirm that the peak area of cyanocobalamin obtained with 20 μL of this solution is equivalent to 7 to 13% of that with 20 μL of the solution for system suitability test.

System performance: Perform this procedure quickly after the solution is prepared. To 25 mg of cyanocobalamin add 10 mL of water, and warm, if necessary, to dissolve. After cooling, add 0.5 mL of sodium toluenesulfonchloramide TS, 0.5 mL of 0.05 mol/L hydrochloric acid TS and water to make 25 mL, mix, and allow the solution to stand for 5 minutes. To 1 mL of the solution add the mobile phase to make 10 mL. When the procedure is run with 20 μL of the solution under the above operating conditions, two principal peaks appear with the resolution between these peaks being not less than 2.5.

System repeatability: When the test is repeated 6 times with 20 μL of the solution for system suitability test under the above operating conditions, the relative standard deviation of the peak area of cyanocobalamin is not more than 3.0%.

Loss on drying *<2.41>* Not more than 12% (50 mg, in vacuum at a pressure not exceeding 0.67 kPa, phosphorus (V) oxide, 100°C, 4 hours).

Assay Weigh accurately about 20 mg each of Cyanocobalamin and Cyanocobalamin RS (previously determine the loss on drying ⟨*2.41*⟩ under the same conditions as Cyanocobalamin), dissolve in water to make exactly 1000 mL, respectively, and use these solutions as the sample solution and the standard solution. Determine the absorbances, A_T and A_S, of the sample solution and standard solution, at 361 nm as directed under Ultraviolet-visible Spectrophotometry ⟨*2.24*⟩.

Amount (mg) of cyanocobalamin ($C_{63}H_{88}CoN_{14}O_{14}P$)
$= M_S \times A_T/A_S$

M_S: Amount (mg) of Cyanocobalamin RS taken, calculated on the dried basis

Containers and storage Containers—Tight containers.
Storage—Light-resistant.

Cyanocobalamin Injection

Vitamin B_{12} Injection

シアノコバラミン注射液

Cyanocobalamin Injection is an aqueous injection.
It contains not less than 95.0% and not more than 115.0% of the labeled amount of cyanocobalamin ($C_{63}H_{88}CoN_{14}O_{14}P$: 1355.37).

Method of preparation Prepare as directed under Injections, with Cyanocobalamin.

Description Cyanocobalamin Injection is a clear, light red to red liquid.

Identification Determine the absorption spectrum of the sample solution obtained in the Assay as directed under Ultraviolet-visible Spectrophotometry ⟨*2.24*⟩: it exhibits maxima between 277 nm and 279 nm, between 360 nm, and 362 nm and between 548 nm and 552 nm. Determine the absorbances, A_1 and A_2, of this solution at the wavelengths of maximum absorption between 360 nm and 362 nm, and between 548 nm and 552 nm, respectively: the ratio A_2/A_1 is not less than 0.29 and not more than 0.32.

Bacterial endotoxins ⟨*4.01*⟩ Less than 0.30 EU/μg.

Extractable volume ⟨*6.05*⟩ It meets the requirement.

Foreign insoluble matter ⟨*6.06*⟩ Perform the test according to Method 1: it meets the requirement.

Insoluble particulate matter ⟨*6.07*⟩ It meets the requirement.

Sterility ⟨*4.06*⟩ Perform the test according to the Membrane filtration method: it meets the requirement.

Assay Measure exactly a volume of Cyanocobalamin Injection, equivalent to about 2 mg of cyanocobalamin ($C_{63}H_{88}CoN_{14}O_{14}P$), add water to make exactly 100 mL, and use this solution as the sample solution. Separately, weigh accurately about 20 mg of Cyanocobalamin RS (previously determine the loss on drying ⟨*2.41*⟩ under the same conditions as Cyanocobalamin), add water to make exactly 1000 mL, and use this solution as the standard solution. Then, proceed as directed in the Assay under Cyanocobalamin.

Amount (mg) of cyanocobalamin ($C_{63}H_{88}CoN_{14}O_{14}P$)
$= M_S \times A_T/A_S \times 1/10$

M_S: Amount (mg) of Cyanocobalamin RS taken, calculated on the dried basis

Containers and storage Containers—Hermetic containers, and colored containers may be used.
Storage—Light-resistant.

Cyclopentolate Hydrochloride

シクロペントラート塩酸塩

OH CH3 • HCl H O CH3 and enantiomer

$C_{17}H_{25}NO_3.HCl$: 327.85
2-(Dimethylamino)ethyl (2*RS*)-2-(1-hydroxycyclopentyl)phenylacetate monohydrochloride
[*5870-29-1*]

Cyclopentolate Hydrochloride, when dried, contains not less than 98.5% of cyclopentolate hydrochloride ($C_{17}H_{25}NO_3.HCl$).

Description Cyclopentolate Hydrochloride occurs as a white crystalline powder. It is odorless, or has a characteristic odor.

It is very soluble in water, freely soluble in ethanol (95), in acetic acid (100) and in chloroform, sparingly soluble in acetic anhydride, and practically insoluble in diethyl ether.

Identification **(1)** To 1 mL of a solution of Cyclopentolate Hydrochloride (1 in 100) add 1 mL of Reinecke salt TS: a light red precipitate is formed.

(2) Dissolve 0.2 g of Cyclopentolate Hydrochloride in 2 mL of water, add 2 mL of sodium hydroxide TS, and boil for 1 minute. After cooling, add 2 drops of nitric acid: a phenylacetic acid-like odor is perceptible.

(3) Determine the infrared absorption spectrum of Cyclopentolate Hydrochloride, previously dried, as directed in the potassium chloride disk method under Infrared Spectrophotometry ⟨*2.25*⟩, and compare the spectrum with the Reference Spectrum: both spectra exhibit similar intensities of absorption at the same wave numbers.

(4) A solution of Cyclopentolate Hydrochloride (1 in 50) responds to Qualitative Tests ⟨*1.09*⟩ for chloride.

pH ⟨*2.54*⟩ Dissolve 0.20 g of Cyclopentolate Hydrochloride in 20 mL of water: the pH of this solution is between 4.5 and 5.5.

Melting point ⟨*2.60*⟩ 135 – 138°C

Purity **(1)** Clarity and color of solution—Dissolve 1.0 g of Cyclopentolate Hydrochloride in 10 mL of water: the solution is clear and colorless.

(2) Heavy metals ⟨*1.07*⟩—Proceed with 1.0 g of Cyclopentolate Hydrochloride according to Method 1, and perform the test. Prepare the control solution with 2.0 mL of Standard Lead Solution (not more than 20 ppm).

(3) Related substances—Dissolve 0.20 g of Cyclopentolate Hydrochloride in 10 mL of chloroform, and use this solution as the sample solution. Pipet 1 mL of the sample solution, and add chloroform to make exactly 20 mL. Pipet 1 mL of this solution, add chloroform to make exactly 10 mL, and use this solution as the standard solution. Perform the test with these solutions as directed under Thin-layer Chromatography <2.03>. Spot 10 μL each of the sample solution and standard solution on a plate of silica gel for thin-layer chromatography. Develop the plate with a mixture of 2-propanol, *n*-butyl acetate, water and ammonia solution (28) (100:60:23:17) to a distance of about 10 cm, and air-dry the plate. Spray evenly a solution of sulfuric acid in ethanol (99.5) (1 in 10) on the plate, and heat the plate at 120°C for 30 minutes. Examine under ultraviolet light (main wavelength: 254 nm): the spots other than the principal spot obtained from the sample solution are not more intense than the spot from the standard solution.

Loss on drying <2.41> Not more than 0.5% (1 g, 105°C, 4 hours).

Residue on ignition <2.44> Not more than 0.05% (1 g).

Assay Weigh accurately about 0.5 g of Cyclopentolate Hydrochloride, previously dried, dissolve in 50 mL of a mixture of acetic anhydride and acetic acid (100) (4:1), and titrate <2.50> with 0.1 mol/L perchloric acid VS until the color of the solution changes from purple through blue-green to yellow-green (indicator: 2 drops of crystal violet TS). Perform a blank determination in the same manner, and make any necessary correction.

Each mL of 0.1 mol/L perchloric acid VS
= 32.79 mg of $C_{17}H_{25}NO_3.HCl$

Containers and storage Containers—Tight containers.

Cyclophosphamide Hydrate

シクロホスファミド水和物

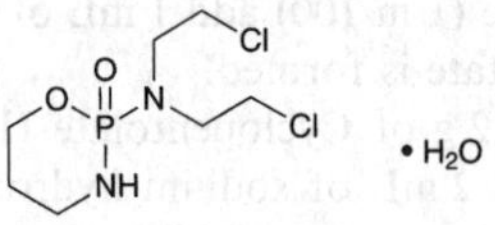

$C_7H_{15}Cl_2N_2O_2P.H_2O$: 279.10
N,*N*-Bis(2-chloroethyl)-3,4,5,6-tetrahydro-2*H*-1,3,2-oxazaphosphorin-2-amine 2-oxide monohydrate
[*6055-19-2*]

Cyclophosphamide Hydrate contains not less than 97.0% of cyclophosphamide hydrate ($C_7H_{15}Cl_2N_2O_2P.H_2O$).

Description Cyclophosphamide Hydrate occurs as white, crystals or crystalline powder. It is odorless.

It is very soluble in acetic acid (100), freely soluble in ethanol (95), in acetic anhydride and in chloroform, and soluble in water and in diethyl ether.

Melting point: 45 - 53°C

Identification (1) Dissolve 0.1 g of Cyclophosphamide Hydrate in 10 mL of water, and add 5 mL of silver nitrate TS: no precipitate is produced. Then boil this solution: a white precipitate is produced. Collect the precipitate, and add dilute nitric acid to a portion of this precipitate: it does not dissolve. Add excess ammonia TS to another portion of the precipitate: it dissolves.

(2) Add 1 mL of diluted sulfuric acid (1 in 25) to 0.02 g of Cyclophosphamide Hydrate, and heat until white fumes are evolved. After cooling, add 5 mL of water, and shake. Neutralize with ammonia TS, then acidify with dilute nitric acid: this solution responds to Qualitative Tests <1.09> (2) for phosphate.

Purity (1) Clarity and color of solution—Dissolve 0.20 g of Cyclophosphamide Hydrate in 10 mL of water: the solution is clear and colorless.

(2) Chloride <1.03>—Perform the test with 0.40 g of Cyclophosphamide Hydrate at a temperature not exceeding 20°C. Prepare the control solution with 0.40 mL of 0.01 mol/L hydrochloric acid VS (not more than 0.036%).

(3) Heavy metals <1.07>—Proceed with 1.0 g of Cyclophosphamide Hydrate according to Method 1, and perform the test. Prepare the control solution with 2.0 mL of Standard Lead Solution (not more than 20 ppm).

Water <2.48> 5.5 - 7.0% (0.5 g, volumetric titration, direct titration).

Assay Weigh accurately about 0.3 g of Cyclophosphamide Hydrate, add 15 mL of hydrogen chloride-ethanol TS, and heat in a water bath under a reflux condenser for 3.5 hours while protecting from moisture. Distil the ethanol under reduced pressure. Dissolve the residue in 40 mL of a mixture of acetic anhydride and acetic acid (100) (7:3), and titrate <2.50> with 0.1 mol/L perchloric acid-dioxane VS (indicator: 2 drops of crystal violet TS) until the color of the solution changes from blue through green to yellow. Perform a blank determination in the same manner, and make any necessary correction.

Each mL of 0.1 mol/L perchloric acid-dioxane VS
= 13.96 mg of $C_7H_{15}Cl_2N_2O_2P.H_2O$

Containers and storage Containers—Tight containers.
Storage—Not exceeding 30°C.

Cyclophosphamide Tablets

シクロホスファミド錠

Cyclophosphamide Tablets contain not less than 93.0% and not more than 107.0% of the labeled amount of cyclophosphamide hydrate ($C_7H_{15}Cl_2N_2O_2P.H_2O$: 279.10).

Method of preparation Prepare as directed under Tablets, with Cyclophosphamide Hydrate.

Identification To Cyclophosphamide Tablets add 1 mL of water for every 53 mg of Cyclophosphamide Hydrate, shake vigorously for 5 minutes, add 6 mL of methanol for every 53 mg of Cyclophosphamide Hydrate, and shake vigorously for 10 minutes. To this solution add methanol so that each mL contains about 5.3 mg of Cyclophosphamide Hydrate, and centrifuge. Filter the supernatant liquid through a membrane filter with a pore size not exceeding 0.45 μm. Discard not less than 3 mL of the first filtrate, and use the subsequent filtrate as the sample solution. Separately, dissolve 53 mg of cyclophosphamide hydrate for assay in 10 mL of a mixture of methanol and water (9:1), and use this solution as the standard solution. Perform the test with these solutions as directed under Thin-layer Chromatography <2.03>. Spot 2 μL each of the sample solution and standard solution on a plate of silica gel for thin-layer chromatography. Develop the plate with a mixture of 1-propanol and water (8:1) to a distance of about 10 cm, and air-dry the plate. Heat the plate at 130°C for 15 minutes. After cooling, spray evenly ninhydrin-butanol TS on the plate, and after air-drying heat at 130°C for 10 minutes: the principal spot obtained from the sample solution and the spot from the standard solution show a red-purple color and the same *Rf* value.

Uniformity of dosage units <*6.02*> Perform the test according to the following method: it meets the requirement of the Content uniformity test.

To 1 tablet of Cyclophosphamide Tablets add 3V/5 mL of a mixture of water and methanol (3:2), and shake vigorously to homogenously disperse the tablet. To this solution add a mixture of water and methanol (3:2) to make exactly V mL so that each mL contains about 1.1 mg of cyclophosphamide hydrate ($C_7H_{15}Cl_2N_2O_2P.H_2O$), and centrifuge. Filter the supernatant liquid through a membrane filter with a pore size not exceeding 0.45 μm. Discard the first 3 mL of the filtrate, and use the subsequent filtrate as the sample solution. Then, proceed as directed in the Assay.

Amount (mg) of cyclophosphamide hydrate ($C_7H_{15}Cl_2N_2O_2P.H_2O$)
$= M_S \times A_T/A_S \times V/50$

M_S: Amount (mg) of cyclophosphamide hydrate for assay taken

Dissolution <*6.10*> When the test is performed at 100 revolutions per minute according to the Basket method, using 900 mL of water as the dissolution medium, the dissolution rate in 45 minutes of Cyclophosphamide Tablets is not less than 80%.

Start the test with 1 tablet of Cyclophosphamide Tablets, withdraw not less than 20 mL of the medium at the specified minute after starting the test, and filter through a membrane filter with a pore size not exceeding 0.45 μm. Discard not less than 10 mL of the first filtrate, pipet V mL of the subsequent filtrate, add water to make exactly V' mL so that each mL contains about 59 μg of cyclophosphamide hydrate ($C_7H_{15}Cl_2N_2O_2P.H_2O$) and use this solution as the sample solution. Separately, weigh accurately about 30 mg of cyclophosphamide hydrate for assay, and dissolve in water to make exactly 50 mL. Pipet 2 mL of this solution, add water to make exactly 20 mL, and use this solution as the standard solution. Perform the test with exactly 50 μL each of the sample solution and standard solution as directed under Liquid Chromatography <*2.01*> according to the following conditions and determine the peak areas, A_T and A_S, of cyclophosphamide in each solution.

Dissolution rate (%) with respect to the labeled amount of cyclophosphamide hydrate ($C_7H_{15}Cl_2N_2O_2P.H_2O$)
$= M_S \times A_T/A_S \times V'/V \times 1/C \times 180$

M_S: Amount (mg) of cyclophosphamide hydrate for assay taken

C: Labeled amount (mg) of cyclophosphamide hydrate ($C_7H_{15}Cl_2N_2O_2P.H_2O$) in 1 tablet

Operating conditions—

Proceed as directed in the operating conditions in the Assay.

System suitability—

System performance: When the procedure is run with 50 μL of the standard solution under the above operating conditions, the number of theoretical plates and the symmetry factor of the peak of clophosphamide are not less than 5000 and not more than 1.5, respectively.

System repeatability: When the test is repeated 6 times with 50 μL of the standard solution under the above operating conditions, the relative standard deviation of the peak area of clophosphamide is not more than 2.0%.

Assay To 10 tablets of Cyclophosphamide Tablets add 13V/20 mL of a mixture of water and methanol (3:2), and shake vigorously to homogenously disperse the tablets. To this solution add a mixture of water and methanol (3:2) to make exactly V mL so that each mL contains about 2.7 mg of cyclophosphamide hydrate ($C_7H_{15}Cl_2N_2O_2P.H_2O$), and centrifuge. Filter the supernatant liquid through a membrane filter with a pore size not exceeding 0.45 μm. Discard the first 3 mL of the filtrate, pipet 4 mL of the subsequent filtrate, add a mixture of water and methanol (3:2) to make exactly 10 mL, and use this solution as the sample solution. Separately, weigh accurately about 53 mg of cyclophosphamide hydrate for assay, dissolve in a mixture of water and methanol (3:2) to make exactly 50 mL, and use this solution as the standard solution. Perform the test with exactly 20 μL each of the sample solution and standard solution as directed under Liquid Chromatography <*2.01*> according to the following conditions, and determine the peak area, A_T and A_S, of cyclophosphamide in each solution.

Amount (mg) of cyclophosphamide hydrate ($C_7H_{15}C_{12}N_2O_2P.H_2O$)
$= M_S \times A_T/A_S \times V/200$

M_S: Amount (mg) of cyclophosphamide hydrate for assay taken

Operating conditions—

Detector: An ultraviolet absorption photometer (wavelength: 205 nm).

Column: A stainless steel column 4.6 mm in inside diameter and 15 cm in length, packed with octadecylsilanized silica gel for liquid chromatography (5 μm in particle diameter).

Column temperature: A constant temperature of about 25°C.

Mobile phase: A mixture of water and methanol (3:2).

Flow rate: Adjust so that the retention time of cyclophosphamide is about 10 minutes.

System suitability—

System performance: When the procedure is run with 20 μL of the standard solution under the above operating conditions, the number of theoretical plates and the symmetry factor of the peak of cyclophosphamide are not less than 4000 and not more than 1.5, respectively.

System repeatability: When the test is repeated 6 times with 20 μL of the standard solution under the above operating conditions, the relative standard deviation of the peak area of cyclophosphamide is not more than 1.0%.

Containers and storage Containers—Tight containers.

Cycloserine

サイクロセリン

$C_3H_6N_2O_2$: 102.09
(4*R*)-4-Aminoisoxazolidin-3-one
[*68-41-7*]

Cycloserine contains not less than 950 μg (potency) and not more than 1020 μg (potency) per mg, calculated on the dried basis. The potency of Cycloserine is expressed as mass (potency) of cycloserine ($C_3H_6N_2O_2$).

Description Cycloserine occurs as white to light yellowwhite, crystals or crystalline powder.

It is soluble in water, and sparingly soluble in ethanol (95).

Identification Determine the infrared absorption spectrum of Cycloserine, previously dried, as directed in the potassium bromide disk method under Infrared Spectrophotometry <*2.25*>, and compare the spectrum with the Reference Spectrum or the spectrum of previously dried Cycloserine RS: both spectra exhibit similar intensities of absorption at the same wave numbers.

Optical rotation <*2.49*> $[\alpha]_D^{20}$: +108 – +114° (2.5 g calculated on the dried basis, 2 mol/L sodium hydroxide TS, 50 mL, 100 mm).

pH <*2.54*> Dissolve 1.0 g of Cycloserine in 20 mL of water: the pH of the solution is between 5.0 and 7.4.

Purity **(1)** Heavy metals <*1.07*>—Proceed with 1.0 g of Cycloserine according to Method 4, and perform the test. Prepare the control solution with 2.0 mL of Standard Lead Solution (not more than 20 ppm).

(2) Condensation products—Dissolve 20 mg of Cycloserine in sodium hydroxide TS to make exactly 50 mL, and determine the absorbance of this solution at 285 nm as directed under Ultraviolet-visible Spectrophotometry <*2.24*>: not more than 0.8.

Loss on drying <*2.41*> Not more than 1.5% (0.5 g, reduced pressure, 60°C, 3 hours).

Residue on ignition <*2.44*> Not more than 0.5% (1 g).

Assay Perform the test according to the Cylinder-plate method as directed under Microbial Assay for Antibiotics <*4.02*> according to the following conditions.

(i) Test organism—*Bacillus subtilis* ATCC 6633

(ii) Culture medium—Use the medium i in 1) Medium for test organism [5] under (1) Agar media for seed and base layer. Adjust the pH of the medium so that it will be 6.0 to 6.1 after sterilization.

(iii) Standard solutions—Weigh accurately an amount of Cycloserine RS, previously dried at 60°C for 3 hours under reduced pressure of not exceeding 0.67 kPa, equivalent to about 40 mg (potency), dissolve in water to make exactly 100 mL, and use this solution as the standard stock solution. Keep the standard stock solution at 5°C or below and use within 24 hours. Take exactly a suitable amount of the standard stock solution before use, and add phosphate buffer solution (pH 6.0) to make solutions so that each mL contains 100 μg (potency) and 50 μg (potency), and use these solutions as the high concentration standard solution and the low concentration standard solution, respectively.

(iv) Sample solutions—Weigh accurately an amount of Cycloserine equivalent to about 40 mg (potency), dissolve in water to make exactly 100 mL. Take exactly a suitable amount of this solution, add phosphate buffer solution (pH 6.0) to make solutions so that each mL contains 100 μg (potency) and 50 μg (potency), and use these solutions as the high concentration sample solution and the low concentration sample solution, respectively.

Containers and storage Containers—Well-closed containers.

Cyproheptadine Hydrochloride Hydrate

シプロヘプタジン塩酸塩水和物

• HCl • 1½H₂O

$C_{21}H_{21}N.HCl.1\frac{1}{2}H_2O$: 350.88
4-(5*H*-Dibenzo[*a*,*d*]cyclohepten-5-ylidene)-1-methylpiperidine monohydrochloride sesquihydrate
[*41354-29-4*]

Cyproheptadine Hydrochloride Hydrate, when dried, contains not less than 98.5% of cyproheptadine hydrochloride ($C_{21}H_{21}N.HCl$: 323.86).

Description Cyproheptadine Hydrochloride Hydrate occurs as a white to pale yellow crystalline powder. It is odorless, and has a slightly bitter taste.

It is freely soluble in methanol and in acetic acid (100), soluble in chloroform, sparingly soluble in ethanol (95), slightly soluble in water, and practically insoluble in diethyl ether.

Identification **(1)** Dissolve 0.1 g of Cyproheptadine Hydrochloride Hydrate in 10 mL of methanol, apply 1 drop of this solution on filter paper, air-dry, and examine under ultraviolet light (main wavelength: 254 nm): the solution shows a pale blue fluorescence.

(2) Weigh 0.1 g of Cyproheptadine Hydrochloride Hydrate, transfer to a separator, dissolve in 5 mL of chloroform, add 4 mL of water and 1 mL of sodium carbonate TS, and shake. Transfer the chloroform layer to another separator, and wash with 4 mL of water by shaking well. Filter the chloroform layer through absorbent cotton moistened previously with chloroform, and evaporate the filtrate to dryness. Dissolve the residue in 8 mL of dilute ethanol by warming at 65°C. Rub the inner wall of the container with a glass rod while cooling until crystallization begins, and allow to stand for 30 minutes. Collect the crystals, and dry at 80°C for 2 hours: the crystals melt <*2.60*> between 111°C and 115°C.

(3) Determine the absorption spectrum of a solution of Cyproheptadine Hydrochloride Hydrate in ethanol (95) (1 in 100,000) as directed under Ultraviolet-visible Spectrophotometry <*2.24*>, and compare the spectrum with the Reference Spectrum: both spectra exhibit similar intensities of absorption at the same wavelengths.

(4) A saturated solution of Cyproheptadine Hydrochloride Hydrate responds to Qualitative Tests <*1.09*> (2) for chloride.

Purity **(1)** Acidity—Dissolve 2.0 g of Cyproheptadine Hydrochloride Hydrate in 25 mL of methanol, and add 1 drop of methyl red TS and 0.30 mL of 0.1 mol/L sodium hydroxide VS: a yellow color develops.

(2) Heavy metals <*1.07*>—Proceed with 1.0 g of Cyproheptadine Hydrochloride Hydrate according to Method 2, and perform the test. Prepare the control solution with 2.0 mL of Standard Lead Solution (not more than 20 ppm).

Loss on drying <*2.41*> 7.0 – 9.0% (1 g, in vacuum at a pressure not exceeding 0.67 kPa, 100°C, 5 hours).

Residue on ignition *<2.44>* Not more than 0.1% (1 g).

Assay Weigh accurately about 0.5 g of Cyproheptadine Hydrochloride Hydrate, previously dried, and dissolve in 20 mL of acetic acid (100) by warming at 50°C. After cooling, add 40 mL of acetic anhydride, and titrate *<2.50>* with 0.1 mol/L perchloric acid VS (potentiometric titration). Perform a blank determination in the same manner, and make any necessary correction.

Each mL of 0.1 mol/L perchloric acid VS
= 32.39 mg of $C_{21}H_{21}N.HCl$

Containers and storage Containers—Well-closed containers.

L-Cysteine

L-システイン

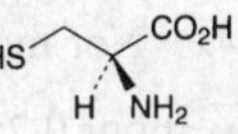

$C_3H_7NO_2S$: 121.16
(2*R*)-2-Amino-3-sulfanylpropanoic acid
[*52-90-4*]

L-Cysteine contains not less than 98.5% and not more than 101.0% of L-cysteine ($C_3H_7NO_2S$), calculated on the dried basis.

Description L-Cysteine occurs as white crystals or a white crystalline powder. It has a characteristic odor and a pungent taste.

It is freely soluble in water, and practically insoluble in ethanol (99.5).

It dissolves in 1 mol/L hydrochloric acid TS.

Identification Determine the infrared absorption spectrum of L-Cysteine as directed in the potassium bromide disk method under Infrared Spectrophotometry *<2.25>*, and compare the spectrum with the Reference Spectrum: both spectra exhibit similar intensities of absorption at the same wave numbers.

Optical rotation *<2.49>* $[\alpha]_D^{20}$: $+8.0 - +10.0°$ (2 g calculated on the dried basis, 1 mol/L hydrochloric acid TS, 25 mL, 100 mm).

pH *<2.54>* The pH of a solution prepared by dissolving 1.25 g of L-Cysteine in 50 mL of water is 4.7 to 5.7.

Purity **(1)** Clarity and color of solution—Dissolve 1.0 g of L-Cysteine in 20 mL of water: the solution is clear and colorless.

(2) Chloride *<1.03>*—Dissolve 0.30 g of L-Cysteine in 10 mL of diluted nitric acid (1 in 4), add 10 mL of hydrogen peroxide (30), heat for 20 minutes in a boiling water bath, cool, and then add water to make 50 mL. Perform the test using this solution as the test solution. Prepare the control solution with 0.35 mL of 0.01 mol/L hydrochloric acid VS (not more than 0.041%).

(3) Sulfate *<1.14>*—Dissolve 0.6 g of L-Cysteine in 30 mL of water and 3 mL of dilute hydrochloric acid, and add water to make 50 mL. Perform the test using this solution as the test solution. Prepare the control solution as follows: To 0.35 mL of 0.005 mol/L sulfuric acid VS add 3 mL of dilute hydrochloric acid and water to make 50 mL. Prepare the test solution and the control solution with 4 mL of barium chloride TS, respectively (not more than 0.028%).

(4) Ammonium *<1.02>*—Perform the test with 0.25 g of L-Cysteine, using the distillation under reduced pressure. Prepare the control solution with 5.0 mL of Standard Ammonium Solution (not more than 0.02%).

(5) Heavy metals *<1.07>*—Proceed with 1.0 g of L-Cysteine according to Method 4, and perform the test. Prepare the control solution with 1.0 mL of Standard Lead Solution (not more than 10 ppm).

(6) Iron *<1.10>*—Prepare the test solution with 1.0 g of L-Cysteine according to Method 1, and perform the test according to Method A. Prepare the control solution with 1.0 mL of Standard Iron Solution (not more than 10 ppm).

(7) Related substances—Dissolve 0.10 g of L-Cysteine in *N*-ethylmaleimide solution (1 in 50) to make exactly 10 mL, leave for 30 minutes, and use this solution as the sample solution. Pipet 1 mL of the sample solution, add water to make exactly 10 mL, pipet 1 mL of this solution, add water to make exactly 50 mL, and use this solution as the standard solution (1). Separately, dissolve 0.10 g of L-cystine in 0.5 mol/L hydrochloric acid TS to make exactly 20 mL. Pipet 1 mL of this solution, add water to make 100 mL, and use this solution as the standard solution (2). Perform the test with these solutions as directed under Thin-layer Chromatography *<2.03>*. Spot 10 μL each of the sample solution and standard solutions (1) and (2) on a plate of silica gel for thin-layer chromatography. Develop the plate with a mixture of 1-butanol, water, and acetic acid (100) (3:1:1) to a distance of about 10 cm, and dry the plate for 30 minutes at 80°C. Spray the plate evenly with a solution of ninhydrin in a mixture of methanol and acetic acid (100) (97:3) (1 in 100), and then heat at 80°C for 10 minutes: the spot obtained from the sample solution corresponding to the spot from the standard solution (2) is not more intense than the spot from the standard solution (2). Also, the spots other than the principal spot and the spots mentioned above from the sample solution are not more intense than the spot from the standard solution (1).

Loss on drying *<2.41>* Not more than 0.5% (1 g, in vacuum, phosphorus (V) oxide, 3 hours).

Residue on ignition *<2.44>* Not more than 0.1% (1 g).

Assay Weigh accurately about 0.2 g of L-Cysteine, place it in a stoppered flask, and dissolve in 20 mL of water. Dissolve 4 g of potassium iodide in this solution, immediately place in ice cold water, add 5 mL of dilute hydrochloric acid and exactly 25 mL of 0.05 mol/L iodine VS, leave in a dark place for 20 minutes, and then titrate *<2.50>* an excess amount of iodine with 0.1 mol/L sodium thiosulfate VS (indicator: starch TS). Perform a blank determination in the same manner.

Each mL of 0.05 mol/L iodine VS = 12.12 mg of $C_3H_7NO_2S$

Containers and storage Containers—Tight containers.

L-Cysteine Hydrochloride Hydrate

L-システイン塩酸塩水和物

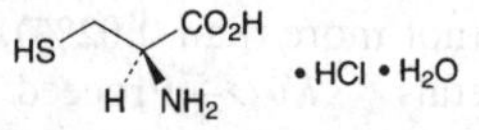

$C_3H_7NO_2S.HCl.H_2O$: 175.63
(2*R*)-2-Amino-3-sulfanylpropanoic acid monohydrochloride monohydrate
[*7048-04-6*]

L-Cysteine Hydrochloride Hydrate contains not less than 98.5% and not more than 101.0% of L-cysteine hydrochloride ($C_3H_7NO_2S.HCl$: 157.62), calculated on the dried basis.

Description L-Cysteine Hydrochloride Hydrate occurs as white, crystals or crystalline powder. It has a characteristic odor and a strong acid taste.

It is very soluble in water, and soluble in ethanol (99.5).

It dissolves in 6 mol/L hydrochloric acid TS.

Identification **(1)** Determine the infrared absorption spectrum of L-Cysteine Hydrochloride Hydrate as directed in the potassium chloride disk method under Infrared Spectrophotometry <*2.25*>, and compare the spectrum with the Reference Spectrum: both spectra exhibit similar intensities of absorption at the same wave numbers.

(2) To 10 mL of a solution of L-Cysteine Hydrochloride Hydrate (1 in 50) add 1 mL of hydrogen peroxide (30), heat on a water bath for 20 minutes, and cool: the solution responds to Qualitative Tests <*1.09*> (2) for chloride.

Optical rotation <*2.49*> $[\alpha]_D^{20}$: +6.0 – +7.5° (2 g, calculated on the dried basis, 6 mol/L hydrochloric acid TS, 25 mL, 100 mm).

pH <*2.54*> The pH of a solution prepared by dissolving 1.0 g of L-Cysteine Hydrochloride Hydrate in 100 mL of water is between 1.3 and 2.3.

Purity **(1)** Clarity and color of solution—A solution obtained by dissolving 1.0 g of L-Cysteine Hydrochloride Hydrate in 10 mL of water is clear and colorless.

(2) Sulfate <*1.14*>—Dissolve 0.8 g of L-Cysteine Hydrochloride Hydrate in 30 mL of water and 3 mL of dilute hydrochloric acid, and add water to make 50 mL. Perform the test using this solution as the test solution. Prepare the control solution as follows: To 0.35 mL of 0.005 mol/L sulfuric acid VS add 3 mL of dilute hydrochloric acid and water to make 50 mL. To both of the test solution and the control solution add 4 mL of barium chloride TS (not more than 0.021%).

(3) Ammonium <*1.02*>—Perform the test with 0.25 g of L-Cysteine Hydrochloride Hydrate using the distillation under reduced pressure. Prepare the control solution with 5.0 mL of Standard Ammonium Solution (not more than 0.02%).

(4) Heavy metals <*1.07*>—Proceed with 1.0 g of L-Cysteine Hydrochloride Hydrate according to Method 4, and perform the test. Prepare the control solution with 1.0 mL of Standard Lead Solution (not more than 10 ppm).

(5) Iron <*1.10*>—Prepare the test solution with 1.0 g of L-Cysteine Hydrochloride Hydrate according to Method 1, and perform the test according to Method A. Prepare the control solution with 1.0 mL of Standard Iron Solution (not more than 10 ppm).

(6) Related substances—Dissolve 0.10 g of L-Cysteine Hydrochloride Hydrate in *N*-ethylmaleimide solution (1 in 50) to make 10 mL, allow to stand for 30 minutes, and use this solution as the sample solution. Pipet 1 mL of the sample solution, add water to make exactly 10 mL. Pipet 1 mL of this solution, add water to make exactly 50 mL, and use this solution as the standard solution. Perform the test with these solutions as directed under Thin-Layer Chromatography <*2.03*>. Spot 5 μL each of the sample solution and standard solution on a plate of silica gel for thin-layer chromatography. Then develop with a mixture of 1-butanol, water and acetic acid (100) (3:1:1) to a distance of about 10 cm, and dry the plate at 80°C for 30 minutes. Spray evenly a solution of ninhydrin in a mixture of methanol and acetic acid (100) (97:3) (1 in 100) on the plate, and then heat at 80°C for 10 minutes: the spot other than the principal spot obtained from the sample solution is not more intense than the spot from the standard solution.

Loss on drying <*2.41*> 8.5 – 12.0% (1 g, in vacuum, phosphorus (V) oxide, 20 hours).

Residue on ignition <*2.44*> Not more than 0.1% (1 g).

Assay Weigh accurately about 0.25 g of L-Cysteine Hydrochloride Hydrate, place in a glass-stoppered flask, and dissolve in 20 mL of water. Dissolve 4 g of potassium iodide in this solution, soak immediately in ice cold water, add 5 mL of dilute hydrochloric acid and exactly 25 mL of 0.05 mol/L iodine VS, allow to stand for 20 minutes in a dark place, titrate <*2.50*> the excess of iodine with 0.1 mol/L sodium thiosulfate VS (indicator: starch TS). Perform a blank determination in the same manner, and make any necessary correction.

Each mL of 0.05 mol/L iodine VS
= 15.76 mg of $C_3H_7NO_2S.HCl$

Containers and storage Containers—Tight containers.

L-Cystine

L-シスチン

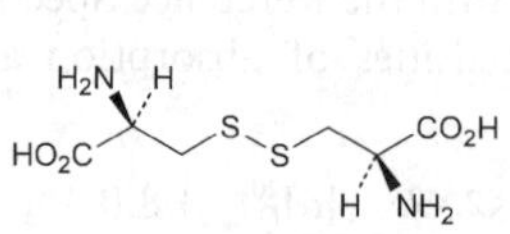

$C_6H_{12}N_2O_4S_2$: 240.30
3,3′-Disulfanediylbis[(2*R*)-2-aminopropanoic acid]
[*56-89-3*]

L-Cystine, when dried, contains not less than 99.0% and not more than 101.0% of L-cystine ($C_6H_{12}N_2O_4S_2$).

Description L-Cystine occurs as white, crystals or crystalline powder.

It is practically insoluble in water and in ethanol (99.5).

It dissolves in 1 mol/L hydrochloric acid TS.

Identification Determine the infrared absorption spectrum of L-Cystine as directed in the potassium bromide disk method under Infrared Spectrophotometry <*2.25*>, and compare the spectrum with the Reference Spectrum: both spectra exhibit similar intensities of absorption at the same wave numbers.

Optical rotation <*2.49*> $[\alpha]_D^{20}$: −215 – −225° (after drying, 1 g, 1 mol/L hydrochloric acid TS, 50 mL, 100 mm).

Purity (1) Clarity and color of solution—A solution obtained by dissolving 1.0 g of L-Cystine in 10 mL of 2 mol/L hydrochloric acid TS is clear and colorless.

(2) Chloride <*1.03*>—Dissolve 0.5 g of L-Cystine in 10 mL of dilute nitric acid, add 10 mL of hydrogen peroxide (30), and heat in a water bath for 10 minutes. After cooling, add water to make 50 mL, and perform the test using this solution as the test solution. Prepare the control solution with 0.30 mL of 0.01 mol/L hydrochloric acid VS (not more than 0.021%).

(3) Sulfate <*1.14*>—Dissolve 0.6 g of L-Cystine in 5 mL of dilute hydrochloric acid, add water to make 45 mL, and perform the test using this solution as the test solution. Prepare the control solution as follows: To 0.35 mL of 0.005 mol/L sulfuric acid VS add 5 mL of dilute hydrochloric acid and water to make 45 mL. To both the test and control solutions add 5 mL of barium chloride TS (not more than 0.028%).

(4) Ammonium <*1.02*>—Perform the test with 0.25 g of L-Cystine, using the distillation under reduced pressure. Prepare the control solution with 5.0 mL of Standard Ammonium Solution (not more than 0.02%).

(5) Heavy metals <*1.07*>—Proceed with 1.0 g of L-Cystine according to Method 4, and perform the test. Prepare the control solution with 1.0 mL of Standard Lead Solution (not more than 10 ppm).

(6) Iron <*1.10*>—Prepare the test solution with 1.0 g of L-Cystine according to Method 3, and perform the test according to Method A. Prepare the control solution with 1.0 mL of Standard Iron Solution (not more than 10 ppm).

(7) Related substances—Dissolve 0.20 g of L-Cystine in 20 mL of 1 mol/L hydrochloric acid TS, and use this solution as the sample solution. Pipet 1 mL of the sample solution, and add water to make exactly 10 mL. Pipet 1 mL of this solution, add water to make exactly 50 mL, and use this solution as the standard solution. Perform the test with these solutions as directed under Thin-layer Chromatography <*2.03*>. Spot 5 μL each of the sample solution and standard solution on a plate of silica gel for thin-layer chromatography. Develop the plate with a mixture of 1-propanol and ammonia solution (28) (67:33) to a distance of about 10 cm, and dry the plate at 80°C for 30 minutes. Spray evenly a solution of ninhydrin in a mixture of methanol and acetic acid (100) (97:3) (1 in 100) on the plate, and heat the plate at 80°C for 10 minutes: the spot other than the principal spot obtained from the sample solution is not more intense than the spot from the standard solution.

Loss on drying <*2.41*> Not more than 0.3% (1 g, 105°C, 3 hours).

Residue on ignition <*2.44*> Not more than 0.1% (1 g).

Assay Weigh accurately about 30 mg of L-Cystine, previously dried, and perform the test as directed under Nitrogen Determination <*1.08*>.

Each mL of 0.005 mol/L sulfuric acid VS
= 1.202 mg of $C_6H_{12}N_2O_4S_2$

Containers and storage Containers—Tight containers.
Storage—Light-resistant.

Cytarabine

シタラビン

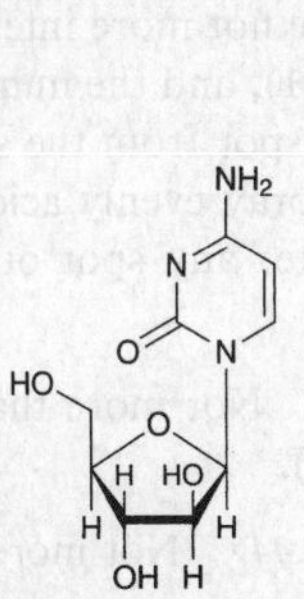

$C_9H_{13}N_3O_5$: 243.22
1-β-D-Arabinofuranosylcytosine
[*147-94-4*]

Cytarabine, when dried, contains not less than 98.5% and not more than 101.0% of cytarabine ($C_9H_{13}N_3O_5$).

Description Cytarabine occurs as white, crystals or crystalline powder.

It is freely soluble in water, soluble in acetic acid (100), and very slightly soluble in ethanol (99.5).

It dissolves in 0.1 mol/L hydrochloric acid TS.

Melting point: about 214°C (with decomposition).

Identification (1) Determine the absorption spectrum of a solution of Cytarabine in 0.1 mol/L hydrochloric acid TS (1 in 100,000) as directed under Ultraviolet-visible Spectrophotometry <*2.24*>, and compare the spectrum with the Reference Spectrum: both spectra exhibit similar intensities of absorption at the same wavelengths.

(2) Determine the infrared absorption spectrum of Cytarabine as directed in the potassium bromide disk method under Infrared Spectrophotometry <*2.25*>, and compare the spectrum with the Reference Spectrum: both spectra exhibit similar intensities of absorption at the same wave numbers.

Optical rotation <*2.49*> $[\alpha]_D^{20}$: +154 – +160° (after drying, 0.1 g, water, 10 mL, 100 mm).

pH <*2.54*> Dissolve 0.20 g of Cytarabine in 20 mL of water: the pH of this solution is between 6.5 and 8.0.

Purity (1) Clarity and color of solution—Dissolve 1.0 g of Cytarabine in 10 mL of water: the solution is clear and colorless.

(2) Chloride <*1.03*>—Perform the test with 1.0 g of Cytarabine. Prepare the control solution with 0.25 mL of 0.01 mol/L hydrochloric acid VS (not more than 0.009%).

(3) Heavy metals <*1.07*>—Proceed with 1.0 g of Cytarabine according to Method 1, and perform the test. Prepare the control solution with 2.0 mL of Standard Lead Solution (not more than 20 ppm).

(4) Related substances—Dissolve 0.10 g of Cytarabine in 10 mL of water, and use this solution as the sample solution. Pipet 1 mL of the sample solution, add water to make exactly 200 mL, and use this solution as the standard solution (1). Pipet 10 mL of the standard solution (1), add water to make exactly 25 mL and use this solution as the standard solution (2). Perform the test with these solutions as directed under Thin-layer Chromatography <*2.03*>. Spot 10 μL each of the sample solution and standard solutions (1) and (2) on a plate of silica gel with fluorescent indicator for thin-layer chromatography. Develop the plate with 1-butanol saturated with water to a distance of about 12 cm, and air-dry the

plate. Examine under ultraviolet light (main wavelength: 254 nm): the spots other than the principal spot obtained from the sample solution are not more intense than the spot from the standard solution (1), and the number of them which are more intense than the spot from the standard solution (2) is not more than two. Spray evenly acidic potassium permanganate TS on the plate: any spot other than the principal spot does not appear.

Loss on drying *<2.41>* Not more than 1.0% (1 g, in vacuum, silica gel, 4 hours).

Residue on ignition *<2.44>* Not more than 0.5% (1 g).

Assay Weigh accurately about 0.2 g of Cytarabine, previously dried, dissolve in 50 mL of acetic acid (100), and titrate *<2.50>* with 0.05 mol/L perchloric acid VS (potentiometric titration). Perform a blank determination in the same manner, and make any necessary correction.

Each mL of 0.05 mol/L perchloric acid VS
= 12.16 mg of $C_9H_{13}N_3O_5$

Containers and storage Containers—Tight containers.

Danazol

ダナゾール

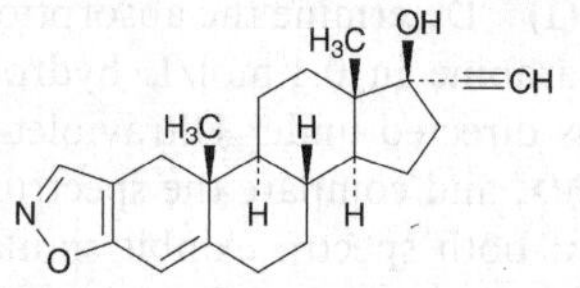

$C_{22}H_{27}NO_2$: 337.46
17α-Pregna-2,4-dien-20-yno[2,3-*d*]isoxazol-17-ol
[*17230-88-5*]

Danazol, when dried, contains not less than 98.5% and not more than 101.0% of danazol ($C_{22}H_{27}NO_2$).

Description Danazol occurs as a white to pale yellow crystalline powder.

It is soluble in acetone, sparingly soluble in ethanol (99.5), and practically insoluble in water.

Melting point: about 225°C (with decomposition).

Identification (1) Determine the absorption spectrum of a solution of Danazol in ethanol (95) (1 in 50,000) as directed under Ultraviolet-visible Spectrophotometry *<2.24>*, and compare the spectrum with the Reference Spectrum or the spectrum of a solution of Danazol RS prepared in the same manner as the sample solution: both spectra exhibit similar intensities of absorption at the same wavelengths.

(2) Determine the infrared absorption spectrum of Danazol as directed in the potassium bromide disk method under Infrared Spectrophotometry *<2.25>*, and compare the spectrum with the Reference Spectrum or the spectrum of Danazol RS: both spectra exhibit similar intensities of absorption at the same wave numbers.

Optical rotation *<2.49>* $[\alpha]_D^{20}$: +8 – +11° (after drying, 0.25 g, ethanol (99.5), 50 mL, 100 mm).

Purity (1) Chloride *<1.03>*—To 2.0 g of Danazol add 80 mL of water, shake well, and boil for 5 minutes. After cooling, add water to make 100 mL, and filter through a glass filter (G4). Discard the first 30 mL of the filtrate, take 40 mL of the subsequent filtrate, and add 6 mL of dilute nitric acid and water to make 50 mL. Perform the test using this solution as the test solution. Prepare the control solution with 0.25 mL of 0.01 mol/L hydrochloric acid VS (not more than 0.011%).

(2) Heavy metals *<1.07>*—Proceed with 2.0 g of Danazol according to Method 2, and perform the test. Prepare the control solution with 2.0 mL of Standard Lead Solution (not more than 10 ppm).

(3) Related substances—Dissolve 0.20 g of Danazol in 4 mL of acetone, and use this solution as the sample solution. Pipet 2 mL of the sample solution, add acetone to make exactly 200 mL. Pipet 4 mL of this solution, add acetone to make exactly 20 mL, and use this solution as the standard solution. Perform the test with these solutions as directed under Thin-layer Chromatography *<2.03>*. Spot 5 μL each of the sample solution and standard solution on a plate of silica gel with fluorescent indicator for thin-layer chromatography. Develop the plate with a mixture of cyclohexane and ethyl acetate (3:2) to a distance of about 15 cm, and air-dry the plate. Examine under ultraviolet light (main wavelength: 254 nm): the spots other than the principal spot and the spot of the starting point obtained from the sample solution are not more intense than the spot from the standard solution.

Loss on drying *<2.41>* Not more than 0.2% (1 g, in vacuum, phosphorous (V) oxide, 60°C, 4 hours).

Residue on ignition *<2.44>* Not more than 0.1% (1 g).

Assay Weigh accurately about 25 mg each of Danazol and Danazol RS, previously dried, dissolve separately in ethanol (95) to make exactly 50 mL. Pipet 2 mL each of these solutions, add ethanol (95) to make exactly 50 mL, and use these solutions as the sample solution and the standard solution, respectively. Perform the test with the sample solution and standard solution as directed under Ultraviolet-visible Spectrophotometry *<2.24>*, and determine the absorbances, A_T and A_S, at 285 nm.

Amount (mg) of danazol ($C_{22}H_{27}NO_2$)
$= M_S \times A_T/A_S$

M_S: Amount (mg) of Danazol RS taken

Containers and storage Containers—Well-closed containers.

Storage—Light-resistant.

Dantrolene Sodium Hydrate

ダントロレンナトリウム水和物

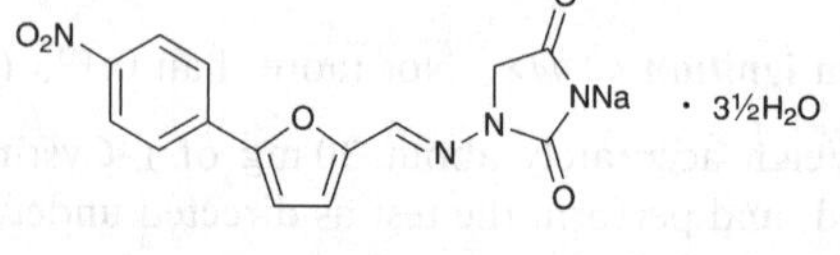

$C_{14}H_9N_4NaO_5.3\frac{1}{2}H_2O$: 399.29
Monosodium 3-[5-(4-nitrophenyl)furan-2-ylmethylene]amino-2,5-dioxo-1,3-imidazolidinate hemiheptahydrate
[*14663-23-1*, anhydride]

Dantrolene Sodium Hydrate contains not less than 98.0% of dantrolene sodium ($C_{14}H_9N_4NaO_5$: 336.23), calculated on the anhydrous basis.

Description Dantrolene Sodium Hydrate occurs as a yellowish orange to deep orange, crystalline powder.

It is soluble in propylene glycol, sparingly soluble in methanol, slightly soluble in ethanol (95), very slightly soluble in water and in acetic acid (100), and practically insoluble in acetone, in tetrahydrofuran and in diethyl ether.

Identification **(1)** Determine the absorption spectrum of a solution of Dantrolene Sodium Hydrate in methanol (1 in 100,000) as directed under Ultraviolet-visible Spectrophotometry 〈*2.24*〉, and compare the spectrum with the Reference Spectrum: both spectra exhibit similar intensities of absorption at the same wavelengths.

(2) Determine the infrared absorption spectrum of Dantrolene Sodium Hydrate as directed in the potassium bromide disk method under Infrared Spectrophotometry 〈*2.25*〉, and compare the spectrum with the Reference Spectrum: both spectra exhibit similar intensities of absorption at the same wave numbers.

(3) To 0.1 g of Dantrolene Sodium Hydrate add 20 mL of water and 2 drops of acetic acid (100), shake well, and filter: the filtrate responds to Qualitative Tests 〈*1.09*〉 (1) for sodium salt.

Purity **(1)** Alkalinity—To 0.7 g of Dantrolene Sodium Hydrate add 10 mL of water, shake well, and centrifuge or filter through a membrane filter. To 5 mL of the supernatant liquid or the filtrate add 45 mL of water, 3 drops of phenolphthalein TS and 0.10 mL of 0.1 mol/L hydrochloric acid VS: a red color is not produced.

(2) Heavy metals 〈*1.07*〉—Proceed with 1.0 g of Dantrolene Sodium Hydrate according to Method 2, and perform the test. Prepare the control solution with 2.0 mL of Standard Lead Solution (not more than 20 ppm).

(3) Related Substances—Dissolve 50 mg of Dantrolene Sodium Hydrate in 20 mL of tetrahydrofuran and 2 mL of acetic acid (100), add ethanol (99.5) to make 100 mL, and use this solution as the sample solution. Pipet 1 mL of the sample solution, add ethanol (99.5) to make exactly 50 mL, and use this solution as the standard solution. Perform the test with exactly 10 μL of the sample solution and standard solution as directed under Liquid Chromatography 〈*2.01*〉 according to the following conditions. Determine each peak area from these solutions by the automatic integration method: the total area of peaks other than dantrolene obtained from the sample solution is not larger than the peak area of dantrolene from the standard solution.

Operating conditions—

Detector: An ultraviolet absorption photometer (wavelength: 300 nm).

Column: A stainless steel column about 4 mm in inside diameter and about 15 cm in length, packed with silica gel for liquid chromatography (5 μm in particle diameter).

Column temperature: A constant temperature of about 30°C.

Mobile phase: A mixture of hexane, acetic acid (100) and ethanol (99.5) (90:10:9).

Flow rate: Adjust so that the retention time of dantrolene is about 8 minutes.

Selection of column: Dissolve 5 mg of Dantrolene Sodium Hydrate and 0.1 g of theophylline in 20 mL of tetrahydrofuran and 2 mL of acetic acid (100), and add ethanol (99.5) to make 100 mL. To 10 mL of this solution add ethanol (99.5) to make 100 mL. Proceed with 10 μL of this solution under the above operating conditions, and calculate the resolution. Use a column giving elution of theophylline and dantrolene in this order with the resolution between these peaks being not less than 6.

Detection sensitivity: Adjust so that the peak height of dantrolene from 10 μL of the standard solution is 10 to 40% of the full scale.

Time span of measurement: About twice as long as the retention time of dantrolene, beginning after the solvent peak.

Water 〈*2.48*〉 14.5 – 17.0% (0.2 g, volumetric titration, direct titration).

Assay Weigh accurately about 0.7 g of Dantrolene Sodium Hydrate, dissolve in 180 mL of a mixture of propylene glycol and acetone (1:1), and titrate 〈*2.50*〉 with 0.1 mol/L perchloric acid VS (potentiometric titration). Perform a blank determination in the same manner, and make any necessary correction.

Each mL of 0.1 mol/L perchloric acid VS
= 33.62 mg of $C_{14}H_9N_4NaO_5$

Containers and storage Containers—Tight containers.

Daunorubicin Hydrochloride

ダウノルビシン塩酸塩

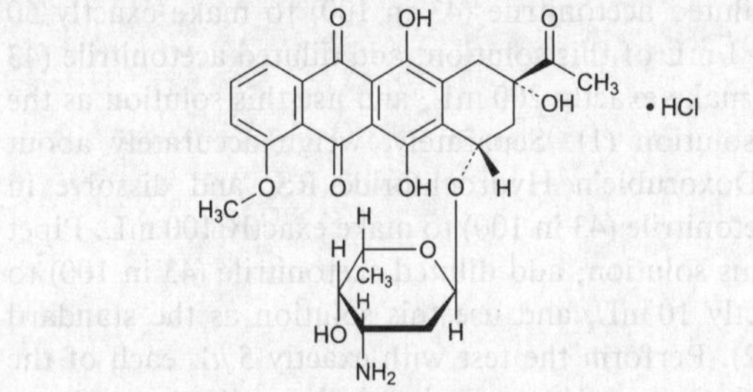

$C_{27}H_{29}NO_{10}.HCl$: 563.98
(2*S*,4*S*)-2-Acetyl-4-(3-amino-2,3,6-trideoxy-α-L-*lyxo*-hexopyranosyloxy)-2,5,12-trihydroxy-7-methoxy-1,2,3,4-tetrahydrotetracene-6,11-dione monohydrochloride
[*23541-50-6*]

Daunorubicin Hydrochloride is the hydrochloride of an anthracycline substance having antitumor activity produced by the growth of *Streptomyces peucetius* or *Streptomyces coeruleorubidus*.

It contains not less than 940 μg (potency) and not more than 1050 μg (potency) per mg, calculated on the dried basis. The potency of Daunorubicin Hydrochloride is expressed as mass (potency) of daunorubicin hydrochloride ($C_{27}H_{29}NO_{10}.HCl$).

Description Daunorubicin Hydrochloride occurs as a red powder.

It is soluble in water and in methanol, and slightly soluble in ethanol (99.5).

Identification **(1)** Determine the absorption spectrum of a solution of Daunorubicin Hydrochloride in methanol (1 in 100,000) as directed under Ultraviolet-visible Spectrophotometry 〈*2.24*〉, and compare the spectrum with the Reference Spectrum or the spectrum of a solution of Daunorubicin Hydrochloride RS prepared in the same manner as the sample solution: both spectra exhibit similar intensities of absorption at the same wavelengths.

(2) Determine the infrared absorption spectrum of Daunorubicin Hydrochloride as directed in the potassium chloride disk method under Infrared Spectrophotometry 〈*2.25*〉, and compare the spectrum with the Reference Spectrum or the spectrum of Daunorubicin Hydrochloride RS: both spectra exhibit similar intensities of absorption at the same wave numbers.

(3) A solution of Daunorubicin Hydrochloride (1 in 50) responds to Qualitative Tests <*1.09*> (2) for chloride.

Optical rotation <*2.49*> $[\alpha]_D^{20}$: +250 – +275° (15 mg calculated on the dried basis, methanol, 10 mL, 100 mm).

pH <*2.54*> Dissolve 0.15 g of Daunorubicin Hydrochloride in 30 mL of water: the pH of the solution is between 4.5 and 6.0.

Purity **(1)** Clarity and color of solution—Dissolve 20 mg of Daunorubicin Hydrochloride in 10 mL of water: the solution is clear and red.

(2) Heavy metals <*1.07*>—Proceed with 1.0 g of Daunorubicin Hydrochloride according to Method 2, and perform the test. Prepare the control solution with 2.0 mL of Standard Lead Solution (not more than 20 ppm).

(3) Related substances—Weigh accurately about 50 mg of Daunorubicin Hydrochloride, dissolve in diluted acetonitrile (43 in 100) to make exactly 50 mL, and use this solution as the sample solution. Separately, weigh accurately about 50 mg of Daunorubicin Hydrochloride RS, and dissolve in diluted acetonitrile (43 in 100) to make exactly 50 mL. Pipet 1 mL of this solution, add diluted acetonitrile (43 in 100) to make exactly 200 mL, and use this solution as the standard solution (1). Separately, weigh accurately about 5 mg of Doxorubicin Hydrochloride RS, and dissolve in diluted acetonitrile (43 in 100) to make exactly 100 mL. Pipet 1 mL of this solution, add diluted acetonitrile (43 in 100) to make exactly 10 mL, and use this solution as the standard solution (2). Perform the test with exactly 5 μL each of the sample solution and standard solutions (1) and (2) as directed under Liquid Chromatography <*2.01*> according to the following conditions. Determine each peak area by the automatic integration method, and calculate the amounts of related substances by the following equations: each amount of each peak, having a relative retention time of about 0.3, about 0.6, about 0.7, about 0.8, about 1.7 and about 2.0 to daunorubicin, is not more than 1.3%, not more than 1.0%, not more than 0.3%, not more than 0.5%, not more than 0.4% and not more than 0.5%, respectively, and the amount of doxorubicin is not more than 0.4%. Furthermore, the total amount of the peaks, other than daunorubicin and the peaks mentioned above, is not more than 0.4%. For the area of the peak, having a relative retention time of about 0.3 to daunorubicin, multiply the correction factor, 0.7.

Each amount (%) of related substances other than doxorubicin
$$= M_{S1}/M_T \times A_T/A_{S1} \times 1/2$$

M_{S1}: Amount (mg) of Daunorubicin Hydrochloride RS taken
M_T: Amount (mg) of Daunorubicin Hydrochloride taken
A_{S1}: Peak area of daunorubicin obtained from the standard solution (1)
A_T: Peak area of each related substance obtained from the sample solution

Amount (%) of doxorubicin $= M_{S2}/M_T \times A_T/A_{S2} \times 5$

M_{S2}: Amount (mg) of Doxorubicin Hydrochloride RS taken
M_T: Amount (mg) of Daunorubicin Hydrochloride taken
A_{S2}: Peak area of doxorubicin obtained from the standard solution (2)
A_T: Peak area of doxorubicin obtained from the sample solution

Operating conditions—

Detector: An ultraviolet absorption photometer (wavelength: 254 nm).

Column: A stainless steel column 4.6 mm in inside diameter and 25 cm in length, packed with octadecylsilanized silica gel for liquid chromatography (5 μm in particle diameter).

Column temperature: A constant temperature of about 25°C.

Mobile phase: Dissolve 2.88 g of sodium lauryl sulfate and 2.25 g of phosphoric acid in water to make 1000 mL. To 570 mL of this solution add 430 mL of acetonitrile.

Flow rate: Adjust so that the retention time of daunorubicin is about 26 minutes.

Time span of measurement: About 2 times as long as the retention time of daunorubicin.

System suitability—

Test for required detectability: To exactly 1 mL of the standard solution (1) add diluted acetonitrile (43 in 100) to make exactly 10 mL. Confirm that the peak area of daunorubicin obtained with 5 μL of this solution is equivalent to 7 to 13% of that with 5 μL of the standard solution (1).

System performance: Dissolve 5 mg each of Daunorubicin Hydrochloride and doxorubicin hydrochloride in 25 mL of diluted acetonitrile (43 in 100). To 1 mL of this solution add diluted acetonitrile (43 in 100) to make 10 mL. When the procedure is run with 5 μL of this solution under the above operating conditions, doxorubicin and daunorubicin are eluted in this order with the resolution between these peaks being not less than 13.

System repeatability: When the test is repeated 6 times with 5 μL of the standard solution (1) under the above operating conditions, the relative standard deviation of the peak area of daunorubicin is not more than 3.0%.

Loss on drying <*2.41*> Not more than 7.5% (0.1 g, reduced pressure not exceeding 0.67 kPa, 60°C, 3 hours).

Assay Weigh accurately an amount of Daunorubicin Hydrochloride and Daunorubicin Hydrochloride RS, equivalent to about 20 mg (potency), dissolve each in a suitable amount of the mobile phase, add exactly 4 mL of the internal standard solution and the mobile phase to make 20 mL, and use these solutions as the sample solution and the standard solution, respectively. Perform the test with 5 μL each of the sample solution and standard solution as directed under Liquid Chromatography <*2.01*> according to the following conditions, and calculate the ratios, Q_T and Q_S, of the peak area of daunorubicin to that of the internal standard.

Amount [μg (potency)] of daunorubicin hydrochloride ($C_{27}H_{29}NO_{10}.HCl$)
$$= M_S \times Q_T/Q_S \times 1000$$

M_S: Amount [mg (potency)] of Daunorubicin Hydrochloride RS taken

Internal standard solution—A solution of 2-naphthalenesulfonic acid in the mobile phase (1 in 100).

Operating conditions—

Detector: An ultraviolet absorption photometer (wavelength: 254 nm).

Column: A stainless steel column 4.6 mm in inside diameter and 30 cm in length, packed with octadecylsilanized silica gel for liquid chromatography (10 μm in particle diameter).

Column temperature: A constant temperature of about 25°C.

Mobile phase: Adjust the pH of a mixture of water and

acetonitrile (31:19) to 2.2 with phosphoric acid.

Flow rate: Adjust so that the retention time of daunorubicin is about 9 minutes.

System suitability—

System performance: When the procedure is run with 5 μL of the standard solution under the above operating conditions, the internal standard and daunorubicin are eluted in this order with the resolution between these peaks being not less than 2.0.

System repeatability: When the test is repeated 6 times with 5 μL of the standard solution under the above operating conditions, the relative standard deviation of the ratios of the peak area of daunorubicin to that of the internal standard is not more than 2.0%.

Containers and storage Containers—Tight containers.

Deferoxamine Mesilate

デフェロキサミンメシル酸塩

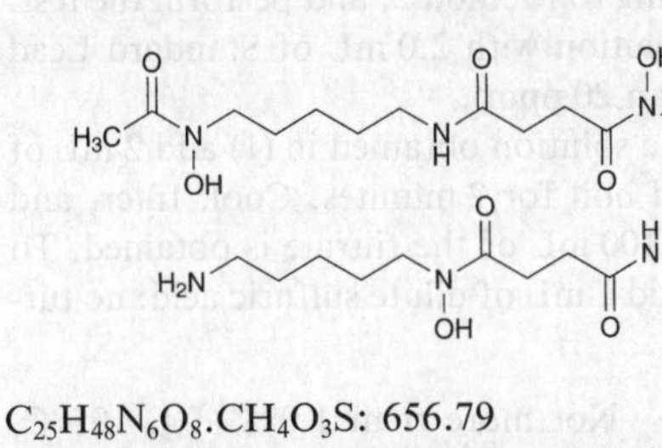

$C_{25}H_{48}N_6O_8.CH_4O_3S$: 656.79

N-[5-(Acetylhydroxyamino)pentyl]-*N′*-(5-{3-[(5-aminopentyl)hydroxycarbamoyl]propanoylamino}pentyl)-*N′*-hydroxysuccinamide monomethanesulfonate

[*138-14-7*]

Deferoxamine Mesilate contains not less than 98.0% and not more than 102.0% of deferoxamine mesilate ($C_{25}H_{48}N_6O_8.CH_4O_3S$), calculated on the anhydrous basis.

Description Deferoxamine Mesilate occurs as a white to pale yellow-white crystalline powder.

It is freely soluble in water, and practically insoluble in ethanol (99.5), in 2-propanol and in diethyl ether.

Melting point: about 147°C (with decomposition).

Identification **(1)** To 5 mL of a solution of Deferoxamine Mesilate (1 in 500) add 1 drop of iron (III) chloride TS: a deep red color develops.

(2) A 50 mg portion of Deferoxamine Mesilate responds to Qualitative Tests <*1.09*> (1) for mesilate.

(3) Determine the infrared absorption spectrum of Deferoxamine Mesilate as directed in the potassium bromide disk method under Infrared Spectrophotometry <*2.25*>, and compare the spectrum with the Reference Spectrum or the spectrum of Deferoxamine Mesilate RS: both spectra exhibit similar intensities of absorption at the same wave numbers.

pH <*2.54*> Dissolve 1.0 g of Deferoxamine Mesilate in 10 mL of water: the pH of this solution is between 3.5 and 5.5.

Purity **(1)** Clarity and color of solution—Dissolve 1.0 g of Deferoxamine Mesilate in 10 mL of water: the solution is clear and colorless to pale yellow.

(2) Chloride <*1.03*>—Perform the test with 1.0 g of Deferoxamine Mesilate. Prepare the control solution with 0.90 mL of 0.01 mol/L hydrochloric acid VS (not more than 0.032%).

(3) Sulfate <*1.14*>—Perform the test with 0.6 g of Deferoxamine Mesilate. Prepare the control solution with 0.50 mL of 0.005 mol/L sulfuric acid VS (not more than 0.040%).

(4) Heavy metals <*1.07*>—Proceed with 2.0 g of Deferoxamine Mesilate according to Method 4, and perform the test. Prepare the control solution with 2.0 mL of Standard Lead Solution (not more than 10 ppm).

(5) Arsenic <*1.11*>—Prepare the test solution with 1.0 g of Deferoxamine Mesilate according to Method 3, and perform the test. Use a solution of magnesium nitrate hexahydrate in ethanol (95) (1 in 10) (not more than 2 ppm).

(6) Related substances—Dissolve 50 mg of Deferoxamine Mesilata in 50 mL of the mobile phase, and use this solution as the sample solution. Pipet 3 mL of the sample solution, add the mobile phase to make exactly 50 mL, and use this solution as the standard solution. Perform the test with exactly 20 μL each of the sample solution and standard solution as directed under Liquid Chromatography <*2.01*> according to the following conditions. Determine each peak area of both solutions by the automatic integration method: the total area of peaks other than deferoxamine obtained from the sample solution is not larger than the peak area of deferoxamine from the standard solution.

Operating conditions—

Detector: An ultraviolet absorption photometer (wavelength: 230 nm).

Column: A stainless steel column 4 mm in inside diameter and 20 cm in length, packed with octadecylsilanized silica gel for liquid chromatography (10 μm in particle diameter).

Column temperature: A constant temperature of about 40°C.

Mobile phase: Dissolve 1.32 g of diammonium hydrogen phosphate, 0.37 g of disodium dihydrogen ethylenediamine tetraacetate dihydrate and 1.08 g of sodium 1-heptanesulfonate in 950 mL of water, and adjust the pH of this solution to 2.8 with phosphoric acid. To 800 mL of this solution add 100 mL of 2-propanol.

Flow rate: Adjust so that the retention time of deferoxamine is about 15 minutes.

Time span of measurement: About two times as long as the retention time of deferoxamine, beginning after the solvent peak.

System suitability—

Test for required detectability: To exactly 2 mL of the standard solution add the mobile phase to make exactly 100 mL. Confirm that the peak area of deferoxamine obtained with 20 μL of this solution is equivalent to 1.5 to 2.5% of that with 20 μL of the standard solution.

System performance: Dissolve 16 mg of Deferoxamine Mesilate and 4 mg of methyl parahydroxybenzoate in 50 mL of the mobile phase. When the procedure is run with 20 μL of this solution under the above operating conditions, deferoxamine and methyl parahydroxybenzoate are eluted in this order with the resolution between these peaks being not less than 4.

System repeatability: When the test is repeated 6 times with 20 μL of the standard solution under the above operating conditions, the relative standard deviation of the peak areas of deferoxamine is not more than 3.0%.

Water <*2.48*> Not more than 2.0% (0.2 g, volumetric titration, direct titration).

Residue on ignition <*2.44*> Not more than 0.1% (1 g).

Assay Weigh accurately about 60 mg of Deferoxamine Mesilate and Deferoxamine Mesilate RS (previously determine the water <*2.48*> in the same manner as Deferoxamine

Mesilate), dissolve each in 20 mL of water, add exactly 10 mL of 0.05 mol/L sulfuric acid TS, and add water to make exactly 50 mL. Pipet 5 mL each of these solutions, add exactly 5 mL of 0.05 mol/L sulfuric acid TS and exactly 0.2 mL of iron (III) chloride TS, then add water to make exactly 50 mL, and use these solutions as the sample solution and the standard solution, respectively. Perform the test with these solutions as directed under Ultraviolet-visible Spectrophotometry <2.24>, using a solution prepared by adding 0.05 mol/L sulfuric acid TS to 0.2 mL of iron (III) chloride TS to make exactly 50 mL as the blank, and determine the absorbances, A_T and A_S, of each solution from the sample solution and the standard solution at 430 nm.

Amount (mg) of deferoxamine mesilate ($C_{25}H_{48}N_6O_8.CH_4O_3S$)
$= M_S \times A_T/A_S$

M_S: Amount (mg) of Deferoxamine Mesilate RS taken, calculated on the anhydrous basis

Containers and storage Containers—Tight containers.

Dehydrocholic Acid

デヒドロコール酸

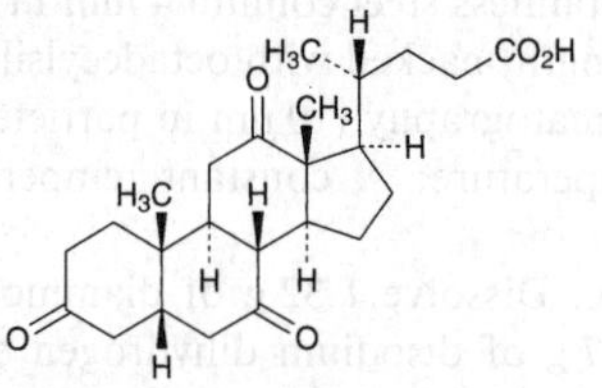

$C_{24}H_{34}O_5$: 402.52
3,7,12-Trioxo-5β-cholan-24-oic acid
[*81-23-2*]

Dehydrocholic Acid, when dried, contains not less than 98.5% of dehydrocholic acid ($C_{24}H_{34}O_5$).

Description Dehydrocholic Acid occurs as a white crystalline powder. It is odorless, and has a bitter taste.

It is sparingly soluble in acetone, slightly soluble in ethanol (95), and practically insoluble in water.

It dissolves in sodium hydroxide TS.

Identification **(1)** Dissolve 5 mg of Dehydrocholic Acid in 1 mL of sulfuric acid and 1 drop of formaldehyde solution, and allow to stand for 5 minutes. Add 5 mL of water to the solution: the solution shows a yellow color and a blue-green fluorescence.

(2) To 0.02 g of Dehydrocholic Acid add 1 mL of ethanol (95), shake, add 5 drops of 1,3-dinitrobenzene TS and 0.5 mL of a solution of sodium hydroxide (1 in 8), and allow to stand: a purple to red-purple color develops, and gradually changes to brown.

Optical rotation <2.49> $[\alpha]_D^{25}$: +20 – +26° (after drying, 0.2 g, acetone, 10 mL, 100 mm).

Melting point <2.60> 233 – 242°C

Purity **(1)** Odor—To 2.0 g of Dehydrocholic Acid add 100 mL of water, and boil for 2 minutes: the solution is odorless.

(2) Clarity and color of solution—To 0.10 g of Dehydrocholic Acid, previously powdered in a mortar, add 30 mL of ethanol (95), and dissolve by shaking for 10 minutes: the solution is clear and colorless.

(3) Chloride <1.03>—To 2.0 g of Dehydrocholic Acid add 100 mL of water, shake for 5 minutes and filter, and use this filtrate as the sample solution. To 25 mL of the sample solution add 6 mL of dilute nitric acid, heat in a water bath for 6 minutes, filter after cooling, and collect the clear filtrate. Wash the residue with 10 mL of water, combine the washings and the filtrate, dilute with water to 50 mL, and perform the test using this solution as the test solution. Prepare the control solution with 0.30 mL of 0.01 mol/L hydrochloric acid VS (not more than 0.021%).

(4) Sulfate <1.14>—Add 1 mL of dilute hydrochloric acid to 25 mL of the sample solution obtained in (3), heat in a water bath for 6 minutes, filter after cooling, and collect the clear filtrate. Wash the residue with 10 mL of water, combine the washings and the filtrate, dilute with water to 50 mL, and perform the test using this solution as the test solution. Prepare the control solution with 0.50 mL of 0.005 mol/L sulfuric acid VS (not more than 0.048%).

(5) Heavy metals <1.07>—Proceed with 1.0 g of Dehydrocholic Acid according to Method 2, and perform the test. Prepare the control solution with 2.0 mL of Standard Lead Solution (not more than 20 ppm).

(6) Barium—To the solution obtained in (1) add 2 mL of hydrochloric acid, and boil for 2 minutes. Cool, filter, and wash with water until 100 mL of the filtrate is obtained. To 10 mL of the filtrate add 1 mL of dilute sulfuric acid: no turbidity is produced.

Loss on drying <2.41> Not more than 1.0% (1 g, 105°C, 2 hours).

Residue on ignition <2.44> Not more than 0.2% (1 g).

Assay Weigh accurately about 0.5 g of Dehydrocholic Acid, previously dried, add 40 mL of neutralized ethanol and 20 mL of water, and dissolve by warming. Add 2 drops of phenolphthalein TS, titrate <2.50> with 0.1 mol/L sodium hydroxide VS, adding 100 mL of freshly boiled and cooled water as the end point is approached, and continue the titration.

Each mL of 0.1 mol/L sodium hydroxide VS
= 40.25 mg of $C_{24}H_{34}O_5$

Containers and storage Containers—Well-closed containers.

Purified Dehydrocholic Acid

精製デヒドロコール酸

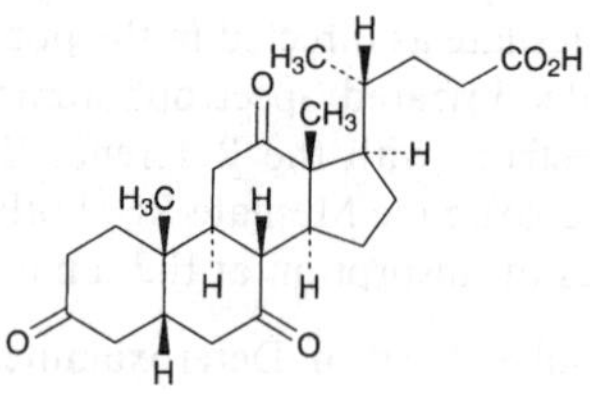

$C_{24}H_{34}O_5$: 402.52
3,7,12-Trioxo-5β-cholan-24-oic acid
[*81-23-2*]

Purified Dehydrocholic Acid, when dried, contains not less than 99.0% of dehydrocholic acid ($C_{24}H_{34}O_5$).

Description Purified Dehydrocholic Acid occurs as a white crystalline powder. It is odorless, and has a bitter taste.

It is sparingly soluble in acetone, slightly soluble in ethanol (95), and practically insoluble in water.

It dissolves in sodium hydroxide TS.

Identification **(1)** Dissolve 5 mg of Purified Dehydrocholic Acid in 1 mL of sulfuric acid and 1 drop of formaldehyde solution, and allow to stand for 5 minutes. Add 5 mL of water to the solution: the solution shows a yellow color and blue-green fluorescence.

(2) To 0.02 g of Purified Dehydrocholic Acid add 1 mL of ethanol (95), shake, add 5 drops of 1,3-dinitrobenzene TS and 0.5 mL of a solution of sodium hydroxide (1 in 8), and allow to stand: a purple to red-purple color develops, and gradually changes to brown.

Optical rotation <*2.49*> $[\alpha]_D^{25}$: +20 – +26° (after drying, 0.2 g, acetone, 10 mL, 100 mm).

Melting point <*2.60*> 237 – 242°C

Purity **(1)** Odor—To 2.0 g of Purified Dehydrocholic Acid add 100 mL of water, and boil for 2 minutes: the solution is odorless.

(2) Clarity and color of solution—Dissolve 0.10 g of Purified Dehydrocholic Acid, previously powdered in a mortar, in 30 mL of ethanol (95) by shaking for 10 minutes: the solution is clear and colorless.

(3) Chloride <*1.03*>—To 2.0 g of Purified Dehydrocholic Acid add 100 mL of water, shake for 5 minutes and filter, and use this filtrate as the sample solution. To 25 mL of the sample solution add 6 mL of dilute nitric acid, heat in a water bath for 6 minutes, filter after cooling, and collect the clear filtrate. Wash the residue with 10 mL of water, combine the washings and the filtrate, dilute with water to 50 mL, and perform the test using this solution as the test solution. Prepare the control solution with 0.30 mL of 0.01 mol/L hydrochloric acid VS (not more than 0.021%).

(4) Sulfate <*1.14*>—Add 1 mL of dilute hydrochloric acid to 25 mL of the sample solution obtained in (3), heat in a water bath for 6 minutes, filter after cooling, and collect the clear filtrate. Wash the residue with 10 mL of water, combine the washings and the filtrate, dilute with water to 50 mL, and perform the test using this solution as the test solution. Prepare the control solution with 0.50 mL of 0.005 mol/L sulfuric acid VS (not more than 0.048%).

(5) Heavy metals <*1.07*>—Proceed with 1.0 g of Purified Dehydrocholic Acid according to Method 2, and perform the test. Prepare the control solution with 2.0 mL of Standard Lead Solution (not more than 20 ppm).

(6) Barium—To the solution obtained in (1) add 2 mL of hydrochloric acid, and boil for 2 minutes, cool, filter, and wash the filter with water until 100 mL of the filtrate is obtained. To 10 mL of the filtrate add 1 mL of dilute sulfuric acid: no turbidity is produced.

Loss on drying <*2.41*> Not more than 1.0% (1 g, 105°C, 2 hours).

Residue on ignition <*2.44*> Not more than 0.2% (1 g).

Assay Weigh accurately about 0.5 g of Purified Dehydrocholic Acid , previously dried, add 40 mL of neutralized ethanol and 20 mL of water, and dissolve by warming. Add 2 drops of phenolphthalein TS, then titrate <*2.50*> with 0.1 mol/L sodium hydroxide VS, adding 100 mL of freshly boiled and cooled water as the end point is approached, and continue the titration.

Each mL of 0.1 mol/L sodium hydroxide VS
= 40.25 mg of $C_{24}H_{34}O_5$

Containers and storage Containers—Well-closed containers.

Dehydrocholic Acid Injection

デヒドロコール酸注射液

Dehydrocholic Acid Injection is an aqueous injection.

It contains not less than 95.0% and not more than 105.0% of the labeled amount of dehydrocholic acid ($C_{24}H_{34}O_5$: 402.52).

Method of preparation Dissolve Purified Dehydrocholic Acid in a solution of Sodium Hydroxide, and prepare as directed under Injections.

Description Dehydrocholic Acid Injection is a clear, colorless to light yellow liquid, and has a bitter taste.

pH: 9 – 11

Identification Transfer a volume of Dehydrocholic Acid Injection, equivalent to 0.1 g of Purified Dehydrocholic Acid, to a separator, and add 10 mL of water and 1 mL of dilute hydrochloric acid: a white precipitate is produced. Extract the mixture with three 15-mL portions of chloroform, combine all the chloroform extracts, evaporate the chloroform on a water bath, and dry the residue at 105°C for 1 hour: the residue so obtained melts <*2.60*> between 235°C and 242°C.

Purity Heavy metals <*1.07*>—Evaporate a volume of Dehydrocholic Acid Injection, equivalent to 1.0 g of Purified Dehydrocholic Acid, on a water bath to dryness. Proceed with the residue according to Method 2, and perform the test. Prepare the control solution with 2.0 mL of Standard Lead Solution (not more than 20 ppm).

Bacterial endotoxins <*4.01*> Less than 0.30 EU/mg.

Extractable volume <*6.05*> It meets the requirement.

Foreign insoluble matter <*6.06*> Perform the test according to Method 1: it meets the requirement.

Insoluble particulate matter <*6.07*> It meets the requirement.

Sterility <*4.06*> Perform the test according to the Membrane filtration method: it meets the requirement.

Assay Transfer an exactly measured volume of Dehydrocholic Acid Injection, equivalent to about 0.5 g of dehydrocholic acid ($C_{24}H_{34}O_5$), to a 100-mL separator, and add, if necessary, water to make 25 mL. Add 2 mL of hydrochloric acid, and extract with 25-mL, 20-mL and 15-mL portions of chloroform successively. Combine the chloroform extracts, wash with cold water until the washings become negative to acid, and evaporate the chloroform on a water bath. Dissolve the residue in 40 mL of neutralized ethanol and 20 mL of water by warming. Add 2 drops of phenolphthalein TS to this solution, titrate <*2.50*> with 0.1 mol/L sodium hydroxide VS, adding 100 mL of freshly boiled and cooled water as the end point is approached, and continue the titration.

Each mL of 0.1 mol/L sodium hydroxide VS
= 40.25 mg of $C_{24}H_{34}O_5$

Containers and storage Containers—Hermetic containers, and colored containers may be used.

Storage—Light-resistant.

Demethylchlortetracycline Hydrochloride

デメチルクロルテトラサイクリン塩酸塩

$C_{21}H_{21}ClN_2O_8.HCl$: 501.31
(4*S*,4a*S*,5a*S*,6*S*,12a*S*)-7-Chloro-4-dimethylamino-3,6,10,12,12a-pentahydroxy-1,11-dioxo-1,4,4a,5,5a,6,11,12a-octahydrotetracene-2-carboxamide monohydrochloride
[*64-73-3*]

Demethylchlortetracycline Hydrochloride is the hydrochloride of a tetracycline substance having antibacterial activity produced by the growth of the mutant of *Streptomyces aureofaciens*.

It contains not less than 900 μg (potency) and not more than 1010 μg (potency) per mg, calculated on the dried basis. The potency of Demethylchlortetracycline Hydrochloride is expressed as mass (potency) of demethylchlortetracycline hydrochloride ($C_{21}H_{21}ClN_2O_8.HCl$).

Description Demethylchlortetracycline Hydrochloride occurs as a yellow crystalline powder.

It is soluble in water, and slightly soluble in ethanol (99.5).

Identification (1) Dissolve 40 mg of Demethylchlortetracycline Hydrochloride in 250 mL of water. To 10 mL of this solution add 85 mL of water and 5 mL of a solution of sodium hydroxide (1 in 5). Determine the absorption spectrum of this solution as directed under Ultraviolet-visible Spectrophotometry *<2.24>*, and compare the spectrum with the Reference Spectrum or the spectrum of a solution of Demethylchlortetracycline Hydrochloride RS prepared in the same manner as the sample solution: both spectra exhibit similar intensities of absorption at the same wavelengths.

(2) Determine the infrared absorption spectrum of Demethylchlortetracycline Hydrochloride as directed in the potassium chloride disk method under Infrared Spectrophotometry *<2.25>*, and compare the spectrum with the Reference Spectrum or the spectrum of Demethylchlortetracycline Hydrochloride RS: both spectra exhibit similar intensities of absorption at the same wave numbers.

(3) A solution of Demethylchlortetracycline Hydrochloride (1 in 100) responds to Qualitative Tests *<1.09>* (2) for chloride.

Optical rotation *<2.49>* $[\alpha]_D^{20}$: −248 − −263° (0.25 g calculated on the dried basis, 0.1 mol/L hydrochloric acid TS, 25 mL, 100 mm).

pH *<2.54>* Dissolve 1.0 g of Demethylchlortetracycline Hydrochloride in 100 mL of water: the pH of the solution is between 2.0 and 3.0.

Purity (1) Heavy metals *<1.07>*—Proceed with 1.0 g of Demethylchlortetracycline Hydrochloride according to Method 2, and perform the test. Prepare the control solution with 2.0 mL of Standard Lead Solution (not more than 20 ppm).

(2) Related substances—Dissolve 25 mg of Demethylchlortetracycline Hydrochloride in 50 mL of 0.01 mol/L hydrochloric acid TS, and use this solution as the sample solution. Pipet 5 mL of the sample solution, add 0.01 mol/L hydrochloric acid TS to make exactly 100 mL, and use this solution as the standard solution. Perform the test with exactly 20 μL each of the sample solution and standard solution as directed under Liquid Chromatography *<2.01>* according to the following conditions. Determine each peak area by the automatic integration method: the area of the peak other than demethylchlortetracycline obtained from the sample solution is not larger than 1.2 times the peak area of demethylchlortetracycline from the standard solution, and the total area of the peaks other than demethylchlortetracycline from the sample solution is not larger than 2 times the peak area of demethylchlortetracycline from the standard solution.

Operating conditions—

Detector, column, column temperature, mobile phase, and flow rate: Proceed as directed in the operating conditions in the Assay.

Time span of measurement: About 2 times as long as the retention time of demethylchlortetracycline, beginning after the solvent peak.

System suitability—

System performance: Proceed as directed in the system suitability in the Assay.

Test for required detectability: To 10 mL of the standard solution add 0.01 mol/L hydrochloric acid TS to make 50 mL, and use this solution as the solution for system suitability test. Pipet 5 mL of the solution for system suitability test, and add 0.01 mol/L hydrochloric acid TS to make exactly 50 mL. Confirm that the peak area of demethylchlortetracycline obtained with 20 μL of this solution is equivalent to 7 to 13% of that with 20 μL of the solution for system suitability test.

System repeatability: When the test is repeated 6 times with 20 μL of the standard solution under the above operating conditions, the relative standard deviation of the peak area of demethylchlortetracycline is not more than 1.0%.

Loss on drying *<2.41>* Not more than 2.0% (1 g, in vacuum, 60°C, 3 hours).

Residue on ignition *<2.44>* Not more than 0.2% (1 g).

Assay Weigh accurately an amount of Demethylchlortetracycline Hydrochloride and Demethylchlortetracycline Hydrochloride RS, equivalent to about 25 mg (potency), dissolve each in 0.01 mol/L hydrochloric acid TS to make exactly 50 mL, and use these solutions as the sample solution and the standard solution, respectively. Perform the test with exactly 20 μL each of the sample solution and standard solution as directed under Liquid Chromatography *<2.01>* according to the following conditions, and determine the peak areas, A_T and A_S, of demethylchlortetracycline in each solution.

Amount [μg (potency)] of demethylchlortetracycline hydrochloride ($C_{21}H_{21}ClN_2O_8.HCl$)
$= M_S \times A_T/A_S \times 1000$

M_S: Amount [mg (potency)] of Demethylchlortetracycline Hydrochloride RS taken

Operating conditions—

Detector: An ultraviolet absorption photometer (wavelength: 254 nm).

Column: A stainless steel column 4.1 mm in inside diameter and 25 cm in length, packed with styrene-divinylbenzene copolymer for liquid chromatography (10 μm in particle diameter).

Column temperature: A constant temperature of about 60°C.

Mobile phase: Dissolve 3.5 g of dipotassium hydrogen phosphate, 1.5 g of tetrabutylammonium hydrogensulfate and 0.4 g of disodium dihydrogen ethylenediamine tetraacetate dihydrate in 300 mL of water, and adjust the pH to 8.5 with sodium hydroxide TS. To this solution add 75.0 g of *t*-butanol and water to make 1000 mL.

Flow rate: Adjust so that the retention time of demethylchlortetracycline is about 8 minutes.

System suitability—

System performance: Heat 10 mL of the standard solution on a water bath for 60 minutes. When the procedure is run with 20 μL of this solution so obtained under the above operating conditions, 4-epidemethylchlortetracycline and demethylchlortetracycline are eluted in this order with the resolution between these peaks being not less than 3. The relative retention time of 4-epidemethylchlortetracycline to demethylchlortetracycline is about 0.7.

System repeatability: When the test is repeated 6 times with 20 μL of the standard solution under the above operating conditions, the relative standard deviation of the peak area of demethylchlortetracycline is not more than 1.0%.

Containers and storage Containers—Tight containers.

Storage—Light-resistant.

Deslanoside

デスラノシド

$C_{47}H_{74}O_{19}$: 943.08

3β-[β-D-Glucopyranosyl-(1→4)-2,6-dideoxy-β-D-*ribo*-hexopyranosyl-(1→4)-2,6-dideoxy-β-D-*ribo*-hexopyranosyl-(1→4)-2,6-dideoxy-β-D-*ribo*-hexopyranosyloxy]-12β,14-dihydroxy-5β,14β-card-20(22)-enolide

[*17598-65-1*]

Deslanoside, when dried, contains not less than 90.0% and not more than 102.0% of deslanoside ($C_{47}H_{74}O_{19}$).

Description Deslanoside occurs as colorless or white crystals or a white, crystalline powder. It is odorless.

It is freely soluble in dehydrated pyridine, sparingly soluble in methanol, slightly soluble in ethanol (95), and practically insoluble in water and in diethyl ether.

It is hygroscopic.

Identification Transfer 1 mg of Deslanoside to a small test tube about 10 mm in inside diameter, dissolve in 1 mL of a solution of iron (III) chloride hexahydrate in acetic acid (100) (1 in 1000), and underlay gently with 1 mL of sulfuric acid: at the zone of contact of two liquids a brown ring is produced, and the color of the upper layer near to the contact zone changes gradually to blue through purple, and the entire acetic acid layer shows a blue-green color through a deep blue color.

Purity (1) Clarity and color of solution—Dissolve 20 mg of Deslanoside in 10 mL of ethanol (95) and 3 mL of water by warming, cool, and dilute to 100 mL with water: the solution is clear and colorless.

(2) Related substances—Dissolve 10 mg of Deslanoside in exactly 5 mL of methanol, and use this solution as the sample solution. Dissolve 1.0 mg of Deslanoside RS in exactly 5 mL of methanol, and use this solution as the standard solution. Perform the test with these solutions as directed under Thin-layer Chromatography 〈*2.03*〉. Spot 20 μL each of the sample solution and standard solution on a plate of silica gel for thin-layer chromatography. Develop the plate with a mixture of dichloromethane, methanol and water (84:15:1) to a distance of about 13 cm, and air-dry the plate. Spray evenly dilute sulfuric acid on the plate, and heat the plate at 110°C for 10 minutes: the spots other than the principal spot obtained from the sample solution are not larger and not more intense than the spot from the standard solution.

Optical rotation 〈*2.49*〉 $[\alpha]_D^{20}$: +6.5 – +8.5° (after drying, 0.5 g, dehydrated pyridine, 25 mL, 100 mm).

Loss on drying 〈*2.41*〉 Not more than 8.0% (0.5 g, in vacuum, phosphorus (V) oxide, 60°C, 4 hours).

Residue on ignition 〈*2.44*〉 Not more than 0.5% (0.1 g).

Assay Dissolve about 12 mg each of Deslanoside and Deslanoside RS, previously dried and accurately weighed, in 20 mL each of methanol, add water to make exactly 100 mL, and use these solutions as the sample solution and the standard solution, respectively. Pipet 5 mL each of these solutions, transfer to light-resistant, 25-mL volumetric flasks, shake well with 5 mL each of 2,4,6-trinitrophenol TS and 0.5 mL each of a solution of sodium hydroxide (1 in 10), add diluted methanol (1 in 4) to make 25 mL, and allow to stand at a temperature between 18°C and 22°C for 25 minutes. Determine the absorbances, A_T and A_S, of the subsequent solutions of the sample solution and the standard solution, respectively, at 485 nm as directed under Ultraviolet-visible Spectrophotometry 〈*2.24*〉, using a solution prepared with 5 mL of diluted methanol (1 in 5) in the same manner as the blank.

Amount (mg) of deslanoside ($C_{47}H_{74}O_{19}$) = $M_S \times A_T/A_S$

M_S: Amount (mg) of Deslanoside RS taken

Containers and storage Containers—Tight containers.

Deslanoside Injection

デスラノシド注射液

Deslanoside Injection is an aqueous injection.

It contains not less than 90.0% and not more than 110.0% of the labeled amount of deslanoside ($C_{47}H_{74}O_{19}$: 943.08).

Method of preparation Dissolve Deslanoside in 10 vol% ethanol and prepare as directed under Injections. It may contain Glycerin. It may be prepared with a suitable amount of Ethanol and Water for Injection or Sterile Water for Injection in Containers.

Description Deslanoside Injection is a clear and colorless liquid.

pH: 5.0 – 7.0

Identification **(1)** Place a volume of Deslanoside Injection, equivalent to 2 mg of Deslanoside, in a separator, add sodium chloride in the ratio of 0.2 g to each mL of this solution, and extract with three 10-mL portions of chloroform. Combine the chloroform extracts, mix uniformly, pipet 15 mL of this solution, and evaporate the chloroform under reduced pressure. Proceed with the residue as directed in the Identification under Deslanoside.

(2) Evaporate the remaining chloroform extract obtained in (1) under reduced pressure, dissolve the residue in 5 mL of methanol, and use this solution as the sample solution. Separately, dissolve 1 mg of Deslanoside RS in 5 mL of methanol, and use this solution as the standard solution. Perform the test with these solutions as directed under Thin-layer Chromatography <*2.03*>. Spot 20 μL each of these solutions on a plate of silica gel for thin-layer chromatography. Develop the plate with a mixture of dichloromethane, methanol and water (84:15:1) to a distance of about 13 cm, and air-dry the plate. Spray evenly dilute sulfuric acid upon the plate, and heat the plate at 110°C for 10 minutes: the spots from the sample solution and standard solution show a black color and have the same *R*f value.

Bacterial endotoxins <*4.01*> Less than 500 EU/mg.

Extractable volume <*6.05*> It meets the requirement.

Foreign insoluble matter <*6.06*> Perform the test according to Method 1: it meets the requirement.

Insoluble particulate matter <*6.07*> It meets the requirement.

Sterility <*4.06*> Perform the test according to the Membrane filtration method: it meets the requirement.

Assay Measure exactly a volume of Deslanoside Injection, equivalent to about 3 mg of deslanoside ($C_{47}H_{74}O_{19}$). Add 5 mL of methanol and water to make exactly 25 mL. Use this solution as the sample solution, and proceed as directed in the Assay under Deslanoside.

$$\text{Amount (mg) of deslanoside } (C_{47}H_{74}O_{19}) = M_S \times A_T/A_S \times 1/4$$

M_S: Amount (mg) of Deslanoside RS taken

Containers and storage Containers—Hermetic containers.

Storage—Light-resistant.

Dexamethasone

デキサメタゾン

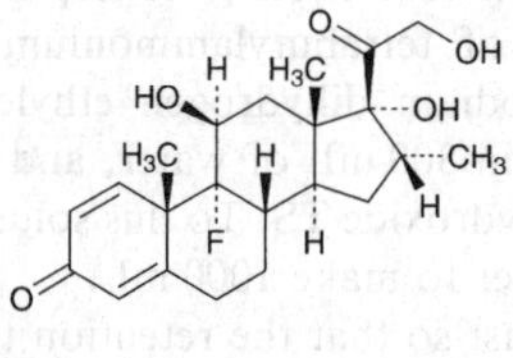

$C_{22}H_{29}FO_5$: 392.46

9-Fluoro-11*β*,17,21-trihydroxy-16*α*-methylpregna-1,4-diene-3,20-dione

[*50-02-2*]

Dexamethasone, when dried, contains not less than 97.0% and not more than 102.0% of dexamethasone ($C_{22}H_{29}FO_5$).

Description Dexamethasone occurs as white to pale yellow, crystals or crystalline powder.

It is sparingly soluble in methanol, in ethanol (95) and in acetone, slightly soluble in acetonitrile, and practically insoluble in water.

Melting point: about 245°C (with decomposition).

It shows crystal polymorphism.

Identification **(1)** Proceed with 10 mg of Dexamethasone as directed under Oxygen Flask Combustion Method <*1.06*>, using a mixture of 0.5 mL of 0.01 mol/L sodium hydroxide TS and 20 mL of water as the absorbing liquid: the solution obtained responds to Qualitative Tests <*1.09*> for fluoride.

(2) Dissolve 1 mg of Dexamethasone in 10 mL of ethanol (95). Mix 2 mL of the solution with 10 mL of phenylhydrazinium chloride TS, heat in a water bath at 60°C for 20 minutes, and cool the solution. Determine the absorption spectrum of the solution as directed under Ultraviolet-visible Spectrophotometry <*2.24*>, using as the blank the solution prepared with 2 mL of ethanol (95) in the same manner as the former solution, and compare the spectrum with the Reference Spectrum or the spectrum of a solution of Dexamethasone RS prepared in the same manner as the former solution: both spectra exhibit similar intensities of absorption at the same wavelengths.

(3) Determine the infrared absorption spectrum of Dexamethasone, previously dried, as directed in the potassium bromide disk method under Infrared Spectrophotometry <*2.25*>, and compare the spectrum with the Reference Spectrum or the spectrum of previously dried Dexamethasone RS: both spectra exhibit similar intensities of absorption at the same wave numbers. If any difference appears between the spectra, dissolve Dexamethasone and Dexamethasone RS in acetone, respectively, then evaporate the acetone to dryness, and repeat the test on the residues.

Optical rotation <*2.49*> $[\alpha]_D^{20}$: +86 – +94° (after drying, 0.1 g, methanol, 10 mL, 100 mm).

Purity **(1)** Heavy metals <*1.07*>—Proceed with 1.0 g of Dexamethasone according to Method 2, and perform the test. Prepare the control solution with 3.0 mL of Standard Lead Solution (not more than 30 ppm).

(2) Related substances—Dissolve 0.18 g of Dexamethasone in 100 mL of acetonitrile. To 33 mL of this solution add a solution, prepared by dissolving 1.32 g of ammonium formate in water to make 1000 mL and adjusted to pH 3.6 with formic acid, to make 100 mL, and use this solution as the sample solution. To exactly 1 mL of the sample solution add the mobile phase to make exactly 100 mL, and use this solution as the standard solution. Perform the test with exactly 10 μL each of the sample solution and standard solution as directed under Liquid Chromatography *<2.01>* according to the following conditions, and determine each peak area by the automatic integration method: each peak area other than dexamethasone obtained from the sample solution is not larger than the peak area of dexamethasone from the standard solution, and the total area of the peaks other than dexamethasone from the sample solution is not larger than 2 times the peak area of dexamethasone from the standard solution.

Operating conditions—

Detector: An ultraviolet absorption photometer (wavelength: 254 nm).

Column: A stainless steel column 4.6 mm in inside diameter and 25 cm in length, packed with phenylsilanized silica gel for liquid chromatography (5 μm in particle diameter).

Column temperature: A constant temperature of about 25°C.

Mobile phase: Dissolve 1.32 g of ammonium formate in 1000 mL of water, and adjust the pH to 3.6 with formic acid. To 670 mL of this solution add 330 mL of acetonitrile.

Flow rate: Adjust so that the retention time of dexamethasone is about 13 minutes.

Time span of measurement: About 4 times as long as the retention time of dexamethasone, beginning after the solvent peak.

System suitability—

Test for required detectability: To exactly 1 mL of the standard solution add the mobile phase to make exactly 10 mL. Confirm that the peak area of dexamethasone obtained with 10 μL of this solution is equivalent to 8 to 12% of that with 10 μL of the standard solution.

System performance: When the procedure is run with 10 μL of the standard solution under the above operating conditions, the number of theoretical plates and the symmetry factor of the peak of dexamethasone are not less than 5000 and not more than 1.5, respectively.

System repeatability: When the test is repeated 6 times with 10 μL of the standard solution under the above operating conditions, the relative standard deviation of the peak area of dexamethasone is not more than 1.0%.

Loss on drying *<2.41>* Not more than 0.5% (0.2 g, 105°C, 3 hours).

Residue on ignition *<2.44>* Not more than 0.1% (0.2 g, platinum crucible).

Assay Dissolve about 10 mg each of Dexamethasone and Dexamethasone RS, previously dried and accurately weighed, in 70 mL each of diluted methanol (1 in 2), add exactly 5 mL each of the internal standard solution, then add diluted methanol (1 in 2) to make 100 mL, and use these solutions as the sample solution and standard solution. Perform the test with 10 μL each of the sample solution and standard solution as directed under Liquid Chromatography *<2.01>* according to the following conditions, and calculate the ratios, Q_T and Q_S, of the peak area of dexamethasone to that of the internal standard.

$$\text{Amount (mg) of dexamethasone } (C_{22}H_{29}FO_5) = M_S \times Q_T/Q_S$$

M_S: Amount (mg) of Dexamethasone RS taken

*Internal standard solution—*A solution of propyl parahydroxybenzoate in diluted methanol (1 in 2) (1 in 1000).

Operating conditions—

Detector: An ultraviolet absorption photometer (wavelength: 254 nm).

Column: A stainless steel column 4 mm in inside diameter and 30 cm in length, packed with octadecylsilanized silica gel for liquid chromatography (10 μm in particle diameter).

Column temperature: A constant temperature of about 25°C.

Mobile phase: A mixture of water and acetonitrile (2:1).

Flow rate: Adjust so that the retention time of dexamethasone is about 6 minutes.

System suitability—

System performance: When the procedure is run with 10 μL of the standard solution under the above operating conditions, dexamethasone and the internal standard are eluted in this order with the resolution between these peaks being not less than 6.

System repeatability: When the test is repeated 6 times with 10 μL of the standard solution under the above operating conditions, the relative standard deviation of the ratio of the peak area of dexamethasone to that of the internal standard is not more than 1.0%.

Containers and storage Containers—Tight containers.

Storage—Light-resistant.

Dextran 40

デキストラン40

Dextran 40 is a product obtained by partial decomposition of polysaccharide, which is produced by fermentation of sucrose with *Leuconostoc mesenteroides* van Tieghem (*Lactobacillaceae*), and the average molecular mass is about 40,000.

When dried, it contains not less than 98.0% and not more than 102.0% of dextran 40.

Manufacture Dextran 40 is produced by the manufacturing method to eliminate or minimize impurities having a possible antigenicity. The manufacturing method is verified to meet the antigenicity test.

Antigenicity Dissolve 10.0 g of Dextran 40 in isotonic sodium chloride solution to make 100 mL, sterilize, and use this solution as the sample solution. Inject 1.0 mL of the sample solution on 3 occasions at intervals of 2 days intraperitoneally to each of 4 well-nourished, healthy guinea pigs weighing 250 to 300 g. Inject 0.10 mL of horse serum intraperitoneally to each of 4 guinea pigs of another group as a control. Inject 0.20 mL of the sample solution intravenously to each of 2 guinea pigs of the first group 14 days after the first intraperitoneal injection and into each of the remaining 2 guinea pigs 21 days after the injection, and inject 0.20 mL of horse serum intravenously in the same manner into each guinea pig of the second group. Observe the signs of respiratory distress, collapse or death of the animals for 30 minutes after each intravenous injection and 24 hours later: the animals of the first group exhibit no signs mentioned above.

All the animals of the second group exhibit symptoms of respiratory distress or collapse and not less than 3 animals are killed.

Description Dextran 40 occurs as a white, amorphous powder. It is odorless and tasteless.

It is practically insoluble in ethanol (95) and in diethyl

ether.

It dissolves gradually in water.

It is hygroscopic.

Identification To 1 mL of a solution of Dextran 40 (1 in 3000) add 2 mL of anthrone TS: a blue-green color develops and turns gradually dark blue-green. Then to this solution add 1 mL of diluted sulfuric acid (1 in 2) or 1 mL of acetic acid (100): the solution does not change in color.

pH <*2.54*> Dissolve 1.0 g of Dextran 40 in 10 mL of water: the pH of this solution is between 5.0 and 7.0.

Purity **(1)** Clarity and color of solution—Dissolve 1.0 g of Dextran 40 in 10 mL of water by warming: the solution is clear and colorless.

(2) Chloride <*1.03*>—Perform the test with 2.0 g of Dextran 40. Prepare the control solution with 1.0 mL of 0.01 mol/L hydrochloric acid VS (not more than 0.018%).

(3) Heavy metals <*1.07*>—Proceed with 1.0 g of Dextran 40 according to Method 1, and perform the test. Prepare the control solution with 2.0 mL of Standard Lead Solution (not more than 20 ppm).

(4) Arsenic <*1.11*>—Prepare the test solution with 1.5 g of Dextran 40 according to Method 1, and perform the test (not more than 1.3 ppm).

(5) Nitrogen—Weigh accurately about 2 g of Dextran 40, previously dried, and perform the test as directed under Nitrogen Determination <*1.08*>, where 10 mL of sulfuric acid is used for decomposition, and 45 mL of a solution of sodium hydroxide (2 in 5) is added: the amount of nitrogen (N: 14.01) is not more than 0.010%.

(6) Reducing substances—Weigh exactly 3.00 g of Dextran 40, previously dried, dissolve in water to make exactly 50 mL, and use this solution as the sample solution. Separately, weigh exactly 0.450 g of glucose, previously dried, dissolve in water to make exactly 500 mL, and use this solution as the control solution. Pipet 5 mL each of the sample solution and the control solution, and add water to make exactly 50 mL, respectively. Pipet 5 mL each of these solutions, add 5 mL of alkaline copper TS, exactly measured, and heat for 15 minutes in a water bath. After cooling, add 1 mL of a solution of potassium iodine (1 in 40) and 1.5 mL of dilute sulfuric acid, and titrate <*2.50*> with 0.005 mol/L sodium thiosulfate VS (indicator: 2 mL of starch TS).

The titrant consumed for the sample solution is not less than that for the control solution.

Loss on drying <*2.41*> Not more than 5.0% (1 g, 105°C, 6 hours).

Residue on ignition <*2.44*> Not more than 0.1% (1 g).

Bacterial endotoxins <*4.01*> Less than 2.5 EU/g.

Viscosity <*2.53*> **(1)** Dextran 40—Weigh accurately 0.2 to 0.5 g of Dextran 40, previously dried, dissolve in water to make exactly 100 mL, and use this solution as the sample solution. Perform the test with the sample solution and with water as directed in Method 1 at 25°C : the intrinsic viscosity is between 0.16 and 0.19.

(2) High-molecular fraction—Weigh accurately about 6 g of Dextran 40, previously dried, dissolve in water to make exactly 100 mL, and transfer to a flask. Add slowly enough methanol to get 7% to 10% of the precipitate (usually 80 to 90 mL) at 25 ± 1°C with stirring. Dissolve the precipitate at 35°C in a water bath with occasional shaking, and allow to stand for more than 15 hours at 25 ± 1°C. Remove the supernatant liquid by decantation, and heat the precipitate of the lower layer to dryness on a water bath. Dry the residue, and determine the intrinsic viscosity of the dried substance as directed in (1): the value is not more than 0.27.

(3) Low-molecular fraction—Weigh accurately about 6 g of Dextran 40, previously dried, dissolve in water to make exactly 100 mL, and transfer to a flask. Add slowly enough methanol to get 90% to 93% of the precipitate (usually 115 to 135 mL) at 25 ± 1°C with stirring, centrifuge at 25°C, and evaporate the supernatant liquid to dryness on a water bath. Dry the residue, and determined the intrinsic viscosity of the dried substance as directed in (1): the value is not less than 0.09.

Assay Weigh accurately about 3 g of Dextran 40, previously dried, dissolve in water to make exactly 50 mL, and use this solution as the sample solution. Determine the optical rotation α_D with the sample solution as directed under Optical Rotation Determination <*2.49*> in a 100-mL cell at 20 ± 1°C.

$$\text{Amount (mg) of dextran 40} = \alpha_D \times 253.8$$

Containers and storage Containers—Tight containers.

Dextran 40 Injection

デキストラン40注射液

Dextran 40 Injection is an aqueous injection.

It contains not less than 9.5 w/v% and not more than 10.5 w/v% of dextran 40.

Method of preparation

Dextran 40	10 g
Isotonic Sodium Chloride Solution	a sufficient quantity
To make	100 mL

Prepare as directed under Injections, with the above ingredients.

No preservative is added.

Description Dextran 40 Injection is a clear and colorless liquid. It is slightly viscous.

Identification **(1)** Dilute 1 mL of Dextran 40 Injection with water to 200 mL, and to 1 mL of the diluted solution add 2 mL of anthrone TS: a blue-green color develops and turns gradually dark blue-green. Add 1 mL of diluted sulfuric acid (1 in 2) or 1 mL of acetic acid (100) to this solution: the solution does not change in color.

(2) Dextran 40 Injection responds to Qualitative Tests <*1.09*> for sodium salt and for chloride.

pH <*2.54*> 4.5 – 7.0

Bacterial endotoxins <*4.01*> Less than 0.50 EU/mL.

Extractable volume <*6.05*> It meets the requirement.

Viscosity <*2.53*> To 2 to 5 mL of Dextran 40 Injection add isotonic sodiumchloride solution to make exactly 100 mL, and use this solution as the sample solution. Perform the test with the sample solution and with isotonic sodium chloride solution as directed in Method 1 at 25°C: the intrinsic viscosity is between 0.16 and 0.19. Calculate the concentration of the sample solution (g/100 mL) as directed in the Assay.

Assay To exactly 30 mL of Dextran 40 Injection add water to make exactly 50 mL, and use this solution as the sample solution. Determine the optical rotation α_D with the sample solution as directed under Optical Rotation Determination *<2.49>* in a 100-mm cell at 20 ± 1°C.

Amount (mg) of dextran 40 in 100 mL of Dextran 40 Injection
$= \alpha_D \times 846.0$

Containers and storage Containers—Hermetic containers. Plastic containers for aqueous injections may be used.

Storage—Avoid exposure to undue fluctuations in temperature.

Dextran 70

デキストラン 70

Dextran 70 is a product obtained by partial decomposition of polysaccharide, which is produced by fermentation of sucrose with *Leuconostoc mesenteroides* van Tieghem (*Lactobacillaceae*), and the average molecular mass is about 70,000.

When dried, it contains not less than 98.0% and not more than 102.0% of dextran 70.

Description Dextran 70 occurs as a white, amorphous powder. It is odorless and tasteless.

It is practically insoluble in ethanol (95) and in diethyl ether.

It dissolves gradually in water.

It is hygroscopic.

Identification To 1 mL of a solution of Dextran 70 (1 in 3000) add 2 mL of anthrone TS: a blue-green color develops and turns gradually dark blue-green. Then to this solution add 1 mL of diluted sulfuric acid (1 in 2) or 1 mL of acetic acid (100): the solution does not change in color.

pH *<2.54>* Dissolve 3.0 g of Dextran 70 in 50 mL of water: the pH of this solution is between 5.0 and 7.0.

Purity **(1)** Clarity and color of solution—Dissolve 1.0 g of Dextran 70 in 10 mL of water with warming: the solution is clear and colorless.

(2) Chloride *<1.03>*—With 2.0 g of Dextran 70, perform the test. Prepare the control solution with 1.0 mL of 0.01 mol/L hydrochloric acid VS (not more than 0.018%).

(3) Heavy metals *<1.07>*—Proceed with 1.0 g of Dextran 70 according to Method 1, and perform the test. Prepare the control solution with 2.0 mL of Standard Lead Solution (not more than 20 ppm).

(4) Arsenic *<1.11>*—Prepare the test solution with 1.5 g of Dextran 70 according to Method 1, and perform the test (not more than 1.3 ppm).

(5) Nitrogen—Weigh accurately about 2 g of Dextran 70, previously dried, perform the test as directed under Nitrogen Determination *<1.08>*, where 10 mL of sulfuric acid is used for decomposition, and 45 mL of a solution of sodium hydroxide (2 in 5) is added: the amount of nitrogen (N: 14.007) is not more than 0.010%.

(6) Reducing substances—Weigh exactly 3.00 g of Dextran 70, previously dried, dissolve in water to make exactly 50 mL, and use this solution as the sample solution. Separately, weigh exactly 0.300 g of glucose, previously dried, dissolve in water to make exactly 500 mL, and use this solution as the control solution. Pipet 5 mL each of the sample solution and the control solution, and add water to make exactly 50 mL, respectively. Pipet 5 mL of these diluted solutions, add exactly 5 mL of alkaline copper TS, and heat for 15 minutes in a water bath. After cooling, add 1 mL of a solution of potassium iodide (1 in 40) and 1.5 mL of dilute sulfuric acid, and titrate *<2.50>* with 0.005 mol/L sodium thiosulfate VS (indicator: 2 mL of starch TS).

The titrant consumed for the sample solution is not less than that for the control solution.

Loss on drying *<2.41>* Not more than 5.0% (1 g, 105°C, 6 hours).

Residue on ignition *<2.44>* Not more than 0.1% (1 g).

Viscosity *<2.53>* **(1)** Dextran 70—Weigh accurately 0.2 to 0.5 g of Dextran 70, previously dried, dissolve in water to make exactly 100 mL, and use this solution as the sample solution. Perform the test with the sample solution and with water as directed in Method 1 at 25°C : the intrinsic viscosity is between 0.21 and 0.26.

(2) High-molecular fraction—Weigh accurately about 6 g of Dextran 70, previously dried, dissolve in water to make exactly 100 mL, and transfer to a flask. Add slowly enough methanol to get 7% to 10% of the precipitate (usually, 75 to 85 mL) at 25 ± 1°C with stirring. Dissolve the precipitate in a water bath at 35°C with occasional shaking, and allow to stand for more than 15 hours at 25 ± 1°C. Remove the supernatant liquid by decantation, and heat the precipitate of the lower layer on a water bath to dryness. Dry the residue, and determine the intrinsic viscosity of the dried residue as directed in (1): the value is not more than 0.35.

(3) Low-molecular fraction—Weigh accurately about 6 g of Dextran 70, previously dried, dissolve in water to make exactly 100 mL, and transfer to a flask. Add slowly enough methanol to get 90% to 93% of the precipitate (usually 110 to 130 mL) at 25 ± 1°C with stirring, centrifuge at 25°C, and evaporate the supernatant liquid to dryness on a water bath. Dry the residue, and determine the intrinsic viscosity of the dried residue as directed in (1): the value is not less than 0.10.

Antigenicity Dissolve 6.0 g of Dextran 70 in isotonic sodium chloride solution to make 100 mL, sterilize, and use this solution as the sample solution. Inject 1.0 mL of the sample solution on 3 occasions at intervals of 2 days intraperitoneally to each of 4 well-nourished, healthy guinea pigs weighing 250 to 300 g. Separately, inject 0.10 mL of horse serum intraperitoneally to each of 4 guinea pigs of another group as a control. Inject 0.20 mL of the sample solution intravenously to each of 2 guinea pigs of the first group 14 days after the first intraperitoneal injection and into each of the remaining 2 guinea pigs 21 days after the injection, and inject 0.20 mL of horse serum intravenously in the same manner into each guinea pigs of the second group. Observe the signs of respiratory distress, collapse or death of the animals for 30 minutes after each intravenous injection and 24 hours later: the animals of the first group exhibit no signs mentioned above.

All the animals of the second group exhibit symptoms of respiratory distress or collapse and not less than 3 animals are killed.

Pyrogen *<4.04>* Dissolve 6.0 g of Dextran 70 in isotonic sodium chloride solution to make 100 mL, and perform the test: this solution meets the requirement.

Assay Weigh accurately about 3 g of Dextran 70, previously dried, dissolve in water to make exactly 50 mL, and use this solution as the sample solution. Determine the optical rotation α_D as directed under Optical Rotation Determination *<2.49>* in a 100-mm cell at 20 ± 1°C.

Amount (mg) of dextran 70 × α_D = 253.8

Containers and storage Containers—Tight containers.

Dextran Sulfate Sodium Sulfur 5

デキストラン硫酸エステルナトリウム イオウ5

Dextran Sulfate Sodium Sulfur 5 is a sodium salt of sulfate ester obtained by sulfation of partial decomposition products of dextran, which is produced by fermentation of sucrose with *Leuconostoc mesenteroides* Van Tieghem (*Lactobacillaceae*).

Description Dextran Sulfate Sodium Sulfur 5 occurs as a white to light yellow-white powder. It is odorless, and has a saline taste.

It is freely soluble in water and practically insoluble in ethanol (95) and in diethyl ether.

It is hygroscopic.

Identification (1) To 10 mL of a solution of toluidine blue (1 in 100,000) add 0.05 mL of a solution of Dextran Sulfate Sodium Sulfur 5 (3 in 50) dropwise: a color of the solution changes from blue to red-purple.

(2) To 1 mL of a solution of Dextran Sulfate Sodium Sulfur 5 (1 in 1500) add 2 mL of anthrone TS: a blue-green color develops, which turns dark blue-green gradually. Then, add 1 mL of diluted sulfuric acid (1 in 2) or 1 mL of acetic acid (100) to this solution: the solution remains dark blue-green.

(3) A solution of Dextran Sulfate Sodium Sulfur 5 (1 in 100) responds to Qualitative Tests 〈*1.09*〉 (1) for sodium salt.

Optical rotation 〈*2.49*〉 $[\alpha]_D^{20}$: +135.0 – +155.0° (1.5 g calculated on the dried basis, water, 25 mL, 100 mm).

Viscosity 〈*2.53*〉 Weigh accurately about 1.5 g of Dextran Sulfate Sodium Sulfur 5, calculated on the dried basis, dissolve in a solution of sodium chloride (29 in 500) to make exactly 100 mL, and use this solution as the sample solution. Perform the test with the sample solution and a solution of sodium chloride (29 in 500) at 25 ± 0.02°C as directed: the intrinsic viscosity is between 0.030 and 0.040.

pH 〈*2.54*〉 Dissolve 1.0 g of Dextran Sulfate Sodium Sulfur 5 in 20 mL of water: the pH of this solution is between 5.5 and 7.5.

Purity (1) Clarity and color of solution—Dissolve 2.5 g of Dextran Sulfate Sodium Sulfur 5 in 50 mL of water: the solution is clear. And, determine the absorbance of the solution at 420 nm as directed under Ultraviolet-visible Spectrophotometry 〈*2.24*〉: not more than 0.090.

(2) Chloride 〈*1.03*〉—Perform the test with 0.10 g of Dextran Sulfate Sodium Sulfur 5. Prepare the control solution with 0.30 mL of 0.01 mol/L hydrochloric acid VS (not more than 0.106%).

(3) Sulfate 〈*1.14*〉—Dissolve 0.10 g of Dextran Sulfate Sodium Sulfur 5 in 6 mL of water, add 0.6 mL of barium chloride TS, and heat in a water bath for 4 minutes. After cooling, add 1 mL of dilute hydrochloric acid and water to make 50 mL, allow to stand for 10 minutes, and observe: the turbidity of the solution is not more intense than that of the control solution. Prepare the control solution as follows: to 0.50 mL of 0.005 mol/L sulfuric acid VS add 6 mL of water, and proceed in the same manner (not more than 0.240%).

(4) Heavy metals 〈*1.07*〉—Proceed with 1.0 g of Dextran Sulfate Sodium Sulfur 5 according to Method 2, and perform the test. Prepare the control solution with 2.0 mL of Standard Lead Solution (not more than 20 ppm).

(5) Arsenic 〈*1.11*〉—Prepare the test solution with 1.0 g of Dextran Sulfate Sodium Sulfur 5 according to Method 3, and perform the test (not more than 2 ppm).

Sulfur content Weigh accurately about 1.0 g of Dextran Sulfate Sodium Sulfur 5, dissolve in 5 mL of water, add 1.5 mL of hydrochloric acid, and heat in a water bath for 1 hour. After cooling, add water to make exactly 100 mL, and use this solution as the sample solution. To exactly 10 mL of the sample solution add exactly 20 mL of 0.02 mol/L barium chloride VS, add 5 mL of methanol, and heat in a water bath for 30 minutes. After cooling, neutralize with sodium hydroxide TS, and add 70 mL of water, 10 mL of a solution of zinc disodium ethylenediamine tetraacetate tetrahydrate (1 in 20), 3 mL of ammonium chloride TS and 7 mL of strong ammonium water, and titrate 〈*2.50*〉 with 0.02 mol/L disodium dihydrogen ethylenediamine tetraacetate VS until the color of the solution changes from red to light blue (indicator: 5 drops of eriochrome black T TS). Perform a blank determination in the same manner. Amount of sulfur (S: 32.07), calculated on the dried basis, is between 3.0 and 6.0%.

Each mL of 0.02 mol/L barium chloride VS
= 0.6414 mg of S

Loss on drying 〈*2.41*〉 Not more than 10.0% (0.5 g, in vacuum, phosphorus (V) oxide, 60°C, 4 hours).

Containers and storage Containers—Tight containers.

Dextran Sulfate Sodium Sulfur 18

デキストラン硫酸エステルナトリウム イオウ18

Dextran Sulfate Sodium Sulfur 18 is a sodium salt of sulfate ester obtained by sulfation of partial decomposition products of dextran, which is produced by fermentation of sucrose with *Leuconostoc mesenteroides* Van Tieghem (*Lactobacillaceae*).

Description Dextran Sulfate Sodium Sulfur 18 occurs as a white to light yellow-white powder. It is odorless, and has a saline taste.

It is freely soluble in water and practically insoluble in ethanol (95) and in diethyl ether.

It is hygroscopic.

Identification (1) To 10 mL of a solution of toluidine blue (1 in 100,000) add 0.05 mL of a solution of Dextran Sulfate Sodium Sulfur 18 (3 in 50) dropwise: a color of the solution changes from blue to red-purple.

(2) To 1 mL of a solution of Dextran Sulfate Sodium Sulfur 18 (1 in 1500) add 2 mL of anthrone TS: a blue-green color develops, which turns dark blue-green gradually. Then, add 1 mL of diluted sulfuric acid (1 in 2) or 1 mL of acetic acid (100) to this solution: the solution remains dark blue-green.

(3) A solution of Dextran Sulfate Sodium Sulfur 18 (1 in 100) responds to Qualitative Tests 〈*1.09*〉 (1) for sodium salt.

Optical rotation 〈*2.49*〉 $[\alpha]_D^{20}$: +90.0 – +110.0° (1.5 g calculated on the dried basis, water, 25 mL, 100 mm).

Viscosity 〈*2.53*〉 Weigh accurately about 1.5 g of Dextran Sulfate Sodium Sulfur 18, calculated on the dried basis, dissolve in a solution of sodium chloride (29 in 500) to make exactly 100 mL, and use this solution as the sample solution.

Perform the test with the sample solution and a solution of sodium chloride (29 in 500) at 25 ± 0.02°C as directed: the intrinsic viscosity is between 0.020 and 0.032.

pH ⟨*2.54*⟩ Dissolve 1.0 g of Dextran Sulfate Sodium Sulfur 18 in 20 mL of water: the pH of this solution is between 5.5 and 7.5.

Purity **(1)** Chloride ⟨*1.03*⟩—Perform the test with 0.10 g of Dextran Sulfate Sodium Sulfer 18. Prepare the control solution with 0.30 mL of 0.01 mol/L hydrochloric acid VS (not more than 0.106%).

(2) Sulfate ⟨*1.14*⟩—Dissolve 0.10 g of Dextran Sulfate Sodium Sulfur 18 in 6 mL of water, add 0.6 mL of barium chloride TS, and heat in a water bath for 4 minutes. After cooling, add 1 mL of dilute hydrochloric acid and water to make 50 mL, allow to stand for 10 minutes, and observe: the turbidity of the solution is not more intense than that of the control solution. Prepare the control solution as follows: to 1.0 mL of 0.005 mol/L sulfuric acid VS add 6 mL of water, and proceed in the same manner (not more than 0.480%).

(3) Heavy metals ⟨*1.07*⟩—Proceed with 1.0 g of Dextran Sulfate Sodium Sulfur 18 according to Method 2, and perform the test. Prepare the control solution with 2.0 mL of Standard Lead Solution (not more than 20 ppm).

(4) Arsenic ⟨*1.11*⟩—Prepare the test solution with 1.0 g of Dextran Sulfate Sodium Sulfur 18 according to Method 3, and perform the test (not more than 2 ppm).

Sulfur content Weigh accurately about 0.5 g of Dextran Sulfate Sodium Sulfur 18, dissolve in 5 mL of water, add 1.5 mL of hydrochloric acid, and heat in a water bath for 1 hour. After cooling, add water to make exactly 100 mL, and use this solution as the sample solution. To exactly 10 mL of the sample solution add exactly 20 mL of 0.02 mol/L barium chloride VS, add 5 mL of methanol, and heat in a water bath for 30 minutes. After cooling, neutralize with sodium hydroxide TS, and add 70 mL of water, 10 mL of a solution of zinc disodium ethylenediamine tetraacetate tetrahydrate (1 in 20), 3 mL of ammonium chloride TS and 7 mL of strong ammonium water, and titrate ⟨*2.50*⟩ with 0.02 mol/L disodium dihydrogen ethylenediamine tetraacetate VS until the color of the solution changes from red to light blue (indicator: 5 drops of eriochrome black T TS). Perform a blank determination in the same manner. Amount of sulfur (S: 32.07), calculated on the dried basis, is between 15.0 and 20.0%.

Each mL of 0.02 mol/L barium chloride VS
= 0.6414 mg of S

Loss on drying ⟨*2.41*⟩ Not more than 10.0% (0.5 g, in vacuum, phosphorus (V) oxide, 60°C, 4 hours).

Containers and storage Containers—Tight containers.

Dextrin

デキストリン

Description Dextrin occurs as a white or light yellow, amorphous powder or granules. It has a slight, characteristic odor and a sweet taste. It does not irritate the tongue.

Dextrin is freely soluble in boiling water, soluble in water, and practically insoluble in ethanol (95) and in diethyl ether.

Identification To 0.1 g of Dextrin add 100 mL of water, shake, and filter if necessary. To 5 mL of the filtrate add 1 drop of iodine TS: a light red-brown or light red-purple color develops.

Purity **(1)** Clarity and color of solution—Take 2.0 g of Dextrin in a Nessler tube, add 40 mL of water, dissolve by heating, cool, and add water to make 50 mL: the solution is colorless or light yellow. It is clear, and even if turbid, the turbidity is not more than that of the following control solution.

Control solution: To 1.0 mL of 0.005 mol/L sulfuric acid VS add 1 mL of dilute hydrochloric acid, 46 mL of water and 2 mL of barium chloride TS, allow to stand for 10 minutes, and shake before use.

(2) Acidity—To 1.0 g of Dextrin add 5 mL of water, dissolve by heating, cool, and add 1 drop of phenolphthalein TS and 0.50 mL of 0.1 mol/L sodium hydroxide VS: a red color develops.

(3) Chloride ⟨*1.03*⟩—To 2.0 g of Dextrin add 80 mL of water, dissolve by heating, cool, add water to make 100 mL, and filter. Take 40 mL of the filtrate, and add 6 mL of dilute nitric acid and water to make 50 mL. Perform the test using this solution as the test solution. Prepare the control solution with 0.30 mL of 0.01 mol/L hydrochloric acid VS (not more than 0.013%).

(4) Sulfate ⟨*1.14*⟩—To 45 mL of the filtrate obtained in (3) add 1 mL of dilute hydrochloric acid and water to make 50 mL, and perform the test using this solution as the test solution. Prepare the control solution with 0.35 mL of 0.005 mol/L sulfuric acid VS (not more than 0.019%).

(5) Oxalate—To 1.0 g of Dextrin add 20 mL of water, dissolve by heating, cool, add 1 mL of acetic acid (31), and filter. To 5 mL of the filtrate add 5 drops of calcium chloride TS: no turbidity is produced immediately.

(6) Calcium—To a 5-mL portion of the filtrate obtained in (5) add 5 drops of ammonium oxalate TS: no turbidity is immediately produced.

(7) Heavy metals ⟨*1.07*⟩—Proceed with 0.5 g of Dextrin according to Method 2, and perform the test. Prepare the control solution with 2.5 mL of Standard Lead Solution (not more than 50 ppm).

Loss on drying ⟨*2.41*⟩ Not more than 10% (0.5 g, 105°C, 4 hours).

Residue on ignition ⟨*2.44*⟩ Not more than 0.5% (0.5 g).

Containers and storage Containers—Well-closed containers.

Dextromethorphan Hydrobromide Hydrate

デキストロメトルファン臭化水素酸塩水和物

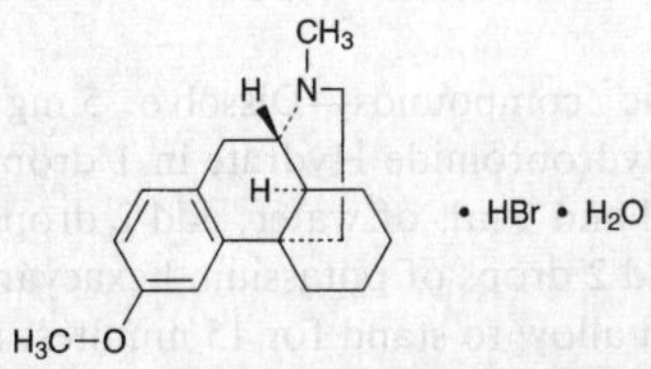

• HBr • H_2O

$C_{18}H_{25}NO.HBr.H_2O$: 370.32
(9*S*,13*S*,14*S*)-3-Methoxy-17-methylmorphinan monohydrobromide monohydrate
[6700-34-1]

Dextromethorphan Hydrobromide Hydrate contains not less than 98.0% of dextromethorphan hydrobromide ($C_{18}H_{25}NO.HBr$: 352.31), calculated on the anhydrous basis.

Description Dextromethorphan Hydrobromide Hydrate occurs as white, crystals or crystalline powder.

It is very soluble in methanol, freely soluble in ethanol (95) and in acetic acid (100), and sparingly soluble in water.

Melting point: about 126°C (Insert the capillary tube into the bath preheated to 116°C, and continue the heating so that the temperature rises at a rate of about 3°C per minute.)

Identification (1) Determine the absorption spectrum of a solution of Dextromethorphan Hydrobromide Hydrate (1 in 10,000) as directed under Ultraviolet-visible Spectrophotometry *<2.24>*, and compare the spectrum with the Reference Spectrum: both spectra exhibit similar intensities of absorption at the same wavelengths.

(2) Determine the infrared absorption spectrum of Dextromethorphan Hydrobromide Hydrate as directed in the potassium bromide disk method under Infrared Spectrophotometry *<2.25>*, and compare the spectrum with the Reference Spectrum: both spectra exhibit similar intensities of absorption at the same wave numbers.

(3) To 50 mL of a solution of Dextromethorphan Hydrobromide Hydrate (1 in 100) add 2 drops of phenolphalein TS and sodium hydroxide TS until a red color develops. Add 50 mL of chloroform, shake, and add 5 mL of dilute nitric acid to 40 mL of the water layer. This solution responds to Qualitative Tests *<1.09>* for bromide.

Optical rotation *<2.49>* $[\alpha]_D^{20}$: +26 – +30° (0.34 g calculated on the anhydrous basis, water, 20 mL, 100 mm).

pH *<2.54>* Dissolve 1.0 g of Dextromethorphan Hydrobromide Hydrate in 100 mL of water: the pH of this solution is between 5.2 and 6.5.

Purity (1) Clarity and color of solution—Dissolve 0.20 g of Dextromethorphan Hydrobromide Hydrate in 20 mL of water: the solution is clear and colorless.

(2) *N,N*-dimethylaniline—To 0.50 g of Dextromethorphan Hydrobromide Hydrate add 20 mL of water, and dissolve by heating on a water bath. After cooling, add 2 mL of dilute acetic acid, 1 mL of sodium nitrite TS and water to make 25 mL: the solution has no more color than the following control solution.

Control solution: Dissolve 0.10 g of *N,N*-dimethylaniline in 400 mL of water by warming on a water bath, cool, and add water to make 500 mL. Pipet 5 mL of this solution, and add water to make 200 mL. To 1.0 mL of this solution add 2 mL of dilute acetic acid, 1 mL of sodium nitrite TS and water to make 25 mL.

(3) Heavy metals *<1.07>*—Proceed with 1.0 g of Dextromethorphan Hydrobromide Hydrate according to Method 4, and perform the test. Prepare the control solution with 2.0 mL of Standard Lead Solution (not more than 20 ppm).

(4) Phenolic compounds—Dissolve 5 mg of Dextromethorphan Hydrobromide Hydrate in 1 drop of dilute hydrochloric acid and 1 mL of water, add 2 drops of iron (III) chloride TS and 2 drops of potassium hexacyanoferrate (III) TS, shake, and allow to stand for 15 minutes: no blue-green color develops.

(5) Related substances—Dissolve 0.25 g of Dextromethorphan Hydrobromide Hydrate in 10 mL of methanol, and use this solution as the sample solution. Pipet 1 mL of the sample solution, add methanol to make exactly 200 mL, and use this solution as the standard solution. Perform the test with these solutions as directed under Thin-layer Chromatography *<2.03>*. Spot 5 μL each of the sample solution and standard solution on a plate of silica gel for thin-layer chromatography. Develop the plate with a mixture of toluene, ethyl acetate, methanol, dichloromethane and 13.5 mol/L ammonia TS (55:20:13:10:2) to a distance of about 15 cm, and air-dry the plate. Spray evenly bismuth potassium iodide TS on the plate, and then spray evenly hydrogen peroxide TS on the plate: the spots other than the principal spot obtained from the sample solution are not more intense than the spot from the standard solution.

Water *<2.48>* 4.0 – 5.5% (0.2 g, volumetric titration, back titration).

Residue on ignition *<2.44>* Not more than 0.1% (1 g).

Assay Weigh accurately about 0.5 g of Dextromethorphan Hydrobromide Hydrate, dissolve in 10 mL of acetic acid (100) and add 40 mL of acetic anhydride. Titrate *<2.50>* with 0.1 mol/L perchloric acid VS (potentiometric titration). Perform a blank determination, and make any necessary correction.

Each mL of 0.1 mol/L perchloric acid VS
= 35.23 mg of $C_{18}H_{25}NO.HBr$

Containers and storage Containers—Well-closed containers.

Diastase

ジアスターゼ

Diastase is an enzyme drug mainly prepared from malt. It has amylolytic activity.

It contains not less than 440 starch saccharifying activity units per g.

It is usually diluted with suitable diluents.

Description Diastase occurs as a light yellow to light brown powder.

It is hygroscopic.

Purity Rancidity—Diastase has no unpleasant or rancid odor, and has no unpleasant or rancid taste.

Loss on drying *<2.41>* Not more than 4.0% (1 g, 105°C, 5 hours).

Assay (i) Substrate solution—Use potato starch TS for amylolytic activity test.

(ii) Sample solution—Weigh accurately about 0.1 g of Diastase, and dissolve in water to make exactly 100 mL.

(iii) Procedure—Proceed as directed in 1.1. Measurement of starch saccharifying activity of 1. Assay for starch digestive activity under Digestion Test *<4.03>*.

Containers and storage Containers—Tight containers.

Storage—Not exceeding 30°C.

Diastase and Sodium Bicarbonate Powder

ジアスターゼ・重曹散

Method of preparation

Diastase	200 g
Sodium Bicarbonate	300 g
Precipitated Calcium Carbonate	400 g
Magnesium Oxide	100 g
To make	1000 g

Prepare before use as directed under Powders, with the above ingredients.

Description Diastase and Sodium Bicarbonate Powder occurs as a light yellow powder. It has a characteristic, salty taste.

Containers and storage Containers—Well-closed containers.

Compound Diastase and Sodium Bicarbonate Powder

複方ジアスターゼ・重曹散

Method of preparation

Diastase	200 g
Sodium Bicarbonate	600 g
Magnesium Oxide	150 g
Powdered Gentian	50 g
To make	1000 g

Prepare before use as directed under Powders, with the above ingredients.

Description Compound Diastase and Sodium Bicarbonate Powder occurs as a slightly brownish, light yellow powder. It has a characteristic odor and a bitter taste.

Containers and storage Containers—Well-closed containers.

Diazepam

ジアゼパム

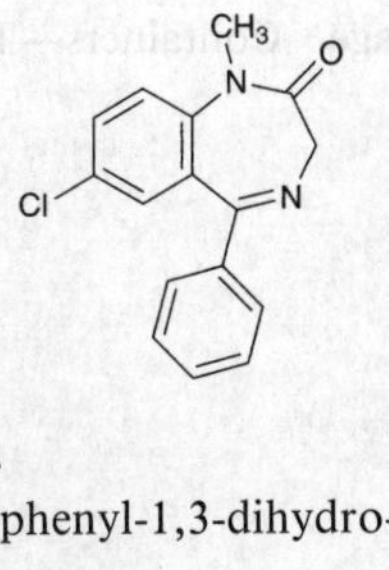

$C_{16}H_{13}ClN_2O$: 284.74
7-Chloro-1-methyl-5-phenyl-1,3-dihydro-2*H*-1,4-benzodiazepin-2-one
[439-14-5]

Diazepam, when dried, contains not less than 98.0% of diazepam ($C_{16}H_{13}ClN_2O$).

Description Diazepam occurs as a white to light yellow crystalline powder. It is odorless, and has a slightly bitter taste.

It is freely soluble in acetone, soluble in acetic anhydride and in ethanol (95), sparingly soluble in diethyl ether, slightly soluble in ethanol (99.5), and practically insoluble in water.

Identification (1) Dissolve 10 mg of Diazepam in 3 mL of sulfuric acid, and observe under ultraviolet light (main wavelength: 365 nm): the solution shows a yellow-green fluorescence.

(2) Dissolve 2 mg of Diazepam in 200 mL of a solution of sulfuric acid in ethanol (99.5) (3 in 1000). Determine the absorption spectrum of the solution as directed under Ultraviolet-visible Spectrophotometry ⟨*2.24*⟩, and compare the spectrum with the Reference Spectrum: both spectra exhibit similar intensities of absorption at the same wavelengths.

(3) Determine the infrared absorption spectrum of Diazepam, previously dried, as directed in the potassium bromide disk method under Infrared Spectrophotometry ⟨*2.25*⟩, and compare the spectrum with the Reference Spectrum: both spectra exhibit similar intensities of absorption at the same wave numbers.

(4) Perform the test with Diazepam as directed under Flame Coloration Test ⟨*1.04*⟩ (2): a blue to blue-green color appears.

Melting point ⟨*2.60*⟩ 130 – 134°C

Purity (1) Clarity of solution—Dissolve 0.10 g of Diazepam in 20 mL of ethanol (95): the solution is clear.

(2) Chloride ⟨*1.03*⟩—To 1.0 g of Diazepam add 50 mL of water, allow to stand for 1 hour, with occasional shaking, and filter. To 25 mL of the filtrate add 6 mL of dilute nitric acid and water to make 50 mL. Perform the test using this solution as the test solution. Prepare the control solution with 0.20 mL of 0.01 mol/L hydrochloric acid VS (not more than 0.014%).

(3) Heavy metals ⟨*1.07*⟩—Proceed with 1.0 g of Diazepam according to Method 2, and perform the test. Prepare the control solution with 2.0 mL of Standard Lead Solution (not more than 20 ppm).

(4) Related substances—Dissolve 1.0 g of Diazepam in 10 mL of acetone, and use this solution as the sample solution. Pipept 1 mL of the sample solution, and add acetone to make exactly 100 mL. Pipet 1 mL of this solution, add acetone to make exactly 10 mL, and use this solution as the standard solution. Perform the test with these solutions as directed under Thin-layer Chromatography ⟨*2.03*⟩. Spot 5 μL each of the sample solution and standard solution on a plate of silica gel with fluorescent indicator for thin-layer chromatography. Develop the plate with a mixture of ethyl acetate and hexane (1:1) to a distance of about 12 cm, and air-dry the plate. Examine under ultraviolet light (main wavelength: 254 nm): the spots other than the principal spot obtained from the sample solution are not more intense than the spot from the standard solution.

Loss on drying ⟨*2.41*⟩ Not more than 0.5% (1 g, 105°C, 2 hours).

Residue on ignition ⟨*2.44*⟩ Not more than 0.1% (1 g).

Assay Weigh accurately about 0.6 g of Diazepam, previously dried, dissolve in 60 mL of acetic anhydride, and titrate ⟨*2.50*⟩ with 0.1 mol/L perchloric acid VS (potentiometric titration). Perform a blank determination in the same manner, and make any necessary correction.

Each mL of 0.1 mol/L perchloric acid VS
= 28.47 mg of $C_{16}H_{13}ClN_2O$

Containers and storage Containers—Tight containers.
Storage—Light-resistant.

Diazepam Tablets

ジアゼパム錠

Diazepam Tablets contain not less than 95.0% and not more than 105.0% of the labeled amount of diazepam ($C_{16}H_{13}ClN_2O$: 284.74).

Method of preparation Prepare as directed under Tablets, with Diazepam.

Identification To a portion of the powdered Diazepam Tablets, equivalent to 50 mg of Diazepam, add 50 mL of acetone, shake, and filter. Evaporate 1 mL of the filtrate on a water bath to dryness, and dissolve the residue with 100 mL of a solution of sulfuric acid in ethanol (99.5) (3 in 1000). Determine the absorption spectrum of this solution as directed under Ultraviolet-visible Spectrophotometry <*2.24*>: it exhibits maxima between 240 nm and 244 nm, between 283 nm and 287 nm, and between 360 nm and 370 nm.

Uniformity of dosage units <*6.02*> Perform the test according to the following method: it meets the requirement of the Content uniformity test.

To 1 tablet of Diazepam Tablets add 5 mL of water, and disintegrate the tablet by shaking. Then add 30 mL of methanol, shake for 10 minutes, add methanol to make exactly 50 mL, and centrifuge. Pipet V mL of the supernatant liquid, equivalent to 0.4 mg of diazepam ($C_{16}H_{13}ClN_2O$), add exactly 5 mL of the internal standard solution, then add methanol to make 20 mL, and use this solution as the sample solution. Separately, weigh accurately about 20 mg of diazepam for assay, previously dried at 105°C for 2 hours, and dissolve in methanol to make exactly 100 mL. Pipet 2 mL of this solution, add exactly 5 mL of the internal standard solution and add methanol to make 20 mL, and use this solution as the standard solution. Perform the test with 10 µL each of the sample solution and standard solution as directed under Liquid Chromatography <*2.01*> under the following conditions, and calculate the ratios, Q_T and Q_S, of the peak area of diazepam to that of the internal standard.

Amount (mg) of diazepam ($C_{16}H_{13}ClN_2O$)
$= M_S \times Q_T/Q_S \times 1/V$

M_S: Amount (mg) of diazepam for assay taken

Internal standard solution—A solution of ethyl parahydroxybenzoate in methanol (1 in 25,000).

Operating conditions—

Proceed as directed in the operating conditions in the Assay.

System suitability—

System performance: When the procedure is run with 10 µL of the standard solution under the above operating conditions, the internal standard and diazepam are eluted in this order with the resolution between these peaks being not less than 6.

System repeatability: When the test is repeated 6 times with 10 µL of the standard solution under the above operating conditions, the relative standard deviation of the ratio of the peak area of diazepam to that of the internal standard is not more than 1.0%.

Dissolution Being specified separately when the drug is granted approval based on the Law.

Assay Weigh accurately the mass of not less than 20 Diazepam Tablets, and powder. Weigh accurately a portion of the powder, equivalent to about 50 mg of diazepam ($C_{16}H_{13}ClN_2O$), add 10 mL of water, shake, then add 60 mL of methanol, shake for 10 minutes, add methanol to make exactly 100 mL, and centrifuge. Pipet 5 mL of the supernatant liquid, add exactly 5 mL of the internal standard solution, then add methanol to make 100 mL, and use this solution as the sample solution. Separately, weigh accurately about 50 mg of diazepam for assay, previously dried at 105°C for 2 hours, and dissolve in 10 mL of water and add methanol to make exactly 100 mL. Pipet 5 mL of this solution, add exactly 5 mL of the internal standard solution and add methanol to make 100 mL, and use this solution as the standard solution. Perform the test with 10 µL each of the sample solution and standard solution as directed under Liquid Chromatography <*2.01*> according to the following conditions, and calculate the ratios, Q_T and Q_S, of the peak area of diazepam to that of the internal standard.

Amount (mg) of diazepam ($C_{16}H_{13}ClN_2O$)
$= M_S \times Q_T/Q_S$

M_S: Amount (mg) of diazepam for assay taken

Internal standard solution—A solution of ethyl parahydroxybenzoate in methanol (1 in 5000).

Operating conditions—

Detector: An ultraviolet absorption photometer (wavelength: 254 nm).

Column: A stainless steel column 4 mm in inside diameter and 15 cm in length, packed with octadecylsilanized silica gel for liquid chromatography (5 µm in particle diameter).

Column temperature: A constant temperature of about 40°C.

Mobile phase: A mixture of methanol and water (13:7).

Flow rate: Adjust so that the retention time of diazepam is about 10 minutes.

System suitability—

System performance: When the procedure is run with 10 µL of the standard solution under the above operating conditions, the internal standard and diazepam are eluted in this order with the resolution between these peaks being not more than 6.

System repeatability: When the test is repeated 6 times with 10 µL of the standard solution under the above operating conditions, the relative standard deviation of the ratio of the peak area of diazepam to that of the internal standard is not more than 1.0%.

Containers and storage Containers—Tight containers.

Dibekacin Sulfate

ジベカシン硫酸塩

$C_{18}H_{37}N_5O_8.xH_2SO_4$
3-Amino-3-deoxy-α-D-glucopyranosyl-(1→6)-[2,6-diamino-2,3,4,6-tetradeoxy-α-D-*erythro*-hexopyranosyl-(1→4)]-2-deoxy-D-streptamine sulfate
[*58580-55-5*]

Dibekacin Sulfate is the sulfate of a derivative of bekanamycin.

It contains not less than 640 μg (potency) and not more than 740 μg (potency) per mg, calculated on the dried basis. The potency of Dibekacin Sulfate is expressed as mass (potency) of dibekacin ($C_{18}H_{37}N_5O_8$: 451.52).

Description Dibekacin Sulfate occurs as a white to yellow-white powder.

It is very soluble in water, and practically insoluble in ethanol (99.5).

Identification **(1)** Dissolve 20 mg each of Dibekacin Sulfate and Dibekacin Sulfate RS in 1 mL of water, and use these solutions as the sample solution and standard solution. Perform the test with these solutions as directed under Thin-layer Chromatography *<2.03>*. Spot 5 μL each of the sample solution and standard solution on a plate of silica gel for thin-layer chromatography. Develop the plate with a mixture of ammonia solution (28) and methanol (1:1) to a distance of about 10 cm, and air-dry the plate. Spray evenly 0.2% ninhydrin-water saturated 1-butanol TS, and heat at 100°C for 10 minutes: the principal spots obtained from the sample solution and the spot from the standard solution show a purple-brown color and the same *R*f value.

(2) To 5 mL of a solution of Dibekacin Sulfate (1 in 50) add 1 drop of barium chloride TS: a white precipitate is produced.

Optical rotation *<2.49>* $[\alpha]_D^{20}$: +96 – +106° (0.25 g calculated on the dried basis, water, 25 mL, 100 mm).

pH *<2.54>* The pH of a solution obtained by dissolving 1.0 g of Dibekacin Sulfate in 20 mL of water is between 6.0 and 8.0.

Purity **(1)** Clarity and color of solution—Dissolve 3.0 g of Dibekacin Sulfate in 10 mL of water: the solution is clear. Determine the absorbance of this solution at 400 nm as directed under Ultraviolet-visible Spectrophotometry *<2.24>*: not more than 0.15.

(2) Heavy metals *<1.07>*—Proceed with 1.0 g of Dibekacin Sulfate according to Method 1, and perform the test. Prepare the control solution with 2.0 mL of Standard Lead Solution (not more than 20 ppm).

Loss on drying *<2.41>* Not more than 5.0% (1 g, reduced pressure not exceeding 0.67 kPa, 60°C, 3 hours).

Assay Perform the test according to the Cylinder-plate method as directed under Microbial Assay for Antibiotics *<4.02>* according to the following conditions.

(i) Test organism—*Bacillus subtilis* ATCC 6633

(ii) Culture medium—Use the medium i in 1) under (1) Agar media for seed and base layer having pH 6.5 to 6.6 after sterilization.

(iii) Standard solutions—Weigh accurately an amount of Dibekacin Sulfate RS, previously dried, equivalent to about 20 mg (potency), dissolve in diluted phosphate buffer solution (pH 6.0) (1 in 2) to make exactly 50 mL, and use this solution as the standard stock solution. Keep the standard stock solution at 5 to 15°C and use within 30 days. Take exactly a suitable amount of the standard stock solution before use, add 0.1 mol/L phosphate buffer solution (pH 8.0) to make solutions so that each mL contains 20 μg (potency) and 5 μg (potency), and use these solutions as the high concentration standard solution and the low concentration standard solution, respectively.

(iv) Sample solutions—Weigh accurately an amount of Dibekacin Sulfate, equivalent to about 20 mg (potency), and dissolve in water to make exactly 50 mL. Take exactly a suitable amount of this solution, add 0.1 mol/L phosphate buffer solution (pH 8.0) to make solutions so that each mL contains 20 μg (potency) and 5 μg (potency), and use these solutions as the high concentration sample solution and the low concentration sample solution, respectively.

Containers and storage Containers—Tight containers.

Dibekacin Sulfate Ophthalmic Solution

ジベカシン硫酸塩点眼液

Dibekacin Sulfate Ophthalmic Solution is an aqueous ophthalmic preparation.

It contains not less than 90.0% and not more than 110.0% of the labeled potency of dibekacin ($C_{18}H_{37}N_5O_8$: 451.52).

Method of preparation Prepare as directed under Ophthalmic Liquids and Solutions, with Dibekacin Sulfate.

Description Dibekacin Sulfate Ophthalmic Solution is a clear, colorless liquid.

Identification To a volume of Dibekacin Sulfate Ophthalmic Solution add water so that each mL contains about 2.5 mg (potency) of Dibekacin Sulfate, and use this solution as the sample solution. Separately, dissolve an amount of Dibekacin Sulfate RS, equivalent to 5 mg (potency), in 2 mL of water, and use this solution as the standard solution. Perform the test with these solutions as directed under Thin-layer Chromatography *<2.03>*. Spot 10 μL each of the sample solution and standard solution on a plate of silica gel for thin-layer chromatography. Proceed as directed in the Identification (1) under Dibekacin Sulfate.

pH *<2.54>* 6.5 – 7.5

Foreign insoluble matter *<6.11>* It meets the requirement.

Insoluble particulate matter *<6.08>* It meets the requirement.

Sterility <*4.06*> Perform the test according to the Membrane filtration method: it meets the requirement.

Assay Perform the test according to the Cylinder-plate method as directed under Microbial Assay for Antibiotics <*4.02*> according to the following conditions.

(i) Test organism, culture medium and standard solutions—Proceed as directed in the Assay under Dibekacin Sulfate.

(ii) Sample solutions—Pipet a volume of Dibekacin Sulfate Ophthalmic Solution, equivalent to about 12 mg (potency), and add water to make exactly 30 mL. Pipet a suitable volume of this solution, add 0.1 mol/L phosphate buffer solution (pH 8.0) to make solutions so that each mL contains 20 μg (potency) and 5 μg (potency), and use these solutions as the high concentration sample solution and the low concentration sample solution, respectively.

Containers and storage Containers—Tight containers.

Dibucaine Hydrochloride

Cinchocaine Hydrochloride

ジブカイン塩酸塩

$C_{20}H_{29}N_3O_2.HCl$: 379.92
2-Butyloxy-*N*-(2-diethylaminoethyl)-4-quinolinecarboxamide monohydrochloride
[*61-12-1*]

Dibucaine Hydrochloride, when dried, contains not less than 98.0% of dibucaine hydrochloride ($C_{20}H_{29}N_3O_2.HCl$).

Description Dibucaine Hydrochloride occurs as white, crystals or crystalline powder.

It is very soluble in water, in ethanol (95) and in acetic acid (100), freely soluble in acetic anhydride, and practically insoluble in diethyl ether.

It is hygroscopic.

Identification **(1)** Determine the absorption spectrum of a solution of Dibucaine Hydrochloride in 1 mol/L hydrochloric acid TS (1 in 100,000) as directed under Ultraviolet-visible Spectrophotometry <*2.24*>, and compare the spectrum with the Reference Spectrum: both spectra exhibit similar intensities of absorption at the same wavelengths.

(2) Determine the infrared absorption spectrum of Dibucaine Hydrochloride, previously dried, as directed in the potassium bromide disk method under Infrared Spectrophotometry <*2.25*>, and compare the spectrum with the Reference Spectrum: both spectra exhibit similar intensities of absorption at the same wave numbers.

(3) A solution of Dibucaine Hydrochloride (1 in 10) responds to Qualitative Tests <*1.09*> for chloride.

pH <*2.54*> Dissolve 1.0 g of Dibucaine Hydrochloride in 50 mL of water: the pH of this solution is between 5.0 and 6.0.

Melting point <*2.60*> 95 – 100°C Charge Dibucaine Hydrochloride into a capillary tube for melting point determination, and dry in vacuum over phosphorus (V) oxide at 80°C for 5 hours. Seal immediately the open end of the tube, and determine the melting point.

Purity **(1)** Clarity and color of solution—Dissolve 1.0 g of Dibucaine Hydrochloride in 20 mL of water: the solution is clear and colorless. Determine the absorbance of this solution at 430 nm as directed under Ultraviolet-visible Spectrophotometry <*2.24*>, using water as the blank: it is not more than 0.03.

(2) Sulfate <*1.14*>—Perform the test with 0.30 g of Dibucaine Hydrochloride. Prepare the control solution with 0.35 mL of 0.005 mol/L sulfuric acid VS (not more than 0.056%).

(3) Heavy metals <*1.07*>—Proceed with 1.0 g of Dibucaine Hydrochloride according to Method 1, and perform the test. Prepare the control solution with 2.0 mL of Standard Lead Solution (not more than 20 ppm).

(4) Related substances—Dissolve 0.20 g of Dibucaine Hydrochloride in 5 mL of ethanol (95), and use this solution as the sample solution. Pipet 1 mL of the sample solution, add ethanol (95) to make exactly 20 mL, then pipet 2 mL of this solution, add ethanol (95) to make exactly 20 mL, and use this solution as the standard solution. Perform the test with these solutions as directed under Thin-layer Chromatography <*2.03*>. Spot 5 μL each of the sample solution and standard solution on a plate of silica gel for thin-layer chromatography. Develop the plate with a mixture of ethyl acetate, water and acetic acid (100) (3:1:1) to a distance of about 10 cm, and air-dry the plate. Examine under ultraviolet (main wavelength: 254 nm): the spots other than the principal spot obtained from the sample solution are not more intense than the spot from the standard solution.

Loss on drying <*2.41*> Not more than 2.0% (1 g, in vacuum, phosphorus (V) oxide, 80°C, 5 hours).

Residue on ignition <*2.44*> Not more than 0.1% (1 g).

Assay Weigh accurately about 0.3 g of Dibucaine Hydrochloride, previously dried, dissolve in 50 mL of a mixture of acetic anhydride and acetic acid (100) (7:3), and titrate <*2.50*> with 0.1 mol/L perchloric acid VS (potentiometric titration). Perform a blank determination in the same manner, and make any necessary correction.

Each mL of 0.1 mol/L perchloric acid VS
= 19.00 mg of $C_{20}H_{29}N_3O_2.HCl$

Containers and storage Containers—Tight containers.

Diclofenac Sodium

ジクロフェナクナトリウム

$C_{14}H_{10}Cl_2NNaO_2$: 318.13
Monosodium 2-(2,6-dichlorophenylamino)phenylacetate
[*15307-79-6*]

Diclofenac Sodium, when dried, contains not less than 98.5% of dichlofenac sodium ($C_{14}H_{10}Cl_2NNaO_2$).

Description Diclofenac Sodium occurs as white to pale yellow-white, crystals or crystalline powder.

It is freely soluble in methanol and in ethanol (95), sparingly soluble in water and in acetic acid (100), and practically insoluble in diethyl ether.

It is hygroscopic.

Identification **(1)** To 1 mL of a solution of Diclofenac Sodium in methanol (1 in 250) add 1 mL of nitric acid: a dark red color develops.

(2) Perform the test with 5 mg of Diclofenac Sodium as directed under Flame Coloration Test <*1.04*> (2): a light green color appears.

(3) Determine the infrared absorption spectrum of Diclofenac Sodium, previously dried, as directed in the potassium bromide disk method under Infrared Spectrophotometry <*2.25*>, and compare the spectrum with the Reference Spectrum: both spectra exhibit similar intensities of absorption at the same wave numbers.

(4) A solution of Diclofenac Sodium (1 in 100) responds to Qualitative Tests <*1.09*> for sodium salt.

Purity **(1)** Heavy metals <*1.07*>—Proceed with 2.0 g of Diclofenac Sodium according to Method 2, and perform the test. Prepare the control solution with 2.0 mL of Standard Lead Solution (not more than 10 ppm).

(2) Arsenic <*1.11*>—Prepare the test solution with 1.0 g of Diclofenac Sodium according to Method 3, and perform the test (not more than 2 ppm).

(3) Related substances—Dissolve 0.05 g of Diclofenac Sodium in 50 mL of the mobile phase, and use this solution as the sample solution. Pipet 2 mL of the sample solution, and add the mobile phase to make exactly 50 mL. Pipet 5 mL of this solution, add the mobile phase to make exactly 100 mL, and use this solution as the standard solution. Perform the test with exactly 20 μL each of these solutions as directed under Liquid Chromatography <*2.01*> according to the following conditions. Determine each peak area of these solutions by the automatic integration method: the area of each peak other than diclofenac obtained from the sample solution is not larger than the peak area of diclofenac from the standard solution.

Operating conditions—

Detector: An ultraviolet absorption photometer (wavelength: 240 nm).

Column: A stainless steel column 4.6 mm in inside diameter and 25 cm in length, packed with octadecylsilanized silica gel for liquid chromatography (7 μm in particle diameter).

Column temperature: A constant temperature of about 40°C.

Mobile phase: A mixture of methanol and diluted acetic acid (100) (3 in 2500) (4:3).

Flow rate: Adjust so that the retention time of diclofenac is about 20 minutes.

Time span of measurement: About twice as long as the retention time of diclofenac, beginning after the solvent peak.

System suitability—

System performance: Dissolve 35 mg of ethyl parahydroxybenzoate and 0.05 g of propyl parahydroxybenzoate in 100 mL of the mobile phase. To 1 mL of this solution add the mobile phase to make 50 mL. When the procedure is run with 20 μL of this solution under the above operating conditions, ethyl parahydroxybenzoate and propyl parahydroxybenzoate are eluted in this order with the resolution between these peaks being not less than 5.

System repeatability: When the test is repeated 6 times with 20 μL of the standard solution under the above operating conditions, the relative standard deviation of the peak areas of diclofenac is not more than 2.0%.

Loss on drying <*2.41*> Not more than 0.5% (1 g, 105°C, 3 hours).

Assay Weigh accurately about 0.5 g of Diclofenac Sodium, previously dried, dissolve in 40 mL of water in a separator, add 2 mL of dilute hydrochloric acid, and extract the precipitate formed with 50 mL of chloroform. Extract again with two 20-mL portions of chloroform, and filter the extract each time through a pledget of absorbent cotton moistened with chloroform. Wash the tip of the separator and the absorbent cotton with 15 mL of chloroform, combine the washing with the extracts, add 10 mL of a solution of 1 mol/L hydrochloric acid TS in ethanol (99.5) (1 in 100), and titrate <*2.50*> with 0.1 mol/L potassium hydroxide-ethanol VS from the first equivalent point to the second equivalent point (potentiometric titration).

Each mL of 0.1 mol/L potassium hydroxide-ethanol VS
= 31.81 mg of $C_{14}H_{10}Cl_2NNaO_2$

Containers and storage Containers—Tight containers.

Diclofenac Sodium Suppositories

ジクロフェナクナトリウム坐剤

Diclofenac Sodium Suppositories contain not less than 93.0% and not more than 107.0% of the labeled amount of diclofenac sodium ($C_{14}H_{10}Cl_2NNaO_2$: 318.13).

Method of preparation Prepare as directed under Suppositories for Rectal Application, with Diclofenac Sodium.

Identification To an amount of Diclofenac Sodium Suppositories, equivalent to 25 mg of Diclofenac Sodium, add 200 mL of a mixture of methanol and 0.01 mol/L sodium hydroxide TS (99:1), and dissolve by warming. Cool while shaking, add a mixture of methanol and 0.01 mol/L sodium hydroxide TS (99:1) to make 250 mL, and filter through a pledget of absorbent cotton if necessary. To 10 mL of this solution add a mixture of methanol and 0.01 mol/L sodium hydroxide TS (99:1) to make 100 mL. Determine the absorption spectrum of this solution as directed under Ultraviolet-visible Spectrophotometry <*2.24*>: it exhibits a maximum between 280 nm and 284 nm.

Uniformity of dosage unit <*6.02*> Perform the test according to the following method: it meets the requirement of the Content uniformity test.

To 1 suppository of Diclofenac Sodium Suppositories add 5 mL of tetrahydrofuran, and sonicate to dissolve. Add a mixture of methanol and water (3:2) to make exactly 100 mL, shake, and filter through a membrane filter with a pore size not exceeding 0.5 μm. Discard the first 5 mL of the filtrate, pipet V mL of the subsequent filtrate, add a mixture of methanol and water (3:2) to make exactly V' mL so that each mL contains about 0.125 mg of diclofenac sodium ($C_{14}H_{10}Cl_2NNaO_2$), and use this solution as the sample solution. Then, proceed as directed in the Assay.

Amount (mg) of diclofenac sodium ($C_{14}H_{10}Cl_2NNaO_2$)
$= M_S \times A_T/A_S \times V'/V \times 1/4$

M_S: Amount (mg) of diclofenac sodium for assay taken

Melting behavior of suppositories Perform the test according to Method 2 under Melting Point Determination <*2.60*>:

the melting range is between 33°C and 36°C.

Assay Weigh accurately the mass of not less than 20 Diclofenac Sodium Suppositories, cut into small pieces carefully, and mix uniformly. Weigh accurately a portion of the pieces, equivalent to about 25 mg of diclofenac sodium ($C_{14}H_{10}Cl_2NNaO_2$), add 5 mL of tetrahydrofuran, and sonicate to dissolve. Add a mixture of methanol and water (3:2) to make exactly 100 mL, shake, and filter through a membrane filter with a pore size not exceeding 0.5 μm. Discard the first 5 mL of the filtrate, pipet 10 mL of the subsequent filtrate, add a mixture of methanol and water (3:2) to make exactly 20 mL, and use this solution as the sample solution. Separately, weigh accurately about 50 mg of diclofenac sodium for assay, previously dried, and dissolve in a mixture of methanol and water (3:2) to make exactly 100 mL. Pipet 5 mL of this solution, add a mixture of methanol and water (3:2) to make exactly 20 mL, and use this solution as the standard solution. Perform the test with exactly 20 μL each of the sample solution and standard solution as directed under Liquid Chromatography <2.01> according to the following conditions, and determine the peak areas, A_T and A_S, of diclofenac in each solution.

Amount (mg) of diclofenac sodium ($C_{14}H_{10}Cl_2NNaO_2$)
$= M_S \times A_T/A_S \times 1/2$

M_S: Amount (mg) of diclofenac sodium for assay taken

Operating conditions—

Detector: An ultraviolet absorption photometer (wavelength: 254 nm).

Column: A stainless steel column 4.0 mm in inside diameter and 12.5 cm in length, packed with octadecylsilanized silica gel for liquid chromatography (5 μm in particle diameter).

Column temperature: A constant temperature of about 25°C.

Mobile phase: Dissolve 13.6 g of sodium acetate trihydrate in water to make 1000 mL. To 200 mL of this solution add 300 mL of methanol.

Flow rate: Adjust so that the retention time of diclofenac is about 3.5 minutes.

System suitability—

System performance: When the procedure is run with 20 μL of the standard solution under the above operating conditions, the number of theoretical plates and the symmetry factor of the peak of diclofenac are not less than 2000 and 0.7 to 1.5, respectively.

System repeatability: When the test is repeated 6 times with 20 μL of the standard solution under the above operating conditions, the relative standard deviation of the peak area of diclofenac is not more than 1.0%.

Containers and storage Containers—Tight containers.
Storage—In a cold place.

Dicloxacillin Sodium Hydrate

ジクロキサシリンナトリウム水和物

$C_{19}H_{16}Cl_2N_3NaO_5S.H_2O$: 510.32
Monosodium (2*S*,5*R*,6*R*)-6-{[3-(2,6-dichlorophenyl)-5-methylisoxazole-4-carbonyl]amino}-3,3-dimethyl-7-oxo-4-thia-1-azabicyclo[3.2.0]heptane-2-carboxylate monohydrate
[13412-64-1]

Dicloxacillin Sodium Hydrate contains not less than 910 μg (potency) and not more than 1020 μg (potency) per mg, calculated on the anhydrous basis. The potency of Dicloxacillin Sodium Hydrate is expressed as mass (potency) of dicroxacillin ($C_{19}H_{17}Cl_2N_3O_5S$: 470.33).

Description Dicloxacillin Sodium Hydrate occurs as a white to light yellow-white crystalline powder.

It is freely soluble in water and in methanol, and soluble in ethanol (95).

Identification **(1)** Determine the absorption spectrum of a solution of Dicloxacillin Sodium Hydrate (1 in 2500) as directed under Ultraviolet-visible Spectrophotometry <2.24>, and compare the spectrum with the Reference Spectrum or the spectrum of a solution of Dicloxacillin Sodium RS prepared in the same manner as the sample solution: both spectra exhibit similar intensities of absorption at the same wavelengths.

(2) Determine the infrared absorption spectrum of Dicloxacillin Sodium Hydrate as directed in the potassium bromide disk method under Infrared Spectrophotometry <2.25>, and compare the spectrum with the Reference Spectrum or the spectrum of Dicloxacillin Sodium RS: both spectra exhibit similar intensities of absorption at the same wave numbers.

(3) Dicloxacillin Sodium Hydrate responds to Qualitative Tests <1.09> (1) for sodium salt.

Water <2.48> Not less than 3.0% and not more than 4.5% (0.1 g, volumetric titration, direct titration).

Assay Perform the test according to the Cylinder-plate method as directed under Microbial Assay for Antibiotics <4.02> according to the following conditions.

(i) Test organism—*Bacillus subtilis* ATCC 6633

(ii) Culture medium—Use the medium i in 1) under (1) Agar media for seed and base layer. Adjust the pH of the medium so that it will be 6.5 to 6.6 after sterilization.

(iii) Standard solutions—Weigh accurately an amount of Dicloxacillin Sodium RS equivalent to about 50 mg (potency), dissolve in phosphate buffer solution (pH 6.0) to make exactly 50 mL, and use this solution as the standard stock solution. Keep the standard stock solution at 5°C or below and use within 24 hours. Take exactly a suitable amount of the standard stock solution before use, add phosphate buffer solution (pH 6.0) to make solutions so that each mL contains 10 μg (potency) and 2.5 μg (potency), and use these solutions as the high concentration standard solution and the low concentration standard solution, respectively.

(iv) Sample solutions—Weigh accurately an amount of Dicloxacillin Sodium Hydrate equivalent to about 50 mg (potency), dissolve in phosphate buffer solution (pH 6.0) to make exactly 50 mL. Take exactly a suitable amount of the solution, add phosphate buffer solution (pH 6.0) to make solutions so that each mL contains 10 μg (potency) and 2.5 μg (potency), and use these solutions as the high concentration sample solution and the low concentration sample solution, respectively.

Containers and storage Containers—Tight containers.

Diethylcarbamazine Citrate

ジエチルカルバマジンクエン酸塩

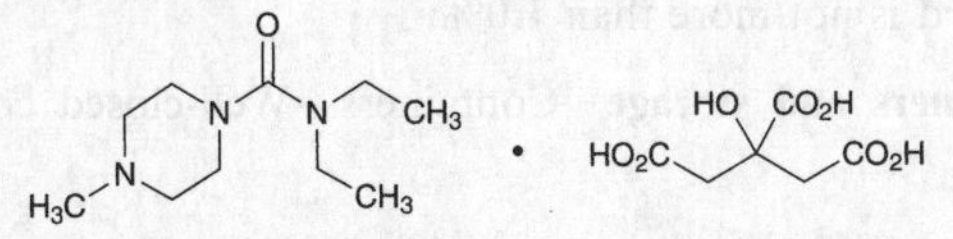

$C_{10}H_{21}N_3O.C_6H_8O_7$: 391.42
N,*N*-Diethyl-4-methylpiperazine-1-carboxamide monocitrate
[*1642-54-2*]

Diethylcarbamazine Citrate, when dried, contains not less than 98.0% of diethylcarbamazine citrate ($C_{10}H_{21}N_3O.C_6H_8O_7$).

Description Diethylcarbamazine Citrate occurs as a white, crystalline powder. It is odorless, and has an acid and bitter taste.

It is very soluble in water, soluble in ethanol (95), and practically insoluble in acetone, in chloroform and in diethyl ether.

A solution of Diethylcarbamazine Citrate (1 in 20) is acid.

Diethylcarbamazine Citrate is hygroscopic.

Identification **(1)** Dissolve 0.5 g of Diethylcarbamazine Citrate in 2 mL of water, add 10 mL of sodium hydroxide TS, and extract with four 5-mL portions of chloroform. Wash the combined chloroform extracts with 10 mL of water, and evaporate the chloroform on a water bath. Add 1 mL of iodoethane to the residue, and boil gently under a reflux condenser for 5 minutes. Evaporate the excess iodoethane with the aid of a current of air, and dissolve the residue in 4 mL of ethanol (95). Cool the ethanol solution in an ice bath, with continuous stirring, add diethyl ether until precipitates are formed, and stir until crystallization is evident. Allow to stand in the ice bath for 30 minutes, and collect the precipitate. Dissolve the precipitate in 4 mL of ethanol (95), repeat the recrystallization in the same manner, then dry at 105°C for 4 hours: the crystals so obtained melt <*2.60*> between 151°C and 155°C.

(2) Neutralize the remaining aqueous layer obtained in (1) with dilute sulfuric acid: the solution responds to Qualitative Tests <*1.09*> (2) and (3) for citrate.

Melting point <*2.60*> 135.5 – 138.5°C

Purity Heavy metals <*1.07*>—Proceed with 2.0 g of Diethylcarbamazine Citrate according to Method 4, and perform the test. Prepare the control solution with 4.0 mL of Standard Lead Solution (not more than 20 ppm).

Loss on drying <*2.41*> Not more than 1.0% (2 g, 105°C, 4 hours).

Residue on ignition <*2.44*> Not more than 0.1% (1 g).

Assay Weigh accurately about 0.75 g of Diethylcarbamazine Citrate, previously dried, dissolve in 50 mL of acetic acid (100) by warming, cool, and titrate <*2.50*> with 0.1 mol/L perchloric acid VS (potentiometric titration). Perform a blank determination in the same manner, and make any necessary correction.

Each mL of 0.1 mol/L perchloric acid VS
= 39.14 mg of $C_{10}H_{21}N_3O.C_6H_8O_7$

Containers and storage Containers—Tight containers.

Diethylcarbamazine Citrate Tablets

ジエチルカルバマジンクエン酸塩錠

Diethylcarbamazine Citrate Tablets contain not less than 95.0% and not more than 105.0% of the labeled amount of diethylcarbamazine citrate ($C_{10}H_{21}N_3O \cdot C_6H_8O_7$: 391.42).

Method of preparation Prepare as directed under Tablets, with Diethylcarbamazine Citrate.

Identification To a quantity of the powdered Diethylcarbamazine Citrate Tablets, equivalent to 0.1 g of Diethylcarbamazine Citrate, add 10 mL of water, shake well, and filter. To the filtrate add 1 mL of Reinecke salt TS: a light red precipitate is formed.

Uniformity of dosage units <*6.02*> Perform the Mass variation test, or the Content uniformity test according to the following method: it meets the requirement.

To 1 tablet of Diethylcarbamazine Citrate Tablets add 70 mL of the mobile phase, shake vigorously for 10 minutes, add the mobile phase to make exactly 100 mL, and filter through a membrane filter with a pore size not exceeding 0.45 μm. Discard the first 3 mL of the filtrate, pipet *V* mL of the subsequent filtrate, equivalent to about 2.5 mg of diethylcarbamazine citrate ($C_{10}H_{21}N_3O.C_6H_8O_7$), add exactly 5 mL of the internal standard solution, add the mobile phase to make 50 mL, and use this solution as the sample solution. Proceed as directed in the Assay.

Amount (mg) of diethylcarbamazine citrate
($C_{10}H_{21}N_3O.C_6H_8O_7$)
$= M_S \times Q_T/Q_S \times 10/V$

M_S: Amount (mg) of Diethylcarbamazine Citrate RS taken

Internal standard solution—A solution of 2-aminobenzimidazol in the mobile phase (1 in 12,500).

Dissolution <*6.10*> When the test is performed at 50 revolutions per minute according to the Paddle method, using 900 mL of water as the dissolution medium, the dissolution rate in 45 minutes of Diethylcarbamazine Citrate Tablets is not less than 80%.

Start the test with 1 tablet of Diethylcarbamazine Citrate Tablets, withdraw not less than 20 mL of the medium at the specified minute after starting the test, and filter through a membrane filter with a pore size not exceeding 0.45 μm. Discard not less than 10 mL of the first filtrate, pipet *V* mL of the subsequent filtrate, add water to make exactly *V′* mL so that each mL contains about 56 μg of diethylcarbamazine citrate ($C_{10}H_{21}N_3O.C_6H_8O_7$), and use this solution as the sample solution. Separately, weigh accurately about 22 mg of Diethylcarbamazine Citrate RS, previously dried at 105°C for 4 hours, and dissolve in water to make exactly 100 mL.

Pipet 25 mL of this solution, add water to make exactly 100 mL, and use this solution as the standard solution. Perform the test with exactly 20 μL each of the sample solution and standard solution as directed under Liquid Chromatography <*2.01*> according to the following conditions, and determine the peak areas, A_T and A_S, of diethylcarbamazine in each solution.

Dissolution rate (%) with respect to the labeled amount of diethylcarbamazine citrate ($C_{10}H_{21}N_3O.C_6H_8O_7$)
$= M_S \times A_T/A_S \times V'/V \times 1/C \times 225$

M_S: Amount (mg) of Diethylcarbamazine Citrate RS taken
C: Labeled amount (mg) of diethylcarbamazine citrate ($C_{10}H_{21}N_3O.C_6H_8O_7$) in 1 tablet

Operating conditions—

Detector, column, column temperature, mobile phase, and flow rate: Proceed as directed in the operating conditions in the Assay.

System suitability—

System performance: When the procedure is run with 20 μL of the standard solution under the above operating conditions, the number of theoretical plates and the symmetry factor of the peak of diethylcarbamazine are not less than 5000 and not more than 1.5, respectively.

System repeatability: When the test is repeated 6 times with 20 μL of the standard solution under the above operating conditions, the relative standard deviation of the peak area of diethylcarbamazine is not more than 2.0%.

Assay Weigh accurately the mass of not less than 20 Diethylcarbamazine Citrate Tablets, and powder. Weigh accurately a portion of the powder, equivalent to about 50 mg of diethylcarbamazine citrate ($C_{10}H_{21}N_3O.C_6H_8O_7$), add 70 mL of the mobile phase, shake vigorously for 10 minutes, add the mobile phase to make exactly 100 mL, and filter through a membrane filter with a pore size not exceeding 0.45 μm. Discard the first 3 mL of the filtrate, pipet 5 mL of the subsequent filtrate, add exactly 5 mL of the internal standard solution, add the mobile phase to make 50 mL, and use this solution as the sample solution. Separately, weigh accurately about 25 mg of Diethylcarbamazine Citrate RS, previously dried at 105°C for 4 hours, dissolve in the mobile phase to make exactly 50 mL. Pipet 5 mL of this solution, add exactly 5 mL of the internal standard solution, add the mobile phase to make 50 mL, and use this solution as the standard solution. Perform the test with 20 μL each of the sample solution and standard solution as directed under Liquid Chromatography <*2.01*> according to the following conditions, and calculate the ratios, Q_T and Q_S, of the peak area of diethylcarbamazine to that of the internal standard.

Amount (mg) of diethylcarbamazine citrate ($C_{10}H_{21}N_3O.C_6H_8O_7$)
$= M_S \times Q_T/Q_S \times 2$

M_S: Amount (mg) of Diethylcarbamazine Citrate RS taken

*Internal standard solution—*A solution of 2-aminobenzimidazole in the mobile phase (1 in 12,500).

Operating conditions—

Detector: An ultraviolet absorption photometer (wavelength: 220 nm).

Column: A stainless steel column 4.6 mm in inside diameter and 15 cm in length, packed with octadecylsilanized silica gel for liquid chromatography (5 μm in particle diameter).

Column temperature: A constant temperature of about 40°C.

Mobile phase: To 0.05 mol/L potassium dihydrogen phosphate TS add phosphoric acid to adjust the pH to 2.5. To 950 mL of this solution add 50 mL of methanol.

Flow rate: Adjust so that the retention time of diethylcarbamazine is about 14 minutes.

System suitability—

System performance: When the procedure is run with 20 μL of the standard solution under the above operating conditions, diethylcarbamazine and the internal standard are eluted in this order with the resolution between these peaks being not less than 2.5.

System repeatability: When the test is repeated 6 times with 20 μL of the standard solution under the above operating conditions, the relative standard deviation of the ratio of the peak area of diethylcarbamazine to that of the internal standard is not more than 1.0%.

Containers and storage Containers—Well-closed containers.

Difenidol Hydrochloride

ジフェニドール塩酸塩

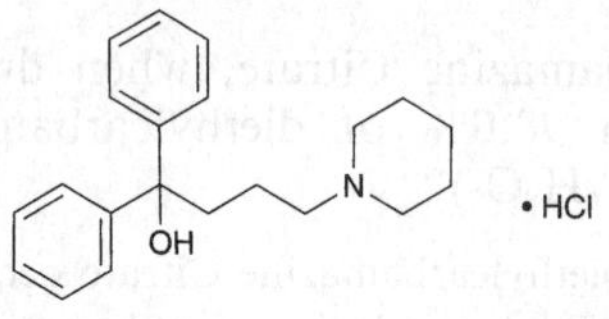

$C_{21}H_{27}NO.HCl$: 345.91
1,1-Diphenyl-4-piperidin-1-ylbutan-1-ol monohydrochloride
[*3254-89-5*]

Difenidol Hydrochloride, when dried, contains not less than 98.5% of difenidol hydrochloride ($C_{21}H_{27}NO.HCl$).

Description Difenidol Hydrochloride occurs as white, crystals or crystalline powder. It is odorless.

It is freely soluble in methanol, soluble in ethanol (95), sparingly soluble in water and in acetic acid (100), and practically insoluble in diethyl ether.

Melting point: about 217°C (with decomposition).

Identification **(1)** Dissolve 0.01 g of Difenidol Hydrochloride in 1 mL of sulfuric acid: an orange-red color develops. To this solution add carefully 3 drops of water: the solution becomes yellowish brown, and colorless on the addition of 10 mL of water.

(2) To 5 mL of a solution of Difenidol Hydrochloride (1 in 100) add 2 mL of Reinecke salt TS: a light red precipitate is formed.

(3) To 10 mL of a solution of Difenidol Hydrochloride (1 in 100) add 2 mL of sodium hydroxide TS, and extract with two 15-mL portions of chloroform. Combine the extracts, wash with three 10-mL portions of water, evaporate the chloroform on a water bath, and dry the residue in a desiccator (in vacuum, silica gel, 55°C) for 5 hours: the residue melts <*2.60*> between 103°C and 106°C.

(4) A solution of Difenidol Hydrochloride (1 in 100) responds to Qualitative Tests <*1.09*> for chloride.

pH <*2.54*> Dissolve 1.0 g of Difenidol Hydrochloride in 100 mL of freshly boiled and cooled water: the pH of this solution is between 4.7 and 6.5.

Purity (1) Clarity and color of solution—Dissolve 1.0 g of Difenidol Hydrochloride in 10 mL of methanol: the solution is clear and colorless.

(2) Heavy metals <*1.07*>—Proceed with 1.0 g of Difenidol Hydrochloride according to Method 2, and perform the test. Prepare the control solution with 2.0 mL of Standard Lead Solution (not more than 20 ppm).

(3) Arsenic <*1.11*>—Prepare the test solution with 2.0 g of Difenidol Hydrochloride according to Method 3, and perform the test (not more than 1 ppm).

(4) Related substances—Dissolve 0.10 g of Difenidol Hydrochloride in methanol to make exactly 10 mL, and use this solution as the sample solution. Separately, dissolve 10 mg of 1,1-diphenyl-4-piperidino-1-butene hydrochloride for thin-layer chromatography in methanol to make exactly 20 mL, pipet 1 mL of this solution, add methanol to make exactly 10 mL, and use this solution as the standard solution. Perform the test with these solutions as directed under Thin-layer Chromatography <*2.03*>. Spot 5 μL each of the sample solution and standard solution on a plate of silica gel with fluorescent indicator for thin-layer chromatography. Develop the plate with a mixture of toluene, methanol and acetic acid (100) (10:2:1) to a distance of about 15 cm, and air-dry the plate. Examine under ultraviolet light (main wavelength: 254 nm): the spots other than the principal spot obtained from the sample solution are not more intense than the spot from the standard solution.

Loss on drying <*2.41*> Not more than 0.5% (1 g, in vacuum, silica gel, 5 hours).

Residue on ignition <*2.44*> Not more than 0.1% (1 g).

Assay Weigh accurately about 0.35 g of Difenidol Hydrochloride, previously dried, dissolve in 30 mL of acetic acid (100) by warming if necessary, cool, add 30 mL of acetic anhydride, and titrate <*2.50*> with 0.05 mol/L perchloric acid VS (potentiometric titration). Perform a blank determination in the same manner, and make any necessary correction.

Each mL of 0.05 mol/L perchloric acid VS
= 17.30 mg of $C_{21}H_{27}NO.HCl$

Containers and storage Containers—Well-closed containers.

Diflorasone Diacetate

ジフロラゾン酢酸エステル

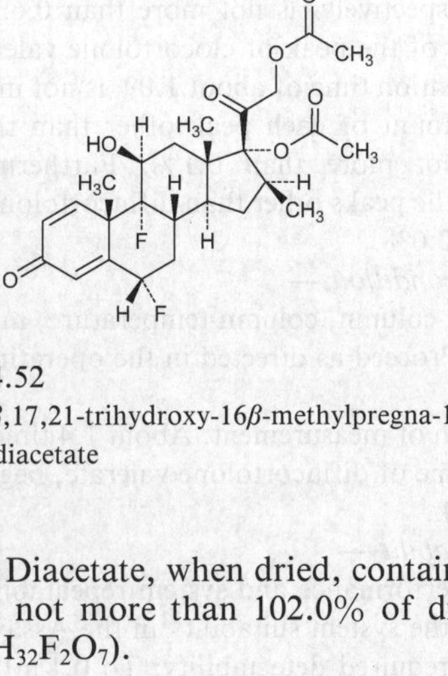

$C_{26}H_{32}F_2O_7$: 494.52
6α,9-Difluoro-11β,17,21-trihydroxy-16β-methylpregna-1,4-diene-3,20-dione 17,21-diacetate
[*33564-31-7*]

Diflorasone Diacetate, when dried, contains not less than 97.0 and not more than 102.0% of diflorasone diacetate ($C_{26}H_{32}F_2O_7$).

Description Diflorasone Diacetate occurs as a white to pale yellow, crystals or crystalline powder.

It is soluble in acetonitrile, slightly soluble in ethanol (99.5), and practically insoluble in water.

Melting point: about 222°C (with decomposition).

Identification (1) Determine the infrared absorption spectrum of Diflorasone Diacetate, previously dried, as directed in the potassium bromide disk method under Infrared Spectrophotometry <*2.25*>, and compare the spectrum with the Reference Spectrum or the spectrum of previously dried Diflorasone Diacetate RS: both spectra exhibit similar intensities of absorption at the same wave numbers.

(2) Prepare the test solution with 10 mg of Diflorasone Diacetate as directed under Oxygen Flask Combustion Method <*1.06*>, using 20 mL of diluted 0.01 mol/L sodium hydroxide VS (1 in 40) as the absorbing liquid: the test solution responds to Qualitative Tests <*1.09*> for fluoride.

Optical rotation <*2.49*> $[\alpha]_D^{20}$: + 88 – + 93° (after drying, 0.1 g, acetonitrile, 10 mL, 100 mm).

Purity (1) Heavy metals <*1.07*>—Proceed with 1.0 g of Diflorasone Diacetate according to Method 2, and perform the test. Prepare the control solution with 1.0 mL of Standard Lead Solution (not more than 10 ppm).

(2) Related substances—Dissolve 20 mg of Diflorasone Diacetate in 20 mL of acetonitrile, and use this solution as the sample solution. Pipet 1 mL of the sample solution, add acetonitrile to make exactly 100 mL, and use this solution as the standard solution. Perform the test with exactly 10 μL each of the sample solution and standard solution as directed under Liquid Chromatography <*2.01*> according to the following conditions. Determine each peak area by the automatic integration method: the areas of the peaks, having a relative retention time of about 0.5, about 0.7, about 0.9 and about 1.1 to diflorasone diacetate, obtained from the sample solution are respectively not larger than 1/4 times, 1/4 times, 1/2 times and 3/4 times the peak area of diflorasone diacetate from the standard solution, and the total area of the peaks other than diflorasone diacetate and the peaks mentioned above from the sample solutions is not larger than 1/5 times the peak area of diflorasone diacetate from the standard solution. Furthermore, the total area of the peaks other than diflorasone diacetate from the sample solution is not larger than 1.5 times the peak area of diflorasone diacetate from the standard solution.

Operating conditions—

Detector, column, column temperature, mobile phase, and flow rate: Proceed as directed in the operating conditions in the Assay.

Time span of measurement: About 1.4 times as long as the retention time of diflorasone diacetate, beginning after the solvent peak.

System suitability—

System performance: Proceed as directed in the system suitability in the Assay.

Test for required detectability: Pipet 2 mL of the standard solution, and add acetonitrile to make exactly 20 mL. Confirm that the peak area of diflorasone diacetate obtained with 10 μL of this solution is equivalent to 7 to 13% of that with 10 μL of the standard solution.

System repeatability: When the test is repeated 6 times with 10 μL of the standard solution, the relative standard deviation of the peak area of diflorasone diacetate is not more than 2.0%.

Loss on drying <*2.41*> Not more than 1.0% (0.2 g, in vacuum, phosphorus (V) oxide, 60°C, 4 hours).

Residue on ignition <*2.44*> Not more than 0.2% (0.5 g, platinum crucible).

Assay Weigh accurately about 20 mg each of Diflorasone Diacetate and Diflorasone Diacetate RS, both previously dried, dissolve in exactly 4 mL each of the internal standard solution, add acetonitrile to make them 20 mL, and use these solutions as the sample solution and the standard solution, respectively. Perform the test with 10 μL each of the sample solution and standard solution as directed under Liquid Chromatography <*2.01*> according to the following conditions, and calculate the ratios, Q_T and Q_S, of the peak area of diflorasone diacetate to that of the internal standard.

Amount (mg) of diflorasone diacetate ($C_{26}H_{23}F_2O_7$)
$$= M_S \times Q_T/Q_S$$

M_S: Amount (mg) of Diflorasone Diacetate RS taken

Internal standard solution—A solution of methyl parahydroxybenzoate in acetonitrile (1 in 1000).
Operating conditions—

Detector: An ultraviolet absorption photometer (wavelength: 254 nm).

Column: A stainless steel column 6 mm in inside diameter and 15 cm in length, packed with octadecylsilanized silica gel for liquid chromatography (5 μm in particle diameter).

Column temperature: A constant temperature of about 25°C.

Mobile phase: Dissolve 6.8 g of potassium dihydrogen phosphate in 1000 mL of water, and adjust to pH 4.0 with diluted phosphoric acid (1 in 200). To 550 mL of this solution add 400 mL of acetonitrile and 100 mL of tetrahydrofuran.

Flow rate: Adjust so that the retention time of diflorasone diacetate is about 15 minutes.
System suitability—

System performance: When the procedure is run with 10 μL of the standard solution under the above operating conditions, the internal standard and diflorasone diacetate are eluted in this order with the resolution between these peaks being not less than 9.

System repeatability: When the test is repeated 6 times with 10 μL of the standard solution under the above operating conditions, the relative standard deviation of the ratio of the peak area of diflorasone diacetate to that of the internal standard is not more than 1.0%.

Containers and storage Containers—Tight containers.

Diflucortolone Valerate

ジフルコルトロン吉草酸エステル

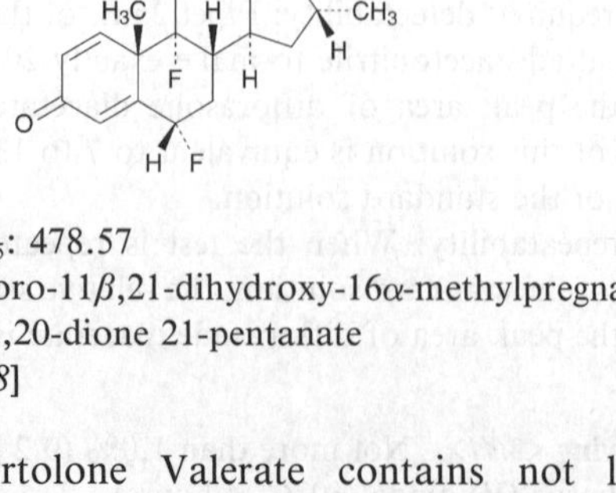

$C_{27}H_{36}F_2O_5$: 478.57
6α,9-Difluoro-11β,21-dihydroxy-16α-methylpregna-1,4-diene-3,20-dione 21-pentanate
[59198-70-8]

Diflucortolone Valerate contains not less than 98.0% and not more than 102.0% of diflucortolone valerate ($C_{27}H_{36}F_2O_5$), calculated on the dried basis.

Description Diflucortolone Valerate occurs as white, crystals or crystalline powder.

It is sparingly soluble in methanol and in ethanol (99.5), and practically insoluble in water.

Identification **(1)** Prepare the test solution by proceeding with 10 mg of Diflucortolone Valerate according to Oxygen Flask Combustion Method <*1.06*>, using a mixture of 0.5 mL of 0.01 mol/L sodium hydroxide TS and 20 mL of water as the absorbing liquid: the test solution responds to Qualitative Tests <*1.09*> for fluoride.

(2) Determine the absorption spectrum of a solution of Diflucortolone Valerate in methanol (3 in 200,000) as directed under Ultraviolet-visible Spectrophotometry <*2.24*>, and compare the spectrum with the Reference Spectrum or the spectrum of a solution of Diflucortolone Valerate RS prepared in the same manner as the sample solution: both spectra exhibit similar intensities of absorption at the same wavelengths.

(3) Determine the infrared absorption spectrum of Diflucortolone Valerate as directed in the potassium bromide disk method under Infrared Spectrophotometry <*2.25*>, and compare the spectrum with the Reference Spectrum or the spectrum of Diflucortolone Valerate RS: both spectra exhibit similar intensities of absorption at the same wave numbers.

Optical rotation <*2.49*> $[\alpha]_D^{20}$: +110 – +115° (0.1 g calculated on the dried basis, ethanol (99.5), 10 mL, 100 mm).

Melting point <*2.60*> 200 – 204°C

Purity **(1)** Heavy metals <*1.07*>—Proceed with 2.0 g of Diflucortolone Valerate in a platinum crucible according to Method 2, and perform the test. Prepare the control solution with 2.0 mL of Standard Lead Solution (not more than 10 ppm). Carbonize and incinerate as directed under Residue on Ignition <*2.44*>.

(2) Related substances—Use the sample solution obtained in the Assay as the sample solution. Perform the test with 10 μL of the sample solution as directed under Liquid Chromatography <*2.01*> according to the following conditions. Determine each peak area of sample solution by the automatic integration method, and calculate the amounts of these peaks by the area percentage method: the amount of each peak of flucortolone valerate, 12α diflucortolone valerate and Δ4 diflucortolone valerate, having the relative retention times of about 0.97, 1.03 and 1.05 to diflucortolone valerate, respectively, is not more than 0.6%, respectively; the amount of the peak of clocortolone valerate, having the relative retention time of about 1.09, is not more than 0.3%; and the amount of each peak other than those mentioned above is not more than 0.1%. Furthermore, the total amount of the peaks other than diflucortolone valerate is not more than 2.0%.
Operating conditions—

Detector, column, column temperature, mobile phase and flow rate: Proceed as directed in the operating conditions in the Assay.

Time span of measurement: About 1.4 times as long as the retention time of diflucortolone valerate, beginning after the solvent peak.
System suitability—

System performance and system repeatability: Proceed as directed in the system suitability in the Assay.

Test for required detectability: To 0.1 mL of the sample

solution, add a mixture of water and acetonitrile (1:1) to make 10 mL, and use this solution as the solution for system suitability test. Pipet 1 mL of the solution for system suitability test, and add a mixture of water and acetonitrile (1:1) to make exactly 20 mL. Confirm that the peak area of diflucortolone valerate obtained with 10 μL of this solution is equivalent to 3.5 to 6.5% of that with 10 μL of the solution for system suitability test.

Loss on drying ⟨*2.41*⟩ Not more than 0.5% (1 g, 105°C, 3 hours).

Residue on ignition ⟨*2.44*⟩ Not more than 0.1% (1 g, platinum crucible).

Assay Weigh accurately about 5 mg each of Diflucortolone Valerate and Diflucortolone Valerate RS (separately, determine the loss on drying ⟨*2.41*⟩ under the same conditions as Diflucortolone Valerate), dissolve each in a mixture of water and acetonitrile (1:1) to make exactly 10 mL, and use these solutions as the sample solution and the standard solution, respectively. Perform the test with exactly 10 μL each of the sample solution and standard solution as directed under Liquid Chromatography ⟨*2.01*⟩ according to the following conditions, and determine the peak areas, A_T and A_S, of diflucortolone valerate in each solution.

Amount (mg) of diflucortolone valerate ($C_{27}H_{36}F_2O_5$)
$= M_S \times A_T/A_S$

M_S: Amount (mg) of Diflucortolone Valerate RS taken, calculated on dried basis

Operating conditions—

Detector: An ultraviolet absorption photometer (wavelength: 238 nm).

Column: A stainless steel column 4.6 mm in inside diameter and 25 cm in length, packed with sulfonamide group bound to hexadecylsilanized silica gel for liquid chromatography (5 μm in particle diameter).

Column temperature: A constant temperature of about 25°C.

Mobile phase A: A mixture of 0.02 mol/L potassium dihydrogen phosphate TS, adjusted to pH 3.0 with phosphoric acid, and acetonitrile for liquid chromatography (11:9).

Mobile phase B: Acetonitrile for liquid chromatography.

Flowing of mobile phase: Control the gradient by mixing the mobile phases A and B as directed in the following table.

Time after injection of sample (min)	Mobile phase A (vol%)	Mobile phase B (vol%)
0 - 10	100 → 90	0 → 10
10 - 25	90	10
25 - 45	90 → 35	10 → 65
45 - 50	35	65

Flow rate: 1.0 mL per minute.

System suitability—

System performance: When the procedure is run with 10 μL of the standard solution under the above operating conditions, the number of theoretical plates and the symmetry factor of the peak of diflucortolone valerate are not less than 10,000 and not more than 1.5, respectively.

System repeatability: When the test is repeated 6 times with 10 μL of the standard solution under the above operating conditions, the relative standard deviation of the peak area of diflucortolone valerate is not more than 1.0%.

Containers and storage Containers—Tight containers.

Digoxin

ジゴキシン

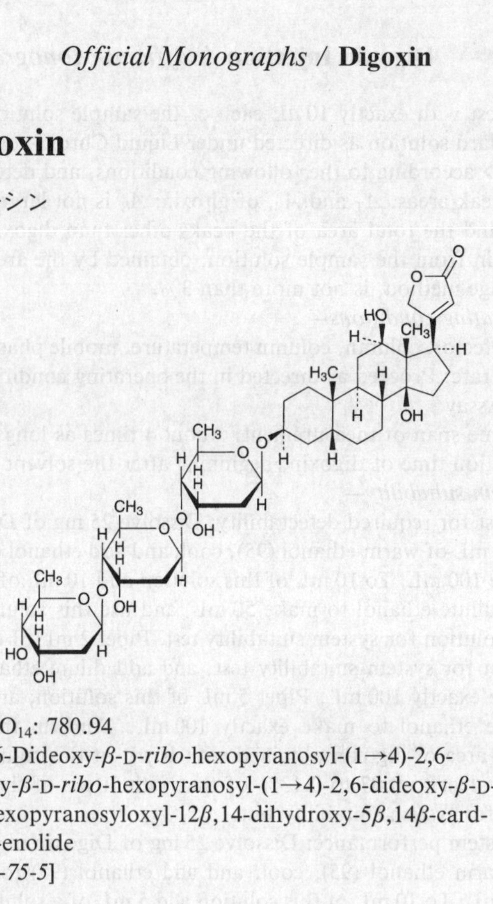

$C_{41}H_{64}O_{14}$: 780.94

3β-[2,6-Dideoxy-β-D-*ribo*-hexopyranosyl-(1→4)-2,6-dideoxy-β-D-*ribo*-hexopyranosyl-(1→4)-2,6-dideoxy-β-D-*ribo*-hexopyranosyloxy]-12β,14-dihydroxy-5β,14β-card-20(22)-enolide

[*20830-75-5*]

Digoxin, when dried, contains not less than 96.0% and not more than 106.0% of digoxin ($C_{41}H_{64}O_{14}$).

Description Digoxin occurs as colorless or white crystals or a white crystalline powder.

It is freely soluble in pyridine, slightly soluble in ethanol (95), very slightly soluble in acetic acid (100), and practically insoluble in water.

Identification **(1)** Transfer 1 mg of Digoxin to a small test tube about 10 mm in inside diameter, dissolve in 1 mL of a solution of iron (III) chloride hexahydrate in acetic acid (100) (1 in 10,000), and underlay gently with 1 mL of sulfuric acid: at the zone of contact of the two liquids a brown ring free from a reddish color is produced, and the color of the upper layer near the contact zone changes to green through purple. Finally the entire acetic acid layer shows a green color through a deep blue color.

(2) Determine the infrared absorption spectrum of Digoxin, previously dried, as directed in the potassium bromide disk method under Infrared Spectrophotometry ⟨*2.25*⟩, and compare the spectrum with the Reference Spectrum: both spectra exhibit similar intensities of absorption at the same wave numbers.

Optical rotation ⟨*2.49*⟩ $[\alpha]_D^{20}$: +10.0 – +13.0° (after drying, 0.20 g, dehydratead pyridine, 10 mL, 100 mm).

Purity **(1)** Clarity and color of solution—Dissolve 0.10 g of Digoxin in 15 mL of diluted ethanol (95) (4 in 5) by warming at 70°C: the solution is clear and colorless.

(2) Related substances—Dissolve 25.0 mg of Digoxin in 50 mL of warm ethanol (95), cool, and add ethanol (95) to make exactly 100 mL. Pipet 10 mL of this solution, add 10 mL of water and dilute ethanol to make exactly 50 mL, and use this solution as the sample solution. Separately, dissolve exactly 5.0 mg of Gitoxin for Purity RS, previously dried under reduced pressure at 105°C for 1 hour, in a mixture of acetonitrile and water (7:3) to make exactly 200 mL. Pipet 2 mL of this solution, add dilute ethanol to make exactly 50 mL, and use this solution as the standard solution. Perform the test with exactly 10 μL each of the sample solution and standard solution as directed under Liquid Chromatography <*2.01*> according to the following conditions, and determine the peak areas, A_T and A_S, of gitoxin: A_T is not larger than A_S, and the total area of the peaks other than digoxin and gitoxin from the sample solution, obtained by the area percentage method, is not more than 3%.

Operating conditions—

Detector, column, column temperature, mobile phase, and flow rate: Proceed as directed in the operating conditions in the Assay.

Time span of measurement: About 4 times as long as the retention time of digoxin, beginning after the solvent peak.

System suitability—

Test for required detectability: Dissolve 25 mg of Digoxin in 50 mL of warm ethanol (95), cool, and add ethanol (95) to make 100 mL. To 10 mL of this solution add 10 mL of water and dilute ethanol to make 50 mL, and use this solution as the solution for system suitability test. Pipet 2 mL of the solution for system suitability test, and add dilute ethanol to make exactly 100 mL. Pipet 5 mL of this solution, and add dilute ethanol to make exactly 100 mL. Confirm that the peak area of digoxin obtained with 10 μL of this solution is equivalent to 0.07 to 0.13% of that with 10 μL of the solution for system suitability test.

System performance: Dissolve 25 mg of Digoxin in 50 mL of warm ethanol (95), cool, and add ethanol (95) to make 100 mL. To 10 mL of this solution add 5 mL of a solution of propyl parahydroxybenzoate in ethanol (95) (1 in 4000), 10 mL of water and dilute ethanol to make 50 mL. When the procedure is run with 10 μL of this solution under the above operating conditions, digoxin and propyl parahydroxybenzoate are eluted in this order with the resolution between these peaks being not less than 5.

System repeatability: When the test is repeated 6 times with 10 μL of the solution for system suitability test under the above operating conditions, the relative standard deviation of the peak area of digoxin is not more than 2.5%.

Loss on drying <*2.41*> Not more than 1.0% (0.5 g, in vacuum, 105°C, 1 hour).

Residue on ignition <*2.44*> Not more than 0.5% (0.1 g).

Assay Weigh accurately about 25 mg each of Digoxin and Digoxin RS, previously dried, dissolve in 50 mL of warm ethanol (95), cool, and add ethanol (95) to make exactly 100 mL. Pipet 10 mL of these solutions, add exactly 5 mL of the internal standard solution, 10 mL of water and dilute ethanol to make 50 mL, and use these solutions as the sample solution and standard solution. Perform the test with 10 μL each of the sample solution and standard solution as directed under Liquid Chromatography <*2.01*> according to the following conditions, and calculate the ratios, Q_T and Q_S, of the peak area of digoxin to that of the internal standard.

$$\text{Amount (mg) of digoxin } (C_{41}H_{64}O_{14}) = M_S \times Q_T/Q_S$$

M_S: Amount (mg) of Digoxin RS taken

*Internal standard solution—*A solution of propyl parahydroxybenzoate in ethanol (95) (1 in 4000).

Operating conditions—

Detector: An ultraviolet absorption photometer (wavelength: 220 nm).

Column: A stainless steel column 4.6 mm in inside diameter and 25 cm in length, packed with octadecylsilanized silica gel for liquid chromatography (5 μm in particle diameter).

Column temperature: A constant temperature of about 30°C.

Mobile phase: A mixture of water and acetonitrile (7:3).

Flow rate: Adjust so that the retention time of digoxin is about 10 minutes.

System suitability—

System performance: When the procedure is run with 10 μL of the standard solution under the above operating conditions, digoxin and the internal standard are eluted in this order with the resolution between these peaks being not less than 5.

System repeatability: When the test is repeated 6 times with 10 μL of the standard solution under the above operating conditions, the relative standard deviation of the ratio of the peak area of digoxin to that of the internal standard is not more than 1.0%.

Containers and storage Containers—Tight containers.

Storage—Light-resistant.

Digoxin Injection

ジゴキシン注射液

Digoxin Injection is an aqueous injection.

It contains not less than 90.0% and not more than 105.0% of the labeled amount of digoxin ($C_{41}H_{64}O_{14}$: 780.94).

Method of preparation Prepare as directed under Injections, with a solution of Digoxin in 10 to 50 vol% ethanol.

Description Digoxin Injection is a clear, colorless liquid.

Identification Dilute Digoxin Injection, if necessary, with methanol so that each mL contains about 0.25 mg of Digoxin, and use this solution as the sample solution. In case where ingredients are suspected to affect the test, remove them by means of a solid-phase extraction. Separately, dissolve 0.5 mg of Digoxin RS in 2 mL of methanol, and use this solution as the standard solution. Perform the test with these solutions as directed under Thin-layer Chromatography <*2.03*>. Spot 10 μL each of the sample solution and standard solution on a plate of octadecylsilanized silica gel for thin-layer chromatography. Develop the plate with a mixture of methanol and water (7:3) to a distance of about 10 cm, and air-dry the plate. Spray evenly a mixture of a solution of trichloroacetic acid in ethanol (99.5) (1 in 4) and a freshly prepared solution of sodium toluenesulfonchloramide trihydrate (3 in 100) (4:1) on the plate, heat at 110°C for 10 minutes, and examine under ultraviolet light (main wavelength: 366 nm): the *R*f values of the principal spots with the sample solution and the standard solution are not different each other.

Alcohol number <*1.01*> 0.8 – 1.2 (Method 1).

Purity Related substances—To a volume of Digoxin Injection, equivalent to about 2.5 mg of Digoxin, add dilute ethanol to make 50 mL, and use this solution as the sample solution. Perform the test with 10 μL of the sample solution as directed under Liquid Chromatography <*2.01*> according to the following conditions. Determine each peak area of the sample solution by the automatic integration method and calculate the amounts of these peaks by the area percentage method: the total amount of the peaks other than digoxin is not more than 5%.

Operating conditions—

Detector, column, column temperature, mobile phase and

flow rate: Proceed as directed in the operating conditions in the Assay.

Time span of measurement: About 4 times as long as the retention time of digoxin, beginning after the solvent peak.

System suitability—

Test for required detectability: Dissolve 25 mg of digoxin in 50 mL of warm ethanol (95), cool, add ethanol (95) to make 100 mL. To 10 mL of this solution add 10 mL of water and dilute ethanol to make 50 mL, and use this solution as the solution for system suitability test. Pipet 2 mL of the solution for system suitability test, and add dilute ethanol to make exactly 100 mL. Pipet 5 mL of this solution, and add dilute ethanol to make exactly 100 mL. Confirm that the peak area of digoxin obtained with 10 μL this solution is equivalent to 0.07 to 0.13% of that with 10 μL of the solution for system suitability test.

System performance: Dissolve 25 mg of digoxin in 50 mL of warm ethanol (95), cool, and add ethanol (95) to make 100 mL. To 10 mL of this solution add 5 mL of a solution of propyl parahydroxybenzoate in ethanol (95) (1 in 4000), 10 mL of water and dilute ethanol to make 50 mL. When the procedure is run with 10 μL of this solution under the above operating conditions, digoxin and propyl parahydroxybenzoate are eluted in this order with the resolution between these peaks being not less than 5.

System repeatability: When the test is repeated 6 times with 10 μL of the solution for system suitability test under the above operating conditions, the relative standard deviation of the peak area of digoxin is not more than 2.5%.

Bacterial endotoxins *<4.01>* Less than 200 EU/mg.

Extractable volume *<6.05>* It meets the requirements.

Foreign insoluble matter *<6.06>* Perform the test according to Method 1: it meets the requirement.

Insoluble particulate matter *<6.07>* Perform the test according to Method 1: it meets the requirement.

Sterility *<4.06>* Perform the test according to the Membrane filtration method: it meets the requirement.

Assay To an exact volume of Digoxin Injection, equivalent to about 2.5 mg of digoxin ($C_{41}H_{64}O_{14}$), add exactly 5 mL of the internal standard solution and dilute ethanol to make 50 mL, and use this solution as the sample solution. Separately, weigh accurately about 25 mg of Digoxin RS, previously dried under reduced pressure at 105°C for 1 hour, dissolve in 50 mL of warm ethanol (95), cool, and add ethanol (95) to make exactly 100 mL. Pipet 10 mL of this solution, add exactly 5 mL of the internal standard solution, 10 mL of water and dilute ethanol to make 50 mL, and use this solution as the standard solution. Perform the test with 10 μL each of the sample solution and standard solution as directed under Liquid Chromatography *<2.01>* according to the following conditions, and calculate the ratios, Q_T and Q_S, of the peak area of digoxin to that of the internal standard.

$$\text{Amount (mg) of digoxin } (C_{41}H_{64}O_{14}) = M_S \times Q_T/Q_S \times 1/10$$

M_S: Amount (mg) of Digoxin RS taken

Internal standard solution—A solution of propyl parahydroxybenzoate in ethanol (95) (1 in 4000).

Operating conditions—

Detector: An ultraviolet absorption photometer (wavelength: 220 nm).

Column: A stainless steel column 4.6 mm in inside diameter and 25 cm in length, packed with octadecylsilanized silica gel for liquid chromatography (5 μm in particle diameter).

Column temperature: A constant temperature of about 30°C.

Mobile phase: A mixture of water and acetonitrile (7:3).

Flow rate: Adjust so that the retention time of digoxin is about 10 minutes.

System suitability—

System performance: When the procedure is run with 10 μL of the standard solution under the above operating conditions, digoxin and the internal standard are eluted in this order with the resolution between these peaks being not less than 5.

System repeatability: When the test is repeated 6 times with 10 μL of the standard solution under the above operating conditions, the relative standard deviation of the ratio of the peak area of digoxin to that of the internal standard is not more than 1.0%.

Containers and storage Containers—Hermetic containers, and colored containers may be used.

Storage—Light-resistant.

Digoxin Tablets

ジゴキシン錠

Digoxin Tablets contain not less than 90.0% and not more than 105.0% of the labeled amount of digoxin ($C_{41}H_{64}O_{14}$: 780.94).

Method of preparation Prepare as directed under Tablets, with Digoxin.

Identification To an amount of powdered Digoxin Tablets, equivalent to 0.5 mg of Digoxin, add 2 mL of methanol, shake for 10 minutes, filter, and use the filtrate as the sample solution. Separately, dissolve 0.5 mg of Digoxin RS in 2 mL of methanol, and use this solution as the standard solution. Perform the test with these solutions as directed under Thin-layer Chromatography *<2.03>*. Spot 10 μL each of the sample solution and standard solution on a plate of octadecylsilanized silica gel for thin-layer chromatography. Develop the plate with a mixture of methanol and water (7:3) to a distance of about 10 cm, and air-dry the plate. Spray evenly a mixture of a solution of trichloroacetic acid in ethanol (99.5) (1 in 4) and a freshly prepared solution of sodium toluenesulfonchloramide trihydrate (3 in 100) (4:1) on the plate, heat at 110°C for 10 minutes, and examine under ultraviolet light (main wavelength: 366 nm): the *R*f values of the principal spots with the sample solution and the standard solution are not different each other.

Purity Related substances—Powder not less than 20 Digoxin Tablets. Weigh a portion of the powder equivalent to 2.5 mg of Digoxin, add 30 mL of dilute ethanol, sonicate for 20 minutes, and shake for 5 minutes. After cooling, add dilute ethanol to make 50 mL, filter, and use the filtrate as the sample solution. Perform the test with 10 μL of the sample solution as directed under Liquid Chromatography *<2.01>* according to the following conditions. Determine each peak area of the sample solution by the automatic integration method and calculate the amount of these peaks by the area percentage method: the total amount of the peaks other than digoxin is not more than 5%.

Operating conditions—

Detector, column, column temperature, mobile phase and flow rate: Proceed as directed in the operating conditions in the Assay.

Time span of measurement: About 4 times as long as the retention time of digoxin, beginning after the solvent peak.

System suitability—

Test for required detectability: Dissolve 25 mg of digoxin in 50 mL of warm ethanol (95), cool, add ethanol (95) to make 100 mL. To 10 mL of this solution add 10 mL of water and dilute ethanol to make 50 mL, and use this solution as the solution for system suitability test. Pipet 2 mL of the solution for system suitability test, and add dilute ethanol to make exactly 100 mL. Pipet 5 mL of this solution, and add dilute ethanol to make exactly 100 mL. Confirm that the peak area of digoxin obtained with 10 μL of this solution is equivalent to 0.07 to 0.13% of that with 10 μL of the solution for system suitability test.

System performance: Dissolve 25 mg of digoxin in 50 mL of warm ethanol (95), cool, and add ethanol (95) to make 100 mL. To 10 mL of this solution add 5 mL of a solution of propyl parahydroxybenzoate in ethanol (95) (1 in 4000), 10 mL of water and dilute ethanol to make 50 mL. When the procedure is run with 10 μL of this solution under the above operating conditions, digoxin and propyl parahydroxybenzoate are eluted in this order with the resolution between these peaks being not less than 5.

System repeatability: When the test is repeated 6 times with 10 μL of the solution for system suitability test under the above operating conditions, the relative standard deviation of the peak area of digoxin is not more than 2.5%.

Uniformity of dosage units <*6.02*> Perform the test according to the following method: it meets the requirement of the Content uniformity test.

To 1 tablet of Digoxin Tablets add 0.5 mL of water to disintegrate, then add exactly 0.5 mL of the internal standard solution, and add *V* mL of dilute ethanol so that each mL contains about 21 μg of digoxin ($C_{41}H_{64}O_{14}$). Sonicate for 20 minutes, shake for 5 minutes, filter, and use the filtrate as the sample solution. Separately, weigh accurately about 25 mg of Digoxin RS, previously dried under reduced pressure at 105°C for 1 hour, dissolve in 50 mL of warm ethanol (95), cool, and add ethanol (95) to make exactly 100 mL. Pipet 10 mL of this solution, and add ethanol (95) to make exactly 20 mL. Pipet 1 mL of this solution, add exactly 0.5 mL of the internal standard solution, then add 1.5 mL of water and $(V - 2)$ mL of dilute ethanol, and use this solution as the standard solution. Proceed with the sample solution and standard solution as directed in the Assay.

$$\text{Amount (mg) of digoxin } (C_{41}H_{64}O_{14}) = M_S \times Q_T/Q_S \times 1/200$$

M_S: Amount (mg) of Digoxin RS taken

Internal standard solution—A solution of propyl parahydroxybenzoate in ethanol (95) (1 in 40,000/*V*).

Dissolution <*6.10*> When the test is performed at 100 revolutions per minute according to the Basket method, using 500 mL of diluted hydrochloric acid (3 in 500) as the dissolution medium, the dissolution rate in 60 minutes of Digoxin Tablets is not less than 65%. No retest requirement is applied to Digoxin Tablets.

Start the test with 1 tablet of Digoxin Tablets, withdraw not less than 20 mL of the medium at the specified minute after starting the test, and filter through a membrane filter with a pore size not exceeding 0.8 μm. Discard not less than 10 mL of the first filtrate, and use the subsequent filtrate as the sample solution. Separately, weigh accurately about 25 mg of Digoxin RS, previously dried in vacuum at 105°C for 1 hour, dissolve in a small portion of ethanol (95), and add a mixture of ethanol (95) and water (4:1) to make exactly 500 mL. Pipet 5 mL of this solution, add the dissolution medium to make exactly 500 mL, and use this solution as the standard solution. Pipet 2 mL each of the sample solution, the standard solution and the dissolution medium, and transfer to brown glass-stoppered test tubes. Add exactly 10 mL of 0.012 g/dL L-ascorbic acid-hydrochloric acid TS to these tubes, and shake. Immediately add exactly 1 mL of dilute hydrogen peroxide TS, shake well, and allow to stand at a constant temperature between 25°C and 30°C for 45 minutes. Determine the fluorescence intensities, F_T, F_S, and F_B, of these solutions at 360 nm of the excitation wavelength and at 485 nm of the fluorescence wavelength as directed under Fluorometry <*2.22*>, respectively.

$$\text{Dissolution rate (\%) with respect to the labeled amount of digoxin } (C_{41}H_{64}O_{14}) = M_S \times (F_T - F_B)/(F_S - F_B) \times 1/C$$

M_S: Amount (mg) of Digoxin RS taken

C: The labeled amount (mg) of digoxin ($C_{41}H_{64}O_{14}$) in 1 tablet

Assay Weigh accurately the mass of not less than 20 Digoxin Tablets, and powder. Weigh accurately a portion of the powder, equivalent to about 2.5 mg of digoxin ($C_{41}H_{64}O_{14}$), add 30 mL of dilute ethanol, sonicate for 20 minutes, and shake for 5 minutes. Add exactly 5 mL of the internal standard solution and dilute ethanol to make 50 mL, centrifuge, and use the supernatant liquid as the sample solution. Separately, weigh accurately about 25 mg of Digoxin RS, previously dried under reduced pressure at 105°C for 1 hour, dissolve in 50 mL of warm ethanol (95), cool, and add ethanol (95) to make exactly 100 mL. Pipet 10 mL of this solution, add exactly 5 mL of the internal standard solution, 10 mL of water and dilute ethanol to make 50 mL, and use this solution as the standard solution. Perform the test with 10 μL each of the sample solution and standard solution as directed under Liquid Chromatography <*2.01*> according to the following conditions, and calculate the ratios, Q_T and Q_S, of the peak area of digoxin to that of the internal standard.

$$\text{Amount (mg) of digoxin } (C_{41}H_{64}O_{14}) = M_S \times Q_T/Q_S \times 1/10$$

M_S: Amount (mg) of Digoxin RS taken

Internal standard solution—A solution of propyl parahydroxybenzoate in ethanol (95) (1 in 4000).

Operating conditions—

Detector: An ultraviolet absorption photometer (wavelength: 220 nm).

Column: A stainless steel column 4.6 mm in inside diameter and 25 cm in length, packed with octadecylsilanized silica gel for liquid chromatography (5 μm in particle diameter).

Column temperature: A constant temperature of about 30°C.

Mobile phase: A mixture of water and acetonitrile (7:3).

Flow rate: Adjust so that the retention time of digoxin is about 10 minutes.

System suitability—

System performance: When the procedure is run with 10 μL of the standard solution under the above operating conditions, digoxin and the internal standard are eluted in this order with the resolution between these peaks being not less than 5.

System repeatability: When the test is repeated 6 times with 10 μL of the standard solution under the above operating conditions, the relative standard deviation of the ratio of the peak area of digoxin to that of the internal standard is not more than 1.0%.

Containers and storage Containers—Tight containers.
Storage—Light-resistant.

Dihydrocodeine Phosphate

ジヒドロコデインリン酸塩

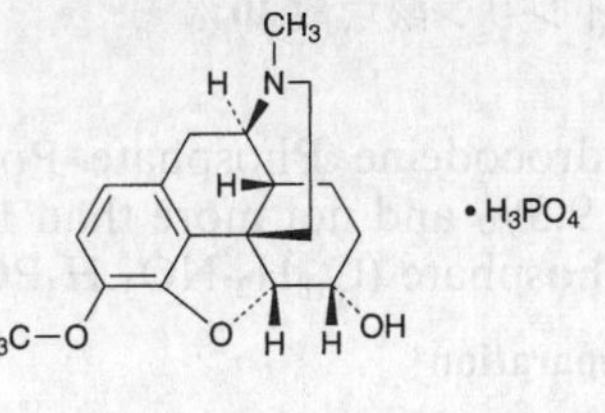

$C_{18}H_{23}NO_3.H_3PO_4$: 399.38
(5*R*,6*S*)-4,5-Epoxy-3-methoxy-17-methylmorphinan-6-ol monophosphate
[*24204-13-5*]

Dihydrocodeine Phosphate contains not less than 98.0% of dihydrocodeine phosphate ($C_{18}H_{23}NO_3.H_3PO_4$), calculated on the dried basis.

Description Dihydrocodeine Phosphate occurs as a white to yellowish white crystalline powder.

It is freely soluble in water and in acetic acid (100), slightly soluble in ethanol (95), and practically insoluble in diethyl ether.

The pH of a solution of 1.0 g of Dihydrocodeine Phosphate in 10 mL of water is between 3.0 and 5.0.

It is affected by light.

Identification **(1)** Determine the absorption spectrum of a solution of Dihydrocodeine Phosphate (1 in 10,000) as directed under Ultraviolet-visible Spectrophotometry <*2.24*>, and compare the spectrum with the Reference Spectrum: both spectra exhibit similar intensities of absorption at the same wavelengths.

(2) Determine the infrared spectrum of Dihydrocodeine Phosphate, previously dried, as directed in the potassium bromide disk method under Infrared Spectrophotometry <*2.25*>, and compare the spectrum with the Reference Spectrum: both spectra exhibit similar intensities of absorption at the same wave numbers.

(3) A solution of Dihydrocodeine Phosphate (1 in 20) responds to Qualitative Tests <*1.09*> (1) for phosphate.

Purity **(1)** Chloride <*1.03*>—Perform the test with 0.5 g of Dihydrocodeine Phosphate. Prepare the control solution with 0.30 mL of 0.01 mol/L hydrochloric acid VS (not more than 0.021%).

(2) Sulfate <*1.14*>—Perform the test with 0.20 g of Dihydrocodeine Phosphate. Prepare the control solution with 1.0 mL of 0.005 mol/L sulfuric acid VS (not more than 0.240%).

(3) Related substances—Dissolve 0.20 g of Dihydrocodeine Phosphate in 10 mL of diluted ethanol (1 in 2), and use this solution as the sample solution. Pipet 1 mL of the sample solution, add diluted ethanol (1 in 2) to make exactly 50 mL, and use this solution as the standard solution. Perform the test with these solutions as directed under Thin-layer Chromatography <*2.03*>. Spot 10 μL of the sample solution and standard solution on a plate of silica gel with fluorescent indicator for thin-chromatography. Develop the plate with a mixture of ethanol (99.5), toluene, acetone and ammonia solution (28) (14:14:7:1) to a distance of about 15 cm, and air-dry the plate. Examine under ultraviolet light (main wavelength: 254 nm): the spots other than the principal spot obtained from the sample solution are not more intense than the spot from the standard solution.

Loss on drying <*2.41*> Not more than 1.0% (0.5 g, 105°C, 4 hours).

Assay Weigh accurately about 0.5 g of Dihydrocodeine Phosphate, dissolve in 70 mL of acetic acid (100), and titrate <*2.50*> with 0.1 mol/L perchloric acid VS until the color of the solution changes from purple through blue to greenish blue (indicator: 3 drops of crystal violet TS). Perform a blank determination in the same manner, and make any necessary correction.

Each mL of 0.1 mol/L perchloric acid VS
= 39.94 mg of $C_{18}H_{23}NO_3.H_3PO_4$

Containers and storage Containers—Tight containers.
Storage—Light-resistant.

1% Dihydrocodeine Phosphate Powder

ジヒドロコデインリン酸塩散1%

1% Dihydrocodeine Phosphate Powder contains not less than 0.90% and not more than 1.10% of dihydrocodeine phosphate ($C_{18}H_{23}NO_3.H_3PO_4$: 399.38).

Method of preparation

Dihydrocodeine Phosphate	10 g
Lactose Hydrate	a sufficient quantity
To make	1000 g

Prepare as directed under Granules or Powders, with the above ingredients.

Identification Determine the absorption spectrum of a solution of 1% Dihydrocodeine Phosphate Powder (1 in 100) as directed under Ultraviolet-visible Spectrophotometry <*2.24*>: it exhibits a maximum between 281 nm and 285 nm.

Dissolution <*6.10*> When the test is performed at 50 revolutions per minute according to the Paddle method, using 900 mL of water as the dissolution medium, the dissolution rate in 15 minutes of 1% Dihydrocodeine Phosphate Powder is not less than 85%.

Start the test with about 1 g of 1% Dihydrocodeine Phosphate Powder, accurately weighed, withdraw not less than 20 mL of the medium at the specified minute after starting the test, and filter through a membrane filter with a pore size not exceeding 0.45 μm. Discard not less than 5 mL of the first filtrate, and use the subsequent filtrate as the sample solution. Separately, weigh accurately about 50 mg of dihydrocodeine phosphate for assay (separately determine the loss on drying <*2.41*> at 105°C for 4 hours), and dissolve in water to make exactly 100 mL. Pipet 2 mL of this solution, add water to make exactly 100 mL, and use this solution as the standard solution. Perform the test with exactly 20 μL each of the sample solution and standard solution as directed under Liquid Chromatography <*2.01*> according to the following conditions, and determine the peak areas, A_T and A_S, of dihydrocodeine in each solution.

Dissolution rate (%) with respect to the labeled amount of dihydrocodeine phosphate ($C_{18}H_{23}NO_3.H_3PO_4$)
$= M_S/M_T \times A_T/A_S \times 9/5$

M_S: Amount (mg) of dihydrocodeine phosphate for assay taken, calculated on the dried basis

M_T: Amount (g) of 1% Dihydrocodeine Phosphate Powder taken

Operating conditions—

Proceed as directed in the operating conditions in the Assay.

System suitability—

System performance: When the procedure is run with 20 μL of the standard solution under the above operating conditions, the number of theoretical plates and the symmetry factor of the peak of dihydrocodeine are not less than 3000 and not more than 2.0, respectively.

System repeatability: When the test is repeated 6 times with 20 μL of the standard solution under the above operating conditions, the relative standard deviation of the peak area of dihydrocodeine is not more than 2.0%.

Assay Weigh accurately about 5 g of 1% Dihydrocodeine Phosphate Powder, dissolve in water to make exactly 100 mL, then pipet 10 mL of this solution, add exactly 10 mL of the internal standard solution, and use this solution as the sample solution. Separately, weigh accurately about 50 mg of dihydrocodeine phosphate for assay (separately determine the loss on drying *<2.41>* at 105°C for 4 hours), dissolve in water to make exactly 100 mL, then pipet 10 mL of this solution, add exactly 10 mL of the internal standard solution, and use this solution as the standard solution. Perform the test with 20 μL each of the sample solution and standard solution as directed under Liquid Chromatography *<2.01>* according to the following conditions, and calculate the ratios, Q_T and Q_S, of the peak area of dihydrocodeine to that of the internal standard.

Amount (mg) of dihydrocodeine phosphate ($C_{18}H_{23}NO_3.H_3PO_4$)
$= M_S \times Q_T/Q_S$

M_S: Amount (mg) of dihydrocodeine phosphate for assay taken, calculated on the dried basis

Internal standard solution—A solution of ethylefurin hydrochloride (3 in 10,000).

Operating conditions—

Detector: An ultraviolet absorption photometer (wavelength: 280 nm).

Column: A stainless steel column 4.6 mm in inside diameter and 15 cm in length, packed with octadecylsilanized silica gel for liquid chromatography (5 μm in particle diameter).

Column temperature: A constant temperature of about 40°C.

Mobile phase: Dissolve 1.0 g of sodium lauryl sulfate in 500 mL of diluted phosphoric acid (1 in 1000), and adjust the pH to 3.0 with sodium hydroxide TS. To 240 mL of this solution add 70 mL of tetrahydrofuran.

Flow rate: Adjust so that the retention time of dihydrocodeine is about 9 minutes.

System suitability—

System performance: When the procedure is run with 20 μL of the standard solution under the above operating conditions, dihydrocodeine and the internal standard are eluted in this order with the resolution between these peaks being not less than 4.

System repeatability: When the test is repeated 5 times with 20 μL of the standard solution under the above operating conditions, the relative standard deviation of the ratios of the peak area of dihydrocodeine to that of the internal standard is not more than 1.0%.

Containers and storage Containers—Tight containers.

10% Dihydrocodeine Phosphate Powder

ジヒドロコデインリン酸塩散10%

10% Dihydrocodeine Phosphate Powder contains not less than 9.3% and not more than 10.7% of dihydrocodeine phosphate ($C_{18}H_{23}NO_3.H_3PO_4$: 399.38).

Method of preparation

Dihydrocodeine Phosphate	100 g
Lactose Hydrate	a sufficient quantity
To make	1000 g

Prepare as directed under Powders, with the above ingredients.

Identification Determine the absorption spectrum of a solution of 10% Dihydrocodeine Phosphate Powder (1 in 1000) as directed under Ultraviolet-visible Spectrophotometry *<2.24>*: it exhibits a maximum between 281 nm and 285 nm.

Dissolution *<6.10>* When the test is performed at 50 revolutions per minute according to the Paddle method, using 900 mL of water as the dissolution medium, the dissolution rate in 15 minutes of 10% Dihydrocodeine Phosphate Powder is not less than 85%.

Start the test with about 0.1 g of 10% Dihydrocodeine Phosphate Powder, accurately weighed, withdraw not less than 10 mL of the medium at the specified minute after starting the test, and filter through a membrane filter with a pore size not exceeding 0.45 μm. Discard not less than 5 mL of the first filtrate, and use the subsequent filtrate as the sample solution. Separately, weigh accurately about 22 mg of dihydrocodeine phosphate for assay (separately determine the loss on drying *<2.41>* at 105°C for 4 hours), and dissolve in water to make exactly 100 mL. Pipet 5 mL of this solution, add water to make exactly 100 mL, and use this solution as the standard solution. Perform the test with exactly 50 μL each of the sample solution and standard solution as directed under Liquid Chromatography *<2.01>* according to the following conditions, and determine the peak areas, A_T and A_S, of dihydrocodeine in each solution.

Dissolution rate (%) with respect to the labeled amount of dihydrocodeine phosphate ($C_{18}H_{23}NO_3.H_3PO_4$)
$= M_S/M_T \times A_T/A_S \times 9/20$

M_S: Amount (mg) of dihydrocodeine phosphate for assay taken, calculated on the dried basis

M_T: Amount (g) of 10% Dihydrocodeine Phosphate Powder taken

Operating conditions—

Proceed as directed in the operating conditions in the Assay.

System suitability—

System performance: When the procedure is run with 50 μL of the standard solution under the above operating conditions, the number of theoretical plates and the symmetry factor of the peak of dihydrocodeine are not less than 3000

and not more than 2.0, respectively.

System repeatability: When the test is repeated 6 times with 50 μL of the standard solution under the above operating conditions, the relative standard deviation of the peak area of dihydrocodeine is not more than 2.0%.

Assay Weigh accurately about 2.5 g of 10% Dihydrocodeine Phosphate Powder, dissolve in water to make exactly 100 mL, then pipet 2 mL of this solution, add exactly 10 mL of the internal standard solution and water to make 20 mL, and use this solution as the sample solution. Separately, weigh accurately about 50 mg of dihydrocodeine phosphate for assay, (separately determine the loss on drying *<2.41>* at 105°C for 4 hours), dissolve in water to make exactly 100 mL, then pipet 10 mL of this solution, add exactly 10 mL of the internal standard solution, and use this solution as the standard solution. Perform the test with 20 μL each of the sample solution and standard solution as directed under Liquid Chromatography *<2.01>* according to the following conditions, and calculate the ratios, Q_T and Q_S, of the peak area of dihydrocodeine to that of the internal standard.

Amount (mg) of dihydrocodeine phosphate ($C_{18}H_{23}NO_3.H_3PO_4$)
$= M_S \times Q_T/Q_S \times 5$

M_S: Amount (mg) of dihydrocodeine phosphate for assay taken, calculated on the dried basis

Internal standard solution—A solution of ethylefrine hydrochloride (3 in 10,000).

Operating conditions—

Detector: An ultraviolet absorption photometer (wavelength: 280 nm).

Column: A stainless steel column 4.6 mm in inside diameter and 15 cm in length, packed with octadecylsilanized silica gel for liquid chromatography (5 μm in particle diameter).

Column temperature: A constant temperature of about 40°C.

Mobile phase: Dissolve 1.0 g of sodium lauryl sulfate in 500 mL of diluted phosphoric acid (1 in 1000), and adjust the pH to 3.0 with sodium hydroxide TS. To 240 mL of this solution add 70 mL of tetrahydrofuran.

Flow rate: Adjust so that the retention time of dihydrocodeine is about 9 minutes.

System suitability—

System performance: When the procedure is run with 20 μL of the standard solution under the above operating conditions, dihydrocodeine and the internal standard are eluted in this order with the resolution between these peaks being not less than 4.

System repeatability: When the test is repeated 5 times with 20 μL of the standard solution under the above operating conditions, the relative standard deviation of the ratios of the peak area of dihydrocodeine to that of the internal standard is not more than 1.0%.

Containers and storage Containers—Tight containers.

Dihydroergotamine Mesilate

ジヒドロエルゴタミンメシル酸塩

$C_{33}H_{37}N_5O_5.CH_4O_3S$: 679.78

(5′*S*,10*R*)-5′-Benzyl-12′-hydroxy-2′-methyl-9,10-dihydroergotaman-3′,6′,18-trione monomethanesulfonate

[*6190-39-2*]

Dihydroergotamine Mesilate contains not less than 97.0% of dihydroergotamine mesilate ($C_{33}H_{37}N_5O_5.CH_4O_3S$), calculated on the dried basis.

Description Dihydroergotamine Mesilate occurs as a white to yellowish white or grayish white to reddish white powder.

It is freely soluble in acetic acid (100), sparingly soluble in methanol and in chloroform, slightly soluble in water and in ethanol (95), and practically insoluble in acetic anhydride and in diethyl ether.

It is gradually colored by light.

Melting point: about 214°C (with decomposition).

Identification (1) Dissolve 1 mg of Dihydroergotamine Mesilate in 5 mL of a solution of L-tartaric acid (1 in 100). To 1 mL of this solution add 2 mL of 4-dimethylaminobenzaldehyde-ferric chloride TS, and shake: a blue color develops.

(2) To 0.1 g of Dihydroergotamine Mesilate add 0.4 g of sodium hydroxide, stir well, and incinerate by gradual ignition. After cooling, add 10 mL of water to the residue, heat to boiling, cool, and filter. To the filtrate add 0.5 mL of hydrochloric acid: the solution responds to Qualitative Tests *<1.09>* for sulfate. Separately, to 0.1 g of Dihydroergotamine Mesilate add 5 mL of dilute hydrochloric acid, shake for 5 minutes, filter, and to the filtrate add 1 mL of barium chloride TS: the solution is clear.

(3) Determine the absorption spectrum of a solution of Dihydroergotamine Mesilate in methanol (1 in 20,000) as directed under Ultraviolet-visible Spectrophotometry *<2.24>*, and compare the spectrum with the Reference Spectrum: both spectra exhibit similar intensities of absorption at the same wavelengths.

(4) Determine the infrared absorption spectrum of Dihydroergotamine Mesilate, previously dried, as directed in the potassium bromide disk method under Infrared Spectrophotometry *<2.25>*, and compare the spectrum with the Reference Spectrum: both spectra exhibit similar intensities of absorption at the same wave numbers.

Optical rotation *<2.49>* $[\alpha]_D^{20}$: −16.7 – −22.7° [0.5 g, calculated on the dried basis, a mixture of ethanol (99.5), chloroform and ammonia solution (28) (10:10:1), 20 mL, 100 mm].

pH *<2.54>* Dissolve 0.05 g of Dihydroergotamine Mesilate in 50 mL of water: the pH of this solution is between 4.4 and 5.4.

Purity (1) Clarity and color of solution—Dissolve 0.10 g of Dihydroergotamine Mesilate in 0.1 mL of a solution of methanesulfonic acid (7 in 100) and 50 mL of water: the solution is clear, and has no more color than the following control solutions [1] or [2].

Control solution [1]: Pipet 0.6 mL of Iron (III) Chloride CS and 0.15 mL of Cobalt (II) Chloride CS, mix, and add diluted hydrochloric acid (1 in 40) to make exactly 100 mL.

Control solution [2]: Pipet 0.6 mL of Iron (III) Chloride CS, 0.25 mL of Cobalt (II) Chloride CS and 0.1 mL of Copper (II) Sulfate CS, mix, and add diluted hydrochloric acid (1 in 40) to make exactly 100 mL.

(2) Related substances—Conduct this procedure without exposure to light, using light-resistant vessels. Dissolve 0.10 g of Dihydroergotamine Mesilate in 5 mL of a mixture of chloroform and methanol (9:1), and use this solution as the sample solution. Pipet 1 mL of the sample solution, add a mixture of chloroform and methanol (9:1) to make exactly 200 mL, and use this solution as the standard solution (1). Pipet 10 mL of the standard solution (1), add a mixture of chloroform and methanol (9:1) to make exactly 25 mL, and use this solution as the standard solution (2). Perform the test with these solutions as directed under Thin-layer Chromatography <*2.03*>. Spot 5 μL each of the sample solution and standard solutions (1) and (2) on a plate of silica gel for thin-layer chromatography. Develop the plate with a mixture of dichloromethane, ethyl acetate, methanol and ammonia solution (28) (50:50:6:1) to a distance of about 15 cm, and dry the plate with cold wind within 1 minute. Develop the plate again immediately with a freshly prepared mixture of dichloromethane, ethyl acetate, methanol and ammonia solution (28) (50:50:6:1) to a distance of about 15 cm, and air-dry the plate. Spray evenly 4-dimethylaminobenzaldehyde TS for spraying on the plate, and dry the plate with warm wind: the spots other than the principal spot obtained from the sample solution are not more intense than the spot from the standard solution (1), and the spots, which are more intense than the spot from the standard solution (2), are not more than two.

Loss on drying <*2.41*> Not more than 4.0% (0.5 g, in vacuum at a pressure not exceeding 0.67 kPa, 100°C, 6 hours).

Assay Weigh accurately about 0.2 g of Dihydroergotamine Mesilate, dissolve in 170 mL of a mixture of acetic anhydride and acetic acid (100) (10:1), and titrate <*2.50*> with 0.02 mol/L perchloric acid VS (potentiometric titration). Perform a blank determination in the same manner, and make any necessary correction.

Each mL of 0.02 mol/L perchloric acid VS
= 13.60 mg of $C_{33}H_{37}N_5O_5.CH_4O_3S$

Containers and storage Containers—Tight containers.
Storage—Light-resistant.

Dihydroergotoxine Mesilate

ジヒドロエルゴトキシンメシル酸塩

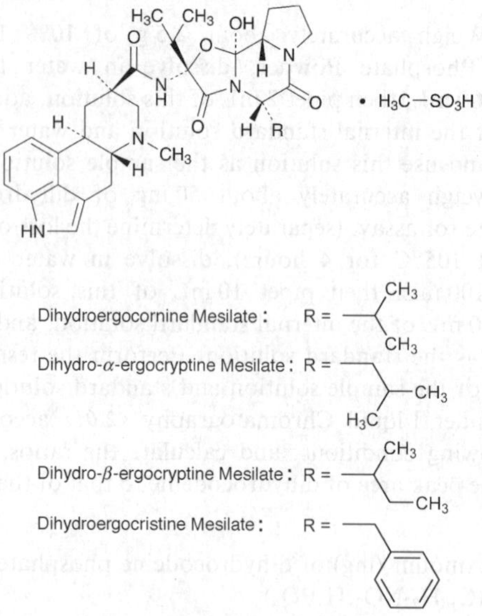

Dihydroergocornine Mesilate
$C_{31}H_{41}N_5O_5.CH_4O_3S$: 659.79
(5′*S*,10*R*)-12′-Hydroxy-2′,5′-bis(1-methylethyl)-9,10-dihydroergotaman-3′,6′,18-trione monomethanesulfonate

Dihydro-α-ergocryptine Mesilate
$C_{32}H_{43}N_5O_5.CH_4O_3S$: 673.82
(5′*S*,10*R*)-12′-Hydroxy-2′-(1-methylethyl)-5′-(2-methylpropyl)-9,10-dihydroergotaman-3′,6′,18-trione monomethanesulfonate

Dihydro-β-ergocryptine Mesilate
$C_{32}H_{43}N_5O_5.CH_4O_3S$: 673.82
(5′*S*,10*R*)-12′-Hydroxy-2′-(1-methylethyl)-5′-(1-methylpropyl)-9,10-dihydroergotaman-3′,6′,18-trione monomethanesulfonate

Dihydroergocristine Mesilate
$C_{35}H_{41}N_5O_5.CH_4O_3S$: 707.84
(5′*S*,10*R*)-5′-Benzyl-12′-hydroxy-2′-(1-methylethyl)-9,10-dihydroergotaman-3′,6′,18-trione monomethanesulfonate

[*8067-24-1*, Dihydroergotoxine Mesilate]

Dihydroergotoxine Mesilate contains not less than 97.0% and not more than 103.0% of dihydroergotoxine mesilate [as a mixture of dihydroergocornine mesilate ($C_{31}H_{41}N_5O_5.CH_4O_3S$), dihydro-α-ergocryptine mesilate ($C_{32}H_{43}N_5O_5.CH_4O_3S$), dihydro-β-ergocryptine mesilate ($C_{32}H_{43}N_5O_5.CH_4O_3S$) and dihydroergocristine mesilate ($C_{35}H_{41}N_5O_5.CH_4O_3S$)], calculated on the anhydrous basis. The relative contents of dihydroergocornine mesilate ($C_{31}H_{41}N_5O_5.CH_4O_3S$), dihydroergocryptine mesilate ($C_{32}H_{43}N_5O_5.CH_4O_3S$) and dihydroergocristine mesilate ($C_{35}H_{41}N_5O_5.CH_4O_3S$) are 30.3–36.3% each, and the content ratio of dihydro-α-ergocryptine mesilate and dihydro-β-ergocryptine mesilate is 1.5–2.5:1.

Description Dihydroergotoxine Mesilate occurs as a white to pale yellow powder.

It is soluble in methanol, sparingly soluble in ethanol (95), slightly soluble in water, in acetonitrile and in chloroform, and practically insoluble in diethyl ether.

Identification Determine the infrared absorption spectrum of Dihydroergotoxine Mesilate as directed in the potassium bromide disk method under Infrared Spectrophotometry <*2.25*>, and compare the spectrum with the Reference Spectrum: both spectra exhibit similar intensities of absorption at the same wave numbers.

Optical rotation <*2.49*> $[\alpha]_D^{20}$: +11.0 – +15.0° (0.2 g calculated on the anhydrous basis, dilute ethanol, 20 mL, 100 mm).

Purity **(1)** Clarity and color of solution—Dissolve 0.10 g of Dihydroergotoxine Mesilate in 20 mL of water: the solution is clear and the color of the solution is not more intense than that of the following control solution.

Control solution: To a mixture of 1.0 mL of Cobalt (II) Chloride CS, 0.4 mL of Copper (II) Sulfate CS and 2.4 mL of Iron (III) Chloride CS add diluted hydrochloric acid (1 in 40) to make exactly 200 mL.

(2) Heavy metals <*1.07*>—Proceed with 1.0 g of Dihydroergotoxine Mesilate according to Method 2, and perform the test. Prepare the control solution with 2.0 mL of Standard Lead Solution (not more than 20 ppm).

(3) Related substances—Weigh accurately 0.100 g of Dihydroergotoxine Mesilate, dissolve it in a mixture of chloroform and methanol (9:1) to make exactly 5 mL, and use this solution as the sample solution. Separately, weigh accurately 10 mg of dihydroergocristine mesilate for thin-layer chromatography, and dissolve in a mixture of chloroform and methanol (9:1) to make exactly 100 mL. Pipet 6 mL, 4 mL and 2 mL of this solution, add a mixture of chloroform and methanol (9:1) to make exactly 10 mL, respectively, and use these solutions as the standard solutions (1), (2) and (3), respectively. Perform the test with these solutions as directed under Thin-layer Chromatography <*2.03*> without putting the filter paper in the developing vessel. Spot 5 μL each of the sample solution and the standard solutions (1), (2) and (3) on a plate of silica gel for thin-layer chromatography. Develop the plate with a mixture of dichloromethane, ethyl acetate, methanol and ammonia solution (28) (50:50:3:1) to a distance of about 15 cm, and dry the plate with the aid of a cool air stream. Immediately after that, develop the plate again with a newly prepared mixture of dichloromethane, ethyl acetate, methanol and ammonia solution (28) (50:50:3:1) to a distance of about 15 cm, and dry the plate within 1 minute with the aid of a cool air stream. Spray evenly *p*-dimethylaminobenzal-dehyde-hydrochloric acid TS on the plate, dry the plate within 2 minutes with the aid of a cool air stream, and heat it at 40°C for 15 minutes: the spots other than the principal spot obtained from the sample solution are not more intense than the spot from the standard solution (1), not more than 2 spots are more intense than that from the standard solution (2), and not more than 4 spots are more intense than that from the standard solution (3).

Water <*2.48*> Not more than 5.0% (0.2 g, volumetric titration, direct titration).

Residue on ignition <*2.44*> Not more than 0.1% (1 g).

Assay **(1)** Dihydroergotoxine mesilate—Weigh accurately about 30 mg each of Dihydroergotoxine Mesilate and Dihydroergotoxine Mesilate RS, and dissolve them separately in a suitable amount of a mixture of water and acetonitrile (3:1). To these solutions add exactly 10 mL of the internal standard solution and an amount of a mixture of water and acetonitrile (3:1) to make 50 mL, and use these solutions as the sample solution and the standard solution. Perform the test with 20 μL of the sample solution and standard solution as directed under Liquid Chromatography <*2.01*> according to the following conditions, and calculate the ratios of the peak areas of dihydroergocornine, dihydro-α-ergocryptine, dihydroergocristine and dihydro-β-ergocryptine to the peak area of the internal standard of these solutions.

$$\text{Amount (mg) of dihydroergotoxine mesilate} = M_S \times (Q_{TA} + Q_{TB} + Q_{TC} + Q_{TD}) / (Q_{SA} + Q_{SB} + Q_{SC} + Q_{SD})$$

M_S: Amount (mg) of Dihydroergotoxine Mesilate RS taken, calculated on the anhydrous basis

Q_{TA}: Ratio of the peak area of dihydroergocornine to that of the internal standard of the sample solution × 659.80

Q_{TB}: Ratio of the peak area of dihydro-α-ergocryptine to that of the internal standard of the sample × 673.83

Q_{TC}: Ratio of the peak area of dihydroergocristine to that of the internal standard of the sample solution × 707.85

Q_{TD}: Ratio of the peak area of dihydro-β-ergocryptine to that of the internal standard of the sample solution × 673.83

Q_{SA}: Ratio of the peak area of dihydroergocornine to that of the internal standard of the standard solution × 659.80

Q_{SB}: Ratio of the peak area of dihydro-α-ergocryptine to that of the internal standard of the standard solution × 673.83

Q_{SC}: Ratio of the peak area of dihydroergocristine to that of the internal standard of the standard solution × 707.85

Q_{SD}: Ratio of the peak area of dihydro-β-ergocryptine to that of the internal standard of the standard solution × 673.83

Internal standard solution—Dissolve 0.04 g of chloramphenicol in a mixture of water and acetonitrile (3:1) to make 250 mL.

Operating conditions—

Detector: An ultraviolet absorption photometer (wavelength: 280 nm).

Column: A stainless steel column 4.6 mm in inside diameter and 15 cm in length, packed with octadecylsilanized silica gel for liquid chromatography (5 μm in particle diameter).

Column temperature: A constant temperature of about 25°C.

Mobile phase: A mixture of water, acetonitrile and triethylamine (30:10:1).

Flow rate: Adjust so that the retention time of chloramphenicol is about 5 minutes.

System suitability—

System performance: When the procedure is run with 20 μL of the standard solution under the above operating conditions, the internal standard, dihydroergocornine, dihydro-α-ergocryptine, dihydroergocristine and dihydro-β-ergocryptine are eluted in this order with the resolution between the peaks of dihydro-α-ergocryptine and dihydroergocristine being not less than 1.5.

System repeatability: When the test is repeated 6 times with 20 μL of the standard solution under the above operating conditions, the relative standard deviation of the ratios of the peak area of dihydroergocornine, dihydro-α-ergocryptine, dihydroergocristine and dihydro-β-ergocryptine to that of the internal standard is not more than 0.5%.

(2) Relative contents of dihydroergocornine mesilate, dihydroergocryptine mesilate and dihydroergocristine mesilate—Calculate the relative amounts of dihydroergocornine mesilate, dihydroergocryptine mesilate (dihydro-α-ergocryptine mesilate and dihydro-β-ergocryptine mesilate) and dihydroergocristine mesilate from the chromatogram obtained in Assay (1) for the sample solution using the following equations:

Relative amount (%) of dihydroergocornine mesilate
$= Q_{TA}/(Q_{TA} + Q_{TB} + Q_{TC} + Q_{TD}) \times 100$

Relative amount (%) of dihydroergocryptine mesilate
$= (Q_{TB} + Q_{TD})/(Q_{TA} + Q_{TB} + Q_{TC} + Q_{TD}) \times 100$

Relative amount (%) of dihydroergocristine mesilate
$= Q_{TC}/(Q_{TA} + Q_{TB} + Q_{TC} + Q_{TD}) \times 100$

(3) Ratio of the content of dihydro-α-ergocryptine mesilate to dihydro-β-ergocryptine mesilate—Calculate the ratio of the amount of dihydro-α-ergocryptine mesilate to dihydro-β-ergocryptine mesilate from the chromatogram obtained in the Assay (1) for the sample solution using the following equations:

Ratio of the content of dihydro-α-ergocryptine mesilate to dihydro-β-ergocryptine mesilate
$= Q_{TB}/Q_{TD}$

Containers and storage Containers—Well-closed containers.

Storage—Light-resistant.

Dilazep Hydrochloride Hydrate

ジラゼプ塩酸塩水和物

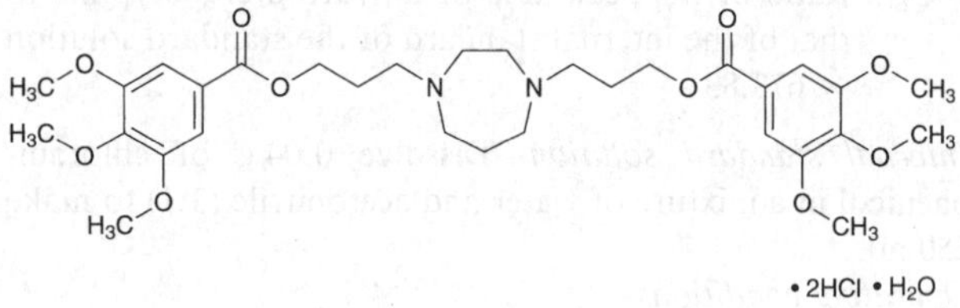

$C_{31}H_{44}N_2O_{10}.2HCl.H_2O$: 695.63
3,3′-(1,4-Diazepane-1,4-diyl)dipropyl bis(3,4,5-trimethoxybenzoate) dihydrochloride monohydrate
[*20153-98-4*, anhydride]

Dilazep Hydrochloride Hydrate contains not less than 98.0% of dilazep hydrochloride ($C_{31}H_{44}N_2O_{10}.2HCl$: 677.62), calculated on the dried basis.

Description Dilazep Hydrochloride Hydrate occurs as a white crystalline powder. It is odorless.

It is freely soluble in acetic acid (100) and in chloroform, soluble in water, slightly soluble in ethanol (95) and in acetic anhydride, and practically insoluble in diethyl ether.

Melting point: 200 – 204°C Immerse the sample in a bath of 110°C, and raise the temperature at the rate of about 3°C per minute from 140°C to 150°C, about 10°C per minute from 160°C to 195°C and about 1°C per minute from 195°C.

Identification **(1)** To 1 mL of a solution of Dilazep Hydrochloride Hydrate (1 in 100) add 0.1 mL of a solution of hydroxylammonium chloride (1 in 10) and 0.1 mL of 8 mol/L potassium hydroxide TS, and warm in a water bath of 70°C for 10 minutes. After cooling, add 0.5 mL of dilute hydrochloric acid and 0.1 mL of iron (III) chloride TS: a purple color develops.

(2) To 5 mL of a solution of Dilazep Hydrochloride Hydrate (3 in 500) add 0.3 mL of Reinecke salt TS: a light red precipitate is formed.

(3) Determine the absorption spectrum of a solution of Dilazep Hydrochloride Hydrate (1 in 50,000) as directed under Ultraviolet-visible Spectrophotometry <*2.24*>, and compare the spectrum with the Reference Spectrum: both spectra exhibit similar intensities of absorption at the same wavelengths.

(4) Determine the infrared absorption spectrum of Dilazep Hydrochloride Hydrate as directed in the potassium chloride disk method under Infrared Spectrophotometry <*2.25*>, and compare the spectrum with the Reference Spectrum: both spectra exhibit similar intensities of absorption at the same wave numbers.

pH <*2.54*> Dissolve 1.0 g of Dilazep Hydrochloride Hydrate in 100 mL of water: the pH of this solution is between 3.0 and 4.0.

Purity **(1)** Clarity and color of solution—Dissolve 1.0 g of Dilazep Hydrochloride Hydrate in 20 mL of water: the solution is clear and colorless.

(2) Sulfate <*1.14*>—Perform the test with 0.5 g of Dilazep Hydrochloride Hydrate. Prepare the control solution with 0.50 mL of 0.005 mol/L sulfuric acid VS (not more than 0.048%).

(3) Heavy metals <*1.07*>—Proceed with 2.0 g of Dilazep Hydrochloride Hydrate according to Method 1, and perform the test. Prepare the control solution with 2.0 mL of Standard Lead Solution (not more than 10 ppm).

(4) Arsenic <*1.11*>—Prepare the test solution with 1.0 g of Dilazep Hydrochloride Hydrate according to Method 3, and perform the test (not more than 2 ppm).

(5) Related substances—Dissolve 0.40 g of Dilazep Hydrochloride Hydrate in 10 mL of chloroform, and use this solution as the sample solution. Pipet 1 mL of the sample solution, add chloroform to make exactly 200 mL, and use this solution as the standard solution. Perform the test with these solutions as directed under Thin-layer Chromatography <*2.03*>. Spot 5 μL each of the sample solution and standard solution on a plate of silica gel for thin-layer chromatography. Develop the plate with a mixture of methanol, ethyl acetate, dichloromethane and hydrochloric acid (500:200:100:1) to a distance of about 10 cm, and air-dry the plate. Spray evenly Dragendorff's TS for spraying on the plate: the spots other than the principal spot obtained from the sample solution are not more intense than the spot from the standard solution.

Loss on drying <*2.41*> 2.0 – 3.0% (1 g, 105°C, 3 hours).

Residue on ignition <*2.44*> Not more than 0.1% (1 g).

Assay Weigh accurately about 0.3 g of Dilazep Hydrochloride Hydrate, dissolve in 40 mL of a mixture of acetic anhydride and acetic acid (100) (7:3), and titrate <*2.50*> with 0.1 mol/L perchloric acid VS (potentiometric titration). Perform a blank determination in the same manner, and make any necessary correction.

Each mL of 0.1 mol/L perchloric acid VS
$= 33.88$ mg of $C_{31}H_{44}N_2O_{10}.2HCl$

Containers and storage Containers—Tight containers.

Diltiazem Hydrochloride

ジルチアゼム塩酸塩

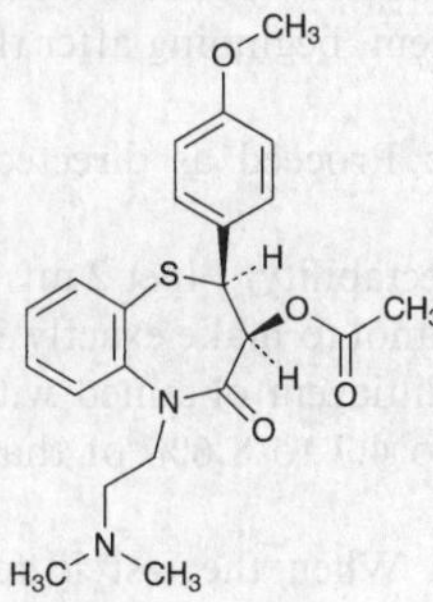

$C_{22}H_{26}N_2O_4S.HCl$: 450.98
(2*S*,3*S*)-5-[2-(Dimethylamino)ethyl]-2-(4-methoxyphenyl)-4-oxo-2,3,4,5-tetrahydro-1,5-benzothiazepin-3-yl acetate monohydrochloride
[*33286-22-5*]

Diltiazem Hydrochloride, when dried, contains not less than 98.5% of diltiazem hydrochloride ($C_{22}H_{26}N_2O_4S.HCl$).

Description Diltiazem Hydrochloride occurs as white, crystals or crystalline powder. It is odorless.

It is very soluble in formic acid, freely soluble in water, in methanol and in chloroform, sparingly soluble in acetonitrile, slightly soluble in acetic anhydride and in ethanol (99.5), and practically insoluble in diethyl ether.

Identification **(1)** Dissolve 0.05 g of Diltiazem Hydrochloride in 1 mL of 1 mol/L hydrochloric acid TS, add 2 mL of ammonium thiocyanate-cobalt (II) nitrate TS and 5 mL of chloroform, shake well, and allow to stand: a blue color develops in the chloroform layer.

(2) Proceed as directed under Oxygen Flask Combustion Method <*1.06*> with 0.03 g of Diltiazem Hydrochloride, using 20 mL of water as the absorbing liquid, and prepare the test solution: the test solution responds to Qualitative Tests <*1.09*> (1) for sulfate.

(3) Dissolve 0.01 g of Diltiazem Hydrchloride in 0.01 mol/L hydrochloric acid TS to make 100 mL. To 2 mL of the solution add 0.01 mol/L hydrochloric acid TS to make 20 mL. Determine the absorption spectrum of the solution as directed under Ultraviolet-visible Spectrophotometry <*2.24*>, and compare the spectrum with the Reference Spectrum: both spectra exhibit similar intensities of absorption at the same wavelengths.

(4) Determine the infrared absorption spectrum of Diltiazem Hydrochloride, previously dried, as directed in the potassium bromide disk method under Infrared Spectrophotometry <*2.25*>: it exhibits absorption at the wave numbers of about 1741 cm^{-1}, 1678 cm^{-1}, 1252 cm^{-1} and 1025 cm^{-1}.

(5) A solution of Diltiazem Hydrochloride (1 in 50) responds to Qualitative Tests <*1.09*> (2) for chloride.

Optical rotation <*2.49*> $[\alpha]_D^{20}$: +115 – +120° (after drying, 0.20 g, water, 20 mL, 100 mm).

Melting point <*2.60*> 210 – 215°C (with decomposition).

pH <*2.54*> Dissolve 1.0 g of Diltiazem Hydrochloride in 100 mL of water: the pH of this solution is between 4.3 and 5.3.

Purity **(1)** Clarity and color of solution—Dissolve 1.0 g of Diltiazem Hydrochloride in 20 mL of water: the solution is clear and colorless.

(2) Sulfate <*1.14*>—Perform the test with 1.0 g of Diltiazem Hydrochloride. Prepare the control solution with 0.50 mL of 0.005 mol/L sulfuric acid VS (not more than 0.024%).

(3) Heavy metals <*1.07*>—Proceed with 2.0 g of Diltiazem Hydrochloride according to Method 2, and perform the test. Prepare the control solution with 2.0 mL of Standard Lead Solution (not more than 10 ppm).

(4) Arsenic <*1.11*>—Place 1.0 g of Diltiazem Hydrochloride in a decomposition flask, add 5 mL of nitric acid and 2 mL of sulfuric acid, put a small funnel on the neck of the flask, and heat cautiously until white fumes are evolved. After cooling, add 2 mL of nitric acid, heat, and repeat this procedure twice, add several 2-mL portions of hydrogen peroxide (30), and heat until the solution becomes colorless to pale yellow. After cooling, add 2 mL of saturated solution of ammonium oxalate monohydrate, and heat again until white fumes are evolved. After cooling, add water to make 5 mL, use this solution as the test solution, and perform the test: the test solution has no more color than the following control solution (not more than 2 ppm).

Control solution: Proceed in the same manner as the test solution without Diltiazem Hydrochloride, add 2.0 mL of Standard Arsenic Solution and water to make 5 mL, and proceed in the same manner as the test solution.

(5) Related substances—Dissolve 50 mg of Diltiazem Hydrochloride in 50 mL of diluted ethanol (4 in 5), and use this solution as the sample solution. Measure exactly 1 mL of the sample solution, add diluted ethanol (4 in 5) to make exactly 200 mL, and use this solution as the standard solution. Perform the test with exactly 20 μL each of the sample solution and standard solution as directed under Liquid Chromatography <*2.01*> according to the following conditions. Determine each peak area of both solutions by automatic integration method: the total area of peaks other than the peak of diltiazem obtained from the sample solution is not larger than 3/5 times the peak area of diltiazem from the standard solution.

Operating conditions—

Detector: An ultraviolet absorption photometer (wavelength: 240 nm).

Column: A stainless steel column 4.6 mm in inside diameter and 15 cm in length, packed with octadecylsilanized silica gel for liquid chromatography (5 μm in particle diameter).

Column temperature: A constant temperature of about 50°C.

Mobile phase: Dissolve 8 g of sodium acetate trihydrate and 1.5 g of *d*-camphorsulfonic acid in 500 mL of water, and filter using a membrane filter (0.4 μm in pore size). Add 250 mL each of acetonitrile and methanol to the filtrate.

Flow rate: Adjust so that the retention time of diltiazem is about 9 minutes.

Time span of measurement: About twice as long as the retention time of diltiazem, beginning after the solvent peak.

System suitability—

Test for required detectability: To exactly 2 mL of the standard solution add diluted ethanol (4 in 5) to make exactly 10 mL. Confirm that the peak area of diltiazem obtained with 20 μL of this solution is equivalent to 15 to 25% of that with 20 μL of the standard solution.

System performance: Dissolve 0.03 g of Diltiazem Hydrochloride, 0.02 g of *d*-3-hydroxy-*cis*-2,3-dihydro-5-[2-(dimethylamino)ethyl]-2-(4-methoxyphenyl)-1,5-benzothiazepin-4-(5*H*)-one hydrochloride (hereinafter referred to as de-acetyl substance) and 0.02 g of phenylbenzoate in 160 mL of ethanol (99.5), and add water to make 200 mL. When the procedure is run with 20 μL of this solution under the above operating conditions, de-acetyl substance, diltiazem and phenyl benzoate are eluted in this order with the resolutions between the peaks of de-acetyl substance and diltiazem and between the peaks of diltiazem and phenyl benzoate being not less than 2.5, respectively.

System repeatability: When the test is repeated 6 times with 20 μL of the standard solution under the above operating conditions, the relative standard deviation of the peak area of diltiazem is not more than 2.0%.

Loss on drying *<2.41>* Not more than 0.5% (1 g, 105°C, 2 hours).

Residue on ignition *<2.44>* Not more than 0.1% (1 g).

Assay Weigh accurately about 0.7 g of Diltiazem Hydrochloride, previously dried, dissolve in 2.0 mL of formic acid, add 60 mL of acetic anhydride, and titrate *<2.50>* with 0.1 mol/L perchloric acid VS (potentiometric titration). Perform a blank determination in the same manner, and make any necessary correction.

Each mL of 0.1 mol/L perchloric acid VS
= 45.10 mg of $C_{22}H_{26}N_2O_4S.HCl$

Containers and storage Containers—Tight containers.
Storage—Light-resistant.

Diltiazem Hydrochloride Extended-release Capsules

ジルチアゼム塩酸塩徐放カプセル

Diltiazem Hydrochloride Extended-release Capsules contain not less than 95.0% and not more than 105.0% of the labeled amount of diltiazem hydrochloride ($C_{22}H_{26}N_2O_4S.HCl$: 450.98).

Method of preparation Prepare as directed under Capsules, with Diltiazem Hydrochloride.

Identification Take out the content of Diltiazem Hydrochloride Extended-release Capsules, and powder. To a portion of the powder, equivalent to 0.1 g of Diltiazem Hydrochloride, add 100 mL of 0.01 mol/L hydrochloric acid TS, shake thoroughly, and filter. To 1 mL of the filtrate add 0.01 mol/L hydrochloric acid TS to make 100 mL, and determine the absorption spectrum of this solution as directed under Ultraviolet-visible Spectrophotometry *<2.24>*: it exhibits a maximum between 234 nm and 238 nm.

Purity Related substances—Take out the content of Diltiazem Hydrochloride Extended-release Capsules, and powder. To a portion of the powder, equivalent to 50 mg of Diltiazem Hydrochloride, add 30 mL of methanol, shake vigorously for 20 minutes, then add methanol to make 50 mL, filter through a membrane filter with a pore size not exceeding 0.45 μm. Discard the first 10 mL of the filtrate, and use the subsequent filtrate as the sample solution. Pipet 3 mL of the sample solution, add methanol to make exactly 200 mL, and use this solution as the standard solution. Perform the test with exactly 20 μL each of the sample solution and standard solution as directed under Liquid Chromatography *<2.01>* according to the following conditions, and determine each peak area by the automatic integration method: the total area of the peaks other than diltiazem obtained from the sample solution is not larger than the peak area of diltiazem from the standard solution.

Operating conditions—

Detector, column, column temperature, mobile phase, and flow rate: Proceed as directed in the operating conditions in the Assay.

Time span of measurement: About 2 times as long as the retention time of diltiazem, beginning after the solvent peak.

System suitability—

System performance: Proceed as directed in the system suitability in the Assay.

Test for required detectability: Pipet 2 mL of the standard solution, and add methanol to make exactly 30 mL. Confirm that the peak area of diltiazem obtained with 20 μL of this solution is equivalent to 4.7 to 8.6% of that with 20 μL of the standard solution.

System repeatability: When the test is repeated 6 times with 20 μL of the standard solution under the above operating conditions, the relative standard deviation of the peak area of diltiazem is not more than 2.0%.

Uniformity of dosage units *<6.02>* Perform the Mass variation test, or the Content uniformity test according to the following method: it meets the requirement.

Take out the content of 1 capsule of Diltiazem Hydrochloride Extended-release Capsules, add $V/2$ mL of methanol, then add exactly $V/10$ mL of the internal standard solution, and shake vigorously for 20 minutes. Add methanol to make V mL so that each mL contains about 1 mg of diltiazem hydrochloride ($C_{22}H_{26}N_2O_4S.HCl$), and filter through a membrane filter with a pore size not exceeding 0.45 μm. Discard the first 5 mL of the filtrate, pipet 3 mL of the subsequent filtrate, add methanol to make 20 mL, and use this solution as the sample solution. Then, proceed as directed in the Assay.

Amount (mg) of diltiazem hydrochloride
($C_{22}H_{26}N_2O_4S.HCl$)
$= M_S \times Q_T/Q_S \times V/100$

M_S: Amount (mg) of diltiazem hydrochloride for assay taken

Internal standard solution—A solution of phenyl benzoate in methanol (3 in 400).

Dissolution Being specified separately when the drug is granted approval based on the Law.

Assay Take out the content of not less than 20 Diltiazem Hydrochloride Extended-release Capsules, weigh the mass of the content accurately, and powder. Weigh accurately a portion of the powder, equivalent to about 0.1 g of diltiazem hydrochloride ($C_{22}H_{26}N_2O_4S.HCl$), add 50 mL of methanol, then add exactly 10 mL of the internal standard solution, shake vigorously for 20 minutes, and add methanol to make 100 mL. Filter this solution through a membrane filter with a pore size not exceeding 0.45 μm, discard the first 5 mL of the filtrate, to 3 mL of the subsequent filtrate add methanol to make 20 mL, and use this solution as the sample solution. Separately, weigh accurately about 0.1 g of diltiazem hydrochloride for assay, previously dried at 105°C for 2 hours, dissolve in 50 mL of methanol, add exactly 10 mL of the internal standard solution, and add methanol to make 100 mL. To 3 mL of this solution add methanol to make 20 mL, and use this solution as the standard solution. Perform the test with 20 μL each of the sample solution and standard solution as directed under Liquid Chromatography *<2.01>* according to the following conditions, and calculate the ratios, Q_T and Q_S, of the peak area of diltiazem to that of the internal standard.

Amount (mg) of diltiazem hydrochloride ($C_{22}H_{26}N_2O_4S.HCl$)
$= M_S \times Q_T/Q_S$

M_S: Amount (mg) of diltiazem hydrochloride for assay taken

Internal standard solution—A solution of phenyl benzoate in methanol (3 in 400).

Operating conditions—

Detector: An ultraviolet absorption photometer (wavelength: 240 nm).

Column: A stainless steel column 4.6 mm in inside diameter and 15 cm in length, packed with octadecylsilanized silica gel for liquid chromatography (5 μm in particle diameter).

Column temperature: A constant temperature of about 50°C.

Mobile phase: Dissolve 8 g of sodium acetate trihydrate and 1.5 g of *d*-camphorsulfonic acid in 500 mL of water, and filter through a membrane filter with a pore size not exceeding 0.45 μm. To the filtrate add 250 mL of acetonitrile and 250 mL of methanol.

Flow rate: Adjust so that the retention time of diltiazem is about 9 minutes.

System suitability—

System performance: Dissolve 30 mg of diltiazem hydrochloride, 20 mg of *d*-3-hydroxy-*cis*-2,3-dihydro-5-[2-(dimethylamino)ethyl]-2-(4-methoxyphenyl)-1,5-benzothiazepin-4(5*H*)-on hydrochloride (hereinafter referred to as de-acetyl substance) and 20 mg of phenyl benzoate in methanol to make 200 mL. When the procedure is run with 20 μL of this solution under the above operating conditions, de-acetyl substance, diltiazem and phenyl benzoate are eluted in this order and the resolutions between the peaks of de-acetyl substance and diltiazem and the peaks of diltiazem and phenyl benzoate are not less than 2.5, respectively.

System repeatability: When the test is repeated 6 times with 20 μL of the standard solution under the above operating conditions, the relative standard deviation of the ratio of the peak area of diltiazem to that of the internal standard is not more than 1.0%.

Containers and storage Containers—Tight containers.

Dimemorfan Phosphate

ジメモルファンリン酸塩

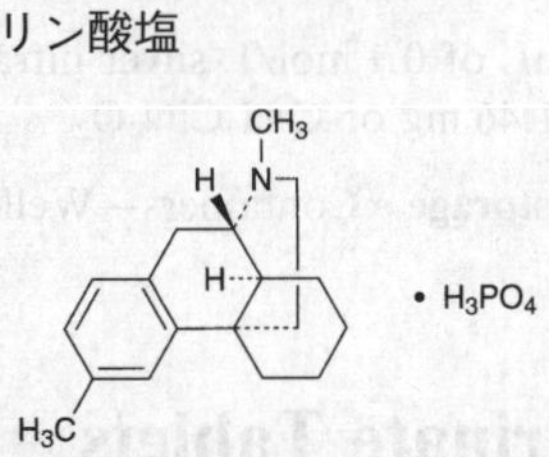

$C_{18}H_{25}N.H_3PO_4$: 353.39
(9*S*,13*S*,14*S*)-3,17-Dimethylmorphinan monophosphate
[*36304-84-4*]

Dimemorfan Phosphate, when dried, contains not less than 98.5% of dimemorfan phosphate ($C_{18}H_{25}N.H_3PO_4$).

Description Dimemorfan Phosphate occurs as white to pale yellow-white, crystals or crystalline powder.

It is freely soluble in acetic acid (100), sparingly soluble in water and in methanol, slightly soluble in ethanol (95), and practically insoluble in diethyl ether.

Melting point: about 265°C (with decomposition).

Identification (1) Determine the absorption spectrum of a solution of Dimemorfan Phosphate (1 in 5000) as directed under Ultraviolet-visible Spectrophotometry <*2.24*>, and compare the spectrum with the Reference Spectrum: both spectra exhibit similar intensities of absorption at the same wavelengths.

(2) Determine the infrared absorption spectrum of Dimemorfan Phosphate, previously dried, as directed in the potassium bromide disk method under Infrared Spectrophotometry <*2.25*>, and compare the spectrum with the Reference Spectrum: both spectra exhibits similar intensities of absorption at the same wave numbers.

(3) To 2 mL of a solution of Dimemorfan Phosphate (1 in 100) add 2 to 3 drops of silver nitrate TS: a yellow precipitate is formed, and it dissolves on the addition of dilute nitric acid.

Optical rotation <*2.49*> $[\alpha]_D^{20}$: +25 – +27° (after drying, 1 g, methanol, 100 mL, 100 mm).

pH <*2.54*> Dissolve 1.0 g of Dimemorfan Phosphate in 100 mL of water: the pH of this solution is between 4.0 and 5.0.

Purity (1) Heavy metals <*1.07*>—Proceed with 1.0 g of Dimemorfan Phosphate according to Method 1, and perform the test. Prepare the control solution with 2.0 mL of Standard Lead Solution (not more than 20 ppm).

(2) Arsenic <*1.11*>—Prepare the test solution with 1.0 g of Dimemorfan Phosphate according to Method 3, and perform the test. Use 10 mL of a solution of magnesium nitrate hexahydrate in ethanol (95) (1 in 10) (not more than 2 ppm).

(3) Related substances—Dissolve 0.10 g of Dimemorfan Phosphate in 10 mL of methanol, and use this solution as the sample solution. Pipet 1 mL of the sample solution, add methanol to make exactly 100 mL, and use this solution as the standard solution. Perform the test with these solutions as directed under Thin-layer Chromatography <*2.03*>. Spot 10 μL each of the sample solution and standard solution on a plate of silica gel for thin-layer chromatography. Develop the plate with a mixture of methanol, chloroform and ammonia solution (28) (150:150:1) to a distance of about 10 cm, and air-dry the plate. Spray evenly the plate with Dragendorff's TS for spraying: the spots other than the principal spot obtained from the sample solution are not more intense than the spot from the standard solution.

Loss on drying <*2.41*> Not more than 0.5% (1 g, 105°C, 3 hours).

Assay Weigh accurately about 0.6 g of Dimemorfan Phosphate, previously dried, dissolve in 100 mL of acetic acid (100), and titrate <*2.50*> with 0.1 mol/L perchloric acid VS (potentiometric titration). Perform a blank determination in the same manner, and make any necessary correction.

Each mL of 0.1 mol/L perchloric acid VS
= 35.34 mg of $C_{18}H_{25}N.H_3PO_4$

Containers and storage Containers—Tight containers.

The JP Drugs are to be tested according to the provisions given in the pertinent monographs, General Notices, General Rules for Crude Drugs, General Rules for Preparations, and General Tests for their conformity to the Japanese Pharmacopoeia. (See the General Notices 5.)

Dimenhydrinate

ジメンヒドリナート

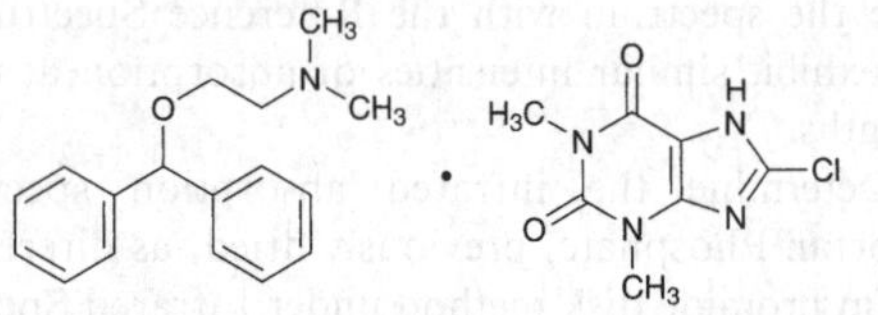

$C_{17}H_{21}NO.C_7H_7ClN_4O_2$: 469.96
2-(Diphenylmethoxy)-*N*,*N*-dimethylethylamine—
8-chloro-1,3-dimethyl-1*H*-purine-2,6(3*H*,7*H*)-dione (1/1)
[*523-87-5*]

Dimenhydrinate, when dried, contains not less than 53.0% and not more than 55.5% of diphenhydramine ($C_{17}H_{21}NO$: 255.36), and not less than 44.0% and not more than 47.0% of 8-chlorotheophylline ($C_7H_7ClN_4O_2$: 214.61).

Description Dimenhydrinate occurs as a white crystalline powder. It is odorless, and has a bitter taste.

It is very soluble in chloroform, freely soluble in ethanol (95), and slightly soluble in water and in diethyl ether.

Identification **(1)** Dissolve 0.5 g of Dimenhydrinate in 30 mL of dilute ethanol, add 30 mL of water, and use this solution as the sample solution. Transfer 30 mL of the sample solution to a separator, and add 2 mL of ammonia solution (28). Extract with two 10-mL portions of diethyl ether, combine the diethyl ether extracts, wash the combined extracts with 5 mL of water, and then extract the combined extracts with 15 mL of diluted hydrochloric acid (1 in 100). With this acid extract perform the following tests.

(i) To 5 mL of this acid extract add 5 drops of Reinecke salt TS: a light red precipitate is produced.

(ii) To 10 mL of this acid extract add 10 mL of 2,4,6-trinitrophenol TS dropwise, and allow to stand for 30 minutes. Collect the precipitate by filtrating, recrystallize from dilute ethanol, and dry at 105°C for 30 minutes: the crystals melt 〈*2.60*〉 between 128°C and 133°C.

(2) To 30 mL of the sample solution obtained in (1) add 2 mL of dilute sulfuric acid, and cool for 30 minutes. Scratch the inside wall of the container frequently to facilitate crystallization. Filter, and wash the white crystals with a small amount of ice-cooled water. Dry the crystals for 1 hour at 105°C: the crystals melt 〈*2.60*〉 between 300°C and 305°C with decomposition.

(3) To 0.01 g of the crystals obtained in (2) add 10 drops of hydrogen peroxide TS and 1 drop of hydrochloric acid, and evaporate on a water bath to dryness: the residue shows a yellow-red color. When the dish containing the residue is held over a vessel containing 2 to 3 drops of ammonia TS, the color changes to red-purple, which is discharged on the addition of 2 to 3 drops of sodium hydroxide TS.

(4) Mix well 0.05 g of the crystals obtained in (2) with 0.5 g of sodium peroxide in a nickel crucible, and heat until the mass melts. Cool, dissolve the melted mass in 20 mL of water, and acidify with dilute nitric acid: the solution responds to Qualitative Tests 〈*1.09*〉 for chloride.

Melting point 〈*2.60*〉 102 – 107°C

Purity **(1)** Chloride 〈*1.03*〉—Transfer 50 mL of the filtrate obtained in the Assay (2) to a Nessler tube, add 1 mL of nitric acid, and allow to stand for 5 minutes: the turbidity of the solution is not greater than that of the following control solution (not more than 0.044%).

Control solution: Dilute 0.25 mL of 0.01 mol/L hydrochloric acid VS with 6 mL of dilute nitric acid and with water to make 50 mL, add 1 mL of silver nitrate TS, and allow to stand for 5 minutes.

(2) Bromide and iodide—Place 0.10 g of Dimenhydrinate in a glass-stoppered test tube, and add 0.05 g of sodium nitrite, 10 mL of chloroform and 10 mL of dilute hydrochloric acid. Stopper, shake well, and allow to stand: the chloroform layer remains colorless.

Loss on drying 〈*2.41*〉 Not more than 0.5% (3 g, in vacuum, phosphorus (V) oxide, 24 hours).

Residue on ignition 〈*2.44*〉 Not more than 0.3% (1 g).

Assay **(1)** Diphenhydramine—Weigh accurately about 0.5 g of Dimenhydrinate, previously dried, transfer to a 250-mL separator, and add 50 mL of water, 3 mL of ammonia TS and 10 g of sodium chloride. Extract with six 15-mL portions of diethyl ether with shaking, combine the diethyl ether extracts, and wash the combined diethyl ether extracts with three 50-mL portions of water. To the diethyl ether extracts add exactly 25 mL of 0.05 mol/L sulfuric acid VS, and add 25 mL of water. Shake thoroughly, and evaporate the diethyl ether gently. Cool, and titrate the excess sulfuric acid with 0.1 mol/L sodium hydroxide VS (indicator: 3 drops of methyl red TS). Perform a blank determination in the same manner, and make any necessary correction.

Each mL of 0.05 mol/L sulfuric acid VS
= 25.54 mg $C_{17}H_{21}NO$

(2) 8-Chlorotheophylline—Weigh accurately about 0.8 g of Dimenhydrinate, previously dried, transfer to a 200-mL volumetric flask, add 50 mL of water, 3 mL of ammonia TS and 6 mL of a solution of ammonium nitrate (1 in 10), and heat on a water bath for 5 minutes. Add exactly 25 mL of 0.1 mol/L silver nitrate VS, heat on a water bath for 15 minutes with occasional shaking, cool, and add water to make exactly 200 mL. Allow to stand overnight to settle the precipitate, and filter through a dry filter paper, discarding the first 20 mL of the filtrate. Measure exactly 100 mL of the subsequent filtrate, acidify with nitric acid, add 3 mL of nitric acid, and titrate the excess silver nitrate with 0.1 mol/L ammonium thiocyanate VS (indicator: 2 mL of ammonium iron (III) sulfate TS). Perform a blank determination in the same manner, and make any necessary correction.

Each mL of 0.1 mol/L silver nitrate VS
= 21.46 mg of $C_7H_7ClN_4O_2$

Containers and storage Containers—Well-closed containers.

Dimenhydrinate Tablets

ジメンヒドリナート錠

Dimenhydrinate Tablets contain not less than 95.0% and not more than 105.0% of the labeled amount of dimenhydrinate ($C_{17}H_{21}NO.C_7H_7ClN_4O_2$: 469.96).

Method of preparation Prepare as directed under Tablets, with Dimenhydrinate.

Identification **(1)** Triturate a quantity of powdered Dimenhydrinate Tablets, equivalent to 0.5 g of Dimenhydrinate, with 25 mL of warm ethanol (95), and filter.

Dilute the filtrate with 40 mL of water, and filter again. Use the filtrate as the sample solution. Transfer 30 mL of the sample solution to a separator, and proceed as directed in the Identification (1) under Dimenhydrinate.

(2) With 30 mL of the sample solution obtained in (1), proceed as directed in the Identification (2), (3) and (4) under Dimenhydrinate.

Dissolution <*6.10*> When the test is performed at 50 revolutions per minute according to the Paddle method, using 900 mL of water as the dissolution medium, the dissolution rate in 15 minutes of Dimenhydrinate Tablets is not less than 85%.

Start the test with 1 tablet of Dimenhydrinate Tablets, withdraw not less than 20 mL of the medium at the specified minute after starting the test, and filter through a membrane filter with a pore size not exceeding 0.45 μm. Discard not less than 10 mL of the first filtrate, pipet V mL of the subsequent filtrate, add water to make exactly V' mL so that each mL contains about 28 μg of dimenhydrinate ($C_{17}H_{21}NO.C_7H_7ClN_4O_2$), and use this solution as the sample solution. Separately, weigh accurately about 28 mg of dimenhydrinate for assay, previously dried in vacuum using phosphorous (V) oxide as the desiccant for 24 hours, and dissolve in water to make exactly 50 mL. Pipet 5 mL of this solution, add water to make exactly 100 mL, and use this solution as the standard solution. Determine the absorbances, A_T and A_S, of the sample solution and standard solution at 276 nm as directed under Ultraviolet-visible Spectrophotometry <*2.24*>.

Dissolution rate (%) with respect to the labeled amount of dimenhydrinate ($C_{17}H_{21}NO.C_7H_7ClN_4O_2$)
$= M_S \times A_T/A_S \times V'/V \times 1/C \times 90$

M_S: Amount (mg) of dimenhydrinate for assay taken
C: Labeled amount (mg) of dimenhydrinate ($C_{17}H_{21}NO.C_7H_7ClN_4O_2$) in 1 tablet

Assay Weigh accurately, and powder not less than 20 Dimenhydrinate Tablets. Weigh accurately a portion of the powder, equivalent to about 0.5 g of dimenhydrinate ($C_{17}H_{21}NO.C_7H_7ClN_4O_2$), transfer to a flask, add 40 mL of ethanol (95), and heat with swirling on a water bath until the solution just boils. Continue to heat for 30 seconds, and filter through a glass filter (G4). Wash the filter with warm ethanol (95), transfer the filtrate and washings to a flask, and evaporate the ethanol on a water bath to make 5 mL. Add 50 mL of water, 3 mL of ammonia TS and 6 mL of a solution of ammonium nitrate (1 in 10), heat the mixture on a water bath for 5 minutes, add exactly 25 mL of 0.1 mol/L silver nitrate VS, and heat on a water bath for 15 minutes with occasional shaking. Transfer the mixture to a 200-mL volumetric flask, using water to rinse the flask, cool, add water to make exactly 200 mL, and proceed as directed in the Assay (2) under Dimenhydrinate.

Each mL of 0.1 mol/L silver nitrate VS
$= 47.00$ mg of $C_{17}H_{21}NO.C_7H_7ClN_4O_2$

Containers and storage Containers—Well-closed containers.

Dimercaprol

ジメルカプロール

HS, H SH, OH and enantiomer

$C_3H_8OS_2$: 124.23
(2*RS*)-2,3-Disulfanylpropan-1-ol
[*59-52-9*]

Dimercaprol contains not less than 98.5% and not more than 101.5% of dimercaprol ($C_3H_8OS_2$).

Description Dimercaprol is a colorless or pale yellow liquid. It has a mercaptan-like, disagreeable odor.

It is miscible with methanol and with ethanol (99.5)

It is soluble in peanut oil, and sparingly soluble in water.

It shows no optical rotation.

Identification **(1)** Add 1 drop of Dimercaprol to a mixture of 1 drop of a solution of cobalt (II) chloride hexahydrate (1 in 200) and 5 mL of water: a yellow-brown color develops.

(2) Determine the infrared absorption spectrum of Dimercaprol as directed in the liquid film method under Infrared Spectrophotometry <*2.25*>, and compare the spectrum with the Reference Spectrum: both spectra exhibit similar intensities of absorption at the same wave numbers.

Refractive index <*2.45*> n_D^{20}: 1.570 – 1.575

Specific gravity <*2.56*> d_{20}^{20}: 1.238 – 1.248

Purity **(1)** Clarity and color of solution—Dissolve 1.0 mL of Dimercaprol in 20 mL of peanut oil: the solution is clear and colorless to pale yellow.

(2) Bromide—To 2.0 g of Dimercaprol add 25 mL of dilute potassium hydroxide-ethanol TS, and heat in a water bath under a reflux condenser for 2 hours. Evaporate the ethanol in a current of warm air, add 20 mL of water, and cool. Add a mixture of 10 mL of hydrogen peroxide (30) and 40 mL of water, boil gently under a reflux condenser for 10 minutes, and filter rapidly after cooling. Wash the residue with two 10-mL portions of water, combine the washings with the filtrate, add 10 mL of dilute nitric acid and exactly 5 mL of 0.1 mol/L silver nitrate VS, and titrate <*2.50*> the excess silver nitrate with 0.1 mol/L ammonium thiocyanate VS (indicator: 2 mL of ammonium iron (III) sulfate TS). Perform a blank determination in the same manner: not more than 1.0 mL of 0.1 mol/L silver nitrate VS is consumed.

(3) Heavy metals <*1.07*>—Proceed with 1.0 g of Dimercaprol according to Method 2, and perform the test. Prepare the control solution with 2.0 mL of Standard Lead Solution (not more than 20 ppm).

Assay Weigh accurately about 0.15 g of Dimercaprol into a glass-stoppered flask, dissolve in 10 mL of methanol, and titrate <*2.50*> immediately with 0.05 mol/L iodine VS until a pale yellow color is produced. Perform a blank determination in the same manner, and make any necessary correction.

Each mL of 0.05 mol/L iodine VS = 6.212 mg of $C_3H_8OS_2$

Containers and storage Containers—Tight containers.

Storage—Not exceeding 5°C.

Dimercaprol Injection

ジメルカプロール注射液

Dimercaprol Injection is an oily solution for injection.

It contains not less than 95.0% and not more than 105.0% of the labeled amount of dimercaprol ($C_3H_8OS_2$: 124.23).

Method of preparation Prepare as directed under Injections, with Dimercaprol. Benzyl Benzoate or Benzyl Alcohol may be added to increase the solubility.

Description Dimercaprol Injection is a clear, colorless or light yellow liquid. It has an unpleasant odor.

Identification Measure a volume of Dimercaprol Injection, equivalent to 30 mg of Dimercaprol, and proceed as directed in the Identification (1) under Dimercaprol.

Extractable volume ⟨*6.05*⟩ It meets the requirement.

Foreign insoluble matter ⟨*6.06*⟩ Perform the test according to Method 1: it meets the requirement.

Insoluble particulate matter ⟨*6.07*⟩ Perform the test according to Method 2: it meets the requirement.

Sterility ⟨*4.06*⟩ Perform the test according to the Membrane filtration method: it meets the requirement.

Assay Pipet a volume of Dimercaprol Injection, equivalent to about 0.1 g of dimercaprol ($C_3H_8OS_2$), into a flask, and rinse the pipet several times with a mixture of methanol and diethyl ether (3:1), adding the rinsings to the flask. Add the mixture of methanol and diethyl ether (3:1) to make 50 mL, and titrate ⟨*2.50*⟩ with 0.05 mol/L iodine VS until a yellow color persists. Perform a blank determination in the same manner, and make any necessary correction.

Each mL of 0.05 mol/L iodine VS
= 6.212 mg of $C_3H_8OS_2$

Containers and storage Containers—Hermetic containers.
Storage—In a cold place.

Dimorpholamine

ジモルホラミン

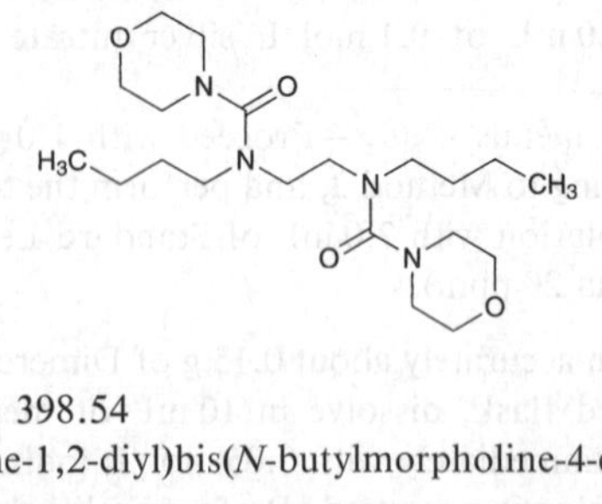

$C_{20}H_{38}N_4O_4$: 398.54
N,*N*′-(Ethane-1,2-diyl)bis(*N*-butylmorpholine-4-carboxamide)
[*119-48-2*]

Dimorpholamine, when dried, contains not less than 98.0% and not more than 101.0% of dimorpholamine ($C_{20}H_{38}N_4O_4$).

Description Dimorpholamine is a white to light yellow, crystalline powder, masses or syrupy liquid.

It is very soluble in ethanol (99.5) and in acetic anhydride, and soluble in water.

The pH of a solution prepared by dissolving 1.0 g of Dimorpholamine in 10 mL of water is between 6.0 and 7.0.

It is hygroscopic.

Identification (1) Determine the absorption spectrum of a solution of Dimorpholamine (1 in 50,000) as directed under Ultraviolet-visible Spectrophotometry ⟨*2.24*⟩, and compare the spectrum with the Reference Spectrum: both spectra exhibit similar intensities of absorption at the same wavelengths.

(2) Determine the infrared absorption spectrum of Dimorpholamine, previously dried, as directed in the potassium bromide disk method under the Infrared Spectrophotometry ⟨*2.25*⟩, and compare the spectrum with the Reference Spectrum: both spectra exhibit similar intensities of absorption at the same wave numbers.

Purity (1) Clarity and color of solution—Dissolve 1.0 g of Dimorpholamine in 50 mL of water: the solution is clear and colorless to pale yellow.

(2) Chloride ⟨*1.03*⟩—To 20 mL of the solution obtained in (1) add 6 mL of dilute nitric acid and water to make 50 mL. Perform the test using this solution as the test solution. Prepare the control solution with 0.40 mL of 0.01 mol/L hydrochloric acid VS (not more than 0.036%).

(3) Sulfate ⟨*1.14*⟩—To 10 mL of the solution obtained in (1) add 1 mL of dilute hydrochloric acid and water to make 50 mL. Perform the test using this solution as the test solution. Prepare the control solution with 0.40 mL of 0.005 mol/L sulfuric acid VS (not more than 0.096%).

(4) Heavy metals ⟨*1.07*⟩—Proceed with 2.0 g of Dimorpholamine according to Method 2, and perform the test. Prepare the control solution with 2.0 mL of Standard Lead Solution (not more than 10 ppm).

(5) Related substances—Dissolve 0.20 g of Dimorpholamine in 10 mL of ethanol (99.5), and use this solution as the sample solution. Pipet 1 mL of the sample solution, add ethanol (99.5) to make exactly 100 mL, and use this solution as the standard solution. Perform the test with these solutions as directed under Thin-layer Chromatography ⟨*2.03*⟩. Spot 10 μL each of the sample solution and standard solution on a plate of silica gel for thin-layer chromatography. Develop the plate with a mixture of ethanol (99.5) and water (4:1) to a distance of about 10 cm, and air-dry the plate. Allow the plate to stand in iodine vapor for 10 minutes: the spot other than the principal spot obtained from the sample solution is not more intense than the spot from the standard solution.

Loss on drying ⟨*2.41*⟩ Not more than 0.5% (1 g, in vacuum, phosphorus (V) oxide, 8 hours).

Residue on ignition ⟨*2.44*⟩ Not more than 0.1% (1 g).

Assay Weigh accurately about 0.6 g of Dimorpholamine, previously dried, dissolve in 50 mL of acetic anhydride, and titrate ⟨*2.50*⟩ with 0.1 mol/L perchloric acid VS (potentiometric titration). Perform a blank determination in the same manner, and make any necessary correction.

Each mL of 0.1 mol/L perchloric acid VS
= 39.85 mg of $C_{20}H_{38}N_4O_4$

Containers and storage Containers—Tight containers.
Storage—Light-resistant.

Dimorpholamine Injection

ジモルホラミン注射液

Dimorpholamine Injection is an aqueous injection.

It contains not less than 95.0% and not more than 105.0% of the labeled amount of dimorpholamine ($C_{20}H_{38}N_4O_4$: 398.54).

Method of preparation Prepare as directed under Injections, with Dimorpholamine.

Description Dimorpholamine Injection is a clear, colorless liquid.

pH: 3.0 – 5.5

Identification **(1)** To a volume of Dimorpholamine Injection, equivalent to 0.1 g of Dimorpholamine, add 3 drops of Dragendorff's TS: an orange color develops.

(2) To a volume of Dimorpholamine Injection, equivalent to 50 mg of Dimorpholamine, add 1 mL of dilute hydrochloric acid, and evaporate on a water bath to dryness. Dissolve the residue in 2 mL of hydrochloric acid, boil for 10 minutes under a reflux condenser, and evaporate to dryness on a water bath. Dissolve the residue with 1 mL of water, neurtralize with sodium hydroxide TS, and add 0.2 mL of a solution of acetaldehyde (1 in 20), 0.1 mL of sodium pentacyanonitrosyl ferrate (III) TS and 0.5 mL of sodium carbonate TS: a blue color develops.

Bacterial endotoxins *<4.01>* Less than 5.0 EU/mg. Perform the test with the sample diluted to 0.15 w/v% with water for bacterial endotoxins test.

Extractable volume *<6.05>* It meets the requirement.

Foreign insoluble matter *<6.06>* Perform the test according to Method 1: it meets the requirement.

Insoluble particulate matter *<6.07>* It meets the requirement.

Sterility *<4.06>* Perform the test according to the Membrane filtration method: it meets the requirement.

Assay Pipet a volume of Dimorpholamine Injection, equivalent to about 30 mg of dimorpholamine ($C_{20}H_{38}N_4O_4$), and add water to make exactly 200 mL. Pipet 1 mL of this solution, shake with exactly 4 mL of the internal standard solution for 5 minutes, and use this solution as the sample solution. Separately, weigh accurately about 0.15 g of dimorpholamine for assay, previously dried in a desiccator (in vacuum, phosphorus (V) oxide) for 8 hours, and dissolve in water to make exactly 1000 mL. Pipet 1 mL of this solution, shake with exactly 4 mL of the internal standard solution for 5 minutes, and use this solution as the standard solution. Perform the test with 10 μL each of the sample solution and standard solution as directed under Liquid Chromatography *<2.01>* according to the following conditions, and calculate the ratios, Q_T and Q_S, of the peak area of dimorpholamine to that of the internal standard.

Amount (mg) of dimorpholamine ($C_{20}H_{38}N_4O_4$)
$= M_S \times Q_T/Q_S \times 1/5$

M_S: Amount (mg) of dimorpholamine for assay taken

Internal standard solution—A solution of butyl parahydroxybenzoate in acetonitrile (1 in 25,000).

Operating conditions—

Detector: An ultraviolet absorption photometer (wavelength: 216 nm).

Column: A stainless steel column 4.6 mm in inside diameter and 15 cm in length, packed with octadecylsilanized silica gel for liquid chromatography (5 μm in particle diameter).

Column temperature: A constant temperature of about 40°C.

Mobile phase: A mixture of water and acetonitrile (1:1).

Flow rate: Adjust so that the retention time of dimorpholamine is about 4 minutes.

System suitability—

System performance: When the procedure is run with 10 μL of the standard solution under the above operating conditions, dimorpholamine and the internal standard are eluted in this order with the resolution between these peaks being not less than 2.0.

System repeatability: When the test is repeated 6 times with 10 μL of the standard solution under the above operating conditions, the relative standard deviation of the ratio of the peak area of dimorpholamine to that of the internal standard is not more than 1.0%.

Containers and storage Containers—Hermetic containers.

Dinoprost

ジノプロスト

$C_{20}H_{34}O_5$: 354.48

(5*Z*)-7-{(1*R*,2*R*,3*R*,5*S*)-3,5-Dihydroxy-2-[(1*E*,3*S*)-3-hydroxyoct-1-en-1-yl]cyclopentyl}hept-5-enoic acid

[551-11-1]

Dinoprost contains not less than 98.5% of dinoprost ($C_{20}H_{34}O_5$), calculated on the anhydrous basis.

Description Dinoprost occurs as white, waxy masses or powder, or a clear, colorless to light yellow and viscous liquid. It is odorless.

It is very soluble in *N*,*N*-dimethylformamide, freely soluble in methanol, in ethanol (99.5) and in diethyl ether, and very slightly soluble in water.

Identification **(1)** To 5 mg of Dinoprost add 2 mL of sulfuric acid, and dissolve by shaking for 5 minutes: a dark red color develops. To this solution add 30 mL of sulfuric acid: an orange color develops with a green fluorescence.

(2) Dissolve 1 mg of Dinoprost in 50 mL of diluted sulfuric acid (7 in 10), and warm in a water bath warmed at 50°C for 40 minutes. After cooling, determine the absorption spectrum of the solution as directed under Ultraviolet-visible Spectrophotometry *<2.24>*, and compare the spectrum with the Reference Spectrum: both spectra exhibit similar intensities of absorption at the same wavelengths.

(3) Warm Dinoprost at 40°C to effect a liquid, and determine the infrared absorption spectrum of the liquid as directed in the liquid film method under Infrared Spectrophotometry *<2.25>*, and compare the spectrum with the Reference Spectrum: both spectra exhibits similar intensities of absorption at the same wave numbers.

Optical rotation *<2.49>* $[\alpha]_D^{20}$: +24 – +31° (0.2 g, ethanol (99.5), 10 mL, 100 mm).

Purity (1) Clarity and color of solution—Dissolve 0.20 g of Dinoprost in 5 mL of ethanol (99.5): the solution is clear and colorless to pale yellow.

(2) Related substances—Dissolve 10 mg of Dinoprost in 2 mL of methanol, add water to make 10 mL, and use this solution as the sample solution. Pipet 3 mL of the sample solution, add diluted methanol (1 in 5) to make exactly 100 mL, and use this solution as the standard solution. Perform the test with exactly 10 μL each of the sample solution and standard solution as directed under Liquid Chromatography <*2.01*> according to the following conditions. Determine each peak area of these solutions by the automatic integration method: the total area of the peaks other than dinoprost obtained from the sample solution is not larger than the peak area of dinoprost from the standard solution.

Operating conditions—

Detector: An ultraviolet absorption photometer (wavelength: 205 nm).

Column: A stainless steel column about 5 mm in inside diameter and about 15 cm in length, packed with octadecylsilanized silica gel for liquid chromatography (5 μm in particle diameter).

Column temperature: A constant temperature of about 25°C.

Mobile phase: A mixture of 0.02 mol/L potassium dihydrogenphosphate TS and acetonitrile (5:2).

Flow rate: Adjust so that the retention time of dinoprost is about 20 minutes.

Selection of column: Dissolve 0.01 g each of isopropyl parahydroxybenzoate and propyl parahydroxybenzoate in 2 mL of methanol, and add water to make 10 mL. To 1 mL of this solution add diluted methanol (1 in 5) to make 30 mL, proceed with 10 μL of this solution under the above operating conditions, and calculate the resolution. Use a column giving elution of isopropyl parahydroxybenzoate and propyl parahydroxybenzoate in this order with the resolution between these peaks being not less than 2.5.

Detection sensitivity: Adjust the detection sensitivity so that the peak height of dinoprost from the standard solution composes 5% to 15% of the full scale.

Time span of measurement: About 1.5 times as long as the retention time of dinoprost, beginning after the solvent peak.

Water <*2.48*> Not more than 0.5% (0.3 g, volumetric titration, direct titration).

Assay Weigh accurately about 50 mg of Dinoprost, dissolve in 30 mL of *N,N*-dimethylformamide, and titrate <*2.50*> with 0.02 mol/L tetramethylammonium hydroxide VS under a stream of nitrogen (potentiometric titration). Perform a blank determination in the same manner, and make any necessary correction.

Each mL of 0.02 mol/L tetramethylammonium hydroxide VS
= 7.090 mg of $C_{20}H_{34}O_5$

Containers and storage Containers—Tight containers.

Storage—Light-resistant, and in a place not exceeding 5°C.

Diphenhydramine

ジフェンヒドラミン

$C_{17}H_{21}NO$: 255.35
2-(Diphenylmethoxy)-*N,N*-dimethylethylamine
[*58-73-1*]

Diphenhydramine contains not less than 96.0% of diphenhydramine ($C_{17}H_{21}NO$).

Description Diphenhydramine is a clear, light yellow to yellow liquid. It has a characteristic odor, and has a burning taste at first, followed by a slight sensation of numbness on the tongue.

It is miscible with acetic anhydride, with acetic acid (100), with ethanol (95) and with diethyl ether.

It is very slightly soluble in water.

It is gradually affected by light.

Refractive index n_D^{20}: about 1.55

Boiling point: about 162°C (in vacuum, 0.67 kPa).

Identification (1) To 50 mg of Diphenhydramine add 2 mL of sulfuric acid: an orange-red precipitate is produced immediately, and its color changes to red-brown on standing. Add carefully 2 mL of water to this solution: the intensity of the color changes, but the color tone does not change.

(2) Dissolve 0.1 g of Diphenhydramine in 10 mL of dilute ethanol, add an excess of a saturated solution of 2,4,6-trinitrophenol in dilute ethanol with stirring, and cool in ice. Collect the produced crystals, recrystallize from dilute ethanol, and dry at 105°C for 30 minutes: the crystals melt <*2.60*> between 128°C and 133°C.

Specific gravity <*2.56*> d_{20}^{20}: 1.013 – 1.020

Purity (1) β-Dimethylaminoethanol—Dissolve 1.0 g of Diphenhydramine in 20 mL of diethyl ether, and extract with two 10-mL portions of water with thorough shaking. Combine the water extracts, and add 2 drops of phenolphthalein TS and 1.0 mL of 0.05 mol/L sulfuric acid VS: no red color develops.

(2) Benzohydrol—Transfer 1.0 g of Diphenhydramine to a separator, dissolve in 20 mL of diethyl ether, and extract with two 25-mL portions of diluted hydrochloric acid (1 in 15) with thorough shaking. Separate the diethyl ether layer, evaporate slowly on a water bath, and dry in a desiccator (in vacuum, silica gel) for 2 hours: the mass of the residue is not more than 20 mg.

(3) Heavy metals <*1.07*>—Proceed with 1.0 g of Diphenhydramine according to Method 2, and perform the test. Prepare the control solution with 2.0 mL of Standard Lead Solution (not more than 20 ppm).

Residue on ignition <*2.44*> Not more than 0.1% (1 g).

Assay Weigh accurately about 0.5 g of Diphenhydramine, dissolve in 50 mL of a mixture of acetic anhydride and acetic acid (100) (7:3), and titrate <*2.50*> with 0.1 mol/L perchloric acid VS (potentiometric titration). Perform a blank determination in the same manner, and make any necessary correction.

Each mL of 0.1 mol/L perchloric acid VS
= 25.54 mg of $C_{17}H_{21}NO$

Containers and storage Containers—Tight containers.
Storage—Light-resistant, and almost well-filled.

Diphenhydramine Hydrochloride

ジフェンヒドラミン塩酸塩

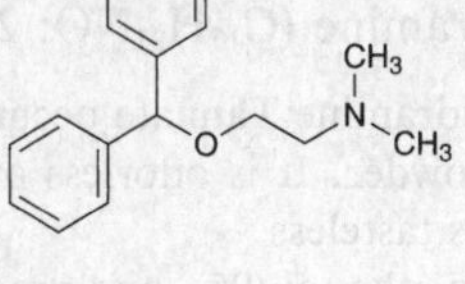

$C_{17}H_{21}NO.HCl$: 291.82
2-(Diphenylmethoxy)-*N*,*N*-dimethylethylamine monohydrochloride
[*147-24-0*]

Diphenhydramine Hydrochloride, when dried, contains not less than 98.0% of diphenhydramine hydrochloride ($C_{17}H_{21}NO.HCl$).

Description Diphenhydramine Hydrochloride occurs as white, crystals or crystalline powder. It is odorless, and has a bitter taste, followed by a sensation of numbness on the tongue.

It is very soluble in methanol and in acetic acid (100), freely soluble in water and in ethanol (95), sparingly soluble in acetic anhydride, and practically insoluble in diethyl ether.

It is gradually affected by light.

Identification **(1)** Determine the absorption spectrum of a solution of Diphenhydramine Hydrochloride in methanol (1 in 2000) as directed under Ultraviolet-visible Spectrophotometry 〈*2.24*〉, and compare the spectrum with the Reference Spectrum: both spectra exhibit similar intensities of absorption at the same wavelengths.

(2) Determine the infrared absorption spectrum of Dipenhydramine Hydrochloride as directed in the potassium chloride disk method under Infrared Spectrophotometry 〈*2.25*〉, and compare the spectrum with the Reference Spectrum: both spectra exhibit similar intensities of absorption at the same wave numbers.

(3) A solution of Diphenhydramine Hydrochloride (1 in 50) responds to Qualitative Tests 〈*1.09*〉 for chloride.

pH 〈*2.54*〉 Dissolve 1.0 g of Diphenhydramine Hydrochloride in 10 mL of water: the pH of this solution is between 4.0 and 5.0.

Melting point 〈*2.60*〉 166 – 170°C

Purity **(1)** Clarity and color of solution—Dissolve 1.0 g of Diphenhydramine Hydrochloride in 10 mL of water: the solution is clear and colorless.

(2) Heavy metals 〈*1.07*〉—Proceed with 1.0 g of Diphenhydramine Hydrochloride according to Method 4, and perform the test. Prepare the control solution with 2.0 mL of Standard Lead Solution (not more than 20 ppm).

(3) Related substances—Dissolve 0.20 g of Diphenhydramine Hydrochloride in 10 mL of methanol, and use this solution as the sample solution. Pipet 1 mL of the sample solution, add methanol to make exactly 200 mL, and use this solution as the standard solution. Perform the test with these solutions as directed under Thin-layer Chromatography 〈*2.03*〉. Spot 5 μL each of the sample solution and standard solution on a plate of silica gel for thin-layer chromatography. Develop the plate with a mixture of hexane, ethyl acetate, methanol and ammonia solution (28) (10:4:2:1) to a distance of about 10 cm, and air-dry the plate. Spray evenly iodine TS on the plate: the spots other than the principal spot and the spot on the original point from the sample solution are not more intense than the spot from the standard solution.

Loss on drying 〈*2.41*〉 Not more than 0.5% (2 g, 105°C, 3 hours).

Residue on ignition 〈*2.44*〉 Not more than 0.1% (1 g).

Assay Weigh accurately about 0.4 g of Diphenhydramine Hydrochloride, previously dried, dissolve in 50 mL of a mixture of acetic anhydride and acetic acid (100) (7:3). Titrate 〈*2.50*〉 with 0.1 mol/L perchloric acid VS (potentiometric titration). Perform a blank determination in the same manner, and make any necessary correction.

Each mL of 0.1 mol/L perchloric acid VS
= 29.18 mg of $C_{17}H_{21}NO.HCl$

Containers and storage Containers—Tight containers.
Storage—Light-resistant.

Diphenhydramine and Bromovalerylurea Powder

ジフェンヒドラミン・バレリル尿素散

Method of preparation

Diphenhydramine Tannate	90 g
Bromovalerylurea	500 g
Starch, Lactose Hydrate, or their mixture	a sufficient quantity
To make	1000 g

Prepare as directed under Powders, with the above ingredients.

Description Diphenhydramine and Bromovalcrylurea Powder occurs as a slightly grayish white powder.

Identification **(1)** To 0.1 g of Diphenhydramine and Bromovalerylurea Powder add 5 mL of dilute hydrochloric acid, 1 mL of ethanol (95) and 10 mL of water, shake, and filter. To the filtrate add 10 mL of sodium hydroxide TS, and extract with 10 mL of chloroform. Separate the chloroform layer, add 1 mL of bromophenol blue TS, and shake: a yellow color develops in the chloroform layer (diphenhydramine tannate).

(2) Shake 0.02 g of Diphenhydramine and Bromovalerylurea Powder with 10 mL of diethyl ether, filter, and evaporate the filtrate on a water bath. Dissolve the residue in 2 mL of sodium hydroxide TS, and add 5 mL of dimethylglyoxime-thiosemicarbazide TS, and heat on a water bath for 30 minutes: a red color develops (bromovalerylurea).

(3) Shake 0.3 g of Diphenhydramine and Bromovalerylurea Powder with 5 mL of methanol, filter, and use the filtrate as the sample solution. Dissolve 0.15 of bromovalerylurea and 0.03 g of diphenhydramine tannate in 5 mL each of methanol, and use the solutions as the standard solution (1) and standard solution (2). Perform the test with these solutions as directed under Thin-layer Chromatography 〈*2.03*〉. Spot 5 μL each of the sample solution and standard solutions (1) and (2) on a plate of silica gel with fluorescent indicator for thin-layer chromatography. Develop the plate in a mixture of ethyl acetate, ethanol (99.5) and ammonia solution (28) (50:5:1) to a distance of about 10 cm. Air-dry the plate, and examine under ultraviolet light (main wavelength: 254 nm): 3 spots obtained from the sample solution and the corresponding spot from standard solutions (1) and (2) show the same *Rf* value. Spray Dragendorff's TS for spraying evenly on the plate: the spot from the standard solution (2) and the corresponding spot from the sample solution reveal an orange color.

Containers and storage Containers—Well-closed containers.

Diphenhydramine, Phenol and Zinc Oxide Liniment

ジフェンヒドラミン･フェノール･亜鉛華リニメント

Method of preparation

Diphenhydramine	20 g
Phenol and Zinc Oxide Liniment	980 g
To make	1000 g

Dissolve and mix the above ingredients.

Description Diphenhydramine, Phenol and Zinc Oxide Liniment is a white to whitish, pasty mass. It has a slight odor of phenol.

Identification **(1)** To 3 g of Diphenhydramine, Phenol and Zinc Oxide Liniment add 20 mL of hexane, shake well, and separate the hexane layer. Shake thoroughly the hexane solution with 10 mL of 0.2 mol/L hydrochloric acid. Separate the aqueous layer, and adjust with sodium hydroxide TS to a pH of 4.6. Add 1 mL of bromophenol blue-potassium biphthalate TS and 10 mL of chloroform, and shake: a yellow color develops in the chloroform layer (diphenhydramine).

(2) Place 1 g of Diphenhydramine, Phenol and Zinc Oxide Liniment in a porcelain crucible, gradually raise the temperature by heating until the mass is charred, and ignite strongly: a yellow color is produced, and disappears on cooling. To the residue add 10 mL of water and 5 mL of dilute hydrochloric acid, shake well, and filter. Add 2 to 3 drops of potassium hexacyanoferrate (II) TS to the filtrate: a white precipitate is produced (zinc oxide).

(3) Shake 0.5 g of Diphenhydramine, Phenol and Zinc Oxide Liniment with 1 mL of water and 5 mL of chloroform, filter, and use the filtrate as the sample solution. Dissolve 0.01 g each of diphenhydramine and phenol in 5 mL each of chloroform, and use these solutions as the standard solution (1) and standard solution (2). Perform the test with these solutions as directed under Thin-layer Chromatography *<2.03>*. Spot 5 μL each of the sample solution and standard solutions (1) and (2) on a plate of silica gel for thin-layer chromatography. Develop the plate with a mixture of ethyl acetate, ethanol (99.5) and ammonia solution (28) (50:5:1) to a distance of about 10 cm, and air-dry the plate. Allow the plate to stand in iodine vapor: two spots obtained from the sample solution and each spot from the standard solution (1) and (2) show the same *Rf* value. Sublime iodine, and spray Dragendorff's TS evenly upon the plate: the spot from standard solution (1) and the corresponding spot from the sample solution reveal an orange color.

Containers and storage Containers—Tight containers. Storage—Light-resistant.

Diphenhydramine Tannate

タンニン酸ジフェンヒドラミン

Diphenhydramine Tannate is a compound of diphenhydramine and tannic acid.

It contains not less than 25.0% and not more than 35.0% of diphenhydramine ($C_{17}H_{21}NO$: 255.35).

Description Diphenhydramine Tannate occurs as a grayish white to light brown powder. It is odorless or has a slight, characteristic odor. It is tasteless.

It is slightly soluble in ethanol (95), and practically insoluble in water and in diethyl ether.

Identification **(1)** To 1 g of Diphenhydramine Tannate add 15 mL of water and 0.3 mL of dilute hydrochloric acid, shake thoroughly for 1 minute, filter, and use this filtrate as the sample solution. Transfer 10 mL of the sample solution to a separator, extract with two 20-mL portions of chloroform, combine the chloroform extracts, and evaporate on a water bath to dryness. To 5 mL of a solution of the residue (1 in 100) add 5 drops of Reinecke salt TS: a light red precipitate is produced.

(2) To 10 mL of a solution of the residue obtained in (1) (1 in 100) add 10 mL of 2,4,6-trinitrophenol TS dropwise, and allow to stand for 30 minutes. Collect the precipitate by filtration, recrystallize from dilute ethanol, and dry at 105°C for 30 minutes: the crystals melt *<2.60>* between 128°C and 133°C.

(3) To 1 mL of the sample solution obtained in (1) add 1 drop of iron (III) chloride TS: a dark blue-purple color develops.

Purity Heavy metals *<1.07>*—Proceed with 1.0 g of Diphenhydramine Tannate according to Method 2, and perform the test. Prepare the control solution with 2.0 mL of Standard Lead Solution (not more than 20 ppm).

Loss on drying *<2.41>* Not more than 7.0% (1 g, 105°C, 5 hours).

Residue on ignition *<2.44>* Not more than 1.0% (1 g).

Assay Transfer about 1.7 g of Diphenhydramine Tannate, accurately weighed, to a separator, dissolve in 20 mL of water and 3.0 mL of dilute hydrochloric acid with thorough shaking, add 20 mL of a solution of sodium hydroxide (1 in 10) and exactly 25 mL of isooctane, shake vigorously for 5 minutes, dissolve 2 g of sodium chloride with shaking, and allow to stand. To 20 mL of the isooctane layer add exactly 80 mL of acetic acid (100), and titrate *<2.50>* with 0.1 mol/L perchloric acid VS (potentiometric titration). Perform a blank determination in the same manner, and make any necessary correction.

Each mL of 0.1 mol/L perchloric acid VS
= 25.54 mg of $C_{17}H_{21}NO$

Containers and storage Containers—Tight containers. Storage—Light-resistant.

Freeze-dried Diphtheria Antitoxin, Equine

乾燥ジフテリアウマ抗毒素

Freeze-dried Diphtheria Antitoxin, Equine, is a preparation for injection which is dissolved before use.

It contains diphtheria antitoxin in immunoglobulin of horse origin.

It conforms to the requirements of Freeze-dried Diphtheria Antitoxin, Equine, in the Minimum Requirements for Biological Products.

Description Freeze-dried Diphtheria Antitoxin, Equine, becomes a colorless or light yellow-brown, clear liquid or a slightly whitish turbid liquid on addition of solvent.

Diphtheria Toxoid

ジフテリアトキソイド

Diphtheria Toxoid is a liquid for injection containing diphtheria toxoid prepared by treating diphtheria toxin with formaldehyde by a method involving no appreciable loss of the immunogenicity.

It conforms to the requirements of Diphtheria Toxoid in the Minimum Requirements for Biological Products.

Description Diphtheria Toxoid is a clear, colorless to light yellow-brown liquid.

Adsorbed Diphtheria Toxoid for Adult Use

成人用沈降ジフテリアトキソイド

Adsorbed Diphtheria Toxoid for Adult Use is a liquid for injection containing diphtheria toxoid prepared by treating diphtheria toxin with formaldehyde by a method involving no appreciable loss of the immunogenicity and very few antigenic substances other than toxoid, and rendered insoluble with aluminum salt.

It conforms to the requirements of Adsorbed Diphtheria Toxoid for Adult Use in the Minimum Requirements of Biological Products.

Description Adsorbed Diphtheria Toxoid for Adult Use becomes a homogeneous, whitish turbid liquid on shaking.

Adsorbed Diphtheria-Purified Pertussis-Tetanus Combined Vaccine

沈降精製百日せきジフテリア破傷風混合ワクチン

Adsorbed Diphtheria-Purified Pertussis-Tetanus Combined Vaccine is a liquid for injection consisting of a liquid containing the protective antigen of *Bordetella pertussis*, Diphtheria Toxoid and a liquid containing tetanus toxoid obtained by detoxifying the tetanus toxin with formaldehyde solution without impairing its immunogenicity, to which aluminum is added to make the antigen and the toxoids insoluble.

It conforms to the requirements of Adsorbed Diphtheria-Purified Pertussis-Tetanus Combined Vaccine in the Minimum Requirements for Biological Products.

Description Adsorbed Diphtheria-Purified Pertussis-Tetanus Combined Vaccine becomes a homogeneous, white turbid liquid on shaking.

Adsorbed Diphtheria-Tetanus Combined Toxoid

沈降ジフテリア破傷風混合トキソイド

Adsorbed Diphtheria-Tetanus Combined Toxoid is a liquid for injection containing diphtheria toxoid and tetanus toxoid which are prepared by treating diphtheria toxin and tetanus toxin, respectively, with formaldehyde by a method involving no appreciable loss of the immunogenicity and rendered insoluble by adding aluminum salt.

It conforms to the requirements of Adsorbed Diphtheria-Tetanus Combined Toxoid in the Minimum Requirements for Biological Products.

Description Adsorbed Diphtheria-Tetanus Combined Toxoid becomes a homogeneous, whitish turbid liquid on shaking.

Dipyridamole

ジピリダモール

$C_{24}H_{40}N_8O_4$: 504.63
2,2′,2″,2‴-{[4,8-Di(piperidin-1-yl)pyrimido[5,4-*d*]pyrimidine-2,6-diyl]dinitrilo}tetraethanol
[*58-32-2*]

Dipyridamole, when dried, contains not less than 98.5% of dipyridamole ($C_{24}H_{40}N_8O_4$).

Description Dipyridamole occurs as yellow, crystals or crystalline powder. It is odorless, and has a slightly bitter taste.

It is freely soluble in chloroform, sparingly soluble in methanol and in ethanol (99.5), and practically insoluble in water and in diethyl ether.

Identification **(1)** Dissolve 5 mg of Dipyridamole in 2 mL of sulfuric acid, add 2 drops of nitric acid, and shake: a deep purple color develops.

(2) Determine the absorption spectrum of a solution of Dipyridamole in a mixture of methanol and hydrochloric acid (99:1) (1 in 100,000) as directed under Ultraviolet-visible Spectrophotometry <*2.24*>, and compare the spectrum with the Reference Spectrum: both spectra exhibit similar intensities of absorption at the same wavelengths.

(3) Determine the infrared absorption spectrum of Dipyridamole, previously dried, as directed in the potassium bromide disk method under Infrared Spectrophotometry <*2.25*>, and compare the spectrum with the Reference Spectrum: both spectra exhibit similar intensities of absorption at the same wave numbers.

Melting point <*2.60*> 165 – 169°C

Purity **(1)** Clarity and color of solution—Dissolve 0.5 g of Dipyridamole in 10 mL of chloroform: the solution is clear, and shows a yellow color.

(2) Heavy metals <*1.07*>—Proceed with 2.0 g of Dipyridamole according to Method 2, and perform the test. Prepare the control solution with 2.0 mL of Standard Lead Solution (not more than 10 ppm).

(3) Arsenic <*1.11*>—Prepare the test solution with 1.0 g of Dipyridamole according to Method 3, and perform the test (not more than 2 ppm).

(4) Related substances—Dissolve 50 mg of Dipyridamole in 50 mL of the mobile phase, and use this solution as the sample solution. Pipet 0.5 mL of the sample solution, add the mobile phase to make exactly 100 mL, and use this solution as the standard solution. Perform the test with exactly 20 μL each of the sample solution and standard solution as directed under Liquid Chromatography <*2.01*> according to the following conditions, and determine each peak area by the automatic integration method: the total area of the peaks other than dipyridamole obtained from the sample solution is not larger than the peak area of dipyridamole from the standard solution.

Operating conditions—

Detector: An ultraviolet absorption photometer (wavelength: 280 nm).

Column: A stainless steel column 4 mm in inside diameter and 15 cm in length, packed with octylsilanized silica gel for liquid chromatography (5 μm in particle diameter).

Column temperature: A constant temperature of about 40°C.

Mobile phase: Dissolve 0.2 g of potassium dihydrogen phosphate in 200 mL of water, and add 800 mL of methanol.

Flow rate: Adjust so that the retention time of dipyridamole is about 4 minutes.

Time span of measurement: About 5 times as long as the retention time of dipyridamole.

System suitability—

Test for required detectability: To exactly 5 mL of the standard solution add the mobile phase to make exactly 25 mL. Confirm that the peak area of dipyridamole obtained with 20 μL of this solution is equivalent to 15 to 25% of that with 20 μL of the standard solution.

System performance: Dissolve 7 mg of Dipyridamole and 3 mg of terphenyl in 50 mL of methanol. When the procedure is run with 20 μL of this solution under the above operating conditions, dipyridamole and terphenyl are eluted in this order with the resolution between these peaks being not less than 5.

System repeatability: When the test is repeated 6 times with 20 μL of the standard solution under the above operating conditions, the relative standard deviation of the peak area of dipyridamole is not more than 1.0%.

Loss on drying <*2.41*> Not more than 0.2% (1 g, 105°C, 3 hours).

Residue on ignition <*2.44*> Not more than 0.1% (1 g).

Assay Weigh accurately about 0.6 g of Dipyridamole, previously dried, dissolve in 70 mL of methanol, and titrate <*2.50*> with 0.1 mol/L perchloric acid VS (potentiometric titration). Perform a blank determination in the same manner, and make any necessary correction.

Each mL of 0.1 mol/L perchloric acid VS
= 50.46 mg of $C_{24}H_{40}N_8O_4$

Containers and storage Containers—Well-closed containers.

Storage—Light-resistant.

Disopyramide

ジソピラミド

$C_{21}H_{29}N_3O$: 339.47
(2*RS*)-4-Bis(1-methylethyl)amino-2-phenyl-2-(pyridin-2-yl)butanamide
[*3737-09-5*]

Disopyramide contains not less than 98.5% of disopyramide ($C_{21}H_{29}N_3O$), calculated on the dried basis.

Description Disopyramide occurs as white, crystals or crystalline powder.

It is very soluble in methanol and in ethanol (95), freely soluble in acetic anhydride, in acetic acid (100) and in diethyl ether, and slightly soluble in water.

Identification (1) To 1 mL of a solution of Disopyramide in ethanol (95) (1 in 20) add 10 mL of 2,4,6-trinitrophenol TS, and warm: a yellow precipitate is formed. Filter this precipitate, wash with water, and dry at 105°C for 1 hour: the residue melts ⟨*2.60*⟩ between 172°C and 176°C.

(2) Determine the absorption spectrum of a solution of Disopyramide in 0.05 mol/L sulfuric acid-methanol TS (1 in 25,000) as directed under Ultraviolet-visible Spectrophotometry ⟨*2.24*⟩, and compare the spectrum with the Reference Spectrum: both spectra exhibit similar intensities of absorption at the same wavelengths.

(3) Determine the infrared absorption spectrum of Disopyramide, previously dried, as directed in the potassium bromide disk method under Infrared Spectrophotometry ⟨*2.25*⟩, and compare the spectrum with the Reference Spectrum: both spectra exhibit similar intensities of absorption at the same wave numbers.

Absorbance ⟨*2.24*⟩ $E^{1\%}_{1\,\mathrm{cm}}$ (269 nm): 194 – 205 (10 mg, 0.05 mol/L sulfuric acid-methanol TS, 500 mL).

Purity (1) Heavy metals ⟨*1.07*⟩—Dissolve 1.0 g of Disopyramide in 10 mL of ethanol (95), and add 2 mL of dilute acetic acid and water to make 50 mL. Perform the test using this solution as the test solution. Prepare the control solution as follows: to 2.0 mL of Standard Lead Solution add 10 mL of ethanol (95), 2 mL of dilute acetic acid and water to make 50 mL (not more than 20 ppm).

(2) Arsenic ⟨*1.11*⟩—Prepare the test solution with 1.0 g of Disopyramide according to Method 3, and perform the test (not more than 2 ppm).

(3) Related substances—Dissolve 0.40 g of Disopyramide in 10 mL of methanol, and use this solution as the sample solution. Pipet 1 mL of the sample solution, add methanol to make exactly 400 mL, and use this solution as the standard solution. Perform the test with these solutions as directed under Thin-layer Chromatography ⟨*2.03*⟩. Spot 10 μL each of the sample solution and standard solution on a plate of silica gel with fluorescent indicator for thin-layer chromatography. Develop the plate with a mixture of 1-butanol, water and ammonia solution (28) (45:4:1) to a distance of about 10 cm, and air-dry the plate. Examine under ultraviolet light (main wavelength: 254 nm): the spots other than the principal spot obtained from the sample solution are not more intense than the spot from the standard solution.

Loss on drying ⟨*2.41*⟩ Not more than 0.5% (0.5 g, in vacuum, 80°C, 2 hours).

Residue on ignition ⟨*2.44*⟩ Not more than 0.2% (1 g).

Assay Weigh accurately about 0.25 g of Disopyramide, dissolve in 30 mL of acetic acid (100), and titrate ⟨*2.50*⟩ with 0.1 mol/L perchloric acid VS (potentiometric titration). Perform a blank determination in the same manner, and make any necessary correction.

Each mL of 0.1 mol/L perchloric acid VS
= 16.97 mg of $C_{21}H_{29}N_3O$

Containers and storage Containers—Tight containers.

Distigmine Bromide

ジスチグミン臭化物

$C_{22}H_{32}Br_2N_4O_4$: 576.32
3,3′-[Hexane-1,6-diylbis(methyliminocarbonyloxy)]bis(1-methylpyridinium) dibromide
[*15876-67-2*]

Distigmine Bromide contains not less than 98.5% of distigmine bromide ($C_{22}H_{32}Br_2N_4O_4$), calculated on the anhydrous basis.

Description Distigmine Bromide occurs as a white crystalline powder.

It is very soluble in water, freely soluble in methanol, in ethanol (95) and in acetic acid (100), and slightly soluble in acetic anhydride.

The pH of a solution of Distigmine Bromide (1 in 100) is between 5.0 and 5.5.

It is slightly hygroscopic.

It is gradually colored by light.

Melting point: about 150°C (with decomposition).

Identification (1) Determine the absorption spectrum of a solution of Distigmine Bromide (1 in 25,000) as directed under Ultraviolet-visible Spectrophotometry ⟨*2.24*⟩, and compare the spectrum with the Reference Spectrum: both spectra exhibit similar intensities of absorption at the same wavelengths.

(2) Determine the infrared absorption spectrum of Distigmine Bromide as directed in the potassium bromide disk method under Infrared Spectrophotometry ⟨*2.25*⟩, and compare the spectrum with the Reference Spectrum: both spectra exhibit similar intensities of absorption at the same wave numbers.

(3) To 5 mL of a solution of Distigmine Bromide (1 in 10) add 2 mL of dilute nitric acid: the solution responds to Qualitative Tests ⟨*1.09*⟩ (1) for bromide.

Purity (1) Clarity and color of solution—Dissolve 0.25 g of Distigmine Bromide in 5 mL of water: the solution is clear and colorless.

(2) Sulfate ⟨*1.14*⟩—Perform the test with 0.40 g of Dis-

tigmine Bromide. Prepare the control solution with 0.40 mL of 0.005 mol/L sulfuric acid VS (not more than 0.048%).

(3) Heavy metals *<1.07>*—Proceed with 2.0 g of Distigmine Bromide according to Method 2, and perform the test. Prepare the control solution with 2.0 mL of Standard Lead Solution (not more than 10 ppm).

(4) Related substances—Dissolve 40 mg of Distigmine Bromide in 10 mL of methanol, and use this solution as the sample solution. Pipet 1 mL of the sample solution, add methanol to make exactly 200 mL, and use this solution as the standard solution. Perform the test with these solutions as directed under Thin-layer Chromatography *<2.03>*. Spot 10 μL each of the sample solution and standard solution on a plate of cellulose with fluorescent indicator for thin-layer chromatography. Develop the plate with a mixture of 1-butanol, water, ethanol (99.5) and acetic acid (100) (8:3:2:1) to a distance of about 13 cm, and air-dry the plate. Examine under ultraviolet light (main wavelength: 254 nm): the spots other than the principal spot from the sample solution are not more intense than the spot from the standard solution. Spray evenly Dragendorff's TS for spraying on the plate: the spots other than the principal spot obtained from the sample solution are not more intense than the spot from the standard solution.

Water *<2.48>* Not more than 1.0% (1 g, volumetric titration, direct titration).

Residue on ignition *<2.44>* Not more than 0.1% (1 g).

Assay Weigh accurately about 0.4 g of Distigmine Bromide, dissolve in 60 mL of a mixture of acetic anhydride and acetic acid (100) (8:1), and titrate *<2.50>* with 0.1 mol/L perchloric acid VS (potentiometric titration with platinum electrode). Perform a blank determination in the same manner, and make any necessary correction.

Each mL of 0.1 mol/L perchloric acid VS
= 28.82 mg of $C_{22}H_{32}Br_2N_4O_4$

Containers and storage Containers—Tight containers.
Storage—Light-resistant.

Distigmine Bromide Tablets

ジスチグミン臭化物錠

Distigmine Bromide Tablets contain not less than 95.0% and not more than 105.0% of the labeled amount of distigmine bromide ($C_{22}H_{32}Br_2N_4O_4$: 576.32).

Method of preparation Prepare as directed under Tablets, with Distigmine Bromide.

Identification Determine the absorption spectrum of the sample solution obtained in the Assay, as directed under Ultraviolet-visible Spectrophotometry *<2.24>*: it exhibits a maximum between 268 nm and 272 nm, and a minimum between 239 nm and 243 nm.

Uniformity of dosage units *<6.02>* Perform the test according to the following method: it meets the requirement of the Content uniformity test.

To 1 tablet of Distigmine Bromide Tablets add 30 mL of 0.1 mol/L hydrochloric acid TS, shake for 1 hour, add 0.1 mol/L hydrochloric acid TS to make exactly 50 mL, and filter. Discard the first 20 mL of the filtrate, pipet V mL of the subsequent filtrate, and add 0.1 mol/L hydrochloric acid TS to make exactly V' mL so that each mL contains about 30 μg of distigmine bromide ($C_{22}H_{32}Br_2N_4O_4$), and use this solution as the sample solution. Proceed as directed in the Assay.

Amount (mg) of distigmine bromide ($C_{22}H_{32}Br_2N_4O_4$)
$= M_S \times (A_{T2} - A_{T1})/(A_{S2} - A_{S1}) \times V'/V \times 1/20$

M_S: Amount (mg) of distigmine bromide for assay taken, calculated on the anhydrous basis

Dissolution *<6.10>* When the test is performed at 75 revolutions per minute according to the Paddle method, using 500 mL of water as the dissolution medium, the dissolution rate in 30 minutes of Distigmine Bromide Tablets is not less than 80%.

Start the test with 1 tablet of Distigmine Bromide Tablets, withdraw not less than 20 mL of the medium at the specified minute after starting the test, and filter through a membrane filter with a pore size not exceeding 0.8 μm. Discard not less than 10 mL of the first filtrate, pipet V mL of the subsequent filtrate, add water to make exactly V' mL so that each mL contains about 10 μg of distigmine bromide ($C_{22}H_{32}Br_2N_4O_4$), and use this solution as the sample solution. Separately, weigh accurately about 50 mg of distigmine bromide for assay (separately determine the water *<2.48>* in the same manner as Distigmine Bromide), and dissolve in water to make exactly 100 mL. Pipet 10 mL of this solution, add water to make exactly 500 mL, and use this solution as the standard solution. Perform the test with the sample solution and standard solution as directed under Ultraviolet-visible Spectrophotometry *<2.24>*, and determine the absorbances, A_{T1} and A_{S1}, at 270 nm, and A_{T2} and A_{S2}, at 350 nm.

Dissolution rate (%) with respect to the labeled amount of distigmine bromide ($C_{22}H_{32}Br_2N_4O_4$)
$= M_S \times (A_{T1} - A_{T2})/(A_{S1} - A_{S2}) \times V'/V \times 1/C \times 10$

M_S: Amount (mg) of distigmine bromide for assay taken, calculated on the anhydrous basis
C: Labeled amount (mg) of distigmine bromide ($C_{22}H_{32}Br_2N_4O_4$) in 1 tablet

Assay Weigh accurately and powder not less than 20 tablets of Distigmine Bromide Tablets. Weigh accurately a portion of the powder, equivalent to about 15 mg of Distigmine Bromide ($C_{22}H_{32}Br_2N_4O_4$), add 30 mL of 0.1 mol/L hydrochloric acid TS, shake for 1 hour, add 0.1 mol/L hydrochloric acid TS to make exactly 50 mL, and filter. Discard the first 20 mL of the filtrate, pipet 10 mL of the subsequent filtrate, add 0.1 mol/L hydrochloric acid TS to make exactly 100 mL, and use this solution as the sample solution. Separately, weigh accurately about 30 mg of distigmine bromide for assay (previously determine the water *<2.48>* in the same manner as Distigmine Bromide), and dissolve in 0.1 mol/L hydrochloric acid TS to make exactly 100 mL. Pipet 10 mL of this solution, add 0.1 mol/L hydrochloric acid TS to make exactly 100 mL, and use this solution as the standard solution. Determine the absorbances of the sample solution and standard solution, A_{T2} and A_{S2}, at 270 nm and, A_{T1} and A_{S1}, at 241 nm as directed under Ultraviolet-visible Spectrophotometry *<2.24>*, respectively.

Amount (mg) of distigmine bromide ($C_{22}H_{32}Br_2N_4O_4$)
$= M_S \times (A_{T2} - A_{T1})/(A_{S2} - A_{S1}) \times 1/2$

M_S: Amount (mg) of distigmine bromide for assay taken, calculated on the anhydrous basis

Containers and storage Containers—Tight containers.

Disulfiram

ジスルフィラム

$C_{10}H_{20}N_2S_4$: 296.54

Tetraethylthiuram disulfide

[97-77-8]

Disulfiram, when dried, contains not less than 99.0% of disulfiram ($C_{10}H_{20}N_2S_4$).

Description Disulfiram occurs as white to yellowish white, crystals or crystalline powder.

It is freely soluble in acetone and in toluene, sparingly soluble in methanol and in ethanol (95), and practically insoluble in water.

Identification **(1)** Determine the absorption spectrum of a solution of Disulfiram in ethanol (95) (1 in 100,000) as directed under Ultraviolet-visible Spectrophotometry <*2.24*>, and compare the spectrum with the Reference Spectrum: both spectra exhibit similar intensities of absorption at the same wavelengths.

(2) Determine the infrared absorption spectrum of Disulfiram, previously dried, as directed in the potassium bromide disk method under Infrared Spectrophotometry <*2.25*>, and compare the spectrum with the Reference Spectrum: both spectra exhibit similar intensities of absorption at the same wave numbers.

Melting point <*2.60*> 70 – 73°C

Purity **(1)** Heavy metals <*1.07*>—Proceed with 2.0 g of Disulfiram according to Method 2, and perform the test. Prepare the control solution with 2.0 mL of Standard Lead Solution (not more than 10 ppm).

(2) Arsenic <*1.11*>—Prepare the test solution with 1.0 g of Disulfiram according to Method 4, and perform the test (not more than 2 ppm).

(3) Diethyldithiocarbamic acid—Dissolve 0.10 g of Disulfiram in 10 mL of toluene, and shake with 10 mL of diluted sodium carbonate TS (1 in 20). Discard the toluene layer, wash the water layer with 10 mL of toluene, shake with 5 drops of a solution of cupric sulfate (1 in 250) and 2 mL of toluene, and allow to stand: no light yellow color develops in the toluene layer.

(4) Related substances—Dissolve 50 mg of Disulfiram in 40 mL of methanol, add water to make 50 mL, and use this solution as the sample solution. Pipet 1 mL of the sample solution, add the mobile phase to make exactly 200 mL, and use this solution as the standard solution. Perform the test with exactly 10 μL each of the sample solution and the standard solution as directed under Liquid Chromatography <*2.01*> according to the following conditions. Determine each peak area of both solutions by the automatic integration method: the total area of the peaks other than disulfiram obtained from the sample solution is not larger than the peak area of disulfiram from the standard solution.

Operating conditions—

Detector: An ultraviolet absorption photometer (wavelength: 210 nm).

Column: A stainless steel column about 5 mm in inside diameter and about 15 cm in length, packed with octadecylsilanized silica gel for liquid chromatography (5 μm in particle diameter).

Column temperature: A constant temperature of about 25°C.

Mobile phase: A mixture of methanol and water (7:3).

Flow rate: Adjust so that the retention time of disulfiram is about 8 minutes.

Selection of column: Dissolve 50 mg of Disulfiram and 50 mg of benzophenone in 40 mL of methanol, and add water to make 50 mL. To 1 mL of this solution add the mobile phase to make 200 mL. Proceed with 10 μL of this solution under the above operating conditions, and calculate the resolution. Use a column giving elution of benzophenone and disulfiram in this order with the resolution between these peaks being not less than 4.

Detection sensitivity: Adjust so that the peak height of disulfiram obtained from 10 μL of the standard solution is 15 – 30 mm.

Time span of measurement: About 3.5 times of the retention time of disulfiram.

Loss on drying <*2.41*> Not more than 0.20% (2 g, silica gel, 24 hours).

Residue on ignition <*2.44*> Not more than 0.1% (2 g).

Assay Weigh accurately about 0.2 g of Disulfiram, previously dried, in an iodine bottle, dissolve in 20 mL of acetone, add 1.5 mL of water and 1.0 g of potassium iodide, and dissolve by shaking thoroughly. To this solution add 3.0 mL of hydrochloric acid, stopper the bottle tightly, shake, and allow to stand in a dark place for 3 minutes. Add 70 mL of water, and titrate <*2.50*> with 0.1 mol/L sodium thiosulfate VS (potentiometric titration). Perform a blank determination in the same manner, and make any necessary correction.

Each mL of 0.1 mol/L sodium thiosulfate VS
= 14.83 mg of $C_{10}H_{20}N_2S_4$

Containers and storage Containers—Tight containers.

Dobutamine Hydrochloride

ドブタミン塩酸塩

$C_{18}H_{23}NO_3.HCl$: 337.84

4-{2-[(1*RS*)-3-(4-Hydroxyphenyl)-1-methylpropylamino]ethyl}benzene-1,2-diol monohydrochloride

[49745-95-1]

Dobutamine Hydrochloride, when dried, contains not less than 98.0% of dobutamine hydrochloride ($C_{18}H_{23}NO_3.HCl$).

Description Dobutamine Hydrochloride occurs as white to very pale orange, crystalline powder or grains.

It is freely soluble in methanol, sparingly soluble in water and in ethanol (95), and practically insoluble in diethyl ether.

A solution of Dobutamine Hydrochloride (1 in 100) shows no optical rotation.

Identification **(1)** Determine the infrared absorption spec-

tra of Dobutamine Hydrochloride, previously dried, as directed in the potassium bromide disk method under Infrared Spectrophotometry <*2.25*>, and compare the spectrum with the Reference Spectrum or the spectrum of dried Dobutamine Hydrochloride RS: both spectra exhibit similar intensities of absorption at the same wave numbers.

(2) A solution of Dobutamine Hydrochloride (1 in 50) responds to Qualitative Tests <*1.09*> (2) for chloride.

pH <*2.54*> Dissolve 1.0 g of Dobutamine Hydrochloride in 100 mL of water: the pH of this solution is between 4.0 and 5.5.

Melting point <*2.60*> 188 – 192°C

Purity **(1)** Clarity and color of solution—Dissolve 0.5 g of Dobutamine Hydrochloride in 30 mL of water: the solution is clear and colorless.

(2) Heavy metals <*1.07*>—Dissolve 1.0 g of Dobutamine Hydrochloride in 40 mL of water by warming, cool, and add 2 mL of dilute acetic acid and water to make 50 mL. Perform the test using this solution as the test solution. Prepare the control solution as follows: to 2.0 mL of Standard Lead Solution add water to make 50 mL (not more than 20 ppm).

(3) Related substances—Dissolve 0.10 g of Dobutamine Hydrochloride in 10 mL of methanol, and use this solution as the sample solution. Pipet 1 mL of the sample solution, add methanol to make exactly 200 mL, and use this solution as the standard solution. Perform the test with these solutions as directed under Thin-layer Chromatography <*2.03*>. Spot 10 μL each of the sample solution and standard solution on a plate of silica gel for thin-layer chromatography. Develop the plate with a mixture of chloroform, methanol and formic acid (78:22:5) to a distance of about 12 cm, and air-dry the plate. Allow the plate to stand for 5 minutes in iodine vapor: the spots other than the principal spot obtained from the sample solution are not more intense than the spot from the standard solution.

Loss on drying <*2.41*> Not more than 0.30% (1 g, 105°C, 3 hours).

Residue on ignition <*2.44*> Not more than 0.1% (1 g).

Assay Weigh accurately about 0.1 g each of Dobutamine Hydrochloride and Dobutamine Hydrochloride RS, each previously dried, dissolve separately in exactly 10 mL of the internal standard solution, add diluted methanol (1 in 2) to make 50 mL, and use these solutions as the sample solution and the standard solution, respectively. Perform the test with 5 μL each of the sample solution and standard solution as directed under Liquid Chromatography <*2.01*> according to the following conditions, and calculate the ratios, Q_T and Q_S, of the peak area of dobutamine to that of the internal standard, respectively.

Amount (mg) of dobutamine hydrochloride ($C_{18}H_{23}NO_3.HCl$)
$= M_S \times Q_T/Q_S$

M_S: Amount (mg) of Dobutamine Hydrochloride RS taken

Internal standard solution—A solution of salicylamide in diluted methanol (1 in 2) (1 in 125).

Operating conditions—

Detector: An ultraviolet absorption photometer (wavelength: 280 nm).

Column: A stainless steel column 4.0 mm in inside diameter and 15 cm in length, packed with octadecylsilanized silica gel for liquid chromatography (7 μm in particle diameter).

Column temperature: A constant temperature of about 25°C.

Mobile phase: A mixture of tartrate buffer solution (pH 3.0) and methanol (7:3).

Flow rate: Adjust so that the retention time of dobutamine is about 7 minutes.

System suitability—

System performance: When the procedure is run with 5 μL of the standard solution under the above operating conditions, dobutamine and internal standard are eluted in this order with the resolution between these peaks being not less than 5.

System repeatability: When the test is repeated 6 times with 5 μL of the standard solution under the above operating conditions, the relative standard deviation of the ratios of the peak area of dobutamine to that of the internal standard is not more than 1.0%.

Containers and storage Containers—Tight containers.

Docetaxel Hydrate

ドセタキセル水和物

$C_{43}H_{53}NO_{14}.3H_2O$: 861.93
(1*S*,2*S*,3*R*,4*S*,5*R*,7*S*,8*S*,10*R*,13*S*)-4-Acetoxy-2-benzoyloxy-5,20-epoxy-1,7,10-trihydroxy-9-oxotax-11-en-13-yl (2*R*,3*S*)-3-(1,1-dimethylethyl)oxycarbonylamino-2-hydroxy-3-phenylpropanoate trihydrate
[*148408-66-6*]

Docetaxel Hydrate contains not less than 97.5% and not more than 102.0% of docetaxel ($C_{43}H_{53}NO_{14}$: 807.88), calculated on the anhydrous and residual solvent-free basis.

Description Docetaxel Hydrate occurs as a white crystalline powder.

It is freely soluble in *N*,*N*-dimethylformamide and in ethanol (99.5), soluble in methanol and in dichloromethane, and practically insoluble in water.

It decomposes on exposure to light.

Identification **(1)** Determine the absorption spectrum of a solution of Docetaxel Hydrate in methanol (1 in 50,000) as directed under Ultraviolet-visible Spectrophotometry <*2.24*>, and compare the spectrum with the Reference Spectrum or the spectrum of a solution of Docetaxel Hydrate RS prepared in the same manner as the sample solution: both spectra exhibit similar intensities of absorption at the same wavelengths.

(2) Dissolve 60 mg of Docetaxel Hydrate in 1 mL of dichloromethane. Perform the test with this solution as directed in the solution method under Infrared Spectrophotometry <*2.25*> using a fixed cell composed of potassium bromide optical plates with the cell length of 0.1 mm, and compare the spectrum with the Reference Spectrum or the spectrum of Docetaxel Hydrate RS: both spectra exhibit similar intensities of absorption at the same wave numbers.

Optical rotation <2.49> $[\alpha]_D^{20}$: −39 – −41° (0.2 g calculated on the anhydrous and residual solvent-free basis, methanol, 20 mL, 100 mm).

Purity (1) Heavy metals <1.07>—Proceed with 1.0 g of Docetaxel Hydrate according to Method 2, and perform the test. Prepare the control solution with 2.0 mL of Standard Lead Solution (not more than 20 ppm).

(2) Related substances—Perform the test with 10 μL of the sample solution obtained in the Assay, as directed under Liquid Chromatography <2.01> according to the following conditions. Determine each peak area by the automatic integration method, and calculate the amount of them by the area percentage method: the amount of each peak, having the relative retention time of about 0.97, about 1.08, and about 1.13 to docetaxel, is not more than 0.50%, not more than 0.30%, and not more than 0.30%, respectively, the amount of each peak other than docetaxel and the peaks mentioned above is not more than 0.10%, and the total amount of the peaks other than docetaxel is not more than 1.0%. For the area of the peak, having the relative retention time of about 0.97 to docetaxel, multiply the correction factor 1.6.

Operating conditions—

Detector, column, column temperature, mobile phase, and flow rate: Proceed as directed in the operating conditions in the Assay.

Time span of measurement: For 39 minutes after injection, beginning after the solvent peak.

System suitability—

Test for required detectability: To 1 mL of the sample solution add a mixture of water, acetonitrile for liquid chromatography and acetic acid (100) (1000:1000:1) to make 100 mL. To 1 mL of this solution add a mixture of water, acetonitrile for liquid chromatography and acetic acid (100) (1000:1000:1) to make 10 mL, and use this solution as the solution for system suitability test. Pipet 5 mL of the solution for system suitability test, add a mixture of water, acetonitrile for liquid chromatography and acetic acid (100) (1000:1000:1) to make exactly 10 mL. Confirm that the peak area of docetaxel obtained with 10 μL of this solution is equivalent to 35 to 65% of that with 10 μL of the solution for system suitability test.

System performance: When the procedure is run with 10 μL of the solution for system suitability test under the above operating conditions, the number of theoretical plates and the symmetry factor of the peak of docetaxel are not less than 100,000 and not more than 2.0, respectively.

System repeatability: When the test is repeated 6 times with 10 μL of the solution for system suitability test under the above operating conditions, the relative standard deviation of the peak area of docetaxel is not more than 2.0%.

Water <2.48> 5.0 – 7.0% (50 mg, coulometric titration).

Residue on ignition <2.44> Not more than 0.1% (1 g).

Assay Weigh accurately about 50 mg each of Docetaxel Hydrate and Docetaxel RS (separately determine the water <2.48> and the residual solvent in the same manner as Docetaxel Hydrate), dissolve them separately in 2.5 mL of ethanol (99.5), add a mixture of water, acetonitrile for liquid chromatography and acetic acid (100) (1000:1000:1) to make exactly 50 mL, and use these solutions as the sample solution and the standard solution, respectively. Perform the test with exactly 10 μL each of the sample solution and standard solution as directed under Liquid Chromatography <2.01> according to the following conditions, and determine the peak areas, A_T and A_S, of docetaxel in each solution.

Amount (mg) of docetaxel ($C_{43}H_{53}NO_{14}$) = $M_S \times A_T/A_S$

M_S: Amount (mg) of Docetaxel RS taken, calculated on the anhydrous and residual solvent-free basis

Operating conditions—

Detector: An ultraviolet absorption photometer (wavelength: 232 nm).

Column: A stainless steel column 4.6 mm in inside diameter and 15 cm in length, packed with octadecylsilanized silica gel for liquid chromatography (3.5 μm in particle diameter).

Column temperature: A constant temperature of about 45°C.

Mobile phase A: Water.

Mobile phase B: Acetonitrile for liquid chromatography.

Flowing of mobile phase: Control the gradient by mixing the mobile phases A and B as directed in the following table.

Time after injection of sample (min)	Mobile phase A (vol%)	Mobile phase B (vol%)
0 – 9	72	28
9 – 39	72 → 28	28 → 72

Flow rate: 1.2 mL per minute.

System suitability—

System performance: When the procedure is run with 10 μL of the standard solution under the above operating conditions, the number of theoretical plates and the symmetry factor of the peak of docetaxel are not less than 100,000 and not more than 2.0, respectively.

System repeatability: When the test is repeated 6 times with 10 μL of the standard solution under the above operating conditions, the relative standard deviation of the peak area of docetaxel is not more than 1.0%.

Containers and storage Containers—Tight containers.

Storage—Light-resistant.

Docetaxel Injection

ドセタキセル注射液

Docetaxel Injection is a hydrophilic injection.

It contains not less than 93.0% and not more than 105.0% of the labeled amount of docetaxel ($C_{43}H_{53}NO_{14}$: 807.88).

Method of preparation Prepare as directed under Injections, with Docetaxel Hydrate.

Description Docetaxel Injection occurs as a clear and pale yellow to orange-yellow, liquid.

Identification To a volume of Docetaxel Injection, equivalent to 20 mg of docetaxel ($C_{43}H_{53}NO_{14}$), add 50 mL of methanol, and use this solution as the sample solution. Separately, dissolve 4 mg of docetaxel hydrate in 10 mL of methanol, and use this solution as the standard solution. Perform the test with these solutions as directed under Thin-layer Chromatography <2.03>. Spot 10 μL each of the sample solution and standard solution on a plate of silica gel with fluorescent indicator for thin-layer chromatography. Then develop the plate with a mixture of ethyl acetate, heptane and ethanol (99.5) (12:3:1) to a distance of about 10 cm, and air-dry the plate. Examine under ultraviolet light (main wavelength: 254 nm): the *Rf* value of the spot from the sample solution and the standard solution is the same.

pH Being specified separately when the drug is granted approval based on the Law.

Purity Related substances—Perform the test with 20 μL of the sample solution obtained in the Assay, as directed under Liquid Chromatography <2.01> according to the following conditions. Determine each peak area by the automatic integration method, and calculate the amount of them by the area percentage method: the amount of each peak, having the relative retention time of about 0.27, about 1.05, about 1.08, about 1.13, and about 1.18 to docetaxel, is not more than 0.30%, not more than 1.3%, not more than 1.5%, not more than 0.50%, and not more than 0.50%, respectively, the amount of each peak other than docetaxel, the peak having the relative retention time of about 0.97 and the peaks mentioned above is not more than 0.20%, and the total amount of the peaks other than docetaxel and the peak having the relative retention time of about 0.97 is not more than 3.5%. For the area of the peak, having the relative retention time of about 0.27 to docetaxel, multiply the correction factor 0.67.

Operating conditions—

Detector, column, column temperature, mobile phase, and flow rate: Proceed as directed in the operating conditions in the Assay under Docetaxel Hydrate.

Time span of measurement: For 39 minutes after injection, beginning after the solvent peak.

System suitability—

Test for required detectability: To 1 mL of the sample solution add a mixture of water, acetonitrile for liquid chromatography and acetic acid (100) (1000:1000:1) to make 100 mL, and use this solution as the solution for system suitability test. Pipet 5 mL of the solution for system suitability test, add a mixture of water, acetonitrile for liquid chromatography and acetic acid (100) (1000:1000:1) to make exactly 100 mL. Confirm that the peak area of docetaxel obtained with 20 μL of this solution is equivalent to 3.5 to 6.5% of that with 20 μL of the solution for system suitability test.

System performance: When the procedure is run with 20 μL of the solution for system suitability test under the above operating conditions, the number of theoretical plates and the symmetry factor of the peak of docetaxel are not less than 100,000 and not more than 2.0, respectively.

System repeatability: When the test is repeated 6 times with 20 μL of the solution for system suitability test under the above operating conditions, the relative standard deviation of the peak area of docetaxel is not more than 2.0%.

Bacterial endotoxins <4.01> Less than 2.5 EU/mg.

Extractable volume <6.05> It meets the requirement.

Foreign insoluble matter <6.06> Perform the test according to Method 1: it meets the requirement.

Insoluble particulate matter <6.07> It meets the requirement.

Sterility <4.06> Perform the test according to the Membrane filtration method: it meets the requirement.

Assay To exactly a volume of Docetaxel Injection, equivalent to about 20 mg of docetaxel ($C_{43}H_{53}NO_{14}$), add 5 mL of ethanol (99.5), further add a mixture of water, acetonitrile for liquid chromatography and acetic acid (100) (1000:1000:1) to make exactly 100 mL, and use this solution as the sample solution. Separately, weigh accurately about 40 mg of Docetaxel RS (separately determine the water <2.48> and the residual solvent in the same manner as Docetaxel Hydrate), dissolve in 20 mL of ethanol (99.5), add a mixture of water, acetonitrile for liquid chromatography and acetic acid (100) (1000:1000:1) to make exactly 200 mL, and use this solution as the standard solution. Perform the test with exactly 20 μL each of the sample solution and standard solution as directed under Liquid Chromatography <2.01> according to the following conditions, and determine the peak areas, A_T and A_S, of docetaxel in each solution.

$$\text{Amount (mg) of docetaxel } (C_{43}H_{53}NO_{14}) = M_S \times A_T/A_S \times 1/2$$

M_S: Amount (mg) of Docetaxel RS taken, calculated on the anhydrous and residual solvent-free basis

Operating conditions—

Proceed as directed in the operating conditions in the Assay under Docetaxel Hydrate.

System suitability—

System performance: When the procedure is run with 20 μL of the standard solution under the above operating conditions, the number of theoretical plates and the symmetry factor of the peak of docetaxel are not less than 100,000 and not more than 2.0, respectively.

System repeatability: When the test is repeated 6 times with 20 μL of the standard solution under the above operating conditions, the relative standard deviation of the peak area of docetaxel is not more than 1.0%.

Containers and storage Containers—Hermetic containers. Storage—Light-resistant.

Docetaxel for Injection

注射用ドセタキセル

Docetaxel for Injection is a preparation for injection which is dissolved before use.

It contains not less than 93.0% and not more than 105.0% of the labeled amount of docetaxel ($C_{43}H_{53}NO_{14}$: 807.88).

Method of preparation Prepare as directed under Injections, with Docetaxel Hydrate.

Description Docetaxel for Injection occurs as a clear and yellow to orange-yellow, viscous liquid.

Identification To an amount of Docetaxel for Injection, equivalent to 20 mg of docetaxel ($C_{43}H_{53}NO_{14}$), add 50 mL of methanol, and use this solution as the sample solution. Separately, dissolve 4 mg of docetaxel hydrate in 10 mL of methanol, and use this solution as the standard solution. Perform the test with these solutions as directed under Thin-layer Chromatography <2.03>. Spot 10 μL each of the sample solution and standard solution on a plate of silica gel with fluorescent indicator for thin-layer chromatography. Then develop the plate with a mixture of ethyl acetate, heptane and ethanol (99.5) (12:3:1) to a distance of about 10 cm, and air-dry the plate. Examine under ultraviolet light (main wavelength: 254 nm): the Rf value of the spot obtained from the sample solution and the standard solution is the same.

pH Being specified separately when the drug is granted approval based on the Law.

Purity Related substances—Perform the test with 20 μL of the sample solution obtained in the Assay, as directed under Liquid Chromatography <2.01> according to the following conditions. Determine each peak area by the automatic integration method, and calculate the amount of them by the area percentage method: the amount of each peak, having the relative retention time of about 0.27, about 1.05, about 1.08, about 1.13, and about 1.18 to docetaxel, is not more than 0.30%, not more than 1.3%, not more than 1.5%, not more than 0.50%, and not more than 0.50%, respectively, the amount of each peak other than docetaxel, the peak having the relative retention time of about 0.97 and the peaks mentioned above is not more than 0.20%, and the total amount of the peaks other than docetaxel and the peak having the relative retention time of about 0.97 is not more than 3.5%. For the area of the peak, having the relative retention time of about 0.27 to docetaxel, multiply the correction factor 0.67.

Operating conditions—

Detector, column, column temperature, mobile phase, and flow rate: Proceed as directed in the operating conditions in the Assay under Docetaxel Hydrate.

Time span of measurement: For 39 minutes after injection, beginning after the solvent peak.

System suitability—

Test for required detectability: To 1 mL of the sample solution add a mixture of water, acetonitrile for liquid chromatography and acetic acid (100) (1000:1000:1) to make 100 mL, and use this solution as the solution for system suitability test. Pipet 5 mL of the solution for system suitability test, add a mixture of water, acetonitrile for liquid chromatography and acetic acid (100) (1000:1000:1) to make exactly 100 mL. Confirm that the peak area of docetaxel obtained with 20 μL of this solution is equivalent to 3.5 to 6.5% of that with 20 μL of the solution for system suitability test.

System performance: When the procedure is run with 20 μL of the solution for system suitability test under the above operating conditions, the number of theoretical plates and the symmetry factor of the peak of docetaxel are not less than 100,000 and not more than 2.0, respectively.

System repeatability: When the test is repeated 6 times with 20 μL of the solution for system suitability test under the above operating conditions, the relative standard deviation of the peak area of docetaxel is not more than 2.0%.

Bacterial endotoxins <*4.01*> Less than 2.5 EU/mg.

Uniformity of dosage units <*6.02*> It meets the requirement of the Mass variation test. (*T*: 120.0%).

Foreign insoluble matter <*6.06*> Perform the test according to Method 2: it meets the requirement.

Insoluble particulate matter <*6.07*> It meets the requirement.

Sterility <*4.06*> Perform the test according to the Membrane filtration method: it meets the requirement.

Assay Weigh accurately an amount of Docetaxel for Injection, equivalent to about 20 mg of docetaxel ($C_{43}H_{53}NO_{14}$), add 5 mL of ethanol (99.5), further add a mixture of water, acetonitrile for liquid chromatography and acetic acid (100) (1000:1000:1) to make exactly 100 mL, and use this solution as the sample solution. Separately, weigh accurately about 40 mg of Docetaxel RS (separately determine the water <*2.48*> and the residual solvent in the same manner as Docetaxel Hydrate), dissolve in 20 mL of ethanol (99.5), add a mixture of water, acetonitrile for liquid chromatography and acetic acid (100) (1000:1000:1) to make exactly 200 mL, and use this solution as the standard solution. Perform the test with exactly 20 μL each of the sample solution and standard solution as directed under Liquid Chromatography <*2.01*> according to the following conditions, and determine the peak areas, A_T and A_S, of docetaxel in each solution.

Amount (mg) of docetaxel ($C_{43}H_{53}NO_{14}$) in 1 mL of Docetaxel for Injection

$$= M_S/M_T \times A_T/A_S \times d \times 1/2$$

M_S: Amount (mg) of Docetaxel RS taken, calculated on the anhydrous and residual solvent-free basis

M_T: Amount (mg) of Docetaxel for Injection taken

d: Density (g/mL) of Docetaxel for Injection

Operating conditions—

Proceed as directed in the operating conditions in the Assay under Docetaxel Hydrate.

System suitability—

System performance: When the procedure is run with 20 μL of the standard solution under the above operating conditions, the number of theoretical plates and the symmetry factor of the peak of docetaxel are not less than 100,000 and not more than 2.0, respectively.

System repeatability: When the test is repeated 6 times with 20 μL of the standard solution under the above operating conditions, the relative standard deviation of the peak area of docetaxel is not more than 1.0%.

Containers and storage Containers—Hermetic containers. Storage—Light-resistant.

Domperidone

ドンペリドン

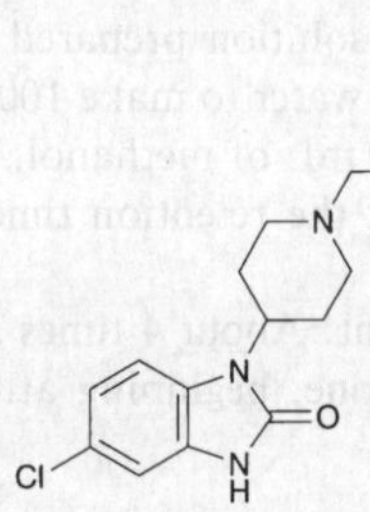

$C_{22}H_{24}ClN_5O_2$: 425.91

5-Chloro-1-{1-[3-(2-oxo-2,3-dihydro-1*H*-benzimidazol-1-yl)propyl]piperidin-4-yl}-1,3-dihydro-2*H*-benzimidazol-2-one

[*57808-66-9*]

Domperidone, when dried, contains not less than 99.0% and not more than 101.0% of domperidone ($C_{22}H_{24}ClN_5O_2$).

Description Domperidone occurs as a white to pale yellow, crystalline powder or powder.

It is freely soluble in acetic acid (100), slightly soluble in methanol and in ethanol (99.5), very slightly soluble in 2-propanol, and practically insoluble in water.

Melting point: about 243°C (with decomposition).

Identification **(1)** Determine the absorption spectrum of a solution of Domperidone in a mixture of 2-propanol and 0.1 mol/L hydrochloric acid TS (9:1) (1 in 50,000) as directed under Ultraviolet-visible Spectrophotometry <*2.24*>, and compare the spectrum with the Reference Spectrum: both spectra exhibit similar intensities of absorption at the same wavelengths.

(2) Determine the infrared absorption spectrum of Domperidone as directed in the potassium bromide disk method under Infrared Spectrophotometry <*2.25*>, and compare the spectrum with the Reference Spectrum: both spectra exhibit similar intensities of absorption at the same wave numbers.

Purity (1) Heavy metals *<1.07>*—Proceed with 2.0 g of Domperidone according to Method 2, and perform the test. Prepare the control solution with 2.0 mL of Standard Lead Solution (not more than 10 ppm).

(2) Related substances—Dissolve 30 mg of Domperidone in 100 mL of methanol, and use this solution as the sample solution. Pipet 1 mL of the sample solution, add methanol to make exactly 200 mL, and use this solution as the standard solution. Perform the test with exactly 10 μL each of the sample solution and standard solution as directed under Liquid Chromatography *<2.01>* according to the following conditions, and determine each peak area of each solution by the automatic integration method: the area of each peak other than domperidone obtained from the sample solution is not larger than 1/2 times the peak area of domperidone from the standard solution. Furthermore, the total area of the peaks other than domperidone is not larger than the peak area of domperidone from the standard solution.

Operating conditions—

Detector: An ultraviolet absorption photometer (wavelength: 287 nm).

Column: A stainless steel column 4.6 mm in inside diameter and 25 cm in length, packed with octylsilanized silica gel for liquid chromatography (5 μm in particle diameter).

Column temperature: A constant temperature of about 35°C.

Mobile phase: Dissolve 2.72 g of potassium dihydrogen phosphate in water to make 1000 mL, and adjust the pH to 3.5 of this solution with a solution prepared by dissolving 2.31 g of phosphoric acid in water to make 1000 mL. To 500 mL of this solution add 500 mL of methanol.

Flow rate: Adjust so that the retention time of domperidone is about 9 minutes.

Time span of measurement: About 4 times as long as the retention time of domperidone, beginning after the solvent peak.

System suitability—

Test for required detectability: Pipet 2 mL of the standard solution, and add methanol to make exactly 5 mL. Confirm that the peak area of domperidone obtained with 10 μL of this solution is equivalent to 30 to 50% of that with 10 μL of the standard solution.

System performance: Dissolve 10 mg of Domperidone and 20 mg of ethyl parahydroxybenzoate in 100 mL of methanol. When the procedure is run with 10 μL of this solution under the above operating conditions, domperidone and ethyl parahydroxybenzoate are eluted in this order with the resolution between these peaks being not less than 1.5.

System repeatability: When the test is repeated 6 times with 10 μL of the standard solution under the above operating conditions, the relative standard deviation of the peak area of domperidone is not more than 3.0%.

Loss on drying *<2.41>* Not more than 0.5% (1 g, 105°C, 4 hours).

Residue on ignition *<2.44>* Not more than 0.1% (1 g).

Assay Weigh accurately about 0.5 g of Domperidone, previously dried, dissolve in 50 mL of acetic acid (100), and titrate *<2.50>* with 0.1 mol/L perchloric acid VS (potentiometric titration). Perform a blank determination in the same manner, and make any necessary correction.

Each mL of 0.1 mol/L perchloric acid VS
= 42.59 mg of $C_{22}H_{24}ClN_5O_2$

Containers and storage Containers—Well-closed containers.

Storage—Light-resistant.

Donepezil Hydrochloride

ドネペジル塩酸塩

and enantiomer

$C_{24}H_{29}NO_3.HCl$: 415.95

(2*RS*)-2-[(1-Benzylpiperidin-4-yl)methyl]-5,6-dimethoxy-2,3-dihydro-1*H*-inden-1-one monohydrochloride

[*120011-70-3*]

Donepezil Hydrochloride contains not less than 98.0% and not more than 102.0% of donepezil hydrochloride ($C_{24}H_{29}NO_3.HCl$), calculated on the anhydrous basis.

Description Donepezil Hydrochloride occurs as a white crystalline powder.

It is soluble in water, and slightly soluble in ethanol (99.5).

A solution of Donepezil Hydrochloride (1 in 100) shows no optical rotation.

Donepezil Hydrochloride shows crystal polymorphism.

Identification (1) Determine the absorption spectrum of a solution of Donepezil Hydrochloride (1 in 50,000) as directed under Ultraviolet-visible Spectrophotometry *<2.24>*, and compare the spectrum with the Reference Spectrum or the spectrum of a solution of Donepezil Hydrochloride RS prepared in the same manner as the sample solution: both spectra exhibit similar intensities of absorption at the same wavelengths.

(2) Determine the infrared absorption spectrum of Donepezil Hydrochloride as directed in the potassium bromide disk method under Infrared Spectrophotometry *<2.25>*, and compare the spectrum with the Reference Spectrum or the spectrum of Donepezil Hydrochloride RS: both spectra exhibit similar intensities of absorption at the same wave numbers. If any difference appears between the spectra, recrystallize the sample and the RS according to the method otherwise specified, filter and dry the crystals, and perform the test with the crystals.

(3) A solution of Donepezil Hydrochloride (1 in 50) responds to Qualitative Tests *<1.09>* (2) for chloride.

Purity (1) Heavy metals *<1.07>*—To 1.0 g of Donepezil Hydrochloride in a porcelain or platinum crucible add 5 mL of sulfuric acid, incinerate by heating gradually, then incinerate by ignition between 500 and 600°C. If a carbonized residue still retains, moisten the residue with a little amount of sulfuric acid, and incinerate again by ignition between 500 and 600°C. After cooling, dissolve the residue with 3 mL of hydrochloric acid, then evaporate to dryness on a water bath or hot plate, and dissolve the residue with 10 mL of water by warming. Then, proceed as directed in Method 4, and perform the test. Prepare the control solution with 1.0 mL of Standard Lead Solution (not more than 10 ppm).

(2) Related substances—Dissolve 50 mg of Donepezil Hydrochloride in 25 mL of the mobile phase. To 10 mL of this solution add the mobile phase to make 50 mL, and use this solution as the sample solution. Pipet 2 mL of the sample solution, and add the mobile phase to make exactly 100

mL. Pipet 5 mL of this solution, add the mobile phase to make exactly 100 mL, and use this solution as the standard solution. Perform the test with exactly 20 μL each of the sample solution and standard solution as directed under Liquid Chromatography <2.01> according to the following conditions, and determine each peak area by the automatic integration method: the area of the peak other than donepezil obtained from the sample solution is not larger than the peak area of donepezil from the standard solution.

Operating conditions—

Detector, column, column temperature, mobile phase, and flow rate: Proceed as directed in the operating conditions in the Assay.

Time span of measurement: About 2 times as long as the retention time of donepezil, beginning after the solvent peak.

System suitability—

System performance: When the procedure is run with 20 μL of the standard solution under the above operating conditions, the number of theoretical plates and the symmetry factor of the peak of donepezil are not less than 5000 and not more than 1.5, respectively.

System repeatability: When the test is repeated 6 times with 20 μL of the standard solution under the above operating conditions, the relative standard deviation of the peak area of donepezil is not more than 2.0%.

Water <2.48> Not more than 0.2% (0.2 g, coulometric titration).

Residue on ignition <2.44> Not more than 0.1% (1 g).

Assay Weigh accurately about 50 mg each of Donepezil Hydrochloride and Donepezil Hydrochloride RS (separately determine the water <2.48> in the same manner as Donepezil Hydrochloride), dissolve them in the mobile phase to make exactly 25 mL. Pipet 10 mL each of these solutions, add the mobile phase to make exactly 50 mL, and use these solutions as the sample solution and the standard solution, respectively. Perform the test with exactly 20 μL each of the sample solution and standard solution as directed under Liquid Chromatography <2.01> according to the following conditions, and determine the peak areas, A_T and A_S, of donepezil in each solution.

Amount (mg) of donepezil hydrochloride ($C_{24}H_{29}NO_3.HCl$)
$= M_S \times A_T/A_S$

M_S: Amount (mg) of Donepezil Hydrochloride RS taken, calculated on the anhydrous basis

Operating conditions—

Detector: An ultraviolet absorption photometer (wavelength: 271 nm).

Column: A stainless steel column 4.6 mm in inside diameter and 15 cm in length, packed with octadecylsilanized silica gel for liquid chromatography (5 μm in particle diameter).

Column temperature: A constant temperature of about 35°C.

Mobile phase: Dissolve 2.5 g of sodium 1-decansulfonate in 650 mL of water, and add 350 mL of acetonitrile and 1 mL of perchloric acid.

Flow rate: Adjust so that the retention time of donepezil is about 11 minutes.

System suitability—

System performance: When the procedure is run with 20 μL of the standard solution under the above operating conditions, the number of theoretical plates and the symmetry factor of the peak of donepezil are not less than 5000 and not more than 1.5, respectively.

System repeatability: When the test is repeated 6 times with 20 μL of the standard solution under the above operating conditions, the relative standard deviation of the peak area of donepezil is not more than 1.0%.

Containers and storage Containers—Well-closed containers.

Donepezil Hydrochloride Fine Granules

ドネペジル塩酸塩細粒

Donepezil Hydrochloride Fine Granules contain not less than 95.0% and not more than 105.0% of the labeled amount of donepezil hydrochloride ($C_{24}H_{29}NO_3.HCl$: 415.95).

Method of preparation Prepare as directed under Granules, with Donepezil Hydrochloride.

Identification To 2.5 mL of the sample solution obtained in the Assay add water to make 100 mL. Determine the absorption spectrum of this solution as directed under Ultraviolet-visible Spectrophotometry <2.24>: it exhibits maxima between 228 nm and 232 nm, between 269 nm and 273 nm, and between 313 nm and 317 nm.

Uniformity of dosage units <6.02> Perform the test according to the following method: the Donepezil Hydrochloride Fine Granules in single-dose packages meet the requirement of the Content uniformity test.

To the total amount of the content of 1 package of Donepezil Hydrochloride Fine Granule add exactly V mL of 0.1 mol/L hydrochloric acid TS so that each mL contains about 0.2 mg of donepezil hydrochloride ($C_{24}H_{29}NO_3.HCl$), disperse the particles by sonicating with occasional shaking, and sonicate for a further 10 minutes. Centrifuge this solution, and use the supernatant liquid as the sample solution. Separately, weigh accurately about 50 mg of Donepezil Hydrochloride RS, (separately determine the water <2.48> in the same manner as Donepezil Hydrochloride), dissolve in a mixture of methanol and 0.1 mol/L hydrochloric acid TS (3:1) to make exactly 25 mL. Pipet 5 mL of this solution, add 0.1 mol/L hydrochloric acid TS to make exactly 50 mL, and use this solution as the standard solution. Perform the test with exactly 20 μL each of the sample solution and standard solution as directed under Liquid Chromatography <2.01> according to the following conditions, and determine the peak areas, A_T and A_S, of donepezil in each solution.

Amount (mg) of donepezil hydrochloride ($C_{24}H_{29}NO_3.HCl$)
$= M_S \times A_T/A_S \times V/250$

M_S: Amount (mg) of Donepezil Hydrochloride RS taken, calculated on the anhydrous basis

Operating conditions—

Proceed as directed in the operating conditions in the Assay under Donepezil Hydrochloride.

System suitability—

System performance: When the procedure is run with 20 μL of the standard solution under the above operating conditions, the number of theoretical plates and the symmetry factor of the peak of donepezil are not less than 4000 and not more than 1.5, respectively.

System repeatability: When the test is repeated 6 times with 20 μL of the standard solution under the above operating conditions, the relative standard deviation of the peak

area of donepezil is not more than 1.0%.

Dissolution <*6.10*> When the test is performed at 50 revolutions per minute according to the Paddle method, using 900 mL of 2nd fluid for dissolution test as the dissolution medium, the dissolution rate in 15 minutes of Donepezil Hydrochloride Fine Granules is not less than 80%.

Start the test with an accurately weighed amount of Donepezil Hydrochloride Fine Granules, equivalent to about 3 mg of donepezil hydrochloride ($C_{24}H_{29}NO_3.HCl$), withdraw not less than 20 mL of the medium at the specified minute after starting the test, and filter through a membrane filter with a pore size not exceeding 0.45 μm. Discard not less than 10 mL of the first filtrate, and use the subsequent filtrate as the sample solution. Separately, weigh accurately about 55 mg of Donepezil Hydrochloride RS (separately determine the water <*2.48*> in the same manner as Donepezil Hydrochloride), and dissolve in a mixture of methanol and 0.1 mol/L hydrochloric acid (3:1) to make exactly 50 mL. Pipet 5 mL of this solution, add the dissolution medium to make exactly 50 mL. Pipet 3 mL of this solution, add the dissolution medium to make exactly 100 mL, and use this solution as the standard solution. Perform the test with exactly 50 μL each of the sample solution and standard solution as directed under Liquid Chromatography <*2.01*> according to the following conditions, and determine the peak areas, A_T and A_S, of donepezil in each solution.

Dissolution rate (%) with respect to the labeled amount of donepezil hydrochloride ($C_{24}H_{29}NO_3.HCl$)
$= M_S/M_T \times A_T/A_S \times 1/C \times 27/5$

M_S: Amount (mg) of Donepezil Hydrochloride RS taken, calculated on the anhydrous basis
M_T: Amount (mg) of Donepezil Hydrochloride Fine Granules taken
C: Labeled amount (mg) of donepezil hydrochloride ($C_{24}H_{29}NO_3.HCl$) in 1 g

Operating conditions—

Detector, column, and column temperature: Proceed as directed in the operating conditions in the Assay under Donepezil Hydrochloride.

Mobile phase: A mixture of water, acetonitrile and perchloric acid (650:350:1).

Flow rate: Adjust so that the retention time of donepezil is about 4 minutes.

System suitability—

System performance: When the procedure is run with 50 μL of the standard solution under the above operating conditions, the number of throretical plates and the symmetry factor of the peak of donepezil are not less than 5000 and not more than 1.5, respectively.

System repeatability: When the test is repeated 6 times with 50 μL of the standard solution under the above operating conditions, the relative standard deviation of the peak area of donepezil is not more than 1.0%.

Assay Powder Donepezil Hydrochloride Fine Granules, if necessary. Weigh accurately a portion of the powder, equivalent to about 20 mg of donepezil hydrochloride ($C_{24}H_{29}NO_3.HCl$), add 30 mL of 0.1 mol/L hydrochloric acid TS, disperse into the fine particles by sonicating with occasional shaking, and sonicate for a further 15 minutes. Add 0.1 mol/L hydrochloric acid TS to make exactly 50 mL. Centrifuge this solution, and use the supernatant liquid as the sample solution. Separately, weigh accurately about 50 mg of Donepezil Hydrochloride RS (separately determine the water <*2.48*> in the same manner as Donepezil Hydrochloride), and dissolve in a mixture of methanol and 0.1 mol/L hydrochloric acid TS (3:1) to make exactly 25 mL. Pipet 10 mL of this solution, add 0.1 mol/L hydrochloric acid TS to make exactly 50 mL, and use this solution as the standard solution. Perform the test with exactly 20 μL each of the sample solution and standard solution as directed under Liquid Chromatography <*2.01*> according to the following conditions, and determine the peak areas, A_T and A_S, of donepezil in each solution.

Amount (mg) of donepezil hydrochloride ($C_{24}H_{29}NO_3.HCl$)
$= M_S \times A_T/A_S \times 2/5$

M_S: Amount (mg) of Donepezil Hydrochloride RS taken, calculated on the anhydrous basis

Operating conditions—

Proceed as directed in the operating conditions in the Assay under Donepezil Hydrochloride.

System suitability—

System performance: When the procedure is run with 20 μL of the standard solution under the above operating conditions, the number of theoretical plates and the symmetry factor of the peak of donepezil are not less than 5000 and not more than 1.5, respectively.

System repeatability: When the test is repeated 6 times with 20 μL of the standard solution under the above operating conditions, the relative standard deviation of the peak area of donepezil is not more than 1.0%.

Containers and storage Containers—Well-closed containers.

Storage—Light-resistant.

Donepezil Hydrochloride Tablets

ドネペジル塩酸塩錠

Donepezil Hydrochloride Tablets contain not less than 95.0% and not more than 105.0% of the labeled amount of donepezil hydrochloride ($C_{24}H_{29}NO_3.HCl$: 415.95).

Method of preparation Prepare as directed under Tablets, with Donepezil Hydrochloride.

Identification To 2.5 mL of the sample solution obtained in the Assay add water to make 100 mL. Determine the absorption spectrum of this solution as directed under Ultraviolet-visible Spectrophotometry <*2.24*>: it exhibits maxima between 228 nm and 232 nm, between 269 nm and 273 nm, and between 313 nm and 317 nm.

Uniformity of dosage units <*6.02*> Perform the test according to the following method: it meets the requirement of the Content uniformity test.

To 1 tablet of Donepezil Hydrochloride Tablets add exactly *V* mL of a mixture of methanol and 0.1 mol/L hydrochloric acid TS (3:1) so that each mL contains about 0.2 mg of donepezil hydrochloride ($C_{24}H_{29}NO_3.HCl$), disperse by sonicating. Shake until the tablet is disintegrated, and sonicate for a further 10 minutes. Centrifuge this solution, and use the supernatant liquid as the sample solution. Separately, weigh accurately about 50 mg of Donepezil Hydrochloride RS (separately, determine the water <*2.48*> in the same manner as Donepezil Hydrochloride), dissolve in a mixture of methanol and 0.1 mol/L hydrochloric acid TS (3:1) to make exactly 25 mL. Pipet 5 mL of this solution, add a mixture of methanol and 0.1 mol/L hydrochloric acid TS (3:1) to make exactly 50 mL, and use this solution as the standard solution. Perform the test with exactly 20 μL each of the sample solution and standard solution as directed under Liquid Chromatography <*2.01*> according to the following conditions, and determine the peak areas, A_T and A_S, of donepezil in each solution.

Amount (mg) of donepezil hydrochloride ($C_{24}H_{29}NO_3.HCl$)
$= M_S \times A_T/A_S \times V/250$

M_S: Amount (mg) of Donepezil Hydrochloride RS taken, calculated on the anhydrous basis

Operating conditions—

Proceed as directed in the operating conditions in the Assay under Donepezil Hydrochloride.

System suitability—

System performance: When the procedure is run with 20 μL of the standard solution under the above operating conditions, the number of theoretical plates and the symmetry factor of the peak of donepezil are not less than 4000 and not more than 1.5, respectively.

System repeatability: When the test is repeated 6 times with 20 μL of the standard solution under the above operating conditions, the relative standard deviation of the peak area of donepezil is not more than 1.0%.

Dissolution <*6.10*> When the test is performed at 50 revolutions per minute according to the Paddle method, using 900 mL of 2nd fluid for dissolution test as the dissolution medium, the dissolution rate in 15 minutes of Donepezil Hydrochloride Tablets is not less than 80%.

Start the test with 1 tablet of Donepezil Hydrochloride Tablets, withdraw not less than 20 mL of the medium at the specified minute after starting the test, and filter through a membrane filter with a pore size not exceeding 0.45 μm. Discard not less than 10 mL of the first filtrate, pipet V mL of the subsequent filtrate, add the dissolution medium to make exactly V' mL so that each mL contains about 3.3 μg of donepezil hydrochloride ($C_{24}H_{29}NO_3.HCl$), and use this solution as the sample solution. Separately, weigh accurately about 55 mg of Donepezil Hydrochloride RS (separately determine the water <*2.48*> in the same manner as Donepezil Hydrochloride), and dissolve in a mixture of methanol and 0.1 mol/L hydrochloric acid TS (3:1) to make exactly 50 mL. Pipet 5 mL of this solution, and add the dissolution medium to make exactly 50 mL. Further, pipet 3 mL of this solution, add the dissolution medium to make exactly 100 mL, and use this solution as the standard solution. Perform the test with exactly 50 μL each of the sample solution and standard solution as directed under Liquid Chromatography <*2.01*> according to the following conditions, and determine the peak areas, A_T and A_S, of donepezil in each solution.

Dissolution rate (%) with respect to the labeled amount of donepezil hydrochloride ($C_{24}H_{29}NO_3.HCl$)
$= M_S \times A_T/A_S \times V'/V \times 1/C \times 27/5$

M_S: Amount (mg) of Donepezil Hydrochloride RS taken, calculated on the anhydrous basis

C: Labeled amount (mg) of donepezil hydrochloride ($C_{24}H_{29}NO_3.HCl$) in 1 tablet

Operating conditions—

Detector, column, and column temperature: Proceed as directed in the operating conditions in the Assay under Donepezil Hydrochloride.

Mobil phase: A mixture of water, acetonitrile and perchloric acid (650:350:1).

Flow rate: Adjust so that the retention time of donepezil is about 4 minutes.

System suitability—

System performance: When the procedure is run with 50 μL of the standard solution under the above operating conditions, the number of theoretical plates and the symmetry factor of the peak of donepezil are not less than 5000 and not more than 1.5, respectively.

System repeatability: When the test is repeated 6 times with 50 μL of the standard solution under the above operating conditions, the relative standard deviation of the peak area of donepezil is not more than 1.0%.

Assay Accurately weigh the mass of not less than 20 Donepezil Hydrochloride Tablets and powder. Weigh accurately a portion of the powder, equivalent to about 20 mg of donepezil hydrochloride ($C_{24}H_{29}NO_3.HCl$), add 30 mL of a mixture of methanol and 0.1 mol/L hydrochloric acid TS (3:1), disperse by sonicating, and add a mixture of methanol and 0.1 mol/L hydrochloric acid TS (3:1) to make exactly 50 mL. Centrifuge this solution, and use the supernatant liquid as the sample solution. Separately, weigh accurately about 50 mg of Donepezil Hydrochloride RS (separately, determine the water <*2.48*> in the same manner as Donepezil Hydrochloride), dissolve in a mixture of methanol and 0.1 mol/L hydrochloric acid TS (3:1) to make exactly 25 mL. Pipet 10 mL of this solution, add a mixture of methanol and 0.1 mol/L hydrochloric acid TS (3:1) to make exactly 50 mL, and use this solution as the standard solution. Perform the test with exactly 20 μL each of the sample solution and standard solution as directed under Liquid Chromatography <*2.01*> according to the following conditions, and determine the peak areas, A_T and A_S, of donepezil in each solution.

Amount (mg) of donepezil hydrochloride ($C_{24}H_{29}NO_3.HCl$)
$= M_S \times A_T/A_S \times 2/5$

M_S: Amount (mg) of Donepezil Hydrochloride RS taken, calculated on the anhydrous basis

Operating conditions—

Proceed as directed in the operating conditions in the Assay under Donepezil Hydrochloride.

System suitability—

System performance: When the procedure is run with 20 μL of the standard solution under the above operating conditions, the number of theoretical plates and the symmetry factor of the peak of donepezil are not less than 5000 and not more than 1.5, respectively.

System repeatability: When the test is repeated 6 times with 20 μL of the standard solution under the above operating conditions, the relative standard deviation of the peak area of donepezil is not more than 1.0%.

Containers and storage Containers—Well-closed containers.

Dopamine Hydrochloride

ドパミン塩酸塩

$C_8H_{11}NO_2.HCl$: 189.64
4-(2-Aminoethyl)benzene-1,2-diol monohydrochloride
[62-31-7]

Dopamine Hydrochloride, when dried, contains not less than 98.5% of dopamine hydrochloride ($C_8H_{11}NO_2.HCl$).

Description Dopamine Hydrochloride occurs as white, crystals or crystalline powder.

It is freely soluble in water and in formic acid, and sparingly soluble in ethanol (95).

Melting point: about 248°C (with decomposition).

Identification (1) Determine the absorption spectrum of a solution of Dopamine Hydrochloride in 0.1 mol/L hydrochloric acid TS (1 in 25,000) as directed under Ultraviolet-visible Spectrophotometry *<2.24>*, and compare the spectrum with the Reference Spectrum: both spectra exhibit similar intensities of absorption at the same wavelengths.

(2) Determine the infrared absorption spectrum of Dopamine Hydrochloride as directed in the potassium chloride disk method under Infrared Spectrophotometry *<2.25>*, and compare the spectrum with the Reference Spectrum: both spectra exhibit similar intensities of absorption at the same wave numbers.

(3) A solution of Dopamine Hydrochloride (1 in 50) responds to Qualitative Tests *<1.09>* (1) for chloride.

pH *<2.54>* Dissolve 1.0 g of Dopamine Hydrochloride in 50 mL of water: the pH of this solution is between 4.0 and 5.5.

Purity (1) Clarity and color of solution—Dissolve 1.0 g of Dopamine Hydrochloride in 10 mL of water: the solution is clear and colorless.

(2) Sulfate *<1.14>*—Perform the test with 0.8 g of Dopamine Hydrochloride. Prepare the control solution with 0.35 mL of 0.005 mol/L sulfuric acid VS (not more than 0.021%).

(3) Heavy metals *<1.07>*—Proceed with 1.0 g of Dopamine Hydrochloride according to Method 1, and perform the test. Prepare the control solution with 2.0 mL of Standard Lead Solution (not more than 20 ppm).

(4) Arsenic *<1.11>*—Prepare the test solution with 1.0 g of Dopamine Hydrochloride according to Method 1, and perform the test (not more than 2 ppm).

(5) Related substances—Dissolve 0.1 g of Dopamine Hydrochloride in 10 mL of water, and use this solution as the sample solution. Pipet 1 mL of the sample solution, add water to make exactly 250 mL, and use this solution as the standard solution. Perform the test with these solutions as directed under Thin-layer Chromatography *<2.03>*. Spot 5 μL each of the sample solution and standard solution on a plate of cellulose with fluorescent indicator for thin-layer chromatography. Develop the plate with a mixture of 1-propanol, water and acetic acid (100) (16:8:1) to a distance of about 10 cm, and air-dry the plate. Spray evenly a solution of ninhydrin in acetone (1 in 50) on the plate, and heat the plate at 90°C for 10 minutes: the spots other than the principal spot obtained from the sample solution are not more intense than the spot from the standard solution.

Loss on drying *<2.41>* Not more than 0.5% (1 g, 105°C, 3 hours).

Residue on ignition *<2.44>* Not more than 0.1% (1 g).

Assay Weigh accurately about 0.2 g of Dopamine Hydrochloride, previously dried, dissolve in 5 mL of formic acid, add exactly 15 mL of 0.1 mol/L perchloric acid VS, and heat on a water bath for 15 minutes. After cooling, add 50 mL of acetic acid (100), and titrate *<2.50>* the excess perchloric acid with 0.1 mol/L sodium acetate VS (potentiometric titration). Perform a blank determination in the same manner.

Each mL of 0.1 mol/L perchloric acid VS
= 18.96 mg of $C_8H_{11}NO_2.HCl$

Containers and storage Containers—Tight containers.

Dopamine Hydrochloride Injection

ドパミン塩酸塩注射液

Dopamine Hydrochloride Injection is an aqueous injection.

It contains not less than 97.0% and not more than 103.0% of the labeled amount of dopamine hydrochloride ($C_8H_{11}NO_2.HCl$: 189.64).

Method of preparation Prepare as directed under Injections, with Dopamine Hydrochloride.

Description Dopamine Hydrochloride Injection occurs as a clear, colorless liquid.

Identification To a volume of Dopamine Hydrochloride Injection, equivalent to 0.04 g of Dopamine Hydrochloride, add 0.1 mol/L hydrochloric acid TS to make 100 mL. To 5 mL of this solution add 0.1 mol/L hydrochloric acid TS to make 50 mL. Determine the absorption spectrum of this solution as directed under Ultraviolet-visible Spectrophotometry *<2.24>*: it exhibits a maximum between 278 nm and 282 nm.

pH *<2.54>* 3.0 – 5.0

Bacterial endotoxins *<4.01>* Less than 4.2 EU/mg.

Extractable volume *<6.05>* It meets the requirement.

Foreign insoluble matter *<6.06>* Perform the test according to Method 1: it meets the requirement.

Insoluble particulate matter *<6.07>* It meets the requirement.

Sterility *<4.06>* Perform the test according to the Membrane filtration method: it meets the requirement.

Assay To an exact volume of Dopamine Hydrochloride Injection, equivalent to about 30 mg of dopamine hydrochloride ($C_8H_{11}NO_2.HCl$), add the mobile phase to make exactly 50 mL. Pipet 2.5 mL of this solution, add exactly 2.5 mL of the internal standard solution and the mobile phase to make 20 mL, and use this solution as the sample solution. Separately, weigh accurately about 30 mg of dopamine hydrochloride for assay, previously dried at 105°C for 3 hours, dissolve in the mobile phase to make exactly 50 mL. Pipet 2.5 mL of this solution, add exactly 2.5 mL of the internal standard solution and the mobile phase to make 20 mL, and use this solution as the standard solution. Perform the test with 10 μL each of the sample solution and standard solution as directed under Liquid Chromatography <*2.01*> according to the following conditions, and calculate the ratios, Q_T and Q_S, of the peak area of dopamine to that of the internal standard.

Amount (mg) of dopamine hydrochloride ($C_8H_{11}NO_2.HCl$)
$= M_S \times Q_T/Q_S$

M_S: Amount (mg) of dopamine hydrochloride for assay taken

Internal standard solution—A solution of uracil in the mobile phase (3 in 10,000).

Operating conditions—

Detector: An ultraviolet absorption photometer (wavelength: 280 nm).

Column: A stainless steel column 4.6 mm in inside diameter and 25 cm in length, packed with octadecylsilanized silica gel for liquid chromatography (5 μm in particle diameter).

Column temperature: A constant temperature of about 25°C.

Mobile phase: Disodium hydrogen phosphate-citric acid buffer solution (pH 3.0).

Flow rate: Adjust so that the retention time of dopamine is about 10 minutes.

System suitability—

System performance: When the procedure is run with 10 μL of the standard solution under the above operating conditions, the internal standard and dopamine are eluted in this order with the resolution between these peaks being not less than 10.

System repeatability: When the test is repeated 6 times with 10 μL of the standard solution under the above operating conditions, the relative standard deviation of the ratios of peak area of dopamine to that of the internal standard is not more than 1.0%.

Containers and storage Containers—Hermetic containers. Plastic containers for aqueous injections may be used.

Doripenem Hydrate

ドリペネム水和物

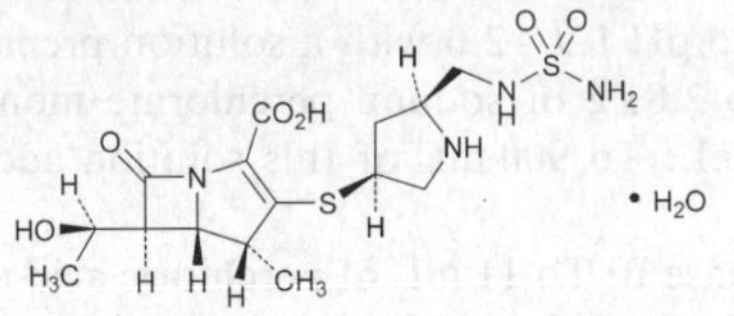

$C_{15}H_{24}N_4O_6S_2.H_2O$: 438.52

(4*R*,5*S*,6*S*)-6-[(1*R*)-1-Hydroxyethyl]-4-methyl-7-oxo-3-{(3*S*,5*S*-5-[(sulfamoylamino)methyl]pyrrolidin-3-ylsulfanyl}-1-azabicyclo[3.2.0]hept-2-ene-2-carboxylic acid monohydrate

[*364622-82-2*]

Doripenem Hydrate contains not less than 970 μg (potency) and not more than 1020 μg (potency) per mg, calculated on the anhydrous basis. The potency of Doripenem Hydrate is expressed as mass (potency) of doripenem ($C_{15}H_{24}N_4O_6S_2$: 420.50).

Description Doripenem Hydrate occurs as a white to pale yellow-brown-white crystalline powder.

It is sparingly soluble in water, slightly soluble in methanol, and practically insoluble in ethanol (99.5).

It is gradually colored to pale yellow-brown-white by light.

Identification (1) Determine the absorption spectrum of a solution of Doripenem Hydrate (1 in 50,000) as directed under Ultraviolet-visible Spectrophotometry <*2.24*>, and compare the spectrum with the Reference Spectrum or the spectrum of a solution of Doripenem RS prepared in the same manner as the sample solution: both spectra exhibit similar intensities of absorption at the same wavelengths.

(2) Determine the infrared absorption spectrum of Doripenem Hydrate as directed in the potassium bromide disk method under Infrared Spectrophotometry <*2.25*>, and compare the spectrum with the Reference Spectrum or the spectrum of Doripenem RS: both spectra exhibit similar intensities of absorption at the same wave numbers.

Optical rotation <*2.49*> $[\alpha]_D^{20}$: +33 – +38° (0.25 g calculated on the anhydrous basis, water, 25 mL, 100 mm).

pH <*2.54*> Dissolve 0.3 g of Doripenem Hydrate in 30 mL of water: the pH of the solution is between 4.5 and 6.0.

Purity (1) Clarity and color of solution—Dissolve 0.2 g of Doripenem Hydrate in 20 mL of water, and perform the test with this solution as directed under Turbidity Measurement <*2.61*>: the solution is clear. Perform the test with this solution according to Method 2 under Methods for Color Matching <*2.65*>: the solution is not more colored than Matching Fluid Y4.

(2) Heavy metals <*1.07*>—Moisten 1.0 g of Doripenem Hydrate with sulfuric acid, cover loosely, and heat gently to carbonize. Then proceed according to Method 2, and perform the test. Prepare the control solution with 2.0 mL of Standard Lead Solution (not more than 20 ppm).

(3) Related substances (i)—Dissolve 20 mg of Doripenem Hydrate in 10 mL of water, and use this solution as the sample solution. Pipet 1 mL of the sample solution, add water to make exactly 100 mL, and use this solution as the standard solution. Perform the test with exactly 20 μL each of the sample solution and standard solution as directed under Liquid Chromatography <*2.01*> according to the following conditions. Determine each peak area by the automatic integration method: the peak areas of related substance A, having the relative retention time of about 2.2 to doripenem, related substance B, having the relative retention time of about 2.5, and related substance C, having the relative retention time of about 3.2, obtained from the sample solution, are not larger than 1/10 times the peak area of doripenem from the standard solution, and the area of the peak other than doripenem, the peaks mentioned above and the peak having the relative retention time of about 2.1, from the sample solution, is not larger than 1/20 times the peak area of doripenem from the standard solution. Furthermore, the total area of the peaks other than doripenem and the peak having the relative retention time of about 2.1 from the sample solution is not larger than 1/2 times the peak area of doripenem from the standard solution.

Operating conditions—

Detector: An ultraviolet absorption photometer (wavelength: 230 nm).

Column: A stainless steel column 4.6 mm in inside diameter and 15 cm in length, packed with octadecylsilanized silica gel for liquid chromatography (5 μm in particle diameter).

Column temperature: A constant temperature of about 30°C.

Mobile phase A: Dissolve 2.04 g of potassium dihydrogen phosphate in water to make 1000 mL, and adjust to pH 5.6 – 5.7 with a solution prepared by dissolving 2.61 g of dipotassium hydrogen phosphate in water to make 1000 mL. To 970 mL of this solution add 30 mL of acetonitrile for liquid chromatography.

Mobile phase B: Dissolve 2.04 g of potassium dihydrogen phosphate in water to make 1000 mL, and adjust to pH 5.6 - 5.7 with a solution prepared by dissolving 2.61 g of dipotassium hydrogen phosphate in water to make 1000 mL. To 700 mL of this solution add 300 mL of acetonitrile for liquid chromatography.

Flowing of mobile phase: Control the gradient by mixing the mobile phases A and B as directed in the following table.

Time after injection of sample (min)	Mobile phase A (vol%)	Mobile phase B (vol%)
0 - 15	100	0
15 - 45	100 → 50	0 → 50
45 - 50	50 → 0	50 → 100
50 - 55	0	100

Flow rate: 1.0 mL per minute.

Time span of measurement: For 55 minutes after injection, beginning after the peak having the relative retention time of about 0.2 to doripenem.

System suitability—

Test for required detectability: Pipet 1.5 mL of the standard solution, and add water to make exactly 50 mL. Confirm that the peak area of doripenem obtained with 20 μL of this solution is equivalent to 2.1 to 3.9% of that with 20 μL of the standard solution.

System performance: When the procedure is run with 20 μL of the standard solution under the above operating conditions, the number of theoretical plates and the symmetry factor of the peak of doripenem are not less than 5000 and not more than 1.3, respectively.

System repeatability: When the test is repeated 3 times with 20 μL of the standard solution under the above operating conditions, the relative standard deviation of the peak area of doripenem is not more than 0.95%.

(ii) Dissolve 20 mg of Doripenem Hydrate in 10 mL of water, and use this solution as the sample solution. Pipet 1 mL of the sample solution, and add water to make exactly 100 mL, and use this solution as the standard solution. Perform the test with exactly 20 μL each of the sample solution and standard solution as directed under Liquid Chromatography <*2.01*> according to the following conditions. Determine each peak area by the automatic integration method: the peak area of related substance D, having the relative retention time of about 0.5 to doripenem, obtained from the sample solution is not larger than 2/5 times the peak area of doripenem from the standard solution.

Operating conditions—

Detector: An ultraviolet absorption photometer (wavelength: 215 nm).

Column: A stainless steel column 4.6 mm in inside diameter and 15 cm in length, packed with octadecyl-strong anion exchange-silanized silica gel for liquid chromatography (5 μm in particle diameter).

Column temperature: A constant temperature of about 40°C.

Mobile phase: To 9 mL of phosphoric acid add 200 mL of water, add 20 mL of triethylamine, and add water to make 2000 mL. Adjust to pH 5.7 - 5.9 with phosphoric acid. To 950 mL of this solution add 50 mL of acetonitrile for liquid chromatography.

Flow rate: Adjust so that the retention time of doripenem is about 10 minutes.

System suitability—

Test for required detectability: Pipet 2 mL of the standard solution, and add water to make exactly 20 mL. Confirm that the peak area of doripenem obtained with 20 μL of this solution is equivalent to 7 to 13% of that with 20 μL of the standard solution.

System performance: To 1 mL of the sample solution add 1 mL of 0.1 mol/L hydrochloric acid TS, allow to stand at 25 ± 5°C for 15 minutes, and add water to make 100 mL. When the procedure is run with 20 μL of this solution under the above operating conditions, related substance D and doripenem are eluted in this order with the resolution between these peaks being not less than 5. The number of theoretical plates and the symmetry factor of the peak of related substance D are not less than 300 and 0.7 to 1.3, respectively, and those of the peak of doripenem are not less than 5000 and 0.7 to 1.3, respectively.

System repeatability: When the test is repeated 6 times with 20 μL of the standard solution under the above operating conditions, the relative standard deviation of the peak area of doripenem is not more than 2.0%.

(iii) Dissolve 20 mg of Doripenem Hydrate in 10 mL of water, and use this solution as the sample solution. Pipet 1 mL of the sample solution, add water to make exactly 100 mL, and use this solution as the standard solution. Perform the test with exactly 20 μL each of the sample solution and standard solution as directed under Liquid Chromatography <*2.01*> according to the following conditions. Determine each peak area by the automatic integration method: the areas of the peaks, having the relative retention time of about 1.8, about 2.2 and about 2.3 to doripenem, obtained from the sample solution are not larger than 1/20, 7/100 and 1/20 times the peak area of doripenem from the standard solution, respectively.

Operating conditions—

Detector: An ultraviolet absorption photometer (wavelength: 310 nm).

Column: A stainless steel column 4.6 mm in inside diameter and 25 cm in length, packed with octadecylsilanized silica gel for liquid chromatography (3 μm in particle diameter).

Column temperature: A constant temperature of about 30°C.

Mobile phase A: To 11 mL of perchloric acid add water to make 500 mL. To 100 mL of this solution add water to make 1000 mL. To 600 mL of this solution add 100 mL of water, and adjust to pH 1.9 - 2.0 with a solution prepared by adding water to 2.81 g of sodium perchlorate monohydrate to make 1000 mL. To 900 mL of this solution add 100 mL of acetonitrile.

Mobile phase B: To 11 mL of perchloric acid add water to make 500 mL. To 100 mL of this solution add water to make 1000 mL. To 600 mL of this solution add 100 mL of water, and adjust to pH 1.9 - 2.0 with a solution prepared by adding water to 2.81 g of sodium perchlorate monohydrate to make 1000 mL. To 300 mL of this solution add 200 mL of acetonitrile.

Flowing of mobile phase: Control the gradient by mixing the mobile phases A and B as directed in the following table.

Time after injection of sample (min)	Mobile phase A (vol%)	Mobile phase B (vol%)
0 - 25	100	0
25 - 55	100 → 0	0 → 100
55 - 60	0	100

Flow rate: 0.8 mL per minute.

System suitability—

Test for required detectability: Pipet 2.5 mL of the standard solution, and add water to make exactly 50 mL. Confirm that the peak area of doripenem obtained with 20 μL of this solution is equivalent to 3.5 to 6.5% of that with 20 μL of the standard solution.

System performance: When the procedure is run with 20 μL of the standard solution under the above operating conditions, the number of theoretical plates and the symmetry factor of the peak of doripenem are not less than 15,000 and not more than 1.3, respectively.

System repeatability: When the test is repeated 3 times with 20 μL of the standard solution under the above operating conditions, the relative standard deviation of the peak area of doripenem is not more than 0.95%.

Water <2.48> 4.0 – 5.0% (0.3 g, volumetric titration, back titration).

Residue on ignition <2.44> Not more than 0.1% (1 g).

Assay Weigh accurately amounts of Doripenem Hydrate and Doripenem RS (separately determine the water <2.48> in the same manner as Doripenem Hydrate), equivalent to about 25 mg (potency), dissolve each in water to make exactly 200 mL, and use these solutions as the sample solution and the standard solution, respectively. Perform the test with exactly 10 μL each of the sample solution and standard solution as directed under Liquid Chromatography <2.01> according to the following conditions, and determine the peak areas, A_T and A_S, of doripenem in each solution.

Amount [μg (potency)] of doripenem ($C_{15}H_{24}N_4O_6S_2$)
$= M_S \times A_T/A_S \times 1000$

M_S: Amount [mg (potency)] of Doripenem RS taken, calculated on the anhydrous basis

Operating conditions—

Detector: An ultraviolet absorption photometer (wavelength: 300 nm).

Column: A stainless steel column 4.6 mm in inside diameter and 15 cm in length, packed with octadecylsilanized silica gel for liquid chromatography (5 μm in particle diameter).

Column temperature: A constant temperature of about 25°C.

Mobile phase: Adjust the pH of 90 mL of 0.02 mol/L potassium dihydrogen phosphate TS to pH 5.6 – 5.7 with a solution prepared by dissolving 3.48 g of dipotassium hydrogen phosphate in water to make 1000 mL. To 100 mL of this solution add water to make exactly 1000 mL. To 970 mL of this solution add 30 mL of acetonitrile.

Flow rate: Adjust so that the retention time of doripenem is about 15 minutes.

System suitability—

System performance: When the procedure is run with 10 μL of the standard solution under the above operating conditions, the number of theoretical plates and the symmetry factor of the peak of doripenem are not less than 5000 and not more than 1.3, respectively.

System repeatability: When the test is repeated 6 times with 10 μL of the standard solution under the above operating conditions, the relative standard deviation of the peak area of doripenem is not more than 1.0%.

Containers and storage Containers—Tight containers.

Storage—At a temperature between 2°C and 8°C.

Others

Related substance A:
(4*R*,5*S*,6*S*)-3-{(3*S*,5*S*)-5-[({*N*-(*E*)-(Dimethylamino)methylene]sulfamoyl}amino)methyl]pyrrolidin-3-ylsulfanyl}-6-[(1*R*)-1-hydroxyethyl]-4-methyl-7-oxo-1-azabicyclo[3.2.0]hept-2-ene-2-carboxylic acid

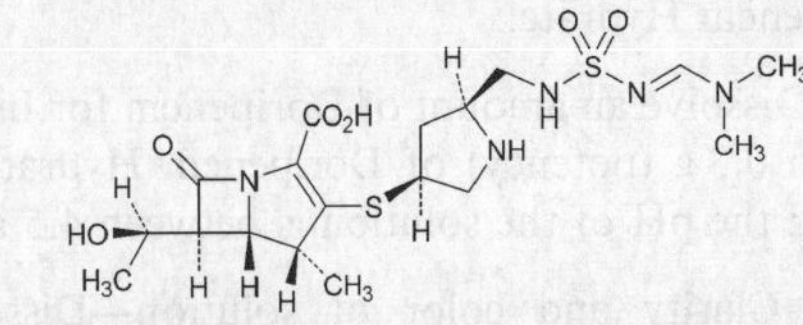

Related substance B:
(1*S*,4*S*,5*S*,6*R*)-4-[(1*R*)-1-Hydroxyethyl]-8-[(4*R*,5*S*,6*S*)-6-[(1*R*)-1-hydroxyethyl]-4-methyl-7-oxo-3-{(3*S*,5*S*)-5-[(sulfamoylamino)methyl]pyrrolidin-3-ylsulfanyl}-1-azabicyclo[3.2.0]hept-2-ene-2-carbonyl]-6-methyl-3-oxo-7-{(3*S*,5*S*)-5-[(sulfamoylamino)methyl]pyrrolidin-3-ylsulfanyl}-2-oxa-8-azabicyclo[3.2.1]octane-1-carboxylic acid

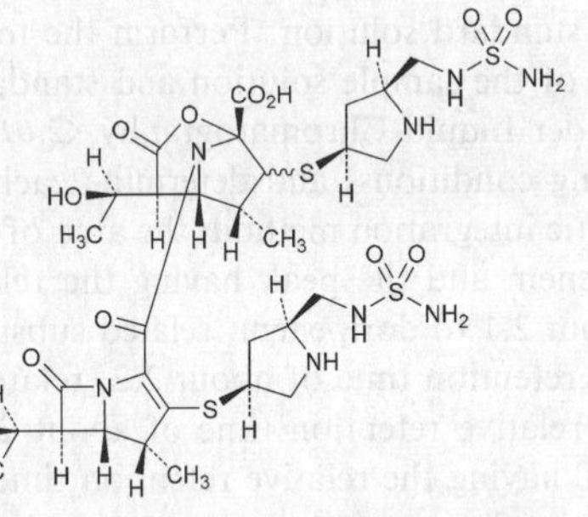

Related substance C:
(4*R*,5*S*,6*S*)-3-[(3*S*,5*S*)-5-({[*N*-(1,1-Dimethylethyl)sulfamoyl]amino}methyl)pyrrolidin-3-ylsulfanyl]-6-[(1*R*)-1-hydroxyethyl]-4-methyl-7-oxo-1-azabicyclo[3.2.0]hept-2-ene-2-carboxylic acid

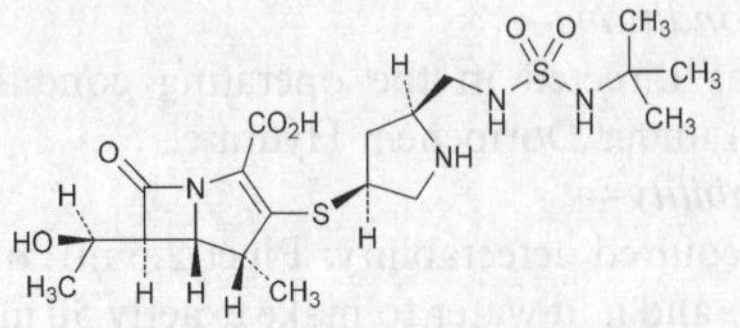

Related substance D:
(2*S*,3*R*,4*S*)-2-[(1*S*,2*R*)-1-Carboxy-2-hydroxypropyl]-3-methyl-4-{(3*S*,5*S*)-5-[(sulfamoylamino)methyl]pyrrolidin-3-ylsulfanyl}-3,4-dihydro-2*H*-pyrrole-5-carboxylic acid

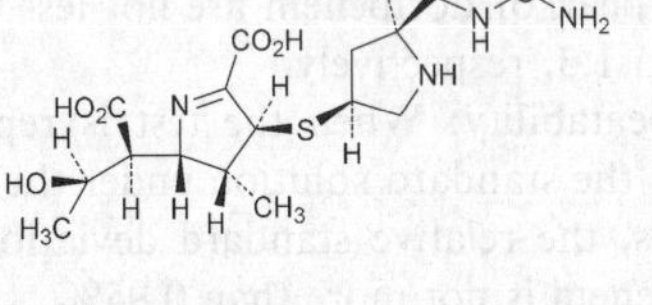

Doripenem for Injection

注射用ドリペネム

Doripenem for Injection is a preparation for injection, which is dissolved before use.

It contains not less than 95.0% and not more than 105.0% of the labeled potency of doripenem ($C_{15}H_{24}N_4O_6S_2$: 420.50).

Method of preparation Prepare as directed under Injections, with Doripenem Hydrate.

Description Doripenem for Injection occurs as a white to pale yellow-brown-white crystalline powder.

Identification Proceed as directed in the Identification (2) under Doripenem Hydrate.

pH <*2.54*> Dissolve an amount of Doripenem for Injection, equivalent to 0.3 g (potency) of Doripenem Hydrate, in 30 mL of water: the pH of the solution is between 4.5 and 6.0.

Purity **(1)** Clarity and color of solution—Dissolve an amount of Doripenem for Injection, equivalent to 0.2 g (potency) of Doripenem Hydrate in 20 mL of water, and proceed as directed in the Purity (1) under Doripenem Hydrate.

(2) Related substances—(i) Dissolve an amount of Doripenem for Injection, equivalent to 20 mg (potency) of Doripenem Hydrate, in 10 mL of water, and use this solution as the sample solution. Pipet 1 mL of the sample solution, add water to make exactly 100 mL, and use this solution as the standard solution. Perform the test with exactly 20 μL each of the sample solution and standard solution as directed under Liquid Chromatography <*2.01*> according to the following conditions, and determine each peak area by the automatic integration method: the area of the peak other than doripenem and the peak having the relative retention time of about 2.1 to doripenem, related substance A having the relative retention time of about 2.2, related substance B having the relative retention time of about 2.5 and related substance C having the relative retention time of about 3.2, obtained from the sample solution, is not larger than 1/10 times the peak area of doripenem from the standard solution, and the total area of the peaks other than doripenem and the peak mentioned above from the sample solution is not larger than 1/2 times the peak area of doripenem from the standard solution.

Operating conditions—

Proceed as directed in the operating conditions in the Purity (3) (i) under Doripenem Hydrate.

System suitability—

Test for required detectability: Pipet 2.5 mL of the standard solution, and add water to make exactly 50 mL. Confirm that the peak area of doripenem obtained with 20 μL of this solution is equivalent to 3.5 to 6.5% of that with 20 μL of the standard solution.

System performance: When the procedure is run with 20 μL of the standard solution under the above operating conditions, the number of theoretical plates and the symmetry factor of the peak of doripenem are not less than 5000 and not more than 1.3, respectively.

System repeatability: When the test is repeated 3 times with 20 μL of the standard solution under the above operating conditions, the relative standard deviation of the peak area of doripenem is not more than 0.95%.

(ii) Dissolve an amount of Doripenem for Injection, equivalent to 20 mg (potency) of Doripenem Hydrate, in 10 mL of water, and use this solution as the sample solution. Pipet 1 mL of the sample solution, add water to make exactly 100 mL, and use this solution as the standard solution. Perform the test with exactly 20 μL each of the sample solution and standard solution as directed under Liquid Chromatography <*2.01*> according to the following conditions. Determine each peak area by the automatic integration method: the peak area of related substance D, having the relative retention time of about 0.5 to doripenem, obtained from the sample solution is not larger than the peak area of doripenem from the standard solution.

Operating conditions—

Proceed as directed in the operating conditions in the Purity (3) (ii) under Doripenem Hydrate.

System suitability—

System performance: To 1 mL of the sample solution add 1 mL of 0.1 mol/L hydrochloric acid TS, allow to stand at 25 ± 5°C for 15 minutes, and add water to make 100 mL. When the procedure is run with 20 μL of this solution under the above operating conditions, related substance D and doripenem are eluted in this order with the resolution between these peaks being not less than 5. The number of theoretical plates and the symmetry factor of the peak of related substance D are not less than 300 and 0.7 to 1.3, respectively, and those of the peak of doripenem are not less than 5000 and 0.7 to 1.3, respectively.

System repeatability: When the test is repeated 6 times with 20 μL of the standard solution under the above operating conditions, the relative standard deviation of the peak area of doripenem is not more than 2.0%.

Water <*2.48*> 4.0 - 5.0% (0.3 g, volumetric titration, back titration).

Bacterial endotoxins <*4.01*> Less than 0.25 EU/mg (potency).

Uniformity of dosage units <*6.02*> It meets the requirement of the Mass variation test.

Foreign insoluble matter <*6.06*> Perform the test according to Method 2: it meets the requirement.

Insoluble particulate matter <*6.07*> It meets the requirement.

Sterility <*4.06*> Perform the test according to the Membrane filtration method: it meets the requirement.

Assay Weigh accurately the mass of the contents of not less than 10 containers of Doripenem for Injection. Weigh accurately an amount of the contents, equivalent to about 25 mg (potency) of Doripenem Hydrate, dissolve in water to make exactly 200 mL, and use this solution as the sample solution. Separately, weigh accurately about 25 mg (potency) of Doripenem RS (separately determine the water <*2.48*> in the same manner as Doripenem Hydrate), dissolve in water to make exactly 200 mL, and use this solution as the standard solution. Then, proceed as directed in the Assay under Doripenem Hydrate.

$$\text{Amount [}\mu\text{g (potency)] of doripenem } (C_{15}H_{24}N_4O_6S_2) = M_S \times A_T/A_S \times 1000$$

M_S: Amount [mg (potency)] of Doripenem RS taken, calculated on the anhydrous basis

Containers and storage Containers—Hermetic containers. Plastic containers for aqueous injections may be used.

Others

Related substances A, B, C and D: Refer to them described in Doripenem Hydrate.

Dorzolamide Hydrochloride

ドルゾラミド塩酸塩

$C_{10}H_{16}N_2O_4S_3.HCl$: 360.90
(4*S*,6*S*)-4-Ethylamino-6-methyl-5,6-dihydro-4*H*-thieno[2,3-*b*]thiopyran-2-sulfonamide 7,7-dioxide monohydrochloride
[*130693-82-2*]

Dorzolamide Hydrochloride contains not less than 99.0% and not more than 101.0% of dorzolamide hydrochloride ($C_{10}H_{16}N_2O_4S_3.HCl$), calculated on the anhydrous basis.

Description Dorzolamide Hydrochloride occurs as a white crystalline powder.

It is soluble in water, sparingly soluble in methanol, and very slightly soluble in ethanol (99.5).

It dissolves in diluted ammonia solution (28) (13 in 400).

Optical rotation $[\alpha]^{25}_{404.7}$: −16.0 − −17.5° (0.25 g calculated on the anhydrous basis, water, 25 mL, 100 mm).

Dorzolamide Hydrochloride shows crystal polymorphism.

Identification (1) Determine the absorption spectrum of a solution of Dorzolamide Hydrochloride in a solution of hydrochloric acid in methanol (9 in 1000) (3 in 200,000) as directed under Ultraviolet-visible Spectrophotometry ⟨*2.24*⟩, and compare the spectrum with the Reference Spectrum or the spectrum of a solution of Dorzolamide Hydrochloride RS prepared in the same manner as the sample solution: both spectra exhibit similar intensities of absorption at the same wavelengths.

(2) Determine the infrared absorption spectrum of Dorzolamide Hydrochloride as directed in the potassium bromide disk method under Infrared Spectrophotometry ⟨*2.25*⟩, and compare the spectrum with the Reference Spectrum or the spectrum of Dorzolamide Hydrochloride RS: both spectra exhibit similar intensities of absorption at the same wave numbers.

(3) A solution of Dorzolamide Hydrochloride (1 in 100) responds to Qualitative Tests ⟨*1.09*⟩ for chloride.

Purity (1) Heavy metals ⟨*1.07*⟩—Proceed with 2.0 g of Dorzolamide Hydrochloride according to Method 2, and perform the test. Prepare the control solution with 2.0 mL of Standard Lead Solution (not more than 10 ppm).

(2) Related substances—Dissolve 30 mg of Dorzolamide Hydrochloride in 50 mL of a mixture of water and methanol (4:1), and use this solution as the sample solution. Perform the test with 10 μL of the sample solution as directed under Liquid Chromatography ⟨*2.01*⟩ according to the following conditions. Determine each peak area by the automatic integration method, and calculate their amounts by the area percentage method: the amount of the peaks other than dorzolamide is not more than 0.1%.

Operating conditions—

Detector, column, column temperature, and flow rate: Proceed as directed in the operating conditions in the Assay.

Mobile phase A: Adjust to pH 4.5 of a mixture of water and acetic acid (100) (1000:1) with triethylamine.

Mobile phase B: Acetonitrile.

Flowing of mobile phase: Control the gradient by mixing the mobile phases A and B as directed in the following table.

Time after injection of sample (min)	Mobile phase A (vol%)	Mobile phase B (vol%)
0 – 10	100	0
10 – 30	100 → 50	0 → 50

Time span of measurement: About 3 times as long as the retention time of dorzolamide, beginning after the solvent peak.

System suitability—

Test for required detectability: Pipet 2 mL of the sample solution, and add a mixture of water and methanol (4:1) to make exactly 100 mL. Pipet 1 mL of this solution, add a mixture of water and methanol (4:1) to make exactly 20 mL, and use this solution as the solution for system suitability test. Confirm that the peak area of dorzolamide obtained with 10 μL of the solution for system suitability test is equivalent to 0.07 to 0.13% of that with 10 μL of the sample solution.

System performance: To 1 mL of the sample solution add 2 mL of a mixture of water and methanol (4:1). When the procedure is run with 10 μL of this solution under the above operating conditions, the number of theoretical plates and the symmetry factor of the peak of dorzolamide are not less than 4000 and not more than 1.5, respectively.

System repeatability: When the test is repeated 6 times with 10 μL of the solution for system suitability test under the above operating conditions, the relative standard deviation of the peak area of dorzolamide is not more than 7%.

(3) Enantiomer—Dissolve 20 mg of Dorzolamide Hydrochloride in 4 mL of diluted ammonia solution (28) (13 in 400), and extract this solution with two 4-mL portions of ethyl acetate. Combine the extracts, and evaporate the ethyl acetate at 50°C under a current of nitrogen. Dissolve the residue in 3 mL of acetonitrile, add 3 drops of (*S*)-1-phenylethyl isocyanate, and allow to stand at 50°C for 10 minutes. Evaporate at 50°C under a current of nitrogen, dissolve the residue in 10 mL of a mixture of *tert*-butylmethyl ether, acetic acid (100) and acetonitrile (873:100:27), and use this solution as the sample solution. Perform the test with 5 μL of the sample solution as directed under Liquid Chromatography ⟨*2.01*⟩ according to the following conditions, and determine the peak areas of dorzolamide, A_2, and that of the enantiomer, having the relative retention time of about 1.5 to dorzolamide, A_1, by the automatic integration method: the result of $A_1/(A_1 + A_2)$ is not more than 0.005.

Operating conditions—

Detector: An ultraviolet absorption photometer (wavelength: 254 nm).

Column: A stainless steel column 4.6 mm in inside diameter and 25 cm in length, packed with silica gel for liquid chromatography (5 μm in particle diameter).

Column temperature: A constant temperature of about 25°C.

Mobile phase: To a mixture of 30 mL of acetonitrile and 3 mL of water add *tert*-butylmethyl ether to make 1000 mL. To 650 mL of this solution add 350 mL of heptane.

Flow rate: Adjust so that the retention time of dorzolamide is about 8 minutes.

System suitability—

Test for required detectability: Pipet 1 mL of the sample solution, add a mixture of *tert*-butylmethyl ether, acetic acid

(100) and acetonitrile (873:100:27) to make exactly 200 mL, and use this solution as the solution for system suitability test. Confirm that the peak area of dorzolamide obtained with 5 μL of the solution for system suitability test is equivalent to 0.4 to 0.6% of that with 5 μL of the sample solution.

System performance: When the procedure is run with 5 μL of the sample solution under the above operating conditions, the number of theoretical plates and the symmetry factor of the peak of dorzolamide are not less than 4000 and not more than 1.4, respectively.

System repeatability: When the test is repeated 6 times with 5 μL of the solution for system suitability test under the above operating conditions, the relative standard deviation of the peak area of dorzolamide is not more than 7%.

Water <*2.48*> Not more than 0.5% (0.5 g, coulometric titration).

Residue on ignition <*2.44*> Not more than 0.1% (1 g).

Assay Weigh accurately about 20 mg each of Dorzolamide Hydrochloride and Dorzolamide Hydrochloride RS (separately, determine the water <*2.48*> in the same manner as Dorzolamide Hydrochloride), dissolve in a mixture of water and methanol (4:1) to make exactly 100 mL, and use these solutions as the sample solution and the standard solution, respectively. Perform the test with exactly 10 μL each of the sample solution and standard solution as directed under Liquid Chromatography <*2.01*> according to the following conditions, and determine the peak areas, A_T and A_S, of dorzolamide in each solution.

Amount (mg) of dorzolamide hydrochloride ($C_{10}H_{16}N_2O_4S_3.HCl$)
$= M_S \times A_T/A_S$

M_S: Amount (mg) of Dorzolamide Hydrochloride RS taken, calculated on the anhydrous basis

Operating conditions—

Detector: An ultraviolet absorption photometer (wavelength: 254 nm).

Column: A stainless steel column 4.6 mm in inside diameter and 8.3 cm in length, packed with octylsilanized silica gel for liquid chromatography (3 μm in particle diameter).

Column temperature: A constant temperature of about 25°C.

Mobile phase: Adjust to pH 4.5 of a mixture of water and acetic acid (100) (1000:1) with triethylamine.

Flow rate: Adjust so that the retention time of dorzolamide is about 9 minutes.

System suitability—

System performance: When the procedure is run with 10 μL of the standard solution under the above operating conditions, the number of theoretical plates and the symmetry factor of the peak of dorzolamide are not less than 4000 and not more than 1.5, respectively.

System repeatability: When the test is repeated 6 times with 10 μL of the standard solution under the above operating conditions, the relative standard deviation of the peak area of dorzolamide is not more than 1.0%.

Containers and storage Containers—Well-closed containers.

Dorzolamide Hydrochloride Ophthalmic Solution

ドルゾラミド塩酸塩点眼液

Dorzolamide Hydrochloride Ophthalmic Solution is an aqueous ophthalmic preparation.

It contains not less than 95.0% and not more than 107.0% of the labeled amount of dorzolamide ($C_{10}H_{16}N_2O_4S_3$: 324.44).

Method of preparation Prepare as directed under Ophthalmic Liquids and Solutions, with Dorzolamide Hydrochloride.

Description Dorzolamide Hydrochloride Ophthalmic Solution occurs as a clear and colorless liquid.

Identification To a volume of Dorzolamide Hydrochloride Ophthalmic Solution, equivalent to about 1.2 mg of dorzolamide ($C_{10}H_{16}N_2O_4S_3$), add 0.1 mol/L hydrochloric acid TS to make 100 mL. Determine the absorption spectrum of this solution as directed under Ultraviolet-visible Spectrophotometry <*2.24*>: it exhibits a maximum between 252 nm and 256 nm.

pH Being specified separately when the drug is granted approval based on the Law.

Purity cis-Isomer—Use the sample solution obtained in the Assay as the sample solution. Perform the test with 20 μL of the sample solution as directed under Liquid Chromatography <*2.01*> according to the following conditions, and determine the peak area of dorzolamide, A_2, and that of cis-isomer, having the relative retention time of about 1.1 to dorzolamide, A_1, by the automatic integration method: $A_1/(A_1 + A_2)$ is not larger than 0.020.

Diluting solution: To 2 mL of phosphoric acid add 900 mL of water, adjust to pH 3.0 with triethylamine, then add water to make 1000 mL.

Operating conditions—

Proceed as directed in the operating conditions in the Assay.

System suitability—

System performance: Proceed as directed in the system suitability in the Assay.

Test for required detectability: To exactly 2 mL of the sample solution add the diluting solution to make exactly 100 mL. Pipet 1 mL of this solution, add the diluting solution to make exactly 20 mL, and use this solution as the solution for system suitability test. Confirm that the peak area of dorzolamide obtained with 20 μL of the solution for system suitability test is equivalent to 0.07 to 0.13% of that with 20 μL of the sample solution.

System repeatability: When the test is repeated 6 times with 20 μL of the solution for system suitability test under the above operating conditions, the relative standard deviation of the peak area of dorzolamide is not more than 7%.

Foreign insoluble matter <*6.11*> It meets the requirement.

Insoluble particulate matter <*6.08*> It meets the requirement.

Sterility <*4.06*> Perform the test according to the Direct inoculation method, using the culture medium containing 0.7% polysorbate 80 and 0.1% of lecithin: it meets the requirement.

Assay Weigh accurately a portion of Dorzolamide Hydrochloride Ophthalmic Solution, equivalent to about 5 mg of dorzolamide ($C_{10}H_{16}N_2O_4S_3$), add the diluting solution to make exactly 50 mL, and use this solution as the sample solution. Separately, weigh accurately about 20 mg of Dorzolamide Hydrochloride RS (separately determine the water <*2.48*> in the same manner as Dorzolamide Hydrochloride), dissolve in the diluting solution to make exactly 200 mL, and use this solution as the standard solution. Perform the test with exactly 20 μL each of the sample solution and standard solution as directed under Liquid Chromatography <*2.01*> according to the following conditions, and determine the peak areas, A_T and A_S, of dorzolamide in each solution.

Diluting solution: To 2 mL of phosphoric acid add 900 mL of water, adjust to pH 3.0 with triethylamine, then add water to make 1000 mL.

Amount (mg/mL) of dorzolamide ($C_{10}H_{16}N_2O_4S_3$)
$= M_S/M_T \times A_T/A_S \times 1/4 \times d \times 0.899$

M_S: Amount (mg) of Dorzolamide Hydrochloride RS taken, calculated on the anhydrous basis

M_T: Amount (g) of Dorzolamide Hydrochloride Ophthalmic Solution taken

d: Density (g/mL) of Dorzolamide Hydrochloride Ophthalmic Solution

Operating conditions—

Detector: An ultraviolet absorption photometer (wavelength: 253 nm).

Column: A stainless steel column 4.6 mm in inside diameter and 25 cm in length, packed with octylsilanized silica gel for liquid chromatography (5 μm in particle diameter).

Column temperature: A constant temperature of about 25°C.

Mobile phase: A mixture of the diluting solution and acetonitrile (19:1).

Flow rate: Adjust so that the retention time of dorzolamide is about 10 minutes.

System suitability—

System performance: When the procedure is run with 20 μL of the standard solution under the above operating conditions, the number of theoretical plates and the symmetry factor of the peak of dorzolamide are not less than 6000 and not more than 1.8, respectively.

System repeatability: When the test is repeated 6 times with 20 μL of the standard solution under the above operating conditions, the relative standard deviation of the peak area of dorzolamide is not more than 1.0%.

Containers and storage Containers—Tight containers.

Dorzolamide Hydrochloride and Timolol Maleate Ophthalmic Solution

ドルゾラミド塩酸塩·チモロールマレイン酸塩点眼液

Dorzolamide Hydrochloride and Timolol Maleate Ophthalmic Solution contains not less than 93.0% and not more than 107.0% of the labelled amount of dorzolamide ($C_{10}H_{16}N_2O_4S_3$: 324.44), and not less than 93.0% and not more than 110.0% of the labelled amount of timolol ($C_{13}H_{24}N_4O_3S$: 316.42).

Method of Preparation Prepare as directed under Ophthalmic Liquids and Solutions, with Dorzolamide Hydrochloride and Timolol Maleate.

Description Dorzolamide Hydrochloride and Timolol Maleate Ophthalmic Solution is a clear, colorless, and slightly viscous liquid.

Identification **(1)** Perform the test with 20 μL each of the sample solution and the standard solution obtained in the Assay (1) as directed under Liquid Chromatography <*2.01*> according to the conditions described in the Assay (1): the retention times of the peak of dorzolamide in the chromatograms obtained from the sample solution and the standard solution are the same.

(2) Perform the test with 20 μL each of the sample solution and the standard solution obtained in the Assay (2) as directed under Liquid Chromatography <*2.01*> according to the conditions described in the Assay (2): the retention times of the peak of timolol in the chromatograms obtained from the sample solution and the standard solution are the same.

Osmotic pressure ratio Being specified separately when the drug is granted approval based on the Law.

Viscosity Being specified separately when the drug is granted approval based on the Law.

pH Being specified separately when the drug is granted approval based on the Law.

Purity **(1)** Related substance 1—Use the sample solution obtained in the Assay (1) as the sample solution. Pipet 1 mL of the sample solution, add a mixture of diluted phosphoric acid (1 in 500) and acetonitrile (19:1) to make exactly 100 mL, and use this solution as the standard solution. Perform the test with exactly 20 μL each of the sample solution and standard solution as directed under Liquid Chromatography <*2.01*> according to the following conditions, and determine each peak area by the automatic integration method: the peak area of related substance OA having the relative retention time of about 0.8 to dorzolamide obtained from the sample solution is not larger than 1/5 times the peak area of dorzolamide from the standard solution, and the peak area of related substance OB having the relative retention time of about 1.2 to dorzolamide from the sample solution is not larger than 2.4 times the peak area of dorzolamide from the standard solution. The area of the peak other than dorzolamide and the peaks mentioned above from the sample solution is not larger than 1/5 times the peak area of dorzolamide from the standard solution. Furthermore, the total area of the peaks other than dorzolamide from the sample solution is not larger than 2.5 times the peak area of dorzolamide from the standard solution.

Operating conditions—

Detector, column, column temperature, mobile phase, and flow rate: Proceed as directed in the operating conditions in the Assay (1).

Time span of measurement: For 18 minutes after injection of the sample solution.

System suitability—

System performance: Proceed as directed in the system suitability in the Assay (1).

Test for required detectability: Pipet 2 mL of the standard solution, add a mixture of diluted phosphoric acid (1 in 500 mL) and acetonitrile (19:1) to make exactly 20 mL. Confirm that the peak area of dorzolamide obtained with 20 μL of this solution is equivalent to 7 to 13% of that with 20 μL of the standard solution.

System repeatability: When the test is repeated 6 times with 20 μL of the standard solution under the above operating conditions, the relative standard deviation of the peak

area of dorzolamide is not more than 5.0%.

(2) Related substance 2—Use the sample solution obtained in the Assay (2) as the sample solution. Pipet 2 mL of the sample solution, add the mobile phase to make exactly 200 mL, and use this solution as the standard solution. Perform the test with exactly 20 μL each of the sample solution and standard solution as directed under Liquid Chromatography <*2.01*> according to the following conditions, and determine each peak area by the automatic integration method: the area of the peak other than timolol and the peak having the relative retention time of about 0.49 to timolol obtained from the sample solution is not larger than 2/5 times the peak area of timolol from the standard solution. Furthermore, the total area of the peaks other than timolol and the peak having the relative retention time of about 0.49 to timolol, from the sample solution is not larger than 1/2 times the peak area of timolol from the standard solution.

Operating conditions—

Detector, column, column temperature, mobile phase, and flow rate: Proceed as directed in the operating conditions in the Assay (2).

Time span of measurement: For 10 minutes after injection of the sample solution.

System suitability—

System performance and system repeatability: Proceed as directed in the system suitability in the Assay (2).

Test for required detectability: Pipet 10 mL of the standard solution, add the mobile phase to make exactly 100 mL. Confirm that the peak area of timolol obtained with 20 μL of this solution is equivalent to 7 to 13% of that with 20 μL of the standard solution.

Foreign insoluble matter <*6.11*> It meets the requirement.

Insoluble particulate matter <*6.08*> It meets the requirement.

Sterility <*4.06*> It meets the requirement.

Assay (1) Dorzolamide hydrochloride—Pipet a volume of Dorzolamide Hydrochloride and Timolol Maleate Ophthalmic Solution, equivalent to about 2.5 mg of dorzolamide ($C_{10}H_{16}N_2O_4S_3$), add a mixture of diluted phosphoric acid (1 in 500) and acetonitrile (19:1) to make exactly 25 mL, and use this solution as the sample solution. Separately, weigh accurately about 22 mg of Dorzolamide Hydrochloride RS (separately determine the water <*2.48*> in the same manner as Dorzolamide Hydrochloride), dissolve in a mixture of diluted phosphoric acid (1 in 500) and acetonitrile (19:1) to make exactly 200 mL, and use this solution as the standard solution. Perform the test with exactly 20 μL each of the sample solution and standard solution as directed under Liquid Chromatography <*2.01*> according to the following conditions, and determine the peak areas, A_T and A_S, of dorzolamide in each solution.

Amount (mg) of dorzolamide ($C_{10}H_{16}N_2O_4S_3$) in 1 mL of Dorzolamide Hydrochloride and Timolol Maleate Ophthalmic Solution

$$= M_S/M_T \times A_T/A_S \times 1/8 \times d \times 0.899$$

M_S: Amount (mg) of Dorzolamide Hydrochloride RS taken, calculated on the anhydrous basis

M_T: Amount (g) of Dorzolamide Hydrochloride and Timolol Maleate Ophthalmic Solution taken

d: Density (g/mL) of Dorzolamide Hydrochloride and Timolol Maleate Ophthalmic Solution

Operating conditions—

Detector: An ultraviolet absorption photometer (wavelength: 253 nm).

Column: A stainless steel column 4.6 mm in inside diameter and 25 cm in length, packed with octylsilanized silica gel for liquid chromatography (5 μm in particle diameter).

Column temperature: A constant temperature of about 25°C.

Mobile phase A: A mixture of diluted phosphoric acid (1 in 500) and acetonitrile (19:1).

Mobile phase B: A mixture of acetonitrile and diluted phosphoric acid (1 in 500) (19:1).

Flowing of mobile phase: Control the gradient by mixing the mobile phases A and B as directed in the following table.

Time after injection of sample (min)	Mobile phase A (vol%)	Mobile phase B (vol%)
0 – 15.0	100	0
15.0 – 15.1	100 → 0	0 → 100
15.1 – 20.0	0	100

Flow rate: 1.2 mL per minute.

System suitability—

System performance: When the procedure is run with 20 μL of the standard solution, the number of theoretical plates and the symmetry factor of the peak of dorzolamide are not less than 5000 and not more than 3.0, respectively.

System repeatability: When the test is repeated 6 times with 20 μL of the standard solution, the relative standard deviation of the peak area of dorzolamide is not more than 2.0%.

(2) Timolol maleate—Pipet a volume of Dorzolamide Hydrochloride and Timolol Maleate Ophthalmic Solution, equivalent to about 6.5 mg of timolol ($C_{13}H_{24}N_4O_3S$), add the mobile phase to make exactly 25 mL, and use this solution as the sample solution. Separately, weigh accurately about 34 mg of Timolol Maleate RS, previously dried at 100°C under reduced pressure for 3 hours, dissolve in the mobile phase to make exactly 100 mL, and use this solution as the standard solution. Perform the test with exactly 20 μL each of the sample solution and standard solution as directed under Liquid Chromatography <*2.01*> according to the following conditions, and determine the peak areas, A_T and A_S, of timolol in each solution.

Amount (mg) of timolol ($C_{13}H_{24}N_4O_3S$) in 1 mL of Dorzolamide Hydrochloride and Timolol Maleate Ophthalmic Solution

$$= M_S/M_T \times A_T/A_S \times 1/4 \times d \times 0.732$$

M_S: Amount (mg) of Timolol Maleate RS taken

M_T: Amount (g) of Dorzolamide Hydrochloride and Timolol Maleate Ophthalmic Solution taken

d: Density (g/mL) of Dorzolamide Hydrochloride and Timolol Maleate Ophthalmic Solution

Operating conditions—

Detector: An ultraviolet absorption photometer (wavelength: 295 nm).

Column: A stainless steel column 4.6 mm in inside diameter and 25 cm in length, packed with octadecylsilanized silica gel for liquid chromatography (5 μm in particle diameter).

Column temperature: A constant temperature of about 40°C.

Mobile phase: Dissolve 25 g of sodium dihydrogen phosphate dihydrate in water to make 2000 mL, and adjust to pH 2.8 with phosphoric acid. To 600 mL of this solution add 400 mL of methanol.

Flow rate: 1.0 mL per minute.

System suitability—

System performance: Dissolve 44 mg of Timolol Maleate RS in 4 mL of sodium hydroxide solution (1 in 250), warm at 70°C for 15 hours, and add the mobile phase to make 25 mL. To 5 mL of this solution, add 28 mg of Dorzolamide Hydrochloride RS to dissolve, add the mobile phase to make 25 mL, and use this solution as the solution for system suitability test. When the procedure is run with 20 μL of the solution for system suitability test according to the above operating conditions, the number of theoretical plates and the symmetry factor of the peak of timolol are not less than 3000 and not more than 2.0, respectively. The resolution between the co-eluting peak of dorzolamide and maleate, having the relative retention time of about 0.49 to timolol, and the peak, having the relative retention time of about 0.58 to timolol, is not less than 1.5, and the resolution between the peaks having the relative retention times of about 0.58 and about 0.70 to timolol is not less than 1.5.

System repeatability: When the test is repeated 6 times with 20 μL of the solution for system suitability test, the relative standard deviation of the peak area of timolol is not more than 2.0%.

Containers and storage Containers—Tight containers.

Storage—Light-resistant.

Others

Related substance OA:
(4*S*,6*S*)-4-Amino-6-methyl-5,6-dihydro-4*H*-thieno[2,3-*b*]thiopyran-2-sulfonamide 7,7-dioxide

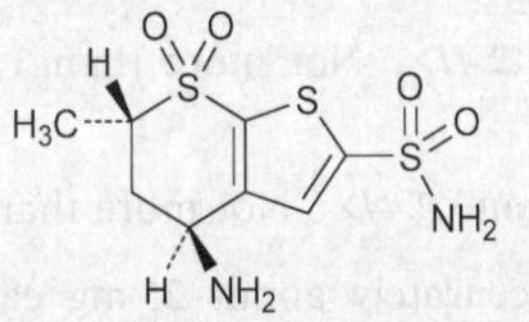

Related substance OB:
(4*RS*,6*SR*)-4-Ethylamino-6-methyl-5,6-dihydro-4*H*-thieno[2,3-*b*]thiopyran-2-sulfonamide 7,7-dioxide

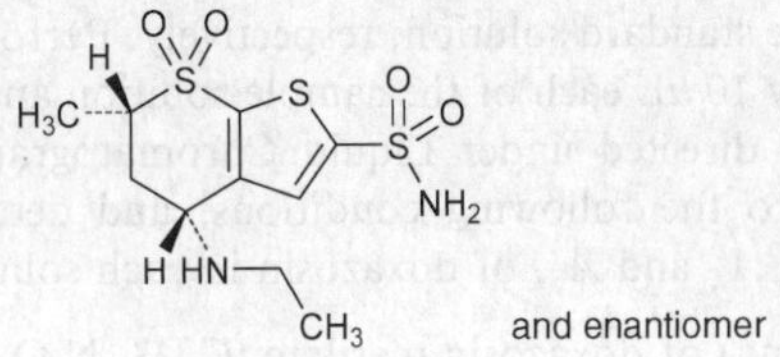

and enantiomer

Doxapram Hydrochloride Hydrate

ドキサプラム塩酸塩水和物

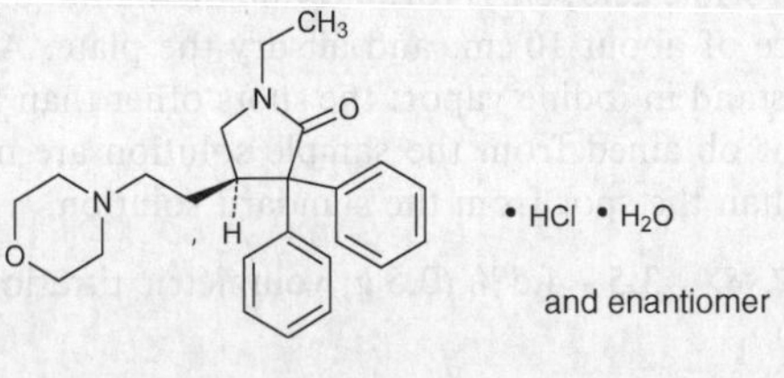

and enantiomer

$C_{24}H_{30}N_2O_2.HCl.H_2O$: 432.98
(4*RS*)-1-Ethyl-4-[2-(morpholin-4-yl)ethyl]-3,3-diphenylpyrrolidin-2-one monohydrochloride monohydrate
[*7081-53-0*]

Doxapram Hydrochloride Hydrate contains not less than 98.0% of doxapram hydrochloride ($C_{24}H_{30}N_2O_2.HCl$: 414.97), calculated on the anhydrous basis.

Description Doxapram Hydrochloride Hydrate occurs as white, crystals or crystalline powder.

It is freely soluble in methanol and in acetic acid (100), sparingly soluble in water, in ethanol (95) and in acetic anhydride, and practically insoluble in diethyl ether.

Identification **(1)** Determine the absorption spectrum of a solution of Doxapram Hydrochloride Hydrate (1 in 2500) as directed under Ultraviolet-visible Spectrophotometry <*2.24*>, and compare the spectrum with the Reference Spectrum: both spectra exhibit similar intensities of absorption at the same wavelengths.

(2) Determine the infrared absorption spectrum of Doxapram Hydrochloride Hydrate as directed in the potassium bromide disk method under Infrared Spectrophotometry <*2.25*>, and compare the spectrum with the Reference Spectrum: both spectra exhibit similar intensities of absorption at the same wave numbers.

(3) A solution of Doxapram Hydrochloride Hydrate (1 in 50) responds to Qualitative Tests <*1.09*> for chloride.

pH <*2.54*> Dissolve 1.0 g of Doxapram Hydrochloride Hydrate in 50 mL of water: the pH of this solution is between 3.5 and 5.0.

Melting point <*2.60*> 218 – 222°C

Purity **(1)** Clarity and color of solution—Dissolve 1.0 g of Doxapram Hydrochloride Hydrate in 50 mL of water: the solution is clear and colorless.

(2) Sulfate <*1.14*>—Perform the test with 1.0 g of Doxapram Hydrochloride Hydrate. Prepare the control solution with 0.50 mL of 0.005 mol/L sulfuric acid VS (not more than 0.024%).

(3) Heavy metals <*1.07*>—Proceed with 2.0 g of Doxapram Hydrochloride Hydrate according to Method 2, and perform the test. Prepare the control solution with 2.0 mL of Standard Lead Solution (not more than 10 ppm).

(4) Arsenic <*1.11*>—Prepare the test solution with 1.0 g of Doxapram Hydrochloride Hydrate according to Method 3, and perform the test (not more than 2 ppm).

(5) Related substances—Dissolve 0.5 g of Doxapram Hydrochloride Hydrate in 10 mL of methanol, and use this solution as the sample solution. Pipet 3 mL of the sample solution, and add methanol to make exactly 100 mL. Pipet 5 mL of this solution, add methanol to make exactly 50 mL, and use this solution as the standard solution. Perform the test with these solutions as directed under Thin-layer Chromatography <2.03>. Spot 6 μL each of the sample solution and standard solution on a plate of silica gel for thin-layer chromatography. Develop the plate with a mixture of chloroform, formic acid, ethyl formate and methanol (8:3:3:2) to a distance of about 10 cm, and air-dry the plate. Allow the plate to stand in iodine vapor: the spots other than the principal spot obtained from the sample solution are not more intense than the spot from the standard solution.

Water <2.48> 3.5 – 4.5% (0.5 g, volumetric titration, direct titration).

Residue on ignition <2.44> Not more than 0.3% (1 g).

Assay Weigh accurately about 0.8 g of Doxapram Hydrochloride Hydrate, dissolve in 50 mL of a mixture of acetic anhydride and acetic acid (100) (7:3), and titrate <2.50> with 0.1 mol/L perchloric acid VS (potentiometric titration). Perform a blank determination in the same manner, and make any necessary correction.

Each mL of 0.1 mol/L perchloric acid VS
= 41.50 mg of $C_{24}H_{30}N_2O_2.HCl$

Containers and storage Containers—Tight containers.

Doxazosin Mesilate

ドキサゾシンメシル酸塩

$C_{23}H_{25}N_5O_5.CH_4O_3S$: 547.58
1-(4-Amino-6,7-dimethoxyquinazolin-2-yl)-4-{[(2*RS*)-2,3-dihydro-1,4-benzodioxin-2-yl]carbonyl}piperazine monomethanesulfonate
[*77883-43-3*]

Doxazosin Mesilate, when dried, contains not less than 98.0% and not more than 102.0% of doxazosin mesilate ($C_{23}H_{25}N_5O_5.CH_4O_3S$).

Description Doxazosin Mesilate occurs as a white to yellowish white crystalline powder.

It is freely soluble in dimethylsulfoxide, slightly soluble in water and in methanol, and very slightly soluble in ethanol (99.5).

A solution of Doxazosin Mesilate in dimethylsulfoxide solution (1 in 20) shows no optical rotation.

Melting point: about 272°C (with decomposition).

Identification (1) Determine the absorption spectrum of a solution of Doxazosin Mesilate in 0.01 mol/L hydrochloric acid-methanol TS (1 in 200,000) as directed under Ultraviolet-visible Spectrophotometry <2.24>, and compare the spectrum with the Reference Spectrum or the spectrum of a solution of Doxazosin Mesilate RS prepared in the same manner as the sample solution: both spectra exhibit similar intensities of absorption at the same wavelengths.

(2) Determine the infrared absorption spectrum of Doxazosin Mesilate as directed in the potassium bromide disk method under Infrared Spectrophotometry <2.25>, and compare the spectrum with the Reference Spectrum or the spectrum of Doxazosin Mesilate RS: both spectra exhibit similar intensities of absorption at the same wave numbers.

(3) 30 mg of Doxazosin Mesilate responds to Qualitative Tests <1.09> (2) for mesilate.

Purity (1) Heavy metals <1.07>—Proceed with 1.0 g of Doxazosin Mesilate according to Method 2, and perform the test. Prepare the control solution with 2.0 mL of Standard Lead Solution (not more than 20 ppm).

(2) Related substances—Dissolve 20 mg of Doxazosin Mesilate in 5 mL of a mixture of methanol and acetic acid (100) (1:1), and use this solution as the sample solution. Pipet 1 mL of the sample solution, add a mixture of methanol and acetic acid (100) (1:1) to make exactly 100 mL. Pipet 5 mL of this solution, add a mixture of methanol and acetic acid (100) (1:1) to make exactly 10 mL, and use this solution as the standard solution. Perform the test with these solutions as directed under Thin-layer Chromatography <2.03>. Spot 5 μL each of the sample solution and standard solution on a plate of silica gel with fluorescent indicator for thin-layer chromatography. Develop the plate with an upper layer of a mixture, prepared by adding 1 volume of water and 1 volume of acetic acid (100) to 2 volumes of 4-methyl-2-pentanon and shaking, to a distance of about 10 cm, and air-dry the plate. Examine under ultraviolet light (main wavelength: 254 nm): the spot at the *R*f value about 0.15 obtained from the sample solution is not more intense than the spot from the standard solution, and no spots other than the principal spot and other than the spots mentioned above appear from the sample solution.

Loss on drying <2.41> Not more than 1.0% (1 g, 105°C, 4 hours).

Residue on ignition <2.44> Not more than 0.2% (1 g).

Assay Weigh accurately about 25 mg each of Doxazosin Mesilate and Doxazosin Mesilate RS, previously dried, dissolve separately in methanol to make exactly 50 mL. Pipet 3 mL each of these solutions, add the mobile phase to make exactly 100 mL, and use these solutions as the sample solution and the standard solution, respectively. Perform the test with exactly 10 μL each of the sample solution and standard solution as directed under Liquid Chromatography <2.01> according to the following conditions, and determine the peak areas, A_T and A_S, of doxazosin in each solution.

Amount (mg) of doxazosin mesilate ($C_{23}H_{25}N_5O_5.CH_4O_3S$)
$= M_S \times A_T/A_S$

M_S: Amount (mg) of Doxazosin Mesilate RS taken

Operating conditions—

Detector: An ultraviolet absorption photometer (wavelength: 246 nm).

Column: A stainless steel column 3.9 mm in inside diameter and 15 cm in length, packed with octadecylsilanized silica gel for liquid chromatography (4 μm in particle diameter).

Column temperature: A constant temperature of about 25°C.

Mobile phase: A mixture of 0.05 mol/L potassium dihydrogen phosphate TS (pH 3.0), methanol and acetonitrile (12:8:3).

Flow rate: Adjust so that the retention time of doxazosin is about 5 minutes.

System suitability—

System performance: When the procedure is run with 10 μL of the standard solution under the above operating conditions, the number of theoretical plates and the symmetry factor of the peak of doxazosin are not less than 2000 and

not more than 2.0, respectively.

System repeatability: When the test is repeated 6 times with 10 μL of the standard solution under the above operating conditions, the relative standard deviation of the peak area of doxazosin is not more than 1.0%.

Containers and storage Containers—Tight containers.

Doxazosin Mesilate Tablets

ドキサゾシンメシル酸塩錠

Doxazosin Mesilate Tablets contain not less than 95.0% and not more than 105.0% of the labeled amount of doxazosin ($C_{23}H_{25}N_5O_5$: 451.48).

Method of preparation Prepare as directed under Tablets, with Doxazosin Mesilate.

Identification To a quantity of powdered Doxazosin Mesilate Tablets, equivalent to 5 mg of doxazosin ($C_{23}H_{25}N_5O_5$), add 100 mL of 0.01 mol/L hydrochloric acid-methanol TS, shake vigorously, and centrifuge. To 4 mL of the supernatant liquid add 0.01 mol/L hydrochloric acid-methanol TS to make 50 mL, and determine the absorption spectrum of this solution as directed under Ultraviolet-visible Spectrophotometry <*2.24*>: it exhibits a maximum between 244 nm and 248 nm.

Uniformity of dosage units <*6.02*> Perform the test according to the following method: it meets the requirement of the Content uniformity test.

To 1 tablet of Doxazosin Mesilate Tablets add 1 mL of water, disintegrate the tablet by shaking, add 0.01 mol/L hydrochloric acid-methanol TS to make exactly 100 mL, and shake for 30 minutes. Centrifuge, pipet V mL of the supernatant liquid, add 0.01 mol/L hydrochloric acid-methanol TS to make exactly V' mL so that each mL contains about 5 μg of doxazosin ($C_{23}H_{25}N_5O_5$), and use this solution as the sample solution. Separately, weigh accurately about 30 mg of Doxazosin Mesilate RS, previously dried at 105°C for 4 hours, and dissolve in 0.01 mol/L hydrochloric acid-methanol TS to make exactly 100 mL. Pipet 2 mL of this solution, add 0.01 mol/L hydrochloric acid-methanol TS to make exactly 100 mL, and use this solution as the standard solution. Then, proceed as directed in the Assay.

Amount (mg) of doxazosin ($C_{23}H_{25}N_5O_5$)
$= M_S \times A_T/A_S \times V'/V \times 1/50 \times 0.825$

M_S: Amount (mg) of Doxazosin Mesilate RS taken

Dissolution <*6.10*> When the test is performed at 75 revolutions per minute according to the Paddle method, using 900 mL of 0.05 mol/L acetic acid-sodium acetate buffer solution (pH 4.0) as the dissolution medium, the dissolution rate in 15 minutes of Doxazosin Mesilate Tablets is not less than 75%.

Start the test with 1 tablet of Doxazosin Mesilate Tablets, withdraw not less than 20 mL of the medium at the specified minute after starting the test, and filter through a membrane filter with a pore size not exceeding 0.45 μm. Discard not less than 10 mL of the first filtrate, pipet V mL of the subsequent filtrate, and add the dissolution medium to make exactly V' mL so that each mL contains about 0.56 μg of doxazosin ($C_{23}H_{25}N_5O_5$). Pipet 5 mL of this solution, add exactly 5 mL of methanol, and use this solution as the sample solution. Separately, weigh accurately about 21 mg of Doxazosin Mesilate RS, previously dried at 105°C for 4 hours, and dissolve in methanol to make exactly 50 mL. Pipet 2 mL of this solution, add methanol to make exactly 50 mL. Then, pipet 2 mL of this solution, add methanol to make exactly 50 mL. Pipet 5 mL of this solution, add exactly 5 mL of the dissolution medium, and use this solution as the standard solution. Perform the test with exactly 20 μL each of the sample solution and standard solution as directed under Liquid Chromatography <*2.01*> according to the following conditions, and determine the peak areas, A_T and A_S, of doxazosin in each solution.

Dissolution rate (%) with respect to the labeled amount of doxazosin ($C_{23}H_{25}N_5O_5$)
$= M_S \times A_T/A_S \times V'/V \times 1/C \times 72/25 \times 0.825$

M_S: Amount (mg) of Doxazosin Mesilate RS taken
C: Labeled amount (mg) of doxazosin ($C_{23}H_{25}N_5O_5$) in 1 tablet

Operating conditions—

Detector: An ultraviolet absorption photometer (wavelength: 246 nm).

Column: A stainless steel column 4.6 mm in inside diameter and 15 cm in length, packed with octadecylsilanized silica gel for liquid chromatography (5 μm in particle diameter).

Column temperature: A constant temperature of about 35°C.

Mobile phase: Dissolve 3.4 g of potassium dihydrogen phosphate in 500 mL of water, and adjust to pH 3.0 with diluted phosphoric acid (1 in 10). To 450 mL of this solution add 550 mL of methanol.

Flow rate: Adjust so that the retention time of doxazosin is about 5 minutes.

System suitability—

System performance: When the procedure is run with 20 μL of the standard solution under the above operating conditions, the number of theoretical plates and the symmetry factor of the peak of doxazosin are not less than 2000 and not more than 2.0, respectively.

System repeatability: When the test is repeated 6 times with 20 μL of the standard solution under the above operating conditions, the relative standard deviation of the peak area of doxazosin is not more than 2.0%.

Assay Weigh accurately the mass of not less than 20 Doxazosin Mesilate Tablets, and powder. Weigh accurately a portion of the powder, equivalent to about 5 mg of doxazosin ($C_{23}H_{25}N_5O_5$), add 0.01 mol/L hydrochloric acid-methanol TS to make exactly 100 mL, and stir for 30 minutes. Centrifuge, pipet 4 mL of the supernatant liquid, add 0.01 mol/L hydrochloric acid-methanol TS to make exactly 50 mL, and use this solution as the sample solution. Separately, weigh accurately about 24 mg of Doxazosin Mesilate RS, previously dried at 105°C for 4 hours, dissolve in 0.01 mol/L hydrochloric acid-methanol TS to make exactly 100 mL. Pipet 2 mL of this solution, add 0.01 mol/L hydrochloric acid-methanol TS to make exactly 100 mL, and use this solution as the standard solution. Determine the absorbances, A_T and A_S, of the sample solution and standard solution at 246 nm as directed under Ultraviolet-visible Spectrophotometry <*2.24*>.

Amount (mg) of doxazosin ($C_{23}H_{25}N_5O_5$)
$= M_S \times A_T/A_S \times 1/4 \times 0.825$

M_S: Amount (mg) of Doxazosin Mesilate RS taken

Containers and storage Containers—Well-closed containers.

Doxifluridine

ドキシフルリジン

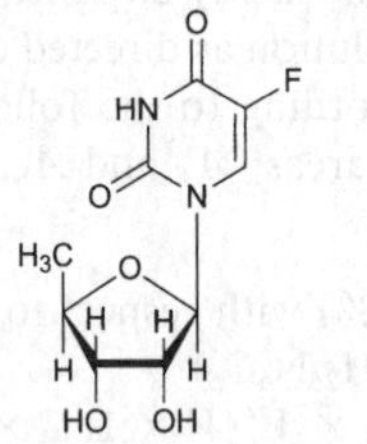

$C_9H_{11}FN_2O_5$: 246.19
5′-Deoxy-5-fluorouridine
[*3094-09-5*]

Doxifluridine, when dried, contains not less than 98.5% and not more than 101.0% of doxifluridine ($C_9H_{11}FN_2O_5$).

Description Doxifluridine occurs as a white crystalline powder.

It is freely soluble in *N,N*-dimethylformamide, soluble in water and in methanol, and slightly soluble in ethanol (99.5).

It dissolves in 0.1 mol/L hydrochloric acid TS and in 0.01 mol/L sodium hydroxide TS.

Melting point: about 191°C (with decomposition).

Identification **(1)** Determine the absorption spectrum of a solution of Doxifluridine in 0.1 mol/L hydrochloric acid TS (1 in 50,000) as directed under Ultraviolet-visible Spectrophotometry *<2.24>*, and compare the spectrum with the Reference Spectrum: both spectra exhibit similar intensities of absorption at the same wavelengths.

(2) Determine the infrared absorption spectrum of Doxifluridine, previously dried, as directed in the potassium bromide disk method under Infrared Spectrophotometry *<2.25>*, and compare the spectrum with the Reference Spectrum: both spectra exhibit similar intensities of absorption at the same wave numbers.

Optical rotation *<2.49>* $[\alpha]_{365}^{20}$: +160 – +174° (after drying, 0.1 g, water, 10 mL, 100 mm).

pH *<2.54>* The pH of a solution obtained by dissolving 0.10 g of Doxifluridine in 10 mL of water is between 4.2 and 5.2.

Purity **(1)** Fluoride—Dissolve 0.10 g of Doxifluridine in 10.0 mL of diluted 0.01 mol/L sodium hydroxide TS (1 in 20). Transfer 5.0 mL of this solution into a 20-mL volumetric flask, add 5 mL of a mixture of acetone and lanthanum-alizarin complexone TS (2:1) and water to make 20 mL, allow to stand for 1 hour, and use this solution as the sample solution. Separately, put 1.0 mL of Standard Fluorine Solution in a 20-mL volumetric flask, add 5.0 mL of diluted 0.01 mol/L sodium hydroxide TS (1 in 20) and 5 mL of the mixture of acetone and alizarin complexone TS (2:1), then proceed in the same manner as for preparation of the sample solution, and use the solution so obtained as the standard solution. Determine the absorbances, A_T and A_S, of the sample solution and standard solution at 620 nm as directed under Ultraviolet-visible Spectrophotometry *<2.24>*, using a solution obtained in the same way with 5.0 mL of diluted 0.01 mol/L sodium hydroxide TS (1 in 20) as a blank: A_T is not larger than A_S.

(2) Chloride *<1.03>*—Perform the test with 0.30 g of Doxifluridine. Prepare the control solution with 0.30 mL of 0.01 mol/L hydrochloric acid VS (not more than 0.035%).

(3) Heavy metals *<1.07>*—Proceed with 1.0 g of Doxifluridine according to Method 1, and perform the test. Prepare the control solution with 2.0 mL of Standard Lead Solution (not more than 20 ppm).

(4) Related substances—Dissolve 20 mg of Doxifluridine in 2 mL of methanol, and use this solution as the sample solution. Pipet 1 mL of the sample solution, and add methanol to make exactly 25 mL. Pipet 5 mL of this solution, add methanol to make exactly 50 mL, and use this solution as the standard solution. Perform the test with these solutions as directed under Thin-layer Chromatography *<2.03>*. Spot 10 μL each of the sample solution and standard solution on a plate of silica gel with fluorescent indicator for thin-layer chromatography. Develop the plate with a mixture of ethyl acetate, acetic acid (100) and water (17:2:1) to a distance of about 12 cm, and air-dry the plate. Examine under ultraviolet light (main wavelength: 254 nm): the number of the spot other than the principal spot obtained from the sample solution is not more than three, and they are not more intense than the spot from the standard solution.

Loss on drying *<2.41>* Not more than 0.5% (1 g, 105°C, 4 hours).

Residue on ignition *<2.44>* Not more than 0.1% (1 g, platinum crucible).

Assay Weigh accurately about 0.25 g of Doxifluridine, previously dried, dissolve in 50 mL of *N,N*-dimethylformamide, and titrate *<2.50>* with 0.1 mol/L tetramethylammonium hydroxide VS (potentiometric titration). Perform a blank determination in the same manner, and make any necessary correction.

Each mL of 0.1 mol/L tetramethylammonium hydroxide VS
= 24.62 mg of $C_9H_{11}FN_2O_5$

Containers and storage Containers—Tight containers.

Doxifluridine Capsules

ドキシフルリジンカプセル

Doxifluridine Capsules contain not less than 95.0% and not more than 105.0% of the labeled amount of doxifluridine ($C_9H_{11}FN_2O_5$: 246.19).

Method of preparation Prepare as directed under Capsules, with Doxifluridine.

Identification **(1)** Dissolve an amount of the contents of Doxifluridine Capsules, equivalent to 20 mg of Doxifluridine, in 0.1 mol/L hydrochloric acid TS to make 100 mL, and filter. To 1 mL of the filtrate add 0.1 mol/L hydrochloric acid TS to make 20 mL, and determine the absorption spectrum of this solution as directed under Ultraviolet-visible Spectrophotometry *<2.24>*, using 0.1 mol/L hydrochloric acid TS as the blank: it exhibits a maximum between 267 nm and 271 nm.

(2) To an amount of powdered contents of Doxifluridine Capsules, equivalent to 20 mg of Doxifluridine, add 2 mL of methanol, shake, centrifuge, and use the supernatant liquid as the sample solution. Separately, dissolve 20 mg of doxifluridine in 2 mL of methanol, and use this solution as the standard solution. Perform the test with these solutions as directed under Thin-layer Chromatography *<2.03>*. Spot 10 μL each of the sample solution and standard solution on a plate of silica gel with fluorescent indicator for thin-layer chromatography. Develop the plate with a mixture of ethyl acetate, acetic acid (100) and water (17:2:1) to a distance of about 12 cm, and air-dry the plate. Examine under ultraviolet light (main wavelength: 254 nm): the principal spot obtained from the sample solution and the spot from the standard solution show a dark purple color and these *Rf* values are the same.

Uniformity of dosage units <*6.02*> It meets the requirement of the Mass variation test.

Dissolution <*6.10*> When the test is performed at 50 revolutions per minute according to the Paddle method using the sinker, using 900 mL of water as the dissolution medium, the dissolution rate in 30 minutes of Doxifluridine Capsules is not less than 85%.

Start the test with 1 capsule of Doxifluridine Capsules, withdraw not less than 20 mL of the medium at the specified minute after starting the test, and filter through a membrane filter with a pore size not exceeding 0.45 μm. Discard not less than 10 mL of the first filtrate, pipet *V* mL of the subsequent filtrate, add water to make exactly *V′* mL so that each mL contains about 13 μg of doxifluridine ($C_9H_{11}FN_2O_5$), and use this solution as the sample solution. Separately, weigh accurately about 26 mg of doxifluridine for assay, previously dried at 105°C for 4 hours, and dissolve in water to make exactly 100 mL. Pipet 5 mL of this solution, add water to make exactly 100 mL, and use this solution as the standard solution. Determine the absorbances, A_T and A_S, of the sample solution and standard solution at 269 nm as directed under Ultraviolet-visible Spectrophotometry <*2.24*>.

Dissolution rate (%) with respect to the labeled amount of doxifluridine ($C_9H_{11}FN_2O_5$)

$$= M_S \times A_T/A_S \times V'/V \times 1/C \times 45$$

M_S: Amount (mg) of doxifluridine for assay taken

C: Labeled amount (mg) of doxifluridine ($C_9H_{11}FN_2O_5$) in 1 capsule

Assay Weigh accurately the mass and powder the contents of not less than 20 Doxifluridine Capsules. Weigh accurately a portion of the powder, equivalent to about 50 mg of doxifluridine ($C_9H_{11}FN_2O_5$), add 40 mL of water, shake for 10 minutes, add water to make exactly 50 mL, and filter. Discard the first 10 mL of the filtrate, pipet 5 mL of the subsequent filtrate, add exactly 10 mL of the internal standard solution, then add a mixture of water and methanol (5:3) to make 100 mL, and use this solution as the sample solution. Separately, weigh accurately about 50 mg of doxifluridine for assay, previously dried at 105°C for 4 hours, and dissolve in water to make exactly 50 mL. Pipet 5 mL of this solution, add exactly 10 mL of the internal standard solution, then add the mixture of water and methanol (5:3) to make exactly 100 mL, and use this solution as the standard solution. Perform the test with 10 μL each of the sample solution and standard solution as directed under Liquid Chromatography <*2.01*> according to the following conditions, and calculate the ratios, Q_T and Q_S, of the peak height of doxifluridine to that of the internal standard.

Amount (mg) of doxifluridine ($C_9H_{11}FN_2O_5$)

$$= M_S \times Q_T/Q_S$$

M_S: Amount (mg) of doxifluridine for assay taken

Internal standard solution—A solution of anhydrous caffeine (1 in 1000).

Operating conditions—

Detector: An ultraviolet absorption photometer (wavelength: 254 nm).

Column: A stainless steel column 6 mm in inside diameter and 15 cm in length, packed with octadecylsilanized silica gel for liquid chromatography (5 μm in particle diameter).

Column temperature: A constant temperature of about 25°C.

Mobile phase: A mixture of water and methanol (13:7).

Flow rate: Adjust so that the retention time of doxifluridine is about 2.5 minutes.

System suitability—

System performance: When the procedure is run with 10 μL of the standard solution under the above operating conditions, doxifluridine and the internal standard are eluted in this order with the resolution between these peaks being not less than 5.

System repeatability: When the test is repeated 6 times with 10 μL of the standard solution under the above operating conditions, the relative standard deviation of the ratio of the peak height of doxifluridine to that of the internal standard is not more than 1.0%.

Containers and storage Containers—Tight containers.

Doxorubicin Hydrochloride

ドキソルビシン塩酸塩

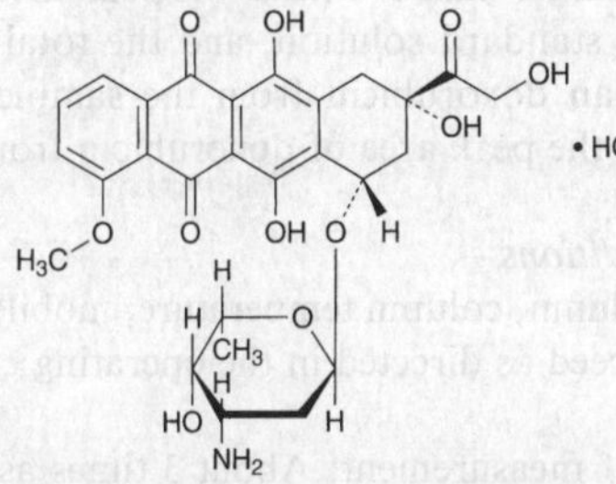

$C_{27}H_{29}NO_{11}$.HCl: 579.98

(2*S*,4*S*)-4-(3-Amino-2,3,6-trideoxy-α-L-*lyxo*-hexopyranosyloxy)-2,5,12-trihydroxy-2-hydroxyacetyl-7-methoxy-1,2,3,4-tetrahydrotetracene-6,11-dione monohydrochloride

[*25316-40-9*]

Doxorubicin Hydrochloride is the hydrochloride of a derivative of daunorubicin.

It contains not less than 980 μg (potency) and not more than 1080 μg (potency) per mg, calculated on the anhydrous basis. The potency of Doxorubicin Hydrochloride is expressed as mass (potency) of doxorubicin hydrochloride ($C_{27}H_{29}NO_{11}$.HCl).

Description Doxorubicin Hydrochloride occurs as a red-orange crystalline powder.

It is sparingly soluble in water, slightly soluble in methanol, very slightly soluble in ethanol (99.5), and practically insoluble in acetonitrile.

Identification **(1)** Determine the absorption spectrum of a solution of Doxorubicin Hydrochloride in methanol (1 in 100,000) as directed under Ultraviolet-visible Spectrophotometry <*2.24*>, and compare the spectrum with the Reference Spectrum or the spectrum of a solution of Doxorubicin Hydrochloride RS prepared in the same manner as the sample solution: both spectra exhibit similar intensities of absorption at the same wavelengths.

(2) Determine the infrared absorption spectrum of Doxorubicin Hydrochloride as directed in the potassium chloride disk method under Infrared Spectrophotometry

<2.25>, and compare the spectrum with the Reference Spectrum or the spectrum of Doxorubicin Hydrochloride RS: both spectra exhibit similar intensities of absorption at the same wave numbers.

(3) A solution of Doxorubicin Hydrochloride (1 in 200) responds to Qualitative Tests <1.09> (1) for chloride.

Optical rotation <2.49> $[\alpha]_D^{20}$: +240 – +290° (20 mg calculated on the anhydrous basis, methanol, 20 mL, 100 mm).

pH <2.54> The pH of a solution obtained by dissolving 50 mg of Doxorubicin Hydrochloride in 10 mL of water is between 4.0 and 5.5.

Purity **(1)** Clarity and color of solution—Dissolve 50 mg of Doxorubicin Hydrochloride in 10 mL of water: the solution is clear and red.

(2) Related substances—Dissolve 25 mg of Doxorubicin Hydrochloride in 100 mL of the mobile phase, and use this solution as the sample solution. Pipet 2 mL of the sample solution, add the mobile phase to make exactly 100 mL, and use this solution as the standard solution. Perform the test with exactly 20 μL each of the sample solution and standard solution as directed under Liquid Chromatography <2.01> according to the following conditions, and determine each peak area by the automatic integration method: the area of the peak other than doxorubicin obtained from the sample solution is not larger than 1/4 times the peak area of doxorubicin from the standard solution, and the total area of the peaks other than doxorubicin from the sample solution is not larger than the peak area of doxorubicin from the standard solution.

Operating conditions—

Detector, column, column temperature, mobile phase, and flow rate: Proceed as directed in the operating conditions in the Assay.

Time span of measurement: About 3 times as long as the retention time of doxorubicin.

System suitability—

Test for required detectability: Pipet 1 mL of the standard solution, and add the mobile phase to make exactly 20 mL. Confirm that the peak area of doxorubicin obtained with 20 μL of this solution is equivalent to 3.5 to 6.5% of that with 20 μL of the standard solution.

System performance: Dissolve 5 mg of Doxorubicin Hydrochloride in 20 mL of water, add 1.5 mL of phosphoric acid, and allow to stand at room temperature for 30 minutes. Adjust the pH of this solution to 2.5 with 2 mol/L sodium hydroxide TS. When the procedure is run with 20 μL of this solution under the above operating conditions, doxorubicinone, having the relative retention time of about 0.6 to doxorubicin, and doxorubicin are eluted in this order with the resolution between these peaks being not less than 5.

System repeatability: When the test is repeated 6 times with 20 μL of the standard solution under the above operating conditions, the relative standard deviation of the peak area of doxorubicin is not more than 2.0%.

Water <2.48> Not more than 3.0% (0.3 g, volumetric titration, direct titration).

Assay Weigh accurately amounts of Doxorubicin Hydrochloride and Doxorubicin Hydrochloride RS, equivalent to about 10 mg (potency), add exactly 5 mL of the internal standard solution to each, dissolve each in the mobile phase to make 100 mL, and use these solutions as the sample solution and the standard solution, respectively. Perform the test with 10 μL each of the sample solution and standard solution as directed under Liquid Chromatography <2.01> according to the following conditions, and calculate the ratios, Q_T and Q_S, of the peak area of doxorubicin to that of the internal standard.

Amount [μg (potency)] of doxorubicin hydrochloride ($C_{27}H_{29}NO_{11}.HCl$)
$= M_S \times Q_T/Q_S \times 1000$

M_S: Amount [mg (potency)] of Doxorubicin Hydrochloride RS taken

Internal standard solution—A solution of butyl parahydroxybenzoate in the mobile phase (1 in 1000).

Operating conditions—

Detector: An ultraviolet absorption photometer (wavelength: 254 nm).

Column: A stainless steel column 4.6 mm in inside diameter and 25 cm in length, packed with octadecylsilanized silica gel for liquid chromatography (5 μm in particle diameter).

Column temperature: A constant temperature of about 25°C.

Mobile phase: Dissolve 3 g of sodium lauryl sulfate in 1000 mL of diluted phosphoric acid (7 in 5000), and add 1000 mL of acetonitrile.

Flow rate: Adjust so that the retention time of doxorubicin is about 8 minutes.

System suitability—

System performance: When the procedure is run with 10 μL of the standard solution under the above operating conditions, doxorubicin and the internal standard are eluted in this order with the resolution between these peaks being not less than 5, and the symmetry factor of the peak of doxorubicin is 0.8 to 1.2.

System repeatability: When the test is repeated 6 times with 10 μL of the standard solution under the above operating conditions, the relative standard deviation of the ratio of the peak area of doxorubicin to that of the internal standard is not more than 1.0%.

Containers and storage Containers—Tight containers.

Doxorubicin Hydrochloride for Injection

注射用ドキソルビシン塩酸塩

Doxorubicin Hydrochloride for Injection is a preparation for injection, which is dissolved before use.

It contains not less than 90.0% and not more than 110.0% of the labeled potency of doxorubicin hydrochloride ($C_{27}H_{29}NO_{11}.HCl$: 579.98).

Method of preparation Prepare as directed under Injections, with Doxorubicin Hydrochloride.

Description Doxorubicin Hydrochloride for Injection occurs as a red-orange, powder or masses.

Identification Dissolve an amount of Doxorubicin Hydrochloride for Injection, equivalent to 10 mg (potency) of Doxorubicin Hydrochloride, in methanol to make 100 mL. To 5 mL of this solution add methanol to make 50 mL, and determine the absorption spectrum of the solution as directed under Ultraviolet-visible Spectrophotometry <2.24>: it exhibits maxima between 231 nm and 235 nm, between 250 nm and 254 nm, between 477 nm and 481 nm, and between 493 nm and 497 nm, and exhibits a shoulder between 528 nm and 538 nm.

pH ⟨*2.54*⟩ The pH of a solution, prepared by dissolving an amount of Doxorubicin Hydrochloride for Injection equivalent to 10 mg (potency) of Doxorubicin Hydrochloride, in 2 mL of water, is 5.0 to 6.0.

Purity Clarity and color of solution—Dissolve an amount of Doxorubicin Hydrochloride for Injection, equivalent to 50 mg (potency) of Doxorubicin Hydrochloride, in 10 mL of water: the solution is clear and red.

Water ⟨*2.48*⟩ Not more than 4.0% (0.25 g, volumetric titration, direct titration).

Bacterial endotoxins ⟨*4.01*⟩ Less than 2.50 EU/mg (potency).

Uniformity of dosage units ⟨*6.02*⟩ It meets the requirement of the Mass variation test.

Foreign insoluble matter ⟨*6.06*⟩ Perform the test according to Method 2: it meets the requirement.

Insoluble particulate matter ⟨*6.07*⟩ It meets the requirement.

Sterility ⟨*4.06*⟩ Perform the test according to the Membrane filtration method: it meets the requirement.

Assay Weigh accurately the mass of the contents of not less than 10 containers of Doxorubicin Hydrochloride for Injection. Weigh accurately an amount of the contents, equivalent to about 10 mg (potency) of Doxorubicin Hydrochloride, add exactly 5 mL of the internal standard solution and the mobile phase to make 100 mL, and use the solution as the sample solution. Separately, weigh accurately an amount of Doxorubicin Hydrochloride RS, equivalent to 10 mg (potency), add exactly 5 mL of the internal standard solution and the mobile phase to make 100 mL, and use this solution as the standard solution. Perform the test with 10 μL each of the sample solution and standard solution as directed under Liquid Chromatography ⟨*2.01*⟩, and calculate the ratios, Q_T and Q_S, of the peak area of doxorubicin to that of the internal standard.

Amount [mg (potency)] of doxorubicin hydrochloride ($C_{27}H_{29}NO_{11}$.HCl)
$= M_S \times Q_T/Q_S$

M_S: Amount [mg (potency)] of Doxorubicin Hydrochloride RS taken

Internal standard solution—A solution of butyl parahydroxybenzoate in the mobile phase (1 in 1000).

Operating conditions—

Detector: An ultraviolet absorption photometer (wavelength: 254 nm).

Column: A stainless steel column 4.6 mm in inside diameter and 25 cm in length, packed with octadecylsilanized silica gel for liquid chromatography (5 μm in particle diameter).

Column temperature: A constant temperature of about 25°C.

Mobile phase: Dissolve 3 g of sodium lauryl sulfate in 1000 mL of diluted phosphoric acid (7 in 5000). To this solution add 1000 mL of acetonitrile.

Flow rate: Adjust so that the retention time of doxorubicin is about 8 minutes.

System suitability—

System performance: When the procedure is run with 10 μL of the standard solution under the above operating conditions, doxorubicin and the internal standard are eluted in this order with the resolution between these peaks being not less than 5, and the symmetry factor of the peak of doxorubicin is between 0.8 and 1.2.

System repeatability: When the test is repeated 6 times with 10 μL of the standard solution under the above operating conditions, the relative standard deviation of the ratio of the peak area of doxorubicin to that of the internal standard is not more than 1.0%.

Containers and storage Containers—Hermetic containers.

Doxycycline Hydrochloride Hydrate

ドキシサイクリン塩酸塩水和物

$C_{22}H_{24}N_2O_8$.HCl.½C_2H_6O.½H_2O: 512.94
(4*S*,4a*R*,5*S*,5a*R*,6*R*,12a*S*)-4-Dimethylamino-3,5,10,12,12a-pentahydroxy-6-methyl-1,11-dioxo-1,4,4a,5,5a,6,11,12a-octahydrotetracene-2-carboxamide monohydrochloride hemiethanolate hemihydrate
[*564-25-0*, Doxycycline]

Doxycycline Hydrochloride Hydrate is the hydrochloride of a derivative of oxytetracycline.

It contains not less than 880 μg (potency) and not more than 943 μg (potency) per mg, calculated on the anhydrous and residual ethanol-free basis. The potency of Doxycycline Hydrochloride Hydrate is expressed as mass (potency) of doxycycline ($C_{22}H_{24}N_2O_8$: 444.43).

Description Doxycycline Hydrochloride Hydrate occurs as yellow to dark yellow, crystals or crystalline powder.

It is freely soluble in water and in methanol, and slightly soluble in ethanol (99.5).

Identification **(1)** Determine the absorption spectrum of a solution of Doxycycline Hydrochloride Hydrate in 0.01 mol/L hydrochloric acid-methanol TS (1 in 74,000) as directed under Ultraviolet-visible Spectrophotometry ⟨*2.24*⟩, and compare the spectrum with the Reference Spectrum or the spectrum of a solution of Doxycycline Hydrochloride RS prepared in the same manner as the sample solution: both spectra exhibit similar intensities of absorption at the same wavelengths.

(2) Determine the infrared absorption Spectrum of Doxycycline Hydrochloride Hydrate as directed in the potassium bromide disk method under Infrared Spectrophotometry ⟨*2.25*⟩, and compare the spectrum with the Reference Spectrum or the spectrum of Doxycycline Hydrochloride RS: both spectra exhibit similar intensities of absorption at the same wave numbers.

(3) Dissolve 10 mg of Doxycycline Hydrochloride Hydrate in 10 mL of water, and add silver nitrate TS: a white turbidity is produced.

Absorbance ⟨*2.24*⟩ $E^{1\%}_{1\,cm}$ (349 nm): 285 – 315 (10 mg, 0.01 mol/L hydrochloric acid-methanol TS, 500 mL).

Optical rotation ⟨*2.49*⟩ $[\alpha]^{20}_D$: −105 – −120° (0.25 g calculated on the anhydrous and residual ethanol-free basis, 0.01 mol/L hydrochloric acid-methanol TS, 25 mL, 100 mm).

Determine within 5 minutes after the sample solution is prepared.

Purity (1) Heavy metals <*1.07*>—Proceed with 1.0 g of Doxycycline Hydrochloride Hydrate according to Method 2, and perform the test. Prepare the control solution with 5.0 mL of Standard Lead Solution (not more than 50 ppm).

(2) Related substance—Dissolve 20 mg of Doxycycline Hydrochloride Hydrate in 0.01 mol/L hydrochloric acid TS to make exactly 25 mL, and use this solution as the sample solution. Separately, dissolve 20 mg of 6-epidoxycycline hydrochloride in 0.01 mol/L hydrochloric acid TS to make exactly 25 mL, and use this solution as the 6-epidoxycycline hydrochloride stock solution. Separately, dissolve 20 mg of metacycline hydrochloride in 0.01 mol/L hydrochloric acid TS to make exactly 25 mL, and use this solution as the metacycline hydrochloride stock solution. Pipet 2 mL each of the 6-epidoxycycline hydrochloride stock solution and the metacycline hydrochloride stock solution, add 0.01 mol/L hydrochloric acid TS to make exactly 100 mL, and use this solution as the standard solution. Perform the test with exactly 20 μL each of the sample solution and standard solution as directed under Liquid Chromatography <*2.01*> according to the following conditions, and determine each peak area by the automatic integration method: the peak areas of metacycline and 6-epidoxycycline obtained from the sample solution are not larger than the peak areas of them from the standard solution, respectively, and the areas of the two peaks, appeared between the solvent peak and metacycline and behind of doxycycline, from the sample solution are not larger than 1/4 times the peak area of 6-epidoxycycline from the standard solution, and the total area of the peaks other than doxycycline from the sample solution is not larger than 1.5 times the peak area of 6-epidoxycycline from the standard solution.

Operating conditions—

Detector: An ultraviolet absorption photometer (wavelength: 254 nm).

Column: A stainless steel column 4.6 mm in inside diameter and 25 cm in length, packed with styrene-divinylbenzene copolymer for liquid chromatography (8 μm in particle diameter).

Column temperature: A constant temperature of about 60°C.

Mobile phase: To 125 mL of 0.2 mol/L potassium dihydrogen phosphate TS and 117 mL of 0.2 mol/L sodium hydroxide TS add water to make 500 mL. To 400 mL of this solution add 50 mL of a solution of tetrabutylammonium hydrogensulfate (1 in 100), 10 mL of a solution of disodium dihydrogen ethylenediamine tetraacetate dihydrate (1 in 25), 60 g of *t*-butyl alcohol and 200 mL of water, adjust to pH 8.0 with 2 mol/L sodium hydroxide TS, and add water to make 1000 mL.

Flow rate: Adjust so that the retention time of doxycycline is about 19 minutes.

Time span of measurement: About 2.4 times as long as the retention time of doxycycline, beginning after the solvent peak.

System suitability—

Test for required detectability: Pipet 1 mL of the standard solution, and add 0.01 mol/L hydrochloric acid TS to make exactly 20 mL. Confirm that the peak areas of 6-epidoxycycline and metacycline obtained with 20 μL of this solution are equivalent to 3.5 to 6.5% of them with 20 μL of the standard solution, respectively.

System performance: To 8 mL of the sample solution, 3 mL of the 6-epidoxycycline hydrochloride stock solution and 2 mL of the metacycline hydrochloride stock solution add 0.01 mol/L hydrochloric acid TS to make 50 mL. When the procedure is run with 20 μL of this solution under the above operating conditions, metacycline, 6-epidoxycycline and doxycycline are eluted in this order with the resolutions between the peaks, metacycline and 6-epidoxycycline, and 6-epidoxycycline and doxycycline, being not less than 1.3 and not less than 2.0, respectively, and the symmetry factor of the peak of doxycycline is not more than 1.3.

System repeatability: When the test is repeated 6 times with 20 μL of the standard solution under the above operating conditions, the relative standard deviations of the peak areas of metacycline and 6-epidoxycycline are not more than 3.0% and not more than 2.0%, respectively.

Ethanol Weigh accurately about 0.1 g of Doxycycline Hydrochloride Hydrate, dissolve in the internal standard solution to make exactly 10 mL, and use this solution as the sample solution. Separately, weigh accurately about 0.4 g of ethanol (99.5), and add the internal standard solution to make exactly 100 mL. Pipet 1 mL of this solution, add the internal standard solution to make exactly 10 mL, and use this solution as the standard solution. Perform the test with 1 μL each of the sample solution and standard solution as directed under Gas Chromatography <*2.02*> according to the following conditions, and calculate the ratios, Q_T and Q_S, of the peak area of ethanol to that of the internal standard: the amount of ethanol is not less than 4.3% and not more than 6.0%.

$$\text{Amount (\%) of ethanol} = M_S/M_T \times Q_T/Q_S$$

M_S: Amount (mg) of ethanol (99.5) taken

M_T: Amount (mg) of Doxycycline Hydrochloride Hydrate taken

Internal standard solution—A solution of 1-propanol (1 in 2000).

Operating conditions—

Detector: A hydrogen flame-ionization detector.

Column: A glass column 3.2 mm in inside diameter and 1.5 m in length, packed with porous ethylvinylbenzene-divinylbenzene copolymer for gas chromatography (0.0075 μm in average pore size, 500 – 600 m^2/g in specific surface area) (150 – 180 μm in particle diameter).

Column temperature: A constant temperature of about 135°C.

Carrier gas: Nitrogen.

Flow rate: Adjust so that the retention time of ethanol is about 5 minutes.

System suitability—

System performance: When the procedure is run with 1 μL of the standard solution under the above operating conditions, ethanol and the internal standard are eluted in this order with the resolution between these peaks being not less than 2.0.

System repeatability: When the test is repeated 5 times with 1 μL of the standard solution under the above operating conditions, the relative standard deviation of the ratios of the peak area of ethanol to that of the internal standard is not more than 2.0%.

Water <*2.48*> Not less than 1.4% and not more than 2.8% (0.6 g, volumetric titration, direct titration).

Residue on ignition <*2.44*> Not more than 0.3% (1 g).

Assay Weigh accurately an amount of Doxycycline Hydrochloride Hydrate and Doxycycline Hydrochloride RS, equivalent to about 50 mg (potency), dissolve each in water to make exactly 50 mL, and use these solutions as the sample solution and standard solution. Perform the test with exactly 10 μL each of the sample solution and standard solution as directed under Liquid Chromatography <*2.01*> according to the following conditions, and determine the peak areas, A_T and A_S, of doxycycline in each solution.

Amount [μg (potency)] of doxycycline ($C_{22}H_{24}N_2O_8$)
$= M_S \times A_T/A_S \times 1000$

M_S: Amount [mg (potency)] of Doxycycline Hydrochloride RS taken

Operating conditions—

Detector: An ultraviolet absorption photometer (wavelength: 280 nm).

Column: A stainless steel column 3.9 mm in inside diameter and 30 cm in length, packed with octadecylsilanized silica gel for liquid chromatography (10 μm in particle diameter).

Column temperature: A constant temperature of about 30°C.

Mobile phase: Dissolve 7.0 g of sodium dihydrogen phosphate dihydrate in 450 mL of water, add 553 mL of a mixture of methanol and *N*,*N*-dimethyl-*n*-octylamine (550:3), and adjust the pH to 8.0 with a solution of sodium hydroxide (43 in 200).

Flow rate: Adjust so that the retention time of doxycycline is about 6 minutes.

System suitability—

System performance: When the procedure is run with 10 μL of the standard solution under the above operating conditions, the theoretical plates and the symmetry factor of the peak of doxycycline are not less than 1000 and not more than 2.0, respectively.

System repeatability: When the test is repeated 6 times with 10 μL of the standard solution under the above operating conditions, the relative standard deviation of the peak area of doxycycline is not more than 1.0%.

Containers and storage Containers—Tight containers.

Storage—Light-resistant.

Doxycycline Hydrochloride Tablets

ドキシサイクリン塩酸塩錠

Doxycycline Hydrochloride Tablets contain not less than 93.0% and not more than 107.0% of the labeled potency of doxycycline ($C_{22}H_{24}N_2O_8$: 444.43).

Method of preparation Prepare as directed under Tablets, with Doxycycline Hydrochloride Hydrate.

Identification Weigh a portion of powdered Doxycycline Hydrochloride Tablets, equivalent to 1 mg (potency) of Doxycycline Hydrochloride Hydrate, add 100 mL of 0.01 mol/L hydrochloric acid-methanol TS, shake thoroughly, and filter. Determine the absorption spectrum of this filtrate as directed under Ultraviolet-visible Spectrophotometry <*2.24*>: it exhibits maxima between 266 nm and 271 nm and between 347 nm and 353 nm.

Purity 4-Epidoxycycline—Use the sample solution obtained in the Assay as the sample solution. Pipet 2 mL of the sample solution, add 0.01 mol/L hydrochloric acid TS to make exactly 200 mL, and use this solution as the standard solution. Perform the test with exactly 10 μL each of the sample solution and standard solution as directed under Liquid Chromatography <*2.01*> according to the following conditions, and determine each peak area by the automatic integration method: the area of the peak, having a relative retention time of about 0.6 to doxycycline, obtained from the sample solution is not larger than 1.5 times the peak area of doxycycline from the standard solution.

Operating conditions—

Proceed as directed in the operating conditions in the Assay.

System suitability—

Test for required detectability: To exactly 2 mL of the standard solution add 0.01 mol/L hydrochloric acid TS to make exactly 20 mL. Confirm that the peak area of doxycycline obtained with 10 μL of this solution is equivalent to 7 to 13% of the peak area of doxycycline with 10 μL of the standard solution.

System performance: When the procedure is run with 10 μL of the standard solution under the above operating conditions, the number of theoretical plates and symmetry factor of the peak of doxycycline are not less than 2200 and not more than 1.6, respectively.

System repeatability: When the test is repeated 6 times with 10 μL of the standard solution under the above operating conditions, the relative standard deviations of the peak area of doxycycline is not more than 2.0%.

Uniformity of dosage units <*6.02*> Perform the Mass variation test, or the Content uniformity test according to the following method: it meets the requirement.

To 1 tablet of Doxycycline Hydrochloride Tablets add 0.01 mol/L hydrochloric acid TS, disperse the tablet by sonicating, shake for 15 minutes, then add 0.01 mol/L hydrochloric acid TS to make exactly *V* mL so that each mL contains about 1 mg (potency) of Doxycycline Hydrochloride Hydrate. Centrifuge this solution, filter the supernatant liquid through a membrane filter with a pore size not exceeding 0.45 μm, discard the first 10 mL of the filtrate, and use the subsequent filtrate as the sample solution. Then, proceed as directed in the Assay.

Amount [mg (potency)] of doxycycline ($C_{22}H_{24}N_2O_8$)
$= M_S \times A_T/A_S \times V/20$

M_S: Amount [mg (potency)] of Doxycycline Hydrochloride RS taken

Dissolution <*6.10*> When the test is performed at 50 revolutions per minute according to the Paddle method, using 900 mL of water as the dissolution medium, the dissolution rate in 30 minutes of Doxycycline Hydrochloride Tablets is not less than 85%.

Start the test with 1 tablet of Doxycycline Hydrochloride Tablets, withdraw not less than 20 mL of the medium at the specified minute after starting the test, and filter through a membrane filter with a pore size not exceeding 0.45 μm. Discard not less than 10 mL of the first filtrate, pipet *V* mL of the subsequent filtrate, add water to make exactly *V′* mL so that each mL contains about 11 μg (potency) of Doxycycline Hydrochloride Hydrate, and use this solution as the sample solution. Separately, weigh accurately about 22 mg (potency) of Doxycycline Hydrochloride RS, dissolve in water to make exactly 100 mL. Pipet 5 mL of this solution, add water to make exactly 100 mL, and use this solution as the standard solution. Determine the absorbances, A_T and A_S, at 274 nm of the sample solution and standard solution as directed under Ultraviolet-visible Spectrophotometry <*2.24*>.

Dissolution rate (%) with respect to the labeled amount of doxycycline ($C_{22}H_{24}N_2O_8$)
$= M_S \times A_T/A_S \times V'/V \times 1/C \times 45$

M_S: Amount [mg (potency)] of Doxycycline Hydrochloride RS taken

C: Labeled amount [mg(potency)] of doxycycline ($C_{22}H_{24}N_2O_8$) in 1 tablet

Assay To 10 Doxycycline Hydrochloride Tablets add 0.01 mol/L hydrochloric acid TS, disperse them by sonicating, shake for 15 minutes, and add 0.01 mol/L hydrochloric acid TS to make exactly V mL so that each mL contains about 2 mg (potency) of Doxycycline Hydrochloride Hydrate. Centrifuge, if necessary, pipet 10 mL of the supernatant liquid, add 0.01 mol/L hydrochloric acid TS to make exactly 20 mL. Filter this solution through a membrane filter with a pore size not exceeding 0.45 μm, discard the first 10 mL of the filtrate, and use the subsequent filtrate as the sample solution. Separately, weigh accurately about 20 mg (potency) of Doxycycline Hydrochloride RS, dissolve in 0.01 mol/L hydrochloric acid TS to make exactly 20 mL, and use this solution as the standard solution. Perform the test with exactly 10 μL of the sample solution and standard solution as directed under Liquid Chromatography *<2.01>* according to the following conditions, and determine the peak areas, A_T and A_S, of doxycycline in each solution.

Amount [mg (potency)] of doxycycline ($C_{22}H_{24}N_2O_8$) in 1 tablet
$= M_S \times A_T/A_S \times V/100$

M_S: Amount [mg (potency)] of Doxycycline Hydrochloride RS taken

Operating conditions—

Detector: An ultraviolet absorption photometer (wavelength: 270 nm).

Column: A stainless steel column 4.6 mm in inside diameter and 15 cm in length, packed with octadecylsilanized silica gel for liquid chromatography (5 μm in particle diameter).

Column temperature: A constant temperature of about 30°C.

Mobile phase: Dissolve 7.0 g of sodium dihydrogen phosphate dihydrate in 450 mL of water. Add to this solution 553 mL of a mixture of methanol and *N,N*-dimethyl-*n*-octylamine (550:3), and adjust to pH 8.0 with sodium hydroxide solution (43 in 200).

Flow rate: Adjust so that the retention time of doxycycline is about 6 minutes.

System suitability—

System performance: When the procedure is run with 10 μL of the standard solution under the above operating conditions, the number of theoretical plates and symmetry factor of the peak of doxycycline are not less than 2200 and not more than 1.6, respectively.

System repeatability: When the test is repeated 6 times with 10 μL of the standard solution under the above operating conditions, the relative standard deviation of the peak area of doxycycline is not more than 1.0%.

Containers and storage Containers—Tight containers.

Droperidol

ドロペリドール

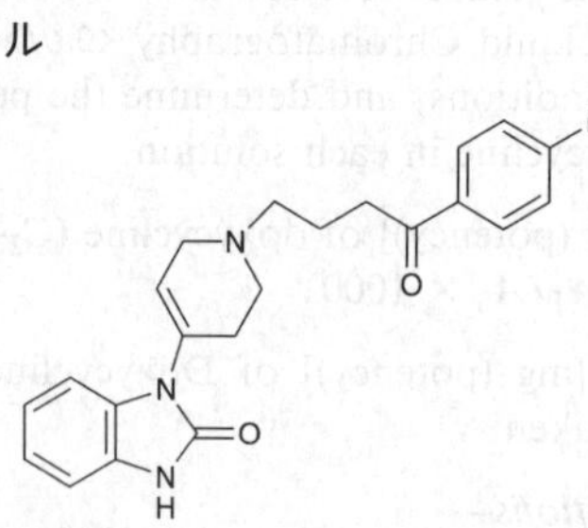

$C_{22}H_{22}FN_3O_2$: 379.43
1-{1-[4-(4-Fluorophenyl)-4-oxobutyl]-1,2,3,6-tetrahydropyridin-4-yl}-1,3-dihydro-2*H*-benzimidazol-2-one
[548-73-2]

Droperidol, when dried, contains not less than 98.0% of droperidol ($C_{22}H_{22}FN_3O_2$).

Description Droperidol occurs as a white to light yellow powder.

It is freely soluble in acetic acid (100), soluble in dichloromethane, slightly soluble in ethanol (99.5), and practically insoluble in water.

It is gradually colored by light.

It shows crystal polymorphism.

Identification **(1)** Put 30 mg of Droperidol in a brown volumetric flask, and dissolve in 10 mL of 0.1 mol/L hydrochloric acid TS and ethanol (95) to make 100 mL. Transfer 5 mL of the solution to a brown volumetric flask, and add 10 mL of 0.1 mol/L hydrochloric acid TS and ethanol (95) to make 100 mL. Determine the absorption spectrum of the solution as directed under Ultraviolet-visible Spectrophotometry *<2.24>*, and compare the spectrum with the Reference Spectrum: both spectra exhibit similar intensities of absorption at the same wavelengths.

(2) Determine the infrared absorption spectrum of Droperidol, previously dried, as directed in the potassium bromide disk method under Infrared Spectrophotometry *<2.25>*, and compare the spectrum with the Reference Spectrum: both spectra exhibit similar intensities of absorption at the same wave numbers. If any difference appears between the spectra, dissolve Droperidol in acetone, evaporate the acetone, dry the residue in a desiccator (in vacuum, silica gel, 70°C) for 4 hours, and perform the test with the residue.

Purity **(1)** Heavy metals *<1.07>*—Proceed with 1.0 g of Droperidol in a platinum crucible according to Method 2, and perform the test. Prepare the control solution with 2.0 mL of Standard Lead Solution (not more than 20 ppm).

(2) Related substances—Conduct this procedure without exposure to light, using light-resistant vessels. Dissolve 50 mg of Droperidol in 5 mL of dichloromethane, and use this solution as the sample solution. Pipet 1 mL of the sample solution, add dichloromethane to make exactly 100 mL, and use this solution as the standard solution. Perform the test with these solutions as directed under Thin-layer Chromatography *<2.03>*. Spot 10 μL each of the sample solution and standard solution on a plate of silica gel with fluorescent indicator for thin-layer chromatography. Develop the plate with a mixture of ethyl acetate, chloroform, methanol and acetic acid-sodium acetate buffer solution (pH 4.7) (54:23:18:5) to a distance of about 15 cm, and air-dry the plate. Examine under ultraviolet light (main wavelength: 254

nm): the spots other than the principal spot obtained from the sample solution are not more intense than the spot from the standard solution.

Loss on drying *<2.41>* Not more than 3.0% (0.5 g, in vacuum, silica gel, 70°C, 4 hours).

Residue on ignition *<2.44>* Not more than 0.2% (1 g, platinum crucible).

Assay Weigh accurately about 0.5 g of Droperidol, previously dried, dissolve in 50 mL of acetic acid (100), and titrate *<2.50>* with 0.1 mol/L perchloric acid VS (potentiometric titration). Perform a blank determination in the same manner, and make any necessary correction.

Each mL of 0.1 mol/L perchloric acid VS
= 37.94 mg of $C_{22}H_{22}FN_3O_2$

Containers and storage Containers—Tight containers.
Storage—Light-resistant.

Droxidopa

ドロキシドパ

$C_9H_{11}NO_5$: 213.19
(2*S*,3*R*)-2-Amino-3-(3,4-dihydroxyphenyl)-3-hydroxypropanoic acid
[*23651-95-8*]

Droxidopa, when dried, contains not less than 99.0% and not more than 101.0% of droxidopa ($C_9H_{11}NO_5$).

Description Droxidopa occurs as white to light brown, crystals or crystalline powder.

It is slightly soluble in water and practically insoluble in ethanol (99.5).

It dissolves in 0.1 mol/L hydrochloric acid TS.

Identification **(1)** Determine the absorption spectrum of a solution of Droxidopa in 0.1 mol/L hydrochloric acid TS (1 in 25,000) as directed under Ultraviolet-visible Spectrophotometry *<2.24>*, and compare the spectrum with the Reference Spectrum: both spectra exhibit similar intensities of absorption at the same wavelengths.

(2) Determine the infrared absorption spectrum of Droxidopa as directed in the potassium bromide disk method under Infrared Spectrophotometry *<2.25>*, and compare the spectrum with the Reference Spectrum: both spectra exhibit similar intensities of absorption at the same wave numbers.

Optical rotation *<2.49>* $[\alpha]_D^{20}$: −38 – −43° (after drying, 0.1 g, 0.1 mol/L hydrochloric acid TS, 20 mL, 100 mm).

Purity **(1)** Chloride *<1.03>*—Dissolve 0.40 g of Droxidopa in 6 mL of dilute nitric acid, and add water to make 50 mL. Perform the test using this solution as the test solution. Prepare the control solution with 0.40 mL of 0.01 mol/L hydrochloric acid VS (not more than 0.036%).

(2) Heavy metals *<1.07>*—Proceed with 2.0 g of Droxidopa according to Method 2, and perform the test. Prepare the control solution with 2.0 mL of Standard Lead Solution (not more than 10 ppm).

(3) Arsenic *<1.11>*—Prepare the test solution with 1.0 g of Droxidopa according to Method 3, and perform the test (not more than 2 ppm).

(4) Related substances—To 0.10 g of Droxidopa add 50 mL of 0.1 mol/L hydrochloric acid TS, dissolve by shaking while cooling in an ice bath, and use this solution as the sample solution. Pipet 1 mL of the sample solution, add 0.1 mol/L hydrochloric acid TS to make exactly 100 mL. Pipet 5 mL of this solution, add 0.1 mol/L hydrochloric acid TS to make 50 mL, and use this solution as the standard solution. Perform the test with exactly 10 μL each of the sample solution and standard solution as directed under Liquid Chromatography *<2.01>* according to the following conditions. Determine each peak area of both solutions by the automatic integration method: the area of each peak other than droxidopa obtained from the sample solution is not larger than the peak area of droxidopa from the standard solution.

Operating conditions—

Detector: An ultraviolet absorption photometer (wavelength: 220 nm).

Column: A stainless steel column 4.6 mm in inside diameter and 15 cm in length, packed with octadecylsilanized silica gel for liquid chromatography (3 μm in particle diameter).

Column temperature: A constant temperature of about 25°C.

Mobile phase: Dissolve 1.0 g of sodium 1-heptanesulfonate and 1.36 g of potassium dihydrogen phosphate in 1000 mL of water, and adjust the pH to 2.0 with phosphoric acid. To 930 mL of this solution add 70 mL of acetonitrile.

Flow rate: Adjust so that the retention time of droxidopa is about 5 minutes.

Time span of measurement: About 12 times as long as the retention time of droxidopa, beginning after the solvent peak.

System suitability—

System performance: When the procedure is run with 10 μL of the standard solution under the above operating conditions, the number of theoretical plates and the symmetry factor of the peak of droxidopa are not less than 10,000 and not more than 1.5, respectively.

System repeatability: When the test is repeated 6 times with 10 μL of the standard solution under the above operating conditions, the relative standard deviation of the peak area of droxidopa is not more than 2.0%.

Loss on drying *<2.41>* Not more than 0.1% (1 g, in vacuum, 60°C, 3 hours).

Residue on ignition *<2.44>* Not more than 0.2% (1 g).

Assay Weigh accurately about 0.3 g of Droxidopa, previously dried, dissolve in exactly 20 mL of 0.1 mol/L perchloric acid VS, add 50 mL of acetic acid (100), and titrate *<2.50>* the excess perchloric acid with 0.1 mol/L sodium acetate VS (potentiometric titration). Perform a blank determination in the same manner, and make any necessary correction.

Each mL of 0.1 mol/L perchloric acid VS
= 21.32 mg of $C_9H_{11}NO_5$

Containers and storage Containers—Well-closed containers.

Droxidopa Capsules

ドロキシドパカプセル

Droxidopa Capsules contain not less than 93.0% and not more than 107.0% of the labeled amount of droxidopa ($C_9H_{11}NO_5$: 213.19).

Method of preparation Prepare as directed under Capsules, with Droxidopa.

Identification **(1)** To an amount of the contents of Droxidopa Capsules, equivalent to 50 mg of Droxidopa, add 50 mL of water, shake for 10 minutes, and filter. To 5 mL of the filtrate add 1 mL of ninhydrin TS, and heat in a water bath for 3 minutes: a blue-purple color develops.

(2) To an amount of the contents of Droxidopa Capsules, equivalent to 20 mg of Droxidopa, add 20 mL of diluted acetic acid (100) (1 in 500), shake for 10 minutes, and filter. To 1 mL of the filtrate add 4 mL of water and 1 drop of iron (III) chloride TS: a deep green color is produced, and it gradually changes to light brown.

(3) To an amount of the contents of Droxidopa Capsules, equivalent to 50 mg of Droxidopa, add 50 mL of 0.1 mol/L hydrochloric acid TS, shake well, add 0.1 mol/L hydrochloric acid TS to make 100 mL, and filter. Discard the first 10 mL of the filtrate, and to 2 mL of the subsequent filtrate add 0.1 mol/L hydrochloric acid TS to make 25 mL. Determine the absorption spectrum of this solution as directed under Ultraviolet-visible Spectrophotometry <*2.24*>: it exhibits a maximum between 278 nm and 282 nm.

Uniformity of dosage units <*6.02*> Perform the Mass variation test, or the Content uniformity test according to the following method: it meets the requirement.

To the contents of 1 capsule of Droxidopa Capsules, add 100 mL of 0.1 mol/L hydrochloric acid TS, shake well, and add 0.1 mol/L hydrochloric acid TS to make exactly V mL so that each mL contains about 0.5 mg of droxidopa ($C_9H_{11}NO_5$). Filter this solution, discard the first 10 mL of the filtrate, pipet 2 mL of the subsequent filtrate, add 0.1 mol/L hydrochloric acid TS to make exactly 25 mL, and use this solution as the sample solution. Separately, weigh accurately about 50 mg of droxidopa for assay, previously dried in vacuum at 60°C for 3 hours, dissolve in 0.1 mol/L hydrochloric acid TS to make exactly 100 mL. Pipet 2 mL of this solution, add 0.1 mol/L hydrochloric acid TS to make exactly 25 mL, and use this solution as the standard solution. Perform the test with the sample solution and standard solution as directed under Ultraviolet-visible Spectrophotometry <*2.24*>, and determine the absorbances, A_T and A_S, at 280 nm.

$$\text{Amount (mg) of droxidopa } (C_9H_{11}NO_5) = M_S \times A_T/A_S \times V/100$$

M_S: Amount (mg) of droxidopa for assay taken

Dissolution <*6.10*> When the test is performed at 75 revolutions per minute according to the Paddle method using the sinker, using 900 mL of water as the dissolution medium, the dissolution rate in 90 minutes of Droxidopa Capsules is not less than 70%.

Start the test with 1 capsule of Droxidopa Capsules, withdraw not less than 20 mL of the medium at the specified minute after starting the test, and filter through a membrane filter with a pore size not exceeding 0.45 µm. Discard not less than 10 mL of the first filtrate, pipet V mL of the subsequent filtrate, add water to make exactly V' mL so that each mL contains about 56 µg of droxidopa ($C_9H_{11}NO_5$), and use this solution as the sample solution. Separately, weigh accurately about 28 mg of droxidopa for assay, previously dried in vacuum at 60°C for 3 hours, dissolve in water to make exactly 100 mL. Pipet 4 mL of this solution, add water to make exactly 20 mL, and use this solution as the standard solution. Perform the test with the sample solution and standard solution as directed under Ultraviolet-visible Spectrophotometry <*2.24*>, and determine the absorbances, A_{T1} and A_{S1}, at 280 nm, and A_{T2} and A_{S2}, at 350 nm.

Dissolution rate (%) with respect to the labeled amount of droxidopa ($C_9H_{11}NO_5$)

$$= M_S \times (A_{T1} - A_{T2})/(A_{S1} - A_{S2}) \times V'/V \times 1/C \times 180$$

M_S: Amount (mg) of droxidopa for assay taken
C: Labeled amount (mg) of droxidopa ($C_9H_{11}NO_5$) in 1 capsule

Assay Take out the contents of not less than 20 Droxidopa Capsules, weigh accurately the mass of the contents, and mix uniformly. Weigh accurately an amount equivalent to about 50 mg of droxidopa ($C_9H_{11}NO_5$), add 50 mL of 0.1 mol/L hydrochloric acid TS, shake well, add 0.1 mol/L hydrochloric acid TS to make exactly 100 mL, and filter. Discard the first 10 mL of the filtrate, pipet 2 mL of the subsequent filtrate, add 0.1 mol/L hydrochloric acid TS to make exactly 25 mL, and use this solution as the sample solution. Separately, weigh accurately about 50 mg of droxidopa for assay, previously dried in vacuum at 60°C for 3 hours, dissolve in 0.1 mol/L hydrochloric acid TS to make exactly 100 mL. Pipet 2 mL of this solution, add 0.1 mol/L hydrochloric acid TS to make exactly 25 mL, and use this solution as the standard solution. Perform the test with the sample solution and standard solution as directed under Ultraviolet-visible Spectrophotometry <*2.24*>, and determine the absorbances, A_T and A_S, at 280 nm.

$$\text{Amount (mg) of droxidopa } (C_9H_{11}NO_5) = M_S \times A_T/A_S$$

M_S: Amount (mg) of droxidopa for assay taken

Containers and storage Containers—Tight containers.

Droxidopa Fine Granules

ドロキシドパ細粒

Droxidopa Fine Granules contain not less than 93.0% and not more than 107.0% of the labeled amount of droxidopa ($C_9H_{11}NO_5$: 213.19).

Method of preparation Prepare as directed under Granules, with Droxidopa.

Identification **(1)** To a quantity of powdered Droxidopa Fine Granules, equivalent to 50 mg of Droxidopa, add 50 mL of water, shake for 10 minutes, and filter. To 5 mL of the filtrate add 1 mL of ninhydrin TS, heat in a water bath for 3 minutes: a blue-purple color develops.

(2) To a quantity of powdered Droxidopa Fine Granules, equivalent to 20 mg of Droxidopa, add 20 mL of diluted acetic acid (100) (1 in 500), shake for 10 minutes, and filter. To 1 mL of the filtrate add 4 mL of water and 1 drop of iron (III) chloride TS: a deep green color is produced, and it gradually changes to light brown.

(3) To a quantity of powdered Droxidopa Fine Granules,

equivalent to 50 mg of Droxidopa, add 50 mL of 0.1 mol/L hydrochloric acid TS, shake well, add 0.1 mol/L hydrochloric acid TS to make 100 mL, and filter. Discard the first 10 mL of the filtrate, to 2 mL of the subsequent filtrate add 0.1 mol/L hydrochloric acid TS to make 25 mL. Determine the absorption spectrum of this solution as directed under Ultraviolet-visible Spectrophotometry <*2.24*>: it exhibits a maximum between 278 nm and 282 nm.

Dissolution <*6.10*> When the test is performed at 75 revolutions per minute according to the Paddle method, using 900 mL of water as the dissolution medium, the dissolution rate in 45 minutes of Droxidopa Fine Granules is not less than 70%.

Start the test with an accurately weighed amount of Droxidopa Fine Granules, equivalent to about 0.1 g of droxidopa ($C_9H_{11}NO_5$), withdraw not less than 20 mL of the medium at the specified minute after starting the test, and filter through a membrane filter with a pore size not exceeding 0.45 μm. Discard not less than 10 mL of the first filtrate, pipet 5 mL of the subsequent filtrate, add exactly 5 mL of water, and use this solution as the sample solution. Separately, weigh accurately about 28 mg of droxidopa for assay, previously dried in vacuum at 60°C for 3 hours, dissolve in water to make exactly 100 mL. Pipet 4 mL of this solution, add water to make exactly 20 mL, and use this solution as the standard solution. Perform the test with the sample solution and standard solution as directed under Ultraviolet-visible Spectrophotometry <*2.24*>, and determine the absorbances, A_{T1} and A_{S1}, at 280 nm, and A_{T2} and A_{S2}, at 350 nm.

Dissolution rate (%) with respect to the labeled amount of droxidopa ($C_9H_{11}NO_5$)
$= M_S/M_T \times (A_{T1} - A_{T2})/(A_{S1} - A_{S2}) \times 1/C \times 360$

M_S: Amount (mg) of droxidopa for assay taken
M_T: Amount (g) of Droxidopa Fine Granules taken
C: Labeled amount (mg) of droxidopa ($C_9H_{11}NO_5$) in 1 g

Assay Powder not less than 20 g of Droxidopa Fine Granules. Weigh accurately a portion of the powder, equivalent to about 50 mg of droxidopa ($C_9H_{11}NO_5$), add 50 mL of 0.1 mol/L hydrochloric acid TS, shake well, add 0.1 mol/L hydrochloric acid TS to make exactly 100 mL, and filter. Discard the first 10 mL of the filtrate, pipet 2 mL of the subsequent filtrate, add 0.1 mol/L hydrochloric acid TS to make exactly 25 mL, and use this solution as the sample solution. Separately, weigh accurately about 50 mg of droxidopa for assay, previously dried in vacuum at 60°C for 3 hours, dissolve in 0.1 mol/L hydrochloric acid TS to make exactly 100 mL. Pipet 2 mL of this solution, add 0.1 mol/L hydrochloric acid TS to make exactly 25 mL, and use this solution as the standard solution. Perform the test with the sample solution and standard solution as directed under Ultraviolet-visible Spectrophotometry <*2.24*>, and determine the absorbances, A_T and A_S, at 280 nm.

Amount (mg) of droxidopa ($C_9H_{11}NO_5$)
$= M_S \times A_T/A_S$

M_S: Amount (mg) of droxidopa for assay taken

Containers and storage Containers—Tight containers.

Dydrogesterone

ジドロゲステロン

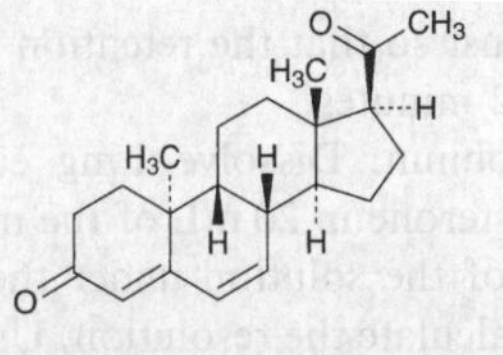

$C_{21}H_{28}O_2$: 312.45
9β,10α-Pregna-4,6-diene-3,20-dione
[*152-62-5*]

Dydrogesterone, when dried, contains not less than 98.0% and not more than 102.0% of dydrogesterone ($C_{21}H_{28}O_2$).

Description Dydrogesterone occurs as white to light yellow-white, crystals or crystalline powder. It is odorless.

It is freely soluble in chloroform, soluble in acetonitrile, sparingly soluble in methanol and in ethanol (95), slightly soluble in diethyl ether, and practically insoluble in water.

Identification (1) To 5 mg of Dydrogesterone add 5 mL of 4-methoxybenzaldehyde-acetic acid TS and 2 to 3 drops of sulfuric acid, and heat in a water bath for 2 minutes: an orange-red color develops.

(2) Determine the absorption spectrum of a solution of Dydrogesterone in methanol (1 in 200,000) as directed under Ultraviolet-visible Spectrophotometry <*2.24*>, and compare the spectrum with the Reference Spectrum: both spectra exhibit similar intensities of absorption at the same wavelengths.

(3) Determine the infrared absorption spectrum of Dydrogesterone, previously dried, as directed in the potassium bromide disk method under Infrared Spectrophotometry <*2.25*>, and compare the spectrum with the Reference Spectrum: both spectra exhibit similar intensities of absorption at the same wave numbers.

Optical rotation <*2.49*> $[\alpha]_D^{20}$: -470 – -500° (after drying, 0.1 g, chloroform, 10 mL, 100 mm).

Melting point <*2.60*> 167 – 171°C

Purity (1) Heavy metals <*1.07*>—Proceed with 1.0 g of Dydrogesterone according to Method 2, and perform the test. Prepare the control solution with 2.0 mL of Standard Lead Solution (not more than 20 ppm).

(2) Related substances—Dissolve 10 mg of Dydrogesterone in 200 mL of the mobile phase, and use this solution as the sample solution. Pipet 1 mL of the sample solution, add the mobile phase to make exactly 100 mL, and use this solution as the standard solution. Perform the test with exactly 10 μL each of the sample solution and standard solution as directed under Liquid Chromatography <*2.01*> according to the following conditions. Determine each peak area of these solutions by the automatic integration method: the total area of peaks other than dydrogesterone obtained from the sample solution is not larger than the peak area of dydrogesterone from the standard solution.

Operating conditions—

Detector: An ultraviolet absorption photometer (wavelength: 280 nm).

Column: A stainless steel column about 4 mm in inside diameter and about 15 cm in length, packed with octadecylsilanized silica gel for liquid chromatography (3 μm in particle diameter).

Column temperature: A constant temperature of about 40°C.

Mobile phase: A mixture of water, ethanol (95) and acetonitrile (53:26:21).

Flow rate: Adjust so that the retention time of dydrogesterone is about 12 minutes.

Selection of column: Dissolve 1 mg each of Dydrogesterone and progesterone in 20 mL of the mobile phase. Proceed with 10 μL of the solution under the above operating conditions, and calculate the resolution. Use a column giving elution of dydrogesterone and progesterone in this order with the resolution between these peaks being not less than 8. Wavelength is 265 nm.

Detection sensitivity: Adjust the detection sensitivity so that the peak height of dydrogesterone obtained with 10 μL of the standard solution is between 5 mm and 10 mm.

Time span of measurement: About twice as long as the retention time of dydrogesterone, beginning after the solvent peak.

Loss on drying *<2.41>* Not more than 0.5% (0.5 g, in vacuum, phosphorus (V) oxide, 24 hours).

Residue on ignition *<2.44>* Not more than 0.1% (1 g).

Assay Weigh accurately about 50 mg of Dydrogesterone, previously dried, and dissolve in methanol to make exactly 100 mL. Pipet 1 mL of this solution, and add methanol to make exactly 100 mL. Determine the absorbance A of this solution at the wavelength of maximum absorption at about 286 nm as directed under Ultraviolet-visible Spectrophotometry *<2.24>*.

$$\text{Amount (mg) of dydrogesterone } (C_{21}H_{28}O_2) = A/845 \times 100{,}000$$

Containers and storage Containers—Tight containers.

Dydrogesterone Tablets

ジドロゲステロン錠

Dydrogesterone Tablets contain not less than 95.0% and not more than 105.0% of the labeled amount of dydrogesterone ($C_{21}H_{28}O_2$: 312.45).

Method of preparation Prepare as directed under Tablets, with Dydrogesterone.

Identification **(1)** To a quantity of powdered Dydrogesterone Tablets, equivalent to 0.05 g of Dydrogesterone, add 50 mL of methanol, shake well, and filter. Evaporate 5 mL of the filtrate on a water bath to dryness. Proceed with the residue as directed in the Identification (1) under Dydrogesterone.

(2) To 1 mL of the filtrate obtained in (1) add methanol to make 200 mL. Determine the absorption spectrum of this solution as directed under Ultraviolet-visible Spectrophotometry *<2.24>*: it exhibits a maximum between 284 nm and 288 nm.

Uniformity of dosage units *<6.02>* Perform the test according to the following method: it meets the requirement of the Content uniformity test.

Crush 1 tablet of Dydrogesterone Tablets, and add methanol to make exactly 100 mL. Shake until the tablet is completely disintegrated, and filter through a membrane filter with a pore size not exceeding 0.45 μm. Discard the first 20 mL of the filtrate, pipet V mL of the subsequent filtrate, add methanol to make exactly V' mL so that each mL contains about 5 μg of dydrogesterone ($C_{21}H_{28}O_2$), and use this solution as the sample solution. Then, proceed as directed in the Assay.

$$\text{Amount (mg) of dydrogesterone } (C_{21}H_{28}O_2) = M_S \times A_T/A_S \times V'/V \times 1/20$$

M_S: Amount (mg) of dydrogesterone for assay taken

Dissolution *<6.10>* When the test is performed at 50 revolutions per minute according to the Paddle method, using 900 mL of water as the dissolution medium, the dissolution rate in 30 minutes of Dydrogesterone Tablets is not less than 80%.

Start the test with 1 tablet of Dydrogesterone Tablets, withdraw not less than 20 mL of the medium at the specified minute after starting the test, and filter. Discard not less than 10 mL of the first filtrate, pipet V mL of the subsequent filtrate, add water to make exactly V' mL so that each mL contains about 56 μg of dydrogesterone ($C_{21}H_{28}O_2$), and use this solution as the sample solution. Separately, weigh accurately about 50 mg of dydrogesterone for assay, previously dried in a desiccator (in vacuum, phosphorus (V) oxide) for 24 hours, and dissolve in methanol to make exactly 100 mL. Pipet 1 mL of this solution, add water to make exactly 100 mL, and use this solution as the standard solution. Determine the absorbances, A_T and A_S, of the sample solution and standard solution at 296 nm as directed under Ultraviolet-visible Spectrophotometry *<2.24>*, using water as the control.

$$\text{Dissolution rate (\%) with respect to the labeled amount of dydrogesterone } (C_{21}H_{28}O_2) = M_S \times A_T/A_S \times V'/V \times 1/C \times 9$$

M_S: Amount (mg) of dydrogesterone for assay taken
C: Labeled amount (mg) of dydrogesterone ($C_{21}H_{28}O_2$) in 1 tablet.

Assay Weigh accurately and powder not less than 20 Dydrogesterone Tablets. Weigh accurately a portion of the powder, equivalent to about 10 mg of dydrogesterone ($C_{21}H_{28}O_2$), shake with 50 mL of methanol, and add methanol to make exactly 100 mL, and filter through a membrane filter with a pore size not exceeding 0.45 μm. Discard the first 20 mL of the filtrate, pipet 5 mL of the subsequent filtrate, add methanol to make exactly 100 mL, and use this solution as the sample solution. Separately, weigh accurately about 10 mg of dydrogesterone for assay, previously dried in vacuum for 24 hours using phosphorus (V) oxide as a dessicant, and dissolve in methanol to make exactly 100 mL. Pipet 5 mL of this solution, add methanol to make exactly 100 mL, and use the solution as the standard solution. Determine the absorbances, A_T and A_S, of the sample solution and standard solution at 286 nm as directed under Ultraviolet-visible Spectrophotometry *<2.24>*.

$$\text{Amount (mg) of dydrogesterone } (C_{21}H_{28}O_2) = M_S \times A_T/A_S$$

M_S: Amount (mg) of dydrogesterone for assay taken

Containers and storage Containers—Tight containers.

Ebastine

エバスチン

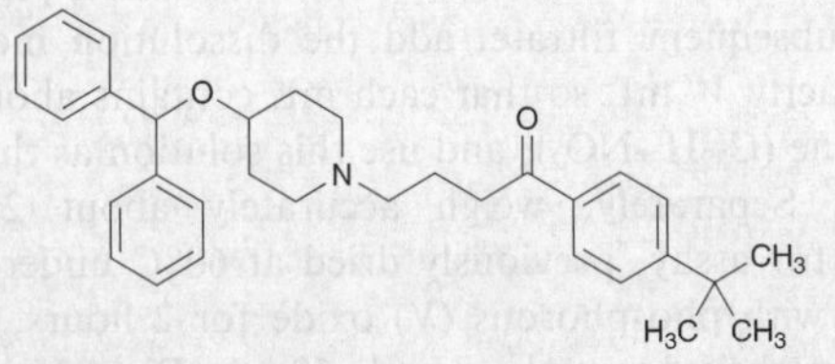

$C_{32}H_{39}NO_2$: 469.66
1-[4-(1,1-Dimethylethyl)phenyl]-
4-[4-(diphenylmethoxy)piperidin-1-yl]butan-1-one
[*90729-43-4*]

Ebastine, when dried, contains not less than 99.0% and not more than 101.0% of ebastine ($C_{32}H_{39}NO_2$).

Description Ebastine occurs as white, crystals or crystalline powder.

It is freely soluble in acetic acid (100), soluble in methanol, sparingly soluble in ethanol (95), and practically insoluble in water.

It gradually becomes yellowish white on exposure to light.

Identification **(1)** Dissolve 20 mg of Ebastine in 5 mL of ethanol (95), add 2 mL of 1,3-dinitrobenzene TS and 2 mL of sodium hydroxide TS, and allow to stand: the color of the solution is purple to red-purple, which gradually changes to blown.

(2) Determine the absorption spectrum of a solution of Ebastine in methanol (1 in 100,000) as directed under Ultraviolet-visible Spectrophotometry 〈*2.24*〉, and compare the spectrum with the Reference Spectrum: both spectra exhibit similar intensities of absorption at the same wavelengths.

(3) Determine the infrared absorption spectrum of Ebastine as directed in the potassium bromide disk method under Infrared Spectrophotometry 〈*2.25*〉, and compare the spectrum with the Reference Spectrum: both spectra exhibit similar intensities of absorption at the same wave numbers.

Melting point 〈*2.60*〉 84 – 87°C

Purity **(1)** Heavy metals 〈*1.07*〉—Proceed with 1.0 g of Ebastine according to Method 2, and perform the test. Prepare the control solution with 2.0 mL of Standard Lead Solution (not more than 20 ppm). A platinum crucible may be used.

(2) Related substances—Dissolve 0.10 g of Ebastine in 50 mL of the mobile phase, and use this solution as the sample solution. Pipet 5 mL of the sample solution, and add the mobile phase to make exactly 100 mL. Pipet 2 mL of this solution, add the mobile phase to make exactly 100 mL, and use this solution as the standard solution. Perform the test with exactly 10 μL each of the sample solution and standard solution as directed under Liquid Chromatography 〈*2.01*〉 according to the following conditions, and determine each peak area by the automatic integration method: each peak area other than ebastine obtained from the sample solution is not larger than the peak area of ebastine from the standard solution, and the total area of the peaks other than ebastine from the sample solution is not larger than 4 times the peak area of ebastine from the standard solution.

Operating conditions—

Detector: An ultraviolet absorption photometer (wavelength: 220 nm).

Column: A stainless steel column 4.6 mm in inside diameter and 15 cm in length, packed with octadecylsilanized silica gel for liquid chromatography (5 μm in particle diameter).

Column temperature: A constant temperature of about 40°C.

Mobile phase: Dissolve 7.8 g of sodium dihydrogen phosphate dihydrate in 900 mL of water, adjust to pH 3.0 with diluted phosphoric acid (1 in 5), and add water to make 1000 mL. To 375 mL of this solution add 625 mL of acetonitrile for liquid chromatography, and dissolve 0.72 g of sodium lauryl sulfate in this solution.

Flow rate: Adjust so that the retention time of ebastine is about 9 minutes.

Time span of measurement: About 2 times as long as the retention time of ebastine, beginning after the solvent peak.

System suitability—

Test for required detectability: Pipet 5 mL of the standard solution, and add the mobile phase to make exactly 10 mL. Confirm that the peak area of ebastine obtained with 10 μL of this solution is equivalent to 35 to 65% of that with 10 μL of the standard solution.

System performance: When the procedure is run with 10 μL of the standard solution under the above operating conditions, the number of theoretical plates and the symmetry factor of the peak of ebastine are not less than 6000 and not more than 1.5, respectively.

System repeatability: When the test is repeated 6 times with 10 μL of the standard solution under the above operating conditions, the relative standard deviation of the peak area of ebastine is not more than 2.0%.

Loss on drying 〈*2.41*〉 Not more than 0.5% (1 g, in vacuum, phosphorus (V) oxide, 60°C, 2 hours).

Residue on ignition 〈*2.44*〉 Not more than 0.1% (1 g).

Assay Weigh accurately about 0.5 g of Ebastine, previously dried, dissolve in 60 mL of acetic acid (100), and titrate 〈*2.50*〉 with 0.1 mol/L perchloric acid VS (potentiometric titration). Perform a blank determination in the same manner, and make any necessary correction.

Each mL of 0.1 mol/L perchloric acid VS
= 46.97 mg of $C_{32}H_{39}NO_2$

Containers and storage Containers—Well-closed containers.

Storage—Light-resistant.

Ebastine Orally Disintegrating Tablets

エバスチンロ腔内崩壊錠

Ebastine Orally Disintegrating Tablets contain not less than 95.0% and not more than 105.0% of the labeled amount of ebastine ($C_{32}H_{39}NO_2$: 469.66).

Method of preparation Prepare as directed under Tablets, with Ebastine.

Identification Powder Ebastine Orally Disintegrating Tablets. To a portion of the powder, equivalent to 30 mg of Ebastine, add 70 mL of methanol, shake for 10 minutes, then add methanol to make 100 mL, and centrifuge. To 5 mL of the supernatant liquid add methanol to make 100 mL. Determine the absorption spectrum of this solution as directed under Ultraviolet-visible Spectrophotometry 〈*2.24*〉: it exhibits a maximum between 251 nm and 255 nm.

The JP Drugs are to be tested according to the provisions given in the pertinent monographs, General Notices, General Rules for Crude Drugs, General Rules for Preparations, and General Tests for their conformity to the Japanese Pharmacopoeia. (See the General Notices 5.)

Purity Related substances—Powder Ebastine Orally Disintegrating Tablets. To a portion of the powder, equivalent to 50 mg of Ebastine, add 30 mL of methanol for liquid chromatography, shake for 10 minutes, and add the mobile phase to make 50 mL. Centrifuge this solution, and use the supernatant liquid as the sample solution. Pipet 1 mL of the sample solution, add the mobile phase to make exactly 200 mL, and use this solution as the standard solution. Perform the test with exactly 10 μL each of the sample solution and standard solution as directed under Liquid Chromatography <*2.01*> according to the following conditions, and determine each peak area by the automatic integration method: the area of the peak other than ebastine obtained from the sample solution is not larger than the peak area of ebastine from the standard solution, and the total area of the peaks other than ebastine from the sample solution is not larger than 2 times the peak area of ebastine from the standard solution.

Operating conditions—

Column, column temperature, mobile phase, and flow rate: Proceed as directed in the operating conditions in the Assay.

Detector: An ultraviolet absorption photometer (wavelength: 220 nm).

Time span of measurement: About 3 times as long as the retention time of ebastine, beginning after the solvent peak.

System suitability—

Test for required detectability: Pipet 10 mL of the standard solution, and add the mobile phase to make exactly 50 mL. Confirm that the peak area of ebastine obtained with 10 μL of this solution is equivalent to 15 to 25% of that with 10 μL of the standard solution.

System performance: When the procedure is run with 10 μL of the standard solution under the above operating conditions, the number of theoretical plates and the symmetry factor of the peak of ebastine are not less than 6000 and not more than 1.5, respectively.

System repeatability: When the test is repeated 6 times with 10 μL of the standard solution under the above operating conditions, the relative standard deviation of the peak area of ebastine is not more than 2.0%.

Uniformity of dosage units <*6.02*> Perform the test according to the following method: it meets the requirement of the Content uniformity test.

To 1 tablet of Ebastine Orally Disintegrating Tablets add V/10 mL of 0.1 mol/L hydrochloric acid TS, and disperse the particles by sonicating with occasional shaking. Add $3V/5$ mL of methanol, shake for 10 minutes, then add methanol to make exactly V mL so that each mL contains about 0.1 mg of ebastine ($C_{32}H_{39}NO_2$), and centrifuge. Pipet 5 mL of the supernatant liquid, add exactly 5 mL of the internal standard solution, and use this solution as the sample solution. Then, proceed as directed in the Assay.

$$\text{Amount (mg) of ebastine } (C_{32}H_{39}NO_2) = M_S \times Q_T/Q_S \times V/500$$

M_S: Amount (mg) of ebastine for assay taken

Internal standard solution—A solution of diphenyl in the mobile phase (1 in 40,000).

Disintegration Being specified separately when the drug is granted approval based on the Law.

Dissolution <*6.10*> When the test is performed at 50 revolutions per minute according to the Paddle method, using 900 mL of 1st fluid for dissolution test as the dissolution medium, the dissolution rate in 15 minutes of Ebastine Orally Disintegrating Tablets is not less than 80%.

Start the test with 1 tablet of Ebastine Orally Disintegrating Tablets, withdraw not less than 20 mL of the medium at the specified minute after starting the test, and filter through a membrane filter with a pore size not exceeding 0.45 μm. Discard not less than 10 mL of the first filtrate, pipet V mL of the subsequent filtrate, add the dissolution medium to make exactly V' mL so that each mL contains about 5.6 μg of ebastine ($C_{32}H_{39}NO_2$), and use this solution as the sample solution. Separately, weigh accurately about 28 mg of ebastine for assay, previously dried at 60°C under reduced pressure with phosphorous (V) oxide for 2 hours, and dissolve in methanol to make exactly 50 mL. Pipet 1 mL of this solution, add the dissolution medium to make exactly 100 mL, and use this solution as the standard solution. Determine the absorbances, A_T and A_S, of the sample solution and standard solution at 258 nm as directed under Ultraviolet-visible Spectrophotometry <*2.24*>, using the dissolution medium as the blank.

$$\text{Dissolution rate (\%) with respect to the labeled amount of ebastine } (C_{32}H_{39}NO_2) = M_S \times A_T/A_S \times V'/V \times 1/C \times 18$$

M_S: Amount (mg) of ebastine for assay taken

C: Labeled amount (mg) of ebastine ($C_{32}H_{39}NO_2$) in 1 tablet

Assay Weigh accurately the mass of not less than 20 Ebastine Orally Disintegrating Tablets, and powder. Weigh accurately a portion of the powder, equivalent to about 20 mg of ebastine ($C_{32}H_{39}NO_2$), add 20 mL of 0.1 mol/L hydrochloric acid TS, and disperse the particles by sonicating. Add 120 mL of methanol, shake for 10 minutes, add methanol to make exactly 200 mL, and centrifuge. Pipet 5 mL of the supernatant liquid, add exactly 5 mL of the internal standard solution, and use this solution as the sample solution. Separately, weigh accurately about 50 mg of ebastine for assay, previously dried at 60°C under reduced pressure with phosphorous (V) oxide for 2 hours, and dissolve in methanol to make exactly 50 mL. Pipet 5 mL of this solution, add 5 mL of 0.1 mol/L hydrochloric acid TS, and add methanol to make exactly 50 mL. Pipet 5 mL of this solution, add exactly 5 mL of the internal standard solution, and use this solution as the standard solution. Perform the test with 10 μL each of the sample solution and standard solution as directed under Liquid Chromatography <*2.01*> according to the following conditions, and calculate the ratios, Q_T and Q_S, of the peak area of ebastine to that of the internal standard.

$$\text{Amount (mg) of ebastine } (C_{32}H_{39}NO_2) = M_S \times Q_T/Q_S \times 2/5$$

M_S: Amount (mg) of ebastine for assay taken

Internal standard solution—A solution of diphenyl in the mobile phase (1 in 40,000).

Operating conditions—

Detector: An ultraviolet absorption photometer (wavelength: 254 nm).

Column: A stainless steel column 4.6 mm in inside diameter and 15 cm in length, packed with octadecylsilanized silica gel for liquid chromatography (5 μm in particle diameter).

Column temperature: A constant temperature of about 40°C.

Mobile phase: Dissolve 7.8 g of sodium dihydrogen phosphate dihydrate in 900 mL of water, adjust to pH 3.0 with diluted phosphoric acid (1 in 5), and add water to make 1000 mL. To 375 mL of this solution add 625 mL of acetonitrile for liquid chromatography, and dissolve 0.72 g of sodium lauryl sulfate in this solution.

Flow rate: Adjust so that the retention time of ebastine is about 9 minutes.

System suitability—

System performance: When the procedure is run with 10 μL of the standard solution under the above operating conditions, the internal standard and ebastine are eluted in this order with the resolution between these peaks being not less than 5.

System repeatability: When the test is repeated 6 times with 10 μL of the standard solution under the above operating conditions, the relative standard deviation of the ratio of the peak area of ebastine to that of the internal standard is not more than 1.0%.

Containers and storage Containers—Tight containers.

Storage—Light-resistant.

Ebastine Tablets

エバスチン錠

Ebastine Tablets contain not less than 95.0% and not more than 105.0% of the labeled amount of ebastine ($C_{32}H_{39}NO_2$: 469.66).

Method of preparation Prepare as directed under Tablets, with Ebastine.

Identification Powder Ebastine Tablets. To a portion of the powder, equivalent to 30 mg of Ebastine, add 70 mL of methanol, shake for 10 minutes, then add methanol to make 100 mL, and centrifuge. To 5 mL of the supernatant liquid add methanol to make 100 mL. Determine the absorption spectrum of this solution as directed under Ultraviolet-visible Spectrophotometry *<2.24>*: it exhibits a maximum between 251 nm and 255 nm.

Purity Related substances—Powder Ebastine Tablets. To a portion of the powder, equivalent to 50 mg of Ebastine, add 30 mL of methanol for liquid chromatography, shake for 10 minutes, and add the mobile phase to make 50 mL. Centrifuge this solution, and use the supernatant liquid as the sample solution. Pipet 1 mL of the sample solution, add the mobile phase to make exactly 200 mL, and use this solution as the standard solution. Perform the test with exactly 10 μL each of the sample solution and standard solution as directed under Liquid Chromatography *<2.01>* according to the following conditions, and determine each peak area by the automatic integration method: the area of the peak other than ebastine obtained from the sample solution is not larger than the peak area of ebastine from the standard solution, and the total area of the peaks other than ebastine from the sample solution is not larger than 2 times the peak area of ebastine from the standard solution.

Operating conditions—

Column, column temperature, mobile phase, and flow rate: Proceed as directed in the operating conditions in the Assay.

Detector: An ultraviolet absorption photometer (wavelength: 220 nm).

Time span of measurement: About 3 times as long as the retention time of ebastine, beginning after the solvent peak.

System suitability—

Test for required detectability: Pipet 10 mL of the standard solution, and add the mobile phase to make exactly 50 mL. Confirm that the peak area of ebastine obtained with 10 μL of this solution is equivalent to 15 to 25% of that obtained with 10 μL of the standard solution.

System performance: When the procedure is run with 10 μL of the standard solution under the above operating conditions, the number of theoretical plates and the symmetry factor of the peak of ebastine are not less than 6000 and not more than 1.5, respectively.

System repeatability: When the test is repeated 6 times with 10 μL of the standard solution under the above operating conditions, the relative standard deviation of the peak area of ebastine is not more than 2.0%.

Uniformity of dosage units *<6.02>* Perform the test according to the following method: it meets the requirement of the Content uniformity test.

To 1 tablet of Ebastine Tablets add $V/10$ mL of 0.1 mol/L hydrochloric acid TS, and disperse the particles by sonicating with occasional shaking. Add $3V/5$ mL of methanol, shake for 10 minutes, then add methanol to make exactly V mL so that each mL contains about 0.1 mg of ebastine ($C_{32}H_{39}NO_2$), and centrifuge. Pipet 5 mL of the supernatant liquid, add exactly 5 mL of the internal standard solution, and use this solution as the sample solution. Then, proceed as directed in the Assay.

Amount (mg) of ebastine ($C_{32}H_{39}NO_2$)
$= M_S \times Q_T/Q_S \times V/500$

M_S: Amount (mg) of ebastine for assay taken

*Internal standard solution—*A solution of diphenyl in the mobile phase (1 in 40,000).

Dissolution *<6.10>* When the test is performed at 50 revolutions per minute according to the Paddle method, using 900 mL of 1st fluid for dissolution test as the dissolution medium, the dissolution rate in 30 minutes of Ebastine Tablets is not less than 75%.

Start the test with 1 tablet of Ebastine Tablets, withdraw not less than 20 mL of the medium at the specified minute after starting the test, and filter through a membrane filter with a pore size not exceeding 0.45 μm. Discard not less than 10 mL of the first filtrate, pipet V mL of the subsequent filtrate, add the dissolution medium to make exactly V' mL so that each mL contains about 5.6 μg of ebastine ($C_{32}H_{39}NO_2$), and use this solution as the sample solution. Separately, weigh accurately about 28 mg of ebastine for assay, previously dried at 60°C under reduced pressure with phosphorous (V) oxide for 2 hours, and dissolve in methanol to make exactly 50 mL. Pipet 1 mL of this solution, add the dissolution medium to make exactly 100 mL, and use this solution as the standard solution. Determine the absorbances, A_T and A_S, of the sample solution and standard solution at 258 nm as directed under Ultraviolet-visible Spectrophotometry *<2.24>*, using the dissolution medium as the blank.

Dissolution rate (%) with respect to the labeled amount of ebastine ($C_{32}H_{39}NO_2$)
$= M_S \times A_T/A_S \times V'/V \times 1/C \times 18$

M_S: Amount (mg) of ebastine for assay taken
C: Labeled amount (mg) of ebastine ($C_{32}H_{39}NO_2$) in 1 tablet

Assay Weigh accurately the mass of not less than 20 Ebastine Tablets, and powder. Weigh accurately a portion of the powder, equivalent to about 20 mg of ebastine ($C_{32}H_{39}NO_2$), add 20 mL of 0.1 mol/L hydrochloric acid TS, and disperse the particles by sonicating. Add 120 mL of methanol, shake for 10 minutes, add methanol to make exactly 200 mL, and centrifuge. Pipet 5 mL of the supernatant liquid, add exactly 5 mL of the internal standard solution, and use this solution as the sample solution. Separately, weigh accurately about 50 mg of ebastine for assay, previously dried at 60°C under reduced pressure with phosphorous (V) oxide for 2 hours, and dissolve in methanol to make exactly 50 mL. Pipet 5 mL of this solution, add 5 mL of 0.1 mol/L hydrochloric acid TS, and add methanol to make exactly 50 mL. Pipet 5 mL of this solution, add exactly 5 mL of the internal standard solution, and use this solution as the standard solution. Perform the test with 10 μL each of the sample solution and standard solution as directed under Liquid Chromatography *<2.01>* according to the following conditions, and calculate the ratios, Q_T and Q_S, of the peak area of ebastine to that of the internal standard.

$$\text{Amount (mg) of ebastine } (C_{32}H_{39}NO_2) = M_S \times Q_T/Q_S \times 2/5$$

M_S: Amount (mg) of ebastine for assay taken

Internal standard solution—A solution of diphenyl in the mobile phase (1 in 40,000).

Operating conditions—

Detector: An ultraviolet absorption photometer (wavelength: 254 nm).

Column: A stainless steel column 4.6 mm in inside diameter and 15 cm in length, packed with octadecylsilanized silica gel for liquid chromatography (5 μm in particle diameter).

Column temperature: A constant temperature of about 40°C.

Mobile phase: Dissolve 7.8 g of sodium dihydrogen phosphate dihydrate in 900 mL of water, adjust to pH 3.0 with diluted phosphoric acid (1 in 5), and add water to make 1000 mL. To 375 mL of this solution add 625 mL of acetonitrile for liquid chromatography, and dissolve 0.72 g of sodium lauryl sulfate in this solution.

Flow rate: Adjust so that the retention time of ebastine is about 9 minutes.

System suitability—

System performance: When the procedure is run with 10 μL of the standard solution under the above operating conditions, the internal standard and ebastine are eluted in this order with the resolution between these peaks being not less than 5.

System repeatability: When the test is repeated 6 times with 10 μL of the standard solution under the above operating conditions, the relative standard deviation of the ratio of the peak area of ebastine to that of the internal standard is not more than 1.0%.

Containers and storage Containers—Tight containers.

Ecabet Sodium Hydrate

エカベトナトリウム水和物

NaO3S CH3 CH3 H3C H • 5H2O H3C CO2H

$C_{20}H_{27}NaO_5S.5H_2O$: 492.56

(1*R*,4a*S*,10a*R*)-1,4a-Dimethyl-7-(1-methylethyl)-6-sodiosulfonato-1,2,3,4,4a,9,10,10a-octahydrophenanthrene-1-carboxylic acid pentahydrate

[219773-47-4]

Ecabet Sodium Hydrate contains not less than 98.5% and not more than 101.5% of ecabet sodium ($C_{20}H_{27}NaO_5S$: 402.48), calculated on the anhydrous basis.

Description Ecabet Sodium Hydrate is white crystals.

It is freely soluble in methanol, and slightly soluble in water and in ethanol (99.5).

It dissolves in sodium hydroxide TS.

Dissolve 1.0 g of Ecabet Sodium Hydrate in 200 mL of water: the pH of the solution is about 3.5.

Identification **(1)** Determine the absorption spectrum of a solution of Ecabet Sodium Hydrate in dilute sodium hydroxide TS (3 in 10,000) as directed under Ultraviolet-visible Spectrophotometry *<2.24>*, and compare the spectrum with the Reference Spectrum: both spectra exhibit similar intensities of absorption at the same wavelengths.

(2) Determine the infrared absorption spectrum of Ecabet Sodium Hydrate as directed in the potassium bromide disk method under Infrared Spectrophotometry *<2.25>*, and compare the spectrum with the Reference Spectrum: both spectra exhibit similar intensities of absorption at the same wave numbers.

(3) Place 1 g of Ecabet Sodium Hydrate in a porcelain crucible, and carbonize. After cooling, add 0.5 mL of nitric acid, heat gradually to incinerate, and dissolve the residue in 10 mL of water: the solution responds to Qualitative Tests *<1.09>* for sodium salt.

Optical rotation *<2.49>* $[\alpha]_D^{20}$: +69 – +76° (0.25 g calculated on the anhydrous basis, methanol, 25 mL, 100 mm).

Purity **(1)** Heavy metals *<1.07>*—Proceed with 2.0 g of Ecabet Sodium Hydrate according to Method 2, and perform the test. Prepare the control solution with 2.0 mL of Standard Lead Solution (not more than 10 ppm).

(2) Related substances—Dissolve 10 mg of Ecabet Sodium Hydrate in 10 mL of the mobile phase, and use this solution as the sample solution. Pipet 2 mL of the sample solution, add the mobile phase to make exactly 20 mL. Pipet 1 mL of this solution, add the mobile phase to make exactly 100 mL, and use this solution as the standard solution. Perform the test with exactly 20 μL each of the sample solution and standard solution as directed under Liquid Chromatography *<2.01>* according to the following conditions. Determine each peak area by the automatic integration method: the area of each peak other than ecabet obtained from the sample solution is not larger than the peak area of ecabet from the standard solution.

Operating conditions—

Detector: An ultraviolet absorption photometer (wavelength: 225 nm).

Column: A stainless steel column 4.6 mm in inside diameter and 15 cm in length, packed with octadecylsilanized silica gel for liquid chromatography (5 μm in particle diameter).

Column temperature: A constant temperature of about 40°C.

Mobile phase: To 0.1 mol/L potassium dihydrogen phosphate TS add phosphoric acid to adjust the pH to 3.0. To 730 mL of this solution add 270 mL of acetonitrile.

Flow rate: Adjust so that the retention time of ecabet is about 8 minutes.

Time span of measurement: About 2 times as long as the retention time of ecabet, beginning after the solvent peak.

System suitability—

System performance: When the procedure is run with 20 μL of the standard solution under the above operating conditions, the number of theoretical plates and the symmetry factor of the peak of ecabet are not less than 5000 and not more than 1.5, respectively.

System repeatability: When the test is repeated 6 times with 20 μL of the standard solution under the above operating conditions, the relative standard deviation of the peak area of ecabet is not more than 2.0%.

Water *<2.48>* 17.3 – 19.2% (0.2 g, volumetric titration, direct titration).

Assay Weigh accurately about 1.2 g of Ecabet Sodium Hydrate, dissolve in 30 mL of methanol, add 30 mL of water, and titrate *<2.50>* with 0.1 mol/L sodium hydroxide VS (indicator: 4 drops of phenolphthalein TS). Perform a blank determination in the same manner, and make any necessary correction.

Each mL of 0.1 mol/L sodium hydroxide VS
= 40.25 mg of $C_{20}H_{27}NaO_5S$

Containers and storage Containers—Well-closed containers.

Ecabet Sodium Granules

エカベトナトリウム顆粒

Ecabet Sodium Granules contain not less than 95.0% and not more than 105.0% of the labeled amount of ecabet sodium hydrate ($C_{20}H_{27}NaO_5S.5H_2O$: 492.56).

Method of preparation Prepare as directed under Granules, with Ecabet Sodium Hydrate.

Identification To a quantity of Ecabet Sodium Granules, equivalent to 50 mg of Ecabet Sodium Hydrate, add 25 mL of dilute sodium hydroxide TS, shake, and filter. Discard the first 10 mL of the filtrate, and to 3 mL of the subsequent filtrate add dilute sodium hydroxide TS to make 20 mL. Determine the absorption spectrum of this solution as directed under Ultraviolet-visible Spectrophotometry *<2.24>*: it exhibits maxima between 269 nm and 273 nm, and between 278 nm and 282 nm.

Uniformity of dosage units *<6.02>* Perform the test according to the following method: Ecabet Sodium Granules in single-dose packages meet the requirement of the Content uniformity test.

Take out the total amount of the content of 1 package of Ecabet Sodium Granules, add 70 mL of dilute sodium hydroxide TS, sonicate for 5 minutes with occasional shaking, add dilute sodium hydroxide TS to make exactly *V* mL so that each mL contains about 10 mg of ecabet sodium hydrate ($C_{20}H_{27}NaO_5S.5H_2O$), and filter. Discard the first 10 mL of the filtrate, pipet 2 mL of the subsequent filtrate, add water to make exactly 50 mL, and use this solution as the sample solution. Separately, weigh accurately about 20 mg of ecabet sodium hydrate for assay (separately, determine the water *<2.48>* in the same manner as Ecabet Sodium Hydrate), dissolve in 2 mL of dilute sodium hydroxide TS, add water to make exactly 50 mL, and use this solution as the standard solution. Determine the absorbances, A_T and A_S, of the sample solution and standard solution at 271 nm as directed under Ultraviolet-visible Spectrophotometry *<2.24>*, using water as the blank.

Amount (mg) of ecabet sodium hydrate ($C_{20}H_{27}NaO_5S.5H_2O$)
$= M_S \times A_T/A_S \times V/2 \times 1.224$

M_S: Amount (mg) of ecabet sodium hydrate for assay taken, calculated on the anhydrous basis

Dissolution *<6.10>* When the test is performed at 50 revolutions per minute according to the Paddle method, using 900 mL of water as the dissolution medium, the dissolution rate in 30 minutes of Ecabet Sodium Granules is not less than 80%.

Start the test with an accurately weighed amount of Ecabet Sodium Granules, equivalent to about 1 g of Ecabet Sodium Hydrate, withdraw not less than 20 mL of the medium at the specified minute after starting the test, and filter through a membrane filter with a pore size not exceeding 0.45 μm. Discard not less than 10 mL of the first filtrate, pipet 2 mL of the subsequent filtrate, add water to make exactly 10 mL, and use this solution as the sample solution. Separately, weigh accurately about 22 mg of ecabet sodium hydrate for assay (separately, determine the water *<2.48>* in the same manner as Ecabet Sodium Hydrate), dissolve in 1 mL of methanol, add water to make exactly 100 mL, and use this solution as the standard solution. Determine the absorbances, A_T and A_S, at 271 nm of the sample solution and standard solution as directed under Ultraviolet-visible Spectrophotometry *<2.24>*, using water as the blank.

Dissolution rate (%) with respect to the labeled amount of ecabet sodium hydrate ($C_{20}H_{27}NaO_5S.5H_2O$)
$= M_S/M_T \times A_T/A_S \times 1/C \times 4500 \times 1.224$

M_S: Amount (mg) of ecabet sodium hydrate for assay taken, calculated on the anhydrous basis
M_T: Amount (g) of Ecabet Sodium Granules taken
C: Labeled amount (mg) of ecabet sodium hydrate ($C_{20}H_{27}NaO_5S.5H_2O$) in 1 g

Assay Weigh accurately an amount of Ecabet Sodium Granules, equivalent to about 30 mg of ecabet sodium hydrate ($C_{20}H_{27}NaO_5S.5H_2O$), add exactly 5 mL of the internal standard solution, add 25 mL of diluted methanol (1 in 2), shake vigorously for 20 minutes, and filter through a membrane filter with a pore size not exceeding 0.45 μm. Discard the first 5 mL of the filtrate, to 3 mL of the subsequent filtrate add the mobile phase to make 50 mL, and use this solution as the sample solution. Separately, weigh accurately about 30 mg of ecabet sodium hydrate for assay (separately, determine the water *<2.48>* in the same manner as Ecabet Sodium Hydrate), add exactly 5 mL of the internal standard solution, and dissolve in dilute methanol (1 in 2) to make 30 mL. To 3 mL of this solution add the mobile phase to make

50 mL, and use this solution as the standard solution. Perform the test with 20 μL each of the sample solution and standard solution as directed under Liquid Chromatography *<2.01>* according to the following conditions, and calculate the ratios, Q_T and Q_S, of the peak area of ecabet to that of the internal standard.

Amount (mg) of ecabet sodium hydrate ($C_{20}H_{27}NaO_5S.5H_2O$)
$$= M_S \times Q_T/Q_S \times 1.224$$

M_S: Amount (mg) of ecabet sodium hydrate for assay taken, calculated on the anhydrous basis

Internal standard solution—A solution of ethyl parahydroxybenzoate in diluted methanol (1 in 2) (3 in 400).

Operating conditions—

Detector: An ultraviolet absorption photometer (wavelength: 225 nm).

Column: A stainless steel column 4.6 mm in inside diameter and 15 cm in length, packed with octadecylsilanized silica gel for liquid chromatography (5 μm in particle diameter).

Column temperature: A constant temperature of about 40°C.

Mobile phase: To 0.1 mol/L potassium dihydrogen phosphate TS add phosphoric acid to adjust the pH to 3.0. To 730 mL of this solution add 270 mL of acetonitrile.

Flow rate: Adjust so that the retention time of ecabet is about 8 minutes.

System suitability—

System performance: When the procedure is run with 20 μL of the standard solution under the above operating conditions, ecabet and the internal standard are eluted in this order with the resolution between these peaks being not less than 6.

System repeatability: When the test is repeated 6 times with 20 μL of the standard solution under the above operating conditions, the relative standard deviation of the ratio of the peak area of ecabet to that of the internal standard is not more than 1.0%.

Containers and storage Containers—Well-closed containers.

Ecothiopate Iodide

エコチオパートヨウ化物

$C_9H_{23}INO_3PS$: 383.23
2-(Diethoxyphosphorylsulfanyl)-*N*,*N*,*N*-trimethylethylaminium iodide
[*513-10-0*]

Ecothiopate Iodide contains not less than 95.0% of ecothiopate iodide ($C_9H_{23}INO_3PS$), calculated on the dried basis.

Description Ecothiopate Iodide occurs as white, crystals or crystalline powder.

It is very soluble in water, freely soluble in methanol, slightly soluble in ethanol (95), and practically insoluble in diethyl ether.

Identification (1) Dissolve 0.1 g of Ecothiopate Iodide in 2 mL of water, and add 1 mL of nitric acid: a brown precipitate is formed. To 1 drop of the turbid solution containing this precipitate add 1 mL of hexane, and shake: a light red color develops in the hexane layer.

(2) Heat the suspension of the precipitate obtained in (1) until it becomes colorless, cool, add 10 mL of water, and use this solution as the sample solution. Two mL of the sample solution responds to Qualitative Tests *<1.09>* (2) for phosphate.

(3) Two mL of the sample solution obtained in (2) responds to Qualitative Tests *<1.09>* for sulfate.

pH *<2.54>* Dissolve 0.1 g of Ecothiopate Iodide in 40 mL of water: the pH of this solution is between 3.0 and 5.0.

Melting point *<2.60>* 116 – 122°C

Purity (1) Clarity and color of solution—Dissolve 0.5 g of Ecothiopate Iodide in 5 mL of water: the solution is clear and colorless.

(2) Heavy metals *<1.07>*—To 1.0 g of Ecothiopate Iodide in a Kjeldahl flask add 5 mL of nitric acid and 2 mL of sulfuric acid, put a small funnel on the mouth of the flask, and heat carefully until white fumes are evolved. After cooling, add 2 mL of nitric acid, and heat. Repeat this procedure twice, add several 2-mL portions of hydrogen peroxide (30), and heat until the solution becomes colorless, and white fumes are evolved. After cooling, transfer the solution together with a small quantity of water to a Nessler tube, and add water to make about 20 mL. Adjust the solution with ammonia solution (28) and ammonia TS to a pH between 3.0 and 3.5, add water to make 50 mL, and use this solution as the test solution. Prepare the control solution as follows: proceed in the same manner as the preparation of the test solution, and add 2.0 mL of Standard Lead Solution and water to make 50 mL (not more than 20 ppm).

(3) Related substances—Dissolve 0.20 g of Ecothiopate Iodide in 10 mL of methanol, and use this solution as the sample solution. Pipet 3 mL of the sample solution, add methanol to make exactly 200 mL, and use this solution as the standard solution. Perform the test with these solutions as directed under Thin-layer Chromatography *<2.03>*. Spot 10 μL each of the sample solution and standard solution on a plate of cellulose for thin-layer chromatography. Develop the plate with a mixture of 1-butanol, water and acetic acid (100) (4:2:1) to a distance of about 10 cm, and air-dry the plate. Spray evenly Dragendorff's TS for spraying on the plate: the spots other than the principal spot obtained from the sample solution are not more intense than the spot from the standard solution.

Loss on drying *<2.41>* Not more than 1.0% (1 g, in vacuum, phosphorus (V) oxide, 50°C, 3 hours).

Assay Weigh accurately about 0.125 g of Ecothiopate Iodide, and dissolve in water to make exactly 100 mL. Pipet 10 mL of of this solution, add 30 mL of water, then add exactly 10 mL of phosphate buffer solution (pH 12), stopper the container, and allow to stand at 25 ± 3°C for 20 minutes. To this solution add quickly 2 mL of acetic acid (100), and titrate *<2.50>* with 0.002 mol/L iodine VS (potentiometric titration). Perform the test in the same manner without phosphate buffer solution (pH 12), and make any necessary correction.

Each mL of 0.002 mol/L iodine VS
= 1.533 mg of $C_9H_{23}INO_3PS$

Containers and storage Containers—Tight containers.
Storage—Light-resistant, and not exceeding 0°C.

Edaravone

エダラボン

$C_{10}H_{10}N_2O$: 174.20
5-Methyl-2-phenyl-2,4-dihydro-3*H*-pyrazol-3-one
[*89-25-8*]

Edaravone, when dried, contains not less than 99.0% and not more than 101.0% of edaravone ($C_{10}H_{10}N_2O$).

Description Edaravone occurs as white to pale yellow-white, crystals or crystalline powder.

It is freely soluble in ethanol (99.5) and in acetic acid (100), and slightly soluble in water.

Identification **(1)** Determine the absorption spectrum of a solution of Edaravone (1 in 200,000) as directed under Ultraviolet-visible Spectrophotometry ⟨*2.24*⟩, and compare the spectrum with the Reference Spectrum: both spectra exhibit similar intensities of absorption at the same wavelengths.

(2) Determine the infrared absorption spectrum of Edaravone, previously dried, as directed in the potassium bromide disk method under Infrared Spectrophotometry ⟨*2.25*⟩, and compare the spectrum with the Reference Spectrum: both spectra exhibit similar intensities of absorption at the same wave numbers.

pH ⟨*2.54*⟩ The pH of a solution obtained by dissolving 20 mg of Edaravone in 20 mL of water is between 4.5 and 5.5.

Melting point ⟨*2.60*⟩ 127 – 131°C

Purity **(1)** Heavy metals ⟨*1.07*⟩—Proceed with 2.0 g of Edaravone according to Method 2, and perform the test. Prepare the control solution with 2.0 mL of Standard Lead Solution (not more than 10 ppm).

(2) Related substances—Dissolve 50 mg of Edaravone in 25 mL of the mobile phase, and use this solution as the sample solution. Pipet 1 mL of the sample solution, and add the mobile phase to make exactly 50 mL. Pipet 1 mL of this solution, add the mobile phase to make exactly 20 mL, and use this solution as the standard solution. Perform the test with exactly 10 μL each of the sample solution and standard solution as directed under Liquid Chromatography ⟨*2.01*⟩ according to the following conditions. Determine each peak area by the automatic integration method: the area of the peak other than edaravone obtained from the sample solution is not larger than the peak area of edaravone from the standard solution.

Operating conditions—

Detector: An ultraviolet absorption photometer (wavelength: 240 nm).

Column: A stainless steel column 4.6 mm in inside diameter and 15 cm in length, packed with octadecylsilanized silica gel for liquid chromatography (5 μm in particle diameter).

Column temperature: A constant temperature of about 40°C.

Mobile phase: A mixture of water, methanol and acetic acid (100) (100:100:1).

Flow rate: Adjust so that the retention time of edaravone is about 4 minutes.

Time span of measurement: About 7 times as long as the retention time of edaravone, beginning after the solvent peak.

System suitability—

System performance: When the procedure is run with 10 μL of the standard solution under the above operating conditions, the number of theoretical plates and the symmetry factor of the peak of edaravone are not less than 1500 and not more than 1.4, respectively.

System repeatability: When the test is repeated 6 times with 10 μL of the standard solution under the above operating conditions, the relative standard deviation of the peak area of edaravone is not more than 2.0%.

Loss on drying ⟨*2.41*⟩ Not more than 0.1% (1 g, in vacuum, phosphorus (V) oxide, 3 hours).

Residue on ignition ⟨*2.44*⟩ Not more than 0.1% (1 g).

Assay Weigh accurately about 0.2 g of Edaravone, previously dried, dissolve in 40 mL of acetic acid (100), and titrate ⟨*2.50*⟩ with 0.1 mol/L perchloric acid VS (potentiometric titration). Perform a blank determination in the same manner, and make any necessary correction.

Each mL of 0.1 mol/L perchloric acid VS
= 17.42 mg of $C_{10}H_{10}N_2O$

Containers and storage Containers—Well-closed containers.

Edaravone Injection

エダラボン注射液

Edaravone Injection is an aqueous injection.

It contains not less than 95.0% and not more than 105.0% of the labeled amount of edaravone ($C_{10}H_{10}N_2O$: 174.20).

Method of preparation Prepare as directed under Injections, with Edaravone.

Description Edaravone Injection occurs as a clear and colorless liquid.

Identification To a volume of Edaravone Injection, equivalent to 1.5 mg of Edaravone, add water to make 50 mL. To 5 mL of this solution add water to make 25 mL. Determine the absorption spectrum of this solution as directed under Ultraviolet-visible Spectrophotometry ⟨*2.24*⟩: it exhibits a maximum between 238 nm and 242 nm.

pH Being specified separately when the drug is granted approval based on the Law.

Purity Related substance—(i) Perform the following test 1). For preparations to which the test 2) can be applied, the test 2) may be performed instead of 1).

1) To a suitable amount of Edaravone Injection add the mobile phase so that each mL contains 0.3 mg of edaravone ($C_{10}H_{10}N_2O$), and use this solution as the sample solution. Pipet 1 mL of the sample solution, and add the mobile phase to make exactly 50 mL. Pipet 1 mL of this solution, add the mobile phase to make exactly 20 mL, and use this solution as the standard solution. Perform the test with exactly 50 μL each of the sample solution and standard solution as directed under Liquid Chromatography ⟨*2.01*⟩ according to the following conditions. Determine each peak area by the automatic integration method: the area of the peak other than

edaravone obtained from the sample solution is not larger than 2 times the peak area of edaravone from the standard solution.

Operating conditions—

Detector, column, column temperature, mobile phase, and flow rate: Proceed as directed in the operating conditions in the Purity (2) under Edaravone.

Time span of measurement: About 7 times as long as the retention time of edaravone, beginning after the peak of edaravone.

System suitability—

System performance: When the procedure is run with 50 μL of the standard solution under the above operating conditions, the number of theoretical plates and the symmetry factor of the peak of edaravone are not less than 1500 and not more than 1.4, respectively.

System repeatability: When the test is repeated 6 times with 50 μL of the standard solution under the above operating conditions, the relative standard deviation of the peak area of edaravone is not more than 2.0%.

2) Use Edaravone Injection as the sample solution. Pipet 1 mL of the sample solution, and add the mobile phase to make exactly 50 mL. Pipet 1 mL of this solution, add the mobile phase to make exactly 20 mL, and use this solution as the standard solution. Perform the test with exactly 10 μL each of the sample solution and standard solution as directed under Liquid Chromatography <*2.01*> according to the following conditions. Determine each peak area by the automatic integration method: the area of the peak other than edaravone obtained from the sample solution is not larger than 2 times the peak area of edaravone from the standard solution.

Operating conditions—

Detector, column, column temperature, mobile phase, and flow rate: Proceed as directed in the operating conditions in the Purity (2) under Edaravone.

Time span of measurement: About 7 times as long as the retention time of edaravone, beginning after the peak of edaravone.

System suitability—

System performance: When the procedure is run with 10 μL of the standard solution under the above operating conditions, the number of theoretical plates and the symmetry factor of the peak of edaravone are not less than 1500 and not more than 1.4, respectively.

System repeatability: When the test is repeated 6 times with 10 μL of the standard solution under the above operating conditions, the relative standard deviation of the peak area of edaravone is not more than 2.0%.

(ii) Perform the following test 1). For preparations to which the test 2) can be applied, the test 2) may be performed instead of 1).

1) To a suitable amount of Edaravone Injection add the mobile phase so that each mL contains 0.3 mg of edaravone ($C_{10}H_{10}N_2O$), and use this solution as the sample solution. Pipet 1 mL of the sample solution, and add the mobile phase to make exactly 50 mL. Pipet 1 mL of this solution, add the mobile phase to make exactly 20 mL, and use this solution as the standard solution. Perform the test with exactly 50 μL each of the sample solution and standard solution as directed under Liquid Chromatography <*2.01*> according to the following conditions. Determine each peak area by the automatic integration method: the area of the peak, having the relative retention time of about 0.3 to edaravone, obtained from the sample solution is not larger than 4 times the peak area of edaravone from the standard solution, the area of the peak, having the relative retention time of about 0.4, obtained from the sample solution is not larger than the peak area of edaravone from the standard solution, and the area of the peak other than edaravone and the peaks mentioned above from the sample solution is not larger than 2 times the peak area of edaravone from the standard solution.

Operating conditions—

Detector, column, and mobile phase: Proceed as directed in the operating conditions in the Assay 1).

Column temperature: A constant temperature of about 40°C.

Flow rate: Adjust so that the retention time of edaravone is about 11 minutes.

Time span of measurement: About 2.5 times as long as the retention time of edaravone, beginning after the solvent peak.

System suitability—

System performance: When the procedure is run with 50 μL of the standard solution under the above operating conditions, the number of theoretical plates and the symmetry factor of the peak of edaravone are not less than 2000 and not more than 1.4, respectively.

System repeatability: When the test is repeated 6 times with 50 μL of the standard solution under the above operating conditions, the relative standard deviation of the peak area of edaravone is not more than 2.0%.

2) Use Edaravone Injection as the sample solution. Pipet 1 mL of the sample solution, and add the mobile phase to make exactly 50 mL. Pipet 1 mL of this solution, add the mobile phase to make exactly 20 mL, and use this solution as the standard solution. Perform the test with exactly 10 μL each of the sample solution and standard solution as directed under Liquid Chromatography <*2.01*> according to the following conditions. Determine each peak area by the automatic integration method: the area of the peak, having the relative retention time of about 0.3 to edaravone, obtained from the sample solution is not larger than 4 times the peak area of edaravone from the standard solution, the area of the peak, having the relative retention time of about 0.4, from the sample solution is not larger than the peak area of edaravone from the standard solution, and the area of the peak other than edaravone and the peaks mentioned above from the sample solution is not larger than 2 times the peak area of edaravone from the standard solution.

Operating conditions—

Detector, column, and mobile phase: Proceed as directed in the operating conditions in the Assay 1).

Column temperature: A constant temperature of about 40°C.

Flow rate: Adjust so that the retention time of edaravone is about 11 minutes.

Time span of measurement: About 2.5 times as long as the retention time of edaravone, beginning after the solvent peak.

System suitability—

System performance: When the procedure is run with 10 μL of the standard solution under the above operating conditions, the number of theoretical plates and the symmetry factor of the peak of edaravone are not less than 2000 and not more than 1.4, respectively.

System repeatability: When the test is repeated 6 times with 10 μL of the standard solution under the above operating conditions, the relative standard deviation of the peak area of edaravone is not more than 2.0%.

Bacterial endotoxins <*4.01*> Less than 5.0 EU/mg.

Extractable volume <*6.05*> It meets the requirement.

Foreign insoluble matter <6.06> Perform the test according to Method 1: it meets the requirement.

Insoluble particulate matter <6.07> It meets the requirement.

Sterility <4.06> Perform the test according to the Membrane filtration method: it meets the requirement.

Assay Perform the following test 1). For preparations to which the test 2) can be applied, the test 2) may be performed instead of 1).

1) To exactly V mL of Edaravone Injection add methanol to make exactly V' mL so that each mL contains about 0.3 mg of edaravone ($C_{10}H_{10}N_2O$). Pipet 2 mL of this solution, add exactly 10 mL of the internal standard solution, then add methanol to make 20 ml, and use this solution as the sample solution. Separately, weigh accurately about 30 mg of edaravone for assay, previously dried in vacuum using phosphorus (V) oxide as a desiccant for 3 hours, and dissolve in methanol to make exactly 100 mL. Pipet 2 mL of this solution, add exactly 10 mL of the internal standard solution, then add methanol to make 20 mL, and use this solution as the standard solution. Perform the test with 10 μL each of the sample solution and standard solution as directed under Liquid Chromatography <2.01> according to the following conditions, and calculate the ratios, Q_T and Q_S, of the peak area of edaravone to that of the internal standard.

$$\text{Amount (mg) of edaravone } (C_{10}H_{10}N_2O) = M_S \times Q_T/Q_S \times V'/V \times 1/100$$

M_S: Amount (mg) of edaravone for assay taken

Internal standard solution—A solution of ethyl aminobenzoate in methanol (1 in 2500).

Operating conditions—

Detector: An ultraviolet absorption photometer (wavelength: 240 nm).

Column: A stainless steel column 4.6 mm in inside diameter and 15 cm in length, packed with octadecylsilanized silica gel for liquid chromatography (5 μm in particle diameter).

Column temperature: A constant temperature of about 50°C.

Mobile phase: A mixture of diluted dilute acetic acid (1 in 100) and methanol (3:1), adjusted to pH 5.5 with diluted ammonia solution (28) (1 in 20).

Flow rate: Adjust so that the retention time of edaravone is about 8 minutes.

System suitability—

System performance: When the procedure is run with 10 μL of the standard solution under the above operating conditions, edaravone and the internal standard are eluted in this order with the resolution between these peaks being not less than 7.

System repeatability: When the test is repeated 6 times with 10 μL of the standard solution under the above operating conditions, the relative standard deviation of the ratio of the peak area of edaravone to that of the internal standard is not more than 1.0%.

2) To an exact volume of Edaravone Injection, equivalent to about 3 mg of edaravone ($C_{10}H_{10}N_2O$) add exactly 10 mL of the internal standard solution, add methanol to make 20 mL, and use this solution as the sample solution. Separately, weigh accurately about 75 mg of edaravone for assay, previously dried in vacuum using phosphorus (V) oxide as a desiccant for 3 hours, and dissolve in methanol to make exactly 50 mL. Pipet 2 mL of this solution, add exactly 10 mL of the internal standard solution, add methanol to make 20 mL, and use this solution as the standard solution. Perform the test with 2 μL each of the sample solution and standard solution as directed under Liquid Chromatography <2.01> according to the following conditions, and calculate the ratios, Q_T and Q_S, of the peak area of edaravone to that of the internal standard.

$$\text{Amount (mg) of edaravone } (C_{10}H_{10}N_2O) = M_S \times Q_T/Q_S \times 1/25$$

M_S: Amount (mg) of edaravone for assay taken

Internal standard solution—A solution of ethyl aminobenzoate in methanol (1 in 500).

Operating conditions—

Proceed as directed in the operating conditions in the Assay 1).

System suitability—

System performance: When the procedure is run with 2 μL of the standard solution under the above operating conditions, edaravone and the internal standard are eluted in this order with the resolution between these peaks being not less than 7.

System repeatability: When the test is repeated 6 times with 2 μL of the standard solution under the above operating conditions, the relative standard deviation of the ratio of the peak area of edaravone to that of the internal standard is not more than 1.0%.

Containers and storage Containers—Hermetic containers. Plastic containers for aqueous injections may be used.

Edrophonium Chloride

エドロホニウム塩化物

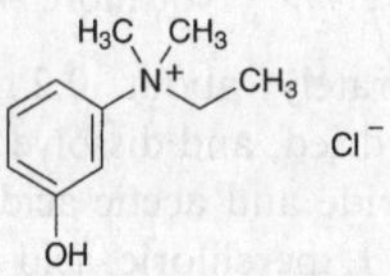

$C_{10}H_{16}ClNO$: 201.69

N-Ethyl-3-hydroxy-*N*,*N*-dimethylanilinium chloride

[116-38-1]

Edrophonium Chloride, when dried, contains not less than 98.0% of edrophonium chloride ($C_{10}H_{16}ClNO$).

Description Edrophonium Chloride occurs as white, crystals or crystalline powder. It is odorless.

It is very soluble in water, freely soluble in ethanol (95) and in acetic acid (100), and practically insoluble in acetic anhydride and in diethyl ether.

It is hygroscopic.

It is gradually colored by light.

Identification **(1)** To 5 mL of a solution of Edrophonium Chloride (1 in 100) add 1 drop of iron (III) chloride TS: a light red-purple color develops.

(2) Determine the absorption spectrum of a solution of Edrophonium Chloride in 0.1 mol/L hydrochloric acid TS (1 in 20,000) as directed under Ultraviolet-visible Spectrophotometry <2.24>, and compare the spectrum with the Reference Spectrum or the spectrum of a solution of Edrophonium Chloride RS prepared in the same manner as the sample solution: both spectra exhibit similar intensities of absorption at the same wavelengths.

(3) A solution of Edrophonium Chloride (1 in 50) responds to Qualitative Tests <1.09> for chloride.

pH <*2.54*> Dissolve 1.0 g of Edrophonium Chloride in 10 mL of water: the pH of this solution is between 3.5 and 5.0.

Melting point <*2.60*> 166 – 171°C (with decomposition).

Purity **(1)** Clarity and color of solution—Dissolve 1.0 g of Edrophonium Chloride in 10 mL of water: the solution is clear and colorless.

(2) Heavy metals <*1.07*>—Proceed with 1.0 g of Edrophonium Chloride according to Method 1, and perform the test. Prepare the control solution with 2.0 mL of Standard Lead Solution (not more than 20 ppm).

(3) Arsenic <*1.11*>—Prepare the test solution with 1.0 g of Edrophonium Chloride according to Method 1, and perform the test (not more than 2 ppm).

(4) Related substances—Dissolve 0.50 g of Edrophonium Chloride in 10 mL of ethanol (95), and use this solution as the sample solution. Pipet 1 mL of the sample solution, and add ethanol (95) to make exactly 100 mL. Pipet 3 mL of this solution, add ethanol (95) to make exactly 10 mL, and use this solution as the standard solution. Perform the test with these solutions as directed under Thin-layer Chromatography <*2.03*>. Spot 10 μL each of the sample solution and standard solution on a plate of silica gel with fluorescent indicator for thin-layer chromatography. Develop the plate with a mixture of methanol, chloroform and ammonia solution (28) (16:4:1) to a distance of about 10 cm, and air-dry the plate. Examine under ultraviolet light (main wavelength: 254 nm): the spots other than the principal spot obtained from the sample solution are not more intense than the spot from the standard solution.

Loss on drying <*2.41*> Not more than 0.20% (1 g, in vacuum, phosphorus (V) oxide, 3 hours).

Residue on ignition <*2.44*> Not more than 0.1% (1 g).

Assay Weigh accurately about 0.2 g of Edrophonium Chloride, previously dried, and dissolve in 100 mL of a mixture of acetic anhydride and acetic acid (100) (7:3). Titrate <*2.50*> with 0.1 mol/L perchloric acid VS (potentiometric titration). Perform a blank determination in the same manner, and make any necessary correction.

Each mL of 0.1 mol/L perchloric acid VS
= 20.17 mg of $C_{10}H_{16}ClNO$

Containers and storage Containers—Tight containers.
Storage—Light-resistant.

Edrophonium Chloride Injection

エドロホニウム塩化物注射液

Edrophonium Chloride Injection is an aqueous injection.

It contains not less than 95.0% and not more than 105.0% of the labeled amount of edrophonium chloride ($C_{10}H_{16}ClNO$: 201.69).

Method of preparation Prepare as directed under Injections, with Edrophonium Chloride.

Description Edrophonium Chloride Injection is a clear and colorless liquid.

Identification **(1)** To a volume of Edrophonium Chloride Injection, equivalent to 0.04 g of Edrophonium Chloride, add 4 mL of barium nitrate TS, shake, and filter. Proceed with the filtrate as directed in the Identification (1) under Edrophonium Chloride.

(2) Determine the absorption spectrum of the sample solution obtained in the Assay as directed under Ultraviolet-visible Spectrophotometry <*2.24*>: it exhibits a maximum between 272 nm and 276 nm.

pH <*2.54*> 6.5 – 8.0

Bacterial endotoxins <*4.01*> Less than 15 EU/mg.

Extractable volume <*6.05*> It meets the requirement.

Foreign insoluble matter <*6.06*> Perform the test according to Method 1: it meets the requirement.

Insoluble particulate matter <*6.07*> It meets the requirement.

Sterility <*4.06*> Perform the test according to the Membrane filtration method: it meets the requirement.

Assay Conduct this procedure without exposure to light, using light-resistant vessels. Measure exactly a volume of Edrophonium Chloride Injection, equivalent to about 50 mg of edrophonium chloride ($C_{10}H_{16}ClNO$), place in a chromatographic column prepared by pouring 10 mL of weakly basic DEAE-bridged dextran anion exchanger (Cl type) (50 to 150 μm in particle diameter) into a chromatographic tube about 2 cm in inside diameter and about 10 cm in length, add 25 mL of water, and elute at the flow rate of 1 to 2 mL per minute. Wash the column with two 25-mL portions of water at the flow rate of 1 to 2 mL per minute. Combine the washings with above effluent solutions, and add water to make exactly 100 mL. Measure exactly 10 mL of this solution, and add 10 mL of phosphate buffer solution (pH 8.0) and 5 g of sodium chloride. Wash this solution with four 20-mL portions of a mixture of diethyl ether and hexane (1:1), collect the water layer, add 0.1 mol/L hydrochloric acid TS to make exactly 100 mL, and use this solution as the sample solution. Separately, weigh accurately about 50 mg of Edrophonium Chloride RS, previously dried in a desiccator (in vacuum, phosphorus (V) oxide) for 3 hours, and dissolve in water to make exactly 100 mL. Measure exactly 10 mL of this solution, and prepare the standard solution in the same manner as the sample solution. Determine the absorbances, A_T and A_S, of the sample solution and standard solution at 273 nm as directed under Ultraviolet-visible Spectrophotometry <*2.24*>.

Amount (mg) of edrophonium chloride ($C_{10}H_{16}ClNO$)
$= M_S \times A_T/A_S$

M_S: Amount (mg) of Edrophonium Chloride RS taken

Containers and storage Containers—Hermetic containers, and colored containers may be used.
Storage—Light-resistant.

Elcatonin

エルカトニン

Ser-Asn-Leu-Ser-Thr—N—Val-Leu-Gly-Lys-Leu-Ser-Gln-Glu-Leu-

His-Lys-Leu-Gln-Thr-Tyr-Pro-Arg-Thr-Asp-Val-Gly-Ala-Gly-Thr-Pro-NH_2

$C_{148}H_{244}N_{42}O_{47}$: 3363.77
[60731-46-6]

Elcatonin contains not less than 5000 Elcatonin Units and not more than 7000 Elcatonin Units per mg of peptide, calculated on the anhydrous and residual acetic acid-free basis.

Description Elcatonin is a white powder.

It is very soluble in water, freely soluble in ethanol (95), and practically insoluble in acetonitrile.

It is hygroscopic.

The pH of a solution of Elcatonin (1 in 500) is between 4.5 and 7.0.

Identification Dissolve 5 mg of Elcatonin in 5 mL of water. Determine the absorption spectrum of the solution as directed under Ultraviolet-visible Spectrophotometry <*2.24*>, and compare the spectrum with the Reference Spectrum: both spectra exhibit similar intensities of absorption at the same wavelengths.

Constituent amino acids Put about 1 mg of Elcatonin in a test tube for hydrolysis, add phenol-hydrochloric acid TS to dissolve, replace the air inside with Nitrogen, seal the tube under reduced pressure, and heat at 110 ± 2°C for 24 hours. After cooling, open the tube, evaporate the hydrolyzate to dryness under reduced pressure, dissolve the residue in about 1 mL of 0.02 mol/L hydrochloric acid TS, and use this solution as the sample solution. Separately, weigh exactly 1.33 mg of L-aspartic acid, 1.19 mg of L-threonine, 1.05 mg of L-serine, 1.47 mg of L-glutamic acid, 1.15 mg of L-proline, 0.75 mg of glycine, 0.89 mg of L-alanine, 1.17 mg of L-valine, 1.89 mg of L-2-aminosuberic acid, 1.31 mg of L-leucine, 1.81 mg of L-tyrosine, 1.83 mg of L-lysine hydrochloride, 2.10 mg of L-histidine hydrochloride monohydrate and 2.11 mg of L-arginine hydrochloride, dissolve them in 0.02 mol/L hydrochloric acid TS to make exactly 50 mL, and use this solution as the standard solution. Perform the test with exactly 10 μL each of the sample solution and standard solution as directed under Liquid Chromatography <*2.01*> according to the following conditions: 14 peaks of amino acids appear on the chromatogram obtained from the sample solution, and their respective molar ratios against alanine are 1.7 – 2.2 for aspartic acid, 3.5 – 4.2 for threonine, 2.4 – 3.0 for serine, 2.7 – 3.2 for glutamic acid, 1.7 – 2.2 for proline, 2.7 – 3.2 for glycine, 1.6 – 2.2 for valine, 0.8 – 1.2 for 2-aminosuberic acid, 4.5 – 5.2 for leucine, 0.7 – 1.2 for tyrosine, 1.7 – 2.2 for lysine, 0.8 – 1.2 for histidine and 0.7 – 1.2 for arginine.

Operating conditions—

Detector: A visible spectrophotometer (wavelength: 440 nm and 570 nm).

Column: A stainless steel column about 4 mm in inside diameter and about 8 cm in length, packed with strongly acidic ion-exchange resin for liquid chromatography composed with a sulfonated styrene-divinylbenzene copolymer (3 μm in particle diameter).

Column temperature: Varied between 50°C and 65°C.

Chemical reaction vessel temperature: A constant temperature of about 130°C.

Color developing time: About 1 minute.

Mobile phase: Buffer solutions A, B, C and D, with sodium ion concentrations of 0.10 mol/L, 0.135 mol/L, 1.26 mol/L and 0.20 mol/L, respectively. The ion concentration of the mobile phase is changed stepwise from 0.10 mol/L to 1.26 mol/L by using these buffer solutions.

Components of buffer solutions

Buffer solution:	A	B	C	D
Citric acid monohydrate	8.85 g	7.72 g	6.10 g	—
Trisodium citrate dihydrate	3.87 g	10.05 g	26.67 g	—
Sodium hydroxide	—	—	2.50 g	8.00 g
Sodium chloride	3.54 g	1.87 g	54.35 g	—
Ethanol (95)	60.0 mL	—	—	60.0 mL
Thiodiglycol	5.0 mL	5.0 mL	—	—
Purified water	a sufficient amount	a sufficient amount	a sufficient amount	a sufficient amount
Total amount	1000 mL	1000 mL	1000 mL	1000 mL

Reaction reagent: Mix 407 g of lithium acetate dihydrate, 245 mL of acetic acid (100) and 801 mL of 1-methoxy-2-propanol, add water to make 2000 mL, stir for about 20 minutes while passing Nitrogen, and use this solution as solution A. Separately, to 1957 mL of 1-methoxy-2-propanol add 77 g of ninhydrin and 0.134 g of sodium borohydride, stir for about 20 minutes while passing Nitrogen, and use this solution as solution B. Mix solution A and solution B before use.

Flow rate of mobile phase: Adjust so that the retention time of arginine is about 75 minutes.

Flow rate of reaction reagent: About 0.2 mL per minute.

Selection of column: Proceed with 10 μL of the standard solution under the above operating conditions. Use a column from which aspartic acid, threonine, serine, glutamic acid, proline, glycine, alanine, valine, 2-aminosuberic acid, leucine, tyrosine, lysine, histidine and arginine are eluted in this order, with complete separation of each peak.

Purity (1) Acetic acid—Weigh accurately 3 – 6 mg of Elcatonin quickly under conditions of 25 ± 2°C and 50 ± 5% relative humidity, add exactly 1 mL of the internal standard solution to dissolve it, and use this solution as the sample solution. Separately, weigh accurately about 0.5 g of acetic acid (100), and add the internal standard solution to make exactly 100 mL. Pipet 5 mL of this solution, add the internal standard solution to make exactly 100 mL, and use this solution as the standard solution. Perform the test with 20 μL each of the sample solution and standard solution as directed under Liquid Chromatography <*2.01*> according to the following conditions, and calculate the ratios, Q_T and Q_S, of the peak area of acetic acid to that of the internal standard: the amount of acetic acid is not more than 7.0%.

$$\text{Amount (\%) of acetic acid } (CH_3COOH) = M_{ST}/M_{SA} \times Q_T/Q_S \times 50$$

M_{ST}: Amount (g) of acetic acid (100) taken
M_{SA}: Amount (mg) of Elcatonin taken

Internal standard solution—A solution of citric acid monohydrate (1 in 4000).

Operating conditions—

Detector: An ultraviolet absorption photometer (wavelength: 210 nm).

Column: A stainless steel column about 4 mm in inside diameter and about 15 cm in length, packed with octadecylsilanized silica gel for liquid chromatography (5 μm in particle diameter).

Column temperature: A constant temperature of about 25°C.

Mobile phase: Dissolve 13.2 g of diammonium hydrogen phosphate in 900 mL of water, add phosphoric acid to adjust the pH to 2.5, and add water to make 1000 mL.

Flow rate: Adjust so that the retention time of acetic acid is about 4 minutes.

Selection of column: Proceed with 20 μL of the standard solution under the above operating conditions. Use a column from which acetic acid and citric acid are eluted in this order with the resolution between their peaks being not less than 2.0.

(2) Related substances—Dissolve 1.0 mg of Elcatonin in 1 mL of a mixture of trifluoroacetic acid TS and acetonitrile (2:1), and use this solution as the sample solution. Take exactly 0.3 mL of the sample solution, add a mixture of trifluoroacetic acid TS and acetonitrile (2:1) to make exactly 10 mL, and use this solution as the standard solution. Perform the test with exactly 10 μL each of the sample solution and standard solution as directed under Liquid Chromatography <*2.01*> according to the following conditions, and determine each peak area by the automatic integration method: each peak area other than elcatonin obtained from the sample solution is not larger than 1/3 times the peak area of elcatonin from the standard solution, and the total of the peak areas other than elcatonin is not larger than the peak area of elcatonin from the standard solution.

Operating conditions—

Detector: An ultraviolet absorption photometer (wavelength: 225 nm).

Column: A stainless steel column about 4 mm in inside diameter and about 15 cm in length, packed with octadecylsilanized silica gel for liquid chromatography (5 μm in particle diameter).

Column temperature: A constant temperature of about 40°C.

Mobile phase: A mixture of trifluoroacetic acid TS and acetonitrile (change the ratio linearly from 85:15 to 55:45 in 30 minutes).

Flow rate: Adjust so that the retention time of elcatonin is about 25 minutes.

Selection of column: Dissolve 2 mg of Elcatonin in 200 μL of trypsin TS for test of elcatonin, warm at 37°C for 1 hour, then add 1 drop of acetic acid (100), and heat at 95°C for 1 minute. To 10 μL of this solution add 50 μL of the sample solution, and mix. Proceed with 10 μL of this solution under the above operating conditions, and calculate the resolution. Use a column such that the resolution between the peak of elcatonin and the peak which appears immediately before the peak of elcatonin is not less than 2.0, and the retention time of elcatonin is about 25 minutes.

Detection sensitivity: Adjust the detection sensitivity so that the peak height of elcatonin from 10 μL of the standard solution is between 50 mm and 200 mm.

Time span of measurement: Continue measurement until the regularly changing base-line of the chromatogram disappears, beginning after the solvent peak.

Water <*2.48*> Weigh accurately 1 - 3 mg of Elcatonin quickly under conditions of 25 ± 2°C and 50 ± 5% relative humidity, and perform the test as directed in Coulometric titration: not more than 8.0%.

Nitrogen content Weigh accurately 0.015 - 0.02 g of Elcatonin quickly under conditions of 25 ± 2°C and 50 ± 5% relative humidity, and perform the test as directed under Nitrogen Determination <*1.08*>: it contains not less than 16.1% and not more than 18.7% of nitrogen (N: 14.01) in the peptide, calculated on the anhydrous and residual acetic acid-free basis.

Assay (i) Animals: Select healthy male Sprague-Dawley rats each weighing between 90 g and 110 g. Keep the rats for not less than 3 days before use, providing an appropriate uniform diet and water.

(ii) Diluent for elcatonin: Dissolve 2.72 g of sodium acetate trihydrate in water to make 200 mL, add 0.2 g of bovine serum albumin, and adjust the pH to 6.0 with acetic acid (100). Prepare before use.

(iii) Standard solution: Dissolve Elcatonin RS in the diluent for elcatonin to make two standard solutions, one to contain exactly 0.075 Unit in each mL which is designated as the high-dose standard solution, S_H, and the other to contain exactly 0.0375 Unit in each mL which is designated as the low-dose standard solution, S_L.

(iv) Sample solution: Weigh accurately 0.5 - 2.0 mg of Elcatonin quickly under conditions of 25 ± 2°C and 50 ± 5% relative humidity, and dissolve in the diluent for elcatonin to make two sample solutions, the high-dose sample solution, T_H, which contains the Units per mL equivalent to S_H and the low-dose sample solution, T_L, which contains the Units per mL equivalent to S_L.

(v) Deproteinizing solution for elcatonin: Dissolve 160 g of trichloroacetic acid and 30.6 g of strontium chloride in water to make 3600 mL.

(vi) Procedure: Divide the animals into 4 equal groups of not less than 10 animals each. Withhold all food, but not water, for 18 to 24 hours before the injections, and withhold water during the assay until the final blood sample is taken. Handle the animals with care in order to avoid undue excitement.

Inject exactly 0.2 mL each of the standard solutions and the sample solutions into the tail vein of each animal as indicated in the following design:

First group	S_H	Third group	T_H
Second group	S_L	Fourth group	T_L

At 1 hour after the injection, take a sufficient blood sample to perform the test from the carotid artery and vein of each animal under ether anesthesia, centrifuge the blood samples to separate serum, and determine the serum calcium according to the following (vii).

(vii) Serum calcium determination: Take exactly 0.3 mL of the serum, add the deproteinizing solution for elcatonin to make exactly 3 mL, mix well, centrifuge, and use the supernatant liquid as the sample solution for calcium determination. Separately, pipet 1 mL of Standard Calcium Solution for Atomic Absorption Spectrophotometry, and add a solution of sodium chloride (17 in 2000) to make exactly 10 mL. Pipet 5 mL of this solution, add the deproteinizing solution for elcatonin to make exactly 50 mL, and use this solution as the standard solution for calcium determination. Determine the absorbances, A_T and A_S, of the sample solution and standard solution as directed under Atomic Absorption Spectrophotometry <*2.23*> according to the following conditions. Determine the absorbance, A_0, of a solution obtained in the same manner used for preparation of the standard solution, but with 1 mL of water instead of the standard solution.

Amount (mg) of calcium (Ca) in 100 mL of the serum
$= 0.01 \times (A_T - A_0)/(A_S - A_0) \times 10 \times 100$

Gas: Combustible gas—Acetylene.
Supporting gas—Air.
Lamp: Calcium hollow-cathode lamp.
Wavelength: 422.7 nm.

(viii) Calculation: Amounts of calcium in 100 mL of the serum obtained with S_H, S_L, T_H and T_L in (vii) are symbolized as y_1, y_2, y_3 and y_4, respectively. Sum up individual y_1, y_2, y_3 and y_4 to obtain Y_1, Y_2, Y_3 and Y_4, respectively.

Units per mg of peptide, calculated on the anhydrous and residual acetic acid-free basis
$= \text{antilog } M \times \text{units per mL of } S_H \times b/a$

$$M = 0.3010 \times Y_a/Y_b$$

$$Y_a = -Y_1 - Y_2 + Y_3 + Y_4$$
$$Y_b = Y_1 - Y_2 + Y_3 - Y_4$$

a: Amount (mg) of Elcatonin taken
× [100 − {water content (%) + acetic acid content (%)}/100]

b: Total volume (mL) of the high-dose sample solution prepared by dissolving Elcatonin with diluent for elcatonin

F' computed by the following equation should be smaller than F shown in the table against n with which s^2 is calculated. Calculate L (P = 0.95) by use of the following equation: L should be not more than 0.20. If F' exceeds F, or if L exceeds 0.20, repeat the test, increasing the number of animals or arranging the assay conditions so that F' is not more than F and L is not more than 0.20.

$$F' = (-Y_1 + Y_2 + Y_3 - Y_4)^2/4fs^2$$

f: Number of the animals of each group

$$s^2 = \{\Sigma y^2 - (Y/f)\}/n$$

Σy^2: The sum of squares of y_1, y_2, y_3 and y_4 in each group
$Y = Y_1^2 + Y_2^2 + Y_3^2 + Y_4^2$
$n = 4(f - 1)$

$$L = 2\sqrt{(C - 1)(CM^2 + 0.09062)}$$
$$C = Y_b^2/(Y_b^2 - 4fs^2t^2)$$

t^2: Value shown in the following table against n used to calculate s^2

n	$t^2 = F$	n	$t^2 = F$	n	$t^2 = F$
1	161.45	13	4.667	25	4.242
2	18.51	14	4.600	26	4.225
3	10.129	15	4.543	27	4.210
4	7.709	16	4.494	28	4.196
5	6.608	17	4.451	29	4.183
6	5.987	18	4.414	30	4.171
7	5.591	19	4.381	40	4.085
8	5.318	20	4.351	60	4.001
9	5.117	21	4.325	120	3.920
10	4.965	22	4.301	∞	3.841
11	4.844	23	4.279		
12	4.747	24	4.260		

Containers and storage Containers—Tight containers.
Storage—Not exceeding 8°C.

Emedastine Fumarate

エメダスチンフマル酸塩

$C_{17}H_{26}N_4O.2C_4H_4O_4$: 534.56
1-(2-Ethoxyethyl)-2-(4-methyl-1,4-diazepan-1-yl)-1*H*-benzimidazole difumarate
[87233-62-3]

Emedastine Fumarate, when dried, contains not less than 98.5% and not more than 101.0% of emedastine fumarate ($C_{17}H_{26}N_4O.2C_4H_4O_4$).

Description Emedastine Fumarate occurs as a white to pale yellow crystalline powder.

It is freely soluble in water, soluble in methanol, sparingly soluble in ethanol (99.5), and slightly soluble in acetic acid (100).

It shows crystal polymorphism.

Identification (1) Dissolve 10 mg of Emedastine Fumarate in 10 mL of water. To 2 mL of this solution add 1 mol/L hydrochloric acid TS to make 100 mL. Determine the absorption spectrum of this solution as directed under Ultraviolet-visible Spectrophotometry <2.24>, and compare the spectrum with the Reference Spectrum: both spectra exhibit similar intensities of absorption at the same wavelengths.

(2) Determine the infrared absorption spectrum of Emedastine Fumarate as directed in the paste method under Infrared Spectrophotometry <2.25>, and compare the spectrum with the Reference Spectrum: both spectra exhibit similar intensities of absorption at the same wave numbers.

(3) Dissolve 30 mg of Emedastine Fumarate in 5 mL of methanol, and use this solution as the sample solution. Separately, dissolve 10 mg of fumaric acid for thin-layer chromatography in 5 mL of methanol, and use this solution as the standard solution. Perform the test with these solutions as directed under Thin-layer Chromatography <2.03>. Spot 5 μL each of the sample solution and standard solution on a plate of silica gel with fluorescent indicator for thin-layer chromatography. Develop the plate with a mixture of isopropyl ether, formic acid and water (90:7:3) to a distance of about 10 cm, and air-dry the plate. Examine under ultraviolet light (main wavelength: 254 nm): the spots other than the spot on the starting point obtained from the sample solution and the spot from the standard solution show the same *Rf* value.

Melting point <2.60> 149 – 152°C

Purity (1) Heavy metals <1.07>—Proceed with 2.0 g of Emedastine Fumarate according to Method 4, and perform the test. Prepare the control solution with 2.0 mL of Standard Lead Solution (not more than 10 ppm).

(2) Related substances—Dissolve 10 mg of Emedastine Fumarate in 10 mL of the mobile phase, and use this solution as the sample solution. Pipet 1 mL of the sample solution, and add the mobile phase to make exactly 100 mL. Pipet 1 mL of this solution, add the mobile phase to make exactly 10 mL, and use this solution as the standard solution. Perform the test with exactly 10 μL each of the sample solu-

tion and standard solution as directed under Liquid Chromatography *<2.01>* according to the following conditions. Determine each peak area by the automatic integration method: the area of the peak other than emedastine and fumaric acid obtained from the sample solution is not larger than the peak area of emedastine from the standard solution.

Operating conditions—

Detector: An ultraviolet absorption photometer (wavelength: 280 nm).

Column: A stainless steel column 6.0 mm in inside diameter and 15 cm in length, packed with octadecylsilanized silica gel for liquid chromatography (5 μm in particle diameter).

Column temperature: A constant temperature of about 40°C.

Mobile phase: Dissolve 3.9 g of sodium dihydrogen phosphate dihydrate and 2.5 g of sodium lauryl sulfate in 1000 mL of water, and adjust to pH 2.4 with phosphoric acid. To 550 mL of this solution add 450 mL of acetonitrile.

Flow rate: Adjust so that the retention time of emedastine is about 18 minutes.

Time span of measurement: About 2 times as long as the retention time of emedastine, beginning after the solvent peak.

System suitability—

System performance: When the procedure is run with 10 μL of the standard solution under the above operating conditions, the number of theoretical plates and the symmetry factor of the peak of emedastine are not less than 10,000 and not more than 1.2, respectively.

System repeatability: When the test is repeated 6 times with 10 μL of the standard solution under the above operating conditions, the relative standard deviation of the peak area of emedastine is not more than 2.0%.

Loss on drying *<2.41>* Not more than 0.5% (0.5 g, 105°C, 3 hours).

Residue on ignition *<2.44>* Not more than 0.1% (1 g).

Assay Weigh accurately about 0.2 g of Emedastine Fumarate, previously dried, dissolve in 80 mL of acetic acid (100), and titrate *<2.50>* with 0.1 mol/L perchloric acid VS (potentiometric titration). Perform a blank determination in the same manner, and make any necessary correction.

Each mL of 0.1 mol/L perchloric acid VS
= 26.73 mg of $C_{17}H_{26}N_4O.2C_4H_4O_4$

Containers and storage Containers—Tight containers.

Emedastine Fumarate Extended-release Capsules

エメダスチンフマル酸塩徐放カプセル

Emedastine Fumarate Extended-release Capsules contain not less than 95.0% and not more than 105.0% of the labeled amount of emedastine fumarate ($C_{17}H_{26}N_4O.2C_4H_4O_4$: 534.56).

Method of preparation Prepare as directed under Capsules, with Emedastine Fumarate.

Identification (1) Powder the content of Emedastine Fumarate Extended-release Capsules. To a portion of the powder, equivalent to 10 mg of Emedastine Fumarate, add 10 mL of water, shake thoroughly, and filter. Spot 1 drop of the filtrate on a filter paper, and spray Dragendorff's TS for spraying on the filter: the spot shows an orange color.

(2) To 2 mL of the filtrate obtained in (1) add 1 mol/L hydrochloric acid TS to make 100 mL. Determine the absorption spectrum of this solution as directed under Ultraviolet-visible Spectrophotometry *<2.24>*: it exhibits maxima between 278 nm and 282 nm, and between 284 nm and 288 nm.

Uniformity of dosage units *<6.02>* Perform the test according to the following method: it meets the requirement of the Content uniformity test.

To 1 tablet of Emedastine Fumarate Extended-release Capsules add 40 mL of the mobile phase, sonicate for 30 minutes while occasional vigorous shaking, and add the mobile phase to make exactly V mL so that each mL contains about 20 μg of emedastine fumarate ($C_{17}H_{26}N_4O.2C_4H_4O_4$). Centrifuge this solution, pipet 10 mL of the supernatant liquid, add exactly 5 mL of the internal standard solution, and use this solution as the sample solution. Then, proceed as directed in the Assay.

Amount (mg) of emedastine fumarate
($C_{17}H_{26}N_4O.2C_4H_4O_4$)
$= M_S \times Q_T/Q_S \times V/1000$

M_S: Amount (mg) of emedastine fumarate for assay taken

*Internal standard solution—*A solution of 4-methyl-benzophenone in the mobile phase (1 in 40,000).

Dissolution Being specified separately when the drug is granted approval based on the Law.

Assay Weigh accurately the content of not less than 20 Emedastine Fumarate Extended-release Capsules, and powder. Weigh accurately a portion of the powder, equivalent to about 2 mg of emedastine fumarate ($C_{17}H_{26}N_4O.2C_4H_4O_4$), add 10 mL of the mobile phase, sonicate for 30 minutes while occasional vigorous shaking, and add the mobile phase to make exactly 100 mL. Centrifuge this solution, pipet 10 mL of the supernatant liquid, add exactly 5 mL of the internal standard solution, and use this solution as the sample solution. Separately, weigh accurately about 20 mg of emedastine fumarate for assay, previously dried at 105°C for 3 hours, and dissolve in the mobile phase to make 100 mL. Pipet 5 mL of this solution, and add the mobile phase to make exactly 50 mL. Then, pipet 10 mL of this solution, add exactly 5 mL of the internal standard solution, and use this solution as the standard solution. Perform the test with 10 μL each of the sample solution and standard solution as directed under Liquid Chromatography *<2.01>*, according to the following conditions, and calculate the ratios, Q_T and Q_S, of the peak area of emedastine to that of the internal standard.

Amount (mg) of emedastine fumarate
($C_{17}H_{26}N_4O.2C_4H_4O_4$)
$= M_S \times Q_T/Q_S \times 1/10$

M_S: Amount (mg) of emedastine fumarate for assay taken

*Internal standard solution—*A solution of 4-methylbenzophenone in the mobile phase (1 in 40,000).

Operating conditions—

Detector: An ultraviolet absorption photometer (wavelength: 280 nm).

Column: A stainless steel column 4.6 mm in inside diameter and 15 cm in length, packed with octadecylsilanized silica gel for liquid chromatography (5 μm in particle diameter).

Column temperature: A constant temperature of about 40°C.

Mobile phase: Dissolve 3.9 g of sodium dihydrogen phosphate dihydrate and 2.5 g of sodium lauryl sulfate in 1000 mL of water, and adjust to pH 2.4 with phosphoric acid. To 500 mL of this solution add 500 mL of acetonitrile.

Flow rate: Adjust so that the retention time of emedastine is about 6 minutes.

System suitability—

System performance: When the procedure is run with 10 μL of the standard solution under the above operating conditions, emedastine and the internal standard are eluted in this order with the resolution between these peaks being not less than 6.

System repeatability: When the test is repeated 6 times with 10 μL of the standard solution under the above operating conditions, the relative standard deviation of the ratio of the peak area of emedastine to that of the internal standard is not more than 1.0%.

Containers and storage Containers—Tight containers.

Emorfazone

エモルファゾン

$C_{11}H_{17}N_3O_3$: 239.27

4-Ethoxy-2-methyl-5-(morpholin-4-yl)pyridazin-3(2*H*)-one

[38957-41-4]

Emorfazone, when dried, contains not less than 98.5% and not more than 101.0% of emorfazone ($C_{11}H_{17}N_3O_3$).

Description Emorfazone occurs as colorless crystals or a white to light yellow crystalline powder.

It is very soluble in ethanol (99.5), and freely soluble in water and in acetic anhydride.

It dissolves in 1 mol/L hydrochloric acid TS.

It gradually turns yellow and decomposes on exposure to light.

Identification **(1)** Dissolve 20 mg of Emorfazone in 2 mL of 1 mol/L hydrochloric acid TS, and add 5 drops of Reinecke's TS: light red floating matters are formed.

(2) Determine the absorption spectrum of a solution of Emorfazone (1 in 100,000) as directed under Ultraviolet-visible Spectrophotometry *<2.24>*, and compare the spectrum with the Reference Spectrum: both spectra exhibit similar intensities of absorption at the same wavelengths.

(3) Determine the infrared absorption spectrum of Emorfazone as directed in the potassium bromide disk method under Infrared Spectrophotometry *<2.25>*, and compare the spectrum with the Reference Spectrum: both spectra exhibit similar intensities of absorption at the same wave numbers.

Melting point *<2.60>* 89 - 92°C (after drying).

Purity **(1)** Chloride *<1.03>*—Perform the test with 1.0 g of Emorfazone. Prepare the control solution with 0.50 mL of 0.01 mol/L hydrochloric acid VS (not more than 0.018%).

(2) Heavy metals *<1.07>*—Proceed with 2.0 g of Emorfazone according to Method 2, and perform the test. Prepare the control solution with 2.0 mL of Standard Lead Solution (not more than 10 ppm).

(3) Arsenic *<1.11>*—Prepare the test solution with 2.0 g of Emorfazone according to Method 3, and perform the test (not more than 1 ppm).

(4) Related substances—Conduct this procedure using light-resistant vessels. Dissolve 0.5 g of Emorfazone in 50 mL of the mobile phase, and use this solution as the sample solution. Pipet 1 mL of the sample solution, add the mobile phase to make exactly 100 mL, and use this solution as the standard solution. Perform the test with exactly 20 μL each of the sample solution and standard solution as directed under Liquid Chromatography *<2.01>* according to the following conditions, and determine each peak area by the automatic integration method: each peak area other than emorfazone obtained from the sample solution is not larger than 1/10 times the peak area of emorfazone from the standard solution, and the total area of the peaks other than emorfazone from the sample solution is not larger than 1/2 times the peak area of emorfazone from the standard solution.

Operating conditions—

Detector: An ultraviolet absorption photometer (wavelength: 254 nm).

Column: A stainless steel column 4.6 mm in inside diameter and 15 cm in length, packed with octadecylsilanized silica gel for liquid chromatography (5 μm in particle diameter).

Column temperature: A constant temperature of about 25°C.

Mobile phase: A mixture of water and methanol (11:10).

Flow rate: Adjust so that the retention time of emorfazone is about 5 minutes.

Time span of measurement: About 2.5 times as long as the retention time of emorfazone, beginning after the solvent peak.

System suitability—

Test for required detectability: Pipet 1 mL of the standard solution, add the mobile phase to make exactly 20 mL. Confirm that the peak area of emorfazone obtained with 20 μL of this solution is equivalent to 3.5 to 6.5% of that with 20 μL of the standard solution.

System performance: Dissolve 16 mg of Emorfazone and 30 mg of 2,4-dinitrophenylhydrazine in 100 mL of methanol. When the procedure is run with 20 μL of this solution under the above operating conditions, emorfazone and 2,4-dinitrophenylhydrazine are eluted in this order with the resolution between these peaks being not less than 2.5.

System repeatability: When the test is repeated 6 times with 20 μL of the standard solution under the above operating conditions, the relative standard deviation of the peak area of emorfazone is not more than 1.0%.

Loss on drying *<2.41>* Not more than 0.5% (1 g, in vacuum, 60°C, 4 hours).

Residue on ignition *<2.44>* Not more than 0.1% (1 g).

Assay Weigh accurately about 0.2 g of Emorfazone, previously dried, dissolve in 60 mL of acetic anhydride, and titrate *<2.50>* with 0.1 mol/L perchloric acid VS (potentiometric titration). Perform a blank determination in the same manner, and make any necessary correction.

Each mL of 0.1 mol/L perchloric acid VS
= 23.93 mg of $C_{11}H_{17}N_3O_3$

Containers and storage Containers—Tight containers.

Storage—Light-resistant.

Emorfazone Tablets

エモルファゾン錠

Emorfazone Tablets contain not less than 95.0% and not more than 105.0% of the labeled amount of emorfazone ($C_{11}H_{17}N_3O_3$: 239.27).

Method of preparation Prepare as directed under Tablets, with Emorfazone.

Identification To a quantity of powdered Emorfazone Tablets, equivalent to 0.1 g of Emorfazone, add 100 mL of water, shake well, and centrifuge. Filter the supernatant liquid, and to 1 mL of the filtrate add water to make 100 mL. Determine the absorption spectrum of this solution as directed under Ultraviolet-visible Spectrophotometry <2.24>: it exhibits maxima between 237 nm and 241 nm, and between 310 nm and 314 nm, and a shoulder between 288 nm and 298 nm.

Uniformity of dosage units <6.02> Perform the test according to the following method: it meets the requirement of the Content uniformity test.

To 1 tablet of Emorfazone Tablets add methanol to make exactly *V* mL so that each mL contains about 4 mg of emorfazone ($C_{11}H_{17}N_3O_3$), and shake well to disintegrate. Centrifuge this solution, pipet 2 mL of the supernatant liquid, add exactly 10 mL of the internal standard solution, add methanol to make 50 mL, and use this solution as the sample solution. Proceed as directed in the Assay.

$$\text{Amount (mg) of emorfazone } (C_{11}H_{17}N_3O_3) = M_S \times Q_T/Q_S \times V/5$$

M_S: Amount (mg) of emorfazone for assay taken

Internal standard solution—A solution of 2,4-dinitrophenylhidrazine in methanol (3 in 2000). Prepare before use.

Dissolution <6.10> When the test is performed at 50 revolutions per minute according to the Paddle method, using 900 mL of water as the dissolution medium, the dissolution rate in 45 minutes of Emorfazone Tablets is not less than 80%.

Start the test with 1 tablet of Emorfazone Tablets, withdraw not less than 20 mL of the medium at the specified minute after starting the test, and filter through a membrane filter with a pore size not exceeding 0.45 μm. Discard not less than 10 mL of the first filtrate, pipet *V* mL of the subsequent filtrate, add water to make exactly *V′* mL so that each mL contains about 11 μg of emorfazone ($C_{11}H_{17}N_3O_3$), and use this solution as the sample solution. Separately, weigh accurately about 28 mg of emorfazone for assay, previously dried in vacuum at 60°C for 4 hours, and dissolve in water to make exactly 100 mL. Pipet 4 mL of this solution, add water to make exactly 100 mL, and use this solution as the standard solution. Determine the absorbances, A_T and A_S, of the sample solution and standard solution at 239 nm as directed under Ultraviolet-visible Spectrophotometry <2.24>.

$$\text{Dissolution rate (\%) with respect to the labeled amount of emorfazone } (C_{11}H_{17}N_3O_3) = M_S \times A_T/A_S \times V'/V \times 1/C \times 36$$

M_S: Amount (mg) of emorfazone for assay taken
C: Labeled amount (mg) of emorfazone ($C_{11}H_{17}N_3O_3$) in 1 tablet

Assay To 10 tablets of Emorfazone Tablets add 200 mL of methanol, shake well to disintegrate, add methanol to make exactly 250 mL, and centrifuge. Pipet a volume of the supernatant liquid, equivalent to about 8 mg of emorfazone ($C_{11}H_{17}N_3O_3$), add exactly 10 mL of the internal standard solution, add methanol to make 50 mL, and use this solution as the sample solution. Separately, weigh accurately about 20 mg of emorfazone for assay, previously dried in vacuum at 60°C for 4 hours, and dissolve in methanol to make exactly 25 mL. Pipet 10 mL of this solution, add exactly 10 mL of the internal standard solution, add methanol to make 50 mL, and use this solution as the standard solution. Perform the test with 20 μL each of the sample solution and standard solution as directed under Liquid Chromatography <2.01> according to the following conditions, and calculate the ratios, Q_T and Q_S, of the peak area of emorfazone to that of the internal standard.

$$\text{Amount (mg) of emorfazone } (C_{11}H_{17}N_3O_3) = M_S \times Q_T/Q_S \times 2/5$$

M_S: Amount (mg) of emorfazone for assay taken

Internal standard solution—A solution of 2,4-dinitrophenylhidrazine in methanol (3 in 2000). Prepare before use.
Operating conditions—

Detector: An ultraviolet absorption photometer (wavelength: 313 nm).

Column: A stainless steel column 4.6 mm in inside diameter and 15 cm in length, packed with octadecylsilanized silica gel for liquid chromatography (5 μm in particle diameter).

Column temperature: A constant temperature of about 25°C.

Mobile phase: A mixture of water and methanol (11:10).

Flow rate: Adjust so that the retention time of emorfazone is about 5 minutes.

System suitability—

System performance: When the procedure is run with 20 μL of the standard solution under the above operating conditions, emorfazone and the internal standard are eluted in this order with the resolution between these peaks being not less than 2.5.

System repeatability: When the test is repeated 6 times with 20 μL of the standard solution under the above operating conditions, the relative standard deviation of the ratio of the peak area of emorfazone to that of the internal standard is not more than 1.0%.

Containers and storage Containers—Tight containers.
Storage—Light-resistant.

Enalapril Maleate

エナラプリルマレイン酸塩

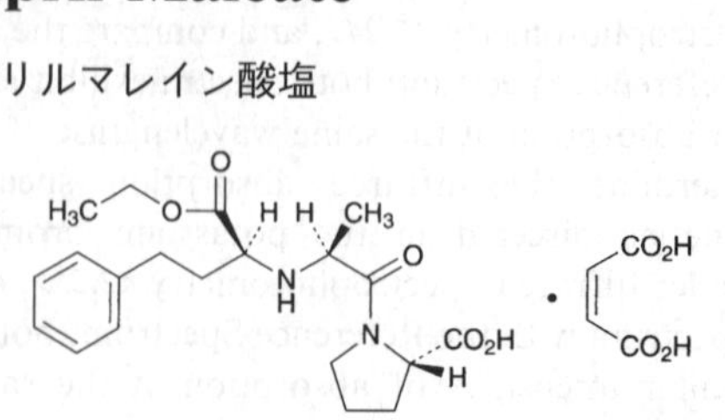

$C_{20}H_{28}N_2O_5.C_4H_4O_4$: 492.52
(2*S*)-1-{(2*S*)-2-[(1*S*)-1-Ethoxycarbonyl-3-phenylpropylamino]propanoyl}pyrrolidine-2-carboxylic acid monomaleate
[*76095-16-4*]

Enalapril Maleate, when dried, contains not less than 98.0% and not more than 102.0% of enalapril maleate ($C_{20}H_{28}N_2O_5.C_4H_4O_4$).

The JP Drugs are to be tested according to the provisions given in the pertinent monographs, General Notices, General Rules for Crude Drugs, General Rules for Preparations, and General Tests for their conformity to the Japanese Pharmacopoeia. (See the General Notices 5.)

Description Enalapril Maleate occurs as white, crystals or crystalline powder.

It is freely soluble in methanol, sparingly soluble in water and in ethanol (99.5), and slightly soluble in acetonitrile.

Melting point: about 145°C (with decomposition).

Identification **(1)** Determine the infrared absorption spectra of Enalapril Maleate as directed in the potassium bromide disc method under Infrared Spectrophotometry ⟨*2.25*⟩, and compare the spectrum with the Reference Spectrum or the spectrum of Enalapril Maleate RS: both spectra exhibit similar intensities of absorption at the same wave numbers.

(2) To 20 mg of Enalapril Maleate add 5 mL of 1 mol/L hydrochloric acid TS, shake, add 5 mL of diethyl ether, and shake for 5 minutes. Take 3 mL of the upper layer, distil off the diethyl ether on a water bath, add 5 mL of water to the residue with shaking, and add 1 drop of potassium permanganate TS: the red color of the test solution immediately disappears.

Optical rotation ⟨*2.49*⟩ $[\alpha]_D^{20}$: $-41.0 - -43.5°$ (after drying, 0.25 g, methanol, 25 mL, 100 mm).

Purity **(1)** Heavy metals ⟨*1.07*⟩—Proceed with 2.0 g of Enalapril Maleate according to Method 2, and perform the test. Prepare the control solution with 2.0 mL of Standard Lead Solution (not more than 10 ppm).

(2) Related substances—Dissolve 30 mg of Enalapril Maleate in 100 mL of a mixture of sodium dihydrogen phosphate TS (pH 2.5) and acetonitrile (19:1), and use this solution as the sample solution. Pipet 1 mL of the sample solution, add the mixture of sodium dihydrogen phosphate TS (pH 2.5) and acetonitrile (19:1) to make exactly 100 mL, and use this solution as the standard solution. Perform the test with exactly 50 μL each of the sample solution and standard solution as directed under Liquid Chromatography ⟨*2.01*⟩ acccording to the following conditions, and determine each peak area of these solutions by the automatic integration method: the area of the peak other than maleic acid and enalapril obtained from the sample solution is not larger than the peak area of enalapril from the standard solution. Furthermore, the total area of the peaks other than maleic acid and enalapril from the sample solution is not larger than 2 times the peak area of enalapril from the standard solution.

Operating conditions—

Detector, column, column temperature, mobile phases, flowing of mobile phase, and flow rate: Proceed as directed in the operating conditions in the Assay.

Time span of measurement: About 2 times as long as the retention time of enalapril, beginning after the peak of maleic acid.

System suitability—

Test for required detectability: Pipet 1 mL of the standard solution, and add a mixture of sodium dihydrogen phosphate TS (pH 2.5) and acetonitrile (19:1) to make exactly 10 mL. Confirm that the peak area of enalapril obtained with 50 μL of this solution is equivalent to 7 to 13% of that with 50 μL of the standard solution.

System performance: When the procedure is run with 50 μL of the standard solution under the above operating conditions, the number of theoretical plates and the symmetry factor of the peak of enalapril are not less than 3000 and not more than 2.0, respectively.

System repeatability: When the test is repeated 6 times with 50 μL of the standard solution under the above operating conditions, the relative standard deviation of the peak area of enalapril is not more than 2.0%.

Loss on drying ⟨*2.41*⟩ Not more than 1.0% (1 g, in vacuum, 60°C, 2 hours).

Residue on ignition ⟨*2.44*⟩ Not more than 0.2% (1 g).

Assay Weigh accurately about 30 mg each of Enalapril Maleate and Enalapril Maleate RS, both previously dried, and dissolve in a mixture of sodium dihydrogen phosphate TS (pH 2.5) and acetonitrile (19:1) to make exactly 100 mL, and use these solutions as the sample solution and standard solution. Perform the test with exactly 50 μL each of the sample solution and standard solution as directed under Liquid Chromatography ⟨*2.01*⟩ according to the following conditions, and determine the peak areas, A_T and A_S, of enalapril in each solution.

Amount (mg) of enalapril maleate ($C_{20}H_{28}N_2O_5.C_4H_4O_4$)
$= M_S \times A_T/A_S$

M_S: Amount (mg) of Enalapril Maleate RS taken

Operating conditions—

Detector: An ultraviolet absorption photometer (wavelength: 215 nm).

Column: A stainless steel column 4.1 mm in inside diameter and 15 cm in length, packed with porous styrene-divinylbenzene copolymer for liquid chromatography (5 μm in particle diameter).

Column temperature: A constant temperature of about 70°C.

Mobile phase A: Dissolve 3.1 g of sodium dihydrogen phosphate dihydrate in 900 mL of water, adjust the pH to 6.8 with a solution of sodium hydroxide (1 in 4), and add water to make 1000 mL. To 950 mL of this solution, add 50 mL of acetonitrile for liquid chromatography.

Mobile phase B: Dissolve 3.1 g of sodium dihydrogen phosphate dihydrate in 900 mL of water, adjust the pH to 6.8 with a solution of sodium hydroxide (1 in 4), and add water to make 1000 mL. To 340 mL of this solution, add 660 mL of acetonitrile for liquid chromatography.

Flowing of mobile phase: Control the concentration gradient by changing the ratio of the mobile phases A and B as follows.

Time after injection of sample (min)	Mobile phase A (vol%)	Mobile phase B (vol%)
0	95	5
0 – 20	95 → 40	5 → 60
20 – 25	40	60

Flow rate: 1.4 mL per minute.

System suitability—

System performance: When the procedure is run with 50 μL of the standard solution under the above operating conditions, the number of theoretical plates and the symmetry factor of the peak of enalapril are not less than 3000 and not more than 2.0, respectively.

System repeatability: When the test is repeated 6 times with 50 μL of the standard solution under the above operating conditions, the relative standard deviation of the peak area of enalapril is not more than 1.0%.

Containers and storage Containers—Well-closed containers.

Enalapril Maleate Tablets

エナラプリルマレイン酸塩錠

Enalapril Maleate Tablets contain not less than 93.0% and not more than 107.0% of the labeled amount of enalapril maleate ($C_{20}H_{28}N_2O_5.C_4H_4O_4$: 492.52).

Method of preparation Prepare as directed under Tablets, with Enalapril Maleate.

Identification To a quantity of powdered Enalapril Maleate Tablets, equivalent to 50 mg of Enalapril Maleate, add 20 mL of methanol, shake, centrifuge, and then use the supernatant liquid as the sample solution. Separately, dissolve 25 mg of enalapril maleate in 10 mL of methanol, and use this solution as the standard solution. Perform the test with these solutions as directed under Thin-Layer Chromatography <*2.03*>. Spot 20 μL each of the sample solution and standard solution on a plate of silica gel with fluorescent indicator for thin-layer chromatography. Develop the plate with a mixture of water, acetone, 1-butanol, acetic acid (100) and toluene (1:1:1:1:1) to a distance of about 10 cm, and air-dry the plate. Examine under ultraviolet light (main wavelength: 254 nm): the *Rf* values of the 2 spots obtained from the sample solution and the 2 spots from the standard solution are equivalent.

Purity Enalaprilat and enalapril diketopiperazine—Use the sample solution obtained in the Assay as the sample solution. Pipet 1 mL of the sample solution, add sodium dihydrogen phosphate TS (pH 2.2) to make exactly 100 mL, and use this solution as the standard solution. Perform the test with exactly 50 μL each of the sample solution and standard solution as directed under Liquid Chromatography <*2.01*> according to the following conditions, and determine each peak area of both solutions by the automatic integration method: the peak area of enalaprilat, having the relative retention time of about 0.5 to enalapril obtained from the sample solution, is not larger than 2 times the peak area of enalapril from the standard solution. Also, the peak area of enalapril diketopiperazine, having the relative retention time of about 1.5 to enalapril, from the sample solution is not larger than the peak area of enalapril from the standard solution.

Operating conditions—

Proceed as directed in the operating conditions in the Assay.

System suitability—

System performance: Proceed as directed in the system suitability in the Assay.

Test for required detectability: Pipet 1 mL of the standard solution, and add sodium dihydrogen phosphate TS (pH 2.2) to make exactly 10 mL. Confirm that the peak area of enalapril obtained with 50 μL of this solution is equivalent to 7 to 13% of that with 50 μL of the standard solution.

System repeatability: When the test is repeated 6 times with 50 μL of the standard solution under the above operating conditions, the relative standard deviation of the peak area of enalapril is not more than 2.0%.

Uniformity of dosage units <*6.02*> Perform the test according to the following method: it meets the requirement of the Content uniformity test.

Take 1 tablet of Enalapril Maleate Tablets, add $V/2$ mL of sodium dihydrogen phosphate TS (pH 2.2), sonicate for 15 minutes, shake for 30 minutes, and add sodium dihydrogen phosphate TS (pH 2.2) to make exactly V mL so that each mL contains about 0.1 mg of enalapril maleate ($C_{20}H_{28}N_2O_5.C_4H_4O_4$). Sonicate this solution for 15 minutes, filter through a membrane filter with a pore size not exceeding 0.45 μm, and use the filtrate as the sample solution. Then, proceed as directed in the Assay.

Amount (mg) of enalapril maleate ($C_{20}H_{28}N_2O_5.C_4H_4O_4$)
$= M_S \times A_T/A_S \times V/200$

M_S: Amount (mg) of Enalapril Maleate RS taken

Dissolution <*6.10*> When the test is performed at 50 revolutions per minute according to the Paddle method, using 900 mL of water as the dissolution medium, the dissolution rates in 15 minutes of a 2.5- and 5-mg tablet and in 30 minutes of a 10-mg tablet are not less than 85%, respectively.

Start the test with 1 tablet of Enalapril Maleate Tablets, withdraw not less than 20 mL of the medium at the specified minute after starting the test, and filter through a membrane filter with a pore size not exceeding 0.45 μm. Discard not less than 10 mL of the first filtrate, pipet V mL of the subsequent filtrate, add water to make exactly V' mL so that each mL contains about 2.8 μg of enalapril maleate ($C_{20}H_{28}N_2O_5.C_4H_4O_4$), and use this solution as the sample solution. Separately, weigh accurately about 14 mg of Enalapril Maleate RS, previously dried in vacuum at 60°C for 2 hours, and dissolve in water to make exactly 500 mL. Pipet 5 mL of this solution, add water to make exactly 50 mL, and use this solution as the standard solution. Perform the test with exactly 50 μL each of the sample solution and standard solution as directed under Liquid Chromatography <*2.01*> according to the following conditions, and determine the peak areas, A_T and A_S, of enalapril in each solution.

Dissolution rate (%) with respect to the labeled amount of enalapril maleate ($C_{20}H_{28}N_2O_5.C_4H_4O_4$)
$= M_S \times A_T/A_S \times V'/V \times 1/C \times 18$

M_S: Amount (mg) of Enalapril Maleate RS taken
C: Labeled amount (mg) of enalapril maleate ($C_{20}H_{28}N_2O_5.C_4H_4O_4$) in 1 tablet

Operating conditions—

Detector, column, column temperature, and flow rate: Proceed as directed in the operating conditions in the Assay.

Mobile phase: Dissolve 1.88 g of sodium dihydrogen phosphate dihydrate in 900 mL of water, adjust the pH to 2.2 with phosphoric acid, and add water to make 1000 mL. To 750 mL of this solution add 250 mL of acetonitrile.

System suitability—

System performance: When the procedure is run with 50 μL of the standard solution under the above operating conditions, the number of theoretical plates and the symmetry factor of the peak of enalapril are not less than 300 and not more than 2.0, respectively.

System repeatability: When the test is repeated 6 times with 50 μL of the standard solution under the above operating conditions, the relative standard deviation of the peak area of enalapril is not more than 2.0%.

Assay Weigh accurately not less than 20 Enalapril Maleate Tablets, and powder. Weigh accurately a portion of the powder, equivalent to about 10 mg of enalapril maleate ($C_{20}H_{28}N_2O_5.C_4H_4O_4$), add 50 mL of sodium dihydrogen phosphate TS (pH 2.2), sonicate for 15 minutes, shake for 30 minutes, and then add sodium dihydrogen phosphate TS (pH 2.2) to make exactly 100 mL. Sonicate this solution for 15 minutes, filter through a membrane filter with a pore size not exceeding 0.45 μm, and use the filtrate as the sample solution. Separately, weigh accurately about 20 mg of Enalapril Maleate RS, previously dried in vacuum at 60°C for 2 hours, dissolve in sodium dihydrogen phosphate TS (pH 2.2) to make exactly 200 mL, and use this solution as the standard solution. Perform the test with exactly 50 μL each of the sample solution and standard solution as directed under Liquid Chromatography *<2.01>* according to the following conditions, and determine the peak areas, A_T and A_S, of enalapril in each solution.

Amount (mg) of enalapril maleate ($C_{20}H_{28}N_2O_5.C_4H_4O_4$)
$= M_S \times A_T/A_S \times 1/2$

M_S: Amount (mg) of Enalapril Maleate RS taken

Operating conditions—

Detector: An ultraviolet absorption photometer (wavelength: 215 nm).

Column: A stainless steel column 4.6 mm in inside diameter and 25 cm in length, packed with octylsilanized silica gel for liquid chromatography (5 μm in particle diameter).

Column temperature: A constant temperature of about 50°C.

Mobile phase: A mixture of sodium dihydrogen phosphate TS (pH 2.2) and acetonitrile (3:1).

Flow rate: Adjust so that the retention time of enalapril is about 5 minutes.

System suitability—

System performance: Heat to fusion about 20 mg of enalapril maleate. After cooling, add 50 mL of acetonitrile, and sonicate to dissolve. To 1 mL of this solution, add the standard solution to make 50 mL, and use this solution as the solution for system suitability test. When the procedure is run with 50 μL of the solution for system suitability test under the above operaring conditions, enalapril and enalapril diketopiperazine, which has a relative retention time of about 1.5 to enalapril, are eluted in this order with the resolution between these peaks being not less than 2.0.

System repeatability: When the test is repeated 6 times with 50 μL of the solution for system suitability test under the above operating conditions, the relative standard deviation of the peak area of enalapril is not more than 1.0%.

Containers and storage Containers—Well-closed containers.

Enflurane

エンフルラン

and enantiomer

$C_3H_2ClF_5O$: 184.49
(2*RS*)-2-Chloro-1-(difluoromethoxy)-1,1,2-trifluoroethane
[13838-16-9]

Description Enflurane is a clear, colorless liquid.

It is slightly soluble in water.

It is miscible with ethanol (95) and with diethyl ether.

It is a volatile, and not an inflammable.

It shows no optical rotation.

Boiling point: 54 – 57°C

Identification **(1)** Take 50 μL of Enflurane, and prepare the test solution as directed to the Oxygen Flask Combustion Method *<1.06>* using 40 mL of water as the absorbing liquid. The test solution responds to Qualitative Tests *<1.09>* for chloride and fluoride.

(2) Determine the infrared absorption spectrum of Enflurane as directed in the liquid film method under Infrared Spectrophotometry *<2.25>*, and compare the spectrum with the Reference Spectrum: both spectra exhibit similar intensities of absorption at the same wave numbers.

Refractive index *<2.45>* n_D^{20}: 1.302 – 1.304

Specific gravity *<2.56>* d_{20}^{20}: 1.520 – 1.540

Purity **(1)** Acidity or alkalinity—To 60 mL of Enflurane add 60 mL of freshly boiled and cooled water, shake for 3 minutes, separate the water later, and use the layer as the sample solution. To 20 mL of the sample solution add one drop of bromocresol purple TS and 0.10 mL of 0.01 mol/L sodium hydroxide VS: the color of the solution is purple. To 20 mL of the sample solution add one drop of bromocresol purple TS and 0.06 mL of 0.01 mol/L hydrochloric acid VS: the color of the solution is yellow.

(2) Chloride *<1.03>*—To 20 g of Enflurane add 20 mL of water, shake well, and separate the water layer. Take 10 mL of the water layer add 6 mL of dilute nitric acid and water to make 50 mL, and perform the test using this solution as the test solution. Prepare the control solution with 0.30 mL of 0.01 mol/L hydrochloric acid VS (not more than 0.001%).

(3) Related substances—Proceed the test with 5 μL of Enflurane as directed under Gas chromatography *<2.02>* according to the following conditions. Determine each peak area other than the peak of air which appears soon after injection of the sample by the automatic integration method, and calculate the amount of each peak by the area percentage method: the amount of the substances other than enflurane is not more than 0.10%.

Operating conditions—

Detector: A thermal conductivity detector.

Column: A column 3 mm in inside diameter and 3 m in length, packed with siliceous earth for gas chromatography, 180 to 250 μm in particle diameter, coated with diethylene glycol succinate ester for gas chromatography in the ratio of 20%.

Column temperature: A constant temperature of about 80°C.

Carrier gas: Helium.

Flow rate: Adjust so that the retention time of enflurane is about 3 minutes.

Time span of measurement: About 3 times as long as the retention time of enflurane.

System suitability—

Test for required detectability: To exactly 1 mL of enflurane add 2-propanol to make exactly 100 mL. To exactly 2 mL of this solution add 2-propanol to make exactly 10 mL, and use this solution as the solution for system suitability test. Pipet 1 mL of the solution for system suitability test, and add 2-propanol to make exactly 10 mL. Confirm that the peak area of enflurane obtained with 5 μL of this solution is equivalent to 7 to 13% of that with 5 μL of the solution for system suitability test.

System performance: Mix 5 mL of Enflurane and 5 mL of 2-propanol. When the procedure is run with 5 μL of this mixture under the above operating conditions, enflurane and 2-propanol are eluted in this order with the resolution between these peaks being not less than 2.0.

System repeatability: When the test is repeated 6 times with 5 μL of the solution for system suitability test under the above operating conditions, the relative standard deviation of the peak area of enflurane is not more than 2.0%.

(4) Nonvolatile residue—Evaporate exactly 65 mL of Enflurane on a water bath to dryness, and dry the residue at 105°C for 1 hour: the residue is not more than 1.0 mg.

Water <*2.48*> Not more than 0.10% (10 g, volumetric titration, direct titration).

Containers and storage Containers—Tight containers.
Storage—Not exceeding 30°C.

Enoxacin Hydrate

エノキサシン水和物

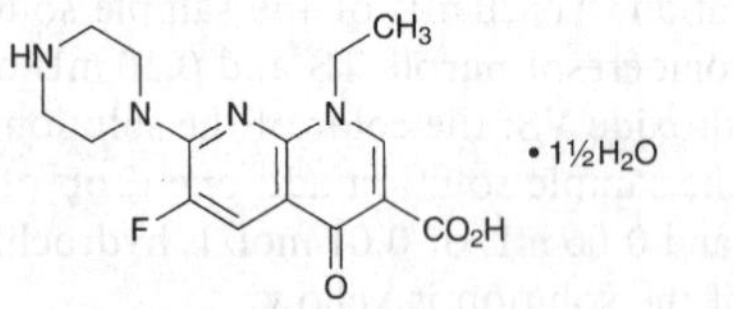

$C_{15}H_{17}FN_4O_3.1\frac{1}{2}H_2O$: 347.34
1-Ethyl-6-fluoro-4-oxo-7-(piperazin-1-yl)-1,4-dihydro-1,8-naphthyridine-3-carboxylic acid sesquihydrate
[84294-96-2]

Enoxacin Hydrate, when dried, contains not less than 98.5% of enoxacin ($C_{15}H_{17}FN_4O_3$: 320.32).

Description Enoxacin Hydrate occurs as white to pale yellow-brown, crystals or crystalline powder.

It is freely soluble in acetic acid (100), slightly soluble in methanol, very slightly soluble in chloroform, and practically insoluble in water, in ethanol (95) and in diethyl ether.

It dissolves in dilute sodium hydroxide TS.

It is gradually colored by light.

Identification **(1)** Place 0.02 g of Enoxacin Hydrate and 0.05 g of sodium in a test tube, and heat gradually to ignition with precaution. After cooling, add 0.5 mL of methanol and then 5 mL of water, and heat to boiling. To this solution add 2 mL of dilute acetic acid, and filter: the filtrate responds to Qualitative Tests <*1.09*> (2) for fluoride.

(2) Dissolve 0.05 g of Enoxacin Hydrate in dilute sodium hydroxide TS to make 100 mL. To 1 mL of the solution add water to make 100 mL. Determine the absorption spectrum of the solution as directed under Ultraviolet-visible Spectrophotometry <*2.24*>, and compare the spectrum with the Reference Spectrum: both spectra exhibit similar intensities of absorption at the same wavelengths.

(3) Determine the infrared absorption spectrum of Enoxacin Hydrate as directed in the potassium bromide disk method under Infrared Spectrophotometry <*2.25*>, and compare the spectrum with the Reference Spectrum: both spectra exhibit similar intensities of absorption at the same wave numbers.

Melting point <*2.60*> 225 – 229°C (after drying).

Purity **(1)** Sulfate <*1.14*>—Dissolve 1.0 g of Enoxacin Hydrate in 50 mL of dilute sodium hydroxide TS, shake with 10 mL of dilute hydrochloric acid, and centrifuge. Filter the supernatant liquid, and to 30 mL of the filtrate add water to make 50 mL. Perform the test using this solution as the test solution. Prepare the control solution as follows: to 0.50 mL of 0.005 mol/L sulfuric acid VS add 25 mL of dilute sodium hydroxide TS, 5 mL of dilute hydrochloric acid TS and water to make 50 mL (not more than 0.048%).

(2) Heavy metals <*1.07*>—Proceed with 1.0 g of Enoxacin Hydrate according to Method 2, and perform the test. Prepare the control solution with 2.0 mL of Standard Lead Solution (not more than 20 ppm).

(3) Arsenic <*1.11*>—Prepare the test solution with 1.0 g of Enoxacin Hydrate according to Method 3, and perform the test (not more than 2 ppm).

(4) Related substances—Dissolve 50 mg of Enoxacin Hydrate in 25 mL of a mixture of chloroform and methanol (7:3), and use this solution as the sample solution. Pipet 1 mL of the sample solution, add a mixture of chloroform and methanol (7:3) to make exactly 200 mL, and use this solution as the standard solution. Perform the test with these solutions as directed under Thin-layer Chromatography <*2.03*>. Spot 5 μL each of the sample solution and standard solution on a plate of silica gel with fluorescent indicator for thin-layer chromatography. Develop the plate with a mixture of 1-butanol, water and acetic acid (100) (3:1:1) to a distance of about 10 cm, and air-dry the plate. Examine under ultraviolet light (main wavelength: 254 nm): the spots other than the principal spot obtained from the sample solution are not more intense than the spot from the standard solution.

Loss on drying <*2.41*> 7.0 – 9.0% (1 g, 105°C, 3 hours).

Residue on ignition <*2.44*> Not more than 0.1% (1 g, platinum crucible).

Assay Weigh accurately about 0.3 g of Enoxacin Hydrate, previously dried, dissolve in 30 mL of acetic acid (100), and titrate <*2.50*> with 0.1 mol/L perchloric acid VS (potentiometric titration). Perform a blank determination in the same manner, and make any necessary correction.

Each mL of 0.1 mol/L perchloric acid VS
= 32.03 mg of $C_{15}H_{17}FN_4O_3$

Containers and storage Containers—Tight containers.
Storage—Light-resistant.

Entacapone

エンタカポン

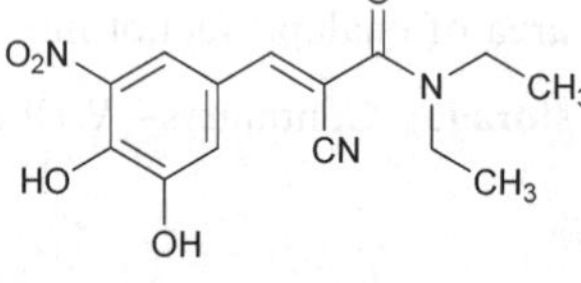

$C_{14}H_{15}N_3O_5$: 305.29
(2*E*)-2-Cyano-3-(3,4-dihydroxy-5-nitrophenyl)-*N*,*N*-diethylprop-2-enamide
[130929-57-6]

Entacapone contains not less than 98.0% and not more than 102.0% of entacapone ($C_{14}H_{15}N_3O_5$), calculated on the dried basis.

Description Entacapone occurs as a yellow to greenish yellow crystalline powder.

It is sparingly soluble in methanol, slightly soluble in ethanol (99.5), and practically insoluble in water.

It shows crystal polymorphism.

Identification **(1)** Dissolve 35 mg of Entacapone in 200 mL of methanol. To 7 mL of this solution add 0.1 mol/L hydrochloric acid TS to make 100 mL. Determine the absorption spectrum of this solution as directed under Ultraviolet-visible Spectrophotometry <*2.24*>, using a solution prepared by adding 0.1 mol/L hydrochloric acid TS to 7 mL of methanol to make 100 mL as the blank, and compare the spectrum with the Reference Spectrum or the spectrum of a solution of Entacapone RS prepared in the same manner as the sample solution: both spectra exhibit similar intensities of absorption at the same wavelengths.

(2) Determine the infrared absorption spectrum of Entacapone as directed in the potassium bromide disk method under Infrared Spectrophotometry <*2.25*>, and compare the spectrum with the Reference Spectrum or the spectrum of Entacapone RS: both spectra exhibit similar intensities of absorption at the same wave numbers.

Purity (1) Heavy metals—Dissolve 1.0 g of Entacapone in 20 mL of a mixture of methanol and *N*,*N*-dimethylformamide (3:1), and use this solution as the sample solution. Separately, weigh exactly 0.400 g of lead (II) nitrate, dissolve in water to make exactly 250 mL. Before use, dilute this solution with water to make exactly 10 times the initial volume, then dilute this solution with water to make exactly 10 times the initial volume. Pipet 1 mL of this solution, add a mixture of methanol and *N*,*N*-dimethylformamide (3:1) to make exactly 20 mL, and use this solution as the standard solution. To each of the sample solution and standard solution add 2 mL of acetate buffer solution (pH 3.5), mix, add 1.2 mL of thioacetamide TS, and mix immediately. Allow them to stand for 2 minutes, filter separately all the amount of each solution through a membrane filter with a pore size of 0.45 μm, wash the membrane filters with not less than 20 mL of methanol, and compare the colors on the membrane filters: the color obtained from the sample solution is not darker than that obtained from the standard solution (not more than 10 ppm).

(2) Halide—Being specified separately when the drug is granted approval based on the Law.

(3) Related substances—Dissolve 50 mg of Entacapone in 50 mL of a mixture of methanol and tetrahydrofuran (7:3), and use this solution as the sample solution. Pipet 5 mL of the sample solution, and add a mixture of methanol and tetrahydrofuran (7:3) to make exactly 50 mL. Pipet 5 mL of this solution, and add a mixture of methanol and tetrahydrofuran (7:3) to make exactly 50 mL. Pipet 1 mL of this solution, add a mixture of methanol and tetrahydrofuran (7:3) to make exactly 10 mL, and use this solution as the standard solution. Perform the test with exactly 10 μL each of the sample solution and standard solution as directed under Liquid Chromatography <*2.01*> according to the following conditions. Determine each peak area by the automatic integration method: the peak area of the related substance A, having the relative retention time of about 0.8 to entacapone, obtained from the sample solution is not larger than 1.5 times the peak area of entacapone from the standard solution, the area of the peak other than entacapone and the peak mentioned above from the sample solution is not larger than the peak area of entacapone from the standard solution, and the total area of the peaks other than entacapone and the related substance A, having the relative retention time of about 0.8 to entacapone, from the sample solution is not larger than 2 times the peak area of entacapone from the standard solution. For the areas of the peaks of related substances B and C, having the relative retention times of about 0.6 and about 1.4 to entacapone, multiply their correction factors, 1.7 and 2.5, respectively.

Operating conditions—

Detector, column, column temperature, mobile phase and flow rate: Proceed as directed in the operating conditions in the Assay.

Time span of measurement: About 2.5 times as long as the retention time of entacapone, beginning after the solvent peak.

System suitability—

System performance: Proceed as directed in the system suitability in the Assay.

Test for required detectability: Pipet 5 mL of the standard solution, add a mixture of methanol and tetrahydrofuran (7:3) to make exactly 10 mL. Confirm that the peak area of entacapone obtained with 10 μL of this solution is equivalent to 35 to 65% of that obtained with 10 μL of the standard solution.

System repeatability: When the test is repeated 5 times with 10 μL of the standard solution under the above operating conditions, the relative standard deviation of the peak area of entacapone is not more than 5%.

Loss on drying <*2.41*> Not more than 0.5% (1 g, in vacuum, 60°C, 3 hours).

Residue on ignition <*2.44*> Not more than 0.1% (1 g).

Assay Weigh accurately about 50 mg each of Entacapone and Entacapone RS (separately determine the loss on drying <*2.41*> under the same conditions as Entacapone), dissolve each in a mixture of methanol and tetrahydrofuran (7:3) to make exactly 50 mL. Pipet 5 mL each of these solutions, add a mixture of methanol and tetrahydrofuran (7:3) to make exactly 50 mL, and use these solutions as the sample solution and the standard solution, respectively. Perform the test with exactly 10 μL each of the sample solution and standard solution as directed under Liquid Chromatography <*2.01*> according to the following conditions, and determine the peak areas, A_T and A_S, of entacapone in each solution.

$$\text{Amount (mg) of entacapone } (C_{14}H_{15}N_3O_5) = M_S \times A_T/A_S$$

M_S: Amount (mg) of Entacapone RS taken, calculated on the dried basis

Operating conditions—

Detector: An ultraviolet absorption photometer (wavelength: 300 nm).

Column: A stainless steel column 4.6 mm in inside diameter and 25 cm in length, packed with phenylated silica gel for liquid chromatography (5 μm in particle diameter).

Column temperature: A constant temperature of about 25°C.

Mobile phase: Dissolve 2.34 g of sodium dihydrogen phosphate dihydrate in water to make 1000 mL, and adjust to pH 2.1 with phosphoric acid. To 540 mL of this solution add 440 mL of methanol and 20 mL of tetrahydrofuran.

Flow rate: 1 mL per minute.

System suitability—

System performance: Dissolve 5 mg of Entacapone Related Substance A for System Suitability RS in a mixture of methanol and tetrahydrofuran (7:3) to make 25 mL. To 1 mL of this solution add a mixture of methanol and tetrahydrofuran (7:3) to make 20 mL, and use this solution as the solution for system suitability test. Separately, to 5 mL of the standard solution add a mixture of methanol and tetrahydrofuran (7:3) to make 50 mL. To 1 mL of this solution and 1 mL of the solution for system suitability test add a mixture of methanol and tetrahydrofuran (7:3) to make 10 mL. When the procedure is run with 10 μL of this solution under the above operating conditions, the related substance A and entacapone are eluted in this order with the resolution between these peaks being not less than 3.

System repeatability: When the test is repeated 6 times with 10 μL of the standard solution under the above operating conditions, the relative standard deviation of the peak

area of entacapone is not more than 1.0%.

Containers and storage Containers—Well-closed containers.

Others

Related substance A:
(2*Z*)-2-Cyano-3-(3,4-dihydroxy-5-nitrophenyl)-*N*,*N*-diethylprop-2-enamide

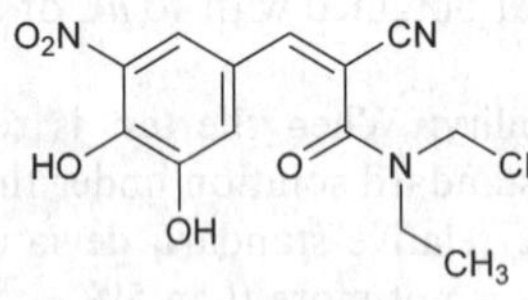

Related substance B:
(2*E*)-2-Cyano-3-(3,4-dihydroxyphenyl)-*N*,*N*-diethylprop-2-enamide

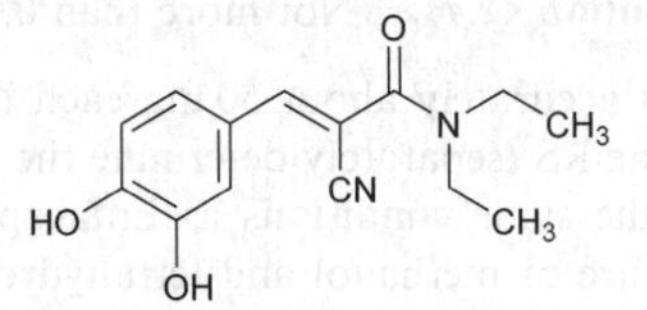

Related substance C:
(2*E*)-3-(3-Bromo-4,5-dihydroxyphenyl)-2-cyano-*N*,*N*-diethylprop-2-enamide

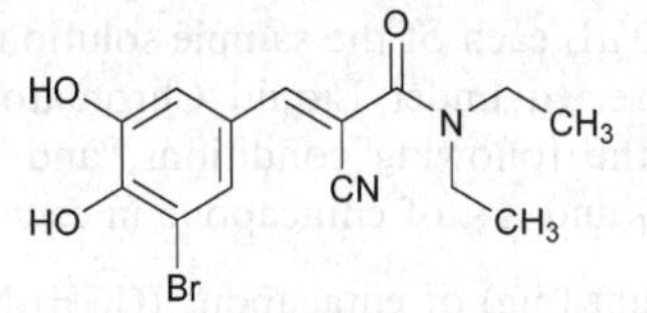

Entacapone Tablets

エンタカポン錠

Entacapone Tablets contain not less than 95.0% and not more than 105.0% of the labeled amount of entacapone ($C_{14}H_{15}N_3O_5$: 305.29).

Method of preparation Prepare as directed under Tablets, with Entacapone.

Identification To 1 mL of the sample solution obtained in the Assay add methanol to make 50 mL. Determine the absorption spectrum of this solution as directed under Ultraviolet-visible Spectrophotometry <*2.24*>: it exhibits a maximum between 301 nm and 305 nm.

Uniformity of dosage units <*6.02*> Perform the Mass variation test, or the Content uniformity test according to the following method: it meets the requirement.

Conduct this procedure using light-resistant vessels. To 1 tablet of Entacapone Tablets add 70 mL of methanol, shake for 5 minutes, and add 60 mL of tetrahydrofuran. Sonicate for 3 minutes, shake for 5 minutes, and add methanol to make exactly 200 mL. Centrifuge this solution, pipet *V* mL of the supernatant liquid, add methanol to make exactly *V′* mL so that each mL contains about 0.5 mg of entacapone ($C_{14}H_{15}N_3O_5$), and use this solution as the sample solution. Then, proceed as directed in the Assay.

Amount (mg) of entacapone ($C_{14}H_{15}N_3O_5$)
$= M_S \times A_T/A_S \times V'/V \times 2$

M_S: Amount (mg) of Entacapone RS taken, calculated on the dried basis

Dissolution <*6.10*> When the test is performed at 50 revolutions per minute according to the Paddle method, using 900 mL of 0.05 mol/L potassium dihydrogen phosphate TS, adjusted to pH 5.5 with sodium hydroxide TS, as the dissolution medium, the dissolution rate in 30 minutes of Entacapone Tablets is not less than 80%.

Start the test with 1 tablet of Entacapone Tablets, withdraw not less than 15 mL of the medium at the specified minute after starting the test, and filter through a membrane filter with a pore size not exceeding 0.45 μm. Discard not less than 5 mL of the first filtrate, pipet *V* mL of the subsequent filtrate, add the dissolution medium to make exactly *V′* mL so that each mL contains about 11 μg of entacapone ($C_{14}H_{15}N_3O_5$), and use this solution as the sample solution. Separately, weigh accurately about 22 mg of Entacapone RS (separately determine the loss on drying <*2.41*> under the same conditions as Entacapone), add 4 mL of methanol, dissolve by sonicating, and add the dissolution medium to make exactly 200 mL. Pipet 5 mL of this solution, add the dissolution medium to make exactly 50 mL, and use this solution as the standard solution. Determine the absorbances, A_T and A_S, of the sample solution and standard solution at 313 nm as directed under Ultraviolet-visible Spectrophotometry <*2.24*>, using the dissolution medium as the blank.

Dissolution rate (%) with respect to the labeled amount of entacapone ($C_{14}H_{15}N_3O_5$)
$= M_S \times A_T/A_S \times V'/V \times 1/C \times 45$

M_S: Amount (mg) of Entacapone RS taken, calculated on the dried basis

C: Labeled amount (mg) of entacapone ($C_{14}H_{15}N_3O_5$) in 1 tablet

Assay Conduct this procedure using light-resistant vessels. Weigh accurately the mass of not less than 20 Entacapone Tablets, and powder. Weigh accurately a portion of the powder, equivalent to about 0.1 g of entacapone ($C_{14}H_{15}N_3O_5$), add 60 mL of tetrahydrofuran, and sonicate for 3 minutes. Add 60 mL of methanol, shake for 5 minutes, and add methanol to make exactly 200 mL. Centrifuge this solution, and use the supernatant liquid as the sample solution. Separately, weigh accurately about 50 mg of Entacapone RS (separately determine the loss on drying <*2.41*> under the same conditions as Entacapone), dissolve in 30 mL of tetrahydrofuran, add methanol to make exactly 100 mL, and use this solution as the standard solution. Perform the test with exactly 10 μL each of the sample solution and standard solution as directed under Liquid Chromatography <*2.01*> according to the following conditions, and determine the peak areas, A_T and A_S, of entacapone in each solution.

Amount (mg) of entacapone ($C_{14}H_{15}N_3O_5$)
$= M_S \times A_T/A_S \times 2$

M_S: Amount (mg) of Entacapone RS taken, calculated on the dried basis

Operating conditions—

Detector: An ultraviolet absorption photometer (wavelength: 300 nm).

Column: A stainless steel column 4.6 mm in inside diameter and 25 cm in length, packed with phenylated silica gel for liquid chromatography (5 μm in particle diameter).

Column temperature: A constant temperature of about 25°C.

Mobile phase: Dissolve 2.34 g of sodium dihydrogen phosphate dihydrate in water, add 2 mL of phosphoric acid, and add water to make 1000 mL. To 540 mL of this solution add 440 mL of methanol and 20 mL of tetrahydrofuran.

Flow rate: Adjust so that the retention time of entacapone is about 12 minutes.

System suitability—

System performance: To 20 mL of the standard solution add a mixture of methanol and tetrahydrofuran (7:3) to make 50 mL, and use this solution as the solution for system suitability test. Separately, dissolve 5 mg of Entacapone Related Substance A for System Suitability RS in a mixture of methanol and tetrahydrofuran (7:3) to make 25 mL. To 15 mL of this solution and 15 mL of the solution for system suitability test add a mixture of methanol and tetrahydrofuran (7:3) to make 100 mL. When the procedure is run with 10 μL of this solution under the above operating conditions, the related substance A, having the relative retention time of about 0.8 to entacapone, and entacapone are eluted in this order with the resolution between these peaks being not less than 2.0.

System repeatability: When the test is repeated 6 times with 10 μL of the standard solution under the above operating conditions, the relative standard deviation of the peak area of entacapone is not more than 1.0%.

Containers and storage Containers—Tight containers.

Others

Related substance A: refer to it described in Entacapone.

Enviomycin Sulfate

エンビオマイシン硫酸塩

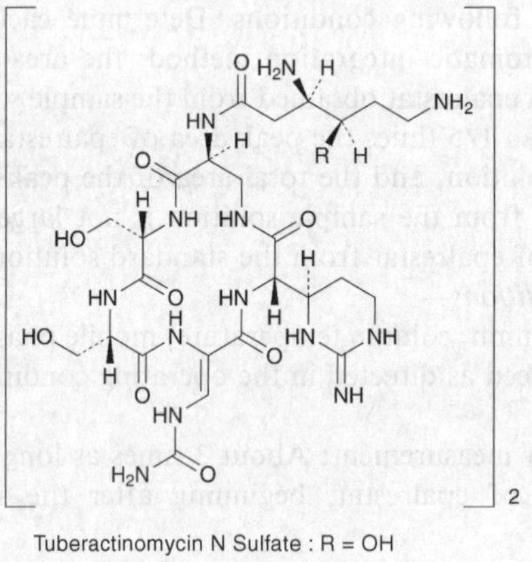

Tuberactinomycin N Sulfate : R = OH
Tuberactinomycin O Sulfate : R = H

Tuberactinomycin N Sulfate
$(C_{25}H_{43}N_{13}O_{10})_2.3H_2SO_4$: 1665.62

Tuberactinomycin O Sulfate
$(C_{25}H_{43}N_{13}O_9)_2.3H_2SO_4$: 1633.62

Tuberactinomycin N Sulfate
(3*R*,4*R*)-*N*-[(3*S*,9*S*,12*S*,15*S*)-9,12-Bis(hydroxymethyl)-3-[(4*R*)-2-iminohexahydropyrimidin-4-yl]-2,5,8,11,14-pentaoxo-6-(*Z*)-ureidomethylene-1,4,7,10,13-pentaazacyclohexadec-15-yl]-3,6-diamino-4-hydroxyhexanamide sesquisulfate
[*33103-22-9*, Tuberactinomycin N]

Tuberactinomycin O Sulfate
(3*S*)-*N*-[(3*S*,9*S*,12*S*,15*S*)-9,12-Bis(hydroxymethyl)-3-[(4*R*)-2-iminohexahydropyrimidin-4-yl]-2,5,8,11,14-pentaoxo-6-(*Z*)-ureidomethylene-1,4,7,10,13-pentaazacyclohexadec-15-yl]-3,6-diaminohexanamide sesquisulfate
[*33137-73-4*, Tuberactinomycin O]

Enviomycin Sulfate is the sulfate of a mixture of peptide substances having antibacterial activity produced by the growth of *Streptomyces griseoverticillatus* var. *tuberacticus*.

It contains not less than 770 μg (potency) and not more than 920 μg (potency) per mg, calculated on the dried basis. The potency of Enviomycin Sulfate is expressed as mass (potency) of tuberactinomycin N ($C_{25}H_{43}N_{13}O_{10}$: 685.69).

Description Enviomycin Sulfate occurs as a white powder.

It is very soluble in water, and practically insoluble in ethanol (99.5).

Identification **(1)** To 5 mL of a solution of Enviomycin Sulfate (1 in 200) add 1.5 mL of sodium hydroxide TS, and add 1 drop of a mixture of 0.01 mol/L citric acid TS and copper (II) sulfate TS (97:3) : a blue-purple color develops.

(2) Determine the absorption spectrum of a solution of Enviomycin Sulfate (1 in 100,000) as directed under Ultraviolet-visible Spectrophotometry <2.24>, and compare the spectrum with the Reference Spectrum: both spectra exhibit similar intensities of absorption at the same wavelengths.

(3) To 2 mL of a solution of Enviomycin Sulfate (1 in 20) add 1 drop of barium chloride TS: a white precipitate is produced.

Optical rotation <2.49> $[\alpha]_D^{20}$: $-16 - -22°$ (0.5 g calculated on the dried basis, water, 50 mL, 100 mm).

pH <2.54> The pH of a solution obtained by dissolving 2.0 g of Enviomycin Sulfate in 20 mL of water is between 5.5 and 7.5.

Content ratio of the active principle Dissolve 0.1 g of Enviomycin Sulfate in water to make 100 mL, and use this solution as the sample solution. Perform the test with 3 μL of the sample solution as directed under Liquid Chromatography <2.01> according to the following conditions, and determine the peak areas, A_{T1} and A_{T2}, of tuberactinomycin N and tuberactinomycin O, having the relative retention time, 1.4 ± 0.4, to tuberactinomycin N, by the automatic integration method: $A_{T2}/(A_{T1} + A_{T2})$ is between 0.090 and 0.150.

Operating conditions—

Detector: An ultraviolet absorption photometer (wavelength: 254 nm).

Column: A stainless steel column 4.6 mm in inside diameter and 15 cm in length, packed with silica gel for liquid chromatography (5 μm in particle diameter).

Column temperature: A constant temperature of about 25°C.

Mobile phase: A mixture of ammonium acetate TS, 1,4-dioxane, tetrahydrofuran, water and ammonia solution (28) (100:75:50:23:2).

Flow rate: Adjust so that the retention time of tuberactinomycin N is about 9 minutes.

System suitability—

System performance: When the procedure is run with 3 μL of the sample solution under the above operating conditions, tuberactinomycin N and tuberactinomycin O are eluted in this order with the resolution between these peaks being not less than 1.5.

System repeatability: When the test is repeated 6 times with 3 μL of the sample solution under the above operating conditions, the relative standard deviation of the peak area of tuberactinomycin N is not more than 2.0%.

Purity **(1)** Clarity and color of solution—Dissolve 1.0 g of Enviomycin Sulfate in 10 mL of water: the solution is clear and colorless.

(2) Heavy metals <*1.07*>—Proceed with 2.0 g of Enviomycin Sulfate according to Method 1, and perform the test. Prepare the control solution with 2.0 mL of Standard Lead Solution (not more than 10 ppm).

(3) Arsenic <*1.11*>—Prepare the test solution with 2.0 g of Enviomycin Sulfate according to Method 1, and perform the test (not more than 1 ppm).

Loss on drying <*2.41*> Not more than 4.0% (0.2 g, in vacuum, phosphorus (V) oxide, 60°C, 3 hours).

Assay Perform the test according to the Cylinder-plate method as directed under Microbial Assay for Antibiotics <*4.02*> according to the following conditions.

(i) Test organism—*Bacillius subtilis* ATCC 6633

(ii) Culture medium—Use the medium i in 1) Medium for test organism [5] under (1) Agar media for seed and base layer.

(iii) Standard solutions—Weigh accurately an amount of Enviomycin Sulfate RS, equivalent to about 20 mg (potency), dissolve in water to make exactly 20 mL, and use this solution as the standard stock solution. Keep the standard stock solution at a temperature not exceeding 5°C and use within 10 days. Take exactly a suitable amount of the standard stock solution before use, add 0.1 mol/L phosphate buffer solution (pH 8.0) to make solutions so that each mL contains 400 μg (potency) and 100 μg (potency), and use these solutions as the high concentration standard solution and the low concentration standard solution, respectively.

(iv) Sample solutions—Weigh accurately an amount of Enviomycin Sulfate, equivalent to about 20 mg (potency), and dissolve in water to make exactly 20 mL. Take exactly a suitable amount of this solution, add 0.1 mol/L phosphate buffer solution (pH 8.0) to make solutions so that each mL contains 400 μg (potency) and 100 μg (potency), and use these solutions as the high concentration sample solution and the low concentration sample solution, respectively.

Containers and storage Containers—Tight containers.

Epalrestat

エパルレスタット

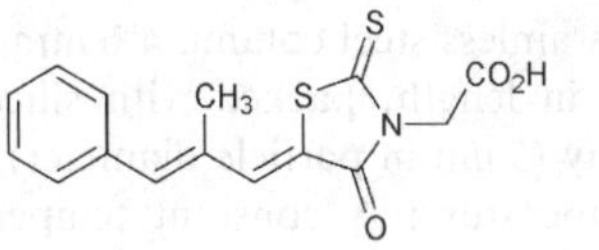

$C_{15}H_{13}NO_3S_2$: 319.40
2-{(5*Z*)-5-[(2*E*)-2-Methyl-3-phenylprop-2-en-1-ylidene]-4-oxo-2-thioxothiazolidin-3-yl}acetic acid
[*82159-09-9*]

Epalrestat, when dried, contains not less than 98.0% and not more than 102.0% of epalrestat ($C_{15}H_{13}NO_3S_2$).

Description Epalrestat occurs as yellow to orange, crystals or crystalline powder.

It is soluble in *N,N*-dimethylformamide, slightly soluble in methanol and in ethanol (99.5), and practically insoluble in water.

It gradually fades the color and decomposes on exposure to light.

It shows crystal polymorphism.

Identification **(1)** Determine the absorption spectrum of a solution of Epalrestat in methanol (1 in 200,000) as directed under Ultraviolet-visible Spectrophotometry <*2.24*>, and compare the spectrum with the Reference Spectrum or the spectrum of a solution of Epalrestat RS prepared in the same manner as the sample solution: both spectra exhibit similar intensities of absorption at the same wavelengths.

(2) Determine the infrared absorption spectrum of Epalrestat as directed in the potassium bromide disk method under Infrared Spectrophotometry <*2.25*>, and compare the spectrum with the Reference Spectrum or the spectrum of Epalrestat RS: both spectra exhibit similar intensities of absorption at the same wave numbers. If any difference appears between the spectra, proceed as follows, using a light-resistant vessel. To 0.1 g of Epalrestat add 40 mL of methanol, dissolve the sample by warming in a water bath, and filter while hot, and cool in ice. Collect the crystals formed, dry, and perform the test.

Melting point <*2.60*> 222 – 227°C

Purity **(1)** Heavy metals <*1.07*>—Proceed with 2.0 g of Epalrestat according to Method 2, and perform the test. Prepare the control solution with 2.0 mL of Standard Lead Solution (not more than 10 ppm).

(2) Related substances—Conduct this procedure using light-resistant vessels. Dissolve about 20 mg of Epalrestat in 8 mL of *N,N*-dimethylformamide, and use this solution as the sample solution. Pipet 1 mL of the sample solution, add *N,N*-dimethylformamide to make exactly 100 mL, and use this solution as the standard solution. Perform the test with exactly 3 μL each of the sample solution and standard solution as directed under Liquid Chromatography <*2.01*> according to the following conditions. Determine each peak area by the automatic integration method: the area of the peak other than epalrestat obtained from the sample solution is not larger than 1/5 times the peak area of epalrestat from the standard solution, and the total area of the peaks other than epalrestat from the sample solution is not larger than the peak area of epalrestat from the standard solution.

Operating conditions—

Detector, column, column temperature, mobile phase, and flow rate: Proceed as directed in the operating conditions in the Assay.

Time span of measurement: About 3 times as long as the retention time of epalrestat, beginning after the solvent peak.

System suitability—

Test for required detectability: Pipet 1 mL of the standard solution, and add *N,N*-dimethylformamide to make exactly 10 mL. Confirm that the peak area of epalrestat obtained with 3 μL of this solution is equivalent to 7 to 13% of that with 3 μL of the standard solution.

System performance: When the procedure is run with 3 μL of the standard solution under the above operating conditions, the number of theoretical plates and the symmetry factor of the peak of epalrestat are not less than 6000 and not more than 1.5, respectively.

System repeatability: When the test is repeated 6 times with 3 μL of the standard solution under the above operating conditions, the relative standard deviation of the peak area of epalrestat is not more than 2.0%.

Loss on drying <*2.41*> Not more than 0.2% (1 g, in vacuum, silica gel, 60°C, 3 hours).

Residue on ignition <*2.44*> Not more than 0.1% (1 g).

Assay Conduct this procedure using light-resistant vessels. Weigh accurately about 20 mg each of Epalrestat and Epalrestat RS, both previously dried, and separately dissolve in 8 mL of *N,N*-dimethylformamide, and add exactly 2 mL of the internal standard solution. To 2 mL each of these solutions add *N,N*-dimethylformamide to make 20 mL, and use these solutions as the sample solution and the standard solution, respectively. Perform the test with 3 μL each of the sample solution and standard solution as directed under Liquid Chromatography <*2.01*> according to the following conditions, and calculate the ratios, Q_T and Q_S, of the peak area of epalrestat to that of the internal standard.

Amount (mg) of epalrestat ($C_{15}H_{13}NO_3S_2$) = $M_S \times Q_T/Q_S$

M_S: Amount (mg) of Epalrestat RS taken

Internal standard solution—A solution of propyl parahydroxybenzoate in *N,N*-dimethylformamide (1 in 100).
Operating conditions—

Detector: An ultraviolet absorption photometer (wavelength: 280 nm).

Column: A stainless steel column 4.6 mm in inside diameter and 15 cm in length, packed with octadecylsilanized silica gel for liquid chromatography (5 μm in particle diameter).

Column temperature: A constant temperature of about 25°C.

Mobile phase: To 0.05 mol/L potassium dihydrogen phosphate TS add 0.05 mol/L disodium hydrogen phosphate TS so that the pH of this mixture is 6.5. To 2 volumes of this mixture add 1 volume of acetonitrile.

Flow rate: Adjust so that the retention time of epalrestat is about 12 minutes.
System suitability—

System performance: When the procedure is run with 3 μL of the standard solution under the above operating conditions, epalrestat and the internal standard are eluted in this order with the resolution between these peaks being not less than 2.0.

System repeatability: When the test is repeated 6 times with 3 μL of the standard solution under the above operating conditions, the relative standard deviation of the ratio of the peak area of epalrestat to that of the internal standard is not more than 1.0%.

Containers and storage Containers—Tight containers.
Storage—Light-resistant.

Epalrestat Tablets

エパルレスタット錠

Epalrestat Tablets contain not less than 95.0% and not more than 105.0% of the labeled amount of epalrestat ($C_{15}H_{13}NO_3S_2$: 319.40).

Method of preparation Prepare as directed under Tablets, with Epalrestat.

Identification **(1)** Powder Epalrestat Tablets. To a portion of the powder, equivalent to 50 mg of Epalrestat, add 100 mL of methanol, shake thoroughly, and filter. To 1 mL of the filtrate add methanol to make 100 mL. Determine the absorption spectrum of this solution as directed under Ultraviolet-visible Spectrophotometry <*2.24*>: it exhibits maxima between 235 nm and 239 nm, between 290 nm and 294 nm, and between 387 nm and 391 nm.

Uniformity of dosage units <*6.02*> Perform the Mass variation test, or the Content uniformity test according to the following method: it meets the requirement.

Conduct this procedure using light-resistant vessels. To 1 tablet of Epalrestat Tablets add exactly 30 mL of *N,N*-dimethylformamide, shake thoroughly to completely disintegrate the tablet, and centrifuge. Pipet 1 mL of the supernatant liquid, and add *N,N*-dimethylformamide to make exactly 100 mL. Pipet *V* mL of this solution, add exactly *V′* mL of *N,N*-dimethylformamide so that each mL contains about 4.2 μg of epalrestat ($C_{15}H_{13}NO_3S_2$), and use this solution as the sample solution. Separately, weigh accurately about 50 mg of Epalrestat RS, previously dried in vacuum at 60°C for 3 hours with silica gel as a desiccant, and dissolve in exactly 30 mL of *N,N*-dimethylformamide. Pipet 1 mL of this solution, add *N,N*-dimethylformamide to make exactly 100 mL. Pipet 5 mL of this solution, add *N,N*-dimethylformamide to make exactly 20 mL, and use this solution as the standard solution. Determine the absorbances, A_T and A_S, at 392 nm of the sample solution and standard solution as directed under Ultraviolet-visible Spectrophotometry <*2.24*>.

$$\text{Amount (mg) of epalrestat } (C_{15}H_{13}NO_3S_2) = M_S \times A_T/A_S \times V'/V \times 1/4$$

M_S: Amount (mg) of Epalrestat RS taken

Dissolution <*6.10*> When the test is performed at 50 revolutions per minute according to the Paddle method, using 900 mL of 2nd fluid for dissolution test as the dissolution medium, the dissolution rate in 45 minutes of Epalrestat Tablets is not less than 70%.

Conduct this procedure using light-resistant vessels. Start the test with 1 tablet of Epalrestat Tablets, withdraw not less than 20 mL of the medium at the specified minute after starting the test, and filter through a membrane filter with a pore size not exceeding 0.45 μm. Discard not less than 10 mL of the first filtrate, pipet *V* mL of the subsequent filtrate, add the dissolution medium to make exactly *V′* mL so that each mL contains about 5.6 μg of epalrestat ($C_{15}H_{13}NO_3S_2$), and use this solution as the sample solution. Separately, weigh accurately about 22 mg of Epalrestat RS, previously dried in vacuum at 60°C for 3 hours with silica gel as a desiccant, dissolve in 10 mL of *N,N*-dimethylformamide, and add the dissolution medium to make exactly 100 mL. Pipet 5 mL of this solution, add the dissolution medium to make exactly 200 mL, and use this solution as the standard solution. Determine the absorbances, A_T and A_S, at 398 nm of the sample solution and standard solution as directed under Ultraviolet-visible Spectrophotometry <*2.24*>, using the dissolution medium as the control.

$$\text{Dissolution rate (\%) with respect to the labeled amount of epalrestat } (C_{15}H_{13}NO_3S_2) = M_S \times A_T/A_S \times V'/V \times 1/C \times 45/2$$

M_S: Amount (mg) of Epalrestat RS taken
C: Labeled amount (mg) of epalrestat ($C_{15}H_{13}NO_3S_2$) in 1 tablet

Assay Conduct this procedure using light-resistant vessels. Weigh accurately the mass of not less than 20 Epalrestat Tablets, and powder. Weigh accurately a portion of the powder, equivalent to about 50 mg of epalrestat ($C_{15}H_{13}NO_3S_2$), add 20 mL of *N,N*-dimethylformamide, add exactly 5 mL of the internal standard solution, shake, and centrifuge. To 2 mL of the supernatant liquid add *N,N*-dimethylformamide to make 20 mL, and use this solution as the sample solution. Separately, weigh accurately about 20 mg of Epalrestat RS, previously dried in vacuum at 60°C for 3 hours with silica gel as a desiccant, dissolve in 8 mL of *N,N*-dimethylformamide, add exactly 2 mL of the internal standard solution, and shake. To 2 mL of this solution add

N,*N*-dimethylformamide to make 20 mL, and use this solution as the standard solution. Then, proceed as directed in the Assay under Epalrestat.

$$\text{Amount (mg) of epalrestat } (C_{15}H_{13}NO_3S_2) = M_S \times Q_T/Q_S \times 5/2$$

M_S: Amount (mg) of Epalrestat RS taken

Internal standard solution—A solution of propyl parahydroxybenzoate in *N*,*N*-dimethylformamide (1 in 100).

Containers and storage Containers—Tight containers.

Eperisone Hydrochloride

エペリゾン塩酸塩

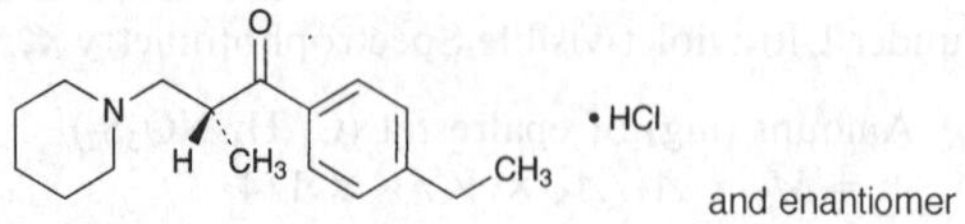

• HCl and enantiomer

$C_{17}H_{25}NO.HCl$: 295.85
(2*RS*)-1-(4-Ethylphenyl)-2-methyl-3-piperidin-1-ylpropan-1-one monohydrochloride
[*56839-43-1*]

Eperisone Hydrochloride contains not less than 98.5% and not more than 101.0% of eperisone hydrochloride ($C_{17}H_{25}NO.HCl$), calculated on the anhydrous basis.

Description Eperisone Hydrochloride occurs as a white crystalline powder.

It is freely soluble in water, in methanol and in acetic acid (100), and soluble in ethanol (99.5).

Melting point: about 167°C (with decomposition).

A solution of Eperisone Hydrochloride in methanol (1 in 100) shows no optical rotation.

Identification (1) Determine the absorption spectrum of a solution of Eperisone Hydrochloride in methanol (1 in 100,000) as directed under Ultraviolet-visible Spectrophotometry *<2.24>*, and compare the spectrum with the Reference Spectrum: both spectra exhibit similar intensities of absorption at the same wavelengths.

(2) Determine the infrared absorption spectrum of Eperisone Hydrochloride as directed in the potassium chloride disk method under Infrared Spectrophotometry *<2.25>*, and compare the spectrum with the Reference Spectrum: both spectra exhibit similar intensities of absorption at the same wave numbers.

(3) A solution of Eperisone Hydrochloride (1 in 50) responds to Qualitative Tests *<1.09>* for chloride.

Purity (1) Heavy metals *<1.07>*—Proceed with 1.0 g of Eperisone Hydrochloride according to Method 1, and perform the test. Prepare the control solution with 2.0 mL of Standard Lead Solution (not more than 20 ppm).

(2) Piperidine hydrochloride—Dissolve 1.0 g of Eperisone Hydrochloride in 20 mL of water, add 2.0 mL of diluted hydrochloric acid (1 in 2), 2.0 mL of a solution of copper (II) sulfate pentahydrate (1 in 20) and 1.5 mL of ammonia solution (28), and use this solution as the sample solution. Separately, to 2.0 mL of a solution of piperidine hydrochloride (1 in 1000) add 18 mL of water, 2.0 mL of diluted hydrochloric acid (1 in 2), 2.0 mL of a solution of copper (II) sulfate pentahydrate (1 in 20) and 1.5 mL of ammonia solution (28), and use this solution as the standard solution. To each of the sample solution and standard solution add 10 mL of a mixture of isopropylether and carbon disulfide (3:1), shake for 30 seconds, allow them to stand for 2 minutes, and compare the color of the upper layer: the color obtained from the sample solution is not more darker than that obtained from the standard solution.

(3) Related substances—Dissolve 0.1 g of Eperisone Hydrochloride in 100 mL of the mobile phase, and use this solution as the sample solution. Pipet 1 mL of the sample solution, add the mobile phase to make exactly 100 mL, and use this solution as the standard solution. Perform the test with exactly 10 μL each of the sample solution and standard solution as directed under Liquid Chromatography *<2.01>* according to the following conditions, and determine each peak area by the automatic integration method: the total area of the peaks other than eperisone obtained from the sample solution is not larger than 1/5 times the peak area of eperisone from the standard solution.

Operating conditions—

Detector: An ultraviolet absorption photometer (wavelength: 254 nm).

Column: A stainless steel column 4.6 mm in inside diameter and 15 cm in length, packed with octadecylsilanized silica gel for liquid chromatography (5 μm in particle diameter).

Column temperature: A constant temperature of about 30°C.

Mobile phase: A mixture of methanol, 0.0375 mol/L sodium 1-decanesulfonate TS and perchloric acid (600:400:1).

Flow rate: Adjust so that the retention time of eperisone is about 17 minutes.

Time span of measurement: About 2 times as long as the retention time of eperisone.

System suitability—

Test for required detectability: Pipet 1 mL of the standard solution, and add the mobile phase to make exactly 10 mL. Confirm that the peak area of eperisone obtained with 10 μL of this solution is equivalent to 7 to 13% of that with 10 μL of the standard solution.

System performance: When the procedure is run with 10 μL of the standard solution under the above operating conditions, the number of theoretical plates and the symmetry factor of the peak of eperisone are not less than 4000 and not more than 2.0, respectively.

System repeatability: When the test is repeated 6 times with 10 μL of the standard solution under the above operating conditions, the relative standard deviation of the peak area of eperisone is not more than 3.0%.

Water *<2.48>* Not more than 0.20% (0.1 g, coulometric titration).

Residue on ignition *<2.44>* Not more than 0.2% (1 g).

Assay Weigh accurately about 0.6 g of Eperisone Hydrochloride, dissolve in 20 mL of acetic acid (100), add 80 mL of acetic anhydride, and titrate *<2.50>* with 0.1 mol/L perchloric acid VS (potentiometric titration). Perform a blank determination in the same manner, and make any necessary correction.

$$\text{Each mL of 0.1 mol/L perchloric acid VS} = 29.59 \text{ mg of } C_{17}H_{25}NO.HCl$$

Containers and storage Containers—Well-closed containers.

Ephedrine Hydrochloride

エフェドリン塩酸塩

$C_{10}H_{15}NO.HCl$: 201.69
(1*R*,2*S*)-2-Methylamino-1-phenylpropan-1-ol monohydrochloride
[*50-98-6*]

Ephedrine Hydrochloride, when dried, contains not less than 99.0% of ephedrine hydrochloride ($C_{10}H_{15}NO.HCl$).

Description Ephedrine Hydrochloride occurs as white, crystals or crystalline powder.

It is freely soluble in water, soluble in ethanol (95), slightly soluble in acetic acid (100), and practically insoluble in acetonitrile and in acetic anhydride.

Identification **(1)** Determine the absorption spectrum of a solution of Ephedrine Hydrochloride (1 in 2000) as directed under Ultraviolet-visible Spectrophotometry *<2.24>*, and compare the spectrum with the Reference Spectrum: both spectra exhibit similar intensities of absorption at the same wavelengths.

(2) Determine the infrared absorption spectrum of Ephedrine Hydrochloride, previously dried, as directed in the potassium chloride disk method under Infrared Spectrophotometry *<2.25>*, and compare the spectrum with the Reference Spectrum: both spectra exhibit similar intensities of absorption at the same wave numbers.

(3) A solution of Ephedrine Hydrochloride (1 in 15) responds to Qualitative Tests *<1.09>* for chloride.

Optical rotation *<2.49>* $[\alpha]_D^{20}$: −33.0 – −36.0° (after drying, 1 g, water, 20 mL, 100 mm).

pH *<2.54>* Dissolve 1.0 g of Ephedrine Hydrochloride in 20 mL of water: the pH of this solution is between 4.5 and 6.5.

Melting point *<2.60>* 218 – 222°C

Purity **(1)** Clarity and color of solution—Dissolve 0.5 g of Ephedrine Hydrochloride in 10 mL of water: the solution is clear and colorless.

(2) Sulfate—Dissolve 0.05 g of Ephedrine Hydrochloride in 40 mL of water, add 1 mL of dilute hydrochloric acid and 1 mL of barium chloride TS, and allow to stand for 10 minutes: no turbidity is produced.

(3) Heavy metals *<1.07>*—Proceed with 1.0 g of Ephedrine Hydrochloride according to Method 2, and perform the test. Prepare the control solution with 1.0 mL of Standard Lead Solution (not more than 10 ppm).

(4) Related substances—Dissolve 0.05 g of Ephedrine Hydrochloride in 50 mL of the mobile phase, and use this solution as the sample solution. Pipet 1 mL of the sample solution, add the mobile phase to make exactly 100 mL, and use this solution as the standard solution. Perform the test with exactly 10 μL each of the sample solution and standard solution as directed under Liquid Chromatography *<2.01>* according to the following conditions, and determine the areas of each peak by the automatic integration method: the total area of the peaks other than ephedrine obtained from the sample solution is not larger than the peak area of ephedrine from the standard solution.

Operating conditions—

Detector: An ultraviolet absorption photometer (wavelength: 210 nm).

Column: A stainless steel column 4.6 mm in inside diameter and 15 cm in length, packed with octadecylsilanized silica gel for liquid chromatography (5 μm in particle diameter).

Column temperature: A constant temperature of about 45°C.

Mobile phase: A mixture of a solution of sodium lauryl sulfate (1 in 128), acetonitrile and phosphoric acid (640:360:1).

Flow rate: Adjust so that the retention time of ephedrine is about 14 minutes.

Time span of measurement: About 3 times as long as the retention time of ephedrine, beginning after the solvent peak.

System suitability—

Test for required detectability: To exactly 1 mL of the standard solution add the mobile phase to make exactly 20 mL. Confirm that the peak area of ephedrine obtained with 10 μL of this solution is equivalent to 4 to 6% of that with 10 μL of the standard solution.

System performance: Dissolve 1 mg of ephedrine hydrochloride for assay and 4 mg of atropine sulfate hydrate in 100 mL of diluted methanol (1 in 2). When the procedure is run with 10 μL of this solution under the above operating conditions, ephedrine and atropine are eluted in this order with the resolution between these peaks being not less than 1.5.

System repeatability: When the test is repeated 6 times with 10 μL of the standard solution under the above operating conditions, the relative standard deviation of the peak areas of ephedrine is not more than 2.0%.

Loss on drying *<2.41>* Not more than 0.5% (1 g, 105°C, 3 hours).

Residue on ignition *<2.44>* Not more than 0.1% (1 g).

Assay Weigh accurately about 0.4 g of Ephedrine Hydrochloride, previously dried, and dissolve in 50 mL of a mixture of acetic anhydride and acetic acid (100) (7:3) by warming. Cool, and titrate *<2.50>* with 0.1 mol/L perchloric acid VS (potentiometric titration). Perform a blank determination in the same manner, and make any necessary correction.

Each mL of 0.1 mol/L perchloric acid VS
= 20.17 mg of $C_{10}H_{15}NO.HCl$

Containers and storage Containers—Well-closed containers.

Ephedrine Hydrochloride Injection

エフェドリン塩酸塩注射液

Ephedrine Hydrochloride Injection is an aqueous injection.

It contains not less than 95.0% and not more than 105.0% of the labeled amount of ephedrine hydrochloride ($C_{10}H_{15}NO.HCl$: 201.69).

Method of preparation Prepare as directed under Injections, with Ephedrine Hydrochloride.

Description Ephedrine Hydrochloride Injection is a clear, colorless liquid.

pH: 4.5 – 6.5

Identification To a volume of Ephedrine Hydrochloride Injection, equivalent to 0.05 g of Ephedrine Hydrochloride, add water to make 100 mL, and determine the absorption spectrum of this solution as directed under Ultraviolet-visible Spectrophotometry <*2.24*>: it exhibits maxima between 249 nm and 253 nm, between 255 nm and 259 nm, and between 261 nm and 265 nm.

Bacterial endotoxins <*4.01*> Less than 7.5 EU/mg.

Extractable volume <*6.05*> It meets the requirement.

Foreign insoluble matter <*6.06*> Perform the test according to Method 1: it meets the requirement.

Insoluble particulate matter <*6.07*> It meets the requirement.

Sterility <*4.06*> Perform the test according to the Membrane filtration method: it meets the requirement.

Assay To an exact volume of Ephedrine Hydrochloride Injection, equivalent to about 40 mg of ephedrine hydrochloride ($C_{10}H_{15}NO.HCl$), add exactly 10 mL of the internal standard solution and water to make 200 mL, and use this solution as the sample solution. Separately, weigh accurately about 40 mg of ephedrine hydrochloride for assay, previously dried at 105°C for 3 hours, add exactly 10 mL of the internal standard solution to dissolve, add water to make 200 mL, and use this solution as the standard solution. Perform the test with 10 μL each of the sample solution and standard solution as directed under Liquid Chromatography <*2.01*> according to the following conditions, and calculate the ratios, Q_T and Q_S, of the peak area of ephedrine to that of the internal standard.

Amount (mg) of ephedrine hydrochloride ($C_{10}H_{15}NO.HCl$)
$= M_S \times Q_T/Q_S$

M_S: Amount (mg) of ephedrine hydrochloride for assay taken

Internal standard solution—A solution of etilefrine hydrochloride (1 in 500).

Operating conditions—

Detector, column, column temperature, mobile phase, and flow rate: Proceed as directed in the operating conditions in the Purity (4) under Ephedrine Hydrochloride.

System suitability—

System performance: When the procedure is run with 10 μL of the standard solution under the above operating conditions, the internal standard and ephedrine are eluted in this order with the resolution between these peaks being not less than 15.

System repeatability: When the test is repeated 6 times with 10 μL of the standard solution under the above operating conditions, the relative standard deviation of the ratios of the peak area of ephedrine to that of the internal standard is not more than 1.0%.

Containers and storage Containers—Hermetic containers.
Storage—Light-resistant.

10% Ephedrine Hydrochloride Powder

エフェドリン塩酸塩散 10%

10% Ephedrine Hydrochloride Powder contains not less than 9.3% and not more than 10.7% of ephedrine hydrochloride ($C_{10}H_{15}NO.HCl$: 201.69).

Method of preparation

Ephedrine Hydrochloride	100 g
Starch, Lactose Hydrate or their mixture	a sufficient quantity
	To make 1000 g

Prepare as directed under Granules or Powders, with the above ingredients.

Identification To 0.5 g of 10% Ephedrine Hydrochloride Powder add 100 mL of water, shake for 20 minutes, and filter. Determine the absorption spectrum of the filtrate as directed under Ultraviolet-visible Spectrophotometry <*2.24*>: it exhibits maxima between 249 nm and 253 nm, between 255 nm and 259 nm, and between 261 nm and 265 nm.

Dissolution <*6.10*> When the test is performed at 50 revolutions per minute according to the Paddle method, using 900 mL of water as the dissolution medium, the dissolution rate in 15 minutes of 10% Ephedrine Hydrochloride Powder is not less than 85%.

Start the test with about 0.25 g of 10% Ephedrine Hydrochloride Powder, accurately weighed, withdraw not less than 20 mL of the medium at the specified minute after starting the test, and filter through a membrane filter with a pore size not exceeding 0.45 μm. Discard not less than 10 mL of the first filtrate, and use the subsequent filtrate as the sample solution. Separately, weigh accurately about 28 mg of ephedrine hydrochloride for assay, previously dried at 105°C for 3 hours, and dissolve in water to make exactly 100 mL. Pipet 5 mL of this solution, add water to make exactly 50 mL, and use this solution as the standard solution. Perform the test with exactly 10 μL each of the sample solution and standard solution as directed under Liquid Chromatography <*2.01*> according to the following conditions, and determine the peak areas, A_T and A_S, of ephedrine in each solution.

Dissolution rate (%) with respect to the labeled amount of ephedrine hydrochloride ($C_{10}H_{15}NO.HCl$)
$= M_S/M_T \times A_T/A_S \times 9/10$

M_S: Amount (mg) of ephedrine hydrochloride for assay taken

M_T: Amount (g) of 10% Ephedrine Hydrochloride Powder taken

Operating conditions—

Detector, column, column temperature, mobile phase, and flow rate: Proceed as directed in the operating conditions in the Purity (4) under Ephedrin Hydrochloride.

System suitability—

System performance: When the procedure is run with 10 μL of the standard solution under the above operating conditions, the number of theoretical plates and the symmetry factor of the peak of ephedrine are not less than 10,000 and not more than 2.0, respectively.

System repeatability: When the test is repeated 6 times with 10 μL of the standard solution under the above operat-

ing conditions, the relative standard deviation of the peak area of ephedrine is not more than 2.0%.

Assay Weigh accurately about 0.4 g of 10% Ephedrine Hydrochloride Powder, add 150 mL of water, and extract by sonicating for 10 minutes with occasional shaking. Shake more for 10 minutes, then add exactly 10 mL of the internal standard solution and water to make 200 mL, centrifuge, and use the supernatant liquid as the sample solution. Separately, weigh accurately about 40 mg of ephedrine hydrochloride for assay, previously dried at 105°C for 3 hours, add exactly 10 mL of the internal standard solution to dissolve, add water to make 200 mL, and use this solution as the standard solution. Perform the test with 10 μL each of the sample solution and standard solution as directed under Liquid Chromatography <2.01> according to the following conditions, and calculate the ratios, Q_T and Q_S, of the peak area of ephedrine to that of the internal standard.

Amount (mg) of ephedrine hydrochloride ($C_{10}H_{15}NO.HCl$)
$= M_S \times Q_T/Q_S$

M_S: Amount (mg) of ephedrine hydrochloride for assay taken

Internal standard solution—A solution of etilefrine hydrochloride (1 in 500).

Operating conditions—

Detector, column, column temperature, mobile phase and flow rate: Perform as directed in the operating conditions in the Purity (4) under Ephedrine Hydrochloride.

System suitability—

System performance: When the procedure is run with 10 μL of the standard solution under the above operating conditions, the internal standard and ephedrine are eluted in this order with the resolution between these peaks being not less than 15.

System repeatability: When the test is repeated 6 times with 10 μL of the standard solution under the above operating conditions, the relative standard deviation of the ratios of the peak area of ephedrine to that of the internal standard is not more than 1.0%.

Containers and storage Containers—Well-closed containers.

Ephedrine Hydrochloride Tablets

エフェドリン塩酸塩錠

Ephedrine Hydrochloride Tablets contain not less than 93.0% and not more than 107.0% of the labeled amount of ephedrine hydrochloride ($C_{10}H_{15}NO.HCl$: 201.69).

Method of preparation Prepare as directed under Tablets, with Ephedrine Hydrochloride.

Identification To an amount of powdered Ephedrine Hydrochloride Tablets, equivalent to 0.05 g of Ephedrine Hydrochloride, add 100 mL of water, shake for 20 minutes, and filter. Determine the absorption spectrum of the filtrate as directed under Ultraviolet-visible Spectrophotometry <2.24>: it exhibits maxima between 249 nm and 253 nm, between 255 nm and 259 nm, and between 261 nm and 265 nm.

Uniformity of dosage units <6.02> Perform the test according to the following method: it meets the requirement of the Content uniformity test.

To 1 tablet of Ephedrine Hydrochloride Tablets add V mL of water so that each mL contains about 0.25 mg of ephedrine hydrochloride ($C_{10}H_{15}NO.HCl$), then add exactly V/4 mL of the internal standard solution, disperse the tablet into small particles by sonicating, then sonicate for a further 10 minutes. Shake this solution for 10 minutes, centrifuge, and use the supernatant liquid as the sample solution. Separately, weigh accurately about 25 mg of ephedrine hydrochloride for assay, previously dried at 105°C for 3 hours, dissolve in water to make exactly 100 mL. Pipet 20 mL of this solution, add exactly 5 mL of the internal standard solution, and use this solution as the standard solution. Then, proceed as directed in the Assay.

Amount (mg) of ephedrine hydrochloride ($C_{10}H_{15}NO.HCl$)
$= M_S \times Q_T/Q_S \times V/100$

M_S: Amount (mg) of ephedrine hydrochloride for assay taken

Internal standard solution—A solution of etilefrine hydrochloride (1 in 2000).

Dissolution <6.10> When the test is performed at 50 revolutions per minute according to the Paddle method, using 900 mL of water as the dissolution medium, the dissolution rate in 30 minutes of Ephedrine Hydrochloride Tablets is not less than 80%.

Start the test with 1 tablet of Ephedrine Hydrochloride Tablets, withdraw not less than 20 mL of the medium at the specified minute after starting the test, and filter through a membrane filter with a pore size not exceeding 0.45 μm. Discard not less than 10 mL of the first filtrate, and use the subsequent filtrate as the sample solution. Separately, weigh accurately about 28 mg of ephedrine hydrochloride for assay, previously dried at 105°C for 3 hours, and dissolve in water to make exactly 100 mL. Pipet 5 mL of this solution, add water to make exactly 50 mL, and use this solution as the standard solution. Perform the test with exactly 10 μL each of the sample solution and standard solution as directed under Liquid Chromatography <2.01> according to the following conditions, and determine the peak areas, A_T and A_S, of ephedrine in each solution.

Dissolution rate (%) with respect to the labeled amount of ephedrine hydrochloride ($C_{10}H_{15}NO.HCl$)
$= M_S \times A_T/A_S \times 1/C \times 90$

M_S: Amount (mg) of ephedrine hydrochloride for assay taken

C: Labeled amount (mg) of ephedrine hydrochloride ($C_{10}H_{15}NO.HCl$) in 1 tablet

Operating conditions—

Detector, column, column temperature, mobile phase and flow rate: Proceed as directed in the operating conditions in the Purity (4) under Ephedrine Hydrochloride.

System suitability—

System performance: When the procedure is run with 10 μL of the standard solution under the above operating conditions, the number of theoretical plates and the symmetry factor of the peak of ephedrine are not less than 10,000 and not more than 2.0, respectively.

System repeatability: When the test is repeated 6 times with 10 μL of the standard solution under the above operating conditions, the relative standard deviation of the peak area of ephedrine is not more than 2.0%.

Assay Weigh accurately not less than 20 tablets of Ephedrine Hydrochloride Tablets, and powder. Weigh accurately an amount of the powder, equivalent to about 40 mg of ephedrine hydrochloride ($C_{10}H_{15}NO.HCl$), add 150 mL of water, and extract by sonicating for 10 minutes with occasional shaking. Shake more for 10 minutes, then add exactly 10 mL of the internal standard solution and water to make 200 mL, centrifuge, and use the supernatant liquid as the sample solution. Separately, weigh accurately about 40 mg of ephedrine hydrochloride for assay, previously dried at 105 °C for 3 hours, add exactly 10 mL of the internal standard solution to dissolve, add water to make 200 mL, and use this solution as the standard solution. Perform the test with 10 μL each of the sample solution and standard solution as directed under Liquid Chromatography *<2.01>* according to the following conditions, and calculate the ratios, Q_T and Q_S, of the peak area of ephedrine to that of the internal standard.

Amount (mg) of ephedrine hydrochloride ($C_{10}H_{15}NO.HCl$)
$= M_S \times Q_T/Q_S$

M_S: Amount (mg) of ephedrine hydrochloride for assay taken

Internal standard solution—A solution of etilefrine hydrochloride (1 in 500).
Operating conditions—

Detector, column, column temperature, mobile phase, and flow rate: Proceed as directed in the operating conditions in the Purity (4) under Ephedrine Hydrochloride.
System suitability—

System performance: When the procedure is run with 10 μL of the standard solution under the above operating conditions, the internal standard and ephedrine are eluted in this order with the resolution between these peaks being not less than 15.

System repeatability: When the test is repeated 6 times with 10 μL of the standard solution under the above operating conditions, the relative standard deviation of the ratios of the peak area of ephedrine to that of the internal standard is not more than 1.0%.

Containers and storage Containers—Well-closed containers.

Epirizole

エピリゾール

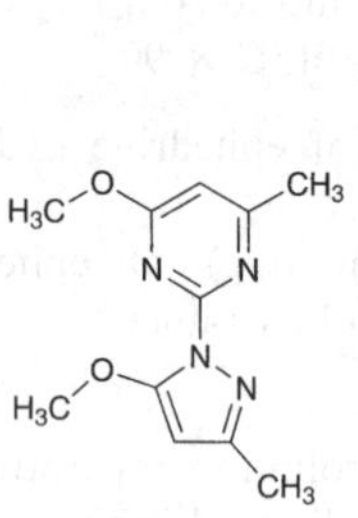

$C_{11}H_{14}N_4O_2$: 234.25
4-Methoxy-2-(5-methoxy-3-methyl-1*H*-pyrazol-1-yl)-6-methylpyrimidine
[18694-40-1]

Epirizole, when dried, contains not less than 99.0% of epirizole ($C_{11}H_{14}N_4O_2$).

Description Epirizole occurs as white, crystals or crystalline powder. It is odorless, and has a bitter taste.

It is very soluble in methanol and in acetic acid (100), freely soluble in ethanol (95), and sparingly soluble in water and in diethyl ether.

It dissolves in dilute hydrochloric acid and in sulfuric acid.

The pH of a solution of 1.0 g of Epirizole in 100 mL of water is between 6.0 and 7.0.

Identification (1) To 0.1 g of Epirizole add 0.1 g of vanillin, 5 mL of water and 2 mL of sulfuric acid, and mix with shaking for a while: a yellow precipitate is formed.

(2) Dissolve 0.1 g of Epirizole in 10 mL of water, and add 10 mL of 2,4,6-trinitrophenol TS: a yellow precipitate is produced. Collect the precipitate by filtration, wash with 50 mL of water, and dry at 105°C for 1 hour: it melts *<2.60>* between 163°C and 169°C.

(3) Determine the absorption spectrum of a solution of Epirizole in 0.1 mol/L hydrochloric acid TS (1 in 200,000) as directed under Ultraviolet-visible Spectrophotometry *<2.24>*, and compare the spectrum with the Reference Spectrum: both spectra exhibit similar intensities of absorption at the same wavelengths.

Melting point *<2.60>* 88 – 91°C

Purity (1) Clarity and color of solution—Dissolve 0.20 g of Epirizole in 20 mL of water: the solution is clear and colorless.

(2) Chloride *<1.03>*—Add 0.5 g of Epirizole to a ground mixture of 0.7 g of potassium nitrate and 1.2 g of anhydrous sodium carbonate, mix well, transfer little by little to a platinum crucible, previously heated, and heat until the reaction is completed. After cooling, add 15 mL of dilute sulfuric acid and 5 mL of water to the residue, boil for 5 minutes, filter, wash the insoluble matter with 10 mL of water, and to the combined filtrate and washings add 6 mL of dilute nitric acid and water to make 50 mL. Perform the test with this solution as the test solution. Prepare the control solution as follows: proceed with the same quantities of the same reagents as directed for the preparation of the test solution, and add 0.25 mL of 0.01 mol/L hydrochloric acid VS and water to make 50 mL (not more than 0.018%).

(3) Heavy metals *<1.07>*—Proceed with 2.0 g of Epirizole according to Method 2, and perform the test. Prepare the control solution with 2.0 mL of Standard Lead Solution (not more than 10 ppm).

(4) Arsenic *<1.11>*—Prepare the test solution with 1.0 g of Epirizole according to Method 3, and perform the test (not more than 2 ppm).

(5) Related substances—Dissolve 1.0 g of Epirizole in 10 mL of methanol, and use this solution as the sample solution. Pipet 1 mL of the sample solution, and add methanol to make exactly 50 mL. Pipet 1 mL of this solution, add methanol to make exactly 10 mL, and use this solution as the standard solution. Perform the test with these solutions as directed under Thin-layer Chromatography *<2.03>*. Spot 2 μL each of the sample solution and standard solution on a plate of silica gel with fluorescent indicator for thin-layer chromatography. Develop the plate with a mixture of isopropyl ether, ethanol (95) and water (23:10:2) to a distance of about 10 cm, and air-dry the plate. Examine under ultraviolet light (main wavelength: 254 nm): the spots other than the principal spot obtained from the sample solution are not more intense than the spot from the standard solution. Place this plate in a chamber filled with iodine vapor: the spots other than the principal spot from the sample solution are not more intense than the spot from the standard solution.

(6) Readily carbonizable substances *<1.15>*—Perform the test with 0.10 g of Epirizole: the solution has no more color than Matching Fluid A.

Loss on drying *<2.41>* Not more than 0.5% (1 g, silica gel, 4 hours).

Residue on ignition *<2.44>* Not more than 0.1% (1 g).

Assay Weigh accurately about 0.5 g of Epirizole, previously dried, dissolve in 40 mL of acetic acid (100) and titrate *<2.50>* with 0.1 mol/L perchloric acid VS (indicator: 2 drops of crystal violet TS) until the color of the solution changes from purple through blue-green to green.

Perform a blank determination in the same manner, and make any necessary correction.

Each mL of 0.1 mol/L perchloric acid VS
= 23.43 mg of $C_{11}H_{14}N_4O_2$

Containers and storage Containers—Well-closed containers.

Epirubicin Hydrochloride

エピルビシン塩酸塩

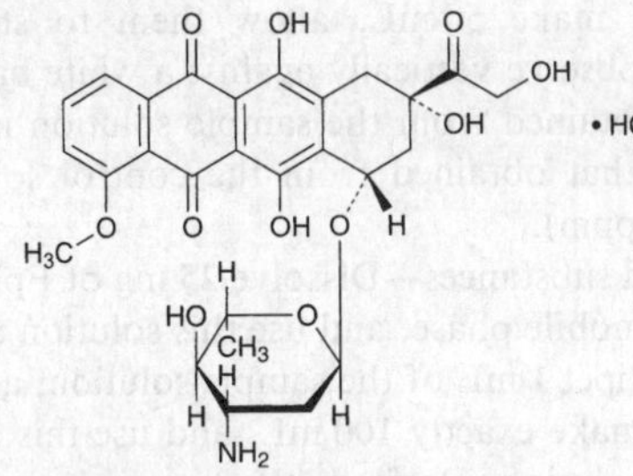

$C_{27}H_{29}NO_{11}$.HCl: 579.98
(2*S*,4*S*)-4-(3-Amino-2,3,6-trideoxy-α-L-*arabino*-hexopyranosyloxy)-2,5,12-trihydroxy-2-hydroxyacetyl-7-methoxy-1,2,3,4-tetrahydrotetracene-6,11-dione monohydrochloride
[*56390-09-1*]

Epirubicin Hydrochloride is the hydrochloride of a derivative of daunorubicin.

It contains not less than 970 μg (potency) and not more than 1020 μg (potency) per mg, calculated on the anhydrous and residual solvent-free basis. The potency of Epirubicin Hydrochloride is expressed as mass (potency) of epirubicin hydrochloride ($C_{27}H_{29}NO_{11}$.HCl).

Description Epirubicin Hydrochloride occurs as a pale yellowish red to brownish red powder.

It is soluble in water and in methanol, slightly soluble in ethanol (95), and practically insoluble in acetonitrile.

It is hygroscopic.

Identification **(1)** Determine the absorption spectrum of a solution of Epirubicin Hydrochloride in methanol (3 in 200,000) as directed under Ultraviolet-visible Spectrophotometry *<2.24>*, and compare the spectrum with the Reference Spectrum: both spectra exhibit similar intensities of absorption at the same wavelengths.

(2) Determine the infrared absorption spectrum of Epirubicin Hydrochloride and Epirubicin Hydrochloride RS as directed in the potassium bromide disk method under Infrared Spectrophotometry *<2.25>*, and compare these spectra: both spectra exhibit similar intensities of absorption at the same wave numbers.

Optical rotation *<2.49>* $[\alpha]_D^{20}$: +310 – +340° (10 mg calculated on the anhydrous and residual solvent-free basis, methanol, 20 mL, 100 mm).

pH *<2.54>* Dissolve 10 mg of Epirubicin Hydrochloride in 2 mL of water: the pH of the solution is between 4.0 and 5.5.

Purity **(1)** Clarity and color of solution—Dissolve 50 mg of Epirubicin Hydrochloride in 5 mL of water: the solution is clear and dark red.

(2) Heavy metals *<1.07>*—Proceed with 1.0 g of Epirubicin Hydrochloride according to Method 2, and perform the test. Prepare the control solution with 2.0 mL of Standard Lead Solution (not more than 20 ppm).

(3) Related substances—Perform the test with 10 μL of the sample solution obtained in the Assay as directed under Liquid Chromatography *<2.01>* according to the following conditions, determine each peak area by the automatic integration method, and calculate the total amount of the peaks other than epirubicin and 2-naphthalenesulfonic acid by the area percentage method: not more than 5.0%.

Operating conditions—

Detector, column, column temperature, mobile phase, and flow rate: Proceed as directed in the operating conditions in the Assay.

Time span of measurement: About 3 times as long as the retention time of epirubicin, beginning after the solvent peak.

System suitability—

System performance, and system repeatability: Proceed as directed in the system suitability in the Assay.

Test for required detectability: To 1 mL of the sample solution add the mobile phase to make 100 mL, and use this solution as the solution for system suitability test. Pipet 1 mL of the solution for system suitability test, and add the mobile phase to make exactly 10 mL. Confirm that the peak area of epirubicin obtained with 10 μL of this solution is equivalent to 7 to 13% of that with 10 μL of the solution for system suitability test.

Water *<2.48>* Not more than 8.0% (0.1 g, volumetric titration, direct titration).

Residue on ignition *<2.44>* Not more than 0.5% (0.1 g).

Assay Weigh accurately an amount of Epirubicin Hydrochloride and Epirubicin Hydrochloride RS, equivalent to about 50 mg (potency), dissolve each in the internal standard solution to make exactly 50 mL, and use these solutions as the sample solution and the standard solution, respectively. Perform the test with 10 μL each of the sample solution and standard solution as directed under Liquid Chromatography *<2.01>* according to the following conditions, and calculate the ratios, Q_T and Q_S, of the peak area of epirubicin to that of the internal standard.

Amount [μg (potency)] of epirubicin hydrochloride ($C_{27}H_{29}NO_{11}$.HCl)
$= M_S \times Q_T/Q_S \times 1000$

M_S: Amount [mg (potency)] of Epirubicin Hydrochloride RS taken

Internal standard solution—A solution of sodium 2-naphthalene sulfonate in a mixture of water, acetonitrile, methanol and phosphoric acid (540:290:170:1) (1 in 2000).

Operating conditions—

Detector: An ultraviolet absorption photometer (wavelength: 254 nm).

Column: A stainless steel column 4 mm in inside diameter and 25 cm in length, packed with trimethylsilanized silica gel for liquid chromatography (6 μm in particle diameter).

Column temperature: A constant temperature of about 35°C.

Mobile phase: Dissolve 2 g of sodium lauryl sulfate in a

mixture of water, acetonitrile, methanol and phosphoric acid (540:290:170:1) to make 1000 mL.

Flow rate: Adjust so that the retention time of epirubicin is about 9.5 minutes.

System suitability—

System performance: When the procedure is run with 10 μL of the standard solution under the above operating conditions, the internal standard and epirubicin are eluted in this order with the resolution between these peaks being not less than 20.

System repeatability: When the test is repeated 5 times with 10 μL of the standard solution under the above operating conditions, the relative standard deviation of the ratios of the peak area of epirubicin to that of the internal standard is not more than 1.0%.

Containers and storage Containers—Tight containers.

Storage—At a temperature between 0°C and 5°C.

Eplerenone

エプレレノン

$C_{24}H_{30}O_6$: 414.49
9,11α-Epoxy-7α-(methoxycarbonyl)-3-oxo-17α-pregn-4-ene-21,17-carbolactone
[*107724-20-9*]

Eplerenone contains not less than 98.0% and not more than 102.0% of eplerenone ($C_{24}H_{30}O_6$), calculated on the dried basis.

Description Eplerenone occurs as a white crystalline powder.

It is freely soluble in acetonitrile, sparingly soluble in methanol, and very slightly soluble in water and in ethanol (99.5).

It shows crystal polymorphism.

Identification **(1)** Determine the absorption spectrum of a solution of Eplerenone in methanol (1 in 77,000) as directed under Ultraviolet-visible Spectrophotometry <*2.24*>, and compare the spectrum with the Reference Spectrum or the spectrum of a solution of Eplerenone RS prepared in the same manner as the sample solution: both spectra exhibit similar intensities of absorption at the same wavelengths.

(2) Determine the infrared absorption spectrum of Eplerenone as directed in the potassium bromide disk method under Infrared Spectrophotometry <*2.25*>, and compare the spectrum with the Reference Spectrum or the spectrum of Eplerenone RS: both spectra exhibit similar intensities of absorption at the same wave numbers.

Optical rotation <*2.49*> $[\alpha]_D^{20}$: −14.0 – −16.0° (0.25 g calculated on the dried basis, acetonitrile, 25 mL, 100 mm).

Purity **(1)** Heavy metals—Take 1.0 g of Eplerenone in a crucible, wet the sample with a suitable amount of sulfuric acid, cover loosely, and heat gently to carbonize. After cooling, add 2 mL of nitric acid, and 5 drops of sulfuric acid to the carbonized residue, and heat gently until white fumes are no longer evolved. Then, incinerate by ignition at 500 – 600°C. After cooling, add 4 mL of 6 mol/L hydrochloric acid TS, cover the crucible, warm on a water bath for 15 minutes, then remove the cover from the crucible, and slowly evaporate to dryness on a water bath. Wet the residue with 1 drop of hydrochloric acid, add 10 mL of hot water, and warm for 2 minutes. After cooling, add ammonia TS until the solution shows alkalinity to litmus paper, add 15 mL of water, and adjust to pH 3.0 – 4.0 with dilute acetic acid. Filter, if necessary, wash the crucible and filter paper with 10 mL of water, put the filtrate and the washings in a Nessler tube, add water to make 40 mL, and use this solution as the sample solution. Separately, take 2.0 mL of Standard Lead Solution in a Nessler tube, and add water to make 25 mL. Adjust to pH 3.0 – 4.0 of this solution with dilute acetic acid or ammonia TS, add water to make 40 mL, and use this solution as the control solution. To the sample solution and the control solution add 2 mL of acetate buffer solution (pH 3.5) and 1.2 mL of thioacetamide-alkaline glycerin TS, then add water to make 50 mL, allow them to stand for 2 minutes, and observe vertically against a white background: the solution obtained from the sample solution is not more colored than that obtained from the control solution (not more than 20 ppm).

(2) Related substances—Dissolve 25 mg of Eplerenone in 50 mL of the mobile phase, and use this solution as the sample solution. Pipet 1 mL of the sample solution, add the mobile phase to make exactly 100 mL, and use this solution as the standard solution. Perform the test with exactly 20 μL each of the sample solution and standard solution as directed under Liquid Chromatography <*2.01*> according to the following conditions, and determine each peak area by the automatic integration method: the area of the peak, having a relative retention time of about 0.58, about 0.85, about 0.90, about 1.2 and about 1.6 to eplerenone, obtained from the sample solution is respectively not larger than 1/5, 3/10, 3/10, 3/10 and 3/10 times the peak area of eplerenone from the standard solution, and the area of the peak other than eplerenone and the peak mentioned above from the sample solution is not larger than 7/50 times the peak area of eplerenone from the standard solution. Furthermore, the total area of the peaks other than eplerenone from the sample solution is not larger than 1.2 times the peak area of eplerenone from the standard solution. For the area of the peak, having the relative retention time of about 0.85 to eplerenon, multiply the correction factor 0.6.

Operating conditions—

Detector, column, column temperature, mobile phase, and flow rate: Proceed as directed in the operating conditions in the Assay.

Time span of measurement: About 4 times as long as the retention time of eplerenone, beginning after the solvent peak.

System suitability—

Test for required detectability: Pipet 1 mL of the standard solution, add the mobile phase to make exactly 10 mL. Confirm that the peak area of eplerenone obtained with 20 μL of this solution is equivalent to 7 to 13% of that with 20 μL of the standard solution.

System performance: When the procedure is run with 20 μL of the standard solution under the above operating conditions, the number of theoretical plates and the symmetry factor of the peak of eplerenone are not less than 15,000 and not more than 1.5, respectively.

System repeatability: When the test is repeated 6 times with 20 μL of the standard solution under the above operating conditions, the relative standard deviation of the peak

area of eplerenone is not more than 2.0%.

Loss on drying <*2.41*> Not more than 0.5% (0.5 g, 105°C, 4 hours).

Residue on ignition <*2.44*> Not more than 0.1% (1 g).

Assay Weigh accurately about 25 mg each of Eplerenone and Eplerenone RS (separately determine the loss on drying <*2.41*> under the same conditions as Eplerenone), separately dissolve in the mobile phase to make exactly 50 mL, and use these solutions as the sample solution and the standard solution, respectively. Perform the test with exactly 20 μL each of the sample solution and standard solution as directed under Liquid Chromatography <*2.01*> according to the following conditions, and determine the peak areas, A_T and A_S, of eplerenone in each solution.

Amount (mg) of eplerenone ($C_{24}H_{30}O_6$) = $M_S \times A_T/A_S$

M_S: Amount (mg) of Eplerenone RS taken, calculated on the dried basis

Operating conditions—

Detector: An ultraviolet absorption photometer (wavelength: 210 nm).

Column: A stainless steel column 4.6 mm in inside diameter and 25 cm in length, packed with octadecylsilanized silica gel for liquid chromatography (5 μm in particle diameter).

Column temperature: A constant temperature of about 35°C.

Mobile phase: Dissolve 1.4 g of potassium dihydrogen phosphate in 1000 mL of water, and adjust to pH 3.0 with phosphoric acid. To 580 mL of this solution add 360 mL of acetonitrile for liquid chromatography and 60 mL of methanol.

Flow rate: Adjust so that the retention time of eplerenone is about 12 minutes.

System suitability—

System performance: When the procedure is run with 20 μL of the standard solution under the above operating conditions, the number of theoretical plates and the symmetry factor of the peak of eplerenone are not less than 15,000 and not more than 1.5, respectively.

System repeatability: When the test is repeated 6 times with 20 μL of the standard solution under the above operating conditions, the relative standard deviation of the peak area of eplerenone is not more than 1.0%.

Containers and storage Containers—Well-closed containers.

Eplerenone Tablets

エプレレノン錠

Eplerenone Tablets contain not less than 95.0% and not more than 105.0% of the labeled amount of eplerenone ($C_{24}H_{30}O_6$: 414.49).

Method of preparation Prepare as directed under Tablets, with Eplerenone.

Identification Determine the absorption spectrum of the sample solution obtained in the Uniformity of dosage units as directed under Ultraviolet-visible Spectrophotometry <*2.24*>: it exhibits a maximum between 240 nm and 244 nm.

Uniformity of dosage units <*6.02*> Perform the Mass variation test, or the Content uniformity test according to the following method: it meets the requirement.

To 1 tablet of Eplerenone Tablets add a suitable amount of a mixture of acetonitrile and water (3:2), shake, disintegrate the tablet by sonicating, add a mixture of acetonitrile and water (3:2) to make exactly 100 mL, and centrifuge. Take exactly V mL of the supernatant liquid, add a mixture of acetonitrile and water (3:2) to make exactly V' mL so that each mL contains about 25 μg of eplerenone ($C_{24}H_{30}O_6$), and use this solution as the sample solution. Separately, weigh accurately about 25 mg of Eplerenone RS (separately determine the loss on drying <*2.41*> under the same conditions as Eplerenone), and dissolve in a mixture of acetonitrile and water (3:2) to make exactly 50 mL. Pipet 5 mL of this solution, add a mixture of acetonitrile and water (3:2) to make exactly 100 mL, and use this solution as the standard solution. Determine the absorbances, A_T and A_S, at 243 nm of the sample solution and standard solution as directed under Ultraviolet-visible Spectrophotometry <*2.24*>.

Amount (mg) of eplerenone ($C_{24}H_{30}O_6$)
$= M_S \times A_T/A_S \times V'/V \times 1/10$

M_S: Amount (mg) of Eplerenone RS taken, calculated on the dried basis

Dissolution <*6.10*> When the test is performed at 50 revolutions per minute according to the Paddle method, using 900 mL of 1st fluid for dissolution test as the dissolution medium, the dissolution rate in 30 minutes of Eplerenone Tablets is not less than 75%.

Start the test with 1 tablet of Eplerenone Tablets, withdraw not less than 20 mL of the medium at the specified minute after starting the test, and filter through a membrane filter with a pore size not exceeding 0.45 μm. Discard not less than 5 mL of the first filtrate, pipet V mL of the subsequent filtrate, add the dissolution medium to make exactly V' mL so that each mL contains about 11 μg of eplerenone ($C_{24}H_{30}O_6$), and use this solution as the sample solution. Separately, weigh accurately about 25 mg of Eplerenone RS (separately determine the loss on drying <*2.41*> under the same conditions as Eplerenone), dissolve in 5 mL of acetonitrile, and add the dissolution medium to make exactly 500 mL. Pipet 10 mL of this solution, add the dissolution medium to make exactly 50 mL, and use this solution as the standard solution. Determine the absorbances, A_T and A_S, at 243 nm of the sample solution and standard solution as directed under Ultraviolet-visible Spectrophotometry <*2.24*> using the dissolution medium as the blank.

Dissolution rate (%) with respect to the labeled amount of eplerenone ($C_{24}H_{30}O_6$)
$= M_S \times A_T/A_S \times V'/V \times 1/C \times 36$

M_S: Amount (mg) of Eplerenone RS taken, calculated on the dried basis

C: Labeled amount (mg) of eplerenone ($C_{24}H_{30}O_6$) in 1 tablet

Assay Weigh accurately the mass of not less than 20 Eplerenone Tablets, and powder. Weigh accurately a portion of the powder, equivalent to about 50 mg of eplerenone ($C_{24}H_{30}O_6$), add a suitable amount of a mixture of acetonitrile and water (3:2), sonicate to disperse the particles, and add a mixture of acetonitrile and water (3:2) to make exactly 100 mL. Centrifuge this solution, and use the supernatant liquid as the sample solution. Separately, weigh accurately about 25 mg of Eplerenone RS (separately determine the loss on drying <*2.41*> under the same conditions as Eplerenone), dissolve in a mixture of acetonitrile and water (3:2) to make exactly 50 mL, and use this solution as the standard solution.

Perform the test with exactly 15 μL each of the sample solution and standard solution as directed under Liquid Chromatography ⟨*2.01*⟩ according to the following conditions, and determine the peak areas, A_T and A_S, of eplerenone in each solution.

$$\text{Amount (mg) of eplerenone } (C_{24}H_{30}O_6) = M_S \times A_T/A_S \times 2$$

M_S: Amount (mg) of Eplerenone RS taken, calculated on the dried basis

Operating conditions—

Detector: An ultraviolet absorption photometer (wavelength: 243 nm).

Column: A stainless steel column 4.6 mm in inside diameter and 15 cm in length, packed with octadecylsilanized silica gel for liquid chromatography (4 μm in particle diameter).

Column temperature: A constant temperature of about 25°C.

Mobile phase: Dissolve 1.4 g of potassium dihydrogen phosphate in 1000 mL of water, and adjust to pH 3.0 with phosphoric acid. To 550 mL of this solution add 360 mL of methanol and 90 mL of acetonitrile.

Flow rate: Adjust so that the retention time of eplerenone is about 12 minutes.

System suitability—

System performance: When the procedure is run with 15 μL of the standard solution under the above operating conditions, the number of theoretical plates and the symmetry factor of the peak of eplerenone are not less than 3000 and not more than 2.0, respectively.

System repeatability: When the test is repeated 6 times with 15 μL of the standard solution under the above operating conditions, the relative standard deviation of the peak area of eplerenone is not more than 1.0%.

Containers and storage Containers—Well-closed containers.

Epoetin Alfa (Genetical Recombination)

エポエチン　アルファ(遺伝子組換え)

Protein moiety

```
APPRLICDSR VLERYLLEAK EAENITTGCA EHCSLNENIT VPDTKVNFYA
WKRMEVGQQA VEVWQGLALL SEAVLRGQAL LVNSSQPWEP LQLHVDKAVS
GLRSLTTLLR ALGAQKEAIS PPDAASAAPL RTITADTFRK LFRVYSNFLR
GKLKLYTGEA CRTGD
```

N24, N38, N83 and S126 : glycosylation

Carbohydrate moiety (structure of major glycans)

N24, N38 and N83

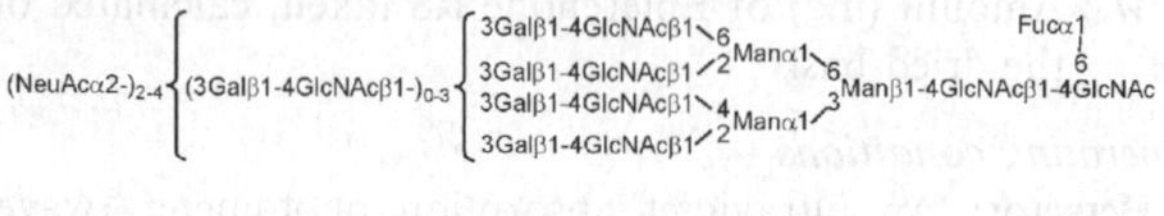

```
                                                  3Galβ1-4GlcNAcβ1↘6                Fucα1
                                                                    Manα1↘6             |
                                                  3Galβ1-4GlcNAcβ1↗2                    6
(NeuAcα2-)2-4 { (3Galβ1-4GlcNAcβ1-)0-3 {                               Manβ1-4GlcNAcβ1-4GlcNAc
                                                  3Galβ1-4GlcNAcβ1↘4                 3
                                                                    Manα1↗
                                                  3Galβ1-4GlcNAcβ1↗2
```

S126

```
               (NeuAcα2)0,1
                     |
                     6
(NeuAcα2-)0,13Galβ1-3GalNAc
```

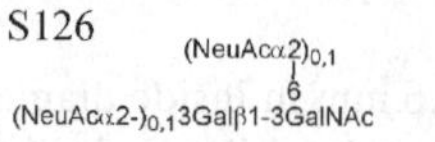

$C_{809}H_{1301}N_{229}O_{240}S_5$: 18235.70 (Protein moiety)
[*113427-24-0*]

Epoetin Alfa (Genetical Recombination) is an aqueous solution in which a desired product is a recombinant human erythropoietin produced in Chinese hamster ovary cells. It is a glycoprotein (molecular mass: ca. 37,000 to 42,000) consisting of 165 amino acid residues.

It contains not less than 1.1 mg and not more than 1.5 mg of protein per mL, and not less than 1.5 × 10^5 units per mg of protein.

Description Epoetin Alfa (Genetical Recombination) occurs as a clear and colorless liquid.

Identification (1) Dilute a suitable volume of Epoetin Alfa (Genetical Recombination) and Epoetin Alfa RS with water. To 3 volume of these solutions add 1 volume each of buffer solution for epoetin alfa sample, heat at 100°C for 5 minutes, and use these solutions as the sample solution and the standard solution, respectively. Transfer a volume of the sample solution and the standard solution, equivalent to 0.7 μg of protein, into each sample well of the polyacrylamide gel for epoetin alfa, and start the SDS-polyacrylamide gel electrophoresis using a vertical discontinuous buffer solution system. After the electrophoresis, immerse the gel, a polyvinylidene fluoride membrane and a filter paper in the blotting TS. Set them on a semi-dry blotting apparatus, and transcribe for about 1 hour with a constant electric current of 0.7 – 0.9 mA/cm² depending on the dimension of the filter paper. Then, immerse the polyvinylidene fluoride membrane in the blocking TS for epoetin alfa for more than 1 hour while shaking, remove the blocking TS for epoetin alfa and add the primary antibody TS, then shake for a night or allow to stand at 4°C for 3 nights. Remove the primary antibody TS, wash the membrane with phosphate-buffered sodium chloride TS, add the secondary antibody TS, and shake for more than 1 hour. Remove the secondary antibody TS, wash the membrane with phosphate-buffered sodium chloride TS, add the avidin-biotin TS, and shake for more than 1 hour. Remove the avidin-biotin TS, wash the membrane with phosphate-buffered sodium chloride TS, and add the substrate TS for epoetin alfa for developing the color image: the main stained bands obtained from the sample solution appear as similar migrating image as those from the standard solution.

(2) Evaporate to dryness under reduced pressure a volume of Epoetin Alfa (Genetical Recombination) and Epoetin Alfa RS, equivalent to about 35 μg of protein, and dissolve these residues in 100 μL of 0.1 mol/L tris buffer solution (pH 7.3). To these solutions add 5 μL of trypsin TS for epoetin alfa, warm at 37°C for 6 hours, then cool in ice, and use these solutions as the sample solution and the standard solution, respectively. Perform the test with 45 μL each of the sample solution and standard solution as directed under Liquid Chromatography <*2.01*> according to the following conditions, and compare the chromatograms obtained from these solutions: both chromatograms show the similar peaks at the corresponding retention time.

Operating conditions—

Detector: An ultraviolet absorption photometer (wavelength: 214 nm).

Column: A stainless steel column 3.9 mm in inside diameter and 15 cm in length, packed with octylsilanized silica gel for liquid chromatography (5 μm in particle diameter).

Column temperature: A constant temperature of about 45°C.

Mobile phase A: A mixture of water and trifluoroacetic acid (5000:3).

Mobile phase B: A mixture of acetonitrile, water and trifluoroacetic acid (4000:1000:3).

Flowing of mobile phase: Control the gradient by mixing the mobile phases A and B as directed in the following table.

Time after injection of sample (min)	Mobile phase A (vol%)	Mobile phase B (vol%)
0 – 5	98	2
5 – 95	98 → 35	2 → 65

Flow rate: 0.75 mL per minute.

System suitability—

System performance: When the procedure is run with 45 μL of the standard solution under the above conditions, the chromatogram shows the similar pattern with the chromatogram of Epoetin Alfa RS obtained in the Peptide mapping.

Sialic acid content To an exact volume of Epoetin Alfa (Genetical Recombination), equivalent to about 1 nmol of protein, add water to make exactly 45 μL. Add exactly 5 μL of sodium hydroxide TS, allow to stand in ice water for 90 minutes, and add exactly 5 μL of dilute acetic acid. Add exactly 45 μL of water and exactly 100 μL of a mixture of water and acetic acid (100) (27:8), and warm at 80°C for 210 minutes. After cooling, add exactly 200 μL of the fluorescence TS, and warm at 60°C for 2 hours avoiding exposure to light. After cooling, add exactly 200 μL of sodium hydroxide TS, and use this solution as the sample solution. Separately, just before starting the test, to exactly 250 μL of 0.4 mmol/L *N*-acetylneuraminic acid TS add exactly 20 μL of 0.1 mmol/L *N*-glycolylneuraminic acid TS and exactly 180 μL of water. Proceed with exactly 45 μL of this solution in the same manner as for the sample solution, and use the solution so obtained as the standard solution. Perform the test with exactly 20 μL each of the sample solution and standard solution as directed under Liquid Chromatography <*2.01*> according to the following conditions, determine the peak areas of *N*-acetylneuraminic acid and *N*-glycolylneuraminic acid, A_{T1} and A_{T2}, obtained from the sample solution, and the peak areas of those, A_{S1} and A_{S2}, from the standard solution. Calculate the content of sialic acid in Epoetin Alfa (Genetical Recombination) by the following equation: between 10 mol/mol and 12 mol/mol.

$$\text{Content (mol/mol) of sialic acid} = (A_{T1}/A_{S1} \times 10 + A_{T2}/A_{S2} \times 1/5)/a$$

a: Number (nmol) of moles of Epoetin Alfa (Genetical Recombination)

where, molar concentration (mmol/L) of Epoetin Alfa (Genetical Recombination) is calculated by the following equation, using the absorbance *A* at 280 nm obtained in the Assay (1).

$$\text{Molar concentration (mmol/L) of Epoetin Alfa (Genetical Recombination)} = A \times 10^3/22{,}430$$

22,430: Molar absorbance coefficient ε

Operating conditions—

Detector: A fluorophotometer (excitation wavelength: 373 nm, fluorescence wavelength: 448 nm).

Column: A stainless steel column 3.9 mm in inside diameter and 15 cm in length, packed with octadecylsilanized silica gel for liquid chromatography (5 μm in particle diameter).

Column temperature: A constant temperature of about 25°C.

Mobile phase A: A mixture of water, acetonitrile and methanol (84:9:7).

Mobile phase B: A mixture of water and methanol (1:1).

Flowing of mobile phase: Control the gradient by mixing the mobile phases A and B as directed in the following table.

Time after injection of sample (min)	Mobile phase A (vol%)	Mobile phase B (vol%)
0 – 20	100	0
20 – 20.1	100 → 0	0 → 100
20.1 – 27	0	100

Flow rate: 0.6 mL per minute.

System suitability—

System performance: When the procedure is run with 20 μL of the standard solution under the above operating conditions, *N*-glycolylneuraminic acid and *N*-acetylneuraminic acid are eluted in this order with the resolution between these peaks being not less than 3.

System repeatability: When the test is repeated 6 times with 20 μL of the standard solution under the above operating conditions, the relative standard deviations of the peak area of *N*-glycolylneuraminic acid and *N*-acetylneuraminic acid are not more than 2.0%, respectively.

Oligosaccharide profile Being specified separately when the drug is granted approval based on the Law.

Molecular mass Use the sample solution obtained in the Identification (1) as the sample solution. Separately, to 20 μL of molecular mass standard stock solution add 6.7 μL of the buffer solution for epoetin alfa sample, heat at 100°C for 5 minutes, and use this solution as the molecular mass standard solution. Transfer a volume of the sample solution, equivalent to 3.5 μg of protein and the total volume of the molecular mass standard solution into each sample well of the vertical discontinuous buffer solution system SDS-polyacrylamide gel, composed with resolving and stacking gels, and perform the electrophoresis. After the electrophoresis, immerse the gel in a solution of Coomassie brilliant blue R-250, containing 1.25 g in a mixture of 450 mL of methanol, 100 mL of acetic acid (100) and sufficient amount of water making up to 1000 mL. Determine the relative mobilities of the stained bands of egg albumin (molecular mass: about 45,000), carbonic anhydrase (molecular mass: about 31,000), soybean trypsin inhibitor (molecular mass: about 21,500) and lysozyme (molecular mass: 14,400), and prepare a calibration curve by linear regression against the logarithm of the molecular masses. Determine the relative mobility of the center of the main band obtained from the sample solution, and calculate the molecular mass of Epoetin Alfa (Genetical Recombination) from the calibration curve: it is between 37,000 and 42,000.

pH <*2.54*> 5.7 – 6.7

Purity **(1)** Multimers—Perform the test with a volume of Epoetin Alfa (Genetical Recombination), equivalent to 50 μg of protein, as directed under Liquid Chromatography <*2.01*> according to the following conditions. Determine each peak area by the automatic integration method, and calculate their amounts by the area percentage method: the total amount of the peaks other than epoetin alfa is not more than 2%.

Operating conditions—

Detector: An ultraviolet absorption photometer (wavelength: 215 nm).

Column: A stainless steel column 7.5 mm in inside diameter and 60 cm in length, packed with hydrophilic silica gel for liquid chromatography.

Column temperature: A constant temperature of about 25°C.

Mobile phase: Dissolve 91 mg of disodium hydrogen phosphate dodecahydrate, 0.27 g of sodium dihydrogen phosphate dihydrate and 8.77 g of sodium chloride in water to make 1000 mL.

Flow rate: Adjust so that the retention time of epoetin alfa is about 16 minutes.

Time span of measurement: From the retention time corresponding to the exclusion volume of the size-exclusion column until the elution of epoetin alfa is finished.

System suitability—

Test for required detectability: To 1 volume of Epoetin Alfa (Genetical Recombination) add 49 volumes of the mobile phase, and use this solution as the solution for system suitability test. Confirm that the peak area of epoetin alfa obtained with a volume, equivalent to 1 μg of protein, of the solution for system suitability test is equivalent to 1.5 to 2.5% of that with the same volume of Epoetin Alfa (Genetical Recombination).

System performance: Dissolve 40 mg of bovine serum albumin for gel filtration molecular mass marker and 20 mg of chymotrypsinogen for gel filtration molecular mass marker in 100 mL of the mobile phase. When the procedure is run with 50 μL of this solution under the above operating conditions, bovine serum albumin and chymotrypsinogen are eluted in this order with the resolution between these peaks being not less than 4.

System repeatability: When the test is repeated 6 times with a volume of Epoetin Alfa (Genetical Recombination), equivalent to 50 μg of protein, under the above operating conditions, the relative standard deviation of the area of the principal peak of epoetin alfa is not more than 2.0%.

(2) Host cell proteins—Being specified separately when the drug is granted approval based on the Law.

(3) Host cell DNA—Being specified separately when the drug is granted approval based on the Law.

Assay **(1)** Protein content—Take a suitable amount of Epoetin Alfa (Genetical Recombination), dilute with phosphate buffer solution for epoetin alfa, if necessary, so that each mL contains 0.5 – 0.8 mg protein and use the solution as the sample solution. Determine the absorbance, A, at 280 nm of the sample solution as directed under Ultraviolet-visible Spectrophotometry <*2.24*>, using the phosphate buffer solution for epoetin alfa as the blank.

Amount (mg) of protein in 1 mL of Epoetin Alfa (Genetical Recombination)

$$= A \times d \times 0.909$$

d: Dilution factor for the sample solution

0.909: Reciprocal number of absorption coefficient ($E^{0.1\%}_{1\,\mathrm{cm}}$) of epoetin alfa protein

(2) Specific activity

(i) Animals: Select healthy 6 to 8 weeks female mice (B6D2F1, etc.). Keep the mice for not less than a week before use, providing an appropriate uniform diet and water.

(ii) Standard solutions: To Epoetin Alfa RS add the bovine serum albumin-saline solution so that each mL contains exactly 10 – 40 units, and designate this solution as the high-dose standard solution, S_H. Dilute S_H exactly 4 times with the bovine serum albumin-saline solution, and designate this solution as the low-dose standard solution, S_L.

(iii) Sample solutions: To Epoetin Alfa (Genetical Recombination) add the bovine serum albumin-saline solution to make two sample solutions, the high-dose sample solution, T_H, which contains the Units per mL equivalent to S_H and the low-dose sample solution, T_L, which contains the Units per mL equivalent to S_L.

(iv) Procedure: Divide the animals into 4 equal groups of not less than 5 animals each. On the 1st, 2nd and 3rd days, inject exactly 0.2 mL each of the standard solutions and the sample solutions into each animal subcutaneously as indicated in the following design:

First group	S_H	Third group	T_H
Second group	S_L	Fourth group	T_L

On the 4th day, take a sufficient blood sample to perform the test from each animal. To 10 mL of the dilution fluid for particle counter add exactly 20 μL of the blood sample, mix, add 100 μL of the appropriate hemolysis agent, stir for 5 minutes, and determine the count of particles derived from hemolytic-resistant erythroid cells.

(v) Calculation: Logarithmic converted counts of the fine particles obtained with S_H, S_L, T_H and T_L in (iv) are symbolized as y_1, y_2, y_3 and y_4, respectively. Sum up individual y_1, y_2, y_3 and y_4 to obtain Y_1, Y_2, Y_3 and Y_4, respectively.

Specific activity (unit/mg protein) of Epoetin Alfa (Genetical Recombination)

= activity (unit/mL) of Epoetin Alfa (Genetical Recombination)/C

Activity (unit/mL) of Epoetin Alfa (Genetical Recombination)

= antilog M × unit in 1 mL of S_H × d

$$M = \log 4 \times Y_a/Y_b$$
$$Y_a = -Y_1 - Y_2 + Y_3 + Y_4$$
$$Y_b = Y_1 - Y_2 + Y_3 - Y_4$$

d: Dilution factor for T_H

C: Concentration (mg/mL) of protein obtained in Assay (1)

F' computed by the following equation should be smaller

than F shown in the table against n with which s^2 is calculated. Calculate L (p = 0.95) by use of the following equation: L should be not more than 0.3. If F' exceeds F, or if L exceeds 0.3, repeat the test, arranging the assay conditions.

$$F' = (Y_1 - Y_2 - Y_3 + Y_4)^2/4fs^2$$

f: Number of animals per group, which should be the same for each group and not less than 5.

$$s^2 = (\Sigma y^2 - Y/f)/n$$

Σy^2: The sum of the squares of each y_1, y_2, y_3 and y_4.
$Y = Y_1^2 + Y_2^2 + Y_3^2 + Y_4^2$
$n = 4\ (f - 1)$

$$L = 2\sqrt{(C - 1)\{CM^2 + (\log 4)^2\}}$$

$$C = Y_b^2/(Y_b^2 - 4fs^2t^2)$$

F (= t^2) values against n

n	$t^2 = F$	n	$t^2 = F$	n	$t^2 = F$
1	161.45	13	4.667	25	4.242
2	18.51	14	4.600	26	4.225
3	10.129	15	4.543	27	4.210
4	7.709	16	4.494	28	4.196
5	6.608	17	4.451	29	4.183
6	5.987	18	4.414	30	4.171
7	5.591	19	4.381	40	4.085
8	5.318	20	4.351	60	4.001
9	5.117	21	4.325	120	3.920
10	4.965	22	4.301	∞	3.841
11	4.844	23	4.279		
12	4.747	24	4.260		

Containers and storage Containers—Tight containers.

Storage—Not exceeding $-70°C$.

Epoetin Beta (Genetical Recombination)

エポエチン　ベータ(遺伝子組換え)

Protein moiety

```
APPRLICDSR VLERYLLEAK EAENITTGCA EHCSLNENIT VPDTKVNFYA
WKRMEVGQQA VEVWQGLALL SEAVLRGQAL LVNSSQPWEP LQLHVDKAVS
GLRSLTTLLR ALGAQKEAIS PPDAASAAPL RTITADTFRK LFRVYSNFLR
GKLKLYTGEA CRTGD
```

N24, N38, N83 and S126: glycosylation

Carbohydrate moiety (structure of major glycans)

N24, N38 and N83

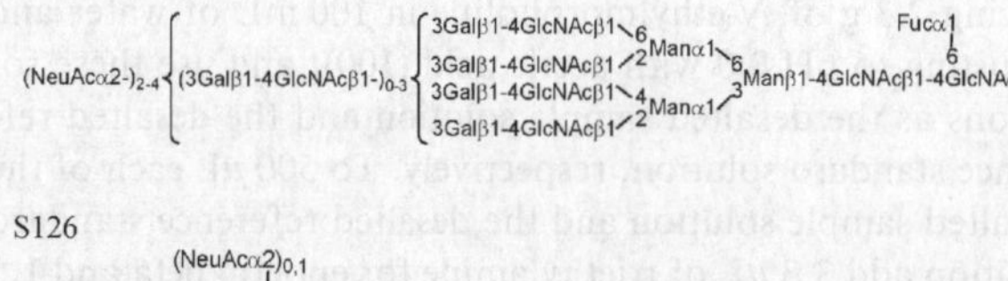

S126

(NeuAcα2)0,1
6
(NeuAcα2-)0,1 3Galβ1-3GalNAc

$C_{809}H_{1301}N_{229}O_{240}S_5$: 18235.70 (Protein moiety)
[*122312-54-3*]

Epoetin Beta (Genetical Recombination) is an aqueous solution in which a desired product is a recombinant human erythropoietin produced in Chinese hamster ovary cells. It is a glycoprotein (molecular mass: ca. 30,000) consisting of 165 amino acid residues.

It contains not less than 0.5 mg and not more than 1.5 mg of protein per mL, and not less than 1.5×10^5 units per mg of protein.

Description Epoetin Beta (Genetical Recombination) occurs as a clear and colorless liquid.

Identification **(1)** Use Epoetin Beta (Genetical Recombination) and Epoetin Beta RS as the sample solution and the standard solution, respectively. When perform a capillary electrophoresis with the sample solution and standard solution according to the following conditions, the mobility of each peak obtained from both solutions is the same and their migrating images are similar each other.

Operating conditions—

Detector: An ultraviolet absorption photometer (wavelength: 200 nm).

Column: A silica capillary tube 50 μm in inside diameter and about 50 cm in length, chemically coated inner surface with amino groups (about 40 cm in effective length).

Electrolyte solution: Dissolve 32.8 g of sodium dihydrogen phosphate dihydrate in water to make 1000 mL, and adjust to pH 4.5 with a solution, prepared by dissolving 75.2 g of disodium hydrogen phosphate dodecahydrate in water to make 1000 mL. To 19 volumes of this solution add 1 volume of ethanol (99.5).

Running temperature: A constant temperature of about 20°C.

Running conditions: Migration current (a constant current of about 45 μA), migration time (30 minutes).

Injection of sample and standard solutions: 5 seconds (pressurization: 0.5 psi).

Time span of measurement: From 10 minutes to 30 minutes after injection (excluding the peak of solvent origin).

System suitability—

System performance: When the procedure is run with the standard solution under the above operating conditions, more than 4 major peaks of epoetin beta are detected, and the resolution between the first and second eluted major peaks is not less than 0.8.

System repeatability: When the test is repeated 3 times with the standard solution under the above operating conditions, the relative standard deviation of the migration time of the first eluted major peak is not more than 2.0%.

(2) Desalt a volume each of Epoetin Beta (Genetical Recombination) and Epoetin Beta RS, equivalent to 600 μg of protein, by a suitable method, and term them as the desalted sample and the desalted reference standard, respectively. Dissolve the desalted sample and the desalted reference standard in 600 μL each of a solution, prepared by dissolving 2.3 g of *N*-ethylmorpholine in 100 mL of water and adjusting to pH 8.0 with acetic acid (100), and use these solutions as the desalted sample solution and the desalted reference standard solution, respectively. To 500 μL each of the desalted sample solution and the desalted reference standard solution add 3.3 μL of triethylamine for epoetin beta and 1.5 μL of 2-mercaptoethanol for epoetin beta, and react at 37°C for 1 hour. After cooling, add 5.5 μL of 4-vinylpyridine to them, and react at 25°C for 1 hour. To these solutions add 50 μL of diluted trifluoroacetic acid for epoetin beta (1 in 10) to stop the reaction, remove the reagents by a suitable method, and use the substances so obtained as the pyridylethylated sample and the pyridylethylated reference substance, respectively. Dissolve the pyridylethylated sample and the pyridylethylated reference substance separately in 500 μL of sodium hydrogen carbonate solution (21 in 2500). To 400 μL each of these solutions add 16 μL of a solution of lysyl endopeptidase in sodium hydrogen carbonate solution (21 in 2500) (1 in 50,000), and react at 37°C for 24 hours. While this reaction, additional two 16-μL portions of a solution of lysyl endopeptidase in sodium hydrogen carbonate (21 in 2500) (1 in 50,000) are added at 4 hours and 20 hours after starting the reaction. Then, stop the reaction by adding 100 μL of diluted trifluoroacetic acid for epoetin beta (1 in 10), and use these solutions as the sample solution and the standard solution, respectively. Perform the test with 100 μL each of the sample solution and standard solution as directed under Liquid Chromatography <*2.01*> according to the following conditions, and compare the chromatograms obtained from these solutions: both chromatograms show the similar peaks at the corresponding retention times.

Operating conditions—

Detector: An ultraviolet absorption photometer (wavelength: 214 nm).

Column: A stainless steel column 4.6 mm in inside diameter and 25 cm in length, packed with octadecylsilanized silica gel for liquid chromatography (5 μm in particle diameter).

Column temperature: A constant temperature of about 25°C.

Mobile phase A: A mixture of water and trifluoroacetic acid for epoetin beta (1000:1).

Mobile phase B: A mixture of acetonitrile for liquid chromatography, water, and trifluoroacetic acid for epoetin beta (900:100:1).

Flowing of mobile phase: Control the gradient by mixing the mobile phases A and B as directed in the following table.

Time after injection of sample (min)	Mobile phase A (vol%)	Mobile phase B (vol%)
0 – 10	90	10
10 – 30	90 → 80	10 → 20
30 – 50	80	20
50 – 130	80 → 40	20 → 60
130 – 140	40 → 10	60 → 90
140 – 150	10	90

Flow rate: Adjust so that the retention time of the first peak, which appears after the solvent peak, is about 17 minutes.

System suitability—

System performance: When the procedure is run with the standard solution under the above operating conditions, 9 major peptide peaks are appeared after the solvent peak, and the resolution between the peaks eluted at the fifth and the sixth is not less than 3.

Sialic acid content To exactly 100 μL of Epoetin Beta (Genetical Recombination) add 1 mL of resorcinol-copper (II) sulfate TS, and heat on a water bath for 30 minutes. After ice-cooling, add 2 mL of a mixture of *n*-butyl acetate and 1-butanol (4:1), shake vigorously, and use the upper layer as the sample solution. Separately, dissolve *N*-acetylneuraminic acid in water to make three solutions, containing 0.1 mg, 0.2 mg and 0.3 mg of *N*-acetylneuraminic acid in each mL, and use these solutions as the standard stock solution (1), the standard stock solution (2) and the standard stock solution (3), respectively. Pipet 100 μL each of these standard stock solutions, add 1 mL of resorcinol-copper (II) sulfate TS to them, then proceed in the same way as for the sample solution, and use these solutions so obtained as the standard solution (1), the standard solution (2) and the standard solution (3), respectively. Determine the absorbances of the sample solution and the standard solutions (1), (2) and (3) at 625 nm as directed under Ultraviolet-visible Spectrophotometry <*2.24*>. Calculate the amount of sialic acid (mg/mL) in the sample solution, by using the calibration curve obtained from the standard solutions, and calculate the amount of sialic acid in Epoetin Beta (Genetical Recombination) by the following equation: between 10 mol/mol and 13 mol/mol.

Amount of sialic acid (mol/mol of epoetin beta protein)
$= A/C \times 18{,}236/309.27$

A: Amount (mg/mL) of sialic acid in the sample solution
C: Amount (mg/mL) of protein in Epoetin Beta (Genetical Recombination)
18,236: Molecular mass of protein moiety of epoetin beta
309.27: Molecular mass of *N*-acetylneuraminic acid

Oligosaccharide profile Being specified separately when the drug is granted approval based on the Law.

pH <*2.54*> 7.0 – 8.0

Purity **(1)** Related substances—Perform the test with 20 μL of Epoetin Beta (Genetical Recombination) as directed under Liquid Chromatography <*2.01*> according to the following conditions. Determine each peak area by the automatic integration method, and calculate the amount of these peaks other than the solvent peak by the area percentage method: the total area of the peaks other than epoetin beta is not more than 1.0%.

Operating conditions—

Detector: An ultraviolet absorption photometer (wave-

length: 214 nm).

Column: A stainless steel column 7.5 mm in inside diameter and 60 cm in length, packed with porous silica gel for liquid chromatography (10 μm in particle diameter).

Column temperature: A constant temperature of about 25°C.

Mobile phase: Dissolve 1.6 g of sodium dihydrogen phosphate dihydrate and 16.1 g of sodium sulfate decahydrate in water to make 1000 mL, and adjust to pH 6.8 with a solution, prepared by dissolving 16.1 g of sodium sulfate decahydrate in 0.01 mol/L sodium hydroxide TS to make 1000 mL.

Flow rate: Adjust so that the retention time of epoetin beta is about 18 minutes.

Time span of measurement: About 2 times as long as the retention time of epoetin beta.

System suitability—

Test for required detectability: When the procedure is run with 20 μL of diluted Epoetin Beta RS with water containing 0.05 vol% polysorbate 20 for epoetin beta (1 in 1000) under the above conditions, the peak of epoetin beta is detectable.

System performance: When the procedure is run with Epoetin Beta RS under the above conditions, the number of theoretical plates of the peak of epoetin beta is not less than 600.

System repeatability: When the test is repeated 6 times with 20 μL of Epoetin Beta RS under the above operating conditions, the relative standard deviation of the peak area of epoetin beta is not more than 1.0%.

(2) Host cell proteins—Being specified separately when the drug is granted approval based on the Law.

(3) Host cell DNA—Being specified separately when the drug is granted approval based on the Law.

Assay **(1)** Protein content—Use Epoetin Beta (Genetical Recombination) and Epoetin Beta RS as the sample solution and the standard solution, respectively. Perform the test with exactly 15 μL each of the sample solution and standard solution as directed under Liquid Chromatography <2.01> according to the following conditions, and determine the total area, A_T and A_S, of the main peak and the sub-peak of epoetin beta in each solution.

Amount (mg) of protein in 1 mL of Epoetin Beta (Genetical Recombination)
$= C_S \times A_T/A_S$

C_S: Protein concentration (mg/mL) of Epoetin Beta RS

Operating conditions—

Detector: An ultraviolet absorption photometer (wavelength: 214 nm).

Column: A stainless steel column 4.6 mm in inside diameter and 25 cm in length, packed with butylsilanized silica gel for liquid chromatography (5 μm in particle diameter).

Column temperature: A constant temperature of about 25°C.

Mobile phase A: A mixture of water, acetonitrile for liquid chromatography and trifluoroacetic acid for epoetin beta (400:100:1).

Mobile phase B: A mixture of acetonitrile for liquid chromatography, water and trifluoroacetic acid for epoetin beta (400:100:1).

Flowing of mobile phase: Control the gradient by mixing the mobile phases A and B as directed in the following table.

Time after injection of sample (min)	Mobile phase A (vol%)	Mobile phase B (vol%)
0 – 18	65 → 50	35 → 50
18 – 33	50 → 0	50 → 100
33 – 43	0	100

Flow rate: Adjust so that the retention time of the main peak of epoetin beta is about 22 minutes.

System suitability—

System performance: When the procedure is run with 15 μL of the standard solution under the above operating conditions, the main peak and the sub-peak of epoetin beta are eluted in this order, and the number of theoretical plates of the main peak is not less than 600.

System repeatability: When the test is repeated 6 times with 15 μL of the standard solution under the above operating conditions, the relative standard deviation of the total area of the main peak and the sub-peak of epoetin beta is not more than 4.0%.

(2) Specific activity—To Epoetin Beta (Genetical Recombination) add 0.1 w/v% bovine serum albumin-sodium chloride-phosphate buffer solution to make three solutions so that each mL contains epoetin beta equivalent to 5, 10 and 20 units (estimate), and use these solutions as the sample solutions (1), (2) and (3), respectively. Separately, to Epoetin Beta RS add 0.1 w/v% bovine serum albumin-sodium chloride-phosphate buffer solution to make three solutions so that each mL contains epoetin beta equivalent to 5, 10 and 20 units, and use these solutions as the standard solutions (1), (2) and (3), respectively. Divide ICR strain mice into 6 equal groups of not less than 5 mice. Inject exactly 0.2 mL each of the sample solutions and the standard solutions to ICR strain mice of each group subcutaneously on the 1st, 2nd and 3rd days. On the 4th day, collect the blood from the mice, put 20 μL each of the collected blood in 9.94 mL of blood dilution liquid, mix, and use these mixtures as the dilute blood solution. To each of the dilute blood solution add 100 μL of a hemolytic agent, mix gently to hemolyze, and count the particles of hemolytic agent-resistant red cell by using a particle counter.

Determine the potency ratio (P_r) of the sample solution to the standard solution, and calculate the unit per mg protein of Epoetin Beta (Genetical Recombination) by the following equation.

$P_r = 10^M$

$M = 4/3 \times \mathrm{i} \times T_a/T_b$

$\mathrm{i} = \log 2$

$T_a = -S_1 - S_2 - S_3 + U_1 + U_2 + U_3$

$T_b = -S_1 + S_3 - U_1 + U_3$

U_1: Sum of the responses obtained from the sample solution (1)

U_2: Sum of the responses obtained from the sample solution (2)

U_3: Sum of the responses obtained from the sample solution (3)

S_1: Sum of the responses obtained from the standard solution (1)

S_2: Sum of the responses obtained from the standard solution (2)

S_3: Sum of the responses obtained from the standard solution (3)

Specific activity (unit/mg of protein) of Epoetin Beta (Genetical Recombination)

$$= S \times P_r \times D_T/D_S/C$$

S: Potency (unit/mL) of Epoetin Beta RS
D_T: Dilution factor for the sample solution (3)
D_S: Dilution factor for the standard solution (3)
C: Protein amount (mg/mL) of Epoetin Beta (Genetical Recombination)

Containers and storage Containers—Tight containers.
Storage—Not exceeding −20°C.

Ergocalciferol

Vitamin D_2

エルゴカルシフェロール

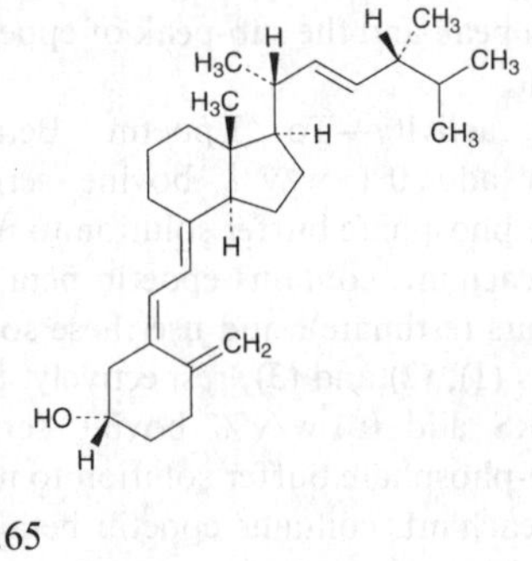

$C_{28}H_{44}O$: 396.65
(3*S*,5*Z*,7*E*,22*E*)-9,10-Secoergosta-5,7,10(19),22-tetraen-3-ol
[*50-14-6*]

Ergocalciferol contains not less than 97.0% and not more than 103.0% of ergocalciferol ($C_{28}H_{44}O$).

Description Ergocalciferol occurs as white crystals. It is odorless, or has a faint, characteristic odor.

It is freely soluble in ethanol (95), in diethyl ether and in chloroform, sparingly soluble in isooctane, and practically insoluble in water.

It is affected by air and by light.

Melting point: 115 – 118°C Transfer Ergocalciferol to a capillary tube, and dry for 3 hours in a desiccator (in vacuum at a pressure not exceeding 2.67 kPa). Immediately fire-seal the capillary tube, put it in a bath fluid, previously heated to a temperature about 10°C below the expected melting point, and heat at a rate of rise of about 3°C per minute, and read the melting point.

Identification (1) Dissolve 0.5 mg of Ergocalciferol in 5 mL of chloroform, add 0.3 mL of acetic anhydride and 0.1 mL of sulfuric acid, and shake: a red color is produced, and rapidly changes through purple and blue to green.

(2) Determine the infrared absorption spectrum of Ergocalciferol as directed in the potassium bromide disk method under Infrared Spectrophotometry *<2.25>*, and compare the spectrum with the Reference Spectrum or the spectrum of Ergocalciferol RS: both spectra exhibit similar intensities of absorption at the same wave numbers.

Absorbance *<2.24>* $E^{1\%}_{1\,cm}$ (265 nm): 445 – 485 (10 mg, ethanol (95), 100 mL).

Optical rotation *<2.49>* $[\alpha]^{20}_{D}$: +102 – +107° (0.3 g, ethanol (95), 20 mL, 100 mm). Prepare the solution of Ergocalciferol within 30 minutes after the container has been opened, and determine the rotation within 30 minutes after the solution has been prepared.

Purity Ergosterol—Dissolve 10 mg of Ergocalciferol in 2.0 mL of diluted ethanol (9 in 10), add a solution of 20 mg of digitonin in 2.0 mL of diluted ethanol (9 in 10), and allow the mixture to stand for 18 hours: no precipitate is formed.

Assay Weigh accurately about 30 mg each of Ergocalciferol and Ergocalciferol RS, and dissolve each in isooctane to make exactly 50 mL. Pipet 10 mL each of these solutions, add exactly 3 mL each of the internal standard solution, then add the mobile phase to make 50 mL, and use these solutions as the sample solution and the standard solution, respectively. Perform the test with 10 to 20 μL each of the sample solution and standard solution as directed under Liquid Chromatography *<2.01>* according to the following conditions, and calculate the ratios, Q_T and Q_S, of the peak area of ergocalciferol to that of the internal standard. Perform the procedure rapidly avoiding contact with air or other oxidizing agents and using light-resistant containers.

Amount (mg) of ergocalciferol ($C_{28}H_{44}O$) = $M_S \times Q_T/Q_S$

M_S: Amount (mg) of Ergocalciferol RS taken

Internal standard solution—A solution of dimethyl phthalate in isooctane (1 in 100).

Operating conditions—

Detector: An ultraviolet absorption photometer (wavelength: 254 nm).

Column: A stainless steel column 4.6 mm in inside diameter and 25 cm in length, packed with a silica gel for liquid chromatography (10 μm particle diameter).

Column temperature: A constant temperature of about 20°C.

Mobile phase: A mixture of hexane and *n*-amylalcohol (997:3).

Flow rate: Adjust so that the retention time of ergocalciferol is about 25 minutes.

System suitability—

System performance: Dissolve 15 mg of Ergocalciferol RS in 25 mL of isooctane. Transfer this solution to a flask, heat in an oil bath under a reflux condenser for 2 hours, and cool immediately to room temperature. Transfer the solution to a quartz test tube, and irradiate with a short-wave lamp (main wavelength: 254 nm) and a long-wave lamp (main wavelength: 365 nm) for 3 hours. To 10 mL of this solution add the mobile phase to make 50 mL. When the procedure is run with 10 μL of this solution under the above operating conditions, the ratios of the retention time of previtamin D_2, trans-vitamin D_2 and tachysterol$_2$ to that of ergocalciferol are about 0.5, about 0.6 and about 1.1, respectively, and the resolution between previtamin D_2 and trans-vitamin D_2 is not less than 0.7, and that between ergocalciferol and tachysterol$_2$ is not less than 1.0.

System repeatability: When the test is repeated 6 times with 10 μL of the standard solution under the above operating conditions, the relative standard deviation of the ratios of the peak area of ergocalciferol to that of the internal standard is not more than 1.0%.

Containers and storage Containers—Hermetic containers.

Storage—Light-resistant, under Nitrogen atmosphere, and in a cold place.

Ergometrine Maleate

エルゴメトリンマレイン酸塩

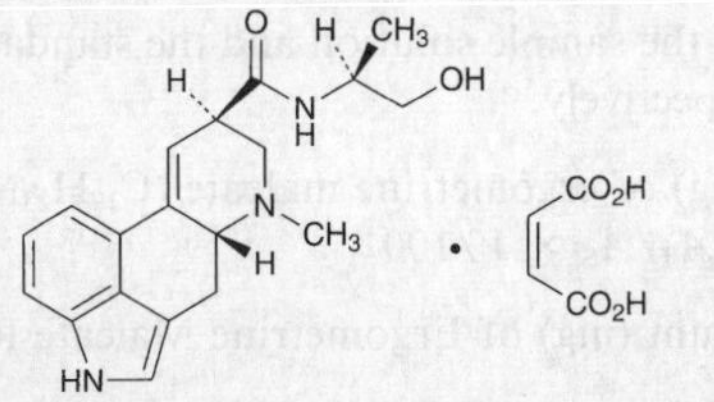

$C_{19}H_{23}N_3O_2.C_4H_4O_4$: 441.48
(8*R*)-*N*-[(2*S*)-1-Hydroxypropan-2-yl]-6-methyl-9,10-didehydroergoline-8-carboxamide monomaleate
[*129-51-1*]

Ergometrine Maleate, when dried, contains not less than 98.0% of ergometrine maleate ($C_{19}H_{23}N_3O_2.C_4H_4O_4$).

Description Ergometrine Maleate occurs as a white to pale yellow crystalline powder. It is odorless.

It is sparingly soluble in water, slightly soluble in methanol and in ethanol (95), and practically insoluble in diethyl ether.

It gradually changes to yellow in color on exposure to light.

Melting point: about 185°C (with decomposition).

Identification **(1)** Prepare a solution of Ergometrine Maleate (1 in 50): the solution shows a blue fluorescence.

(2) Dissolve 1 mg of Ergometrine Maleate in 5 mL of water. To 1 mL of this solution add 2 mL of 4-dimethylaminobenzaldehyde-ferric chloride TS, shake, and allow to stand for 5 to 10 minutes: a deep blue color develops.

(3) To 5 mL of a solution of Ergometrine Maleate (1 in 500) add 1 drop of potassium permanganate TS: the red color of the solution disappears immediately.

Optical rotation ⟨*2.49*⟩ $[\alpha]_D^{20}$ +48 – +57° (after drying, 0.25 g, water, 25 mL, 100 mm).

pH ⟨*2.54*⟩ Dissolve 0.10 g of Ergometrine Maleate in 10 mL of water. The pH of the solution is between 3.0 and 5.0.

Purity **(1)** Clarity and color of solution—Dissolve 0.10 g of Ergometrine Maleate in 10 mL of water: the solution is clear and colorless to light yellow.

(2) Ergotamine and ergotoxine—To 0.02 g of Ergometrine Maleate add 2 mL of a solution of sodium hydroxide (1 in 10), and heat to boiling: the gas evolved does not change moistened red litmus paper to blue.

(3) Related substances—Dissolve 5.0 mg each of Ergometrine Maleate and Ergometrine Maleate RS in 1.0 mL of methanol, and use these solutions as the sample solution and the standard solution, respectively. Perform the test with these solutions as directed under Thin-layer Chromatography ⟨*2.03*⟩. Spot 10 μL each of the sample solution and standard solution on a plate, prepared with silica gel for thin-layer chromatography and dilute sodium hydroxide TS. Develop the plate with a mixture of chloroform and methanol (4:1) to a distance of about 10 cm, and air-dry the plate. Spray evenly 4-dimethylaminobenzaldehyde TS on the plate: the spots obtained from the sample solution and the standard solution show a red-purple color and the same *R*f value, and any spot from the sample solution other than that corresponding to the spot from the standard solution does not appear.

Loss on drying ⟨*2.41*⟩ Not more than 2.0% (0.2 g, silica gel, 4 hours).

Assay Weigh accurately about 10 mg each of Ergometrine Maleate and Ergometrine Maleate RS, previously dried in a desiccator (silica gel) for 4 hours, dissolve in water to make exactly 250 mL, and use these solutions as the sample solution and the standard solution, respectively. Pipet 2 mL of each solution into a separate brown glass-stoppered tube. To each tube add 4 mL of 4-dimethylaminobenzaldehyde-iron (III) chloride TS, exactly measured, while cooling in an ice bath, then warm at 45°C for 10 minutes. Allow to stand at room temperature for 20 minutes, and perform the test with these solutions as directed under Ultraviolet-visible Spectrophotometry ⟨*2.24*⟩, using a solution, prepared with 2 mL of water in the same manner, as the blank. Determine the absorbances, A_T and A_S, of the subsequent solutions of the sample solution and the standard solution at 550 nm, respectively.

Amount (mg) of ergometrine maleate ($C_{19}H_{23}N_3O_2.C_4H_4O_4$)
$= M_S \times A_T/A_S$

M_S: Amount (mg) of Ergometrine Maleate RS taken

Containers and storage Containers—Tight containers.
Storage—Light-resistant.

Ergometrine Maleate Injection

エルゴメトリンマレイン酸塩注射液

Ergometrine Maleate Injection is an aqueous injection.

It contains not less than 90.0% and not more than 110.0% of the labeled amount of ergometrine maleate ($C_{19}H_{23}N_3O_2.C_4H_4O_4$: 441.48).

Method of preparation Prepare as directed under Injections, with Ergometrine Maleate.

Description Ergometrine Maleate Injection is a clear, colorless to pale yellow liquid.

pH: 2.7 – 3.5

Identification **(1)** Measure a volume of Ergometrine Maleate Injection, equivalent to 3 mg of Ergometrine Maleate, if necessary, dilute with water or evaporate on a water bath to make 15 mL, and use this solution as the sample solution. The sample solution shows a blue fluorescence.

(2) To 1 mL of the sample solution obtained in (1) add 1 mL of ammonia TS, and extract with 20 mL of diethyl ether. To the diethyl ether extract add 1 mL of dilute sulfuric acid, shake, and warm to remove diethyl ether in a water bath. Cool, to the residue obtained add 2 mL of 4-dimethylamino-benzaldehyde-iron (III) chloride TS, and allow to stand for 5 to 10 minutes: a deep blue color develops.

(3) To 5 mL of the sample solution obtained in (1) add 1 drop of potassium permanganate TS: a red color disappears immediately.

Bacterial endotoxins ⟨*4.01*⟩ Less than 1500 EU/mg.

Extractable volume ⟨*6.05*⟩ It meets the requirement.

Foreign insoluble matter ⟨*6.06*⟩ Perform the test according to Method 1: it meets the requirement.

Insoluble particulate matter ⟨*6.07*⟩ It meets the requirement.

Sterility <4.06> Perform the test according to the Membrane filtration method: it meets the requirement.

Assay Transfer an exactly measured volume of Ergometrine Maleate Injection, equivalent to about 2 mg of ergometrine maleate ($C_{19}H_{23}N_3O_2.C_4H_4O_4$), and add sodium chloride in a ratio of 0.3 g to 1 mL of the solution. To this mixture add 20 mL of diethyl ether and 2 mL of ammonia TS, shake, and extract. Further, extract with three 15-mL portions of diethyl ether, combine all the extracts, add 5 g of anhydrous sodium sulfate, filter through a pledget of absorbent cotton, and wash with three 5-mL portions of diethyl ether. Add the washings to the filtrate, shake with 5 mL of dilute sulfuric acid, evaporate the diethyl ether by warming in a current of nitrogen, to the remaining solution add water to make exactly 50 mL, and use this solution as the sample solution. Separately, weigh accurately about 2 mg of Ergometrine Maleate RS, previously dried in a desiccator (silica gel) for 4 hours, add water to make exactly 50 mL, and use this solution as the standard solution. Transfer 2 mL each of the sample solution and standard solution, accurately measured, to separate glass-stoppered test tubes, and proceed as directed in the Assay under Ergometrine Maleate.

Amount (mg) of ergometrine maleate ($C_{19}H_{23}N_3O_2.C_4H_4O_4$)
$= M_S \times A_T/A_S$

M_S: Amount (mg) of Ergometrine Maleate RS taken

Containers and storage Containers—Hermetic containers, and colored containers may be used.

Storage—Light-resistant, and in a cold place.

Ergometrine Maleate Tablets

エルゴメトリンマレイン酸塩錠

Ergometrine Maleate Tablets contain not less than 90.0% and not more than 110.0% of the labeled amount of ergometrine maleate ($C_{19}H_{23}N_3O_2.C_4H_4O_4$: 441.48).

Method of preparation Prepare as directed under Tablets, with Ergometrine Maleate.

Identification To a quantity of powdered Ergometrine Maleate Tablets, equivalent to 3 mg of Ergometrine Maleate, add 15 mL of warm water, shake, and filter: the filtrate shows a blue fluorescence. Proceed with this solution as directed in the Identification (2) and (3) under Ergometrine Maleate.

Uniformity of dosage units <6.02> Perform the test according to the following method: it meets the requirement of the Content uniformity test.

Transfer 1 tablet of Ergometrine Maleate Tablets to a brown glass-stoppered centrifuge tube, and add exactly V mL of a solution of L-tartaric acid (1 in 100) so that each mL contains about 40 μg of ergometrine maleate ($C_{19}H_{23}N_3O_2.C_4H_4O_4$). Stopper the tube, shake for 30 minutes vigorously, centrifuge, and use the supernatant liquid as the sample solution. Separately, weigh accurately about 4 mg of Ergometrine Maleate RS, previously dried in a desiccator (silica gel) for 4 hours, dissolve in water to make exactly 100 mL, and use this solution as the standard solution. Pipet 4 mL each of the sample solution and standard solution into separate brown glass-stoppered test tubes, add exactly 8 mL each of 4-dimethylaminobenzaldehyde-iron (III) chloride TS while cooling in an ice bath, after shaking, and allow to stand for 1 hour at ordinary temperature. Perform the test with these solutions as directed under Ultraviolet-visible Spectrophotometry <2.24>, using a solution, prepared with 4 mL of water in the same manner, as the blank. Determine the absorbances, A_T and A_S, of the subsequent solutions of the sample solution and the standard solution at 550 nm, respectively.

Amount (mg) of ergometrine maleate ($C_{19}H_{23}N_3O_2.C_4H_4O_4$)
$= M_S \times A_T/A_S \times V/100$

M_S: Amount (mg) of Ergometrine Maleate RS taken

Assay Weigh accurately, and powder not less the 20 Ergometrine Maleate Tablets. Weigh accurately a portion of the powder, equivalent to about 2 mg of ergometrine maleate ($C_{19}H_{23}N_3O_2.C_4H_4O_4$), transfer to a glass filter (G4), add 10 mL of a solution of L-tartaric acid (1 in 100), and filter with thorough shaking. Repeat the procedures 3 times, combine the filtrates, add a solution of L-tartaric acid (1 in 100) to make exactly 50 mL, and use this solution as the sample solution. Separately, weigh accurately about 2 mg of Ergometrine Maleate RS, previously dried in a desiccator (silica gel) for 4 hours, dissolve in a solution of L-tartaric acid (1 in 100) to make exactly 50 mL, and use this solution as the standard solution. Pipet 2 mL each of the sample solution and standard solution, and proceed as directed in the Assay under Ergometrine Maleate.

Amount (mg) of ergometrine maleate ($C_{19}H_{23}N_3O_2.C_4H_4O_4$)
$= M_S \times A_T/A_S$

M_S: Amount (mg) of Ergometrine Maleate RS taken

Containers and storage Containers—Well-closed containers.

Storage—Light-resistant.

Ergotamine Tartrate

エルゴタミン酒石酸塩

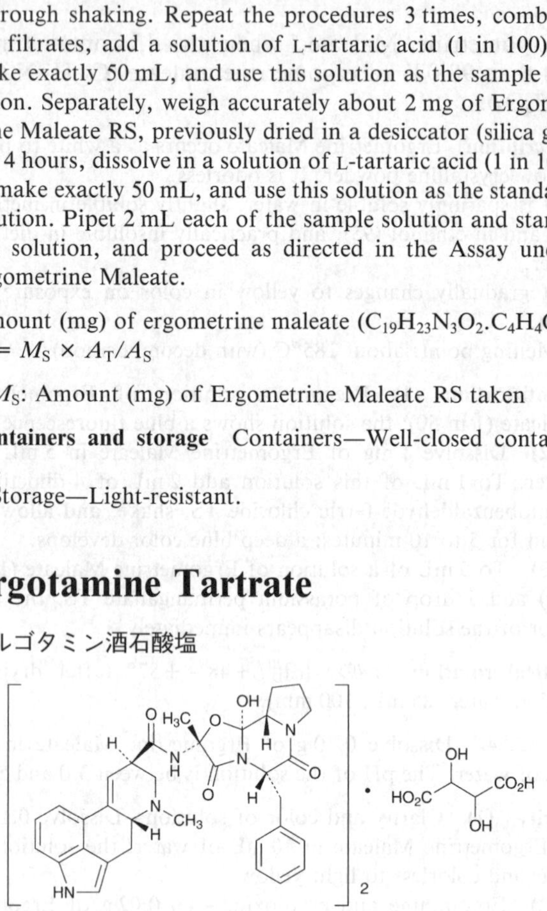

$(C_{33}H_{35}N_5O_5)_2.C_4H_6O_6$: 1313.41
(5′S)-5′-Benzyl-12′-hydroxy-2′-methylergotaman-3′,6′,18-trione hemitartrate
[379-79-3]

Ergotamine Tartrate contains not less than 98.0% of ergotamine tartrate [$(C_{33}H_{35}N_5O_5)_2.C_4H_6O_6$], calculated on the dried basis.

Description Ergotamine Tartrate occurs as colorless crystals, or a white to pale yellow-white or grayish white crystalline powder.

It is slightly soluble in water and in ethanol (95).

Melting point: about 180°C (with decomposition).

Identification (1) Dissolve 1 mg of Ergotamine Tartrate in 10 mL of a mixture of acetic acid (100) and ethyl acetate (1:1). To 0.5 mL of this solution add slowly 0.5 mL of sulfuric acid, with shaking in cold water, and allow to stand: a purple color develops. To this solution add 0.1 mL of diluted iron (III) chloride TS (1 in 12): the color of the solution changes to blue to blue-purple.

(2) Dissolve 1 mg of Ergotamine Tartrate in 5 mL of a solution of L-tartaric acid (1 in 100). To 1 mL of this solution add 2 mL of 4-dimethylaminobenzaldehyde-iron (III) chloride TS, and shake: a blue color develops.

Optical rotation <*2.49*> Ergotamine base $[\alpha]_D^{20}$: −155 – −165°. Dissolve 0.35 g of Ergotamine Tartrate in 25 mL of a solution of L-tartaric acid (1 in 100), add 0.5 g of sodium hydrogen carbonate, shake gently and sufficiently, and extract with four 10-mL portions of ethanol-free chloroform. Filter the extracts successively through a small filter paper, moistened with ethanol-free chloroform, into a 50-mL volumetric flask. Allow the flask to stand in a water bath at 20°C for 10 minutes, and determine the optical rotation in a 100-mm cell. Separately, pipet 25 mL of this solution, evaporate to dryness under reduced pressure at a temperature not higher than 45°C, dissolve the residue in 25 mL of acetic acid (100), and titrate <*2.50*> with 0.05 mol/L perchloric acid VS (indicator: 1 drop of crystal violet TS). Perform a blank determination in the same manner, and make any necessary correction. Calculate the specific rotation of the ergotamine base from the consumed volume of 0.05 mol/L perchloric acid VS and the optical rotation.

Each mL of 0.05 mol/L perchloric acid VS
= 29.08 mg of $C_{33}H_{35}N_5O_5$

Purity Related substances—Conduct this procedure without exposure to light, using light-resistant vessels. To 40 mg of Ergotamine Tartrate add 10 mL of a solution of L-tartaric acid in diluted methanol (1 in 2) (1 in 1000), dissolve with thorough shaking, and use this solution as the sample solution. Pipet 1 mL of the sample solution, add a solution of L-tartaric acid in diluted methanol (1 in 2) (1 in 1000) to make exactly 50 mL, and use this solution as the standard solution. Perform the test with these solutions as directed under Thin-layer Chromatography <*2.03*>. Spot 10 μL each of the sample solution and standard solution on a plate of silica gel for thin-layer chromatography. Develop the plate with a mixture of chloroform and methanol (9:1) to a distance of about 10 cm, and air-dry the plate. Spray evenly 4-dimethylaminobenzaldehyde TS on the plate: the spots other than the principal spot obtained from the sample solution are not more intense than the spot from the standard solution.

Loss on drying <*2.41*> Not more than 5.0% (0.1 g, in vacuum, 60°C, 4 hours).

Assay Weigh accurately about 0.2 g of Ergotamine Tartrate, dissolve in 15 mL of a mixture of acetic acid (100) and acetic anhydride (50:3), and titrate <*2.50*> with 0.05 mol/L perchloric acid VS (indicator: 1 drop of crystal violet TS). Perform a blank determination in the same manner, and make any necessary correction.

Each mL of 0.05 mol/L perchloric acid VS
= 32.84 mg of $(C_{33}H_{35}N_5O_5)_2.C_4H_6O_6$

Containers and storage Containers—Tight containers.

Storage—Light-resistant, and almost well-filled, or under nitrogen atmosphere, and not exceeding 5°C.

Eribulin Mesilate

エリブリンメシル酸塩

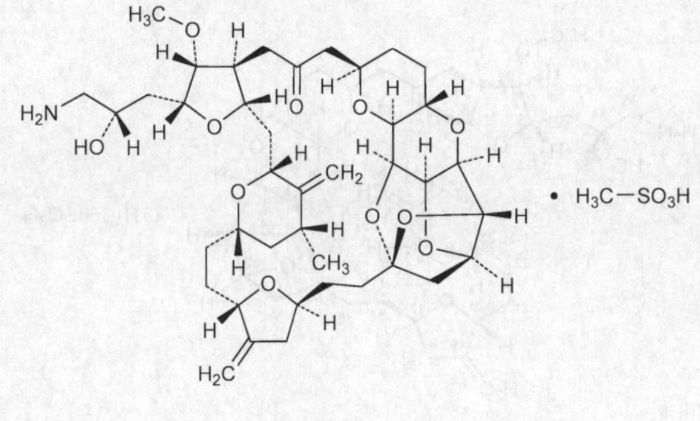

$C_{40}H_{59}NO_{11}.CH_4O_3S$: 826.00

(2*R*,3*R*,3a*S*,7*R*,8a*S*,9*S*,10a*R*,11*S*,12*R*,13a*R*,13b*S*,15*S*,18*S*,21*S*,24*S*,26*R*,28*R*,29a*S*)-2-[(2*S*)-3-Amino-2-hydroxypropyl]-3-methoxy-26-methyl-20,27-dimethylidenehexacosahydro-11,15:18,21:24,28-triepoxy-7,9-ethano-12,15-methano-9*H*,15*H*-furo[3,2-*i*]furo[2′,3′:5,6]pyrano[4,3-*b*][1,4]dioxacyclopentacosin-5(4*H*)-one monomethanesulfonate

[441045-17-6]

Eribulin Mesilate contains not less than 95.0% and not more than 102.0% of eribulin mesilate ($C_{40}H_{59}NO_{11}.CH_4O_3S$), and not less than 9.8% and not more than 12.2% of methanesulfonic acid (CH_4O_3S), calculated on the anhydrous basis.

Manufacture Eribulin Mesilate has 19 chiral carbons, and its purity tests can not estimate all isomers derived from them. Therefore, based on sound science and the understanding of the product and the manufacturing process, control and manage the isomers and related substances during manufacturing process, and ensure the three-dimensional structure of eribulin mesilate. In the quality control strategy of Eribulin Mesilate, control the related substances including the principal isomers in the drug substance or starting materials and intermediates in upstream process. The acceptance values are not more than 0.22% and not more than 0.68% for the related substances B and C, which are the isomers at position C34 and controlled in the drug substance, and are not more than the identification threshold (0.10%) for the related substances including other isomers. When Eribulin Mesilate is manufactured through the compounds 1 and 2, control as follows.

In the compound 1, control so that the isomers at positions C3 and C11, C12 *cis*-olefin, and other related substances are not more than the identification threshold (0.10%). In the compound 2, control so that the isomers at positions C17 and C29 are not more than 0.30%, and the isomer at position C20 is not more than 0.50%, the isomer at position C25 is not more than 0.40%, and the isomers at positions C23, C27, C34 and C18/C19 *endo*-olefin and the other related substances are not more than the identification threshold (0.10%).

Furthermore, ensure that the isomers at positions C17, C20, C25 and C29 are not more than the identification threshold (0.10%) in the processes after the compounds 1 and 2, and the other related substances are not more than the qualification threshold (0.15%).

When manufactured without reaction using the compounds 1 and 2, perform the control based on the control mentioned above.

The position numbers of eribulin mesilate used in this Manufacture are as follows. The numbers are used commonly for the related substances, but are not related to the position numbers prescribed by the chemical names.

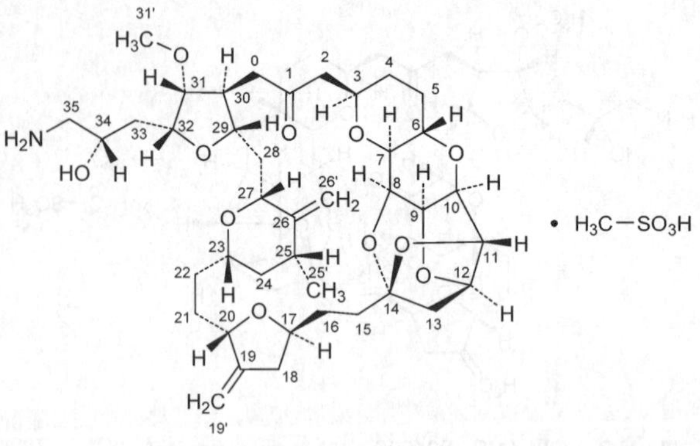

Position numbers of Eribulin Mesilate in Manufacture

Description Eribulin Mesilate occurs as a white powder.

It is freely soluble in water, in methanol, in ethanol (99.5) and in dimethylsulfoxide.

It is hygroscopic.

Identification (1) Determine the ^1H spectrum of a solution of Eribulin Mesilate in deuterated methanol for nuclear magnetic resonance spectroscopy (1 in 200), as directed under Nuclear Magnetic Resonance Spectroscopy *<2.21>*, using light hydrogen contaminated in deuterated methanol for nuclear magnetic resonance spectroscopy as an internal reference compound and the chemical shift of methyl group of deuterated methanol as δ 3.3 ppm: it exhibits a doublet signal A at around δ 1.1 ppm, a multiplet signal B at around δ 2.7 ppm and a singlet signal C at around δ 2.7 ppm, a singlet signal D at around δ 3.4 ppm, a doublet signal E at around δ 3.7 ppm, a doublet signal F at around δ 4.5 ppm, a triplet signal G at around δ 4.6 ppm, and a triplet signal H at around δ 4.7 ppm. The ratio of integrated intensity of these signals, A:B + C:D:E:F:G:H, is about 3:5:3:1:1:1:1. (When measured with a nuclear magnetic resonance spectrometer having ^1H resonance frequency of not less than or equal to 400 MHz.)

(2) Perform the test with 15 μL each of the sample solution and standard solution obtained in the Assay (2) as directed under Liquid Chromatography *<2.01>* according to the following conditions: the retention times of the peaks of methanesulfonic acid in the chromatograms obtained from the sample solution and standard solution are the same.

Operating conditions—

Proceed as directed in the operating conditions in the Assay (2).

System suitability—

Proceed as directed in the system suitability in the Assay (2).

Optical rotation *<2.49>* $[\alpha]_{365}^{20}$: -160 – $-210°$ (50 mg calculated on the anhydrous and solvent-free basis, dimethylsulfoxide, 10 mL, 100 mm).

Purity (1) Heavy metals—Being specified separately when the drug is granted approval based on the Law.

(2) Related substances—Weigh accurately about 20 mg of Eribulin Mesilate, dissolve in the dissolving solution to make exactly 5 mL, and use this solution as the sample solution. Separately, weigh accurately about 20 mg of Eribulin Mesilate RS (separately determine the water *<2.48>* in the same manner as Eribulin Mesilate), dissolve in the dissolving solution to make exactly 5 mL. Pipet 1 mL of this solution, add the dissolving solution to make exactly 100 mL, and use this solution as the standard solution. Perform the test with exactly 5 μL each of the sample solution and standard solution as directed under Liquid Chromatography *<2.01>* according to the following conditions. Determine each peak area, A_T, of the related substances in the sample solution and the peak area, A_S, of eribulin in the standard solution by the automatic integration method, and calculate the amounts of the related substances by the following formula: the amounts of related substance A having the relative retention time of about 0.29 to eribulin, related substance B having the relative retention time of about 0.87, related substance C having the relative retention time of about 1.07, related substance D having the relative retention time of about 1.29, related substance E having the relative retention time of about 1.37, and related substance F having the relative retention time of about 1.67, are not more than 0.15%, 0.22%, 0.68%, 0.50%, 0.15%, and 0.19%, respectively, and other related substances are not more than 0.10%. Furthermore, the total amount of these related substances is not more than 3.0%.

$$\text{Amount (\%) of related substance} = M_S/M_T \times A_T/A_S$$

M_S: Amount (mg) of Eribulin Mesilate RS taken, calculated on the anhydrous basis

M_T: Amount (mg) of Eribulin Mesilate taken, calculated on the anhydrous basis

Dissolving solution—A mixture of water, acetonitrile for liquid chromatography and phosphoric acid (6500:3500:7) adjusted to pH 6.9 – 7.1 with diluted ammonium water (28) (1 in 5) or 1 mol/L hydrochloric acid TS.

Operating conditions—

Detector, column, column temperature, mobile phase, and flow rate: Proceed as directed in the operating conditions in the Assay (1).

Time span of measurement: For 85 minutes after injection, beginning after the solvent peak.

System suitability—

System performance: Proceed as directed in the system suitability in the Assay (1).

Test for required detectability: Pipet 1 mL of the standard solution, and add the dissolving solution to make exactly 20 mL. Confirm that the peak area of eribulin obtained with 5 μL of this solution is equivalent to 3.5 to 6.5% of that with 5 μL of the standard solution.

System repeatability: When the test is repeated 5 times with 5 μL of the solution for system suitability test obtained in the Assay (1) under the above operating conditions, the relative standard deviation of the peak area of eribulin is not more than 1.0%.

(3) Residual solvent—Being specified separately when the drug is granted approval based on the Law.

Water *<2.48>* Not more than 3.0% (Weigh accurately 15-25 mg of Eribulin Mesilate, dissolve in 2.5 mL of methanol for water determination, and perform the test with exactly 1 mL of this solution; coulometric titration).

Assay (1) Eribulin Mesilate—Weigh accurately about 20 mg each of Eribulin Mesilate and Eribulin Mesilate RS (separately determine the water *<2.48>* in the same manner as Eribulin Mesilate), dissolve each in the dissolving solution to make exactly 5 mL, and use these solutions as the sample solution and the standard solution. Perform the test with exactly 5 μL each of the sample solution and standard solution as directed under Liquid Chromatography *<2.01>* according to the following conditions, and determine the peak areas,

A_T and A_S, of eribulin in each solution.

Amount (mg) of eribulin mesilate ($C_{40}H_{59}NO_{11}.CH_4O_3S$)
$= M_S \times A_T/A_S$

M_S: Amount (mg) of Eribulin Mesilate RS taken, calculated on the anhydrous basis

Dissolving solution—A mixture of water, acetonitrile for liquid chromatography and phosphoric acid (6500:3500:7) adjusted to pH 6.9 - 7.1 with diluted ammonia water (28) (1 in 5) or 1 mol/L hydrochloric acid TS.

Operating conditions—

Detector: An ultraviolet absorption photometer (wavelength: 200 nm).

Column: A stainless steel column 3 mm in inside diameter and 15 cm in length, packed with octadecylsilanized silica gel for liquid chromatography (3 μm in particle diameter).

Column temperature: A constant temperature of about 40°C.

Mobile phase A: Dissolve 7.0 g of ammonium trifluoromethanesulfonate in 760 mL of water, add 3.0 mL of a solution of tetrabutylammonium dihydrogen phosphate (17 in 50) and 240 mL of acetonitrile for liquid chromatography, and adjust to pH 6.9 - 7.1 with diluted ammonium water (28) (1 in 5) or 1 mol/L hydrochloric acid TS.

Mobile phase B: Dissolve 7.0 g of ammonium trifluoromethanesulfonate in 300 mL of water, add 3.0 mL of a solution of tetrabutylammonium dihydrogen phosphate (17 in 50), 700 mL of acetonitrile for liquid chromatography and 20 mL of 2-propanol for liquid chromatography, and adjust to pH 6.9 - 7.1 with diluted ammonium water (28) (1 in 5) or 1 mol/L hydrochloric acid TS.

Flowing of mobile phase: Control the gradient by mixing the mobile phases A and B as directed in the following table.

Time after injection of sample (min)	Mobile phase A (vol%)	Mobile phase B (vol%)
0 - 55	100	0
55 - 75	100 → 0	0 → 100
75 - 85	0	100
85 - 86	0 → 100	100 → 0
86 - 105	100	0

Flow rate: Control the flow rate as directed in the following table.

Time after injection of sample (min)	Flow rate (mL/minute)
0 - 55	0.50
55 - 75	0.50 → 0.63
75 - 105	0.63

System suitability—

System performance: Dissolve 2 mg of Eribulin Mesilate Related Substance C for System Suitability RS in the dissolving solution to make exactly 50 mL. To 0.2 mL of this solution add 4 mg of Eribulin Mesilate RS, dissolve in the dissolving solution to make exactly 1 mL, and use this solution as the solution for system suitability test. When the procedure is run with 5 μL of the solution for system suitability test under the above operating conditions, eribulin and the related substance C are eluted in this order with the resolution between these peaks being not less than 1.5. The number of theoretical plates and the symmetry factor of the peak of eribulin are not less than 13,500 and not more than 1.5, respectively.

System repeatability: When the test is repeated 5 times with 5 μL of the solution for system suitability test under the above operating conditions, the relative standard deviation of the peak area of eribulin is not more than 1.0%.

(2) Methanesulfonic acid—Weigh accurately about 50 mg of Eribulin Mesilate, dissolve in a mixture of the mobile phase and acetonitrile for liquid chromatography (13:7) to make exactly 10 mL, and use this solution as the sample solution. Separately, weigh accurately about 50 mg of methanesulfonic acid, dissolve in a mixture of the mobile phase and acetonitrile for liquid chromatography (13:7) to make exactly 100 mL, and use this solution as the standard solution. Perform the test with 15 μL each of the sample solution and standard solution as directed under Liquid Chromatography <*2.01*> according to the following conditions, and determine the peak areas, A_T and A_S, of methanesulfonic acid in each solution. Calculate the content of methanesulfonic acid by the following formula.

Content (%) of methanesulfonic acid (CH_4O_3S)
$= M_S \times A_T/A_S \times 1/10$

M_S: Amount (mg) of methanesulfonic acid taken

Operating conditions—

Detector: An electric conductivity detector.

Column: A stainless steel column 4.6 mm in inside diameter and 25 cm in length, packed with aminopropylsilanized silica gel for liquid chromatography (5 μm in particle diameter).

Column temperature: A constant temperature of about 40°C.

Mobile phase: Dissolve 2.8 g of sodium dihydrogen phosphate monohydrate in 950 mL of water, add 11 μL of phosphoric acid, adjust to pH 4.2 - 4.3 with phosphoric acid if necessary, and add 50 mL of acetonitrile for liquid chromatography.

Flow rate: Adjust so that the retention time of methanesulfonic acid is about 6.5 minutes.

System suitability—

System performance: When the procedure is run with 15 μL of the standard solution under the above operating conditions, the number of theoretical plates and the symmetry factor of the peak of methanesulfonic acid are not less than 12,000 and not more than 0.7 - 1.5, respectively.

System repeatability: When the test is repeated 6 times with 15 μL of the standard solution under the above operating conditions, the relative standard deviation of the peak area of methanesulfonic acid is not more than 3.0%.

Containers and storage Containers—Tight containers.

Storage—Light-resistant, at a temperature not exceeding −65°C.

Others

Compound 1:
Methyl{(2*R*,4a*S*,6*S*,7*R*,8*S*,8a*S*)-7,8-bis{[(1,1-dimethylethyl)dimethylsilyl]oxy}-6-[(1*S*,2*E*)-1-{[(1,1-dimethylethyl)dimethylsilyl]oxy}-3-iodoprop-2-en-1-yl]octahydropyrano[3,2-*b*]pyran-2-yl}acetate

Compound 2:
3-[(2*S*,5*S*)-5-{2-[(2*S*,4*R*,6*R*)-6-({(2*S*,3*S*,4*R*,5*R*)-5-[(2*S*)-2,3-Bis{[(1,1-dimethylethyl)dimethylsilyl]oxy}propyl]-4-methoxy-3-[(phenylsulfonyl)methyl]tetrahydrofuran-2-yl}methyl)-4-methyl-5-methylidenetetrahydro-2*H*-pyran-2-yl]ethyl}-4-methylidenetetrahydrofuran-2-yl]propan-1-ol

Related substance A:
(1*R*,3*S*,8*S*,11*S*,14*S*,16*R*,18*R*,20*S*,22*R*,23*R*,24*S*,28*R*,31*S*,33*S*,34*R*,35*S*,37*S*)-22-[(2*S*)-3-Amino-2-hydroxypropyl]-34,37-dihydroxy-23-methoxy-16-methyl-10,17-dimethylidene-2,21,32,36,38,39-hexaoxaheptacyclo[26.6.2.1^{3,33}.1^{8,11}.1^{14,18}.0^{20,24}.0^{31,35}]nonatriacontane-5,26-dione

Related substance B:
(2*R*,3*R*,3a*S*,7*R*,8a*S*,9*S*,10a*R*,11*S*,12*R*,13a*R*,13b*S*,15*S*,18*S*,21*S*,24*S*,26*R*,28*R*,29a*S*)-2-[(2*R*)-3-Amino-2-hydroxypropyl]-3-methoxy-26-methyl-20,27-dimethylidenehexacosahydro-11,15:18,21:24,28-triepoxy-7,9-ethano-12,15-methano-9*H*,15*H*-furo[3,2-*i*]furo[2′,3′:5,6]pyrano[4,3-*b*][1,4]dioxacyclopentacosin-5(4*H*)-one

Related substance C:
(2*R*,3*R*,3a*S*,7*R*,8a*S*,9*S*,10a*R*,11*S*,12*R*,13a*R*,13b*S*,15*S*,18*S*,21*S*,24*S*,26*R*,28*R*,29a*S*)-2-[(2*R*)-2-Amino-3-hydroxypropyl]-3-methoxy-26-methyl-20,27-dimethylidenehexacosahydro-11,15:18,21:24,28-triepoxy-7,9-ethano-12,15-methano-9*H*,15*H*-furo[3,2-*i*]furo[2′,3′:5,6]pyrano[4,3-*b*][1,4]dioxacyclopentacosin-5(4*H*)-one

Related substance D:
(1*R*,2*S*,3*S*,4*S*,5*S*,6*R*,11*S*,14*S*,17*S*,19*R*,21*R*,23*S*,25*R*,26*R*,27*S*,31*R*,34*S*)-25-[(2*S*)-3-Amino-2-hydroxypropyl]-2,5-dihydroxy-26-methoxy-19-methyl-13,20-dimethylidene-24,35,36,37,38,39-hexaoxaheptacyclo[29.3.1.1^{3,6}.1^{4,34}.1^{11,14}.1^{17,21}.0^{23,27}]nonatriacontane-8,29-dione

Related substance E:
(1*R*,2*S*,3*S*,4*S*,5*S*,6*S*,11*S*,14*S*,17*S*,19*R*,21*R*,23*S*,25*R*,26*R*,27*S*,31*R*,34*S*)-25-[(2*S*)-3-Amino-2-hydroxypropyl]-2,5-dihydroxy-26-methoxy-19-methyl-13,20-dimethylidene-24,35,36,37,38,39-hexaoxaheptacyclo[29.3.1.1^{3,6}.1^{4,34}.1^{11,14}.1^{17,21}.0^{23,27}]nonatriacontane-8,29-dione

Related substance F:
(2*R*,3*R*,3a*S*,7*R*,8a*S*,9*S*,10a*R*,11*S*,12*R*,13a*R*,13b*S*,15*S*,18*S*,21*S*,24*S*,26*R*,28*R*,29a*S*)-2-[(2*S*)-2,3-Dihydroxypropyl]-3-methoxy-26-methyl-20,27-dimethylidenehexacosahydro-

11,15:18,21:24,28-triepoxy-7,9-ethano-12,15-methano-9*H*,15*H*-furo[3,2-*i*]furo[2′,3′:5,6]pyrano[4,3-*b*][1,4]dioxacyclopentacosin-5(4*H*)-one

Erythromycin

エリスロマイシン

$C_{37}H_{67}NO_{13}$: 733.93
(2*R*,3*S*,4*S*,5*R*,6*R*,8*R*,10*R*,11*R*,12*S*,13*R*)-5-(3,4,6-Trideoxy-3-dimethylamino-β-D-*xylo*-hexopyranosyloxy)-3-(2,6-dideoxy-3-*C*-methyl-3-*O*-methyl-α-L-*ribo*-hexopyranosyloxy)-6,11,12-trihydroxy-2,4,6,8,10,12-hexamethyl-9-oxopentadecan-13-olide
[*114-07-8*]

Erythromycin is a macrolide substance having antibacterial activity produced by the growth of *Saccharopolyspora erythraea*.

It contains not less than 930 μg (potency) and not more than 1020 μg (potency) per mg, calculated on the anhydrous basis. The potency of Erythromycin is expressed as mass (potency) of erythromycin ($C_{37}H_{67}NO_{13}$).

Description Erythromycin occurs as a white to light yellow-white powder.

It is freely soluble in methanol and in ethanol (95), and very slightly soluble in water.

Identification **(1)** Determine the infrared absorption spectrum of Erythromycin as directed in the potassium bromide disk method under Infrared Spectrophotometry *<2.25>*, and compare the spectrum with the Reference Spectrum or the spectrum of Erythromycin RS: both spectra exhibit similar intensities of absorption at the same wave numbers.

(2) Dissolve 10 mg each of Erythromycin and Erythromycin RS in 1 mL of methanol, and use these solutions as the sample solution and standard solution. Perform the test with these solutions as directed under Thin-layer Chromatography *<2.03>*. Spot 5 μL each of the sample solution and standard solution on a plate of silica gel for thin-layer chromatography. Develop the plate with a mixture of methanol and ammonia solution (28) (50:1) to a distance of about 10 cm, and air-dry the plate. Spray evenly 4-methoxybenzaldehyde-sulfuric acid TS on the plate, and heat at 100°C for 15 minutes: the principal spot from the sample solution and the spot from the standard solution are dark purple in color, and their *Rf* values are the same.

Optical rotation *<2.49>* $[\alpha]_D^{20}$: −71 − −78° (1 g calculated on the anhydrous basis, ethanol (95), 50 mL, 100 mm).

Purity **(1)** Heavy metals *<1.07>*—Proceed with 1.0 g of Erythromycin according to Method 4, and perform the test. Prepare the control solution with 2.0 mL of Standard Lead Solution (not more than 20 ppm).

(2) Related substances—Dissolve 40 mg of Erythromycin in 2 mL of methanol, add a mixture of phosphate buffer solution (pH 7.0) and methanol (15:1) to make exactly 10 mL, and use this solution as the sample solution. Separately, dissolve 16 mg of Erythromycin RS in 2 mL of methanol, add a mixture of phosphate buffer solution (pH 7.0) and methanol (15:1) to make exactly 10 mL, and use this solution as the standard stock solution. Dissolve 5 mg each of erythromycin B and erythromycin C in 2 mL of methanol, add exactly 2 mL of the standard stock solution, add a mixture of phosphate buffer solution (pH 7.0) and methanol (15:1) to make exactly 25 mL, and use this solution as the standard solution. Perform the test with exactly 100 μL each of the sample solution and standard solution as directed under Liquid Chromatography *<2.01>* according to the following conditions, and determine each peak area by the automatic integration method: the peak areas of erythromycin B and erythromycin C obtained from the sample solution are not larger than those of erythromycin B and erythromycin C from the standard solution, respectively, and the area of the peaks other than erythromycin, erythromycin B and erythromycin C from the sample solution is not larger than the peak area of erythromycin from the standard solution.

Operating conditions—

Detector: An ultraviolet absorption photometer (wavelength: 215 nm).

Column: A stainless steel column 4.6 mm in inside diameter and 25 cm in length, packed with styrene-divinylbenzene copolymer for liquid chromatography (8 μm in particle diameter).

Column temperature: A constant temperature of about 70°C.

Mobile phase: Dissolve 3.5 g of dipotassium hydrogen phosphate in water to make 100 mL, and adjust the pH to 9.0 with diluted phosphoric acid (1 in 10). To 50 mL of this solution add 190 mL of *t*-butyl alcohol, 30 mL of acetonitrile and water to make 1000 mL.

Flow rate: Adjust so that the retention time of erythromycin is about 20 minutes.

Time span of measurement: About 4 times as long as the retention time of erythromycin, beginning after the solvent peak.

System suitability—

System performance: Dissolve 2 mg of *N*-demethylerythromycin in 10 mL of the standard solution. When the procedure is run with 100 μL of this solution under the above operating conditions, *N*-demethylerythromycin, erythromycin C, erythromycin and erythromycin B are eluted in this order, with the resolution between the peaks of *N*-demethylerythromycin and erythromycin C being not less than 0.8 and with the resolution between the peaks of *N*-demethylerythromycin and erythromycin being not less than 5.5.

System repeatability: When the test is repeated 3 times with 100 μL of the standard solution under the above operat-

ing conditions, the relative standard deviation of the peak area of erythromycin is not more than 3.0%.

Water <*2.48*> Not more than 10.0% (0.2 g, volumetric titration, direct titration).

Residue on ignition <*2.44*> Not more than 0.2% (1 g).

Assay Perform the test according to the Cylinder-plate method as directed under Microbial Assay for Antibiotics <*4.02*> according to the following conditions.

(i) Test organism—*Staphylococcus aureus* ATCC 6538 P

(ii) Culture medium—Use the medium i in 3) Medium for other organisms under (1) Agar media for seed and base layer. Adjust the pH of the medium so that it will be 7.8 to 8.0 after sterilization.

(iii) Standard solutions—Weigh accurately an amount of Erythromycin RS, equivalent to about 25 mg (potency), dissolve in 25 mL of methanol, add 0.1 mol/L phosphate buffer solution (pH 8.0) to make exactly 100 mL, and use this solution as the standard stock solution. Keep the standard stock solution at 5°C or below, and use within 7 days. Take exactly a suitable amount of the standard stock solution before use, add 0.1 mol/L phosphate buffer solution (pH 8.0) to make solutions so that each mL contains 20 μg (potency) and 5 μg (potency), and use these solutions as the high concentration standard solution and the low concentration standard solution, respectively.

(iv) Sample solutions—Weigh accurately an amount of Erythromycin, equivalent to about 25 mg (potency), dissolve in 25 mL of methanol, and add 0.1 mol/L phosphate buffer solution (pH 8.0) to make exactly 100 mL. Take exactly a suitable amount of this solution, add 0.1 mol/L phosphate buffer solution (pH 8.0) to make solutions so that each mL contains 20 μg (potency) and 5 μg (potency), and use these solutions as the high concentration sample solution and the low concentration sample solution, respectively.

Containers and storage Containers—Well-closed containers.

Erythromycin Delayed-release Tablets

エリスロマイシン腸溶錠

Erythromycin Delayed-release Tablets contain not less than 90.0% and not more than 110.0% of the labeled potency of erythromycin ($C_{37}H_{67}NO_{13}$: 733.93).

Method of preparation Prepare as directed under Tablets, with Erythromycin.

Identification To a quantity of powdered Erythromycin Delayed-release Tablets, equivalent to 10 mg (potency) of Erythromycin, add 1 mL of methanol, shake well, filter, and use the filtrate as the sample solution. Separately, dissolve 10 mg of Erythromycin RS in 1 mL of methanol, and use this solution as the standard solution. Then, proceed as directed in the Identification (2) under Erythromycin.

Loss on drying <*2.41*> Not more than 10.0% (0.2 g, in vacuum not exceeding 0.67 kPa, 60°C, 3 hours).

Uniformity of dosage units <*6.02*> It meets the requirement of the Mass variation test.

Disintegration <*6.09*> It meets the requirement. For the test with 2nd fluid for disintegration test, use the disk.

Assay Perform the test according to the Cylinder-plate method as directed under Microbial Assay for Antibiotics <*4.02*> according to the following conditions.

(i) Test organism, culture medium, and standard solutions—Proceed as directed in the Assay under Erythromycin.

(ii) Sample solutions—Weigh accurately the mass of not less than 20 Erythromycin Delayed-release Tablets, and powder. Weigh accurately a portion of the powder, equivalent to about 25 mg (potency) of Erythromycin, add 25 mL of methanol, shake vigorously, add 0.1 mol/L phosphate buffer solution (pH 8.0) to make exactly 100 mL, and filter. Take exactly an appropriate volume of the filtrate, add 0.1 mol/L phosphate buffer solution (pH 8.0) to prepare solutions containing 20 μg (potency) and 5 μg (potency) per mL, and use these solutions as the high and the low concentration sample solutions, respectively.

Containers and storage Containers—Well-closed containers.

Erythromycin Ethylsuccinate

エリスロマイシンエチルコハク酸エステル

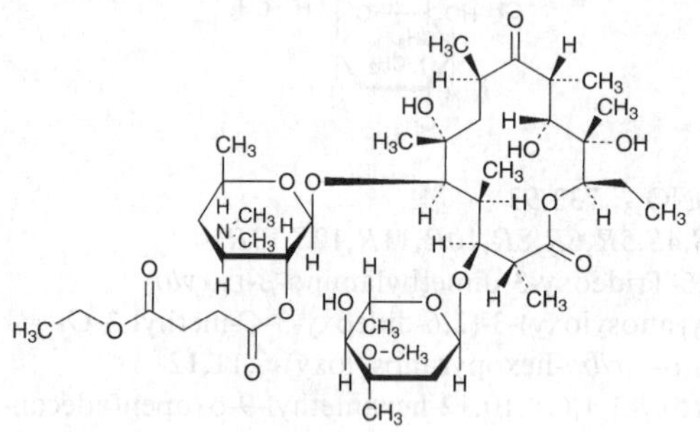

$C_{43}H_{75}NO_{16}$: 862.05
(2*R*,3*S*,4*S*,5*R*,6*R*,8*R*,10*R*,11*R*,12*S*,13*R*)-5-[3,4,6-Trideoxy-2-*O*-(3-ethoxycarbonylpropanoyl)-3-dimethylamino-*β*-D-*xylo*-hexopyranosyloxy]-3-(2,6-dideoxy-3-*C*-methyl-3-*O*-methyl-*α*-L-*ribo*-hexopyranosyloxy)-6,11,12-trihydroxy-2,4,6,8,10,12-hexamethyl-9-oxopentadecan-13-olide
[*41342-53-4*]

Erythromycin Ethylsuccinate is a derivative of erythromycin.

It contains not less than 780 μg (potency) and not more than 900 μg (potency) per mg, calculated on the anhydrous basis. The potency of Erythromycin Ethylsuccinate is expressed as mass (potency) of erythromycin ($C_{37}H_{67}NO_{13}$: 733.93).

Description Erythromycin Ethylsuccinate occurs as a white powder.

It is freely soluble in methanol and in acetone, soluble in ethanol (95), and practically insoluble in water.

Identification **(1)** Dissolve 3 mg of Erythromycin Ethylsuccinate in 2 mL of acetone, and add 2 mL of hydrochloric acid: an orange color develops and is immediately changed to red to deep purple.

(2) Determine the infrared absorption spectrum of Erythromycin Ethylsuccinate, previously dried in a desiccator (reduced pressure, silica gel) for 24 hours, as directed in the potassium bromide disk method under Infrared Spectrophotometry <2.25>, and compare the spectrum with the Reference Spectrum: both spectra exhibit similar intensities of absorption at the same wave numbers.

Water <2.48> Not more than 5.0% (0.5 g, volumetric titration, direct titration).

Assay Perform the test according to the Cylinder-plate method as directed under Microbial Assay for Antibiotics <4.02> according to the following conditions.

(i) Test organism—*Staphylococcus aureus* ATCC 6538 P

(ii) Culture medium—Use the medium i in 3) Medium for other organisms under (1) Agar media for seed and base layer. Adjust the pH of the medium so that it will be 7.8 to 8.0 after sterilization.

(iii) Standard solutions—Weigh accurately an amount of Erythromycin RS, equivalent to about 50 mg (potency), dissolve in 50 mL of methanol, add 0.1 mol/L phosphate buffer solution (pH 8.0) to make exactly 100 mL, and use this solution as the standard stock solution. Keep the standard stock solution at 5°C or below and use within 7 days. Take exactly a suitable amount of the standard stock solution before use, add 0.1 mol/L phosphate buffer solution (pH 8.0) to make solutions so that each mL contains 20 μg (potency) and 5 μg (potency), and use these solutions as the high concentration standard solution and the low concentration standard solution, respectively.

(iv) Sample solutions—Weigh accurately an amount of Erythromycin Ethylsuccinate, equivalent to about 50 mg (potency), dissolve in 50 mL of methanol, and add 0.1 mol/L phosphate buffer solution (pH 8.0) to make exactly 100 mL. Take exactly a suitable amount of the solution, add 0.1 mol/L phosphate buffer solution (pH 8.0) to make solutions so that each mL contains 20 μg (potency) and 5 μg (potency), and use these solutions as the high concentration sample solution and the low concentration sample solution, respectively.

Containers and storage Containers—Tight containers.

Erythromycin Lactobionate

エリスロマイシンラクトビオン酸塩

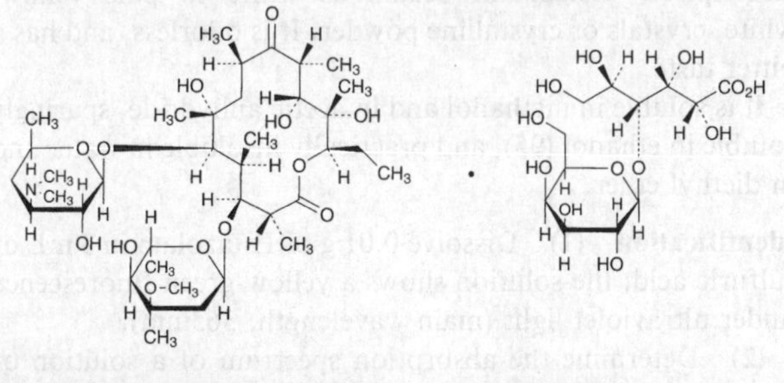

$C_{37}H_{67}NO_{13}.C_{12}H_{22}O_{12}$: 1092.22
(2*R*,3*S*,4*S*,5*R*,6*R*,8*R*,10*R*,11*R*,12*S*,13*R*)-5-(3,4,6-Trideoxy-3-dimethylamino-*β*-D-*xylo*-hexopyranosyloxy)-3-(2,6-dideoxy-3-*C*-methyl-3-*O*-methyl-*α*-L-*ribo*-hexopyranosyloxy)-6,11,12-trihydroxy-2,4,6,8,10,12-hexamethyl-9-oxopentadecan-13-olide mono(4-*O*-*β*-D-galactopyranosyl-D-gluconate)
[*3847-29-8*]

Erythromycin Lactobionate is the lactobionate of erythromycin.

It contains not less than 590 μg (potency) and not more than 700 μg (potency) per mg, calculated on the anhydrous basis. The potency of Erythromycin Lactobionate is expressed as mass (potency) of erythromycin ($C_{37}H_{67}NO_{13}$: 733.93).

Description Erythromycin Lactobionate occurs as a white powder.

It is freely soluble in water, in methanol and in ethanol (99.5), and very slightly soluble in acetone.

Identification **(1)** To 3 mg of Erythromycin Lactobionate add 2 mL of acetone, and add 2 mL of hydrochloric acid: an orange color is produced, and it changes immediately to red to deep purple.

(2) Transfer about 0.3 g of Erythromycin Lactobionate to a separator, add 15 mL of ammonia TS and 15 mL of chloroform, shake, and take the separated aqueous layer. Wash the aqueous layer with three 15-mL portions of chloroform, and evaporate the aqueous liquid on a water bath to dryness. Dissolve the residue in 10 mL of a mixture of methanol and water (3:2), and use this solution as the sample solution. Separately, dissolve 0.10 g of lactobionic acid in 10 mL of a mixture of methanol and water (3:2), and use this solution as the standard solution. Perform the test with these solutions as directed under Thin-layer Chromatography <2.03>. Spot 10 μL each of the sample solution and standard solution on a plate of silica gel for thin-layer chromatography. Develop the plate with the upper layer obtained from a mixture of water, 1-butanol and acetic acid (100) (3:3:1) to a distance of about 10 cm, and air-dry the plate. Spray evenly dilute sulfuric acid, and heat at 105°C for 20 minutes: the principal spot obtained from the sample solution shows a deep brown and the *R*f value which are the same as those of the principal spot from the standard solution.

pH <2.54> The pH of a solution obtained by dissolving 0.5 g of Erythromycin Lactobionate in 10 mL of water is between 5.0 and 7.5.

Water <2.48> Not more than 5.0% (0.5 g, volumetric titration, direct titration).

Assay Perform the test according to the Cylinder-plate method as directed under Microbial Assay for Antibiotics <4.02> according to the following conditions.

(i) Test organism—*Staphylococcus aureus* ATCC 6538 P

(ii) Culture medium—Use the medium i in 3) Medium for other organisms under (1) Agar media for seed and base layer. Adjust the pH of the medium so that it will be 7.8 to 8.0 after sterilization.

(iii) Standard solutions—Weigh accurately an amount of Erythromycin RS, equivalent to about 50 mg (potency), dissolve in 50 mL of methanol, add 0.1 mol/L phosphate buffer solution (pH 8.0) to make exactly 100 mL, and use this solution as the standard stock solution. Keep the standard stock solution at not exceeding 5°C and use within 7 days. Take exactly a suitable amount of the standard stock solution before use, add 0.1 mol/L phosphate buffer solution (pH 8.0) to make solutions so that each mL contains 20 μg (potency) and 5 μg (potency), and use these solutions as the high concentration standard solution and the low concentration standard solution, respectively.

(iv) Sample solutions—Weigh accurately an amount of Erythromycin Lactobionate, equivalent to about 50 mg (potency), dissolve in 50 mL of methanol, and add 0.1 mol/L phosphate buffer solution (pH 8.0) to make exactly 100 mL. Take exactly a suitable amount of this solution, add 0.1 mol/L phosphate buffer solution (pH 8.0) to make solutions so that each mL contains 20 μg (potency) and 5 μg (potency), and use these solutions as the high concentration sample solution and the low concentration sample solution, respectively.

Containers and storage Containers—Tight containers.

Erythromycin Stearate

エリスロマイシンステアリン酸塩

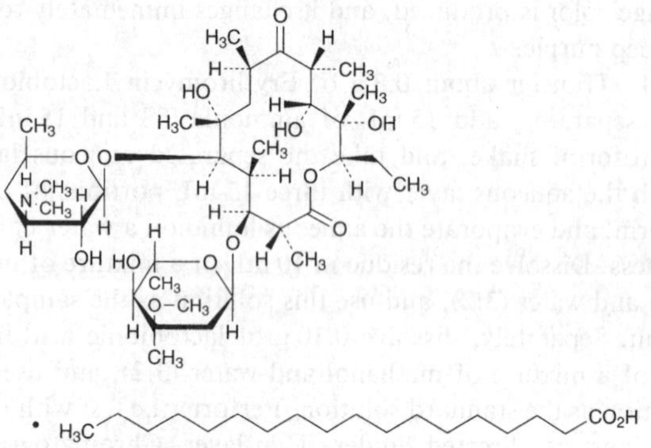

$C_{37}H_{67}NO_{13}.C_{18}H_{36}O_2$: 1018.40
(2*R*,3*S*,4*S*,5*R*,6*R*,8*R*,10*R*,11*R*,12*S*,13*R*)-5-(3,4,6-Trideoxy-3-dimethylamino-*β*-D-*xylo*-hexopyranosyloxy)-3-(2,6-dideoxy-3-*C*-methyl-3-*O*-methyl-*α*-L-*ribo*-hexopyranosyloxy)-6,11,12-trihydroxy-2,4,6,8,10,12-hexamethyl-9-oxopentadecan-13-olide monostearate
[*643-22-1*]

Erythromycin Stearate is the stearate of erythromycin.

It contains not less than 600 *μ*g (potency) and not more than 720 *μ*g (potency) per mg, calculated on the anhydrous basis. The potency of Erythromycin Stearate is expressed as mass (potency) of erythromycin ($C_{37}H_{67}NO_{13}$: 733.93).

Description Erythromycin Stearate occurs as a white powder.

It is freely soluble in ethanol (95) and in acetone, soluble in methanol, and practically insoluble in water.

Identification **(1)** Dissolve 3 mg of Erythromycin Stearate in 2 mL of acetone, and add 2 mL of hydrochloric acid: an orange color develops and is immediately changed to red to deep purple.

(2) Determine the infrared absorption spectrum of Erythromycin Stearate, previously dried in a desiccator (reduced pressure, silica gel) for 24 hours, as directed in the potassium bromide disk method under Infrared Spectrophotometry <*2.25*>, and compare the spectrum with the Reference Spectrum: both spectra exhibit similar intensities of absorption at the same wave numbers.

Water <*2.48*> Not more than 5.0% (0.5 g, volumetric titration, direct titration).

Assay Perform the test according to the Cylinder-plate method as directed under Microbial Assay for Antibiotics <*4.02*> according to the following conditions.

(i) Test organism—*Staphylococcus aureus* ATCC 6538 P

(ii) Culture medium—Use the medium i in 3) Medium for other organisms under (1) Agar media for seed and base layer. Adjust the pH of the medium so that it will be 7.8 to 8.0 after sterilization.

(iii) Standard solutions—Weigh accurately an amount of Erythromycin RS equivalent to about 50 mg (potency), dissolve in 50 mL of methanol, add 0.1 mol/L phosphate buffer solution (pH 8.0) to make exactly 100 mL, and use this solution as the standard stock solution. Keep the standard stock solution at 5°C or below and use within 7 days. Take exactly a suitable amount of the standard stock solution before use, add 0.1 mol/L phosphate buffer solution (pH 8.0) to make solutions so that each mL contains 20 *μ*g (potency) and 5 *μ*g (potency), and use these solutions as the high concentration standard solution and the low concentration standard solution, respectively.

(iv) Sample solutions—Weigh accurately an amount of Erythromycin Stearate equivalent to about 50 mg (potency), dissolve in 50 mL of methanol, and add 0.1 mol/L phosphate buffer solution (pH 8.0) to make exactly 100 mL. Take exactly a suitable amount of the solution, add 0.1 mol/L phosphate buffer solution (pH 8.0) to make solutions so that each mL contains 20 *μ*g (potency) and 5 *μ*g (potency), and use these solutions as the high concentration sample solution and the low concentration sample solution, respectively.

Containers and storage Containers—Tight containers.

Estazolam

エスタゾラム

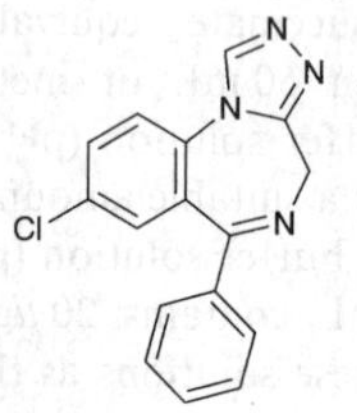

$C_{16}H_{11}ClN_4$: 294.74
8-Chloro-6-phenyl-4*H*-[1,2,4]triazolo[4,3-*a*][1,4]benzodiazepine
[*29975-16-4*]

Estazolam, when dried, contains not less than 98.5% of estazolam ($C_{16}H_{11}ClN_4$).

Description Estazolam occurs as white to pale yellow-white, crystals or crystalline powder. It is odorless, and has a bitter taste.

It is soluble in methanol and in acetic anhydride, sparingly soluble in ethanol (95), and practically insoluble in water and in diethyl ether.

Identification **(1)** Dissolve 0.01 g of Estazolam in 3 mL of sulfuric acid: the solution shows a yellow-green fluorescence under ultraviolet light (main wavelength: 365 nm).

(2) Determine the absorption spectrum of a solution of Estazolam in 1 mol/L hydrochloric acid TS (1 in 100,000) as directed under Ultraviolet-visible Spectrophotometry <*2.24*>, and compare the spectrum with the Reference Spectrum: both spectra exhibit similar intensities of absorption at the same wavelengths.

(3) Perform the test with Estazolam as directed under Flame Coloration Test <*1.04*> (2): a green color appears.

Melting point <*2.60*> 229 – 233°C

Purity **(1)** Clarity and color of solution—Dissolve 0.10 g of Estazolam in 10 mL of ethanol (95): the solution is clear and colorless.

(2) Chloride <*1.03*>—Dissolve 1.0 g of Estazolam in 10 mL of ethanol (95) by heating, add 40 mL of water, cool with shaking in ice water, allow to stand to attain ordinary temperature, and filter. To 30 mL of the filtrate add 6 mL of dilute nitric acid and water to make 50 mL, and perform the test using this solution as the test solution. Prepare the control solution with 0.25 mL of 0.01 mol/L hydrochloric acid VS and 6 mL of ethanol (95) (not more than 0.015%).

(3) Heavy metals ⟨*1.07*⟩—Proceed with 1.0 g of Estazolam according to Method 2, and perform the test. Prepare the control solution with 2.0 mL of Standard Lead Solution (not more than 20 ppm).

(4) Arsenic ⟨*1.11*⟩—Prepare the test solution with 1.0 g of Estazolam according to Method 3, and perform the test (not more than 2 ppm).

(5) Related substances—Dissolve 0.20 g of Estazolam in 10 mL of methanol, and use this solution as the sample solution. Pipet 1 mL of the sample solution, add methanol to make exactly 200 mL, and use this solution as the standard solution. Perform the test with these solutions as directed under Thin-layer Chromatography ⟨*2.03*⟩. Spot 10 μL each of the sample solution and standard solution on a plate of silica gel with fluorescent indicator for thin-layer chromatography. Develop the plate with a mixture of hexane, chloroform and methanol (5:3:1) to a distance of about 10 cm, and air-dry the plate. Examine the plate under ultraviolet light (main wavelength: 254 nm): the spots other than the principal spot obtained from the sample solution are not more intense than the principal spot from the standard solution.

Loss on drying ⟨*2.41*⟩ Not more than 1.0% (1 g, 105°C, 4 hours).

Residue on ignition ⟨*2.44*⟩ Not more than 0.1% (2 g).

Assay Weigh accurately about 0.25 g of Estazolam, previously dried, dissolve in 100 mL of acetic anhydride, and titrate ⟨*2.50*⟩ with 0.1 mol/L perchloric acid VS (potentiometric titration), until the solution changes to the second equivalence point. Perform a blank determination in the same manner, and make any necessary correction.

Each mL of 0.1 mol/L perchloric acid VS
= 14.74 mg of $C_{16}H_{11}ClN_4$

Containers and storage Containers—Well-closed containers.

Estradiol Benzoate

エストラジオール安息香酸エステル

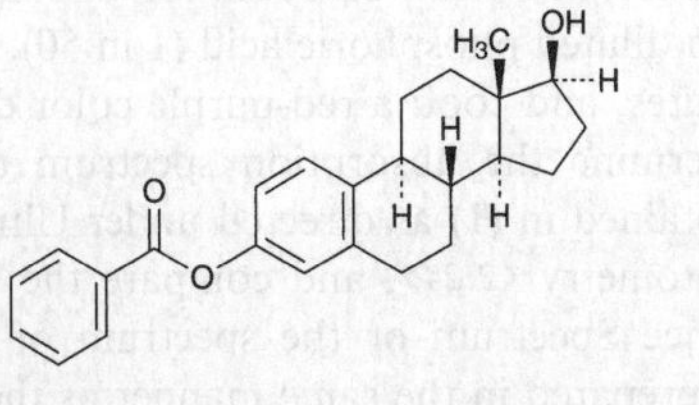

$C_{25}H_{28}O_3$: 376.49
Estra-1,3,5(10)-triene-3,17*β*-diol 3-benzoate
[*50-50-0*]

Estradiol Benzoate, when dried, contains not less than 97.0% of estradiol benzoate ($C_{25}H_{28}O_3$).

Description Estradiol Benzoate occurs as a white crystalline powder. It is odorless.

It is sparingly soluble in acetone, slightly soluble in methanol, in ethanol (95) and in diethyl ether, and practically insoluble in water.

Identification **(1)** To 2 mg of Estradiol Benzoate add 2 mL of sulfuric acid: a yellowish green color with a blue fluorescence is produced, and the color of the solution changes to light orange on the careful addition of 2 mL of water.

(2) Determine the infrared absorption spectrum of Estradiol Benzoate, previously dried, as directed in the potassium bromide disk method under Infrared Spectrophotometry ⟨*2.25*⟩, and compare the spectrum with the Reference Spectrum or the spectrum of dried Estradiol Benzoate RS: both spectra exhibit similar intensities of absorption at the same wave numbers.

Optical rotation ⟨*2.49*⟩ $[\alpha]_D^{20}$: +54 – +58° (after drying, 0.1 g, acetone, 10 mL, 100 mm).

Melting point ⟨*2.60*⟩ 191 – 198°C

Purity **(1)** 3,17*α*-Estradiol—Dissolve 5.0 mg each of Estradiol Benzoate and Estradiol Benzoate RS in acetone to make exactly 100 mL, and use these solutions as the sample solution and the standard solution, respectively. Place exactly 2 mL each of the sample solution and standard solution in separate glass-stoppered test tube, add boiling stones, evaporate the acetone by heating in a water bath, and dry the residue in a desiccator (in vacuum, phosphorus (V) oxide) for 1 hour. Add 1.0 mL of dilute iron-phenol TS to each test tube. Stopper the test tubes loosely, heat for 30 seconds in a water bath, shake in a water bath for several seconds, and heat for 2 minutes. Cool the solutions in ice for 2 minutes, add 4.0 mL of diluted sulfuric acid (7 in 20), and mix well: the solution obtained from the sample solution has no more color than that from the standard solution.

(2) Related substances—Dissolve 40 mg of Estradiol Benzoate in 2 mL of acetone, and use this solution as the sample solution. Pipet 1 mL of the sample solution, add acetone to make exactly 100 mL, and use this solution as the standard solution. Perform the test with these solutions as directed under Thin-layer Chromatography ⟨*2.03*⟩. Spot 10 μL each of the sample solution and standard solution on a plate of silica gel with fluorescent indicator for thin-layer chromatography. Develop the plate with a mixture of chloroform and diethylamine (19:1) to a distance of about 15 cm, and air-dry the plate. Examine under ultraviolet light (main wavelength: 254 nm): the spots other than the principal spot obtained from the sample solution are not more intense than the spot from the standard solution.

Loss on drying ⟨*2.41*⟩ Not more than 0.5% (0.5 g, in vacuum, phosphorus (V) oxide, 4 hours).

Residue on ignition ⟨*2.44*⟩ Not more than 0.2% (0.1 g).

Assay Weigh accurately about 10 mg each of Estradiol Benzoate and Estradiol Benzoate RS, previously dried, and dissolve each in methanol to make exactly 20 mL. Pipet 5 mL each of these solutions, add 5 mL of the internal standard solution, then add methanol to make 20 mL, and use these solutions as the sample solution and the standard solution, respectively. Perform the test with 5 μL of the sample solution and standard solution as directed under Liquid Chromatography ⟨*2.01*⟩ according to the following conditions, and calculate the ratios, Q_T and Q_S, of the peak area of estradiol benzoate to that of the internal standard.

Amount (mg) of estradiol benzoate ($C_{25}H_{28}O_3$)
$= M_S \times Q_T/Q_S$

M_S: Amount (mg) of Estradiol Benzoate RS taken

Internal standard solution—A solution of progesterone in methanol (13 in 80,000).

Operating conditions—

Detector: An ultraviolet absorption photometer (wavelength: 230 nm).

Column: A stainless steel column 4.6 mm in inside diameter and 15 cm in length, packed with octadecylsilanized silica gel for liquid chromatography (5 μm in particle diameter).

Column temperature: A constant temperature of about 35°C.

Mobile phase: A mixture of acetonitrile and water (7:3).

Flow rate: Adjust so that the retention time of estradiol benzoate is about 10 minutes.

System suitability—

System performance: When the procedure is run with 5 μL of the standard solution under the above operating conditions, the internal standard and estradiol benzoate are eluted in this order with the resolution between these peaks being not less than 9.

System repeatability: When the test is repeated 6 times with 5 μL of the standard solution under the above operating conditions, the relative standard deviation of the ratios of the peak area of estradiol benzoate to that of the internal standard is not more than 1.0%.

Containers and storage Containers—Tight containers.

Storage—Light-resistant.

Estradiol Benzoate Injection (Aqueous Suspension)

エストラジオール安息香酸エステル水性懸濁注射液

Estradiol Benzoate Injection (Aqueous Suspension) is an aqueous suspension for injection.

It contains not less than 90.0% and not more than 110.0% of the labeled amount of estradiol benzoate ($C_{25}H_{28}O_3$: 376.49).

Method of preparation Prepare as directed under Injection, with Estradiol Benzoate.

Description Estradiol Benzoate Injection (Aqueous Suspension) produces a white turbidity on shaking.

Identification Extract a volume of Estradiol Benzoate Injection (Aqueous Suspension), equivalent to 1 mg of Estradiol Benzoate, with 5 mL of chloroform, and use this extract as the sample solution. Separately, dissolve 1 mg of Estradiol Benzoate RS in 5 mL of chloroform, and use this solution as the standard solution. Perform the test with these solutions as directed under Thin-layer Chromatography <*2.03*>. Spot 50 μL each of the sample solution and standard solution on a plate of silica gel with fluorescent indicator for thin-layer chromatography. Develop the plate with a mixture of chloroform and methanol (99:1) to a distance of about 15 cm, and air-dry the plate. Examine under ultraviolet light (main wavelength: 254 nm): the principal spot obtained from the sample solution and the spot from the standard solution show the same *R*f value.

Extractable volume <*6.05*> It meets the requirement.

Foreign insoluble matter <*6.06*> Perform the test according to Method 1: it meets the requirement.

Sterility <*4.06*> Perform the test according to the Direct inoculation method: it meets the requirement.

Assay Measure exactly a volume of well-mixed Estradiol Benzoate Injection (Aqueous Suspension), equivalent to about 2 mg of estradiol benzoate ($C_{25}H_{28}O_3$), dissolve the crystals with an appropriate quantity of methanol, and add methanol to make exactly 20 mL. Pipet 10 mL of this solution, add exactly 10 mL of the internal standard solution, add methanol to make 100 mL, and use this solution as the sample solution. Separately, weigh accurately about 10 mg of Estradiol Benzoate RS, previously dried in desiccator (reduced pressure, phosphorus (V) oxide) for 4 hours, and dissolve in methanol to make exactly 100 mL. Pipet 10 mL of this solution, add exactly 10 mL of the internal standard solution and methanol to make 100 mL, and use this solution as the standard solution. Proceed with these solutions as directed in the Assay under Estradiol Benzoate.

Amount (mg) of estradiol benzoate ($C_{25}H_{28}O_3$)
$= M_S \times Q_T/Q_S \times 1/5$

M_S: Amount (mg) of Estradiol Benzoate RS taken

Internal standard solution—A solution of progesterone in methanol (13 in 100,000).

Containers and storage Containers—Hermetic containers.

Estriol

エストリオール

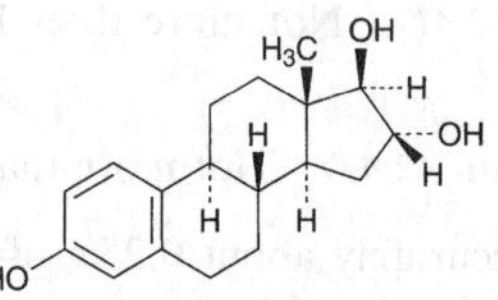

$C_{18}H_{24}O_3$: 288.38
Estra-1,3,5(10)-triene-3,16α,17β-triol
[50-27-1]

Estriol, when dried, contains not less than 97.0% and not more than 102.0% of estriol ($C_{18}H_{24}O_3$).

Description Estriol occurs as a white crystalline powder. It is odorless.

It is sparingly soluble in methanol, slightly soluble in ethanol (99.5), and practically insoluble in water.

Identification **(1)** Dissolve 0.01 g of Estriol in 100 mL of ethanol (95) by warming, and use this solution as the sample solution. Evaporate 1 mL of the sample solution on a water bath to dryness, add 5 mL of a solution of sodium *p*-phenolsulfonate in diluted phosphoric acid (1 in 50), heat at 150°C for 10 minutes, and cool: a red-purple color develops.

(2) Determine the absorption spectrum of the sample solution obtained in (1) as directed under Ultraviolet-visible Spectrophotometry <*2.24*>, and compare the spectrum with the Reference Spectrum or the spectrum of a solution of Estriol RS prepared in the same manner as the sample solution: both spectra exhibit similar intensities of absorption at the same wavelengths.

(3) Determine the infrared absorption spectrum of Estriol, previously dried, as directed in the potassium bromide disk method under Infrared Spectrophotometry <*2.25*>, and compare the spectrum with the Reference Spectrum or the spectrum of previously dried Estriol RS: both spectra exhibit similar intensities of absorption at the same wave numbers.

Optical rotation <*2.49*> $[\alpha]_D^{25}$: +55 – +65° (after drying, 40 mg, ethanol (99.5), 10 mL, 100 mm).

Melting point *<2.60>* 281 - 286°C

Purity **(1)** Heavy metals *<1.07>*—Proceed with 1.0 g of Estriol according to Method 2, and perform the test. Prepare the control solution with 2.0 mL of Standard Lead Solution (not more than 20 ppm).

(2) Related substances—Dissolve 40 mg of Estriol in 10 mL of ethanol (95) by warming, and use this solution as the sample solution. Pipet 1 mL of the sample solution, add ethanol (95) to make exactly 100 mL, and use this solution as the standard solution. Perform the test with these solutions as directed under Thin-layer Chromatography *<2.03>*. Spot 5 μL each of the sample solution and standard solution on a plate of silica gel for thin-layer chromatography. Develop the plate with a mixture of chloroform, methanol, acetone and acetic acid (100) (18:1:1:1) to a distance of about 15 cm, and air-dry the plate. Spray evenly diluted sulfuric acid (1 in 2) on the plate, and heat at 105°C for 15 minutes: the spots other than the principal spot obtained from the sample solution are not more intense than the spot from the standard solution.

Loss on drying *<2.41>* Not more than 0.5% (0.5 g, 105°C, 3 hours).

Residue on ignition *<2.44>* Not more than 0.1% (0.5 g).

Assay Weigh accurately about 25 mg each of Estriol and Estriol RS, previously dried, and dissolve each in methanol to make exactly 50 mL. Pipet 10 mL each of these solutions, add exactly 5 mL of the internal standard solution, add methanol to make 100 mL, and use these solutions as the sample solution and the standard solution, respectively. Perform the test with 10 μL each of the sample solution and standard solution as directed under Liquid Chromatography *<2.01>* according to the following conditions, and calculate the ratios, Q_T and Q_S, of the peak area of estriol to that of the internal standard.

$$\text{Amount (mg) of estriol } (C_{18}H_{24}O_3) = M_S \times Q_T/Q_S$$

M_S: Amount (mg) of Estriol RS taken

Internal standard solution—A solution of methyl benzoate for estriol test in methanol (1 in 1000).

Operating conditions—

Detector: An ultraviolet absorption photometer (wavelength: 280 nm).

Column: A stainless steel column 4.6 mm in inside diameter and 15 cm in length, packed with octadecylsilanized silica gel for liquid chromatography (5 μm in particle diameter).

Column temperature: A constant temperature of about 25°C.

Mobile phase: A mixture of water and methanol (51:49).

Flow rate: Adjust so that the retention time of estriol is about 10 minutes.

System suitability—

System performance: When the procedure is run with 10 μL of the standard solution under the above operating conditions, estriol and the internal standard are eluted in this order with the resolution between these peaks being not less than 8.

System repeatability: When the test is repeated 6 times with 10 μL of the standard solution under the above operating conditions, the relative standard deviation of the ratios of the peak area of estriol to that of the internal standard is not more than 1.0%.

Containers and storage Containers—Tight containers.

Estriol Injection (Aqueous Suspension)

エストリオール水性懸濁注射液

Estriol Injection (Aqueous Suspension) is an aqueous suspension for injection.

It contains not less than 90.0% and not more than 110.0% of the labeled amount of estriol ($C_{18}H_{24}O_3$: 288.38).

Method of preparation Prepare as directed under Injections, with Estriol.

Description Shake Estriol Injection (Aqueous Suspension): a white turbidity is produced.

Identification **(1)** Shake well, take a volume of Estriol Injection (Aqueous Suspension), equivalent to 2 mg of Estriol, add ethanol (95) to make 20 mL, and use this solution as the sample solution. Proceed with the sample solution as directed in the Identification (1) under Estriol.

(2) Determine the absorption spectrum of the sample solution obrtained in (1) as directed under Ultraviolet-visible Spectrophotometry *<2.24>*: it exhibits a maximum between 279 nm and 283 nm.

Extractable volume *<6.05>* It meets the requirement.

Foreign insoluble matter *<6.06>* Perform the test according to Method 1: it meets the requirement.

Sterility *<4.06>* Perform the test according to the Direct inoculation method: it meets the requirement.

Assay Shake well, pipet a volume of Estriol Injection (Aqueous Suspension), equivalent to about 5 mg of estriol ($C_{18}H_{24}O_3$), and dissolve in methanol to make exactly 20 mL. Pipet 4 mL of this solution, add exactly 5 mL of the internal standard solution, then add methanol to make 50 mL, and use this solution as the sample solution. Separately, weigh accurately about 25 mg of Estriol RS, previously dried at 105°C for 3 hours, and dissolve in methanol to make exactly 100 mL. Pipet 4 mL of this solution, add exactly 5 mL of the internal standard solution, then add methanol to make 50 mL, and use this solution as the standard solution. Proceed as directed in the Assay under Estriol.

$$\text{Amount (mg) of estriol } (C_{18}H_{24}O_3) = M_S \times Q_T/Q_S \times 1/5$$

M_S: Amount (mg) of Estriol RS taken

Internal standard solution—A solution of methyl benzoate for estriol test in ethanol (95) (1 in 5000).

Containers and storage Containers—Hermetic containers.

Estriol Tablets

エストリオール錠

Estriol Tablets contain not less than 90.0% and not more than 110.0% of the labeled amount of estriol ($C_{18}H_{24}O_3$: 288.38).

Method of preparation Prepare as directed under Tablets, with Estriol.

Identification **(1)** Weigh a portion of powdered Estriol

Tablets, equivalent to 2 mg of Estriol, add 20 mL of ethanol (95), shake for 10 minutes, centrifuge, and use the supernatant liquid as the sample solution. Proceed with the sample solution as directed in the Identification (1) under Estriol.

(2) Determine the absorption spectrum of the sample solution obtained in (1) as directed under Ultraviolet-visible Spectrophotometry *<2.24>*: it exhibits a maximum between 279 nm and 283 nm.

Uniformity of dosage units *<6.02>* Perform the test according to the following method: it meets the requirement of the Content uniformity test.

To 1 tablet of Estriol Tablets add exactly 5 mL of water, disperse the fine particles by sonicating, add exactly 15 mL of methanol, and shake for 15 minutes. Centrifuge this solution for 10 minutes, pipet a definite amount of the supernatant liquid, and add methanol to make exactly a definite amount of solution so that each ml of the solution contains about 5 μg of estriol ($C_{18}H_{24}O_3$). Pipet 5 mL of this solution, add exactly 1 mL of the internal standard solution, and use this solution as the sample solution. Proceed with 20 μL of the sample solution as directed in the Assay under Estriol. Use a solution of methyl benzoate for estriol test in methanol (1 in 40,000) as the internal standard solution. Calculate the mean value from each ratio of peak areas of 10 samples: the samples conform to the requirements if the deviation (%) of the mean value and each ratio of peak areas is within 15%. If the deviation (%) exceeds 15%, and 1 sample shows deviation within 25%, repeat the test with 20 samples. Calculate the deviation (%) of the mean value from each ratio of peak areas of the 30 samples used in the 2 tests and each ratio of peak areas: the samples conform to the requirements if the deviation exceeds 15%, not more than 1 sample shows deviation within 25%, and no sample shows deviation exceeding 25%.

Dissolution *<6.10>* When the test is performed at 50 revolutions per minute according to the Paddle method, using 900 mL of water as the dissolution medium, the dissolution rate in 30 minutes of Estriol Tablets is not less than 80%.

Start the test with 1 tablet of Estriol Tablets, withdraw not less than 20 mL of the medium at the specified minute after starting the test, and filter through a membrane filter with a pore size not exceeding 0.8 μm. Discard not less than 10 mL of the first filtrate, pipet V mL of the subsequent filtrate, add water to make exactly V' mL so that each mL contains about 0.1 μg of estriol ($C_{18}H_{24}O_3$), and use this solution as the sample solution. Separately, weigh accurately about 10 mg of Estriol RS, previously dried at 105°C for 3 hours, dissolve in methanol to make exactly 100 mL, then pipet 5 mL of this solution, and add water to make exactly 100 mL. Pipet 2 mL of this solution, add water to make exactly 100 mL, and use this solution as the standard solution. Perform the test with exactly 100 μL each of the sample solution and standard solution as directed under Liquid chromatography *<2.01>* according to the following conditions, and determine the peak areas, A_T and A_S, of estriol.

Dissolution rate (%) with respect to the labeled amount of estriol ($C_{18}H_{24}O_3$)
$$= M_S \times A_T/A_S \times V'/V \times 1/C \times 9/10$$

M_S: Amount (mg) of Estriol RS taken
C: Labeled amount (mg) of estriol ($C_{18}H_{24}O_3$) in 1 tablet

Operating conditions—

Proceed as directed in the operating conditions in the Assay under Estriol.

System suitability—

Proceed as directed in the system suitability in the Assay under Estriol.

Assay Weigh accurately and powder not less than 20 Estriol Tablets. Weigh accurately a portion of the powder, equivalent to about 1 mg of estriol ($C_{18}H_{24}O_3$), add exactly 5 mL of water, disperse the fine particles by sonicating, shake with 25 mL of methanol for 10 minutes, centrifuge, and take the supernatant liquid. Add 25 mL of methanol, repeat the above procedure twice, combine the supernatant liquid, add exactly 5 mL of the internal standard solution, then add methanol to make 100 mL, and use this solution as the sample solution. Separately, weigh accurately about 25 mg of Estriol RS, previously dried at 105°C for 3 hours, and dissolve in methanol to make exactly 100 mL. Pipet 4 mL of this solution, add exactly 5 mL of the internal standard solution, then add methanol to make 100 mL, and use this solution as the standard solution. Proceed with 20 μL each of the sample solution and standard solution as directed in the Assay under Estriol.

Amount (mg) of estriol ($C_{18}H_{24}O_3$)
$$= M_S \times Q_T/Q_S \times 1/25$$

M_S: Amount (mg) of Estriol RS taken

*Internal standard solution—*A solution of methyl benzoate for estriol test in methanol (1 in 5000).

Containers and storage Containers—Tight containers.

Etacrynic Acid

エタクリン酸

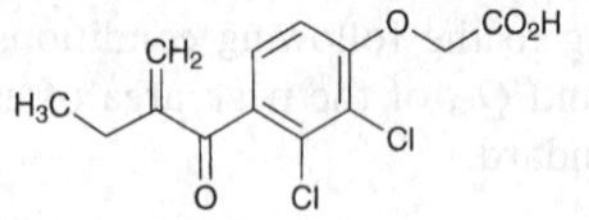

$C_{13}H_{12}Cl_2O_4$: 303.14
[2,3-Dichloro-4-(2-ethylacryloyl)phenoxy]acetic acid
[58-54-8]

Etacrynic Acid, when dried, contains not less than 98.0% of etacrynic acid ($C_{13}H_{12}Cl_2O_4$).

Description Etacrynic Acid occurs as a white crystalline powder. It is odorless, and has a slightly bitter taste.

It is very soluble in methanol, freely soluble in ethanol (95), in acetic acid (100) and in diethyl ether, and very slightly soluble in water.

Identification **(1)** Dissolve 0.2 g of Etacrynic Acid in 10 mL of acetic acid (100), and to 5 mL of this solution add 0.1 mL of bromine TS: the color of the test solution disappears. To the remaining 5 mL of the solution add 0.1 mL of potassium permanganate TS: the color of the test solution changes to light orange immediately.

(2) To 0.01 g of Etacrynic Acid add 1 mL of sodium hydroxide TS, and heat in a water bath for 3 minutes. After cooling, add 1 mL of chromotropic acid TS, and heat in a water bath for 10 minutes: a deep purple color develops.

(3) Determine the absorption spectrum of a solution of Etacrynic Acid in methanol (1 in 20,000) as directed under Ultraviolet-visible Spectrophotometry *<2.24>*, and compare the spectrum with the Reference Spectrum: both spectra exhibit similar intensities of absorption at the same wavelengths.

(4) Perform the test with Etacrynic Acid as directed under Flame Coloration Test <*1.04*> (2): a green color appears.

Melting point <*2.60*> 121 – 125°C

Purity **(1)** Clarity and color of solution—Dissolve 1.0 g of Etacrynic Acid in 10 mL of methanol: the solution is clear and colorless.

(2) Heavy metals <*1.07*>—Proceed with 1.0 g of Etacrynic Acid according to Method 4, and perform the test. Prepare the control solution with 2.0 mL of Standard Lead Solution (not more than 20 ppm).

(3) Arsenic <*1.11*>—Prepare the test solution with 1.0 g of Etacrynic Acid according to Method 3, and perform the test. Add 10 mL of a solution of magnesium nitrate hexahydrate in ethanol (95) (1 in 50), then add 1.5 mL of hydrogen peroxide (30), and fire to burn (not more than 2 ppm).

(4) Related substances—Dissolve 0.20 g of Etacrynic Acid in 10 mL of ethanol (95), and use this solution as the sample solution. Pipet 3 mL of the sample solution, add ethanol (95) to make exactly 200 mL, and use this solution as the standard solution. Perform the test with these solutions as directed under Thin-layer Chromatography <*2.03*>. Spot 10 μL each of the sample solution and standard solution on a plate of silica gel with fluorescent indicator for thin-layer chromatography. Develop the plate with a mixture of chloroform, ethyl acetate and acetic acid (100) (6:5:2) to a distance of about 15 cm, and air-dry the plate. Examine under ultraviolet light (main wavelength: 254 nm): the spots other than the principal spot obtained from the sample solution are not more intense than the spot from the standard solution.

Loss on drying <*2.41*> Not more than 0.25% (1 g, in vacuum, 60°C, 2 hours).

Residue on ignition <*2.44*> Not more than 0.1% (1 g).

Assay Weigh accurately about 0.1 g of Etacrynic Acid, previously dried, place in an iodine bottle, dissolve in 20 mL of acetic acid (100), and add exactly 20 mL of 0.05 mol/L bromine VS. To this solution add 3 mL of hydrochloric acid, stopper tightly at once, shake, and allow to stand in a dark place for 60 minutes. Add carefully 50 mL of water and 15 mL of potassium iodide TS, stopper tightly at once, shake well, and titrate <*2.50*> the liberated iodine with 0.1 mol/L sodium thiosulfate VS (indicator: 1 mL of starch TS). Perform a blank determination in the same manner.

Each mL of 0.05 mol/L bromine VS
= 15.16 mg of $C_{13}H_{12}Cl_2O_4$

Containers and storage Containers—Well-closed containers.

Etacrynic Acid Tablets

エタクリン酸錠

Etacrynic Acid Tablets contain not less than 90.0% and not more than 110.0% of the labeled amount of etacrynic acid ($C_{13}H_{12}Cl_2O_4$: 303.14).

Method of preparation Prepare as directed under Tablets, with Etacrynic Acid.

Identification **(1)** Weigh a quantity of powdered Etacrynic Acid Tablets, equivalent to 0.3 g of Etacrynic Acid, add 25 mL of 0.1 mol/L hydrochloric acid TS, and extract with 50 mL of dichloromethane. Filter the dichloromethane extract, and evaporate the filtrate on a water bath to dryness. Proceed with the residue as directed in the Identification (1), (2) and (4) under Etacrynic Acid.

(2) Prepare a solution of the residue obtained in (1), equivalent to a solution of Etacrynic Acid in methanol (1 in 20,000), and determine the absorption spectrum of this solution as directed under Ultraviolet-visible Spectrophotometry <*2.24*>: it exhibits a maximum between 268 nm and 272 nm.

Dissolution <*6.10*> When the test is performed at 50 revolutions per minute according to the Paddle method, using 900 mL of water as the dissolution medium, the dissolution rate in 45 minutes of Etacrynic Acid Tablets is not less than 70%.

Start the test with 1 tablet of Etacrynic Acid Tablets, withdraw not less than 20 mL of the medium at the specified minute after starting the test, and filter through a membrane filter with a pore size not exceeding 0.8 μm. Discard not less than 10 mL of the first filtrate, pipet V mL of the subsequent filtrate, add water to make exactly V' mL so that each mL contains about 28 μg of etacrynic acid ($C_{13}H_{12}Cl_2O_4$), and use this solution as the sample solution. Separately, weigh accurately about 55 mg of etacrynic acid for assay, previously dried in vacuum at 60°C for 2 hours, dissolve in 10 mL of methanol, and add water to make exactly 100 mL. Pipet 5 mL of this solution, add water to make exactly 100 mL, and use this solution as the standard solution. Determine the absorbances, A_T and A_S, at 277 nm of the sample solution and standard solution as directed under Ultraviolet-visible Spectrophotometry <*2.24*>, using water as the blank.

Dissolution rate (%) with respect to the labeled amount of etacrynic acid ($C_{13}H_{12}Cl_2O_4$)
$= M_S \times A_T/A_S \times V'/V \times 1/C \times 45$

M_S: Amount (mg) of etacrynic acid for assay taken
C: Labeled amount (mg) of etacrynic acid ($C_{13}H_{12}Cl_2O_4$) in 1 tablet

Assay Weigh accurately and powder not less than 20 Etacrynic Acid Tablets. Weigh accurately a portion of the powder, equivalent to about 0.1 g of etacrynic acid ($C_{13}H_{12}Cl_2O_4$), add 25 mL of 0.1 mol/L hydrochloric acid TS, and extract with three 30-mL portions of dichloromethane. Filter the dichloromethane extracts through a pledget of absorbent cotton into an iodine bottle. Wash the pledget of absorbent cotton with a small amount of dichloromethane, and combine the washing with the extracts. Evaporate this solution on a water bath to dryness in a current of air, to the residue add 20 mL of acetic acid (100), and proceed as directed in the Assay under Etacrynic Acid.

Each mL of 0.05 mol/L bromine VS
= 15.16 mg of $C_{13}H_{12}Cl_2O_4$

Containers and storage Containers—Well-closed containers.

Ethambutol Hydrochloride

エタンブトール塩酸塩

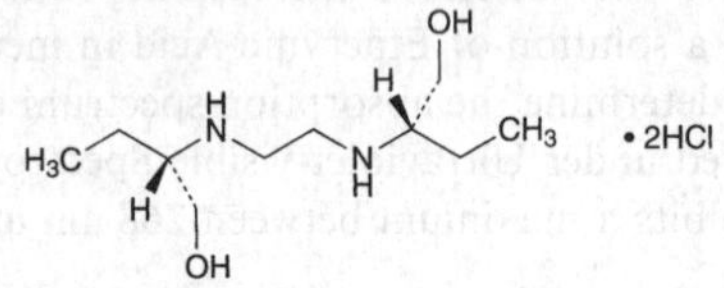

$C_{10}H_{24}N_2O_2.2HCl$: 277.23
(2*S*,2′*S*)-2,2′-(Ethane-1,2-diyldiimino)bis(butan-1-ol) dihydrochloride
[*1070-11-7*]

Ethambutol Hydrochloride, when dried, contains not less than 98.5% of ethambutol hydrochloride ($C_{10}H_{24}N_2O_2.2HCl$).

Description Ethambutol Hydrochloride occurs as white, crystals or crystalline powder. It is odorless, and has a bitter taste.

It is very soluble in water, soluble in methanol and in ethanol (95), and practically insoluble in diethyl ether.

The pH of a solution prepared by dissolving 1.0 g of Ethambutol Hydrochloride in 20 mL of water is between 3.4 and 4.0.

Identification **(1)** To 10 mL of a solution of Ethambutol Hydrochloride (1 in 100) add 0.5 mL of copper (II) sulfate TS and 2 mL of sodium hydroxide TS: a deep blue color is produced.

(2) Dissolve 0.1 g of Ethambutol Hydrochloride in 40 mL of water, add 20 mL of 2,4,6-trinitrophenol TS, and allow to stand for 1 hour. Collect the precipitate, wash with 50 mL of water, and dry at 105°C for 2 hours: the precipitate melts <*2.60*> between 193°C and 197°C.

(3) A solution of Ethambutol Hydrochloride (1 in 30) responds to Qualitative Tests <*1.09*> for chloride.

Optical rotation <*2.49*> $[\alpha]_D^{20}$: +5.5 – +6.1° (after drying, 5 g, water, 50 mL, 200 mm).

Melting point <*2.60*> 200 – 204°C

Purity **(1)** Clarity and color of solution—Dissolve 1.0 g of Ethambutol Hydrochloride in 10 mL of water: the solution is clear and colorless.

(2) Heavy metals <*1.07*>—Proceed with 2.0 g Ethambutol Hydrochloride according to Method 1, and perform the test. Prepare the control solution with 2.0 mL of Standard Lead Solution (not more than 10 ppm).

(3) Arsenic <*1.11*>—Prepare the test solution with 1.0 g of Ethambutol Hydrochloride according to Method 1, and perform the test (not more than 2 ppm).

(4) 2-Aminobutanol—Dissolve 5.0 g of Ethambutol Hydrochloride in methanol to make exactly 100 mL, and use this solution as the sample solution. Separately, dissolve 0.05 g of 2-amino-1-butanol in methanol to make exactly 100 mL, and use this solution as the standard solution. Perform the test with these solutions as directed under Thin-layer Chromatography <*2.03*>. Spot 2 μL each of the sample solution and standard solution on a plate of silica gel for thin-layer chromatography. Develop the plate with a mixture of ethyl acetate, acetic acid (100), hydrochloric acid and water (11:7:1:1) to a distance of about 10 cm, air-dry the plate, and heat at 105°C for 5 minutes. Cool, spray evenly ninhydrin-L-ascorbic acid TS upon the plate, air-dry the plate, and heat at 105°C for 5 minutes: the spot obtained from the sample solution, corresponding to that from the standard solution, has no more color than that from the standard solution.

Loss on drying <*2.41*> Not more than 0.5% (1 g, 105°C, 3 hours).

Residue on ignition <*2.44*> Not more than 0.1% (1 g).

Assay Weigh accurately about 0.2 g of Ethambutol Hydrochloride, previously dried, dissolve in 20 mL of water, and add 1.8 mL of copper (II) sulfate TS. To the solution add 7 mL of sodium hydroxide TS with shaking, add water to make exactly 50 mL, and centrifuge. Pipet 10 mL of the supernatant liquid, add 10 mL of ammonia-ammonium chloride buffer solution (pH 10.0) and 100 mL of water, and titrate <*2.50*> with 0.01 mol/L disodium dihydrogen ethylenediamine tetraacetate VS until the color of the solution changes from blue-purple through light red to light yellow (indicator: 0.15 mL of Cu-PAN TS). Perform a blank determination in the same manner, and make any necessary correction.

Each mL of 0.01 mol/L disodium dihydrogen ethylenediamine tetraacetate VS
= 2.772 mg of $C_{10}H_{24}N_2O_2.2HCl$

Containers and storage Containers—Tight containers.

Ethanol

Alcohol

エタノール

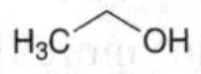

C_2H_6O: 46.07
Ethanol
[*64-17-5*]

This monograph is harmonized with the European Pharmacopoeia and the U.S. Pharmacopeia.

The parts of the text that are not harmonized are marked with symbols (◆ ◆).

Information on the harmonization with the European Pharmacopoeia and the U.S. Pharmacopeia is available on the website of the Pharmaceuticals and Medical Devices Agency.

Ethanol contains not less than 95.1 vol% and not more than 96.9 vol% (by specific gravity) of ethanol (C_2H_6O) at 15°C.

◆**Description** Ethanol is a clear, colorless liquid.

It is miscible with water.

It is flammable and burns with a light blue flame on ignition.

It is volatile.◆

Identification Determine the infrared absorption spectrum of Ethanol as directed in the liquid film method under Infrared Spectrophotometry <*2.25*>, and compare the spectrum with the Reference Spectrum: both spectra exhibit similar intensities of absorption at the same wave numbers.

Specific gravity <*2.56*> d_{15}^{15}: 0.80872 – 0.81601

Purity **(1)** Clarity and color of solution—Ethanol is clear and colorless. To 1.0 mL of Ethanol add water to make 20 mL, and allow to stand for 5 minutes: the resulting liquid is clear.

Control solution: water.

(2) Acidity or alkalinity—To 20 mL of Ethanol add 20 mL of freshly boiled and cooled water and 0.1 mL of a solution prepared by addition of 7.0 mL of ethanol (95) and 2.0 mL of water to 1.0 mL of phenolphthalein TS : no color develops. Add 1.0 mL of 0.01 mol/L sodium hydroxide VS to this solution: a pink color develops.

(3) Volatile impurities—Pipet 500 mL of Ethanol, add 150 μL of 4-methylpentan-2-ol, and use this solution as the sample solution. Separately, to 100 μL of anhydrous methanol add Ethanol to make exactly 50 mL. Pipet 5 mL of this solution, add Ethanol to make exactly 50 mL, and use this solution as the standard solution (1). Separately, to 50 μL each of anhydrous methanol and acetaldehyde add Ethanol to make exactly 50 mL. To 100 μL of this solution add Ethanol to make exactly 10 mL, and use this solution as the standard solution (2). Separately, to 150 μL of acetal add Ethanol to make exactly 50 mL. To 100 μL of this solution add Ethanol to make exactly 10 mL, and use this solution as the standard solution (3). Separately, to 100 μL of benzene add Ethanol to make exactly 100 mL. To 100 μL of this solution add Ethanol to make exactly 50 mL, and use this solution as the standard solution (4). Perform the test with exactly 1 μL each of Ethanol, the sample solution and standard solutions (1), (2), (3) and (4) as directed under Gas Chromatography *<2.02>* according to the following conditions, and determine the peak areas of acetaldehyde, A_E, benzene, B_E and acetal, C_E obtained with Ethanol, and the peak area of methanol with the standard solution (1), the peak area of acetaldehyde, A_T with the standard solution (2), the peak area of acetal, C_T with the standard solution (3) and the peak area of benzene, B_T with the standard solution (4) by the automatic integration method: the peak area of methanol obtained with Ethanol is not larger than 1/2 times the peak area of methanol with the standard solution (1). When calculate the amounts of the volatile impurities by the following equation, the total amount of acetaldehyde and acetal is not more than 10 vol ppm as acetaldehyde, and the amount of benzene is not more than 2 vol ppm. The total area of the peaks other than the peak mentioned above with the sample solution is not larger than the peak area of 4-methylpentan-2-ol. For this calculation the peak having the area not more than 3% of that of 4-methylpentan-2-ol is excluded.

$$\text{Total amount (vol ppm) of acetaldehyde and acetal} = (10 \times A_E)/(A_T - A_E) + (30 \times C_E \times 44.05)/\{(C_T - C_E) \times 118.2\}$$

$$\text{Amount (vol ppm) of benzene} = 2B_E/(B_T - B_E)$$

If necessary, identify the peak of benzene by using a different stationary liquid phase and suitable chromatographic conditions.

Operating conditions—

Detector: A hydrogen flame-ionization detector.

Column: A fused silica column 0.32 mm in inside diameter and 30 m in length, coated with 6% cyanopropyl phenyl-94% dimethyl silicone polymer for gas chromatography in 1.8 μm thickness.

Column temperature: Inject at a constant temperature of about 40°C, maintain the temperature for 12 minutes, then raise to 240°C at a rate of 10°C per minute, and maintain at a constant temperature of about 240°C for 10 minutes.

Injection port temperature: 200°C.

Detector temperature: 280°C.

Carrier gas: Helium.

Flow rate: 35 cm per second.

Split ratio: 1:20.

System suitability—

System performance: When the procedure is run with 1 μL of the standard solution (2) under the above operating conditions, acetaldehyde and methanol are eluted in this order with the resolution between these peaks being not less than 1.5.

(4) Other impurities (absorbance)—Determine the absorption spectrum of Ethanol between 235 nm and 340 nm as directed under Ultraviolet-visible Spectrophotometry *<2.24>*, in a 5-cm cell using water as a blank: the absorbances at 240 nm, between 250 nm and 260 nm and between 270 nm and 340 nm are not more than 0.40, 0.30, and 0.10, respectively, and the spectrum shows a steadily descending curve with no observable peaks or shoulders.

(5) Residue on evaporation—Evaporate 100 mL of Ethanol, exactly measured, in a tared dish on a water bath, and dry at 105°C for 1 hour: the mass of the residue does not exceed 2.5 mg.

Containers and storage ◆Containers—Tight containers.◆

Storage—Without exposure to light.

◆**Shelf life** In not glass containers: Unless otherwise specified, 24 months after preparation.◆

Anhydrous Ethanol

Dehydrated Alcohol

無水エタノール

H_3C–CH_2–OH

C_2H_6O: 46.07

Ethanol

[64-17-5]

This monograph is harmonized with the European Pharmacopoeia and the U.S. Pharmacopeia.

The parts of the text that are not harmonized are marked with symbols (◆ ◆).

Information on the harmonization with the European Pharmacopoeia and the U.S. Pharmacopeia is available on the website of the Pharmaceuticals and Medical Devices Agency.

Anhydrous Ethanol contains not less than 99.5 vol% (by specific gravity) of ethanol (C_2H_6O) at 15°C.

◆**Description** Anhydrous Ethanol is a clear, colorless liquid.

It is miscible with water.

It is flammable and burns with a light blue flame on ignition.

It is volatile.

Boiling point: 78 – 79°C◆

Identification Determine the infrared absorption spectrum of Anhydrous Ethanol as directed in the liquid film method under Infrared Spectrophotometry *<2.25>*, and compare the spectrum with the Reference Spectrum: both spectra exhibit similar intensities of absorption at the same wave numbers.

Specific gravity *<2.56>* d_{15}^{15}: 0.79422 – 0.79679

Purity **(1)** Clarity and color of solution—Anhydrouse Ethanol is clear and colorless. To 1.0 mL of Anhydrous Ethanol add water to make 20 mL, and allow to stand for 5 minutes: the resulting liquid is clear.

Control solution: water

(2) Acidity or alkalinity—To 20 mL of Anhydrous Ethanol add 20 mL of freshly boiled and cooled water and 0.1 mL of a solution obtained by addition of 7.0 mL of ethanol (95) and 2.0 mL of water to 1.0 mL of phenolphthalein TS: no color develops. Add 1.0 mL of 0.01 mol/L sodium hydroxide VS to this solution: pink color develops.

(3) Volatile impurities—Pipet 500 mL of Anhydrous Ethanol, add 150 μL of 4-methylpentan-2-ol, and use this solution as the sample solution. Separately, to 100 μL of anhydrous methanol add Anhydrous Ethanol to make exactly 50 mL. Pipet 5 mL of this solution, add Anhydrous Ethanol to make exactly 50 mL, and use this solution as the standard solution (1). Separately, to 50 μL each of anhydrous methanol and acetaldehyde add Anhydrous Ethanol to make exactly 50 mL. To 100 μL of this solution add Anhydrous Ethanol to make exactly 10 mL, and use this solution as the standard solution (2). Separately, to 150 μL of acetal add Anhydrous Ethanol to make exactly 50 mL. To 100 μL of this solution add Anhydrous Ethanol to make exactly 10 mL, and use this solution as the standard solution (3). Separately, to 100 μL of benzene add Anhydrous Ethanol to make exactly 100 mL. To 100 μL of this solution add Anhydrous Ethanol to make exactly 50 mL, and use this solution as the standard solution (4). Perform the test with exactly 1 μL each of Anhydrous Ethanol, the sample solution and standard solutions (1), (2), (3) and (4) as directed under Gas Chromatography <*2.02*> according to the following conditions, and determine the peak areas of acetaldehyde, A_E, benzene, B_E and acetal, C_E obtained with Anhydrous Ethanol, and the peak area of methanol with the standard solution (1), the peak area of acetaldehyde, A_T with the standard solution (2), the peak area of acetal, C_T with the standard solution (3) and the peak area of benzene, B_T with the standard solution (4) by the automatic integration method: the peak area of methanol obtained with Anhydrous Ethanol is not larger than 1/2 times the peak area of methanol with the standard solution (1). When calculate the amounts of the volatile impurities by the following equation, the total amount of acetaldehyde and acetal is not more than 10 vol ppm as acetaldehyde, and the amount of benzene is not more than 2 vol ppm. The total area of the peaks other than the peak mentioned above with the sample solution is not larger than the peak area of 4-methylpentan-2-ol. For this calculation the peak having the area not more than 3% of that of 4-methylpentan-2-ol is excluded.

$$\text{Total amount (vol ppm) of acetaldehyde and acetal} = (10 \times A_E)/(A_T - A_E) + (30 \times C_E \times 44.05)/\{(C_T - C_E) \times 118.2\}$$

$$\text{Amount (vol ppm) of benzene} = 2B_E/(B_T - B_E)$$

If necessary, identify the peak of benzene by using a different stationary liquid phase and suitable chromatographic conditions.

Operating conditions—

Detector: A hydrogen flame-ionization detector.

Column: A fused silica column 0.32 mm in inside diameter and 30 m in length, coated with 6% cyanopropyl phenyl-94% dimethyl silicone polymer for gas chromatography in 1.8 μm thickness.

Column temperature: Inject at a constant temperature of about 40°C, maintain the temperature for 12 minutes, then raise to 240°C at a rate of 10°C per minute, and maintain at a constant temperature of about 240°C for 10 minutes.

Injection port temperature: 200°C.

Detector temperature: 280°C.

Carrier gas: Helium.

Flow rate: 35 cm per second.

Split ratio: 1:20.

System suitability—

System performance: When the procedure is run with 1 μL of the standard solution (2) under the above operating conditions, acetaldehyde and methanol are eluted in this order with the resolution between these peaks being not less than 1.5.

(4) Other impurities (absorbance)—Determine the absorption spectrum of Anhydrous Ethanol between 235 nm and 340 nm as directed under Ultraviolet-visible Spectrophotometry <*2.24*>, in a 5-cm cell using water as a blank: the absorbances at 240 nm, between 250 nm and 260 nm and between 270 nm and 340 nm are not more than 0.40, 0.30, and 0.10, respectively, and the spectrum shows a steadily descending curve with no observable peaks or shoulders.

(5) Residue on evaporation—Evaporate 100 mL of Anhydrous Ethanol, exactly measured, in a tared dish on a water bath, and dry at 105°C for 1 hour: the mass of the residue does not exceed 2.5 mg.

Containers and storage ◆Containers—Tight containers.◆

Storage—Without exposure to light.

◆**Shelf life** In not glass containers: Unless otherwise specified, 24 months after preparation.◆

Ethanol for Disinfection

Alcohol for Disinfection

消毒用エタノール

Ethanol for Disinfection contains not less than 76.9 vol% and not more than 81.4 vol% (by specific gravity) of ethanol (C_2H_6O: 46.07) at 15°C.

Method of preparation

Ethanol	830 mL
Purified Water or Purified Water in Containers	a sufficient quantity
To make	1000 mL

Prepare by mixing the above ingredients.

Description Ethanol for Disinfection is a colorless, clear liquid.

It is miscible with water.

It burns with a light blue flame on ignition.

It is volatile.

Identification **(1)** To 1 mL of Ethanol for Disinfection add 2 mL of iodine TS and 1 mL of sodium hydroxide TS, and mix: light yellow precipitates appear.

(2) To 1 mL of Ethanol for Disinfection add 1 mL of acetic acid (100) and 3 drops of sulfuric acid, and heat: the odor of ethyl acetate is produced.

Specific gravity <*2.56*> d^{15}_{15}: 0.86027 – 0.87264

Purity Proceed as directed in the Purity under Ethanol, with the exeption of (4), which is changed as follows.

(4) Other impurities (absorbance)—Perform the test with Ethanol for Disinfection as directed under Ultraviolet-visible Spectorophotometry <*2.24*>: the absorbances at 240 nm, between 250 nm and 260 nm and between 270 nm and 340 nm are not more than 0.40, 0.30, and 0.10, respectively. The absorption spectrum determined in a 5-cm cell using water as a blank shows a smooth absorption curve between 235 nm and 340 nm.

Containers and storage Containers—Tight containers.
Storage—Light-resistant.

Ethenzamide

エテンザミド

$C_9H_{11}NO_2$: 165.19
2-Ethoxybenzamide
[*938-73-8*]

Ethenzamide, when dried, contains not less than 98.0% of ethenzamide ($C_9H_{11}NO_2$).

Description Ethenzamide occurs as white, crystals or crystalline powder.

It is soluble in methanol, in ethanol (95), and in acetone, and practically insoluble in water.

It begins to sublime slightly at about 105°C.

Identification **(1)** Determine the absorption spectrum of a solution of Ethenzamide in methanol (1 in 100,000) as directed under Ultraviolet-visible Spectrophotometry <*2.24*>, and compare the spectrum with the Reference Spectrum or the spectrum of a solution of Ethenzamide RS prepared in the same manner as the sample solution: both spectra exhibit similar intensities of absorption at the same wavelengths.

(2) Determine the infrared absorption spectrum of Ethenzamide, previously dried, as directed in the potassium bromide disk method under Infrared Spectrophotometry <*2.25*>, and compare the spectrum with the Reference Spectrum or the spectrum of Ethenzamide RS: both spectra exhibit similar intensities of absorption at the same wave numbers.

Melting point <*2.60*> 131 – 134°C

Purity **(1)** Chloride <*1.03*>—Dissolve 0.5 g of Ethenzamide in 30 mL of acetone, add 6 mL of dilute nitric acid, and dilute with water to make 50 mL. Perform the test using this solution as the test solution. Prepare the control solution as follows: to 0.7 mL of 0.01 mol/L hydrochloric acid VS add 30 mL of acetone and 6 mL of dilute nitric acid, and dilute with water to make 50 mL (not more than 0.050%).

(2) Sulfate <*1.14*>—Dissolve 0.5 g of Ethenzamide in 30 mL of acetone, add 1 mL of dilute hydrochloric acid, and dilute with water to 50 mL. Perform the test using this solution as the test solution. Prepare the control solution as follows: to 0.50 mL of 0.005 mol/L sulfuric acid VS add 30 mL of acetone and 1 mL of dilute hydrochloric acid, and dilute with water to 50 mL (not more than 0.048%).

(3) Heavy metals <*1.07*>—Proceed with 2.0 g of Ethenzamide according to Method 2, and perform the test. Prepare the control solution with 2.0 mL of Standard Lead Solution (not more than 10 ppm).

(4) Arsenic <*1.11*>—To 0.40 g of Ethenzamide add 0.3 g of potassium nitrate and 0.5 g of anhydrous sodium carbonate, mix thoroughly, ignite the mixture gradually, and cool. Dissolve the residue in 10 mL of dilute sulfuric acid, and heat the solution until white fumes begin to evolve. After cooling, add water carefully to make 5 mL, use this solution as the test solution, and perform the test (not more than 5 ppm).

(5) Salicylamide—Dissolve 0.20 g of Ethenzamide in 15 mL of diluted ethanol (95) (2 in 3), and add 2 to 3 drops of dilute iron (III) chloride TS: no purple color develops.

Loss on drying <*2.41*> Not more than 1.0% (1 g, silica gel, 3 hours).

Residue on ignition <*2.44*> Not more than 0.1% (1 g).

Assay Weigh accurately about 20 mg each of Ethenzamide and Ethenzamide RS, previously dried, and dissolve each in 70 mL of ethanol (95) by warming, and after cooling, add ethanol (95) to make exactly 100 mL. Pipet 5 mL each of these solutions, add ethanol (95) to make exactly 50 mL, and use these solutions as the sample solution and the standard solution, respectively. Determine the absorbances, A_T and A_S, of the sample solution and standard solution at 290 nm as directed under Ultraviolet-visible Spectrophotometry <*2.24*>, using ethanol (95) as the blank.

Amount (mg) of ethenzamide ($C_9H_{11}NO_2$) = $M_S \times A_T/A_S$

M_S: Amount (mg) of Ethenzamide RS taken

Containers and storage Containers—Well-closed containers.

Ether

エーテル

$C_4H_{10}O$: 74.12
Diethyl ether
[*60-29-7*]

Ether contains not less than 96% and not more than 98% (by specific gravity) of ether ($C_4H_{10}O$).

It contains a small quantity of ethanol and water.

It cannot be used for anesthesia.

Description Ether is a colorless, clear, mobile liquid, having a characteristic odor.

It is miscible with ethanol (95).

It is soluble in water.

It is highly volatile and flammable.

It is slowly oxidized by the action of air and light, with the formation of peroxides.

Its vapor, when mixed with air and ignited, may explode violently.

Boiling point: 35 – 37°C

Specific gravity <*2.56*> d^{20}_{20}: 0.718 – 0.721

Purity **(1)** Foreign odor—Place 10 mL of Ether in an evaporating dish, and allow it to evaporate spontaneously to a volume of about 1 mL: no foreign odor is perceptible. Drop this residue onto a piece of clean, odorless filter paper to evaporate the ether: no foreign odor is perceptible.

(2) Acidity—Place 10 mL of diluted ethanol (95) (4 in 5) and 0.5 mL of phenolphthalein TS in a 50-mL glass-stoppered flask, and add 0.02 mol/L sodium hydroxide VS dropwise to produce a red color which persists after shaking for 30 seconds. Add 25 mL of Ether, stopper the flask, shake gently, and add 0.40 mL of 0.02 mol/L sodium hydroxide VS with shaking: a red color develops.

(3) Aldehyde—Place 10 mL of Ether in a Nessler tube, add 1 mL of potassium hydroxide TS, and allow the mixture to stand for 2 hours, protecting from light, with occasional shaking: no color is produced in the ether layer and the aqueous layer.

(4) Peroxide—Place 10 mL of Ether in a Nessler tube, add 1 mL of a freshly prepared solution of potassium iodide (1 in 10), shake for 1 minute, then add 1 mL of starch TS, and shake well: no color is produced in the ether layer and in the aqueous layer.

(5) Residue on evaporation—Evaporate 140 mL of Ether, and dry the residue at 105°C for 1 hour: the mass of the residue is not more than 1.0 mg.

Containers and storage Containers—Tight containers.

Storage—Without fill up, light-resistant, remote from fire, and not exceeding 25°C.

Anesthetic Ether

麻酔用エーテル

H_3C–CH_2–O–CH_2–CH_3

$C_4H_{10}O$: 74.12
Diethyl ether
[60-29-7]

Anesthetic Ether contains not less than 96% and not more than 98% (by specific gravity) of ether ($C_4H_{10}O$).

It contains small quantities of ethanol and water. Suitable stabilizers may be added.

It is not to be used for anesthesia if it has been removed from the original container for more than 24 hours.

Description Anesthetic Ether occurs as a colorless, clear, mobile liquid, having a characteristic odor.

It is miscible with ethanol (95).

It is soluble in water.

It is highly volatile and flammable.

It is slowly oxidized by the action of air and light, with the formation of peroxides.

Its vapor, when mixed with air and ignited, may explode violently.

Boiling point: 35 – 37°C

Specific gravity *<2.56>* d^{20}_{20}: 0.718 – 0.721

Purity **(1)** Foreign odor—Place 10 mL of Anesthetic Ether in an evaporating dish, and allow it to evaporate spontaneously to a volume of about 1 mL: no foreign odor is perceptible. Drop this residue onto a piece of clean, odorless filter paper to evaporate the ether: no foreign odor is perceptible.

(2) Acidity—Place 10 mL of diluted ethanol (95) (4 in 5) and 0.5 mL of phenolphthalein TS in a 50-mL glass-stoppered flask, and add 0.02 mol/L sodium hydroxide VS dropwise to produce a red color which persists after shaking for 30 seconds. Add 25 mL of Anesthetic Ether, stopper the flask, shake gently, and add 0.40 mL of 0.02 mol/L sodium hydroxide VS with shaking: a red color develops.

(3) Aldehyde—To 100 mL of water in a 200-mL glass-stoppered flask add 10 mL of Anesthetic Ether and 1 mL of a solution of sodium hydrogen sulfite (1 in 1000), stopper tightly, shake vigorously for 10 seconds, and allow the mixture to stand in a cool place for 30 minutes, protected from light. Add 2 mL of starch TS, and add dropwise 0.01 mol/L iodine VS until a pale blue color develops. Shake with about 2 g of sodium hydrogen carbonate to decolorize the solution, and add 1 mL of diluted 0.01 mol/L iodine VS (9 in 40): a blue color develops. Keep the temperature of the solution below 18°C during the procedure.

(4) Peroxide—Place 10 mL of Anesthetic Ether in a Nessler tube, add 1 mL of a freshly prepared solution of potassium iodide (1 in 10), shake occasionally for 1 hour, protecting from light, then add 1 mL of starch TS, and shake well: no color is produced and in the aqueous layer and in the ether layer.

(5) Residue on evaporation—Evaporate 50 mL of Anesthetic Ether, and dry the residue at 105°C for 1 hour: the mass of the residue is not more than 1.0 mg.

Containers and storage Containers—Tight containers.

Storage—Without fill up, light-resistant, remote from fire, and not exceeding 25°C.

Ethinylestradiol

エチニルエストラジオール

$C_{20}H_{24}O_2$: 296.40
19-Nor-17α-pregna-1,3,5(10)-triene-20-yne-3,17-diol
[57-63-6]

Ethinylestradiol, when dried, contains not less than 98.0% of ethinylestradiol ($C_{20}H_{24}O_2$).

Description Ethinylestradiol occurs as white to pale yellow, crystals or crystalline powder. It is odorless.

It is freely soluble in pyridine and in tetrahydrofuran, soluble in ethanol (95) and in diethyl ether, and practically insoluble in water.

It dissolves in sodium hydroxide TS.

Identification **(1)** Dissolve 2 mg of Ethinylestradiol in 1 mL of a mixture of sulfuric acid and ethanol (95) (1:1): a purplish red color develops with a yellow-green fluorescence. Add carefully 2 mL of water to this solution: the color of the solution changes to red-purple.

(2) Transfer 0.02 g of Ethinylestradiol to a glass-stoppered test tube, dissolve in 10 mL of a solution of potassium hydroxide (1 in 20), add 0.1 g of benzoyl chloride, and shake. Collect the resulting precipitate, recrystallize from methanol, and dry in a desiccator (in vacuum, phosphorus (V) oxide): the precipitate melts *<2.60>* between 200°C and 202°C.

Optical rotation *<2.49>* $[\alpha]^{20}_{D}$: −26 – −31° (after drying, 0.1 g, pyridine, 25 mL, 100 mm).

Melting point *<2.60>* 180 – 186°C or 142 – 146°C

Purity Estrone—Dissolve 5 mg of Ethinylestradiol in 0.5 mL of ethanol (95), and add 0.05 g of 1,3-dinitrobenzene. Add 0.5 mL of freshly prepared dilute potassium hydroxide-ethanol TS, allow to stand in a dark place for 1 hour, and add 10 mL of ethanol (95): the solution has no more color than the following control solution.

Control solution: Proceed in the same manner as mentioned above, omitting Ethinylestradiol.

Loss on drying *<2.41>* Not more than 0.5% (0.5 g, in vacuum, phosphorus (V) oxide, 4 hours).

Residue on ignition <*2.44*> Not more than 0.1% (0.5 g).

Assay Weigh accurately about 0.2 g of Ethinylestradiol, previously dried, and dissolve in 40 mL of tetrahydrofuran. Add 10 mL of a solution of silver nitrate (1 in 20), and titrate <*2.50*> with 0.1 mol/L sodium hydroxide VS (potentiometric titration).

Each mL of 0.1 mol/L sodium hydroxide VS
$= 29.64$ mg of $C_{20}H_{24}O_2$

Containers and storage Containers—Tight containers.
Storage—Light-resistant.

Ethinylestradiol Tablets

エチニルエストラジオール錠

Ethinylestradiol Tablets contain not less than 90.0% and not more than 110.0% of the labeled amount of ethinylestradiol ($C_{20}H_{24}O_2$: 296.40).

Method of preparation Prepare as directed under Tablets, with Ethinylestradiol.

Identification **(1)** Evaporate to dryness 5 mL of the sample solution obtained in Assay, and add 2 mL of a mixture of sulfuric acid and ethanol (95) (2:1) to the residue: a light red color with a yellow fluorescence develops. To the solution add carefully 4 mL of water: the color of the solution changes to red-purple.

(2) Evaporate to dryness 10 mL of the sample solution obtained in Assay, add 0.2 mL of acetic acid (31) and 2 mL of phosphoric acid to the residue, and heat on a water bath for 5 minutes: a red color with a yellow-green fluorescence develops.

Uniformity of dosage units <*6.02*> Perform the test according to the following method: it meets the requirement of the Content uniformity test.

Place 1 tablet of Ethinylestradiol Tablets in a separator, add 10 mL of 2nd fluid for disintegration test, and shake until the tablet is disintegrated. Add 10 mL of dilute sulfuric acid and 20 mL of chloroform, shake vigorously for 5 minutes, and filter the chloroform layer into a conical flask through filter paper on which 5 g of anhydrous sodium sulfate is placed. Extract the aqueous layer with two 20-mL portions of chloroform, proceed with the extracts in the same manner as before, and combine the filtrates with the previous one. Evaporate gently the combined filtrate on a water bath with the aid of a current of nitrogen, dissolve the residue in exactly 100 mL of methanol, and centrifuge, if necessary. Pipet x mL of the supernatant liquid, add methanol to make exactly V mL of a solution containing about 40 ng of ethinylestradiol ($C_{20}H_{24}O_2$) per mL, and use this solution as the sample solution. Separately, weigh accurately about 10 mg of Ethinylestradiol RS, previously dried in a desiccator (in vacuum, phosphorus (V) oxide) for 4 hours, dissolve in methanol, dilute to a volume containing about 40 ng of ethinylestradiol ($C_{20}H_{24}O_2$) per mL, and use this solution as the standard solution. Pipet 4 mL each of sulfuric acid-methanol TS into three glass-stoppered test tubes, T, S and B, cool in ice, to each tube add exactly 1 mL each of the sample solution, the standard solution and methanol, shake immediately, and allow to stand in a water bath at 30°C for 40 minutes, then allow to stand in a water bath at 20°C for 5 minutes. Perform the test with these solutions as directed under Fluorometry <*2.22*>. Determine the fluorescence intensities, F_T, F_S and F_B, of these solutions using the fluorophotometer, at about 460 nm of the excitation and at about 493 nm of the fluorescence.

$$\text{Amount (mg) of ethinylestradiol } (C_{20}H_{24}O_2) = M_S \times (F_T - F_B)/(F_S - F_B) \times V/2500 \times 1/x$$

M_S: Amount (mg) of Ethinylestradiol RS taken

Dissolution Being specified separately when the drug is granted approval based on the Law.

Assay (i) Chromatographic tube: Pack a pledget of glass wool in the bottom of a tube 25 mm in inside diameter and 300 mm in length, and place 5 g of anhydrous sodium sulfate on the glass wool.

(ii) Chromatographic column: Place 5 g of siliceous earth for chromatography in a 200-mL beaker, soak well in 4 mL of 1 mol/L hydrochloric acid TS, and mix uniformly. Put the siliceous earth into the chromatographic tube in small portions to make 60 to 80 mm in height in proper hardness with a tamping rod.

(iii) Standard solution: Weigh accurately about 10 mg of Ethinylestradiol RS, previously dried in a desiccator (in vacuum, phosphorus (V) oxide) for 4 hours, and dissolve in chloroform to make exactly 100 mL. Pipet 5 mL of this solution, and add chloroform to make exactly 100 mL.

(iv) Sample: Weigh accurately not less than 20 Ethinylestradiol Tablets, and powder. Weigh accurately a portion of the powder, equivalent to about 0.5 mg of ethinylestradiol ($C_{20}H_{24}O_2$), place in a 50-mL beaker, add 2 mL of water, shake well, add 3 mL of chloroform, and shake well again. Add 4 g of siliceous earth for chromatography, mix well until the contents do not stick to the inner wall of the beaker, and use the substance as the sample.

(v) Procedure: To the chromatographic column add the sample with a funnel, and pack in proper hardness. Mix well the sample sticking to the beaker with 0.5 g of siliceous earth for chromatography, and place in the chromatographic tube. Wipe off the sample solution sticking to the beaker and the tamping rod with glass wool, and place it in the chromatographic tube. Push down the sample, and press lightly on the chromatographic column to make the height of the column 110 mm to 130 mm. Take 70 mL of chloroform, rinse the inner wall of the chromatographic tube with a portion of the chloroform, and transfer the remaining portion to the chromatographic tube. Collect the effluent solution at a flow rate not more than 0.8 mL per minute. After completing the elution, rinse the lower end of the chromatographic tube with a small quantity of chloroform, add chloroform to make exactly 100 mL, and use this solution as the sample solution. Transfer 6 mL each of the sample solution and standard solution to each separators, and add 20 mL each of isooctane. Add exactly 10 mL of a mixture of sulfuric acid and methanol (7:3), shake vigorously for 5 minutes, allow to stand in a dark place for 15 minutes, and centrifuge. Perform the test with the resulting color solutions as directed under Ultraviolet-visible Spectrophotometry <*2.24*>, using a solution, prepared with 6 mL of chloroform in the same manner, as the blank. Determine the absorbances, A_T and A_S, of the subsequent solutions obtained from the sample solution and standard solution at 540 nm, respectively.

$$\text{Amount (mg) of ethinylestradiol } (C_{20}H_{24}O_2) = M_S \times A_T/A_S \times 1/20$$

M_S: Amount (mg) of Ethinylestradiol RS taken

Containers and storage Coniners—Well-closed containers.

Ethionamide

エチオナミド

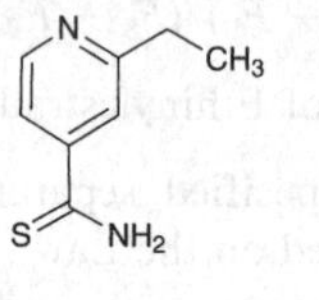

$C_8H_{10}N_2S$: 166.24
2-Ethylpyridine-4-carbothioamide
[*536-33-4*]

Ethionamide, when dried, contains not less than 98.5% and not more than 101.0% of ethionamide ($C_8H_{10}N_2S$).

Description Ethionamide occurs as yellow, crystals or crystalline powder, having a characteristic odor.

It is soluble in methanol and in acetic acid (100), sparingly soluble in ethanol (99.5) and in acetone, and practically insoluble in water.

Identification **(1)** Determine the absorption spectrum of a solution of Ethionamide in methanol (3 in 160,000) as directed under Ultraviolet-visible Spectrophotometry *<2.24>*, and compare the spectrum with the Reference Spectrum: both spectra exhibit similar intensities of absorption at the same wavelengths.

(2) Determine the infrared absorption spectrum of Ethionamide as directed in the potassium bromide disk method under Infrared Spectrophotometry *<2.25>*, and compare the spectrum with the Reference Spectrum: both spectra exhibit similar intensities of absorption at the same wave numbers.

Melting point *<2.60>* 161 – 165°C

Purity **(1)** Acidity—Dissolve 3.0 g of Ethionamide in 30 mL of methanol by warming, add 90 mL of water, allow to stand in ice water for 1 hour, and filter. To 80 mL of the filtrate add 0.8 mL of cresol red TS and 0.20 mL of 0.1 mol/L sodium hydroxide VS: a red color develops.

(2) Heavy metals *<1.07>*—Proceed with 1.0 g of Ethionamide according to Method 2, and perform the test. Prepare the control solution with 2.0 mL of Standard Lead Solution (not more than 20 ppm).

(3) Arsenic *<1.11>*—Prepare the test solution with 1.0 g of Ethionamide according to Method 3. Add 10 mL of a solution of magnesium nitrate hexahydrate in ethanol (95) (1 in 50), then add 1.5 mL of hydrogen peroxide (30), and fire to burn (not more than 2 ppm).

(4) Related substances—Conduct this procedure without exposure to light, using light-resistant vessels. Dissolve 0.20 g of Ethionamide in 10 mL of acetone, and use this solution as the sample solution. Pipet 0.5 mL of the sample solution, add acetone to make exactly 100 mL, and use this solution as the standard solution (1). Separately, pipet exactly 0.2 mL of the sample solution, add acetone to make exactly 100 mL, and use this solution as the standard solution (2). Perform the test with these solutions as directed under Thin-layer Chromatography *<2.03>*. Spot 10 μL each of the sample solution and standard solutions (1) and (2) on a plate of silica gel with fluorescent indicator for thin-layer chromatography, develop with a mixture of ethyl acetate, hexane and methanol (6:2:1) to a distance of about 15 cm, and air-dry the plate. Examine under ultraviolet light (main wavelength: 254 nm): the spot other than the principal spot obtained from the sample solution is not more intense than the spot from the standard solution (1), and number of the spot other than the principal spot from the sample solution which is more intense than the spot from the standard solution (2) is not more than one.

Loss on drying *<2.41>* Not more than 0.5% (1 g, 105°C, 3 hours).

Residue on ignition *<2.44>* Not more than 0.1% (1 g).

Assay Weigh accurately about 0.3 g of Ethionamide, previously dried, dissolve in 50 mL of acetic acid (100), and titrate *<2.50>* with 0.1 mol/L perchloric acid VS until the color of the solution changes from orange-red to dark orange-brown (indicator: 2 mL of *p*-naphtholbenzein TS). Perform a blank determination in the same manner, and make any necessary correction.

Each mL of 0.1 mol/L perchloric acid VS
= 16.62 mg of $C_8H_{10}N_2S$

Containers and storage Containers—Well-closed containers.

Ethosuximide

エトスクシミド

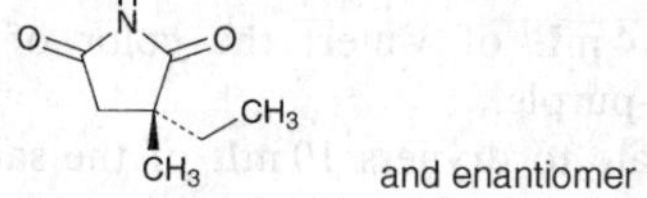

and enantiomer

$C_7H_{11}NO_2$: 141.17
(2*RS*)-2-Ethyl-2-methylsuccinimide
[*77-67-8*]

Ethosuximide contains not less than 98.5% of ethosuximide ($C_7H_{11}NO_2$), calculated on the anhydrous basis.

Description Ethosuximide occurs as a white, paraffin-like solid or powder. It is odorless or has a slight, characteristic odor.

It is very soluble in methanol, in ethanol (95), in diethyl ether, and in *N,N*-dimethylformamide, and freely soluble in water.

Melting point: about 48°C

Identification **(1)** To 0.2 g of Ethosuximide add 10 mL of sodium hydroxide TS, and boil: the gas evolved turns a moistened red litmus paper blue.

(2) Dissolve 0.05 g of Ethosuximide in 1 mL of ethanol (95), add 3 drops of a solution of copper (II) acetate monohydrate (1 in 100), warm slightly, and add 1 to 2 drops of sodium hydroxide TS: a purple color is produced.

(3) Determine the absorption spectrum of a solution of Ethosuximide in ethanol (95) (1 in 2000) as directed under Ultraviolet-visible Spectrophotometry *<2.24>*, and compare the spectrum with the Reference Spectrum: both spectra exhibit similar intensities of absorption at the same wavelengths.

Purity **(1)** Clarity and color of solution—Dissolve 1.0 g of Ethosuximide in 10 mL of water: the solution is clear and colorless.

(2) Chloride *<1.03>*—With 1.0 g of Ethosuximide, perform the test. Prepare the control solution with 0.30 mL of 0.01 mol/L hydrochloric acid VS (not more than 0.011%).

(3) Heavy metals *<1.07>*—Proceed with 1.0 g of Ethosuximide according to Method 1, and perform the test. Prepare the control solution with 2.0 mL of Standard Lead Solution (not more than 20 ppm).

(4) Arsenic *<1.11>*—Prepare the test solution with 1.0 g of Ethosuximide, according to Method 1, and perform the test (not more than 2 ppm).

(5) Acid anhydride—Dissolve 0.50 g of Ethosuximide in 1 mL of ethanol (95), add 1 mL of hydroxylammonium chloride-iron (III) chloride TS, and allow to stand for 5 minutes. Add 3 mL of water, mix, and allow to stand for 5 minutes: the red to red-purple color of this solution is not more intense than that of the following control solution.

Control solution: Dissolve 70 mg of succinic anhydride in ethanol (95) to make exactly 100 mL. To 1.0 mL of this solution add 1 mL of hydroxylammonium chloride-iron (III) chloride TS, and proceed in the same manner.

(6) Cyanide—Dissolve 1.0 g of Ethosuximide in 10 mL of ethanol (95), and add 3 drops of iron (II) sulfate TS, 1 mL of sodium hydroxide TS and 2 to 3 drops of iron (III) chloride TS. Warm gently, and acidify with dilute sulfuric acid: not a blue precipitate and a blue color are produced within 15 minutes.

Water *<2.48>* Not more than 0.5% (2 g, volumetric titration, direct titration).

Residue on ignition *<2.44>* Not more than 0.1% (1 g).

Assay Weigh accurately about 0.2 g of Ethosuximide, dissolve in 20 mL of *N*,*N*-dimethylformamide, and titrate *<2.50>* with 0.1 mol/L tetramethylammonium hydroxide VS (potentiometric titration). Perform a blank determination in the same manner, and make any necessary correction.

Each mL of 0.1 mol/L tetramethylammonium hydroxide VS
= 14.12 mg of $C_7H_{11}NO_2$

Containers and storage Containers—Tight containers.

Ethyl Aminobenzoate

Anesthamine
Benzocaine

アミノ安息香酸エチル

$C_9H_{11}NO_2$: 165.19
Ethyl 4-aminobenzoate
[94-09-7]

Ethyl Aminobenzoate, when dried, contains not less than 99.0% of ethyl aminobenzoate ($C_9H_{11}NO_2$).

Description Ethyl Aminobenzoate occurs as white, crystals or crystalline powder. It is odorless. It has a slightly bitter taste, numbing the tongue.

It is freely soluble in ethanol (95) and in diethyl ether, and very slightly soluble in water.

It dissolves in dilute hydrochloric acid.

Identification **(1)** Dissolve 10 mg of Ethyl Aminobenzoate in 1 mL of dilute hydrochloric acid and 4 mL of water. This solution responds to Qualitative Tests *<1.09>* for primary aromatic amines.

(2) Dissolve 0.1 g of Ethyl Aminobenzoate in 5 mL of water with the aid of dilute hydrochloric acid added dropwise, and add iodine TS dropwise: a brown precipitate is produced.

(3) Warm 50 mg of Ethyl Aminobenzoate with 2 drops of acetic acid (31) and 5 drops of sulfuric acid: the odor of ethyl acetate is perceptible.

Melting point *<2.60>* 89 - 91°C

Purity **(1)** Acidity—Dissolve 1.0 g of Ethyl Aminobenzoate in 10 mL of neutralized ethanol, and add 10 mL of water, 2 drops of phenolphthalein TS and 0.50 mL of 0.01 mol/L sodium hydroxide VS: a red color is produced.

(2) Chloride—Dissolve 0.20 g of Ethyl Aminobenzoate in 5 mL of ethanol (95), add 2 to 3 drops each of dilute nitric acid and of silver nitrate TS: no change occurs immediately.

(3) Heavy metals *<1.07>*—Dissolve 2.0 g of Ethyl Aminobenzoate in 20 mL of ethanol (95), add 2 mL of dilute acetic acid and ethanol (95) to make 50 mL, and perform the test using this solution as the test solution. Prepare the control solution as follows: to 2.0 mL of Standard Lead Solution add 2 mL of dilute acetic acid and sufficient ethanol (95) to make 50 mL (not more than 10 ppm).

(4) Readily carbonizable substances *<1.15>*—Perform the test with 0.5 g of Ethyl Aminobenzoate: the solution has no more color than Matching Fluid A.

Loss on drying *<2.41>* Not more than 1.0% (1 g, silica gel, 3 hours).

Residue on ignition *<2.44>* Not more than 0.1% (1 g).

Assay Weigh accurately about 0.25 g of Ethyl Aminobenzoate, previously dried, dissolve in 10 mL of hydrochloric acid and 70 mL of water, add 10 mL of a solution of potassium bromide (3 in 10), and cool to a temperature below 15°C. Then titrate *<2.50>* with 0.1 mol/L sodium nitrite VS by the potentiometric titration or the amperometric titration.

Each mL of 0.1 mol/L sodium nitrite VS
= 16.52 mg of $C_9H_{11}NO_2$

Containers and storage Containers—Well-closed containers.

Ethylcellulose

エチルセルロース

[9004-57-3]

This monograph is harmonized with the European Pharmacopoeia and the U. S. Pharmacopeia.

The corresponding part of the attributes/provisions which are agreed as non-harmonized within the scope of the harmonization is marked with symbols (◆ ◆), and the corresponding parts which are agreed as the JP local requirement other than the scope of the harmonization are marked with symbols (◇ ◇).

Information on the harmonization with the European Pharmacopoeia and the U.S. Pharmacopeia is available on the website of the Pharmaceuticals and Medical Devices Agency.

Ethylcellulose is a partly *O*-ethylated cellulose.

It contains not less than 44.0% and not more than 51.0% of ethoxy group ($-OC_2H_5$: 45.06), calculated on the dried basis.

It may contain a suitable antioxidant.

The viscosity of Ethylcellulose is shown in millipascal second (mPa·s) on the label.

◆**Description** Ethylcellulose occurs as a white to yellowish white, amorphous powder or grains.

It is soluble in dichloromethane.

It forms a slightly white-turbid or white-turbid, viscous liquid upon addition of ethanol (95).

To 1 g of Ethylcellulose add 100 mL of hot water, shake to become turbid, cool to room temperature, and add freshly boiled and cooled water to make 100 mL: the solution is neutral.◆

Identification Spread 2 drops of a solution of Ethylcellulose in dichloromethane (1 in 25) between sodium chloride plates, then remove one of the plates to evaporate the solvent, and determine the infrared absorption spectrum of the plate as directed in the film method under Infrared Spectrophotometry *<2.25>*, and compare the spectrum with the Reference Spectrum: both spectra exhibit similar intensities of absorption at the same wave numbers.

Viscosity *<2.53>* Weigh exactly a quantity of Ethylcellulose, equivalent to 5.00 g calculated on the dried basis, add 95 g of a mixture of 80 g of toluene and 20 g of ethanol (95), and shake to dissolve. Perform the test with this solution at 25°C as directed in Method I: not less than 80.0% and not more than 120.0% of the labeled viscosity for a nominal viscosity more than 6 mPa·s, and not less than 75.0% and not more than 140.0% of the labeled viscosity for a nominal viscosity not more than 6 mPa·s.

Purity **(1)** Acidity or alkalinity—To 0.5 g of Ethylcellulose add 25 mL of freshly boiled and cooled water, shake for 15 minutes, filter through a glass filter (G3), and use the filtrate as the sample solution. To 10 mL of the sample solution add 0.1 mL of dilute phenolphthalein TS and 0.5 mL of 0.01 mol/L sodium hydroxide VS: a light red color develops. To 10 mL of the sample solution add 0.1 mL of methyl red-sodium hydroxide TS and 0.5 mL of 0.01 mol/L hydrochloric acid VS: a red color develops.

(2) Chloride—Disperse 0.250 g of Ethylcellulose in 50 mL of water, and boil with occasional shaking. Allow to cool, and filter. Discard the first 10 mL of the filtrate, to 10 mL of the subsequent filtrate add water to make 15 mL, and use this solution as the sample solution. Separately, to 10 mL of Standard Chloride Solution add 5 mL of water, and use this solution as the control solution. To 15 mL each of the sample solution and control solution add 1 mL of 2 mol/L nitric acid TS, transfer to test tubes containing 1 mL of a solution of silver nitrate (17 in 1000), allow to stand for 5 minutes protecting from light, and compare the opalescence developed in the both solutions against a black background by viewing transversely: the opalescence developed in the sample solution is not more intense than that of the control solution (not more than 0.1%).

◇**(3)** Heavy metal *<1.07>*—Proceed with 1.0 g of Ethylcellulose according to Method 2, and perform the test. Prepare the control solution with 4.0 mL of Standard Lead Solution (not more than 40 ppm).◇

(4) Acetaldehyde—Introduce 3.0 g of Ethylcellulose into a 250-mL glass-stoppered conical flask, add 10 mL of water, and stir for 1 hour. Allow to stand for 24 hours, filter, add water to the filtrate to make 100 mL, and use this solution as the sample solution. Separately, dissolve 1.0 g of acetaldehyde for assay in water to make 100 mL. To 5 mL of this solution add water to make 500 mL. To 3 mL of this solution add water to make 100 mL, and use this solution as the control solution. Transfer 5 mL each of the sample solution and control solution to 25-mL volumetric flasks, add 5 mL of a solution of 3-methyl-2-benzothiazolonehydrazone hydrochloride monohydrate (1 in 2000), and heat in a water bath at 60°C for 5 minutes. Add 2 mL of iron (III) chloride-amidosulfuric acid TS, and warm again at 60°C for 5 minutes. After cooling, add water to make 25 mL, and compare the color of these solutions: the sample solution is not more intensely colored than the control solution (not more than 100 ppm).

Loss on drying *<2.41>* Not more than 3.0% (1 g, 105°C, 2 hours).

Residue on Ignition *<2.44>* Not more than 0.5% (1 g).

Assay Weigh accurately about 30 mg of Ethylcellulose, transfer to a 5-mL pressure-tight serum vial, add exactly 60 mg of adipic acid, 2 mL of the internal standard solution and 1 mL of hydroiodic acid, seal the vial immediately with a septum coated with fluororesin and an aluminum cap or any other sealing system providing a sufficient air-tightness, and weigh accurately the vial. Take care not to mix the contents in the vial before heating. Place the vial in an oven or heat in a suitable heater with continuous stirring, maintaining an internal temperature of about 115 ± 2°C for 70 min. Allow to cool, and weigh accurately the vial. If the difference of the mass between before heating and after heating is more than 10 mg, prepare a new sample solution. If the difference of the mass between before heating and after heating is not more than 10 mg, after phase separation, pierce through the septum of the vial with a cooled syringe, and withdraw a sufficient volume of the upper phase as the sample solution. Separately, place exactly 60 mg of adipic acid, 2 mL of the internal standard solution and 1 mL of hydroiodic acid in another serum vial, and seal immediately. Weigh accurately the vial, inject 25 μL of iodoethane for assay through the septum in the vial, and weigh again accurately. Shake thoroughly, after phase separation, pierce through the septum of the vial with a cooled syringe, withdraw a sufficient volume of the upper phase, and use this solution as the standard solution. Perform the test with 1 μL each of the sample solution and standard solution as directed under Gas Chromatography *<2.02>* according to the following conditions, and calculate the ratios, Q_T and Q_S, of the peak area of iodoethane to that of the internal standard.

$$\text{Amount (\%) of ethoxy group } (C_2H_5O) = M_S/M_T \times Q_T/Q_S \times 28.89$$

M_S: Amount (mg) of iodoethane for assay taken

M_T: Amount (mg) of Ethylcellulose taken, calculated on the dried basis

Internal standard solution—A solution of *n*-octane in *o*-xylene (1 in 200).

Operating conditions—

Detector: A hydrogen flame-ionization detector.

Column: A fused silica column 0.53 mm in inside diameter and 30 m in length, coated with dimethylpolysiloxane for gas chromatography in 3 μm thickness.

Column temperature: Maintain the temperature at 50°C for 3 minutes, raise to 100°C at a rate of 10°C per minute, then to 250°C at a rate of 35°C per minute, and maintain at 250°C for 8 minutes.

Injection port temperature: A constant temperature of about 250°C.

Detector temperature: A constant temperature of about 280°C.

Carrier gas: Helium.

Flow rate: 4.2 mL per minute (the retention time of the internal standard is about 10 minutes).

Split ratio: 1:40.

System suitability—

System performance: When the procedure is run with 1 μL of the standard solution under the above operating conditions, iodoethane and the internal standard are eluted in this order with the relative retention time of iodoethane to the internal standard being about 0.6, and with the resolution between these peaks being not less than 5.0.

System repeatability: When the test is repeated 6 times with 1 μL of the standard solution under the above operating conditions, the relative standard deviation of the ratio of the peak area of iodoethane to that of the internal standard is not more than 2.0%.

◆**Containers and storage** Containers—Well-closed containers.◆

Ethyl L-Cysteine Hydrochloride

L-エチルシステイン塩酸塩

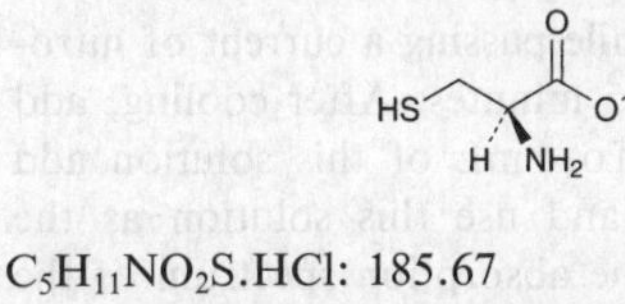

$C_5H_{11}NO_2S.HCl$: 185.67
Ethyl (2*R*)-2-amino-3-sulfanylpropanoate monohydrochloride
[868-59-7]

Ethyl L-Cysteine Hydrochloride, when dried, contains not less than 98.5% of ethyl cysteine hydrochloride ($C_5H_{11}NO_2S.HCl$).

Description Ethyl L-Cysteine Hydrochloride occurs as white, crystals or crystalline powder. It has a characteristic odor, and has a bitter taste at first with a burning aftertaste.

It is very soluble in water, and freely soluble in ethanol (95).

Melting point: about 126°C (with decomposition).

Identification **(1)** Determine the infrared absorption spectrum of Ethyl L-Cysteine Hydrochloride as directed in the potassium bromide disk method under Infrared Spectrophotometry *<2.25>*, and compare the spectrum with the Reference Spectrum: both spectra exhibit similar intensities of absorption at the same wave numbers.

(2) A solution of Ethyl L-Cysteine Hydrochloride (1 in 20) responds to Qualitative Tests *<1.09>* (1) for chloride.

Optical rotation *<2.49>* $[\alpha]_D^{20}$: −10.0 – −13.0° (after drying, 2.0 g, 1 mol/L hydrochloric acid TS, 25 mL, 100 mm).

Purity **(1)** Sulfate *<1.14>*—Perform the test with 0.6 g of Ethyl L-Cysteine Hydrochloride. Prepare the the control solution with 0.35 mL of 0.005 mol/L sulfuric acid VS (not more than 0.028%).

(2) Heavy metals *<1.07>*—Proceed with 1.0 g of Ethyl L-Cysteine Hydrochloride according to Method 1, and perform the test. Prepare the control solution with 1.0 mL of Standard Lead Solution (not more than 10 ppm).

(3) Related substances—Conduct this procedure rapidly. Dissolve 0.05 g each of Ethyl L-Cysteine Hydrochloride and *N*-ethylmaleimide in 5 mL of mobile phase, allow to stand for 30 minutes, and use this solution as the sample solution. Pipet 3 mL of the sample solution, add the mobile phase to make exactly 200 mL, and use this solution as the standard solution. Perform the test with exactly 2 μL each of the sample solution and standard solution as directed under Liquid Chromatography *<2.01>* according to the following conditions. Determine each peak area of these solutions by the automatic integration method: a peak area obtained from the sample solution with the relative retention time to ethyl L-cysteine-*N*-ethylmaleimide complex from the standard solution being about 0.7 is not larger than the peak area of ethyl L-cysteine-*N*-ethylmaleimide complex from the standard solution. Each area of all peaks other than ethyl L-cysteine-*N*-ethylmaleimide complex and *N*-ethylmaleimide from the sample solution is not larger than 1/3 times the peak area of ethyl L-cysteine *N*-ethylmaleimide complex from the standard solution.

Operating conditions—

Detector: An ultraviolet absorption photometer (wavelength: 250 nm).

Column: A stainless steel column about 6 mm in inside diameter and about 15 cm in length, packed with octadecylsilanized silica gel for liquid chromatography (5 μm in particle diameter).

Column temperature: A constant temperature of about 25°C.

Mobile phase: A mixture of 0.02 mol/L potassium dihydrogenphoshate TS and acetonitrile (2:1).

Flow rate: Adjust so that the retention time of ethyl L-cysteine-*N*-ethylmaleimide complex is about 4 minutes.

Selection of column: Dissolve 0.05 g of Ethyl L-Cysteine Hydrochloride, 0.01 g of L-cysteine hydrochloride and 0.05 g of *N*-ethylmaleimide in 25 mL of the mobile phase, and allow to stand for 30 minutes. Proceed with 2 μL of this solution under the above operating conditions, and calculate the resolution. Use a column giving elution of L-cysteine-*N*-ethylmaleimide complex, ethyl L-cysteine-*N*-ethylmaleimide complex and *N*-ethylmaleimide in this order, complete resolution of each component, and the resolution of the peaks of L-cysteine-*N*-ethylmaleimide complex and ethyl L-cysteine-*N*-ethylmaleimide complex being not less than 3.

Detection sensitivity: Adjust the detection sensitivity so that the peak height of ethyl L-cysteine-*N*-ethylmaleimide complex obtained from 2 μL of the standard solution is between 10 mm and 20 mm.

Time span of measurement: About 3 times as long as the retention time of ethyl L-cysteine-*N*-ethylmaleimide complex.

Loss on drying *<2.41>* Not more than 0.5% (1 g, in vacuum, phosphorus oxide (V), 5 hours).

Residue on ignition *<2.44>* Not more than 0.1% (1 g).

Assay Weigh accurately about 0.25 g of Ethyl L-Cysteine Hydrochloride, previously dried, transfer into a glass-stoppered flask, and dissolve in 10 mL of water previously freshly boiled and cooled to a temperature not exceeding 5°C in a stream of nitrogen. Add exactly 20 mL of 0.05 mol/L iodine VS, previously cooled to a temperature not exceeding 5°C, and allow to stand for 30 seconds, then titrate *<2.50>* with 0.1 mol/L sodium thiosulfate VS, on cooling below 5°C (indicator: 1 mL of starch TS). Perform a blank determination in the same manner, and make any necessary correction.

Each mL of 0.05 mol/L iodine VS
= 18.57 mg of $C_5H_{11}NO_2S.HCl$

Containers and storage Containers—Tight containers.

Ethylenediamine

エチレンジアミン

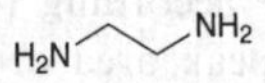

$C_2H_8N_2$: 60.10
Ethane-1,2-diamine
[107-15-3]

Ethylenediamine contains not less than 97.0% of ethylenediamine ($C_2H_8N_2$).

Description Ethylenediamine is a clear, colorless to pale yellow liquid. It has an ammonia-like odor.

It is miscible with water, with ethanol (95) and with diethyl ether.

It has a caustic nature and an irritating property.

It is gradually affected by air.

Specific gravity d^{20}_{20}: about 0.898

Identification **(1)** A solution of Ethylenediamine (1 in 500) is alkaline.

(2) To 2 mL of copper (II) sulfate TS add 2 drops of Ethylenediamine: a blue-purple color develops.

(3) To 0.04 g of Ethylenediamine add 6 drops of benzoyl chloride and 2 mL of a solution of sodium hydroxide (1 in 10), warm for 2 to 3 minutes with occasional shaking, collect the white precipitate formed, and wash with water. Dissolve the precipitate in 8 mL of ethanol (95) by warming, promptly add 8 mL of water, cool, filter the crystals, wash with water, and dry at 105°C for 1 hour: it melts *<2.60>* between 247°C and 251°C.

Purity **(1)** Heavy metals *<1.07>*—Place 1.0 g of Ethylenediamine in a porcelain crucible, evaporate to dryness on a water bath, cover loosely, ignite at a low temperature until charred, proceed according to Method 2, and perform the test. Prepare the control solution with 2.0 mL of Standard Lead Solution (not more than 20 ppm).

(2) Residue on evaporation—Pipet 5 mL of Ethylenediamine, heat on a water bath to dryness, and dry to constant mass at 105°C: the mass of the residue does not exceed 3.0 mg.

Distilling range *<2.57>* 114 – 119°C, not less than 95 vol%.

Assay Weigh accurately about 0.7 g of Ethylenediamine in a glass-stoppered conical flask, add 50 mL of water, and titrate *<2.50>* with 1 mol/L hydrochloric acid VS (indicator: 3 drops of bromophenol blue TS).

Each mL of 1 mol/L hydrochloric acid VS
= 30.05 mg of $C_2H_8N_2$

Containers and storage Containers—Tight containers.

Storage—Light-resistant, and almost well-filled.

Ethyl Icosapentate

イコサペント酸エチル

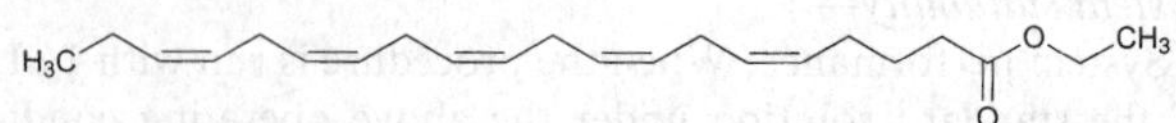

$C_{22}H_{34}O_2$: 330.50
Ethyl (5*Z*,8*Z*,11*Z*,14*Z*,17*Z*)-icosa-5,8,11,14,17-pentaenoate
[86227-47-6]

Ethyl Icosapentate contains not less than 96.5% and not more than 101.0% of ethyl icosapentate ($C_{22}H_{34}O_2$).

It may contain a suitable antioxidant.

Description Icosapentate is a colorless or pale yellow, clear liquid. It has a faint, characteristic odor.

It is miscible with ethanol (99.5), with acetic acid (100) and with hexane. It is practically insoluble in water and in ethylene glycol.

Identification **(1)** To 20 mg of Ethyl Icosapentate add 3 mL of a solution of potassium hydroxide in ethylene glycol (21 in 100), stopper tightly while passing a current of nitrogen, and heat at 180°C for 15 minutes. After cooling, add methanol to make 100 mL. To 4 mL of this solution add methanol to make 100 mL, and use this solution as the sample solution. Determine the absorption spectrum of the sample solution as directed under Ultraviolet-visible Spectrophotometry *<2.24>*, using a solution, prepared in the same manner as the sample solution with 3 mL of the solution of potassium hydroxide in ethylene glycol (21 in 100), as a control, and compare the spectrum with the Reference Spectrum or the spectrum of a solution of Ethyl Icosapentate RS prepared in the same manner as the sample solution: both spectra exhibit similar intensities of absorption at the same wavelengths.

(2) Determine the infrared absorption spectrum of Ethyl Icosapentate as directed in the liquid film method under Infrared Spectrophotometry *<2.25>*, and compare the spectrum with the Reference Spectrum or the spectrum of Ethyl Icosapentate RS: both spectra exhibit similar intensities of absorption at the same wave numbers.

Refractive index *<2.45>* n^{20}_{D}: 1.481 – 1.491

Specific gravity *<2.56>* d^{20}_{20}: 0.905 – 0.915

Acid value *<1.13>* Not more than 0.5.

Saponification value *<1.13>* 165 – 175

Iodine value *<1.13>* 365 – 395 Perform the test with 20 mg of Ethyl Icosapentate.

Purity **(1)** Heavy metals *<1.07>*—Mix 1.0 g of Ethyl Icosapentate with ethanol (99.5), and add 2 mL of dilute acetic acid and ethanol (99.5) to make 50 mL. Perform the test with this solution as the test solution.

Control solution: To 1.0 mL of Standard Lead Solution add 2 mL of dilute acetic acid and ethanol (99.5) to make 50 mL (not more than 10 ppm).

(2) Arsenic *<1.11>*—Prepare the test solution with 1.0 g of Ethyl Icosapentate according to Method 3, and perform the test (not more than 2 ppm).

(3) Related substances—To 0.40 g of Ethyl Icosapentate add hexane to make 50 mL, and use this solution as the sample solution. Perform the test with 1.5 μL of the sample solution as directed under Gas Chromatography <2.02> according to the following conditions. Determine each peak area by the automatic integration method, and calculate the amounts of these peaks by the area percentage method: the amount of the peak, having the relative retention time of about 0.53 to ethyl icosapentate, is not more than 0.5%, the amount of each peak, having the relative retention time of about 0.80 and 0.93, is not more than 1.0%, the amount of each peak other than the principal peak and the peak mentioned above is not more than 1.0%, and the total amount of these peaks other than the principal peak is not more than 3.5%.

Operating conditions—

Detector, column, column temperature, carrier gas and flow rate: Proceed as directed in the operating conditions in the Assay.

Time span of measurement: About 2.5 times as long as the retention time of ethyl icosapentate, beginning after the solvent peak.

System suitability—

System performance: Proceed as directed in the system suitability in the Assay.

Test for required detectability: To exactly 1 mL of the sample solution add hexane to make exactly 100 mL, and use this solution as the solution for system suitability test. Pipet 1 mL of the solution for system suitability test, and add hexane to make exactly 10 mL. Confirm that the peak area of ethyl icosapentate obtained with 1.5 μL of this solution is equivalent to 7 to 13% of that with 1.5 μL of the solution for system suitability test.

System repeatability: When the test is repeated 6 times with 1.5 μL of the solution for system suitability test under the above operating conditions, the relative standard deviation of the peak area of ethyl icosapentate is not more than 2.0%.

(4) Peroxide—Weigh accurately about 1 g of Ethyl Icosapentate, put in a 200-mL glass-stoppered conical flask, add 25 mL of a mixture of acetic acid (100) and chloroform (3:2), and dissolve by gentle shaking. Add 1 mL of saturated potassium iodide solution TS, immediately stopper tightly, shake gently, and allow to stand in a dark place for 10 minutes. Then add 30 mL of water, shake vigorously for 5 to 10 seconds, and titrate <2.50> with 0.01 mol/L sodium thiosulfate VS until the blue color of the solution disappears after addition of 1 mL of starch TS. Calculate the amount of peroxide by the following equation: not more than 2 mEq/kg.

$$\text{Amount (mEq/kg) of peroxide} = V/M \times 10$$

V: Volume (mL) of 0.01 mol/L sodium thiosulfate VS consumed

M: Amount (g) of Ethyl Icosapentate taken

Residue on ignition <2.44> Not more than 0.1% (1 g).

Assay Weigh accurately about 0.4 g of Ethyl Icosapentate, and add hexane to make exactly 50 mL. Pipet 2 mL of this solution, add exactly 2 mL of the internal standard solution, and use this solution as the sample solution. Separately, weigh accurately about 80 mg of Ethyl Icosapentate RS, and add hexane to make exactly 10 mL. Pipet 2 mL of this solution, add exactly 2 mL of the internal standard solution, and use this solution as the standard solution. Perform the test with 3 μL each of the sample solution and standard solution as directed under Gas Chromatography <2.02> according to the following conditions, and calculate the ratios, Q_T and Q_S, of the peak area of ethyl icosapentate to that of the internal standard.

$$\text{Amount (mg) of ethyl icosapentate } (C_{22}H_{34}O_2) = M_S \times Q_T/Q_S \times 5$$

M_S: Amount (mg) of Ethyl Icosapentate RS taken

*Internal standard solution—*A solution of methyl docosanate in hexane (1 in 125).

Operating conditions—

Detector: A hydrogen flame-ionization detector.

Column: A glass column in 4 mm inside diameter and 1.8 m in length, packed with siliceous earth for gas chromatography (175 to 246 μm in particle diameter), coated with diethylene glycol succinate polyester for gas chromatography in the ratio of 25%.

Column temperature: A constant temperature of about 190°C.

Carrier gas: Nitrogen.

Flow rate: Adjust so that the retention time of ethyl icosapentate is about 30 minutes.

System suitability—

System performance: When the procedure is run with 3 μL of the standard solution under the above operating conditions, the internal standard and ethyl icosapentate are eluted in this order with the resolution between these peaks being not less than 3.

System repeatability: When the test is repeated 6 times with 3 μL of the standard solution under the above operating conditions, the relative standard deviation of the ratio of the peak area of ethyl icosapentate to that of the internal standard is not more than 1.0%.

Containers and storage Containers—Tight containers.

Storage—Being fully filled, or replacing the air with Nitrogen.

Ethyl Icosapentate Capsules

イコサペント酸エチルカプセル

Ethyl Icosapentate Capsules contain not less than 95.0% and not more than 105.0% of the labeled amount of ethyl icosapentate ($C_{22}H_{34}O_2$: 330.50).

Method of preparation Prepare as directed under Capsules, with Ethyl Icosapentate.

Identification Take out the content of Ethyl Icosapentate Capsules, to a quantity of the contents, equivalent to 20 mg of Ethyl Icosapentate, add 3 mL of a solution of potassium hydroxide in ethylene glycol (21 in 100), stopper the vessel tightly while passing a current of nitrogen, and heat at 180°C for 15 minutes. After cooling, add methanol to make 100 mL. To 1 mL of this solution add methanol to make 25 mL, and determine the absorption spectrum of this solution as directed under Ultraviolet-visible Spectrophotometry <2.24> using a solution, obtained by proceeding as above with 3 mL of a solution of potassium hydroxide in ethylene glycol (21 in 100), as a blank: it exhibits maxima between 298 nm and 302 nm, between 311 nm and 315 nm, between 325 nm and 329 nm, and between 343 nm and 347 nm.

Purity Peroxide—Take out the content of Ethyl Icosapentate Capsules. Weigh accurately about 1 g of the content, dissolve in 25 mL of a mixture of acetic acid (100) and isooctane (3:2), replace the air of the inside gently with Nitrogen, then add 1 mL of saturated potassium iodide TS under a current of Nitrogen, stopper immediately and shake gently, and allow to stand in a dark place for 10 minutes. Then, add

30 mL of water, shake vigorously, and titrate <*2.50*> with 0.01 mol/L sodium thiosulfate VS (indicator: 1 mL of starch TS). Perform a blank determination in the same manner, and make any necessary correction. The amount of peroxide calculated by the following formula is not more than 20 mEq/kg.

$$\text{Amount (mEq/kg) of peroxide} = V/M \times 10$$

V: Amount (mL) of 0.01 mol/L sodium thiosulfate VS consumed
M: Amount (g) of Ethyl Icosapentate Capsules taken

Uniformity of dosage units <*6.02*> It meets the requirement of the Mass variation test.

Disintegration <*6.09*> Perform the test using the disk: it meets the requirement. However, for the preparations in single-dose packages, carry out the test for 10 minutes.

Assay Weigh accurately the mass of an amount of not less than 20 Ethyl Icosapentate Capsules, then open the capsules and take out the contents. Wash the empty capsules with a little amount of hexane, volatilize the hexane by allowing them to stand at the room temperature, and weigh the mass of the total empty capsules accurately. Weigh accurately a portion of the content, equivalent to about 0.4 g of ethyl icosapentate ($C_{22}H_{34}O_2$), add exactly 40 mL of the internal standard solution, then add hexane to make 200 mL, and use this solution as the sample solution. For the preparations in single-dose packages, weigh accurately the mass of the total capsules of not less than 20 packages, and mix them well. Weigh accurately a portion of the capsules, equivalent to about 0.4 g of ethyl icosapentate ($C_{22}H_{34}O_2$), add 15 mL of hexane, then extract the content by opening the capsules. Separate the hexane extract from the residual solids, wash the residues with three 10-mL portions of hexane, combine the washings and the hexane extract, add exactly 40 mL of the internal standard solution, then add hexane to make 200 mL, and use this solution as the sample solution. Separately, weigh accurately about 50 mg of Ethyl Icosapentate RS, add exactly 5 mL of the internal standard solution, then add hexane to make 25 mL, and use this solution as the standard solution. Perform the test with 4 μL each of the sample solution and standard solution as directed under Gas Chromatography <*2.02*> according to the following conditions, and calculate the ratios, Q_T and Q_S, of the peak area of ethyl icosapentate to that of the internal standard.

$$\text{Amount (mg) of ethyl icosapentate } (C_{22}H_{34}O_2) = M_S \times Q_T/Q_S \times 8$$

M_S: Amount (mg) of Ethyl Icosapentate RS taken

Internal standard solution—A solution of methyl docosanate in hexane (1 in 200).
Operating conditions—

Proceed as directed in the operating conditions in the Assay under Ethyl Icosapentate.
System suitability—

System performance: When the procedure is run with 4 μL of the standard solution under the above operating conditions, the internal standard and ethyl icosapentate are eluted in this order with the resolution between these peaks being not less than 3.

System repeatability: When the test is repeated 6 times with 4 μL of the standard solution under the above operating conditions, the relative standard deviation of the ratio of the peak area of ethyl icosapentate to that of the internal standard is not more than 1.0%.

Containers and storage Containers—Tight containers.

Ethyl Loflazepate

ロフラゼプ酸エチル

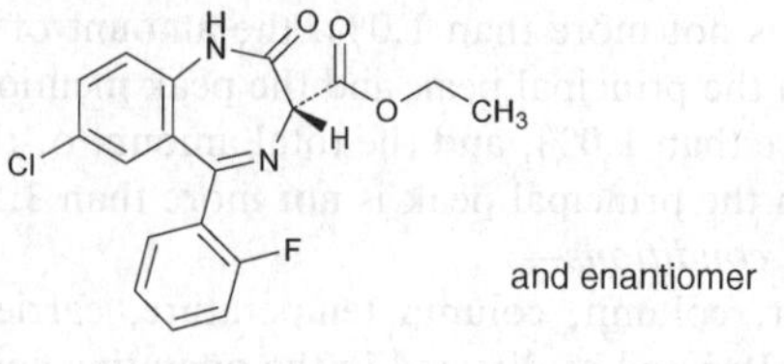

$C_{18}H_{14}ClFN_2O_3$: 360.77
Ethyl (3*RS*)-7-chloro-5-(2-fluorophenyl)-2-oxo-2,3-dihydro-1*H*-1,4-benzodiazepine-3-carboxylate
[*29177-84-2*]

Ethyl Loflazepate, when dried, contains not less than 98.5% and not more than 102.0% of ethyl loflazepate ($C_{18}H_{14}ClFN_2O_3$).

Description Ethyl Loflazepate occurs as a white crystalline powder.

It is freely soluble in dimethylsulfoxide, sparingly soluble in acetonitrile, slightly soluble in ethanol (99.5), and practically insoluble in water.

A solution of Ethyl Loflazepate in dimethylsulfoxide (1 in 50) shows no optical rotation.

Melting point: about 199°C (with decomposition).

Identification **(1)** Determine the absorption spectrum of a solution of Ethyl Loflazepate in acetonitrile (1 in 100,000) as directed under Ultraviolet-visible Spectrophotometry <*2.24*>, and compare the spectrum with the Reference Spectrum or the spectrum of a solution of Ethyl Loflazepate RS prepared in the same manner as the sample solution: both spectra exhibit similar intensities of absorption at the same wavelengths.

(2) Determine the infrared absorption spectrum of Ethyl Loflazepate, previously dried, as directed in the potassium bromide disk method under Infrared Spectrophotometry <*2.25*>, and compare the spectrum with the Reference Spectrum or the spectrum of dried Ethyl Loflazepate RS: both spectra exhibit similar intensities of absorption at the same wave numbers.

Purity **(1)** Soluble halides—To 1.0 g of Ethyl Loflazepate add 50 mL of water, allow to stand for 1 hour with occasional shaking, and filter. Discard the first 10 mL of the filtrate, transfer 25 mL of the subsequent filtrate to a Nessler tube, add 6 mL of dilute nitric acid and water to make 50 mL, and use this solution as the test solution. Proceed as directed under Chloride Limit Test <*1.03*>. Prepare the control solution as follows: to 0.20 mL of 0.01 mol/L hydrochloric acid VS add 6 mL of dilute nitric acid and water to make 50 mL.

(2) Heavy metals <*1.07*>—Proceed with 1.0 g of Ethyl Loflazepate according to Method 2, and perform the test. Prepare the control solution with 2.0 mL of Standard Lead Solution (not more than 20 ppm).

(3) Arsenic <*1.11*>—Prepare the test solution with 1.0 g of Ethyl Loflazepate according to Method 3, and perform the test (not more than 2 ppm).

(4) Related substances—Dissolve 20 mg of Ethyl Loflazepate in 20 mL of the mobile phase, and use this solution as the sample solution. Pipet 1 mL of the sample solution, add the mobile phase to make exactly 100 mL, and use this solution as the standard solution. Perform the test with exactly 5 μL each of the sample solution and standard solution as directed under Liquid Chromatography <2.01> according to the following conditions, and determine each peak area by the automatic integration method: the peak area of the related substance A, having the relative retention time of about 1.15 to ethyl loflazepate, obtained from the sample solution is not larger than 1/5 times the peak area of ethyl loflazepate from the standard solution, the peak area of the related substance B, having the relative retention time of about 1.38, from the sample solution is not larger than 7/10 times the peak area of ethyl loflazepate from the standard solution, and the area of the peak other than ethyl loflazepate and the peaks mentioned above from the sample solution is not larger than 1/10 times the peak area of ethyl loflazepate from the standard solution. Furthermore, the total area of the peaks other than ethyl loflazepate from the sample solution is not larger than the peak area of ethyl loflazepate from the standard solution.

Operating conditions—

Detector: An ultraviolet absorption photometer (wavelength: 254 nm).

Column: A stainless steel column 4.6 mm in inside diameter and 15 cm in length, packed with octadecylsilanized silica gel for liquid chromatography (5 μm in particle diameter).

Column temperature: A constant temperature of about 25°C.

Mobile phase: Dissolve 3.9 g of sodium dihydrogen phosphate dihydrate in water to make 1000 mL, and adjust to pH 6.0 with a solution prepared by dissolving 9.0 g of disodium hydrogen phosphate dodecahydrate in water to make 1000 mL. To 500 mL of this solution add 500 mL of acetonitrile for liquid chromatography.

Flow rate: Adjust so that the retention time of ethyl loflazepate is about 10 minutes.

Time span of measurement: About 3 times as long as the retention time of ethyl loflazepate.

System suitability—

Test for required detectability: Pipet 1 mL of the standard solution, and add the mobile phase to make exactly 20 mL. Confirm that the peak area of ethyl loflazepate obtained with 5 μL of this solution is equivalent to 4 to 6% of that with 5 μL of the standard solution.

System performance: When the procedure is run with 5 μL of the standard solution under the above operating conditions, the number of theoretical plates and the symmetry factor of the peak of ethyl loflazepate are not less than 2500 and not more than 2.0, respectively.

System repeatability: When the test is repeated 6 times with 5 μL of the standard solution under the above operating conditions, the relative standard deviation of the peak area of ethyl loflazepate is not more than 2.0%.

Loss on drying <2.41> Not more than 0.2% (0.2 g, 105°C, 3 hours).

Residue on ignition <2.44> Not more than 0.1% (0.5 g, platinum crucible).

Assay Weigh accurately about 10 mg each of Ethyl Loflazepate and Ethyl Loflazepate RS, both previously dried, add the internal standard solution to dissolve to make exactly 100 mL, and use these solutions as the sample solution and the standard solution, respectively. Perform the test with 10 μL each of the sample solution and standard solution as directed under Liquid Chromatography <2.01> according to the following conditions, and calculate the ratios, Q_T and Q_S, of the peak area of ethyl loflazepate to that of the internal standard.

$$\text{Amount (mg) of ethyl loflazepate } (C_{18}H_{14}ClFN_2O_3) = M_S \times Q_T/Q_S$$

M_S: Amount (mg) of Ethyl Loflazepate RS taken

Internal standard solution—A solution of methyl parahydroxybenzoate in acetonitrile for liquid chromatography (1 in 3000).

Operating conditions—

Detector: An ultraviolet absorption photometer (wavelength: 229 nm).

Column: A stainless steel column 4.0 mm in inside diameter and 25 cm in length, packed with octadecylsilanized silica gel for liquid chromatography (7 μm in particle diameter).

Column temperature: A constant temperature of about 25°C.

Mobile phase: A mixture of water, acetonitrile for liquid chromatography and ethanol (95) (2:1:1).

Flow rate: Adjust so that the retention time of ethyl loflazepate is about 13 minutes.

System suitability—

System performance: When the procedure is run with 10 μL of the standard solution under the above operating conditions, the internal standard and ethyl loflazepate are eluted in this order with the resolution between these peaks being not less than 6.

System repeatability: When the test is repeated 6 times with 10 μL of the standard solution under the above operating conditions, the relative standard deviation of the ratio of the peak area of ethyl loflazepate to that of the internal standard is not more than 1.0%.

Containers and storage Containers—Tight containers.

Others

Related substance A:
Ethyl 7-chloro-2-oxo-5-phenyl-2,3-dihydro-1*H*-1,4-benzodiazepine-3-carboxylate

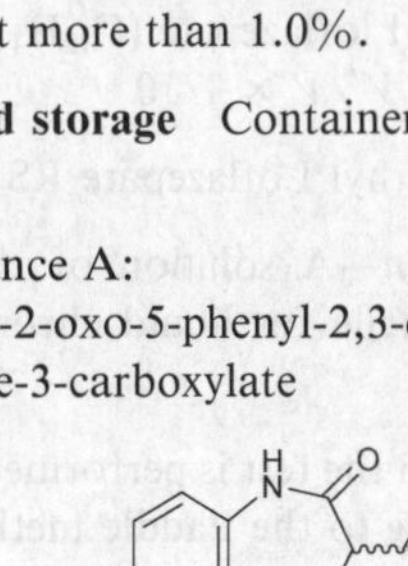

Related substance B:
Propyl 7-chloro-5-(2-fluorophenyl)-2-oxo-2,3-dihydro-1*H*-1,4-benzodiazepine-3-carboxylate

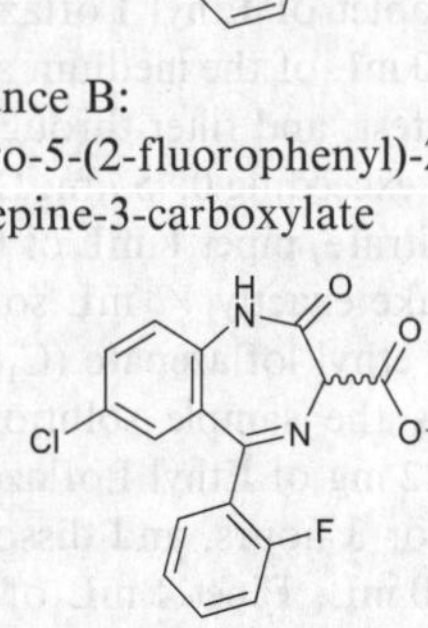

Ethyl Loflazepate Tablets

ロフラゼプ酸エチル錠

Ethyl Loflazepate Tablets contain not less than 93.0% and not more than 107.0% of the labeled amount of ethyl loflazepate ($C_{18}H_{14}ClFN_2O_3$: 360.77).

Method of preparation Prepare as directed under Tablets, with Ethyl Loflazepate.

Identification To a quantity of powdered Ethyl Loflazepate Tablets, equivalent to 1 mg of Ethyl Loflazepate, add 10 mL of acetonitrile, shake for 15 minutes, and centrifuge. To 1 mL of the supernatant liquid add acetonitrile to make 10 mL. Determine the absorption spectrum of this solution as directed under Ultraviolet-visible Spectrophotometry <*2.24*>: it exhibits a maximum between 227 nm and 231 nm.

Uniformity of dosage units <*6.02*> Perform the test according to the following method: it meets the requirement of the Content uniformity test.

To 1 tablet of Ethyl Loflazepate Tablets add exactly 0.5 mL of water, sonicate to disintegrate the tablet, add exactly 10 mL of the internal standard solution, shake for 20 minutes, and centrifuge. Pipet V mL of the supernatant liquid, add water so that each mL contains 48 μL of water, add the internal standard solution to make exactly V' mL so that each mL contains about 95 μg of ethyl loflazepate ($C_{18}H_{14}ClFN_2O_3$), and use this solution as the sample solution. Then, proceed as directed in the Assay.

Amount (mg) of ethyl loflazepate ($C_{18}H_{14}ClFN_2O_3$)
$= M_S \times Q_T/Q_S \times V'/V \times 1/10$

M_S: Amount (mg) of Ethyl Loflazepate RS taken

Internal standard solution—A solution of methyl parahydroxybenzoate in acetonitrile for liquid chromatography (1 in 3000).

Dissolution <*6.10*> When the test is performed at 50 revolutions per minute according to the Paddle method, using 900 mL of water as the dissolution medium, the dissolution rate in 30 minutes of Ethyl Loflazepate Tablets is not less than 80%.

Start the test with 1 tablet of Ethyl Loflazepate Tablets, withdraw not less than 20 mL of the medium at the specified minute after starting the test, and filter through a membrane filter with a pore size not exceeding 0.45 μm. Discard not less than 10 mL of the first filtrate, pipet V mL of the subsequent filtrate, add water to make exactly V' mL so that each mL contains about 1.1 μg of ethyl loflazepate ($C_{18}H_{14}ClFN_2O_3$), and use this solution as the sample solution. Separately, weigh accurately about 22 mg of Ethyl Loflazepate RS, previously dried at 105°C for 3 hours, and dissolve in ethanol (95) to make exactly 100 mL. Pipet 1 mL of this solution, add water to make exactly 200 mL, and use this solution as the standard solution. Perform the test with exactly 10 μL each of the sample solution and standard solution as directed under Liquid Chromatography <*2.01*> according to the following conditions, and determine the peak areas, A_T and A_S, of ethyl loflazepate in each solution.

Dissolution rate (%) with respect to the labeled amount of ethyl loflazepate ($C_{18}H_{14}ClFN_2O_3$)
$= M_S \times A_T/A_S \times V'/V \times 1/C \times 9/2$

M_S: Amount (mg) of Ethyl Loflazepate RS taken
C: Labeled amount (mg) of ethyl loflazepate ($C_{18}H_{14}ClFN_2O_3$) in 1 tablet

Operating conditions—

Detector: An ultraviolet absorption photometer (wavelength: 230 nm).

Column: A stainless steel column 4.0 mm in inside diameter and 15 cm in length, packed with octadecylsilanized silica gel for liquid chromatography (5 μm in particle diameter).

Column temperature: A constant temperature of about 25°C.

Mobile phase: A mixture of water, acetonitrile and ethanol (99.5) (2:1:1).

Flow rate: Adjust so that the retention time of ethyl loflazepate is about 7 minutes.

System suitability—

System performance: When the procedure is run with 10 μL of the standard solution under the above operating conditions, the number of theoretical plates and the symmetry factor of the peak of ethyl loflazepate are not less than 1500 and not more than 1.5, respectively.

System repeatability: When the test is repeated 6 times with 10 μL of the standard solution under the above operating conditions, the relative standard deviation of the peak area of ethyl loflazepate is not more than 3.0%.

Assay Weigh accurately the mass of not less than 20 tablets of Ethyl Loflazepate Tablets, and powder. Weigh accurately a portion of the powder, equivalent to about 1 mg of ethyl loflazepate ($C_{18}H_{14}ClFN_2O_3$), add 0.5 mL of water, and sonicate. Add exactly 10 mL of the internal standard, shake, centrifuge, and use the supernatant liquid as the sample solution. Separately, weigh accurately about 10 mg of Ethyl Loflazepate RS, previously dried at 105°C for 3 hours, and add the internal standard solution to make exactly 100 mL. To 10 mL of this solution add 0.5 mL of water, and use this solution as the standard solution. Perform the test with exactly 10 μL each of the sample solution and standard solution as directed under Liquid Chromatography <*2.01*> according to the following conditions, and calculate the ratios, Q_T and Q_S, of the peak area of ethyl loflazepate to that of the internal standard.

Amount (mg) of ethyl loflazepate ($C_{18}H_{14}ClFN_2O_3$)
$= M_S \times Q_T/Q_S \times 1/10$

M_S: Amount (mg) of Ethyl Loflazepate RS taken

Internal standard solution—A solution of methyl parahydroxybenzoate in acetonitrile for liquid chromatography (1 in 3000).

Operating conditions—

Detector: An ultraviolet absorption photometer (wavelength: 229 nm).

Column: A stainless steel column 4.6 mm in inside diameter and 25 cm in length, packed with octadecylsilanized silica gel for liquid chromatography (5 μm in particle diameter).

Column temperature: A constant temperature of about 25°C.

Mobile phase: A mixture of water, acetonitrile for liquid chromatography and ethanol (95) (2:1:1).

Flow rate: Adjust so that the retention time of ethyl loflazepate is about 13 minutes.

System suitability—

System performance: When the procedure is run with 10 μL of the standard solution under the above operating conditions, the internal standard and ethyl loflazepate are eluted in this order with the resolution between these peaks being not less than 6.

System repeatability: When the test is repeated 6 times

with 10 μL of the standard solution under the above operating conditions, the relative standard deviation of the ratio of the peak area of ethyl loflazepate to that of the internal standard is not more than 1.0%.

Containers and storage Containers—Well-closed containers.

Ethylmorphine Hydrochloride Hydrate

エチルモルヒネ塩酸塩水和物

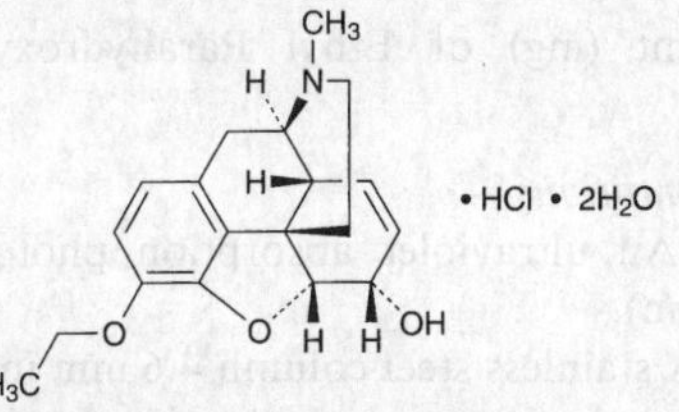

$C_{19}H_{23}NO_3.HCl.2H_2O$: 385.88
(5*R*,6*S*)-4,5-Epoxy-3-ethoxy-17-methyl-7,8-didehydromorphinan-6-ol monohydrochloride dihydrate
[*125-30-4*, anhydride]

Ethylmorphine Hydrochloride Hydrate contains not less than 98.0% of ethylmorphine hydrochloride ($C_{19}H_{23}NO_3.HCl$: 349.85), calculated on the anhydrous basis.

Description Ethylmorphine Hydrochloride Hydrate occurs as white to pale yellow, crystals or crystalline powder.

It is very soluble in methanol and in acetic acid (100), freely soluble in water, soluble in ethanol (95), sparingly soluble in acetic anhydride, and practically insoluble in diethyl ether.

It is affected by light.

Melting point: about 123°C (with decomposition).

Identification **(1)** Determine the absorption spectrum of a solution of Ethylmorphine Hydrochloride Hydrate (1 in 10,000) as directed under Ultraviolet-visible Spectrophotometry <*2.24*>, and compare the spectrum with the Reference Spectrum: both spectra exhibit similar intensities of absorption at the same wavelengths.

(2) Determine the infrared absorption spectrum of Ethylmorphine Hydrochloride Hydrate as directed in the potassium bromide disk method under Infrared Spectrophotometry <*2.25*>, and compare the spectrum with the Reference Spectrum: both spectra exhibit similar intensities of absorption at the same wave numbers.

(3) A solution of Ethylmorphine Hydrochloride Hydrate (1 in 50) responds to Qualitative Tests <*1.09*> (2) for chloride.

Optical rotation <*2.49*> $[\alpha]_D^{20}$: $-103 - -106°$ (0.4 g calculated on the anhydrous basis, water, 20 mL, 100 mm).

pH <*2.54*> Dissolve 0.10 g of Ethylmorphine Hydrochloride Hydrate in 10 mL of water: the pH of this solution is between 4.0 and 6.0.

Purity Related substances—Dissolve 0.20 g of Ethylmorphine Hydrochloride Hydrate in 10 mL of diluted ethanol (1 in 2), and use this solution as the sample solution. Pipet 0.5 mL of the sample solution, add diluted ethanol (1 in 2) to make exactly 100 mL, and use this solution as the standard solution. Perform the test with these solutions as directed under Thin-layer Chromatography <*2.03*>. Spot 10 μL each of the sample solution and standard solution on a plate of silica gel with fluorescent indicator for thin-layer chromatography. Develop the plate with a mixture of ethanol (99.5), toluene, acetone and ammonia solution (28) (14:14:7:1) to a distance of about 10 cm, and air-dry the plate. Examine under ultraviolet light (main wavelength: 254 nm): the spots other than the principal spot obtained from the sample solution are not more intense than the spot from the standard solution.

Water <*2.48*> 8.0 - 10.0% (0.25 g, volumetric titration, direct titration).

Residue on ignition <*2.44*> Not more than 0.1% (0.5 g).

Assay Weigh accurately about 0.5 g of Ethylmorphine Hydrochloride Hydrate, and dissolve in 50 mL of a mixture of acetic anhydride and acetic acid (100) (7:3), and titrate <*2.50*> with 0.1 mol/L perchloric acid VS (potentiometric titration). Perform a blank determination in the same manner, and make any necessary correction.

Each mL of 0.1 mol/L perchloric acid VS
= 34.99 mg of $C_{19}H_{23}NO_3.HCl$

Containers and storage Containers—Tight containers.
Storage—Light-resistant.

Ethyl Parahydroxybenzoate

パラオキシ安息香酸エチル

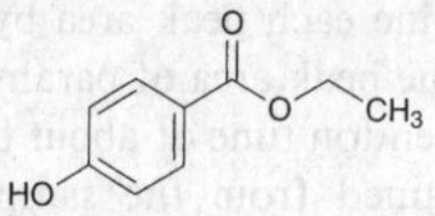

$C_9H_{10}O_3$: 166.17
Ethyl 4-hydroxybenzoate
[*120-47-8*]

This monograph is harmonized with the European Pharmacopoeia and the U.S. Pharmacopeia.

The parts of the text that are not harmonized are marked with symbols (◆ ◆).

Information on the harmonization with the European Pharmacopoeia and the U.S. Pharmacopeia is available on the website of the Pharmaceuticals and Medical Devices Agency.

Ethyl Parahydroxybenzoate contains not less than 98.0% and not more than 102.0% of ethyl parahydroxybenzoate ($C_9H_{10}O_3$).

◆**Description** Ethyl Parahydroxybenzoate occurs as colorless crystals or a white crystalline powder.

It is freely soluble in methanol, in ethanol (95) and in acetone, and very slightly soluble in water.◆

Identification Determine the infrared absorption spectrum of Ethyl Parahydroxybenzoate as directed in the potassium bromide disk method under Infrared Spectrophotometry <*2.25*>, and compare the spectrum with the Reference Spectrum or the spectrum of Ethyl Parahydroxybenzoate RS: both spectra exhibit similar intensities of absorption at the same wave numbers.

Melting point <*2.60*> 115 - 118°C

Purity **(1)** Clarity and color of solution—Dissolve 1.0 g of Ethyl Parahydroxybenzoate in ethanol (95) to make 10 mL: the solution is clear and not more intensely colored than the following control solution.

Control solution: To 5.0 mL of Cobalt (II) Chloride CS, 12.0 mL of Iron (III) Chloride CS and 2.0 mL of Copper (II) Sulfate CS add diluted dilute hydrochloric acid (1 in 10) to make 1000 mL.

(2) Acidity—To 2 mL of the solution of Ethyl Parahydroxybenzoate obtained in (1) add 3 mL of ethanol (95), add 5 mL of freshly boiled and cooled water and 0.1 mL of bromocresol green-sodium hydroxide-ethanol TS, then add 0.1 mol/L sodium hydroxide VS until the solution shows a blue color: the volume of 0.1 mol/L sodium hydroxide VS used does not exceed 0.1 mL.

◆**(3)** Heavy metals *<1.07>*—Dissolve 1.0 g of Ethyl Parahydroxybenzoate in 25 mL of acetone, add 2 mL of dilute acetic acid and water to make 50 mL, and perform the test using this solution as the test solution. Prepare the control solution as follows: to 2.0 mL of Standard Lead Solution add 25 mL of acetone, 2 mL of dilute acetic acid, and water to make 50 mL (not more than 20 ppm).◆

(4) Related substances—Dissolve 50.0 mg of Ethyl Parahydroxybenzoate in 2.5 mL of methanol, and add the mobile phase to make exactly 50 mL. Pipet 10 mL of this solution, add the mobile phase to make exactly 100 mL, and use this solution as the sample solution. Pipet 1 mL of the sample solution, and add the mobile phase to make exactly 20 mL. Pipet 1 mL of this solution, add the mobile phase to make exactly 10 mL, and use this solution as the standard solution. Perform the test with exactly 10 μL each of the sample solution and standard solution as directed under Liquid Chromatography *<2.01>* according to the following conditions, and determine each peak area by the automatic integration method: the peak area of parahydroxybenzoic acid having a relative retention time of about 0.5 to ethyl parahydroxybenzoate obtained from the sample solution is not larger than the peak area of ethyl parahydroxybenzoate from the standard solution (0.5%). For the peak area of parahydroxybenzoic acid, multiply its correction factor, 1.4. Furthermore, the area of the peak other than ethyl parahydroxybenzoate and parahydroxybenzoic acid from the sample solution is not larger than the peak area of ethyl parahydroxybenzoate from the standard solution (0.5%), and the total area of the peaks other than ethyl parahydroxybenzoate is not larger than 2 times the peak area of ethyl parahydroxybenzoate from the standard solution (1.0%). For this calculation the peak area not larger than 1/5 times the peak area of ethyl parahydroxybenzoate from the standard solution is excluded (0.1%).

Operating conditions—

Detector, column, column temperature, mobile phase, and flow rate: Proceed as directed in the operating conditions in the Assay.

Time span of measurement: About 4 times as long as the retention time of ethyl parahydroxybenzoate.

System suitability—

System performance: Proceed as directed in the system suitability in the Assay.

◆Test for required detectability: To exactly 2 mL of the standard solution add the mobile phase to make exactly 10 mL. Confirm that the peak area of ethyl parahydroxybenzoate obtained with 10 μL of this solution is equivalent to 14 to 26% of that with 10 μL of the standard solution.◆

◆System repeatability: When the test is repeated 6 times with 10 μL of the standard solution under the above operating conditions, the relative standard deviation of the peak area of ethyl parahydroxybenzoate is not more than 2.0%.◆

Residue on ignition *<2.44>* Not more than 0.1% (1 g).

Assay Weigh accurately about 50.0 mg each of Ethyl Parahydroxybenzoate and Ethyl Parahydroxybenzoate RS, dissolve separately in 2.5 mL each of methanol, and add the mobile phase to make exactly 50 mL. Pipet 10 mL each of these solutions, add the mobile phase to make exactly 100 mL, and use these solutions as the sample solution and the standard solution, respectively. Perform the test with exactly 10 μL each of the sample solution and standard solution as directed under Liquid Chromatography *<2.01>* according to the following conditions, and determine the peak areas, A_T and A_S, of ethyl parahydroxybenzoate in each solution.

Amount (mg) of ethyl parahydroxybenzoate ($C_9H_{10}O_3$)
$= M_S \times A_T/A_S$

M_S: Amount (mg) of Ethyl Parahydroxybenzoate RS taken

Operating conditions—

Detector: An ultraviolet absorption photometer (wavelength: 272 nm).

Column: A stainless steel column 4.6 mm in inside diameter and 15 cm in length, packed with octadecylsilanized silica gel for liquid chromatography (5 μm in particle diameter).

Column temperature: A constant temperature of about 35°C.

Mobile phase: A mixture of methanol and potassium dihydrogen phosphate solution (17 in 2500) (13:7).

Flow rate: 1.3 mL per minute.

System suitability—

System performance: Dissolve 5 mg each of Ethyl Parahydroxybenzoate, methyl parahydroxybenzoate and parahydroxybenzoic acid in the mobile phase to make exactly 100 mL. Pipet 1 mL of this solution, and add the mobile phase to make exactly 10 mL. When the procedure is run with 10 μL of this solution under the above operating conditions, parahydroxybenzoic acid, methyl parahydroxybenzoate and ethyl parahydroxybenzoate are eluted in this order, the relative retention times of parahydroxybenzoic acid and methyl parahydroxybenzoate to ethyl parahydroxybenzoate are about 0.5 and about 0.8, respectively, and the resolution between the peaks of methyl parahydroxybenzoate and ethyl parahydroxybenzoate is not less than 2.0.

System repeatability: When the test is repeated 6 times with 10 μL of the standard solution under the above operating conditions, the relative standard deviation of the peak area of ethyl parahydroxybenzoate is not more than 0.85%.

◆**Containers and storage** Containers—Well-closed containers.◆

Etidronate Disodium

エチドロン酸二ナトリウム

H_3C, PO_3HNa, HO, PO_3HNa

$C_2H_6Na_2O_7P_2$: 249.99
Disodium dihydrogen 1-hydroxyethane-1,1-diyldiphosphonate
[7414-83-7]

Etidronate Disodium, when dried, contains not less than 98.0% and not more than 101.0% of etidronate disodium ($C_2H_6Na_2O_7P_2$).

Description Etidronate Disodium occurs as a white powder.

It is freely soluble in water, and practically insoluble in

ethanol (99.5).

The pH of a solution prepared by dissolving 0.10 g of Etidronate Disodium in 10 mL of water is between 4.4 and 5.4.

It is hygroscopic.

Identification (1) To 5 mL of a solution of Etidronate Disodium (1 in 100) add 1 mL of copper (II) sulfate TS, and mix for 10 minutes: a blue precipitate is formed.

(2) Determine the infrared absorption spectrum of Etidronate Disodium, previously dried, as directed in the potassium bromide disk method under Infrared Spectrophotometry <2.25>, and compare the spectrum with the Reference Spectrum: both spectra exhibit similar intensities of absorption at the same wave numbers.

(3) A solution of Etidronate Disodium (1 in 100) responds to Qualitative Tests <1.09> for sodium salt.

Purity (1) Heavy metals <1.07>—Proceed with 1.0 g of Etidronate Disodium according to Method 4, and perform the test using the supernatant liquid obtained by centrifuging after addition of 2 mL of dilute acetic acid. Prepare the control solution with 2.0 mL of Standard Lead Solution (not more than 20 ppm).

(2) Arsenic <1.11>—Prepare the test solution with 1.0 g of Etidronate Disodium according to Method 1, and perform the test (not more than 2 ppm).

(3) Phosphite—Weigh accurately about 3.5 g of Etidronate Disodium, dissolve in 100 mL of 0.1 mol/L sodium dihydrogen phosphate TS adjusted the pH to 8.0 with sodium hydroxide TS, add exactly 20 mL of 0.05 mol/L iodine VS, and immediately stopper tightly. Allow to stand in a dark place for 30 minutes, add 1 mL of acetic acid (100), and titrate <2.50> the excess of iodine with 0.1 mol/L sodium thiosulfate VS (indicator: 1 mL of starch TS). Perform a blank determination in the same manner. The amount of phosphite (NaH_2PO_3) is not more than 1.0%.

Each mL of 0.05 mol/L iodine VS = 5.199 mg of NaH_2PO_3

(4) Methanol—Weigh accurately about 0.5 g of Etidronate Disodium, dissolve in water to make exactly 5 mL, and use this solution as the sample solution. Separately, pipet 1 mL of methanol, and add water to make exactly 100 mL. Pipet 1 mL of this solution, add water to make exactly 100 mL, and use this solution as the standard solution. Perform the test with exactly 1 μL each of the sample solution and standard solution as directed under Gas Chromatography <2.02> according to the following conditions, and determine the peak areas, A_T and A_S, of methanol in each solution and determine the amount of methanol (CH_4O) by the following equation: not more than 0.1%.

$$\text{Amount (\%) of methanol } (CH_4O) = 1/M \times A_T/A_S \times 1/20 \times 0.79$$

M: Amount (g) of Etidronate Disodium taken
0.79: Density (g/mL) of methanol

Operating conditions—

Detector: A hydrogen flame-ionization detector.

Column: A glass column 3 mm in inside diameter and 2 m in length, packed with porous copolymer beads for gas chromatography (180 - 250 μm in particle diameter).

Column temperature: A constant temperature of about 130°C.

Carrier gas: Nitrogen.

Flow rate: Adjust so that the retention time of methanol is about 2 minutes.

System suitability—

System performance: To 1 mL of methanol and 1 mL of ethanol (99.5) add water to make 100 mL. To 1 mL of this solution add water to make 100 mL. When the procedure is run with 1 μL of this solution under the above operating conditions, methanol and ethanol are eluted in this order with the resolution between these peaks being not less than 2.0.

System repeatability: When the test is repeated 6 times with 1 μL of the standard solution under the above operating conditions, the relative standard deviation of the peak area of methanol is not more than 5.0%.

Loss on drying <2.41> Not more than 5.0% (0.5 g, 210°C, 2 hours).

Assay Weigh accurately about 0.5 g of Etidronate Disodium, previously dried, and dissolve in water to make exactly 50 mL. Transfer exactly 15 mL of this solution to a chromatographic column of 10 mm in internal diameter containing 5 mL of strongly acidic ion exchange resin for column chromatography (H type), allow to flow at a flow rate of about 1.5 mL per minute, and wash the column with two 25-mL portions of water. Combine the eluate and the washings, and titrate <2.50> with 0.1 mol/L sodium hydroxide VS (potentiometric titration). Perform a blank determination in the same manner, and make any necessary correction.

Each mL of 0.1 mol/L sodium hydroxide VS
= 12.50 mg of $C_2H_6Na_2O_7P_2$

Containers and storage Containers—Tight containers.

Etidronate Disodium Tablets

エチドロン酸二ナトリウム錠

Etidronate Disodium Tablets contain not less than 93.0% and not more than 107.0% of the labeled amount of etidronate disodium ($C_2H_6Na_2O_7P_2$: 249.99).

Method of preparation Prepare as directed under Tablets, with Etidronate Disodium.

Identification (1) Shake an amount of powdered Etidronate Disodium Tablets, equivalent to 0.2 g of Etidronate Disodium, with 20 mL of water, and filter. Proceed with the filtrate as directed in the Identification (1) under Etidronate Disodium.

(2) Shake an amount of powdered Etidronate Disodium Tablets, equivalent to 0.4 g of Etidronate Disodium, with 10 mL of water, and filter. Evaporate total amount of the filtrate to dryness under reduced pressure, shake the residue with 15 mL of ethanol (99.5), centrifuge, and dry the precipitate at 150°C for 4 hours. Determine the infrared absorption spectrum of the precipitate as directed in the potassium bromide disk method under Infrared Spectrophotometry <2.25>: it exhibits absorption at the wave numbers of about 1170 cm^{-1}, 1056 cm^{-1}, 916 cm^{-1} and 811 cm^{-1}.

Uniformity of dosage units <6.02> It meets the requirement of the Mass variation test.

Dissolution <6.10> When the test is performed at 50 revolutions per minute according to the Paddle method, using 900 mL of water as the dissolution medium, the dissolution rate in 60 minutes of Etidronate Disodium Tablets is not less than 85%.

Start the test with 1 tablet of Etidronate Disodium Tablets, withdraw not less than 20 mL of the medium at the specified minute after starting the test, and filter through a membrane filter with a pore size not exceeding 0.45 μm. Discard not less than 10 mL of the first filtrate, take exactly V mL of the subsequent filtrate, add water to make exactly V' mL so that each mL contains about 0.22 mg of etidronate disodium ($C_2H_6Na_2O_7P_2$), and use this solution as the sample solution. Separately, weigh accurately about 30 mg of etidronate disodium for assay, previously dried at 210°C for 2 hours, and dissolve in water to make exactly 100 mL. Dilute exactly a suitable amount of this solution with water to make solutions so that each mL contains about 0.12 mg, about 0.21 mg and about 0.24 mg of etidronate disodium ($C_2H_6Na_2O_7P_2$), and use these solutions as the standard solutions. Pipet 2 mL each of the sample solution and standard solutions, add exactly 2 mL of a solution of copper (II) sulfate (7 in 10,000) and water to make exactly 10 mL. Determine the absorbances of these solutions at 233 nm as directed under Ultraviolet-visible Spectrophotometry *<2.24>*, using a solution prepared by diluting exactly 2 mL of the solution of copper (II) sulfate (7 in 10,000) with water to make exactly 10 mL as the control. From the calibration curve obtained with the standard solutions calculate the concentration of etidronate disodium, C_T, in the sample solution.

Dissolution rate (%) with respect to the labeled amount of etidronate disodium ($C_2H_6Na_2O_7P_2$)
$= C_T \times V'/V \times 1/C \times 90$

C_T: Concentration (μg/mL) of etidronate disodium ($C_2H_6Na_2O_7P_2$) in the sample solution
C: Labeled amount (mg) of etidronate disodium ($C_2H_6Na_2O_7P_2$) in 1 tablet

Assay Weigh accurately and powder not less than 20 Etidronate Disodium Tablets. Weigh accurately a portion of the powder, equivalent to about 0.5 g of etidronate disodium ($C_2H_6Na_2O_7P_2$), add 30 mL of water, shake vigorously for 10 minutes, add water to make exactly 50 mL, and filter. Proceed with exactly 15 mL of the filtrate as directed in the Assay under Etidronate Disodium.

Containers and storage Containers—Tight containers.

Etilefrine Hydrochloride

エチレフリン塩酸塩

$C_{10}H_{15}NO_2.HCl$: 217.69
(1*RS*)-2-Ethylamino-1-(3-hydroxyphenyl)ethanol monohydrochloride
[*943-17-9*]

Etilefrine Hydrochloride, when dried, contains not less than 98.0% and not more than 101.0% of etilefrine hydrochloride ($C_{10}H_{15}NO_2.HCl$).

Description Etilefrine Hydrochloride occurs as white, crystals or crystalline powder.

It is very soluble in water, freely soluble in ethanol (99.5), and sparingly soluble in acetic acid (100).

It is gradually colored to yellow-brown by light.

A solution of Etilefrine Hydrochloride (1 in 20) shows no optical rotation.

Identification (1) Dissolve 5 mg of Etilefrine Hydrochloride in 100 mL of diluted hydrochloric acid (1 in 1000). Determine the absorption spectrum of the solution as directed under Ultraviolet-visible Spectrophotometry *<2.24>*, and compare the spectrum with the Reference Spectrum: both spectra exhibit similar intensities of absorption at the same wavelengths.

(2) Determine the infrared absorption spectrum of Etilefrine Hydrochloride, previously dried, as directed in the potassium chloride disk method under Infrared Spectrophotometry *<2.25>*, and compare the spectrum with the Reference Spectrum: both spectra exhibit similar intensities of absorption at the same wave numbers.

(3) A solution of Etilefrine Hydrochloride (1 in 1000) responds to Qualitative Tests *<1.09>* (2) for chloride.

Melting point *<2.60>* 118 – 122°C

Purity (1) Clarity and color of solution—Dissolve 0.5 g of Etilefrine Hydrochloride in 10 mL of water: the solution is clear and colorless.

(2) Acidity or alkalinity—To 10 mL of a solution of Etilefrine Hydrochloride (1 in 50) add 0.1 mL of methyl red TS for acid or alkali test and 0.2 mL of 0.01 mol/L sodium hydroxide VS: a yellow color develops, and the necessary volume of 0.01 mol/L hydrochloric acid VS to change the color to red is not more than 0.4 mL.

(3) Sulfate *<1.14>*—Perform the test with 0.85 g of Etilefrine Hydrochloride. Prepare the control solution with 0.35 mL of 0.005 mol/L sulfuric acid VS (not more than 0.020%).

(4) Heavy metals *<1.07>*—Dissolve 1.0 g of Etilefrine Hydrochloride in 30 mL of water and 2 mL of acetic acid (100), adjust with sodium hydroxide TS to a pH of 3.3, add water to make 50 mL, and perform the test. Prepare the control solution with 2.0 mL of Standard Lead Solution (not more than 20 ppm).

Loss on drying *<2.41>* Not more than 0.5% (1 g, 105°C, 4 hours).

Residue on ignition *<2.44>* Not more than 0.1% (1 g).

Assay Weigh accurately about 0.15 g of Etilefrine Hydrochloride, previously dried, dissolve in 20 mL of acetic acid (100), add 50 mL of acetic anhydride, and titrate *<2.50>* with 0.1 mol/L perchloric acid VS (potentiometric titration). Perform a blank determination in the same manner, and make any necessary correctoin.

Each mL of 0.1 mol/L perchloric acid VS
$= 21.77$ mg of $C_{10}H_{15}NO_2.HCl$

Containers and storage Containers—Tight containers.
Storage—Light-resistant.

Etilefrine Hydrochloride Tablets

エチレフリン塩酸塩錠

Etilefrine Hydrochloride Tablets contain not less than 93.0% and not more than 107.0% of the labeled amount of etilefrine hydrochloride ($C_{10}H_{15}NO_2.HCl$: 217.69).

Method of preparation Prepare as directed under Tablets, with Etilefrine Hydrochloride.

Identification To a quantity of powdered Etilefrine Hydrochloride Tablets, equivalent to 5 mg of Etilefrine Hydrochloride, add 60 mL of diluted hydrochloric acid (1 in 1000), shake well, add 40 mL of diluted hydrochloric acid (1 in 1000), and filter. Determine the absorption spectrum of the filtrate as directed under Ultraviolet-visible Spectrophotometry *<2.24>*, using diluted hydrochloric acid (1 in 1000) as the blank: it exhibits a maximum between 271 nm and 275 nm.

Uniformity of dosage units *<6.02>* Perform the test according to the following method: it meets the requirements of the Content uniformity test.

To 1 tablet of Etilefrine Hydrochloride Tablets add 60 mL of diluted hydrochloric acid (1 in 1000), and proceed as directed in the Assay.

Amount (mg) of etilefrine hydrochloride ($C_{10}H_{15}NO_2.HCl$)
$= M_S \times A_T/A_S \times 1/10$

M_S: Amount (mg) of etilefrine hydrochloride for assay taken

Dissolution *<6.10>* When the test is performed at 50 revolutions per minute according to the Paddle method, using 900 mL of water as the dissolution medium, the dissolution rate in 30 minutes of Etilefrine Hydrochloride Tablets is not less than 70%.

Start the test with 1 tablet of Etilefrine Hydrochloride Tablets, withdraw not less than 20 mL of the medium at the specified minute after starting the test, and filter through a membrane filter with a pore size not exceeding 0.45 μm. Discard not less than 10 mL of the first filtrate, pipet V mL of the subsequent filtrate, add water to make exactly V' mL so that each mL contains about 5 μg of etilefrine hydrochloride ($C_{10}H_{15}NO_2.HCl$), and use this solution as the sample solution. Separately, weigh accurately about 25 mg of etilefrine hydrochloride for assay, previously dried at 105°C for 4 hours, and dissolve in water to make exactly 50 mL. Pipet 1 mL of this solution, add water to make exactly 100 mL, and use this solution as the standard solution. Perform the test with exactly 20 μL each of the sample solution and standard solution as directed under Liquid Chromatography *<2.01>* according to the following conditions, and determine the peak areas, A_T and A_S, of etilefrine in each solution.

Dissolution rate (%) with respect to the labeled amount of etilefrine hydrochloride ($C_{10}H_{15}NO_2.HCl$)
$= M_S \times A_T/A_S \times V'/V \times 1/C \times 18$

M_S: Amount (mg) of etilefrine hydrochloride for assay taken

C: Labeled amount (mg) of etilefrine hydrochloride ($C_{10}H_{15}NO_2.HCl$) in 1 tablet.

Operating conditions—

Proceed as directed in the operating conditions in the Assay.

System suitability—

System performance: When the procedure is run with 20 μL of the standard solution under the above operating conditions, the number of theoretical plates and the symmetry factor of the peak of etilefrine are not less than 8000 and 0.9 - 1.2, respectively.

System repeatability: When the test is repeated 6 times with 20 μL of the standard solution under the above operating conditions, the relative standard deviation of the peak area of etilefrine is not more than 2.0%.

Assay Weigh accurately the mass of not less than 20 Etilefrine Hydrochloride Tablets, and powder. Weigh accurately a portion of the powder, equivalent to about 5 mg of etilefrine hydrochloride ($C_{10}H_{15}NO_2.HCl$), add 60 mL of diluted hydrochloric acid (1 in 1000), shake for 10 minutes, add diluted hydrochloric acid (1 in 1000) to make exactly 100 mL, and filter. Discard the first 20 mL of the filtrate, and use the subsequent filtrate as the sample solution. Separately, weigh accurately about 50 mg of etilefrine hydrochloride for assay, previously dried at 105°C for 4 hours, and dissolve in diluted hydrochloric acid (1 in 1000) to make exactly 100 mL. Pipet 10 mL of this solution, add diluted hydrochloric acid (1 in 1000) to make exactly 100 mL, and use this solution as the standard solution. Perform the test with exactly 20 μL each of the sample solution and standard solution as direct under Liquid Chromatography *<2.01>* according to the following conditions, and determine the peak areas, A_T and A_S, of etilefrine in each solution.

Amount (mg) of etilefrine hydrochloride ($C_{10}H_{15}NO_2.HCl$)
$= M_S \times A_T/A_S \times 1/10$

M_S: Amount (mg) of etilefrine hydrochloride for assay taken

Operating conditions—

Detector: An ultraviolet absorption photometer (wavelength: 220 nm).

Column: A stainless steel column 4.6 mm in inside diameter and 25 cm in length, packed with octylsilanized silica gel for liquid chromatography (5 μm in particle diameter).

Column temperature: A constant temperature of about 40°C.

Mobile phase: Dissolve 5 g of sodium lauryl sulfate in 940 mL of water and 500 mL of acetonitrile, and adjust the pH to 2.3 with phosphoric acid.

Flow rate: Adjust so that the retention time of etilefrine is about 6 minutes.

System suitability—

System performance: Dissolve 4 mg of bamethan sulfate and 4 mg of etilefrine hydrochloride in the mobile phase to make 50 mL. When the procedure is run with 20 μL of this solution under the above operating conditions, etilefrine and bamethan are eluted in this order with the resolution between these peaks being not less than 5.

System repeatability: When the test is repeated 6 times with 20 μL of the standard solution under the above operating conditions, the relative standard deviation of the peak area of etilefrine is not more than 1.0%.

Containers and storage Containers—Tight containers.

Storage—Light-resistant.

Etizolam

エチゾラム

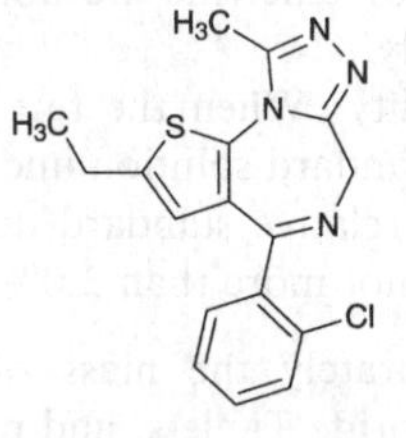

$C_{17}H_{15}ClN_4S$: 342.85
4-(2-Chlorophenyl)-2-ethyl-9-methyl-6*H*-thieno[3,2-*f*][1,2,4]triazolo[4,3-*a*][1,4]diazepine
[40054-69-1]

Etizolam, when dried, contains not less than 98.5% and not more than 101.0% of etizolam ($C_{17}H_{15}ClN_4S$).

Description Etizolam occurs as a white to pale yellow-white crystalline powder.

It is soluble in ethanol (99.5), sparingly soluble in acetonitrile and in acetic anhydride, and practically insoluble in water.

Identification **(1)** Determine the absorption spectrum of a solution of Etizolam in ethanol (99.5) (1 in 100,000) as directed under Ultraviolet-visible Spectrophotometry <*2.24*>, and compare the spectrum with the Reference Spectrum: both spectra exhibit similar intensities of absorption at the same wavelengths.

(2) Determine the infrared absorption spectrum of Etizolam as directed in the potassium bromide disk method under Infrared Spectrophotometry <*2.25*>, and compare the spectrum with the Reference Spectrum: both spectra exhibit similar intensities of absorption at the same wave numbers.

Melting point <*2.60*> 147 – 151°C

Purity **(1)** Heavy metals <*1.07*>—Proceed with 2.0 g of Etizolam according to Method 2, and perform the test. Prepare the control solution with 2.0 mL of Standard Lead Solution (not more than 10 ppm).

(2) Related substances—Dissolve 20 mg of Etizolam in 50 mL of acetonitrile, and use this solution as the sample solution. Pipet 1 mL of the sample solution, and add acetonitrile to make exactly 20 mL. Pipet 1 mL of this solution, add acetonitrile to make exactly 50 mL, and use this solution as the standard solution. Perform the test with exactly 10 μL each of the sample solution and standard solution as directed under Liquid Chromatography <*2.01*> according to the following conditions, and determine each peak area by the automatic integration method: the area of the peak other than etizolam obtained from the sample solution is not larger than the peak area of etizolam from the standard solution.

Operating conditions—

Detector: An ultraviolet absorption photometer (wavelength: 240 nm).

Column: A stainless steel column 4.6 mm in inside diameter and 15 cm in length, packed with octadecylsilanized silica gel for liquid chromatography (5 μm in particle diameter).

Column temperature: A constant temperature of about 35°C.

Mobile phase: Dissolve 1.36 g of potassium dihydrogen phosphate in water to make 1000 mL, and adjust the pH to 3.5 with diluted phosphoric acid (1 in 10). To 550 mL of this solution add 450 mL of acetonitrile.

Flow rate: Adjust so that the retention time of etizolam is about 6 minutes.

Time span of measurement: About 5 times as long as the retention time of etizolam, beginning after the solvent peak.

System suitability—

Test for required detectability: Measure exactly 2 mL of the standard solution, and add acetonitrile to make exactly 20 mL. Confirm that the peak area of etizolam obtained with 10 μL of this solution is equivalent to 8 to 12% of that with 10 μL of the standard solution.

System performance: Dissolve 0.02 g each of Etizolam and ethyl parahydroxybenzoate in the mobile phase to make 50 mL. To 1 mL of this solution add the mobile phase to make 50 mL. When the procedure is run with 10 μL of this solution under the above operating conditions, ethyl parahydroxybenzoate and etizolam are eluted in this order with the resolution between these peaks being not less than 3.

System repeatability: When the test is repeated 6 times with 10 μL of the standard solution under the above operating conditions, the relative standard deviation of the peak area of etizolam is not more than 2%.

Loss on drying <*2.41*> Not more than 0.5% (1 g, 105°C, 3 hours).

Residue on ignition <*2.44*> Not more than 0.1% (1 g).

Assay Weigh accurately about 0.3 g of Etizolam, previously dried, dissolve in 70 mL of a mixture of acetic anhydride and acetic acid (100) (7:3), and titrate <*2.50*> with 0.1 mol/L perchloric acid VS (potentiometric titration). The end point is the second equivalent point. Perform a blank determination in the same manner, and make any necessary correction.

Each mL of 0.1 mol/L perchloric acid VS
= 17.14 mg of $C_{17}H_{15}ClN_4S$

Containers and storage Containers—Tight containers.
Storage—Light-resistant.

Etizolam Fine Granules

エチゾラム細粒

Etizolam Fine Granules contain not less than 93.0% and not more than 107.0% of the labeled amount of etizolam ($C_{17}H_{15}ClN_4S$: 342.85).

Method of preparation Prepare as directed under Granules, with Etizolam.

Identification **(1)** To a quantity of powdered Etizolam Fine Granules, equivalent to 5 mg of Etizolam, add 10 mL of methanol, shake, and filter through a membrane filter with a pore size not exceeding 0.45 μm. Evaporate the filtrate to dryness on a water bath, cool, and then dissolve the residue in 2 mL of sulfuric acid. The solution gives off a light yellow-green fluorescent when exposed to ultraviolet light (main wavelength: 365 nm).

(2) To a quantity of powdered Etizolam Fine Granules, equivalent to 1 mg of Etizolam, add 80 mL of 0.1 mol/L hydrochloric acid TS, shake, and then filter. Determine the absorption spectrum of the filtrate as directed under Ultraviolet-visible Spectrophotometry <*2.24*>: it exhibits absorption maxima between 249 nm and 253 nm, and between 292 nm and 296 nm, when perform the measurement within 10 minutes.

Uniformity of dosage units <6.02> The Granules in single-dose packages meet the requirement of the Mass variation test.

Dissolution <6.10> When the test is performed at 50 revolutions per minute according to the Paddle method, using 900 mL of water as the dissolution medium, the dissolution rate in 30 minutes of Etizolam Fine Granules is not less than 75%.

Start the test with an accurately weighed amount of Etizolam Fine Granules, equivalent to about 1 mg of etizolam ($C_{17}H_{15}ClN_4S$), withdraw not less than 20 mL of the medium at the specified minute after starting the test, and filter through a membrane filter with a pore size not exceeding 0.45 μm. Discard not less than 10 mL of first filtrate, pipet 2 mL of the subsequent filtrate, add exactly 2 mL of acetonitrile, and use this solution as the sample solution. Separately, weigh accurately about 28 mg of etizolam for assay, previously dried at 105°C for 3 hours, and dissolve in methanol to make exactly 50 mL. Pipet 5 mL of this solution, and add water to make exactly 100 mL. Pipet 4 mL of this solution, and add water to make exactly 100 mL. Pipet 2 mL of this solution, add exactly 2 mL of acetonitrile, and use this solution as the standard solution. Perform the test with exactly 50 μL each of the sample solution and standard solution as directed under Liquid Chromatography <2.01> according to the following conditions, and determine the peak areas, A_T and A_S, of etizolam in each solution.

Dissolution rate (%) with respect to the labeled amount of etizolam ($C_{17}H_{15}ClN_4S$)

$$= M_S/M_T \times A_T/A_S \times 1/C \times 18/5$$

M_S: Amount (mg) of etizolam for assay taken
M_T: Amount (g) of Etizolam Fine Granules taken
C: Labeled amount (mg) of etizolam ($C_{17}H_{15}ClN_4S$) in 1 g

Operating conditions—

Detector: An ultraviolet absorption photometer (wavelength: 243 nm).

Column: A stainless steel column 4.6 mm in inside diameter and 15 cm in length, packed with octadecylsilanized silica gel for liquid chromatography (5 μm in particle diameter).

Column temperature: A constant temperature of about 30°C.

Mobile phase: A mixture of water and acetonitrile (1:1).

Flow rate: Adjust so that the retention time of etizolam is about 7 minutes.

System suitability—

System performance: When the procedure is run with 50 μL of the standard solution under the above operating conditions, the number of theoretical plates and the symmetry factor of the peak of etizolam are not less than 3000 and not more than 2.0, respectively.

System repeatability: When the test is repeated 6 times with 50 μL of the standard solution under the above operating conditions, the relative standard deviation of the peak area of etizolam is not more than 2.0%.

Assay Weigh accurately an amount of powdered Etizolam Fine Granules, equivalent to about 4 mg of etizolam ($C_{17}H_{15}ClN_4S$), add 30 mL of water, and stir. Add 60 mL of methanol, stir for 20 minutes, add methanol to make exactly 100 mL, and centrifuge. Pipet 5 mL of the supernatant liquid, add exactly 10 mL of the internal standard solution, add diluted methanol (7 in 10) to make 25 mL, and use this solution as the sample solution. Separately, weigh accurately about 0.1 g of etizolam for assay, previously dried at 105°C for 3 hours, and dissolve in diluted methanol (7 in 10) to make exactly 100 mL. Pipet 2 mL of this solution, and add diluted methanol (7 in 10) to make exactly 100 mL. Pipet 10 mL of this solution, add exactly 10 mL of the internal standard solution, add diluted methanol (7 in 10) to make 25 mL, and use this solution as the standard solution. Perform the test with 10 μL each of the sample solution and standard solution as directed under Liquid Chromatography <2.01> according to the following conditions, and calculate the ratios, Q_T and Q_S, of the peak area of etizolam to that of the internal standard.

Amount (mg) of etizolam ($C_{17}H_{15}ClN_4S$)

$$= M_S \times Q_T/Q_S \times 1/25$$

M_S: Amount (mg) of etizolam for assay taken

*Internal standard solution—*A solution of ethyl parahydroxybenzoate in diluted methanol (7 in 10) (1 in 50,000).

Operating conditions—

Detector: An ultraviolet absorption photometer (wavelength: 240 nm).

Column: A stainless steel column 4.6 mm in inside diameter and 15 cm in length, packed with octadecylsilanized silica gel for liquid chromatography (5 μm in particle diameter).

Column temperature: A constant temperature of about 35°C.

Mobile phase: Dissolve 1.36 g of potassium dihydrogen phosphate in water to make 1000 mL, and adjust the pH to 3.5 with diluted phosphoric acid (1 in 10). To 550 mL of this solution add 450 mL of acetonitrile.

Flow rate: Adjust so that the retention time of etizolam is about 6 minutes.

System suitability—

System performance: When the procedure is run with 10 μL of the standard solution under the above operating conditions, the internal standard and etizolam are eluted in this order with the resolution between these peaks being not less than 3.

System repeatability: When the test is repeated 6 times with 10 μL of the standard solution under the above operating conditions, the relative standard deviation of the ratio of the peak area of etizolam to that of the internal standard is not more than 1.0%.

Containers and storage Containers—Tight containers.
Storage—Light-resistant.

Etizolam Tablets

エチゾラム錠

Etizolam Tablets contain not less than 93.0% and not more than 107.0% of the labeled amount of etizolam ($C_{17}H_{15}ClN_4S$: 342.85).

Method of preparation Prepare as directed under Tablets, with Etizolam.

Identification **(1)** To a quantity of powdered Etizolam Tablets, equivalent to 5 mg of Etizolam, add 10 mL of methanol, shake, and filter. Evaporate the filtrate to dryness on a water bath, and dissolve the residue in 2 mL of sulfuric acid. The solution gives off a light yellow-green fluorescence when exposed to ultraviolet light (main wavelength: 365 nm).

(2) To a quantity of powdered Etizolam Tablets, equivalent to 1 mg of Etizolam, add 80 mL of 0.1 mol/L hydrochloric acid TS, shake, and then filter through a membrane filter with a pore size not exceeding 0.45 μm. Determine the absorption spectrum of this filtrate as directed under Ultraviolet-visible Spectrophotometry <2.24>: it exhibits absorption maxima between 249 nm and 253 nm, and between 292 nm and 296 nm when perform the measurement within 10 minutes.

Uniformity of dosage units <6.02> Perform the test according to the following method: it meets the requirement of the Content uniformity test.

To 1 tablet of Etizolam Tablets add 2.5 mL of water, and stir until the tablet is disintegrated. Add 20 mL of methanol, stir for 20 minutes, add methanol to make exactly 25 mL, and centrifuge. Pipet V mL of the supernatant liquid, add exactly 2 mL of the internal standard solution, add diluted methanol (9 in 10) to make 25 mL so that each mL contains about 8 μg of etizolam ($C_{17}H_{15}ClN_4S$), and use this solution as the sample solution. Then, proceed as directed in the Assay.

$$\text{Amount (mg) of etizolam } (C_{17}H_{15}ClN_4S) = M_S \times Q_T/Q_S \times 1/V \times 1/20$$

M_S: Amount (mg) of etizolam for assay taken

Internal standard solution—A solution of ethyl parahydroxybenzoate in diluted methanol (9 in 10) (1 in 10,000).

Dissolution <6.10> When the test is performed at 50 revolutions per minute according to the Paddle method, using 900 mL of water as the dissolution medium, the dissolution rate in 30 minutes of Etizolam Tablets is not less than 70%.

Start the test with 1 tablet of Etizolam Tablets, withdraw not less than 20 mL of the medium at the specified minute after starting the test, and filter through a membrane filter with a pore size not exceeding 0.45 μm. Discard not less than 10 mL of the first filtrate, pipet V mL of the subsequent filtrate, add water to make exactly V' mL so that each mL contains about 0.28 μg of etizolam ($C_{17}H_{15}ClN_4S$). Pipet 2 mL of this solution, add exactly 2 mL of acetonitrile, and use this solution as the sample solution. Separately, weigh accurately about 28 mg of etizolam for assay, previously dried at 105°C for 3 hours, dissolve in 50 mL of methanol, and add water to make exactly 100 mL. Pipet 5 mL of this solution, add water to make exactly 100 mL. Pipet 2 mL of this solution, add water to make exactly 100 mL. Pipet 2 mL of this solution, add exactly 2 mL of acetonitrile, and use this solution as the standard solution. Perform the test with exactly 100 μL each of the sample solution and standard solution as directed under Liquid Chromatography <2.01> according to the following conditions, and determine the peak areas, A_T and A_S, of etizolam in each solution.

$$\text{Dissolution rate (\%) with respect to the labeled amount of etizolam } (C_{17}H_{15}ClN_4S) = M_S \times A_T/A_S \times V'/V \times 1/C \times 9/10$$

M_S: Amount (mg) of etizolam for assay taken
C: Labeled amount (mg) of etizolam ($C_{17}H_{15}ClN_4S$) in 1 tablet

Operating conditions—

Detector: An ultraviolet absorption photometer (wavelength: 243 nm).

Column: A stainless steel column 4.6 mm in inside diameter and 15 cm in length, packed with octadecylsilanized silica gel for liquid chromatography (5 μm in particle diameter).

Column temperature: A constant temperature of about 30°C.

Mobile phase: A mixture of water and acetonitrile (1:1).

Flow rate: Adjust so that the retention time of etizolam is about 7 minutes.

System suitability—

System performance: When the procedure is run with 100 μL of the standard solution under the above operating conditions, the number of theoretical plates and the symmetry factor of the peak of etizolam are not less than 3000 and not more than 2.0, respectively.

System repeatability: When the test is repeated 6 times with 100 μL of the standard solution under the above operating conditions, the relative standard deviation of the peak area of etizolam is not more than 2.0%.

Assay To 20 Etizolam Tablets add 50 mL of water, and stir until they disintegrate. Add 400 mL of methanol, stir for 20 minutes, add methanol to make exactly 500 mL, and centrifuge. Pipet an amount of the supernatant liquid, equivalent to about 0.2 mg of etizolam ($C_{17}H_{15}ClN_4S$), add exactly 2 mL of the internal standard solution, add diluted methanol (9 in 10) to make 25 mL, and use this solution as the sample solution. Separately, weigh accurately about 100 mg of etizolam for assay, previously dried at 105°C for 3 hours, and dissolve in diluted methanol (9 in 10) to make exactly 100 mL. Pipet 2 mL of this solution, and add diluted methanol (9 in 10) to make exactly 100 mL. Pipet 10 mL of this solution, add exactly 2 mL of the internal standard solution, add diluted methanol (9 in 10) to make 25 mL, and use this solution as the standard solution. Perform the test with 10 μL each of the sample solution and standard solution as directed under Liquid Chromatography <2.01> according to the following conditions, and calculate the ratios, Q_T and Q_S, of the peak area of etizolam to that of the internal standard.

$$\text{Amount (mg) of etizolam } (C_{17}H_{15}ClN_4S) = M_S \times Q_T/Q_S \times 1/500$$

M_S: Amount (mg) of etizolam for assay taken

Internal standard solution—A solution of ethyl parahydroxybenzoate in diluted methanol (9 in 10) (1 in 10,000).

Operating conditions—

Detector: An ultraviolet absorption photometer (wavelength: 240 nm).

Column: A stainless steel column 4.6 mm in inside diameter and 15 cm in length, packed with octadecylsilanized silica gel for liquid chromatography (5 μm in particle diameter).

Column temperature: A constant temperature of about 35°C.

Mobile phase: Dissolve 1.36 g of potassium dihydrogen phosphate in water to make 1000 mL, and adjust the pH to 3.5 with diluted phosphoric acid (1 in 10). To 550 mL of this solution add 450 mL of acetonitrile.

Flow rate: Adjust so that the retention time of etizolam is about 6 minutes.

System suitability—

System performance: When the procedure is run with 10 μL of the standard solution under the above operating conditions, the internal standard and etizolam are eluted in this order with the resolution between these peaks being not less than 3.

System repeatability: When the test is repeated 6 times with 10 μL of the standard solution under the above operating conditions, the relative standard deviation of the ratio of the peak area of etizolam to that of the internal standard is not more than 1.0%.

Containers and storage Containers—Tight containers.

Storage—Light-resistant.

Etodolac

エトドラク

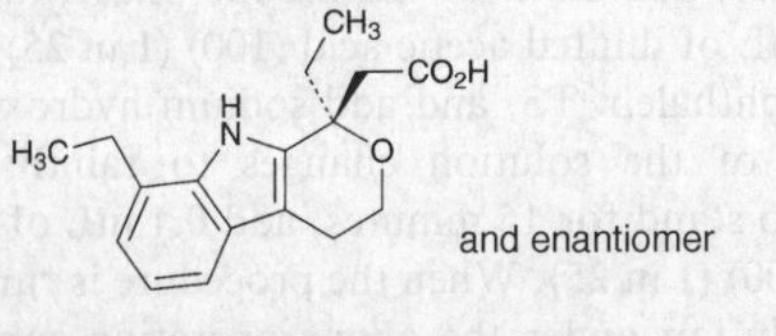

and enantiomer

$C_{17}H_{21}NO_3$: 287.35
2-[(1*RS*)-1,8-Diethyl-1,3,4,9-tetrahydropyrano[3,4-*b*]indol-1-yl]acetic acid
[*41340-25-4*]

Etodolac, when dried, contains not less than 98.5% and not more than 101.0% of etodolac ($C_{17}H_{21}NO_3$).

Description Etodolac occurs as white to pale yellow, crystals or crystalline powder.

It is freely soluble in methanol and in ethanol (99.5), and practically insoluble in water.

A solution of Etodolac in methanol (1 in 50) shows no optical rotation.

Melting point: about 147°C (with decomposition).

Identification (1) Determine the absorption spectrum of a solution of Etodolac in ethanol (99.5) (3 in 200,000) as directed under Ultraviolet-visible Spectrophotometry <*2.24*>, and compare the spectrum with the Reference Spectrum: both spectra exhibit similar intensities of absorption at the same wavelengths.

(2) Determine the infrared absorption spectrum of Etodolac as directed in the potassium bromide disk method under Infrared Spectrophotometry <*2.25*>, and compare the spectrum with the Reference Spectrum: both spectra exhibit similar intensities of absorption at the same wave numbers.

Purity (1) Heavy metals <*1.07*>—Proceed with 2.0 g of Etodolac according to Method 2, and perform the test. Prepare the control solution with 2.0 mL of Standard Lead Solution (not more than 10 ppm).

(2) Related substances—Dissolve 0.5 g of Etodolac in 10 mL of methanol, and use this solution as the sample solution. Pipet 2 mL of the sample solution, and add methanol to make exactly 100 mL. Pipet 5 mL of this solution, add methanol to make exactly 20 mL, and use this solution as the standard solution (1). Pipet 4 mL of the standard solution (1), add methanol to make exactly 10 mL, and use this solution as the standard solution (2). Perform the test with these solutions as directed under Thin-layer Chromatography <*2.03*>. Previously develop a plate of silica gel with fluorescent indicator for thin-layer chromatography in a developing container containing 2 cm depth of a solution of L-ascorbic acid in a mixture of methanol and water (4:1) (1 in 200 mL) to the distance of 3 cm, and air-dry for 30 minutes. Spot 10 μL each of the sample solution and standard solutions (1) and (2) on the plate 2.5 cm away from the bottom of the plate, then immediately develop with a mixture of toluene, ethanol (95) and acetic acid (100) (140:60:1) to a distance of about 15 cm, and air-dry the plate. Examine under ultraviolet light (main wavelength: 254 nm): any spot other than the principal spot obtained with the sample solution is not more intense than the spot with the standard solution (1), and the number of spots which are more intense than the spot with the standard solution (2) is not more than 2.

Loss on drying <*2.41*> Not more than 0.5% (1 g, in vacuum, 60°C, 4 hours).

Residue on ignition <*2.44*> Not more than 0.1% (1 g).

Assay Weigh accurately about 0.3 g of Etodolac, previously dried, dissolve in 50 mL of ethanol (99.5), and titrate <*2.50*> with 0.1 mol/L sodium hydroxide VS (potentiometric titration). Perform a blank determination in the same manner, and make any necessary correction.

Each mL of 0.1 mol/L sodium hydroxide VS
= 28.74 mg of $C_{17}H_{21}NO_3$

Containers and storage Containers—Tight containers.
Storage—Light-resistant.

Etoposide

エトポシド

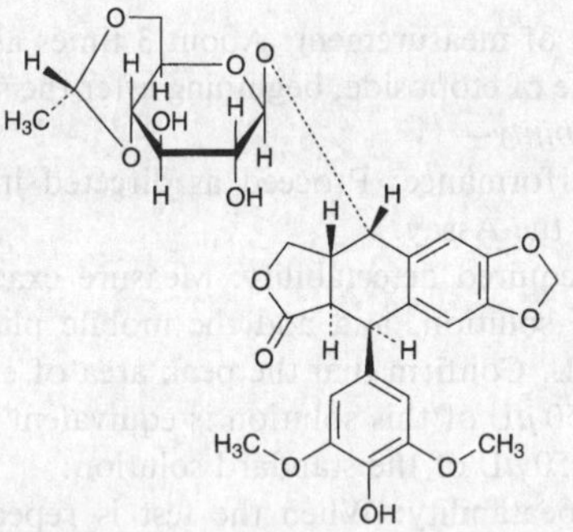

$C_{29}H_{32}O_{13}$: 588.56
(5*R*,5a*R*,8a*R*,9*S*)-9-{[4,6-*O*-(1*R*)-Ethylidene-β-D-glucopyranosyl]oxy}5-(4-hydroxy-3,5-dimethoxyphenyl)-5,8,8a,9-tetrahydrofuro[3′,4′:6,7]naphtho[2,3-*d*]-1,3-dioxol-6(5a*H*)-one
[*33419-42-0*]

Etoposide contains not less than 98.0% and not more than 102.0% of etoposide ($C_{29}H_{32}O_{13}$), calculated on the anhydrous basis.

Description Etoposide occurs as white, crystals or crystalline powder.

It is sparingly soluble in methanol, slightly soluble in ethanol (99.5), and very slightly soluble in water.

Melting point: about 260°C (with decomposition).

Identification (1) Determine the absorption spectrum of a solution of Etoposide in methanol (1 in 10,000) as directed under Ultraviolet-visible Spectrophotometry <*2.24*>, and compare the spectrum with the Reference Spectrum or the spectrum of a solution of Etoposide RS prepared in the same manner as the sample solution: both spectra exhibit similar intensities of absorption at the same wavelengths.

(2) Determine the infrared absorption spectrum of Etoposide as directed in the potassium bromide disk method under Infrared Spectrophotometry <*2.25*>, and compare the spectrum with the Reference Spectrum or the spectrum of Etoposide RS: both spectra exhibit similar intensities of absorption at the same wave numbers.

Optical rotation <*2.49*> $[\alpha]_D^{20}$: −100 − −105° (0.1 g calculated on the anhydrous basis, methanol, 20 mL, 100 mm).

Purity (1) Heavy metals <*1.07*>—Proceed with 2.0 g of Etoposide according to Method 2, and perform the test. Prepare the control solution with 2.0 mL of Standard Lead So-

lution (not more than 10 ppm).

(2) Related substances—Dissolve 50 mg of Etoposide in 10 mL of methanol, add the mobile phase to make 50 mL, and use this solution as the sample solution. Pipet 2 mL of the sample solution, add the mobile phase to make exactly 200 mL, and use this solution as the standard solution. Perform the test with exactly 50 μL each of the sample solution and standard solution as directed under Liquid Chromatography *<2.01>* according to the following conditions, and determine each peak area by the automatic integration method: the area of the peak other than etoposide obtained from the sample solution is not larger than 1/5 times the peak area of etoposide from the standard solution, and the total area of the peaks other than etoposide is not larger than 1/2 times the peak area of etoposide from the standard solution.

Operating conditions—

Detector, column, column temperature, mobile phase, and flow rate: Proceed as directed in the operating conditions in the Assay.

Time span of measurement: About 3 times as long as the retention time of etoposide, beginning after the solvent peak.

System suitability—

System performance: Proceed as directed in the system suitability in the Assay.

Test for required detectability: Measure exactly 1 mL of the standard solution, and add the mobile phase to make exactly 10 mL. Confirm that the peak area of etoposide obtained with 50 μL of this solution is equivalent to 7 to 13% of that with 50 μL of the standard solution.

System repeatability: When the test is repeated 6 times with 50 μL of the standard solution under the above operating conditions, the relative standard deviation of the peak area of etoposide is not more than 2.0%.

Water *<2.48>* Not more than 4.0% (0.5 g, volumetric titration, direct titration).

Residue on ignition *<2.44>* Not more than 0.1% (1 g).

Assay Weigh accurately about 25 mg each of Etoposide and Etoposide RS (previously determined the water *<2.48>* in the same manner as Etoposide) dissolve separately in methanol to make exactly 25 mL. Pipet 10 mL each of these solutions, add exactly 5 mL of the internal standard solution and the mobile phase to make 50 mL, and use these solutions as the sample solution and standard solution. Perform the test with 50 μL each of the sample solution and standard solution as directed under Liquid Chromatography *<2.01>* according to the following conditions, and calculate the ratios, Q_T and Q_S, of the peak area of etoposide to that of the internal standard.

Amount (mg) of etoposide ($C_{29}H_{32}O_{13}$) $= M_S \times Q_T/Q_S$

M_S: Amount (mg) of Etoposide RS taken, calculated on the anhydrous basis

Internal standard solution—A solution of 2,6-dichlorophenol in methanol (3 in 2500).

Operating conditions—

Detector: An ultraviolet absorption photometer (wavelength: 290 nm).

Column: A stainless steel column 3.9 mm in inside diameter and 30 cm in length, packed with phenylsilanized silica gel for liquid chromatography (10 μm in particle diameter).

Column temperature: A constant temperature of about 35°C.

Mobile phase: Dissolve 6.44 g of sodium sulfate decahydrate in diluted acetic acid (100) (1 in 100) to make 1000 mL, and add 250 mL of acetonitrile.

Flow rate: Adjust so that the retention time of etoposide is about 20 minutes.

System suitability—

System performance: Dissolve 10 mg of Etoposide in 2 mL of methanol, add 8 mL of the mobile phase, and mix well. Add 0.1 mL of diluted acetic acid (100) (1 in 25) and 0.1 mL of phenolphthalein TS, and add sodium hydroxide TS until the color of the solution changes to faintly red. After allowing to stand for 15 minutes, add 0.1 mL of diluted acetic acid (100) (1 in 25). When the procedure is run with 10 μL of this solution under the above operating conditions, the resolution between the peak of etoposide and the peak having the relative retention time of about 1.3 to etoposide is not less than 3.

System repeatability: When the test is repeated 6 times with 50 μL of the standard solution under the above operating conditions, the relative standard deviation of the ratio of the peak area of etoposide to that of the internal standard is not more than 1.0%.

Containers and storage Containers—Tight containers.

Storage—Light-resistant.

Famotidine

ファモチジン

$C_8H_{15}N_7O_2S_3$: 337.45

N-Aminosulfonyl-3-{[2-(diaminomethyleneamino)-1,3-thiazol-4-yl]methylsulfanyl}propanimidamide

[76824-35-6]

Famotidine, when dried, contains not less than 98.5% of famotidine ($C_8H_{15}N_7O_2S_3$).

Description Famotidine occurs as white to yellowish white crystals.

It is freely soluble in acetic acid (100), slightly soluble in ethanol (95), and very slightly soluble in water.

It dissolves in 0.5 mol/L hydrochloric acid TS.

It is gradually colored by light.

Melting point: about 164°C (with decomposition).

Identification **(1)** Determine the absorption spectrum of a solution of Famotidine in 0.05 mol/L potassium dihydrogen phosphate TS (1 in 50,000) as directed under Ultraviolet-visible Spectrophotometry *<2.24>*, and compare the spectrum with the Reference Spectrum: both spectra exhibit similar intensities of absorption at the same wavelengths.

(2) Determine the infrared absorption spectrum of Famotidine, previously dried, as directed in the potassium bromide disk method under Infrared Spectrophotometry *<2.25>*, and compare the spectrum with the Reference Spectrum: both spectra exhibit similar intensities of absorption at the same wave numbers.

Purity **(1)** Clarity and color of solution—Dissolve 0.5 g of Famotidine in 10 mL of 0.5 mol/L hydrochloric acid TS: the solution is clear and colorless to pale yellow.

(2) Heavy metals *<1.07>*—Proceed with 2.0 g of Famotidine according to Method 2, and perform the test. Prepare the control solution with 2.0 mL of Standard Lead Solution (not more than 10 ppm).

(3) Related substances—Dissolve 0.20 g of Famotidine in

10 mL of acetic acid (100), and use this solution as the sample solution. Pipet 1 mL of the sample solution, and add acetic acid (100) to make exactly 100 mL. Pipet 1 mL, 2 mL and 3 mL of this solution, add acetic acid (100) to make exactly 10 mL, respectively, and use these solutions as the standard solution (1), the standard solution (2) and the standard solution (3). Perform the test with these solutions as directed under Thin-layer Chromatography <2.03>. Spot 5 μL each of the sample solution and standard solutions (1), (2) and (3) on a plate of silica gel (5 to 7 μm) with fluorescent indicator for thin-layer chromatography, and dry in a stream of nitrogen. Develop the plate with a mixture of ethyl acetate, methanol, toluene and ammonia solution (28) (40:25:20:2) to a distance of about 8 cm, and air-dry the plate. Examine under ultraviolet light (main wavelength: 254 nm): the spots other than the principal spot and the spot of the starting point obtained from the sample solution are not more intense than the spot from the standard solution (3). Total intensity of the spots other than the principal spot and the spot of the starting point from the sample solution is not more than 0.5% calculated on the basis of intensities of the spots from the standard solution (1) and the standard solution (2).

Loss on drying <2.41> Not more than 0.5% (1 g, in vacuum, phosphorus (V) oxide, 80°C, 4 hours).

Residue on ignition <2.44> Not more than 0.1% (1 g).

Assay Weigh accurately about 0.3 g of Famotidine, previously dried, dissolve in 50 mL of acetic acid (100), and titrate <2.50> with 0.1 mol/L perchloric acid VS (potentiometric titration). Perform a blank determination in the same manner, and make any necessary correction.

Each mL of 0.1 mol/L perchloric acid VS
= 16.87 mg of $C_8H_{15}N_7O_2S_3$

Containers and storage Containers—Tight containers.
Storage—Light-resistant.

Famotidine Injection

ファモチジン注射液

Famotidine Injection is an aqueous injection.

It contains not less than 92.0% and not more than 108.0% of the labeled amount of famotidine ($C_8H_{15}N_7O_2S_3$: 337.45).

Method of preparation Prepare as directed under Injections, with Famotidine.

Description Famotidine Injection is a colorless or light yellow, clear liquid.

Identification To an amount of Famotidine Injection, equivalent to 10 mg of Famotidine, add water to make 100 mL. Run 1 mL of this solution on a column prepared by filling about 1 cm inside diameter chromatography tube with about 0.4 g of 55 – 105 μm octadecylsilanized silica gel for pretreatment. Wash the column with 15 mL of water, followed by elution with 5 mL of methanol. To the eluate add methanol to make 10 mL. Determine the absorption spectrum of this solution as directed under Ultraviolet-visible Spectrophotometry <2.24>: it exhibits a maximum between 285 nm and 289 nm.

Osmotic pressure ratio Being specified separately when the drug is granted approval based on the Law.

pH Being specified separately when the drug is granted approval based on the Law.

Purity Related substances—To an exact amount of Famotidine Injection, equivalent to 25 mg of Famotidine, add the mobile phase to make exactly 50 mL, and use this solution as the sample solution. Separately, weigh accurately about 10 mg of famotidine for assay, dissolve in methanol, and add methanol to make exactly 100 mL. Pipet 5 mL of this solution, add the mobile phase to make exactly 100 mL, and use this solution as the standard solution. Perform the test with exactly 20 μL each of the sample solution and standard solution as directed under Liquid Chromatography <2.01> according to the following conditions. Determine the peak area of each solution by the automatic integration method, and calculate the amounts of the related substances by the following equation: the amounts of related substances, having the relative retention time about 1.3 and about 1.5 to famotidine are not more than 3.0% respectively, and the amount of other related substances except the above substances is not more than 0.5%, and the total amount of the related substances is not more than 5.0%.

Amount (%) of related substance = $M_S \times A_T/A_S \times 1/10$
Total amount (%) of related substances
= $M_S \times \Sigma A_T/A_S \times 1/10$

M_S: Amount (mg) of famotidine for assay taken
A_S: Peak area of famotidine in the standard solution
A_T: Peak area of related substances in the sample solution
ΣA_T: Total peak area of the related substances in the sample solution

Operating conditions—

Detector, column and column temperature: Proceed as directed in the operating conditions in the Assay.

Mobile phase: Dissolve 1.74 g of sodium 1-pentane sulfonate in 900 mL of water, adjust to pH 4.0 with diluted acetic acid (100) (1 in 10), and add water to make 1000 mL. To 840 mL of this solution add 80 mL of methanol and 40 mL of acetonitrile.

Flow rate: Adjust so that the retention time of famotidine is about 17 minutes.

Time span of measurement: About 4 times as long as the retention time of famotidine, beginning after the solvent peak.

System suitability—

Test for required detectability: Pipet 5 mL of the standard solution, add the mobile phase to make exactly 50 mL. Confirm that the peak area of famotidine obtained with 20 μL of this solution is equivalent to 8 to 12% of that with 20 μL of the standard solution.

System performance: To 20 mg of famotidine for assay add 2 mL of a solution of methyl parahydroxybenzoate in acetonitrile (1 in 500), and add methanol to make 20 mL. To 5 mL of this solution add the mobile phase to make 50 mL. When the procedure is run with 10 μL of this solution under the above operating conditions, famotidine and methyl parahydroxybenzoate are eluted in this order with the resolution between these peaks being not less than 19.

System repeatability: When the test is repeated 6 times with 20 μL of the standard solution under the above operations conditions, the relative standard deviation of the peak area of famotidine is not more than 2.0%.

Bacterial endotoxins <4.01> Less than 15 EU/mg.

Extractable volume <6.05> It meets the requirement.

Foreign insoluble matter <6.06> Perform the test according to Method I: it meets the requirement.

Insoluble particulate matter ⟨*6.07*⟩ It meets the requirement.

Sterility ⟨*4.06*⟩ Perform the test according to Membrane filtration method: it meets the requirement.

Assay To an exactly measured volume of Famotidine Injection, equivalent to about 25 mg of famotidine ($C_8H_{15}N_7O_2S_3$), add exactly 2.5 mL of the internal standard solution, and add the mobile phase to make 50 mL. Pipet 10 mL of this solution, add the mobile phase to make 50 mL, and use this solution as the sample solution. Separately, weigh accurately about 50 mg of famotidine for assay, previously dried in vacuum with phosphorus (V) oxide at 80°C for 4 hours, dissolve in methanol, add exactly 5 mL of the internal standard solution, and add methanol to make 50 mL. Pipet 5 mL of this solution, add the mobile phase to make 50 mL, and use this solution as the standard solution. Perform the test with 10 μL each of the sample solution and standard solution as directed under Liquid Chromatography ⟨*2.01*⟩ according to the following conditions. Calculate the ratios, Q_T and Q_S of the peak area of famotidine to that of the internal standard.

$$\text{Amount (mg) of famotidine } (C_8H_{15}N_7O_2S_3) = M_S \times Q_T/Q_S \times 1/2$$

M_S: Amount (mg) of famotidine for assay taken

Internal standard solution—A solution of methyl parahydroxybenzoate in acetonitrile (1 in 500).

Operating conditions—

Ditector: An ultraviolet absorption photometer (Wavelength: 254 nm).

Column: A stainless steel column 4.6 mm in inside diameter and 15 cm in length, packed with octadecylsilanized silica gel for liquid chromatography (5 μm in particle diameter).

Column temperature: A constant temperature of about 40°C.

Mobile phase: Dissolve 1.74 g of sodium 1-pentane sulfonate in 900 mL of water, adjust to pH 4.0 with diluted acetic acid (100) (1 in 10), and add water to make 1000 mL. To 750 mL of this solution add 200 mL of methanol and 50 mL of acetonitrile.

Flow rate: Adjust so that the retention time of famotidine is about 4 minutes.

System suitability—

System performance: When the procedure is run with 10 μL of the standard solution under the above operating conditions, famotidine and the internal standard are eluted in this order with the resolution between these peaks being not less than 26.

System repeatability: When the test is repeated 5 times with 10 μL of the standard solution under the above operating conditions, the relative standard deviation of the ratio of the peak area of famotidine to that of the internal standard is not more than 1.0%.

Containers and storage Containers—Hermetic containers.

Famotidine for Injection

注射用ファモチジン

Famotidine for Injection is a preparation for injection which is dissolved before use.

It contains not less than 94.0% and not more than 106.0% of the labeled amount of famotidine ($C_8H_{15}N_7O_2S_3$: 337.45).

Method of preparation Prepare as directed under Injection, with Famotidine.

Description Famotidine for Injection occurs as white, porous masses or powder.

Identification Dissolve an amount of Famotidine for Injection, equivalent to 0.01 g of Famotidine, in 50 mL of 0.05 mol/L potassium dihydrogen phosphate TS. To 5 mL of this solution add 0.05 mol/L potassium dihydrogen phosphate TS to make 50 mL, and determine the absorption spectrum of this solution as directed under Ultraviolet-visible Spectrophotometry ⟨*2.24*⟩: it exhibits a maximum between 263 nm and 267 nm.

pH ⟨*2.54*⟩ Dissolve an amount of Famotidine for Injection, equivalent to 0.02 g of Famotidine, in 1 mL of water: the pH of this solution is between 4.9 and 5.5.

Purity **(1)** Clarity and color of solution—Dissolve an amount of Famotidine for Injection, equivalent to 0.02 g of Famotidine, in 1 mL of water: the solution is clear and colorless.

(2) Related substances—Take a number of Famotidine for Injection, equivalent to about 0.1 g of famotidine ($C_8H_{15}N_7O_2S_3$), dissolve each content in water, wash the inside of the container with water, combine the solutions of the contents with the washings, add water to the combined solution to make exactly 100 mL, and use this solution as the sample solution. Pipet 1 mL of the sample solution, add water to make exactly 100 mL, and use this solution as the standard solution. Perform the test with exactly 5 μL each of the sample solution and standard solution as directed under Liquid Chromatography ⟨*2.01*⟩ according to the following conditions, and determine each peak area of these solutions by the automatic integration method: the total area of the peaks other than famotidine obtained from the sample solution is not larger than peak area of famotidine from the standard solution.

Operating conditions—

Detector, column, column temperature, mobile phase, and flow rate: Proceed as directed in the operating conditions in the Assay.

Time span of measurement: About 2 times as long as the retention time of famotidine, beginning after the solvent peak.

System suitability—

System performance: Proceed as directed in the system suitability in the Assay.

Test for required detectability: To exactly 2 mL of the standard solution add the water to make exactly 20 mL. Confirm that the peak area of famotidine obtained with 5 μL of this solution is equivalent to 8 to 12% of that with 5 μL of the standard solution.

System repeatability: When the test is repeated 6 times with 5 μL of the standard solution under the above operating conditions, the relative standard deviation of the peak area of famotidine is not more than 2.0%.

Water <2.48> Not more than 1.5% (0.1 g, coulometric titration).

Bacterial endotoxins <4.01> Not more than 15 EU/mg.

Uniformity of dosage units <6.02> It meets the requirement of the Mass variation test.

Foreign insoluble matter <6.06> Perform the test according to Method 2: it meets the requirement.

Insoluble particulate matter <6.07> It meets the requirement.

Sterility <4.06> Perform the test according to the Membrane filtration method: it meets the requirement.

Assay Take a number of Famotidine for Injection, equivalent to about 0.1 g of famotidine ($C_8H_{15}N_7O_2S_3$), dissolve each content in water, wash the inside of each container with water, combine the solutions of the contents with the washings, add water to the combined solution to make exactly 100 mL. Pipet 5 mL of this solution, add exactly 5 mL of the internal standard solution, add the mobile phase to make 50 mL, and use this solution as the sample solution. Separately, weigh accurately about 50 mg of famotidine for assay, previously dried in vacuum with phosphorus (V) oxide at 80°C for 4 hours, dissolve in the mobile phase to make exactly 50 mL. Pipet 5 mL of this solution, add exactly 5 mL of the internal standard solution, add the mobile phase to make 50 mL, and use this solution as the standard solution. Perform the test with 5 μL each of the sample solution and standard solution as directed under Liquid Chromatography <2.01> according to the following conditions, and calculate the ratios, Q_T and Q_S, of the peak area of famotidine to that of the internal standard.

Amount (mg) of famotidine ($C_8H_{15}N_7O_2S_3$)
$= M_S \times Q_T/Q_S \times 2$

M_S: Amount (mg) of famotidine for assay taken

Internal standard solution—To 5 mL of a solution of methyl parahydroxybenzoate in methanol (1 in 500) add water to make 50 mL.

Operating conditions—

Detector: An ultraviolet absorption photometer (wavelength: 254 nm).

Column: A stainless steel column 4.6 mm in inside diameter and 15 cm in length, packed with octadecylsilanized silica gel for liquid chromatography (5 μm in particle diameter).

Column temperature: A constant temperature of about 25°C.

Mobile phase: Dissolve 2 g of sodium 1-heptane sulfonate in 900 mL of water, adjust to pH 3.0 with acetic acid (100), and add water to make 1000 mL. To this solution add 240 mL of acetonitrile and 40 mL of methanol.

Flow rate: Adjust so that the retention time of famotidine is about 6 minutes.

System suitability—

System performance: When the procedure is run with 5 μL of the standard solution under the above operating conditions, famotidine and the internal standard are eluted in this order with the resolution between these peaks being not less than 11.

System repeatability: When the test is repeated 6 times with 5 μL of the standard solution under the above operating conditions, the relative standard deviation of the ratios of the peak area of famotidine to that of the internal standard is not more than 1.0%.

Containers and storage Containers—Hermetic containers.

Famotidine Powder

ファモチジン散

Famotidine Powder contains not less than 94.0% and not more than 106.0% of the labeled amount of famotidine ($C_8H_{15}N_7O_2S_3$: 337.45).

Method of preparation Prepare as directed under Granules or Powders, with Famotidine.

Identification Weigh a portion of Famotidine Powder, equivalent to 0.01 g of Famotidine, add 50 mL of 0.05 mol/L potassium dihydrogen phosphate TS, shake well, and centrifuge. To 5 mL of the supernatant liquid add 0.05 mol/L potassium dihydrogen phosphate TS to make 50 mL, and determine the absorption spectrum of this solution as directed under Ultraviolet-visible Spectrophotometry <2.24>: it exhibits a maximum between 263 nm and 267 nm.

Uniformity of dosage units <6.02> Perform the test according to the following method: Famotidine Powder in single-dose packages meets the requirement of the Content uniformity test.

Take out the total content of 1 package of Famotidine Powder, add 10 mL of water per 10 mg of famotidine ($C_8H_{15}N_7O_2S_3$), shake well, add 10 mL of methanol, shake well, add methanol to make exactly V mL so that each mL contains about 0.4 mg of famotidine ($C_8H_{15}N_7O_2S_3$), and centrifuge. Pipet 5 mL of the supernatant liquid, add exactly 2 mL of the internal standard solution, add the mobile phase to make 20 mL, and use this solution as the sample solution. Proceed as directed in the Assay.

Amount (mg) of famotidine ($C_8H_{15}N_7O_2S_3$)
$= M_S \times Q_T/Q_S \times V/250$

M_S: Amount (mg) of famotidine for assay taken

Internal standard solution—To 5 mL of a solution of methyl parahydroxybenzoate in methanol (1 in 500) add water to make 50 mL.

Dissolution <6.10> When the test is performed at 50 revolutions per minute according to the Paddle method, using 900 mL of 0.05 mol/L acetic acid-sodium acetate buffer solution (pH 4.0) as the dissolution medium, the dissolution rates in 15 minutes of a 20-mg/g powder and a 100-mg/g powder are not less than 80% and not less than 85%, respectively.

Start the test with an accurately weighed amount of Famotidine Powder, equivalent to about 20 mg of famotidine ($C_8H_{15}N_7O_2S_3$), withdraw not less than 20 mL of the medium at the specified minute after starting the test, and filter through a membrane filter with a pore size not exceeding 0.5 μm. Discard not less than 10 mL of the first filtrate, and use the subsequent filtrate as the sample solution. Separately, weigh accurately about 40 mg of famotidine for assay, previously dried in vacuum on phosphorus (V) oxide at 80°C for 4 hours, dissolve in the dissolution medium to make exactly 100 mL. Pipet 5 mL of this solution, add the dissolution medium to make exactly 100 mL, and use this solution as the standard solution. Determine the absorbances, A_T and A_S, of the sample solution and standard solution at 266 nm as directed under Ultraviolet-visible Spectrophotometry <2.24>.

Dissolution rate (%) with respect to the labeled amount of famotidine ($C_8H_{15}N_7O_2S_3$)
$= M_S/M_T \times A_T/A_S \times 1/C \times 45$

M_S: Amount (mg) of famotidine for assay taken

M_T: Amount (g) of Famotidine Powder taken

C: Labeled amount (mg) of famotidine ($C_8H_{15}N_7O_2S_3$) in 1 g

Assay Weigh accurately a portion of Famotidine Powder, equivalent to about 20 mg of famotidine ($C_8H_{15}N_7O_2S_3$), add 20 mL of water, and shake well. Add 20 mL of methanol, then shake well, add methanol to make exactly 50 mL, and centrifuge. Pipet 5 mL of the supernatant liquid, add exactly 2 mL of the internal standard solution, add the mobile phase to make 20 mL, and use this solution as the sample solution. Separately, weigh accurately about 0.1 g of famotidine for assay, previously dried in vacuum with phosphorus (V) oxide at 80°C for 4 hours, dissolve in methanol to make exactly 50 mL. Pipet 10 mL of this solution, and add methanol to make exactly 50 mL. Pipet 5 mL of this solution, add exactly 2 mL of the internal standard solution, add the mobile phase to make 20 mL, and use this solution as the standard solution. Perform the test with 5 μL each of the sample solution and standard solution as directed under Liquid Chromatography <2.01> according to the following conditions, and calculate the ratios, Q_T and Q_S, of the peak area of famotidine to that of the internal standard.

$$\text{Amount (mg) of famotidine } (C_8H_{15}N_7O_2S_3) = M_S \times Q_T/Q_S \times 1/5$$

M_S: Amount (mg) of famotidine for assay taken

Internal standard solution—To 5 mL of a solution of methyl parahydroxybenzoate in methanol (1 in 500) add water to make 50 mL.

Operating conditions—

Detector: An ultraviolet absorption photometer (wavelength: 254 nm).

Column: A stainless steel column 4.6 mm in inside diameter and 15 cm in length, packed with octadecylsilanized silica gel for liquid chromatography (5 μm in particle diameter).

Column temperature: A constant temperature of about 25°C.

Mobile phase: Dissolve 2 g of sodium 1-heptane sulfonate in 900 mL of water, adjust to pH 3.0 with acetic acid (100), and add water to make 1000 mL. To this solution add 240 mL of acetonitrile and 40 mL of methanol.

Flow rate: Adjust so that the retention time of famotidine is about 6 minutes.

System suitability—

System performance: When the procedure is run with 5 μL of the standard solution under the above operating conditions, famotidine and the internal standard are eluted in this order with the resolution between these peaks being not less than 11.

System repeatability: When the test is repeated 6 times with 5 μL of the standard solution under the above operating conditions, the relative standard deviation of the ratios of the peak area of famotidine to that of the internal standard is not more than 1.0%.

Containers and storage Containers—Tight containers.

Famotidine Tablets

ファモチジン錠

Famotidine Tablets contain not less than 94.0% and not more than 106.0% of the labeled amount of famotidine ($C_8H_{15}N_7O_2S_3$: 337.45).

Method of preparation Prepare as directed under Tablets, with Famotidine.

Identification Weigh a portion of powdered Famotidine Tablets, equivalent to 0.01 g of Famotidine, add 50 mL of 0.05 mol/L potassium dihydrogen phosphate TS, shake well, and centrifuge. To 5 mL of the supernatant liquid add 0.05 mol/L potassium dihydrogen phosphate TS to make 50 mL, and determine the absorption spectrum of this solution as directed under Ultraviolet-visible Spectrophotometry <2.24>: it exhibits a maximum between 263 nm and 267 nm.

Uniformity of dosage units <6.02> Perform the test according to the following method: it meets the requirement of the Content uniformity test.

To 1 tablet of Famotidine Tablets add 2 mL of water, shake to disintegrate, then add a suitable amount of methanol, and shake well. Add methanol to make exactly V mL of a solution containing about 0.2 mg of famotidine ($C_8H_{15}N_7O_2S_3$) per mL, and centrifuge. Pipet 10 mL of the supernatant liquid, add exactly 2 mL of the internal standard solution, add the mobile phase to make 20 mL, and use this solution as the sample solution. Separately, weigh accurately about 0.1 g of famotidine for assay, previously dried in vacuum with phosphorus (V) oxide at 80°C for 4 hours, dissolve in methanol to make exactly 100 mL. Pipet 10 mL of this solution, and add methanol to make exactly 50 mL. Pipet 10 mL of this solution, add exactly 2 mL of the internal standard solution, add the mobile phase to make 20 mL, and use this solution as the standard solution. Perform the test with 5 μL each of the sample solution and standard solution as directed under Liquid Chromatography <2.01> according to the operating conditions described in the Assay, and calculate the ratios, Q_T and Q_S, of the peak area of famotidine to that of the internal standard.

$$\text{Amount (mg) of famotidine } (C_8H_{15}N_7O_2S_3) = M_S \times Q_T/Q_S \times V/500$$

M_S: Amount (mg) of famotidine for assay taken

Internal standard solution—To 5 mL of a solution of methyl paraphydroxybenzoate in methanol (1 in 500) add water to make 50 mL.

Dissolution Being specified separately when the drug is granted approval based on the Law.

Assay Take a number of Famotidine Tablets, equivalent to 0.2 g of famotidine ($C_8H_{15}N_7O_2S_3$), add 50 mL of water, and disintegrate by shaking well. Add 100 mL of methanol, then shake well, add methanol to make exactly 200 mL, and centrifuge. Pipet 5 mL of the supernatant liquid, add exactly 5 mL of the internal standard solution, add the mobile phase to make 50 mL, and use this solution as the sample solution. Separately, weigh accurately about 0.1 g of famotidine for assay, previously dried in vacuum with phosphorus (V) oxide at 80°C for 4 hours, dissolve in methanol to make exactly 100 mL. Pipet 5 mL of this solution, add exactly 5 mL of the internal standard solution, add the mobile phase to make 50 mL, and use this solution as the standard solution. Perform

The JP Drugs are to be tested according to the provisions given in the pertinent monographs, General Notices, General Rules for Crude Drugs, General Rules for Preparations, and General Tests for their conformity to the Japanese Pharmacopoeia. (See the General Notices 5.)

the test with 5 μL each of the sample solution and standard solution as directed under Liquid Chromatography <2.01> according to the following conditions, and calculate the ratios, Q_T and Q_S, of the peak area of famotidine to that of the internal standard.

Amount (mg) of famotidine ($C_8H_{15}N_7O_2S_3$)
$$= M_S \times Q_T/Q_S \times 2$$

M_S: Amount (mg) of famotidine for assay taken

Internal standard solution—To 5 mL of a solution of methyl parahydroxybenzoate in methanol (1 in 500) add water to make 50 mL.

Operating conditions—

Detector: An ultraviolet absorption photometer (wavelength: 254 nm).

Column: A stainless steel column 4.6 mm in inside diameter and 15 cm in length, packed with octadecylsilanized silica gel for liquid chromatography (5 μm in particle diameter).

Column temperature: A constant temperature of about 25°C.

Mobile phase: Dissolve 2 g of sodium 1-heptane sulfonate in 900 mL of water, adjust to pH 3.0 with acetic acid (100), and add water to make 1000 mL. To this solution add 240 mL of acetonitrile and 40 mL of methanol.

Flow rate: Adjust so that the retention time of famotidine is about 6 minutes.

System suitability—

System performance: When the procedure is run with 5 μL of the standard solution under the above operating conditions, famotidine and the internal standard are eluted in this order with the resolution between these peaks being not less than 11.

System repeatability: When the test is repeated 6 times with 5 μL of the standard solution under the above operating conditions, the relative standard deviation of the ratios of the peak area of famotidine to that of the internal standard is not more than 1.0%.

Containers and storage Containers—Tight containers.

Faropenem Sodium Hydrate

ファロペネムナトリウム水和物

$C_{12}H_{14}NNaO_5S.2\frac{1}{2}H_2O$: 352.34

Monosodium (5*R*,6*S*)-6-[(1*R*)-1-hydroxyethyl]-7-oxo-3-[(2*R*)-tetrahydrofuran-2-yl]-4-thia-1-azabicyclo[3.2.0]hept-2-ene-2-carboxylate hemipentahydrate

[*122547-49-3*, anhydride]

Faropenem Sodium Hydrate contains not less than 870 μg (potency) and not more than 943 μg (potency) per mg, calculated on the anhydrous basis. The potency of Faropenem Sodium Hydrate is expressed as mass (potency) of faropenem ($C_{12}H_{15}NO_5S$: 285.32).

Description Faropenem Sodium Hydrate occurs as white to light yellow, crystals or crystalline powder.

It is freely soluble in water and in methanol, slightly soluble in ethanol (95), and practically insoluble in diethyl ether.

Identification (1) Dissolve 5 mg of Faropenem Sodium Hydrate in 1 mL of hydroxylammonium chloride-ethanol TS, allow to stand for 3 minutes, add 1 mL of acidic ammonium iron (III) sulfate TS, and shake: a red-brown to brown color develops.

(2) Determine the absorption spectra of solutions of Faropenem Sodium Hydrate and Faropenem Sodium RS (1 in 20,000) as directed under Ultraviolet-visible Spectrophotometry <2.24>, and compare the spectra: both spectra exhibit similar intensities of absorption at the same wavelengths.

(3) Determine the infrared absorption spectra of Faropenem Sodium Hydrate and Faropenem Sodium RS as directed in the potassium bromide disk method under Infrared Spectrophotometry <2.25>, and compare the spectra: both spectra exhibit similar intensities of absorption at the same wave numbers.

Optical rotation <2.49> $[\alpha]_D^{20}$: +145 – +150° (0.5 g calculated as the anhydrous basis, water, 50 mL, 100 mm).

Purity (1) Heavy metals <1.07>—Proceed with 2.0 g of Faropenem Sodium Hydrate according to Method 4, and perform the test. Prepare the control solution with 2.0 mL of Standard Lead Solution (not more than 10 ppm).

(2) Related substances—Dissolve a quantity of Faropenem Sodium Hydrate equivalent to 0.10 g (potency) in 200 mL of water, and use this solution as the sample solution. Pipet 2 mL of the sample solution, add water to make exactly 200 mL, and use this solution as the standard solution. Perform the test with exactly 20 μL each of the sample solution and standard solution as directed under Liquid Chromatography <2.01> according to the following conditions, and determine each peak area by the automatic integration method: the peak area of the epimer, having the relative retention time of about 1.1 to faropenem, obtained from the sample solution is not larger than 3/10 times the peak area of faropenem from the standard solution, and the total area of the peaks other than faropenem from the sample solution is not larger than 1/2 times the peak area of faropenem from the standard solution.

Operating conditions—

Column, column temperature, mobile phase, and flow rate: Proceed as directed in the operating conditions in the Assay.

Detector: An ultraviolet absorption photometer (wavelength: 240 nm).

Time span of measurement: About 6 times as long as the retention time of faropenem, beginning after the solvent peak.

System suitability—

Test for required detectability: To exactly 2 mL of the standard solution add water to make exactly 20 mL. Confirm that the peak area of faropenem obtained with 20 μL of this solution is equivalent to 7 to 13% of that with 20 μL of the standard solution.

System performance: When the procedure is run with 20 μL of the standard solution obtained in the Assay under the above operating conditions, the internal standard and faropenem are eluted in this order with the resolution between these peaks being not less than 1.5.

System repeatability: When the test is repeated 6 times with 20 μL of the standard solution under the above operating conditions, the relative standard deviation of the peak area of faropenem is not more than 2.0%.

Water <2.48> Not less than 12.6% and not more than 13.1% (20 mg, coulometric titration).

Assay Weigh accurately an amount of Faropenem Sodium

Hydrate and Faropenem Sodium RS, equivalent to about 25 mg (potency), add exactly 10 mL each of the internal standard solution, add water to make 50 mL, and use these solutions as the sample solution and the standard solution, respectively. Perform the test with 20 μL of the sample solution and standard solution as directed under Liquid Chromatography *<2.01>* according to the following conditions, and calculate the ratios, Q_T and Q_S, of the peak area of faropenem to that of the internal standard.

Amount [μg (potency)] of faropenem ($C_{12}H_{15}NO_5S$)
$= M_S \times Q_T/Q_S \times 1000$

M_S: amount [mg (potency)] of Faropenem Sodium RS taken

Internal standard solution—Dissolve 0.5 g of *m*-hydroxyacetophenone in 20 mL of acetonitrile, and add water to make 200 mL.

Operating conditions—

Detector: An ultraviolet absorption photometer (wavelength: 305 nm).

Column: A stainless steel column 4.6 mm in inside diameter and 25 cm in length, packed with octadecylsilanized silica gel for liquid chromatography (5 μm in particle diameter).

Column temperature: A constant temperature of about 40°C.

Mobile phase: Dissolve 4.8 g of potassium dihydrogen phosphate, 5.4 g of disodium hydrogen phosphate dodecahydrate and 1.0 g of tetra *n*-butyl ammonium bromide in water to make 1000 mL. To 870 mL of this solution add 130 mL of acetonitrile.

Flow rate: Adjust so that the retention time of faropenem is about 11 minutes.

System suitability—

System performance: When the procedure is run with 20 μL of the standard solution under the above operating conditions, the internal standard and faropenem are eluted in this order with the resolution between these peaks being not less than 1.5.

System repeatability: When the test is repeated 6 times with 20 μL of the standard solution under the above operating conditions, the relative standard deviation of the ratios of the peak area of faropenem to that of the internal standard is not more than 1.0%.

Containers and storage Containers—Tight containers.

Faropenem Sodium for Syrup

シロップ用ファロペネムナトリウム

Faropenem Sodium for Syrup is a preparation for syrup, which is dissolved before use.

It contains not less than 93.0% and not more than 106.0% of the labeled potency of faropenem ($C_{12}H_{15}NO_5S$: 285.32).

Method of preparation Prepare as directed under Preparations for Syrups, with Faropenem Sodium Hydrate.

Identification Dissolve an amount of powdered Faropenem Sodium for Syrup, equivalent to 25 mg (potency) of Faropenem Sodium Hydrate, in water to make 50 mL. To 5 mL of this solution add water to make 50 mL, filter, if necessary, and determine the absorption spectrum of the solution so obtained as directed under Ultraviolet-visible Spectrophotometry *<2.24>*: it exhibits maxima between 254 nm and 258 nm, and between 304 nm and 308 nm.

Purity Related substances—Powder Faropenem Sodium for Syrup, if necessary. To a part of the powder, equivalent to about 25 mg (potency) of Faropenem Sodium Hydrate, add about 10 mL of water, shake well, then add water to make exactly 50 mL, and filter. Discard the first 10 mL of the filtrate, and use the subsequent filtrate as the sample solution. Pipet 2 mL of the sample solution, add water to make exactly 200 mL, and use this solution as the standard solution. Perform the test with exactly 20 μL each of the sample solution and standard solution as directed under Liquid Chromatography *<2.01>* according to the following conditions, and determine each peak area of both solutions by the automatic integration method: the area of the peak of cleaved derivative, having the relative retention time of about 0.71 to faropenem, obtained from the sample solution is not larger than 1.5 times the peak area of faropenem from the standard solution, and the total area of the peaks other than faropenem from the sample solution is not larger than 2 times the peak area of faropenem from the standard solution. For the area of the peak, having the relative retention time of about 0.71 to faropenem, multiply its correction factor 0.37.

Operating conditions—

Detector: An ultraviolet absorption photometer (wavelength: 240 nm).

Column: A stainless steel column 4 mm in inside diameter and 25 cm in length, packed with octadecylsilanized silica gel for liquid chromatography (5 μm in particle diameter).

Column temperature: A constant temperature of about 40°C.

Mobile phase A: Dissolve 6.12 g of potassium dihydrogen phosphate, 1.79 g of disodium hydrogen phosphate dodecahydrate and 1.61 g of tetra *n*-butylammonium bromide in water to make 1000 mL.

Mobile phase B: A mixture of the mobile phase A and acetonitrile (1:1).

Flowing of mobile phase: Control the gradient by mixing the mobile phases A and B as directed in the following table.

Time after injection of sample (min)	Mobile phase A (vol%)	Mobile phase B (vol%)
0 – 54	84 → 30	16 → 70

Flow rate: 1.5 mL per minute.

Time span of measurement: 2.5 times as long as the retention time of faropenem, beginning after the solvent peak.

System suitability—

Test for required detectability: To exactly 2 mL of the standard solution add water to make exactly 20 mL. Confirm that the peak area of faropenem obtained with 20 μL of this solution is equivalent to 7 to 13% of that with 20 μL of the standard solution.

System performance: When the procedure is run with 20 μL of the standard solution obtained in the Assay under the above operating conditions, the internal standard and faropenem are eluted in this order with the resolution between these peaks being not less than 11.

System repeatability: When the test is repeated 6 times with 20 μL of the standard solution under the above operating conditions, the relative standard deviation of the peak area of faropenem is not more than 3.0%.

Water *<2.48>* Not less than 1.5% and not more than 2.1% (80 mg, coulometric titration).

Uniformity of dosage units ⟨*6.02*⟩ Faropenem Sodium for Syrup in single-dose packages meet the requirement of the Mass variation test.

Assay Powder, if necessary, and weigh accurately an amount of Faropenem Sodium for Syrup, equivalent to about 25 mg (potency) of faropenem ($C_{12}H_{15}NO_5S$), add exactly 10 mL of the internal standard solution and a suitable amount of water, shake well, and add water to make 50 mL. Filter, discard the first 10 mL of the filtrate, and use the subsequent filtrate as the sample solution. Separately, weigh accurately about 25 mg (potency) of Faropenem Sodium RS, add exactly 10 mL of the internal standard solution and water to make 50 mL, and use this solution as the standard solution. Preceed as directed in the Assay under Faropenem Sodium Hydrate.

Amount [mg (potency)] of faropenem ($C_{12}H_{15}NO_5S$)
$= M_S \times Q_T/Q_S$

M_S: Amount [mg (potency)] of Faropenem Sodium RS taken

Internal standard solution—Dissolve 0.5 g of *m*-hydroxyacetophenone in 20 mL of acetonitrile, and add water to make 200 mL.

Containers and storage Containers—Tight containers.
Storage—Light-resistant.

Faropenem Sodium Tablets

ファロペネムナトリウム錠

Faropenem Sodium Tablets contain not less than 94.0% and not more than 106.0% of the labeled potency of faropenem ($C_{12}H_{15}NO_5S$: 285.32).

Method of preparation Prepare as directed under Tablets, with Faropenem Sodium Hydrate.

Identification To powdered Faropenem Sodium Tablets, equivalent to 70 mg (potency) of Faropenem Sodium Hydrate, add water to make 100 mL. To 5 mL of this solution add water to make 100 mL, filter, if necessary, and determine the absorption spectrum of this solution as directed under Ultraviolet-visible Spectrophotometry ⟨*2.24*⟩: it exhibits maxima between 254 nm and 258 nm and between 304 nm and 308 nm.

Purity Related substances—Powder not less than 5 Faropenem Sodium Tablets. To a part of the powder, equivalent to about 25 mg (potency) of Faropenem Sodium Hydrate, add about 10 mL of water, shake well, then add water to make exactly 50 mL, and filter. Discard the first 10 mL of the filtrate, and use the subsequent filtrate as the sample solution. Pipet 2 mL of the sample solution, add water to make exactly 200 mL, and use this solution as the standard solution. Perform the test with exactly 20 μL each of the sample solution and standard solution as directed under Liquid Chromatography ⟨*2.01*⟩ according to the following conditions, and determine each peak area of both solutions by the automatic integration method: the area of the peak of cleaved derivative, having the relative retention time of about 0.71 to faropenem, obtained from the sample solution is not larger than 1.5 times the peak area of faropenem from the standard solution, and the total area of the peaks other than faropenem from the sample solution is not larger than 2.5 times the peak area of faropenem from the standard solution. For the area of the peak, having the relative retention time of about 0.71 to faropenem, multiply its correction factor 0.37.

Operating conditions—

Detector: An ultraviolet absorption photometer (wavelength: 240 nm).

Column: A stainless steel column 4 mm in inside diameter and 25 cm in length, packed with octadecylsilanized silica gel for liquid chromatography (5 μm in particle diameter).

Column temperature: A constant temperature of about 40°C.

Mobile phase A: Dissolve 6.12 g of potassium dihydrogen phosphate, 1.79 g of disodium hydrogen phosphate dodecahydrate and 1.61 g of tetra *n*-butylammonium bromide in water to make 1000 mL.

Mobile phase B: A mixture of the mobile phase A and acetonitrile (1:1).

Flowing of mobile phase: Control the gradient by mixing the mobile phases A and B as directed in the following table.

Time after injection of sample (min)	Mobile phase A (vol%)	Mobile phase B (vol%)
0 – 54	84 → 30	16 → 70

Flow rate: 1.5 mL per minute.

Time span of measurement: About 2.5 times as long as the retention time of faropenem, beginning after the solvent peak.

System suitability—

Test for required detectability: To exactly 2 mL of the standard solution add water to make exactly 20 mL. Confirm that the peak area of faropenem obtained with 20 μL of this solution is equivalent to 7 to 13% of that with 20 μL of the standard solution.

System performance: When the procedure is run with 20 μL of the standard solution obtained in the Assay under the above operating conditions, the internal standard and faropenem are eluted in this order with the resolution between these peaks being not less than 11.

System repeatability: When the test is repeated 6 times with 20 μL of the standard solution under the above operating conditions, the relative standard deviation of the peak area of faropenem is not more than 3.0%.

Uniformity of dosage units ⟨*6.02*⟩ Perform the Mass variation test, or the Content uniformity test according to the following method: it meets the requirement.

To 1 tablet of Faropenem Sodium Tablets add 130 mL of water, shake vigorously until the tablets are disintegrated, and add water to make exactly *V* mL so that each mL contains about 1 mg (potency) of Faropenem Sodium Hydrate. Pipet 5 mL of this solution, add water to make exactly 100 mL, and filter. Discard the first 10 mL of the filtrate, and use the subsequent filtrate as the sample solution. Separately, weigh accurately about 25 mg (potency) of Faropenem Sodium RS, and dissolve in water to make exactly 50 mL. Pipet 10 mL of this solution, add water to make exactly 100 mL, and use this solution as the standard solution. Determine the absorbances, A_{T275}, A_{T305}, A_{T354}, A_{S275}, A_{S305} and A_{S354}, of the sample solution and standard solution at 275 nm, 305 nm and 354 nm as directed under Ultraviolet-visible Spectrophotometry ⟨*2.24*⟩, and calculate A_T and A_S, using the following equations.

$$A_T = A_{T305} - (49 \times A_{T275} + 30 \times A_{T354})/79$$

$$A_S = A_{S305} - (49 \times A_{S275} + 30 \times A_{S354})/79$$

$$\text{Amount [mg (potency)] of faropenem } (C_{12}H_{15}NO_5S) = M_S \times A_T/A_S \times V/25$$

M_S: Amount [mg (potency)] of Faropenem Sodium RS taken

Dissolution ⟨*6.10*⟩ When the test is performed at 50 revolutions per minute according to the Paddle method, using 900 mL of water as the dissolution medium, the dissolution rate in 30 minutes of Faropenem Sodium Tablets is not less than 85%.

Start the test with 1 tablet of Faropenem Sodium Tablets, withdraw not less than 20 mL of the medium at the specified minute after starting the test, and filter through a membrane filter with a pore size not exceeding 0.45 μm. Discard not less than 10 mL of the first filtrate, pipet V mL of the subsequent filtrate, add water to make exactly V' mL so that each mL contains about 56 μg (potency) of Faropenem Sodium Hydrate, and use this solution as the sample solution. Separately, weigh accurately an amount of Faropenem Sodium RS, equivalent to about 18 mg (potency), and dissolve in water to make exactly 100 mL. Pipet 5 mL of this solution, add water to make exactly 20 mL, and use this solution as the standard solution. Perform the test with the sample solution and standard solution as directed under Ultraviolet-visible Spectrophotometry ⟨*2.24*⟩, and determine the absorbances, A_T and A_S, at 306 nm.

$$\text{Dissolution rate (\%) with respect to the labeled amount of faropenem } (C_{12}H_{15}NO_5S) = M_S \times A_T/A_S \times V'/V \times 1/C \times 225$$

M_S: Amount [mg (potency)] of Faropenem Sodium RS taken

C: Labeled amount [mg (potency)] of faropenem ($C_{12}H_{15}NO_5S$) in 1 tablet

Assay Weigh accurately the mass of not less than 5 Faropenem Sodium Tablets, and powder. Weigh accurately a portion of the powder, equivalent to about 25 mg (potency) of faropenem ($C_{12}H_{15}NO_5S$), add exactly 10 mL of the internal standard solution, shake well, and add water to make 50 mL. Filter, discard the first 10 mL of the filtrate, and use the subsequent filtrate as the sample solution. Separately, weigh accurately about 25 mg (potency) of Faropenem Sodium RS, add exactly 10 mL of the internal standarad solution and water to make 50 mL, and use this solution as the standard solution. Proceed as directed in the Assay under Faropenem Sodium Hydrate.

$$\text{Amount [mg (potency)] of faropenem } (C_{12}H_{15}NO_5S) = M_S \times Q_T/Q_S$$

M_S: Amount [mg (potency)] of Faropenem Sodium RS taken

Internal standard solution—Dissolve 0.5 g of *m*-hydorxyacetophenone in 20 mL of acetonitrile, and add water to make 200 mL.

Containers and storage Containers—Tight containers.

Felbinac

フェルビナク

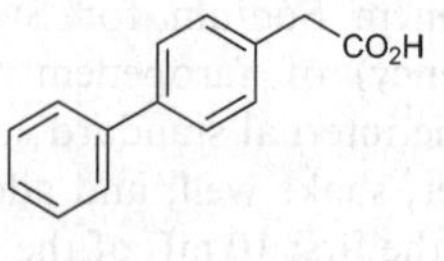

$C_{14}H_{12}O_2$: 212.24

Biphenyl-4-ylacetic acid

[5728-52-9]

Felbinac, when dried, contains not less than 98.5% and not more than 101.0% of felbinac ($C_{14}H_{12}O_2$).

Description Felbinac occurs as white to pale yellow-white, crystals or crystalline powder.

It is soluble in methanol and in acetone, sparingly soluble in ethanol (95), and practically insoluble in water.

Identification **(1)** Determine the absorption spectrum of a solution of Felbinac in ethanol (95) (1 in 200,000) as directed under Ultraviolet-visible Spectrophotometry ⟨*2.24*⟩, and compare the spectrum with the Reference Spectrum: both spectra exhibit similar intensities of absorption at the same wavelengths.

(2) Determine the infrared absorption spectrum of Felbinac as directed in the potassium bromide disc method under Infrared Spectrophotometry ⟨*2.25*⟩, and compare the spectrum with the Reference Spectrum: both spectra exhibit similar intensities of absorption at the same wave numbers.

Melting point ⟨*2.60*⟩ 163 – 166°C

Purity **(1)** Chloride ⟨*1.03*⟩—Dissolve 1.0 g of Felbinac in 40 mL of acetone, add 6 mL of dilute nitric acid and water to make 50 mL. Perform the test using this solution as the test solution. Prepare the control solution by combining 0.30 mL of 0.01 mol/L hydrochloric acid VS, 40 mL of acetone and 6 mL of dilute nitric acid, and add water to make 50 mL (not more than 0.011%).

(2) Heavy metals ⟨*1.07*⟩—Proceed with 1.0 g of Felbinac according to Method 2, and perform the test. Prepare the control solution with 1.0 mL of Standard Lead Solution (not more than 10 ppm).

(3) Related substances—Dissolve 0.10 g of Felbinac in 10 mL of acetone, and use this solution as the sample solution. Pipet 2 mL of the sample solution, and add acetone to make exactly 100 mL. Pipet 5 mL of the sample solution, add acetone to make exactly 50 mL, and use this solution as the standard solution. Perform the test with these solutions as directed under Thin-layer Chromatography ⟨*2.03*⟩. Spot 10 μL each of the sample solution and standard solution on a plate of silica gel with fluorescent indicator for thin-layer chromatography. Develop the plate with a mixture of heptane, acetone, and acetic acid (100) (50:25:1) to a distance of about 12 cm, and air-dry the plate. Examine the plate under ultraviolet light (main wavelength: 254 nm): spots other than the principal spot obtained from the sample solution are not more intense than the spot from the standard solution.

Loss on drying ⟨*2.41*⟩ Not more than 0.3% (1 g, 105°C, 3 hours).

Residue on ignition ⟨*2.44*⟩ Not more than 0.1% (1 g).

Assay Weigh accurately about 0.5 g of Felbinac, previously dried, dissolve in 50 mL of methanol, add 15 mL of water, and titrate ⟨*2.50*⟩ with 0.1 mol/L sodium hydroxide VS (potentiometric titration). Perform a blank determination in the same manner, and make any necessary correction.

Each mL of 0.1 mol/L sodium hydroxide VS
= 21.22 mg of $C_{14}H_{12}O_2$

Containers and storage Containers—Tight containers.

Felbinac Cataplasm

フェルビナクパップ

Felbinac Cataplasm contains not less than 90.0% and not more than 110.0% of the labeled amount of felbinac ($C_{14}H_{12}O_2$: 212.24).

Method of preparation Prepare as directed under Cataplasms/Gel Patches, with Felbinac.

Identification Weigh a quantity of Felbinac Cataplasm, equivalent to 10 mg of Felbinac, cut into minute pieces, add 20 mL of methanol, shake for 30 minutes, filter, and use the filtrate as the sample solution. Separately, dissolve 1 mg of felbinac for assay in 2 mL of methanol, and use this solution as the standard solution. Perform the test with these solutions as directed under Thin-layer Chromatography *<2.03>*. Spot 10 μL each of the sample solution and standard solution on a plate of silica gel with fluorescent indicator for thin-layer chromatography. Develop the plate with a mixture of hexane, acetone and acetic acid (100) (50:25:1) to a distance of about 10 cm, and air-dry the plate. Examine under ultraviolet light (main wavelength: 254 nm): the *R*f value of the principal spot obtained from the sample solution and the spot from the standard solution is the same.

pH Being specified separately when the drug is granted approval based on the Law.

Adhesiveness Being specified separately when the drug is granted approval based on the Law.

Drug release Being specified separately when the drug is granted approval based on the Law.

Assay Take exactly a quantity of Felbinac Cataplasm, equivalent to 70 mg of felbinac ($C_{14}H_{12}O_2$), cut into minute pieces, add 150 mL of methanol, and heat under a reflux condenser. After cooling, separate the extraction liquid, add 20 mL of water to the residue, heat in a water bath at 75°C for 10 minutes, then add 150 mL of methanol, and heat under a reflux condenser. After cooling, separate the extraction liquid, add 150 mL of methanol to the residue, and heat under a reflux condenser. After cooling, separate the extraction liquid, wash the residue and vessels with a small amount of methanol, combine the extraction liquids and washings, and add methanol to make exactly 500 mL. Pipet 6 mL of this solution, add exactly 3 mL of the internal standard solution, add methanol to make 50 mL, and use this solution as the sample solution. Separately, weigh accurately about 35 mg of felbinac for assay, previously dried at 105°C for 3 hours, and dissolve in methanol to make exactly 250 mL. Pipet 6 mL of this solution, add exactly 3 mL of the internal standard solution, add methanol to make 50 mL, and use this solution as the standard solution. Perform the test with 10 μL each of the sample solution and standard solution as directed under Liquid Chromatography *<2.01>* according to the following conditions, and calculate the ratios, Q_T and Q_S, of the peak area of felbinac to that of the internal standard.

$$\text{Amount (mg) of felbinac } (C_{14}H_{12}O_2) = M_S \times Q_T/Q_S \times 2$$

M_S: Amount (mg) of felbinac for assay taken

Internal standard solution—A solution of indometacin in methanol (1 in 1250).

Operating conditions—

Detector: An ultraviolet absorption photometer (wavelength: 254 mn).

Column: A stainless steel column 4.6 mm in inside diameter and 15 cm in length, packed with octadecylsilanized silica gel for liquid chromatography (5 μm in particle diameter).

Column temperature: A constant temperature of about 40°C.

Mobile phase: To 1.5 mL of phosphoric acid add 300 mL of water, then dissolve 5 g of sodium lauryl sulfate, and add water to make 500 mL. To this solution add 500 mL of acetonitrile.

Flow rate: Adjust so that the retention time of felbinac is about 6 minutes.

System suitability—

System performance: When the procedure is run with 10 μL of the standard solution under the above operating conditions, felbinac and the internal standard are eluted in this order with the resolution between these peaks being not less than 6.

System repeatability: When the test is repeated 6 times with 10 μL of the standard solution under the above operating conditions, the relative standard deviation of the ratio of the peak area of felbinac to that of the internal standard is not more than 1.0%.

Containers and storage Containers—Tight containers.

Felbinac Tape

フェルビナクテープ

Felbinac Tape contains not less than 90.0% and not more than 110.0% of the labeled amount of felbinac ($C_{14}H_{12}O_2$: 212.24).

Method of preparation Prepare as directed under Tapes/Plasters, with Felbinac.

Identification Cut up a quantity of Felbinac Tape, equivalent to 5 mg of Felbinac, add 30 mL of ethanol (95), and heat under a reflux condenser. After cooling, separate the ethanol extract, add ethanol (95) to make 50 mL, and filter. To 5 mL of the filtrate add ethanol (95) to make 100 mL, and determine the absorption spectrum of this solution as directed under Ultraviolet-visible Spectrophotometry *<2.24>*: it exhibits a maximum between 251 nm and 255 nm.

Adhesiveness Being specified separately when the drug is granted approval based on the Law.

Drug release Being specified separately when the drug is granted approval based on the Law.

Assay Take exactly a quantity of Felbinac Tape, equivalent to 35 mg of felbinac ($C_{14}H_{12}O_2$), cut up them, add 60 mL of acetone, sonicate, and heat under a reflux condenser. After cooling, separate the acetone extract, and repeat the extraction twice more with 60 mL each of acetone by heating under a reflux condenser. After cooling, separate the extract, wash the residue and vessel with a small volume of acetone, combine the washings and the extracts, and add acetone to make exactly 250 mL. Pipet 6 mL of this solution, add exactly 2 mL of the internal standard solution and the mobile phase to make 50 mL, and use this solution as the sample solution. Separately, weigh accurately about 14 mg of felbinac for assay, previously dried at 105°C for 3 hours, and dissolve in acetone to make exactly 100 mL. Pipet 6 mL of this solution, add exactly 2 mL of the internal standard solution and the mobile phase to make 50 mL, and use this solution as the standard solution. Perform the test with 20 μL each of the sample solution and standard solution as directed under Liquid Chromatography ⟨*2.01*⟩ according to the following conditions, and calculate the ratios, Q_T and Q_S, of the peak area of felbinac to that of the internal standard.

$$\text{Amount (mg) of felbinac } (C_{14}H_{12}O_2) = M_S \times Q_T/Q_S \times 5/2$$

M_S: Amount (mg) of felbinac for assay taken

Internal standard solution—A solution of indomethacin in acetone (1 in 1250).

Operating conditions—

Detector: An ultraviolet absorption photometer (wavelength: 254 nm).

Column: A stainless steel column 4.6 mm in inside diameter and 25 cm in length, packed with octadecylsilanized silica gel for liquid chromatography (5 μm in particle diameter).

Column temperature: A constant temperature of about 40°C.

Mobile phase: A mixture of water, acetonitrile and phosphoric acid (500:500:1).

Flow rate: Adjust so that the retention time of felbinac is about 7 minutes.

System suitability—

System performance: When the procedure is run with 20 μL of the standard solution under the above operating conditions, felbinac and the internal standard are eluted in this order with the resolution between these peaks being not less than 3.

System repeatability: When the test is repeated 6 times with 20 μL of the standard solution under the above operating conditions, the relative standard deviation of the ratio of the peak area of felbinac to that of the internal standard is not more than 1.0%.

Containers and storage Containers—Well-closed containers.

Felodipine

フェロジピン

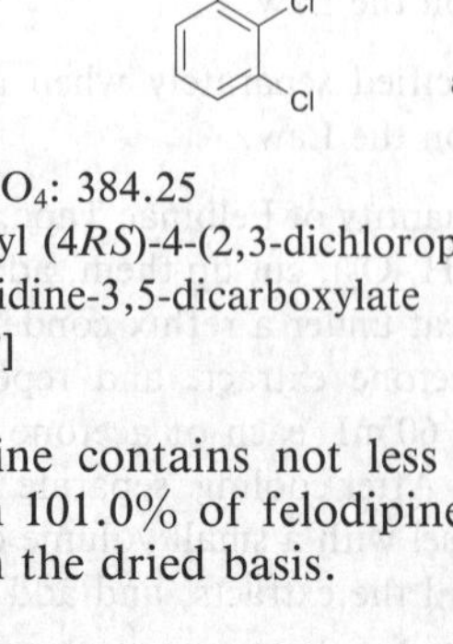

$C_{18}H_{19}Cl_2NO_4$: 384.25

Ethyl methyl (4*RS*)-4-(2,3-dichlorophenyl)-2,6-dimethyl-1,4-dihydropyridine-3,5-dicarboxylate

[*72509-76-3*]

Felodipine contains not less than 99.0% and not more than 101.0% of felodipine ($C_{18}H_{19}Cl_2NO_4$), calculated on the dried basis.

Description Felodipine occurs as pale yellow-white to light yellow-white, crystals or crystalline powder.

It is freely soluble in methanol and in ethanol (99.5), and practically insoluble in water.

A solution of Felodipine in methanol (1 in 20) shows no optical rotation.

Identification **(1)** Determine the absorption spectrum of a solution of Felodipine in methanol (1 in 62,500) as directed under Ultraviolet-visible Spectrophotometry ⟨*2.24*⟩, and compare the spectrum with the Reference Spectrum: both spectra exhibit similar intensities of absorption at the same wavelengths.

(2) Determine the infrared absorption spectrum of Felodipine as directed in the potassium bromide disk method under Infrared Spectrophotometry ⟨*2.25*⟩, and compare the spectrum with the Reference Spectrum: both spectra exhibit similar intensities of absorption at the same wave numbers.

Purity **(1)** Heavy metals—Being specified separately when the drug is granted approval based on the Law.

(2) Related substances—Dissolve 25 mg of Felodipine in 50 mL of the mobile phase, and use this solution as the sample solution. Pipet 1 mL of the sample solution, and add the mobile phase to make exactly 100 mL. Pipet 1 mL of this solution, add the mobile phase to make exactly 10 mL, and use this solution as the standard solution. Perform the test with exactly 20 μL each of the sample solution and standard solution as directed under Liquid Chromatography ⟨*2.01*⟩ according to the following conditions. Determine each peak area by the automatic integration method: the area of the peak other than felodipine, related substance B having the relative retention time of about 0.7 to felodipine, and related substance C having the relative retention time of about 1.4 obtained from the sample solution is not larger than the peak area of felodipine from the standard solution. Furthermore, the total area of the peaks of related substances B and C from the sample solution is not larger than 10 times the peak area of felodipine from the standard solution, and the total area of the peaks other than felodipine and related substances mentioned above from the sample solution is not larger than 3 times the peak area of felodipine from the standard solution. For this calculation the peak area less than 1/5 times the peak area of felodipine from the standard solution is excluded.

Operating conditions—

Detector: An ultraviolet absorption photometer (wavelength: 254 nm).

Column: A stainless steel column 4.6 mm in inside diameter and 15 cm in length, packed with octadecylsilanized silica gel for liquid chromatography (5 μm in particle diameter).

Column temperature: A constant temperature of about 25°C.

Mobile phase: Dissolve 3.2 g of sodium dihydrogen phosphate dihydrate in 400 mL of water, adjust to pH 3.0 with phosphoric acid, and add 200 mL of methanol and 400 mL of acetonitrile.

Flow rate: Adjust so that the retention time of felodipine is about 12 minutes.

Time span of measurement: About 2 times as long as the retention time of felodipine, beginning after the solvent peak.

System suitability—

Test for required detectability: When the procedure is run with 20 μL of the standard solution under the above operating conditions, the SN ratio of the peak of felodipine is not less than 30.

System performance: When the procedure is run with 20

μL of the standard solution under the above operating conditions, the number of theoretical plates and the symmetry factor of the peak of felodipine are not less than 5000 and not more than 1.5, respectively.

System repeatability: When the test is repeated 6 times with 20 μL of the standard solution under the above operating conditions, the relative standard deviation of the peak area of felodipine is not more than 2.0%.

Loss on drying ⟨*2.41*⟩ Not more than 0.2% (1 g, 105°C, 3 hours).

Residue on ignition ⟨*2.44*⟩ Not more than 0.1% (1 g).

Assay Weigh accurately about 0.16 g of Felodipine, dissolve in 25 mL of t-butyl alcohol and 25 mL of diluted perchloric acid (17 in 200), and titrate ⟨*2.50*⟩ with 0.1 mol/L cerium (IV) sulfate VS (indicator: 50 μL of 1,10-phenanthroline TS) until the color of the solution changes from orange to colorless. Perform a blank determination in the same manner, and make any necessary correction.

Each mL of 0.1 mol/L cerium (IV) sulfate VS
$= 19.21$ mg of $C_{18}H_{19}Cl_2NO_4$

Containers and storage Containers—Well-closed containers.

Others
Related substance B:
Dimethyl 4-(2,3-dichlorophenyl)-2,6-dimethyl-1,4-dihydropyridine-3,5-dicarboxylate

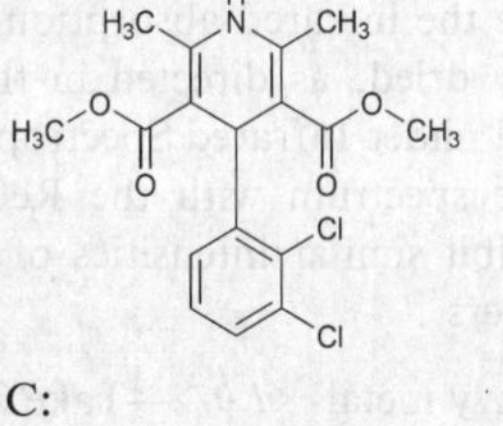

Related substance C:
Diethyl 4-(2,3-dichlorophenyl)-2,6-dimethyl-1,4-dihydropyridine-3,5-dicarboxylate

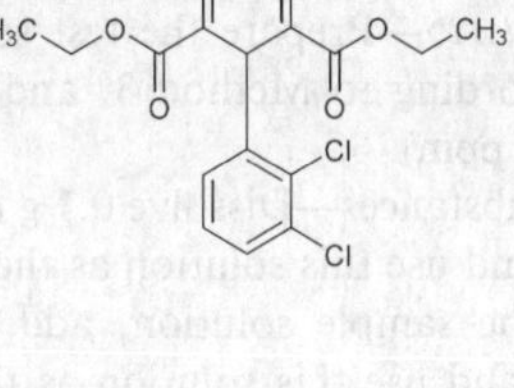

Felodipine Tablets

フェロジピン錠

Felodipine Tablets contain not less than 95.0% and not more than 105.0% of the labeled amount of felodipine ($C_{18}H_{19}Cl_2NO_4$: 384.25).

Method of preparation Prepare as directed under Tablets, with Felodipine.

Identification To a quantity of powdered Felodipine Tablets, equivalent to 4 mg of Felodipine, add 200 mL of methanol, shake thoroughly, add methanol to make 250 mL, and centrifuge. Determine the absorption spectrum of the supernatant liquid as directed under Ultraviolet-visible Spectrophotometry ⟨*2.24*⟩: it exhibits maxima between 235 nm and 239 nm, and between 357 nm and 363 nm.

Uniformity of dosage units ⟨*6.02*⟩ Perform the Mass variation test, or the Content uniformity test according to the following method: it meets the requirement.

To 1 tablet of Felodipine Tablets add 1 mL of water per 2.5 mg of felodipine ($C_{18}H_{19}Cl_2NO_4$), and shake thoroughly until the tablet is completely disintegrated. Add exactly 1 mL of the internal standard solution per 2.5 mg of felodipine ($C_{18}H_{19}Cl_2NO_4$), and add methanol to make V mL so that each mL contains about 0.25 mg of felodipine ($C_{18}H_{19}Cl_2NO_4$). Centrifuge this solution, filter the supernatant liquid, and use this filtrate as the sample solution. Separately, weigh accurately about 25 mg of felodipine for assay (separately determine the loss on drying ⟨*2.41*⟩ in the same conditions as Felodipine), add 10 mL of water, and add exactly 10 mL of the internal standard solution. Add methanol to make 100 mL, and use this solution as the standard solution. Then, proceed as directed in the Assay.

Amount (mg) of felodipine ($C_{18}H_{19}Cl_2NO_4$)
$= M_S \times Q_T/Q_S \times V/100$

M_S: Amount (mg) of felodipine for assay taken, calculated on the dried basis

Internal standard solution—A solution of butyl parahydroxybenzoate in methanol (1 in 3000).

Dissolution ⟨*6.10*⟩ When the test is performed at 50 revolutions per minute according to the Paddle method, using 900 mL of a solution prepared by dissolving 1 g of polysorbate 80 in water to make 5000 mL, as the dissolution medium, the dissolution rates in 45 minutes of a 2.5-mg tablet and a 5-mg tablet are not less than 80% and not less than 75%, respectively.

Start the test with 1 tablet of Felodipine Tablets, withdraw not less than 20 mL of the medium at the specified minute after starting the test, and filter through a membrane filter with a pore size not exceeding 0.45 μm. Discard not less than 10 mL of the first filtrate, pipet V mL of the subsequent filtrate, add the dissolution medium to make exactly V' mL so that each mL contains about 2.8 μg of felodipine ($C_{18}H_{19}Cl_2NO_4$), and use this solution as the sample solution. Separately, weigh accurately about 28 mg of felodipine for assay (separately determine the loss on drying ⟨*2.41*⟩ in the same conditions as Felodipine), and dissolve in methanol to make exactly 200 mL. Pipet 2 mL of this solution, add the dissolution medium to make exactly 100 mL, and use this solution as the standard solution. Perform the test with exactly 50 μL each of the sample solution and standard solution as directed under Liquid Chromatography ⟨*2.01*⟩ according to the following conditions, and determine the peak areas, A_T and A_S, of felodipine in each solution.

Dissolution rate (%) with respect to the labeled amount of felodipine ($C_{18}H_{19}Cl_2NO_4$)
$= M_S \times A_T/A_S \times V'/V \times 1/C \times 9$

M_S: Amount (mg) of felodipine for assay taken, calculated on the dried basis
C: Labeled amount (mg) of felodipine ($C_{18}H_{19}Cl_2NO_4$) in 1 tablet

Operating conditions—

Column, column temperature, mobile phase and flow rate: Proceed as directed in the operating conditions in the Assay.

Detector: An ultraviolet absorption photometer (wavelength: 238 nm).

System suitability—

System performance: When the procedure is run with 50 μL of the standard solution under the above operating conditions, the number of theoretical plates and the symmetry

factor of the peak of felodipine are not less than 3000 and not more than 1.5, respectively.

System repeatability: When the test is repeated 6 times with 50 μL of the standard solution under the above operating conditions, the relative standard deviation of the peak area of felodipine is not more than 2.0%.

Assay Weigh accurately the mass of not less than 20 Felodipine Tablets, and powder. Weigh accurately a portion of the powder, equivalent to about 10 mg of felodipine ($C_{18}H_{19}Cl_2NO_4$), add 20 mL of water, add exactly 4 mL of the internal standard solution, add methanol to make 100 mL and shake. Centrifuge this solution, filter the supernatant liquid through a membrane filter with a pore size not exceeding 0.45 μm, and use the filtrate as the sample solution. Separately, weigh accurately about 10 mg of felodipine for assay (separately determine the loss on drying *<2.41>* in the same conditions as Felodipine), add 20 mL of water, add exactly 4 mL of the internal standard solution, add methanol to make 100 mL, and use this solution as the standard solution. Perform the test with 20 μL each of the sample solution and standard solution as directed under Liquid Chromatography *<2.01>* according to the following conditions, and calculate the ratios, Q_T and Q_S, of the peak area of felodipine to that of the internal standard.

Amount (mg) of felodipine ($C_{18}H_{19}Cl_2NO_4$) $= M_S \times Q_T/Q_S$

M_S: Amount (mg) of felodipine for assay taken, calculated on the dried basis

Internal standard solution—A solution of butyl parahydroxybenzoate in methanol (1 in 6000).

Operating conditions—

Detector: An ultraviolet absorption photometer (wavelength: 264 nm).

Column: A stainless steel column 4.6 mm in inside diameter and 15 cm in length, packed with octadecylsilanized silica gel for liquid chromatography (5 μm in particle diameter).

Column temperature: A constant temperature of about 25°C.

Mobile phase: A mixture of methanol, water, a solution of sodium perchlorate monohydrate (281 in 2000) and diluted perchloric acid (17 in 200) (65:25:8:2).

Flow rate: Adjust so that the retention time of felodipine is about 12 minutes.

System suitability—

System performance: When the procedure is run with 20 μL of the standard solution under the above operating conditions, the internal standard and felodipine are eluted in this order with the resolution between these peaks being not less than 5.

System repeatability: When the test is repeated 6 times with 20 μL of the standard solution under the above operating conditions, the relative standard deviation of the peak area of felodipine is not more than 1.0%.

Containers and storage Containers—Tight containers.

Fenbufen

フェンブフェン

$C_{16}H_{14}O_3$: 254.28

4-(Biphenyl-4-yl)-4-oxobutanoic acid

[36330-85-5]

Fenbufen, when dried, contains not less than 98.0% of fenbufen ($C_{16}H_{14}O_3$).

Description Fenbufen occurs as a white crystalline powder. It has a bitter taste.

It is sparingly soluble in acetone, slightly soluble in methanol, in ethanol (95) and in diethyl ether, and practically insoluble in water.

Melting point: about 188°C (with decomposition).

Identification **(1)** Determine the absorption spectrum of a solution of Fenbufen in ethanol (95) (1 in 200,000) as directed under Ultraviolet-visible Spectrophotometry *<2.24>*, and compare the spectrum with the Reference Spectrum: both spectra exhibit similar intensities of absorption at the same wavelengths.

(2) Determine the infrared absorption spectrum of Fenbufen, previously dried, as directed in the potassium bromide disk method under Infrared Spectrophotometry *<2.25>*, and compare the spectrum with the Reference Spectrum: both spectra exhibit similar intensities of absorption at the same wave numbers.

Purity **(1)** Heavy metals *<1.07>*—Take 2.0 g of Fenbufen, add 2 mL of sulfuric acid, and carbonize by gentle heating, proceed according to Method 2, and perform the test. Prepare the control solution with 2.0 mL of Standard Lead Solution (not more than 10 ppm).

(2) Arsenic *<1.11>*—Prepare the test solution with 1.0 g of Fenbufen according to Method 3, and perform the test (not more than 2 ppm).

(3) Related substances—Dissolve 0.1 g of Fenbufen in 20 mL of acetone, and use this solution as the sample solution. Pipet 1 mL of the sample solution, add acetone to make exactly 100 mL, and use this solution as the standard solution. Perform the test with these solutions as directed under Thin-layer Chromatography *<2.03>*. Spot 10 μL each of the sample solution and standard solution on a plate of silica gel with fluorescent indicator for thin-layer chromatography. Develop the plate with a mixture of dichloromethane, methanol and water (80:20:3) to a distance of about 10 cm, and air-dry the plate. Examine under ultraviolet light (main wavelength: 254 nm): the spots other than the principal spot obtained from the sample solution are not more intense than the spot from the standard solution.

Loss on drying *<2.41>* Not more than 0.3% (1 g, 105°C, 3 hours).

Residue on ignition *<2.44>* Not more than 0.1% (1 g).

Assay Weigh accurately about 0.2 g of Fenbufen, previously dried, dissolve in 100 mL of ethanol (99.5), and titrate *<2.50>* with 0.1 mol/L potassium hydroxide-ethanol VS (potentiometric titration). Perform a blank determination in the same manner, and make any necessary correction.

Each mL of 0.1 mol/L potassium hydroxide-ethanol VS
= 25.43 mg of $C_{16}H_{14}O_3$

Containers and storage Containers—Tight containers.

Fenofibrate

フェノフィブラート

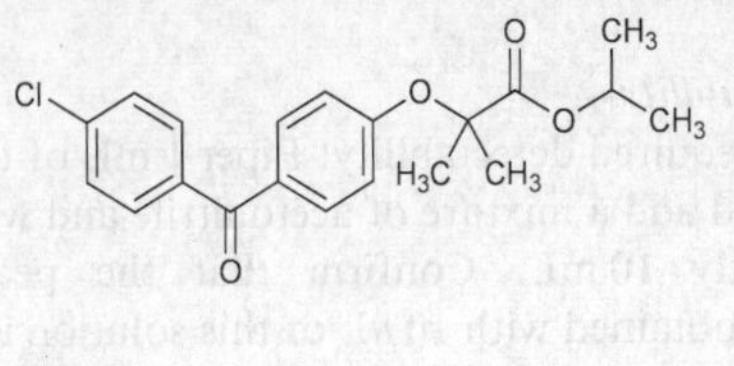

$C_{20}H_{21}ClO_4$: 360.83

1-Methylethyl 2-[4-(4-chlorobenzoyl)phenoxy]-2-methylpropanoate

[49562-28-9]

Fenofibrate, when dried, contains not less than 98.5% and not more than 101.0% of fenofibrate ($C_{20}H_{21}ClO_4$).

Description Fenofibrate occurs as a white to pale yellow-white crystalline powder.

It is soluble in ethanol (99.5), and practically insoluble in water.

It shows crystal polymorphism.

Identification **(1)** Determine the absorption spectrum of a solution of Fenofibrate in ethanol (99.5) (1 in 80,000) as directed under Ultraviolet-visible Spectrophotometry <*2.24*>, and compare the spectrum with the Reference Spectrum or the spectrum of a solution of Fenofibrate RS prepared in the same manner as the sample solution: both spectra exhibit similar intensities of absorption at the same wavelengths.

(2) Determine the infrared absorption spectrum of Fenofibrate, previously dried, as directed in the potassium bromide disk method under Infrared Spectrophotometry <*2.25*>, and compare the spectrum with the Reference Spectrum or the spectrum of dried Fenofibrate RS: both spectra exhibit similar intensities of absorption at the same wave numbers.

(3) Perform the test with Fenofibrate as directed under Flame Coloration Test <*1.04*>: a green color appears.

Melting point <*2.60*> 80 – 83°C

Purity **(1)** Heavy metals <*1.07*>—Proceed with 1.0 g of Fenofibrate according to Method 4, and perform the test. Prepare the control solution with 2.0 mL of Standard Lead Solution (not more than 20 ppm).

(2) Related substances—Conduct this procedure using light-resistant vessels. Dissolve 0.10 g of Fenofibrate in a mixture of acetonitrile and water (7:3) to make 100 mL. To 5 mL of this solution add a mixture of acetonitrile and water (7:3) to make 25 mL, and use this solution as the sample solution. Pipet 3 mL of the sample solution, add a mixture of acetonitrile and water (7:3) to make exactly 50 mL. Pipet 2.5 mL of this solution, add a mixture of acetonitrile and water (7:3) to make exactly 50 mL, and use this solution as the standard solution. Perform the test with exactly 20 μL each of the sample solution and standard solution as directed under Liquid Chromatography <*2.01*> according to the following conditions, and determine each peak area by the automatic integration method: the peak area of related substance A having the relative retention time of about 1.4 to fenofibrate, obtained from the sample solution is not larger than 4/5 times the peak area of fenofibrate from the standard solution, and the total area of the peaks other than fenofibrate from the sample solution is not larger than the peak area of fenofibrate from the standard solution.

Operating conditions—

Detector, column, column temperature, mobile phase, and flow rate: Proceed as directed in the operating conditions in the Assay.

Time span of measurement: About 2 times as long as the retention time of fenofibrate, beginning after the solvent peak.

System suitability—

Test for required detectability: Pipet 5 mL of the standard solution, and add a mixture of acetonitrile and water (7:3) to make exactly 25 mL. Confirm that the peak area of fenofibrate obtained with 20 μL of this solution is equivalent to 15 to 25% of that with 20 μL of the standard solution.

System performance: Dissolve 0.10 g each of Fenofibrate and 4-chlorobenzophenon in 100 mL of a mixture of acetonitrile and water (7:3). To 2 mL of this solution add a mixture of acetonitrile and water (7:3) to make 50 mL. To 1 mL of this solution add a mixture of acetonitrile and water (7:3) to make 50 mL. When the procedure is run with 20 μL of this solution under the above operating conditions, 4-chlorobenzophenon and fenofibrate are eluted in this order with the resolution between these peaks being not less than 10.

System repeatability: When the test is repeated 6 times with 20 μL of the standard solution under the above operating conditions, the relative standard deviation of the peak area of fenofibrate is not more than 5%.

Loss on drying <*2.41*> Not more than 0.5% (1 g, in vacuum, phosphorus (V) oxide, 60°C, 4 hours).

Residue on ignition <*2.44*> Not more than 0.1% (1 g).

Assay Conduct this procedure using light-resistant vessels. Weigh accurately about 50 mg each of Fenofibrate and Fenofibrate RS, both previously dried, dissolve each in a mixture of acetonitrile and water (7:3) to make exactly 50 mL. Pipet 2 mL each of these solutions, add exactly 2 mL of the internal standard solution to each, add a mixture of acetonitrile and water (7:3) to make 50 mL, and use these solutions as the sample solution and the standard solution, respectively. Perform the test with 20 μL each of the sample solution and standard solution as directed under Liquid Chromatography <*2.01*> according to the following conditions, and calculate the ratios, Q_T and Q_S, of the peak area of fenofibrate to the internal standard.

$$\text{Amount (mg) of fenofibrate } (C_{20}H_{21}ClO_4) = M_S \times Q_T/Q_S$$

M_S: Amount (mg) of Fenofibrate RS taken

*Internal standard solution—*A solution of 4-chlorobenzophenon in a mixture of acetonitrile and water (7:3) (11 in 10,000).

Operating conditions—

Detector: An ultraviolet absorption photometer (wavelength: 286 nm).

Column: A stainless steel column 4.6 mm in inside diameter and 15 cm in length, packed with octadecylsilanized silica gel for liquid chromatography (5 μm in particle diameter).

Column temperature: A constant temperature of about 40°C.

Mobile phase: A mixture of acetonitrile and 0.02 mol/L phosphate buffer solution (pH 3.0) (7:3).

Flow rate: Adjust so that the retention time of fenofibrate

is about 8 minutes.

System suitability—

System performance: When the procedure is run with 20 μL of the standard solution under the above operating conditions, the internal standard and fenofibrate are eluted in this order with the resolution between these peaks being not less than 10.

System repeatability: When the test is repeated 6 times with 20 μL of the standard solution under the above operating conditions, the relative standard deviation of the ratio of the peak area of fenofibrate to that of the internal standard is not more than 1.0%.

Containers and storage Containers—Tight containers.

Storage—Light-resistant.

Others

Related substance A:

2-Methyl-1-(1-methylethoxy)-1-oxopropan-2-yl 2-[4-(4-chlorobenzoyl)phenoxy]-2-methylpropanoate

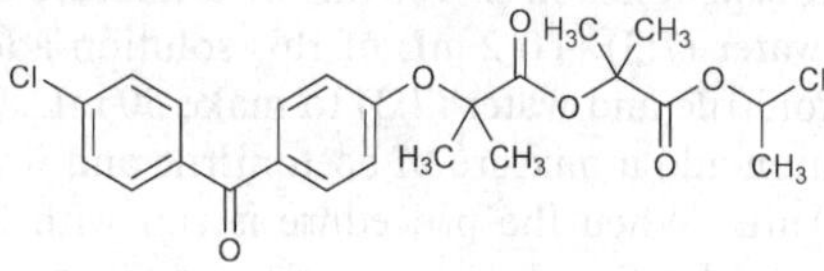

Fenofibrate Tablets

フェノフィブラート錠

Fenofibrate Tablets contain not less than 95.0% and not more than 105.0% of the labeled amount of fenofibrate ($C_{20}H_{21}ClO_4$: 360.83).

Method of preparation Prepare as directed under Tablets, with Fenofibrate.

Identification To a quantity of powdered Fenofibrate Tablets, equivalent to 10 mg of Fenofibrate, add 10 mL of a mixture of acetonitrile and water (7:3), shake, and centrifuge. To 1 mL of the supernatant liquid add a mixture of acetonitrile and water (7:3) to make 100 mL. Determine the absorption spectrum of this solution as directed under Ultraviolet-visible Spectrophotometry <*2.24*>: it exhibits a maximum between 285 nm and 289 nm.

Purity Related substances—Conduct this procedure using light-resistant vessels. To 4 mL of the supernatant liquid obtained in the Assay add a mixture of acetonitrile and water (7:3) to make 10 mL, and use this solution as the sample solution. Pipet 1 mL of this solution, and add a mixture of acetonitrile and water (7:3) to make exactly 20 mL. Pipet 5 mL of this solution, add a mixture of acetonitrile and water (7:3) to make exactly 50 mL, and use this solution as the standard solution. Perform the test with exactly 10 μL each of the sample solution and standard solution as directed under Liquid Chromatography <*2.01*> according to the following conditions, and determine each peak area by the automatic integration method: the area of the peak other than fenofibrate and related substance A having the relative retention time of about 1.4 to fenofibrate obtained from the sample solution, is not larger than 2/5 times the peak area of fenofibrate from the standard solution, and the total area of the peaks other than fenofibrate from the sample solution is not larger than the peak area of fenofibrate from the standard solution.

Operating conditions—

Detector, column temperature, and mobile phase: Proceed as directed in the operating conditions in the Assay under Fenofibrate.

Column: A stainless steel column 4.6 mm in inside diameter and 25 cm in length, packed with octadecylsilanized silica gel for liquid chromatography (5 μm in particle diameter).

Flow rate: Adjust so that the retention time of fenofibrate is about 21 minutes.

Time span of measurement: About 2 times as long as the retention time of fenofibrate, beginning after the solvent peak.

System suitability—

Test for required detectability: Pipet 1 mL of the standard solution, and add a mixture of acetonitrile and water (7:3) to make exactly 10 mL. Confirm that the peak area of fenofibrate obtained with 10 μL of this solution is equivalent to 7 to 13% of that with 10 μL of the standard solution.

System performance: When the procedure is run with 10 μL of the standard solution under the above operating conditions, the number of theoretical plates and the symmetry factor of the peak of fenofibrate are not less than 10,000 and 0.8 to 1.5, respectively.

System repeatability: When the test is repeated 6 times with 10 μL of the standard solution under the above operating conditions, the relative standard deviation of the peak area of fenofibrate is not more than 3.0%.

Uniformity of dosage units <*6.02*> Perform the Mass variation test, or the Content uniformity test according to the following method: it meets the requirement.

Conduct this procedure using light-resistant vessels. To 1 tablet of Fenofibrate Tablets add exactly 20 mL of a mixture of acetonitrile and water (7:3), and shake until the tablet is disintegrated. Centrifuge this solution, pipet *V* mL of the supernatant liquid, equivalent to about 20 mg of fenofibrate ($C_{20}H_{21}ClO_4$), and add a mixture of acetonitrile and water (7:3) to make exactly 20 mL. Pipet 2 mL of this solution, add exactly 2 mL of the internal standard solution, add a mixture of acetonitrile and water (7:3) to make 50 mL, and use this solution as the sample solution. Then, proceed as directed in the Assay.

$$\text{Amount (mg) of fenofibrate } (C_{20}H_{21}ClO_4) = M_S \times Q_T/Q_S \times 8/V$$

M_S: Amount (mg) of Fenofibrate RS taken

Dissolution <*6.10*> When the test is performed at 50 revolutions per minute according to the Paddle method, using 900 mL of a solution prepared by dissolving 1 g of polysorbate 80 in water to make 100 mL as the dissolution medium, the dissolution rate in 30 minutes of Fenofibrate Tablets is not less than 75%.

Conduct this procedure using light-resistant vessels. Start the test with 1 tablet of Fenofibrate Tablets, withdraw not less than 10 mL of the medium at the specified minute after starting the test, and filter through a membrane filter with a pore size not exceeding 0.45 μm. Discard not less than 5 mL of the first filtrate, pipet *V* mL of the subsequent filtrate, add the dissolution medium to make exactly *V′* mL so that each mL contains about 59 μg of fenofibrate ($C_{20}H_{21}ClO_4$), and use this solution as the sample solution. Separately, weigh accurately about 12 mg of Fenofibrate RS, previously dried in vacuum over phosphorus (V) oxide at 60°C for 4 hours, and dissolve in a mixture of acetonitrile and water (7:3) to make exactly 20 mL. Pipet 2 mL of this solution add the dissolution medium to make exactly 20 mL, and use this solution as the standard solution. Perform the test with exactly 10 μL each of the sample solution and standard solution as directed under Liquid Chromatography <2.01> according to the following conditions, and determine the peak areas, A_T and A_S, of fenofibrate in each solution.

Dissolution rate (%) with respect to the labeled amount of fenofibrate ($C_{20}H_{21}ClO_4$)
$= M_S \times A_T/A_S \times V'/V \times 1/C \times 450$

M_S: Amount (mg) of Fenofibrate RS taken
C: Labeled amount (mg) of fenofibrate ($C_{20}H_{21}ClO_4$) in 1 tablet

Operating conditions—

Detector, column, and column temperature: Proceed as directed in the operating conditions in the Assay under Fenofibrate.

Mobile phase: A mixture of acetonitrile and 0.02 mol/L phosphate buffer solution (pH 3.0) (4:1).

Flow rate: Adjust so that the retention time of fenofibrate is about 4 minutes.

System suitability—

System performance: When the procedure is run with 10 μL of the standard solution under the above operating conditions, the number of theoretical plates and the symmetry factor of the peak of fenofibrate are not less than 4000 and not more than 2.0, respectively.

System repeatability: When the test is repeated 6 times with 10 μL of the standard solution under the above operating conditions, the relative standard deviation of the peak area of fenofibrate is not more than 2.0%.

Assay Conduct this procedure using light-resistant vessels. Weigh accurately the mass of not less than 20 tablets of Fenofibrate Tablets, and powder. Weigh accurately a portion of the powder, equivalent to about 50 mg of fenofibrate ($C_{20}H_{21}ClO_4$), add 30 mL of a mixture of acetonitrile and water (7:3), shake thoroughly, and add a mixture of acetonitrile and water (7:3) to make exactly 50 mL. Centrifuge this solution, pipet 2 mL of the supernatant liquid, add exactly 2 mL of the internal standard solution, add a mixture of acetonitrile and water (7:3) to make 50 mL, and use this solution as the sample solution. Separately, weigh accurately about 50 mg of Fenofibrate RS, previously dried in vacuum over phosphorus (V) oxide at 60°C for 4 hours, and dissolve in a mixture of acetonitrile and water (7:3) to make exactly 50 mL. Pipet 2 mL of this solution, add exactly 2 mL of the internal standard solution, add a mixture of acetonitrile and water (7:3) to make 50 mL, and use this solution as the standard solution. Perform the test with 20 μL each of the sample solution and standard solution as directed under Liquid Chromatography <2.01> according to the following conditions, and calculate the ratios, Q_T and Q_S, of the peak area of fenofibrate to that of the internal standard.

Amount (mg) of fenofibrate ($C_{20}H_{21}ClO_4$)
$= M_S \times Q_T/Q_S$

M_S: Amount (mg) of Fenofibrate RS for assay taken

*Internal standard solution—*A solution of 4-chlorobenzophenon in a mixture of acetonitrile and water (7:3) (11 in 10,000).

Operating conditions—

Proceed as directed in the operating conditions in the Assay under Fenofibrate.

System suitability—

Proceed as directed in the system suitability in the Assay under Fenofibrate.

Containers and storage Containers—Tight containers.

Storage—Light-resistant.

Others

Related substance A: Refer to it described in Fenofibrate.

Fentanyl Citrate

フェンタニルクエン酸塩

$C_{22}H_{28}N_2O.C_6H_8O_7$: 528.59
N-(1-Phenethylpiperidin-4-yl)-*N*-phenylpropanamide monocitrate
[*990-73-8*]

Fentanyl Citrate contains not less than 98.0% of fentanyl citrate ($C_{22}H_{28}N_2O.C_6H_8O_7$), calculated on the dried basis.

Description Fentanyl Citrate occurs as white, crystals or crystalline powder.

It is freely soluble in methanol and in acetic acid (100), sparingly soluble in water and in ethanol (95), and very slightly soluble in diethyl ether.

Identification **(1)** Dissolve 0.05 g of Fentanyl Citrate in 10 mL of 0.1 mol/L hydrochloric acid TS and ethanol (95) to make 100 mL. Determine the absorption spectrum of the solution as directed under Ultraviolet-visible Spectrophotometry <2.24>, and compare the spectrum with the Reference Spectrum: both spectra exhibit similar intensities of absorption at the same wavelengths.

(2) Determine the infrared absorption spectrum of Fentanyl Citrate, previously dried, as directed in the potassium bromide disk method under Infrared Spectrophotometry <2.25>, and compare the spectrum with the Reference Spectrum: both spectra exhibit similar intensities of absorption at the same wave numbers.

(3) A solution of Fentanyl Citrate (1 in 100) responds to Qualitative Tests <1.09> (1) for citrate.

pH <2.54> Dissolve 0.10 g of Fentanyl Citrate in 10 mL of water: the pH of this solution is between 3.0 and 5.0.

Melting point <2.60> 150 – 154°C

Purity **(1)** Heavy metals <1.07>—Proceed with 0.5 g of Fentanyl Citrate according to Method 2, and perform the test. Prepare the control solution with 1.0 mL of Standard Lead Solution (not more than 20 ppm).

(2) Related substances—Dissolve 0.10 g of Fentanyl Citrate in 5 mL of methanol, and use this solution as the sample solution. Pipet 1 mL of the sample solution, add methanol to make exactly 100 mL, and use this solution as the standard solution. Perform the test with these solutions as directed under Thin-layer Chromatography <2.03>. Spot 5 μL each of the sample solution and standard solution on a plate of silica gel for thin-layer chromatography. Develop the plate with a mixture of 1-butanol, water and acetic acid (100) (3:1:1) to a distance of about 10 cm, and air-dry the plate. Spray evenly Dragendorff's TS for spraying on the plate: the spots other than the principal spot obtained from the sample solution are not more intense than the spot from the standard solution.

Loss on drying *<2.41>* Not more than 0.5% (0.2 g, in vacuum, silica gel, 60°C, 2 hours).

Residue on ignition *<2.44>* Not more than 0.2% (0.5 g).

Assay Weigh accurately about 75 mg of Fentanyl Citrate, dissolve in 50 mL of acetic acid (100), and titrate *<2.50>* with 0.02 mol/L perchloric acid VS (potentiometric titration). Perform a blank determination in the same manner, and make any necessary correction.

Each mL of 0.02 mol/L perchloric acid VS
= 10.57 mg of $C_{22}H_{28}N_2O.C_6H_8O_7$

Containers and storage Containers—Tight containers.
Storage—Light-resistant.

Ferrous Sulfate Hydrate

硫酸鉄水和物

$FeSO_4.7H_2O$: 278.01

Ferrous Sulfate Hydrate contains not less than 98.0% and not more than 104.0% of ferrous sulfate hydrate ($FeSO_4.7H_2O$).

Description Ferrous Sulfate Hydrate occurs as pale green, crystals or crystalline powder. It is odorless, and has an astringent taste.

It is freely soluble in water, and practically insoluble in ethanol (95) and in diethyl ether.

It is efflorescent in dry air, and its surface becomes yellowish brown in moist air.

Identification A solution of Ferrous Sulfate Hydrate (1 in 10) responds to Qualitative Tests *<1.09>* for ferrous salt and for sulfate.

Purity **(1)** Clarity of solution—Dissolve 1.0 g of Ferrous Sulfate Hydrate in 20 mL of water and 1 mL of dilute sulfuric acid: the solution is clear.

(2) Acidity—To 5.0 g of powdered Ferrous Sulfate Hydrate add 50 mL of ethanol (95), shake well for 2 minutes, and filter the mixture. To 25 mL of the filtrate add 50 mL of water, 3 drops of bromothymol blue TS and 0.5 mL of dilute sodium hydroxide TS: a blue color develops.

(3) Heavy metals *<1.07>*—Take 1.0 g of Ferrous Sulfate Hydrate in a porcelain dish, add 3 mL of aqua regia, and dissolve. Then evaporate on a water bath to dryness. To the residue add 5 mL of 6 mol/L hydrochloric acid TS, and dissolve. Transfer this solution to a separator. Wash the porcelain dish with two 5-mL portions of 6 mol/L hydrochloric acid TS, and combine the washings and the solution in the separator. Pour two 40-mL portions and one 20-mL portion of diethyl ether in the separator, shaking each time to mix. Allow to stand, and discard each separated diethyl ether layer. To the aqueous layer add 0.05 g of hydroxylammonium chloride, dissolve, and heat on a water bath for 10 minutes. Cool, adjust the solution to a pH of 3 to 4 by dropping ammonia solution (28), add water to make 50 mL, and perform the test using this solution as the test solution. Prepare the control solution as follows: take 2.5 mL of Standard Lead Solution in a porcelain dish, add 3 mL of aqua regia, and proceed as directed for the preparation of the test solution (not more than 25 ppm).

(4) Arsenic *<1.11>*—Prepare the test solution with 1.0 g of Ferrous Sulfate Hydrate according to Method 1, and perform the test (not more than 2 ppm).

Assay Dissolve about 0.7 g of Ferrous Sulfate Hydrate, accurately weighed, in a mixture of 20 mL of water and 20 mL of dilute sulfuric acid, add 2 mL of phosphoric acid, and immediately titrate *<2.50>* with 0.02 mol/L potassium permanganate VS.

Each mL of 0.02 mol/L potassium permanganate VS
= 27.80 mg of $FeSO_4.7H_2O$

Containers and storage Containers—Tight containers.

Fexofenadine Hydrochloride

フェキソフェナジン塩酸塩

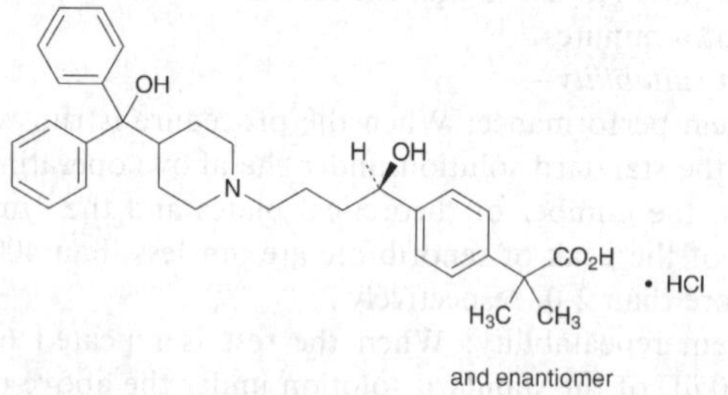

and enantiomer

$C_{32}H_{39}NO_4.HCl$: 538.12
2-(4-{(1*RS*)-1-Hydroxy-4-[4-(hydroxydiphenylmethyl)piperidin-1-yl]butyl}phenyl)-2-methylpropanoic acid monohydrochloride
[*153439-40-8*]

Fexofenadine Hydrochloride contains not less than 98.0% and not more than 102.0% of fexofenadine hydrochloride ($C_{32}H_{39}NO_4.HCl$), calculated on the anhydrous basis.

Description Fexofenadine Hydrochloride occurs as a white crystalline powder.

It is very soluble in methanol, soluble in ethanol (99.5), and slightly soluble in water.

A solution of Fexofenadine Hydrochloride in methanol (3 in 100) shows no optical rotation.

Fexofenadine Hydrochloride shows crystal polymorphism.

Identification **(1)** Determine the absorption spectrum of a solution of Fexofenadine Hydrochloride in methanol (1 in 2500) as directed under Ultraviolet-visible Spectrophotometry *<2.24>*, and compare the spectrum with the Reference Spectrum or the spectrum of a solution of Fexofenadine Hydrochloride RS prepared in the same manner as the sample solution: both spectra exhibit similar intensities of absorption at the same wavelengths.

(2) Determine the infrared absorption spectrum of Fexofenadine Hydrochloride as directed in the potassium bromide disk method under Infrared Spectrophotometry *<2.25>*, and compare the spectrum with the Reference Spectrum or the spectrum of Fexofenadine Hydrochloride RS: both spectra exhibit similar intensities of absorption at the same wave numbers. If any difference appears between the spectra, recrystallize the sample and the RS according to the method otherwise specified, filter and dry the crystals, and perform the test with the crystals.

(3) A solution of Fexofenadine Hydrochloride in a mixture of water and methanol (1:1) (3 in 200) responds to Qualitative Tests *<1.09>* (2) for chloride.

Purity (1) Heavy metals <1.07>—Proceed with 2.0 g of Fexofenadine Hydrochloride according to Method 4, and perform the test. Prepare the control solution with 2.0 mL of Standard Lead Solution (not more than 10 ppm).

(2) Related substances—Dissolve 7.51 g of sodium dihydrogen phosphate dihydrate and 0.84 g of sodium perchlorate in 1000 mL of water, and adjust to pH 2.0 with phosphoric acid. In a mixture of this solution and acetonitrile for liquid chromatography (1:1) dissolve 25 mg of Fexofenadine Hydrochloride to make 25 mL, and use this solution as the sample solution. Pipet 1 mL of the sample solution, and add the mobile phase to make exactly 100 mL. Pipet 1 mL of this solution, add the mobile phase to make exactly 10 mL, and use this solution as the standard solution. Perform the test with exactly 20 μL each of the sample solution and standard solution as directed under Liquid Chromatography <2.01> according to the following conditions, and determine each peak area of both solutions by the automatic integration method: the area of the peak other than fexofenadine obtained from the sample solution is not larger than the peak area of fexofenadine from the standard solution. For the areas of the peaks, having the relative retention time of about 1.8 and about 3.3 to fexofenadine, multiply their correction factor, 1.5 and 0.9, respectively.

Operating conditions—

Detector, column, column temperature, mobile phase, and flow rate: Proceed as directed in the operating conditions in the Assay.

Time span of measurement: About 6 times as long as the retention time of fexofenadine, beginning after the solvent peak.

System suitability—

System performance: When the procedure is run with 20 μL of the standard solution under the above operating conditions, the number of theoretical plates and the symmetry factor of the peak of fexofenadine are not less than 8000 and not more than 2.0, respectively.

System repeatability: When the test is repeated 6 times with 20 μL of the standard solution under the above operating conditions, the relative standard deviation of the peak area of fexofenadine is not more than 2.0%.

Water <2.48> Not more than 0.5% (0.25 g, coulometric titration).

Residue on ignition <2.44> Not more than 0.1% (1 g).

Assay Dissolve 7.51 g of sodium dihydrogen phosphate dihydrate and 0.84 g of sodium perchlorate in 1000 mL of water, and adjust to pH 2.0 with phosphoric acid. In a mixture of this solution and acetonitrile for liquid chromatography (1:1) dissolve accurately weighed about 25 mg each of Fexofenadine Hydrochloride and Fexofenadine Hydrochloride RS (separately determine the water <2.48> in the same manner as Fexofenadine Hydrochloride), to make exactly 25 mL each. Pipet 3 mL each of these solutions, add the mobile phase to make exactly 50 mL, and use these solutions as the sample solution and the standard solution, respectively. Perform the test with exactly 20 μL each of the sample solution and standard solution as directed under Liquid Chromatography <2.01> according to the following conditions, and determine the peak areas, A_T and A_S, of fexofenadine in each solution.

Amount (mg) of fexofenadine hydrochloride ($C_{32}H_{39}NO_4.HCl$)
$$= M_S \times A_T/A_S$$

M_S: Amount (mg) of Fexofenadine Hydrochloride RS taken, calculated on the anhydrous basis

Operating conditions—

Detector: An ultraviolet absorption photometer (wavelength: 220 nm).

Column: A stainless steel column 4.6 mm in inside diameter and 25 cm in length, packed with phenylated silica gel for liquid chromatography (5 μm in particle diameter).

Column temperature: A constant temperature of about 25°C.

Mobile phase: To 650 mL of a solution, prepared by dissolving 7.51 g of sodium dihydrogen phosphate dihydrate and 0.84 g of sodium perchlorate in 1000 mL of water and adjusting to pH 2.0 with phosphoric acid, add 350 mL of acetonitrile for liquid chromatography and 3 mL of triethylamine.

Flow rate: Adjust so that the retention time of fexofenadine is about 9 minutes.

System suitability—

System performance: When the procedure is run with 20 μL of the standard solution under the above operating conditions, the number of theoretical plates and the symmetry factor of the peak of fexofenadine are not less than 8000 and not more than 2.0, respectively.

System repeatability: When the test is repeated 6 times with 20 μL of the standard solution under the above operating conditions, the relative standard deviation of the peak area of fexofenadine is not more than 1.0%.

Containers and storage Containers—Well-closed containers.

Fexofenadine Hydrochloride Tablets

フェキソフェナジン塩酸塩錠

Fexofenadine Hydrochloride Tablets contain not less than 95.0% and not more than 105.0% of the labeled amount of fexofenadine hydrochloride ($C_{32}H_{39}NO_4.HCl$: 538.12).

Method of preparation Prepare as directed under Tablets, with Fexofenadine Hydrochloride.

Identification To an amount of powdered Fexofenadine Hydrochloride Tablets, equivalent to 40 mg of Fexofenadine Hydrochloride, add 100 mL of methanol, and shake well. Filter, discard the first 10 mL of the filtrate, and determine the absorption spectrum of the subsequent filtrate as directed under Ultraviolet-visible Spectrophotometry <2.24>: it exhibits a maximum between 257 nm and 261 nm.

Uniformity of dosage units <6.02> Perform the Mass variation test, or the Content uniformity test according to the following method: it meets the requirement.

To 1 tablet of Fexofenadine Hydrochloride Tablets add $V/5$ mL of diluted acetic acid (100) (17 in 10,000), shake until the tablet is disintegrated. Add $3V/5$ mL of acetonitrile for liquid chromatography, shake well, add a mixture of acetonitrile for liquid chromatography and diluted acetic acid (100) (17 in 10,000) (3:1) to make exactly V mL so that each mL contains about 0.3 mg of fexofenadine hydrochloride ($C_{32}H_{39}NO_4.HCl$). Pipet 5 mL of this solution, add the mobile phase to make exactly 100 mL, and filter this solution through a membrane filter with a pore size not exceeding 0.45 μm. Discard the first 2 mL of the filtrate, and use the subsequent filtrate as the sample solution. Separately, weigh accurately about 50 mg of Fexofenadine Hydrochloride RS (separately determine the water <*2.48*> in the same manner as Fexofenadine Hydrochloride), and dissolve in a mixture of acetonitrile for liquid chromatography and diluted acetic acid (100) (17 in 10,000) (3:1) to make exactly 200 mL. Pipet 6 mL of this solution, add the mobile phase to make exactly 100 mL, and use this solution as the standard solution. Then, proceed as directed in the Assay.

Amount (mg) of fexofenadine hydrochloride ($C_{32}H_{39}NO_4.HCl$)
$= M_S \times A_T/A_S \times 3V/500$

M_S: Amount (mg) of Fexofenadine Hydrochloride RS taken, calculated on the anhydrous basis

Dissolution <*6.10*> When the test is performed at 50 revolutions per minute according to the Paddle method, using 900 mL of water as the dissolution medium, the dissolution rate in 30 minutes of Fexofenadine Hydrochloride Tablets is not less than 80%.

Start the test with 1 tablet of Fexofenadine Hydrochloride Tablets, withdraw not less than 20 mL of the medium at the specified minute after starting the test, and filter through a membrane filter with a pore size not exceeding 0.45 μm. Discard not less than 10 mL of the first filtrate, pipet V mL of the subsequent filtrate, add water to make exactly V' mL so that each mL contains about 30 μg of fexofenadine hydrochloride ($C_{32}H_{39}NO_4.HCl$), and use this solution as the sample solution. Separately, weigh accurately about 30 mg of Fexofenadine Hydrate RS (separately determine the water <*2.48*> in the same manner as Fexofenadine Hydrochloride), dissolve in 5 mL of methanol, add water to make exactly 100 mL. Pipet 5 mL of this solution, and add water to make exactly 50 mL, and use this solution as the standard solution. Perform the test with exactly 50 μL each of the sample solution and standard solution as directed under Liquid Chromatography <*2.01*> according to the following conditions, and determine the peak areas, A_T and A_S, of fexofenadine in each solution.

Dissolution rate (%) with respect to the labeled amount of fexofenadine hydrochloride ($C_{32}H_{39}NO_4.HCl$)
$= M_S \times A_T/A_S \times V'/V \times 1/C \times 90$

M_S: Amount (mg) of Fexofenadine Hydrochloride RS taken, calculated on the anhydrous basis
C: Labeled amount (mg) of fexofenadine hydrochloride ($C_{32}H_{39}NO_4.HCl$) in 1 tablet

Operating conditions—

Detector: An ultraviolet absorption photometer (wavelength: 220 nm).

Column: A stainless steel column 4.6 mm in inside diameter and 10 cm in length, packed with octadecylsilanized silica gel for liquid chromatography (5 μm in particle diameter).

Column temperature: A constant temperature of about 25°C.

Mobile phase: Dissolve 1.1 g of sodium dihydrogen phosphate dihydrate, 0.3 mL of phosphoric acid and 0.5 g of sodium perchlorate in 300 mL of water, add 700 mL of acetonitrile for liquid chromatography.

Flow rate: Adjust so that the retention time of fexofenadine is about 3.5 minutes.

System suitability—

System performance: When the procedure is run with 50 μL of the standard solution under the above operating conditions, the number of theoretical plates and the symmetry factor of the peak of fexofenadine are not less than 3000 and not more than 2.0, respectively.

System repeatability: When the test is repeated 6 times with 50 μL of the standard solution under the above operating conditions, the relative standard deviation of the peak area of fexofenadine is not more than 2.0%.

Assay To 20 Fexofenadine Hydrochloride Tablets add $V/5$ mL of diluted acetic acid (100) (17 in 10,000), and shake until the tablets are disintegrated. Then, add $3V/5$ mL of acetonitrile for liquid chromatography, shake well, and add a mixture of acetonitrile for liquid chromatography and diluted acetic acid (100) (17 in 10,000) (3:1) to make exactly V mL so that each mL contains about 1.2 mg of fexofenadine hydrochloride ($C_{32}H_{39}NO_4.HCl$). Pipet 15 mL of this solution, and add the mobile phase to make exactly 50 mL. Pipet 5 mL of this solution, add the mobile phase to make exactly 100 mL, and filter through a membrane filter with a pore size not exceeding 0.45 μm. Discard the first 2 mL of the filtrate, and use the subsequent filtrate as the sample solution. Separately, weigh accurately about 45 mg of Fexofenadine Hydrochloride RS (separately determine the water <*2.48*> in the same manner as Fexofenadine Hydrochloride), and dissolve in a mixture of acetonitrile for liquid chromatography and diluted acetic acid (100) (17 in 10,000) (3:1) to make exactly 200 mL. Pipet 20 mL of this solution, add the mobile phase to make exactly 250 mL, and use this solution as the standard solution. Perform the test with exactly 20 μL each of the sample solution and standard solution as directed under Liquid Chromatography <*2.01*> according to the following conditions, and determine the peak areas, A_T and A_S, of fexofenadine in each solution.

Amount (mg) of fexofenadine hydrochloride ($C_{32}H_{39}NO_4.HCl$) in 1 tablet
$= M_S \times A_T/A_S \times V/750$

M_S: Amount (mg) of Fexofenadine Hydrochloride RS taken, calculated on the anhydrous basis

Operating conditions—

Detector: An ultraviolet absorption photometer (wavelength: 220 nm).

Column: A stainless steel column 4.6 mm in inside diameter and 25 cm in length, packed with phenylated silica gel for liquid chromatography (5 μm in particle diameter).

Column temperature: A constant temperature of about 35°C.

Mobile phase: To 1000 mL of diluted acetic acid (100) (17 in 10,000) add 15 mL of a mixture of triethylamine and acetonitrile for liquid chromatography (1:1), and adjust to pH 5.25 with phosphoric acid. To 16 volumes of this solution add 9 volumes of acetonitrile for liquid chromatography.

Flow rate: Adjust so that the retention time of fexofenadine is about 6 minutes.

System suitability—

System performance: When the procedure is run with 20 μL of the standard solution under the above operating conditions, the number of theoretical plates and the symmetry factor of the peak of fexofenadine are not less than 7000 and not more than 2.0, respectively.

System repeatability: When the test is repeated 6 times with 20 μL of the standard solution under the above operating conditions, the relative standard deviation of the peak area of fexofenadine is not more than 1.0%.

Containers and storage Containers—Tight containers.

Filgrastim (Genetical Recombination)

フィルグラスチム(遺伝子組換え)

```
MTPLGPASSL PQSFLLKCLE QVRKIQGDGA ALQEKLCATY KLCHPEELVL
LGHSLGIPWA PLSSCPSQAL QLAGCLSQLH SGLFLYQGLL QALEGISPEL
GPTLDTLQLD VADFATTIWQ QMEELGMAPA LQPTQGAMPA FASAFQRRAG
GVLVASHLQS FLEVSYRVLR HLAQP
```

$C_{845}H_{1339}N_{223}O_{243}S_9$: 18798.61
[121181-53-1]

Filgrastim (Genetical Recombination) is an aqueous solution in which a desired product is a recombinant *N*-methionyl human granulocyte colony-stimulating factor consisting of 175 amino acid residues.

It contains not less than 0.45 mg and not more than 0.55 mg of protein per mL, and not less than 1.0 × 10^8 units per mg of protein.

Description Filgrastim (Genetical Recombination) occurs as a clear and colorless liquid.

Identification **(1)** Take a volume of Filgrastim (Genetical Recombination), equivalent to 5 to 10 µg of protein depending on the size of polyacrylamide gel for filgrastim, and add 10 µL of water. To 3 volumes of this solution add 1 volume of buffer solution for filgrastim sample, and use this solution as the sample solution. Separately, take a volume of Filgrastim RS which contains equal amount of protein to Filgrastim (Genetical Recombination) used above, proceed as directed for the sample solution, and use the solution so obtained as the standard solution. Set a polyacrylamide gel for filgrastim up to the electrophoresis apparatus, and put a necessary amount of buffer solution for SDS-polyacrylamide gel electrophoresis in the upper and lower reservoirs. Pipet the all amount of the sample solution and standard solution into each well of the gel, and start the electrophoresis setting the electrode of the lower reservoir as the anode. Stop the electrophoresis when the bromophenol blue band has been migrated to about the lower end of the gel. When stain the gel with a staining solution, which is prepared by dissolving 1.25 g of Coomassie brilliant blue R250 in a mixture of 450 mL of methanol, 100 mL of acetic acid (100) and water to make 1000 mL, stained bands obtained from the sample solution appear as similar migrating image at the same position as those from the standard solution.

(2) Take a volume of Filgrastim (Genetical Recombination) and Filgrastim RS, equivalent to about 80 µg of protein, add 200 µL of the buffer solution for enzyme digestion, and add water to make 390 µL. To each of these solution add 10 µL of a solution containing 50 µg of V8 protease in 250 µL of water, incubate at 25°C for 17 to 19 hours, then add 18 µL of a mixture of water and trifluoroacetic acid (19:1) to stop the reaction, and use these solutions as the sample solution and the standard solution, respectively. Perform the test with 70 µL each of the sample solution and standard solution as directed under Liquid Chromatography *<2.01>* according to the following conditions. When the chromatograms obtained from these solutions are compared, both chromatograms show the similar peaks at the same retention time.

Operating conditions—

Detector: An ultraviolet absorption photometer (wavelength: 214 nm).

Column: A stainless steel column 2.1 mm in inside diameter and 25 cm in length, packed with butylsilanized silica gel for liquid chromatography (5 µm in particle diameter).

Column temperature: A constant temperature of about 40°C.

Mobile phase A: A mixture of water and trifluoroacetic acid (1000:1).

Mobile phase B: A mixture of acetonitrile, water and trifluoroacetic acid (9000:1000:9).

Flowing of mobile phase: Control the gradient by mixing the mobile phases A and B as directed in the following table.

Time after injection of sample (min)	Mobile phase A (vol%)	Mobile phase B (vol%)
0 – 2	98	2
2 – 30	98 → 70	2 → 30
30 – 85	70 → 50	30 → 50
85 – 90	50 → 2	50 → 98
90 – 100	2	98

Flow rate: 0.20 mL per minute.

System suitability—

System performance: When the procedure is run with 70 µL of the standard solution under the above operating conditions, the resolutions between each adjacent peakpair of the major 8 peaks, which are eluted after the solvent peak appeared within 10 minutes, are not less than 1.5.

pH *<2.54>* 3.7 – 4.3

Purity **(1)** Multimers—Perform the test with 250 µL of Filgrastim (Genetical Recombination) as directed under Liquid Chromatography *<2.01>* according to the following conditions, and determine each peak area by the automatic integration method. Calculate their amounts of the peaks by the area percentage method; the total amount of the peaks other than filgrastim is not more than 2%.

Operating conditions—

Detector: An ultraviolet absorption photometer (wavelength: 280 nm).

Column: A stainless steel column 7.5 mm in inside diameter and 60 cm in length, packed with hydrophilic silica gel for liquid chromatography.

Column temperature: A constant temperature of about 25°C.

Mobile phase: Dissolve 5.8 g of sodium chloride in 10 mL of dilute acetic acid and 900 mL of water, adjust to pH 5.5 with sodium hydroxide TS, then add 250 mg of sodium lauryl sulfate, and add water to make 1000 mL.

Flow rate: Adjust so that the retention time of filgrastim is about 17 minutes.

Time span of measurement: From the retention time corresponding to the exclusion volume of the size-exclusion column to the time when the elution of filgrastim is completed.

System suitability—

Test for required detectability: Measure exactly 10 µL of Filgrastim (Genetical Recombination), and add the mobile phase to make exactly 1000 µL. Confirm that the peak area of filgrastim obtained with 250 µL of this solution is 0.7 to 1.3% of that with 250 µL of Filgrastim (Genetical Recombination).

System performance: When the procedure is run with 10 µL of a solution containing 12.5 mg of egg albumin and 12.5 mg of myoglobin in 5 mL of water under the above operating conditions, egg albumin and myoglobin are eluted in this order with the resolution between these peaks being not less than 1.7.

System repeatability: When the test is repeated 6 times with 250 μL of Filgrastim (Genetical Recombination) under the above operating conditions, the relative standard deviation of the peak area of filgrastim is not more than 2.5%.

(2) Charge isomer—Perform the test with 100 μL of Filgrastim (Genetical Recombination) as directed under Liquid Chromatography <*2.01*> according to the following conditions, and determine the each peak area by the automatic integration method. Calculate their amounts of the peaks by the area percentage method; the amount of charge isomer, having the relative retention time of about 0.87 to filgrastim, is not more than 3%.

Operating conditions—

Detector: An ultraviolet absorption photometer (wavelength: 280 nm).

Column: A stainless steel column 4.6 mm in inside diameter and 35 mm in length, packed with strongly acidic ion-exchange non-porous resin for liquid chromatography (2.5 μm in particle diameter).

Column temperature: A constant temperature of about 25°C.

Mobile phase A: To 900 mL of water add 1.14 mL of acetic acid (100), adjust to pH 5.4 with sodium hydroxide TS, and add water to make 1000 mL.

Mobile phase B: Dissolve 5.84 g of sodium chloride in 1.14 mL of acetic acid (100) and 900 mL of water, adjust to pH 5.4 with sodium hydroxide TS, and add water to make 1000 mL.

Flowing of mobile phase: Control the gradient by mixing the mobile phases A and B as directed in the following table.

Time after injection of sample (min)	Mobile phase A (vol%)	Mobile phase B (vol%)
0 – 2	100	0
2 – 10	100 → 40	0 → 60
10 – 11	40 → 100	60 → 0
11 – 20	100	0

Flow rate: Adjust so that the retention time of filgrastim is about 14 minutes.

Time span of measurement: From 6 minutes to 17 minutes.

System suitability—

Test for required detectability: Confirm that when perform the test with 100 μL of the system suitability test solution for filgrastim under the above operating conditions, the content of charge isomer is between 1.4 to 2.6%.

System performance: When the procedure is run with 100 μL of the system suitability test solution for filgrastim under the above operating conditions, charge isomer peak and filgrastim are eluted in this order with the resolution between these peaks being not less than 1.5.

System repeatability: When the test is repeated 6 times with 100 μL of Filgrastim (Genetical Recombination) under the above operating conditions, the relative standard deviation of the peak area of filgrastim is not more than 2.5%.

(3) Host cell proteins—Being specified separately when the drug is granted approval based on the Law.

(4) Host cell DNA—Being specified separately when the drug is granted approval based on the Law.

Bacterial endotoxins <*4.01*> Less than 0.25 EU/mL.

Assay **(1)** Protein content—Perform the test with exactly 200 μL each of Filgrastim (Genetical Recombination) and Filgrastim RS as directed under Liquid Chromatography <*2.01*> according to the following conditions, and determine the peak areas, A_T and A_S, of filgrastim.

$$\text{Amount (mg) of protein in 1 mL of Filgrastim (Genetical Recombination)} = C \times A_T/A_S$$

C: Protein concentration (mg/mL) of Filgrastim RS

Operating conditions—

Detector: An ultraviolet absorption photometer (wavelength: 280 nm).

Column: A stainless steel column 4.6 mm in inside diameter and 25 cm in length, packed with octylsilanized silica gel for liquid chromatography (10 μm in particle diameter).

Column temperature: A constant temperature of about 25°C.

Mobile phase A: A mixture of water, 1-propanol and trifluoroacetic acid (699:300:1).

Mobile phase B: A mixture of 1-propanol, water and trifluoroacetic acid (800:199:1).

Flowing of mobile phase: Control the gradient by mixing the mobile phases A and B as directed in the following table.

Time after injection of sample (min)	Mobile phase A (vol%)	Mobile phase B (vol%)
0 – 2	90	10
2 – 13	90 → 70	10 → 30
13 – 15	70 → 0	30 → 100
15 – 18	0	100

Flow rate: Adjust so that the retention time of filgrastim is about 15 minutes.

System suitability—

System performance: When the procedure is run with 200 μL of a solution prepared by dissolving 1 mg of uracil and 2 mg of diphenyl in 100 mL of a mixture of water, 1-propanol and trifluoroacetic acid (649:350:1) under the above operating conditions, uracil and diphenyl are eluted in this order with the resolution between these peaks being not less than 8.

System repeatability: When the test is repeated 6 times with 200 μL of Filgrastim RS under the above operating conditions, the relative standard deviation of the peak area of filgrastim is not more than 2.5%.

(2) Specific activity—

(i) Test cell: 32D clone3 cell.

(ii) Sample dilution solution for assay: To Iscove's modified Dulbecco's fluid medium for filgrastim add 200 mmol/L L-glutamine solution and fetal calf serum to make 1 vol% and 5 vol% solution, respectively, and sterilize by filtration.

(iii) Standard solutions Dilute Filgrastim RS by the sample dilution solution for assay to prepare not less than 5 serial dilutions started from any concentration S_H so that all of their protein concentrations are within the range of 0.5 to 6 ng/mL, and use them as the standard solutions.

(iv) Sample solutions Dilute Filgrastim (Genetical Recombination) by the sample dilution solution for assay to prepare not less than 5 serial dilutions in equal ratio started from any concentration U_H so that all of their protein concentrations are within the range of 0.5 to 6 ng/mL, and use them as the sample solutions.

(v) Procedure The procedure before stopping the incubation should be performed under aseptic condition.

Transfer exactly 100 μL of each concentration of the standard solutions and sample solutions to the wells of 96-well flat bottom microplates. Not less than three plates are prepared for both standard solutions and sample solutions. Add exactly 100 μL of a test cell suspension containing 1×10^5 cells per mL in the sample dilution solution for assay to each well, and incubate under atmosphere of 5% carbon dioxide at 37 ± 2°C for 21 to 27 hours. After incubation, add 40 μL of fluorogenic substrate TS to each well, incubate under the same conditions as above for 21 to 51 hours, and measure fluorescence intensities at excitation wavelength 530 to 560 nm and at measurement wavelength 590 nm, using fluorescence microplate reader. Use the data from at least 3 plates and not less than 3 concentrations of the standard solution and sample solution for the calculation.

(vi) Calculation Transform each concentration of the sample solutions and standard solutions to common logarithm, and name them as x_U and x_S, respectively, and their totals are named as X_U and X_S, respectively. The fluorescence intensities obtained from the sample solution and the standard solution are named as y_U and y_S, and their totals are named as Y_U and Y_S, respectively. The numbers of the concentrations of the sample solution and the standard solution are named as n_U and n_S, respectively, the number of the plate is r. Calculate the specific activity of Filgrastim (Genetical Recombination) by the following equation, using the protein content (mg/mL) obtained in (1).

Specific activity (unit/mg) of Filgrastim (Genetical Recombination)

$$= \text{antilog } M \times \text{biological activity of Filgrastim RS (unit/mL)} \times \frac{\text{dilution factor for U}_H}{\text{dilution factor for S}_H} \times \frac{U_H}{S_H} \times \frac{1}{\text{protein content (mg/mL) obtained in the Assay (1)}}$$

$$M = X_S/n_S - X_U/n_U - (\Sigma Y_S/n_S r - \Sigma Y_U/n_U r)/b$$
$$b = (Sxy_S + Sxy_U)/(Sxx_S + Sxx_U)$$
$$Sxy_S = \Sigma x_S Y_S - X_S \Sigma Y_S/n_S$$
$$Sxy_U = \Sigma x_U Y_U - X_U \Sigma Y_U/n_U$$
$$Sxx_S = r\Sigma x_S^2 - rX_S^2/n_S$$
$$Sxx_U = r\Sigma x_U^2 - rX_U^2/n_U$$

The necessary requirements for validity of the test are following three items:

1) F'_S is not less than F_1 against $m = n_S\ (r - 1)$ shown in the table below, and F'_U is not less than F_1 against $m = n_U$ $(r - 1)$ shown in the table.

$$F'_S = V_{RS}/V_{ES}$$
$$V_{RS} = Sxy_S^2/Sxx_S$$
$$V_{ES} = \{\Sigma y_S^2 - \Sigma(Y_S^2/r)\}/\{n_S(r - 1)\}$$
$$F'_U = V_{RU}/V_{EU}$$
$$V_{RU} = Sxy_U^2/Sxx_U$$
$$V_{EU} = \{\Sigma y_U^2 - \Sigma(Y_U^2/r)\}/\{n_U(r - 1)\}$$

2) F' is smaller than F_1 against $m = (n_S + n_U)(r - 1)$ shown in the table below.

$$F' = V_P/V_E$$
$$V_P = Sxy_S^2/Sxx_S + Sxy_U^2/Sxx_U - (Sxy_S + Sxy_U)^2/(Sxx_S + Sxx_U)$$
$$V_E = \{\Sigma y_S^2 + \Sigma y_U^2 - \Sigma(Y_S^2/r) - \Sigma(Y_U^2/r)\}/\{(n_S + n_U)(r - 1)\}$$

3) $L \leqq 0.3$

$$L = 2/b(1 - g)\sqrt{V_E F_1\{(1 - g)(1/n_S r + 1/n_U r) + (\Sigma Y_S/n_S r - \Sigma Y_U/n_U r)^2/b^2(Sxx_S + Sxx_U)\}}$$

F_1: Value against $m = (n_S + n_U)(r - 1)$ shown in the table.

$$g = V_E F_1/b^2(Sxx_S + Sxx_U)$$

Value of F_1 against m

m	F_1	m	F_1	m	F_1
1	161.45	13	4.667	25	4.242
2	18.51	14	4.600	26	4.225
3	10.129	15	4.543	27	4.210
4	7.709	16	4.494	28	4.196
5	6.608	17	4.451	29	4.183
6	5.987	18	4.414	30	4.171
7	5.591	19	4.381	40	4.085
8	5.318	20	4.351	60	4.001
9	5.117	21	4.325	120	3.920
10	4.965	22	4.301	∞	3.841
11	4.844	23	4.279		
12	4.747	24	4.260		

Containers and storage Containers—Hermetic containers.
Storage—Not exceeding 10°C, avoiding freezing.

Filgrastim (Genetical Recombination) Injection

フィルグラスチム(遺伝子組換え)注射液

Filgrastim (Genetical Recombination) Injection is an aqueous injection.

It contains not less than 90.0% and not more than 110.0% of the labeled amount of filgrastim (genetical recombination) ($C_{845}H_{1339}N_{223}O_{243}S_9$: 18798.61).

Method of preparation Prepare as directed under Injections, with Filgrastim (Genetical Recombination).

Description Filgrastim (Genetical Recombination) Injection is a clear and colorless liquid.

Identification Take a volume of Filgrastim (Genetical Recombination) Injection, equivalent to 5 to 10 μg of Filgrastim (Genetical Recombination) depending on the size of polyacrylamide gel for filgrastim, and add 0 to 16 μL of water. To 3 volumes of this solution add 1 volume of buffer solution for filgrastim sample so that each mL contains about 0.19 mg of protein, and use this solution as the sample solution. Then, proceed as directed in the Identification (1) under Filgrastim (Genetical Recombination).

Osmotic pressure ratio Being specified separately when the drug is granted approval based on the Law.

pH Being specified separately when the drug is granted approval based on the Law.

Purity Multimers—Proceed as directed in the Purity (1) under Filgrastim (Genetical Recombination) using a volume of Filgrastim (Genetical Recombination) Injection, equivalent to about 125 μg of Filgrastim (Genetical Recombination). Where, the test for required detectability and the system repeatability under the system suitability are tested using Filgrastim RS.

Bacterial endotoxins <*4.01*> Less than 0.25 EU/mL.

Extractable volume <*6.05*> It meets the requirement.

Foreign insoluble matter <*6.06*> Perform the test according to Method 1: it meets the requirement.

Insoluble particulate matter <*6.07*> It meets the requirement.

Sterility <*4.06*> Perform the test according to the Membrane filtration method: it meets the requirement.

Biological activity Calculate the biological activity in 1 ampoule or syringe of Filgrastim (Genetical Recombination) Injection by the following equation, using the biological actively in 1 mL of Filgrastim (Genetical Recombination) Injection determined as directed in the Assay (2) under Filgrastim (Genetical Recombination) and the labeled volume of Filgrastim (Genetical Recombination) Injection: it is not less than 70% and not more than 140% of the target biological activity (unit).

Biological activity (unit) in 1 ampoule or syringe of Filgrastim (Genetical Recombination) Injection
= antilog M × biological activity (unit/mL) of Filgrastim RS × dilution factor for U_H/dilution factor for S_H × U_H/S_H × labeled volume (mL) of Filgrastim (Genetical Recombination) Injection

where, the target biological activity (unit) is calculated by the following formula.

Target biological activity (unit)
= 1.5×10^8 (unit/mg) × labeled amount (mg) of Filgrastim (Genetical Recombination) in labeled volume (mL)

Assay Perform the test with an exact volume each of Filgrastim (Genetical Recombination) Injection and Filgrastim RS, equivalent to about 100 μg of Filgrastim (Genetical Recombination), as directed in the Assay (1) under Filgrastim (Genetical Recombination).

Calculate the amount of filgrastim in 1 mL of Filgrastim (Genetical Recombination) Injection by following formula.

$$\text{Amount (mg) of filgrastim in 1 mL} = C \times A_T/A_S \times V_S/V_T$$

C: Protein concentration (mg/mL) of Filgrastim RS
V_S: Amount (μL) of Filgrastim RS taken
V_T: Amount (μL) of Filgrastim (Genetical Recombination) Injection taken

Containers and storage Containers—Hermetic containers.
Storage—Light-resistant, not exceeding 10°C avoiding freezing.

Flavin Adenine Dinucleotide Sodium

フラビンアデニンジヌクレオチドナトリウム

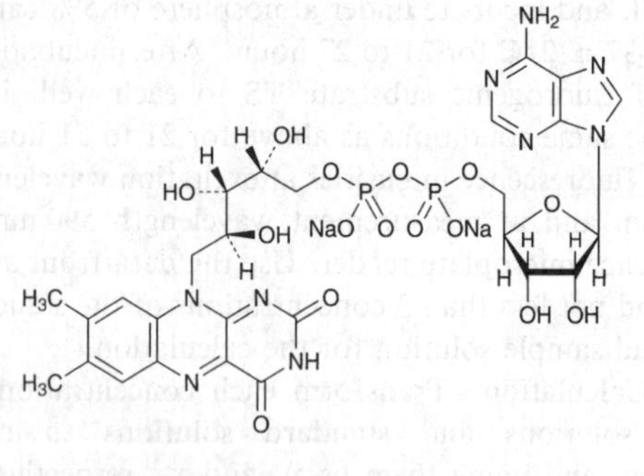

$C_{27}H_{31}N_9Na_2O_{15}P_2$: 829.51
Disodium adenosine 5′-[(2*R*,3*S*,4*S*)-5-(7,8-dimethyl-2,4-dioxo-3,4-dihydrobenzo[*g*]pteridin-10(2*H*)-yl)-2,3,4-trihydroxypentyl diphosphate]
[*84366-81-4*]

Flavin Adenine Dinucleotide Sodium contains not less than 93.0% of flavin adenine dinucleotide sodium ($C_{27}H_{31}N_9Na_2O_{15}P_2$), calculated on the anhydrous basis.

Description Flavin Adenine Dinucleotide Sodium occurs as an orange-yellow to light yellow-brown powder. It is odorless or has a slight, characteristic odor, and has a slightly bitter taste.

It is freely soluble in water, and practically insoluble, in methanol, in ethanol (95), in ethyleneglycol and in diethyl ether.

It is hygroscopic.

It is decomposed by light.

Identification **(1)** A solution of Flavin Adenine Dinucleotide Sodium (1 in 100,000) is light yellow-green in color, and shows a strong yellow-green fluorescence. To 5 mL of the solution add 0.02 g of hydrosulfite sodium: the color and the fluorescence of the solution disappear, and gradually reappear when the solution is shaken in air. Add dilute hydrochloric acid or sodium hydroxide TS dropwise: the fluorescence of the solution disappears.

(2) Determine the infrared absorption spectrum of Flavin Adenine Dinucleotide Sodium as directed in the potassium bromide disk method under Infrared Spectrophotometry <*2.25*>, and compare the spectrum with the Reference Spectrum: both spectra exhibit similar intensities of absorption at the same wave numbers.

(3) To 0.1 g of Flavin Adenine Dinucleotide Sodium add 10 mL of nitric acid, evaporate on a water bath to dryness, and ignite. To the residue add 10 mL of diluted nitric acid (1 in 50), boil for 5 minutes, and after cooling, neutralize with ammonia TS, then filter the solution if necessary: the solution responds to Qualitative Tests <*1.09*> for sodium salt and Qualitative Tests <*1.09*> (1) and (3) for phosphate.

Optical rotation <*2.49*> $[\alpha]_D^{20}$: −21.0 – −25.5° (0.3 g, calculated on the anhydrous basis, water, 20 mL, 100 mm).

pH <*2.54*> Dissolve 1.0 g of Flavin Adenine Dinucleotide Sodium in 100 mL of water: the pH of this solution is between 5.5 and 6.5.

Purity **(1)** Clarity and color of solution—Dissolve 0.20 g of Flavin Adenine Dinucleotide Sodium in 10 mL of water:

the solution is clear and orange-yellow in color.

(2) Free phosphoric acid—Weigh accurately about 0.02 g of Flavin Adenine Dinucleotide Sodium, dissolve in 10 mL of water, and use this solution as the sample solution. Separately, measure exactly 2 mL of Standard Phosphoric Acid Solution, add 10 mL of water, and use this solution as the standard solution. To each of the sample solution and standard solution add 2 mL of diluted perchloric acid (100 in 117), then add 1 mL of hexaammonium heptamolybdate TS and 2 mL of 2,4-diaminophenol dihydrochloride TS, respectively, shake, add water to make exactly 25 mL, and allow to stand at 20±1°C for 30 minutes. Perform the test with these solutions as directed under Ultraviolet-visible Spectrophotometry <*2.24*>, using a solution prepared in the same manner with 2 mL of water, as the blank, and determine the absorbances, A_T and A_S, of the subsequent solutions of the sample solution and the standard solution at 730 nm, respectively: the amount of free phosphoric acid is less than 0.25%.

$$\text{Amount (\%) of free phosphoric acid } (H_3PO_4) = 1/M \times A_T/A_S \times 5.16$$

M: Amount (mg) of flavin adenine dinucleotide sodium taken, calculated on the anhydrous basis

(3) Heavy metals <*1.07*>—Proceed with 1.0 g of Flavin Adenine Dinucleotide Sodium according to Method 2, and perform the test. Prepare the control solution with 2.0 mL of Standard Lead Solution (not more than 20 ppm).

(4) Arsenic <*1.11*>—Prepare the test solution with 2.0 g of Flavin Adenine Dinucleotide Sodium according to Method 3, and perform the test (not more than 1 ppm).

(5) Related substances—Dissolve 0.10 g of Flavin Adenine Dinucleotide Sodium in 200 mL of the mobile phase, and use this solution as the sample solution. Perform the test with 20 μL of the sample solution as directed under Liquid Chromatography <*2.01*> according to the following conditions. Determine the peak area, *A*, of flavin adenine dinucleotide and the total area, *S*, of peaks other than flavin adenine dinucleotide by the automatic integration method: $S/(A + S)$ is not more than 0.10.

Operating conditions—

Column, column temperature, mobile phase, flow rate, and time span of measurement: Proceed as directed in the operating conditions in the Procedure (ii) under the Assay (1).

Detector: An ultraviolet absorption photometer (wavelength: 260 nm).

System suitability—

System performance: Proceed as directed in the system suitability in the Procedure (ii) under the Assay (1).

Test for required detectability: To exactly 2 mL of the sample solution add the mobile phase to make exactly 20 mL, and use this solution as the solution for system suitability test. Confirm that the peak area of flavin adenine dinucleotide obtained with 20 μL of the solution for system suitability test is equivalent to 8 to 12% of that with 20 μL of the sample solution.

System repeatability: When the test is repeated 6 times with 20 μL of the solution for system suitability test under the above operating conditions, the relative standard deviation of the peak area of flavin adenine dinucleotide is not more than 1.0%.

Water <*2.48*> Take 50 mL of a mixture of methanol for water determination and ethyleneglycol for water determination (1:1) into a dry titration flask, and titrate with Karl Fischer TS for water determination until end point. Weigh accurately about 0.1 g of Flavin Adenine Dinucleotide Sodium, transfer quickly to the titration flask, add an excess and constant volume of Karl Fischer TS for water determination, dissolve by stirring for 10 minutes, and perform the test: the water content is not more than 10.0%.

Assay **(1)** Procedure (i) Total flavin content—Conduct this procedure without exposure to light, using light-resistant vessels. Weigh accurately about 0.1 g of Flavin Adenine Dinucleotide Sodium, and dissolve in water to make exactly 200 mL. Pipet 5 mL of this solution, add 5 mL of zinc chloride TS, and heat in a water bath for 30 minutes. After cooling, add water to make exactly 100 mL, and use this solution as the sample solution. Separately, weigh accurately about 50 mg of Riboflavin RS, previously dried at 105°C for 2 hours, dissolve in 200 mL of diluted acetic acid (100) (1 in 100) by warming, cool, add water to make exactly 500 mL. Pipet 10 mL of this solution, add water to make exactly 100 mL, and use this solution as the standard solution. Determine the absorbances, A_T and A_S, of the sample solution and standard solution at 450 nm as directed under Ultraviolet-visible Spectrophotometry <*2.24*>, using water as the blank.

$$\text{Total amout (mg) of flavin} = M_S \times A_T/A_S \times 4/5$$

M_S: Amount (mg) of Riboflavin RS taken

(ii) Peak area ratio of flavin adenine dinucleotide—Dissolve 0.1 g of Flavin Adenine Dinucleotide Sodium in 200 mL of water, and use this solution as the sample solution. Perform the test with 5 μL of the sample solution as directed under the Liquid Chromatography <*2.01*> according to the following conditions. Determine the peak area, *A* of flavin adenine dinucleotide, and the total area, *S*, of the peaks other than flavin adenine dinucleotide by the automatic integration method.

$$\text{Peak area ratio of flavin adenine dinucleotide} = 1.08A/(1.08A + S)$$

Operating conditions—

Detector: A visible spectrophotometer (wavelength: 450 nm).

Column: A stainless steel column 4 mm in inside diameter and 15 cm in length, packed with octadecylsilanized silica gel for liquid chromatography (5 μm in particle diameter).

Column temperature: A constant temperature of about 35°C.

Mobile phase: A mixture of a solution of potassium dihydrogen phosphate (1 in 500) and methanol (4:1).

Flow rate: Adjust so that the retention time of flavin adenine dinucleotide is about 10 minutes.

Time span of measurement: About 4.5 times as long as the retention time of flavin adenine dinucleotide.

System suitability—

Test for required detectability: To exactly 2 mL of the sample solution add water to make exactly 20 mL, and use this solution as the solution for system suitability test. Pipet 2 mL of the solution for system suitability test, and add water to make exactly 20 mL. Confirm that the peak area of flavin adenine dinucleotide obtained with 5 μL of this solution is equivalent to 8 to 12% of that with 5 μL of the solution for system suitability test.

System performance: Dissolve 20 mg each of Flavin Adenine Dinucleotide Sodium and riboflavin sodium phosphate in 100 mL of water. When the procedure is run with 5 μL of this solution under the above operating conditions, flavin adenine dinucleotide and riboflavin phosphate are eluted in this order with the resolution between these peaks being not less than 2.0.

System repeatability: When the test is repeated 6 times with 5 μL of the solution for system suitability test under the above operating conditions, the relative standard deviation of the peak area of flavin adenine dinucleotide is not more than 1.0%.

(2) Calculation

Amount (mg) of flavin adenine dinucleotide sodium ($C_{27}H_{31}N_9Na_2O_{15}P_2$)
$= f_T \times f_R \times 2.2040$

f_T: Total amount (mg) of flavin in Flavin Adenine Dinucleotide Sodium obtained from the procedure (i)
f_R: Peak area ratio of flavin adenine dinucleotide in Flavin Adenine Dinucleotide Sodium obtained from the procedure (ii)

Containers and storage Containers—Tight containers.
Storage—Light-resistant.

Flavoxate Hydrochloride

フラボキサート塩酸塩

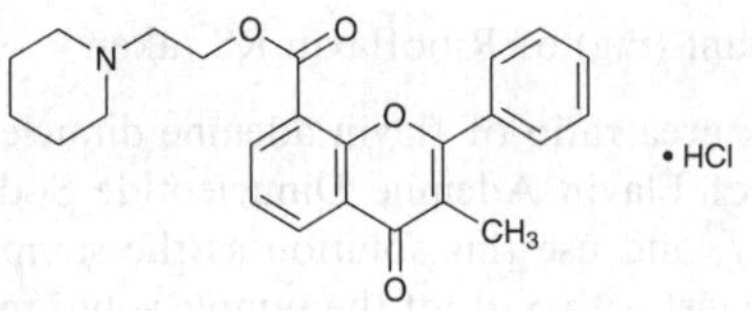

$C_{24}H_{25}NO_4.HCl$: 427.92
2-(Piperidin-1-yl)ethyl 3-methyl-4-oxo-2-phenyl-4*H*-chromene-8-carboxylate monohydrochloride
[*3717-88-2*]

Flavoxate Hydrochloride, when dried, contains not less than 99.0% of flavoxate hydrochloride ($C_{24}H_{25}NO_4.HCl$).

Description Flavoxate Hydrochloride occurs as white, crystals or crystalline powder.

It is sparingly soluble in acetic acid (100) and in chloroform, slightly soluble in water and in ethanol (95), and practically insoluble in acetonitrile and in diethyl ether.

Identification **(1)** Determine the absorption spectrum of a solution of Flavoxate Hydrochloride in 0.01 mol/L hydrochloric acid TS (1 in 50,000) as directed under Ultraviolet-visible Spectrophotometry *<2.24>*, and compare the spectrum with the Reference Spectrum: both spectra exhibit similar intensities of absorption at the same wavelengths.

(2) Determine the infrared absorption spectrum of Flavoxate Hydrochloride, previously dried, as directed in the potassium bromide disk method under Infrared Spectrophotometry *<2.25>*, and compare the spectrum with the Reference Spectrum: both spectra exhibit similar intensities of absorption at the same wave numbers.

(3) A solution of Flavoxate Hydrochloride (1 in 100) responds to Qualitative Tests *<1.09>* for chloride.

Purity **(1)** Heavy metals *<1.07>*—Proceed with 2.0 g of Flavoxate Hydrochloride according to Method 2, and perform the test. Prepare the control solution with 2.0 mL of Standard Lead Solution (not more than 10 ppm).

(2) Arsenic *<1.11>*—Prepare the test solution with 2.0 g of Flavoxate Hydrochloride according to Method 4, and perform the test (not more than 1 ppm).

(3) Related substances—Dissolve 80 mg of Flavoxate Hydrochloride in 10 mL of chloroform, and use this solution as the sample solution. Pipet 1 mL of the sample solution, add chloroform to make exactly 20 mL, then pipet 1 mL of this solution, add chloroform to make exactly 20 mL, and use this solution as the standard solution. Perform the test with these solutions as directed under Thin-layer Chromatography *<2.03>*. Spot 5 μL each of the sample solution and standard solution on a plate of silica gel with fluorescent indicator for thin-layer chromatography. Develop the plate with a mixture of 1-butanol, water and acetic acid (100) (3:1:1) to a distance of about 12 cm, and air-dry the plate. Examine under ultraviolet light (main wavelength: 254 nm): the spots other than the principal spot obtained from the sample solution are not more intense than the spot from the standard solution.

Loss on drying *<2.41>* Not more than 1.0% (1 g, reduced pressure, silica gel, 2 hours).

Residue on ignition *<2.44>* Not more than 0.1% (1 g).

Assay Weigh accurately about 0.6 g of Flavoxate Hydrochloride, previously dried, add 10 mL of acetic acid (100) and 40 mL of acetonitrile to dissolve, add 50 mL of acetic anhydride, and titrate *<2.50>* with 0.1 mol/L perchloric acid VS (potentiometric titration). Perform a blank determination in the same manner, and make any necessary correction.

Each mL of 0.1 mol/L perchloric acid VS
= 42.79 mg of $C_{24}H_{25}NO_4.HCl$

Containers and storage Containers—Tight containers.

Flecainide Acetate

フレカイニド酢酸塩

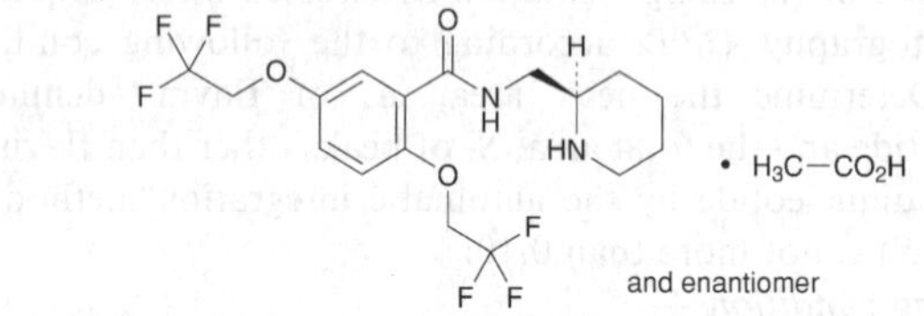

and enantiomer

$C_{17}H_{20}F_6N_2O_3.C_2H_4O_2$: 474.39
N-[(2*RS*)-Piperidin-2-ylmethyl]-2,5-bis(2,2,2-trifluoroethoxy)benzamide monoacetate
[*54143-56-5*]

Flecainide Acetate, when dried, contains not less than 98.0% and not more than 101.0% of flecainide acetate ($C_{17}H_{20}F_6N_2O_3.C_2H_4O_2$).

Description Flecainide Acetate occurs as a white crystalline powder, having slightly a characteristic or acetic acid like odor.

It is freely soluble in methanol, in ethanol (95) and in acetic acid (100), and sparingly soluble in water.

A solution of Flecainide Acetate in methanol (1 in 25) shows no optical rotation.

Melting point: about 150°C (with decomposition).

Identification **(1)** Dissolve 20 mg of Flecainide Acetate in 1 mL of water, add 1 mL of a solution of acetaldehyde (1 in 20), and shake. To this solution add dropwise at the same time 1 - 2 drops each of sodium pentacyanonitrosylferrate (III) dihydrate solution (1 in 10) and sodium hydrogen carbonate TS: a blue precipitate is formed.

(2) Determine the absorption spectrum of a solution of Flecainide Acetate in ethanol (95) (13 in 100,000) as directed under Ultraviolet-visible Spectrophotometry <2.24>, and compare the spectrum with the Reference Spectrum: both spectra exhibit similar intensities of absorption at the same wavelengths.

(3) Determine the infrared absorption spectrum of Flecainide Acetate as directed in the potassium bromide disk method under Infrared Spectrophotometry <2.25>, and compare the spectrum with the Reference Spectrum: both spectra exhibit similar intensities of absorption at the same wave numbers.

(4) Flecainide Acetate responds to Qualitative Tests <1.09> (1) for acetate.

pH <2.54> The pH of a solution of 0.5 g of Flecainide Acetate in 20 mL of water is 6.7 to 7.1.

Purity **(1)** Clarity and color of solution—Dissolve 0.25 g of Flecainide Acetate in 10 mL of water: the solution is clear and colorless.

(2) Heavy metals <1.07>—Transfer 1.0 g of Flecainide Acetate in a porcelain crucible, and heat gentry to carbonize. After cooling, add 2 mL of sulfuric acid, heat carefully until white fumes are no longer evolved, then proceed according to Method 2 to prepare the test solution, and perform the test. Prepare the control solution as follows: Place 2 mL each of sulfuric acid and hydrochloric acid in a porcelain crucible, evaporate on a water bath, then evaporate to dryness on a sand bath, add to the residue 3 drops of hydrochloric acid, then proceed in the same manner as for the test solution, and add 2.0 mL of Standard Lead Solution and water to make 50 mL (not more than 20 ppm).

(3) 2-Aminomethylpiperidine—Dissolve exactly 0.25 g of Flecainide Acetate in exactly 5 mL of methanol, and use this solution as the sample solution. Separately, dissolve exactly 50 mg of 2-aminomethylpiperidine in methanol to make exactly 100 mL. Pipet 2 mL of this solution, add methanol to make exactly 10 mL, and use this solution as the standard solution. Perform the test with these solutions as directed under Thin-layer Chromatography <2.03>. Spot 5 μL each of the sample solution and standard solution on a plate of silica gel for thin-layer chromatography. Develop the plate with a mixture of acetone and ammonia solution (28) (20:1) to a distance of about 10 cm, and air-dry the plate. Spray evenly a solution of ninhydrin in methanol (1 in 500), and heat at 105°C for 2 to 5 minutes: the spot obtained from the sample solution, corresponding to the spot obtained from the standard solution, is not more intense than the spot from the standard solution.

(4) Related substances—Dissolve 0.25 g of Flecainide Acetate in 25 mL of a mixture of water and acetonitrile (71:29), and use this solution as the sample solution. Pipet 1 mL of the sample solution, and add a mixture of water and acetonitrile (71:29) to make exactly 50 mL. Pipet 1 mL of this solution, add a mixture of water and acetonitrile (71:29) to make exactly 10 mL, and use this solution as the standard solution. Perform the test with exactly 20 μL each of the sample solution and standard solution as directed under Liquid Chromatography <2.01> according to the following conditions. Determine each peak area of these solutions by the automatic integration method: the area of the peak other than flecainide obtained from the sample solution is not larger than the peak area of flecainide obtained from the standard solution, and the total area of the peaks other than flecainide from the sample solution is not larger than 2.5 times the peak area of flecainide from the standard solution. For the areas of the peaks, having the relative retention time of about 1.5 and about 2.9 to flecainide, multiply their correction factors, 0.3 and 1.7, respectively.

Operating conditions—

Detector: An ultraviolet absorption photometer (wavelength: 254 nm).

Column: A stainless steel column 4 mm in inside diameter and 15 cm in length, packed with octylsilanized silica gel for liquid chromatography (5 μm in particle diameter).

Column temperature: A constant temperature of about 40°C.

Mobile phase: A mixture of water, acetonitrile, acetic acid (100) and tetrabutylammonium hydroxide-methanol TS (142:58:2:1), adjusted to pH 5.8 with ammonia solution (28).

Flow rate: Adjust so that the retention time of flecainide is about 4 minutes.

Time span of measurement: About 5 times as long as the retention time of flecainide, beginning after the solvent peak.

System suitability—

Test for required detectability: To exactly 1 mL of the standard solution add a mixture of water and acetonitrile (71:29) to make exactly 10 mL. Confirm that the peak area of flecainide obtained with 20 μL of this solution is equivalent to 7 - 13% of that with 20 μL of the standard solution.

System performance: When the procedure is run with 20 μL of the standard solution under the above operating conditions, the number of theoretical plates and the symmetry factor of the peak of flecainide are not less than 4000 and not more than 2.0, respectively.

System repeatability: When the test is repeated 6 times with 20 μL of the standard solution under the above operating conditions, the relative standard deviation of the peak area of flecainide is not more than 2.0%.

Loss on drying <2.41> Not more than 0.5% (1 g, reduced pressure not exceeding 0.67 kPa, 60°C, 2 hours).

Residue on ignition <2.44> Not more than 0.2% (1 g).

Assay Weigh accurately about 0.6 g of Flecainide Acetate, previously dried, dissolve in 100 mL of acetic acid (100), and titrate <2.50> with 0.1 mol/L perchloric acid VS (potentiometric titration). Perform the blank determination in the same manner, and make any necessary correction.

Each mL of 0.1 mol/L perchloric acid VS
= 47.44 mg of $C_{17}H_{20}F_6N_2O_3.C_2H_4O_2$

Containers and storage Containers—Tight containers.
Storage—Light-resistant.

Flecainide Acetate Tablets

フレカイニド酢酸塩錠

Flecainide Acetate Tablets contain not less than 93.0% and not more than 107.0% of the labeled amount of flecainide acetate ($C_{17}H_{20}F_6N_2O_3.C_2H_4O_2$: 474.39).

Method of preparation Prepare as directed under Tablets, with Flecainide Acetate.

Identification To an amount of powdered Flecainide Acetate Tablets, equivalent to 0.2 g of Flecainide Acetate, add 4 mL of methanol, shake for 20 minutes, then centrifuge and use the supernatant liquid as the sample solution. Separately, dissolve 0.1 g of flecainide acetate in 2 mL of methanol, and use this solution as the standard solution. Perform the test with these solutions as directed under Thin-layer Chromatography <2.03>. Spot 5 μL each of the sample solution and standard solution on a plate of silica gel with fluorescent indicator for thin-layer chromatography. Develop the plate with a mixture of acetone and ammonia solution (28) (20:1) to a distance of about 10 cm, and air-dry the plate. Examine under ultraviolet light (main wavelength: 254 nm): the principal spot obtained from the sample solution and the spot from standard solution show the same *Rf* value.

Uniformity of dosage units <*6.02*> Perform the Mass variation test, or the Content uniformity test according to the following method: it meets the requirement.

Completely disintegrate 1 tablet of Flecainide Acetate Tablets in $4V/5$ mL of a solution of lactic acid (1 in 500) by sonicating. After allowing to stand for 30 minutes while swirling occasionally, add a solution of lactic acid (1 in 500) to make exactly V mL so that each mL contains about 1 mg of flecainide acetate ($C_{17}H_{20}F_6N_2O_3.C_2H_4O_2$), and filter. Discard the first 10 mL of the filtrate, pipet 5 mL of the subsequent filtrate, add a solution of lactic acid (1 in 500) to make exactly 50 mL, and use this solution as the sample solution. Then, proceed as directed in the Assay.

Amount (mg) of flecainide acetate ($C_{17}H_{20}F_6N_2O_3.C_2H_4O_2$)
$= M_S \times A_T/A_S \times V/25$

M_S: Amount (mg) of flecainide acetate for assay taken

Dissolution <*6.10*> When the test is performed at 50 revolutions per minute according to the Paddle method, using 900 mL of water as the dissolution medium, the dissolution rate in 30 minutes of Flecainide Acetate Tablets is not less than 70%.

Start the test with 1 tablet of Flecainide Acetate Tablets, withdraw not less than 20 mL of the medium at the specified minute after starting the test, and filter through a membrane filter with a pore size not exceeding 0.5 μm. Discard not less than 10 mL of the first filtrate, pipet V mL of the subsequent filtrate, add water to make exactly V' mL so that each mL contains about 56 μg of flecainide acetate ($C_{17}H_{20}F_6N_2O_3.C_2H_4O_2$), and use this solution as the sample solution. Separately, weigh accurately about 28 mg of flecainide acetate for assay, previously dried under reduced pressure not exceeding 0.67 kPa at 60°C for 2 hours, and dissolve in water to make exactly 50 mL. Pipet 2 mL of this solution, add water to make exactly 20 mL, and use this solution as the standard solution. Determine the absorbances, A_T and A_S, of the sample solution and standard solution at 296 nm as directed under Ultraviolet-visible Spectrophotometry <*2.24*>.

Dissolution rate (%) with respect to the labeled amount of flecainide acetate ($C_{17}H_{20}F_6N_2O_3.C_2H_4O_2$)
$= M_S \times A_T/A_S \times V'/V \times 1/C \times 180$

M_S: Amount (mg) of flecainide acetate for assay taken
C: Labeled amount (mg) of flecainide acetate ($C_{17}H_{20}F_6N_2O_3.C_2H_4O_2$) in 1 tablet

Assay Accurately weigh the mass of not less than 20 Flecainide Acetate Tablets, and powder. Weigh accurately a portion of the powder, equivalent to about 0.1 g of flecainide acetate ($C_{17}H_{20}F_6N_2O_3.C_2H_4O_2$), add 80 mL of a solution of lactic acid (1 in 500), sonicate for 5 minutes, then add a solution of lactic acid (1 in 500) to make exactly 100 mL, and filter. Discard the first 10 mL of the filtrate, pipet 5 mL of the subsequent filtrate, add a solution of lactic acid (1 in 500) to make exactly 50 mL, and use this solution as the sample solution. Separately, weigh accurately about 25 mg of flecainide acetate for assay, previously dried under reduced pressure not exceeding 0.67 kPa at 60°C for 2 hours, dissolve in a solution of lactic acid (1 in 500) to make exactly 50 mL. Pipet 10 mL of this solution, add a solution of lactic acid (1 in 500) to make exactly 50 mL, and use this solution as the standard solution. Determine the absorbances, A_T and A_S, of the sample solution and standard solution at 296 nm as directed under Ultraviolet-visible Spectrophotometry <*2.24*>.

Amount (mg) of flecainide acetate ($C_{17}H_{20}F_6N_2O_3.C_2H_4O_2$)
$= M_S \times A_T/A_S \times 4$

M_S: Amount (mg) of flecainide acetate for assay taken

Containers and storage Containers—Tight containers.

Flomoxef Sodium

フロモキセフナトリウム

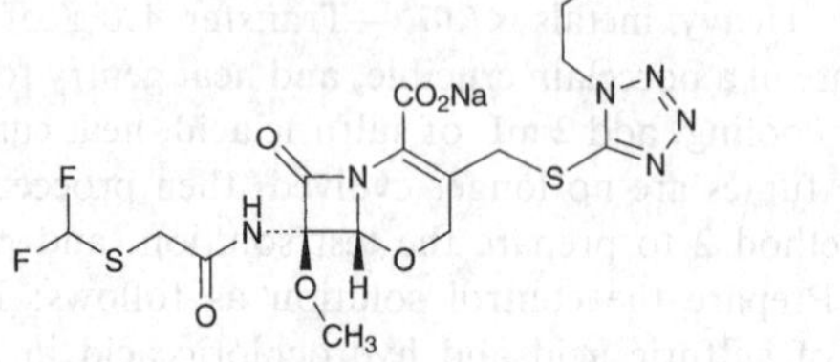

$C_{15}H_{17}F_2N_6NaO_7S_2$: 518.45
Monosodium (6*R*,7*R*)-7-{[(difluoromethylsulfanyl)acetyl]amino}-3-[1-(2-hydroxyethyl)-1*H*-tetrazol-5-ylsulfanylmethyl]-7-methoxy-8-oxo-5-oxa-1-azabicyclo[4.2.0]oct-2-ene-2-carboxylate
[*92823-03-5*]

Flomoxef Sodium contains not less than 870 μg (potency) and not more than 985 μg (potency) per mg, calculated on the anhydrous basis. The potency of Flomoxef Sodium is expressed as mass (potency) of flomoxef ($C_{15}H_{18}F_2N_6O_7S_2$: 496.47).

Description Flomoxef Sodium occurs as white to light yellow-white, powder or masses.

It is very soluble in water, freely soluble in methanol, and sparingly soluble in ethanol (99.5).

Identification **(1)** Decompose 0.01 g of Flomoxef Sodium as directed under Oxygen Flask Combustion Method <*1.06*>, using a mixture of 0.5 mL of 0.01 mol/L sodium hydroxide TS and 20 mL of water as the absorbing liquid. To 2 mL of the test solution so obtained add 1.5 mL of a mixture of alizarin complexone TS, acetic acid-potassium acetate buffer solution (pH 4.3) and cerium (III) nitrate TS (1:1:1): blue-purple color develops.

(2) Determine the absorption spectrum of a solution of Flomoxef Sodium (3 in 100,000) as directed under Ultraviolet-visible Spectrophotometry <*2.24*>, and compare the spectrum with the Reference Spectrum: both spectra exhibit similar intensities of absorption at the same wavelengths.

(3) Determine the infrared absorption spectrum of Flomoxef Sodium as directed in the potassium bromide disk method under Infrared Spectrophotometry <*2.25*>, and compare the spectrum with the Reference Spectrum: both spectra exhibit similar intensities of absorption at the same wave numbers.

(4) Determine the ^1H spectrum of a solution of Flomoxef Sodium in heavy water for nuclear magnetic resonance spectroscopy (1 in 10) as directed under Nuclear Magnetic Resonance Spectroscopy <*2.21*>, using sodium 3-trimethylsilylpropanesulfonate for nuclear magnetic resonance spectroscopy as an internal reference compound: it exhibits a single signal A at around δ 3.5 ppm, a single signal or a sharp multiple signal B at around δ 3.7 ppm, and a single signal C at around δ 5.2 ppm. The ratio of the integrated intensity of these signals, A:B:C, is about 3:2:1.

(5) Flomoxef Sodium responds to Qualitative Tests <*1.09*> (1) for sodium salt.

Optical rotation <*2.49*> $[\alpha]_D^{20}$: $-8 - -13°$ (1 g calculated on the anhydrous basis, a mixture of water and ethanol (99.5) (4:1), 50 mL, 100 mm).

pH <*2.54*> The pH of a solution obtained by dissolving 0.5 g of Flomoxef Sodium in 5 mL of water is between 4.0 and 5.5.

Purity **(1)** Clarity and color of solution—Dissolve 1.0 g of Flomoxef Sodium in 10 mL of water: the solution is clear and has no more color than the following control solution.

Control solution: To a mixture of 3.0 mL of Cobalt (II) Chloride CS and 12 mL of Iron (III) Chloride CS add 35 mL of diluted dilute hydrochloric acid (1 in 10). To 5.0 mL of this solution add 5.0 mL of diluted dilute hydrochloric acid (1:10).

(2) Heavy metals <*1.07*>—Proceed with 1.0 g of Flomoxef Sodium in a quartz crucible according to Method 2, and perform the test. Prepare the control solution with 2.0 mL of Standard Lead Solution (not more than 20 ppm).

(3) Arsenic <*1.11*>—To 1.0 g of Flomoxef Sodium 5 mL of sulfuric acid and 5 mL of nitric acid, heat carefully until the solution changes to colorless to light yellow with occasional addition of 2 mL of nitric acid. After cooling, add 10 mL of ammonium oxalate TS, heat until white fumes evolve, and concentrate to 2 to 3 mL. After cooling, add water to make 10 mL, and perform the test using this solution as the test solution: the color is not darker than that of the control solution.

Control solution: Proceed to prepare a solution in the same manner as the test solution without Flomoxef Sodium, and transfer 10 mL of the solution so obtained to the generator bottle, add exactly 2 mL of Standard Arsenic Solution, and proceed in the same manner as the test solution (not more than 2 ppm).

(4) 1-(2-Hydroxyethyl)-1*H*-tetrazol-5-thiol—Use the sample solution obtained in the Assay as the sample solutions. Weigh accurately about 20 mg of 1-(2-hydroxyethyl)-1*H*-tetrazol-5-thiol, and dissolve in water to make exactly 100 mL. Pipet 5 mL of this solution, add exactly 25 mL of the internal standard solution and water to make 50 mL, and use this solution as the standard solution. Perform the test with 5 μL each of the sample solution and standard solution as directed under Liquid Chromatography <*2.01*> according to the following conditions, and calculate the ratios, Q_T and Q_S, of the peak area of 1-(2-hydroxyethyl)-1*H*-tetrazol-5-thiol to that of the internal standard: the amount of 1-(2-hydroxyethyl)-1*H*-tetrazol-5-thiol is not more than 1.0% of the amount of Flomoxef Sodium calculated on the anhydrous basis.

Amount (mg) of 1-(2-hydroxyethyl)-1*H*-tetrazol-5-thiol ($C_3H_6N_4OS$)
$= M_S \times Q_T/Q_S \times 1/10$

M_S: Amount (mg) of 1-(2-hydroxyethyl)-1*H*-tetrazol-5-thiol taken

Internal standard solution—A solution of *m*-cresol (3 in 1000).

Operating conditions—

Proceed as directed in the operating conditions in the Assay.

System suitability—

Test for required detectability: Pipet 1 mL of the standard solution, and add water to make exactly 20 mL. Confirm that the peak area of 1-(2-hydroxyethyl)-1*H*-tetrazol-5-thiol obtained with 5 μL of this solution is equivalent to 3.5 to 6.5% of that with 5 μL of the standard solution.

System performance: When the procedure is run with 5 μL of the standard solution under the above operating conditions, 1-(2-hydroxyethyl)-1*H*-tetrazol-5-thiol and the internal standard are eluted in this order with the resolution between these peaks being not less than 20.

System repeatability: When the test is repeated 3 times with 5 μL of the standard solution under the above operating conditions, the relative standard deviation of the ratio of the peak area of 1-(2-hydroxyethyl)-1*H*-tetrazol-5-thiol to that of the internal standard is not more than 1.0%.

Water <*2.48*> Not more than 1.5% (0.5 g, volumetric titration, back titration).

Assay Weigh accurately an amount of Flomoxef Sodium and Flomoxef Triethylammonium RS, equivalent to about 50 mg (potency), and dissolve each in exactly 50 mL of the internal standard solution, add water to make 100 mL, and use these solutions as the sample solution and standard solution. Perform the test with 5 μL each of the sample solution and standard solution as directed under Liquid Chromatography <*2.01*> according to the following conditions, and calculate the ratios, Q_T and Q_S, of the peak area of flomoxef to that of the internal standard.

Amount [μg (potency)] of flomoxef ($C_{15}H_{18}F_2N_6O_7S_2$)
$= M_S \times Q_T/Q_S \times 1000$

M_S: Amount [mg (potency)] of Flomoxef Triethylammonium RS taken

Internal standard solution—A solution of *m*-cresol (3 in 1000).

Operating conditions—

Detector: An ultraviolet absorption photometer (wavelength: 246 nm).

Column: A stainless steel column 4 mm in inside diameter and 20 cm in length, packed with octadecylsilanized silica gel for liquid chromatography (5 – 10 μm in particle diameter).

Column temperature: A constant temperature of about 25°C.

Mobile phase: Dissolve 6.94 g of potassium dihydrogen phosphate, 3.22 g of disodium hydrogen phosphate dodecahydrate and 1.60 g of tetra-*n*-butylammonium bromide in water to make 1000 mL. To 750 mL of this solution add 250 mL of methanol.

Flow rate: Adjust so that the retention time of flomoxef is about 9 minutes.

System suitability—

System performance: When the procedure is run with 5 μL of the standard solution under the above operating conditions, flomoxef and the internal standard are eluted in this order with the resolution between these peaks being not less than 10.

System repeatability: When the test is repeated 3 times with 5 μL of the standard solution under the above operating conditions, the relative standard deviation of the ratios of the peak area of flomoxef to that of the internal standard is not more than 1.0%.

Containers and storage Containers—Tight containers.

Storage—Not exceeding 5°C.

Flomoxef Sodium for Injection

注射用フロモキセフナトリウム

Flomoxef Sodium for Injection is a preparation for injection which is dissolved before use.

It contains not less than 90.0% and not more than 110.0% of the labeled potency of flomoxef ($C_{15}H_{18}F_2N_6O_7S_2$: 496.47).

Method of preparation Prepare as directed under Injections, with Flomoxef Sodium.

Description Flomoxef Sodium for Injection occurs as white to light yellow-white, friable masses or powder.

Identification Proceed as directed in the Identification (3) under Flomoxef Sodium.

pH <*2.54*> The pH of a solution obtained by dissolving an amount of Flomoxef Sodium for Injection, equivalent to 0.5 g (potency) of Flomoxef Sodium, in 5 mL of water is between 4.0 and 5.5.

Purity **(1)** Clarity and color of solution—Dissolve an amount of Flomoxef Sodium for Injection, equivalent to 1.0 g (potency) of Flomoxef Sodium, in 10 mL of water: the solution is clear and colorless or pale yellow.

(2) 1-(2-Hydroxyethyl)-1*H*-tetrazol-5-thiol—Use the sample solution obtained in the Assay as the sample solution. Weigh accurately about 20 mg of 1-(2-hydroxyethyl)-1*H*-tetrazol-5-thiol, and dissolve in water to make exactly 100 mL. Pipet 5 mL of this solution, add exactly 25 mL of the internal standard solution and water to make 50 mL, and use this solution as the standard solution. Perform the test with 5 μL each of the sample solution and standard solution as directed under Liquid Chromatography <*2.01*> according to the following conditions, and calculate the ratios, Q_T and Q_S, of the peak area of 1-(2-hydroxyethyl)-1*H*-tetrazol-5-thiol to that of the internal standard. Calculate the amount of 1-(2-hydroxyethyl)-1*H*-tetrazol-5-thiol per 1 g (potency) of Flomoxef Sodium for Injection by the following formula: not more than 10 mg.

Amount (mg) of 1-(2-hydroxyethyl)-1*H*-tetrazol-5-thiol ($C_3H_6N_4OS$)
$= M_S \times Q_T/Q_S \times 1/10$

M_S: Amount (mg) of 1-(2-hydroxyethyl)-1*H*-tetrazol-5-thiol taken

Internal standard solution—A solution of *m*-cresol (3 in 1000).

Operating conditions—

Proceed as directed in the operating conditions in the Assay under Flomoxef Sodium.

System suitability—

Test for required detectability: Pipet 1 mL of the standard solution, and add water to make exactly 20 mL. Confirm that the peak area of 1-(2-hydroxyethyl)-1*H*-tetrazol-5-thiol obtained with 5 μL of this solution is equivalent to 3.5 – 6.5% of that with 5 μL of the standard solution.

System performance: When the procedure is run with 5 μL of the standard solution under the above operating conditions, 1-(2-hydroxyethyl)-1*H*-tetrazol-5-thiol and the internal standard are eluted in this order with the resolution between these peaks being not less than 20.

System repeatability: When the test is repeated 3 times with 5 μL of the standard solution under the above operating conditions, the relative standard deviation of the ratio of the peak area of 1-(2-hydroxyethyl)-1*H*-tetrazol-5-thiol to that of the internal standard is not more than 1.0%.

Water <*2.48*> Not more than 1.5% (0.5 g, volumetric titration, back titration).

Bacterial endotoxins <*4.01*> Less than 0.025 EU/mg (potency).

Uniformity of dosage units <*6.02*> It meets the requirement of the Mass variation test.

Foreign insoluble matter <*6.06*> Perform the test according to Method 2: it meets the requirement.

Insoluble particulate matter <*6.07*> It meets the requirement.

Sterility <*4.06*> Perform the test according to the Membrane filtration method: it meets the requirement.

Assay Weigh accurately the mass of the contents of not less than 10 Flomoxef Sodium for Injection, and calculate the average mass of the content. Spread out thinly about 1 g of the content in a petri dish, allow the dish to stand in a desiccator containing a saturated solution of magnesium bromide without light exposure to equilibrate the sample to constant water content. Determine the water content, separately, with about 0.1 g of the sample according to the method described in Water. Weigh accurately an amount of the sample, equivalent to about 50 mg (potency) of Flomoxef Sodium, add exactly 50 mL of the internal standard solution to dissolve, add water to make 100 mL, and use this solution as the sample solution. Separately weigh accurately about 50 mg (potency) of Flomoxef Triethylammonium RS, add exactly 50 mL of the internal standard solution to dissolve, add water to make 100 mL, and use this solution as the standard solution. Proceed as directed in the Assay under Flomoxef Sodium.

Amount [μg (potency)] of flomoxef ($C_{15}H_{18}F_2N_6O_7S_2$)
$= M_S \times Q_T/Q_S \times 1000$

M_S: Amount [mg (potency)] of Flomoxef Triethylammonium RS taken

Internal standard solution—A solution of *m*-cresol (3 in 1000).

Containers and storage Containers—Hermetic containers. Plastic containers for aqueous injection may be used.

Flopropione

フロプロピオン

$C_9H_{10}O_4$: 182.17
1-(2,4,6-Trihydroxyphenyl)propan-1-one
[2295-58-1]

Flopropione contains not less than 98.0% and not more than 101.0% of flopropione ($C_9H_{10}O_4$), calculated on the anhydrous basis.

Description Flopropione occurs as a white to pale yellow-brown crystalline powder.

It is very soluble in *N,N*-dimethylformamide, freely soluble in methanol and in ethanol (99.5), and practically insoluble in water.

Identification (1) Determine the absorption spectrum of a solution of Flopropione in ethanol (99.5) (1 in 200,000) as directed under Ultraviolet-visible Spectrophotometry *<2.24>*, and compare the spectrum with the Reference Spectrum: both spectra exhibit similar intensities of absorption at the same wavelengths.

(2) Determine the infrared absorption spectrum of Flopropione as directed in the potassium bromide disk method under Infrared Spectrophotometry *<2.25>*, and compare the spectrum with the Reference Spectrum: both spectra exhibit similar intensities of absorption at the same wave numbers.

Melting point *<2.60>* 177 – 181°C

Purity (1) Heavy metals *<1.07>*—Proceed with 1.0 g of Flopropione according to Method 4, and perform the test. Prepare the control solution with 2.0 mL of Standard Lead Solution (not more than 20 ppm).

(2) Related substances—Dissolve 50 mg of Flopropione in 50 mL of the mobile phase, and use this solution as the sample solution. Pipet 1 mL of the sample solution, add the mobile phase to make exactly 100 mL, and use this solution as the standard solution. Perform the test with exactly 20 μL each of the sample solution and standard solution as directed under Liquid Chromatography *<2.01>* according to the following conditions. Determine each peak area of both solutions by the automatic integration method: the area of each peak other than flopropione obtained from the sample solution is not larger than 1/10 times the peak area of flopropione from the standard solution.

Operating conditions—

Detector: An ultraviolet absorption photometer (wavelength: 267 nm).

Column: A stainless steel column 4.6 mm in inside diameter and 15 cm in length, packed with octadecylsilanized silica gel for liquid chromatography (5 μm in particle diameter).

Column temperature: A constant temperature of about 35°C.

Mobile phase: A mixture of acetonitrile, water and phosphoric acid (114:86:1).

Flow rate: Adjust so that the retention time of flopropione is about 3 minutes.

Time span of measurement: About 7 times as long as the retention time of flopropione.

System suitability—

Test for required detectability: Pipet 1 mL of the standard solution, and add the mobile phase to make exactly 10 mL. Confirm that the peak area of flopropione obtained with 20 μL of this solution is equivalent to 7 to 13% of that with from 20 μL of the standard solution.

System performance: Dissolve 25 mg of ethyl parahydroxybenzoate in 30 mL of acetonitrile, and add the mobile phase to make 50 mL. To 2.5 mL of this solution add 2 mL of the sample solution and the mobile phase to make 50 mL. When the procedure is run with 20 μL of this solution under the above operating conditions, flopropione and ethyl parahydroxybenzoate are eluted in this order with the resolution between these peaks being not less than 2.0.

System repeatability: When the test is repeated 6 times with 20 μL of the standard solution under the above operating conditions, the relative standard deviation of the peak area of flopropione is not more than 1.0%.

Water *<2.48>* Not more than 4.0% (0.5 g, volumetric titration, direct titration).

Residue on ignition *<2.44>* Not more than 0.1% (1 g).

Assay Weigh accurately about 0.3 g of Flopropione, dissolve in 30 mL of *N,N*-dimethylformamide, and titrate *<2.50>* with 0.1 mol/L tetramethylammonium hydroxide VS (potentiometric titration). Perform a blank determination in the same manner, and make any necessary correction.

Each mL of 0.1 mol/L tetramethylammonium hydroxide VS
= 18.22 mg of $C_9H_{10}O_4$

Containers and storage Containers—Tight containers.
Storage—Light-resistant.

Flopropione Capsules

フロプロピオンカプセル

Flopropione Capsules contain not less than 93.0% and not more than 107.0% of the labeled amount of flopropione ($C_9H_{10}O_4$: 182.17).

Method of preparation Prepare as directed under the Capsules, with Flopropione.

Identification (1) Powder the contents of Flopropione Capsules. To a portion of the powder, equivalent to 60 mg of Flopropione, add 40 mL of water, shake well, and filter. To 5 mL of the filtrate add 1 mL of iron (III) nitrate TS: a red-purple color appears.

(2) Powder the contents of Flopropione Capsules. To a portion of the powder, equivalent to 90 mg of Flopropione, add 100 mL of ethanol (99.5), shake well, and filter. To 5 mL of the filtrate add ethanol (99.5) to make 50 mL. To 5 mL of this solution add ethanol (99.5) to make 100 mL, and use this solution as the sample solution. Determine the absorption spectrum of the sample solution as directed under Ultraviolet-visible Spectrophotometry *<2.24>*: it exhibits a maximum between 283 nm and 287 nm.

Uniformity of dosage units *<6.02>* Perform the test according to the following method: it meets the requirement of the Content uniformity test.

To 1 capsule of Flopropione Capsules add 43 mL of a mixture of water and phosphoric acid (86:1), and disintegrate the capsule in a water bath at 50°C. After cooling, add a suitable amount of acetonitrile to make exactly V mL of a solution containing about 0.4 mg of flopropione ($C_9H_{10}O_4$) per mL. Stir the solution for 10 minutes, centrifuge a part of the solution at 3000 rpm for 5 minutes, and use the supernatant liquid as the sample solution. Proceed as directed in the Assay.

$$\text{Amount (mg) of flopropione } (C_9H_{10}O_4) = M_S \times A_T/A_S \times V/100$$

M_S: Amount (mg) of flopropione for assay taken, calculated on the anhydrous basis

Dissolution <*6.10*> When the test is performed at 100 revolutions per minute according to the Paddle method using the sinker, using 900 mL of water as the dissolution medium, the dissolution rate in 45 minutes of Flopropione Capsules is not less than 80%.

Start the test with 1 capsule of Flopropione Capsules, withdraw not less than 20 mL of the medium at the specified minute after starting the test, and filter through a membrane filter with a pore size not exceeding 0.45 μm. Discard not less than 10 mL of the first filtrate, pipet V mL of the subsequent filtrate, add 0.1 mol/L hydrochloric acid TS to make exactly V' mL so that each mL contains about 8.8 μg of flopropione ($C_9H_{10}O_4$), and use this solution as the sample solution. Separately, weigh accurately about 22 mg of flopropione for assay (separately determine the water <*2.48*> in the same manner as Flopropione), and dissolve in methanol to make exactly 50 mL. Pipet 2 mL of this solution, add 0.1 mol/L hydrochloric acid TS to make exactly 100 mL, and use this solution as the standard solution. Determine the absorbances, A_T and A_S, at 284 nm of the sample solution and standard solution as directed under Ultraviolet-visible Spectrophotometry <*2.24*>, using 0.1 mol/L hydrochloric acid TS as the blank.

$$\text{Dissolution rate (\%) with respect to the labeled amount of flopropione } (C_9H_{10}O_4) = M_S \times A_T/A_S \times V'/V \times 1/C \times 36$$

M_S: Amount (mg) of flopropione for assay taken, calculated on the anhydrous basis
C: Labeled amount (mg) of flopropione ($C_9H_{10}O_4$) in 1 capsule

Assay Take out the contents of not less than 20 Flopropione Capsules, weigh accurately the mass of the contents, and power. Weigh accurately a part of the powder, equivalent to about 40 mg of flopropione ($C_9H_{10}O_4$), and add the mobile phase to make exactly 100 mL. Stir the solution for 10 minutes, centrifuge a part of this solution for 5 minutes at 3000 rpm, and use the supernatant liquid as the sample solution. Separately, weigh accurately about 40 mg of flopropione for assay (previously determine the water <*2.48*> in the same manner as Flopropione), add 70 mL of the mobile phase, and dissolve by sonicating for 10 minutes. Add the mobile phase to make exactly 100 mL, and use this solution as the standard solution. Perform the test with exactly 5 μL each of the sample solution and standard solution as directed under Liquid chromatography <*2.01*> according to the following conditions, and determine the peak areas, A_T and A_S, of flopropione in each solution.

$$\text{Amount (mg) of flopropione } (C_9H_{10}O_4) = M_S \times A_T/A_S$$

M_S: Amount (mg) of flopropione for assay taken, calculated on the anhydrous basis

Operating conditions—

Detector: An ultraviolet absorption photometer (wavelength: 267 nm).

Column: A stainless steel column 4.6 mm in inside diameter and 15 cm in length, packed with octadecylsilanized silica gel for liquid chromatography (5 μm in particle diameter).

Column temperature: A constant temperature of about 35°C.

Mobile phase: A mixture of acetonitrile, water and phosphoric acid (114:86:1).

Flow rate: Adjust so that the retention time of flopropione is about 3 minutes.

System suitability—

System performance: Dissolve 50 mg of flopropione in 50 mL of the mobile phase. To 20 mL of the solution add 25 mL of a solution prepared by dissolving 25 mg of ethyl parahydroxybenzoate in 30 mL of acetonitrile and add water to make 50 mL, and then add the mobile phase to make 50 mL. When the procedure is run with 5 μL of this solution under the above operating conditions, Flopropione and ethyl parahydroxybenzoate are eluted in this order with the resolution between these peaks being not less than 2.0.

System repeatability: When the test is repeated 6 times with 5 μL of the standard solution under the above operating conditions, the relative standard deviation of the peak area of flopropione is not more than 1.0%.

Containers and storage Containers—Tight containers.

Fluconazole

フルコナゾール

$C_{13}H_{12}F_2N_6O$: 306.27
2-(2,4-Difluorophenyl)-1,3-bis(1*H*-1,2,4-triazol-1-yl)propan-2-ol
[*86386-73-4*]

Fluconazole, when dried, contains not less than 99.0% and not more than 101.0% of fluconazole ($C_{13}H_{12}F_2N_6O$).

Description Fluconazole occurs as a white to pale yellowwhite crystalline powder.

It is soluble in ethanol (99.5), and slightly soluble in water.

It dissolves in dilute hydrochloric acid.

Identification **(1)** Dissolve 0.1 g of Fluconazole in 10 mL of dilute hydrochloric acid, and add 1 mL of Reinecke's salt TS: a light red precipitate is formed.

(2) Determine the absorption spectrum of a solution of Fluconazole in 0.01 mol/L hydrochloric acid-methanol TS (1 in 4000) as directed under Ultraviolet-visible Spectrophotometry <*2.24*>, and compare the spectrum with the Reference Spectrum: both spectra exhibit similar intensities of absorption at the same wavelengths.

(3) Determine the infrared absorption spectrum of Fluconazole as directed in the potassium bromide disk method under Infrared Spectrophotometry <*2.25*>, and compare the spectrum with the Reference Spectrum: both spectra exhibit similar intensities of absorption at the same wave numbers.

Melting point ⟨*2.60*⟩ 137 – 141°C

Purity (1) Clarity and color of solution—A solution obtained by dissolving 0.10 g of Fluconazole in 50 mL of water is clear and colorless.

(2) Heavy metals ⟨*1.07*⟩—Proceed with 1.0 g of Fluconazole according to Method 4, and perform the test. Prepare the control solution with 2.0 mL of Standard Lead Solution (not more than 20 ppm).

(3) Related substances—Dissolve 30 mg of Fluconazole in 10 mL of the mobile phase, and use this solution as the sample solution. Pipet 1 mL of the sample solution, add the mobile phase to make exactly 100 mL. Pipet 1 mL of this solution, add the mobile phase to make exactly 10 mL, and use this solution as the standard solution. Perform the test with exactly 20 μL each of the sample solution and standard solution as directed under Liquid Chromatography ⟨*2.01*⟩ according to the following conditions, and determine each peak area of both solutions by the automatic integration method: the peak area of related substance I, having the relative retention time about 0.60 to fluconazole obtained from the sample solution is not larger than 6 times the peak area of fluconazole from the standard solution, the area of the peak other than fluconazole and the related substance I from the sample solution is not larger than the peak area of fluconazole from the standard solution, and the total area of the peaks other than fluconazole from the sample solution is not larger than 8 times the peak area of fluconazole from the standard solution.

Operating conditions—

Detector: An ultraviolet absorption photometer (wavelength: 260 nm).

Column: A stainless steel column 4.6 mm in inside diameter and 15 cm in length, packed with octadecylsilanized silica gel for liquid chromatography (5 μm in particle diameter).

Column temperature: A constant temperature of about 40°C.

Mobile phase: A mixture of water and acetonitrile (4:1).

Flow rate: Adjust so that the retention time of fluconazole is about 10 minutes.

Time span of measurement: About 3 times as long as the retention time of fluconazole, beginning after the solvent peak.

System suitability—

Test for required detectability: Pipet 5 mL of the standard solution, and add the mobile phase to make exactly 10 mL. Confirm that the peak area of fluconazole obtained with 20 μL of this solution is equivalent to 35 to 65% of that with 20 μL of the standard solution.

System performance: When the procedure is run with 20 μL of the standard solution under the above operating conditions, the number of theoretical plates and the symmetry factor of the peak of fluconazole are not less than 4000 and not more than 2.0, respectively.

System repeatability: When the test is repeated 6 times with 20 μL of the standard solution under the above operating conditions, the relative standard deviation of the peak area of fluconazole is not more than 2.0%.

Loss on drying ⟨*2.41*⟩ Not more than 1.0% (1 g, 105°C, 4 hours).

Residue on ignition ⟨*2.44*⟩ Not more than 0.2% (1 g).

Assay Weigh accurately about 0.25 g of Fluconazole, previously dried, dissolve in 100 mL of a mixture of acetic anhydride and acetic acid (100) (7:3), and titrate ⟨*2.50*⟩ with 0.1 mol/L perchloric acid VS (potentiometric titration). Perform the blank determination in the same manner, and make any necessary correction.

Each mL of 0.1 mol/L perchloric acid VS
= 15.31 mg of $C_{13}H_{12}F_2N_6O$

Containers and storage Containers—Tight containers.

Fluconazole Capsules

フルコナゾールカプセル

Fluconazole Capsules contain not less than 93.0% and not more than 107.0% of the labeled amount of fluconazole ($C_{13}H_{12}F_2N_6O$: 306.27).

Method of preparation Prepare as directed under Capsules, with Fluconazole.

Identification To an amount of powdered contents of Fluconazole Capsules, equivalent to 25 mg of Fluconazole, add 0.01 mol/L hydrochloric acid-methanol TS to make 100 mL, shake for 30 minutes, and filter. Determine the absorption spectrum of the filtrate as directed under Ultraviolet-visible Spectrophotometry ⟨*2.24*⟩: it exhibits maxima between 259 nm and 263 nm and between 265 nm and 269 nm.

Uniformity of dosage units ⟨*6.02*⟩ Perform the Mass variation test, or the Content uniformity test according to the following method: it meets the requirement.

To the total amount of the content of 1 capsule of Fluconazole Capsules add the mobile phase to make exactly 100 mL. Disperse the particles by sonicating, stir for 30 minutes, and filter through a membrane filter with a pore size not exceeding 0.45 μm. Discard the first 10 mL of the filtrate, pipet V mL of the subsequent filtrate, add the mobile phase to make exactly V' mL so that each mL contains about 50 μg of fluconazole ($C_{13}H_{12}F_2N_6O$), and use this solution as the sample solution. Then, proceed as directed in the Assay.

$$\text{Amount (mg) of fluconazole } (C_{13}H_{12}F_2N_6O) = M_S \times A_T/A_S \times V'/V \times 1/5$$

M_S: Amount (mg) of fluconazole for assay taken

Dissolution ⟨*6.10*⟩ When the test is performed at 50 revolutions per minute according to the Paddle method using the sinker, using 900 mL of water as the dissolution medium, the dissolution rates in 90 minutes of 50-mg capsule and 100-mg capsule are not less than 80% and not less than 70%, respectively.

Start the test with 1 capsule of Fluconazole Capsules, withdraw not less than 20 mL of the medium at the specified minute after starting the test, and filter through a membrane filter with a pore size not exceeding 0.45 μm. Discard not less than 10 mL of the first filtrate, pipet V mL of the subsequent filtrate, add the mobile phase to make exactly V' mL so that each mL contains about 28 μg of fluconazole ($C_{13}H_{12}F_2N_6O$), and use this solution as the sample solution. Separately, weigh accurately about 28 mg of fluconazole for assay, previously dried at 105°C for 4 hours, and dissolve in the mobile phase to make exactly 50 mL. Pipet 5 mL of this solution, add the mobile phase to make exactly 100 mL, and use this solution as the standard solution. Perform the test with exactly 20 μL each of the sample solution and standard solution as directed under Liquid Chromatography ⟨*2.01*⟩ according to the following conditions, and determine the peak areas, A_T and A_S, of fluconazole in each solution.

Dissolution rate (%) with respect to the labeled amount of fluconazole ($C_{13}H_{12}F_2N_6O$)

$$= M_S \times A_T/A_S \times V'/V \times 1/C \times 90$$

M_S: Amount (mg) of fluconazole for assay taken
C: Labeled amount (mg) of fluconazole ($C_{13}H_{12}F_2N_6O$) in 1 capsule

Operating conditions—

Proceed as directed in the operating conditions in the Assay.

System suitability—

System performance: When the procedure is run with 20 μL of the standard solution under the above operating conditions, the number of theoretical plates and the symmetry factor of the peak of fluconazole are not less than 3000 and not more than 1.5, respectively.

System repeatability: When the test is repeated 6 times with 20 μL of the standard solution under the above operating conditions, the relative standard deviation of the peak area of fluconazole is not more than 1.0%.

Assay Take out the contents from not less than 20 Fluconazole Capsules, weigh accurately, and powder, if necessary. Weigh accurately a quantity of the contents, equivalent to about 50 mg of fluconazole ($C_{13}H_{12}F_2N_6O$), and add the mobile phase to make exactly 100 mL. Disperse the particles by sonicating, stir for 30 minutes, and filter through a membrane filter with a pore size not exceeding 0.45 μm. Discard the first 10 mL of the filtrate, pipet 5 mL of the subsequent filtrate, add the mobile phase to make exactly 50 mL, and use this solution as the sample solution. Separately, weigh accurately about 25 mg of fluconazole for assay, previously dried at 105°C for 4 hours, and dissolve in the mobile phase to make exactly 50 mL. Pipet 5 mL of this solution, add the mobile phase to make exactly 50 mL, and use this solution as the standard solution. Perform the test with exactly 20 μL each of the sample solution and standard solution as directed under Liquid Chromatography <*2.01*> according to the following conditions, and determine the peak areas, A_T and A_S, of fluconazole in each solution.

$$\text{Amount (mg) of fluconazole } (C_{13}H_{12}F_2N_6O) = M_S \times A_T/A_S \times 2$$

M_S: Amount (mg) of fluconazole for assay taken

Operating conditions—

Detector: An ultraviolet absorption photometer (wavelength: 261 nm).

Column: A stainless steel column 3.9 mm in inside diameter and 15 cm in length, packed with octadecylsilanized silica gel for liquid chromatography (4 μm in particle diameter).

Column temperature: A constant temperature of about 35°C.

Mobile phase: Dissolve 0.82 g of anhydrous sodium acetate in 1000 mL of water, and adjust to pH 5.0 with acetic acid (100). To 700 mL of this solution add 200 mL of methanol and 100 mL of acetonitrile.

Flow rate: Adjust so that the retention time of fluconazole is about 4 minutes.

System suitability—

System performance: When the procedure is run with 20 μL of the standard solution under the above operating conditions, the number of theoretical plates and the symmetry factor of the peak of fluconazole are not less than 3000 and not more than 1.5, respectively.

System repeatability: When the test is repeated 6 times with 20 μL of the standard solution under the above operating conditions, the relative standard deviation of the peak area of fluconazole is not more than 1.0%.

Containers and storage Containers—Tight containers.

Fluconazole Injection

フルコナゾール注射液

Fluconazole Injection is an aqueous injection.

It contains not less than 95.0% and not more than 105.0% of the labeled amount of fluconazole ($C_{13}H_{12}F_2N_6O$: 306.27).

Method of preparation Prepare as directed under Injections, with Fluconazole.

Description Fluconazole Injection occurs as a clear and colorless liquid.

Identification **(1)** Take a volume of Fluconazole Injection, equivalent to 0.1 g of Fluconazole, and evaporate to dryness on a water bath. To the residue add 10 mL of dilute hydrochloric acid, shake, and filter. Add 1 mL of Reinecke salt TS to the filtrate: a light red precipitate is produced.

(2) Determine the absorption spectrum of the sample solution obtained in the Assay as directed under Ultraviolet-visible Spectrophotometry <*2.24*>: it exhibits maxima between 259 nm and 263 nm, and between 264 nm and 268 nm.

pH Being specified separately when the drug is granted approval based on the Law.

Bacterial endotoxins <*4.01*> Less than 0.75 EU/mg.

Extractable volume <*6.05*> It meets the requirement.

Foreign insoluble matter <*6.06*> Perform the test according to Method 1: it meets the requirement.

Insoluble particulate matter <*6.07*> It meets the requirement.

Sterility <*4.06*> Perform the test according to the Membrane filtration method: it meets the requirement.

Assay Pipet a volume of Fluconazole Injection, equivalent to 10 mg of fluconazole ($C_{13}H_{12}F_2N_6O$), add water to make exactly 50 mL, and use this solution as the sample solution. Separately, weigh accurately about 50 mg of fluconazole for assay, previously dried at 105°C for 4 hours, dissolve in a solution of sodium chloride (9 in 1000) to make exactly 50 mL. Pipet 10 mL of this solution, add water to make exactly 50 mL, and use this solution as the standard solution. Determine the absorbances, A_T and A_S, of the sample solution and standard solution at 261 nm as directed under Ultraviolet-visible Spectrophotometry <*2.24*>.

$$\text{Amount (mg) of fluconazole } (C_{13}H_{12}F_2N_6O) = M_S \times A_T/A_S \times 1/5$$

M_S: Amount (mg) of fluconazole for assay taken

Containers and storage Containers—Hermetic containers.

Flucytosine

フルシトシン

$C_4H_4FN_3O$: 129.09
5-Fluorocytosine
[2022-85-7]

Flucytosine, when dried, contains not less than 98.5% of flucytosine ($C_4H_4FN_3O$), and not less than 14.0% and not more than 15.5% of fluorine (F: 19.00).

Description Flucytosine occurs as a white crystalline powder. It is odorless.

It is sparingly soluble in water, slightly soluble in methanol, in ethanol (95), in acetic anhydride and in acetic acid (100), and practically insoluble in diethyl ether.

It dissolves in 0.1 mol/L hydrochloric acid TS.

The pH of a solution of 1.0 g of Flucytosine in 100 mL of water is between 5.5 and 7.5.

It is slightly hygroscopic.

Melting point: about 295°C (with decomposition).

Identification **(1)** Add 0.2 mL of bromine TS to 5 mL of a solution of Flucytosine (1 in 500): a yellow-brown color of bromine TS is immediately discharged. Further add 2 mL of barium hydroxide TS: a purple precipitate is formed.

(2) Proceed with 0.1 g of Flucytosine as directed under Oxygen Flask Combustion Method ⟨*1.06*⟩, using a mixture of 0.5 mL of 0.01 mol/L sodium hydroxide TS and 20 mL of water as the absorbing liquid. The solution responds to Qualitative Tests ⟨*1.09*⟩ (2) for fluoride.

(3) Determine the absorption spectrum of a solution of Flucytosine in 0.1 mol/L hydrochloric acid TS (1 in 125,000) as directed under Ultraviolet-visible Spectrophotometry ⟨*2.24*⟩, and compare the spectrum with the Reference Spectrum: both spectra exhibit similar intensities of absorption at the same wavelengths.

Purity **(1)** Clarity and color of solution—Dissolve 1.0 g of Flucytosine in 100 mL of water: the solution is clear and colorless.

(2) Chloride ⟨*1.03*⟩—Dissolve 1.0 g of Flucytosine in 80 mL of water by heating on a water bath. After cooling, to 40 mL of this solution add 6 mL of dilute nitric acid and water to make 50 mL. Perform the test using this solution as the test solution. Prepare the control solution with 0.20 mL of 0.01 mol/L hydrochloric acid VS (not more than 0.014%).

(3) Fluoride—Dissolve 0.10 g of Flucytosine in 10.0 mL of diluted 0.01 mol/L sodium hydroxide TS (1 in 20). Transfer 5.0 mL of this solution to a 20-mL volumetric flask, add 10 mL of a mixture of alizarin complexone TS, acetic acid-potassium acetate buffer solution (pH 4.3) and cerrous nitrate TS (1:1:1), and add water to make 20 mL. Allow the mixture to stand for 1 hour, and use this solution as the sample solution. Separately, transfer 4.0 mL of Standard Fluorine Solution to a 20-mL volumetric flask, add 5.0 mL of diluted 0.01 mol/L sodium hydroxide TS (1 in 20), add 10 mL of a mixture of alizarin complexone TS, acetic acid-potassium acetate buffer solution (pH 4.3) and cerrous nitrate TS (1:1:1). Proceed in the same manner as directed in the preparation of the sample solution, and use this solution as the standard solution. Transfer 5.0 mL of diluted 0.01 mol/L sodium hydroxide TS (1 in 20) to a 20-mL volumetric flask, proceed in the same manner as directed in the preparation of the standard solution, and use this solution as the blank solution. Determine the absorbances, A_T and A_S, of the sample solution and standard solution at 600 nm, using the blank solution as the control as directed under Ultraviolet-visible Spectrophotometry ⟨*2.24*⟩: A_T is not larger than A_S (not more than 0.048%).

(4) Heavy metals ⟨*1.07*⟩—Proceed with 1.0 g of Flucytosine according to Method 2, and perform the test. Prepare the control solution with 2.0 mL of Standard Lead Solution (not more than 20 ppm).

(5) Arsenic ⟨*1.11*⟩—Prepare the test solution with 1.0 g of Flucytosine according to Method 2, and perform the test (not more than 2 ppm).

(6) Related substances—Dissolve 50 mg of Flucytosine in 5 mL of diluted methanol (1 in 2), and use this solution as the sample solution. Measure accurately 1 mL of the sample solution, add diluted methanol (1 in 2) to make exactly 25 mL. Measure accurately 1 mL of this solution, add diluted methanol (1 in 2) to make exactly 20 mL, and use this solution as the standard solution. Perform the test with these solutions as directed under Thin-layer Chromatography ⟨*2.03*⟩. Spot 20 μL each of the sample solution and standard solution on a plate of silica gel with fluorescent indicator for thin-layer chromatography. Develop the plate with a mixture of ethyl acetate, methanol and water (5:3:2) to a distance of about 12 cm, air-dry the plate, and observe the spots under ultraviolet light (main wavelength: 254 nm): the spots other than the principal spot obtained from the sample solution are not more intense than the spot from the standard solution.

Loss on drying ⟨*2.41*⟩ Not more than 1.0% (1 g, 105°C, 4 hours).

Residue on ignition ⟨*2.44*⟩ Not more than 0.1% (1 g).

Assay **(1)** Flucytosine—Weigh accurately about 0.2 g of Flucytosine, previously dried, dissolve in 40 mL of acetic acid (100), add 100 mL of acetic anhydride, and titrate ⟨*2.50*⟩ with 0.1 mol/L perchloric acid VS (potentiometric titration). Perform a blank determination in the same manner, and make any necessary correction.

Each mL of 0.1 mol/L perchloric acid VS
= 12.91 mg of $C_4H_4FN_3O$

(2) Fluorine—Weigh accurately about 10 mg of Flucytosine, previously dried, and proceed as directed in the determination of fluorine under Oxygen Flask Combustion Method ⟨*1.06*⟩, using a mixture of 0.5 mL of 0.01 mol/L sodium hydroxide VS and 20 mL of water as the absorbing liquid.

Containers and storage Containers—Tight containers.

Storage—Light-resistant.

Fludiazepam

フルジアゼパム

$C_{16}H_{12}ClFN_2O$: 302.73
7-Chloro-5-(2-fluorophenyl)-1-methyl-1,3-dihydro-2*H*-1,4-benzodiazepin-2-one
[*3900-31-0*]

Fludiazepam, when dried, contains not less than 99.0% of fludiazepam ($C_{16}H_{12}ClFN_2O$).

Description Fludiazepam occurs as white to light yellow, crystals or crystalline powder.

It is very soluble in chloroform, freely soluble in methanol, in ethanol (95), in acetic acid (100) and in diethyl ether, and practically insoluble in water.

Identification (1) Prepare the test solution with 0.01 g of Fludiazepam as directed under Oxygen Flask Combustion Method 〈*1.06*〉, using a mixture of 0.5 mL of 0.01 mol/L sodium hydroxide TS and 20 mL of water as the absorbing liquid: the test solution responds to Qualitative Tests 〈*1.09*〉 (2) for fluoride.

(2) Determine the absorption spectrum of a solution of Fludiazepam in methanol (1 in 200,000) as directed under Ultraviolet-visible Spectrophotometry 〈*2.24*〉, and compare the spectrum with the Reference Spectrum 1: both spectra exhibit similar intensities of absorption at the same wavelengths. Separately, determine the absorption spectrum of a solution of Fludiazepam in methanol (1 in 20,000) as directed under Ultraviolet-visible Spectrophotometry 〈*2.24*〉, and compare the spectrum with the Reference Spectrum 2: both spectra exhibit similar intensities of absorption at the same wavelengths.

(3) Determine the infrared absorption spectrum of Fludiazepam, previously dried, as directed in the potassium bromide disk method under Infrared Spectrophotometry 〈*2.25*〉, and compare the spectrum with the Reference Spectrum: both spectra exhibit similar intensities of absorption at the same wave numbers.

(4) Perform the test with Fludiazepam as directed under Flame Coloration Test 〈*1.04*〉 (2): a green color appears.

Melting point 〈*2.60*〉 91 - 94°C

Purity (1) Chloride 〈*1.03*〉—Dissolve 1.0 g of Fludiazepam in 50 mL of diethyl ether, add 50 mL of water, and shake. Separate the water layer, wash it with two 20-mL portions of diethyl ether, and filter the water layer. To 20 mL of the filtrate add 6 mL of dilute nitric acid and water to make 50 mL. Perform the test using this solution as the test solution. Prepare the control solution with 0.40 mL of 0.01 mol/L hydrochloric acid VS (not more than 0.036%).

(2) Heavy metals 〈*1.07*〉—Proceed with 2.0 g of Fludiazepam according to Method 2, and perform the test. Prepare the control solution with 2.0 mL of Standard Lead Solution (not more than 10 ppm).

(3) Related substances—Dissolve 0.10 g of Fludiazepam in 20 mL of chloroform, and use this solution as the sample solution. Pipet 1 mL of the sample solution, and add chloroform to make exactly 50 mL. Pipet 2 mL of this solution, add chloroform to make exactly 20 mL, and use this solution as the standard solution. Perform the test with these solutions as directed under Thin-layer Chromatography 〈*2.03*〉. Spot 20 μL each of the sample solution and standard solution on a plate of silica gel with fluorescent indicator for thin-layer chromatography. Develop the plate with a mixture of chloroform and ethyl acetate (10:7) to a distance of about 12 cm, and air-dry the plate. Examine under ultraviolet light (main wavelength: 254 nm): the spots other than the principal spot obtained from the sample solution are not more intense than the spot from the standard solution.

Loss on drying 〈*2.41*〉 Not more than 0.30% (1 g, in vacuum, 60°C, 3 hours).

Residue on ignition 〈*2.44*〉 Not more than 0.1% (1 g, platinum crucible).

Assay Weigh accurately about 0.5 g of Fludiazepam, previously dried, dissolve in 50 mL of acetic acid (100), and titrate 〈*2.50*〉 with 0.1 mol/L perchloric acid VS (potentiometric titration). Perform a blank determination in the same manner, and make any necessary correction.

Each mL of 0.1 mol/L perchloric acid VS
= 30.28 mg of $C_{16}H_{12}ClFN_2O$

Containers and storage Containers—Tight containers.

Fludiazepam Tablets

フルジアゼパム錠

Fludiazepam Tablets contain not less than 93.0% and not more than 107.0% of the labeled amount of fludiazepam ($C_{16}H_{12}ClFN_2O$: 302.73).

Method of preparation Prepare as directed under Tablets, with Fludiazepam.

Identification To a quantity of powdered Fludiazepam Tablets, equivalent to 2 mg of Fludiazepam, add 40 mL of methanol, shake for 20 minutes, and filter. Determine the absorption spectrum of the filtrate as directed under Ultraviolet-visible Spectrophotometry 〈*2.24*〉: it exhibits a maximum between 315 nm and 319 nm. Therefore, to 5 mL of the filtrate add methanol to make 50 mL. Determine the absorption spectrum of this solution as directed under Ultraviolet-visible Spectrophotometry 〈*2.24*〉: it exhibits a maximum between 229 nm and 233 nm.

Uniformity of dosage units 〈*6.02*〉 Perform the test according to the following method: it meets the requirement of the Content uniformity test.

To 1 tablet of Fludiazepam Tablets add $2V/25$ mL of water, disintegrate the fine particles by sonicating, add $3V/25$ mL of acetonitrile, and shake for 10 minutes. Add a mixture of acetonitrile and water (3:2) to make exactly V mL so that each mL contains about 5 μg of fludiazepam ($C_{16}H_{12}ClFN_2O$), centrifuge, and use the supernatant liquid as the sample solution. Then, proceed as directed in the Assay.

Amount (mg) of fludiazepam ($C_{16}H_{12}ClFN_2O$)
$= M_S \times A_T/A_S \times V/5000$

M_S: Amount (mg) of fludiazepam for assay taken

Dissolution 〈*6.10*〉 When the test is performed at 50 revolutions per minute according to the Paddle method, using 900 mL of water as the dissolution medium, the dissolution rate in 15 minutes of Fludiazepam Tablets is not less than 80%.

Start the test with 1 tablet of Fludiazepam Tablets, withdraw not less than 20 mL of the medium at the specified minute after starting the test, and filter through a membrane filter with a pore size not exceeding 0.45 μm. Discard not less than 10 mL of the first filtrate, pipet V mL of the subsequent filtrate, add water to make exactly V' mL so that each mL contains about 0.28 μg of fludiazepam ($C_{16}H_{12}ClFN_2O$), and use this solution as the sample solution. Separately, weigh accurately about 28 mg of fludiazepam for assay, previously dried at 60°C for 3 hours under reduced pressure, and dissolve in methanol to make exactly 100 mL. Pipet 5 mL of this solution, and add water to make exactly 100 mL. Then, pipet 2 mL of this solution, and add water to make exactly 100 mL, and use this solution as the standard solution. Perform the test with exactly 50 μL each of the sample solution and standard solution as directed under Liquid Chromatography *<2.01>* according to the following conditions, and determine the peak areas, A_T and A_S, of fludiazepam in each solution.

Dissolution rate (%) with respect to the labeled amount of fludiazepam ($C_{16}H_{12}ClFN_2O$)
$= M_S \times A_T/A_S \times V'/V \times 1/C \times 9/10$

M_S: Amount (mg) of fludiazepam for assay taken
C: Labeled amount (mg) of fludiazepam ($C_{16}H_{12}ClFN_2O$) in 1 tablet

Operating conditions—

Detector, column temperature and flow rate: Proceed as directed in the operating conditions in the Assay.

Column: A stainless steel column 3.9 mm in inside diameter and 15 cm in length, packed with octadecylsilanized silica gel for liquid chromatography (5 μm in particle diameter).

Mobile phase: A mixture of water and acetonitrile (1:1).

System suitability—

System performance: When the procedure is run with 50 μL of the standard solution under the above operating conditions, the number of theoretical plates and the symmetry factor of the peak of fludiazepam are not less than 3000 and not more than 2.0, respectively.

System repeatability: When the test is repeated 6 times with 50 μL of the standard solution under the above operating conditions, the relative standard deviation of the peak area of fludiazepam is not more than 2.0%.

Assay Weigh accurately the mass of not less than 20 tablets of Fludiazepam Tablets, and powder. Weigh accurately a portion of the powder, equivalent to about 0.25 mg of fludiazepam ($C_{16}H_{12}ClFN_2O$), add 4 mL of water, disperse the fine particles by sonicating, add 6 mL of acetonitrile, and shake for 10 minutes. To this solution add a mixture of acetonitrile and water (3:2) to make exactly 50 mL, centrifuge, and use the supernatant liquid as the sample solution. Separately, weigh accurately about 25 mg of fludiazepam for assay, previously dried at 60°C for 3 hours under reduced pressure, dissolve in a mixture of acetonitrile and water (3:2) to make exactly 50 mL. Pipet 5 mL of this solution, add a mixture of acetonitrile and water (3:2) to make exactly 50 mL. Then, pipet 5 mL of this solution, add a mixture of acetonitrile and water (3:2) to make exactly 50 mL, and use this solution as the standard solution. Perform the test with exactly 20 μL each of the sample solution and standard solution as directed under Liquid Chromatography *<2.01>* according to the following conditions, and determine the peak areas, A_T and A_S, of fludiazepam in each solution.

Amount (mg) of fludiazepam ($C_{16}H_{12}ClFN_2O$)
$= M_S \times A_T/A_S \times 1/100$

M_S: Amount (mg) of fludiazepam for assay taken

Operating conditions—

Detector: An ultraviolet absorption photometer (wavelength: 232 nm).

Column: A stainless steel column 4.6 mm in inside diameter and 15 cm in length, packed with octadecylsilanized silica gel for liquid chromatography (5 μm in particle diameter).

Column temperature: A constant temperature of about 25°C.

Mobile phase: A mixture of methanol and water (3:2).

Flow rate: Adjust so that the retention time of fludiazepam is about 10 minutes.

System suitability—

System performance: When the procedure is run with 20 μL of the standard solution under the above operating conditions, the number of theoretical plates and the symmetry factor of the peak of fludiazepam are not less than 6000 and not more than 2.0, respectively.

System repeatability: When the test is repeated 6 times with 20 μL of the standard solution under the above operating conditions, the relative standard deviation of the peak area of fludiazepam is not more than 1.0%.

Containers and storage Containers—Tight containers.

Fludrocortisone Acetate

フルドロコルチゾン酢酸エステル

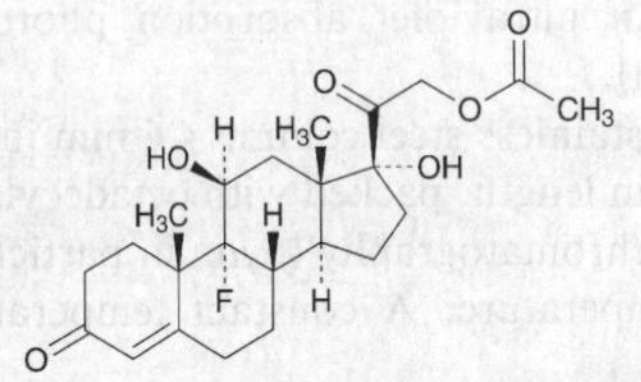

$C_{23}H_{31}FO_6$: 422.49
9-Fluoro-11β,17,21-trihydroxypregn-4-ene-3,20-dione 21-acetate
[514-36-3]

Fludrocortisone Acetate, when dried, contains not less than 97.5% and not more than 102.5% of fludrocortisone acetate ($C_{23}H_{31}FO_6$).

Description Fludrocortisone Acetate occurs as a white to pale yellow, crystals or crystalline powder.

It is soluble in acetone, sparingly soluble in ethanol (95), and practically insoluble in water.

Melting point: about 220°C (with decomposition).

Identification **(1)** Prepare the test solution by proceeding with 10 mg of Fludrocortisone Acetate according to the Oxygen Flask Combustion Method *<1.06>*, using a mixture of 0.5 mL of 0.01 mol/L sodium hydroxide VS and 20 mL of water as the absorbing liquid: the test solution responds to Qualitative Tests *<1.09>* for fluoride.

(2) Determine the absorption spectrum of a solution of Fludrocortisone Acetate in ethanol (95) (1 in 100,000) as directed under Ultraviolet-visible Spectrophotometry *<2.24>*, and compare the spectrum with the Reference Spectrum or the spectrum of a solution of Fludrocortisone Acetate RS prepared in the same manner as the sample solution: both spectra exhibit similar intensities of absorption at the same wavelengths.

(3) Determine the infrared absorption spectrum of Fludrocortisone Acetate, previously dried, as directed in the potassium bromide disk method under Infrared Spectrophotometry *<2.25>*, and compare the spectrum with the Reference Spectrum or the spectrum of previously dried Fludrocortisone Acetate RS: both spectra exhibit similar intensities of absorption at the same wave numbers.

Optical rotation *<2.49>* $[\alpha]_D^{25}$: +131 – +138° (after drying, 0.1 g, acetone, 20 mL, 100 mm).

Purity **(1)** Heavy metals *<1.07>*—Proceed with 0.5 g of Fludrocortisone Acetate according to Method 2, and perform the test. Prepare the control solution with 1.5 mL of Standard Lead Solution (not more than 30 ppm).

(2) Related substances—Dissolve 20 mg of Fludrocortisone Acetate in 10 mL of the mobile phase, and use this solution as the sample solution. Pipet 1 mL of the sample solution, add the mobile phase to make exactly 50 mL, and use this solution as the standard solution. Perform the test with exactly 20 μL each of the sample solution and standard solution as directed under Liquid Chromatography *<2.01>* according to the following conditions. Determine each peak area of both solutions by the automatic integration method: the area of each peak other than fludrocortisone acetate obtained from the sample solution is not larger than 1/4 times the peak area of fludrocortisone acetate from the standard solution, and the total area of the peaks other than fludrocortisone acetate from the sample solution is not larger than 1/2 times the peak area of fludrocortisone acetate from the standard solution.

Operating conditions—

Detector: An ultraviolet absorption photometer (wavelength: 254 nm).

Column: A stainless steel column 4.6 mm in inside diameter and 20 cm in length, packed with octadecylsilanized silica gel for liquid chromatography (5 μm in particle diameter).

Column temperature: A constant temperature of about 25°C.

Mobile phase: A mixture of water and tetrahydrofuran (13:7).

Flow rate: Adjust so that the retention time of fludrocortisone acetate is about 10 minutes.

Time span of measurement: About 2 times as long as the retention time of fludrocortisone acetate, beginning after the solvent peak.

System suitability—

Test for required detectability: Pipet 5 mL of the standard solution, and add the mobile phase to make exactly 100 mL. Confirm that the peak area of fludrocortisone acetate obtained with 20 μL of this solution is equivalent to 4.0 to 6.0% of that with 20 μL of the standard solution.

System performance: Dissolve 2 mg each of Fludrocortisone Acetate and hydrocortisone acetate in 50 mL of the mobile phase. When the procedure is run with 20 μL of this solution under the above operating conditions, hydrocortisone acetate and fludrocortisone acetate are eluted in this order with the resolution between these peaks being not less than 1.5.

System repeatability: When the test is repeated 6 times with 20 μL of the standard solution under the above operating conditions, the relative standard deviation of the peak area of fludrocortisone acetate is not more than 2.0%.

Loss on drying *<2.41>* Not more than 1.0% (1 g, in vacuum, 100°C, 2 hours).

Residue on ignition *<2.44>* Not more than 0.1% (1 g, platinum crucible).

Assay Weigh accurately about 25 mg each of Fludrocortisone Acetate and Fludrocortisone Acetate RS, previously dried, and dissolve separately in ethanol (95) to make exactly 100 mL. Pipet 4 mL each of these solutions, add ethanol (95) to make exactly 100 mL, and use these solutions as the sample solution and the standard solution, respectively. Perform the test with the sample solution and standard solution as directed under Ultraviolet-visible Spectrophotometry *<2.24>*, and determine the absorbances, A_T and A_S, at 238 nm.

Amount (mg) of fludrocortisone acetate ($C_{23}H_{31}FO_6$)
$= M_S \times A_T/A_S$

M_S: Amount (mg) of Fludrocortisone Acetate RS taken

Containers and storage Containers—Well-closed containers.

Storage—Light-resistant.

Flunitrazepam

フルニトラゼパム

$C_{16}H_{12}FN_3O_3$: 313.28
5-(2-Fluorophenyl)-1-methyl-7-nitro-1,3-dihydro-2*H*-1,4-benzodiazepin-2-one
[*1622-62-4*]

Flunitrazepam, when dried, contains not less than 99.0% of flunitrazepam ($C_{16}H_{12}FN_3O_3$).

Description Flunitrazepam occurs as a white to pale yellow crystalline powder.

It is freely soluble in acetic acid (100), soluble in acetic anhydride and in acetone, slightly soluble in ethanol (99.5) and in diethyl ether, and practically insoluble in water.

Identification **(1)** Determine the absorption spectrum of a solution of Flunitrazepam in ethanol (99.5) (1 in 100,000) as directed under Ultraviolet-visible Spectrophotometry *<2.24>*, and compare the spectrum with the Reference Spectrum: both spectra exhibit similar intensities of absorption at the same wavelengths.

(2) Determine the infrared absorption spectrum of Flunitrazepam, previously dried, as directed in the potassium bromide disk method under Infrared Spectrophotometry *<2.25>*, and compare the spectrum with the Reference Spectrum: both spectra exhibit similar intensities of absorption at the same wave numbers.

Melting point *<2.60>* 168 – 172°C

Purity **(1)** Chloride *<1.03>*—To 1.0 g of Flunitrazepam add 50 mL of water, allow to stand for 1 hour with occasional stirring, and filter. To 20 mL of the filtrate add 6 mL of dilute nitric acid and water to make 50 mL, and perform the test with this solution. Prepare the control solution with 0.25 mL of 0.01 mol/L hydrochloric acid VS (not more than 0.022%).

(2) Heavy metals *<1.07>*—Proceed with 2.0 g of Flunitrazepam according to Method 4 using a platinum crucible, and perform the test. Prepare the control solution with 2.0 mL of Standard Lead Solution (not more than 10 ppm).

(3) Related substances—Dissolve 50 mg of Flunitrazepam in 10 mL of acetone, and use this solution as the sample solution. Pipet 2 mL of the sample solution, and add acetone to make exactly 20 mL. Pipet 1 mL of this solution, add acetone to make exactly 25 mL, and use this solution as the standard solution. Perform the test with these solutions as directed under Thin-layer Chromatography <*2.03*>. Spot 10 μL each of the sample solution and standard solution on a plate of silica gel with fluorescent indicator for thin-layer chromatography. Develop the plate with a mixture of 1,2-dichloroethane, diethyl ether and ammonia solution (28) (200:100:3) to a distance of about 12 cm, and air-dry the plate. Examine under ultraviolet light (main wavelength: 254 nm): number of the spots other than the principal spot obtained from the sample solution is not more than 2, and they are not more intense than the spot from the standard solution.

Loss on drying <*2.41*> Not more than 0.5% (1 g, 105°C, 4 hours).

Residue on ignition <*2.44*> Not more than 0.1% (1 g, platinum crucible).

Assay Weigh accurately about 0.5 g of Flunitrazepam, previously dried, dissolve in 20 mL of acetic acid (100), add 50 mL of acetic anhydride, and titrate <*2.50*> with 0.1 mol/L perchloric acid VS (potentiometric titration). Perform a blank determination in the same manner, and make any necessary correction.

Each mL of 0.1 mol/L perchloric acid VS
= 31.33 mg of $C_{16}H_{12}FN_3O_3$

Containers and storage Containers—Tight containers.

Storage—Light-resistant.

Fluocinolone Acetonide

フルオシノロンアセトニド

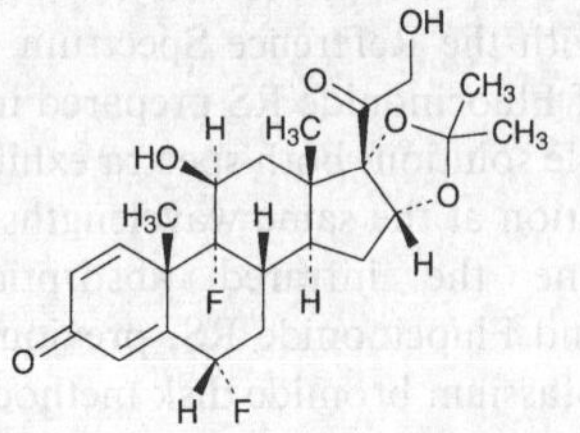

$C_{24}H_{30}F_2O_6$: 452.49

6α,9-Difluoro-11β,21-dihydroxy-16α,17-(1-methylethylidenedioxy)pregna-1,4-diene-3,20-dione

[67-73-2]

Fluocinolone Acetonide, when dried, contains not less than 97.0% and not more than 102.0% of fluocinolone acetonide ($C_{24}H_{30}F_2O_6$).

Description Fluocinolone Acetonide occurs as white, crystals or crystalline powder.

It is freely soluble in acetic acid (100) and in acetone, soluble in ethanol (99.5), sparingly soluble in methanol, and practically insoluble in water.

Melting point: 266 – 274°C (with decomposition).

It shows crystal polymorphism.

Identification (1) To 2 mg of Fluocinolone Acetonide add 2 mL of sulfuric acid: a yellow color is produced.

(2) Dissolve 0.01 g of Fluocinolone Acetonide in 1 mL of methanol, add 1 mL of Fehling's TS, and heat: a red precipitate is produced.

(3) Proceed with 0.01 g of Fluocinolone Acetonide as directed under Oxygen Flask Combustion Method <*1.06*>, using a mixture of 0.5 mL of 0.01 mol/L sodium hydroxide TS and 20 mL of water as the absorbing liquid: the test solution responds to Qualitative Tests <*1.09*> for fluoride.

(4) Determine the infrared absorption spectrum of Fluocinolone Acetonide, previously dried, as directed in the potassium bromide disk method under Infrared Spectrophotometry <*2.25*>, and compare the spectrum with the Reference Spectrum or the spectrum of previously dried Fluocinolone Acetonide RS: both spectra exhibit similar intensities of absorption at the same wave numbers. If any difference appears between the spectra, dissolve Fluocinolone Acetonide and Fluocinolone Acetonide RS in acetone, respectively, then evaporate the acetone to dryness, and repeat the test on the residues.

Optical rotation <*2.49*> $[\alpha]_D^{20}$: +98 – +108° (after drying, 0.1 g, methanol, 10 mL, 100 mm).

Purity Related substances—Dissolve 15 mg of Fluocinolone Acetonide in 25 mL of the mobile phase, and use this solution as the sample solution. Pipet 2 mL of the sample solution, add the mobile phase to make exactly 100 mL, and use this solution as the standard solution. Perform the test with exactly 20 μL each of the sample solution and standard solution as directed under Liquid Chromatography <*2.01*> according to the following conditions. Determine each peak area of each solution by the automatic integration method: the total area of the peaks other than fluocinolone acetonide obtained from the sample solution is not larger than the peak area of fluocinolone acetonide from the standard solution.

Operating conditions—

Detector: An ultraviolet absorption photometer (wavelength: 254 nm).

Column: A stainless steel column 4.6 mm in inside diameter and 15 cm in length, packed with silica gel for liquid chromatography (5 μm in particle diameter).

Column temperature: A constant temperature of about 30°C.

Mobile phase: A mixture of water-saturated chloroform, methanol and acetic acid (100) (200:3:2).

Flow rate: Adjust so that the retention time of fluocinolone acetonide is about 12 minutes.

Time span of measurement: About 2 times as long as the retention time of fluocinolone acetonide, beginning after the solvent peak.

System suitability—

Test for required detectability: To exactly 5 mL of the standard solution add the mobile phase to make exactly 100 mL. Confirm that the peak area of fluocinolone acetonide obtained with 20 μL of this solution is equivalent to 4 to 6% of that with 20 μL of the standard solution.

System performance: Dissolve 15 mg each of Fluocinolone Acetonide and triamcinolone acetonide in 25 mL of the mobile phase. To 5 mL of this solution add the mobile phase to make 20 mL. When the procedure is run with 20 μL of this solution under the above operating conditions, triamcinolone acetonide and fluocinolone acetonide are eluted in this order with the resolution between these peaks being not less than 1.9.

System repeatability: When the test is repeated 6 times with 20 μL of the standard solution under the above operating conditions, the relative standard deviation of the peak

areas of fluocinolone acetonide is not more than 1.0%.

Loss on drying ⟨*2.41*⟩ Not more than 1.0% (0.2 g, in vacuum, 105°C, 3 hours).

Residue on ignition ⟨*2.44*⟩ Not more than 0.1% (0.2 g, platinum crucible).

Assay Weigh accurately about 20 mg each of Fluocinolone Acetonide and Fluocinolone Acetonide RS, previously dried, and dissolve in 40 mL each of methanol, add exactly 10 mL each of the internal standard solution, then add water to make 100 mL, and use these solutions as the sample solution and standard solution. Perform the test with 20 μL each of the sample solution and standard solution as directed under Liquid Chromatography ⟨*2.01*⟩ according to the following conditions, and calculate the ratios, Q_T and Q_S, of the peak area of fluocinolone acetonide to that of the internal standard.

Amount (mg) of fluocinolone acetonide ($C_{24}H_{30}F_2O_6$)
$= M_S \times Q_T/Q_S$

M_S: Amount (mg) of Fluocinolone Acetonide RS taken

Internal standard solution—A solution of ethyl parahydroxybenzoate (1 in 2500).

Operating conditions—

Detector: An ultraviolet absorption photometer (wavelength: 254 nm).

Column: A stainless steel column 4.6 mm in inside diameter and 25 cm in length, packed with octadecylsilanized silica gel for liquid chromatography (5 μm in particle diameter).

Column temperature: A constant temperature of about 40°C.

Mobile phase: A mixture of water and acetonitrile (7:3).

Flow rate: Adjust so that the retention time of fluocinolone acetonide is about 20 minutes.

System suitability—

System performance: Dissolve 5 mg each of isopropyl parahydroxybenzoate and propyl parahydroxybenzoate in 50 mL of acetonitrile, and add water to make 100 mL. When the procedure is run with 20 μL of this solution under the above operating conditions, isopropyl parahydroxybenzoate and propyl parahydroxybenzoate are eluted in this order with the resolution between these peaks being not less than 1.9.

System repeatability: When the test is repeated 6 times with 20 μL of the standard solution under the above operating conditions, the relative standard deviation of the ratios of the peak area of fluocinolone acetonide to that of the internal standard is not more than 1.0%.

Containers and storage Containers—Tight containers.

Storage—Light-resistant.

Fluocinonide

フルオシノニド

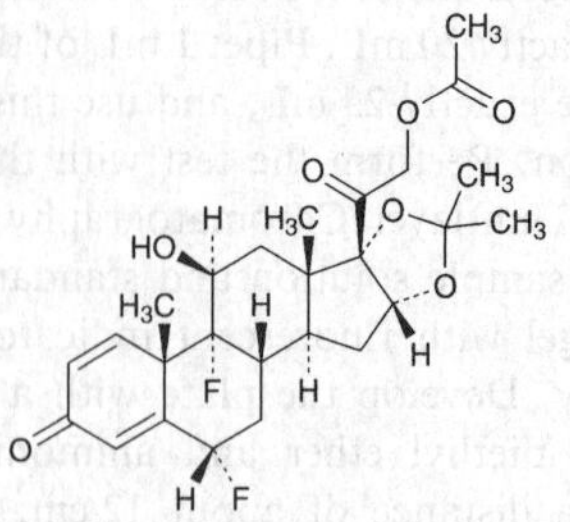

$C_{26}H_{32}F_2O_7$: 494.52

6α,9-Difluoro-11β,21-dihydroxy-16α,17-(1-methylethylidenedioxy)pregna-1,4-diene-3,20-dione 21-acetate

[356-12-7]

Fluocinonide, when dried, contains not less than 97.0% and not more than 103.0% of fluocinonide ($C_{26}H_{32}F_2O_7$).

Description Fluocinonide occurs as white, crystals or crystalline powder.

It is sparingly soluble in chloroform, slightly soluble in acetonitrile, in methanol, in ethanol (95) and in ethyl acetate, and practically insoluble in water.

It shows crystal polymorphism.

Identification **(1)** To 0.01 g of Fluocinonide add 4 mL of water and 1 mL of Fehling's TS, and heat: a red precipitate is formed.

(2) Prepare the test solution with 0.01 g of Fluocinonide as directed under Oxygen Flask Combustion Method ⟨*1.06*⟩, using a mixture of 0.5 mL of 0.01 mol/L sodium hydroxide TS and 20 mL of water as an absorbing liquid: the test solution responds to Qualitative Tests ⟨*1.09*⟩ for fluoride.

(3) Determine the absorption spectrum of a solution of Fluocinonide in methanol (1 in 100,000) as directed under Ultraviolet-visible Spectrophotometry ⟨*2.24*⟩, and compare the spectrum with the Reference Spectrum or the spectrum of a solution of Fluocinonide RS prepared in the same manner as the sample solution: both spectra exhibit similar intensities of absorption at the same wavelengths.

(4) Determine the infrared absorption spectra of Fluocinonide and Fluocinonide RS, previously dried, as directed in the potassium bromide disk method under Infrared Spectrophotometry ⟨*2.25*⟩, and compare both spectra: both spectra exhibit similar intensities of absorption at the same wave numbers. If any difference appears in the absorption spectra, dissolve the sample and the RS in ethyl acetate, respectively, evaporate the ethyl acetate, and perform the test with the residue in the same manner.

Optical rotation ⟨*2.49*⟩ $[\alpha]_D^{20}$: +81 – +89° (after drying, 0.2 g, chloroform, 20 mL, 100 mm).

Purity Related substances—Dissolve 10 mg of Fluocinonide in 2 mL of chloroform, and use this solution as the sample solution. Pipet 1 mL of the sample solution, add chloroform to make exactly 100 mL, and use this solution as the standard solution. Perform the test with these solutions as directed under Thin-layer Chromatography ⟨*2.03*⟩. Spot 10 μL each of the sample solution and standard solution on a plate of silica gel for thin-layer chromatography. Develop the plate with a mixture of chloroform and methanol (97:3) to a distance of about 12 cm, and air-dry the plate. Spray evenly alkaline blue tetrazolium TS on the plate: the spots other than the principal spot obtained from the sample solution are not more intense than the spot from the standard solution.

Loss on drying *<2.41>* Not more than 1.0% (0.5 g, 105°C, 3 hours).

Residue on ignition *<2.44>* Not more than 0.1% (0.5 g, platinum crucible).

Assay Weigh accurately about 20 mg each of Fluocinonide and Fluocinonide RS, previously dried, dissolve each in 50 mL of acetonitrile, to each add exactly 8 mL of the internal standard solution and water to make 100 mL, and use these solutions as the sample solution and the standard solution, respectively. Perform the test with 20 μL each of the sample solution and standard solution as directed under Liquid Chromatography *<2.01>* according to the following conditions, and calculate the ratios, Q_T and Q_S, of the peak area of fluocinonide to that of the internal standard, respectively.

$$\text{Amount (mg) of fluocinonide } (C_{26}H_{32}F_2O_7) = M_S \times Q_T/Q_S$$

M_S: Amount (mg) of Fluocinonide RS taken

Internal standard solution—A solution of propyl benzoate in acetonitrile (1 in 100).

Operating conditions—

Detector: An ultraviolet absorption photometer (wavelength: 254 nm).

Column: A stainless steel column 4.6 mm in inside diameter and 25 cm in length, packed with octadecylsilanized silica gel for liquid chromatography (5 μm in particle diameter).

Column temperature: A constant temperature of about 40°C.

Mobile phase: A mixture of water and acetonitrile (1:1).

Flow rate: Adjust so that the retention time of fluocinonide is about 8 minutes.

System suitability—

System performance: When the procedure is run with 20 μL of the standard solution under the above operating conditions, fluocinonide and the internal standard are eluted in this order with the resolution between these peaks being not less than 6.

System repeatability: When the test is repeated 6 times with 20 μL of the standard solution under the above operating conditions, the relative standard deviation of the ratios of the peak area of fluocinonide to that of the internal standard is not more than 1.0%.

Containers and storage Containers—Well-closed containers.

Fluorescein Sodium

フルオレセインナトリウム

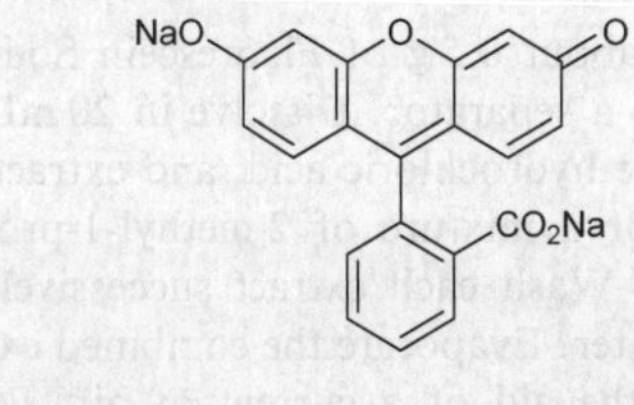

$C_{20}H_{10}Na_2O_5$: 376.27

Disodium 2-(6-oxido-3-oxo-3*H*-xanthen-9-yl)benzoate

[*518-47-8*]

Fluorescein Sodium contains not less than 98.5% of fluorescein sodium ($C_{20}H_{10}Na_2O_5$), calculated on the dried basis.

Description Fluorescein Sodium occurs as an orange powder. It is odorless, and tasteless.

It is freely soluble in water, in methanol and in ethanol (95), and practically insoluble in diethyl ether.

It is hygroscopic.

Identification **(1)** To a solution of Fluorescein Sodium (1 in 100) having a strong green fluorescence, add a large quantity of water: the fluorescence remains. Acidify the solution with hydrochloric acid: the fluorescence disappears. Then render the solution alkaline with sodium hydroxide TS: the fluorescence reappears.

(2) Place 1 drop of a solution of Fluorescein Sodium (1 in 2000) on a piece of filter paper: a yellow spot develops. Expose the spot, while moist, to the vapor of bromine for 1 minute and then to ammonia vapor: the yellow color of the spot changes to red.

(3) Char 0.5 g of Fluorescein Sodium by ignition, cool, mix the residue with 20 mL of water, and filter: the filtrate responds to Qualitative Tests *<1.09>* for sodium salt.

Purity **(1)** Clarity and color of solution—Dissolve 1 g of Fluorescein Sodium in 10 mL of water: the solution is clear, and shows a red color.

(2) Chloride *<1.03>*—Dissolve 0.15 g of Fluorescein Sodium in 20 mL of water, add 6 mL of dilute nitric acid and water to make 30 mL, and filter. To 20 mL of the filtrate add 2 mL of dilute nitric acid and water to make 50 mL. Perform the test using this solution as the test solution. Prepare the control solution with 1.0 mL of 0.01 mol/L hydrochloric acid VS (not more than 0.355%).

(3) Sulfate *<1.14>*—Dissolve 0.20 g of Fluorescein Sodium in 30 mL of water, add 2.5 mL of dilute hydrochloric acid and water to make 40 mL, and filter. To 20 mL of the filtrate add water to make 50 mL. Perform the test using this solution as the test solution. Prepare the control solution with 1.0 mL of 0.005 mol/L sulfuric acid VS (not more than 0.480%).

(4) Zinc—Dissolve 0.10 g of Fluorescein Sodium in 10 mL of water, add 2 mL of hydrochloric acid, and filter. To the filtrate add 0.1 mL of potassium hexacyanoferrate (II) TS: no turbidity is produced immediately.

(5) Related substances—Dissolve 0.20 g of Fluorescein Sodium in exactly 10 mL of methanol, and use this solution as the sample solution. Perform the test with this solution as directed under Thin-layer Chromatography *<2.03>*. Spot 5 μL of the sample solution on a plate of silica gel for thin-layer chromatography. Develop the plate with a mixture of chloroform, methanol and ammonia solution (28) (30:15:1) to a distance of about 10 cm, and air-dry the plate: any colored spot other than the principal spot does not appear.

Loss on drying *<2.41>* Not more than 10.0% (1 g, 105°C, constant mass).

Assay Transfer about 0.5 g of Fluorescein Sodium, accurately weighed, to a separator. Dissolve in 20 mL of water, add 5 mL of dilute hydrochloric acid, and extract with four 20-mL portions of a mixture of 2-methyl-1-propanol and chloroform (1:1). Wash each extract successively with the same 10 mL of water. Evaporate the combined extracts on a water bath with the aid of a current of air. Dissolve the residue in 10 mL of ethanol (99.5), evaporate the solution on a water bath to dryness, dry the residue at 105°C for 1 hour, and weigh as fluorescein ($C_{20}H_{12}O_5$: 332.31).

Amount (mg) of fluorescein sodium ($C_{20}H_{10}Na_2O_5$)
= amount (mg) of fluorescein ($C_{20}H_{12}O_5$) × 1.132

Containers and storage Containers—Tight containers.

Fluorometholone

フルオロメトロン

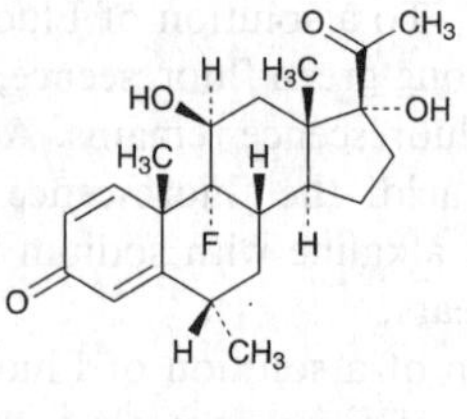

$C_{22}H_{29}FO_4$: 376.46
9-Fluoro-11β,17-dihydroxy-6α-methylpregna-1,4-diene-3,20-dione
[*426-13-1*]

Fluorometholone, when dried, contains not less than 97.0% and not more than 103.0% of fluorometholone ($C_{22}H_{29}FO_4$).

Description Fluorometholone occurs as a white to light yellow-white crystalline powder. It is odorless.

It is freely soluble in pyridine, slightly soluble in methanol, in ethanol (99.5) and in tetrahydrofuran, and practically insoluble in water and in diethyl ether.

Identification **(1)** Proceed with 7 mg of Fluorometholone as directed under Oxygen Flask Combustion Method *<1.06>*, using a mixture of 0.5 mL of 0.01 mol/L sodium hydroxide TS and 20 mL of water as an absorbing liquid: the liquid responds to Qualitative Tests *<1.09>* (2) for fluoride.

(2) Determine the absorption spectrum of a solution of Fluorometholone in methanol (1 in 100,000) as directed under Ultraviolet-visible Spectrophotometry *<2.24>*, and compare the spectrum with the Reference Spectrum or the spectrum of a solution of Fluorometholone RS prepared in the same manner as the sample solution: both spectra exhibit similar intensities of absorption at the same wavelengths.

(3) Determine the infrared absorption spectrum of Fluorometholone, previously dried, as directed in the potassium bromide disk method under Infrared Spectrophotometry *<2.25>*, and compare the spectrum with the Reference Spectrum or the spectrum of previously dried Fluorometholone RS: both spectra exhibit similar intensities of absorption at the same wave numbers.

Optical rotation *<2.49>* $[\alpha]_D^{20}$: +52 – +60° (after drying, 0.1 g, pyridine, 10 mL, 100 mm).

Purity **(1)** Heavy metals *<1.07>*—Proceed with 1.0 g of Fluorometholone according to Method 3, and perform the test. Prepare the control solution with 2.0 mL of Standard Lead Solution (not more than 20 ppm).

(2) Related substances—Dissolve 20 mg of Fluorometholone in 10 mL of tetrahydrofuran, and use this solution as the sample solution. Pipet 1 mL of the sample solution, add tetrahydrofuran to make exactly 100 mL, and use this solution as the standard solution. Perform the test with these solutions as directed under Thin-layer chromatography *<2.03>*. Spot 25 μL each of the sample solution and standard solution on a plate of silica gel with fluorescent indicator for thin-layer chromatography. Develop the plate with a mixture of dichloromethane, acetone and methanol (45:5:1) to a distance of about 12 cm, and air-dry the plate. Examine under ultraviolet light (main wavelength: 254 nm): the spots other than the principal spot obtained from the sample solution are not more intense than the spot from the standard solution.

Loss on drying *<2.41>* Not more than 1.0% (0.2 g, in vacuum, phosphorus (V) oxide, 60°C, 3 hours).

Residue on ignition *<2.44>* Not more than 0.2% (0.2 g, platinum crucible).

Assay Weigh accurately about 0.1 g each of Fluorometholone and Fluorometholone RS, previously dried, and dissolve each in methanol to make exactly 100 mL. Pipet 5 mL each of these solutions, and add diluted methanol (7 in 10) to make exactly 50 mL. Pipet 10 mL each of these solutions, add exactly 10 mL of the internal standard solution and diluted methanol (7 in 10) to make 100 mL, and use these solutions as the sample solution and the standard solution, respectively. Perform the test with 20 μL each of the sample solution and standard solution as directed under Liquid Chromatography *<2.01>* according to the following conditions and calculate the ratios, Q_T and Q_S, of the peak area of fluorometholone to that of the internal standard.

Amount (mg) of fluorometholone ($C_{22}H_{29}FO_4$)
$= M_S \times Q_T/Q_S$

M_S: Amount (mg) of Fluorometholone RS taken

Internal standard solution—A solution of butyl parahydroxybenzoate in methanol (1 in 10,000).
Operating conditions—

Detector: An ultraviolet absorption photometer (wavelength: 254 nm).

Column: A stainless steel column about 4 mm in inside diameter and 25 to 30 cm in length, packed with octadecylsilanized silica gel for liquid chromatography (5 μm in particle diameter).

Column temperature: A constant temperature of about 35°C.

Mobile phase: Diluted methanol (7 in 10).

Flow rate: Adjust so that the retention time of fluorometholone is about 8 minutes.

Selection of column: Proceed with 20 μL of the standard solution under the above operating conditions, and calculate the resolution. Use a column giving elution of fluorometholone and the internal standard in this order with the resolution between these peaks being not less than 4.

Containers and storage Containers—Well-closed containers.

Storage—Light-resistant.

Fluorouracil

フルオロウラシル

$C_4H_3FN_2O_2$: 130.08
5-Fluorouracil
[*51-21-8*]

Fluorouracil, when dried, contains not less than 98.5% of fluorouracil ($C_4H_3FN_2O_2$), and not less than 13.1% and not more than 16.1% of fluorine (F: 19.00).

Description Fluorouracil occurs as white, crystals or crystalline powder. It is odorless.

It is freely soluble in *N,N*-dimethylformamide, sparingly soluble in water, slightly soluble in ethanol (95), and practically insoluble in diethyl ether.

Melting point: about 282°C (with decomposition).

Identification **(1)** Add 0.2 mL of bromine TS to 5 mL of a solution of Fluorouracil (1 in 500): the color of bromine TS is discharged. Further add 2 mL of barium hydroxide TS: a purple precipitate is formed.

(2) Proceed with 0.01 g of Fluorouracil as directed under Oxygen Flask Combustion Method 〈*1.06*〉, using a mixture of 0.5 mL of 0.01 mol/L sodium hydroxide TS and 20 mL of water as the absorbing liquid: the test solution responds to Qualitative Tests 〈*1.09*〉 for fluoride.

(3) Determine the absorption spectrum of a solution of Fluorouracil in 0.1 mol/L hydrochloric acid TS (1 in 100,000) as directed under Ultraviolet-visible Spectrophotometry 〈*2.24*〉, and compare the spectrum with the Reference Spectrum: both spectra exhibit similar intensities of absorption at the same wavelengths.

Purity **(1)** Clarity and color of solution—Add 20 mL of water to 0.20 g of Fluorouracil, and dissolve by warming: the solution is clear and colorless.

(2) Fluoride—Dissolve 0.10 g of Fluorouracil in 10.0 mL of diluted 0.01 mol/L sodium hydroxide TS (1 in 20). Transfer 5.0 mL of this solution to a 20-mL volumetric flask, add 10 mL of a mixture of alizarin complexone TS, acetic acid-potassium acetate buffer solution (pH 4.3) and cerium (III) nitrate TS (1:1:1), and add water to make 20 mL. Allow to stand for 1 hour, and use this solution as the sample solution. Separately, transfer 1.0 mL of Standard Fluorine Solution to a 20-mL volumetric flask, add 5.0 mL of diluted 0.01 mol/L sodium hydroxide TS (1 in 20), and add 10 mL of a mixture of alizarin complexone TS, acetic acid-potassium acetate buffer solution (pH 4.3) and cerium (III) nitrate TS (1:1:1). Proceed in the same manner as directed for the preparation of the sample solution, and use this solution as the standard solution. Perform the test as directed under Ultraviolet-visible Spectrophotometry 〈*2.24*〉, using a solution, prepared with 5.0 mL of diluted 0.01 mol/L sodium hydroxide TS (1 in 20) in the same manner, as the blank: the absorbance of the sample solution at 600 nm is not larger than that of the standard solution (not more than 0.012%).

(3) Heavy metals 〈*1.07*〉—Proceed with 1.0 g of Fluorouracil according to Method 2, and perform the test. Prepare the control solution with 2.0 mL of Standard Lead Solution (not more than 20 ppm).

(4) Arsenic 〈*1.11*〉—To 1.0 g of Fluorouracil in a crucible add 10 mL of a solution of magnesium nitrate hexahydrate in ethanol (95) (1 in 10), ignite the ethanol to burn, and incinerate by strong heating at 750°C to 850°C. If a carbonized substance remains in this method, moisten with a small amount of nitric acid, and incinerate by strong heating. Cool, add 10 mL of dilute hydrochloric acid to the residue, dissolve it by warming on a water bath, use this solution as the test solution, and perform the test (not more than 2 ppm).

(5) Related substances—Dissolve 0.10 g of Fluorouracil in 10 mL of water, and use this solution as the sample solution. Measure exactly 1 mL of the sample solution, add water to make exactly 200 mL, and use this solution as the standard solution. Perform the test with these solutions as directed under Thin-layer Chromatography 〈*2.03*〉. Spot 10 μL each of the sample solution and standard solution on a plate of silica gel with fluorescent indicator for thin-layer chromatography. Develop the plate with a mixture of ethyl acetate, acetone and water (7:4:1) to a distance of about 12 cm, air-dry the plate, and examine under ultraviolet light (main wavelength: 254 nm): the spots other than the principal spot obtained from the sample solution are not more intense than the spot from the standard solution.

Loss on drying 〈*2.41*〉 Not more than 0.5% (1 g, in vacuum, 80°C, 4 hours).

Residue on ignition 〈*2.44*〉 Not more than 0.1% (1 g).

Assay **(1)** Fluorouracil—Weigh accurately about 0.2 g of Fluorouracil, previously dried, dissolve in 20 mL of *N,N*-dimethylformamide, and titrate 〈*2.50*〉 with 0.1 mol/L tetramethylammonium hydroxide VS until the color of the solution changes from yellow through blue-green to blue (indicator: 3 drops of thymol blue-dimethylformamide TS). Perform a blank determination in the same manner, and make any necessary correction.

Each mL of 0.1 mol/L tetramethylammonium hydroxide VS
= 13.01 mg of $C_4H_3FN_2O_2$

(2) Fluorine—Weigh accurately about 4 mg of Fluorouracil, previously dried, and proceed as directed in the determination of fluorine under Oxygen Flask Combustion Method 〈*1.06*〉, using a mixture of 0.5 mL of 0.01 mol/L sodium hydroxide TS and 20 mL of water as the absorbing liquid.

Containers and storage Containers—Tight containers.

Fluphenazine Enanthate

フルフェナジンエナント酸エステル

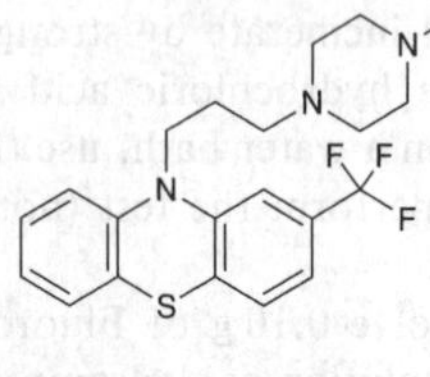

$C_{29}H_{38}F_3N_3O_2S$: 549.69
2-(4-{3-[2-(Trifluoromethyl)-10*H*-phenothiazin-10-yl]propyl}piperazin-1-yl)ethyl heptanoate
[*2746-81-8*]

Fluphenazine Enanthate, when dried, contains not less than 98.5% of fluphenazine enanthate ($C_{29}H_{38}F_3N_3O_2S$).

Description Fluphenazine Enanthate is a light yellow to yellowish orange viscous liquid. It is generally clear, and can be opaque by producing crystals.

It is freely soluble in methanol and in diethyl ether, soluble in ethanol (95) and in acetic acid (100), and practically insoluble in water.

Identification **(1)** Prepare the test solution with 0.01 g of Fluphenazine Enanthate as directed under Oxygen Flask Combustion Method ⟨*1.06*⟩, using a mixture of 0.5 mL of 0.01 mol/L sodium hydroxide TS and 20 mL of water as the absorbing liquid: the test solution responds to Qualitative Tests ⟨*1.09*⟩ for fluoride.

(2) Dissolve 2 mg of Fluphenazine Enanthate in 200 mL of a solution of hydrochloric acid in methanol (17 in 2000). Determine the absorption spectrum of the solution as directed under Ultraviolet-visible Spectrophotometry ⟨*2.24*⟩, and compare the spectrum with the Reference Spectrum: both spectra exhibit similar intensities of absorption at the same wavelengths.

(3) Determine the infrared absorption spectrum of Fluphenazine Enanthate as directed in the liquid firm method under Infrared Spectrophotometry ⟨*2.25*⟩, and compare the spectrum with the Reference Spectrum: both spectra exhibit similar intensities of absorption at the same wave numbers.

Purity **(1)** Heavy metals ⟨*1.07*⟩—Proceed with 1.0 g of Fluphenazine Enanthate according to Method 2, and perform the test. Prepare the control solution with 3.0 mL of Standard Lead Solution (not more than 30 ppm).

(2) Related substances—Dissolve 0.25 g of Fluphenazine Enanthate in 10 mL of methanol, and use this solution as the sample solution. Pipet 1 mL of the sample solution, add methanol to make exactly 100 mL, and use this solution as the standard solution. Perform the test with these solutions as directed under Thin-layer Chromatography ⟨*2.03*⟩. Spot 20 μL each of the sample solution and standard solution on a plate of silica gel with fluorescent indicator for thin-layer chromatography. Develop the plate with a mixture of acetone, hexane and ammonia solution (28) (16:6:1) to a distance of about 15 cm, and air-dry the plate. Examine under ultraviolet light (main wavelength: 254 nm): the spots other than the principal spot from the sample solution are not more intense than the spot from the standard solution. Then spray evenly diluted sulfuric acid (1 in 2) on the plate: the spots other than the principal spot obtained from the sample solution are not more intense than the spot from the standard solution.

Loss on drying ⟨*2.41*⟩ Not more than 1.0% (1 g, in vacuum, 60°C, 3 hours).

Residue on ignition ⟨*2.44*⟩ Not more than 0.2% (1 g).

Assay Weigh accurately about 0.5 g of Fluphenazine Enanthate, previously dried, dissolve in 50 mL of acetic acid (100), and titrate ⟨*2.50*⟩ with 0.1 mol/L perchloric acid VS (indicator: 2 drops of crystal violet TS). Perform a blank determination in the same manner, and make any necessary correction.

Each mL of 0.1 mol/L perchloric acid VS
= 27.49 mg of $C_{29}H_{38}F_3N_3O_2S$

Containers and storage Containers—Tight containers.
Storage—Light-resistant.

Flurazepam Hydrochloride

フルラゼパム塩酸塩

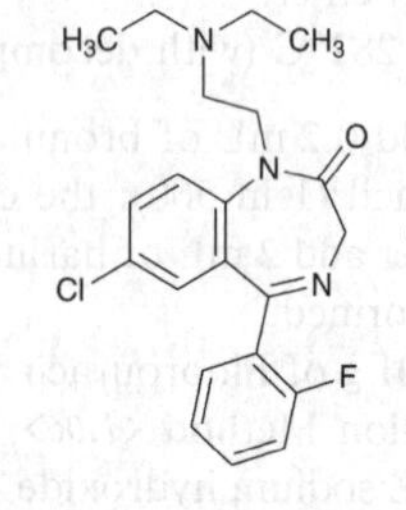

$C_{21}H_{23}ClFN_3O.HCl$: 424.34
7-Chloro-1-[2-(diethylamino)ethyl]-5-(2-fluorophenyl)-1,3-dihydro-2*H*-1,4-benzodiazepin-2-one monohydrochloride
[*36105-20-1*]

Flurazepam Hydrochloride, when dried, contains not less than 99.0% of flurazepam hydrochloride ($C_{21}H_{23}ClFN_3O.HCl$).

Description Flurazepam Hydrochloride occurs as white to yellowish white, crystals or crystalline powder.

It is freely soluble in water, in ethanol (95), in ethanol (99.5) and in acetic acid (100).

Melting point: about 197°C (with decomposition).

Identification **(1)** Determine the absorption spectrum of a solution of Flurazepam Hydrochloride in sulfuric acid-ethanol TS (1 in 100,000) as directed under Ultraviolet-visible Spectrophotometry ⟨*2.24*⟩, and compare the spectrum with the Reference Spectrum: both spectra exhibit similar intensities of absorption at the same wavelengths.

(2) Determine the infrared absorption spectrum of Flurazepam Hydrochloride, previously dried, as directed in the potassium chloride disk method under Infrared Spectrophotometry ⟨*2.25*⟩, and compare the spectrum with the Reference Spectrum: both spectra exhibit similar intensities of absorption at the same wave numbers.

(3) A solution of Flurazepam Hydrochloride (1 in 20) responds to Qualitative Tests ⟨*1.09*⟩ for chloride.

pH ⟨*2.54*⟩ Dissolve 1.0 g of Flurazepam Hydrochloride in 20 mL of water: the pH of this solution is between 5.0 and 6.0.

Purity **(1)** Clarity and color of solution—Dissolve 1.0 g of Flurazepam Hydrochloride in 10 mL of water: the solution is clear and colorless to pale yellow.

(2) Sulfate <*1.14*>—Perform the test with 1.5 g of Flurazepam Hydrochloride. Prepare the control solution with 0.35 mL of 0.005 mol/L sulfuric acid VS (not more than 0.011%).

(3) Heavy metals <*1.07*>—Proceed with 1.0 g of Flurazepam Hydrochloride in a platinum crucible according to Method 2, and perform the test. Prepare the control solution with 2.0 mL of Standard Lead Solution (not more than 20 ppm).

(4) Related substances—Dissolve 0.05 g of Flurazepam Hydrochloride in 5 mL of ethanol (95), and use this solution as the sample solution. Pipet 1 mL of the sample solution, add ethanol (95) to make exactly 50 mL. Pipet 1 mL of this solution, add ethanol (95) to make exactly 10 mL, and use this solution as the standard solution. Perform the test with these solutions as directed under Thin-layer Chromatography <*2.03*>. Spot 20 μL each of the sample solution and standard solution on a plate of silica gel with fluorescent indicator for thin-layer chromatography. Place the plate in a chamber filled with ammonia vapor, allow to stand for about 15 minutes, and immediately develop the plate with a mixture of diethyl ether and diethylamine (39:1) to a distance of about 12 cm, and air-dry the plate. Examine under ultraviolet light (main wavelength: 254 nm): not more than 3 spots other than the principal spot and the spot on the starting point obtained from the sample solution appear, and are not more intense than the spot from the standard solution.

Loss on drying <*2.41*> Not more than 0.5% (1 g, 105°C, 4 hours).

Residue on ignition <*2.44*> Not more than 0.1% (1 g).

Assay Weigh accurately about 0.3 g of Flurazepam Hydrochloride, previously dried, dissolve in 10 mL of acetic acid (100), add 40 mL of acetic anhydride, and titrate <*2.50*> with 0.1 mol/L perchloric acid VS (potentiometric titration). Perform a blank determination in the same manner, and make any necessary correction.

Each mL of 0.1 mol/L perchloric acid VS
= 21.22 mg of $C_{21}H_{23}ClFN_3O.HCl$

Containers and storage Containers—Tight containers.

Flurbiprofen

フルルビプロフェン

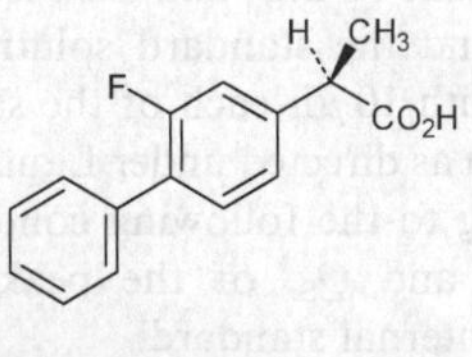

and enantiomer

$C_{15}H_{13}FO_2$: 244.26
(2*RS*)-2-(2-Fluorobiphenyl-4-yl)propanoic acid
[*5104-49-4*]

Flurbiprofen, when dried, contains not less than 98.0% of flurbiprofen ($C_{15}H_{13}FO_2$).

Description Flurbiprofen occurs as a white crystalline powder. It has a slightly irritating odor.

It is freely soluble in methanol, in ethanol (95), in acetone and in diethyl ether, soluble in acetonitrile, and practically insoluble in water.

A solution of Flurbiprofen in ethanol (95) (1 in 50) shows no optical rotation.

Identification **(1)** Determine the absorption spectrum of a solution of Flurbiprofen in methanol (1 in 200,000) as directed under Ultraviolet-visible Spectrophotometry <*2.24*>, and compare the spectrum with the Reference Spectrum: both spectra exhibit similar intensities of absorption at the same wavelengths.

(2) Determine the infrared absorption spectrum of Flurbiprofen, previously dried, as directed in the potassium bromide disk method under Infrared Spectrophotometry <*2.25*>, and compare the spectrum with the Reference Spectrum: both spectra exhibit similar intensities of absorption at the same wave numbers.

Melting point <*2.60*> 114 - 117°C

Purity **(1)** Chloride <*1.03*>—Dissolve 0.6 g of Flurbiprofen in 40 mL of acetone, and add 6 mL of dilute nitric acid and water to make 50 mL. Perform the test using this solution as the test solution. Prepare the control solution as follows: to 0.25 mL of 0.01 mol/L hydrochloric acid VS add 40 mL of acetone, 6 mL of dilute nitric acid and water to make 50 mL (not more than 0.015%).

(2) Heavy metals <*1.07*>—Dissolve 2.0 g of Flurbiprofen in 30 mL of acetone, and add 2 mL of dilute acetic acid and water to make 50 mL. Perform the test using this solution as the test solution. Prepare the control solution as follows: to 2.0 mL of Standard Lead Solution add 30 mL of acetone, 2 mL of dilute acetic acid and water to make 50 mL (not more than 10 ppm).

(3) Related substances—Dissolve 20 mg of Flurbiprofen in 10 mL of a mixture of water and acetonitrile (11:9), and use this solution as the sample solution. Pipet 1 mL of the sample solution, and add a mixture of water and acetonitrile (11:9) to make exactly 200 mL, and use this solution as the standard solution. Perform the test with exactly 20 μL each of the sample solution and standard solution as directed under Liquid Chromatography <*2.01*> according to the following conditions. Determine each peak area of both solutions by the automatic integration method: the area of the peak other than flurbiprofen obtained from the sample solution is not larger than the peak area of flurbiprofen from the standard solution, and the total area of these peaks is not larger than 2 times the peak area of flurbiprofen from the standard solution.

Operating conditions—

Detector: An ultraviolet absorption photometer (wavelength: 254 nm).

Column: A stainless steel column 4.6 mm in inside diameter and 15 cm in length, packed with octadecylsilanized silica gel for liquid chromatography (5 μm in particle diameter).

Column temperature: A constant temperature of about 30°C.

Mobile phase: A mixture of water, acetonitrile and acetic acid (100) (12:7:1).

Flow rate: Adjust so that the retention time of flurbiprofen is about 20 minutes.

Time span of measurement: About twice as long as the retention time of flurbiprofen, beginning after the solvent peak.

System suitability—

Test for required detectability: To exactly 5 mL of the standard solution add a mixture of water and acetonitrile (11:9) to make exactly 25 mL. Confirm that the peak area of flurbiprofen obtained with 20 μL of this solution is equivalent to 16 to 24% of that with 20 μL of the standard solution.

System performance: Dissolve 0.04 g of flurbiprofen and 0.02 g of butyl parahydroxybenzoate in 100 mL of a mixture of water and acetonitrile (11:9). To 5 mL of this solution add a mixture of water and acetonitrile (11:9) to make 50 mL. When the procedure is run with 20 μL of this solution under the above operating conditions, butyl parahydroxybenzoate and flurbiprofen are eluted in this order with the resolution between these peaks being not less than 12.

System repeatability: When the test is repeated 6 times with 20 μL of the standard solution under the above operating conditions, the relative standard deviation of the peak area of flurbiprofen is not more than 2.0%.

Loss on drying *<2.41>* Not more than 0.10% (1 g, in vacuum at a pressure not exceeding 0.67 kPa, silica gel, 4 hours).

Residue on ignition *<2.44>* Not more than 0.1% (1 g, platinum crucible).

Assay Weigh accurately about 0.6 g of Flurbiprofen, previously dried, dissolve in 50 mL of ethanol (95), and titrate *<2.50>* with 0.1 mol/L sodium hydroxide VS (indicator: 3 drops of phenolphthalein TS). Perform a blank determination in the same manner, and make any necessary correction.

Each mL of 0.1 mol/L sodium hydroxide VS
= 24.43 mg of $C_{15}H_{13}FO_2$

Containers and storage Containers—Well-closed containers.

Flutamide

フルタミド

$C_{11}H_{11}F_3N_2O_3$: 276.21
2-Methyl-*N*-[4-nitro-3-(trifluoromethyl)phenyl]propanamide
[13311-84-7]

Flutamide, when dried, contains not less than 98.5% and not more than 101.5% of flutamide ($C_{11}H_{11}F_3N_2O_3$).

Description Flutamide occurs as a light yellow crystalline powder.

It is freely soluble in methanol and in ethanol (95), and practically insoluble in water.

Identification **(1)** Determine the absorption spectrum of a solution of Flutamide in ethanol (95) (1 in 50,000) as directed under Ultraviolet-visible Spectrophotometry *<2.24>*, and compare the spectrum with the Reference Spectrum or the spectrum of a solution of Flutamide RS prepared in the same manner as the sample solution: both spectra exhibit similar intensities of absorption at the same wavelengths.

(2) Determine the infrared absorption spectrum of Flutamide as directed in the potassium bromide disk method under Infrared Spectrophotometry *<2.25>*, and compare the spectrum with the Reference Spectrum or the spectrum of Flutamide RS: both spectra exhibit similar intensities of absorption at the same wave numbers.

Melting point *<2.60>* 109 – 113°C

Purity **(1)** Heavy metals *<1.07>*—Proceed with 2.0 g of Flutamide according to Method 2, and perform the test. Prepare the control solution with 2.0 mL of Standard Lead Solution (not more than 10 ppm).

(2) Related substances—Dissolve 40 mg of Flutamide in 50 mL of methanol, and use this solution as the sample solution. Perform the test with 10 μL of the sample solution as directed under Liquid Chromatography *<2.01>* according to the following conditions. Determine each peak area of the sample solution by the automatic integration method and calculate the amounts of them by the area percentage method: the amount of each peak other than flutamide is not more than 0.3%, and the total amount of the peaks other than flutamide is not more than 0.5%.

Operating conditions—

Column, column temperature, mobile phase and flow rate: Proceed as directed in the operating conditions in the Assay.

Detector: An ultraviolet absorption photometer (wavelength: 230 nm).

Time span of measurement: About 2 times as long as the retention time of flutamide, beginning after the solvent peak.

System suitability—

System performance: Proceed as directed in the system suitability in the Assay.

Test for required detectability: To 1 mL of the sample solution, add methanol to make 100 mL, and use this solution as the solution for system suitability test. Pipet 2 mL of the solution for system suitability test, and add methanol to make exactly 20 mL. Confirm that the peak area of flutamide obtained with 10 μL of this solution is equivalent to 7 to 13% of that with 10 μL of the solution for system suitability test.

System repeatability: When the test is repeated 6 times with 10 μL of the solution for system suitability test under the above operating conditions, the relative standard deviation of the peak area of flutamide is not more than 2.0%.

Loss on drying *<2.41>* Not more than 0.5% (0.5 g, in vacuum, phosphorus (V) oxide, 60°C, 3 hours).

Residue on ignition *<2.44>* Not more than 0.1% (1 g, platinum crucible).

Assay Weigh accurately about 40 mg each of Flutamide and Flutamide RS, previously dried, and dissolve separately in methanol to make exactly 25 mL. Pipet 5 mL each of these solutions, add exactly 5 mL of the internal standard solution, add methanol to make 50 mL, and use these solutions as the sample solution and the standard solution, respectively. Perform the test with 10 μL each of the sample solution and standard solution as directed under Liquid Chromatography *<2.01>* according to the following conditions, and calculate the ratios, Q_T and Q_S, of the peak height of flutamide to that of the internal standard.

Amount (mg) of flutamide ($C_{11}H_{11}F_3N_2O_3$)
$= M_S \times Q_T/Q_S$

M_S: Amount (mg) of Flutamide RS taken

Internal standard solution—A solution of testosterone in methanol (9 in 10,000).

Operating conditions—

Detector: An ultraviolet absorption photometer (wavelength: 254 nm).

Column: A stainless steel column 3.9 mm in inside diameter and 30 cm in length, packed with octadecylsilanized silica gel for liquid chromatography (10 μm in particle diameter).

Column temperature: A constant temperature of about

25°C.

Mobile phase: A mixture of methanol and 0.05 mol/L potassium dihydrogen phosphate TS (7:4).

Flow rate: Adjust so that the retention time of flutamide is about 12 minutes.

System suitability—

System performance: When the procedure is run with 10 μL of the standard solution under the above operating conditions, flutamide and the internal standard are eluted in this order with the resolution between these peaks being not less than 2.0.

System repeatability: When the test is repeated 6 times with 10 μL of the standard solution under the above operating conditions, the relative standard deviation of the peak area of flutamide is not more than 1.0%.

Containers and storage Containers—Tight containers.

Flutoprazepam

フルトプラゼパム

$C_{19}H_{16}ClFN_2O$: 342.79
7-Chloro-1-cyclopropylmethyl-5-(2-fluorophenyl)-1,3-dihydro-2*H*-1,4-benzodiazepin-2-one
[25967-29-7]

Flutoprazepam, when dried, contains not less than 99.0% and not more than 101.0% of flutoprazepam ($C_{19}H_{16}ClFN_2O$).

Description Flutoprazepam occurs as a white to light yellow, crystals or crystalline powder.

It is freely soluble in ethyl acetate, soluble in ethanol (99.5) and in acetic anhydride, and practically insoluble in water.

Identification **(1)** Dissolve 2 mg of Flutoprazepam in 200 mL of a solution of sulfuric acid in ethanol (99.5) (3 in 1000). Determine the absorption spectrum of this solution as directed under Ultraviolet-visible Spectrophotometry *<2.24>*, and compare the spectrum with the Reference Spectrum: both spectra exhibit similar intensities of absorption at the same wavelengths.

(2) Determine the infrared absorption spectrum of Flutoprazepam as directed in the potassium bromide disk method under Infrared Spectrophotometry *<2.25>*, and compare the spectrum with the Reference Spectrum: both spectra exhibit similar intensities of absorption at the same wave numbers.

(3) Perform the test with Flutoprazepam as directed under Flame Coloration Test *<1.04>* (2): a green color appears.

Melting point *<2.60>* 118 – 122°C

Purity **(1)** Chloride *<1.03>*—To 1.0 g of Flutoprazepam add 50 mL of water, allow to stand for 1 hour with occasional shaking, and filter. To 20 mL of the filtrate add 6 mL of dilute nitric acid and water to make 50 mL. Perform the test using this solution as the test solution. Prepare the control solution with 0.40 mL of 0.01 mol/L hydrochloric acid VS (not more than 0.036%).

(2) Heavy metals *<1.07>*—Proceed with 1.0 g of Flutoprazepam according to Method 2, and perform the test. Prepare the control solution with 1.0 mL of Standard Lead Solution (not more than 10 ppm).

(3) Related substances—Dissolve 0.10 g of Flutoprazepam in 20 mL of ethyl acetate, and use this solution as the sample solution. Pipet 1 mL of the sample solution, and add ethyl acetate to make exactly 50 mL. Pipet 1 mL of this solution, add ethyl acetate to make exactly 20 mL, and use this solution as the standard solution. Perform the test with these solutions as directed under Thin-layer Chromatography *<2.03>*. Spot 10 μL each of the sample solution and standard solution on a plate of silica gel with fluorescent indicator for thin-layer chromatography. Develop the plate with a mixture of ethyl acetate and hexane (3:2) to a distance of about 12 cm, and air-dry the plate. Examine under ultraviolet light (main wavelength: 254 nm): the spots other than the principal spot obtained from the sample solution are not more intense than the spot from the standard solution.

Loss on drying *<2.41>* Not more than 0.20% (1 g, 105°C, 2 hours).

Residue on ignition *<2.44>* Not more than 0.1% (1 g, platinum crucible).

Assay Weigh accurately about 0.5 g of Flutoprazepam, previously dried, dissolve in 70 mL of acetic anhydride, and titrate *<2.50>* with 0.1 mol/L perchloric acid VS (potentiometric titration). Perform a blank determination in the same manner, and make any necessary correction.

Each mL of 0.1 mol/L perchloric acid VS
= 34.28 mg of $C_{19}H_{16}ClFN_2O$

Containers and storage Containers—Well-closed containers.

Flutoprazepam Tablets

フルトプラゼパム錠

Flutoprazepam Tablets contain not less than 93.0% and not more than 107.0% of the labeled amount of flutoprazepam ($C_{19}H_{16}ClFN_2O$: 342.79).

Method of preparation Prepare as directed under Tablets, with Flutoprazepam.

Identification To a quantity of powdered Flutoprazepam Tablets, equivalent to 10 mg of Flutoprazepam, add 20 mL of a solution of sulfuric acid in ethanol (99.5) (3 in 1000), shake well, and add a solution of sulfuric acid in ethanol (99.5) (3 in 1000) to make 100 mL. Centrifuge this solution, to 10 mL of the supernatant liquid add a solution of sulfuric acid in ethanol (99.5) (3 in 1000) to make 100 mL. Determine the absorption spectrum of this solution as directed under Ultraviolet-visible Spectrophotometry *<2.24>*: it exhibits maxima between 240 nm and 244 nm, between 279 nm and 285 nm, and between 369 nm and 375 nm.

Uniformity of dosage units *<6.02>* Perform the test according to the following method: it meets the requirement of the Content uniformity test.

To 1 tablet of Flutoprazepam Tablets add 60 mL of the mobile phase, shake for 15 minutes to disintegrate, disperse the particle by sonicating, and add the mobile phase to make exactly V mL so that each mL contains about 20 μg of flutoprazepam ($C_{19}H_{16}ClFN_2O$). Filter this solution through a membrane filter with a pore size not exceeding 0.45 μm, discard the first 5 mL of the filtrate, and use the subsequent filtrate as the sample solution. Proceed as directed in the Assay.

Amount (mg) of flutoprazepam ($C_{19}H_{16}ClFN_2O$)
$= M_S \times A_T/A_S \times V/1000$

M_S: Amount (mg) of flutoprazepam for assay taken

Dissolution <*6.10*> When the test is performed at 50 revolutions per minute according to the Paddle method, using 900 mL of water as the dissolution medium, the dissolution rate in 90 minutes of Flutoprazepam Tablets is not less than 70%.

Start the test with 1 tablet of Flutoprazepam Tablets, withdraw not less than 20 mL of the medium at the specified minute after starting the test, and filter through a membrane filter with a pore size not exceeding 0.45 μm. Discard not less than 10 mL of the first filtrate, pipet V mL of the subsequent filtrate, add water to make exactly V' mL so that each mL contains about 2.2 μg of flutoprazepam ($C_{19}H_{16}ClFN_2O$), and use this solution as the sample solution. Separately, weigh accurately about 22 mg of flutoprazepam for assay, previously dried at 105°C for 2 hours, and dissolve in methanol to make exactly 100 mL. Pipet 1 mL of this solution, add water to make exactly 100 mL, and use this solution as the standard solution. Perform the test with exactly 20 μL each of the sample solution and standard solution as directed under Liquid Chromatography <*2.01*> according to the following conditions, and determine the peak areas, A_T and A_S, of flutoprazepam in each solution.

Dissolution rate (%) with respect to the labeled amount of flutoprazepam ($C_{19}H_{16}ClFN_2O$)
$= M_S \times A_T/A_S \times V'/V \times 1/C \times 9$

M_S: Amount (mg) of flutoprazepam for assay taken
C: Labeled amount (mg) of flutoprazepam ($C_{19}H_{16}ClFN_2O$) in 1 tablet

Operating conditions—

Proceed as directed in the operating conditions in the Assay.

System suitability—

System performance: When the procedure is run with 20 μL of the standard solution under the above operating conditions, the number of theoretical plates and the symmetry factor of the peak of flutoprazepam are not less than 4000 and not more than 1.5, respectively.

System repeatability: When the test is repeated 6 times with 20 μL of the standard solution under the above operating conditions, the relative standard deviation of the peak area of flutoprazepam is not more than 1.0%.

Assay Weigh accurately not less than 20 Flutoprazepam Tablets, and powder. Weigh accurately a portion of the powder, equivalent to about 2 mg of flutoprazepam ($C_{19}H_{16}ClFN_2O$), add 60 mL of the mobile phase, shake for 15 minutes, and add the mobile phase to make exactly 100 mL. Filter this solution through a membrane filter with a pore size not exceeding 0.45 μm. Discard the first 5 mL of the filtrate, and use the subsequent filtrate as the sample solution. Separately, weigh accurately about 20 mg of flutoprazepam for assay, previously dried at 105°C for 2 hours, and dissolve in the mobile phase to make exactly 100 mL. Pipet 2 mL of this solution, add the mobile phase to make exactly 20 mL, and use this solution as the standard solution. Perform the test with exactly 20 μL each of the sample solution and standard solution as directed under Liquid Chromatography <*2.01*> according to the following conditions, and determine the peak areas, A_T and A_S, of flutoprazepam in each solution.

Amount (mg) of flutoprazepam ($C_{19}H_{16}ClFN_2O$)
$= M_S \times A_T/A_S \times 1/10$

M_S: Amount (mg) of flutoprazepam for assay taken

Operating conditions—

Detector: An ultraviolet absorption photometer (wavelength: 230 nm).

Column: A stainless steel column 4.6 mm in inside diameter and 15 cm in length, packed with octadecylsilanized silica gel for liquid chromatography (5 μm in particle diameter).

Column temperature: A constant temperature of about 40°C.

Mobile phase: A mixture of methanol and water (3:1).

Flow rate: Adjust so that the retention time of flutoprazepam is about 5 minutes.

System suitability—

System performance: When the procedure is run with 20 μL of the standard solution under the above operating conditions, the number of theoretical plates and the symmetry factor of the peak of flutoprazepam are not less than 4000 and not more than 1.5, respectively.

System repeatability: When the test is repeated 6 times with 20 μL of the standard solution under the above operating conditions, the relative standard deviation of the peak area of flutoprazepam is not more than 1.0%.

Containers and storage Containers—Well-closed containers.

Fluvoxamine Maleate

フルボキサミンマレイン酸塩

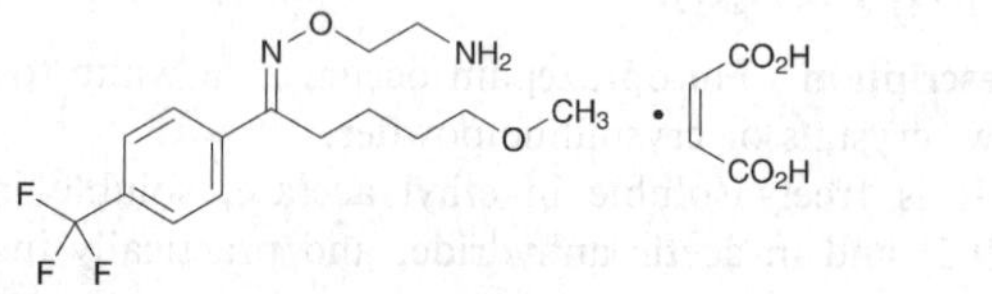

$C_{15}H_{21}F_3N_2O_2.C_4H_4O_4$: 434.41
5-Methoxy-1-[4-(trifluoromethyl)phenyl]pentan-1-one (*E*)-*O*-(2-aminoethyl)oxime monomaleate
[*61718-82-9*]

Fluvoxamine Maleate contains not less than 98.0% and not more than 101.0% of fluvoxamine maleate ($C_{15}H_{21}F_3N_2O_2.C_4H_4O_4$), calculated on the dried basis.

Description Fluvoxamine Maleate occurs as a white crystalline powder.

It is freely soluble in ethanol (99.5), and sparingly soluble in water.

Identification **(1)** Dissolve 10 mg of Fluvoxamine Maleate in 5 mL of water, neutralize with dilute sodium hydroxide TS, then add 1 mL of ninhydrin TS, and heat in a water bath at 60 – 70°C for 5 minutes: a blue-purple color develops.

(2) Determine the absorption spectrum of a solution of Fluvoxamine Maleate (1 in 50,000) as directed under Ultraviolet-visible Spectrophotometry <*2.24*>, and compare the spectrum with the Reference Spectrum or the spectrum of a solution of Fluvoxamine Maleate RS prepared in the same manner as the sample solution: both spectra exhibit similar intensities of absorption at the same wavelengths.

(3) Determine the infrared absorption spectrum of Fluvoxamine Maleate as directed in the potassium bromide disk method under Infrared Spectrophotometry <*2.25*>, and compare the spectrum with the Reference Spectrum or the spectrum of Fluvoxamine Maleate RS: both spectra exhibit similar intensities of absorption at the same wave numbers.

(4) To 5 mL of a solution of Fluvoxamine Maleate (1 in 500) add 1 drop of potassium permanganate TS: the red color of the TS disappears immediately.

Melting point <*2.60*> 120 – 124°C

Purity **(1)** Clarity and color of solution—A solution obtained by dissolving 0.5 g of Fluvoxamine Maleate in 50 mL of water is clear and colorless.

(2) Chloride <*1.03*>—Perform the test with 1.0 g of Fluvoxamine Maleate. Prepare the control solution with 0.25 mL of 0.01 mol/L hydrochloric acid VS (not more than 0.009%).

(3) Sulfate <*1.14*>—Perform the test with 1.0 g of Fluvoxamine Maleate. Prepare the control solution with 0.35 mL of 0.005 mol/L sulfuric acid VS (not more than 0.017%).

(4) Heavy metals <*1.07*>—Proceed with 1.0 g of Fluvoxamine Maleate according to Method 2, using alumina ceramic crucible, and perform the test. Prepare the control solution with 2.0 mL of Standard Lead Solution (not more than 20 ppm).

(5) Related substances—Dissolve 20 mg of Fluvoxamine Maleate in 20 mL of a mixture of methanol for liquid chromatography and water (7:3), and use this solution as the sample solution. Pipet 1 mL of the sample solution, add a mixture of methanol for liquid chromatography and water (7:3) to make exactly 100 mL, and use this solution as the standard solution. Perform the test with exactly 10 μL each of the sample solution and standard solution as directed under Liquid Chromatography <*2.01*> according to the following conditions, and determine each peak area by the automatic integration method: the areas of the peaks, having the relative retention time of about 0.76, about 0.82, about 0.89, about 1.58 and about 1.66 to fluvoxamine, obtained from the sample solution are not larger than 1/5 times, 3/10 times, 7/10 times, 1/10 times and 1/10 times the peak area of fluvoxamine from the standard solution, respectively, and the total area of the peaks other than fluvoxamine from the sample solution is not larger than 1.5 times the peak area of fluvoxamine from the standard solution. For the areas of the peaks, having the relative retention times of about 0.76, about 0.89, about 1.58 and about 1.66 to fluvoxamine, multiply their correction factors, 0.87, 2.00, 0.67 and 2.76, respectively.

Operating conditions—

Detector: An ultraviolet absorption photometer (wavelength: 254 nm).

Column: A stainless steel column 4.6 mm in inside diameter and 25 cm in length, packed with octylsilanized silica gel for liquid chromatography (5 μm in particle diameter).

Column temperature: A constant temperature of about 25°C.

Mobile phase: Dissolve 12.67 g of diammonium hydrogen phosphate and 0.85 g of sodium 1-heptanesulfonate in 900 mL of water, adjust to pH 2.0 with phosphoric acid, and add water to make 1000 mL. To 300 mL of this solution add 700 mL of methanol for liquid chromatography.

Flow rate: Adjust so that the retention time of fluvoxamine is about 9 minutes.

Time span of measurement: About 2 times as long as the retention time of fluvoxamine, beginning after the peak of maleic acid.

System suitability—

Test for required detectability: Pipet 1 mL of the standard solution, add a mixture of methanol for liquid chromatography and water (7:3) to make exactly 20 mL. Confirm that the peak area of fluvoxamine obtained with 10 μL of this solution is equivalent to 3.5 to 6.5% of that with 10 μL of the standard solution.

System performance: When the procedure is run with 10 μL of the standard solution under the above operating conditions, the number of theoretical plates and the symmetry factor of the peak of fluvoxamine are not less than 5000 and not more than 2.0, respectively.

System repeatability: When the test is repeated 6 times with 10 μL of the standard solution under the above operating conditions, the relative standard deviation of the peak area of fluvoxamine is not more than 2.0%.

Loss on drying <*2.41*> Not more than 0.1% (1 g, in vacuum, 50°C, 4 hours).

Residue on ignition <*2.44*> Not more than 0.1% (1 g, platinum crucible).

Assay Weigh accurately about 20 mg each of Fluvoxamine Maleate and Fluvoxamine Maleate RS (separately determine the loss on drying <*2.41*> under the same condition as Fluvoxamine Maleate), dissolve each in 10 mL of the mobile phase, add exactly 5 mL of the internal standard solution, then add the mobile phase to make 100 mL, and use these solutions as the sample solution and the standard solution, respectively. Perform the test with 20 μL each of the sample solution and standard solution as directed under Liquid Chromatography <*2.01*> according to the following conditions, and calculate the ratios, Q_T and Q_S, of the peak area of fluvoxamine to that of the internal standard.

$$\text{Amount (mg) of fluvoxamine maleate } (C_{15}H_{21}F_3N_2O_2.C_4H_4O_4) = M_S \times Q_T/Q_S$$

M_S: Amount (mg) of Fluvoxamine Maleate RS taken, calculated on the dried basis

*Internal standard solution—*A solution of diphenylamine in methanol (7 in 2000).

Operating conditions—

Detector: An ultraviolet absorption photometer (wavelength: 254 nm).

Column: A stainless steel column 4.6 mm in inside diameter and 25 cm in length, packed with octylsilanized silica gel for liquid chromatography (5 μm in particle diameter).

Column temperature: A constant temperature of about 25°C.

Mobile phase: Dissolve 3.8 g of diammonium hydrogen phosphate and 0.8 g of sodium 1-heptanesulfonate in water to make 300 mL, add 700 mL of methanol, and adjust to pH 3.5 with phosphoric acid.

Flow rate: Adjust so that the retention time of fluvoxamine is about 9 minutes.

System suitability—

System performance: When the procedure is run with 20 μL of the standard solution under the above operating conditions, fluvoxamine and the internal standard are eluted in this order with the resolution between these peaks being not less than 8.

System repeatability: When the test is repeated 6 times

with 20 μL of the standard solution under the above operating conditions, the relative standard deviation of the ratio of the peak area of fluvoxamine to that of the internal standard is not more than 1.0%.

Containers and storage Containers—Well-closed containers.

Fluvoxamine Maleate Tablets

フルボキサミンマレイン酸塩錠

Fluvoxamine Maleate Tablets contain not less than 95.0% and not more than 105.0% of the labeled amount of fluvoxamine maleate ($C_{15}H_{21}F_3N_2O_2.C_4H_4O_4$: 434.41).

Method of preparation Prepare as directed under Tablets, with Fluvoxamine Maleate.

Identification Powder Fluvoxamine Maleate Tablets. To a portion of the powder, equivalent to 0.1 g of Fluvoxamine Maleate, add 50 mL of water, shake, then allow to stand, and filter the supernatant liquid through a membrane filter with a pore size not exceeding 0.45 μm. To 0.5 mL of the filtrate add 50 mL of water, and determine the absorption spectrum of this solution as directed under Ultraviolet-visible Spectrophotometry <2.24>: it exhibits a maximum between 243 nm and 247 nm.

Uniformity of dosage units <6.02> Perform the Mass variation test, or the Content uniformity test according to the following method: it meets the requirement.

To 1 tablet of Fluvoxamine Maleate Tablets add 4 mL of water, disintegrate the tablet by sonicating, add a mixture of methanol for liquid chromatography and water (7:3) to make exactly 50 mL, and filter. Pipet *V* mL of the filtrate, equivalent to about 6 mg of fluvoxamine maleate ($C_{15}H_{21}F_3N_2O_2.C_4H_4O_4$), add exactly 2 mL of the internal standard solution, then add a mixture of methanol for liquid chromatography and water (7:3) to make 50 mL, and use this solution as the sample solution. Then, proceed as directed in the Assay.

Amount (mg) of fluvoxamine maleate ($C_{15}H_{21}F_3N_2O_2.C_4H_4O_4$)
$= M_S \times Q_T/Q_S \times 6/V$

M_S: Amount (mg) of Fluvoxamine Maleate RS taken, calculated on the dried basis

Internal standard solution—A solution of diphenylamine in methanol for liquid chromatography (3 in 1000).

Dissolution <6.10> When the test is performed at 50 revolutions per minute according to the Paddle method, using 900 mL of water as the dissolution medium, the dissolution rate in 20 minutes of Fluvoxamine Maleate Tablets is not less than 80%.

Start the test with 1 tablet of Fluvoxamine Maleate Tablets, withdraw not less than 20 mL of the medium at the specified minute after starting the test, and filter through a membrane filter with a pore size not exceeding 0.45 μm. Discard not less than 10 mL of the first filtrate, pipet *V* mL of the subsequent filtrate, add water to make exactly *V′* mL so that each mL contains about 20 μg of fluvoxamine maleate ($C_{15}H_{21}F_3N_2O_2.C_4H_4O_4$), and use this solution as the sample solution. Separately, weigh accurately about 20 mg of Fluvoxamine Maleate RS (separately determine the loss on drying <2.41> under the same condition as Fluvoxamine Maleate), and dissolve in water to make exactly 100 mL. Pipet 5 mL of this solution, add water to make exactly 50 mL, and use this solution as the standard solution. Determine the absorbances, A_T and A_S, at 245 nm of the sample solution and standard solution as directed under Ultraviolet-visible Spectrophotometry <2.24>.

Dissolution rate (%) with respect to the labeled amount of fluvoxamine maleate ($C_{15}H_{21}F_3N_2O_2.C_4H_4O_4$)
$= M_S \times A_T/A_S \times V'/V \times 1/C \times 90$

M_S: Amount (mg) of Fluvoxamine Maleate RS taken, calculated on the dried basis
C: Labeled amount (mg) of fluvoxamine maleate ($C_{15}H_{21}F_3N_2O_2.C_4H_4O_4$) in 1 tablet

Assay To 10 Fluvoxamine Maleate Tablets add 20 mL of water, disintegrate the tablets by sonicating, then add a mixture of methanol for liquid chromatography and water (7:3) to make exactly 250 mL, and filter. Pipet *V* mL of the filtrate, equivalent to about 6 mg of fluvoxamine maleate ($C_{15}H_{21}F_3N_2O_2.C_4H_4O_4$), add exactly 2 mL of the internal standard solution, then add a mixture of methanol for liquid chromatography and water (7:3) to make 50 mL, and use this solution as the sample solution. Separately, weigh accurately about 50 mg of Fluvoxamine Maleate RS (separately determine the loss on drying <2.41> under the same condition as Fluvoxamine Maleate), and dissolve in a mixture of methanol for liquid chromatography and water (7:3) to make exactly 25 mL. Pipet 3 mL of this solution, add exactly 2 mL of the internal standard solution, then add a mixture of methanol for liquid chromatography and water (7:3) to make exactly 50 mL, and use this solution as the standard solution. Perform the test with 20 μL each of the sample solution and standard solution as directed under Liquid Chromatography <2.01> according to the following conditions, and calculate the ratios, Q_T and Q_S, of the peak area of fluvoxamine to that of the internal standard.

Amount (mg) of fluvoxamine maleate ($C_{15}H_{21}F_3N_2O_2.C_4H_4O_4$) in 1 tablet
$= M_S \times Q_T/Q_S \times 3/V$

M_S: Amount (mg) of Fluvoxamine Maleate RS taken, calculated on the dried basis

Internal standard solution—A solution of diphenylamine in methanol for liquid chromatography (3 in 1000).

Operating conditions—

Proceed as directed in the operating conditions in the Assay under Fluvoxamine Maleate.

System suitability—

System performance: When the procedure is run with 20 μL of the standard solution under the above operating conditions, fluvoxamine and the internal standard are eluted in this order with the resolution between these peaks being not less than 8.

System repeatability: When the test is repeated 6 times with 20 μL of the standard solution under the above operating conditions, the relative standard deviation of the ratio of the peak area of fluvoxamine to that of the internal standard is not more than 1.0%.

Containers and storage Containers—Tight containers.

Folic Acid

葉酸

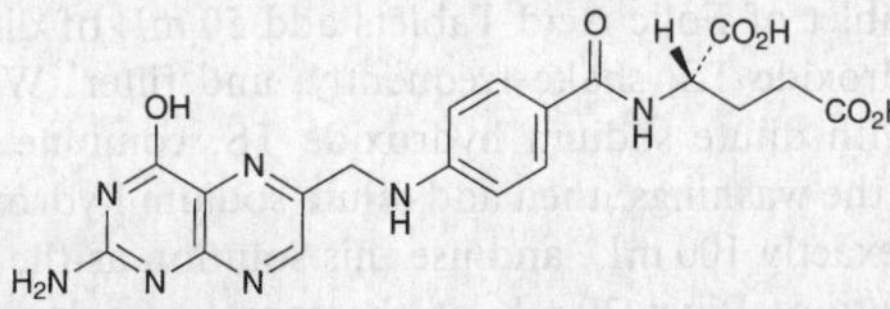

$C_{19}H_{19}N_7O_6$: 441.40
N-{4-[(2-Amino-4-hydroxypteridin-6-ylmethyl)amino]benzoyl}-L-glutamic acid
[*59-30-3*]

Folic Acid contains not less than 98.0% and not more than 102.0% of folic acid ($C_{19}H_{19}N_7O_6$), calculated on the anhydrous basis.

Description Folic Acid occurs as a yellow to orange-yellow crystalline powder. It is odorless.

It is practically insoluble in water, in methanol, in ethanol (95), in pyridine and in diethyl ether.

It dissolves in hydrochloric acid, in sulfuric acid, in dilute sodium hydroxide TS and in a solution of sodium carbonate decahydrate (1 in 100), and these solutions are yellow in color.

It is slowly affected by light.

Identification **(1)** Dissolve 1.5 mg of Folic Acid in dilute sodium hydroxide TS to make 100 mL. Determine the absorption spectrum of the solution as directed under Ultraviolet-visible Spectrophotometry <*2.24*>, and compare the spectrum with the Reference Spectrum or the spectrum of a solution of Folic Acid RS prepared in the same manner as the sample solution: both spectra exhibit similar intensities of absorption at the same wavelengths.

(2) To 10 mL of the solution obtained in (1) add 1 drop of potassium permanganate TS, and mix well until the color changes to blue, and immediately observe under ultraviolet light (main wavelength: 365 nm): a blue fluorescence is produced.

Purity **(1)** Clarity and color of solution—Dissolve 0.10 g of Folic Acid in 10 mL of dilute sodium hydroxide TS : the solution is clear and yellow in color.

(2) Free amines—Pipet 30 mL of the sample solution obtained in the Assay, add 20 mL of dilute hydrochloric acid and water to make exactly 100 mL, and use this solution as the sample solution. Separately, weigh accurately about 50 mg of *p*-Aminobenzoyl Glutamic Acid for Purity RS, previously dried in a desiccator (in vacuum, silica gel) for 4 hours, dissolve in diluted ethanol (2 in 5) to make exactly 100 mL. Pipet 3 mL of this solution, add water to make exactly 1000 mL, and use this solution as the standard solution. Pipet 4 mL each of the sample solution and standard solution, proceed as directed in the Assay, and perform the test as directed under Ultraviolet-visible Spectrophotometry <*2.24*>. Determine the absorbances, A_T and A_S, of subsequent solutions of the sample solution and standard solution at 550 nm: the content of free amines is not more than 1.0%.

$$\text{Content (\%) of free amines} = M_S/M_T \times A_T/A_S$$

M_S: Amount (mg) of *p*-Aminobenzoyl Glutamic Acid for Purity RS taken
M_T: Amount (mg) of Folic Acid taken, calculated on the anhydrous basis

Water <*2.48*> Not more than 8.5% (10 mg, coulometric titration).

Residue on ignition <*2.44*> Not more than 0.5% (1 g).

Assay Weigh accurately about 50 mg each of Folic Acid and Folic Acid RS (separately, determine the water <*2.48*> in the same manner as Folic Acid). To each add 50 mL of dilute sodium hydroxide TS, mix well to dissolve, add dilute sodium hydroxide TS to make exactly 100 mL, and use these solutions as the sample solution and standard solution. To 30 mL each of these solutions, accurately measured, add 20 mL of dilute hydrochloric acid and water to make exactly 100 mL. Pipet 60 mL each of these solutions add 0.5 g of zinc powder, and allow to stand with frequent shaking for 20 minutes. Filter each mixture through a dry filter paper, and discard the first 10 mL of the filtrate. Pipet 10 mL each of the subsequent filtrate, and add water to make exactly 100 mL. To 4 mL each of solutions, accurately measured, add 1 mL of water, 1 mL of dilute hydrochloric acid and 1 mL of a solution of sodium nitrite (1 in 1000), mix well, and allow to stand for 2 minutes. To each solution add 1 mL of a solution of ammonium amidosulfate (1 in 200), mix thoroughly, and allow to stand for 2 minutes. To each of these solutions, add 1 mL of a solution of *N*-(1-naphthyl)-*N'*-diethylethylenediamine oxalate (1 in 1000), shake, allow to stand for 10 minutes, and add water to make exactly 20 mL. Separately, to 30 mL of the sample solution, accurately measured, add 20 mL of dilute hydrochloric acid and water to make exactly 100 mL. Pipet 10 mL of this solution, add 18 mL of dilute hydrochloric acid and water to make exactly 100 mL. Pipet 4 mL of this solution, and prepare the blank solution in the same manner as the sample solution. Perform the test with these solutions as directed under Ultraviolet-visible Spectrophotometry <*2.24*>, using a solution prepared with 4 mL of water in the same manner as a blank. Determine the absorbances, A_T, A_S and A_C, of the subsequent solution of the sample solution, the standard solution and the blank solution at 550 nm.

$$\text{Amount (mg) of folic acid } (C_{19}H_{19}N_7O_6) = M_S \times (A_T - A_C)/A_S$$

M_S: Amount (mg) of Folic Acid RS taken, calculated on the anhydrous basis

Containers and storage Containers—Tight containers.
Storage—Light-resistant.

Folic Acid Injection

葉酸注射液

Folic Acid Injection is an aqueous injection.

It contains not less than 95.0% and not more than 115.0% of the labeled amount of folic acid ($C_{19}H_{19}N_7O_6$: 441.40).

Method of preparation Dissolve Folic Acid in water with the aid of Sodium Hydroxide or Sodium Carbonate, and prepare as directed under Injections.

Description Folic Acid Injection is a yellow to orange-yellow, clear liquid.

pH: 8.0 – 11.0

Identification **(1)** To a volume of Folic Acid Injection, equivalent to 1.5 mg of Folic Acid, add dilute sodium hydroxide TS to make 100 mL. Proceed as directed in the Identification (2) under Folic Acid, using this solution as the sample solution.

(2) Determine the absorption spectrum of the sample solution obtained in (1) as directed under Ultraviolet-visible Spectrophotometry <2.24>: it exhibits maxima between 255 nm and 257 nm, between 281 nm and 285 nm and between 361 nm and 369 nm. Separately, determine the maximal absorbances of the sample solution, A_1 and A_2, between 255 nm and 257 nm and between 361 nm and 369 nm, respectively: the ratio of A_1/A_2 is between 2.80 and 3.00.

(3) Folic Acid Injection responds to Qualitative Tests <1.09> (1) for sodium salt.

Extractable volume <6.05> It meets the requirement.

Foreign insoluble matter <6.06> Perform the test according to Method 1: it meets the requirement.

Insoluble particulate matter <6.07> It meets the requirement.

Sterility <4.06> Perform the test according to the Membrane filtration method: it meets the requirement.

Assay To an exactly measured volume of Folic Acid Injection, equivalent to about 50 mg of folic acid ($C_{19}H_{19}N_7O_6$) add dilute sodium hydroxide TS to make exactly 100 mL, and use this solution as the sample solution. Separately, weigh accurately about 50 mg of Folic Acid RS (separately, determine the water <2.48> in the same manner as Folic Acid), dissolve in dilute sodium hydroxide TS to make exactly 100 mL, and use this solution as the standard solution. Proceed with exactly 30 mL each of the sample solution and standard solution as directed in the Assay under Folic Acid.

$$\text{Amount (mg) of folic acid } (C_{19}H_{19}N_7O_6) = M_S \times (A_T - A_C)/A_S$$

M_S: Amount (mg) of Folic Acid RS taken, calculated on the anhydrous basis

Containers and storage Containers—Hermetic containers, and colored containers may be used.

Storage—Light-resistant.

Folic Acid Tablets

葉酸錠

Folic Acid Tablets contain not less than 90.0% and not more than 115.0% of the labeled amount of folic acid ($C_{19}H_{19}N_7O_6$: 441.40).

Method of preparation Prepare as directed under Tablets, with Folic Acid.

Identification **(1)** Take a quantity of powdered Folic Acid Tablets, equivalent to 1.5 mg of Folic Acid, add 100 mL of dilute sodium hydroxide TS, shake, and filter. Discard the first 10 mL of the filtrate, use the subsequent filtrate as the sample solution, and proceed as directed in the Identification (2) under Folic Acid.

(2) Determine the absorption spectrum of the filtrate obtained in (1) as directed under Ultraviolet-visible Spectrophotometry <2.24>: it exhibits maxima between 255 nm and 257 nm, between 281 nm and 285 nm and between 361 nm and 369 nm. Separately, determine the maximal absorbances of the filtrate, A_1 and A_2, between 255 nm and 257 nm and between 361 nm and 369 nm, respectively: the ratio of A_1/A_2 is between 2.80 and 3.00.

Uniformity of dosage units <6.02> Perform the test according to the following method: it meets the requirement of the Content uniformity test.

To 1 tablet of Folic Acid Tablets add 50 mL of dilute sodium hydroxide TS, shake frequently, and filter. Wash the residue with dilute sodium hydroxide TS, combine the filtrate and the washings, then add dilute sodium hydroxide TS to make exactly 100 mL, and use this solution as the sample stock solution. Pipet 30 mL of the sample stock solution, add 20 mL of dilute hydrochloric acid and water to make exactly 100 mL. Pipet 60 mL of this solution, add 0.5 g of zinc powder, shake frequently, allow to stand for 20 minutes, and filter the solution through a dried filter paper. Discard the first 10 mL of the filtrate, pipet V mL of the subsequent filtrate, add water to make exactly V' mL so that each mL contains about 15 μg of folic acid ($C_{19}H_{19}N_7O_6$), and use this solution as the sample solution. Separately, weigh accurately about 50 mg of Folic Acid RS (separately determine the water <2.48> in the same manner as Folic Acid), and dissolve in dilute sodium hydroxide TS to make exactly 100 mL. Pipet 30 mL of this solutions, add 20 mL of dilute hydrochloric acid and water to make exactly 100 mL. Pipet 60 mL of this solution, add 0.5 g of zinc powder, shake frequently, allow to stand for 20 minutes, and filter the solution through a dried filter paper. Discard the first 10 mL of the filtrate, pipet 10 mL of the subsequent filtrate, add water to make exactly 100 mL, and use this solution as the standard solution. Pipet 4 mL each of the sample solution and standard solution, add 1 mL of water, 1 mL of dilute hydrochloric acid and 1 mL of sodium nitrite solution (1 in 1000) to them, mix, and allow to stand for 2 minutes. To these solutions add 1 mL of a solution of ammonium amidosulfate (1 in 200), shake, and allow them to stand for 2 minutes. To these solutions add 1 mL of a solution of *N,N*-diethyl-*N'*-1-naphthylethylenediamine oxalate (1 in 1000), shake, allow to stand for 10 minutes, and add water to make exactly 20 mL. Separately, pipet 30 mL of the sample stock solution, add 20 mL of dilute hydrochloric acid, and add water to make exactly 100 mL. Pipet V mL of this solution, and add water to make exactly V' mL so that each mL contains about 15 μg of folic acid ($C_{19}H_{19}N_7O_6$). With exactly 4 mL of this solution perform the same procedure described above for obtaining the sample solution, and use the solution so obtained as the blank solution. Determine the absorbances at 550 nm, A_T, A_S and A_C, of the solutions obtained from the sample solution and standard solution, and the blank solution as directed under Ultraviolet-visible Spectrophotometry <2.24>, using a control solution obtained with 4 mL of water in the same manner as described above.

$$\text{Amount (mg) of folic acid } (C_{19}H_{19}N_7O_6) = M_S \times (A_T - A_C)/A_S \times V'/V \times 1/10$$

M_S: Amount (mg) of Folic Acid RS taken, calculated on the anhydrous basis

Dissolution <6.10> When the test is performed at 50 revolutions per minute according to the Paddle method, using 900 mL of water as the dissolution medium, the dissolution rate in 45 minutes of Folic Acid Tablets is not less than 75%.

Start the test with 1 tablet of Folic Acid Tablets, withdraw not less than 20 mL of the medium at the specified minute after starting the test, and filter through a membrane filter with a pore size not exceeding 0.45 μm. Discard not less than 10 mL of the first filtrate, pipet V mL of the subsequent filtrate, add water to make exactly V' mL so that each mL contains about 5.6 μg of folic acid ($C_{19}H_{19}N_7O_6$), and use this solution as the sample solution. Separately, weigh accurately about 20 mg of Folic Acid RS (separately determine the water <*2.48*> in the same manner as Folic Acid), and dissolve in the 2nd fluid for dissolution test to make exactly 100 mL. Pipet 2.5 mL of this solution, add the 2nd fluid for dissolution test to make exactly 100 mL, and use this solution as the standard solution. Determine the absorbances, A_T and A_S, at 280 nm of the sample solution and standard solution as directed under Ultraviolet-visible Spectrophotometry <*2.24*>, using water as the blank.

Dissolution rate (%) with respect to the labeled amount of folic acid ($C_{19}H_{19}N_7O_6$)
$= M_S \times A_T/A_S \times V'/V \times 1/C \times 45/2$

M_S: Amount (mg) of Folic Acid RS taken, calculated on the anhydrous basis
C: Labeled amount (mg) of folic acid ($C_{19}H_{19}N_7O_6$) in 1 tablet

Assay Weigh accurately and powder not less than 20 Folic Acid Tablets. Weigh accurately a portion of the powder, equivalent to about 50 mg of folic acid ($C_{19}H_{19}N_7O_6$). Add 50 mL of dilute sodium hydroxide TS, shake frequently, then filter into a 100-mL volumetric flask, and wash with dilute sodium hydroxide TS. To the combined filtrate and washings add dilute sodium hydroxide TS to make exactly 100 mL, and use this solution as the sample solution. Separately, weigh accurately about 50 mg of Folic Acid RS (separately, determine the water <*2.48*> in the same manner as Folic Acid), dissolve in dilute sodium hydroxide TS to make exactly 100 mL, and use this solution as the standard solution. Proceed with exactly 30 mL each of the sample solution and standard solution as directed in the Assay under Folic Acid.

Amount (mg) of folic acid ($C_{19}H_{19}N_7O_6$)
$= M_S \times (A_T - A_C)/A_S$

M_S: Amount (mg) of Folic Acid RS taken, calculated on the anhydrous basis

Containers and storage Containers—Well-closed containers.
Storage—Light-resistant.

Formalin

ホルマリン

Formalin contains not less than 35.0% and not more than 38.0% of formaldehyde (CH_2O: 30.03.)
It contains 5% to 13% of methanol to prevent polymerization.

Description Formalin is a clear, colorless liquid. Its vapor is irritating to the mucous membrane.
It is miscible with water and with ethanol (95).
When stored for a long time, especially in a cold place, it may become cloudy.

Identification **(1)** Dilute 2 mL of Formalin with 10 mL of water in a test tube, and add 1 mL of silver nitrate-ammonia TS: a gray precipitate is produced, or a silver mirror is formed on the wall of the test tube.
(2) To 5 mL of sulfuric acid in which 0.1 g of salicylic acid has been dissolved add 2 drops of Formalin, and warm the solution: a persistent, dark red color develops.

Purity Acidity—Dilute 20 mL of Formalin with 20 mL of water, and add 5.0 mL of 0.1 mol/L sodium hydroxide VS and 2 drops of bromothymol blue TS: a blue color develops.

Residue on ignition <*2.44*> Not more than 0.06 w/v% (5 mL, after evaporation).

Assay Weigh accurately a weighing bottle containing 5 mL of water, add about 1 g of Formalin, and weigh accurately again. Add water to make exactly 100 mL. Pipet 10 mL of this solution, add exactly 50 mL of 0.05 mol/L iodine VS and 20 mL of potassium hydroxide TS, and allow to stand for 15 minutes at an ordinary temperature. To this mixture add 15 mL of dilute sulfuric acid, and titrate <*2.50*> the excess iodine with 0.1 mol/L sodium thiosulfate VS (indicator: 1 mL of starch TS). Perform a blank determination in the same manner.

Each mL of 0.05 mol/L iodine VS = 1.501 mg of CH_2O

Containers and storage Containers—Tight containers.
Storage—Light-resistant.

Formalin Water

ホルマリン水

Formalin Water contains not less than 0.9 w/v% and not more than 1.1 w/v% of formaldehyde (CH_2O: 30.03).

Method of preparation

Formalin	30 mL
Water, Purified Water or Purified Water in Containers	a sufficient quantity
To make	1000 mL

Prepare by mixing the above ingredients.

Description Formalin Water is a clear, colorless liquid. It has a slight odor of formaldehyde.
It is almost neutral.

Assay Transfer 20 mL of Formalin Water, measured exactly, to a 100-mL volumetric flask containing 2.5 mL of 1 mol/L sodium hydroxide VS, and add water to make 100 mL. Pipet 10 mL of this solution, and proceed as directed in the Assay under Formalin.

Each mL of 0.05 mol/L iodine VS = 1.501 mg of CH_2O

Containers and storage Containers—Tight containers.

Formoterol Fumarate Hydrate

ホルモテロールフマル酸塩水和物

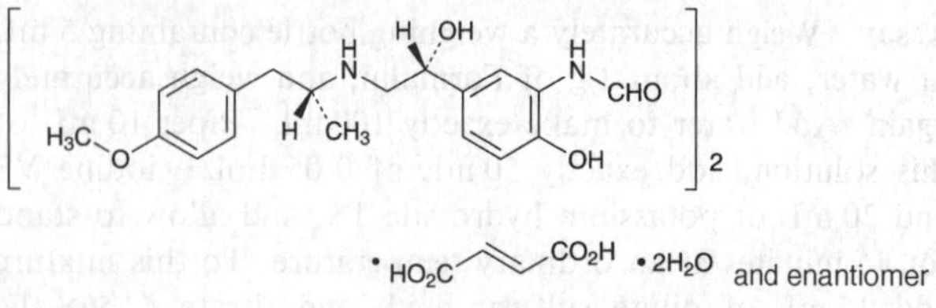

and enantiomer

$(C_{19}H_{24}N_2O_4)_2.C_4H_4O_4.2H_2O$: 840.91
N-(2-Hydroxy-5-{(1*RS*)-1-hydroxy-2-[(1*RS*)-2-(4-methoxyphenyl)-1-methylethylamino]ethyl}phenyl)formamide hemifumarate monohydrate
[*43229-80-7*, anhydride]

Formoterol Fumarate Hydrate contains not less than 98.5% of formoterol fumarate [$(C_{19}H_{24}N_2O_4)_2.C_4H_4O_4$: 804.88], calculated on the anhydrous basis.

Description Formoterol Fumarate Hydrate occurs as a white to yellowish white crystalline powder.

It is freely soluble in acetic acid (100), soluble in methanol, very slightly soluble in water and in ethanol (95), and practically insoluble in diethyl ether.

A solution of Formoterol Fumarate Hydrate in methanol (1 in 100) shows no optical rotation.

Melting point: about 138°C (with decomposition).

Identification **(1)** Dissolve 0.5 g of Formoterol Fumarate Hydrate in 20 mL of 0.5 mol/L sulfuric acid TS, and extract with three 25-mL portions of diethyl ether. Wash the combined diethyl ether extracts with 10 mL of 0.5 mol/L sulfuric acid TS, and evaporate the ether layer under reduced pressure, and dry the residue at 105°C for 3 hours: the residue melts *<2.60>* at about 290°C (with decomposition, in a sealed tube).

(2) Determine the absorption spectrum of a solution of Formoterol Fumarate Hydrate in methanol (1 in 40,000) as directed under Ultraviolet-visible Spectrophotometry *<2.24>*, and compare the spectrum with the Reference Spectrum: both spectra exhibit similar intensities of absorption at the same wavelengths.

(3) Determine the infrared absorption spectrum of Formoterol Fumarate Hydrate as directed in the potassium bromide disk method under Infrared Spectrophotometry *<2.25>*, and compare the spectrum with the Reference Spectrum: both spectra exhibit similar intensities of absorption at the same wave numbers.

Purity **(1)** Heavy metals *<1.07>*—Proceed with 1.0 g of Formoterol Fumarate Hydrate according to Method 2, and perform the test. Prepare the control solution with 2.0 mL of Standard Lead Solution (not more than 20 ppm).

(2) Related Substances—Dissolve 0.20 g of Formoterol Fumarate Hydrate in 10 mL of methanol, and use this solution as the sample solution. Pipet 1 mL of the sample solution, add methanol to make exactly 200 mL, and use this solution as the standard solution. Perform the test with these solutions as directed under Thin-layer Chromatography *<2.03>*. Spot 5 μL each of the sample solution and standard solution on a plate of silica gel for thin-layer chromatography. Develop the plate with a mixture of chloroform, 1,4-dioxane, ethanol (99.5) and ammonia solution (28) (20:20:10:3) to a distance of about 12 cm, and air-dry the plate. Allow the plate to stand for 5 minutes in iodine vapor: the spots other than the principal spot obtained from the sample solution are not more intense than the spot from the standard solution.

Water *<2.48>* 4.0 – 5.0% (0.5 g, volumetric titration, direct titration).

Residue on ignition *<2.44>* Not more than 0.1% (1 g).

Assay Weigh accurately about 0.7 g of Formoterol Fumarate Hydrate, dissolve in 50 mL of acetic acid (100), and titrate *<2.50>* with 0.1 mol/L perchloric acid VS (potentiometric titration). Perform a blank determination in the same manner, and make any necessary correction.

Each mL of 0.1 mol/L perchloric acid VS
= 40.24 mg of $(C_{19}H_{24}N_2O_4)_2.C_4H_4O_4$

Containers and storage Containers—Tight containers.

Fosfomycin Calcium Hydrate

ホスホマイシンカルシウム水和物

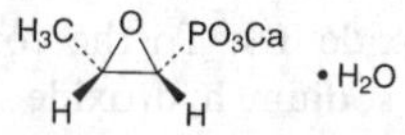

$C_3H_5CaO_4P.H_2O$: 194.14
Monocalcium (2*R*,3*S*)-3-methyloxiran-2-ylphosphonate monohydrate
[*26016-98-8*]

Fosfomycin Calcium Hydrate is the calcium salt of a substance having antibacterial actively produced by the growth of *Streptomyces fradiae* or by the chemical synthesis.

It contains not less than 725 μg (potency) and not more than 805 μg (potency) per mg, calculated on the anhydrous basis. The potency of Fosfomycin Calcium Hydrate is expressed as mass (potency) of fosfomycin ($C_3H_7O_4P$: 138.06).

Description Fosfomycin Calcium Hydrate occurs as a white crystalline powder.

It is slightly soluble in water, and practically insoluble in methanol and in ethanol (99.5).

Identification **(1)** Determine the infrared absorption spectrum of Fosfomycin Calcium Hydrate as directed in the potassium bromide disk method under Infrared Spectrophotometry *<2.25>*, and compare the spectrum with the Reference Spectrum: both spectra exhibit similar intensities of absorption at the same wave numbers.

(2) Determine the ^{1}H spectrum of a solution of Fosfomycin Calcium Hydrate in heavy water for nuclear magnetic resonance spectroscopy (1 in 300), using sodium 3-trimethylsilylpropanesulfonate for nuclear magnetic resonance spectroscopy as an internal reference compound, as directed under Nuclear Magnetic Resonance Spectroscopy *<2.21>*: it exhibits a double signal at around δ 1.5 ppm, a duple double signal at around δ 2.9 ppm, a multiple signal at around δ 3.3 ppm, and no signal at around δ 1.4 ppm.

(3) A solution of Fosfomycin Calcium Hydrate (1 in 500) responds to Qualitative Tests *<1.09>* (3) for calcium salt.

Optical rotation *<2.49>* $[\alpha]_D^{20}$: −2.5 – −5.4° (0.5 g calculated on the anhydrous bases, 0.4 mol/L disodium dihydrogen ethylenediamine tetraacetate TS (pH 8.5), 10 mL, 100 mm).

Phosphorus Content Weigh accurately about 0.1 g of Fosfomycin Calcium Hydrate, add 40 mL of sodium periodate (107 in 10,000) and 2 mL of perchloric acid, and heat in a water bath for 1 hour. After cooling, add water to make exactly 200 mL. Pipet 10 mL of this solution, and add 1 mL of potassium iodide TS. To this solution add sodium thiosulfate TS until the solution is colorless, add water to make exactly 100 mL, and use this solution as the sample stock solution. Separately, weigh accurately about 70 mg of potassium dihydrogen phosphate, proceed with this solution in the same manner as directed for the preparation of the sample stock solution, and use the solution so obtained as the standard stock solution. Proceed and prepare a solution in the same manner for the preparation of the sample stock solution without using Fosfomycin Calcium Hydrate, and use the solution so obtained as the blank stock solution. Pipet 5 mL each of the sample stock solution, the standard stock solution, and the blank stock solution, add 2.5 mL of ammonium molybdate-sulfuric acid TS and 1 mL of 1-amino-2-naphthol-4-sulfonic acid TS, mix, and add water to make exactly 25 mL, and use these solutions as the sample solution, the standard solution, and the blank solution, respectively. After allowing these solutions to stand at 20 ± 1°C for 30 minutes, perform the test with these solutions as directed under Ultraviolet-visible Spectrophotometry <2.24>, using water as a blank, and determine the absorbances at 740 nm, A_T, A_S and A_B, of the sample solution, the standard solution and the blank solution: the content of phosphorus is 15.2 – 16.7%.

$$\text{Amount (mg) of phosphorus (P)} = M_S \times (A_T - A_B)/(A_S - A_B) \times 0.228$$

M_S: Amount (mg) of potassium dihydrogen phosphate taken

Calcium Content Weigh accurately about 0.2 g of Fosfomycin Calcium Hydrate, add 4 mL of 1 mol/L Hydrochloric acid TS, and shake well until the sample is completely dissolved. To this solution add 100 mL of water, 9 mL of sodium hydroxide TS and 0.1 g of methylthymol blue-sodium chloride indicator, and titrate <2.50> with 0.05 mol/L disodium dihydrogen ethylenediamine tetraacetate VS until the color of the solution changes from clear blue to gray or gray-purple: calcium content is 19.6 – 21.7%. Perform a blank determination in the same manner, and make any necessary correction.

Each mL of 0.05 mol/L disodium dihydrogen ethylenediamine tetraacetate VS = 2.004 mg of Ca

Purity (1) Heavy metals <1.07>—To 1.0 g of Fosfomycin Calcium Hydrate add 40 mL of 0.25 mol/L acetic acid TS and water to make 50 mL. Proceed with this solution according to Method 1, and perform the test. Prepare the control solution with 2.0 mL of Standard Lead Solution (not more than 20 ppm).

(2) Arsenic <1.11>—Prepare the test solution with 1.0 g of Fosfomycin Calcium Hydrate according to Method 3, and perform the test (not more than 2 ppm).

(3) Glycol substance—Weigh accurately about 0.2 g of Fosfomycin Calcium Hydrate, transfer into a 250-mL iodine flask, add 100 mL of water, and dissolve by sonicating while cooling in ice. Add exactly 50 mL of phthalate buffer solution (pH 5.8) and exactly 5 mL of sodium periodate solution (107 in 100,000), stopper, stir, and add 1 mL of water in the receiving part. Avoid exposure to light, allow to stand in a water bath at 30°C for 60 minutes, add exactly 10 mL of a solution of potassium iodide (2 in 5) without haste, and titrate <2.50> with 0.01 mol/L sodium thiosulfate VS (indicator: 2 mL of starch TS). Perform a blank determination in the same manner, and make any necessary correction: amount of glycol substance ($C_3H_7CaO_5P$) is not more than 1.5%.

Each mL of 0.01 mol/L sodium thiosulfate VS = 0.4854 mg of $C_3H_7CaO_5P$

Water <2.48> Not more than 12.0% (0.1 g, volumetric titration, direct titration. Use a mixture of formamide for water determination and methanol for water determination (2:1) instead of methanol for water determination).

Assay Perform the test according to the Cylinder-plate method as directed under Microbial Assay for Antibiotics <4.02> according to the following conditions.

(i) Test organism—*Proteus* sp. (MB838)

(ii) Culture medium—Dissolve 5.0 g of peptone, 3.0 g of meat extract, 2.0 g of yeast extract, and 15 g of agar in 1000 mL of water, sterilize, and use as the agar media for base layer and seed layer with the pH of between 6.5 and 6.6 after sterilization.

(iii) Seeded agar layer—Incubate the test organism on the slant of the agar medium for transferring test organisms at 37°C for 40 – 48 hours. Subcultures at least 3 times. Inoculate the grown organisms onto the surface of 300 mL of the agar medium for transferring test organisms in a Roux bottle, incubate at 37°C for 40 – 48 hours, and suspend the grown organisms in about 30 mL of water. To the suspension add water, and use this as the stock suspension of test organism. The amount of the water to be added is adjust so that the percent transmission at 560 nm of the suspension diluted ten times with water is 17%. Keep the stock suspension at 10°C or below and use within 7 days. Add 1.0 – 2.0 mL of the stock suspension of test organism to 100 mL of the agar medium for seed layer previously kept at 48°C, mix thoroughly, and use this as the deeded agar layer.

(iv) Standard solutions—Weigh accurately an amount of Fosfomycin Phenethylammonium RS equivalent to about 20 mg (potency), dissolve in 0.05 mol/L tris buffer solution (pH 7.0) to make exactly 50 mL, and use this solution as the standard stock solution. Keep the standard stock solution at 5°C or below and use within 7 days. Take exactly a suitable amount of the standard stock solution before use, add 0.05 mol/L tris buffer solution (pH 7.0) to make solutions so that each mL contains 10 μg (potency) and 5 μg (potency), and use these solutions as the high concentration standard solution and the low concentration standard solution, respectively.

(v) Sample solutions—Weigh accurately an amount of Fosfomycin Calcium Hydrate equivalent to about 20 mg (potency), and dissolve in 0.05 mol/L tris buffer solution (pH 7.0) to make exactly 50 mL. To exactly a suitable amount of this solution add 0.05 mol/L tris buffer solution (pH 7.0) to make solutions so that each mL contains 10 μg (potency) and 5 μg (potency), and use these solutions as the high concentration sample solution and the low concentration sample solution, respectively.

Containers and storage Containers—Tight containers.

Fosfomycin Calcium for Syrup

シロップ用ホスホマイシンカルシウム

Fosfomycin Calcium for Syrup is a preparation for syrups which is suspended before use.

It contains not less than 90.0% and not more than 110.0% of the labeled potency of fosfomycin ($C_3H_7O_4P$: 138.06).

Method of preparation Prepare as directed under Syrups, with Fosfomycin Calcium Hydrate.

Identification **(1)** To an amount of Fosfomycin Calcium for Syrup, equivalent to 40 mg (potency) of Fosfomycin Calcium Hydrate, add 10 mL of warm water, shake for 10 to 20 minutes, and collect the insoluble substances by filtration. Dissolve the substances in 3 mL of a solution of perchloric acid (1 in 4), add 1 mL of 0.1 mol/L sodium periodate solution, and warm in a water bath at 60°C for 30 minutes. After cooling, add 50 mL of water, neutralize the solution with a saturated solution of sodium hydrogen carbonate, and add 1 mL of potassium iodide TS: the solution does not show a red color.

(2) To an amount of Fosfomycin Calcium for Syrup, equivalent to 40 mg (potency) of Fosfomycin Calcium Hydrate, add 10 mL of warm water, shake for 10 to 20 minutes, and collect the insoluble substances by filtration. Dissolve the substances in 3 mL of a solution of perchloric acid (1 in 4), add 2 mL of 0.1 mol/L sodium periodate solution, and heat in a water bath for 10 minutes. After cooling, add 1 mL of hexaammonium heptamolybdate-sulfuric acid TS and 1 mL of 1-amino-2-naphthol-4-sulfonic acid TS, and allow to stand for 30 minutes: the solution shows a blue color.

(3) To an amount of Fosfomycin Calcium for Syrup, equivalent to 40 mg (potency) of Fosfomycin Calcium Hydrate, add 10 mL of warm water, shake for 10 to 20 minutes, and collect the insoluble substances by filtration. Dissolve the substances in 25 mL of water: the solution responds to Qualitative Tests <*1.09*> (3) for calcium salt.

Loss on drying <*2.41*> Not more than 3.0% (2 g, reduced pressure not exceeding 0.67 kPa, 60°C, 3 hours).

Uniformity of dosage units <*6.02*> Fosfomycin Calcium for Syrup in single-dose packages meets the requirement of the Mass variation test.

Dissolution <*6.10*> When the test is performed at 50 revolutions per minute according to the Paddle method, using 900 mL of water as the dissolution medium, the dissolution rate in 15 minutes of Fosfomycin Calcium for Syrup is not less than 80%.

Start the test with an accurately weighed amount of Fosfomycin Calcium for Syrup, equivalent to about 0.5 g (potency) of Fosfomycin Calcium Hydrate, withdraw not less than 20 mL of the medium at the specified minute after starting the test, and filter through a membrane filter with a pore size not exceeding 0.45 µm. Discard not less than 10 mL of the first filtrate, and use the subsequent filtrate as the sample solution. Separately, weigh accurately an amount of Fosfomycin Phenethylammonium RS, equivalent to about 28 mg (potency), dissolve in water to make exactly 50 mL, and use this solution as the standard solution. Perform the test with exactly 10 µL each of the sample solution and standard solution as directed under Liquid Chromatography <*2.01*> according to the following conditions, and determine the peak areas, A_T and A_S, of fosfomycin in each solution.

Dissolution rate (%) with respect to the labeled amount of fosfomycin ($C_3H_7O_4P$)

$$= M_S/M_T \times A_T/A_S \times 1/C \times 1800$$

M_S: Amount [mg (potency)] of Fosfomycin Phenethylammonium RS taken

M_T: Amount (g) of Fosfomycin Calcium for Syrup taken

C: Labeled amount [mg (potency)] of fosfomycin ($C_3H_7O_4P$) in 1 g

Operating conditions—

Detector: A conductivity detector.

Column: A polyetheretherketone column 4.6 mm in inside diameter and 7.5 cm in length, packed with quaternary ammonium group introducing hydrophilic vinyl polymer gel for liquid chromatography (6 µm in particle diameter).

Column temperature: A constant temperature of about 30°C.

Mobile phase: Dissolve 10.5 g of citric acid monohydrate in water to make 1000 mL. To 800 mL of this solution add 200 mL of acetonitrile.

Flow rate: Adjust so that the retention time of fosfomycin is about 8 minutes.

System suitability—

System performance: When the procedure is run with 10 µL of the standard solution under the above operating conditions, the number of theoretical plates and the symmetry factor of the peak of fosfomycin are not less than 2000 and not more than 2.0, respectively.

System repeatability: When the test is repeated 6 times with 10 µL of the standard solution under the above operating conditions, the relative standard deviation of the peak area of fosfomycin is not more than 2.0%.

Assay Perform the test according to the Cylinder-plate method as directed under Microbial Assay for Antibiotics <*4.02*> according to the following conditions.

(i) Test organism, culture medium, agar media for seed and base layer, and standard solutions—Proceed as directed in the Assay under Fosfomycin Calcium Hydrate.

(ii) Sample solutions—Weigh accurately an amount of Fosfomycin Calcium for Syrup, equivalent to about 0.1 g (potency) of Fosfomycin Calcium Hydrate, dissolve in 0.05 mol/L tris buffer solution (pH 7.0) to make exactly 200 mL. Take exactly a suitable amount of this solution, add exactly 0.05 mol/L tris buffer solution (pH 7.0) to make solutions so that each mL contains 10 µg (potency) and 5 µg (potency), and use these solutions as the high concentration sample solution and the low concentration sample solution, respectively.

Containers and storage Containers—Tight containers.

Fosfomycin Sodium

ホスホマイシンナトリウム

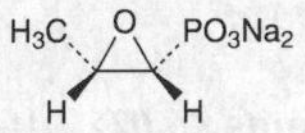

$C_3H_5Na_2O_4P$: 182.02
Disodium (2*R*,3*S*)-3-methyloxiran-2-ylphosphonate
[*26016-99-9*]

Fosfomycin Sodium is the sodium salt of a substance having antibacterial activity produced by the growth of *Streptomyces fradiae* or by the chemical synthesis.

It contains not less than 725 μg (potency) and not more than 770 μg (potency) per mg, calculated on the anhydrous basis. The potency of Fosfomycin Sodium is expressed as mass (potency) of fosfomycin ($C_3H_7O_4P$: 138.06).

Description Fosfomycin Sodium occurs as a white crystalline powder.

It is very soluble in water, sparingly soluble in methanol, and practically insoluble in ethanol (99.5).

Identification **(1)** Determine the infrared absorption spectrum of Fosfomycin Sodium as directed in the potassium bromide disk method under Infrared Spectrophotometry <*2.25*>, and compare the spectrum with the Reference Spectrum: both spectra exhibit similar intensities of absorption at the same wave numbers.

(2) Determine the ^1H spectrum of a solution of Fosfomycin Sodium in heavy water for nuclear magnetic resonance spectroscopy (1 in 300), using sodium 3-trimethylsilylpropanesulfonate for nuclear magnetic resonance spectroscopy as an internal reference compound, as directed under Nuclear Magnetic Resonance Spectroscopy <*2.21*>: it exhibits a double signal at around δ 1.5 ppm, a duple double signal at around δ 2.8 ppm, a multiple signal at around δ 3.3 ppm, and no signal at around δ 1.3 ppm.

(3) A solution of Fosfomycin Sodium (1 in 500) responds to Qualitative Tests <*1.09*> (1) for sodium salt.

Optical rotation <*2.49*> $[\alpha]_D^{20}$: −3.5 − −5.5° (0.5 g calculated on the anhydrous bases, water, 10 mL, 100 mm).

pH <*2.54*> Dissolve 0.70 g of Fosfomycin Sodium in 10 mL of water: the pH of the solution is between 8.5 and 10.5.

Phosphorus Content Weigh accurately about 0.1 g of Fosfomycin Sodium, add 40 mL of a solution of sodium periodate (107 in 10,000) and 2 mL of perchloric acid, and heat in a water bath for 1 hour. After cooling, add water to make exactly 200 mL. Pipet 10 mL of this solution, and add 1 mL of potassium iodide TS. To this solution add sodium thiosulfate TS until the solution is colorless, add water to make exactly 100 mL, and use this solution as the sample stock solution. Separately, weigh accurately about 70 mg of potassium dihydrogen phosphate, proceed with this solution in the same manner as directed for the preparation of the sample stock solution, and use the solution so obtained as the standard stock solution. Proceed and prepare a solution in the same manner for the preparation of the sample stock solution without using Fosfomycin Sodium, and use the solution so obtained as the blank stock solution. Pipet 5 mL each of the sample stock solution, the standard stock solution, and the blank stock solution, add 2.5 mL of ammonium molybdate-sulfuric acid TS and 1 mL of 1-amino-2-naphthol-4-sulfonic acid TS, mix, and add water to make exactly 25 mL, and use these solutions as the sample solution, the standard solution, and the blank solution, respectively. After allowing these solutions to stand for 30 minutes at 20 ± 1°C, perform the test with these solutions as directed under Ultraviolet-visible Spectrophotometry <*2.24*>, using water as a blank, and determine the absorbances at 740 nm, A_T, A_S and A_B, of the sample solution, the standard solution and the blank solution: the content of phosphorus is 16.2 − 17.9%.

$$\text{Amount (mg) of phosphorus (P)} = M \times (A_T - A_B)/(A_S - A_B) \times 0.228$$

M: Amount (mg) of potassium dihydrogen phosphate taken

Purity **(1)** Clarity and color of solution—Dissolve 1.0 g of Fosfomycin Sodium in 10 mL of water: the solution is clear and colorless.

(2) Heavy metals <*1.07*>—Proceed with 1.0 g of Fosfomycin Sodium according to Method 1, and perform the test. Prepare the control solution with 2.0 mL Standard Lead Solution (not more than 20 ppm).

(3) Arsenic <*1.11*>—Prepare the test solution with 1.0 g of Fosfomycin Sodium according to Method 3, and perform the test (not more than 2 ppm).

(4) Glycol substance—Weigh accurately about 0.2 g of Fosfomycin Sodium, and dissolve in 100 mL of water in a 250-mL iodine flask. Add exactly 50 mL of phthalate buffer solution (pH 5.8) and exactly 5 mL of sodium periodate solution (107 in 100,000), stopper, stir, and add 1 mL of water in the receiving part. Allow to stand in a dark place for 90 minutes, add exactly 10 mL of a solution of potassium iodide (2 in 5) without haste, and titrate <*2.50*> with 0.01 mol/L sodium thiosulfate VS (indicator: 2 mL of starch TS). Perform a blank determination in the same manner, and make any necessary correction: amount of glycol substance ($C_3H_7Na_2O_5P$) is not more than 0.5%.

$$\text{Each mL of 0.01 mol/L sodium thiosulfate VS} = 0.5001 \text{ mg of } C_3H_7Na_2O_5P$$

Water <*2.48*> Not more than 3.0% (0.2 g, volumetric titration, direct titration).

Assay Perform the test according to the Cylinder-plate method as directed under Microbial Assay for Antibiotics <*4.02*> according to the following conditions.

(i) Test organism—*Proteus* sp. (MB838)

(ii) Culture medium—Mix 5.0 g of peptone, 3.0 g of meat extract, 2.0 g of yeast extract, and 15 g of agar in 1000 mL of water, sterilize, and use as the agar media for base layer and seed layer with the pH of between 6.5 and 6.6 after sterilization.

(iii) Seeded agar layer—Incubate the test organism on the slant of the agar medium for transferring test organisms at 37°C for 40 − 48 hours. Subcultures at least 3 times. Inoculate the grown organisms onto the surface of 300 mL of the agar medium for transferring test organisms in a Roux bottle, incubate at 37°C for 40 − 48 hours, and suspend the grown organisms in about 30 mL of water. To the suspension add water, and use this as the stock suspension of test organism. The amount of the water to be added is adjust so that the percent transmission at 560 nm of the suspension diluted ten times with water is 17%. Keep the stock suspension at 10°C or below and use within 7 days. Add 1.0 − 2.0 mL of the stock suspension of test organism to 100 mL of the agar medium for seed layer previously kept at 48°C, mix thoroughly, and use this as the deeded agar layer.

(iv) Standard solutions—Weigh accurately an amount of Fosfomycin Phenethylammonium RS equivalent to about 20 mg (potency), dissolve in 0.05 mol/L tris buffer solution (pH 7.0) to make exactly 50 mL, and use this solution as the standard stock solution. Keep the standard stock solution at 5°C or below and use within 7 days. Take exactly a suitable amount of the standard stock solution before use, add 0.05 mol/L tris buffer solution (pH 7.0) to make solutions so that each mL contains 10 μg (potency) and 5 μg (potency), and use these solutions as the high concentration standard solution and the low concentration standard solution, respectively.

(v) Sample solutions—Weigh accurately an amount of Fosfomycin Sodium equivalent to about 20 mg (potency), and dissolve in 0.05 mol/L tris buffer solution (pH 7.0) to make exactly 50 mL. To exactly a suitable amount of this solution add 0.05 mol/L tris buffer solution (pH 7.0) to make solutions so that each mL contains 10 μg (potency) and 5 μg (potency), and use these solutions as the high concentration sample solution and the low concentration sample solution, respectively.

Containers and storage Containers—Hermetic containers.

Fosfomycin Sodium for Injection

注射用ホスホマイシンナトリウム

Fosfomycin Sodium for Injection is a preparation for injection which is dissolved before use.

It contains not less than 90.0% and not more than 110.0% of the labeled potency of fosfomycin ($C_3H_7O_4P$: 138.06).

Method of preparation Prepare as directed under Injections, with Fosfomycin Sodium.

Description Fosfomycin Sodium for Injection occurs as a white crystalline powder.

Identification **(1)** Dissolve about 0.1 g of Fosfomycin Sodium for Injection in 3 mL of a solution of perchloric acid (1 in 4), add 1 mL of 0.1 mol/L sodium periodate solution, and heat in a water bath at 60°C for 30 minutes. After cooling, add 50 mL of water, neutralize with saturated sodium hydrogen carbonate solution, and add 1 mL of potassium iodide TS; the solution does not reveal a red color, while the blank solution reveals a red color.

(2) To 2 mL of a solution of Fosfomycin Sodium for Injection (1 in 250) add 1 mL of perchloric acid and 2 mL of 0.1 mol/L sodium periodate solution, and heat in a water bath for 10 minutes. After cooling, add 1 mL of hexaammonium heptamolybdate-sulfuric acid TS and 1 mL of 1-amino-2-naphtol-4-sulfonic acid TS, and allow to stand for 30 minutes: a blue color develops.

(3) Dissolve an amount of Fosfomycin Sodium for Injection, equivalent to 0.1 g (potency) of Fosfomycin Sodium, in 50 mL of water. Perform the test with this solution as directed in the Identification (3) under Fosfomycin Sodium.

pH <*2.54*> The pH of a solution prepared by dissolving an amount of Fosfomycin Sodium for Injection, equivalent to 1.0 g (potency) of Fosfomycin Sodium, in 20 mL of water is between 6.5 and 8.5.

Purity Clarity and color of solution—Dissolve an amount of Fosfomycin Sodium for Injection, equivalent to 1.0 g (potency) of Fosfomycin Sodium, in 10 mL of water: the solution is clear and colorless.

Water <*2.48*> Not more than 4.0% (0.1 g, coulometric titration).

Bacterial endotoxins <*4.01*> Less than 0.025 EU/mg (potency).

Uniformity of dosage units <*6.02*> It meets the requirement of the Mass variation test.

Foreign insoluble matter <*6.06*> Perform the test according to the Method 2: it meets the requirement.

Insoluble particulate matter <*6.07*> It meets the requirement.

Sterility <*4.06*> Perform the test according to the Membrane filtration method: it meets the requirement.

Assay Perform the test according to the Cylinder-plate method as directed under Microbial Assay for Antibiotics <*4.02*> according to the following conditions.

(i) Test organism, culture medium, seeded agar layer, and standard solutions—Proceed as directed in the Assay under Fosfomycin Sodium.

(ii) Sample solutions—Weigh accurately the mass of the contents of not less than 10 Fosfomycin Sodium for Injection. Weigh accurately an amount of the content, equivalent to about 20 mg (potency) of Fosfomycin Sodium, and dissolve in 0.05 mol/L tris buffer solution (pH 7.0) to make exactly 50 mL. Take exactly a suitable amount of this solution, add 0.05 mol/L tris buffer solution (pH 7.0) to make solutions so that each mL contains 10 μg (potency) and 5 μg (potency), and use these solutions as the high concentration sample solution and the low concentration sample solution, respectively.

Containers and storage Containers—Hermetic containers. Plastic containers for aqueous injections may be used.

Fradiomycin Sulfate

Neomycin Sulfate

フラジオマイシン硫酸塩

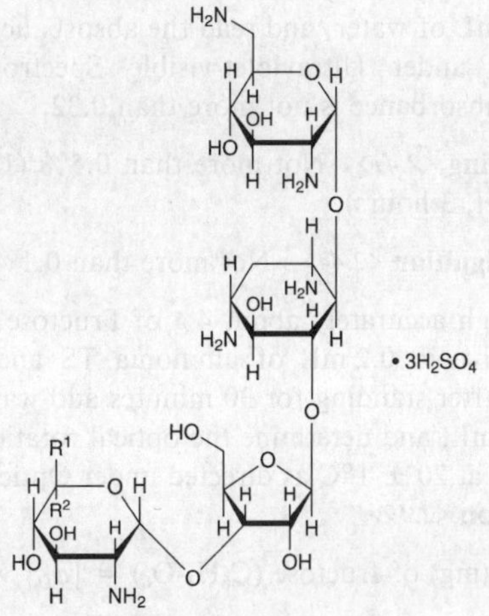

Fradiomycin B Sulfate : R^1=H R^2=CH_2NH_2

Fradiomycin C Sulfate : R^1=CH_2NH_2 R^2=H

$C_{23}H_{46}N_6O_{13}.3H_2SO_4$: 908.88

Fradiomycin B Sulfate

2,6-Diamino-2,6-dideoxy-*α*-D-glucopyranosyl-(1→4)-[2,6-diamino-2,6-dideoxy-*β*-L-idopyranosyl-(1→3)-*β*-D-ribofuranosyl-(1→5)]-2-deoxy-D-streptamine trisulfate

[*119-04-0*, Neomycin B]

Fradiomycin C Sulfate

2,6-Diamino-2,6-dideoxy-*α*-D-glucopyranosyl-(1→4)-[2,6-diamino-2,6-dideoxy-*α*-D-glucopyranosyl-(1→3)-*β*-D-ribofuranosyl-(1→5)]-2-deoxy-D-streptamine trisulfate

[*66-86-4*, Neomycin C]

[*1405-10-3*, Neomycin Sulfate]

Fradiomycin Sulfate is the sulfate of a mixture of aminoglycoside substances having antibacterial activity produced by the growth of *Streptomyces fradiae*.

It, when dried, contains not less than 623 μg (potency) and not more than 740 μg (potency) per mg. The potency of Fradiomycin Sulfate is expressed as mass (potency) of fradiomycin ($C_{23}H_{46}N_6O_{13}$: 614.64).

Description Fradiomycin Sulfate occurs as a white to light yellow powder.

It is freely soluble in water, and practically insoluble in ethanol (95).

It is hygroscopic.

Identification **(1)** Dissolve 50 mg each of Fradiomycin Sulfate and Fradiomycin Sulfate RS in 1 mL of water, and use these solutions as the sample solution and the standard solution. Perform the test with these solutions as directed under Thin-layer Chromatography <*2.03*>. Spot 2 μL each of the sample solution and standard solution on a plate of silica gel for thin-layer chromatography. Develop the plate with a mixture of methanol, ammonia solution (28) and dichloromethane (3:2:1) to a distance of about 10 cm, and air-dry the plate. Spray evenly a solution of ninhydrin in acetone (1 in 50) on the plate, and heat at 110°C for 15 minutes: the principal spot obtained from the sample solution and the spot from the standard solution show the same *R*f value.

(2) A solution of Fradiomycin Sulfate (1 in 20) responds to Qualitative Tests <*1.09*> (1) for sulfate.

Optical rotation <*2.49*> $[\alpha]_D^{20}$: +53.5 – +59.0° (1 g calculated on the dried basis, water, 10 mL, 100 mm).

pH <*2.54*> The pH of a solution obtained by dissolving 1.0 g of Fradiomycin Sulfate in 10 mL of water is between 5.0 and 7.5.

Purity **(1)** Heavy metals <*1.07*>—Proceed with 1.0 g of Fradiomycin Sulfate according to Method 2, and perform the test. Prepare the control solution with 2.0 mL of Standard Lead Solution (not more than 20 ppm).

(2) Arsenic <*1.11*>—Prepare the test solution with 1.0 g of Fradiomycin Sulfate according to Method 1, and perform the test (not more than 2 ppm).

(3) Related substances—Dissolve 0.63 g of Fradiomycin Sulfate in 5 mL of water, and use this solution as the sample solution. Pipet 1 mL of the sample solution, add water to make exactly 50 mL, and use this solution as the standard solution. Perform the test with these solutions as directed under Thin-layer Chromatography <*2.03*>. Spot 1 μL each of the sample solution and standard solution on a plate of silica gel for thin-layer chromatography. Develop the plate with a mixture of methanol, ammonia solution (28) and dichloromethane (3:2:1) to a distance of about 10 cm, and air-dry the plate. Spray evenly a solution of ninhydrin in acetone (1 in 50) on the plate, and heat the plate at 110°C for 15 minutes: the spot at around *R*f value 0.4 obtained from the sample solution is not more intense than the spot from the standard solution.

Loss on drying <*2.41*> Not more than 8.0% (0.2 g, in vacuum, 60°C, 3 hours).

Residue on ignition <*2.44*> Not more than 0.3% (1 g).

Assay Perform the test according to the Cylinder-plate method as directed under Microbial Assay for Antibiotics <*4.02*> according to the following conditions.

(i) Test organism—*Staphylococcus aureus* ATCC 6538 P

(ii) Agar medium for seed and base layer

Glucose	1.0 g
Peptone	6.0 g
Meat extract	1.5 g
Yeast extract	3.0 g
Sodium chloride	2.5 g
Agar	15.0 g
Water	1000 mL

Mix all the ingredients and sterilize. Adjust the pH after sterilization to 7.8 – 8.0 with sodium hydroxide TS.

(iii) Standard solutions—Weigh accurately an amount of Fradiomycin Sulfate RS, previously dried, equivalent to about 50 mg (potency), dissolve in 0.1 mol/L phosphate buffer solution for antibiotics (pH 8.0) to make exactly 50 mL, and use this solution as the standard stock solution. Keep the standard stock solution at 5°C or below and use within 14 days. Take exactly a suitable amount of the standard stock solution before use, add 0.1 mol/L phosphate buffer solution for antibiotics (pH 8.0) to make solutions so that each mL contains 80 μg (potency) and 20 μg (potency), and use these solutions as the high concentration standard solution and the low concentration standard solution, respectively.

(iv) Sample solutions—Weigh accurately an amount of Fradiomycin Sulfate, previously dried, equivalent to about 50 mg (potency), dissolve in 0.1 mol/L phosphate buffer solution for antibiotics (pH 8.0) to make exactly 50 mL. Take exactly a suitable amount of this solution, add 0.1 mol/L phosphate buffer solution for antibiotics (pH 8.0) to make solutions so that each mL contains 80 μg (potency) and 20 μg (potency), and use these solutions as the high concentration sample solution and the low concentration sample solution, respectively.

Containers and storage Containers—Tight containers.
Storage—Light-resistant.

Fructose

果糖

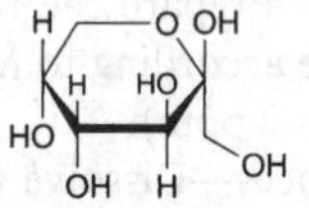

$C_6H_{12}O_6$: 180.16
β-D-Fructopyranose
[*57-48-7*]

Fructose, when dried, contains not less than 98.0% of fructose ($C_6H_{12}O_6$).

Description Fructose occurs as colorless to white, crystals or crystalline powder. It is odorless and has a sweet taste.

It is very soluble in water, sparingly soluble in ethanol (95) and practically insoluble in diethyl ether.

It is hygroscopic.

Identification **(1)** Add 2 to 3 drops of a solution of Fructose (1 in 20) to 5 mL of boiling Fehling's TS: a red precipitate is produced.

(2) Determine the infrared absorption spectrum of Fructose as directed in the paste method under Infrared Spectrophotometry 〈*2.25*〉, and compare the spectrum with the Reference Spectrum: both spectra exhibit similar intensities of absorption at the same wave numbers.

pH 〈*2.54*〉 Dissolve 4.0 g of Fructose in 20 mL of water: the pH of the solution is between 4.0 and 6.5.

Purity **(1)** Clarity and color of solution—Dissolve 25.0 g of Fructose in 50 mL of water: the solution is clear and has no more color than the following control solution.

Control solution: To a mixture of 1.0 mL of Cobalt (II) Chloride CS, 3.0 mL of Iron (III) Chloride CS and 2.0 mL of Copper (II) Sulfate CS, and add water to make 10.0 mL. To 3.0 mL of the solution add water to make 50 mL.

(2) Acidity—Dissolve 5.0 g of Fructose in 50 mL of freshly boiled and cooled water, and add 3 drops of phenolphthalein TS and 0.60 mL of 0.01 mol/L sodium hydroxide VS: a red color develops.

(3) Chloride 〈*1.03*〉—Perform the test with 2.0 g of Fructose. Prepare the control solution with 1.0 mL of 0.01 mol/L hydrochloric acid VS (not more than 0.018%).

(4) Sulfate 〈*1.14*〉—Perform the test with 2.0 g of Fructose. Prepare the control solution with 1.0 mL of 0.005 mol/L sulfuric acid VS (not more than 0.024%).

(5) Sulfite—Dissolve 0.5 g of Fructose in 5 mL of water, and add 0.25 mL of 0.02 mol/L iodine: the color of the solution is yellow.

(6) Heavy metals 〈*1.07*〉—Proceed with 5.0 g of Fructose according to Method 2, and perform the test. Prepare the control solution with 2.0 mL of Standard Lead Solution (not more than 4 ppm).

(7) Calcium—Dissolve 0.5 g of Fructose in 5 mL of water, add 2 to 3 drops of ammonia TS and 1 mL of ammonium oxalate TS, and allow to stand for 1 minute: the solution is clear.

(8) Arsenic 〈*1.11*〉—Dissolve 1.5 g of Fructose in 5 mL of water, heat with 5 mL of dilute sulfuric acid and 1 mL of bromine TS on a water bath for 5 minutes, concentrate to 5 mL, and cool. Perform the test with this solution as the test solution (not more than 1.3 ppm).

(9) 5-Hydroxymethylfurfurals—Dissolve 5.0 g of Fructose in 100 mL of water, and read the absorbance at 284 nm as directed under Ultraviolet-visible Spectrophotometry 〈*2.24*〉: the absorbance is not more than 0.32.

Loss on drying 〈*2.41*〉 Not more than 0.5% (1 g, in vacuum, silica gel, 3 hours).

Residue on ignition 〈*2.44*〉 Not more than 0.1% (1 g).

Assay Weigh accurately about 4 g of Fructose, previously dried, dissolve in 0.2 mL of ammonia TS and 80 mL of water, and after standing for 30 minutes add water to make exactly 100 mL, and determine the optical rotation, α_D, in a 100-mm cell at 20 ± 1°C as directed under Optical Rotation Determination 〈*2.49*〉.

$$\text{Amount (mg) of fructose } (C_6H_{12}O_6) = |\alpha_D| \times 1087.0$$

Containers and storage Containers—Tight containers.

Fructose Injection

果糖注射液

Fructose Injection is an aqueous injection.

It contains not less than 95.0% and not more than 105.0% of the labeled amount of fructose ($C_6H_{12}O_6$: 180.16).

Method of preparation Prepare as directed under Injections, with Fructose. No preservative is added.

Description Fructose Injection is a colorless to pale yellow, clear liquid. It has a sweet taste.

Identification **(1)** Take a volume of Fructose Injection, equivalent to 1 g of Fructose, dilute with water or concentrate on a water bath to 20 mL, if necessary, and use this solution as the sample solution. Add 2 to 3 drops of the sample solution to 5 mL of boiling Fehling's TS: a red precipitate is produced.

(2) To 10 mL of the sample solution obtained in (1) add 0.1 g of resorcinol and 1 mL of hydrochloric acid, and warm in a water bath for 3 minutes: a red color develops.

pH 〈*2.54*〉 3.0 – 6.5 In the case where the labeled concentration of the injection exceeds 5%, dilute to 5% with water before the test.

Purity **(1)** Heavy metals 〈*1.07*〉—Take a volume of Fructose Injection, equivalent to 5.0 g of Fructose, and evaporate on a water bath to dryness. With the residue, proceed according to Method 2, and perform the test. Prepare the control solution with 2.0 mL of Standard Lead Solution.

(2) Arsenic 〈*1.11*〉—Take a volume of Fructose Injection, equivalent to 1.5 g of Fructose, dilute with water or concentrate on a water bath to 5 mL, if necessary, and add 5 mL of dilute sulfuric acid and 1 mL of bromine TS. Proceed as directed in the purity (8) under Fructose.

Residue on ignition 〈*2.44*〉 Measure exactly a volume of Fructose Injection, equivalent to 2 g of Fructose, evaporate on a water bath to dryness, and perform the test: the residue weighs not more than 2 mg.

Bacterial endotoxins ⟨*4.01*⟩ Less than 0.5 EU/mL.

Extractable volume ⟨*6.05*⟩ It meets the requirement.

Foreign insoluble matter ⟨*6.06*⟩ Perform the test according to Method 1: it meets the requirement.

Insoluble particulate matter ⟨*6.07*⟩ It meets the requirement.

Sterility ⟨*4.06*⟩ Perform the test according to the Membrane filtration method: it meets the requirement.

Assay Measure exactly a volume of Fructose Injection, equivalent to about 4 g of fructose ($C_6H_{12}O_6$), add 0.2 mL of ammonia TS, dilute with water to make exactly 100 mL, shake well, and after allowing to stand for 30 minutes, determine the optical rotation, α_D, in a 100-mm cell at 20 ± 1°C as directed under Optical Rotation Determination ⟨*2.49*⟩.

$$\text{Amount (mg) of fructose } (C_6H_{12}O_6) = |\alpha_D| \times 1087.0$$

Containers and storage Containers—Hermetic containers. Plastic containers for aqueous injections may be used.

Fudosteine

フドステイン

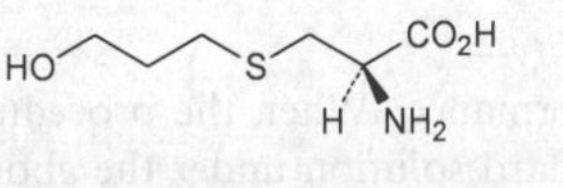

$C_6H_{13}NO_3S$: 179.24
(2*R*)-2-Amino-3-(3-hydroxypropylsulfanyl)propanoic acid
[*13189-98-5*]

Fudosteine, when dried, contains not less than 99.0% and not more than 101.0% of fudosteine ($C_6H_{13}NO_3S$).

Description Fudosteine occurs as white, crystals or crystal- [illegible] soluble in acetic acid [illegible]

Melting point: about 200°C (with decomposition).

Identification (1) To 5 mL of a solution of fudosteine (1 in 1000) add 2 mL of sodium hydroxide TS, shake well, add 0.3 mL of sodium pentacyanonitrosylferrate (III) TS, and shake well again. After allowing to stand at 40°C for 10 minutes, cool the solution in an ice bath for 2 minutes, add 2 mL of dilute hydrochloric acid, and shake: a red-orange color develops.

(2) Determine the infrared absorption spectrum of Fudosteine as directed in the potassium bromide disk method under Infrared Spectrophotometry ⟨*2.25*⟩, and compare the spectrum with the Reference Spectrum: both spectra exhibit similar intensities of absorption at the same wave numbers.

Optical rotation ⟨*2.49*⟩ $[\alpha]_D^{20}$: −7.4 − −8.9° (after drying, 1 g, 6 mol/L hydrochloric acid TS, 25 mL, 100 mm).

Purity (1) Chloride ⟨*1.03*⟩—Dissolve 0.20 g of Fudosteine in 10 mL of water and 20 mL of nitric acid, and add water to make 50 mL. Perform the test using this solution as the test solution. Prepare the control solution as follows: to 0.25 mL of 0.01 mol/L hydrochloric acid VS add 20 mL of nitric acid and water to make 50 mL (not more than 0.044%).

(2) Heavy metals ⟨*1.07*⟩—Proceed with 2.0 g of Fudosteine according to Method 2, and perform the test. Prepare the control solution with 2.0 mL of Standard Lead solution (not more than 10 ppm).

(3) Arsenic ⟨*1.11*⟩—Prepare the test solution with 2.0 g of Fudosteine according to Method 3, and perform the test (not more than 1 ppm).

(4) L-Cystine—Dissolve exactly 0.25 g of Fudosteine in the mobile phase to make exactly 50 mL, and use this solution as the sample solution. Separately, dissolve exactly 25 mg of L-cystine in 2 mL of 1 mol/L hydrochloric acid TS, then add the mobile phase to make exactly 50 mL. Pipet 2.5 mL of this solution, add the mobile phase to make exactly 50 mL, and use this solution as the standard solution. Perform the test with exactly 10 μL each of the sample solution and standard solution as directed under Liquid Chromatography ⟨*2.01*⟩ according to the following conditions. Determine each peak area by the automatic integration method: the peak area of L-cystine obtained from the sample solution is not larger than the peak area of L-cystine from the standard solution.

Operating conditions—

Detector: An ultraviolet absorption photometer (wavelength: 210 nm).

Column: A stainless steel column 4.6 mm in inside diameter and 15 cm in length, packed with octadecylsilanized silica gel for liquid chromatography (5 μm in particle diameter).

Column temperature: A constant temperature of about 50°C.

Mobile phase: A solution of sodium 1-hexanesulfonate in diluted phosphoric acid (1 in 1000) (1 in 1250).

Flow rate: Adjust so that the retention time of fudosteine is about 8 minutes.

System suitability—

System performance: Dissolve 25 mg of L-cystine in 2 mL of 1 mol/L hydrochloric acid TS, add 25 mg of Fudosteine, and add the mobile phase to make 50 mL. Take 2.5 mL of this solution, add the mobile phase to make 50 mL. When the procedure is run with 10 μL of this solution under the above operating conditions, L-cystine and fudosteine are eluted in this order with the resolution between these peaks being not less than 10.

System repeatability: When the test is repeated 6 times with 10 μL of the standard solution under the above operating conditions, the relative standard deviation of the peak area of L-cystine is not more than 2.0%.

(5) Related substances—Dissolve 0.25 g of Fudosteine in the mobile phase to make 50 mL, and use this solution as the sample solution. Pipet 2 mL of the sample solution, add the mobile phase to make exactly 100 mL, pipet 2.5 mL of this solution, add the mobile phase to make exactly 50 mL, and use this solution as the standard solution. Perform the test with exactly 10 μL each of the sample solution and standard solution as directed under Liquid Chromatography ⟨*2.01*⟩ according to the following conditions. Determine each peak area by the automatic integration method: the area of the peak other than fudosteine obtained from the sample solution is not larger than the peak area of fudosteine from the standard solution.

Operating conditions—

Detector: An ultraviolet absorption photometer (wavelength: 210 nm).

Column: A stainless steel column 4.6 mm in inside diameter and 25 cm in length, packed with octadecylsilanized silica gel for liquid chromatography (5 μm in particle diameter).

Column temperature: A constant temperature of about 55°C.

Mobile phase: Diluted phosphoric acid (1 in 1000).

Flow rate: Adjust so that the retention time of fudosteine is about 3 minutes.

Time span of measurement: About 10 times as long as the retention time of fudosteine, beginning after the peak of fudosteine.

System suitability—

System performance: When the procedure is run with 10 μL of the standard solution under the above operating conditions, the number of theoretical plates and the symmetry factor of the peak of fudosteine are not less than 5000 and not more than 1.5, respectively.

System repeatability: When the test is repeated 6 times with 10 μL of the standard solution under the above operating conditions, the relative standard deviation of the peak area of fudosteine is not more than 2.0%.

Loss on drying *<2.41>*—Not more than 0.5% (1 g, 105°C, 3 hours).

Residue on ignition *<2.44>*—Not more than 0.1% (1 g).

Assay Weigh accurately about 0.3 g of Fudosteine, previously dried, dissolve in 50 mL of acetic acid (100), and titrate *<2.50>* with 0.1 mol/L perchloric acid VS (potentiometric titration). Perform a blank determination in the same manner, and make any necessary correction.

Each mL of 0.1 mol/L perchloric acid VS
= 17.92 mg of $C_6H_{13}NO_3S$

Containers and storage Containers—Well-closed containers.

Fudosteine Tablets

フドステイン錠

Fudosteine Tablets contain not less than 95.0% and not more than 105.0% of the labeled amount of fudosteine ($C_6H_{13}NO_3S$: 179.24).

Method of preparation Prepare as directed under Tablets, with Fudosteine.

Identification Powder Fudostine Tablets. To a portion of the powder, equivalent to 88 mg of Fudosteine, add 10 mL of a mixture of water and methanol (1:1), shake, centrifuge, and use the supernatant liquid as the sample solution. Separately, dissolve 90 mg of fudosteine for assay in 10 mL of a mixture of water and methanol (1:1), and use this solution as the standard solution. Perform the test with these solutions as directed under Thin-layer Chromatography *<2.03>*. Spot 2.5 μL each of the sample solution and standard solution on a plate of silica gel for thin-layer chromatography. Develop the plate with a mixture of 1-butanol, water and acetic acid (100) (3:2:1) to a distance of about 10 cm, and air-dry the plate. Spray evenly a solution of ninhydrin in acetone (1 in 50) on the plate, and heat at 80°C for 5 minutes: the principal spot obtained from the sample solution and the spot from the standard solution show a red-purple color and have the same *R*f value.

Uniformity of dosage units *<6.02>* It meets the requirement of the Mass variation test.

Dissolution *<6.10>* When the test is performed at 75 revolutions per minute according to the Paddle method, using 900 mL of water as the dissolution medium, the dissolution rate in 20 minutes of Fudosteine Tablets is not less than 85%.

Start the test with 1 tablet of Fudosteine Tablets, withdraw not less than 20 mL of the medium at the specified minute after starting the test, and filter through a membrane filter with a pore size not exceeding 0.45 μm. Discard not less than 5 mL of the first filtrate, pipet *V* mL of the subsequent filtrate, add the mobile phase to make exactly *V′* mL so that each mL contains about 55.6 μg of fudosteine ($C_6H_{13}NO_3S$), and use this solution as the sample solution. Separately, weigh accurately about 50 mg of fudosteine for assay, previously dried at 105°C for 3 hours, dissolve in the mobile phase to make exactly 50 mL. Pipet 5 mL of this solution, add the mobile phase to make exactly 100 mL, and use this solution as the standard solution. Perform the test with exactly 20 μL each of the sample solution and standard solution as directed under Liquid Chromatography *<2.01>* according to the following conditions, and determine the peak areas, A_T and A_S, of fudosteine in each solution.

Dissolution rate (%) with respect to the labeled amount of fudosteine ($C_6H_{13}NO_3S$)
$= M_S \times A_T/A_S \times V'/V \times 1/C \times 90$

M_S: Amount (mg) of fudosteine for assay taken
C: Labeled amount (mg) of fudosteine ($C_6H_{13}NO_3S$) in 1 tablet

Operating conditions—

Proceed as directed in the operating conditions in the Assay.

System suitability—

System performance: When the procedure is run with 20 μL of the standard solution under the above operating conditions, the number of theoretical plates and the symmetry factor of the peak of fudosteine are not less than 5000 and not more than 1.5, respectively.

System repeatability: When the test is repeated 6 times with 20 μL of the standard solution under the above operating conditions, the relative standard deviation of the peak area of fudosteine is not more than 2.0%.

Assay Weigh accurately the mass of not less than 20 Fudosteine Tablets, and powder. Weigh accurately a portion of the powder, equivalent to about 0.5 g of fudosteine ($C_6H_{13}NO_3S$), add 70 mL of the mobile phase, shake vigorously for 15 minutes, add the mobile phase to make exactly 100 mL, and centrifuge. Pipet 10 mL of the supernatant liquid, and add the mobile phase to make exactly 50 mL. Pipet 5 mL of this solution, add exactly 5 mL of the internal standard solution, add the mobile phase to make 50 mL, and use this solution as the sample solution. Separately, weigh accurately about 50 mg of fudosteine for assay, previously dried at 105°C for 3 hours, and dissolve in the mobile phase to make exactly 50 mL. Pipet 5 mL of this solution, add exactly 5 mL of the internal standard solution, add the mobile phase to make 50 mL, and use this solution as the standard solution. Perform the test with 20 μL each of the sample solution and standard solution as directed under Liquid Chromatography *<2.01>* according to the following conditions, and calculate the ratios, Q_T and Q_S, of the peak area of fudosteine to that of the internal standard.

Amount (mg) of fudosteine ($C_6H_{13}NO_3S$)
$= M_S \times Q_T/Q_S \times 10$

M_S: Amount (mg) of fudosteine for assay taken

Internal standard solution—A solution of L-methionine in the mobile phase (1 in 1000).

Operating conditions—

Detector: An ultraviolet absorption photometer (wavelength: 210 nm).

Column: A stainless steel column 4.6 mm in inside diameter and 15 cm in length, packed with octadecylsilanized silica gel for liquid chromatography (5 μm in particle diameter).

Column temperature: A constant temperature of about 50°C.

Mobile phase: A solution of sodium 1-hexanesulfonate in diluted phosphoric acid (1 in 1000) (1 in 1250).

Flow rate: Adjust so that the retention time of fudosteine is about 8 minutes.

System suitability—

System performance: When the procedure is run with 20 μL of the standard solution under the above operating conditions, fudosteine and the internal standard are eluted in this order with the resolution between these peaks being not less than 12.

System repeatability: When the test is repeated 6 times with 20 μL of the standard solution under the above operating conditions, the relative standard deviation of the ratio of the peak area of fudosteine to that of the internal standard is not more than 1.0%.

Containers and storage containers—Tight containers.

Furosemide

フロセミド

$C_{12}H_{11}ClN_2O_5S$: 330.74

4-Chloro-2-[(furan-2-ylmethyl)amino]-5-sulfamoylbenzoic acid

[54-31-9]

Furosemide, when dried, contains not less than 98.0% and not more than 101.0% of furosemide ($C_{12}H_{11}ClN_2O_5S$).

Description Furosemide occurs as white, crystals or crystalline powder.

It is freely soluble in *N,N*-dimethylformamide, soluble in methanol, sparingly soluble in ethanol (99.5), slightly soluble in acetonitrile and in acetic acid (100), and practically insoluble in water.

It dissolves in dilute sodium hydroxide TS.

It is gradually colored by light.

Melting point: about 205°C (with decomposition).

Identification **(1)** Dissolve 25 mg of Furosemide in 10 mL of methanol. To 1 mL of this solution add 10 mL of 2 mol/L hydrochloric acid TS. Heat the solution under a reflux condenser on a water bath for 15 minutes, cool, and add 18 mL of sodium hydroxide TS to make weakly acidic: the solution responds to Qualitative Tests <*1.09*> for primary aromatic amines, producing a red to red-purple color.

(2) Determine the absorption spectrum of a solution of Furosemide in dilute sodium hydroxide TS (1 in 125,000) as directed under Ultraviolet-visible Spectrophotometry <*2.24*>, and compare the spectrum with the Reference Spectrum or the spectrum of a solution of Furosemide RS prepared in the same manner as the sample solution: both spectra exhibit similar intensities of absorption at the same wavelengths.

(3) Determine the infrared absorption spectrum of Furosemide as directed in the potassium bromide disk method under Infrared Spectrophotometry <*2.25*>, and compare the spectrum with the Reference Spectrum or the spectrum of Furosemide RS: both spectra exhibit similar intensities of absorption at the same wave numbers.

Purity **(1)** Clarity and color of solution—Dissolve 0.5 g of Furosemide in 10 mL of a solution of sodium hydroxide (1 in 50): the solution is clear and colorless.

(2) Chloride <*1.03*>—Dissolve 2.6 g of Furosemide in 90 mL of dilute sodium hydroxide TS, add 2 mL of nitric acid, and filter. To 25 mL of the filtrate add 6 mL of dilute nitric acid and water to make 50 mL, and perform the test using this solution as the test solution. Prepare the control solution as follows: To 0.40 mL of 0.01 mol/L hydrochloric acid VS add 6 mL of dilute nitric acid and water to make 50 mL (not more than 0.020%).

(3) Sulfate <*1.14*>—To 20 mL of the filtrate obtained in (2) add 1 mL of dilute hydrochloric acid and water to make 50 mL, and perform the test using this solution as the test solution. Prepare the control solution as follows: To 0.35 mL of 0.005 mol/L sulfuric acid VS add 1 mL of dilute hydrochloric acid and water to make 50 mL (not more than 0.030%).

(4) Heavy metals <*1.07*>—Proceed with 2.0 g of Furosemide according to Method 2, and perform the test. Prepare the control solution with 2.0 mL of Standard Lead Solution (not more than 10 ppm).

(5) Related substances—Dissolve 25 mg of Furosemide in 25 mL of the dissolving solution, and use this solution as the sample solution. Pipet 1 mL of the sample solution, add the dissolving solution to make exactly 200 mL, and use this solution as the standard solution. Perform the test with exactly 20 μL each of the sample solution and standard solution as directed under Liquid Chromatography <*2.01*> according to the following conditions, and determine each peak area by the automatic integration method: the area of each peak appeared ahead of the peak of furosemide obtained from sample solution is not larger than 2/5 times the peak area of furosemide from the standard solution, the area of each peak appeared behind the peak of furosemide is not larger than 1/4 times the peak area of furosemide from the standard solution, and the total area of these peaks is not larger than 2 times the peak area of furosemide from the standard solution.

Dissolving solution—To 22 mL of acetic acid (100) add a mixture of water and acetonitrile (1:1) to make 1000 mL.

Operating conditions—

Detector: An ultraviolet absorption photometer (wavelength: 272 nm).

Column: A stainless steel column 4.6 mm in inside diameter and 25 cm in length, packed with octadecylsilanized silica gel for liquid chromatography (5 μm in particle diameter).

Column temperature: A constant temperature of about 25°C.

Mobile phase: A mixture of water, tetrahydrofuran and acetic acid (100) (70:30:1).

Flow rate: Adjust so that the retention time of furosemide is about 18 minutes.

Time span of measurement: About 2.5 times as long as the retention time of furosemide, beginning after the solvent peak.

System suitability—

Test for required detectability: Measure exactly 2 mL of the standard solution, and add the dissolving solution to make exactly 50 mL. Confirm that the peak area of furosemide obtained with 20 μL of this solution is equivalent to 3.2 to 4.8% of that with 20 μL of the standard solution.

System performance: When the procedure is run with 20 μL of the standard solution under the above operating conditions, the number of theoretical plates and the symmetry factor of the peak of furosemide is not less than 7000 and not more than 1.5, respectively.

System repeatability: When the test is repeated 6 times with 20 μL of the standard solution under the above operating conditions, the relative standard deviation of the peak area of furosemide is not more than 2.0%.

Loss on drying <*2.41*> Not more than 0.5% (1 g, 105°C, 4 hours).

Residue on ignition <*2.44*> Not more than 0.1% (1 g).

Assay Weigh accurately about 0.5 g of Furosemide, previously dried, dissolve in 50 mL of *N*,*N*-dimethylformamide, and titrate <*2.50*> with 0.1 mol/L sodium hydroxide VS until the color of the solution changes from yellow to blue (indicator: 3 drops of bromothymol blue TS). Perform a blank determination with a mixture of 50 mL of *N*,*N*-dimethylformamide and 15 mL of water in the same manner, and make any necessary correction.

Each mL of 0.1 mol/L sodium hydroxide VS
= 33.07 mg of $C_{12}H_{11}ClN_2O_5S$

Containers and storage Containers—Tight containers.
Storage—Light-resistant.

Furosemide Injection

フロセミド注射液

Furosemide Injection is an aqueous injection.

It contains not less than 95.0% and not more than 105.0% of the labeled amount of furosemide ($C_{12}H_{11}ClN_2O_5S$: 330.74).

Method of preparation Prepare as directed under Injection, with Furosemide.

Description Furosemide Injection is a colorless, clear liquid.

Identification **(1)** To a volume of Furosemide Injection, equivalent to 2.5 mg of Furosemide, add 10 mL of 2 mol/L hydrochloric acid TS, heat under a reflux condenser on a water bath for 15 minutes. After cooling, render the solution slightly acid with 18 mL of sodium hydroxide TS: the solution responds to Qualitative Tests <*1.09*> for primary aromatic amines. The color of the solution is red to red-purple.

(2) To a volume of Furosemide Injection, equivalent to 20 mg of Furosemide, add water to make 100 mL. To 2 mL of this solution add 0.01 mol/L sodium hydroxide TS to make 50 mL. Determine the absorption spectrum of this solution as directed under Ultraviolet-visible Spectrophotometry <*2.24*>: it exhibits maxima between 227 nm and 231 nm, between 269 nm and 273 nm, and between 330 nm and 336 nm.

Osmotic pressure ratio Being specified separately when the drug is granted approval based on the Law.

pH Being specified separately when the drug is granted approval based on the Law.

Purity Pipet a volume of Furosemide Injection, equivalent to 40 mg of Furosemide, add 30 mL of acetone, shake well, and add acetone to make exactly 50 mL. Centrifuge this solution, to 1.0 mL of the supernatant liquid add 3.0 mL of water, cool in a ice bath, add 3.0 mL of dilute hydrochloric acid and 0.15 mL of sodium nitrite TS, shake, and allow to stand for 1 minute. To this solution add 1.0 mL of ammonium amidosulfate TS, shake well, allow to stand for 3 minutes, add 1.0 mL of *N*,*N*-diethyl-*N*′-1-naphtylethylenediamine oxalate TS, shake well, and allow to stand for 5 minutes. Determine the absorbance of this solution at 530 nm as directed under Ultraviolet-visible Spectrophotometry <*2.24*> using a solution, prepared in the same manner with 1.0 mL of acetone, as the blank: the absorbance is not more than 0.10.

Bacterial endotoxins <*4.01*> Less than 1.25 EU/mg.

Extractable volume <*6.05*> It meets the requirement.

Foreign insoluble matter <*6.06*> Perform the test according to Method 1: it meets the requirement.

Insoluble particulate matter <*6.07*> It meets the requirement.

Sterility <*4.06*> Perform the test according to the Membrane filtration method: it meets the requirement.

Assay To an exactly measured volume of Furosemide Injection, equivalent to about 20 mg of Furosemide ($C_{12}H_{11}ClN_2O_5S$), add water to make exactly 100 mL. Pipet 3 mL of this solution, add 0.01 mol/L sodium hydrochloride TS to make exactly 100 mL, and use this solution as the sample solution. Separately, weigh accurately about 20 mg of Furosemide RS, previously dried at 105°C for 4 hours, add 0.01 mol/L sodium hydroxide TS to make exactly 100 mL. Pipet 3 mL of this solution, add 0.01 mol/L sodium hydroxide TS to make exactly 100 mL, and use this solution as the standard solution. Perform the test with the sample solution and standard solution as directed under Ultraviolet-visible Spectrophotometry <*2.24*>, and determine the absorbances, A_T and A_S, at 271 nm.

Amount (mg) of furosemide ($C_{12}H_{11}ClN_2O_5S$)
$= M_S \times A_T/A_S$

M_S: Amount (mg) of Furosemide RS taken

Containers and storage Containers—Hermetic containers.
Storage—Light-resistant.

Furosemide Tablets

フロセミド錠

Furosemide Tablets contain not less than 95.0% and not more than 105.0% of the labeled amount of furosemide ($C_{12}H_{11}ClN_2O_5S$: 330.74).

Method of preparation Prepare as directed under Tablets, with Furosemide.

Identification **(1)** Shake well a quantity of powdered Furosemide Tablets, equivalent to 0.2 g of Furosemide, with 40 mL of acetone, and filter. To 0.5 mL of the filtrate add 10 mL of 2 mol/L hydrochloric acid TS, and heat under a reflux condenser on a water bath for 15 minutes. After cooling, add 18 mL of sodium hydroxide TS to make the solution slightly acidic: the solution responds to Qualitative Tests <*1.09*> for primary aromatic amines, producing a red to red-purple color.

(2) Determine the absorption spectrum of the sample solution obtained in the Assay as directed under Ultraviolet-visible Spectrophotometry <*2.24*>: it exhibits maxima between 227 nm and 231 nm, between 269 nm and 273 nm, and between 330 nm and 336 nm.

Purity To a quantity of powdered Furosemide Tablets, equivalent to 40 mg of Furosemide, add about 30 mL of acetone, shake well, and add acetone to make exactly 50 mL. Centrifuge the solution, add 3.0 mL of water to 1.0 mL of the supernatant liquid, cool in ice, add 3.0 mL of dilute hydrochloric acid and 0.15 mL of sodium nitrite TS, shake, and allow to stand for 1 minute. Add 1.0 mL of ammonium amidosulfate TS, shake well, allow to stand for 3 minutes, add 1.0 mL of *N*,*N*-diethyl-*N*′-1-naphthylethylenediamine oxalate TS, shake well, and allow to stand for 5 minutes. Perform the test with this solution as directed under Ultraviolet-visible Spectrophotometry <*2.24*>, using a solution prepared in the same manner with 1.0 mL of acetone as the blank: the absorbance at 530 nm is not more than 0.10.

Uniformity of dosage units <*6.02*> Perform the Mass variation test, or the Content uniformity test according to the following method: it meets the requirement.

To 1 tablet of Furosemide Tablets add a suitable amount of 0.05 mol/L sodium hydroxide TS, shake to disintegrate, then add 0.05 mol/L sodium hydroxide TS to make exactly *V* mL so that each mL contains about 0.4 mg of furosemide ($C_{12}H_{11}ClN_2O_5S$). Filter the solution, discard the first 10 mL of the filtrate, pipet 2 mL of the subsequent filtrate, add 0.05 mol/L sodium hydroxide TS to make exactly 100 mL, and use this solution as the sample solution. Proceed as directed in the Assay.

Amount (mg) of furosemide ($C_{12}H_{11}ClN_2O_5S$)
$= M_S \times A_T/A_S \times V/50$

M_S: Amount (mg) of Furosemide RS taken

Dissolution <*6.10*> When the test is performed at 50 revolutions per minute according to the Paddle method, using 900 mL of 2nd fluid for dissolution test as the dissolution medium, the dissolution rates of a 20-mg tablet in 15 minutes and a 40-mg tablet in 30 minutes are not less than 80%.

Start the test with 1 tablet of Furosemide Tablets, withdraw not less than 30 mL of the medium at the specified minute after starting the test, and filter through a membrane filter with a pore size not exceeding 0.45 μm. Discard not less than 10 mL of the first filtrate, pipet *V* mL of the subsequent filtrate, add the dissolution medium to make exactly *V*′ mL so that each mL contains about 10 μg of furosemide ($C_{12}H_{11}ClN_2O_5S$), and use this solution as the sample solution. Separately, weigh accurately about 20 mg of Furosemide RS, previously dried at 105°C for 4 hours, and dissolve in 5 mL of methanol, and add the dissolution medium to make exactly 100 mL. Pipet 5 mL of this solution, add the dissolution medium to make exactly 100 mL, and use this solution as the standard solution. Determine the absorbances, A_T and A_S, of the sample solution and standard solution at 277 nm as directed under Ultraviolet-visible Spectrophotometry <*2.24*>.

Dissolution rate (%) with respect to the labeled amount of furosemide ($C_{12}H_{11}ClN_2O_5S$)
$= M_S \times A_T/A_S \times V'/V \times 1/C \times 45$

M_S: Amount (mg) of Furosemide RS taken
C: Labeled amount (mg) of furosemide ($C_{12}H_{11}ClN_2O_5S$) in 1 tablet

Assay Weigh accurately the mass of not less than 20 Furosemide Tablets, and powder. Weigh accurately a portion of the powder, equivalent to about 40 mg of furosemide ($C_{12}H_{11}ClN_2O_5S$), add about 70 mL of 0.05 mol/L sodium hydroxide TS, shake well, and add 0.05 mol/L sodium hydroxide TS to make exactly 100 mL. Filter, discard the first 10 mL of the filtrate, pipet 2 mL of the subsequent filtrate, add 0.05 mol/L sodium hydroxide TS to make exactly 100 mL, and use this solution as the sample solution. Separately, weigh accurately about 20 mg of Furosemide RS, previously dried at 105°C for 4 hours, and dissolve in 0.05 mol/L sodium hydroxide TS to make exactly 50 mL. Pipet 2 mL of this solution, add 0.05 mol/L sodium hydroxide TS to make exactly 100 mL, and use this solution as the standard solution. Determine the absorbances, A_T and A_S, of the sample solution and standard solution at 271 nm as directed under the Ultraviolet-visible Spectrophotometry <*2.24*>.

Amount (mg) of furosemide ($C_{12}H_{11}ClN_2O_5S$)
$= M_S \times A_T/A_S \times 2$

M_S: Amount (mg) of Furosemide RS taken

Containers and storage Containers—Tight containers.
Storage—Light-resistant.

Fursultiamine Hydrochloride

フルスルチアミン塩酸塩

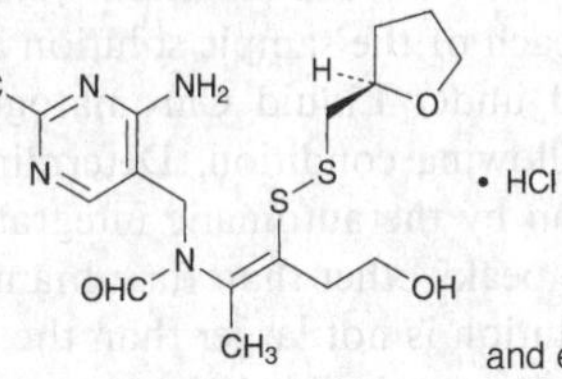

and enantiomer

$C_{17}H_{26}N_4O_3S_2.HCl$: 435.00
N-(4-Amino-2-methylpyrimidin-5-ylmethyl)-*N*-{(1*Z*)-4-hydroxy-1-methyl-2-[(2*RS*)-tetrahydrofuran-2-ylmethyldisulfanyl]but-1-en-1-yl}formamide monohydrochloride
[*804-30-8*, Fursultiamine]

Fursultiamine Hydrochloride contains not less than 98.5% of fursultiamine hydrochloride ($C_{17}H_{26}N_4O_3S_2.HCl$), calculated on the anhydrous basis.

Description Fursultiamine Hydrochloride occurs as white, crystals or crystalline powder. It is odorless or has a characteristic odor, and has a bitter taste.

It is freely soluble in water, in methanol and in ethanol (95).

It shows crystal polymorphism.

Identification **(1)** Dissolve 5 mg of Fursultiamine Hydrochloride in 6 mL of 0.1 mol/L hydrochloric acid TS, add 0.1 g of zinc powder, allow to stand for several minutes, and filter. To 3 mL of the filtrate, add 3 mL of sodium hydroxide TS and 0.5 mL of potassium hexacyanoferrate (III) TS, then add 5 mL of 2-methyl-1-propanol, shake vigorously for 2 minutes, allow to stand to separate the 2-methyl-1-propanol layer, and examine under ultraviolet light (main wavelength: 365 nm): the 2-methyl-1-propanol layer shows a blue-purple fluorescence. The fluorescence disappears by acidifying, and appears again by alkalifying.

(2) Determine the infrared absorption spectrum of Fursultiamine Hydrochloride, previously dried in a desiccator (in vacuum, phosphorus (V) oxide) for 24 hours, as directed in the potassium bromide disk method under Infrared Spectrophotometry <*2.25*>, and compare the spectrum with the Reference Spectrum or the spectrum of Fursultiamine Hydrochloride RS, previously dried in a desiccator (in vacuum, phosphorus (V) oxide) for 24 hours: both spectra exhibit similar intensities of absorption at the same wave numbers. If any differences appear, dissolve the Fursultiamine Hydrochloride in water, evaporate the water, and dry the residue in a desiccator (in vacuum, phosphorus (V) oxide) for 24 hours, and repeat the test.

(3) A solution of Fursultiamine Hydrochloride (1 in 50) responds to Qualitative Tests <*1.09*> (2) for chloride.

Purity **(1)** Clarity and color of solution—Dissolve 1.0 g of Fursultiamine Hydrochloride in 20 mL of water: the solution is clear and colorless.

(2) Sulfate <*1.14*>—Proceed with 1.5 g of Fursultiamine Hydrochloride, and perform the test. Prepare the control solution with 0.35 mL of 0.005 mol/L sulfuric acid VS (not more than 0.011%).

(3) Heavy metals <*1.07*>—Proceed with 1.0 g of Fursultiamine Hydrochloride according to Method 2, and perform the test. Prepare the control solution with 2.0 mL of Standard Lead Solution (not more than 20 ppm).

(4) Related substances—Dissolve 0.10 g of Fursultiamine Hydrochloride in 100 mL of the mobile phase, and use this solution as the sample solution. Pipet 1 mL of the sample solution, add the mobile phase to make exactly 100 mL, and use this solution as the standard solution. Perform the test with exactly 10 μL each of the sample solution and standard solution as directed under Liquid Chromatography <*2.01*> according to the following condition. Determine each peak area of each solution by the automatic integration method: the total area of the peaks other than fursultiamine obtained from the sample solution is not larger than the peak area of fursultiamine from the standard solution.

Operating conditions—

Detector, column, column temperature, mobile phase, flow rate, and selection of column: Proceed as directed in the operating conditions in the Assay.

Detection sensitivity: Adjust the detection sensitivity so that the peak height of fursultiamine from 10 μL of the standard solution is between 20 mm and 30 mm.

Time span of measurement: About 3 times as long as the retention time of fursultiamine.

Water <*2.48*> Not more than 5.0% (0.3 g, volumetric titration, direct titration).

Residue on ignition <*2.44*> Not more than 0.1% (1 g).

Assay Weigh accurately about 55 mg each of Fursultiamine Hydrochloride and Fursultiamine Hydrochloride RS (previously determined the water <*2.48*> in the same manner as Fursultiamine Hydrochiloride) and dissolve each in 50 mL of water, and add exactly 10 mL each of the internal standard solution, then add water to make exactly 100 mL. To 8 mL each of the solution add water to make 50 mL, and use these solutions as the sample solution and the standard solution, respectively. Perform the test with 10 μL each of the sample solution and standard solution as directed under Liquid Chromatography <*2.01*> according to the following conditions, and calculate the ratios, Q_T and Q_S, of the peak area of fursultiamine to that of the internal standard.

Amount (mg) of fursultiamine hydrochloride ($C_{17}H_{26}N_4O_3S_2.HCl$)
$= M_S \times Q_T/Q_S$

M_S: Amount (mg) of Fursultiamine Hydrochloride RS taken, calculated on the anhydrous basis

Internal standard solution—A solution of isopropyl 4-aminobenzoate in ethanol (95) (3 in 400).

Operating conditions—

Detector: An ultraviolet absorption photometer (wavelength: 254 nm).

Column: A stainless steel column about 4 mm in inside diameter and about 15 cm in length, packed with octadecylsilanized silica gel for liquid chromatography (5 μm in particle diameter).

Column temperature: A constant temperature of about 50°C.

Mobile phase: Dissolve 1.01 g of sodium 1-heptane sulfonate in 1000 mL of diluted acetic acid (100) (1 in 100). To 675 mL of this solution add 325 mL of a mixture of methanol and acetonitrile (3:2).

Flow rate: Adjust so that the retention time of Fursultiamine is about 9 minutes.

Selection of column: Proceed with 10 μL of the standard solution under the above operating conditions and calculate the resolution. Use a column giving elution of fursultiamine and the internal standard in this order with the resolution between these peaks being not less than 10.

Containers and storage Containers—Tight containers.

Gabexate Mesilate

ガベキサートメシル酸塩

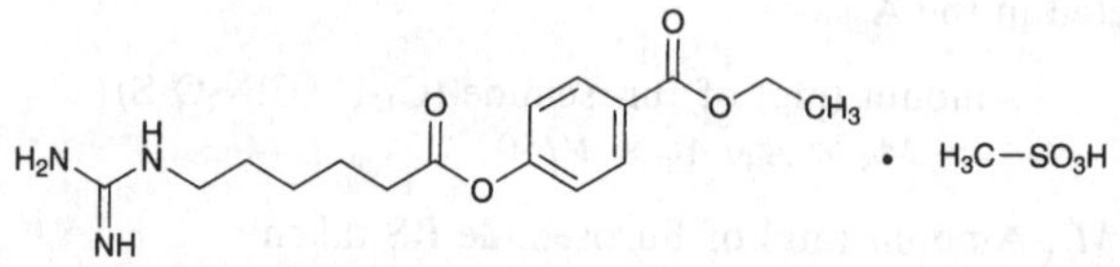

$C_{16}H_{23}N_3O_4.CH_4O_3S$: 417.48
Ethyl 4-(6-guanidinohexanoyloxy)benzoate monomethanesulfonate
[*56974-61-9*]

Gabexate Mesilate, when dried, contains not less than 98.5% and not more than 101.0% of gabexate mesilate ($C_{16}H_{23}N_3O_4.CH_4O_3S$).

Description Gabexate Mesilate occurs as white, crystals or crystalline powder.

It is very soluble in water, freely soluble in ethanol (95).

Identification **(1)** To 4 mL of a solution of Gabexate Mesilate (1 in 2000) add 2 mL of 1-naphthol TS and 1 mL of diacetyl TS, and allow to stand for 10 minutes: a red color develops.

(2) Dissolve 1 g of Gabexate Mesilate in 5 mL of water, add 2 mL of sodium hydroxide TS, and heat in a water bath for 5 minutes. After cooling, add 2 mL of dilute nitric acid and 5 mL of ethanol (95), shake, add 5 drops of iron (III) chloride TS, and shake: a purple color develops.

(3) Determine the absorption spectrum of a solution of Gabexate Mesilate (1 in 100,000) as directed under Ultraviolet-visible Spectrophotometry <*2.24*>, and compare the spectrum with the Reference Spectrum or the spectrum of a solution of Gabexate Mesilate RS prepared in the same manner as the sample solution: both spectra exhibit similar intensities of absorption at the same wavelengths.

(4) A 0.1 g portion of Gabexate Mesilate responds to Qualitative Tests <*1.09*> (1) for mesilate.

pH <*2.54*> Dissolve 1.0 g of Gabexate Mesilate in 10 mL of water: the pH of the solution is between 4.7 and 5.7.

Melting point <2.60> 90 - 93°C

Purity (1) Clarity and color of solution—Dissolve 1.0 g of Gabexate Mesilate in 10 mL of water: the solution is clear and colorless.

(2) Heavy metals <1.07>—Proceed with 2.0 g of Gabexate Mesilate according to Method 1, and perform the test. Prepare the control solution with 2.0 mL of Standard Lead Solution (not more than 10 ppm).

(3) Arsenic <1.11>—Dissolve 2.0 g of Gabexate Mesilate in 20 mL of 1 mol/L hydrochloric acid TS by heating in a water bath, and continue the heating for 20 minutes. After cooling, centrifuge, and use 10 mL of the supernatant liquid as the test solution. Perform the test (not more than 2 ppm).

(4) Ethyl parahydroxybenzoate—Weigh 50 mg of Gabexate Mesilate, previously dried, and dissolve in dilute ethanol to make exactly 100 mL. Pipet 5 mL of this solution, add exactly 5 mL of the internal standard solution, and use this solution as the sample solution. Separately, dissolve 5.0 mg of ethyl parahydroxybenzoate in dilute ethanol to make exactly 100 mL. Pipet 1 mL of this solution, and add dilute ethanol to make exactly 20 mL. To exactly 5 mL of this solution add exactly 5 mL of the internal standard solution, and use this solution as the standard solution. Perform the test with 3 μL each of the sample solution and standard solution as directed under Liquid Chromatography <2.01> according to the following conditions, and calculate the ratios, Q_T and Q_S, of the peak area of ethyl parahydroxybenzoate to that of the internal standard: Q_T is not larger than Q_S.

Internal standard solution—A solution of butyl parahydroxybenzoate in dilute ethanol (1 in 5000).

Operating conditions—

Proceed as directed in the operating conditions in the Assay.

System suitability—

Proceed as directed in the system suitability in the Assay.

(5) Related substances—Dissolve 0.20 g of Gabexate Mesilate in 5 mL of ethanol (95), and use this solution as the sample solution. Pipet 1 mL of the sample solution, add ethanol (95) to make exactly 100 mL, and use this solution as the standard solution. Perform the test with these solutions as directed under Thin-layer Chromatography <2.03>. Spot 5 μL each of the sample solution and standard solution on a plate of silica gel for thin-layer chromatography. Develop the plate with a mixture of ethyl acetate, water and acetic acid (100) (3:1:1) to a distance of about 10 cm, and air-dry the plate until it has no acetic odor. Spray evenly a solution of 8-quinolinol in acetone (1 in 1000) on the plate, and after air-drying, spray evenly bromine-sodium hydroxide TS: the spots other than the principal spot obtained from the sample solution are not more intense than the spot from the standard solution.

Loss on drying <2.41> Not more than 0.30% (1 g, in vacuum, silica gel, 4 hours).

Residue on ignition <2.44> Not more than 0.1% (1 g).

Assay Weigh accurately about 50 mg each of Gabexate Mesilate and Gabexate Mesilate RS, previously dried, and dissolve each in dilute ethanol to make exactly 100 mL. Pipet 5 mL each of these solutions, add exactly 5 mL each of the internal standard solution, and use these solutions as the sample solution and the standard solution, respectively. Perform the test with 3 μL each of the sample solution and standard solution as directed under Liquid Chromatography <2.01> according to the following conditions, and calculate the ratios, Q_T and Q_S, of the peak area of gabexate to that of the internal standard.

Amount (mg) of gabexate mesilate ($C_{16}H_{23}N_3O_4.CH_4O_3S$)
$= M_S \times Q_T/Q_S$

M_S: Amount (mg) of Gabexate Mesilate RS taken

Internal standard solution—A solution of butyl parahydroxybenzoate in dilute ethanol (1 in 5000).

Operating conditions—

Detector: An ultraviolet absorption photometer (wavelength: 245 nm).

Column: A stainless steel column 4.6 mm in inside diameter and 15 cm in length, packed with octadecylsilanized silica gel for liquid chromatography (5 μm in particle diameter).

Column temperature: A constant temperature of about 25°C.

Mobile phase: A mixture of methanol, a solution of sodium lauryl sulfate (1 in 1000), a solution of sodium 1-heptane sulfonate (1 in 200) and acetic acid (100) (540:200:20:1).

Flow rate: Adjust so that the retention time of gabexate is about 13 minutes.

System suitability—

System performance: When the procedure is run with 3 μL of the standard solution under the above operating conditions, the internal standard and gabexate are eluted in this order with the resolution between these peaks being not less than 5.

System repeatability: When the test is repeated 6 times with 3 μL of the standard solution under the above operating conditions, the relative standard deviation of the ratios of the peak area of gabexate to that of the internal standard is not more than 1.0%.

Containers and storage Containers—Tight containers.

β-Galactosidase (Aspergillus)

β-ガラクトシダーゼ（アスペルギルス）

[9031-11-2]

β-Galactosidase (Aspergillus) contains an enzyme produced by *Aspergillus oryzae*. It is an enzyme drug having lactose decomposition activity.

It contains 8,000 to 12,000 units per g.

Usually, it is diluted with a mixture of Maltose Hydrate and Dextrin, Maltose Hydrate and D-Mannitol, or Maltose Hydrate, Dextrin and D-Mannitol.

Description β-Galactosidase (Aspergillus) occurs as a white to light yellow powder.

It is slightly soluble in water with a turbidity, and practically insoluble in ethanol (95) and in diethyl ether.

Identification (1) Dissolve 25 mg of β-Galactosidase (Aspergillus) in 100 mL of water, then to 1 mL of this solution add 9 mL of lactose substrate TS, and stand at 30°C for 10 minutes. To 1 mL of this solution add 6 mL of glucose detection TS, and stand at 30°C for 10 minutes: a red to red-purple color develops.

(2) Dissolve 0.1 g of β-Galactosidase (Asperigillus) in 100 mL of water, and filter the solution if necessary. Determine the absorption spectrum of the solution as directed under Ultraviolet-visible Spectrophotometry <2.24>, and compare the spectrum with the Reference Spectrum: both spectra exhibit similar intensities of absorption at the same wavelengths.

Purity (1) Odor—β-Galactosidase (Aspergillus) has no

any rancid odor.

(2) Heavy metals 〈*1.07*〉—Proceed with 1.0 g of *β*-Galactosidase (Aspergillus) according to Method 2, and perform the test. Prepare the control solution with 2.0 mL of Standard Lead Solution (not more than 20 ppm).

(3) Arsenic 〈*1.11*〉—Prepare the test solution with 1.0 g of *β*-Galactosidase (Aspergillus) according to Method 3, and perform the test (not more than 2 ppm).

Loss on drying 〈*2.41*〉 Not more than 9.0% (0.5 g, in vacuum, 80°C, 4 hours).

Residue on ignition 〈*2.44*〉 Not more than 3% (0.5 g).

Nitrogen content Weigh accurately about 70 mg of *β*-Galactosidase (Aspergillus), and perform the test as directed under Nitrogen Determination 〈*1.08*〉: the amount of nitrogen (N: 14.01) is between 0.5% and 5.0%, calculated on the dried basis.

Assay (i) Substrate solution—Dissolve 0.172 g of 2-nitrophenyl-*β*-D-galactopyranoside in disodium hydrogenphosphate-citric acid buffer solution (pH 4.5) to make 100 mL.

(ii) Procedure—Weigh accurately about 25 mg of *β*-Galactosidase (Aspergillus), dissolve in water to make exactly 100 mL, then pipet 2 mL of this solution, add water to make exactly 50 mL, and use this solution as the sample solution. Take exactly 3.5 mL of the substrate solution, stand at 30 ± 0.1°C for 5 minutes, add exactly 0.5 mL of the sample solution, immediately mix, and stand at 30 ± 0.1°C for exactly 10 minutes, then add exactly 1 mL of sodium carbonate TS and mix immediately. Perfoum the test as directed under Ultraviolet-visible Spectrophotometry 〈*2.24*〉, and determine the absorbance, A_1, of this solution at 420 nm using water as the control. Separately, take exactly 3.5 mL of the substrate solution, add exactly 1 mL of sodium carbonate TS and mix, then add exactly 0.5 mL of the sample solution and mix. Determine the absorbance, A_2, of this solution in the same manner as above.

Units per g of *β*-Galactosidase (Aspergillus)
$= 1/M \times (A_1 - A_2)/0.917 \times 1/0.5 \times 1/10$

0.917: Absorbance of 1 *μ*mol/5 mL of *o*-nitrophenol
M: Amount (g) of *β*-Galactosidase (Aspergillus) in the sample solution per mL
Unit: One unit indicates an amount of the enzyme which decomposes 1 *μ*mol of 2-nitrophenyl-*β*-D-galactopyranoside in 1 minute under the above conditions.

Containers and storage Containers—Tight containers.
Storage—In a cold place.

β-Galactosidase (Penicillium)

β-ガラクトシダーゼ（ペニシリウム）

[*9031-11-2*]

β-Galactosidase (Penicillium) contains an enzyme, having lactose decomposition activity, produced by *Penicillium multicolor*.

It contains not less than 8500 units and not more than 11,500 units in each g.

Usually, it is diluted with D-Mannitol.

Description *β*-Galactosidase (Penicillium) occurs as a white to pale yellow-white, crystalline powder or powder.

It is soluble in water with a turbidity, and practically insoluble in ethanol (95).

It is hygroscopic.

Identification **(1)** Dissolve 0.05 g of *β*-Galactosidase (Penicillium) in 100 mL of water, then to 0.2 mL of this solution add 0.2 mL of lactose substrate TS for *β*-galactosidase (penicillium), and allow to stand at 30°C for 10 minutes. To this solution add 3 mL of glucose detection TS for penicillium origin *β*-galactosidase, and allow to stand at 30°C for 10 minutes: a red to red-purple color develops.

(2) Dissolve 0.15 g of *β*-Galactosidase (Penicillium) in 100 mL of water, filter if necessary, and determine the absorption spectrum of this solution as directed under Ultraviolet-visible Spectrophotometry 〈*2.24*〉: it exhibits a maximum between 278 nm and 282 nm.

Purity **(1)** Odor—*β*-Galactosidase (Penicillium) has no any rancid odor.

(2) Heavy metals 〈*1.07*〉—Proceed with 1.0 g of *β*-Galactosidase (Penicillium) according to Method 2, and perform the test. Prepare the control solution with 2.0 mL of Standard Lead Solution (not more than 20 ppm).

(3) Arsenic 〈*1.11*〉—Prepare the test solution with 1.0 g of *β*-Galactosidase (Penicillium) according to Method 3, and perform the test (not more than 2 ppm).

(4) Nitrogen—Weigh accurately about 0.1 g of *β*-Galactosidase (Penicillium), and perform the test as directed under Nitrogen Determination 〈*1.08*〉: not more than 3 mg of nitrogen (N: 14.01) is found for each labeled 1000 Units.

(5) Protein contaminants—Dissolve 0.15 g of *β*-Galactosidase (Penicillium) in 4 mL of water, and use this solution as the sample solution. Perform the test with 15 *μ*L of the sample solution as directed under Liquid Chromatography 〈*2.01*〉 according to the following conditions, and determine each peak area by the automatic integration method: the total area of the peaks other than the peak having retention time of about 19 minutes is not more than 75% of the total area of all peaks, and the areas of peaks other than the peaks having retention times of about 3, 16 and 19 minutes are not more than 15% of the total area of all peaks.

Operating conditions—

Detector: An ultraviolet absorption photometer (wavelength: 280 nm).

Column: A stainless steel column about 7.5 mm in inside diameter and about 75 mm in length, packed with strongly acidic ion-exchange resin for liquid chromatography of sulfopropyl group-binding hydrophilic polymer (10 *μ*m in particle diameter).

Column temperature: A constant temperature of about 20°C.

Mobile phase: A solution obtained by dissolving 2.83 g of sodium acetate in 1000 mL of water, and adjusting to pH 4.5 with acetic acid (100) (mobile phase A), and a solution obtained by dissolving 29.2 g of sodium chloride in 1000 mL of mobile phase A (mobile phase B).

Flow system: Adjust a linear concentration gradient from the mobile phase A to the mobile phase B immediately after injection of the sample so that the retention times of non-retaining protein and the enzyme protein are about 3 minutes and 19 minutes, respectively, when the flow runs 0.8 mL per minute, and then continue the running of the mobile phase B.

Selection of column: Dissolve 15 mg of *β*-lactoglobulin in 4.5 mL of water, add 0.5 mL of a solution of cytosine (1 in 5000), and use this solution as the column-selecting solution. Proceed with 15 *μ*L of the column-selecting solution under the above operating conditions, and calculate the resolution. Use a column giving elution of cytosine and β-lactoglobulin in this order with the resolution between these peaks being not less than 4.

Detection sensitivity: Adjust the detection sensitivity so that the peak height of β-lactoglobulin from 15 μL of the column-selecting solution is between 5 cm and 14 cm.

Time span of measurement: About 1.4 times as long as the retention time of β-lactoglobulin.

Loss on drying ⟨*2.41*⟩ Not more than 5.0% (0.5 g, in vacuum, phosphorus (V) oxide, 4 hours).

Residue on ignition ⟨*2.44*⟩ Not more than 2% (1 g).

Assay (i) Substrate solution—Dissolve 0.603 g of 2-nitrophenyl-β-D-galactopyranoside in disodium hydrogen phosphate-citric acid buffer solution for penicillium origin β-galactosidase (pH 4.5) to make 100 mL.

(ii) Procedure—Weigh accurately about 0.15 g of β-Galactosidase (Penicillium), dissolve in water with thorough shaking to make exactly 100 mL, and allow to stand at room temperature for an hour. Pipet 2 mL of this solution, add disodium hydrogen phosphate-citric acid buffer solution for penicillium origin β-galactosidase (pH 4.5) to make exactly 100 mL, and use this solution as the sample solution. Transfer exactly 0.5 mL of the sample solution to a test tube, stand at 30 ± 0.1°C for 10 minutes, add exactly 0.5 mL of the substrate solution previously kept at 30 ± 0.1°C, then mix immediately, and stand at 30 ± 0.1°C for exactly 10 minutes. Then add exactly 1 mL of sodium carbonate TS, mix immediately to stop the reaction. To this solution add exactly 8 mL of water, mix, and use as the colored sample solution. Separately, pipet 0.5 mL of disodium hydrogen phosphate-citric acid buffer solution for penicillium origin β-galactosidase (pH 4.5), then proceed in the same manner as the sample solution, and use the solution so obtained as the colored blank solution. Perform the test with the colored sample solution and the colored blank solution as directed under Ultraviolet-visible Spectrophotometry ⟨*2.24*⟩, using water as the blank, and determine the absorbances, A_T and A_B, at 420 nm.

$$\text{Units per g of } \beta\text{-Galactosidase (Penicillium)} = 1/M \times (A_T - A_B)/0.459 \times 1/10$$

0.459: Absorbance of 1 μmol/10 mL of *o*-nitrophenol
M: Amount (g) of β-Galactosidase (Penicillium) in 0.5 mL of the sample solution
Unit: One unit indicates an amount of the enzyme which decomposes 1 μmol of 2-nitrophenyl-β-D-galactopyranoside in 1 minute under the above conditions.

Containers and storage Containers—Tight containers.

Gallium (^{67}Ga) Citrate Injection

クエン酸ガリウム（^{67}Ga）注射液

Gallium (^{67}Ga) Citrate Injection is an aqueous injection containing gallium-67 (^{67}Ga) in the form of gallium citrate.

It conforms to the requirements of Gallium (^{67}Ga) Citrate Injection in the Minimum Requirements for Radiopharmaceuticals.

Test for Extractable volume of Parenteral Preparations and Insoluble Particulate Matter Test for Injections are not applied to this injection.

Description Gallium (^{67}Ga) Citrate Injection is a clear, colorless or light red liquid.

Gatifloxacin Hydrate

ガチフロキサシン水和物

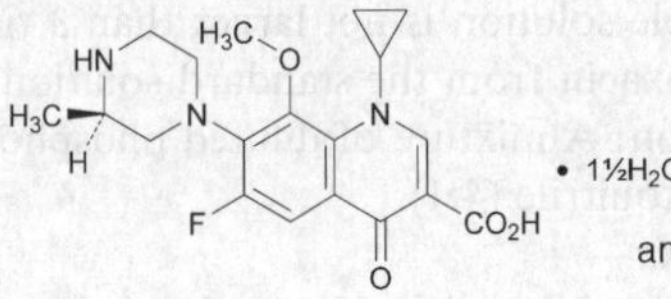

$C_{19}H_{22}FN_3O_4.1\frac{1}{2}H_2O$: 402.42
1-Cyclopropyl-6-fluoro-8-methoxy-7-[(3*RS*)-3-methylpiperazin-1-yl]-4-oxo-1,4-dihydroquinoline-3-carboxylic acid sesquihydrate
[*180200-66-2*]

Gatifloxacin Hydrate contains not less than 98.5% and not more than 101.5% of gatifloxacin ($C_{19}H_{22}FN_3O_4$: 375.39), calculated on the anhydrous basis.

Description Gatifloxacin Hydrate occurs as white to pale yellow, crystals or crystalline powder.

It is slightly soluble in methanol and in ethanol (99.5), and very slightly soluble in water.

It dissolves in sodium hydroxide TS.

It is gradually colored to pale yellow by light.

A solution of Gatifloxacin Hydrate in dilute sodium hydroxide TS (1 in 100) shows no optical rotation.

Identification (1) Determine the absorption spectrum of a solution of Gatifloxacin Hydrate in dilute sodium hydroxide TS (1 in 100,000) as directed under Ultraviolet-visible Spectrophotometry ⟨*2.24*⟩, and compare the spectrum with the Reference Spectrum or the spectrum of a solution of Gatifloxacin RS prepared in the same manner as the sample solution: both spectra exhibit similar intensities of absorption at the same wavelengths.

(2) Determine the infrared absorption spectrum of Gatifloxacin Hydrate as directed in the potassium bromide disk method under Infrared Spectrophotometry ⟨*2.25*⟩, and compare the spectrum with the Reference Spectrum or the spectrum of Gatifloxacin RS: both spectra exhibit similar intensities of absorption at the same wave numbers.

Purity (1) Clarity and color of solution—Dissolve 1.0 g of Gatifloxacin Hydrate in 10 mL of sodium hydroxide TS: the solution is clear. Perform the test with the solution as directed under Methods for Color Matching ⟨*2.65*⟩: the solution is not more colored than diluted Matching Fluid O (1 in 5).

(2) Heavy metals ⟨*1.07*⟩—Proceed with 1.0 g of Gatifloxacin Hydrate according to Method 4, and perform the test. Prepare the control solution with 2.0 mL of Standard Lead Solution (not more than 20 ppm).

(3) Related substances—Dissolve 20 mg of Gatifloxacin Hydrate in 50 mL of the dissolving solution, and use this solution as the sample solution. Pipet 1 mL of the sample solution, and add the dissolving solution to make exactly 100 mL. Pipet 2 mL of this solution, add the dissolving solution to make exactly 20 mL, and use this solution as the standard solution. Perform the test with exactly 20 μL each of the sample solution and standard solution as directed under Liquid Chromatography ⟨*2.01*⟩ according to the following con-

ditions. Determine each peak area by the automatic integration method: the peak area of the related substance A, having the relative retention time of about 1.2 to gatifloxacin, obtained from the sample solution is not larger than 2 times the peak area of gatifloxacin from the standard solution, and the area of the peak other than gatifloxacin and the peak mentioned above from the sample solution is not larger than the peak area of gatifloxacin from the standard solution. Furthermore, the total area of the peaks other than gatifloxacin from the sample solution is not larger than 3 times the peak area of gatifloxacin from the standard solution.

Dissolving solution: A mixture of diluted phosphoric acid (1 in 1000) and acetonitrile (4:1).

Operating conditions—

Detector: An ultraviolet absorption photometer (wavelength: 325 nm).

Column: A stainless steel column 4.6 mm in inside diameter and 15 cm in length, packed with octadecylsilanized silica gel for liquid chromatography (5 μm in particle diameter).

Column temperature: A constant temperature of about 35°C.

Mobile phase A: A mixture of diluted triethylamine (1 in 100), adjusted to pH 4.3 with phosphoric acid, and acetonitrile (22:3).

Mobile phase B: A mixture of diluted triethylamine (1 in 100), adjusted to pH 4.3 with phosphoric acid, and acetonitrile (1:1).

Flowing of mobile phase: Control the gradient by mixing the mobile phases A and B as directed in the following table.

Time after injection of sample (min)	Mobile phase A (vol%)	Mobile phase B (vol%)
0 – 15	100	0
15 – 30	100 → 0	0 → 100
30 – 40	0	100

Flow rate: 1.0 mL per minute (the retention time of gatifloxacin is about 16 minutes).

Time span of measurement: About 2.5 times as long as the retention time of gatifloxacin, beginning after the solvent peak.

System suitability—

Test for required detectability: Pipet 5 mL of the standard solution, and add the dissolving solution to make exactly 10 mL. Confirm that the peak area of gatifloxacin obtained with 20 μL of this solution is equivalent to 40 to 60% of that with 20 μL of the standard solution.

System performance: Dissolve 20 mg of methyl 4-aminobenzoate in 50 mL of the dissolving solution. To 5 mL of this solution add 1 mL of the sample solution and the dissolving solution to make 100 mL. When the procedure is run with 20 μL of this solution under the above operating conditions, gatifloxacin and methyl 4-aminobenzoate are eluted in this order with the resolution between these peaks being not less than 4.

System repeatability: When the test is repeated 6 times with 20 μL of the standard solution under the above operating conditions, the relative standard deviation of the peak area of gatifloxacin is not more than 3.0%.

Water <*2.48*> 6.0 – 9.0% (0.1 g, volumetric titration, direct titration).

Residue on ignition <*2.44*> Not more than 0.1% (1 g).

Assay Weigh accurately about 50 mg of Gatifloxacin Hydrate and Gatifloxacin RS (separately determine the water <*2.48*> in the same manner as Gatifloxacin Hydrate), and dissolve each in the dissolving solution to make exactly 100 mL. Pipet 2 mL each of these solution, add exactly 2 mL of the internal standard solution to them, add the dissolving solution to make 25 mL, and use these solutions as the sample solution and standard solutions. Perform the test with 20 μL each of the sample solution and standard solution as directed under Liquid Chromatography <*2.01*> according to the following conditions, and calculate the ratios, Q_T and Q_S, of the peak area of gatifloxacin to that of the internal standard.

$$\text{Amount (mg) of gatifloxacin } (C_{19}H_{22}FN_3O_4) = M_S \times Q_T/Q_S$$

M_S: Amount (mg) of Gatifloxacin RS taken, calculated on the anhydrous basis

*Internal standard solution—*A solution of methyl 4-aminobenzoate in the dissolving solution (1 in 4000).

Dissolving solution: A mixture of diluted phosphoric acid (1 in 1000) and acetonitrile (4:1).

Operating conditions—

Detector: An ultraviolet absorption photometer (wavelength: 280 nm).

Column: A stainless steel column 4 mm in inside diameter and 12.5 cm in length, packed with octadecylsilanized silica gel for liquid chromatography (5 μm in particle diameter).

Column temperature: A constant temperature of about 40°C.

Mobile phase: A mixture of diluted triethylamine (1 in 100), adjusted to pH 4.5 with phosphoric acid, and acetonitrile (87:13).

Flow rate: Adjust so that the retention time of gatifloxacin is about 5 minutes.

System suitability—

System performance: When the procedure is run with 20 μL of the standard solution under the above operating conditions, gatifloxacin and the internal standard are eluted in this order with the resolution between these peaks being not less than 4.

System repeatability: When the test is repeated 6 times with 20 μL of the standard solution under the above operating conditions, the relative standard deviation of the ratio of the peak area of gatifloxacin to that of the internal standard is not more than 1.0%.

Containers and storage Containers—Tight containers.

Storage—Light-resistant.

Others

Related substance A:

1-Cyclopropyl-6-fluoro-8-methoxy-7-[(2*RS*)-2-methylpiperazin-1-yl]-4-oxo-1,4-dihydroquinoline-3-carboxylic acid

and enantiomer

Gatifloxacin Ophthalmic Solution

ガチフロキサシン点眼液

Gatifloxacin Ophthalmic Solution is an aqueous ophthalmic preparation.

It contains not less than 95.0% and not more than 107.0% of the labeled amount of gatifloxacin ($C_{19}H_{22}FN_3O_4$: 375.39).

Method of preparation Prepare as directed under Ophthalmic Liquids and Solutions, with Gatifloxacin Hydrate.

Description Gatifloxacin Ophthalmic Solution is a clear, pale yellow liquid.

Identification To a volume of Gatifloxacin Ophthalmic Solution, equivalent to 6 mg of gatifloxacin ($C_{19}H_{22}FN_3O_4$), add diluted sodium hydroxide TS (1 in 10) to make 30 mL. To 1 mL of this solution add diluted sodium hydroxide TS (1 in 10) to make 20 mL, and determine the absorption spectrum of this solution as directed under Ultraviolet-visible Spectrophotometry *<2.24>*: it exhibits maxima between 238 nm and 242 nm, between 287 nm and 291 nm, and between 336 nm and 340 nm.

Osmotic pressure ratio Being specified separately when the drug is granted approval based on the Law.

pH Being specified separately when the drug is granted approval based on the Law.

Purity Related substance—To a volume of Gatifloxacin Ophthalmic Solution, equivalent to 6 mg of gatifloxacin ($C_{19}H_{22}FN_3O_4$), add the diluting solution to make 30 mL, and use this solution as the sample solution. Pipet 1 mL of the sample solution, add the diluting solution to make exactly 100 mL. Pipet 2 mL of this solution, add the diluting solution to make exactly 20 mL, and use this solution as the standard solution. Perform the test with exactly 40 μL each of the sample solution and standard solution as directed under Liquid Chromatography *<2.01>* according to the following conditions. Determine each peak area by the automatic integration method: the peak area of the related substance A, having the relative retention time of about 1.2 to gatifloxacin, obtained from the sample solution is not larger than 2 times the peak area of gatifloxacin from the standard solution, and the area of the peak other than gatifloxacin and the peak mentioned above from the sample solution is not larger than the peak area of gatifloxacin from the standard solution. Furthermore, the total area of the peaks other than gatifloxacin from the sample solution is not larger than 3 times the peak area of gatifloxacin from the standard solution.

Diluting solution: A mixture of diluted phosphoric acid (1 in 1000) and acetonitrile (4:1).

Operating conditions—

Detector: An ultraviolet absorption photometer (wavelength: 325 nm).

Column: A stainless steel column 4.6 mm in inside diameter and 15 cm in length, packed with octadecylsilanized silica gel for liquid chromatography (5 μm in particle diameter).

Column temperature: A constant temperature of about 40°C.

Mobile phase A: A mixture of diluted triethylamine (1 in 100) and acetonitrile (22:3), adjusted to pH 4.3 with phosphoric acid.

Mobile phase B: A mixture of diluted triethylamine (1 in 100) and acetonitrile (1:1), adjusted to pH 4.3 with phosphoric acid.

Flowing of mobile phase: Control the gradient by mixing the mobile phases A and B as directed in the following table.

Time after injection of sample (min)	Mobile phase A (vol%)	Mobile phase B (vol%)
0 – 15	100	0
15 – 30	100 → 0	0 → 100
30 – 40	0	100

Flow rate: 0.9 mL per minute (the retention time of gatifloxacin is about 16 minutes).

Time span of measurement: For 40 minutes after injection, beginning after the solvent peak.

System suitability—

Test for required detectability: Pipet 5 mL of the standard solution, and add the diluting solution to make exactly 10 mL. Confirm that the peak area of gatifloxacin obtained with 40 μL of this solution is equivalent to 40 to 60% of that with 40 μL of the standard solution.

System performance: Dissolve 20 mg of methyl 4-aminobenzoate in 100 mL of the diluting solution. To 5 mL of this solution and 1 mL of the sample solution add the diluting solution to make 100 mL. When the procedure is run with 40 μL of this solution under the above operating conditions, gatifloxacin and methyl 4-aminobenzoate are eluted in this order with the resolution between these peaks being not less than 4.

System repeatability: When the test is repeated 6 times with 40 μL of the standard solution under the above operating conditions, the relative standard deviation of the peak area of gatifloxacin is not more than 3.0%.

Foreign insoluble matter *<6.11>* It meets the requirement.

Insoluble particulate matter *<6.08>* It meets the requirement.

Sterility *<4.06>* Perform the test according to the Membrane filtration method: it meets the requirement.

Assay Pipet a volume of Gatifloxacin Ophthalmic Solution, equivalent to about 6 mg of gatifloxacin ($C_{19}H_{22}FN_3O_4$), and add the diluting solution to make exactly 30 mL. Pipet 2 mL of this solution, add exactly 3 mL of the internal standard solution, add the diluting solution to make 20 mL, and use this solution as the sample solution. Separately, weigh accurately about 22 mg of Gatifloxacin RS (separately determine the water *<2.48>* in the same manner as Gatifloxacin Hydrate), and dissolve in the diluting solution to make exactly 100 mL. Pipet 2 mL of this solution, add exactly 3 mL of the internal standard solution, add the diluting solution to make 20 mL, and use this solution as the standard solution. Perform the test with 20 μL each of the sample solution and standard solution as directed under Liquid Chromatography *<2.01>* according to the following conditions, and calculate the ratios, Q_T and Q_S, of the peak area of gatifloxacin to that of the internal standard.

$$\text{Amount (mg) of gatifloxacin } (C_{19}H_{22}FN_3O_4) = M_S \times Q_T/Q_S \times 3/10$$

M_S: Amount (mg) of Gatifloxacin RS taken, calculated on the anhydrous basis

Internal standard solution—A solution of methyl 4-aminobenzoate in the diluting solution (1 in 10,000).

Diluting solution: A mixture of diluted phosphoric acid (1

in 1000) and acetonitrile (4:1).

Operating conditions—

Detector: An ultraviolet absorption photometer (wavelength: 280 nm).

Column: A stainless steel column 4.6 mm in inside diameter and 15 cm in length, packed with octadecylsilanized silica gel for liquid chromatography (5 μm in particle diameter).

Column temperature: A constant temperature of about 40°C.

Mobile phase: A mixture of water, acetonitrile and triethylamine (81:18:1), adjusted to pH 4.5 with phosphoric acid.

Flow rate: Adjust so that the retention time of gatifloxacin is about 6 minutes.

System suitability—

System performance: When the procedure is run with 20 μL of the standard solution under the above operating conditions, gatifloxacin and the internal standard are eluted in this order with the resolution between these peaks being not less than 10.

System repeatability: When the test is repeated 6 times with 20 μL of the standard solution under the above operating conditions, the relative standard deviation of the ratio of the peak area of gatifloxacin to that of the internal standard is not more than 1.0%.

Containers and storage Containers—Tight containers.

Others

Related substances A: Refer to it described in Gatifloxacin Hydrate.

Gefarnate

ゲファルナート

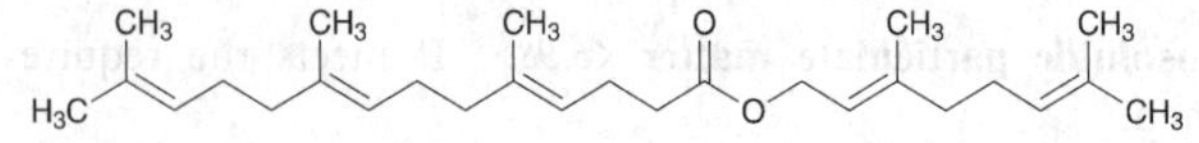

$C_{27}H_{44}O_2$: 400.64

(2*E*)-3,7-Dimethylocta-2,6-dienyl(4*E*,8*E*)-5,9,13-trimethyltetradeca-4,8,12-trienoate

[*51-77-4*, 4*E* isomer]

Gefarnate is a mixture of 4*E* geometrical isomer.

It contains not less than 98.0% and not more than 101.0% of gefarnate ($C_{27}H_{44}O_2$).

Description Gefarnate is a light yellow to yellow, clear oily liquid.

It is miscible with acetonitrile, with ethanol (99.5) and with cyclohexane.

It is practically insoluble in water.

Identification Determine the infrared absorption spectrum of Gefarnate as directed in the liquid film method under Infrared Spectrophotometry <*2.25*>, and compare the spectrum with the Reference Spectrum or the spectrum of Gefarnate RS: both spectra exhibit similar intensities of absorption at the same wave numbers.

Specific gravity <*2.56*> d^{20}_{20}: 0.906 – 0.914

Purity (1) Acidity—To 1.0 g of Gefarnate add 30 mL of neutralized ethanol. To this solution add 1 drop of phenolphthalein TS and 0.40 mL of 0.1 mol/L sodium hydroxide VS: a red color develops.

(2) Heavy metals <*1.07*>—Proceed with 2.0 g of Gefarnate according to Method 2, and perform the test. Prepare the control solution with 2.0 mL of Standard Lead Solution (not more than 10 ppm).

(3) Related substances—Use a solution of Gefarnate in acetonitrile (1 in 500) as the sample solution. Pipet 2 mL of the sample solution, add acetonitrile to make exactly 100 mL, and use this solution as the standard solution. Perform the test with exactly 2 μL each of the sample solution and standard solution as directed under Liquid Chromatography <*2.01*> according to the following conditions. Determine each peak area of both solutions by the automatic integration method: the area of each peak other than the peak of gefarnate obtained from the sample solution is not larger than 1/2 times the peak area of gefarnate from the standard solution, and the total area of the peaks other than the peak of gefarnate from the sample solution is not larger than the peak area of gefarnate from the standard solution.

Operating conditions—

Detector, column, column temperature, mobile phase and flow rate: Proceed as directed in the operating conditions in the Assay.

Time span of measurement: About 2 times as long as the retention time of gefarnate, beginning after the solvent peak.

System suitability—

Test for required detectability: Pipet 2 mL of the standard solution, add acetonitrile to make exactly 20 mL. Confirm that the peak area of gefarnate obtained with 2 μL of this solution is equivalent to 7 to 13% of that of gefarnate with 2 μL of the standard solution.

System performance: When the procedure is run with 2 μL of the standard solution under the above operating conditions, the number of theoretical plates and the symmetry factor of the peak of gefarnate are not less than 4000, and between 0.9 and 1.2, respectively.

System repeatability: When the test is repeated 6 times with 2 μL of the standard solution under the above operating conditions, the relative standard deviation of the peak area of gefarnate is not more than 1.0%.

Isomer ratio To 1 mL of Gefarnate add 100 mL of ethanol (99.5), and use this solution as the sample solution. Perform the test with 4 μL of the sample solution as directed under Gas Chromatography <*2.02*> according to the following conditions. Determine the areas of two adjacent peaks, A_a and A_b, having the retention time of about 37 minutes, where A_a is the peak area of shorter retention time and A_b is the peak area of longer retention time: $A_a/(A_a + A_b)$ is between 0.2 and 0.3.

Operating conditions—

Detector: A hydrogen flame-ionization detector.

Column: A glass column 3 mm in inside diameter and 160 cm in length, packed with polyethylene glycol 20M for gas chromatography coated at the ratio of 5% on acid-treated and silanized siliceous earth for gas chromatography (149 to 177 μm in particle diameter).

Column temperature: A constant temperature of about 210°C.

Carrier gas: Nitrogen.

Flow rate: Adjust so that the reaction time of the peak showing earlier elution of the two peaks of gefarnate is about 35 minutes.

System suitability—

System performance: When the procedure is run with 4 μL of the sample solution under the above conditions: the resolution between the two peaks of gefarnate is not less than 1.0.

System repeatability: When the test is repeated 6 times with 4 μL of the sample solution under the above operating conditions: the relative standard deviation of the peak area of gefarnate with the shorter retention time of the two peaks of gefarnate is not more than 2.0%.

Assay Weigh accurately about 50 mg each of Gefarnate and Gefarnate RS, add exactly 5 mL of the internal standard solution and 20 mL of acetonitrile, and use these solutions as the sample solution and standard solution. Perform the test with 2 μL each of the sample solution and standard solution as directed under Liquid Chromatography ⟨*2.01*⟩ according to the following conditions, and calculate the ratios, Q_T and Q_S, of the peak area of gefarnate to that of the internal standard.

$$\text{Amount (mg) of gefarnate } (C_{27}H_{44}O_2) = M_S \times Q_T/Q_S$$

M_S: Amount (mg) of Gefarnate RS taken

Internal standard solution—A solution of tris (4-*t*-butylphenyl) phosphate in acetonitrile (1 in 400).

Operating conditions—

Detector: An ultraviolet absorption photometer (wavelength: 220 nm).

Column: A stainless steel column 4 mm in inside diameter and 30 cm in length, packed with phenylsilanized silica gel for liquid chromatography (10 μm in particle diameter).

Column temperature: A constant temperature of about 40°C.

Mobile phase: A mixture of acetonitrile for liquid chromatography, water and phosphoric acid (700:300:1).

Flow rate: Adjust so that the retention time of gefarnate is about 19 minutes.

System suitability—

System performance: When the procedure is run with 2 μL of the standard solution under the above operating conditions, the internal standard and gefarnate are eluted in this order with the resolution between these peaks being not less than 2.0.

System repeatability: When the test is repeated 6 times with 2 μL of the standard solution under the above operating conditions, the relative standard deviation of the ratio of the peak area of gefarnate to that of the internal standard is not more than 1.0%.

Containers and storage Containers—Tight containers.

Storage—Light-resistant, and under nitrogen atmosphere.

Gefitinib

ゲフィチニブ

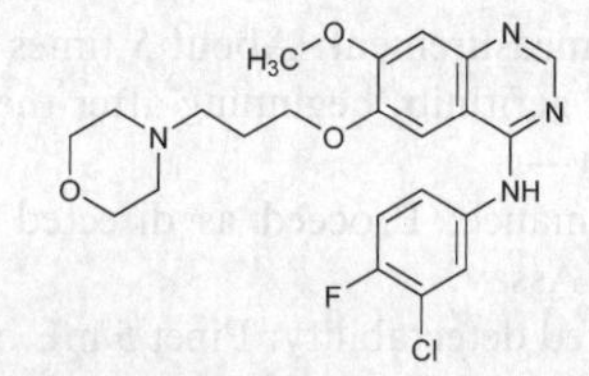

$C_{22}H_{24}ClFN_4O_3$: 446.90

N-(3-Chloro-4-fluorophenyl)-7-methoxy-6-[3-(morpholin-4-yl)propoxy]quinazolin-4-amine

[*184475-35-2*]

Gefitinib contains not less than 98.0% and not more than 102.0% of gefitinib ($C_{22}H_{24}ClFN_4O_3$), calculated on the anhydrous basis.

Description Gefitinib occurs as a white powder.

It is slightly soluble in ethanol (99.5), and practically insoluble in water.

Identification (1) Determine the absorption spectrum of a solution of Gefitinib in a mixture of trifluoroacetic acid solution (1 in 500) and acetonitrile (3:2) (1 in 100,000) as directed under Ultraviolet-visible Spectrophotometry ⟨*2.24*⟩, and compare the spectrum with the Reference Spectrum or the spectrum of a solution of Gefitinib RS prepared in the same manner as the sample solution: both spectra exhibit similar intensities of absorption at the same wavelengths.

(2) Determine the infrared absorption spectrum of Gefitinib as directed in the potassium bromide disk method under Infrared Spectrometry ⟨*2.25*⟩, and compare the spectrum with the Reference Spectrum or the spectrum of Gefitinib RS: both spectra exhibit similar intensities of absorption at the same wave numbers. Or, perform the test by the diffuse reflectance method, and compare the spectrum with the spectrum of Gefitinib RS: both spectra exhibit similar intensities of absorption at the same wave numbers.

Purity (1) Heavy metals—Being specified separately when the drug is granted approval based on the Law.

(2) Related substances—Use the sample solution obtained in the Assay as the sample solution. Pipet 1 mL of the sample solution, add a mixture of trifluoroacetic acid solution (1 in 500) and acetonitrile (3:2) to make exactly 100 mL. Pipet 1 mL of this solution, and add a mixture of trifluoroacetic acid solution (1 in 500) and acetonitrile (3:2) to make exactly 10 mL, and use this solution as the standard solution. Perform the test with exactly 5 μL each of the sample solution and standard solution as directed under Liquid Chromatography ⟨*2.01*⟩ according to the following conditions, and determine each peak area by the automatic integration method: the peak area of related substance A having the relative retention time of about 0.13 to gefitinib obtained from the sample solution is not larger than the peak area of gefitinib from the standard solution, the peak area of related substance B having the relative retention time of about 1.3 from the sample solution is not larger than 2 times the peak area of gefitinib from the standard solution, and the area of the peak other than gefitinib and the peaks mentioned above from the sample solution is not larger than the peak area of gefitinib from the standard solution. Furthermore, the total area of the peaks other than gefitinib from the sample solution is not larger than 4 times the peak area of gefitinib from

the standard solution.

Operating conditions—

Detector, column, column temperature, mobile phase, and flow rate: Proceed as directed in the operating conditions in the Assay.

Time span of measurement: About 5 times as long as the retention time of gefitinib, beginning after the solvent peak.

System suitability—

System performance: Proceed as directed in the system suitability in the Assay.

Test for required detectability: Pipet 5 mL of the standard solution, and add a mixture of trifluoroacetic acid solution (1 in 500) and acetonitrile (3:2) to make exactly 10 mL. When the procedure is run with 5 μL of this solution under the above operating conditions, the SN ratio of the peak of gefitinib is not less than 10.

System repeatability: When the test is repeated 6 times with 5 μL of the standard solution under the above operating conditions, the relative standard deviation of the peak area of gefitinib is not more than 2.0%.

Water *<2.48>* Not more than 0.4% (0.1 g, coulometric titration).

Residue on ignition *<2.44>* Not more than 0.2% (1.0 g, platinum crucible).

Assay Weigh accurately about 35 mg each of Gefitinib and Gefitinib RS (separately determine the water *<2.48>* in the same manner as Gefitinib), add 85 mL of a mixture of trifluoroacetic acid solution (1 in 500) and acetonitrile (3:2) to each, sonicate to dissolve, add a mixture of trifluoroacetic acid solution (1 in 500) and acetonitrile (3:2) to make exactly 100 mL, and use these solutions as the sample solution and the standard solution, respectively. Perform the test with exactly 5 μL each of the sample solution and standard solution as directed under Liquid Chromatography *<2.01>* according to the following conditions, and determine the peak areas, A_T and A_S, of gefitinib in each solution.

Amount (mg) of gefitinib ($C_{22}H_{24}ClFN_4O_3$)
$= M_S \times A_T/A_S$

M_S: Amount (mg) of Gefitinib RS taken, calculated on the anhydrous basis

Operating conditions—

Detector: An ultraviolet absorption photometer (wavelength: 247 nm).

Column: A stainless steel column 3 mm in inside diameter and 10 cm in length, packed with octadesylsilanized silica gel for liquid chromatography (3 μm in particle diameter).

Column temperature: A constant temperature of about 60°C.

Mobile phase: A mixture of ammonium acetate solution (3 in 310) and acetonitrile (31:19).

Flow rate: 0.9 mL per minute (the retention time of gefitinib is about 5.5 minutes).

System suitability—

System performance: Dissolve 15 mg of 3,4-dichloroaniline in 60 mL of the standard solution. When the procedure is run with 5 μL of this solution under the above operating conditions, 3,4-dichloroaniline and gefitinib are eluted in this order with the resolution between these peaks being not less than 5.

System repeatability: When the test is repeated 6 times with 5 μL of the standard solution under the above operating conditions, the relative standard deviation of the peak area of gefitinib is not more than 1.0%.

Containers and storage Containers—Tight containers.

Others

Related substance A:
7-Methoxy-6-[3-(morpholin-4-yl)propoxy]quinazolin-4(3*H*)-one

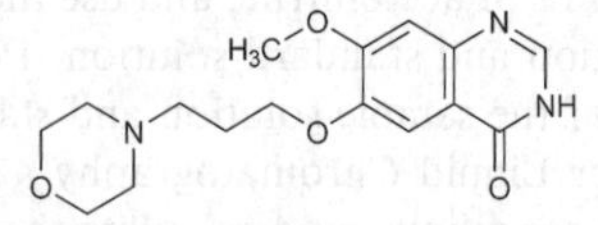

Related substance B:
N-(4-Chloro-3-fluorophenyl)-7-methoxy-6-[3-(morpholin-4-yl)propoxy]quinazolin-4-amine

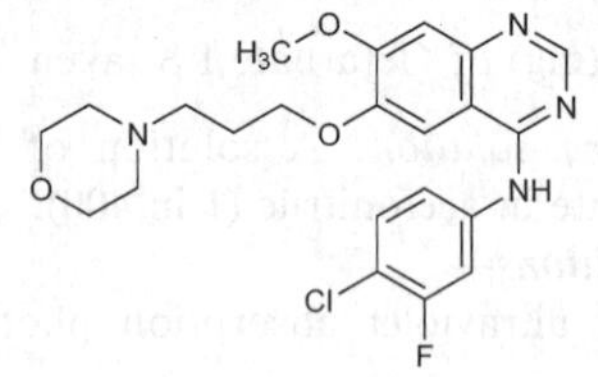

Gelatin

ゼラチン

This monograph is harmonized with the European Pharmacopoeia and the U.S. Pharmacopeia.

The corresponding part of the attributes/provisions which are agreed as non-harmonized within the scope of the harmonization is marked with symbols (◆ ◆), and the corresponding parts which are agreed as the JP local requirement other than the scope of the harmonization are marked with symbols (◇ ◇).

Information on the harmonization with the European Pharmacopoeia and the U.S. Pharmacopeia is available on the website of the Pharmaceuticals and Medical Devices Agency.

Gelatin is a purified protein obtained from collagen of animals by partial alkaline and/or acid hydrolysis, and/or enzymatic hydrolysis or by thermal hydrolysis. The hydrolysis leads to gelling or non-gelling grades.

The label states the gel strength (Bloom value) for the gelling grade, and that it is a non-gelling grade for the non-gelling grade.

◆**Description** Gelatin occurs as colorless or white to light yellow-brown sheets, shreds, granules or powder.

It is freely soluble in hot water, and practically insoluble in ethanol (95).

The gelling grade does not dissolve in water, but slowly swells and softens when immersed in it, gradually absorbing water 5 to 10 times its own mass.

The gelling grade derived from an acid-treated collagen exhibits an isoelectric point between pH 7.0 and 9.0, and the gelling grade derived from an alkali-treated collagen exhibits an isoelectric point between pH 4.5 and 5.0.

The non-gelling grade is freely soluble in water.◆

Identification **(1)** Dissolve 1.00 g of Gelatin in freshly boiled and cooled water at about 55°C to make 100 mL, and use this solution as the sample solution. To 2 mL of the sample solution keeping at about 55°C add 0.05 mL of copper (II) sulfate TS. Mix and add 0.5 mL of 2 mol/L sodium hydroxide TS: a violet color is produced.

(2) In a test tube about 15 mm in internal diameter, place

0.5 g of Gelatin, add 10 mL of water, and allow to stand for 10 minutes. Heat at 60°C for 15 minutes, then keep the tube upright at 2 to 8°C for 6 hours, and invert the tube: the contents do not flow out immediately for the gelling grade. In case of the non-gelling grade the contents flow out immediately.

(3) Apply to the non-gelling grade. Place 0.5 g of Gelatin in a 250-mL flask and add 10 mL of water and 5 mL of sulfuric acid. Cover with a watch glass or other instrument, avoiding complete closure, and heat at 105°C for 4 hours. Cool, add 200 mL of water, and then adjust to pH 6.0 to 8.0 with a sodium hydroxide solution (1 in 5). In a test tube, place 2 mL of this solution, add 2 mL of the oxidizing reagent, shake, and allow to stand for 20 minutes. Add 2 mL of the colored solution, shake, and warm in a water bath of 60°C for about 15 minutes: a red to purple color develops.

Oxidizing reagent: Dissolve 5.53 g of disodium hydrogen phosphate dodecahydrate and 0.48 g of citric acid monohydrate in water to make 100 mL. Dissolve 1.4 g of sodium toluenesulfonchloramide trihydrate in this solution. Prepare before use.

Colored solution: Dissolve 1.0 g of 4-dimethylaminobenzaldehyde in 3.5 mL of a solution of perchloric acid (1 in 2) and add slowly 6.5 mL of 2-propanol. Prepare before use.

Gel strength (Bloom value) Apply to the gelling grade. Determine the mass (g) necessary to produce the force which, applied to a plunger 12.7 mm in diameter, makes a depression 4 mm deep in a gel having a concentration of 6.67% and matured at 10°C.

(i) Apparatus: Texture analyzer or gelometer with a cylindrical piston 12.7 ± 0.1 mm in diameter with a plane pressure surface and a sharp bottom edge, and with a bottle 59 ± 1 mm in internal diameter and 85 mm high (jelly cup).

(ii) Procedure: Place 7.5 g of Gelatin in a jelly cup, add 105 mL of water, close the cup, and allow to stand for 1 to 4 hours. Heat in a water bath at 65 ± 2°C for 15 minutes. While heating, stir gently with a glass rod. Ensure that the solution is uniform and any condensed water on the inner walls of the cup is incorporated. Allow to cool at room temperature for 15 minutes and transfer the cup to a thermostatically controlled bath at 10.0 ± 0.1°C, and fitted with a device to ensure that the platform on which the cup stands is perfectly horizontal. Close the cup, and allow to stand for 17 ± 1 hours. Remove the sample cup from the bath and quickly wipe the water from the exterior of the cup. Center the cup on the platform of the apparatus so that the plunger contacts the sample as nearly at its midpoint as possible, and start the measurement with 4 mm depression distance and 0.5 mm per second test speed: 80 to 120% of the labeled nominal value.

pH <*2.54*> pH at 55°C of the sample solution obtained in Identification (1) is 3.8 - 7.6.

Purity ◇**(1)** Heavy metals <*1.07*>—Proceed with 0.5 g of Gelatin according to Method 2, and perform the test. Prepare the control solution with 2.5 mL of Standard Lead Solution (not more than 50 ppm).◇

(2) Iron—To 5.00 g of Gelatin, in a glass-stoppered flask, add 10 mL of hydrochloric acid, close the flask, and heat in a water bath at 75 - 80°C for 2 hours. If necessary for proper solubilization, the gelatin may be allowed to swell after addition of the acid and before heating, the heating time may be prolonged and a higher temperature may be used. After cooling, adjust the content of the flask to 100.0 g with water, and use this solution as the sample solution. Separately, place 5.00 g each of Gelatin in three glass-stoppered flasks, proceed with them in the same manner as the sample solution, then add 10 mL, 20 mL and 30 mL of Standard Iron Solution (2) for Atomic Absorption Spectrophotometry exactly to each flask separately. Adjust the content of these flasks to 100.0 g each with water, and use these solutions as the standard solutions. The amount of the standard solution to be added may be adjusted according to the sensitivity of the instrument to be used. Perform the test with the sample solution and standard solutions as directed in the standard addition method under Atomic Absorption Spectrophotometry <*2.23*> according to the following conditions, and determine the content of iron: not more than 30 ppm.

Gas: Combustible gas—Acetylene.
Supporting gas—Air.
Lamp: Iron hollow cathode lamp.
Wavelength: 248.3 nm.

(3) Chromium—Use the sample solution obtained in (2) as the sample solution. Separately, place 5.00 g each of Gelatin in three glass-stoppered flasks, proceed with them in the same manner as the sample solution, then add 0.25 mL, 0.50 mL and 0.75 mL of Standard Chromium Solution for Atomic Absorption Spectrophotometry exactly to each flask separately. Adjust the content of these flasks to 100.0 g each with water, and use these solutions as the standard solutions. The amount of the standard solution to be added may be adjusted according to the sensitivity of the instrument to be used. Perform the test with the sample solution and standard solutions as directed in the standard addition method under Atomic Absorption Spectrophotometry <*2.23*> according to the following conditions, and determine the content of chromium: not more than 10 ppm.

Gas: Combustible gas—Acetylene.
Supporting gas—Air.
Lamp: Chromium hollow cathode lamp.
Wavelength: 357.9 nm.

(4) Zinc—Use the sample solution obtained in (2) as the sample solution. Separately, place 5.00 g each of Gelatin in three glass-stoppered flasks, proceed with them in the same manner as the sample solution, then add 7.5 mL, 15 mL and 22.5 mL of Standard Zinc Solution for Atomic Absorption Spectrophotometry exactly to each flask separately. Adjust the content of these flasks to 100.0 g each with water, and use these solutions as the standard solutions. The amount of the standard solution to be added may be adjusted according to the sensitivity of the instrument to be used. Perform the test with the sample solution and standard solutions as directed in the standard addition method under Atomic Absorption Spectrophotometry <*2.23*> according to the following conditions, and determine the content of zinc: not more than 30 ppm.

Gas: Combustible gas—Acetylene.
Supporting gas—Air.
Lamp: Zinc hollow cathode lamp.
Wavelength: 213.9 nm.

◇**(5)** Arsenic <*1.11*>—Take 15.0 g of Gelatin in a flask, add 60 mL of diluted hydrochloric acid (1 in 5), and dissolve by heating. Add 15 mL of bromine TS, heat until the excess of bromine is expelled, neutralize with ammonia TS, add 1.5 g of disodium hydrogen phosphate dodecahydrate, and allow to cool. To this solution add 30 mL of magnesia TS, allow to stand for 1 hour, and collect the precipitates. Wash the precipitates with five 10-mL portions of diluted ammonia TS (1 in 4), and dissolve in diluted hydrochloric acid (1 in 4) to make exactly 50 mL. Perform the test with 5 mL of this solution: the solution has no more color than the following color standard.

Color standard: Proceed with 15 mL of Standard Arsenic

Solution, instead of Gelatin, in the same manner (not more than 1 ppm).◇

(6) Peroxides—

(i) Enzyme reaction: Peroxidase transfers oxygen from peroxides to an organic redox indicator which is converted to a blue oxidation product. The intensity of the color obtained is proportional to the quantity of peroxide and can be compared with a color scale provided with the test strips, to determine the peroxide concentration.

(ii) Procedure: Weigh 20.0 ± 0.1 g of Gelatin in a beaker, add 80.0 ± 0.2 mL of water, and stir to moisten all the gelatin. Allow to stand at room temperature for 1 - 3 hours. Cover the beaker with a watch-glass, and heat the beaker for 20 ± 5 minutes in a water bath at 65 ± 2°C for dissolving the sample. Stir the contents of the beaker with a glass rod to achieve a homogeneous solution, and use this as the sample solution. Dip a peroxide test strip for 1 second into the sample solution, such that the reaction zone is properly wetted. Remove the test strip, shake off excess liquid, and compare the reaction zone after 15 seconds with the color scale provided. Multiply the concentration read from the color scale by a factor of 5 to calculate the concentration of peroxide in the test substance: not more than 10 ppm.

(iii) Suitability test: To exactly 10 mL of Standard Hydrogen Peroxide Solution add water to make exactly 300 mL. Pipet 2 mL of this solution, add water to make exactly 1000 mL (2 ppm). Dip a peroxide test strip for 1 second into this solution, such that the reaction zone is properly wetted. Remove the test strip, shake off excess liquid and compare the color of the reaction zone after 15 seconds with the color scale: the color of the zone is equivalent to 2 ppm of the color scale.

(7) Sulfur dioxide—

(i) Apparatus: Use as shown in the figure.

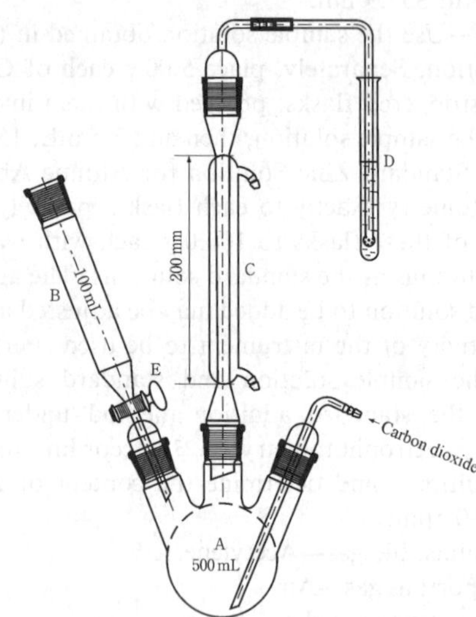

A: Three-necked round-bottomed flask (500 mL)
B: Cylindrical dropping funnel (100 mL)
C: Condenser
D: Test tube
E: Tap

(ii) Procedure: Introduce 150 mL of water into the three-necked round-bottomed flask and pass carbon dioxide through the whole system at a rate of 100 mL per minute. Place 10 mL of hydrogen peroxide-sodium hydroxide TS in the test tube. After 15 minutes, remove the cylindrical dropping funnel without interrupting the stream of carbon dioxide, and introduce through the opening into the three-necked round-bottomed flask about 25.0 g of Gelatin with the aid of 100 mL of water. Pour 80 mL of 2 mol/L hydrochloric acid TS into the funnel, open the tap to introduce the hydrochloric acid into the three-necked round-bottomed flask ◇and close the tap while several mL of the hydrochloric acid remains, in order to avoid losing sulfur dioxide◇, and boil the mixture for 1 hour. Transfer the contents of the test tube with the aid of a little water to a 200 mL wide-necked conical flask. Heat the flask in a water bath for 15 minutes and cool. Add 0.1 mL of bromophenol blue TS and titrate <2.50> with 0.1 mol/L sodium hydroxide VS until the color changes from yellow to violet-blue lasting for at least 20 seconds. Perform a blank determination in the same manner, and make any necessary correction. Calculate the amount of sulfur dioxide from the following expression: it is not more than 50 ppm.

$$\text{Amount (ppm) of sulfur dioxide} = V/M \times 1000 \times 3.203$$

M: Amount (g) of Gelatin taken
V: Amount (mL) of 0.1 mol/L sodium hydroxide VS consumed

Conductivity *<2.51>* Perform the test at 30 ± 1.0°C with the sample solution obtained in Identification (1), without temperature compensation: not more than 1 $\text{mS}\cdot\text{cm}^{-1}$.

Loss on drying *<2.41>* Not more than 15.0% (5 g, 105°C, 16 hours).

Microbial limit *<4.05>* The acceptance criteria of TAMC and TYMC are 10^3 CFU/g and 10^2 CFU/g, respectively. *Escherichia coli* and *Salmonella* are not observed.

Containers and storage ◇Containers—Tight containers.◇
Storage—Protect from heat and moisture.

Purified Gelatin

精製ゼラチン

Purified Gelatin is a purified protein obtained from collagen of animals by partial alkaline and/or acid hydrolysis, and/or enzymatic hydrolysis, or by thermal hydrolysis. The hydrolysis leads to gelling or non-gelling grades.

The label states the gel strength (Bloom value) for the gelling grade, and that it is a non-gelling grade for the non-gelling grade.

Description Purified Gelatin occurs as colorless or white to light yellow-brown sheets, shreds, granules or powder.

It is very soluble in hot water, and practically insoluble in ethanol (95).

The gelling grade does not dissolve in water. It slowly swells and softens when immersed in water, and absorbs water 5 to 10 times its own mass. The non-gelling grade is freely soluble in water.

Identification **(1)** To 5 mL of a solution of Purified Gelatin (1 in 100) add 2,4,6-trinitrophenol TS dropwise: a precipitate is formed.

(2) To 5 mL of a solution of Purified Gelatin (1 in 5000) add tannic acid TS dropwise: the solution becomes turbid.

(3) In a test tube about 15 mm in internal diameter, place 0.5 g of Purified Gelatin, add 10 mL of water, and allow to stand for 10 minutes. Heat at 60°C for 15 minutes, then keep the tube upright at 2 to 8°C for 6 hours, and invert the tube: the contents do not flow out immediately for the gelling grade. In case of the non-gelling grade the contents flow out immediately.

Gel strength (Bloom value) Apply to the gelling grade. Determine the mass (g) necessary to produce the force which, applied to a plunger 12.7 mm in diameter, makes a depression 4 mm deep in the surface of the gel having a concentration of 6.67% and matured at 10°C.

(i) Apparatus, instruments: Texture analyzer or gelometer with a cylindrical piston 12.7 ± 0.1 mm in diameter with a plane bottom and a sharp bottom edge, and with a cup 59 ± 1 mm in internal diameter and 85 mm high (jelly cup).

(ii) Procedure: Place 7.5 g of Purified Gelatin in a jelly cup, add 105 mL of water, close the cup, and allow to stand for 1 to 4 hours. Heat in a water bath at 65 ± 2°C for 15 minutes. While heating, stir gently with a glass rod. Incorporate any condensed water on the inner wall of the cup into the solution, and ensure that the solution is uniform. Allow to cool at room temperature for 15 minutes and transfer the cup to a thermostatically controlled bath at 10.0 ± 0.1°C, and fitted with a device to ensure that the platform on which the cup stands is perfectly horizontal. Close the cup, and allow to stand for 17 ± 1 hours. Remove the sample cup from the bath and quickly wipe the water from the exterior of the cup. Put the cup on the platform of the apparatus so that the tip of plunger contacts the sample as nearly at its midpoint as possible, and start the measurement with 4 mm depression distance and 0.5 mm per second test speed: 80 to 120% of the labeled nominal value.

pH *<2.54>* Dissolve 1.00 g of Purified Gelatin in freshly boiled water and kept at about 55°C, to make 100 mL. pH at 55°C of this solution is 3.8 - 9.0.

Purity **(1)** Heavy metals*<1.07>*—Proceed with 1.0 g of Purified Gelatin according to Method 2, and perform the test. Prepare the control solution with 2.0 mL of Standard Lead Solution (not more than 20 ppm).

(2) Iron—To 5.00 g of Purified Gelatin, in a glass-stoppered flask, add 10 mL of hydrochloric acid, close the flask, and place in a water bath at 75 - 80°C for 2 hours. If necessary for proper solubilization, the gelatin may be allowed to swell after addition of the acid and the heating time may be prolonged or a higher temperature may be used. After cooling, adjust the content of the flask to 100.0 g with water, and use this solution as the sample solution. Separately, place 5.00 g each of Purified Gelatin in three glass-stoppered flasks, proceed with them in the same manner as the sample solution, then add exactly 10 mL, 20 mL and 30 mL of Standard Iron Solution (2) for Atomic Absorption Spectrophotometry to each flask, respectively. Adjust the content of these flasks to 100.0 g each with water, and use these solutions as the standard solutions. The volume of Standard Iron Solution may be adjusted appropriately according to the sensitivity of the instrument to be used. Perform the test with the sample solution and standard solutions as directed in the standard addition method under Atomic Absorption Spectrophotometry*<2.23>* according to the following conditions, and determine the content of iron: not more than 30 ppm.

Gas: Combustible gas—Acetylene.
Supporting gas—Air.
Lamp: Iron hollow cathode lamp.
Wavelength: 248.3 nm.

(3) Chromium—Use the sample solution obtained in (2) as the sample solution. Separately, place 5.00 g each of Purified Gelatin in three glass-stoppered flasks, proceed with them in the same manner as the sample solution, then add exactly 0.25 mL, 0.50 mL and 0.75 mL of Standard Chromium Solution for Atomic Absorption Spectrophotometry to each flask, respectively. Adjust the content of these flasks to 100.0 g each with water, and use these solutions as the standard solutions. The volume of Standard Iron Solution may be adjusted appropriately according to the sensitivity of the instrument to be used. Perform the test with the sample solution and standard solutions as directed in the standard addition method under Atomic Absorption Spectrophotometry *<2.23>* according to the following conditions, and determine the content of chromium: not more than 10 ppm.

Gas: Combustible gas—Acetylene.
Supporting gas—Air.
Lamp: Chromium hollow cathode lamp.
Wavelength: 357.9 nm.

(4) Zinc—Use the sample solution obtained in (2) as the sample solution. Separately, place 5.00 g each of Purified Gelatin in three glass-stoppered flasks, proceed with them in the same manner as the sample solution, then add exactly 7.5 mL, 15 mL and 22.5 mL of Standard Zinc Solution for Atomic Absorption Spectrophotometry to each flask, respectively. Adjust the content of these flasks to 100.0 g each with water, and use these solutions as the standard solutions. The volume of Standard Iron Solution may be adjusted appropriately according to the sensitivity of the instrument to be used. Perform the test with the sample solution and standard solutions as directed in the standard addition method under Atomic Absorption Spectrophotometry *<2.23>* according to the following conditions, and determine the content of zinc: not more than 30 ppm.

Gas: Combustible gas—Acetylene.
Supporting gas—Air.
Lamp: Zinc hollow cathode lamp.
Wavelength: 213.9 nm.

(5) Arsenic*<1.11>*—Place 15.0 g of Purified Gelatin in a flask, add 60 mL of diluted hydrochloric acid (1 in 5), and dissolve by heating. Add 15 mL of bromine TS, heat until the excess of bromine is expelled, neutralize with ammonia TS, add 1.5 g of disodium hydrogen phosphate dodecahydrate, and allow to cool. To this solution add 30 mL of magnesia TS, allow to stand for 1 hour, and collect the precipitates. Wash the precipitates with five 10-mL portions of diluted ammonia TS (1 in 4), and dissolve in diluted hydrochloric acid (1 in 4) to make exactly 50 mL. Perform the test with 5 mL of this solution: the solution has no more color than the following color standard.

Color Standard: Proceed with 12 mL of Standard Arsenic Solution, instead of Purified Gelatin, in the same manner (not more than 0.8 ppm).

(6) Peroxides—

(i) Enzyme reaction: Peroxidase transfers oxygen atom at on from peroxides to an organic redox indicator which is converted to a blue oxidized form. The intensity of the color obtained is proportional to the quantity of peroxide. The peroxide concentration can be determined by comparing it with the color scale provided with the test strips employing this reaction.

(ii) Procedure: Weigh 20.0 ± 0.1 g of Purified Gelatin in a beaker, add 80.0 ± 0.2 mL of water, and stir to moisten all the gelatin. Allow to stand at room temperature for 1—3 hours. Cover the beaker with a watch-glass, and heat the beaker for 20 ± 5 minutes in a water bath at 65 ± 2°C to dissolve the sample. Stir the contents of the beaker with a glass rod to achieve a homogeneous solution, and use this as the sample solution. Dip a peroxide test strip for 1 second into the sample solution, such that the reaction zone is properly wetted. Remove the test strip, shake off excess liquid, and compare the reaction zone after 15 seconds with the color scale provided. Multiply the concentration read from the color scale by a factor of 5 to calculate the concentration of peroxide in the test substance: not more than 10 ppm.

(iii) Sensitivity: To exactly 10 mL of Standard Hydrogen Peroxide Solution add water to make exactly 300 mL. Pipet exactly 2 mL of this solution, add water to make exactly 1000 mL (2 ppm). Dip a peroxide test strip for 1 second into this solution, such that the reaction zone is properly wetted. Remove the test strip, shake off excess liquid and compare the color of the reaction zone after 15 seconds with the color scale: the color of the zone is equivalent to 2 ppm of the color scale.

(7) Sulfur dioxide—

(i) Apparatus: Use as shown in the figure.

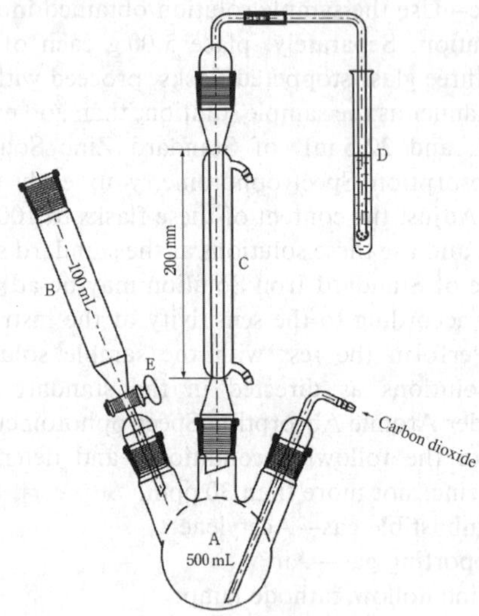

A: Three-necked round-bottomed flask (500 mL)
B: Cylindrical dropping funnel (100 mL)
C: Condenser
D: Test tube
E: Tap

(ii) Procedure: Introduce 150 mL of water into the three-necked round-bottomed flask and pass carbon dioxide through the whole system at a rate of 100 mL per minute. Place 10 mL of hydrogen peroxide-sodium hydroxide TS in the test tube. After 15 minutes, remove the cylindrical dropping funnel from the flask without interrupting the stream of carbon dioxide, and introduce through the opening into the flask about 25.0 g of Purified Gelatin with the aid of 100 mL of water. Pour 80 mL of 2 mol/L hydrochloric acid TS into the funnel, open the tap to introduce the hydrochloric acid into the flask and close the tap while several mL of the hydrochloric acid remains, in order to avoid losing sulfur dioxide, and boil the mixture for 1 hour. Remove the test tube, and transfer the contents of the test tube to a 200-mL wide-necked conical flask, wash the test tube with a small amount of water, and add the washing to the conical flask. Heat the flask in a water bath for 15 minutes and cool. Add 0.1 mL of bromophenol blue TS, and titrate <2.50> with 0.1 mol/L sodium hydroxide VS until the color changes from yellow to violet-blue lasting for at least 20 seconds. Perform a blank determination in the same manner and make any necessary correction. Calculate the amount of sulfur dioxide from the following expression: it is not more than 20 ppm.

Amount (ppm) of sulfur dioxide = $V/M \times 1000 \times 3.203$

M: Amount (g) of Purified Gelatin taken
V: Amount (mL) of 0.1 mol/L sodium hydroxide VS consumed

Conductivity <*2.51*> Dissolve 1.00 g of Purified Gelatin in freshly boiled water and kept at about 55°C, to make 100 mL. Perform the test at 30 ± 1.0°C with this solution, without temperature compensation: not more than 1 mS·cm^{-1}.

Loss on drying <*2.41*> Not more than 15.0% (5 g, 105°C, 16 hours).

Microbial limit <*4.05*> The acceptance criteria of TAMC and TYMC are 10^3 CFU/g and 10^2 CFU/g, respectively. *Escherichia coli* and *Salmonella* are not observed.

Containers and storage Containers—Tight containers.
Storage—Protect from heat and moisture.

Gentamicin Sulfate

ゲンタマイシン硫酸塩

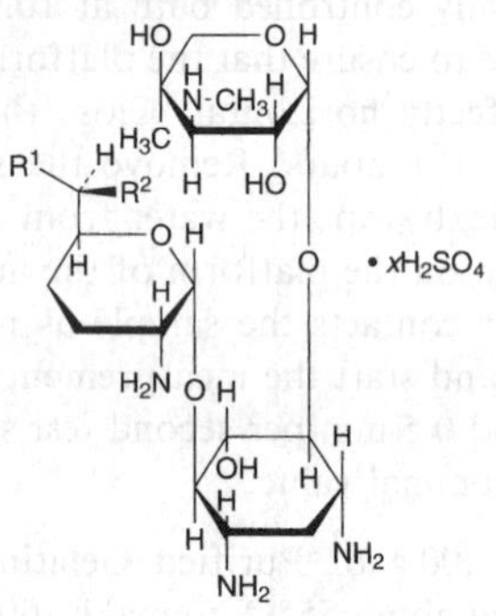

Gentamicin C_1 Sulfate : $R^1 = CH_3$ $R^2 = NHCH_3$
Gentamicin C_2 Sulfate : $R^1 = CH_3$ $R^2 = NH_2$
Gentamicin C_{1a} Sulfate : $R^1 = H$ $R^2 = NH_2$

Gentamicin C_1 Sulfate
(6*R*)-2-Amino-2,3,4,6-tetradeoxy-6-methylamino-6-methyl-α-D-*erythro*-hexopyranosyl-(1→4)-[3-deoxy-4-*C*-methyl-3-methylamino-β-L-arabinopyranosyl-(1→6)]-2-deoxy-D-streptamine sulfate

Gentamicin C_2 Sulfate
(6*R*)-2,6-Diamino-2,3,4,6-tetradeoxy-6-methyl-α-D-*erythro*-hexopyranosyl-(1→4)-[3-deoxy-4-*C*-methyl-3-methylamino-β-L-arabinopyranosyl-(1→6)]-2-deoxy-D-streptamine sulfate

Gentamicin C_{1a} Sulfate
2,6-Diamino-2,3,4,6-tetradeoxy-α-D-*erythro*-hexopyranosyl-(1→4)-[3-deoxy-4-*C*-methyl-3-methylamino-β-L-arabinopyranosyl-(1→6)]-2-deoxy-D-streptamine sulfate

[*1405-41-0*, Gentamicin Sulfate]

Gentamicin Sulfate is the sulfate of a mixture of aminoglycoside substances having antibacterial activity produced by the growth of *Micromonospora purpurea* or *Micromonospora echinospora*.

It contains not less than 590 μg (potency) and not more than 775 μg (potency) per mg, calculated on the dried basis. The potency of Gentamicin Sulfate is expressed as mass (potency) of gentamicin C_1 ($C_{21}H_{43}N_5O_7$: 477.60).

Description Gentamicin Sulfate occurs as a white to light yellow-white powder.

It is very soluble in water, and practically insoluble in ethanol (99.5).

It is hygroscopic.

Identification **(1)** Dissolve 50 mg each of Gentamicin Sulfate and Gentamicin Sulfate RS in 10 mL of water, and use these solutions as the sample solution and standard solution. Perform the test with these solutions as directed under Thin-layer Chromatography <2.03>. Spot 20 μL of the sample solution and standard solution on a plate of silica gel for thin-layer chromatography. Separately, shake a mixture of chloroform, ammonia solution (28) and methanol (2:1:1) in a separator, and allow the mixture to stand for more than 1 hour. To 20 mL of the lower layer so obtained add 0.5 mL of methanol, and use this as the developing solvent. Develop the plate with the developing solvent to a distance of about 17 cm in a developing container with a cover, having an opening of about 20 mm^2, and without putting a filter paper in the container, and air-dry the plate. Allow the plate to stand in iodine vapors: three principal spots obtained from the sample solution are the same with the corresponding spots from the standard solution in color tone and the *R*f value, respectively.

(2) Dissolve 50 mg of Gentamicin Sulfate in 5 mL of water, and add 0.5 mL of barium chloride TS: a white precipitate is formed.

Optical rotation *<2.49>* $[\alpha]_D^{25}$: +107 – +121° (0.25 g calculated on the dried basis, water, 25 mL, 100 mm).

pH *<2.54>* The pH of a solution obtained by dissolving 0.20 g of Gentamicin Sulfate in 5 mL of water is between 3.5 and 5.5.

Content ratio of the active principle Dissolve 50 mg of Gentamicin Sulfate in water to make 10 mL, and use this solution as the sample solution. Perform the test with the sample solution as directed under Thin-layer Chromatography *<2.03>*. Spot 20 μL of the sample solution on a plate of silica gel for thin-layer chromatography. Separately, shake a mixture of chloroform, ammonia solution (28) and methanol (2:1:1) in a separator, and allow the mixture to stand for more than 1 hour. To 20 mL of the lower layer so obtained add 0.5 mL of methanol, and use this as the developing solvent. Develop the plate with the developing solvent to a distance of about 17 cm in a developing container with a cover, having an opening of about 20 mm^2, without putting a filter paper in the container, and air-dry the plate. Allow the plate to stand in iodine vapor. Determine the integral absorbances, A_a, A_b and A_c, of the colored spots of gentamicin C_1 (*R*f value: about 0.3), gentamicin C_2 (*R*f value: about 0.2) and gentamicin C_{1a} (*R*f value: about 0.1), respectively, by a densitometer (wavelength: 450 nm) while covering the plate with a glass plate, and calculate these amounts by the following formulae: gentamicin C_1 is between 25% and 55%, gentamicin C_2 is between 25% and 50%, and gentamicin C_{1a} is between 5% and 30%.

$$\text{Amount (\%) of gentamicin } C_1 = A_a/(A_a + 1.35A_b + A_c) \times 100$$

$$\text{Amount (\%) of gentamicin } C_2 = 1.35A_b/(A_a + 1.35A_b + A_c) \times 100$$

$$\text{Amount (\%) of gentamicin } C_{1a} = A_c/(A_a + 1.35A_b + A_c) \times 100$$

Purity **(1)** Clarity and color of solution—Dissolve 1.0 g of Gentamicin Sulfate in 10 mL of water: the solution is clear and its absorbance at 400 nm determined as directed under Ultraviolet-visible Spectrophotometry *<2.24>* is not more than 0.08.

(2) Heavy metals *<1.07>*—Proceed with 2.0 g of Gentamicin Sulfate according to Method 4, and perform the test. Prepare the control solution with 2.0 mL of Standard Lead Solution (not more than 10 ppm).

(3) Related substances—Dissolve 50 mg of Gentamicin Sulfate in 10 mL of water, and use this solution as the sample solution. Pipet 1 mL of the sample solution, add water to make exactly 50 mL, and use this solution as the standard solution. Perform the test with these solutions as directed under Thin-layer Chromatography *<2.03>*. Spot 20 μL of the sample solution and standard solution on a plate of silica gel for thin-layer chromatography. Separately, shake a mixture of chloroform, ammonia solution (28) and methanol (2:1:1) in a separator, and allow the mixture to stand for more than 1 hour. To 20 mL of the lower layer so obtained add 0.5 mL of methanol, and use this as the developing solvent. Develop the plate with the developing solvent to a distance of about 17 cm in a developing container with a cover, having an opening of about 20 mm^2, without putting a filter paper in the container, and air-dry the plate. Allow the plate to stand in iodine vapor, and compare the colored spots while covering with a glass plate: the spots other than the spots of gentamicin C_1 (*R*f value: about 0.3), gentamicin C_2 (*R*f value: about 0.2) and gentamicin C_{1a} (*R*f value: about 0.1) obtained from the sample solution are not more intense than the spot of gentamicin C_2 from the standard solution.

Loss on drying *<2.41>* Not more than 18.0% (0.15 g, reduced pressure not exceeding 0.67 kPa, 110°C, 3 hours). Handle the sample avoiding absorption of moisture.

Residue on ignition *<2.44>* Not more than 1.0% (1 g).

Assay Perform the test according to the Cylinder-plate method as directed under Microbial Assay for Antibiotics *<4.02>* according to the following conditions.

(i) Test organism—*Staphylococcus epidermidis* ATCC 12228

(ii) Agar media for seed and base layer—

Glucose	1.0 g
Peptone	6.0 g
Meat extract	1.5 g
Yeast extract	3.0 g
Sodium chloride	10.0 g
Agar	15.0 g
Water	1000 mL

Mix all the ingredients, and sterilize. Adjust the pH of the solution so that it will be 7.8 to 8.0 after sterilization.

(iii) Agar medium for transferring test organisms—Use the medium ii in 2) Medium for other organisms under (2) Agar media for transferring test organisms.

(iv) Standard solutions—Weigh accurately an amount of Gentamicin Sulfate RS, equivalent to about 25 mg (potency), dissolve in 0.1 mol/L phosphate buffer solution (pH 8.0) to make exactly 25 mL, and use this solution as the standard stock solution. Keep the standard stock solution at 15°C or lower, and use within 30 days. Take exactly a suitable amount of the standard stock solution before use, add 0.1 mol/L phosphate buffer solution (pH 8.0) to make solutions so that each mL contains 4 μg (potency) and 1 μg (potency), and use these solutions as the high concentration standard solution and the low concentration standard solution, respectively.

(v) Sample solutions—Weigh accurately an amount of Gentamicin Sulfate, equivalent to about 25 mg (potency), and dissolve in 0.1 mol/L phosphate buffer solution (pH 8.0) to make exactly 25 mL. Take exactly a suitable amount of this solution, add 0.1 mol/L phosphate buffer solution (pH 8.0) to make solutions so that each mL contains 4 μg (potency) and 1 μg (potency), and use these solutions as the high concentration sample solution and the low concentration sample solution, respectively.

Containers and storage Containers—Tight containers.

Gentamicin Sulfate Injection

ゲンタマイシン硫酸塩注射液

Gentamicin Sulfate Injection is an aqueous injection.

It contains not less than 90.0% and not more than 110.0% of the labeled potency of gentamicin C_1 ($C_{21}H_{43}N_5O_7$: 477.60).

Method of preparation Prepare as directed under Injections, with Gentamicin Sulfate.

Description Gentamicin Sulfate Injection is a clear and colorless liquid.

Identification To a volume of Gentamicin Sulfate Injection, equivalent to 40 mg (potency) of Gentamicin Sulfate, add water to make 10 mL, and use this solution as the sample solution. Separately, dissolve an amount of Gentamicin Sulfate RS, equivalent to 20 mg (potency), in 5 mL of water, and use this solution as the standard solution. Perform the test with these solutions as directed under Thin-layer Chromatography <*2.03*>. Spot 5 μL each of the sample solution and standard solution on a plate of silica gel for thin-layer chromatography. Develop the plate with the lower layer of a mixture of chloroform, ammonia solution (28) and methanol (2:1:1) to a distance of about 15 cm, and air-dry the plate. Spray evenly 0.2% ninhydrin-water saturated 1-butanol TS on the plate, and heat the plate at 100°C for 10 minutes: three principal spots obtained from the sample solution are the same with the corresponding spots from the standard solution in color tone and the *R*f value, respectively.

Osmotic pressure ratio Being specified separately when the drug is granted approval based on the Law.

pH <*2.54*> 4.0 – 6.0

Bacterial endotoxins <*4.01*> Less than 0.50 EU/mg (potency).

Extractable volume <*6.05*> It meets the requirement.

Foreign insoluble matter <*6.06*> Perform the test according to Method 1: it meets the requirement.

Insoluble particulate matter <*6.07*> It meets the requirement.

Sterility <*4.06*> Perform the test according to the Membrane filtration method: it meets the requirement.

Assay Perform the test according to the Cylinder-plate method as directed under Microbial Assay for Antibiotics <*4.02*> according to the following conditions.

(i) Test organism, agar media for base and seed layer, agar medium for transferring test organisms, and standard solutions—Proceed as directed in the Assay under Gentamicin Sulfate.

(ii) Sample solutions—Pipet a volume of Gentamicin Sulfate Injection, equivalent to about 40 mg (potency) of Gentamicin Sulfate, add 0.1 mol/L phosphate buffer solution (pH 8.0) to make exactly 200 mL. Pipet a suitable volume of this solution, add 0.1 mol/L phosphate buffer solution (pH 8.0) to make solutions so that each mL contains 4 μg (potency) and 1 μg (potency), and use these solutions as the high concentration sample solution and the low concentration sample solution, respectively.

Containers and storage Containers—Hermetic containers.

Gentamicin Sulfate Ointment

ゲンタマイシン硫酸塩軟膏

Gentamicin Sulfate Ointment contains not less than 90.0% and not more than 110.0% of the labeled potency of gentamicin C_1 ($C_{21}H_{43}N_5O_7$: 477.60).

Method of preparation Prepare as directed under Ointments, with Gentamicin Sulfate.

Identification To an amount of Gentamicin Sulfate Ointment, equivalent to 5 mg (potency) of Gentamicin Sulfate, add 10 mL of diethyl ether, and shake in lukewarm water, if necessary, to dissolve. Add 5 mL of water, shake for 10 minutes, centrifuge, and use the water layer as the sample solution. Separately, dissolve an amount of Gentamicin Sulfate RS, equivalent to 10 mg (potency), in 10 mL of water, and use this solution as the standard solution. Perform the test with these solutions as directed under Thin-layer Chromatography <*2.03*>. Spot 10 μL each of the sample solution and standard solution on a plate of silica gel for thin-layer chromatography. Develop the plate with the lower layer of a mixture of chloroform, ammonia solution (28) and methanol (2:1:1) to a distance of about 15 cm, and air-dry the plate. Spray evenly 0.2% ninhydrin-water saturated 1-butanol TS on the plate, and heat the plate at 100°C for 10 minutes: three principal spots obtained from the sample solution are the same with the corresponding spots from the standard solution in color tone and the *R*f value, respectively.

Assay Perform the test according to the Cylinder-plate method as directed under Microbial Assay for Antibiotics <*4.02*> according to the following conditions.

(i) Test organism, agar media for base and seed layer, agar medium for transferring test organisms, and standard solutions—Proceed as directed in the Assay under Gentamicin Sulfate.

(ii) Sample solutions—Weigh accurately an amount of Gentamicin Sulfate Ointment, equivalent to about 1 mg (potency) of Gentamicin Sulfate, transfer to a separator, add 50 mL of diethyl ether, and shake until the solution becomes uniform. Add 25 mL of 0.1 mol/L phosphate buffer solution (pH 8.0), shake, and collect the water layer. Repeat the same procedure with 25 mL of 0.1 mol/L phosphate buffer solution (pH 8.0), and combine the water layers. To this solution add 0.1 mol/L phosphate buffer solution (pH 8.0) to make exactly 100 mL. Pipet a suitable volume of this solution, add 0.1 mol/L phosphate buffer solution (pH 8.0) to make solutions so that each mL contains 4 μg (potency) and 1 μg (potency), and use these solutions as the high concentration sample solution and the low concentration sample solution, respectively.

Containers and storage Containers—Tight containers.

Gentamicin Sulfate Ophthalmic Solution

ゲンタマイシン硫酸塩点眼液

Gentamicin Sulfate Ophthalmic Solution is an aqueous ophthalmic preparation.

It contains not less than 90.0% and not more than 110.0% of the labeled potency of expressed as mass of gentamicin C_1 ($C_{21}H_{43}N_5O_7$: 477.60).

Method of preparation Prepare as directed under Ophthalmic Liquids and Solutions, with Gentamicin Sulfate.

Description Gentamicin Sulfate Ophthalmic Solution is a clear, colorless or pale yellow liquid.

Identification To a volume of Gentamicin Sulfate Ophthalmic Solution, equivalent to 10 mg (potency) of Gentamicin Sulfate, add water to make 5 mL, and use this solution as the sample solution. Separately, dissolve an amount of Gentamicin Sulfate RS, equivalent to 10 mg (potency), in 5 mL of water, and use this solution as the standard solution. Perform the test with these solutions as directed under Thin-layer Chromatography *<2.03>*. Spot 5 μL each of the sample solution and standard solution on a plate of silica gel for thin-layer chromatography. Develop the plate with the lower layer of a mixture of chloroform, ammonia solution (28) and methanol (2:1:1) to a distance of about 15 cm, and air-dry the plate. Spray evenly 0.2% ninhydrin-water saturated 1-butanol TS on the plate, and heat the plate at 100°C for 5 minutes: three principal spots obtained from the sample solution are the same with the corresponding spots from the standard solution in color tone and the *R*f value, respectively.

pH *<2.54>* 5.5 – 7.5

Foreign insoluble matter *<6.11>* It meets the requirement.

Insoluble particulate matter *<6.08>* It meets the requirement.

Sterility *<4.06>* Perform the test according to the Membrane filtration method: it meets the requirement.

Assay Perform the test according to the Cylinder-plate method as directed under Microbial Assay for Antibiotics *<4.02>* according to the following conditions.

(i) Test organism, agar media for seed and base layer, agar medium for transferring test organism, and standard solutions—Proceed as directed in the Assay under Gentamicin Sulfate.

(ii) Sample solutions—Pipet a volume of Gentamicin Sulfate Ophthalmic Solution, equivalent to about 12 mg (potency) of Gentamicin Sulfate, add 0.1 mol/L phosphate buffer solution (pH 8.0) to make a solution so that each mL contains about 1 mg (potency). Pipet a suitable volume of this solution, add 0.1 mol/L phosphate buffer solution (pH 8.0) to make solutions so that each mL contains 4 μg (potency) and 1 μg (potency), and use these solutions as the high concentration sample solution and the low concentration sample solution, respectively.

Containers and storage Containers—Tight containers.

Shelf life 24 months after preparation.

Glibenclamide

グリベンクラミド

$C_{23}H_{28}ClN_3O_5S$: 494.00
4-[2-(5-Chloro-2-methoxybenzoylamino)ethyl]-*N*-(cyclohexylcarbamoyl)benzenesulfonamide
[*10238-21-8*]

Glibenclamide, when dried, contains not less than 98.5% of glibenclamide ($C_{23}H_{28}ClN_3O_5S$).

Description Glibenclamide occurs as white to pale yellowish white, crystals or crystalline powder.

It is freely soluble in dimethylformamide, sparingly soluble in chloroform, slightly soluble in methanol and in ethanol (95), and practically insoluble in water.

Identification **(1)** Determine the absorption spectrum of a solution of Glinbenclamide in methanol (1 in 10,000) as directed under Ultraviolet-visible Spectrophotometry *<2.24>*, and compare the spectrum with the Reference Spectrum: both spectra exhibit similar intensities of absorption at the same wavelengths.

(2) Determine the infrared absorption spectrum of Glibenclamide, previously dried, as directed in the potassium bromide disk method under Infrared Spectrophotometry *<2.25>*, and compare the spectrum with the Reference Spectrum: both spectra exhibit similar intensities of absorption at the same wave numbers.

(3) Perform the test with Glibenclamide as directed under Flame Coloration Test *<1.04>* (2): a green color appears.

Melting point *<2.60>* 169 – 174°C

Purity **(1)** Heavy metals *<1.07>*—Proceed with 1.0 g of Glibenclamide according to Method 2, and perform the test. Prepare the control solution with 2.0 mL of Standard Lead Solution (not more than 20 ppm).

(2) Related substances—Dissolve 0.20 g of Glibenclamide in 20 mL of chloroform, and use this solution as the sample solution. Pipet 1 mL of the sample solution, and add chloroform to make exactly 20 mL. Pipet 1 mL of this solution, add chloroform to make exactly 10 mL, and use this solution as the standard solution. Perform the test with these solutions as directed under Thin-layer Chromatography *<2.03>*. Spot 10 μL each of the sample solution and standard solution on a plate of silica gel with fluorescent indicator for thin-layer chromatography. Develop the plate with a mixture of 1-propanol, chloroform and diluted ammonia TS (4 in 5) (11:7:2) to a distance of about 12 cm, and air-dry the plate. Examine under ultraviolet light (main wavelength: 254 nm): the spots other than the principal spot obtained from the sample solution are not more intense than the spot from the standard solution.

Loss on drying *<2.41>* Not more than 0.5% (1 g, 105°C, 4 hours).

Assay Weigh accurately about 0.9 g of Glibenclamide, previously dried, dissolve in 50 mL of *N*,*N*-dimethylformamide, and titrate 〈*2.50*〉 with 0.1 mol/L sodium hydroxide VS (indicator: 3 drops of phenolphthalein TS). Perform a blank determination in the same manner with a solution prepared by adding 18 mL of water to 50 mL of *N,N*-dimethylformamide, and make any necessary correction.

Each mL of 0.1 mol/L sodium hydroxide VS
= 49.40 mg of $C_{23}H_{28}ClN_3O_5S$

Containers and storage Containers—Tight containers.

Gliclazide

グリクラジド

$C_{15}H_{21}N_3O_3S$: 323.41
1-(Hexahydrocyclopenta[c]pyrrol-2(1*H*)-yl)-
3-[(4-methylphenyl)sulfonyl]urea
[21187-98-4]

Gliclazide, when dried, contains not less than 98.5% and not more than 101.0% of gliclazide ($C_{15}H_{21}N_3O_3S$).

Description Gliclazide is a white crystalline powder.

It is sparingly soluble in acetonitrile and in methanol, slightly soluble in ethanol (99.5) and practically insoluble in water.

Identification **(1)** Determine the absorption spectrum of a solution of Gliclazide in methanol (1 in 62,500) as directed under Ultraviolet-visible Spectrophotometry 〈*2.24*〉, and compare the spectrum with the Reference Spectrum: both spectra exhibit similar intensities of absorption at the same wavelengths.

(2) Determine the infrared absorption spectrum of Gliclazide, previously dried, as directed in the potassium bromide disk method under Infrared Spectrophotometry 〈*2.25*〉, and compare the spectrum with the Reference Spectrum: both spectra exhibit similar intensities of absorption at the same wave numbers.

Melting point 〈*2.60*〉 165 – 169°C

Purity **(1)** Heavy metals 〈*1.07*〉—Proceed with 2.0 g of Gliclazide according to Method 2, and perform the test. Prepare the control solution with 2.0 mL of Standard Lead Solution (not more than 10 ppm).

(2) Related substances—Conduct this procedure within 2 hours after preparation of the sample solution. Dissolve 50 mg of Gliclazide in 23 mL of acetonitrile, add water to make 50 mL, and use this solution as the sample solution. Pipet 1 mL of the sample solution, and add a mixture of water and acetonitrile (11:9) to make exactly 100 mL. Pipet 10 mL of this solution, add a mixture of water and acetonitrile (11:9) to make exactly 100 mL, and use this solution as the standard solution. Perform the test with exactly 20 μL each of the sample solution and standard solution as directed under Liquid Chromatography 〈*2.01*〉 according to the following conditions. Determine each peak area of both solutions by the automatic integration method: the area of each peak other than gliclazide obtained from the sample solution is not larger than the peak area of gliclazide from the standard solution, and the total area of the peaks other than the peak of gliclazide from the sample solution is not larger than 3 times the peak area of gliclazide from the standard solution. For the area of the peak, having the relative retention time of about 0.9 to gliclazide, multiply the correction factor 5.65.

Operating conditions—

Detector: An ultraviolet absorption photometer (wavelength: 235 nm).

Column: A stainless steel column 4.0 mm in inside diameter and 25 cm in length, packed with octylsilanized silica gel for liquid chromatography (4 μm in particle diameter).

Column temperature: A constant temperature of about 25°C.

Mobile phase: A mixture of water, acetonitrile, triethylamine and trifluoroacetic acid (550:450:1:1).

Flow rate: Adjust so that the retention time of gliclazide is about 14 minutes.

Time span of measurement: About 2 times as long as the retention time of gliclazide, beginning after the solvent peak.

System suitability—

Test for required detectability: Pipet 4 mL of the standard solution, and add a mixture of water and acetonitrile (11:9) to make exactly 20 mL. Confirm that the peak area of gliclazide obtained with 20 μL of this solution is equivalent to 10 to 30% of that of gliclazide with 20 μL of the standard solution.

System performance: When the procedure is run with 20 μL of the standard solution under the above operating conditions, the number of theoretical plates and the symmetry factor of the peak of gliclazide are not less than 8000 and not more than 1.5, respectively.

System repeatability: When the test is repeated 6 times with 20 μL of the standard solution under the above operating conditions, the relative standard deviation of the peak area of gliclazide is not more than 2.0%.

Loss on drying 〈*2.41*〉 Not more than 0.5% (1 g, 105°C, 2 hours).

Residue on ignition 〈*2.44*〉 Not more than 0.1% (1 g).

Assay Weigh accurately about 0.3 g of Gliclazide, previously dried, dissolve in 30 mL of a mixture of acetic anhydride and acetic acid (100) (7:3), and titrate 〈*2.50*〉 with 0.1 mol/L perchloric acid VS (potentiometric titration). Perform a blank determination in the same manner, and make any necessary correction.

Each mL of 0.1 mol/L perchloric acid VS
= 32.34 mg of $C_{15}H_{21}N_3O_3S$

Containers and storage Containers—Well-closed containers.

Glimepiride

グリメピリド

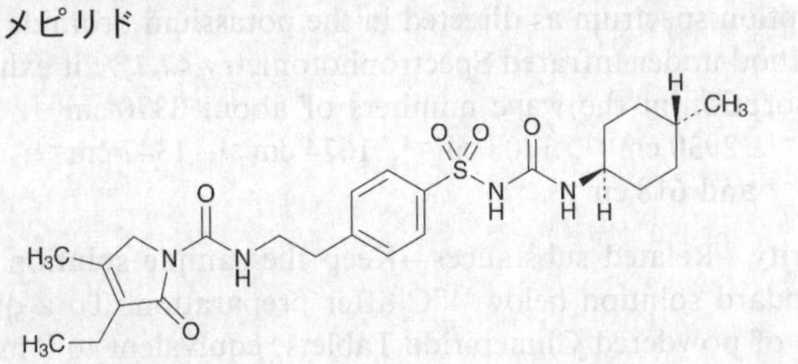

$C_{24}H_{34}N_4O_5S$: 490.62
1-(4-{2-[(3-Ethyl-4-methyl-2-oxo-3-pyrroline-1-carbonyl)amino]ethyl}phenylsulfonyl)-3-(*trans*-4-methylcyclohexyl)urea
[93479-97-1]

Glimepiride contains not less than 98.0% and not more than 102.0% of glimepiride ($C_{24}H_{34}N_4O_5S$), calculated on the anhydrous basis.

Description Glimepiride occurs as a white crystalline powder.

It is slightly soluble in dichloromethane, very slightly soluble in methanol and in ethanol (99.5), and practically insoluble in water.

Melting point: about 202°C (with decomposition).

Identification **(1)** Determine the absorption spectrum of a solution of Glimepiride in methanol (1 in 125,000) as directed under Ultraviolet-visible Spectrophotometry <*2.24*>, and compare the spectrum with the Reference Spectrum or the spectrum of a solution of Glimepiride RS prepared in the same manner as the sample solution: both spectra exhibit similar intensities of absorption at the same wavelengths.

(2) Determine the infrared absorption spectrum of Glimepiride as directed in the potassium bromide disk method under Infrared Spectrophotometry <*2.25*>, and compare the spectrum with the Reference Spectrum or the spectrum of Glimepiride RS: both spectra exhibit similar intensities of absorption at the same wave numbers.

Purity **(1)** Heavy metals <*1.07*>—Proceed with 2.0 g of Glimepiride according to Method 2, and perform the test. Prepare the control solution with 2.0 mL of Standard Lead Solution (not more than 10 ppm).

(2) *cis*-Isomer—Dissolve 10 mg of Glimepiride in 5 mL of dichloromethane, add the mobile phase to make 20 mL, and use this solution as the sample solution. Pipet 1 mL of the sample solution, add the mobile phase to make exactly 100 mL, and use this solution as the standard solution. Perform the test with exactly 10 μL each of the sample solution and standard solution as directed under Liquid Chromatography <*2.01*> according to the following conditions. Determine each peak area of both solutions by the automatic integration method: the area of the peak, having the relative retention time of about 0.9 to glimepiride, obtained from the sample solution is not larger than 3/4 times the peak area of glimepiride from the standard solution.

Operating conditions—

Detector: An ultraviolet absorption photometer (wavelength: 228 nm).

Column: A stainless steel column 3 mm in inside diameter and 15 cm in length, packed with diol silica gel for liquid chromatography (5 μm in particle diameter).

Column temperature: A constant temperature of about 25°C.

Mobile phase: A mixture of heptane for liquid chromatography, 2-propanol for liquid chromatography, and acetic acid (100) (900:100:1).

Flow rate: Adjust so that the retention time of glimepiride is about 14 minutes.

System suitability—

Test for required detectability: Pipet 5 mL of the standard solution, and add the mobile phase to make exactly 10 mL. Confirm that the peak area of glimepiride obtained with 10 μL of this solution is equivalent to 35 to 65% of that with 10 μL of the standard solution.

System performance: When the procedure is run with 10 μL of the standard solution under the above operating conditions, the number of theoretical plates and the symmetry factor of the peak of glimepiride are not less than 3000 and not more than 1.5, respectively.

System repeatability: When the test is repeated 6 times with 10 μL of the standard solution under the above operating conditions, the relative standard deviation of the peak area of glimepiride is not more than 2.0%.

(3) Related substances—Keep the sample solution and standard solution below 4°C after preparing. Dissolve 20 mg of Glimepiride in 100 mL of a mixture of acetonitrile for liquid chromatography and water (4:1), and use this solution as the sample solution. Pipet 1 mL of the sample solution, and add the mobile phase to make exactly 100 mL. Pipet 1 mL of this solution, add the mobile phase to make exactly 10 mL, and use this solution as the standard solution. Perform the test with exactly 20 μL each of the sample solution and standard solution as directed under Liquid Chromatography <*2.01*> according to the following conditions. Determine each peak area of both solutions by the automatic integration method: the area of the peak, having the relative retention time of about 0.25 to glimepiride, obtained from the sample solution is not larger than 4 times the peak area of glimepiride from the standard solution, the area of the peak, having the relative retention time of about 1.1, is not larger than 2 times the peak area of glimepiride from the standard solution, the area of the peak, having the relative retention time of about 0.32, is not larger than 1.5 times the peak area of glimepiride from the standard solution, the area of peak other than glimepiride and above mentioned peak from the sample solution is not larger than the peak of glimepiride from the standard solution, and the total area of the peaks other than glimepiride and the peak, having the relative retention time of about 0.25, from the sample solution is not larger than 5 times the peak area of glimepiride from the standard solution.

Operating conditions—

Detector, column, column temperature, mobile phase, and flow rate: Proceed as directed in the operating conditions in the Assay.

Time span of measurement: About 2.5 times as long as the retention time of glimepiride, beginning after the solvent peak.

System suitability—

Test for required detectability: Pipet 5 mL of the standard solution, and add the mobile phase to make exactly 10 mL. Confirm that the peak area of glimepiride obtained with 20 μL of this solution is equivalent to 35 to 65% of that with 20 μL of the standard solution.

System performance: When the procedure is run with 20 μL of the standard solution under the above operating conditions, the number of theoretical plates and the symmetry factor of the peak of glimepiride are not less than 9000 and not more than 1.5, respectively.

System repeatability: When the test is repeated 6 times

with 20 μL of the standard solution under the above operating conditions, the relative standard deviation of the peak area of glimepiride is not more than 2.0%.

Water <*2.48*> Not more than 0.5% (0.25 g, coulometric titration).

Residue on ignition <*2.44*> Not more than 0.2% (1 g).

Assay Weigh accurately about 20 mg each of Glimepiride and Glimepiride RS (separately determine the water <*2.48*> in the same manner as Glimepiride), dissolve each substance in a mixture of acetonitrile for liquid chromatography and water (4:1) to make exactly 100 mL, and use these solutions as the sample solution and the standard solution, respectively. Perform the test with exactly 20 μL each of the sample solution and standard solution as directed under Liquid Chromatography <*2.01*> according to the following conditions, and determine the peak areas, A_T and A_S, of glimepiride in each solution.

$$\text{Amount (mg) of glimepiride } (C_{24}H_{34}N_4O_5S) = M_S \times A_T/A_S$$

M_S: Amount (mg) of Glimepiride RS taken, calculated on the anhydrous basis

Operating conditions—

Detector: An ultraviolet absorption photometer (wavelength: 228 nm).

Column: A stainless steel column 4 mm in inside diameter and 25 cm in length, packed with octadecylsilanized silica gel for liquid chromatography (4 μm in particle diameter).

Column temperature: A constant temperature of about 25°C.

Mobile phase: Dissolve 0.5 g of sodium dihydrogen phosphate dihydrate in 500 mL of water, adjust to pH 2.5 with phosphoric acid, and add 500 mL of acetonitrile for liquid chromatography.

Flow rate: Adjust so that the retention time of glimepiride is about 17 minutes.

System suitability—

System performance: When the procedure is run with 20 μL of the standard solution under the above operating conditions, the number of theoretical plates and the symmetry factor of the peak of glimepiride are not less than 9000 and not more than 1.5, respectively.

System repeatability: When the test is repeated 6 times with 20 μL of the standard solution under the above operating conditions, the relative standard deviation of the peak area of glimepiride is not more than 1.0%.

Containers and storage Containers—Well-closed containers.

Glimepiride Tablets

グリメピリド錠

Glimepiride Tablets contain not less than 93.0% and not more than 107.0% of the labeled amount of glimepiride ($C_{24}H_{34}N_4O_5S$: 490.62).

Method of preparation Prepare as directed under Tablets, with Glimepiride.

Identification To a quantity of powdered Glimepiride Tablets, equivalent to 20 mg of Glimepiride, add 40 mL of acetonitrile, shake for 15 minutes, and centrifuge. Evaporate the supernatant liquid on a water bath under reduced pressure, suspend the residue with 1 mL of water, and filter under reduced pressure. Wash the residue with 1 mL of water, dry at 105°C for 1 hour. Determine the infrared absorption spectrum as directed in the potassium bromide disk method under Infrared Spectrophotometry <*2.25*>: it exhibits absorption at the wave numbers of about 3370 cm^{-1}, 3290 cm^{-1}, 2930 cm^{-1}, 1708 cm^{-1}, 1674 cm^{-1}, 1347 cm^{-1}, 1156 cm^{-1} and 618 cm^{-1}.

Purity Related substances—Keep the sample solution and standard solution below 4°C after preparation. To a quantity of powdered Glimepiride Tablets, equivalent to 9 mg of Glimepiride, wet with 0.5 mL of water, add a mixture of acetonitrile for liquid chromatography and water (4:1) to make 50 mL, shake, centrifuge, and use the supernatant liquid as the sample solution. Pipet 1 mL of the sample solution, add a mixture of acetonitrile for liquid chromatography and water (4:1) to make exactly 100 mL, and use this solution as the standard solution. Perform the test with exactly 5 μL each of the sample solution and standard solution as directed under Liquid Chromatography <*2.01*> according to the following conditions. Determine each peak area of both solutions by the automatic integration method: the area of the peak, having the relative retention time of about 0.3 to glimepiride, obtained from the sample solution is not larger than 2.6 times the peak area of glimepiride from the standard solution, the area of the peak other than glimepiride and the peak mentioned above from the sample solution is not larger than 3/10 times the peak area of glimepiride from the standard solution, and the total area of the peaks other than glimepiride and the peak mentioned above from the sample solution is not larger than the peak area of glimepiride from the standard solution, and the total area of the peaks other than glimepiride from the sample solution is not larger than 3 times the peak area of glimepiride from the standard solution.

Operating conditions—

Detector, column, column temperature, and mobile phase: Proceed as directed in the operating conditions in the Assay.

Flow rate: Adjust so that the retention time of glimepiride is about 12 minutes.

Time span of measurement: About 2 times as long as the retention time of glimepiride.

System suitability—

Test for required detectability: Pipet 2 mL of the standard solution, and add the mobile phase to make exactly 20 mL. Confirm that the peak area of glimepiride obtained with 5 μL of this solution is equivalent to 7 to 13% of that with 5 μL of the standard solution.

System performance: When the procedure is run with 5 μL of the standard solution under the above operating conditions, the number of theoretical plates and the symmetry factor of the peak of glimepiride are not less than 6000 and not more than 1.5, respectively.

System repeatability: When the test is repeated 6 times with 5 μL of the standard solution under the above operating conditions, the relative standard deviation of the peak area of glimepiride is not more than 2.0%.

Uniformity of dosage units <*6.02*> Perform the test according to the following method: it meets the requirement of the Content uniformity test.

To 1 tablet of Glimepiride Tablets add $V/10$ mL of water, disintegrate, add $V/2$ mL of a mixture of acetonitrile for liquid chromatography and water (4:1), and shake. To this solution add exactly $V/5$ mL of the internal standard solution, add a mixture of acetonitrile for liquid chromatography and water (4:1) to make V mL so that each mL contains about

100 μg of glimepiride ($C_{24}H_{34}N_4O_5S$), and centrifuge. To 2.5 mL of the supernatant liquid add a mixture of acetonitrile for liquid chromatography and water (4:1) to make 5 mL, and use this solution as the sample solution. Separately, weigh accurately about 20 mg of Glimepiride RS (separately determine the water <*2.48*> in the same manner as Glimepiride), and dissolve in a mixture of acetonitrile for liquid chromatography and water (4:1) to make exactly 100 mL. Pipet 5 mL of this solution, add exactly 2 mL of the internal standard solution, add a mixture of acetonitrile for liquid chromatography and water (4:1) to make 20 mL, and use this solution as the standard solution. Then, proceed as directed in the Assay.

$$\text{Amount (mg) of glimepiride } (C_{24}H_{34}N_4O_5S) = M_S \times Q_T/Q_S \times V/200$$

M_S: Amount (mg) of Glimepiride RS taken, calculated on the anhydrous basis

Internal standard solution—A solution of butyl parahydroxybenzoate in a mixture of acetonitrile for liquid chromatography and water (4:1) (1 in 1000).

Dissolution <*6.10*> When the test is performed at 50 revolutions per minute according to the Paddle method, using 900 mL of disodium hydrogen phosphate-citric acid buffer solution (pH 7.5) as the dissolution medium, the dissolution rate in 15 minutes of 0.5-mg and 1-mg tablets is not less than 75%, and that in 30 minutes of 3-mg tablet is not less than 70%.

Start the test with 1 tablet of Glimepiride Tablets, withdraw not less than 20 mL of the medium at the specified minute after starting the test, and filter through a membrane filter with a pore size not exceeding 0.45 μm. Discard not less than 10 mL of the first filtrate, pipet V mL of the subsequent filtrate, add the dissolution medium to make exactly V' mL so that each mL contains about 0.56 μg of glimepiride ($C_{24}H_{34}N_4O_5S$), and use this solution as the sample solution. Separately, weigh accurately about 22 mg of Glimepiride RS (separately determine the water <*2.48*> in the same manner as Glimepiride), and dissolve in acetonitrile for liquid chromatography to make exactly 100 mL. Pipet 2 mL of this solution, add 8 mL of acetonitrile for liquid chromatography, and add the dissolution medium to make exactly 200 mL. Pipet 5 mL of this solution, add the dissolution medium to make exactly 20 mL, and use this solution as the standard solution. Perform the test with exactly 50 μL each of the sample solution and standard solution as directed under Liquid Chromatography <*2.01*> according to the following conditions, and determine the peak areas, A_T and A_S, of glimepiride in each solution.

$$\text{Dissolution rate (\%) with respect to the labeled amount of glimepiride } (C_{24}H_{34}N_4O_5S) = M_S \times A_T/A_S \times V'/V \times 1/C \times 9/4$$

M_S: Amount (mg) of Glimepiride RS taken, calculated on the anhydrous basis

C: Labeled amount (mg) of glimepiride ($C_{24}H_{34}N_4O_5S$) in 1 tablet

Operating conditions—

Detector, column temperature, mobile phase, and flow rate: Proceed as directed in the operating conditions in the Assay.

Column: A stainless steel column 4.6 mm in inside diameter and 15 cm in length, packed with octadecylsilanized silica gel for liquid chromatography (5 μm in particle diameter).

System suitability—

System performance: When the procedure is run with 50 μL of the standard solution under the above operating conditions, the number of theoretical plates and the symmetry factor of the peak of glimepiride are not less than 3000 and not more than 1.5, respectively.

System repeatability: When the test is repeated 6 times with 50 μL of the standard solution under the above operations conditions, the relative standard deviation of the peak area of glimepiride is not more than 1.5%.

Assay Weigh accurately the mass of not less than 20 Glimepiride Tablets, and powder. Weigh accurately a portion of the powder, equivalent to about 3 mg of glimepiride ($C_{24}H_{34}N_4O_5S$), add 3 mL of water, and shake with 30 mL of a mixture of acetonitrile for liquid chromatography and water (4:1). Add exactly 6 mL of the internal standard solution, and add a mixture of acetonitrile for liquid chromatography and water (4:1) to make 50 mL, centrifuge, and use the supernatant liquid as the sample solution. Separately, weigh accurately about 20 mg of Glimepiride RS, (separately, determine the water <*2.48*> in the same manner as Glimepiride), dissolve in a mixture of acetonitrile for liquid chromatography and water (4:1) to make exactly 100 mL. Pipet 15 mL of this solution, add exactly 6 mL of the internal standard solution, add a mixture of acetonitrile for liquid chromatography and water (4:1) to make 50 mL, and use this solution as the standard solution. Perform the test with 10 μL each of the sample solution and standard solution as directed under Liquid Chromatography <*2.01*> according to the following conditions, and calculate the ratios, Q_T and Q_S, of the peak area of glimepiride to that of the internal standard.

$$\text{Amount (mg) of glimepiride } (C_{24}H_{34}N_4O_5S) = M_S \times Q_T/Q_S \times 3/20$$

M_S: Amount (mg) of Glimepiride RS taken, calculated on the anhydrous basis

Internal standard solution—A solution of butyl parahydroxybenzoate in a mixture of acetonitrile for liquid chromatography and water (4:1) (1 in 1000).

Operating conditions—

Detector: An ultraviolet spectrophotometer (wavelength: 228 nm).

Column: A stainless steel column 4 mm in inside diameter and 12.5 cm in length, packed with octadecylsilanized silica gel for liquid chromatography (5 μm in particle diameter).

Column temperature: A constant temperature of about 25°C.

Mobile phase: Dissolve 0.5 g of sodium dihydrogen phosphate dihydrate in 500 mL of water, add 500 mL of acetonitrile for liquid chromatography, and adjust to pH 3.5 with diluted phosphoric acid (1 in 5).

Flow rate: Adjust so that the retention time of glimepiride is about 10 minutes.

System suitability—

System performance: When the procedure is run with 10 μL of the standard solution under the above operating conditions, the internal standard and glimepiride are eluted in this order with the resolution between these peaks being not less than 6.

System repeatability: When the test is repeated 6 times with 10 μL of the standard solution under the above operating conditions, the relative standard deviation of the ratio of the peak area of glimepiride to that of the internal standard is not more than 1.0%.

Containers and storage Containers—Tight containers.

Glucagon (Genetical Recombination)

グルカゴン(遺伝子組換え)

```
HSQGTFTSDY SKYLDSRRAQ DFVQWLMNT
```

$C_{153}H_{225}N_{43}O_{49}S$: 3482.75
[*16941-32-5*]

Glucagon (Genetical Recombination) is a recombinant human glucagon, and is a peptide consisting of 29 amino acid residues.

It contains not less than 92.5% and not more than 105.0% of glucagon, calculated on the anhydrous basis.

Manufacture Glucagon (Genetical Recombination) is manufactured by the process that has been properly validated to be able to manufacture the drug substance having predefined biological activity. When the residual amount of host cell proteins is determined by enzyme immunoassay as in-process tests, the amount should be not more than the control value. In addition, Glucagon (Genetical Recombination) is purified by the process that has been validated that the residual amount of host cell DNA is not more than the control value.

Description Glucagon (Genetical Recombination) occurs as a white lyophilized powder.

It is practically insoluble in water and in ethanol (99.5).

It is hygroscopic.

Identification **(1)** Dissolve 5 mg of Glucagon (Genetical Recombination) in 1 mL of 0.01 mol/L hydrochloric acid TS. To 200 μL of this solution add 800 μL of 0.1 mol/L ammonium hydrogen carbonate TS and 25 μL of enzyme TS for glucagon, react at 37°C for 2 hours, add 120 μL of acetic acid (100) to stop the reaction, and use this solution as the sample solution. Separately, dissolve a suitable amount of Glucagon RS in 0.1 mol/L ammonium hydrogen carbonate TS so that each mL contains 1 mg of glucagon. To 1000 μL of this solution add 25 μL of enzyme TS for glucagon, react at 37°C for 2 hours, add 120 μL of acetic acid (100) to stop the reaction, and use this solution as the standard solution. Perform the test with 20 μL each of the sample solution and standard solution as directed under Liquid Chromatography <*2.01*> according to the following conditions, and compare the chromatograms obtained from these solutions: both chromatograms show the similar peaks at the same retention time.

Operating conditions—

Detector: An ultraviolet absorption photometer (wavelength: 215 nm).

Column: A stainless steel column 4 mm in inside diameter and 50 mm in length, packed with octadecylsilanized silica gel for liquid chromatography (5 μm in particle diameter).

Column temperature: A constant temperature of about 22°C.

Mobile phase A: To 0.5 mL of trifluoroacetic acid add 1000 mL of water.

Mobile phase B: To 0.5 mL of trifluoroacetic acid add 600 mL of ethanol (99.5) and 400 mL of water.

Flowing of mobile phase: Control the gradient by mixing the mobile phases A and B as directed in the following table.

Time after injection of sample (min)	Mobile phase A (vol%)	Mobile phase B (vol%)
0 – 35	100 → 53	0 → 47
35 – 45	53 → 0	47 → 100

Flow rate: 1.0 mL per minute.

System suitability—

System performance: When the procedure is run with 20 μL of the standard solution under the above operating conditions, the peaks 1, 2, 3, 4 and 5 are eluted in this order, and the resolution between the peak 2 and the peak 3 is not less than 1.5.

(2) Perform the test with 15 μL each of the sample solution and standard solution obtained in the Assay as directed under Liquid chromatography <*2.01*> according to the conditions described in the Assay: the retention times of the principal peaks obtained from the sample solution and the standard solution are the same.

Purity Related substances and desamido substances—Conduct this procedure at a temperature between 2°C and 8°C. Dissolve 50 mg of Glucagon (Genetical Recombination) in 100 mL of 0.01 mol/L hydrochloric acid TS, and use this solution as the sample solution. Perform the test with 15 μL of the sample solution as directed under Liquid Chromatography <*2.01*> according to the following conditions. Determine each peak area by the automatic integration method, and calculate the amounts of them by the area percentage method: the total amount of desamido substance 1 having the relative retention time of about 1.1 to glucagon, desamido substance 2 having the relative retention time of about 1.2, desamido substance 3 having the relative retention time of about 1.3 and desamido substance 4 having the relative retention time of about 1.4 is not more than 0.8%, and the total amount of peaks other than glucagon is not more than 2.0%.

Operating conditions—

Detector, column, column temperature, mobile phases A and B, flowing of mobile phase, and flow rate: Proceed as directed in the operating conditions in the Assay.

Time span of measurement: For 37 minutes after injection, beginning after the solvent peak.

System suitability—

System performance: Proceed as directed in the system suitability in the Assay.

Test for required detectability: When the procedure is run with 15 μL of the standard solution obtained in the Assay under the above operating conditions, the peak corresponding to the desamido substance 2 is detected.

Water <*2.48*> Not more than 10% (50 mg, coulometric titration).

Assay Conduct this procedure at a temperature between 2°C and 8°C. Weigh accurately about 50 mg of Glucagon (Genetical Recombination), dissolve in 100 mL of 0.01 mol/L hydrochloric acid TS, and use this solution as the sample solution. Separately dissolve Glucagon RS in 0.01 mol/L hydrochloric acid TS so that each mL contains about 0.5 mg of glucagon, and use this solution as the standard solution. Perform the test with exactly 15 μL each of the sample solution and standard solution as directed under Liquid Chromatography <*2.01*> according to the following conditions, and determine the peak areas, A_T and A_S, of glucagon in each solution.

$$\text{Amount (\%) of glucagon} = A_T/A_S \times C_S/C_T \times 100$$

C_S: Concentration (mg/mL) of the standard solution
C_T: Concentration (mg/mL) of the sample solution

The calculated amount (%) of glucagon is corrected by the water content to obtain the amount (%) of glucagon on the anhydrous basis.

Operating conditions—

Detector: An ultraviolet absorption photometer (wavelength: 214 nm).

Column: A stainless steel column 3 mm in inside diameter and 150 mm in length, packed with octadecylsilanized silica gel for liquid chromatography (3 μm in particle diameter).

Column temperature: A constant temperature of about 45°C.

Mobile phase A: Dissolve 16.3 g of potassium dihydrogen phosphate in 750 mL of water, adjust to pH 2.7 with phosphoric acid, add water to make 800 mL, and add 200 mL of acetonitrile for liquid chromatography.

Mobile phase B: A mixture of water and acetonitrile (3:2).

Flowing of mobile phase: Control the gradient by mixing the mobile phases A and B as directed in the following table.

Time after injection of sample (min)	Mobile phase A (vol%)	Mobile phase B (vol%)
0 – 25*	61	39
25 – 29	61 → 12	39 → 88
29 – 30	12	88
30 – 31	12 → 61	88 → 39
31 – 37	61	39

* Adjust the time for the isocratic condition so that the gradient starts after the desamido substance 4 is eluted.

Flow rate: 0.5 mL per minute.

System suitability—

System performance: Dissolve Glucagon RS in 0.01 mol/L hydrochloric acid TS to make a solution so that each mL contains 0.5 mg of glucagon. Warm this solution at 50°C for 48 hours, and use this solution as the solution for system suitability test. When the procedure is run with 15 μL of the solution for system suitability test under the above operating conditions, four peaks corresponding to the desamido substances 1, 2, 3 and 4 eluted after the principal peak are clearly detected, the total amount of these peaks is not less than 7%, and the resolution between glucagon and the desamido substance 1 is not less than 1.5. Furthermore, when the procedure is run with 15 μL of the standard solution under the above operating conditions, the symmetry factor of the principal peak is not more than 1.8.

System repeatability: When the test is repeated 5 times with the standard solution under the above operating conditions, the relative standard deviation of the peak area of glucagon is not more than 2.0%.

Containers and storage Containers—Tight containers.

Storage—Light-resistant, and not exceeding −15°C.

Glucose

ブドウ糖

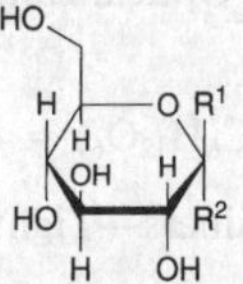

α-D-Glucopyranose : R^1=H, R^2=OH
β-D-Glucopyranose : R^1=OH, R^2=H

$C_6H_{12}O_6$: 180.16
D-Glucopyranose
[50-99-7]

Glucose is α-D-glucopyranose, β-D-glucopyranose, or a mixture of them.

It, when dried, contains not less than 99.5% of glucose [D-glucopyranose ($C_6H_{12}O_6$)].

Description Glucose occurs as white, crystals or crystalline powder. It is odorless, and has a sweet taste.

It is freely soluble in water, slightly soluble in ethanol (95), and practically insoluble in diethyl ether.

Identification Add 2 to 3 drops of a solution of Glucose (1 in 20) to 5 mL of boiling Fehling's TS: a red precipitate is produced.

Purity (1) Clarity and color of solution—Add 25 g of Glucose to 30 mL of water in a Nessler tube, warm at 60°C in a water bath until solution is effected, cool, and add water to make 50 mL: the solution is clear and has no more color than the following control solution.

Control solution: To a mixture of 1.0 mL of Cobalt (II) Chloride CS, 3.0 mL of Iron (III) Chloride CS, and 2.0 mL of Copper (II) Sulfate CS, add water to make 10.0 mL. To 3.0 mL of this solution add water to make 50 mL.

(2) Acidity—Dissolve 5.0 g of Glucose in 50 mL of freshly boiled and cooled water, and add 3 drops of phenolphthalein TS and 0.60 mL of 0.01 mol/L sodium hydroxide VS: a red color develops.

(3) Chloride *<1.03>*—Perform the test with 2.0 g of Glucose. Prepare the control solution with 1.0 mL of 0.01 mol/L hydrochloric acid VS (not more than 0.018%).

(4) Sulfate *<1.14>*—Perform the test with 2.0 g of Glucose. Prepare the control solution with 1.0 mL of 0.005 mol/L sulfuric acid VS (not more than 0.024%).

(5) Heavy metals *<1.07>*—Proceed with 5.0 g of Glucose according to Method 2, and perform the test. Prepare the control solution with 2.0 mL of Standard Lead Solution (not more than 4 ppm).

(6) Arsenic *<1.11>*—Dissolve 1.5 g of Glucose in 5 mL of water, add 5 mL of dilute sulfuric acid and 1 mL of bromine TS, heat on a water bath for 5 minutes, and concentrate to 5 mL. After cooling, perform the test with this solution as the test solution (not more than 1.3 ppm).

(7) Dextrin—To 1.0 g of Glucose add 20 mL of ethanol (95), and boil under a reflux condenser: the solution is clear.

(8) Soluble starch and sulfite—Dissolve 1.0 g of Glucose in 10 mL of water, and add 1 drop of iodine TS: a yellow color develops.

Loss on drying *<2.41>* Not more than 1.0% (1 g, 105°C, 6 hours).

Residue on ignition *<2.44>* Not more than 0.1% (2 g).

Assay Weigh accurately about 10 g of Glucose, previously dried, dissolve in 0.2 mL of ammonia TS and water to make exactly 100 mL, allow to stand for 30 minutes, and determine the optical rotation, α_D, of this solution at 20 ± 1°C in a 100-mm cell as directed under Optical Rotation Determination *<2.49>*.

Amount (mg) of glucose ($C_6H_{12}O_6$) = α_D × 1895.4

Containers and storage Containers—Tight containers.

Glucose Hydrate

ブドウ糖水和物

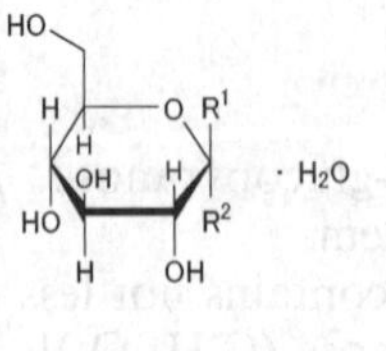

α-D-glucopyranose monohydrate: $R^1 = H$, $R^2 = OH$
β-D-glucopyranose monohydrate: $R^1 = OH$, $R^2 = H$

$C_6H_{12}O_6.H_2O$: 198.17
D-Glucopyranose monohydrate
[77938-63-7]

This monograph is harmonized with the European Pharmacopoeia and the U.S. Pharmacopeia.

The corresponding part of the attributes/provisions which are agreed as non-harmonized within the scope of the harmonization is marked with symbols (◆ ◆), and the corresponding parts which are agreed as the JP local requirement other than the scope of the harmonization are marked with symbols (◇ ◇).

Information on the harmonization with the European Pharmacopoeia and the U.S. Pharmacopeia is available on the website of the Pharmaceuticals and Medical Devices Agency.

Glucose Hydrate is the monohydrate of D-glucopyranose derived from starch.

It contains not less than 97.5% and not more than 102.0% of glucose [D-glucopyranose ($C_6H_{12}O_6$: 180.16)], calculated on the anhydrous basis.

◆**Description** Glucose Hydrate occurs as white, crystals or crystalline powder, and has a sweet taste.

It is freely soluble in water, sparingly soluble in methanol, and slightly soluble in ethanol (95).◆

Identification ◇**(1)** Add 2 to 3 drops of a solution of Glucose Hydrate (1 in 20) to 5 mL of boiling Fehling's TS: a red precipitate is produced.◇

(2) Perform the test with 20 μL each of the sample solution and standard solution obtained in the Assay as directed under Liquid Chromatography *<2.01>* according to the following conditions: the principal peak in the chromatogram obtained from the sample solution is similar in retention time and size to the principal peak in the chromatogram from the standard solution.

Operating conditions—

Proceed as directed in the operating conditions in the Assay.

System suitability—

Proceed as directed in the system suitability in the Assay.

Purity **(1)** Clarity and color of solution—Dissolve 10.0 g of Glucose Hydrate in 15 mL of water, and use this solution as the test solution. Perform the test with the test solution as directed under Turbidity Measurement *<2.61>*: the solution is clear. Perform the test with the test solution according to Method 2 under Methods for Color Matching *<2.65>*: the solution is not more colored than Matching Fluid BY7.

◆**(2)** Heavy metals *<1.07>*—Proceed with 5.0 g of Glucose Hydrate according to Method 2, and perform the test. Prepare the control solution with 2.0 mL of Standard Lead Solution (not more than 4 ppm).◆

(3) Related substances—Use the sample solution obtained in the Assay as the sample solution. Pipet 1 mL of the sample solution, add water to make exactly 250 mL, and use this solution as the standard solution (1). Pipet 25 mL of the standard solution (1), add water to make exactly 200 mL, and use this solution as the standard solution (2). Perform the test with exactly 20 μL each of the sample solution, the standard solution (1) and the standard solution (2) as directed under Liquid Chromatography *<2.01>* according to the following conditions. Determine each peak area by the automatic integration method: the total area of the peaks of maltose and isomaltose, having the relative retention time of about 0.8 to glucose, obtained from the sample solution, is not larger than the peak area of glucose from the standard solution (1) (not more than 0.4%), and the peak area of maltotriose, having the relative retention time of about 0.7 from the sample solution, is not larger than 1/2 times the peak area of glucose from the standard solution (1) (not more than 0.2%), and the peak area of fructose, having the relative retention time of about 1.3 from the sample solution, is not larger than 3 times the peak area of glucose from the standard solution (2) (not more than 0.15%), and the area of the peak other than glucose and the peaks mentioned above from the sample solution is not larger than 2 times the peak area of glucose from the standard solution (2) (not more than 0.10%). Furthermore, the total area of the peaks other than glucose from the sample solution is not larger than 1.25 times the peak area of glucose from the standard solution (1) (not more than 0.5%). For these calculations the peak areas not larger than the peak area of glucose from the standard solution (2) are excluded (disregard limit: 0.05%).

Operating conditions—

Detector, column, column temperature, mobile phase and flow rate: Proceed as directed in the operating conditions in the Assay.

Time span of measurement: About 1.5 times as long as the retention time of glucose.

System suitability—

System performance: Proceed as directed in the system suitability in the Assay.

◇Test for required detectability: Confirm that the peak area of glucose obtained with 20 μL of the standard solution (2) is equivalent to 8.8 to 16.3% of that with 20 μL of the standard solution (1).

System repeatability: When the test is repeated 6 times with 20 μL of the standard solution (1) under the above operating conditions, the relative standard deviation of the peak area of glucose is not more than 1.0%.◇

(4) Dextrin—To 1.0 g of powdered Glucose Hydrate add 20 mL of ethanol (95), and boil under a reflux condenser: the solution is clear.

(5) Soluble starch and sulfite—To 7.4 g of Glucose Hydrate add 15 mL of water, dissolve by heating on a water bath, cool, and add 25 μL of 0.05 mol/L iodine VS: a yellow color develops (not more than 15 ppm as SO_3).

Conductivity 〈*2.51*〉 Dissolve 20.0 g of Glucose Hydrate in a fleshly boiled and cooled distilled water to make 100 mL, and use this solution as the sample solution. Measure the conductivity of the sample solution at 25 ± 0.1°C while gently stirring with a magnetic stirrer: not more than 20 μS·cm^{-1}.

Water 〈*2.48*〉 7.5 – 9.5% (0.25 g, volumetric titration, direct titration).

Assay Weigh accurately about 0.33 g of Glucose Hydrate and 0.3 g of ◆Glucose RS◆ (separately determine the water 〈*2.48*〉 in the same manner as Purified Glucose), dissolve separately in water to make exactly 10 mL, and use these solutions as the sample solution and the standard solution, respectively. Perform the test with exactly 20 μL each of the sample solution and standard solution as directed under Liquid Chromatography 〈*2.01*〉 according to the following conditions, and determine the peak areas, A_T and A_S, of glucose in each solution.

Amount (g) of glucose ($C_6H_{12}O_6$) = $M_S \times A_T/A_S$

M_S: Amount (g) of Glucose RS taken, calculated on the anhydrous basis

Operating conditions—

Detector: A differential refractometer maintained at a constant temperature (40°C for example).

Column: A stainless steel column 7.8 mm in inside diameter and 30 cm in length, packed with strongly acidic ion-exchange resin for liquid chromatography (Ca type) composed with a sulfonated polystyrene cross-linked with divinylbenzene (degree of cross-linkage: 8%) (9 μm in particle diameter).

Column temperature: A constant temperature of about 85°C.

Mobile phase: Water.

Flow rate: 0.3 mL per minute (the retention time of glucose is about 21 minutes).

System suitability—

System performance: Dissolve 5 mg of maltose, 5 mg of maltotriose and 5 mg of fructose in 50 mL of water, and use this solution as the solution for system suitability test. When the procedure is run with 20 μL each of the solution for system suitability test and the standard solution (2) in Purity (3) under the above operating conditions, maltotriose, maltose, glucose and fructose are eluted in this order, the relative retention times of maltotriose, maltose, isomaltose and fructose to glucose are about 0.7, about 0.8, about 0.8 and about 1.3, respectively, and the resolution between the peaks of maltotriose and maltose is not less than 1.3.

◇System repeatability: When the test is repeated 6 times with 20 μL of the standard solution under the above operating conditions, the relative standard deviation of the peak area of glucose is not more than 1.0%.◇

◆**Containers and storage** Containers—Tight containers.◆

Purified Glucose

精製ブドウ糖

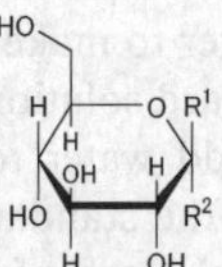

α-D-glucopyranose: R^1 = H, R^2 = OH
β-D-glucopyranose: R^1 = OH, R^2 = H

$C_6H_{12}O_6$: 180.16

D-Glucopyranose

[*50-99-7*]

This monograph is harmonized with the European Pharmacopoeia and the U.S. Pharmacopeia.

The corresponding part of the attributes/provisions which are agreed as non-harmonized within the scope of the harmonization is marked with symbols (◆ ◆), and the corresponding parts which are agreed as the JP local requirement other than the scope of the harmonization are marked with symbols (◇ ◇).

Information on the harmonization with the European Pharmacopoeia and the U.S. Pharmacopeia is available on the website of the Pharmaceuticals and Medical Devices Agency.

Purified Glucose is D-glucopyranose derived from starch.

It contains not less than 97.5% and not more than 102.0% of glucose [D-glucopyranose ($C_6H_{12}O_6$)], calculated on the anhydrous basis.

◆**Description** Purified Glucose occurs as white, crystals or crystalline powder, and has a sweet taste.

It is freely soluble in water, and slightly soluble in methanol and in ethanol (95).◆

Identification ◇**(1)** Add 2 to 3 drops of a solution of Purified Glucose (1 in 20) to 5 mL of boiling Fehling's TS: a red precipitate is produced.◇

(2) Perform the test with 20 μL each of the sample solution and standard solution obtained in the Assay as directed under Liquid Chromatography 〈*2.01*〉 according to the following conditions: the principal peak in the chromatogram obtained from the sample solution is similar in retention time and size to the principal peak in the chromatogram from the standard solution.

Operating conditions—

Proceed as directed in the operating conditions in the Assay.

System suitability—

Proceed as directed in the system suitability in the Assay.

Purity **(1)** Clarity and color of solution—Dissolve 10.0 g of Purified Glucose in 15 mL of water by heating on a water bath, and allow to cool to room temperature, and use this solution as the test solution. Perform the test with the test solution as directed under Turbidity Measurement 〈*2.61*〉: the solution is clear. Perform the test with the test solution according to Method 2 under Methods for Color Matching 〈*2.65*〉: the solution is not more colored than Matching Fluid BY7.

◆**(2)** Heavy metals 〈*1.07*〉—Proceed with 5.0 g of Purified Glucose according to Method 2, and perform the test. Prepare the control solution with 2.0 mL of Standard Lead Solution (not more than 4 ppm).◆

(3) Related substances—Use the sample solution obtained in the Assay as the sample solution. Pipet 1 mL of the sample solution, add water to make exactly 250 mL, and use this solution as the standard solution (1). Pipet 25 mL of the standard solution (1), add water to make exactly 200 mL, and use this solution as the standard solution (2). Perform the test with exactly 20 μL each of the sample solution, the standard solution (1) and the standard solution (2) as directed under Liquid Chromatography *<2.01>* according to the following conditions. Determine each peak area by the automatic integration method: the total area of the peaks of maltose and isomaltose, having the relative retention time of about 0.8 to glucose, obtained from the sample solution, is not larger than the peak area of glucose from the standard solution (1) (not more than 0.4%), and the peak area of maltotriose, having the relative retention time of about 0.7 from the sample solution, is not larger than 1/2 times the peak area of glucose from the standard solution (1) (not more than 0.2%), and the peak area of fructose, having the relative retention time of about 1.3 from the sample solution, is not larger than 3 times the peak area of glucose from the standard solution (2) (not more than 0.15%), and the area of the peak other than glucose and the peaks mentioned above from the sample solution is not larger than 2 times the peak area of glucose from the standard solution (2) (not more than 0.10%). Furthermore, the total area of the peaks other than glucose from the sample solution is not larger than 1.25 times the peak area of glucose from the standard solution (1) (not more than 0.5%). For these calculations the peak areas not larger than the peak area of glucose from the standard solution (2) are excluded (disregard limit: 0.05%).

Operating conditions—

Detector, column, column temperature, mobile phase and flow rate: Proceed as directed in the operating conditions in the Assay.

Time span of measurement: About 1.5 times as long as the retention time of glucose.

System suitability—

System performance: Proceed as directed in the system suitability in the Assay.

◇Test for required detectability: Confirm that the peak area of glucose obtained with 20 μL of the standard solution (2) is equivalent to 8.8 to 16.3% of that with 20 μL of the standard solution (1).

System repeatability: When the test is repeated 6 times with 20 μL of the standard solution (1) under the above operating conditions, the relative standard deviation of the peak area of glucose is not more than 1.0%.◇

(4) Dextrin—To 1.0 g of powdered Purified Glucose add 20 mL of ethanol (95), and boil under a reflux condenser: the solution is clear.

(5) Soluble starch and sulfite—To 6.7 g of Purified Glucose add 15 mL of water, dissolve by heating on a water bath, cool, and add 25 μL of 0.05 mol/L iodine VS: a yellow color develops (not more than 15 ppm as SO_3).

Conductivity *<2.51>* Dissolve 20.0 g of Purified Glucose in a fleshly boiled and cooled distilled water to make 100 mL, and use this solution as the sample solution. Measure the conductivity of the sample solution at 25 ± 0.1°C while gently stirring with a magnetic stirrer: not more than 20 μS·cm^{-1}.

Water *<2.48>* Not more than 1.0% (0.5 g, volumetric titration, direct titration).

Assay Weigh accurately about 0.3 g each of Purified Glucose and ◆Glucose RS◆ (separately determine the water *<2.48>* in the same manner as Purified Glucose), dissolve separately in water to make exactly 10 mL, and use these solutions as the sample solution and the standard solution, respectively. Perform the test with exactly 20 μL each of the sample solution and standard solution as directed under Liquid Chromatography *<2.01>* according to the following conditions, and determine the peak areas, A_T and A_S, of glucose in each solution.

$$\text{Amount (g) of glucose } (C_6H_{12}O_6) = M_S \times A_T/A_S$$

M_S: Amount (g) of Glucose RS taken, calculated on the anhydrous basis

Operating conditions—

Detector: A differential refractometer maintained at a constant temperature (40°C for example).

Column: A stainless steel column 7.8 mm in inside diameter and 30 cm in length, packed with strongly acidic ion-exchange resin for liquid chromatography (Ca type) composed with a sulfonated polystyrene cross-linked with divinylbenzene (degree of cross-linkage: 8%) (9 μm in particle diameter).

Column temperature: A constant temperature of about 85°C.

Mobile phase: Water.

Flow rate: 0.3 mL per minute (the retention time of glucose is about 21 minutes).

System suitability—

System performance: Dissolve 5 mg of maltose, 5 mg of maltotriose and 5 mg of fructose in 50 mL of water, and use this solution as the solution for system suitability test. When the procedure is run with 20 μL each of the solution for system suitability test and the standard solution (2) in Purity (3) under the above operating conditions, maltotriose, maltose, glucose and fructose are eluted in this order, the relative retention times of maltotriose, maltose, isomaltose and fructose to glucose are about 0.7, about 0.8, about 0.8 and about 1.3, respectively, and the resolution between the peaks of maltotriose and maltose is not less than 1.3.

◇System repeatability: When the test is repeated 6 times with 20 μL of the standard solution under the above operating conditions, the relative standard deviation of the peak area of glucose is not more than 1.0%.◇

◆**Containers and storage** Containers—Tight containers.◆

Glucose Injection

ブドウ糖注射液

Glucose Injection is an aqueous injection.

It contains not less than 95.0% and not more than 105.0% of the labeled amount of glucose ($C_6H_{12}O_6$: 180.16).

Method of preparation Prepare as directed under Injections, with Purified Glucose or Glucose Hydrate.

No preservative is added.

Description Glucose Injection is a clear, colorless liquid. It has a sweet taste. It occurs as a colorless to pale yellow, clear liquid when its labeled concentration exceeds 40%.

Identification Measure a volume of Glucose Injection, equivalent to 0.1 g of glucose ($C_6H_{12}O_6$), and, if necessary, add water or evaporate on a water bath to make 2 mL. Add

2 to 3 drops of the solution to 5 mL of boiling Fehling's TS: a red precipitate is produced.

pH <*2.54*> 3.5 – 6.5 In the case where the labeled concentration of the injection exceeds 5%, dilute to 5% with water before the test.

Purity 5-Hydroxymethylfurfural and related substances—Pipet a volume of Glucose Injection, equivalent to 2.5 g of glucose ($C_6H_{12}O_6$), and add water to make exactly 100 mL. Determine the absorbance of this solution at 284 nm as directed under Ultraviolet-visible Spectrophotometry <*2.24*>: it is not more than 0.80.

Bacterial endotoxins <*4.01*> Less than 0.50 EU/mL.

Extractable volume <*6.05*> It meets the requirement.

Foreign insoluble matter <*6.06*> Perform the test according to Method 1: it meets the requirement.

Insoluble particulate matter <*6.07*> It meets the requirement.

Sterility <*4.06*> Perform the test according to the Membrane filtration method: it meets the requirement.

Assay Measure accurately a volume of Glucose Injection, equivalent to about 4 g of glucose ($C_6H_{12}O_6$), and add 0.2 mL of ammonia TS and water to make exactly 100 mL. Shake the solution well, allow to stand for 30 minutes, and determine the optical rotation, α_D, at 20 ± 1°C in a 100-mm cell as directed under Optical Rotation Determination <*2.49*>.

$$\text{Amount (mg) of glucose } (C_6H_{12}O_6) = \alpha_D \times 1895.4$$

Containers and storage Containers—Hermetic containers. Plastic containers for aqueous injections may be used.

L-Glutamic Acid

L-グルタミン酸

$C_5H_9NO_4$: 147.13
(2*S*)-2-Aminopentanedioic acid
[*56-86-0*]

L-Glutamic Acid contains not less than 99.0% and not more than 101.0% of L-glutamic acid ($C_5H_9NO_4$), calculated on the dried basis.

Description L-Glutamic acid occurs as white, crystals or crystalline powder. It has a slight characteristic and acid taste.

It is slightly soluble in water, and practically insoluble in ethanol (99.5).

It dissolves in 2 mol/L hydrochloric acid TS.

It shows crystal polymorphism.

Identification Determine the infrared absorption spectrum of L-Glutamic Acid as directed in the potassium bromide disk method under Infrared Spectrophotometry <*2.25*>, and compare the spectrum with the Reference Spectrum: both spectra exhibit similar intensities of absorption at the same wave numbers. If any difference appears between the spectra, dissolve L-Glutamic Acid in a small amount of water, evaporate water at 60°C under reduced pressure, and perform the test in the same manner with the dried residue.

Optical rotation <*2.49*> $[\alpha]_D^{20}$: +31.5 – +32.5° (2.5 g calculated on the dried basis, 2 mol/L hydrochloric acid TS, 25 mL, 100 mm).

pH <*2.54*> The pH of a solution prepared by dissolving 0.7 g of L-Glutamic Acid in 100 mL of water by warming and then cooling is 2.9 to 3.9.

Purity (1) Clarity and color of solution—Dissolve 1.0 g of L-Glutamic Acid in 10 mL of 2 mol/L hydrochloric acid TS: the solution is clear and colorless.

(2) Chloride <*1.03*>—Dissolve 0.5 g of L-Glutamic Acid in 6 mL of dilute nitric acid and 20 mL of water, and add water to make 50 mL. Perform the test using this solution as the test solution. Prepare the control solution with 0.30 mL of 0.01 mol/L hydrochloric acid VS (not more than 0.021%).

(3) Sulfate <*1.14*>—Dissolve 0.6 g of L-Glutamic Acid in 5 mL of dilute hydrochloric acid and 30 mL of water, and add water to make 45 mL. Perform the test using this solution as the test solution. Prepare the control solution from 0.35 mL of 0.005 mol/L sulfuric acid VS and 5 mL of dilute hydrochloric acid, and dilute with water to 45 mL. Prepare the test solution and the control solution with 5 mL of barium chloride TS, respectively (not more than 0.028%).

(4) Ammonium <*1.02*>—Perform the test with 0.25 g of L-Glutamic Acid. Prepare the control solution with 5.0 mL of Standard Ammonium Solution (not more than 0.02%).

(5) Heavy metals <*1.07*>—Dissolve 1.0 g of L-Glutamic Acid in 20 mL of water and 7 mL of a solution of sodium hydroxide (1 in 25) by warming, cool, and add 2 mL of dilute acetic acid and water to make 50 mL. Perform the test using this solution as the test solution. Prepare the control solution from 1.0 mL of Standard Lead Solution and 2 mL of dilute acetic acid, and dilute with water to 50 mL (not more than 10 ppm).

(6) Iron <*1.10*>—Prepare the test solution with 1.0 g of L-Glutamic Acid according to Method 1, and perform the test according to Method A. Prepare the control solution with 1.0 mL of Standard Iron Solution (not more than 10 ppm).

(7) Related substances—Weigh accurately about 0.5 g of L-Glutamic Acid, and dissolve in 0.5 mL of hydrochloric acid and water to make exactly 100 mL. Pipet 10 mL of this solution, add 0.02 mol/L hydrochloric acid TS to make exactly 50 mL, and use this solution as the sample solution. Separately, weigh accurately an amount, equivalent to 2.5 mmol, of L-aspartic acid, L-threonine, L-serine, L-glutamic acid, glycine, L-alanine, L-cystine, L-valine, L-methionine, L-isoleucine, L-leucine, L-tyrosine, L-phenylalanine, L-lysine hydrochloride, ammonium chloride, L-histidine and L-arginine, dissolve them in 0.1 mol/L hydrochloric acid TS to make exactly 1000 mL, and use this solution as the standard stock solution. Pipet 5 mL of the standard stock solution, and add 0.02 mol/L hydrochloric acid TS to make exactly 100 mL. Pipet 6 mL of this solution, add 0.02 mol/L hydrochloric acid TS to make exactly 50 mL, and use this solution as the standard solution. Perform the test with exactly 20 μL each of the sample solution and standard solution as directed under Liquid Chromatography <*2.01*> according to the following conditions, and calculate the mass percentage of each amino acid, using the mass of amino acid other than glutamic acid in 1 mL of the sample solution obtained from the height of the peaks obtained from the sample solution and standard solution: the amount of each amino acid other than glutamic acid is not more than 0.2%, and the total amount of these amino acids is not more than 0.6%.

Operating conditions—

Detector: A visible absorption photometer (wavelength:

570 nm).

Column: A stainless steel column 4.6 mm in inside diameter and 8 cm in length, packed with strongly acidic ion-exchange resin for liquid chromatography (Na type) composed with a sulfonated polystyrene (3 μm in particle diameter).

Column temperature: A constant temperature of about 57°C.

Chemical reaction bath temperature: A constant temperature of about 130°C.

Reaction time: About 1 minute.

Mobile phase: Prepare the mobile phases A, B, C, D and E according to the following table, and add 0.1 mL each of caprylic acid.

Mobile phase	A	B	C	D	E
Citric acid monohydrate	19.80 g	22.00 g	12.80 g	6.10 g	—
Trisodium citrate dihydrate	6.19 g	7.74 g	13.31 g	26.67 g	—
Sodium chloride	5.66 g	7.07 g	3.74 g	54.35 g	—
Sodium hydroxide	—	—	—	—	8.00 g
Ethanol (99.5)	130 mL	20 mL	4 mL	—	100 mL
Thiodiglycol	5 mL	5 mL	5 mL	—	—
Benzyl alcohol	—	—	—	5 mL	—
Lauromacrogol solution (1 in 4)	4 mL	4 mL	4 mL	4 mL	4 mL
Water	a sufficient amount	a sufficient amount	a sufficient amount	a sufficient amount	a sufficient amount
Total amount	1000 mL	1000 mL	1000 mL	1000 mL	1000 mL

Changing of mobile phase: Switch the mobile phases A, B, C, D and E sequentially so that when proceed with 20 μL of the standard solution under the above conditions, aspartic acid, threonine, serine, glutamic acid, glycine, alanine, cystine, valine, methionine, isoleucine, leucine, tyrosine, phenylalanine, lysine, ammonia, histidine and arginine are eluted in this order with the resolution between the peaks of isoleucine and leucine being not less than 1.2.

Reaction reagent: Dissolve 204 g of lithium acetate dihydrate in an appropriate amount of water, add 123 mL of acetic acid (100), 401 mL of 1-methoxy-2-propanol and water to make 1000 mL, introduce nitrogen for 10 minutes, and use this solution as Solution (I). Separately, to 979 mL of 1-methoxy-2-propanol add 39 g of ninhydrin, introduce nitrogen for 5 minutes, add 81 mg of sodium borohydride, introduce nitrogen for 30 minutes, and use this solution as Solution (II). Prepare a mixture with an equal volume of the Solution (I) and Solution (II) (Prepare before use).

Flow rate of mobile phase: 0.20 mL per minute.

Flow rate of reaction regent: 0.24 mL per minute.

System suitability—

System performance: When the test is run with 20 μL of the standard solution under the above operating conditions, the resolution between the peaks of glycine and L-alanine is not less than 1.2.

System repeatability: When the test is repeated 6 times with 20 μL of the standard solution under the above operating conditions, the relative standard deviation of the peak height of each amino acid in the standard solution is not more than 5.0%, and the relative standard deviation of the retention time of them is not more than 1.0%.

Loss on drying *<2.41>* Not more than 0.3% (1 g, 105°C, 3 hours).

Residue on ignition *<2.44>* Not more than 0.1% (1 g).

Assay Weigh accurately about 0.12 g of L-Glutamic Acid, dissolve in 40 mL of water by warming, cool, and titrate *<2.50>* with 0.1 mol/L sodium hydroxide VS (potentiometric titration). Perform a blank determination in the same manner, and make any necessary correction.

Each mL of 0.1 mol/L sodium hydroxide VS
= 14.71 mg of $C_5H_9NO_4$

Containers and storage Containers—Tight containers.

L-Glutamine

L-グルタミン

$C_5H_{10}N_2O_3$: 146.14
(2*S*)-2,5-Diamino-5-oxopentanoic acid
[56-85-9]

L-Glutamine, when dried, contains not less than 99.0% and not more than 101.0% of L-glutamine ($C_5H_{10}N_2O_3$).

Description L-Glutamine occurs as white, crystals or a crystalline powder. It has a slight characteristic taste.

It is freely soluble in formic acid, soluble in water, and practically insoluble in ethanol (99.5).

Identification Determine the infrared absorption spectrum of L-Glutamine as directed in the potassium bromide disk method under Infrared Spectrophotometry *<2.25>*, and compare the spectrum with the Reference Spectrum: both spectra exhibit similar intensities of absorption at the same wave numbers.

Optical rotation *<2.49>* $[\alpha]_D^{20}$: +6.3 – +7.3° Weigh accurately about 2 g of L-Glutamine, previously dried, add 45 mL of water, warm to 40°C to dissolve, and after cooling, add water to make exactly 50 mL. Determine the optical rotation of this solution in a 100-mm cell, within 60 minutes.

pH *<2.54>* The pH of a solution prepared by dissolving 1.0 g of L-Glutamine in 50 mL of water is between 4.5 and 6.0.

Purity **(1)** Clarity and color of solution—A solution obtained by dissolving 0.5 g of L-Glutamine in 20 mL of water is clear and colorless.

(2) Chloride *<1.03>*—Perform the test with 0.5 g of L-Glutamine. Prepare the control solution with 0.30 mL of 0.01 mol/L hydrochloric acid VS (not more than 0.021%).

(3) Sulfate *<1.14>*—Perform the test with 0.6 g of L-Glutamine. Prepare the control solution with 0.35 mL of 0.005 mol/L sulfuric acid VS (not more than 0.028%).

(4) Ammonium *<1.02>*—Perform the test with 0.10 g of L-Glutamine, using the distillation under reduced pressure. Prepare the control solution with 10.0 mL of Standard Ammonium Solution. The temperature of the water bath is 45°C (not more than 0.1%).

(5) Heavy metals *<1.07>*—Proceed with 1.0 g of L-Glutamine according to Method 1, and perform the test. Prepare the control solution with 1.0 mL of Standard Lead Solution (not more than 10 ppm).

(6) Iron *<1.10>*—Prepare the test solution with 1.0 g of

L-Glutamine according to Method 1, and perform the test according to Method A. Prepare the control solution with 1.0 mL of Standard Iron Solution (not more than 10 ppm).

(7) Related substances—Dissolve 0.10 g of L-Glutamine in 10 mL of water, and use this solution as the sample solution. Pipet 1 mL of the sample solution, add water to make exactly 10 mL. Pipet 1 mL of this solution, add water to make exactly 50 mL, and use this solution as the standard solution. Perform the test with these solutions as directed under Thin-layer Chromatography *<2.03>*. Spot 5 μL each of the sample solution and standard solution on a plate of silica gel for thin-layer chromatography. Then develop with a mixture of 1-butanol, water and acetic acid (100) (3:1:1) to a distance of about 10 cm, and dry the plate at 80°C for 30 minutes. Spray evenly a solution of ninhydrin in a mixture of methanol and acetic acid (100) (97:3) (1 in 100) on the plate, and heat the plate at 80°C for 10 minutes: the spot other than the principal spot obtained from the sample solution is not more intense than the spot from the standard solution.

Loss on drying *<2.41>* Not more than 0.3% (1 g, 105°C, 3 hours).

Residue on Ignition *<2.44>* Not more than 0.1% (1 g).

Assay Weigh accurately about 0.15 g of L-Glutamine, previously dried, dissolve in 3 mL of formic acid, add 50 mL of acetic acid (100), and titrate *<2.50>* with 0.1 mol/L perchloric acid VS (potentiometric titration). Perform a blank determination in the same manner, and make any necessary correction.

Each mL of 0.1 mol/L perchloric acid VS
= 14.61 mg of $C_5H_{10}N_2O_3$

Containers and storage Containers—Tight containers.

Glutathione

グルタチオン

$C_{10}H_{17}N_3O_6S$: 307.32
(2*S*)-2-Amino-4-[1-(carboxymethyl)carbamoyl-(2*R*)-2-sulfanylethylcarbamoyl]butanoic acid
[70-18-8]

Glutathione, when dried, contains not less than 98.0% and not more than 101.0% of glutathione ($C_{10}H_{17}N_3O_6S$).

Description Glutathione occurs as a white crystalline powder.

It is freely soluble in water, and practically insoluble in ethanol (99.5).

Melting point: about 185°C (with decomposition).

Identification Determine the infrared absorption spectrum of Glutathione, previously dried, as directed in the potassium bromide disk method under Infrared Spectrophotometry *<2.25>*, and compare the spectrum with the Reference Spectrum: both spectra exhibit similar intensities of absorption at the same wave numbers.

Optical rotation *<2.49>* $[\alpha]_D^{20}$: −15.5 – −17.5° (after drying, 2 g, water, 50 mL, 100 mm).

Purity **(1)** Clarity and color of solution—Dissolve 1.0 g of Glutathione in 10 mL of water: the solution is clear and colorless.

(2) Heavy metals *<1.07>*—Proceed with 2.0 g of Glutathione according to Method 2, and perform the test. Prepare the control solution with 2.0 mL of Standard Lead Solution (not more than 10 ppm).

(3) Arsenic *<1.11>*—Prepare the test solution with 1.0 g of Glutathione according to Method 1, and perform the test (not more than 2 ppm).

(4) Related substances—Dissolve 50 mg of Glutathione in 100 mL of the mobile phase, and use this solution as the sample solution. Pipet 2 mL of the sample solution, add the mobile phase to make exactly 100 mL, and use this solution as the standard solution. Perform the test with exactly 10 μL each of the sample solution and standard solution as directed under Liquid Chromatography *<2.01>* according to the following conditions, and determine each peak area by the automatic integration method: the area of the peak having the relative retention time of about 4 to glutathione obtained from the sample solution is not larger than 3/4 times the peak area of glutathione from the standard solution, and the total area of the peaks other than glutathione is not larger than the peak area of glutathione from the standard solution.

Operating conditions—

Detector: An ultraviolet absorption photometer (wavelength: 210 nm).

Column: A stainless steel column 4.6 mm in inside diameter and 15 cm in length, packed with octadecylsilanized silica gel for liquid chromatography (5 μm in particle diameter).

Column temperature: A constant temperature of about 30°C.

Mobile phase: Dissolve 6.8 g of potassium dihydrogen phosphate and 2.02 g of sodium 1-heptane sulfonate in 1000 mL of water, and adjust the pH to 3.0 with phosphoric acid. To 970 mL of this solution add 30 mL of methanol.

Flow rate: Adjust so that the retention time of glutathione is about 5 minutes.

Time span of measurement: About 6 times as long as the retention time of glutathione, beginning after the solvent peak.

System suitability—

Test for required detectability: Pipet 10 mL of the standard solution, and add the mobile phase to make exactly 100 mL. Confirm that the peak area of glutathione obtained with 10 μL of this solution is equivalent to 8 to 12% of that with 10 μL of the standard solution.

System performance: Dissolve 50 mg of glutathione, 10 mg of D-phenylglycine and 50 mg of ascorbic acid in 100 mL of water. When the procedure is run with 10 μL of this solution under the above operating conditions, ascorbic acid, glutathione and D-phenylglycine are eluted in this order, and the resolutions between the peaks of ascorbic acid and glutathione and between the peaks of glutathione and D-phenylglycine are not less than 5, respectively.

System repeatability: When the test is repeated 6 times with 10 μL of the standard solution under the above operating conditions, the relative standard deviation of the peak area of glutathione is not more than 1.5%.

Loss on drying *<2.41>* Not more than 0.5% (1 g, 105°C, 3 hours).

Residue on ignition *<2.44>* Not more than 0.1% (1 g).

Assay Weigh accurately about 0.5 g of Glutathione, previously dried, dissolve in 50 mL of a solution of metaphosphoric acid (1 in 50), and titrate <2.50> with 0.05 mol/L iodine VS (indicator: 1 mL of starch TS). Perform a blank determination in the same manner, and make any necessary correction.

Each mL of 0.05 mol/L iodine VS
= 30.73 mg of $C_{10}H_{17}N_3O_6S$

Containers and storage Containers—Tight containers.

Glycerin

Glycerol

グリセリン

$C_3H_8O_3$: 92.09

Glycerin contains not less than 84.0% and not more than 87.0% of glycerin ($C_3H_8O_3$).

Description Glycerin is a clear, colorless, viscous liquid. It has a sweet taste.

It is miscible with water and with ethanol (99.5).

It is hygroscopic.

Identification Determine the infrared absorption spectrum of Glycerin as directed in the liquid film method under Infrared Spectrophotometry <2.25>, and compare the spectrum with the Reference Spectrum: both spectra exhibit similar intensities of absorption at the same wave numbers.

Refractive index <2.45> n_D^{20}: 1.449 – 1.454

Specific gravity <2.56> d_{20}^{20}: 1.221 – 1.230

Purity (1) Color—Place 50 mL of Glycerin in a Nessler tube, and observe downward: the solution has no more color than the following control solution.

Control solution: Place 0.40 mL of Iron (III) Chloride CS in a Nessler tube, and add water to make 50 mL.

(2) Acidity or alkalinity—To 2 mL of Glycerin add 8 mL of water and mix: the solution is neutral.

(3) Chloride <1.03>—Take 10.0 g of Glycerin, and perform the test: Prepare the control solution with 0.30 mL of 0.01 mol/L hydrochloric acid VS (not more than 0.001%).

(4) Sulfate <1.14>—Take 10.0 g of Glycerin, and perform the test. Prepare the control solution with 0.40 mL of 0.005 mol/L sulfuric acid VS (not more than 0.002%).

(5) Ammonium—To 5 mL of Glycerin add 5 mL of a solution of sodium hydroxide (1 in 10), and boil: the gas evolved does not change moistened red litmus paper to blue.

(6) Heavy metals <1.07>—Proceed with 5.0 g of Glycerin according to Method 1, and perform the test: Prepare the control solution with 2.5 mL of Standard Lead Solution (not more than 5 ppm).

(7) Calcium—To 5 mL of the solution obtained in (2) add 3 drops of ammonium oxalate TS: the solution remains unchanged.

(8) Arsenic <1.11>—Prepare the test solution with 1.0 g of Glycerin according to Method 1, and perform the test (not more than 2 ppm).

(9) Acrolein, glucose, and other reducing substances—To 1.0 g of Glycerin add 1 mL of ammonia TS, mix, and warm in a water bath at 60°C for 5 minutes: no yellow color is produced. Take the solution out of the water bath, add 3 drops of silver nitrate TS immediately, and allow to stand in a dark place for 5 minutes: the color of the solution does not change, and no turbidity is produced.

(10) Fatty acids and esters—Mix 50 g of Glycerin with 50 mL of freshly boiled and cooled water, add exactly 10 mL of 0.1 mol/L sodium hydroxide VS, boil the mixture for 15 minutes, cool, and titrate <2.50> the excess sodium hydroxide with 0.1 mol/L hydrochloric acid VS: 0.1 mol/L sodium hydroxide VS consumed is not more than 3.0 mL (indicator: 3 drops of phenolphthalein TS). Perform a blank determination in the same manner.

(11) Ethylene glycol, diethylene glycol and related substances—Weigh accurately about 5.88 g of Glycerin, mix with methanol to make exactly 100 mL, and use this solution as the sample solution. Separately, weigh accurately about 0.1 g each of ethylene glycol and diethylene glycol, mix with methanol to make exactly 100 mL. Pipet 5 mL of this solution and transfer into a 100-mL volumetric flask. Separately, weigh 5.0 g of glycerin for gas chromatography, mix with a suitable amount of methanol and put in the volumetric flask, add methanol to make exactly 100 mL, and use this solution as the standard solution. Perform the test with exactly 1 μL each of the sample solution and standard solution as directed under Gas Chromatography <2.02> according to the following conditions, and determine the peak areas, A_{T1} and A_{S1}, of ethylene glycol and, A_{T2} and A_{S2}, of diethylene glycol by the automatic integration method. The amounts of ethylene glycol and diethylene glycol, calculated by the following equations, are not more than 0.1%, respectively. The amount of the peak other than glycerin, ethylene glycol and diethylene glycol obtained from the sample solution, calculated by the area percentage method, is not more than 0.1%, and the total amount of the peaks other than glycerin is not more than 1.0%.

$$\text{Amount (\%) of ethylene glycol} = M_{S1}/M_T \times A_{T1}/A_{S1} \times 5$$

$$\text{Amount (\%) of diethylene glycol} = M_{S2}/M_T \times A_{T2}/A_{S2} \times 5$$

M_{S1}: Amount (g) of ethylene glycol taken
M_{S2}: Amount (g) of diethylene glycol taken
M_T: Amount (g) of Glycerin taken

Operating conditions—

Detector: A hydrogen flame-ionization detector.

Column: A fused-silica column 0.32 mm in inside diameter and 30 m in length, coated the inner surface with 14% cyanopropylphenyl-86% dimethyl silicone polymer for gas chromatography 1 μm in thickness.

Column temperature: Inject at a constant temperature of about 100°C, raise the temperature at the rate of 7.5°C per minute to 220°C, and maintain at a constant temperature of about 220°C.

Injection port temperature: A constant temperature of about 220°C.

Detector temperature: A constant temperature of about 250°C.

Carrier gas: Helium.

Flow rate: about 38 cm per second.

Split ratio: 1:20.

Time span of measurement: About 3 times as long as the retention time of glycerin, beginning after the solvent peak.

System suitability—

System performance: Mix 50 mg each of ethylene glycol, diethylene glycol and glycerin for gas chromatography with 100 mL of methanol. When the procedure is run with 1 μL of this solution under the above operating conditions, ethylene glycol, diethylene glycol and glycerin are eluted in this order, and the resolution between the peaks of ethylene glycol and diethylene glycol is not less than 40, and between the peaks of diethylene glycol and glycerin is not less than 10.

System repeatability: When the test is repeated 6 times with 1 μL of the standard solution under the above operating conditions, the relative standard deviations of the peak area of ethylene glycol and diethylene glycol are not more than 10%, respectively.

(12) Readily carbonizable substances—To 5 mL of Glycerin add carefully 5 mL of sulfuric acid for readily carbonizable substances, mix gently at a temperature between 18°C and 20°C, and allow to stand for 1 hour between 15°C and 25°C: the solution has not more color than Matching Fluid H.

Water <*2.48*> 13 - 17% (0.1 g, volumetric titration, direct titration).

Residue on ignition <*2.44*> Weigh accurately about 10 g of Glycerin in a tared crucible, heat to boiling, and fire to burn immediately. After cooling, moisten the residue with 1 to 2 drops of sulfuric acid, and ignite cautiously to constant mass: the mass of the residue is not more than 0.01%.

Assay Weigh accurately about 0.2 g of Glycerin, transfer into a glass-stoppered flask, add 50 mL of water, mix, add exactly 50 mL of sodium periodate TS, shake, and allow to stand in a dark place at a room temperature for about 30 minutes. Add 10 mL of a mixture of water and ethylene glycol (1:1), allow to stand for about 20 minutes, add 100 mL of water, and titrate <*2.50*> with 0.1 mol/L sodium hydroxide VS (indicator: 2 drops of phenolphthalein TS). Perform a blank determination in the same manner, and make the necessary correction.

Each mL of 0.1 mol/L sodium hydroxide VS
= 9.209 mg of $C_3H_8O_3$

Containers and storage Containers—Tight containers.

Concentrated Glycerin

Concentrated Glycerol

濃グリセリン

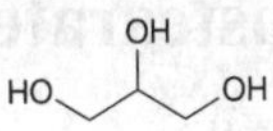

$C_3H_8O_3$: 92.09
Propane-1,2,3-triol
[*56-81-5*]

Concentrated Glycerin contains not less than 98.0% and not more than 101.0% of glycerin ($C_3H_8O_3$), calculated of the anhydrous basis.

Description Concentrated Glycerin is a clear, colorless and viscous liquid. It has a sweet taste.

It is miscible with water and with ethanol (99.5).

It is hygroscopic.

Identification Determine the infrared absorption spectrum of Concentrated Glycerin as directed in the liquid film method under Infrared Spectrophotometry <*2.25*>, and compare the spectrum with the Reference Spectrum: both spectra exhibit similar intensities of absorption at the same wave numbers.

Refractive index <*2.45*> n_D^{20}: Not less than 1.470.

Specific gravity <*2.56*> d_{20}^{20}: Not less than 1.258.

Purity **(1)** Color—Place 50 mL of Concentrated Glycerin in a Nessler tube, and observe downward: the solution has no more color than the following control solution.

Control solution: Pipet 0.40 mL of Iron (III) Chloride CS into a Nessler tube, and add water to make 50 mL.

(2) Acidity or alkalinity—To 2 mL of Concentrated Glycerin add 8 mL of water and mix: the solution is neutral.

(3) Chloride <*1.03*>—Take 10.0 g of Concentrated Glycerin, and perform the test. Prepare the control solution with 0.30 mL of 0.01 mol/L hydrochloric acid VS (not more than 0.001%).

(4) Sulfate <*1.14*>—Take 10.0 g of Concentrated Glycerin, and perform the test. Prepare the control solution with 0.40 mL of 0.005 mol/L sulfuric acid VS (not more than 0.002%).

(5) Ammonium—To 5 mL of Concentrated Glycerin add 5 mL of a solution of sodium hydroxide (1 in 10), and boil: the gas evolved does not change moistened red litmus paper to blue.

(6) Heavy metals <*1.07*>—Proceed with 5.0 g of Concentrated Glycerin according to Method 1, and perform the test. Prepare the control solution with 2.5 mL of Standard Lead Solution (not more than 5 ppm).

(7) Calcium—To 5 mL of the solution obtained in (2) add 3 drops of ammonium oxalate TS: the solution remains unchanged.

(8) Arsenic <*1.11*>—Prepare the test solution with 1.0 g of Concentrated Glycerin according to Method 1, and perform the test (not more than 2 ppm).

(9) Acrolein, glucose, or other reducing substances—To 1.0 g of Concentrated Glycerin add 1 mL of ammonia TS, mix, and warm in a water bath at 60°C for 5 minutes: no yellow color is produced. Take the solution out of the water bath, add 3 drops of silver nitrate TS immediately, and allow to stand in a dark place for 5 minutes: the color of the solution does not change, and no turbidity is produced.

(10) Fatty acids and esters—Mix 50 g of Concentrated Glycerin with 50 mL of freshly boiled and cooled water, add 10 mL of 0.1 mol/L sodium hydroxide VS, accurately measured, boil the mixture for 15 minutes, cool, and titrate <*2.50*> the excess sodium hydroxide with 0.1 mol/L hydrochloric acid VS: not more than 3.0 mL of 0.1 mol/L sodium hydroxide VS is consumed (indicator: 3 drops of phenolphthalein TS). Perform a blank determination in the same manner.

(11) Ethylene glycol, diethylene glycol and related substances—Weigh accurately about 5 g of Concentrated Glycerin, mix with methanol to make exactly 100 mL, and use this solution as the sample solution. Separately, weigh accurately about 0.1 g each of ethylene glycol and diethylene glycol, mix with methanol to make exactly 100 mL. Pipet 5 mL of this solution and transfer into a 100-mL volumetric flask. Separately, weigh 5.0 g of glycerin for gas chromatography, mix with a suitable amount of methanol and put in the volumetric flask, add methanol to make exactly 100 mL, and use this solution as the standard solution. Perform the test with exactly 1 μL each of the sample solution and standard solution as directed under Gas Chromatography <*2.02*> according to the following conditions, and determine the peak areas, A_{T1} and A_{S1}, of ethylene glycol and, A_{T2} and A_{S2}, of diethylene glycol by the automatic integration method. The amounts of ethylene glycol and diethylene glycol, calculated by the following equations, are not more than 0.1%, respectively. The amount of the peak other than glycerin, ethylene glycol and diethylene glycol obtained from the sample solution, calculated by the area percentage method, is not more than 0.1%, and the total amount of the peaks other than glycerin is not more than 1.0%.

Amount (%) of ethylene glycol
$= M_{S1}/M_T \times A_{T1}/A_{S1} \times 5$

Amount (%) of diethylene glycol
$= M_{S2}/M_T \times A_{T2}/A_{S2} \times 5$

M_{S1}: Amount (g) of ethylene glycol taken
M_{S2}: Amount (g) of diethylene glycol taken
M_T: Amount (g) of Concentrated Glycerin taken

Operating conditions—

Detector: A hydrogen flame-ionization detector.

Column: A fused-silica column 0.32 mm in inside diameter and 30 m in length, coated the inner surface with 14% cyanopropylphenyl-86% dimethyl silicone polymer for gas chromatography 1 μm in thickness.

Column temperature: Inject at a constant temperature of about 100°C, raise the temperature at the rate of 7.5°C per minute to 220°C, and maintain at a constant temperature of about 220°C.

Injection port temperature: A constant temperature of about 220°C.

Detector temperature: A constant temperature of about 250°C.

Carrier gas: Helium.

Flow rate: about 38 cm per second.

Split ratio: 1:20.

Time span of measurement: About 3 times as long as the retention time of glycerin, beginning after the solvent peak.

System suitability—

System performance: Mix 50 mg each of ethylene glycol, diethylene glycol and glycerin for gas chromatography with 100 mL of methanol. When the procedure is run with 1 μL of this solution under the above operating conditions, ethylene glycol, diethylene glycol and glycerin are eluted in this order, and the resolution between the peaks of ethylene glycol and diethylene glycol is not less than 40, and between the peaks of diethylene glycol and glycerin is not less than 10.

System repeatability: When the test is repeated 6 times with 1 μL of the standard solution under the above operating conditions, the relative standard deviations of the peak area of ethylene glycol and diethylene glycol are not more than 10%, respectively.

(12) Readily carbonizable substances—To 5 mL of Concentrated Glycerin add carefully 5 mL of sulfuric acid for readily carbonizable substances, mix gently at a temperature between 18°C and 20°C, and allow to stand for 1 hour between 15°C and 25°C: the solution has no more color than Matching Fluid H.

Water <*2.48*> Not more than 2.0% (6 g, volumetric titration, direct titration).

Residue on ignition <*2.44*> Weigh accurately about 10 g of Concentrated Glycerin in a tared crucible, heat to boiling, and fire to burn immediately. Cool, moisten the residue with 1 to 2 drops of sulfuric acid, and ignite cautiously to constant mass: the mass of the residue is not more than 0.01%.

Assay Weigh accurately about 0.2 g of Concentrated Glycerin, transfer into a glass-stoppered flask, add 50 mL of water, mix, add exactly 50 mL of sodium periodate TS, shake, and allow to stand in a dark place at a room temperature for about 30 minutes. Add 10 mL of a mixture of water and ethylene glycol (1:1), allow to stand for about 20 minutes, add 100 mL of water, and titrate <*2.50*> with 0.1 mol/L sodium hydroxide VS (indicator: 2 drops of phenolphthalein TS). Perform a blank determination in the same manner, and make the necessary correction.

Each mL of 0.1 mol/L sodium hydroxide VS
$= 9.209$ mg of $C_3H_8O_3$

Containers and storage Containers—Tight containers.

Glycerin and Potash Solution

グリセリンカリ液

Method of preparation

Potassium Hydroxide	3 g
Glycerin	200 mL
Ethanol	250 mL
Aromatic substance	a suitable quantity
Water, Purified Water or Purified Water in Containers	a sufficient quantity
To make	1000 mL

Dissolve Potassium Hydroxide in a portion of Water, Purified Water or Purified Water in Containers, add Glycerin, Ethanol, a suitable quantity of aromatic substance and another portion of Water, Purified Water or Purified Water in Containers to volume, and filter. Concentrated Glycerin may be used in place of Glycerin.

Description Glycerin and Potash Solution is a clear, colorless liquid, having an aromatic odor.

The pH of a solution of Glycerin and Potash Solution (1 in 5) is about 12.

Specific gravity d^{20}_{20}: about 1.02

Identification **(1)** A solution of Glycerin and Potash Solution (1 in 2) is alkaline (potassium hydroxide).

(2) Place 10 mL of a solution of Glycerin and Potash Solution (1 in 10) in a glass-stoppered test tube, add 2 mL of sodium hydroxide TS and 1 mL of copper (II) sulfate TS, and shake: a blue color is produced (glycerin).

(3) Glycerin and Potash Solution responds to Qualitative Tests <*1.09*> for potassium salt.

Containers and storage Containers—Tight containers.

Glyceryl Monostearate

モノステアリン酸グリセリン

Glyceryl Monostearate is a mixture of α- and β-glyceryl monostearate and other fatty acid esters of glycerin.

Description Glyceryl Monostearate occurs as white to light yellow, waxy masses, thin flakes, or granules. It has a characteristic odor and taste.

It is very soluble in hot ethanol (95), soluble in chloroform, sparingly soluble in diethyl ether, and practically insoluble in water and in ethanol (95).

It is slowly affected by light.

Identification **(1)** Heat 0.2 g of Glyceryl Monostearate with 0.5 g of potassium hydrogen sulfate until thoroughly charred: the irritative odor of acrolein is perceptible.

(2) Dissolve 0.1 g of Glyceryl Monostearate in 2 mL of ethanol (95) by warming, heat with 5 mL of dilute sulfuric acid in a water bath for 30 minutes, and cool: a white to yellow solid is produced. This separated solid dissolves when shaken with 3 mL of diethyl ether.

Melting point ⟨*1.13*⟩ Not below 55°C.

Acid value ⟨*1.13*⟩ Not more than 15.

Saponification value ⟨*1.13*⟩ 157 – 170

Iodine value ⟨*1.13*⟩ Not more than 3.0. Use chloroform instead of cyclohexane.

Purity ⟨*1.13*⟩ Acidity or alkalinity—To 1.0 g of Glyceryl Monostearate add 20 mL of boiling water, and cool with swirling: the solution is neutral.

Residue on ignition ⟨*2.44*⟩ Not more than 0.1% (1 g).

Containers and storage Containers—Tight containers.
Storage—Light-resistant.

Glycine

グリシン

H_2N–CH_2–CO_2H

$C_2H_5NO_2$: 75.07
Aminoacetic acid
[*56-40-6*]

Glycine, when dried, contains not less than 98.5% of glycine ($C_2H_5NO_2$).

Description Glycine occurs as white, crystals or crystalline powder. It has a sweet taste.

It is freely soluble in water and in formic acid, and practically insoluble in ethanol (95).

It shows crystal polymorphism.

Identification Determine the infrared absorption spectrum of Glycine, previously dried, as directed in the potassium bromide disk method under Infrared Spectrophotometry ⟨*2.25*⟩, and compare the spectrum with the Reference Spectrum: both spectra exhibit similar intensities of absorption at the same wave numbers. If any difference appears between the spectra, dissolve Glycine in water, evaporate the water to dryness, and repeat the test with the residue.

pH ⟨*2.54*⟩ Dissolve 1.0 g of Glycine in 20 mL of water: the pH of the solution is between 5.6 and 6.6.

Purity **(1)** Clarity and color of solution—Dissolve 1.0 g of Glycine in 10 mL of water: the solution is clear and colorless.

(2) Chloride ⟨*1.03*⟩—Perform the test with 0.5 g of Glycine. Prepare the control solution with 0.30 mL of 0.01 mol/L hydrochloric acid VS (not more than 0.021%).

(3) Sulfate ⟨*1.14*⟩—Perform the test with 0.6 g of Glycine. Prepare the control solution with 0.35 mL of 0.005 mol/L sulfuric acid VS (not more than 0.028%).

(4) Ammonium⟨*1.02*⟩—Perform the test using 0.25 g of Glycine. Prepare the control solution with 5.0 mL of Standard Ammonium Solution (not more than 0.02%).

(5) Heavy metals ⟨*1.07*⟩—Proceed with 1.0 g of Glycine according to Method 1, and perform the test. Prepare the control solution with 2.0 mL of Standard Lead Solution (not more than 20 ppm).

(6) Arsenic ⟨*1.11*⟩—Prepare the test solution with 1.0 g of Glycine according to Method 1, and perform the test (not more than 2 ppm).

(7) Related substances—Dissolve 0.10 g of Glycine in 25 mL of water and use this solution as the sample solution. Pipet 1 mL of the sample solution, add water to make exactly 50 mL. Pipet 5 mL of this solution, add water to make exactly 20 mL, and use this solution as the standard solution. Perform the test with these solutions as directed under Thin-layer Chromatography ⟨*2.03*⟩. Spot 5 μL each of the sample solution and standard solution on a plate of silica gel for thin-layer chromatography. Develop the plate with a mixture of 1-butanol, water and acetic acid (100) (3:1:1) to a distance of about 10 cm, and dry the plate at 80°C for 30 minutes. Spray evenly a solution of ninhydrin in acetone (1 in 50), and heat at 80°C for 5 minutes: the spots other than the principal spot from the sample solution are not more intense than the spot from the standard solution.

Loss on drying ⟨*2.41*⟩ Not more than 0.30% (1 g, 105°C, 3 hours).

Residue on ignition ⟨*2.44*⟩ Not more than 0.1% (1 g).

Assay Weigh accurately about 80 mg of Glycine, previously dried, dissolve in 3 mL of formic acid, add 50 mL of acetic acid (100), and titrate ⟨*2.50*⟩ with 0.1 mol/L perchloric acid VS (potentiometric titration). Perform a blank determination in the same manner, and make any necessary correction.

Each mL of 0.1 mol/L perchloric acid VS
= 7.507 mg of $C_2H_5NO_2$

Containers and storage Containers—Well-closed containers.

Gonadorelin Acetate

ゴナドレリン酢酸塩

His-Trp-Ser-Tyr-Gly-Leu-Arg-Pro-Gly-NH_2 • $[H_3C-CO_2H]_2$

$C_{55}H_{75}N_{17}O_{13}.2C_2H_4O_2$: 1302.39
5-Oxo-L-prolyl-L-histidyl-L-tryptophyl-L-seryl-L-tyrosyl-glycyl-L-leucyl-L-arginyl-L-prolyl-glycinamide diacetate
[*34973-08-5*]

Gonadorelin Acetate contains not less than 96.0% and not more than 102.0% of gonadorelin acetate ($C_{55}H_{75}N_{17}O_{13}.2C_2H_4O_2$), calculated on the anhydrous basis.

Description Gonadorelin Acetate occurs as a white to pale yellow powder. It is odorless or has a slight, acetic odor.

It is freely soluble in water, in methanol and in acetic acid (100), and sparingly soluble in ethanol (95).

It is hygroscopic.

Identification **(1)** Determine the absorption spectrum of a solution of Gonadorelin Acetate in methanol (1 in 10,000) as directed under Ultraviolet-visible Spectrophotometry ⟨*2.24*⟩, and compare the spectrum with the Reference Spectrum: both spectra exhibit similar intensities of absorption at the same wavelengths.

(2) Determine the infrared absorption spectrum of Gonadorelin Acetate as directed in the potassium bromide disk method under Infrared Spectrophotometry ⟨*2.25*⟩, and compare the spectrum with the Reference Spectrum or the spectrum of Gonadorelin Acetate RS: both spectra exhibit similar intensities of absorption at the same wave numbers.

(3) Dissolve 20 mg of Gonadorelin Acetate in 0.5 mL of

ethanol (99.5), add 1 mL of sulfuric acid, and heat: the odor of ethyl acetate is perceptible.

Optical rotation ⟨*2.49*⟩ $[\alpha]_D^{20}$: −53.0 − −57.0° (0.1 g calculated on the anhydrous basis, diluted acetic acid (100) (1 in 100), 10 mL, 100 mm).

pH ⟨*2.54*⟩ Dissolve 0.10 g of Gonadorelin Acetate in 10 mL of water: the pH of this solution is between 4.8 and 5.8.

Constituent amino acids Put 10 mg of Gonadorelin Acetate in a test tube for hydrolysis, add 0.5 mL of hydrochloric acid and 0.5 mL of a solution of mercaptoacetic acid (2 in 25), seal the tube under reduced pressure, and heat at 110°C for 5 hours. After cooling, open the tube, transfer the hydrolyzate into a beaker, and evaporate to dryness on a water bath. Add exactly 100 mL of 0.02 mol/L hydrochloric acid TS to dissolve the residue, and use this solution as the sample solution. Separately, weigh exactly 0.105 g of L-serine, 0.147 g of L-glutamic acid, 0.115 g of L-proline, 75 mg of glycine, 0.131 g of L-leucine, 0.181 g of L-tyrosine, 0.210 g of L-histidine hydrochloride monohydrate, 0.204 g of L-tryptophan and 0.211 g of L-arginine hydrochloride, which are all previously dried at 105°C for 3 hours, add 50 mL of 1 mol/L hydrochloric acid TS to dissolve them, and add water to make exactly 1000 mL. Pipet 10 mL of this solution, add 0.02 mol/L hydrochloric acid TS to make exactly 200 mL, and use this solution as the standard solution. Perform the test with 50 μL each of the sample solution and standard solution as directed under Liquid Chromatography ⟨*2.01*⟩ according to the following conditions: the peaks of nine constituent amino acids are observed on the chromatogram obtained from the sample solution, and their respective molar ratios to arginine are 0.7 − 1.0 for serine and tryptophan, 0.8 − 1.2 for proline, 0.9 − 1.1 for glutamic acid, leucine, tyrosine and histidine, respectively, and 1.8 − 2.2 for glycine.

Operating conditions—

Detector: A visible spectrophotometer (wavelength: 440 nm for proline and 570 nm for others).

Column: A stainless steel column 4 mm in inside diameter and 8 cm in length, packed with strongly acidic ion-exchange resin for liquid chromatography composed with a sulfonated polystyrene copolymer (5 μm in particle diameter).

Column temperature: A constant temperature of about 57°C.

Chemical reaction bath temperature: A constant temperature of about 130°C.

Mobile phase: Prepare the mobile phases A, B, C and D according to the following table.

Mobile phase	A	B	C	D
Trisodium citrate dihydrate	6.19 g	7.74 g	26.67 g	—
Sodium hydroxide	—	—	—	8.00 g
Sodium chloride	5.66 g	7.07 g	54.35 g	—
Citric acid monohydrate	19.80 g	22.00 g	6.10 g	—
Ethanol (99.5)	130 mL	20 mL	—	100 mL
Benzyl alcohol	—	—	5 mL	—
Thiodiglycol	5 mL	5 mL	—	—
Lauromacrogol solution in diethyl ether (1 in 4)	4 mL	4 mL	4 mL	4 mL
Caprylic acid	0.1 mL	0.1 mL	0.1 mL	0.1 mL
Water	a sufficient amount	a sufficient amount	a sufficient amount	a sufficient amount
Total volume	1000 mL	1000 mL	1000 mL	1000 mL

Flowing of mobile phase: Control the gradient by mixing the mobile phases A, B, C and D as directed in the following table.

Time after injection of sample (min)	Mobile phase A (vol%)	Mobile phase B (vol%)	Mobile phase C (vol%)	Mobile phase D (vol%)
0 ~ 9	100	0	0	0
9 ~ 25	0	100	0	0
25 ~ 61	0	100 → 0	0 → 100	0
61 ~ 76	0	0	100	0
76 ~ 96	0	0	0	100

Reaction reagent: Dissolve 204 g of lithium acetate dihydrate in 336 mL of water, add 123 mL of acetic acid (100) and 401 mL of 1-methoxy-2-propanol, and use as Solution A. Separately, dissolve 39 g of ninhydrin and 81 mg of sodium borohydride in 979 mL of 1-methoxy-2-propanol, and use as Solution B. Mix the same volume of Solution A and Solution B before use.

Flow rate of mobile phase: 0.25 mL per minute.

Flow rate of reaction reagent: 0.3 mL per minute.

System suitability—

System performance: When the procedure is run with 50 μL of the standard solution under the above operating conditions, serine, glutamic acid, proline, glycine, leucine, tyrosine, histidine, tryptophan and arginine are eluted in this order with enough separation between these peaks.

Purity (1) Clarity and color of solution—A solution obtained by dissolving 0.10 g of Gonadorelin Acetate in 10 mL of water is clear, and the absorbance of this solution at 350 nm determined as directed under Ultraviolet-visible Spectrophotometry ⟨*2.24*⟩ is not more than 0.10.

(2) Related substances—Dissolve 50 mg of Gonadorelin Acetate in 100 mL of the mobile phase, and use this solution as the sample solution. Pipet 1 mL of the sample solution, add the mobile phase to make exactly 20 mL, and use this solution as the standard solution. Perform the test with exactly 10 μL each of the sample solution and standard solution as directed under Liquid Chromatography ⟨*2.01*⟩ according to the following conditions, and determine each peak area by the automatic integration method: the area of the peak other than gonadorelin from the sample solution is not larger than 1/5 times the peak area of gonadorelin from the standard solution, and the total area of the peaks other than gonadorelin from the sample solution is not larger than 3/5 times the peak area of gonadorelin from the standard solution.

Operating conditions—

Detector, column, column temperature, mobile phase, and flow rate: Proceed as directed in the operating conditions in the Assay.

Time span of measurement: About 2.5 times as long as the retention time of gonadorelin, beginning after the solvent peak.

System suitability—

Test for required detectability: To exactly 2 mL of the standard solution add the mobile phase to make exactly 100 mL. Confirm that the peak area of gonadorelin obtained with 10 μL of this solution is equivalent to 1 to 3% of that with 10 μL of the standard solution.

System performance: Dissolve 4 mg of Gonadorelin Acetate in a suitable amount of the mobile phase, add 5 mL of a solution of phenacetin in acetonitrile (1 in 1000) and the mobile phase to make 50 mL. When the procedure is run with 10 μL of this solution under the above operating conditions, gonadorelin and phenacetin are eluted in this order with the resolution between these peaks being not less than 3.

System repeatability: When the test is repeated 6 times with 10 μL of the standard solution under the above operat-

ing conditions, the relative standard deviation of the peak area of gonadorelin is not more than 5%.

Water <*2.48*> Not more than 8.0% (0.15 g, volumetric titration, direct titration).

Residue on ignition <*2.44*> Not more than 0.2% (0.1 g).

Assay Weigh accurately about 20 mg of Gonadorelin Acetate and Gonadorelin Acetate RS (separately determine the water <*2.48*> in the same manner as Gonadorelin Acetate) and dissolve in diluted acetic acid (100) (1 in 1000) to make exactly 25 mL each. Pipet 5 mL each of these solutions, add exactly 5 mL of the internal standard solution and add water to make 25 mL, and use these solutions as the sample solution and standard solution. Perform the test with 10 μL each of the sample solution and standard solution as directed under Liquid Chromatography <*2.01*> according to the following conditions, and calculate the ratios, Q_T and Q_S, of the peak area of gonadorelin to that of the internal standard.

Amount (mg) of gonadorelin acetate ($C_{55}H_{75}N_{17}O_{13}.2C_2H_4O_2$)
$= M_S \times Q_T/Q_S$

M_S: Amount (mg) of Gonadorelin Acetate RS taken, calculated on the anhydrous basis

Internal standard solution—A solution of phenacetin in a mixture of water and acetonitrile (3:2) (1 in 1000).
Operating conditions—

Detector: An ultraviolet absorption photometer (wavelength: 220 nm).

Column: A stainless steel column 4.6 mm in inside diameter and 15 cm in length, packed with octadecylsilanized silica gel for liquid chromatography (5 μm in particle diameter).

Column temperature: A constant temperature of about 40°C.

Mobile phase: A mixture of 0.05 mol/L potassium dihydrogen phosphate TS (pH 3.0) and acetonitrile (90:17).

Flow rate: Adjust so that the retention time of gonadorelin is about 13 minutes.

System suitability—

System performance: When the procedure is run with 10 μL of the standard solution under the above operating conditions, gonadorelin and the internal standard are eluted in this order with the resolution between these peaks being not less than 3.

System repeatability: When the test is repeated 6 times with 10 μL of the standard solution under the above operating conditions, the relative standard deviation of the ratio of the peak area of gonadorelin to that of the internal standard is not more than 1.5%.

Containers and storage Containers—Tight containers.
Storage—Light-resistant.

Human Chorionic Gonadotrophin

Chorionic Gonadotrophin

ヒト絨毛性性腺刺激ホルモン

Human Chorionic Gonadotrophin is a dried preparation of gonad-stimulating hormone obtained from the urine of healthy pregnant women after the manufacturing process to remove or inactivate the virus.

It contains not less than 2500 human chorionic gonadotrophin Units per mg, and contains not less than 3000 chorionic gonadotrophin Units per mg protein.

It contains not less than 80% and not more than 125% of the labeled human chorionic gonadotrophin Units.

Description Human Chorionic Gonadotrophin occurs as a white to light yellow-brown powder.

It is freely soluble in water.

Identification Calculate b by the following equation, using Y_3 and Y_4 obtained in the Assay: b is not more than 120.

$b = E/I$

$E = (Y_3 - Y_4)/f$

f: Number of test animals per group

$I = \log (T_H/T_L)$

Purity (1) Clarity and color of solution—Dissolve 0.05 g of Human Chorionic Gonadotrophin in 5 mL of isotonic sodium chloride solution: the solution is clear and colorless or light yellow.

(2) Estrogen—Inject subcutaneously into each of three female albino rats or albino mice ovariectomized at least two weeks before the test, single dose of 100 units according to the labeled Units dissolved in 0.5 mL of isotonic sodium chloride solution. Take vaginal smear twice daily, on the third, fourth and fifth day. Place the smear thinly on a slide glass, dry, stain with Giemsa's TS, wash with water, and again dry: no estrus figure is shown microscopically.

Loss on drying <*2.41*> Not more than 5.0% (0.1 g, in vacuum, phosphorus (V) oxide, 4 hours).

Bacterial endotoxins <*4.01*> Less than 0.03 EU/unit.

Abnormal toxicity Dilute Human Chorionic Gonadotrophin with isotonic sodium chloride solution so that each mL of the solution contains 120 Units, and use this solution as the sample solution. Inject 5.0 mL of the sample solution into the peritoneal cavity of each of 2 or more of well-nourished, healthy guinea pigs weighing about 350 g, and observe the conditions of the animals for more than 7 days: all the animals exhibit no abnormalities.

Specific activity When calculate from the results obtained by the Assay and the following test, the specific activity is not less than 3000 human chorionic gonadotrophin Units per mg protein.

(i) Sample solution—To an exactly amount of Human Chorionic Gonadotrophin add water to make a solution so that each mL contains about 500 Units of human chorionic gonadotrophin.

(ii) Standard solution—Weigh accurately about 10 mg of bovine serum albumin, and dissolve in water to make exactly 20 mL. To a suitable volume of this solution add water to make four solutions containing exactly 300, 200, 100 and 50 μg of the albumin per mL, respectively.

(iii) Procedure—Pipet 0.5 mL each of the sample solution and standard solutions, put them in glass test tubes about 18 mm in inside diameter and about 130 mm in length, add exactly 5 mL of alkaline copper TS, mix, and allow the tubes to stand in a water bath at 30°C for 10 minutes. Then add exactly 0.5 mL of diluted Folin's TS (1 in 2), mix, and warm in a water bath at 30°C for 20 minutes. Determine the absorbances of these solutions at 750 nm as directed under Ultraviolet-visible Spectrophotometry <*2.24*> using a solution obtained in the same manner with 0.5 mL of water as the blank.

Plot the absorbances of the standard solutions on the vertical axis and their protein concentrations on the horizontal axis to prepare a calibration curve, and determine the protein content of the sample solution from its absorbance by using this curve. Then calculate the amount of the protein in the sample.

Assay (i) Test animals—Select healthy female albino rats weighing about 45 to 65 g.

(ii) Standard solution—Dissolve a quantity of Human Chorionic Gonadotrophin RS in bovine serum albumin-isotonic sodium chloride solution to prepare four kinds of solutions, having 7.5, 15, 30 and 60 Units per 2.5 mL, respectively. Inject these solutions into four groups consisting of five test animals each, and weigh their ovaries, as directed in procedure of (iv). Inject bovine serum albumin-isotonic sodium chloride solution to another group, and use this group as the control group. According to the result of this test, designate the concentration of the reference standard which will increase the masses of the ovaries about 2.5 times the mass of the ovaries of the control group as a low-dose concentration of the standard solution, and the concentration 1.5 to 2.0 times the low-dose concentration as a high-dose concentration. Dissolve a quantity of Human Chorionic Gonadotrophin RS, in bovine serum albumin-isotonic sodium chloride solution, and prepare a high-dose standard solution S_H and a low-dose standard solution S_L whose concentrations are equal to those determined by the above test.

(iii) Sample solution—According to the labeled units, weigh accurately a suitable quantity of Human Chorionic Gonadotrophin, dissolve in bovine serum albumin-isotonic sodium chloride solution, and prepare a high-dose sample solution T_H and a low-dose sample solution T_L having Units equal to the standard solutions in equal volumes.

(iv) Procedure—Divide the test animals at random into 4 groups, A, B, C and D, with not less than 10 animals and equal numbers in each group. Inject subcutaneously 0.5 mL of S_H, S_L, T_H and T_L in each group for 5 days. On the sixth day, excise the ovaries, remove the fat and other unwonted tissues attached to the ovaries, and remove the adhering water by lightly pressing between filter paper, and immediately weigh the ovaries.

(v) Calculation—Designate the mass of ovaries by S_H, S_L, T_H and T_L as y_1, y_2, y_3 and y_4, respectively. Sum up y_1, y_2, y_3 and y_4 on each set to obtain Y_1, Y_2, Y_3 and Y_4.

Units per mg of Human Chorionic Gonadotrophin
$= \text{antilog}\, M \times$ units per mL of $S_H \times b/a$

$$M = IY_a/Y_b$$
$$I = \log(S_H/S_L) = \log(T_H/T_L)$$
$$Y_a = -Y_1 - Y_2 + Y_3 + Y_4$$
$$Y_b = Y_1 - Y_2 + Y_3 - Y_4$$

a: Mass (mg) of Human Chorionic Gonadotrophin taken

b: Total volume (mL) of the high dose of the test solution prepared by diluting with bovine serum albumin-isotonic sodium chloride solution

F' computed by the following equation should be smaller than F_1 against n when s^2 is calculated. And compute L (P = 0.95) by the following equation: L should be not more than 0.3. If F' exceeds F_1, or if L exceeds 0.3, repeat the test increasing the number of the test animals or arranging the assay method in a better way until F' is smaller than F_1 or L is not more than 0.3.

$$F' = (Y_1 - Y_2 - Y_3 + Y_4)^2/(4fs^2)$$

f: Number of test animals per group

$$s^2 = \{\Sigma y^2 - (Y/f)\}/n$$

Σy^2: The sum of the squares of each y_1, y_2, y_3 and y_4

$$Y = Y_1^2 + Y_2^2 + Y_3^2 + Y_4^2$$
$$n = 4(f-1)$$

$$L = 2\sqrt{(C-1)(CM^2 + I^2)}$$
$$C = Y_b^2/(Y_b^2 - 4fs^2t^2)$$

t^2: Value shown in the following table against n used to calculate s^2

n	$t^2 = F_1$	n	$t^2 = F_1$	n	$t^2 = F_1$
1	161.45	13	4.667	25	4.242
2	18.51	14	4.600	26	4.225
3	10.129	15	4.543	27	4.210
4	7.709	16	4.494	28	4.196
5	6.608	17	4.451	29	4.183
6	5.987	18	4.414	30	4.171
7	5.591	19	4.381	40	4.085
8	5.318	20	4.351	60	4.001
9	5.117	21	4.325	120	3.920
10	4.965	22	4.301	∞	3.841
11	4.844	23	4.279		
12	4.747	24	4.260		

Containers and storage Containers—Tight containers.
Storage—Light-resistant, and in a cold place.

Human Chorionic Gonadotrophin for Injection

Chorionic Gonadotrophin for Injection

注射用ヒト絨毛性性腺刺激ホルモン

Human Chorionic Gonadotrophin for Injection is a preparation for injection which is dissolved before use.

It contains not less than 80% and not more than 125% of the labeled human chorionic gonadotrophin Units.

Method of preparation Prepare as directed under Injections with Human Chorionic Gonadotrophin.

Description Human Chorionic Gonadotrophin for Injection occurs as a white to light yellow-brown powder or masses.

Identification Proceed as directed in the Identification under Human Chorionic Gonadotrophin.

pH <*2.54*> Prepare a solution so that each mL of isotonic sodium chloride solution contains 2 mg of Human Chorionic Gonadotorophin for Injection: the pH of this solution is between 5.0 and 7.0.

Loss on drying <*2.41*> Not more than 5.0% (0.1 g, in vacuum, phosphorus (V) oxide, 4 hours).

Bacterial endotoxins <*4.01*> Less than 0.03 EU/unit.

Uniformity of dosage units <*6.02*> It meets the requirement of the Mass variation test, when calculate the acceptance value using the mean of estimated contents of the units tested as M.

Foreign insoluble matter <6.06> Perform the test according to the Method 2: it meets the requirement.

Insoluble particulate matter <6.07> It meets the requirement.

Sterility <4.06> Perform the test according to the Membrane filtration method: it meets the requirement.

Assay Proceed as directed in the Assay under Human Chorionic Gonadotrophin. The ratio of the assayed Units to the labeled Units should be calculated by the following equation.

The ratio of the assayed Units to the labeled Units
$= \text{antilog } M$

Containers and storage Containers—Hermetic containers.
Storage—Light-resistant, and in a cold place.

Human Menopausal Gonadotrophin

ヒト下垂体性性腺刺激ホルモン

Human Menopausal Gonadotrophin is a dried preparation of gonad-stimulating hormone obtained from the urine of postmenopausal healthy women, after processing for virus removal or inactivation. It has follicle-stimulating hormonal action and luteinizing hormonal action.

It contains not less than 40 follicle-stimulating hormone Units per mg.

Description Human Menopausal Gonadotrophin occurs as a white to pale yellow powder.

It is soluble in water.

Ratio of interstitial cell-stimulating hormone to follicle-stimulating hormone Perform the test according to the following method: the ratio of the unit of interstitial cell-stimulating hormone (luteinizing hormone) to that of follicle-stimulating hormone is not more than 1.

(i) Test animals—Select healthy male albino rats weighing about 45 to 65 g.

(ii) Standard solutions—Dissolve Menopausal Gonadotrophin RS in bovine serum albumin-sodium chloride-phosphate buffer solution (pH 7.2) to prepare three kinds of solutions, containing 10, 20 and 40 interstitial cell-stimulating hormone (luteinizing hormone) units per 1.0 mL, respectively. Inject these solutions into three groups consisting of five test animals each, and weigh their seminal vesicles as directed in (iv). According to the result of the test, designate the concentration of the reference standard, which will make the mass of the seminal vesicle 20 to 35 mg, as the high-dose standard solution, S_H. Dilute the S_H to 1.5 to 2.0 times the initial volume with the bovine serum albumin-sodium chloride-phosphate buffer solution (pH 7.2) and designate this solution as the low-dose standard solution, S_L.

(iii) Sample solutions—Weigh accurately a suitable amount of Human Menopausal Gonadotrophin, and dissolve in the bovine serum albumin-sodium chloride-phosphate buffer solution (pH 7.2) to prepare the high-dose sample solution, T_H and the low-dose sample solution, T_L, so that their concentrations are similar to those of the corresponding standard solutions, respectively. Store these solutions at 2 - 8°C.

(iv) Procedure—Divide the test animals at random into 4 groups, A, B, C and D, with not less than 10 animals and equal numbers in each group. Inject subcutaneously once every day 0.2 mL each of S_H, S_L, T_H and T_L to each animal in the respective groups for five days. On the sixth day, excise the seminal vesicles, remove extraneous tissue, remove fluid adhering to the vesicles and the contents of the vesicles by lightly pressing between filter papers, and weigh the vesicles.

(v) Calculation—Proceed as directed in (v) in the Assay by changing the mass of ovaries to the mass of seminal vesicles and the unit of follicle-stimulating hormone to the unit of interstitial cell-stimulating hormone to read.

Water <2.48> Not more than 5.0% (0.2 g, volumetric titration, direct titration).

Bacterial endotoxins <4.01> Dissolve Human Menopausal Gonadotrophin in water for bacterial endotoxins test to prepare a solution containing 75 follicle-stimulating hormone Units per mL, and perform the test: less than 0.66 EU/follicle-stimulating hormone Unit.

Specific activity Perform the test with Human Menopausal Gonadotrophin according to the following method, and calculate the specific activity using the amount (Unit) obtained in the Assay: it is not less than 50 follicle-stimulating hormone Units per 1 mg of protein.

(i) Sample solution—Weigh accurately about 10 mg of Human Menopausal Gonadotrophin, dissolve in water so that each mL contains exactly 200 μg, and use this solution as the sample solution.

(ii) Standard solutions—Weigh accurately about 10 mg of bovine serum albumin, and dissolve in water to make exactly 20 mL. To this solution add water to make four solutions containing exactly 300 μg, 200 μg, 100 μg and 50 μg of the albumin per mL, respectively, and use these solutions as the standard solutions.

(iii) Procedure—To glass test tubes, about 18 mm in inside diameter and about 130 mm in height, add separately exactly 0.5 mL each of the sample solution and the standard solutions. To these tubes add exactly 5 mL of alkaline copper TS, warm in a water bath at 30°C for 10 minutes, then add exactly 0.5 mL of diluted Folin's TS (1 in 2), and warm in a water bath at 30°C for 20 minutes. Perform the test with these solutions as directed under Ultraviolet-visible Spectrometry <2.24>, and determine the absorbances at 750 nm, using a liquid obtained with 0.5 mL of water in the same manner as above as a blank.

Prepare a calibration curve from the absorbances of the standard solutions, with absorbance on the vertical axis and concentration on the horizontal axis. Calculate the amount of protein in the sample solution from the absorbance of the sample solution using the curve, and calculate the protein content of the sample.

Assay

(i) Test animals—Select healthy female albino rats weighing about 45 to 65 g.

(ii) Standard solutions—Dissolve Human Menopausal Gonadotrophin RS in human chorionic gonadotrophin TS to prepare three solutions which contain 0.75, 1.5 and 3.0 follicle-stimulating hormone Units per 1.0 mL, respectively. Inject these solutions into three groups consisting of five test animals each, and weigh their ovaries, as directed in (iv). According to the result of the test, designate the concentration of the reference standard, which will make the mass of the ovary about 120 to 160 mg, as the high-dose standard solution, S_H. Dilute the S_H to 1.5 to 2.0 times the initial volume with the human chorionic gonadotrophin TS, and designate the solution as the low-dose standard solution, S_L.

(iii) Sample solutions—Weigh accurately a suitable amount of Human Menopausal Gonadotrophin, dissolve in human chorionic gonadotrophin TS, and prepare the high-dose sample solution, T_H, and the low-dose sample solution, T_L, which have similar numbers of units to those of corresponding standard solutions in equal volume, respectively.

(iv) Procedure—Divide the test animals at random into 4 groups, A, B, C and D, with not less than 10 animals and equal numbers in each group. Inject subcutaneously 0.2 mL each of S_H, S_L, T_H and T_L into the animals in each group, once in the afternoon on the first day, three times in the morning, noon and afternoon on the second day, and two times in the morning and afternoon on the third day. On the fifth day, excise the ovaries, remove the fat and extraneous tissue, remove fluid adhering to the ovaries by lightly pressing between filter papers, and immediately weigh the ovaries.

(v) Calculation—Designate the mass of ovaries by S_H, S_L, T_H and T_L as y_1, y_2, y_3 and y_4, respectively. Sum up y_1, y_2, y_3 and y_4 on each set to obtain Y_1, Y_2, Y_3 and Y_4.

Units of follicle-stimulating hormone per mg of Human Menopausal Gonadotrophin

$$= \text{antilog } M \times (\text{units per mL of } S_H) \times b/a$$

$$M = IY_a/Y_b$$
$$I = \log (S_H/S_L) = \log (T_H/T_L)$$
$$Y_a = -Y_1 - Y_2 + Y_3 + Y_4$$
$$Y_b = Y_1 - Y_2 + Y_3 - Y_4$$

a: Mass (mg) of Human Menopausal Gonadotrophin taken

b: Total volume (mL) of the high dose of the test solution prepared by diluting with human chorionic gonadotrophin TS

F' computed by the following equation should be smaller than F_1 against n when s^2 is calculated. And compute L ($P = 0.95$) by the following equation: L should be not more than 0.3. If F' exceeds F_1, or if L exceeds 0.3, repeat the test increasing the number of the test animals or arranging the assay method in a better way until F' is smaller than F_1 or L is not more than 0.3.

$$F' = (Y_1 - Y_2 - Y_3 + Y_4)^2/(4fs^2)$$

f: Number of test animals per group

$$s^2 = \{\Sigma y^2 - (Y/f)\}/n$$

Σy^2: The sum of the squares of each y_1, y_2, y_3 and y_4

$$Y = Y_1^2 + Y_2^2 + Y_3^2 + Y_4^2$$
$$n = 4(f - 1)$$
$$L = 2\sqrt{(C-1)(CM^2 + I^2)}$$
$$C = Y_b^2/(Y_b^2 - 4fs^2t^2)$$

t^2: Value shown in the following table against n used to calculate s^2

n	$t^2 = F_1$	n	$t^2 = F_1$	n	$t^2 = F_1$
1	161.45	13	4.667	25	4.242
2	18.51	14	4.600	26	4.225
3	10.129	15	4.543	27	4.210
4	7.709	16	4.494	28	4.196
5	6.608	17	4.451	29	4.183
6	5.987	18	4.414	30	4.171
7	5.591	19	4.381	40	4.085
8	5.318	20	4.351	60	4.001
9	5.117	21	4.325	120	3.920
10	4.965	22	4.301	∞	3.841
11	4.844	23	4.279		
12	4.747	24	4.260		

Containers and storage Containers—Tight containers.
Storage—Light-resistant, and in a cold place.

Guaifenesin

グアイフェネシン

and enantiomer

$C_{10}H_{14}O_4$: 198.22
(2*RS*)-3-(2-Methoxyphenoxy)propane-1,2-diol
[93-14-1]

Guaifenesin, when dried, contains not less then 98.0% and not more than 102.0% of guaifenesin ($C_{10}H_{14}O_4$).

Description Guaifenesin occurs as white, crystals or crystalline powder.

It is freely soluble in ethanol (95), and sparingly soluble in water.

A solution of ethanol (95) (1 in 20) shows no optical rotation.

Identification **(1)** Determine the absorption spectrum of a solution of Guaifenesin (1 in 50,000) as directed under Ultraviolet-visible Spectrophotometry *<2.24>*, and compare the spectrum with the Reference Spectrum or the spectrum of a solution of Guaifenesin RS prepared in the same manner as the sample solution: both spectra exhibit similar intensities of absorption at the same wavelengths.

(2) Determine the infrared absorption spectrum of Guaifenesin, previously dried, as directed in the potassium bromide disk method under Infrared Spectrophotometry *<2.25>*, and compare the spectrum with the Reference Spectrum or the spectrum of previously dried Guaifenesin RS: both spectra exhibit similar intensities of absorption at the same wave numbers.

pH *<2.54>* Dissolve 1.0 g of Guaifenesin in 100 mL of water: the pH of the solution is between 5.0 and 7.0.

Melting point *<2.60>* 80 – 83°C

Purity **(1)** Clarity and color of solution—Dissolve 0.20 g of Guaifenesin in 10 mL of water: the solution is clear and colorless.

(2) Chloride *<1.03>*—Dissolve 0.7 g of Guaifenesin in 25 mL of water by warming. Cool, add 6 mL of dilute nitric acid and water to make 50 mL, and perform the test using this solution as the test solution. Prepare the control solution with 0.40 mL of 0.01 mol/L hydrochloric acid VS (not more than 0.020%).

(3) Heavy metals <*1.07*>—Dissolve 2.0 g of Guaifenesin in 25 mL of water by warming. Cool, add 2 mL of dilute acetic acid and water to make 50 mL, and perform the test using this solution as the test solution. Prepare the control solution with 2.0 mL of Standard Lead Solution (not more than 10 ppm).

(4) Arsenic <*1.11*>—Prepare the test solution with 1.0 g of Guaifenesin according to Method 3, and perform the test (not more than 2 ppm).

(5) Free guaiacol—To 1.0 g of Guaifenesin add exactly 25 mL of water, dissolve by warming, cool, and use this solution as the sample solution. Separately, dissolve 0.100 g of guaiacol in water to make exactly 1000 mL. Pipet 3 mL of this solution, add exactly 22 mL of water, and use this solution as the standard solution. To each of the sample solution and standard solution add 1.0 mL of potassium hexacyanoferrate (III) TS and 5.0 mL of a solution of 4-aminoantipyrine (1 in 200), and immediately after shaking for exactly 5 seconds add a solution of sodium hydrogen carbonate (1 in 1200) to make exactly 100 mL. Determine the absorbances of these solutions at 500 nm exactly 15 minutes after the addition of the 4-aminoantipyrine solution as directed under Ultraviolet-visible Spectrophotometry <*2.24*>, using a solution, prepared in the same manner with 25 mL of water, as the blank: the absorbance of the solution obtained from the sample solution is not more than that from the standard solution.

(6) Related substances—Dissolve 1.0 g of Guaifenesin in 100 mL of ethanol (95), and use this solution as the sample solution. Pipet 1 mL of the sample solution, add water to make exactly 200 mL, and use this solution as the standard solution. Perform the test with these solutions as directed under Thin-layer Chromatography <*2.03*>. Spot 10 μL each of the sample solution and standard solution on a plate of silica gel for thin-layer chromatography. Develop the plate with a mixture of diethyl ether, ethanol (95), and ammonia solution (28) (40:10:1) to a distance of about 10 cm, and air-dry the plate. Spray evenly 4-dimethylaminobenzaldehyde TS for spraying on the plate, and heat the plate at 110°C for 10 minutes: the spots other than the principal spot obtained from the sample solution are not more intense than the spot from the standard solution.

Loss on drying <*2.41*> Not more than 0.5% (1 g, in vacuum, 60°C, 3 hours).

Residue on ignition <*2.44*> Not more than 0.1% (1 g).

Assay Weigh accurately about 60 mg of Guaifenesin and Guaifenesin RS, previously dried, and dissolve each then in water to make exactly 100 mL. Pipet 5 mL of these solutions, and add water to make exactly 100 mL, and use these solutions as the sample solution and standard solution. Determine the absorbances, A_T and A_S, of the sample solution and standard solution at 273 nm as directed under Ultraviolet-visible Spectrophotometry <*2.24*>.

Amount (mg) of guaifenesin ($C_{10}H_{14}O_4$) = $M_S \times A_T/A_S$

M_S: Amount (mg) of Guaifenesin RS taken

Containers and storage Containers—Tight containers.

Guanabenz Acetate

グアナベンズ酢酸塩

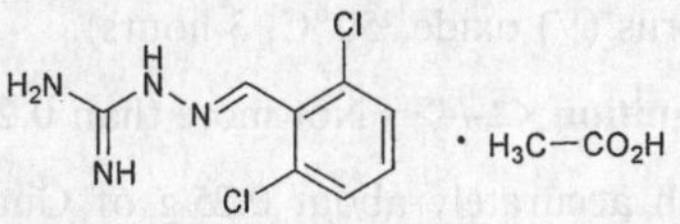

$C_8H_8Cl_2N_4.C_2H_4O_2$: 291.13

(*E*)-1-(2,6-Dichlorobenzylideneamino)guanidine monoacetate

[*23256-50-0*]

Guanabenz Acetate, when dried, contains not less than 98.5% of guanabenz acetate ($C_8H_8Cl_2N_4.C_2H_4O_2$).

Description Guanabenz Acetate occurs as white, crystals or crystalline powder.

It is freely soluble in acetic acid (100), soluble in methanol and in ethanol (95), slightly soluble in water, and practically insoluble in diethyl ether.

It is gradually affected by light.

Melting point: about 190°C (with decomposition).

Identification **(1)** To 5 mL of a solution of Guanabenz Acetate (1 in 1000) add 0.5 mL of a diluted ethanol (95) (5 in 6) which contains 16 g of urea and 0.2 g of 1-naphthol in 100 mL, and add 1 mL of *N*-bromosuccinimide TS: a purple color develops.

(2) Determine the absorption spectrum of a solution of Guanabenz Acetate in methanol (1 in 100,000) as directed under Ultraviolet-visible Spectrophotometry <*2.24*>, and compare the spectrum with the Reference Spectrum: both spectra exhibit similar intensities of absorption at the same wavelengths.

(3) Determine the infrared absorption spectrum of Guanabenz Acetate, previously dried, as directed in the potassium bromide disk method under Infrared Spectrophotometry <*2.25*>, and compare the spectrum with the Reference Spectrum: both spectra exhibit similar intensities of absorption at the same wave numbers.

(4) To 0.1 g of Guanabenz Acetate add 5 mL of water and 1 mL of ammonia TS, shake, filter, and neutralize the filtrate with dilute hydrochloric acid: the solution responds to Qualitative Tests <*1.09*> (3) for acetate.

Purity **(1)** Heavy metals <*1.07*>—Proceed with 2.0 g of Guanabenz Acetate according to Method 2, and perform the test. Prepare the control solution with 2.0 mL of Standard Lead Solution (not more than 10 ppm).

(2) Related substances—Conduct this procedure without exposure to light, using light-resistant vessels. Dissolve 0.05 g of Guanabenz Acetate in 5 mL of methanol, and use this solution as the sample solution. Pipet 1 mL of the sample solution, add methanol to make exactly 10 mL, then pipet 1 mL of this solution, add methanol to make exactly 20 mL, and use this solution as the standard solution. Perform the test with these solutions as directed under Thin-layer Chromatography <*2.03*>. Spot 5 μL each of the sample solution and standard solution on a plate of silica gel with fluorescent indicator for thin-layer chromatography. Develop the plate with a mixture of chloroform, methanol and ammonia solution (28) (80:20:1) to a distance of about 10 cm, and air-dry the plate. Examine under ultraviolet light (main wavelength: 254 nm): the spots other than the principal spot obtained from the sample solution are not more intense than the spot from the standard solution. Place the plate in a chamber filled with iodine vapor for 10 minutes: the spots other than the principal spot from the sample solution are not more intense than the spot from the standard solution.

Loss on drying *<2.41>* Not more than 0.5% (1 g, in vacuum, phosphorus (V) oxide, 50°C, 3 hours).

Residue on ignition *<2.44>* Not more than 0.2% (1 g).

Assay Weigh accurately about 0.25 g of Guanabenz Acetate, previously dried, dissolve in 50 mL of acetic acid (100), and titrate *<2.50>* with 0.1 mol/L perchloric acid VS (potentiometric titration). Perform a blank determination in the same manner, and make any necessary correction.

Each mL of 0.1 mol/L perchloric acid VS
= 29.11 mg of $C_8H_8Cl_2N_4.C_2H_4O_2$

Containers and storage Containers—Tight containers.
Storage—Light-resistant.

Guanethidine Sulfate

グアネチジン硫酸塩

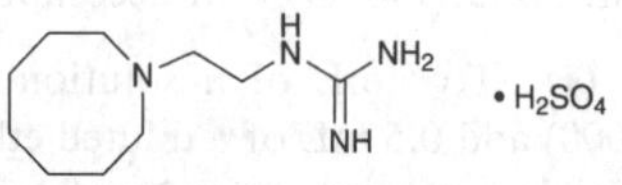

$\cdot H_2SO_4$

$C_{10}H_{22}N_4.H_2SO_4$: 296.39
1-[2-(Hexahydroazocin-1(2*H*)-yl)ethyl]guanidine monosulfate
[645-43-2]

Guanethidine Sulfate, when dried, contains not less than 98.5% of guanethidine sulfate ($C_{10}H_{22}N_4.H_2SO_4$).

Description Guanethidine Sulfate occurs as white, crystals or crystalline powder. It is odorless or has a slight, characteristic odor and a bitter taste.

It is very soluble in formic acid, freely soluble in water, and practically insoluble in ethanol (95) and in diethyl ether.

Melting point: 251 - 256°C (an evacuated sealed capillary tube, with decomposition).

Identification (1) To 4 mL of a solution of Guanethidine Sulfate (1 in 4000) add 2 mL of 1-naphthol TS, 1 mL of diacetyl TS and 15 mL of water, and allow to stand for 30 minutes: a red color develops.

(2) Determine the infrared absorption spectrum of Guanethidine Sulfate, previously dried, as directed in the potassium bromide disk method under Infrared Spectrophotometry *<2.25>*, and compare the spectrum with the Reference Spectrum: both spectra exhibit similar intensities of absorption at the same wave numbers.

(3) A solution of Guanethidine Sulfate (1 in 10) responds to Qualitative Tests *<1.09>* for sulfate.

pH *<2.54>* Dissolve 1.0 g of Guanethidine Sulfate in 50 mL of water: the pH of the solution is between 4.7 and 5.7.

Purity (1) Clarity and color of solution—Dissolve 1.0 g of Guanethidine Sulfate in 50 mL of water: the solution is clear and colorless.

(2) Methylisothiourea sulfate—Dissolve 2.0 g of Guanethidine Sulfate in 80 mL of sodium hydroxide TS, and allow to stand for 10 minutes. Add 60 mL of hydrochloric acid, 2 g of sodium bromide and water to make 200 mL. Then, to this solution add 0.70 mL of 1/60 mol/L potassium bromate VS and 2 mL of zinc iodide-starch TS: a blue color develops.

(3) Heavy metals *<1.07>*—Proceed with 2.0 g of Guanethidine Sulfate according to Method 4, and perform the test. Prepare the control solution with 2.0 mL of Standard Lead Solution (not more than 10 ppm).

Loss on drying *<2.41>* Not more than 0.5% (1 g, 105°C, 4 hours).

Residue on ignition *<2.44>* Not more than 0.2% (1 g).

Assay Weigh accurately about 0.5 g of Guanethidine Sulfate, previously dried, dissolve in 2 mL of formic acid, add 70 mL of a mixture of acetic anhydride and acetic acid (100) (6:1), and titrate *<2.50>* with 0.1 mol/L perchloric acid VS (potentiometric titration). Perform a blank determination in the same manner, and make any necessary correction.

Each mL of 0.1 mol/L perchloric acid VS
= 29.64 mg of $C_{10}H_{22}N_4.H_2SO_4$

Containers and storage Containers—Tight containers.
Storage—Light-resistant.

Freeze-dried Habu Antivenom, Equine

乾燥はぶウマ抗毒素

Freeze-dried Habu Antivenom, Equine, is a preparation for injection which is dissolved before use.

It contains *Trimeresurus flavoviridis* antivenom in immunoglobulin of horse origin.

It conforms to the requirements of Freeze-dried Habu Anti-venom, Equine, in the Minimum Requirements for Biological Products.

Description Freeze-dried Habu Antivenom, Equine, becomes colorless or light yellow-brown, clear liquid or a slightly white turbid liquid on addition of solvent.

Haloperidol

ハロペリドール

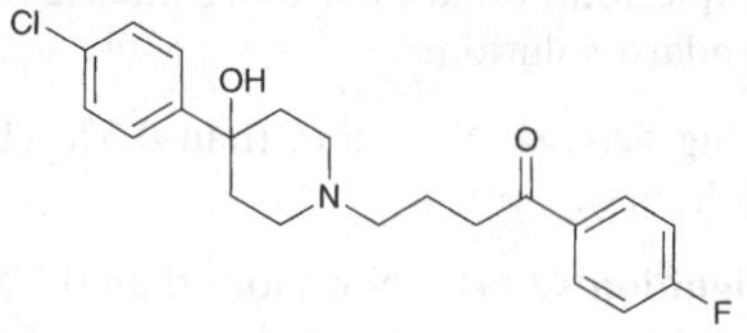

$C_{21}H_{23}ClFNO_2$: 375.86
4-[4-(4-Chlorophenyl)-4-hydroxypiperidin-1-yl]-1-(4-fluorophenyl)butan-1-one
[52-86-8]

Haloperidol, when dried, contains not less than 99.0% and not more than 101.0% of haloperidol ($C_{21}H_{23}ClFNO_2$).

Description Haloperidol occurs as white to pale yellow, crystals or powder.

It is freely soluble in acetic acid (100), sparingly soluble in methanol, slightly soluble in 2-propanol and in ethanol (99.5), and practically insoluble in water.

Identification (1) Dissolve 30 mg of Haloperidol in 100 mL of 2-propanol. To 5 mL of the solution add 10 mL of 0.1 mol/L hydrochloric acid TS and 2-propanol to make 100 mL. Determine the absorption spectrum of the solution as directed under Ultraviolet-visible Spectrophotometry *<2.24>*, and compare the spectrum with the Reference Spectrum: both spectra exhibit similar intensities of absorption at the same wavelengths.

(2) Determine the infrared absorption spectrum of Haloperidol as directed in the potassium bromide disk method under Infrared Spectrophotometry *<2.25>*, and compare the spectrum with the Reference Spectrum: both spectra exhibit similar intensities of absorption at the same wave numbers.

Melting point *<2.60>* 150 - 154°C

Purity **(1)** Sulfate *<1.14>*—To 1.0 g of Haloperidol add 50 mL of water, shake, and filter. To 25 mL of the filtrate add 1 mL of dilute hydrochloric acid and water to make 50 mL, and perform the test using this solution as the test solution. Prepare the control solution with 0.50 mL of 0.005 mol/L sulfuric acid VS (not more than 0.048%).

(2) Heavy metals *<1.07>*—Proceed with 1.0 g of Haloperidol according to method 2, and perform the test. Prepare the control solution with 2.0 mL of Standard Lead Solution (not more than 20 ppm).

(3) Related substances—Dissolve 25 mg of Haloperidol in 50 mL of the mobile phase, and use this solution as the sample solution. Pipet 1 mL of the sample solution, add the mobile phase to make exactly 200 mL, and use this solution as the standard solution. Perform the test with exactly 10 μL each of the sample solution and standard solution as directed under Liquid Chromatography *<2.01>* according to the following conditions, and determine each peak area by the automatic integration method: the area of the peak other than haloperidol obtained from the sample solution is not larger than the peak area of haroperidol from the standard solution, and the total area of these peaks is not larger than 2 times the peak area of haloperidol from the standard solution. For the areas of the peaks, having the relative retention time of about 0.5, about 1.2 and about 2.6 to haloperidol, multiply their correction factors, 0.75, 1.47 and 0.76, respectively.

Operating conditions—

Detector: An ultraviolet absorption photometer (wavelength: 220 nm).

Column: A stainless steel column 4.6 mm in inside diameter and 15 cm in length, packed with octadecylsilanized silica gel for liquid chromatography (5 μm in particle diameter).

Column temperature: A constant temperature of about 40°C.

Mobile phase: Dissolve 2.95 g of trisodium citrate dihydrate in 900 mL of water, adjust to pH 3.5 with dilute hydrochloric acid, and add water to make 1000 mL. To 300 mL of this solution add 700 mL of methanol and 1.0 g of sodium lauryl sulfate.

Flow rate: Adjust so that the retention time of haloperidol is about 9 minutes.

Time span of measurement: About 3 times as long as the retention time of haloperidol, beginning after the solvent peak.

System suitability—

Test for required detectability: To exactly 5 mL of the standard solution add the mobile phase to make exactly 25 mL. Confirm that the peak area of haloperidol obtained with 10 μL of this solution is equivalent to 15 to 25% of that with 10 μL of the standard solution.

System performance: When the procedure is run with 10 μL of the standard solution under the above operating conditions, the number of theoretical plates and the symmetry factor of the peak of haloperidol are not less than 4000 and not more than 2.0, respectively.

System repeatability: When the test is repeated 6 times with 10 μL of the standard solution under the above operating conditions, the relative standard deviation of the peak area of haloperidol is not more than 2.0%.

Loss on drying *<2.41>* Not more than 0.5% (1 g, in vacuum, 60°C, phosphorus (V) oxide, 3 hours).

Residue on ignition *<2.44>* Not more than 0.1% (1 g).

Assay Weigh accurately about 0.6 g of haloperidol, previously dried, and dissolve in 40 mL of acetic acid (100), and titrate *<2.50>* with 0.1 mol/L perchloric acid VS (indicator: 1 drop of crystal violet TS). Perform a blank determination in the same manner.

Each mL of 0.1 mol/L perchloric acid VS
= 37.59 mg of $C_{21}H_{23}ClFNO_2$

Containers and storage Containers—Tight containers.
Storage—Light-resistant.

Haloperidol Fine Granules

ハロペリドール細粒

Haloperidol Fine Granules contain not less than 95.0% and not more than 105.0% of the labeled amount of haloperidol ($C_{21}H_{23}ClFNO_2$: 375.86).

Method of preparation Prepare as directed under Granules, with Haloperidol.

Identification Powder Haloperidol Fine Granules. To a portion of the powder, equivalent to 6 mg of Haloperidol, add 70 mL of 2-propanol, and heat to boiling on a water bath while shaking. After cooling, add 2-propanol to make 100 mL, and centrifuge. To 5 mL of the supernatant liquid add 2 mL of 0.1 mol/L hydrochloric acid TS and 2-propanol to make 20 mL. Determine the absorption spectrum of this solution as directed under Ultraviolet-visible Spectrophotometry *<2.24>*: it exhibits maxima between 219 nm and 223 nm and between 243 nm and 247 nm.

Dissolution *<6.10>* When the test is performed at 50 revolutions per minute according to the Paddle method, using 900 mL of water as the dissolution medium, the dissolution rate in 60 minutes of Haloperidol Fine Granules is not less than 70%.

Start the test with an accurately weighed amount of Haloperidol Fine Granules, equivalent to about 3 mg of haloperidol ($C_{21}H_{23}ClFNO_2$), withdraw not less than 20 mL of the medium at the specified minute after starting the test, and filter through a membrane filter with a pore size not exceeding 0.45 μm. Discard not less than 10 mL of the first filtrate, pipet 5 mL of the subsequent filtrate, add water to make exactly 20 mL, and use this solution as the sample solution. Separately, weigh accurately about 17 mg of haloperidol for assay, previously dried in vacuum at 60°C for 3 hours using phosphorus (V) oxide as a desiccant, and dissolve in methanol to make exactly 200 mL. Pipet 2 mL of this solution, add water to make exactly 200 mL, and use this solution as the standard solution. Perform the test with exactly 100 μL each of the sample solution and standard solution as directed under Liquid Chromatography *<2.01>*, and determine the peak areas, A_T and A_S, of haloperidol in each solution.

Dissolution rate (%) with respect to the labeled amount of haloperidol ($C_{21}H_{23}ClFNO_2$)

$$= M_S/M_T \times A_T/A_S \times 1/C \times 18$$

M_S: Amount (mg) of haloperidol for assay taken
M_T: Amount (g) of Haloperidol Fine Granules taken
C: Labeled amount (mg) of haloperidol ($C_{21}H_{23}ClFNO_2$) in 1 g

Operating conditions—

Column, column temperature, mobile phase, and flow rate: Proceed as detected in the operating conditions in the Assay.

Detector: An ultraviolet absorption photometer (wavelength: 245 nm).

System suitability—

System performance: When the procedure is run with 100 μL of the standard solution under the above operating conditions, the number of theoretical plates and the symmetry factor of the peak of haloperidol are not less than 4000 and not more than 2.0, respectively.

System repeatability: When the test is repeated 6 times with 100 μL of the standard solution under the above operating conditions, the relative standard deviation of the peak area of haloperidol is not more than 2.0%.

Assay Powder Haloperidol Fine Granules. Weigh accurately a portion of the powder, equivalent to about 10 mg of haloperidol ($C_{21}H_{23}ClFNO_2$), add 10 mL of water, disperse the particle by sonicating, add exactly 20 mL of the internal standard solution, sonicate, extract for 30 minutes with occasional shaking, and add the mobile phase to make 100 mL. Centrifuge after shaking for more 30 minutes, and use the supernatant liquid as the sample solution. Separately, weigh accurately about 25 mg of haloperidol for assay, previously dried in vacuum at 60°C for 3 hours on phosphorus (V) oxide, and dissolve in methanol to make exactly 25 mL. Pipet 10 mL of this solution, add exactly 20 mL of the internal standard solution and the mobile phase to make 100 mL, and use this solution as the standard solution. Perform the test with 10 μL each of the sample solution and standard solution as directed under Liquid Chromatography <2.01> according to the following conditions, and calculate the ratios, Q_T and Q_S, of the peak area of haloperidol to that of the internal standard.

Amount (mg) of haloperidol ($C_{21}H_{23}ClFNO_2$)

$$= M_S \times Q_T/Q_S \times 2/5$$

M_S: Amount (mg) of haloperidol for assay taken

*Internal standard solution—*A solution of diphenyl in methanol (1 in 2000).

Operating conditions—

Detector: An ultraviolet absorption photometer (wavelength: 220 nm).

Column: A stainless steel column 4.6 mm in inside diameter and 15 cm in length, packed with octadecylsilanized silica gel for liquid chromatography (5 μm in particle diameter).

Column temperature: A constant temperature of about 40°C.

Mobile phase: Dissolve 2.95 g of trisodium citrate dihydrate in 900 mL of water, adjust to pH 3.5 with dilute hydrochloric acid, and add water to make 1000 mL. To 250 mL of this solution add 750 mL of methanol and 1.0 g of sodium lauryl sulfate, and mix to dissolve.

Flow rate: Adjust so that the retention time of haloperidol is about 9 minutes.

System suitability—

System performance: When the procedure is run with 10 μL of the standard solution under the above operating conditions, haloperidol and diphenyl are eluted in this order with the resolution between these peaks being not less than 5.

System repeatability: When the test is repeated 6 times with 10 μL of the standard solution under the above operating conditions, the relative standard deviation of the ratio of the peak area of haloperidol to that of the internal standard is not more than 1.0%.

Containers and storage Containers—Tight containers.
Storage—Light-resistant.

Haloperidol Injection

ハロペリドール注射液

Haloperidol Injection is an aqueous injection.

It contains not less than 95.0% and not more than 105.0% of the labeled amount of haloperidol ($C_{21}H_{23}ClFNO_2$: 375.86).

Method of preparation Prepare as directed under Injections, with Haloperidol.

Description Haloperidol Injection occurs as a colorless to pale yellow, clear liquid.

Identification To a volume of Haloperidol Injection, equivalent to 5 mg of Haloperidol, add 2-propanol to make 100 mL. To 5 mL of this solution add 2 mL of 0.1 mol/L hydrochloric acid TS and 2-propanol to make 20 mL. Determine the absorption spectrum of this solution as directed under Ultraviolet-visible Spectrophotometry <2.24>: it exhibits maxima between 219 nm and 223 nm and between 243 nm and 247 nm.

Osmotic pressure ratio Being specified separately when the drug is granted approval based on the Law.

pH Being specified separately when the drug is granted approval based on the Law.

Bacterial endotoxins <4.01> Less than 60 EU/mg.

Extractable volume <6.05> It meets the requirement.

Foreign insoluble matter <6.06> Perform the test according to Method 1: it meets the requirement.

Insoluble particulate matter <6.07> It meets the requirement.

Sterility <4.06> Perform the test according to the Membrane filtration method: it meets the requirement.

Assay Pipet a volume of Haloperidol Injection, equivalent to about 10 mg of haloperidol ($C_{21}H_{23}ClFNO_2$), add the mobile phase to make exactly 100 mL, and use this solution as the sample solution. Separately, weigh accurately about 25 mg of haloperidol for assay, previously dried in vacuum at 60°C using phosphorus (V) oxide as a desiccant for 3 hours, dissolve in methanol to make exactly 25 mL. Pipet 10 mL of this solution, add the mobile phase to make exactly 100 mL, and use this solution as the standard solution. Perform the test with exactly 10 μL each of the sample solution and standard solution as directed under Liquid Chromatography <2.01> according to the following conditions, and determine the peak areas, A_T and A_S, of haloperidol in each solution.

Amount (mg) of haloperidol ($C_{21}H_{23}ClFNO_2$)

$$= M_S \times A_T/A_S \times 2/5$$

M_S: Amount (mg) of haloperidol for assay taken

Operating conditions—

Detector: An ultraviolet absorption photometer (wavelength: 220 nm).

Column: A stainless steel column 4.6 mm in inside diameter and 15 cm in length, packed with octadecylsilanized silica gel for liquid chromatography (5 μm in particle diameter).

Column temperature: A constant temperature of about 40°C.

Mobile phase: Dissolve 2.95 g of trisodium citrate dihydrate in 900 mL of water, adjust to pH 3.5 with dilute hydrochloric acid, and add water to make 1000 mL. To 250 mL of this solution add 750 mL of methanol, and add 1.0 g of sodium lauryl sulfate to dissolve.

Flow rate: Adjust so that the retention time of haloperidol is about 9 minutes.

System suitability—

System performance: When the procedure is run with 10 μL of the standard solution under the above operating conditions, the number of theoretical plates and the symmetry factor of the peak of haloperidol are not less than 4000 and not more than 1.5, respectively.

System repeatability: When the test is repeated 6 times with 10 μL of the standard solution under the above operating conditions, the relative standard deviation of the peak area of haloperidol is not more than 1.0%.

Containers and storage Containers—Hermetic containers. Colored containers may be used.

Storage—Light-resistant.

Haloperidol Tablets

ハロペリドール錠

Haloperidol Tablets contain not less than 93.0% and not more than 107.0% of the labeled amount of haloperidol ($C_{21}H_{23}ClFNO_2$: 375.86).

Method of preparation Prepare as directed under Tablets, with Haloperidol.

Identification To powdered Haloperidol Tablets, equivalent to 6 mg of Haloperidol, add 70 mL of 2-propanol, and heat on a water bath until to boiling while shaking. After cooling, add 2-propanol to make 100 mL, and centrifuge. To 5 mL of the supernatant liquid add 2 mL of 0.1 mol/L hydrochloric acid TS and 2-propanol to make 20 mL. Determine the absorption spectrum of the solution as directed under Ultraviolet-visible Spectrophotometry <*2.24*>: it exhibits maxima between 219 nm and 223 nm and between 243 nm and 247 nm.

Uniformity of dosage units <*6.02*> Perform the test according to the following method: it meets the requirement of the Content uniformity test.

To 1 tablet of Haloperidol Tablets add 5 mL of the mobile phase, disperse the particle by sonicating, add 30 mL of the mobile phase, sonicate, and extract for 30 minutes with occasional shaking. Shake for more 30 minutes, and add the mobile phase to make exactly 50 mL. Centrifuge the solution, pipet V mL of the supernatant liquid, equivalent to about 0.3 mg of haloperidol ($C_{21}H_{23}ClFNO_2$), add exactly 2 mL of the internal standard solution and the mobile phase to make 25 mL, and use this solution as the sample solution. Separately, weigh accurately about 20 mg of haloperidol for assay, previously dried in vacuum at 60°C for 3 hours on phosphorus (V) oxide, and dissolve in the mobile phase to make exactly 100 mL. Pipet 15 mL of this solution, and add the mobile phase to make exactly 50 mL. Pipet 5 mL of this solution, add exactly 2 mL of the internal standard solution and the mobile phase to make 25 mL, and use this solution as the standard solution. Perform the test with 10 μL each of the sample solution and standard solution as directed under Liquid Chromatography <*2.01*> according the following conditions, and calculate the ratios, Q_T and Q_S, of the peak area of haloperidol to that of the internal standard.

$$\text{Amount (mg) of haloperidol } (C_{21}H_{23}ClFNO_2) = M_S \times Q_T/Q_S \times 1/V \times 3/4$$

M_S: Amount (mg) of haloperidol for assay taken

*Internal standard solution—*A solution of diphenyl in the mobile phase (1 in 6700).

Operating conditions—

Proceed as detected in the operating condition in the Assay.

System suitability—

System performance: When the procedure is run with 10 μL of the standard solution under the above operating conditions, haloperidol and diphenyl are eluted in this order with the resolution between these peaks being not less than 5.

System repeatability: When the test is repeated 6 times with 10 μL of the standard solution under the above operating conditions, the relative standard deviation of the ratio of the peak area of haloperidol to that of the internal standard is not more than 1.0%.

Dissolution Being specified separately when the drug is granted approval based on the Law.

Assay Weigh accurately, and powder not less than 20 Haloperidol Tablets. Weigh accurately a portion of the powder, equivalent to about 10 mg of haloperidol ($C_{21}H_{23}ClFNO_2$), add 10 mL of water, disperse the particle by sonicating, add exactly 20 mL of the internal standard solution, sonicate, extract for 30 minutes with occasional shaking, and add the mobile phase to make 100 mL. Centrifuge after shaking for more 30 minutes, and use the supernatant liquid as the sample solution. Separately, weigh accurately about 25 mg of haloperidol for assay, previously dried in vacuum at 60°C for 3 hours on phosphorus (V) oxide, and dissolve in methanol to make exactly 25 mL. Pipet 10 mL of this solution, add exactly 20 mL of the internal standard solution and the mobile phase to make exactly 100 mL, and use this solution as the standard solution. Perform the test with 10 μL each of the sample solution and standard solution as directed under Liquid Chromatography <*2.01*> according to the following conditions, and calculate the ratios, Q_T and Q_S, of the peak area of haloperidol to that of the internal standard.

$$\text{Amount (mg) of haloperidol } (C_{21}H_{23}ClFNO_2) = M_S \times Q_T/Q_S \times 2/5$$

M_S: Amount (mg) of haloperidol for assay taken

*Internal standard solution—*A solution of diphenyl in methanol (1 in 2000).

Operating conditions—

Detector: An ultraviolet absorption photometer (wavelength: 220 nm).

Column: A stainless steel column 4.6 mm in inside diameter and 15 cm in length, packed with octadecylsilanized silica gel for liquid chromatography (5 μm in particle diameter).

Column temperature: A constant temperature of about 40°C.

Mobile phase: Dissolve 2.95 g of trisodium citrate dihydrate in 900 mL of water, adjust to pH 3.5 with dilute hydrochloric acid, and add water to make 1000 mL. To 250 mL of this solution add 750 mL of methanol and 1.0 g of sodium lauryl sulfate, and mix to dissolve.

Flow rate: Adjust so that the retention time of haloperidol is about 9 minutes.

System suitability—

System performance: When the procedure is run with 10 μL of the standard solution under the above operating conditions, haloperidol and diphenyl are eluted in this order with the resolution between these peaks being not less than 5.

System repeatability: When the test is repeated 6 times with 10 μL of the standard solution under the above operating conditions, the relative standard deviation of the ratio of the peak area of haloperidol to that of the internal standard is not more than 1.0%.

Containers and storage Containers—Tight containers.

Storage—Light-resistant for the tablets without coating.

Halothane

ハロタン

and enantiomer

$C_2HBrClF_3$: 197.38

(2*RS*)-2-Bromo-2-chloro-1,1,1-trifluoroethane

[*151-67-7*]

Halothane contains not less than 0.008% and not more than 0.012% of Thymol as a stabilizer.

Description Halothane is a clear, colorless, and mobile liquid.

It is miscible with ethanol (95), with diethyl ether and with isooctane.

It is slightly soluble in water.

It is a volatile, nonflammable liquid, and setting fire to its heated vapor does not support combustion.

It is affected by light.

Refractive index n_D^{20}: 1.369 – 1.371

Identification Transfer about 3 μL of Halothane to a gas cell having light path 10 cm in length, and determine the infrared absorption spectrum as directed in the gas sampling method under Infrared Spectrophotometry <*2.25*>, and compare the spectrum with the Reference Spectrum: both spectra exhibit similar intensities of absorption at the same wave numbers.

Specific gravity <*2.56*> d_{20}^{20}: 1.872 – 1.877

Purity (1) Acidity or alkalinity—Shake 60 mL of Halothane with 60 mL of freshly boiled and cooled water vigorously for 3 minutes. Separate the water layer, and use this as the sample solution. To 20 mL of the sample solution add 1 drop of bromocresol purple TS and 0.10 mL of 0.01 mol/L sodium hydroxide VS: a red-purple color develops. To 20 mL of the sample solution add 1 drop of bromocresol purple TS and 0.6 mL of 0.01 mol/L hydrochloric acid VS: a yellow color is produced.

(2) Halide and halogen—To 5 mL of the sample solution obtained in (1) add 1 drop of nitric acid and 0.20 mL of silver nitrate TS: no turbidity is produced. To 10 mL of the sample solution obtained in (1) add 1 mL of potassium iodide TS and 2 drops of starch TS, and allow to stand for 5 minutes: no blue color develops.

(3) Phosgene—Transfer 50 mL of Halothane to a dried 300-mL conical flask, suspend a strip of phosgene test paper vertically inside the flask with the lower end about 10 mm above the surface of the liquid, insert the stopper, and allow to stand at a dark place for 20 to 24 hours: the test paper shows no yellow color.

(4) Residue on evaporation—Pipet 50 mL of Halothane, evaporate on a water bath, and dry the residue at 105°C for 2 hours: the mass of the residue is not more than 1.0 mg.

(5) Volatile related substances—To 100 mL of Halothane add exactly 5.0 μL of the internal standard, and use this solution as the sample solution. Perform the test with 5 μL of the sample solution as directed under Gas Chromatography <*2.02*>, and determine each peak area by the automatic integration method: the total area of the peaks other than halothane and the internal standard is not larger than the peak area of the internal standard.

Internal standard—1,1,2-Trichloro-1,2,2-trifluoroethane

Operating conditions—

Detector: A hydrogen flame-ionization detector.

Column: A column about 3 mm in inside diameter and 3 m in length, at the first 2 m from the injection port, having macrogol 400 coated in the ratio of 30% on siliceous earth for gas chromatography (180 to 250 μm in particle diameter), and at the remaining 1 m, having dinonyl phthalate coated in the ratio of 30% on siliceous earth for gas chromatography (180 to 250 μm in particle diameter).

Column temperature: A constant temperature of about 50°C.

Carrier gas: Nitrogen.

Flow rate: Adjust so that the retention time of the internal standard is 2 to 3 minutes.

Selection of column: Mix 3 mL of Halothane and 1 mL of the internal standard. Proceed with 1 μL of this solution under the above operating conditions, and calculate the resolution. Use a column giving elution of the internal standard and halothane in this order with the resolution between these peaks being not less than 10.

Detection sensitivity: Adjust the detection sensitivity so that the peak height of the internal standard obtained with 5 μL of the sample solution composes 30 to 70% of the full scale.

Time span of measurement: About 3 times as long as the retention time of halothane.

Distilling range <*2.57*> Not less than 95 vol% distils within a 1°C range between 49°C and 51°C.

Thymol To 0.50 mL of Halothane add 5.0 mL of isooctane and 5.0 mL of titanium (IV) oxide TS, shake vigorously for 30 seconds, and allow to stand: the separated upper layer has more color than the following control solution A, and has no more color than the following control solution B.

Control solution: Dissolve 0.225 g of thymol for assay in isooctane to make exactly 100 mL. To 10 mL each of this solution, accurately measured, add isooctane to make exactly 150 mL and 100 mL, respectively. Proceed with 0.50 mL each of these solutions in the same manner as Halothane, and use the separated upper layers so obtained as the control solution A and B, respectively.

Containers and storage Containers—Tight containers.

Storage—Light-resistant, and not exceeding 30°C.

Haloxazolam

ハロキサゾラム

and enantiomer

$C_{17}H_{14}BrFN_2O_2$: 377.21
(11b*RS*)-10-Bromo-11b-(2-fluorophenyl)-2,3,7,11b-tetrahydro[1,3]oxazolo[3,2-*d*][1,4]benzodiazepin-6(5*H*)-one
[*59128-97-1*]

Haloxazolam, when dried, contains not less than 99.0% of haloxazolam ($C_{17}H_{14}BrFN_2O_2$).

Description Haloxazolam occurs as white, crystals or crystalline powder. It is odorless and tasteless.

It is freely soluble in acetic acid (100), sparingly soluble in acetonitrile, in methanol and in ethanol (99.5), slightly soluble in diethyl ether, and practically insoluble in water.

Melting point: about 183°C (with decomposition).

Identification (1) Dissolve 10 mg of Haloxazolam in 10 mL of methanol, add 1 drop of hydrochloric acid: the solution shows a yellow-green fluorescence under ultraviolet light (main wavelength: 365 nm). To this solution add 1 mL of sodium hydroxide TS: the fluorescence disappears immediately.

(2) Prepare the test solution with 50 mg of Haloxazolam as directed under Oxygen Flask Combustion Method <*1.06*>, using a mixture of 20 mL of dilute sodium hydroxide TS and 1 mL of hydrogen peroxide (30) as an absorbing liquid: the test solution responds to Qualitative Tests <*1.09*> for bromide and for fluoride.

(3) Determine the absorption spectrum of a solution of Haloxazolam in methanol (1 in 100,000) as directed under Ultraviolet-visible Spectrophotometry <*2.24*>, and compare the spectrum with the Reference Spectrum: both spectra exhibit similar intensities of absorption at the same wavelengths.

(4) Determine the infrared absorption spectrum of Haloxazolam, previously dried, as directed in the potassium bromide disk method under Infrared Spectrophotometry <*2.25*>, and compare the spectrum with the Reference Spectrum: both spectra exhibit similar intensities of absorption at the same wave numbers.

Absorbance <*2.24*> $E^{1\%}_{1\,cm}$ (247 nm): 390 – 410 (10 mg, methanol, 1000 mL).

Purity (1) Clarity and color of solution—Dissolve 0.10 g of Haloxazolam in 20 mL of ethanol (99.5): the solution is clear and colorless.

(2) Soluble halides—To 1.0 g of Haloxazolam add 50 mL of water, allow to stand for 1 hour with occasional shaking, and filter. To 25 mL of the filtrate add 6 mL of dilute nitric acid and water to make 50 mL. Perform the test with this solution as directed under Chloride Limit Test <*1.03*>. Prepare the control solution with 0.10 mL of 0.01 mol/L hydrochloric acid VS.

(3) Heavy metals <*1.07*>—Proceed with 1.0 g of Haloxazolam according to Method 2, and perform the test. Prepare the control solution with 2.0 mL of Standard Lead Solution (not more than 20 ppm).

(4) Arsenic <*1.11*>—To 1.0 g of Haloxazolam in a decomposition flask add 5 mL of nitric acid and 2 mL of sulfuric acid, place a small funnel on the mouth of the flask, and heat carefully until white fumes are evolved. After cooling, add 2 mL of nitric acid, heat, repeat this procedure twice, add several 2-mL portions of hydrogen peroxide (30), and heat until the solution is colorless to pale yellow. After cooling, add 2 mL of a saturated solution of ammonium oxalate monohydrate, and heat until white fumes are evolved. After cooling, add water to make 5 mL, and perform the test with this solution: the solution has no more color than the following control solution (not more than 2 ppm).

Control solution: Proceed in the same manner as above without using Haloxazolam, add 2.0 mL of Standard Arsenic Solution and water to make 5 mL, and proceed in the same manner as the test solution.

(5) Related substances—Dissolve 0.10 g of Haloxazolam in 100 mL of acetonitrile, and use this solution as the sample solution. Pipet 1 mL of the sample solution, add acetonitrile to make exactly 100 mL, and use this solution as the standard solution. Perform the test with exactly 10 μL each of the sample solution and standard solution as directed under Liquid Chromatography <*2.01*> according to the following conditions. Determine each peak area of both solutions by the automatic integration method: the total area of all peaks other than haloxazolam from the sample solution is not larger than the peak area of the haloxazolam from the standard solution.

Operating conditions—

Detector: An ultraviolet absorption photometer (wavelength: 250 nm).

Column: A stainless steel column 4.6 mm in inside diameter and 15 cm in length, packed with octadecylsilanized silica gel for liquid chromatography (5 μm in particle diameter).

Column temperature: A constant temperature of about 25°C.

Mobile phase: Dissolve 6.2 g of boric acid and 7.5 g of potassium chloride in 900 mL of water, adjust the pH with triethylamine to 8.5, and add water to make 1000 mL. To 300 mL of this solution add 200 mL of acetonitrile.

Flow rate: Adjust so that the retention time of haloxazolam is about 10 minutes.

Time span of measurement: About 3 times as long as the retention time of haloxazolam, beginning after the solvent peak.

System suitability—

Test for required detectability: To exactly 5 mL of the standard solution add acetonitrile to make exactly 50 mL. Confirm that the peak area of haloxazolam obtained with 10 μL of this solution is equivalent to 8 to 12% of that with 10 μL of the standard solution.

System performance: Dissolve 10 mg each of Haloxazolam and cloxazolam in 200 mL of acetonitrile. When the procedure is run with 10 μL of this solution under the above operating conditions, haloxazolam and cloxazolam are eluted in this order with the resolution between these peaks being not less than 1.5.

System repeatability: When the test is repeated 6 times with 10 μL of the standard solution under the above operating conditions, the relative standard deviation of the peak area of haloxazolam is not more than 1.0%.

Loss on drying <*2.41*> Not more than 0.5% (1 g, 105°C, 3 hours).

Residue on ignition <*2.44*> Not more than 0.1% (1 g, platinum crucible).

Assay Weigh accurately about 0.5 g of Haloxazolam, previously dried, dissolve in 50 mL of acetic acid (100), and titrate <2.50> with 0.1 mol/L perchloric acid VS (potentiometric titration). Perform a blank determination in the same manner, and make any necessary correction.

Each mL of 0.1 mol/L perchloric acid VS
= 37.72 mg of $C_{17}H_{14}BrFN_2O_2$

Containers and storage Containers—Tight containers.
Storage—Light-resistant.

Heparin Calcium

ヘパリンカルシウム

$R^1, R^3, R^4 = SO_3^-$ or H or $COCH_3$
$R^2 = SO_3^-$ or $COCH_3$
$R^5 = CO_2^-$, $R^6 = H$
or
$R^5 = H$, $R^6 = CO_2^-$
$\cdot\, x Ca^{2+}$

[*37270-89-6*]

Heparin Calcium is the calcium salt of sulfated glycosaminoglycans composed of disaccharide units of D-glucosamine and uronic acid (L-iduronic acid or D-glucuronic acid) obtained from the intestinal mucosa of healthy edible swine.

It contains not less than 180 Heparin Units (anti-factor IIa activity) per mg and not less than 8.0% and not more than 12.0% of calcium (Ca: 40.08), calculated on the dried basis.

Description Heparin Calcium occurs as a white to grayish brown, powder or grains.

It is freely soluble in water, and practically insoluble in ethanol (99.5).

It is hygroscopic.

Identification (1) Dissolve 10 mg of Heparin Calcium in 5 mL of water, and add 0.1 mL of 1 mol/L hydrochloric acid TS and 5 mL of toluidine blue O solution (1 in 20,000): a purple to red-purple color develops.

(2) Dissolve 1 mg each of Heparin Calcium and Heparin Sodium for Identification RS in 1 mL of water, and use these solutions as the sample solution and the standard solution, respectively. Perform the test with 20 μL each of the sample solution and standard solution as directed under Liquid Chromatography <2.01> according to the following conditions: the retention time for the major peak from the sample solution and standard solution is identical.

Operating conditions—

Detector, column, column temperature, mobile phases A and B, flowing of mobile phase and flow rate: Proceed as directed under the operating conditions in Purity (9).

System suitability—

System performance: Dissolve 1.0 mg of Heparin Sodium for Identification RS in 0.60 mL of water. Dissolve 0.10 mg of Over-sulfated Chondroitin Sulfate for System Suitability RS in 0.20 mL of water. Dissolve 1.0 mg of dermatan sulfate in 2.0 mL of water. To 90 μL of the solution of Heparin Sodium for Identification RS add 30 μL each of the solutions of Over-sulfated Chondroitin Sulfate for System Suitability RS and dermatan sulfate, and mix. When the procedure is run with 20 μL of the mixture under the above operating conditions, dermatan sulfate, heparin and over-sulfated chondroitin sulfate are eluted in this order with the resolution between the peaks of dermatan sulfate and heparin being not less than 1.0 and that between the peaks of heparin and over-sulfated chondroitin sulfate being not less than 1.5.

(3) A solution of 50 mg of Heparin Calcium in 5 mL of water responds to Qualitative Tests <1.09> for calcium salt.

pH <2.54> Dissolve 1.0 g of Heparin Calcium in 100 mL of water: the pH of the solution is between 6.0 and 8.0.

Purity (1) Clarity and color of solution—Dissolve 0.5 g of Heparin Calcium in 20 mL of water: the solution is clear. Determine the absorbance of this solution at 400 nm as directed under Ultraviolet-visible Spectrophotometry <2.24>: the absorbance is not more than 0.05.

(2) Chloride <1.03>—Perform the test with 0.5 g of Heparin Calcium. Prepare the control solution with 0.30 mL of 0.01 mol/L hydrochloric acid VS (not more than 0.021%).

(3) Heavy metals <1.07>—Proceed with 0.5 g of Heparin Calcium according to Method 2, and perform the test. Prepare the control solution with 1.5 mL of Standard Lead Solution (not more than 30 ppm).

(4) Barium—Dissolve 30 mg of Heparin Calcium in 3.0 mL of water, and use this solution as the sample solution. To 1.0 mL of the sample solution add 3 drops of dilute sulfuric acid, and allow to stand for 10 minutes: no turbidity is produced.

(5) Total nitrogen—Weigh accurately about 0.1 g of Heparin Calcium, previously dried, and perform the test as directed under Nitrogen Determination <1.08>: the amount of nitrogen (N: 14.01) is not more than 3.0%.

(6) Protein—(i) Sodium carbonate solution: To 4 volumes of a mixture of sodium hydroxide solution (1 in 100) and anhydrous sodium carbonate solution (1 in 20) (1:1) add 1 volume of water.

(ii) Copper sulfate solution: To 4 volumes of a mixture of copper (II) sulfate pentahydrate solution (1 in 80) and sodium tartrate dihydrate solution (149 in 5000) (1:1) add 1 volume of water.

(iii) Alkaline copper solution for heparin: Mix 50 volumes of the sodium carbonate solution and 1 volume of the copper sulfate solution. Prepare before using.

(iv) Procedure: Use a solution of Heparin Calcium (1 in 200) as the sample solution. Use a solution of bovine serum albumin (1 in 40,000) as the standard solution. To exactly 1 mL each of the sample solution and standard solution add exactly 5 mL of the alkaline copper solution for heparin, mix, and allow them to stand at room temperature for 10 minutes. To each of these solutions add exactly 0.5 mL of diluted Folin's TS (1 in 2), shake, allow them to stand at room temperature for 30 minutes, and centrifuge at room temperature. Determine the absorbances at 750 nm of the supernatant liquids as directed under Ultraviolet-visible Spectrophotometry <2.24> using water as the blank: the absorbance of the solution obtained from the sample solution is not more than that of the solution from the standard solution.

(7) Nucleic acid—Dissolve 40 mg of Heparin Calcium in 10 mL of a solution of disodium dihydrogen ethylenediamine tetraacetate dihydrate (93 in 50,000), and determine

the absorbance of this solution at 260 nm as directed under Ultraviolet-visible Spectrophotometry <*2.24*>: the absorbance is not more than 0.15.

(8) Over-sulfated chondroitin sulfate—Dissolve 20 mg of Heparin Calcium in 0.60 mL of a solution of sodium 3-trimethylsilylpropionate-d_4 for nuclear magnetic resonance spectroscopy in heavy water for nuclear magnetic resonance spectroscopy (1 in 10,000). Determine the spectrum of this solution as directed under Nuclear Magnetic Resonance Spectroscopy <*2.21*> (^{1}H) in accordance with the following conditions, using sodium 3-trimethylsilylpropionate-d_4 for nuclear magnetic resonance spectroscopy as an internal reference compound: it exhibits no signal corresponding to *N*-acetyl proton of over-sulfated chondroitin sulfate at δ 2.18 ± 0.05 ppm, or the signal disappears when determining the spectrum of the sample solutions as directed under ^{1}H with ^{13}C-decoupling.

Operating conditions—

Spectrometer: 1.1. FT-NMR, Not less than 400 MHz.

Temperature: 25°C.

Spinning: off.

Number of data points: 32,768.

Spectral range: Signal of DHO ± 6.0 ppm.

Flip angle: 90°.

Delay time: 20 seconds.

Dummy scans: 4.

Number of scans: SN ratio of the signal of *N*-acetyl proton of heparin is not less than 1000.

Window function: Exponential function (Line broadening factor = 0.2 Hz).

System suitability—

System performance: Dissolve 20 mg of Heparin Calcium in 0.40 mL of a solution of sodium 3-trimethylsilylpropionate-d_4 for nuclear magnetic resonance spectroscopy in heavy water for nuclear magnetic resonance spectroscopy (1 in 10,000). Dissolve 0.10 mg of Over-sulfated Chondroitin Sulfate for System Suitability RS in 1.0 mL of a solution of sodium 3-trimethylsilylpropionate-d_4 for nuclear magnetic resonance spectroscopy in heavy water for nuclear magnetic resonance spectroscopy (1 in 10,000). To the solution of heparin calcium add 0.20 mL of the solution of Over-sulfated Chondroitin Sulfate for System Suitability RS. When determining the spectrum of this solution under the above operating conditions, it exhibits the signal of *N*-acetyl proton of heparin and the signal of *N*-acetyl proton of over-sulfated chondroitin sulfate at δ 2.04 ± 0.02 ppm and δ 2.18 ± 0.05 ppm, respectively.

(9) Related substances—Dissolve 2.0 mg of Heparin Calcium in 0.1 mL of water, and perform the test with exactly 20 μL of this solution as directed under Liquid Chromatography <*2.01*> according to the following conditions: it exhibits no peaks after the heparin peak.

Operating conditions—

Detector: An ultraviolet absorption photometer (wavelength: 202 nm).

Column: A stainless steel column 2.0 mm in inside diameter and 7.5 cm in length, packed with synthetic polymer for liquid chromatography to which diethylaminoethyl group binds (10 μm in particle diameter).

Column temperature: A constant temperature of about 35°C.

Mobile phase A: Dissolve 0.4 g of sodium dihydrogen phosphate dihydrate in 1000 mL of water, and adjust to pH 3.0 with diluted phosphoric acid (1 in 10).

Mobile phase B: Dissolve 0.4 g of sodium dihydrogen phosphate dihydrate and 106.4 g of lithium perchlorate in 1000 mL of water, and adjust to pH 3.0 with diluted phosphoric acid (1 in 10).

Flowing of mobile phase: Control the gradient by mixing the mobile phases A and B as directed in the following table.

Time after injection of sample (min)	Mobile phase A (vol%)	Mobile phase B (vol%)
0 – 3	90	10
3 – 15	90 → 0	10 → 100

Flow rate: 0.2 mL per minute.

Time span of measurement: About 2 times as long as the retention time of heparin, beginning after the solvent peak.

System suitability—

Test for required detectability: Dissolve 10 mg of Heparin Sodium for Identification RS in 0.40 mL of water, and use this solution as the heparin sodium standard stock solution. Separately, dissolve 0.10 mg of Over-sulfated Chondroitin Sulfate for System Suitability RS in 0.20 mL of water, and use this solution as the over-sulfated chondroitin sulfate standard solution. To 60 μL of the heparin sodium standard stock solution add 3 μL of the over-sulfated chondroitin sulfate standard solution and 12 μL of water, and mix. When the procedure is run with 20 μL of the mixture under the above operating conditions, it exhibits an over-sulfated chondroitin sulfate peak.

System performance: To 120 μL of the heparin sodium standard stock solution add 30 μL of the over-sulfated chondroitin sulfate standard solution, mix and use this solution as the solution for system suitability test. When the procedure is run with 20 μL of the solution for system suitability test under the above operating conditions, heparin and over-sulfated chondroitin sulfate are eluted in this order with the resolution between these peaks being not less than 1.5.

System repeatability: When the test is repeated 6 times with 20 μL of the solution for system suitability test under the above operating conditions, the relative standard deviation of the peak area of over-sulfated chondroitin sulfate is not more than 2.0%.

Loss on drying <*2.41*> Not more than 8% (50 mg, in vacuum, 60°C, 3 hours).

Bacterial endotoxins <*4.01*> Less than 0.0030 EU/heparin Unit.

Anti-factor Xa activity to anti-factor IIa activity ratio The ratio of the anti-factor Xa activity determined by the following method to the anti-factor IIa activity obtained in the Assay, calculated by dividing the former with the later, is 0.9 – 1.1.

Anti-factor Xa activity determination

(i) Substrate solution: Dissolve 25 mg of *N*-benzoyl-L-isoleucyl-L-glutamyl(γ-OR)-glycyl-L-arginyl-*p*-nitroanilide hydrochloride in 33.3 mL of water.

(ii) Anti-thrombin solution: Dissolve human anti-thrombin in water so that each mL contains 1 IU. To 150 μL of this solution add 2250 μL of buffer solution.

(iii) Factor Xa solution: To 1200 μL of factor Xa TS add 1200 μL of buffer solution.

(iv) Buffer solution: Proceed as directed in the Assay (1).

(v) Stopping solution: Proceed as directed in the Assay (1).

(vi) Heparin standard solutions: Proceed as directed in the Assay (1). However, the standard solutions are prepared based on anti-factor Xa activity Unit instead of Heparin Unit.

(vii) Heparin sample solutions: Proceed as directed in

the Assay (1). However, the sample solutions are prepared based on anti-factor Xa activity Unit instead of Heparin Unit.

(viii) Procedure: Transfer separately two 50-μL portions of each different dilution of the heparin standard solutions and the heparin sample solutions and five 50-μL portions of buffer solution as the blank to 1.5-mL tubes. Warm these 21 tubes, anti-thrombin solution, factor Xa solution and substrate solution at 37°C all together. Start the following procedure at 2 minutes after warming in the order: buffer solution, S_1, S_2, S_3, S_4, buffer solution, T_1, T_2, T_3, T_4, buffer solution, T_1, T_2, T_3, T_4, buffer solution, S_1, S_2, S_3, S_4, and buffer solution. To each tube add 50 μL of anti-thrombin solution, mix, and warm at 37°C for exactly 4 minutes, add 100 μL of factor Xa solution, mix, and incubate for exactly 12 minutes. Then, add 100 μL of substrate solution, mix, incubate for exactly 4 minutes, add 50 μL of stopping solution to each tube, and mix immediately. Separately, to 50 μL of stopping solution add 100 μL of substrate solution, 100 μL of factor Xa solution, 50 μL of anti-thrombin solution and 50 μL of buffer solution, mix, and use this solution as a control. Determine the absorbance of each solution at 405 nm against the control. Confirm that the relative standard deviation of the reading of the blank is not more than 10%.

(ix) Calculations: When the regression expression, $y = I_c + Ax_S + Bx_T$, is obtained using y as log of the absorbance values, x_S as the concentration of the heparin standard solutions and x_T as the concentration of the heparin sample solutions, the potency ratio R is B/A.

I_c: Common intercept

A: Slope of regression expression of the heparin standard solution

B: Slope of regression expression of the heparin sample solution

Calculate anti-factor Xa activity per mg of Heparin Calcium by the following formula.

$$\text{Anti-factor Xa activity per mg of Heparin Calcium} = 100 \times R \times V/M$$

V: Total volume (mL) of the solution (the sample stock solution) prepared as containing about 100 anti-factor Xa activity Units per mL

M: Amount (mg) of Heparin Calcium taken for the sample stock solution

However, when a 90% confidence interval of D of the regression expression $y = I'_c + A'x_S + B'x_T + D$, where D is a constant term showing the difference between the blank and the intercept assumed from the two lines, is not in the range of between -0.2 and 0.2, analyze by excluding the measurements of the blank.

The criteria for the test suitability are performed as directed in the Assay (1). When these criteria are not satisfied, repeat the test after changing the dilution rate so that the potency ratio becomes about 1 using the obtained potency as reference.

Assay **(1)** Heparin

(i) Substrate solution: Dissolve 25 mg of *H*-D-phenylalanyl-L-pipecolyl-L-arginyl-*p*-nitroanilide dihydrochloride in 32.0 mL of water.

(ii) Anti-thrombin solution (for heparin assay): Dissolve human anti-thrombin in water so that each mL contains 1 IU. Dilute this solution to an appropriate dilution factor of approximately more than 16 times with the buffer solution, and designate this solution as the anti-thrombin solution (for heparin assay). The dilution factor with the buffer solution is adjusted so that the absorbance of reaction solution with the blank solution (average of five tubes) is not more than 2.0, and that of reaction solution with S_4 (0.020 Unit/mL heparin standard solution) (average of two tubes) is not less than 0.2 and not more than 1.0 when the test is performed according to the Assay. The absorbance is measured with 1 cm light path in length.

(iii) Factor IIa solution: Add an equivalent volume of water to the buffer solution, and use this solution as the factor IIa diluent. Dissolve factor IIa in the factor IIa diluent to make a solution so that each mL contains 20 IU. Dilute this solution to an appropriate dilution factor of approximately less than 4 times with the factor IIa diluent, and designate this solution as the factor IIa solution. Adjust the dilution factor with the factor IIa diluent so that the absorbance of reaction solution with the blank solution (average of five tubes) is not more than 2.0, and that of reaction solution with S_4 (0.020 Unit/mL heparin standard solution) (average of two tubes) is not less than 0.2 and not more than 1.0 when the test is performed according to the Assay. The absorbance is measured with 1 cm light path in length.

(iv) Buffer solution: Dissolve 6.1 g of 2-amino-2-hydroxymethyl-1,3-propanediol, 10.2 g of sodium chloride, 2.8 g of disodium dihydrogen ethylenediamine tetraacetate dihydrate and 1.0 g of polyethylene glycol 6000 in 800 mL of water, adjust to pH 8.4 with 1 mol/L hydrochloric acid TS, and add water to make 1000 mL.

(v) Stopping solution: To 2 mL of acetic acid (100) add water to make 10 mL.

(vi) Heparin standard solutions: Dissolve Heparin Sodium RS in water so that each mL contains 100 Heparin Units, and use this solution as the standard stock solution. Dilute the standard stock solution with buffer solution so that each mL contains exactly 0.1 Heparin Units, and use this solution as the standard solution. Make heparin standard solutions S_1, S_2, S_3 and S_4 respectively by adding the standard solution to buffer solution as directed in the following table.

Heparin standard solution		Buffer solution (μL)	Standard solution (μL)
No.	Heparin concentration (Unit/mL)		
S_1	0.005	950	50
S_2	0.010	900	100
S_3	0.015	850	150
S_4	0.020	800	200

(vii) Heparin sample solutions: Weigh accurately an appropriate amount of Heparin Calcium, dissolve in water so that each mL contains about 100 Heparin Units, and use this solution as the sample stock solution. Dilute exactly the sample stock solution with buffer solution so that each mL contains 0.1 Heparin Units, and use this solution as the sample solution. Make heparin sample solutions T_1, T_2, T_3 and T_4 respectively by adding the sample solution to buffer solution as directed in the following table.

Heparin sample solution			
No.	Heparin concentration (Unit/mL)	Buffer solution (μL)	Sample solution (μL)
T_1	0.005	950	50
T_2	0.010	900	100
T_3	0.015	850	150
T_4	0.020	800	200

(viii) Procedure: Transfer separately two 50-μL portions of each dilution of the heparin standard solutions and the heparin sample solutions and five 50-μL portions of buffer solution as the blank to 1.5-mL tubes. Warm these 21 tubes, anti-thrombin solution (for heparin assay), factor IIa solution and substrate solution at 37°C all together. Start the following procedure at 2 minutes after warming in the order: buffer solution, S_1, S_2, S_3, S_4, buffer solution, T_1, T_2, T_3, T_4, buffer solution, T_1, T_2, T_3, T_4, buffer solution, S_1, S_2, S_3, S_4, and buffer solution. To each tube add 100 μL of anti-thrombin solution (for heparin assay), mix, and warm at 37°C for exactly 4 minutes, add 25 μL of factor IIa solution, mix, and incubate for exactly 4 minutes. Then, add 50 μL of substrate solution, mix, incubate for exactly 4 minutes, add 50 μL of stopping solution to each tube, and mix. Separately, to 50 μL of stopping solution add 50 μL of substrate solution, 25 μL of factor IIa solution, 100 μL of anti-thrombin solution (for heparin assay) and 50 μL of buffer solution, mix, and use this solution as a control. Determine the absorbance of each solution at 405 nm against the control. Confirm that the relative standard deviation of the reading of the blank is not more than 10%.

(ix) Calculations: When the regression expression, $y = I_c + A_{Xs} + B_{Xt}$, is obtained using y as log of the absorbance values, $_{Xs}$ as the concentration of the heparin standard solutions and $_{Xt}$ as the concentration of the heparin sample solutions, the potency ratio R is B/A.

I_c: Common intercept
A: Slope of regression expression of the heparin standard solution
B: Slope of regression expression of the heparin sample solution

Calculate Heparin Unit (anti-factor IIa activity) per mg of Heparin Calcium by the following formula.

Heparin Unit (anti-factor IIa activity) per mg of Heparin Calcium

$$= 100 \times R \times V/M$$

V: Total volume (mL) of the solution (the sample stock solution) prepared as containing about 100 Heparin Units (anti-factor IIa activity) per mL
M: Amount (mg) of Heparin Calcium taken for the sample stock solution

However, when a 90% confidence interval of D of the regression expression $y = I'_c + A'_{Xs} + B'_{Xt} + D$, where D is a constant term showing the difference between the blank and the intercept assumed from the two lines, is not in the range of between -0.2 and 0.2, analyze by excluding the measurements of the blank.

The criteria for the test suitability are the following 3 items, (1), (2) and (3).

(1) Judgment on consistence of the intercept assumed from the two lines

When the regression expression, $y = I_s + A''_{Xs} + B''_{Xt} + I_{t\text{-}s}$, is obtained from the data of the heparin standard solutions and the heparin sample solutions except of the blank solution, a 90% confidence interval of the constant term, $I_{t\text{-}s}$, is between -0.2 and 0.2.

I_s: Intercept of the regression expression of the heparin standard solution
$I_{t\text{-}s}$: Difference of the intercepts assumed from the two lines

(2) Judgment on linearity

When the regression expression, $y = I_c + A'''_{Xs} + B'''_{Xt} + Q_{sXs}{}^2 + Q_{tXt}{}^2$, is obtained from the data of the heparin standard solutions and the heparin sample solutions, a 90% confidence interval of the secondary coefficients, Q_s and Q_t, is between -1000 and 1000.

Q_s: Secondary coefficient of the regression expression of the heparin standard solution
Q_t: Secondary coefficient of the regression expression of the heparin sample solution

(3) Judgment by checking if the relative potency obtained is within the range previously validated on this test method

The potency ratio obtained is not less than 0.8 and not more than 1.2.

When these criteria are not satisfied, repeat the test after changing the dilution rate so that the potency ratio becomes about 1 using the obtained potency as reference.

(2) Calcium: Weigh accurately about 50 mg of Heparin Calcium, dissolve in 20 mL of water, add 2 mL of 8 mol/L potassium hydroxide TS, allow to stand for 3 to 5 minutes with occasional shaking, add 0.1 g of NN indicator, and immediately titrate <2.50> with 0.01 mol/L disodium dihydrogen ethylenediamine tetraacetate VS until the color of the solution changes from red-purple to blue.

Each mL of 0.01 mol/L disodium dihydrogen ethylenediamine tetraacetate VS
= 0.4008 mg of Ca

Containers and storage Containers—Tight containers.

Heparin Sodium

ヘパリンナトリウム

R^1, R^3, R^4 = SO_3Na or H

R^2 = SO_3Na or $COCH_3$

R^5 = CO_2Na, R^6 = H
or
R^5 = H, R^6 = CO_2Na

[9041-08-1]

Heparin Sodium is a sodium salt of sulfated glycosaminoglycans composed of disaccharide units of D-glucosamine and uronic acid (L-iduronic acid or D-glucuronic acid) obtained from the intestinal mucosa of healthy edible swine.

It contains not less than 180 Heparin Units (anti-factor IIa activity) per mg, calculated on the dried basis.

Description Heparin Sodium occurs as a white to grayish brown, powder or grains. It is odorless.

It is soluble in water, and practically insoluble in ethanol (95) and in diethyl ether.

It is hygroscopic.

Identification Dissolve 1 mg each of Heparin Sodium and Heparin Sodium for Identification RS in 1 mL of water, and use these solutions as the sample solution and the standard solution, respectively. Perform the test with 20 μL each of the sample solution and standard solution as directed under Liquid Chromatography <*2.01*> according to the following conditions: the retention time for the major peak from the sample solution and standard solution is identical.

Operating conditions—

Detector, column, column temperature, mobile phases A and B, flowing of mobile phase and flow rate: Proceed as directed under the operating conditions in Purity (7).

System suitability—

System performance: Dissolve 1.0 mg of Heparin Sodium for Identification RS in 0.60 mL of water. Dissolve 0.10 mg of Over-sulfated Chondroitin Sulfate for System Suitability RS in 0.20 mL of water. Dissolve 1.0 mg of dermatan sulfate in 2.0 mL of water. To 90 μL of the solution of Heparin Sodium for Identification RS add 30 μL each of the solutions of Over-sulfated Chondroitin Sulfate for System Suitability RS and dermatan sulfate, and mix. When the procedure is run with 20 μL of the mixture under the above operating conditions, dermatan sulfate, heparin and over-sulfated chondroitin sulfate are eluted in this order with the resolution between the peaks of dermatan sulfate and heparin being not less than 1.0 and that between the peaks of heparin and over-sulfated chondroitin sulfate being not less than 1.5.

pH <*2.54*> The pH of a solution of 1.0 g of Heparin Sodium in 100 mL of water is between 6.0 and 8.0.

Purity (1) Clarity and color of solution—Dissolve 0.5 g of Heparin Sodium in 20 mL of water: the solution is clear and colorless to light yellow.

(2) Barium—Dissolve 30 mg of Heparin Sodium in 3.0 mL of water, and use this solution as the sample solution. To 1.0 mL of the sample solution add 3 drops of dilute sulfuric acid, and allow to stand for 10 minutes: no turbidity is produced.

(3) Total nitrogen—Weigh accurately about 0.1 g of Heparin Sodium, previously dried at 60°C for 3 hours under reduced pressure, and perform the test as directed under Nitrogen Determination <*1.08*>: the amount of nitrogen (N: 14.01) is not more than 3.0%.

(4) Protein—(i) Sodium carbonate solution: To 4 volumes of a mixture of sodium hydroxide solution (1 in 100) and anhydrous sodium carbonate solution (1 in 20) (1:1) add 1 volume of water.

(ii) Copper sulfate solution: To 4 volumes of a mixture of copper (II) sulfate pentahydrate solution (1 in 80) and sodium tartrate dihydrate solution (149 in 5000) (1:1) add 1 volume of water.

(iii) Alkaline copper solution for heparin: Mix 50 volumes of the sodium carbonate solution and 1 volume of the copper sulfate solution. Prepare before using.

(iv) Procedure: Use a solution of Heparin Sodium (1 in 200) as the sample solution. Use a solution of bovine serum albumin (1 in 40,000) as the standard solution. To exactly 1 mL each of the sample solution and standard solution add exactly 5 mL of the alkaline copper solution for heparin, mix, and allow them to stand at room temperature for 10 minutes. To each of these solutions add exactly 0.5 mL of diluted Folin's TS (1 in 2), shake, and allow them to stand at room temperature for 30 minutes. Determine the absorbances at 750 nm of these solutions as directed under Ultraviolet-visible Spectrophotometry <*2.24*> using water as the blank: the absorbance of the solution obtained from the sample solution is not more than that of the solution from the standard solution.

(5) Nucleic acid—Dissolve 40 mg of Heparin Sodium in 10 mL of water, and determine the absorbance of this solution at 260 nm as directed under Ultraviolet-visible Spectrophotometry <*2.24*>: the absorbance is not more than 0.15.

(6) Over-sulfated chondroitin sulfate—Dissolve 20 mg of Heparin Sodium in 0.60 mL of a solution of sodium 3-trimethylsilylpropionate-d_4 for nuclear magnetic resonance spectroscopy in heavy water for nuclear magnetic resonance spectroscopy (1 in 10,000). Determine the spectrum of this solution as directed under Nuclear Magnetic Resonance Spectroscopy <*2.21*> (^{1}H) in accordance with the following conditions, using sodium 3-trimethylsilylpropionate-d_4 for nuclear magnetic resonance spectroscopy as an internal reference compound: it exhibits no signal corresponding to *N*-acetyl proton of over-sulfated chondroitin sulfate at δ 2.15 ± 0.02 ppm, or the signal disappears when determining the spectrum of the sample solutions as directed under ^{1}H with ^{13}C-decoupling.

Operating conditions—

Spectrometer: 1.1. FT-NMR, Not less than 400 MHz.
Temperature: 25°C.
Spinning: off.
Number of data points: 32,768.
Spectral range: Signal of DHO ± 6.0 ppm.
Flip angle: 90°.
Delay time: 20 seconds.
Dummy scans: 4.
Number of scans: SN ratio of the signal of *N*-acetyl proton of heparin is not less 1000.

Window function: Exponential function (Line broadening factor = 0.2 Hz).

System suitability—

System performance: Dissolve 20 mg of Heparin Sodium for Identification RS in 0.40 mL of a solution of sodium 3-trimethylsilylpropionate-d_4 for nuclear magnetic resonance spectroscopy in heavy water for nuclear magnetic resonance spectroscopy (1 in 10,000). Dissolve 0.10 mg of Over-sulfated Chondroitin Sulfate for System Suitability RS in 1.0 mL of a solution of sodium 3-trimethylsilylpropionate-d_4 for nuclear magnetic resonance spectroscopy in heavy water for nuclear magnetic resonance spectroscopy (1 in 10,000). To the solution of Heparin Sodium for Identification RS add 0.20 mL of the solution of Over-sulfated Chondroitin Sulfate for System Suitability RS. When determining the spectrum of this solution under the above operating conditions, it exhibits the signal of *N*-acetyl proton of heparin and the signal of *N*-acetyl proton of over-sulfated chondroitin sulfate at δ 2.04 ± 0.02 ppm and δ 2.15 ± 0.02 ppm, respectively.

(7) Related substances—Dissolve 2.0 mg of Heparin Sodium in 0.1 mL of water and perform the test with exactly 20 μL of this solution as directed under Liquid Chromatography <*2.01*> according to the following conditions: it exhibits no peaks after the heparin peak.

Operating conditions—

Detector: An ultraviolet absorption photometer (wavelength: 202 nm).

Column: A stainless steel column 2.0 mm in inside diameter and 7.5 cm in length, packed with synthetic polymer for liquid chromatography to which diethylaminoethyl group binds (10 μm in particle diameter).

Column temperature: A constant temperature of about 35°C.

Mobile phase A: Dissolve 0.4 g of sodium dihydrogen phosphate dihydrate in 1000 mL of water, and adjust to pH 3.0 with diluted phosphoric acid (1 in 10).

Mobile phase B: Dissolve 0.4 g of sodium dihydrogen phosphate dihydrate and 106.4 g of lithium perchlorate in 1000 mL of water, and adjust to a pH of 3.0 with diluted phosphoric acid (1 in 10).

Flowing of mobile phase: Control the gradient by mixing the mobile phases A and B as directed in the following table.

Time after injection of sample (min)	Mobile phase A (vol%)	Mobile phase B (vol%)
0 – 3	90	10
3 – 15	90 → 0	10 → 100

Flow rate: 0.2 mL per minute.

Time span of measurement: About 2 times as long as the retention time of heparin, beginning after the solvent peak.

System suitability—

Test for required detectability: Dissolve 10 mg of Heparin Sodium for Identification RS in 0.40 mL of water, and use this solution as the heparin sodium standard stock solution. Separately, dissolve 0.10 mg of Over-sulfated Chondroitin Sulfate for System Suitability RS in 0.20 mL of water, and use this solution as the over-sulfated chondroitin sulfate standard solution. To 60 μL of the heparin sodium standard stock solution add 3 μL of the over-sulfated chondroitin sulfate standard solution and 12 μL of water, and mix. When the procedure is run with 20 μL of the mixture under the above operating conditions, it exhibits a peak for over-sulfated chondroitin sulfate.

System performance: To 120 μL of the heparin sodium standard stock solution add 30 μL of the over-sulfated chondroitin sulfate standard solution, mix and use this solution as the solution for system suitability test. When the procedure is run with 20 μL of the solution for system suitability test under the above operating conditions, heparin and over-sulfated chondroitin sulfate are eluted in this order with the resolution between these peaks being not less than 1.5.

System repeatability: When the test is repeated 6 times with 20 μL of the solution for system suitability test under the above operating conditions, the relative standard deviation of the peak area of over-sulfated chondroitin sulfate is not more than 2.0%.

(8) Galactosamine—Dissolve 2.4 mg of Heparin Sodium in 1.0 mL of a mixture of water and hydrochloric acid (7:5), and use this solution as the heparin sodium stock solution. Dissolve 8.0 mg of D-glucosamine hydrochloride in a mixture of water and hydrochloric acid (7:5) to make exactly 10 mL. Dissolve 8.0 mg of D-galactosamine hydrochloride in a mixture of water and hydrochloric acid (7:5) to make exactly 10 mL. To 99 volumes of the solution of D-glucosamine add 1 volume of the solution of D-galactosamine, and use this solution as the standard stock solution. Transfer 500 μL each of the heparin sodium stock solution and the standard stock solution to a glass-stoppered test tube, stopper tightly, and heat at 100°C for 6 hours. After cooling to room temperature, evaporate 100 μL each of the reaction solutions to dryness. Add 50 μL of methanol to each of the residues and evaporate to dryness at room temperature. Dissolve each of the residues in 10 μL of water, add 40 μL of aminobenzoate derivatization TS, and heat at 80°C for 1 hour. After cooling to room temperature, evaporate the reaction solutions to dryness. Add 200 μL of each of water and ethyl acetate to each of the residues, shake vigorously, and then centrifuge. After remove the upper layers, add 200 μL of ethyl acetate to each of the lower layers, shake vigorously, and then centrifuge. These lower layers are used as the sample solution and the standard solution. Perform the test with 5 μL each of the sample solution and standard solution as directed under Liquid Chromatography <*2.01*> according to the following conditions: the peak area ratio of galactosamine to glucosamine of the sample solution is not larger than that of the standard solution.

Operating conditions—

Detector: A fluorescence photometer (excitation wavelength: 305 nm; emission wavelength: 360 nm).

Column: A stainless steel column 4.6 mm in inside diameter and 15 cm in length, packed with octadecylsilanized silica gel for liquid chromatography (3 μm in particle diameter).

Column temperature: A constant temperature of about 45°C.

Mobile phase: To 100 mL of a mixture of water and trifluoroacetic acid (1000:1) add 100 mL of acetonitrile. Add 140 mL of the solution to 860 mL of a mixture of water and trifluoroacetic acid (1000:1).

Flow rate: 1.0 mL per minute.

Time span of measurement: About 50 minutes after injected.

System suitability—

Test for required detectability: Dissolve 8.0 mg of D-mannosamine hydrochloride in 10 mL of a mixture of water and hydrochloric acid (7:5), and use this solution as the mannosamine standard solution. Transfer 500 μL of a mixture of the standard stock solution and the mannosamine standard solution (100:1) to a glass-stoppered test tube, stopper tightly, and heat at 100°C for 6 hours. After cooling this solution to room temperature, evaporate 100 μL of the reaction solution to dryness. Add 50 μL of methanol to the residue and evaporate to dryness at room temperature. Dissolve the residue in 10 μL of water, add 40 μL of aminobenzoate derivatization TS, and heat at 80°C for 1 hour. After cooling to room temperature, evaporate the reaction solution to dryness. Add 200 μL each of water and ethyl acetate to the residue, shake vigorously, and then centrifuge. After removing the upper layer, add 200 μL of ethyl acetate to the lower layer, shake vigorously, and then centrifuge. The lower layer is used as the solution for system suitability test. When the procedure is run with 5 μL of the solution for system suitability test under the above operating conditions, the ratio of the peak area of galactosamine to that of glucosamine is 0.7 – 2.0%.

System performance: When the procedure is run with 5 μL of the solution for system suitability test under the above operating conditions, glucosamine, mannosamine and galactosamine are eluted in this order with the resolutions between the peaks of glucosamine and mannosamine and between the peaks of mannosamine and galactosamine being not less than 1.5, respectively.

System repeatability: When the test is repeated 6 times with 5 μL of the solution for system suitability test under the above operating conditions, the relative standard deviation of the ratio of the peak area of galactosamine to that of glucosamine is not more than 4.0%.

Loss on drying <*2.41*> Not more than 10% (20 mg, in vacuum, 60°C, 3 hours).

Residue on ignition <*2.44*> Not more than 40% (after drying, 20 mg).

Bacterial endotoxins <*4.01*> Less than 0.0030 EU/Heparin Unit.

Anti-factor Xa activity to anti-factor IIa activity ratio The ratio of the anti-factor Xa activity determined by the following method to the anti-factor IIa activity obtained in the Assay, calculated by dividing the former with the later, is 0.9 – 1.1.

Anti-factor Xa activity determination

(i) Substrate solution: Dissolve 25 mg of *N*-benzoyl-L-isoleucyl-L-glutamyl(γ-OR)-glycyl-L-arginyl-*p*-nitroanilide hydrochloride in 33.3 mL of water.

(ii) Anti-thrombin solution: Dissolve human anti-thrombin in water so that each mL contains 1 IU. To 150 μL of this solution add 2250 μL of buffer solution

(iii) Factor Xa solution: To 1200 μL of factor Xa TS add 1200 μL of buffer solution.

(iv) Buffer solution: Proceed as directed in the Assay.

(v) Stopping solution: Proceed as directed in the Assay.

(vi) Heparin standard solutions: Proceed as directed in the Assay. However, the standard solutions are prepared based on anti-factor Xa activity Unit instead of Heparin Unit.

(vii) Heparin sample solutions: Proceed as directed in the Assay. However, the sample solutions are prepared based on anti-factor Xa activity Unit instead of Heparin Unit.

(viii) Procedure: Transfer separately two 50-μL portions of each dilution of the heparin standard solutions and the heparin sample solutions and five 50-μL portions of buffer solution as the blank to 1.5 mL-tubes. Warm these 21 tubes, anti-thrombin solution, factor Xa solution and substrate solution at 37°C all together. Start the following procedure at 2 minutes after warming in the order: buffer solution, S_1, S_2, S_3, S_4, buffer solution, T_1, T_2, T_3, T_4, buffer solution, T_1, T_2, T_3, T_4, buffer solution, S_1, S_2, S_3, S_4, and buffer solution. To each tube add 50 μL of anti-thrombin solution, mix, and warm at 37°C for exactly 4 minutes, add 100 μL of factor Xa solution, mix, and incubate for exactly 12 minutes. Then, add 100 μL of substrate solution, mix, incubate for exactly 4 minutes, add 50 μL of stopping solution to each tube, and mix immediately. Separately, to 50 μL of stopping solution add 100 μL of substrate solution, 100 μL of factor Xa solution, 50 μL of anti-thrombin solution and 50 μL of buffer solution, mix, and use this solution as a control. Determine the absorbance of each solution at 405 nm against the control. Confirm that the relative standard deviation of the reading of the blank is not more than 10%.

(ix) Calculations: When the regression expression, $y = I_c + Ax_s + Bx_t$, is obtained using y as log of the absorbance values, x_s as the concentration of the heparin standard solutions and x_t as the concentration of the heparin sample solutions, the potency ratio R is B/A.

I_c: Common intercept
A: Slope of regression expression of the heparin standard solution
B: Slope of regression expression of the heparin sample solution

Calculate anti-factor Xa activity per mg of Heparin Sodium by the following formula.

Anti-factor Xa activity per mg of Heparin Sodium
$= 100 \times R \times V/M$

V: Total volume (mL) of the solution (the sample stock solution) prepared as containing about 100 anti-factor Xa activity Units per mL
M: Amount (mg) of Heparin Sodium taken for the sample stock solution

However, when a 90% confidence interval of D of the regression expression $y = I'_c + A'x_s + B'x_t + D$, where D is a constant term showing the difference between the blank and the intercept assumed from the two lines, is not in a range of between −0.2 and 0.2, analyze by excluding the measurements of the blank.

The criteria for the test suitability are performed as directed in the Assay. When these criteria are not satisfied, repeat the test after changing the dilution rate so that the potency ratio becomes about 1 using the obtained potency as reference.

Assay

(i) Substrate solution: Dissolve 25 mg of *H*-D-phenylalanyl-L-pipecolyl-L-arginyl-*p*-nitroanilide dihydrochloride in 32.0 mL of water.

(ii) Anti-thrombin solution (for heparin assay): Dissolve human anti-thrombin in water so that each mL contains 1 IU. Dilute this solution to an appropriate dilution factor of approximately more than 16 times with the buffer solution, and designate this solution as the anti-thrombin solution (for heparin assay). The dilution factor with the buffer solution is adjusted so that the absorbance of reaction solution with the blank solution (average of five tubes) is not more than 2.0, and that of reaction solution with S_4 (0.020 Unit/mL heparin standard solution) (average of two tubes) is not less than 0.2 and not more than 1.0 when the test is performed according to the Assay. The absorbance is measured with 1 cm light path in length.

(iii) Factor IIa solution: Add an equivalent volume of water to the buffer solution, and use this solution as the factor IIa diluent. Dissolve factor IIa in the factor IIa diluent to make a solution so that each mL contains 20 IU. Dilute this solution to an appropriate dilution factor of approximately less than 4 times with the factor IIa diluent, and designate this solution as the factor IIa solution. Adjust the dilution factor with the factor IIa diluent so that the absorbance of reaction solution with the blank solution (average of five tubes) is not more than 2.0, and that of reaction solution with S_4 (0.020 Unit/mL heparin standard solution) (average of two tubes) is not less than 0.2 and not more than 1.0 when the test is performed according to the Assay. The absorbance is measured with 1 cm light path in length.

(iv) Buffer solution: Dissolve 6.1 g of 2-amino-2-hydroxymethyl-1,3-propanediol, 10.2 g of sodium chloride, 2.8 g of disodium dihydrogen ethylenediamine tetraacetate dihydrate and 1.0 g of polyethylene glycol 6000 in 800 mL of water, adjust to pH 8.4 with 1 mol/L hydrochloric acid TS, and add water to make 1000 mL.

(v) Stopping solution: To 2 mL of acetic acid (100) add water to make 10 mL.

(vi) Heparin standard solutions: Dissolve Heparin Sodium RS in water so that each mL contains 100 Heparin Units, and use this solution as the standard stock solution. Dilute the standard stock solution with buffer solution so that each mL contains exactly 0.1 Heparin Units, and use this solution as the standard solution. Make heparin standard solutions S_1, S_2, S_3 and S_4 respectively by adding the standard solution to buffer solution as directed in the following table.

Heparin standard solution		Buffer solution (μL)	Standard solution (μL)
No.	Heparin concentration (Unit/mL)		
S_1	0.005	950	50
S_2	0.010	900	100
S_3	0.015	850	150
S_4	0.020	800	200

(vii) Heparin sample solutions: Weigh accurately an appropriate amount of Heparin Sodium, dissolve in water so that each mL contains about 100 Heparin Units, and use this solution as the sample stock solution. Dilute exactly the sample stock solution with buffer solution so that each mL contains 0.1 Heparin Units, and use this solution as the sample solution. Make heparin sample solutions T_1, T_2, T_3 and T_4 respectively by adding the sample solution to buffer solution as directed in the following table.

Heparin sample solution		Buffer solution (μL)	Sample solution (μL)
No.	Heparin concentration (Unit/mL)		
T_1	0.005	950	50
T_2	0.010	900	100
T_3	0.015	850	150
T_4	0.020	800	200

(viii) Procedure: Transfer separately two 50-μL portions of each dilution of the heparin standard solutions and the heparin sample solutions and five 50-μL portions of buffer solution as the blank to 1.5 mL-tubes. Warm these 21 tubes, anti-thrombin solution (for heparin assay), factor IIa solution and substrate solution at 37°C all together. Start the following procedure at 2 minutes after warming in the order: buffer solution, S_1, S_2, S_3, S_4, buffer solution, T_1, T_2, T_3, T_4, buffer solution, T_1, T_2, T_3, T_4, buffer solution, S_1, S_2, S_3, S_4, and buffer solution. To each tube add 100 μL of anti-thrombin solution (for heparin assay), mix, and warm at 37°C for exactly 4 minutes, add 25 μL of factor IIa solution, mix, and incubate for exactly 4 minutes. Then, add 50 μL of substrate solution, mix, incubate for exactly 4 minutes, add 50 μL of stopping solution to each tube, and mix. Separately, to 50 μL of stopping solution add 50 μL of substrate solution, 25 μL of factor IIa solution, 100 μL of anti-thrombin solution (for heparin assay) and 50 μL of buffer solution, mix, and use this solution as a control. Determine the absorbance of each solution at 405 nm against the control. Confirm that the relative standard deviation of the reading of the blank is not more than 10%.

(ix) Calculations: When the regression expression, $y = I_c + A_{X_S} + B_{X_T}$, is obtained using y as log of the absorbance values, $_{X_S}$ as the concentration of the heparin standard solutions and $_{X_T}$ as the concentration of the heparin sample solutions, the potency ratio R is B/A.

I_c: Common intercept

A: Slope of regression expression of the heparin standard solution

B: Slope of regression expression of the heparin sample solution

Calculate Heparin Unit (anti-factor IIa activity) per mg of Heparin Sodium by the following formula.

Heparin Unit (anti-factor IIa activity) per mg of Heparin Sodium
$= 100 \times R \times V/M$

V: Total volume (mL) of the solution (the sample stock solution) prepared as containing about 100 Heparin Units (anti-factor IIa activity) per mL

M: Amount (mg) of Heparin Sodium taken for the sample stock solution

However, when a 90% confidence interval of D of the regression expression $y = I'_c + A'_{X_S} + B'_{X_T} + D$, where D is a constant term showing the difference between the blank and the intercept assumed from the two lines, is not in the range of between −0.2 and 0.2, analyze by excluding the measurements of the blank.

The criteria for the test suitability are the following 3 items, (1), (2) and (3).

(1) Judgment on consistence of the intercept assumed from the two lines

When the regression expression, $y = I_s + A''_{X_S} + B''_{X_T} + I_{t\text{-}s}$, is obtained from the data of the heparin standard solution and the heparin sample solution except of the blank solution, a 90% confidence interval of the constant term, $I_{t\text{-}s}$, is between −0.2 and 0.2.

I_s: Intercept of the regression expression of the heparin standard solution

$I_{t\text{-}s}$: Difference of the intercepts assumed from the two lines

(2) Judgment on linearity

When the regression expression, $y = I_c + A'''_{X_S} + B'''_{X_T} + Q_{s}{X_S}^2 + Q_{t}{X_T}^2$, is obtained from the data of the heparin standard solution and the heparin sample solution, a 90% confidence interval of the secondary coefficients, Q_s and Q_t, is between −1000 and 1000.

Q_s: Secondary coefficient of the regression expression of the heparin standard solution

Q_t: Secondary coefficient of the regression expression of the heparin sample solution

(3) Judgment by checking if the relative potency obtained is within the range previously validated on this test method

The potency ratio obtained is not less than 0.8 and not more than 1.2.

When these criteria are not satisfied, repeat the test after changing the dilution rate so that the potency ratio becomes about 1 using the obtained potency as reference.

Containers and storage Containers—Tight containers.

Heparin Sodium Injection

ヘパリンナトリウム注射液

Heparin Sodium Injection is an aqueous injection.

It contains not less than 90% and not more than 110% of the labeled heparin Units.

Method of preparation Dissolve Heparin Sodium in Isotonic Sodium Chloride Solution and prepare as directed under Injections.

Description Heparin Sodium Injection is a clear, colorless to light yellow liquid.

pH <*2.54*> 5.5 – 8.0

Purity Barium—Measure exactly a volume of Heparin Sodium Injection, equivalent to 3000 Units of Heparin Sodium, add water to make 3.0 mL and use this solution as the sample solution. To 1.0 mL of the sample solution add 3 drops of dilute sulfuric acid, and allow to stand for 10 minutes: no turbidity is produced.

Bacterial endotoxins <*4.01*> Less than 0.0030 EU/unit.

Extractable volume <*6.05*> It meets the requirement.

Foreign insoluble matter <*6.06*> Perform the test according to Method 1: it meets the requirement.

Insoluble particulate matter <*6.07*> It meets the requirement.

Sterility <*4.06*> Perform the test according to the Membrane filtration method: it meets the requirement.

Assay Proceed as directed in the Assay under Heparin Sodium, replacing (vii) Heparin sample solutions and (ix) Calculations with the following.

(vii) Heparin sample solutions: Take exactly an appropriate amount of Heparin Sodium Injection, dilute exactly with buffer solution so that each mL contains 0.1 Heparin Units, and use this solution as the sample solution. Make heparin sample solutions T_1, T_2, T_3 and T_4 respectively by adding the sample solution to buffer solution as directed in the following table.

Heparin sample solution			
No.	Heparin concentration (Unit/mL)	Buffer solution (μL)	Sample solution (μL)
T_1	0.005	950	50
T_2	0.010	900	100
T_3	0.015	850	150
T_4	0.020	800	200

(ix) Calculations: When the regression expression, $y = I_c + A_{Xs} + B_{Xt}$, is obtained using y as log of the absorbance values, $_{Xs}$ as the concentration of the heparin standard solutions and $_{Xt}$ as the concentration of the heparin sample solutions, the potency ratio R is B/A.

I_c: Common intercept

A: Slope of regression expression of the heparin standard solution

B: Slope of regression expression of the heparin sample solution

Calculate Heparin Units (anti-factor IIa activity) in 1 mL of Heparin Sodium Injection by the following formula.

Heparin Units (anti-factor IIa activity) in 1 mL of Heparin Sodium Injection

$= 0.1 \times R \times V/a$

V: Total volume (mL) of the sample solution prepared as containing 0.1 Heparin Units (anti-factor IIa activity) per mL

a: Amount (mL) of Heparin Sodium Injection taken for the sample solution

However, when a 90% confidence interval of D of the regression expression $y = I'_c + A'_{Xs} + B'_{Xt} + D$, where D is a constant term showing the difference between the intercepts assumed from the measurement of the blank and the two lines, is not in the range of between −0.2 and 0.2, analyze by excluding the measurements of the blank.

The criteria for the test suitability are followed as directed in the Assay under Heparin Sodium. When these criteria are not satisfied, repeat the test after changing the dilution rate so that the potency ratio becomes about 1 using the obtained potency as reference.

Containers and storage Containers—Hermetic containers.
Storage—Light-resistant.

Heparin Sodium Lock Solution

ロック用ヘパリンナトリウム液

Heparin Sodium Lock Solution is a preparation used to prevent blood coagulation in intravenous indwelling routes.

It contains not less than 90% and not more than 110% of the labeled Heparin Units.

Method of preparation Prepare as directed under Injections, with Heparin Sodium.

Description Heparin Sodium Lock Solution is a clear, colorless to light yellow liquid.

Osmotic pressure ratio: 0.9 – 1.1

pH <2.54> 5.5 – 8.0

Bacterial endotoxins <4.01> Less than 0.0030 EU/unit.

Extractable volume <6.05> It meets the requirement.

Foreign insoluble matter <6.06> Perform the test according to Method 1: it meets the requirement.

Insoluble particulate matter <6.07> It meets the requirement.

Sterility <4.06> Perform the test according to the Membrane filtration method: it meets the requirement.

Assay Proceed as directed in the Assay under Heparin Sodium, replacing (vii) Heparin sample solutions and (ix) Calculations with the following.

(vii) Heparin sample solutions: Pipet a suitable volume of Heparin Sodium Lock Solution, dilute exactly with the buffer solution so that each mL contains 0.1 Heparin Units, and use this solution as the sample solution. Prepare heparin sample solutions T_1, T_2, T_3 and T_4 respectively by adding the sample solution to the buffer solution as directed in the following table.

Heparin sample solution		Buffer solution (μL)	Sample solution (μL)
No.	Heparin concentration (Unit/mL)		
T_1	0.005	950	50
T_2	0.010	900	100
T_3	0.015	850	150
T_4	0.020	800	200

(ix) Calculations: When the regression expression, $y = I_c + A_{X_s} + B_{X_t}$, is obtained using y as log of the absorbance values, x_s as the concentration of the heparin standard solutions and x_t as the concentration of the heparin sample solutions, the potency ratio R is B/A.

I_c: Common intercept
A: Slope of regression expression of the heparin standard solution
B: Slope of regression expression of the heparin sample solution

Calculate Heparin Units (anti-factor IIa activity) in 1 mL of Heparin Sodium Lock Solution by the following formula.

Heparin Units (anti-factor IIa activity) in 1 mL of Heparin Sodium Lock Solution
$= 0.1 \times R \times V/a$

V: Total volume (mL) of the sample solution prepared as containing 0.1 Heparin Units (anti-factor IIa activity) per mL
a: Amount (mL) of Heparin Sodium Lock Solution taken

However, when a 90% confidence interval of D of the regression expression $y = I'_c + A'_{X_s} + B'_{X_t} + D$, where D is a constant term showing the difference between the intercepts assumed from the measurement of the blank and the two lines, is not in the range of between −0.2 and 0.2, analyze by excluding the measurements of the blank.

The criteria for the test suitability are followed as directed in the Assay under Heparin Sodium. When these criteria are not satisfied, repeat the test after changing the dilution rate so that the potency ratio becomes about 1 using the obtained potency as reference.

Containers and storage Containers—Hermetic containers. Plastic containers for aqueous injections may be used.

Heparin Sodium Solution for Dialysis

透析用ヘパリンナトリウム液

Heparin Sodium Solution for Dialysis is a preparation used to prevent coagulation of perfused blood during hemodialysis.

It contains not less than 90% and not more than 110% of the labeled Heparin Unit.

Method of preparation Prepare as directed under Injections, with Heparin Sodium.

Description Heparin Sodium Solution for Dialysis is a clear, colorless to light yellow liquid.

Osmotic pressure ratio: 0.9 – 1.1

pH <2.54> 5.5 – 8.0

Bacterial endotoxins <4.01> Less than 0.0030 EU/unit.

Extractable volume <6.05> It meets the requirement.

Foreign insoluble matter <6.06> Perform the test according to Method 1: it meets the requirement.

Insoluble particulate matter <6.07> It meets the requirement.

Sterility <4.06> Perform the test according to the Membrane filtration method: it meets the requirement.

Assay Proceed as directed in the Assay under Heparin Sodium, replacing (vii) Heparin sample solutions and (ix) Calculations with the following.

(vii) Heparin sample solutions: Pipet a suitable volume of Heparin Sodium Solution for Dialysis, dilute exactly with the buffer solution so that each mL contains 0.1 Heparin Units, and use this solution as the sample solution. Prepare heparin sample solutions T_1, T_2, T_3 and T_4 respectively by adding the sample solution to the buffer solution as directed in the following table.

Heparin sample solution		Buffer solution (μL)	Sample solution (μL)
No.	Heparin concentration (Unit/mL)		
T_1	0.005	950	50
T_2	0.010	900	100
T_3	0.015	850	150
T_4	0.020	800	200

(ix) Calculations: When the regression expression, $y = I_c + A_{X_s} + B_{X_t}$, is obtained using y as log of the absorbance values, x_s as the concentration of the heparin standard solutions and x_t as the concentration of the heparin sample solutions, the potency ratio R is B/A.

I_c: Common intercept
A: Slope of regression expression of the heparin standard solution

B: Slope of regression expression of the heparin sample solution

Calculate Heparin Units (anti-factor IIa activity) in 1 mL of Heparin Sodium Solution for Dialysis by the following formula.

Heparin Units (anti-factor IIa activity) in 1 mL of Heparin Sodium Solution for Dialysis
$= 0.1 \times R \times V/a$

V: Total volume (mL) of the sample solution prepared as containing 0.1 Heparin Units (anti-factor IIa activity) per mL
a: Amount (mL) of Heparin Sodium Solution for Dialysis taken

However, when a 90% confidence interval of *D* of the regression expression $y = I'_c + A'_{X_s} + B'_{X_t} + D$, where *D* is a constant term showing the difference between the intercepts assumed from the measurement of the blank and the two lines, is not in the range of between −0.2 and 0.2, analyze by excluding the measurements of the blank.

The criteria for the test suitability are followed as directed in the Assay under Heparin Sodium. When these criteria are not satisfied, repeat the test after changing the dilution rate so that the potency ratio becomes about 1 using the obtained potency as reference.

Containers and storage Containers—Hermetic containers. Plastic containers for aqueous injections may be used.

Adsorbed Hepatitis B Vaccine

沈降B型肝炎ワクチン

Adsorbed Hepatitis B Vaccine is a liquid for injection prepared by adding an aluminum salt to a liquid containing a surface antigen of hepatitis B virus to make the HBs antigen insoluble.

It conforms to the requirements of Adsorbed Hepatitis B Vaccine in the Minimum Requirements for Biological Products.

Description Adsorbed Hepatitis B Vaccine becomes a homogeneous, whitish turbid liquid on shaking.

L-Histidine

L-ヒスチジン

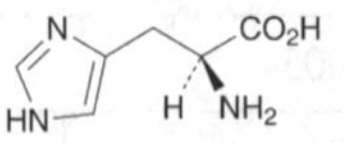

$C_6H_9N_3O_2$: 155.15
(2*S*)-2-Amino-3-(1*H*-imidazol-4-yl)propanoic acid
[*71-00-1*]

L-Histidine contains not less than 99.0% and not more than 101.0% of L-histidine ($C_6H_9N_3O_2$), calculated on the dried basis.

Description L-Histidine occurs as white, crystals or crystalline powder, having a slight bitter taste.

It is freely soluble in formic acid, and soluble in water, and practically insoluble in ethanol (99.5).

It dissolves in 6 mol/L hydrochloric acid TS.

It shows crystal polymorphism.

Identification Determine the infrared absorption spectrum of L-Histidine as directed in the potassium bromide disk method under Infrared Spectrophotometry <*2.25*>, and compare the spectrum with the Reference Spectrum: both spectra exhibit similar intensities of absorption at the same wave numbers. If any difference appears between the spectra, dissolve the sample with a little amount of water, evaporate the water at 60°C under reduced pressure, dry the residue, and perform the test.

Optical rotation <*2.49*> $[\alpha]_D^{20}$: +11.8 – +12.8° (5.5 g calculated on the dried basis, 6 mol/L hydrochloric acid TS, 50 mL, 100 mm).

pH <*2.54*> The pH of a solution of 1.0 g of L-Histidine in 50 mL of water is between 7.0 and 8.5.

Purity (1) Clarity and color of solution—A solution of 0.40 g of L-Histidine in 20 mL of water is clear and colorless.

(2) Chloride <*1.03*>—Perform the test with 0.5 g of L-Histidine. Prepare the control solution with 0.30 mL of 0.01 mol/L hydrochloric acid VS (not more than 0.021%).

(3) Sulfate <*1.14*>—Perform the test with 0.6 g of L-Histidine. Prepare the control solution with 0.35 mL of 0.005 mol/L sulfuric acid VS (not more than 0.028%).

(4) Ammonium <*1.02*>—Perform the test with 0.25 g of L-Histidine. Prepare the control solution with 5.0 mL of Standard Ammonium Solution (not more than 0.02%).

(5) Heavy metals <*1.07*>—Dissolve 1.0 g of L-Histidine in 30 mL of water by warming. To this solution add 2.4 mL of dilute hydrochloric acid, 2 mL of dilute acetic acid and water to make 50 mL. Perform the test using this solution as the test solution. Prepare the control solution as follows: To 1.0 mL of Standard Lead Solution add 2 mL of dilute acetic acid and water to make 50 mL (not more than 10 ppm).

(6) Iron <*1.10*>—Prepare the test solution with 1.0 g of L-Histidine according to Method 1, and perform the test according to Method A. Prepare the control solution with 1.0 mL of Standard Iron Solution (not more than 10 ppm).

(7) Related substances—Dissolve 0.10 g of L-Histidine in 10 mL of water, and use this solution as the sample solution. Pipet 1 mL of the sample solution, add water to make exactly 10 mL. Pipet 1 mL of this solution, add water to make exactly 50 mL, and use this solution as the standard solution. Perform the test with these solutions as directed under Thin-layer Chromatography <*2.03*>. Spot 5 µL each of the sample solution and standard solution on a plate of silica gel for thin-layer chromatography, develop the plate with a mixture of 1-propanol and ammonia solution (28) (67:33) to a distance of about 10 cm, and dry the plate at 80°C for 30 minutes. Spray evenly a solution of ninhydrin in a mixture of methanol and acetic acid (100) (97:3) (1 in 100) to the plate, and heat at 80°C for 10 minutes: the spot other than the principal spot obtained from the sample solution is not more intense than the spot from the standard solution.

Loss on drying <*2.41*> Not more than 0.3% (1 g, 105°C, 3 hours).

Residue on ignition <*2.44*> Not more than 0.1% (1 g).

Assay Weigh accurately about 0.15 g of L-Histidine, dissolve in 2 mL of formic acid, add 50 mL of acetic acid (100), and titrate <*2.50*> with 0.1 mol/L perchloric acid VS (potentiometric titration). Perform a blank determination in the same manner, and make any necessary correction.

Each mL of 0.1 mol/L perchloric acid VS
= 15.52 mg of $C_6H_9N_3O_2$

Containers and storage Containers—Tight containers.

L-Histidine Hydrochloride Hydrate

L-ヒスチジン塩酸塩水和物

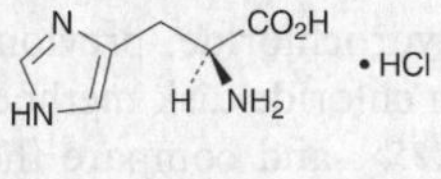

$C_6H_9N_3O_2.HCl.H_2O$: 209.63
(2*S*)-2-Amino-3-(1*H*-imidazol-4-yl)propanoic acid monohydrochloride monohydrate
[*5934-29-2*]

L-Histidine Hydrochloride Hydrate contains not less than 99.0% and not more than 101.0% of L-histidine hydrochloride ($C_6H_9N_3O_2.HCl$: 191.62), calculated on the anhydrous basis.

Description L-Histidine Hydrochloride Hydrate occurs as white crystals or a white crystalline powder. It has an acid taste at first, and a slight bitter taste later.

It is freely soluble in water and in formic acid, and practically insoluble in ethanol (99.5).

It dissolves in 6 mol/L hydrochloric acid TS.

Identification **(1)** Determine the infrared absorption spectrum of L-Histidine Hydrochloride Hydrate as directed in the potassium chloride disk method under Infrared Spectrophotometry *<2.25>*, and compare the spectrum with the Reference Spectrum: both spectra exhibit similar intensities of absorption at the same wave numbers.

(2) A solution of L-Histidine Hydrochloride Hydrate (1 in 10) responds to Qualitative Tests *<1.09>* for chloride.

Optical rotation *<2.49>* $[\alpha]_D^{20}$: $+9.2 - +10.6°$ (5.5 g calculated on the anhydrous basis, 6 mol/L hydrochloric acid TS, 50 mL, 100 mm).

pH *<2.54>* The pH of a solution of 1.0 g of L-Histidine Hydrochloride Hydrate in 10 mL of water is between 3.5 and 4.5.

Purity **(1)** Clarity and color of solution—A solution of 1.0 g of L-Histidine Hydrochloride Hydrate in 10 mL of water is clear and colorless.

(2) Sulfate *<1.14>*—Perform the test with 0.6 g of L-Histidine Hydrochloride Hydrate. Prepare the control solution with 0.35 mL of 0.005 mol/L sulfuric acid VS (not more than 0.028%).

(3) Ammonium *<1.02>*—Perform the test with 0.25 g of L-Histidine Hydrochloride Hydrate. Prepare the control solution with 5.0 mL of Standard Ammonium Solution (not more than 0.02%).

(4) Heavy metals *<1.07>*—Proceed with 1.0 g of L-Histidine Hydrochloride Hydrate according to Method 1, and perform the test. Prepare the control solution with 1.0 mL of Standard Lead Solution (not more than 10 ppm).

(5) Iron *<1.10>*—Prepare the test solution with 1.0 g of L-Histidine Hydrochloride Hydrate according to Method 1, and perform the test according to Method A. Prepare the control solution with 1.0 mL of Standard Iron Solution (not more than 10 ppm).

(6) Related substances—Dissolve 0.10 g of L-Histidine Hydrochloride Hydrate in 10 mL of water, and use this solution as the sample solution. Pipet 1 mL of the sample solution, add water to make exactly 10 mL. Pipet 1 mL of this solution, add water to make exactly 50 mL, and use this solution as the standard solution. Perform the test with these solutions as directed under Thin-layer Chromatography *<2.03>*. Spot 5 μL each of the sample solution and standard solution on a plate of silica gel for thin-layer chromatography, develop the plate with a mixture of 1-propanol and ammonia solution (28) (67:33) to a distance of about 10 cm, and dry the plate at 80°C for 30 minutes. Spray evenly a solution of ninhydrin in a mixture of methanol and acetic acid (100) (97:3) (1 in 100) to the plate, and heat the plate at 80°C for 10 minutes: the spot other than the principal spot obtained from the sample solution is not more intense than the spot from the standard solution.

Water *<2.48>* 7.2 – 10.0% (0.12 g, volumetric titration, direct titration, using a mixture of methanol for water determination and formamide for water determination (2:1) instead of methanol for water determination).

Residue on ignition *<2.44>* Not more than 0.1% (1 g).

Assay Weigh accurately about 0.1 g of L-Histidine Hydrochloride Hydrate, dissolve in 3 mL of formic acid, add exactly 15 mL of 0.1 mol/L perchloric acid VS, and heat on a water bath for 30 minutes. After cooling, add 45 mL of acetic acid (100), and titrate *<2.50>* the excess of perchloric acid with 0.1 mol/L sodium acetate VS (potentiometric titration). Perform a blank determination in the same manner.

Each mL of 0.1 mol/L perchloric acid VS
= 9.581 mg of $C_6H_9N_3O_2.HCl$

Containers and storage Containers—Tight containers.

Homatropine Hydrobromide

ホマトロピン臭化水素酸塩

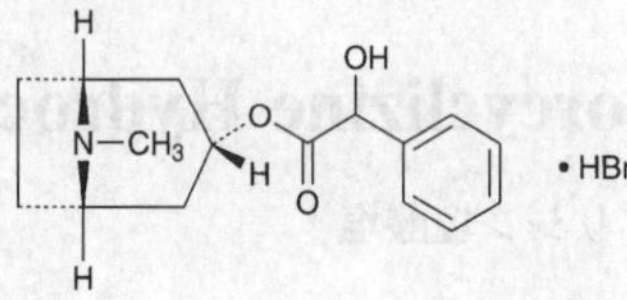

$C_{16}H_{21}NO_3.HBr$: 356.25
(1*R*,3*r*,5*S*)-8-Methyl-8-azabicyclo[3.2.1]oct-3-yl [(2*RS*)-2-hydroxy-2-phenyl]acetate monohydrobromide
[*51-56-9*]

Homatropine Hydrobromide contains not less than 99.0% of homatropine hydrobromide ($C_{16}H_{21}NO_3.HBr$), calculated on the dried basis.

Description Homatropine Hydrobromide occurs as white, crystals or crystalline powder. It is odorless.

It is freely soluble in water, sparingly soluble in ethanol (95), slightly soluble in acetic acid (100), very slightly soluble in acetic anhydride, and practically insoluble in diethyl ether.

It is affected by light.

Melting point: about 214°C (with decomposition).

Identification **(1)** To 5 mL of a solution of Homatropine Hydrobromide (1 in 20) add 2 to 3 drops of iodine TS: a brown precipitate is produced.

(2) Dissolve 0.05 g of Homatropine Hydrobromide in 5 mL of water, and add 3 mL of 2,4,6-trinitrophenol TS: a yellow precipitate is produced. Filter the precipitate, wash with five 10-mL portions of water, and dry at 105°C for 2 hours: it melts *<2.60>* between 184°C and 187°C.

(3) A solution of Homatropine Hydrobromide (1 in 20) responds to Qualitative Tests *<1.09>* for bromide.

Purity **(1)** Acidity—Dissolve 1.0 g of Homatropine

Hydrobromide in 20 mL of water, and add 0.40 mL of 0.01 mol/L sodium hydroxide VS and 1 drop of methyl red-methylene blue TS: a green color develops.

(2) Atropine, hyoscyamine and scopolamine—To 10 mg of Homatropine Hydrobromide add 5 drops of nitric acid, evaporate on a water bath to dryness, and cool. Dissolve the residue in 1 mL of *N*,*N*-dimethylformamide, and add 5 to 6 drops of tetraethylammonium hydroxide TS: no red-purple color is produced.

(3) Related substances—Dissolve 0.15 g of Homatropine Hydrobromide in 3 mL of water, and use this solution as the sample solution.

(i) To 1 mL of the sample solution add 2 to 3 drops of tannic acid TS: no precipitate is produced.

(ii) To 1 mL of the sample solution add 2 to 3 drops each of dilute hydrochloric acid and platinic chloride TS: no precipitate is produced.

Loss on drying <*2.41*> Not more than 1.5% (0.5 g, 105°C, 2 hours).

Residue on ignition <*2.44*> Not more than 0.2% (0.2 g).

Assay Dissolve by warming about 0.4 g of Homatropine Hydrobromide in 60 mL of a mixture of acetic anhydride and acetic acid (100) (7:3). Cool, and titrate <*2.50*> with 0.1 mol/L perchloric acid VS (potentiometric titration). Perform a blank determination in the same manner, and make any necessary correction.

Each mL of 0.1 mol/L perchloric acid VS
= 35.63 mg of $C_{16}H_{21}NO_3.HBr$

Containers and storage Containers—Tight containers.
Storage—Light-resistant.

Homochlorcyclizine Hydrochloride

ホモクロルシクリジン塩酸塩

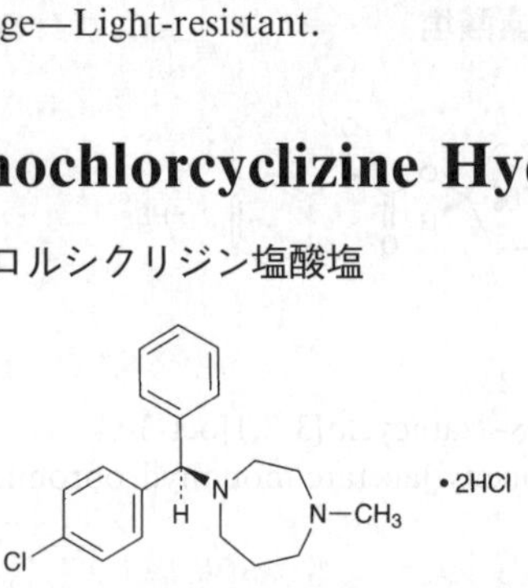

•2HCl

and enantiomer

$C_{19}H_{23}ClN_2.2HCl$: 387.77
1-[(*RS*)-(4-Chlorophenyl)(phenyl)methyl]-4-methylhexahydro-1*H*-1,4-diazepine dihydrochloride
[*1982-36-1*]

Homochlorcyclizine Hydrochloride, when dried, contains not less than 98.0% of homochlorcyclizine hydrochloride ($C_{19}H_{23}ClN_2.2HCl$).

Description Homochlorcyclizine Hydrochloride occurs as white to pale brown, crystals or powder.

It is very soluble in water, freely soluble in acetic acid (100), slightly soluble in ethanol (99.5), and very slightly soluble in acetonitrile and in acetic anhydride.

It dissolves in 0.1 mol/L hydrochloric acid TS.

It is hygroscopic.

It is colored slightly by light.

A solution of Homochlorcyclizine Hydrochloride (1 in 10) shows no optical rotation.

Melting point: about 227°C (with decomposition).

Identification **(1)** Determine the absorption spectrum of a solution of Homochlorcyclizine Hydrochloride in 0.1 mol/L hydrochloric acid TS (1 in 100,000) as directed under Ultraviolet-visible Spectrophotometry <*2.24*>, and compare the spectrum with the Reference Spectrum: both spectra exhibit similar intensities of absorption at the same wavelengths.

(2) Determine the infrared absorption spectrum of Homochlorcyclizine Hydrochloride, previously dried, as directed in the potassium chloride disk method under Infrared Spectrophotometry <*2.25*>, and compare the spectrum with the Reference Spectrum: both spectra exhibit similar intensities of absorption at the same wave numbers.

(3) A solution of Homochlorcyclizine Hydrochloride (1 in 100) responds to Qualitative Tests <*1.09*> for chloride.

Purity **(1)** Heavy metals <*1.07*>—Proceed with 1.0 g of Homochlorcyclizine Hydrochloride according to Method 2, and perform the test. Prepare the control solution with 2.0 mL of Standard Lead Solution (not more than 20 ppm).

(2) Related substances—Dissolve 0.10 g of Homochlorcyclizine Hydrochloride in 100 mL of the mobile phase, and use this solution as the sample solution. Measure exactly 1 mL of the sample solution, add the mobile phase to make exactly 100 mL, and use this solution as the standard solution. Perform the test with exactly 10 μL each of the sample solution and standard solution as directed under Liquid Chromatography <*2.01*> according to the following conditions, and determine the peak areas by the automatic integration method: the areas of the peaks other than homochlorcyclizine obtained from the sample solution are not larger than 1/2 times the peak area of homochlorcyclizine from the standard solution, and the total area of the peaks other than homochlorcyclizine from the sample solution is not larger than the peak area of homochlorcyclizine from the standard solution.

Operating conditions—

Detector: An ultraviolet absorption photometer (wavelength: 223 nm).

Column: A stainless steel column 4.6 mm in inside diameter and 25 cm in length, packed with octadecylsilanized silica gel for liquid chromatography (5 μm in particle diameter).

Column temperature: A constant temperature of about 40°C.

Mobile phase: A mixture of water, acetonitrile and perchloric acid (134:66:1).

Flow rate: Adjust so that the retention time of homochlorcyclizine is about 10 minutes.

Time span of measurement: About 2 times as long as the retention time of homochlorcyclizine.

System suitability—

Test for required detectability: To exactly 5 mL of the standard solution add the mobile phase to make exactly 50 mL. Confirm that the peak area of homochlorcyclizine obtained with 10 μL of this solution is equivalent to 7 to 13% of that with 10 μL of the standard solution.

System performance: Dissolve 5 mg each of Homochlorcyclizine Hydrochloride and methyl parahydroxybenzoic acid in 100 mL of the mobile phase. When the procedure is run with 10 μL of this solution under the above operating conditions, methyl parahydroxybenzoic acid and homochlorcyclizine are eluted in this order with the resolution between these peaks being not less than 5.

System repeatability: When the test is repeated 6 times with 10μL of the standard solution under the above operating conditions, the relative standard deviation of the peak area of homochlorcyclizine is not more than 1.0%.

Loss on drying <*2.41*> Not more than 2.0% (1 g, 110°C, 4 hours).

Residue on ignition <*2.44*> Not more than 0.2% (1 g).

Assay Weigh accurately about 0.3 g of Homochlorcyclizine Hydrochloride, previously dried, dissolve in 50 mL of a mixture of acetic anhydride and acetic acid (100) (7:3), and titrate <*2.50*> with 0.1 mol/L perchloric acid VS (potentiometric titration). Perform a blank determination in the same manner, and make any necessary correction.

Each mL of 0.1 mol/L perchloric acid VS
= 19.39 mg of $C_{19}H_{23}ClN_2.2HCl$

Containers and storage Containers—Tight containers.
Storage—Light-resistant.

Human Normal Immunoglobulin

人免疫グロブリン

Human Normal Immunoglobulin is a liquid for injection containing immunoglobulin G in serum globulins of humans.

It conforms to the requirements of Human Normal Immunoglobulin in the Minimum Requirements for Biological Products.

Description Human Normal Immunoglobulin is a clear, colorless or yellow-brown liquid.

Hydralazine Hydrochloride

ヒドララジン塩酸塩

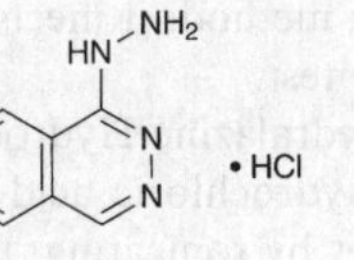

$C_8H_8N_4.HCl$: 196.64
Phthalazin-1-ylhydrazine monohydrochloride
[*304-20-1*]

Hydralazine Hydrochloride, when dried, contains not less than 98.0% of hydralazine hydrochloride ($C_8H_8N_4.HCl$).

Description Hydralazine Hydrochloride occurs as a white crystalline powder. It is odorless, and has a bitter taste.

It is soluble in water, slightly soluble in ethanol (95), and practically insoluble in diethyl ether.

Melting point: about 275°C (with decomposition).

Identification **(1)** Determine the absorption spectrum of a solution of Hydralazine Hydrochloride (1 in 100,000) as directed under Ultraviolet-visible Spectrophotometry <*2.24*>, and compare the spectrum with the Reference Spectrum: both spectra exhibit similar intensities of absorption at the same wavelengths.

(2) Determine the infrared absorption spectrum of Hydralazine Hydrochloride, previously dried, as directed in the potassium bromide disk method under Infrared Spectrophotometry <*2.25*>, and compare the spectrum with the Reference spectrum: both spectra exhibit similar intensities of absorption at the same wave numbers.

(3) A solution of Hydralazine Hydrochloride (1 in 50) responds to Qualitative Tests <*1.09*> for chloride.

pH <*2.54*> Dissolve 1.0 g of Hydralazine Hydrochloride in 50 mL of water: the pH of the solution is between 3.5 and 4.5.

Purity **(1)** Clarity and color of solution—Dissolve 1.0 g of Hydralazine Hydrochloride in 50 mL of water: the solution is clear, and colorless or pale yellow.

(2) Heavy metals <*1.07*>—Proceed with 1.0 g of Hydralazine Hydrochloride according to Method 2, and perform the test. Prepare the control solution with 2.0 mL of Standard Lead Solution (not more than 20 ppm).

Loss on drying <*2.41*> Not more than 0.5% (0.5 g, in vacuum, phosphorus (V) oxide, 8 hours).

Residue on ignition <*2.44*> Not more than 0.1% (1 g).

Assay Weigh accurately about 0.15 g of Hydralazine Hydrochloride, previously dried, transfer it to a glass-stoppered flask, dissolve in 25 mL of water, add 25 mL of hydrochloric acid, cool to room temperature, add 5 mL of chloroform, and titrate <*2.50*> with 0.05 mol/L potassium iodate VS while shaking until the purple color of the chloroform layer disappears. The end point is reached when the red-purple color no more reappears in the chloroform layer within 5 minutes after the layer has been decolorized.

Each mL of 0.05 mol/L potassium iodate VS
= 9.832 mg of $C_8H_8N_4.HCl$

Containers and storage Containers—Tight containers.

Hydralazine Hydrochloride for Injection

注射用ヒドララジン塩酸塩

Hydralazine Hydrochloride for Injection is a preparation for injection which is dissolved before use.

It contains not less than 99.0% and not more than 113.0% of the labeled amount of hydralazine hydrochloride ($C_8H_8N_4.HCl$: 196.64).

Method of preparation Prepare as directed under Injections, with Hydralazine Hydrochloride.

Description Hydralazine Hydrochloride for Injection occurs as a white to pale yellow powder or mass. It is odorless, and has a bitter taste.

Identification Determine the absorption spectrum of a solution of Hydralazine Hydrochloride for Injection (1 in 100,000) as directed under Ultraviolet-visible Spectrophotometry <*2.24*>: it exhibits maxima between 238 nm and 242 nm, between 258 nm and 262 nm, between 301 nm and 305 nm, and between 313 nm and 317 nm.

pH <*2.54*> Dissolve 1.0 g of Hydralazine Hydrochloride for Injection in 50 mL of water: the pH of this solution is between 3.5 and 4.5.

Bacterial endotoxins <*4.01*> Less than 5.0 EU/mg.

Uniformity of dosage units <*6.02*> It meets the requirement of the Mass variation test. (*T*: 106.0%)

Foreign insoluble matter <*6.06*> Perform the test according to Method 2: it meets the requirement.

Insoluble particulate matter <*6.07*> It meets the requirement.

Sterility <*4.06*> Perform the test according to the Mem-

brane filtration method: it meets the requirement.

Assay Weigh accurately the contents of not less than 10 samples of Hydralazine Hydrochloride for Injection. Weigh accurately about 0.15 g of the contents, transfer it to a glass-stoppered flask, dissolve in 25 mL of water, add 25 mL of hydrochloric acid, cool to room temperature, and proceed as directed in the Assay under Hydralazine Hydrochloride.

Each mL of 0.05 mol/L potassium iodate VS
= 9.832 mg of $C_8H_8N_4.HCl$

Containers and storage Containers—Hermetic containers.

Hydralazine Hydrochloride Powder

ヒドララジン塩酸塩散

Hydralazine Hydrochloride Powder contains not less than 95.0% and not more than 105.0% of the labeled amount of hydralazine hydrochloride ($C_8H_8N_4.HCl$: 196.64).

Method of preparation Prepare as directed under Granules or Powders, with Hydralazine Hydrochloride.

Identification Weigh a portion of Hydralazine Hydrochloride Powder, equivalent to 25 mg of Hydralazine Hydrochloride, add 100 mL of water, shake well, and filter, if necessary. Add water to 2 mL of this solution to make 50 mL and determine the absorption spectrum of this solution as directed under Ultraviolet-visible Spectrophotometry <*2.24*>: it exhibits maxima between 238 nm and 242 nm, between 258 nm and 262 nm, between 301 nm and 305 nm, and between 313 nm and 317 nm.

Dissolution <*6.10*> When the test is performed at 50 revolutions per minute according to the Paddle method, using 900 mL of water as the dissolution medium, the dissolution rate in 15 minutes of Hydralazine Hydrochloride Powder is not less than 85%.

Start the test with an accurately weighed amount of Hydralazine Hydrochloride Powder, equivalent to about 50 mg of hydralazine hydrochloride ($C_8H_8N_4.HCl$), withdraw not less than 10 mL of the medium at the specified minute after starting the test, and filter through a membrane filter with a pore size not exceeding 0.5 μm. Discard not less than 5 mL of the first filtrate, pipet 4 mL of the subsequent filtrate, add water to make exactly 20 mL, and use this solution as the sample solution. Separately, weigh accurately about 28 mg of hydralazine hydrochloride for assay, previously dried at 105°C for 3 hours, and dissolve in water to make exactly 50 mL. Pipet 2 mL of this solution, add water to make exactly 100 mL, and use this solution as the standard solution. Determine the absorbances, A_T and A_S, at 260 nm of the sample solution and standard solution as directed under Ultraviolet-visible Spectrophotometry <*2.24*>.

Dissolution rate (%) with respect to the labeled amount of hydralazine hydrochloride ($C_8H_8N_4.HCl$)
$= M_S/M_T \times A_T/A_S \times 1/C \times 180$

M_S: Amount (mg) of hydralazine hydrochloride for assay taken
M_T: Amount (g) of the Hydralazine Hydrochloride Powder taken
C: Labeled amount (mg) of hydralazine hydrochloride ($C_8H_8N_4.HCl$) in 1 g

Assay Weigh accurately a portion of Hydralazine Hydrochloride Powder, equivalent to about 0.15 g of hydralazine hydrochloride ($C_8H_8N_4.HCl$), transfer it to a glass-stoppered flask, add 25 mL of water, shake well, add 25 mL of hydrochloric acid, cool to room temperature, and proceed as directed in the Assay under Hydralazine Hydrochloride.

Each mL of 0.05 mol/L potassium iodate VS
= 9.832 mg of $C_8H_8N_4.HCl$

Containers and storage Containers—Tight containers.

Hydralazine Hydrochloride Tablets

ヒドララジン塩酸塩錠

Hydralazine Hydrochloride Tablets contain not less than 95.0% and not more than 105.0% of the labeled amount of hydralazine hydrochloride ($C_8H_8N_4.HCl$: 196.64).

Method of preparation Prepare as directed under Tablets, with Hydralazine Hydrochloride.

Identification Weigh a quantity of powdered Hydralazine Hydrochloride Tablets, equivalent to 25 mg of Hydralazine Hydrochloride, add 100 mL of water, mix well, and filter if necessary. To 2 mL of this solution add water to make 50 mL, and determine the absorption spectrum of this solution as directed under Ultraviolet-visible Spectrophotometry <*2.24*>: it exhibits maxima between 238 nm and 242 nm, between 258 nm and 262 nm, between 301 nm and 305 nm and between 313 nm and 317 nm.

Uniformity of dosage units <*6.02*> Perform the test according to the following method: it meets the requirement of the Content uniformity test.

To 1 tablet of Hydralazine Hydrochloride Tablets add 25 mL of 0.1 mol/L hydrochloric acid TS, disperse the tablet into a small particles by sonicating, then shake well, add 0.1 mol/L hydrochloric acid TS to make exactly 50 mL, and centrifuge. Pipet V mL of the supernatant liquid, add 0.1 mol/L hydrochloric acid TS to make exactly V' mL so that each mL contains about 10 μg of hydralazine hydrochloride ($C_8H_8N_4.HCl$), and use this solution as the sample solution. Separately, weigh accurately about 25 mg of hydralazine hydrochloride for assay, previously dried at 105°C for 3 hours, dissolve in 0.1 mol/L hydrochloric acid TS to make exactly 50 mL. Pipet 2 mL of this solution, add 0.1 mol/L hydrochloric acid TS to make exactly 100 mL, and use this solution as the standard solution. Determine the absorbances at 260 nm, A_{T1} and A_{S1}, and at 350 nm, A_{T2} and A_{S2}, of the sample solution and standard solution as directed under Ultraviolet-visible Spectrophotometry <*2.24*>.

Amount (mg) of hydralazine hydrochloride ($C_8H_8N_4.HCl$)
$= M_S \times (A_{T1} - A_{T2})/(A_{S1} - A_{S2}) \times V'/V \times 1/50$

M_S: Amount (mg) of hydralazine hydrochloride for assay taken

Dissolution <*6.10*> When the test is performed at 50 revolutions per minute according to the Paddle method, using 900 mL of water as the dissolution medium, the dissolution rate in 45 minutes of Hydralazine Hydrochloride Tablets is not less than 80%.

Start the test with 1 tablet of Hydralazine Hydrochloride Tablets, withdraw not less than 20 mL of the medium at the specified minute after starting the test, and filter through a membrane filter with a pore size not exceeding 0.8 μm.

Discard not less than 10 mL of the first filtrate, pipet V mL of the subsequent filtrate, add water to make exactly V' mL so that each mL contains about 11 μg of hydralazine hydrochloride ($C_8H_8N_4.HCl$), and use this solution as the sample solution. Separately, weigh accurately about 50 mg of hydralazine hydrochloride for assay, previously dried at 105°C for 3 hours, and dissolve in water to make exactly 50 mL. Pipet 1 mL of this solution, add water to make exactly 100 mL, and use this solution as the standard solution. Determine the absorbances, A_T and A_S, of the sample solution and standard solution at 260 nm as directed under Ultraviolet-visible Spectrophotometry <2.24>.

Dissolution rate (%) with respect to the labeled amount of hydralazine hydrochloride ($C_8H_8N_4.HCl$)
$= M_S \times A_T/A_S \times V'/V \times 1/C \times 18$

M_S: Amount (mg) of hydralazine hydrochloride for assay taken
C: Labeled amount (mg) of hydralazine hydrochloride ($C_8H_8N_4.HCl$) in 1 tablet

Assay Weigh accurately not less than 20 Hydralazine Hydrochloride Tablets, and powder. Weigh accurately a portion of the powder, equivalent to about 0.15 g of hydralazine hydrochloride ($C_8H_8N_4.HCl$), transfer it to a glass-stoppered flask, and proceed as directed in the Assay under Hydralazine Hydrochloride.

Each mL of 0.05 mol/L potassium iodate VS
= 9.832 mg of $C_8H_8N_4.HCl$

Containers and storage Containers—Tight containers.

Hydrochloric Acid

塩酸

Hydrochloric Acid contains not less than 35.0% and not more than 38.0% of hydrogen chloride (HCl: 36.46).

Description Hydrochloric Acid is a colorless liquid having a pungent odor.

It is fuming but ceases to fume when it is diluted with 2 volumes of water.

Specific gravity d^{20}_{20}: about 1.18.

Identification (1) Allow a glass stick wet with ammonia TS to come near the surface of Hydrochloric Acid: a remarkable white smoke evolves.

(2) A solution of Hydrochloric Acid (1 in 100) changes blue litmus paper to red, and responds to Qualitative Tests <1.09> for chloride.

Purity (1) Sulfate <1.14>—To 15 mL of Hydrochloric Acid add water to make 50 mL, and use this solution as the sample solution. To 3.0 mL of the sample solution add 5 mL of water and 5 drops of barium chloride TS, and allow to stand for 1 hour: no turbidity is produced.

(2) Sulfite—To 3.0 mL of the sample solution obtained in (1) add 5 ml of water and 1 drop of iodine TS: the color of iodine TS does not disappear.

(3) Bromide or iodide—Place 10 mL of the sample solution obtained in (1) in a glass-stoppered test tube, add 1 mL of chloroform and 1 drop of 0.002 mol/L potassium permanganate VS, and shake well: the chloroform layer remains colorless.

(4) Bromine or chlorine—Place 10 mL of the sample solution obtained in (1) in a glass-stoppered test tube, add 5 drops of potassium iodide TS and 1 mL of chloroform, and shake for 1 minute: the chloroform layer remains free from a purple color.

(5) Heavy metals <1.07>—Evaporate 5 mL of Hydrochloric Acid on a water bath to dryness, and add 2 mL of dilute acetic acid and water to the residue to make 50 mL. Perform the test using this solution as the test solution. Prepare the control solution as follows: to 3.0 mL of Standard Lead Solution add 2 mL of dilute acetic acid and water to make 50 mL (not more than 5 ppm).

(6) Arsenic <1.11>—Prepare the test solution with 1.7 mL of Hydrochloric Acid according to Method 1, and perform the test (not more than 1 ppm).

(7) Mercury—Dilute 20 mL of Hydrochloric Acid with water to make exactly 100 mL, and use the solution as the sample solution. Perform the test with the sample solution as directed under Atomic Absorption Spectrophotometry <2.23> (cold vapor type). Place the sample solution in a sample bottle of the atomic absorption spectrophotometer, add 10 mL of tin (II) chloride-sulfuric acid TS, connect the bottle immediately to the spectrophotometer, circulate air, and determine the absorbance A_T of the sample solution after the recorder reading has risen rapidly, and becomes constant at a wavelength of 253.7 nm. On the other hand, to 8 mL of Standard Mercury Solution add water to make exactly 100 mL, and determine the absorbance A_S of the solution obtained by the same procedure as used for the sample solution: A_T is smaller than A_S (not more than 0.04 ppm).

Residue on ignition <2.44> Pipet 10 mL of Hydrochloric Acid, add 2 drops of sulfuric acid, evaporate to dryness, and ignite: not more than 1.0 mg of residue remains.

Assay Weigh accurately a glass-stoppered flask containing 20 mL of water, add about 3 mL of Hydrochloric Acid, and weigh accurately again. Dilute with 25 mL of water, and titrate <2.50> with 1 mol/L sodium hydroxide VS (indicator: 2 to 3 drops of methyl red TS).

Each mL of 1 mol/L sodium hydroxide VS
= 36.46 mg of HCl

Containers and storage Containers—Tight containers.

Dilute Hydrochloric Acid

希塩酸

Dilute Hydrochloric Acid contains not less than 9.5 w/v% and not more than 10.5 w/v% of hydrogen chloride (HCl: 36.46).

Description Dilute Hydrochloric Acid is a colorless liquid. It is odorless and has a strong acid taste.

Specific gravity d^{20}_{20}: about 1.05.

Identification A solution of Dilute Hydrochloric Acid (1 in 30) changes blue litmus paper to red and responds to Qualitative Tests <1.09> for chloride.

Purity (1) Sulfate—To 3.0 mL of Dilute Hydrochloric Acid add 5 mL of water and 5 drops of barium chloride TS, and allow to stand for 1 hour: no turbidity is produced.

(2) Sulfite—To 3.0 mL of Dilute Hydrochloric Acid add 5 mL of water and 1 drop of iodine TS: the color of iodine TS does not disappear.

(3) Bromide or iodide—Place 10 mL of Dilute Hydrochloric Acid in a glass-stoppered test tube, add 1 mL of chlo-

roform and 1 drop of 0.002 mol/L potassium permanganate VS, and shake well: the chloroform layer remains colorless.

(4) Bromine or chlorine—Place 10 mL of Dilute Hydrochloric Acid in a glass-stoppered test tube, add 5 drops of potassium iodide TS and 1 mL of chloroform, and shake for 1 minute: the chloroform layer remains free from a purple color.

(5) Heavy metals *〈1.07〉*—Evaporate 9.5 mL of Dilute Hydrochloric Acid on a water bath to dryness, add 2 mL of dilute acetic acid and water to make 50 mL, and perform the test using this solution as the test solution. Prepare the control solution as follows: to 3.0 mL of Standard Lead Solution add 2 mL of dilute acetic acid and water to make 50 mL (not more than 3 ppm).

(6) Arsenic *〈1.11〉*—Prepare the test solution with 4.0 mL of Dilute Hydrochloric Acid according to Method 1, and perform the test (not more than 0.5 ppm).

(7) Mercury—Dilute 80 mL of Dilute Hydrochloric Acid with water to make exactly 100 mL, and use this solution as the sample solution. Perform the test with the sample solution as directed under Atomic Absorption Spectrophotometry *〈2.23〉* (cold vapor type). Place the sample solution in a sample bottle of the atomic absorption spectrophotometer, add 10 mL of tin (II) chloride-sulfuric acid TS, connect the bottle immediately to the spectrophotometer, circulate air, and determine the absorbance A_T of the sample solution after the recorder reading has risen rapidly and become constant at a wavelength of 253.7 nm. On the other hand, to 8 mL of Standard Mercury Solution add water to make exactly 100 mL, and determine the absorbance A_S of the solution obtained by the same procedure as used for the sample solution: A_T is smaller than A_S (not more than 0.01 ppm).

Residue on ignition *〈2.44〉* Pipet 10 mL of Dilute Hydrochloric Acid, add 2 drops of sulfuric acid, evaporate to dryness, and ignite: the mass of the residue is not more than 1.0 mg.

Assay Measure exactly 10 mL of Dilute Hydrochloric Acid, and dilute with 20 mL of water. Titrate *〈2.50〉* with 1 mol/L sodium hydroxide VS (indicator: 2 to 3 drops of methyl red TS).

Each mL of 1 mol/L sodium hydroxide VS
= 36.46 mg of HCl

Containers and storage Containers—Tight containers.

Hydrochloric Acid Lemonade

塩酸リモナーデ

Method of preparation

Dilute Hydrochloric Acid	5 mL
Simple Syrup	80 mL
Purified Water or Purified Water in Containers	a sufficient quantity
	To make 1000 mL

Prepare before use as directed under Lemonades, with the above ingredients.

Description Hydrochloric Acid Lemonade is a clear, colorless liquid. It has a sweet, cool, acid taste.

Containers and storage Containers—Tight containers.

Hydrochlorothiazide

ヒドロクロロチアジド

$C_7H_8ClN_3O_4S_2$: 297.74
6-Chloro-3,4-dihydro-2*H*-1,2,4-benzothiadiazine-7-sulfonamide 1,1-dioxide
[*58-93-5*]

Hydrochlorothiazide, when dried, contains not less than 99.0% of hydrochlorothiazide ($C_7H_8ClN_3O_4S_2$).

Description Hydrochlorothiazide occurs as white, crystals or crystalline powder. It is odorless, and has a slightly bitter taste.

It is freely soluble in acetone, sparingly soluble in acetonitrile, very slightly soluble in water and in ethanol (95), and practically insoluble in diethyl ether.

It dissolves in sodium hydroxide TS.

Melting point: about 267°C (with decomposition).

Identification **(1)** To 5 mg of Hydrochlorothiazide add 5 mL of chromotropic acid TS, and allow to stand for 5 minutes: a purple color develops.

(2) Fuse a mixture of 0.1 g of Hydrochlorothiazide and 0.5 g of sodium carbonate decahydrate cautiously: the gas evolved changes moistened red litmus paper to blue. After cooling, crush with a glass rod, add 10 mL of water, stir, and filter. To 4 mL of the filtrate add 2 drops of hydrogen peroxide (30), 5 mL of diluted hydrochloric acid (1 in 5) and 2 to 3 drops of barium chloride TS: a white precipitate is produced.

(3) To 4 mL of the filtrate obtained in (2) add 5 mL of dilute nitric acid and 3 drops of silver nitrate TS: a white precipitate is produced.

(4) Dissolve 12 mg of Hydrochlorothiazide in 100 mL of sodium hydroxide TS. Dilute 10 mL of the solution with water to make 100 mL. Determine the absorption spectrum of the solution as directed under Ultraviolet-visible Spectrophotometry *〈2.24〉*, and compare the spectrum with the Reference Spectrum or the spectrum of a solution of Hydrochlorothiazide RS prepared in the same manner as the sample solution: both spectra exhibit similar intensities of absorption at the same wavelengths.

Purity **(1)** Chloride *〈1.03〉*—Dissolve 1.0 g of Hydrochlorothiazide in 30 mL of acetone, add 6 mL of dilute nitric acid and water to make 50 mL, and perform the test using this solution as the test solution. Prepare the control solution as follows: to 1.0 mL of 0.01 mol/L hydrochloric acid VS add 30 mL of acetone, 6 mL of dilute nitric acid and water to make 50 mL (not more than 0.036%).

(2) Sulfate *〈1.14〉*—Dissolve 1.0 g of Hydrochlorothiazide in 30 mL of acetone, add 1 mL of dilute hydrochloric acid and water to make 50 mL, and perform the test using this solution as the test solution. Prepare the control solution as follows: to 1.0 mL of 0.005 mol/L sulfuric acid VS add 30 mL of acetone, 1 mL of dilute hydrochloric acid and water to make 50 mL (not more than 0.048%).

(3) Heavy metals *〈1.07〉*—Proceed with 1.0 g of Hydrochlorothiazide according to Method 2, and perform the test. Prepare the control solution with 2.0 mL of Standard Lead Solution (not more than 20 ppm).

(4) Primary aromatic amines—Dissolve 80 mg of Hydrochlorothiazide in acetone to make exactly 100 mL. Measure exactly 1 mL of the solution, add 3.0 mL of dilute hydrochloric acid, 3.0 mL of water and 0.15 mL of sodium nitrite TS, shake, and allow to stand for 1 minute. Shake this solution with 1.0 mL of ammonium amidosulfate TS, allow to stand for 3 minutes, then add 1.0 mL of *N,N*-diethyl-*N′*-1-naphthylenediamine oxalate TS, shake, and allow to stand for 5 minutes. Perform the test with this solution as directed under Ultraviolet-visible Spectrophotometry <2.24>, using a solution prepared with 1.0 mL of acetone in the same manner as the blank: the absorbance at 525 nm is not more than 0.10.

Loss on drying <2.41> Not more than 1.0% (1 g, 105°C, 2 hours).

Residue on ignition <2.44> Not more than 0.1% (1 g).

Assay Weigh accurately about 30 mg each of Hydrochlorothiazide and Hydrochlorothiazide RS, previously dried, and dissolve in 150 mL of the mobile phase, add exactly 10 mL each of the internal standard solution, then add the mobile phase to make 200 mL, and use these solutions as the sample solution and the standard solution, respectively. Perform the test with 20 μL each of the sample solution and standard solution as directed under Liquid Chromatography <2.01> according to the following conditions, and calculate the ratios, Q_T and Q_S, of the peak area of hydrochlorothiazide to that of the internal standard.

Amount (mg) of hydrochlorothiazide ($C_7H_8ClN_3O_4S_2$)
$= M_S \times Q_T/Q_S$

M_S: Amount (mg) of Hydrochlorothiazide RS taken

Internal standard solution—A solution of 4-aminoacetophenone in acetonitrile (9 in 2000).

Operating conditions—

Detector: An ultraviolet absorption photometer (wavelength: 254 nm).

Column: A stainless steel column 4.6 mm in inside diameter and 25 cm in length, packed with octadecylsilanized silica gel for liquid chromatography (5 μm in particle diameter).

Column temperature: A constant temperature of about 25°C.

Mobile phase: A mixture of 0.1 mol/L sodium dihydrogen phosphate TS (pH 3.0) and acetonitrile (9:1).

Flow rate: Adjust so that the retention time of hydrochlorothiazide is about 10 minutes.

System suitability—

System performance: When the procedure is run with 20 μL of the standard solution under the above operating conditions, hydrochlorothiazide and the internal standard are eluted in this order with the resolution between these peaks being not less than 4.

System repeatability: When the test is repeated 6 times with 20 μL of the standard solution under the above operating conditions, the relative standard deviation of the ratios of the peak area of hydrochlorothiazide to that of the internal standard is not more than 1.0%.

Containers and storage Containers—Well-closed containers.

Hydrocortisone

ヒドロコルチゾン

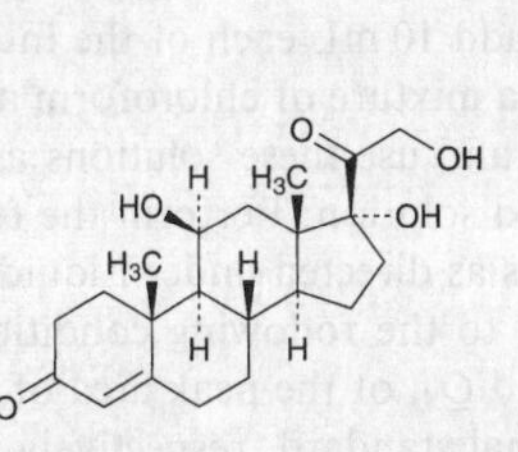

$C_{21}H_{30}O_5$: 362.46
11β,17,21-Trihydroxypregn-4-ene-3,20-dione
[50-23-7]

Hydrocortisone, when dried, contains not less than 97.0% and not more than 102.0% of hydrocortisone ($C_{21}H_{30}O_5$).

Description Hydrocortisone occurs as a white crystalline powder.

It is sparingly soluble in methanol and in ethanol (99.5), and very slightly soluble in water.

Melting point: 212 – 220°C (with decomposition).

It shows crystal polymorphism.

Identification **(1)** Add 2 mL of sulfuric acid to 2 mg of Hydrocortisone: the solution shows a yellow-green fluorescence immediately, and the color of the solution changes gradually from orange to dark red. Dilute carefully the solution with 10 mL of water: the color changes through yellow to orange-yellow with green fluorescence, and a small amount of a flocculent precipitate is formed.

(2) Dissolve 0.01 g of Hydrocortisone in 1 mL of methanol, add 1 mL of Fehling's TS, and heat: a red precipitate is formed.

(3) Determine the infrared absorption spectrum of Hydrocortisone, previously dried, as directed in the potassium bromide disk method under Infrared Spectrophotometry <2.25>, and compare the spectrum with the Reference Spectrum or the spectrum of previously dried Hydrocortisone RS: both spectra exhibit similar intensities of absorption at the same wave numbers. If any difference appears between the spectra, dissolve Hydrocortisone and Hydrocortisone RS in ethanol (95), respectively, then evaporate the ethanol to dryness, and repeat the test on the residues.

Optical rotation <2.49> $[\alpha]_D^{25}$: +160 – +170° (after drying, 0.1 g, ethanol (99.5), 10 mL, 100 mm).

Purity Related substances—Dissolve 20 mg of Hydrocortisone in 10 mL of a mixture of chloroform and methanol (9:1), and use this solution as the sample solution. Pipet 1 mL of the sample solution, add a mixture of chloroform and methanol (9:1) to make exactly 50 mL, and use this solution as the standard solution. Perform the test with these solutions as directed under Thin-layer Chromatography <2.03>. Spot 10 μL each of the sample solution and standard solution on a plate of silica gel with fluorescent indicator for thin-layer chromatography. Develop the plate with a mixture of chloroform and ethanol (95) (17:3) to a distance of about 10 cm, and air-dry the plate. Examine under ultraviolet light (main wavelength: 254 nm): the spots other than the principal spot obtained from the sample solution are not more intense than the spot from the standard solution.

Loss on drying <2.41> Not more than 1.0% (0.5 g, 105°C, 3 hours).

Residue on ignition <2.44> Not more than 0.1% (0.5 g).

Assay Dissolve about 20 mg each of Hydrocortisone and Hydrocortisone RS, previously dried and accurately weighed, in 20 mL each of a mixture of chloroform and methanol (9:1), add 10 mL each of the internal standard solution, then add a mixture of chloroform and methanol (9:1) to make 50 mL, and use these solutions as the sample solution and standard solution. Perform the test with 5 μL each of these solutions as directed under Liquid Chromatography <*2.01*> according to the following conditions, and calculate the ratios, Q_T and Q_S, of the peak area of hydrocortisone to that of the internal standard, respectively.

Amount (mg) of hydrocortisone ($C_{21}H_{30}O_5$) = $M_S \times Q_T/Q_S$

M_S: Amount (mg) of Hydrocortisone RS taken

Internal standard solution—A solution of prednisone in a mixture of chloroform and methanol (9:1) (9 in 10,000).

Operating conditions—

Detector: An ultraviolet absorption photometer (wavelength: 254 nm).

Column: A stainless steel column 4.6 mm in inside diameter and 25 cm in length, packed with silica gel for liquid chromatography (5 μm in particle diameter).

Column temperature: A constant temperature of about 20°C.

Mobile phase: A mixture of chloroform, methanol and acetic acid (100) (1000:20:1).

Flow rate: Adjust so that the retention time of hydrocortisone is about 15 minutes.

System suitability—

System performance: When the procedure is run with 5 μL of the standard solution under the above operating conditions, the internal standard and hydrocortisone are eluted in this order with the resolution between these peaks being not less than 7.

System repeatability: When the test is repeated 6 times with 5 μL of the standard solution under the above operating conditions, the relative standard deviation of the ratios of the peak area of hydrocortisone to that of the internal standard is not more than 1.0%.

Containers and storage Containers—Tight containers.

Hydrocortisone Acetate

ヒドロコルチゾン酢酸エステル

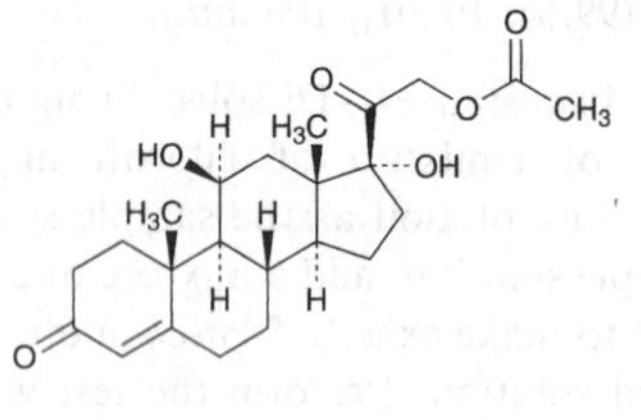

$C_{23}H_{32}O_6$: 404.50

11β,17,21-Trihydroxypregn-4-ene-3,20-dione 21-acetate

[*50-03-3*]

Hydrocortisone Acetate, when dried, contains not less than 97.0% and not more than 102.0% of hydrocortisone acetate ($C_{23}H_{32}O_6$).

Description Hydrocortisone Acetate occurs as white, crystals or crystalline powder.

It is freely soluble in dimethylsulfoxide, slightly soluble in methanol and in ethanol (95), and practically insoluble in water.

Melting point: about 220°C (with decomposition).

It shows crystal polymorphism.

Identification **(1)** Add 2 mL of sulfuric acid to 2 mg of Hydrocortisone Acetate: the solution shows a yellowish green fluorescence immediately, and the color of the solution gradually changes through orange-yellow to dark red. This solution shows a strong light green fluorescence under ultraviolet light. Add carefully 10 mL of water to this solution: the color changes from yellow to orange-yellow with a light green fluorescence, and a yellow-brown, flocculent precipitate is formed.

(2) Dissolve 0.01 g of Hydrocortisone Acetate in 1 mL of methanol by warming, add 1 mL of Fehling's TS, and heat: an orange to red precipitate is formed.

(3) To 0.05 g of Hydrocortisone Acetate add 2 mL of potassium hydroxide-ethanol TS, and heat on a water bath for 5 minutes. Cool, add 2 mL of diluted sulfuric acid (2 in 7), and boil gently for 1 minute: the odor of ethyl acetate is perceptible.

(4) Determine the infrared absorption spectra of Hydrocortisone Acetate and Hydrocortisone Acetate RS, previously dried, as directed in the potassium bromide disk method under Infrared Spectrophotometry <*2.25*>: both the sample and the RS exhibit similar intensities of absorption at the same wave numbers. If any difference appears, dissolve the sample and the Reference Standard in ethanol (95), respectively, evaporate to dryness, and repeat the test on the residues.

Optical rotation <*2.49*> $[\alpha]_D^{25}$: +154 – +164° (after drying, 50 mg, dimethylsulfoxide, 10 mL, 100 mm).

Purity Related substances—Dissolve 40 mg of Hydrocortisone Acetate in 25 mL of a mixture of chloroform and methanol (9:1), and use this solution as the sample solution. Pipet 2 mL of the sample solution, add a mixture of chloroform and methanol (9:1) to make exactly 100 mL, and use this solution as the standard solution. Perform the test with these solutions as directed under Thin-layer Chromatography <*2.03*>. Spot 5 μL each of the sample solution and standard solution on a plate of silica gel for thin-layer chromatography. Develop the plate with a mixture of dichloromethane, diethyl ether, methanol and water (160:30:8:1) to a distance of about 12 cm, and air-dry the plate. Spray evenly alkaline blue tetrazolium TS on the plate: the spots other than the principal spot obtained from the sample solution are not more intense than the spot from the standard solution.

Loss on drying <*2.41*> Not more than 1.0% (0.5 g, 105°C, 3 hours).

Residue on ignition <*2.44*> Not more than 0.1% (0.5 g).

Assay Dissolve about 20 mg each of Hydrocortisone Acetate and Hydrocortisone Acetate RS, previously dried and accurately weighed, in methanol, add exactly 10 mL each of the internal standard solution, then add methanol to make 100 mL, and use these solutions as the sample solution and standard solution. Perform the test with 20 μL each of the sample solution and standard solution as directed under Liquid Chromatography <*2.01*> according to the following conditions, and calculate the ratios, Q_T and Q_S, of the peak area of hydrocortisone acetate to that of the internal standard, respectively.

Amount (mg) of hydrocortisone acetate ($C_{23}H_{32}O_6$)
= $M_S \times Q_T/Q_S$

M_S: Amount (mg) of Hydrocortisone Acetate RS taken

Internal standard solution—A solution of benzyl parahydroxybenzoate in methanol (1 in 1000).

Operating conditions—

Detector: An ultraviolet absorption photometer (wavelength: 254 nm).

Column: A stainless steel column 3.9 mm in inside diameter and 30 cm in length, packed with octadecylsilanized silica gel for liquid chromatography (10 μm in particle diameter).

Column temperature: A constant temperature of about 25°C.

Mobile phase: A mixture of water and acetonitrile (13:7).

Flow rate: Adjust so that the retention time of hydrocortisone acetate is about 8 minutes.

System suitability—

System performance: When the procedure is run with 20 μL of the standard solution under the above operating conditions, hydrocortisone acetate and the internal standard are eluted in this order with the resolution between these peaks being not less than 4.

System repeatability: When the test is repeated 6 times with 20 μL of the standard solution under the above operating conditions, the relative standard deviation of the ratios of the peak area of hydrocortisone acetate to that of the internal standard is not more than 1.0%.

Containers and storage Containers—Tight containers.

Hydrocortisone and Diphenhydramine Ointment

ヒドロコルチゾン·ジフェンヒドラミン軟膏

Method of preparation

Hydrocortisone Acetate	5 g
Diphenhydramine	5 g
White Petrolatum	a sufficient quantity
To make	1000 g

Prepare as directed under Ointments, with the above ingredients.

Description Hydrocortisone and Diphenhydramine Ointment is white to pale yellow in color.

Identification **(1)** To 1 g of Hydrocortisone and Diphenhydramine Ointment add 10 mL of ethanol (95), heat on a water bath for 5 minutes with occasional shaking, cool, and filter. Take 5 mL of the filtrate, distill off the ethanol, and to the residue add 2 mL of sulfuric acid: the solution shows a yellow-green fluorescence immediately and the color of the solution gradually changes through yellow to yellow-brown. Add carefully 10 mL of water to this solution: the color changes to yellow with green fluorescence, and a light yellow, flocculent precipitate is formed (hydrocortisone acetate).

(2) To 1 mL of the filtrate obtained in (1) add 5 mL of potassium hydrogen phthalate buffer solution (pH 4.6) and 2 mL of bromophenol blue TS, and add further 5 mL of chloroform. Shake well, and allow to stand: a yellow color develops in the chloroform layer (diphenhydramine).

(3) To 0.2 g of Hydrocortisone and Diphenhydramine Ointment add 0.5 mL of methanol, warm, and shake. After cooling, separate the methanol layer, and use this layer as the sample solution. Dissolve 10 mg each of hydrocortisone acetate and diphenhydramine in 10 mL each of methanol, and use these solutions as standard solutions (1) and (2). Perform the test with these solutions as directed under Thin-layer Chromatography <*2.03*>. Spot 5 μL each of the sample solution and standard solutions (1) and (2) on a plate of silica gel with fluorescent indicator for thin-layer chromatography. Develop the plate with a mixture of ethyl acetate and diethyl ether (4:1) to a distance of about 5 cm, and air-dry the plate. Examine under ultraviolet light (main wavelength: 254 nm): two spots obtained from the sample solution show the same *Rf* value as the corresponding spots from standard solutions (1) and (2).

Containers and storage Containers—Tight containers.

Storage—Light-resistant.

Hydrocortisone Butyrate

ヒドロコルチゾン酪酸エステル

$C_{25}H_{36}O_6$: 432.55

11β,17,21-Trihydroxypregn-4-ene-3,20-dione 17-butanoate

[*13609-67-1*]

Hydrocortisone Butyrate, when dried, contains not less than 96.0% and not more than 104.0% of hydrocortisone butyrate ($C_{25}H_{36}O_6$).

Description Hydrocortisone Butyrate occurs as a white powder. It is odorless.

It is freely soluble in chloroform, soluble in methanol, sparingly soluble in ethanol (99.5) and practically insoluble in water.

Melting point: about 200°C (with decomposition).

Identification **(1)** Add 2 mL of sulfuric acid to 2 mg of Hydrocortisone Butyrate: the solution shows a yellowish green fluorescence immediately, and the color of the solution gradually changes through orange-yellow to dark red. This solution shows a strong light green fluorescence under ultraviolet light (main wavelength: 254 nm). Add carefully 10 mL of water to this solution: the color changes from yellow to orange-yellow with a light green fluorescence, and a yellow-brown, flocculent precipitate is formed.

(2) Dissolve 0.01 g of Hydrocortisone Butyrate in 1 mL of methanol by warming, add 1 mL of Fehling's TS, and heat: an orange to red precipitate is formed.

(3) To 50 mg of Hydrocortisone Butyrate add 2 mL of potassium hydrox-ide-ethanol TS, and heat on a water bath for 5 minutes. Cool, add 2 mL of diluted sulfuric acid (2 in 7), and boil gently for 1 minute: the odor of ethyl butyrate is perceptible.

(4) Determine the infrared absorption spectrum of Hydrocortisone Butyrate, previously dried, as directed in the potassium bromide disk method under Infrared Spectrophotometry <*2.25*>, and compare the spectrum with the Reference Spectrum: both spectra exhibit similar intensities of absorption at the same wave numbers.

Optical rotation <*2.49*> $[\alpha]_D^{25}$: +48 – +52° (after drying, 0.1 g, chloroform, 10 mL, 100 mm).

Purity **(1)** Heavy metals <*1.07*>—Proceed with 1.0 g of

Hydrocortisone Butyrate according to Method 2, and perform the test. Prepare the control solution with 2.0 mL of Standard Lead Solution (not more than 20 ppm).

(2) Related substances—Dissolve 50 mg of Hydrocortisone Butyrate in 50 mL of a mixture of acetonitrile and the mobile phase A (4:1), and use this solution as the sample solution. Pipet 1 mL of the sample solution, add a mixture of acetonitrile and the mobile phase A (4:1) to make exactly 100 mL, and use this solution as the standard solution. Perform the test with exactly 5 μL each of the sample solution and standard solution as directed under Liquid Chromatography <*2.01*> according to the following conditions. Determine each peak area by the automatic integration method: the area of the peak other than hydrocortisone butyrate obtained from the sample solution is not larger than the peak area of hydrocortisone butyrate from the standard solution, and the total area of the peaks other than hydrocortisone butyrate from the sample solution is not larger than 2 times the peak area of hydrocortisone butyrate from the standard solution.

Operating conditions—

Detector: An ultraviolet absorption photometer (wavelength: 254 nm).

Column: A stainless steel column 4.6 mm in inside diameter and 10 cm in length, packed with octadecylsilanized silica gel for liquid chromatography (3 μm in particle diameter).

Column temperature: A constant temperature of about 25°C.

Mobile phase A: Dissolve 1 g of potassium dihydrogen phosphate in 1000 mL of water, and adjust to pH 5.5 with potassium hydroxide TS.

Mobile phase B: Acetonitrile.

Flowing of mobile phase: Control the gradient by mixing the mobile phases A and B as directed in the following table.

Time after injection of sample (min)	Mobile phase A (vol%)	Mobile phase B (vol%)
0 – 12.5	80 → 35	20 → 65
12.5 – 15.5	35	65

Flow rate: 2.0 mL per minute.

Time span of measurement: For 15.5 minutes after injection, beginning after the solvent peak.

System suitability—

Test for required detectability: Pipet 1 mL of the standard solution, and add a mixture of acetonitrile and the mobile phase A (4:1) to make exactly 20 mL. Confirm that the peak area of hydrocortisone butyrate obtained with 5 μL of this solution is equivalent to 3.5 to 6.5% of that with 5 μL of the standard solution.

System performance: When the procedure is run with 5 μL of the standard solution under the above operating conditions, the number of theoretical plates and the symmetry factor of the peak of hydrocortisone butyrate are not less than 10,000 and not more than 1.5, respectively.

System repeatability: When the test is repeated 6 times with 5 μL of the standard solution under the above operating conditions, the relative standard deviation of the peak area of hydrocortisone butyrate is not more than 2.0%.

Loss on drying <*2.41*> Not more than 1.0% (1 g, 105°C, 3 hours).

Residue on ignition <*2.44*> Not more than 0.1% (1 g).

Assay Weigh accurately about 50 mg of Hydrocortisone Butyrate, previously dried, and dissolve in ethanol (99.5) to make exactly 100 mL. Pipet 2 mL of this solution, and add ethanol (99.5) to make exactly 50 mL. Determine the absorbance A of this solution at the wavelength of maximum absorption at about 241 nm as directed under Ultraviolet-visible Spectrophotometry <*2.24*>.

Amount (mg) of hydrocortisone butyrate ($C_{25}H_{36}O_6$)
$= A/375 \times 25{,}000$

Containers and storage Containers—Tight containers.

Hydrocortisone Sodium Phosphate

ヒドロコルチゾンリン酸エステルナトリウム

$C_{21}H_{29}Na_2O_8P$: 486.40
11β,17,21-Trihydroxypregn-4-ene-3,20-dione 21-(disodium phosphate)
[*6000-74-4*]

Hydrocortisone Sodium Phosphate contains not less than 96.0% and not more than 102.0% of hydrocortisone sodium phosphate ($C_{21}H_{29}Na_2O_8P$), calculated on the anhydrous basis.

Description Hydrocortisone Sodium Phosphate occurs as a white to light yellow powder.

It is freely soluble in water, sparingly soluble in methanol, and very slightly soluble in ethanol (95).

It is hygroscopic.

It shows crystal polymorphism.

Identification (1) To 2 mg of Hydrocortisone Sodium Phosphate add 2 mL of sulfuric acid: a yellowish green fluorescence is exhibited initially, then gradually changes through orange-yellow to dark red. Examine the solution under ultraviolet light (main wavelength: 254 nm): an intense, light green fluorescence is exhibited. To this solution add carefully 10 mL of water: the color changes from yellow to orange-yellow with a light green fluorescence and a yellow-brown, flocculent floating substance is formed.

(2) Determine the infrared absorption spectrum of Hydrocortisone Sodium Phosphate as directed in the paste method under Infrared Spectrophotometry <*2.25*>, and compare the spectrum with the Reference Spectrum or the spectrum of Hydrocortisone Sodium Phosphate RS: both spectra exhibit similar intensities of absorption at the same wave numbers. If any difference appears between the spectra, dissolve Hydrocortisone Sodium Phosphate and Hydrocortisone Sodium Phosphate RS in methanol, respectively, then evaporate the methanol to dryness, and repeat the test on the residues.

(3) Moisten 1.0 g of Hydrocortisone Sodium Phosphate with a small quantity of sulfuric acid, and incinerate by gradual heating. After cooling, dissolve the residue in 10 mL of dilute nitric acid, and heat in a water bath for 30 minutes. After cooling, filter if necessary. This solution responds to Qualitative Tests <*1.09*> for sodium salt and for phosphate.

Optical rotation <*2.49*> $[\alpha]_D^{20}$: +123 – +131° (1 g calculated on the anhydrous basis, phosphate buffer solution (pH 7.0), 100 mL, 100 mm).

pH 〈2.54〉 Dissolve 1.0 g of Hydrocortisone Sodium Phosphate in 100 mL of water: the pH of this solution is between 7.5 and 9.5.

Purity **(1)** Clarity and color of solution—Dissolve 1.0 g of Hydrocortisone Sodium Phosphate in 10 mL of water: the solution is clear and colorless to pale yellow.

(2) Chloride 〈1.03〉—Dissolve 0.30 g of Hydrocortisone Sodium Phosphate in 20 mL of water, and add 6 mL of dilute nitric acid and water to make 100 mL. To 5 mL of this solution add water to make 50 mL. Perform the test using this solution as the test solution. Prepare the control solution with 0.25 mL of 0.01 mol/L hydrochloric acid VS (not more than 0.600%).

(3) Heavy metals 〈1.07〉—Proceed with 0.5 g of Hydrocortisone Sodium Phosphate according to Method 2, and perform the test. Prepare the control solution with 2.0 mL of Standard Lead Solution (not more than 40 ppm).

(4) Arsenic 〈1.11〉—Prepare the test solution with 1.0 g of Hydrocortisone Sodium Phosphate according to Method 3, and perform the test (not more than 2 ppm).

(5) Free phosphoric acid—Weigh accurately about 0.25 g of Hydrocortisone Sodium Phosphate, dissolve in water to make exactly 100 mL, and use this solution as the sample solution. Pipet 5 mL each of the sample solution and Standard Phosphoric Acid Solution into separate 25-mL volumetric flasks, add 2.5 mL of hexaammonium heptamolybdate-sulfuric acid TS and 1 mL of 1-amino-2-naphthol-4-sulfonic acid TS, shake, add water to make exactly 25 mL, and allow to stand at 20 ± 1°C for 30 minutes. Perform the test with these solutions as directed under Ultraviolet-visible Spectrophotometry 〈2.24〉, using a solution prepared with 5 mL of water in the same manner as the blank. Determine the absorbances, A_T and A_S, at 740 nm of the sample solution and Standard Phosphoric Acid Solution: the amount of free phosphoric acid is not more than 1.0%.

Content (%) of free phosphoric acid (H_3PO_4)
$= 1/M \times A_T/A_S \times 258.0$

M: Amount (mg) of Hydrocortisone Sodium Phosphate taken, calculated on the anhydrous basis

(6) Free hydrocortisone—Dissolve 25 mg of Hydrocortisone Sodium Phosphate in the mobile phase to make exactly 20 mL, and use this solution as the sample solution. Separately, weigh 25 mg of Hydrocortisone RS, previously dried at 105°C for 3 hours, and dissolve in the mobile phase to make exactly 100 mL. Pipet 10 mL of this solution, add the mobile phase to make exactly 200 mL, and use this solution as the standard solution. Perform the test with exactly 20 μL each of the sample solution and standard solution as directed under Liquid Chromatography 〈2.01〉 according to the following conditions. Determine the peak areas, A_T and A_S, of hydrocortisone in each solution: A_T is not larger than A_S.

Operating conditions—

Proceed as directed in the operating conditions in the Assay.

System suitability—

System performance: Proceed as directed in the system suitability in the Assay.

System repeatability: When the test is repeated 6 times with 20 μL of the standard solution under the above operating conditions, the relative standard deviation of the peak area of hydrocortisone is not more than 1.0%.

Water 〈2.48〉 Not more than 5.0% (30 mg, coulometric titration).

Assay Weigh accurately about 20 mg each of Hydrocortisone Sodium Phosphate and Hydrocortisone Sodium Phosphate RS (previously determine the water 〈2.48〉 in the same manner as Hydrocortisone Sodium Phosphate), dissolve each in 50 mL of the mobile phase, add exactly 10 mL of the internal standard solution, then add the mobile phase to make 200 mL, and use these solutions as the sample solution and the standard solution, respectively. Perform the test with 20 μL each of the sample solution and standard solution as directed under Liquid Chromatography 〈2.01〉 according to the following conditions, and calculate the ratios, Q_T and Q_S, of the peak area of hydrocortisone phosphate to that of the internal standard, respectively.

Amount (mg) of hydrocortisone sodium phosphate
($C_{21}H_{29}Na_2O_8P$)
$= M_S \times Q_T/Q_S$

M_S: Amount (mg) of Hydrocortisone Sodium Phosphate RS taken, calculated on the anhydrous basis

Internal standard solution—A solution of isopropyl parahydroxybenzoate in the mobile phase (3 in 5000).

Operating conditions—

Detector: An ultraviolet absorption photometer (wavelength: 254 nm).

Column: A stainless steel column 4.6 mm in inside diameter and 25 cm in length, packed with octadecylsilanized silica gel for liquid chromatography (7 μm in particle diameter).

Column temperature: A constant temperature of about 25°C.

Mobile phase: A mixture of 0.05 mol/L sodium dihydrogen phosphate TS (pH 2.6) and methanol (1:1).

Flow rate: Adjust so that the retention time of hydrocortisone phosphate is about 10 minutes.

System suitability—

System performance: When the procedure is run with 20 μL of the standard solution under the above operating conditions, hydrocortisone phosphate and the internal standard are eluted in this order with the resolution between these peaks being not less than 8.

System repeatability: When the test is repeated 6 times with 20 μL of the standard solution under the above operating conditions, the relative standard deviation of the ratios of the peak area of hydrocortisone phosphate to that of the internal standard is not more than 1.0%.

Containers and storage Containers—Tight containers.

Hydrocortisone Sodium Succinate

ヒドロコルチゾンコハク酸エステルナトリウム

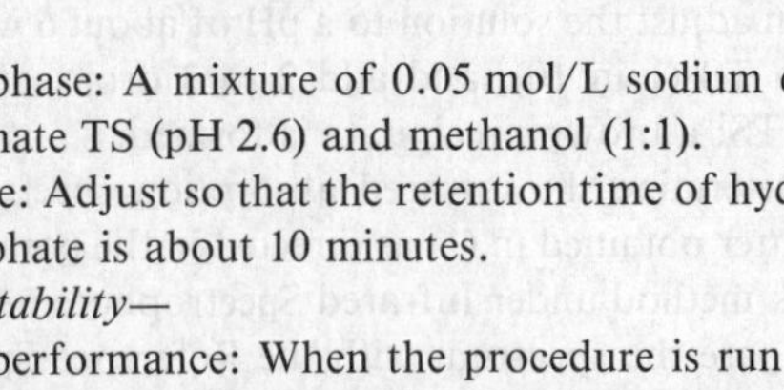

$C_{25}H_{33}NaO_8$: 484.51

Monosodium 11β,17,21-trihydroxypregn-4-ene-3,20-dione 21-succinate

[125-04-2]

Hydrocortisone Sodium Succinate, calculated on the dried basis, contains not less than 97.0% and not more than 103.0% of hydrocortisone sodium succinate ($C_{25}H_{33}NaO_8$).

Description Hydrocortisone Sodium Succinate occurs as a white, powder or masses.

It is freely soluble in water, in methanol and in ethanol (95).

It is hygroscopic.

It is gradually colored by light.

It shows crystal polymorphism.

Identification **(1)** Dissolve 0.2 g of Hydrocortisone Sodium Succinate in 20 mL of water, and add 0.5 mL of dilute hydrochloric acid with stirring: a white precipitate is formed. Collect the precipitate, wash it with two 10-mL portions of water, and dry at 105°C for 3 hours. To 3 mg of this dried matter add 2 mL of sulfuric acid: the solution shows a yellowish green fluorescence immediately, and the color of the solution gradually changes through orange-yellow to dark red. This solution shows a strong light green fluorescence under ultraviolet light. Add carefully 10 mL of water to this solution: the color changes from yellow to orange-yellow with a light green fluorescence, and a yellow-brown flocculent precipitate is formed.

(2) Dissolve 10 mg of the dried matter obtained in (1) in 1 mL of methanol, add 1 mL of Fehling's TS, and heat: an orange to red precipitate is formed.

(3) To 0.1 g of the dried matter obtained in (1) add 2 mL of sodium hydroxide TS, and allow to stand for 10 minutes. Filter the solution to remove the precipitate formed, mix the filtrate with 1 mL of dilute hydrochloric acid, filter if necessary, then adjust the solution to a pH of about 6 with diluted ammonia TS (1 in 10), and add 2 to 3 drops of iron (III) chloride TS: a brown precipitate is formed.

(4) Determine the infrared absorption spectrum of the dried matter obtained in (1) as directed in the potassium bromide disk method under Infrared Spectrophotometry *<2.25>*, and compare the spectrum with the Reference Spectrum or the spectrum of previously dried Hydrocortisone Succinate RS: both spectra exhibit similar intensities of absorption at the same wave numbers. If any difference appears between the spectra, dissolve Hydrocortisone Sodium Succinate and Hydrocortisone Succinate RS in methanol, respectively, then evaporate the methanol to dryness, and repeat the test on the residues.

(5) Hydrocortisone Sodium Succinate responds to Qualitative Tests *<1.09>* (1) for sodium salt.

Optical rotation *<2.49>* $[\alpha]_D^{20}$: +135 – +145° (0.1 g calculated on the dried basis, ethanol (95), 10 mL, 100 mm).

Purity **(1)** Clarity and color of solution—Dissolve 0.5 g of Hydrocortisone Sodium Succinate in 5 mL of water: the solution is clear and colorless.

(2) Related substances—Dissolve 25 mg of Hydrocortisone Sodium Succinate in methanol to make exactly 10 mL, and use this solution as the sample solution. Separately, dissolve 25 mg of hydrocortisone in methanol to make exactly 10 mL. Pipet 1 mL of this solution, add methanol to make exactly 20 mL, and use this solution as the standard solution (1). Pipet 6 mL of the standard solution (1), add methanol to make exactly 10 mL, and use this solution as the standard solution (2). Perform the test with these solutions as directed under Thin-layer Chromatography *<2.03>*. Spot 3 μL each of the sample solution and standard solutions (1) and (2) on a plate of silica gel with fluorescent indicator for thin-layer chromatography. Develop the plate with a mixture of chloroform, ethanol (99.5) and formic acid (150:10:1) to a distance of about 10 cm, and air-dry the plate. Examine under ultraviolet light (main wavelength: 254 nm): the spot obtained from the sample solution corresponding to the spot from the standard solution (1) is not more intense than the spot from the standard solution (1). Any spot other than the principal spot and the above spot from the sample solution is not more than one, and is not more intense than the spot from the standard solution (2).

Loss on drying *<2.41>* Not more than 2.0% (0.5 g, 105°C, 3 hours).

Assay Weigh accurately about 10 mg of Hydrocortisone Sodium Succinate, and dissolve in methanol to make exactly 100 mL. Pipet 5 mL of this solution, add methanol to make exactly 50 mL, and use this solution as the sample solution. Separately, weigh accurately about 10 mg of Hydrocortisone Succinate RS, previously dried at 105°C for 3 hours, proceed in the same manner as directed for the sample solution, and use this solution as the standard solution. Determine the absorbances, A_T and A_S, of the sample solution and standard solution at 240 nm as directed under Ultraviolet-visible Spectrophotometry *<2.24>*.

Amount (mg) of hydrocortisone sodium succinate ($C_{25}H_{33}NaO_8$)

$$= M_S \times A_T/A_S \times 1.048$$

M_S: Amount (mg) of Hydrocortisone Succinate RS taken

Containers and storage Containers—Tight containers.

Storage—Light-resistant.

Hydrocortisone Succinate

ヒドロコルチゾンコハク酸エステル

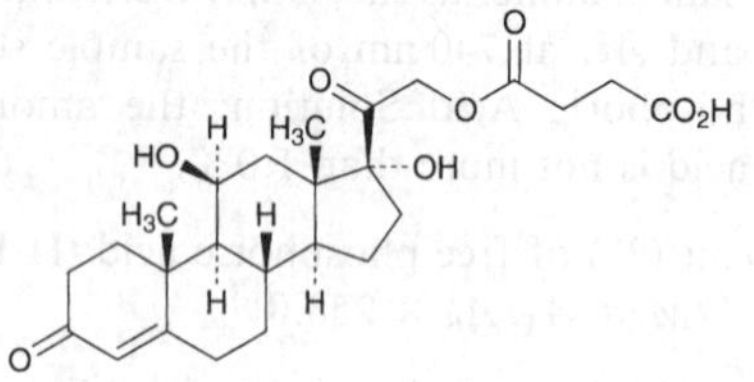

$C_{25}H_{34}O_8$: 462.53

11*β*,17,21-Trihydroxypregn-4-ene-3,20-dione 21-(hydrogen succinate)

[*2203-97-6*]

Hydrocortisone Succinate, when dried, contains not less than 97.0% and not more than 103.0% of hydrocortisone succinate ($C_{25}H_{34}O_8$).

Description Hydrocortisone Succinate occurs as a white crystalline powder.

It is very soluble in methanol, freely soluble in ethanol (99.5), and practically insoluble in water.

It shows crystal polymorphism.

Identification **(1)** To 3 mg of Hydrocortisone Succinate add 2 mL of sulfuric acid: the solution shows a yellowish green fluorescence immediately, and the color of the solution gradually changes through orange-yellow to dark red. This solution shows a strong light green fluorescence under ultraviolet light. Add carefully 10 mL of water to this solution: the color changes from yellow to orange-yellow with a light green fluorescence, and a yellow-brown flocculent precipitate is formed.

(2) Determine the infrared absorption spectrum of Hydrocortisone Succinate, previously dried, as directed in the potassium bromide disk method under Infrared Spectrophotometry *<2.25>*, and compare the spectrum with the Reference Spectrum or the spectrum of previously dried Hydrocortisone Succinate RS: both spectra exhibit similar intensities of absorption at the same wave numbers. If any difference appears between the spectra, dissolve Hydrocortisone Succinate and Hydrocortisone Succinate RS in methanol, respectively, then evaporate the methanol to dryness, and repeat the test on the residues.

Optical rotation ⟨*2.49*⟩ $[\alpha]_D^{20}$: +147 – +153° (after drying, 0.1 g, ethanol (99.5), 10 mL, 100 nm).

Purity Related substances—Dissolve 25 mg of Hydrocortisone Succinate in exactly 10 mL of methanol, and use this solution as the sample solution. Separately, dissolve 25 mg of hydrocortisone in exactly 10 mL of methanol. Pipet 1 mL of this solution, dilute with methanol to exactly 50 mL, and use this solution as the standard solution. Perform the test with these solutions as directed under Thin-layer Chromatography ⟨*2.03*⟩. Spot 3 μL each of the sample solution and standard solution on a plate of silica gel with fluorescent indicator for thin-layer chromatography. Develop the plate with a mixture of chloroform, ethanol (99.5) and formic acid (150:10:1) to a distance of about 10 cm, and air-dry the plate. Examine under ultraviolet light (main wavelength: 254 nm): the spots other than the principal spot obtained from the sample solution are not more intense than the spot from the standard solution.

Loss on drying ⟨*2.41*⟩ Not more than 2.0% (0.5 g, 105°C, 3 hours).

Residue on ignition ⟨*2.44*⟩ Not more than 0.1% (0.5 g).

Assay Weigh accurately about 50 mg each of Hydrocortisone Succinate and Hydrocortisone Succinate RS, previously dried, and dissolve in methanol to make exactly 50 mL. Pipet 5 mL each of these solutions, add exactly 5 mL each of the internal standard solution, then add methanol to make 50 mL, and use these solutions as the sample solution and standard solution. Perform the test with 10 μL each of the sample solution and standard solution as directed under Liquid Chromatography ⟨*2.01*⟩ according to the following operating conditions, and calculate the ratios, Q_T and Q_S, of the peak area of hydrocortisone succinate to that of the internal standard, respectively.

Amount (mg) of hydrocortisone succinate ($C_{25}H_{34}O_8$)
$= M_S \times Q_T/Q_S$

M_S: Amount (mg) of Hydrocortisone Succinate RS taken

Internal standard solution—A solution of butyl parahydroxy benzoate in methanol (1 in 2500).
Operating conditions—

Detector: An ultraviolet absorption photometer (wavelength: 254 nm).

Column: A stainless steel column 4 mm in inside diameter and 30 cm in length, packed with octadecylsilanized silica gel (10 μm in particle diameter).

Column temperature: A constant temperature of about 25°C.

Mobile phase: A mixture of acetic acid-sodium acetate buffer solution (pH 4.0) and acetonitrile (3:2).

Flow rate: Adjust so that the retention time of hydrocortisone succinate is about 5 minutes.
System suitability—

System performance: When the procedure is run with 10 μL of the standard solution under the above operating conditions, hydrocortisone succinate and the internal standard are eluted in this order with the resolution between these peaks being not less than 9.

System repeatability: When the test is repeated 6 times with 10 μL of the standard solution under the above operating conditions, the relative standard deviation of the ratios of the peak area of hydrocortisone succinate to that of the internal standard is not more than 1.0%.

Containers and storage Containers—Tight containers.
Storage—Light-resistant.

Hydrocotarnine Hydrochloride Hydrate

ヒドロコタルニン塩酸塩水和物

$C_{12}H_{15}NO_3.HCl.H_2O$: 275.73
4-Methoxy-6-methyl-5,6,7,8-tetrahydro[1,3]dioxolo[4,5-*g*]isoquinoline monohydrochloride monohydrate
[*5985-55-7*, anhydride]

Hydrocotarnine Hydrochloride Hydrate, when dried, contains not less than 98.0% of hydrocotarnine-hydrochloride ($C_{12}H_{15}NO_3.HCl$: 257.72).

Description Hydrocotarnine Hydrochloride Hydrate occurs as white to pale yellow, crystals or crystalline powder.

It is freely soluble in water, sparingly soluble in ethanol (95) and in acetic acid (100), and slightly soluble in acetic anhydride.

Identification **(1)** Determine the absorption spectrum of a solution of Hydrocotarnine Hydrochloride Hydrate (1 in 10,000) as directed under Ultraviolet-visible Spectrophotometry ⟨*2.24*⟩, and compare the spectrum with the Reference Spectrum: both spectra exhibit similar intensities of absorption at the same wavelengths.

(2) Determine the infrared absorption spectrum of Hydrocotarnine Hydrochloride Hydrate as directed in the potassium bromide disk method under Infrared Spectrophotometry ⟨*2.25*⟩, and compare the spectrum with the Reference Spectrum: both spectra exhibit similar intensities of absorption at the same wave numbers.

(3) A solution of Hydrocotarnine Hydrochloride Hydrate (1 in 50) responds to Qualitative Tests ⟨*1.09*⟩ (2) for chloride.

pH ⟨*2.54*⟩ Dissolve 1.0 g of Hydrocotarnine Hydrochloride Hydrate in 20 mL of water: the pH of the solution is between 4.0 and 6.0.

Purity **(1)** Clarity and color of solution—Dissolve 0.5 g of Hydrocotarnine Hydrochloride Hydrate in 10 mL of water: the solution is clear, and when perform the test with this solution as directed under Ultraviolet-visible Spectrophotometry ⟨*2.24*⟩, using water as the blank, the absorbance at 400 nm is not more than 0.17.

(2) Heavy metals ⟨*1.07*⟩—Proceeds with 1.0 g of Hydrocotarnine Hydrochloride Hydrate according to Method 1, and perform the test. Prepare the control solution with 2.0 mL of Standard Lead Solution (not more than 20 ppm).

(3) Related substances—Dissolve 0.10 g of Hydrocotarnine Hydrochloride Hydrate in 10 mL of diluted ethanol

(99.5) (1 in 2), and use this solution as the sample solution. Pipet 1 mL of the sample solution, add diluted ethanol (99.5) (1 in 2) to make exactly 100 mL, and use this solution as the standard solution. Perform the test with these solutions as directed under Thin-layer Chromatography <*2.03*>. Spot 10 μL each of the sample solution and standard solution on a plate of silica gel with fluorescent indicator for thin-layer chromatography. Develop the plate with a mixture of acetone, toluene, ethanol (99.5) and ammonia water (28) (20:20:3:1) to a distance of about 15 cm, and air-dry the plate. Examine under ultraviolet light (main wavelength: 365 nm): the spots other than the principal spot obtained from the sample solution are not more intense than the spot from the standard solution.

Loss on drying <*2.41*> Not more than 7.0% (1 g, 105°C, 3 hours).

Residue on ignition <*2.44*> Not more than 0.2% (1 g).

Assay Weigh accurately about 0.5 g of Hydrocotarnine Hydrochloride Hydrate, previously dried. Dissolve in 50 mL of a mixture of acetic anhydride and acetic acid (100) (7:3) by warming. Cool, and titrate <*2.50*> with 0.1 mol/L perchloric acid VS (potentiometric titration). Perform a blank determination in the same manner, and make any necessary correction.

Each mL of 0.1 mol/L perchloric acid VS
= 25.77 mg of $C_{12}H_{15}NO_3.HCl$

Containers and storage Containers—Tight containers.

Hydrogenated Oil

硬化油

Hydrogenated Oil is the fat obtained by hydrogenation of fish oil or of other oils originating from animal or vegetable.

Description Hydrogenated Oil occurs as a white mass or powder and has a characteristic odor and a mild taste.

It is freely soluble in diethyl ether, very slightly soluble in ethanol (95), and practically insoluble in water.

The oil obtained by hydrogenation of castor oil is slightly soluble in diethyl ether, very slightly soluble in ethanol (95), and practically insoluble in water.

Acid value <*1.13*> Not more than 2.0.

Purity **(1)** Moisture and coloration—Hydrogenated Oil (5.0 g), melted by heating on a water bath, forms a clear liquid, from which no water separates. In a 10-mm thick layer of the liquid, it is colorless or slightly yellow.

(2) Alkalinity—To 2.0 g of Hydrogenated Oil add 10 mL of water, melt by heating on a water bath, and shake vigorously. After cooling, add 1 drop of phenolphthalein TS to the separated water layer: no color develops.

(3) Chloride—To 1.5 g of Hydrogenated Oil add 30 mL of ethanol (95), boil for 10 minutes under a reflux condenser, and filter after cooling. To 20 mL of the filtrate add 5 drops of a solution of silver nitrate in ethanol (95) (1 in 50): the turbidity of the solution does not exceed that of the following control solution.

Control solution: To 1.0 mL of 0.01 mol/L hydrochloric acid VS add ethanol (95) to make 20 mL, then add 5 drops of a solution of silver nitrate in ethanol (95) (1 in 50).

(4) Heavy metals—Heat 2.0 g of Hydrogenated Oil with 5 mL of dilute hydrochloric acid and 10 mL of water on a water bath for 5 minutes with occasional shaking. After cooling, filter, and make 5 mL of the filtrate weakly alkaline with ammonia TS, then add 3 drops of sodium sulfide TS: the solution remains unchanged.

(5) Nickel—Place 5.0 g of Hydrogenated Oil in a quartz or porcelain crucible, heat slightly with caution at the beginning, and, after carbonization, incinerate by strong heating (500 ± 20°C). Cool, add 1 mL of hydrochloric acid, evaporate on a water bath to dryness, dissolve the residue in 3 mL of dilute hydrochloric acid, and add 7 mL of water. Then add 1 mL of bromine TS and 1 mL of a solution of citric acid monohydrate (1 in 5), make alkaline with 5 mL of ammonia TS, and cool in running water. To this solution add 1 mL of dimethylglyoxime TS, add water to make 20 mL, and use this solution as the test solution. Allow to stand for 5 minutes: the solution has no more color than the following control solution.

Control solution: Evaporate 1 mL of hydrochloric acid on a water bath to dryness, add 1 mL of Standard Nickel Solution and 3 mL of dilute hydrochloric acid, and add 6 mL of water. Then proceed as directed in the test solution, add water to make 20 mL, and allow to stand for 5 minutes.

Residue on ignition <*2.44*> Not more than 0.1% (5 g).

Containers and storage Containers—Well-closed containers.

Hydroxocobalamin Acetate

ヒドロキソコバラミン酢酸塩

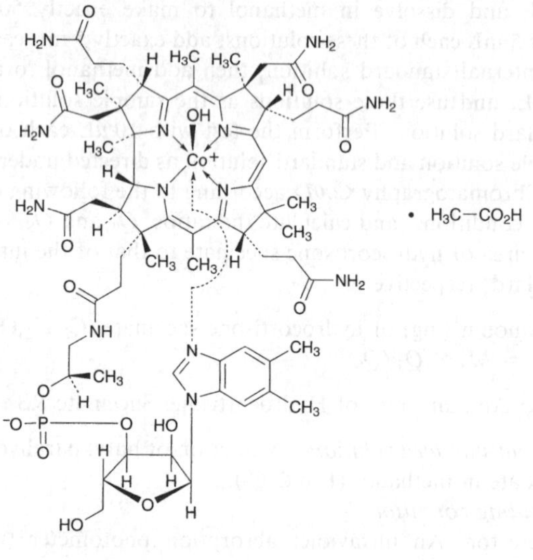

$C_{62}H_{89}CoN_{13}O_{15}P.C_2H_4O_2$: 1406.41
Coα-[*α*-(5,6-Dimethyl-1*H*-benzimidazol-1-yl)]-*Coβ*-hydroxocobamide monoacetate
[*13422-51-0*, Hydroxocobalamin]

Hydroxocobalamin Acetate contains not less than 96.0% and not more than 101.0% of hydroxocobalamin acetate ($C_{62}H_{89}CoN_{13}O_{15}P.C_2H_4O_2$), calculated on the anhydrous and residual solvent-free basis.

Description Hydroxocobalamin Acetate occurs as dark red, crystals or powder. It is odorless.

It is freely soluble in water and in methanol, slightly soluble in ethanol (95), and practically insoluble in diethyl ether.

It is hygroscopic.

Identification **(1)** Determine the absorption spectrum of a solution of Hydroxocobalamin Acetate in acetic acid-sodium acetate buffer solution (pH 4.5) (1 in 50,000) as directed under Ultraviolet-visible Spectrophotometry *<2.24>*, and compare the spectrum with the Reference Spectrum: both spectra exhibit similar intensities of absorption at the same wavelengths.

(2) Mix 1 mg of Hydroxocobalamin Acetate with 50 mg of potassium hydrogen sulfate, and fuse by igniting. Cool, break up the mass with a glass rod, add 3 mL of water, and dissolve by boiling. Add 1 drop of phenolphthalein TS, and add dropwise sodium hydroxide TS until the solution develops a light red. Then add 0.5 g of sodium acetate trihydrate, 0.5 mL of dilute acetic acid and 0.5 mL of a solution of disodium 1-nitroso-2-naphthol-3,6-disulfonate (1 in 500): a red to orange-red color develops immediately. Then add 0.5 mL of hydrochloric acid, and boil for 1 minute: the red color does not disappear.

(3) Add 0.5 mL of ethanol (99.5) and 1 mL of sulfuric acid to 20 mg of Hydroxocobalamin Acetate, and heat the mixture: the odor of ethyl acetate is perceptible.

Purity Conduct this procedure using light-resistant vessels. Dissolve 75 mg of Hydroxocobalamin Acetate in 100 mL of the dissolving solution, and use this solution as the sample solution. Pipet 1 mL of the sample solution, add the dissolving solution to make exactly 20 mL, and use this solution as the standard solution. Perform the test with exactly 20 μL each of the sample solution and standard solution as directed under Liquid Chromatography *<2.01>* according to the following conditions, and determine each peak area by the automatic integration method: the total area of the peaks other than hydroxocobalamin obtained from the sample solution is not larger than the peak area of hydroxocobalamin from the standard solution.

Dissolving solution: A mixture of water, mobile phase C and methanol (41:5:4).

Operating conditions—

Detector: An ultraviolet absorption photometer (wavelength: 351 nm).

Column: Connect two columns which are 4.6 mm in inside diameter and 10 cm in length, composed of octadecylsilanized monolithic silica for liquid chromatography, having a bimodal pore structure with 2 μm macropore and 13 nm mesopore, coated with polyether ether ketone.

Column temperature: A constant temperature of about 30°C.

Mobile phase A: Water.

Mobile phase B: Methanol.

Mobile phase C: Dissolve 15.6 g of sodium dihydrogen phosphate dihydrate in 1000 mL of water, and adjust to pH 3 with diluted phosphoric acid (1 in 100).

Flowing of mobile phase: Control the gradient by mixing the mobile phase A, B and C as directed in the following table.

Time after injection of sample (min)	Mobile phase A (vol%)	Mobile phase B (vol%)	Mobile phase C (vol%)
0 – 20	82	8	10
20 – 40	82 → 50	8 → 40	10

Flow rate: 2 mL per minute.

Time span of measurement: For 40 minutes after injection of the sample solution.

System suitability—

Test for required detectability: Pipet 1 mL of the standard solution, add the dissolving solution to make exactly 50 mL. Confirm that the peak area of hydroxocobalamin obtained with 20 μL of this solution is equivalent to 1.4 to 2.6% of that with 20 μL of the standard solution.

System performance: When the procedure is run with 20 μL of the standard solution under the above operating conditions, the number of theoretical plates and the symmetry factor of the peak of hydroxocobalamin are not less than 4000 and not more than 2.4, respectively.

System repeatability: When the test is repeated 6 times with 20 μL of the standard solution under the above operating conditions, the relative standard deviation of the peak area of hydroxocobalamin is not more than 2.0%.

Water *<2.48>* 8.0 – 12.0% (50 mg, volumetric titration, direct titration).

Assay Weigh accurately about 0.1 g of Hydroxocobalamin Acetate, and dissolve in water to make exactly 500 mL. Pipet 5 mL of this solution, and add acetic acid-sodium acetate buffer solution (pH 4.5) to make exactly 25 mL. Determine the absorbance, *A*, of this solution at 351 nm as directed under Ultraviolet-visible Spectrophotometry *<2.24>*.

Amount (mg) of hydroxocobalamin acetate
$(C_{62}H_{89}CoN_{13}O_{15}P.C_2H_4O_2)$
$= A/187 \times 25{,}000$

Containers and storage Containers—Tight containers.
Storage—Light-resistant, and in a cold place.

Hydroxyethylcellulose

ヒドロキシエチルセルロース

[9004-62-0]

This monograph is harmonized with the European Pharmacopoeia and the U. S. Pharmacopeia.

The corresponding part of the attributes/provisions which are agreed as non-harmonized within the scope of the harmonization is marked with symbols (◆ ◆), and the corresponding parts which are agreed as the JP local requirement other than the scope of the harmonization are marked with symbols (◇ ◇).

Information on the harmonization with the European Pharmacopoeia and the U.S. Pharmacopeia is available on the website of the Pharmaceuticals and Medical Devices Agency.

Hydroxyethylcellulose is partly *O*-(2-hydroxyethylated) cellulose.

It contains not less than 30.0% and not more than 70.0% of hydroxyethoxy group ($-OC_2H_4OH$: 61.06), calculated on the dried basis.

It may contain suitable pH-adjusting agents such as phosphates.

◆The viscosity is shown in millipascal second (mPa·s) on the label.◆

◆**Description** Hydroxyethylcellulose occurs as a white to yellowish white, powder or grains.

It is practically insoluble in ethanol (95).

It forms a viscous liquid upon addition of water.

It is hygroscopic.◆

Identification **(1)** Determine the infrared absorption spec-

trum of Hydroxyethylcellulose as directed in the ATR method under Infrared Spectrophotometry <2.25> and compare the spectrum with the spectrum of Hydroxyethylcellulose for Identification RS: both spectra exhibit similar intensities of absorption at the same wave numbers.

(2) Disperse 1.0 g of Hydroxyethylcellulose, calculated on the dried basis, in 50 mL of freshly boiled and cooled water. After 10 minutes, add freshly boiled and cooled water to make 100 mL, stir to dissolve completely, and use this solution as the sample solution. Boil 10 mL of the sample solution: the solution is clear.

◆**Viscosity** <2.53> Weigh exactly a quantity of Hydroxyethylcellulose, equivalent to 10.00 g calculated on the dried basis, add 400 mL of water, stir to dissolve, and add water to make exactly 500.0 g. Remove air bubbles, and use this solution as the sample solution. Perform the test with the sample solution at 20 ± 0.1°C as directed in Method II under Viscosity Determination, using a beaker with an inside diameter of not less than 70 mm and a single cylinder-type rotational viscometer, according to the following operating conditions: not less than 75% and not more than 140% of the labeled viscosity.

Operating conditions—

Apparatus: Brookfield type viscometer LV or RV model.

Rotor No., rotation frequency and calculation multiplier: According to the following table, depending on the labeled viscosity.

Labeled viscosity (mPa·s)	Model	Rotor No.	Rotation frequency /min	Calculation multiplier
less than 200	LV	1	30	2
Not less than 200 and less than 4000	LV	3	30	40
〃 4000 〃 10,000	LV	4	30	200
〃 10,000 〃 50,000	RV	6	20	500
〃 50,000	RV	7	20	2000

Procedure of apparatus: Read a value after 2 minutes of rotation, and stop the rotation for at least 2 minutes. Repeat this procedure more two times, and average the three observed values.◆

pH <2.54> The pH of the sample solution obtained in the Identification (2) is between 5.5 and 8.5.

Purity **(1)** Chloride—To 1 mL of the sample solution obtained in the Identification (2) add water to make 30 mL, and use this solution as the sample solution. Separately, to 10 mL of Standard Chloride Solution add 5 mL of water, and use this solution as the control solution. To 15 mL each of the sample solution and control solution add 1 mL of diluted nitric acid (1 in 5), transfer to test tubes containing 1 mL of a solution of silver nitrate (17 in 1000), allow to stand for 5 minutes protecting from light, and compare the opalescence developed in the both solutions against a black background by viewing transversely: the opalescence developed in the sample solution is not more intense than that of the control solution (not more than 1.0%).

(2) Nitrate—Prepare the solutions before use. Dissolve 0.50 g of Hydroxyethylcellulose in the diluting solution to make exactly 100 mL, and use this solution as the sample solution. Separately, dissolve 0.8154 g of potassium nitrate in the diluting solution to make 1000 mL, and use this solution as the standard nitrate stock solution. If the viscosity of Hydroxyethylcellulose is not more than 1000 mPa·s, pipet 10 mL, 20 mL and 40 mL of the standard nitrate stock solution, add the diluting solution to each to make exactly 100 mL, and use these solutions as the standard solutions. If the viscosity of Hydroxyethylcellulose is more than 1000 mPa·s, pipet 1 mL, 2 mL and 4 mL of the standard nitrate stock solution, add the diluting solution to each to make exactly 100 mL, and use these solutions as the standard solutions. Perform the test with the sample solution and standard solutions using a nitrate-selective electrode as an indicator electrode, a silver-silver chloride electrode as a reference electrode and diluted ammonium sulfate TS (1 in 30) as reference electrolyte. Calculate the concentration of nitrates in the sample solution using a calibration curve obtained from the potential differences of the standard solutions: not more than 3.0%, calculated on the dried basis, if Hydroxyethylcellulose has a viscosity of not more than 1000 mPa·s, and not more than 0.2%, calculated on the dried basis, if Hydroxyethylcellulose has a viscosity of more than 1000 mPa·s.

Diluting solution: To a mixture of 50 mL of 1 mol/L sulfuric acid TS and 800 mL of water add 135 g of potassium dihydrogen phosphate, and add water to make 1000 mL. To this solution add water to make exactly 25 times the initial volume.

In order to determine the applicable limit, determine the viscosity using the following procedure.

Introduce a quantity of Hydroxyethylcellulose, equivalent to 2.00 g calculated on the dried basis, into 50 g of water, stir, add water to make 100 g, and stir to dissolve completely. Determine the viscosity using a rotating viscometer at 25°C and at a shear rate of 100 s^{-1} for substances with an expected viscosity less than 100 mPa·s, at a shear rate of 10 s^{-1} for substances with an expected viscosity not less than 100 mPa·s and not more than 20,000 mPa·s, and at a shear rate of 1 s^{-1} for substances with an expected viscosity more than 20,000 mPa·s. If it is impossible to obtain a shear rate of exactly 10 s^{-1} or 100 s^{-1} respectively, use a rate slightly higher and a rate slightly lower and interpolate.

◇**(3)** Heavy metal <1.07>—Proceed with 1.0 g of Hydroxyethylcellulose according to Method 2, and perform the test. Prepare the control solution with 2.0 mL of Standard Lead Solution (not more than 20 ppm).◇

(4) Aldehydes—Introduce 1.0 g of Hydroxyethylcellulose into a glass-stoppered test tube, add 10 mL of ethanol (99.5), stopper the tube tightly, and stir for 30 minutes. Centrifuge, and use the supernatant liquid as the sample solution. Use Standard Glyoxal Solution as the control solution. Pipet 2 mL each of the sample solution and control solution, to each add 5 mL of a solution prepared by dissolving 4 g of 3-methyl-2-benzothiazolonehydrazone hydrochloride monohydrate in diluted acetic acid (100) (4 in 5) to make 1000 mL, shake to homogenize, and allow to stand for 2 hours. Compare the color of these solutions: the sample solution is not more intensely colored than the control solution (not more than 20 ppm).

Loss on drying <2.41> Not more than 10.0% (1 g, 105°C, 3 hours).

Residue on Ignition <2.44> Not more than 4.0% if the viscosity of Hydroxyethylcellulose is not more than 1000 mPa·s, and not more than 1.0% if the viscosity of Hydroxyethylcellulose is more than 1000 mPa·s (1 g). In order to determine the applicable limit, determine the viscosity according to the method in the Purity (2).

Assay Weigh accurately about 30 mg of Hydroxyethylcellulose, transfer to a 5-mL pressure-tight serum vial, add exactly 60 mg of adipic acid, 2 mL of the internal standard solution and 1 mL of hydroiodic acid, seal the vial immediately with a septum coated with fluororesin and an aluminum cap or any other sealing system providing a sufficient air-tightness, and weigh accurately the vial. Take care not to mix the content of the vial before heating. Place the vial in an oven or heat in a suitable heater with continuous stirring, maintaining the internal temperature of about 165 ± 2°C for 2.5 hours. Allow to cool and weigh accurately the vial. If the difference of the mass between before heating and after heating is more than 10 mg, prepare a new sample solution. If the difference of the mass between before heating and after heating is not more than 10 mg, after phase separation, pierce through the septum of the vial with a cooled syringe, and withdraw a sufficient volume of the upper phase as the sample solution. Separately, place exactly 60 mg of adipic acid, 2 mL of the internal standard solution and 1 mL of hydroiodic acid in another serum vial, and seal immediately. Weigh accurately the vial, inject 55 μL of iodoethane for assay through the septum in the vial, and weigh again accurately. Shake thoroughly, after phase separation, pierce through the septum of the vial with a cooled syringe, and withdraw a sufficient volume of the upper phase as the standard solution. Perform the test with 1 μL each of the sample solution and standard solution as directed under Gas Chromatography <2.02> according to the following conditions, and calculate the ratios, Q_T and Q_S, of the peak area of iodoethane to that of the internal standard.

Amount (%) of hydroethoxy group ($C_2H_5O_2$)
$$= M_S/M_T \times Q_T/Q_S \times 39.15$$

M_S: Amount (mg) of iodoethane for assay taken
M_T: Amount (mg) of Hydroxyethylcellulose taken, calculated on the dried basis

Internal standard solution—A solution of *n*-octane in *o*-xylene (1 in 200).

Operating conditions—

Detector: A hydrogen flame-ionization detector.

Column: A fused silica column 0.53 mm in inside diameter and 30 m in length, coated with dimethylpolysiloxane for gas chromatography in 3 μm thickness.

Column temperature: Maintain the temperature at 50°C for 3 minutes, raise to 100°C at a rate of 10°C per minute, then raise to 250°C at a rate of 35°C per minute, and maintain at 250°C for 8 minutes.

Injection port temperature: A constant temperature of about 250°C.

Detector temperature: A constant temperature of about 280°C.

Carrier gas: Helium.

Flow rate: 4.2 mL per minutes (the retention time of the internal standard is about 10 minutes).

Split ratio: 1:40.

System suitability—

System performance: When the procedure is run with 1 μL of the standard solution under the above operating conditions, iodoethane and the internal standard are eluted in this order with the relative retention time of iodoethane to the internal standard being about 0.6 and the resolution between these peaks being not less than 5.0.

System repeatability: When the test is repeated 6 times with 1 μL of the standard solution under the above operating conditions, the relative standard deviation of the ratio of the peak area of iodoethane to that of the internal standard is not more than 2.0%.

◆**Containers and storage** Containers—Tight containers.◆

Hydroxypropylcellulose

ヒドロキシプロピルセルロース

[*9004-64-2*]

This monograph is harmonized with the European Pharmacopoeia and the U. S. Pharmacopeia.

The corresponding part of the attributes/provisions which are agreed as non-harmonized within the scope of the harmonization is marked with symbols (◆ ◆), and the corresponding parts which are agreed as the JP local requirement other than the scope of the harmonization are marked with symbols (◇ ◇).

Information on the harmonization with the European Pharmacopoeia and the U.S. Pharmacopeia is available on the website of the Pharmaceuticals and Medical Devices Agency.

Hydroxypropylcellulose is partially *O*-(2-hydroxypropylated) cellulose.

It contains not less than 53.4% and not more than 80.5% of hydroxypropoxy group (-OC_3H_6OH: 75.09), calculated on the dried basis.

It may contain silicon dioxide as anti-caking agent.

◆The label states the addition in the case where silicon dioxide is added as anti-caking agent.◆

◆**Description** Hydroxypropylcellulose occurs as a white to yellowish white powder.

It forms a viscous liquid upon addition of water or ethanol (95).◆

Identification **(1)** Dissolve 1 g of Hydroxypropylcellulose in 100 mL of water, transfer 1 mL of the solution to a glass plate, and allow the water to evaporate: a thin film is formed.

(2) Determine the infrared absorption spectrum of Hydroxypropylcellulose as directed in the potassium bromide disk method under Infrared Spectrophotometry <2.25>, and compare the spectrum with the Reference Spectrum: both spectra exhibit similar intensities of absorption at the same wave numbers. If there are an absorption at about 1719 cm^{-1}, disregard the absorption.

pH <2.54> Disperse evenly 1.0 g of Hydroxypropylcellulose in 100 mL of freshly boiled water, and allow to cool the mixture while stirring with a magnetic stirrer: the pH of the solution is between 5.0 and 8.0.

Purity

◇**(1)** Heavy metals <1.07>—Proceed with 1.0 g of Hydroxypropylcellulose according to Method 2 and perform the test. Prepare the control solution with 2.0 mL of Standard Lead Solution (not more than 20 ppm).◇

(2) Silicon dioxide—Apply to Hydroxypropylcellulose, if the addition of silicon dioxide is stated on the label and if more than 0.2% residue is found in the Residue on ignition test. Weigh accurately the crucible containing the residue tested in the Residue on ignition of Hydroxypropylcellulose (*a* (g)). Moisten the residue with water, and add 5 mL of hydrofluoric acid, in small portions. Evaporate it on a steam bath to dryness and cool. Add 5 mL of hydrofluoric acid and 0.5 mL of sulfuric acid, and evaporate to dryness. Slowly increase the temperature until all the acids have been volatilized, and ignite at 1000 ± 25°C. Cool the crucible in a desiccator, and weigh (*b* (g)). Calculate the amount of silicon dioxide by the following equation: not more than 0.6%.

Amount (%) of silicon dioxide (SiO_2)
$= (a - b)/M \times 100$

M: Amount (g) of Hydroxypropylcellulose used for residue on ignition test

Loss on drying *<2.41>* Not more than 5.0% (1 g, 105°C, 4 hours).

Residue on ignition *<2.44>* Not more than 0.8% (1 g, platinum crucible).

Assay Weigh accurately about 30 mg of Hydroxypropylcellulose, transfer to a reaction vial, add exactly 60 mg of adipic acid, 2 mL of the internal standard solution and 1 mL of hydriodic acid, stopper the vial tightly, and weigh accurately. Place the vial in an oven or heat by a suitable heater with continuous stirring, maintaining the internal temperature of 115 ± 2°C for 70 minutes. Allow the vial to cool and weigh accurately. If the difference of the mass between before heating and after heating is more than 10 mg, prepare a new test solution. If the difference of the mass between before heating and after heating is not more than 10 mg, after phase separation by allowing the vial to stand, pierce through the septum of the vial with a cooled syringe, and withdraw a sufficient volume of the upper phase as the sample solution. Separately, place exactly 60 mg of adipic acid, 2 mL of internal standard solution and 1 mL of hydriodic acid in an another reaction vial, stopper tightly, and weigh accurately. Inject 25 μL of isopropyl iodide for assay through the septum, and again weigh accurately. Shake the vial thoroughly, and after phase separation by allowing the vial to stand, pierce through the septum of the vial with a cooled syringe, and withdraw a sufficient volume of the upper phase as the standard solution. Perform the test with 2 μL each of the sample solution and standard solution as directed under Gas Chromatography *<2.02>* according to the following conditions, and calculate the ratios, Q_T and Q_S, of the peak area of isopropyl iodide to that of the internal standard.

Amount (%) of hydroxypropoxy group ($C_3H_7O_2$)
$= M_S/M_T \times Q_T/Q_S \times 1.15 \times 44.17$

M_S: Amount (mg) of isopropyl iodide for assay taken
M_T: Amount (mg) of Hydroxypropylcellulose taken, calculated on the dried basis
1.15: Correction factor

Internal standard solution—A solution of methylcyclohexan in *o*-xylene (1 in 50).

Operating conditions—

Detector: A hydrogen flame-ionization detector.

Column: A fused silica tube 0.53 mm in diameter and 30 m in length, coated with methylsilicone polymer for gas chromatography in 3 μm thickness.

Column Temperature: Maintain the temperature at 40°C for 3 minutes, raise to 100°C at a rate of 10°C per minute, then raise to 250°C at a rate of 50°C per minute, and maintain at 250°C for 3 minutes.

Injection port temperature: A constant temperature of about 180°C.

Detector temperature: A constant temperature of about 280°C.

Carrier gas: Helium.

Flow rate: 52 cm per second (the retention time of the internal standard is about 8 minutes).

Split ratio: 1:50.

System suitability—

System performance: When the procedure is run with 2 μL of the standard solution under the above operating conditions, isopropyl iodide and the internal standard are eluted in this order with the relative retention time of isopropyl iodide to the internal standard being about 0.8, and with the resolution between these peaks being not less than 2.0.

System repeatability: When the test is repeated 6 times with 2 μL of the standard solution under the above operating conditions, the relative standard deviation of the ratio of the peak area of isopropyl iodide to that of the internal standard is not more than 2.0%.

◆**Containers and storage** Containers—Well-closed containers.◆

Low Substituted Hydroxypropylcellulose

低置換度ヒドロキシプロピルセルロース

[*9004-64-2*, Hydroxypropylcellulose]

This monograph is harmonized with the European Pharmacopoeia and the U.S. Pharmacopeia.

The corresponding part of the attributes/provisions which are agreed as non-harmonized within the scope of the harmonization is marked with symbols (◆ ◆), and the corresponding parts which are agreed as the JP local requirement other than the scope of the harmonization are marked with symbols (◇ ◇).

Information on the harmonization with the European Pharmacopoeia and the U.S. Pharmacopeia is available on the website of the Pharmaceuticals and Medical Devices Agency.

Low Substituted Hydroxypropylcellulose is a low substituted hydroxypropyl ether of cellulose.

It contains not less than 5.0% and not more than 16.0% of hydroxypropoxy group ($-OC_3H_6OH$: 75.09), calculated on the dried basis.

◆**Description** Low Substituted Hydroxypropylcellulose occurs as a white to yellowish white, powder or granules.

It is practically insoluble in ethanol (99.5).

It dissolves in a solution of sodium hydroxide (1 in 10), and produces a viscous solution.

It swells in water, in sodium carbonate TS and in 2 mol/L hydrochloric acid TS.◆

Identification

(1) Shake thoroughly 0.1 g of Low Substituted Hydroxypropylcellulose with 10 mL of water: it does not dissolve.

(2) To the dispersed solution obtained in (1) add 1 g of sodium hydroxide, and shake until the solution becomes uniform. Transfer 5 mL of this solution to a suitable vessel, add 10 mL of a mixture of acetone and methanol (4:1), and shake: a white, flocculent precipitate is formed.

(3) Determine the infrared absorption spectrum of Low Substituted Hydroxypropylcellulose as directed in the potassium bromide disk method under Infrared Spectrophotometry *<2.25>*, and compare the spectrum with the Reference Spectrum: both spectra exhibit similar intensities of absorption at the same wave numbers.

pH *<2.54>* To 1.0 g of Low Substituted Hydroxypropylcellulose add 100 mL of freshly boiled and cooled water, and shake: the pH of the solution is between 5.0 and 7.5.

Purity ◇Heavy metals *<1.07>*—Proceed with 2.0 g of Low Substituted Hydroxypropylcellulose according to Method 2, and perform the test. Prepare the control solution with 2.0 mL of Standard Lead Solution (not more than 10 ppm).◇

Loss on drying ⟨*2.41*⟩ Not more than 5.0% (1 g, 105°C, 1 hour).

Residue on ignition ⟨*2.44*⟩ Not more than 0.8% (1 g).

Assay (i) Apparatus—Reaction vial: A 5-mL pressure-tight serum vial, 20 mm in outside diameter and 50 mm in height, 20 mm in outside diameter and 13 mm in inside diameter at the neck, equipped with a septum made of butyl-rubber whose surface is processed with fluoroplastics, which can be fixed to the vial and stoppered tightly with an aluminum cap or another system providing an equivalent air-tightness.

Heater: A square-shaped aluminum block, having holes 20 mm in diameter and 32 mm in depth, adopted to the reaction vial. Capable of stirring the content of the reaction vial by means of a magnetic stirrer or of a reciprocal shaker about 100 times per minute.

(ii) Procedure—Weigh accurately about 65 mg of Low Substituted Hydroxypropylcellulose, transfer to a reaction vial, add 0.06 to 0.10 g of adipic acid, 2.0 mL of the internal standard solution and 2.0 mL of hydroiodic acid, immediately stopper the vial tightly, and weigh accurately. Using a magnetic stirrer equipped in the heating module, or using a shaker, mix for 60 minutes while heating so that the temperature of the vial content is 130 ± 2°C. In the case when a magnetic stirrer or shaker is not available, heat for 30 minutes with repeated shaking at 5-minutes intervals by hand, and continue heating for an additional 30 minutes. Allow the vial to cool, and again weigh accurately. If the mass loss is less than 26 mg and there is no evidence of a leak of the content, use the upper layer of the mixture as the sample solution. Separately, put 0.06 to 0.10 g of adipic acid, 2.0 mL of the internal standard solution and 2.0 mL of hydroiodic acid in a reaction vial, immediately stopper the vial tightly, and weigh accurately. Add 15 to 22 μL of isopropyl iodide for assay through the septum using a microsyringe, and weigh accurately. Shake the reaction vial thoroughly, and use the upper layer of the content as the standard solution. Perform the test with 1 to 2 μL each of the sample solution and standard solution as directed under Gas Chromatography ⟨*2.02*⟩ according to the following conditions, and calculate the ratios, Q_T and Q_S, of the peak area of isopropyl iodide to that of the internal standard.

Amount (%) of hydroxypropoxy group ($C_3H_7O_2$)
$= M_S/M_T \times Q_T/Q_S \times 44.17$

M_S: Amount (mg) of isopropyl iodide for assay taken
M_T: Amount (mg) of Low Substituted Hydroxypropylcellulose taken, calculated on the dried basis

Internal standard solution—A solution of *n*-octane in *o*-xylene (3 in 100).

Operating conditions—

Detector: A thermal conductivity detector or hydrogen flame-ionization detector.

Column: A fused silica column 0.53 mm in inside diameter and 30 m in length, coated with dimethylpolysiloxane for gas chromatography in 3 μm thickness. Use a guard column if necessary.

Column temperature: Maintain the temperature at 50°C for 3 minutes after injection, raise to 100°C at a rate of 10°C per minute, then to 250°C at a rate of 35°C per minute and maintain at 250°C for 8 minutes.

Injection port temperature: 250°C.

Detector temperature: 280°C.

Carrier gas: Helium.

Flow rate: 4.3 mL per minute (the retention time of the internal standard is about 10 minutes).

Split ratio: 1:40.

System suitability—

System performance: When the procedure is run with 1 to 2 μL of the standard solution under the above operating conditions, isopropyl iodide and the interal standard are eluted in this order with the resolution between these peaks being not less than 5.

System repeatability: When the test is repeated 6 times with 1 to 2 μL of the standard solution under the above operating conditions, the relative standard deviation of the ratio of the peak area of isopropyl iodide to that of the internal standard is not more than 2.0%.

Containers and storage Containers—Tight containers.

Hydroxyzine Hydrochloride

ヒドロキシジン塩酸塩

and enantiomer

$C_{21}H_{27}ClN_2O_2.2HCl$: 447.83
2-(2-{4-[(*RS*)-(4-Chlorophenyl)(phenyl)methyl]piperazin-1-yl}ethoxy)ethanol dihydrochloride
[*2192-20-3*]

Hydroxyzine Hydrochloride, when dried, contains not less than 98.5% of hydroxyzine hydrochloride ($C_{21}H_{27}ClN_2O_2.2HCl$).

Description Hydroxyzine Hydrochloride occurs as a white crystalline powder. It is odorless, and has a bitter taste.

It is very soluble in water, freely soluble in methanol, in ethanol (95) and in acetic acid (100), very slightly soluble in acetic anhydride, and practically insoluble in diethyl ether.

Melting point: about 200°C (with decomposition).

Identification (1) To 5 mL of a solution of Hydroxyzine Hydrochloride (1 in 100) add 2 to 3 drops of ammonium thiocyanate-cobalt (II) nitrate TS: a blue precipitate is formed.

(2) Determine the absorption spectrum of a solution of Hydroxyzine Hydrochloride in methanol (1 in 100,000) as directed under Ultraviolet-visible Spectrophotometry ⟨*2.24*⟩, and compare the spectrum with the Reference Spectrum: both spectra exhibit similar intensities of absorption at the same wavelengths.

(3) A solution of Hydroxyzine Hydrochloride (1 in 10) responds to Qualitative Tests ⟨*1.09*⟩ for chloride.

pH ⟨*2.54*⟩ Dissolve 1.0 g of Hydroxyzine Hydrochloride in 20 mL of water: the pH of this solution is between 1.3 and 2.5.

Purity (1) Clarity and color of solution—Dissolve 1.0 g of Hydroxyzine Hydrochloride in 10 mL of water: the solution is clear and colorless.

(2) Heavy metals ⟨*1.07*⟩—Proceed with 1.0 g of Hydroxyzine Hydrochloride according to Method 2, and perform the test. Prepare the control solution with 2.0 mL of Standard Lead Solution (not more than 20 ppm).

(3) Related substances—Dissolve 0.20 g of Hydroxyzine Hydrochloride in 10 mL of methanol, and use this solution as the sample solution. Pipet 1 mL of the sample solution, add methanol to make exactly 200 mL, and use this solution as the standard solution. Perform the test with these solutions as directed under Thin-layer Chromatography *<2.03>*. Spot 5 μL each of the sample solution and standard solution on a plate of silica gel for thin-layer chromatography. Develop the plate with a mixture of ethyl acetate, ethanol (95) and ammonia solution (28) (150:95:1) to a distance of about 10 cm, and air-dry the plate. Allow the plate to stand in iodine vapor: the spots other than the principal spot obtained from the sample solution are not more intense than the spot obtained from the standard solution.

Loss on drying *<2.41>* Not more than 3.0% (1 g, 105°C, 2 hours).

Residue on ignition *<2.44>* Not more than 0.2% (1 g).

Assay Weigh accurately about 0.1 g of Hydroxyzine Hydrochloride, previously dried, dissolve in 60 mL of a mixture of acetic anhydride and acetic acid (100) (7:3), and titrate *<2.50>* with 0.1 mol/L perchloric acid VS (potentiometric titration). Perform a blank determination in the same manner, and make any necessary correction.

Each mL of 0.1 mol/L perchloric acid VS
= 22.39 mg of $C_{21}H_{27}ClN_2O_2.2HCl$

Containers and storage Containers—Tight containers.

Hydroxyzine Pamoate

ヒドロキシジンパモ酸塩

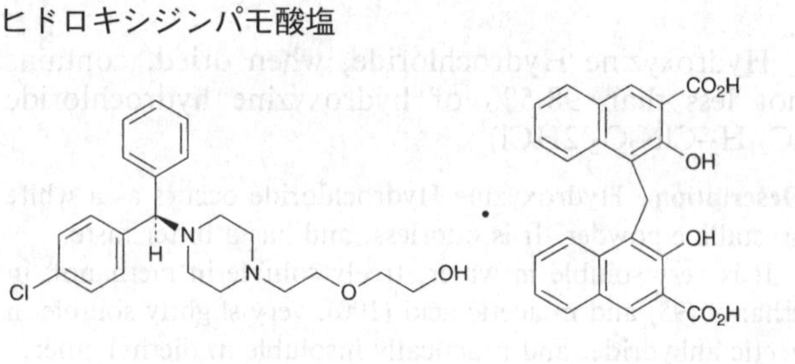

and enantiomer

$C_{21}H_{27}ClN_2O_2.C_{23}H_{16}O_6$: 763.27
2-(2-{4-[(*RS*)-(4-Chlorophenyl)(phenyl)methyl]piperazin-1-yl}ethoxy)ethanol mono[4,4′-methylenebis(3-hydroxy-2-naphthoate)]
[*10246-75-0*]

Hydroxyzine Pamoate contains not less than 98.0% of hydroxyzine pamoate ($C_{21}H_{27}ClN_2O_2.C_{23}H_{16}O_6$), calculated on the anhydrous basis.

Description Hydroxyzine Pamoate occurs as a light yellow crystalline powder. It is odorless, and has a slightly bitter taste.

It is freely soluble in *N*,*N*-dimethylformamide, slightly soluble in acetone, and practically insoluble in water, in methanol, in ethanol (95) and in diethyl ether.

Identification **(1)** To 0.1 g of Hydroxyzine Pamoate add 25 mL of sodium hydroxide TS, and shake well. Extract with 20 mL of chloroform, and use the chloroform layer as the sample solution. Use the water layer for test (4). To 5 mL of the sample solution add 2 mL of ammonium thiocyanate-cobalt (II) nitrate TS, shake well, and allow to stand: a blue color is produced in the chloroform layer.

(2) Evaporate 2 mL of the sample solution obtained in (1) on a water bath to dryness, and dissolve the residue in 0.1 mol/L hydrochloric acid TS to make 500 mL. Determine the absorption spectrum of the solution as directed under Ultraviolet-visible Spectrophotometry *<2.24>*, and compare the spectrum with the Reference Spectrum: both spectra exhibit similar intensities of absorption at the same wavelengths.

(3) Perform the test with Hydroxyzine Pamoate as directed under Flame Coloration Test *<1.04>* (2): a green color appears.

(4) To 1 mL of the water layer obtained in (1), add 2 mL of 1 mol/L hydrochloric acid TS: a yellow precipitate is produced. Collect the precipitate, dissolve the precipitate in 5 mL of methanol, and add 1 drop of iron (III) chloride TS: a green color is produced.

Purity **(1)** Clarity and color of solution—Dissolve 1.0 g of Hydroxyzine Pamoate in 10 mL of *N*,*N*-dimethylformamide: the solution is clear, and shows a slightly greenish, light yellow-brown color.

(2) Chloride *<1.03>*—To 0.3 g of Hydroxyzine Pamoate add 6 mL of dilute nitric acid and 10 mL of water, shake for 5 minutes, and filter. Wash the residue with two 10-mL portions of water, combine the washings with the filtrate, and add water to make 50 mL. Perform the test using this solution as the test solution. Prepare the control solution with 0.80 mL of 0.01 mol/L hydrochloric acid VS (not more than 0.095%).

(3) Heavy metals *<1.07>*—Proceed with 1.0 g of Hydroxyzine Pamoate according to Method 2, and perform the test. Prepare the control solution with 2.0 mL of Standard Lead Solution (not more than 20 ppm).

(4) Arsenic *<1.11>*—Prepare the test solution with 2.0 g of Hydroxyzine Pamoate according to Method 3, and perform the test (not more than 1 ppm).

(5) Related substances—Dissolve 0.40 g of Hydroxyzine Pamoate in 10 mL of a mixture of sodium hydroxide TS and acetone (1:1), and use the solution as the sample solution. Pipet 1 mL of the sample solution, add a mixture of sodium hydroxide TS and acetone (1:1) to make exactly 20 mL. Pipet 5 mL of this solution, add a mixture of sodium hydroxide TS and acetone (1:1) to make exactly 50 mL, and use the solution as the standard solution. Perform the test with these solutions as directed under Thin-layer Chromatography *<2.03>*. Spot 5 μL each of the sample solution and standard solution on a plate of silica gel for thin-layer chromatography. Develop the plate with a mixture of ethyl acetate, ethanol (95) and ammonia TS (150:95:1) to a distance of about 10 cm, and air-dry the plate. Spray evenly hydrogen hexachloroplatinate (IV)-potassium iodide TS on the plate: the spots other than hydroxyzine and pamoic acid obtained from the sample solution are not more intense than the spot from the standard solution.

Water *<2.48>* Not more than 3.0% (1 g, volumetric titration, direct titration).

Residue on ignition *<2.44>* Not more than 0.5% (1 g).

Assay Weigh accurately about 0.6 g of Hydroxyzine Pamoate, add 25 mL of sodium hydroxide TS, shake well, and extract with six 25-mL portions of chloroform. Filter each extract through 5 g of anhydrous sodium sulfate on a pledget of absorbent cotton. Combine the chloroform extracts, and evaporate the combined chloroform extracts on a water bath to about 30 mL. Add 30 mL of acetic acid (100), and titrate *<2.50>* with 0.1 mol/L perchloric acid VS until the color of the solution changes from purple through blue to blue-green (indicator: 2 drops of crystal violet TS). Perform a blank determination in the same manner, and make any necessary correction.

Each mL of 0.1 mol/L perchloric acid VS
= 38.16 mg of $C_{21}H_{27}ClN_2O_2.C_{23}H_{16}O_6$

Containers and storage Containers—Tight containers.

Hymecromone

ヒメクロモン

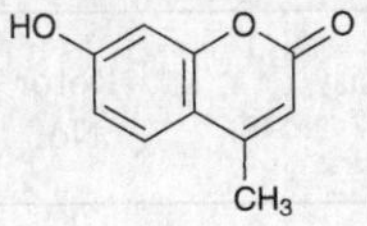

$C_{10}H_8O_3$: 176.17
7-Hydroxy-4-methylchromen-2-one
[*90-33-5*]

Hymecromone, when dried, contains not less than 98.0% of hymecromone ($C_{10}H_8O_3$).

Description Hymecromone occurs as white, crystals or crystalline powder. It is odorless and tasteless.

It is freely soluble in *N*,*N*-dimethylformamide, sparingly soluble in ethanol (95), in ethanol (99.5) and in acetone, slightly soluble in diethyl ether, and practically insoluble in water.

Identification (1) Dissolve 2 mg of Hymecromone in 5 mL of ammonia-ammonium chloride buffer solution (pH 11.0): the solution shows an intense blue-purple fluorescence.

(2) Dissolve 25 mg of Hymecromone in 5 mL of diluted ethanol (95) (1 in 2), and add 1 drop of iron (III) chloride TS: initially a blackish brown color develops, and when allowed to stand the color changes to yellow-brown.

(3) Determine the absorption spectrum of a solution of Himecromone in ethanol (99.5) (1 in 250,000) as directed under Ultraviolet-visible Spectrophotometry <*2.24*>, and compare the spectrum with the Reference Spectrum: both spectra exhibit similar intensities of absorption at the same wavelengths.

(4) Determine the infrared absorption spectrum of Himecromone, previously dried, as directed in the potassium bromide disk method under Infrared Spectrophotometry <*2.25*>, and compare the spectrum with the Reference Spectrum: both spectra exhibit similar intensities of absorption at the same wave numbers.

Melting point <*2.60*> 187 – 191°C

Purity (1) Chloride <*1.03*>—Dissolve 0.8 g of Hymecromone in 40 mL of a mixture of acetone and water (2:1), and add 6 mL of dilute nitric acid and a mixture of acetone and water (2:1) to make 50 mL. Perform the test using this solution as the test solution. Prepare the control solution as follows: to 0.25 mL of 0.01 mol/L hydrochloric acid VS add 6 mL of dilute nitric acid and a mixture of acetone and water (2:1) to make 50 mL (not more than 0.011%).

(2) Sulfate <*1.14*>—Dissolve 0.8 g of Hymecromone in 40 mL of a mixture of acetone and water (2:1), and add 1 mL of dilute hydrochloric acid and a mixture of acetone and water (2:1) to make 50 mL. Perform the test using this solution as the test solution. Prepare the control solution as follows: to 0.40 mL of 0.005 mol/L sulfuric acid VS add 1 mL of dilute hydrochloric acid and a mixture of acetone and water (2:1) to make 50 mL (not more than 0.024%).

(3) Heavy metals <*1.07*>—Proceed with 2.0 g of Hymecromone according to Method 2, and perform the test. Prepare the control solution with 2.0 mL of Standard Lead Solution (not more than 10 ppm).

(4) Arsenic <*1.11*>—Prepare the test solution with 1.0 g of Hymecromone according to Method 3, and perform the test (not more than 2 ppm).

(5) Related substances—Dissolve 80 mg of Hymecromone in 10 mL of ethanol (95), and use this solution as the sample solution. Pipet 1 mL of the sample solution, and add ethanol (95) to make exactly 50 mL. Pipet 1 mL of this solution, add ethanol (95) to make exactly 20 mL, and use this solution as the standard solution. Perform the test with these solutions as directed under Thin-layer Chromatography <*2.03*>. Spot 10 μL each of the sample solution and standard solution on a plate of silica gel for thin-layer chromatography. Develop the plate with a mixture of chloroform and ethanol (95) (10:1) to a distance of about 10 cm, and air-dry the plate. Allow the plate to stand in iodine vapor for 5 minutes: the spots other than the principal spot obtained from the sample solution are not more intense than the spot from the standard solution.

Loss on drying <*2.41*> Not more than 0.5% (1 g, 105°C, 4 hours).

Residue on ignition <*2.44*> Not more than 0.1% (1 g).

Assay Weigh accurately about 0.25 g of Hymecromone, previously dried, dissolve in 90 mL of *N*,*N*-dimethylformamide, and titrate <*2.50*> with 0.1 mol/L tetramethylammonium hydroxide VS (potentiometric titration). Separately, perform a blank determination in the same manner with a solution prepared by adding 14 mL of water to 90 mL of *N*,*N*-dimethylformamide, and make any necessary correction.

Each mL of 0.1 mol/L tetramethylammonium hydroxide VS
= 17.62 mg of $C_{10}H_8O_3$

Containers and storage Containers—Tight containers.

Hypromellose

ヒプロメロース

[*9004-65-3*]

This monograph is harmonized with the European Pharmacopoeia and the U.S. Pharmacopeia.

The corresponding part of the attributes/provisions which are agreed as non-harmonized within the scope of the harmonization is marked with symbols (◆ ◆), and the corresponding parts which are agreed as the JP local requirement other than the scope of the harmonization are marked with symbols (◇ ◇).

Information on the harmonization with the European Pharmacopoeia and the U.S. Pharmacopeia is available on the website of the Pharmaceuticals and Medical Devices Agency.

Hypromellose is a methyl and hydroxypropyl mixed ether of cellulose.

There are four substitution types of Hypromellose, 1828, 2208, 2906 and 2910. They contain methoxy ($-OCH_3$: 31.03) and hydroxypropoxy ($-OC_3H_6OH$:

75.09) groups conforming to the limits for the types of Hypromellose shown in the table below, calculated on the dried basis.

The viscosity is shown in millipascal second (mPa·s) on the label, together with the substitution type.

Substitution Type	Methoxy Group (%)		Hydroxypropoxy Group (%)	
	Min.	Max.	Min.	Max.
1828	16.5	20.0	23.0	32.0
2208	19.0	24.0	4.0	12.0
2906	27.0	30.0	4.0	7.5
2910	28.0	30.0	7.0	12.0

◆**Description** Hypromellose occurs as a white to yellowish white, powder or grains.

It is practically insoluble in ethanol (99.5).

It swells with water and becomes a clear or slightly turbid, viscous solution.◆

Identification (1) Disperse evenly 1.0 g of Hypromellose over the surface of 100 mL of water in a beaker, while gently tapping the top of the beaker, if necessary, and allow the beaker to stand: it aggregates on the surface of water.

(2) Add 1.0 g of Hypromellose to 100 mL of hot water, and stir: it becomes a suspension. Cool the suspension to 10°C, and stir: the resulting liquid is a clear or a slightly cloudy, viscous fluid.

(3) To 0.1 mL of the viscous fluid obtained in (2) add 9 mL of diluted sulfuric acid (9 in 10), shake, heat in a water bath for exactly 3 minutes, and immediately cool in ice water. Add carefully 0.6 mL of ninhydrin TS, shake, and allow to stand at 25°C: the solution shows a red color first, then changes to purple color within 100 minutes.

(4) Pour and spread out 2 to 3 mL of the viscous fluid obtained in (2) onto a glass plate, and allow the water to evaporate: a transparent film results.

(5) Pipet 50 mL of water, add exactly 50 mL of the viscous fluid obtained in (2), and warm to raise the temperature at a rate of 2 to 5°C per minute while stirring: the temperature, when a white turbidity of the solution starts to increase, is not less than 50°C.

Viscosity *<2.53>* (i) Method I: Apply to Hypromellose having a labeled viscosity of less than 600 mPa·s. Put an exact amount of Hypromellose, equivalent to 4.000 g calculated on the dried basis, in a tared, wide-mouth bottle, add water (between 90°C and 99°C) to make 200 g, stopper the bottle, stir by mechanical means at 350 to 450 revolutions per minute for 10 to 20 minutes to get a homogeneous dispersion. If necessary, take off the sample attached on the walls of the bottle, put them in the dispersed solution, and dissolve by continuing the stirring in a water bath at not exceeding 10°C for 20 to 40 minutes. Add cold water, if necessary, to make 200 g, and use this solution as the sample solution. Centrifuge the solution if necessary to expel any entrapped air bubbles. Perform the test with the sample solution at 20 ± 0.1°C as directed in Method I under Viscosity Determination: not less than 80% and not more than 120% of the labeled viscosity.

(ii) Method II: Apply to Hypromellose having a labeled viscosity of not less than 600 mPa·s. Put an exact amount of Hypromellose, equivalent to 10.00 g calculated on the dried basis, in a tared, wide-mouth bottle, add water (between 90°C and 99°C) to make 500 g, and prepare the sample solution in the same manner as directed in Method I. Perform the test with the sample solution at 20 ± 0.1°C as directed in Method II under Viscosity Determination, using a single cylinder-type rotational viscometer, according to the following operating conditions: not less than 75% and not more than 140% of the labeled viscosity.

Operating conditions—

Apparatus: Brookfield type viscometer LV model or an equivalent apparatus.

Rotor No., rotation frequency, and calculation multiplier: According to the following table, depending on the labeled viscosity.

Labeled viscosity (mPa·s)	Rotor No.	Rotation frequency /min	Calculation multiplier
Not less than 600 and less than 1400	3	60	20
〃 1400 〃 3500	3	12	100
〃 3500 〃 9500	4	60	100
〃 9500 〃 99,500	4	6	1000
〃 99,500	4	3	2000

Procedure of apparatus: Read the value after 2 minutes of rotation, and stop the rotation for at least 2 minutes. Repeat this procedure more two times, and average the three observed values.

pH *<2.54>* The pH of the sample solution obtained in the Viscosity, measured after 5 minutes immersing the electrode in the sample solution, is between 5.0 and 8.0.

◇**Purity** Heavy metals—Put 1.0 g of Hypromellose in a 100-mL Kjeldahl flask, add a sufficient amount of a mixture of nitric acid and sulfuric acid (5:4) to wet the sample, and heat gently. Repeat this procedure until to use totally 18 mL of the mixture of nitric acid and sulfuric acid (5:4). Then boil gently until the solution changes to black. After cooling, add 2 mL of nitric acid, and heat until the solution changes to black. Repeat this procedure until the solution no longer changes to black, and heat strongly until dense white fumes are evolved. After cooling, add 5 mL of water, boil gently until dense white fumes are evolved, then heat until the volume of the solution becomes to 2 to 3 mL. After cooling, if the solution reveals yellow color by addition of 5 mL of water, add 1 mL of hydrogen peroxide (30), and heat until the volume of the solution becomes to 2 to 3 mL. After cooling, dilute the solution with 2 to 3 mL of water, transfer to a Nessler tube, add water to make 25 mL, and use this solution as the sample solution. Separately, put 2.0 mL of Standard Lead Solution in a 100-mL Kjeldahl flask, add 18 mL of the mixture of nitric acid and sulfuric acid (5:4) and an amount of nitric acid equal to that used for preparation of the sample solution, and heat until white fumes are evolved. After cooling, add 10 mL of water. In the case where hydrogen peroxide (30) is added for the preparation of the sample solution, add the same amount of hydrogen peroxide (30), then proceed in the same manner for preparation of the sample solution, and use so obtained solution as the control solution. Adjust the sample solution and the control solution to pH 3.0 to 4.0 with ammonia solution (28), and add water to make 40 mL, respectively. To these solutions add 1.2 mL of thioacetamide-alkaline glycerin TS, 2 mL of acetate buffer solution (pH 3.5) and water to make 50 mL, separately. After allowing to stand for 5 minutes, observe vertically both tubes on a white background: the color obtained with the sample solution is not more intense than that with the control solution (not more than 20 ppm).◇

Loss on drying *<2.41>* Not more than 5.0% (1 g, 105°C,

1 hour).

Residue on ignition <*2.44*> Not more than 1.5% (1 g).

Assay (i) Apparatus—Reaction vial: A 5-mL pressure-tight serum vial, having 20 mm in outside diameter and 50 mm in height, the neck 20 mm in outside diameter and 13 mm in inside diameter, equipped with a septum of butyl-rubber processed the surface with fluoroplastics, which can be fixed tightly to vial with aluminum cap, or equivalent.

Heater: A square-shaped aluminum block, having holes 20 mm in diameter and 32 mm in depth, adopted to the reaction vial. Capable of stirring the content of the reaction vial by means of magnetic stirrer or of reciprocal shaker about 100 times per minute.

(ii) Procedure—Weigh accurately about 65 mg of Hypromellose, transfer to a reaction vial, add 60 to 100 mg of adipic acid, 2.0 mL of the internal standard solution and 2.0 mL of hydroiodic acid, immediately stopper the vial tightly, and weigh accurately. Using a magnetic stirrer equipped in the heating module, or using a shaker, stir for 60 minutes while heating so that the temperature of the vial content is 130 ± 2°C. In the case when a magnetic stirrer or shaker is not available, heat for 30 minutes with repeated shaking at 5-minute intervals by hand, and continue heating for an additional 30 minutes. Allow the vial to cool, and again weigh accurately. If the mass loss is less than 26 mg and there is no evidence of a leak of the content, use the upper layer of the mixture as the sample solution. Separately, put 60 to 100 mg of adipic acid, 2.0 mL of the internal standard solution and 2.0 mL of hydroiodic acid in a reaction vial, immediately stopper the vial tightly, and weigh accurately. Add 45 μL of iodomethane for assay and 15 to 22 μL of isopropyl iodide for assay through the septum using a micro-syringe with weighing accurately every time, shake thoroughly, and use the upper layer of the content as the standard solution. Perform the test with 1 to 2 μL each of the sample solution and standard solution as directed under Gas Chromatography <*2.02*> according to the following conditions, and calculate the ratios, Q_{Ta} and Q_{Tb}, of the peak area of iodomethane and isopropyl iodide to that of the internal standard obtained from the sample solution, and Q_{Sa} and Q_{Sb}, of the peak area of iodomethane and isopropyl iodide to that of the internal standard from the standard solution.

Content (%) of methoxy group (CH_3O)
$$= M_{Sa}/M \times Q_{Ta}/Q_{Sa} \times 21.86$$

Content (%) of hydroxypropoxy group ($C_3H_7O_2$)
$$= M_{Sb}/M \times Q_{Tb}/Q_{Sb} \times 44.17$$

M_{Sa}: Amount (mg) of iodomethane for assay taken
M_{Sb}: Amount (mg) of isopropyl iodide for assay taken
M: Amount (mg) of Hypromellose taken, calculated on the dried basis

Internal standard solution—A solution of *n*-octane in *o*-xylene (3 in 100).
Operating conditions—

Detector: A thermal conductivity detector or hydrogen flame-ionization detector.

Column: A fused silica column 0.53 mm in inside diameter and 30 m in length, coated with dimethylpolysiloxane for gas chromatography in 3 μm thickness. Use a guard column, if necessary.

Column temperature: Maintain the temperature at 50°C for 3 minutes, raise to 100°C at a rate of 10°C per minute, then raise to 250°C at a rate of 35°C per minute, and maintain at 250°C for 8 minutes.

Injection port temperature: A constant temperature of about 250°C.

Detector temperature: A constant temperature of about 280°C.

Carrier gas: Helium.

Flow rate: 4.3 mL per minute (the retention time of the internal standard is about 10 minutes).

Split ratio: 1:40.

System suitability—

System performance: When the procedure is run with 1 – 2 μL of the standard solution under the above operating conditions, iodomethane, isopropyl iodide and the internal standard are eluted in this order with the resolution between these peaks being not less than 5.

System repeatability: When the test is repeated 6 times with 1 – 2 μL of the standard solution under the above operating conditions, the relative standard deviations of the ratio of the peak area of iodomethane and isopropyl iodide to that of the internal standard are not more than 2.0%, respectively.

◆**Containers and storage** Containers—Well-closed containers.◆

Hypromellose Acetate Succinate

ヒプロメロース酢酸エステルコハク酸エステル

[*71138-97-1*]

Hypromellose Acetate Succinate is an acetic acid and monosuccinic acid mixed ester of hypromellose.

It contains not less than 12.0% and not more than 28.0% of methoxy group (-OCH_3: 31.03), not less than 4.0 and not more than 23.0% of hydroxypropoxy group (-OC_3H_6OH: 75.09), not less than 2.0% and not more than 16.0% of acetyl group (-$COCH_3$: 43.04), and not less than 4.0% and not more than 28.0% of succinyl group (-COC_2H_4COOH: 101.08), calculated on the dried basis.

Its viscosity is expressed in millipascal second (mPa·s).

Description Hypromellose Acetate Succinate occurs as a white to yellowish white, powder or granules.

It is practically insoluble in water and in ethanol (99.5).

It dissolves in sodium hydroxide TS.

It is hygroscopic.

Identification Determine the infrared absorption spectrum of Hypromellose Acetate Succinate as directed in the ATR method under Infrared Spectrophotometry <*2.25*>: it exhibits absorption at the wave numbers of about 2840 cm^{-1}, 1737 cm^{-1}, 1371 cm^{-1}, 1231 cm^{-1} and 1049 cm^{-1}.

Viscosity <*2.53*> To 2.00 g of Hypromellose Acetate Succinate, previously dried, add dilute sodium hydroxide TS to make 100.0 g, stopper tightly, and dissolve by shaking for 30 minutes. Perform the test with this solution at 20°C according to Method 1: 80 – 120% of the labeled viscosity.

Purity **(1)** Heavy metals <*1.07*>—Proceed with 2.0 g of Hypromellose Acetate Succinate according to Method 2, and perform the test. Prepare the control solution with 2.0 mL of Standard Lead Solution (not more than 10 ppm).

(2) Free acetic acid and free succinic acid—Weigh accurately about 0.1 g of Hypromellose Acetate Succinate, add exactly 4 mL of 0.02 mol/L phosphate buffer solution (pH

7.5), stopper tightly, and stir for 2 hours. Then add exactly 4 mL of diluted phosphoric acid (1 in 500), turn the test tube upside down several times, centrifuge, and use the supernatant liquid as the sample solution. Separately, place 20 mL of water in a 100-mL volumetric flask, weigh the mass of the flask accurately, then add 2.0 mL of acetic acid (100), weigh the mass of the flask to calculate the accurate mass of added acetic acid, and dilute with water to volume. Pipet 6 mL of this solution, add water to make exactly 100 mL, and use this solution as the acetic acid stock solution. Separately, weigh accurately about 0.13 g of succinic acid, dissolve in water to make exactly 100 mL, and use this solution as the succinic acid stock solution. Pipet exactly 4 mL each of the acetic acid stock solution and the succinic acid stock solution, add the mobile phase to make exactly 25 mL, and use this solution as the standard solution. Perform the test with exactly 10 μL each of the sample solution and standard solution as directed under Liquid Chromatography <2.01> according to the following conditions. Determine the peak areas of acetic acid and succinic acid of both solutions, A_{TA}, A_{TS} and A_{SA}, A_{SS}, and calculate the amount of free acetic acid and free succinic acid by the following expressions: the total amount is not more than 1.0%.

Amount (%) of free acetic acid ($C_2H_4O_2$)

$$= M_{SA}/M_T \times A_{TA}/A_{SA} \times 48/625$$

Amount (%) of free succinic acid ($C_4H_6O_4$)

$$= M_{SS}/M_T \times A_{TS}/A_{SS} \times 32/25$$

M_{SA}: Amount (mg) of acetic acid (100) taken
M_{SS}: Amount (mg) of succinic acid taken
M_T: Amount (mg) of Hypromellose Acetate Succinate taken, calculated on the dried basis

Operating conditions—

Proceed as directed in the operating conditions in the Assay (1).

System suitability—

System performance and system repeatability: Proceed as directed in the system suitability in the Assay (1).

Test for required detectability: To 3 mL of the standard solution add the mobile phase to make 10 mL, and use this solution as the solution for system suitability test. Pipet 1 mL of the solution for system suitability test, and add the mobile phase to make exactly 10 mL. Confirm that the peak areas of acetic acid and succinic acid obtained with 10 μL of this solution are equivalent to 7 to 13% of corresponding those with 10 μL of the solution for system suitability test.

Loss on drying <2.41> Not more than 5.0% (1 g, 105°C, 1 hour).

Residue on ignition <2.44> Not more than 0.2% (1 g).

Assay **(1)** Acetyl group and succinyl group—Weigh accurately about 30 mg of Hypromellose Acetate Succinate, add exactly 10 mL of sodium hydroxide TS, stopper tightly, and stir for 4 hours. Add exactly 10 mL of diluted phosphoric acid (17 in 200), turn the test tube upside down several times, and filter the solution through a membrane filter with a pore size 0.22 μm. Discard the first 1 mL of the filtrate, and use the subsequent filtrate as the sample solution. Separately, place 20 mL of water in a 100-mL volumetric flask, weigh the mass of the flask accurately, then add 2.0 mL of acetic acid (100), weigh the mass of the flask to calculate the accurate mass of added acetic acid, and dilute with water to volume. Pipet 6 mL of this solution, add water to make exactly 100 mL, and use this solution as the acetic acid stock solution. Separately, weigh accurately about 0.13 g of succinic acid, dissolve in water to make exactly 100 mL, and use this solution as the succinic acid stock solution. Pipet 4 mL each of the acetic acid stock solution and the succinic acid stock solution, add the mobile phase to make exactly 25 mL, and use this solution as the standard solution. Perform the test with exactly 10 μL each of the sample solution and standard solution as directed under Liquid Chromatography <2.01> according to the following conditions, and determine the peak areas, A_{TA}, A_{TS} and A_{SA}, A_{SS}, of acetic acid and succinic acid in each solution.

Amount (%) of acetyl group (C_2H_3O)

$$= (M_{SA}/M_T \times A_{TA}/A_{SA} \times 24/125 - A_{free}) \times 0.717$$

Amount (%) of succinyl group ($C_4H_5O_3$)

$$= (M_{SS}/M_T \times A_{TS}/A_{SS} \times 16/5 - S_{free}) \times 0.856$$

M_{SA}: Amount (mg) of acetic acid (100) taken
M_{SS}: Amount (mg) of succinic acid taken
M_T: Amount (mg) of Hypromellose Acetate Succinate taken, calculated on the dried basis
A_{free}: Amount (%) of free acetic acid obtained in the Purity (2)
S_{free}: Amount (%) of free succinic acid obtained in the Purity (2)

Operating conditions—

Detector: An ultraviolet absorption photometer (wavelength: 215 nm).

Column: A stainless steel column 4.6 mm in inside diameter and 15 cm in length, packed with octadecylsilanized silica gel for liquid chromatography (5 μm in particle diameter).

Column temperature: A constant temperature of about 25°C.

Mobile phase: 0.02 mol/L potassium dihydrogen phosphate TS, adjusted to pH 2.8 with phosphoric acid.

Flow rate: Adjust so that the retention time of succinic acid is about 7 minutes.

System suitability—

System performance: When the procedure is run with 10 μL of the standard solution under the above operating conditions, acetic acid and succinic acid are eluted in this order with the resolution between these peaks being not less than 5.

System repeatability: When the test is repeated 6 times with 10 μL of the standard solution under the above operating conditions, the relative standard deviation of the peak areas of acetic acid and succinic acid is not more than 2.0%.

(2) Methoxy group and hydroxypropoxy group

(i) Apparatus—Reaction bottle: A 5 mL pressure-tight glass vial, having 20 mm in outside diameter, 50 mm in height, the neck 20 mm in outside diameter and 13 mm in inside diameter, equipped with a septum of butyl rubber processed the surface with fluoroplastics, which can be fixed tightly to vial with aluminum cap, or equivalent.

Heater: A square-shaped aluminum block, having holes 20 mm in inside diameter and 32 mm in depth, adopted to the reaction bottle. Capable of stirring the content of the bottle by means of magnetic stirrer or reciprocal shaker about 100 times per minute.

(ii) Procedure—Weigh accurately about 65 mg of Hypromellose Acetate Succinate, place in the reaction bottle, add 0.06 to 0.10 g of adipic acid, 2.0 mL of the internal standard solution and 2.0 mL of hydriodic acid, stopper the bottle immediately, and weigh accurately. Stir or shake for 60 minutes while heating so that the temperature of the bottle content is 130 ± 2°C. In a case where the magnetic stirrer or shaker is not available, heat for 30 minutes with repeated shaking at 5 minute intervals by hand, and continue heating for additional 30 minutes. Allow the bottle to cool, and again weigh accurately. If the mass loss is less than 0.50% or there is no evidence of a leak, use the upper layer of the mixture as the sample solution. Separately, put 0.06 to 0.10 g of adipic acid, 2.0 mL of the internal standard solution and 2.0 mL of hydriodic acid in a reaction bottle, stopper the bottle immediately, and weigh accurately. Add 45 μL of iodomethane for assay and 15 to 22 μL of isopropyl iodide for assay through the septum using a micro-syringe with weighing accurately every time, stir thoroughly, and use the upper layer of the mixture as the standard solution. Perform the test with 1 to 2 μL each of the sample solution and standard solution as directed under Gas Chromatography <*2.02*> according to the following conditions, and calculate the ratios of the peak areas of iodomethane and isopropyl iodide to the peak area of the internal standard, Q_{Ta}, Q_{Tb} and Q_{Sa}, Q_{Sb}.

Amount (%) of methoxy group (CH_3O)
$= M_{Sa}/M_T \times Q_{Ta}/Q_{Sa} \times 21.86$

Amount (%) of hydroxypropoxy group ($C_3H_7O_2$)
$= M_{Sb}/M_T \times Q_{Tb}/Q_{Sb} \times 44.17$

M_{Sa}: Amount (mg) of iodomethane for assay taken
M_{Sb}: Amount (mg) of isopropyl iodide for assay taken
M_T: Amount (mg) of Hypromellose Acetate Succinate taken, calculated on the dried basis

Internal standard solution—A solution of *n*-octane in *o*-xylene (3 in 100).

Operating conditions—

Detector: A thermal conductivity detector or hydrogen flame-ionization detector.

Column: A glass tube 3 - 4 mm in inside diameter and 1.8 - 3 m in length, packed with siliceous earth for gas chromatography, 120 to 150 μm in diameter coated with methyl silicon polymer for gas chromatography in 10 - 20%.

Column temperature: A constant temperature of about 100°C.

Carrier gas: Helium for the thermal conductivity detector, or Helium or Nitrogen for the hydrogen flame-ionization detector.

Flow rate: Adjust so that the retention time of the internal standard is about 10 minutes.

System suitability—

System performance: When the procedure is run with 1 - 2 μL of the standard solution under the above operating conditions, iodomethane, isopropyl iodide and the internal standard are eluted in this order with the resolution between each peak being not less than 5.

System repeatability: When the test is repeated 6 times with 1 - 2 μL of the standard solution under the above operating conditions, the relative standard deviations of the ratio of the peak area of iodomethane and isopropyl iodide to that of the internal standard are not more than 2.0%, respectively.

Containers and storage Containers—Tight containers.

Hypromellose Phthalate

ヒプロメロースフタル酸エステル

[*9050-31-1*]

This monograph is harmonized with the European Pharmacopoeia and the U.S. Pharmacopeia.

The parts of the text that are not harmonized are marked with symbols (◆ ◆).

Information on the harmonization with the European Pharmacopoeia and the U.S. Pharmacopeia is available on the website of the Pharmaceuticals and Medical Devices Agency.

Hypromellose Phthalate is a monophthalic acid ester of hypromellose.

It contains methoxy group ($-OCH_3$: 31.03), hydroxypropoxy group ($-OCH_2CHOHCH_3$: 75.09), and carboxybenzoyl group ($-COC_6H_4COOH$: 149.12).

It contains not less than 21.0% and not more than 35.0% of carboxybenzoyl group, calculated on the anhydrous basis.

◆Its substitution type and its viscosity in millipascal second (mPa·s) are shown on the label.

Substitution Type	Carboxybenzoyl group (%) Min.	Max.
200731	27.0	35.0
220824	21.0	27.0

◆**Description** Hypromellose Phthalate occurs as white, powder or granules.

It is practically insoluble in water, in acetonitrile and in ethanol (99.5).

It becomes a viscous liquid when a mixture of methanol and dichloromethane (1:1) or a mixture of ethanol (99.5) and acetone (1:1) is added.

It dissolves in sodium hydroxide TS.◆

◆**Identification** Determine the infrared absorption spectrum of Hypromellose Phthalate as directed in the potassium bromide disk method under Infrared Spectrophotometry <*2.25*>, and compare the spectrum with the Reference Spectrum: both spectra exhibit similar intensities of absorption at the same wave numbers.◆

Viscosity <*2.53*> To 10 g of Hypromellose Phthalate, previously dried at 105°C for 1 hour, add 90 g of a mixture of methanol and dichloromethane in equal mass ratio, and stir to dissolve. Determine the viscosity at 20 ± 0.1°C as directed in Method 1 under Viscosity Determination: the viscosity is not less than 80% and not more than 120% of the labeled unit.

Purity (1) Chloride <*1.03*>—Dissolve 1.0 g of Hypromellose Phthalate in 40 mL of 0.2 mol/L sodium hydroxide VS, add 1 drop of phenolphthalein TS, and add dilute nitric acid dropwise with vigorous stirring until the red color is discharged. Further add 20 mL of dilute nitric acid with stirring. Heat on a water bath with stirring until the gelatinous precipitate formed turns to granular particles. After cooling, centrifuge, and take off the supernatant liquid. Wash the precipitate with three 20-mL portions of water by centrifuging each time, combine the supernatant liquid and the washings, add water to make 200 mL, and filter. Perform the test with 50 mL of the filtrate. Control solution: To 0.50 mL of 0.01 mol/L hydrochloric acid VS add 10 mL of 0.2 mol/L sodium hydroxide VS and 7 mL of dilute nitric acid, and add water to make 50 mL (not more than 0.07%).

◆**(2)** Heavy metals ⟨*1.07*⟩—Proceed with 2.0 g of Hypromellose Phthalate according to Method 2, and perform the test. Prepare the control solution with 2.0 mL of Standard Lead Solution (not more than 10 ppm).◆

(3) Phthalic acid—Weigh accurately about 0.2 g of Hypromellose Phthalate, add about 50 mL of acetonitrile to dissolve partially with the aid of ultrasonic waves, add 10 mL of water, and dissolve further with the ultrasonic waves. After cooling, add acetonitrile to make exactly 100 mL, and use this solution as the sample solution. Separately, weigh accurately about 12.5 mg of phthalic acid, dissolve in about 125 mL of acetonitrile by mixing, add 25 mL of water, then add acetonitrile to make exactly 250 mL, and use this solution as the standard solution. Perform the test with exactly 10 μL each of the sample solution and standard solution as directed under Liquid Chromatography ⟨*2.01*⟩ according to the following conditions, and determine the peak areas, A_T and A_S, of phthalic acid in each solution: amount of phthalic acid ($C_8H_6O_4$: 166.13) is not more than 1.0%.

Amount (%) of phthalic acid = $M_S/M_T \times A_T/A_S \times 40$

M_S: Amount (mg) of phthalic acid taken

M_T: Amount (mg) of Hypromellose Phthalate taken, calculated on the anhydrous basis

Operating conditions—

Detector: An ultraviolet absorption photometer (wavelength: 235 nm).

Column: A stainless steel column about 4.6 mm in inside diameter and 25 cm in length, packed with octadecylsilanized silica gel for liquid chromatography (3 to 10 μm in particle diameter).

Column temperature: A constant temperature of about 20°C.

Mobile phase: A mixture of 0.1% trifluoroacetic acid and acetonitrile (9:1).

Flow rate: About 2.0 mL per minute.

System suitability—

◆System performance: When the procedure is run with 10 μL of the standard solution under the above operating conditions, the number of theoretical plates and the symmetry factor of the peak of phthalic acid are not less than 2500 and not more than 1.5, respectively.◆

System repeatability: When repeat the test 6 times with 10 μL of the standard solution under the above operating conditions, the relative standard deviation of the peak area of phthalic acid is not more than 1.0%.

Water ⟨*2.48*⟩ Not more than 5.0% (1 g, volumetric titration, direct titration, using a mixture of ethanol (99.5) and dichloromethane (3:2) instead of methanol for water determination).

Residue on ignition ⟨*2.44*⟩ Not more than 0.2% (1 g).

Assay Weigh accurately about 1 g of Hypromellose Phthalate, dissolve in 50 mL of a mixture of ethanol (95), acetone and water (2:2:1), and titrate ⟨*2.50*⟩ with 0.1 mol/L sodium hydroxide VS (indicator: 2 drops of phenolphthalein TS). Perform a blank determination in the same manner, and make any necessary correction.

Amount (%) of carboxybenzoyl group ($C_8H_5O_3$)
$= \{(0.01 \times 149.1 \times V)/M\} - \{(2 \times 149.1 \times P)/166.1\}$

P: Amount (%) of phthalic acid obtained in the Purity (3)

V: Amount (mL) of 0.1 mol/L sodium hydroxide VS consumed

M: Amount (g) of Hypromellose Phthalate taken, calculated on the anhydrous basis

Containers and storage Containers—Tight containers.

Ibudilast

イブジラスト

$C_{14}H_{18}N_2O$: 230.31
1-[2-(1-Methylethyl)pyrazolo[1,5-*a*]pyridin-3-yl]-2-methylpropan-1-one
[*50847-11-5*]

Ibudilast, when dried, contains not less than 98.5% and not more than 101.0% of ibudilast ($C_{14}H_{18}N_2O$).

Description Ibudilast occurs as a white crystalline powder.

It is very soluble in methanol, freely soluble in ethanol (99.5) and in acetic anhydride, and very slightly soluble in water.

Identification **(1)** Determine the absorption spectrum of a solution of Ibudilast in methanol (1 in 250,000) as directed under Ultraviolet-visible Spectrophotometry ⟨*2.24*⟩, and compare the spectrum with the Reference Spectrum: both spectra exhibit similar intensities of absorption at the same wavelengths.

(2) Determine the infrared absorption spectrum of Ibudilast as directed in the potassium bromide disk method under Infrared Spectrophotometry ⟨*2.25*⟩, and compare the spectrum with the Reference Spectrum: both spectra exhibit similar intensities of absorption at the same wave numbers.

Melting point ⟨*2.60*⟩ 54 – 58°C

Purity **(1)** Heavy metals ⟨*1.07*⟩—Proceed with 1.0 g of Ibudilast according to Method 2, and perform the test. Prepare the control solution with 2.0 mL of Standard Lead Solution (not more than 20 ppm).

(2) Related substances—Dissolve 50 mg of Ibudilast in 50 mL of the mobile phase, and use this solution as the sample solution. Pipet 1 mL of the sample solution, and add the mobile phase to make exactly 50 mL. Pipet 1 mL of this solution, add the mobile phase to make exactly 20 mL, and use this solution as the standard solution. Perform the test with exactly 10 μL each of the sample solution and standard solution as directed under Liquid Chromatography ⟨*2.01*⟩ according to the following conditions, and determine each peak area by the automatic integration method: each peak area other than ibudilast obtained from the sample solution is not larger than the peak area of ibudilast from the standard solution, and the total area of the peaks other than ibudilast is not larger than 3 times the peak area of ibudilast from the standard solution.

Operating conditions—

Detector: An ultraviolet absorption photometer (wave-

length: 292 nm).

Column: A stainless steel column 2.6 mm in inside diameter and 15 cm in length, packed with silica gel for liquid chromatography (5 μm in particle diameter).

Column temperature: A constant temperature of about 25°C.

Mobile phase: A mixture of hexane and ethyl acetate (50:1).

Flow rate: Adjust so that the retention time of ibudilast is about 9 minutes.

Time span of measurement: About 4 times as long as the retention time of ibudilast, beginning after the solvent peak.

System suitability—

Test for required detectability: To exactly 5 mL of the standard solution add the mobile phase to make exactly 10 mL. Confirm that the peak area of ibudilast obtained with 10 μL of this solution is equivalent to 40 to 60% of that with 10 μL of the standard solution.

System performance: To 5 mL of the sample solution add the mobile phase to make 50 mL. To 2 mL of this solution add the mobile phase to make 20 mL. When the procedure is run with 10 μL of this solution under the above operating conditions, the number of theoretical plates and the symmetry factor of the peak of ibudilast are not less than 3500 and not more than 2.0, respectively.

System repeatability: When the test is repeated 6 times with 10 μL of the standard solution under the above operating conditions, the relative standard deviation of the peak area of ibudilast is not more than 3.0%.

Loss on drying *<2.41>* Not more than 0.3% (1 g, in vacuum, 4 hours).

Residue on ignition *<2.44>* Not more than 0.1% (1 g).

Assay Weigh accurately about 0.2 g of Ibudilast, previously dried, dissolve in 50 mL of acetic anhydride, and titrate *<2.50>* with 0.1 mol/L perchloric acid VS (potentiometric titration). Perform a blank determination in the same manner, and make any necessary correction.

Each mL of 0.1 mol/L perchloric acid VS
= 23.03 mg of $C_{14}H_{18}N_2O$

Containers and storage Containers—Tight containers.

Ibuprofen

イブプロフェン

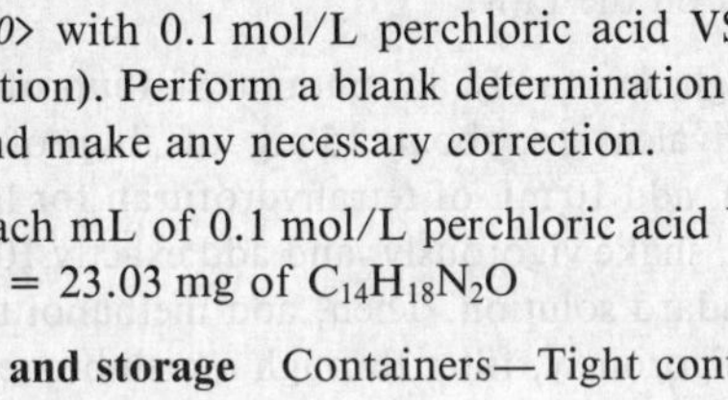

and enantiomer

$C_{13}H_{18}O_2$: 206.28
(2*RS*)-2-[4-(2-Methylpropyl)phenyl]propanoic acid
[15687-27-1]

Ibuprofen, when dried, contains not less than 98.5% of ibuprofen ($C_{13}H_{18}O_2$).

Description Ibuprofen occurs as a white crystalline powder.

It is freely soluble in ethanol (95) and in acetone, and practically insoluble in water.

It dissolves in dilute sodium hydroxide TS.

Identification **(1)** Determine the absorption spectrum of a solution of Ibuprofen in dilute sodium hydroxide TS (3 in 20,000) as directed under Ultraviolet-visible Spectrophotometry *<2.24>*, and compare the spectrum with the Reference Spectrum: both spectra exhibit similar intensities of absorption at the same wavelengths.

(2) Determine the infrared absorption spectrum of Ibuprofen, previously dried, as directed in the potassium bromide disk method under Infrared Spectrophotometry *<2.25>*, and compare the spectrum with the Reference Spectrum: both spectra exhibit similar intensities of absorption at the same wave numbers.

Melting point *<2.60>* 75 – 77°C

Purity **(1)** Heavy metals *<1.07>*—Proceed with 3.0 g of Ibuprofen according to Method 2, and perform the test. Prepare the control solution with 3.0 mL of Standard Lead Solution (not more than 10 ppm).

(2) Arsenic *<1.11>*—Prepare the test solution with 1.0 g of Ibuprofen according to Method 3, and perform the test (not more than 2 ppm).

(3) Related substances—Dissolve 0.50 g of Ibuprofen in 5 mL of acetone , and use this solution as the sample solution. Pipet 1 mL of the sample solution, add acetone to make exactly 100 mL, and use this solution as the standard solution. Perform the test with these solutions as directed under Thin-layer Chromatography *<2.03>*. Spot 5 μL each of the sample solution and standard solution on a plate of silica gel with fluorescent indicator for thin-layer chromatography. Develop the plate with a mixture of hexane, ethyl acetate and acetic acid (100) (15:5:1) to a distance of about 10 cm, and air-dry the plate. Examine the plate under ultraviolet light (main wavelength: 254 nm): the spots other than the principal spot obtained from the sample solution are not more intense than the spot from the standard solution.

Loss on drying *<2.41>* Not more than 0.5% (1 g, reduced pressure not exceeding 0.67 kPa, phosphorus (V) oxide, 4 hours).

Residue on ignition *<2.44>* Not more than 0.1% (1 g).

Assay Weigh accurately about 0.5 g of Ibuprofen, previously dried, dissolve in 50 mL of ethanol (95), and titrate *<2.50>* with 0.1 mol/L sodium hydroxide VS (indicator: 3 drops of phenolphthalein TS). Perform a blank determination in the same manner, and make any necessary correction.

Each mL of 0.1 mol/L sodium hydroxide VS
= 20.63 mg of $C_{13}H_{18}O_2$

Containers and storage Containers—Well-closed containers.

Ibuprofen Piconol

イブプロフェンピコノール

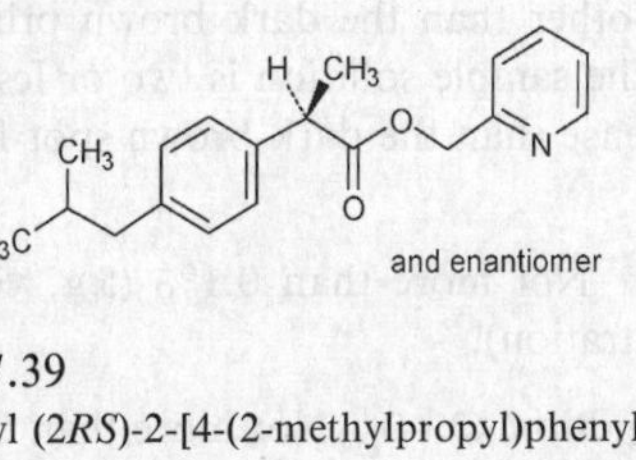

and enantiomer

$C_{19}H_{23}NO_2$: 297.39
Pyridin-2-ylmethyl (2*RS*)-2-[4-(2-methylpropyl)phenyl]propanoate
[64622-45-3]

Ibuprofen Piconol contains not less than 98.5% and not more than 101.0% of ibuprofen piconol ($C_{19}H_{23}NO_2$), calculated on the anhydrous basis.

Description Ibuprofen Piconol occurs as a clear, colorless to pale yellow liquid. It is odorless or has a slight characteristic odor.

It is miscible with methanol, with ethanol (95), with acetone and with acetic acid (100).

It is practically insoluble in water.

It decomposes on exposure to light.

It shows no optical rotation.

Identification **(1)** Dissolve 10 mg of Ibuprofen Piconol in 250 mL of ethanol (95). Determine the absorption spectrum of this solution as directed under Ultraviolet-visible Spectrophotometry *<2.24>*, and compare the spectrum with the Reference Spectrum: both spectra exhibit similar intensities of absorption at the same wavelengths.

(2) Determine the infrared absorption spectrum of Ibuprofen Piconol as directed in the liquid film method under Infrared Spectrophotometry *<2.25>*, and compare the spectrum with the Reference Spectrum: both spectra exhibit similar intensities of absorption at the same wave numbers.

Refractive index *<2.45>* n_D^{20}: 1.529 – 1.532

Specific gravity *<2.56>* d_{20}^{20}: 1.046 – 1.050

Purity **(1)** Chloride *<1.03>*—Dissolve 0.5 g of Ibuprofen Piconol in 20 mL of acetone, add 6 mL of dilute nitric acid and water to make 50 mL. Perform the test using this solution as the test solution. Prepare the control solution as follows: to 0.30 mL of 0.01 mol/L hydrochloric acid VS add 20 mL of acetone, 6 mL of dilute nitric acid and water to make 50 mL (not more than 0.021%).

(2) Sulfate *<1.14>*—Dissolve 0.5 g of Ibuprofen Piconol in 20 mL of acetone, add 1 mL of dilute hydrochloric acid and water to make 50 mL. Perform the test using this solution as the test solution. Prepare the control solution as follows: to 0.40 mL of 0.005 mol/L sulfuric acid VS add 20 mL of acetone, 1 mL of dilute hydrochloric acid and water to make 50 mL (not more than 0.038%).

(3) Heavy metals *<1.07>*—Proceed with 4.0 g of Ibuprofen Piconol according to Method 2, and perform the test. Prepare the control solution with 2.0 mL of Standard Lead Solution (not more than 5 ppm).

(4) Related substances—Dissolve 0.10 g of Ibuprofen Piconol in 5 mL of methanol, and use this solution as the sample solution. Pipet 1 mL of the sample solution, add methanol to make exactly 200 mL, and use this solution as the standard solution. Perform the test with these solutions as directed under Thin-layer Chromatography *<2.03>*. Spot 10 μL each of the sample solution and standard solution on a plate of silica gel for thin-layer chromatography. Develop the plate with a mixture of hexane, ethyl acetate, acetic acid (100) and methanol (30:10:2:1) to a distance of about 10 cm, and air-dry the plate. Spray evenly a solution of phosphomolybdic acid *n*-hydrate in ethanol (95) (1 in 10) on the plate, and heat the plate at 170°C for 10 minutes: the number of spots other than the dark brown principal spot obtained from the sample solution is two or less, and they are not more intense than the dark brown spot from the standard solution.

Water *<2.48>* Not more than 0.1% (5 g, volumetric titration, direct titration).

Residue on ignition *<2.44>* Not more than 0.1% (1 g).

Assay Weigh accurately about 0.6 g of Ibuprofen Piconol, dissolve in 50 mL of acetic acid (100), and titrate *<2.50>* with 0.1 mol/L perchloric acid VS (potentiometric titration). Perform a blank determination in the same manner, and make any necessary correction.

Each mL of 0.1 mol/L perchloric acid VS
= 29.74 mg of $C_{19}H_{23}NO_2$

Containers and storage Containers—Tight containers.

Storage—Light-resistant.

Ibuprofen Piconol Cream

イブプロフェンピコノールクリーム

Ibuprofen Piconol Cream contains not less than 95.0% and not more than 105.0% of the labeled amount of ibuprofen piconol ($C_{19}H_{23}NO_2$: 297.39).

Method of preparation Prepare as directed under Creams, with Ibuprofen Piconol.

Identification To an amount of Ibuprofen Piconol Cream, equivalent to 50 mg of Ibuprofen Piconol, add 10 mL of methanol, warm in a water bath, mix well, filter after cooling, and use the filtrate as the sample solution. Separately, dissolve 50 mg of ibuprofen piconol in 10 mL of methanol, and use this solution as the standard solution. Perform the test with these solutions as directed under Thin-layer Chromatography *<2.03>*. Spot 10 μL each of the sample solution and standard solution on a plate of silica gel with fluorescent indicator for thin-layer chromatography. Develop the plate with a mixture of hexane, ethyl acetate and acetic acid (100) (15:5:1) to a distance of about 13 cm, and air-dry the plate. Examine under ultraviolet light (main wavelength: 254 nm): the principal spot obtained from the sample solution and the spot from the standard solution show the same *R*f value.

pH Being specified separately when the drug is granted approval based on the Law.

Assay Weigh accurately an amount of Ibuprofen Piconol Cream, equivalent to about 15 mg of ibuprofen piconol ($C_{19}H_{23}NO_2$), add 10 mL of tetrahydrofuran for liquid chromatography, shake vigorously, and add exactly 10 mL of the internal standard solution. Then, add methanol to make 30 mL, shake vigorously, filter through a membrane filter with a pore size not exceeding 0.45 μm, and use the filtrate as the sample solution. Separately, weigh accurately about 0.15 g of ibuprofen piconol for assay (separately determine the water *<2.48>* in the same manner as Ibuprofen Piconol), and dissolve in tetrahydrofuran for liquid chromatography to make exactly 100 mL. Pipet 10 mL of this solution, add exactly 10 mL of the internal standard solution, add methanol to make 30 mL, and use this solution as the standard solution. Perform the test with 5 μL each of the sample solution and standard solution as directed under Liquid Chromatography *<2.01>* according to the following conditions, and calculate the ratios, Q_T and Q_S, of the peak area of ibuprofen piconol to that of the internal standard.

$$\text{Amount (mg) of ibuprofen piconol } (C_{19}H_{23}NO_2) = M_S \times Q_T/Q_S \times 1/10$$

M_S: Amount (mg) of ibuprofen piconol for assay taken, calculated on the anhydrous basis

Internal standard solution—A solution of triphenylmethane in methanol (1 in 200).

Operating conditions—

Detector: An ultraviolet absorption photometer (wavelength: 254 nm).

Column: A stainless steel column 4.6 mm in inside diame-

ter and 15 cm in length, packed with octadecylsilanized silica gel for liquid chromatography (5 μm in particle diameter).

Column temperature: A constant temperature of about 40°C.

Mobile phase: A mixture of methanol and acetic acid-sodium acetate buffer solution (pH 4.0) (3:1).

Flow rate: Adjust so that the retention time of ibuprofen piconol is about 6.5 minutes.

System suitability—

System performance: When the procedure is run with 5 μL of the standard solution under the above operating conditions, ibuprofen piconol and the internal standard are eluted in this order with the resolution between these peaks being not less than 8.

System repeatability: When the test is repeated 6 times with 5 μL of the standard solution under the above operating conditions, the relative standard deviation of the ratio of the peak area of ibuprofen piconol to that of the internal standard is not more than 1.0%.

Containers and storage Containers—Tight containers.

Storage—Light-resistant.

Ibuprofen Piconol Ointment

イブプロフェンピコノール軟膏

Ibuprofen Piconol Ointment contains not less than 95.0% and not more than 105.0% of the labeled amount of ibuprofen piconol ($C_{19}H_{23}NO_2$: 297.39).

Method of preparation Prepare as directed under Ointments, with Ibuprofen Piconol.

Identification To an amount of Ibuprofen Piconol Ointment, equivalent to 50 mg of Ibuprofen Piconol, add 10 mL of methanol, warm at 60°C in a water bath, mix well, and filter after cooling. Use the filtrate as the sample solution. Separately, dissolve 50 mg of ibuprofen piconol in 10 mL of methanol, and use this solution as the standard solution. Perform the test with these solutions as directed under Thin-layer Chromatography <*2.03*>. Spot 10 μL each of the sample solution and standard solution on a plate of silica gel with fluorescent indicator for thin-layer chromatography. Develop the plate with a mixture of hexane, ethyl acetate and acetic acid (100) (15:5:1) to a distance of about 13 cm, and air-dry the plate. Examine under ultraviolet light (main wavelength: 254 nm): the principal spot obtained from the sample solution and the spot from the standard solution show the same *R*f value.

Assay Weigh accurately an amount of Ibuprofen Piconol Ointment, equivalent to about 15 mg of ibuprofen piconol ($C_{19}H_{23}NO_2$), add 10 mL of tetrahydrofuran for liquid chromatography, shake vigorously, and add exactly 10 mL of the internal standard solution. Then, add methanol to make 30 mL, shake vigorously, filter through a membrane filter with a pore size not exceeding 0.45 μm, and use the filtrate as the sample solution. Separately, weigh accurately about 0.15 g of ibuprofen piconol for assay (separately determine the water <*2.48*> in the same manner as Ibuprofen Piconol), and dissolve in tetrahydrofuran for liquid chromatography to make exactly 100 mL. Pipet 10 mL of this solution, add exactly 10 mL of the internal standard solution, add methanol to make exactly 30 mL, and use this solution as the standard solution. Perform the test with 5 μL each of the sample solution and standard solution as directed under Liquid Chromatography <*2.01*> according to the following conditions, and calculate the ratios, Q_T and Q_S, of the peak area of ibuprofen piconol to that of the internal standard.

$$\text{Amount (mg) of ibuprofen piconol } (C_{19}H_{23}NO_2) = M_S \times Q_T/Q_S \times 1/10$$

M_S: Amount (mg) of ibuprofen piconol for assay taken, calculated on the anhydrous basis

*Internal standard solution—*A solution of triphenylmethane in methanol (1 in 200).

Operating conditions—

Detector: An ultraviolet absorption photometer (wavelength: 254 nm).

Column: A stainless steel column 4.6 mm in inside diameter and 15 cm in length, packed with octadecylsilanized silica gel for liquid chromatography (5 μm in particle diameter).

Column temperature: A constant temperature of about 40°C.

Mobile phase: A mixture of methanol and acetic acid-sodium acetate buffer solution (pH 4.0) (3:1).

Flow rate: Adjust so that the retention time of ibuprofen piconol is about 6.5 minutes.

System suitability—

System performance: When the procedure is run with 5 μL of the standard solution under the above operating conditions, ibuprofen piconol and the internal standard are eluted in this order with the resolution between these peaks being not less than 8.

System repeatability: When the test is repeated 6 times with 5 μL of the standard solution under the above operating conditions, the relative standard deviation of the ratio of the peak area of ibuprofen piconol to that of the internal standard is not more than 1.0%.

Containers and storage Containers—Tight containers.

Storage—Light-resistant.

Ichthammol

イクタモール

Ichthammol, calculated on the dried basis, contains not less than 2.5% of ammonia (NH_3: 17.03), not more than 8.0% of ammonium sulfate [$(NH_4)_2SO_4$: 132.14], and not less than 10.0% of total sulfur (as S: 32.07).

Description Ichthammol is a red-brown to black-brown, viscous fluid. It has a characteristic odor.

It is miscible with water.

It is partially soluble in ethanol (95) and in diethyl ether.

Identification **(1)** To 4 mL of a solution of Ichthammol (3 in 10) add 8 mL of hydrochloric acid: a yellow-brown to blackish brown, oily or resinous mass is produced. Cool the mass with ice to solidify, and discard the water layer. Wash the residue with diethyl ether: a part of the mass dissolves but it does not dissolve completely even when it is washed until almost no color develops in the washing. Perform the following tests with this residue.

(i) To 0.1 g of the residue add 1 mL of a mixture of ethanol (95) and diethyl ether (1:1): it dissolves.

(ii) To 0.1 g of the residue add 2 mL of water: it dissolves. To 1 mL of this solution add 0.4 mL of hydrochloric acid: a yellow-brown to blackish brown oily or resinous substance is produced.

(iii) To 1 mL of the solution obtained in (ii) add 0.3 g of sodium chloride: a yellow-brown or blackish brown oily or resinous substance is produced.

(2) Boil 2 mL of a solution of Ichthammol (1 in 10) with 2 mL of sodium hydroxide TS: the gas evolved changes moistened red litmus paper to blue.

Loss on drying <*2.41*> Not more than 50% (0.5 g, 105°C, 6 hours).

Residue on ignition <*2.44*> Not more than 0.5% (1 g).

Assay **(1)** Ammonia—Weigh accurately about 5 g of Ichthammol, transfer to a Kjeldahl flask, and add 60 mL of water, 1 mL of 1-octanol and 4.5 mL of a solution of sodium hydroxide (2 in 5). Connect the flask to a distilling tube with a spray trap and a condenser, and immerse the lower outlet of the condenser in the receiver containing exactly 30 mL of 0.25 mol/L sulfuric acid VS. Distil slowly, collect about 50 mL of the distillate, and titrate <*2.50*> the excess sulfuric acid with 0.5 mol/L sodium hydroxide VS (indicator: 3 drops of methyl red TS). Perform a blank determination in the same manner.

Each mL of 0.25 mol/L sulfuric acid VS
= 8.515 mg of NH_3

(2) Ammonium sulfate—Weigh accurately about 1 g of Ichthammol, add 25 mL of ethanol (95), stir thoroughly, and filter. Wash with a mixture of ethanol (95) and diethyl ether (1:1) until the washings are clear and colorless. Dry the filter paper and the residue in air, dissolve the residue in 200 mL of hot water acidified slightly with hydrochloric acid, and filter. Boil the filtrate, add 30 mL of barium chloride TS slowly, heat for 30 minutes on a water bath, and filter. Wash the precipitate with water, dry, and ignite to constant mass. Weigh the residue as barium sulfate ($BaSO_4$: 233.39).

Amount (mg) of ammonium sulfate [$(NH_4)_2SO_4$]
= amount (mg) of barium sulfate ($BaSO_4$) × 0.566

(3) Total sulfur—Weigh accurately about 0.6 g of Ichthammol, transfer to a 200-mL Kjeldahl flask, and add 30 mL of water and 5 g of potassium chlorate, then add slowly 30 mL of nitric acid, and evaporate the mixture to about 5 mL. Transfer the residue to a 300-mL beaker with the aid of 25 mL of hydrochloric acid, and evaporate again to 5 mL. Add 100 mL of water, boil, filter, and wash with water. Heat the combined filtrate and washings to boil, add gradually 30 mL of barium chloride TS, heat the mixture on a water bath for 30 minutes, and filter. Wash the precipitate with water, dry, and ignite to constant mass. Weigh the residue as barium sulfate ($BaSO_4$).

Amount (mg) of total sulfur (S)
= amount (mg) of barium sulfate ($BaSO_4$) × 0.13739

Containers and storage Containers—Tight containers.

Idarubicin Hydrochloride

イダルビシン塩酸塩

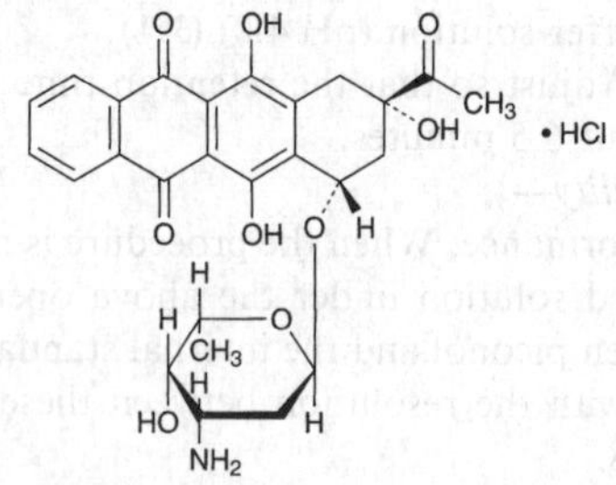

$C_{26}H_{27}NO_9$.HCl: 533.95
(2*S*,4*S*)-2-Acetyl-4-(3-amino-2,3,6-trideoxy-α-L-*lyxo*-hexopyranosyloxy)-2,5,12-trihydroxy-1,2,3,4-tetrahydrotetracene-6,11-dione monohydrochloride
[*57852-57-0*]

Idarubicin Hydrochloride contains not less than 960 μg (potency) and not more than 1030 μg (potency) per mg, calculated on the anhydrous basis. The potency of Idarubicin Hydrochloride is expressed as mass (potency) of idarubicin hydrochloride ($C_{26}H_{27}NO_9$.HCl).

Description Idarubicin Hydrochloride occurs as a yellow-red powder.

It is sparingly soluble in methanol, slightly soluble in water and in ethanol (95), and practically insoluble in acetonitrile and in diethyl ether.

Identification **(1)** Determine the absorption spectra of a solution of Idarubicin Hydrochloride in methanol (1 in 100,000) as directed under Ultraviolet-visible Spectrophotometry <*2.24*>, and compare the spectrum with the Reference Spectrum or the spectrum of a solution of Idarubicin Hydrochloride RS prepared in the same manner as the sample solution: both spectra exhibit similar intensities of absorption at the same wavelengths.

(2) Determine the infrared absorption spectra of Idarubicin Hydrochloride and Idarubicin Hydrochloride RS as directed in the potassium bromide disk method under Infrared Spectrophotometry <*2.25*>, and compare these spectra: both spectra exhibit similar intensities of absorption at the same wave numbers.

(3) Dissolve 2 mg of Idarubicin Hydrochloride in 3 mL of water, and add 1 mL of dilute nitric acid and 3 drops of silver nitrate TS: a white turbidity is produced.

Optical rotation <*2.49*> $[\alpha]_D^{20}$: +188 – +201° (20 mg calculated on the anhydrous basis, methanol, 20 mL, 100 mm).

pH <*2.54*> Dissolve 10 mg of Idarubicin Hydrochloride in 10 mL of water: the pH of the solution is between 5.0 and 6.5.

Purity **(1)** Clarity and color of solution—Dissolve 10 mg of Idarubicin Hydrochloride in 10 mL of water: the solution is clear and yellow-red in color.

(2) Silver— Dissolve exactly 0.10 g of Idarubicin Hydrochloride in diluted nitric acid (1 in 200) to make exactly 20 mL, and use this solution as the sample solution. Separately, to exactly 5 mL of Standard Silver Solution for Atomic Absorption Spectrophotometry add diluted nitric acid (1 in 200) to make exactly 50 mL. Pipet a suitable amount of this solution, dilute exactly it with diluted nitric acid (1 in 200) so that each mL contains 0.05 μg, 0.075 μg, 0.1 μg and 0.2 μg of silver (Ag: 107.87), and use this solution as the standard solution. Perform the test with the sample solution and standard solution as directed under Atomic Absorption Spectrophotometry <2.23> according to the following conditions, and calculate the amount of silver in the sample solution using the calibration curve obtained with the absorbances of the standard solution: not more than 20 ppm.

Gas: Combustible gas—Acetylene.
Supporting gas—Air.

Lamp: Silver hollow-cathode lamp.
Wavelength: 328.1 nm.

(3) Related substances—Conduct this procedure using light-resistant vessels. Perform the test with 20 μL of the sample solution obtained in the Assay as directed under Liquid Chromatography <2.01> according to the following conditions, determine each peak area by the automatic integration method, and calculate their amounts by the area percentage method: the amount of the peak other than idarubicin is not more than 1.0%, and the total amount of the peaks other than idarubicin is not more than 2.0%.

Operating conditions—

Detector, column, column temperature, mobile phase, and flow rate: Proceed as directed in the operating conditions in the Assay.

Time span of measurement: About 3.3 times as long as the retention time of idarubicin, beginning after the solvent peak.

System suitability—

Test for required detectability: To 1 mL of the sample solution add the mobile phase without sodium lauryl sulfate to make exactly 100 mL, and use this solution as the standard solution for system suitability test. Pipet 2 mL of the solution for system suitability test, and add the mobile phase without sodium lauryl sulfate to make exactly 20 mL. Confirm that the peak area of idarubicin obtained with 20 μL of this solution is equivalent to 7 to 13% of that with 20 μL of the solution for system suitability test.

System performance: When the procedure is run with 20 μL of the solution for system suitability test under the above operating conditions, the number of theoretical plates and the symmetry factor of the peak of idarubicin are not less than 3000 and 0.8 to 1.2, respectively.

System repeatability: When the test is repeated 6 times with 20 μL of the solution for system suitability test under the above operating conditions, the relative standard deviation of the peak area of idarubicin is not more than 2.0%.

Water <2.48> Not more than 5.0% (0.1 g, coulometric titration).

Residue on ignition <2.44> Not more than 0.5% (2 g).

Assay Weigh accurately an amount of Idarubicin Hydrochloride and Idarubicin Hydrochloride RS, equivalent to about 10 mg (potency), dissolve each in the mobile phase prepared without addition of sodium lauryl sulfate to make exactly 50 mL, and use these solutions as the sample solution and the standard solution, respectively. Perform the test with exactly 20 μL each of the sample solution and standard solution as directed under Liquid Chromatography <2.01> according to the following conditions, and determine the peak areas, A_T and A_S, of idarubicin in each solution.

Amount [μg (potency)] of idarubicin hydrochloride ($C_{26}H_{27}NO_9.HCl$)
$= M_S \times A_T/A_S \times 1000$

M_S: Amount [mg (potency)] of Idarubicin Hydrochloride RS taken

Operating conditions—

Detector: An ultraviolet absorption photometer (wavelength: 254 nm).

Column: A stainless steel column 3.9 mm in inside diameter and 15 cm in length, packed with octadecylsilanized silica gel for liquid chromatography (4 μm in particle diameter).

Column temperature: A constant temperature of about 35°C.

Mobile phase: Dissolve 10.2 g of potassium dihydrogenphosphate in a suitable amount of water, add 1 mL of phosphoric acid and water to make 750 mL, and add 250 mL of tetrahydrofuran. To 500 mL of this solution add 0.72 g of sodium lauryl sulfate and 0.5 mL of *N,N*-dimethyl-*n*-octylamine, and adjust to pH 4 with 2 mol/L sodium hydroxide TS.

Flow rate: Adjust so that the retention time of idarubicin is about 15 minutes.

System suitability—

System performance: When the procedure is run with 20 μL of the standard solution under the above operating conditions, the number of theoretical plates of the peak of idarubicin is not less than 3000.

System repeatability: When the test is repeated 6 times with 20 μL of the standard solution under the above operating conditions, the relative standard deviation of the peak areas of idarubicin is not more than 2.0%.

Containers and storage Containers—Tight containers.

Idarubicin Hydrochloride for Injection

注射用イダルビシン塩酸塩

Idarubicin Hydrochloride for Injection is a preparation for injection, which is dissolved before use.

It contains not less than 90.0% and not more than 110.0% of the labeled amount of idarubicin hydrochloride ($C_{26}H_{27}NO_9.HCl$: 533.95).

Method of preparation Prepare as directed under Injections, with Idarubicin Hydrochloride.

Description Idarubicin Hydrochloride for Injection occurs as yellow-red masses.

Identification **(1)** Dissolve an amount of Idarubicin Hydrochloride for Injection, equivalent to 2 mg (potency) of Idarubicin Hydrochloride, in 5 mL of sodium hydroxide TS: the solution shows a blue-purple color.

(2) Dissolve an amount of Idarubicin Hydrochloride for Injection, equivalent to 1 mg (potency) of Idarubicin Hydrochloride, in 1 mL of water, and add methanol to make 100 mL. Determine the absorption spectrum of the solution as directed under Ultraviolet-visible Spectrophotometry <2.24>: it exhibits maxima between 250 nm and 254 nm, between 285 nm and 289 nm, between 480 nm and 484 nm, and between 510 nm and 520 nm.

pH <2.54> The pH of a solution prepared by dissolving an amount of Idarubicin Hydrochloride for Injection, equivalent to 5 mg (potency) of Idarubicin Hydrochloride, in 5 mL of water is between 5.0 and 7.0.

Purity Clarity and color of solution—Dissolve an amount of Idarubicin Hydrochloride for Injection, equivalent to 5 mg (potency) of Idarubicin Hydrochloride, in 5 mL of water: the solution is clear and yellow-red.

Water <*2.48*> Weigh accurately the mass of 1 Idarubicin Hydrochloride for Injection, add 5 mL of methanol for water determination using a syringe, dissolve with thorough shaking, and perform the test with 4 mL of this solution as directed in the Volumetric titration (direct titration). Use 4 mL of methanol for water determination as the blank. Determine the mass of the content from the difference between the mass of 1 Idarubicin Hydrochloride for Injection obtained above and the mass of its bottle and rubber stopper, which are weighed accurately after washing with water then with ethanol (95), drying at 105°C for 1 hour and allowing to cool to room temperature in a desiccator (not more than 4.0%).

Bacterial endotoxins <*4.01*> Less than 8.9 EU/mg (potency).

Uniformity of dosage units <*6.02*> Perform the test according to the following method: it meets the requirement of the Content uniformity test.

To 1 Idarubicin Hydrochloride for Injection add the mobile phase prepared without addition of sodium lauryl sulfate to make exactly *V* mL so that each mL contains 0.2 mg (potency) of idarubicin hydrochloride ($C_{26}H_{27}NO_9.HCl$), and use this solution as the sample solution. Separately, weigh accurately an amount of Idarubicin Hydrochloride RS, equivalent to about 10 mg (potency), dissolve in the mobile phase without sodium lauryl sulfate to make exactly 50 mL, and use this solution as the standard solution. Proceed as directed in the Assay under Idarubicin Hydrochloride.

Amount [mg (potency)] of idarubicin hydrochloride ($C_{26}H_{27}NO_9.HCl$)
$= M_S \times A_T/A_S \times V/50$

M_S: Amount [mg (potency)] of Idarubicin Hydrochloride RS taken

Foreign insoluble matter <*6.06*> Perform the test according to the Method 2: it meets the requirement.

Insoluble particulate matter <*6.07*> It meets the requirement.

Sterility <*4.06*> Perform the test according to the Membrane filtration method: it meets the requirement.

Assay Weigh accurately the mass of the contents of not less than 10 Idarubicin Hydrochloride for Injection. Weigh accurately an amount of the content, equivalent to about 5 mg (potency), dissolve in the mobile phase prepared without addition of sodium lauryl sulfate to make exactly 25 mL, and use this solution as the sample solution. Separately, weigh accurately an amount of Idarubicin Hydrochloride RS, equivalent to about 10 mg (potency), dissolve in the mobile phase without sodium lauryl sulfate to make exactly 50 mL, and use this solution as the standard solution. Proceed as directed in the Assay under Idarubicin Hydrochloride.

Amount [mg (potency)] of idarubicin hydrochloride ($C_{26}H_{27}NO_9.HCl$)
$= M_S \times A_T/A_S \times 1/2$

M_S: Amount [mg (potency)] of Idarubicin Hydrochloride RS taken

Containers and storage Containers—Hermetic containers.

Idoxuridine

イドクスウリジン

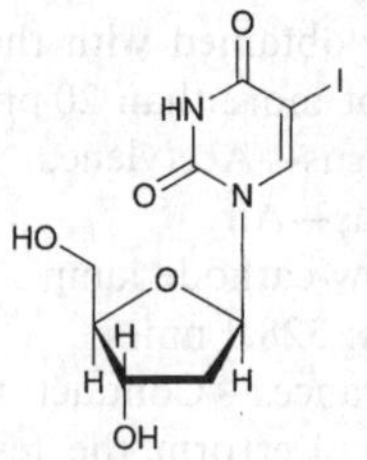

$C_9H_{11}IN_2O_5$: 354.10
5-Iodo-2′-deoxyuridine
[54-42-2]

Idoxuridine, when dried, contains not less than 98.0% of idoxuridine ($C_9H_{11}IN_2O_5$).

Description Idoxuridine occurs as colorless, crystals or a white, crystalline powder. It is odorless.

It is freely soluble in dimethylamide, slightly soluble in water, very slightly soluble in ethanol (95), and practically insoluble in diethyl ether.

It dissolves in sodium hydroxide TS.

Melting point: about 176°C (with decomposition).

Identification **(1)** Dissolve 0.01 g of Idoxuridine in 5 mL of water by warming, add 5 mL of diphenylamine-acetic acid TS, and heat for 5 minutes: a blue color develops.

(2) Heat 0.1 g of Idoxuridine: a purple gas evolves.

(3) Dissolve 2 mg of Idoxuridine in 50 mL of 0.01 mol/L sodium hydroxide. Determine the absorption spectrum of the solution as directed under Ultraviolet-visible Spectrophotometry <*2.24*>, and compare the spectrum with the Reference Spectrum or the spectrum of a solution of Idoxuridine RS prepared in the same manner as the sample solution: both spectra exhibit similar intensities of absorption at the same wavelengths.

Optical rotation <*2.49*> $[\alpha]_D^{20}$: +28 – +31° (after drying, 0.2 g, sodium hydroxide TS, 20 mL, 100 mm).

Purity **(1)** Clarity and color of solution—Dissolve 0.20 g of Idoxuridine in 5 mL of a solution of sodium hydroxide (1 in 200): the solution is clear and colorless.

(2) Heavy metals <*1.07*>—Proceed with 2.0 g of Idoxuridine according to Method 2, and perform the test. Prepare the control solution with 2.0 mL of Standard Lead Solution (not more than 10 ppm).

(3) Related substances—Dissolve 0.10 g of Idoxuridine in exactly 10 mL of a mixture of dilute ethanol and ammonia solution (28) (99:1), and use this solution as the sample solution. Perform the test with the sample solution as directed under Thin-layer Chromatography <*2.03*>. Spot 50 μL of the sample solution on a plate of silica gel with fluorescent indicator for thin-layer chromatography. Develop the plate with a mixture of ethyl acetate and diluted 2-propanol (2 in 3) (4:1) to a distance of about 10 cm, and air-dry the plate. Then develop two-dimensionally at right angles to the first, and air-dry the plate. Examine under ultraviolet light (main wavelength: 254 nm): any spot other than the principal spot does not appear.

(4) Iodine and iodide—Dissolve 0.10 g of Idoxuridine in 20 mL of water and 5 mL of sodium hydroxide TS, and add immediately 5 mL of dilute sulfuric acid under ice-cooling. Allow to stand for 10 minutes with occasional shaking, and filter. Transfer the filtrate into a Nessler tube, add 10 mL of chloroform and 3 drops of a solution of potassium iodate (1 in 100), shake for 30 seconds, and allow to stand: the chloroform layer has no more color than the following control solution.

Control solution: Weigh accurately 0.111 g of potassium iodide, and dissolve in water to make 1000 mL. To exactly 1 mL of this solution add 19 mL of water, 5 mL of sodium hydroxide TS and 5 mL of dilute sulfuric acid, mix, and filter. Transfer the filtrate to a Nessler tube, and proceed in the same manner.

Loss on drying <*2.41*> Not more than 0.5% (2 g, in vacuum, 60°C, 3 hours).

Residue on ignition <*2.44*> Not more than 0.3% (1 g).

Assay Weigh accurately about 0.7 g of Idoxuridine, previously dried, dissolve in 80 mL of *N*,*N*-dimethylformamide, and titrate <*2.50*> with 0.1 mol/L tetramethylammonium hydroxide VS until the color of the solution changes from yellow through yellow-green to blue (indicator: 5 drops of thymol blue-dimethylformamide TS). Perform a blank determination, and make any necessary correction in the same manner.

Each mL of 0.1 mol/L tetramethylammonium hydroxide VS
= 35.41 mg of $C_9H_{11}IN_2O_5$

Containers and storage Containers—Tight containers.
Storage—Light-resistant.

Idoxuridine Ophthalmic Solution

イドクスウリジン点眼液

Idoxuridine Ophthalmic Solution contains not less than 90.0% and not more than 110.0% of the labeled amount of idoxuridine ($C_9H_{11}IN_2O_5$: 354.10).

Method of preparation Prepare as directed under Ophthalmic Liquids and Solutions, with Idoxuridine.

Description Idoxuridine Ophthalmic Solution is a clear, colorless liquid.

Identification **(1)** To a volume of Idoxuridine Opthalmic Solution, equivalent to 5 mg of Idoxuridine, add 5 mL of diphenylamine-acetic acid TS, and heat for 20 minutes: a light blue color develops.

(2) Place a volume of Idoxuridine Ophthalmic Solution, equivalent to 5 mg of Idoxuridine, in a porcelain crucible, add 0.1 g of anhydrous sodium carbonate, heat slowly, evaporate to dryness and ignite until the residue is incinerated. Dissolve the residue in 5 mL of water, acidify with hydrochloric acid, and add 2 to 3 drops of sodium nitrite TS: a yellow-brown color develops. Then add 2 to 3 drops of starch TS: a deep blue color develops.

(3) To a volume of Idoxuridine Ophthalmic Solution, equivalent to 2 mg of Idoxuridine, add 0.01 mol/L sodium hydroxide TS to make 50 mL. Determine the absorption spectrum of this solution as directed under Ultraviolet-visible Spectrophotometry <*2.24*>: it exhibits a maximum between 277 nm and 281 nm.

pH <*2.54*> 4.5 – 7.0

Purity 5-Iodouracil and 2′-deoxyuridine—To a volume of Idoxuridine Ophthalmic Solution, equivalent to 4.0 mg of Idoxuridine, add water to make exactly 5 mL, and use this solution as the sample solution. Separately, dissolve 12.0 mg of 5-iodouracil for liquid chromatography and 4.0 mg of 2′-deoxyuridine for liquid chromatography in water to make exactly 200 mL. Measure exactly 5 mL of this solution, add water to make exactly 25 mL, and use this solution as the standard solution. Perform the test with exactly 10 μL each of the sample solution and standard solution as directed under Liquid Chromatography <*2.01*> according to the following conditions, and determine the peak areas of 5-iodouracil and 2′-deoxyuridine: the peak areas of 5-iodouracil and 2′-deoxyuridine of the sample solution are not larger than the peak areas of 5-iodouracil and 2′-deoxyuridine of the standard solution.

Operating conditions—

Detector: An ultraviolet absorption photometer (wavelength: 254 nm).

Column: A stainless steel column 3.9 mm in inside diameter and 30 cm in length, packed with octadecylsilanized silica gel for liquid chromatography (10 μm in particle diameter).

Column temperature: A constant temperature of about 25°C.

Mobile phase: A mixture of water and methanol (24:1).

Flow rate: Adjust so that the retention time of 2′-deoxyuridine is about 6 minutes.

System suitability—

System performance: When the procedure is run with 10 μL of the standard solution under the above operating conditions, 2′-deoxyuridine and 5-iodouracil are eluted in this order with the resolution between these peaks being not less than 2.0.

System repeatability: When the test is repeated 6 times with 10 μL of the standard solution under the above operating conditions, the relative standard deviation of the peak area of 2′-deoxyuridine is not more than 1.0%.

Foreign insoluble matter <*6.11*> It meets the requirement.

Insoluble particulate matter <*6.08*> It meets the requirement.

Sterility <*4.06*> Perform the test according to the Membrane filtration method: it meets the requirement.

Assay Measure exactly a volume of Idoxuridine Ophthalmic Solution, equivalent to 3 mg of idoxuridine ($C_9H_{11}IN_2O_5$), add exactly 2 mL of the internal standard solution, then add water to make 10 mL, and use this solution as the sample solution. Separately weigh accurately about 10 mg of Idoxuridine RS, previously dried at 60°C for 3 hours, dissolve in water to make exactly 10 mL. Measure exactly 3 mL of this solution, add exactly 2 mL of the internal standard solution, then add water to make 10 mL, and use this solution as the standard solution. Perform the test with 10 μL each of the sample solution and standard solution as directed under Liquid Chromatography <*2.01*> according to the following conditions, and calculate the ratios, Q_T and Q_S, of the peak area of idoxuridine to that of the internal standard, respectively.

Amount (mg) of idoxuridine ($C_9H_{11}IN_2O_5$)
$= M_S \times Q_T/Q_S \times 3/10$

M_S: Amount (mg) of Idoxuridine RS taken

Internal standard solution—A solution of sulfathiazole in the mobile phase (1 in 4000).

Operating conditions—

Detector: An ultraviolet absorption photometer (wavelength: 254 nm).

Column: A stainless steel column 3.9 mm in inside diameter and 30 cm in length, packed with octadecylsilanized silica gel for liquid chromatography (10 μm in particle diameter).

Column temperature: A constant temperature of about 25°C.

Mobile phase: A mixture of water and methanol (87:13).

Flow rate: Adjust so that the retention time of idoxuridine is about 9 minutes.

System suitability—

System performance: When the procedure is run with 10 μL of the standard solution under the above operating conditions, idoxuridine and the internal standard are eluted in this order with the resolution between these peaks being not less than 2.0.

System repeatability: When the test is repeated 6 times with 10 μL of the standard solution under the above operating conditions, the relative standard deviation of the ratios of the peak area of idoxuridine to that of the internal standard is not more than 1.0%.

Containers and storage Containers—Tight containers.

Storage—Light-resistant, in a cold place, and avoid freezing.

Ifenprodil Tartrate

イフェンプロジル酒石酸塩

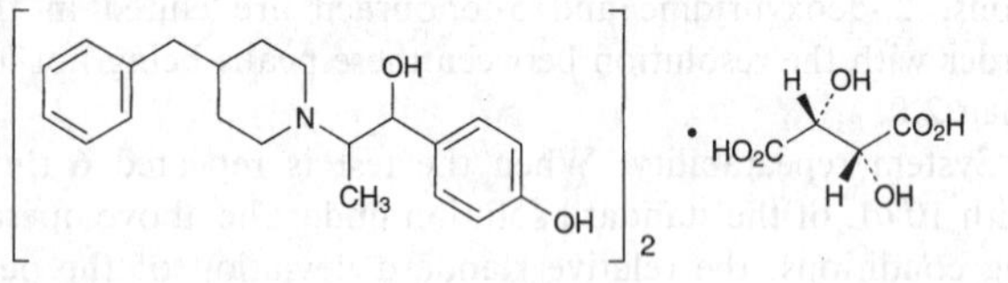

$(C_{21}H_{27}NO_2)_2.C_4H_6O_6$: 800.98

(1*RS*,2*SR*)-4-[2-(4-Benzylpiperidin-1-yl)-1-hydroxypropyl]phenol hemi-(2*R*,3*R*)-tartrate

[23210-58-4]

Ifenprodil Tartrate contains not less than 98.5% of ifenprodil tartrate [$(C_{21}H_{27}NO_2)_2.C_4H_6O_6$], calculated on the anhydrous basis.

Description Ifenprodil Tartrate occurs as a white crystalline powder. It is odorless.

It is freely soluble in acetic acid (100), soluble in ethanol (95), slightly soluble in water and in methanol, and practically insoluble in diethyl ether.

Optical rotation $[\alpha]_D^{20}$: +11 – +15° (1 g calculated on the anhydrous basis, ethanol (95), 20 mL, 100 mm).

Melting point: about 148°C (with decomposition).

Identification **(1)** Determine the absorption spectrum of a solution of Ifenprodil Tartrate in methanol (1 in 10,000) as directed under Ultraviolet-visible Spectrophotometry *<2.24>*, and compare the spectrum with the Reference Spectrum: both spectra exhibit similar intensities of absorption at the same wavelengths.

(2) Determine the infrared absorption spectrum of Ifenprodil Tartrate as directed in the potassium bromide disk method under Infrared Spectrophotometry *<2.25>*, and compare the spectrum with the Reference Spectrum: both spectra exhibit similar intensities of absorption at the same wave numbers.

(3) Dissolve 0.4 g of Ifenprodil Tartrate in 40 mL of water by warming. After cooling, add 0.5 mL of ammonia TS to this solution, extract with two 40-mL portions of chloroform, and collect the water layer. Evaporate 30 mL of the water layer on a water bath to dryness, and after cooling, dissolve the residue in 6 mL of water: the solution responds to Qualitative Tests *<1.09>* for tartrate.

Purity **(1)** Heavy metals *<1.07>*—Proceed with 2.0 g of Ifenprodil Tartrate according to Method 2, and perform the test. Prepare the control solution with 2.0 mL of Standard Lead Solution (not more than 10 ppm).

(2) Related substances—Dissolve 0.30 g of Ifenprodil Tartrate in 10 mL of diluted ethanol (95) (3 in 4), and use this solution as the sample solution. Pipet 1 mL of the sample solution, add diluted ethanol (95) (3 in 4) to make exactly 200 mL, and use this solution as the standard solution. Perform the test with these solutions as directed under Thin-layer Chromatography *<2.03>*. Spot 10 μL each of the sample solution and standard solution on a plate of silica gel for thinlayer chromatography. Develop the plate with a mixture of ethyl acetate, hexane, 1-butanol and ammonia solution (28) (140:40:20:1) to a distance of about 10 cm, and air-dry the plate. Spray hydrogen hexachloroplatinate (IV)-potassium iodide TS evenly on the plate: the spots other than the principal spot obtained from the sample solution are not more intense than the spot from the standard solution.

Water *<2.48>* Not more than 4.0% (0.5 g, volumetric titration, direct titration).

Residue on ignition *<2.44>* Not more than 0.1% (1 g).

Assay Weigh accurately about 0.5 g of Ifenprodil Tartrate, dissolve in 50 mL of acetic acid (100), and titrate *<2.50>* with 0.1 mol/L perchloric acid VS (potentiometric titration). Perform a blank determination in the same manner, and make any necessary correction.

Each mL of 0.1 mol/L perchloric acid VS
= 40.05 mg of $(C_{21}H_{27}NO_2)_2.C_4H_6O_6$

Containers and storage Containers—Well-closed containers.

Storage—Light-resistant.

Ifenprodil Tartrate Fine Granules

イフェンプロジル酒石酸塩細粒

Ifenprodil Tartrate Fine Granules contain not less than 95.0% and not more than 105.0% of the labeled amount of ifenprodil tartrate [$(C_{21}H_{27}NO_2)_2.C_4H_6O_6$: 800.98].

Method of preparation Prepare as directed under Granules, with Ifenprodil Tartrate.

Identification Determine the absorption spectrum of the sample solution obtained in the Assay as directed under Ultraviolet-visible Spectrophotometry *<2.24>*: it exhibits a maximum between 274 nm and 278 nm.

Uniformity of dosage units *<6.02>* Perform the test according to the following method: Ifenprodil Tartrate Fine Granules in single-dose packages meet the requirement of the Content uniformity test.

To the total amount of the content of 1 package of Ifenprodil Tartrate Fine Granules, add 10 mL of water and a suitable amount of a mixture of ethanol (99.5) and water (3:1), shake thoroughly, and add a mixture of ethanol (99.5) and water (3:1) to make exactly V mL so that each mL contains about 0.1 mg of ifenprodil tartrate

$[(C_{21}H_{27}NO_2)_2.C_4H_6O_6]$. Filter through a membrane filter with a pore size not exceeding 0.45 μm, discard the first 10 mL of the filtrate, and use the subsequent filtrate as the sample solution. Then, proceed as directed in the Assay.

Amount (mg) of ifenprodil tartrate $[(C_{21}H_{27}NO_2)_2.C_4H_6O_6]$
$= M_S \times A_T/A_S \times V/200$

M_S: Amount (mg) of ifenprodil tartrate for assay taken, calculated on the anhydrous basis

Dissolution Being specified separately when the drug is granted approval based on the Law.

Assay Powder Ifenprodil Tartrate Fine Granules, and weigh accurately a portion of the powder, equivalent to about 10 mg of ifenprodil tartrate $[(C_{21}H_{27}NO_2)_2.C_4H_6O_6]$, add 5 mL of water and a suitable amount of a mixture of ethanol (99.5) and water (3:1), shake thoroughly, and add a mixture of ethanol (99.5) and water (3:1) to make exactly 100 mL. Filter through a membrane filter with a pore size not exceeding 0.45 μm. Discard the first 10 mL of the filtrate, and use the subsequent filtrate as the sample solution. Separately, weigh accurately about 20 mg of ifenprodil tartrate for assay (separately determine the water <*2.48*> in the same manner as Ifenprodil Tartrate), add 10 mL of water and a mixture of ethanol (99.5) and water (3:1) to make exactly 200 mL, and use this solution as the standard solution. Perform the test with exactly 20 μL each of the sample solution and standard solution as directed under Liquid Chromatography <*2.01*> according to the following conditions, and determine the peak areas, A_T and A_S, of ifenprodil in each solution.

Amount (mg) of ifenprodil tartrate $[(C_{21}H_{27}NO_2)_2.C_4H_6O_6]$
$= M_S \times A_T/A_S \times 1/2$

M_S: Amount (mg) of ifenprodil tartrate for assay taken, calculated on the anhydrous basis

Operating conditions—

Detector: An ultraviolet absorption photometer (wavelength: 224 nm).

Column: A stainless steel column 4.6 mm in inside diameter and 15 cm in length, packed with octadecylsilanized silica gel for liquid chromatography (5 μm in particle diameter).

Column temperature: A constant temperature of about 25°C.

Mobile phase: Dissolve 6.8 g of potassium dihydrogen phosphate in 900 mL of water, adjust to pH 6.5 with potassium hydroxide TS, and add water to make 1000 mL. To 420 mL of this solution add 320 mL of methanol for liquid chromatography and 260 mL of acetonitrile for liquid chromatography.

Flow rate: Adjust so that the retention time of ifenprodil is about 10 minutes.

System suitability—

System performance: When the procedure is run with 20 μL of the standard solution under the above operating conditions, the number of theoretical plates and the symmetry factor of the peak of ifenprodil are not less than 3000 and not more than 2.0, respectively.

System repeatability: When the test is repeated 6 times with 20 μL of the standard solution under the above operating conditions, the relative standard deviation of the peak area of ifenprodil is not more than 1.0%.

Containers and storage Containers—Tight containers.
Storage—Light-resistant.

Ifenprodil Tartrate Tablets

イフェンプロジル酒石酸塩錠

Ifenprodil Tartrate Tablets contain not less than 95.0% and not more than 105.0% of the labeled amount of ifenprodil tartrate $[(C_{21}H_{27}NO_2)_2.C_4H_6O_6$: 800.98].

Method of preparation Prepare as directed under Tablets, with Ifenprodil Tartrate.

Identification Determine the absorption spectrum of the sample solution obtained in the Assay as directed under Ultraviolet-visible Spectrophotometry <*2.24*>: it exhibits a maximum between 274 nm and 278 nm.

Uniformity of dosage units <*6.02*> Perform the test according to the following method: it meets the requirement of the Content uniformity test.

To 1 tablet of Ifenprodil Tartrate Tablets, add $V/20$ mL of water, and shake until the tablet is completely disintegrated. Then, add $7V/10$ mL of a mixture of ethanol (99.5) and water (3:1), shake thoroughly, and add a mixture of ethanol (99.5) and water (3:1) to make exactly V mL so that each mL contains about 0.1 mg of ifenprodil tartrate $[(C_{21}H_{27}NO_2)_2.C_4H_6O_6]$. Filter through a membrane filter with a pore size not exceeding 0.45 μm, discard the first 10 mL of the filtrate, and use the subsequent filtrate as the sample solution. Then, proceed as directed in the Assay.

Amount (mg) of ifenprodil tartrate $[(C_{21}H_{27}NO_2)_2.C_4H_6O_6]$
$= M_S \times A_T/A_S \times V/200$

M_S: Amount (mg) of ifenprodil tartrate for assay taken, calculated on the anhydrous basis

Dissolution Being specified separately when the drug is granted approval based on the Law.

Assay Weigh accurately the mass of not less than 20 Ifenprodil Tartrate Tablets, and powder. Weigh accurately a portion of the powder, equivalent to about 10 mg of ifenprodil tartrate $[(C_{21}H_{27}NO_2)_2C_4H_6O_6]$, add 5 mL of water and a suitable amount of a mixture of ethanol (99.5) and water (3:1), shake thoroughly, and add a mixture of ethanol (99.5) and water (3:1) to make exactly 100 mL. Filter through a membrane filter with a pore size not exceeding 0.45 μm. Discard the first 10 mL of the filtrate, and use the subsequent filtrate as the sample solution. Separately, weigh accurately about 20 mg of ifenprodil tartrate for assay (separately determine the water <*2.48*> in the same manner as Ifenprodil Tartrate), add 10 mL of water and a mixture of ethanol (99.5) and water (3:1) to make exactly 200 mL, and use this solution as the standard solution. Perform the test with 20 μL each of the sample solution and standard solution as directed under Liquid Chromatography <*2.01*> according to the following conditions, and determine the peak areas, A_T and A_S, of ifenprodil tartrate in each solution.

Amount (mg) of ifenprodil tartrate $[(C_{21}H_{27}NO_2)_2.C_4H_6O_6]$
$= M_S \times A_T/A_S \times 1/2$

M_S: Amount (mg) of ifenprodil tartrate for assay taken, calculated on the anhydrous basis

Operating conditions—

Detector: An ultraviolet absorption photometer (wavelength: 224 nm).

Column: A stainless steel column 4.6 mm in inside diame-

ter and 15 cm in length, packed with octadecylsilanized silica gel for liquid chromatography (5 μm in particle diameter).

Column temperature: A constant temperature of about 25°C.

Mobile phase: Dissolve 6.8 g of potassium dihydrogen phosphate in 900 mL of water, adjust to pH 6.5 with potassium hydroxide TS, and add water to make 1000 mL. To 420 mL of this solution, add 320 mL of methanol for liquid chromatography and 260 mL of acetonitrile for liquid chromatography.

Flow rate: Adjust so that the retention time of ifenprodil is about 10 minutes.

System suitability—

System performance: When the procedure is run with 20 μL of the standard solution under the above operating conditions, the number of theoretical plates and the symmetry factor of the peak of ifenprodil are not less than 3000 and not more than 2.0, respectively.

System repeatability: When the test is repeated 6 times with 20 μL of the standard solution under the above operating conditions, the relative standard deviation of the peak area of ifenprodil is not more than 1.0%.

Containers and storage containers—Tight containers.

Imidapril Hydrochloride

イミダプリル塩酸塩

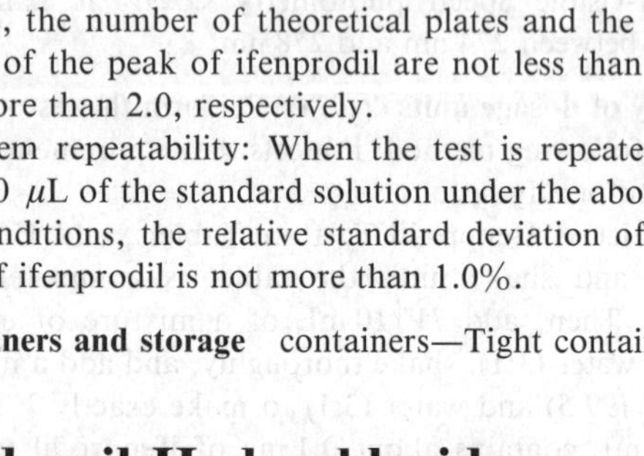

$C_{20}H_{27}N_3O_6.HCl$: 441.91

(4*S*)-3-{(2*S*)-2-[(1*S*)-1-Ethoxycarbonyl-3-phenylpropylamino]propanoyl}-1-methyl-2-oxoimidazolidine-4-carboxylic acid monohydrochloride

[*89396-94-1*]

Imidapril Hydrochloride, when dried, contains not less than 98.5% and not more than 101.0% of imidapril hydrochloride ($C_{20}H_{27}N_3O_6.HCl$).

Description Imidapril Hydrochloride occurs as white crystals.

It is freely soluble in methanol, soluble in water, and sparingly soluble in ethanol (99.5).

Dissolve 1.0 g of Imidapril Hydrochloride in 100 mL of water: the pH of the solution is about 2.

Melting point: about 203°C (with decomposition).

Identification **(1)** To 3 mL of a solution of Imidapril Hydrochloride (1 in 50) add 5 drops of Reinecke salt TS: a light red precipitate is formed.

(2) Determine the infrared absorption spectrum of Imidapril Hydrochloride as directed in the potassium chloride disk method under Infrared Spectrophotometry <*2.25*>, and compare the spectrum with the Reference Spectrum: both spectra exhibit similar intensities of absorption at the same wave numbers.

(3) A solution of Imidapril Hydrochloride (1 in 50) responds to Qualitative Tests <*1.09*> for chloride.

Optical rotation <*2.49*> $[\alpha]_D^{20}$: −65.0 − −69.0° (after drying, 0.1 g, methanol, 10 mL, 100 mm).

Purity **(1)** Heavy metals <*1.07*>—Proceed with 2.0 g of Imidapril Hydrochloride according to Method 4, and perform the test. Prepare the control solution with 2.0 mL of Standard Lead Solution (not more than 10 ppm).

(2) Related substances—Dissolve 25 mg of Imidapril Hydrochloride in 50 mL of the mobile phase, and use this solution as the sample solution. Pipet 1 mL of the sample solution, add the mobile phase to make exactly 100 mL, and use this solution as the standard solution. Perform the test with exactly 20 μL each of the sample solution and standard solution as directed under Liquid Chromatography <*2.01*> according to the following conditions. Determine each peak area of both solutions by the automatic integration method: the area of the peak having the relative retention time of about 0.45 to imidapril, obtained from the sample solution, is not larger than 2/5 times the peak area of imidapril from the standard solution, and the area of each peak other than imidapril and the peak mentioned above from the sample solution is not larger than 1/5 times the peak area of imidapril from the standard solution. Furthermore, the total area of the peaks other than imidapril from the sample solution is not larger than 1/2 times the peak area of imidapril from the standard solution.

Operating conditions—

Detector: An ultraviolet absorption photometer (wavelength: 215 nm).

Column: A stainless steel column 4.6 mm in inside diameter and 15 cm in length, packed with octylsilanized silica gel for liquid chromatography (5 μm in particle diameter).

Column temperature: A constant temperature of about 40°C.

Mobile phase: Dissolve 1.36 g of potassium dihydrogen phosphate in 1000 mL of water, and adjust the pH to 2.7 with phosphoric acid. To 600 mL of this solution add 400 mL of methanol.

Flow rate: Adjust so that the retention time of imidapril is about 8 minutes.

Time span of measurement: About 2 times as long as the retention time of imidapril, beginning after the solvent peak.

System suitability—

Test for required detectability: Pipet 2 mL of the standard solution, and add the mobile phase to make exactly 20 mL. Confirm that the peak area of imidapril obtained with 20 μL of this solution is equivalent to 7 to 13% of that with 20 μL of the standard solution.

System performance: When the procedure is run with 20 μL of the standard solution under the above operating conditions, the number of theoretical plates and the symmetry factor of the peak of imidapril are not less than 5000 and not more than 1.5, respectively.

System repeatability: When the test is repeated 6 times with 20 μL of the standard solution under the above operating conditions, the relative standard deviation of the peak area of imidapril is not more than 2.0%.

Loss on drying <*2.41*> Not more than 0.5% (1 g, 105°C, 3 hours).

Residue on ignition <*2.44*> Not more than 0.1% (1 g).

Assay Weigh accurately about 0.4 g of Imidapril Hydrochloride, previously dried, dissolve in 70 mL of water, and titrate <*2.50*> with 0.1 mol/L sodium hydroxide VS from the first equivalent point to the second equivalent point (potentiometric titration).

Each mL of 0.1 mol/L sodium hydroxide VS
= 44.19 mg of $C_{20}H_{27}N_3O_6.HCl$

Containers and storage Containers—Well-closed containers.

Imidapril Hydrochloride Tablets

イミダプリル塩酸塩錠

Imidapril Hydrochloride Tablets contain not less than 95.0% and not more than 105.0% of the labeled amount of Imidapril Hydrochloride ($C_{20}H_{27}N_3O_6.HCl$: 441.91).

Method of preparation Prepare as directed under Tablets, with Imidapril Hydrochloride.

Identification Weigh accurately an amount of powdered Imidapril Hydrochloride Tablets, equivalent to 25 mg of Imidapril Hydrochloride, add 5 mL of ethanol (99.5), shake well, filter, and use the filtrate as the sample solution. Separately, dissolve 25 mg of imidapril hydrochloride in 5 mL of ethanol (99.5), and use this solution as the standard solution. Perform the test with these solutions as directed under Thin-layer Chromatography <*2.03*>. Spot 10 μL each of the sample solution and standard solution on a plate of silica gel with fluorescent indicator for thin-layer chromatography. Develop the plate with a mixture of 1-butanol, ethyl acetate, water, ethanol (99.5) and acetic acid (100) (16:16:7:2:2) to a distance of about 13 cm, and air-dry the plate. Examine under ultraviolet light (main wavelength: 254 nm): the principal spot obtained from the sample solution has the same *R*f value as the spot from the standard solution.

Purity Related substances—To a quantity of powdered Imidapril Hydrochloride Tablets, equivalent to 25 mg of Imidapril Hydrochloride, add 40 mL of diluted methanol (2 in 5), shake vigorously for 10 minutes, add diluted ethanol (2 in 5) to make 50 mL, and filter through a membrane filter with a pore size not exceeding 0.45 μm. Discard the first 2 mL of the filtrate, and use the subsequent filtrate as the sample solution. Pipet 1 mL of the sample solution, add diluted methanol (2 in 5) to make exactly 100 mL, and use this solution as the standard solution. Perform the test with exactly 20 μL each of the sample solution and standard solution as directed under Liquid Chromatography <*2.01*> according to the following conditions. Determine each peak area of both solutions by the automatic integration method: the area of the peak having the relative retention time of about 0.45 to imidapril, obtained from the sample solution, is not larger than the peak area of imidapril from the standard solution, the area of the peak having the relative retention time of about 0.8 to imidapril from the sample solution is not larger than 7/10 times the peak area of imidapril from the standard solution, and the area of each peak other than imidapril and the peaks mentioned above from the sample solution is not larger than 3/10 times the peak area of imidapril from the standard solution. Furthermore, the total area of the peaks other than imidapril from the sample solution is not larger than 1.5 times the peak area of imidapril from the standard solution.

Operating conditions—

Detector, column, column temperature, mobile phase and flow rate: Proceed as directed in the operating conditions in the Assay.

Time span of measurement: About 2 times as long as the retention time of imidapril, beginning after the solvent peak.

System suitability—

Test for required detectability: Pipet 2 mL of the standard solution, and add diluted methanol (2 in 5) to make exactly 20 mL. Confirm that the peak area of imidapril obtained with 20 μL of this solution is equivalent to 7 to 13% of that with 20 μL of the standard solution.

System performance: When the procedure is run with 20 μL of the standard solution under the above operating conditions, the number of theoretical plates and the symmetry factor of the peak of imidapril are not less than 5000 and not more than 1.5, respectively.

System repeatability: When the test is repeated 6 times with 20 μL of the standard solution under the above operating conditions, the relative standard deviation of the peak area of imidapril is not more than 2.0%.

Uniformity of dosage units <*6.02*> Perform the test according to the following method: it meets the requirement of the Content uniformity test.

To 1 tablet of Imidapril Hydrochloride Tablets add $2V/5$ mL of water, shake vigorously for 10 minutes, add diluted methanol (2 in 3) to make exactly V mL so that each mL contains about 0.1 mg of imidapril hydrochloride ($C_{20}H_{27}N_3O_6.HCl$), filter through a membrane filter with a pore size not exceeding 0.45 μm. Discard the first 2 mL of the filtrate, and use the subsequent filtrate as the sample solution. Separately, weigh accurately about 10 mg of imidapril for assay, previously dried at 105°C for 3 hours, dissolve in diluted methanol (2 in 5) to make exactly 100 mL, and use this solution as the standard solution. Perform the test with exactly 20 μL each of the sample solution and standard solution as directed under Liquid Chromatography <*2.01*> according to the following conditions, and determine the peak areas, A_T and A_S, of imidapril in each solution.

Amount (mg) of imidapril hydrochloride ($C_{20}H_{27}N_3O_6.HCl$)
$= M_S \times A_T/A_S \times V/100$

M_S: Amount (mg) of imidapril hydrochloride for assay taken

Operating conditions—

Proceed as directed in the operating conditions in the Assay.

System suitability—

System performance: When the procedure is run with 20 μL of the standard solution under the above operating conditions, the number of theoretical plates and the symmetry factor of the peak of imidapril are not less than 5000 and not more than 1.5, respectively.

System repeatability: When the test is repeated 6 times with 20 μL of the standard solution under the above operating conditions, the relative standard deviation of the peak area of imidapril is not more than 1.0%.

Dissolution <*6.10*> When the test is performed at 50 revolutions per minute according to the Paddle method, using 900 mL of water as the dissolution medium, the dissolution rate in 45 minutes of Imidapril Hydrochloride Tablets is not less than 85%.

Start the test with 1 tablet of Imidapril Hydrochloride Tablets, withdraw not less than 20 mL of the medium at the specified minute after starting the test, and filter through a membrane filter with a pore size not exceeding 0.45 μm. Discard not less than 10 mL of the first filtrate, pipet V mL of the subsequent filtrate, add water to make exactly V' mL so that each mL contains about 2.8 μg of imidapril hydrochloride ($C_{20}H_{27}N_3O_6.HCl$), and use this solution as the sample solution. Separately, weigh accurately about 28 mg of imidapril hydrochloride for assay, previously dried at 105°C for 3 hours, and dissolve in water to make exactly 100 mL. Pipet 2 mL of this solution, add water to make exactly 200 mL, and use this solution as the standard solution. Perform the test with exactly 50 μL each of the sample solution and standard solution as directed under Liquid Chromatography ‹*2.01*› according to the following conditions, and determine the peak areas, A_T and A_S, of imidapril in each solution.

Dissolution rate (%) with respect to the labeled amount of imidapril hydrochloride ($C_{20}H_{27}N_3O_6.HCl$)
$= M_S \times A_T/A_S \times V'/V \times 1/C \times 9$

M_S: Amount (mg) of imidapril hydrochloride for assay taken
C: Labeled amount (mg) of imidapril hydrochloride ($C_{20}H_{27}N_3O_6.HCl$) in 1 tablet

Operating conditions—
Proceed as directed in the operating conditions in the Assay.
System suitability—
System performance: When the procedure is run with 50 μL of the standard solution under the above operating conditions, the number of theoretical plates and the symmetry factor of the peak of imidapril are not less than 5000 and not more than 1.5, respectively.
System repeatability: When the test is repeated 6 times with 50 μL of the standard solution under the above operating conditions, the relative standard deviation of the peak area of imidapril is not more than 2.0%.

Assay Weigh accurately not less than 20 Imidapril Hydrochloride Tablets, and powder. Weigh accurately a portion of the powder, equivalent to about 20 mg of imidapril hydrochloride ($C_{20}H_{27}N_3O_6.HCl$), add 30 mL of diluted methanol (2 in 5) and exactly 5 mL of the internal standard solution, shake vigorously for 10 minutes, add diluted methanol (2 in 5) to make 50 mL, and filter through a membrane filter with a pore size not exceeding 0.45 μm. Discard the first 2 mL of the filtrate, pipet 5 mL of the subsequent filtrate, add diluted methanol (2 in 5) to make 20 mL, and use this solution as the sample solution. Separately, weigh accurately about 20 mg of imidapril hydrochloride for assay, previously dried at 105°C for 3 hours, dissolve in exactly 5 mL of the internal standard solution, add diluted methanol (2 in 5) to make 50 mL. Pipet 5 mL of this solution, add diluted methanol (2 in 5) to make 20 mL, and use this solution as the standard solution. Perform the test with 20 μL each of the sample solution and standard solution as directed under Liquid Chromatography ‹*2.01*› according to the following conditions, and calculate the ratios, Q_T and Q_S, of the peak area of imidapril to that of the internal standard.

Amount (mg) of imidapril hydrochloride ($C_{20}H_{27}N_3O_6.HCl$)
$= M_S \times Q_T/Q_S$

M_S: Amount (mg) of imidapril hydrochloride for assay taken

*Internal standard solution—*A solution of ethyl parahydroxybenzoate in diluted methanol (2 in 5) (1 in 500).
Operating conditions—
Detector: An ultraviolet absorption photometer (wavelength: 215 nm).
Column: A stainless steel column 4.6 mm in inside diameter and 15 cm in length, packed with octylsilanized silica gel for liquid chromatography (5 μm in particle diameter).
Column temperature: A constant temperature of about 40°C.
Mobile phase: Dissolve 1.36 g of potassium dihydrogen phosphate in 1000 mL of water, and adjust the pH to 2.7 with phosphoric acid. To 600 mL of this solution add 400 mL of methanol.
Flow rate: Adjust so that the retention time of imidapril is about 8 minutes.
System suitability—
System performance: When the procedure is run with 20 μL of the standard solution under the above operating conditions, imidapril and the internal standard are eluted in this order with the resolution between these peaks being not less than 4.
System repeatability: When the test is repeated 6 times with 20 μL of the standard solution under the above operating conditions, the relative standard deviation of the ratio of the peak area of imidapril to that of the internal standard is not more than 1.0%.

Containers and storage Containers—Tight containers.

Imipenem Hydrate

イミペネム水和物

$C_{12}H_{17}N_3O_4S.H_2O$: 317.36
(5*R*,6*S*)-3-[2-(Formimidoylamino)ethylsulfanyl]-6-[(1*R*)-1-hydroxyethyl]-7-oxo-1-azabicyclo[3.2.0]hept-2-ene-2-carboxylic acid monohydrate
[*74431-23-5*]

Imipenem Hydrate contains not less than 980 μg (potency) and not more than 1010 μg (potency) per mg, calculated on the anhydrous basis. The potency of Imipenem Hydrate is expressed as mass (potency) of imipenem ($C_{12}H_{17}N_3O_4S$: 299.35).

Description Imipenem Hydrate occurs as a white to light yellow crystalline powder.
It is sparingly soluble in water, and practically insoluble in ethanol (99.5).

Identification (1) Determine the absorption spectrum of a solution of Imipenem Hydrate in 0.1 mol/L 3-(*N*-morpholino)propanesulfonic acid buffer solution (pH 7.0) (1 in 50,000) as directed under Ultraviolet-visible Spectrophotometry ‹*2.24*›, and compare the spectrum with the Reference Spectrum or the spectrum of a solution of Imipenem RS prepared in the same manner as the sample solution: both spectra exhibit similar intensities of absorption at the same wavelengths.

(2) Determine the infrared absorption spectrum of Imipenem Hydrate as directed in the potassium bromide disk method under Infrared Spectrophotometry ‹*2.25*›, and compare the spectrum with the Reference Spectrum or the spectrum of Imipenem RS: both spectra exhibit similar intensities of absorption at the same wave numbers.

Optical rotation ‹*2.49*› $[\alpha]_D^{20}$: +89 – +94° (50 mg calculated on the anhydrous basis, 0.1 mol/L 3-(*N*-morpholino)propanesulfonic acid buffer solution (pH 7.0), 10 mL, 100 mm).

pH <2.54> The pH of a solution obtained by dissolving 1.0 g of Imipenem Hydrate in 200 mL of water is between 4.5 and 7.0.

Purity **(1)** Heavy metals <1.07>—Proceed with 1.0 g of Imipenem Hydrate according to Method 2, and perform the test. Prepare the control solution with 2.0 mL of Standard Lead Solution (not more than 20 ppm).

(2) Arsenic <1.11>—Put 2.0 g of Imipenem Hydrate in a crucible, add 5 mL of nitric acid and 1 mL of sulfuric acid, and heat carefully until white fumes evolve. After cooling, add 2 mL of nitric acid, heat, and repeat this procedure once more. Then add 2 mL of hydrogen peroxide (30), heat, and repeat this procedure several times until the color of the solution changes to colorless to pale yellow. After cooling, heat again until white fumes evolve. After cooling, add water to make 5 mL, and perform the test with this solution as the test solution (not more than 1 ppm).

(3) Related substances—Dissolve 50 mg of Imipenem Hydrate in 50 mL of 0.1 mol/L 3-(*N*-morpholino)propanesulfonic acid buffer solution (pH 7.0) and use this solution as the sample solution. Pipet 1 mL of the sample solution, add 0.1 mol/L 3-(*N*-morpholino)propanesulfonic acid buffer solution (pH 7.0) to make exactly 100 mL, and use this solution as the standard solution. Perform the test with exactly 10 μL each of the sample solution and standard solution as directed under Liquid Chromatography <2.01> according to the following conditions, and determine each peak area by the automatic integration method: the peak area of thienamycin, having the relative retention time of about 0.8 to imipenem, obtained from the sample solution is not larger than 1.4 times the peak area of imipenem from the standard solution, the area of the peak other than imipenem and thienamycin from the sample solution is not larger than 1/3 times the peak area of imipenem from the standard solution, and the total area of the peaks other than imipenem and thienamycin from the sample solution is not larger than the peak area of imipenem from the standard solution.

Operating conditions—

Detector, column, column temperature, mobile phase, and flow rate: Proceed as directed in the operating conditions in the Assay.

Time span of measurement: About 2 times as long as the retention time of imipenem.

System suitability—

System performance: Proceed as directed in the system suitability in the Assay.

Test for required detectability: Measure exactly 5 mL of the standard solution, add 0.1 mol/L 3-(*N*-morpholino)propanesulfonic acid buffer solution (pH 7.0) to make exactly 50 mL. Confirm that the peak area of imipenem obtained with 10 μL of this solution is equivalent to 7 to 13% of that with the standard solution.

System repeatability: When the test is repeated 6 times with 10 μL of the standard solution under the above operating conditions, the relative standard deviation of the peak area of imipenem is not more than 2.0%.

Water <2.48> Not less than 5.0% and not more than 8.0% (20 mg, coulometric titration, water evaporation temperature: 140°C).

Residue on ignition <2.44> Not more than 0.2% (1 g).

Assay Perform the procedure within 30 minutes after preparation of the sample solution and standard solution. Weigh accurately an amount of Imipenem Hydrate and Imipenem RS, equivalent to about 50 mg (potency), dissolve each in 0.1 mol/L 3-(*N*-morpholino)-propanesulfonic acid buffer solution (pH 7.0) to make exactly 50 mL, and use these solutions as the sample solution and standard solution. Perform the test with exactly 10 μL each of the sample solution and standard solution, within 30 minutes after preparation of these solutions, as directed under Liquid Chromatography <2.01> according to the following conditions, and determine the peak areas, A_T and A_S, of imipenem in each solution.

$$\text{Amount [}\mu\text{g (potency)] of imipenem } (C_{12}H_{17}N_3O_4S) = M_S \times A_T/A_S \times 1000$$

M_S: Amount [mg (potency)] of Imipenem RS taken

Operating conditions—

Detector: An ultraviolet absorption photometer (wavelength: 280 nm).

Column: A stainless steel column 3.9 mm in inside diameter and 30 cm in length, packed with octadecylsilanized silica gel for liquid chromatography (10 μm in particle diameter).

Column temperature: A constant temperature of about 25°C.

Mobile phase: A mixture of 0.1 mol/L 3-(*N*-morpholino)propanesulfonic acid buffer solution (pH 7.0) and acetonitrile (100:1).

Flow rate: Adjust so that the retention time of imipenem is about 6 minutes.

System suitability—

System performance: Dissolve 50 mg of Imipenem Hydrate and 75 mg of resorcinol in 50 mL of 0.1 mol/L 3-(*N*-morpholino)propanesulfonic acid buffer solution (pH 7.0). When the procedure is run with 10 μL of this solution under the above operating conditions, imipenem and resorcinol are eluted in this order with the resolution between these peaks being not less than 4.

System repeatability: When the test is repeated 5 times with 10 μL of the standard solution under the above operating conditions, the relative standard deviation of the peak area of imipenem is not more than 0.80%.

Containers and storage Containers—Hermetic containers.

Imipenem and Cilastatin Sodium for Injection

注射用イミペネム·シラスタチンナトリウム

Imipenem and Cilastatin Sodium for Injection is a preparation for injection which is dissolved or suspended before use.

It contains not less than 93.0% and not more than 115.0% of the labeled potency of imipenem ($C_{12}H_{17}N_3O_4S$: 299.35) and an amount of cilastatin sodium ($C_{16}H_{25}N_2NaO_5S$: 380.43), equivalent to not less than 93.0% and not more than 115.0% of the labeled amount of cilastatin ($C_{16}H_{26}N_2O_5S$: 358.45).

Method of preparation Prepare as directed under Injections, with Imipenem Hydrate and Cilastatin Sodium.

Description Imipenem and Cilastatin Sodium for Injection occurs as a white to light yellow-white powder.

Identification **(1)** To 1 mL of a solution of Imipenem and Cilastatin Sodium for Injection (1 in 100) add 1 mL of ninhydrin TS, heat in a water bath for 5 minutes: a purple color appears (cilastatin).

(2) To 2 mL of a solution of Imipenem and Cilastatin

Sodium for Injection (1 in 1000) add 0.1 mol/L 3-(*N*-morpholino)propanesulfonic acid buffer solution (pH 7.0) to make 50 mL, and determine the absorption spectrum of the solution as directed under Ultraviolet-visible Spectrophotometry ⟨*2.24*⟩: it exhibits a maximum between 296 nm and 300 nm (imipenem).

pH ⟨*2.54*⟩ The pH of a solution prepared by dissolving an amount of Imipenem and Cilastatin Sodium for Injection, equivalent to 0.5 g (potency) of Imipenem Hydrate, in 100 mL of isotonic sodium chloride solution is between 6.5 and 8.0. The pH of the Injection intended for intramuscular use is between 6.0 and 7.5.

Purity Clarity and color of solution—Dissolve an amount of Imipenem and Cilastatin Sodium for Injection, equivalent to 0.5 g (potency) of Imipenem Hydrate, in 100 mL of isotonic sodium chloride solution: the solution is clear and colorless or pale yellow.

Loss on drying ⟨*2.41*⟩ Not more than 3.0% (1 g, in vacuum, 60°C, 3 hours).

Bacterial endotoxins ⟨*4.01*⟩ Less than 0.25 EU/mg (potency).

Uniformity of dosage units ⟨*6.02*⟩ Perform the test according to the following method: it meets the requirement of the Content uniformity test (*T*: 104.0%).

Dissolve the total amount of the content of 1 Imipenem and Cilastatin Sodium for Injection in isotonic sodium chloride solution to make exactly 100 mL. Measure exactly *V* mL of this solution, equivalent to about 25 mg (potency) of Imipenem Hydrate, add 0.1 mol/L 3-(*N*-morpholino)propanesulfonic acid buffer solution (pH 7.0) to make exactly 50 mL, and use this solution as the sample solution. Proceed hereafter as directed in the Assay.

Amount [mg (potency)] of imipenem ($C_{12}H_{17}N_3O_4S$)
$= M_{SI} \times A_{TI}/A_{SI} \times 100/V$

Amount (mg) of cilastatin ($C_{16}H_{26}N_2O_5S$)
$= M_{SC} \times A_{TC}/A_{SC} \times 100/V \times 0.955$

M_{SI}: Amount [mg (potency)] of Imipenem RS taken
M_{SC}: Amount (mg) of cilastatin ammonium for assay taken, calculated on anhydrous and ethanol-free basis

Foreign insoluble matter ⟨*6.06*⟩ Perform the test according to Method 2: It meets the requirement.

Insoluble particulate matter ⟨*6.07*⟩ Perform the test according to the Method 1: the Injection which is dissolved before use meets the requirement.

Sterility ⟨*4.06*⟩ Perform the test according to the Membrane filtration method: it meets the requirement.

Assay Weigh accurately the mass of the contents of not less than 10 Imipenem and Cilastatin Sodium for Injections. Weigh accurately an amount of the content, equivalent to 1 Imipenem and Cilastatin Sodium for Injection, dissolve in isotonic sodium chloride solution to make exactly 100 mL. Measure exactly an amount of this solution, equivalent to about 25 mg (potency) of imipenem, add 0.1 mol/L 3-(*N*-morpholino)propanesulfonic acid buffer solution (pH 7.0) to make exactly 50 mL, and use this as the sample solution. Separately, weigh accurately an amount of Imipenem RS, equivalent to about 25 mg (potency), and weigh accurately about 25 mg of cilastatin ammonium for assay, dissolve in 10 mL of isotonic sodium chloride solution, add 0.1 mol/L 3-(*N*-morpholino)propanesulfonic acid buffer solution (pH 7.0) to make exactly 50 mL, and use this solution as the standard solution. Perform the test with exactly 10 µL each of the sample solution and standard solution as directed under Liquid Chromatography ⟨*2.01*⟩ according to the following conditions, and determine the peak areas, A_{TI} and A_{SI} of imipenem, and those, A_{TC} and A_{SC} of cilastatin in each solution.

Amount [mg (potency)] of imipenem ($C_{12}H_{17}N_3O_4S$)
$= M_{SI} \times A_{TI}/A_{SI}$

Amount (mg) of cilastatin ($C_{16}H_{26}N_2O_5S$)
$= M_{SC} \times A_{TC}/A_{SC} \times 0.955$

M_{SI}: Amount [mg (potency)]of Imipenem RS taken
M_{SC}: Amount (mg) of cilastatin ammonium for assay taken, calculated on anhydrous and ethanol-free basis

Operating conditions—

Detector: An ultraviolet absorption photometer (wavelength: 250 nm).

Column: A stainless steel column 4.6 mm in inside diameter and 20 cm in length, packed with octylsilanized silica gel for liquid chromatography (10 µm in particle diameter).

Column temperature: A constant temperature of about 50°C.

Mobile phase: Dissolve 0.836 g of 3-(*N*-morpholino)propanesulfonic acid, 1.0 g of sodium 1-hexane sulfonate and 50 mg of disodium dihydrogen ethylenediamine tetraacetate dihydrate in 800 mL of water, adjust to pH 7.0 with 0.1 mol/L sodium hydrate TS, and add water to make 1000 mL.

Flow rate: Adjust so that the retention time of imipenem is about 3 minutes.

System suitability—

System performance: When the procedure is run with 10 µL of the standard solution under the above operating conditions, imipenem and cilastatin are eluted in this order with the resolution between these peaks being not less than 2.0, and the symmetry factors of the peak of imipenem and cilastatin are not more than 2.0, respectively.

System repeatability: When the test is repeated 6 times with 10 µL of the standard solution under the above operating conditions, the relative standard deviations of the peak area of imipenem and cilastatin are not more than 2.0%, respectively.

Containers and storage Containers—Hermetic containers. Plastic containers for aqueous injections may be used.

Imipramine Hydrochloride

イミプラミン塩酸塩

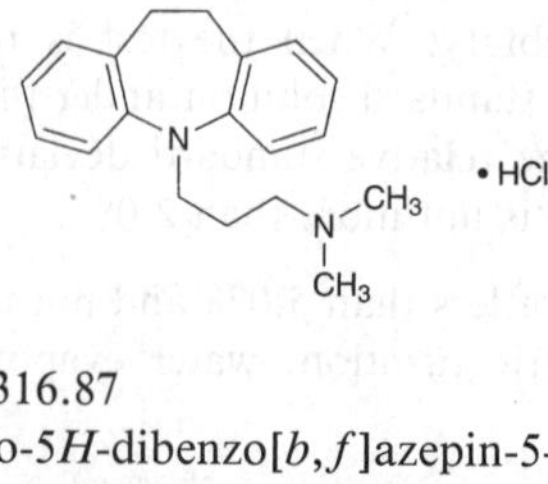

$C_{19}H_{24}N_2.HCl$: 316.87
3-(10,11-Dihydro-5*H*-dibenzo[*b*,*f*]azepin-5-yl)-*N*,*N*-dimethylpropylamine monohydrochloride
[*113-52-0*]

Imipramine Hydrochloride, when dried, contains not less than 98.5% of imipramine hydrochloride ($C_{19}H_{24}N_2.HCl$).

Description Imipramine Hydrochloride occurs as a white to pale yellow-white crystalline powder. It is odorless.

It is freely soluble in water and in ethanol (95), and practically insoluble in diethyl ether.

The pH of a solution of 0.1 g of Imipramine Hydrochloride in 10 mL of water is between 4.2 and 5.2.

It is gradually colored by light.

Identification **(1)** Dissolve 5 mg of Imipramine Hydrochloride in 2 mL of nitric acid: a deep blue color develops.

(2) Dissolve 5 mg of Imipramine Hydrochloride in 250 mL of 0.01 mol/L hydrochloric acid TS. Determine the absorption spectrum of the solution as directed under Ultraviolet-visible Spectrophotometry <*2.24*>, and compare the spectrum with the Reference Spectrum or the spectrum of a solution of Imipramine Hydrochloride RS prepared in the same manner as the sample solution: both spectra exhibit similar intensities of absorption at the same wavelengths.

(3) Dissolve 0.05 g of Imipramine Hydrochloride in 5 mL of water, add 1 mL of ammonia TS, allow to stand for 5 minutes, filter, and acidify the filtrate with dilute nitric acid: it responds to Qualitative Tests <*1.09*> (2) for chloride.

Melting point <*2.60*> 172 – 176°C (with decomposition).

Purity **(1)** Clarity and color of solution—Dissolve 1.0 g of Imipramine Hydrochloride in 10 mL of water: the solution is clear, and has no more color than the following control solution.

Control solution: Take exactly 1.0 mL of Cobalt (II) Chloride CS, 2.4 mL of Iron (III) Chloride CS, 0.4 mL of Copper (II) Sulfate CS and 6.2 mL of diluted hydrochloric acid (1 in 40), and mix them. Pipet 0.5 mL of this solution, and add exactly 9.5 mL of water.

(2) Iminodibenzyl—Dissolve 50 mg of Imipramine Hydrochloride in 10 mL of a mixture of hydrochloric acid and ethanol (95) (1:1) in a 25-mL brown volumetric flask. Cool the flask in ice water, add 5 mL of an ethanol (95) solution of furfural (1 in 250) and 5 mL of hydrochloric acid, and allow to stand at 25°C for 3 hours. Add a mixture of hydrochloric acid and ethanol (95) (1:1) to make 25 mL, and determine the absorbance of this solution at 565 nm as directed under Ultraviolet-visible Spectrophotometry <*2.24*>: it is not more than 0.16.

(3) Related substances—Dissolve 0.20 g of Imipramine Hydrochloride in 10 mL of ethanol (95), and use this solution as the sample solution. Pipet 1 mL of the sample solution, and add ethanol (95) to make exactly 50 mL. Pipet 5 mL of this solution, add ethanol (95) to make exactly 50 mL, and use this solution as the standard solution. Perform the test with these solutions as directed under Thin-layer Chromatography <*2.03*>. Spot 5 μL each of the sample solution and standard solution on a plate of silica gel for thin-layer chromatography. Develop the plate with a mixture of ethyl acetate, acetic acid (100), hydrochloric acid and water (11:7:1:1) to a distance of about 12 cm, and air-dry the plate. Spray evenly potassium dichromate-sulfuric acid TS on the plate: the spots other than the principal spot obtained from the sample solution are not more intense than the spot from the standard solution.

Loss on drying <*2.41*> Not more than 0.5% (1 g, 105°C, 2 hours).

Residue on ignition <*2.44*> Not more than 0.1% (1 g).

Assay Weigh accurately about 0.3 g of Imipramine Hydrochloride, previously dried, and dissolve in 20 mL of water. Add 5 mL of sodium hydroxide TS, and extract with three 20-mL portions of chloroform. Filter each extract through a pledget of absorbent cotton on which a small quantity of anhydrous sodium sulfate is placed. Combine the chloroform extracts, and titrate <*2.50*> with 0.1 mol/L perchloric acid VS until the yellow solution changes to red-purple (indicator: 10 drops of metanil yellow TS). Perform a blank determination in the same manner, and make any necessary correction.

Each mL of 0.1 mol/L perchloric acid VS
= 31.69 mg of $C_{19}H_{24}N_2.HCl$

Containers and storage Containers—Tight containers.

Storage—Light-resistant.

Imipramine Hydrochloride Tablets

イミプラミン塩酸塩錠

Imipramine Hydrochloride Tablets contain not less than 93.0% and not more than 107.0% of the labeled amount of imipramine hydrochloride ($C_{19}H_{24}N_2.HCl$: 316.87).

Method of preparation Prepare as directed under Tablets, with Imipramine Hydrochloride.

Identification **(1)** Weigh a quantity of powdered Imipramine Hydrochloride Tablets, equivalent to 0.25 g of Imipramine Hydrochloride, add 25 mL of chloroform, shake thoroughly, and filter. Evaporate the filtrate on a water bath, and proceed with the residue as directed in the Identification (1) under Imipramine Hydrochloride.

(2) Dissolve an amount of the residue obtained in (1), equivalent to 5 mg of Imipramine Hydrochloride, in 250 mL of 0.01 mol/L hydrochloric acid TS, and determine the absorption spectrum as directed under Ultraviolet-visible Spectrophotometry <*2.24*>: it exhibits a maximum between 249 nm and 253 nm, and a shoulder between 270 nm and 280 nm.

Uniformity of dosage units <*6.02*> Perform the test according to the following method: it meets the requirement of the Content uniformity test.

To 1 tablet of Imipramine Hydrochloride Tablets add exactly 40 mL of 0.01 mol/L hydrochloric acid TS, disperse the tablet into a small particles by sonicating, then shake well. Centrifuge the solution, pipet V mL of the supernatant liquid, add water to make exactly V' mL so that each mL contains about 20 μg of imipramine hydrochloride ($C_{19}H_{24}N_2.HCl$), and use this solution as the sample solution. Separately, weigh accurately about 25 mg of Imipramine Hydrochloride RS, previously dried at 105°C for 2 hours, dissolve in 0.01 mol/L hydrochloric acid TS to make exactly 100 mL. Pipet 2 mL of this solution, add water to make exactly 25 mL, and use this solution as the standard solution. Determine the absorbances at 251 nm, A_{T1} and A_{S1}, and at 330 nm, A_{T2} and A_{S2}, of the sample solution and standard solution as directed under Ultraviolet-visible Spectrophotometry <*2.24*>.

Amount (mg) of imipramine hydrochloride ($C_{19}H_{24}N_2.HCl$)
$= M_S \times (A_{T1} - A_{T2})/(A_{S1} - A_{S2}) \times V'/V \times 4/125$

M_S: Amount (mg) of Imipramine Hydrochloride RS taken

Dissolution <*6.10*> When the test is performed at 75 revolutions per minute according to the Paddle method, using 900 mL of 2nd fluid for dissolution test as the dissolution medium, the dissolution rate in 60 minutes of Imipramine Hydrochloride Tablets is not less than 75%.

Start the test with 1 tablet of Imipramine Hydrochloride Tablets, withdraw not less than 20 mL of the medium at the specified minute after starting the test, and filter through a membrane filter with a pore size not exceeding 0.8 μm. Discard not less than 10 mL of the first filtrate, pipet V mL of the subsequent filtrate, add the dissolution medium to make exactly V' mL so that each mL of the filtrate contains about 10 μg of imipramine hydrochloride ($C_{19}H_{24}N_2.HCl$), and use this solution as the sample solution. Separately, weigh accurately about 25 mg of Imipramine Hydrochloride RS, previously dried at 105°C for 2 hours, dissolve in the dissolution medium to make exactly 100 mL. Pipet 4 mL of this solution, add the dissolution medium to make exactly 100 mL, and use this solution as the standard solution. Determine the absorbances, A_T and A_S, of the sample solution and the standard solution at 250 nm as directed under Ultraviolet-visible Spectrophotometry <*2.24*>.

Dissolution rate (%) with respect to the labeled amount of imipramine hydrochloride ($C_{19}H_{24}N_2.HCl$)
$= M_S \times A_T/A_S \times V'/V \times 1/C \times 36$

M_S: Amount (mg) of Imipramine Hydrochloride RS taken
C: Labeled amount (mg) of imipramine hydrochloride ($C_{19}H_{24}N_2.HCl$) in 1 tablet

Assay Take 20 Imipramine Hydrochloride Tablets, add exactly 200 mL of 0.01 mol/L hydrochloric acid TS, and shake well until the tablets are completely disintegrated. After centrifuging the solution, pipet a volume of the supernatant liquid, equivalent to about 25 mg of imipramine hydrochloride ($C_{19}H_{24}N_2.HCl$), add 0.01 mol/L hydrochloric acid TS to make exactly 100 mL, and use this solution as the sample solution. Separately, weigh accurately about 25 mg of Imipramine Hydrochloride RS, previously dried at 105°C for 2 hours, dissolve in 0.01 mol/L hydrochloric acid TS to make exactly 100 mL, and use this solution as the standard solution. Pipet 3 mL each of these solutions into separators which contain 15 mL of potassium hydrogen phthalate buffer solution (pH 5.6), 8 mL of bromocresol green-sodium hydroxide TS and 30 mL of chloroform, and shake. Filter the chloroform layer through a pledget of absorbent cotton into a 100-mL volumetric flask. Repeat the extraction with two 30-mL portions of chloroform, combine the chloroform layers in the 100-mL volumetric flask, and add chloroform to make exactly 100 mL. Perform the test with these solutions as directed under Ultraviolet-visible Spectrophotometry <*2.24*>, using a solution obtained by proceeding with 3 mL of 0.01 mol/L hydrochloric acid TS in the same manner as the blank. Determine the absorbances, A_T and A_S, of these solutions at 416 nm.

Amount (mg) of imipramine hydrochloride ($C_{19}H_{24}N_2.HCl$)
$= M_S \times A_T/A_S$

M_S: Amount (mg) of Imipramine Hydrochloride RS taken

Containers and storage Containers—Tight containers.

Indapamide

インダパミド

and enantiomer

$C_{16}H_{16}ClN_3O_3S$: 365.83
4-Chloro-*N*-[(2*RS*)-2-methyl-2,3-dihydro-1*H*-indol-1-yl]-3-sulfamoylbenzamide
[*26807-65-8*]

Indapamide contains not less than 98.5% and not more than 101.5% of indapamide ($C_{16}H_{16}ClN_3O_3S$), calculated on the dried basis.

Description Indapamide occurs as a white crystalline powder.

It is freely soluble in ethanol (99.5), and practically insoluble in water.

A solution of Indapamide in ethanol (99.5) (1 in 10) shows no optical rotation.

Identification **(1)** Determine the absorption spectrum of a solution of Indapamide in ethanol (99.5) (1 in 100,000) as directed under Ultraviolet-visible Spectrophotometry <*2.24*>, and compare the spectrum with the Reference Spectrum or the spectrum of a solution of Indapamide RS prepared in the same manner as the sample solution: both spectra exhibit similar intensities of absorption at the same wavelengths.

(2) Determine the infrared absorption spectrum of Indapamide as directed in the potassium bromide disk method under Infrared Spectrophotometry <*2.25*>, and compare the spectrum with the Reference Spectrum or the spectrum of Indapamide RS: both spectra exhibit similar intensities of absorption at the same wave numbers.

(3) Perform the test with Indapamide as directed under Flame Coloration Test <*1.04*> (2): a green color appears.

Melting point <*2.60*> 167 – 171°C

Purity **(1)** Chloride <*1.03*>—To 1.5 g of Indapamide add 50 mL of water, shake for 15 minutes, allow to stand in an ice bath for 30 minutes, and filter. To 30 mL of the filtrate add 6 mL of dilute nitric acid and water to make 50 mL. Perform the test using this solution as the test solution. Prepare the control solution with 0.25 mL of 0.01 mol/L hydrochloric acid VS (not more than 0.01%).

(2) Heavy metals <*1.07*>—Proceed with 2.0 g of Indapamide according to Method 2, and perform the test. Prepare the control solution with 2.0 mL of Standard Lead Solution (not more than 10 ppm).

(3) Related substances—Conduct this procedure using light-resistant vessels. Dissolve 0.10 g of Indapamide in 5 mL of ethanol (99.5), and use this solution as the sample solution. Pipet 1 mL of the sample solution, add ethanol (99.5) to make exactly 200 mL, and use this solution as the standard solution (1). Pipet 5 mL of the standard solution (1), add ethanol (99.5) to make exactly 10 mL, and use this solution as the standard solution (2). Perform the test with these solutions as directed under Thin-layer Chromatography <*2.03*>. Spot 10 μL each of the sample solution and standard solutions (1) and (2) on a plate of silica gel with fluorescent indicator for thin-layer chromatography. Immediately develop the plate with a mixture of ethyl acetate, cyclohexane and acetic acid (100) (100:80:1) to a distance of about 10 cm, and air-dry the plate. Examine under ultraviolet light (main wavelength: 254 nm): the spots other than the principal spot obtained from the sample solution are not more intense than the spot from the standard solution (1), and the total amount of these related substances, calculated by comparison with the spots from the standard solutions (1) and (2), is not more than 2.0%.

Loss on drying <*2.41*> Not more than 3.0% (0.5 g, reduced pressure not exceeding 0.67 kPa, phosphorus (V) oxide, 110°C, 2 hours).

Residue on ignition <*2.44*> Not more than 0.1% (1 g).

Assay Weigh accurately about 20 mg each of Indapamide and Indapamide RS (separately, determine the loss on drying <*2.41*> under the same condition as Indapamide), and dissolve each in a mixture of water and ethanol (99.5) (1:1) to make exactly 100 mL. Pipet 10 mL each of these solutions, add exactly 2 mL of the internal standard solution and a mixture of water and ethanol (99.5) (1:1) to make 20 mL, and use these solutions as the sample solution and the standard solution, respectively. Perform the test with 10 μL each of the sample solution and standard solution as directed under Liquid Chromatography <*2.01*> according to the following conditions, and calculate the ratios, Q_T and Q_S, of the peak area of indapamide to that of the internal standard.

$$\text{Amount (mg) of indapamide } (C_{16}H_{16}ClN_3O_3S) = M_S \times Q_T/Q_S$$

M_S: Amount (mg) of Indapamide RS taken, calculated on the dried basis

Internal standard solution—A solution of isopropyl parahydroxybenzoate in a mixture of water and ethanol (99.5) (1:1) (3 in 1000).

Operating conditions—

Detector: An ultraviolet absorption photometer (wavelength: 287 nm).

Column: A stainless steel column 4.6 mm in inside diameter and 15 cm in length, packed with octadecylsilanized silica gel for liquid chromatography (5 μm in particle diameter).

Column temperature: A constant temperature of about 40°C.

Mobile phase: A mixture of diluted phosphoric acid (1 in 1000), acetonitrile and methanol (6:3:1).

Flow rate: Adjust so that the retention time of indapamide is about 6 minutes.

System suitability—

System performance: When the procedure is run with 10 μL of the standard solution under the above operating conditions, indapamide and the internal standard are eluted in this order with the resolution between these peaks being not less than 4.

System repeatability: When the test is repeated 6 times with 10 μL of the standard solution under the above operating conditions, the relative standard deviation of the peak area of indapamide is not more than 1.0%.

Containers and storage Containers—Tight containers.

Storage—Light-resistant.

Indapamide Tablets

インダパミド錠

Indapamide Tablets contain not less than 93.0% and not more than 103.0% of the labeled amount of indapamide ($C_{16}H_{16}ClN_3O_3S$: 365.83).

Method of preparation Prepare as directed under Tablets, with Indapamide.

Identification To an amount of powdered Indapamide Tablets, equivalent to 10 mg of Indapamide, add 5 mL of ethyl acetate, shake for 10 minutes, centrifuge, and use the supernatant liquid as the sample solution. Separately, dissolve 10 mg of Indapamide RS in 5 mL of ethyl acetate, and use this solution as the standard solution. Perform the test with these solutions as directed under Thin-layer Chromatography <*2.03*>. Spot 10 μL each of the sample solution and standard solution on a plate of silica gel with fluorescent indicator for thin-layer chromatography. Develop the plate with a mixture of ethyl acetate, cyclohexane and acetic acid (100) (100:80:1) to a distance of about 10 cm, and air-dry the plate. Examine under ultraviolet light (main wavelength: 254 nm): the principal spot obtained from the sample solution and the spot from the standard solution show a blue-purple color and the same *R*f value.

Uniformity of dosage units <*6.02*> Perform the test according to the following method: it meets the requirement of the Content uniformity test.

To 1 tablet of Indapamide Tablets add exactly *V*/10 mL of the internal standard solution, and add a mixture of water and ethanol (99.5) (1:1) to make *V* mL so that each mL contains about 0.1 mg of indapamide ($C_{16}H_{16}ClN_3O_3S$), shake to disintegrate, sonicate for 10 minutes, shake again for 10 minutes, centrifuge, and use the supernatant liquid as the sample solution. Proceed as directed in the Assay.

$$\text{Amount (mg) of indapamide } (C_{16}H_{16}ClN_3O_3S) = M_S \times Q_T/Q_S \times V/200$$

M_S: Amount (mg) of Indapamide RS taken, calculated on the dried basis

Internal standard solution—A solution of isopropyl parahydroxybenzoate in a mixture of water and ethanol (99.5) (1:1) (3 in 1000).

Dissolution <*6.10*> When the test is performed at 50 revolutions per minute according to the Paddle method, using 900 mL of water as the dissolution medium, the dissolution rates in 45 minutes of 1-mg tablet and in 90 minutes of 2-mg tablet are not less than 70%, respectively.

Start the test with 1 tablet of Indapamide Tablets, withdraw not less than 20 mL of the medium at the specified minute after starting the test, and filter through a membrane filter with a pore size not exceeding 0.45 μm. Discard not less than 10 mL of the first filtrate, pipet *V* mL of the subsequent filtrate, add water to make exactly *V′* mL so that each mL contains about 1.1 μg of indapamide ($C_{16}H_{16}ClN_3O_3S$), and use this solution as the sample solution. Separately, weigh accurately about 20 mg of Indapamide RS (separately, determine the loss on drying <*2.41*> under the same condition as Indapamide), and dissolve in ethanol (99.5) to make exactly 50 mL. Pipet 5 mL of this solution, and add water to make exactly 100 mL. Pipet 5 mL of this solution, add water to make exactly 100 mL, and use this solution as the standard solution. Perform the test with exactly 50 μL each of the sample solution and standard solution as directed under Liquid Chromatography <2.01> according to the following conditions, and determine the peak areas, A_T and A_S, of indapamide in each solution.

Dissolution rate (%) with respect to the labeled amount of indapamide ($C_{16}H_{16}ClN_3O_3S$)
$= M_S \times A_T/A_S \times V'/V \times 1/C \times 9/2$

M_S: Amount (mg) of Indapamide RS taken, calculated on the dried basis

C: Labeled amount (mg) of indapamide ($C_{16}H_{16}ClN_3O_3S$) in tablet

Operating conditions—

Proceed as directed in the operating conditions in the Assay under Indapamide.

System suitability—

System performance: When the procedure is run with 50 µL of the standard solution under the above operating conditions, the number of theoretical plates and the symmetry factor of the peak of indapamide are not less than 3500 and not more than 1.5, respectively.

System repeatability: When the test is repeated 6 times with 50 µL of the standard solution under the above operating conditions, the relative standard deviation of the peak area of indapamide is not more than 1.5%.

Assay To 20 Indapamide Tablets add 80 mL of a mixture of water and ethanol (99.5) (1:1), shake well to disintegrate, and sonicate for 10 minutes. Shake the solution for 10 minutes, and add a mixture of water and ethanol (99.5) (1:1) to make exactly 100 mL. Pipet a volume of indapamide ($C_{16}H_{16}ClN_3O_3S$), equivalent to about 2 mg, and add exactly 2 mL of the internal standard solution and a mixture of water and ethanol (99.5) (1:1) to make 20 mL. Centrifuge this solution, and use the supernatant liquid as the sample solution. Separately, weigh accurately about 20 mg of Indapamide RS (separately, determine the loss on drying <2.41> under the same condition as Indapamide), and dissolve in a mixture of water and ethanol (99.5) (1:1) to make exactly 100 mL. Pipet 10 mL of this solution, add exactly 2 mL of the internal standard solution and a mixture of water and ethanol (99.5) (1:1) to make 20 mL, and use this solution as the standard solution. Proceed as directed in the Assay under Indapamide.

Amount (mg) of indapamide ($C_{16}H_{16}ClN_3O_3S$)
$= M_S \times Q_T/Q_S \times 1/10$

M_S: Amount [mg (potency)] of Indapamide RS taken, calculated on the dried basis

Internal standard solution—A solution of isopropyl parahydroxybenzoate in a mixture of water and ethanol (99.5) (1:1) (3 in 1000).

Containers and storage Containers—Tight containers.

Indenolol Hydrochloride

インデノロール塩酸塩

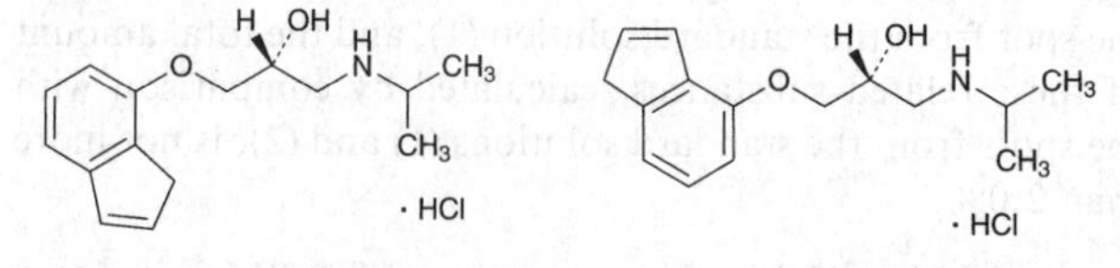

and enantiomer and enantiomer

$C_{15}H_{21}NO_2.HCl$: 283.79
(2*RS*)-1-(3*H*-Inden-4-yloxy)-3-(1-methylethyl)aminopropan-2-ol monohydrochloride
(2*RS*)-1-(3*H*-Inden-7-yloxy)-3-(1-methylethyl)aminopropan-2-ol monohydrochloride
[68906-88-7]

Indenolol Hydrochloride is a mixture of (2*RS*)-1-(3*H*-Inden-4-yloxy)-3-(1-methylethyl)aminopropan-2-ol monohydrochloride and (2*RS*)-1-(3*H*-Inden-7-yloxy)-3-(1-methylethyl)aminopropan-2-ol monohydrochloride.

When dried, it contains not less than 98.5% of indenolol hydrochloride ($C_{15}H_{21}NO_2.HCl$).

Description Indenolol Hydrochloride occurs as white to pale yellow, crystals or crystalline powder.

It is freely soluble in water and in acetic acid (100), soluble in ethanol (95) and in chloroform, slightly soluble in acetic anhydride, very slightly soluble in ethyl acetate, and practically insoluble in diethyl ether.

The pH of a solution of 1.0 g of Indenolol Hydrochloride in 10 mL of water is between 3.5 and 5.5.

It is colored by light.

Identification **(1)** Dissolve 0.1 g of Indenolol Hydrochloride in 1 to 2 drops of dilute hydrochloric acid and 5 mL of water, and add 1 mL of Reinecke salt TS: a red-purple precipitate is formed.

(2) Determine the absorption spectrum of a solution of Indenolol Hydrochloride (1 in 50,000) as directed under Ultraviolet-visible Spectrophotometry <2.24>, and compare the spectrum with the Reference Spectrum 1: both spectra exhibit similar intensities of absorption at the same wavelengths. Separately, determine the absorption spectrum of a solution of Indenolol Hydrochloride (1 in 10,000) as directed under Ultraviolet-visible Spectrophotometry <2.24>, and compare the spectrum with the Reference Spectrum 2: both spectra exhibit similar intensities of absorption at the same wavelengths.

(3) Determine the infrared absorption spectrum of Indenolol Hydrochloride, previously dried, as directed in the potassium chloride disk method under Infrared Spectrophotometry <2.25>, and compare the spectrum with the Reference Spectrum: both spectra exhibit similar intensities of absorption at the same wave numbers.

(4) A solution of Indenolol Hydrochloride (1 in 10) responds to Qualitative Tests <1.09> for chloride.

Absorbance <2.24> $E^{1\%}_{1\,cm}$ (250 nm): 330 – 340 (after drying, 10 mg, water, 1000 mL).

Melting point <2.60> 140 – 143°C

Purity **(1)** Clarity and color of solution—Dissolve 1.0 g of Indenolol Hydrochloride in 10 mL of water: the solution is clear and colorless to pale yellow.

(2) Heavy metals <1.07>—Proceed with 1.0 g of Indenolol Hydrochloride according to Method 2, and perform the test. Prepare the control solution with 2.0 mL of Standard Lead Solution (not more than 20 ppm).

(3) Arsenic *<1.11>*—Prepare the test solution with 1.0 g of Indenolol Hydrochloride according to Method 1, and perform the test (not more than 2 ppm).

(4) Related substances—Dissolve 0.20 g of Indenolol Hydrochloride in 10 mL of chloroform, and use this solution as the sample solution. Pipet 1 mL of the sample solution, add chloroform to make exactly 200 mL, and use this solution as the standard solution. Perform the test with these solutions as directed under Thin-layer Chromatography *<2.03>*. Spot 10 μL each of the sample solution and standard solution on a plate of silica gel with fluorescent indicator for thin-layer chromatography. Develop the plate with a mixture of 1,2-dichloroethane, ethanol (99.5) and ammonia solution (28) (70:15:2) to a distance of about 12 cm, and air-dry the plate. Examine under ultraviolet light (main wavelength: 254 nm): the spots other than the principal spot obtained from the sample solution are not more intense than the spot from the standard solution.

Loss on drying *<2.41>* Not more than 0.5% (1 g, in vacuum, phosphorus (V) oxide, 4 hours).

Residue on ignition *<2.44>* Not more than 0.1% (1 g).

Isomer ratio Dissolve 5 mg of Indenolol Hydrochloride in 1.0 mL of a mixture of ethyl acetate and trifluoroacetic anhydride for gas chromatography (9:1), and use this solution as the sample solution. Perform the test with 2 μL of the sample solution as directed under Gas Chromatography *<2.02>* according to the following conditions. Determine the areas of two adjacent peaks, A_a and A_b, having the retention times of about 16 minutes, where A_a is the peak area of shorter retention time and A_b is the peak area of longer retention time: the ratio $A_a/(A_a + A_b)$ is between 0.6 and 0.7.

Operating conditions—

Detector: A hydrogen flame-ionization detector.

Column: A glass column about 2 mm in inside diameter and about 2 m in length, packed with siliceous earth for gas chromatography (150 to 180 μm in particle diameter) coated with 65% phenyl-methyl silicon polymer for gas chromatography at the ratio of 2%.

Column temperature: A constant temperature between 150°C and 170°C.

Carrier gas: Helium.

Flow rate: Adjust so that the retention time of the peak showing earlier elution of the two peaks of indenolol hydrochloride is about 16 minutes.

Selection of column: Proceed with 2 μL of the sample solution under the above operating conditions, and calculate the resolution. Use a column with the resolution between the two peaks being not less than 1.1.

Assay Weigh accurately about 0.5 g of Indenolol Hydrochloride, previously dried, dissolve in 50 mL of a mixture of acetic anhydride and acetic acid (100) (4:1), and titrate *<2.50>* with 0.1 mol/L perchloric acid VS until the color of the solution changes from purple through blue to green (indicator: 3 drops of crystal violet TS). Perform a blank determination in the same manner, and make any necessary correction.

Each mL of 0.1 mol/L perchloric acid VS
= 28.38 mg of $C_{15}H_{21}NO_2.HCl$

Containers and storage Containers—Well-closed containers.

Storage—Light-resistant.

Indigocarmine

インジゴカルミン

$C_{16}H_8N_2Na_2O_8S_2$: 466.35
Disodium 3,3′-dioxo-[$\Delta^{2,2'}$-biindoline]-5,5′-disulfonate
[860-22-0]

Indigocarmine, when dried, contains not less than 95.0% of indigocarmine ($C_{16}H_8N_2Na_2O_8S_2$).

Description Indigocarmine occurs as a blue to dark blue, powder or granules. It is odorless.

It is sparingly soluble in water, and practically insoluble in ethanol (95) and in diethyl ether.

It is hygroscopic.

When compressed, it has a coppery luster.

Identification **(1)** A solution of Indigocarmine (1 in 100) is dark blue in color. Perform the following tests with this solution as the sample solution: the dark blue color of each solution disappears.

(i) Add 1 mL of nitric acid to 2 mL of the sample solution;

(ii) Add 1 mL of bromine TS to 2 mL of the sample solution;

(iii) Add 1 mL of chlorine TS to 2 mL of the sample solution;

(iv) Add 2 mL of sodium hydroxide TS and 0.2 g of zinc powder to 2 mL of the sample solution, and warm.

(2) Dissolve 0.1 g of Indigocarmine in 100 mL of a solution of ammonium acetate (1 in 650). To 1 mL of the solution add a solution of ammonium acetate (1 in 650) to make 100 mL. Determine the absorption spectrum of the solution as directed under Ultraviolet-visible Spectrophotometry *<2.24>*, and compare the spectrum with the Reference Spectrum: both spectra exhibit similar intensities of absorption at the same wavelengths.

(3) Ignite 1 g of Indigocarmine to carbonize. After cooling, add 20 mL of water to the residue, shake, and filter the mixture: the filtrate responds to Qualitative Tests *<1.09>* for sodium salt and for sulfate.

pH *<2.54>* Dissolve 0.10 g of Indigocarmine in 20 mL of water: the pH of the solution is between 5.0 and 6.0.

Purity **(1)** Water-insoluble substances—To 1.00 g of Indigocarmine add 200 mL of water, shake, and filter through a tared glass filter (G4). Wash the residue with water until the blue color of the filtrate becomes practically colorless, and dry the residue at 105°C for 4 hours: the mass of the residue does not exceed 5.0 mg.

(2) Arsenic *<1.11>*—Place 0.8 g of Indigocarmine in a Kjeldahl flask, add 5 mL of sulfuric acid and 5 mL of nitric acid, and ignite gently. Repeat the addition of 2 to 3 mL of nitric acid occasionally, and continue to heat until a colorless to light yellow solution is obtained. After cooling, add 15 mL of a saturated ammonium oxalate solution, heat the solution until dense white fumes are evolved, and concentrate to 2 to 3 mL. After cooling, dilute with water to 10 mL, and perform the test with 5 mL of this solution as the test solution (not more than 5 ppm).

Loss on drying ⟨*2.41*⟩ Not more than 10.0% (1 g, 105°C, 2 hours).

Residue on ignition ⟨*2.44*⟩ Not less than 28% and not more than 38% (after drying, 1 g).

Assay Weigh accurately about 0.5 g of Indigocarmine, previously dried, add 15 g of sodium hydrogen tartrate monohydrate, and dissolve in 200 mL of water, boil with bubbling of a stream of carbon dioxide, and titrate ⟨*2.50*⟩, while being hot, with 0.1 mol/L titanium (III) chloride VS until the color of the solution changes from blue through yellow to orange.

Each mL of 0.1 mol/L titanium (III) chloride VS
= 23.32 mg of $C_{16}H_8N_2Na_2O_8S_2$

Containers and storage Containers—Tight containers.
Storage—Light-resistant.

Indigocarmine Injection

インジゴカルミン注射液

Indigocarmine Injection is an aqueous injection.

It contains not less than 95.0% and not more than 105.0% of the labeled amount of indigocarmine ($C_{16}H_8N_2Na_2O_8S_2$: 466.35).

Method of preparation Prepare as directed under Injection, with Indigocarmine.

Description Indigocarmine Injection is a dark blue liquid.
pH: 3.0 – 5.0

Identification **(1)** To a volume of Indigocarmine Injection, equivalent to 20 mg of Indigocarmine, add 1 mL of nitric acid: the dark blue color of the liquid disappears, and a yellow-brown color develops.

(2) To a volume of Indigocarmine Injection, equivalent to 20 mg of Indigocarmine, add 1 mL of bromine TS: the dark blue color disappears, and a yellow-brown color develops.

(3) To a volume of Indigocarmine Injection, equivalent to 20 mg of Indigocarmine, add 1 mL of chlorine TS: the dark blue color disappears, and a yellow-brown color develops.

(4) To a volume of Indigocarmine Injection, equivalent to 10 mg of Indigocarmine, add ammonium acetate solution (1 in 650) to make 1000 mL, and determine the absorbance of the solution as directed under Ultraviolet-visible Spectrophotometry ⟨*2.24*⟩: it exhibits a maximum between 610 nm and 614 nm.

Bacterial endotoxins ⟨*4.01*⟩ Less than 7.5 EU/mg.

Extractable volume ⟨*6.05*⟩ It meets the requirement.

Foreign insoluble matter ⟨*6.06*⟩ Perform the test according to Method 1: it meets the requirement.

Insoluble particulate matter ⟨*6.07*⟩ Perform the test according to Method 2: it meets the requirement.

Sterility ⟨*4.06*⟩ Perform the test according to the Membrane filtration method: it meets the requirement.

Assay Measure exactly a volume of Indigocarmine Injection, equivalent to about 0.2 g of indigocarmine ($C_{16}H_8N_2Na_2O_8S_2$), add 6 g of sodium hydrogen tartrate monohydrate, and dissolve in water to make 200 mL. Then boil under a carbon dioxide stream, and proceed as directed in the Assay under Indigocarmine.

Each mL of 0.1 mol/L titanium (III) chloride VS
= 23.32 mg of $C_{16}H_8N_2Na_2O_8S_2$

Containers and storage Containers—Hermetic containers, and colored containers may be used.
Storage—Light-resistant.

Indium (^{111}In) Chloride Injection

塩化インジウム (**^{111}In**) 注射液

Indium (^{111}In) Chloride Injection is an aqueous injection.

It contains indium-111 (^{111}In) in the form of indium chloride.

It conforms to the requirements of Indium (^{111}In) Chloride Injection in the Minimum Requirements for Radiopharmaceuticals.

Test for Extractable Volume of Parenteral Preparations and Insoluble Particulate Matter Test for Injections are not applied to this injection.

Description Indium (^{111}In) Chloride Injection is a clear, colorless liquid.

Indometacin

インドメタシン

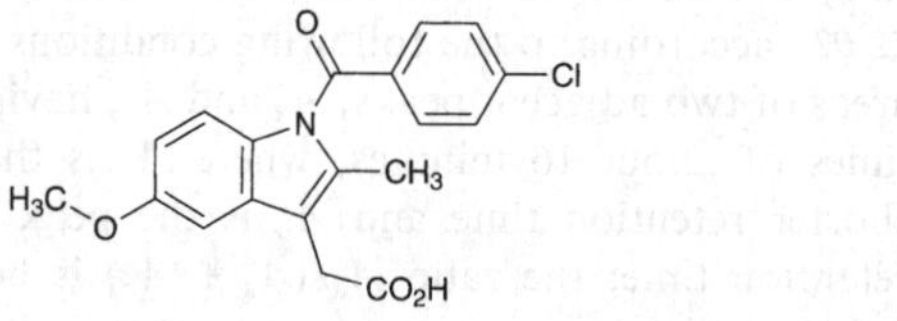

$C_{19}H_{16}ClNO_4$: 357.79
[1-(4-Chlorobenzoyl)-5-methoxy-2-methyl-1*H*-indol-3-yl]acetic acid
[*53-86-1*]

Indometacin, when dried, contains not less than 98.0% of indometacin ($C_{19}H_{16}ClNO_4$).

Description Indometacin occurs as a white to light yellow, fine, crystalline powder.

It is sparingly soluble in methanol, in ethanol (95) and in diethyl ether, and practically insoluble in water.

It dissolves in sodium hydroxide TS.

It is colored by light.

Melting point: 155 – 162°C

It shows crystal polymorphism.

Identification **(1)** Dissolve 2 mg of Indometacin in 100 mL of methanol. Determine the absorption spectrum of the solution as directed under Ultraviolet-visible Spectrophotometry ⟨*2.24*⟩, and compare the spectrum with the Reference Spectrum or the spectrum of a solution of Indometacin RS prepared in the same manner as the sample solution: both spectra exhibit similar intensities of absorption at the same wavelengths.

(2) Determine the infrared absorption spectrum of Indometacin, previously dried, as directed in the potassium bromide disk method under Infrared Spectrophotometry ⟨*2.25*⟩, and compare the spectrum with the Reference Spectrum or the spectrum of dried Indometacin RS: both spectra exhibit similar intensities of absorption at the same wave numbers.

If any difference appears between the spectra, recrystallize the sample and the RS with diethyl ether, filter and dry the crystals, and perform the test with the crystals.

(3) Perform the test with Indometacin as directed under Flame Coloration Test <*1.04*> (2): a green color appears.

Purity **(1)** Acidity—To 1.0 g of Indometacin add 50 mL of water, shake for 5 minutes, and filter. To the filtrate add 0.20 mL of 0.1 mol/L sodium hydroxide VS and 1 drop of phenolphthalein TS: a red color develops.

(2) Heavy metals <*1.07*>—Proceed with 1.0 g of Indometacin according to Method 2, and perform the test. Prepare the control solution with 2.0 mL of Standard Lead Solution (not more than 20 ppm).

(3) Arsenic <*1.11*>—Prepare the test solution with 1.0 g of Indometacin according to Method 3, and perform the test (not more than 2 ppm).

(4) Related substances—Dissolve 0.10 g of Indometacin in 10 mL of methanol, and use this solution as the sample solution. Pipet 1 mL of the sample solution, and add methanol to make exactly 50 mL. Pipet 5 mL of this solution, add methanol to make exactly 20 mL, and use this solution as the standard solution. Perform the test with these solutions as directed under Thin-layer Chromatography <*2.03*>. Spot 25 μL each of the sample solution and standard solution on a plate of silica gel with fluorescent indicator for thin-layer chromatography. Develop the plate with a mixture of dehydrated diethyl ether and acetic acid (100) (100:3) to a distance of about 10 cm, and air-dry the plate. Examine under ultraviolet light (main wavelength: 254 nm): the spots other than the principal spot obtained from the sample solution are not more intense than the spot from the standard solution.

Loss on drying <*2.41*> Not more than 0.5% (1 g, 105°C, 4 hours).

Residue on ignition <*2.44*> Not more than 0.1% (1 g).

Assay Weigh accurately about 0.7 g of Indometacin, previously dried, dissolve in 60 mL of methanol, add 30 mL of water, and titrate <*2.50*> with 0.1 mol/L sodium hydroxide VS (indicator: 3 drops of phenolphthalein TS). Perform a blank determination in the same manner, and make any necessary correction.

Each mL of 0.1 mol/L sodium hydroxide VS
= 35.78 mg of $C_{19}H_{16}ClNO_4$

Containers and storage Containers—Tight containers.
Storage—Light-resistant.

Indometacin Capsules

インドメタシンカプセル

Indometacin Capsules contain not less than 90.0% and not more than 110.0% of the labeled amount of indometacin ($C_{19}H_{16}ClNO_4$: 357.79).

Method of preparation Prepare as directed under Capsules, with Indometacin.

Identification Powder the contents of Indometacin Capsules. To a quantity of the powder, equivalent to 0.1 g of Indometacin, add 20 mL of chloroform, shake well, and centrifuge. Filter the supernatant liquid, and evaporate the filtrate to dryness. After cooling, dissolve the residue in 20 mL of methanol. To 10 mL of this solution add methanol to make 50 mL, then to 2 mL of this solution add methanol to make 100 mL, and use this solution as the sample solution. Determine the absorption spectrum of the sample solution as directed under Ultraviolet-visible Spectrophotometry <*2.24*>: it exhibits a maximum between 317 nm and 321 nm.

Purity Related substances—Powder the content of Indometacin Capsules. To a quantity of the powder, equivalent to 0.10 g of Indometacin, add exactly 10 mL of methanol, shake well, filter, and use the filtrate as the sample solution. Dissolve 25 mg of Indometacin RS in methanol to make exactly 50 mL. Pipet 1 mL of the solution, add methanol to make exactly 10 mL, and use this solution as the standard solution. Proceed as directed in the Purity (4) under Indometacin.

Uniformity of dosage units <*6.02*> Perform the test according to the following method: it meets the requirement of the Content uniformity test.

Take out the content of 1 capsule of Indometacin Capsules, and dissolve in methanol to make exactly *V* mL so that each mL contains about 1 mg of indometacin ($C_{19}H_{16}ClNO_4$). Filter the solution, discard the first 10 mL of the filtrate, pipet 5 mL of the subsequent filtrate, add exactly 3 mL of the internal standard solution, then add the mobile phase to make 100 mL, and use this solution as the sample solution. Separately, weigh accurately about 25 mg of Indometacin RS, previously dried at 105°C for 4 hours, dissolve in methanol to make exactly 25 mL. Pipet 5 mL of this solution, add exactly 3 mL of the internal standard solution, then add the mobile phase to make 100 mL, and use this solution as the standard solution. Then, proceed as directed in the Assay.

$$\text{Amount (mg) of indometacin } (C_{19}H_{16}ClNO_4) = M_S \times Q_T/Q_S \times V/25$$

M_S: Amount (mg) of Indometacin RS taken

Internal standard solution—A solution of butyl parahydroxybenzoate in methanol (1 in 1000).

Dissolution <*6.10*> When the test is performed at 100 revolutions per minute according to the Basket method, using 900 mL of a mixture of water and phosphate buffer solution (pH 7.2) (4:1) as the dissolution medium, the dissolution rate in 20 minutes of Indometacin Capsules is not less than 75%.

Start the test with 1 capsule of Indometacin Capsules, withdraw not less than 20 mL of the medium at the specified minute after starting the test, and filter through a membrane filter with a pore size not exceeding 0.8 μm. Discard not less than 10 mL of the first filtrate, pipet *V* mL of the subsequent filtrate, add the dissolution medium to make exactly *V′* mL so that each mL contains about 28 μg of indometacin ($C_{19}H_{16}ClNO_4$), and use this solution as the sample solution. Separately, weigh accurately about 30 mg of Indometacin RS, previously dried at 105°C for 4 hours, dissolve in the dissolution medium to make exactly 1000 mL, and use this solution as the standard solution. Determine the absorbances, A_T and A_S, of the sample solution and the standard solution at 320 nm as directed under Ultraviolet-visible Spectrophotometry <*2.24*>.

$$\text{Dissolution rate (\%) with respect to the labeled amount of indometacin } (C_{19}H_{16}ClNO_4) = M_S \times A_T/A_S \times 1/C \times 90$$

M_S: Amount (mg) of Indometacin RS taken
C: Labeled amount (mg) of indometacin ($C_{19}H_{16}ClNO_4$) in 1 capsule

Assay Weigh accurately the contents of not less than 20 Indometacin Capsules. Powder the combined contents, and weigh accurately a portion of the powder, equivalent to about 50 mg of indometacin ($C_{19}H_{16}ClNO_4$). Dissolve in 40 mL of methanol, and add methanol to make exactly 50 mL. Filter this solution, discarding the first 10-mL portion of the filtrate. Pipet 5 mL of the subsequent filtrate, add exactly 3 mL of the internal standard solution, add the mobile phase to make 100 mL, and use this solution as the sample solution. Separately, weigh accurately about 50 mg of Indometacin RS, previously dried at 105°C for 4 hours, and dissolve in methanol to make exactly 50 mL. Pipet 5 mL of the solution, add exactly 3 mL of the internal standard solution, add the mobile phase to make 100 mL, and use this solution as the standard solution. Perform the test with 20 μL each of the sample solution and standard solution as directed under Liquid Chromatography <2.01> according to the following conditions, and calculate the ratios, Q_T and Q_S, of the peak area of indometacin to that of the internal standard, respectively.

$$\text{Amount (mg) of indometacin } (C_{19}H_{16}ClNO_4) = M_S \times Q_T/Q_S$$

M_S: Amount (mg) of Indometacin RS taken

Internal standard solution—A solution of butyl parahydroxybenzoate in methanol (1 in 1000).

Operating conditions—

Detector: An ultraviolet absorption photometer (wavelength: 254 nm).

Column: A stainless steel column 4.6 mm in inside diameter and 25 cm in length, packed with octadecylsilanized silica gel for liquid chromatography (7 μm in particle diameter).

Column temperature: A constant temperature of about 25°C.

Mobile phase: A mixture of methanol and diluted phosphoric acid (1 in 1000) (7:3).

Flow rate: Adjust so that the retention time of indometacin is about 8 minutes.

System suitability—

System performance: Dissolve 50 mg of 4-chlorobenzoic acid, 30 mg of butyl parahydroxybenzoate and 50 mg of indometacin in 50 mL of methanol. To 5 mL of this solution add the mobile phase to make 100 mL. When the procedure is run with 20 μL of this solution under the above operating conditions, 4-chlorobenzoic acid, butyl parahydroxybenzoate and indometacin are eluted in this order, with the resolution between the peaks of 4-chlorobenzoic acid and butyl parahydroxybenzoate being not less than 2.0, and between the peaks of butyl parahydroxybenzoate and indometacin being not less than 5.

System repeatability: When the test is repeated 6 times with 20 μL of the standard solution under the above operating conditions, the relative standard deviation of the ratios of the peak area of indometacin to that of the internal standard is not more than 1.0%.

Containers and storage Containers—Tight containers.

Indometacin Suppositories

インドメタシン坐剤

Indometacin Suppositories contain not less than 90.0% and not more than 110.0% of the labeled amount of indometacin ($C_{19}H_{16}ClNO_4$: 357.79).

Method of preparation Prepare as directed under Suppositories, with Indometacin.

Identification Dissolve a quantity of Indometacin Suppositories, equivalent to 50 mg of Indometacin, in 20 mL of methanol by warming, add methanol to make 50 mL, and filter if necessary. To 2 mL of this solution add methanol to make 100 mL, and use this solution as the sample solution. Determine the absorption spectrum of the sample solution as directed under Ultraviolet-visible Spectrophotometry <2.24>: it exhibits a maximum between 317 nm and 321 nm.

Uniformity of dosage units <6.02> Perform the test according to the following method: it meets the requirement of the Content uniformity test.

To 1 suppository of Indometacin Suppositories add 80 mL of a mixture of methanol and acetic acid (100) (200:1), dissolve by warming, add a mixture of methanol and acetic acid (100) (200:1) to make exactly 100 mL. Pipet V mL of this solution, equivalent to about 2 mg of indometacin ($C_{19}H_{16}ClNO_4$), add a mixture of methanol and acetic acid (100) (200:1) to make exactly 50 mL, and use this solution as the sample solution. Separately, weigh accurately about 0.1 g of Indometacin RS, previously dried at 105°C for 4 hours, and dissolve in a mixture of methanol and acetic acid (100) (200:1) to make exactly 100 mL. Pipet 4 mL of this solution, add a mixture of methanol and acetic acid (100) (200:1) to make exactly 100 mL, and use this solution as the standard solution. Perform the test with the sample solution and standard solution as directed under Ultraviolet-visible Spectrophotometry <2.24>, and determine the absorbances, A_T and A_S, at 320 nm.

$$\text{Amount (mg) of indometacin } (C_{19}H_{16}ClNO_4) = M_S \times A_T/A_S \times 2/V$$

M_S: Amount (mg) of Indometacin RS taken

Assay Weigh accurately not less than 20 Indometacin Suppositories, cut into small pieces carefully, and mix well. Weigh accurately a portion of the mass, equivalent to about 50 mg of indometacin ($C_{19}H_{16}ClNO_4$), add 40 mL of tetrahydrofuran, warm at 40°C, dissolve by shaking, cool, and add tetrahydrofuran to make exactly 50 mL. Filter the solution, discard the first 10 mL of the filtrate, pipet 5 mL of the subsequent filtrate, add exactly 3 mL of the internal standard solution, and add the mobile phase to make 100 mL. Allow the solution to stand for 30 minutes, filter through a membrane filter (0.5 μm pore size), discard the first 10 mL of the filtrate, and use the subsequent filtrate as the sample solution. Separately, weigh accurately about 50 mg of Indometacin RS, previously dried at 105°C for 4 hours, and dissolve in tetrahydrofuran to make exactly 50 mL. Pipet 5 mL of the solution, proceed in the same manner as the sample solution, and use this solution as the standard solution. Perform the test with 20 μL each of the sample solution and standard solution as directed under Liquid Chromatography <2.01> according to the following conditions, and calculate the ratios, Q_T and Q_S, of the peak area of indometacin to that of the internal standard, respectively.

Amount (mg) of indometacin ($C_{19}H_{16}ClNO_4$)
$= M_S \times Q_T/Q_S$

M_S: Amount (mg) of Indometacin RS taken

Internal standard solution—A solution of butyl parahydroxybenzoate in methanol (1 in 1000).

Operating conditions—

Detector: An ultraviolet absorption photometer (wavelength: 254 nm).

Column: A stainless steel column 4.0 mm in inside diameter and 25 cm in length, packed with octadecylsilanized silica gel for liquid chromatography (7 μm in particle diameter).

Column temperature: A constant temperature of about 25°C.

Mobile phase: A mixture of methanol and diluted phosphoric acid (1 in 1000) (7:3).

Flow rate: Adjust so that the retention time of indometacin is about 8 minutes.

System suitability—

System performance: Dissolve 50 mg of 4-chlorobenzoic acid, 30 mg of butyl parahydroxybenzoate and 50 mg of indometacin in 50 mL of methanol. To 5 mL of this solution add the mobile phase to make 100 mL. When the procedure is run with 20 μL of this solution under the above operating conditions, 4-chlorobenzoic acid, butyl parahydroxybenzoate and indometacin are eluted in this order with the resolution between the peaks of 4-chlorobenzoic acid and butyl parahydroxybenzoate being not less than 2.0 and between the peaks of parahydroxybenzoate and indometacin being not less than 5.

System repeatability: When the test is repeated 6 times with 20 μL of the standard solution under the above operating conditions, the relative standard deviation of the ratios of the peak area of indometacin to that of the internal standard is not more than 1.0%.

Containers and storage Containers—Well-closed containers.

Storage—Light-resistant, and in a cold place.

Influenza HA Vaccine

インフルエンザ**HA**ワクチン

Influenza HA Vaccine is a liquid for injection containing hemagglutinin of influenza virus.

It conforms to the requirements of Influenza HA Vaccine in the Minimum Requirements for Biological Products.

Description Influenza HA Vaccine is a clear liquid or a slightly whitish turbid liquid.

Insulin Human (Genetical Recombination)

インスリン ヒト(遺伝子組換え)

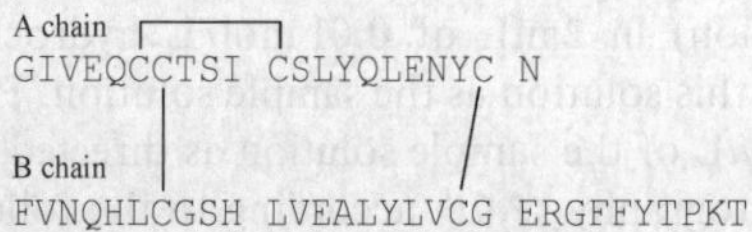

$C_{257}H_{383}N_{65}O_{77}S_6$: 5807.57 (two chains)
A chain $C_{99}H_{153}N_{25}O_{35}S_4$: 2381.68
B chain $C_{158}H_{234}N_{40}O_{42}S_2$: 3429.92
[11061-68-0]

Insulin Human (Genetical Recombination) is a recombinant human insulin. It is a peptide composed of A chain consisting of 21 amino acid residues and B chain consisting of 30 amino acid residues.

It contains not less than 27.5 Insulin Units per mg, calculated on the dried basis.

Description Insulin Human (Genetical Recombination) occurs as a white powder.

It is practically insoluble in water and in ethanol (95).

It dissolves in 0.01 mol/L hydrochloric acid TS and in sodium hydroxide TS with decomposition.

It is hygroscopic.

Identification Weigh accurately a suitable amount of Insulin Human (Genetical Recombination), and dissolve in 0.01 mol/L hydrochloric acid TS to make a solution so that each mL contains 2.0 mg. Transfer 500 μL of this solution into a clean test tube, add 2.0 mL of HEPES buffer solution (pH 7.5) and 400 μL of V8-protease TS, incubate at 25°C for 6 hours, then add 2.9 mL of ammonium sulfate buffer solution to stop the reaction, and use this solution as the sample solution. Separately, proceed with Insulin Human RS in the same manner as above, and use this solution as the standard solution. Perform the test with 50 μL each of the sample solution and standard solution as directed under Liquid Chromatography <2.01> according to the following conditions, and compare the chromatograms obtained from these solutions: a similar peak is observed at the same retention time in the both chromatograms.

Operating conditions—

Detector: An ultraviolet absorption photometer (wavelength: 214 nm).

Column: A stainless steel column 4.6 mm in inside diameter and 10 cm in length, packed with octadecylsilanized silica gel for liquid chromatography (3 μm in particle diameter).

Column temperature: A constant temperature of about 40°C.

Mobile phase A: A mixture of water, ammonium sulfate buffer solution and acetonitrile (7:2:1).

Mobile phase B: A mixture of water, acetonitrile and ammonium sulfate buffer solution (2:2:1).

Flowing of mobile phase: Change the mixing ratio of the mobile phase A and B linearly from 9:1 to 3:7 in 60 minutes after sample injection, further change to 0:10 linearly in 5 minutes, and then flow the mobile phase B only for 5 minutes.

Flow rate: 1.0 mL per minute.

System suitability—

System performance: When the procedure is run with 50 μL of the standard solution under the above operating con-

ditions, the symmetry factor of the two larger peaks which appear next to the first peak just after the solvent peak are not more than 1.5 respectively, and the resolution between these peaks is not less than 3.4.

Purity **(1)** Related substances—Perform this procedure rapidly. Dissolve 7.5 mg of Insulin Human (Genetical Recombination) in 2 mL of 0.01 mol/L hydrochloric acid TS, and use this solution as the sample solution. Perform the test with 20 μL of the sample solution as directed under Liquid Chromatography <*2.01*> according to the following conditions, and determine the peak area of human insulin, A_1, the peak area of the desamido substance having the relative retention time of about 1.3 to human insulin, A_D, and the total area of the peaks other than the solvent peak, A_T: the amounts of the desamido substance and related substances other than the desamido substance are not more than 2.0%, respectively. Previously, perform the test with 0.01 mol/L hydrochloric acid TS in the same manner to confirm the solvent peak.

Amount (%) of the desamido substance = $A_D/A_T \times 100$

Amount (%) of related substances other than the desamido substance
$= [\{A_T - (A_1 + A_D)\}/A_T] \times 100$

Operating conditions—

Detector: An ultraviolet absorption photometer (wavelength: 214 nm).

Column: A stainless steel column 4.6 mm in inside diameter and 25 cm in length, packed with octadecylsilanized silica gel for liquid chromatography (5 μm in particle diameter).

Column temperature: A constant temperature of about 40°C.

Mobile phase A: A mixture of phosphoric acid-sodium sulfate buffer solution (pH 2.3) and acetonitrile for liquid chromatography (41:9).

Mobile phase B: A mixture of phosphoric acid-sodium sulfate buffer solution (pH 2.3) and acetonitrile for liquid chromatography (1:1).

Flowing of mobile phase: Flow a mixture of the mobile phase A and B (78:22) for 36 minutes before and after the sample injection, then change the mixing ratio to 33:67 linearly in 25 minutes, and maintain this ratio for 6 minutes. Then flow the first mixture (78:22) for the next 15 minutes. Adjust the mixing ratio of the first mixture so that the retention time of human insulin is about 25 minutes.

Flow rate: 1.0 mL per minute.

Time span of measurement: For about 75 minutes after the sample is injected.

System suitability—

Test for required detectability: Confirm that the peak height of the desamido substance obtained with 20 μL of human insulin desamido substance-containing TS is between 30% and 70% of the full scale.

System performance: When the procedure is run with 20 μL of human insulin desamido substance-containing TS under the above operating conditions, human insulin and human insulin desamido substance are eluted in this order with the resolution between these peaks being not less than 2.0, and the symmetry factor of the peak of human insulin is not more than 1.8.

(2) High-molecular mass proteins—Dissolve 4 mg of Insulin Human (Genetical Recombination) in 1 mL of 0.01 mol/L hydrochloric acid TS. Perform the test with 100 μL of this solution as directed under Liquid Chromatography <*2.01*> according to the following conditions, and calculate each peak area: the total of areas of the peaks having smaller retention time than human insulin is not more than 1.0% of the total area of all peaks.

Operating conditions—

Detector: An ultraviolet absorption photometer (wavelength: 276 nm).

Column: A stainless steel column 7.5 mm in inside diameter and 30 cm in length, packed with hydrophilic silica gel for liquid chromatography.

Column temperature: A constant temperature of about 25°C.

Mobile phase: A mixture of a solution of L-arginine (1 in 1000), acetonitrile and acetic acid (100) (13:4:3).

Flow rate: Adjust so that the retention time of human insulin is about 20 minutes.

Time span of measurement: Until the peak of human insulin monomer has appeared.

System suitability—

Test for required detectability: Confirm that the peak height of the dimer obtained with 100 μL of human insulin dimer-containing TS is between 10% and 50% of the full scale.

System performance: When the procedure is run with 100 μL of human insulin dimer-containing TS under the above operating conditions, polymer, dimer and monomer are eluted in this order, and the ratio, H_1/H_2, of the peak height of the dimer H_1 to the height of the bottom between the peaks of the dimer and the monomer H_2 is not less than 2.0.

(3) Product related impurities—Being specified separately when the drug is granted approval based on the Law.

(4) Process related impurities—Being specified separately when the drug is granted approval based on the Law.

Loss on drying <*2.41*> Not more than 10.0% (0.2 g, 105°C, 24 hours).

Bacterial endotoxins <*4.01*> Less than 10 EU/mg.

Zinc content Weigh accurately about 50 mg of Insulin Human (Genetical Recombination), and dissolve in 0.01 mol/L hydrochloric acid TS to make exactly 25 mL. If necessary, dilute with 0.01 mol/L hydrochloric acid TS to make a solution so that each mL contains between 0.4 μg and 1.6 μg of zinc (Zn: 65.38), and use this solution as the sample solution. Separately, take exactly a suitable amount of Standard Zinc Solution for Atomic Absorption Spectrophotometry, dilute with 0.01 mol/L hydrochloric acid TS to make solutions containing 0.40 μg, 0.80 μg, 1.20 μg and 1.60 μg of zinc (Zn: 65.38) in each mL, respectively, and use these solutions as the standard solutions. Perform the test with the sample solution and standard solutions as directed under Atomic Absorption Spectrophotometry <*2.23*>, and calculate the amount of zinc (Zn: 65.38) in the sample solution by using a calibration curve obtained from the absorbances of the standard solutions: not more than 1.0%, calculated on the dried basis.

Gas: Combustible gas—Acetylene.
Supporting gas—Air.

Lamp: Zinc hollow cathode lamp.

Wavelength: 213.9 nm.

Assay Perform this procedure quickly. Weigh accurately about 7.5 mg of Insulin Human (Genetical Recombination), dissolve in 0.01 mol/L hydrochloric acid TS to make exactly 5 mL, and use this solution as the sample solution. Separately, weigh accurately a suitable amount of Insulin Human RS, dissolve exactly in 0.01 mol/L hydrochloric acid TS to make a solution so that each mL contains about 40 Insulin Units, and use this solution as the standard solution. Perform the test with exactly 20 μL each of the sample solution and standard solution as directed under Liquid Chromatography <*2.01*> according to the following conditions, and determine the peak areas of human insulin, A_{TI} and A_{SI}, and the peak areas of the desamido substance having the relative retention time of 1.3 to human insulin, A_{TD} and A_{SD}, respectively, of these solutions.

Amount (Insulin Unit/mg) of human insulin ($C_{257}H_{383}N_{65}O_{77}S_6$)
$= (M_S \times F)/D \times (A_{TI} + A_{TD})/(A_{SI} + A_{SD}) \times 5/M_T$

F: Labeled unit (Insulin Unit/mg) of Insulin Human RS
D: Volume (mL) of 0.01 mol/L hydrochloric acid TS used to dissolve the reference standard
M_T: Amount (mg) of Insulin Human (Genetical Recombination) taken, calculated on the dried basis
M_S: Amount (mg) of Insulin Human RS taken

Operating conditions—

Detector: An ultraviolet absorption photometer (wavelength: 214 nm).

Column: A stainless steel column 4.6 mm in inside diameter and 15 cm in length, packed with octadecylsilanized silica gel for liquid chromatography (5 μm in particle diameter).

Column temperature: A constant temperature of about 40°C.

Mobile phase: A mixture of phosphoric acid-sodium sulfate buffer solution (pH 2.3) and acetonitrile for liquid chromatography (3:1). Adjust the mixing ratio of the component of the mobile phase so that the retention time of human insulin is between 10 minutes and 17 minutes.

Flow rate: 1.0 mL per minute.

System suitability—

System performance: When the procedure is run with 20 μL of human insulin desamido substance-containing TS under the above operating conditions, human insulin and human insulin desamido substance are eluted in this order with the resolution between these peaks being not less than 2.0, and the symmetry factor of the peak of human insulin is not more than 1.8.

System repeatability: When the test is repeated 6 times with 20 μL of the standard solution under the above operating conditions, the relative standard deviation of the peak areas of human insulin is not more than 1.6%.

Containers and storage Containers—Tight containers.
Storage—Not exceeding −20°C.

Insulin Human (Genetical Recombination) Injection

インスリン ヒト(遺伝子組換え)注射液

Insulin Human (Genetical Recombination) Injection is an aqueous injection.

It contains not less than 95.0% and not more than 105.0% of the labeled Insulin Unit of insulin human (genetical recombination) ($C_{257}H_{383}N_{65}O_{77}S_6$: 5807.57).

Method of preparation Prepare as directed under Injections, with Insulin Human (Genetical Recombination) suspended in Water for Injection then dissolved by addition of Hydrochloric Acid or Sodium Hydroxide.

Description Insulin Human (Genetical Recombination) Injection occurs as a clear, colorless liquid, and slightly a fine precipitate may be observable upon storage.

Identification Insulin Human (Genetical Recombination) Injection forms a precipitate when adjusted to pH 5.3 – 5.5 by addition of dilute hydrochloric acid, and the precipitate disappears when adjusted to pH 2.5 – 3.5 by further addition of the acid.

Osmotic pressure ratio Being specified separately when the drug is granted approval based on the Law.

pH Being specified separately when the drug is granted approval based on the Law.

Purity **(1)** Desamido substance—Perform the test with 20 μL of the sample solution obtained in the Assay as directed under Liquid Chromatography <*2.01*> according to the following conditions. Determine each peak area by the automatic integration method, and calculate their amounts by the area percentage method: the amount of the peak, having the relative retention time of about 1.3 to human insulin, is not more than 1.5%.

Operating conditions—

Proceed as directed in the operating conditions in the Assay under Insulin Human (Genetical Recombination).

System suitability—

System performance: Proceed as directed in the system suitability in the Assay under Insulin Human (Genetical Recombination).

Test for required detectability: Pipet 1 mL of the sample solution, and add 0.01 mol/L hydrochloric acid TS to make exactly 50 mL. Confirm that the peak area of human insulin obtained with 20 μL of this solution is equivalent to 1.4 to 2.6% of that with 20 μL of the sample solution.

System repeatability: Dissolve Insulin Human RS in 0.01 mol/L hydrochloric acid TS so that each mL contains about 4 Insulin Units. When the test is repeated 6 times with 20 μL of this solution under the above operating conditions, the relative standard deviation of the peak area of human insulin is not more than 2.0%.

(2) High-molecular mass proteins—For each mL of Insulin Human (Genetical Recombination) Injection add 4 μL of 6 mol/L hydrochloric acid TS, and use this solution as the sample solution. Perform the test with 100 μL of the sample solution as directed under Liquid Chromatography <*2.01*> according to the following conditions. Determine each peak area by the automatic integration method, and calculate the amount of them by the area percentage method: the total amount of the peaks other than human insulin is not more than 2.0%.

Operating conditions—

Detector, column temperature, mobile phase, and flow rate: Proceed as directed in the operating conditions in the Purity (2) under Insulin Human (Genetical Recombination).

Column: A stainless steel column 7.8 mm in inside diameter and 30 cm in length, packed with hydrophilic silica gel for liquid chromatography.

Time span of measurement: From the retention time corresponding to the exclusion volume of the size-exclusion column to the completion of the elution of human insulin.

System suitability—

System performance: Proceed as directed in the system suitability in the Purity (2) under Insulin Human (Genetical Recombination).

Test for required detectability: Pipet 1 mL of the sample solution, and add 0.01 mol/L hydrochloric acid TS to make exactly 50 mL. Confirm that the peak area of human insulin obtained with 100 μL of this solution is equivalent to 1.4 to 2.6% of that with 100 μL of the sample solution.

Bacterial endotoxins <*4.01*> Less than 0.80 EU/Insulin

Unit. Apply to the preparations intended for intravenous administration.

Extractable volume <*6.05*> It meets the requirement.

Foreign insoluble matter <*6.06*> Perform the test according to Method1: it meets the requirement.

Insoluble particulate matter <*6.07*> It meets the requirement.

Sterility <*4.06*> Perform the test according to the Membrane filtration method: it meets the requirement.

Zinc content To an exact volume of Insulin Human (Genetical Recombination) Injection, equivalent to 300 Insulin Units, add 0.01 mol/L hydrochloric acid TS to make exactly 50 mL. If necessary, further dilute with 0.01 mol/L hydrochloric acid TS to make exactly 100 mL, and use this solution as the sample solution. Separately, take exactly a suitable amount of Standard Zinc Solution for Atomic Absorption Spectrophotometry, dilute with 0.01 mol/L hydrochloric acid TS to make three solutions containing 0.20 μg, 0.60 μg and 1.20 μg of zinc (Zn: 65.38) in each mL, respectively, and use these solutions as the standard solutions. Perform the test with the sample solution and standard solutions as directed under Atomic Absorption Spectrophotometry <*2.23*> according to the following conditions, using the 0.01 mol/L hydrochloric acid TS as the blank, and calculate the amount of zinc in the sample solution by using a calibration curve obtained from the absorbances of the standard solutions: 10 – 40 μg of zinc (Zn: 65.38) per 100 Insulin Units.

Gas: Combustible gas—Acetylene.
 Supporting gas—Air.
Lamp: Zinc hollow cathode lamp.
Wavelength: 213.9 nm.

Assay To exactly 10 mL of Insulin Human (Genetical Recombination) Injection add exactly 40 μL of 6 mol/L hydrochloric acid TS. Pipet 2 mL of this solution, add 0.01 mol/L hydrochloric acid TS to make exactly 5 mL, and use this solution as the sample solution. Then, proceed as directed in the Assay under Insulin Human (Genetical Recombination).

Amount (Insulin Unit) of human insulin ($C_{257}H_{383}N_{65}O_{77}S_6$) in 1 mL

$$= M_S \times F/D \times (A_{T1}+A_{TD})/(A_{S1}+A_{SD}) \times 1.004 \times 5/2$$

M_S: Amount (mg) of Insulin Human RS taken
F: Labeled unit (Insulin Unit/mg) of Insulin Human RS
D: Volume (mL) of 0.01 mol/L hydrochloric acid TS used to dissolve Insulin Human RS

Containers and storage Containers—Hermetic containers.
 Storage—Light-resistant, at a temperature of 2 – 8°C avoiding freezing.

Isophane Insulin Human (Genetical Recombination) Injectable Aqueous Suspension

イソフェンインスリン ヒト(遺伝子組換え)水性懸濁注射液

Isophane Insulin Human (Genetical Recombination) Injectable Aqueous Suspension is an aqueous suspension for injection.

It contains not less than 95.0% and not more than 105.0% of the labeled Insulin Unit of insulin human (genetical recombination) ($C_{257}H_{383}N_{65}O_{77}S_6$: 5807.57). It contains not less than 10 μg and not more than 40 μg of zinc (Zn: 65.38) per the labeled 100 Insulin Units.

Method of preparation Prepare as directed under Injections, with Insulin Human (Genetical Recombination) and Protamine Sulfate.

Description Isophane Insulin Human (Genetical Recombination) Injectable Aqueous Suspension is a white aqueous suspension. When allowed to stand, it separates into a white precipitate and colorless supernatant liquid, and the precipitate returns to the suspension state on gentle shaking.

When it is examined microscopically, the precipitate mostly consists of fine, oblong crystals of 1 to 30 μm in major axis, and does not contain amorphous substances or large aggregates.

Identification Adjust Isophane Insulin Human (Genetical Recombination) Injectable Aqueous Suspension to pH between 2.5 and 3.0 with dilute hydrochloric acid: the precipitate dissolves, and the solution is clear and colorless.

pH Being specified separately when the drug is granted approval based on the Law.

Purity (1) Desamido substance—Perform the test with 20 μL of the sample solution obtained in the Assay (1) as directed under Liquid Chromatography <*2.01*> according to the following conditions. Determine each peak area by the automatic integration method, and calculate the amount of them by the area percentage method: the amount of the peak, having the relative retention time of about 1.3 to insulin human, is not more than 1.5%.

Operating conditions—

Proceed as directed in the operating conditions in the Assay (1).

System suitability—

System performance: Proceed as directed in the system suitability in the Assay (1).

Test for required detectability: Pipet 1 mL of the sample solution, add 0.01 mol/L hydrochloric acid TS to make exactly 50 mL. Confirm that the peak area of insulin human obtained with 20 μL of this solution is equivalent to 1.4 to 2.6% of that with 20 μL of the sample solution.

System repeatability: Dissolve Insulin Human RS in 0.01 mol/L hydrochloric acid TS so that each mL contains about 4 Insulin Units. When the test is repeated 6 times with 20 μL of this solution under the above operating conditions, the relative standard deviation of the peak area of insulin human is not more than 2.0%.

(2) Dissolved insulin human—Centrifuge Isophane Insulin Human (Genetical Recombination) Injectable Aqueous Suspension, and use the supernatant liquid as the sample solution. Separately, dissolve exactly Insulin Human RS in 0.01 mol/L hydrochloric acid TS to make a solution so that each mL contains about 1.0 Insulin Units, and use this solution as the standard solution. Perform the test with exactly 20 μL each of the sample solution and standard solution as directed under Liquid Chromatography <*2.01*> according to the following conditions. Determine the peak areas, A_T and A_S, of insulin human by the automatic integration method, and calculate the amount of dissolved insulin human by the following equation: not more than 0.5 Insulin Units per mL.

Amount (mg) of dissolved insulin human (Insulin Unit /mL)

$$= (M_S \times F)/D \times A_T/A_S$$

M_S: Amount (mg) of Insulin Human RS taken

F: Labeled unit (Insulin Unit /mg) of Insulin Human RS
D: Volume (mL) of 0.01 mol/L hydrochloric acid TS used to dissolve Insulin Human RS

Operating conditions—

Proceed as directed in the operating conditions in the Assay (1).

System suitability—

System performance: When the procedure is run with 20 μL of insulin human desamido substance-containing TS under the above operating conditions, insulin human and insulin human desamido substance are eluted in this order with the resolution between these peaks being not less than 2.0, and the symmetry factor of the peak of insulin human is not more than 1.6.

System repeatability: When the test is repeated 4 times with 20 μL of the standard solution under the above operating conditions, the relative standard deviation of the peak area of insulin human is not more than 6.0%.

(3) High-molecular mass protein—Take a suitable volume of gently shaken Isophane Insulin Human (Genetical Recombination) Injectable Aqueous Suspension, add 4 μL of 6 mol/L hydrochloric acid TS for each mL of the suspension, and mix until the solution becomes clear. Perform the test with 100 μL of this solution as directed under Liquid Chromatography <*2.01*> according to the following conditions. Determine each peak area by the automatic integration method, and calculate the amount of them by the area percentage method: the total amount of the peaks other than insulin human is not more than 2.5%.

Operating conditions—

Detector, column temperature, mobile phase and flow rate: Proceed as directed in the operating conditions in the Purity (2) under Insulin Human (Genetical Recombination).

Column: A stainless steel column 7.8 mm in inside diameter and 30 cm in length, packed with hydrophilic silica gel for liquid chromatography.

Time span of measurement: From the retention time corresponding to the exclusion volume of the size-exclusion column to the completion of the elution of insulin human.

System suitability—

System performance: Proceed as directed in the system suitability in the Purity (2) under Insulin Human (Genetical Recombination).

Test for required detectability: Pipet 1 mL of the sample solution, and add 0.01 mol/L hydrochloric acid TS to make exactly 50 mL. Confirm that the peak area of insulin human obtained with 100 μL of this solution is equivalent to 1.4 to 2.6% of that with 100 μL of the sample solution.

Extractable volume <*6.05*> It meets the requirement.

Foreign insoluble matter <*6.06*> Perform the test according to Method 1: it meets the requirement.

Sterility <*4.06*> Perform the test according to the Membrane filtration method: it meets the requirement.

Assay **(1)** Insulin human—Pipet 10 mL of gently shaken Isophane Insulin Human (Genetical Recombination) Injectable Aqueous Suspension, and add exactly 40 μL of 6 mol/L hydrochloric acid TS. Pipet 2 mL of this solution, add 0.01 mol/L hydrochloric acid TS to make exactly 5 mL, and use this solution as the sample solution. Then, proceed as directed in the Assay under Insulin Human (Genetical Recombination).

Amount (Insulin Unit) of insulin human ($C_{257}H_{383}N_{65}O_{77}S_6$) in 1 mL

$$= (M_S \times F)/D \times (A_{TI} + A_{TD})/(A_{SI} + A_{SD}) \times 1.004 \times 5/2$$

M_S: Amount (mg) of Insulin Human RS taken
F: Labeled unit (Insulin Unit /mg) of Insulin Human RS
D: Volume (mL) of 0.01 mol/L hydrochloric acid TS used to dissolve Insulin Human RS

(2) Zinc—Pipet a volume of gently shaken Isophane Insulin Human (Genetical Recombination) Injectable Aqueous Suspension, equivalent to 300 Insulin Units, and add 0.01 mol/L hydrochloric acid TS to make exactly 50 mL. If necessary, further add 0.01 mol/L hydrochloric acid TS to make exactly 100 mL, and use this solution as the sample solution. Separately, pipet a suitable volume of Standard Zinc Solution for Atomic Absorption Spectroscopy, dilute with 0.01 mol/L hydrochloric acid TS to make three solutions containing 0.20 μg, 0.60 μg and 1.20 μg of zinc (Zn: 65.38) in each mL, respectively, and use these solutions as the standard solutions. Perform the test with the sample solution and standard solutions as directed under Atomic Absorption Spectroscopy <*2.23*> according to the following conditions, using 0.01 mol/L hydrochloric acid TS as the blank, and calculate the content of zinc in the sample solution by using the calibration curve obtained from the absorbances of the standard solutions.

Gas: Combustible gas—Acetylene.
Supporting gas—Air.
Lamp: Zinc hollow cathode lamp.
Wavelength: 213.9 nm.

Containers and storage Containers—Hermetic containers.

Storage—Light-resistant, at a temperature between 2°C and 8°C avoiding freezing.

Biphasic Isophane Insulin Human (Genetical Recombination) Injectable Aqueous Suspension

二相性イソフェンインスリン ヒト(遺伝子組換え)水性懸濁注射液

Biphasic Isophane Insulin Human (Genetical Recombination) Injectable Aqueous Suspension is an aqueous suspension for injection.

It contains not less than 95.0% and not more than 105.0% of the labeled Insulin Unit of insulin human (genetical recombination) ($C_{257}H_{383}N_{65}O_{77}S_6$: 5807.57). It contains not less than 10 μg and not more than 40 μg of zinc (Zn: 65.38) per the labeled 100 Insulin Units.

Method of preparation Prepare as directed under Injections, with Insulin Human (Genetical Recombination) Injection and Isophane Insulin Human (Genetical Recombination) Injectable Aqueous Suspension.

Description Biphasic Isophane Insulin Human (Genetical Recombination) Injectable Aqueous Suspension is a white aqueous suspension. When allowed to stand, it separates into a white precipitate and colorless supernatant liquid, and the precipitate returns to the suspension state on gentle shaking.

When it is examined microscopically, the precipitate mostly consists of fine, oblong crystals of 1 to 30 μm in major axis, and does not contain amorphous substances or large aggregates.

Identification Adjust Biphasic Isophane Insulin Human (Genetical Recombination) Injectable Aqueous Suspension to pH between 2.5 and 3.0 with dilute hydrochloric acid: the precipitate dissolves, and the solution is clear and colorless.

pH Being specified separately when the drug is granted approval based on the Law.

Purity **(1)** Desamido substance—Perform the test with 20 μL of the sample solution obtained in the Assay (1) as directed under Liquid Chromatography <*2.01*> according to the following conditions. Determine each peak area by the automatic integration method, and calculate the amount of them by the area percentage method: the amount of the peak, having the relative retention time of about 1.3 to insulin human, is not more than 1.5%.

Operating conditions—

Proceed as directed in the operating conditions in the Assay (1).

System suitability—

System performance: Proceed as directed in the system suitability in the Assay (1).

Test for required detectability: Pipet 1 mL of the sample solution, add 0.01 mol/L hydrochloric acid TS to make exactly 50 mL. Confirm that the peak area of insulin human obtained with 20 μL of this solution is equivalent to 1.4 to 2.6% of that with 20 μL of the sample solution.

System repeatability: Dissolve Insulin Human RS in 0.01 mol/L hydrochloric acid TS so that each mL contains about 4 Insulin Units. When the test is repeated 6 times with 20 μL of this solution under the above operating conditions, the relative standard deviation of the peak area of insulin human is not more than 2.0%.

(2) High-molecular mass protein—Take a suitable volume of gently shaken Biphasic Isophane Insulin Human (Genetical Recombination) Injectable Aqueous Suspension, add 4 μL of 6 mol/L hydrochloric acid TS for each mL of the suspension, and mix until the solution becomes clear. Perform the test with 100 μL of this solution as directed under Liquid Chromatography <*2.01*> according to the following conditions. Determine each peak area by the automatic integration method, and calculate the amount of them by the area percentage method: the total amount of the peaks other than insulin human is not more than 2.0%.

Operating conditions—

Detector, column temperature, mobile phase and flow rate: Proceed as directed in the operating conditions in the Purity (2) under Insulin Human (Genetical Recombination).

Column: A stainless steel column 7.8 mm in inside diameter and 30 cm in length, packed with hydrophilic silica gel for liquid chromatography.

Time span of measurement: From the retention time corresponding to the exclusion volume of the size-exclusion column to the completion of the elution of insulin human.

System suitability—

System performance: Proceed as directed in the system suitability in the Purity (2) under Insulin Human (Genetical Recombination).

Test for required detectability: Pipet 1 mL of the sample solution, and add 0.01 mol/L hydrochloric acid TS to make exactly 50 mL. Confirm that the peak area of insulin human obtained with 100 μL of this solution is equivalent to 1.4 to 2.6% of that with 100 μL of the sample solution.

Extractable volume <*6.05*> It meets the requirement.

Foreign insoluble matter <*6.06*> Perform the test according to Method 1: it meets the requirement.

Sterility <*4.06*> Perform the test according to the Membrane filtration method: it meets the requirement.

Soluble Insulin Human Being specified separately when the drug is granted approval based on the Law.

Assay **(1)** Insulin human—Pipet 10 mL of gently shaken Biphasic Isophane Insulin Human (Genetical Recombination) Injectable Aqueous Suspension, and add exactly 40 μL of 6 mol/L hydrochloric acid TS. Pipet 2 mL of this solution, add 0.01 mol/L hydrochloric acid TS to make exactly 5 mL, and use this solution as the sample solution. Then, proceed as directed in the Assay under Insulin Human (Genetical Recombination).

Amount (Insulin Unit) of insulin human ($C_{257}H_{383}N_{65}O_{77}S_6$) in 1 mL

$$= (M_S \times F)/D \times (A_{TI} + A_{TD})/(A_{SI} + A_{SD}) \times 1.004 \times 5/2$$

M_S: Amount (mg) of Insulin Human RS taken

F: Labeled unit (Insulin Unit /mg) of Insulin Human RS

D: Volume (mL) of 0.01 mol/L hydrochloric acid TS used to dissolve Insulin Human RS

(2) Zinc—Pipet a volume of gently shaken Biphasic Isophane Insulin Human (Genetical Recombination) Injectable Aqueous Suspension, equivalent to 300 Insulin Units, and add 0.01 mol/L hydrochloric acid TS to make exactly 50 mL. If necessary, further add 0.01 mol/L hydrochloric acid TS to make exactly 100 mL, and use this solution as the sample solution. Separately, pipet a suitable volume of Standard Zinc Solution for Atomic Absorption Spectroscopy, dilute with 0.01 mol/L hydrochloric acid TS to make three solutions containing 0.20 μg, 0.60 μg and 1.20 μg of zinc (Zn: 65.38) in each mL, respectively, and use these solutions as the standard solutions. Perform the test with the sample solution and standard solutions as directed under Atomic Absorption Spectroscopy <*2.23*> according to the following conditions, using 0.01 mol/L hydrochloric acid TS as the blank, and calculate the content of zinc in the sample solution by using the calibration curve obtained from the absorbances of the standard solutions.

Gas: Combustible gas—Acetylene.
Supporting gas—Air.
Lamp: Zinc hollow cathode lamp.
Wavelength: 213.9 nm.

Containers and storage Containers—Hermetic containers.

Storage—Light-resistant, at a temperature between 2°C and 8°C avoiding freezing.

Insulin Aspart (Genetical Recombination)

インスリン　アスパルト(遺伝子組換え)

```
A chain
GIVEQCCTSI CSLYQLENYC N

B chain
FVNQHLCGSH LVEALYLVCG ERGFFYTDKT
```

$C_{256}H_{381}N_{65}O_{79}S_6$: 5825.54 (two chains)
A chain $C_{99}H_{153}N_{25}O_{35}S_4$: 2381.68
B chain $C_{157}H_{232}N_{40}O_{44}S_2$: 3447.89
[*116094-23-6*]

Insulin Aspart (Genetical Recombination) is a recombinant human insulin analogue, in which proline residue at 28th of B chain is substituted with aspartic acid. It is a peptide composed of A chain consisting of 21 amino acid residues and B chain consisting of 30 amino acid residues.

It contains not less than 92.6% and not more than 109.5% of insulin aspart (genetical recombination) ($C_{256}H_{381}N_{65}O_{79}S_6$), calculated on the dried and residue on ignition-free basis.

0.0350 mg of Insulin Aspart (Genetical Recombination) is equivalent to 1 Insulin Unit.

Description Insulin Aspart (Genetical Recombination) occurs as a white powder.

It is practically insoluble in water and in ethanol (95).

It dissolves in 0.01 mol/L hydrochloric acid TS.

It is hygroscopic.

Identification Weigh a suitable amount of Insulin Aspart (Genetical Recombination), and dissolve in 0.01 mol/L hydrochloric acid TS to make a solution so that each mL contains 2.0 mg. Separately, dissolve Insulin Aspart RS in 0.01 mol/L hydrochloric acid TS to make a solution so that each mL contains 2.0 mg. Transfer 25 μL each of these solutions into clean test tubes, add 100 μL of HEPES buffer solution (pH 7.5) and 20 μL of V8-protease TS, and allow to react at 25°C for 6 hours. Then add 145 μL of ammonium sulfate buffer solution to stop the reaction, and use these solutions as the sample solution and the standard solution, respectively. Perform the test with exactly 50 μL each of the sample solution and standard solution as directed under Liquid Chromatography *<2.01>* according to the following conditions, and compare the peak (peak 1) eluted just after the peak of the solvent and the succeeding three peaks (peaks 2, 3 and 4) with apparently higher peak height in the chromatograms obtained from these solutions: the similar peaks are observed at the same retention times.

Operating conditions—

Detector: An ultraviolet absorption photometer (wavelength: 214 nm).

Column: A stainless steel column 4.6 mm in inside diameter and 10 cm in length, packed with octadecylsilanized silica gel for liquid chromatography (not exceeding 5 μm in particle diameter).

Column temperature: A constant temperature of about 40°C.

Mobile phase A: A mixture of water, ammonium sulfate buffer solution and acetonitrile for liquid chromatography (7:2:1).

Mobile phase B: A mixture of water, acetonitrile for liquid chromatography and ammonium sulfate buffer solution (2:2:1).

Flowing of mobile phase: Control the gradient by mixing the mobile phases A and B as directed in the following table.

Time after injection of sample (min)	Mobile phase A (vol%)	Mobile phase B (vol%)
0 – 60	90 → 30	10 → 70
60 – 65	30 → 0	70 → 100
65 – 70	0	100

Flow rate: 1 mL per minute.

System suitability—

System performance: When the procedure is run with 50 μL of the standard solution under the above operating conditions, the symmetry factors of the peaks 2 and 3 are not more than 1.5, respectively, and the resolution between these peaks is not less than 8.

Purity **(1)** Related substances—Perform the test with 10 μL of the sample solution obtained in the Assay as directed under Liquid Chromatography *<2.01>* according to the following conditions. Determine each peak area by the automatic integration method, and calculate the amounts of them by the area percentage method: the amount of the peak of B28isoAsp insulin aspart, having the relative retention time of about 0.9 to insulin aspart, is not more than 0.3%, the total amount of the peak of A21Asp insulin aspart and B3Asp insulin aspart, having the relative retention times of about 1.3, and the peak of B3isoAsp insulin aspart, having the relative retention time of about 1.5, is not more than 1.0%, and the total amount of the peaks other than the peaks mentioned above is not more than 0.5%.

Operating conditions—

Detector, column, column temperature, mobile phase A, mobile phase B, flowing of mobile phase and flow rate: Proceed as directed in the operating conditions in the Assay.

Time span of measurement: From 4 minutes to 50 minutes after injection of the sample solution.

System suitability—

System performance and system repeatability: Proceed as directed in the system suitability in the Assay.

Test for required detectability: Pipet 5 mL of the solution for system suitability test obtained in the Assay, add 0.01 mol/L hydrochloric acid TS to make exactly 10 mL. Confirm that the area percentage of the peak of B28isoAsp insulin aspart obtained with 10 μL of this solution is equivalent to 80 to 120% of that with 10 μL of the solution for system suitability test.

(2) High-molecular proteins—Store the sample solution at a temperature between 2°C and 8°C, and use within 48 hours after preparation. Dissolve 4 mg of Insulin Aspart (Genetical Recombination) in 1 mL of 0.01 mol/L hydrochloric acid TS, and use this solution as the sample solution. Perform the test with 100 μL of the sample solution as directed under Liquid Chromatography *<2.01>* according to the following conditions, determine each peak area by the automatic integration method, and calculate the amounts of them by the area percentage method: the total amount of the peaks other than insulin aspart is not more than 0.3%.

Operating conditions—

Detector: An ultraviolet absorption photometer (wavelength: 276 nm).

Column: A stainless steel column 7.8 mm in inside diameter and 30 cm in length, packed with hydrophilic silica gel for liquid chromatography (5 to 10 μm in particle diameter).

Column temperature: A constant temperature of about 20°C.

Mobile phase: A mixture of a solution of L-arginine (1 in 1000), acetonitrile for liquid chromatography and acetic acid (100) (13:4:3).

Flow rate: 0.5 mL per minute.

Time span of measurement: From the retention time corresponding to the exclusion volume of the size-exclusion column to the completion of the elution of insulin aspart.

System suitability—

Test for required detectability: Allow Insulin Aspart (Genetic Recombination) to stand at ordinary temperature for about 10 days, which results in containing about 0.4% of high-molecular proteins, dissolve in 0.01 mol/L hydrochloride TS so that each mL contains about 4 mg of insulin aspart, and use this solution as the solution for system suitability test. Store the solution for system suitability test at a temperature between 2°C and 8°C, and use within 7 days. Pipet 5 mL of the solution for system suitability test, and add 0.01 mol/L hydrochloric acid TS to make exactly 10 mL. Confirm that the area percentage of the peak of insulin aspart dimer obtained with 100 μL of this solution is equivalent to 80 to 120% of that with 100 μL of the solution for system suitability test.

System performance: When the procedure is run with 100 μL of the solution for system suitability test under the above operating conditions, insulin aspart polymer (retention time: 13 to 17 minutes), insulin aspart dimer (retention time: about 17.5 minutes) and insulin aspart (retention time: 18 to 20 minutes) are eluted in this order, and determine the peak height of the dimer and the height of the bottom between the peaks of the dimer and the monomer: the peak-valley ratio is not less than 2.0.

System repeatability: When the test is repeated 6 times with 100 μL of the solution for system suitability test under the above operating conditions, the relative standard deviation of the peak area of insulin aspart is not more than 2.0%.

(3) Host cell proteins—Being specified separately when the drug is granted approval based on the Law.

(4) Host cell DNA—Being specified separately when the drug is granted approval based on the Law.

Loss on drying 〈*2.41*〉 Not more than 10.0% (0.2 g, 105°C, 24 hours).

Residue on ignition 〈*2.44*〉 Not more than 6.0% (0.2 g).

Assay Store the sample solution and the standard solution at a temperature between 2°C and 8°C, use the sample solution within 24 hours after preparation, and use the standard solution within 48 hours after preparation. Weigh accurately a suitable amount of Insulin Aspart (Genetical Recombination), dissolve in 0.01 mol/L hydrochloric acid TS so that each mL contains 4.0 mg, and use this solution as the sample solution. Separately, dissolve Insulin Aspart RS in 0.01 mol/L hydrochloric acid TS so that each mL contains 4.0 mg, and use this solution as the standard solution. Perform the test with exactly 10 μL each of the sample solution and standard solution as directed under Liquid Chromatography 〈*2.01*〉 according to the following conditions, and determine the total areas, A_T and A_S, of the peak of B28isoAsp insulin aspart (relative retention time to insulin aspart: about 0.9), the peak of insulin aspart (retention time: 20 to 24 minutes), the peak of A21Asp insulin aspart and B3Asp insulin aspart (usually eluted together having the relative retention time of about 1.3) and the peak of B3isoAsp insulin aspart (relative retention time: about 1.5) in each solution.

Amount (mg) of insulin aspart ($C_{256}H_{381}N_{65}O_{79}S_6$)
$= M_S \times A_T/A_S$

M_S: Total amount (mg) of insulin aspart, B28isoAsp insulin aspart, A21Asp insulin aspart and B3Asp insulin aspart, and B3isoAsp insulin aspart in 1 mL of the standard solution

Operating conditions—

Detector: An ultraviolet absorption photometer (wavelength: 214 nm).

Column: A stainless steel column 4.0 mm in inside diameter and 25 cm in length, packed with octadecylsilanized silica gel for liquid chromatography (not exceeding 5 μm in particle diameter).

Column temperature: A constant temperature of about 40°C.

Mobile phase A: Dissolve 142.0 g of anhydrous sodium sulfate in water, add 13.5 mL of phosphoric acid, and add water to make 5 L. Adjust to pH 3.6 with sodium hydroxide TS. To 4500 mL of this solution add 500 mL of acetonitrile for liquid chromatography.

Mobile phase B: A mixture of water and acetonitrile for liquid chromatography (1:1).

Flowing of mobile phase: Control the gradient by mixing the mobile phases A and B as directed in the following table.

Time after injection of sample (min)	Mobile phase A (vol%)	Mobile phase B (vol%)
0 – 35	58	42
35 – 40	58 → 20	42 → 80
40 – 45	20	80
45 – 46	20 → 58	80 → 42
46 – 60	58	42

Flow rate: 1 mL per minute.

System suitability—

System performance: Dissolve Insulin Aspart (Genetical Recombination) in 0.01 mol/L sodium dihydrogen phosphate TS (pH 7.5) so that each mL contains 8 mg, and allow to stand at ordinary temperature for 10 to 15 days. To 1 mL of this solution add 1 mL of 0.01 mol/L hydrochloric acid TS, allow to stand at ordinary temperature for 1 to 3 days, and use this solution as the solution for system suitability test. The solution for system suitability test contains 0.1 to 2.2% of B28isoAsp insulin aspart, and not less than 1% of B3Asp insulin aspart and A21Asp insulin aspart. Store the solution for system suitability test at a temperature between 2°C and 8°C, and use within 72 hours. When the procedure is run with 10 μL of the solution for system suitability test under the above operating conditions, B28isoAsp insulin aspart, insulin aspart, A21Asp insulin aspart and B3Asp insulin aspart, and B3isoAsp insulin aspart are eluted in this order with the resolution between the peak of insulin aspart and the peak of A21Asp insulin aspart and B3Asp insulin aspart being not less than 2.0.

System repeatability: When the test is repeated 5 times with 10 μL of the standard solution under the above operating conditions, the relative standard deviation of A_S is not more than 1.5%.

Containers and storage Containers—Tight containers.

Storage—Not exceeding −18°C.

Insulin Glargine (Genetical Recombination)

インスリン　グラルギン(遺伝子組換え)

```
A chain
GIVEQCCTSI CSLYQLENYC G

B chain
FVNQHLCGSH LVEALYLVCG ERGFFYTPKT RR
```

$C_{267}H_{404}N_{72}O_{78}S_6$: 6062.89 (two chains)
A chain $C_{97}H_{150}N_{24}O_{34}S_4$: 2324.63
B chain $C_{170}H_{258}N_{48}O_{44}S_2$: 3742.29
[*160337-95-1*]

Insulin Glargine (Genetical Recombination) is a recombinant human insulin analogue, being substituted asparagine residue with glycine residue at 21st of A chain and added two arginine residues at C-terminal of B chain. It is a peptide composed with A chain consisting of 21 amino acid residues and B chain consisting of 32 amino acid residues.

It contains not less than 94.0% and not more than 105.0% of insulin glargine (genetical recombination) ($C_{267}H_{404}N_{72}O_{78}S_6$), calculated on the anhydrous basis.

0.0364 mg of Insulin Glargine (Genetical Recombination) is equivalent to 1 Insulin Unit.

Description Insulin Glargine (Genetical Recombination) occurs as a white powder.

It is practically insoluble in water and in ethanol (99.5).

It is sparingly soluble in 0.01 mol/L hydrochloric acid TS.

It is hygroscopic.

It is gradually decomposed by light.

Identification Keep the sample solution and standard solution at 2 - 8°C. Weigh a suitable amount of Insulin Glargine (Genetical Recombination) and Insulin Glargine RS, and dissolve separately in 0.01 mol/L hydrochloric acid TS so that each mL contains 10.0 mg. Transfer 5 μL of these solutions into clean test tubes, add 1 mL of 1 mol/L tris buffer solution (pH 7.5) and 100 μL of a solution of V8 protease for insulin glargine in 1 mol/L tris buffer solution (pH 7.5) (20 units/mL), allow to react at 35 - 37°C for 3 hours, then add 2 μL of phosphoric acid to stop the reaction, and use these solutions as the sample solution and the standard solution, respectively. Perform the test with exactly 50 μL each of the sample solution and standard solution as directed under Liquid Chromatography <*2.01*> according to the following conditions, and compare the chromatograms obtained from these solutions: The similar peaks appear at the same retention times.

Operating conditions—

Detector: An ultraviolet absorption photometer (wavelength: 214 nm).

Column: A stainless steel column 3 mm in inside diameter and 12.5 cm in length, packed with octadecylsilanized silica gel for liquid chromatography (4 μm in particle diameter).

Column temperature: A constant temperature of about 35°C.

Mobile phase A: To 930 mL of a solution, prepared by dissolving 11.6 g of phosphoric acid and 42.1 g of sodium perchloric acid in 1600 mL of water, adjusting to pH 2.3 with triethylamine and adding water to make 2000 mL, add 70 mL of acetonitrile for liquid chromatography.

Mobile phase B: To 430 mL of a solution, prepared by dissolving 11.6 g of phosphoric acid and 42.1 g of sodium perchloric acid in 1600 mL of water, adjusting to pH 2.3 with triethylamine and adding water to make 2000 mL, add 570 mL of acetonitrile for liquid chromatography.

Flowing of mobile phase: Control the gradient by mixing the mobile phases A and B as follows.

Time after injection of sample (min)	Mobile phase A (vol%)	Mobile phase B (vol%)
0 – 30	90 → 20	10 → 80
30 – 35	20	80

Flow rate: 0.55 mL per minute.

System suitability—

System performance: When the procedure is run with 50 μL of the standard solution under the above operating conditions, the symmetry factors of the two larger peaks, which appear next to the first peak just after the solvent peak, are not more than 1.5, respectively, and the resolution between these peaks is not less than 3.4.

Purity (1) Related substances—Perform the test with 5 μL of the sample solution obtained in the Assay as directed under Liquid Chromatography <*2.01*> according to the following conditions. Determine each peak area by the automatic integration method, and calculate the amount of these peaks by the area percentage method: the amount of the peak other than insulin glargine is not more than 0.4%, and the total amount of the peaks other than insulin glargine is not more than 1.0%.

Operating conditions—

Detector, column, column temperature, mobile phases A and B, flowing of mobile phase, and flow rate: Proceed as directed in the operating conditions in the Assay.

Time span of measurement: For 40 minutes after injection, beginning after the solvent peak.

System suitability—

Test for required detectability: Pipet 1 mL of the sample solution, add 0.01 mol/L hydrochloric acid TS to make exactly 100 mL, and use this solution as the solution for system suitability test. Pipet 1 mL of the solution for system suitability test, add 0.01 mol/L hydrochloric acid TS to make exactly 10 mL. Confirm that the peak area of insulin glargine obtained with 5 μL of this solution is equivalent to 5 to 15% of that with 5 μL of the solution for system suitability test.

System performance: When the procedure is run with 5 μL of the standard solution obtained in the Assay under the above operating conditions, the number of theoretical plates and the symmetry factor of the peak of insulin glargine are not less than 20,000 and not more than 1.8, respectively.

System repeatability: When the test is repeated 6 times with 5 μL of the standard solution obtained in the Assay under the above operating conditions, the relative standard deviation of the peak area of insulin glargine is not more than 2.0%.

(2) High-molecular mass proteins—Keep the sample solution at 2 - 8°C. Dissolve 15 mg of Insulin Glargine (Genetical Recombination) in 1.5 mL of 0.01 mol/L hydrochloric acid TS, add water to make 10 mL, and use this solution as the sample solution. Perform the test with 100 μL of the sample solution as directed under Liquid Chromatography <*2.01*> according to the following conditions. Determine each peak area by the automatic integration method, and calculate the amount of them by the area percentage method: the total amount of the peaks other than insulin glargine is not more than 0.3%.

Operating conditions—

Detector: An ultraviolet absorption photometer (wavelength: 276 nm).

Column: Two stainless steel columns connected in series of 8 mm in inside diameter and 30 cm in length, packed with hydrophilic silica gel for liquid chromatography (5 μm in particle diameter).

Column temperature: A constant temperature of about 25°C.

Mobile phase: To 400 mL of water add 300 mL of acetonitrile for liquid chromatography and 200 mL of acetic acid (100), adjust to pH 3.0 with ammonia solution (28), and add water to make 1000 mL.

Flow rate: Adjust so that the retention time of insulin glargine is about 35 minutes.

Time span of measurement: From the retention time corresponding to the exclusion volume of the size-exclusion

column to the completion of the elution of insulin glargine.
System suitability—

Test for required detectability: To 1 mL of the sample solution add 0.01 mol/L hydrochloric acid TS to make 50 mL, and use this solution as the solution for system suitability test. Pipet 1 mL of the solution for system suitability test, add 0.01 mol/L hydrochloric acid TS to make exactly 10 mL. Confirm that the peak area of insulin glargine obtained with 100 μL of this solution is equivalent to 5 to 15% of that with 100 μL of the solution for system suitability test.

System performance: Heat 15 mg of Insulin Glargine (Genetical Recombination) at 100°C for 1.5 - 3 hours, then dissolve in 1.5 mL of 0.01 mol/L hydrochloric acid TS, and add water to make exactly 10 mL. When the procedure is run with 100 μL of this solution under the above operating conditions, the high-molecular mass protein and insulin glargine are eluted in this order with the resolution between these peaks is not less than 1.5.

System repeatability: When the test is repeated 6 times with 100 μL of the solution for system suitability test under the above operating conditions, the relative standard deviation of the peak area of insulin glargine is not more than 2.0%.

(3) Other product-related impurities—Being specified separately when the drug is granted approval based on the Law.

(4) Host cell proteins—Being specified separately when the drug is granted approval based on the Law.

(5) Host cell DNA—Being specified separately when the drug is granted approval based on the Law.

Water <*2.48*> Not more than 8.0% (90 mg, coulometric titration).

Bacterial endotoxins <*4.01*> Less than 10 EU/mg.

Zinc content Weigh accurately about 45 mg of Insulin Glargine (Genetical Recombination), dissolve in 0.01 mol/L hydrochloric acid TS to make exactly 50 mL. Pipet 10 mL of this solution, add 0.01 mol/L hydrochloric acid TS to make exactly 100 mL, and use this solution as the sample solution. Separately, take exactly a suitable amount of Standard Zinc Solution for Atomic Absorption Spectrophotometry, dilute with 0.01 mol/L hydrochloric acid TS to make three solutions containing 0.20 μg, 0.40 μg and 0.60 μg of zinc (Zn: 65.38) in each mL, respectively, and use these solutions as the standard solutions. Perform the test with the sample solution and standard solutions as directed under Atomic Absorption Spectrophotometry <*2.23*> according to the following conditions, and calculate the amount of zinc in the sample solution using a calibration curve obtained from the absorbances of the standard solutions: not more than 0.80% of zinc (Zn: 65.38), calculated on the anhydrous basis.

Gas: Combustible gas—Acetylene.
Supporting gas—Air.

Lamp: Zinc hollow-cathode lamp.

Wavelength: 213.9 nm.

Assay Keep the sample solution and standard solution at 2 - 8°C. Weigh accurately about 15 mg of Insulin Glargine (Genetical Recombination), dissolve in 1.5 mL of 0.01 mol/L hydrochloric acid TS, add water to make exactly 10 mL, and use this solution as the sample solution. Separately, dissolve Insulin Glargine RS in 0.01 mol/L hydrochloric acid TS so that each mL contains about 10 mg of insulin glargine, then exactly dilute with water so that each mL contains about 1.5 mg of insulin glargine, and use this solution as the standard solution. Perform the test with exactly 5 μL each of the sample solution and standard solution as directed under Liquid Chromatography <*2.01*> according to the following conditions, and determine the peak areas, A_T and A_S, of insulin glargine in each solution.

$$\text{Amount (mg) of insulin glargine } (C_{267}H_{404}N_{72}O_{78}S_6) = M_S \times A_T/A_S$$

M_S: Amount (mg) of insulin glargine in 1 mL of the standard solution

Operating conditions—

Detector: An ultraviolet absorption photometer (wavelength: 214 nm).

Column: A stainless steel column 3 mm in inside diameter and 25 cm in length, packed with octadecylsilanized silica gel for liquid chromatography (4 μm in particle diameter).

Column temperature: A constant temperature of about 35°C.

Mobile phase A: Dissolve 20.7 g of anhydrous sodium dihydrogen phosphate in 900 mL of water, adjust to pH 2.5 with phosphoric acid, and add water to make 1000 mL. To 250 mL of this solution add 250 mL of acetonitrile for liquid chromatography, dissolve 18.4 g of sodium chloride in this solution, and add water to make 1000 mL.

Mobile phase B: Dissolve 20.7 g of anhydrous sodium dihydrogen phosphate in 900 mL of water, adjust to pH 2.5 with phosphoric acid, and add water to make 1000 mL. To 250 mL of this solution add 650 mL of acetonitrile for liquid chromatography, dissolve 3.2 g of sodium chloride in this solution, and add water to make 1000 mL.

Flowing of mobile phase: Control the gradient by mixing the mobile phases A and B as directed in the following table.

Time after injection of sample (min)	Mobile phase A (vol%)	Mobile phase B (vol%)
0 - 20	96 → 83	4 → 17
20 - 30	83 → 63	17 → 37
30 - 40	63 → 96	37 → 4

Flow rate: 0.55 mL per minute (the retention time of insulin glargine is about 21 minutes).

System suitability—

System performance: When the procedure is run with 5 μL of the standard solution under the above operating conditions, the number of theoretical plates and the symmetry factor of the peak of insulin glargine are not less than 20,000 and not more than 1.8, respectively.

System repeatability: When the test is repeated 6 times with 5 μL of the standard solution under the above operating conditions, the relative standard deviation of the peak area of insulin glargine is not more than 2.0%.

Containers and storage Containers—Tight containers.
Storage—Not exceeding −15°C.

Insulin Glargine (Genetical Recombination) Injection

インスリン　グラルギン(遺伝子組換え)注射液

Insulin Glargine (Genetical Recombination) Injection is an aqueous injection.

It contains not less than 95.0% and not more than 105.0% of the labeled Insulin Unit of insulin glargine (genetical recombination) ($C_{267}H_{404}N_{72}O_{78}S_6$: 6062.89).

Method of preparation Prepare as directed under Injections, with Insulin Glargine (Genetical Recombination).

Description Insulin Glargine (Genetical Recombination) Injection occurs as a clear, colorless liquid.

Identification **(1)** Insulin Glargine (Genetical Recombination) Injection forms a precipitate when adjusted to pH 5.7 – 6.5 with dilute sodium hydroxide TS, and the precipitate disappears when adjusted to pH 3.5 – 4.5 with 0.1 mol/L hydrochloric acid TS.

(2) Perform the test with 5 μL each of the sample solution and the standard solution obtained in the Assay as directed under Liquid Chromatography <*2.01*> according to the conditions described in the Assay: the retention times of the principal peaks obtained from the sample solution and standard solution are the same.

pH Being specified separately when the drug is granted approval based on the Law.

Purity **(1)** Related substances—Keep the sample solution at 2 – 8°C. Perform the test with 5 μL of the sample solution obtained in the Assay as directed under Liquid Chromatography <*2.01*> according to the following conditions. Determine each peak area by the automatic integration method, and calculate their amounts by the area percentage method: the amount of the peak other than insulin glargine is not more than 0.5%, and the total amount of the peaks other than insulin glargine is not more than 2.0%.

Operating conditions—

Detector, column, column temperature, mobile phases A and B, flowing of mobile phase, and flow rate: Proceed as directed in the operating conditions in the Assay under Insulin Glargine (Genetical Recombination).

Time span of measurement: For 40 minutes after injection, beginning after the solvent peak.

System suitability—

Test for required detectability: Pipet 1 mL of the sample solution, add 0.01 mol/L hydrochloric acid TS to make exactly 100 mL, and use this solution as the solution for system suitability test. Pipet 1 mL of the solution for system suitability test, and add 0.01 mol/L hydrochloric acid TS to make exactly 10 mL. Confirm that the peak area of insulin glargine obtained with 5 μL of this solution is equivalent to 5 to 15% of that with 5 μL of the solution for system suitability test.

System performance: When the procedure is run with 5 μL of the standard solution obtained in the Assay under the above operating conditions, the number of theoretical plates and the symmetry factor of the peak of insulin glargine are not less than 20,000 and not more than 1.8, respectively.

System repeatability: When the test is repeated 6 times with 5 μL of the standard solution obtained in the Assay under the above operating conditions, the relative standard deviation of the peak area of insulin glargine is not more than 2.0%.

(2) High-molecular mass proteins—To a suitable amount of Insulin Glargine (Genetical Recombination) Injection add water so that each mL contains 40 Insulin Units, and use this solution as the sample solution. Then, proceed as directed in the Purity (2) under Insulin Glargine (Genetical Recombination).

Extractable volume <*6.05*> It meets the requirement.

Foreign insoluble matter <*6.06*> Perform the test according to Method 1: it meets the requirement.

Insoluble particulate matter <*6.07*> It meets the requirement.

Sterility <*4.06*> Perform the test according to the Membrane filtration method: it meets the requirement.

Zinc content Being specified separately when the drug is granted approval based on the Law.

Assay To a suitable amount of Insulin Glargine (Genetical Recombination) Injection add exactly water so that each mL contains 40 Insulin Units, and use this solution as the sample solution. Then, proceed as directed in the Assay under Insulin Glargine (Genetical Recombination).

Amount (Insulin Unit) of insulin glargine ($C_{267}H_{404}N_{72}O_{78}S_6$) in 1 mL

$= M_S \times A_T/A_S \times d \times 1/0.0364$

M_S: Amount (mg) of insulin glargine in 1 mL of the standard solution

d: Dilution factor of the sample solution

0.0364: Mass (mg) of insulin glargine equivalent to 1 Insulin Unit

Containers and storage Containers—Hermetic containers.

Storage—Light-resistant, at a temperature of 2 – 8°C avoiding freezing.

Interferon Alfa (NAMALWA)

インターフェロン　アルファ(NAMALWA)

Interferon Alfa (NAMALWA) is essentially a human interferon alfa, which is a glycoprotein (molecular mass: 17,000 – 30,000) produced by the human lymphoblast NAMALWA cell induced by Sendai virus. It is an aqueous solution. It possesses the antiviral activity.

It contains not less than 50 μg and not more than 500 μg of protein per mL, and not less than 1.0×10^8 Units per mg of the protein.

Description Interferon Alfa (NAMALWA) occurs as a clear and colorless liquid.

Identification **(1)** To Interferon Alfa (NAMALWA) add Eagle's minimum essential medium containing bovine serum so that each mL contains 5000 Units, and use this solution as the sample stock solution. To anti-interferon alfa antiserum add an amount of Eagle's minimum essential medium containing bovine serum so that each mL contains an amount of anti-interferon alfa antiserum which neutralizes 10,000 Units of interferon alfa. To this solution add an equal volume of the sample stock solution, stir, and use this solution as the sample solution. Separately, to the sample stock solution add an equal volume of Eagle's minimum essential medium containing bovine serum, stir, and use this solution as the control solution. Determine the remained potency of the sample solution and control solution after allowing to stand at 37 ± 1°C for 1 hour, according to the Assay. When the antiviral activity of Interferon Alfa (NAMALWA) is neutralized by anti-interferon alfa antiserum, it meets the requirement. Not detection of the remaining potency of the sample solution is a criterion of neutralization.

(2) Soak polyvinylidene fluoride membrane in methanol for 10 – 20 seconds, then soak additionally in phosphate-buffered sodium chloride TS for more than 30 minutes. To the well in the dot blot apparatus mounted the polyvinylidene fluoride membrane, add a volume of Interferon Alfa (NAMALWA), corresponding to about 20 μg protein, allow to stand for 15 minutes, and aspirate. After repeating twice to aspirate with a 0.2-mL portion of phosphate-buffered sodium chloride TS, take out the polyvinylidene fluoride membrane, soak in 0.01 mol/L tris buffer solution-sodium chloride TS (pH 7.4), and stir gently for 10 minutes. Replace the liquid, and repeat this operation two more times. Remove 0.01 mol/L tris buffer solution-sodium chloride TS (pH 7.4), add elderberry lectin TS, and stir gently for 2 hours. Remove the elderberry lectin TS, add 0.01 mol/L tris buffer solution-sodium chloride TS (pH 7.4), and stir gently for 10 minutes. Replace the liquid, and repeat this operation two more times. Remove 0.01 mol/L tris buffer solution-sodium chloride TS (pH 7.4), add the peroxidase-labeled avidin TS, and stir gently for 15 minutes. Remove the peroxidase-labeled avidin TS, add 0.01 mol/L tris buffer solution-sodium chloride TS (pH 7.4), and stir gently for 10 minutes. Replace the liquid, and repeat this operation two more times. Remove 0.01 mol/L tris buffer solution-sodium chloride TS (pH 7.4), add substrate TS for interferon alfa identification, and allow to develop the color: a brown dot is observed.

Constituent amino acids When perform the test by Method 2 of 2. Methodologies of Amino Acid Analysis after hydrolyzing by Method 1 (but not containing phenol) of 1. Hydrolysis of Protein and Peptide under Amino Acid Analysis of Proteins <*2.04*>, the molar ratios of each constituent amino acid are 8 – 11 for aspartic acid, 4 – 7 for threonine, 7 – 10 for serine, 16 – 19 for glutamic acid, 2 – 4 for glycine and tyrosine, 5 – 7 for alanine, phenylalanine and lysine, 3 – 6 for valine, 2 – 5 for methionine, 4 – 6 for isoleucine, 12 – 15 for leucine, 1 – 3 for histidine and 6 – 9 for arginine.

(i) Hydrolysis—To Interferon Alfa (NAMALWA) add tris-glycine buffer solution (pH 6.8) so that each mL contains 6,000,000 Units. Pass 3 mL of the solution through a column 4 mm in internal diameter, packed with 0.145 g of ethylsilanized silica gel for column chromatography and previously washed with 5 mL of a mixture of water, acetonitrile and diluted trifluoroacetic acid (1 in 50) (13:6:1). Then, after washing with not less than 10 mL of a mixture of water, acetonitrile and diluted trifluoroacetic acid (1 in 50) (13:6:1), elute interferon alfa with 0.5 mL of a mixture of acetonitrile and diluted trifluoroacetic acid (1 in 50) (19:1), and use the eluate as the sample stock solution. To 0.45 mL of the sample stock solution add 50 μL of the internal standard solution, and stir. Transfer 0.1 mL each of this solution into two glass vessels for hydrolysis, and evaporate to dryness under reduced pressure. Add 20 μL of a solution which is prepared by adding 10 μL of mercapto acetic acid to 1 mL of 6 mol/L hydrochloric acid TS for amino acid automatic analysis, and 0.18 mL of 6 mol/L hydrochloric acid TS for amino acid automatic analysis to the bottom of the glass vessels, replace the air in the vessels with nitrogen, close the vessels tightly under reduced pressure, and heat at 110 ± 2°C for 24 hours for one of the vessels and for 72 hours for another. After cooling, open the vessels, evaporate the hydrolyzate to dryness under reduced pressure, dissolve the residue in 20 μL of water, and evaporate to dryness under reduced pressure. Dissolve the residues with 0.1 mL each of diluted 6 mol/L hydrochloric acid TS for amino acid automatic analysis (31 in 10,000), and use these solutions as the sample solutions (1) and (2), respectively. Separately, weigh exactly a suitable amount each of L-lysine hydrochloride, L-histidine hydrochloride monohydrate, L-arginine, L-aspartic acid, L-threonine, L-serine, L-glutamic acid, glycine, L-alanine, L-valine, L-methionine, L-isoleucine, L-leucine, L-tyrosine, L-phenylalanine and L-norleucine, dissolve in diluted 6 mol/L hydrochloric acid TS for amino acid automatic analysis (31 in 10,000) so that each mL contains a certain concentration of about 20 nmol for each amino acid, and use this solution as the standard solution.

(ii) Amino acid analysis—When perform the test with 15 μL each of the sample solutions (1) and (2) and 10 μL of the standard solution as directed under Liquid Chromatography <*2.01*> according to the following conditions, either chromatogram obtained from the sample solutions shows the peaks corresponding to the peaks obtained from the standard solution. The molar ratios of each constituent amino acids are calculated. When calculate the molar ratios of each constituent amino acid, for threonine and serine the molar value is corrected by extrapolation to 0 hour-heating based on the values obtained from the sample solutions (1) and (2), for isoleucine and valine use the value from the sample solution (2), and for the other amino acids use the value from the sample solution (1). The molar ratios of cystine, proline and tryptophan are excluded from calculation.

Internal standard solution—To exactly 32.81 mg of L-norleucine add diluted 6 mol/L hydrochloric acid TS for amino acid automatic analysis (31 in 10,000) to make exactly 100 mL. Pipet 4 mL of this solution, add diluted 6 mol/L hydrochloric acid TS for amino acid automatic analysis (31 in 10,000) to make exactly 100 mL.

Operating conditions—

Detector: A fluorophotometer (excitation wavelength: 340 nm, fluorescence wavelength: 450 nm).

Column: A stainless steel column 5 mm in inside diameter and 8 cm in length, packed with strongly acidic ion-exchange resin (Na type) for liquid chromatography composed with a sulfonated styrene-divinylbenzene copolymer (3 μm in particle diameter).

Column temperature: Inject the sample at 50 ± 1°C, maintain the temperature for 11 minutes, change to 40 ± 1°C and maintain for 23 minutes, then change to 65 ± 1°C and maintain for 56 minutes, and change to 45 ± 1°C.

Reaction vessel temperature: A constant temperature of about 51°C.

Mobile phase: Prepare the mobile phases A, B, C and D according to the following table.

	Mobile phase A	Mobile phase B	Mobile phase C	Mobile phase D
Citric acid monohydrate	15.93 g	8.40 g	6.10 g	—
Sodium citrate hydrate	6.97 g	10.00 g	26.67 g	—
Sodium chloride	6.36 g	2.34 g	54.35 g	—
Sodium hydroxide	—	—	2.0 g	8.0 g
Ethanol (99.5)	54 mL	—	—	—
Lauromacrogol solution (1 in 4)	4 mL	4 mL	4 mL	4 mL
Benzyl alcohol	—	2 mL	5 mL	—
Caprylic acid	0.1 mL	0.1 mL	0.1 mL	0.1 mL
Water	a suitable quantity	a suitable quantity	a suitable quantity	a suitable quantity
Total amount	1000 mL	1000 mL	1000 mL	1000 mL

Flowing of mobile phase: Control the gradient by mixing the mobile phases A, B, C and D as directed in the following table.

Time after injection of sample (min)	Mobile phase A (vol%)	Mobile phase B (vol%)	Mobile phase C (vol%)	Mobile phase D (vol%)
0 – 11	100	0	0	0
11 – 12	100 → 0	0 → 100	0	0
12 – 34	0	100	0	0
34 – 39.1	0	100 → 0	0 → 100	0
39.1 – 71	0	0	100	0
71 – 86	0	0	0	100

Reaction reagent: Prepare the reaction reagents A, B and C according to the following table.

	Reaction reagent A	Reaction reagent B	Reaction reagent C
Sodium hydroxide	24.0 g	—	—
Boric acid	—	21.60 g	21.60 g
o-Phthalaldehyde in ethanol (99.5) solution (2 in 25)	—	—	10 mL
Lauromacrogol solution (1 in 4)	—	—	4 mL
2-Mercaptoethanol	—	—	2 mL
10% Sodium hypochlorite TS	—	0.1 mL	—
Water	a suitable quantity	a suitable quantity	a suitable quantity
Total amount	1000 mL	1000 mL	1000 mL

Flow rate of mobile phase: Adjust so that the retention times of aspartic acid, glutamic acid and methionine are about 12, 20 and 42 minutes, respectively.

Flow rate of reaction reagent: About 0.2 mL per minute for each of reagent A, B, and C.

System suitability—

System performance: When the procedure is run with 10 μL of the standard solution under the above operating conditions, the resolutions between the peaks of threonine and serine, glycine and alanine, and isoleucine and leucine are not less than 0.6, not less than 0.8 and not less than 1.2, respectively.

System repeatability: When the test is repeated 3 times with 10 μL of the standard solution under the above operating conditions, the relative standard deviations of the peak area of aspartic acid, proline, valine, and arginine are not more than 2.5%, respectively.

Molecular mass To a suitable amount of Interferon Alfa (NAMALWA) add tris-glycine buffer solution (pH 6.8) so that each mL contains 6,000,000 Units. To 3 volumes of this solution add 1 volume of reduction liquid for molecular mass determination, heat on a water bath for 90 seconds, and use this solution as the sample solution. Separately, to 3 volumes of molecular mass marker for interferon alfa add 1 volume of reduction liquid for molecular mass determination, heat on a water bath for 90 seconds, and use this solution as the standard solution. After performing the electrophoresis with 40 μL of the sample solution and 15 μL of the standard solution using tris buffer solution (pH 8.3) and polyacrylamide gel for interferon alfa, fix the gel by immersing for 1 hour in a solution of trichloroacetic acid (3 in 20). Then, stain the gel by immersing for more than 2 hours in a solution, prepared by dissolving 1.0 g of Coomassie brilliant blue R-250 in 450 mL of methanol and 100 mL of acetic acid (100) and adding water to make 1000 mL, and destain by immersing the gel in 1000 mL of a mixture of water, methanol and acetic acid (100) (33:4:3). Determine the relative mobility of each band obtained from the standard solution, and prepare a calibration curve by linear regression against the logarithm of molecular mass. Determine the relative mobility of the center of the main band obtained from the sample solution, and calculate the molecular mass of Interferon Alfa (NAMALWA) from the calibration curve: at least 4 bands are observed between 17,000 and 30,000 of molecular mass.

Purity **(1)** Egg albumin, Sendai virus coat protein, other foreign proteins, and other process-related impurities—Being specified separately when the drug is granted approval based on the Law.

(2) Nucleic acids—Perform the test according to the following method: the amount of nucleic acids is not more than 1.0 pg as DNA per 1,000,000 Units of interferon alfa (NAMALWA).

(i) DNA standard solutions: To the DNA standard stock solution for interferon alfa (NAMALWA) add salmon sperm DNA solution (1 in 10,000,000) so that each mL contains exactly 20 ng DNA. Hereinafter, the concentration of DNA is the concentration of DNA for interferon alfa (NAMALWA). To this solution add tris-glycine buffer solution (pH 6.8) exactly so that each mL contains 10 ng DNA. Then, dilute serially by adding tris-glycine buffer solution (pH 6.8). Dilute exactly with a mixture of tris-glycine buffer solution (pH 6.8) and 1 mol/L tris buffer solution (pH 8.0) (40:1) so that each mL contains 128, 64, 32, 16, 8, and 4 pg of DNA, respectively, and use these solutions as DNA standard solutions.

(ii) Procedure: Use Interferon Alfa (NAMALWA) as the sample solution. Place 0.11 mL each of DNA standard solutions, a mixture of tris-glycine buffer solution (pH 6.8) and 1 mol/L tris buffer solution (pH 8.0) (43:1), and the sample solution into tubes separately. Heat these solutions in an aluminum block thermostat bath at 98°C for 10 minutes. After ice-cooling, centrifuge, and transfer 50 μL each of the supernatants to new tubes. In separate wells of a PCR microplate place 6 μL each of DNA standard solutions which have been treated by heating for DNA extraction, a mixture of tris-glycine buffer solution (pH 6.8) and 1 mol/L tris buffer solution (pH 8.0) (43:1), and the sample solution. Then, add 20 μL each of a mixture of 2-fold PCR reaction solution containing SYBR Green, nuclease free water, primer F TS and primer R TS (167:70:10:10) into each well. Seal with plate film, and centrifuge. After centrifugation, attach the plate to a real-time PCR system, repeat 40 cycles of 15 seconds at 95°C and 1 minute at 60°C, and measure the fluorescence intensity of each well in every PCR cycle. Plot the fluorescent amount on the vertical axis and the PCR cycle number on the horizontal axis, and determine the PCR cycle number at which the fluorescence of each well is greater than a certain value. Further, make a calibration curve by plotting the number of PCR cycles on the vertical axis and the logarithm of the concentration of DNA standard solution on the horizontal axis to calculate the concentration of DNA in the sample solution.

System suitability—

Test for required detectability: The PCR cycle number obtained with 4 pg/mL DNA standard solution is not greater than that obtained with a mixture of tris-glycine buffer solution (pH 6.8) and tris buffer solution (pH 8.0) (43:1).

System performance: When the procedure is run with each DNA standard solution under the above conditions, the correlation coefficient of the calibration curve obtained is 0.990 or more.

(3) Infective virus test—Inject 0.2 mL each of Interferon Alfa (NAMALWA) into the allantoic cavity of not less than 6 embryonated eggs, allow them to stand at 36 ± 1°C for 3 days, and then allow to stand at 4°C for a night. Collect more than 1 mL of the allantoic fluid from each egg. To 50 μL of the allantoic fluid add 50 μL of 0.5 vol% chicken erythrocyte suspension, mix, and allow to stand at room temperature for 1 hour. Examine the presence of the aggregation. When the aggregation is not found, inject 0.2 mL each of this allantoic fluid into the allantoic cavity of the embryonated eggs, and repeat the same procedure as above: the test is met when the aggregation is not found. As a positive control, inoculate the Sendai virus 1.6×10^{-4} to 6.4×10^{-4} HA value per embryonated chicken egg into the allantoic cavity, and perform the test at the same time.

Assay (1) Protein content—

(i) Sample solution: Dilute Interferon Alfa (NAMALWA) with isotonic sodium chloride solution so that each mL contains 3,000,000 to 4,000,000 Units, and use this solution as the sample solution.

(ii) Standard solution: Weigh accurately about 50 mg of bovine serum albumin, and dissolve in isotonic sodium chloride solution to make exactly 50 mL. Determine the absorbance of this solution at 280 nm as directed under Ultraviolet-visible Spectrophotometry <*2.24*>. Calculate the protein concentration based on $E^{1\%}_{1\,\mathrm{cm}}$ (280 nm) = 6.6. To this solution add isotonic sodium chloride solution so that each mL contains exactly 50, 25, 12.5, 6.25, and 3.13 μg of the bovine serum albumin, and use these solutions as the standard solutions.

(iii) Procedure: To exactly 0.25 mL each of the sample solution and the standard solutions add exactly 0.25 mL of Coomassie brilliant blue TS for interferon alfa, and allow to stand at room temperature for exactly 30 seconds. Determine the absorbance of these solutions at 614 nm as directed under Ultraviolet-visible Spectrophotometry <*2.24*> using water as the blank. Plot the absorbance of the standard solutions on the vertical axis and their protein concentrations on the horizontal axis to prepare a calibration curve. Determine the protein content of the sample solution from its absorbance using the calibration curve, and calculate the amount of protein per mL of the sample solution. Perform a blank determination in the same manner with isotonic sodium chloride solution, and make any necessary correction.

(2) Specific activity—To each well of a flat-bottom microplate add 45,000 to 60,000 cells of FL cell, prepared with Eagle's minimum essential medium containing bovine serum, and incubate at 37 ± 1°C for 18 to 22 hours in an incubator filled with 5% carbon dioxide. Dilute Interferon Alfa (NAMALWA) and Interferon Alfa RS separately with Eagle's minimum essential medium containing bovine serum so that each mL contains about 30 Units, and use these solutions as the sample solution (1) and the standard solution (1), respectively. To 200 μL each of these solutions add 117 μL of Eagle's minimum essential medium containing bovine serum, and use these solutions as the sample solution (2) and the standard solution (2), respectively. Repeat this operation, and prepare the sample solutions and standard solutions with log dilutions of 8 serials (dilution ratio per stage is 0.2 $\log_{10}$ fold). Repeat to prepare the sample solutions three or more times. Add each sample solution or standard solution into each well of the cell culture, and incubate at 37 ± 1°C for 6 hours. Discard the culture medium, add 1×10^5 to 1×10^6 PFU of Sindbis virus per well, and incubate at 37 ± 1°C for 38 to 42 hours. Discard the culture medium, add neutral red-Eagle's minimum essential medium containing bovine serum, and incubate at 37 ± 1°C for 45 to 75 minutes. Discard the culture medium, and add 0.01 mol/L phosphate buffer solution. Discard the liquid. Repeat this operation. Elute the neutral red that is taken up by the cells by adding sodium dihydrogen phosphate-ethanol TS. Determine the absorbance at 540 nm, prepare the dose-response curves by plotting the absorbances on the vertical axis and the logarithm of the dilution ratio on the horizontal axis with the absorbances obtained from the sample solution and standard solution. On the dose-response curves of the sample solution and standard solution, calculate the relative potency of the sample solution (n = 3 or more), obtained independently, to the standard solution by comparing the points where the intermediate of absorbances in cells infected with virus and cells not infected with virus, and calculate the average value of them as the potency of Interferon Alfa (NAMALWA) in 1 mL. Calculate the specific activity by dividing the obtained potency by the amount of protein content.

When all of the following conditions are satisfied, the test is valid.

Absorbance obtained from cells not infected with virus is 0.8 to 1.2.

Absorbance obtained from the cells infected with virus is not more than 0.1.

Standard deviation of the (log) potency of Interferon Alfa (NAMALWA) in 1 mL obtained from the sample solution prepared three or more times independently is not more than 0.06.

Containers and storage Containers—Tight containers.

Storage—Light-resistant, and at a temperature not exceeding 5°C, avoiding freezing.

Interferon Alfa (NAMALWA) Injection

インターフェロン　アルファ(NAMALWA)注射液

Interferon Alfa (NAMALWA) Injection is an aqueous injection.

It contains not less than 70% and not more than 150% of the labelled amount of interferon alfa (NAMALWA).

Method of preparation Prepare as directed under Injections, with Interferon Alfa (NAMALWA).

Description Interferon Alfa (NAMALWA) Injection is a clear and colorless liquid.

Identification To Interferon Alfa (NAMALWA) Injection add Eagle's minimum essential medium containing bovine serum so that each mL contains 5000 Units, and use this solution as the sample stock solution. To anti-interferon alfa antiserum add an amount of Eagle's minimum essential medium containing bovine serum so that each mL contains an amount of anti-interferon alfa antiserum which neutralizes 10,000 Units of interferon alfa. To this solution add an equal volume of the sample stock solution, stir, and use this solution as the sample solution. Separately, to the sample stock solution add an equal volume of Eagle's minimum essential medium containing bovine serum, stir, and use this solution as the control solution. Determine the remained potency of the sample solution and control solution after allowing to stand at 37 ± 1°C for 1 hour, according to the Assay. When neutralized the antiviral activity of Interferon Alfa (NAMALWA) by anti-interferon alfa antiserum, it meets the requirement. Not detection of the remaining potency of the sample solution is the criterion of neutralization.

Osmotic pressure ratio Being specified separately when the drug is granted approval based on the Law.

pH Being specified separately when the drug is granted approval based on the Law.

Purity Multimers—To a suitable amount of Interferon Alfa (NAMALWA) Injection add tris-glycine buffer solution (pH 6.8) so that each mL contains 3,000,000 Units, and use this as the sample solution. Perform the test with 200 μL of the sample solution as directed under Liquid Chromatography <*2.01*> according to the following conditions. Determine each peak area by the automatic integration method, and calculate their amounts by the area percentage method: the total amount of the peaks, having the retention time smaller than that of interferon alfa monomer, is not more than 3.0%.

Operating conditions—

Detector: An ultraviolet absorption photometer (wavelength: 220 nm).

Column: A glass column 10 mm in inside diameter and 30 cm in length, packed with dextran-highly cross-linked agarose gel filtration carrier for liquid chromatography.

Column temperature: A constant temperature of about 25°C.

Mobile phase: Dissolve 1.15 g of anhydrous disodium hydrogen phosphate, 0.2 g of potassium dihydrogen phosphate, 8.0 g of sodium chloride and 0.2 g of potassium chloride in water to make 1000 mL. To 950 mL of this solution add 50 mL of a solution prepared by dissolving 10 g of sodium lauryl sulfate in 100 mL of water, and mix gently.

Flow rate: 1 mL per minute.

Time span of measurement: Until the elution of interferon alfa monomer is completed.

System suitability—

Test for required detectability: Pipet 50 μL of the sample solution, add tris-glycine buffer solution (pH 6.8) to make exactly 2 mL. Confirm that the peak area of the main peak obtained with 200 μL of this solution is equivalent to 2.0 to 3.0% of that with 200 μL of the sample solution.

System performance: Dissolve 15 mg of egg albumin for gel filtration molecular mass marker and 15 mg of ribonuclease A for gel filtration molecular mass marker in 100 mL of tris-glycine buffer solution (pH 6.8). When the procedure is run with 20 μL of this solution under the above conditions, egg albumin and ribonuclease A are eluted in this order with the resolution between these peaks being not less than 2.0.

System repeatability: When the test is repeated 6 times with 200 μL of the sample solution under the above operating conditions, the relative standard deviation of the area of the main peak is not more than 2.0%.

Bacterial endotoxins <*4.01*> Less than 0.25 EU per 600,000 Units.

Extractable volume <*6.05*> It meets the requirement.

Foreign insoluble matter <*6.06*> Perform the test according to Method1: it meets the requirement.

Insoluble particulate matter <*6.07*> It meets the requirement.

Sterility <*4.06*> Perform the test according to the Membrane filtration method: it meets the requirement.

Assay To each well of a flat-bottom microplate add 45,000 to 60,000 cells of FL cell, prepared with Eagle's minimum essential medium containing bovine serum, and incubate at 37 ± 1°C for 18 to 22 hours in an incubator filled with 5% carbon dioxide. Dilute Interferon Alfa (NAMALWA) Injection and Interferon Alfa RS separately with Eagle's minimum essential medium containing bovine serum so that each mL contains about 30 Units, and use these solutions as the sample solution (1) and the standard solution (1), respectively. To 200 μL each of these solutions add 117 μL of Eagle's minimum essential medium containing bovine serum, and use these solutions as the sample solution (2) and the standard solution (2), respectively. Repeat this operation, and prepare the sample solutions and standard solutions with logarithm dilutions of 8 serials (dilution ratio per stage is 0.2 $\log_{10}$ fold). Repeat to prepare the sample solutions three or more times. Add each sample solution or each standard solution into each well of the cell culture, and incubate at 37 ± 1°C for 6 hours. Discard the culture medium, add 1×10^5 to 1×10^6 PFU of Sindbis virus per well, and incubate at 37 ± 1°C for 38 to 42 hours. Discard the culture medium, add neutral red-Eagle's minimum essential medium containing bovine serum, and incubate at 37 ± 1°C for 45 to 75 minutes. Discard the culture medium, and add 0.01 mol/L phosphate buffer solution. Discard the liquid. Repeat this operation. Elute the neutral red that is taken up by the cells by adding sodium dihydrogen phosphate-ethanol TS. Determine the absorbance at 540 nm, prepare the dose-response curves by plotting the absorbances on the vertical axis and the logarithm of the dilution ratio on the horizontal axis with the absorbances obtained from the sample solution and standard solution. On the dose-response curves of the sample solution and standard solution, calculate the relative potency of the sample solution (n = 3 or more), prepared independently, to the standard solution by comparing the points where the intermediate of absorbances in cells infected with virus and cells not infected with virus, and calculate the average value of them as the potency of Interferon Alfa (NAMALWA) in 1 mL.

When all of the following conditions are satisfied, the test is valid.

Absorbance obtained from cells not infected with virus is 0.8 to 1.2.

Absorbance obtained from the cells infected with virus is not more than 0.1.

Standard deviation of the (log) potency of Interferon Alfa (NAMALWA) Injection in 1 mL obtained from the sample solution prepared three or more times independently is not more than 0.06.

Containers and storage Containers—Hermetic containers.

Storage—Light-resistant, and at a temperature not exceeding 10°C, avoiding freezing.

Iodinated (^{131}I) Human Serum Albumin Injection

ヨウ化人血清アルブミン (^{131}I) 注射液

Iodinated (^{131}I) Human Serum Albumin Injection is an aqueous injection containing normal human serum albumin iodinated by iodine-131 (^{131}I).

It conforms to the requirements of Iodinated (^{131}I) Human Serum Albumin Injection in the Minimum Requirements for Radiopharmaceuticals.

Test for Extractable Volume of Parenteral Preparations and Insoluble Particulate Matter Test for Injections are not applied to this injection.

Description Iodinated (^{131}I) Human Serum Albumin Injection is a clear, colorless or light yellow liquid.

Iodine

ヨウ素

I: 126.90

Iodine contains not less than 99.5% of iodine (I).

Description Iodine occurs as grayish black, plates or granular, heavy crystals, having a metallic luster and a characteristic odor.

It is freely soluble in diethyl ether, soluble in ethanol (95), sparingly soluble in chloroform, and very slightly soluble in water.

It dissolves in potassium iodide TS.

It sublimes at room temperature.

Identification **(1)** A solution of Iodine in ethanol (95) (1 in 50) shows a red-brown color.

(2) A solution of Iodine in chloroform (1 in 1000) shows a red-purple to purple color.

(3) Add 0.5 mL of starch TS to 10 mL of a saturated solution of Iodine: a dark blue color is produced. When the mixture is boiled, the color disappears, and it reappears on cooling.

Purity **(1)** Non-volatile residue—Sublime 2.0 g of Iodine on a water bath, and dry the residue at 105°C for 1 hour: the mass of the residue is not more than 1.0 mg.

(2) Chloride or bromide—Mix 1.0 g of finely powdered Iodine with 20 mL of water, and filter the mixture. To 10 mL of the filtrate add dropwise diluted sulfurous acid solution (1 in 5) until the yellow color disappears. Add 1 mL of ammonia TS, followed by 1 mL of silver nitrate TS in small portions, and add water to make 20 mL. Shake well, filter, and after discarding the first 2 mL of the filtrate, take 10 mL of the subsequent filtrate. To the filtrate add 2.0 mL of nitric acid and water to make 20 mL: the solution so obtained has no more turbidity than the following control solution.

Control solution: To 0.20 mL of 0.01 mol/L hydrochloric acid VS add 5 mL of water, 2.5 mL of ammonia TS, 1 mL of silver nitrate TS, 2.0 mL of nitric acid and water to make 20 mL.

Assay Place 1 g of potassium iodide and 1 mL of water in a glass-stoppered flask, weigh accurately, add about 0.3 g of Iodine to the flask, and weigh accurately again. Dissolve the iodine by gentle shaking, add 20 mL of water and 1 mL of dilute hydrochloric acid, and titrate <*2.50*> with 0.1 mol/L sodium thiosulfate VS (indicator: 1 mL of starch TS).

Each mL of 0.1 mol/L sodium thiosulfate VS
= 12.69 mg of I

Containers and storage Containers—Tight containers.

Iodine Tincture

ヨードチンキ

Iodine Tincture contains not less than 5.7 w/v% and not more than 6.3 w/v% of iodine (I: 126.90), and not less than 3.8 w/v% and not more than 4.2 w/v% of potassium iodide (KI: 166.00).

Method of preparation

Iodine	60 g
Potassium Iodide	40 g
70 vol% Ethanol	a sufficient quantity
To make	1000 mL

Prepare as directed under Spirits, with the above ingredients. It may be prepared with an appropriate quantity of Ethanol or Ethanol for Disinfection and Purified Water or Purified Water in Containers in place of 70 vol% Ethanol.

Description Iodine Tincture is a dark red-brown liquid, and has a characteristic odor.

Specific gravity d^{20}_{20}: about 0.97

Identification **(1)** To a mixture of 1 mL of starch TS and 9 mL of water add 1 drop of Iodine Tincture: a dark blue-purple color develops.

(2) Evaporate 3 mL of Iodine Tincture to dryness on a water bath, and heat gently over a free flame: a white residue is formed which responds to Qualitative Tests <*1.09*> for potassium salt and iodide.

Alcohol number <*1.01*> Not less than 6.6 (Method 2). Perform the pretreatment (ii) in the Method 1.

Assay **(1)** Iodine—Pipet 5 mL of Iodine Tincture, add 0.5 g of potassium iodide, 20 mL of water and 1 mL of dilute hydrochloric acid, and titrate <*2.50*> with 0.1 mol/L sodium thiosulfate VS (indicator: 2 mL of starch TS).

Each mL of 0.1 mol/L sodium thiosulfate VS
= 12.69 mg of I

(2) Potassium iodide—Pipet 5 mL of Iodine Tincture into an iodine flask, add 20 mL of water, 50 mL of hydrochloric acid and 5 mL of chloroform. Cool to room temperature, and titrate <*2.50*> with 0.05 mol/L potassium iodate VS until the red-purple color disappears from the chloroform layer, with agitating the mixture vigorously and continuously. After the chloroform layer has been decolorized, allow the mixture to stand for 5 minutes. If the color reappears, the mixture should be titrated <*2.50*> further with 0.05 mol/L potassium iodate VS. Calculate the amount (mg) of potassium iodide from the number of mL (*a*) of 0.05 mol/L potassium iodate VS used as above and the number of mL (*b*) of 0.1 mol/L sodium thiosulfate VS used in the titration under the Assay (1).

$$\text{Amount (mg) of potassium iodide (KI)} = 16.60 \times \{a - (b/2)\}$$

Containers and storage Containers—Tight containers.

Dilute Iodine Tincture

希ヨードチンキ

Dilute Iodine Tincture contains not less than 2.8 w/v% and not more than 3.2 w/v% of iodine (I: 126.90), and not less than 1.9 w/v% and not more than 2.1 w/v% of potassium iodide (KI: 166.00).

Method of preparation

Iodine	30 g
Potassium Iodide	20 g
70 vol% Ethanol	a sufficient quantity
To make	1000 mL

Prepare as directed under Spirits, with the above ingredients. It may be prepared with an appropriate quantity of Ethanol or Ethanol for Disinfection and Purified Water or Purified Water in Containers in place of 70 vol% Ethanol. It may also be prepared by adding 70 vol% Ethanol to 500 mL of Iodine Tincture to make 1000 mL.

Description Dilute Iodine Tincture is a dark red-brown liquid, and has a characteristic odor.

Specific gravity d_{20}^{20}: about 0.93

Identification **(1)** To a mixture of 1 mL of starch TS and 9 mL of water add 1 drop of Dilute Iodine Tincture: a dark blue-purple color develops.

(2) Evaporate 3 mL of Diluted Iodine Tincture to dryness on a water bath, and heat gently over a free flame: a white residue is formed which responds to the Qualitative Tests <*1.09*> for potassium salt and iodide.

Alcohol number <*1.01*> Not less than 6.7 (Method 2). Perform the pretreatment (ii) in the Method 1.

Assay **(1)** Iodine—Pipet exactly 10 mL of Dilute Iodine Tincture, add 0.5 g of potassium iodide, 20 mL of water and 1 mL of dilute hydrochloric acid, and titrate <*2.50*> with 0.1 mol/L sodium thiosulfate VS (indicator: 2 mL of starch TS).

Each mL of 0.1 mol/L sodium thiosulfate VS
= 12.69 mg of I

(2) Potassium iodide—Pipet 10 mL of Dilute Iodine Tincture into an iodine flask, add 20 mL of water, 50 mL of hydrochloric acid and 5 mL of chloroform. Cool to room temperature, and titrate <*2.50*> with 0.05 mol/L potassium iodate VS until the red-purple color in the chloroform layer disappears while agitating vigorously and continuously. After the chloroform layer has been decolorized, allow the mixture to stand for 5 minutes. If the color reappears, the mixture should be titrated <*2.50*> further with 0.05 mol/L potassium iodate VS. Calculate the amount (mg) of potassium iodide from the volume (a mL) of 0.05 mol/L potassium iodate VS consumed as above and the volume (b mL) of 0.1 mol/L sodium thiosulfate VS consumed in the titration under Assay (1).

Amount (mg) of potassium iodide (KI)
$= 16.60 \times \{a - (b/2)\}$

Containers and storage Containers—Tight containers.

Compound Iodine Glycerin

複方ヨード・グリセリン

Compound Iodine Glycerin contains not less than 1.1 w/v% and not more than 1.3 w/v% of iodine (I: 126.90), not less than 2.2 w/v% and not more than 2.6 w/v% of potassium iodide (KI: 166.00), not less than 2.7 w/v% and not more than 3.3 w/v% of total iodine (as I), and not less than 0.43 w/v% and not more than 0.53 w/v% of phenol (C_6H_6O: 94.11).

Method of preparation

Iodine	12 g
Potassium Iodide	24 g
Glycerin	900 mL
Mentha Water	45 mL
Liquefied Phenol	5 mL
Purified Water or Purified Water in Containers	a sufficient quantity
To make	1000 mL

Dissolve Potassium Iodide and Iodine in about 25 mL of Purified Water or Purified Water in Containers. After adding Glycerin, add Mentha Water, Liquefied Phenol and sufficient Purified Water or Purified Water in Containers to make 1000 mL, mixing thoroughly. It may be prepared with an appropriate quantity of Concentrated Glycerin and Purified Water or Purified Water in Containers in place of Glycerin, and with an appropriate quantity of Phenol and Purified Water or Purified Water in Containers in place of Liquefied Phenol.

Description Compound Iodine Glycerin is a red-brown, viscous liquid. It has a characteristic odor.

Specific gravity d_{20}^{20}: about 1.23

Identification **(1)** The colored solution obtained in the Assay (1) acquires a red color. Determine the absorption spectrum of this solution as directed under Ultraviolet-visible Spectrophotometry <*2.24*>: it exhibits a maximum between 510 nm and 514 nm (iodine).

(2) The colored solution obtained in the Assay (2) acquires a red color. Determine the absorption spectrum of this solution as directed under Ultraviolet-visible Spectrophotometry <*2.24*>: it exhibits a maximum between 510 nm and 514 nm (potassium iodide).

(3) The colored solution obtained in the Assay (4) has a yellow color. Determine the absorption spectrum of this solution as directed under Ultraviolet-visible Spectrophotometry <*2.24*>: it exhibits a maximum between 401 nm and 405 nm (phenol).

(4) Take 1 mL of Compound Iodine Glycerin in a glass-stoppered test tube, add 10 mL of ethanol (95), and mix. Then add 2 mL of sodium hydroxide TS, add 1 mL of a solution of copper (II) chloride dihydrate in ethanol (95) (1 in 10), and shake: a blue color develops (glycerin).

Assay **(1)** Iodine—Measure the specific gravity of Compound Iodine Glycerin according to Method 2 under Determination of Specific gravity and density <*2.56*>. Weigh exactly about 7 mL of it, add ethanol (95) to make exactly 200 mL, and use this solution as the sample solution. On the other hand, weigh accurately about 80 mg of iodine for assay and about 0.17 g of potassium iodide for assay, previously dried at 105°C for 4 hours, dissolve in ethanol (95) to make exactly 200 mL, and use this solution as the standard solution. Pipet 3 mL each of the sample solution and the standard solution into 50-mL separators, to each add exactly 10 mL of a mixture of chloroform and hexane (2:1) and 15 mL of water successively, and shake immediately and vigorously. Separate the chloroform-hexane layers [use the water layers in (2)], and filter through a pledget of cotton. Determine the absorbances of the filtrates, A_T and A_S, at 512 nm as directed under Ultraviolet-visible Spectrophotometry <*2.24*>, using a mixture of chloroform and hexane (2:1) as the blank.

Amount (mg) of iodine (I) = $M_S \times A_T/A_S$

M_S: Amount (mg) of iodine for assay taken

(2) Potassium iodide—Separate the water layers of the sample solution and the standard solution obtained in (1), pipet 10 mL of each of the water layers, and to each add 1 mL of diluted dilute hydrochloric acid (1 in 2), 1 mL of sodium nitrite TS and exactly 10 mL of a mixture of chloroform and hexane (2:1). Shake immediately and vigorously, separate the chloroform-hexane layers, and filter through a pledget of cotton. Determine the absorbances, A_T and A_S, of both solutions at 512 nm as directed under Ultraviolet-visible Spectrophotometry <*2.24*>, using a mixture of chloroform and hexane (2:1) as the blank.

Amount (mg) of potassium iodide (KI) = $M_S \times A_T/A_S$

M_S: Amount (mg) of potassium iodide for assay taken

(3) Total iodine—Measure the specific gravity of Compound Iodine Glycerin according to Method 2 under Determination of Specific gravity and density <*2.56*>. Weigh exactly about 5 mL of it, and add water to make exactly 50 mL. Pipet 5 mL of this solution into a 50-mL flask, and add 0.5 g of zinc powder and 5 mL of acetic acid (100). Shake until the color of iodine disappears, and heat under a reflux condenser on a water bath for 30 minutes. Wash the condenser with 10 mL of hot water, and filter through a glass filter (G3). Wash the flask with two 10-mL portions of warm water, and combine the filtrate and the washings. After cooling, add water to make exactly 50 mL, and use this solution as the sample solution. On the other hand, dissolve about 0.2 g of potassium iodide for assay, previously dried at 105°C for 4 hours and accurately weighed, in water to make exactly 50 mL. Pipet 5 mL of this solution, add 5 mL of acetic acid (100) and water to make exactly 50 mL, and use this solution as the standard solution. Pipet 4 mL each of the sample solution and standard solution into 30-mL separators, and to each add 5 mL of water, 1 mL of diluted dilute hydrochloric acid (1 in 2), 1 mL of sodium nitrite TS and 10 mL of a mixture of chloroform and hexane (2:1). Shake well immediately, and proceed as directed in (2).

Amount (mg) of total iodine (I) = $M_S \times A_T/A_S \times 0.764$

M_S: Amount (mg) of potassium iodide for assay taken

(4) Phenol—Measure the specific gravity of Compound Iodine Glycerin according to Method 2 under Determination of Specific gravity and density <*2.56*>. Weigh exactly about 2 mL of it, add 3 mL of 0.1 mol/L sodium thiosulfate VS, and shake. Add 2 mL of dilute hydrochloric acid, and shake with two 10-mL portions of chloroform. Separate the chloroform layer, and shake with two 10-mL portions of 0.5 mol/L sodium hydroxide TS. Separate the water layer, add water to make exactly 500 mL, and use this solution as the sample solution. Dissolve about 0.5 g of phenol for assay, accurately weighed, in ethanol (95) to make exactly 100 mL, pipet 2 mL of this solution, proceed in the same manner as the sample solution, and use so obtaind solution as the standard solution. Pipet 3 mL each of the sample solution and standard solution, to each add 2 mL of dilute hydrochloric acid, and place in a water bath at 30°C. Allow to stand for 10 minutes, and add exactly 2 mL of a solution of sodium nitrite (1 in 100), shake, and allow to stand at 30°C for 60 minutes. Add dilute potassium hydroxide-ethanol TS to make exactly 25 mL, and determine the absorbances of these solutions, A_T and A_S, at 403 nm as directed under Ultraviolet-visible Spectrophotometry <*2.24*>, using the solution prepared in the same manner with 3 mL of water instead of the sample solution as the blank.

Amount (mg) of phenol (C_6H_6O)
= $M_S \times A_T/A_S \times 1/50$

M_S: Amount (mg) of phenol for assay taken

Containers and storage Containers—Tight containers.
Storage—Light-resistant.

Dental Iodine Glycerin

歯科用ヨード・グリセリン

Dental Iodine Glycerin contains not less than 9.0 w/v% and not more than 11.0 w/v% of iodine (I: 126.90), not less than 7.2 w/v% and not more than 8.8 w/v% of potassium iodide (KI: 166.00), and not less than 0.9 w/v% and not more than 1.1 w/v% of zinc sulfate hydrate ($ZnSO_4.7H_2O$: 287.55).

Method of preparation

Iodine	10 g
Potassium Iodide	8 g
Zinc Sulfate Hydrate	1 g
Glycerin	35 mL
Purified Water or Purified Water in Containers	a sufficient quantity
To make	100 mL

Dissolve and mix the above ingredients.

Description Dental Iodine Glycerin is a dark red-brown liquid, having the odor of iodine.

Identification **(1)** The colored solution obtained in the Assay (1) acquires a red color. Determine the absorption spectrum of this solution as directed under Ultraviolet-visible Spectrophotometry <*2.24*>: it exhibits a maximum between 510 nm and 514 nm (iodine).

(2) The colored solution obtained in the Assay (2) acquires a red color. Determine the absorption spectrum of this solution as directed under Ultraviolet-visible Spectrophotometry <*2.24*>: it exhibits a maximum between 510 nm and 514 nm (potassium iodide).

(3) Put 1 mL of Dental Iodine Glycerin in a glass-stoppered, test tube, add 10 mL of ethanol (95), and mix. Then add 2 mL of sodium hydroxide TS, add 1 mL of a solution of copper (II) chloride dihydrate in ethanol (95) (1 in 10), and shake: a blue color develops (glycerin).

(4) The colored solution obtained in the Assay (3) acquires a red-purple to purple color. Determine the absorption spectrum of this solution as directed under Ultraviolet-visible Spectrophotometry <*2.24*>: it exhibits a maximum between 618 nm and 622 nm (zinc sulfate hydrate).

Assay **(1)** Iodine—Pipet 5 mL of Dental Iodine Glycerin, and add diluted ethanol (3 in 10) to make exactly 50 mL. Pipet 5 mL of this solution, add water to make exactly 200 mL, and use this solution as the sample solution. On the other hand, weigh accurately about 0.5 g of iodine for assay and about 0.4 g of potassium iodide for assay, previously dried at 105°C for 4 hours, and dissolve in diluted ethanol (3 in 10) to make exactly 50 mL. Pipet 5 mL of this solution, add water to make exactly 200 mL, and use this solution as the standard solution. Pipet 10 mL each of the sample solution and standard solution, to each add exactly 20 mL of a mixture of chloroform and hexane (2:1), shake immediately, and separate the chloroform-hexane layer [use the water layer in (2)]. Filter through a pledget of cotton. Determine the absorbances, A_T and A_S, of the filtrates obtained from the sample solution and standard solution, respectively, at 512 nm as directed under Ultraviolet-visible Spectrophotometry <2.24>, using a mixture of chloroform and hexane (2:1) as the blank.

$$\text{Amount (mg) of iodine (I)} = M_S \times A_T/A_S$$

M_S: Amount (mg) of iodine for assay taken

(2) Potassium iodide—Separate the water layers of the sample solution and standard solution obtained in (1), pipet 7 mL each of the water layers, and to each add exactly 1 mL of diluted hydrochloric acid (1 in 2), 1 mL of sodium nitrite TS and 10 mL of a mixture of chloroform and hexane (2:1), and shake immediately. Separate the chloroform-hexane layer, and filter through a pledget of cotton. Determine the absorbances, A_T and A_S, of the filtrates obtained from the sample solution and standard solution, respectively, at 512 nm as directed under Ultraviolet-visible Spectrophotometry, using a mixture of chloroform and hexane (2:1) as the blank.

$$\text{Amount (mg) of potassium iodide (KI)} = M_S \times A_T/A_S$$

M_S: Amount (mg) of potassium iodide for assay taken

(3) Zinc sulfate hydrate—Pipet 5 mL of Dental Iodine Glycerin, and add diluted ethanol (3 in 10) to make exactly 50 mL. Pipet 5 mL of this solution, add water to make exactly 100 mL, and use this solution as the sample solution. On the other hand, pipet 10 mL of Standard Zinc Stock Solution, add diluted ethanol (3 in 200) to make exactly 1000 mL, and use this solution as the standard solution. Pipet 10 mL each of the sample solution and standard solution, to each add 10 mL of a mixture of chloroform and hexane (2:1), shake, and allow to stand. Pipet 3 mL each of the water layers, and to each add 2 mL of boric acid-potassium chloride-sodium hydroxide buffer solution (pH 10.0), 2 mL of zincon TS and water to make exactly 25 mL. Determine the absorbances, A_T and A_S, obtained from the sample solution and standard solution, respectively, at 620 nm as directed under Ultraviolet-visible Spectrophotometry <2.24>, using the solution prepared in the same manner with 3 mL of water as the blank.

$$\text{Amount (mg) of zinc sulfate hydrate } (ZnSO_4.7H_2O) = M_S \times A_T/A_S \times 4.398$$

M_S: Amount (mg) of zinc in 10 mL of Standard Zinc Stock Solution

Containers and storage Containers—Tight containers.
Storage—Light-resistant.

Iodine, Salicylic Acid and Phenol Spirit

ヨード・サリチル酸・フェノール精

Iodine, Salicylic Acid and Phenol Spirit contains not less than 1.08 w/v% and not more than 1.32 w/v% of iodine (I: 126.90), not less than 0.72 w/v% and not more than 0.88 w/v% of potassium iodide (KI: 166.00), not less than 4.5 w/v% and not more than 5.5 w/v% of salicylic acid ($C_7H_6O_3$: 138.12), not less than 1.8 w/v% and not more than 2.2 w/v% of phenol (C_6H_6O: 94.11), and not less than 7.2 w/v% and not more than 8.8 w/v% of benzoic acid ($C_7H_6O_2$: 122.12).

Method of preparation

Iodine Tincture	200 mL
Salicylic Acid	50 g
Phenol	20 g
Benzoic Acid	80 g
Ethanol for Disinfection	a sufficient quantity
To make	1000 mL

Prepare as directed under Spirits, with the above ingredients. It may be prepared with an appropiate quantity of Ethanol and Purified Water or Purified Water in Containers in place of Ethanol for Disinfection.

Description Iodine, Salicylic Acid and Phenol Spirit is a dark red-brown liquid, having the odor of phenol.

Identification **(1)** To a mixture of 1 mL of starch TS and 9 mL of water add 1 drop of Iodine, Salicylic Acid and Phenol Spirit: a dark blue-purple color develops (iodine).

(2) To 1 mL of Iodine, Salicylic Acid and Phenol Spirit add 5 mL of ethanol (95) and water to make 50 mL. To 1 mL of this solution add hydrochloric acid-potassium chloride buffer solution (pH 2.0) to make 50 mL, and to 15 mL of this solution add 5 mL of a solution of iron (III) nitrate enneahydrate (1 in 200): a red-purple color is produced (salicylic acid).

(3) Shake 1 mL of Iodine, Salicylic Acid and Phenol Spirit with 1 mL of sodium thiosulfate TS, add 20 mL of water and 5 mL of dilute hydrochloric acid, and extract with 25 mL of diethyl ether. Wash the diethyl ether extract with two 25-mL portions of sodium hydrogen carbonate TS, and extract with 10 mL of dilute sodium hydroxide TS. Shake 1 mL of the extract with 1 mL of sodium nitrite TS and 1 mL of dilute hydrochloric acid, and add 3 mL of sodium hydroxide TS: a yellow color is developed (phenol).

(4) Shake 1 mL of Iodine, Salicylic Acid and Phenol Spirit with 1 mL of sodium thiosulfate TS, add 20 mL of water and 5 mL of dilute hydrochloric acid, extract with 10 mL of diethyl ether, and use the diethyl ether extract as the sample solution. Dissolve 25 mg of salicylic acid, 10 mg of phenol and 40 mg of benzoic acid in 5 mL each of diethyl ether, respectively, and use these solutions as the standard solutions (1), (2) and (3). Perform the test with these solutions as directed under Thin-layer Chromatography <2.03>. Spot 5 μL each of the sample solution and standard solutions (1), (2) and (3) on a plate of silica gel with fluorescent indicator for thin-layer chromatography. Develop the plate with a mixture of chloroform, acetone and acetic acid (100) (45:5:1) to a distance of about 10 cm, and air-dry the plate. Examine under ultraviolet light (main wavelength: 254 nm): the 3 spots from the sample solution show the same Rf value as the corresponding spots of the standard solutions (1), (2) and (3). Spray evenly iron (III) chloride TS on the plate: the spot from standard solution (1) and the corresponding spot from the sample solution acquires a purple color.

Assay **(1)** Iodine—Pipet 4 mL of Iodine, Salicylic Acid and Phenol Spirit, add ethanol (95) to make exactly 50 ml, and use this solution as the sample solution. On the other hand, weigh accurately about 1.2 g of iodine for assay and about 0.8 g of potassium iodide for assay, previously dried at 105°C for 4 hours, and dissolve in ethanol (95) to make exactly 100 ml. Pipet 4 ml of this solution, add ethanol (95) to make exactly 50 ml, and use this solution as the standard solution. Pipet 3 ml each of the sample solution and standard solution, to each add exactly 25 ml of a mixture of chloroform and hexane (2:1), and shake. Further add exactly 10 ml of water, shake and separate the chloroform-hexane layers [use the water layers in (2)]. Filter through a pledget of absorbent cotton, and determine the absorbances of the filtrates from the sample solution and standard solution, respectively, A_T and A_S, at 512 nm as directed under Ultraviolet-visible Spectrophotometry <*2.24*>, using a mixture of chloroform and hexane (2:1) as the blank.

$$\text{Amount (mg) of iodine (I)} = M_S \times A_T/A_S \times 1/25$$

M_S: Amount (mg) of iodine for assay taken

(2) Potassium iodide—Separate the water layers of the sample solution and standard solution obtained in the Assay (1), pipet 8 ml each of the water layers, and add 1 ml of diluted dilute hydrochloric acid (1 in 2) and 1 ml of sodium nitrite TS. Immediately after shaking, add exactly 10 ml of a mixture of chloroform and hexane (2:1), shake, and proceed in the same manner as for the Assay (1).

$$\text{Amount (mg) of potassium iodide (KI)} = M_S \times A_T/A_S \times 1/25$$

M_S: Amount (mg) of potassium iodide for assay taken

(3) Salicylic acid, phenol and benzoic acid—Pipet 2 mL of Iodine, Salicylic Acid and Phenol Spirit, add 20 mL of diluted methanol (1 in 2) and 0.1 mol/L sodium thiosulfate VS until the color of iodine disappears, add exactly 20 mL of the internal standard solution, then add diluted methanol (1 in 2) to make 200 mL, and use this solution as the sample solution. Weigh accurately about 0.2 g of salicylic acid for assay, previously dried in a desiccator (silica gel) for 3 hours, about 80 mg of phenol for assay, and 0.32 g of benzoic acid, previously dried in a desiccator (silica gel) for 3 hours, dissolve in diluted methanol (1 in 2) to make exactly 50 mL. Pipet 25 mL of this solution, add exactly 20 mL of the internal standard solution and diluted methanol (1 in 2) to make 200 mL, and use this solution as the standard solution. Perform the test with 3 μL of the sample solution and standard solution as directed under Liquid Chromatography <*2.01*> according to the following conditions. Calculate the ratios, Q_{Ta}, Q_{Tb} and Q_{Tc}, of the peak areas of salicylic acid, phenol and benzoic acid to those of the internal standard of the sample solution, and the ratios, Q_{Sa}, Q_{Sb} and Q_{Sc}, of the peak areas of salicylic acid, phenol and benzoic acid to those of the internal standard of the standard solution.

$$\text{Amount (mg) of salicylic acid } (C_7H_6O_3) = M_{Sa} \times Q_{Ta}/Q_{Sa} \times 1/2$$

$$\text{Amount (mg) of phenol } (C_6H_6O) = M_{Sb} \times Q_{Tb}/Q_{Sb} \times 1/2$$

$$\text{Amount (mg) of benzoic acid } (C_7H_6O_2) = M_{Sc} \times Q_{Tc}/Q_{Sc} \times 1/2$$

M_{Sa}: Amount (mg) of salicylic acid for assay taken
M_{Sb}: Amount (mg) of phenol for assay taken
M_{Sc}: Amount (mg) of benzoic acid taken

Internal standard solution—A solution of theophylline in methanol (1 in 1000).

Operating conditions—

Detector: An ultraviolet absorption photometer (wavelength: 270 nm).

Column: A stainless steel column about 4 mm in inside diameter and 25 to 30 cm in length, packed with octadecylsilanized silica gel for liquid chromatography (5 μm in particle diameter).

Column temperature: Room temperature.

Mobile phase: A mixture of 0.1 mol/L phosohate buffer solution (pH 7.0) and methanol (3:1).

Flow rate: Adjust so that the retention time of salicylic acid is about 6 minutes.

Selection of column: Dissolve 0.2 g of benzoic acid, 0.2 g of salicylic acid and 50 mg of theophylline in 100 mL of diluted ethanol (1 in 2). To 10 mL of this solution add 90 mL of diluted methanol (1 in 2). Proceed with 10 μL of this solution under the above operating conditions. Use a column giving elution of benzoic acid, salicylic acid and theophylline in this order, and clearly dividing each peak.

Containers and storage Containers—Tight containers.
Storage—Light-resistant.

Iodoform

ヨードホルム

CHI_3: 393.73
Triiodomethane
[*75-47-8*]

Iodoform, when dried, contains not less than 99.0% of iodoform (CHI_3).

Description Iodoform occurs as lustrous, yellow crystals or crystalline powder. It has a characteristic odor.

It is freely soluble in diethyl ether, sparingly soluble in ethanol (95), and practically insoluble in water.

It is slightly volatile at ordinary temperature.

Melting point: about 120°C (with decomposition).

Identification Heat 0.1 g of Iodoform: a purple gas is evolved.

Purity **(1)** Water-soluble colored substances and acidity or alkalinity—Shake well 2.0 g of Iodoform, previously powdered, with 5 mL of water for 1 minute, allow to stand, and filter the supernatant liquid: the filtrate is colorless and neutral.

(2) Chloride <*1.03*>—Shake well 3.0 g of Iodoform, previously powdered, with 75 mL of water for 1 minute, allow to stand, and filter the supernatant liquid. To 25 mL of the filtrate add 6 mL of dilute nitric acid and water to make 50 mL, and perform the test using this solution as the test solution. Prepare the control solution with 0.30 mL of 0.01 mol/L hydrochloric acid VS (not more than 0.011%).

(3) Sulfate <*1.14*>—To 25 mL of the filtrate obtained in

(2) add 1 mL of dilute hydrochloric acid and water to make 50 mL, and perform the test using this solution as the test solution. Prepare the control solution with 0.35 mL of 0.005 mol/L sulfuric acid VS (not more than 0.017%).

Loss on drying ⟨*2.41*⟩ Not more than 0.5% (1 g, silica gel, 24 hours).

Residue on ignition ⟨*2.44*⟩ Not more than 0.1% (1 g).

Assay Weigh accurately about 0.2 g of Iodoform, previously dried, in a 500-mL glass-stoppered flask, and dissolve it in 20 mL of ethanol (95). Add exactly 30 mL of 0.1 mol/L silver nitrate VS and 10 mL of nitric acid, stopper the flask, shake well, and allow to stand in a dark place over 16 hours. Add 150 mL of water, and titrate ⟨*2.50*⟩ the excess silver nitrate with 0.1 mol/L ammonium thiocyanate VS (indicator: 5 mL of ammonium iron (III) sulfate TS). Perform a blank determination in the same manner.

Each mL of 0.1 mol/L silver nitrate VS
= 13.12 mg of CHI_3

Containers and storage Containers—Tight containers.
Storage—Light-resistant.

Iohexol

イオヘキソール

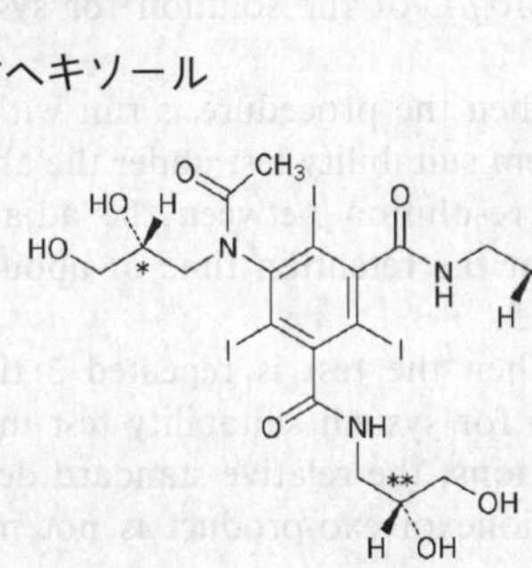

and epimers at C* and C**, and their enantiomers

$C_{19}H_{26}I_3N_3O_9$: 821.14
5-{Acetyl[(2*RS*)-2,3-dihydroxypropyl]amino}-*N*,*N'*-bis[(2*RS*)-2,3-dihydroxypropyl]-2,4,6-triiodobenzene-1,3-dicarboxamide
5-{Acetyl[(2*RS*)-2,3-dihydroxypropyl]amino}-*N*-[(2*RS*)-2,3-dihydroxypropyl]-*N'*-[(2*SR*)-2,3-dihydroxypropyl]-2,4,6-triiodobenzene-1,3-dicarboxamide
5-{Acetyl[(2*RS*)-2,3-dihydroxypropyl]amino}-*N*,*N'*-bis[(2*SR*)-2,3-dihydroxypropyl]-2,4,6-triiodobenzene-1,3-dicarboxamide
[*66108-95-0*]

Iohexol is a mixture of endo- and exo-products of iohexol.

It contains not less than 98.5% and not more than 101.0% of iohexol ($C_{19}H_{26}I_3N_3O_9$), calculated on the anhydrous basis.

Description Iohexol occurs as a white powder.

It is very soluble in water, freely soluble in methanol and sparingly soluble in ethanol (99.5).

It dissolves in a solution of sodium hydroxide (1 in 20).

A solution of Iohexol (1 in 20) shows no optical rotation.

Identification **(1)** Determine the absorption spectrum of a solution of Iohexol (13 in 1,000,000) as directed under Ultraviolet-visible Spectrophotometry ⟨*2.24*⟩, and compare the spectrum with the Reference Spectrum: both spectra exhibit similar intensities of absorption at the same wavelengths.

(2) Determine the infrared absorption spectrum of Iohexol, previously dried at 105°C for 6 hours, as directed in the potassium bromide disk method under Infrared Spectrophotometry ⟨*2.25*⟩, and compare the spectrum with the Reference Spectrum: both spectra exhibit similar intensities of absorption at the same wave numbers.

(3) Dissolve 0.1 g of Iohexol in 10 mL of methanol, and use this solution as the sample solution. Perform the test with the sample solution as directed under Thin-layer Chromatography ⟨*2.03*⟩. Spot 10 μL of the sample solution on a plate of silica gel with fluorescent indicator for thin-layer chromatography. Develop the plate with a mixture of 1-butanol, water and acetic acid (100) (50:25:11) to a distance of about 12 cm, and air-dry the plate. Examine under ultraviolet light (main wavelength: 254 nm): the number of principal spots obtained from the sample solutions is two, and their *R*f values are about 0.2 and about 0.3, respectively.

Purity **(1)** Clarity and color of solution—A solution obtained by dissolving 1.0 g of Iohexol in 5 mL of water is clear and colorless.

(2) Aromatic primary amine—Conduct this procedure using light-resistant vessels. Dissolve 0.20 g of Iohexol in 15 mL of water, cool in ice for 5 minutes, add 1.5 mL of 6 mol/L hydrochloric acid TS and 1 mL of a solution of sodium nitrite (1 in 50), prepared before use, stir, and cool in ice for 4 minutes. Add 1 mL of a solution of amidosulfuric acid (standard reagent) (1 in 25), stir, and cool in ice for 1 minute. Then, add 0.5 mL of a solution, prepared by dissolving 0.3 g of *N*-1-naphthylethylenediamine dihydrochloride in diluted propylene glycol (7 in 10) to make 100 mL, and add water to make exactly 25 mL. Perform the test with this solution as directed under Ultraviolet-visible Spectrophotometry ⟨*2.24*⟩ within 20 minutes, using a solution prepared in the same manner with 15 mL of water as the blank: the absorbance at 495 nm is not more than 0.21.

(3) Chloride ⟨*1.03*⟩—Perform the test with 2.0 g of Iohexol. Prepare the control solution with 0.40 mL of 0.01 mol/L hydrochloric acid VS (not more than 0.007%).

(4) Iodine and iodide—Dissolve 1.0 g of Iohexol in 4 mL of water, add 1 mL of dilute sulfuric acid, and allow to stand for 10 minutes while occasional shaking. Add 5 mL of chloroform, shake well, and allow to stand: the chloroform layer is colorless. Then, add 1 mL of sodium nitrite solution (1 in 50), prepared before use, shake, allow to stand, and determine the absorbance of collected chloroform layer as directed under Ultraviolet-visible Spectrophotometry ⟨*2.24*⟩, using a chloroform layer prepared in the same manner with 4.0 mL of water as the blank: the absorbance at 510 nm is not larger than that of chloroform layer obtained from the following control solution.

Control solution: Dissolve exactly 0.131 g of potassium iodide in water to make exactly 100 mL. Pipet 1 mL of this solution, and add water to make exactly 100 mL. Pipet 3 mL of this solution, add 1 mL of water and 1 mL of dilute sulfuric acid, then proceed in the same manner.

(5) Heavy metals ⟨*1.07*⟩—Proceed with 2.0 g of Iohexol according to Method 1, and perform the test. Prepare the control solution with 2.0 mL of Standard Lead Solution (not more than 10 ppm).

(6) 3-Chloro-1,2-propanediol—To exactly 1.0 g of Iohexol, add exactly 2 mL of diethyl ether, and sonicate for 10 minutes under cooling. Centrifuge, and use the diethyl ether layer as the sample solution. Separately, dissolve exactly 0.50 g of 3-chloro-1,2-propanediol in diethyl ether to make exactly 50 mL. Pipet 1 mL of this solution, and add diethyl ether to make exactly 100 mL. Pipet 5 mL of this solution, add diethyl ether to make exactly 25 mL, and use this solution as the standard solution. Perform the test with exactly 5 μL each of the sample solution and standard solution as directed under Gas Chromatography <2.02>, and determine the peak areas, A_T and A_S, of 3-chloro-1,2-propanediol in each solution: A_T is not larger than 2.5 times A_S.

Operating conditions—

Detector: A hydrogen flame-ionization detector.

Column: A fused silica column 0.25 mm in inside diameter and 30 m in length, coated the inside surface with a layer about 0.25 μm thick of 5% diphenyl-95% dimethylpolysiloxane for gas chromatography.

Column temperature: A constant temperature of about 70°C.

Injection port and detector temperature: A constant temperature of about 230°C.

Carrier gas: Helium.

Flow rate: Adjust so that the retention time of 3-chloro-1,2-propanediol is about 7 minutes.

Split ratio: 1:40.

System suitability—

System performance: To 1 mL of a solution of 3-chloro-1,2-propanediol in diethyl ether (1 in 200) and 1 mL of a solution of 1-hexanol in diethyl ether (1 in 800) add diethyl ether to make 200 mL. When the procedure is run with 5 μL of this solution under the above operating conditions, 1-hexanol and 3-chloro-1,2-propanediol are eluted in this order with the resolution between these peaks being not less than 20.

System repeatability: When the test is repeated 6 times with 5 μL of the standard solution under the above operating conditions, the relative standard deviation of the peak area of 3-chloro-1,2-propanediol is not more than 15%.

(7) Related substance—(i) Dissolve 1.0 g of Iohexol in 10 mL of methanol, and use this solution as the sample solution. Pipet 1 mL of the sample solution, and add methanol to make exactly 25 mL. Pipet 1 mL of this solution, add the methanol to make exactly 20 mL, and use this solution as the standard solution. Perform the test with these solutions as directed under Thin-layer Chromatography <2.03>. Spot 10 μL each of the sample solution and standard solution on a plate of silica gel with fluorescent indicator for thin-layer chromatography. Develop the plate with a mixture of acetone, 2-propanol, ammonia solution (28) and methanol (10:7:4:4) to a distance about 14 cm, and air-dry the plate. Examine under ultraviolet light (main wavelength: 254 nm): a spot, other than the principal spot obtained from the sample solution, having the relative *R*f value of 1.4 to the spot from the standard solution, is not more intense than the spot from the standard solution.

(ii) Dissolve 0.15 g of Iohexol in water to make 100 mL, and use this solution as the sample solution. Perform the test with 10 μL of the sample solution as directed under Liquid Chromatography <2.01> according to the following conditions. Determine the peak area by the automatic integration method, and calculate the amounts by the area percentage method: the total amount of *O*-alkyl substances, having the relative retention time between 1.2 and 1.5 to the second principal peak (having bigger retention time) among the two principal peaks of iohexol, is not more than 0.6%, the amount of the peaks, which are eluted after the peak of iohexol and other than *O*-alkyl substances, is not more than 0.1%, respectively, and the total amount of the peaks, which are eluted after iohexol and other than *O*-alkyl substances, is not more than 0.3%.

Operating conditions—

Detector: An ultraviolet absorption photometer (wavelength: 254 nm).

Column: A stainless steel column 4.6 mm in inside diameter and 25 cm in length, packed with octadecylsilanized silica gel for liquid chromatography (5 μm in particle diameter).

Column temperature: A constant temperature of about 25°C.

Mobile phase A: Acetonitrile.

Mobile phase B: Water.

Flowing of mobile phase: Control the gradient by mixing the mobile phases A and B as directed in the following table.

Time after injection of sample (min)	Mobile phase A (vol%)	Mobile phase B (vol%)
0 – 1	1	99
1 – 46	1 → 10	99 → 90

Flow rate: Adjust so that the retention time of the second principal peak (iohexol exo-product) is about 19 minutes.

Time span of measurement: About 2 times as long as the retention time of iohexol exo-product.

System suitability—

Test for required detectability: To 1 mL of the sample solution add water to make 50 mL, and use this solution as the solution for system suitability test. Pipet 1 mL of the solution for system suitability test, and add water to make exactly 20 mL. Confirm that the peak area of iohexol exo-product obtained with 10 μL of this solution is equivalent to 3.5 to 6.5% of that with 10 μL of the solution for system suitability test.

System performance: When the procedure is run with 10 μL of the solution for system suitability test under the above operating conditions, the resolution between the adjacent two peaks, which appear at the retention time of about 18 minutes, is not less than 1.5.

System repeatability: When the test is repeated 3 times with 10 μL of the solution for system suitability test under the above operating conditions, the relative standard deviation of the peak area of iohexol exo-product is not more than 3.0%.

Water <2.48> Not more than 4.0% (0.3 g, volumetric titration, direct titration).

Residue on ignition <2.44> Not more than 0.1% (1 g).

Assay Weigh accurately about 0.5 g of Iohexol, dissolve in 25 mL of a solution of sodium hydroxide (1 in 20), add 0.5 g of zinc powder, boil under a reflux condenser for 30 minutes, and filter after cooling. Wash the flask and filter paper with 200 mL of water, combine the washings and filter, add 5 mL of acetic acid (100), and titrate <2.50> with 0.1 mol/L silver nitrate VS (indicator: 1 mL of tetrabromophenolphthalein ethyl ester TS) until the color of the precipitate changes from yellow to green.

Each mL of 0.1 mol/L silver nitrate VS
= 27.37 mg of $C_{19}H_{26}I_3N_3O_9$

Containers and storage Containers—Tight containers.

Iohexol Injection

イオヘキソール注射液

Iohexol Injection is an aqueous injection.

It contains not less than 95.0% and not more than 105.0% of the labeled amount of iohexol ($C_{19}H_{26}I_3N_3O_9$: 821.14).

Method of preparation Prepare as directed under Injections, with Iohexol.

Description Iohexol Injection is a clear and colorless liquid.

Identification To a volume of Iohexol Injection, equivalent to 0.65 g of Iohexol, add water to make 500 mL. To 1 mL of this solution add water to make 100 mL, and determine the absorption spectrum of this solution as directed under Ultraviolet-visible Spectrophotometry <2.24>: it exhibits a maximum between 243 nm and 247 nm.

pH Being specified separately when the drug is granted approval based on the Law.

Purity (1) Aromatic primary amine—Conduct this procedure using light-resistant vessels. To a volume of Iohexol Injection, equivalent to 0.20 g of Iohexol add 15 mL of water, cool in ice for 5 minutes, add 1.5 mL of 6 mol/L hydrochloric acid TS and 1 mL of solution of sodium nitrite (1 in 50), prepared before use, shake, and cool in ice for 4 minutes. Then, proceed as directed in the Purity (2) under Iohexol: the absorbance of a solution so obtained is not more than 0.23.

(2) Iodine and iodide—To a volume of Iohexol Injection, equivalent to 1.0 g of Iohexol, add 4 mL of water and 1 mL of dilute sulfuric acid, and allow to stand for 10 minutes while occasional shaking. Then, proceed as directed in the Purity (4) under Iohexol: the absorbance of a chloroform layer so obtained is not more than 0.14.

Bacterial endotoxins <4.01> Less than 0.47 EU/mL.

Extractable volume <6.05> It meets the requirement.

Foreign insoluble matter <6.06> Perform the test according to Method 1: it meets the requirement.

Insoluble particulate matter <6.07> It meets the requirement.

Sterility <4.06> Perform the test according to the Membrane filtration method: it meets the requirement.

Assay To an exactly measured volume of Iohexol Injection, equivalent to about 1.5 g of iohexol ($C_{19}H_{26}I_3N_3O_9$), add water to make exactly 25 mL. Pipet 10 mL of this solution, add 25 mL of a solution of sodium hydroxide (1 in 20) and 0.5 g of zinc powder, and boil under a reflux condenser for 30 minutes. After cooling, wash down the inside of the condenser with 20 mL of water, and filter. Then, proceed as directed in the Assay under Iohexol.

Each mL of 0.1 mol/L silver nitrate VS
= 27.37 mg of $C_{19}H_{26}I_3N_3O_9$

Containers and storage Containers—Hermetic containers. Colored containers and plastic containers for aqueous injections may be used.

Iopamidol

イオパミドール

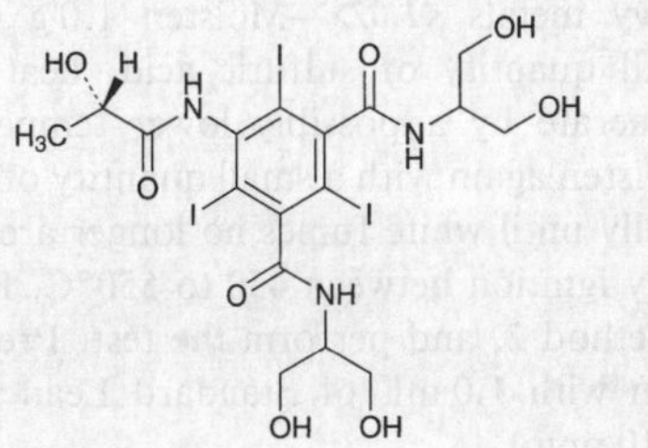

$C_{17}H_{22}I_3N_3O_8$: 777.09
N,N'-Bis[2-hydroxy-1-(hydroxymethyl)ethyl]-5-[(2*S*)-2-hydroxypropanoylamino]-2,4,6-triiodoisophthalamide
[62883-00-5]

Iopamidol, when dried, contains not less than 99.0% of iopamidol ($C_{17}H_{22}I_3N_3O_8$).

Description Iopamidol occurs as a white crystalline powder.

It is very soluble in water, sparingly soluble in methanol, and very slightly soluble in ethanol (99.5).

Identification (1) To 50 mg of Iopamidol add 5 mL of hydrochloric acid, heat for 10 minutes in a water bath: the test solution responds to Qualitative Tests <1.09> for primary aromatic amines.

(2) Heat 0.1 g of Iopamidol over a flame: a purple gas is evolved.

(3) Determine the infrared absorption spectrum of Iopamidol, previously dried, as directed in the potassium bromide disk method under Infrared Spectrophotometry <2.25>, and compare the spectrum with the Reference Spectrum: both spectra exhibit similar intensities of absorption at the same wave numbers.

Optical rotation <2.49> $[\alpha]_{436}^{20}$: −4.6 − −5.2° (after drying, 4 g, water, warm, after cooling, 10 mL, 100 mm).

Purity (1) Clarity and color of solution—Dissolve 1.0 g of Iopamidol in 10 mL of water: the solution is clear and colorless.

(2) Primary aromatic amines—Dissolve 0.60 g of Iopamidol in 8 mL of water, add 1 mL of a solution of sodium nitrite (1 in 50) and 12 mL of 2 mol/L hydrochloric acid TS, shake, and allow to stand for 2 minutes. Add 1 mL of a solution of ammonium amidosulfate (1 in 10), shake well, allow to stand for 1 minute, and add 1 mL of naphthylethylenediamine TS and water to make exactly 50 mL. Determine the absorbance of this solution at 495 nm as directed under Ultraviolet-visible Spectrophotometry <2.24> using a solution, prepared in the same manner, as the blank: the absorbance is not more than 0.12 (not more than 0.020%).

(3) Iodine—Dissolve 2.0 g of Iopamidol in 25 mL of water, add 5 mL of 1 mol/L sulfuric acid TS and 5 mL of toluene, shake well, and allow to stand: the toluene layer is colorless.

(4) Free iodine ion—Weigh accurately about 5 g of Iopamidol, dissolve in 70 mL of water, and adjust the pH to about 4.5 with dilute acetic acid. To this solution add 2 mL of 0.1 mol/L sodium chloride TS, and titrate <2.50> with 0.001 mol/L silver nitrate VS (potentiometric titration).

Each mL of 0.001 mol/L silver nitrate VS
= 0.1269 mg of I

Content of iodine ion in Iopamidol is not more than 0.001%.

(5) Heavy metals *<1.07>*—Moisten 1.0 g of Iopamidol with a small quantity of sulfuric acid, heat gradually to almost incinerate by a possibly lower temperature. After cooling, moisten again with a small quantity of sulfuric acid, heat gradually until white fumes no longer are evolved, and incinerate by ignition between 450 to 550°C. Proceed as directed in Method 2, and perform the test. Prepare the control solution with 1.0 mL of Standard Lead Solution (not more than 10 ppm).

(6) Related substances—Dissolve 0.10 g of Iopamidol in water to make exactly 10 mL, and use this solution as the sample solution. Separately, dissolve 10 mg of *N,N′*-bis[2-hydroxy-1-(hydroxymethyl)ethyl]-5-hydroxyacetylamino-2,4,6-triiodoisophthalamide in water to make exactly 100 mL. Pipet 5 mL of this solution, add water to make exactly 50 mL, and use this solution as the standard solution. Perform the test with exactly 20 μL each of the sample solution and standard solution as directed under Liquid Chromatography *<2.01>* according to the following conditions, and determine each peak area of the both solutions by the automatic integration method: each area of the peaks other than the peak of iopamidol from the sample solution is not larger than the peak area of the standard solution, and the total of these areas is not larger than 2.5 times of the peak area of the standard solution.

Operating conditions—

Detector: An ultraviolet absorption photometer (wavelength: 240 nm).

Column: A stainless steel column 4.6 mm in inside diameter and 25 cm in length, packed with octadecylsilanized silica gel for liquid chromatography (5 μm in particle diameter).

Column temperature: A constant temperature of about 35°C.

Mobile phase A: Water.

Mobile phase B: A mixture of water and methanol (3:1).

Flowing of mobile phase: Control the gradient by mixing the mobile phase A and B as directed in the following table.

Time after injection of sample (min)	Mobile phase A (vol%)	Mobile phase B (vol%)
0 – 6	92	8
6 – 18	92 → 65	8 → 35
18 – 30	65 → 8	35 → 92
30 – 34	8	92

Flow rate: 1.5 mL per minute.

Time span of measurement: About 4.3 times as long as the retention time of iopamidol.

System suitability—

System performance: Dissolve 1 mL of the sample solution and 10 mg of *N,N′*-bis[2-hydroxy-1-(hydroxymethyl)ethyl]-5-hydroxyacetylamino-2,4,6-triiodoisophthalamide in water to make 100 mL. When the procedure is run with 20 μL of this solution under the above operating conditions, *N,N′*-bis[2-hydroxy-1-(hydroxymethyl)ethyl]-5-hydroxyacetylamino-2,4,6-triiodoisophthalamide and iopamidol are eluted in this order with the resolution between these peaks being not less than 7.

System repeatability: When the test is repeated 6 times with 20 μL of the standard solution under the above operating conditions, the relative standard deviation of the peak areas of *N,N′*-bis[2-hydroxy-1-(hydroxymethyl)ethyl]-5-hydroxyacetylamino-2,4,6-triiodoisophthalamide is not more than 1.0%.

Loss on drying *<2.41>* Not more than 0.30% (1 g, 105°C, 3 hours).

Residue on ignition *<2.44>* Not more than 0.1% (1 g).

Assay Weigh accurately about 0.5 g of Iopamidol, previously dried, transfer to a saponification flask, dissolve in 40 mL of sodium hydroxide TS, add 1 g of zinc powder, boil for 30 minutes under a reflux condenser, cool, and filter. Wash the flask and the filter paper with 50 mL of water, and combine the washing with the filtrate. Add 5 mL of acetic acid (100) to this solution, and titrate *<2.50>* with 0.1 mol/L silver nitrate VS (potentiometric titration).

Each mL of 0.1 mol/L sliver nitrate VS
= 25.90 mg of $C_{17}H_{22}I_3N_3O_8$

Containers and storage Containers—Well-closed containers.

Storage—Light-resistant.

Iopamidol Injection

イオパミドール注射液

Iopamidol Injection is an aqueous injection.

It contains not less than 95.0% and not more than 105.0% of the labeled amount of iopamidol ($C_{17}H_{22}I_3N_3O_8$: 777.09).

Method of preparation Prepare as directed under Injections, with Iopamidol.

Description Iopamidol Injection occurs as a clear, colorless or faint yellow, liquid, having slight viscosity.

It is gradually colored to faint yellow by light.

Identification **(1)** To a volume of Iopamidol Injection, equivalent to 0.3 g of Iopamidol, add 0.2 mL of sulfuric acid, and mix. When heat the solution over a flame, the color of the solution changes from colorless to purplish brown, and a purple gas is evolved.

(2) To a volume of Iopamidol Injection, equivalent to 0.6 g of Iopamidol, add water to make 100 mL, and use this solution as the sample solution. Separately, dissolve 60 mg of iopamidol for assay in 10 mL of water, and use this solution as the standard solution. Perform the test with these solutions as directed under Thin-layer Chromatography *<2.03>*. Spot 4 μL each of the sample solution and standard solution on a plate of silica gel with fluorescent indicator for thin-layer chromatography. Develop the plate with a mixture of 2-propanol, 2-butanone and ammonia solution (28) (2:2:1) to a distance of about 15 cm, and air-dry the plate. Examine under ultra-violet light (main wavelength: 254 nm): the *Rf* value of the principal spot obtained from the sample solution is the same as that from the standard solution.

pH Being specified separately when the drug is granted approval based on the Law.

Purity **(1)** Primary aromatic amines—To a volume of Iopamidol Injection, equivalent to 0.18 g of Iopamidol, add 6 mL of water and mix. Add 1 mL of a solution of sodium nitrite (1 in 50) and 12 mL of 2 mol/L hydrochloric acid TS, shake the solution and allow to stand for 2 minutes. Add 1 mL of a solution of ammonium amidosulfate (1 in 10), shake well, and allow to stand for 1 minute. Add 1 mL of naphthylethylenediamine TS and water to make exactly 50 mL. Determine the absorbance of this solution at 495 nm as directed under Ultraviolet-visible Spectrophotometry <*2.24*> using a solution prepared in the same manner as the blank: the absorbance is not more than 0.18.

(2) Iodine—Take a volume of Iopamidol Injection, equivalent to 2.0 g of Iopamidol, and add 2 mL of 1 mol/L sulfuric acid TS and 1 mL of toluene. Then shake well and allow to stand: the toluene layer is colorless.

(3) Free iodine ion—To exactly 10 mL of Iopamidol Injection add a suitable amount of water, and adjust the pH to about 4.5 with diluted 0.25 mol/L sulfuric acid TS (1 in 10). Titrate <*2.50*> with 0.001 mol/L silver nitrate VS (potentiometric titration): the amount of iodine ion contained in Iopamidol Injection is not more than 40 μg per mL.

Each mL of 0.001 mol/L silver nitrate VS = 0.1269 mg of I

Bacterial endotoxins <*4.01*> Less than 1.5 EU/mL.

Extractable volume <*6.05*> It meets the requirement.

Foreign insoluble matter <*6.06*> Perform the test according to Method 1: it meets the requirement.

Insoluble particulate matter <*6.07*> It meets the requirement.

Sterility <*4.06*> Perform the test according to the Membrane filtration method: it meets the requirement.

Assay To exactly 1 mL of Iopamidol Injection add water to make exactly 200 mL. Take exactly V mL of this solution, add water to make exactly V' mL so that each mL contains about 80 μg of iopamidol ($C_{17}H_{22}I_3N_3O_8$), and use this solution as the sample solution. Separately, weigh accurately about 20 mg of iopamidol for assay, previously dried at 105°C for 3 hours, and dissolve in water to make exactly 10 mL. Pipet 4 mL of this solution, add water to make exactly 100 mL, and use this solution as the standard solution. Perform the test with exactly 20 μL each of the sample solution and standard solution as directed under Liquid Chromatography <*2.01*> according to the following conditions, and determine the peak areas, A_T and A_S, of iopamidol in each solution.

Amount (mg) of iopamidol ($C_{17}H_{22}I_3N_3O_8$)
$= M_S \times A_T/A_S \times V'/V \times 4/5$

M_S: Amount (mg) of iopamidol for assay taken

Operating conditions—

Detector: An ultraviolet absorption photometer (wavelength: 240 nm).

Column: A stainless steel column 4.6 mm in inside diameter and 25 cm in length, packed with octadecylsilanized silica gel for liquid chromatography (5 μm in particle diameter).

Column temperature: A constant temperature of about 35°C.

Mobile phase A: Water.

Mobile phase B: A mixture of water and methanol (3:1).

Flowing of mobile phase: Control the gradient by mixing the mobile phases A and B as directed in the following table.

Time after injection of sample (min)	Mobile phase A (vol%)	Mobile phase B (vol%)
0 – 6	92	8
6 – 18	92 → 65	8 → 35
18 – 30	65 → 8	35 → 92
30 – 34	8	92

Flow rate: 1.5 mL per minute.

System suitability—

System performance: Dissolve 1 mg each of iopamidol for assay and N,N'-bis[2-hydroxy-1-(hydroxymethyl)ethyl]-5-hydroxyacetylamino-2,4,6-triiodoisophthalamide in water to make 100 mL. When the procedure is run with 20 μL of this solution under the above operating conditions, N,N'-bis[2-hydroxy-1-(hydroxymethyl)ethyl]-5-hydroxyacetylamino-2,4,6-triiodoisophthalamide and iopamidol are eluted in this order with the resolution between these peaks being not less than 7.

System repeatability: When the test is repeated 6 times with 20 μL of the standard solution under the above operating conditions, the relative standard deviation of the peak area of iopamidol is not more than 1.0%.

Containers and storage Containers—Hermetic containers. Plastic containers for aqueous injections may be used.

Storage—Light-resistant.

Iotalamic Acid

イオタラム酸

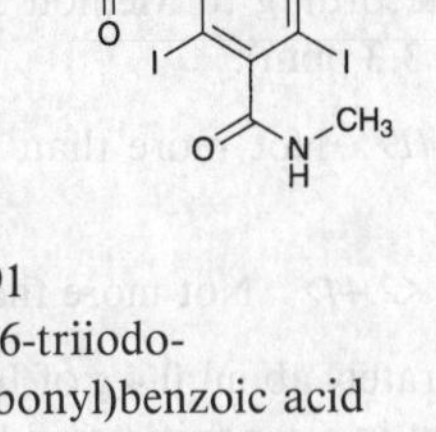

$C_{11}H_9I_3N_2O_4$: 613.91
3-Acetylamino-2,4,6-triiodo-
5-(methylaminocarbonyl)benzoic acid
[2276-90-6]

Iotalamic Acid, when dried, contains not less than 99.0% of iotalamic acid ($C_{11}H_9I_3N_2O_4$).

Description Iotalamic Acid occurs as a white powder. It is odorless.

It is sparingly soluble in ethanol (95), very slightly soluble in water, and practically insoluble in diethyl ether.

It dissolves in sodium hydroxide TS.

It gradually colored by light.

Identification **(1)** Heat 0.1 g of Iotalamic Acid over a flame: a purple gas is evolved.

(2) Determine the infrared spectrum of Iotalamic Acid, previously dried, as directed in the potassium bromide disk method under Infrared Spectrophotometry <*2.25*>, and compare the spectrum with the Reference Spectrum: both spectra exhibit similar intensities of absorption at the same wave numbers.

Purity **(1)** Clarity and color of solution—Dissolve 2.0 g of Iotalamic Acid in 10 mL of sodium hydroxide TS: the solution is clear and colorless.

(2) Primary aromatic amines—To 0.50 g of Iotalamic

Acid add 15 mL of water, and dissolve it in 1 mL of sodium hydroxide TS while ice-cooling. Add 4 mL of a solution of sodium nitrite (1 in 100) to the solution, immediately add 12 mL of 1 mol/L hydrochloric acid TS, and shake gently. Then allow the mixture to stand for exactly 2 minutes, add 8 mL of ammonium amidosulfate TS, and shake occasionally for 5 minutes. Add 3 drops of a solution of 1-naphthol in ethanol (95) (1 in 10), allow to stand for 1 minute, add 3.5 mL of ammonia-ammonium chloride buffer solution (pH 10.7), mix, and immediately add water to make 50 mL. Determine within 20 minutes the absorbance of this solution at 485 nm as directed under Ultraviolet-visible Spectrophotometry <*2.24*>, using a solution, prepared in the same manner, as the blank: the absorbance is not more than 0.25.

(3) Soluble halides—Dissolve 0.5 g of Iotalamic Acid in 20 mL of diluted ammonia TS (1 in 40), add 6 mL of dilute nitric acid, shake, allow to stand for 5 minutes, and filter. Transfer the filtrate to a Nessler tube, wash the residue with 20 mL of water, combine the filtrate and the washings, and add water to make 50 mL. Proceed as directed for Chloride Limit Test <*1.03*> using this solution as the test solution. Prepare the control solution as follows: to 0.10 mL of 0.01 mol/L hydrochloric acid VS and add 20 mL of diluted ammonia TS (1 in 40), 6 mL of dilute nitric acid and water to make 50 mL.

(4) Iodine—Dissolve 0.20 g of Iotalamic Acid in 2.0 mL of sodium hydroxide TS, add 2.5 mL of 0.5 mol/L sulfuric acid TS, and allow to stand for 10 minutes with occasional shaking. Add 5 mL of chloroform, shake well, and allow to stand: the chloroform layer remains colorless.

(5) Heavy metals <*1.07*>—Proceed with 1.0 g of Iotalamic Acid according to Method 2, and perform the test. Prepare the control solution with 2.0 mL of Standard Lead Solution (not more than 20 ppm).

(6) Arsenic <*1.11*>—Prepare the test solution with 0.6 g of Iotalamic Acid according to Method 3, and perform the test (not more than 3.3 ppm).

Loss on drying <*2.41*> Not more than 0.5% (1 g, 105°C, 4 hours).

Residue on ignition <*2.44*> Not more than 0.1% (1 g).

Assay Weigh accurately about 0.4 g of Iotalamic Acid, previously dried, place it in a saponification flask, dissolve in 40 mL of sodium hydroxide TS, add 1 g of zinc powder, and heat for 30 minutes under a reflux condenser. Cool, filter, wash the flask and the filter paper with 50 mL of water, and combine the washings and the filtrate. Add 5 mL of acetic acid (100) to this solution, and titrate <*2.50*> with 0.1 mol/L silver nitrate VS, until the color of the precipitate changes from yellow to green (indicator: 1 mL of tetrabromophenolphthalein ethyl ester TS).

Each mL of 0.1 mol/L silver nitrate VS
= 20.46 mg of $C_{11}H_9I_3N_2O_4$

Containers and storage Containers—Tight containers.
Storage—Light-resistant.

Iotroxic Acid

イオトロクス酸

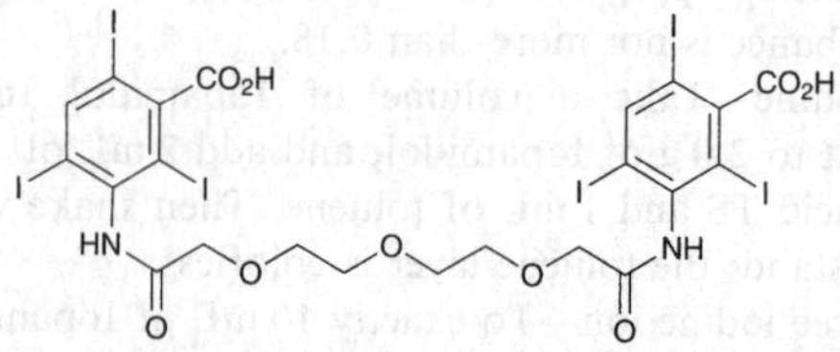

$C_{22}H_{18}I_6N_2O_9$: 1215.81
3,3′-(3,6,9-Trioxaundecanedioyl)diiminobis(2,4,6-triiodobenzoic acid)
[*51022-74-3*]

Iotroxic Acid contains not less than 98.5% of iotroxic acid ($C_{22}H_{18}I_6N_2O_9$), calculated on the anhydrous basis.

Description Iotroxic Acid occurs as a white crystalline powder.

It is soluble in methanol, slightly soluble in ethanol (95), and practically insoluble in water and in diethyl ether.

It is gradually colored by light.

Identification **(1)** Heat 0.1 g of Iotroxic Acid over a flame: a purple gas evolves.

(2) Dissolve a suitable amount of Iotroxic Acid in a suitable amount of methanol, evaporate the methanol under reduced pressure, and determine the infrared absorption spectrum of the residue so obtained as directed in the potassium bromide disk method under Infrared Spectrophotometry <*2.25*>, and compare the spectrum with the Reference Spectrum: both spectra exhibit similar intensities of absorption at the same wave numbers.

Purity **(1)** Clarity and color of solution—Dissolve 1.0 g of Iotroxic Acid in 10 mL of diluted sodium hydroxide TS (1 in 5): the solution is clear and colorless.

(2) Primary aromatic amines—Dissolve 0.20 g of Iotroxic Acid in 5 mL of water and 1 mL of sodium hydroxide TS, add 4 mL of a solution of sodium nitrite (1 in 100) and 10 mL of 1 mol/L hydrochloric acid TS, mix, and allow to stand for 2 minutes. Add 5 mL of ammonium amidosulfate TS, shake well, allow to stand for 1 minute, then add 0.4 mL of a solution of α-naphthol in ethanol (95) (1 in 10), 15 mL of sodium hydroxide TS and water to make exactly 50 mL. Read the absorbance of this solution at 485 nm as directed under Ultraviolet-visible Spectrophotometry <*2.24*>, using a blank solution obtained in the same manner as above: the absorbance is not more than 0.22.

(3) Iodine—Dissolve 0.20 g of Iotroxic Acid in 2.0 mL of sodium hydrogen carbonate TS, add 5 mL of toluene, mix well, and allow to stand: the toluene layer is colorless.

(4) Free iodine ion—Weigh accurately about 5.0 g of Iotroxic Acid, dissolve in 12 mL of a solution of meglumine (3 in 20), add water to make 70 mL, and adjust the pH to about 4.5 with acetic acid (100). To this solution add 2 mL of 0.1 mol/L sodium chloride TS, and titrate <*2.50*> with 0.001 mol/L silver nitrate VS (potentiometric titration).

Each mL of 0.001 mol/L silver nitrate
= 0.1269 mg of I

Content of iodine ion in Iotroxic Acid, calculated on the anhydrous basis, is not more than 0.004%.

(5) Heavy metals <*1.07*>—Heat strongly 1.0 g of Iotroxic

Acid as directed under Residue on Ignition Test <2.44>, then proceed according to Method 2, and perform the test. Prepare the control solution with 1.0 mL of Standard Lead Solution (not more than 10 ppm).

(6) Related substances—Dissolve 0.15 g of Iotroxic Acid in 10 mL of methanol, and use this solution as the sample solution. Pipet 1 mL of the sample solution, add methanol to make exactly 200 mL, and use this solution as the standard solution. Perform the test with these solutions as directed under Thin-layer Chromatography <2.03>. Spot 10 μL each of the sample solution and standard solution on a plate of silica gel with fluorescent indicator for thin-layer chromatography. Develop the plate with a mixture of toluene, acetone and formic acid (6:4:1) to a distance of about 15 cm, and air-dry the plate. Examine under ultraviolet light (main wavelength: 254 nm): the spots other than the principal spot obtained from the sample solution are not more intense than the spot from the standard solution.

Water <2.48> 1.0 – 2.0% (0.5 g, volumetric titration, direct titration).

Residue on ignition <2.44> Not more than 0.1% (1 g).

Assay Weigh accurately about 0.5 g of Iotroxic Acid, dissolve in 40 mL of sodium hydroxide TS in a saponification flask, add 1 g of zinc powder, and boil for 30 minutes under a reflux condenser. After cooling, filter, wash the flask and the filter paper with 50 mL of water, and combine the washings to the filtrate. To this solution add 5 mL of acetic acid (100), and titrate <2.50> with 0.1 mol/L silver nitrate VS (potentiometric titration).

Each mL of 0.1 mol/L silver nitrate VS
= 20.26 mg of $C_{22}H_{18}I_6N_2O_9$

Containers and storage Containers—Tight containers.
Storage—Light-resistant.

Ipratropium Bromide Hydrate

イプラトロピウム臭化物水和物

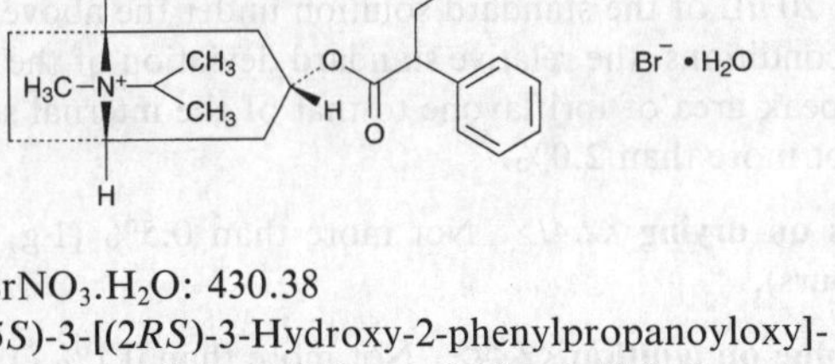

$C_{20}H_{30}BrNO_3.H_2O$: 430.38
(1*R*,3*r*,5*S*)-3-[(2*RS*)-3-Hydroxy-2-phenylpropanoyloxy]-8-methyl-8-(1-methylethyl)-8-azoniabicyclo[3.2.1]octane bromide monohydrate
[66985-17-9]

Ipratropium Bromide Hydrate, when dried, contains not less than 99.0% of ipratropium bromide ($C_{20}H_{30}BrNO_3$: 412.36).

Description Ipratropium Bromide Hydrate occurs as a white crystalline powder.

It is freely soluble in water, soluble in ethanol (99.5), slightly soluble in acetonitrile and in acetic acid (100), and practically insoluble in diethyl ether.

The pH of a solution of 1.0 g of Ipratropium Bromide Hydrate in 20 mL of water is between 5.0 and 7.5.

Melting point: about 223°C (with decomposition, after drying).

Identification **(1)** To 5 mg of Ipratropium Bromide Hydrate add 0.5 mL of fuming nitric acid, and evaporate on a water bath to dryness. After cooling, dissolve the residue in 5 mL of acetone, and add 2 drops of potassium hydroxide-ethanol TS: a purple color develops.

(2) Determine the absorption spectrum of a solution of Ipratropium Bromide Hydrate in 0.01 mol/L hydrochloric acid TS (3 in 2000) as directed under Ultraviolet-visible Spectrophotometry <2.24>, and compare the spectrum with the Reference Spectrum: both spectra exhibit similar intensities of absorption at the same wavelengths.

(3) Determine the infrared absorption spectrum of Ipratropium Bromide Hydrate as directed in the potassium bromide disk method under Infrared Spectrophotometry <2.25>, and compare the spectrum with the Reference Spectrum: both spectra exhibit similar intensities of absorption at the same wave numbers.

(4) The solution of Ipratropium Bromide Hydrate (1 in 100) responds to Qualitative Tests <1.09> for bromide.

Purity **(1)** Clarity and color of solution—Dissolve 1.0 g of Ipratropium Bromide Hydrate in 20 mL of water: the solution is clear and colorless.

(2) Sulfate <1.14>—Perform the test with 1.0 g of Ipratropium Bromide Hydrate. Prepare the control solution with 0.50 mL of 0.005 mol/L sulfuric acid VS (not more than 0.024%).

(3) Heavy metals <1.07>—Proceed with 2.0 g of Ipratropium Bromide Hydrate according to Method 4, and perform the test. Prepare the control solution with 2.0 mL of Standard Lead Solution (not more than 10 ppm).

(4) Arsenic <1.11>—Prepare the test solution with 2.0 g of Ipratropium Bromide Hydrate according to Method 3, and perform the test. Use a solution of magnesium nitrate hexahydrate in ethanol (95) (1 in 10) (not more than 1 ppm).

(5) Isopropylatropine bromide—Dissolve 25 mg of Ipratropium Bromide Hydrate in the mobile phase to make exactly 100 mL, and use this solution as the sample solution. Perform the test with 25 μL of the sample solution as directed under Liquid Chromatography <2.01> according to the following conditions. Determine the peak area, A_a, of ipratropium and the peak area, A_b, having the relative retention time to ipratropium about 1.3 by the automatic integration method: $A_b/(A_a + A_b)$ is not more than 0.01, and no peak other than the peak of ipratropium and the peak having the relative retention time to ipratropium about 1.3 appears within about 14 minutes of the retention time after the solvent peak.

Operating conditions—

Detector: An ultraviolet absorption photometer (wavelength: 210 nm).

Column: A stainless steel column about 4 mm in inside diameter and 10 to 15 cm in length, packed with octylsilanized silica gel for liquid chromatography (5 μm in particle diameter).

Column temperature: Room temperature.

Mobile phase: A mixture of diluted phosphoric acid (1 in 200), acetonitrile and methanesulfonic acid (1000:120:1).

Flow rate: Adjust so that the retention time of ipratropium is about 7 minutes.

Selection of column: Heat a solution of Ipratropium Bromide Hydrate in 1 mol/L hydrochloric acid TS (1 in 100) at 100°C for 1 hour, and cool. To 2.5 mL of this solution add the mobile phase to make 100 mL. Proceed with 25 μL of this solution under the above operating conditions, and calculate the resolution. Use a column showing a resolution not less than 3 between the peak of ipratropium and the peak having the relative retention time to ipratropium about 0.6.

Detection sensitivity: Adjust so that the peak height of ipratropium obtained with 25 μL of the sample solution composes 50 to 80% of the full scale.

(6) Apo-compounds—Dissolve 0.14 g of Ipratropium Bromide Hydrate in 0.01 mol/L hydrochloric acid TS to make 100 mL. Perform the test with this solution as directed under Ultraviolet-visible Spectrophotometry *<2.24>*, and determine the absorbances, A_1 and A_2, at 246 nm and 263 nm, respectively: A_1/A_2 is not more than 0.91.

Loss on drying *<2.41>* 3.9 - 4.4% (1 g, 105°C, 4 hours).

Residue on ignition *<2.44>* Not more than 0.1% (1 g).

Assay Weigh accurately about 0.3 g of Ipratropium Bromide Hydrate, previously dried, dissolve in 40 mL of acetic acid (100), add 40 mL of 1,4-dioxane and 2.5 mL of bismuth nitrate TS, and titrate *<2.50>* with 0.1 mol/L perchloric acid VS (potentiometric titration). Perform a blank determination in the same manner, and make any necessary correction.

Each mL of 0.1 mol/L perchloric acid VS
= 41.24 mg of $C_{20}H_{30}BrNO_3$

Containers and storage Containers—Tight containers.

Ipriflavone

イプリフラボン

$C_{18}H_{16}O_3$: 280.32
7-(1-Methylethyl)oxy-3-phenyl-4*H*-chromen-4-one
[35212-22-7]

Ipriflavone, when dried, contains not less than 98.5% and not more than 101.0% of ipriflavone ($C_{18}H_{16}O_3$).

Description Ipriflavone occurs as white to yellowish white, crystals or crystalline powder.

It is soluble in acetonitrile, sparingly soluble in methanol and in ethanol (99.5), and practically insoluble in water.

It gradually turns yellow on exposure to light.

Identification **(1)** Determine the absorption spectrum of a solution of Ipriflavone in methanol (1 in 200,000) as directed under Ultraviolet-visible Spectrophotometry *<2.24>*, and compare the spectrum with the Reference Spectrum or the spectrum of a solution of Ipriflavone RS prepared in the same manner as the sample solution: both spectra exhibit similar intensities of absorption at the same wavelengths.

(2) Determine the infrared absorption spectrum of Ipriflavone as directed in the potassium bromide disk method under Infrared Spectrophotometry *<2.25>*, and compare the spectrum with the Reference Spectrum or the spectrum of Ipriflavone RS: both spectra exhibit similar intensities of absorption at the same wave numbers.

Melting point *<2.60>* 116 - 119°C

Purity **(1)** Heavy metals *<1.07>*—Proceed with 1.0 g of Ipriflavone according to Method 2, and perform the test. Prepare the control solution with 1.0 mL of Standard Lead Solution (not more than 10 ppm).

(2) Arsenic *<1.11>*—Prepare the test solution with 1.0 g of Ipriflavone according to Method 4, and perform the test. Prepare the test solution with 10 mL of dilute hydrochloric acid instead of using 3 mL of hydrochloric acid. Prepare the standard color with 1.0 mL of Standard Arsenic Solution (not more than 1 ppm).

(3) Related substances—Dissolve 30 mg of Ipriflavone in 50 mL of acetonitrile. To 5 mL of this solution add acetonitrile to make 50 mL, and use this solution as the sample solution. Pipet 1 mL of this solution, add acetonitrile to make exactly 100 mL, and use this solution as the standard solution. Perform the test with exactly 20 μL each of the sample solution and standard solution as directed under Liquid Chromatography *<2.01>* according to the following conditions. Determine each peak area of both solutions by the automatic integration method: the area of each peak other than the peak of ipriflavone obtained from the sample solution is not larger than 1/2 times the peak area of ipriflavone from the standard solution, and the total area of the peaks other than the peak of ipriflavone from the sample solution is not larger than the peak area of ipriflavone from the standard solution.

Operating conditions—

Detector, column, column temperature, mobile phase and flow rate: Proceed as directed in the operating conditions in the Assay.

Time span of measurement: About 2 times as long as the retention time of ipriflavone, beginning after the solvent peak.

System suitability—

Test for required detectability: Pipet 2 mL of the standard solution, and add acetonitrile to make exactly 20 mL. Confirm that the peak area of ipriflavone obtained with 20 μL of this solution is equivalent to 7 to 13% of that with 20 μL of the standard solution.

System performance: When the procedure is run with 20 μL of the standard solution under the above operating conditions, the number of theoretical plates and the symmetry factor of the peak of ipriflavone are not less than 2000 and not more than 1.5, respectively.

System repeatability: When the test is repeated 6 times with 20 μL of the standard solution under the above operating conditions, the relative standard deviation of the ratio of the peak area of ipriflavone to that of the internal standard is not more than 2.0%.

Loss on drying *<2.41>* Not more than 0.5% (1 g, 105°C, 2 hours).

Residue on ignition *<2.44>* Not more than 0.1% (1 g).

Assay Weigh accurately about 30 mg each of Ipriflavone and Ipriflavone RS, previously dried, dissolve separately in acetonitrile to make exactly 50 mL. Pipet 5 mL each of these solutions, add exactly 5 mL of the internal standard solution and acetonitrile to make 50 mL, and use these solutions as the sample solution and the standard solution, respectively. Perform the test with 20 μL each of the sample solution and standard solution as directed under Liquid Chromatography *<2.01>* according to the following conditions, and calculate the ratios, Q_T and Q_S, of the peak area of ipriflavone to that of the internal standard.

Amount (mg) of ipriflavone ($C_{18}H_{16}O_3$)
$= M_S \times Q_T/Q_S$

M_S: Amount (mg) of Ipriflavone RS taken

Internal standard solution—A solution of di-*n*-butyl phthalate in acetonitrile (1 in 100).

Operating conditions—

Detector: An ultraviolet absorption photometer (wavelength: 280 nm).

Column: A stainless steel column 4 mm in inside diameter and 15 cm in length, packed with octylsilanized silica gel for liquid chromatography (5 μm in particle diameter).

Column temperature: A constant temperature of about 25°C.

Mobile phase: A mixture of acetonitrile and water (3:2).

Flow rate: Adjust so that the retention time of ipriflavone is about 6 minutes.

System suitability—

System performance: When the procedure is run with 20 μL of the standard solution under the above operating conditions, ipriflavone and the internal standard are eluted in this order with the resolution between these peaks being not less than 3.

System repeatability: When the test is repeated 6 times with 20 μL of the standard solution under the above operating conditions, the relative standard deviation of the ratio of the peak area of ipriflavone to that of the internal standard is not more than 1.0%.

Containers and storage Containers—Tight containers.

Storage—Light-resistant.

Ipriflavone Tablets

イプリフラボン錠

Ipriflavone Tablets contain not less than 95.0% and not more than 105.0% of the labeled amount of ipriflavone ($C_{18}H_{16}O_3$: 280.32).

Method of preparation Prepare as directed under Tablets, with Ipriflavone.

Identification To a quantity of powdered Ipriflavone Tablets, equivalent to 11 mg of Ipriflavone, add 100 mL of methanol, shake vigorously for 10 minutes, and centrifuge. To 5 mL of the supernatant liquid add methanol to make 100 mL. Determine the absorption spectrum of this solution as directed under Ultraviolet-visible Spectrophotometry *<2.24>*: it exhibits maxima between 247 nm and 251 nm, and between 297 nm and 301 nm.

Uniformity of dosage units *<6.02>* It meets the requirement of the Mass variation test.

Dissolution Being specified separately when the drug is granted approval based on the Law.

Assay Weigh accurately the mass of not less than 20 Ipriflavone Tablets, and powder. Weigh accurately a portion of the powder, equivalent to about 30 mg of ipriflavone ($C_{18}H_{16}O_3$), add 30 mL of acetonitrile, shake vigorously for 15 minutes, add acetonitrile to make exactly 50 mL, and centrifuge. Pipet 5 mL of the supernatant liquid, add exactly 5 mL of the internal standard solution, and add acetonitrile to make 50 mL, and use this solution as the sample solution. Separately, weigh accurately about 30 mg of Ipriflavone RS, previously dried at 105°C for 2 hours, and dissolve in acetonitrile to make exactly 50 mL. Pipet 5 mL of this solution, add exactly 5 mL of the internal standard solution, and add acetonitrile to make 50 mL, and use this solution as the standard solution. Proceed as directed in the Assay under Ipriflavone.

Amount (mg) of ipriflavone ($C_{18}H_{16}O_3$)
$= M_S \times Q_T/Q_S$

M_S: Amount (mg) of Ipriflavone RS taken

Internal standard solution—A solution of di-*n*-butyl phthalate in acetonitrile (1 in 100).

Containers and storage Containers—Tight containers.

Storage—Light-resistant.

Irbesartan

イルベサルタン

$C_{25}H_{28}N_6O$: 428.53

2-Butyl-3-{[2′-(1*H*-tetrazol-5-yl)biphenyl-4-yl]methyl}-1,3-diazaspiro[4.4]non-1-en-4-one

[*138402-11-6*]

Irbesartan contains not less than 99.0% and not more than 101.0% of irbesartan ($C_{25}H_{28}N_6O$), calculated on the anhydrous basis.

Description Irbesartan occurs as a white crystalline powder.

It is freely soluble in acetic acid (100), sparingly soluble in methanol, slightly soluble in ethanol (99.5) and practically insoluble in water.

It shows crystal polymorphism.

Identification (1) Determine the absorption spectrum of a solution of Irbesartan in methanol (1 in 100,000) as directed under Ultraviolet-visible Spectrophotometry *<2.24>*, and compare the spectrum with the Reference Spectrum: both spectra exhibit similar intensities of absorption at the same wavelengths.

(2) Determine the infrared absorption spectrum of Irbesartan as directed in the potassium bromide disk method under Infrared Spectrophotometry *<2.25>*, and compare the spectrum with the Reference Spectrum: both spectra exhibit similar intensities of absorption at the same wave numbers. If any difference appears between the spectra, dissolve the Irbesartan in methanol, evaporate the solvent, dry the residue, and perform the test using the residue.

Purity (1) Heavy metals *<1.07>*—Proceed with 1.0 g of Irbesartan according to Method 4, and perform the test. Prepare the control solution with 2.0 mL of Standard Lead Solution (not more than 20 ppm).

(2) Related substances—Dissolve 50 mg of Irbesartan in 50 mL of methanol, and use this solution as the sample solution. Pipet 1 mL of the sample solution, and add methanol to make exactly 20 mL. Pipet 1 mL of this solution, add methanol to make exactly 50 mL, and use this solution as the standard solution. Perform the test with exactly 10 μL each of the sample solution and standard solution as directed under Liquid Chromatography *<2.01>* according to the following conditions. Determine each peak area by the automatic integration method: the area of the peak, having a relative retention time of about 0.8 to irbesartan, obtained from the sample solution is not larger than 1.5 times the

peak area of irbesartan from the standard solution, the area of the peak other than irbesartan and the peak mentioned above from the sample solution is not larger than the peak area of irbesartan from the standard solution, and the total area of the peaks other than irbesartan from the sample solutions is not larger than 2 times the peak area of irbesartan from the standard solution.

Operating conditions—

Detector: An ultraviolet absorption photometer (wavelength: 220 nm).

Column: A stainless steel column 4.0 mm in inside diameter and 25 cm in length, packed with octadecylsilanized silica gel for liquid chromatography (5 μm in particle diameter).

Column temperature: A constant temperature of about 25°C.

Mobile phase: To 5.5 mL of phosphoric acid add 950 mL of water, and adjust to pH 3.2 with triethylamine. To 670 mL of this solution add 330 mL of acetonitrile for liquid chromatography.

Flow rate: 1.0 mL per minute.

Time span of measurement: About 1.4 times as long as the retention time of irbesartan, beginning after the solvent peak.

System suitability—

Test for required detectability: Pipet 5 mL of the standard solution, and add methanol to make exactly 10 mL. Confirm that the peak area of irbesartan obtained with 10 μL of this solution is equivalent to 35 to 65% of that with 10 μL of the standard solution.

System performance: When the procedure is run with 10 μL of the standard solution under the above operating conditions, the number of theoretical plates and the symmetry factor of the peak of irbesartan are not less than 5000 and not more than 1.5, respectively.

System repeatability: When the test is repeated 6 times with 10 μL of the standard solution under the above operating conditions, the relative standard deviation of the peak area of irbesartan is not more than 3.0%.

(3) Azides—Being specified separately when the drug is granted approval based on the Law.

Water <*2.48*> Not more than 0.5% (1 g, volumetric titration, back titration).

Residue on ignition <*2.44*> Not more than 0.1% (1 g).

Assay Weigh accurately about 0.3 g of Irbesartan, dissolve in 50 mL of acetic acid (100), and titrate <*2.50*> with 0.1 mol/L perchloric acid VS (potentiometric titration). Perform a blank determination in the same manner, and make any necessary correction.

Each mL of 0.1 mol/L perchloric acid VS
= 42.85 mg of $C_{25}H_{28}N_6O$

Containers and storage Containers—Tight containers.

Irbesartan Tablets

イルベサルタン錠

Irbesartan Tablets contain not less than 95.0% and not more than 105.0% of the labeled amount of irbesartan ($C_{25}H_{28}N_6O$: 428.53).

Method of preparation Prepare as directed under Tablets, with Irbesartan.

Identification To a quantity of powdered Irbesartan Tablets, equivalent to about 25 mg of Irbesartan, add 2 mL of acetone, shake, and filter through a membrane filter with a pore size not exceeding 0.45 μm. Evaporate the filtrate to dryness, and determine the infrared absorption spectrum of the residue as directed in the potassium bromide disk method under Infrared Spectrophotometry <*2.25*>: it exhibits absorptions at the wave numbers of about 1733 cm^{-1}, 1617 cm^{-1}, 1435 cm^{-1} and 758 cm^{-1}.

Uniformity of dosage unit <*6.02*> Perform the Mass variation test, or the Content uniformity test according to the following method: it meets the requirement.

To 1 tablet of Irbesartan Tablets add 1.5 mL of water, shake vigorously to disintegrate, and add 15 mL of methanol. Shake vigorously for 15 minutes, add methanol to make exactly 20 mL, and centrifuge. Pipet V mL of the supernatant liquid, equivalent to about 20 mg of irbesartan ($C_{25}H_{28}N_6O$), and add a mixture of water and acetonitrile for liquid chromatography (3:2) to make exactly 20 mL. Pipet 2.5 mL of this solution, add a mixture of water and acetonitrile for liquid chromatography (3:2) to make exactly 20 mL, and use this solution as the sample solution. Then, proceed as directed in the Assay.

$$\text{Amount (mg) of irbesartan } (C_{25}H_{28}N_6O) = M_S \times A_T/A_S \times 16/V$$

M_S: Amount (mg) of irbesartan for assay taken, calculated on the anhydrous basis

Dissolution <*6.10*> When the test is performed at 50 revolutions per minute according to the Paddle method, using 900 mL of 2nd fluid for dissolution test as the dissolution medium, the dissolution rate in 45 minutes of 50-mg and 100-mg tablets is not less than 85%, respectively, and that in 60 minutes of a 200-mg tablet is not less than 70%.

Start the test with 1 tablet of Irbesartan Tablets, withdraw not less than 10 mL of the medium at the specified minute after starting the test, and filter through a membrane filter with a pore size not exceeding 0.45 μm. Discard not less than 3 mL of the first filtrate, pipet V mL of the subsequent filtrate, add the dissolution medium to make exactly V' mL so that each mL contains about 22 μg of irbesartan ($C_{25}H_{28}N_6O$), and use this solution as the sample solution. Separately, weigh accurately about 44 mg of irbesartan for assay (separately determine the water <*2.48*> in the same manner as Irbesartan), and dissolve in methanol to make exactly 20 mL. Pipet 2 mL of this solution, add the dissolution medium to make exactly 200 mL, and use this solution as the standard solution. Determine the absorbances, A_T and A_S, of the sample solution and standard solution at 244 nm as directed under Ultraviolet-visible Spectrophotometry <*2.24*>, using the dissolution medium as the control.

$$\text{Dissolution rate (\%) with respect to the labeled amount of irbesartan } (C_{25}H_{28}N_6O) = M_S \times A_T/A_S \times V'/V \times 1/C \times 45$$

M_S: Amount (mg) of irbesartan for assay taken, calculated on the anhydrous basis

C: Labeled amount (mg) of irbesartan ($C_{25}H_{28}N_6O$) in 1 tablet

Assay To 10 Irbesartan Tablets add 15 mL of water, shake vigorously to disintegrate, and add 150 mL of methanol. Shake vigorously for 15 minutes, add methanol to make exactly 200 mL, and centrifuge. Pipet V mL of the supernatant liquid, equivalent to about 20 mg of irbesartan ($C_{25}H_{28}N_6O$), and add a mixture of water and acetonitrile for liquid chromatography (3:2) to make exactly 20 mL. Pipet

2.5 mL of this solution, add a mixture of water and acetonitrile for liquid chromatography (3:2) to make exactly 20 mL, and use this solution as the sample solution. Separately, weigh accurately about 25 mg of irbesartan for assay (separately determine the water <*2.48*> in the same manner as Irbesartan), and dissolve in methanol to make exactly 10 mL. Pipet 2.5 mL of this solution, add a mixture of water and acetonitrile for liquid chromatography (3:2) to make exactly 50 mL, and use this solution as the standard solution. Perform the test with exactly 15 μL each of the sample solution and standard solution as directed under Liquid Chromatography <*2.01*> according to the following conditions, and determine the peak areas, A_T and A_S, of irbesartan in each solution.

Amount (mg) of irbesartan ($C_{25}H_{28}N_6O$) in 1 tablet
$= M_S \times A_T/A_S \times 16/V$

M_S: Amount (mg) of irbesartan for assay taken, calculated on the anhydrous basis

Operating conditions—

Detector: An ultraviolet absorption photometer (wavelength: 220 nm).

Column: A stainless steel column 4.6 mm in inside diameter and 25 cm in length, packed with octadecylsilanized silica gel for liquid chromatography (5 μm in particle diameter).

Column temperature: A constant temperature of about 25°C.

Mobile phase: To 5.5 mL of phosphoric acid add 950 mL of water, adjust to pH 3.0 with triethylamine, and add water to make 1000 mL. To 3 volume of this solution add 2 volume of acetonitrile for liquid chromatography.

Flow rate: Adjust so that the retention time of irbesartan is about 13 minutes.

System suitability—

System performance: When the procedure is run with 15 μL of the standard solution under the above operating conditions, the number of theoretical plates and the symmetry factor of the peak of irbesartan are not less than 10,000 and not more than 1.5, respectively.

System repeatability: When the test is repeated 6 times with 15 μL of the standard solution under the above operating conditions, the relative standard deviation of the peak area of irbesartan is not more than 1.0%.

Containers and storage Containers—Tight containers.

Irbesartan and Amlodipine Besilate Tablets

イルベサルタン·アムロジピンベシル酸塩錠

Irbesartan and Amlodipine Besilate Tablets contain not less than 95.0% and not more than 105.0% of the labeled amount of irbesartan ($C_{25}H_{28}N_6O$: 428.53) and amlodipine besilate ($C_{20}H_{25}ClN_2O_5.C_6H_6O_3S$: 567.05).

Method of preparation Prepare as directed under Tablets, with Irbesartan and Amlodipine Besilate.

Identification **(1)** Perform the test with 5 μL each of the sample solution and standard solution obtained in the Assay (1) as directed under Liquid Chromatography <*2.01*> according to the following conditions: the retention time of the peak of irbesartan in the chromatogram from the sample solution is the same with that of the principal peak in the chromatogram from the standard solution, and both absorption spectra of these peaks exhibit similar intensities of absorption at the same wavelengths.

Operating conditions—

Column, column temperature, mobile phase and flow rate: Proceed as directed in the operating conditions in the Assay (1).

Detector: A photodiode array detector (wavelength: 237 nm, spectrum range of measurement: 210 – 400 nm).

System suitability—

System performance: Proceed as directed in the system suitability in the Assay (1).

(2) Perform the test with 5 μL each of the sample solution and standard solution obtained in the Assay (2) as directed under Liquid Chromatography <*2.01*> according to the following conditions: the retention time of the peak of amlodipine in the chromatogram from the sample solution is the same with that of the principal peak in the chromatogram from the standard solution, and both absorption spectra of these peaks exhibit similar intensities of absorption at the same wavelengths.

Operating conditions—

Column, column temperature, mobile phase and flow rate: Proceed as directed in the operating conditions in the Assay (1).

Detector: A photodiode array detector (wavelength: 237 nm, spectrum range of measurement: 210 – 400 nm).

System suitability—

System performance: Proceed as directed in the system suitability in the Assay (2).

Uniformity of dosage unit <*6.02*> **(1)** Irbesartan—Perform the Mass variation test, or the Content uniformity test according to the following method: it meets the requirement.

To 1 tablet of Irbesartan and Amlodipine Besilate Tablets add 4 mL of 0.02 mol/L phosphate buffer solution (pH 3.0), and sonicate. Add 16 mL of methanol, shake vigorously until the tablet is disintegrated completely, and add the mobile phase to make exactly 100 mL. Pipet *V* mL of this solution, add the mobile phase to make exactly *V′* mL so that each mL contains about 1 mg of irbesartan ($C_{25}H_{28}N_6O$), and filter through a membrane filter with a pore size not exceeding 0.45 μm. Discard the first 5 mL of the filtrate, and use the subsequent filtrate as the sample solution. Then, proceed as directed under the Assay (1).

Amount (mg) of irbesartan ($C_{25}H_{28}N_6O$)
$= M_S \times A_T/A_S \times V'/V \times 2$

M_S: Amount (mg) of irbesartan for assay taken, calculated on the anhydrous basis

(2) Amlodipine besilate—Perform the test according to the following method: it meets the requirement of the Content uniformity test.

To 1 tablet of Irbesartan and Amlodipine Besilate Tablets add 4 mL of 0.02 mol/L phosphate buffer solution (pH 3.0), and sonicate. Add 16 mL of methanol, shake vigorously until the tablet is disintegrated completely, and add the mobile phase to make exactly 100 mL. Pipet *V* mL of this solution, add the mobile phase to make exactly *V′* mL so that each mL contains about 69 μg of amlodipine besilate ($C_{20}H_{25}ClN_2O_5.C_6H_6O_3S$), and filter through a membrane filter with a pore size not exceeding 0.45 μm. Discard the first 5 mL of the filtrate, and use the subsequent filtrate as the sample solution. Then, proceed as directed under the Assay (2).

Amount (mg) of amlodipine besilate
($C_{20}H_{25}ClN_2O_5.C_6H_6O_3S$)
$= M_S \times A_T/A_S \times V'/V \times 1/5$

M_S: Amount (mg) of Amlodipine Besilate RS taken, calculated on the anhydrous basis

Dissolution <*6.10*> **(1)** Irbesartan—When the test is performed at 50 revolutions per minute according to the Paddle method, using 900 mL of 2nd fluid for dissolution test as the dissolution medium, the dissolution rate in 30 minutes of Irbesartan and Amlodipine Besilate Tablets is not less than 70%.

Start the test with 1 tablet of Irbesartan and Amlodipine Besilate Tablets, withdraw not less than 15 mL of the medium at the specified minute after starting the test, and filter through a membrane filter with a pore size not exceeding 0.45 μm. Discard not less than 10 mL of the first filtrate, pipet V mL of the subsequent filtrate, and add the mobile phase to make exactly V' mL so that each mL contains about 0.11 mg of irbesartan ($C_{25}H_{28}N_6O$). Pipet 2 mL of this solution, add exactly 2 mL of the mobile phase, and use this solution as the sample solution. Separately, weigh accurately about 20 mg of irbesartan for assay (separately determine the water <*2.48*> in the same manner as Irbesartan), dissolve in the mobile phase to make exactly 25 mL, and use this solution as the irbesartan standard stock solution. Pipet 7 mL of the irbesartan standard stock solution, and add the mobile phase to make exactly 50 mL. Pipet 5 mL of this solution, add exactly 5 mL of the dissolution medium, and use this solution as the standard solution. Perform the test with exactly 10 μL each of the sample solution and standard solution as directed under Liquid Chromatography <*2.01*> according to the following conditions, and determine the peak areas, A_T and A_S, of irbesartan in each solution.

Dissolution rate (%) with respect to the labeled amount of irbesartan ($C_{25}H_{28}N_6O$)
$= M_S \times A_T/A_S \times V'/V \times 1/C \times 504$

M_S: Amount (mg) of irbesartan for assay taken, calculated on the anhydrous basis
C: Labeled amount (mg) of irbesartan ($C_{25}H_{28}N_6O$) in 1 tablet

Operating conditions—

Proceed as directed in the operating conditions in the Assay (1).

System suitability—

System performance: To 7 mL of the irbesartan standard stock solution and 5 mL of the amlodipine besilate standard stock solution obtained in (2) add the mobile phase to make 50 mL. To 5 mL of this solution add 5 mL of the dissolution medium. When the procedure is run with 10 μL of this solution under the above operating conditions, amlodipine and irbesartan are eluted in this order with the resolution between these peaks being not less than 5.

System repeatability: When the test is repeated 6 times with 10 μL of the standard solution under the above operating conditions, the relative standard deviation of the peak area of irbesartan is not more than 2.0%.

(2) Amlodipine besilate—When the test is performed at 50 revolutions per minute according to the Paddle method, using 900 mL of 2nd fluid for dissolution test as the dissolution medium, the dissolution rate in 30 minutes of Irbesartan and Amlodipine Besilate Tablets is not less than 75%.

Start the test with 1 tablet of Irbesartan and Amlodipine Besilate Tablets, withdraw not less than 15 mL of the medium at the specified minute after starting the test, and filter through a membrane filter with a pore size not exceeding 0.45 μm. Discard not less than 10 mL of the first filtrate, pipet V mL of the subsequent filtrate, and add the mobile phase to make exactly V' mL so that each mL contains about 7.7 μg of amlodipine besilate ($C_{20}H_{25}ClN_2O_5.C_6H_6O_3S$). Pipet 2 mL of this solution, add exactly 2 mL of the mobile phase, and use this solution as the sample solution. Separately, weigh accurately about 26 mg of Amlodipine Besilate RS (separately determine the water <*2.48*> in the same manner as Amlodipine Besilate), and dissolve in the mobile phase to make exactly 50 mL. Pipet 15 mL of this solution, add the mobile phase to make exactly 100 mL, and use this solution as the amlodipine besilate standard stock solution. Pipet 5 mL of the amlodipine besilate standard stock solution, and add the mobile phase to make exactly 50 mL. Pipet 5 mL of this solution, add exactly 5 mL of the dissolution medium, and use this solution as the standard solution. Perform the test with exactly 10 μL each of the sample solution and standard solution as directed under Liquid Chromatography <*2.01*> according to the following conditions, and determine the peak areas, A_T and A_S, of amlodipine in each solution.

Dissolution rate (%) with respect to the labeled amount of amlodipine besilate ($C_{20}H_{25}ClN_2O_5.C_6H_6O_3S$)
$= M_S \times A_T/A_S \times V'/V \times 1/C \times 27$

M_S: Amount (mg) of Amlodipine Besilate RS taken, calculated on the anhydrous basis
C: Labeled amount (mg) of amlodipine besilate ($C_{20}H_{25}ClN_2O_5.C_6H_6O_3S$) in 1 tablet

Operating conditions—

Proceed as directed in the operating conditions in the Assay (1).

System suitability—

System performance: To 7 mL of the irbesartan standard stock solution obtained in (1) and 5 mL of the amlodipine besilate standard stock solution add the mobile phase to make 50 mL. To 5 mL of this solution add 5 mL of the dissolution medium. When the procedure is run with 10 μL of this solution under the above operating conditions, amlodipine and irbesartan are eluted in this order with the resolution between these peaks being not less than 5.

System repeatability: When the test is repeated 6 times with 10 μL of the standard solution under the above operating conditions, the relative standard deviation of the peak area of amlodipine is not more than 2.0%.

Assay **(1)** Irbesartan—To 10 tablets of Irbesartan and Amlodipine Besilate Tablets add 20 mL of 0.02 mol/L phosphate buffer solution (pH 3.0), and sonicate. Add 120 mL of methanol, shake vigorously until the tablets are disintegrated completely, and add the mobile phase to make exactly 200 mL. Pipet V mL of this solution, add the mobile phase to make exactly V' mL so that each mL contains about 1 mg of irbesartan ($C_{25}H_{28}N_6O$), and filter through a membrane filter with a pore size not exceeding 0.45 μm. Discard the first 5 mL of the filtrate, and use the subsequent filtrate as the sample solution. Separately, weigh accurately about 50 mg of irbesartan for assay (separately determine the water <*2.48*> in the same manner as Irbesartan), dissolve in methanol to make exactly 25 mL, and use this solution as the irbesartan standard stock solution. Pipet 10 mL of the irbesartan standard stock solution, add 2 mL of methanol, add 0.02 mol/L phosphate buffer solution (pH 3.0) to make exactly 20 mL, and use this solution as the standard solution. Perform the test with exactly 5 μL each of the sample solution and standard solution as directed under Liquid Chromatography <*2.01*> according to the following conditions, and determine the peak areas, A_T and A_S, of irbesartan in each solution.

Amount (mg) of irbesartan ($C_{25}H_{28}N_6O$) in 1 tablet
$= M_S \times A_T/A_S \times V'/V \times 2/5$

M_S: Amount (mg) of irbesartan for assay taken, calculated on the anhydrous basis

Operating conditions—

Detector: An ultraviolet absorption photometer (wavelength: 237 nm).

Column: A stainless steel column 3.0 mm in inside diameter and 75 mm in length, packed with octadecylsilanized silica gel for liquid chromatography (2.2 μm in particle diameter).

Column temperature: A constant temperature of about 40°C.

Mobile phase: A mixture of methanol and 0.02 mol/L phosphate buffer solution (pH 3.0) (3:2).

Flow rate: Adjust so that the retention time of irbesartan is about 3 minutes.

System suitability—

System performance: To 10 mL of the irbesartan standard stock solution and 2 mL of the amlodipine besilate standard stock solution obtained in (2) add 0.02 mol/L phosphate buffer solution (pH 3.0) to make 20 mL. When the procedure is run with 5 μL of this solution under the above operating conditions, amlodipine and irbesartan are eluted in this order with the resolution between these peaks being not less than 5.

System repeatability: When the test is repeated 6 times with 5 μL of the standard solution under the above operating conditions, the relative standard deviation of the peak area of irbesartan is not more than 1.0%.

(2) Amlodipine besilate—To 10 tablets of Irbesartan and Amlodipine Besilate Tablets add 20 mL of 0.02 mol/L phosphate buffer solution (pH 3.0), and sonicate. Add 120 mL of methanol, shake vigorously until the tablets are disintegrated completely, and add the mobile phase to make exactly 200 mL. Pipet *V* mL of this solution, add the mobile phase to make exactly *V′* mL so that each mL contains about 69 μg of amlodipine besilate ($C_{20}H_{25}ClN_2O_5.C_6H_6O_3S$), and filter through a membrane filter with a pore size not exceeding 0.45 μm. Discard the first 5 mL of the filtrate, and use the subsequent filtrate as the sample solution. Separately, weigh accurately about 35 mg of Amlodipine Besilate RS (separately determine the water <*2.48*> in the same manner as Amlodipine Besilate), dissolve in methanol to make exactly 50 mL, and use this solution as the amlodipine besilate standard stock solution. Pipet 2 mL of the amlodipine besilate standard stock solution, add 10 mL of methanol, add 0.02 mol/L phosphate buffer solution (pH 3.0) to make exactly 20 mL, and use this solution as the standard solution. Perform the test with exactly 5 μL each of the sample solution and standard solution as directed under Liquid Chromatography <*2.01*> according to the following conditions, and determine the peak areas, A_T and A_S, of amlodipine in each solution.

Amount (mg) of amlodipine besilate ($C_{20}H_{25}ClN_2O_5.C_6H_6O_3S$) in 1 tablet
$$= M_S \times A_T/A_S \times V'/V \times 1/25$$

M_S: Amount (mg) of Amlodipine Besilate RS taken, calculated on the anhydrous basis

Operating conditions—

Proceed as directed in the operating conditions in (1).

System suitability—

System performance: To 10 mL of the irbesartan standard stock solution obtained in (1) and 2 mL of the amlodipine besilate standard stock solution add 0.02 mol/L phosphate buffer solution (pH 3.0) to make 20 mL. When the procedure is run with 5 μL of this solution under the above operating conditions, amlodipine and irbesartan are eluted in this order with the resolution between these peaks being not less than 5.

System repeatability: When the test is repeated 6 times with 5 μL of the standard solution under the above operating conditions, the relative standard deviation of the peak area of amlodipine is not more than 1.0%.

Containers and storage Containers—Tight containers.

Irinotecan Hydrochloride Hydrate

イリノテカン塩酸塩水和物

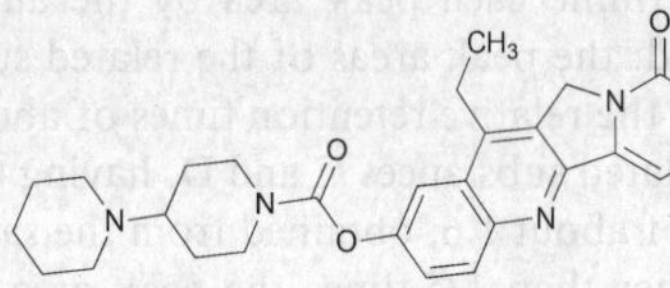

$C_{33}H_{38}N_4O_6.HCl.3H_2O$: 677.18

(4*S*)-4,11-Diethyl-4-hydroxy-3,14-dioxo-3,4,12,14-tetrahydro-1*H*-pyrano[3′,4′:6,7]indolizino[1,2-*b*]quinolin-9-yl [1,4′-bipiperidine]-1′-carboxylate monohydrochloride trihydrate
[*136572-09-3*]

Irinotecan Hydrochloride Hydrate contains not less than 99.0% and not more than 102.0% of irinotecan hydrochloride ($C_{33}H_{38}N_4O_6.HCl$: 623.14), calculated on the anhydrous basis.

Description Irinotecan Hydrochloride Hydrate occurs as pale yellow to light yellow, crystals or crystalline powder.

It is sparingly soluble in methanol, and slightly soluble in water and in ethanol (99.5).

It is gradually colored to yellow-brown and decomposed by light.

Melting point: about 255°C (with decomposition).

It shows crystal polymorphism.

Identification (1) Determine the absorption spectrum of a solution of Irinotecan Hydrochloride Hydrate in methanol (1 in 100,000) as directed under Ultraviolet-visible Spectrophotometry <*2.24*>, and compare the spectrum with the Reference Spectrum: both spectra exhibit similar intensities of absorption at the same wavelengths.

(2) Determine the infrared absorption spectrum of Irinotecan Hydrochloride Hydrate as directed in the potassium bromide disk method under Infrared Spectrophotometry <*2.25*>, and compare the spectrum with the Reference Spectrum: both spectra exhibit similar intensities of absorption at the same wave numbers.

(3) To 1 g of Irinotecan Hydrochloride Hydrate add 50 mL of water, dissolve by heating, and cool: the solution responds to Qualitative Tests <*1.09*> (2) for chloride.

Optical rotation <*2.49*> $[\alpha]_D^{20}$: + 64 – + 69° (0.5 g calculated on the anhydrous basis, water, heat, after cooling, 50 mL, 100 mm).

pH <*2.54*> Dissolve 1 g of Irinotecan Hydrochloride Hydrate in 50 mL of water by heating, and cool: the pH of this solution is between 3.5 and 4.5.

Purity (1) Heavy metals <*1.07*>—Proceed with 2.0 g of Irinotecan Hydrochloride Hydrate according to Method 2, and perform the test. Prepare the control solution with 2.0 mL of Standard Lead Solution (not more than 10 ppm).

(2) Related substances—Dissolve 50 mg of Irinotecan

Hydrochloride Hydrate in a suitable amount of a mixture of diluted 0.1 mol/L potassium dihydrogen phosphate TS (1 in 10), methanol and acetonitrile (6:4:3) and 1 mL of 1 mol/L hydrochloric acid TS, and add a mixture of diluted 0.1 mol/L potassium dihydrogen phosphate TS (1 in 10), methanol and acetonitrile (6:4:3) to make 20 mL, and use this solution as the sample solution. Pipet 1 mL of the sample solution, add a mixture of diluted 0.1 mol/L potassium dihydrogen phosphate TS (1 in 10), methanol and acetonitrile (6:4:3) to make exactly 100 mL, and use this solution as the standard solution. Perform the test with exactly 20 μL each of the sample solution and standard solution as directed under Liquid Chromatography <*2.01*> according to the following conditions. Determine each peak area by the automatic integration method: the peak areas of the related substances A and B, having the relative retention times of about 0.8 to irinotecan, and related substances C and D, having the relative retention times of about 1.6, obtained from the sample solution are not larger than 1/5 times the peak area of irinotecan from the standard solution, and the area of the peak other than irinotecan and the peaks mentioned above from the sample solution is not larger than 1/10 times the peak area of irinotecan from the standard solution. Furthermore, the total area of the peaks other than irinotecan from the sample solution is not larger than 4/5 times the peak area of irinotecan from the standard solution.

Operating conditions—

Detector: An ultraviolet absorption photometer (wavelength: 254 nm).

Column: A stainless steel column 4.6 mm in inside diameter and 25 cm in length, packed with octadecylsilanized silica gel for liquid chromatography (5 μm in particle diameter).

Column temperature: A constant temperature of about 40°C.

Mobile phase: Dissolve 1.22 g of sodium 1-decanesulfonate in a mixture of diluted 0.1 mol/L potassium dihydrogen phosphate TS (1 in 10), methanol and acetonitrile (6:4:3) to make 1000 mL.

Flow rate: Adjust so that the retention time of irinotecan is about 12 minutes.

Time span of measurement: About 3 times as long as the retention time of irinotecan.

System suitability—

Test for required detectability: Pipet 1 mL of the standard solution, and add a mixture of diluted 0.1 mol/L potassium dihydrogen phosphate TS (1 in 10), methanol and acetonitrile (6:4:3) to make exactly 20 mL. Confirm that the peak area of irinotecan obtained with 20 μL of this solution is equivalent to 3.5 to 6.5% of that with 20 μL of the standard solution.

System performance: When the procedure is run with 20 μL of the standard solution under the above operating conditions, the number of theoretical plates and the symmetry factor of the peak of irinotecan are not less than 6000 and not more than 2.0, respectively.

System repeatability: When the test is repeated 6 times with 20 μL of the standard solution under the above operating conditions, the relative standard deviation of the peak area of irinotecan is not more than 2.0%.

(3) Enantiomer—Being specified separately when the drug is granted approval based on the Law.

Water <*2.48*> 7.5 – 9.5% (0.1 g, volumetric titration, direct titration).

Residue on ignition <*2.44*> Not more than 0.1% (1 g).

Assay Weigh accurately about 0.44 g of Irinotecan Hydrochloride Hydrate, dissolve in 120 mL of a mixture of acetic anhydride and acetic acid (100) (7:3), and titrate <*2.50*> with 0.1 mol/L perchloric acid VS (potentiometric titration). Perform a blank determination in the same manner, and make any necessary correction.

Each mL of 0.1 mol/L perchloric acid VS
= 31.16 mg of $C_{33}H_{38}N_4O_6$.HCl

Containers and storage Containers—Tight containers.
Storage—Light-resistant.

Others

Related substance A:
(4*S*)-4,11-Diethyl-4,12-dihydroxy-3,14-dioxo-3,4,12,14-tetrahydro-1*H*-pyrano[3′,4′:6,7]indolizino[1,2-*b*]quinolin-9-yl [1,4′-bipiperidine]-1′-carboxylate

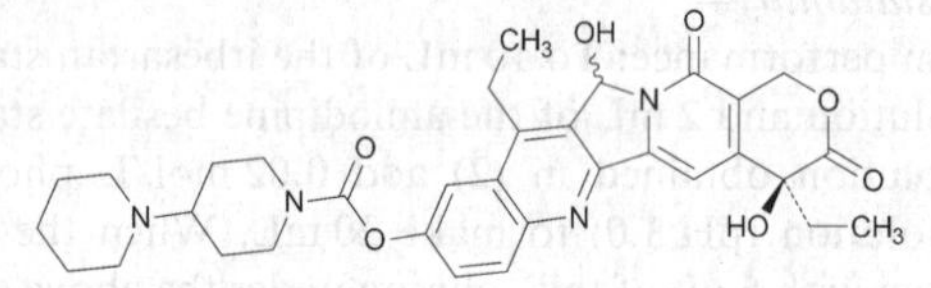

Related substance B:
(4*S*)-4,11-Diethyl-4-hydroxy-3,14-dioxo-3,4,12,14-tetrahydro-1*H*-pyrano[3′,4′:6,7]indolizino[1,2-*b*]quinolin-9-yl 2′-hydroxy-[1,4′-bipiperidine]-1′-carboxylate

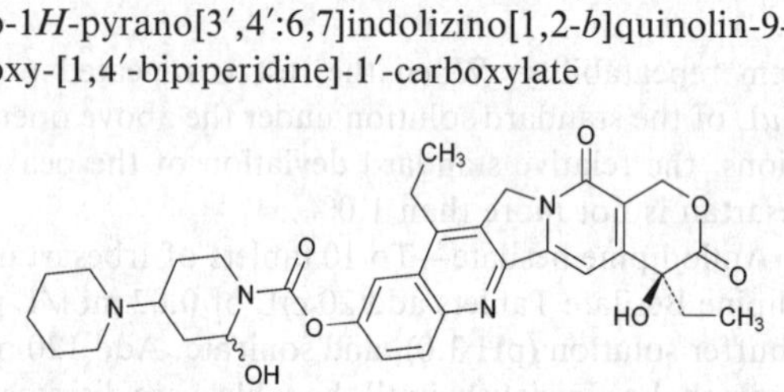

Related substance C:
(4*S*)-4,8,11-Triethyl-4-hydroxy-3,14-dioxo-3,4,12,14-tetrahydro-1*H*-pyrano[3′,4′:6,7]indolizino[1,2-*b*]quinolin-9-yl [1,4′-bipiperidine]-1′-carboxylate

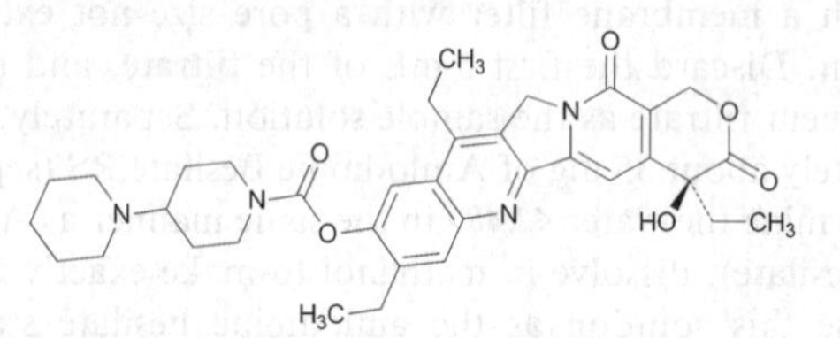

Related substance D:
(4*S*)-4,11-Diethyl-4-hydroxy-3,14-dioxo-3,4,12,14-tetrahydro-1*H*-pyrano[3′,4′:6,7]indolizino[1,2-*b*]quinolin-9-yl 2′-ethoxy-[1,4′-bipiperidine]-1′-carboxylate

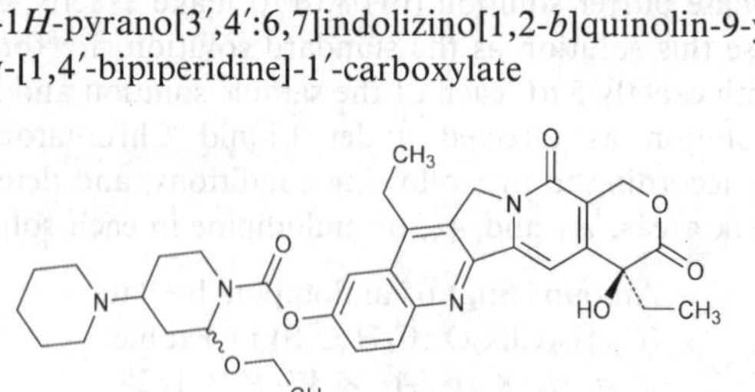

Irinotecan Hydrochloride Injection

イリノテカン塩酸塩注射液

Irinotecan Hydrochloride Injection is an aqueous injection.

It contains not less than 95.0% and not more than 105.0% of the labeled amount of irinotecan hydrochloride hydrate ($C_{33}H_{38}N_4O_6.HCl.3H_2O$: 677.18).

Method of preparation Prepare as directed under Injections, with Irinotecan Hydrochloride Hydrate.

Description Irinotecan Hydrochloride Injection is a clear and pale yellow liquid.

It is gradually decomposed by light.

Identification To a volume of Irinotecan Hydrochloride Injection, equivalent to 20 mg of Irinotecan Hydrochloride Hydrate, add water to make 10 mL. To 1 mL of this solution add water to make 100 mL. Determine the absorption spectrum of this solution as directed under Ultraviolet-visible Spectrophotometry <2.24>: it exhibits maxima between 253 nm and 257 nm, between 354 nm and 358 nm, and between 368 nm and 372 nm.

pH Being specified separately when the drug is granted approval based on the Law.

Purity Related substances—To a volume of Irinotecan Hydrochloride Injection, equivalent to 40 mg of Irinotecan Hydrochloride Hydrate, add a mixture of diluted 0.1 mol/L potassium dihydrogen phosphate TS (1 in 10), methanol and acetonitrile (6:4:3) and 1 mL of 1 mol/L hydrochloric acid TS to make 20 mL, and use this solution as the sample solution. Pipet 1 mL of this solution, add a mixture of diluted 0.1 mol/L potassium dihydrogen phosphate TS (1 in 10), methanol and acetonitrile (6:4:3) to make exactly 100 mL, and use this solution as the standard solution. Perform the test with exactly 25 μL each of the sample solution and standard solution as directed under Liquid Chromatography <2.01> according to the following conditions. Determine each peak area by the automatic integration method: the area of related substance IA, having the relative retention time of about 0.3 to irinotecan, obtained from the sample solution is not larger than 1/2 times the peak area of irinotecan from the standard solution, the areas of related substances A and B, having the relative retention time of about 0.8, from the sample solution are not larger than 3/10 times the peak area of irinotecan from the standard solution, the area of related substance IB, having the relative retention time of about 1.3, from the sample solution is not larger than 1/3 times the peak area of irinotecan from the standard solution, the areas of related substances C and D, having the relative retention time of about 1.6, and the related substance IC, having the relative retention time of about 2.2, from the sample solution are not larger than 1/5 times the peak area of irinotecan from the standard solution, and the area of the peak other than irinotecan and the peaks mentioned above from the sample solution is not larger than 1/10 times the peak area of irinotecan from the standard solution. Furthermore, the total area of the peaks other than irinotecan from the sample solution is not larger than 1.5 times the peak area of irinotecan from the standard solution.

Operating conditions—

Proceed as directed in the operating conditions in the Purity (2) under Irinotecan Hydrochloride Hydrate.

System suitability—

Test for required detectability: Pipet 1 mL of the standard solution, add a mixture of diluted 0.1 mol/L potassium dihydrogen phosphate TS (1 in 10), methanol and acetonitrile (6:4:3) to make exactly 20 mL. Confirm that the peak area of irinotecan obtained with 25 μL of this solution is equivalent to 3.5 to 6.5% of that with 25 μL of the standard solution.

System performance: When the procedure is run with 25 μL of the standard solution under the above operating conditions, the number of theoretical plates and the symmetry factor of the peak of irinotecan are not less than 6000 and not more than 2.0, respectively.

System repeatability: When the test is repeated 6 times with 25 μL of the standard solution under the above operating conditions, the relative standard deviation of the peak area of irinotecan is not more than 2.0%.

Bacterial endotoxins <4.01> Less than 1.8 EU/mg.

Extractable volume <6.05> It meets the requirement.

Foreign insoluble matter <6.06> Perform the test according to Method 1: it meets the requirement.

Insoluble particulate matter <6.07> It meets the requirement.

Sterility <4.06> Perform the test according to the Membrane filtration method: it meets the requirement.

Assay Pipet a volume of Irinotecan Hydrochloride Injection, equivalent to about 20 mg of irinotecan hydrochloride hydrate ($C_{33}H_{38}N_4O_6.HCl.3H_2O$), and add a mixture of methanol and acetic acid-sodium acetate buffer solution (pH 4.0) (11:9) to make exactly 50 mL. Pipet 10 mL of this solution, add the internal standard solution to make exactly 100 mL, and use this solution as the sample solution. Separately, weigh accurately about 20 mg of irinotecan hydrochloride hydrate for assay (separately determine the water <2.48> in the same manner as Irinotecan Hydrochloride Hydrate), dissolve in a mixture of methanol and acetic acid-sodium acetate buffer solution (pH 4.0) (11:9) to make exactly 50 mL. Pipet 10 mL of this solution, add the internal standard solution to make exactly 100 mL, and use this solution as the standard solution. Perform the test with 10 μL each of the sample solution and standard solution as directed under Liquid Chromatography <2.01> according to the following conditions, and calculate the ratios, Q_T and Q_S, of the peak area of irinotecan to that of the internal standard.

Amount (mg) of irinotecan hydrochloride hydrate ($C_{33}H_{38}N_4O_6.HCl.3H_2O$)
$= M_S \times Q_T/Q_S \times 1.087$

M_S: Amount (mg) of irinotecan hydrochloride hydrate for assay taken, calculated on the anhydrous basis

Internal standard solution—Dissolve 33.3 mg of propyl parahydroxybenzoate in a mixture of methanol and acetic acid-sodium acetate buffer solution (pH 4.0) (11:9) to make 1000 mL.

Operating conditions—

Detector: An ultraviolet absorption photometer (wavelength: 254 nm).

Column: A stainless steel column 6 mm in inside diameter and 15 cm in length, packed with octadecylsilanized silica gel for liquid chromatography (5 μm in particle diameter).

Column temperature: A constant temperature of about 40°C.

Mobile phase: Dissolve 1.01 g of sodium 1-heptanesulfonate in a mixture of methanol and acetic acid-sodium acetate buffer solution (pH 4.0) (11:9) to make 1000 mL.

Flow rate: Adjust so that the retention time of irinotecan is about 7 minutes.

System Suitability—

System performance: When the procedure is run with 10 µL of the standard solution under the above operating conditions, irinotecan and the internal standard are eluted in this order with the resolution between these peaks being not less than 6.

System repeatability: When the test is repeated 6 times with 10 µL of the standard solution under the above operating conditions, the relative standard deviation of the ratios of the peak area of irinotecan to that of the internal standard is not more than 1.0%.

Containers and storage Containers—Hermetic containers.

Storage—Light-resistant.

Others

Related substances A, B, C and D: refer to them described in Irinotecan Hydrochloride Hydrate.

Related substances IA:

6-{[1,4′-Bipiperidine]-1′-carbonyloxy}-4-ethyl-2-[(4*S*)-4-ethyl-4-hydroxy-3,8-dioxo-3,4,7,8-tetrahydro-1*H*-pyrano[3,4-*c*]pyridin-6-yl]quinoline-3-carboxylic acid

Related substances IB:

3,10-Diethyl-1,13-dioxo-1,3,11,13-tetrahydrofuro[3′,4′:6,7]indolizino[1,2-*b*]quinolin-8-yl [1,4′-bipiperidine]-1′-carboxylate

Related substances IC:

12-Ethyl-8-methyl-9-oxo-7-propionyl-9,11-dihydroindolizino[1,2-*b*]quinolin-2-yl[1,4′-bipiperidine]-1′-carboxylate

Irsogladine Maleate

イルソグラジンマレイン酸塩

$C_9H_7Cl_2N_5.C_4H_4O_4$: 372.16

6-(2,5-Dichlorophenyl)-1,3,5-triazine-2,4-diamine monomaleate

[*84504-69-8*]

Irsogladine Maleate, when dried, contains not less than 99.0% and not more than 101.0% of irsogladine maleate ($C_9H_7Cl_2N_5.C_4H_4O_4$).

Description Irsogladine Maleate occurs as white, crystals or crystalline powder. It has a slightly bitter taste.

It is sparingly soluble in acetic acid (100) and in ethylene-glycol, slightly soluble in methanol and in ethanol (99.5), and practically insoluble in water.

Identification **(1)** Dissolve 20 mg of Irsogladine Maleate in methanol to make 20 mL. Take 2 mL of this solution, and add water to make 20 mL. To 2 mL of this solution add water to make 50 mL. Determine the absorption spectrum of this solution as directed under Ultraviolet-visible Spectrophotometry <*2.24*>, and compare the spectrum with the Reference Spectrum: both spectra exhibit similar intensities of absorption at the same wavelengths.

(2) Determine the infrared absorption spectrum of Irsogladine Maleate as directed in the potassium bromide disk method under Infrared Spectrophotometry <*2.25*>, and compare the spectrum with the Reference Spectrum: both spectra exhibit similar intensities of absorption at the same wave numbers.

(3) Dissolve 10 mg of Irsogladine Maleate in 1 mL of dilute hydrochloric acid and 4 mL of water, and add 3 drops of potassium permanganate TS: the color of the solution is discharged immediately.

Purity **(1)** Heavy metals <*1.07*>—Proceed with 2.0 g of Irsogladine Maleate according to Method 4, and perform the test. Prepare the control solution with 2.0 mL of Standard Lead Solution (not more than 10 ppm).

(2) Related substances—Dissolve 50 mg of Irsogladine Maleate in 10 mL of ethylene glycol, and use this solution as the sample solution. Pipet 1 mL of the sample solution, add ethylene glycol to make exactly 100 mL, and use this solution as the standard solution. Perform the test with exactly 5 µL each of the sample solution and standard solution as directed under Liquid Chromatography <*2.01*> according to the following conditions. Determine each peak area of both solutions by the automatic integration method: the area of each peak other than the peaks of maleic acid and irsogladine obtained from the sample solution is not larger than 1/10 times the peak area of irsogladine from the standard solution.

Operating conditions—

Detector: An ultraviolet absorption photometer (wavelength: 250 nm).

Column: A stainless steel column 4.6 mm in inside diameter and 7.5 cm in length, packed with octadecylsilanized silica gel for liquid chromatography (3 µm in particle diameter).

Column temperature: A constant temperature of about 40°C.

Mobile phase: A mixture of methanesulfonic acid solution (1 in 1000) and methanol (4:1).

Flow rate: Adjust so that the retention time of irsogladine is about 8 minutes.

Time span of measurement: About 3 times as long as the retention time of irsogladine, beginning after the solvent peak.

System suitability—

Test for required detectability: Pipet 1 mL of the standard solution, and add ethylene glycol to make exactly 10 mL. Confirm that the peak area of irsogladine obtained with 5 μL of this solution is equivalent to 7 to 13% of that with 5 μL of the standard solution.

System performance: When the procedure is run with 5 μL of the standard solution under the above operating conditions, the number of theoretical plates and the symmetry factor of the peak of irsogladine are not less than 3000 and not more than 1.5, respectively.

System repeatability: When the test is repeated 6 times with 5 μL of the standard solution under the above operating conditions, the relative standard deviation of the peak area of irsogladine is not more than 2.0%.

Loss on drying <*2.41*> Not more than 0.5% (1 g, 105°C, 4 hours).

Residue on ignition <*2.44*> Not more than 0.1% (1 g).

Assay Weigh accurately about 0.3 g of Irsogladine Maleate, previously dried, dissolve in 25 mL of acetic acid (100), add 25 mL of acetic anhydride, and titrate <*2.50*> with 0.05 mol/L perchloric acid VS (potentiometric titration). Perform a blank determination in the same manner, and make any necessary correction.

Each mL of 0.05 mol/L perchloric acid VS
= 18.61 mg of $C_9H_7Cl_2N_5.C_4H_4O_4$

Containers and storage Containers—Well-closed containers.

Irsogladine Maleate Fine Granules

イルソグラジンマレイン酸塩細粒

Irsogladine Maleate Fine Granules contain not less than 93.0% and not more than 107.0% of the labeled amount of irsogladine maleate ($C_9H_7Cl_2N_5.C_4H_4O_4$: 372.16).

Method of preparation Prepare as directed under Granules, with Irsogladine Maleate.

Identification To a quantity of powdered Irsogladine Maleate Fine Granules, equivalent to 2 mg of Irsogladine Maleate, add 5 mL of methanol, shake for 10 minutes, centrifuge, and use the supernatant liquid as the sample solution. Separately, dissolve 2 mg of irsogladine maleate in 5 mL of methanol, and use this solution as the standard solution. Perform the test with these solutions as directed under Thin-layer Chromatography <*2.03*>. Spot 10 μL each of the sample solution and standard solution on a plate of silica gel with fluorescent indicator for thin-layer chromatography. Develop the plate with a mixture of petroleum ether, acetone and acetic acid (100) (12:4:1) to a distance of about 10 cm, and air-dry the plate. Examine under ultraviolet light (main wavelength: 254 nm): the spot from the sample solution has the same *R*f value as the spot from the standard solution.

Uniformity of dosage units <*6.02*> Perform the test according to the following method: Irsogladine Maleate Fine Granules in single-dose packages meet the requirement of the Content uniformity test.

Take out the total contents of 1 package of Irsogladine Maleate Fine Granules, add 2 mL of water, add 2 mL methanol per mg of irsogladine maleate ($C_9H_7Cl_2N_5.C_4H_4O_4$), sonicate for 10 minutes with occasional shaking, and add water to make exactly *V* mL so that each mL contains about 40 μg of irsogladine maleate ($C_9H_7Cl_2N_5.C_4H_4O_4$). Centrifuge this solution, pipet 1 mL of the supernatant liquid, and add water to make exactly 20 mL. Filter this solution through a membrane filter with a pore size not exceeding 0.5 μm, discard the first 10 mL of the filtrate, and use the subsequent filtrate as the sample solution. Separately, weigh accurately about 20 mg of irsogladine maleate for assay, previously dried at 105°C for 4 hours, dissolve in methanol to make exactly 20 mL. Pipet 2 mL of this solution, add water to make exactly 20 mL. Pipet 2 mL of this solution, add water to make exactly 100 mL, and use this solution as the standard solution. Perform the test with the sample solution and standard solution as directed under Ultraviolet-visible Spectrophotometry <*2.24*>, using water as the blank, and determine the absorbances, A_T and A_S, at 210 nm.

Amount (mg) of irsogladine maleate ($C_9H_7Cl_2N_5.C_4H_4O_4$)
$= M_S \times A_T/A_S \times V/500$

M_S: Amount (mg) of irsogladine maleate for assay taken

Dissolution <*6.10*> When the test is performed at 50 revolutions per minute according to the Paddle method, using 900 mL of water as the dissolution medium, the dissolution rate in 30 minutes of Irsogladine Maleate Fine Granules is not less than 70%.

Start the test with an accurately weighed amount of Irsogladine Maleate Fine Granules, equivalent to about 4 mg of irsogladine maleate ($C_9H_7Cl_2N_5.C_4H_4O_4$), withdraw not less than 20 mL of the medium at the specified minute after starting the test, and filter through a membrane filter with a pore size not exceeding 0.5 μm. Discard not less than 10 mL of the first filtrate, and use the subsequent filtrate as the sample solution. Separately, weigh accurately about 40 mg of irsogladine maleate for assay, previously dried at 105°C for 4 hours, and dissolve in methanol to make exactly 20 mL. Pipet 2 mL of this solution, and add water to make exactly 20 mL. Pipet 2 mL of this solution, add water to make exactly 100 mL, and use this solution as the standard solution. Perform the test with the sample solution and standard solution as directed under Ultraviolet-visible Spectrophotometry <*2.24*>, using water as the blank, and determine the absorbances, A_T and A_S, at 210 nm.

Dissolution rate (%) with respect to the labeled amount of irsogladine maleate ($C_9H_7Cl_2N_5.C_4H_4O_4$)
$= M_S/M_T \times A_T/A_S \times 1/C \times 9$

M_S: Amount (mg) of irsogladine maleate for assay taken
M_T: Amount (g) of Irsogladine Maleate Fine Granules taken
C: Labeled amount (mg) of irsogladine maleate ($C_9H_7Cl_2N_5.C_4H_4O_4$) in 1 g

Assay Weigh accurately an amount of powdered Irsogladine Maleate Fine Granules, equivalent to about 5 mg of irsogladine maleate ($C_9H_7Cl_2N_5.C_4H_4O_4$), add exactly 5 mL of the internal standard solution, shake until it is dispersed, and add 5 mL of water. To the solution add 25 mL of ethylene glycol, sonicate for 10 minutes with occasional shaking, and add ethylene glycol to make 50 mL. Filter this solution through a membrane filter with a pore size not exceeding 0.5 μm, discard the first 10 mL of the filtrate, and use the subsequent filtrate as the sample solution. Separately, weigh accurately about 25 mg of irsogladine maleate for assay, previously dried at 105°C for 4 hours, and dissolve in ethylene glycol to make exactly 25 mL. Pipet 5 mL of this solution, add exactly 5 mL of the internal standard solution, add 5 mL of water and ethylene glycol to make 50 mL, and use this solution as the standard solution. Perform the test with 5 μL each of the sample solution and standard solution as directed under Liquid Chromatography <*2.01*> according to the following conditions, and calculate the ratios, Q_T and Q_S, of the peak area of irsogladine to that of the internal standard.

Amount (mg) of irsogladine maleate ($C_9H_7Cl_2N_5.C_4H_4O_4$)
$= M_S \times Q_T/Q_S \times 1/5$

M_S: Amount (mg) of irsogladine maleate for assay taken

Internal standard solution—A solution of ethyl parahydroxybenzoate in methanol (1 in 2500).

Operating conditions—

Detector: An ultraviolet absorption photometer (wavelength: 250 nm).

Column: A stainless steel column 4.6 mm in inside diameter and 15 cm in length, packed with octadecylsilanized silica gel for liquid chromatography (5 μm in particle diameter).

Column temperature: A constant temperature of about 25°C.

Mobile phase: A mixture of water, acetonitrile and acetic acid (100) (750:250:3).

Flow rate: Adjust so that the retention time of irsogladine is about 9 minutes.

System suitability—

System performance: When the procedure is run with 5 μL of the standard solution under the above operating conditions, irsogladine and the internal standard are eluted in this order with the resolution between these peaks being not less than 10.

System repeatability: When the test is repeated 6 times with 5 μL of the standard solution under the above operating conditions, the relative standard deviation of the ratio of the peak area of irsogladine to that of the internal standard is not more than 1.0%.

Containers and storage Containers—Tight containers.

Irsogladine Maleate Tablets

イルソグラジンマレイン酸塩錠

Irsogladine Maleate Tablets contain not less than 93.0% and not more than 107.0% of the labeled amount of irsogladine maleate ($C_9H_7Cl_2N_5.C_4H_4O_4$: 372.16).

Method of preparation Prepare as directed under Tablets, with Irsogladine Maleate.

Identification To a quantity of powdered Irsogladine Maleate Tablets, equivalent 2 mg of Irsogladine Maleate, add 5 mL of methanol, shake for 10 minutes, centrifuge, and use the supernatant liquid as the sample solution. Separately, dissolve 2 mg of irsogladine maleate in 5 mL of methanol, and use this solution as the standard solution. Perform the test with these solutions as directed under Thin-layer Chromatography <*2.03*>. Spot 10 μL each of the sample solution and standard solution on a plate of silica gel with fluorescent indicator for thin-layer chromatography. Develop the plate with a mixture of petroleum ether, acetone and acetic acid (100) (12:4:1) to a distance of about 10 cm, and air-dry the plate. Examine under ultraviolet light (main wavelength: 254 nm): the spot from the sample solution has the same *R*f value as the spot from the standard solution.

Uniformity of dosage units <*6.02*> Perform the test according to the following method: it meets the requirement of the Content uniformity test.

To 1 tablet of Irsogladine Maleate Tablets add 2 mL of water, add 2 mL of methanol per mg of irsogladine maleate ($C_9H_7Cl_2N_5.C_4H_4O_4$), sonicate for 10 minutes with occasional shaking, add water to make exactly V mL so that each mL contains about 40 μg of irsogladine maleate ($C_9H_7Cl_2N_5.C_4H_4O_4$). Centrifuge this solution, pipet 1 mL of the supernatant liquid, and add water to make exactly 20 mL. Filter this solution through a membrane filter with a pore size not exceeding 0.5 μm, discard the first 10 mL of the filtrate, and use the subsequent filtrate as the sample solution. Separately, weigh accurately about 20 mg of irsogladine maleate for assay, previously dried at 105°C for 4 hours, and dissolve in methanol to make exactly 20 mL. Pipet 2 mL of this solution, and add water to make exactly 20 mL. Pipet 2 mL of this solution, add water to make exactly 100 mL, and use this solution as the standard solution. Perform the test with the sample solution and standard solution as directed under Ultraviolet-visible Spectrophotometry <*2.24*>, using water as the blank, and determine the absorbances, A_T and A_S, at 210 nm.

Amount (mg) of irsogladine maleate ($C_9H_7Cl_2N_5.C_4H_4O_4$)
$= M_S \times A_T/A_S \times V/500$

M_S: Amount (mg) of irsogladine maleate for assay taken

Dissolution <*6.10*> When the test is performed at 50 revolutions per minute according to the Paddle method, using 900 mL of water as the dissolution medium, the dissolution rate in 30 minutes of Irsogladine Maleate Tablets is not less than 80%.

Start the test with 1 tablet of Irsogladine Maleate Tablets, withdraw not less than 20 mL of the medium at the specified minute after starting the test, and filter through a membrane filter with a pore size not exceeding 0.5 μm. Discard not less than 10 mL of the first filtrate, pipet V mL of the subsequent filtrate, add water to make exactly V' mL so that each mL contains about 2.2 μg of irsogladine maleate ($C_9H_7Cl_2N_5.C_4H_4O_4$), and use this solution as the sample solution. Separately, weigh accurately about 20 mg of irsogladine maleate for assay, previously dried at 105°C for 4 hours, and dissolve in methanol to make exactly 20 mL. Pipet 2 mL of this solution, and add water to make exactly 20 mL. Pipet 2 mL of this solution, add water to make exactly 100 mL, and use this solution as the standard solution. Perform the test with the sample solution and standard solution as directed under Ultraviolet-visible Spectrophotometry <*2.24*>, using water as the blank, and determine the absorbances, A_T and A_S, at 210 nm.

Dissolution rate (%) with respect to the labeled amount of irsogladine maleate ($C_9H_7Cl_2N_5.C_4H_4O_4$)
$= M_S \times A_T/A_S \times V'/V \times 1/C \times 9$

M_S: Amount (mg) of irsogladine maleate for assay taken
C: Labeled amount (mg) of irsogladine maleate ($C_9H_7Cl_2N_5.C_4H_4O_4$) in 1 tablet

Assay Weigh accurately the mass of not less than 20 Irsogladine Maleate Tablets, and powder. Weigh accurately a portion of the powder, equivalent to about 5 mg of irsogladine maleate ($C_9H_7Cl_2N_5.C_4H_4O_4$), add exactly 5 mL of the internal standard solution, shake until it is dispersed, and add 5 mL of water. To this solution add 25 mL of ethylene glycol, sonicate for 10 minutes with occasional shaking, and add ethylene glycol to make 50 mL. Filter this solution through a membrane filter with a pore size not exceeding 0.5 μm, discard the first 10 mL of the filtrate, and use the subsequent filtrate as the sample solution. Separately, weigh accurately about 25 mg of irsogladine maleate for assay, previously dried at 105°C for 4 hours, and dissolve in ethylene glycol to make exactly 25 mL. Pipet 5 mL of this solution, add exactly 5 mL of the internal standard solution, add 5 mL of water and ethylene glycol to make 50 mL, and use this solution as the standard solution. Perform the test with 5 μL each of the sample solution and standard solution as directed under Liquid Chromatography <2.01> according to the following conditions, and calculate the ratios, Q_T and Q_S, of the peak area of irsogladine to that of the internal standard.

Amount (mg) of irsogladine maleate ($C_9H_7Cl_2N_5.C_4H_4O_4$)
$= M_S \times Q_T/Q_S \times 1/5$

M_S: Amount (mg) of irsogladine maleate for assay taken

Internal standard solution—A solution of ethyl parahydroxybenzoate in methanol (1 in 2500).

Operating conditions—

Detector: An ultraviolet absorption photometer (wavelength: 250 nm).

Column: A stainless steel column 4.6 mm in inside diameter and 15 cm in length, packed with octadecylsilanized silica gel for liquid chromatography (5 μm in particle diameter).

Column temperature: A constant temperature of about 25°C.

Mobile phase: A mixture of water, acetonitrile and acetic acid (100) (750:250:3).

Flow rate: Adjust so that the retention time of irsogladine is about 9 minutes.

System suitability—

System performance: When the procedure is run with 5 μL of the standard solution under the above operating conditions, irsogladine and the internal standard are eluted in this order with the resolution between these peaks being not less than 10.

System repeatability: When the test is repeated 6 times with 5 μL of the standard solution under the above operating conditions, the relative standard deviation of the ratio of the peak area of irsogladine to that of the internal standard is not more than 1.0%.

Containers and storage Containers—Tight containers.

Isepamicin Sulfate

イセパマイシン硫酸塩

$C_{22}H_{43}N_5O_{12}.xH_2SO_4$

6-Amino-6-deoxy-α-D-glucopyranosyl-(1→4)-[3-deoxy-4-*C*-methyl-3-methylamino-β-L-arabinopyranosyl-(1→6)]-2-deoxy-1-*N*-[(2*S*)-3-amino-2-hydroxypropanoyl]-D-streptamine sulfate

[*67814-76-0*]

Isepamicin Sulfate is the sulfate of a derivative of gentamycin B, an aminoglycoside substance, having antibacterial activity produced by the growth of *Micromonospora purpurea.*

It contains not less than 680 μg (potency) and not more than 780 μg (potency) per mg, calculated on the anhydrous basis. The potency of Isepamicin Sulfate is expressed as mass (potency) of isepamicin ($C_{22}H_{43}N_5O_{12}$: 569.60).

Description Isepamicin Sulfate occurs as a white to pale yellow-white powder.

It is very soluble in water, and practically insoluble in methanol and in ethanol (95).

It is hygroscopic.

Identification (1) Dissolve 20 mg of Isepamicun Sulfate in 1 mL of water, add 3 mL of anthrone TS, shake, and allow to stand: a blue-purple color develops.

(2) Dissolve 10 mg each of Isepamicin Sulfate and Isepamicin Sulfate RS in 5 mL of water, and use these solutions as the sample solution and standard solution. Perform the test with these solutions as directed under Thin-layer chromatography <2.03>. Spot 5 μL each of the sample solution and standard solution on a plate of silica gel for thin-layer chromatography. Develop the plate with a mixture of ammonia water (28), ethanol (99.5), 1-butanol and chloroform (5:5:4:2) to a distance of about 15 cm, and air-dry the plate. Spray evenly 0.2% ninhydrin-water saturated 1-butanol TS on the plate, and heat the plate at about 100°C for about 10 minutes: the principal spots from the sample solution and the spot from the standard solution exhibit a red-brown color and show the same *R*f value.

(3) Dissolve 10 mg of Isepamicin Sulfate in 1 mL of water, and add 1 drop of barium chloride TS: a white precipitate is produced.

Optical rotation <2.49> $[\alpha]_D^{20}$: +100 – +120° (0.25 g calculated on the anhydrous bases, water, 25 mL, 100 mm).

pH <2.54> Dissolve 0.5 g of Isepamicin Sulfate in 5 mL of water: the pH of the solution is between 5.5 and 7.5.

Purity (1) Clarity and color of solution—Dissolve 1.0 g

of Isepamicin Sulfate in 10 mL of water: the solution is clear and colorless.

(2) Heavy metals <*1.07*>—Proceed with 1.0 g of Isepamicin Sulfate according to Method 4, and perform the test. Prepare the control solution with 1.0 mL Standard Lead Solution (not more than 10 ppm).

(3) Related substances—Use the sample solution obtained in the Assay as the sample solution. Perform the test with 5 μL of the sample solution as directed under Liquid Chromatography <*2.01*> according to the following conditions. Determine each peak area of the sample solution by the automatic integration method, and calculate the amounts of their peaks by the area percentage method: the amount of HAPA-gentamine-B equivalent to about 0.4 of the relative retention time to isepamicin is not more than 5.0%, and gentamicin B equivalent to about 1.3 of that is not more than 3.0%. For the peak area of gentamicin B, multiply the correction factor, 1.11.

Operating conditions—

Apparatus, detector, column, column temperature, reaction coil, mobile phase, reagent, reaction temperature, flow rate of mobile phase, and flow rate of reagent: Proceed as directed in the operating conditions in the Assay.

Time span of measurement: About 2 times as long as the retention time of isepamicin.

System suitability—

System performance and system repeatability: Proceed as directed in the system suitability in the Assay.

Test for required detectability: To 1 mL of the sample solution, add water to make 10 mL, and use this solution as the solution for system suitability test. Pipet 1 mL of the solution for system suitability test, and add water to make exactly 10 mL. Confirm that the peak area of isepamicin obtained with 5 μL of this solution is equivalent to 7 to 13% of that with 5 μL of the solution for system suitability test.

Water <*2.48*> Not more than 12.0% (0.2 g, volumetric titration, direct titration. Use a mixture of formamide for water determination and methanol for water determination (2:1) instead of methanol for water determination).

Residue on ignition <*2.44*> Not more than 1.0% (1 g).

Assay Weigh accurately an amount of Isepamicin Sulfate and Isepamicin Sulfate RS, equivalent to about 20 mg (potency), dissolve each in water to make exactly 100 mL, and use these solutions as the sample solution and the standard solution, respectively. Perform the test with exactly 5 μL each of the sample solution and standard solution as directed under Liquid Chromatography <*2.01*> according to the following conditions, and determine the peak areas, A_T and A_S, of isepamicin in each solution.

Amount [μg (potency)] of isepamicin ($C_{22}H_{43}N_5O_{12}$)
$= M_S \times A_T/A_S \times 1000$

M_S: Amount [mg (potency)] of Isepamicin Sulfate RS taken

Operating conditions—

Apparatus: Consist of two pumps for the mobile phase and the reagent transport, inject port, column, reaction coil, detector and recorder. Use a reaction coil with thermostat.

Detector: A fluorophotometer (excitation wavelength: 360 nm, detection wavelength: 440 nm).

Column: A stainless steel column 4 mm in inside diameter and 15 cm in length, packed with octadecylsilanized silica gel for liquid chromatography (5 μm in particle diameter).

Column temperature: A constant temperature of about 25°C.

Reaction coil: A column 0.25 mm in inside diameter and 5 m in length.

Mobile phase: Dissolve 28.41 g of anhydrous sodium sulfate and 5.23 g of sodium 1-pentane sulfonate in 900 mL of water, add 1 mL of acetic acid (100), and add water to make exactly 1000 mL.

Reagent: To 500 mL of boric acid-potassium chloride-sodium hydroxide buffer solution (pH 10.0) add 5 mL of a solution of *o*-phthalaldehyde in ethanol (95) (2 in 25), 1 mL of 2-mercaptoethanol and 2 mL of a solution of lauromacrogol (1 in 4).

Reaction temperature: A constant temperature of about 45°C.

Flow rate of mobile phase: About 0.6 mL per minute.

Flow rate of reagent: About 0.5 mL per minute.

System suitability—

System performance: Dissolve 2 mg of gentamicin B in 10 mL of the standard solution. When the procedure is run with 5 μL of this solution under the above operating conditions, isepamicin and gentamicin B are eluted in this order with the resolution between these peaks being not less than 1.0.

System repeatability: When the test is repeated 5 times with 5 μL of the standard solution under the above operating conditions, the relative standard deviation of the peak areas of isepamicin is not more than 3.0%.

Containers and storage Containers—Tight containers.

Isepamicin Sulfate Injection

イセパマイシン硫酸塩注射液

Isepamicin Sulfate Injection is an aqueous injection.

It contains not less than 90.0% and not more than 110.0% of the labeled potency of isepamicin ($C_{22}H_{43}N_5O_{12}$: 569.60).

Method of preparation Prepare as directed under Injections, with Isepamicin Sulfate.

Description Isepamicin Sulfate Injection is a clear, colorless liquid.

Identification To a volume of Isepamicin Sulfate Injection, equivalent to 20 mg (potency) of Isepamicin Sulfate, add water to make 10 mL, and use this solution as the sample solution. Separately, dissolve an amount of Isepamicin Sulfate RS, equivalent to 20 mg (potency) in 10 mL of water, and use this solution as the standard solution. Proceed with these solutions as directed in the Identification (2) under Isepamicin Sulfate.

Osmotic pressure ratio Being specified separately when the drug is granted approval based on the Law.

pH <*2.54*> 5.5 – 7.5.

Purity Related substances—Use the sample solution obtained in the Assay as the sample solution. Perform the test with 5 μL of the sample solution as directed under Liquid Chromatography <*2.01*> according to the following conditions. Determine each peak area of the sample solution by the automatic integration method and calculate the amounts of their peaks by the area percentage method: the amount of isoserine, having the relative retention time of about 0.3 to isepamicin, is not more than 2.0%, and the amount of gentamicin B, having the relative retention time of about 1.3, is not more than 4.0%. For the peak area of gentamicin B, multiply the correction factor, 1.11.

Operating conditions—

Apparatus, detector, column, column temperature, reaction coil, mobile phase, reaction reagent, reaction temperature, flow rate of mobile phase, and flow rate of reaction reagent: Proceed as directed in the operating conditions in the Assay under Isepamicin Sulfate.

Time span of measurement: About 2 times as long as the retention time of isepamicin.

System suitability—

System performance and system repeatability: Proceed as directed in the Assay under Isepamicin Sulfate.

Test for required detectability: To 1 mL of the sample solution add water to make 10 mL, and use this solution as the solution for system suitability test. Pipet 1 mL of the solution for system suitability test, and add water to make exactly 10 mL. Confirm that the peak area of isepamicin obtained with 5 μL of this solution is equivalent to 7 to 13% of that with 5 μL of the solution for system suitability test.

Bacterial endotoxins <*4.01*> Less than 0.50 EU/mg (potency).

Extractable volume <*6.05*> It meets the requirement.

Foreign insoluble matter <*6.06*> Perform the test according to Method 1: it meets the requirement.

Insoluble particulate matter <*6.07*> It meets the requirement.

Sterility <*4.06*> Perform the test according to the Membrane filtration method: it meets the requirement.

Assay Pipet a volume of Isepamicin Sulfate Injection, equivalent to about 0.2 g (potency) of Isepamicin Sulfate, add water to make exactly 100 mL. Pipet 10 mL of this solution, add water to make exactly 100 mL, and use this solution as the sample solution. Separately, weigh accurately an amount of Isepamicin Sulfate RS, equivalent to about 20 mg (potency), dissolve in water to make exactly 100 mL, and use this solution as the standard solution. Proceed as directed in the Assay under Isepamicin Sulfate.

Amount [mg (potency)] of isepamicin ($C_{22}H_{43}N_5O_{12}$)
$= M_S \times A_T/A_S \times 10$

M_S: Amount [mg (potency)] of Isepamicin Sulfate RS taken

Containers and storage Containers—Hermetic containers.

Shelf life 24 months after preparation.

Isoflurane

イソフルラン

and enantiomer

$C_3H_2ClF_5O$: 184.49
(2*RS*)-2-Chloro-2-(difluoromethoxy)-1,1,1-trifluoroethane
[*26675-46-7*]

Isoflurane contains not less than 99.0% and not more than 101.0% of isoflurane ($C_3H_2ClF_5O$), calculated on the anhydrous basis.

Description Isoflurane occurs as a clear, colorless fluid liquid.

It is miscible with ethanol (99.5), with methanol and with *o*-xylene.

It is slightly soluble in water.

It is volatile, and has no inflammability.

It shows no optical rotation.

Refractive index n_D^{20}: about 1.30

Boiling point: about 47 - 50°C

Identification **(1)** The test solution obtained by Oxygen Flask Combustion Method <*1.06*> with 50 μL of Isoflurane, using 40 mL of water as the absorbing liquid, responds to Qualitative Tests <*1.09*> for chloride and fluoride.

(2) Determine the infrared absorption spectrum of Isoflurane as directed in the liquid film method under Infrared Spectrophotometry <*2.25*>, and compare the spectrum with the Reference Spectrum or the spectrum of Isoflurane RS: both spectra exhibit similar intensities of absorption at the same wave numbers.

Specific gravity <*2.56*> d_{20}^{20}: 1.500 - 1.520

Purity **(1)** Acidity or alkalinity—To 10 mL of Isoflurane add 5 mL of freshly boiled and cooled water, and shake for 1 minute: the water layer is neutral.

(2) Soluble chloride—To 60 g of Isoflurane add 40 mL of water, shake thoroughly, and separate the water layer. To 20 mL of the layer add 6 mL of dilute nitric acid and water to make 50 mL. Perform the test with this solution as directed under Chloride Limit Test <*1.03*>. Prepare the control solution with 0.25 mL of 0.01 mol/L hydrochloric acid VS (not more than 3 ppm).

(3) Soluble fluoride—To 6 g of Isoflurane add 12 mL of diluted 0.01 mol/L sodium hydroxide TS (1 in 20), and shake for 10 minutes. Transfer 4.0 mL of the water layer into a Nessler tube, add 30 mL of a mixture of alizarin complexone TS, acetic acid-potassium acetate buffer solution (pH 4.3) and cerium (III) nitrate TS (1:1:1), add water to make 50 mL, allow to stand for 60 minutes, and use this solution as the sample solution. Separately, to 0.4 mL of the fluorine standard solution and 4.0 mL of diluted 0.01 mol/L sodium hydroxide TS (1 in 20) in a Nessler tube add 30 mL of the mixture of alizarin complexone TS, acetic acid-potassium acetate buffer solution (pH 4.3) and cerium (III) nitrate TS (1:1:1), then proceed in the same manner as for the preparation of the sample solution, and use the solution so obtained as the standard solution. Determine the absorbances of the sample solution and standard solution at 600 nm as directed under Ultraviolet-visible Spectrophotometry <*2.24*>, using a solution, obtained by proceeding in the same manner as above with 4.0 mL of diluted 0.01 mol/L sodium hydroxide TS (1 in 20), as the blank: the absorbance of the sample solution is not more than that of the standard solution (not more than 2 ppm).

Fluorine standard solution: Dissolve exactly 2.21 g of sodium fluoride in water to make exactly 1000 mL. Pipet 10 mL of this solution, and add water to make exactly 1000 mL. Each mL of this solution contains 0.01 mg of fluorine (F).

(4) Related substances—Use Isoflurane as the sample solution. To exactly 1 mL of the sample solution add *o*-xylene to make exactly 100 mL. Pipet 1 mL of this solution, add *o*-xylene to make exactly 100 mL, and use this solution as the standard solution. Perform the test with exactly 5 μL each of the sample solution and standard solution as directed under Gas Chromatography <*2.02*> according to the following conditions, and determine each peak area by the automatic integration method: the area of the peak other than isoflurane from sample solution is not larger than the peak area of isoflurane from the standard solution, and the total area of the peaks other than isoflurane from the sample solution is not larger than 3 times the peak area of isoflurane from the standard solution.

Operating conditions—

Detector, column, column temperature, carrier gas, and flow rate: Proceed as directed in the operating conditions in the Assay.

Time span of measurement: About 5 times as long as the retention time of isoflurane.

System suitability—

System performance and system repeatability: Proceed as directed in the system suitability in the Assay.

Test for required detectability: To exactly 1 mL of the standard solution add *o*-xylene to make exactly 2 mL. Confirm that the peak area of isoflurane obtained with 5 μL of this solution is equivalent to 35 to 65% of that with 5 μL of the standard solution.

(5) Peroxide—Take 10 mL of Isoflurane in a Nessler tube add 1 mL of a freshly prepared solution of potassium iodide (1 in 10), shake vigorously, and allow to stand in a dark place for 1 hour: the water layer is not yellow.

(6) Residue on evaporation—Pipet 65 mL of Isoflurane, evaporate on a water bath, and dry the residue at 105°C for 1 hour: not more than 1.0 mg.

Water *<2.48>* Not more than 0.1% (2 g, Coulometric titration).

Assay To exactly 5 mL each of Isoflurane and Isoflurane RS (separately determined the water *<2.48>* in the same manner as Isoflurane), add exactly 3 mL of ethyl acetate as the internal standard, then add *o*-xylene to make 50 mL each. To 5 mL each of these solutions add *o*-xylene to make 50 mL, and use these solutions as the sample solution and the standard solution, respectively. Perform the test with 2 μL each of the sample solution and standard solution as directed under Gas Chromatography *<2.02>* according to the following conditions, and calculate the ratios, Q_T and Q_S, of the peak area of isoflurane to that of the internal standard.

Amount (mg) of isoflurane ($C_3H_2ClF_5O$) in 5 mL of Isoflurane
$= V_S \times Q_T/Q_S \times 1000 \times 1.506$

V_S: Amount (mL) of Isoflurane RS taken, calculated on the anhydrous basis
1.506: Specific gravity (d^{20}_{20}) of isoflurane

Operating conditions—

Detector: A hydrogen flame-ionization detector.

Column: A stainless steel column 3 mm in inside diameter and 3.5 m in length, packed with siliceous earth for gas chromatography (125 – 149 μm in particle diameter), coated in 10% with nonylphenoxypoly(ethyleneoxy)ethanol for gas chromatography and in 15% with polyalkylene glycol for gas chromatography.

Column temperature: A constant temperature of about 80°C.

Carrier gas: Nitrogen.

Flow rate: Adjust so that the retention time of isoflurane is about 7 minutes.

System suitability—

System performance: When the procedure is run with 2 μL of the standard solution under the above operating conditions, isoflurane and the internal standard are eluted in this order with the resolution between these peaks being not less than 3.

System repeatability: When the test is repeated 6 times with 2 μL of the standard solution under the above operating conditions, the relative standard deviation of the peak area of isoflurane is not more than 1.0%.

Containers and storage Containers—Tight containers.
Storage—At a temperature not exceeding 30°C.

L-Isoleucine

L-イソロイシン

$C_6H_{13}NO_2$: 131.17
(2*S*,3*S*)-2-Amino-3-methylpentanoic acid
[*73-32-5*]

L-Isoleucine, when dried, contains not less than 98.5% of L-isoleucine ($C_6H_{13}NO_2$).

Description L-Isoleucine occurs as white, crystals or crystalline powder. It is odorless or has a faint characteristic odor, and has a slightly bitter taste.

It is freely soluble in formic acid, sparingly soluble in water, and practically insoluble in ethanol (95).

It dissolves in dilute hydrochloric acid.

Identification Determine the infrared absorption spectrum of L-Isoleucine, previously dried, as directed in the potassium bromide disk method under Infrared Spectrophotometry *<2.25>*, and compare the spectrum with the Reference Spectrum: both spectra exhibit similar intensities of absorption at the same wave numbers.

Optical rotation *<2.49>* $[\alpha]^{20}_D$: +39.5 – +41.5° (after drying, 1 g, 6 mol/L hydrochloric acid TS, 25 mL, 100 mm).

pH *<2.54>* Dissolve 1.0 g of L-Isoleucine in 100 mL of water: the pH of this solution is between 5.5 and 6.5.

Purity **(1)** Clarity and color of solution—Dissolve 0.5 g of L-Isoleucine in 10 mL of 1 mol/L hydrochloric acid TS: the solution is clear and colorless.

(2) Chloride *<1.03>*—Perform the test with 0.5 g of L-Isoleucine. Prepare the control solution with 0.30 mL of 0.01 mol/L hydrochloric acid VS (not more than 0.021%).

(3) Sulfate *<1.14>*—Perform the test with 0.6 g of L-Isoleucine. Prepare the control solution with 0.35 mL of 0.005 mol/L sulfuric acid VS (not more than 0.028%).

(4) Ammonium *<1.02>*—Perform the test with 0.25 g of L-Isoleucine. Prepare the control solution with 5.0 mL of Standard Ammonium Solution (not more than 0.02%).

(5) Heavy metals *<1.07>*—Dissolve 1.0 g of L-Isoleucine in 40 mL of water and 2 mL of dilute acetic acid by warming, cool, and add water to make 50 mL. Perform the test using this solution as the test solution. Prepare the control solution as follows: to 2.0 mL of Standard Lead Solution add 2 mL of dilute acetic acid and water to make 50 mL (not more than 20 ppm).

(6) Arsenic *<1.11>*—Prepare the test solution with 1.0 g of L-Isoleucine according to Method 2, and perform the test (not more than 2 ppm).

(7) Related substances—Dissolve 0.10 g of L-Isoleucine in 25 mL of water, and use this solution as the sample solution. Pipet 1 mL of the sample solution, and add water to make exactly 50 mL. Pipet 5 mL of this solution, add water to make exactly 20 mL, and use this solution as the standard solution. Perform the test with these solutions as directed under Thin-layer Chromatography <2.03>. Spot 5 μL each of the sample solution and standard solution on a plate of silica gel for thin-layer chromatography. Develop the plate with a mixture of 1-butanol, water and acetic acid (100) (3:1:1) to a distance of about 10 cm, and dry the plate at 80°C for 30 minutes. Spray evenly the plate with a solution of ninhydrin in acetone (1 in 50), and heat the plate at 80°C for 5 minutes: the spots other than the principal spot obtained from the sample solution are not more intense than the spot from the standard solution.

Loss on drying <2.41> Not more than 0.30% (1 g, 105°C, 3 hours).

Residue on ignition <2.44> Not more than 0.1% (1 g).

Assay Weigh accurately about 0.13 g of L-Isoleucine, previously dried, and dissolve in 3 mL of formic acid, add 50 mL of acetic acid (100), and titrate <2.50> with 0.1 mol/L perchloric acid VS (potentiometric titration). Perform a blank determination in the same manner, and make any necessary correction.

Each mL of 0.1 mol/L perchloric acid VS
= 13.12 mg of $C_6H_{13}NO_2$

Containers and storage Containers—Tight containers.

L-Isoleucine, L-Leucine and L-Valine Granules

イソロイシン・ロイシン・バリン顆粒

L-Isoleucine, L-Leucine and L-Valine Granules contain not less than 93.0% and not more than 107.0% of the labeled amount of L-isoleucine ($C_6H_{13}NO_2$: 131.17), L-leucine ($C_6H_{13}NO_2$: 131.17) and L-valine ($C_5H_{11}NO_2$: 117.15).

Method of preparation Prepare as directed under Granules, with L-Isoleucine, L-Leucine and L-Valine.

Identification Dissolve an amount of powdered L-Isoleucine, L-Leucine and L-Valine Granules, equivalent to about 92 mg of L-Isoleucine, in the mobile phase to make 100 mL, and use this solution as the sample solution. Separately, dissolve 0.46 g of L-isoleucine, 0.92 g of L-leucine and 0.55 g of L-valine in the mobile phase to make 100 mL. Take 10 mL of this solution, add the mobile phase to make 50 mL, and use this solution as the standard solution. Perform the test with 20 μL each of the sample solution and the standard solution as directed under Liquid Chromatography <2.01> according to the following conditions: the retention times of the peak in the chromatograms obtained from the sample solution and the standard solution are the same.

Operating conditions—

Detector: An ultraviolet absorption photometer (wavelength: 210 nm).

Column: A stainless steel column 4.6 mm in inside diameter and 15 cm in length, packed with octadecylsilanized silica gel for liquid chromatography (3 μm in particle diameter).

Column temperature: A constant temperature of about 40°C.

Mobile phase: Dissolve 31.2 g of sodium dihydrogen phosphate dihydrate in 1000 mL of water, and adjust to pH 2.8 with phosphoric acid. To 970 mL of this solution add 30 mL of acetonitrile.

Flow rate: Adjust so that the retention time of L-valine is about 2.5 minutes.

System suitability—

System performance: When the procedure is run with 20 μL of the standard solution under the above operating conditions, valine, isoleucine and leucine are eluted in this order, and the resolution between the peaks of isoleucine and leucine is not less than 1.5.

System repeatability: When the test is repeated 6 times with 20 μL of the standard solution under the above operating conditions, the relative standard deviations of the retention time of isoleucine, leucine and valine are not more than 1.0%, respectively.

Uniformity of dosage units <6.02> Perform the test according to the following method: the Granules in single-dose package meets the requirement of the Content uniformity test.

To the total content of 1 package of L-Isoleucine, L-Leucine and L-Valine Granules add exactly V/25 mL of the internal standard solution, and add 0.1 mol/L hydrochloric acid TS to make V mL so that each mL contains about 3.8 mg of L-isoleucine ($C_6H_{13}NO_2$). To 2 mL of this solution add 0.02 mol/L hydrochloric acid TS to make 200 mL, and use this solution as the sample solution. Then, proceed as directed in the Assay.

Amount (mg) of L-isoleucine ($C_6H_{13}NO_2$)
$= M_{Sa} \times Q_{Ta}/Q_{Sa} \times V/50$

Amount (mg) of L-leucine ($C_6H_{13}NO_2$)
$= M_{Sb} \times Q_{Tb}/Q_{Sb} \times V/50$

Amount (mg) of L-valine ($C_5H_{11}NO_2$)
$= M_{Sc} \times Q_{Tc}/Q_{Sc} \times V/50$

M_{Sa}: Amount (mg) of L-isoleucine for assay taken
M_{Sb}: Amount (mg) of L-leucine for assay taken
M_{Sc}: Amount (mg) of L-valine for assay taken

Internal standard solution—A solution of glycine in 0.1 mol/L hydrochloric acid TS (1 in 20).

Disintegration <6.09> It meets the requirement. Carry out the test for 15 minutes.

Assay Powder the total amount of the content of not less than ten packages of L-Isoleucine, L-Leucine and L-Valine Granules. Weigh accurately a portion of the powder, equivalent to about 0.95 g of L-isoleucine ($C_6H_{13}NO_2$), add exactly 10 mL of the internal standard solution, dissolve in 0.1 mol/L hydrochloric acid TS to make 250 mL. To 2 mL of this solution add 0.02 mol/L hydrochloric acid TS to make 200 mL, and use this solution as the sample solution. Separately, weigh accurately about 0.2 g of L-isoleucine for assay, about 0.4 g of L-leucine for assay and about 0.24 g of L-valine for assay, previously these are dried at 105°C for 3 hours, add exactly 2 mL of the internal standard solution, dissolve in 0.1 mol/L hydrochloric acid TS to make 100 mL. To 2 mL of this solution add 0.02 mol/L hydrochloric acid TS to make 100 mL, and use this solution as the standard solution. Perform the test with 20 μL each of the sample solution and standard solution as directed under Liquid Chromatography <2.01> according to the following conditions. Calculate the ratios, Q_{Ta}, Q_{Tb} and Q_{Tc} of the peak area of L-isoleucine, L-leucine and L-valin to that of the internal standard obtained from the sample solution, and the ratios, Q_{Sa}, Q_{Sb} and Q_{Sc} of the peak area of L-isoleucine, L-leucine and L-valin to that of the internal standard from the standard solution.

Amount (mg) of L-isoleucine ($C_6H_{13}NO_2$)
$= M_{Sa} \times Q_{Ta}/Q_{Sa} \times 5$
Amount (mg) of L-leucine ($C_6H_{13}NO_2$)
$= M_{Sb} \times Q_{Tb}/Q_{Sb} \times 5$
Amount (mg) of L-valine ($C_5H_{11}NO_2$)
$= M_{Sc} \times Q_{Tc}/Q_{Sc} \times 5$

M_{Sa}: Amount (mg) of L-isoleucine for assay taken
M_{Sb}: Amount (mg) of L-leucine for assay taken
M_{Sc}: Amount (mg) of L-valine for assay taken

Internal standard solution—A solution of glycine in 0.1 mol/L hydrochloric acid TS (1 in 20).

Operating conditions—

Detector: A visible absorption photometer (wavelength: 570 nm).

Column: A stainless steel column 4.6 mm in inside diameter and 6 cm in length, packed with strongly acidic ion-exchange resin for liquid chromatography composed with a sulfonated polystyrene (3 μm in particle diameter) (sodium type).

Column temperature: A constant temperature of about 57°C.

Reaction vessel temperature: A constant temperature of about 130°C.

Reaction time: About 1 minute.

Mobile phase: After prepare the mobile phases A, B, C, D and E according to the following table, add 0.1 mL caprylic acid to each mobile phase.

	Mobile phase A	Mobile phase B	Mobile phase C	Mobile phase D	Mobile phase E
Citric acid monohydrate	19.80 g	22.00 g	12.80 g	6.10 g	—
Trisodium citrate dihydrate	6.19 g	7.74 g	13.31 g	26.67 g	—
Sodium chloride	5.66 g	7.07 g	3.74 g	54.35 g	—
Sodium hydroxide	—	—	—	—	8.00 g
Ethanol (99.5)	130 mL	20 mL	4 mL	—	100 mL
Thiodiglycol	5 mL	5 mL	5 mL	—	—
Benzyl alcohol	—	—	—	5 mL	—
Lauromacrogol solution (1 in 4)	4 mL	4 mL	4 mL	4 mL	4 mL
Water	a sufficient amount	a sufficient amount	a sufficient amount	a sufficient amount	a sufficient amount
Total amount	1000 mL	1000 mL	1000 mL	1000 mL	1000 mL

Switching of mobile phase: Switch the mobile phases A, B, C, D and E sequentially so that when proceed with 20 μL of the standard solution under the conditions above, the internal standard, valine, isoleucine and leucine are eluted in this order with the resolution between the peaks of isoleucine and leucine being not less than 1.2.

Reaction reagent: Dissolve 407 g of lithium acetate dihydrate in an appropriate amount of water, add 245 mL of acetic acid (100), 801 mL of 1-methoxy-2-propanol and water to make 2000 mL, pass nitrogen for 10 minutes, and use this solution as Solution (I). Separately, to 1957 mL of 1-methoxy-2-propanol add 77 g of ninhydrin, pass nitrogen for 5 minutes, add 0.161 g of sodium borohydride, and pass nitrogen for 30 minutes. To this solution add an equal volume of the Solution (I). Prepare before use.

Flow rate of mobile phase: 0.40 mL per minute.

Flow rate of reaction regent: 0.35 mL per minute.

System suitability—

System performance: When the test is run with 20 μL of the standard solution under the above operating conditions, the internal standard, valine, isoleucine and leucine are eluted in this order with the resolution between the peaks of isoleucine and leucine being not less than 1.2.

System repeatability: When the test is repeated 6 times with 20 μL of the standard solution under the above operating conditions, the relative standard deviations of the ratio of the peak area of isoleucine, leucine and valine to that of the internal standard are not more than 1.0%, respectively.

Containers and storage Containers—Tight containers.

Isomalt Hydrate

Isomalt

イソマル水和物

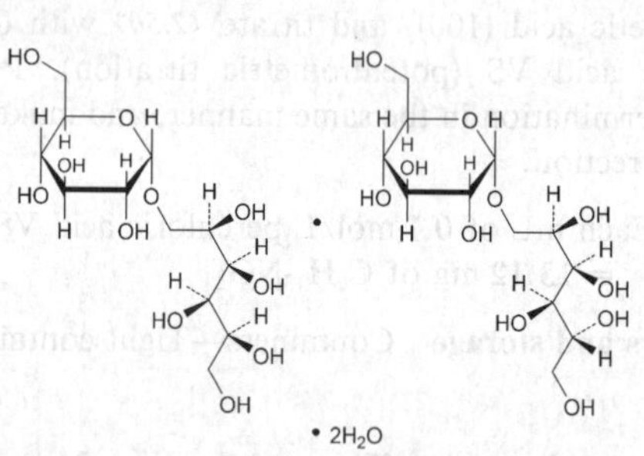

$\cdot 2H_2O$

6-*O*-α-D-Glucopyranosyl-D-glucitol $C_{12}H_{24}O_{11}$: 344.31
1-*O*-α-D-Glucopyranosyl-D-mannitol dihydrate
$C_{12}H_{24}O_{11}.2H_2O$: 380.34
6-*O*-α-D-Glucopyranosyl-D-glucitol—1-*O*-α-D-glucopyranosyl-D-mannitol dihydrate
[64519-82-0]

This monograph is harmonized with the European Pharmacopoeia and the U.S. Pharmacopeia.

The corresponding part of the attributes/provisions which are agreed as non-harmonized within the scope of the harmonization is marked with symbols (◆ ◆), and the corresponding parts which are agreed as the JP local requirement other than the scope of the harmonization are marked with symbols (◇ ◇).

Information on the harmonization with the European Pharmacopoeia and the U.S. Pharmacopeia is available on the website of the Pharmaceuticals and Medical Devices Agency.

Isomalt Hydrate is a mixture of 6-*O*-α-D-glucopyranosyl-D-sorbitol and 1-*O*-α-D-glucopyranosyl-D-mannitol.

It contains not less than 98.0% and not more than 102.0% as the mixture of 6-*O*-α-D-glucopyranosyl-D-sorbitol ($C_{12}H_{24}O_{11}$) and 1-*O*-α-D-glucopyranosyl-D-mannitol ($C_{12}H_{24}O_{11}$), calculated on the anhydrous basis, and the amount of each component is not less than 3.0%, respectively.

The label states the contents (%) of 6-*O*-α-D-glucopyranosyl-D-sorbitol and 1-*O*-α-D-glucopyranosyl-D-mannitol.

◆**Description** Isomalt Hydrate occurs as a white, powder or grains.

It is freely soluble in water, and practically insoluble in ethanol (95).

Optical rotation $[\alpha]_D^{20}$: about + 92° (1 g calculated on the anhydrous basis, water, 100 mL, 100 mm).◆

The JP Drugs are to be tested according to the provisions given in the pertinent monographs, General Notices, General Rules for Crude Drugs, General Rules for Preparations, and General Tests for their conformity to the Japanese Pharmacopoeia. (See the General Notices 5.)

Identification ◇**(1)** To 1 mL of a solution of Isomalt Hydrate (1 in 100) add 1 mL of a solution of catechol (1 in 10) prepared before use, shake thoroughly, add 2 mL of sulfuric acid rapidly, and shake: a reddish purple to red-purple color develops.◇

(2) Perform the test with 20 μL each of the sample solution and standard solution obtained in the Assay as directed under Liquid Chromatography <*2.01*> according to the following conditions, and compare the chromatograms obtained from these solutions: the two principal peaks in the chromatogram obtained from the sample solution are similar in retention time to respective two peaks from the standard solution.

Operating conditions—

Proceed as directed in the operating conditions in the Assay.

System suitability—

Proceed as directed in the system suitability in the Assay.

Purity ◇**(1)** Heavy metals <*1.07*>—Proceed with 2.0 g of Isomalt Hydrate according to Method 1, and perform the test. Prepare the control solution with 2.0 mL of Standard Lead Solution (not more than 10 ppm).◇

(2) Nickel—Weigh exactly an amount of Isomalt Hydrate, equivalent to 10.0 g calculated on the anhydrous basis, dissolve in 30 mL of 2 mol/L acetic acid TS, and add water to make exactly 100 mL. Add exactly 2 mL of a solution of ammonium pyrrolidinedithiocarbamate (1 in100) and exactly 10 mL of water-saturated 4-methyl-2-pentanone, and shake for 30 seconds protected from light. Allow the layers to separate, and use the 4-methyl-2-pentanone layer as the sample solution. Separately, take in three vessels three exact portions of Isomalt Hydrate, each equivalent to 10.0 g calculated on the anhydrous basis, dissolve in 30 mL of 2 mol/L acetic acid TS, then add exactly 0.5 mL, 1.0 mL and 1.5 mL respectively of Standard Nickel Solution for Atomic Absorption Spectrophotometry, and add water to make them exactly 100 mL. Then, proceed in the same manner as the sample solution, and use the solutions so obtained as the standard solutions. Separately, prepare 4-methyl-2-pentanone layer by proceeding in the same manner as the sample solution but omitting the substance to be examined, and use this solution as the blank solution. Perform the test with the sample solution and standard solution as directed in the standard addition method under Atomic Absorption Spectrophotometry <*2.23*> according to the following conditions. The blank solution is used to set the zero of the instrument, and to ascertain that the readings return to zero after rinsing the sample introduction system with water between each measurement: the amount of nickel is not more than 1 ppm.

Gas: Combustible gas—Acetylene.

Supporting gas—Air.

Lamp: Nickel hollow-cathode lamp.

Wavelength: 232.0 nm.

(3) Related substances—Weigh exactly 0.20 g of Isomalt Hydrate, dissolve in water to make exactly 10 mL, and use this solution as the sample solution. Separately, weigh exactly 10.0 mg of D-sorbitol and 10.0 mg of D-mannitol, dissolve in water to make exactly 100 mL, and use this solution as the standard solution. Perform the test with exactly 20 μL each of the sample solution and standard solution as directed under Liquid Chromatography <*2.01*> according to the following conditions, and determine each peak area by the automatic integration method: the peak areas of D-mannitol, having the relative retention time of about 1.6 to 1-*O*-α-D-glucopyranosyl-D-mannitol, and D-sorbitol, having the relative retention time of about 2.0, obtained from the sample solution are not larger than the area of the corresponding peak from the standard solution (not more than 0.5%), and the area of the peak other than 1-*O*-α-D-glucopyranosyl-D-mannitol and 6-*O*-α-D-glucopyranosyl-D-sorbitol having the relative retention time of about 1.2 and the peaks mentioned above from the sample solution is not larger than the peak area of D-sorbitol from the standard solution (not more than 0.5%). In addition, the total area of the peaks other than 1-*O*-α-D-glucopyranosyl-D-mannitol and 6-*O*-α-D-glucopyranosyl-D-sorbitol from the sample solution is not larger than 4 times the peak area of D-sorbitol from the standard solution (not more than 2.0%). However, the peaks which area is not larger than 1/5 times the peak area of D-sorbitol from the standard solution are disregarded (not more than 0.1%).

Operating conditions—

Detector, column, column temperature, mobile phase, and flow rate: Proceed as directed in the operating conditions in the Assay.

Time span of measurement: About 2.5 times as long as the retention time of 1-*O*-α-D-glucopyranosyl-D-mannitol.

System suitability—

System performance: Proceed as directed in the system suitability in the Assay.

◇Test for required detectability: Pipet 2 mL of the standard solution, and add water to make exactly 10 mL. Confirm that the peak area of D-sorbitol obtained with 20 μL of this solution is equivalent to 14 to 26% of that with 20 μL the standard solution.◇

◇System repeatability: When the test is repeated 6 times with 20 μL of the standard solution under the above operating conditions, the relative standard deviations of the peak area of D-mannitol and D-sorbitol are not more than 2.0%, respectively.◇

(4) Reducing sugars—Dissolve 3.3 g of Isomalt Hydrate in 10 mL of water with the aid of gentle heat, cool, and add 20 mL of copper (II) citrate TS. Add a few amount of boiling chips, heat so that the boiling begins after 4 minutes, and maintain boiling for 3 minutes. Cool rapidly, add 100 mL of a solution of acetic acid (100) (3 in 125) and exactly 20 mL of 0.025 mol/L iodine VS. With continuous shaking, add 25 mL of a mixture of water and hydrochloric acid (47:3). When the precipitate has dissolved, titrate <*2.50*> the excess of iodine with 0.05 mol/L sodium thiosulfate VS, until the blue color due to 1 mL of soluble starch TS added at near of the end point disappears: not less than 12.8 mL of 0.05 mol/L sodium thiosulfate VS is required (not more than 0.3% as glucose).

Conductivity <*2.51*> Dissolve 20 g of Isomalt Hydrate in a suitable amount of freshly boiled and cooled water with the aid of gentle heat at 40 - 50°C, cool, add the same water to make exactly 100 mL, and use this solution as the sample solution. Measure the conductivity (25°C) of the sample solution at 25 ± 0.1°C while gently stirring with a magnetic stirrer: not more than 20 $\mu S \cdot cm^{-1}$.

Water <*2.48*> Not more than 7.0% (0.3 g, volumetric titration, direct titration. Use a mixture of methanol for water determination and formamide for water determination (1:1) heated at 50 ± 5°C instead of methanol for water determination).

Assay Weight accurately about 0.2 g of Isomalt Hydrate, dissolve in water to make exactly 10 mL, and use this solution as the sample solution. Separately, weigh accurately about 0.2 g of Isomalt RS (separately determine the water <*2.48*> in the same manner as Isomalt Hydrate), dissolve in water to make exactly 10 mL, and use this solution as the standard solution. Perform the test with exactly 20 μL each of the sample solution and standard solution as directed under Liquid Chromatography <2.01> according to the following conditions, and determine the peak areas, A_{Ta} and A_{Tb}, and A_{Sa} and A_{Sb}, of 1-*O*-α-D-glucopyranosyl-D-mannitol and 6-*O*-α-D-glucopyranosyl-D-sorbitol in each solution.

Amount (g) of 1-*O*-α-D-glucopyranosyl-D-mannitol ($C_{12}H_{24}O_{11}$)
$= M_S \times K_a/100 \times A_{Ta}/A_{Sa}$

Amount (g) of 6-*O*-α-D-glucopyranosyl-D-sorbitol ($C_{12}H_{24}O_{11}$)
$= M_S \times K_b/100 \times A_{Tb}/A_{Sb}$

M_S: Amount (g) of Isomalt RS taken, calculated on the anhydrous basis
K_a: Content (%) of 1-*O*-α-D-glucopyranosyl-D-mannitol ($C_{12}H_{24}O_{11}$) in Isomalt RS
K_b: Content (%) of 6-*O*-α-D-glucopyranosyl-D-sorbitol ($C_{12}H_{24}O_{11}$) in Isomalt RS

Operating conditions—

Detector: A differential refractometer maintained at a constant temperature (40°C for example).

Column: Two stainless steel columns, 4.6 mm in inside diameter and 3 cm in length, and 7.8 mm in inside diameter and 30 cm in length, both packed with strongly acidic ion-exchange resin (Ca type) for liquid chromatography with sulfonic acid groups attached to a polymer lattice consisting of polystyrene cross-linked with divinylbenzene (degree of cross-linkage: 8%) (9 μm in particle diameter). These are used as the pre-column and the separation column, respectively.

Column temperature: 80 ± 3°C.

Mobile phase: Water.

Flow rate: 0.5 mL per minute (retention time of 1-*O*-α-D-glucopyranosyl-D-mannitol is about 12 minutes).

System suitability—

System performance: When the procedure is run with 20 μL of the standard solution under the above operating conditions, 1-*O*-α-D-glucopyranosyl-D-mannitol and 6-*O*-α-D-glucopyranosyl-D-sorbitol are eluted in this order with the resolution between these peaks being not less than 2.0.

◇System repeatability: When the test is repeated 6 times with 20 μL of the standard solution under the above operating conditions, the relative standard deviations of the peak area of 1-*O*-α-D-glucopyranosyl-D-mannitol and 6-*O*-α-D-glucopyranosyl-D-sorbitol are not more than 2.0%, respectively.◇

◆**Containers and storage** Containers—Well-closed containers.◆

Isoniazid

イソニアジド

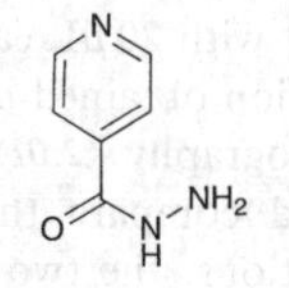

$C_6H_7N_3O$: 137.14
Pyridine-4-carbohydrazide
[54-85-3]

Isoniazid, when dried, contains not less than 98.5% of isoniazid ($C_6H_7N_3O$).

Description Isoniazid occurs as colorless crystals or a white crystalline powder. It is odorless.

It is freely soluble in water and in acetic acid (100), sparingly soluble in ethanol (95), slightly soluble in acetic anhydride, and very slightly soluble in diethyl ether.

Identification (1) Dissolve about 20 mg of Isoniazid in water to make 200 mL. To 5 mL of the solution add 1 mL of 0.1 mol/L hydrochloric acid TS and water to make 50 mL. Determine the absorption spectrum of the solution as directed under Ultraviolet-visible Spectrophotometry <2.24>, and compare the spectrum with the Reference Spectrum: both spectra exhibit similar intensities of absorption at the same wavelengths.

(2) Determine the infrared absorption spectrum of Isoniazid, previously dried, as directed in the potassium bromide disk method under Infrared Spectrophotometry <2.25>, and compare the spectrum with the Reference Spectrum: both spectra exhibit similar intensities of absorption at the same wave numbers.

pH <2.54> Dissolve 1.0 g of Isoniazid in 10 mL of freshly boiled and cooled water: the pH of this solution is between 6.5 and 7.5.

Melting point <2.60> 170 – 173°C

Purity (1) Clarity and color of solution—Dissolve 1.0 g of Isoniazid in 20 mL of water: the solution is clear and colorless.

(2) Heavy metals <1.07>—Proceed with 1.0 g of Isoniazid according to Method 2, and perform the test. Prepare the control solution with 2.0 mL of Standard Lead Solution (not more than 20 ppm).

(3) Arsenic <1.11>—Prepare the test solution with 0.40 g of Isoniazid according to Method 3, and perform the test. In this case, add 10 mL of a solution of magnesium nitrate hexahydrate in ethanol (95) (1 in 50), then add 1.5 mL of hydrogen peroxide (30), and ignite the ethanol to burn (not more than 5 ppm).

(4) Hydrazine—Dissolve 0.10 g of Isoniazid in 5 mL of water, add 0.1 mL of a solution of salicylaldehyde in ethanol (95) (1 in 20), shake immediately, and allow to stand for 5 minutes: no turbidity is produced.

Loss on drying <2.41> Not more than 0.5% (1 g, 105°C, 2 hours).

Residue on ignition <2.44> Not more than 0.1% (1 g).

Assay Weigh accurately about 0.3 g of Isoniazid, previously dried, dissolve in 50 mL of acetic acid (100) and 10 mL of acetic anhydride, and titrate <2.50> with 0.1 mol/L perchloric acid VS until the color of the solution changes from yellow to green (indicator: 0.5 mL of *p*-naphtholbenzein TS). Perform a blank determination in the same manner, and make any necessary correction.

Each mL of 0.1 mol/L perchloric acid VS
= 13.71 mg of $C_6H_7N_3O$

Containers and storage Containers—Tight containers.
Storage—Light-resistant.

Isoniazid Injection

イソニアジド注射液

Isoniazid Injection is an aqueous injection.

It contains not less than 95.0% and not more than 105.0% of the labeled amount of isoniazid ($C_6H_7N_3O$: 137.14).

Method of preparation Prepare as directed under Injections, with Isoniazid.

Description Isoniazid Injection occurs as a clear, colorless liquid.

pH: 6.5 – 7.5

Identification To a volume of Isoniazid Injection, equivalent to 20 mg of Isoniazid, and add water to make 200 mL. To 5 mL of the solution add 1 mL of 0.1 mol/L hydrochloric acid TS and water to make 50 mL. Determine the absorption spectrum of this solution as directed under Ultraviolet-visible Spectrophotometry <*2.24*>: it exhibits a maximum between 264 nm and 268 nm.

Bacterial endotoxins <*4.01*> Less than 0.50 EU/mg.

Extractable volume <*6.05*> It meets the requirement.

Foreign insoluble matter <*6.06*> Perform the test according to Method 1: it meets the requirement.

Insoluble particulate matter <*6.07*> It meets the requirement.

Sterility <*4.06*> Perform the test according to the Membrane filtration method: it meets the requirement.

Assay To an exactly measured volume of Isoniazid Injection, equivalent to about 50 mg of isoniazid ($C_6H_7N_3O$), add water to make exactly 100 mL. Pipet 5 mL of the solution, add exactly 5 mL of the internal standard solution and the mobile phase to make 50 mL, and use this solution as the sample solution. Separately, weigh accurately about 50 mg of isoniazid for assay, previously dried at 105°C for 2 hours, and dissolve in water to make exactly 100 mL. Pipet 5 mL of this solution, add exactly 5 mL of the internal standard solution and the mobile phase to make 50 mL, and use this solution as the standard solution. Perform the test with 5 μL each of the sample solution and standard solution as directed under Liquid Chromatography <*2.01*> according to the following conditions, and calculate the ratios, Q_T and Q_S, of the peak area of isoniazid to that of the internal standard.

Amount (mg) of isoniazid ($C_6H_7N_3O$) = $M_S \times Q_T/Q_S$

M_S: Amount (mg) of isoniazid for assay taken

Internal standard solution—A solution of propyl parahydroxybenzoate (1 in 4000).

Operating conditions—

Detector: An ultraviolet absorption photometer (wavelength: 265 nm).

Column: A stainless steel column 4.6 mm in inside diameter and 15 cm in length, packed with octadecylsilanized silica gel for liquid chromatography (5 μm in particle diameter).

Column temperature: A constant temperature of about 40°C.

Mobile phase: Dissolve 6.80 g of potassium dihydrogen phosphate in water to make 1000 mL. Separately, to 5.76 g of phosphoric acid add water to make 1000 mL. Mix these solutions to make a solution having pH 2.5. To 500 mL of this solution add 500 mL of methanol, and add 2.86 g of sodium tridecanesulfonate to dissolve.

Flow rate: Adjust so that the retention time of isoniazid is about 5 minutes.

System suitability—

System performance: When the procedure is run with 5 μL of the standard solution under the above operating conditions, isoniazid and the internal standard are eluted in this order with the resolution between these peaks being not less than 10.

System repeatability: When the test is repeated 6 times with 5 μL of the standard solution under the above operating conditions, the relative standard deviation of the ratios of the peak area of isoniazid to that of the internal standard is not more than 1.3%.

Containers and storage Containers—Hermetic containers, and colored containers may be used.

Storage—Light-resistant.

Isoniazid Tablets

イソニアジド錠

Isoniazid Tablets contain not less than 95.0% and not more than 105.0% of the labeled amount of isoniazid ($C_6H_7N_3O$: 137.14).

Method of preparation Prepare as directed under Tablets, with Isoniazid.

Identification Take a quantity of powdered Isoniazid Tablets, equivalent to 20 mg of Isoniazid, add 200 mL of water, shake well, and filter. To 5 mL of the filtrate add 1 mL of 0.1 mol/L hydrochloric acid TS and water to make 50 mL, and determine the absorption spectrum of this solution as directed under Ultraviolet-visible Spectrophotometry <*2.24*>: it exhibits a maximum between 264 nm and 268 nm.

Uniformity of dosage units <*6.02*> Perform the test according to the following method: it meets the requirement of the Content uniformity test.

To 1 tablet of Isoniazid Tablets add water to make exactly *V* mL so that each mL contains about 0.5 mg of isoniazid ($C_6H_7N_3O$), and shake well to disintegrate. Filter this solution, discard the first 10 mL of the filtrate, pipet 5 mL of the subsequent filtrate, add the mobile phase to make exactly 50 mL, and use this solution as the sample solution. Proceed as directed in the Assay.

Amount (mg) of isoniazid ($C_6H_7N_3O$)
= $M_S \times A_T/A_S \times V/100$

M_S: Amount (mg) of isoniazid for assay taken

Dissolution <*6.10*> When the test is performed at 50 revolutions per minute according to the Paddle method, using 900 mL of water as the dissolution medium, the dissolution rate in 20 minutes of Isoniazid Tablets is not less than 75%.

Start the test with 1 tablet of Isoniazid Tablets, withdraw not less than 20 mL of the medium at the specified minute after starting the test, and filter through a membrane filter with a pore size of not more than 0.45 μm. Discard not less than 10 mL of the first filtrate, pipet 5 mL of the subsequent filtrate, add water to make exactly 50 mL, and use this solution as the sample solution. Separately, weigh accurately about 0.1 g of isoniazid for assay, previously dried at 105°C for 2 hours, dissolve in water to make exactly 100 mL, then pipet 5 mL of this solution, add water to make exactly 50 mL, and then pipet 5 mL of this solution, add water to make exactly 50 mL, and use this solution as the standard solution. Determine the absorbances, A_T and A_S, of the sample solution and standard solution at 267 nm as directed under Ultraviolet-visible Spectrophotometry <*2.24*>.

Dissolution rate (%) with respect to the labeled amount of isoniazid ($C_6H_7N_3O$)
$= M_S \times A_T/A_S \times 1/C \times 90$

M_S: Amount (mg) of isoniazid for assay taken
C: Labeled amount (mg) of isoniazid ($C_6H_7N_3O$) in 1 tablet

Assay Weigh accurately and powder not less than 20 Isoniazid Tablets. Weigh accurately a quantity of the powder, equivalent to about 0.1 g of isoniazid ($C_6H_7N_3O$), add 150 mL of water, shake for 30 minutes, then add water to make exactly 200 mL, and filter. Discard the first 10 mL of the filtrate, pipet 5 mL of the subsequent filtrate, add the mobile phase to make exactly 50 mL, and use this solution as the sample solution. Separately, weigh accurately about 50 mg of isoniazid for assay, previously dried at 105°C for 2 hours, dissolve in water to make exactly 100 mL. Pipet 5 mL of this solution, add the mobile phase to make exactly 50 mL, and use this solution as the standard solution. Perform the test with exactly 10 μL each of the sample solution and standard solution as directed under Liquid Chromatography <*2.01*> according to the following conditions. Determine the peak areas, A_T and A_S, of isoniazid in each solution.

Amount (mg) of isoniazid ($C_6H_7N_3O$)
$= M_S \times A_T/A_S \times 2$

M_S: Amount (mg) of isoniazid for assay taken

Operating conditions—

Detector: An ultraviolet absorption photometer (wavelength: 265 nm).

Column: A stainless steel column 4.6 mm in inside diameter and 25 cm in length, packed with octadecylsilanized silica gel for liquid chromatography (5 μm in particle diameter).

Column temperature: A constant temperature of about 40°C.

Mobile phase: Dissolve 6.80 g of potassium dihydrogen phosphate in water to make 1000 mL. Separately, to 5.76 g of phosphoric acid add water to make 1000 mL. Mix these solutions to adjust the pH to 2.5. To 400 mL of this solution add 600 mL of methanol, and add 2.86 g of sodium tridecanesulfonate to dissolve.

Flow rate: Adjust so that the retention time of isoniazid is about 5 minutes.

System suitability—

System performance: Dissolve 5 mg of Isoniazid and 5 mg of isonicotinic acid in 100 mL of the mobile phase. When the procedure is run with 10 μL of this solution under the above operating conditions, isonicotinic acid and isoniazid are eluted in this order with the resolution between these peaks being not less than 1.5.

System repeatability: When the test is repeated 6 times with 10 μL of the standard solution under the above operating conditions, the relative standard deviation of the peak area of isoniazid is not more than 1.0%.

Containers and storage Containers—Tight containers.
Storage—Light-resistant.

l-Isoprenaline Hydrochloride

l-イソプレナリン塩酸塩

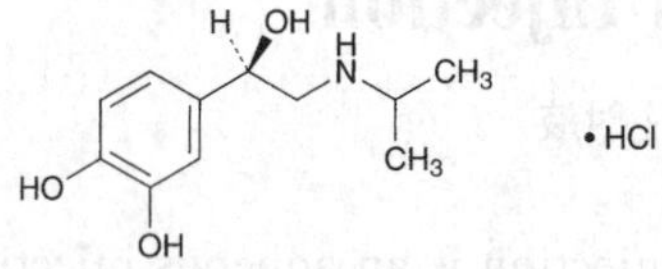

$C_{11}H_{17}NO_3.HCl$: 247.72
4-{(1*R*)-1-Hydroxy-2-[(1-methylethyl)amino]ethyl}benzene-1,2-diol monohydrochloride
[*5984-95-2*]

l-Isoprenaline Hydrochloride, when dried, contains not less than 98.0% of *l*-isoprenaline hydrochloride ($C_{11}H_{17}NO_3.HCl$).

Description *l*-Isoprenaline Hydrochloride occurs as a white, crystalline powder. It is odorless.

It is freely soluble in water, sparingly soluble in ethanol (95), and practically insoluble in acetic acid (100), in acetic anhydride, in diethyl ether and in chloroform.

It gradually changes in color by air and by light.

Identification **(1)** Dissolve 10 mg of *l*-Isoprenaline Hydrochloride in 5 mL of water, and add 1 drop of iron (III) chloride TS: a deep green color develops, and changes through yellow-green to brown on standing.

(2) Dissolve 1 mg each of *l*-Isoprenaline Hydrochloride in 1 mL of water in the test tubes A and B. Add 10 mL of potassium hydrogen phthalate buffer solution (pH 3.5) to A, and add 10 mL of phosphate buffer solution (pH 6.5) to B. To each of the test tubes add 1 mL of iodine TS, allow to stand for 5 minutes, and add 2 mL each of sodium thiosulfate TS: a red color develops in the test tube A, and a deep red color develops in the test tube B.

(3) Dissolve 10 mg of *l*-Isoprenaline Hydrochloride in 1 mL of water, and add 1 mL of phosphotungstic acid TS: a light brown precipitate is produced.

(4) Determine the absorption spectrum of a solution of *l*-Isoprenaline Hydrochloride in 0.1 mol/L hydrochloric acid TS (1 in 20,000) as directed under Ultraviolet-visible Spectrophotometry <*2.24*>, and compare the spectrum with the Reference Spectrum: both spectra exhibit similar intensities of absorption at the same wavelengths.

(5) A solution of *l*-Isoprenaline Hydrochloride (1 in 10) responds to Qualitative Tests <*1.09*> (2) for chloride.

Optical rotation <*2.49*> $[\alpha]_D^{20}$: −36 – −41° (after drying, 0.25 g, water, 25 mL, 100 mm).

pH <*2.54*> Dissolve 0.10 g of *l*-Isoprenaline Hydrochloride in 10 mL of water: the pH of the solution is between 4.5 and 5.5.

Purity **(1)** Clarity and color of solution—Dissolve 1.0 g of *l*-Isoprenaline Hydrochloride in 20 mL of 0.1 mol/L hydrochloric acid TS: the solution is clear and colorless.

(2) Sulfate <*1.14*>—Perform the test with 0.10 g of *l*-

Isoprenaline Hydrochloride. Prepare the control solution with 0.40 mL of 0.005 mol/L sulfuric acid VS (not more than 0.192%).

(3) Heavy metals <*1.07*>—Proceed with 1.0 g of *l*-Isoprenaline Hydrochloride according to Method 1, and perform the test. Prepare the control solution with 2.0 mL of Standard Lead Solution (not more than 20 ppm).

(4) Isoproterenone—Dissolve 50 mg of *l*-Isoprenaline Hydrochloride in 0.01 mol/L hydrochloric acid TS to make exactly 25 mL, and determine the absorbance of the solution at 310 nm as directed under Ultraviolet-visible Spectrophotometry <*2.24*>: not more than 0.040.

Loss on drying <*2.41*> Not more than 0.5% (1 g, in vacuum, silica gel, 4 hours).

Residue on ignition <*2.44*> Not more than 0.2% (1 g).

Assay Weigh accurately about 0.5 g of *l*-Isoprenaline Hydrochloride, previously dried, dissolve in 100 mL of a mixture of acetic acid (100) and acetic anhydride (3:2) by warming, cool, and titrate <*2.50*> with 0.1 mol/L perchloric acid VS (potentiometric titration). Perform a blank determination in the same manner, and make any necessary correction.

Each mL of 0.1 mol/L perchloric acid VS
= 24.77 mg of $C_{11}H_{17}NO_3.HCl$

Containers and storage Containers—Tight containers.
Storage—Light-resistant.

Isopropanol

Isopropyl Alcohol

イソプロパノール

C_3H_8O: 60.10
Propan-2-ol
[*67-63-0*]

Description Isopropanol is a clear, colorless liquid. It has a characteristic odor.

It is miscible with water, with methanol, with ethanol (95), and with diethyl ether.

It is flammable and volatile.

Identification **(1)** To 1 mL of Isopropanol add 2 mL of iodine TS and 2 mL of sodium hydroxide TS, and shake: a light yellow precipitate is formed.

(2) To 5 mL of Isopropanol add 20 mL of potassium dichromate TS and 5 mL of sulfuric acid with caution, and warm gently on a water bath: the produced gas has the odor of acetone, and the gas turns the filter paper, previously wetted with a solution of salicylaldehyde in ethanol (95) (1 in 10) and with a solution of sodium hydroxide (3 in 10), to red-brown.

Specific gravity <*2.56*> d^{20}_{20}: 0.785 – 0.788

Purity **(1)** Clarity of solution—To 2.0 mL of Isopropanol add 8 mL of water, and shake: the solution is clear.

(2) Acidity—To 15.0 mL of Isopropanol add 50 mL of freshly boiled and cooled water and 2 drops of phenolphthalein TS, and add 0.40 mL of 0.01 mol/L sodium hydroxide VS: a red color develops.

(3) Residue on evaporation—Evaporate 20.0 mL of Isopropanol on a water bath to dryness, and dry at 105°C for 1 hour: the mass of the residue is not more than 1.0 mg.

Water <*2.48*> Not more than 0.75 w/v% (2 mL, volumetric titration, direct titration).

Distilling range <*2.57*> 81 – 83°C, not less than 94 vol%.

Containers and storage Containers—Tight containers.
Storage—Remote from fire.

Isopropylantipyrine

Propyphenazone

イソプロピルアンチピリン

$C_{14}H_{18}N_2O$: 230.31
1,5-Dimethyl-4-(1-methylethyl)-2-phenyl-1,2-dihydro-3*H*-pyrazol-3-one
[*479-92-5*]

Isopropylantipyrine, when dried, contains not less than 98.0% of isopropylantipyrine ($C_{14}H_{18}N_2O$).

Description Isopropylantipyrine occurs as white, crystals or crystalline powder. It is odorless, and has a slightly bitter taste.

It is very soluble in acetic acid (100), freely soluble in ethanol (95) and in acetone, soluble in diethyl ether, and slightly soluble in water.

Identification **(1)** To 2 mL of a solution of Isopropylantipyrine (1 in 500) add 1 drop of iron (III) chloride TS: a light red color develops. Further add 3 drops of sulfuric acid to this solution: the color changes to pale yellow.

(2) Add 5 mL of a solution of Isopropylantipyrine (1 in 500) to a mixture of 5 mL of potassium hexacyanoferrate (III) TS and 1 to 2 drops of iron (III) chloride TS: a dark green color gradually develops.

(3) To 2 mL of a solution of Isopropylantipyrine (1 in 500) add 2 to 3 drops of tannic acid TS: a white precipitate is produced.

Melting point <*2.60*> 103 – 105°C

Purity **(1)** Chloride <*1.03*>—Dissolve 1.0 g of Isopropylantipyrine in 30 mL of dilute ethanol, and add 6 mL of dilute nitric acid and water to make 50 mL. Perform the test using this solution as the test solution. Prepare the control solution as follows: to 0.40 mL of 0.01 mol/L hydrochloric acid VS add 6 mL of dilute nitric acid, 30 mL of dilute ethanol and water to make 50 mL (not more than 0.014%).

(2) Sulfate <*1.14*>—Dissolve 1.0 g of Isopropylantipyrine in 30 mL of dilute ethanol, and add 1 mL of dilute hydrochloric acid and water to make 50 mL. Perform the test using this solution as the test solution. Prepare the control solution as follows: to 0.40 mL of 0.005 mol/L sulfuric acid VS add 1 mL of dilute hydrochloric acid and 30 mL of dilute ethanol, and dilute with water to make 50 mL (not more than 0.019%).

(3) Heavy metals <*1.07*>—Dissolve 1.0 g of Isopropylantipyrine in 25 mL of acetone, add 2 mL of dilute acetic acid and water to make 50 mL, and perform the test using this solution as the test solution. Prepare the control solution as follows: to 2.0 mL of Standard Lead Solution add 2 mL of dilute acetic acid, 25 mL of acetone, and dilute with water to make 50 mL (not more than 20 ppm).

(4) Arsenic *<1.11>*—Prepare the test solution with 1.0 g of Isopropylantipyrine according to Method 3, and perform the test (not more than 2 ppm).

(5) Antipyrine—Dissolve 1.0 g of Isopropylantipyrine in 10 mL of dilute ethanol, and add 1 mL of sodium nitrite TS and 1 mL of dilute sulfuric acid: no green color develops.

Loss on drying *<2.41>* Not more than 0.5% (1 g, in vacuum, silica gel, 5 hours).

Residue on ignition *<2.44>* Not more than 0.1% (1 g).

Assay Weigh accurately about 0.4 g of Isopropylantipyrine, previously dried, dissolve in 60 mL of a mixture of acetic acid (100) and acetic anhydride (2:1), and titrate *<2.50>* with 0.1 mol/L perchloric acid VS (potentiometric titration). Perform a blank determination in the same manner, and make any necessary correction.

Each mL of 0.1 mol/L perchloric acid VS
= 23.03 mg of $C_{14}H_{18}N_2O$

Containers and storage Containers—Tight containers.

Isosorbide

イソソルビド

$C_6H_{10}O_4$: 146.14
1,4:3,6-Dianhydro-D-glucitol
[652-67-5]

Isosorbide contains not less than 98.5% of isosorbide ($C_6H_{10}O_4$), calculated on the anhydrous basis.

Description Isosorbide occurs as white, crystals or masses. It is odorless, or has a faint, characteristic odor, and has a bitter taste.

It is very soluble in water and in methanol, freely soluble in ethanol (95), and slightly soluble in diethyl ether.

It is hygroscopic.

Identification **(1)** To 0.1 g of Isosorbide add 6 mL of diluted sulfuric acid (1 in 2), and dissolve by heating in a water bath. After cooling, shake well with 1 mL of a solution of potassium permanganate (1 in 30), and heat in a water bath until the color of potassium permanganate disappears. To this solution add 10 mL of 2,4-dinitrophenylhydrazine TS, and heat in a water bath: an orange precipitate is formed.

(2) To 2 g of Isosorbide add 30 mL of pyridine and 4 mL of benzoyl chloride, boil under a reflux condenser for 50 minutes, cool, and pour gradually the solution into 100 mL of cold water. Filter the formed precipitate by suction through a glass filter (G3), wash with water, recrystallize twice from ethanol (95), and dry in a desiccator (in vacuum, silica gel) for 4 hours: it melts *<2.60>* between 102°C and 103°C.

(3) Determine the infrared absorption spectrum of Isosorbide as directed in the potassium bromide disk method under Infrared Spectrophotometry *<2.25>*, and compare the spectrum with the Reference Spectrum: both spectra exhibit similar intensities of absorption at the same wave numbers.

Optical rotation *<2.49>* $[\alpha]_D^{20}$: +45.0 – +46.0° (5 g calculated on the anhydrous basis, water, 50 mL, 100 mm).

Purity **(1)** Clarity and color of solution—Take 25 g of Isosorbide in a Nessler tube, and dissolve in 50 mL of water: the solution is clear, and has no more color than the following control solution.

Control solution: To a mixture of 1.0 mL of Cobalt (II) Chloride CS, 3.0 mL of Iron (III) Chloride CS and 2.0 mL of Copper (II) Sulfate CS add water to make 10.0 mL. To 3.0 mL of this solution add water to make 50 mL.

(2) Sulfate *<1.14>*—Perform the test with 2.0 g of Isosorbide. Prepare the control solution with 1.0 mL of 0.005 mol/L sulfuric acid VS (not more than 0.024%).

(3) Heavy metals *<1.07>*—Proceed with 5.0 g of Isosorbide according to Method 1, and perform the test. Prepare the control solution with 2.5 mL of Standard Lead Solution (not more than 5 ppm).

(4) Arsenic *<1.11>*—Prepare the test solution with 1.0 g of Isosorbide according to Method 1, and perform the test (not more than 2 ppm).

(5) Related substances—Dissolve 0.10 g of Isosorbide in 10 mL of methanol, and use this solution as the sample solution. Pipet 2 mL of the sample solution, add methanol to make exactly 100 mL, and use this solution as the standard solution. Perform the test with these solutions as directed under Thin-layer Chromatography *<2.03>*. Spot 10 μL each of the sample solution and standard solution on a plate of silica gel for thin-layer chromatography. Develop the plate with a mixture of ethanol (95) and cyclohexane (1:1) to a distance of about 10 cm, and air-dry the plate. Spray evenly a mixture of ethanol (95) and sulfuric acid (9:1) on the plate, and heat the plate at 150°C for 30 minutes: the spots other than the principal spot obtained from the sample solution are not more intense than the spot from the standard solution.

Water *<2.48>* Not more than 1.5% (2 g, volumetric titration, direct titration).

Residue on ignition *<2.44>* Not more than 0.1% (1 g).

Assay Weigh accurately about 10 g of Isosorbide, calculated on the anhydrous basis, and dissolve in water to make exactly 100 mL. Determine the optical rotation *<2.49>*, α_D, of this solution at 20 ± 1°C in a 100-mm cell.

Amount (g) of isosorbide ($C_6H_{10}O_4$) = $\alpha_D \times 2.1978$

Containers and storage Containers—Tight containers.

Isosorbide Dinitrate

硝酸イソソルビド

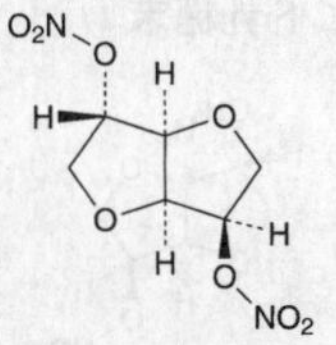

$C_6H_8N_2O_8$: 236.14
1,4:3,6-Dianhydro-D-glucitol dinitrate
[87-33-2]

Isosorbide Dinitrate contains not less than 95.0% of isosorbide dinitrate ($C_6H_8N_2O_8$), calculated on the anhydrous basis.

Description Isosorbide Dinitrate occurs as white, crystals or crystalline powder. It is odorless or has a faint odor like that of nitric acid.

It is very soluble in *N,N*-dimethylformamide and in acetone, freely soluble in chloroform and in toluene, soluble in methanol, in ethanol (95) and in diethyl ether, and practically insoluble in water.

It explodes if heated quickly or subjected to percussion.

Identification **(1)** Dissolve 10 mg of Isosorbide Dinitrate in 1 mL of water, and dissolve by adding 2 mL of sulfuric acid cautiously. After cooling, superimpose 3 mL of iron (II) sulfate TS, and allow to stand for 5 to 10 minutes: a brown ring is produced at the zone of contact.

(2) Dissolve 0.1 g of Isosorbide Dinitrate in 6 mL of diluted sulfuric acid (1 in 2) by heating in a water bath. After cooling, add 1 mL of a solution of potassium permanganate (1 in 30), stir well, and heat in a water bath until the color of potassium permanganate disappears. Add 10 mL of 2,4-dinitro-phenylhydrazine TS, and heat in a water bath: an orange precipitate is produced.

Optical rotation 〈*2.49*〉 $[\alpha]_D^{20}$: +134 – +139° (1 g calculated on the anhydrous basis, ethanol (95), 100 mL, 100 mm).

Purity **(1)** Clarity and color of solution—Dissolve 1.0 g of Isosorbide Dinitrate in 10 mL of acetone: the solution is clear and colorless.

(2) Sulfate 〈*1.14*〉—Dissolve 1.5 g of Isosorbide Dinitrate in 15 mL of *N,N*-dimethylformamide, add 60 mL of water, cool, and filter. Wash the filter paper with three 20-mL portions of water, combine the washings with the filtrate, and add water to make 150 mL. To 40 mL of this solution add 1 mL of dilute hydrochloric acid and water to make 50 mL. Perform the test using this solution as the test solution. Prepare the control solution with 0.40 mL of 0.005 mol/L sulfuric acid VS (not more than 0.048%).

(3) Nitrate—Dissolve 50 mg of Isosorbide Dinitrate in 30 mL of toluene, and extract with three 20-mL portions of water. Combine the aqueous layers, and wash with two 20-mL portions of toluene. To the aqueous layer add water to make 100 mL, and use this solution as the sample solution. Pipet 5.0 mL of Standard Nitric Acid Solution and 25 mL of the sample solution in each Nessler tube, and add water to make 50 mL, respectively. To each of them add 60 mg of Griss-Romijin's nitric acid reagent, stir well, allow to stand for 30 minutes, and observe from the side of the Nessler tube: the sample solution has no more color than the standard solution.

(4) Heavy metals 〈*1.07*〉—Dissolve 1.0 g of Isosorbide Dinitrate in 30 mL of acetone, and add 2 mL of dilute acetic acid and water to make 50 mL. Perform the test using this solution as the test solution. Prepare the control solution as follows: to 2.0 mL of Standard Lead Solution add 30 mL of acetone, 2 mL of dilute acetic acid and water to make 50 mL (not more than 20 ppm).

Water 〈*2.48*〉 Not more than 1.5% (0.3 g, volumetric titration, direct titration).

Assay Weigh accurately about 0.1 g of Isosorbide Dinitrate in a Kjeldahl flask as described under the Nitrogen Determination 〈*1.08*〉, dissolve in 10 mL of methanol, add 3 g of Devarda's alloy and 50 mL of water, and connect the flask with the distillation apparatus as described under the Nitrogen Determination 〈*1.08*〉. Measure exactly 25 mL of 0.05 mol/L sulfuric acid VS in an absorption flask, add 5 drops of bromocresol green-methyl red TS, and immerse the lower end of the condenser tube in it. Add 15 mL of a solution of sodium hydroxide (1 in 2) through the funnel, cautiously rinse the funnel with 20 mL of water, immediately close the clamp attached to the rubber tubing, then begin the distillation with steam gradually, and continue the distillation until the distillate measures 100 mL. Remove the absorption flask, rinse the end of the condenser tube with a small quantity of water, and titrate 〈*2.50*〉 the distillate and the rinsings with 0.1 mol/L sodium hydroxide VS until the color of the solution changes from red through light red-purple to light blue-green. Perform a blank determination in the same manner, and make any necessary correction.

Each mL of 0.05 mol/L sulfuric acid VS
= 11.81 mg of $C_6H_8N_2O_8$

Containers and storage Containers—Tight containers.
Storage—Light-resistant, and in a cold place.

Isosorbide Dinitrate Tablets

硝酸イソソルビド錠

Isosorbide Dinitrate Tablets contain not less than 93.0% and not more than 107.0% of the labeled amount of isosorbide dinitrate ($C_6H_8N_2O_8$: 236.14).

Method of preparation Prepare as directed under Tablets, with Isosorbide Dinitrate.

Identification Weigh a quantity of powdered Isosorbide Dinitrate Tablets, equivalent to 0.1 g of Isosorbide Dinitrate, add 50 mL of diethyl ether, shake well, and filter. Measure 5 mL of the filtrate, evaporate to dryness cautiously, add 1 mL of water to the residue, and dissolve by adding 2 mL of sulfuric acid cautiously. After cooling, superimpose 3 mL of iron (II) sulfate TS, and allow to stand for 5 to 10 minutes: a brown ring is produced at the zone of contact.

Purity Nitrate—Weigh accurately a quantity of powdered Isosorbide Dinitrate Tablets, equivalent to 50 mg of Isosorbide Dinitrate, transfer to a separator, add 30 mL of toluene, shake thoroughly, extract with three 20-mL portions of water, and proceed as directed in Purity (3) under Isosorbide Dinitrate.

Uniformity of dosage units 〈*6.02*〉 Perform the test according to the following method: it meets the requirement of the Content uniformity test.

To 1 tablet of Isosorbide Dinitrate Tablets add 1 mL of

water, and shake to disintegrate. To this solution add a mixture of water and methanol (1:1) to make exactly V mL so that each mL contains about 0.1 mg of isosorbide dinitrate ($C_6H_8N_2O_8$), and shake for 10 minutes. Centrifuge this solution, and use the supernatant liquid as the sample solution. Proceed as directed in the Assay.

$$\text{Amount (mg) of isosorbide dinitrate } (C_6H_8N_2O_8) = M_S \times A_T/A_S \times V \times 1/500$$

M_S: Amount (mg) of isosorbide dinitrate for assay taken, calculated on the anhydrous basis

Disintegration <*6.09*> It meets the requirement.

For Sublingual Tablets, the time limit of the test is 2 minutes, and omit the use of the disk.

Assay Weigh accurately the mass of not less than 20 tablets of Isosorbide Dinitrate Tablets, and powder. Weigh accurately a portion of the powder, equivalent to about 5 mg of isosorbide dinitrate ($C_6H_8N_2O_8$), add a mixture of water and methanol (1:1) to make exactly 50 mL, and shake for 10 minutes. Centrifuge this solution, and use the supernatant liquid as the sample solution. Separately, weigh accurately about 50 mg of isosorbide dinitrate for assay (separately, determine the water <*2.48*> in the same manner as Isosorbide Dinitrate), dissolve in a mixture of water and methanol (1:1) to make exactly 100 mL. Pipet 10 mL of this solution, add a mixture of water and methanol (1:1) to make exactly 50 mL, and use this solution as the standard solution. Perform the test with exactly 10 μL each of the sample solution and standard solution as directed under Liquid Chromatography <*2.01*> according to the following conditions, and determine the peak areas, A_T and A_S, of isosorbide dinitrate in each solution.

$$\text{Amount (mg) of isosorbide dinitrate } (C_6H_8N_2O_8) = M_S \times A_T/A_S \times 1/10$$

M_S: Amount (mg) of isosorbide dinitrate for assay taken, calculated on the anhydrous basis

Operating conditions—

Detector: An ultraviolet absorption photometer (wavelength: 220 nm).

Column: A stainless steel column 4.6 mm in inside diameter and 15 cm in length, packed with octadecylsilanized silica gel for liquid chromatography (5 μm in particle diameter).

Column temperature: A constant temperature of about 40°C.

Mobile phase: A mixture of water and methanol (11:9).

Flow rate: Adjust so that the retention time of isosorbide dinitrate is about 6 minutes.

System suitability—

System performance: When the procedure is run with 10 μL of the standard solution under the above operating conditions, the number of theoretical plates and the symmetry factor of the peak of isosorbide dinitrate are not less than 3000 and not more than 1.5, respectively.

System repeatability: When the test is repeated 6 times with 10 μL of the standard solution under the above operating conditions, the relative standard deviation of the peak area of isosorbide dinitrate is not more than 1.0%.

Containers and storage Containers—Tight containers.

Isosorbide Mononitrate 70%/Lactose 30%

70%一硝酸イソソルビド乳糖末

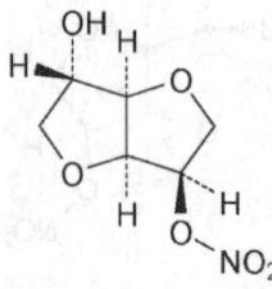

$C_6H_9NO_6$: 191.14
1,4:3,6-Dianhydro-D-glucitol 5-nitrate
[*16051-77-7*, Isosorbide mononitrate]

Isosorbide Mononitrate 70%/Lactose 30%, when dried, contains not less than 68.0% and not more than 72.0% of isosorbide mononitrate ($C_6H_9NO_6$).

Description Isosorbide Mononitrate 70%/Lactose 30% occurs as a white, powder, crystalline powder, or masses.

It is freely soluble in water, and practically insoluble in ethanol (99.5).

Identification (1) Shake thoroughly 1 g of Isosorbide Mononitrate 70%/Lactose 30% with 30 mL of ethyl acetate, and filter. Wash the residue with a small quantity of ethyl acetate, combine the filtrate and the washings, evaporate to dryness on a water bath, then dry in vacuum at room temperature for 4 hours. Determine the infrared absorption spectrum of the crystals obtained as directed in the potassium bromide disk method under Infrared Spectrophotometry <*2.25*>, and compare the spectrum with the Reference Spectrum of isosorbide mononitrate: both spectra exhibit similar intensities of absorption at the same wave numbers.

(2) Dry the residue obtained in (1) at 80°C for 2 hours. Determine the infrared absorption spectrum of the residue as directed in the potassium bromide disk method under Infrared Spectrophotometry <*2.25*>, and compare the spectrum with the Reference Spectrum of Lactose Hydrate or the spectrum of Lactose for Identification RS: both spectra exhibit similar intensities of absorption at the same wave numbers.

Optical rotation <*2.49*> $[\alpha]_D^{20}$: +116 – +124° (after drying, 1 g, water, 100 mL, 100 mm).

Purity (1) Nitrate—Dissolve an exact quantity of Isosorbide Mononitrate 70%/Lactose 30%, equivalent to 50 mg of isosorbide mononitrate ($C_6H_9NO_6$), in water to make exactly 100 mL. Pipet 25 mL of this solution, add water to make exactly 50 mL, and use this solution as the sample solution. Separately, to exactly 5 mL of Standard Nitric Acid Solution add water to make exactly 150 mL. Pipet 25 mL of this solution, add water to make exactly 150 mL, and use this solution as the standard solution. Perform the test with exactly 100 μL each of the sample solution and standard solution as directed under Liquid Chromatography <*2.01*> according to the following conditions, and determine the peak area of nitric acid of each solution by the automatic integration method: the peak area of nitric acid obtained from the sample solution is not larger than the peak area of nitric acid from the standard solution.

Operating conditions—

Detector: An ultraviolet absorption photometer (wavelength: 214 nm).

Column: A stainless steel column 4.6 mm in inside diameter and 5 cm in length, packed with gel type strong basic ion-exchange resin for liquid chromatography (10 μm in particle diameter).

Column temperature: A constant temperature of about 35°C.

Mobile phase: Dissolve 16.0 g of sodium gluconate, 18.0 g of boric acid, 25.0 g of sodium tetraborate decahydrate, and 250 mL of glycerin in water to make 1000 mL. To 20 mL of this solution add 20 mL of 1-butanol, 120 mL of acetonitrile, and add water to make 1000 mL.

Flow rate: Adjust so that the retention time of nitric acid is about 5.3 minutes.

System suitability—

System performance: When the procedure is run with 100 μL of the standard solution under the above operating conditions, the number of theoretical plates and the symmetry factor of the peak of nitric acid are not less than 800 and not more than 1.5, respectively.

System repeatability: When the test is repeated 6 times with 100 μL of the standard solution under the above operating conditions, the relative standard deviation of the peak area of nitric acid is not more than 2.0%.

(2) Heavy metals <*1.07*>—Proceed with 1.0 g of Isosorbide Mononitrate 70%/Lactose 30% according to Method 1, and perform the test. Prepare the control solution with 1.0 mL of Standard Lead Solution (not more than 10 ppm).

(3) Isosorbide—To an amount of Isosorbide Mononitrate 70%/Lactose 30%, equivalent to 1.0 g of isosorbide mononitrate ($C_6H_9NO_6$), add 10 mL of acetone, shake well, centrifuge, and filter the supernatant liquid through a membrane filter with a pore size not exceeding 0.5 μm. To the residue add 2 mL of acetone and proceed in the same manner, and combine the filtrates. Evaporate the combined filtrate to dryness on a water bath, and further dry the residue in vacuum for 30 minutes. Dissolve the residue in the mobile phase to make 10 mL, and use this solution as the sample solution. Pipet 1 mL of the sample solution, and add the mobile phase to make exactly 20 mL. Pipet 1 mL of this solution, add the mobile phase to make exactly 25 mL, and use this solution as the standard solution. Perform the test with exactly 20 μL each of the sample solution and standard solution as directed under Liquid Chromatography <*2.01*> according to the following conditions, and determine the peak areas by the automatic integration method: the peak area of isosorbide, having the relative retention time of about 0.2 to isosorbide mononitrate, obtained from the sample solution is not larger than the peak area of isosorbide mononitrate from the standard solution.

Operating conditions—

Detector: A differential refractometer.

Column: A stainless steel column 4.6 mm in inside diameter and 25 cm in length, packed with octadecylsilanized silica gel for liquid chromatography (5 μm in particle diameter).

Column temperature: A constant temperature of about 25°C.

Mobile phase: A mixture of water and methanol (9:1).

Flow rate: Adjust so that the retention time of isosorbide mononitrate is about 16 minutes.

System suitability—

System performance: When the procedure is run with 20 μL of the standard solution under the above operating conditions, the number of theoretical plates and the symmetry factor of the peak of isosorbide mononitrate are not less than 5000 and not more than 2.0, respectively.

System repeatability: When the test is repeated 6 times with 20 μL of the standard solution under the above operating conditions, the relative standard deviation of the peak area of isosorbide mononitrate is not more than 4.0%.

(4) Related substances—Dissolve an amount of Isosorbide Mononitrate 70%/Lactose 30%, equivalent to 50 mg of isosorbide mononitrate ($C_6H_9NO_6$), in 5 mL of water, and use this solution as the sample solution. Pipet 1 mL of the sample solution, add water to make exactly 100 mL, and use this solution as the standard solution. Perform the test with exactly 10 μL each of the sample solution and standard solution as directed under Liquid Chromatography <*2.01*> according to the following conditions. Determine each peak area by the automatic integration method: the area of the peak other than isosorbide mononitrate obtained from the sample solution is not larger than 1/2 times the peak area of isosorbide mononitrate from the standard solution, and the total area of the peaks other than isosorbide mononitrate from the sample solution is not larger than the peak area of isosorbide mononitrate from the standard solution. For the area of the peak, having the relative retention time of about 4.5 to isosorbide mononitrate, multiply the correction factor, 0.62.

Operating conditions—

Detector, column, column temperature, mobile phase, and flow rate: Proceed as directed in the operating conditions in the Assay.

Time span of measurement: About 5 times as long as the retention time of isosorbide mononitrate, beginning after the solvent peak.

System suitability—

System performance: Proceed as directed in the system suitability in the Assay.

Test for required detectability: Pipet 1 mL of the standard solution, and add water to make exactly 10 mL. Confirm that the peak area of isosorbide mononitrate obtained with 10 μL of this solution is equivalent to 7 to 13% of that with 10 μL of the standard solution.

System repeatability: When the test is repeated 6 times with 10 μL of the standard solution under the above operating conditions, the relative standard deviation of the peak area of isosorbide mononitrate is not more than 2.0%.

Loss on drying <*2.41*> Not more than 0.5% (1 g, in vacuum, silica gel, 4 hours).

Water <*2.48*> Between 1.0% and 2.0% (0.4 g, volumetric titration, direct titratioin. Use a mixture of methanol for water determination and formamide for water determination (2:1) instead of methanol for water determination).

Residue on ignition <*2.44*> Not more than 0.1% (0.5 g).

Assay Weigh accurately an amount of Isosorbide Mononitrate 70%/Lactose 30%, previously dried, equivalent to about 0.2 g of isosorbide mononitrate ($C_6H_9NO_6$), and dissolve in water to make exactly 50 mL. Pipet 10 mL of this solution, add exactly 20 mL of the internal standard solution, then add water to make 100 mL, and use this solution as the sample solution. Separately, weigh accurately about 40 mg of isosorbide mononitrate for assay, previously dried, and dissolve in 60 mL of water, add exactly 20 mL of the internal standard solution, then, add water to make 100 mL, and use this solution as the standard solution. Perform the test with 10 μL each of the sample solution and standard solution as directed under Liquid Chromatography <*2.01*> according to the following conditions, and calculate the ratios, Q_T and Q_S, of the peak area of isosorbide mononitrate to that of the internal standard.

Amount (mg) of isosorbide mononitrate ($C_6H_9NO_6$)
$= M_S \times Q_T/Q_S \times 5$

M_S: Amount (mg) of isosorbide mononitrate for assay taken

Internal standard solution—A solution of benzyl alcohol (1 in 1000).

Operating conditions—

Detector: An ultraviolet absorption photometer (wavelength: 214 nm).

Column: A stainless steel column 4.6 mm in inside diameter and 15 cm in length, packed with octadecylsilanized silica gel for liquid chromatography (5 μm in particle diameter).

Column temperature: A constant temperature of about 40°C.

Mobile phase: A mixture of diluted phosphoric acid (1 in 1000) and methanol (4:1).

Flow rate: Adjust so that the retention time of isosorbide mononitrate is about 4.5 minutes.

System suitability—

System performance: When the procedure is run with 10 μL of the standard solution under the above operating conditions, isosorbide mononitrate and the internal standard are eluted in this order with the resolution between these peaks being not less than 10.

System repeatability: When the test is repeated 6 times with 10 μL of the standard solution under the above operating conditions, the relative standard deviation of the ratio of the peak area of isosorbide mononitrate to that of the internal standard is not more than 1.0%.

Containers and storage Containers—Tight containers.

Isosorbide Mononitrate Tablets

一硝酸イソソルビド錠

Isosorbide Mononitrate Tablets contain not less than 95.0% and not more than 105.0% of the labeled amount of isosorbide mononitrate ($C_6H_9NO_6$: 191.14).

Method of preparation Prepare as directed under Tablets, with Isosorbide Mononitrate 70%/Lactose 30%.

Identification Shake well a portion of powdered Isosorbide Mononitrate Tablets, equivalent to 50 mg of isosorbide mononitrate ($C_6H_9NO_6$), with 5 mL of acetone, centrifuge, and use the supernatant liquid as the sample solution. Separately, dissolve 10 mg of isosorbide mononitrate for assay in 1 mL of acetone, and use this solution as the standard solution. Perform the test with these solutions as directed under Thin-layer Chromatography *<2.03>*. Spot 20 μL each of the sample solution and standard solution on a plate of silica gel for thin-layer chromatography. Develop the plate with a mixture of ethyl acetate and hexane (2:1) to a distance of about 15 cm, and air-dry the plate. Spray evenly a solution of potassium permanganate in potassium hydroxide TS (1 in 50), and allow to stand for about 50 minutes: the principal spot obtained with the sample solution and the spot from the standard solution are yellow, and their *Rf* values are the same.

Uniformity of dosage units *<6.02>* Perform the test according to the following method: it meets the requirement of the Content uniformity test.

To 1 tablet of Isosorbide Mononitrate Tablets add 30 mL of water, allow standing to disintegrate the tablet, and disperse the fine particles by sonicating. Add exactly V/10 mL of the internal standard solution, and add water to make V mL so that each mL contains about 0.2 mg of isosorbide mononitrate ($C_6H_9NO_6$). Centrifuge this solution, filter the supernatant liquid through a membrane filter with a pore size not exceeding 0.45 μm, discard the first 10 mL of the filtrate, and use the subsequent filtrate as the sample solution. Separately, weigh accurately about 20 mg of isosorbide mononitrate for assay, previously dried in vacuum (silica gel) for 4 hours, add 30 mL of water and exactly 10 mL of the internal standard solution, then add water to make 100 mL, and use this solution as the standard solution. Then, proceed as directed in the Assay.

$$\text{Amount (mg) of isosorbide mononitrate } (C_6H_9NO_6) = M_S \times Q_T/Q_S \times V/100$$

M_S: Amount (mg) of isosorbide mononitrate for assay taken

Internal standard solution—A solution of benzyl alcohol (1 in 1000).

Dissolution *<6.10>* When the test is performed at 50 revolutions per minute according to the Paddle method, using 900 mL of water as the dissolution medium, the dissolution rate in 15 minutes of Isosorbide Mononitrate Tablets is not less than 85%.

Start the test with 1 tablet of Isosorbide Mononitrate Tablets, withdraw not less than 20 mL of the medium at the specified minute after starting the test, and filter through a membrane filter with a pore size not exceeding 0.45 μm. Discard not less than 10 mL of the first filtrate, pipet V mL of the subsequent filtrate, add water to make exactly V' mL so that each mL contains about 11 μg of isosorbide mononitrate ($C_6H_9NO_6$), and use this solution as the sample solution. Separately, weigh accurately about 22 mg of isosorbide mononitrate for assay, previously dried in vacuum (silica gel) for 4 hours, and dissolve in water to make exactly 100 mL. Pipet 5 mL of this solution, add water to make exactly 100 mL, and use this solution as the standard solution. Perform the test with exactly 15 μL each of the sample solution and standard solution as directed under Liquid Chromatography *<2.01>* according to the following conditions, and determine the peak areas, A_T and A_S, of isosorbide mononitrate in each solution.

$$\text{Dissolution rate (\%) with respect to the labeled amount of isosorbide mononitrate } (C_6H_9NO_6) = M_S \times A_T/A_S \times V'/V \times 1/C \times 45$$

M_S: Amount (mg) of isosorbide mononitrate for assay taken

C: Labeled amount (mg) of isosorbide mononitrate ($C_6H_9NO_6$) in 1 tablet

Operating conditions—

Proceed as directed in the operating conditions in the Assay.

System suitability—

System performance: When the procedure is run with 15 μL of the standard solution under the above operating conditions, the number of theoretical plates and the symmetry factor of the peak of isosorbide mononitrate are not less than 2000 and not more than 1.5, respectively.

System repeatability: When the test is repeated 6 times with 15 μL of the standard solution under the above operating conditions, the relative standard deviation of the peak area of isosorbide mononitrate is not more than 2.0%.

Assay Weigh accurately the mass of not less than 20 Isosorbide Mononitrate Tablets, and powder. Weigh accurately a portion of the powder, equivalent to about 20 mg of isosorbide mononitrate ($C_6H_9NO_6$), add 30 mL of water, and disperse the fine particles by sonicating. Add exactly 10 mL of the internal standard solution and water to make 50 mL.

Centrifuge this solution, and filter the supernatant liquid through a membrane filter with a pore size not exceeding 0.45 μm. Discard the first 10 mL of the filtrate, and use the subsequent filtrate as the sample solution. Separately, weigh accurately about 20 mg of isosorbide mononitrate for assay, previously dried, and dissolve in 30 mL of water, add exactly 10 mL of the internal standard solution, then, add water to make 50 mL, and use this solution as the standard solution. Perform the test with 10 μL each of the sample solution and standard solution as directed under Liquid Chromatography <2.01> according to the following conditions, and calculate the ratios, Q_T and Q_S, of the peak area of isosorbide mononitrate to that of the internal standard.

Amount (mg) of isosorbide mononitrate ($C_6H_9NO_6$)
$= M_S \times Q_T/Q_S$

M_S: Amount (mg) of isosorbide mononitrate for assay taken

Internal standard solution—A solution of benzyl alcohol (1 in 1000).

Operating conditions—

Detector: An ultraviolet absorption photometer (wavelength: 214 nm).

Column: A stainless steel column 4.6 mm in inside diameter and 15 cm in length, packed with octadecylsilanized silica gel for liquid chromatography (5 μm in particle diameter).

Column temperature: A constant temperature of about 40°C.

Mobile phase: A mixture of diluted phosphoric acid (1 in 1000) and methanol (4:1).

Flow rate: Adjust so that the retention time of isosorbide mononitrate is about 4.5 minutes.

System suitability—

System performance: When the procedure is run with 10 μL of the standard solution under the above operating conditions, isosorbide mononitrate and the internal standard are eluted in this order with the resolution between these peaks being not less than 10.

System repeatability: When the test is repeated 6 times with 10 μL of the standard solution under the above operating conditions, the relative standard deviation of the ratio of the peak area of isosorbide mononitrate to that of the internal standard is not more than 1.0%.

Containers and storage Containers—Tight containers.

Isoxsuprine Hydrochloride

イソクスプリン塩酸塩

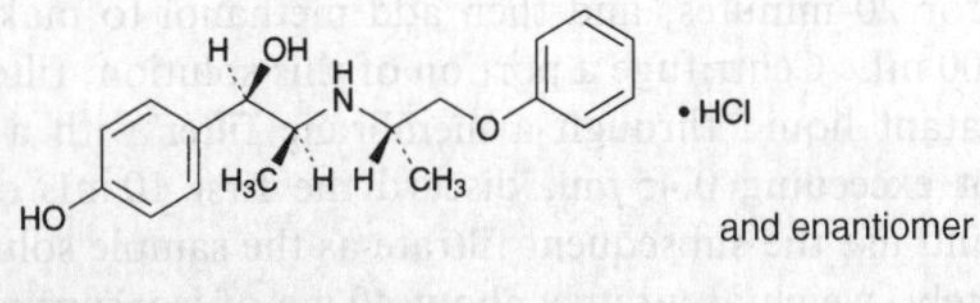

and enantiomer

$C_{18}H_{23}NO_3.HCl$: 337.84
(1*RS*,2*SR*)-1-(4-Hydroxyphenyl)-2-{[(2*SR*)-1-phenoxypropan-2-yl]amino}propan-1-ol monohydrochloride
[*579-56-6*]

Isoxsuprine Hydrochloride, when dried, contains not less than 99.0% and not more than 101.0% of isoxsuprine hydrochloride ($C_{18}H_{23}NO_3.HCl$).

Description Isoxsuprine Hydrochloride occurs as a white, powder or crystalline powder.

It is soluble in formic acid and in methanol, and slightly soluble in water and in ethanol (99.5).

Melting point: about 204°C (with decomposition).

A solution of Isoxsuprine Hydrochloride in methanol (1 in 50) shows no optical rotation.

Identification (1) Determine the absorption spectrum of a solution of Isoxsuprine Hydrochloride (1 in 20,000) as directed under Ultraviolet-visible Spectrophotometry <2.24>, and compare the spectrum with the Reference Spectrum: both spectra exhibit similar intensities of absorption at the same wavelengths.

(2) Determine the infrared absorption spectrum of Isoxsuprine Hydrochloride as directed in the potassium chloride disk method under Infrared Spectrophotometry <2.25>, and compare the spectrum with the Reference Spectrum: both spectra exhibit similar intensities of absorption at the same wave numbers.

(3) Dissolve 0.5 g of Isoxsuprine Hydrochloride in 50 mL of water by warming, and cool: the solution responds to Qualitative Tests <1.09> (2) for chloride.

pH <2.54> Dissolve 0.5 g of Isoxsuprine Hydrochloride in 50 mL of water by warming, and cool: the pH of the solution is between 4.5 and 6.0.

Purity (1) Clarity and color of solution—Dissolve 0.1 g of Isoxsuprine Hydrochloride in 10 mL of water, warm if necessary, and cool: the solution is clear and colorless.

(2) Heavy metals <1.07>—Proceed with 1.0 g of Isoxsuprine Hydrochloride according to Method 2, and perform the test. Prepare the control solution with 2.0 mL of Standard Lead Solution (not more than 20 ppm).

(3) Related substances—Dissolve 20 mg of Isoxsuprine Hydrochloride in 20 mL of the mobile phase, and use this solution as the sample solution. Pipet 1 mL of the sample solution, add the mobile phase to make exactly 100 mL, and use this solution as the standard solution. Perform the test with exactly 10 μL each of the sample solution and standard solution as directed under Liquid Chromatography <2.01> according to the following conditions. Determine each peak area by the automatic integration method: each peak area other than isoxsuprine obtained from the sample solution is not larger than the peak area of isoxsuprine from the standard solution, and the total area of the peaks other than the peak of isoxsuprine from the sample solution is not larger than 2 times the peak area of isoxsuprine from the standard solution.

Operating conditions—

Detector: An ultraviolet absorption photometer (wavelength: 269 nm).

Column: A stainless steel column 4.6 mm in inside diameter and 25 cm in length, packed with octadecylsilanized silica gel for liquid chromatography (5 μm in particle diameter).

Column temperature: A constant temperature of about 40°C.

Mobile phase: Dissolve 4.3 g of diammonium hydrogen phosphate and 3.2 g of sodium 1-pentane sulfonate in water to make 1000 mL, and adjust to pH 2.5 with phosphoric acid. To 770 mL of this solution add 230 mL of acetonitrile.

Flow rate: Adjust so that the retention time of isoxsuprine is about 18 minutes.

Time span of measurement: About 3 times as long as the retention time of isoxsuprine, beginning after the solvent peak.

System suitability—

Test for required detectability: Pipet 1 mL of the standard

solution, and add the mobile phase to make exactly 10 mL. Confirm that the peak area of isoxsuprine obtained with 10 μL of this solution is equivalent to 7 to 13% of that with 10 μL of the standard solution.

System performance: To 1 mL of the sample solution add 2.5 mL of a solution of methyl parahydroxybenzoate (1 in 25,000) and the mobile phase to make 50 mL. When the procedure is run with 10 μL of this solution under the above operating conditions, methyl parahydroxybenzoate and isoxsuprine are eluted in this order with the resolution between these peaks being not less than 4.

System repeatability: When the test is repeated 6 times with 10 μL of the standard solution under the above operating conditions, the relative standard deviation of the peak area of isoxsuprine is not more than 2.5%.

Loss on drying *<2.41>* Not more than 0.5% (1 g, 105°C, 1 hour).

Residue on ignition *<2.44>* Not more than 0.2% (1 g).

Assay Weigh accurately about 0.3 g of Isoxsuprine Hydrochloride, previously dried, dissolve in 5 mL of formic acid, add 50 mL of a mixture of acetic anhydride and acetic acid (100) (7:3), and titrate *<2.50>* with 0.1 mol/L perchloric acid VS (potentiometric titration). Perform a blank determination in the same manner, and make any necessary correction.

Each mL of 0.1 mol/L perchloric acid VS
= 33.78 mg of $C_{18}H_{23}NO_3.HCl$

Containers and storage Containers—Well-closed containers.

Isoxsuprine Hydrochloride Tablets

イソクスプリン塩酸塩錠

Isoxsuprine Hydrochloride Tablets contain not less than 95.0% and not more than 105.0% of the labeled amount of isoxsuprine hydrochloride ($C_{18}H_{23}NO_3.HCl$: 337.84).

Method of preparation Prepare as directed under Tablets, with Isoxsuprine Hydrochloride.

Identification To a quantity of powdered Isoxsuprine Hydrochloride Tablets, equivalent to 10 mg of Isoxsuprine Hydrochloride, add 150 mL of water, shake, and then add water to make 200 mL. Centrifuge this solution, filter the supernatant liquid through a membrane filter with a pore size not exceeding 0.45 μm, discard the first 10 mL of filtrate, and determine the absorption spectrum of the subsequent filtrate as directed under Ultraviolet-visible Spectrophotometry *<2.24>*: it exhibits maxima between 267 nm and 271 nm, and between 272 nm and 276 nm.

Uniformity of dosage units *<6.02>* Perform the test according to the following method: it meets the requirement of the Content uniformity test.

Add methanol to 1 tablet of Isoxsuprine Hydrochloride Tablets, and shake to disintegrate. Add methanol to make exactly *V* mL so that each mL contains about 0.4 mg of isoxsuprine hydrochloride ($C_{18}H_{23}NO_3.HCl$). Centrifuge this solution, and use the supernatant liquid as the sample solution. Then, proceed as directed in the Assay.

Amount (mg) of isoxsuprine hydrochloride ($C_{18}H_{23}NO_3.HCl$)
$= M_S \times A_T/A_S \times V \times 1/100$

M_S: Amount (mg) of isoxsuprine hydrochloride for assay taken

Dissolution *<6.10>* When the test is performed at 50 revolutions per minute according to the Paddle method, using 900 mL of water as the dissolution medium, the dissolution rate in 15 minutes of Isoxsuprine Hydrochloride Tablets is not less than 80%.

Start the test with 1 tablet of Isoxsuprine Hydrochloride Tablets, withdraw not less than 20 mL of the medium at the specified minute after starting the test, and filter through a membrane filter with a pore size not exceeding 0.45 μm. Discard not less than 10 mL of the first filtrate, pipet *V* mL of the subsequent filtrate, add water to make exactly *V′* mL so that each mL contains about 11 μg of isoxsuprine hydrochloride ($C_{18}H_{23}NO_3.HCl$), and use this solution as the sample solution. Separately, weigh accurately about 28 mg of isoxsuprine hydrochloride for assay, previously dried at 105°C for 1 hour, and dissolve in water to make exactly 100 mL. Pipet 4 mL of this solution, add water to make exactly 100 mL, and use this solution as the standard solution. Perform the test with exactly 10 μL each of the sample solution and standard solution as directed under Liquid Chromatography *<2.01>* according to the following conditions, and determine the peak areas, A_T and A_S, of isoxsuprine in each solution.

Dissolution rate (%) with respect to the labeled amount of isoxsuprine hydrochloride ($C_{18}H_{23}NO_3.HCl$)
$= M_S \times A_T/A_S \times V'/V \times 1/C \times 36$

M_S: Amount (mg) of isoxsuprine hydrochloride for assay taken
C: Labeled amount (mg) of isoxsuprine hydrochloride ($C_{18}H_{23}NO_3.HCl$) in 1 tablet

Operating conditions—

Proceed as directed in the operating conditions in the Assay.

System suitability—

System performance: When the procedure is run with 10 μL of the standard solution under the above operating conditions, the number of theoretical plates and the symmetry factor of the peak of isoxsuprine are not less than 2000 and not more than 2.0, respectively.

System repeatability: When the test is repeated 6 times with 10 μL of the standard solution under the above operating conditions, the relative standard deviation of the peak area of isoxsuprine is not more than 2.0%.

Assay Weigh accurately not less than 20 Isoxsuprine Hydrochloride Tablets, and powder. Weigh accurately a portion of the powder, equivalent to about 40 mg of isoxsuprine hydrochloride ($C_{18}H_{23}NO_3.HCl$), add 60 mL of methanol, shake for 20 minutes, and then add methanol to make exactly 100 mL. Centrifuge a portion of this solution, filter the supernatant liquid through a membrane filter with a pore size not exceeding 0.45 μm, discard the first 10 mL of filtrate, and use the subsequent filtrate as the sample solution. Separately, weigh accurately about 40 mg of isoxsuprine hydrochloride for assay, previously dried at 105°C for 1 hour, and dissolve in methanol to make exactly 100 mL. Filter through a membrane filter with a pore size not exceeding 0.45 μm, discard the first 10 mL of the filtrate, and use the subsequent filtrate as the standard solution. Perform the test with exactly 10 μL each of the sample solution and standard solution as directed under Liquid Chromatography *<2.01>* according to the following conditions, and determine the peak areas, A_T and A_S, of isoxsuprine in each solution.

Amount (mg) of isoxsuprine hydrochloride ($C_{18}H_{23}NO_3.HCl$)
$= M_S \times A_T/A_S$

M_S: Amount (mg) of isoxsuprine hydrochloride for assay taken

Operating conditions—

Detector: An ultraviolet absorption photometer (wavelength: 269 nm).

Column: A stainless steel column 4.6 mm in inside diameter and 15 cm in length, packed with octadecylsilanized silica gel for liquid chromatography (5 μm in particle diameter).

Column temperature: A constant temperature of about 40°C.

Mobile phase: Dissolve 4.3 g of diammonium hydrogen phosphate and 3.2 g of sodium 1-pentane sulfonate in water to make 1000 mL, and adjust to pH 2.5 with phosphoric acid. To 600 mL of this solution add 400 mL of methanol.

Flow rate: Adjust so that the retention time of isoxsuprine is about 9 minutes.

System suitability—

System performance: To exactly 1 mL of the standard solution add the mobile phase to make exactly 50 mL. When the procedure is run with 10 μL of this solution under the above operating conditions, the number of theoretical plates and the symmetry factor of the peak of isoxsuprine are not less than 2000 and not more than 2.0, respectively.

System repeatability: When the test is repeated 6 times with 10 μL of the standard solution under the above operating conditions, the relative standard deviation of the peak area of isoxsuprine is not more than 1.0%.

Containers and storage Containers—Well-closed containers.

Itraconazole

イトラコナゾール

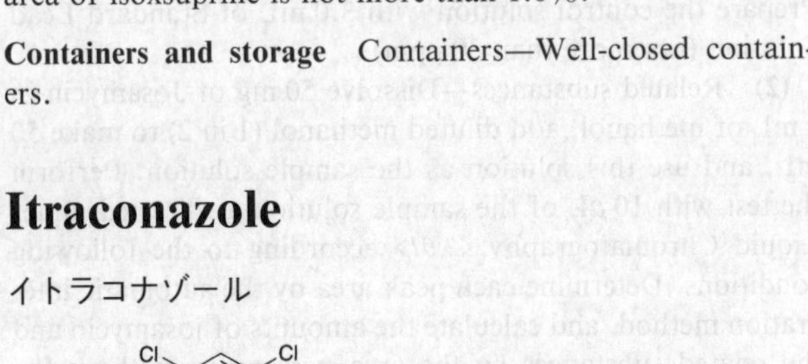

and enantiomer

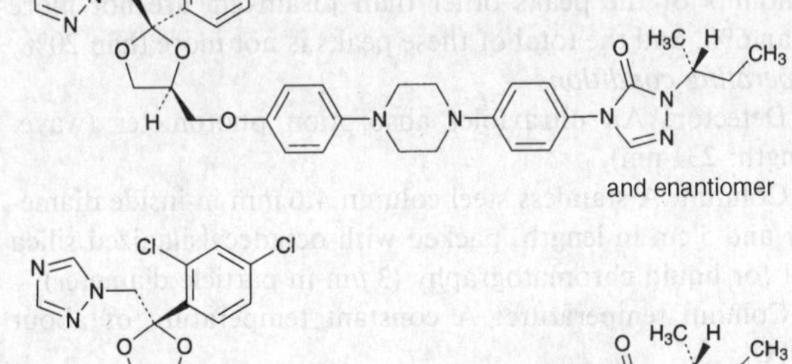

and enantiomer

$C_{35}H_{38}Cl_2N_8O_4$: 705.63
4-(4-{4-[4-({(2*RS*,4*SR*)-2-(2,4-Dichlorophenyl)-2-[(1*H*-1,2,4-triazol-1-yl)methyl]-1,3-dioxolan-4-yl}methoxy)phenyl]piperazin-1-yl}phenyl)-2-[(1*RS*)-1-methylpropyl]-2,4-dihydro-3*H*-1,2,4-triazol-3-one
4-(4-{4-[4-({(2*SR*,4*RS*)-2-(2,4-Dichlorophenyl)-2-[(1*H*-1,2,4-triazol-1-yl)methyl]-1,3-dioxolan-4-yl}methoxy)phenyl]piperazin-1-yl}phenyl)-2-[(1*RS*)-1-methylpropyl]-2,4-dihydro-3*H*-1,2,4-triazol-3-one
[84625-61-6]

Itraconazole contains not less than 98.5% and not more than 101.0% of itraconazole ($C_{35}H_{38}Cl_2N_8O_4$), calculated on the dried basis.

Description Itraconazole occurs as a white powder.

It is soluble in *N*,*N*-dimethylformamide, very slightly soluble in ethanol (99.5), and practically insoluble in water and in 2-propanol.

A solution of Itraconazole in *N*,*N*-dimethylformamide (1 in 100) shows no optical rotation.

Identification **(1)** Determine the absorption spectrum of a solution of Itraconazole in 2-propanol (1 in 100,000) as directed under Ultraviolet-visible Spectrophotometry <*2.24*>, and compare the spectrum with the Reference Spectrum: both spectra exhibit similar intensities of absorption at the same wavelengths.

(2) Determine the infrared absorption spectrum of Itraconazole, previously dried, as directed in the potassium bromide disk method under Infrared Spectrophotometry <*2.25*>, and compare the spectrum with the Reference Spectrum: both spectra exhibit similar intensities of absorption at the same wave numbers.

(3) Perform the test with Itraconazole as directed under Flame Coloration Test <*1.04*> (2): a green color appears.

Melting point <*2.60*> 166 – 170°C

Purity **(1)** Heavy metals <*1.07*>—Proceed with 1.0 g of Itraconazole according to Method 2, and perform the test. Prepare the control solution with 2.0 mL of Standard Lead Solution (not more than 20 ppm).

(2) Related substances—Dissolve 0.10 g of Itraconazole in 10 mL of a mixture of methanol and tetrahydrofuran (1:1), and use this solution as the sample solution. Pipet 1 mL of the sample solution, add the mixture of methanol and tetrahydrofuran (1:1) to make exactly 100 mL. Pipet 5 mL of this solution, add the mixture of methanol and tetrahydrofuran (1:1) to make exactly 10 mL, and use this solution as the standard solution. Perform the test with exactly 10 μL each of the sample solution and standard solution as directed under Liquid Chromatography <*2.01*> according to the following conditions. Determine each peak area of each solution by the automatic integration method: the area of each peak other than itraconazole obtained from the sample solution is not larger than the peak area of itraconazole from the standard solution. Furthermore, the total area of the peaks other than itraconazole from the sample solution is not larger than 2.5 times the peak area of itraconazole from the standard solution.

Operating conditions—

Detector: An ultraviolet absorption photometer (wavelength: 225 nm).

Column: A stainless steel column 4.6 mm in inside diameter and 10 cm in length, packed with octadecylsilanized silica gel for liquid chromatography (3 μm in particle diameter).

Column temperature: A constant temperature of about 30°C.

Mobile phase A: A solution of tetrabutylammonium hydrogensulfate (17 in 625).

Mobile phase B: Acetonitrile.

Flowing of mobile phase: Control the gradient by mixing the mobile phases A and B as directed in the following table.

Time after injection of sample (min)	Mobile phase A (vol%)	Mobile phase B (vol%)
0 – 20	80 → 50	20 → 50
20 – 25	50	50

Flow rate: 1.5 mL per minute.

Time span of measurement: About 2 times as long as the retention time of itraconazole, beginning after the solvent peak.

System suitability—

Test for required detectability: To exactly 1 mL of the standard solution add the mixture of methanol and tetrahydrofuran (1:1) to make exactly 10 mL. Confirm that the peak area of itraconazole obtained with 10 μL of this solution is equivalent to 7 to 13% of that with 10 μL of the standard solution.

System performance: Dissolve 1 mg of Itraconazole and 1 mg of miconazole nitrate in 20 mL of the mixture of methanol and tetrahydrofuran (1:1). When the procedure is run with 10 μL of this solution under the above operating conditions, miconazole and itraconazole are eluted in this order with the resolution between these peaks being not less than 2.0.

System repeatability: When the test is repeated 6 times with 10 μL of the standard solution under the above operating conditions, the relative standard deviation of the peak area of itraconazole is not more than 2.0%.

Loss on drying *<2.41>* Not more than 0.5% (1 g, 105°C, 4 hours).

Residue on ignition *<2.44>* Not more than 0.1% (1 g).

Assay Weigh accurately about 0.3 g of Itraconazole, dissolve in 70 mL of a mixture of 2-butanone and acetic acid (100) (7:1), and titrate *<2.50>* with 0.1 mol/L perchloric acid VS (potentiometric titration). Perform a blank determination in the same manner, and make any necessary correction.

Each mL of 0.1 mol/L perchloric acid VS
= 35.28 mg of $C_{35}H_{38}Cl_2N_8O_4$

Containers and storage Containers—Tight containers.

Josamycin

ジョサマイシン

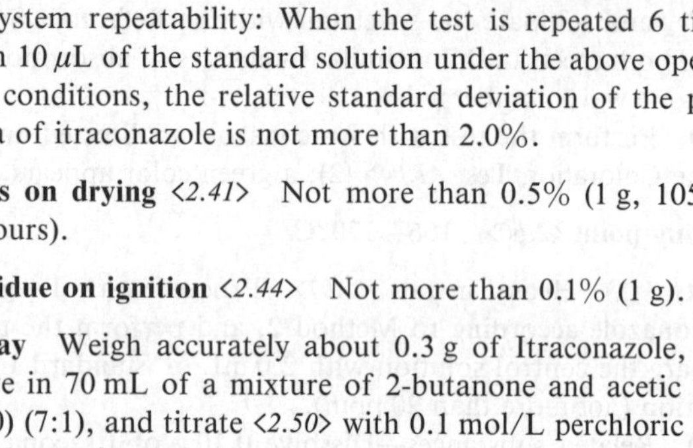

$C_{42}H_{69}NO_{15}$: 827.99
(3*R*,4*S*,5*S*,6*R*,8*R*,9*R*,10*E*,12*E*,15*R*)-3-Acetoxy-5-[2,6-dideoxy-4-*O*-(3-methylbutanoyl)-3-*C*-methyl-α-L-*ribo*-hexopyranosyl-(1→4)-3,6-dideoxy-3-dimethylamino-β-D-glucopyranosyloxy]-6-formylmethyl-9-hydroxy-4-methoxy-8-methylhexadeca-10,12-dien-15-olide
[*16846-24-5*]

Josamycin is a macrolide substance having antibacterial activity produced by the growth of *Streptomyces narbonensis* var. *josamyceticus*.

It contains not less than 900 μg (potency) and not more than 1100 μg (potency) per mg, calculated on the dried basis. The potency of Josamycin is expressed as mass (potency) of josamycin ($C_{42}H_{69}NO_{15}$).

Description Josamycin occurs as a white to yellowish white powder.

It is very soluble in methanol and in ethanol (99.5), and very slightly soluble in water.

Identification **(1)** Determine the absorption spectrum of a solution of Josamycin in methanol (1 in 100,000) as directed under Ultraviolet-visible Spectrophotometry *<2.24>*, and compare the spectrum with the Reference Spectrum or the spectrum of a solution of Josamycin RS prepared in the same manner as the sample solution: both spectra exhibit similar intensities of absorption at the same wavelengths.

(2) Dissolve 5 mg each of Josamycin and Josamycin RS in 1 mL of methanol, add diluted methanol (1 in 2) to make 100 mL, and use these solutions as the sample solution and the standard solution, respectively. Perform the test with 10 μL each of the sample solution and standard solution as directed under Liquid Chromatography *<2.01>* according to the following conditions, and compare the chromatograms obtained from these solutions: the retention time of the main peak from the sample solution is the same as that of the peak of josamycin from the standard solution.

Operating conditions—

Detector, column, column temperature, mobile phase, and flow rate: Proceed as directed in the operating conditions in the Purity (2).

Purity **(1)** Heavy metals *<1.07>*—Proceed with 1.0 g of Josamycin according to Method 2, and perform the test. Prepare the control solution with 3.0 mL of Standard Lead Solution (not more than 30 ppm).

(2) Related substances—Dissolve 50 mg of Josamycin in 5 mL of methanol, add diluted methanol (1 in 2) to make 50 mL, and use this solution as the sample solution. Perform the test with 10 μL of the sample solution as directed under Liquid Chromatography *<2.01>* according to the following conditions. Determine each peak area by the automatic integration method, and calculate the amounts of josamycin and the related substances by the area percentage method: the amounts of the peaks other than josamycin are not more than 6%, and the total of these peaks is not more than 20%.

Operating conditions—

Detector: An ultraviolet absorption photometer (wavelength: 231 nm).

Column: A stainless steel column 4.6 mm in inside diameter and 5 cm in length, packed with octadecylsilanized silica gel for liquid chromatography (3 μm in particle diameter).

Column temperature: A constant temperature of about 40°C.

Mobile phase: Dissolve 119 g of sodium perchlorate monohydrate in water to make 1000 mL, and adjust the pH to 2.5 with 1 mol/L hydrochloric acid TS. To 600 mL of this solution add 400 mL of acetonitrile.

Flow rate: Adjust so that the retention time of josamycin is about 10 minutes.

Time span of measurement: About 4 times as long as the retention time of josamycin, beginning after the solvent peak.

System suitability—

Test for required detectability: Measure 3 mL of the sample solution, add diluted methanol (1 in 2) to make 50 mL, and use this solution as the solution for system suitability test. Measure exactly 2 mL of the solution for system suitability test, and add diluted methanol (1 in 2) to make exactly 20 mL. Confirm that the peak area of josamycin obtained with 10 μL of this solution is equivalent to 8 to 12% of that with 10 μL of the solution for system suitability test.

System performance: Dissolve about 0.05 g of Josamycin in 50 mL of 0.1 mol/L potassium dihydrogen phosphate TS (pH 2.0) and allow to stand at 40°C for 3 hours. Adjust the pH of this solution to 6.8 to 7.2 with 2 mol/L sodium hydroxide TS, and add 50 mL of methanol. When the procedure is run with 10 μL of this solution under the above operating conditions, the resolution between the peaks of josamycin S_1, which relative retention time to josamycin is about 0.9, and josamycin is not less than 1.5.

System repeatability: When the test is repeated 6 times with 10 μL of the solution for system suitability test under the above operating conditions, the relative standard deviation of the peak areas of josamycin is not more than 1.5%.

Loss on drying *<2.41>* Not more than 1.0% (0.5 g, in vacuum, phosphorus (V) oxide, 60°C, 3 hours).

Residue on ignition *<2.44>* Not more than 0.1% (1 g).

Assay Perform the test according to the Cylinder-plate method as directed under Microbial Assay for Antibiotics *<4.02>* according to the following conditions.

(i) Test organism—*Bacillus subtilis* ATCC 6633

(ii) Culture medium—Use the medium ii in 3) Medium for other organisms under (1) Agar media for seed and base layer. Adjust the pH of the medium so that it will be 7.9 to 8.1 after sterilization.

(iii) Standard solutions—Weigh accurately an amount of Josamycin RS, equivalent to about 30 mg (potency), dissolve in 5 mL of methanol, add water to make exactly 100 mL, and use this solution as the standard stock solution. Keep the standard stock solution at 5°C or below, and use within 7 days. Take exactly a suitable amount of the standard stock solution before use, add water to make solutions so that each mL contains 30 μg (potency) and 7.5 μg (potency), and use these solutions as the high concentration standard solution and the low concentration standard solution, respectively.

(iv) Sample solutions—Weigh accurately an amount of Josamycin, equivalent to about 30 mg (potency), dissolve in 5 mL of methanol, and add water to make exactly 100 mL. Take exactly a suitable amount of this solution, add water to make solutions so that each mL contains 30 μg (potency) and 7.5 μg (potency), and use these solutions as the high concentration sample solution and the low concentration sample solution, respectively.

Containers and storage Containers—Tight containers.

Storage—Light-resistant.

Josamycin Tablets

ジョサマイシン錠

Josamycin Tablets contain not less than 90.0% and not more than 110.0% of the labeled potency of josamycin ($C_{42}H_{69}NO_{15}$: 827.99).

Method of preparation Prepare as directed under Tablets, with Josamycin.

Identification To a quantity of powdered Josamycin Tablets, equivalent to 10 mg (potency) of Josamycin, add 100 mL of methanol, shake vigorously, and centrifuge. To 5 mL of the supernatant liquid, add methanol to make 50 mL, and determine the absorption spectrum of this solution as directed under Ultraviolet-visible Spectrophotometry *<2.24>*: it exhibits a maximum between 229 nm and 233 nm.

Loss on drying *<2.41>* Not more than 5.0% (0.5 g, in vacuum, 60°C, 3 hours).

Uniformity of dosage units *<6.02>*—Perform the test according to the following method: it meets the requirement of the Content uniformity test.

Take 1 tablet of Josamycin Tablets, add 5 mL of water, and shake vigorously to disintegrate the tablet. Add methanol and sonicate to disperse the particles, add methanol to make exactly V mL so that each mL contains about 2 mg (potency) of Josamycin, and centrifuge. Pipet 3 mL of the supernatant liquid, and add methanol to make exactly 100 mL. Pipet 10 mL of this solution, add methanol to make exactly 50 mL, and use this solution as the sample solution. Separately, accurately weigh about 50 mg (potency) of Josamycin RS, dissolve in 5 mL of water and methanol to make exactly 25 mL. Pipet 3 mL of this solution, and add methanol to make exactly 100 mL. Pipet 10 mL of this solution, add methanol to make exactly 50 mL, and use this solution as the standard solution. Determine the absorbances, A_T and A_S, of the sample solution and standard solution at 231 nm as directed under Ultraviolet-visible Spectrophotometry *<2.24>*. However, $\bar{X}$ in the formula for calculation of acceptance value is the result of the assay.

$$\text{Amount [mg (potency)] of josamycin } (C_{42}H_{69}NO_{15}) = M_S \times A_T/A_S \times V/25$$

M_S: Amount [mg (potency)] of Josamycin RS taken

Disintegration *<6.09>* Perform the test using the disk: it meets the requirement.

Assay Perform the test according to the Cylinder-plate method as directed under Microbial Assay for Antibiotics *<4.02>* according to the following conditions.

(i) Test organism, culture medium, and standard solutions—Proceed as directed in the Assay under Josamycin.

(ii) Sample solutions—Weigh accurately the mass of not less than 20 Josamycin Tablets and powder. Weigh accurately a portion of the powder, equivalent to about 0.3 g (potency) of Josamycin, add 50 mL of methanol, shake vigorously, and add water to make exactly 1000 mL. Take exactly an appropriate amount of this solution, add water to prepare solutions containing 30 μg (potency) and 7.5 μg (potency) per mL, and use these solutions as the high and the low concentration sample solutions, respectively.

Containers and storage Containers—Tight containers.

Josamycin Propionate

ジョサマイシンプロピオン酸エステル

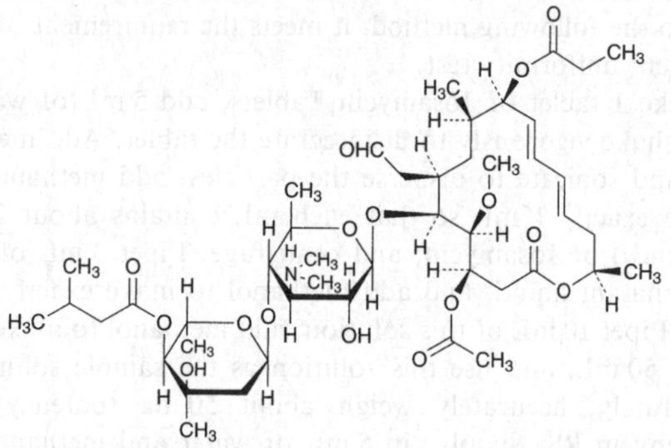

$C_{45}H_{73}NO_{16}$: 884.06
(3*R*,4*S*,5*S*,6*R*,8*R*,9*R*,10*E*,12*E*,15*R*)-3-Acetoxy-5-[2,6-dideoxy-4-*O*-(3-methylbutanoyl)-3-*C*-methyl-α-L-*ribo*-hexopyranosyl-(1→4)-3,6-dideoxy-3-dimethylamino-*β*-D-glucopyranosyloxy]-6-formylmethyl-4-methoxy-8-methyl-9-propanoyloxyhexadeca-10,12-dien-15-olide
[*16846-24-5*, Josamycin]

Josamycin Propionate is a derivative of josamycin.

It contains not less than 843 μg (potency) and not more than 1000 μg (potency) per mg, calculated on the dried basis. The potency of Josamycin Propionate is expressed as mass (potency) of josamycin ($C_{42}H_{69}NO_{15}$: 827.99).

Description Josamycin Propionate occurs as a white to light yellow-white crystalline powder.

It is very soluble in acetonitrile, freely soluble in methanol and in ethanol (99.5), and practically insoluble in water.

Identification **(1)** Determine the absorption spectrum of a solution of Josamycin Propionate in methanol (1 in 100,000) as directed under Ultraviolet-visible Spectrophotometry <*2.24*>, and compare the spectrum with the Reference Spectrum or the spectrum of a solution of Josamycin Propionate RS prepared in the same manner as the sample solution: both spectra exhibit similar intensities of absorption at the same wavelengths.

(2) Dissolve 5 mg each of Josamycin Propionate and Josamycin Propionate RS in 50 mL of diluted acetonitrile (1 in 2), and use these solutions as the sample solution and the standard solution, respectively. Perform the test with 10 μL each of the sample solution and standard solution as directed under Liquid Chromatography <*2.01*> according to the following conditions, and compare the chromatograms obtained from these solutions: the retention time of the peak of josamycin propionate from the sample solution is the same with that of the peak of josamycin propionate from the standard solution.

Operating conditions—

Detector, column, column temperature, mobile phase, and flow rate: Proceed as directed in the operating conditions in the Purity (2).

Purity **(1)** Heavy metals <*1.07*>—Proceed with 1.0 g of Josamycin Propionate according to Method 2, and perform the test. Prepare the control solution with 3.0 mL of Standard Lead Solution (not more than 30 ppm).

(2) Related substances—Dissolve 50 mg of Josamycin Propionate in the mobile phase to make 50 mL, and use this solution as the sample solution. Perform the test with 10 μL of the sample solution as directed under Liquid Chromatography <*2.01*> according to the following conditions. Determine each peak area by the automatic integration method, and calculate the amounts of each peak other than josamycin propionate by the area percentage method: the amount of any peak other than josamycin is not more than 6%, and the total of these peaks is not more than 22%.

Operating conditions—

Detector: An ultraviolet absorption photometer (wavelength: 234 nm).

Column: A stainless steel column 6 mm in inside diameter and 15 cm in length, packed with octadecylsilanized silica gel for liquid chromatography (5 μm in particle diameter).

Column temperature: A constant temperature of about 40°C.

Mobile phase: To 10 mL of triethylamine add water to make 1000 mL, and adjust the pH to 4.3 with acetic acid (100). To 500 mL of this solution add 500 mL of acetonitrile.

Flow rate: Adjust so that the retention time of josamycin propionate is about 24 minutes.

Time span of measurement: About 3.5 times as long as the retention time of josamycin propionate, beginning after the solvent peak.

System suitability—

Test for required detectability: Measure 3 mL of the sample solution, add the mobile phase to make 50 mL, and use this solution as the solution for system suitability test. Measure exactly 2 mL of the solution for system suitability test, and add the mobile phase to make exactly 20 mL. Confirm that the peak area of josamycin propionate obtained with 10 μL of this solution is equivalent to 8 to 12% of that with 10 μL of the solution for system suitability test.

System performance: Dissolve 5 mg of Josamycin Propionate and 2 mg of josamycin in 50 mL of the mobile phase. When the procedure is run with 10 μL of this solution under the above operating conditions, josamycin and josamycin propionate are eluted in this order with the resolution between these peaks being not less than 25.

System repeatability: When the test is repeated 6 times with 10 μL of the solution for system suitability test under the above operating conditions, the relative standard deviation of the peak area of josamycin propionate is not more than 1.5%.

Loss on drying <*2.41*> Not more than 1.0% (1 g, in vacuum, phosphorus (V) oxide, 60°C, 3 hours).

Residue on ignition <*2.44*> Not more than 0.1% (1 g).

Assay Perform the test according to the Cylinder-plate method as directed under Microbial Assay for Antibiotics <*4.02*> according to the following conditions.

(i) Test organism—*Bacillus subtilis* ATCC 6633

(ii) Culture medium—Use the medium ii in 3) Medium for other organisms under (1) Agar media for seed and base layer. Adjust the pH of the medium so that it will be 7.9 to 8.1 after sterilization.

(iii) Standard solutions—Weigh accurately an amount of Josamycin Propionate RS, equivalent to about 20 mg (potency), dissolve in 10 mL of methanol, add 1/15 mol/L phosphate buffer solution (pH 5.6) to make exactly 50 mL, and use this solution as the standard stock solution. Keep the standard stock solution at 5°C or below, and use within 3 days. Take exactly a suitable amount of the standard stock solution before use, add 1/15 mol/L phosphate buffer solution (pH 5.6) to make solutions so that each mL contains 80 μg (potency) and 20 μg (potency), and use these solutions as the high concentration standard solution and the low concentration standard solution, respectively.

(iv) Sample solutions—Weigh accurately an amount of Josamycin Propionate, equivalent to about 20 mg (potency), dissolve in 10 mL of methanol, add 1/15 mol/L phosphate buffer solution (pH 5.6) to make exactly 50 mL. Take exactly a suitable amount of this solution, add 1/15 mol/L phosphate buffer solution (pH 5.6) to make solutions so that each mL contains 80 μg (potency) and 20 μg (potency), and use these solutions as the high concentration sample solution and the low concentration sample solution, respectively.

Containers and storage Containers—Tight containers.

Storage—Light-resistant.

Kainic Acid Hydrate

カイニン酸水和物

$C_{10}H_{15}NO_4.H_2O$: 231.25
(2*S*,3*S*,4*S*)-3-(Carboxymethyl)-4-(1-methylethenyl)pyrrolidine-2-carboxylic acid monohydrate
[*487-79-6*, anhydride]

Kainic Acid Hydrate, when dried, contains not less than 99.0% of kainic acid ($C_{10}H_{15}NO_4$: 213.23).

Description Kainic Acid Hydrate occurs as white, crystals or crystalline powder. It is odorless, and has an acid taste.

It is sparingly soluble in water and in warm water, very slightly soluble in acetic acid (100) and in ethanol (95), and practically insoluble in diethyl ether.

It dissolves in dilute hydrochloric acid and in sodium hydroxide TS.

The pH of a solution of 1.0 g of Kainic Acid Hydrate in 100 mL of water is between 2.8 and 3.5.

Melting point: about 252°C (with decomposition).

Identification **(1)** To 5 mL of a solution of Kainic Acid Hydrate (1 in 5000) add 1 mL of ninhydrin TS, and warm in a water bath at a temperature between 60°C and 70°C for 5 minutes: a yellow color is produced.

(2) Dissolve 50 mg of Kainic Acid Hydrate in 5 mL of acetic acid (100), and add 0.5 mL of bromine TS: the color of bromine disappears immediately.

Optical rotation <*2.49*> $[\alpha]_D^{20}$: −13 – −17° (0.5 g, water, 50 mL, 200 mm).

Purity **(1)** Clarity and color of solution—Dissolve 0.10 g of Kainic Acid Hydrate in 10 mL of water: the solution is clear and colorless.

(2) Chloride <*1.03*>—Take 0.5 g of Kainic Acid Hydrate in a platinum crucible, dissolve in 5 mL of sodium carbonate TS, and evaporate on a water bath to dryness. Heat the crucible slowly at first, and then ignite until the sample is almost incinerated. After cooling, add 12 mL of dilute nitric acid to the residue, dissolve by warming, and filter. Wash the residue with 15 mL of water, combine the washings and the filtrate, and add water to make 50 mL. Perform the test using this solution as the test solution.

Control solution: Add 5 mL of sodium carbonate TS to 0.30 mL of 0.01 mol/L hydrochloric acid VS, and proceed as directed above (not more than 0.021%).

(3) Sulfate <*1.14*>—Dissolve 0.5 g of Kainic Acid Hydrate in 40 mL of water by warming. Cool, add 1 mL of dilute hydrochloric acid and water to make 50 mL, and perform the test using this solution as the test solution. Prepare the control solution with 0.30 mL of 0.005 mol/L sulfuric acid VS (not more than 0.028%).

(4) Ammonium <*1.02*>—Take 0.25 g of Kainic Acid Hydrate, and perform the test. Prepare the control solution with 5.0 mL of Standard Ammonium Solution (not more than 0.02%).

(5) Heavy metals <*1.07*>—Proceed with 1.0 g of Kainic Acid Hydrate according to Method 2, and perform the test. Prepare the control solution with 2.0 mL of Standard Lead Solution (not more than 20 ppm).

(6) Arsenic <*1.11*>—Dissolve 1.0 g of Kainic Acid Hydrate in 5 mL of dilute hydrochloric acid, and perform the test with this solution as the test solution (not more than 2 ppm).

(7) Amino acid and other imino acid—Dissolve 0.10 g of Kainic Acid Hydrate in 10 mL of water, and use this solution as the sample solution. Pipet 2 mL of the sample solution, and add water to make exactly 100 mL. Pipet 1 mL of this solution, add water to make exactly 20 mL, and use this solution as the standard solution. Perform the test as directed under Thin-layer Chromatography <*2.03*> with these solutions. Spot 10 μL each of the sample solution and standard solution on a plate of silica gel for thin-layer chromatography. Develop the plate with the supernatant liquid of a mixture of water, 1-butanol and acetic acid (100) (5:4:1) to a distance of about 10 cm, and air-dry the plate. Spray evenly a solution of ninhydrin in acetone (1 in 50) on the plate, and dry the plate at 80°C for 5 minutes: the spots other than the principal spot from the sample solution are not more intense than the spot from the standard solution.

Loss on drying <*2.41*> 6.5 – 8.5% (1 g, 105°C, 4 hours).

Residue on ignition <*2.44*> Not more than 0.1% (0.5 g).

Assay Weigh accurately about 0.4 g of Kainic Acid Hydrate, previously dried, and dissolve in 50 mL of warm water, cool and titrate <*2.50*> with 0.1 mol/L sodium hydroxide VS (indicator: 10 drops of bromothymol blue TS).

Each mL of 0.1 mol/L sodium hydroxide VS
= 21.32 mg of $C_{10}H_{15}NO_4$

Containers and storage Containers—Tight containers.

Kainic Acid and Santonin Powder

カイニン酸・サントニン散

Kainic Acid and Santonin Powder contains not less than 9.0% and not more than 11.0% of santonin ($C_{15}H_{18}O_3$: 246.30), and not less than 1.80% and not more than 2.20% of kainic acid hydrate ($C_{10}H_{15}NO_4.H_2O$: 231.25).

Method of preparation

Santonin	100 g
Kainic Acid Hydrate	20 g
Starch, Lactose Hydrate or their mixture	a sufficient quantity
To make	1000 g

Prepare as directed under Powders, with the above ingredients.

Description Kainic Acid and Santonin Powder occurs as a white powder.

Identification (1) Shake 1 g of Kainic Acid and Santonin Powder with 10 mL of chloroform, and filter [use the residue for the test (2)]. Distil off the chloroform of the filtrate, and dissolve the residue in 2 mL of potassium hydroxide-ethanol TS: a red color is produced (santonin).

(2) Shake the residue obtained in (1) with 20 mL of warm water, filter, and to 1 mL of the filtrate add 10 mL of water and 1 mL of ninhydrin-L-ascorbic acid TS. Warm in a water bath between 60°C and 70°C for 5 minutes: a yellow color is produced (kainic acid).

Assay (1) Santonin—Weigh accurately about 0.25 g of Kainic Acid and Santonin Powder and about 25 mg of santonin for assay, add 20 mL each of ethanol (95), shake thoroughly for 5 minutes, and filter. Wash the residue with three 10-mL portions of ethanol (95), and filter. Combine the filtrate and the washings, and add ethanol (95) to make exactly 50 mL. Pipet 2 mL each of these solutions, add ethanol (95) to make exactly 100 mL, and use these solutions as the sample solution and the standard solution, respectively. Determine the absorbances, A_T and A_S, of the sample solution and standard solution at 240 nm as directed under Ultraviolet-visible Spectrophotometry <2.24>.

$$\text{Amount (mg) of santonin } (C_{15}H_{18}O_3) = M_S \times A_T/A_S$$

M_S: Amount (mg) of santonin for assay taken

(2) Kainic acid—Weigh accurately about 1.25 g of Kainic Acid and Santonin Powder, add 20 mL of diluted pyridine (1 in 10), shake thoroughly for 5 minutes, and filter. Wash the residue with three 10-mL portions of diluted pyridine (1 in 10), and filter. Combine the filtrate and the washings, and add diluted pyridine (1 in 10) to make exactly 50 mL. Pipet 2 mL of this solution, add diluted pyridine (1 in 10) to make exactly 25 mL, and use this solution as the sample solution. Separately, dissolve about 25 mg of kainic acid hydrate for assay, previously dried at 105°C for 4 hours and accurately weighed, in diluted pyridine (1 in 10) to make exactly 50 mL. Pipet 2 mL of this solution, add diluted pyridine (1 in 10) to make exactly 25 mL, and use this solution as the standard solution. Pipet 2 mL each of the sample solution and standard solution, add 2 mL of ninhydrin-L-ascorbic acid TS, and heat on a water bath for 30 minutes. After cooling immediately, shake vigorously for 2 minutes, add water to make exactly 20 mL, and allow to stand for 15 minutes. Determine the absorbances, A_T and A_S, of these solutions at 425 nm as directed under Ultraviolet-visible Spectrophotometry <2.24>, using the solution prepared in the same manner with 2 mL of diluted pyridine (1 in 10) instead of the sample solution as the blank.

$$\text{Amount (mg) of kainic acid hydrate } (C_{10}H_{15}NO_4.H_2O) = M_S \times A_T/A_S \times 1.085$$

M_S: Amount (mg) of kainic acid hydrate for assay taken

Containers and storage Containers—Well-closed containers.

Storage—Light-resistant.

Kallidinogenase

カリジノゲナーゼ

[*9001-01-8*]

Kallidinogenase is an enzyme obtained from healthy porcine pancreas, and has kinin-releasing activity based on cleavage of kininogen.

It contains not less than 25 Kallidinogenase Units per mg. Usually, it is diluted with Lactose Hydrate or the like.

Kallidinogenase contains not less than 90% and not more than 110% of the labeled Units.

Description Kallidinogenase occurs as a white to light brown powder. It is odorless or has a faint, characteristic odor.

It is freely soluble in water, and practically insoluble in ethanol (95) and in diethyl ether.

The pH of a solution of Kallidinogenase (1 in 300) is between 5.5 and 7.5.

Identification (1) Weigh accurately an appropriate amount of Kallidinogenase according to the labeled Units, and dissolve in 0.05 mol/L phosphate buffer solution (pH 7.0) to prepare a solution containing 10 Kallidinogenase Units per mL. Pipet 5 mL of this solution, and add exactly 1 mL of trypsin inhibitor TS and 0.05 mol/L phosphate buffer solution (pH 7.0) to make exactly 10 mL. Pipet 4 mL each of this solution into two separate test tubes, add exactly 1 mL each of aprotinin TS and 0.05 mol/L phosphate buffer solution (pH 7.0) separately to each test tube, allow them to stand at room temperature for 20 minutes, and use these solutions as the sample solutions 1 and 2. Separately, pipet 1 mL of trypsin inhibitor TS, and add 0.05 mol/L phosphate buffer solution (pH 7.0) to make exactly 10 mL. Pipet 4 mL each of this solution into two separate test tubes, add exactly 1 mL each of aprotinin TS and 0.05 mol/L phosphate buffer solution (pH 7.0) separately to each tube, allow them to stand at room temperature for 20 minutes, and use these solutions as the sample solutions 3 and 4. Then, pipet 2.5 mL of substrate TS for kallidinogenase assay (1), previously warmed at 30.0 ± 0.5°C for 5 minutes, place in a 1-cm cell, add exactly 0.5 mL of the sample solution 1 warmed at 30.0 ± 0.5°C for 5 minutes, and start simultaneously a chronograph. Perform the test at 30.0 ± 0.5°C as directed under Ultraviolet-visible Spectrophotometry <2.24> using water as the blank, and determine the absorbances at 405 nm, $A_{1\text{-}2}$ and $A_{1\text{-}6}$, of this solution, after having allowed it to stand for exactly 2 and 6 minutes. Perform the same test with the sample solutions 2, 3 and 4, and determine the absorbances, $A_{2\text{-}2}$, $A_{2\text{-}6}$, $A_{3\text{-}2}$, $A_{3\text{-}6}$, $A_{4\text{-}2}$ and $A_{4\text{-}6}$, of these solutions. Calculate I by using the following equation: the value of I does not exceed 0.2.

$$I = \frac{(A_{1\text{-}6} - A_{1\text{-}2}) - (A_{3\text{-}6} - A_{3\text{-}2})}{(A_{2\text{-}6} - A_{2\text{-}2}) - (A_{4\text{-}6} - A_{4\text{-}2})}$$

(2) Pipet 2.9 mL of substrate TS for kallidinogenase assay (2), previously warmed at 30.0 ± 0.5°C for 5 minutes, place in a 1-cm cell, add exactly 0.1 mL of the sample solution obtained in the Assay, and start simultaneously a chronograph. Perform the test at 30.0 ± 0.5°C as directed under Ultraviolet-visible Spectrophotometry <2.24>, and determine the change of the absorbance at 253 nm for 4 to 6 minutes. Separately, pipet 1 mL of trypsin inhibitor TS, and add 0.05 mol/L phosphate buffer solution (pH 7.0) to make

exactly 10 mL. Add exactly 0.1 mL of this solution to exactly 2.9 mL of substrate TS for kallidinogenase assay (2), previously warmed at 30.0 ± 0.5°C for 5 minutes, and use this solution as the blank. If the rate of change in the absorbance remains constant, determine the change of absorbance per 1 minute, A, and calculate R by using the following equation: the value of R is between 0.12 and 0.16.

$$R = A/0.0383 \times 1/(a \times b)$$

a: Amount (mg) of Kallidinogenase in 1 mL of the sample solution

b: Amount (Unit) of kallidinogenase in 1 mg of Kallidinogenase obtained in the Assay

Specific activity Perform the test with Kallidinogenase as directed under Nitrogen Determination <*1.08*> to determine the nitrogen content, convert 1mg of nitrogen (N:14.01) into 6.25 mg of protein, and calculate the specific activity using the amount (Units) of Kallidinogenase obtained in the Assay: it is not less than 100 Kallidinogenase Units per 1mg of protein.

Purity (1) Fat—To 1.0 g of Kallidinogenase add 20 mL of diethyl ether, extract with occasional shaking for 30 minutes, and filter. Wash the residue with 10 mL of diethyl ether, combine the washing with the filtrate, evaporate the diethyl ether, and dry the residue at 105°C for 2 hours: the mass of the residue is not more than 1 mg.

(2) Kininase—

(i) Bradykinin solution: Weigh an appropriate amount of bradykinin, and dissolve in gelatin-phosphate buffer solution (pH 7.4) to prepare a solution containing 0.200 μg of bradykinin per mL.

(ii) Kallidinogenase solution: Weigh accurately a suitable amount of Kallidinogenase according to the labeled unit, dissolve in gelatin-phosphate buffer solution (pH 7.4) to make a solution containing 1 unit of kallidinogenase per mL.

(iii) Sample solution: Pipet 0.5 mL of bradykinin solution, warm at 30 ± 0.5°C for 5 minutes, then add exactly 0.5 mL of kallidinogenase solution previously warmed at 30 ± 0.5°C for 5 minutes, and mix immediately. After allowing this solution to stand at 30 ± 0.5°C for exactly 150 seconds, add exactly 0.2 mL of a solution of trichloroacetic acid (1 in 5), and shake. Boil for 3 minutes, then cool in ice immediately, centrifuge, and allow to stand at a room temperature for 15 minutes. Pipet 0.5 mL of the supernatant liquid, add exactly 0.5 mL of gelatin-tris buffer solution (pH 8.0), and shake. Pipet 0.1 mL of this solution, add exactly 0.9 mL of trichloroacetic acid-gelatin-tris buffer solution, and mix. Pipet 0.2 mL of this solution, add exactly 0.6 mL of trichloroacetic acid-gelatin-tris buffer solution, shake, and use this solution as the sample solution.

(iv) Control solution: Proceed with 0.5 mL of gelatin-phosphate buffer solution (pH 7.4) as described in (iii), and use the solution so obtained as the control solution.

(v) Procedure: Add 0.1 mL of anti-bradykinin antibody TS to goat anti-rabbit IgG antibody-coated wells of a 96-well microplate, shake, and allow to stand at a constant temperature of about 25°C for 1 hour. Remove the anti-bradykinin antibody TS, add 0.3 mL of phosphate buffer solution for microplate washing to the wells, then remove. Repeat this procedure 3 times, take off the washings thoroughly, then add 100 μL each of the sample solution and control solution, and 50 μL of gelatin-phosphate buffer solution (pH 7.0), shake, and allow to stand at a constant temperature of about 25°C for 1 hour. Then add 50 μL of peroxidase-labeled bradykinin TS, shake, and allow to stand in a cold place for a night. Take off the reaction solution, add 0.3 mL of phosphate buffer solution for microplate washing, and remove. Repeat this procedure more 4 times, take off the washings thoroughly, add 100 μL of substrate solution for peroxidase determination, and allow to stand at a constant temperature of about 25°C for exactly 30 minutes while protecting from light. Then add 100 μL of diluted sulfuric acid (23 in 500), shake, and determine the absorbance at 490 – 492 nm. Separately, dissolve a suitable amount of bradykinin in gelatin-phosphate buffer solution (pH 7.0) to make solutions containing exactly 100 ng, 25 ng, 6.25 ng, 1.56 ng, 0.39 ng and 0.098 ng of bradykinin per mL, and use these solutions as the standard solution (1), the standard solution (2), the standard solution (3), the standard solution (4), the standard solution (5) and the standard solution (6), respectively. Use 1 mL of gelatin-phosphate buffer solution (pH 7.0) as the standard solution (7). To each of the well add 50 μL each of the standard solutions and 100 μL of trichloroacetic acid-gelatin-tris buffer solution, and proceed in the same manner as for the sample solution and for the control solution.

Prepare the calibration curve from the amounts of bradykinin in the standard solutions and their absorbances, and calculate the amounts of bradykinin, B_T (pg) and B_S (pg), of the sample solution and the control solution.

(vi) Judgment: The value R calculated by the following equation is not less than 0.8.

$$R = B_T/B_S$$

(3) Trypsin-like substances—Pipet 4 mL of the sample stock solution prepared for the Assay, add exactly 1 mL of trypsin inhibitor TS and 0.05 mol/L phosphate buffer solution (pH 7.0) to make exactly 10 mL, and use this solution as the sample solution. Pipet 2.5 mL of substrate TS for kallidinogenase assay (1), previously warmed at 30 ± 0.5°C for 5 minutes, place in a 1-cm cell, add exactly 0.5 mL of the sample solution, warmed at 30 ± 0.5°C for 5 minutes, and start simultaneously a chronograph. Perform the test at 30 ± 0.5°C as directed under Ultraviolet-visible Spectrophotometry <*2.24*> using water as the blank, and determine the absorbances at 405 nm, A_2 and A_6, of this solution after having allowed it to stand for exactly 2 and 6 minutes. Separately, pipet 4 mL of the sample stock solution prepared for the Assay, add 0.05 mol/L phosphate buffer solution (pH 7.0) to make exactly 10 mL, and use this solution as the control solution. Perform the same test with the control solution, and determine the absorbances, A_2' and A_6'. Calculate T by using the following equation: the value of T does not exceed 0.05.

$$T = \{(A_6' - A_2') - (A_6 - A_2)\}/(A_6' - A_2')$$

(4) Protease—Weigh accurately an appropriate amount of Kallidinogenase according to the labeled Units, dissolve in 0.05 mol/L phosphate buffer solution (pH 7.0) to prepare a solution containing 1 Kallidinogenase Unit per mL, and use this solution as the sample solution. Pipet 1 mL of the sample solution, place in a test tube, and allow to stand at 35 ± 0.5°C for 5 minutes. Then, pipet 5 mL of substrate TS for kallidinogenase assay (3), previously warmed to 35 ± 0.5°C, add quickly to the sample solution in the test tube, and allow to stand at 35 ± 0.5°C for exactly 20 minutes. Then add exactly 5 mL of trichloroacetic acid TS, shake well, allow to stand at room temperature for 1 hour, and filter through a membrane filter (5 μm in pore size). Discard the first 3 mL of the filtrate, and determine the absorbance, A, of the subsequent filtrate at 280 nm within 2 hours as directed under Ultraviolet-visible Spectrophotometry <*2.24*>, using water as the blank. Separately, pipet 1 mL of the sample solution, add exactly 5 mL of trichloroacetic acid TS, shake well, and

add exactly 5 mL of the substrate TS for kallidinogenase assay (3). Proceed in the same manner as described for the sample solution, and determine the absorbance, A_0, of this solution. Calculate the value of $(A\text{–}A_0)$: it is not more than 0.2.

Loss on drying <*2.41*> Not more than 2.0% (0.5 g, in vacuum, phosphorus (V) oxide, 4 hours).

Residue on ignition <*2.44*> Not more than 3% (0.5 g, 650 – 750°C).

Kinin-releasing activity

(i) Kallidinogenase solution: Weigh accurately a suitable amount of Kallidinogenase, according to the labeled unit, dissolve in 0.02 mol/L phosphate buffer solution (pH 8.0) to make a solution containing 0.1 unit of kallidinogenase per mL. Perform this procedure by using glassware.

(ii) Sample solution: Pipet 0.5 mL of kininogen TS, warm at 30 ± 0.5°C for 5 minutes, then add exactly 0.5 mL of kallidinogenase solution previously warmed at 30 ± 0.5°C for 5 minutes, and mix immediately. After allow this solution to stand at 30 ± 0.5°C for exactly 2 minutes, add exactly 0.2 mL of a solution of trichloroacetic acid (1 in 5), and shake. Boil for 3 minutes, then cool in ice immediately, centrifuge, and allow to stand at a room temperature for 15 minutes. Pipet 0.5 mL of the supernatant liquid, add exactly 0.5 mL of gelatin-tris buffer solution (pH 8.0), and shake. Pipet 0.1 mL of this solution, add exactly 1.9 mL of trichloroacetic acid-gelatin-tris buffer solution, shake, and use this solution as the sample solution.

(iii) Procedure: Perform the test with the sample solution as directed in the Purity (2), and determine the amount, B (pg), of kinin per well. The kinin-releasing activity per 1 unit of Kallidinogenase calculated by the following equation is not less than 500 ng bradykinin equivalent/minute/unit.

Kinin-releasing activity (ng bradykinin equivalent/minute/unit) per 1 unit of Kallidinogenase = $B \times 4.8$

Assay Weigh accurately an appropriate amount of Kallidinogenase according to the labeled Units, dissolve in 0.05 mol/L phosphate buffer solution (pH 7.0) to prepare a solution containing about 10 Kallidinogenase Units per mL, and use this solution as the sample stock solution. Pipet 4 mL of the sample stock solution, add exactly 1 mL of trypsin inhibitor TS and 0.05 mol/L phosphate buffer solution (pH 7.0) to make exactly 10 mL, and use this solution as the sample solution. Pipet 2.5 mL of substrate TS for kallidinogenase assay (1), previously warmed at 30 ± 0.5°C for 5 minutes, place in a 1-cm cell, add exactly 0.5 mL of the sample solution, warmed at 30 ± 0.5°C for 5 minutes, and start simultaneously a chronograph. Perform the test at 30 ± 0.5°C as directed under the Ultraviolet-visible Spectrophotometry <*2.24*> using water as the blank, and determine the absorbances at 405 nm, A_{T2} and A_{T6}, of this solution after allowing to stand for exactly 2 and 6 minutes. Separately, dissolve Kallidinogenase RS in 0.05 mol/L phosphate buffer solution (pH 7.0) to make a solutin so that each mL contains exactly 10 Units, and use this solution as the standard stock solution. Pipet 4 mL of the stock solution, add exactly 1 mL of trypsin inhibitor TS and 0.05 mol/L phosphate buffer solution (pH 7.0) to make exactly 10 mL, and use this solution as the standard solution. Take exactly 0.5 mL of the standard solution, perform the test in the same manner as described for the sample solution, and determine the absorbances, A_{S2} and A_{S6}, of the solution after allowing to stand for exactly 2 and 6 minutes. Separately, take exactly 1 mL of the trypsin inhibitor TS, and add 0.05 mol/L phosphate buffer solution (pH 7.0) to make exactly 10 mL. Pipet 0.5 mL of this solution, perform the test in the same manner as described for the sample solution, and determine the absorbances, A_{O2} and A_{O6}, of the solution after allowing to stand for exactly 2 and 6 minutes.

Units per 1 mg of Kallidinogenase

$$= \frac{(A_{T6} - A_{T2}) - (A_{O6} - A_{O2})}{(A_{S6} - A_{S2}) - (A_{O6} - A_{O2})} \times \frac{M_S}{a} \times \frac{1}{b}$$

M_S: Amount (Units) of Kallidinogenase RS taken
a: Volume (mL) of the standard stock solution
b: Amount (mg) of Kallidinogenase in 1 mL of the sample stock solution

Containers and storage Containers—Tight containers.

Kanamycin Monosulfate

カナマイシン一硫酸塩

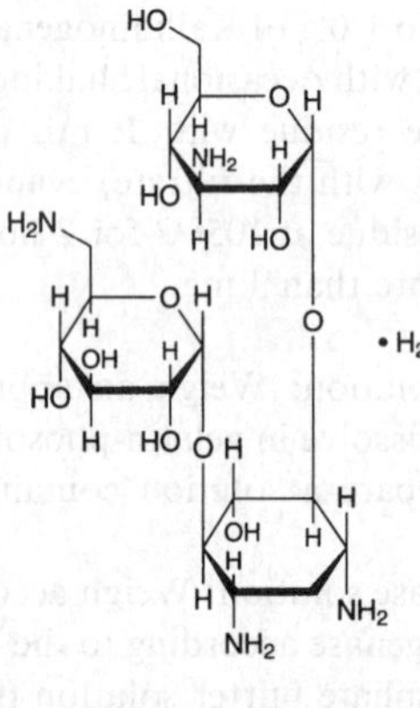

$C_{18}H_{36}N_4O_{11}.H_2SO_4$: 582.58
3-Amino-3-deoxy-α-D-glucopyranosyl-(1→6)-[6-amino-6-deoxy-α-D-glucopyranosyl-(1→4)]-2-deoxy-D-streptamine monosulfate
[*25389-94-0*]

Kanamycin Monosulfate is the sulfate of an aminoglycoside substance having antibacterial activity produced by the growth of *Streptomyces kanamyceticus*.

It contains not less than 750 μg (potency) and not more than 832 μg (potency) per mg, calculated on the dried basis. The potency of Kanamycin Monosulfate is expressed as mass (potency) of kanamycin ($C_{18}H_{36}N_4O_{11}$: 484.50).

Description Kanamycin Monosulfate occurs as a white crystalline powder.

It is freely soluble in water, and practically insoluble in ethanol (99.5).

Identification **(1)** Dissolve 50 mg of Kanamycin Monosulfate in 3 mL of water, and add 6 mL of anthrone TS: a blue-purple color develops.

(2) Dissolve 20 mg each of Kanamycin Monosulfate and Kanamycin Monosulfate RS in 1 mL of water, and use these solutions as the sample solution and standard solution. Perform the test with these solutions as directed under Thin-layer Chromatography <*2.03*>. Spot 5 μL each of the sample solution and standard solution on a plate of silica gel for thin-layer chromatography. Develop the plate with the supernatant layer of a mixture of chloroform, ammonia solution (28) and methanol (2:1:1) to a distance of about 10 cm, and air-dry the plate. Spray evenly a solution of 0.2% ninhydrin-water saturated 1-butanol TS on the plate, and heat the plate at 100°C for 10 minutes: the principal spot obtained from the sample solution and the spot from the standard solution show a purple-brown color and the same *R*f value.

(3) To a solution of Kanamycin Monosulfate (1 in 5) add 1 drop of barium chloride TS: a white precipitate is formed.

Optical rotation <*2.49*> $[\alpha]_D^{20}$: +112 – +123° (0.2 g calculated on the dried basis, water, 20 mL, 100 mm).

Sulfuric acid Weigh accurately about 0.25 g of Kanamycin Monosulfate, dissolve in 100 mL of water, adjust the pH to 11.0 with ammonia solution (28), add exactly 10 mL of 0.1 mol/L barium chloride VS, and titrate <*2.50*> with 0.1 mol/L disodium dihydrogen ethylenediamine tetraacetate VS until the color of the solution, blue-purple, disappears (indicator: 0.5 mg of phthalein purple). At a near of the end-point add 50 mL of ethanol (99.5). Perform a blank determination in the same manner. The amount of sulfuric acid (SO_4) is not less than 15.0% and not more than 17.0%, calculated on the dried basis.

Each mL of 0.1 mol/L barium chloride VS
= 9.606 mg of SO_4

Purity **(1)** Heavy metals <*1.07*>—Proceed with 2.0 g of Kanamycin Monosulfate according to Method 4, and perform the test. Prepare the control solution with 2.0 mL of Standard Lead Solution (not more than 10 ppm).

(2) Arsenic <*1.11*>—Prepare the test solution with 2.0 g of Kanamycin Monosulfate according to Method 4, and perform the test (not more than 1 ppm).

(3) Related substances—Dissolve 0.30 g of Kanamycin Monosulfate in water to make exactly 10 mL, and use this solution as the sample solution. Separately, dissolve 45 mg of Kanamycin Monosulfate RS in water to make exactly 50 mL, and use this solution as the standard solution. Perform the test with these solutions as directed under Thin-layer Chromatography <*2.03*>. Spot 1 μL each of the sample solution and standard solution on a plate of silica gel for thin-layer chromatography. Develop the plate with a solution of potassium dihydrogen phosphate (3 in 40) to a distance of about 10 cm, and air-dry the plate. Spray evenly a solution of ninhydrin in 1-butanol (1 in 100) on the plate, and heat the plate at 110°C for 10 minutes: the spot other than the principal spot obtained from the sample solution is not more intense than the spot from the standard solution.

Loss on drying <*2.41*> Not more than 4.0% (5 g, reduced pressure not exceeding 0.67 kPa, 60°C, 3 hours).

Residue on ignition <*2.44*> Not more than 0.5% (1 g).

Assay Perform the test according to the Cylinder-plate method as directed under Microbial Assay for Antibiotics <*4.02*> according to the following conditions.

(i) Test organism—*Bacillus subtilis* ATCC 6633

(ii) Culture medium—Use the medium i in 1) under (1) Agar media for seed and base layer.

(iii) Standard solutions—Weigh accurately an amount of Kanamycin Monosulfate RS, previously dried, equivalent to about 20 mg (potency), dissolve in diluted phosphate buffer solution (pH 6.0) (1 in 2) to make exactly 50 mL, and use this solution as the standard stock solution. Keep the standard stock solution between 5 and 15°C and use within 30 days. Take exactly a suitable amount of the standard stock solution before use, add 0.1 mol/L phosphate buffer solution (pH 8.0) to make solutions so that each mL contains 20 μg (potency) and 5 μg (potency), and use these solutions as the high concentration standard solution and the low concentration standard solution, respectively.

(iv) Sample solutions—Weigh accurately an amount of Kanamycin Monosulfate, equivalent to about 20 mg (potency), and dissolve in water to make exactly 50 mL. Take exactly a suitable amount of this solution, add 0.1 mol/L phosphate buffer solution (pH 8.0) to make solutions so that each mL contains 20 μg (potency) and 5 μg (potency), and use these solutions as the high concentration sample solution and the low concentration sample solution, respectively.

Containers and storage Containers—Well-closed containers.

Kanamycin Sulfate

カナマイシン硫酸塩

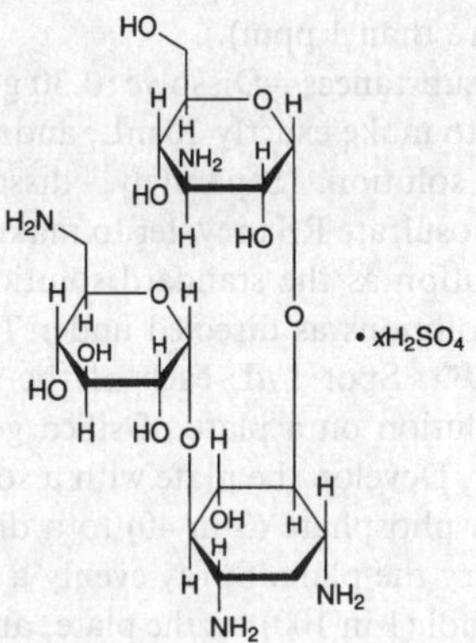

$C_{18}H_{36}N_4O_{11}.xH_2SO_4$
3-Amino-3-deoxy-α-D-glucopyranosyl-(1→6)-[6-amino-6-deoxy-α-D-glucopyranosyl-(1→4)]-2-deoxy-D-streptamine sulfate
[*133-92-6*]

Kanamycin Sulfate is the sulfate of an aminoglycoside substance having antibacterial activity produced by the growth of *Streptomyces kanamyceticus*.

It contains not less than 690 μg (potency) and not more than 740 μg (potency) per mg, calculated on the dried basis. The potency of Kanamycin Sulfate is expressed as mass (potency) of kanamycin ($C_{18}H_{36}N_4O_{11}$: 484.50).

Description Kanamycin Sulfate occurs as a white to yellow-white powder.

It is very soluble in water, and practically insoluble in ethanol (99.5).

Identification **(1)** Dissolve 20 mg each of Kanamycin Sulfate and Kanamycin Monosulfate RS in 1 mL of water, and use these solutions as the sample solution and standard solution. Perform the test with these solutions as directed under Thin-layer Chromatography <*2.03*>. Spot 5 μL each of the sample solution and standard solution on a plate of silica gel for thin-layer chromatography. Develop the plate with a mixture of chloroform, ammonia solution (28) and methanol (2:1:1) to a distance of about 10 cm, and air-dry the plate. Spray evenly 0.2% ninhydrin-water saturated 1-butanol TS on the plate, and heat the plate at 100°C for 10 minutes: the principal spot obtained from the sample solution and the spot from the standard solution show a purple-brown color and the same *R*f value.

(2) A solution of Kanamycin Sulfate (1 in 10) responds

to Qualitative Test <*1.09*> (1) for sulfate.

Optical rotation <*2.49*> $[\alpha]_D^{20}$: + 103 – + 115° (0.5 g calculated on the dried basis, water, 50 mL, 100 mm).

pH <*2.54*> The pH of a solution obtained by dissolving 1.0 g of Kanamycin Sulfate in 20 mL of water is between 6.0 and 7.5.

Purity (1) Clarity and color of solution—Dissolve 1.5 g of Kanamycin Sulfate in 5 mL of water: the solution is clear. Determine the absorbance of this solution at 400 nm as directed under Ultraviolet-visible Spectrophotometry <*2.24*>: not more than 0.15.

(2) Heavy metals <*1.07*>—Proceed with 1.0 g of Kanamycin Sulfate according to Method 4, and perform the test. Prepare the control solution with 3.0 mL of Standard Lead Solution (not more than 30 ppm).

(3) Arsenic <*1.11*>—Prepare the test solution with 2.0 g of Kanamycin Sulfate according to Method 3, and perform the test (not more than 1 ppm).

(4) Related substances—Dissolve 0.30 g of Kanamycin Sulfate in water to make exactly 10 mL, and use this solution as the sample solution. Separately, dissolve 9.0 mg of Kanamycin Monosulfate RS in water to make exactly 10 mL, and use this solution as the standard solution. Perform the test with these solutions as directed under Thin-layer Chromatography <*2.03*>. Spot 1 μL each of the sample solution and standard solution on a plate of silica gel for thin-layer chromatography. Develop the plate with a solution of potassium dihydrogen phosphate (3 in 40) to a distance of about 10 cm, and air-dry the plate. Spray evenly a solution of ninhydrin in 1-butanol (1 in 100) on the plate, and heat the plate at 110°C for 10 minutes: the spot other than the principal spot obtained from the sample solution is not more intense than the spot from the standard solution.

Loss on drying <*2.41*> Not more than 5.0% (0.5 g, reduced pressure not exceeding 0.67 kPa, 60°C, 3 hours).

Assay Perform the test according to the Cylinder-plate method as directed under Microbial Assay for Antibiotics <*4.02*> according to the following conditions.

(i) Test organism—*Bacillus subtilis* ATCC 6633

(ii) Culture medium—Use the medium i in 1) under (1) Agar media for seed and base layer having pH 7.8 to 8.0 after sterilization.

(iii) Standard solutions—Weigh accurately an amount of Kanamycin Monosulfate RS, previously dried, equivalent to about 20 mg (potency), dissolve in diluted phosphate buffer solution (pH 6.0) (1 in 2) to make exactly 50 mL, and use this solution as the standard stock solution. Keep the standard stock solution at 5 to 15°C and use within 30 days. Take exactly a suitable amount of the standard stock solution before use, add 0.1 mol/L phosphate buffer solution (pH 8.0) to make solutions so that each mL contains 20 μg (potency) and 5 μg (potency), and use these solutions as the high concentration standard solution and the low concentration standard solution, respectively.

(iv) Sample solutions—Weigh accurately an amount of Kanamycin Sulfate, equivalent to about 20 mg (potency), and dissolve in water to make exactly 50 mL. Take exactly a suitable amount of this solution, add 0.1 mol/L phosphate buffer solution (pH 8.0) to make solutions so that each mL contains 20 μg (potency) and 5 μg (potency), and use these solutions as the high concentration sample solution and the low concentration sample solution, respectively.

Containers and storage Containers—Tight containers.

Kaolin

カオリン

Kaolin is a native, hydrous aluminum silicate.

Description Kaolin occurs as white or nearly white, fragmentary masses or powder. It has a slightly clay-like odor.

It is practically insoluble in water, in ethanol (99.5) and in diethyl ether.

It is insoluble in dilute hydrochloric acid and in sodium hydroxide TS.

When moistened with water, it darkens and becomes plastic.

Identification (1) Heat 1 g of Kaolin with 10 mL of water and 5 mL of sulfuric acid in a porcelain dish, and evaporate the mixture nearly to dryness. Cool, add 20 mL of water, boil for 2 to 3 minutes, and filter: the color of the residue is gray.

(2) The filtrate obtained in (1) responds to Qualitative Tests <*1.09*> (1), (2) and (4) for aluminum salt.

Purity (1) Acid or alkali—Add 25 mL of water to 1.0 g of Kaolin, agitate thoroughly, and filter: the pH <*2.54*> of the filtrate is between 4.0 and 7.5.

(2) Acid-soluble substances—Add 20 mL of dilute hydrochloric acid to 1.0 g of Kaolin, agitate for 15 minutes, and filter. Evaporate 10 mL of the filtrate to dryness, and heat strongly between 450°C and 550°C to constant mass: the mass of the ignited residue is not more than 10 mg.

(3) Carbonate—Stir 1.0 g of Kaolin with 5 mL of water, then add 10 mL of diluted sulfuric acid (1 in 2): no effervescence occurs.

(4) Heavy metals <*1.07*>—Boil 1.5 g of Kaolin gently with 50 mL of water and 5 mL of hydrochloric acid for 20 minutes with frequent agitation, cool, centrifuge, and separate the supernatant liquid. Wash the precipitate twice with 10 mL of water, centrifuge each time, and combine the supernatant liquid and the washings. Add dropwise ammonia solution (28) to this solution until a slight precipitate occurs, then add dilute hydrochloric acid dropwise while agitating strongly to complete solution. Add 0.45 g of hydroxylammonium chloride, and heat. Cool, add 0.45 g of sodium acetate trihydrate and 6 mL of dilute acetic acid, filter if necessary, and wash with 10 mL of water. Combine the filtrate and the washings, and add water to make 150 mL. Perform the test using 50 mL of this solution as the test solution. To 2.5 mL of Standard Lead Solution add 0.15 g of hydroxylammonium chloride, 0.15 g of sodium acetate trihydrate, 2 mL of dilute acetic acid and water to make 50 mL, and use this solution as the control solution (not more than 50 ppm).

(5) Iron <*1.10*>—Add 10 mL of dilute hydrochloric acid to 40 mg of Kaolin, and heat for 10 minutes with shaking in a water bath. After cooling, add 0.5 g of L-tartaric acid, dissolve with shaking, prepare the test solution with this solution according to Method 2, and perform the test according to Method B. Prepare the control solution with 2.0 mL of Standard Iron Solution (not more than 500 ppm).

(6) Arsenic <*1.11*>—Add 5 mL of water and 1 mL of sulfuric acid to 1.0 g of Kaolin, and heat on a sand bath until white fumes begin to evolve. Cool, and add water to make 5 mL. Perform the test with this solution as the test solution (not more than 2 ppm).

(7) Foreign matter—Place 5 g of Kaolin in a beaker, add 100 mL of water, stir, and decant to leave sand. Repeat this procedure several times with 100-mL portions of water: no sandy residue remains.

Loss on ignition ‹*2.43*› Not more than 15.0% (1 g, 600°C, 5 hours).

Plasticity Add 7.5 mL of water to 5.0 g of Kaolin, and agitate thoroughly: the resultant mass has no remarkable fluidity.

Containers and storage Containers—Well-closed containers.

Ketamine Hydrochloride

ケタミン塩酸塩

and enantiomer

$C_{13}H_{16}ClNO.HCl$: 274.19
(2*RS*)-2-(2-Chlorophenyl)-2-(methylamino)cyclohexanone monohydrochloride
[*1867-66-9*]

Ketamine Hydrochloride, when dried, contains not less than 99.0% of ketamine hydrochloride ($C_{13}H_{16}ClNO.HCl$).

Description Ketamine Hydrochloride occurs as white, crystals or crystalline powder.

It is very soluble in formic acid, freely soluble in water and in methanol, sparingly soluble in ethanol (95) and in acetic acid (100), and practically insoluble in acetic anhydride and in diethyl ether.

A solution of Ketamine Hydrochloride (1 in 10) shows no optical rotation.

Melting point: about 258°C (with decomposition).

Identification **(1)** Determine the absorption spectrum of a solution of Ketamine Hydrochloride in 0.1 mol/L hydrochloric acid TS (1 in 3000) as directed under Ultraviolet-visible Spectrophotometry ‹*2.24*›, and compare the spectrum with the Reference Spectrum: both spectra exhibit similar intensities of absorption at the same wavelengths.

(2) Determine the infrared absorption spectrum of Ketamine Hydrochloride, previously dried, as directed in the potassium bromide disk method under Infrared Spectrophotometry ‹*2.25*›, and compare the spectrum with the Reference Spectrum: both spectra exhibit similar intensities of absorption at the same wave numbers.

(3) A solution of Ketamine Hydrochloride (1 in 10) responds to Qualitative Tests ‹*1.09*› (2) for chloride.

Absorbance ‹*2.24*› $E^{1\%}_{1\,cm}$ (269 nm): 22.0 – 24.5 (after drying, 30 mg, 0.1 mol/L hydrochloric acid TS, 100 mL).

pH ‹*2.54*› Dissolve 1.0 g of Ketamine Hydrochloride in 10 mL of freshly boiled and cooled water: the pH of the solution is between 3.5 and 4.5.

Purity **(1)** Clarity and color of solution—Dissolve 1.0 g of Ketamine Hydrochloride in 5 mL of water: the solution is clear and colorless.

(2) Heavy metals ‹*1.07*›—Proceed with 1.0 g of Ketamine Hydrochloride according to Method 1, and perform the test. Prepare the control solution with 2.0 mL of Standard Lead Solution (not more than 20 ppm).

(3) Arsenic ‹*1.11*›—Prepare the test solution with 1.0 g of Ketamine Hydrochloride, according to Method 1, and perform the test (not more than 2 ppm).

(4) Related substances—Dissolve 0.5 g of Ketamine Hydrochloride in 10 mL of methanol and use this solution as the sample solution. Pipet 1 mL of the sample solution, add methanol to make exactly 200 mL, and use this solution as the standard solution. Perform the test with these solutions as directed under Thin-layer Chromatography ‹*2.03*›. Spot 2 μL each of the sample solution and standard solution on a plate of silica gel for thin-layer chromatography. Develop the plate with a mixture of cyclohexane and isopropylamine (49:1) to a distance of about 10 cm, and air-dry the plate. Spray evenly Dragendorff's TS for spraying on the plate, dry the plate, and then spray evenly hydrogen peroxide TS: the spots other than the principal spot obtained from the sample solution is not more intense than the spot from the standard solution.

Loss on drying ‹*2.41*› Not more then 0.5% (1 g, 105°C, 3 hours).

Residue on ignition ‹*2.44*› Not more than 0.1% (1 g).

Assay Weigh accurately about 0.5 g of Ketamine Hydrochloride, previously dried, dissolve in 1 mL of formic acid, add 70 mL of a mixture of acetic anhydride and acetic acid (100) (6:1), and titrate ‹*2.50*› with 0.1 mol/L perchloric acid VS (potentiometric titration). Perform a blank determination in the same manner, and make any necessary correction.

Each mL of 0.1 mol/L perchloric acid VS
= 27.42 mg of $C_{13}H_{16}ClNO.HCl$

Containers and storage Containers—Tight containers.

Ketoconazole

ケトコナゾール

and enantiomer

$C_{26}H_{28}Cl_2N_4O_4$: 531.43
1-Acetyl-4-(4-{[(2*RS*,4*SR*)-2-(2,4-dichlorophenyl)-2-(1*H*-imidazol-1-ylmethyl)-1,3-dioxolan-4-yl]methoxy}phenyl)piperazine
[*65277-42-1*]

Ketoconazole, when dried, contains not less than 99.0% and not more than 101.0% of ketoconazole ($C_{26}H_{28}Cl_2N_4O_4$).

Description Ketoconazole occurs as a white to light yellowwhite powder.

It is soluble in methanol, sparingly soluble in ethanol (99.5), and practically insoluble in water.

A solution of Ketoconazole in methanol (1 in 20) shows no optical rotation.

Identification **(1)** Determine the absorption spectrum of a solution of Ketoconazole in methanol (3 in 100,000) as directed under Ultraviolet-visible Spectrophotometry ‹*2.24*›, and compare the spectrum with the Reference Spectrum:

both spectra exhibit similar intensities of absorption at the same wavelengths.

(2) Determine the infrared absorption spectrum of Ketoconazole as directed in the potassium bromide disk method under Infrared Spectrophotometry <*2.25*>, and compare the spectrum with the Reference Spectrum: both spectra exhibit similar intensities of absorption at the same wave numbers.

(3) Perform the test with Ketoconazole as directed under Flame Coloration Test <*1.04*> (2): a green color appears.

Melting point <*2.60*> 148 – 152°C

Purity **(1)** Heavy metals <*1.07*>—Proceed with 1.0 g of Ketoconazole according to Method 2, and perform the test. Prepare the control solution with 1.0 mL of Standard Lead Solution (not more than 10 ppm).

(2) Related Substances—Dissolve 0.10 g of Ketoconazole in 10 mL of methanol, and use this solution as the sample solution. Pipet 5 mL of the sample solution, and add methanol to make exactly 100 mL. Pipet 1 mL of this solution, add methanol to make exactly 10 mL, and use this solution as the standard solution. Perform the test with exactly 10 μL each of the sample solution and standard solution as directed under Liquid Chromatography <*2.01*> according to the following conditions. Determine each peak area of both solutions by the automatic integration method: the area of the peak other than ketoconazole obtained from the sample solution is not larger than 2/5 times the peak area of ketoconazole from the standard solution, and the total area of the peaks other than ketoconazole from the sample solution is not larger than the peak area of ketoconazole from the standard solution.

Operating conditions—

Detector: An ultraviolet absorption photometer (wavelength: 220 nm).

Column: A stainless steel column 4.6 mm in inside diameter and 10 cm in length, packed with octadecylsilanized silica gel for liquid chromatography (3 μm in particle diameter).

Column temperature: A constant temperature of about 25°C.

Mobile phase A: Acetonitrile for liquid chromatography.

Mobile phase B: A solution of tetrabutylammonium hydrogensulfate (17 in 5000).

Flowing of mobile phase: Control the gradient by mixing the mobile phases A and B as directed in the following table.

Time after injection of sample (min)	Mobile phase A (vol%)	Mobile phase B (vol%)
0 – 10	5 → 50	95 → 50
10 – 15	50	50

Flow rate: 2.0 mL per minute.

Time span of measurement: For 15 minutes after injection, beginning after the solvent peak.

System suitability—

Test for required detectability: Pipet 2 mL of the standard solution, and add methanol to make exactly 20 mL. Confirm that the peak area of ketoconazole obtained with 10 μL of this solution is equivalent to 7 to 13% of that with 10 μL of the standard solution.

System performance: When the procedure is run with 10 μL of the standard solution under the above operating conditions, the number of theoretical plates and the symmetry factor of the peak of ketoconazole are not less than 40,000 and not more than 1.5, respectively.

System repeatability: When the test is repeated 6 times with 10 μL of the standard solution under the above operating conditions, the relative standard deviation of the peak area of ketoconazole is not more than 2.5%.

Loss on drying <*2.41*> Not more than 0.5% (1 g, 105°C, 4 hours).

Residue on ignition <*2.44*> Not more than 0.1% (1 g).

Assay Weigh accurately about 0.2 g of Ketoconazole, previously dried, dissolve in 70 mL of a mixture of 2-butanone and acetic acid (100) (7:1), and titrate <*2.50*> with 0.1 mol/L perchloric acid VS (potentiometric titration). Perform a blank determination in the same manner, and make any necessary correction.

Each mL of 0.1 mol/L perchloric acid VS
= 26.57 mg of $C_{26}H_{28}Cl_2N_4O_4$

Containers and storage Containers—Tight containers.
Storage—Light-resistant.

Ketoconazole Cream

ケトコナゾールクリーム

Ketoconazole Cream contains not less than 95.0% and not more than 105.0% of the labeled amount of ketoconazole ($C_{26}H_{28}Cl_2N_4O_4$: 531.43).

Method of preparation Prepare as directed under Creams, with Ketoconazole.

Identification To a quantity of Ketoconazole Cream, equivalent to 0.1 g of Ketoconazole, add 20 mL of 2-propanol, shake for 20 minutes, centrifuge, and use the supernatant liquid as the sample solution. Separately, dissolve 25 mg of ketoconazole in 5 mL of 2-propanol, and use this solution as the standard solution. Perform the test with these solutions as directed under Thin-layer Chromatography <*2.03*>. Spot 5 μL each of the sample solution and standard solution on a plate of silica gel with fluorescent indicator for thin-layer chromatography. Develop the plate with a mixture of ethyl acetate, hexane, methanol, water and ammonia solution (28) (40:40:25:2:1) to a distance of about 12 cm, and air-dry the plate. Examine under ultraviolet light (main wavelength: 254 nm): the principal spot obtained from the sample solution has the same *R*f value as the spot from the standard solution.

Assay Weigh accurately an amount of Ketoconazole Cream, equivalent to about 25 mg of ketoconazole ($C_{26}H_{28}Cl_2N_4O_4$), dissolve in methanol to make exactly 100 mL. Pipet 10 mL of this solution, add exactly 4 mL of the internal standard solution, add methanol to make 50 mL, and use this solution as the sample solution. Separately, weigh accurately about 25 mg of ketoconazole for assay, previously dried at 105°C for 4 hours, and dissolve in methanol to make exactly 50 mL. Pipet 5 mL of this solution, add exactly 4 mL of the internal standard solution, add methanol to make 50 mL, and use this solution as the standard solution. Perform the test with 10 μL each of the sample solution and standard solution as directed under Liquid Chromatography <*2.01*> according to the following conditions, and calculate the ratios, Q_T and Q_S, of the peak area of ketoconazole to that of the internal standard.

Amount (mg) of ketoconazole ($C_{26}H_{28}Cl_2N_4O_4$)
$= M_S \times Q_T/Q_S$

M_S: Amount (mg) of ketoconazole for assay taken

Internal standard solution—A solution of xanthone in methanol (1 in 10,000).

Operating conditions—

Detector: An ultraviolet absorption photometer (wavelength: 230 nm).

Column: A stainless steel column 4.6 mm in inside diameter and 15 cm in length, packed with octadecylsilanized silica gel for liquid chromatography (5 μm in particle diameter).

Column temperature: A constant temperature of about 40°C.

Mobile phase: To ammonium acetate solution (1 in 200) add acetic acid (100) to adjust the pH to 5.0. To 250 mL of this solution add 750 mL of methanol.

Flow rate: Adjust so that the retention time of ketoconazole is about 8 minutes.

System suitability—

System performance: When the procedure is run with 10 μL of the standard solution under the above operating conditions, the internal standard and ketoconazole are eluted in this order with the resolution between these peaks being not less than 5.

System repeatability: When the test is repeated 6 times with 10 μL of the standard solution under the above operating conditions, the relative standard deviation of the ratio of the peak area of ketoconazole to that of the internal standard is not more than 1.0%.

Containers and storage Containers—Tight containers.

Ketoconazole Lotion

ケトコナゾールローション

Ketoconazole Lotion is an emulsion lotion.

It contains not less than 93.0% and not more than 107.0% of the labeled amount of ketoconazole ($C_{26}H_{28}Cl_2N_4O_4$: 531.43).

Method of preparation Prepare as directed under Lotions, with Ketoconazole.

Description Ketoconazole Lotion occurs as a white emulsion.

Identification Shake well and take an amount of Ketoconazole Lotion, equivalent to 0.1 g of Ketoconazole, add 20 mL of 2-propanol, shake for 20 minutes, centrifuge, and use the supernatant liquid as the sample solution. Separately, dissolve 25 mg of ketoconazole in 5 mL of 2-propanol, and use this solution as the standard solution. Perform the test with these solutions as directed under Thin-layer Chromatography <*2.03*>. Spot 5 μL each of the sample solution and standard solution on a plate of silica gel with fluorescent indicator for thin-layer chromatography. Develop the plate with a mixture of ethyl acetate, hexane, methanol, water and ammonia solution (28) (40:40:25:2:1) to a distance of about 12 cm, and air-dry the plate. Examine under ultraviolet light (main wavelength: 254 nm): the principal spot obtained from the sample solution has the same *R*f value as the spot from the standard solution.

Assay Shake well and weigh accurately an amount of Ketoconazole Lotion, equivalent to about 25 mg of ketoconazole ($C_{26}H_{28}Cl_2N_4O_4$), dissolve in methanol to make exactly 100 mL. Pipet 10 mL of this solution, add exactly 4 mL of the internal standard solution, add methanol to make 50 mL, and use this solution as the sample solution. Separately, weigh accurately about 25 mg of ketoconazole for assay, previously dried at 105°C for 4 hours, dissolve in methanol to make exactly 50 mL. Pipet 5 mL of this solution, add exactly 4 mL of the internal standard solution, add methanol to make 50 mL, and use this solution as the standard solution. Perform the test with 10 μL each of the sample solution and standard solution as directed under Liquid Chromatography <*2.01*> according to the following conditions, and calculate the ratios, Q_T and Q_S, of the peak area of ketoconazole to that of the internal standard.

$$\text{Amount (mg) of ketoconazole } (C_{26}H_{28}Cl_2N_4O_4) = M_S \times Q_T/Q_S$$

M_S: Amount (mg) of ketoconazole for assay taken

Internal standard solution—A solution of xanthone in methanol (1 in 10,000).

Operating conditions—

Detector: An ultraviolet absorption photometer (wavelength: 230 nm).

Column: A stainless steel column 4.6 mm in inside diameter and 15 cm in length, packed with octadecylsilanized silica gel for liquid chromatography (5 μm in particle diameter).

Column temperature: A constant temperature of about 40°C.

Mobile phase: To ammonium acetate solution (1 in 200) add acetic acid (100) to adjust the pH to 5.0. To 250 mL of this solution add 750 mL of methanol.

Flow rate: Adjust so that the retention time of ketoconazole is about 8 minutes.

System suitability—

System performance: When the procedure is run with 10 μL of the standard solution under the above operating conditions, the internal standard and ketoconazole are eluted in this order with the resolution between these peaks being not less than 5.

System repeatability: When the test is repeated 6 times with 10 μL of the standard solution under the above operating conditions, the relative standard deviation of the ratio of the peak area of ketoconazole to that of the internal standard is not more than 1.0%.

Containers and storage Containers—Tight containers.

Ketoconazole Solution

ケトコナゾール液

Ketoconazole Solution is a liquid for external use.

Ketoconazole Solution contains not less than 95.0% and not more than 105.0% of the labeled amount of ketoconazole ($C_{26}H_{28}Cl_2N_4O_4$: 531.43).

Method of preparation Prepare as directed under Liquids and Solutions for Cutaneous Application, with Ketoconazole.

Description Ketoconazole Solution is a clear liquid.

Identification To a volume of Ketoconazole Solution, equivalent to 10 mg of Ketoconazole, add methanol to make 10 mL, and use this solution as the sample solution. Separately, dissolve 10 mg of ketoconazole in 10 mL of methanol, and use this solution as the standard solution. Perform the test with these solutions as directed under Thin-layer Chromatography <*2.03*>. Spot 5 μL each of the sample solution and standard solution on a plate of silica gel with fluorescent indicator for thin-layer chromatography. Develop the plate with a mixture of ethyl acetate, hexane, methanol, water and ammonia solution (28) (40:40:30:2:1) to a distance of about 10 cm, and air-dry the plate. Examine under ultraviolet light (main wavelength: 254 nm): the principal spot obtained from the sample solution has the same *R*f value as the spot from the standard solution.

pH Being specified separately when the drug is granted approval based on the Law.

Assay To an exact amount of Ketoconazole Solution, equivalent to about 10 mg of ketoconazole ($C_{26}H_{28}Cl_2N_4O_4$), add exactly 5 mL of the internal standard solution, and add 15 mL of methanol. To 1 mL of this solution add methanol to make 25 mL, and use this solution as the sample solution. Separately, weigh accurately about 50 mg of ketoconazole for assay, previously dried at 105°C for 4 hours, and dissolve in methanol to make exactly 50 mL. Pipet 10 mL of this solution, add exactly 5 mL of the internal standard solution, add methanol to make 20 mL. Take 1 mL of this solution, add methanol to make 25 mL, and use this solution as the standard solution. Perform the test with 20 μL each of the sample solution and standard solution as directed under Liquid Chromatography <*2.01*> according to the following conditions, and calculate the ratios, Q_T and Q_S, of the peak area of ketoconazole to that of the internal standard.

Amount (mg) of ketoconazole ($C_{26}H_{28}Cl_2N_4O_4$)
$= M_S \times Q_T/Q_S \times 1/5$

M_S: Amount (mg) of ketoconazole for assay taken

Internal standard solution—A solution of bifonazole in methanol (3 in 2000).

Operating conditions—

Detector: An ultraviolet absorption photometer (wavelength: 240 nm).

Column: A stainless steel column 4.6 mm in inside diameter and 25 cm in length, packed with octadecylsilanized silica gel for liquid chromatography (5 μm in particle diameter).

Column temperature: A constant temperature of about 40°C.

Mobile phase: A mixture of a solution of diisopropylamine in methanol (1 in 500), ammonium acetate solution (1 in 200) and acetic acid (100) (1800:600:1).

Flow rate: Adjust so that the retention time of ketoconazole is about 11 minutes.

System suitability—

System performance: When the procedure is run with 20 μL of the standard solution under the above operating conditions, ketoconazole and the internal standard are eluted in this order with the resolution between these peaks being not less than 3.

System repeatability: When the test is repeated 6 times with 20 μL of the standard solution under the above operating conditions, the relative standard deviation of the ratio of the peak area of ketoconazole to that of the internal standard is not more than 1.0%.

Containers and storage Containers—Tight containers.

Ketoprofen

ケトプロフェン

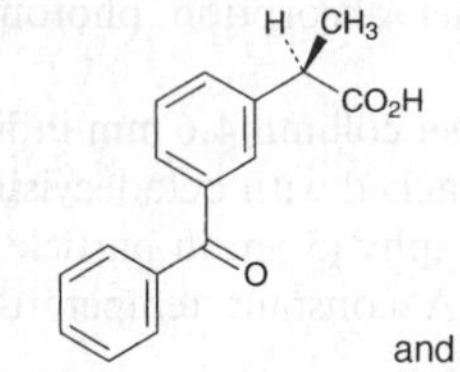

and enantiomer

$C_{16}H_{14}O_3$: 254.28
(2*RS*)-2-(3-Benzoylphenyl)propanoic acid
[*22071-15-4*]

Ketoprofen, when dried, contains not less than 99.0% and not more than 100.5% of ketoprofen ($C_{16}H_{14}O_3$).

Description Ketoprofen occurs as a white crystalline powder.

It is very soluble in methanol, freely soluble in ethanol (95) and in acetone, and practically insoluble in water.

A solution of Ketoprofen in ethanol (99.5) (1 in 100) shows no optical rotation.

It is colored to pale yellow by light.

Identification **(1)** Determine the absorption spectrum of a solution of Ketoprofen in methanol (1 in 200,000) as directed under Ultraviolet-visible Spectrophotometry <*2.24*>, and compare the spectrum with the Reference Spectrum: both spectra exhibit similar intensities of absorption at the same wavelengths.

(2) Determine the infrared absorption spectrum of Ketoprofen, previously dried, as directed in the potassium bromide disk method under Infrared Spectrophotometry <*2.25*>, and compare the spectrum with the Reference Spectrum: both spectra exhibit similar intensities of absorption at the same wave numbers.

Melting point <*2.60*> 94 – 97°C

Purity **(1)** Clarity and color of solution—Dissolve 1.0 g of Ketoprofen in 10 mL of acetone: the solution is clear, and has no more color than the following control solution.

Control solution: To a mixture of 0.6 mL of Cobalt (II) Chloride CS and 2.4 mL of Iron (III) Chloride CS add diluted hydrochloric acid (1 in 10) to make 10 mL. To 5.0 mL of this solution add diluted hydrochloric acid (1 in 10) to make 100 mL.

(2) Heavy metals <*1.07*>—Proceed with 2.0 g of Ketoprofen according to Method 2, and perform the test. Prepare the control solution with 2.0 mL of Standard Lead Solution (not more than 10 ppm).

(3) Related substances—Conduct this procedure with a minimum of exposure to light, using light-resistant vessels. Dissolve 20 mg of Ketoprofen in 20 mL of the mobile phase, and use this solution as the sample solution. Pipet 1 mL of the sample solution, and add the mobile phase to make exactly 50 mL. Pipet 1 mL of this solution, add the mobile phase to make exactly 10 mL, and use this solution as the standard solution. Perform the test with exactly 20 μL each of the sample solution and standard solution as directed under Liquid Chromatography <*2.01*> according to the following conditions, and determine each peak area by the automatic integration method: the areas of the peaks, having the relative retention time of about 1.5 and about 0.3 to ketoprofen obtained from the sample solution, are not larger than 4.5 times and not larger than 2 times the peak area of ketoprofen from the standard solution, respectively, the area of the peak other than ketoprofen and the peaks mentioned above from the sample solution is not larger than the peak area of ketoprofen from the standard solution, and the total area of these peaks is not larger than 2 times the peak area of ketoprofen from the standard solution.

Operating conditions—

Detector: An ultraviolet absorption photometer (wavelength: 233 nm).

Column: A stainless steel column 4.6 mm in inside diameter and 15 cm in length, packed with octadecylsilanized silica gel for liquid chromatography (5 μm in particle diameter).

Column temperature: A constant temperature of about 25°C.

Mobile phase: Dissolve 68.0 g of potassium dihydrogen phosphate in water to make 1000 mL, and adjust the pH to 3.5 with phosphoric acid. To 20 mL of this solution add 430 mL of acetonitrile and 550 mL of water.

Flow rate: Adjust so that the retention time of ketoprofen is about 7 minutes.

Time span of measurement: About 7 times as long as the retention time of ketoprofen.

System suitability—

Test for required detectability: To exactly 1 mL of the standard solution add the mobile phase to make exactly 10 mL. Confirm that the peak area of ketoprofen obtained with 20 μL of this solution is equivalent to 9 to 11% of that with 20 μL of the standard solution.

System performance: When the procedure is run with 20 μL of the standard solution under the above operating conditions, the number of theoretical plates and the symmetry factor of the peak of ketoprofen are not less than 8000 and not more than 1.5, respectively.

System repeatability: When the test is repeated 6 times with 20 μL of the standard solution under the above operating conditions, the relative standard deviation of the peak area of ketoprofen is not more than 2.0%.

Loss on drying <*2.41*> Not more than 0.5% (0.5 g, in vacuum, 60°C, 24 hours).

Residue on ignition <*2.44*> Not more than 0.1% (1 g).

Assay Weigh accurately about 0.3 g of Ketoprofen, previously dried, dissolve in 25 mL of ethanol (95), add 25 mL of water, and titrate <*2.50*> with 0.1 mol/L sodium hydroxide VS (potentiometric titration). Perform a blank determination in the same manner, and make any necessary correction.

Each mL of 0.1 mol/L sodium hydroxide VS
= 25.43 mg of $C_{16}H_{14}O_3$

Containers and storage Containers—Tight containers.

Storage—Light-resistant.

Ketotifen Fumarate

ケトチフェンフマル酸塩

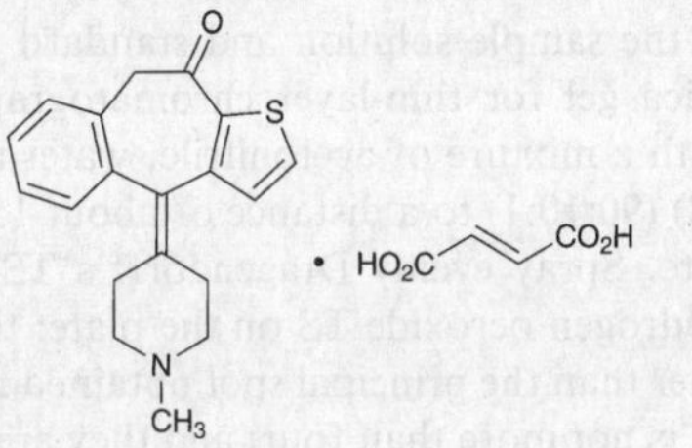

$C_{19}H_{19}NOS.C_4H_4O_4$: 425.50

4-(1-Methylpiperidin-4-ylidene)-4*H*-benzo[4,5]cyclohepta[1,2-*b*]thiophen-10(9*H*)-one monofumarate

[34580-14-8]

Ketotifen Fumarate, when dried, contains not less than 99.0% and not more than 101.0% of ketotifen fumarate ($C_{19}H_{19}NOS.C_4H_4O_4$).

Description Ketotifen Fumarate occurs as a white to light yellow-white crystalline powder.

It is sparingly soluble in methanol and in acetic acid (100), and slightly soluble in water, in ethanol (99.5) and in acetic anhydride.

Melting point: about 190°C (with decomposition).

Identification **(1)** Prepare the test solution with 30 mg of Ketotifen Fumarate as directed under Oxygen Flask Combustion Method <*1.06*> using 20 mL of water as the absorbing liquid: the test solution responds to Qualitative Tests <*1.09*> for sulfate.

(2) Determine the absorption spectrum of a solution of Ketotifen Fumarate in methanol (1 in 50,000) as directed under Ultraviolet-visible Spectrophotometry <*2.24*>, and compare the spectrum with the Reference Spectrum: both spectra exhibit similar intensities of absorption at the same wavelengths.

(3) Determine the infrared absorption spectrum of Ketotifen Fumarate, previously dried, as directed in the potassium bromide disk method under Infrared Spectrophotometry <*2.25*>, and compare the spectrum with the Reference Spectrum: both spectra exhibit similar intensities of absorption at the same wave numbers.

Purity **(1)** Chloride <*1.03*>—Dissolve 0.6 g of Ketotifen Fumarate in 2.5 mL of sodium carbonate TS in a crucible, heat on a water bath to dryness, and ignite at about 500°C. Dissolve the residue in 15 mL of water, filter if necessary, neutralize with diluted nitric acid (3 in 10), and add 6 mL of dilute nitric acid and water to make 50 mL. Perform the test using this solution as the test solution. Prepare the control solution as follows: To 0.25 mL of 0.01 mol/L hydrochloric acid VS add 2.5 mL of sodium carbonate TS, the used amount of diluted nitric acid (3 in 10) for the neutralization, 6 mL of dilute nitric acid and water to make 50 mL (not more than 0.015%).

(2) Heavy metals <*1.07*>—Proceed with 1.0 g of Ketotifen Fumarate according to Method 2, and perform the test. Prepare the control solution with 2.0 mL of Standard Lead Solution (not more than 20 ppm).

(3) Related substances—Dissolve 0.10 g of Ketotifen Fumarate in 10 mL of a mixture of methanol and ammonia TS (99:1), and use this solution as the sample solution. Pipet 1 mL of the sample solution, and add a mixture of methanol and ammonia TS (99:1) to make exactly 25 mL. Pipet 1 mL of this solution, add a mixture of methanol and ammonia TS (99:1) to make exactly 20 mL, and use this solution as the standard solution. Perform the test with these solutions as directed under Thin-layer Chromatography <2.03>. Spot 10 μL each of the sample solution and standard solution on a plate of silica gel for thin-layer chromatography. Develop the plate with a mixture of acetonitrile, water and ammonia solution (28) (90:10:1) to a distance of about 15 cm, and air-dry the plate. Spray evenly Dragendorff's TS for spraying and then hydrogen peroxide TS on the plate: the number of the spot other than the principal spot obtained from the sample solution is not more than four, and they are not more intense than the spot from the standard solution.

Loss on drying <2.41> Not more than 0.5% (1 g, 105°C, 4 hours).

Residue on ignition <2.44> Not more than 0.1% (1 g).

Assay Weigh accurately about 0.35 g of Ketotifen Fumarate, previously dried, dissolve in 80 mL of a mixture of acetic anhydride and acetic acid (100) (7:3), and titrate <2.50> with 0.1 mol/L perchloric acid VS (potentiometric titration). Perform a blank determination in the same manner, and make any necessary correction.

Each mL of 0.1 mol/L perchloric acid VS
= 42.55 mg of $C_{19}H_{19}NOS.C_4H_4O_4$

Containers and storage Containers—Tight containers.

Kitasamycin

キタサマイシン

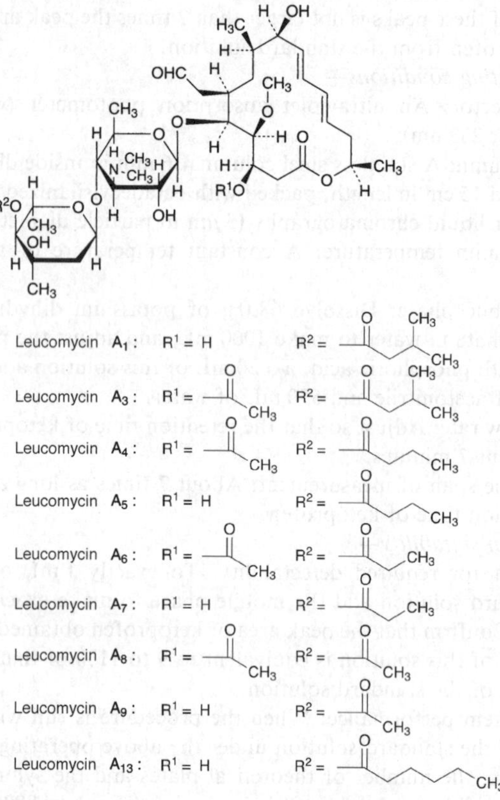

Leucomycin A_1 : R^1 = H
Leucomycin A_3 : R^1 = acetyl
Leucomycin A_4 : R^1 = acetyl
Leucomycin A_5 : R^1 = H
Leucomycin A_6 : R^1 = acetyl
Leucomycin A_7 : R^1 = H
Leucomycin A_8 : R^1 = acetyl
Leucomycin A_9 : R^1 = H
Leucomycin A_{13} : R^1 = H

(Leucomycins A_1, A_5, A_7, A_9 and A_{13})
(3*R*,4*R*,5*S*,6*R*,8*R*,9*R*,10*E*,12*E*,15*R*)-5-[4-*O*-Acyl-2,6-dideoxy-3-*C*-methyl-α-L-*ribo*-hexopyranosyl-(1→4)-3,6-dideoxy-3-dimethylamino-β-D-glucopyranosyloxy]-6-formylmethyl-3,9-dihydroxy-4-methoxy-8-methylhexadeca-10,12-dien-15-olide

Leucomycin A_1 : acyl = 3-methylbutanoyl
Leucomycin A_5 : acyl = butanoyl
Leucomycin A_7 : acyl = propanoyl
Leucomycin A_9 : acyl = acetyl
Leucomycin A_{13}: acyl = hexanoyl

(Leucomycins A_3, A_4, A_6 and A_8)
(3*R*,4*R*,5*S*,6*R*,8*R*,9*R*,10*E*,12*E*,15*R*)-3-Acetoxy-5-[4-*O*-acyl-2,6-dideoxy-3-*C*-methyl-α-L-*ribo*-hexopyranosyl-(1→4)-3,6-dideoxy-3-dimethylamino-β-D-glucopyranosyloxy]-6-formylmethyl-9-hydroxy-4-methoxy-8-methylhexadeca-10,12-dien-15-olide

Leucomycin A_3: acyl = 3-methylbutanoyl
Leucomycin A_4: acyl = butanoyl
Leucomycin A_6: acyl = propanoyl
Leucomycin A_8: acyl = acetyl

[*1392-21-8*, Kitasamycin]

Kitasamycin is a mixture of macrolide substances having antibacterial activity produced by the growth of *Streptomyces kitasatoensis*.

It contains not less than 1450 μg (potency) and not more than 1700 μg (potency) per mg, calculated on the anhydrous basis. The potency of Kitasamycin is expressed as mass (potency) of kitasamycin corresponding to the mass of leucomycin A_5 ($C_{39}H_{65}NO_{14}$: 771.93). One mg (potency) of kitasamycin is equivalent to 0.530 mg of leucomycin A_5 ($C_{39}H_{65}NO_{14}$).

Description Kitasamycin occurs as a white to light yellow-white powder.

It is very soluble in acetonitrile, in methanol and in ethanol (95), and practically insoluble in water.

Identification Determine the absorption spectrum of a solution of Kitasamycin in methanol (1 in 40,000) as directed under Ultraviolet-visible Spectrophotometry <2.24>, and compare the spectrum with the Reference Spectrum: both spectra exhibit similar intensities of absorption at the same wavelengths.

Content ratio of the active principle Dissolve 20 mg of Kitasamycin in diluted acetonitrile (1 in 2) to make 20 mL, and use this solution as the sample solution. Perform the test with 5 μL of the sample solution as directed under Liquid Chromatography <2.01> according to the following conditions, and measure each peak area by the automatic integration method. Calculate the amounts of leucomycin A_5, leucomycin A_4 and leucomycin A_1 by the area percentage method: the amounts of leucomycin A_5, leucomycin A_4 and leucomycin A_1 are 40 to 70%, 5 to 25% and 3 to 12%, respectively. Relative retention times of leucomycin A_4 and leucomycin A_1 to leucomycin A_5 are about 1.2 and about 1.5, respectively.

Operating conditions—

Detector: An ultraviolet absorption photometer (wavelength: 232 nm).

Column: A stainless steel column 4.0 mm in inside diameter and 15 cm in length, packed with octylsilanized silica gel for liquid chromatography (5 μm in particle diameter).

Column temperature: A constant temperature of about 40°C.

Mobile phase: To a volume of a solution of ammonium acetate (77 in 5000) add diluted phosphoric acid (1 in 150) to adjust to pH 5.5. To 370 mL of this solution add 580 mL of methanol and 50 mL of acetonitrile.

Flow rate: Adjust so that the retention time of leucomycin A_5 is about 8 minutes.

Time span of measurement: About 3 times as long as the retention time of leucomycin A_5.

System suitability—

System performance: Dissolve about 20 mg each of Leucomycin A_5 RS and Josamycin RS in 20 mL of diluted acetonitrile (1 in 2). When the procedure is run with 5 μL of this solution under the above operating conditions, leucomycin A_5 and josamycin are eluted in this order with the resolution between these peaks being not less than 5.

System repeatability: When the test is repeated 6 times with 5 μL of the sample solution under the above operating conditions, the relative standard deviation of the peak area of leucomycin A_5 is not more than 1.0%.

Water <2.48> Not more than 3.0% (0.1 g, volumetric titration, direct titration).

Assay Perform the test according to the Cylinder-plate method as directed under Microbial Assay for Antibiotics <4.02> according to the following conditions.

(i) Test organism—*Bacillus subtilis* ATCC 6633

(ii) Culture medium—Use the medium i in 1) under (1) Agar media for seed and base layer.

(iii) Standard solutions—Weigh accurately an amount of Leucomycin A_5 RS equivalent to about 30 mg (potency), dissolve in 10 mL of methanol, add water to make exactly 100 mL, and use this solution as the standard stock solution. Keep the standard stock solution at 5°C or below and use within 3 days. Take exactly a suitable amount of the standard stock solution before use, add phosphate buffer solution (pH 8.0) to make solutions so that each mL contains 30 μg (potency) and 7.5 μg (potency), and use these solutions as the high concentration standard solution and the low concentration standard solution, respectively.

(iv) Sample solutions—Weigh accurately an amount of Kitasamycin equivalent to about 30 mg (potency), dissolve in 10 mL of methanol, and add water to make exactly 100 mL. Take exactly a suitable amount of the solution, add phosphate buffer solution (pH 8.0) to make solutions so that each mL contains 30 μg (potency) and 7.5 μg (potency), and use these solutions as the high concentration sample solution and the low concentration sample solution, respectively.

Containers and storage Containers—Tight containers.

Kitasamycin Acetate

キタサマイシン酢酸エステル

Leucomycin A_1 Acetate: R =

Leucomycin A_3 Acetate: R =

Leucomycin A_4 Acetate: R =

Leucomycin A_5 Acetate: R =

Leucomycin A_6 Acetate: R =

Leucomycin A_7 Acetate: R =

Leucomycin A_1 Acetate
(3*R*,4*R*,5*S*,6*R*,8*R*,9*R*,10*E*,12*E*,15*R*)-3,9-Diacetoxy-5-[4-*O*-3-methylbutanoyl-2,6-dideoxy-3-*C*-methyl-α-L-*ribo*-hexopyranosyl-(1→4)-2-*O*-acetyl-3,6-dideoxy-3-dimethylamino-β-D-glucopyranosyloxy]-6-formylmethyl-4-methoxy-8-methylhexadeca-10,12-dien-15-olide

Leucomycin A_3 Acetate
(3*R*,4*R*,5*S*,6*R*,8*R*,9*R*,10*E*,12*E*,15*R*)-3,9-Diacetoxy-5-[4-*O*-3-methylbutanoyl-2,6-dideoxy-3-*C*-methyl-α-L-*ribo*-hexopyranosyl-(1→4)-2-*O*-acetyl-3,6-dideoxy-3-dimethylamino-β-D-glucopyranosyloxy]-6-formylmethyl-4-methoxy-8-methylhexadeca-10,12-dien-15-olide

Leucomycin A_4 Acetate
(3*R*,4*R*,5*S*,6*R*,8*R*,9*R*,10*E*,12*E*,15*R*)-3,9-Diacetoxy-5-[4-*O*-butanoyl-2,6-dideoxy-3-*C*-methyl-α-L-*ribo*-hexopyranosyl-(1→4)-2-*O*-acetyl-3,6-dideoxy-3-dimethylamino-β-D-glucopyranosyloxy]-6-formylmethyl-4-methoxy-8-methylhexadeca-10,12-dien-15-olide

Leucomycin A_5 Acetate
(3*R*,4*R*,5*S*,6*R*,8*R*,9*R*,10*E*,12*E*,15*R*)-3,9-Diacetoxy-5-[4-*O*-butanoyl-2,6-dideoxy-3-*C*-methyl-α-L-*ribo*-hexopyranosyl-(1→4)-2-*O*-acetyl-3,6-dideoxy-3-dimethylamino-β-D-glucopyranosyloxy]-6-formylmethyl-4-methoxy-8-methylhexadeca-10,12-dien-15-olide

Leucomycin A_6 Acetate
(3*R*,4*R*,5*S*,6*R*,8*R*,9*R*,10*E*,12*E*,15*R*)-3,9-Diacetoxy-5-[4-*O*-propanoyl-2,6-dideoxy-3-*C*-methyl-α-L-*ribo*-hexopyranosyl-(1→4)-2-*O*-acetyl-3,6-dideoxy-3-dimethylamino-β-D-glucopyranosyloxy]-6-formylmethyl-4-methoxy-8-methylhexadeca-10,12-dien-15-olide

Leucomycin A_7 Acetate
(3*R*,4*R*,5*S*,6*R*,8*R*,9*R*,10*E*,12*E*,15*R*)-3,9-Diacetoxy-5-[4-*O*-propanoyl-2,6-dideoxy-3-*C*-methyl-α-L-*ribo*-hexopyranosyl-(1→4)-2-*O*-acetyl-3,6-dideoxy-3-dimethylamino-β-D-glucopyranosyloxy]-6-formylmethyl-4-methoxy-8-methylhexadeca-10,12-dien-15-olide

[*178234-32-7*, Kitasamycin Acetate]

Kitasamycin Acetate is a derivative of kitasamycin.

It contains not less than 680 μg (potency) and not more than 790 μg (potency) per mg, calculated on the anhydrous basis. The potency of Kitasamycin Acetate is expressed as mass (potency) of kitasamycin corresponding to the mass of leucomycin A_5 ($C_{39}H_{65}NO_{14}$: 771.93). One mg (potency) of kitasamycin is equivalent to 0.530 mg of leucomycin A_5 ($C_{39}H_{65}NO_{14}$).

Description Kitasamycin Acetate occurs as a white to light yellow-white powder.

It is very soluble in methanol and in ethanol (95), and practically insoluble in water.

Identification **(1)** Determine the absorption spectrum of a solution of Kitasamycin Acetate in methanol (1 in 40,000) as directed under Ultraviolet-visible Spectrophotometry ⟨*2.24*⟩, and compare the spectrum with the Reference Spectrum: both spectra exhibit similar intensities of absorption at the same wavelengths.

(2) Determine the infrared absorption spectrum of Kitasamycin Acetate as directed in the potassium bromide disk method under Infrared Spectrophotometry ⟨*2.25*⟩, and compare the spectrum with the Reference Spectrum: both spectra exhibit similar intensities of absorption at the same wave numbers.

Water ⟨*2.48*⟩ Not more than 5.0% (0.1 g, volumetric titration, direct titration).

Assay Perform the test according to the Cylinder-plate method as directed under Microbial Assay for Antibiotics ⟨*4.02*⟩ according to the following conditions.

(i) Test organism—*Bacillus subtilis* ATCC 6633

(ii) Culture medium—Use the medium i in 1) under (1) Agar media for seed and base layer.

(iii) Standard solution—Weigh accurately an amount of Leucomycin A_5 RS equivalent to about 30 mg (potency), dissolve in 10 mL of methanol, add water to make exactly 100 mL, and use this solution as the standard stock solution. Keep the standard stock solution at 5°C or below and use within 3 days. Take exactly a suitable amount of the standard stock solution before use, add 0.1 mol/L phosphate buffer solution (pH 8.0) to make solutions so that each mL contains 30 μg (potency) and 7.5 μg (potency), and use these solutions as the high concentration standard solution and the low concentration standard solution, respectively.

(iv) Sample solution—Weigh accurately an amount of Kitasamycin Acetate equivalent to about 30 mg (potency), dissolve in 25 mL of methanol, add water to make exactly 50 mL, shake well, and allow to stand at 37 ± 2°C for 24 hours. Take exactly a suitable amount of the solution, add 0.1 mol/L phosphate buffer solution (pH 8.0) to make solutions so that each mL contains 30 μg (potency) and 7.5 μg (potency), and use these solutions as the high concentration sample solution and the low concentration sample solution, respectively.

Containers and storage Containers—Tight containers.

Kitasamycin Tartrate

キタサマイシン酒石酸塩

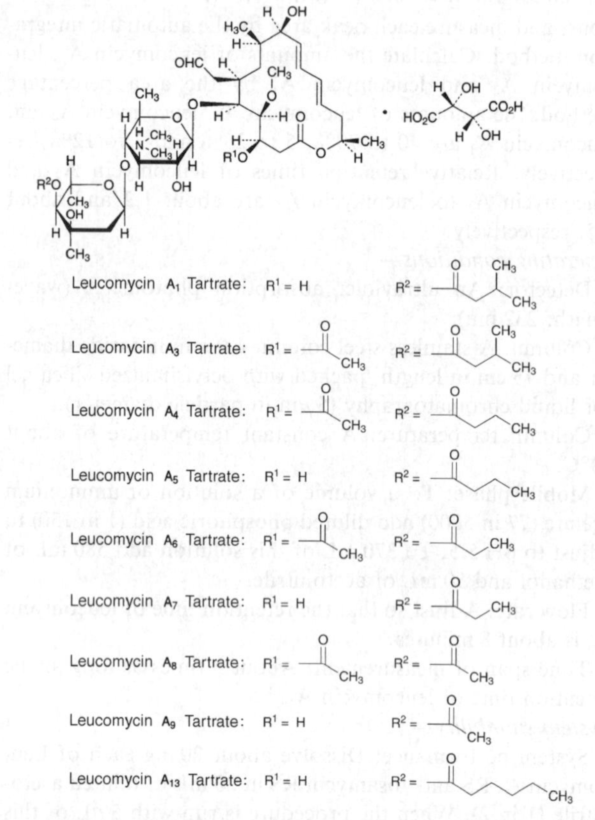

Leucomycin A_1 Tartrate: R^1 = H, R^2 = 3-methylbutanoyl
Leucomycin A_3 Tartrate: R^1 = acetyl, R^2 = 3-methylbutanoyl
Leucomycin A_4 Tartrate: R^1 = acetyl, R^2 = butanoyl
Leucomycin A_5 Tartrate: R^1 = H, R^2 = butanoyl
Leucomycin A_6 Tartrate: R^1 = acetyl, R^2 = propanoyl
Leucomycin A_7 Tartrate: R^1 = H, R^2 = propanoyl
Leucomycin A_8 Tartrate: R^1 = acetyl, R^2 = acetyl
Leucomycin A_9 Tartrate: R^1 = H, R^2 = acetyl
Leucomycin A_{13} Tartrate: R^1 = H, R^2 = hexanoyl

Leucomycin A_1 Tartrate
(3*R*,4*R*,5*S*,6*R*,8*R*,9*R*,10*E*,12*E*,15*R*)-5-[4-*O*-3-Methylbutanoyl-2,6-dideoxy-3-*C*-methyl-α-L-*ribo*-hexopyranosyl-(1→4)-3,6-dideoxy-3-dimethylamino-β-D-glucopyranosyloxy]-6-formylmethyl-3,9-dihydroxy-4-methoxy-8-methylhexadeca-10,12-dien-15-olide mono-(2*R*,3*R*)-tartrate

Leucomycin A_3 Tartrate
(3*R*,4*R*,5*S*,6*R*,8*R*,9*R*,10*E*,12*E*,15*R*)-3-Acetoxy-5-[4-*O*-3-methylbutanoyl-2,6-dideoxy-3-*C*-methyl-α-L-*ribo*-hexopyranosyl-(1→4)-3,6-dideoxy-3-dimethylamino-β-D-glucopyranosyloxy]-6-formylmethyl-9-hydroxy-4-methoxy-8-methylhexadeca-10,12-dien-15-olide mono-(2*R*,3*R*)-tartrate

Leucomycin A_4 Tartrate
(3*R*,4*R*,5*S*,6*R*,8*R*,9*R*,10*E*,12*E*,15*R*)-3-Acetoxy-5-[4-*O*-butanoyl-2,6-dideoxy-3-*C*-methyl-α-L-*ribo*-hexopyranosyl-(1→4)-3,6-dideoxy-3-dimethylamino-β-D-glucopyranosyloxy]-6-formylmethyl-9-hydroxy-4-methoxy-8-methylhexadeca-10,12-dien-15-olide mono-(2*R*,3*R*)-tartrate

Leucomycin A_5 Tartrate
(3*R*,4*R*,5*S*,6*R*,8*R*,9*R*,10*E*,12*E*,15*R*)-5-[4-*O*-Butanoyl-2,6-dideoxy-3-*C*-methyl-α-L-*ribo*-hexopyranosyl-(1→4)-3,6-dideoxy-3-dimethylamino-β-D-glucopyranosyloxy]-6-formylmethyl-3,9-dihydroxy-4-methoxy-8-methylhexadeca-10,12-dien-15-olide mono-(2*R*,3*R*)-tartrate

Leucomycin A_6 Tartrate
(3*R*,4*R*,5*S*,6*R*,8*R*,9*R*,10*E*,12*E*,15*R*)-3-Acetoxy-5-[4-*O*-propanoyl-2,6-dideoxy-3-*C*-methyl-α-L-*ribo*-hexopyranosyl-(1→4)-3,6-dideoxy-3-dimethylamino-β-D-glucopyranosyloxy]-6-formylmethyl-9-hydroxy-4-methoxy-8-methylhexadeca-10,12-dien-15-olide mono-(2*R*,3*R*)-tartrate

Leucomycin A_7 Tartrate
(3*R*,4*R*,5*S*,6*R*,8*R*,9*R*,10*E*,12*E*,15*R*)-5-[4-*O*-Propanoyl-2,6-dideoxy-3-*C*-methyl-α-L-*ribo*-hexopyranosyl-(1→4)-3,6-dideoxy-3-dimethylamino-β-D-glucopyranosyloxy]-6-formylmethyl-3,9-dihydroxy-4-methoxy-8-methylhexadeca-10,12-dien-15-olide mono-(2*R*,3*R*)-tartrate

Leucomycin A_8 Tartrate
(3*R*,4*R*,5*S*,6*R*,8*R*,9*R*,10*E*,12*E*,15*R*)-3-Acetoxy-5-[4-*O*-acetyl-2,6-dideoxy-3-*C*-methyl-α-L-*ribo*-hexopyranosyl-(1→4)-3,6-dideoxy-3-dimethylamino-β-D-glucopyranosyloxy]-6-formylmethyl-9-hydroxy-4-methoxy-8-methylhexadeca-10,12-dien-15-olide mono-(2*R*,3*R*)-tartrate

Leucomycin A_9 Tartrate
(3*R*,4*R*,5*S*,6*R*,8*R*,9*R*,10*E*,12*E*,15*R*)-5-[4-*O*-Acetyl-2,6-dideoxy-3-*C*-methyl-α-L-*ribo*-hexopyranosyl-(1→4)-3,6-dideoxy-3-dimethylamino-β-D-glucopyranosyloxy]-6-formylmethyl-3,9-dihydroxy-4-methoxy-8-methylhexadeca-10,12-dien-15-olide mono-(2*R*,3*R*)-tartrate

Leucomycin A_{13} Tartrate
(3*R*,4*R*,5*S*,6*R*,8*R*,9*R*,10*E*,12*E*,15*R*)-5-[4-*O*-Hexanoyl-2,6-dideoxy-3-*C*-methyl-α-L-*ribo*-hexopyranosyl-(1→4)-3,6-dideoxy-3-dimethylamino-β-D-glucopyranosyloxy]-6-formylmethyl-3,9-dihydroxy-4-methoxy-8-methylhexadeca-10,12-dien-15-olide mono-(2*R*,3*R*)-tartrate

[*37280-56-1*, Kitasamycin Tartrate]

Kitasamycin Tartrate is the tartrate of kitasamycin. It contains not less than 1300 μg (potency) and not more than 1500 μg (potency) per mg, calculated on the anhydrous basis. The potency of Kitasamycin Tartrate is expressed as mass (potency) of kitasamycin based on the amount of leucomycin A_5 ($C_{39}H_{65}NO_{14}$: 771.93). One mg (potency) of Kitasamycin Tartrate is equivalent to 0.530 mg of leucomycin A_5 ($C_{39}H_{65}NO_{14}$).

Description Kitasamycin Tartrate occurs as a white to light yellow-white powder.

It is very soluble in water, in methanol and in ethanol (99.5).

Identification (1) Determine the absorption spectrum of a solution of Kitasamycin Tartrate in methanol (1 in 40,000) as directed under Ultraviolet-visible Spectrophotometry *<2.24>*, and compare the spectrum with the Reference Spectrum: both spectra exhibit similar intensities of absorption at the same wavelengths.

(2) Determine the infrared absorption spectrum of Kitasamycin Tartrate as directed in the potassium bromide disk method under Infrared Spectrophotometry *<2.25>*, and compare the spectrum with the Reference Spectrum: both spectra exhibit similar intensities of absorption at the same wave numbers.

(3) Dissolve 1 g of Kitasamycin Tartrate in 20 mL of water, add 3 mL of sodium hydroxide TS, add 20 mL of *n*-butyl acetate, shake well, and discard the *n*-butyl acetate layer. To the aqueous layer add 20 mL of *n*-butyl acetate, and shake well. The aqueous layer so obtained responds to Qualitative Tests *<1.09>* (1) for tartrate.

pH *<2.54>* Dissolve 3.0 g of Kitasamycin Tartrate in 100 mL of water: the pH of the solution is between 3.0 and 5.0.

Content ratio of the active principle Dissolve 20 mg of Kitasamycin Tartrate in diluted acetonitrile (1 in 2) to make 20 mL, and use this solution as the sample solution. Perform the test with 5 μL of the sample solution as directed under Liquid Chromatography *<2.01>* according to the following conditions, determine the peak areas by the automatic integration method, and calculate the amounts of leucomycin A_5, leucomycin A_4 and leucomycin A_1 by the area percentage method: the amount of leucomycin A_5 is 40 – 70%, leucomycin A_4 is 5 – 25%, and leucomycin A_1 is 3 – 12%. The relative retention times of leucomycin A_4 and leucomycin A_1 to leucomycin A_5 are about 1.2 and about 1.5, respectively.

Operating conditions—

Detector: An ultraviolet absorption photometer (wavelength: 232 nm).

Column: A stainless steel column 4.0 mm in inside diameter and 15 cm in length, packed with octylsilanized silica gel for liquid chromatography (5 μm in particle diameter).

Column temperature: A constant temperature of about 40°C.

Mobile phase: To a suitable amount of a solution of ammonium acetate (77 in 5000) add diluted phosphoric acid (1 in 150) to adjust the pH to 5.5. To 370 mL of this solution add 580 mL of methanol and 50 mL of acetonitrile.

Flow rate: Adjust so that the retention time of leucomycin A_5 is about 8 minutes.

Time span of measurement: About 3 times as long as the retention time of leucomycin A_5.

System suitability—

System performance: Dissolve about 20 mg each of Leucomycin A_5 RS and Josamycin RS in 20 mL of diluted acetonitrile (1 in 2). When the procedure is run with 5 μL of this solution under the above operating conditions, leucomycin A_5 and josamycin are eluted in this order with the resolution between these peaks being not less than 5.

System repeatability: When the test is repeated 6 times with 5 μL of the sample solution under the above operating conditions, the relative standard deviation of the peak area of leucomycin A_5 is not more than 1.0%.

Purity (1) Clarity and color of solution—Dissolve 1.0 g of Kitasamycin Tartrate in 10 mL of water: the solution is clear and colorless or light yellow.

(2) Heavy metals *<1.07>*—Proceed with 1.0 g of Kitasamycin Tartrate according to Method 2, and perform the test. Prepare the control solution with 3.0 mL of Standard Lead Solution (not more than 30 ppm).

Water *<2.48>* Not more than 3.0% (0.1 g, volumetric titration, direct titration).

Assay Perform the test according to the Cylinder-plate method as directed under Microbial Assay for Antibiotics *<4.02>* according to the following conditions.

(i) Test organism—*Bacillus subtilis* ATCC 6633

(ii) Culture medium—Use the medium i in 1) under (1) Agar media for seed and base layer.

(iii) Standard solutions—Weigh accurately an amount of

Leucomycin A_5 RS, equivalent to about 30 mg (potency), dissolve in 10 mL of methanol, add water to make exactly 100 mL, and use this solution as the standard stock solution. Keep the standard stock solution at not exceeding 5°C, and use within 3 days. Take exactly a suitable amount of the standard stock solution before use, add phosphate buffer solution (pH 8.0) to make solutions so that each mL contains 30 μg (potency) and 7.5 μg (potency), and use these solutions as the high concentration standard solution and the low concentration standard solution, respectively.

(iv) Sample solutions—Weigh accurately an amount of Kitasamycin Tartrate, equivalent to about 30 mg (potency), and dissolve in water to make exactly 100 mL. Take exactly a suitable amount of this solution, add phosphate buffer solution (pH 8.0) to make solutions so that each mL contains 30 μg (potency) and 7.5 μg (potency), and use these solutions as the high concentration sample solution and the low concentration sample solution, respectively.

Containers and storage Containers—Tight containers.

Labetalol Hydrochloride

ラベタロール塩酸塩

and enantiomer

and enantiomer

$C_{19}H_{24}N_2O_3$.HCl: 364.87
2-Hydroxy-5-{(1*RS*)-1-hydroxy-2-[(1*RS*)-1-methyl-3-phenylpropylamino]ethyl}benzamide monohydrochloride
2-Hydroxy-5-{(1*RS*)-1-hydroxy-2-[(1*SR*)-1-methyl-3-phenylpropylamino]ethyl}benzamide monohydrochloride
[*32780-64-6*]

Labetalol Hydrochloride, when dried, contains not less than 98.5% and not more than 101.0% of labetalol hydrochloride ($C_{19}H_{24}N_2O_3$.HCl).

Description Labetalol Hydrochloride occurs as a white crystalline powder.

It is freely soluble in methanol, and sparingly soluble in water and in ethanol (99.5).

It dissolves in 0.05 mol/L sulfuric acid TS.

Melting point: about 181°C (with decomposition).

Identification (1) Determine the absorption spectrum of a solution of Labetalol Hydrochloride in 0.05 mol/L sulfuric acid TS (1 in 20,000) as directed under Ultraviolet-visible Spectrophotometry *<2.24>*, and compare the spectrum with the Reference Spectrum: both spectra exhibit similar intensities of absorption at the same wavelengths.

(2) Determine the infrared absorption spectrum of Labetalol Hydrochloride as directed in the potassium chloride disc method under Infrared Spectrophotometry *<2.25>*, and compare the spectrum with the Reference Spectrum: both spectra exhibit similar intensities of absorption at the same wave numbers.

(3) A solution of Labetalol Hydrochloride (1 in 50) responds to Qualitative Tests *<1.09>* for chloride.

pH *<2.54>* The pH of a solution prepared by dissolving 0.5 g of Labetalol Hydrochloride in 50 mL of water is between 4.0 and 5.0.

Purity (1) Heavy metals *<1.07>*—Proceed with 1.0 g of Labetalol Hydrochloride according to Method 2, and perform the test. Prepare the control solution with 2.0 mL of Standard Lead Solution (not more than 20 ppm).

(2) Related substances—Dissolve 0.8 g of Labetalol Hydrochloride in 10 mL of methanol, and use this solution as the sample solution. Pipet 1 mL of the sample solution, add methanol to make exactly 200 mL, and use this solution as the standard solution. Perform the test with these solutions as directed under Thin-layer Chromatography *<2.03>*. Spot 5 μL each of the sample solution and standard solution on a plate of silica gel for thin-layer chromatography. Develop the plate with a mixture of ethyl acetate, 2-propanol, water, and ammonia solution (28) (25:15:8:2) to a distance of about 10 cm, and air-dry the plate. Allow the plate to stand in iodine vapor for 30 minutes: the spots other than the principal spot obtained from the sample solution do not exceed 2 in number and are not more intense than the spot from the standard solution.

Loss on drying *<2.41>* Not more than 1.0% (1 g, 105°C, 3 hours).

Residue on ignition *<2.44>* Not more than 0.1% (1 g).

Isomer ratio Dissolve 5 mg of Labetalol Hydrochloride in 0.7 mL of a solution of *n*-butylboronic acid in dehydrated pyridine (3 in 250), allow to stand for 20 minutes, and use this solution as the sample solution. Perform the test with 2 μL of the sample solution as directed under Gas Chromatography *<2.02>* according to the following conditions. Determine the areas of two adjacent peaks, A_a and A_b, where A_a is the peak area of the shorter retention time and A_b is the peak area of the longer retention time, using the automatic integration method: the ratio $A_b/(A_a + A_b)$ is between 0.45 and 0.55.

Operating conditions—

Detector: A hydrogen flame-ionization detector.

Column: A fused silica column 0.53 mm in inside diameter and 25 m in length, coated inside with methyl silicone polymer for gas chromatography in 5 μm thickness.

Column temperature: A constant temperature of about 290°C.

Injection port temperature: A constant temperature of about 350°C.

Detector temperature: A constant temperature of about 350°C.

Carrier gas: Helium.

Flow rate: Adjust so that the retention time of the peak showing earlier elution of the two peaks of labetalol is about 9 minutes.

System suitability—

System performance: Proceed with 2 μL of the sample solution under the above conditions: the resolution between the two labetalol peaks is not less than 1.5.

System repeatability: Repeat the test 6 times under the above conditions with 2 μL of the sample solution: the relative standard deviation of the ratio of the peak area of labetalol with the shorter retention time to that of the longer retention time is not more than 2.0%.

Assay Weigh accurately about 0.3 g of Labetalol Hydrochloride, previously dried, dissolve in 100 mL of a mixture of acetic anhydride and acetic acid (100) (7:3), and titrate <*2.50*> with 0.1 mol/L perchloric acid VS (potentiometric titration). Perform a blank determination in the same manner, and make any necessary correction.

Each mL of 0.1 mol/L perchloric acid VS
= 36.49 mg of $C_{19}H_{24}N_2O_3.HCl$

Containers and storage Containers—Tight containers.

Labetalol Hydrochloride Tablets

ラベタロール塩酸塩錠

Labetalol Hydrochloride Tablets contain not less than 93.0% and not more than 107.0% of the labeled amount of labetalol hydrochloride ($C_{19}H_{24}N_2O_3.HCl$: 364.87).

Method of preparation Prepare as directed under Tablets, with Labetalol Hydrochloride.

Identification **(1)** To a quantity of powdered Labetalol Hydrochloride Tablets equivalent to 5 mg of Labetalol Hydrochloride, add 100 mL of 0.05 mol/L sulfuric acid TS, shake, and filter. Determine the absorption spectrum of the filtrate as directed under Ultraviolet-visible Spectrophotometry <*2.24*>: it exhibits a maximum between 300 nm and 304 nm.

(2) To a quantity of powdered Labetalol Hydrochloride Tablets equivalent to 0.25 g of Labetalol Hydrochloride, add 25 mL of methanol, shake vigorously for 30 minutes, filter, and use the filtrate as the sample solution. Separately, dissolve 10 mg of labetalol hydrochloride in 1 mL of methanol, and use this solution as the standard solution. Perform the test using these solutions as directed under Thin-layer Chromatography <*2.03*>. Spot 5 μL each of the sample solution and standard solution on a plate of silica gel with fluorescent indicator for thin-layer chromatography. Develop the plate with a mixture of ethyl acetate, 2-propanol, water, and ammonia solution (28) (25:15:8:2) to a distance of about 10 cm, and air-dry the plate. Examine under ultraviolet light (main wavelength: 254 nm): the principal spot obtained from the sample solution and the spot from the standard solution show the same *R*f value.

Uniformity of dosage units <*6.02*> Perform the Mass variation test, or the Content uniformity test according to the following method: it meets the requirement.

To 1 tablet of Labetalol Hydrochloride Tablets add 5 mL of 0.5 mol/L sulfuric acid TS and 30 mL of water, shake vigorously for 30 minutes, add water to make exactly 50 mL, and filter. Discard the first 5 mL of the filtrate, pipet 4 mL of the subsequent filtrate, add 0.05 mol/L sulfuric acid TS to make exactly *V* mL so that each mL contains about 40 μg of labetalol hydrochloride ($C_{19}H_{24}N_2O_3.HCl$), and use this solution as the sample solution. Separately, weigh accurately about 20 mg of labetalol hydrochloride for assay, previously dried at 105°C for 3 hours, and dissolve in 0.05 mol/L sulfuric acid TS to make exactly 50 mL. Pipet 5 mL of this solution, add 0.05 mol/L sulfuric acid TS to make exactly 50 mL, and use this solution as the standard solution. Determine the absorbances, A_T and A_S, of the sample solution and standard solution at 302 nm as directed under Ultraviolet-visible Spectrophotometry <*2.24*>.

Amount (mg) of labetalol hydrochloride ($C_{19}H_{24}N_2O_3.HCl$)
$= M_S \times A_T/A_S \times V/40$

M_S: Amount (mg) of labetalol hydrochloride for assay taken

Dissolution <*6.10*> When the test is performed at 50 revolutions per minute according to the Paddle method, using 900 mL of water as the dissolution medium, the dissolution rate in 30 minutes of Labetalol Hydrochloride Tablets is not less than 75%.

Start the test with 1 tablet of Labetalol Hydrochloride Tablets, withdraw not less than 20 mL of the medium at specified minute after starting the test, and filter through a membrane filter with a pore size not exceeding 0.8 μm. Discard not less than 10 mL of the first filtrate, pipet *V* mL of the subsequent filtrate, and add water to make exactly *V′* mL so that each mL contains about 50 μg of labetalol hydrochloride ($C_{19}H_{24}N_2O_3.HCl$), and use this solution as the sample solution. Separately, weigh accurately about 50 mg of labetalol hydrochloride for assay, previously dried at 105°C for 3 hours, and dissolve in water to make exactly 100 mL. Pipet 10 mL of this solution, add water to make exactly 100 mL, and use this solution as the standard solution. Perform the test with the sample solution and standard solution as directed under Ultraviolet-visible Spectrophotometry <*2.24*>, and determine the absorbances, A_T and A_S, at 302 nm.

Dissolution rate (%) with respect to the labeled amount of labetalol hydrochloride ($C_{19}H_{24}N_2O_3.HCl$)
$= M_S \times A_T/A_S \times V'/V \times 1/C \times 90$

M_S: Amount (mg) of labetalol hydrochloride for assay taken
C: Labeled amount (mg) of labetalol hydrochloride ($C_{19}H_{24}N_2O_3.HCl$) in 1 tablet

Assay Weigh accurately not less than 20 Labetalol Hydrochloride Tablets, and powder. Weigh accurately a portion of the powder, equivalent to about 1 g of labetalol hydrochloride ($C_{19}H_{24}N_2O_3.HCl$), add 100 mL of 0.5 mol/L sulfuric acid TS and 600 mL of water, shake vigorously for 30 minutes, add water to make exactly 1000 mL, and filter. Discard the first 5 mL of the filtrate, pipet 5 mL of the subsequent filtrate, and add 0.05 mol/L sulfuric acid TS to make exactly 25 mL. Pipet 5 mL of this solution, add 0.05 mol/L sulfuric acid TS to make exactly 25 mL, and use this solution as the sample solution. Separately, weigh accurately about 40 mg of labetalol hydrochloride for assay, previously dried at 105°C for 3 hours, and dissolve in 0.05 mol/L sulfuric acid TS to make exactly 100 mL. Pipet 5 mL of this solution, add 0.05 mol/L sulfuric acid TS to make exactly 50 mL, and use this solution as the standard solution. Perform the test with the sample solution and standard solution as directed under Ultraviolet-visible Spectrophotometry <*2.24*>, and determine the absorbances, A_T and A_S, at 302 nm.

Amount (mg) of labetalol hydrochloride ($C_{19}H_{24}N_2O_3.HCl$)
$= M_S \times A_T/A_S \times 25$

M_S: Amount (mg) of labetalol hydrochloride for assay taken

Containers and storage Containers—Tight containers.

Lactic Acid

乳酸

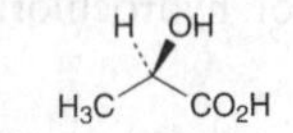

and enantiomer

$C_3H_6O_3$: 90.08
(2*RS*)-2-Hydroxypropanoic acid
[*50-21-5*]

Lactic Acid is a mixture of lactic acid and lactic anhydride.

It contains not less than 85.0% and not more than 92.0% of lactic acid ($C_3H_6O_3$).

Description Lactic Acid occurs as a clear, colorless or light yellow, viscous liquid. It is odorless or has a faint, unpleasant odor.

It is miscible with water, with ethanol (95) and with diethyl ether.

It is hygroscopic.

Specific gravity d_{20}^{20}: about 1.20

Identification A solution of Lactic Acid (1 in 50) changes blue litmus paper to red and responds to Qualitative Tests <*1.09*> for lactate.

Purity **(1)** Chloride <*1.03*>—Perform the test with 1.0 g of Lactic Acid. Prepare the control solution with 1.0 mL of 0.01 mol/L hydrochloric acid VS (not more than 0.036%).

(2) Sulfate <*1.14*>—Perform the test with 2.0 g of Lactic Acid. Prepare the control solution with 0.40 mL of 0.005 mol/L sulfuric acid VS (not more than 0.010%).

(3) Heavy metals <*1.07*>—To 2.0 g of Lactic Acid add 10 mL of water and 1 drop of phenolphthalein TS, and add ammonia TS dropwise until a pale red color appears. Add 2 mL of dilute acetic acid and water to make 50 mL, and perform the test using this solution as the test solution. Prepare the control solution from 2.0 mL of Standard Lead Solution and 2 mL of dilute acetic acid, and dilute with water to 50 mL (not more than 10 ppm).

(4) Iron <*1.10*>—Prepare the test solution with 4.0 g of Lactic Acid according to Method 1, and perform the test according to Method A. Prepare the control solution with 2.0 mL of Standard Iron Solution (not more than 5 ppm).

(5) Sugars—To 1.0 g of Lactic Acid add 10 mL of water, and neutralize with sodium hydroxide TS. Boil the mixture with 10 mL of Fehling's TS for 5 minutes: no red precipitate is produced.

(6) Citric, oxalic, phosphoric and L-tartaric acid—To 1.0 g of Lactic Acid add 1.0 mL of water, followed by 40 mL of calcium hydroxide TS. Boil the mixture for 2 minutes: no change occurs.

(7) Glycerin or mannitol—Shake 10 mL of Lactic Acid with 12 mL of diethyl ether: no turbidity is produced.

(8) Volatile fatty acids—Warm Lactic Acid: it does not produce any acetic acid-like or butyric acid-like odor.

(9) Cyanide—Transfer 1.0 g of Lactic Acid to a Nessler tube, add 10 mL of water and 1 drop of phenolphthalein TS, add dropwise a solution of sodium hydroxide (1 in 10) by shaking until a pale red color develops, add 1.5 mL of a solution of sodium hydroxide (1 in 10) and water to make 20 mL, and heat in a water bath for 10 minutes. Cool, add dropwise dilute acetic acid until a red color of the solution disappears, add 1 drop of dilute acetic acid, add 10 mL of phosphate buffer solution (pH 6.8), and 0.25 mL of sodium toluensulfonchloramide TS, stopper immediately, mix gently, and allow to stand for 5 minutes. To the solution add 15 mL of pyridine-pyrazolone TS and water to make 50 mL, and allow to stand at 25°C for 30 minutes: the solution has no more color than the following control solution.

Control solution: Pipet 1.0 mL of Standard Cyanide Solution, and add water to make exactly 20 mL. Transfer 1.0 mL of this solution to a Nessler tube, add 10 mL of water and 1 drop of phenolphthalein TS, and then proceed as described above.

(10) Readily carbonizable substances—Superimpose slowly 5 mL of Lactic Acid, previously kept at 15°C, upon 5 mL of sulfuric acid for readily carbonizable substances, previously kept at 15°C, and allow to stand at 15°C for 15 minutes: no dark color develops at the zone of contact.

Residue on ignition <*2.44*> Not more than 0.1% (1 g).

Assay Weigh accurately about 3 g of Lactic Acid, transfer in a conical flask, add accurately measured 40 mL of 1 mol/L sodium hydroxide VS, invert a watch glass over the flask, and heat on a water bath for 10 minutes. Titrate <*2.50*> the excess sodium hydroxide with 0.5 mol/L sulfuric acid VS immediately (indicator: 2 drops of phenolphthalein TS). Perform a blank determination in the same manner.

Each mL of 1 mol/L sodium hydroxide VS
= 90.08 mg of $C_3H_6O_3$

Containers and storage Containers—Tight containers.

L-Lactic Acid

L-乳酸

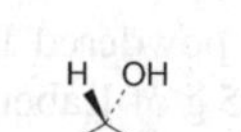

$C_3H_6O_3$: 90.08
(2*S*)-2-Hydroxypropanoic acid
[*79-33-4*]

L-Lactic Acid is a mixture of L-lactic acid and L-lactic anhydride.

It contains not less than 85.0% and not more than 92.0% of L-lactic acid ($C_3H_6O_3$).

Description L-Lactic Acid occurs as a clear, colorless or light yellow, viscous liquid. It is odorless or has a faint, no unpleasant odor.

It is miscible with water, with ethanol (99.5) and with diethyl ether.

It is hygroscopic.

Specific gravity d_{20}^{20}: about 1.20

Identification A solution of L-Lactic Acid (1 in 50) changes the color of blue litmus paper to red, and responds to Qualitative Tests <*1.09*> for lactate.

Optical rotation <*2.49*> $[\alpha]_D^{20}$: −46 − −52° Weigh accurately an amount of L-Lactic Acid, equivalent to about 2 g of L-lactic acid ($C_3H_6O_3$), add exactly 25 mL of 1 mol/L sodium hydroxide VS, cover with a watch glass, and heat on a water bath for 15 minutes. Cool, and adjust to pH 7.0 with 1 mol/L hydrochloric acid VS. Dissolve 5.0 g of hexaammonium heptamolybdate tetrahydrate in this solution, add water to make exactly 50 mL, and determine the optical rotation using a 100-mm cell.

Purity **(1)** Chloride <*1.03*>—Perform the test with 1.0 g of L-Lactic Acid. Prepare the control solution with 1.0 mL of

0.01 mol/L hydrochloric acid VS (not more than 0.036%).

(2) Sulfate <*1.14*>—Perform the test with 2.0 g of L-Lactic Acid. Prepare the control solution with 0.40 mL of 0.005 mol/L sulfuric acid VS (not more than 0.010%).

(3) Heavy metals <*1.07*>—To 2.0 g of L-Lactic Acid add 10 mL of water and 1 drop of phenolphthalein TS, and add ammonia TS dropwise until a pale red color appears. Add 2 mL of dilute acetic acid and water to make 50 mL, and perform the test using this solution as the test solution. Prepare the control solution from 2.0 mL of Standard Lead Solution and 2 mL of dilute acetic acid, and dilute with water to 50 mL (not more than 10 ppm).

(4) Iron <*1.10*>—Prepare the test solution with 4.0 g of L-Lactic Acid according to Method 1, and perform the test according to Method A. Prepare the control solution with 2.0 mL of Standard Iron Solution (not more than 5 ppm).

(5) Sugars—To 1.0 g of L-Lactic Acid add 10 mL of water, and neutralize with sodium hydroxide TS. Boil the mixture with 10 mL of Fehling's TS for 5 minutes: no red precipitate is produced.

(6) Citric, oxalic, phosphoric and L-tartaric acid—To 1.0 g of L-Lactic Acid add 1.0 mL of water, followed by 40 mL of calcium hydroxide TS. Boil the mixture for 2 minutes: no change occurs.

(7) Glycerin or mannitol—Shake 10 mL of L-Lactic Acid with 12 mL of diethyl ether: no turbidity is produced.

(8) Volatile fatty acids—Warm L-Lactic Acid: it does not produce any acetic acid-like or butyric acid-like odor.

(9) Cyanide—Transfer 1.0 g of L-Lactic Acid to a Nessler tube, add 10 mL of water and 1 drop of phenolphthalein TS, add dropwise a solution of sodium hydroxide (1 in 10) while shaking until a pale red color develops, then add 1.5 mL of a solution of sodium hydroxide (1 in 10) and water to make 20 mL, and heat in a water bath for 10 minutes. After cooling, add dropwise dilute acetic acid until a red color of the solution disappears, add 1 drop of dilute acetic acid, 10 mL of phosphate buffer solution (pH 6.8) and 0.25 mL of sodium toluenesulfonchloramide TS, stopper immediately, mix gently, and allow to stand for 5 minutes. To the solution add 15 mL of pyridine-pyrazolone TS and water to make 50 mL, and allow to stand at 25°C for 30 minutes: the solution has no more color than the following control solution.

Control solution: Pipet 1.0 mL of Standard Cyanide Solution, and add water to make 20 mL. Transfer 1.0 mL of this solution to a Nessler tube, add 10 mL of water and 1 drop of phenolphthalein TS, and then proceed as described above.

(10) Readily carbonizable substances—Superimpose slowly 5 mL of L-Lactic Acid, previously kept at 15°C, upon 5 mL of sulfuric acid for readily carbonizable substances, previously kept at 15°C, and allow to stand at 15°C for 15 minutes: no dark color develops at the zone of contact.

Residue on ignition <*2.44*> Not more than 0.1% (1 g).

Assay Weigh accurately about 3 g of L-Lactic Acid, transfer in a conical flask, add accurately measured 40 mL of 1 mol/L sodium hydroxide VS, invert a watch glass over the flask, and heat on a water bath for 10 minutes. Titrate <*2.50*> the excess sodium hydroxide with 0.5 mol/L sulfuric acid VS immediately (indicator: 2 drops of phenolphthalein TS). Perform a blank determination in the same manner.

Each mL of 1 mol/L sodium hydroxide VS
= 90.08 mg of $C_3H_6O_3$

Containers and storage Containers—Tight containers.

Anhydrous Lactose

無水乳糖

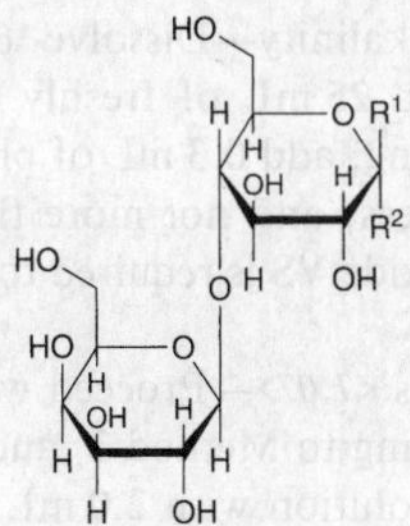

$C_{12}H_{22}O_{11}$: 342.30
β-D-Galactopyranosyl-(1→4)-β-D-glucopyranose (β-lactose)
β-D-Galactopyranosyl-(1→4)-α-D-glucopyranose (α-lactose)
[*63-42-3*, Anhydrous Lactose]

This monograph is harmonized with the European Pharmacopoeia and the U.S. Pharmacopeia.

The corresponding part of the attributes/provisions which are agreed as non-harmonized within the scope of the harmonization is marked with symbols (◆ ◆), and the corresponding parts which are agreed as the JP local requirement other than the scope of the harmonization are marked with symbols (◇ ◇).

Information on the harmonization with the European Pharmacopoeia and the U.S. Pharmacopeia is available on the website of the Pharmaceuticals and Medical Devices Agency.

Anhydrous Lactose is β-lactose or a mixture of β-lactose and α-lactose.

◆The relative quantities of α-lactose and β-lactose in Anhydrous Lactose is labeled as the isomer ratio.◆

◆**Description** Anhydrous Lactose occurs as white, crystals or powder.

It is freely soluble in water, and practically insoluble in ethanol (99.5).◆

Identification Determine the infrared absorption spectrum of Anhydrous Lactose, previously dried, as directed in the potassium bromide disk method under Infrared Spectrophotometry <*2.25*>, and compare the spectrum with the Reference Spectrum or the spectrum of Anhydrous Lactose for Identification RS: both spectra exhibit similar intensities of absorption at the same wave numbers.

Optical rotation <*2.49*> $[\alpha]_D^{20}$: +54.4 – +55.9° Weigh accurately about 10 g of Anhydrous Lactose, calculated on the anhydrous basis, dissolve in 80 mL of water warmed to 50°C, and add 0.2 mL of ammonia TS after cooling. After standing for 30 minutes, add water to make exactly 100 mL, and determine the optical rotation of this solution in a 100-mm cell.

Purity (1) Clarity and color of solution—Dissolve 1.0 g of Anhydrous Lactose in 10 mL of boiling water, and allow to cool: the solution is clear, and colorless or nearly colorless and has no more color than the following control solution. Determine the absorbance at 400 nm of this solution as directed under Ultraviolet-visible Spectrophotometry <*2.24*>, using water as the control solution: not more than 0.04.

Control solution: To a mixture of 2.5 mL of Cobalt (II) Chloride CS, 6.0 mL of Iron (III) Chloride CS and 1.0 mL of Copper (II) Sulfate CS, add diluted dilute hydrochloric acid (1 in 10) to make 1000 mL.

(2) Acidity or alkalinity—Dissolve 6 g of Anhydrous Lactose by heating in 25 mL of freshly boiled and cooled water, and after cooling, add 0.3 mL of phenolphthalein TS: the solution is colorless, and not more than 0.4 mL of 0.1 mol/L sodium hydroxide VS is required to produce a pink or red color.

◇**(3)** Heavy metals 〈*1.07*〉—Proceed with 4.0 g of Anhydrous Lactose according to Method 2, and perform the test. Prepare the control solution with 2.0 mL of Standard Lead Solution (not more than 5 ppm).◇

(4) Proteins and light absorbing substances—Dissolve 1.0 g of Anhydrous Lactose in water to make 100 mL, and use this solution as the sample solution. Determine the absorbances of the sample solution as directed under Ultraviolet-visible Spectrophotometry 〈*2.24*〉, using water as the control solution: not more than 0.25 at between 210 nm and 220 nm, and not more than 0.07 at between 270 nm and 300 nm.

Loss on drying 〈*2.41*〉 Not more than 0.5% (1 g, 80°C, 2 hours).

Water 〈*2.48*〉 Not more than 1.0% (1 g, volumetric titration, direct titration. Use a mixture of methanol for water determination and formamide for water determination (2:1) instead of methanol for water determination).

Residue on ignition 〈*2.44*〉 Not more than 0.1% (1 g).

Microbial limit 〈*4.05*〉 The acceptance criteria of TAMC and TYMC are 10^2 CFU/g and 5×10^1 CFU/g, respectively, and ◇*Salmonella* and◇ *Escherichia coli* are not observed.

Isomer ratio Place 10 mg of Anhydrous Lactose in a screw capped reaction vial for gas chromatography, add 4 mL of a mixture of pyridine, trimethylsilylimidazole and dimethylsulfoxide (117:44:39), stopper, and sonicate at room temperature for 20 minutes. After cooling, transfer 400 μL of this solution into a vial for injection, add 1 mL of pyridine, stopper tightly, mix, and use this fluid as the sample solution. Perform the test with 0.5 μL of the sample solution as directed under Gas Chromatography 〈*2.02*〉 according to the following conditions. Determine the peak areas of α-lactose and β-lactose, A_a and A_b, and calculate the contents (%) of α-lactose and β-lactose in Anhydrous Lactose by the following equations.

$$\text{Content (\%) of } \alpha\text{-lactose} = A_a/(A_a + A_b) \times 100$$

$$\text{Content (\%) of } \beta\text{-lactose} = A_b/(A_a + A_b) \times 100$$

Operating conditions—

Detector: A hydrogen flame-ionization detector.

Column: A fused silica column 0.25 mm in inside diameter and 15 m in length, coated with 5% diphenyl-95% dimethylpolysiloxane in 0.25 μm thickness. Use a middle polar inertness fused silica column 0.53 mm in inside diameter and 2 m in length as a guard column.

Column temperature: Maintain the temperature at 80°C for 1 minute after injection, raise to 150°C at a rate of 35°C per minute, then raise to 300°C at a rate of 12°C per minute, and maintain at 300°C for 2 minutes.

Injection port temperature: A constant temperature of about 275°C, or use cold-on column injection.

Detector temperature: A constant temperature of about 325°C.

Carrier gas: Helium.

Flow rate: 2.8 mL per minute (Retention time of β-lactose is about 12 minutes).

Splitless.

System suitability—

System performance: Prepare a solution with 10 mg of a mixture of α-lactose and β-lactose (1:1) in the same manner as for preparing the sample solution, and proceed with 0.5 μL of this solution under the above operating conditions, and determine the retention times of the peaks of α-lactose and β-lactose: the relative retention time of α-lactose to β-lactose is about 0.9 with the resolution between these peaks being not less than 3.0.

◇System repeatability: When the test is repeated 6 times with 0.5 μL of the solution used in the system performance under the above operating conditions, the relative standard deviation of the peak area of β-lactose is not more than 5.0%.◇

◆**Containers and storage** Containers—Well-closed containers.◆

Lactose Hydrate

乳糖水和物

$C_{12}H_{22}O_{11}.H_2O$: 360.31

β-D-Galactopyranosyl-(1→4)-α-D-glucopyranose monohydrate

[*64044-51-5*, Mixture of α- and β-lactose monohydrate]

This monograph is harmonized with the European Pharmacopoeia and the U.S. Pharmacopeia.

The corresponding part of the attributes/provisions which are agreed as non-harmonized within the scope of the harmonization is marked with symbols (◆ ◆), and the corresponding parts which are agreed as the JP local requirement other than the scope of the harmonization are marked with symbols (◇ ◇).

Information on the harmonization with the European Pharmacopoeia and the U.S. Pharmacopeia is available on the website of the Pharmaceuticals and Medical Devices Agency.

Lactose Hydrate is the monohydrate of β-D-galactopyranosyl-(1→4)-α-D-glucopyranose.

◇It is a disaccharide obtained from milk, consist of one unit of glucose and one unit of galactose.◇

◆The label states the effect where it is the granulated powder.◆

◆**Description** Lactose Hydrate occurs as white, crystals, powder or granulated powder.

It is freely soluble in water, and practically insoluble in ethanol (99.5).◆

Identification Determine the infrared absorption spectrum of Lactose Hydrate, previously dried, as directed in the potassium bromide disk method under Infrared Spectrophotometry <*2.25*>, and compare the spectrum with the Reference Spectrum or the spectrum of Lactose for Identification RS: both spectra exhibit similar intensities of absorption at the same wave numbers.

Optical rotation <*2.49*> $[\alpha]_D^{20}$: +54.4 – +55.9°. Weigh accurately about 10 g of Lactose Hydrate, calculated on the anhydrous basis, dissolve in 80 mL of water warmed to 50°C, and add 0.2 mL of ammonia TS after cooling. After standing for 30 minutes, add water to make exactly 100 mL, and determine the optical rotation of this solution in a 100-mm cell.

Purity **(1)** Clarity and color of solution—Dissolve 1.0 g of Lactose Hydrate in 10 mL of hot water, allow to cool, and determine the turbidity of this solution as directed under Turbidity Measurement <*2.61*>: it is clear, and has no more color than the following control solution. Determine the absorbance at 400 nm of this solution as directed under Ultraviolet-visible Spectrophotometry <*2.24*>, using water as the control solution: not more than 0.04.

Control solution: To 2.5 mL of Cobalt (II) Chloride CS, 6.0 mL of Iron (III) Chloride CS and 1.0 mL of Copper (II) Sulfate CS add diluted dilute hydrochloric acid (1 in 10) to make 1000 mL.

(2) Acidity or alkalinity—Dissolve 6 g of Lactose Hydrate by heating in 25 mL of freshly boiled and cooled water, and after cooling, add 0.3 mL of phenolphthalein TS: the solution is colorless, and not more than 0.4 mL of 0.1 mol/L sodium hydroxide VS is required to produce a pale red color or red color.

◇**(3)** Heavy metals <*1.07*>—Dissolve 4.0 g of Lactose Hydrate in 20 mL of warm water, add 1 mL of 0.1 mol/L hydrochloric acid TS and water to make 50 mL. Proceed with this solution according to Method 1, and perform the test. Prepare the control solution with 2.0 mL of Standard Lead Solution and 1 mL of 0.1 mol/L hydrochloric acid TS (not more than 5 ppm).◇

(4) Proteins and light absorbing substances—Dissolve 1.0 g of Lactose Hydrate in water to make 100 mL, and use this solution as the sample solution. Determine the absorbances of the sample solution as directed under Ultraviolet-visible Spectrophotometry <*2.24*>, using water as the control solution: not more than 0.25 at between 210 nm and 220 nm, and not more than 0.07 at between 270 nm and 300 nm.

Loss on drying <*2.41*> Not more than 0.5%. For the granulated powder, not more than 1.0% (1 g, 80°C, 2 hours).

Water <*2.48*> 4.5 – 5.5%. ◇For the granulated powder, 4.0 – 5.5%◇ (1 g, volumetric titration, direct titration. Use a mixture of methanol for water determination and formamide for water determination (2:1) instead of methanol for water determination).

Residue on ignition <*2.44*> Not more than 0.1% (1 g).

Microbial limit <*4.05*> The acceptance criteria of TAMC and TYMC are 10^2 CFU/g and 5×10^1 CFU/g, respectively. ◇*Salmonella* and◇ *Escherichia coli* are not observed.

◆**Containers and storage** Containers—Well-closed containers.◆

Lactulose

ラクツロース

$C_{12}H_{22}O_{11}$: 342.30

β-D-Galactopyranosyl-(1→4)-D-fructose

[*4618-18-2*]

Lactulose is a solution of lactulose prepared by isomerizing lactose under the existing of alkaline and purified by ion-exchange resin.

It contains not less than 50.0% and not more than 56.0% of lactulose ($C_{12}H_{22}O_{11}$).

Description Lactulose occurs as a clear, colorless or light yellow, viscous liquid. It is odorless, and has a sweet taste.

It is miscible with water and with formamide.

Identification **(1)** To 0.7 g of Lactulose add 10 mL of water, 10 mL of a solution of hexaammonium heptamolybdate tetrahydrate (1 in 25) and 0.2 mL of acetic acid (100), and heat in a water bath for 5 to 10 minutes: a blue color develops.

(2) Mix 0.3 g of Lactulose and 30 mL of water, add 16 mL of 0.5 mol/L iodine TS, then immediately add 2.5 mL of 8 mol/L sodium hydroxide TS, allow to stand for 7 minutes, and add 2.5 mL of diluted sulfuric acid (3 in 20). To this solution add a saturated solution of sodium sulfite heptahydrate until the solution turns light yellow, then add 3 drops of methyl orange TS, neutralize with a solution of sodium hydroxide (4 in 25), and add water to make 100 mL. To 10 mL of this solution add 5 mL of Fehling's TS, and boil for 5 minutes: a red precipitate is produced.

pH <*2.54*> To 2.0 g of Lactulose add 15 mL of water: the pH of the solution is between 3.5 and 5.5.

Specific gravity <*2.56*> d_{20}^{20}: 1.320 – 1.360

Purity **(1)** Heavy metals <*1.07*>—Proceed with 5.0 g of Lactulose according to Method 4, and perform the test. Prepare the control solution with 2.5 mL of Standard Lead Solution (not more than 5 ppm).

(2) Arsenic <*1.11*>—Prepare the test solution with 1.0 g of Lactulose according to Method 1, and perform the test (not more than 2 ppm).

(3) Galactose and lactose—Determine the heights of the peaks corresponding to galactose and lactose respectively, on the chromatogram obtained in Assay from the sample solution and the standard solution, and calculate the ratios of the peak heights of galactose and lactose to that of the internal standard from the sample solution, Q_{Ta} and Q_{Tb}, and then from the standard solution, Q_{Sa} and Q_{Sb}: it contains galactose of not more than 11%, and lactose of not more than 6%.

$$\text{Amount (mg) of galactose } (C_6H_{12}O_6) = M_S \times Q_{Ta}/Q_{Sa}$$

M_S: Amount (mg) of galactose taken

Amount (mg) of lactose ($C_{12}H_{22}O_{11}.H_2O$)
$= M_S \times Q_{Tb}/Q_{Sb}$

M_S: Amount (mg) of lactose hydrate taken

Loss on drying <*2.41*> Not more than 35% (0.5 g, in vacuum, 80°C, 5 hours).

Residue on ignition <*2.44*> Not more than 0.1% (1 g).

Assay Weigh accurately about 1 g of Lactulose, add exactly 10 mL of the internal standard solution and water to make 50 mL, and use this solution as the sample solution. Separately, weigh accurately about 0.5 g of Lactulose RS, about 80 mg of D-galactose and about 40 mg of lactose monohydrate, add exactly 10 mL of the internal standard solution and water to make 50 mL, and use this solution as the standard solution. Perform the test with 20 μL each of the sample solution and standard solution as directed under Liquid Chromatography <*2.01*> according to the following conditions, and calculate the ratios, Q_T and Q_S, of the peak height of lactulose to that of the internal standard.

Amount (mg) of lactulose ($C_{12}H_{22}O_{11}$)
$= M_S \times Q_T/Q_S$

M_S: Amount (mg) of Lactulose RS taken

Internal standard solution—A solution of D-mannitol (1 in 20).

Operating conditions—

Detector: A differential refractometer.

Column: A stainless steel column 8 mm in inside diameter and 50 cm in length, packed with gel type strongly acidic ion-exchange resin for liquid chromatography (degree of crosslinkage: 6%) (11 μm in particle diameter).

Column temperature: A constant temperature of about 75°C.

Mobile phase: Water.

Flow rate: Adjust so that the retention time of lactulose is about 18 minutes.

System suitability—

System performance: When the procedure is run with 10 μL of the standard solution under the above operating conditions, lactulose and the internal standard are eluted in this order with the resolution between these peaks being not less than 8.

System repeatability: When the test is repeated 6 times with 20 μL of the standard solution under the above operating conditions, the relative standard deviation of the ratios of the peak heights of lactulose, galactose and lactose to the height of the internal standard are not more than 2.0%, respectively.

Containers and storage Containers—Tight containers.

Lafutidine

ラフチジン

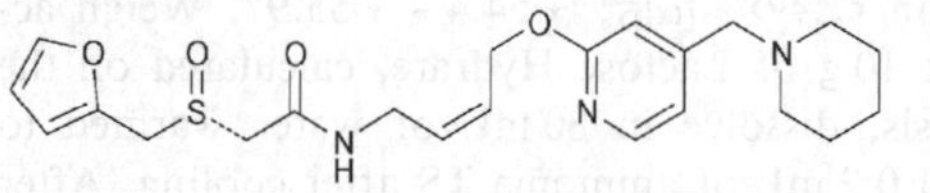

and enantiomer

$C_{22}H_{29}N_3O_4S$: 431.55
2-[(*RS*)-Furan-2-ylmethylsulfinyl]-*N*-{4-[4-(piperidin-1-ylmethyl)pyridin-2-yl]oxy-(2*Z*)-but-2-en-1-yl}acetamide
[*206449-93-6*]

Lafutidine, when dried, contains not less than 99.0% and not more than 101.0% of lafutidine ($C_{22}H_{29}N_3O_4S$).

Description Lafutidine occurs as a white to pale yellow-white crystalline powder.

It is freely soluble in acetic acid (100), soluble in methanol, sparingly soluble in ethanol (99.5), and practically insoluble in water.

A solution of Lafutidine in methanol (1 in 100) shows no optical rotation.

Lafutidine shows crystal polymorphism.

Identification **(1)** Determine the absorption spectrum of a solution of Lafutidine in methanol (1 in 20,000) as directed under Ultraviolet-visible Spectrophotometry <*2.24*>, and compare the spectrum with the Reference Spectrum: both spectra exhibit similar intensities of absorption at the same wavelengths.

(2) Determine the infrared absorption spectrum of Lafutidine, previously dried, as directed in the potassium bromide disk method under Infrared Spectrophotometry <*2.25*>, and compare the spectrum with the Reference Spectrum: both spectra exhibit similar intensities of absorption at the same wave numbers.

Purity **(1)** Heavy metals <*1.07*>—Proceed with 2.0 g of Lafutidine according to Method 2, and perform the test. Prepare the control solution with 2.0 mL of Standard Lead Solution (not more than 10 ppm).

(2) Related substances—Dissolve 0.10 g of Lafutidine in 100 mL of the mobile phase, and use this solution as the sample solution. Pipet 1 mL of the sample solution, add the mobile phase to make exactly 100 mL, and use this solution as the standard solution. Perform the test with exactly 5 μL each of the sample solution and standard solution as directed under Liquid Chromatography <*2.01*> according to the following conditions. Determine each peak area by the automatic integration method: the area of the peak, having the relative retention time of about 0.85 to lafutidine, obtained from the sample solution is not larger than 3/10 times the peak area of lafutidine from the standard solution, the area of the peak other than lafutidine and the peak mentioned above from the sample solution is not larger than 1/10 times the peak area of lafutidine from the standard solution, and the total area of the peaks other than lafutidine from the sample solution is not larger than 2/5 times the peak area of lafutidine from the standard solution.

Operating conditions—

Detector: An ultraviolet absorption photometer (wavelength: 220 nm).

Column: A stainless steel column 6 mm in inside diameter and 15 cm in length, packed with octadecylsilanized silica gel for liquid chromatography (5 μm in particle diameter).

Column temperature: A constant temperature of about 40°C.

Mobile phase: Dissolve 0.87 g of sodium 1-pentanesulfonate in 1000 mL of diluted phosphoric acid (1 in 1000). To 850 mL of this solution add 150 mL of acetonitrile.

Flow rate: Adjust so that the retention time of lafutidine is about 15 minutes.

Time span of measurement: About 6 times as long as the retention time of lafutidine.

System suitability—

Test for required detectability: To exactly 1 mL of the standard solution add the mobile phase to make exactly 20 mL. Confirm that the peak area of lafutidine obtained with 5 μL of this solution is equivalent to 3.5 to 6.5% of that with 5 μL of the standard solution.

System performance: When the procedure is run with 5 μL of the standard solution under the above operating conditions, the number of theoretical plates and the symmetry factor of the peak of lafutidine are not less than 8000 and not more than 1.5, respectively.

System repeatability: When the test is repeated 6 times with 5 μL of the standard solution under the above operating conditions, the relative standard deviation of the peak area of lafutidine is not more than 2.0%.

Loss on drying <*2.41*> Not more than 0.5% (1 g, reduced pressure not exceeding 0.67 kPa, phosphorus (V) oxide, 4 hours).

Residue on ignition <*2.44*> Not more than 0.1% (1 g).

Assay Weigh accurately about 0.3 g of Lafutidine, previously dried, dissolve in 50 mL of acetic acid (100), and titrate <*2.50*> with 0.1 mol/L perchloric acid VS (potentiometric titration). Perform a blank determination in the same manner, and make any necessary correction.

Each mL of 0.1 mol/L perchloric acid VS
= 21.58 mg of $C_{22}H_{29}N_3O_4S$

Containers and storage Containers—Tight containers.

Lafutidine Tablets

ラフチジン錠

Lafutidine Tablets contain not less than 95.0% and not more than 105.0% of the labeled amount of lafutidine ($C_{22}H_{29}N_3O_4S$: 431.55).

Method of preparation Prepare as directed under Tablets, with Lafutidine.

Identification Powder Lafutidine Tablets. To a portion of the powder, equivalent to 10 mg of Lafutidine, add 10 mL of methanol, shake thoroughly, and centrifuge. To 5 mL of the supernatant liquid add methanol to make 100 mL. Determine the absorption spectrum of this solution as directed under Ultraviolet-visible Spectrophotometry <*2.24*>: it exhibits an absorption maximum between 271 nm and 275 nm.

Purity Related substances—To 10 Lafutidine Tablets add $4V/5$ mL of the mobile phase, disintegrate the tablets by sonicating, then shake vigorously for not less than 30 minutes, and add the mobile phase to make V mL so that each mL contains about 1 mg of lafutidine ($C_{22}H_{29}N_3O_4S$). Centrifuge, and use the supernatant liquid as the sample solution. Pipet 1 mL of the sample solution, add the mobile phase to make exactly 100 mL, and use this solution as the standard solution. Perform the test with exactly 5 μL each of the sample solution and standard solution as directed under Liquid Chromatography <*2.01*> according to the following conditions, and determine each peak area by the automatic integration method: the area of the peak, other than lafutidine and the peak having the relative retention time of about 0.85 to lafutidine, obtained from the sample solution is not larger than 1/5 times the peak area of lafutidine from the standard solution, and the total area of the peaks, other than lafutidine and the peak having the relative retention time of about 0.85, from the sample solution is not larger than 3/5 times the peak area of lafutidine from the standard solution.

Operating conditions—

Column, column temperature, mobile phase, and flow rate: Proceed as directed in the operating conditions in the Assay.

Detector: An ultraviolet absorption photometer (wavelength: 220 nm).

Time span of measurement: About 6 times as long as the retention time of lafutidine.

System suitability—

Test for required detectability: To exactly 1 mL of the standard solution add the mobile phase to make exactly 20 mL. Confirm that the peak area of lafutidine obtained with 5 μL of this solution is equivalent to 3.5 to 6.5% of that with 5 μL of the standard solution.

System performance: When the procedure is run with 5 μL of the standard solution under the above operating conditions, the number of theoretical plates and the symmetry factor of the peak of lafutidine are not less than 8000 and not more than 1.5, respectively.

System repeatability: When the test is repeated 6 times with 5 μL of the standard solution under the above operating conditions, the relative standard deviation of the peak area of lafutidine is not more than 2.0%.

Uniformity of dosage units <*6.02*> Perform the test according to the following method: it meets the requirement of the Content uniformity test.

To 1 tablet of Lafutidine Tablets add exactly V mL of the internal standard solution so that each mL contains about 2 mg of lafutidine ($C_{22}H_{29}N_3O_4S$), disintegrate the tablet by sonicating, then shake vigorously for 30 minutes. Centrifuge this solution, filter the supernatant liquid through a membrane filter with a pore size not exceeding 0.45 μm, and use the filtrate as the sample solution. Separately, weigh accurately about 0.1 g of lafutidine for assay, previously dried under a reduced pressure (not exceeding 0.67 kPa) using phosphorus (V) oxide as desiccant for 4 hours, dissolve in exactly 50 mL of the internal standard solution, and use this solution as the standard solution. Then, proceed as directed in the Assay.

Amount (mg) of lafutidine ($C_{22}H_{29}N_3O_4S$)
$= M_S \times Q_T/Q_S \times V/50$

M_S: Amount (mg) of lafutidine for assay taken

*Internal standard solution—*A solution of ethyl aminobenzoate in a mixture of acetonitrile and water (4:1) (3 in 10,000).

Dissolution <*6.10*> When the test is performed at 50 revolutions per minute according to the Paddle method, using 900 mL of 2nd fluid for dissolution test as the dissolution medium, the dissolution rate in 15 minutes of Lafutidine Tablets is not less than 75%.

Start the test with 1 tablet of Lafutidine Tablets, withdraw not less than 20 mL of the medium at the specified minute after starting the test, and filter through a membrane filter with a pore size not exceeding 0.45 μm. Discard not less than 10 mL of the first filtrate, pipet V mL of the subsequent filtrate, add the dissolution medium to make exactly V' mL so that each mL contains about 5.6 μg of lafutidine ($C_{22}H_{29}N_3O_4S$), and use this solution as the sample solution. Separately, weigh accurately about 25 mg of lafutidine for assay, previously dried under a reduced pressure (not exceeding 0.67 kPa) using phosphorus (V) oxide as desiccant for 4 hours, and dissolve in the dissolution medium to make exactly 100 mL. Pipet 2 mL of this solution, add the dissolution medium to make exactly 100 mL, and use this solution as the standard solution. Perform the test with exactly 25 μL each of the sample solution and standard solution as directed under Liquid Chromatography <*2.01*> according to the following conditions, and determine the peak areas, A_T and A_S, of lafutidine in each solution.

Dissolution rate (%) with respect to the labeled amount of lafutidine ($C_{22}H_{29}N_3O_4S$)
$= M_S \times A_T/A_S \times V'/V \times 1/C \times 18$

M_S: Amount (mg) of lafutidine for assay taken
C: Labeled amount (mg) of lafutidine ($C_{22}H_{29}N_3O_4S$) in 1 tablet

Operating conditions—
Proceed as directed in the operating conditions in the Assay.
System suitability—
System performance: When the procedure is run with 25 μL of the standard solution under the above operating conditions, the number of theoretical plates and the symmetry factor of the peak of lafutidine are not less than 7000 and not more than 1.5, respectively.
System repeatability: When the test is repeated 6 times with 25 μL of the standard solution under the above operating conditions, the relative standard deviation of the peak area of lafutidine is not more than 2.0%.

Assay To 20 Lafutidine Tablets add $4V/5$ mL of the internal standard solution, disintegrate the tablets with the aid of ultrasonic waves, then shake vigorously for 30 minutes. Add the internal standard solution to make exactly V mL so that each mL contains about 2 mg of lafutidine ($C_{22}H_{29}N_3O_4S$), centrifuge, filter the supernatant liquid through a membrane filter with a pore size not exceeding 0.45 μm, and use the filtrate as the sample solution. Separately, weigh accurately about 0.1 g of lafutidine for assay, previously dried under a reduced pressure (not exceeding 0.67 kPa) using phosphorus (V) oxide as desiccant for 4 hours, dissolve in the internal standard solution to make exactly 50 mL, and use this solution as the standard solution. Perform the test with 5 μL each of the sample solution and standard solution as directed under Liquid Chromatography <*2.01*> according to the following conditions, and calculate the ratios, Q_T and Q_S, of the peak area of lafutidine to that of the internal standard.

Amount (mg) of lafutidine ($C_{22}H_{29}N_3O_4S$) in 1 tablet
$= M_S \times Q_T/Q_S \times V/1000$

M_S: Amount (mg) of lafutidine for assay taken

Internal standard solution—A solution of ethyl aminobenzoate in a mixture of acetonitrile and water (4:1) (3 in 10,000).
Operating conditions—
Detector: An ultraviolet absorption photometer (wavelength: 275 nm).
Column: A stainless steel column 6 mm in inside diameter and 15 cm in length, packed with octadecylsilanized silica gel for liquid chromatography (5 μm in particle diameter).
Column temperature: A constant temperature of about 40°C.
Mobile phase: Dissolve 0.87 g of sodium 1-pentanesulfonate in 1000 mL of diluted phosphoric acid (1 in 1000). To 850 mL of this solution add 150 mL of acetonitrile.
Flow rate: Adjust so that the retention time of lafutidine is about 15 minutes.
System suitability—
System performance: When the procedure is run with 5 μL of the standard solution under the above operating conditions, lafutidine and the internal standard are eluted in this order with the resolution between these peaks being not less than 6.
System repeatability: When the test is repeated 6 times with 5 μL of the standard solution under the above operating conditions, the relative standard deviation of the ratio of the peak area of lafutidine to that of the internal standard is not more than 1.0%.

Containers and storage Containers—Tight containers.

Lanoconazole

ラノコナゾール

and enantiomer

$C_{14}H_{10}ClN_3S_2$: 319.83
(2*E*)-2-[(4*RS*)-4-(2-Chlorophenyl)-1,3-dithiolan-2-ylidene]-2-(1*H*-imidazol-1-yl)acetonitrile
[*101530-10-3*]

Lanoconazole, when dried, contains not less than 98.0% and not more than 102.0% of lanoconazole ($C_{14}H_{10}ClN_3S_2$).

Description Lanoconazole occurs as white to pale yellow, crystals or crystalline powder.
It is soluble in acetone, sparingly soluble in methanol and in ethanol (99.5), and practically insoluble in water.
It is gradually colored to yellow by light.
A solution of Lanoconazole in acetone (1 in 25) shows no optical rotation.

Identification **(1)** To 0.1 g of Lanoconazole add 0.5 g of sodium hydroxide, heat gradually to melt, and carbonize. After cooling, add 10 mL of dilute hydrochloric acid: the gas evolved darkens moistened lead (II) acetate paper.
(2) Perform the test with Lanoconazole as directed under Flame Coloration Test <*1.04*> (2): a green color appears.
(3) Determine the absorption spectrum of a solution of Lanoconazole in methanol (1 in 100,000) as directed under Ultraviolet-visible Spectrophotometry <*2.24*>, and compare the spectrum with the Reference Spectrum or the spectrum of a solution of Lanoconazole RS prepared in the same manner as the sample solution: both spectra exhibit similar intensities of absorption at the same wavelengths.
(4) Determine the infrared absorption spectrum of Lanoconazole, previously dried, as directed in the potassium bromide disk method under Infrared Spectrophotometry <*2.25*>, and compare the spectrum with the Reference Spectrum or the spectrum of previously dried Lanoconazole RS: both spectra exhibit similar intensities of absorption at the same wave numbers.

Melting point <*2.60*> 141 – 146°C

Purity (1) Heavy metals <*1.07*>—Proceed with 2.0 g of Lanoconazole according to Method 4, and perform the test. Prepare the control solution with 2.0 mL of Standard Lead Solution (not more than 10 ppm).

(2) Related substances—Conduct this procedure using light-resistant vessels. Dissolve 0.10 g of Lanoconazole in 100 mL of methanol, and use this solution as the sample solution. Pipet 1 mL of the sample solution, add methanol to make exactly 50 mL, and use this solution as the standard solution. Perform the test with exactly 5 μL each of the sample solution and standard solution as directed under Liquid Chromatography <*2.01*> according to the following conditions. Determine each peak area by the automatic integration method: the total area of the peaks other than lanoconazole obtained from the sample solution is not larger than 1/2 times the peak area of lanoconazole from the standard solution.

Operating conditions—

Detector, column, and column temperature: Proceed as directed in the operating conditions in the Assay.

Mobile phase: Dissolve 0.576 g of sodium 1-nonanesulfonate in 1000 mL of a mixture of methanol, water and acetic acid (100) (55:44:1).

Flow rate: Adjust so that the retention time of lanoconazole is about 7 minutes.

Time span of measurement: About 3 times as long as the retention time of lanoconazole, beginning after the solvent peak.

System suitability—

Test for required detectability: Pipet 2.5 mL of the standard solution, and add methanol to make exactly 50 mL. Confirm that the peak area of lanoconazole obtained with 5 μL of this solution is equivalent to 3.5 to 6.5% of that with 5 μL of the standard solution.

System performance: Put 20 mL of the sample solution in a colorless vessel, and expose to ultraviolet light (main wavelength: 365 nm) for 30 minutes. When the procedure is run with 5 μL of this solution under the above operating conditions, the resolution between the peak having the relative retention time of about 0.8 to lanoconazole and the peak of lanoconazole is not less than 1.5.

System repeatability: When the test is repeated 6 times with 5 μL of the standard solution under the above operating conditions, the relative standard deviation of the peak area of lanoconazole is not more than 1.0%.

Loss on drying <*2.41*> Not more than 0.4% (1 g, 105°C, 2 hours).

Residue on ignition <*2.44*> Not more than 0.1% (1 g).

Assay Conduct this procedure using light-resistant vessels. Weigh accurately about 50 mg each of Lanoconazole and Lanoconazole RS, both previously dried, and dissolve each in methanol to make exactly 50 mL. Pipet 5 mL each of these solutions, add exactly 5 mL of the internal standard solution, add methanol to make 50 mL, and use these solutions as the sample solution and the standard solution, respectively. Perform the test with 5 μL each of the sample solution and standard solution as directed under Liquid Chromatography <*2.01*> according to the following conditions, and calculate the ratios, Q_T and Q_S, of the peak area of lanoconazole to that of the internal standard.

$$\text{Amount (mg) of lanoconazole } (C_{14}H_{10}ClN_3S_2) = M_S \times Q_T/Q_S$$

M_S: Amount (mg) of Lanoconazole RS taken

Internal standard solution—A solution of diisopropyl 1,3-dithiolan-2-ylidenemalonate in methanol (1 in 1000).

Operating conditions—

Detector: An ultraviolet absorption photometer (wavelength: 295 nm).

Column: A stainless steel column 4.6 mm in inside diameter and 15 cm in length, packed with octadecylsilanized silica gel for liquid chromatography (5 μm in particle diameter).

Column temperature: A constant temperature of about 50°C.

Mobile phase: A mixture of methanol and water (11:9).

Flow rate: Adjust so that the retention time of lanoconazole is about 9 minutes.

System suitability—

System performance: When the procedure is run with 5 μL of the standard solution under the above operating conditions, lanoconazole and the internal standard are eluted in this order with the resolution between these peaks being not less than 3.

System repeatability: When the test is repeated 6 times with 5 μL of the standard solution under the above operating conditions, the relative standard deviation of the ratio of the peak area of lanoconazole to that of the internal standard is not more than 1.0%.

Containers and storage Containers—Well-closed containers.

Storage—Light-resistant.

Lanoconazole Cream

ラノコナゾールクリーム

Lanoconazole Cream contains not less than 95.0% and not more than 105.0% of the labeled amount of lanoconazole ($C_{14}H_{10}ClN_3S_2$: 319.83).

Method of preparation Prepare as directed under Creams, with Lanoconazole.

Identification Warm Lanoconazole Cream to soften, if necessary. To a quantity of Lanoconazole Cream, equivalent to 50 mg of Lanoconazole, add 10 mL of diluted hydrochloric acid (1 in 6) saturated with sodium chloride, previously warmed, shake vigorously for 15 minutes to disperse, and centrifuge. Filter the supernatant liquid, wash the residue with 1.5 mL of diluted hydrochloric acid (1 in 6) saturated with sodium chloride, filter, and combine the washing with the filtrate. To the combined filtrate add 2.5 g of sodium hydrogen carbonate to dissolve, and extract with 10 mL of diethyl ether. Wash the diethyl ether layer with three 10-mL portions of water, and dry under reduced pressure. Dissolve the residue in 15 mL of acetone, and use this solution as the sample solution. Separately, dissolve 10 mg of lanoconazole in 10 mL of acetone, and use this solution as the standard solution. Perform the test with these solutions as directed under Thin-layer Chromatography <*2.03*>. Spot 10 μL each of the sample solution and standard solution on a plate of silica gel with fluorescent indicator for thin-layer chromatography. Develop the plate with a mixture of ethyl acetate, toluene, methanol and ammonia solution (28) (400:400:20:1) to a distance of about 15 cm, and air-dry the plate. Examine under ultraviolet light (main wavelength: 254 nm): the principal spot obtained from the sample solution and the spot from the standard solution show the same *Rf* value.

Assay Conduct this procedure using light-resistant vessels. Weigh accurately a quantity of Lanoconazole Cream, equivalent to about 15 mg of lanoconazole ($C_{14}H_{10}ClN_3S_2$), add 80 mL of methanol, sonicate to disperse, and add exactly 10 mL of the internal standard solution. Add methanol to make 100 mL, filter through a membrane filter with a pore size of 0.45 μm if necessary, and use this solution as the sample solution. Separately, weigh accurately about 15 mg of Lanoconazole RS, previously dried at 105°C for 2 hours, dissolve in methanol, and add exactly 10 mL of the internal standard solution. Add methanol to make 100 mL, and use this solution as the standard solution. Perform the test with 10 μL each of the sample solution and standard solution as directed under Liquid Chromatography <2.01> according to the following conditions, and calculate the ratios, Q_T and Q_S, of the peak area of lanoconazole to that of the internal standard.

$$\text{Amount (mg) of lanoconazole } (C_{14}H_{10}ClN_3S_2) = M_S \times Q_T/Q_S$$

M_S: Amount (mg) of Lanoconazole RS taken

Internal standard solution—A solution of diisopropyl 1,3-dithiolan-2-ylidenemalonate in methanol (1 in 1000).

Operating conditions—

Proceed as directed in the operating conditions in the Assay under Lanoconazole.

System suitability—

System performance: When the procedure is run with 10 μL of the standard solution under the above operating conditions, lanoconazole and the internal standard are eluted in this order with the resolution between these peaks being not less than 3.

System repeatability: When the test is repeated 6 times with 10 μL of the standard solution under the above operating conditions, the relative standard deviation of the ratio of the peak area of lanoconazole to that of the internal standard is not more than 1.0%.

Containers and storage Containers—Tight containers.
Storage—Light-resistant.

Lanoconazole Cutaneous Solution

ラノコナゾール外用液

Lanoconazole Cutaneous Solution is a liquid for external use.

It contains not less than 95.0% and not more than 105.0% of the labeled amount of lanoconazole ($C_{14}H_{10}ClN_3S_2$: 319.83).

Method of preparation Prepare as directed under Liquids and Solutions for Cutaneous Application, with Lanoconazole.

Identification To a volume of Lanoconazole Cutaneous Solution, equivalent to 50 mg of Lanoconazole, add water enough to produce precipitate, and shake vigorously. Filter this solution, rinse the vessel with a suitable amount of water, and collect the precipitates. Wash the precipitates with 100 mL of water, dissolve in acetone, and dry under reduced pressure. If there are water droplets in the residue, dissolve the residue in 40 mL of acetone, and dry again under reduced pressure. Dissolve the residue in 30 mL of acetone, and use this solution as the sample solution. Separately, dissolve 10 mg of lanoconazole in 10 mL of acetone, and use this solution as the standard solution. Perform the test with these solutions as directed under Thin-layer Chromatography <2.03>. Spot 10 μL each of the sample solution and standard solution on a plate of silica gel with fluorescent indicator for thin-layer chromatography. Develop the plate with a mixture of ethyl acetate, toluene, methanol and ammonia solution (28) (400:400:20:1) to a distance of about 15 cm, and air-dry the plate. Examine under ultraviolet light (main wavelength: 254 nm): the principal spot obtained from the sample solution and the spot from the standard solution show the same *R*f value.

Assay Conduct this procedure using light-resistant vessels. Pipet a volume of Lanoconazole Cutaneous Solution, equivalent to about 50 mg of lanoconazole ($C_{14}H_{10}ClN_3S_2$), and add methanol to make exactly 50 mL. Pipet 15 mL of this solution, add exactly 10 mL of the internal standard solution, add methanol to make 100 mL, and use this solution as the sample solution. Separately, weigh accurately about 15 mg of Lanoconazole RS, previously dried at 105°C for 2 hours, dissolve in methanol, and add exactly 10 mL of the internal standard solution. Add methanol to make 100 mL, and use this solution as the standard solution. Perform the test with 10 μL each of the sample solution and standard solution as directed under Liquid Chromatography <2.01> according to the following conditions, and calculate the ratios, Q_T and Q_S, of the peak area of lanoconazole to that of the internal standard.

$$\text{Amount (mg) of lanoconazole } (C_{14}H_{10}ClN_3S_2) = M_S \times Q_T/Q_S \times 10/3$$

M_S: Amount (mg) of Lanoconazole RS taken

Internal standard solution—A solution of diisopropyl 1,3-dithiolan-2-ylidenemalonate in methanol (1 in 1000).

Operating conditions—

Proceed as directed in the operating conditions in the Assay under Lanoconazole.

System suitability—

System performance: When the procedure is run with 10 μL of the standard solution under the above operating conditions, lanoconazole and the internal standard are eluted in this order with the resolution between these peaks being not less than 3.

System repeatability: When the test is repeated 6 times with 10 μL of the standard solution under the above operating conditions, the relative standard deviation of the ratio of the peak area of lanoconazole to that of the internal standard is not more than 1.0%.

Containers and storage Containers—Tight containers.
Storage—Light-resistant.

Lanoconazole Ointment

ラノコナゾール軟膏

Lanoconazole Ointment contains not less than 93.0% and not more than 107.0% of the labeled amount of lanoconazole ($C_{14}H_{10}ClN_3S_2$: 319.83).

Method of preparation Prepare as directed under Ointments, with Lanoconazole.

Identification To a quantity of Lanoconazole Ointment, equivalent to 50 mg of Lanoconazole, add 15 mL of hexane, sonicate to disperse, add 10 mL of methanol, and shake for 10 minutes. Centrifuge this solution, discard the hexane layer, and take the methanol layer. Wash the residue with a small amount of methanol if necessary, and combine the washing with the methanol layer. Dry the combined methanol layer under reduced pressure, dissolve the residue in 40 mL of acetone, and use this solution as the sample solution. Separately, dissolve 10 mg of lanoconazole in 10 mL of acetone, and use this solution as the standard solution. Perform the test with these solutions as directed under Thin-layer Chromatography <*2.03*>. Spot 10 μL each of the sample solution and standard solution on a plate of silica gel with fluorescent indicator for thin-layer chromatography. Develop the plate with a mixture of ethyl acetate, toluene, methanol and ammonia solution (28) (400:400:20:1) to a distance of about 15 cm, and air-dry the plate. Examine under ultraviolet light (main wavelength: 254 nm): the principal spot obtained from the sample solution and the spot from the standard solution show the same *R*f value.

Assay Conduct this procedure using light-resistant vessels. Weigh accurately a quantity of Lanoconazole Ointment, equivalent to about 15 mg of lanoconazole ($C_{14}H_{10}ClN_3S_2$), add 20 mL of tetrahydrofuran, sonicate to disperse, and add exactly 10 mL of the internal standard solution. Add methanol to make 100 mL, and use this solution as the sample solution. Separately, weigh accurately about 15 mg of Lanoconazole RS, previously dried at 105°C for 2 hours, dissolve in methanol, and add exactly 10 mL of the internal standard solution. Add methanol to make 100 mL, and use this solution as the standard solution. Perform the test with 10 μL each of the sample solution and standard solution as directed under Liquid Chromatography <*2.01*> according to the following conditions, and calculate the ratios, Q_T and Q_S, of the peak area of lanoconazole to that of the internal standard.

Amount (mg) of lanoconazole ($C_{14}H_{10}ClN_3S_2$)
$= M_S \times Q_T/Q_S$

M_S: Amount (mg) of Lanoconazole RS taken

Internal standard solution—A solution of diisopropyl 1,3-dithiolan-2-ylidenemalonate in methanol (1 in 1000).
Operating conditions—
Proceed as directed in the operating conditions in the Assay under Lanoconazole.
System suitability—
System performance: When the procedure is run with 10 μL of the standard solution under the above operating conditions, lanoconazole and the internal standard are eluted in this order with the resolution between these peaks being not less than 3.
System repeatability: When the test is repeated 6 times with 10 μL of the standard solution under the above operating conditions, the relative standard deviation of the ratio of the peak area of lanoconazole to that of the internal standard is not more than 1.0%.

Containers and storage Containers—Tight containers.
Storage—Light-resistant.

Lansoprazole

ランソプラゾール

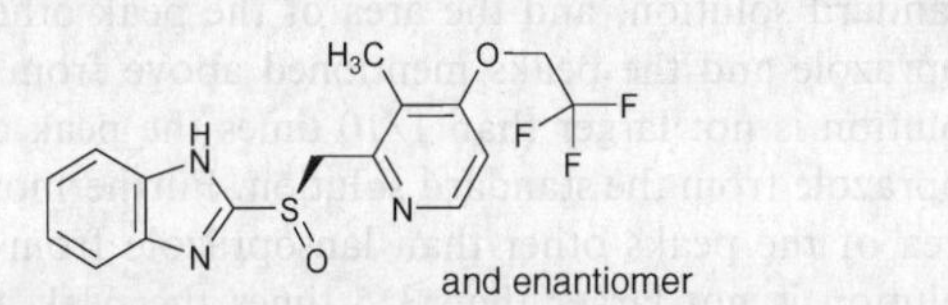

and enantiomer

$C_{16}H_{14}F_3N_3O_2S$: 369.36
(*RS*)-2-({[3-Methyl-4-(2,2,2-trifluoroethoxy)pyridin-2-yl]methyl}sulfinyl)-1*H*-benzimidazole
[*103577-45-3*]

Lansoprazole contains not less than 99.0% and not more than 101.0% of lansoprazole ($C_{16}H_{14}F_3N_3O_2S$), calculated on the anhydrous basis.

Description Lansoprazole occurs as a white to brownish white crystalline powder.

It is freely soluble in *N*, *N*-dimethylformamide, soluble in methanol, sparingly soluble in ethanol (99.5), and practically insoluble in water.

A solution of Lansoprazole in *N*, *N*-dimethylformamide (1 in 10) shows no optical rotation.

Melting point: about 166°C (with decomposition).

It shows crystal polymorphism.

Identification **(1)** Determine the absorption spectrum of a solution of Lansoprazole in methanol (1 in 100,000) as directed under Ultraviolet-visible Spectrophotometry <*2.24*>, and compare the spectrum with the Reference Spectrum or the spectrum of a solution of Lansoprazole RS prepared in the same manner as the sample solution: both spectra exhibit similar intensities of absorption at the same wavelengths.

(2) Determine the infrared absorption spectrum of Lansoprazole as directed in the potassium bromide disk method under Infrared Spectrophotometry <*2.25*>, and compare the spectrum with the Reference Spectrum or the spectrum of Lansoprazole RS: both spectra exhibit similar intensities of absorption at the same wave numbers.

Purity **(1)** Clarity and color of solution—Dissolve 1.0 g of Lansoprazole in 20 mL of *N*, *N*-dimethylformamide: the solution is clear and not more colored than Matching Fluid G.

(2) Heavy metals <*1.07*>—Proceed with 1.0 g of Lansoprazole in a platinum crucible according to Method 2, and perform the test. Prepare the control solution with 1.0 mL of Standard Lead Solution (not more than 10 ppm).

(3) Arsenic <*1.11*>—Prepare the test solution with 1.0 g of Lansoprazole in a platinum crucible according to Method 3, using a solution of magnesium nitrate hexahydrate in ethanol (95) (1 in 5), and perform the test. Prepare the standard color with 1.0 mL of Standard Arsenic Solution (not more than 1 ppm).

(4) Related substances—Dissolve 50 mg of Lansoprazole in a mixture of dilute sodium hydroxide TS and methanol (3:1) to make 20 mL. To 2 mL of this solution add a mixture of dilute sodium hydroxide TS and methanol (3:1) to make 20 mL, and use this solution as the sample solution. Pipet 1 mL of the sample solution, add a mixture of dilute sodium hydroxide TS and methanol (3:1) to make exactly 100 mL, and use this solution as the standard solution. Perform the test with exactly 40 μL each of the sample solution and standard solution as directed under Liquid Chromatography <*2.01*> according to the following conditions, and determine each peak area by the automatic integration method: the area of the peak, having a relative retention time of about 1.1 to lansoprazole, obtained from the sample solution is not larger than 2/5 times the peak area of lansoprazole from the standard solution, and the area of the peak other than lansoprazole and the peaks mentioned above from the sample solution is not larger than 1/10 times the peak area of lansoprazole from the standard solution. Furthermore, the total area of the peaks other than lansoprazole from the sample solution is not larger than 3/5 times the peak area of lansoprazole from the standard solution. For the area of the peaks, having the relative retention time of about 0.8, about 1.1 and about 1.2, multiply their correction factors, 0.8, 1.2, and 1.3, respectively.

Operating conditions—

Detector: An ultraviolet absorption photometer (wavelength: 285 nm).

Column: A stainless steel column 4.6 mm in inside diameter and 15 cm in length, packed with octadecylsilanized silica gel for liquid chromatography (5 μm in particle diameter).

Column temperature: A constant temperature of about 25°C.

Mobile phase A: Water.

Mobile phase B: A mixture of acetonitrile, water and triethylamine (160:40:1), adjusted to pH 7.0 with phosphoric acid.

Flowing of mobile phase: Control the gradient by mixing the mobile phases A and B as directed in the following table.

Time after injection of sample (min)	Mobile phase A (vol%)	Mobile phase B (vol%)
0 - 40	90 → 20	10 → 80
40 - 50	20	80

Flow rate: About 0.8 mL per minute (the retention time of lansoprazole is about 29 minutes).

Time span of measurement: About 1.7 times as long as the retention time of lansoprazole.

System suitability—

Test for required detectability: Pipet 1 mL of the standard solution, and add a mixture of dilute sodium hydroxide TS and methanol (3:1) to make exactly 20 mL. Confirm that the peak area of lansoprazole obtained with 40 μL of this solution is equivalent to 4% to 6% of that with 40 μL of the standard solution.

System performance: When the procedure is run with 40 μL of the standard solution under the above operating conditions, the number of theoretical plates and the symmetry factor of the peak of lansoprazole are not less than 150,000 and not more than 1.5, respectively.

System repeatability: When the test is repeated 6 times with 40 μL of the standard solution under the above operating conditions, the relative standard deviation of the peak area of lansoprazole is not more than 3.0%.

Water *<2.48>* Not more than 0.10% (0.5 g, coulometric titration).

Residue on ignition *<2.44>* Not more than 0.1% (1 g, platinum crucible).

Assay Weigh accurately about 50 mg each of Lansoprazole and Lansoprazole RS (separately determine the water *<2.48>* in the same manner as Lansoprazole), and dissolve each in exactly 10 mL of the internal standard solution. To 1 mL each of both solutions add diluting solution to make 50 mL, and use these solutions as the sample solution and the standard solution, respectively. Perform the test with 10 μL each of the sample solution and standard solution as directed under Liquid Chromatography *<2.01>* according to the following conditions, and calculate the ratios, Q_T and Q_S, of the peak area of lansoprazole to that of the internal standard.

$$\text{Amount (mg) of lansoprazole } (C_{16}H_{14}F_3N_3O_2S) = M_S \times Q_T/Q_S$$

M_S: Amount (mg) of Lansoprazole RS taken, calculated on the anhydrous basis

*Internal standard solution—*A solution of 4′-ethoxyacetophenone in diluting solution (1 in 400).

Diluting solution: A mixture of water, acetonitrile and triethylamine (60:40:1), adjusted to pH 11.0 with phosphoric acid.

Operating conditions—

Detector: An ultraviolet absorption photometer (wavelength: 285 nm).

Column: A stainless steel column 4.6 mm in inside diameter and 25 cm in length, packed with octadecylsilanized silicon polymer coated silica gel for liquid chromatography (5 μm in particle diameter).

Column temperature: A constant temperature of about 25°C.

Mobile phase: A mixture of water, acetonitrile and triethylamine (60:40:1), adjusted to pH 7.0 with phosphoric acid.

Flow rate: Adjust so that the retention time of lansoprazole is about 7 minutes.

System suitability—

System performance: When the procedure is run with 10 μL of the standard solution under the above operating conditions, lansoprazole and the internal standard are eluted in this order with the resolution between these peaks being not less than 10.

System repeatability: When the test is repeated 6 times with 10 μL of the standard solution under the above operating conditions, the relative standard deviation of the ratio of the peak area of lansoprazole to that of the internal standard is not more than 1.0%.

Containers and storage Containers—Tight containers.

Storage—Light-resistant.

Lansoprazole Delayed-release Capsules

ランソプラゾール腸溶カプセル

Lansoprazole Delayed-release Capsules contain not less than 95.0% and not more than 105.0% of the labeled amount of lansoprazole ($C_{16}H_{14}F_3N_3O_2S$: 369.36).

Method of preparation Prepare as directed under Capsules, with Lansoprazole.

Identification Take out the contents of Lansoprazole Delayed-release Capsules, and powder. To a portion of the powder, equivalent to 5 mg of Lansoprazole, add 5 mL of methanol, shake thoroughly, and centrifuge. To 0.1 mL of the supernatant liquid add 10 mL of methanol, and determine the absorption spectrum of this solution as directed under Ultraviolet-visible Spectrophotometry *<2.24>*: it exhibits a maximum between 282 nm and 286 nm.

Uniformity of dosage units <*6.02*> Perform the test according to the following method: it meets the requirement of the Content uniformity test.

Take out the contents of 1 capsule of Lansoprazole Delayed-release Capsules, add $3V/10$ mL of dilute sodium hydroxide TS, and sonicate with occasional stirring to disintegrate the contents completely. Add acetonitrile to make exactly V mL so that each mL contains about 0.15 mg of lansoprazole ($C_{16}H_{14}F_3N_3O_2S$). Centrifuge this solution, filter the supernatant liquid through a membrane filter with a pore size not exceeding 0.5 μm. Discard the first 5 mL of the filtrate, pipet 4 mL of the subsequent filtrate, add a mixture of acetonitrile and dilute sodium hydroxide TS (7:3) to make exactly 50 mL, and use this solution as the sample solution. Separately, weigh accurately about 30 mg of Lansoprazole RS (separately determine the water <*2.48*> in the same manner as Lansoprazole), and dissolve in 60 mL of dilute sodium hydroxide TS, and add acetonitrile to make exactly 200 mL. Pipet 4 mL of this solution, add a mixture of acetonitrile and dilute sodium hydroxide TS (7:3) to make exactly 50 mL, and use this solution as the standard solution. Determine the absorbances, A_T and A_S, at 294 nm of the sample solution and standard solution as directed under Ultraviolet-visible Spectrophotometry <*2.24*>.

$$\text{Amount (mg) of lansoprazole } (C_{16}H_{14}F_3N_3O_2S) = M_S \times A_T/A_S \times V/200$$

M_S: Amount (mg) of Lansoprazole RS taken, calculated on the anhydrous basis

Dissolution Being specified separately when the drug is granted approval based on the Law.

Assay Take out the contents of not less than 20 capsules of Lansoprazole Delayed-release Capsules. Weigh accurately the mass of the contents, and powder. Weigh accurately a portion of the powder, equivalent to about 0.3 g of lansoprazole ($C_{16}H_{14}F_3N_3O_2S$), add 60 mL of dilute sodium hydroxide TS, sonicate, and shake thoroughly. To this solution add 20 mL of acetonitrile and exactly 20 mL of the internal standard solution, shake thoroughly, and centrifuge. To 1 mL of the supernatant liquid add diluting solution to make 30 mL, and filter through a membrane filter with a pore size not exceeding 0.5 μm. Discard not less than 5 mL of the first filtrate, and use the subsequent filtrate as the sample solution. Separately, weigh accurately about 30 mg of Lansoprazole RS (separately determine the water <*2.48*> in the same manner as Lansoprazole), dissolve in 6 mL of dilute sodium hydroxide TS and 2 mL of acetonitrile, and add exactly 2 mL of the internal standard solution. To 1 mL of this solution add diluting solution to make 30 mL, and use this solution as the standard solution. Perform the test with 10 μL each of the sample solution and standard solution as directed under Liquid Chromatography <*2.01*> according to the following conditions, and calculate the ratios, Q_T and Q_S, of the peak area of lansoprazole to that of the internal standard.

$$\text{Amount (mg) of lansoprazole } (C_{16}H_{14}F_3N_3O_2S) = M_S \times Q_T/Q_S \times 10$$

M_S: Amount (mg) of Lansoprazole RS taken, calculated on the anhydrous basis

Internal standard solution—A solution of 4′-ethoxyacetophenone in acetonitrile (3 in 400).

Diluting solution: A mixture of water, acetonitrile and triethylamine (60:40:1), adjusted to pH 11.0 with phosphoric acid.

Operating conditions—

Proceed as directed in the operating conditions in the Assay under Lansoprazole.

System suitability—

System performance: When the procedure is run with 10 μL of the standard solution under the above operating conditions, lansoprazole and the internal standard are eluted in this order with the resolution between these peaks being not less than 10.

System repeatability: When the test is repeated 6 times with 10 μL of the standard solution under the above operating conditions, the relative standard deviation of the ratio of the peak area of lansoprazole to that of the internal standard is not more than 1.0%.

Containers and storage Containers—Tight containers.

Lansoprazole Delayed-release Orally Disintegrating Tablets

ランソプラゾール腸溶性口腔内崩壊錠

Lansoprazole Delayed-release Orally Disintegrating Tablets contain not less than 95.0% and not more than 105.0% of the labeled amount of lansoprazole ($C_{16}H_{14}F_3N_3O_2S$: 369.36).

Method of preparation Prepare as directed under Tablets, with Lansoprazole.

Identification Powder 10 tablets of Lansoprazole Delayed-release Orally Disintegrating Tablets. To a portion of the powder, equivalent to 5 mg of Lansoprazole, add 5 mL of methanol, shake thoroughly, and centrifuge. To 0.1 mL of the supernatant liquid add 10 mL of methanol, and determine the absorption spectrum of this solution as directed under Ultraviolet-visible Spectrophotometry <*2.24*>: it exhibits a maximum between 282 nm and 286 nm.

Purity Related substances—Keep the sample solution and standard solution at not exceeding 5°C, and use them within 12 hours. Powder not less than 10 tablets of Lansoprazole Delayed-release Orally Disintegrating Tablets. To a portion of the powder, equivalent to 25 mg of Lansoprazole, add 10 mL of a mixture of dilute sodium hydroxide TS and methanol (3:1), sonicate, shake thoroughly, and centrifuge. To 2 mL of the supernatant liquid add diluting solution to make 20 mL, filter through a membrane filter with a pore size not exceeding 0.5 μm, and use the filtrate as the sample solution. Pipet 1 mL of the sample solution, add diluting solution to make exactly 100 mL, and use this solution as the standard solution. Perform the test with exactly 40 μL each of the sample solution and standard solution as directed under Liquid Chromatography <*2.01*> according to the following conditions, and determine each peak area by the automatic integration method: the area of the peak, having a relative retention time of about 1.1 to lansoprazole, obtained from the sample solution is not larger than 2/5 times the peak area of lansoprazole from the standard solution, and the area of the peak other than lansoprazole and the peak mentioned above from the sample solution is not larger than 1/5 times the peak area of lansoprazole from the standard solution. Furthermore, the total area of the peaks other than lansoprazole from the sample solution is not larger than 1.6 times the peak area of lansoprazole from the standard solution.

Diluting solution: A mixture of acetonitrile, water and

triethylamine (160:40:1), adjusted to pH 11.0 with phosphoric acid. To 100 mL of this solution add 900 mL of water.

Operating conditions—

Detector, column, column temperature, mobile phase A, mobile phase B, and time span of measurement: Proceed as directed in the operating conditions in the Purity (4) under Lansoprazole.

Flowing of mobile phase: Control the gradient by mixing the mobile phases A and B as directed in the following table.

Time after injection of sample (min)	Mobile phase A (vol%)	Mobile phase B (vol%)
0 – 30	90 → 20	10 → 80
30 – 40	20	80

Flow rate: About 0.8 mL per minute (the retention time of lansoprazole is about 24 minutes).

System suitability—

Test for required detectability: Pipet 1 mL of the standard solution, and add diluting solution to make exactly 20 mL. Confirm that the peak area of lansoprazole obtained with 40 μL of this solution is equivalent to 4 to 6% of that with 40 μL of the standard solution.

System performance: When the procedure is run with 40 μL of the standard solution under the above operating conditions, the number of theoretical plates and the symmetry factor of the peak of lansoprazole are not less than 150,000 and not more than 1.5, respectively.

System repeatability: When the test is repeated 6 times with 40 μL of the standard solution under the above operating conditions, the relative standard deviation of the peak area of lansoprazole is not more than 3.0%.

Uniformity of dosage units <6.02> Perform the test according to the following method: it meets the requirements of the Content uniformity test.

To 1 tablet of Lansoprazole Delayed-release Orally Disintegrating Tablets add $3V/10$ mL of dilute sodium hydroxide TS, and sonicate with occasional stirring to disintegrate the tablet completely. Add acetonitrile to make exactly V mL so that each mL contains about 0.15 mg of lansoprazole ($C_{16}H_{14}F_3N_3O_2S$). Centrifuge this solution, and filter the supernatant liquid through a membrane filter with a pore size not exceeding 0.5 μm. Discard the first 5 mL of the filtrate, pipet 4 mL of the subsequent filtrate, add a mixture of acetonitrile and dilute sodium hydroxide TS (7:3) to make exactly 50 mL, and use this solution as the sample solution. Separately, weigh accurately about 30 mg of Lansoprazole RS (separately determine the water <2.48> in the same manner as Lansoprazole), and dissolve in 60 mL of dilute sodium hydroxide TS, and add acetonitrile to make exactly 200 mL. Pipet 4 mL of this solution, add a mixture of acetonitrile and dilute sodium hydroxide TS (7:3) to make exactly 50 mL, and use this solution as the standard solution. Determine the absorbances, A_T and A_S, at 294 nm of the sample solution and standard solution as directed under Ultraviolet-visible Spectrophotometry <2.24>.

Amount (mg) of lansoprazole ($C_{16}H_{14}F_3N_3O_2S$)
$= M_S \times A_T/A_S \times V/200$

M_S: Amount (mg) of Lansoprazole RS taken, calculated on the anhydrous basis

Disintegration Being specified separately when the drug is granted approval based on the Law.

Dissolution Being specified separately when the drug is granted approval based on the Law.

Assay Weigh accurately the mass of not less than 20 tablets of Lansoprazole Delayed-release Orally Disintegrating Tablets, and powder. Weigh accurately a portion of the powder, equivalent to about 0.3 g of lansoprazole ($C_{16}H_{14}F_3N_3O_2S$), add 60 mL of dilute sodium hydroxide TS, sonicate, and shake thoroughly. To this solution add 20 mL of acetonitrile and exactly 20 mL of the internal standard solution, shake thoroughly, and centrifuge. To 1 mL of the supernatant liquid add diluting solution to make 30 mL, and filter through a membrane filter with a pore size not exceeding 0.5 μm. Discard the first 5 mL of the filtrate, and use the subsequent filtrate as the sample solution. Separately, weigh accurately about 30 mg of Lansoprazole RS (separately determine the water <2.48> in the same manner as Lansoprazole), dissolve in 6 mL of dilute sodium hydroxide TS and 2 mL of acetonitrile, and add exactly 2 mL of the internal standard solution. To 1 mL of this solution add diluting solution to make 30 mL, and use this solution as the standard solution. Perform the test with 10 μL each of the sample solution and standard solution as directed under Liquid Chromatography <2.01> according to the following conditions, and calculate the ratios, Q_T and Q_S, of the peak area of lansoprazole to that of the internal standard.

Amount (mg) of lansoprazole ($C_{16}H_{14}F_3N_3O_2S$)
$= M_S \times Q_T/Q_S \times 10$

M_S: Amount (mg) of Lansoprazole RS taken, calculated on the anhydrous basis

*Internal standard solution—*A solution of 4′-ethoxyacetophenone in acetonitrile (3 in 400).

Diluting solution: A mixture of water, acetonitrile and triethylamine (60:40:1), adjusted to pH 11.0 with phosphoric acid.

Operating conditions—

Proceed as directed in the operating conditions in the Assay under Lansoprazole.

System suitability—

System performance: When the procedure is run with 10 μL of the standard solution under the above operating conditions, lansoprazole and the internal standard are eluted in this order with the resolution between these peaks being not less than 10.

System repeatability: When the test is repeated 6 times with 10 μL of the standard solution under the above operating conditions, the relative standard deviation of the ratio of the peak area of lansoprazole to that of the internal standard is not more than 1.0%.

Containers and storage Containers—Tight containers.

Latamoxef Sodium

ラタモキセフナトリウム

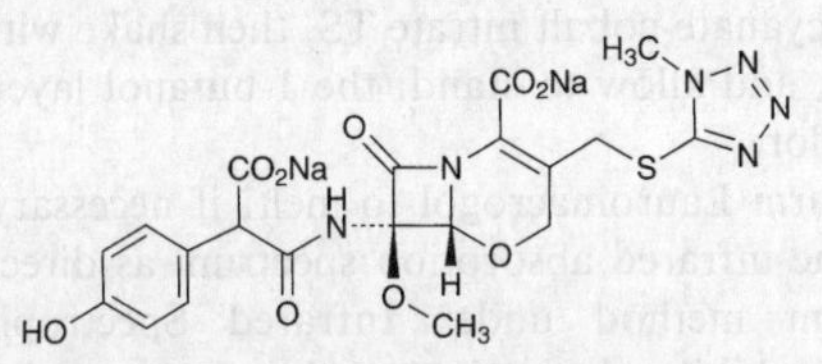

$C_{20}H_{18}N_6Na_2O_9S$: 564.44
Disodium (6*R*,7*R*)-7-[2-carboxylato-2-(4-hydroxyphenyl)acetylamino]-7-methoxy-3-(1-methyl-1*H*-tetrazol-5-ylsulfanylmethyl)-8-oxo-5-oxa-1-azabicyclo[4.2.0]oct-2-ene-2-carboxylate
[*64953-12-4*]

Latamoxef Sodium contains not less than 830 μg (potency) and not more than 940 μg (potency) per mg, calculated on the anhydrous basis. The potency of Latamoxef Sodium is expressed as mass (potency) of latamoxef ($C_{20}H_{20}N_6O_9S$: 520.47).

Description Latamoxef Sodium occurs as white to light yellow-white, powder or masses.

It is very soluble in water, freely soluble in methanol, and slightly soluble in ethanol (95).

Identification **(1)** Determine the absorption spectrum of a solution of Latamoxef Sodium (3 in 100,000) as directed under Ultraviolet-visible Spectrophotometry 〈*2.24*〉, and compare the spectrum with the Reference Spectrum: both spectra exhibit similar intensities of absorption at the same wavelengths.

(2) Determine the infrared absorption spectrum of Latamoxef Sodium as directed in the potassium bromide disk method under Infrared Spectrophotometry 〈*2.25*〉, and compare the spectrum with the Reference Spectrum: both spectra exhibit similar intensities of absorption at the same wave numbers.

(3) Determine the ^1H spectrum of a solution of Latamoxef Sodium in heavy water for nuclear magnetic resonance spectroscopy (1 in 10) as directed under Nuclear Magnetic Resonance Spectroscopy 〈*2.21*〉, using sodium 3-trimethylsilylpropanesulfonate for nuclear magnetic resonance spectroscopy as an internal reference compound: it exhibits single signals, A and B, at around δ 3.5 ppm and at around δ 4.0 ppm. The ratio of the integrated intensity of these signals, A:B, is about 1:1.

(4) Latamoxef Sodium responds to Qualitative Tests 〈*1.09*〉 (1) for sodium salt.

Optical rotation 〈*2.49*〉 $[\alpha]_D^{20}$: −32 − −40° (0.5 g calculated on the anhydrous basis, phosphate buffer solution (pH 7.0), 50 mL, 100 mm).

pH 〈*2.54*〉 The pH of a solution obtained by dissolving 1.0 g of Latamoxef Sodium in 10 mL of water is between 5.0 and 7.0.

Purity **(1)** Clarity and color of solution—Dissolve 1.0 g of Latamoxef Sodium in 10 mL of water: the solution is clear and has no more color than the following control solution.

Control solution: To a mixture of 3.0 mL of Cobalt (II) Chloride CS and 36 mL of Iron (III) Chloride CS add 11 mL of diluted dilute hydrochloric acid (1 in 10). To 2.5 mL of this solution add 7.5 mL of diluted dilute hydrochloric acid (1:10).

(2) Heavy metals 〈*1.07*〉—Carbonize 1.0 g of Latamoxef Sodium by heating gently, previously powdered if it is masses. After cooling, add 10 mL of a solution of magnesium nitrate hexahydrate in ethanol (1 in 10), and burn the ethanol. After cooling, add 1 mL of sulfuric acid. Proceed according to Method 4, and perform the test. Prepare the control solution with 2.0 mL of Standard Lead Solution (not more than 20 ppm).

(3) Arsenic 〈*1.11*〉—Prepare the test solution by dissolving 1.0 g of Latamoxef Sodium in 20 mL of water, and perform the test (not more than 2 ppm).

(4) Related substances—Dissolve 25 mg of Latamoxef Sodium in water to make 50 mL, and use this solution as the sample solution. Pipet 2 mL of the sample solution, add water to make exactly 100 mL, and use this solution as the standard solution. Perform the test with exactly 5 μL each of the sample solution and standard solution as directed under Liquid Chromatography 〈*2.01*〉 according to the following conditions, and determine each peak area by the automatic integration method: the peak area of 1-methyl-1*H*-tetrazole-5-thiol, having the relative retention time of about 0.5 to the first eluted peak of the two peaks of latamoxef, obtained from the sample solution is not larger than the peak area of latamoxef from the standard solution, and the peak area of decarboxylatamoxef, having the relative retention time of about 1.7 to the first peak of the two peaks of latamoxef, is not larger than 2 times that of latamoxef from the standard solution. For the peak area of 1-methyl-1*H*-tetrazole-5-thiol, multiply its correction factor, 0.52.

Operating conditions—

Proceed as directed in the operating conditions in the Assay.

System suitability—

System performance: Proceed as directed in the system suitability in the Assay.

System repeatability: When the test is repeated 6 times with 5 μL of the standard solution under the above operating conditions, the relative standard deviation of the peak area of latamoxef is not more than 2.0%.

Water 〈*2.48*〉 Not more than 5.0% (0.5 g, volumetric titration, back titration).

Isomer ratio Dissolve 25 mg of Latamoxef Sodium in water to make 50 mL, and use this solution as the sample solution. Perform the test with 5 μL of the sample solution as directed under Liquid Chromatography 〈*2.01*〉 according to the following conditions, and determine the areas, A_a and A_b, of the two peaks in order of elution, which appear close to each other at the retention time of about 10 minutes: A_a/A_b is between 0.8 and 1.4.

Operating conditions—

Detector: An ultraviolet absorption photometer (wavelength: 254 nm).

Column: A stainless steel column 4 mm in inside diameter and 15 cm in length, packed with octadecylsilanized silica gel for liquid chromatography (10 μm in particle diameter).

Column temperature: A constant temperature of about 25°C.

Mobile phase: Dissolve 7.7 g of ammonium acetate in water to make 1000 mL. To 950 mL of this solution add 50 mL of methanol.

Flow rate: Adjust so that the retention time of the first eluted peak of latamoxef is about 8 minutes.

System suitability—

System performance: When the procedure is run with 5 μL of the sample solution under the above operating conditions, the resolution between the two peaks of latamoxef is not less than 3.

System repeatability: When the test is repeated 3 times with 5 μL of the sample solution under the above operating conditions, the relative standard deviation of the area of the first eluted peak of latamoxef is not more than 2.0%.

Assay Weigh accurately an amount of Latamoxef Sodium and Latamoxef Ammonium RS, equivalent to about 25 mg (potency) each, dissolve in exactly 5 mL of the internal standard solution, add water to make 50 mL, and use these solutions as the sample solution and standard solution. Perform the test with 5 μL each of the sample solution and standard solution as directed under Liquid Chromatography *<2.01>* according to the following conditions, and calculate the ratios, Q_T and Q_S, of the peak area of latamoxef to that of the internal standard.

Amount [μg (potency)] of latamoxef ($C_{20}H_{20}N_6O_9S$)
$= M_S \times Q_T/Q_S \times 1000$

M_S: Amount [mg (potency)] of Latamoxef Ammonium RS taken

Internal standard solution—A solution of *m*-cresol (3 in 200).

Operating conditions—

Detector: An ultraviolet absorption photometer (wavelength: 254 nm).

Column: A stainless steel column 4 mm in inside diameter and 15 cm in length, packed with octadecylsilanized silica gel for liquid chromatography (10 μm in particle diameter).

Column temperature: A constant temperature of about 25°C.

Mobile phase: Dissolve 6.94 g of potassium dihydrogen phosphate, 3.22 g of disodium hydrogen phosphate dodecahydrate and 1.60 g of tetra-*n*-butylammonium bromide in water to make exactly 1000 mL. To 750 mL of this solution add 250 mL of methanol.

Flow rate: Adjust so that the retention time of latamoxef is about 7 minutes.

System suitability—

System performance: When the procedure is run with 5 μL of the standard solution under the above operating conditions, latamoxef and the internal standard are eluted in this order with the resolution between these peaks being not less than 5.

System repeatability: When the test is repeated 6 times with 5 μL of the standard solution under the above operating conditions, the relative standard deviation of the ratios of the peak area of latamoxef to that of the internal standard is not more than 1.0%.

Containers and storage Containers—Tight containers.

Storage—Not exceeding 5°C.

Lauromacrogol

ラウロマクロゴール

Lauromacrogol is a polyoxyethylene ether prepared by the polymerization of ethylene oxide with laury alcohol.

Description Lauromacrogol is a colorless or light yellow, clear liquid or a white, petrolatum-like or waxy solid. It has a characteristic odor, and a somewhat bitter and slightly irritative taste.

It is very soluble in ethanol (95) and in diethyl ether.

It is freely soluble or dispersed as fine oily drops in water.

Identification **(1)** Shake throughly 0.5 g of Lauromacrogol with 10 mL of water and 5 mL of ammonium thiocyanate-cobalt nitrate TS, then shake with 5 mL of 1-butanol, and allow to stand: the 1-butanol layer becomes blue in color.

(2) Warm Lauromacrogol to melt, if necessary, and determine the infrared absorption spectrum as directed in the liquid film method under Infrared Spectrophotometry *<2.25>*: it exhibits absorption at the wave numbers of between 3500 cm^{-1} and 3400 cm^{-1}, and about 2920 cm^{-1}, 1350 cm^{-1}, 1250 cm^{-1}, and 1115 cm^{-1}.

Purity **(1)** Acidity—Transfer 10.0 g of Lauromacrogol into a flask, and add 50 mL of neutralized ethanol. Heat on a water bath nearly to boil, shaking once or twice while heating. Cool, and add 5.3 mL of 0.1 mol/L sodium hydroxide VS and 5 drops of phenolphthalein TS: a red color develops.

(2) Unsaturated compound—Shake 0.5 g of Lauromacrogol with 10 mL of water, and add 5 drops of bromine TS: the color of the solution does not disappear.

Residue on ignition *<2.44>* Not more than 0.2% (1 g).

Containers and storage Containers—Tight containers.

Lenampicillin Hydrochloride

レナンピシリン塩酸塩

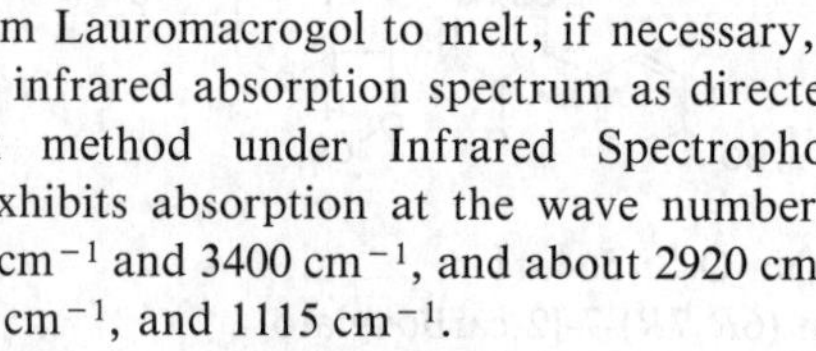

$C_{21}H_{23}N_3O_7S.HCl$: 497.95

5-Methyl-2-oxo[1,3]dioxol-4-ylmethyl (2*S*,5*R*,6*R*)-6-[(2*R*)-2-amino-2-phenylacetylamino]-3,3-dimethyl-7-oxo-4-thia-1-azabicyclo[3.2.0]heptane-2-carboxylate monohydrochloride

[*80734-02-7*]

Lenampicillin Hydrochloride is the hydrochloride of ampicillin methyloxodioxolenylmethyl ester.

It contains not less than 653 μg (potency) and not more than 709 μg (potency) per mg, calculated on the anhydrous basis and corrected by the amount of the residual solvents. The potency of Lenampicillin Hydrochloride is expressed as mass (potency) of ampicillin ($C_{16}H_{19}N_3O_4S$: 349.40).

Description Lenampicillin Hydrochloride occurs as a white to light yellow-white powder.

It is very soluble in water, in methanol and in ethanol (95), and freely soluble in *N*,*N*-dimethylformamide.

Identification **(1)** Determine the infrared absorption spectrum of Lenampicillin Hydrochloride as directed in the potassium chloride disk method under Infrared Spectrophotometry *<2.25>*, and compare the spectrum with the Reference Spectrum or the spectrum of Lenampicillin Hydrochloride RS: both spectra exhibit similar intensities of absorption at the same wave numbers.

(2) To 1 mL of a solution of Lenampicillin Hydrochloride (1 in 100) add 0.5 mL of dilute nitric acid and 1 drop of silver nitrate TS: a white precipitate is formed.

Optical rotation <*2.49*> $[\alpha]_D^{20}$: +174 – +194° (0.2 g calculated on the anhydrous basis and corrected on the amount of residual solvent, ethanol (95), 20 mL, 100 mm).

Purity **(1)** Heavy metals <*1.07*>—Proceed with 2.0 g of Lenampicillin Hydrochloride according to Method 2, and perform the test. Prepare the control solution with 2.0 mL of Standard Lead Solution (not more than 10 ppm).

(2) Arsenic <*1.11*>—Prepare the test solution with 1.0 g of Lenampicillin Hydrochloride according to Method 3, and perform the test (not more than 2 ppm).

(3) Free ampicillin—Weigh accurately about 0.1 g of Lenampicillin Hydrochloridein, dissolve in exactly 10 mL of the internal standard solution, and use this solution as the sample solution. Separately, weigh accurately an amount of Ampicillin RS, equivalent to about 25 mg (potency), and dissolve in water to make exactly 100 mL. Pipet 2 mL of this solution, add exactly 10 mL of the internal standard solution, and use this solution as the standard solution. The sample solution should be used to the following test immediately after the solution is prepared. Perform the test with 10 μL each of the sample solution and standard solution as directed under Liquid Chromatography <*2.01*> according to the following conditions, and calculate the ratios, Q_T and Q_S, of the peak height of ampicillin to that of the internal standard: the amount of ampicillin is not more than 1.0%.

Amount (%) of ampicillin ($C_{16}H_{19}N_3O_4S$)
$$= M_S/M_T \times Q_T/Q_S \times 2$$

M_S: Amount [mg (potency)] of Ampicillin RS taken
M_T: Amount (mg) of Lenampicillin Hydrochloride taken

Internal standard solution—A solution of anhydrous caffeine in the mobile phase (1 in 50,000).

Operating conditions—

Detector: An ultraviolet absorption photometer (wavelength: 230 nm).

Column: A stainless steel column 4 mm in inside diameter and 30 cm in length, packed with octadecylsilanized silica gel for liquid chromatography (10 μm in particle diameter).

Column temperature: A constant temperature of about 25°C.

Mobile phase: Dissolve 1.22 g of potassium dihydrogen phosphate in water to make 900 mL, and add 100 mL of acetonitrile.

Flow rate: Adjust so that the retention time of ampicillin is about 7 minutes.

System suitability—

System performance: When the procedure is run with 10 μL of the standard solution under the above operating conditions, ampicillin and the internal standard are eluted in this order with the resolution between these peaks being not less than 5.

System repeatability: When the test is repeated 6 times with 10 μL of the standard solution under the above operating conditions, the relative standard deviation of the ratios of the peak height of ampicillin to that of the internal standard is not more than 5%.

(4) Penicilloic acid—Weigh accurately about 0.1 g of Lenampicillin Hydrochloride, dissolve in water to make exactly 100 mL, and use this solution as the sample solution. Pipet 10 mL of the sample solution, add 10 mL of potassium hydrogen phthalate buffer solution (pH 4.6) and exactly 10 mL of 0.005 mol/L iodine VS, allow to stand for exactly 15 minutes while protecting from exposure to light, and titrate <*2.50*> with 0.01 mol/L sodium thiosulfate VS (indicator: 1 mL of starch TS). Perform a blank determination in the same manner, and make any necessary correction: the amount of penicilloic acid ($C_{16}H_{21}N_3O_5S$: 367.42) is not more than 3.0%.

Each mL of 0.01 mol/L sodium thiosulfate VS
= 0.45 mg of $C_{16}H_{21}N_3O_5S$

(5) Residual solvent <*2.46*>—Weigh accurately about 0.25 g of Lenampicillin Hydrochloride, dissolve in exactly 1 mL of the internal standard solution, add *N*,*N*-dimethylformamide to make 5 mL, and use this solution as the sample solution. Separately, weigh accurately about 80 mg of 2-propanol and about 0.12 g of ethyl acetate, and add *N*,*N*-dimethylformamide to make exactly 100 mL. Pipet 1 mL and 3 mL of this solution, add exactly 1 mL each of the internal standard solution, add *N*,*N*-dimethylformamide to make 5 mL, and use these solutions as the standard solution (1) and the standard solution (2), respectively. Perform the test with 4 μL each of the sample solution, standard solution (1) and (2) as directed under Gas Chromatography <*2.02*> according to the following conditions, and calculate the ratios, Q_{Ta} and Q_{Tb}, of the peak height of 2-propanol and ethyl acetate to that of the internal standard of the sample solution, the ratios, Q_{Sa1} and Q_{Sb1}, of the peak height of 2-propanol and ethyl acetate to that of the internal standard of the standard solution (1) and the ratios, Q_{Sa2} and Q_{Sb2}, of the peak height of 2-propanol and ethyl acetate to that of the internal standard of the standard solution (2). Calculate the amounts of 2-propanol and ethyl acetate by the following equations: not more than 0.7% and not more than 1.7%, respectively.

Amount (%) of 2-propanol
$$= M_{Sa}/M_T \times (2Q_{Ta} - 3Q_{Sa1} + Q_{Sa2})/(Q_{Sa2} - Q_{Sa1})$$

Amount (%) of ethyl acetate
$$= M_{Sb}/M_T \times (2Q_{Tb} - 3Q_{Sb1} + Q_{Sb2})/(Q_{Sb2} - Q_{Sb1})$$

M_{Sa}: Amount (g) of 2-propanol taken
M_{Sb}: Amount (g) of ethyl acetate taken
M_T: Amount (g) of the Lenampicillin Hydrochloride taken

Internal standard solution—A solution of cyclohexane in *N*,*N*-dimethylformamide (1 in 1000).

Operating conditions—

Detector: A hydrogen flame-ionization detector.

Column: A glass column 3 mm in inside diameter and 3 m in length, packed with siliceous earth for gas chromatography (180 – 250 μm in particle diameter) coated with tetrakishydroxypropylethylenediamine for gas chromatography at the ratio of 10 to 15%.

Column temperature: A constant temperature of about 80°C.

Injection port temperature: A constant temperature of about 160°C.

Carrier gas: Nitrogen.

Flow rate: Adjust so that the retention time of the internal standard is about 1 minute.

System suitability—

System performance: When the procedure is run with 4 μL of the standard solution (2) under the above operating conditions, the internal standard, ethyl acetate and 2-propanol are eluted in this order, and the resolution between the peaks of the internal standard and ethyl acetate is not less than 2.0.

System repeatability: When the test is repeated 3 times with 4 μL of the standard solution (2) under the above operating conditions, the relative standard deviation of the ratios of the peak height of ethyl acetate to that of the internal standard is not more than 5.0%.

Water <*2.48*> Not more than 1.5% (1 g, volumetric titration, direct titration).

Residue on ignition <*2.44*> Not more than 0.2% (1 g).

Assay Weigh accurately an amount of Lenampicillin Hydrochloride and Lenampicillin Hydrochloride RS, equivalent to about 0.1 g (potency), dissolve each in the internal standard solution to make exactly 10 mL, and use these solutions as the sample solution and the standard solution. Perform the test with 5 μL each of the sample solution and standard solution as directed under Liquid Chromatography <*2.01*> according to the following conditions, and calculate the ratios, Q_T and Q_S, of the peak area of lenampicillin to that of the internal standard.

Amount [μg (potency)] of ampicillin ($C_{16}H_{19}N_3O_4S$)
$= M_S \times Q_T/Q_S \times 1000$

M_S: Amount [mg (potency)] of Lenampicillin Hydrochloride RS taken

Internal standard solution—A solution of ethyl aminobenzoate in the mobile phase (1 in 4000).

Operating conditions—

Detector: An ultraviolet absorption photometer (wavelength: 254 nm).

Column: A stainless steel column 6 mm in inside diameter and 15 cm in length, packed with octadecylsilanized silica gel for liquid chromatography (5 μm in particle diameter).

Column temperature: A constant temperature of about 25°C.

Mobile phase: Dissolve 9.53 g of potassium dihydrogen phosphate in water to make exactly 700 mL, and add acetonitrile to make exactly 1000 mL.

Flow rate: Adjust so that the retention time of lenampicillin is about 6 minutes.

System suitability—

System performance: When the procedure is run with 5 μL of the standard solution under the above operating conditions, lenampicillin and the internal standard are eluted in this order with the resolution between these peaks being not less than 10.

System repeatability: When the test is repeated 6 times with 5 μL of the standard solution under the above operating conditions, the relative standard deviation of the ratios of the peak area of lenampicillin to that of the internal standard is not more than 1.0%.

Containers and storage Containers—Tight containers.

Lenograstim (Genetical Recombination)

レノグラスチム(遺伝子組換え)

Protein moiety

```
TPLGPASSLP QSFLLKCLEQ VRKIQGDGAA LQEKLCATYK LCHPEELVLL
GHSLGIPWAP LSSCPSQALQ LAGCLSQLHS GLFLYQGLLQ ALEGISPELG
PTLDTLQLDV ADFATTIWQQ MEELGMAPAL QPTQGAMPAF ASAFQRRAGG
VLVASHLQSF LEVSYRVLRH LAQP
```

T133: glycosylation site

Carbohydrate moiety (structure of major glycans)

```
      (NeuAcα2)0,1
              ⁝
              6
NeuAcα2-3Galβ1-3GalNAc
```

$C_{840}H_{1330}N_{222}O_{242}S_8$: 18667.41 (Protein moiety)
[*135968-09-1*]

Lenograstim (Genetical Recombination) is an aqueous solution in which a desired product is a recombinant human granulocyte colony-stimulating factor produced in Chinese hamster ovary cells. It is a glycoprotein (molecular mass: ca. 20,000) consisting of 174 amino acid residues.

It contains not less than 0.40 mg and not more than 0.60 mg of protein per mL, and not less than 1.02×10^8 units per mg of protein.

Description Lenograstim (Genetical Recombination) occurs as a clear and colorless liquid.

Identification **(1)** Use Lenograstim (Genetical Recombination) and Lenograstim RS as the sample solution and the standard solution, respectively. Perform the test with a volume each of the sample solution and standard solution, equivalent to 20 μg of protein, as directed under Liquid Chromatography <*2.01*> according to the following conditions: the retention times of the two peaks of lenograstim in the chromatogram obtained from the sample solution and of those in the chromatogram obtained from the standard solution are the same.

Operating conditions—

Detector: An ultraviolet absorption photometer (wavelength: 215 nm).

Column: A stainless steel column 7.5 mm in inside diameter and 7.5 cm in length, packed with diethylaminoethyl group binding synthetic polymer for liquid chromatography (10 μm in particle diameter).

Column temperature: A constant temperature of about 25°C.

Mobile phase A: 0.02 mol/L tris buffer solution (pH 7.4).

Mobile phase B: 0.02 mol/L tris buffer solution (pH 7.4) containing 0.5 mol/L sodium chloride.

Flowing of mobile phase: Control the gradient by mixing the mobile phases A and B as directed in the following table.

Time after injection of sample (min)	Mobile phase A (vol%)	Mobile phase B (vol%)
0 - 35	100 → 80	0 → 20
35 - 40	80	20

Flow rate: Adjust so that the retention time of the first appeared peak of lenograstim is about 27 minutes.

System suitability—

System performance: When the procedure is run with a volume of the standard solution, equivalent to 20 μg of protein, under the above operating conditions, the resolution between the two peaks of lenograstim is not less than 4.

(2) Desalt 2 mL each of Lenograstim (Genetical Recombination) and Lenograstim RS by a suitable method, and assign them as the desalted sample and the desalted reference standard, respectively. Add the desalted sample and the desalted reference standard in 100 μL each of a mixture of water and 1-propanol (3:2), add 4 mL of urea-EDTA TS, and allow them to stand at 37°C for 18 hours. Then, add 10 μL of 2-mercaptoethanol to them, and allow to stand at 37°C for 4 hours. To these solutions add a solution of 27 mg of iodoacetic acid in 150 μL of sodium hydroxide TS, and react at 37°C for 15 minutes, avoiding exposure to light. Remove the reagents from these reaction solution by a suitable method, and assign obtained these substances as the reduced carboxymethylated sample and the reduced carboxymethylated reference standard. To these substances add 100 μL each of a mixture of water and 1-propanol (3:2), and add 1 mL of 0.05 mol/L ammonium hydrogen carbonate solution. Add 20 μL each of a solution of V8 protease in 0.05 mol/L ammonium hydrogen carbonate solution (1 in 1000), and react at 37°C for 18 hours. To each reaction solution add 50 μL of diluted trifluoroacetic acid (1 in 10) to stop the reaction, and use these solutions as the sample solution and the standard solution, respectively. Perform the test with 100 μL - 150 μL each of the sample solution and standard solution as directed under Liquid Chromatography <*2.01*> according to the following conditions, and compare the chromatograms from these solutions: both chromatograms show the similar peaks at the corresponding retention time.

Operating conditions—

Detector: An ultraviolet absorption photometer (wavelength: 220 nm).

Column: A stainless steel column 4.6 mm in inside diameter and 25 cm in length, packed with octadecylsilanized silica gel for liquid chromatography (5 μm in particle diameter).

Column temperature: A constant temperature of about 25°C.

Mobile phase A: A mixture of water, acetonitrile for liquid chromatography and trifluoroacetic acid (950:50:1).

Mobile phase B: A mixture of acetonitrile for liquid chromatography, water, and trifluoroacetic acid (800:200:1).

Flowing of mobile phase: Control the gradient by mixing the mobile phases A and B as directed in the following table.

Time after injection of sample (min)	Mobile phase A (vol%)	Mobile phase B (vol%)
0 - 120	100 → 20	0 → 80
120 - 140	20 → 0	80 → 100
140 - 150	0	100

Flow rate: Adjust so that the retention time of the first appeared peak is about 33 minutes.

System suitability—

System performance: When the procedure is run with the standard solution under the above operating conditions, the resolution between the first appeared peak and the second appeared peak is not less than 15.

Monosaccharide composition Put exactly 2 mL of Lenograstim (Genetical Recombination) into a precolumn, packed with 0.36 g of octadecylsilanized silica gel for pretreatment, wash the column with 5 mL of a mixture of water, acetonitrile and trifluoroacetic acid (600:400:1), then elute with a mixture of acetonitrile, water and trifluoroacetic acid (800:200:1), and collect exactly 5 mL of the first eluate. Pipet 1.5 mL of the eluate in a test tube, add exactly 20 μL of the internal standard solution, and lyophilize. Dissolve the lyophilized substance in 250 μL of a mixture of methanol and acetyl chloride (9:1), seal the tube, and heat at 90°C for 2 hours. After cooling, open the tube, and dry the content under reduced pressure. To the residue add 200 μL of methanol, and evaporate to dryness under reduced pressure. Dissolve the residue in 200 μL of a solution of pyridine in methanol (1 in 10) and 50 μL of acetic anhydride, stopper the tube tightly, and allow to stand for 10 minutes. Evaporate the solution to dryness at about 50°C under reduced pressure, add 200 μL of methanol to the residue, and evaporate to dryness at 50°C under reduced pressure. To the residue add 50 μL of a mixture of pyridine, 1,1,1,3,3,3-hexamethyldisilazane and chlorotrimethylsilane (10:2:1), stopper tightly, shake vigorously for 30 seconds, and warm at 50°C for 10 minutes. After cooling, add 300 μL of pentane, stir gently, then add 300 μL of water, and stir gently. Separate the upper layer, evaporate to concentrate to about 10 μL under a stream of nitrogen, and use this as the sample solution. Separately, weigh accurately about 54 mg of D-galactose and about 33 mg of *N*-acetylgalactosamine, dissolve them separately in water to make exactly 20 mL each, and use these solutions as D-galactose solution and *N*-acetylgalactosamine solution, respectively. Weigh accurately about 9.3 mg of *N*-acetylneuraminic acid, add exactly 1 mL of the D-galactose solution and exactly 2 mL of the *N*-acetylgalactosamine solution to dissolve, and add water to make exactly 20 mL. Pipet 1 mL of this solution, add exactly 1 mL of the internal standard solution, and freeze-dry 40 μL of this solution. Dissolve the freeze-dried substance in 250 μL of a mixture of methanol and acetyl chloride (9:1), then proceed in the same manner as the sample solution, and use the solution obtained as the monosaccharide standard solution. Perform the test with 2 μL each of the sample solution and the monosaccharide standard solution as directed under Gas Chromatography <*2.02*> according to the following conditions, and calculate the ratios of each peak area of D-galactose, *N*-acetylgalactosamine and *N*-acetylneuraminic acid to that of the internal standard, Q_T and Q_S. Calculate the amount (mol/mol of lenograstim) of each monosaccharide by the following formula: the amounts of D-galactose, *N*-acetylgalactosamine and *N*-acetylneuraminic acid are between 0.7 and 1.2, between 0.7 and 1.2, and between 1.0 and 2.0, respectively.

Amount (mol/mol of lenograstim) of each monosaccharide
$= M/(M_m \times D_S) \times Q_T/Q_S \times 18{,}667/C \times 5/3$

M: Amount (mg) of each monosaccharide taken
M_m: Molecular mass of each monosaccharide
D-galactose: 180.16
N-acetylgalactosamine: 221.21
N-acetylneuraminic acid: 309.27
D_S: Dilution rate of each monosaccharide
D-galactose: 20,000

N-acetylgalactosamine and: 10,000
N-acetylneuraminic acid: 1000
C: Protein concentration (mg/mL) of Lenograstim (Genetical Recombination)
18,667: Molecular mass of protein moiety of lenograstim

Internal standard solution—Dissolve 48 mg of myoinositol in water to make 50 mL. To 1 mL of this solution add water to make 20 mL.

Operating conditions—

Detector: A hydrogen flame-ionization detector.

Column: A fused silica column 0.25 mm in inside diameter and 30 m in length, coated the inside surface with 7% cyanopropyl-7% phenyl-methyl silicon polymer for gas chromatography 0.25 μm in thickness.

Column temperature: Rise the temperature at a rate of 10°C per minute from 110°C to 185°C, then at a rate of 2°C per minute to 210°C, and to 260°C at a rate of 8°C per minute, and maintain 260°C for 15 minutes.

Carrier gas: Helium.

Flow rate: Adjust so that the retention time of the internal standard is about 24 minutes.

System suitability—

System performance: When the procedure is run with 2 μL of the monosaccharide standard solution under the above operating conditions, D-galactose, the internal standard, *N*-acetylgalactosamine and *N*-acetylneuraminic acid are eluted in this order, and the resolution between the peaks of the internal standard and *N*-acetylgalactosamine is not less than 10.

pH <*2.54*> 7.7 - 8.3

Purity **(1)** Related substances—Perform the test with a volume of Lenograstim (Genetical Recombination), equivalent to 30 μg of protein, as directed under Liquid Chromatography <*2.01*> according to the following conditions. Determine each peak area by the automatic integration method, and calculate the amount of these peaks by the area percentage method excluding the area of the solvent peak: the total amount of the peaks other than lenograstim is not more than 1.0%.

Operating conditions—

Detector: An ultraviolet absorption photometer (wavelength: 215 nm).

Column: A stainless steel column 7.5 mm in inside diameter and 60 cm in length, packed with porous silica gel for liquid chromatography (10 μm in particle diameter).

Column temperature: A constant temperature of about 25°C.

Mobile phase: Dissolve 1.4 g of anhydrous disodium hydrogen phosphate and 5.8 g of sodium chloride in water to make 1000 mL (Solution A). Separately, dissolve 1.6 g of sodium dihydrogen phosphate dihydrate and 5.8 g of sodium chloride in water to make 1000 mL (Solution B). Adjust the pH of Solution A to 7.4 with Solution B.

Flow rate: Adjust so that the retention time of lenograstim is about 21 minutes.

Time span of measurement: About 2 times as long as the retention time of lenograstim.

System suitability—

Test for required detectability: When the procedure is run with 60 μL of diluted Lenograstim RS with the solvent of Lenograstim (Genetical Recombination) containing 0.1 vol% polysorbate 20 (1 in 500) under the above operating conditions, the peak of lenograstim is detectable.

System performance: When the procedure is run using Lenograstim RS under the above operating conditions, the number of theoretical plates of the peak of lenograstim is not less than 2700.

(2) Host cell proteins—Being specified separately when the drug is granted approval based on the Law.

(3) Host cell DNA—Being specified separately when the drug is granted approval based on the Law.

Assay **(1)** Protein—Use Lenograstim (Genetical Recombination) and Lenograstim RS as the sample solution and the standard solution, respectively. Perform the test with exactly 30 μL each of the sample solution and standard solution as directed under Liquid Chromatography <*2.01*> according to the following conditions, and determine the peak areas, A_T and A_S, of lenograstim in each solution.

Amount (mg) of protein in 1 mL of Lenograstim (Genetical Recombination)
$= C_S \times A_T/A_S$

C_S: Concentration (mg/mL) of protein in Lenograstim RS

Operating conditions—

Detector: An ultraviolet absorption photometer (wavelength: 220 nm).

Column: A stainless steel column 4.6 mm in inside diameter and 25 cm in length, packed with octadecylsilanized silica gel for liquid chromatography (5 μm in particle diameter).

Column temperature: A constant temperature of about 25°C.

Mobile phase A: A mixture of water, acetonitrile for liquid chromatography and trifluoroacetic acid (600:400:1).

Mobile phase B: A mixture of acetonitrile for liquid chromatography, water and trifluoroacetic acid (800:200:1).

Flowing of mobile phase: Control the gradient by mixing the mobile phases A and B as directed in the following table.

Time after injection of sample (min)	Mobile phase A (vol%)	Mobile phase B (vol%)
0 - 40	80 → 30	20 → 70

Flow rate: Adjust so that the retention time of lenograstim is about 35 minutes.

System suitability—

System performance: When the procedure is run with 30 μL of the standard solution under the above operating conditions, the number of theoretical plates of the peak of lenograstim is not less than 2900.

System repeatability: When the test is repeated 6 times with 30 μL of the standard solution under the above operating conditions, the relative standard deviation of the peak area of lenograstim is not more than 4.0%.

(2) Specific activity—Dilute Lenograstim (Genetical Recombination) with FBS-IMDM so that each mL contains an estimate amount of 7.69 units, 10.0 units and 13.0 units, and name them as the sample solution (1), the sample solution (2) and the sample solution (3), respectively. Separately, dilute Lenograstim RS with FBS-IMDM so that each mL contains 7.69 units, 10.0 units and 13.0 units, and name them as the standard solution (1), the standard solution (2) and the standard solution (3), respectively. Put exactly 100 μL each of the sample solutions and standard solutions in wells of a sterile disposable multiple well plate, add 50 μL each of NFS-60 cell suspension (prepared by adding FBS-IMDM so the each mL contains about 5×10^5 cells) to each well and mix to make homogenize, and place the plate in a CO_2 incubator at 37°C. After incubation for 22 hours, add 15 μL of resazurin solution to each well, and determine the absorbances at 570 nm, A_{T1} and A_{S1}, and at 600 nm, A_{T2} and A_{S2}. From the reaction values at each concentration of the standard solution and sample solution [deference of absorbance ($A_{S1} - A_{S2}$ and $A_{T1} - A_{T2}$)], determine the rate of potency (Pr) of the sample solution to the standard solution by the parallel assay, and calculate the potency (unit) per 1 mg of protein of Lenograstim (Genetical Recombination).

$Pr = \text{anti} \ln (M)$
$M = (P_T - P_S)/\text{db}$
$P_T = T_1 + T_2 + T_3$
$P_S = S_1 + S_2 + S_3$
$\text{b} = H_L(L_S + L_T)/\text{Inh}$
$H_L = 12\text{n}/(\text{d}^3 - \text{d})$
$L_S = 1S_1 + 2S_2 + 3S_3 - 1/2(\text{d} + 1)P_S$
$L_T = 1T_1 + 2T_2 + 3T_3 - 1/2(\text{d} + 1)P_T$
d = 3
I = ln 1.3
n = 3
h = 2
T_1: Mean of reaction values of the sample solution (1)
T_2: Mean of reaction values of the sample solution (2)
T_3: Mean of reaction values of the sample solution (3)
S_1: Mean of reaction values of the standard solution (1)
S_2: Mean of reaction values of the standard solution (2)
S_3: Mean of reaction values of the standard solution (3)

Specific activity (unit/mg of protein) of lenograstim
$= S \times Pr \times D_T/D_S/C$

S: Potency (unit/mL) of Lenograstim RS
D_T: Dilution rate of the sample solution (3)
D_S: Dilution rate of the standard solution (3)
C: Concentration (mg/mL) of protein of sample

Containers and storage Containers—Tight containers.
Storage—At a temperature not exceeding −20°C.

L-Leucine

L-ロイシン

H_3C CO_2H CH_3 H NH_2

$C_6H_{13}NO_2$: 131.17
(2*S*)-2-Amino-4-methylpentanoic acid
[*61-90-5*]

L-Leucine, when dried, contains not less than 98.5% of L-leucine ($C_6H_{13}NO_2$).

Description L-Leucine occurs as white, crystals or crystalline powder. It is odorless or has a faint characteristic odor, and has a slightly bitter taste.

It is freely soluble in formic acid, sparingly soluble in water, and practically insoluble in ethanol (95).

It dissolves in dilute hydrochloric acid.

Identification Determine the infrared absorption spectrum of L-Leucine, previously dried, as directed in the potassium bromide disk method under Infrared Spectrophotometry <*2.25*>, and compare the spectrum with the Reference Spectrum: both spectra exhibit similar intensities of absorption at the same wave numbers.

Optical rotation <*2.49*> $[\alpha]_D^{20}$: +14.5 – +16.0° (after drying, 1 g, 6 mol/L hydrochloric acid TS, 25 mL, 100 mm).

pH <*2.54*> Dissolve 1.0 g of L-Leucine in 100 mL of water: the pH of this solution is between 5.5 and 6.5.

Purity **(1)** Clarity and color of solution—Dissolve 0.5 g of L-Leucine in 10 mL of 1 mol/L hydrochloric acid TS: the solution is clear and colorless.

(2) Chloride <*1.03*>—Dissolve 0.5 g of L-Leucine in 40 mL of water and 6 mL of dilute nitric acid, and add water to make 50 mL. Perform the test using this solution as the test solution. Prepare the control solution with 0.30 mL of 0.01 mol/L hydrochloric acid VS (not more than 0.021%).

(3) Sulfate <*1.14*>—Dissolve 0.6 g of L-Leucine in 40 mL of water and 1 mL of dilute hydrochloric acid, and add water to make 50 mL. Perform the test using this solution as the test solution. Prepare the control solution with 0.35 mL of 0.005 mol/L sulfuric acid VS (not more than 0.028%).

(4) Ammonium <*1.02*>—Perform the test with 0.25 g of L-Leucine. Prepare the control solution with 5.0 mL of Standard Ammonium Solution (not more than 0.02%).

(5) Heavy metals <*1.07*>—Proceed with 1.0 g of L-Leucine according to Method 4, and perform the test. Prepare the control solution with 2.0 mL of Standard Lead Solution (not more than 20 ppm).

(6) Arsenic <*1.11*>—Prepare the test solution with 1.0 g of L-Leucine according to Method 2, and perform the test (not more than 2 ppm).

(7) Related substances—Dissolve 0.10 g of L-Leucine in water by warming, after cooling, add water to make 25 mL, and use this solution as the sample solution. Pipet 1 mL of the sample solution, and add water to make exactly 50 mL. Pipet 5 mL of this solution, add water to make exactly 20 mL, and use this solution as the standard solution. Perform the test with these solutions as directed under Thin-layer Chromatography <*2.03*>. Spot 5 μL each of the sample solution and standard solution on a plate of silica gel for thin-layer chromatography. Develop the plate with a mixture of 1-butanol, water and acetic acid (100) (3:1:1) to a distance of about 10 cm, and dry the plate at 80°C for 30 minutes. Spray evenly a solution of ninhydrin in acetone (1 in 50) on the plate, and heat the plate at 80°C for 5 minutes: the spots other than the principal spot obtained from the sample solution are not more intense than the spot from the standard solution.

Loss on drying <*2.41*> Not more than 0.30% (1 g, 105°C, 3 hours).

Residue on ignition <*2.44*> Not more than 0.1% (1 g).

Assay Weigh accurately about 0.13 g of L-Leucine, previously dried, and dissolve in 3 mL of formic acid, add 50 mL of acetic acid (100), and titrate <*2.50*> with 0.1 mol/L perchloric acid VS (potentiometric titration). Perform a blank determination in the same manner, and make any necessary correction.

Each mL of 0.1 mol/L perchloric acid VS
$= 13.12$ mg of $C_6H_{13}NO_2$

Containers and storage Containers—Well-closed containers.

Leuprorelin Acetate

リュープロレリン酢酸塩

5-Oxo-Pro-His-Trp-Ser-Tyr-D-Leu-Leu-Arg-Pro-NH-CH$_2$CH$_3$ • H_3C-CO_2H

$C_{59}H_{84}N_{16}O_{12}.C_2H_4O_2$: 1269.45
5-Oxo-L-prolyl-L-histidyl-L-tryptophyl-L-seryl-L-tyrosyl-D-leucyl-L-leucyl-L-arginyl-*N*-ethyl-L-prolinamide monoacetate
[*74381-53-6*]

Leuprorelin Acetate contains not less than 96.0% and not more than 102.0% of leuprorelin ($C_{59}H_{84}N_{16}O_{12}$: 1209.40), calculated on the anhydrous and residual acetic acid-free basis.

Description Leuprorelin Acetate occurs as a white to yellowish white powder.

It is very soluble in water and in acetic acid (100), freely soluble in methanol, and sparingly soluble in ethanol (99.5).

It is hygroscopic.

Identification Determine the infrared absorption spectrum of Leuprorelin Acetate as directed in the potassium bromide disk method under Infrared Spectrophotometry <*2.25*>, and compare the spectrum with the Reference Spectrum or the spectrum of Leuprorelin Acetate RS: both spectra exhibit similar intensities of absorption at the same wave numbers.

Optical rotation <*2.49*> $[\alpha]_D^{20}$: −38 − −41° (0.25 g calculated on the anhydrous and residual acetic acid-free basis, diluted acetic acid (100) (1 in 100), 25 mL, 100 mm).

pH <*2.54*> The pH of a solution of 0.10 g of Leuprorelin Acetate in 10 mL of water is 5.5 to 7.5.

Constituent amino acids When hydrolyzed by Method 1 described in "1. Hydrolysis of Protein and Peptide" and performed the test by Method 1 described in "2. Methodologies of Amino Acid Analysis" under Amino Acid Analysis of Proteins <*2.04*>, histidine, glutamic acid, proline, tyrosine and arginine is 1 and leucine is 2, respectively.

Procedure

(i) Hydrolysis Weigh accurately about 50 mg of Leuprorelin Acetate, and dissolve in 1 mL of water. Put 0.1 mL of this solution in a test tube for hydrolysis, freeze-dry the content, and add 2 mL of a solution of phenol in 6 mol/L hydrochloric acid (1 in 200). Freeze the solution, seal the tube in vacuum, and heat the tube at 110°C for 24 hours. After cooling, open the tube, take out 0.1 mL of the hydrolyzate, add 1 mL of water, and freeze-dry. Dissolve the residue in 7.8 mL of diluting solution, and use this solution as the sample solution. Separately, weigh exactly 0.45 mg of L-alanine, 0.66 mg of L-aspartic acid, 1.05 mg of L-arginine hydrochloride, 0.74 mg of L-glutamic acid, 0.38 mg of glycine, 1.05 mg of L-histidine hydrochloride monohydrate, 0.66 mg of L-isoleucine, 0.66 mg of L-leucine, 0.58 mg of L-proline, 0.53 mg of L-serine, 0.60 mg of L-threonine and 0.91 mg of L-tyrosine, dissolve in diluting solution to make exactly 100 mL, and use this solution as the standard solution (1). Separately, dissolve 1 mg of L-tryptophan and 0.4 mg of ethylamine hydrochloride in diluting solution to make 100 mL, and use this solution as the standard solution (2).

(ii) Amino acid analysis Perform the test with exactly 100 μL each of the sample solution and the standard solutions (1) and (2) as directed under Liquid Chromatography <*2.01*> according to the following conditions: the peaks of histidine, glutamic acid, leucine, proline, tyrosine, arginine, serine and tryptophan appear on the chromatogram obtained from the sample solution. Apart from this, calculate the molar content of each constituent amino acid in 1 mL of the sample solution from the peak area of each amino acid obtained from the sample solution and standard solution (1), and further calculate the number of the constituent amino acids assuming that the sum of each molar content of histidine, glutamic acid, leucine, proline, tyrosine and arginine in 1 mole of leuprorelin acetate is 7.

Diluting solution: Dissolve 6.29 g of lithium hydroxide monohydrate and 10.51 g of citric acid monohydrate in water to make 1000 mL, and adjust to pH 2.2 with hydrochloric acid.

Operating conditions—

Detector: A visible spectrophotometer (wavelength: 440 nm and 570 nm).

Column: A stainless steel column 4.6 mm in inside diameter and 6 cm in length, packed with strongly acidic ion-exchange resin (Na type) for liquid chromatography (3 μm in particle diameter).

Column temperature: Maintain a constant temperature of about 58°C for 18 minutes after injection, then maintain a constant temperature of about 70°C for a further 20 minutes.

Reaction vessel temperature: A constant temperature of about 135°C.

Mobile phase: Prepare the mobile phases A, B, C, D and E according to the following table, then add 0.1 mL of caprylic acid to each mobile phase.

	Mobile phase A	Mobile phase B	Mobile phase C	Mobile phase D	Mobile phase E
Citric acid monohydrate	19.80 g	22.00 g	12.80 g	6.10 g	—
Trisodium citrate dihydrate	6.19 g	7.74 g	13.31 g	26.67 g	—
Sodium chloride	5.66 g	7.07 g	3.74 g	54.35 g	—
Sodium hydroxide	—	—	—	—	8.00 g
Ethanol (99.5)	130 mL	20.0 mL	4.0 mL	—	100 mL
Thiodiglycol	5.0 mL	5.0 mL	5.0 mL	—	—
Benzyl alcohol	—	—	—	5.0 mL	—
Lauromacrogol solution (1 in 4)	4.0 mL	4.0 mL	4.0 mL	4.0 mL	4.0 mL
Water	a sufficient amount	a sufficient amount	a sufficient amount	a sufficient amount	a sufficient amount
Total amount	1000 mL	1000 mL	1000 mL	1000 mL	1000 mL

Flowing of mobile phase: Control the gradient by mixing the mobile phases A, B, C, D and E as directed in the following table.

Time after injection of sample (min)	Mobile phase A (vol%)	Mobile phase B (vol%)	Mobile phase C (vol%)	Mobile phase D (vol%)	Mobile phase E (vol%)
0 – 1.6	100	0	0	0	0
1.6 – 4.5	0	100	0	0	0
4.5 – 13.5	0	0	100	0	0
13.5 – 27.0	0	0	0	100	0
27.0 – 33.0	0	0	0	0	100

Reaction reagent: Dissolve an appropriate amount of lithium acetate dihydrate, acetic acid (100) and 1-methoxy-2-propanol in water to make 1000 mL, and use this solution as solution A. Separately, dissolve an appropriate amount of ninhydrin and sodium borohydride in 1-methoxy-2-propanol to make 1000 mL, and use this solution as solution B. Mix equal parts of solutions A and B before use.

Flow rate of mobile phase: About 0.40 mL per minute.

Flow rate of reaction reagent: About 0.35 mL per minute.

System suitability—

System performance: When the procedure is run with 100 μL of the standard solution (1) under the above operating conditions, the resolutions between the peaks of threonine and serine, glycine and alanine, and isoleucine and leucine are not less than 1.2, respectively.

System repeatability: When the test is repeated 5 times with 100 μL of the standard solution (1) under the above operating conditions, the relative standard deviation of the peak area of arginine, aspartic acid, proline and serine is not more than 4.0%.

Purity Related substances—Dissolve 0.10 g of Leuprorelin Acetate in the mobile phase to make 100 mL, and use this solution as the sample solution. Pipet 1 mL of the sample solution, add the mobile phase to make exactly 100 mL, and use this solution as the standard solution. Perform the test with exactly 20 μL each of the sample solution and standard solution as directed under Liquid Chromatography <2.01> according to the following conditions, and determine each peak area by the automatic integration method: the area of the peaks, having the relative retention time of about 0.65, about 0.77, about 0.78 and about 0.90 to leuprorelin, obtained from the sample solution is not larger than 1/2 times the peak area of leuprorelin from the standard solution, and the total area of the peaks other than leuprorelin from the sample solution is not larger than 2 times the peak area of leuprorelin from the standard solution.

Operating conditions—

Detector, column, column temperature, mobile phase, and flow rate: Proceed as directed in the operating conditions in the Assay.

Time span of measurement: About 2 times as long as the retention time of leuprorelin, beginning after the solvent peak.

System suitability—

System performance and system repeatability: Proceed as directed in the system suitability in the Assay.

Test for required detectability: To exactly 1 mL of the standard solution add the mobile phase to make exactly 20 mL. Confirm that the peak area of leuprorelin obtained with 20 μL of this solution is equivalent to 3.5 to 6.5% of that with 20 μL of the standard solution.

Water <2.48> Not more than 5.0% (0.1 g, coulometric titration).

Residue on ignition <2.44> Not more than 0.2% (0.5 g).

Acetic acid Weigh accurately about 0.1 g of Leuprorelin Acetate, dissolve in the mobile phase to make exactly 10 mL, and use this solution as the sample solution. Separately, weigh accurately about 0.1 g of acetic acid (100), add the mobile phase to make exactly 100 mL, and use this solution as the standard solution. Perform the test with exactly 10 μL each of the sample solution and standard solution as directed under Liquid Chromatography <2.01> according to the following conditions. Determine the peak areas, A_T and A_S, of acetic acid in each solution, and calculate the amount of acetic acid by the following equation: 4.7 – 8.0%.

$$\text{Amount (\%) of acetic acid} = M_S/M_T \times A_T/A_S \times 10$$

M_S: Amount (g) of acetic acid (100) taken

M_T: Amount (g) of Leuprorelin Acetate taken

Operating conditions—

Detector: An ultraviolet absorption photometer (wavelength: 210 nm).

Column: A stainless steel column 4.6 mm in inside diameter and 25 cm in length, packed with octadecylsilanized silica gel for liquid chromatography (5 μm in particle diameter).

Column temperature: A constant temperature of about 25°C.

Mobile phase: To 0.7 mL of phosphoric acid add water to make 1000 mL, and adjust to pH 3.0 with a solution of sodium hydroxide (21 in 50). To 950 mL of this solution add 50 mL of methanol.

Flow rate: Adjust so that the retention time of acetic acid is 3 to 4 minutes.

System suitability—

System performance: When the procedure is run with 10 μL of the standard solution under the above operating conditions, the symmetry factor of the peak of acetic acid is not more than 1.5.

System repeatability: When the test is repeated 6 times with 10 μL of the standard solution under the above operating conditions, the relative standard deviation of the peak area of acetic acid is not more than 2.0%.

Assay Weigh accurately about 0.1 g each of Leuprorelin Acetate and Leuprorelin Acetate RS (separately determine the water <2.48> and acetic acid in the same manner as Leuprorelin Acetate), dissolve separately in the mobile phase to make exactly 100 mL. To exactly 5 mL each of these solutions add the mobile phase to make them exactly 100 mL, and use so obtained solutions as the sample solution and the standard solution, respectively. Perform the test with exactly 20 μL each of the sample solution and standard solution as directed under Liquid Chromatography <2.01> according to the following conditions, and determine the peak areas, A_T and A_S, of leuprorelin in each solution.

$$\text{Amount (mg) of leuprorelin } (C_{59}H_{84}N_{16}O_{12}) = M_S \times A_T/A_S$$

M_S: Amount (mg) of Leuprorelin Acetate RS taken, calculated on the anhydrous and de-acetic acid basis

Operating conditions—

Detector: An ultraviolet absorption photometer (wavelength: 220 nm).

Column: A stainless steel column 4.6 mm in inside diameter and 10 cm in length, packed with octadecylsilanized silica gel for liquid chromatography (3 μm in particle diameter).

Column temperature: A constant temperature of about 25°C.

Mobile phase: Dissolve 15.2 g of triethylamine in 800 mL of water, adjust to pH 3.0 with phosphoric acid, and add water to make 1000 mL. To 850 mL of this solution add 150 mL of a mixture of acetonitrile and 1-propanol (3:2).

Flow rate: Adjust so that the retention time of leuprorelin is 41 to 49 minutes (1.0 - 1.5 mL per minute).

System suitability—

System performance: Dissolve about 0.1 g of Leuprorelin Acetate RS in 100 mL of the mobile phase. To 5 mL of this solution add water to make 50 mL. To 5 mL of this solution add 0.1 mL of sodium hydroxide TS, stopper the vessel, shake vigorously, then heat at 100°C for 60 minutes. After cooling, add 50 μL of 1 mol/L phosphoric acid solution, and shake vigorously. When the procedure is run with 20 μL of this solution under the above operating conditions, a peak having the relative retention time of about 0.90 to leuprorelin and leuprorelin are eluted in this order with the resolution between these peaks being not less than 1.5.

System repeatability: When the test is repeated 5 times with 20 μL of the standard solution under the above operating conditions, the relative standard deviation of the peak area of leuprorelin is not more than 1.5%.

Containers and storage Containers—Hermetic containers.

Levallorphan Tartrate

レバロルファン酒石酸塩

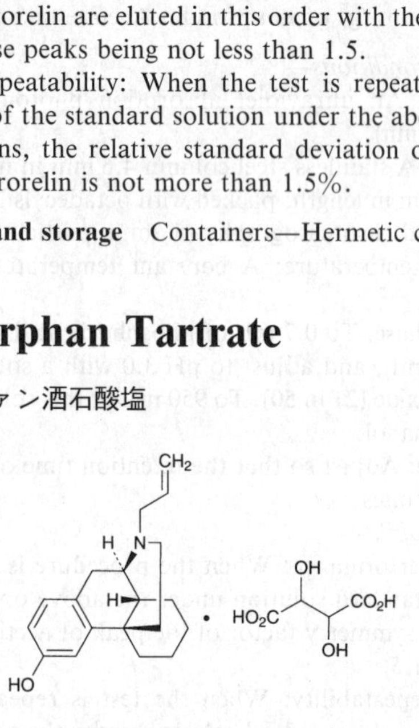

$C_{19}H_{25}NO.C_4H_6O_6$: 433.49

17-Allylmorphinan-3-ol monotartrate

[*71-82-9*]

Levallorphan Tartrate, when dried, contains not less than 98.5% of levallorphan tartrate ($C_{19}H_{25}NO.C_4H_6O_6$).

Description Levallorphan Tartrate occurs as a white to pale yellow crystalline powder. It is odorless.

It is soluble in water and in acetic acid (100), sparingly soluble in ethanol (95), and practically insoluble in diethyl ether.

Identification **(1)** Determine the absorption spectrum of a solution of Levallorphan Tartrate in 0.01 mol/L hydrochloric acid TS (1 in 10,000) as directed under Ultraviolet-visible Spectrophotometry <*2.24*>, and compare the spectrum with the Reference Spectrum: both spectra exhibit similar intensities of absorption at the same wavelengths.

(2) Determine the infrared absorption spectrum of Levallorphan Tartrate, previously dried, as directed in the potassium bromide disk method under Infrared Spectrophotometry <*2.25*>, and compare the spectrum with the Reference Spectrum: both spectra exhibit similar intensities of absorption at the same wave numbers.

(3) A solution of Levallorphan Tartrate (1 in 30) responds to Qualitative Tests <*1.09*> (1) and (2) for tartrate.

Optical rotation <*2.49*> $[\alpha]_D^{20}$: $-37.0 - -39.2°$ (after drying, 0.2 g, water, 10 mL, 100 mm).

pH <*2.54*> Dissolve 0.2 g of Levallorphan Tartrate in 20 mL of water: the pH of this solution is between 3.3 and 3.8.

Melting point <*2.60*> 174 - 178°C

Purity **(1)** Clarity and color of solution—Dissolve 0.2 g of Levallorphan Tartrate in 10 mL of water: the solution is clear and colorless.

(2) Heavy metals <*1.07*>—Proceed with 1.0 g of Levallorphan Tartrate according to Method 4, and perform the test. Prepare the control solution with 2.0 mL of Standard Lead Solution (not more than 20 ppm).

(3) Related substances—Dissolve 0.20 g of Levallorphan Tartrate in 10 mL of water, and use this solution as the sample solution. Pipet 1 mL of the sample solution, add water to make exactly 100 mL, and use this solution as the standard solution. Perform the test with these solutions as directed under Thin-layer Chromatography <*2.03*>. Spot 20 μL each of the sample solution and standard solution on a plate of silica gel for thin-layer chromatography. Develop the plate with a mixture of methanol and ammonia TS (200:3) to a distance of about 10 cm, and air-dry the plate. Spray evenly Dragendorff's TS for spraying on the plate: the spots other than the principal spot obtained from the sample solution are not more intense than the spot from the standard solution.

Loss on drying <*2.41*> Not more than 0.5% (1 g, in vacuum, phosphorus (V) oxide, 80°C, 4 hours).

Residue on ignition <*2.44*> Not more than 0.10% (1 g).

Assay Weigh accurately about 0.5 g of Levallorphan Tartrate, previously dried, dissolve in 30 mL of acetic acid (100), and titrate <*2.50*> with 0.1 mol/L perchloric acid VS (indicator: 2 drops of crystal violet TS). Perform a blank determination in the same manner, and make any necessary correction.

Each mL of 0.1 mol/L perchloric acid VS
= 43.35 mg of $C_{19}H_{25}NO.C_4H_6O_6$

Containers and storage Containers—Well-closed containers.

Levallorphan Tartrate Injection

レバロルファン酒石酸塩注射液

Levallorphan Tartrate Injection is an aqueous injection.

It contains not less than 93.0% and not more than 107.0% of the labeled amount of levallorphan tartrate ($C_{19}H_{25}NO.C_4H_6O_6$: 433.49).

Method of preparation Prepare as directed under Injection, with Levallorphan Tartrate.

Description Levallorphan Tartrate Injection is a clear, colorless liquid.

pH: 3.0 - 4.5

Identification Take an exact volume of Levallorphan Tartrate Injection, equivalent to 3 mg of Levallorphan Tartrate, add 5 mL of water and 2 drops of dilute hydrochloric acid, and wash with five 15-mL portions of diethyl ether by a vigorous shaking. Take the water layer, evaporate the diethyl ether remained by warming on a water bath, and after cooling, add 0.01 mol/L hydrochloric acid TS to make 50 mL. Determine the absorption spectrum of this solution as directed under Ultraviolet-visible Spectrophotometry <*2.24*>: it exhibits a maximum between 277 nm and 281 nm.

Bacterial endotoxins *〈4.01〉* Less than 150 EU/mg.

Extractable volume *〈6.05〉* It meets the requirement.

Foreign insoluble matter *〈6.06〉* Perform the test according to Method 1: it meets the requirement.

Insoluble particulate matter *〈6.07〉* It meets the requirement.

Sterility *〈4.06〉* Perform the test according to the Membrane filtration method: it meets the requirement.

Assay Take exactly a volume of Levallorphan Tartrate Injection, equivalent to about 2 mg of levallorphan tartrate ($C_{19}H_{25}NO.C_4H_6O_6$), add exactly 10 mL of the internal standard solution, and use this solution as the sample solution. Separately, weigh accurately about 0.1 g of levallorphan tartrate for assay, previously dried at 80°C for 4 hours on phosphorus (V) oxide under reduced pressure, and dissolve in water to make exactly 100 mL. Pipet 2 mL of this solution, add exactly 10 mL of the internal standard solution, and use this solution as the standard solution. Perform the test with 10 μL each of the sample solution and standard solution as directed under Liquid Chromatography *〈2.01〉* according to the following conditions, and calculate the ratios, Q_T and Q_S, of the peak area of levallorphan to that of the internal standard:

Amount (mg) of levallorphan tartrate ($C_{19}H_{25}NO.C_4H_6O_6$)
$= M_S \times Q_T/Q_S \times 1/50$

M_S: Amount (mg) of levallorphan tartrate for assay taken

Internal standard solution—Dissolve 0.04 g of isobutyl parahydroxybenzoate in 10 mL of ethanol (95), add water to make 100 mL, and to 10 mL of this solution add water to make 100 mL.

Operating conditions—

Detector: An ultraviolet absorption photometer (wavelength: 280 nm).

Column: A stainless steel column 4.6 mm in inside diameter and 15 cm in length, packed with octadecylsilanized silica gel for liquid chromatography (5 μm in particle diameter).

Column temperature: A constant temperature of about 40°C.

Mobile phase: Dissolve 1.0 g of sodium lauryl sulfate in 500 mL of diluted phosphoric acid (1 in 1000), and adjust the pH to 3.0 with sodium hydroxide TS. To 300 mL of this solution add 200 mL of acetonitrile.

Flow rate: Adjust so that the retention time of levallorphan is about 12 minutes.

System suitability—

System performance: When the procedure is run with 10 μL of the standard solution under the above operating conditions, the internal standard and levallorphan are eluted in this order with the resolution between these peaks being not less than 5.

System repeatability: When the test is repeated 6 times with 10 μL of the standard solution under the above operating conditions, the relative standard deviation of the ratios of the peak area of levallorphan to that of the internal standard is not more than 1.0%.

Containers and storage Containers—Hermetic containers.

Levodopa

レボドパ

$C_9H_{11}NO_4$: 197.19
3-Hydroxy-L-tyrosine
[59-92-7]

Levodopa, when dried, contains not less than 98.5% of levodopa ($C_9H_{11}NO_4$).

Description Levodopa occurs as white or slightly grayish white, crystals or crystalline powder. It is odorless.

It is freely soluble in formic acid, slightly soluble in water, and practically insoluble in ethanol (95).

It dissolves in dilute hydrochloric acid.

The pH of a saturated solution of Levodopa is between 5.0 and 6.5.

Melting point: about 275°C (with decomposition).

Identification **(1)** To 5 mL of a solution of Levodopa (1 in 1000) add 1 mL of ninhydrin TS, and heat for 3 minutes in a water bath: a purple color develops.

(2) To 2 mL of a solution of Levodopa (1 in 5000) add 10 mL of 4-aminoantipyrine TS, and shake: a red color develops.

(3) Dissolve 3 mg of Levodopa in 0.001 mol/L hydrochloric acid TS to make 100 mL. Determine the absorption spectrum of the solution as directed under Ultraviolet-visible Spectrophotometry *〈2.24〉*, and compare the spectrum with the Reference Spectrum: both spectra exhibit similar intensities of absorption at the same wavelengths.

Absorbance *〈2.24〉* $E^{1\%}_{1\,cm}$ (280 nm): 136 – 146 (after drying, 30 mg, 0.001 mol/L hydrochloric acid TS, 1000 mL).

Optical rotation *〈2.49〉* $[\alpha]^{20}_D$: $-11.5 - -13.0°$ (after drying, 2.5 g, 1 mol/L hydrochloric acid TS, 50 mL, 100 mm).

Purity **(1)** Clarity and color of solution—Dissolve 1.0 g of Levodopa in 20 mL of 1 mol/L hydrochloric acid TS: the solution is clear and colorless.

(2) Chloride *〈1.03〉*—Dissolve 0.5 g of Levodopa in 6 mL of dilute nitric acid, and add water to make 50 mL. Perform the test using this solution as the test solution. Prepare the control solution with 0.30 mL of 0.01 mol/L hydrochloric acid VS (not more than 0.021%).

(3) Sulfate *〈1.14〉*—Dissolve 0.40 g of Levodopa in 1 mL of dilute hydrochloric acid and 30 mL of water, and add water to make 50 mL. Perform the test using this solution as the test solution. Prepare the control solution with 0.25 mL of 0.005 mol/L sulfuric acid VS (not more than 0.030%).

(4) Heavy metals *〈1.07〉*—Proceed with 1.0 g of Levodopa according to Method 2, and perform the test. Prepare the control solution with 2.0 mL of Standard Lead Solution (not more than 20 ppm).

(5) Arsenic *〈1.11〉*—Dissolve 1.0 g of Levodopa in 5 mL of dilute hydrochloric acid, and perform the test with this solution as the test solution (not more than 2 ppm).

(6) Related substances—Dissolve 0.10 g of Levodopa in 10 mL of sodium disulfite TS, and use this solution as the sample solution. Pipet 1 mL of the sample solution, add sodium disulfite TS to make exactly 25 mL. Pipet 1 mL of this solution, add sodium disulfite TS to make exactly 20 mL, and use this solution as the standard solution. Perform the test with these solutions as directed under Thin-layer Chromatography <*2.03*>. Spot 5 μL each of the sample solution and standard solution on a plate of cellulose for thin-layer chromatography. Develop the plate with a mixture of 1-butanol, water, acetic acid (100) and methanol (10:5:5:1) to a distance of about 10 cm, and air-dry the plate. Spray evenly a solution of ninhydrin in acetone (1 in 50) on the plate and heat the plate at 90°C for 10 minutes: the spots other than the principal spot obtained from the sample solution are not more intense than the spot from the standard solution.

Loss on drying <*2.41*> Not more than 0.30% (1 g, 105°C, 3 hours).

Residue on ignition <*2.44*> Not more than 0.1% (1 g).

Assay Weigh accurately about 0.3 g of Levodopa, previously dried, dissolve in 3 mL of formic acid, add 80 mL of acetic acid (100), and titrate <*2.50*> with 0.1 mol/L perchloric acid VS until the color of the solution changes from purple through blue-green to green (indicator: 3 drops of crystal violet TS). Perform a blank determination in the same manner, and make any necessary correction.

Each mL of 0.1 mol/L perchloric acid VS
= 19.72 mg of $C_9H_{11}NO_4$

Containers and storage Containers—Tight containers.
Storage—Light-resistant.

Levofloxacin Hydrate

レボフロキサシン水和物

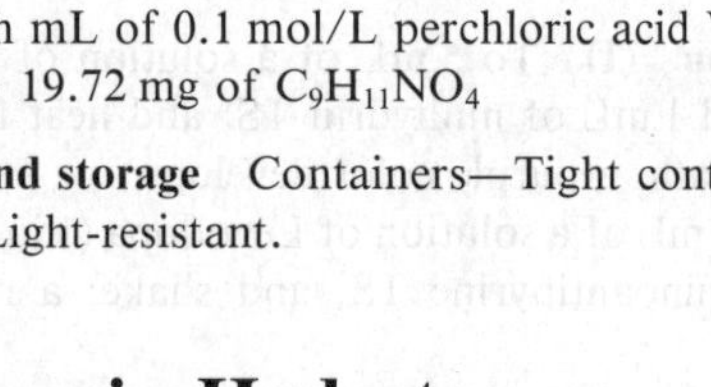

$C_{18}H_{20}FN_3O_4 . \frac{1}{2}H_2O$: 370.38
(3*S*)-9-Fluoro-3-methyl-10-(4-methylpiperazin-1-yl)-7-oxo-2,3-dihydro-7*H*-pyrido[1,2,3-*de*][1,4]benzoxazine-6-carboxylic acid hemihydrate
[*138199-71-0*]

Levofloxacin Hydrate contains not less than 99.0% and not more than 101.0% of levofloxacin ($C_{18}H_{20}FN_3O_4$: 361.37), calculated on the anhydrous basis.

Description Levofloxacin Hydrate occurs as light yellowish white to yellow-white, crystals or crystalline powder.

It is freely soluble in acetic acid (100), sparingly soluble in water and in methanol, and slightly soluble in ethanol (99.5).

It dissolves in 0.1 mol/L hydrochloric acid TS.

It gradually turns dark light yellow-white on exposure to light.

Melting point: about 226°C (with decomposition).

Identification **(1)** Determine the absorption spectrum of a solution of Levofloxacin Hydrate in 0.1 mol/L hydrochloric acid TS (1 in 150,000) as directed under Ultraviolet-visible Spectrophotometry <*2.24*>, and compare the spectrum with the Reference Spectrum: both spectra exhibit similar intensities of absorption at the same wavelengths.

(2) Determine the infrared absorption spectrum of Levofloxacin Hydrate as directed in the potassium bromide disk method under Infrared Spectrophotometry <*2.25*>, and compare the spectrum with the Reference Spectrum: both spectra exhibit similar intensities of absorption at the same wave numbers.

Optical rotation <*2.49*> $[\alpha]_D^{20}$: −92 – −99° (0.1 g calculated on the anhydrous basis, methanol, 10 mL, 100 mm).

Purity **(1)** Heavy metals <*1.07*>—Proceed with 2.0 g of Levofloxacin Hydrate according to Method 4, and perform the test. Prepare the control solution with 2.0 mL of Standard Lead Solution (not more than 10 ppm).

(2) Related substances—Conduct this procedure using light-resistant vessels. Dissolve 50 mg of Levofloxacin Hydrate in 10 mL of a mixture of water and methanol (1:1), and use this solution as the sample solution. Pipet 1 mL of the sample solution, and add a mixture of water and methanol (1:1) to make exactly 10 mL. Pipet 1 mL of this solution, add a mixture of water and methanol (1:1) to make exactly 10 mL, and use this solution as the standard solution. Perform the test with exactly 10 μL each of the sample solution and standard solution as directed under Liquid Chromatography <*2.01*> according to the following conditions. Determine each peak area of both solutions by the automatic integration method: the area of the peak of the enantiomer having the relative retention time of about 1.2 to levofloxacin obtained from the sample solution is not larger than 2/5 times the peak area of levofloxacin from the standard solution, and the area of each peak other than the peaks of levofloxacin and the enantiomer from the sample solution is not larger than 1/5 times the peak area of levofloxacin from the standard solution. Furthermore, the total area of the peaks other than levofloxacin and the peak of the enantiomer from the sample solution is not larger than 3/10 times the peak area of levofloxacin from the standard solution.

Operating conditions—

Detector: An ultraviolet absorption photometer (wavelength: 340 nm).

Column: A stainless steel column 4.6 mm in inside diameter and 15 cm in length, packed with octadecylsilanized silica gel for liquid chromatography (5 μm in particle diameter).

Column temperature: A constant temperature of about 45°C.

Mobile phase: Dissolve 1.76 g of L-valine, 7.71 g of ammonium acetate and 1.25 g of Copper (II) sulfate pentahydrate in water to make 1000 mL. To this solution add 250 mL of methanol.

Flow rate: Adjust so that the retention time of levofloxacin is about 22 minutes.

Time span of measurement: About 2 times as long as the retention time of levofloxacin, beginning after the solvent peak.

System suitability—

Test for required detectability: Pipet 1 mL of the standard solution, and add a mixture of water and methanol (1:1) to make exactly 20 mL. Confirm that the peak area of levofloxacin obtained with 10 μL of this solution is equivalent to 4 to 6% of that with 10 μL of the standard solution.

System performance: Dissolve 10 mg of ofloxacin in 20 mL of a mixture of water and methanol (1:1). To 1 mL of this solution add a mixture of water and methanol (1:1) to make 10 mL. When the procedure is run with 10 μL of this solution under the above operating conditions, the resolution between the peaks of levofloxacin and the enantiomer is not less than 3.

System repeatability: When the test is repeated 6 times with 10 μL of the standard solution under the above operat-

ing conditions, the relative standard deviation of the peak area of levofloxacin is not more than 3.0%.

Water <2.48> 2.1 – 2.7% (0.5 g, volumetric titration, direct titration).

Residue on ignition <2.44> Not more than 0.1% (1 g, platinum crucible).

Assay Weigh accurately about 0.3 g of Levofloxacin Hydrate, dissolve in 100 mL of acetic acid (100), and titrate <2.50> with 0.1 mol/L perchloric acid VS (potentiometric titration). Perform a blank determination in the same manner, and make any necessary correction.

Each mL of 0.1 mol/L perchloric acid VS
$= 36.14$ mg of $C_{18}H_{20}FN_3O_4$

Containers and storage Containers—Tight containers.
Storage—Light-resistant.

Levofloxacin Fine Granules

レボフロキサシン細粒

Levofloxacin Fine Granules contain not less than 93.0% and not more than 107.0% of the labeled amount of levofloxacin ($C_{18}H_{20}FN_3O_4$: 361.37).

Method of preparation Prepare as directed under Granules, with Levofloxacin Hydrate.

Identification To an amount of Levofloxacin Fine Granules, equivalent to 50 mg of levofloxacin ($C_{18}H_{20}FN_3O_4$), add diluted 3 mol/L hydrochloric acid TS (1 in 100) to make 50 mL, and stir for 20 minutes. Filter this solution through a membrane filter with a pore size not exceeding 0.45 μm, discard the first 10 mL of the filtrate, and to 1 mL of the subsequent filtrate add diluted 3 mol/L hydrochloric acid TS (1 in 100) to make 100 mL. Determine the absorption spectrum of this solution as directed under Ultraviolet-visible Spectrophotometry <2.24>: it exhibits maxima between 225 nm and 229 nm and between 292 nm and 296 nm, and a shoulder between 321 nm and 331 nm.

Uniformity of dosage units <6.02> Perform the test according to the following method: the Granules in single-dose packages meet the requirement of the Content uniformity test.

To the total amount of the content of 1 package of Levofloxacin Fine Granules add diluted 3 mol/L hydrochloric acid TS (1 in 100) to make exactly V mL so that each mL contains about 1 mg of levofloxacin ($C_{18}H_{20}FN_3O_4$), and stir for 20 minutes. Filter this solution through a membrane filter with a pore size not exceeding 0.45 μm. Discard the first 10 mL of the filtrate, pipet 1 mL of the subsequent filtrate, add diluted 3 mol/L hydrochloric acid TS (1 in 100) to make exactly 100 mL, and use this solution as the sample solution. Separately, weigh accurately about 25 mg of levofloxacin hydrate for assay (separately determine the water <2.48> in the same manner as Levofloxacin Hydrate), and dissolve in diluted 3 mol/L hydrochloric acid TS (1 in 100) to make exactly 50 mL. Pipet 2 mL of this solution, add diluted 3 mol/L hydrochloric acid TS (1 in 100) to make exactly 100 mL, and use this solution as the standard solution. Determine the absorbances, A_T and A_S, at 327 nm of the sample solution and standard solution as directed under Ultraviolet-visible Spectrophotometry <2.24>.

Amount (mg) of levofloxacin ($C_{18}H_{20}FN_3O_4$)
$= M_S \times A_T/A_S \times V/25$

M_S: Amount (mg) of levofloxacin hydrate for assay taken, calculated on the anhydrous basis

Dissolution <6.10> When the test is performed at 75 revolutions per minute according to the Paddle method, using 900 mL of water as the dissolution medium, the dissolution rate in 90 minutes of Levofloxacin Fine Granules is not less than 70%.

Start the test with an accurately weighed amount of Levofloxacin Fine Granules, equivalent to about 0.1 g of levofloxacin ($C_{18}H_{20}FN_3O_4$), withdraw not less than 20 mL of the medium at the specified minute after starting the test, and filter through a membrane filter with a pore size not exceeding 0.45 μm. Discard not less than 10 mL of the first filtrate, pipet 5 mL of the subsequent filtrate, add water to make exactly 100 mL, and use this solution as the sample solution. Separately, weigh accurately about 28 mg of levofloxacin hydrate for assay (separately determine the water <2.48> in the same manner as Levofloxacin Hydrate), and dissolve in water to make exactly 100 mL. Pipet 2 mL of this solution, add water to make exactly 100 mL, and use this solution as the standard solution. Determine the absorbances, A_T and A_S, at 289 nm of the sample solution and standard solution as directed under Ultraviolet-visible Spectrophotometry <2.24>.

Dissolution rate (%) with respect to the labeled amount of levofloxacin ($C_{18}H_{20}FN_3O_4$)
$= M_S/M_T \times A_T/A_S \times 1/C \times 360$

M_S: Amount (mg) of levofloxacin hydrate for assay taken, calculated on the anhydrous basis
M_T: Amount (g) of Levofloxacin Fine Granules taken
C: Labeled amount (mg) of levofloxacin ($C_{18}H_{20}FN_3O_4$) in 1 g

Assay Weigh accurately an amount of Levofloxacin Fine Granules, powder if necessary, equivalent to about 50 mg of levofloxacin ($C_{18}H_{20}FN_3O_4$), add diluted 3 mol/L hydrochloric acid TS (1 in 100) to make exactly 50 mL, stir for 20 minutes, and filter this solution through a membrane filter with a pore size not exceeding 0.45 μm. Discard the first 10 mL of the filtrate, pipet 5 mL of the subsequent filtrate, add diluted 3 mol/L hydrochloric acid TS (1 in 100) to make exactly 100 mL, and use this solution as the sample solution. Separately, weigh accurately about 50 mg of levofloxacin hydrate for assay (separately determine the water <2.48> in the same manner as Levofloxacin Hydrate), and dissolve in diluted 3 mol/L hydrochloric acid TS (1 in 100) to make exactly 50 mL. Pipet 5 mL of this solution, add diluted 3 mol/L hydrochloric acid TS (1 in 100) to make exactly 100 mL, and use this solution as the standard solution. Perform the test with exactly 10 μL each of the sample solution and standard solution as directed under Liquid Chromatography <2.01> according to the following conditions, and determine the peak areas, A_T and A_S, of levofloxacin in each solution.

Amount (mg) of levofloxacin ($C_{18}H_{20}FN_3O_4$)
$= M_S \times A_T/A_S$

M_S: Amount (mg) of levofloxacin hydrate for assay taken, calculated on the anhydrous basis

Operating conditions—

Detector: An ultraviolet absorption photometer (wavelength: 340 nm).

Column: A stainless steel column 4.6 mm in inside diameter and 15 cm in length, packed with octadecylsilanized silica

gel for liquid chromatography (5 μm in particle diameter).

Column temperature: A constant temperature of about 45°C.

Mobile phase: Dissolve 1.00 g of copper (II) sulfate pentahydrate, 1.41 g of L-valine and 6.17g of ammonium acetate in 800 mL of water, and add 200 mL of methanol.

Flow rate: Adjust so that the retention time of levofloxacin is about 20 minutes.

System suitability—

System performance: Dissolve 10 mg of ofloxacin in 20 mL of diluted 3 mol/L hydrochloric acid TS (1 in 100). To 1 mL of this solution add diluted 3 mol/L hydrochloric acid TS (1 in 100) to make 20 mL. When the procedure is run with 10 μL of this solution under the above operating conditions, levofloxacin and an enantiomer are eluted in this order with the resolution between these peaks being not less than 3.

System repeatability: When the test is repeated 6 times with 10 μL of the standard solution under the above operating conditions, the relative standard deviation of the peak area of levofloxacin is not more than 1.0%.

Containers and storage Containers—Tight containers.
Storage—Light-resistant.

Levofloxacin Injection

レボフロキサシン注射液

Levofloxacin Injection is an aqueous injection.

It contains not less than 95.0% and not more than 105.0% of the labeled amount of levofloxacin ($C_{18}H_{20}FN_3O_4$: 361.37).

Method of preparation Prepare as directed under Injections, with Levofloxacin Hydrate.

Description Levofloxacin Injection is yellow to greenish yellow, clear liquid.

Identification To a volume of Levofloxacin Injection, equivalent to 50 mg of levofloxacin ($C_{18}H_{20}FN_3O_4$), add diluted 1 mol/L hydrochloric acid TS (3 in 100) to make 50 mL. To 1 mL of this solution add diluted 1 mol/L hydrochloric acid TS (3 in 100) to make 100 mL. Determine the absorption spectrum of this solution as directed under Ultraviolet-visible Spectrophotometry *<2.24>*: it exhibits maxima between 225 nm and 229 nm and between 292 nm and 296 nm, and a shoulder between 321 nm and 331 nm.

pH Being specified separately when the drug is granted approval based on the Law.

Bacterial endotoxin *<4.01>* Less than 0.60 EU/mg.

Extractable volume *<6.05>* It meets the requirement.

Foreign insoluble matter *<6.06>* Perform the test according to Method 1: it meets the requirement.

Insoluble particulate matter *<6.07>* It meets the requirement.

Sterility *<4.06>* Perform the test according to the Membrane filtration method: it meets the requirement.

Assay To an exact volume of Levofloxacin Injection, equivalent to about 50 mg of levofloxacin ($C_{18}H_{20}FN_3O_4$), add diluted 1 mol/L hydrochloric acid TS (3 in 100) to make exactly 50 mL. Pipet 5 mL of this solution, add diluted 1 mol/L hydrochloric acid TS (3 in 100) to make exactly 100 mL, and use this solution as the sample solution. Separately, weigh accurately about 50 mg of levofloxacin hydrate for assay (separately determine the water *<2.48>* in the same manner as Levofloxacin Hydrate), and dissolve in diluted 1 mol/L hydrochloric acid TS (3 in 100) to make exactly 50 mL. Pipet 5 mL of this solution, add diluted 1 mol/L hydrochloric acid TS (3 in 100) to make exactly 100 mL, and use this solution as the standard solution. Perform the test with exactly 10 μL each of the sample solution and standard solution as directed under Liquid Chromatography *<2.01>* according to the following conditions, and determine the peak areas, A_T and A_S, of levofloxacin in each solution.

$$\text{Amount (mg) of levofloxacin } (C_{18}H_{20}FN_3O_4) = M_S \times A_T/A_S$$

M_S: Amount (mg) of levofloxacin for assay taken, calculated on the anhydrous basis

Operating conditions—

Detector, column, and column temperature: Proceed as directed in the operating conditions in the Purity (2) under Levofloxacin Hydrate.

Mobile phase: Dissolve 1.00 g of copper (II) sulfate pentahydrate, 1.41 g of L-valine and 6.17 g of ammonium acetate in 800 mL of water, and add 200 mL of methanol.

Flow rate: Adjust so that the retention time of levofloxacin is about 20 minutes.

System suitability—

System performance: Dissolve 10 mg of ofloxacin in 20 mL of diluted 1 mol/L hydrochloric acid TS (3 in 100). To 1 mL of this solution add diluted 1 mol/L hydrochloric acid TS (3 in 100) to make 20 mL. When the procedure is run with 10 μL of this solution under the above operating conditions, levofloxacin and the enantiomer are eluted in this order with the resolution between these peaks being not less than 3.

System repeatability: When the test is repeated 6 times with 10 μL of the standard solution under the above operating conditions, the relative standard deviation of the peak area of levofloxacin is not more than 1.0%.

Containers and storage Containers—Hermetic containers. Plastic containers for aqueous injections may be used.

Levofloxacin Ophthalmic Solution

レボフロキサシン点眼液

Levofloxacin Ophthalmic Solution is an aqueous ophthalmic preparation.

It contains not less than 95.0% and not more than 107.0% of the labeled amount of levofloxacin hydrate ($C_{18}H_{20}FN_3O_4.½H_2O$: 370.38).

Method of preparation Prepare as directed under Ophthalmic Liquids and Solutions, with Levofloxacin Hydrate.

Description Levofloxacin Ophthalmic Solution occurs as a clear, pale yellow to yellow liquid.

Identification (1) To a volume of Levofloxacin Ophthalmic Solution, equivalent to 5 mg of Levofloxacin Hydrate, add 0.01 mol/L hydrochloric acid TS to make 100 mL. To 2 mL of this solution add 0.01 mol/L hydrochloric acid TS to make 20 mL, and use this solution as the sample solution. Determine the absorption spectrum of the sample solution as directed under Ultraviolet-visible Spectrophotometry *<2.24>*: it exhibits maxima between 225 nm and 229 nm, and between 292 nm and 296 nm.

(2) To a volume of Levofloxacin Ophthalmic Solution, equivalent to 5 mg of Levofloxacin Hydrate, add a mixture of water and methanol (1:1) to make 5 mL, and use this solution as the sample solution. Separately, dissolve 10 mg of levofloxacin hydrate for assay in 10 mL of a mixture of water and methanol (1:1), and use this solution as the standard solution. Perform the test with 10 μL each of the sample solution and standard solution as directed under Liquid Chromatography <*2.01*> according to the following conditions: the retention time of the principal peaks in the chromatogram obtained from the sample solution and the standard solution is the same.

Operating conditions—

Detector: An ultraviolet absorption photometer (wavelength: 340 nm).

Column: A stainless steel column 4.6 mm in inside diameter and 15 cm in length, packed with octadecylsilanized silica gel for liquid chromatography (5 μm in particle diameter).

Column temperature: A constant temperature of about 45°C.

Mobile phase: Dissolve 1.25 g of copper (II) sulfate pentahydrate, 1.76 g of L-valine and 7.71 g of ammonium acetate in water to make 1000 mL, and add 250 mL of methanol.

Flow rate: Adjust so that the retention time of levofloxacin is about 22 minutes.

System suitability—

System performance: Dissolve 10 mg of ofloxacin in 20 mL of a mixture of water and methanol (1:1). To 1 mL of this solution add a mixture of water and methanol (1:1) to make 10 mL. When the procedure is run with 10 μL of this solution under the above operating conditions, the resolution between the peak of levofloxacin and the peak having the relative retention time of about 1.2 to levofloxacin is not less than 3.

Osmotic pressure ratio Being specified separately when the drug is granted approval based on the Law.

pH Being specified separately when the drug is granted approval based on the Law.

Foreign insoluble matter <*6.11*> It meets the requirement.

Insoluble particulate matter <*6.08*> It meets the requirement.

Sterility <*4.06*> Perform the test according to the Membrane filtration method: it meets the requirement.

Assay To an exact volume of Levofloxacin Ophthalmic Solution, equivalent to about 5 mg of levofloxacin hydrate ($C_{18}H_{20}FN_3O_4 . ½H_2O$) add exactly 2 mL of the internal standard solution, then add the mobile phase to make 100 mL, and use this solution as the sample solution. Separately, weigh accurately about 25 mg of levofloxacin hydrate for assay (separately determine the water <*2.48*> in the same manner as Levofloxacin Hydrate), and dissolve in water to make exactly 50 mL. Pipet 10 mL of this solution, add exactly 2 mL of the internal standard solution, then add the mobile phase to make 100 mL, and use this solution as the standard solution. Perform the test with 10 μL each of the sample solution and standard solution as directed under Liquid Chromatography <*2.01*> according to the following conditions, and calculate the ratios, Q_T and Q_S, of the peak area of levofloxacin to that of the internal standard.

Amount (mg) of levofloxacin hydrate ($C_{18}H_{20}FN_3O_4 . ½H_2O$)
$= M_S \times Q_T/Q_S \times 1/5 \times 1.025$

M_S: Amount (mg) of levofloxacin hydrate for assay taken, calculated on the anhydrous basis

*Internal standard solution—*A solution of naphazoline hydrochloride in the mobile phase (3 in 500).

Operating conditions—

Detector: An ultraviolet absorption photometer (wavelength: 280 nm).

Column: A stainless steel column 4 mm in inside diameter and 15 cm in length, packed with octadecylsilanized silica gel for liquid chromatography (5 μm in particle diameter).

Column temperature: A constant temperature of about 40°C.

Mobile phase: Dissolve 13.61 g of potassium dihydrogen phosphate and 0.77 g of ammonium acetate in 900 mL of water, adjust to pH 3.0 with 1 mol/L hydrochloric acid TS, and add water to make 1000 mL. To 900 mL of this solution add 100 mL of acetonitrile.

Flow rate: Adjust so that the retention time of levofloxacin is about 17 minutes.

System suitability—

System performance: When the procedure is run with 10 μL of the standard solution under the above operating conditions, levofloxacin and the internal standard are eluted in this order with the resolution between these peaks being not less than 5.

System repeatability: When the test is repeated 6 times with 10 μL of the standard solution under the above operating conditions, the relative standard deviation of the ratio of the peak area of levofloxacin to that of the internal standard is not more than 1.0%.

Containers and storage Containers—Tight containers.
Storage—Light-resistant.

Levofloxacin Tablets

レボフロキサシン錠

Levofloxacin Tablets contain not less than 95.0% and not more than 105.0% of the labeled amount of levofloxacin ($C_{18}H_{20}FN_3O_4$: 361.37).

Method of preparation Prepare as directed under Tablets, with Levofloxacin Hydrate.

Identification To an amount of powdered Levofloxacin Tablets, equivalent to 0.1 g of levofloxacin ($C_{18}H_{20}FN_3O_4$), add diluted 3 mol/L hydrochloric acid TS (1 in 100) to make 100 mL, and stir for 20 minutes. Filter this solution through a membrane filter with a pore size not exceeding 0.45 μm, discard the first 10 mL of the filtrate, and to 1 mL of the subsequent filtrate add diluted 3 mol/L hydrochloric acid TS (1 in 100) to make 100 mL. Determine the absorption spectrum of this solution as directed under Ultraviolet-visible Spectrophotometry <*2.24*>: it exhibits maxima between 225 nm and 229 nm and between 292 nm and 296 nm, and a shoulder between 321 nm and 331 nm.

Uniformity of dosage units <*6.02*> Perform the Mass variation test, or the Content uniformity test according to the following method: it meets the requirement.

To 1 tablet of Levofloxacin Tablets add about 70 mL of diluted 3 mol/L hydrochloric acid TS (1 in 100), sonicate to disintegrate the tablet, add diluted 3 mol/L hydrochloric acid TS (1 in 100) to make exactly 100 mL, and stir for 20 minutes. Pipet V mL the solution, add diluted 3 mol/L hydrochloric acid TS (1 in 100) to make exactly V' mL so that each mL contains about 50 μg of levofloxacin ($C_{18}H_{20}FN_3O_4$), and filter this solution through a membrane filter with a pore size not exceeding 0.45 μm. Discard the first 10 mL of the filtrate, and use the subsequent filtrate as the sample solution. Then, proceed as directed in the Assay.

Amount (mg) of levofloxacin ($C_{18}H_{20}FN_3O_4$)
$= M_S \times A_T/A_S \times V'/V \times 1/5$

M_S: Amount (mg) of levofloxacin hydrate for assay taken, calculated on the anhydrous basis

Dissolution <*6.10*> **(1)** For a 100-mg Tablet When the test is performed at 50 revolutions per minute according to the Paddle method, using 900 mL of water as the dissolution medium, the dissolution rate in 90 minutes is not less than 80%.

Start the test with 1 tablet of Levofloxacin Tablets, withdraw not less than 20 mL of the medium at the specified minute after starting the test, and filter through a membrane filter with a pore size not exceeding 0.45 μm. Discard not less than 10 mL of the first filtrate, pipet 5 mL of the subsequent filtrate, add water to make exactly 100 mL, and use this solution as the sample solution. Separately, weigh accurately about 28 mg of levofloxacin hydrate for assay (separately determine the water <*2.48*> in the same manner as Levofloxacin Hydrate), and dissolve in water to make exactly 100 mL. Pipet 2 mL of this solution, add water to make exactly 100 mL, and use this solution as the standard solution. Determine the absorbances, A_T and A_S, at 289 nm of the sample solution and standard solution as directed under Ultraviolet-visible Spectrophotometry <*2.24*>.

Dissolution rate (%) with respect to the labeled amount of levofloxacin hydrate ($C_{18}H_{20}FN_3O_4.{}^1\!/\!_2H_2O$)
$= M_S \times A_T/A_S \times 18/5 \times 1.025$

M_S: Amount (mg) of levofloxacin hydrate for assay taken, calculated on the anhydrous basis

(2) For a 250-mg Tablet and 500-mg Tablet When the tests are performed at 50 revolutions per minute according to the Paddle method, using 900 mL of 2nd fluid for dissolution test as the dissolution medium, the dissolution rate in 30 minutes is not less than 80%.

Start the test with 1 tablet of Levofloxacin Tablets, withdraw not less than 20 mL of the medium at the specified minute after starting the test, and filter through a membrane filter with a pore size not exceeding 0.45 μm. Discard not less than 10 mL of the first filtrate, pipet V mL of the subsequent filtrate, add the dissolution medium to make exactly V' mL so that each mL contains about 11.2 μg of levofloxacin ($C_{18}H_{20}FN_3O_4$), and use this solution as the sample solution. Separately, weigh accurately about 28 mg of levofloxacin hydrate for assay (separately determine the water <*2.48*> in the same manner as Levofloxacin Hydrate), and dissolve in the dissolution medium to make exactly 50 mL. Pipet 2 mL of this solution, add the dissolution medium to make exactly 100 mL, and use this solution as the standard solution. Determine the absorbances, A_T and A_S, at 287 nm of the sample solution and standard solution as directed under Ultraviolet-visible Spectrophotometry <*2.24*>.

Dissolution rate (%) with respect to the labeled amount of levofloxacin ($C_{18}H_{20}FN_3O_4$)
$= M_S \times A_T/A_S \times V'/V \times 1/C \times 36$

M_S: Amount (mg) of levofloxacin hydrate for assay taken, calculated on the anhydrous basis
C: Amount (mg) of levofloxacin ($C_{18}H_{20}FN_3O_4$) in 1 g

Assay Accurately weigh the mass of not less than 20 Levofloxacin Tablets, and powder them. Weigh accurately a portion of the powder, equivalent to about 1 g of levofloxacin ($C_{18}H_{20}FN_3O_4$), add 150 mL of diluted 3 mol/L hydrochloric acid TS (1 in 100), sonicate for 5 minutes, and add diluted 3 mol/L hydrochloric acid TS (1 in 100) to make exactly 200 mL, and stir for 10 minutes. Pipet 2 mL of this solution, add diluted 3 mol/L hydrochloric acid TS (1 in 100) to make exactly 200 mL, and filter through a membrane filter with a pore size not exceeding 0.45 μm. Discard the first 10 mL of the filtrate, and use the subsequent filtrate as the sample solution. Separately, weigh accurately about 25 mg of levofloxacin hydrate for assay (separately determine the water <*2.48*> in the same manner as Levofloxacin Hydrate), and dissolve in diluted 3 mol/L hydrochloric acid TS (1 in 100) to make exactly 50 mL. Pipet 2 mL of this solution, add diluted 3 mol/L hydrochloric acid TS (1 in 100) to make exactly 20 mL, and use this solution as the standard solution. Perform the test with exactly 10 μL each of the sample solution and standard solution as directed under Liquid Chromatography <*2.01*> according to the following conditions, and determine the peak areas, A_T and A_S, of levofloxacin in each solution.

Amount (mg) of levofloxacin ($C_{18}H_{20}FN_3O_4$)
$= M_S \times A_T/A_S \times 40$

M_S: Amount (mg) of levofloxacin hydrate for assay taken, calculated on the anhydrous basis

Operating conditions—

Detector: An ultraviolet absorption photometer (wavelength: 340 nm).

Column: A stainless steel column 4.6 mm in inside diameter and 15 cm in length, packed with octadecylsilanized silica gel for liquid chromatography (5 μm in particle diameter).

Column temperature: A constant temperature of about 45°C.

Mobile phase: Dissolve 1.00 g of copper (II) sulfate pentahydrate, 1.41 g of L-valine and 6.17g of ammonium acetate in 800 mL of water, and add 200 mL of methanol.

Flow rate: Adjust so that the retention time of levofloxacin is about 20 minutes.

System suitability—

System performance: Dissolve 10 mg of ofloxacin in 20 mL of diluted 3 mol/L hydrochloric acid TS (1 in 100). To 1 mL of this solution add diluted 3 mol/L hydrochloric acid TS (1 in 100) to make 20 mL. When the procedure is run with 10 μL of this solution under the above operating conditions, levofloxacin and an enantiomer are eluted in this order with the resolution between these peaks being not less than 3.

System repeatability: When the test is repeated 6 times with 10 μL of the standard solution under the above operating conditions, the relative standard deviation of the peak area of levofloxacin is not more than 1.0%.

Containers and storage Containers—Tight containers.

Levomepromazine Maleate

レボメプロマジンマレイン酸塩

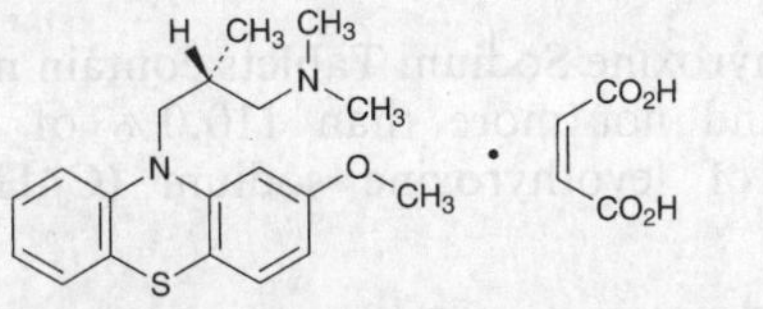

$C_{19}H_{24}N_2OS.C_4H_4O_4$: 444.54
(2*R*)-3-(2-Methoxy-10*H*-phenothiazin-10-yl)-*N*,*N*,2-trimethylpropylamine monomaleate
[*7104-38-3*]

Levomepromazine Maleate, when dried, contains not less than 98.0% of levomepromazine maleate ($C_{19}H_{24}N_2OS.C_4H_4O_4$).

Description Levomepromazine Maleate occurs as white, crystals or crystalline powder. It is odorless, and has a slightly bitter taste.

It is freely soluble in acetic acid (100), soluble in chloroform, sparingly soluble in methanol, slightly soluble in ethanol (95) and in acetone, very slightly soluble in water, and practically insoluble in diethyl ether.

Melting point: 184 – 190°C (with decomposition).

Identification **(1)** Dissolve 5 mg of Levomepromazine Maleate in 5 mL of sulfuric acid: a red-purple color develops, which slowly becomes deep red-purple. To this solution add 1 drop of potassium dichromate TS: a brownish yellow-red color is produced.

(2) To 0.2 g of Levomepromazine Maleate add 5 mL of sodium hydroxide TS and 20 mL of diethyl ether, and shake well. Separate the diethyl ether layer, wash twice with 10-mL portions of water, add 0.5 g of anhydrous sodium sulfate, filter, evaporate the diethyl ether on a water bath, and dry the residue at 105°C for 2 hours: the residue melts <*2.60*> between 124°C and 128°C.

(3) To 0.5 g of Levomepromazine Maleate add 5 mL of water and 2 mL of ammonia solution (28), extract with three 5-mL portions of chloroform, separate and evaporate the water layer to dryness. To the residue add 2 to 3 drops of dilute sulfuric acid and 5 mL of water, and extract with four 25-mL portions of diethyl ether. Combine all the diethyl ether extracts, evaporate the diethyl ether in a water bath at a temperature of about 35°C with the aid of a current of air: the residue melts <*2.60*> between 128°C and 136°C.

Optical rotation <*2.49*> $[\alpha]_D^{20}$: −13.5 – −16.5° (after drying, 0.5 g, chloroform, 20 mL, 200 mm).

Purity **(1)** Clarity and color of solution—To 0.5 g of Levomepromazine Maleate add 10 mL of methanol, and dissolve by warming: the solution is clear, and colorless or pale yellow.

(2) Chloride <*1.03*>—Dissolve 0.5 g of Levomepromazine Maleate in 40 mL of methanol, and add 6 mL of dilute nitric acid and water to make 50 mL. Perform the test using this solution as the test solution. Prepare the control solution with 0.40 mL of 0.01 mol/L hydrochloric acid VS, 40 mL of methanol, 6 mL of dilute nitric acid and water to make 50 mL (not more than 0.028%).

(3) Heavy metals <*1.07*>—Proceed with 2.0 g of Levomepromazine Maleate according to Method 2, and perform the test. Prepare the control solution with 2.0 mL of Standard Lead Solution (not more than 10 ppm).

Loss on drying <*2.41*> Not more than 0.5% (2 g, 105°C, 3 hours).

Residue on ignition <*2.44*> Not more than 0.1% (1 g).

Assay Weigh accurately about 1 g of Levomepromazine Maleate, previously dried, and dissolve in a mixture of 40 mL of acetic acid (100) and 20 mL of acetone for nonaqueous titration. Titrate <*2.50*> with 0.1 mol/L perchloric acid VS until the color of the solution changes from red-purple through blue-purple to blue (indicator: 5 drops of bromocresol green-methylrosaniline chloride TS). Perform a blank determination in the same manner, and make any necessary correction.

Each mL of 0.1 mol/L perchloric acid VS
= 44.45 mg of $C_{19}H_{24}N_2OS.C_4H_4O_4$

Containers and storage Containers—Tight containers.
Storage—Light-resistant.

Levothyroxine Sodium Hydrate

レボチロキシンナトリウム水和物

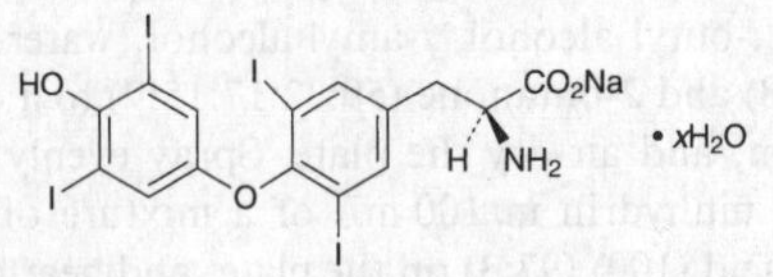

$C_{15}H_{10}I_4NNaO_4.xH_2O$
Monosodium *O*-(4-hydroxy-3,5-diiodophenyl)-3,5-diiodo-L-tyrosinate hydrate
[*25416-65-3*]

Levothyroxine Sodium Hydrate contains not less than 97.0% of levothyroxine sodium ($C_{15}H_{10}I_4NNaO_4$: 798.85), calculated on the dried basis.

Description Levothyroxine Sodium Hydrate occurs as a pale yellow-white to light yellow-brown powder. It is odorless.

It is slightly soluble in ethanol (95), and practically insoluble in water and in diethyl ether.

It dissolves in sodium hydroxide TS.

It is gradually colored by light.

Identification **(1)** Heat 0.1 g of Levothyroxine Sodium Hydrate over a flame: a purple gas evolves.

(2) To 0.5 mg of Levothyroxine Sodium Hydrate add 8 mL of a mixture of water, ethanol (95), hydrochloric acid and sodium hydroxide TS (6:5:2:2), warm in a water bath for 2 minutes, cool, and add 0.1 mL of sodium nitrite TS. Allow to stand in a dark place for 20 minutes, and add 1.5 mL of ammonia solution (28): a yellowish red color is produced.

(3) Determine the absorption spectrum of a solution of Levothyroxine Sodium Hydrate in dilute sodium hydroxide TS (1 in 10,000) as directed under Ultraviolet-visible Spectrophotometry <*2.24*>, and compare the spectrum with the Reference Spectrum: both spectra exhibit similar intensities of absorption at the same wavelengths.

(4) Moisten Levothyroxine Sodium Hydrate with sulfuric acid, and ignite: the residue responds to Qualitative Tests <*1.09*> (1) and (2) for sodium salt.

Optical rotation <*2.49*> $[\alpha]_D^{20}$: −5 – −6° (0.3 g calculated on the dried basis, a mixture of ethanol (95) and sodium hydroxide TS (2:1), 10 mL, 100 mm).

Purity (1) Clarity and color of solution—Dissolve 0.3 g of Levothyroxine Sodium Hydrate in 10 mL of a mixture of ethanol (95) and sodium hydroxide TS (2:1) by warming: the solution is clear and pale yellow to pale yellow-brown in color.

(2) Soluble halides—Dissolve 0.01 g of Levothyroxine Sodium Hydrate in 10 mL of water and 1 drop of dilute nitric acid, shake for 5 minutes, and filter. To the filtrate add water to make 10 mL, then add 3 drops of silver nitrate TS, and mix: the solution has no more opalescence than the following control solution.

Control solution: To 0.20 mL of 0.01 mol/L hydrochloric acid VS add 10 mL of water and 1 drop of dilute nitric acid, and proceed as directed above.

(3) Related substances—Dissolve 20 mg of Levothyroxine Sodium Hydrate in 2 mL of a mixture of ethanol (95) and ammonia solution (28) (14:1), and use this solution as the sample solution. Pipet 1 mL of the sample solution, add a mixture of ethanol (95) and ammonia solution (28) (14:1) to make exactly 50 mL, and use this solution as the standard solution. Perform the test with these solutions as directed under Thin-layer Chromatography <*2.03*>. Spot 5 μL each of the sample solution and standard solution on a plate of silica gel for thin-layer chromatography. Develop the plate with a mixture of *t*-butyl alcohol, *t*-amyl alcohol, water, ammonia solution (28) and 2-butanone (59:32:17:15:7) to a distance of about 12 cm, and air-dry the plate. Spray evenly a solution of 0.3 g of ninhydrin in 100 mL of a mixture of 1-butanol and acetic acid (100) (97:3) on the plate, and heat the plate at 100°C for 3 minutes: the red-purple spots other than the principal spot obtained from the sample solution are not more intense than the spot from the standard solution.

Loss on drying <*2.41*> 7 – 11% (0.5 g, in vacuum, phosphorus (V) oxide, 60°C, 4 hours).

Assay Weigh accurately about 25 mg of Levothyroxine Sodium Hydrate, and proceed as directed under Oxygen Flask Combustion Method <*1.06*>, using a mixture of 10 mL of sodium hydroxide solution (1 in 100) and 1 mL of a freshly prepared sodium bisulfate solution (1 in 100) as the absorbing liquid, and prepare the test solution. Apply a small amount of water to the upper part of apparatus A, pull out C carefully, and wash C, B and the inner wall of A with 40 mL of water. To the test solution add 1 mL of bromine-acetic acid TS, insert the stopper C, and shake vigorously for 1 minute. Remove the stopper, rinse the stopper, the sample holder and the inner wall of the flask with 40 mL of water, and add 0.5 mL of formic acid. Stopper the flask with C, and shake vigorously for 1 minute again. Remove the stopper, and rinse the stopper, the sample holder and the inner wall of the flask with 40 mL of water. Bubble the solution with enough nitrogen gas in the flask to remove the oxygen and excess bromine, add 0.5 g of potassium iodide to the solution, and dissolve. Add immediately 3 mL of dilute sulfuric acid, mix, and allow to stand for 2 minutes. Titrate <*2.50*> the solution with 0.02 mol/L sodium thiosulfate VS (indicator: 3 mL of starch TS). Perform a blank determination in the same manner, and make any necessary correction.

Each mL of 0.02 mol/L sodium thiosulfate VS
= 0.6657 mg of $C_{15}H_{10}I_4NNaO_4$

Containers and storage Containers—Tight containers.
Storage—Light-resistant.

Levothyroxine Sodium Tablets

レボチロキシンナトリウム錠

Levothyroxine Sodium Tablets contain not less than 90.0% and not more than 110.0% of the labeled amount of levothyroxine sodium ($C_{15}H_{10}I_4NNaO_4$: 798.85).

Method of preparation Prepare as directed under Tablets, with Levothyroxine Sodium Hydrate.

Identification (1) Weigh a quantity of powdered Levothyroxine Sodium Tablets, equivalent to 0.5 mg of Levothyroxine Sodium Hydrate, add 8 mL of a mixture of water, ethanol (95), hydrochloric acid and sodium hydroxide TS (6:5:2:2), warm in a water bath for 2 minutes, cool, and filter. To the filtrate add 0.1 mL of sodium nitrite TS, and allow to stand in a dark place for 20 minutes. Add 1.5 mL of ammonia solution (28): a yellowish red color develops.

(2) To a quantity of powdered Levothyroxine Sodium Tablets, equivalent to 1 mg of Levothyroxine Sodium Hydrate, add 10 mL of ethanol (95), shake, filter, and use the filtrate as the sample solution. Dissolve 0.01 g of levothyroxine sodium for thin-layer chromatography in 100 mL of ethanol (95), and use this solution as the standard solution. Perform the test with these solutions as directed under Thin-layer Chromatography <*2.03*>. Spot 20 μL each of the sample solution and standard solution on a plate of silica gel for thin-layer chromatography. Develop the plate with a mixture of *t*-butyl alcohol, *t*-amyl alcohol, water, ammonia solution (28) and 2-butanone (59:32:17:15:7) to a distance of about 12 cm, and air-dry the plate. Spray evenly a solution of 0.3 g of ninhydrin in 100 mL of a mixture of 1-butanol and acetic acid (100) (97:3) on the plate, and heat the plate at 100°C for 3 minutes: the spots obtained from the sample solution and the standard solution show a red-purple color, and has the same *Rf* value.

Purity Soluble halides—Weigh a quantity of powdered Levothyroxine Sodium Tablets, equivalent to 2.5 mg of Levothyroxine Sodium Hydrate, add 25 mL of water, warm to 40°C, shake for 5 minutes, add 3 drops of dilute nitric acid, and filter. To the filtrate add 3 drops of silver nitrate TS, and mix: the solution has no more opalescence than the following control solution.

Control solution: To 0.25 mL of 0.01 mol/L hydrochloric acid VS add 25 mL of water and 3 drops of dilute nitric acid, and proceed as directed above.

Uniformity of dosage units <*6.02*> Perform the test according to the following method: it meets the requirement of the Content uniformity test.

Place 1 tablet of Levothyroxine Sodium Tablets in a glass-stoppered centrifuge tube, add exactly 10 mL of 0.01 mol/L sodium hydroxide TS, warm at 50°C for 15 minutes, and shake vigorously for 20 minutes. Centrifuge this solution, pipet 5 mL of the supernatant liquid, add exactly 1 mL of the internal standard solution, and use this solution as the sample solution. Perform the test with 20 μL of the sample solution as directed under Liquid Chromatography <*2.01*> according to the following conditions, and calculate the ratio of the peak area of levothyroxine to that of the internal standard. Calculate the mean value from the ratios of each peak area of 10 samples: the deviation (%) of the mean value and the ratio of each peak area should be not more than 15%. When the deviation (%) is more than 15%, and 1 sample shows not more than 25%, perform another test with 20 samples. Calculate the deviation (%) of the mean value of the 30 samples used in the 2 tests and the ratio of each peak area: there should be not more than 1 sample with the deviation more than 15% but not more than 25%, and no sample should deviate by more than 25%.

Internal standard solution—A solution of ethinylestradiol in a mixture of acetonitrile and diluted phosphoric acid (1 in 10) (9:1) (3 in 40,000).

Operating conditions—

Detector: An ultraviolet absorption photometer (wavelength: a constant wavelength between 220 nm and 230 nm).

Column: A stainless steel column 4 to 6 mm in inside diameter and 10 to 25 cm in length, packed with octadecylsilanized silica gel (5 μm in particle diameter).

Column temperature: A constant temperature at about 25°C.

Mobile phase: A mixture of methanol, water and phosphoric acid (1340:660:1).

Flow rate: Adjust so that the retention time of levothyroxine is about 9 minutes.

Selection of column: To 5 mL of a solution of levothyroxine sodium in 0.01 mol/L sodium hydroxide TS (1 in 200,000) add 1 mL of the internal standard solution. Proceed with 20 μL of this solution under the above operating conditions, and calculate the resolution. Use a column giving elution of levothyroxine and the internal standard in this order with the resolution between these peaks being not less than 2.0.

Dissolution Being specified separately when the drug is granted approval based on the Law.

Assay Weigh accurately and powder not less than 20 Levothyroxine Sodium Tablets. Weigh accurately a portion of the powder, equivalent to about 3 mg of levothyroxine sodium ($C_{15}H_{10}I_4NNaO_4$), into a crucible, and add potassium carbonate amounting to twice the mass of the powder. In the case that the weighed powder is less than 4 g, add 8 g of potassium carbonate to the crucible. Mix well, and gently tap the crucible on the bench to compact the mixture. Overlay with 10 g of potassium carbonate, and compact again by tapping. Heat the crucible strongly at a temperature between 675°C and 700°C for 25 minutes. Cool, add 30 mL of water, heat gently to boiling, and filter into a flask. To the residue add 30 mL of water, boil, and filter into the same flask. Rinse the crucible and the char on the funnel with hot water until the filtrate measures 300 mL. Add slowly 7 mL of freshly prepared bromine TS and diluted phosphoric acid (1 in 2) in the ratio of 3.5 mL to 1 g of the added potassium carbonate, and boil until starch-potassium iodide paper is no longer colored blue by the evolved gas. Wash the inside of the flask with water, and continue boiling for 5 minutes. During the boiling add water from time to time to maintain a volume of not less than 250 mL. Cool, add 5 mL of a solution of phenol (1 in 20), again rinse the inside of the flask with water, and allow to stand for 5 minutes. Add 2 mL of diluted phosphoric acid (1 in 2) and 5 mL of potassium iodide TS, and titrate 〈*2.50*〉 immediately the liberated iodine with 0.01 mol/L sodium thiosulfate VS (indicator: 3 mL of starch TS). Perform a blank determination in the same manner, and make any necessary correction.

Each mL of 0.01 mol/L sodium thiosulfate VS
= 0.3329 mg of $C_{15}H_{10}I_4NNaO_4$

Containers and storage Containers—Tight containers.
Storage—Light-resistant.

Lidocaine

リドカイン

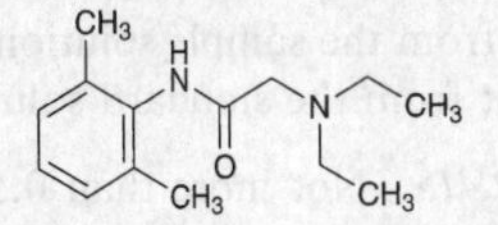

$C_{14}H_{22}N_2O$: 234.34

2-Diethylamino-*N*-(2,6-dimethylphenyl)acetamide

[*137-58-6*]

Lidocaine, when dried, contains not less than 99.0% of lidocaine ($C_{14}H_{22}N_2O$).

Description Lidocaine occurs as white to pale yellow, crystals or crystalline powder.

It is very soluble in methanol and in ethanol (95), soluble in acetic acid (100) and in diethyl ether, and practically insoluble in water.

It dissolves in dilute hydrochloric acid.

Identification **(1)** Dissolve 40 mg of Lidocaine in 10 mL of 1 mol/L hydrochloric acid TS, and add water to make 100 mL. Determine the absorption spectrum of the solution as directed under Ultraviolet-visible Spectrophotometry 〈*2.24*〉, and compare the spectrum with the Reference Spectrum: both spectra exhibit similar intensities of absorption at the same wavelengths.

(2) Determine the infrared absorption spectrum of Lidocaine as directed in the potassium bromide disk method under Infrared Spectrophotometry 〈*2.25*〉, and compare the spectrum with the Reference Spectrum: both spectra exhibit similar intensities of absorption at the same wave numbers.

Melting point 〈*2.60*〉 66 – 69°C

Purity **(1)** Clarity and color of solution—Dissolve 1.0 g of Lidocaine in 2 mL of dilute hydrochloric acid, and add water to make 10 mL: the solution is clear and colorless to light yellow.

(2) Chloride 〈*1.03*〉—Dissolve 0.6 g of Lidocaine in 6 mL of dilute nitric acid, add water to make 50 mL, and perform the test using this solution as the test solution. Prepare the control solution with 0.70 mL of 0.01 mol/L hydrochloric acid VS (not more than 0.041%).

(3) Sulfate 〈*1.14*〉—Dissolve 0.5 g of Lidocaine in 5 mL of dilute hydrochloric acid, add water to make 50 mL, and perform the test using this solution as the test solution. Prepare the control solution with 1.0 mL of 0.005 mol/L sulfuric acid VS, 5 mL of dilute hydrochloric acid and water to make 50 mL (not more than 0.096%).

(4) Heavy metals 〈*1.07*〉—Carbonize 2.0 g of Lidocaine by gentle ignition. After cooling, add 10 mL of a solution of magnesium nitrate hexahydrate in ethanol (95) (1 in 10), and fire the ethanol to burn. After cooling, add 1 mL of sulfuric acid, proceed according to Method 4, and perform the test. Prepare the control solution with 2.0 mL of Standard Lead Solution (not more than 10 ppm).

(5) Related substances—Dissolve 0.10 g of Lidocaine in 2 mL of methanol, and use this solution as the sample solution. Pipet 1 mL of the sample solution, add methanol to make exactly 100 mL, and use this solution as the standard solution. Perform the test with these solutions as directed under Thin-layer Chromatography 〈*2.03*〉. Spot 10 μL each of the sample solution and standard solution on a plate of silica gel with fluorescent indicator for thin-layer chromatography. Develop the plate with a mixture of ethyl acetate, 2-butanone, water and formic acid (5:3:1:1) to a distance of about 10 cm, air-dry the plate, and dry more at 80°C for 30 minutes. After cooling, examine under ultraviolet light (main wavelength: 254 nm): the spots other than the principal spot obtained from the sample solution are not more intense than the spot from the standard solution.

Loss on drying <*2.41*> Not more than 0.5% (1 g, in vacuum, silica gel, 24 hours).

Residue on ignition <*2.44*> Not more than 0.1% (1 g).

Assay Dissolve about 0.5 g of Lidocaine, previously dried and accurately weighed, in 20 mL of acetic acid (100), and titrate <*2.50*> with 0.1 mol/L perchloric acid VS (indicator: 1 drop of crystal violet TS) until the color of the solution changes from purple to blue-green through blue. Perform a blank determination in the same manner, and make any necessary correction.

Each mL of 0.1 mol/L perchloric acid VS
= 23.43 mg of $C_{14}H_{22}N_2O$

Containers and storage Containers—Tight containers.

Lidocaine Injection

リドカイン注射液

Lidocaine Injection is an aqueous injection.

It contains not less than 95.0% and not more than 105.0% of the labeled amount of lidocaine hydrochloride ($C_{14}H_{22}N_2O.HCl$: 270.80).

Method of preparation Prepare as directed under Injections, with Lidocaine and an equivalent amount of Hydrochloric Acid.

No preservative is added in the case of intravenous injections.

Description Lidocaine Injection is a colorless, clear liquid.
pH: 5.0 – 7.0

Identification To a volume of Lidocaine Injection, equivalent to 20 mg of lidocaine hydrochloride ($C_{14}H_{22}N_2O.HCl$), add 1 mL of sodium hydroxide TS, and extract with 20 mL of hexane. To 10 mL of the hexane extract add 20 mL of 1 mol/L hydrochloric acid TS, and shake vigorously. Determine the absorption spectrum of the water layer as directed under Ultraviolet-visible Spectrophotometry <*2.24*>: it exhibits a maximum between 261 nm and 265 nm.

Bacterial endotoxins <*4.01*> Less than 1.0 EU/mg.

Extractable volume <*6.05*> It meets the requirement.

Foreign insoluble matter <*6.06*> Perform the test according to Method 1: it meets the requirement.

Insoluble particulate matter <*6.07*> It meets the requirement.

Sterility <*4.06*> Perform the test according to the Membrane filtration method: it meets the requirement.

Assay To an exactly measured volume of Lidocaine Injection, equivalent to about 0.1 g of lidocaine hydrochloride ($C_{14}H_{22}N_2O.HCl$), add exactly 10 mL of the internal standard solution and 0.001 mol/L hydrochloric acid TS to make 50 mL, and use this solution as the sample solution. Separately, weigh accurately about 85 mg of lidocaine for assay, previously dried in a desiccator (in vacuum, silica gel) for 24 hours, dissolve in 0.5 mL of 1 mol/L hydrochloric acid TS and a suitable volume of 0.001 mol/L hydrochloric acid TS, and add exactly 10 mL of the internal standard solution, then add 0.001 mol/L hydrochloric acid TS to make 50 mL, and use this solution as the standard solution. Perform the test with 5 μL each of the sample solution and standard solution as directed under Liquid Chromatography <*2.01*> according to the following conditions, and calculate the ratios, Q_T and Q_S, of the peak area of lidocaine to that of the internal standard.

Amount (mg) of lidocaine hydrochloride ($C_{14}H_{22}N_2O.HCl$)
$= M_S \times Q_T/Q_S \times 1.156$

M_S: Amount (mg) of lidocaine for assay taken

Internal standard solution—A solution of benzophenone in methanol (1 in 4000).

Operating conditions—

Detector: An ultraviolet absorption photometer (wavelength: 254 nm).

Column: A stainless steel column 4 mm in inside diameter and 15 cm in length, packed with octadecylsilanized silica gel for liquid chromatography (10 μm in particle diameter).

Column temperature: A constant temperature of about 25°C.

Mobile phase: Dissolve 2.88 g of sodium lauryl sulfate in 1000 mL of a mixture of 0.02 mol/L phosphate buffer solution (pH 3.0) and acetonitrile (11:9).

Flow rate: Adjust so that the retention time of lidocaine is about 6 minutes.

System suitability—

System performance: When proceed with 5 μL of the standard solution under the above operating conditions, lidocaine and the internal standard are eluted in this order with the resolution between these peaks being not less than 6.

System repeatability: When the test is repeated 6 times with 5 μL of the standard solution under the above operating conditions, the relative standard deviation of the ratios of the peak area of lidocaine to that of the internal standard is not more than 1.0%.

Containers and storage Containers—Hermetic containers.

Limaprost Alfadex

リマプロスト　アルファデクス

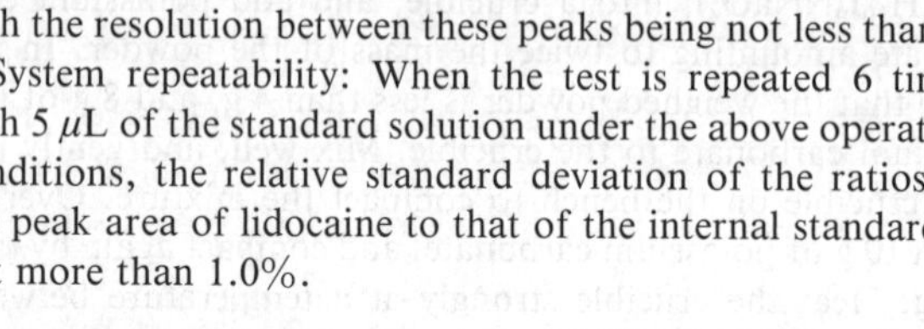

$C_{22}H_{36}O_5 \cdot xC_{36}H_{60}O_{30}$
(2*E*)-7-{(1*R*,2*R*,3*R*)-3-Hydroxy-2-[(1*E*,3*S*,5*S*)-3-hydroxy-5-methylnon-1-en-1-yl]-5-oxocyclopentyl}hept-2-enoic acid-α-cyclodextrin
[*100459-01-6*, limaprost:alfadex = 1:1; clathrate compound]

Limaprost Alfadex is a α-cyclodextrin clathrate compound of limaprost.

It contains not less than 2.8% and not more than 3.2% of limaprost ($C_{22}H_{36}O_5$: 380.52), calculated on the anhydrous basis.

Description Limaprost Alfadex occurs as a white powder.

It is freely soluble in water, slightly soluble in methanol, very slightly soluble in ethanol (99.5), and practically insoluble in ethyl acetate.

It is hygroscopic.

Identification **(1)** Dissolve 20 mg of Limaprost Alfadex in 5 mL of water, add 5 mL of ethyl acetate, shake, centrifuge, and use the upper layer as the sample solution (1). Separately, to 20 mg of Limaprost Alfadex add 5 mL of ethyl acetate, shake, centrifuge, and use the supernatant liquid as the sample solution (2). Evaporate the solvent of the sample solutions (1) and (2) under reduced pressure, add 2 mL of sulfuric acid to each of the residue, and shake them for 5 minutes: the solution obtained from the sample solution (1) develops an orange-yellow color while the solution obtained from the sample solution (2) does not develop any color.

(2) Dissolve 20 mg of Limaprost Alfadex in 5 mL of water, add 5 mL of ethyl acetate, shake, centrifuge, and evaporate the solvent of the upper layer under reduced pressure. Dissolve the residue in 2 mL of ethanol (95), 5 mL of 1,3-dinitrobenzene TS, add 5 mL of a solution of potassium hydroxide in ethanol (95) (17 in 100) while ice-cooling, and allow to stand in a dark place while ice-cooling for 20 minutes: a purple color develops.

(3) To 50 mg of Limaprost Alfadex add 1 mL of iodine TS, dissolve by heating in a water bath, and allow to stand: a dark blue precipitate is formed.

(4) Determine the absorption spectrum of a solution of Limaprost Alfadex in dilute ethanol (3 in 10,000) as directed under Ultraviolet-visible Spectrophotometry *<2.24>*: it does not exhibit a maximum between 200 nm and 400 nm. To 10 mL of this solution add 1 mL of potassium hydroxide-ethanol TS, and allow to stand for 15 minutes. Determine the absorption spectrum of this solution as directed under Ultraviolet-visible Spectrophotometry *<2.24>*, and compare the spectrum with the Reference Spectrum: both spectra exhibit similar intensities of absorption at the same wavelengths.

Optical rotation *<2.49>* $[\alpha]_D^{20}$: +125 – 135° (0.1 g calculated on the anhydrous basis, dilute ethanol, 20 mL, 100 mm).

Purity Related substances—Perform the test immediately after preparation of the sample solution. Dissolve 0.10 g of Limaprost Alfadex in 2 mL of water, add 1 mL of ethanol (95), and use this solution as the sample solution. Pipet 1 mL of the sample solution, add dilute ethanol to make exactly 100 mL, and use this solution as the standard solution (1). Pipet 3 mL of the standard solution (1), add dilute ethanol to make exactly 10 mL, and use this solution as the standard solution (2). Perform the test with exactly 3 μL each of the sample solution and standard solutions (1) and (2) as directed under Liquid Chromatography *<2.01>* according to the following conditions, and determine each peak area by the automatic integration method: the area of the peak of 17-epi-isomer, having the relative retention time of about 1.1 to limaprost, and the area of the peak of 11-deoxy substance, having the relative retention time of about 2.1, obtained from the sample solution are not larger than the peak area of limaprost from the standard solution (2), and the area of the peak other than the principal peak and the peaks mentioned above from the sample solution is not larger than 1/3 times the peak area of limaprost from the standard solution (2). The total area of the peaks other than limaprost from the samples solution is not larger than the peak area of limaprost from the standard solution (1).

Operating conditions—

Detector, column, column temperature, mobile phase and flow rate: Proceed as directed in the operating conditions in the Assay.

Time span of measurement: About 3 times as long as the retention time of limaprost beginning after the solvent peak.

System suitability—

System performance: Proceed as directed in the system suitability in the Assay.

Test for required detectability: To exactly 1 mL of the standard solution (1) add dilute ethanol to make exactly 10 mL. Confirm that the peak area of limaprost obtained with 3 μL of this solution is equivalent to 8 to 12% of that with 3 μL of the standard solution (1).

System repeatability: When the test is repeated 6 times with 3 μL of the standard solution (1) under the above conditions, the relative standard deviation of the peak area of limaprost is not more than 2.0%.

Water *<2.48>* Not more than 6.0% (0.2 g, volumetric titration, direct titration).

Assay Weigh accurately about 0.1 g of Limaprost Afladex, dissolve in 5 mL of water, add exactly 5 mL of the internal standard solution, and use this solution as the sample solution. Separately, weigh accurately about 3 mg of Limaprost RS, dissolve in exactly 5 mL of the internal standard solution, add 5 mL of water, and use this solution as the standard solution. Perform the test with 3 μL each of the sample solution and the standard solution as directed under Liquid Chromatography *<2.01>* according to the following conditions, and calculate the ratios, Q_T and Q_S, of the peak area of limaprost to that of the internal standard.

$$\text{Amount (mg) of limaprost } (C_{22}H_{36}O_5) = M_S \times Q_T/Q_S$$

M_S: Amount (mg) of Limaprost RS taken

*Internal standard solution—*A solution of propyl parahydroxybenzoate in ethanol (95) (1 in 4000).

Operating conditions—

Detector: An ultraviolet absorption photometer (wavelength: 215 nm).

Column: A stainless steel column 4.6 mm in inside diameter and 15 cm in length, packed with octadecylsilanized silica gel for liquid chromatography (5 μm in particle diameter).

Column temperature: A constant temperature of about 25°C.

Mobile phase: A mixture of 0.02 mol/L potassium dihydrogen phosphate TS, acetonitrile for liquid chromatography and 2-propanol for liquid chromatography (9:5:2).

Flow rate: Adjust so that the retention time of limaprost is about 12 minutes.

System suitability—

System performance: When the procedure is run with 3 μL of the standard solution under the above operating conditions, the internal standard and limaprost are eluted in this order with the resolution between these peaks being not less than 7.

System repeatability: When the test is repeated 6 times with 3 μL of the standard solution under the above operating conditions, the relative standard deviation of the ratios of the peak area of limaprost to that of the internal standard is not more than 1.0%.

Containers and storage Containers—Tight containers.

Storage—Light-resistant, at a temperature not exceeding −10°C.

Lincomycin Hydrochloride Hydrate

リンコマイシン塩酸塩水和物

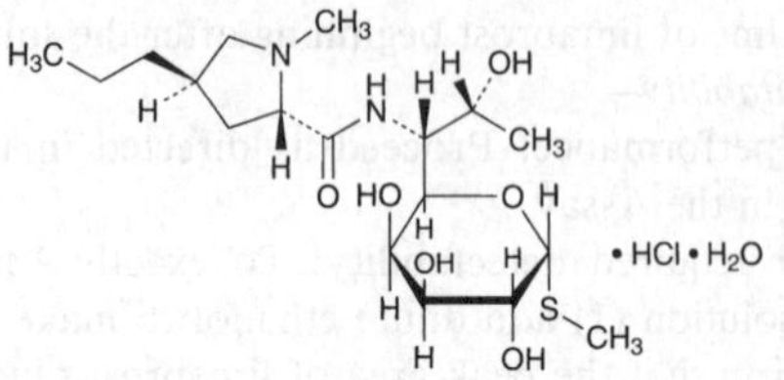

$C_{18}H_{34}N_2O_6S.HCl.H_2O$: 461.01
Methyl 6,8-dideoxy-6-[(2*S*,4*R*)-1-methyl-4-propylpyrrolidine-2-carboxamido]-1-thio-D-*erythro*-α-D-*galacto*-octopyranoside monohydrochloride monohydrate
[*7179-49-9*]

Lincomycin Hydrochloride Hydrate is the hydrochloride of a substance having antibacterial activity produced by the growth of *Streptomyces lincolnensis* var. *lincolnensis*.

It contains not less than 850 μg (potency) and not more than 930 μg (potency) per mg, calculated on the anhydrous basis. The potency of Lincomycin Hydrochloride Hydrate is expressed as mass (potency) of lincomycin ($C_{18}H_{34}N_2O_6S$: 406.54).

Description Lincomycin Hydrochloride Hydrate occurs as white, crystals or crystalline powder.

It is freely soluble in water and in methanol, sparingly soluble in ethanol (95).

Identification **(1)** Determine the infrared absorption spectrum of Lincomycin Hydrochloride Hydrate as directed in the paste method under Infrared Spectrophotometry 〈*2.25*〉, and compare the spectrum with the Reference Spectrum or the spectrum of Lincomycin Hydrochloride RS: both spectra exhibit similar intensities of absorption at the same wave numbers.

(2) A solution of Lincomycin Hydrochloride Hydrate (1 in 100) responds to Qualitative Tests 〈*1.09*〉 (2) for chloride.

Optical rotation 〈*2.49*〉 $[\alpha]_D^{20}$: +135 – +150° (0.5 g, water, 25 mL, 100 mm).

pH 〈*2.54*〉 Dissolve 0.10 g of Lincomycin Hydrochloride Hydrate in 1 mL of water: 3.0 – 5.5.

Purity **(1)** Clarity and color of solution—Dissolve 1.0 g of Lincomycin Hydrochloride Hydrate in 10 mL of water: the solution is clear and colorless.

(2) Heavy metals 〈*1.07*〉—Proceed with 2.0 g of Lincomycin Hydrochloride Hydrate according to Method 4, and perform the test. Prepare the control solution with 1.0 mL of Standard Lead Solution (not more than 5 ppm).

(3) Lincomycin B—Use the sample solution obtained in the Assay as the sample solution. Perform the test with 20 μL of the sample solution as directed under Liquid Chromatography 〈*2.01*〉 according to the following conditions, and determine the peak areas of lincomycin and lincomycin B, having the relative retention time of about 0.5 to lincomycin obtained from the sample solution, by the automatic integration method: the peak area of lincomycin B is not more than 2.0% of the sum of the peak areas of lincomycin and lincomycin B.

Operating conditions—

Proceed as directed in the operating conditions in the Assay.

System suitability—

System performance, and system repeatability: Proceed as directed in the system suitability in the Assay.

Test for required detectability: Measure exactly 1 mL of the sample solution, and add the mobile phase to make exactly 50 mL. Confirm that the peak area of lincomycin obtained from 20 μL of this solution is equivalent to 1.4 to 2.6% of that obtained from 20 μL of the sample solution.

Water 〈*2.48*〉 3.0 – 6.0% (0.5 g, volumetric titration, direct titration).

Assay Weigh accurately an amount of Lincomycin Hydrochloride Hydrate and Lincomycin Hydrochloride RS, equivalent to about 10 mg (potency), dissolve each in the mobile phase to make exactly 10 mL, and use these solutions as the sample solution and standard solution. Perform the test with exactly 20 μL each of the sample solution and standard solution as directed under Liquid Chromatography 〈*2.01*〉 according to the following conditions, and determine the peak areas, A_T and A_S, of lincomycin in each solution.

Amount [μg (potency)] of lincomycin ($C_{18}H_{34}N_2O_6S$)
$= M_S \times A_T/A_S \times 1000$

M_S: Amount [mg (potency)] of Lincomycin Hydrochloride RS taken

Operating conditions—

Detector: An ultraviolet absorption photometer (wavelength: 210 nm).

Column: A stainless steel column 4 mm in inside diameter and 25 cm in length, packed with octylsilanized silica gel for liquid chromatography (5 μm in particle diameter).

Column temperature: A constant temperature of about 46°C.

Mobile phase: To 13.5 mL phosphoric acid add 1000 mL of water, and adjust the pH to 6.0 with ammonia TS. To 780 mL of this solution add 150 mL of acetonitrile and 150 mL of methanol.

Flow rate: Adjust so that the retention time of lincomycin is about 9 minutes.

System suitability—

System performance: When the procedure is run with 20 μL of the standard solution under the above operating conditions, the number of theoretical plates and the symmetry factor of the peak of lincomycin are not less than 4000 and not more than 1.3, respectively.

System repeatability: When the test is repeated 6 times with 20 μL of the standard solution under the above operating conditions, the relative standard deviation of the peak area of lincomycin is not more than 2.0%.

Containers and storage Containers—Tight containers.

Lincomycin Hydrochloride Injection

リンコマイシン塩酸塩注射液

Lincomycin Hydrochloride Injection is an aqueous injection.

It contains not less than 93.0% and not more than 107.0% of the labeled potency of lincomycin ($C_{18}H_{34}N_2O_6S$: 406.54).

Method of preparation Prepare as directed under Injections, with Lincomycin Hydrochloride Hydrate.

Description Lincomycin Hydrochloride Injection is a clear, colorless liquid.

Identification To a volume of Lincomycin Hydrochloride Injection, equivalent to 30 mg (potency) of Lincomycin Hydrochloride Hydrate, add 30 mL of water, and use this solution as the sample solution. Separately, dissolve 10 mg (potency) of Lincomycin Hydrochloride RS in 10 mL of water, and use this solution as the standard solution. Perform the test with these solutions as directed under Thin-layer Chromatography <*2.03*>. Spot 5 μL each of the sample solution and standard solution on a plate of silica gel for thin-layer chromatography. Dissolve 150 g of ammonium acetate in 800 mL of water, adjust the pH to 9.6 with ammonia solution (28), and add water to make 1000 mL. To 80 mL of this solution add 40 mL of 2-propanol and 90 mL of ethyl acetate, shake, develop the plate with the upper layer of this solution to a distance of about 15 cm, and air-dry the plate. Spray evenly a solution of potassium permanganate (1 in 1000) on the plate: the principal spot obtained from the sample solution and the spot from the standard solution show the same *Rf* value.

pH <*2.54*> 3.5 – 5.5

Bacterial endotoxins <*4.01*> Less than 0.50 EU/mg (potency).

Extractable volume <*6.05*> It meets the requirement.

Foreign insoluble matter <*6.06*> Perform the test according to Method 1: it meets the requirement.

Insoluble particulate matter <*6.07*> It meets the requirement.

Sterility <*4.06*> Perform the test according to the Membrane filtration method: it meets the requirement.

Assay Pipet a volume of Lincomycin Hydrochloride Injection, equivalent to about 0.3 g (potency) of Lincomycin Hydrochloride Hydrate, add the mobile phase to make exactly 30 mL. Pipet 2 mL of this solution, add the mobile phase to make exactly 20 mL, and use this solution as the sample solution. Separately, weigh accurately an amount of Lincomycin Hydrochloride RS, equivalent to 20 mg (potency), dissolve in the mobile phase to make exactly 20 mL, and use this solution as the standard solution. Then, proceed as directed in the Assay under Lincomycin Hydrochloride Hydrate.

Amount [mg (potency)] of lincomycin ($C_{18}H_{34}N_2O_6S$)
$= M_S \times A_T/A_S \times 15$

M_S: Amount [mg (potency)] of Lincomycin Hydrochloride RS taken

Containers and storage Containers—Hermetic containers.

Liothyronine Sodium

リオチロニンナトリウム

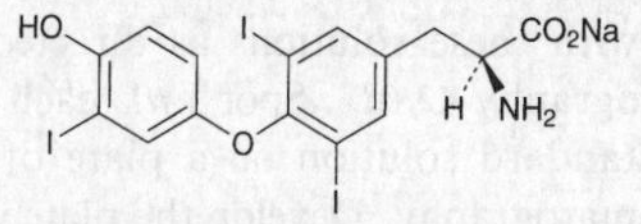

$C_{15}H_{11}I_3NNaO_4$: 672.96
Monosodium *O*-(4-hydroxy-3-iodophenyl)-3,5-diiodo-L-tyrosinate
[*55-06-1*]

Liothyronine Sodium contains not less than 95.0% of liothyronine sodium ($C_{15}H_{11}I_3NNaO_4$), calculated on the dried basis.

Description Liothyronine Sodium occurs as a white to light brown powder. It is odorless.

It is slightly soluble in ethanol (95), and practically insoluble in water and in diethyl ether.

It dissolves in sodium hydroxide TS and in ammonia TS.

Identification **(1)** To 5 mL of a solution of Liothyronine Sodium in ethanol (95) (1 in 1000) add 1 mL of ninhydrin TS, and warm in a water bath for 5 minutes: a purple color develops.

(2) Heat 0.02 g of Liothyronine Sodium with a few drops of sulfuric acid over a flame: a purple gas is evolved.

(3) Determine the absorption spectrum of a solution of Liothyronine Sodium in ethanol (95) (1 in 10,000) as directed under Ultraviolet-visible Spectrophotometry <*2.24*>, and compare the spectrum with the Reference Spectrum: both spectra exhibit similar intensities of absorption at the same wavelengths.

(4) Ignite 0.02 g of Liothyronine Sodium until thoroughly charred. After cooling, add 5 mL of water to the residue, shake, and filter: the filtrate responds to Qualitative Tests <*1.09*> (1) for sodium salt.

Optical rotation <*2.49*> $[\alpha]_D^{20}$: +18 – +22° (0.2 g calculated on the dried basis, a mixture of ethanol (95) and 1 mol/L hydrochloric acid TS (4:1), 10 mL, 100 mm).

Purity **(1)** Soluble halide—To 10 mg of Liothyronine Sodium add 10 mL of water and 1 drop of dilute nitric acid, shake for 5 minutes, and filter. Add water to the filtrate to make 10 mL, and mix with 3 drops of silver nitrate TS: the solution shows no more turbidity than the following control solution.

Control solution: To 0.35 mL of 0.01 mol/L hydrochloric acid VS add 1 drop of dilute nitric acid and water to make 10 mL, and add 3 drops of silver nitrate TS.

(2) Iodine and iodide—Dissolve 0.10 g of Liothyronine Sodium in 10 mL of dilute sodium hydroxide TS and 15 mL of water, add 5 mL of dilute sulfuric acid, and allow to stand for 10 minutes with occasional shaking. Filter the mixture into a Nessler tube, add 10 mL of chloroform and 3 drops of a solution of potassium iodate (1 in 100) to the filtrate, mix for 30 seconds, and allow to stand: the chloroform layer has no more color than the following control solution.

Control solution: Weigh exactly 0.111 g of potassium iodide, and dissolve in water to make 1000 mL. Pipet 1 mL of this solution, add 10 mL of dilute hydroxide TS, 14 mL of water and 5 mL of dilute sulfuric acid, and mix. Filter the mixture into a Nessler tube, and perform the test with the filtrate in the same manner as for the sample.

(3) Related substances—Dissolve 0.15 g of Liothyronine Sodium in 5 mL of diluted ammonia TS (1 in 3), and use this solution as the sample solution. Pipet 1 mL of the sample solution, add diluted ammonia TS (1 in 3) to make exactly 50 mL, and use this solution as the standard solution. Perform the test with these solutions as directed under Thin-layer Chromatography <*2.03*>. Spot 1 μL each of the sample solution and standard solution on a plate of silica gel for thin-layer chromatography. Develop the plate with a mixture of *t*-butyl alcohol, *t*-amyl alcohol, water, ammonia solution (28) and 2-butanone (59:32:17:15:7) to a distance of about 12 cm, and air-dry the plate. Spray evenly a solution of 0.3 g of ninhydrin in 100 mL of a mixture of 1-butanol and acetic acid (100) (97:3) on the plate, and dry the plate at 100°C for 3 minutes: the spots other than the principal spot obtained from the sample solution are not more intense than the spot from the standard solution.

Loss on drying <*2.41*> Not more than 4.0% (0.2 g, 105°C, 2 hours).

Assay Weigh accurately about 25 mg of Liothyronine Sodium, and proceed as directed under Oxygen Flask Combustion Method <*1.06*>, using a mixture of 10 mL of a solution of sodium hydroxide (1 in 100) and 1 mL of a freshly prepared solution of sodium bisulfate (1 in 100) as the absorbing liquid, and prepare the test solution. Apply a small amount of water to the upper part of apparatus A, pull out C carefully, and wash C, B and the inner wall of A with 40 mL of water. To the test solution add 1 mL of bromine-acetic acid TS, insert the stopper C, and shake vigorously for 1 minute. Remove the stopper, rinse the stopper, the sample holder and the inner wall of the flask with 40 mL of water, and add 0.5 mL of formic acid. Stopper the flask with C, and shake vigorously for 1 minute again. Remove the stopper, and rinse the stopper, the sample holder and the inner wall of the flask with 40 mL of water again. Bubble the solution with enough nitrogen gas in the flask to remove the oxygen and excess bromine, add 0.5 g of potassium iodide to the solution, and dissolve. Add immediately 3 mL of dilute sulfuric acid, mix, and allow to stand for 2 minutes. Titrate <*2.50*> the solution with 0.02 mol/L sodium thiosulfate VS (indicator: 3 mL of starch TS). Perform a blank determination in the same manner, and make any necessary correction.

Each mL of 0.02 mol/L sodium thiosulfate VS
= 0.7477 mg of $C_{15}H_{11}I_3NNaO_4$

Containers and storage Containers—Tight containers.
Storage—Light-resistant.

Liothyronine Sodium Tablets

リオチロニンナトリウム錠

Liothyronine Sodium Tablets contain not less than 90.0% and not more than 110.0% of the labeled amount of liothyronine sodium ($C_{15}H_{11}I_3NNaO_4$: 672.96).

Method of preparation Prepare as directed under Tablets, with Liothyronine Sodium.

Identification **(1)** To a glass-stoppered centrifuge tube add a portion of finely powdered Liothyronine Sodium Tablets, equivalent to 0.1 mg of Liothyronine Sodium, add 30 mL of dilute sodium hydroxide TS, shake vigorously, and centrifuge. Transfer the supernatant liquid to a separator, add 10 mL of dilute hydrochloric acid, and extract with two 20-mL portions of ethyl acetate. Filter each extract successively through absorbent cotton previously overlaid with 8 g of anhydrous sodium sulfate. Evaporate the filtrate on a water bath to dryness with the aid of a current of nitrogen. Dissolve the residue in 0.5 mL of methanol, and use this solution as the sample solution. Separately, dissolve 10 mg of liothyronine sodium for thin-layer chromatography in 50 mL of methanol, and use this solution as the standard solution. Perform the test with these solutions as directed under Thin-layer Chromatography <*2.03*>. Spot 20 μL each of the sample solution and standard solution on a plate of silica gel for thin-layer chromatography. Develop the plate with a mixture of *t*-butyl alcohol, *t*-amyl alcohol, water, ammonia solution (28) and 2-butanone (59:32:17:15:7) to a distance of about 12 cm, and air-dry the plate. Spray evenly a solution of 0.3 g of ninhydrin in 100 mL of a mixture of 1-butanol and acetic acid (100) (97:3) on the plate, and dry the plate at 100°C for 3 minutes: the spots obtained from the sample solution and the standard solution show a red-purple color, and has the same *Rf* value.

(2) The colored solution obtained in the Assay is blue in color.

Uniformity of dosage units <*6.02*> Perform the test according to the following method: it meets the requirement of the Content uniformity test.

Place 1 tablet of Liothyronine Sodium Tablets in a glass-stoppered centrifuge tube, add exactly 10 mL of 0.01 mol/L sodium hydroxide TS, warm at 50°C for 15 minutes, and shake vigorously for 20 minutes. Centrifuge for 5 minutes, and filter the supernatant liquid, if necessary. Pipet a definite volume of this solution, and add a volume of 0.01 mol/L sodium hydroxide TS to prepare a definite volume of a solution containing about 0.5 μg of liothyronine sodium ($C_{15}H_{11}I_3NNaO_4$) per mL. Pipet 5 mL of this solution, add exactly 1 mL of the internal standard solution, and use this solution as the sample solution. Perform the test with 200 μL of the sample solution as directed under Liquid Chromatography <*2.01*> according to the following conditions, and calculate the ratio of the peak area of the liothyronine to that of the internal standard. Calculate the mean value of the ratios of each peak area of 10 samples: the deviation (%) of each ratio of the peak area from the mean value should be not more than 15%. When the deviation (%) is more than 15%, and 1 sample shows not more than 25%, perform another test with 20 samples. Calculate the deviation (%) of each ratio of the peak area from the mean value of the 30 samples used in the two tests: there should be not more than 1 sample with the deviation more than 15% but not more than 25%, and no sample should deviate by more than 25%.

Internal standard solution—A solution of propylparahydroxybenzoate in a mixture of methanol and diluted phosphoric acid (1 in 10) (9:1) (1 in 250,000).

Operating conditions—

Detector: An ultraviolet absorption photometer (wavelength: 225 nm).

Column: A stainless steel column 4.6 mm in inside diameter and 15 cm in length, packed with octadecylsylanized silica gel for liquid chromatography (5 μm in particle diameter).

Column temperature: A constant temperature of about 25°C.

Mobile phase: Diluted methanol (57 in 100).

Flow rate: Adjust so that the retention time of liothyronine is about 9 minutes.

System suitability—

System performance: To 5 mL of a solution of liothyronine sodium in 0.01 mol/L sodium hydroxide TS (1 in 2,000,000) add 1 mL of the internal standard solution, and use this solution as the solution for system suitability test. When the procedure is run with 200 μL of this solution under the above operating conditions, the internal standard and liothyronine are eluted in this order with the resolution between these peaks being not less than 2.0.

System repeatability: When the test is repeated 6 times with 200 μL of the solution for system suitability test under the above operating conditions, the relative standard deviation of the ratios of the peak area of liothyronine to that of the internal standard is not more than 1.0%.

Assay Weigh accurately not less than 20 Liothyronine Sodium Tablets, and finely powder. Place an accurately weighed portion of the powder, equivalent to about 50 μg of liothyronine sodium ($C_{15}H_{11}I_3NNaO_4$), in an agate mortar, add 1 g of powdered potassium carbonate, and mix well. Transfer the mixture cautiously to a porcelain crucible, and compact the contents by gently tapping the crucible on a table. Add an additional 1.5 g of powdered potassium carbonate to the same agate mortar, mix well with any content adhering to the mortar, cautiously overlay the mixture on the top of the same porcelain crucible, and compact the charge again in the same manner. Ignite the combined mixture in the crucible between 675°C and 700°C for 30 minutes. Cool, add a few mL of water to the crucible, heat gently to boiling, and filter the contents of the crucible through a glass filter (G4) into a 20-mL volumetric flask. Wash the residue with water, and combine the washings with the filtrate. Cool, add water to make 20 mL, and use this solution as the sample solution. Separately, weigh accurately about 75 mg of potassium iodide for assay, previously dried at 105°C for 4 hours, and dissolve in water to make exactly 200 mL. Measure exactly 5 mL of the solution, and add a solution of potassium carbonate (1 in 8) to make exactly 100 mL. To 2 mL of this solution, exactly measured, add a solution of potassium carbonate (1 in 8) to make exactly 20 mL, and use the solution as the standard solution. Pipet 5 mL each of the sample solution and the standard solution into glass-stoppered test tubes, add 3.0 mL of diluted sulfuric acid (4 in 25) and 2.0 mL of potassium permanganate TS, and heat on a water bath for 15 minutes. Cool, add 1.0 mL of diluted sodium nitrite TS (1 in 10), swirl to mix, and add 1.0 mL of a solution of ammonium amidosulfate (1 in 10). Allow to stand at room temperature for 10 minutes with occasional shaking. Then add 1.0 mL of potato starch TS and 1.0 mL of a freshly prepared, diluted potassium iodide TS (1 in 40), swirl to mix, and transfer each solution to a 20-mL volumetric flask. Rinse the test tube with water, collect the washings in the volumetric flask, add water to make 20 mL, and allow to stand for 10 minutes. Perform the test with these solutions as directed under Ultraviolet-visible Spectrophotometry <2.24>, using a solution prepared with 5 mL of potassium carbonate (1 in 8) in the same manner as the sample solution as the blank. Determine the absorbances, A_T and A_S, of the subsequent solutions of the sample solution and the standard solution at the wavelength of maximum absorption at about 600 nm, respectively.

Amount (mg) of liothyronine sodium ($C_{15}H_{11}I_3NNaO_4$)
$= M_S \times A_T/A_S \times 1/2000 \times 1.351$

M_S: Amount (mg) of potassium iodide for assay taken

Containers and storage Containers—Tight containers.

Storage—Light-resistant.

Lisinopril Hydrate

リシノプリル水和物

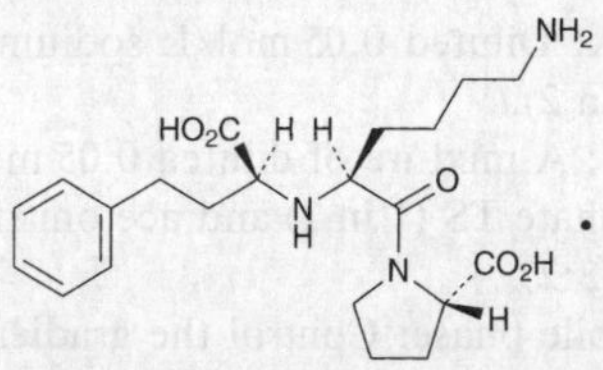

$C_{21}H_{31}N_3O_5 \cdot 2H_2O$: 441.52

(2*S*)-1-{(2*S*)-6-Amino-2-[(1*S*)-1-carboxy-3-phenylpropylamino]hexanoyl}pyrrolidine-2-carboxylic acid dihydrate

[*83915-83-7*]

Lisinopril Hydrate contains not less than 98.5% and not more than 101.0% of lisinopril ($C_{21}H_{31}N_3O_5$: 405.49), calculated on the anhydrous basis.

Description Lisinopril Hydrate occurs as a white crystalline powder, having a slight characteristic odor.

It is soluble in water, sparingly soluble in methanol, and practically insoluble in ethanol (99.5).

Melting point: about 160°C (with decomposition).

Identification (1) Determine the absorption spectrum of a solution of Lisinopril Hydrate in methanol (1 in 1000) as directed under Ultraviolet-visible Spectrophotometry <2.24>, and compare the spectrum with the Reference Spectrum: both spectra exhibit similar intensities of absorption at the same wavelengths.

(2) Determine the infrared absorption spectrum of Lisinopril Hydrate as directed in the paste method under Infrared Spectrophotometry <2.25>, and compare the spectrum with the Reference Spectrum: both spectra exhibit similar intensities of absorption at the same wave numbers.

Optical rotation <2.49> $[\alpha]_D^{25}$: $-43.0 - -47.0°$ (0.25 g calculated on the anhydrous basis, 0.25 mol/L zinc acetate buffer solution (pH 6.4), 25 mL, 100 mm).

Purity (1) Heavy metals <1.07>—Proceed with 2.0 g of Lisinopril Hydrate according to Method 4, and perform the test. Prepare the control solution with 2.0 mL of Standard Lead Solution (not more than 10 ppm).

(2) Related substances—Dissolve about 0.10 g of Lisinopril Hydrate in 50 mL of water, and use this solution as the sample solution. Pipet 3 mL of the sample solution, add water to make exactly 200 mL, and use this solution as the standard solution. Perform the test with exactly 15 μL each of the sample solution and standard solution as directed under Liquid Chromatography <2.01> according to the following conditions, and determine each peak area by the automatic integration method: the area of the peak, having the relative retention time of about 1.2 to lisinopril obtained from the sample solution, is not larger than 1/5 times the peak area of lisinopril from the standard solution, the area of the peak other than lisinopril and the peak mentioned above from the sample solution, is not larger than 2/15 times the peak area of lisinopril from the standard solution, and the total area of the peaks other than lisinopril from the sample solution, is not larger than the peak area of lisinopril from the standard solution.

Operating conditions—

Detector: An ultraviolet absorption photometer (wavelength: 215 nm).

Column: A stainless steel column 4.0 mm in inside diameter and 20 cm in length, packed with octadecylsilanized silica gel for liquid chromatography (7 μm in particle diameter).

Column temperature: A constant temperature of about 60°C.

Mobile phase A: Diluted 0.05 mol/L sodium dihydrogen phosphate TS (1 in 2).

Mobile phase B: A mixture of diluted 0.05 mol/L sodium dihydrogen phosphate TS (1 in 2) and acetonitrile for liquid chromatography (3:2).

Flowing of mobile phase: Control the gradient by mixing the mobile phases A and B as directed in the following table.

Time after injection of sample (min)	Mobile phase A (vol%)	Mobile phase B (vol%)
0 – 10	90 → 50	10 → 50
10 – 25	50	50

Flow rate: About 1.5 mL per minute.

Time span of measurement: About 2.5 times as long as the retention time of lisinopril, beginning after the solvent peak.

System suitability—

Test for required detectability: Measure exactly 2.5 mL of the standard solution, and add water to make exactly 50 mL. Confirm that the peak area of lisinopril obtained with 15 μL of this solution is equivalent to 3.5 to 6.5% of that with 15 μL of the standard solution.

System performance: To 10 mg of lisinopril hydrate and 2 mL of a solution of anhydrous caffeine (1 in 1000) add water to make 200 mL. When the procedure is run with 15 μL of this solution under the above operating conditions, lisinopril and caffeine are eluted in this order with the resolution between these peaks being not less than 6.

System repeatability: When the test is repeated 6 times with 15 μL of the standard solution under the above operating conditions, the relative standard deviation of the peak area of lisinopril is not more than 2.0%.

Water <*2.48*> Not less than 8.0% and not more than 9.5% (0.3 g, volumetric titration, back titration).

Residue on ignition <*2.44*> Not more than 0.1% (1 g).

Assay Weigh accurately about 0.66 g of Lisinopril Hydrate, dissolve in 80 mL of water, and titrate <*2.50*> with 0.1 mol/L sodium hydroxide VS (potentiometric titration). Perform a blank determination in the same manner, and make any necessary correction.

Each mL of 0.1 mol/L sodium hydroxide VS
= 40.55 mg of $C_{21}H_{31}N_3O_5$

Containers and storage Containers—Well-closed containers.

Lisinopril Tablets

リシノプリル錠

Lisinopril Tablets contain not less than 95.0% and not more than 105.0% of the labeled amount of lisinopril ($C_{21}H_{31}N_3O_5$: 405.49).

Method of preparation Prepare as directed under Tablets, with Lisinopril Hydrate.

Identification To an amount of powdered Lisinopril Tablets, equivalent to 10 mg of lisinopril ($C_{21}H_{31}N_3O_5$), add 10 mL of methanol, shake for 20 minutes, filter, and use the filtrate as the sample solution. Separately, dissolve 10 mg of lisinopril in 10 mL of methanol, and use this solution as the standard solution. Perform the test with these solutions as directed under Thin-layer Chromatography <*2.03*>. Spot 30 μL each of the sample solution and standard solution on a plate of silica gel for thin-layer chromatography. Develop the plate with a mixture of acetonitrile, acetic acid (100), water and ethyl acetate (2:2:1:1) to a distance of about 10 cm, and air-dry the plate. Spray evenly ninhydrin TS on the plate, and heat the plate at 120°C: the principal spot obtained from the sample solution and the spot from the standard solution show a red-purple color and their *R*f values are the same.

Purity Related substances—Powder not less than 20 Lisinopril Tablets. Take a portion of the powder, equivalent to about 25 mg of lisinopril ($C_{21}H_{31}N_3O_5$), add 25 mL of water, shake for 20 minutes, filter, and use the filtrate as the sample solution. Pipet 3 mL of the sample solution, add water to make exactly 200 mL, and use this solution as the standard solution. Perform the test with exactly 15 μL each of the sample solution and standard solution as directed under Liquid Chromatography <*2.01*> according to the following conditions, and determine each peak area by the automatic integration method: the peak area of lisinopril diketopiperazine, having the relative retention time of about 2.0 to lisinopril obtained from the sample solution, is not larger than 2/3 times the peak area of lisinopril from the standard solution.

Operating conditions—

Proceed as directed in the operating conditions in the Purity (2) under Lisinopril Hydrate.

System suitability—

System performance: Proceed as directed in the system suitability in the Purity (2) under Lisinopril Hydrate.

Test for required detectability: To exactly 2.5 mL of the standard solution add water to make exactly 50 mL. Confirm that the peak area of lisinopril obtained with 15 μL of this solution is equivalent to 3.5 to 6.5% of that with 15 μL of the standard solution.

System repeatability: When the test is repeated 6 times with 15 μL of the standard solution under the above operating conditions, the relative standard deviation of the peak area of lisinopril is not more than 2.0%.

Uniformity of dosage units <*6.02*> Perform the test according to the following method: it meets the requirement of the Content uniformity test.

To 1 tablet of Lisinopril Tablets add exactly 5 mL of the internal standard solution per 1 mg of lisinopril ($C_{21}H_{31}N_3O_5$), shake for 20 minutes, centrifuge, and use the supernatant liquid as the sample solution. Hereafter, proceed as directed in the Assay.

$$\text{Amount (mg) of lisinopril } (C_{21}H_{31}N_3O_5) = M_S \times Q_T/Q_S \times C/10$$

M_S: Amount (mg) of lisinopril for assay taken, calculated on the anhydrous basis

C: Labeled amount (mg) of lisinopril ($C_{21}H_{31}N_3O_5$) in 1 tablet

Internal standard solution—A solution of anhydrous caffeine (1 in 20,000).

Dissolution <*6.10*> When the test is performed at 50 revolutions per minute according to the Paddle method, using 900 mL of water as the dissolution medium, the dissolution rate of a 5-mg tablet in 60 minutes and that of a 10-mg tablet in 90 minutes is not less than 80%, and that of a 20-mg tablet in 90 minutes is not less than 75%.

Start the test with 1 tablet of Lisinopril Tablets, withdraw not less than 20 mL of the medium at the specified minute after starting the test, and filter through a membrane filter with a pore size not exceeding 0.5 μm. Discard not less than 10 mL of the first filtrate, pipet V mL of the subsequent filtrate, add water to make exactly V' mL so that each mL contains about 5.6 μg of lisinopril ($C_{21}H_{31}N_3O_5$), and use this solution as the sample solution. Separately, weigh accurately about 15 mg of lisinopril for assay (separately determined the water *<2.48>* in the same manner as Lisinopril Hydrate), and dissolve in water to make exactly 100 mL. Pipet 2 mL of this solution, add water to make exactly 50 mL, and use this solution as the standard solution. Perform the test with exactly 50 μL each of the sample solution and standard solution as directed under Liquid Chromatography *<2.01>* according to the following conditions, and determine the peak areas, A_T and A_S, of lisinopril in each solution.

Dissolution rate (%) with respect to the labeled amount of lisinopril ($C_{21}H_{31}N_3O_5$)
$= M_S \times A_T/A_S \times V'/V \times 1/C \times 36$

M_S: Amount (mg) of lisinopril for assay taken, calculated on the anhydrous basis

C: Labeled amount (mg) of lisinopril ($C_{21}H_{31}N_3O_5$) in 1 tablet

Operating conditions—

Detector, column temperature, and mobile phase: Proceed as directed in the operating conditions in the Assay.

Column: A stainless steel column 4.6 mm in inside diameter and 15 cm in length, packed with octadecylsilanized silica gel for liquid chromatography (5 μm in particle diameter).

Flow rate: Adjust so that the retention time of lisinopril is about 7 minutes.

System suitability—

System performance: When the procedure is run with 50 μL of the standard solution under the above operating conditions, the number of theoretical plates and the symmetry factor of the peak of lisinopril are not less than 1000 and not more than 1.5, respectively.

System repeatability: When the test is repeated 6 times with 50 μL of the standard solution under the above operating conditions, the relative standard deviation of the peak area of lisinopril is not more than 2.0%.

Assay Weigh accurately the mass of not less than 20 Lisinopril Tablets, and powder. Weigh accurately a portion of the powder, equivalent to about 5 mg of lisinopril ($C_{21}H_{31}N_3O_5$), add exactly 25 mL of the internal standard solution, shake for 20 minutes, centrifuge, and use the supernatant liquid as the sample solution. Separately, weigh accurately about 10 mg of lisinopril for assay (separately determined the water *<2.48>* in the same manner as Lisinopril Hydrate), add exactly 50 mL of the internal standard solution to dissolve, and use this solution as the standard solution. Perform the test with 10 μL each of the sample solution and standard solution as directed under Liquid Chromatography *<2.01>* according to the following conditions, and calculate the ratios, Q_T and Q_S, of the peak area of lisinopril to that of the internal standard.

Amount (mg) of lisinopril ($C_{21}H_{31}N_3O_5$)
$= M_S \times Q_T/Q_S \times 1/2$

M_S: Amount (mg) of lisinopril for assay taken, calculated on the anhydrous basis

*Internal standard solution—*A solution of anhydrous caffeine (1 in 20,000).

Operating conditions—

Detector: An ultraviolet absorption photometer (wavelength: 215 nm).

Column: A stainless steel column 4.0 mm in inside diameter and 20 cm in length, packed with octadecylsilanized silica gel for liquid chromatography (7 μm in particle diameter).

Column temperature: A constant temperature of about 60°C.

Mobile phase: A mixture of diluted 0.05 mol/L sodium dihydrogen phosphate TS (1 in 2) and acetonitrile for liquid chromatography (19:1).

Flow rate: Adjust so that the retention time of lisinopril is about 6 minutes.

System suitability—

System performance: When the procedure is run with 10 μL of the standard solution under the above operating conditions, lisinopril and the internal standard are eluted in this order with the resolution between these peaks being not less than 7.

System repeatability: When the test is repeated 6 times with 10 μL of the standard solution under the above operating conditions, the relative standard deviation of the ratio of the peak area of lisinopril to that of the internal standard is not more than 1.0%.

Containers and storage Containers—Well-closed containers.

Lithium Carbonate

炭酸リチウム

Li_2CO_3: 73.89

Lithium Carbonate, when dried, contains not less than 99.5% of lithium carbonate (Li_2CO_3).

Description Lithium Carbonate occurs as a white crystalline powder. It is odorless.

It is sparingly soluble in water, slightly soluble in hot water, and practically insoluble in ethanol (95) and in diethyl ether.

It dissolves in dilute acetic acid.

The pH of a solution dissolved 1.0 g of Lithium Carbonate in 100 mL of water is between 10.9 and 11.5.

Identification **(1)** Perform the test as directed under Flame Coloration Test *<1.04>* (1) with Lithium Carbonate: a persistent red color appears.

(2) Dissolve 0.2 g of Lithium Carbonate in 3 mL of dilute hydrochloric acid, and add 4 mL of sodium hydroxide TS and 2 mL of disodium hydrogen phosphate TS: a white precipitate is produced. To the precipitate add 2 mL of dilute hydrochloric acid: it dissolves.

(3) A solution of Lithium Carbonate (1 in 100) responds to Qualitative Tests *<1.09>* for carbonate.

Purity **(1)** Clarity and color of solution—Dissolve 0.10 g of Lithium Carbonate in 10 mL of water by warming: the solution is clear and colorless.

(2) Acetic acid-insoluble substances—Take 1.0 g of Lithium Carbonate, dissolve in 40 mL of dilute acetic acid, filter the insoluble substances using filter paper for quantitative analysis, wash with five 10-mL portions of water, and ignite the insoluble substances together with the filter paper to incinerate: the mass of the residue is not more than 1.5 mg.

(3) Chloride <*1.03*>—To 0.40 g of Lithium Carbonate add 10 mL of water and 7 mL of dilute nitric acid, and dissolve by heating to boil. After cooling, add 6 mL of dilute nitric acid, and dilute with water to make 50 mL. Perform the test using this solution as the test solution. Prepare the control solution with 0.25 mL of 0.01 mol/L hydrochloric acid VS (not more than 0.022%).

(4) Sulfate <*1.14*>—To 0.40 g of Lithium Carbonate add 10 mL of water and 4 mL of dilute hydrochloric acid, and dissolve by heating to boil. After cooling, add 1 mL of dilute hydrochloric acid, and dilute with water to make 50 mL. Perform the test using this solution as the test solution. Prepare the control solution with 0.40 mL of 0.005 mol/L sulfuric acid VS (not more than 0.048%).

(5) Heavy metals <*1.07*>—To 4.0 g of Lithium Carbonate add 5 mL of water, gradually add 10 mL of hydrochloric acid while mixing, and dissolve. Evaporate the solution on a water bath to dryness. To the residue add 10 mL of water, and dissolve. Place the solution in a Nessler tube, add 1 drop of phenolphthalein TS, add ammonia TS until the solution shows a slight red color, then add 2 mL of dilute acetic acid, and dilute with water to make 50 mL. Perform the test using this solution as the test solution. Prepare the control solution as follows: Evaporate 10 mL of hydrochloric acid on a water bath to dryness. To the residue add 10 mL of water, and dissolve. Place the solution in a Nessler tube, add 1 drop of phenolphthalein TS, add ammonia TS until the solution shows a pale red color, then add 2.0 mL of Standard Lead Solution and 2 mL of dilute acetic acid, and dilute with water to make 50 mL (not more than 5 ppm).

(6) Iron <*1.10*>—Prepare the test solution with 1.0 g of Lithium Carbonate according to Method 2 using 11 mL of dilute hydrochloric acid, and perform the test according to Method B. Prepare the control solution with 1.0 mL of Standard Iron Solution (not more than 10 ppm).

(7) Aluminum—To 5.0 g of Lithium Carbonate add 20 mL of water, add gradually 15 mL of hydrochloric acid while stirring, and evaporate to dryness on a water bath. To the residue add 50 mL of water to dissolve, filter if necessary, and assign this solution as solution A. Separately, evaporate 15 mL of hydrochloric acid to dryness on a water bath, then proceed in the same manner, and assign the solution so obtained as solution B. To 10 mL of solution A add 10 mL of water and 5 mL of acetic acid-sodium acetate buffer solution (pH 4.5), and shake. Add 1 mL of a solution of L-ascorbic acid (1 in 100), 2 mL of aluminon TS and water to make 50 mL, shake well, and allow to stand for 10 minutes: the solution has no more color than the following control solution.

Control solution: Dissolve 0.1758 g of aluminum potassium sulfate dodecahydrate in water to make 1000 mL. To 1.0 mL of this solution add 10 mL of solution B and water to make 20 mL, add 5 mL of acetic acid-sodium acetate buffer solution (pH 4.5), and proceed in the same manner.

(8) Barium—To 20 mL of solution A obtained in (7) add 6 mL of water, 0.5 mL of dilute hydrochloric acid, 3 mL of ethanol (95) and 2 mL of potassium sulfate TS, and allow to stand for 1 hour: the solution has no more turbidity than the following control solution.

Control solution: Dissolve 17.8 mg of barium chloride dihydrate in water to make 1000 mL. To 6 mL of this solution add 20 mL of solution B obtained in (7), 0.5 mL of dilute hydrochloric acid and 3 mL of ethanol (95), and proceed in the same manner.

(9) Calcium—Weigh accurately about 5 g of Lithium Carbonate, add 50 mL of water and 15 mL of hydrochloric acid, and dissolve. Remove carbon dioxide from the solution by boiling, add 5 mL of ammonium oxalate TS, then make alkaline with ammonia TS, and allow to stand for 4 hours. Filter the produced precipitate through a glass filter (G4), wash with warm water until the turbidity of the washing is not produced with calcium chloride TS within 1 minute. Transfer the precipitate and the glass filter into a beaker, add water until the glass filter is covered with water, then add 3 mL of sulfuric acid, heat between 70°C and 80°C, and titrate <*2.50*> with 0.02 mol/L potassium permanganate VS until a pale red color persists for 30 seconds: the amount of calcium (Ca: 40.08) is not more than 0.05%.

Each mL of 0.02 mol/L potassium permanganate VS
= 2.004 mg of Ca

(10) Magnesium—To 3.0 mL of solution A obtained in (7) add 0.2 mL of a solution of titan yellow (1 in 1000) and water to make 20 mL, then add 5 mL of sodium hydroxide (3 in 20), and allow to stand for 10 minutes: the solution has no more color than the following control solution.

Control solution: Dissolve 49.5 mg of magnesium sulfate heptahydrate, previously dried at 105°C for 2 hours and heated at 450°C for 3 hours, in water to make 1000 mL. To 6 mL of this solution add 3 mL of solution B obtained in (7), 0.2 mL of a solution of titanium yellow (1 in 1000) and water to make 20 mL, and proceed in the same manner.

(11) Potassium—Dissolve 1.0 g of Lithium Carbonate in water to make 100 mL, and use this solution as the sample solution. To 5 mL of the sample solution add 1.0 mL of dilute acetic acid, shake, add 5 mL of a solution of sodium tetraphenylborate (1 in 30), shake immediately, and allow to stand for 10 minutes: the solution has no more turbidity than the following control solution.

Control solution: Dissolve 9.5 mg of potassium chloride in water to make 1000 mL. To 5 mL of this solution add 1.0 mL of dilute acetic acid, shake, and proceed in the same manner.

(12) Sodium—Weigh accurately about 0.8 g of Lithium Carbonate, dissolve in water to make exactly 100 mL, and use this solution as the sample stock solution. Measure exactly 25 mL of the sample stock solution, add water to make exactly 100 mL, and use this solution as the sample solution (1). Separately, weigh accurately 25.4 mg of sodium chloride, dissolve in water to make exactly 1000 mL, and use this solution as the standard solution. Measure exactly 25 mL of the sample stock solution, add exactly 20 mL of the standard solution, then add water to make exactly 100 mL, and use this solution as the sample solution (2). Determine emission intensities of sodium using a flame photometer with the sample solution (1) and the sample solution (2) under the following conditions. Adjust the wavelength dial to 589 nm, atomize the sample solution (2) into the flame, then adjust the sensitivity so that the emission intensity L_S shows 100 adjustment, and determine emission intensity L_T of the sample solution (1). Then, make the other conditions identical, change the wavelength dial to 580 nm, determine emission intensity L_B of the sample solution (1): the amount of sodium, calculated from the following equation, is not more than 0.05%.

Amount (%) of sodium (Na)
$$= (L_T - L_B)/(L_S - L_T) \times M'/M \times 100$$

M: Amount (mg) of the sample in 25 mL of the sample stock solution

M': Amount (mg) of sodium in 20 mL of the standard solution

(13) Arsenic <*1.11*>—Prepare the test solution with 1.0 g of Lithium Carbonate, add 2 mL of water and 3 mL of hydrochloric acid, and perform the test (not more than 2 ppm).

Loss on drying <*2.41*> Not more than 0.5% (1 g, 105°C, 3 hours).

Assay Weigh accurately about 1 g of Lithium Carbonate, previously dried, add exactly 100 mL of water and 50 mL of 0.5 mol/L sulfuric acid VS, remove carbon dioxide by boiling gently, cool, and titrate <*2.50*> the excess sulfuric acid with 1 mol/L sodium hydroxide VS until the color of the solution changes from red to yellow (indicator: 3 drops of methyl red TS). Perform a blank determination in the same manner.

Each mL of 0.5 mol/L sulfuric acid VS
= 36.95 mg of Li_2CO_3

Containers and storage Containers—Well-closed containers.

Lobenzarit Sodium

ロベンザリットナトリウム

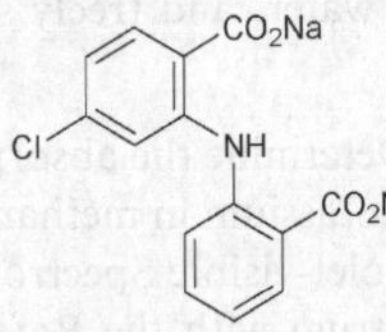

$C_{14}H_8ClNNa_2O_4$: 335.65
Disodium 2-[(2-carboxylatophenyl)amino]-4-chlorobenzoate
[*64808-48-6*]

Lobenzarit Sodium, when dried, contains not less than 98.0% and not more than 101.0% of lobenzarit sodium ($C_{14}H_8ClNNa_2O_4$).

Description Lobenzarit Sodium occurs as a white to pale yellow-white crystalline powder.

It is soluble in water, and practically insoluble in ethanol (99.5).

Identification **(1)** A solution of Lobenzarit Sodium (1 in 50) responds to Qualitative Tests <*1.09*> (1) for chloride.

(2) Determine the absorption spectrum of a solution of Lobenzarit Sodium (1 in 100,000) as directed under Ultraviolet-visible Spectrophotometry <*2.24*>, and compare the spectrum with the Reference Spectrum: both spectra exhibit similar intensities of absorption at the same wavelengths.

(3) Determine the infrared absorption spectrum of Lobenzarit Sodium, previously dried, as directed in the potassium bromide disk method under Infrared Spectrophotometry <*2.25*>, and compare the spectrum with the Reference Spectrum: both spectra exhibit similar intensities of absorption at the same wave numbers.

(4) A solution of Lobenzarit Sodium (1 in 50) responds to Qualitative Tests <*1.09*> (2) for sodium salt.

Purity **(1)** Heavy metals <*1.07*>—Proceed with 1.0 g of Lobenzarit Sodium according to Method 2, and perform the test. Prepare the control solution with 2.0 mL of Standard Lead Solution (not more than 20 ppm).

(2) Arsenic <*1.11*>—Prepare the test solution with 2.0 g of Lobenzarit Sodium according to Method 3, and perform the test (not more than 1 ppm).

(3) Related substances—Dissolve 50 mg of Lobenzarit Sodium in 2.5 mL of water, and use this solution as the sample solution. Pipet 1 mL of the sample solution, and add water to make exactly 100 mL. Pipet 4 mL of this solution, add water to make exactly 20 mL, and use this solution as the standard solution. Perform the test with these solutions as directed under Thin-layer Chromatography <*2.03*>. Spot 5 μL each of the sample solution and standard solution on a plate of silica gel with fluorescent indicator for thin-layer chromatography. Develop the plate with a mixture of tetrahydrofuran, water and triethylamine (50:15:8) to a distance of about 10 cm, and air-dry the plate. Examine under ultraviolet light (main wavelength: 254 nm): the spot other than the principal spot obtained from the sample solution is not more intense than the spot from the standard solution.

Loss on drying <*2.41*> Not more than 1.0% (1 g, 105°C, 2 hours).

Assay Weigh accurately about 0.1 g of Lobenzarit Sodium, previously dried, dissolve in exactly 40 mL of water, add exactly 60 mL of a mixture of diethyl ether and tetrahydrofuran (1:1), and titrate <*2.50*> with 0.1 mol/L hydrochloric acid VS while well shaking (indicator: 10 drops of bromophenol blue TS) until the blue color of the water layer changes to a persistent light blue-green. Perform a blank determination in the same manner, and make any necessary correction.

Each mL of 0.1 mol/L hydrochloric acid VS
= 16.78 mg of $C_{14}H_8ClNNa_2O_4$

Containers and storage Containers—Tight containers.

Lorazepam

ロラゼパム

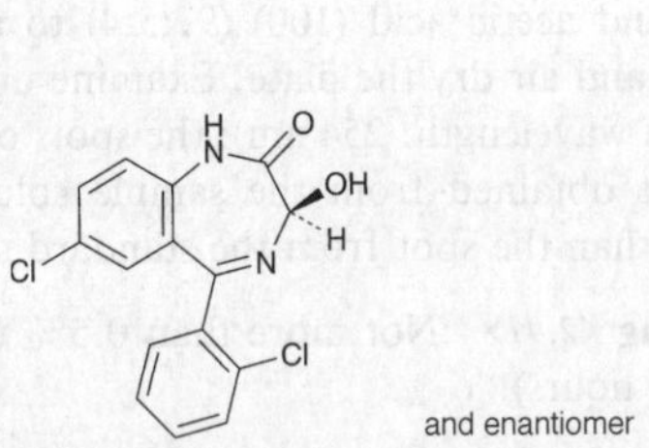

and enantiomer

$C_{15}H_{10}Cl_2N_2O_2$: 321.16
(3*RS*)-7-Chloro-5-(2-chlorophenyl)-3-hydroxy-1,3-dihydro-2*H*-1,4-benzodiazepin-2-one
[*846-49-1*]

Lorazepam, when dried, contains not less than 98.5% of lorazepam ($C_{15}H_{10}Cl_2N_2O_2$).

Description Lorazepam occurs as a white crystalline powder. It is odorless.

It is sparingly soluble in ethanol (95) and in acetone, slightly soluble in diethyl ether, and practically insoluble in water.

It is gradually colored by light.

Identification **(1)** To 0.02 g of Lorazepam add 15 mL of dilute hydrochloric acid, boil for 5 minutes, and cool: the solution responds to Qualitative Tests <*1.09*> for primary aromatic amines.

(2) Determine the absorption spectrum of a solution of Lorazepam in ethanol (95) (1 in 200,000) as directed under Ultraviolet-visible Spectrophotometry <*2.24*>, and compare the spectrum with the Reference Spectrum: both spectra exhibit similar intensities of absorption at the same wavelengths.

(3) Determine the infrared absorption spectrum of

Lorazepam, previously dried, as directed in the potassium bromide disk method under Infrared Spectrophotometry *<2.25>*, and compare the spectrum with the Reference Spectrum: both spectra exhibit similar intensities of absorption at the same wave numbers.

(4) Perform the test with Lorazepam as directed under Flame Coloration Test *<1.04>* (2): a green color appears.

Absorbance *<2.24>* $E^{1\%}_{1\,\mathrm{cm}}$ (229 nm): 1080 – 1126 (after drying, 1 mg, ethanol (95), 200 mL).

Purity **(1)** Chloride *<1.03>*—To 1.0 g of Lorazepam add 50 mL of water, allow to stand for 1 hour with occasional shaking, and filter. To 25 mL of the filtrate add 6 mL of dilute nitric acid and water to make 50 mL. Perform the test using this solution as the test solution. Prepare the control solution with 0.20 mL of 0.01 mol/L hydrochloric acid VS (not more than 0.014%).

(2) Heavy metals *<1.07>*—Proceed with 1.0 g of Lorazepam according to Method 2, and perform the test. Prepare the control solution with 2.0 mL of Standard Lead Solution (not more than 20 ppm).

(3) Arsenic *<1.11>*—Prepare the test solution with 1.0 g of Lorazepam according to Method 3, and perform the test (not more than 2 ppm).

(4) Related substances—Dissolve 0.10 g of Lorazepam in 20 mL of ethanol (95), and use this solution as the sample solution. Pipet 1 mL of the sample solution, add ethanol (95) to make exactly 100 mL, and use this solution as the standard solution. Perform the test with these solutions as directed under Thin-layer Chromatography *<2.03>*. Spot 10 μL each of the sample solution and standard solution on a plate of silica gel with fluorescent indicator for thin-layer chromatography. Develop the plate with a mixture of chloroform, 1,4-dioxane and acetic acid (100) (91:5:4) to a distance of about 15 cm, and air-dry the plate. Examine under ultraviolet light (main wavelength: 254 nm): the spots other than the principal spot obtained from the sample solution are not more intense than the spot from the standard solution.

Loss on drying *<2.41>* Not more than 0.5% (1 g, in vacuum, 105°C, 3 hours).

Residue on ignition *<2.44>* Not more than 0.3% (1 g).

Assay Weigh accurately about 0.4 g of Lorazepam, previously dried, dissolve in 50 mL of acetone, and titrate *<2.50>* with 0.1 mol/L tetrabutylammonium hydroxide VS (potentiometric titration). Perform a blank determination in the same manner, and make any necessary correction.

Each mL of 0.1 mol/L tetrabutylammonium hydroxide VS
= 32.12 mg of $C_{15}H_{10}Cl_2N_2O_2$

Containers and storage Containers—Tight containers.
Storage—Light-resistant.

Losartan Potassium

ロサルタンカリウム

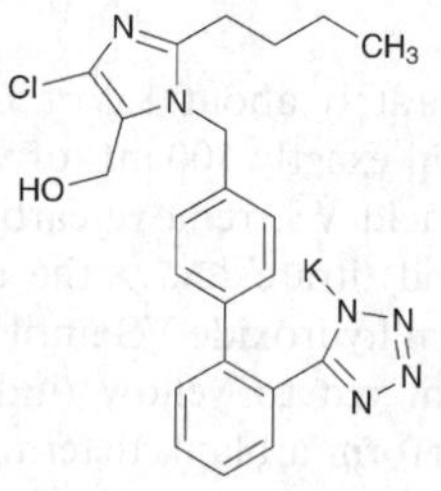

$C_{22}H_{22}ClKN_6O$: 461.00
Monopotassium 5-{[4′-(2-butyl-4-chloro-5-hydroxymethyl-1*H*-imidazol-1-yl)methyl]biphenyl-2-yl}-1*H*-tetrazol-1-ide
[*124750-99-8*]

Losartan Potassium contains not less than 98.5% and not more than 101.0% of losartan potassium ($C_{22}H_{22}ClKN_6O$), calculated on the anhydrous basis.

Description Losartan Potassium occurs as a white crystalline powder.

It is very soluble in water, and freely soluble in methanol and in ethanol (99.5).

Identification **(1)** Determine the absorption spectrum of a solution of Losartan Potassium in methanol (1 in 100,000) as directed under Ultraviolet-visible Spectrophotometry *<2.24>*, and compare the spectrum with the Reference Spectrum or the spectrum of a solution of Losartan Potassium RS prepared in the same manner as the sample solution: both spectra exhibit similar intensities of absorption at the same wavelengths.

(2) Determine the infrared absorption spectrum of Losartan Potassium as directed in the potassium bromide disk method under Infrared Spectrophotometry *<2.25>*, and compare the spectrum with the Reference Spectrum or the spectrum of Losartan Potassium RS: both spectra exhibit similar intensities of absorption at the same wave numbers.

(3) Losartan Potassium responds to Qualitative Tests *<1.09>* (1) for potassium salt.

(4) Perform the test with Losartan Potassium as directed under Flame Coloration Test *<1.04>* (2): a green color appears.

Purity **(1)** Heavy metals *<1.07>*—Proceed with 2.0 g of Losartan Potassium according to Method 2, and perform the test. Prepare the control solution with 2.0 mL of Standard Lead Solution (not more than 10 ppm).

(2) Related substances—Dissolve 30 mg of Losartan Potassium in 100 mL of methanol, and use this solution as the sample solution. Pipet 1 mL of this solution, add methanol to make exactly 100 mL, and use this solution as the standard solution. Perform the test with exactly 10 μL each of the sample solution and standard solution as directed under Liquid Chromatography *<2.01>* according to the following conditions. Determine each peak area of both solutions by the automatic integration method: the area of each peak other than the peaks of solvent and losartan obtained from the sample solution is not larger than 1/10 times the peak area of losartan from the standard solution, and the total area of the peaks other than losartan from the sample solution is not larger than 3/10 times the peak area of losartan from the standard solution.

Operating conditions—

Detector: An ultraviolet absorption photometer (wavelength: 220 nm).

Column: A stainless steel column 4 mm in inside diameter and 25 cm in length, packed with octadecylsilanized silica gel for liquid chromatography (5 μm in particle diameter).

Column temperature: A constant temperature of about 25°C.

Mobile phase A: Diluted phosphoric acid (1 in 1000).

Mobile phase B: Acetonitrile.

Flowing of mobile phase: Control the gradient by mixing the mobile phases A and B as directed in the following table.

Time after injection of sample (min)	Mobile phase A (vol%)	Mobile phase B (vol%)
0 – 25	75 → 10	25 → 90
25 – 35	10	90

Flow rate: 1.0 mL per minute.

Time span of measurement: For 35 minutes after injection of the sample solution.

System suitability—

Test for required detectability: Pipet 1 mL of the standard solution, and add methanol to make exactly 10 mL. Confirm that the peak area of losartan obtained with 10 μL of this solution is equivalent to 7 to 13% of that with 10 μL of the standard solution.

System performance: When the procedure is run with 10 μL of the standard solution under the above operating conditions, the number of theoretical plates and the symmetry factor of the peak of losartan are not less than 10,000 and not more than 1.3, respectively.

System repeatability: When the test is repeated 6 times with 10 μL of the standard solution under the above operating conditions, the relative standard deviation of the peak area of losartan is not more than 2.0%.

Water <2.48> Not more than 0.5% (0.25 g, volumetric titration, direct titration).

Assay Weigh accurately about 25 mg each of Losartan Potassium and Losartan Potassium RS (separately, determine the water <2.48> in the same manner as Losartan Potassium), dissolve separately in methanol to make exactly 100 mL, and use these solutions as the sample solution and the standard solution, respectively. Perform the test with exactly 10 μL each of the sample solution and standard solution as directed under Liquid Chromatography <2.01> according to the following conditions, and determine the peak areas, A_T and A_S, of losartan in each solution.

Amount (mg) of losartan potassium ($C_{22}H_{22}ClKN_6O$)
$= M_S \times A_T/A_S$

M_S: Amount (mg) of Losartan Potassium RS taken, calculated on the anhydrous basis

Operating conditions—

Detector: An ultraviolet absorption photometer (wavelength: 254 nm).

Column: A stainless steel column 4 mm in inside diameter and 25 cm in length, packed with octadecylsilanized silica gel for liquid chromatography (5 μm in particle diameter).

Column temperature: A constant temperature of about 35°C.

Mobile phase: A mixture of diluted phosphoric acid (1 in 1000) and acetonitrile (3:2).

Flow rate: Adjust so that the retention time of losartan is about 6 minutes.

System suitability—

System performance: When the procedure is run with 10 μL of the standard solution under the above operating conditions, the number of theoretical plates and the symmetry factor of the peak of losartan are not less than 5500 and not more than 1.4, respectively.

System repeatability: When the test is repeated 6 times with 10 μL of the standard solution under the above operating conditions, the relative standard deviation of the peak area of losartan is not more than 1.0%.

Containers and storage Containers—Tight containers.

Losartan Potassium Tablets

ロサルタンカリウム錠

Losartan Potassium Tablets contain not less than 95.0% and not more than 105.0% of the labeled amount of losartan potassium ($C_{22}H_{22}ClKN_6O$: 461.00).

Method of preparation Prepare as directed under Tablets, with Losartan Potassium.

Identification To an amount of powdered Losartan Potassium Tablets, equivalent to 25 mg of losartan potassium, add 10 mL of methanol, shake well, and centrifuge. To 5 mL of the supernatant liquid add methanol to make 25 mL, and use this solution as the sample solution. Separately, dissolve 25 mg of losartan potassium in 10 mL of methanol. To 5 mL of this solution add methanol to make 25 mL, and use this solution as the standard solution. Perform the test with these solutions as directed under Thin-layer Chromatography <2.03>. Spot 10 μL each of the sample solution and standard solution on a plate of silica gel with fluorescent indicator for thin-layer chromatography. Develop the plate with a mixture of ethyl acetate, methanol and acetic acid (100) (75:25:1) to a distance of about 10 cm, and air-dry the plate. Examine under ultraviolet light (main wavelength: 254 nm): the principal spot obtained from the sample solution and the spot from the standard solution show the same *R*f value.

Uniformity of dosage units <6.02> Perform the Mass variation test, or the Content uniformity test according to the following method: it meets the requirement.

To 1 tablet of Losartan Potassium Tablets add diluted 0.1 mol/L phosphate buffer solution (pH 8.0) (1 in 10) to make exactly 100 mL, and stir until the tablet is completely disintegrated. Pipet 5 mL of this solution, add diluted 0.1 mol/L phosphate buffer solution (pH 8.0) (1 in 10) to make exactly *V* mL so that each mL contains about 50 μg of losartan potassium ($C_{22}H_{22}ClKN_6O$), centrifuge, and use the supernatant liquid as the sample solution. Then, proceed as directed in the Assay.

Amount (mg) of losartan potassium ($C_{22}H_{22}ClKN_6O$)
$= M_S \times A_T/A_S \times V/25$

M_S: Amount (mg) of Losartan Potassium RS taken, calculated on the anhydrous basis

Dissolution <6.10> When the test is performed at 50 revolutions per minute for 25-mg and 50-mg tablets and at 75 revolutions per minute for 100-mg tablet according to the Paddle method, using 900 mL of water as the dissolution medium, the dissolution rate in 45 minutes of 25-mg and 50-mg tablets, and in 30 minutes of 100-mg tablet are not less than

85%, respectively.

Start the test with 1 tablet of Losartan Potassium Tablets, withdraw not less than 20 mL of the medium at the specified minute after starting the test, and filter through a membrane filter with a pore size not exceeding 0.45 μm. Discard not less than 5 mL of the first filtrate, pipet V mL of the subsequent filtrate, add water to make exactly V' mL so that each mL contains about 22 μg of losartan potassium ($C_{22}H_{22}ClKN_6O$), and use this solution as the sample solution. Separately, weigh accurately about 50 mg of Losartan Potassium RS (separately determine the water <*2.48*> in the same manner as Losartan Potassium), and dissolve in water to make exactly 100 mL. Pipet 5 mL of this solution, add water to make exactly 100 mL, and use this solution as the standard solution. Determine the absorbances, A_T and A_S, at 256 nm of the sample solution and standard solution as directed under Ultraviolet-visible Spectrophotometry <*2.24*>.

Dissolution rate (%) with respect to the labeled amount of losartan potassium ($C_{22}H_{22}ClKN_6O$)
$= M_S \times A_T/A_S \times V'/V \times 1/C \times 45$

M_S: Amount (mg) of Losartan Potassium RS taken, calculated on the anhydrous basis

C: Labeled amount (mg) of losartan potassium ($C_{22}H_{22}ClKN_6O$) in 1 tablet

Assay To 20 Losartan Potassium Tablets add diluted 0.1 mol/L phosphate buffer solution (pH 8.0) (1 in 10) to make exactly 1000 mL, and stir until the tablets are completely disintegrated. Pipet 5 mL of this solution, add diluted 0.1 mol/L phosphate buffer solution (pH 8.0) (1 in 10) to make exactly V mL so that each mL contains about 50 μg of losartan potassium ($C_{22}H_{22}ClKN_6O$), centrifuge, and use the supernatant liquid as the sample solution. Separately, weigh accurately about 25 mg of Losartan Potassium RS (separately determine the water <*2.48*> in the same manner as Losartan Potassium), dissolve in diluted 0.1 mol/L phosphate buffer solution (pH 8.0) (1 in 10) to make exactly 500 mL, and use this solution as the standard solution. Perform the test with exactly 20 μL each of the sample solution and standard solution as directed under Liquid Chromatography <*2.01*> according to the following conditions, and determine the peak areas, A_T and A_S, of losartan in each solution.

Amount (mg) of losartan potassium ($C_{22}H_{22}ClKN_6O$) in 1 tablet
$= M_S \times A_T/A_S \times V/50$

M_S: Amount (mg) of Losartan Potassium RS taken, calculated on the anhydrous basis

Operating conditions—

Detector: An ultraviolet absorption photometer (wavelength: 230 nm).

Column: A stainless steel column 4.6 mm in inside diameter and 25 cm in length, packed with octylsilanized silica gel for liquid chromatography (10 μm in particle diameter).

Column temperature: A constant temperature of about 35°C.

Mobile phase: Dissolve 1.36 g of potassium dihydrogen phosphate in 900 mL of water, adjust to pH 2.5 with phosphoric acid, and add water to make 1000 mL. To 600 mL of this solution add 400 mL of acetonitrile

Flow rate: Adjust so that the retention time of losartan is about 10 minutes.

System suitability—

System performance: When the procedure is run with 20 μL of the standard solution under the above operating conditions, the number of theoretical plates and the symmetry factor of the peak of losartan are not less than 3000 and not more than 1.5, respectively.

System repeatability: When the test is repeated 6 times with 20 μL of the standard solution under the above operating conditions, the relative standard deviation of the peak area of losartan is not more than 1.0%.

Containers and storage Containers—Tight containers.

Losartan Potassium and Hydrochlorothiazide Tablets

ロサルタンカリウム・ヒドロクロロチアジド錠

Losartan Potassium and Hydrochlorothiazide Tablets contain not less than 95.0% and not more than 105.0% of the labeled amount of losartan potassium ($C_{22}H_{22}ClKN_6O$: 461.00) and hydrochlorothiazide ($C_7H_8ClN_3O_4S_2$: 297.74).

Method of preparation Prepare as directed under Tablets, with Losartan Potassium and Hydrochlorothiazide.

Identification **(1)** Shake thoroughly a portion of powdered Losartan Potassium and Hydrochlorothiazide Tablets, equivalent to 50 mg of Losartan Potassium, with 10 mL of methanol, and centrifuge. To 5 mL of the supernatant liquid add methanol to make 50 mL, and use this solution as the sample solution. Separately, dissolve 25 mg of losartan potassium in methanol to make 10 mL. To 5 mL of this solution add methanol to make 25 mL, and use this solution as the standard solution. Perform the test with these solutions as directed under Thin-layer Chromatography <*2.03*>. Spot 20 μL each of the sample solution and standard solution on a plate of silica gel with fluorescent indicator for thin-layer chromatography. Develop the plate with a mixture of ethyl acetate, methanol and acetic acid (100) (75:25:1) to a distance of about 15 cm, and air-dry the plate. Examine under ultraviolet light (main wavelength: 254 nm): one of the two spots obtained from the sample solution and the spot from the standard solution show the same *R*f value.

(2) Shake well a portion of powdered Losartan Potassium and Hydrochlorothiazide Tablets, equivalent to 12.5 mg of Hydrochlorothiazide, with 10 mL of methanol, and centrifuge. To 5 mL of the supernatant liquid add methanol to make 50 mL, and use this solution as the sample solution. Separately, dissolve 25 mg of hydrochlorothiazide in methanol to make 10 mL. To 5 mL of this solution add methanol to make 100 mL, and use this solution as the standard solution. Perform the test with these solutions as directed under Thin-layer Chromatography <*2.03*>. Spot 20 μL each of the sample solution and standard solution on a plate of silica gel with fluorescent indicator for thin-layer chromatography. Develop the plate with a mixture of ethyl acetate, methanol and acetic acid (100) (75:25:1) to a distance of about 15 cm, and air-dry the plate. Examine under ultraviolet light (main wavelength: 254 nm): one of the two spots obtained from the sample solution and the spot from the standard solution show the same *R*f value.

Uniformity of dosage units <*6.02*>

(1) Losartan potassium—Perform the Mass variation test, or the Content uniformity test according to the following method: it meets the requirement.

To 1 tablet of Losartan Potassium and Hydrochlorothiazide Tablets add $V/2$ mL of a mixture of acetonitrile and sodium dihydrogen phosphate TS (pH 2.5) (3:2), and stir for

60 minutes to disintegrate the tablet, add sodium dihydrogen phosphate TS (pH 2.5) to make exactly V mL so that each mL contains about 0.5 mg of losartan potassium ($C_{22}H_{22}ClKN_6O$). Pipet 10 mL of this solution, add 45 mL of a mixture of acetonitrile and sodium dihydrogen phosphate TS (pH 2.5) (3:2), add sodium dihydrogen phosphate TS (pH 2.5) to make exactly 100 mL, and filter through a membrane filter with a pore size not exceeding 0.45 μm. Discard the first 2 mL of the filtrate, and use the subsequent filtrate as the sample solution. Separately, weigh accurately about 46 mg of Losartan Potassium RS (separately determine the water <*2.48*> in the same manner as Losartan Potassium), and dissolve in 50 mL of a mixture of acetonitrile and sodium dihydrogen phosphate TS (pH 2.5) (3:2), add sodium dihydrogen phosphate TS (pH 2.5) to make exactly 100 mL, and use this solution as the losartan potassium standard stock solution. Pipet 12 mL of the losartan potassium standard stock solution, add 44 mL of a mixture of acetonitrile and sodium dihydrogen phosphate TS (pH 2.5) (3:2), add sodium dihydrogen phosphate TS (pH 2.5) to make exactly 100 mL, and use this solution as the standard solution. Perform the test with exactly 20 μL each of the sample solution and standard solution as directed under Liquid Chromatography <*2.01*> according to the following conditions, and determine the peak areas, A_T and A_S, of losartan in each solution.

Amount (mg) of losartan potassium ($C_{22}H_{22}ClKN_6O$)
$= M_S \times A_T/A_S \times 3V/250$

M_S: Amount (mg) of Losartan Potassium RS taken, calculated on the anhydrous basis

Operating conditions—

Detector: An ultraviolet absorption photometer (wavelength: 230 nm).

Column: A stainless steel column 4.6 mm in inside diameter and 25 cm in length, packed with octylsilanized silica gel for liquid chromatography (10 μm in particle diameter).

Column temperature: A constant temperature of about 35°C.

Mobile phase: Dissolve 1.36 g of potassium dihydrogen phosphate in 900 mL of water, adjust to pH 2.5 with phosphoric acid, and add water to make 1000 mL. To 900 mL of this solution add 600 mL of acetonitrile.

Flow rate: Adjust so that the retention time of losartan is about 5 minutes.

System suitability—

System performance: To 12 mL of the losartan potassium standard stock solution and 4 mL of the hydrochlorothiazide standard stock solution obtained in (2), add 42 mL of a mixture of acetonitrile and sodium dihydrogen phosphate TS (pH 2.5) (3:2), and add sodium dihydrogen phosphate TS (pH 2.5) to make 100 mL. When the procedure is run with 20 μL of this solution under the above operating conditions, hydrochlorothiazide and losartan are eluted in this order with the resolution between these peaks being not less than 10.

System repeatability: When the test is repeated 6 times with 20 μL of the standard solution under the above operating conditions, the relative standard deviation of the peak area of losartan is not more than 1.0%.

(2) Hydrochlorothiazide—Perform the test according to the following method: it meets the requirement of the Content uniformity test.

To 1 tablet of Losartan Potassium and Hydrochlorothiazide Tablets add $V/2$ mL of a mixture of acetonitrile and sodium dihydrogen phosphate TS (pH 2.5) (3:2), and stir for 60 minutes to disintegrate the tablet, add sodium dihydrogen phosphate TS (pH 2.5) to make exactly V mL so that each mL contains about 0.125 mg of hydrochlorothiazide ($C_7H_8ClN_3O_4S_2$). Pipet 10 mL of this solution, add 45 mL of a mixture of acetonitrile and sodium dihydrogen phosphate TS (pH 2.5) (3:2), add sodium dihydrogen phosphate TS (pH 2.5) to make exactly 100 mL, and filter through a membrane filter with a pore size not exceeding 0.45 μm. Discard the first 2 mL of the filtrate, and use the subsequent filtrate as the sample solution. Separately, weigh accurately about 35 mg of Hydrochlorothiazide RS (separately determine the loss on drying <*2.41*> under the same conditions as Hydrochlorothiazide), and dissolve in 50 mL of a mixture of acetonitrile and sodium dihydrogen phosphate TS (pH 2.5) (3:2), add sodium dihydrogen phosphate TS (pH 2.5) to make exactly 100 mL, and use this solution as the hydrochlorothiazide standard stock solution. Pipet 4 mL of the hydrochlorothiazide standard stock solution, add 48 mL of a mixture of acetonitrile and sodium dihydrogen phosphate TS (pH 2.5) (3:2), add sodium dihydrogen phosphate TS (pH 2.5) to make exactly 100 mL, and use this solution as the standard solution. Perform the test with exactly 20 μL each of the sample solution and standard solution as directed under Liquid Chromatography <*2.01*> according to the following conditions, and determine the peak areas, A_T and A_S, of hydrochlorothiazide in each solution.

Amount (mg) of hydrochlorothiazide ($C_7H_8ClN_3O_4S_2$)
$= M_S \times A_T/A_S \times V/250$

M_S: Amount (mg) of Hydrochlorothiazide RS taken, calculated on the dried basis

Operating conditions—

Proceed as directed in the operating conditions in (1).

System suitability—

System performance: To 12 mL of the losartan potassium standard stock solution obtained in (1) and 4 mL of the hydrochlorothiazide standard stock solution, add 42 mL of a mixture of acetonitrile and sodium dihydrogen phosphate TS (pH 2.5) (3:2), and add sodium dihydrogen phosphate TS (pH 2.5) to make 100 mL. When the procedure is run with 20 μL of this solution under the above operating conditions, hydrochlorothiazide and losartan are eluted in this order with the resolution between these peaks being not less than 10.

System repeatability: When the test is repeated 6 times with 20 μL of the standard solution under the above operating conditions, the relative standard deviation of the peak area of hydrochlorothiazide is not more than 1.0%.

Dissolution <*6.10*> (1) Losartan potassium—When the test is performed at 100 revolutions per minute according to the Basket method, using 900 mL of water as the dissolution medium, the dissolution rate in 30 minutes of Losartan Potassium and Hydrochlorothiazide Tablets is not less than 85%.

Start the test with 1 tablet of Losartan Potassium and Hydrochlorothiazide Tablets, withdraw not less than 10 mL of the medium at the specified minute after starting the test, and filter through a membrane filter with a pore size not exceeding 0.45 μm. Discard not less than 2 mL of the first filtrate, pipet V mL of the subsequent filtrate, add water to make exactly V' mL so that each mL contains about 56 μg of losartan potassium ($C_{22}H_{22}ClKN_6O$), and use this solution as the sample solution. Separately, weigh accurately about 46 mg of Losartan Potassium RS (separately determine the water <*2.48*> in the same manner as Losartan Potassium), and dissolve in water to make exactly 100 mL, and use this solution as the losartan potassium standard stock solution. Pipet 12 mL of the losartan potassium standard stock solution, add water to make exactly 100 mL, and use this solution as the standard solution. Perform the test with exactly 20 μL each of the sample solution and standard solution as directed under Liquid Chromatography <*2.01*> according to the following conditions, and determine the peak areas, A_T and A_S, of losartan in each solution.

Dissolution rate (%) with respect to the labeled amount of losartan potassium ($C_{22}H_{22}ClKN_6O$)
$= M_S \times A_T/A_S \times V'/V \times 1/C \times 108$

M_S: Amount (mg) of Losartan Potassium RS taken, calculated on the anhydrous basis
C: Labeled amount (mg) of losartan potassium ($C_{22}H_{22}ClKN_6O$) in 1 tablet

Operating conditions—
Proceed as directed in the operating conditions in the Uniformity of dosage units (1).
System suitability—
System performance: To 12 mL of the losartan potassium standard stock solution and 8 mL of the hydrochlorothiazide standard stock solution obtained in (2), add water to make 100 mL. When the procedure is run with 20 μL of this solution under the above operating conditions, hydrochlorothiazide and losartan are eluted in this order with the resolution between these peaks being not less than 10.

System repeatability: When the test is repeated 6 times with 20 μL of the standard solution under the above operating conditions, the relative standard deviation of the peak area of losartan is not more than 1.0%.

(2) Hydrochlorothiazide—When the test is performed at 100 revolutions per minute according to the Basket method, using 900 mL of water as the dissolution medium, the dissolution rate in 45 minutes of Losartan Potassium and Hydrochlorothiazide Tablets is not less than 80%.

Start the test with 1 tablet of Losartan Potassium and Hydrochlorothiazide Tablets, withdraw not less than 10 mL of the medium at the specified minute after starting the test, and filter through a membrane filter with a pore size not exceeding 0.45 μm. Discard not less than 2 mL of the first filtrate, pipet V mL of the subsequent filtrate, add water to make exactly V' mL so that each mL contains about 13.9 μg of hydrochlorothiazide ($C_7H_8ClN_3O_4S_2$), and use this solution as the sample solution. Separately, weigh accurately about 35 mg of Hydrochlorothiazide RS (separately determine the loss on drying <*2.41*> under the same conditions as Hydrochlorothiazide), dissolve in 20 mL of methanol, and add water to make exactly 200 mL, and use this solution as the hydrochlorochiazide standard stock solution. Pipet 8 mL of hydrochlorothiazide standard stock solution, add water to make exactly 100 mL, and use this solution as the standard solution. Perform the test with exactly 20 μL each of the sample solution and standard solution as directed under Liquid Chromatography <*2.01*> according to the following conditions, and determine the peak areas, A_T and A_S, of hydrochlorothiazide in each solution.

Dissolution rate (%) with respect to the labeled amount of hydrochlorothiazide ($C_7H_8ClN_3O_4S_2$)
$= M_S \times A_T/A_S \times V'/V \times 1/C \times 36$

M_S: Amount (mg) of Hydrochlorothiazide RS taken, calculated on the dried basis
C: Labeled amount (mg) of hydrochlorothiazide ($C_7H_8ClN_3O_4S_2$) in 1 tablet

Operating conditions—
Proceed as directed in the operating conditions in the Uniformity of dosage units (1).
System suitability—
System performance: To 12 mL of the losartan potassium standard stock solution obtained in (1) and 8 mL of the hydrochlorothiazide standard stock solution, add water to make 100 mL. When the procedure is run with 20 μL of this solution under the above operating conditions, hydrochlorothiazide and losartan are eluted in this order with the resolution between these peaks being not less than 10.

System repeatability: When the test is repeated 6 times with 20 μL of the standard solution under the above operating conditions, the relative standard deviation of the peak area of hydrochlorothiazide is not more than 1.0%.

Assay (1) Losartan potassium—To 10 Losartan Potassium and Hydrochlorothiazide Tablets add $21V/25$ mL of a mixture of acetonitrile and sodium dihydrogen phosphate TS (pH 2.5) (3:2), stir for 60 minutes to disintegrate the tablets, add sodium dihydrogen phosphate TS (pH 2.5) to make exactly V mL so that each mL contains about 2 mg of losartan potassium ($C_{22}H_{22}ClKN_6O$), and sonicate for 2 minutes. Pipet 10 mL of this solution, add 10 mL of acetonitrile, and add sodium dihydrogen phosphate TS (pH 2.5) to make exactly 50 mL, and filter through a membrane filter with a pore size not exceeding 0.45 μm. Discard the first 2 mL of the filtrate, and use the subsequent filtrate as the sample solution. Separately, weigh accurately about 40 mg of Losartan Potassium RS (separately determine the water <*2.48*> in the same manner as Losartan Potassium), and dissolve in 30 mL of a mixture of acetonitrile and sodium dihydrogen phosphate TS (pH 2.5) (3:2), add sodium dihydrogen phosphate TS (pH 2.5) to make exactly 50 mL, and use this solution as the losartan potassium standard stock solution. Pipet 10 mL of the losartan potassium standard stock solution, add 4 mL of a mixture of acetonitrile and sodium dihydrogen phosphate TS (pH 2.5) (3:2), add sodium dihydrogen phosphate TS (pH 2.5) to make exactly 20 mL, and use this solution as the standard solution. Perform the test with exactly 20 μL each of the sample solution and standard solution as directed under Liquid Chromatography <*2.01*> according to the following conditions, and determine the peak areas, A_T and A_S, of losartan in each solution.

Amount (mg) of losartan potassium ($C_{22}H_{22}ClKN_6O$) in 1 tablet
$= M_S \times A_T/A_S \times V/200$

M_S: Amount (mg) of Losartan Potassium RS taken, calculated on the anhydrous basis

Operating conditions—
Detector: An ultraviolet absorption photometer (wavelength: 280 nm).

Column: A stainless steel column 3.9 mm in inside diameter and 15 cm in length, packed with octylsilanized silica gel for liquid chromatography (5 μm in particle diameter).

Column temperature: A constant temperature of about 35°C.

Mobile phase A: Dissolve 1.25 g of potassium dihydrogen phosphate and 1.5 g of anhydrous disodium hydrogen phosphate in water to make 1000 mL. To 930 mL of this solution add 70 mL of acetonitrile.

Mobile phase B: Acetonitrile.

Flowing of mobile phase: Control the gradient by mixing the mobile phases A and B as directed in the following table.

Time after injection of sample (min)	Mobile phase A (vol%)	Mobile phase B (vol%)
0 – 12	100 → 92	0 → 8
12 – 28	92 → 38	8 → 62

Flow rate: Adjust so that the retention time of losartan is about 20 minutes.

System suitability—

System performance: To 25 mL of the losartan potassium standard stock solution and 10 mL of the hydrochlorothiazide standard stock solution obtained in (2), add sodium dihydrogen phosphate TS (pH 2.5) to make 50 mL. When the procedure is run with 20 μL of this solution under the above operating conditions, hydrochlorothiazide and losartan are eluted in this order, and the number of theoretical plates of the peak of hydrochlorothiazide and the symmetry factor of the peak of losartan are not less than 4000 and not more than 2.5, respectively.

System repeatability: When the test is repeated 6 times with 20 μL of the standard solution under the above operating conditions, the relative standard deviation of the peak area of losartan is not more than 1.0%.

(2) Hydrochlorothiazide—To 10 Losartan Potassium and Hydrochlorothiazide Tablets add 21V/25 mL of a mixture of acetonitrile and sodium dihydrogen phosphate TS (pH 2.5) (3:2), stir for 60 minutes to disintegrate the tablets, add sodium dihydrogen phosphate TS (pH 2.5) to make exactly V mL so that each mL contains about 0.5 mg of hydrochlorothiazide ($C_7H_8ClN_3O_4S_2$), and sonicate for 2 minutes. Pipet 10 mL of this solution, add 10 mL of acetonitrile, and add sodium dihydrogen phosphate TS (pH 2.5) to make exactly 50 mL, and filter through a membrane filter with a pore size not exceeding 0.45 μm. Discard the first 2 mL of the filtrate, and use the subsequent filtrate as the sample solution. Separately, weigh accurately about 25 mg of Hydrochlorothiazide RS (separately determine the loss on drying 〈*2.41*〉 under the same conditions as Hydrochlorothiazide), and dissolve in a mixture of acetonitrile and sodium dihydrogen phosphate TS (pH 2.5) (3:2), to make exactly 50 mL, and use this solution as the hydrochlorothiazide standard stock solution. Pipet 20 mL of the hydrochlorothiazide standard stock solution, add 30 mL of a mixture of acetonitrile and sodium dihydrogen phosphate TS (pH 2.5) (3:2), add sodium dihydrogen phosphate TS (pH 2.5) to make exactly 100 mL, and use this solution as the standard solution. Perform the test with exactly 20 μL each of the sample solution and standard solution as directed under Liquid Chromatography 〈*2.01*〉 according to the following conditions, and determine the peak areas, A_T and A_S, of hydrochlorothiazide in each solution.

Amount (mg) of hydrochlorothiazide ($C_7H_8ClN_3O_4S_2$) in 1 tablet
$= M_S \times A_T/A_S \times V/500$

M_S: Amount (mg) of Hydrochlorothiazide RS taken, calculated on the dried basis

Operating conditions—

Proceed as directed in the operating conditions in (1).

System suitability—

System performance: To 25 mL of the losartan potassium standard stock solution obtained in (1) and 10 mL of the hydrochlorothiazide standard stock solution, add sodium dihydrogen phosphate TS (pH 2.5) to make 50 mL. When the procedure is run with 20 μL of this solution under the above operating conditions, hydrochlorothiazide and losartan are eluted in this order, and the number of theoretical plates of the peak of hydrochlorothiazide and the symmetry factor of the peak of losartan are not less than 4000 and not more than 2.5, respectively.

System repeatability: When the test is repeated 6 times with 20 μL of the standard solution under the above operating conditions, the relative standard deviation of the peak area of hydrochlorothiazide is not more than 1.0%.

Containers and storage Containers—Tight containers.

Loxoprofen Sodium Hydrate

ロキソプロフェンナトリウム水和物

$C_{15}H_{17}NaO_3.2H_2O$: 304.31
Monosodium 2-{4-[(2-oxocyclopentyl)methyl]phenyl}propanoate dihydrate
[80382-23-6]

Loxoprofen Sodium Hydrate contains not less than 98.5% of loxoprofen sodium ($C_{15}H_{17}NaO_3$: 268.28), calculated on the anhydrous basis.

Description Loxoprofen Sodium Hydrate occurs as white to yellowish white, crystals or crystalline powder.

It is very soluble in water and in methanol, freely soluble in ethanol (95), and practically insoluble in diethyl ether.

A solution of Loxoprofen Sodium Hydrate (1 in 20) does not show optical rotation.

The pH of a solution of 1.0 g of Loxoprofen Sodium Hydrate in 20 mL of freshly boiled and cooled water is between 6.5 and 8.5.

Identification **(1)** Determine the absorption spectrum of a solution of Loxoprofen Sodium Hydrate (1 in 55,000) as directed under Ultraviolet-visible Spectrophotometry 〈*2.24*〉, and compare the spectrum with the Reference Spectrum: both spectra exhibit similar intensities of absorption at the same wavelengths.

(2) Determine the infrared absorption spectrum of Loxoprofen Sodium Hydrate as directed in the potassium bromide disk method under the Infrared Spectrophotometry 〈*2.25*〉, and compare the spectrum with the Reference Spectrum: both spectra exhibit similar intensities of absorption at the same wave numbers.

(3) A solution of Loxoprofen Sodium Hydrate (1 in 10) responds to Qualitative Tests 〈*1.09*〉 for sodium salt.

Purity **(1)** Clarity and color of solution—Dissolve 1.0 g of Loxoprofen Sodium Hydrate in 10 mL of water: the solution is clear and colorless or pale yellow. The color is not darker than that of diluted Matching Fluid A (1 in 2).

(2) Heavy metals 〈*1.07*〉—Proceed with 2.0 g of Loxoprofen Sodium Hydrate according to Method 2, and perform the test. Prepare the control solution with 2.0 mL of Standard Lead Solution (not more than 10 ppm).

(3) Related substances—Dissolve 1.0 g of Loxoprofen Sodium Hydrate in 10 mL of methanol, and use this solution as the sample solution. Pipet 1 mL of the sample solution, add methanol to make exactly 200 mL, and use this solution as the standard solution. Perform the test with these solutions as directed under Thin-layer Chromatography <*2.03*>. Spot 10 μL each of the sample solution and standard solution on a plate of silica gel with fluorescent indicator for thin-layer chromatography. Develop the plate with a mixture of 1,2-dichloroethane and acetic acid (100) (9:1) to a distance of about 15 cm, and air-dry the plate. Examine under ultraviolet light (main wavelength: 254 nm): the spots other than the principal spot obtained from the sample solution are not more intense than the spot from the standard solution.

Water <*2.48*> 11.0 – 13.0% (0.2 g, volumetric titration, direct titration).

Assay Weigh accurately about 60 mg of Loxoprofen Sodium Hydrate, and dissolve in diluted methanol (3 in 5) to make exactly 100 mL. Pipet 5 mL of this solution, add exactly 10 mL of the internal standard solution, add diluted methanol (3 in 5) to make 100 mL, and use this solution as the sample solution. Separately, weigh accurately about 50 mg of Loxoprofen RS, previously dried in a desiccator (in vacuum, 60°C) for 3 hours, and dissolve in diluted methanol (3 in 5) to make exactly 100 mL. Pipet 5 mL of this solution, proceed in the same manner as directed for the preparation of the sample solution, and use so obtained solution as the standard solution. Perform the test with 10 μL each of the sample solution and standard solution as directed under Liquid Chromatography <*2.01*> according to the following conditions, and calculate the ratios, Q_T and Q_S, of the peak area of loxoprofen to that of the internal standard.

Amount (mg) of loxoprofen sodium ($C_{15}H_{17}NaO_3$)
$= M_S \times Q_T/Q_S \times 1.089$

M_S: Amount (mg) of Loxoprofen RS taken

Internal standard solution—A solution of ethyl benzoate in diluted methanol (3 in 5) (7 in 50,000).

Operating conditions—

Detector: An ultraviolet absorption photometer (wavelength: 222 nm).

Column: A stainless steel column 4.6 mm in inside diameter and 15 cm in length, packed with octadecylsilanized silica gel for liquid chromatography (5 μm in particle diameter).

Column temperature: A constant temperature of about 40°C.

Mobile phase: A mixture of methanol, water, acetic acid (100) and triethylamine (600:400:1:1).

Flow rate: Adjust so that the retention time of loxoprofen is about 7 minutes.

System suitability—

System performance: When the procedure is run with 10 μL of the standard solution under the above operating conditions, loxoprofen and the internal standard are eluted in this order with the resolution between these peaks being not less than 10.

System repeatability: When the test is repeated 5 times with 10 μL of the standard solution under the above operating conditions, the relative standard deviation of the ratios of the peak area of loxoprofen to that of the internal standard is not more than 1.0%.

Containers and storage Containers—Tight containers.

Loxoprofen Sodium Tablets

ロキソプロフェンナトリウム錠

Loxoprofen Sodium Tablets contain not less than 95.0% and not more than 105.0% of the labeled amount of loxoprofen sodium ($C_{15}H_{17}NaO_3$: 268.28).

Method of preparation Prepare as directed under Tablets, with Loxoprofen Sodium Hydrate.

Identification To a quantity of powdered Loxoprofen Sodium Tablets, equivalent to 60 mg of loxoprofen sodium ($C_{15}H_{17}NaO_3$), add 20 mL of methanol, shake vigorously for 10 minutes, and centrifuge. To 1 mL of the supernatant liquid add methanol to make 20 mL. To 2 mL of this solution add methanol to make 20 mL, and determine the absorption spectrum of this solution as directed under Ultraviolet-visible Spectrophotometry <*2.24*>: it exhibits a maximum between 221 nm and 225 nm.

Uniformity of dosage units <*6.02*> Perform the Mass variation test, or the Content uniformity test according to the following method: it meets the requirement.

To 1 tablet of Loxoprofen Sodium Tablets add exactly V mL of the internal standard solution so that each mL contains about 3 mg of loxoprofen sodium ($C_{15}H_{17}NaO_3$). After sonicating for 10 minutes with occasional shaking, centrifuge the solution. To 2 mL of the supernatant liquid add diluted methanol (3 in 5) to make 100 mL, and use this solution as the sample solution. Then, proceed as directed in the Assay.

Amount (mg) of loxoprofen sodium ($C_{15}H_{17}NaO_3$)
$= M_S \times Q_T/Q_S \times V/10 \times 1.089$

M_S: Amount (mg) of Loxoprofen RS taken

Internal standard solution—A solution of ethyl benzoate in diluted methanol (3 in 5) (3 in 2000).

Dissolution <*6.10*> When the test is performed at 50 revolutions per minute according to the Paddle method, using 900 mL of water as the dissolution medium, the dissolution rate in 30 minutes of Loxoprofen Sodium Tablets is not less than 85%.

Start the test with 1 tablet of Loxoprofen Sodium Tablets, withdraw not less than 20 mL of the medium at the specified minute after starting the test, and filter through a membrane filter with a pore size not exceeding 0.8 μm. Discard not less than 10 mL of the first filtrate, pipet V mL of the subsequent filtrate, and add 2nd fluid for dissolution test to make exactly V' mL so that each mL contains about 13 μg of loxoprofen sodium ($C_{15}H_{17}NaO_3$). Use this solution as the sample solution. Separately, weigh accurately about 31 mg of Loxoprofen RS, previously dried in vacuum at 60°C for 3 hours, dissolve in 5 mL of ethanol (99.5), and add water to make exactly 250 mL. Pipet 5 mL of this solution, add 2nd fluid for dissolution test to make exactly 50 mL, and use this solution as the standard solution. Determine the absorbances, A_T and A_S, of the sample solution and standard solution at 223 nm as directed under Ultraviolet-visible Spectrophotometry <*2.24*>, using water as the control.

Dissolution rate (%) with respect to the labeled amount of loxoprofen sodium ($C_{15}H_{17}NaO_3$)
$= M_S \times A_T/A_S \times V'/V \times 1/C \times 36 \times 1.089$

M_S: Amount (mg) of Loxoprofen RS taken
C: Labeled amount (mg) of loxoprofen sodium

($C_{15}H_{17}NaO_3$) in 1 tablet

Assay Weigh accurately the mass of not less than 20 Loxoprofen Sodium Tablets, and powder. Weigh accurately a portion of the powder, equivalent to about 60 mg of loxoprofen sodium ($C_{15}H_{17}NaO_3$), add exactly 20 mL of the internal standard solution, and shake vigorously for 15 minutes. Centrifuge this solution, and to 2 mL of the supernatant liquid add diluted methanol (3 in 5) to make 100 mL. Use this solution as the sample solution. Separately, weigh accurately about 30 mg of Loxoprofen RS, previously dried in vacuum at 60°C for 3 hours, and dissolve in exactly 10 mL of the internal standard solution. To 2 mL of this solution add diluted methanol (3 in 5) to make 100 mL, and use this solution as the standard solution. Perform the test with 10 μL each of the sample solution and standard solution as directed under Liquid Chromatography 〈2.01〉 according to the following conditions, and calculate the ratios, Q_T and Q_S, of the peak area of loxoprofen to that of the internal standard.

Amount (mg) of loxoprofen sodium ($C_{15}H_{17}NaO_3$)
$= M_S \times Q_T/Q_S \times 2 \times 1.089$

M_S: Amount (mg) of Loxoprofen RS taken

Internal standard solution—A solution of ethyl benzoate in diluted methanol (3 in 5) (3 in 2000).

Operating conditions—

Detector: An ultraviolet absorption photometer (wavelength: 222 nm).

Column: A stainless steel column 6 mm in inside diameter and 15 cm in length, packed with octadecylsilanized silica gel for liquid chromatography (5 μm in particle diameter).

Column temperature: A constant temperature of about 40°C.

Mobile phase: A mixture of methanol, water, acetic acid (100) and triethylamine (600:400:1:1).

Flow rate: Adjust so that the retention time of loxoprofen is about 7 minutes.

System suitability—

System performance: When the procedure is run with 10 μL of the standard solution under the above operating conditions, loxoprofen and the internal standard are eluted in this order with the resolution between these peaks being not less than 10.

System repeatability: When the test is repeated 6 times with 10 μL of the standard solution under the above operating conditions, the relative standard deviation of the ratio of the peak area of loxoprofen to that of the internal standard is not more than 1.0%.

Containers and storage Containers—Tight containers.

L-Lysine Acetate

L-リシン酢酸塩

$C_6H_{14}N_2O_2.C_2H_4O_2$: 206.24
(2*S*)-2,6-Diaminohexanoic acid monoacetate
[*57282-49-2*]

L-Lysine Acetate, when dried, contains not less than 98.5% and not more than 101.0% of L-lysine acetate ($C_6H_{14}N_2O_2.C_2H_4O_2$).

Description L-Lysine Acetate occurs as white, crystals or crystalline powder. It has a characteristic odor and a slightly acid taste.

It is very soluble in water, freely soluble in formic acid, and practically insoluble in ethanol (99.5).

It is deliquescent.

Identification **(1)** Determine the infrared absorption spectrum of L-Lysine Acetate as directed in the potassium bromide disk method under Infrared Spectrophotometry 〈*2.25*〉, and compare the spectrum with the Reference Spectrum: both spectra exhibit similar intensities of absorption at the same wave numbers.

(2) A solution of L-Lysine Acetate (1 in 20) responds to Qualitative Tests 〈*1.09*〉 (2) for acetate.

Optical rotation 〈*2.49*〉 $[\alpha]_D^{20}$: +8.5 – +10.0° (after drying, 2.5 g, water, 25 mL, 100 mm).

pH 〈*2.54*〉 Dissolve 1.0 g of L-Lysine Acetate in 10 mL of water: the pH of the solution is between 6.5 and 7.5.

Purity **(1)** Clarity and color of solution—Dissolve 1.0 g of L-Lysine Acetate in 10 mL of water: the solution is colorless and clear.

(2) Chloride 〈*1.03*〉—Perform the test with 0.5 g of L-Lysine Acetate. Prepare the control solution with 0.30 mL of 0.01 mol/L hydrochloric acid VS (not more than 0.021%).

(3) Sulfate 〈*1.14*〉—Perform the test with 0.6 g of L-Lysine Acetate. Prepare the control solution with 0.35 mL of 0.005 mol/L sulfuric acid VS (not more than 0.028%).

(4) Ammonium 〈*1.02*〉—Perform the test with 0.25 g of L-Lysine Acetate. Prepare the control solution with 5.0 mL of Standard Ammonium Solution (not more than 0.02%).

(5) Heavy metals 〈*1.07*〉—Proceed with 1.0 g of L-Lysine Acetate according to Method 4, and perform the test. Prepare the control solution with 1.0 mL of Standard Lead Solution (not more than 10 ppm).

(6) Iron 〈*1.10*〉—Prepare the test solution with 1.0 g of L-Lysine Acetate according to Method 1, and perform the test according to Method A. Prepare the control solution with 1.0 mL of Standard Iron Solution (not more than 10 ppm).

(7) Related substances—Weigh accurately about 0.5 g of L-Lysine Acetate, dissolve in 0.5 mL of hydrochloric acid and water to make exactly 100 mL. Pipet 10 mL of this solution, add 0.02 mol/L hydrochloric acid to make exactly 50 mL, and use this solution as the sample solution. Separately, weigh accurately 2.5 mmol amounts of L-aspartic acid, L-threonine, L-serine, L-glutamic acid, glycine, L-alanine, L-cystine, L-valine, L-methionine, L-isoleucine, L-leucine, L-tyrosine, L-phenylalanine, L-lysine hydrochloride, ammonium chloride, L-histidine and L-arginine, dissolve in 0.1 mol/L hydrochloric acid TS to make exactly 1000 mL, and use this solution as the standard stock solution. Pipet 5 mL of this solution, add 0.02 mol/L hydrochloric acid to make exactly 100 mL. Pipet 4 mL of this solution, add 0.02 mol/L hydrochloric acid to make exactly 50 mL, and use this solution as the standard solution. Perform the test with exactly 20 μL each of the sample solution and standard solution as directed under Liquid Chromatography 〈*2.01*〉 according to the following conditions. Based on the peak heights of the amino acids obtained from the sample solution and standard solution, determine the mass of the amino acids other than lysine contained in 1 mL of the sample solution, and calculate the mass percent: the amount of each amino acids other than lysine is not more than 0.1%.

Operating conditions—

Detector: A visible spectrophotometer (wavelength: 570 nm).

Column: A stainless steel column 4.6 mm in inside diameter and 8 cm in length, packed with strongly acidic ion-exchange resin for liquid chromatography (Na type) composed with a sulfonated polystyrene copolymer (3 μm in particle diameter).

Column temperature: A constant temperature of about 57°C.

Chemical reaction bath temperature: A constant temperature of about 130°C.

Color developing time: About 1 minute.

Mobile phase: Prepare mobile phases A, B, C, D and E according to the following table, and to each phase add 0.1 mL of capric acid.

	Mobile phase A	Mobile phase B	Mobile phase C	Mobile phase D	Mobile phase E
Citric acid monohydrate	19.80 g	22.00 g	12.80 g	6.10 g	—
Trisodium citrate dihydrate	6.19 g	7.74 g	13.31 g	26.67 g	—
Sodium chloride	5.66 g	7.07 g	3.74 g	54.35 g	—
Sodium hydroxide	—	—	—	—	8.00 g
Ethanol (99.5)	130 mL	20 mL	4 mL	—	100 mL
Thiodiglycol	5 mL	5 mL	5 mL	—	—
Benzyl alcohol	—	—	—	5 mL	—
Lauromacrogol solution (1 in 4)	4 mL	4 mL	4 mL	4 mL	4 mL
Water	Appropriate amount	Appropriate amount	Appropriate amount	Appropriate amount	Appropriate amount
Total volume	1000 mL	1000 mL	1000 mL	1000 mL	1000 mL

Changing mobile phases: Proceed with 20 μL of the standard solution under the above operating conditions: aspartic acid, threonine, serine, glutamic acid, glycine, alanine, cystine, valine, methionine, isoleucine, leucine, tyrosine, phenylalanine, lysine, ammonia, histidine and arginine are eluted in this order. Switchover the mobile phases A, B, C, D and E in sequence so that the resolution between the peaks of isoleucine and leucine is not less than 1.2.

Reaction reagents: Dissolve 204 g of lithium acetate dihydrate in water, and add 123 mL of acetic acid (100), 401 mL of 1-methoxy-2-propanol, and water to make 1000 mL, gas with nitrogen for 10 minutes, and use this solution as the solution (I). Separately, to 979 mL of 1-methoxy-2-propanol add 39 g of ninhydrin, gas with nitrogen for 5 minutes, add 81 mg of sodium borohydride, gas the solution with nitrogen for 30 minutes, and use this solution as solution (II). To 1 volume of the solution (I) add 1 volume of the solution (II). Prepare before use.

Mobile phase flow rate: 0.20 mL per minute.

Reaction reagent flow rate: 0.24 mL per minute.

System suitability—

System performance: When the procedure is run with 20 μL of the standard solution under the above operating conditions, the resolution between the peaks of glycine and alanine is not less than 1.2.

System repeatability: When the test is repeated 6 times with 20 μL of the standard solution under the above operating conditions, the relative standard deviation of the peak height of each amino acid in the standard solution is not more than 5.0%, and the relative standard deviation of the retention time is not more than 1.0%.

Loss on drying <*2.41*> Not more than 0.3% (1 g, 80°C, 3 hours).

Residue on ignition <*2.44*> Not more than 0.1% (1 g).

Assay Weigh accurately about 0.1 g of L-Lysine Acetate, previously dried, dissolve in 3 mL of formic acid, add 50 mL of acetic acid (100), and titrate <*2.50*> with 0.1 mol/L perchloric acid VS (potentiometric titration). Perform a blank determination in the same manner, and make any necessary correction.

Each mL of 0.1 mol/L perchloric acid VS
= 10.31 mg of $C_6H_{14}N_2O_2.C_2H_4O_2$

Containers and storage Containers—Tight containers.

L-Lysine Hydrochloride

L-リシン塩酸塩

$C_6H_{14}N_2O_2.HCl$: 182.65
(2*S*)-2,6-Diaminohexanoic acid monohydrochloride
[*657-27-2*]

L-Lysine Hydrochloride, when dried, contains not less than 98.5% of L-lysine hydrochloride ($C_6H_{14}N_2O_2.HCl$).

Description L-Lysine Hydrochloride occurs as a white powder. It has a slight, characteristic taste.

It is freely soluble in water and in formic acid, and practically insoluble in ethanol (95).

It shows crystal polymorphism.

Identification **(1)** Determine the infrared absorption spectrum of L-Lysine Hydrochloride, previously dried, as directed in the potassium bromide disk method under Infrared Spectrophotometry <*2.25*>, and compare the spectrum with the Reference Spectrum: both spectra exhibit similar intensities of absorption at the same wave numbers. If any difference appears between the spectra, dissolve L-Lysine Hydrochloride in water, evaporate the water to dryness at 60°C, and repeat the test with the residue.

(2) A solution of L-Lysine Hydrochloride (1 in 10) responds to Qualitative Tests <*1.09*> for chloride.

Optical rotation <*2.49*> $[\alpha]_D^{20}$: +19.0 – +21.5° (after drying, 2 g, 6 mol/L hydrochloric acid TS, 25 mL, 100 mm).

pH <*2.54*> Dissolve 1.0 g of L-Lysine Hydrochloride in 10 mL of water: the pH of this solution is between 5.0 and 6.0.

Purity **(1)** Clarity and color of solution—Dissolve 1.0 g of L-Lysine Hydrochloride in 10 mL of water: the solution is clear and colorless.

(2) Sulfate <*1.14*>—Perform the test with 0.6 g of L-Lysine Hydrochloride. Prepare the control solution with 0.35 mL of 0.005 mol/L sulfuric acid VS (not more than 0.028%).

(3) Ammonium <*1.02*>—Perform the test with 0.25 g of L-Lysine Hydrochloride. Prepare the control solution with 5.0 mL of Standard Ammonium Solution (not more than 0.02%).

(4) Heavy metals <*1.07*>—Proceed with 2.0 g of L-Lysine Hydrochloride according to Method 1, and perform the test. Prepare the control solution with 2.0 mL of Standard Lead Solution (not more than 10 ppm).

(5) Arsenic <*1.11*>—Prepare the test solution with 1.0 g of L-Lysine Hydrochloride according to Method 1, and perform the test (not more than 2 ppm).

(6) Related substances—Dissolve 0.10 g of L-Lysine Hydrochloride in 25 mL of water, and use this solution as the sample solution. Pipet 1 mL of the sample solution, add water to make exactly 50 mL, pipet 5 mL of this solution, add water to make exactly 20 mL, and use this solution as the standard solution. Perform the test with these solutions as directed under Thin-layer Chromatography ⟨*2.03*⟩. Spot 5 μL each of the sample solution and standard solution on a plate of silica gel for thin-layer chromatography. Develop the plate with a mixture of 1-propanol and ammonia water (28) (67:33) to a distance of about 10 cm, and dry the plate at 100°C for 30 minutes. Spray evenly the plate with a solution of ninhydrin in acetone (1 in 50) and heat the plate at 80°C for 5 minutes: the spots other than the principal spot obtained from the sample solution are not more intense than the spot from the standard solution.

Loss on drying ⟨*2.41*⟩ Not more than 1.0% (1 g, 105°C, 3 hours).

Residue on ignition ⟨*2.44*⟩ Not more than 0.1% (1 g).

Assay Weigh accurately about 0.1 g of L-Lysine Hydrochloride, previously dried, dissolve in 2 mL of formic acid, add exactly 15 mL of 0.1 mol/L perchloric acid VS, and heat on a water bath for 30 minutes. After cooling, add 45 mL of acetic acid (100), and titrate ⟨*2.50*⟩ the excess perchloric acid with 0.1 mol/L sodium acetate VS (potentiometric titration). Perform a blank determination in the same manner, and make any necessary correction.

Each mL of 0.1 mol/L perchloric acid VS
= 9.132 mg of $C_6H_{14}N_2O_2.HCl$

Containers and storage Containers—Tight containers.

Lysozyme Hydrochloride

リゾチーム塩酸塩

```
KVFGRCELAA AMKRHGLDNY RGYSLGNWVC AAKFESNFNT QATNRNTDGS

TDYGILQINS RWWCNDGRTP GSRNLCNIPC SALLSSDITA SVNCAKKIVS

DGNGMNAWVA WRNRCKGTDV QAWIRGCRL
                                            • xHCl
```

$C_{616}H_{963}N_{193}O_{182}S_{10}.xHCl$
[*12650-88-3*, egg white lysozyme]

Lysozyme Hydrochloride is the hydrochloride of lysozyme obtained from albumen of hen's egg, and is a protein consisting of 129 amino acid residues.

It contains not less than 0.9 mg (potency) of lysozyme per mg, calculated on the dried basis.

Description Lysozyme Hydrochloride occurs as white, crystals, or crystalline or amorphous powder.

It is freely soluble in water, and practically insoluble in ethanol (99.5).

It is hygroscopic.

The pH of a solution of 3 g of Lysozyme Hydrochloride in 200 mL of water is between 3.0 and 5.0.

Identification (1) To 5 mL of a solution of Lysozyme Hydrochloride in acetate buffer solution (pH 5.4) (1 in 500) add 1 mL of ninhydrin TS, and heat for 10 minutes: a blue-purple color develops.

(2) Determine the absorption spectrum of a solution of Lysozyme Hydrochloride in acetate buffer solution (pH 5.4) (1 in 10,000) as directed under Ultraviolet-visible Spectrophotometry ⟨*2.24*⟩, and compare the spectrum with the Reference Spectrum: both spectra exhibit similar intensities of absorption at the same wavelengths.

Purity (1) Clarity of solution—To 5 mL of a solution of Lysozyme Hydrochloride (3 in 200) add, if necessary, dilute hydrochloric acid to adjust the pH to 3: the solution is clear.

(2) Heavy metals ⟨*1.07*⟩—Proceed with 1.0 g of Lysozyme Hydrochloride according to Method 2, and perform the test. Prepare the control solution with 2.0 mL of Standard Lead Solution (not more than 20 ppm).

Loss on drying ⟨*2.41*⟩ Not more than 8.0% (0.1 g, 105°C, 2 hours).

Residue on ignition ⟨*2.44*⟩ Not more than 2.0% (0.5 g).

Nitrogen Perform the test as directed under Nitrogen Determination ⟨*1.08*⟩: the amount of nitrogen (N: 14.01) is between 16.8% and 18.6%, calculated on the dried basis.

Assay Weigh accurately an amount of Lysozyme Hydrochloride, equivalent to about 25 mg (potency), dissolve in phosphate buffer solution (pH 6.2) to make exactly 100 mL. Pipet 2 mL of this solution, add phosphate buffer solution (pH 6.2) to make exactly 50 mL, and use this solution as the sample solution. Separately, weigh accurately an amount of Lysozyme RS (separately determine its loss on drying ⟨*2.41*⟩ under the same condition as Lysozyme Hydrochloride), equivalent to about 25 mg (potency), and dissolve in phosphate buffer solution (pH 6.2) to make exactly 100 mL. Pipet 1 mL and 2 mL of this solution, add phosphate buffer solution (pH 6.2) to them to make exactly 50 mL, and use these solutions as the standard solution (1) and the solution (2), respectively. Keep the sample solution and the standard solutions in an ice-bath. Pipet 4 mL of substrate solution for lysozyme hydrochloride, previously warmed in a water bath of 35°C for about 5 minutes, add exactly 100 μL of the sample solution, previously warmed in a water bath of 35°C for about 3 minutes, and allow to stand at 35°C for exactly 10 minutes, then add exactly 0.5 mL of 1 mol/L hydrochloric acid TS, and immediately shake. Determine the absorbance under Ultraviolet-visible Spectrophotometry ⟨*2.24*⟩, A_T, of this solution at 640 nm, using water as the blank. Determine the absorbances, A_{S1} and A_{S2}, of the solutions obtained with the standard solution (1) and the standard solution (2) in the same manner as the sample solution.

Amount [mg (potency)] of lysozyme per mg, calculated on the dried basis
$= M_S/2M_T \times \{(A_{S1} - A_T)/(A_{S1} - A_{S2}) + 1\}$

M_S: Amount (mg) of Lysozyme RS taken, calculated on the dried basis.
M_T: Amount (mg) of the sample taken, calculated on the dried basis.

Containers and storage Containers—Tight containers.

Macrogol 400

Polyethylene Glycol 400

マクロゴール 400

Macrogol 400 is a polymer of ethylene oxide and water, represented by the formula $HOCH_2(CH_2OCH_2)_nCH_2OH$, in which the value of n ranges from 7 to 9.

Description Macrogol 400 occurs as a clear, colorless and viscous liquid. It has no odor or a slight, characteristic odor.

It is miscible with water, with methanol, with ethanol (95) and with pyridine.

It is soluble in diethyl ether.

It is slightly hygroscopic.

Congealing point: 4 – 8°C

Specific gravity d^{20}_{20}: 1.110 – 1.140

Identification Dissolve 50 mg of Macrogol 400 in 5 mL of dilute hydrochloric acid, add 1 mL of barium chloride TS, shake, and filter, if necessary. To the filtrate add 1 mL of a solution of phosphomolybdic acid n-hydrate (1 in 10): a yellow-green precipitate is formed.

pH <2.54> Dissolve 1.0 g of Macrogol 400 in 20 mL of water: the pH of this solution is between 4.0 and 7.0.

Purity (1) Acidity—Dissolve 5.0 g of Macrogol 400 in 20 mL of neutralized ethanol, and add 2 drops of phenolphthalein TS and 0.20 mL of 0.1 mol/L sodium hydroxide VS: the solution is red in color.

(2) Ethylene glycol and diethylene glycol—Dissolve 4.0 g of Macrogol 400 in water to make exactly 10 mL, and use this solution as the sample solution. Weigh accurately about 50 mg each of ethylene glycol and diethylene glycol, dissolve in water to make exactly 100 mL, and use this solution as the standard solution. Perform the test with exactly 2 μL each of the sample solution and standard solution as directed under Gas Chromatography <2.02> according to the following conditions. Determine the peak heights, H_{Ta} and H_{Sa}, of ethylene glycol of each solution, and the peak heights, H_{Tb} and H_{Sb}, of diethylene glycol, and calculate the amount of ethylene glycol and diethylene glycol: the sum of the contents of ethylene glycol and diethylene glycol is not more than 0.25%.

$$\text{Amount (mg) of ethylene glycol} = M_{Sa} \times H_{Ta}/H_{Sa} \times 1/10$$

$$\text{Amount (mg) of diethylene glycol} = M_{Sb} \times H_{Tb}/H_{Sb} \times 1/10$$

M_{Sa}: Amount (mg) of ethylene glycol taken
M_{Sb}: Amount (mg) of diethylene glycol taken

Operating conditions—

Detector: A hydrogen flame-ionization detector.

Column: A colum about 3 mm in inside diameter and about 1.5 m in length, packed with siliceous earth for gas chromatography, 150 to 180 μm in particle diameter, coated with D-sorbitol for gas chromatography at the ratio of 12%.

Column temperature: A constant temperature of about 165°C.

Carrier gas: Nitrogen or helium.

Flow rate: Adjust so that the retention time of diethylene glycol is about 8 minutes.

Selection of column: Proceed with 2 μL of the standard solution under the above operating conditions, and calculate the resolution. Use a column clearly dividing peaks of ethylene glycol and diethylene glycol in this order.

Detection sensitivity: Adjust the detection sensitivity so that the peak height of diethylene glycol obtained from 2 μL of the standard solution composes about 80% of the full scale.

Average molecular mass Add 42 g of phthalic anhydride to 300 mL of freshly distilled pyridine, exactly measured, in a 1-L light-resistant glass-stoppered bottle. Shake the bottle vigorously to dissolved the solid, and allow to stand for 16 hours or more. Pipet 25 mL of this solution into an about 200-mL glass-stoppered pressure bottle. Add about 1.5 g of Macrogol 400, accurately weighed, stopper the bottle, wrap it securely with strong cloth, and immerse in a water bath, having a temperature of 98 ± 2°C, to the level so that the mixture in the bottle soaks completely in water. Maintain the temperature of the bath at 98 ± 2°C for 30 minutes. Remove the bottle from the bath, and allow to cool in air to room temperature. Add exactly 50 mL of 0.5 mol/L sodium hydroxide VS and 5 drops of a solution of phenolphthalein in pyridine (1 in 100). Titrate <2.50> with 0.5 mol/L sodium hydroxide VS until a light red color remains for not less than 15 seconds. Perform a blank determination in the same manner.

$$\text{Average molecular mass} = (M \times 4000)/(a - b)$$

M: Amount (g) of Macrogol 400 taken
a: Volume (mL) of 0.5 mol/L sodium hydroxide VS used in the blank determination
b: Volume (mL) of 0.5 mol/L sodium hydroxide VS used in the test of the sample

Average molecular mass is between 380 and 420.

Water <2.48> Not more than 1.0% (2 g, volumetric titration, direct titration).

Residue on ignition <2.44> Not more than 0.1% (1 g).

Containers and storage Containers—Tight containers.

Macrogol 1500

Polyethylene Glycol 1500

マクロゴール 1500

Macrogol 1500 is a mixture containing equal amounts of lower and higher polymers of ethylene oxide and water, represented by the formula $HOCH_2(CH_2OCH_2)_nCH_2OH$, in which the value of n is 5 or 6 for the lower polymers and from 28 to 36 for the higher.

Description Macrogol 1500 occurs as a white, smooth petrolatum-like solid. It is odorless or has a faint, characteristic odor.

It is very soluble in water, in pyridine and in diphenyl ether, freely soluble in methanol, sparingly soluble in ethanol (95), very slightly soluble in ethanol (99.5), and practically insoluble in diethyl ether.

Congealing point: 37 – 41°C

Identification Dissolve 50 mg of Macrogol 1500 in 5 mL of dilute hydrochloric acid, add 1 mL of barium chloride TS, shake, and filter, if necessary. To the filtrate add 1 mL of a solution of phosphomolybdic acid n-hydrate (1 in 10): a yellow-green precipitate is formed.

pH ⟨2.54⟩ Dissolve 1.0 g of Macrogol 1500 in 20 mL of water: the pH of the solution is between 4.0 and 7.0.

Purity (1) Clarity and color of solution—Dissolve 5.0 g of Macrogol 1500 in 50 mL of water: the solution is clear and colorless.

(2) Acidity—Dissolve 5.0 g of Macrogol 1500 in 20 mL of neutralized ethanol, and add 2 drops of phenolphthalein TS and 0.20 mL of 0.1 mol/L sodium hydroxide VS: the solution is red in color.

(3) Ethylene glycol and diethylene glycol—Place 50.0 g of Macrogol 1500 in a distilling flask, add 75 mL of diphenyl ether, warm to dissolve if necessary, distil slowly under a reduced pressure of 0.13 to 0.27 kPa and take 25 mL of the distillate in a 100-mL container with 1-mL graduation. To the distillate add exactly 20 mL of water, shake vigorously, cool in ice water, congeal the diphenyl ether, and filtrate into a 25-mL volumetric flask. Wash the residue with 5.0 mL of ice-cold water, combine the washings with the filtrate, warm to room temperature, and add water to make 25 mL. Transfer this solution to a glass-stoppered flask, shake with 25.0 mL of freshly distilled acetonitrile, and use this solution as the sample solution. Separately, to 62.5 mg of diethylene glycol add a mixture of water and freshly distilled acetonitrile (1:1) to make exactly 25 mL, and use this solution as the standard solution. Take exactly 10 mL each of the sample solution and the standard solution, and add to each exactly 15 mL of cerium (IV) diammonium nitrate TS. Perform the test with this solution as directed under Ultraviolet-visible Spectrophotometry ⟨2.24⟩ within 2 to 5 minutes: the absorbance of the solution obtained from the sample solution at the wavelength of maximum absorption at about 450 nm is not larger than the absorbance of the solution obtained from the standard solution.

Water ⟨2.48⟩ Not more than 1.0% (2 g, volumetric titration, direct titration).

Residue on ignition ⟨2.44⟩ Not more than 0.1% (1 g).

Containers and storage Containers—Tight containers.

Macrogol 4000

Polyethylene Glycol 4000

マクロゴール 4000

Macrogol 4000 is a polymer of ethylene oxide and water, represented by the formula $HOCH_2(CH_2OCH_2)_nCH_2OH$, in which the value of n ranges from 59 to 84.

Description Macrogol 4000 is a white, paraffin-like solid, occurring as flakes or powder. It is odorless or has a faint, characteristic odor.

It is very soluble in water, freely soluble in methanol and in pyridine, and practically insoluble in ethanol (99.5) and in diethyl ether.

Congealing point: 53 – 57°C

Identification Dissolve 50 mg of Macrogol 4000 in 5 mL of dilute hydrochloric acid, add 1 mL of barium chloride TS, shake, and filter, if necessary. To the filtrate add 1 mL of a solution of phosphomolybdic acid *n*-hydrate (1 in 10): a yellow-green precipitate is formed.

pH ⟨2.54⟩ Dissolve 1.0 g of Macrogol 4000 in 20 mL of water: the pH of this solution is between 4.0 and 7.5.

Purity (1) Clarity and color of solution—A solution of 5.0 g of Macrogol 4000 in 50 mL of water is clear and colorless.

(2) Acidity—Dissolve 5.0 g of Macrogol 4000 in 20 mL of neutralized ethanol by warming, cool, and add 0.20 mL of 0.1 mol/L sodium hydroxide VS and 1 drop of phenolphthelein TS: the color of the solution is red.

Average molecular mass Weigh accurately about 12.5 g of Macrogol 4000, transfer to an about 200-mL glass-stoppered pressure bottle, add about 25 mL of pyridine, dissolve by warming, and allow to cool. Separately, pipet 300 mL of freshly distilled pyridine into a 1-L light-resistant, glass-stoppered bottle, add 42 g of phthalic anhydride, dissolve with vigorous shaking, and allow to stand for 16 hours or more. Pipet 25 mL of this solution, transfer to the former pressure bottle, stopper the bottle tightly, wrap it securely with strong cloth, and immerse in a water bath, previously heated at 98 ± 2°C, to the level so that the mixture in the bottle soaks completely in water. Maintain the temperature of the bath at 98 ± 2°C for 30 minutes. Remove the bottle from the bath, and allow to cool in air to room temperature. Add exactly 50 mL of 0.5 mol/L sodium hydroxide VS and 5 drops of a solution of phenolphthalein in pyridine (1 in 100). Titrate ⟨2.50⟩ with 0.5 mol/L sodium hydroxide VS until a light red color remains for not less than 15 seconds. Perform a blank determination in the same manner.

$$\text{Average molecular mass} = (M \times 4000)/(a - b)$$

M: Amount (g) of Macrogol 4000 taken
a: Volume (mL) of 0.5 mol/L sodium hydroxide VS consumed in the blank determination
b: Volume (mL) of 0.5 mol/L sodium hydroxide VS consumed in the test of the sample

Average molecular mass is between 2600 and 3800.

Water ⟨2.48⟩ Not more than 1.0% (2 g, volumetric titration, direct titration).

Residue on ignition ⟨2.44⟩ Not more than 0.2% (1 g).

Containers and storage Containers—Well-closed containers.

Macrogol 6000

Polyethylene Glycol 6000

マクロゴール 6000

Macrogol 6000 is a polymer of ethylene oxide and water, represented by the formula $HOCH_2(CH_2OCH_2)_nCH_2OH$, in which the value of n ranges from 165 to 210.

Description Macrogol 6000 is a white, paraffin-like solid, occurring as flakes or powder. It is odorless or has a faint, characteristic odor.

It is very soluble in water, freely soluble in pyridine, and practically insoluble in methanol, in ethanol (95), in ethanol (99.5) and in diethyl ether.

Congealing point: 56 – 61°C

Identification Dissolve 50 mg of Macrogol 6000 in 5 mL of dilute hydrochloric acid, add 1 mL of barium chloride TS, shake, and filter, if necessary. To the filtrate add 1 mL of a solution of phosphomolybdic acid *n*-hydrate (1 in 10): a yellow-green precipitate is formed.

pH <*2.54*> Dissolve 1.0 g of Macrogol 6000 in 20 mL of water: the pH of this solution is between 4.5 and 7.5.

Purity **(1)** Clarity and color of solution—Dissolve 5.0 g of Macrogol 6000 in 50 mL of water: the solution is clear and colorless.

(2) Acidity—Dissolve 5.0 g of Macrogol 6000 in 20 mL of neutralized ethanol by warming, cool, and add 0.20 mL of 0.1 mol/L sodium hydroxide VS and 1 drop of phenolphthalein TS: the color of the solution is red.

Average molecular mass Weigh accurately about 12.5 g of Macrogol 6000, transfer to an about 200-mL glass-stoppered pressure bottle, add about 25 mL of pyridine, dissolve by warming, and allow to cool. Separately, pipet 300 mL of freshly distilled pyridine into a 1-L light-resistant, glass-stoppered bottle, add 42 g of phthalic anhydride, dissolve with vigorous shaking, and allow to stand for 16 hours or more. Pipet 25 mL of this solution, transfer to the former pressure bottle, stopper the bottle tightly, wrap it securely with strong cloth, and immerse in a water bath, previously heated at 98 ± 2°C, to the level so that the mixture in the bottle soaks completely in water. Maintain the temperature of the bath at 98 ± 2°C for 30 minutes. Remove the bottle from the bath, and allow to cool in air to room temperature. Add exactly 50 mL of 0.5 mol/L sodium hydroxide VS and 5 drops of a solution of phenolphthalein in pyridine (1 in 100). Titrate <*2.50*> with 0.5 mol/L sodium hydroxide VS until a light red color remains for not less than 15 seconds. Perform a blank determination in the same manner.

$$\text{Average molecular mass} = (M \times 4000)/(a - b)$$

M: Amount (g) of Macrogol 6000 taken
a: Volume (mL) of 0.5 mol/L sodium hydroxide VS consumed in the blank determination
b: Volume (mL) of 0.5 mol/L sodium hydroxide VS consumed in the test of the sample

Average molecular mass is between 7300 and 9300.

Water <*2.48*> Not more than 1.0% (2 g, volumetric titration, direct titration).

Residue on ignition <*2.44*> Not more than 0.2% (1 g).

Containers and storage Containers—Well-closed containers.

Macrogol 20000

Polyethylene Glycol 20000

マクロゴール 20000

Macrogol 20000 is a polymer of ethylene oxide and water, represented by the formula $HOCH_2(CH_2OCH_2)_nCH_2OH$, in which the value of *n* lies between 340 and 570.

Description Macrogol 20000 occurs as white, paraffin-like flakes or powder. It is odorless or has a faint, characteristic odor.

It is freely soluble in water and in pyridine, and practically insoluble in methanol, in ethanol (95), in petroleum benzine and in macrogol 400.

Congealing point: 56 - 64°C

Identification Dissolve 50 mg of Macrogol 20000 in 5 mL of dilute hydrochloric acid, add 1 mL of barium chloride TS, shake, and filter, if necessary. To the filtrate add 1 mL of a solution of phosphomolybdic acid *n*-hydrate (1 in 10): a yellow-green precipitate is formed.

pH <*2.54*> Dissolve 1.0 g of Macrogol 20000 in 20 mL of water: the pH of this solution is between 4.5 and 7.5.

Purity **(1)** Clarity and color of solution—Dissolve 5.0 g of Macrogol 20000 in 50 mL of water: the solution is clear and colorless.

(2) Acidity—Dissolve 5.0 g of Macrogol 20000 in 20 mL of neutralized ethanol by warming, cool, and add 0.20 mL of 0.1 mol/L sodium hydroxide VS and 1 drop of phenolphthalein TS: the color of the solution is red.

Average molecular mass Weigh accurately about 15 g of Macrogol 20000, transfer to an about 200-mL glass-stoppered pressure bottle, add about 25 mL of pyridine, dissolve by warming, and allow to cool. Separately, pipet 300 mL of freshly distilled pyridine into a 1-L light-resistant glass-stoppered bottle, add 42 g of phthalic anhydride, dissolve with vigorous shaking, and allow to stand for 16 hours or more. Pipet 25 mL of this solution, transfer to the former pressure bottle, stopper the bottle tightly, wrap it securely with strong cloth, and immerse in a water bath, having a temperature of 98 ± 2°C, to the same depth as the mixture in the bottle. Maintain the temperature of the bath at 98 ± 2°C for 60 minutes. Remove the bottle from the bath, and allow to cool in air to room temperature. Add exactly 50 mL of 0.5 mol/L sodium hydroxide VS and 5 drops of a solution of phenolphthalein in pyridine (1 in 100). Titrate <*2.50*> with 0.5 mol/L sodium hydroxide VS until a light red color remains for not less than 15 seconds. Perform a blank determination in the same manner.

$$\text{Average molecular mass} = (M \times 4000)/(a - b)$$

M: Amount (g) of Macrogol 20000 taken
a: Volume (mL) of 0.5 mol/L sodium hydroxide VS used in the blank determination
b: Volume (mL) of 0.5 mol/L sodium hydroxide VS used in the test of the sample

Average molecular mass is between 15000 and 25000.

Water <*2.48*> Not more than 1.0% (2 g, volumetric titration, direct titration).

Residue on ignition <*2.44*> Not more than 0.2% (1 g).

Containers and storage Containers—Well-closed containers.

Macrogol Ointment

Polyethylene Glycol Ointment

マクロゴール軟膏

Method of preparation

Macrogol 4000	500 g
Macrogol 400	500 g
To make	1000 g

Melt Macrogol 4000 and Macrogol 400 by warming on a water bath at 65°C, and mix well until it congeals. Less than

100 g of Macrogol 4000 or Macrogol 400 may be replaced by an equal amount of Macrogol 400 or Macrogol 4000 to prepare 1000 g of a proper soft ointment.

Description Macrogol Ointment is white in color. It has a faint, characteristic odor.

Identification Dissolve 50 mg of Macrogol Ointment in 5 mL of dilute hydrochloric acid, add 1 mL of barium chloride TS, shake, filter if necessary, and add 1 mL of a solution of phosphomolybdic acid *n*-hydrate (1 in 10) to the filtrate: a yellow-green precipitate is formed.

Containers and storage Containers—Tight containers.

Magnesium Aluminosilicate

ケイ酸アルミン酸マグネシウム

Magnesium Aluminosilicate contains not less than 27.0% and not more than 34.3% of aluminum oxide (Al_2O_3: 101.96), not less than 20.5% and not more than 27.7% of magnesium oxide (MgO: 40.30), and not less than 14.4% and not more than 21.7% of silicon dioxide (SiO_2: 60.08), calculated on the dried basis.

Description Magnesium Aluminosilicate occurs as a white, powder or grain.

It is practically insoluble in water and in ethanol (99.5).

When heat 1 g of Magnesium Aluminosilicate with 10 mL of dilute hydrochloric acid, most of it dissolves.

Identification **(1)** To 0.5 g of Magnesium Aluminosilicate add 5 mL of diluted sulfuric acid (1 in 3), heat until white fumes are evolved, cool, add 20 mL of water, and filtrate. Neutralize the filtrate with ammonia TS, and filter the precipitate produced. Dissolve the residue in dilute hydrochloric acid: the solution responds to Qualitative Tests <*1.09*> for aluminum salt.

(2) The filtrate obtained in (1) responds to Qualitative Tests <*1.09*> (2) for magnesium salt.

(3) Wash the residue obtained in (1) with 30 mL of water, add 2 mL of a solution of methylene blue trihydrate (1 in 10,000), and wash with 30 mL of water: the precipitate has a blue color.

Purity **(1)** Soluble salts—To 10.0 g of Magnesium Aluminosilicate add 150 mL of water, boil gently for 15 minutes while shaking thoroughly. After cooling, add water to make 150 mL, and centrifuge. To 75 mL of the supernatant liquid add water to make 100 mL, and use this solution as the sample solution. Evaporate 25 mL of the sample solution on a water bath to dryness, then ignite the residue at 700°C for 2 hours: the mass of the residue is not more than 20 mg.

(2) Alkalinity—To 20 mL of the sample solution obtained in (1), add 2 drops of phenolphthalein TS, and add 0.1 mol/L hydrochloric acid VS until the solution becomes colorless: the consumed volume is not more than 0.50 mL.

(3) Chloride <*1.03*>—To 10 mL of the sample solution obtained in (1), add 6 mL of dilute nitric acid and water to make 50 mL. Perform the test using this solution as the test solution. Prepare the control solution with 0.75 mL of 0.01 mol/L hydrochloric acid VS (not more than 0.053%).

(4) Sulfate <*1.14*>—To 2 mL of the sample solution obtained in (1), add 1 mL of dilute hydrochloric acid and water to make 50 mL. Perform the test using this solution as the test solution. Prepare the control solution with 1.0 mL of 0.005 mol/L sulfuric acid VS (not more than 0.480%).

(5) Heavy metals <*1.07*>—To 2.67 g of Magnesium Aluminosilicate add 20 mL of water and 8 mL of hydrochloric acid, evaporate to dryness on a water bath. To the residue add 5 mL of dilute acetic acid and 20 mL of water, boil for 2 minutes, add 0.4 g of hydroxylammonium chloride, and heat to boiling. After cooling, add water to make exactly 100 mL, and filter. Pipet 25 mL of the filtrate, adjust to pH 3.0 with dilute acetic acid or ammonia TS, and add water to make 50 mL. Perform the test using this solution as the test solution. Prepare the control solution as follows: evaporate 2 mL of hydrochloric acid to dryness on a water bath, add 2.0 mL of Standard Lead Solution, 0.1 g of hydroxylammonium chloride and water to make 25 mL, adjust to pH 3.0 with dilute acetic acid or ammonia TS, and add water to make 50 mL (not more than 30 ppm).

(6) Iron—To 0.11 g of Magnesium Aluminosilicate add 8 mL of 2 mol/L nitric acid TS, boil for 1 minute, cool, add water to make exactly 100 mL, and centrifuge. Pipet 30 mL of the supernatant liquid, add water to make 45 mL, add 2 mL of hydrochloric acid, and shake. Add 50 mg of ammonium peroxodisulfate and 3 mL of a solution of ammonium thiocyanate (3 in 10), and shake: the solution is not more colored than the following control solution (not more than 0.03%).

Control solution: Pipet 1 mL of Standard Iron Solution, add water to make 45 mL, add 2 mL of hydrochloric acid, shake, and proceed in the same manner.

(7) Arsenic <*1.11*>—To 1.0 g of Magnesium Aluminosilicate add 10 mL of water and 1 mL of sulfuric acid, and shake thoroughly. After cooling, perform the test using this solution as the test solution (not more than 2 ppm).

Loss on drying <*2.41*> Not more than 20.0% (1 g, 110°C, 7 hours).

Acid-consuming capacity <*6.04*> Weigh accurately about 0.2 g of Magnesium Aluminosilicate, transfer to a glass-stoppered flask, add exactly 100 mL of 0.1 mol/L hydrochloric acid VS, stopper the flask tightly, shake at 37 ± 2°C for 1 hour, and filter. Pipet 50 mL of the filtrate, and titrate <*2.50*> the excess hydrochloric acid, while stirring thoroughly, with 0.1 mol/L sodium hydroxide VS until the pH of the solution becomes 3.5. Perform a blank determination in the same manner. The consumed volume of 0.1 mol/L hydrochloric acid VS is not less than 250 mL per g of Magnesium Aluminosilicate calculated on the dried basis.

Assay **(1)** Aluminum oxide—Weigh accurately about 1.25 g of Magnesium Aluminosilicate, transfer to a conical flask, add 10 mL of 3 mol/L hydrochloric acid TS and 50 mL of water, and heat on a water bath for 15 minutes. To the solution add 8 mL of hydrochloric acid, heat on a water bath for 10 minutes. After cooling, transfer to a 250-mL volumetric flask, rinse the flask with water, and add water to make 250 mL. Centrifuge the solution, and use the supernatant liquid as the sample solution. Pipet 20 mL of the sample solution, add exactly 20 mL of 0.05 mol/L disodium dihydrogen ethylenediamine tetraacetate VS. To this solution add 15 mL of acetic acid-ammonium acetate buffer solution (pH 4.8) and 20 mL of water, and boil for 5 minutes. After cooling, add 50 mL of ethanol (95), and titrate <*2.50*> with 0.05 mol/L zinc sulfate VS until the color of the solution changes from light dark green to light red (indicator: 2 mL of dithizone TS). Perform a blank determination in the same manner.

Each mL of 0.05 mol/L disodium dihydrogen ethylenediamine tetraacetate VS
= 2.549 mg of Al_2O_3

(2) Magnesium oxide—Pipet 50 mL of the sample solution obtained in (1), add 50 mL of water and 25 mL of a solution of 2,2′,2″-nitrilotriethanol (1 in 2), shake thoroughly, then add 25 mL of ammonia-ammonium chloride buffer solution (pH 10.7), and titrate <*2.50*> with 0.05 mol/L disodium dihydrogen ethylenediamine tetraacetate VS until the color of the solution changes from red-purple to blue lasting for 30 seconds (indicator: 40 mg of eriochrome black T-sodium chloride indicator).

Each mL of 0.05 mol/L disodium dihydrogen ethylenediamine tetraacetate VS
= 2.015 mg of MgO

(3) Silicon dioxide—Weigh accurately about 1 g of Magnesium Aluminosilicate, add 30 mL of dilute hydrochloric acid, and evaporate to dryness on a water bath. Moisten the residue with hydrochloric acid, evaporate to dryness on a water bath. To the residue add 8 mL of hydrochloric acid, stir, then add 25 mL of hot water, and stir again. After allowing to stand, filter the supernatant liquid through a filter paper for quantitative analysis, add 10 mL of hot water to the residue, stir, and decant the supernatant liquid on a filter paper to filter. Then wash the residue with three 10-mL portions of hot water, add 50 mL of water to the residue, and heat on a water bath for 15 minutes. Transfer the residue onto the filter paper, wash the residue with hot water until the last 5 mL of washing yields no precipitate on addition of 1 mL of silver nitrate TS, place the residue and the filter paper in a platinum crucible, ignite to ash, and then ignite at 800 ± 25°C for 1 hour. After cooling, weigh the crucible, and designate the mass as *a* (g). Then add 6 mL of hydrofluoric acid, evaporate to dryness, ignite for 5 minutes, weigh the crucible after cooling, and designate the mass as *b* (g).

Amount (g) of silicon dioxide (SiO_2) = $a - b$

Containers and storage Containers—Well-closed containers.

Magnesium Aluminometasilicate

メタケイ酸アルミン酸マグネシウム

Magnesium Aluminometasilicate contains not less than 29.1% and not more than 35.5% of aluminum oxide (Al_2O_3: 101.96), not less than 11.4% and not more than 14.0% of magnesium oxide (MgO: 40.30), and not less than 29.2% and not more than 35.6% of silicon dioxide (SiO_2: 60.08), calculated on the dried basis.

Description Magnesium Aluminometasilicate occurs as a white, powder or grain.

It is practically insoluble in water and in ethanol (99.5).

When heat 1 g of Magnesium Aluminometasilicate with 10 mL of dilute hydrochloric acid, most of it dissolves.

Identification **(1)** To 0.5 g of Magnesium Aluminometasilicate add 5 mL of diluted sulfuric acid (1 in 3), heat until white fumes are evolved, cool, add 20 mL of water, and filtrate. Neutralize the filtrate with ammonia TS, and filter the precipitate produced. Dissolve the residue in dilute hydrochloric acid: the solution responds to Qualitative Tests <*1.09*> for aluminum salt.

(2) The filtrate obtained in (1) responds to Qualitative Tests <*1.09*> (2) for magnesium salt.

(3) Wash the residue obtained in (1) with 30 mL of water, add 2 mL of a solution of methylene blue trihydrate (1 in 10,000), and wash with 30 mL of water: the precipitate has a blue color.

Purity **(1)** Soluble salts—To 10.0 g of Magnesium Aluminometasilicate add 150 mL of water, boil gently for 15 minutes while shaking thoroughly. After cooling, add water to make 150 mL, and centrifuge. To 75 mL of the supernatant liquid add water to make 100 mL, and use this solution as the sample solution. Evaporate 25 mL of the sample solution on a water bath to dryness, then ignite the residue at 700°C for 2 hours: the mass of the residue is not more than 20 mg.

(2) Alkalinity—To 20 mL of the sample solution obtained in (1), add 2 drops of phenolphthalein TS, and add 0.1 mol/L hydrochloric acid VS until the solution becomes colorless: the consumed volume is not more than 0.50 mL.

(3) Chloride <*1.03*>—To 10 mL of the sample solution obtained in (1), add 6 mL of dilute nitric acid and water to make 50 mL. Perform the test using this solution as the test solution. Prepare the control solution with 0.75 mL of 0.01 mol/L hydrochloric acid VS (not more than 0.053%).

(4) Sulfate <*1.14*>—To 2 mL of the sample solution obtained in (1), add 1 mL of dilute hydrochloric acid and water to make 50 mL. Perform the test using this solution as the test solution. Prepare the control solution with 1.0 mL of 0.005 mol/L sulfuric acid VS (not more than 0.480%).

(5) Heavy metals <*1.07*>—To 2.67 g of Magnesium Aluminometasilicate add 20 mL of water and 8 mL of hydrochloric acid, evaporate to dryness on a water bath. To the residue add 5 mL of dilute acetic acid and 20 mL of water, boil for 2 minutes, add 0.4 g of hydroxylammonium chloride, and heat to boiling. After cooling, add water to make exactly 100 mL, and filter. Pipet 25 mL of the filtrate, adjust to pH 3.0 with dilute acetic acid or ammonia TS, and add water to make 50 mL. Perform the test using this solution as the test solution. Prepare the control solution as follows: evaporate 2 mL of hydrochloric acid to dryness on a water bath, add 2.0 mL of Standard Lead Solution, 0.1 g of hydroxylammonium chloride and water to make 25 mL, adjust to pH 3.0 with dilute acetic acid or ammonia TS, and add water to make 50 mL (not more than 30 ppm).

(6) Iron—To 0.11 g of Magnesium Aluminometasilicate add 8 mL of 2 mol/L nitric acid TS, boil for 1 minute, cool, add water to make exactly 100 mL, and centrifuge. Pipet 30 mL of the supernatant liquid, add water to make 45 mL, add 2 mL of hydrochloric acid, and shake. Add 50 mg of ammonium peroxodisulfate and 3 mL of a solution of ammonium thiocyanate (3 in 10), and shake: the solution is not more colored than the following control solution (not more than 0.03%).

Control solution: Pipet 1 mL of Standard Iron Solution, add water to make 45 mL, add 2 mL of hydrochloric acid, shake, and proceed in the same manner.

(7) Arsenic <*1.11*>—To 1.0 g of Magnesium Aluminometasilicate add 10 mL of water and 1 mL of sulfuric acid, and shake thoroughly. After cooling, perform the test using this solution as the test solution (not more than 2 ppm).

Loss on drying <*2.41*> Not more than 20.0% (1 g, 110°C, 7 hours).

Acid-consuming capacity <*6.04*> Weigh accurately about 0.2 g of Magnesium Aluminometasilicate, transfer to a glass-stoppered flask, add exactly 100 mL of 0.1 mol/L hydrochloric acid VS, stopper the flask tightly, shake at 37 ± 2°C for 1 hour, and filter. Pipet 50 mL of the filtrate, and titrate <2.50> the excess hydrochloric acid, while stirring thoroughly, with 0.1 mol/L sodium hydroxide VS until the pH of the solution becomes 3.5. Perform a blank determination in the same manner. The consumed volume of 0.1 mol/L hydrochloric acid VS is not less than 210 mL per g of Magnesium Aluminometasilicate calculated on the dried basis.

Assay **(1)** Aluminum oxide—Weigh accurately about 1.25 g of Magnesium Aluminometasilicate, transfer to a conical flask, add 10 mL of 3 mol/L hydrochloric acid TS and 50 mL of water, and heat on a water bath for 15 minutes. To the solution add 8 mL of hydrochloric acid, heat on a water bath for 10 minutes. After cooling, transfer to a 250-mL volumetric flask, rinse the flask with water, and add water to make 250 mL. Centrifuge the solution, and use the supernatant liquid as the sample solution. Pipet 20 mL of the sample solution, add exactly 20 mL of 0.05 mol/L disodium dihydrogen ethylenediamine tetraacetate VS. To this solution add 15 mL of acetic acid-ammonium acetate buffer solution (pH 4.8) and 20 mL of water, and boil for 5 minutes. After cooling, add 50 mL of ethanol (95), and titrate <2.50> with 0.05 mol/L zinc sulfate VS until the color of the solution changes from light dark green to light red (indicator: 2 mL of dithizone TS). Perform a blank determination in the same manner.

Each mL of 0.05 mol/L disodium dihydrogen
ethylenediamine tetraacetate VS
= 2.549 mg of Al_2O_3

(2) Magnesium oxide—Pipet 50 mL of the sample solution obtained in (1), add 50 mL of water and 25 mL of a solution of 2,2′,2″-nitrilotriethanol (1 in 2), shake thoroughly, then add 25 mL of ammonia-ammonium chloride buffer solution (pH 10.7), and titrate <2.50> with 0.05 mol/L disodium dihydrogen ethylenediamine tetraacetate VS until the color of the solution changes from red-purple to blue lasting for 30 seconds (indicator: 40 mg of eriochrome black T-sodium chloride indicator).

Each mL of 0.05 mol/L disodium dihydrogen
ethylenediamine tetraacetate VS
= 2.015 mg of MgO

(3) Silicon dioxide—Weigh accurately about 1 g of Magnesium Aluminometasilicate, add 30 mL of dilute hydrochloric acid, and evaporate to dryness on a water bath. Moisten the residue with hydrochloric acid, evaporate to dryness on a water bath. To the residue add 8 mL of hydrochloric acid, stir, then add 25 mL of hot water, and stir again. After allowing to stand, filter the supernatant liquid through a filter paper for quantitative analysis, add 10 mL of hot water to the residue, stir, and decant the supernatant liquid on a filter paper to filter. Then wash the residue with three 10-mL portions of hot water, add 50 mL of water to the residue, and heat on a water bath for 15 minutes. Transfer the residue onto the filter paper, wash the residue with hot water until the last 5 mL of washing yields no precipitate on addition of 1 mL of silver nitrate TS, place the residue and the filter paper in a platinum crucible, ignite to ash, and then ignite at 800 ± 25°C for 1 hour. After cooling, weigh the crucible, and designate the mass as *a* (g). Then add 6 mL of hydrofluoric acid, evaporate to dryness, ignite for 5 minutes, weigh the crucible after cooling, and designate the mass as *b* (g).

Amount (g) of silicon dioxide (SiO_2) = $a - b$

Containers and storage Containers—Well-closed containers.

Magnesium Carbonate

炭酸マグネシウム

Magnesium Carbonate is a basic hydrated magnesium carbonate or a normal hydrated magnesium carbonate.

Magnesium Carbonate contains not less than 40.0% and not more then 44.0% of magnesium oxide (MgO: 40.30).

"Heavy magnesium carbonate" may be used as commonly used name for Magnesium Carbonate which shows the height of the precipitate below the 12.0-mL graduation line in the Precipitation test.

Description Magnesium Carbonate occurs as white, friable masses or powder. It is odorless.

It is practically insoluble in water, in ethanol (95), in 1-propanol and in diethyl ether.

It dissolves in dilute hydrochloric acid with effervescence.

Its saturated solution is alkaline.

Identification **(1)** Dissolve 1 g of Magnesium Carbonate in 10 mL of dilute hydrochloric acid, boil, then cool, neutralize with sodium hydroxide TS, and filter, if necessary: the solution responds to Qualitative Tests <1.09> for magnesium salt.

(2) Magnesium Carbonate responds to Qualitative Tests <1.09> (1) for carbonate.

Purity **(1)** Soluble salts—To 2.0 g of Magnesium Carbonate add 40 mL of 1-propanol and 40 mL of water, heat to boil with constant stirring, cool, and filter. Wash the residue with water, combine the washings with the filtrate, and add water to make exactly 100 mL. Evaporate 50 mL of the solution on a water bath to dryness, and dry at 105°C for 1 hour: the mass of the residue does not exceed 10.0 mg.

(2) Heavy metals <1.07>—Moisten 1.0 g of Magnesium Carbonate with 4 mL of water, dissolve by addition of 10 mL of dilute hydrochloric acid, and evaporate on a water bath to dryness. Dissolve the residue in 35 mL of water, 2 mL of dilute acetic acid, 1 drop of ammonia TS, filter, if necessary, wash the filter paper with water, combine the washings with the filtrate, and add water to make 50 mL, and perform the test using this solution as the test solution. Prepare the control solution as follows: evaporate 10 mL of dilute hydrochloric acid on a water bath to dryness, add 2 mL of dilute acetic acid and 3.0 mL of Standard Lead Solution, and dilute with water to make 50 mL (not more than 30 ppm).

(3) Iron <1.10>—Prepare the test solution with 0.10 g of Magnesium Carbonate according to Method 1, and perform the test according to Method A. Prepare the control solution with 2.0 mL of Standard Iron Solution (not more than 200 ppm).

(4) Arsenic <1.11>—Prepare the test solution with 0.40 g of Magnesium Carbonate, previously moistened with 1.5 mL of water, add 3.5 mL of dilute hydrochloric acid, and perform the test (not more than 5 ppm).

(5) Calcium oxide—Weigh accurately about 0.6 g of Magnesium Carbonate, and dissolve in 35 mL of water and 6 mL of dilute hydrochloric acid. Add 250 mL of water and 5 mL of a solution of L-tartaric acid (1 in 5), then add 10 mL of a solution of 2,2′,2″-nitrilotriethanol (3 in 10) and 10 mL of 8 mol/L potassium hydroxide TS, allow to stand for 5 minutes, and titrate <*2.50*> with 0.01 mol/L disodium dihydrogen ethylenediamine tetraacetate VS until the color of the solution changes form red-purple to blue (indicator: 0.1 g of NN indicator). Perform a blank determination in the same manner, and make any necessary correction.

Each mL of 0.01 mol/L disodium dihydrogen ethylenediamine tetraacetate VS
= 0.5608 mg of CaO

The content of calcium oxide (CaO: 56.08) is not more than 0.6%.

(6) Acid-insoluble substances—Mix 5.0 g of Magnesium Carbonate and 75 mL of water, add 10 mL of hydrochloric acid dropwise while stirring, boil for 5 minutes, and cool. Collect the insoluble residue using filter paper for quantitative analysis, wash well with water until the last washing shows no turbidity with silver nitrate TS, and ignite the residue together with the filter paper: the mass of the residue is not more than 2.5 mg.

Precipitation test Transfer 1.0 g of Magnesium Carbonate, previously sifted through a No. 100 (150 μm) sieve to a glass-stoppered measuring cylinder with a 50-mL graduation line at 150 mm from the bottom, and add water to make 50 mL. Shake vigorously for exactly 1 minute, allow to stand for 15 minutes, and measure the height of the precipitate (in graduation in ml).

Assay Weigh accurately about 0.4 g of Magnesium Carbonate, dissolve in 10 mL of water and 3.5 mL of dilute hydrochloric acid, and add water to make exactly 100 mL. Pipet 25 mL of the solution, add 50 mL of water and 5 mL of ammonia-ammonium chloride buffer solution (pH 10.7) and titrate <*2.50*> with 0.05 mol/L disodium dihydrogen ethylenediamine tetraacetate VS (indicator: 40 mg of eriochrome black T-sodium chloride indicator). Perform a blank determination in the same manner, and make any necessary correction.

From the volume of 0.05 mol/L disodium dihydrogen ethylenediamine tetraacetate VS consumed deduct the volume of 0.05 mol/L disodium dihydrogen ethylenediamine tetraacetate VS corresponding to the content of calcium oxide (CaO) obtained in the Purity (5).

Each mL of 0.05 mol/L disodium dihydrogen ethylenediamine tetraacetate VS
= 2.015 mg of MgO

Each mg of calcium oxide (CaO)
= 0.36 mL of 0.05 mol/L disodium dihydrogen ethylenediamine tetraacetate VS

Containers and storage Containers—Well-closed containers.

Magnesium Oxide

酸化マグネシウム

MgO: 40.30

Magnesium Oxide, when ignited, contains not less than 96.0% of magnesium oxide (MgO).

When 5 g of Magnesium Oxide has a volume not more than 30 mL, it may be labeled heavy magnesium oxide.

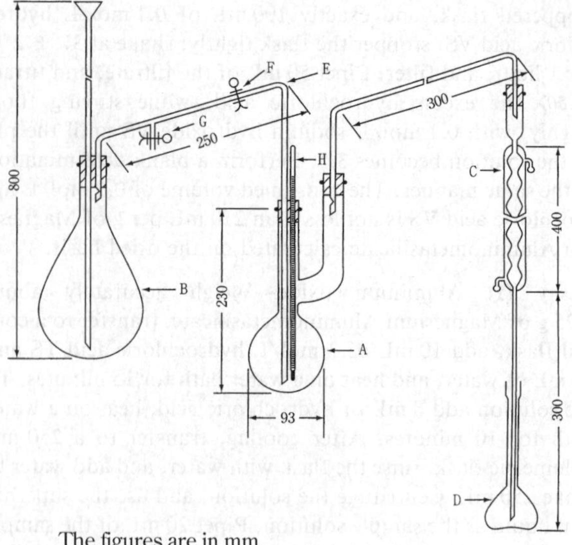

The figures are in mm.

A: Distilling flask of about 300-mL capacity.
B: Steam generator of about 1000-mL capacity, containing a few boiling tips to prevent bumping
C: Condenser
D: Receiver: 200-mL volumetric flask
E: Steam-introducing tube having an internal diameter of about 8 mm
F, G: Rubber tube with a clamp
H: Thermometer

Description Magnesium Oxide occurs as a white, powder or granules. It is odorless.

It is practically insoluble in water, in ethanol (95) and in diethyl ether.

It dissolves in dilute hydrochloric acid.

It absorbs moisture and carbon dioxide in air.

Identification A solution of Magnesium Oxide in dilute hydrochloric acid (1 in 50) responds to Qualitative Tests <*1.09*> for magnesium salt.

Purity **(1)** Alkali and soluble salts—Transfer 2.0 g of Magnesium Oxide to a beaker, add 100 mL of water, cover the beaker with a watch-glass, heat on a water bath for 5 minutes, and filter immediately. After cooling, to 50 mL of the filtrate add 2 drops of methyl red TS and 2.0 mL of 0.05 mol/L sulfuric acid VS: a red color develops. Evaporate 25 mL of the remaining filtrate to dryness, and dry the residue at 105°C for 1 hour: the mass of the residue is not more than 10 mg.

(2) Carbonate—Boil 0.10 g of Magnesium Oxide with 5 mL of water, cool, and add 5 mL of acetic acid (31): almost no effervescence occurs.

(3) Heavy metals <*1.07*>—Dissolve 1.0 g of Magnesium Oxide in 20 mL of dilute hydrochloric acid, and evaporate on a water bath to dryness. Dissolve the residue in 35 mL of water, add 1 drop of phenolphthalein TS, neutralize with ammonia TS, add 2 mL of dilute acetic acid, and filter, if necessary. Wash the filter paper with water, add water to the combined washing and the filtrate to make 50 mL, and perform the test using this solution as the test solution. Prepare the control solution as follows: to 20 mL of dilute hydrochloric acid add 1 drop of phenolphthalein TS, neutralize with ammonia TS, and add 2 mL of dilute acetic acid, 4.0 mL of Standard Lead Solution and water to make 50 mL (not more than 40 ppm).

(4) Iron <*1.10*>—Prepare the test solution with 40 mg of

Magnesium Oxide according to Method 1, and perform the test according to Method A. Prepare the control solution with 2.0 mL of Standard Iron Solution (not more than 500 ppm).

(5) Calcium oxide—Weigh accurately about 0.25 g of Magnesium Oxide, previously ignited, dissolve in 6 mL of dilute hydrochloric acid by heating. Cool, add 300 mL of water and 3 mL of a solution of L-tartaric acid (1 in 5), then add 10 mL of a solution of 2,2′,2″-nitrilotriethanol (3 in 10) and 10 mL of 8 mol/L potassium hydroxide TS, allow to stand for 5 minutes, and titrate *<2.50>* with 0.01 mol/L disodium dihydrogen ethylenediamine tetraacetate VS until the color of the solution changes from red-purple to blue (indicator: 0.1 g of NN indicator). Perform a blank determination in the same manner, and make any necessary correction.

Each mL of 0.01 mol/L disodium dihydrogen ethylenediamine tetraacetate VS
= 0.5608 mg of CaO

The mass of calcium oxide (CaO: 56.08) is not more than 1.5%.

(6) Arsenic *<1.11>*—Dissolve 0.20 g of Magnesium Oxide in 5 mL of dilute hydrochloric acid, and perform the test with this solution as the test solution (not more than 10 ppm).

(7) Acid-insoluble substances—Mix 2.0 g of Magnesium Oxide with 75 mL of water, add 12 mL of hydrochloric acid dropwise, while shaking, and boil for 5 minutes. Collect the insoluble residue using filter paper for quantitative analysis, wash well with water until the last washing shows no turbidity with silver nitrate TS, and ignite the residue together with the filter paper: the mass of the ignited residue does not more than 2.0 mg.

(8) Fluoride—(i) Apparatus: Use a hard glass apparatus as illustrated in the figure. Ground-glass joints may be used.

(ii) Procedure: Transfer 5.0 g of Magnesium Oxide to the distilling flask A with the aid of 20 mL of water, add about 1 g of glass wool and 50 mL of diluted purified sulfuric acid (1 in 2), and connect A to the distillation apparatus, previously washed with steam streamed through the steam introducing tube E. Connect the condenser C with the receiver D containing 10 mL of 0.01 mol/L sodium hydroxide VS and 10 mL of water so that the lower end of C is immersed in the solution. Heat A gradually until the temperature of the solution in A reaches 130°C, then open the rubber tube F, close the rubber tube G, boil water in the steam generator B vigorously, and introduce the generated steam into F. Simultaneously, heat A, and maintain the temperature of the solution in A between 135°C and 145°C. Adjust the distilling rate to about 10 mL per minute. Collect about 170 mL of the distillate, then stop the distillation, wash C with a small quantity of water, combine the washings with the distillate, add water to make exactly 200 mL, and use this solution as the test solution. Perform the test with the test solution as directed in the procedure of determination for fluoride under Oxygen Flask Combustion Method *<1.06>*. No corrective solution is used in this procedure. The content of fluoride (F) is not more than 0.08%.

Amount (mg) of fluoride (F: 19.00) in the test solution
= amount (mg) of fluoride in 5 mL of the standard solution
$\times A_T/A_S \times 200/V$

Loss on ignition *<2.43>* Not more than 10% (0.25 g, 900°C, constant mass).

Assay Ignite Magnesium Oxide to constant mass at 900°C, weigh accurately about 0.2 g of the residue, dissolve in 10 mL of water and 4.0 mL of dilute hydrochloric acid, and add water to make exactly 100 mL. Pipet 25 mL of this solution, add 50 mL of water and 5 mL of ammonia-ammonium chloride buffer solution (pH 10.7) and titrate *<2.50>* with 0.05 mol/L disodium dihydrogen ethylenediamine tetraacetate VS (indicator: 40 mg of eriochrome black T-sodium chloride indicator). Perform a blank determination in the same manner, and make any necessary correction.

From the volume of 0.05 mol/L disodium dihydrogen ethylenediamine tetraacetate VS consumed, deduct the volume of 0.05 mol/L disodium dihydrogen ethylenediamine tetraacetate VS corresponding to the content of calcium oxide (CaO) obtained in the Purity (5).

Each mL of 0.05 mol/L disodium dihydrogen ethylenediamine tetraacetate VS
= 2.015 mg of MgO

Each mg of calcium oxide (CaO)
= 0.36 mL of 0.05 mol/L disodium dihydrogen ethylenediamine tetraacetate VS

Containers and storage Containers—Tight containers.

Magnesium Silicate

ケイ酸マグネシウム

Magnesium Silicate contains not less than 45.0% of silicon dioxide (SiO_2: 60.08) and not less than 20.0% of magnesium oxide (MgO: 40.30), and the ratio of percentage (%) of magnesium oxide to silicon dioxide is not less than 2.2 and not more than 2.5.

Description Magnesium Silicate occurs as a white, fine powder. It is odorless and tasteless.

It is practically insoluble in water, in ethanol (95) and in diethyl ether.

Identification **(1)** Mix 0.5 g of Magnesium Silicate with 10 mL of dilute hydrochloric acid, filter, and neutralize the filtrate with ammonia TS: the solution responds to Qualitative Tests *<1.09>* for magnesium salt.

(2) Prepare a bead by fusing ammonium sodium hydrogenphosphate tetrahydrate on a platinum loop. Place the bead in contact with Magnesium Silicate, and fuse again: an infusible matter appears in the bead, which changes to an opaque bead with a web-like structure upon cooling.

Purity **(1)** Soluble salts—Add 150 mL of water to 10.0 g of Magnesium Silicate, heat on a water bath for 60 minutes with occasional shaking, then cool, dilute with water to 150 mL, and centrifuge. Dilute 75 mL of the resultant transparent liquid with water to 100 mL, and use this solution as the sample solution. Evaporate 25 mL of the sample solution on a water bath to dryness, and ignite the residue at 700°C for 2 hours: the mass of the ignited residue is not more than 0.02 g.

(2) Alkalinity—To 20 mL of the sample solution obtained in (1) add 2 drops of phenolphthalein TS and 1.0 mL of 0.1 mol/L hydrochloric acid VS: no color develops.

(3) Chloride *<1.03>*—Take 10 mL of the sample solution obtained in (1), add 6 mL of dilute nitric acid, dilute with water to 50 mL, and perform the test using this solution as the test solution. Prepare the control solution with 0.75 mL of 0.01 mol/L hydrochloric acid VS (not more than

0.053%).

(4) Sulfate <*1.14*>—To the residue obtained in (1) add about 3 mL of dilute hydrochloric acid, and heat on a water bath for 10 minutes. Add 30 mL of water, filter, wash the residue on the filter with water, combine the washings with the filtrate, and dilute to 50 mL with water. To 4 mL of the solution add 1 mL of dilute hydrochloric acid and water to make 50 mL. Perform the test using this solution as the test solution. Prepare the control solution with 1.0 mL of 0.005 mol/L sulfuric acid VS (not more than 0.480%).

(5) Heavy metals <*1.07*>—To 1.0 g of Magnesium Silicate add 20 mL of water and 3 mL of hydrochloric acid, and boil for 2 minutes. Filter, and wash the residue on the filter with two 5-mL portions of water. Evaporate the combined filtrate and washings on a water bath to dryness, add 2 mL of dilute acetic acid to the residue, warm until solution is complete, filter, if necessary, add water to make 50 mL, and perform the test using this solution as the test solution. Prepare the control solution with 3.0 mL of Standard Lead Solution, 2 mL of dilute acetic acid and water to make 50 mL (not more than 30 ppm).

(6) Arsenic <*1.11*>—To 0.40 g of Magnesium Silicate add 5 mL of dilute hydrochloric acid, heat gently to boiling while shaking well, cool rapidly, and centrifuge. Mix the residue with 5 mL of dilute hydrochloric acid with shaking, centrifuge, then add 10 mL of water to the residue, and repeat the extraction in the same manner. Concentrate the combined extracts on a water bath to 5 mL. Use this solution as the test solution, and perform the test (not more than 5 ppm).

Loss on ignition <*2.43*> Not more than 34% (0.5 g, 850°C, 3 hours).

Acid-consuming capacity <*6.04*> Place about 0.2 g of Magnesium Silicate, accurately weighed, in a glass-stoppered flask, add exactly 30 mL of 0.1 mol/L hydrochloric acid VS and 20 mL of water, shake at 37 ± 2°C for 1 hour, and cool. Pipet 25 mL of the supernatant liquid, and titrate <*2.50*> the excess hydrochloric acid, while stirring well, with 0.1 mol/L sodium hydroxide VS until the pH becomes 3.5.

1 g of Magnesium Silicate, calculated on the anhydrous basis by making allowance for the observed loss on ignition determined as directed in the preceding Loss on ignition, consumes not less than 140 mL and not more than 160 mL of 0.1 mol/L hydrochloric acid VS.

Assay **(1)** Silicon dioxide—Weigh accurately about 0.7 g of Magnesium Silicate, add 10 mL of 0.5 mol/L sulfuric acid TS, evaporate on a water bath to dryness, add 25 mL of water to the residue, and heat on a water bath for 15 minutes with occasional stirring. Filter the supernatant liquid through filter paper for quantitative analysis, add 25 mL of hot water to the residue, stir, and decant the supernatant liquid on the filter paper to filter. Wash the residue in the same manner with two 25-mL portions of hot water, transfer the residue onto the filter paper, and wash with hot water until the last washing does not respond to Qualitative Tests <*1.09*> (1) for sulfate. Place the residue and the filter paper in a platinum crucible, incinerate with strong heating, and ignite between 775°C and 825°C for 30 minutes, then cool, and weigh the residue as a (g). Moisten the residue with water, and add 6 mL of hydrofluoric acid and 3 drops of sulfuric acid. Evaporate to dryness, ignite for 5 minutes, cool, and weigh the residue as b (g).

Content (%) of silicon dioxide (SiO_2)
$= (a - b)/M \times 100$

M: Mass (g) of the Magnesium Silicate taken

(2) Magnesium oxide—Weigh accurately about 0.3 g of Magnesium Silicate, transfer to a 50-mL conical flask, add 10 mL of 0.5 mol/L sulfuric acid VS, and heat on a water bath for 15 minutes. Cool, transfer to a 100-mL volumetric flask, wash the conical flask with water, add the washings to the volumetric flask, dilute with water to 100 mL, and filter. Pipet 50 mL of the filtrate, shake with 50 mL of water and 5 mL of diluted 2,2′,2″-nitrilotriethanol (1 in 2), add 2.0 mL of ammonia TS and 10 mL of ammonia-ammonium chloride buffer solution (pH 10.7) and titrate <*2.50*> with 0.05 mol/L disodium dihydrogen ethylenediamine tetraacetate VS (indicator: 40 mg of eriochrome black T-sodium chloride indicator).

Each mL of 0.05 mol/L disodium dihydrogen ethylenediamine tetraacetate VS
= 2.015 mg of MgO

(3) Ratio of percentage (%) of magnesium oxide (MgO) to silicon dioxide (SiO_2)—Calculate the quotient from the percentages obtained in (1) and (2).

Containers and storage Containers—Well-closed containers.

Magnesium Stearate

ステアリン酸マグネシウム

This monograph is harmonized with the European Pharmacopoeia and the U.S.Pharmacopeia.

The parts of the text that are not harmonized are marked with symbols (◆ ◆).

Information on the harmonization with the European Pharmacopoeia and the U.S. Pharmacopeia is available on the website of the Pharmaceuticals and Medical Devices Agency.

Magnesium Stearate is a compound of magnesium with a mixture of solid fatty acids, and consists chiefly of variable proportions of magnesium stearate and magnesium palmitate obtained from sources of vegetable or animal origin.

It contains not less than 4.0% and not more than 5.0% of magnesium (Mg: 24.31), calculated on the dried basis.

◆**Description** Magnesium Stearate occurs as a white, light, bulky powder.

It is smooth to the touch and sticky to the skin. It has no odor or a faint, characteristic odor.

It is practically insoluble in water and in ethanol (99.5).◆

Identification Mix 5.0 g of Magnesium Stearate with 50 mL of peroxide-free diethyl ether, 20 mL of dilute nitric acid, and 20 mL of water in a round-bottom flask, and heat to dissolve completely under a reflux condenser. After cooling, transfer the contents of the flask to a separator, shake, allow the layers to separate, and transfer the aqueous layer to a flask. Extract the diethyl ether layer with two 4-mL portions of water, and combine these extracts to the main aqueous extract. After washing the combined aqueous extract with 15 mL of peroxide-free diethyl ether, transfer to a 50-mL volumetric flask, add water to make 50 mL, and use this solution as the sample solution. To 1 mL of the sample solution add 1 mL of ammonia TS: A white precipitate is formed that dissolves on addition of 1 mL of ammonium chloride TS. By further addition of 1 mL of a solution of disodium hydrogen phosphate dodecahydrate (4 in 25) a white crystalline precipitate is formed.

Purity **(1)** Acidity or alkalinity—Heat 1.0 g of Magnesium Stearate in 20 mL of freshly boiled and cooled water on a water bath for 1 minute while shaking, cool, and filter. Add 0.05 mL of bromothymol blue TS to 10 mL of the filtrate: not more than 0.05 mL of 0.1 mol/L hydrochloric acid VS or 0.1 mol/L sodium hydroxide VS is required to change the color of the solution.

(2) Chloride *<1.03>*—Perform the test with 10.0 mL of the sample solution obtained in Identification. Prepare the control solution with 1.4 mL of 0.02 mol/L hydrochloric acid VS (not more than 0.1%).

(3) Sulfate *<1.14>*—Perform the test with 6.0 mL of the sample solution obtained in Identification. Prepare the control solution with 3.0 mL of 0.02 mol/L sulfuric acid VS (not more than 1.0%).

◆**(4)** Heavy metals *<1.07>*—Heat 1.0 g of Magnesium Stearate weakly first, then incinerate at about 500 ± 25°C. After cooling, add 2 mL of hydrochloric acid, evaporate on a water bath to dryness, add 20 mL of water and 2 mL of dilute acetic acid to the residue, and heat for 2 minutes. After cooling, filter this solution through a filter paper, wash the filter paper with 15 mL of water, and combine the washing with the filtrate. To the filtrate add water to make 50 mL, and perform the test with this solution as the test solution. Prepare the control solution as follows: evaporate 2 mL of hydrochloric acid on a water bath to dryness, add 2 mL of dilute acetic acid, 2.0 mL of Standard Lead Solution and water to make 50 mL (not more than 20 ppm).◆

Loss on drying *<2.41>* Not more than 6.0% (2 g, 105°C, constant mass).

◆**Microbial limit** *<4.05>* The acceptance criteria of TAMC and TYMC are 10^3 CFU/g and 5×10^2 CFU/g, respectively. *Salmonella* and *Escherichia coli* are not observed.◆

Relative content of stearic acid and palmitic acid Transfer 0.10 g of Magnesium Stearate to a small conical flask fitted with a reflux condenser. Add 5.0 mL of boron trifluoride-methanol TS, mix, and reflux for 10 minutes to dissolve the solids. Add 4 mL of heptane through the condenser, and reflux for 10 minutes. After cooling, add 20 mL of saturated sodium chloride solution, shake, and allow the layers to separate. Pass the heptane layer through about 0.1 g of anhydrous sodium sulfate, previously washed with heptane, into another flask. Transfer 1.0 mL of this solution to a 10-mL volumetric flask, dilute with heptane to volume, and use this solution as the sample solution. Perform the test with 1 μL of the sample solution as directed under Gas chromatography *<2.02>* according to the following conditions, and determine the area, A, of the methyl stearate peak and the sum of the areas, B, of all of the fatty acid ester peaks. Calculate the percentage of stearic acid in the fatty acid fraction of Magnesium Stearate by the following formula.

$$\text{Content (\%) of stearic acid} = A/B \times 100$$

Similarly, calculate the percentage of palmitic acid in the portion of Magnesium Stearate taken. The methyl stearate peak, and the sum of the stearate and palmitate peaks are not less than 40% and not less than 90% of the total area of all fatty acid ester peaks, respectively.

Operating conditions—

Detector: A hydrogen flame-ionization detector.

Column: A fused silica capillary column 0.32 mm in inside diameter and 30 m in length, the inside coated with a 0.5-μm layer of polyethylene glycol 15000-diepoxide for gas chromatography.

Column temperature: Maintain at 70°C for 2 minutes after injection, then program to increase the temperature at the rate of 5°C per minute to 240°C and to maintain 240°C for 5 minutes.

Injection port temperature: A constant temperature of about 220°C.

Detector temperature: A constant temperature of about 260°C.

Carrier gas: Helium.

Flow rate: 2.4 mL per minute.

Splitless.

◆Time span of measurement: For 41 minutes after the solvent peak.◆

System suitability—

◆Test for required detectability:◆ Place about 50 mg each of stearic acid for gas chromatography and palmitic acid for gas chromatography in a small conical flask fitted with a reflux condenser. Add 5.0 mL of boron trifluoride-methanol TS, mix, and proceed in the same manner as directed for the preparation of the sample solution, and use the solution so obtained as the solution for system suitability test. ◆To exactly 1 mL of the solution for system suitability test add heptane to make exactly 10 mL. To exactly 1 mL of this solution add heptane to make exactly 10 mL. Further, to exactly 1 mL of this solution add heptane to make exactly 10 mL. Confirm that the peak area of methyl stearate obtained with 1 μL of this solution is equivalent to 0.05 to 0.15% of that with 1 μL of the solution for system suitability test.◆

System performance: When the procedure is run with 1 μL of the solution for system suitability test under the above operating conditions, the relative retention time of methyl palmitate to methyl stearate is about 0.9, and the resolution between these peaks is not less than 5.0.

System repeatability: When the test is repeated 6 times with the solution for system suitability test under the above operating conditions, the relative standard deviation of the peak areas of methyl palmitate and methyl stearate are not more than 3.0%, respectively, and the relative standard deviation of the ratios of the peak area of methyl palmitate to methyl stearate is not more than 1.0%.

Assay Transfer about 0.5 g of Magnesium Stearate, accurately weighed, to a 250-mL flask, add 50 mL of a mixture of ethanol (99.5) and 1-butanol (1:1), 5 mL of ammonia solution (28), 3 mL of ammonium chloride buffer solution (pH 10), 30.0 mL of 0.1 mol/L disodium dihydrogen ethylenediamine tetraacetate VS and 1 to 2 drops of eriochrome black T TS, and mix. Heat at 45 – 50°C to make the solution clear, and after cooling, titrate *<2.50>* the excess disodium dihydrogen ethylenediamine tetraacetate with 0.1 mol/L zinc sulfate VS until the solution changes from blue to violet in color. Perform a blank determination in the same manner, and make any necessary correction.

Each mL of 0.1 mol/L disodium dihydrogen
ethylenediamine tetraacetate VS
= 2.431 mg of Mg

◆**Containers and storage** Containers—Tight containers.◆

Magnesium Sulfate Hydrate

硫酸マグネシウム水和物

$MgSO_4.7H_2O$: 246.47

Magnesium Sulfate Hydrate, when ignited, contains not less than 99.0% of magnesium sulfate ($MgSO_4$: 120.37).

Description Magnesium Sulfate Hydrate occurs as colorless or white crystals. It has a cooling, saline, bitter taste.

It is very soluble in water, and practically insoluble in ethanol (95).

It dissolves in dilute hydrochloric acid.

Identification A solution of Magnesium Sulfate Hydrate (1 in 40) responds to Qualitative Tests <*1.09*> for magnesium salt and for sulfate.

pH <*2.54*> Dissolve 1.0 g of Magnesium Sulfate Hydrate in 20 mL of water: the pH of this solution is between 5.0 and 8.2.

Purity **(1)** Clarity and color of solution—Dissolve 1.0 g of Magnesium Sulfate Hydrate in 20 mL of water: the solution is clear and colorless.

(2) Chloride <*1.03*>—Perform the test with 1.0 g of Magnesium Sulfate Hydrate. Prepare the control solution with 0.40 mL of 0.01 mol/L hydrochloric acid VS (not more than 0.014%).

(3) Heavy metals <*1.07*>—Proceed with 2.0 g of Magnesium Sulfate Hydrate according to Method 1, and perform the test. Prepare the control solution with 2.0 mL of Standard Lead Solution (not more than 10 ppm).

(4) Zinc—Dissolve 2.0 g of Magnesium Sulfate Hydrate in 20 mL of water, and add 1 mL of acetic acid (31) and 5 drops of potassium hexacyanoferrate (II) TS: no turbidity is produced.

(5) Calcium—Dissolve 1.0 g of Magnesium Sulfate Hydrate in 5.0 mL of dilute hydrochloric acid, add water to make 100 mL, and use this solution as the sample solution. Separately, dissolve 1.0 g of Magnesium Sulfate Hydrate in 2.0 mL of Standard Calcium Solution and 5.0 mL of dilute hydrochloric acid, add water to make exactly 100 mL, and use this solution as the standard solution. Perform the test with the sample solution and standard solution as directed under Atomic Absorption Spectrophotometry <*2.23*> according to the following conditions, and determine the absorbances, A_T and A_S, of both solutions: A_T is smaller than $A_S - A_T$ (not more than 0.02%).

Gas: Combustible gas—Acetylene or hydrogen.
Supporting gas—Air.
Lamp: Calcium hollow-cathod lamp.
Wavelength: 422.7 nm.

(6) Arsenic <*1.11*>—Prepare the test solution with 1.0 g of Magnesium Sulfate Hydrate according to Method 1, and perform the test (not more than 2 ppm).

Loss on ignition <*2.43*> 45.0 – 52.0% (1 g, after drying at 105°C for 2 hours, ignite at 450°C for 3 hours).

Assay Weigh accurately about 0.6 g of Magnesium Sulfate Hydrate, previously ignited at 450°C for 3 hours after drying at 105°C for 2 hours, and dissolve in 2 mL of dilute hydrochloric acid and water to make exactly 100 mL. Pipet 25 mL of this solution, add 50 mL of water and 5 mL of ammonia-ammonium chloride buffer solution (pH 10.7), and titrate <*2.50*> with 0.05 mol/L disodium dihydrogen ethylenediamine tetraacetate VS (indicator: 40 mg of eriochrome black T-sodium chloride indicator). Perform a blank determination in the same manner, and make any necessary correction.

Each mL of 0.05 mol/L disodium dihydrogen ethylenediamine tetraacetate VS
= 6.018 mg of $MgSO_4$

Containers and storage Containers—Well-closed containers.

Magnesium Sulfate Injection

硫酸マグネシウム注射液

Magnesium Sulfate Injection is an aqueous injection.

It contains not less than 95.0% and not more than 105.0% of the labeled amount of magnesium sulfate hydrate ($MgSO_4.7H_2O$: 246.47).

Method of preparation Prepare as directed under Injections, with Magnesium Sulfate Hydrate.

Description Magnesium Sulfate Injection is a clear, colorless liquid.

Identification Measure a volume of Magnesium Sulfate Injection, equivalent to 0.5 g of Magnesium Sulfate Hydrate, and add water to make 20 mL: the solution responds to Qualitative Tests <*1.09*> for magnesium salt and for sulfate.

pH <*2.54*> 5.5 – 7.0 When the labeled concentration exceeds 5%, prepare a solution of 5% with water, and perform the test.

Bacterial endotoxins <*4.01*> Less than 0.09 EU/mg.

Extractable volume <*6.05*> It meets the requirement.

Foreign insoluble matter <*6.06*> Perform the test according to Method 1: it meets the requirement.

Insoluble particulate matter <*6.07*> It meets the requirement.

Sterility <*4.06*> Perform the test according to the Membrane filtration method: it meets the requirement.

Assay Measure exactly a volume of Magnesium Sulfate Injection, equivalent to about 0.3 g of magnesium sulfate hydrate ($MgSO_4.7H_2O$), and add water to make 75 mL. Then add 5 mL of ammonia-ammonium chloride buffer solution (pH 10.7), and proceed as directed in the Assay under Magnesium Sulfate Hydrate.

Each mL of 0.05 mol/L disodium dihydrogen ethylenediamine tetraacetate VS
= 12.32 mg of $MgSO_4.7H_2O$

Containers and storage Containers—Hermetic containers.
Plastic containers for aqueous injections may be used.

Magnesium Sulfate Mixture

硫酸マグネシウム水

Magnesium Sulfate Mixture contains not less than 13.5 w/v% and not more than 16.5 w/v% of magnesium sulfate hydrate ($MgSO_4.7H_2O$: 246.47).

Method of preparation

Magnesium Sulfate Hydrate	150 g
Bitter Tincture	20 mL
Dilute Hydrochloric Acid	5 mL
Purified Water or Purified Water in Containers	a sufficient quantity
To make	1000 mL

Prepare before use, with the above ingredients.

Description Magnesium Sulfate Mixture is a light yellow clear liquid. It has a bitter and acid taste.

Identification (1) Magnesium Sulfate Mixture responds to Qualitative Tests 〈*1.09*〉 for magnesium salt.

(2) Magnesium Sulfate Mixture responds to Qualitative Tests 〈*1.09*〉 (2) for chloride.

Assay Pipet 10 mL of Magnesium Sulfate Mixture, and add water to make exactly 100 mL. Pipet 10 mL of this solution, add 50 mL of water and 5 mL of ammonia-ammonium chloride buffer solution (pH 10.7), and titrate 〈*2.50*〉 with 0.05 mol/L disodium dihydrogen ethylenediamine tetraacetate VS (indicator: 40 mg of eriochrome black T-sodium chloride indicator).

Each mL of 0.05 mol/L disodium dihydrogen ethylenediamine tetraacetate VS
= 12.32 mg of $MgSO_4.7H_2O$

Containers and storage Containers—Tight containers.

Maltose Hydrate

マルトース水和物

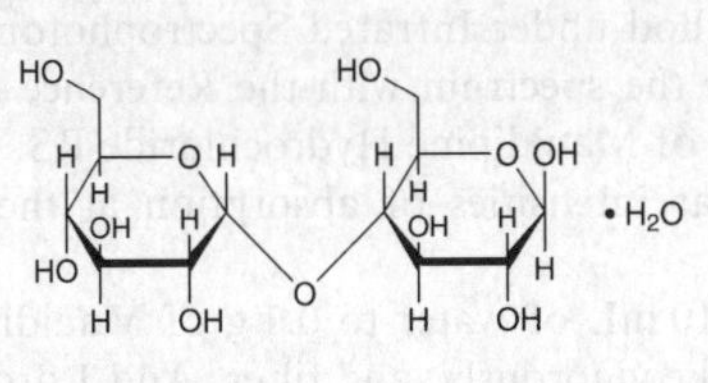

$C_{12}H_{22}O_{11}.H_2O$: 360.31
α-D-Glucopyranosyl-(1→4)-β-D-glucopyranose monohydrate
[*6363-53-7*]

Maltose Hydrate, when dried, contains not less than 98.0% of maltose hydrate ($C_{12}H_{22}O_{11}.H_2O$).

Description Maltose Hydrate occurs as white, crystals or crystalline powder. It has a sweet taste.

It is freely soluble in water, very slightly soluble in ethanol (95), and practically insoluble in diethyl ether.

Identification (1) Dissolve 0.5 g of Maltose Hydrate in 5 mL of water, add 5 mL of ammonia TS, and heat for 5 minutes on a water bath: an orange color develops.

(2) Add 2 to 3 drops of a solution of Maltose Hydrate (1 in 50) to 5 mL of boiling Fehling TS: a red precipitate is formed.

Optical rotation 〈*2.49*〉 $[\alpha]_D^{20}$: +126 – +131° Weigh accurately about 10 g of Maltose Hydrate, previously dried, dissolve in 0.2 mL of ammonia TS and water to make exactly 100 mL, and determine the optical rotation of this solution in a 100-mm cell.

pH 〈*2.54*〉 The pH of a solution of 1.0 g of Maltose Hydrate in 10 mL of water is between 4.5 and 6.5.

Purity (1) Clarity and color of solution—Put 10 g of Maltose Hydrate in 30 mL of water in a Nessler tube, warm at 60°C in a water bath to dissolve, and after cooling, add water to make 50 mL: the solution is clear, and has no more color than the following control solution.

Control solution: Add water to a mixture of 1.0 mL of Cobalt (II) Chloride CS, 3.0 mL of Iron (III) Chloride CS and 2.0 mL of Copper (II) Sulfate CS to make 10.0 mL. To 1.0 mL of this solution add water to make 50 mL.

(2) Chloride 〈*1.03*〉—Perform the test with 2.0 g of Maltose Hydrate. Prepare the control solution with 1.0 mL of 0.01 mol/L hydrochloric acid VS (not more than 0.018%).

(3) Sulfate 〈*1.14*〉—Perform the test with 2.0 g of Maltose Hydrate. Prepare the control solution with 1.0 mL of 0.005 mol/L sulfuric acid VS (not more than 0.024%).

(4) Heavy metals 〈*1.07*〉—Proceed with 5.0 g of Maltose Hydrate according to Method 1, and perform the test. Prepare the control solution with 2.0 mL of Standard Lead Solution (not more than 4 ppm).

(5) Arsenic 〈*1.11*〉—Dissolve 1.5 g of Maltose Hydrate in 5 mL of water, add 5 mL of dilute sulfuric acid and 1 mL of bromine TS, heat on a water bath for 5 minutes, then heat to concentrate to 5 mL, and use this solution as the test solution after cooling. Perform the test (not more than 1.3 ppm).

(6) Dextrin, soluble starch and sulfite—Dissolve 1.0 g of Maltose Hydrate in 10 mL of water, and add 1 drop of iodine TS: a yellow color appears, and the color changes to a blue by adding 1 drop of starch TS.

(7) Nitrogen—Weigh accurately about 2 g of Maltose Hydrate, and perform the test as directed under Nitrogen Determination 〈*1.08*〉 using 10 mL of sulfuric acid for the decomposition and 45 mL of a solution of sodium hydroxide (2 in 5) for the addition: the amount of nitrogen (N: 14.01) is not more than 0.01%.

(8) Related substances—Dissolve 0.5 g of Maltose Hydrate in 10 mL of water, and use this solution as the sample solution. Pipet 1 mL of the sample solution, add water to make exactly 100 mL, and use this solution as the standard solution. Perform the test with exactly 20 μL each of the sample solution and standard solution as directed under Liquid Chromatography 〈*2.01*〉 according to the following operating conditions. Determine the peak areas from both solutions by the automatic integration method: the total area of the peaks which appear before the peak of maltose obtained from the sample solution is not larger than 1.5 times the peak area of maltose from the standard solution, and the total area of the peaks which appear after the peak of maltose from the sample solution is not larger than 1/2 times the peak area of maltose from the standard solution.

Operating conditions—

Detector, column, column temperature, mobile phase, flow rate, and selection of column: Proceed as directed in the operating conditions in the Assay.

Detection sensitivity: Adjust the sensitivity so that the peak height of maltose obtained with 20 μL of the standard solution is about 30 mm.

Time span of measurement: About 2 times as long as the

retention time of maltose.

Loss on drying ⟨*2.41*⟩ Not more than 0.5% (1 g, 80°C, 4 hours).

Residue on ignition ⟨*2.44*⟩ Not more than 0.1% (1 g).

Assay Weigh accurately about 0.1 g each of Maltose Hydrate and Maltose RS, previously dried, dissolve in exactly 10 mL each of the internal standard solution, and use these solutions as the sample solution and the standard solution, respectively. Perform the test with 20 μL each of the sample solution and standard solution as directed under Liquid Chromatography ⟨*2.01*⟩ according to the following operating conditions, and calculate the ratios, Q_T and Q_S, of the peak area of maltose to that of the internal standard.

Amount (mg) of maltose hydrate ($C_{12}H_{22}O_{11}.H_2O$)
$= M_S \times Q_T/Q_S$

M_S: Amount (mg) of Maltose RS taken

Internal standard solution—A solution of ethylene glycol (1 in 50).

Operating conditions—

Detector: A differential refractometer.

Column: A stainless steel column about 8 mm in inside diameter and about 55 cm in length, packed with gel-type strong acid cation-exchange resin for liquid chromatography (degree of cross-linking: 8 %) (10 μm in particle diameter).

Column temperature: A constant temperature of about 50°C.

Mobile phase: Water.

Flow rate: Adjust so that the retention time of maltose is about 18 minutes.

Selection of column: Dissolve 0.25 g of maltose, 0.25 g of glucose and 0.4 g of ethylene glycol in water to make 100 mL. Proceed with 20 μL of this solution under the above operating conditions, and calculate the resolution. Use a column giving elution of maltose, glucose and ethylene glycol in this order with the resolution of between the peaks of maltose and glucose being not less than 4.

Containers and storage Containers—Tight containers.

Freeze-dried Mamushi Antivenom, Equine

乾燥まむしウマ抗毒素

Freeze-dried Mamushi Antivenom, Equine, is a preparation for injection which is dissolved before use.

It contains *Agkistrodon Halys* antivenom in immunoglobulin of horse origin.

It conforms to the requirements of Freeze-dried Mamushi Antivenom, Equine, in the Minimum Requirements for Biological Products.

Description Freeze-dried Mamushi Antivenom, Equine, becomes a colorless or light yellow-brown, clear liquid, or a slightly white-turbid liquid on addition of solvent.

Manidipine Hydrochloride

マニジピン塩酸塩

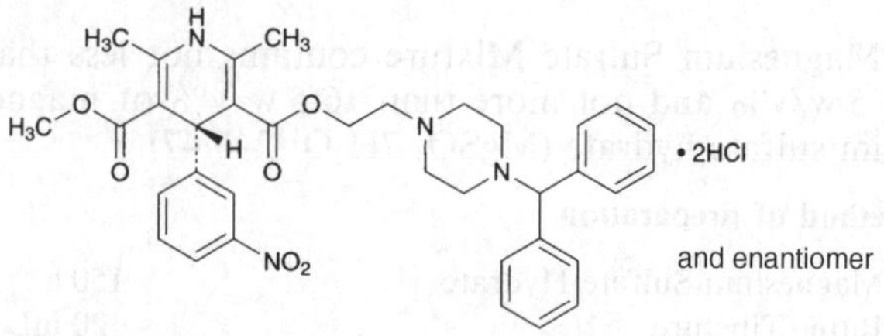

• 2HCl and enantiomer

$C_{35}H_{38}N_4O_6.2HCl$: 683.62
3-{2-[4-(Diphenylmethyl)piperazin-1-yl]ethyl}
5-methyl (4*RS*)-2,6-dimethyl-4-(3-nitrophenyl)-
1,4-dihydropyridine-3,5-dicarboxylate dihydrochloride
[*126229-12-7*]

Manidipine Hydrochloride, when dried, contains not less than 98.5% and not more than 101.0% of manidipine hydrochloride ($C_{35}H_{38}N_4O_6.2HCl$).

Description Manidipine Hydrochloride occurs as white to pale yellow, crystals or crystalline powder.

It is freely soluble in dimethylsulfoxide, sparingly soluble in methanol, slightly soluble in ethanol (99.5), and practically insoluble in water.

A solution of Manidipine Hydrochloride in dimethylsulfoxide (1 in 100) shows no optical rotation.

Manidipine Hydrochloride turns slightly brown-yellowish white on exposure to light.

Melting point: about 207°C (with decomposition).

Identification **(1)** Determine the absorption spectrum of a solution of Manidipine Hydrochloride in methanol (1 in 100,000) as directed under Ultraviolet-visible Spectrophotometry ⟨*2.24*⟩, and compare the spectrum with the Reference Spectrum or the spectrum of a solution of Manidipine Hydrochloride RS prepared in the same manner as the sample solution: both spectra exhibit similar intensities of absorption at the same wavelengths.

(2) Determine the infrared absorption spectrum of Manidipine Hydrochloride as directed in the potassium chloride disc method under Infrared Spectrophotometry ⟨*2.25*⟩, and compare the spectrum with the Reference Spectrum or the spectrum of Manidipine Hydrochloride RS: both spectra exhibit similar intensities of absorption at the same wave numbers.

(3) Add 10 mL of water to 0.1 g of Manidipine Hydrochloride, shake vigorously, and filter. Add 1 drop of ammonia TS to 3 mL of the filtrate, allow to stand 5 minutes, and filter. The filtrate responds to Qualitative Tests ⟨*1.09*⟩ (2) for chlorides.

Purity **(1)** Heavy metals ⟨*1.07*⟩— Proceed with 1.0 g of Manidipine Hydrochloride according to Method 2, and perform the test. Prepare the control solution with 1.0 mL of Standard Lead Solution (not more than 10 ppm).

(2) Arsenic ⟨*1.11*⟩—Prepare the test solution with 2.0 g of Manidipine Hydrochloride according to Method 4, and perform the test (not more than 1 ppm).

(3) Related substances—Dissolve 20 mg of Manidipine Hydrochloride in a mixture of water and acetonitrile (1:1) to make 200 mL, and use this solution as the sample solution. Pipet 1 mL of the sample solution, add the mixture of water and acetonitrile (1:1) to make exactly 100 mL, and use this solution as the standard solution. Perform the test with exactly 20 μL each of the sample solution and standard solution as directed under Liquid Chromatography <2.01> according to the following conditions. Determine each peak area from both solutions by the automatic integration method: the area of the peaks other than manidipine obtained from the sample solution is not larger than 1/5 times the manidipine peak area from the standard solution. Furthermore, the total of the areas of all peaks other than manidipine from the sample solution is not larger than 7/10 times the peak area of manidipine from the standard solution.

Operating conditions—

Detector, column, column temperature, mobile phase, and flow rate: Proceed as directed in the operating conditions in the Assay.

Time span of measurement: About 3.5 times as long as the retention time of manidipine, beginning after the solvent peak.

System suitability—

Test for required detectability: Pipet 10 mL of the standard solution, add a mixture of water and acetonitrile (1:1) to make exactly 100 mL. Confirm that the peak area of manidipine obtained with 20 μL of this solution is equivalent to 8 to 12% of that with 20 μL of the standard solution.

System performance: Dissolve 50 mg of Manidipine Hydrochloride in a mixture of water and acetonitrile (1:1) to make 50 mL. To 10 mL of this solution add 5 mL of a solution of butyl benzoate in acetonitrile (7 in 5000) and the mixture of water and acetonitrile (1:1) to make 100 mL. When the procedure is run with 20 μL of this solution under the above operating conditions, manidipine and butyl benzoate are eluted in this order with the resolution between these peaks being not less than 5.

System repeatability: When the test is repeated 6 times with 20 μL of the standard solution under the above operating conditions, the relative standard deviation of the peak area of manidipine is not more than 2.0%.

Loss on drying <2.41> Not more than 1.5% (1 g, 105°C, 4 hours).

Residue on ignition <2.44> Not more than 0.2% (1 g).

Assay Weigh accurately about 0.1 g of Manidipine Hydrochloride, previously dried, and dissolve in a mixture of water and acetonitrile (1:1) to make exactly 50 mL. Pipet 5 mL of this solution, add exactly 5 mL of the internal standard solution, add the mixture of water and acetonitrile (1:1) to make 100 mL, and use this solution as the sample solution. Separately, weigh accurately about 25 mg of Manidipine Hydrochloride RS, previously dried, and dissolve in the mixture of water and acetonitrile (1:1) to make exactly 50 mL. Pipet 20 mL of this solution, add exactly 5 mL of the internal standard solution, add the mixture of water and acetonitrile (1:1) to make 100 mL, and use this solution as the standard solution. Perform the test with 20 μL each of the sample solution and standard solution as directed under Liquid Chromatography <2.01> according to the following conditions, and calculate the ratios, Q_T and Q_S, of the peak area of manidipine to that of the internal standard.

Amount (mg) of manidipine hydrochloride ($C_{35}H_{38}N_4O_6.2HCl$)
$= M_S \times Q_T/Q_S \times 4$

M_S: Amount (mg) of Manidipine Hydrochloride RS taken

*Internal standard solution—*A solution of butyl benzoate in acetonitrile (7 in 5000).

Operating conditions—

Detector: An ultraviolet absorption photometer (wavelength: 228 nm).

Column: A stainless steel column 4.0 mm in inside diameter and 15 cm in length, packed with octadecylsilanized silica gel for liquid chromatography (5 μm in particle diameter).

Column temperature: A constant temperature of about 25°C.

Mobile phase: Dissolve 13.6 g of potassium dihydrogen phosphate in water to make 1000 mL, and adjust to pH 4.6 with diluted potassium hydroxide TS (1 in 10). To 490 mL of this solution add 510 mL of acetonitrile.

Flow rate: Adjust so that the retention time of manidipine is about 10 minutes.

System suitability—

System performance: When the procedure is run with 20 μL of the standard solution under the above operating conditions, manidipine and the internal standard are eluted in this order with the resolution between these peaks being not less than 5.

System repeatability: When the test is repeated 6 times with 20 μL of the standard solution under the above operating conditions, the relative standard deviation of the ratio of the peak area of manidipine to that of the internal standard is not more than 1.0%.

Containers and storage Containers—Tight containers.
Storage—Light-resistant.

Manidipine Hydrochloride Tablets

マニジピン塩酸塩錠

Manidipine Hydrochloride Tablets contain not less than 92.0% and not more than 108.0% of the labeled amount of manidipine hydrochloride ($C_{35}H_{38}N_4O_6.2HCl$: 683.62).

Method of preparation Prepare as directed under Tablets, with Manidipine Hydrochloride.

Identification To a quantity of powdered Manidipine Hydrochloride Tablets, equivalent to 10 mg of Manidipine Hydrochloride, add 5 mL of methanol, shake vigorously, centrifuge, and use the supernatant liquid as the sample solution. Separately, dissolve 10 mg of Manidipine Hydrochloride RS in 5 mL of methanol, and use this solution as the standard solution. Perform the test with these solutions as directed under Thin-layer Chromatography <2.03>. Spot 5 μL each of the sample solution and standard solution on a plate of silica gel with fluorescent indicator for thin-layer chromatography. Develop the plate with a mixture of ethyl acetate and diethylamine (200:1) to a distance of about 10 cm, and air-dry the plate. Examine under ultraviolet light (main wavelength: 254 nm): the principal spot obtained from the sample solution and the spot from the standard solution show the same *Rf* value.

Uniformity of dosage units <6.02> Perform the test according to the following method: it meets the requirement of the Content uniformity test.

Conduct this procedure using light-resistant vessels. To 1 tablet of Manidipine Hydrochloride Tablets, add exactly 1 mL of the internal standard solution per 1 mg of manidipine hydrochloride ($C_{35}H_{38}N_4O_6.2HCl$), disintegrate by adding a mixture of water and acetonitrile (1:1) to make *V* mL so that each mL contains about 0.1 mg of manidipine hydrochloride

($C_{35}H_{38}N_4O_6.2HCl$), shake vigorously for 10 minutes, and filter through a membrane filter with a pore size not exceeding 0.45 μm. Discard the first 1 mL of the filtrate, and use the subsequent filtrate as the sample solution. Then, proceed as directed in the Assay.

Amount (mg) of manidipine hydrochloride ($C_{35}H_{38}N_4O_6.2HCl$)
$= M_S \times Q_T/Q_S \times V/250$

M_S: Amount (mg) of Manidipine Hydrochloride RS taken

Internal standard solution—A solution of butyl benzoate in acetonitrile (7 in 10,000).

Dissolution *<6.10>* When the test is performed at 50 revolutions per minute according to the Paddle method, using 900 mL of 0.05 mol/L acetic acid-sodium acetate buffer solution (pH 4.0) as the dissolution medium, the dissolution rate in 45 minutes of Manidipine Hydrochloride Tablets is not less than 75%.

Conduct this procedure using light-resistant vessels. Start the test with 1 tablet of Manidipine Hydrochloride Tablets, withdraw not less than 20 mL of the medium at the specified minute after starting the test, and filter through a membrane filter with a pore size not exceeding 0.45 μm. Discard not less than 10 mL of the first filtrate, pipet V mL of the subsequent filtrate, and add the dissolution medium to make exactly V' mL so that each mL contains about 5.6 μg of manidipine hydrochloride ($C_{35}H_{38}N_4O_6.2HCl$). Pipet 2 mL of this solution, add exactly 2 mL of methanol, and use this solution as the sample solution. Separately, weigh accurately about 25 mg of Manidipine Hydrochloride RS, previously dried, dissolve in a mixture of water and acetonitrile (1:1) to make exactly 50 mL. Pipet 1 mL of this solution, and add the dissolution medium to make exactly 100 mL. Pipet 2 mL of this solution, add exactly 2 mL of methanol, and use this solution as the standard solution. Perform the test with exactly 20 μL each of the sample solution and standard solution as directed under Liquid Chromatography *<2.01>* according to the following conditions, and determine the peak areas, A_T and A_S, of manidipine in each solution.

Dissolution rate (%) with respect to the labeled amount of manidipine hydrochloride ($C_{35}H_{38}N_4O_6.2HCl$)
$= M_S \times A_T/A_S \times V'/V \times 1/C \times 18$

M_S: Amount (mg) of Manidipine Hydrochloride RS taken
C: Labeled amount (mg) of manidipine hydrochloride ($C_{35}H_{38}N_4O_6.2HCl$) in 1 tablet

Operating conditions—

Detector: An ultraviolet absorption photometer (wavelength: 228 nm).

Column: A stainless steel column 4.0 mm in inside diameter and 15 cm in length, packed with octadecylsilanized silica gel for liquid chromatography (5 μm in particle diameter).

Column temperature: A constant temperature of about 25°C.

Mobile phase: A mixture of acetonitrile and a solution of potassium dihydrogen phosphate (681 in 100,000) (3:2).

Flow rate: Adjust so that the retention time of manidipine is about 6 minutes.

System suitability—

System performance: When the procedure is run with 20 μL of the standard solution under the above operating conditions, the number of theoretical plates and the symmetry factor of the peak of manidipine are not less than 1500 and not more than 1.5, respectively.

System repeatability: When the test is repeated 6 times with 20 μL of the standard solution under the above operating conditions, the relative standard deviation of the peak area of manidipine is not more than 2.0%.

Assay Conduct this procedure using light-resistant vessels. Weigh accurately not less than 20 Manidipine Hydrochloride Tablets, and powder. Weigh accurately a portion of the powder, equivalent to about 10 mg of manidipine hydrochloride ($C_{35}H_{38}N_4O_6.2HCl$), add exactly 10 mL of the internal standard solution, add a mixture of water and acetonitrile (1:1) to make 100 mL, shake vigorously for 10 minutes, and filter through a membrane filter with a pore size not exceeding 0.45 μm. Discard the first 1 mL of the filtrate, and use the subsequent filtrate as the sample solution. Separately, weigh accurately about 25 mg of Manidipine Hydrochloride RS, previously dried, and dissolve in the mixture of water and acetonitrile (1:1) to make exactly 50 mL. Pipet 20 mL of this solution, add exactly 10 mL of the internal standard solution, add the mixture of water and acetonitrile (1:1) to make 100 mL, and use this solution as the standard solution. Then, proceed as directed in the Assay under Manidipine Hydrochloride.

Amount (mg) of manidipine hydrochloride ($C_{35}H_{38}N_4O_6.2HCl$)
$= M_S \times Q_T/Q_S \times 2/5$

M_S: Amount (mg) of Manidipine Hydrochloride RS taken

Internal standard solution—A solution of butyl benzoate in acetonitrile (7 in 10,000).

Containers and storage Containers—Tight containers.
Storage—Light-resistant.

D-Mannitol

D-マンニトール

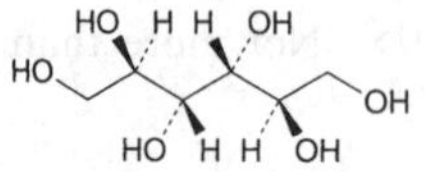

$C_6H_{14}O_6$: 182.17
D-Mannitol
[69-65-8]

This monograph is harmonized with the European Pharmacopoeia and the U.S. Pharmacopeia.

The parts of the text that are not harmonized are marked with symbols (◆ ◆).

Information on the harmonization with the European Pharmacopoeia and the U.S. Pharmacopeia is available on the website of the Pharmaceuticals and Medical Devices Agency.

D-Mannitol contains not less than 97.0% and not more than 102.0% of D-mannitol ($C_6H_{14}O_6$), calculated on the dried basis.

◆**Description** D-Mannitol occurs as white, crystals, powder or grain. It has a sweet taste with a cold sensation.

It is freely soluble in water, and practically insoluble in ethanol (99.5).

It dissolves in sodium hydroxide TS.

It shows crystal polymorphism.◆

Identification Determine the infrared absorption spectrum of D-Mannitol as directed in the potassium bromide disk method under Infrared Spectrophotometry <2.25>, and compare the spectrum with the Reference Spectrum or the spectrum of D-Mannitol RS: both spectra exhibit similar intensities of absorption at the same wave numbers. If any difference appears between the spectra, put 25 mg each of D-Mannitol and D-Mannitol RS in glass vessels, dissolve in 0.25 mL of water without heating, dry them in a 600 - 700 W microwave oven for 20 minutes or in a drying chamber at 100°C for 1 hour, then further dry by gradual reducing pressure, and perform the same test as above with so obtained non-sticky white to pale yellow powders: both spectra exhibit similar intensities of absorption at the same wave numbers.

Melting point <2.60> 165 - 170°C

Purity (1) Clarity and color of solution—Dissolve 5.0 g of D-Mannitol in water to make 50 mL, and use this solution as the test solution. Perform the test with the test solution as directed under Turbidity Measurement <2.61>: the solution is clear. Perform the test with the test solution according to Method 2 under Methods for Color Matching <2.65>: the solution is colorless.

◆(2) Heavy metals <1.07>—Proceed with 5.0 g of D-Mannitol according to Method 1, and perform the test. Prepare the control solution with 2.5 mL of Standard Lead Solution (not more than 5 ppm)◆.

(3) Nickel—Shake 10.0 g of D-Mannitol with 30 mL of 2 mol/L acetic acid TS, and add water to make exactly 100 mL. Add 2.0 mL of a saturated solution of ammonium pyrrolidinedithiocarbamate (about 10 g/L) and 10.0 mL of water-saturated 4-methyl-2-pentanone, and shake for 30 seconds without exposure to light. Allow the layers to separate, and use the 4-methyl-2-pentanone layer as the sample solution. Separately, put 10.0 g each of D-Mannitol in three vessels, add 30 mL of 2 mol/L acetic acid TS to them, shake, add a suitable amount of water and exactly 0.5 mL, 1.0 mL and 1.5 mL respectively of Standard Nickel Solution for Atomic Absorption Spectrophotometry, and add water to make them exactly 100 mL. Then, proceed in the same manner as the sample solution, and use so obtained three 4-methyl-2-pentanone layers as the standard solutions. Additionally, prepare a 4-methyl-2-pentanone layer by proceeding in the same manner as the sample solution without using D-Mannitol, and use this layer as the blank solution. Perform the test with the sample solution and standard solutions as directed in the standard addition method under Atomic Absorption Spectrophotometry <2.23> according to the following conditions. Set the zero of the instrument using the blank solution, and between each measurement, rinse with water and ascertain that the readings return to zero with the blank solution: amount of nickel is not more than 1 ppm.

Gas: Combustible gas—Acetylene.
Supporting gas—Air.
Lamp: Nickel hollow-cathode lamp.
Wavelength: 232.0 nm.

(4) Related substances—Dissolve 0.50 g of D-Mannitol in water to make 10 mL, and use this solution as the sample solution. Pipet 2 mL of the sample solution, add water to make exactly 100 mL, and use this solution as the standard solution (1). Pipet 0.5 mL of the standard solution (1), add water to make exactly 20 mL, and use this solution as the standard solution (2). Perform the test with exactly 20 μL each of the sample solution and standard solutions (1) and (2) as directed under Liquid Chromatography <2.01> according to the following conditions. Determine each peak area by the automatic integration method: the peak area of D-sorbitol, having the relative retention time of about 1.2 to D-mannitol, obtained from the sample solution is not larger than that of D-mannitol from the standard solution (1) (not more than 2.0%), the total peak area of maltitol, having the relative retention time of about 0.69, and isomalt, having the relative retention times of about 0.6 and about 0.73, is not larger than the peak area of D-mannitol from the standard solution (1) (not more than 2.0%), and the area of the peak other than D-mannitol and the peaks mentioned above is not larger than 2 times the peak area of D-mannitol from the standard solution (2) (not more than 0.1%). Furthermore, the total area of the peak other than D-mannitol from the sample solution is not larger than the peak area of D-mannitol from the standard solution (1) (not more than 2.0%). For these calculations exclude the peak which area is not larger than the peak area of D-mannitol from the standard solution (2) (not more than 0.05%).

Operating conditions—

Detector, column, column temperature, mobile phase, and flow rate: Proceed as directed in the operating conditions in the Assay.

Time span of measurement: About 1.5 times as long as the retention time of D-mannitol.

System suitability—

System performance: Proceed as directed in the system suitability in the Assay.

◆Test for required detectability: Confirm that the peak area of D-mannitol obtained with 20 μL of the standard solution (2) is equivalent to 1.75 to 3.25% of that with 20 μL of the standard solution (1).

System repeatability: When the test is repeated 6 times with 20 μL of the standard solution (1) under the above operating conditions, the relative standard deviation of the peak area of D-mannitol is not more than 1.0%.◆

(5) Glucose—To 7.0 g of D-Mannitol add 13 mL of water and 40 mL of Fehling's TS, boil gently for 3 minutes, and allow to stand for 2 minutes to precipitate copper (I) oxide. Separate the supernatant liquid, filter through a sintered glass filter for cupric oxide filtration coated with siliceous earth or a sintered glass filter (G4). Wash the precipitates with 50 - 60°C hot water until the washing no longer alkaline, and filter the washings through the filter described above. Discard all the filtrate at this step. Immediately, dissolve the precipitate with 20 mL of iron (III) sulfate TS, filter through the filter described above in a clean flask, and wash the filter with 15 - 20 mL of water. Combine the filtrate and the washings, heat to 80°C, and titrate <2.50> with 0.02 mol/L potassium permanganate VS until the green color turns to light red and the color persists at least 10 seconds: not more than 3.2 mL is required to change the color of the solution (not more than 0.1% expressed as glucose).

Conductivity <2.51> Dissolve 20.0 g of D-Mannitol in a fleshly boiled and cooled water prepared from distilled water by heating to 40 - 50°C, add the same water to make 100 mL, and use this solution as the sample solution. After cooling, measure the conductivity of the sample solution at 25 ± 0.1°C while gently stirring with a magnetic stirrer: not more than 20 $\mu S \cdot cm^{-1}$.

Loss on drying <2.41> Not more than 0.5% (1 g, 105°C, 4 hours).

Assay Weigh accurately about 0.5 g each of D-Mannitol and D-Mannitol RS (separately determine the loss on drying <2.41> under the same conditions as D-Mannitol), dissolve separately in water to make exactly 10 mL, and use these solutions as the sample solution and the standard solution, respectively. Perform the test with exactly 20 μL each of the sample solution and standard solution as directed under

Liquid Chromatography <2.01> according to the following conditions, and determine the peak areas, A_T and A_S, of D-mannitol in each solution.

Amount (g) of D-mannitol ($C_6H_{14}O_6$) = $M_S \times A_T/A_S$

M_S: Amount (g) of D-Mannitol RS taken, calculated on the dried basis

Operating conditions—

Detector: A differential refractometer maintained at a constant temperature (40°C for example).

Column: A stainless steel column 7.8 mm in inside diameter and 30 cm in length, packed with strongly acidic ion-exchange resin for liquid chromatography (calcium type) composed with a sulfonated polystyrene cross-linked with 8% of divinylbenzene (9 μm in particle diameter).

Column temperature: 85 ± 2°C.

Mobile phase: water.

Flow rate: 0.5 mL per minute (the retention time of D-mannitol is about 20 minutes).

System suitability—

System performance: Dissolve 0.25 g each of D-Mannitol and D-sorbitol in water to make 10 mL, and use this solution as the solution for system suitability test (1). Separately, dissolve 0.5 g each of maltitol and isomalt in water to make 100 mL. To 2 mL of this solution add water to make 10 mL, and use this solution as the solution for system suitability test (2). When proceed with 20 μL each of the solution for system suitability test (1) and the solution for system suitability test (2) as directed under the above operating conditions, isomalt (first peak), maltitol, isomalt (second peak), D-mannitol and D-sorbitol are eluted in this order, the relative retention time of isomalt (first peak), maltitol, isomalt (second peak) and D-sorbitol to D-mannitol is about 0.6, about 0.69, about 0.73 and about 1.2, respectively, and the resolution between the peaks of D-mannitol and D-sorbitol is not less than 2.0. Coelution of maltitol and the second peak of isomalt may be observed.

◆System repeatability: When the test is repeated 6 times with 20 μL of the standard solution under the above operating conditions, the relative standard deviation of the peak area of D-mannitol is not more than 1.0%.◆

◆**Containers and storage** Containers—Well-closed containers.◆

D-Mannitol Injection

D-マンニトール注射液

D-Mannitol Injection is an aqueous injection.

It contains not less than 95.0% and not more than 105.0% of the labeled amount of D-mannitol ($C_6H_{14}O_6$: 182.17).

Method of preparation Prepare as directed under Injections, with D-Mannitol. No preservative is added.

Description D-Mannitol Injection is a clear, colorless liquid. It has a sweet taste.

It may precipitate crystals.

Identification Concentrate D-Mannitol Injection on a water bath to make a saturated solution. To 5 drops of this solution add 1 mL of iron (III) chloride TS and 5 drops of a solution of sodium hydroxide (1 in 5): a yellow precipitate is produced. Shake this solution vigorously: a clear solution is produced. On addition of a solution of sodium hydroxide (1 in 5), no precipitate is produced.

pH <2.54> 4.5 – 7.0

Bacterial endotoxins <4.01> Less than 0.50 EU/mL.

Extractable volume <6.05> It meets the requirement.

Foreign insoluble matter <6.06> Perform the test according to Method 1: it meets the requirement.

Insoluble particulate matter <6.07> It meets the requirement.

Sterility <4.06> Perform the test according to the Membrane filtration method: it meets the requirement.

Assay Measure exactly a volume of D-Mannitol Injection, equivalent to about 5 g of D-mannitol ($C_6H_{14}O_6$), and add water to make exactly 250 mL. To exactly 10 mL of this solution add water to make exactly 100 mL. Measure exactly 10 mL of this solution into an iodine flask, add exactly 50 mL of potassium periodate TS, and heat for 15 minutes in a water bath. After cooling, add 2.5 g of potassium iodide, stopper tightly, and shake well. Allow to stand for 5 minutes in a dark place, and titrate <2.50> with 0.1 mol/L sodium thiosulfate VS (indicator: 1 mL of starch TS). Perform a blank determination in the same manner.

Each mL of 0.1 mol/L sodium thiosulfate VS
= 1.822 mg of $C_6H_{14}O_6$

Containers and storage Containers—Hermetic containers. Plastic containers for aqueous injections may be used.

Maprotiline Hydrochloride

マプロチリン塩酸塩

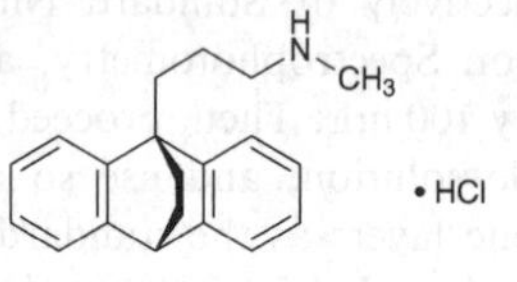

$C_{20}H_{23}N.HCl$: 313.86
3-(9,10-Dihydro-9,10-ethanoanthracen-9-yl)-*N*-methylpropylamine monohydrochloride
[*10347-81-6*]

Maprotiline Hydrochloride, when dried, contains not less than 99.0% of maprotiline hydrochloride ($C_{20}H_{23}N.HCl$).

Description Maprotiline Hydrochloride occurs as a white crystalline powder.

It is soluble in methanol and in acetic acid (100), sparingly soluble in ethanol (99.5), and slightly soluble in water.

Melting point: about 244°C (with decomposition).

It shows crystal polymorphism.

Identification **(1)** Determine the absorption spectrum of a solution of Maprotiline Hydrochloride in methanol (1 in 10,000) as directed under Ultraviolet-visible Spectrophotometry <2.24>, and compare the spectrum with the Reference Spectrum: both spectra exhibit similar intensities of absorption at the same wavelengths.

(2) Determine the infrared absorption spectrum of Maprotiline Hydrochloride, previously dried, as directed in the potassium chloride disk method under Infrared Spectrophotometry <2.25>, and compare the spectrum with the Reference Spectrum: both spectra exhibit similar intensities of absorption at the same wave numbers. If any difference appears between the spectra, recrystallize Maprotiline Hydrochloride with ethanol (99.5), filter, dry the crystals so obtained, and perform the test with the crystals.

(3) To 5 mL of a solution of Maprotiline Hydrochloride (1 in 200) add 2 mL of ammonia TS, heat on a water bath for 5 minutes, cool, and filter. Acidify the filtrate with dilute nitric acid: the solution responds to Qualitative Tests <*1.09*> for chloride.

Purity **(1)** Heavy metals <*1.07*>—Proceed with 2.0 g of Maprotiline Hydrochloride according to Method 2, and perform the test. Prepare the control solution with 2.0 mL of Standard Lead Solution (not more than 10 ppm).

(2) Related substances—Dissolve 0.10 g of Maprotiline Hydrochloride in 5 mL of methanol, and use this solution as the sample solution. Pipet 1 mL of the sample solution, add methanol to make exactly 200 mL, and use this solution as the standard solution. Perform the test with these solutions as directed under Thin-layer Chromatography <*2.03*>. Spot 10 μL each of the sample solution and standard solution on a plate of silica gel with fluorescent indicator for thin-layer chromatography. Develop with a mixture of 2-butanol, diluted ammonia solution (28) (1 in 3) and ethyl acetate (14:5:4) to a distance of about 10 cm, and air-dry the plate. Examine under ultraviolet light (main wavelength: 254 nm): the number of the spot other than the principal spot obtained from the sample solution is not more than 2 and they are not more intense than the spot from the standard solution.

Loss on drying <*2.41*> Not more than 0.5% (1 g, 105°C, 3 hours).

Residue on ignition <*2.44*> Not more than 0.1% (1 g).

Assay Weigh accurately about 0.25 g of Maprotiline Hydrochloride, previously dried, dissolve in 80 mL of acetic acid (100), add 8 mL of a solution of bismuth nitrate pentahydrate in acetic acid (100) (1 in 50), and titrate <*2.50*> with 0.1 mol/L perchloric acid VS (potentiometric titration). Perform a blank determination in the same manner, and make any necessary correction.

Each mL of 0.1 mol/L perchloric acid VS
= 31.39 mg of $C_{20}H_{23}N.HCl$

Containers and storage Containers—Well-closed containers.

Freeze-dried Live Attenuated Measles Vaccine

乾燥弱毒生麻しんワクチン

Freeze-dried Live Attenuated Measles Vaccine is a preparation for injection which is dissolved before use.

It contains live attenuated measles virus.

It conforms to the requirements of Freeze-dried Live Attenuated Measles Vaccine in the Minimum Requirements for Biological Products.

Description Freeze-dried Live Attenuated Measles Vaccine becomes a colorless, yellowish or reddish clear liquid on addition of solvent.

Meclofenoxate Hydrochloride

メクロフェノキサート塩酸塩

$C_{12}H_{16}ClNO_3.HCl$: 294.17
2-(Dimethylamino)ethyl (4-chlorophenoxy)acetate monohydrochloride
[3685-84-5]

Meclofenoxate Hydrochloride contains not less than 98.0% of meclofenoxate hydrochloride ($C_{12}H_{16}ClNO_3.HCl$), calculated on the anhydrous basis.

Description Meclofenoxate Hydrochloride occurs as white, crystals or crystalline powder. It has a faint, characteristic odor and a bitter taste.

It is freely soluble in water and in ethanol (95), sparingly soluble in acetic anhydride, and practically insoluble in diethyl ether.

The pH of a solution of 1.0 g of Meclofenoxate Hydrochloride in 20 mL of water is between 3.5 and 4.5.

Identification **(1)** To 10 mg of Meclofenoxate Hydrochloride add 2 mL of ethanol (95), dissolve by warming if necessary, cool, add 2 drops of a saturated solution of hydroxylammonium chloride in ethanol (95) and 2 drops of a saturated solution of potassium hydroxide in ethanol (95), and heat in a water bath for 2 minutes. After cooling, render the solution slightly acidic with dilute hydrochloric acid, and add 3 drops of iron (III) chloride TS: a red-purple to dark purple color develops.

(2) Dissolve 50 mg of Meclofenoxate Hydrochloride in 5 mL of water, and add 2 drops of Reinecke salt TS: a light red precipitate is formed.

(3) Determine the absorption spectrum of a solution of Meclofenoxate Hydrochloride (1 in 10,000) as directed under Ultraviolet-visible Spectrophotometry <*2.24*>, and compare the spectrum with the Reference Spectrum: both spectra exhibit similar intensities of absorption at the same wavelengths.

(4) A solution of Meclofenoxate Hydrochloride (1 in 100) responds to Qualitative Tests <*1.09*> for chloride.

Melting point <*2.60*> 139 – 143°C

Purity **(1)** Clarity and color of solution—Dissolve 0.5 g of Meclofenoxate Hydrochloride in 10 mL of water: the solution is clear and colorless.

(2) Sulfate <*1.14*>—Perform the test with 1.0 g of Meclofenoxate Hydrochloride. Prepare the control solution with 1.0 mL of 0.005 mol/L sulfuric acid VS (not more than 0.048%).

(3) Heavy metals <*1.07*>—Proceed with 1.0 g of Meclofenoxate Hydrochloride according to Method 1, and perform the test. Prepare the control solution with 2.0 mL of Standard Lead Solution (not more than 20 ppm).

(4) Arsenic <*1.11*>—Prepare the test solution with 1.0 g of Meclofenoxate Hydrochloride according to method 3, and perform the test (not more than 2 ppm).

(5) Organic acids—To 2.0 g of Meclofenoxate Hydrochloride add 50 mL of diethyl ether, shake for 10 minutes, filter through a glass filter (G3), wash the residue with two 5-mL portions of diethyl ether, and combine the washings with the filtrate. To this solution add 50 mL of neutralized ethanol and 5 drops of phenolphthalein TS, and neutralize with 0.1 mol/L sodium hydroxide VS: the volume of 0.1 mol/L sodium hydroxide VS consumed is not more than 0.54 mL.

Water *⟨2.48⟩* Not more than 0.50% (1 g, volumetric titration, dirct titration).

Residue on ignition *⟨2.44⟩* Not more than 0.1% (1 g).

Assay Weigh accurately about 0.4 g of Meclofenoxate Hydrochloride, dissolve in 70 mL of acetic anhydride, and titrate *⟨2.50⟩* with 0.1 mol/L perchloric acid VS until the color of the solution changes from blue-green through yellow-green to pale greenish yellow [indicator: 3 drops of a solution of malachite green oxalate in acetic acid (100) (1 in 100)]. Perform a blank determination in the same manner, and make any necessary correction.

Each mL of 0.1 mol/L perchloric acid VS
= 29.42 mg of $C_{12}H_{16}ClNO_3.HCl$

Containers and storage Containers—Tight containers.

Mecobalamin

メコバラミン

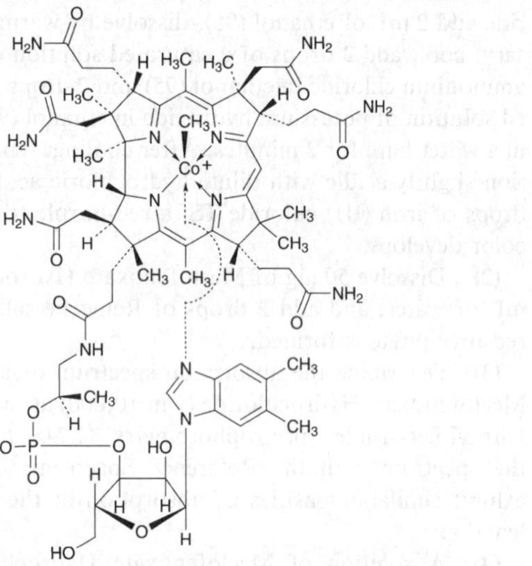

$C_{63}H_{91}CoN_{13}O_{14}P$: 1344.38
Coα-[α-(5,6-Dimethyl-1*H*-benzimidazol-1-yl)]-*Coβ*-methylcobamide
[13422-55-4]

Mecobalamin contains not less than 98.0% and not more than 101.0% of mecobalamin ($C_{63}H_{91}CoN_{13}O_{14}P$), calculated on the anhydrous basis.

Description Mecobalamin occurs as dark red, crystals or crystalline powder.

It is sparingly soluble in water, slightly soluble in ethanol (99.5), and practically insoluble in acetonitrile.

It decomposes on exposure to light.

Identification **(1)** Conduct this procedure without exposure to light, using light-resistant vessels. Determine the absorption spectrum of a solution of Mecobalamin in hydrochloric acid-potassium chloride buffer solution (pH 2.0) (1 in 20,000) as directed under Ultraviolet-visible Spectrophotometry *⟨2.24⟩*, and compare the spectrum with the Reference Spectrum 1 or the spectrum of a solution of Mecobalamin RS prepared in the same manner as the sample solution: both spectra exhibit similar intensities of absorption at the same wavelengths. Separately, determine the absorption spectrum of a solution of Mecobalamin in phosphate buffer solution (pH 7.0) (1 in 20,000) as directed under Ultraviolet-visible Spectrophotometry *⟨2.24⟩*, and compare the spectrum with the Reference Spectrum 2 or the spectrum of a solution of Mecobalamin RS prepared in the same manner as the sample solution: both spectra exhibit similar intensities of absorption at the same wavelengths.

(2) Mix 1 mg of Mecobalamin with 50 mg of potassium bisulfate, and fuse by igniting. Cool, break up the mass with a glass rod, add 3 mL of water, and dissolve by boiling. Add 1 drop of phenolphthalein TS, then add dropwise sodium hydroxide TS until a light red color just develops. Add 0.5 g of sodium acetate, 0.5 mL of dilute acetic acid and 0.5 mL of a solution of disodium 1-nitroso-2-naphthol-3,6-disulfonate (1 in 500): a red to orange-red color is immediately produced. Then add 0.5 mL of hydrochloric acid, and boil for 1 minute: the red color does not disappear.

Purity **(1)** Clarity and color of solution—Dissolve 20 mg of Mecobalamin in 10 mL of water: the solution is clear and red color.

(2) Related substances—Perform the test with 10 μL of the sample solution obtained in the Assay as directed under Liquid Chromatography *⟨2.01⟩* according to the following conditions. Determine each peak area by the automatic integration method: each area of the peaks other than mecobalamin is not more than 0.5% of the peak area of mecobalamin, and the total area of the peaks other than mecobalamin is not more than 2.0%.

Operating conditions—

Detector, column, column temperature, mobile phase, and flow rate: Proceed as directed in the operating conditions in the Assay.

Time span of measurement: About 2.5 times as long as the retention time of mecobalamin.

System suitability—

System performance: Proceed as directed in the system suitability in the Assay.

Test for required detectability: To exactly 1 mL of the sample solution add the mobile phase to make exactly 100 mL, and use this solution as the solution for system suitability test. Pipet 1 mL of the solution for system suitability test, add the mobile phase to make exactly 10 mL. Confirm that the peak area of mecobalamin obtained with 10 μL of this solution is equivalent to 7 to 13% of that with 10 μL of the solution for system suitability test.

System repeatability: When the test is repeated 6 times with 10 μL of the solution for system suitability test under the above operating conditions, the relative standard deviation of the peak areas of mecobalamin is not more than 3.0%.

Water *⟨2.48⟩* Not more than 12% (0.1 g, volumetric titration, direct titration).

Assay Conduct this procedure without exposure to light, using light-resistant vessels. Weigh accurately about 50 mg of Mecobalamin and Mecobalamin RS (separately, determine the water *⟨2.48⟩* in the same manner as Mecobalamin), dissolve each in the mobile phase to make exactly 50 mL, and use these solutions as the sample solution and the standard solution, respectively. Perform the test with exactly 10 μL of each of the sample solution and standard solution as directed under Liquid Chromatography *⟨2.01⟩* according to the following conditions, and determine the peak areas, A_T and A_S, of mecobalamin in each solution.

Amount (mg) of mecobalamin ($C_{63}H_{91}CoN_{13}O_{14}P$)
$= M_S \times A_T/A_S$

M_S: Amount (mg) of Mecobalamin RS taken, calculated on the anhydrous basis

Operating conditions—

Detector: An ultraviolet absorption photometer (wavelength: 266 nm).

Column: A stainless steel column 4.6 mm in inside diameter and 25 cm in length, packed with octadecylsilanized silica gel for liquid chromatography (5 μm in particle diameter).

Column temperature: A constant temperature of about 40°C.

Mobile phase: To 200 mL of acetonitrile add 800 mL of 0.02 mol/L phosphate buffer solution (pH 3.5), then add 3.76 g of sodium 1-hexane sulfonate to dissolve.

Flow rate: Adjust so that the retention time of mecobalamin is about 12 minutes.

System suitability—

System performance: Dissolve 5 mg each of cyanocobalamin and hydroxocobalamin acetate in the mobile phase to make 100 mL. When the procedure is run with 10 μL of this solution under the above operating conditions, cyanocobalamin and hydroxocobalamin are eluted in this order with the resolution between these peaks being not less than 3. And when the procedure is run with 10 μL of the standard solution under the above operating conditions, the number of theoretical plates of the peak of mecobalamin is not less than 6000.

System repeatability: When the test is repeated 6 times with 10 μL of the standard solution under the above operating conditions, the relative standard deviation of the peak areas of mecobalamin is not more than 1.0%.

Containers and storage Containers—Tight containers.

Storage—Light-resistant.

Mecobalamin Tablets

メコバラミン錠

Mecobalamin Tablets contain not less than 92.0% and not more than 108.0% of the labeled amount of mecobalamin ($C_{63}H_{91}CoN_{13}O_{14}P$: 1344.38).

Method of preparation Prepare as directed under Tablets, with Mecobalamin.

Identification **(1)** Conduct this procedure without exposure to light, using light-resistant vessels. To a quantity of powdered Mecobalamin Tablets, equivalent to 1 mg of Mecobalamin, add 10 mL of hydrochloric acid-potassium chloride buffer solution (pH 2.0), sonicate, and add hydrochloric acid-potassium chloride buffer solution (pH 2.0) to make 20 mL. Centrifuge this solution, and filter the supernatant liquid through a membrane filter with a pore size not exceeding 0.8 μm. Determine the absorption spectrum of the filtrate as directed under Ultraviolet-visible Spectrophotometry *<2.24>*: it exhibits maxima between 262 nm and 266 nm, between 303 nm and 307 nm, and between 461 nm and 465 nm.

(2) Conduct this procedure without exposure to light, using light-resistant vessels. To a quantity of powdered Mecobalamin Tablets, equivalent to 1 mg of Mecobalamin, add 10 mL of phosphate buffer solution (pH 7.0), sonicate, and add phosphate buffer solution (pH 7.0) to make 20 mL. Centrifuge this solution, and filter the supernatant liquid through a membrane filter with a pore size not exceeding 0.8 μm. Determine the absorption spectrum of the filtrate as directed under Ultraviolet-visible Spectrophotometry *<2.24>*: it exhibits maxima between 264 nm and 268 nm, between 339 nm and 343 nm, and between 520 nm and 524 nm.

Uniformity of dosage units *<6.02>* Perform the test according to the following method: it meets the requirement of the Content uniformity test.

Conduct this procedure without exposure to light, using light-resistant vessels. Take 1 tablet of Mecobalamin Tablets, and disintegrate the tablet by adding $V/5$ mL of water. Add methanol to make exactly V mL so that each mL contains about 25 μg of mecobalamin ($C_{63}H_{91}CoN_{13}O_{14}P$). After shaking for 5 minutes, allow to stand for not less than 10 minutes. Filter thus obtained supernatant liquid through a membrane filter with a pore size not exceeding 0.45 μm. Discard the first 5 mL of the filtrate, and use the subsequent filtrate as the sample solution. Separately, weigh accurately about 25 mg of Mecobalamin RS (separately determine the water *<2.48>* in the same manner as Mecobalamin), and dissolve in water to make exactly 100 mL. Pipet 5 mL of this solution, add 5 mL of water and methanol to make exactly 50 mL. Use this solution as the standard solution. Perform the test with exactly 10 μL each of the sample solution and standard solution as directed under Liquid Chromatography *<2.01>* according to the following conditions, and determine the peak areas, A_T and A_S, of mecobalamin in each solution.

Amount (mg) of mecobalamin ($C_{63}H_{91}CoN_{13}O_{14}P$)
$= M_S \times A_T/A_S \times V/1000$

M_S: Amount (mg) of Mecobalamin RS taken, calculated on the anhydrous basis

Operating conditions—

Proceed as directed in the operating conditions in the Assay under Mecobalamin.

System suitability—

System performance: When the procedure is run with 10 μL of the standard solution under the above operating conditions, the number of theoretical plates and the symmetry factor of the peak of mecobalamin are not less than 2000 and 0.8 to 1.1, respectively.

System repeatability: When the test is repeated 6 times with 10 μL of the standard solution under the above operating conditions, the relative standard deviation of the peak area of mecobalamin is not more than 1.0%.

Dissolution *<6.10>* When the test is performed at 50 revolutions per minute according to the Paddle method, using 900 mL of water as the dissolution medium, the dissolution rate in 45 minutes of Mecobalamin Tablets is not less than 80%.

Conduct this procedure without exposure to light, using light-resistant vessels. Start the test with 1 tablet of Mecobalamin Tablets, withdraw not less than 20 mL of the medium at the specified minute after starting the test, and filter through a membrane filter with a pore size not exceeding 0.8 μm. Discard not less than 10 mL of the first filtrate, pipet V mL of the subsequent filtrate, and add water to make exactly V' mL so that each mL contains about 0.28 μg of mecobalamin ($C_{63}H_{91}CoN_{13}O_{14}P$). Use this solution as the sample solution. Separately, weigh accurately about 28 mg of Mecobalamin RS (separately determine the water *<2.48>* in the same manner as Mecobalamin), and dissolve in water to make exactly 100 mL. Pipet 5 mL of this solution, add water to make exactly 100 mL. Pipet 2 mL of this solution, add water to make exactly 100 mL, and use this solution as the standard solution. Perform the test with exactly 100 μL each of the sample solution and standard solution as directed under Liquid Chromatography <2.01> according to the following conditions, and determine the peak areas, A_T and A_S, of mecobalamin in each solution.

Dissolution rate (%) with respect to the labeled amount of mecobalamin ($C_{63}H_{91}CoN_{13}O_{14}P$)
$= M_S \times A_T/A_S \times V'/V \times 1/C \times 9/10$

M_S: Amount (mg) of Mecobalamin RS taken, calculated on the anhydrous basis
C: Labeled amount (mg) of mecobalamin ($C_{63}H_{91}CoN_{13}O_{14}P$) in 1 tablet

Operating conditions—

Detector: An ultraviolet absorption photometer (wavelength: 264 nm).

Column: A stainless steel column of 4.6 mm in inside diameter and 15 cm in length, packed with octadecylsilanized silica gel for liquid chromatography (5 μm in particle diameter).

Column temperature: A constant temperature of about 40°C.

Mobile phase: Adjust to pH 3.0 of a solution of 6.0 g of L-tartaric acid in 1000 mL of water with a solution of 14.3 g of disodium hydrogen phosphate dodecahydrate in 1000 mL of water. To 630 mL of this solution add 370 mL of methanol.

Flow rate: Adjust so that the retention time of mecobalamin is about 8 minutes.

System suitability—

System performance: When the procedure is run with 100 μL of the standard solution under the above operating conditions, the number of theoretical plates and the symmetry factor of the peak of mecobalamin are not less than 3000 and not more than 1.5, respectively.

System repeatability: When the test is repeated 6 times with 100 μL of the standard solution under the above operating conditions, the relative standard deviation of the peak area of mecobalamin is not more than 2.0%.

Assay Conduct this procedure without exposure to light, using light-resistant vessels. Disintegrate 20 tablets of Mecobalamin Tablets with V/5 mL of water. Add methanol to make exactly V mL so that each mL contains about 50 μg of mecobalamin ($C_{63}H_{91}CoN_{13}O_{14}P$). After shaking for 5 minutes, allow to stand for not less than 10 minutes. Filter thus obtained supernatant liquid through a membrane filter with a pore size not exceeding 0.45 μm. Discard the first 5 mL of the filtrate, and use the subsequent filtrate as the sample solution. Separately, weigh accurately about 25 mg of Mecobalamin RS (separately determine the water <2.48> in the same manner as Mecobalamin), and dissolve in water to make exactly 100 mL. To exactly 10 mL of this solution add methanol to make exactly 50 mL, and use this solution as the standard solution. Perform the test with exactly 10 μL each of the sample solution and standard solution as directed under Liquid Chromatography <2.01> according to the following conditions, and determine the peak areas, A_T and A_S, of mecobalamin in each solution.

Amount (mg) of mecobalamin ($C_{63}H_{91}CoN_{13}O_{14}P$) in 1 tablet
$= M_S \times A_T/A_S \times V/10000$

M_S: Amount (mg) of Mecobalamin RS taken, calculated on the anhydrous basis

Operating conditions—

Proceed as directed in the operating conditions in the Assay under Mecobalamin.

System suitability—

System performance: When the procedure is run with 10 μL of the standard solution under the above operating conditions, the number of theoretical plates and the symmetry factor of the peak of mecobalamin are not less than 3000 and 0.8 to 1.1, respectively.

System repeatability: When the test is repeated 6 times with 10 μL of the standard solution under the above operating conditions, the relative standard deviation of the peak area of mecobalamin is not more than 1.0%.

Containers and storage Containers—Tight containers.

Storage—Light-resistant.

Medazepam

メダゼパム

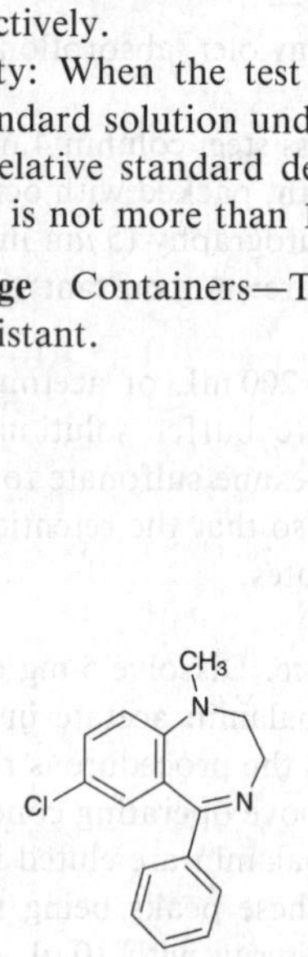

$C_{16}H_{15}ClN_2$: 270.76
7-Chloro-1-methyl-5-phenyl-2,3-dihydro-1*H*-1,4-benzodiazepine
[2898-12-6]

Medazepam, when dried, contains not less than 98.5% and not more than 101.0% of medazepam ($C_{16}H_{15}ClN_2$).

Description Medazepam occurs as white to light yellow, crystals or crystalline powder.

It is freely soluble in methanol, in ethanol (99.5), in acetic acid (100) and in diethyl ether, and practically insoluble in water.

It gradually turns yellow on exposure to light.

Identification **(1)** Dissolve 10 mg of Medazepam in 3 mL of citric acid-acetic acid TS: a deep orange color develops. Heat in a water bath for 3 minutes: the color changes to dark red.

(2) Determine the absorption spectrum of a solution of Medazepam in methanol (1 in 100,000) as directed under Ultraviolet-visible Spectrophotometry <2.24>, and compare the spectrum with the Reference Spectrum: both spectra exhibit similar intensities of absorption at the same wavelengths.

(3) Determine the infrared absorption spectrum of Medazepam as directed in the potassium bromide disk method under Infrared Spectrophotometry <2.25>, and compare the spectrum with the Reference Spectrum: both spectra exhibit similar intensities of absorption at the same wave numbers.

(4) Perform the test with Medazepam as directed under Flame Coloration Test <1.04> (2): a green color appears.

Melting point <2.60> 101 – 104°C

Purity **(1)** Clarity and color of solution—Dissolve 1.0 g of Medazepam in 10 mL of methanol: the solution is clear and light yellow to yellow in color.

(2) Chloride <1.03>—Dissolve 1.5 g of Medazepam in 50

mL of diethyl ether, add 46 mL of water and 4 mL of sodium carbonate TS, shake, and collect the water layer. Wash the water layer with two 20-mL portions of diethyl ether, and filter. To 20 mL of the filtrate add dilute nitric acid to neutralize, add 6 mL of dilute nitric acid and water to make 50 mL, and perform the test using this solution as the test solution. Prepare the control solution with 0.30 mL of 0.01 mol/L hydrochloric acid VS (not more than 0.018%).

(3) Heavy metals <*1.07*>—Proceed with 1.0 g of Medazepam according to Method 2, and perform the test. Prepare the control solution with 2.0 mL of Standard Lead Solution (not more than 20 ppm).

(4) Arsenic <*1.11*>—Prepare the test solution with 1.0 g of Medazepam according to Method 3, and perform the test (not more than 2 ppm).

(5) Related substances—Dissolve 0.25 g of Medazepam in 10 mL of methanol, and use this solution as the sample solution. Pipet 1 mL of the sample solution, and add methanol to make exactly 20 mL. Pipet 2 mL of this solution, add methanol to make exactly 50 mL, and use this solution as the standard solution. Perform the test with these solutions as directed under Thin-layer Chromatography <*2.03*>. Spot 10 μL each of the sample solution and standard solution on a plate of silica gel with fluorescent indicator for thin-layer chromatography. Develop the plate with a mixture of cyclohexane, acetone and ammonia solution (28) (60:40:1) to a distance of about 10 cm, and air-dry the plate. Examine under ultraviolet light (main wavelength: 254 nm): the spots other than the principal spot obtained from the sample solution are not more intense than the spot from the standard solution.

Loss on drying <*2.41*> Not more than 0.5% (1 g, in vacuum, 60°C, 4 hours).

Residue on ignition <*2.44*> Not more than 0.1% (1 g).

Assay Weigh accurately about 0.4 g of Medazepam, previously dried, dissolve in 50 mL of acetic acid (100), and titrate <*2.50*> with 0.1 mol/L perchloric acid VS (potentiometric titration). Perform a blank determination in the same manner, and make any necessary correction.

Each mL of 0.1 mol/L perchloric acid VS
= 27.08 mg of $C_{16}H_{15}ClN_2$

Containers and storage Containers—Tight containers.
Storage—Light-resistant.

Medicinal Carbon

薬用炭

Description Medicinal Carbon occurs as a black, odorless and tasteless powder.

Identification Place 0.5 g of Medicinal Carbon in a test tube, and heat by direct application of flame with the aid of a current of air: it burns without any flame. Pass the evolved gas through calcium hydroxide TS: a white turbidity is produced.

Purity **(1)** Acidity or alkalinity—Boil 3.0 g of Medicinal Carbon with 60 mL of water for 5 minutes, allow to cool, dilute to 60 mL with water, and filter: the filtrate is colorless and neutral.

(2) Chloride <*1.03*>—Take 4.0 mL of the filtrate obtained in (1) in a Nessler tube, add 6 mL of dilute nitric acid and sufficient water to make 50 mL, and perform the test using this solution as the test solution. Prepare the control solution with 0.80 mL of 0.01 mol/L hydrochloric acid VS (not more than 0.142%).

(3) Sulfate <*1.14*>—Take 5 mL of the filtrate obtained in (1) in a Nessler tube, add 1 mL of dilute hydrochloric acid and sufficient water to make 50 mL, and perform the test using this solution as the test solution. Prepare the control solution with 1.0 mL of 0.005 mol/L sulfuric acid VS (not more than 0.192%).

(4) Sulfide—Boil 0.5 g of Medicinal Carbon with a mixture of 15 mL of dilute hydrochloric acid and 10 mL of water: lead (II) acetate paper does not become brown when held in the evolved gas within 5 minutes.

(5) Cyanogen compounds—Place a mixture of 5 g of Medicinal Carbon, 2 g of L-tartaric acid and 50 mL of water in a distilling flask connected to a condenser provided with a tightly fitting adapter, the end of which dips below the surface of a mixture of 2 mL of sodium hydroxide TS and 10 mL of water, contained in a small flask surrounded by ice. Heat the mixture in the distilling flask to boiling, and distil to 25 mL. Dilute the distillate with water to 50 mL. To 25 mL of the diluted distillate add 1 mL of a solution of iron (II) sulfate heptahydrate (1 in 20), heat the mixture almost to boiling, cool, and filter. To the filtrate add 1 mL of hydrochloric acid and 0.5 mL of dilute iron (III) chloride TS: no blue color is produced.

(6) Acid soluble substances—To about 1 g of Medicinal Carbon, accurately weighed, add 20 mL of water and 5 mL of hydrochloric acid, boil for 5 minutes, filter, wash the residue with 10 mL of hot water, and add the washings to the filtrate. Add 5 drops of sulfuric acid to the filtrate, evaporate to dryness, and ignite the residue strongly: the mass of the residue is not more than 3.0%.

(7) Heavy metals <*1.07*>—Proceed with 0.5 g of Medicinal Carbon according to Method 2, and perform the test. Prepare the control solution with 2.5 mL of Standard Lead Solution (not more than 50 ppm).

(8) Zinc—Ignite 0.5 g of Medicinal Carbon to ash, add 5 mL of dilute nitric acid to the residue, boil gently for 5 minutes, filter, wash with 10 mL of water, and combine the washings and the filtrate. Add 3 mL of ammonia TS to the solution, filter again, wash with water, combine the washings and the filtrate, add another washing to make 25 mL, add 1 drop of sodium sulfide TS, and allow to stand for 3 minutes: the liquid produces no turbidity.

(9) Arsenic <*1.11*>—Prepare the test solution with 1.0 g of Medicinal Carbon according to Method 3, and perform the test (not more than 2 ppm).

Loss on drying <*2.41*> Not more than 15.0% (1 g, 105°C, 4 hours).

Residue on ignition <*2.44*> Not more than 4% (1 g).

Adsorptive power **(1)** Add 1.0 g of Medicinal Carbon, previously dried, to 100 mL of water containing 120 mg of quinine sulfate hydrate, shake the mixture vigorously for 5 minutes, filter immediately, and reject the first 20 mL of the filtrate. Add 5 drops of iodine TS to 10 mL of the subsequent filtrate: no turbidity is produced.

(2) Dissolve 250 mg of methylene blue trihydrate, exactly weighed, in water to make exactly 250 mL. Measure two 50-mL portions of this solution into each of two glass-stoppered flasks. To one flask add exactly 250 mg of Medicinal Carbon, previously dried, and shake vigorously for 5 minutes. Filter the contents of each flask, rejecting the first 20 mL of each filtrate. Pipet 25-mL portions of the remaining filtrate into two 250-mL volumetric flasks. To each volumetric flask add 50 mL of a solution of sodium acetate trihydrate (1 in 10), then add exactly 35 mL of 0.05 mol/L iodine VS with swirling. Allow them to stand for 50 minutes, shaking vigorously from time to time. Dilute each mixture to exactly 250 mL with water, allow to stand for 10 minutes, and filter each solution at a temperature not exceeding 20°C, rejecting the first 30 mL of each filtrate. Titrate <*2.50*> the excess iodine in a 100-mL aliquot of each filtrate with 0.1 mol/L sodium thiosulfate VS. The difference between the two titrations is not less than 1.2 mL.

Containers and storage Containers—Well-closed containers.

Medicinal Soap

薬用石ケン

Medicinal Soap is sodium salts of fatty acids.

Description Medicinal Soap occurs as a white to light yellow, powder or granules. It has a characteristic odor free from rancidity.

Medicinal Soap is sparingly soluble in water, and slightly soluble in ethanol (95).

A solution of Medicinal Soap (1 in 100) is alkaline.

Fatty acid Dissolve 25 g of Medicinal Soap in 300 mL of hot water, add 60 mL of dilute sulfuric acid slowly, and warm in a water bath for 20 minutes. After cooling, filter off the precipitate, and wash with warm water until the washing no longer shows acidity to methyl orange TS. Transfer the precipitate to a small beaker, and heat on a water bath to complete separation of water and transparent fatty acids. Filter the fatty acid into a small beaker while warm, dry at 100°C for 20 minutes, and perform the test with this material as directed under Fats and Fatty Oils <*1.13*>. The congealing point of the fatty acid is between 18°C and 28°C. The acid value is 185 - 205. The iodine value is 82 - 92.

Purity **(1)** Acidity or alkalinity—Dissolve 5.0 g of Medicinal Soap in 85 mL of neutralized ethanol by warming on a water bath, filter while hot through absorbent cotton, and wash the filter and the residue with three 5-mL portions of hot neutralized ethanol. Combine the filtrate and the washings, add hot neutralized ethanol to make exactly 100 mL, and perform the following tests quickly using this as the sample solution at 70°C.

(i) Add 3 drops of phenolphthalein TS and 0.20 mL of 0.1 mol/L sodium hydroxide VS to 40 mL of the sample solution: a red color develops.

(ii) Add 3 drops of phenolphthalein TS and 0.20 mL of 0.05 mol/L sulfuric acid VS to 40 mL of the sample solution: no red color develops.

(2) Heavy metals <*1.07*>—Proceed with 1.0 g of Medicinal Soap according to Method 2, and perform the test. Prepare the control solution with 2.0 mL of Standard Lead Solution (not more than 20 ppm).

(3) Ethanol-insoluble substances—Weigh accurately about 2 g of Medicinal Soap, dissolve by warming in 100 mL of neutralized ethanol, filter the solution through a glass filter (G4), wash the residue with 100 mL of hot neutralized ethanol, and dry at 105°C for 4 hours: the mass of the residue is not more than 1.0%.

(4) Water-insoluble substances—Wash thoroughly the dried substances obtained in (3) with 200 mL of water, and dry at 105°C for 4 hours: the mass of the residue is not more than 0.15%.

(5) Alkali carbonates—To the washings obtained in (4) add 3 drops of methyl orange TS and 2 mL of 0.05 mol/L sulfuric acid VS: a red color develops.

Loss on drying Not more than 5.0% in the case of the powder, and not more than 10.0% in the case of the granules.

Weigh accurately about 0.5 g of Medicinal Soap in a tared beaker, add 10 g of sea sand (No. 1), previously dried at 105°C for 1 hour, and again weigh the beaker. Add 10 mL of ethanol (95), evaporate on a water bath to dryness with thorough stirring, and dry at 105°C for 3 hours.

Containers and storage Containers—Well-closed containers.

Medroxyprogesterone Acetate

メドロキシプロゲステロン酢酸エステル

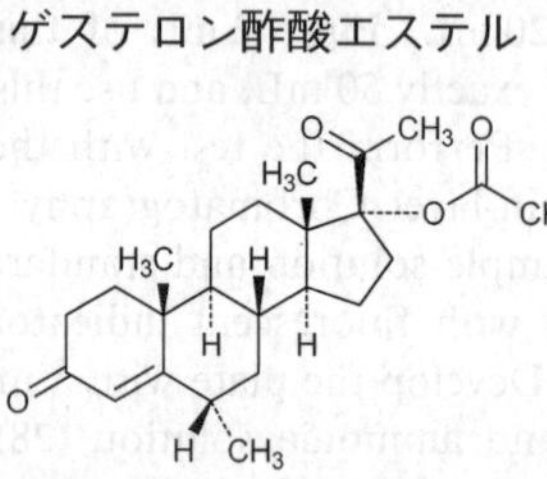

$C_{24}H_{34}O_4$: 386.52
6α-Methyl-3,20-dioxopregn-4-en-17-yl acetate
[*71-58-9*]

Medroxyprogesterone Acetate, when dried, contains not less than 97.0 and not more than 103.0% of medroxyprogesterone acetate ($C_{24}H_{34}O_4$).

Description Medroxyprogesterone Acetate occurs as a white crystalline powder.

It is soluble in acetone, sparingly soluble in acetonitrile, slightly soluble in ethanol (99.5), and practically insoluble in water.

Identification **(1)** Determine the absorption spectrum of a solution of Medroxyprogesterone Acetate in ethanol (99.5) (1 in 100,000) as directed under Ultraviolet-visible Spectrophotometry <*2.24*>, and compare the spectrum with the Reference Spectrum or the spectrum of a solution of Medroxyprogesterone Acetate RS prepared in the same manner as the sample solution: both spectra exhibit similar intensities of absorption at the same wavelengths.

(2) Determine the infrared absorption spectrum of Medroxyprogesterone Acetate, previously dried, as directed in the potassium bromide disk method under Infrared Spectrophotometry <*2.25*>, and compare the spectrum with the Reference Spectrum or the spectrum of dried Medroxyprogesterone Acetate RS: both spectra exhibit similar intensities of absorption at the same wave numbers.

Optical rotation <*2.49*> $[\alpha]_D^{20}$: + 47 – + 53°(after drying, 0.25 g, acetone, 25 mL, 100 mm).

Melting point <*2.60*> 204 - 209°C

Purity **(1)** Heavy metals <*1.07*>—Proceed with 1.0 g of Medroxyprogesterone Acetate according to Method 2, and perform the test. Prepare the control solution with 2.0 mL of Standard Lead Solution (not more than 20 ppm).

(2) Related substances—Use the sample solution obtained in the Assay as the sample solution. Pipet 1 mL of the sample solution, add acetonitrile to make exactly 100 mL, and use this solution as the standard solution. Perform the test with exactly 10 μL each of the sample solution and standard solution as directed under Liquid Chromatography <*2.01*> according to the following conditions. Determine each peak area by the automatic integration method: the area of the peak other than medroxyprogesterone acetate obtained from the sample solution is not larger than the peak area of medroxyprogesterone acetate from the standard solution, and the total area of the peaks other than medroxyprogesterone acetate from the sample solution is not larger than 2 times the peak area of medroxyprogesterone acetate from the standard solution.

Operating conditions—

Detector, column, column temperature, mobile phase, and flow rate: Proceed as directed in the operating conditions in the Assay.

Time span of measurement: About 1.2 times as long as the retention time of medroxyprogesterone acetate, beginning after the solvent peak.

System suitability—

Test for required detectability: Pipet 1 mL of the standard solution, and add acetonitrile to make exactly 10 mL. Confirm that the peak area of medroxyprogesterone acetate obtained with 10 μL of this solution is equivalent to 7 to 13% of that with 10 μL of the standard solution.

System performance: When the procedure is run with 10 μL of the standard solution under the above operating conditions, the number of theoretical plates and the symmetry factor of the peak of medroxyprogesterone acetate are not less than 5000 and not more than 2.0, respectively.

System repeatability: When the test is repeated 6 times with 10 μL of the standard solution, the relative standard deviation of the peak area of medroxyprogesterone acetate is not more than 2.0%.

Loss on drying <*2.41*> Not more than 1.0% (1 g, 105°C, 3 hours).

Residue on ignition <*2.44*> Not more than 0.2% (0.5 g).

Assay Weigh accurately about 25 mg each of Medroxyprogesterone Acetate and Medroxyprogesterone Acetate RS, both previously dried, dissolve in acetonitrile to make them exactly 25 mL, and use these solutions as the sample solution and the standard solution, respectively. Perform the test with exactly 10 μL each of the sample solution and standard solution as directed under Liquid Chromatography <*2.01*> according to the following conditions, and determine the peak areas, A_T and A_S, of medroxyprogesterone acetate in each solution.

Amount (mg) of medroxyprogesterone acetate ($C_{24}H_{34}O_4$)
$= M_S \times A_T/A_S$

M_S: Amount (mg) of Medroxyprogesterone Acetate RS taken

Operating conditions—

Detector: An ultraviolet absorption photometer (wavelength: 254 nm).

Column: A stainless steel column 4.6 mm in inside diameter and 25 cm in length, packed with octadecylsilanized silica gel for liquid chromatography (5 μm in particle diameter).

Column temperature: A constant temperature of about 25°C.

Mobile phase: A mixture of water and acetonitrile (3:2).

Flow rate: Adjust so that the retention time of medroxyprogesterone acetate is about 31 minutes.

System suitability—

System performance: When the procedure is run with 10 μL of the standard solution under the above operating conditions, the number of theoretical plates and the symmetry factor of the peak of medroxyprogesterone acetate are not less than 5000 and not more than 2.0, respectively.

System repeatability: When the test is repeated 6 times with 10 μL of the standard solution, the relative standard deviation of the peak area of medroxyprogesterone acetate is not more than 1.0%.

Containers and storage Containers—Well-closed containers.

Storage—Light-resistant.

Mefenamic Acid

メフェナム酸

$C_{15}H_{15}NO_2$: 241.29

2-(2,3-Dimethylphenylamino)benzoic acid

[*61-68-7*]

Mefenamic Acid, when dried, contains not less than 99.0% of mefenamic acid ($C_{15}H_{15}NO_2$).

Description Mefenamic Acid occurs as a white to light yellow powder. It is odorless and tasteless at first, but leaves a slightly bitter aftertaste.

It is sparingly soluble in diethyl ether, slightly soluble in methanol, in ethanol (95) and in chloroform, and practically insoluble in water.

It dissolves in sodium hydroxide TS.

Melting point: about 225°C (with decomposition).

Identification **(1)** Dissolve 10 mg of Mefenamic Acid in 1 mL of methanol by warming, cool, add 1 mL of a solution of 4-nitrobenzene diazonium fluoroborate (1 in 1000) and 1 mL of sodium hydroxide TS, and mix thoroughly: an orange-red color is produced.

(2) Dissolve 10 mg of Mefenamic Acid in 2 mL of sulfuric acid, and heat: the solution shows a yellow color and a green fluorescence.

(3) Dissolve 7 mg of Mefenamic Acid in a solution of hydrochloric acid in methanol (1 in 1000) to make 500 mL. Determine the absorption spectrum of the solution as directed under Ultraviolet-visible Spectrophotometry <*2.24*>, and compare the spectrum with the Reference Spectrum: both spectra exhibit similar intensities of absorption at the same wavelengths.

Purity **(1)** Chloride <*1.03*>—To 1.0 g of Mefenamic Acid add 20 mL of sodium hydroxide TS, and dissolve by warming. Cool, add 2 mL of acetic acid (100) and water to make 100 mL, and mix well. Remove the produced precipitate by filtration, discard the first 10 mL of the filtrate, and to subsequent 25 mL of the filtrate add 6 mL of dilute nitric acid and water to make 50 mL. Perform the test using this solution as the test solution. Prepare the control solution as follows: to 0.50 mL of 0.01 mol/L hydrochloric acid VS add 5 mL of sodium hydroxide TS, 0.5 mL of acetic acid (100), 6 mL of nitric acid and water to make 50 mL (not more than 0.071%).

(2) Heavy metals *<1.07>*—Proceed with 2.0 g of Mefenamic Acid according to Method 2, and perform the test. Prepare the control solution with 2.0 mL of Standard Lead Solution (not more than 10 ppm).

(3) Arsenic *<1.11>*—Prepare the test solution with 1.0 g of Mefenamic Acid according to Method 3, and perform the test (not more than 2 ppm).

(4) Related substances—Dissolve 0.10 g of Mefenamic Acid, in 5 mL of a mixture of chloroform and methanol (3:1), and use this solution as the sample solution. Pipet 1 mL of the sample solution, add a mixture of chloroform and methanol (3:1) to make exactly 200 mL, pipet 10 mL of this solution, add a mixture of chloroform and methanol (3:1) to make exactly 50 mL, and use this solution as the standard solution. Perform the test with these solutions as directed under Thin-layer Chromatography *<2.03>*. Spot 25 μL each of the sample solution and standard solution on a plate of silica gel with fluorescent indicator for thin-layer chromatography. Develop the plate with a mixture of 2-methyl-1-propanol and ammonia solution (28) (3:1) to a distance of about 10 cm, and air-dry the plate. Examine under ultraviolet light (main wavelength: 254 nm): the spots other than the principal spot obtained from the sample solution are not more intense than the spot from the standard solution.

Loss on drying *<2.41>* Not more than 0.5% (1 g, in vacuum, phosphorus (V) oxide, 4 hours).

Residue on ignition *<2.44>* Not more than 0.1% (1 g).

Assay Weigh accurately about 0.5 g of Mefenamic Acid, previously dried, and dissolve in 100 mL of ethanol (95), previously neutralized to phenol red TS with 0.1 mol/L sodium hydroxide VS, by warming gently. Cool, and titrate *<2.50>* with 0.1 mol/L sodium hydroxide VS until the color of the solution changes from yellow through yellow-red to red-purple (indicator: 2 to 3 drops of phenol red TS). Perform a blank determination in the same manner, and make any necessary correction.

Each mL of 0.1 mol/L sodium hydroxide VS
= 24.13 mg of $C_{15}H_{15}NO_2$

Containers and storage Containers—Well-closed containers.

Mefloquine Hydrochloride

メフロキン塩酸塩

$C_{17}H_{16}F_6N_2O.HCl$: 414.77
(1*RS*)-[2,8-Bis(trifluoromethyl)quinolin-4-yl][(2*SR*)-piperidin-2-yl]methanol monohydrochloride
[51773-92-3]

Mefloquine Hydrochloride contains not less than 99.0% and not more than 101.0% of mefloquine hydrochloride ($C_{17}H_{16}F_6N_2O.HCl$), calculated on the anhydrous basis.

Description Mefloquine Hydrochloride occurs as white crystals or a white crystalline powder.

It is freely soluble in methanol, soluble in ethanol (99.5), and slightly soluble in water.

It dissolves in sulfuric acid.

A solution of Mefloquine Hydrochloride in methanol (1 in 20) shows no optical rotation.

Melting point: about 260°C (with decomposition).

Identification **(1)** Dissolve 2 mg of Mefloquine Hydrochloride in 1 mL of sulfuric acid: the solution shows a blue fluorescence under ultraviolet light (main wavelength: 365 nm).

(2) Determine the absorption spectrum of a solution of Mefloquine Hydrochloride in methanol (1 in 25,000) as directed under Ultraviolet-visible Spectrophotometry *<2.24>*, and compare the spectrum with the Reference Spectrum: both spectra exhibit similar intensities of absorption at the same wavelengths.

(3) Determine the infrared absorption spectrum of Mefloquine Hydrochloride, previously dried at 105°C for 2 hours, as directed in the potassium chloride disk method under Infrared Spectrophotometry *<2.25>*, and compare the spectrum with the Reference Spectrum: both spectra exhibit similar intensities of absorption at the same wave numbers.

(4) To 5 mL of a solution of Mefloquine Hydrochloride (1 in 1000) add 1 mL of dilute nitric acid and 1 mL of silver nitrate TS: a white precipitate is formed, and the separated precipitate dissolves on the addition of an excess amount of ammonia TS.

Purity **(1)** Heavy metals *<1.07>*—Proceed with 1.0 g of Mefloquine Hydrochloride according to Method 2 using a quartz crucible, and perform the test. Prepare the control solution with 2.0 mL of Standard Lead Solution (not more than 20 ppm).

(2) Arsenic *<1.11>*—To 1.0 g of Mefloquine Hydrochloride add 10 mL of a solution of magnesium nitrate hexahydrate in ethanol (95) (1 in 10), burn the ethanol, gradually heat, and incinerate by ignition at 800°C. If a carbonized residue still retains, moisten the residue with a little amount of nitric acid, and ignite again to incinerate. After cooling, to the residue add 3 mL of hydrochloric acid, warm on a water bath to dissolve, and perform the test using this solution as the test solution (not more than 2 ppm).

(3) Related substances—Dissolve 50 mg of Mefloquine Hydrochloride in 50 mL of the mobile phase, and use this solution as the sample solution. Pipet 1 mL of the sample solution, and add the mobile phase to make exactly 50 mL. Pipet 2 mL of this solution, add the mobile phase to make exactly 20 mL, and use this solution as the standard solution. Perform the test with exactly 10 μL each of the sample solution and standard solution as directed under Liquid Chromatography *<2.01>* according to the following conditions, and determine each peak area by the automatic integration method: the area of the peak other than mefloquine and the peak eluted first obtained from the sample solution is not larger than the peak area of mefloquine from the standard solution, and the total area of the peaks other than the peak of mefloquine and the peak eluted first from the sample solution is not larger than 2.5 times the peak area of mefloquine from the standard solution.

Operating conditions—

Detector: An ultraviolet absorption photometer (wavelength: 282 nm).

Column: A stainless steel column 3.9 mm in inside diameter and 30 cm in length, packed with aminopropylsilanized silica gel for liquid chromatography (10 μm in particle diameter).

Column temperature: A constant temperature of about 40°C.

Mobile phase: A mixture of acetonitrile and diluted phosphoric acid (1 in 14) (24:1).

Flow rate: Adjust so that the retention time of mefloquine is about 10 minutes.

Time span of measurement: About 3 times as long as the retention time of mefloquine.

System suitability—

Test for required detectability: To exactly 10 mL of the standard solution add the mobile phase to make exactly 20 mL. Confirm that the peak area of mefloquine obtained with 10 μL of this solution is equivalent to 40 to 60% of that with 10 μL of the standard solution.

System performance: Dissolve 10 mg of mefloquine hydrochloride and 5 mg of diprophylline in 50 mL of the mobile phase. To 2 mL of this solution add the mobile phase to make 20 mL. When the procedure is run with 10 μL of this solution under the above operating conditions, diprophylline and mefloquine are eluted in this order with the resolution between these peaks being not less than 5.

System repeatability: When the test is repeated 6 times with 10 μL of the standard solution under the above operating conditions, the relative standard deviation of the peak area of mefloquine is not more than 2.0%.

Water 〈*2.48*〉 Not more than 3.0% (1 g, volumetric titration, direct titration).

Residue on ignition 〈*2.44*〉 Not more than 0.1% (1 g, platinum crucible).

Assay Weigh accurately about 0.5 g of Mefloquine Hydrochloride, dissolve in 100 mL of a mixture of acetic anhydride and acetic acid (100) (7:3), and titrate 〈*2.50*〉 with 0.1 mol/L perchloric acid VS (potentiometric titration). Perform a blank determination in the same manner, and make any necessary correction.

Each mL of 0.1 mol/L perchloric acid VS
= 41.48 mg of $C_{17}H_{16}F_6N_2O.HCl$

Containers and storage Containers—Well-closed containers.

Mefruside

メフルシド

and enantiomer

$C_{13}H_{19}ClN_2O_5S_2$: 382.88
4-Chloro-*N*-methyl-*N*-[(2*RS*)-2-methyltetrahydrofuran-2-ylmethyl]-3-sulfamoylbenzenesulfonamide
[*7195-27-9*]

Mefruside, when dried, contains not less than 98.5% of mefruside ($C_{13}H_{19}ClN_2O_5S_2$).

Description Mefruside occurs as a white crystalline powder.

It is very soluble in *N,N*-dimethylformamide, freely soluble in acetone, soluble in methanol, sparingly soluble in ethanol (95), and practically insoluble in water.

A solution of Mefruside in *N,N*-dimethylformamide (1 in 10) has no optical rotation.

Identification **(1)** Determine the absorption spectrum of a solution of Mefruside in methanol (1 in 40,000) as directed under Ultraviolet-visible Spectrophotometry 〈*2.24*〉, and compare the spectrum with the Reference Spectrum: both spectra exhibit similar intensities of absorption at the same wavelengths.

(2) Determine the infrared absorption spectrum of Mefruside, previously dried, as directed in the potassium bromide disk method under Infrared Spectrophotometry 〈*2.25*〉, and compare the spectrum with the Reference Spectrum: both spectra exhibit similar intensities of absorption at the same wave numbers.

(3) Perform the test with Mefruside as directed under Flame Coloration Test 〈*1.04*〉 (2): a green color appears.

Melting point 〈*2.60*〉 149 - 152°C

Purity **(1)** Heavy metals 〈*1.07*〉—Dissolve 1.0 g of Mefruside in 30 mL of acetone, and add 2 mL of dilute acetic acid and water to make 50 mL. Perform the test using this solution as the test solution. Prepare the control solution as follows: to 2.0 mL of Standard Lead Solution add 30 mL of acetone, 2 mL of dilute acetic acid and water to make 50 mL (not more than 20 ppm).

(2) Arsenic 〈*1.11*〉—Prepare the test solution with 1.0 g of Mefruside according to Method 3, and perform the test (not more than 2 ppm).

(3) Related substances—Dissolve 0.20 g of Mefruside in 10 mL of acetone, and use this solution as the sample solution. Pipet 1 mL of the sample solution, add acetone to make exactly 200 mL, and use this solution as the standard solution. Perform the test with these solutions as directed under Thin-layer Chromatography 〈*2.03*〉. Spot 10 μL each of the sample solution and standard solution on a plate of silica gel with fluorescent indicator for thin-layer chromatography. Develop the plate with a mixture of chloroform and acetone (5:2) to a distance of about 10 cm, and air-dry the plate. Examine under ultraviolet light (main wavelength: 254 nm): the spots other than the principal spot obtained from the sample solution are not more intense than the spot from the standard solution.

Loss on drying 〈*2.41*〉 Not more than 0.5% (1 g, 105°C, 2 hours).

Residue on ignition 〈*2.44*〉 Not more than 0.1% (1 g).

Assay Weigh accurately about 0.5 g of Mefruside, previously dried, dissolve in 80 mL of *N,N*-dimethylformamide, and titrate 〈*2.50*〉 with 0.1 mol/L tetramethylammonium hydroxide VS (potentiometric titration). Separately, perform a blank determination in the same manner with a solution prepared by adding 13 mL of water to 80 mL of *N,N*-dimethylformamide, and make any necessary correction.

Each mL of 0.1 mol/L tetramethylammonium
hydroxide VS
= 38.29 mg of $C_{13}H_{19}ClN_2O_5S_2$

Containers and storage Containers—Well-closed containers.

Mefruside Tablets

メフルシド錠

Mefruside Tablets contain not less than 95.0% and not more than 105.0% of the labeled amount of mefruside ($C_{13}H_{19}ClN_2O_5S_2$: 382.88).

Method of preparation Prepare as directed under Tablets, with Mefruside.

Identification **(1)** Weigh a quantity of powdered Mefruside Tablets, equivalent to 0.3 g of Mefruside, shake with 15 mL of heated methanol for 20 minutes, and filter. Add 25 mL of water to the filtrate, and allow to stand while ice-cooling for 30 minutes. Filter the white precipitate formed, wash with water, and dry at 105°C for 2 hours: the precipitate melts 〈*2.60*〉 between 149°C and 152°C.

(2) Weigh a quantity of powdered Mefruside Tablets, equivalent to 0.01 g of Mefruside, shake with 70 mL of methanol strongly for 15 minutes, add methanol to make 100 mL, and filter. Determine the absorption spectrum of the filtrate as directed under Ultraviolet-visible Spectrophotometry 〈*2.24*〉: it exhibits maxima between 274 nm and 278 nm, and between 283 nm and 287 nm.

Uniformity of dosage units 〈*6.02*〉 Perform the test according to the following method: it meets the requirement of the Content uniformity test.

To 1 tablet of Mefruside Tablets add 40 mL of methanol, disintegrate the tablet by sonicating with occasional stirring, then further sonicate for 10 minutes, and add methanol to make exactly V mL of a solution containing about 0.5 mg of mefruside ($C_{13}H_{19}ClN_2O_5S_2$) per mL. Centrifuge the solution, pipet 5 mL of the supernatant liquid, add methanol to make exactly 20 mL, and use this solution as the sample solution. Then, proceed as directed in the Assay.

Amount (mg) of mefruside ($C_{13}H_{19}ClN_2O_5S_2$)
$= M_S \times A_T/A_S \times V/125$

M_S: Amount (mg) of mefruside for assay taken

Dissolution 〈*6.10*〉 When the test is performed at 50 revolutions per minute according to the Paddle method, using 900 mL of water as the dissolution medium, the dissolution rate in 45 minutes of Mefruside Tablets is not less than 85%.

Start the test with 1 tablet of Mefruside Tablets, withdraw not less than 20 mL of the medium at the specified minute after starting the test, and filter through a filter paper for quantitative analysis (5C). Discard not less than 5 mL of the first filtrate, pipet V mL of the subsequent filtrate, add water to make exactly V' mL so that each mL contains about 28 μg of mefruside ($C_{13}H_{19}ClN_2O_5S_2$), and use this solution as the sample solution. Separately, weigh accurately about 70 mg of mefruside for assay, previously dried at 105°C for 2 hours, dissolve in methanol to make exactly 50 mL. Pipet 2 mL of this solution, add water to make exactly 100 mL, and use this solution as the standard solution. Determine the absorbances, A_T and A_S, of the sample solution and standard solution at 285 nm in a layer of 5 cm in length as directed under Ultraviolet-visible Spectrophotometry 〈*2.24*〉, using water as the blank.

Dissolution rate (%) with respect to the labeled amount of mefruside ($C_{13}H_{19}ClN_2O_5S_2$)
$= M_S \times A_T/A_S \times V'/V \times 1/C \times 36$

M_S: Amount (mg) of mefruside for assay taken
C: Labeled amount (mg) of mefruside ($C_{13}H_{19}ClN_2O_5S_2$) in 1 tablet

Assay Weigh accurately not less than 20 Mefruside Tablets, and powder. Weigh accurately a portion of the powder, equivalent to about 65 mg of mefruside ($C_{13}H_{19}ClN_2O_5S_2$), shake with 70 mL of methanol for 15 minutes, then add methanol to make exactly 100 mL, and filter. Discard the first 20 mL of the filtrate, take exactly 10 mL of the subsequent filtrate, add methanol to make exactly 50 mL, and use this solution as the sample solution. Separately, weigh accurately about 65 mg of mefruside for assay, previously dried at 105°C for 2 hours, and dissolve in methanol to make exactly 100 mL. Pipet 10 mL of this solution, add methanol to make exactly 50 mL, and use this solution as the standard solution. Determine the absorbances, A_T and A_S, of the sample solution and standard solution at 285 nm as directed under Ultraviolet-visible Spectrophotometry 〈*2.24*〉.

Amount (mg) of mefruside ($C_{13}H_{19}ClN_2O_5S_2$)
$= M_S \times A_T/A_S$

M_S: Amount (mg) of mefruside for assay taken

Containers and storage Containers—Tight containers.

Meglumine

メグルミン

$C_7H_{17}NO_5$: 195.21
1-Deoxy-1-methylamino-D-glucitol
[6284-40-8]

Meglumine, when dried, contains not less than 99.0% of meglumine ($C_7H_{17}NO_5$).

Description Meglumine occurs as a white crystalline powder. It is odorless, and has a slightly bitter taste.

It is freely soluble in water, and slightly soluble in ethanol (95), and practically insoluble in diethyl ether.

The pH of a solution of 1.0 g of Meglumine in 10 mL of water is between 11.0 and 12.0.

Identification **(1)** To 1 mL of a solution of Meglumine (1 in 10) add 1 mL of potassium 1,2-naphthoquinone-4-sulfonate TS: a deep red color develops.

(2) To 2 mL of a solution of Meglumine (1 in 10) add 1 drop of methyl red TS, and add 0.5 mL of dilute sodium hydroxide TS and 0.5 g of boric acid after neutralizing with 0.5 mol/L sulfuric acid TS: a deep red color develops.

(3) Dissolve 0.5 g of Meglumine in 1 mL of diluted hydrochloric acid (1 in 3), and add 10 mL of ethanol (99.5): a white precipitate is produced. Then, rubbing the inside wall of the container with a glass rod, cool with ice and produce more precipitate. Filter the precipitate by suction through a glass filter (G3), wash the precipitate with a small volume of ethanol (99.5), and dry at 105°C for 1 hour: the residue thus obtained melts 〈*2.60*〉 between 149°C and 152°C.

Optical rotation 〈*2.49*〉 $[\alpha]_D^{20}$: $-16.0 - -17.0°$ (after drying, 1 g, water, 10 mL, 100 mm).

Melting point 〈*2.60*〉 128 - 131°C

Purity (1) Clarity and color of solution—Dissolve 1.0 g of Meglumine in 10 mL of water: the solution is clear and colorless.

(2) Chloride <*1.03*>—Dissolve 1.0 g of Meglumine in 30 mL of water, and add 10 mL of dilute nitric acid and water to make 50 mL. Perform the test using this solution as the test solution. Prepare the control solution with 0.25 mL of 0.01 mol/L hydrochloric acid VS (not more than 0.009%).

(3) Sulfate <*1.14*>—Dissolve 1.0 g of Meglumine in 30 mL of water, and add 5 mL of dilute hydrochloric acid and water to make 50 mL. Perform the test using this solution as the test solution. Prepare the control solution with 0.40 mL of 0.005 mol/L sulfuric acid VS (not more than 0.019%).

(4) Heavy metals <*1.07*>—Proceed with 2.0 g of Meglumine according to Method 4, and perform the test. Prepare the control solution with 2.0 mL of Standard Lead Solution (not more than 10 ppm).

(5) Arsenic <*1.11*>—Prepare the test solution with 2.0 g of Meglumine according to Method 3, and perform the test (not more than 1 ppm).

(6) Reducing substances—To 5 mL of a solution of Meglumine (1 in 20) add 5 mL of Fehling's TS, and boil for 2 minutes: no red-brown precipitate is produced.

Loss on drying <*2.41*> Not more than 0.5% (1 g, 105°C, 4 hours).

Residue on ignition <*2.44*> Not more than 0.1% (1 g).

Assay Weigh accurately about 0.4 g of Meglumine, previously dried, dissolve in 25 mL of water, and titrate <*2.50*> with 0.1 mol/L hydrochloric acid VS (indicator: 2 drops of methyl red TS).

Each mL of 0.1 mol/L hydrochloric acid VS
= 19.52 mg of $C_7H_{17}NO_5$

Containers and storage Containers—Tight containers.

Meglumine Iotalamate Injection

イオタラム酸メグルミン注射液

Meglumine Iotalamate Injection is an aqueous injection.

It contains not less than 95.0% and not more than 105.0% of the labeled amount of iotalamic acid ($C_{11}H_9I_3N_2O_4$: 613.91).

Method of preparation

(1)

Iotalamic Acid	227.59 g
Meglumine	72.41 g
Water for Injection or Sterile Water for Injection in Containers	a sufficient quantity
To make	1000 mL

(2)

Iotalamic Acid	455 g
Meglumine	145 g
Water for Injection or Sterile Water for Injection in Containers	a sufficient quantity
To make	1000 mL

Prepare as directed under Injections, with the above ingredients (1) or (2).

Description Meglumine Iotalamate Injection is a clear, colorless to pale yellow, slightly viscous liquid.

It gradually changes in color by light.

Identification (1) To 1 mL of Meglumine Iotalamate Injection add 1 mL of potassium 1,2-naphthoquinone-4-sulfonate TS and 0.2 mL of sodium hydroxide TS: a deep red color develops.

(2) To a volume of Meglumine Iotalamate Injection, equivalent to 1 g of Iotalamic Acid, add 25 mL of water, and add 2.5 mL of dilute hydrochloric acid while shaking: a white precipitate is produced. Filter the precipitate by suction through a glass filter (G4), wash the precipitate with two 10-mL portions of water, and dry at 105°C for 4 hours. Proceed with the precipitate so obtained as directed in the Identification (2) under Iotalamic Acid.

Optical rotation <*2.49*>

Method of preparation (1) α_D^{20}: −1.67 – −1.93° (100 mm).

Method of preparation (2) α_D^{20}: −3.35 – −3.86° (100 mm).

pH <*2.54*> 6.5 – 7.7

Purity (1) Primary aromatic amines—To a volume of Meglumine Iotalamate Injection, equivalent to 0.20 g of Iotalamic Acid, add 15 mL of water, shake, add 4 mL of a solution of sodium nitrite (1 in 100) under ice-cooling, and proceed as directed in the Purity (2) under Iotalamic Acid: the absorbance is not more than 0.17.

(2) Iodine and iodide—Take a volume of Meglumine Iotalamate Injection, equivalent to 1.5 g of Iotalamic Acid, add 20 mL of water and 5 mL of dilute sulfuric acid, shake well, and filter the precipitate by suction throuth a glass filter (G4). To the filtrate add 5 mL of toluene, and shake vigorously: the toluene layer is colorless. Then add 2 mL of a solution of sodium nitrite (1 in 100), and shake vigorously: the toluene layer has no more color than the following control solution.

Control solution: Dissolve 0.25 g of potassium iodide in water to make 1000 mL. To 2.0 mL of this solution add 20 mL of water, 5 mL of dilute sulfuric acid, 5 mL of toluene and 2 mL of a solution of sodium nitrite (1 in 100), and shake vigorously.

Extractable volume <*6.05*> It meets the requirement.

Foreign insoluble matter <*6.06*> Perform the test according to Method 1: it meets the requirement.

Insoluble particulate matter <*6.07*> It meets the requirement.

Sterility <*4.06*> Perform the test according to the Membrane filtration method: it meets the requirement.

Assay To an exactly measured volume of Meglumine Iotalamate Injection, equivalent to about 4 g of iotalamic acid ($C_{11}H_9I_3N_2O_4$), add water to make exactly 200 mL. Pipet 2 mL of this solution, add water to make exactly 200 mL. To exactly 5 mL of this solution add exactly 5 mL of the internal standard solution, add the mobile phase to make 100 mL, and use this solution as the sample solution. Separately, weigh accurately about 0.4 g of iotalamic acid for assay, previously dried at 105°C for 4 hours, dissolve in 100 mL of water and 1 mL of sodium hydroxide TS, and add water to make exactly 200 mL. Pipet 5 mL of this solution, add water to make exactly 50 mL. To exactly 5 mL of this solution add exactly 5 mL of the internal standard solution, add the mobile phase to make 100 mL, and use this solution as the standard solution. Perform the test with 10 μL each of the sample solution and standard solution as directed under Liquid Chromatography <2.01> according to the following conditions, and calculate the ratios, Q_T and Q_S, of the peak area of iotalamic acid to that of the internal standard.

Amount (mg) of iotalamic acid ($C_{11}H_9I_3N_2O_4$)
$= M_S \times Q_T/Q_S \times 10$

M_S: Amount (mg) of iotalamic acid for assay taken

Internal standard solution—A solution of L-tryptophan in the mobile phase (3 in 2500).

Operating conditions—

Detector: An ultraviolet absorption photometer (wavelength: 240 nm).

Column: A stainless steel column 4.6 mm in inside diameter and 15 cm in length, packed with octadecylsilanized silica gel for liquid chromatography (5 μm in particle diameter).

Column temperature: A constant temperature of about 20°C.

Mobile phase: Dissolve 3.9 g of phosphoric acid and 2.8 mL of triethylamine in water to make 2000 mL. To this solution add 100 mL of acetonitrile.

Flow rate: Adjust so that the retention time of iotalamic acid is about 6 minutes.

System suitability—

System performance: When the procedure is run with 10 μL of the standard solution under the above operating conditions, iotalamic acid and the internal standard are eluted in this order with the resolution between these peaks being not less than 5.

System repeatability: When the test is repeated 6 times with 10 μL of the standard solution under the above operating conditions, the relative standard deviation of the ratios of the peak area of iotalamic acid to that of the internal standard is not more than 1.0%.

Containers and storage Containers—Hermetic containers, and colored containers may be used.

Storage—Light-resistant.

Meglumine Sodium Amidotrizoate Injection

アミドトリゾ酸ナトリウムメグルミン注射液

Meglumine Sodium Amidotrizoate Injection is an aqueous injection.

It contains not less than 95.0% and not more than 105.0% of the labeled amount of amidotrizoic acid ($C_{11}H_9I_3N_2O_4$: 613.91).

Method of preparation

(1)

Amidotrizoic Acid (anhydrous)	471.78 g
Sodium Hydroxide	5.03 g
Meglumine	125.46 g
Water for Injection or Sterile Water for Injection in Containers	a sufficient quantity
To make	1000 mL

(2)

Amidotorizoic Acid (anhydrous)	597.30 g
Sodium Hydroxide	6.29 g
Meglumine	159.24 g
Water for Injection or Sterile Water for Injection in Containers	a sufficient quantity
To make	1000 mL

Prepare as directed under Injections, with the above ingredients (1) or (2).

Description Meglumine Sodium Amidotrizoate Injection is a clear, colorless to pale yellow, slightly viscous liquid.

It gradually changes in color by light.

Identification **(1)** To a volume of Meglumine Sodium Amidotrizoate Injection, equivalent to 1 g of Amidotrizoic Acid, add 25 mL of water, and add 2.5 mL of dilute hydrochloric acid with stirring: a white precipitate is produced. Filter the precipitate by suction through a glass filter (G4), wash with two 10-mL portions of water, and dry at 105°C for 1 hour. Proceed with the precipitate so obtained as directed in the Identification (2) under Amidotrizoic Acid.

(2) To 1 mL of Meglumine Sodium Amidotrizoate Injection add 1 mL of potassium 1,2-naphthoquinone-4-sulfonate TS and 0.2 mL of sodium hydroxide TS: a deep red color develops.

(3) Meglumine Sodium Amidotrizoate Injection responds to Qualitative Tests <1.09> (1) for sodium salt.

Optical rotation <2.49>

Method of preparation (1) α_D^{20}: −2.91 – −3.36° (100 mm).

Method of preparation (2) α_D^{20}: −3.69 – −4.27° (100 mm).

pH <2.54> 6.0 – 7.7

Purity **(1)** Primary aromatic amines—To a volume of Meglumine Sodium Amidotrizoate Injection, equivalent to 0.20 g of Amidotrizoic Acid, add 6 mL of water, mix, add 4 mL of a solution of sodium nitrite (1 in 100) and 10 mL of 1 mol/L hydrochloric acid TS, and shake. Proceed as directed in the Purity (2) under Amidotrizoic Acid: the absorbance is not more than 0.19.

(2) Iodine and iodide—To a volume of Meglumine Sodium Amidotrizoate Injection, equivalent to 0.25 g of Amidotrizoic Acid, add water to make 20 mL, add 5 mL of dilute nitric acid, shake well, and filter by suction through a glass filter (G4). Add 5 mL of chloroform to the filtrate, and shake vigorously: no color develops in the chloroform layer. Then add 1 mL of hydrogen peroxide (30), and shake vigorously: the chloroform layer has no more color than the following control solution.

Control solution: Dissolve 0.10 g of potassium iodide in water to make 100 mL. Add 20 mL of water to 0.10 mL of this solution, add 5 mL of dilute nitric acid, 5 mL of chloroform and 1 mL of hydrogen peroxide (30), and shake vigorously.

Extractable volume <6.05> It meets the requirement.

Foreign insoluble matter <6.06> Perform the test according to Method 1: it meets the requirement.

Insoluble particulate matter <6.07> It meets the requirement.

Sterility <4.06> Perform the test according to the Membrane filtration method: it meets the requirement.

Assay To an exactly measured volume of Meglumine Sodium Amidotrizoate Injection, equivalent to about 0.5 g of amidotrizoic acid ($C_{11}H_9I_3N_2O_4$), add water to make exactly 200 mL. Pipet 2 mL of this solution, add exactly 10 mL of the internal standard solution and water to make 100 mL, and use this solution as the sample solution. Separately, weigh accurately about 0.25 g of amidotrizoic acid for assay (separately determine the loss on drying *<2.41>* under the same condition as Amidotrizoic Acid), dissolve in a solution of meglumine (3 in 1000) to make exactly 100 mL, then pipet 2 mL of this solution, add exactly 10 mL of the internal standard solution and water to make 100 mL, and use this solution as the standard solution. Perform the test with 5 μL each of the sample solution and standard solution as directed under Liquid Chromatography *<2.01>* according to the following conditions, and calculate the ratios, Q_T and Q_S, of the peak area of amidotrizoic acid to that of the internal standard.

$$\text{Amount (mg) of amidotrizoic acid } (C_{11}H_9I_3N_2O_4) = M_S \times Q_T/Q_S \times 2$$

M_S: Amount (mg) of amidotrizoic acid for assay taken, calculated on the dried basis

Internal standard solution—Dissolve 0.06 g of acetrizoic acid in a solution of meglumine (3 in 1000) to make 100 mL.

Operating conditions—

Detector: An ultraviolet absorption photometer (wavelength: 254 nm).

Column: A stainless steel column 4.6 mm in inside diameter and 25 cm in length, packed with octadecylsilanized silica gel for liquid chromatography (5 μm in particle diameter).

Column temperature: A constant temperature of about 25°C.

Mobile phase: Dissolve 1.7 g of tetrabutylammonium dihydrogen phosphate and 7.0 g of dipotassium hydrogenphosphate in 750 mL of water, adjust the pH to 7.0 with diluted phosphoric acid (1 in 10), add water to make 800 mL, then add 210 mL of acetonitrile, and mix.

Flow rate: Adjust so that the retention time of amidotrizoic acid is about 5 minutes.

System suitability—

System performance: When the procedure is run with 5 μL of the standard solution under the above operating conditions, amidotrizoic acid and the internal standard are eluted in this order with the resolution between these peaks being not less than 6.

System repeatability: When the test is repeated 6 times with 5 μL of the standard solution under the above operating conditions, the relative standard deviation of the ratios of the peak area of amidotrizoic acid to that of the internal standard is not more than 1.0%.

Containers and storage Containers—Hermetic containers, and colored containers may be used.

Storage—Light-resistant.

Melphalan

メルファラン

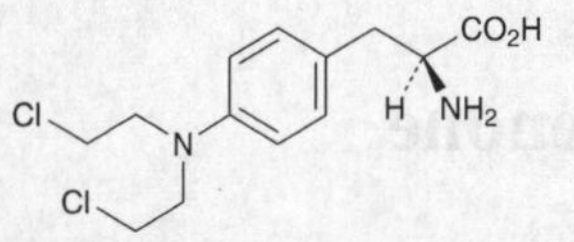

$C_{13}H_{18}Cl_2N_2O_2$: 305.20

4-Bis(2-chloroethyl)amino-L-phenylalanine

[*148-82-3*]

Melphalan contains not less than 93.0% of melphalan ($C_{13}H_{18}Cl_2N_2O_2$), calculated on the dried basis.

Description Melphalan occurs as a white to light yellowish white crystalline powder.

It is slightly soluble in water, in methanol and in ethanol (95), and practically insoluble in diethyl ether.

It dissolves in dilute hydrochloric acid and in dilute sodium hydroxide TS.

It is gradually colored by light.

Optical rotation $[\alpha]_D^{20}$: about −32° (0.5 g calculated on the dried basis, methanol, 100 mL, 100 mm).

Identification **(1)** To 20 mg of Melphalan add 50 mL of methanol, dissolve by warming, add 1 mL of a solution of 4-(4-nitrobenzyl)pyridine in acetone (1 in 20), and evaporate on a water bath to dryness. Dissolve the residue in 1 mL of warmed methanol and add 2 drops of ammonia solution (28): a purple color develops.

(2) Dissolve 0.1 g of Melphalan in 10 mL of dilute sodium hydroxide TS, and heat on a water bath for 10 minutes. After cooling, add dilute nitric acid to acidify, and filter: the filtrate responds to Qualitative Tests *<1.09>* for chloride.

(3) Determine the absorption spectrum of a solution of Melphalan in methanol (1 in 100,000) as directed under Ultraviolet-visible Spectrophotometry *<2.24>*, and compare the spectrum with the Reference Spectrum: both spectra exhibit similar intensities of absorption at the same wavelengths.

Purity **(1)** Ionisable chloride—Weigh accurately about 0.5 g of Melphalan, dissolve in 80 mL of diluted nitric acid (1 in 40), stir for 2 minutes, and titrate *<2.50>* with 0.1 mol/L silver nitrate VS (potentiometric titration): the consumed volume is not more than 1.0 mL to 0.50 g of Melphalan.

(2) Heavy metals *<1.07>*—Proceed with 1.0 g of Melphalan according to Method 4, and perform the test. Prepare the control solution with 2.0 mL of Standard Lead Solution (not more than 20 ppm).

(3) Arsenic *<1.11>*—Prepare the test solution with 1.0 g of Melphalan according to Method 3, and perform the test (not more than 2 ppm).

Loss on drying *<2.41>* Not more than 7.0% (1 g, in vacuum at a pressure not exceeding 0.67 kPa, 105°C, 2 hours).

Residue on ignition *<2.44>* Not more than 0.3% (1 g).

Assay Weigh accurately about 0.25 g of Melphalan, add 20 mL of a solution of potassium hydroxide (1 in 5), and heat under a reflux condenser on a water bath for 2 hours. After cooling, add 75 mL of water and 5 mL of nitric acid, cool, and titrate *<2.50>* with 0.1 mol/L silver nitrate VS (potentiometric titration). Make any necessary correction by using the results obtained in the Purity (1).

Each mL of 0.1 mol/L silver nitrate VS
= 15.26 mg of $C_{13}H_{18}Cl_2N_2O_2$

Containers and storage Containers—Tight containers.
Storage—Light-resistant.

Menatetrenone

メナテトレノン

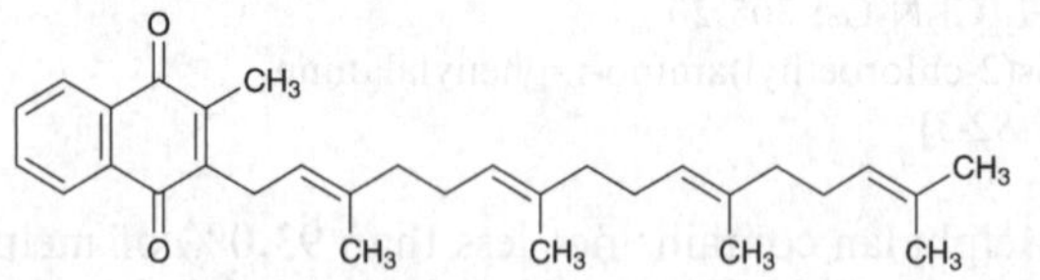

$C_{31}H_{40}O_2$: 444.65
2-Methyl-3-[(2*E*,6*E*,10*E*)-3,7,11,15-tetramethylhexadeca-2,6,10,14-tetraen-1-yl]-1,4-naphthoquinone
[*863-61-6*]

Menatetrenone contains not less than 98.0% of menatetrenone ($C_{31}H_{40}O_2$), calculated on the anhydrous basis.

Description Menatetrenone occurs as yellow, crystals, crystalline powder, waxy mass or oily material.

It is very soluble in hexane, soluble in ethanol (99.5), sparingly soluble in 2-propanol, slightly soluble in methanol, and practically insoluble in water.

It decomposes and the color becomes more intense by light.

Melting point: about 37°C.

Identification **(1)** Dissolve 0.1 g of Menatetrenone in 5 mL of ethanol (99.5) by warming, cool, and add 1 mL of a solution of potassium hydroxide in ethanol (95) (1 in 10): a blue color develops, and upon standing it changes from blue-purple to red-brown through red-purple.

(2) Determine the infrared absorption spectrum of Menatetrenone, after melting by warming if necessary, as directed in the liquid film method under Infrared Spectrophotometry 〈*2.25*〉, and compare the spectrum with the Reference Spectrum or the spectrum of Menatetrenone RS: both spectra exhibit similar intensities of absorption at the same wave numbers.

Purity **(1)** Heavy metals 〈*1.07*〉—Proceed with 1.0 g of Menatetrenone according to Method 4, and perform the test. Prepare the control solution with 2.0 mL of Standard Lead Solution (not more than 20 ppm).

(2) Menadione—To 0.20 g of Menatetrenone add 5 mL of diluted ethanol (1 in 2), shake well, and filter. To 0.5 mL of the filtrate add 1 drop of a solution of 3-methyl-1-phenyl-5-pyrazorone in ethanol (99.5) (1 in 20) and 1 drop of ammonia water (28), and allow to stand for 2 hours: no blue-purple color develops.

(3) *cis* Isomer—Dissolve 0.10 g of Menatetrenone in 10 mL of hexane, and use this solution as the sample solution. Pipet 1 mL of the sample solution, add hexane to make exactly 50 mL, and use this solution as the standard solution. Perform the test with these solutions as directed under Thin-layer Chromatography 〈*2.03*〉. Spot 10 μL each of the sample solution and standard solution on a plate of silica gel with fluorescent indicator for thin-layer chromatography. Develop the chromatogram with a mixture of hexane and di-*n*-butyl ether (17:3) to a distance of about 12 cm, and air-dry the plate. Examine under ultraviolet light (main wavelength: 254 nm): the spot corresponding to relative *Rf* value 1.1 regarding to the principal spot obtained from the sample solution is not more intense than the spot from the standard solution.

(4) Related substances—Conduct this procedure without exposure to light, using a light-resistant vessel. Dissolve 0.10 g of Menatetrenone in 100 mL of ethanol (99.5), and use this solution as the sample solution. Pipet 1 mL of the sample solution, add ethanol (99.5) to make exactly 100 mL, and use this solution as the standard solution. Perform the test with exactly 20 μL each of the sample solution and standard solution as directed under Liquid Chromatography 〈*2.01*〉 according to the following conditions. Determine each peak area of these solutions by the automatic integration method: the total area of peaks other than the peak of menatetrenone obtained from the sample solution is not larger than the peak area of menatetrenone from the standard solution.

Operating conditions—

Detector, column, column temperature, mobile phase, and flow rate: Proceed as directed in the operating conditions in the Assay.

Time span of measurement: About 6 times as long as the retention time of menatetrenone, beginning after the solvent peak.

System suitability—

System performance: Proceed as directed in the system suitability in the Assay.

Test for required detectability: To exactly 5 mL of the standard solution add ethanol (99.5) to make exactly 50 mL. Confirm that the peak area of menatetrenone obtained with 20 μL of this solution is equivalent to 7 to 13% of that with 20 μL of the standard solution.

System repeatability: When the test is repeated 6 times with 20 μL of the standard solution under the above operating conditions, the relative standard deviation of the peak areas of menatetrenone is not more than 1.0%.

Water 〈*2.48*〉 Not more than 0.5% (0.5 g, volumetric titration, direct titration).

Residue on ignition 〈*2.44*〉 Not more than 0.1% (1 g).

Assay Conduct this procedure without exposure to light, using a light-resistant vessel. Weigh accurately about 0.1 g each of Menatetrenone and Menatetrenone RS (separately, determine the water 〈*2.48*〉 in the same manner as Menatetrenone), dissolve each in 50 mL of 2-propanol, and add ethanol (99.5) to make exactly 100 mL. Pipet 10 mL of these solutions, and add ethanol (99.5) to make exactly 100 mL. Pipet 2 mL each of these solutions, add exactly 4 mL each of the internal standard solution, and use these solutions as the sample solution and standard solution. Perform the test with 20 μL each of the sample solution and standard solution as directed under Liquid Chromatography 〈*2.01*〉 according to the following conditions, and calculate the ratios, Q_T and Q_S, of the peak area of menatetrenone to that of the internal standard.

$$\text{Amount (mg) of menatetrenone } (C_{31}H_{40}O_2) = M_S \times Q_T/Q_S$$

M_S: Amount (mg) of Menatetrenone RS taken, calculated on the dehydrated basis

Internal standard solution—A solution of phytonadione in 2-propanol (1 in 20,000).

Operating conditions—

Detector: An ultraviolet absorption photometer (wavelength: 270 nm).

Column: A stainless steel column 4.6 mm in inside diameter and 15 cm in length, packed with octadecylsilanized silica

gel for liquid chromatography (5 μm in particle diameter).

Column temperature: A constant temperature of about 40°C.

Mobile phase: Methanol.

Flow rate: Adjust so that the retention time of menatetrenone is about 7 minutes.

System suitability—

System performance: When the procedure is run with 20 μL of the standard solution under the above operating conditions, menatetrenone and the internal standard are eluted in this order with the resolution between these peaks being not less than 4.

System repeatability: When the test is repeated 6 times with 20 μL of the standard solution under the above operating conditions, the relative standard deviation of the ratios of the peak area of menatetrenone to that of the internal standard is not more than 1.0%.

Containers and storage Containers—Tight containers.

Storage—Light-resistant.

dl-Menthol

dl-メントール

and enantiomer

$C_{10}H_{20}O$: 156.27
(1*RS*,2*SR*,5*RS*)-5-Methyl-2-(1-methylethyl)cyclohexanol
[*89-78-1*]

dl-Menthol contains not less than 98.0% of *dl*-menthol ($C_{10}H_{20}O$).

Description *dl*-Menthol occurs as colorless crystals. It has a characteristic and refreshing odor and a burning taste, followed by a cool taste.

It is very soluble in ethanol (95) and in diethyl ether, and very slightly soluble in water.

It sublimes gradually at room temperature.

Identification **(1)** Triturate *dl*-Menthol with an equal amount of camphor, chloral hydrate or thymol: the mixture liquefies.

(2) Shake 1 g of *dl*-Menthol with 20 mL of sulfuric acid: the mixture becomes turbid with a yellow-red color. Allow to stand for 3 hours: a clear, oily layer possesses no aroma of menthol is separated.

Congealing point <*2.42*> 27 – 28°C

Optical rotation <*2.49*> $[\alpha]_D^{20}$: −2.0 – +2.0° (2.5 g, ethanol (95), 25 mL, 100 mm).

Purity **(1)** Non-volatile residue—Volatilize 2.0 g of *dl*-Menthol on a water bath, and dry the residue at 105°C for 2 hours: the residue weighs not more than 1.0 mg.

(2) Thymol—Add 0.20 g of *dl*-Menthol to a cold mixture of 2 mL of acetic acid (100), 6 drops of sulfuric acid and 2 drops of nitric acid: no green to blue-green color immediately develops.

(3) Nitromethane or nitroethane—To 0.5 g of *dl*-Menthol placed in a flask add 2 mL of a solution of sodium hydroxide (1 in 2) and 1 mL of hydrogen peroxide (30), connect a reflux condenser to the flask, and boil the mixture gently for 10 minutes. After cooling, add water to make exactly 20 mL, and filter. Take 1 mL of the filtrate in a Nessler tube, add water to make 10 mL, neutralize with dilute hydrochloric acid, then add 1 mL of dilute hydrochloric acid, and cool. To the mixture add 1 mL of a solution of sulfanilic acid (1 in 100), allow to stand for 2 minutes, and then add 1 mL of a solution of *N*,*N*-diethyl-*N′*-1-naphthylethylenediamine oxalate (1 in 1000) and water to make 25 mL: no red-purple color immediately develops.

Assay Weigh accurately about 2 g of *dl*-Menthol, add exactly 20 mL of a mixture of dehydrated pyridine and acetic anhydride (8:1), connect a reflux condenser, and heat on a water bath for 2 hours. Wash down the condenser with 20 mL of water, and titrate <*2.50*> with 1 mol/L sodium hydroxide VS (indicator: 5 drops of phenolphthalein TS). Perform a blank determination in the same manner.

Each mL of 1 mol/L sodium hydroxide VS
= 156.3 mg of $C_{10}H_{20}O$

Containers and storage Containers—Tight containers.

Storage—In a cold place.

l-Menthol

l-メントール

$C_{10}H_{20}O$: 156.27
(1*R*,2*S*,5*R*)-5-Methyl-2-(1-methylethyl)cyclohexanol
[*2216-51-5*]

l-Menthol contains not less than 98.0% of *l*-menthol ($C_{10}H_{20}O$).

Description *l*-Menthol occurs as colorless crystals. It has a characteristic and refreshing odor and a burning taste, followed by a cool taste.

It is very soluble in ethanol (95) and in diethyl ether, and very slightly soluble in water.

It sublimes gradually at room temperature.

Identification **(1)** Triturate *l*-Menthol with an equal amount of camphor, chloral hydrate or thymol: the mixture liquefies.

(2) Shake 1 g of *l*-Menthol with 20 mL of sulfuric acid: the mixture becomes turbid with a yellow-red color. Allow to stand for 3 hours: a clear, oily layer which possesses no aroma of menthol is separated.

Optical rotation <*2.49*> $[\alpha]_D^{20}$: −45.0 – −51.0° (2.5 g, ethanol (95), 25 mL, 100 mm).

Melting point <*2.60*> 42 – 44°C

Purity **(1)** Non-volatile residue—Volatilize 2.0 g of *l*-Menthol on a water bath, and dry the residue at 105°C for 2 hours: the residue weighs not more than 1.0 mg.

(2) Thymol—Add 0.20 g of *l*-Menthol to a cold mixture of 2 mL of acetic acid (100), 6 drops of sulfuric acid and 2 drops of nitric acid: no green to blue-green color immediately develops.

(3) Nitromethane or nitroethane—To 0.5 g of *l*-Menthol placed in a flask add 2 mL of a solution of sodium hydroxide (1 in 2) and 1 mL of hydrogen peroxide (30), connect a reflux condenser to the flask, and boil the mixture gently for 10 minutes. After cooling, add water to make exactly 20 mL, and filter. Take 1 mL of the filtrate in a Nessler tube, add water to make 10 mL, neutralize with dilute hydrochloric acid, add 1 mL of dilute hydrochloric acid, and cool. To the mixture add 1 mL of a solution of sulfanilic acid (1 in 100), allow to stand for 2 minutes, and then add 1 mL of a solution of *N*,*N*-diethyl-*N'*-1-naphthylethylenediamine oxalate (1 in 1000) and water to make 25 mL: no red-purple color immediately develops.

Assay Weigh accurately about 2 g of *l*-Menthol, add exactly 20 mL of a mixture of dehydrated pyridine and acetic anhydride (8:1), connect a reflux condenser, and heat on a water bath for 2 hours. Wash the condenser with 20 mL of water, and titrate <2.50> with 1 mol/L sodium hydroxide VS (indicator: 5 drops of phenolphthalein TS). Perform a blank determination in the same manner.

Each mL of 1 mol/L sodium hydroxide VS
= 156.3 mg of $C_{10}H_{20}O$

Containers and storage Containers—Tight containers.
Storage—In a cold place.

Mepenzolate Bromide

メペンゾラート臭化物

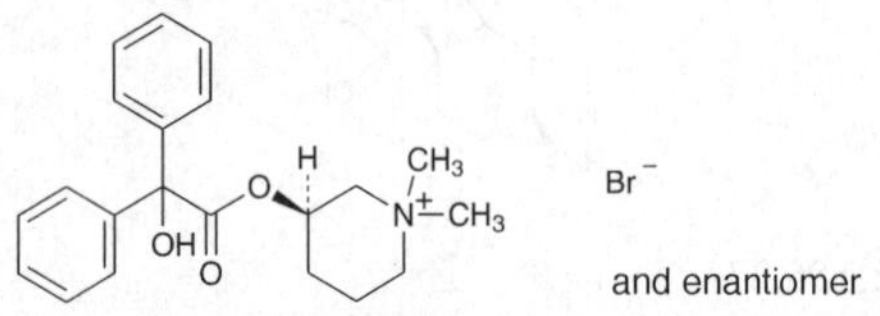

and enantiomer

$C_{21}H_{26}BrNO_3$: 420.34
(3*RS*)-3-[(Hydroxy)(diphenyl)acetoxy]-1,1-dimethylpiperidinium bromide
[*76-90-4*]

Mepenzolate Bromide, when dried, contains not less than 98.5% of mepenzolate bromide ($C_{21}H_{26}BrNO_3$).

Description Mepenzolate Bromide is white to pale yellow, crystals or crystalline powder. It is odorless, and has a bitter taste.

It is very soluble in formic acid, freely soluble in methanol, soluble in hot water, slightly soluble in water and in ethanol (95), very slightly soluble in acetic anhydride, and practically insoluble in diethyl ether.

Melting point: about 230°C (with decomposition).

Identification (1) To 30 mg of Mepenzolate Bromide add 10 drops of sulfuric acid: a red color develops.

(2) Dissolve 10 mg of Mepenzolate Bromide in 20 mL of water and 5 mL of dilute hydrochloric acid, and to 5 mL of this solution add 1 mL of Dragendorff's TS: an orange precipitate is produced.

(3) Determine the absorption spectrum of a solution of Mepenzolate Bromide in 0.01 mol/L hydrochloric acid TS (1 in 2000) as directed under Ultraviolet-visible Spectrophotometry <2.24>, and compare the spectrum with the Reference Spectrum: both spectra exhibit similar intensities of absorption at the same wavelengths.

(4) Dissolve 0.5 g of Mepenzolate Bromide in 50 mL of water and 3 mL of nitric acid by heating. This solution responds to Qualitative Tests <1.09> for Bromide.

Purity (1) Heavy Metals <1.07>—Proceed with 1.0 g of Mepenzolate Bromide according to Method 2, and perform the test. Prepare the control solution with 2.0 mL of Standard Lead Solution (not less than 20 ppm).

(2) Arsenic <1.11>—Prepare the test solution with 1.0 g of Mepenzolate Bromide according to Method 3, and perform the test (not more than 2 ppm).

(3) Related substances—Dissolve 0.40 g of Mepenzolate Bromide in exactly measured 10 mL of methanol, and use this solution as the sample solution. Pipet 1 mL of the sample solution, add methanol to make exactly 200 mL, and use this solution as the standard solution (1). Separately, dissolve 40 mg of benzophenone in methanol to make exactly 100 mL. Pipet 2 mL of this solution, add methanol to make exactly 10 mL, and use this solution as the standard solution (2). Perform the test with these solutions as directed under Thin-layer Chromatography <2.03>. Spot 10 μL each of the sample solution, standard solutions (1) and (2) on a plate of silica gel with fluorecent indicator for thin-layer chromatography. Develop the plate with a mixture of methanol, 1-butanol, water and acetic acid (100) (3:3:2:1) to a distance of about 10 cm, and air-dry the plate and then at 80°C for 30 minutes. Examine under ultraviolet light (main wavelength: 254 nm): the spots other than either the principal spot or the spot corresponding to benzophenone obtained from the sample solution are not more intense than the spot from standard solution (1), and the spot corresponding to benzophenone from the sample solution is not more intense than the spot from standard solution (2). Spray evenly Dragendorff's TS on the plate: the spots other than the principal spot from the sample solution are not more intense than the spot from standard solution (1).

Loss on drying <2.41> Not more than 0.5% (1 g, 105°C, 4 hours).

Residue on ignition <2.44> Not more than 0.1% (1 g).

Assay Weigh accurately about 0.35 g of Mepenzolate Bromide, previously dried, dissolve in 2 mL of formic acid, add 60 mL of acetic anhydride, and titrate <2.50> with 0.1 mol/L perchloric acid VS (potentiometric titration). Perform a blank determination in the same manner, and make any necessary correction.

Each mL of 0.1 mol/L perchloric acid VS
= 42.03 mg of $C_{21}H_{26}BrNO_3$

Containers and storage Containers—Tight containers.

Mepitiostane

メピチオスタン

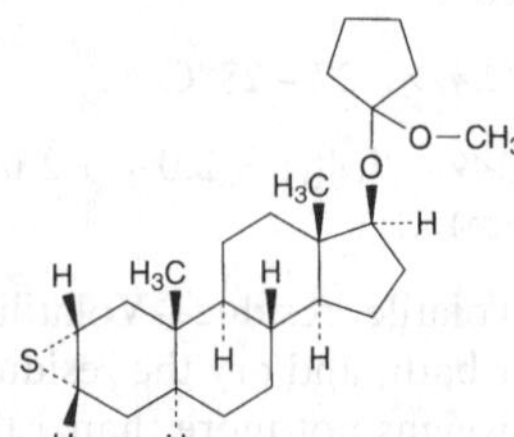

$C_{25}H_{40}O_2S$: 404.65
2α,3α-Epithio-17β-(1-methoxycyclopentyloxy)-5α-androstane
[*21362-69-6*]

Mepitiostane contains not less than 96.0% and not more than 102.0% of mepitiostane ($C_{25}H_{40}O_2S$), calculated on the anhydrous basis.

Description Mepitiostane occurs as white to pale yellow, crystals or crystalline powder.

It is freely soluble in triethylamine, in chloroform, in diethyl ether and in cyclohexane, soluble in diethylene glycol dimethyl ether and in petroleum ether, sparingly soluble in acetone, slightly soluble in methanol and in ethanol (99.5), and practically insoluble in water.

It is hydrolyzed in moist air.

Identification **(1)** Dissolve 1 mg of Mepitiostane in 1 mL of methanol, and add 0.5 mL of palladium (II) chloride TS: an orange precipitate is formed. To this suspension add 1 mL of water and 2 mL of chloroform, shake well, and allow to stand: an orange color develops in the chloroform layer.

(2) Dissolve 0.1 g of Mepitiostane in 2 mL of diethylene glycol dimethyl ether, shake with 1 mL of 1 mol/L hydrochloric acid TS, and filter. To the filtrate add 1.5 mL of 2,4-dinitrophenylhydrazine-diethylene glycol dimethyl ether TS and 1.5 mL of diluted ethanol (95) (2 in 3): an orange-yellow precipitate is formed. Filter the precipitate, recrystallize from ethanol (99.5), and dry in a desiccator (in vacuum, phosphorus (V) oxide) for 4 hours: the crystals melt ⟨*2.60*⟩ between 144°C and 149°C.

(3) Determine the infrared absorption spectrum of Mepitiostane as directed in the potassium bromide disk method under Infrared Spectrophotometry ⟨*2.25*⟩, and compare the spectrum with the Reference Spectrum: both spectra exhibit similar intensities of absorption at the same wave numbers.

Optical rotation ⟨*2.49*⟩ $[\alpha]_D^{20}$: +20 – +23° (0.1 g, chloroform, 10 mL, 100 mm).

Purity **(1)** Clarity and color of solution—Dissolve 0.10 g of Mepitiostane in 4 mL of petroleum ether: the solution is clear and colorless to pale yellow.

(2) Heavy metals ⟨*1.07*⟩—Proceed with 1.0 g of Mepitiostane according to Method 2, and perform the test. Prepare the control solution with 2.0 mL of Standard Lead Solution (not more than 20 ppm).

(3) Related substances—Dissolve 20 mg of Mepitiostane in exactly 5 mL of a mixture of acetone and triethylamine (1000:1), and use this solution as the sample solution. Separately, dissolve 10 mg of Epitiostanol RS in a mixture of acetone and triethylamine (1000:1) to make exactly 10 mL. Pipet 1 mL and 3 mL of this solution, to each add a mixture of acetone and triethylamine (1000:1) to make exactly 25 mL, and use these solutions as the standard solution (1) and the standard solution (2), respectively. Perform the test with these solutions as directed under Thin-layer Chromatography ⟨*2.03*⟩. Spot 5 μL each of the sample solution and standard solutions (1) and (2) on a plate of silica gel with fluorescent indicator for thin-layer chromatography. Develop the plate with a mixture of hexane and acetone (3:1) to a distance of about 10 cm, and air-dry the plate. Spray evenly diluted sulfuric acid (1 in 5) on the plate, heat the plate between 120°C and 130°C for 5 minutes, and examine under ultraviolet light (main wavelength: 365 nm): the spots other than the principal spot obtained from the sample solution showing the same *R*f value as the standard solutions are not more intense than the spot from the standard solution (2), and the remaining spots other than the principal spot are not more intense than the spot from the standard solution (1).

Water ⟨*2.48*⟩ Not more than 0.7% (0.3 g, volumetric titration, back titration).

Residue on ignition ⟨*2.44*⟩ Not more than 0.1% (0.5 g).

Assay Weigh accurately about 0.3 g of Mepitiostane, and dissolve in cyclohexane to make exactly 10 mL. Pipet 2 mL of this solution, add 10 mL of ethanol (99.5), mix with exactly 2 mL each of 0.01 mol/L hydrochloric acid TS and the internal standard solution, add ethanol (99.5) to make 20 mL, allow to stand at ordinary temperature for 30 minutes, and use this solution as the sample solution. Separately, weigh accurately about 45 mg of Epitiostanol RS, dissolve in exactly 2 mL of the internal standard solution, add ethanol (99.5) to make 20 mL, and use this solution as the standard solution. Perform the test with 10 μL each of the sample solution and standard solution as directed under Liquid Chromatography ⟨*2.01*⟩ according to the following conditions, and calculate the ratios, Q_T and Q_S, of the peak area of epitiostanol to that of the internal standard, respectively.

Amount (mg) of mepitiostane ($C_{25}H_{40}O_2S$)
$= M_S \times Q_T/Q_S \times 5 \times 1.320$

M_S: Amount (mg) of Epitiostanol RS taken, calculated on the anhydrous basis

Internal standard solution—A solution of *n*-octylbenzene in ethanol (99.5) (1 in 300).

Operating conditions—

Detector: An ultraviolet absorption photometer (wavelength: 265 nm).

Column: A stainless steel column 4.0 mm in inside diameter and 15 cm in length, packed with octadecylsilanized silica gel for liquid chromatography (10 μm in particle diameter).

Column temperature: A constant temperature of about 25°C.

Mobile phase: A mixture of methanol and water (20:3).

Flow rate: Adjust so that the retention time of epitiostanol is about 6 minutes.

System suitability—

System performance: When the procedure is run with 10 μL of the standard solution under the above operating conditions, epitiostanol and the internal standard are eluted in this order with the resolution between these peaks being not less than 4.

System repeatability: When the test is repeated 6 times with 10 μL of the standard solution under the above operating conditions, the relative standard deviation of the ratios of the peak area of epitiostanol to that of the internal standard is not more than 1.0%.

Containers and storage Containers—Hermetic containers.

Storage—Light-resistant, under Nitrogen atmosphere, and in a cold place.

Mepivacaine Hydrochloride

メピバカイン塩酸塩

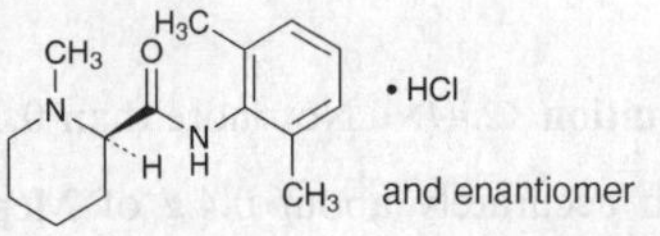

• HCl and enantiomer

$C_{15}H_{22}N_2O.HCl$: 282.81
(2*RS*)-*N*-(2,6-Dimethylphenyl)-1-methylpiperidine-2-carboxamide monohydrochloride
[*1722-62-9*]

Mepivacaine Hydrochloride, when dried, contains not less than 98.5% and not more than 101.0% of mepivacaine hydrochloride ($C_{15}H_{22}N_2O.HCl$).

The JP Drugs are to be tested according to the provisions given in the pertinent monographs, General Notices, General Rules for Crude Drugs, General Rules for Preparations, and General Tests for their conformity to the Japanese Pharmacopoeia. (See the General Notices 5.)

Description Mepivacaine Hydrochloride occurs as white, crystals or crystalline powder.

It is freely soluble in water and in methanol, soluble in acetic acid (100), and sparingly soluble in ethanol (99.5).

A solution of Mepivacaine Hydrochloride (1 in 10) shows no optical rotation.

Melting point: about 256°C (with decomposition).

Identification **(1)** Determine the absorption spectrum of a solution of Mepivacaine Hydrochloride (1 in 2500) as directed under Ultraviolet-visible Spectrophotometry <*2.24*>, and compare the spectrum with the Reference Spectrum: both spectra exhibit similar intensities of absorption at the same wavelengths.

(2) Determine the infrared absorption spectrum of Mepivacaine Hydrochloride as directed in the potassium chloride disk method under Infrared Spectrophotometry <*2.25*>, and compare the spectrum with the Reference Spectrum: both spectra exhibit similar intensities of absorption at the same wave numbers.

(3) A solution of Mepivacaine Hydrochloride (1 in 50) responds to Qualitative Tests <*1.09*> for chloride.

pH <*2.54*> Dissolve 0.2 g of Mepivacaine Hydrochloride in 10 mL of water: the pH of this solution is between 4.0 and 5.0.

Purity **(1)** Clarity and color of solution—Dissolve 1.0 g of Mepivacaine Hydrochloride in 10 mL of water: the solution is clear and colorless.

(2) Sulfate <*1.14*>—Perform the test with 0.5 g of Mepivacaine Hydrochloride. Prepare the control solution with 0.40 mL of 0.005 mol/L sulfuric acid VS (not more than 0.038%).

(3) Heavy metals <*1.07*>—Proceed with 2.0 g of Mepivacaine Hydrochloride according to Method 1, and perform the test. Prepare the control solution with 2.0 mL of Standard Lead Solution (not more than 10 ppm).

(4) Related substances—Dissolve 0.10 g of Mepivacaine Hydrochloride in 5 mL of methanol, and use this solution as the sample solution. Pipet 1 mL of the sample solution, and add methanol to make exactly 20 mL. Pipet 2 mL of this solution, add methanol to make exactly 50 mL, and use this solution as the standard solution. Perform the test with these solutions as directed under Thin-layer Chromatography <*2.03*>. Spot 10 μL each of the sample solution and standard solution on a plate of silica gel for thin-layer chromatography. Develop the plate with a mixture of diethyl ether, methanol and ammonia solution (28) (100:5:1) to a distance of about 10 cm, and air-dry the plate. Spray evenly bismuth nitrate-potassium iodide TS on the plate: the spots other than the principal spot obtained from the sample solution are not more intense than the spot from the standard solution.

Loss on drying <*2.41*> Not more than 1.0% (1 g, 105°C, 3 hours).

Residue on ignition <*2.44*> Not more than 0.1% (1 g).

Assay Weigh accurately about 0.4 g of Mepivacaine Hydrochloride, previously dried, dissolve in 10 mL of acetic acid (100) and add 70 mL of acetic anhydride. Titrate <*2.50*> with 0.1 mol/L perchloric acid VS (potentiometric titration). Perform a blank determination in the same manner, and make any necessary correction.

Each mL of 0.1 mol/L perchloric acid VS
= 28.28 mg of $C_{15}H_{22}N_2O.HCl$

Containers and storage Containers—Tight containers.

Mepivacaine Hydrochloride Injection

メピバカイン塩酸塩注射液

Mepivacaine Hydrochloride Injection is an aqueous injection.

It contains not less than 95.0% and not more than 105.0% of the labeled amount of mepivacaine hydrochloride ($C_{15}H_{22}N_2O.HCl$: 282.81).

Method of preparation Prepare as directed under Injections, with Mepivacaine Hydrochloride.

Description Mepivacaine Hydrochloride Injection is a clear, colorless liquid.

Identification To a volume of Mepivacaine Hydrochloride Injection, equivalent to 20 mg of Mepivacaine Hydrochloride, add 1 mL of sodium hydrochloride TS, and extract with 20 mL of hexane. To 8 mL of the hexane extract add 20 mL of 1 mol/L hydrochloric acid TS, shake vigorously, and determine the absorption spectrum of the water layer separated as directed under Ultraviolet-visible Spectrophotometry <*2.24*>: it exhibits maxima between 261 nm and 265 nm, and between 270 nm and 273 nm.

pH Being specified separately when the drug is granted approval based on the Law.

Bacterial endotoxins <*4.01*> Less than 0.6 EU/mg.

Extractable volume <*6.05*> It meets the requirement.

Foreign insoluble matter <*6.06*> Perform the test according to Method 1: it meets the requirement.

Insoluble particulate matter <*6.07*> It meets the requirement.

Sterility <*4.06*> Perform the test according to the Membrane filtration method: it meets the requirement.

Assay Pipet a volume of Mepivacaine Hydrochloride Injection, equivalent to about 40 mg of mepivacaine hydrochloride ($C_{15}H_{22}N_2O.HCl$), add exactly 4 mL of the internal standard solution and 0.001 mol/L hydrochloric acid TS to make 20 mL, and use this solution as the sample solution. Separately, weigh accurately about 40 mg of mepivacaine hydrochloride for assay, previously dried at 105°C for 3 hours, dissolve in 0.001 mol/L hydrochloric acid TS, add exactly 4 mL of the internal standard solution and 0.001 mol/L hydrochloride TS to make 20 mL, and use this solution as the standard solution. Perform the test with 5 μL each of the sample solution and standard solution as directed under Liquid Chromatography <*2.01*> according to the following conditions, and calculate the ratios, Q_T and Q_S, of the peak area of mepivacaine to that of the internal standard.

Amount (mg) of mepivacaine hydrochloride
($C_{15}H_{22}N_2O.HCl$)
$= M_S \times Q_T/Q_S$

M_S: Amount (mg) of mepivacaine hydrochloride for assay taken

Internal standard solution—A solution of benzophenone in methanol (1 in 4000).

Operating conditions—

Detector: An ultraviolet absorption photometer (wavelength: 254 nm).

Column: A stainless steel column about 4 mm in inside diameter and 15 cm in length, packed with octadecylsilanized silica gel for liquid chromatography (10 μm in particle diameter).

Column temperature: A constant temperature of about 25°C.

Mobile phase: Dissolve 2.88 g of sodium lauryl sulfate in 1000 mL of a mixture of 0.02 mol/L phosphate buffer solution (pH 3.0) and acetonitrile (11:9).

Flow rate: Adjust so that the retention time of mepivacaine is about 6 minutes.

System suitability—

System performance: When the procedure is run with 5 μL of the standard solution under the above operating conditions, mepivacaine and the internal standard are eluted in this order with the resolution between these peaks being not less than 6.

System repeatability: When the test is repeated 6 times with 5 μL of the standard solution under the above operating conditions, the relative standard deviation of the ratio of the peak area of mepivacaine to that of the internal standard is not more than 1.0%.

Containers and storage Containers—Hermetic containers.

Mequitazine

メキタジン

and enantiomer

$C_{20}H_{22}N_2S$: 322.47
10-[(3*RS*)-1-Azabicyclo[2.2.2]oct-3-ylmethyl]-10*H*-phenothiazine
[*29216-28-2*]

Mequitazine contains not less than 98.5% of mequitazine ($C_{20}H_{22}N_2S$), calculated on the dried basis.

Description Mequitazine occurs as white, crystals or crystalline powder.

It is freely soluble in methanol and in acetic acid (100), soluble in ethanol (95), and practically insoluble in water.

It is gradually colored by light.

A solution of Mequitazine in methanol (1 in 50) shows no optical rotation.

Identification **(1)** Determine the absorption spectrum of a solution of Mequitazine in ethanol (95) (1 in 250,000) as directed under Ultraviolet-visible Spectrophotometry <*2.24*>, and compare the spectrum with the Reference Spectrum: both spectra exhibit similar intensities of absorption at the same wavelengths.

(2) Determine the infrared absorption spectrum of Mequitazine, previously dried, as directed in the potassium bromide disk method under Infrared Spectrophotometry <*2.25*>, and compare the spectrum with the Reference Spectrum: both spectra exhibit similar intensities of absorption at the same wave numbers.

Melting point <*2.60*> 146 – 150°C

Purity **(1)** Heavy metals <*1.07*>—Proceed with 1.0 g of Mequitazine according to Method 2, and perform the test. Prepare the control solution with 2.0 mL of Standard Lead Solution (not more than 20 ppm).

(2) Related substances—Conduct this procedure without exposure to light, using light-resistant vessels. Dissolve 50 mg of Mequitazine in 5 mL of methanol, and use this solution as the sample solution. Pipet 1 mL of the sample solution, add methanol to make exactly 50 mL, then pipet 5 mL of this solution, add methanol to make exactly 50 mL, and use this solution as the standard solution. Perform the test with these solutions as directed under Thin-layer Chromatography <*2.03*>. Spot 5 μL each of the sample solution and standard solution on a plate of silica gel with fluorescent indicator for thin-layer chromatography. Develop with a mixture of ethyl acetate, methanol and diethylamine (7:2:2) to a distance of about 10 cm, and air-dry the plate. Examine under ultraviolet light (main wavelength: 254 nm): the number of the spot other than the principal spot obtained from the sample solution is not more than 3 and they are not more intense than the spot from the standard solution.

Loss on drying <*2.41*> Not more than 0.5% (1 g, in vacuum, phosphorus (V) oxide, 60°C, 3 hours).

Residue on ignition <*2.44*> Not more than 0.1% (1 g).

Assay Weigh accurately about 0.25 g of Mequitazine, dissolve in 50 mL of acetic acid (100), titrate <*2.50*> with 0.1 mol/L perchloric acid VS (potentiometric titration). Perform a blank determination in the same manner, and make any necessary correction.

Each mL of 0.1 mol/L perchloric acid VS
= 32.25 mg of $C_{20}H_{22}N_2S$

Containers and storage Containers—Tight containers.

Storage—Light-resistant.

Mequitazine Tablets

メキタジン錠

Mequitazine Tablets contain not less than 95.0% and not more than 105.0% of the labeled amount of mequitazine ($C_{20}H_{22}N_2S$: 322.47).

Method of preparation Prepare as directed under Tablets, with Mequitazine.

Identification Powder Mequitazine Tablets. To a portion of the powder, equivalent to 3 mg of Mequitazine, add 50 mL of ethanol (95), shake thoroughly, and add ethanol (95) to make 100 mL. Centrifuge, if necessary, and filter the supernatant liquid through a membrane filter with a pore size not exceeding 0.5 μm. Discard 10 mL of the first filtrate, to 4 mL of the subsequent filtrate add ethanol (95) to make 25 mL, and determine the absorption spectrum of this solution as directed under Ultraviolet-visible Spectrophotometry <*2.24*>: it exhibits maxima between 253 nm and 257 nm and between 301 nm and 311 nm.

Uniformity of dosage units <*6.02*> Perform the test according to the following method: it meets the requirement of the Content uniformity test.

To 1 tablet of Mequitazine Tablets add 50 mL of a mixture of methanol and water (4:3), and disperse to fine particles by sonicating. Shake this solution thoroughly, and add methanol to make exactly 100 mL. Centrifuge, if necessary, and filter the supernatant liquid through a membrane filter with a pore size not exceeding 0.5 μm. Discard 10 mL of the first filtrate, pipet V mL of the subsequent filtrate, add methanol to make exactly V' mL so that each mL contains about 4.8 μg of mequitazine ($C_{20}H_{22}N_2S$), and use this solution as the sample solution. Then, proceed as directed in the Assay.

Amount (mg) of mequitazine ($C_{20}H_{22}N_2S$)
$= M_S \times A_T/A_S \times V'/V \times 1/50$

M_S: Amount (mg) of mequitazine for assay taken

Dissolution *<6.10>* When the test is performed at 50 revolutions per minute according to the Paddle method, using 900 mL of 2nd fluid for dissolution test as the dissolution medium, the dissolution rate in 45 minutes of Mequitazine Tablets is not less than 70%.

Start the test with 1 tablet of Mequitazine Tablets, withdraw not less than 20 mL of the medium at the specified minute after starting the test, and filter through a membrane filter with a pore size not exceeding 0.5 μm. Discard not less than 10 mL of the first filtrate, pipet V mL of the subsequent filtrate, add the dissolution medium to make exactly V' mL so that each mL contains about 3.3 μg of mequitazine ($C_{20}H_{22}N_2S$), and use this solution as the sample solution. Separately, weigh accurately about 15 mg of mequitazine for assay, previously dried in vacuum at 60°C using phosphorous (V) oxide as the desiccant for 3 hours, dissolve in 50 mL of methanol, and add the dissolution medium to make exactly 100 mL. Pipet 5 mL of this solution, add the dissolution medium to make exactly 200 mL, and use this solution as the standard solution. Determine the absorbances, A_T and A_S, of the sample solution and standard solution at 253 nm as directed under Ultraviolet-visible Spectrophotometry *<2.24>*, using the dissolution medium as the control.

Dissolution rate (%) with respect to the labeled amount of mequitazine ($C_{20}H_{22}N_2S$)
$= M_S \times A_T/A_S \times V'/V \times 1/C \times 45/2$

M_S: Amount (mg) of mequitazine for assay taken
C: Labeled amount (mg) of mequitazine ($C_{20}H_{22}N_2S$) in 1 tablet

Assay Weigh accurately the mass of not less than 20 Mequitazine Tablets, and powder. Weigh accurately a portion of the powder, equivalent to about 3 mg of mequitazine ($C_{20}H_{22}N_2S$), add 50 mL of a mixture of methanol and water (4:3), shake thoroughly, and add methanol to make exactly 100 mL. Centrifuge, if necessary, and filter the supernatant liquid through a membrane filter with a pore size not exceeding 0.5 μm. Discard 10 mL of the first filtrate, pipet 4 mL of the subsequent filtrate, add methanol to make exactly 25 mL, and use this solution as the sample solution. Separately, weigh accurately about 24 mg of mequitazine for assay, previously dried in vacuum at 60°C using phosphorous (V) oxide as the desiccant for 3 hours, and dissolve in methanol to make exactly 50 mL. Pipet 1 mL of this solution, add methanol to make exactly 100 mL, and use this solution as the standard solution. Determine the absorbances, A_T and A_S, of the sample solution and standard solution at 254 nm as directed under Ultraviolet-visible Spectrophotometry *<2.24>*.

Amount (mg) of mequitazine ($C_{20}H_{22}N_2S$)
$= M_S \times A_T/A_S \times 1/8$

M_S: Amount (mg) of mequitazine for assay taken

Containers and storage Containers—Tight containers.

Storage—Light-resistant.

Mercaptopurine Hydrate

メルカプトプリン水和物

$C_5H_4N_4S.H_2O$: 170.19
1,7-Dihydro-6*H*-purine-6-thione monohydrate
[6112-76-1]

Mercaptopurine Hydrate contains not less than 98.0% of mercaptopurine ($C_5H_4N_4S$: 152.18), calculated on the anhydrous basis.

Description Mercaptopurine Hydrate occurs as light yellow to yellow, crystals or crystalline powder. It is odorless.

It is practically insoluble in water, in acetone and in diethyl ether.

It dissolves in sodium hydroxide TS and in ammonia TS.

Identification **(1)** Dissolve 0.6 g of Mercaptopurine Hydrate in 6 mL of sodium hydroxide solution (3 in 100), and add slowly 0.5 mL of iodomethane with vigorous stirring. Stir well for 10 minutes, cool in an ice bath, and adjust the pH with acetic acid (31) to about 5. Collect the separated crystals by filtration, recrystallize from water, and dry at 120°C for 30 minutes: the crystals melt *<2.60>* between 218°C and 222°C (with decomposition).

(2) Determine the absorption spectrum of a solution of Mercaptopurine Hydrate in 0.1 mol/L hydrochloric acid TS (1 in 200,000) as directed under Ultraviolet-visible Spectrophotometry *<2.24>*, and compare the spectrum with the Reference Spectrum: both spectra exhibit similar intensities of absorption at the same wavelengths.

Purity **(1)** Clarity of solution—Dissolve 0.20 g of Mercaptopurine Hydrate in 10 mL of ammonia TS: the solution is clear.

(2) Sulfate *<1.14>*—Dissolve 50 mg of Mercaptopurine Hydrate in 10 mL of dilute hydrochloric acid, add 5 drops of barium chloride TS, and allow to stand for 5 minutes: no turbidity is produced.

(3) Heavy metals *<1.07>*—Proceed with 1.0 g of Mercaptopurine Hydrate according to Method 2, and perform the test. Prepare the control solution with 2.0 mL of Standard Lead Solution (not more than 20 ppm).

(4) Hypoxanthine—Dissolve 50 mg of Mercaptopurine Hydrate in exactly 10 mL of a solution of ammonia solution (28) in methanol (1 in 10), and use this solution as the sample solution. Separately, dissolve 5.0 mg of hypoxanthine in a solution of ammonia solution (28) in methanol (1 in 10) to make exactly 100 mL, and use this solution as the standard solution. Perform the test with these solutions as directed under Thin-layer Chromatography *<2.03>*. Spot 10 μL each of the sample solution and standard solution on a plate of silica gel with fluorescent indicator for thin-layer chromatography. Develop the plate with a mixture of methanol, chloroform, *n*-butyl formate and ammonia solution (28) (8:6:4:1) to a distance of about 10 cm, and air-dry the plate. Examine under ultraviolet light (main wavelength: 254 nm): the spot obtained from the sample solution observed at the same place as that from the standard solution, is not larger and not more intense than that from the standard solution.

(5) Phosphorus—Take 0.20 g of Mercaptopurine Hydrate in a crucible, add 2 mL of diluted sulfuric acid (3 in 7), then heat gently, slowly adding dropwise several 0.5-mL portions of nitric acid, until the liquid becomes colorless. Continue to heat until most of the liquid has evaporated, cool, and dissolve the residue in 10 mL of water. Transfer the solution to a 25-mL volumetric flask, wash the crucible with two 4-mL portions of water, combine the washings with the solution in the volumetric flask, and use this solution as the sample solution. Separately, dissolve 0.4396 g of potassium dihydrogen phosphate in water to make exactly 200 mL. To 2.0 mL of this solution add water to make exactly 100 mL. Transfer 2.0 mL of this solution to a 25-mL volumetric flask, add 16 mL of water, and use this solution as the standard solution. To the sample solution and standard solution add 1 mL of diluted sulfuric acid (3 in 7), 0.5 mL of nitric acid, 0.75 mL of hexaammonium heptamolybdate TS, 1 mL of 1-amino-2-naphthol-4-sulfonic acid TS and water to make 25 mL, and allow to stand for 5 minutes. Perform the test with these solutions as directed under Ultraviolet-visible Spectrophotometry ⟨*2.24*⟩, using water as the blank: the absorbance of the subsequent solution of the sample solution at 750 nm is not larger than that of the subsequent solution of the standard solution.

Water ⟨*2.48*⟩ 10.0 – 12.0% (0.2 g, volumetric titration, back titration).

Residue on ignition ⟨*2.44*⟩ Not more than 0.1% (1 g).

Assay Weigh accurately about 0.25 g of Mercaptopurine Hydrate, dissolve in 90 mL of *N,N*-dimethylformamide, and titrate ⟨*2.50*⟩ with 0.1 mol/L tetramethylammonium hydroxide VS (potentiometric titration). Perform a blank determination in the same manner with a mixture of 90 mL of *N,N*-dimethylformamide and 15 mL of water, and make any necessary correction.

Each mL of 0.1 mol/L tetramethylammonium hydroxide VS
= 15.22 mg of $C_5H_4N_4S$

Containers and storage Containers—Well-closed containers.

Meropenem Hydrate

メロペネム水和物

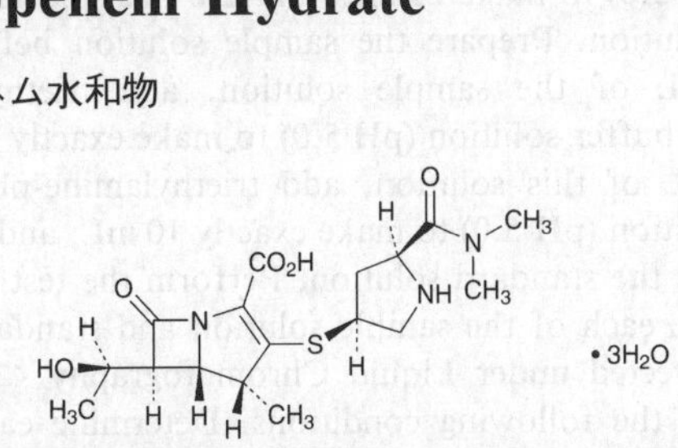

$C_{17}H_{25}N_3O_5S.3H_2O$: 437.51
(4*R*,5*S*,6*S*)-3-[(3*S*,5*S*)-5-(Dimethylcarbamoyl)pyrrolidin-3-ylsulfanyl]-6-[(1*R*)-1-hydroxyethyl]-4-methyl-7-oxo-1-azabicyclo[3.2.0]hept-2-ene-2-carboxylic acid trihydrate
[*119478-56-7*]

Meropenem Hydrate contains not less than 980 μg (potency) and not more than 1010 μg (potency) per mg, calculated on the anhydrous basis. The potency of Meropenem Hydrate is expressed as mass (potency) of meropenem ($C_{17}H_{25}N_3O_5S$: 383.46).

Description Meropenem Hydrate occurs as a white to light yellow crystalline powder.

It is sparingly soluble in water, and practically insoluble in ethanol (95) and in diethyl ether.

It dissolves in sodium hydrogen carbonate TS.

Identification **(1)** Dissolve 10 mg of Meropenem Hydrate in 2 mL of water, add 3 mL of hydroxylammonium chloride-ethanol TS, allow to stand for 5 minutes, add 1 mL of acidic ammonium iron (III) sulfate TS, and shake: a red-brown color develops.

(2) Determine the absorption spectra of solutions of Meropenem Hydrate and Meropenem RS (3 in 100,000) as directed under Ultraviolet-visible Spectrophotometry ⟨*2.24*⟩, and compare the spectra: both spectra exhibit similar intensities of absorption at the same wavelengths.

(3) Determine the infrared absorption spectra of Meropenem Hydrate and Meropenem RS as directed in the potassium bromide disk method under Infrared Spectrophotometry ⟨*2.25*⟩, and compare the spectra: both spectra exhibit similar intensities of absorption at the same wave numbers.

Optical rotation ⟨*2.49*⟩ $[\alpha]_D^{20}$: $-17 - -21°$ (0.22 g calculated on the anhydrous basis, water, 50 mL, 100 mm).

pH ⟨*2.54*⟩ Dissolve 0.2 g of Meropenem Hydrate in 20 mL of water: the pH of the solution is between 4.0 and 6.0.

Purity **(1)** Clarity and color of solution—Dissolve 0.5 g of Meropenem Hydrate in 10 mL of sodium hydrogen carbonate TS: the solution is clear and has no more color than the following control solution.

Control solution: To a mixture of 0.3 mL of Cobalt (II) Chloride CS and 1.2 mL of Iron (III) Chloride CS add 18.5 mL of diluted hydrochloric acid (1 in 40).

(2) Heavy metals ⟨*1.07*⟩—Proceed with 2.0 g of Meropenem Hydrate according to Method 2, and perform the test. Prepare the control solution with 2.0 mL of Standard Lead Solution (not more than 10 ppm).

(3) Related substances—Dissolve 50 mg of Meropenem Hydrate in 10 mL of triethylamine-phosphate buffer solution (pH 5.0), and use this solution as the sample solution. Prepare the sample solution before use. Pipet 1 mL of the sample solution, and add triethylamine-phosphate buffer solution (pH 5.0) to make exactly 100 mL. Pipet 3 mL of this solution, add triethylamine-phosphate buffer solution (pH 5.0) to make exactly 10 mL, and use this solution as the standard solution. Perform the test with exactly 10 μL each of the sample solution and standard solution as directed under Liquid Chromatography ⟨*2.01*⟩ according to the following conditions, and determine each peak area by the automatic integration method: the peak area of ring-opened meropenem, having the relative retention time about 0.5 to meropenem, and the peak area of the dimmer, having the relative retention time about 2.2 to meropenem, obtained from the sample solution are not larger than the peak area of meropenem from the standard solution, the area of the peak other than meropenem and the peaks mentioned above from the sample solution is not larger than 1/3 times the peak area of meropenem from the standard solution, and the total area of the peaks other than meropenem from the sample solution is not larger than 3 times the peak area of meropenem from the standard solution.

Operating conditions—

Detector: An ultraviolet absorption photometer (wavelength: 220 nm).

Column: A stainless steel column 6.0 mm in inside diameter and 15 cm in length, packed with octadecylsilanized silica gel for liquid chromatography (5 μm in particle diameter).

Column temperature: A constant temperature of about 40°C.

Mobile phase: A mixture of triethylamine-phosphate buffer solution (pH 5.0) and acetonitrile (100:7).

Flow rate: Adjust so that the retention time of meropenem is about 6 minutes.

Time span of measurement: About 7 times as long as the retention time of meropenem.

System suitability—

Test for required detectability: Pipet 5 mL of the standard solution, and add triethylamine-phosphate buffer solution (pH 5.0) to make exactly 25 mL. Confirm that the peak area of meropenem obtained with 10 μL of this solution is equivalent to 16 to 24% of that with 10 μL of the standard solution.

System performance: Warm the sample solution at 60°C for 30 minutes. When the procedure is run with 10 μL of this solution under the above operating conditions, the ring-opened meropenem, meropenem and the dimer are eluted in this order, and the resolution between the peaks of the ring-opened meropenem and meropenem is not less than 1.5.

System repeatability: When the test is repeated 6 times with 10 μL of the standard solution under the above operating conditions, the relative standard deviation of the peak area of meropenem is not more than 1.5%.

Water <*2.48*> Not less than 11.4% and not more than 13.4% (0.35 g, volumetric titration, direct titration).

Residue on ignition <*2.44*> Not more than 0.1% (1 g).

Assay Weigh accurately an amount of Meropenem Hydrate and Meropenem RS, equivalent to about 50 mg (potency), dissolve each in exactly 10 mL of the internal standard solution, add triethylamine-phosphate buffer solution (pH 5.0) to make 100 mL, and use these solutions as the sample solution and the standard solution, respectively. Perform the test with 5 μL of the sample solution and standard solution as directed under Liquid Chromatography <*2.01*> according to the following conditions, and calculate the ratios, Q_T and Q_S, of the peak area of meropenem to that of the internal standard.

$$\text{Amount } [\mu\text{g (potency)}] \text{ of meropenem } (C_{17}H_{25}N_3O_5S) = M_S \times Q_T/Q_S \times 1000$$

M_S: Amount [mg (potency)] of Meropenem RS taken

*Internal standard solution—*A solution of benzyl alcohol in triethylamine-phosphate buffer solution (pH 5.0) (1 in 300).

Operating conditions—

Detector: An ultraviolet absorption photometer (wavelength: 220 nm).

Column: A stainless steel column 6.0 mm in inside diameter and 15 cm in length, packed with octadecylsilanized silica gel for liquid chromatography (5 μm in particle diameter).

Column temperature: A constant temperature of about 25°C.

Mobile phase: A mixture of triethylamine-phosphate buffer solution (pH 5.0) and methanol (5:1).

Flow rate: Adjust so that the retention time of meropenem is about 7 minutes.

System suitability—

System performance: When the procedure is run with 5 μL of the standard solution under the above operating conditions, meropenem and the internal standard are eluted in this order with the resolution between these peaks being not less than 20.

System repeatability: When the test is repeated 6 times with 5 μL of the standard solution under the above operating conditions, the relative standard deviation of the ratios of the peak area of meropenem to that of the internal standard is not more than 1.0%.

Containers and storage Containers—Tight containers.

Meropenem for Injection

注射用メロペネム

Meropenem for Injection is a preparation for injection, which is dissolved before use.

It contains not less than 93.0% and not more than 107.0% of the labeled potency of meropenem ($C_{17}H_{25}N_3O_5S$: 383.46).

Method of preparation Prepare as directed under Injections, with Meropenem Hydrate.

Description Meropenem for Injection occurs as a white to light yellow crystalline powder.

Identification Determine the infrared absorption spectrum of Meropenem for Injection as directed in the potassium bromide disk method under Infrared Spectrophotometry <*2.25*>: it exhibits absorption at the wave numbers of about 3410 cm^{-1}, 1750 cm^{-1}, 1655 cm^{-1}, 1583 cm^{-1} and 1391 cm^{-1}.

pH <*2.54*> Dissolve an amount of Meropenem for Injection, equivalent to 0.25 g (potency) of Meropenem Hydrate, in 5 mL of water: the pH of the solution is between 7.3 and 8.3.

Purity (1) Clarity and color of solution—Dissolve an amount of Meropenem for Injection, equivalent to 1.0 g (potency) of Meropenem Hydrate, in 20 mL of water: the solution is clear and is not more intensely colored than the following control solution.

Control solution: To a mixture of 0.3 mL of Cobalt (II) Chloride CS and 1.2 mL of Iron (III) Chloride CS add 18.5 mL of diluted hydrochloric acid (1 in 40).

(2) Related substances—Dissolve an amount of Meropenem for Injection, equivalent to 0.10 g (potency) of Meropenem Hydrate, in triethylamine-phosphate buffer solution (pH 5.0) to make 25 mL, and use this solution as the sample solution. Prepare the sample solution before use. Pipet 1 mL of the sample solution, add triethylamine-phosphate buffer solution (pH 5.0) to make exactly 100 mL. Pipet 5 mL of this solution, add triethylamine-phosphate buffer solution (pH 5.0) to make exactly 10 mL, and use this solution as the standard solution. Perform the test with exactly 10 μL each of the sample solution and standard solution as directed under Liquid Chromatography <*2.01*> according to the following conditions. Determine each peak area by the automatic integration method: the peak area of ring-opened meropenem and meropenem dimer, respectively having the relative retention time of about 0.5 and about 2.2 to meropenem obtained from the sample solution is not larger than the peak area of meropenem from the standard solution, the area of the peak, other than meropenem and the peaks mentioned above, is not larger than 1/5 times the peak area of meropenem from the standard solution, and the total area of the peaks other than meropenem is not larger than 3 times the peak area of meropenem from the standard solution.

Operating conditions—

Proceed as directed in the operating conditions in the

Purity (3) under Meropenem Hydrate.

System suitability—

Test for required detectability: Pipet 5 mL of the standard solution, and add triethylamine-phosphate buffer solution (pH 5.0) to make exactly 25 mL. Confirm that the peak area of meropenem obtained with 10 μL of this solution is equivalent to 16 to 24% of that with 10 μL of the standard solution.

System performance: When the procedure is run with 10 μL of the sample solution, previously allowed to stand at 60°C for 30 minutes, under the above operating conditions, the ring-opened meropenem, meropenem and the meropenem dimer are eluted in this order, and the resolution between the peaks of the ring-opened meropenem and meropenem is not less than 1.5.

System repeatability: When the test is repeated 6 times with 10 μL of the standard solution under the above operating conditions, the relative standard deviation of the peak area of meropenem is not more than 1.5%.

Loss on drying ⟨*2.41*⟩ 9.5 – 12.0% (0.1 g, reduced pressure not exceeding 0.67 kPa, 60°C, 3 hours).

Bacterial endotoxins ⟨*4.01*⟩ Less than 0.12 EU/mg (potency).

Uniformity of dosage units ⟨*6.02*⟩ It meets the requirement of the Mass variation test.

Foreign insoluble matter ⟨*6.06*⟩ Perform the test according to Method 2: it meets the requirement.

Insoluble particulate matter ⟨*6.07*⟩ It meets the requirement.

Sterility ⟨*4.06*⟩ Perform the test according to the Membrane filtration method: it meets the requirement.

Assay Weigh accurately the mass of the contents of not less than 10 containers of Meropenem for Injection. Weigh accurately an amount of the contents, equivalent to about 50 mg (potency) of Meropenem Hydrate, dissolve in exactly 10 mL of the internal standard solution, add triethylamine-phosphate buffer solution (pH 5.0) to make 100 mL, and use this solution as the sample solution. Separately, weigh accurately an amount of Meropenem RS, equivalent to about 50 mg (potency), dissolve in exactly 10 mL of the internal standard solution, add triethylamine-phosphate buffer solution (pH 5.0) to make 100 mL, and use this solution as the standard solution. Then, proceed as directed in the Assay under Meropenem Hydrate.

Amount [mg (potency)] of meropenem ($C_{17}H_{25}N_3O_5S$)
$= M_S \times Q_T/Q_S$

M_S: Amount [mg (potency)] of Meropenem RS taken

*Internal standard solution—*A solution of benzyl alcohol in triethylamine-phosphate buffer solution (pH 5.0) (1 in 300).

Containers and storage Containers—Hermetic containers. Plastic containers for aqueous injections may be used.

Mesalazine

メサラジン

$C_7H_7NO_3$: 153.14

5-Amino-2-hydroxybenzoic acid

[89-57-6]

Mesalazine, when dried, contains not less than 98.5% and not more than 101.0% of mesalazine ($C_7H_7NO_3$).

Description Mesalazine occurs as white, light gray or reddish-white, crystals or crystalline powder.

It is very slightly soluble in water, and practically insoluble in ethanol (99.5).

It dissolves in dilute hydrochloric acid.

Identification **(1)** Determine the absorption spectrum of a solution of Mesalazine in 0.1 mol/L hydrochloric acid TS (1 in 80,000) as directed under Ultraviolet-visible Spectrophotometry ⟨*2.24*⟩, and compare the spectrum with the Reference Spectrum: both spectra exhibit similar intensities of absorption at the same wavelengths.

(2) Determine the infrared absorption spectrum of Mesalazine, previously dried, as directed in the potassium bromide disk method under Infrared Spectrophotometry ⟨*2.25*⟩, and compare the spectrum with the Reference Spectrum: both spectra exhibit similar intensities of absorption at the same wave numbers.

Purity **(1)** Clarity and color of solution—Perform this procedure while keeping the solution at 40°C. A solution obtained by dissolving 0.5 g of Mesalazine in 20 mL of 1 mol/L hydrochloric acid TS is clear, and its absorbance at 440 nm and 650 nm, determined immediately as directed under Ultraviolet-visible Spectrophotometry ⟨*2.24*⟩, is not more than 0.15 and not more than 0.10, respectively.

(2) Chloride ⟨*1.03*⟩—Dissolve 0.30 g of Mesalazine in 6 mL of dilute nitric acid and 40 mL of water, and add water to make 50 mL. Perform the test using this solution as the test solution. Prepare the control solution with 0.80 mL of 0.01 mol/L hydrochloric acid VS (not more than 0.095%).

(3) Sulfate—To 1.0 g of Mesalazine add 20 mL of water, shake for 1 minute, and filter. To 15 mL of the filtrate add 0.5 mL of acetic acid (31), then add 2.5 mL of the following solution A, and use this solution as the test solution. Solution A: To 3 mL of barium chloride TS add 4.5 mL of a solution of potassium sulfate in diluted ethanol (3 in 10) (181 in 10,000,000), shake, and allow to stand for 1 minute. Prepare the control solution by adding 14.7 mL of water and 0.5 mL of acetic acid (31) to 0.31 mL of 0.005 mol/L sulfuric acid VS, and then proceeding in the same manner for the test solution. Compare the test solution and the control solution after allowing to stand for 5 minutes: the turbidity of the test solution is not more intense than that of the control solution (not more than 0.02%).

(4) Heavy metals ⟨*1.07*⟩—Proceed with 0.5 g of Mesalazine according to Method 2, and perform the test. Prepare the control solution with 1.0 mL of Standard Lead Solution (not more than 20 ppm).

(5) Reducing substances—Dissolve 0.10 g of Mesalazine in dilute hydrochloric acid to make 25 mL, add 0.2 mL of starch TS and 0.25 mL of dilute iodine TS, and allow to stand for 2 minutes: a blue or purple-brown color is produced.

(6) 2-Aminophenol and 4-aminophenol—Weigh exactly 50 mg of Mesalazine, dissolve in the mobile phase A to make exactly 50 mL, and use this solution as the sample solution. Separately, weigh exactly 5.0 mg of 2-aminophenol, and dissolve in the mobile phase A to make exactly 100 mL. Pipet 10 mL of this solution, add the mobile phase A to make exactly 100 mL, and use this solution as the 2-aminophenol standard stock solution. Weigh exactly 5.0 mg of 4-aminophenol, dissolve in the mobile phase A to make exactly 250 mL, and use this solution as the 4-aminophenol standard stock solution. Pipet 1 mL each of the 2-aminophenol standard stock solution and 4-aminophenol standard stock solution, add the mobile phase A to make exactly 100 mL, and use this solution as the standard solution. Perform the test with exactly 20 μL each of the sample solution and standard solution as directed under Liquid Chromatography <*2.01*> according to the following conditions, and determine the peak areas of 4-aminophenol and 2-aminophenol: the peak area of 4-aminophenol obtained from the sample solution is not larger than that of 4-aminophenol from the standard solution (not more than 0.02%), and the peak area of 2-aminophenol from the sample solution is not larger than 4 times that of 2-aminophenol from the standard solution (not more than 0.02%).

Operating conditions—

Detector: An ultraviolet absorption photometer (wavelength: 220 nm).

Column: A stainless steel column 4.6 mm in inside diameter and 25 cm in length, packed with octadecylsilanized silica gel for liquid chromatography (3 μm in particle diameter).

Column temperature: A constant temperature of about 25°C.

Mobile phase A: Mix 2.2 g of perchloric acid and 1.0 g of phosphoric acid with water to make 1000 mL.

Mobile phase B: Mix 1.7 g of perchloric acid and 1.0 g of phosphoric acid with acetonitrile for liquid chromatography to make 1000 mL.

Flowing of mobile phase: Control the gradient by mixing the mobile phases A and B as directed in the following table.

Time after injection of sample (min)	Mobile phase A (vol%)	Mobile phase B (vol%)
0 – 10	100	0
10 – 25	100 → 40	0 → 60

Flow rate: About 0.8 mL per minute (the retention time of mesalazine is about 16 minutes).

System suitability—

System performance: To 1 mL of the sample solution add the mobile phase A to make 200 mL. To 5 mL of this solution add 5 mL of the 2-aminophenol standard stock solution. When the procedure is run with 20 μL of this solution under the above operating conditions, 2-aminophenol and mesalazine are eluted in this order with the resolution between these peaks being not less than 3.

System repeatability: When the test is repeated 6 times with 20 μL of the standard solution under the above operating conditions, the relative standard deviation of the peak area of 2-aminophenol is not more than 2.5%.

(7) Aniline—Dissolve exactly 0.10 g of Mesalazine in the mobile phase to make exactly 50 mL, and use this solution as the sample solution. Separately, dissolve exactly 30.5 mg of aniline sulfate in the mobile phase to make exactly 100 mL. Pipet 1 mL of this solution, add the mobile phase to make exactly 100 mL. Pipet 1 mL of this solution, add the mobile phase to make exactly 100 mL, and use this solution as the standard solution. Perform the test with exactly 100 μL each of the sample solution and standard solution as directed under Liquid Chromatography <*2.01*> according to the following conditions, and determine the peak area of aniline in each solution: the peak area of aniline obtained from the sample solution is not larger than that of aniline from the standard solution (not more than 10 ppm).

Operating conditions—

Detector: A fluorophotometer (excitation wavelength: 280 nm, fluorescence wavelength: 340 nm).

Column: A stainless steel column 4.6 mm in inside diameter and 25 cm in length, packed with octadecylsilanized silica gel for liquid chromatography (5 μm in particle diameter).

Column temperature: A constant temperature of about 40°C.

Mobile phase: Dissolve 9.52 g of sodium acetate trihydrate in a suitable amount of water, add 1.72 mL of acetic acid (100), then add water to make 1000 mL, and adjust to pH 5.0 with acetic acid (100) or dilute sodium hydroxide TS. To 500 mL of this solution add 500 mL of acetonitrile for liquid chromatography.

Flow rate: Adjust so that the retention time of aniline is about 5 minutes.

System suitability—

System performance: When the procedure is run with 100 μL of the standard solution under the above operating conditions, the number of theoretical plates and the symmetry factor of the peak of aniline are not less than 3000 and not more than 2.0, respectively.

System repeatability: When the test is repeated 6 times with 100 μL of the standard solution under the above operating conditions, the relative standard deviation of the peak area of aniline is not more than 2.0%.

(8) 3-Aminophenol, 3-aminobenzoic acid, gentisic acid, salicylic acid and other related substances—Weigh exactly 50 mg of Mesalazine, dissolve in the mobile phase A to make exactly 50 mL, and use this solution as the sample solution. Pipet 1 mL of the sample solution, add the mobile phase A to make exactly 100 mL, and use this solution as the standard solution. Separately, weigh exactly 10 mg of 3-aminophenol, and dissolve in the mobile phase A to make exactly 100 mL. Pipet 1 mL of this solution, add the mobile phase A to make exactly 50 mL, and use this solution as the 3-aminophenol standard solution. Weigh exactly 5.0 mg of 3-aminobenzoic acid, dissolve in the mobile phase A to make exactly 100 mL. Pipet 1 mL of this solution, add the mobile phase A to make exactly 50 mL, and use this solution as the 3-aminobenzoic acid standard solution. Weigh exactly 5.0 mg of gentisic acid, dissolve in the mobile phase A to make exactly 100 mL. Pipet 1 mL of this solution, add the mobile phase A to make exactly 50 mL, and use this solution as the gentisic acid standard solution. Weigh exactly 15 mg of salicylic acid, dissolve in the mobile phase A to make exactly 100 mL. Pipet 1 mL of this solution, add the mobile phase A to make exactly 50 mL, and use this solution as the salicylic acid standard solution. Perform the test with exactly 10 μL each of the sample solution, standard solution, 3-aminophenol standard solution, 3-aminobenzoic acid standard solution, gentisic acid standard solution and salicylic acid standard solution as directed under Liquid Chromatography <*2.01*> according to the following conditions, and determine each peak area by the automatic integration method: the peak area of 3-aminophenol obtained from the sample solution is not larger than that from 3-aminophenol standard solution (not more than 0.2%), the peak area of 3-aminobenzoic acid from the sample solution is not larger than that from 3-aminobenzoic acid standard solution (not more than 0.1%), the peak area of gentisic acid from the sample solution is not larger than that from gentisic acid standard solution (not more than 0.1%), and the peak area of salicylic acid from the sample solution is not larger than that from salicylic acid standard solution (not more than 0.3%). The area of the peak other than 3-aminophenol, mesalazine, 3-aminobenzoic acid, gentisic acid and salicylic acid from the sample solution is not larger than 1/10 times the peak area of mesalazine from the standard solution (not more than 0.1%), and the total area of the peaks other than mesalazine from the sample solution is not larger than the peak area of mesalazine from the standard solution (not more than 1.0%).

Operating conditions—

Detector: An ultraviolet absorption photometer (wavelength: 220 nm).

Column: A stainless steel column 4.6 mm in inside diameter and 25 cm in length, packed with octylsilanized silica gel for liquid chromatography (5 μm in particle diameter).

Column temperature: A constant temperature of about 25°C.

Mobile phase A: Mix 2.2 g of perchloric acid and 1.0 g of phosphoric acid with water to make 1000 mL.

Mobile phase B: Mix 1.7 g of perchloric acid and 1.0 g of phosphoric acid with acetonitrile for liquid chromatography to make 1000 mL.

Flowing of mobile phase: Control the gradient by mixing the mobile phases A and B as directed in the following table.

Time after injection of sample (min)	Mobile phase A (vol%)	Mobile phase B (vol%)
0 – 7	100	0
7 – 25	100 → 40	0 → 60

Flow rate: About 1.8 mL per minute (the retention time of mesalazine is about 5 minutes).

Time span of measurement: For 25 minutes after injection of the sample solution.

System suitability—

Test for required detectability: Pipet 1 mL of the standard solution, and add the mobile phase A to make exactly 20 mL. Confirm that the peak area of mesalazine obtained with 10 μL of this solution is equivalent to 3.5 to 6.5% of that with 10 μL of the standard solution.

System performance: To 1 mL of the sample solution and 2 mL of a solution of 3-aminobenzoic acid in the mobile phase A (1 in 20,000) add the mobile phase A to make 100 mL. When the procedure is run with 10 μL of this solution under the above operating conditions, mesalazine and 3-aminobenzoic acid are eluted in this order with the resolution between these peaks being not less than 3.

System repeatability: When the test is repeated 6 times with 10 μL of the standard solution under the above operating conditions, the relative standard deviation of the peak area of mesalazine is not more than 2.0%.

Loss on drying <*2.41*> Not more than 0.5% (1 g, 105°C, 2 hours).

Residue on ignition <*2.44*> Not more than 0.2% (1 g).

Assay Weigh accurately about 50 mg of Mesalazine, previously dried, dissolve in 100 mL of hot water, cool to room temperature quickly, and titrate <*2.50*> with 0.1 mol/L sodium hydroxide VS (potentiometric titration). Perform a blank determination in the same manner, and make any necessary correction.

Each mL of 0.1 mol/L sodium hydroxide VS
= 15.31 mg of $C_7H_7NO_3$

Containers and storage Containers—Well-closed containers.

Storage—Light-resistant.

Mesalazine Extended-release Tablets

メサラジン徐放錠

Mesalazine Extended-release Tablets contain not less than 95.0% and not more than 105.0% of the labeled amount of mesalazine ($C_7H_7NO_3$: 153.14).

Method of preparation Prepare as directed under Tablets, with Mesalazine.

Identification Powder Mesalazine Extended-release Tablets. To a portion of the powder, equivalent to 20 mg of Mesalazine, add 100 mL of diluted phosphoric acid (1 in 1000) and shake vigorously. To 5 mL of this solution add diluted phosphoric acid (1 in 1000) to make 50 mL, filter, and determine the absorbance spectrum of the filtrate as directed under Ultraviolet-visible Spectrophotometry <*2.24*>: it exhibits maxima between 227 nm and 231 nm, and between 298 nm and 302 nm.

Uniformity of dosage units <*6.02*> Perform the Mass variation test, or the Content uniformity test according to the following method: it meets the requirement.

To 1 tablet of Mesalazine Extended-release Tablets add $6V/25$ mL of diluted phosphoric acid (1 in 1000), shake until the tablet is disintegrated, then add $3V/5$ mL of methanol, and sonicate for 30 minutes. Add diluted phosphoric acid (1 in 1000) to make exactly V mL so that each mL contains about 1 mg of mesalazine ($C_7H_7NO_3$), and centrifuge. Pipet 8 mL of the supernatant liquid, add exactly 2 mL of the internal standard solution and 13 mL of methanol, then add diluted phosphoric acid (1 in 1000) to make 50 mL, and use this solution as the sample solution. Then, proceed as directed in the Assay.

Amount (mg) of mesalazine ($C_7H_7NO_3$)
$= M_S \times Q_T/Q_S \times V/40$

M_S: Amount (mg) of mesalazine for assay taken

*Internal standard solution—*A solution of ethyl aminobenzoate in methanol (1 in 800).

Dissolution <*6.10*> When the test is performed at 50 revolutions per minute according to the Paddle method, using 900 mL of 2nd fluid for dissolution test as the dissolution medium, the dissolution rates in 3 hours, in 6 hours and in 24 hours of Mesalazine Extended-release Tablets are 10 to 40%, 30 to 60%, and not less than 80%, respectively.

Start the test with 1 tablet of Mesalazine Extended-release Tablets, withdraw exactly 20 mL of the medium at the specified minutes after starting the test and supply exactly 20 mL of dissolution medium warmed to 37 ± 0.5°C immediately after withdrawing of the medium every time. Filter the withdrawn media through a membrane filter with a pore size not exceeding 0.45 μm. Discard not less than 10 mL of the first filtrate, pipet V mL of the subsequent filtrate, add the dissolution medium to make exactly V' mL so that each mL contains about 56 μg of mesalazine ($C_7H_7NO_3$), and use these solutions as the sample solutions. Separately, weigh accurately about 28 mg of mesalazine for assay, previously dried at 105°C for 2 hours, and dissolve in the dissolution medium to make exactly 100 mL. Pipet 5 mL of this solution, add the dissolution medium to make exactly 25 mL, and use this solution as the standard solution. Determine the absorbances, $A_{T(n)}$ and A_S, of the sample solutions and standard solution at 330 nm as directed under Ultraviolet-visible Spectrophotometry <2.24>.

Dissolution rate (%) with respect to the labeled amount of mesalazine ($C_7H_7NO_3$) on the nth medium withdrawing (n = 1, 2, 3)

$$= M_S \times \left\{\frac{A_{T(n)}}{A_S} + \sum_{i=1}^{n-1}\left(\frac{A_{T(i)}}{A_S} \times \frac{1}{45}\right)\right\} \times \frac{V'}{V} \times \frac{1}{C} \times 180$$

M_S: Amount (mg) of mesalazine for assay taken
C: Labeled amount (mg) of mesalazine ($C_7H_7NO_3$) in 1 tablet

Assay Weigh accurately the mass of not less than 20 Mesalazine Extended-release Tablets, and powder. Weigh accurately a portion of the powder, equivalent to about 40 mg of mesalazine ($C_7H_7NO_3$), add 100 mL of diluted phosphoric acid (1 in 1000), shake vigorously, and sonicate for 5 minutes. Add exactly 10 mL of the internal standard solution, then add 90 mL of methanol and diluted phosphoric acid (1 in 1000) to make 250 mL. Filter this solution through a membrane filter with a pore size 0.45 μm. Discard the first 5 mL of the filtrate, and use the subsequent filtrate as the sample solution. Separately, weigh accurately about 40 mg of mesalazine for assay, previously dried at 105°C for 2 hours, add 100 mL of diluted phosphoric acid (1 in 1000), shake vigorously, and sonicate for 5 minutes to dissolve. Add exactly 10 mL of the internal standard solution, then add 90 mL of methanol and diluted phosphoric acid (1 in 1000) to make 250 mL, and use this solution as the standard solution. Perform the test with 10 μL each of the sample solution and standard solution as directed under Liquid Chromatography <2.01> according to the following conditions, and calculate the ratios, Q_T and Q_S, of the peak area of mesalazine to that of the internal standard.

Amount (mg) of mesalazine ($C_7H_7NO_3$) = $M_S \times Q_T/Q_S$

M_S: Amount (mg) of mesalazine for assay taken

Internal standard solution—A solution of ethyl aminobenzoate in methanol (1 in 800).
Operating conditions—

Detector: An ultraviolet absorption photometer (wavelength: 300 nm).

Column: A stainless steel column 4.0 mm in inside diameter and 10 cm in length, packed with octadecylsilanized silica gel for liquid chromatography (5 μm in particle diameter).

Column temperature: A constant temperature of about 40°C.

Mobile phase: Dissolve 400 mL of methanol, 1 mL of phosphoric acid, 0.865 g of sodium lauryl sulfate and 0.679 g of tetrabutylammonium hydrogensulfate in water to make 1000 mL.

Flow rate: Adjust so that the retention time of mesalazine is about 10 minutes.
System suitability—

System performance: When the procedure is run with 10 μL of the standard solution under the above operating conditions, mesalazine and the internal standard are eluted in this order with the resolution between these peaks being not less than 3.

System repeatability: When the test is repeated 6 times with 10 μL of the standard solution under the above operating conditions, the relative standard deviation of the ratio of the peak area of mesalazine to that of the internal standard is not more than 1.0%.

Containers and storage Containers—Well-closed containers.

Storage—Light-resistant.

Mestranol

メストラノール

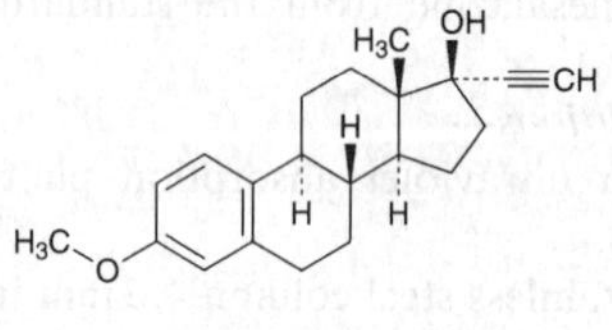

$C_{21}H_{26}O_2$: 310.43
3-Methoxy-19-nor-17α-pregna-1,3,5(10)-trien-20-yn-17-ol
[72-33-3]

Mestranol, when dried, contains not less than 97.0% and not more than 102.0% of mestranol ($C_{21}H_{26}O_2$).

Description Mestranol occurs as a white to pale yellow-white crystalline powder. It is odorless.

It is freely soluble in chloroform, sparingly soluble in ethanol (99.5), and practically insoluble in water.

Identification **(1)** Dissolve 2 mg of Mestranol in 1 mL of a mixture of sulfuric acid and ethanol (99.5) (2:1): a red-purple color develops with a yellow-green fluorescence.

(2) Determine the absorption spectrum of a solution of Mestranol in ethanol (99.5) (1 in 10,000) as directed under Ultraviolet-visible Spectrophotometry <2.24>, and compare the spectrum with the Reference Spectrum or the spectrum of a solution of Mestranol RS prepared in the same manner as the sample solution: both spectra exhibit similar intensities of absorption at the same wavelengths.

(3) Determine the infrared absorption spectrum of Mestranol, previously dried, as directed in the potassium bromide disk method under Infrared Spectrophotometry <2.25>, and compare the spectrum with the Reference Spectrum or the spectrum of previously dried Mestranol RS: both spectra exhibit similar intensities of absorption at the same wave numbers.

Optical rotation <2.49> $[\alpha]_D^{25}$: +1 – +6° (after drying, 0.1 g, ethanol (99.5), 10 mL, 100 mm).

Melting point <2.60> 148 – 154°C

Purity **(1)** Heavy metals <1.07>—Proceed with 1.0 g of Mestranol according to Method 2, and perform the test. Prepare the control solution with 2.0 mL of Standard Lead Solution (not more than 20 ppm).

(2) Arsenic <1.11>—Prepare the test solution with 1.0 g of Mestranol according to Method 3, and perform the test (not more than 2 ppm).

(3) Related substances—Dissolve 0.10 g of Mestranol in 20 mL of chloroform, and use this solution as the sample solution. Pipet 1 mL of the sample solution, add chloroform to make exactly 200 mL, and use this solution as the standard solution. Perform the test with these solutions as directed under Thin-layer Chromatography <2.03>. Spot 10 μL each of the sample solution and standard solution on a plate of silica gel for thin-layer chromatography. Develop the plate with a mixture of chloroform and ethanol (99.5) (29:1) to a distance of about 10 cm, and air-dry the plate. Spray evenly diluted sulfuric acid (1 in 5) on the plate, and heat the plate at 105°C for 15 minutes: the spots other than the principal spot obtained from the sample solution are not more intense than the spot from the standard solution.

Loss on drying *<2.41>* Not more than 0.5% (0.5 g, 105°C, 3 hours).

Residue on ignition *<2.44>* Not more than 0.1% (0.5 g).

Assay Weigh accurately about 10 mg each of Mestranol and Mestranol RS, previously dried, dissolve in ethanol (99.5) to make exactly 100 mL, and use these solutions as the sample solution and the standard solution, respectively. Determine the absorbances, A_T and A_S, of the sample solution and the standard solution at 279 nm as directed under Ultraviolet-visible Spectrophotometry *<2.24>*.

Amount (mg) of mestranol ($C_{21}H_{26}O_2$) = $M_S \times A_T/A_S$

M_S: Amount (mg) of Mestranol RS taken

Containers and storage Containers—Tight containers.
Storage—Light-resistant.

Metenolone Acetate

メテノロン酢酸エステル

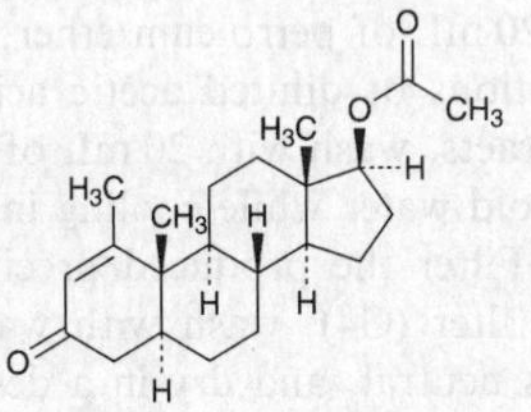

$C_{22}H_{32}O_3$: 344.49
1-Methyl-3-oxo-5α-androst-1-en-17β-yl acetate
[434-05-9]

Metenolone Acetate, when dried, contains not less than 97.0% and not more than 103.0% of metenolone acetate ($C_{22}H_{32}O_3$).

Description Metenolone Acetate occurs as a white to pale yellow-white crystalline powder. It is odorless.

It is freely soluble in acetone, in 1,4-dioxane and in chloroform, soluble in methanol and in ethanol (95), sparingly soluble in diethyl ether and in sesame oil, slightly soluble in hexane and in petroleum ether, and practically insoluble in water.

Identification **(1)** Dissolve 1 mg of Metenolone Acetate in 5 mL of a mixture of sulfuric acid and ethanol (95) (1:1), and heat for 30 minutes in a water bath: a red-brown color develops.

(2) To 10 mg of Metenolone Acetate add 0.5 mL of dilute sodium hydroxide-ethanol TS, and heat for 1 minute on a water bath. After cooling, add 0.5 mL of diluted sulfuric acid (1 in 2), and boil gently for 1 minute: the odor of ethyl acetate is perceptible.

(3) Dissolve 50 mg of Metenolone Acetate in 3 mL of methanol, add 0.3 mL of a solution of potassium carbonate (1 in 6), and boil for 2 hours under a reflux condenser. After cooling, add this solution gradually to 50 mL of cold water, and stir for 15 minutes. Filter the precipitate so obtained by suction through a glass filter (G4), wash with 10 mL of water, and dry at 105°C for 1 hour: it melts *<2.60>* between 157°C and 161°C.

(4) Determine the infrared absorption spectrum of Metenolone Acetate, previously dried, as directed in the potassium bromide disk method under Infrared Spectrophotometry *<2.25>*, and compare the spectrum with the Reference Spectrum: both spectra exhibit similar intensities of absorption at the same wave numbers.

Optical rotation *<2.49>* $[\alpha]_D^{20}$: +39 – +42° (after drying, 0.2 g, chloroform, 10 mL, 100 mm).

Melting point *<2.60>* 141 – 144°C

Purity **(1)** Clarity and color of solution—Dissolve 0.50 g of Metenolone Acetate in 10 mL of 1,4-dioxane: the solution is clear and colorless to pale yellow.

(2) Heavy metals *<1.07>*—Proceed with 2.0 g of Metenolone Acetate according to Method 2, and perform the test. Prepare the control solution with 2.0 mL of Standard Lead Solution (not more than 10 ppm).

(3) Related substances—Dissolve 35 mg of Metenolone Acetate in 20 mL of chloroform, and use this solution as the sample solution. Pipet 1 mL of the sample solution, dilute with chloroform to exactly 250 mL, and use this solution as the standard solution. Perform the test with these solutions as directed under Thin-layer Chromatography *<2.03>*. Spot 10 μL each of the sample solution and standard solution on a plate of silica gel with fluorescent indicator for thin-layer chromatography. Develop the plate with a mixture of ethyl acetate and cyclohexane (1:1) to a distance of about 12 cm, and air-dry the plate. Examine under ultraviolet light (main wavelength: 254 nm): the spots other than the principal spot obtained from the sample solution are not more intense than the spot from the standard solution.

Loss on drying *<2.41>* Not more than 0.5% (0.5 g, 105°C, 3 hours).

Residue on ignition *<2.44>* Not more than 0.1% (0.5 g).

Assay Weigh accurately about 10 mg of Metenolone Acetate, previously dried, and dissolve in methanol to make exactly 100 mL. Pipet 5 mL of this solution, and dilute with methanol to exactly 50 mL. Determine the absorbance A of this solution at the wavelength of maximum absorption at about 242 nm as directed under Ultraviolet-visible Spectrophotometry *<2.24>*.

Amount (mg) of metenolone acetate ($C_{22}H_{32}O_3$)
$= A/391 \times 10{,}000$

Containers and storage Containers—Tight containers.
Storage—Light-resistant.

Metenolone Enanthate

メテノロンエナント酸エステル

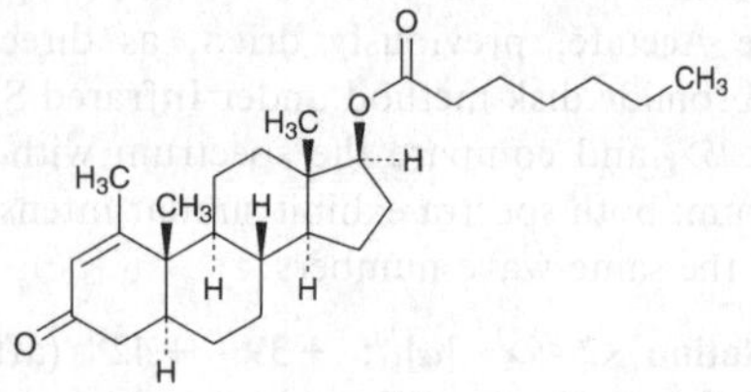

$C_{27}H_{42}O_3$: 414.62
1-Methyl-3-oxo-5α-androst-1-en-17β-yl heptanoate
[*303-42-4*]

Metenolone Enanthate, when dried, contains not less than 97.0% and not more than 103.0% of metenolone enanthate ($C_{27}H_{42}O_3$).

Description Metenolone Enanthate occurs as white, crystals or crystalline powder. It is odorless.

It is very soluble in ethanol (95), in acetone, in 1,4-dioxane and in chloroform, freely soluble in methanol, in ethyl acetate, in diethyl ether, in cyclohexane, in petroleum ether and in toluene, soluble in sesame oil, and practically insoluble in water.

Identification **(1)** Heat 1 mg of Metenolone Enanthate with 5 mL of a mixture of sulfuric acid and ethanol (95) (1:1) on a water bath for 30 minutes: a red-brown color develops.

(2) Dissolve 50 mg of Metenolone Enanthate in 3 mL of methanol, add 0.3 mL of a solution of potassium carbonate (1 in 6), boil under a reflux condenser for 2 hours, cool, add slowly this solution to 50 mL of cold water, and stir for 15 minutes. Filter the produced precipitate by suction through a glass filter (G4), wash with water until the washings become neutral, and dry at 105°C for 1 hour: it melts 〈*2.60*〉 between 156°C and 162°C.

Optical rotation 〈*2.49*〉 $[\alpha]_D^{20}$: +39 – +43° (after drying, 0.2 g, chloroform, 10 mL, 100 mm).

Melting point 〈*2.60*〉 67 – 72°C

Purity **(1)** Clarity and color of solution—Dissolve 0.5 g of Metenolone Enanthate in 10 mL of 1,4-dioxane: the solution is clear and colorless.

(2) Heavy metals 〈*1.07*〉—Proceed with 2.0 g of Metenolone Enanthate according to Method 2, and perform the test. Prepare the control solution with 2.0 mL of Standard Lead Solution (not more than 10 ppm).

(3) Related substances—Dissolve 20 mg of Metenolone Enanthate in exactly 10 mL of chloroform, and use this solution as the sample solution. Perform the test with the sample solution as directed under Thin-layer Chromatography 〈*2.03*〉. Spot 10 μL of the sample solution on a plate of silica gel with fluorescent indicator for thin-layer chromatography. Develop the plate with a mixture of ethyl acetate and cyclohexane (1:1) to a distance of about 15 cm, and air-dry the plate. Examine under ultraviolet light (main wavelength: 254 nm): any spot other than the principal spot does not appear.

Loss on drying 〈*2.41*〉 Not more than 0.5% (0.5 g, in vacuum, phosphorus (V) oxide, 4 hours).

Residue on ignition 〈*2.44*〉 Not more than 0.1% (0.5 g).

Assay Weigh accurately about 0.1 g of Metenolone Enanthate, previously dried, and dissolve in methanol to make exactly 100 mL. Pipet 10 mL of this solution, and dilute with methanol to make exactly 100 mL. Pipet 10 mL of this solution, and dilute again with methanol to make exactly 100 mL. Determine the absorbance, A, of this solution at the wavelength of maximum absorption at about 242 nm as directed under Ultraviolet-visible Spectrophotometry 〈*2.24*〉.

Amount (mg) of metenolone enanthate ($C_{27}H_{42}O_3$)
$= A/325 \times 100{,}000$

Containers and storage Containers—Tight containers.
Storage—Light-resistant.

Metenolone Enanthate Injection

メテノロンエナント酸エステル注射液

Metenolone Enanthate Injection is an oily solution for injection.

It contains not less than 90.0% and not more than 110.0% of the labeled amount of metenolone enanthate ($C_{27}H_{42}O_3$: 414.62).

Method of preparation Prepare as directed under Injections, with Metenolone Enanthate.

Description Metenolone Enanthate Injection is a clear, pale yellow, oily liquid.

Identification **(1)** Measure a volume of Metenolone Enanthate Injection, equivalent to 0.1 g of Metenolone Enanthate, add 20 mL of petroleum ether, and extract with three 20-mL portions of diluted acetic acid (100) (5 in 7). Combine the extracts, wash with 20 mL of petroleum ether, add 300 mL of cold water while cooling in an ice bath, and stir sufficiently. Filter the produced precipitate by suction through a glass filter (G4), wash with water until the last washing becomes neutral, and dry in a desiccator (in vacuum, phosphorus (V) oxide) for 6 hours. With this sample, proceed as directed in the Identification (1) under Metenolone Enanthate.

(2) Measure a volume of Metenolone Enanthate Injection, equivalent to 10 mg of Metenolone Enanthate, dissolve in 10 mL of chloroform, and use this solution as the sample solution. Separately dissolve 10 mg of metenolone enanthate in 10 mL of chloroform, and use this solution as the standard solution. Perform the test with these solutions as directed under Thin-layer Chromatography 〈*2.03*〉. Spot 10 μL each of the sample solution and standard solution on a plate of silica gel with fluorescent indicator for thin-layer chromatography. Develop the plate with toluene to a distance of about 15 cm, and air-dry the plate. Again develop this plate with a mixture of ethyl acetate and cyclohexane (1:1) to a distance of about 15 cm, and air-dry the plate. Examine under ultraviolet light (main wavelength: 254 nm): the principal spot obtained from the sample solution and the spot from the standard solution show the same Rf value.

Extractable volume 〈*6.05*〉 It meets the requirement.

Foreign insoluble matter 〈*6.06*〉 Perform the test according to Method 1: it meets the requirement.

Insoluble particulate matter 〈*6.07*〉 It meets the requirement.

Sterility 〈*4.06*〉 Perform the test according to the Membrane filtration method: it meets the requirement.

Assay To an exactly measured volume of Metenolone Enanthate Injection, equivalent to about 0.1 g of metenolone enanthate ($C_{27}H_{42}O_3$), add chloroform to make exactly 100 mL. Pipet 5 mL of this solution, add chloroform to make exactly 50 mL, and use this solution as the sample solution. Weigh accurately about 0.1 g of metenolone enanthate for assay, previously dried in a desiccator (in vacuum, phosphorus (V) oxide) for 4 hours, and prepare the standard solution in the same manner as directed for the preparation of the sample solution. Pipet 3 mL each of the sample solution and standard solution, add exactly 10 mL of isoniazid TS, add methanol to make exactly 20 mL, and allow to stand for 60 minutes. Determine the absorbances, A_T and A_S, of the solutions from the sample solution and standard solution, respectively, at 384 nm as directed under Ultraviolet-visible Spectrophotometry *<2.24>*, using a solution obtained by proceeding with 3 mL of chloroform as the blank.

Amount (mg) of metenolone enanthate ($C_{27}H_{42}O_3$)
$= M_S \times A_T/A_S$

M_S: Amount (mg) of metenolone enanthate for assay taken

Containers and storage Containers—Hermetic containers.
Storage—Light-resistant.

Metformin Hydrochloride

メトホルミン塩酸塩

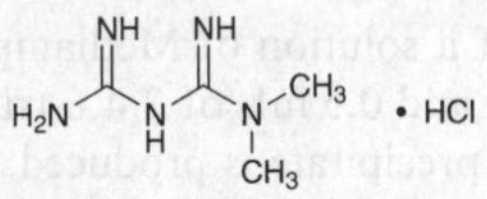

$C_4H_{11}N_5.HCl$: 165.62
1,1-Dimethylbiguanide monohydrochloride
[*1115-70-4*]

Metformin Hydrochloride, when dried, contains not less than 98.5% and not more than 101.0% of metformin hydrochloride ($C_4H_{11}N_5.HCl$).

Description Metformin Hydrochloride occurs as white, crystals or crystalline powder.

It is freely soluble in water, sparingly soluble in acetic acid (100), and slightly soluble in ethanol (99.5).

Melting point: about 221°C (with decomposition).

Identification **(1)** Determine the absorption spectrum of a solution of Metformin Hydrochloride (1 in 100,000) as directed under Ultraviolet-visible Spectrophotometry *<2.24>*, and compare the spectrum with the Reference Spectrum: both spectra exhibit similar intensities of absorption at the same wavelengths.

(2) Determine the infrared absorption spectrum of Metformin Hydrochloride as directed in the potassium chloride disk method under Infrared Spectrophotometry *<2.25>*, and compare the spectrum with the Reference Spectrum: both spectra exhibit similar intensities of absorption at the same wave numbers.

(3) A solution of Metformin Hydrochloride (1 in 50) responds to Qualitative Tests *<1.09>* for chloride.

Purity **(1)** Heavy metals *<1.07>*—Proceed with 2.0 g of Metformin Hydrochloride according to Method 1, and perform the test. Prepare the control solution with 2.0 mL of Standard Lead Solution (not more than 10 ppm).

(2) Related substances—Dissolve 2.5 g of Metformin Hydrochloride in 10 mL of water, and use this solution as the sample solution. Pipet 1 mL of the sample solution, and add water to make exactly 50 mL. Pipet 1 mL of this solution, add water to make exactly 10 mL, and use this solution as the standard solution (1). Pipet 5 mL of the standard solution (1), add water to make exactly 10 mL, and use this solution as the standard solution (2). Separately, to 0.10 g of 1-cyanoguanidine add water to make exactly 50 mL. Pipet 1 mL of this solution, add water to make exactly 20 mL, and use this solution as the standard solution (3). Perform the test with these solutions as directed under Thin-layer Chromatography *<2.03>*. Spot 10 μL each of the sample solution and standard solutions (1), (2) and (3) on a plate of cellulose for thin-layer chromatography. Develop the plate with a mixture of 4-methyl-2-pentanone, 2-methoxyethanol, water and acetic acid (100) (30:20:5:3) to a distance of about 10 cm, air-dry the plate, then dry at 105°C for 10 minutes. Spray evenly sodium pentacyanonitrosylferrate (III)-potassium hexacyanoferrate (III) TS on the plate: the spot other than the principal spot obtained from the sample solution is not more intense than the spot from the standard solution (1), the number of them showing more intense than the spot from the standard solution (2) is not more than two, and the spot from the sample solution appeared at the position corresponding to the spot from the standard solution (3) is not more intense than the spot from the standard solution (3).

Loss on drying *<2.41>* Not more than 0.5% (1 g, 105°C, 3 hours).

Residue on ignition *<2.44>* Not more than 0.1% (1 g).

Assay Weigh accurately about 0.1 g of Metformin Hydrochloride, previously dried, dissolve in 40 mL of acetic acid (100), add 40 mL of acetic anhydride, and titrate *<2.50>* with 0.05 mol/L perchloric acid VS (potentiometric titration). Perform a blank determination in the same manner, and make any necessary correction.

Each mL of 0.05 mol/L perchloric acid VS
= 4.141 mg of $C_4H_{11}N_5.HCl$

Containers and storage Containers—Tight containers.

Metformin Hydrochloride Tablets

メトホルミン塩酸塩錠

Metformin Hydrochloride Tablets contain not less than 95.0% and not more than 105.0% of the labeled amount of metformin hydrochloride ($C_4H_{11}N_5.HCl$: 165.62).

Method of preparation Prepare as directed under Tablets, with Metformin Hydrochloride.

Identification Shake an amount of powdered Metformin Hydrochloride Tablets, equivalent to 250 mg of Metformin Hydrochloride, with 25 mL of 2-propanol, and filter. Evaporate the filtrate under reduced pressure in a water bath at 40°C, and determine the infrared absorption spectrum of the residue as directed in the potassium chloride disk method under Infrared Spectrophotometry *<2.25>*: it exhibits absorption at the wave numbers of about 3370 cm^{-1}, 3160 cm^{-1}, 1627 cm^{-1}, 1569 cm^{-1} and 1419 cm^{-1}.

Uniformity of dosage units *<6.02>* It meets the requirement of the Mass variation test.

Dissolution Being specified separately when the drug is

granted approval based on the Law.

Assay Weigh accurately the mass of not less than 20 Metformin Hydrochloride Tablets, and powder. Weigh accurately a portion of the powder, equivalent to about 0.15 g of metformin hydrochloride ($C_4H_{11}N_5.HCl$), add 70 mL of a mixture of water and acetonitrile (3:2), shake for 10 minutes, add the mixture of water and acetonitrile (3:2) to make exactly 100 mL, and filter through a membrane filter with a pore size not exceeding 0.45 μm. Discard the first 10 mL of the filtrate, pipet 3 mL of the subsequent filtrate, add exactly 3 mL of the internal standard solution and the mixture of water and acetonitrile (3:2) to make 50 mL, and use this solution as the sample solution. Separately, weigh accurately about 0.15 g of metformin hydrochloride for assay, previously dried at 105°C for 3 hours, and dissolve in the mixture of water and acetonitrile (3:2) to make exactly 100 mL. Pipet 3 mL of this solution, add exactly 3 mL of the internal standard solution and the mixture of water and acetonitrile (3:2) to make 50 mL, and use this solution as the standard solution. Perform the test with 5 μL each of the sample solution and standard solution as directed under Liquid Chromatography <*2.01*> according to the following conditions, and calculate the ratios, Q_T and Q_S, of the peak area of metformin to that of the internal standard.

Amount (mg) of metformin hydrochloride ($C_4H_{11}N_5.HCl$)
$= M_S \times Q_T/Q_S$

M_S: Amount (mg) of metformin hydrochloride for assay taken

Internal standard solution—Dissolve 0.3 g of isobutyl parahydroxybenzoate in 100 mL of the mixture of water and acetonitrile (3:2).

Operating conditions—

Detector: An ultraviolet absorption photometer (wavelength: 235 nm).

Column: A stainless steel column 4.6 mm in inside diameter and 15 cm in length, packed with octadecylsilanized silica gel for liquid chromatography (5 μm in particle diameter).

Column temperature: A constant temperature of about 40°C.

Mobile phase: Dissolve 0.8 g of sodium lauryl sulfate in 620 mL of diluted phosphoric acid (1 in 2500), and add 380 mL of acetonitrile.

Flow rate: Adjust so that the retention time of metformin is about 10 minutes.

System suitability—

System performance: When the procedure is run with 5 μL of the standard solution under the above operating conditions, metformin and the internal standard are eluted in this order with the resolution between these peaks being not less than 6.

System repeatability: When the test is repeated 6 times with 5 μL of the standard solution under the above operating conditions, the relative standard deviation of the ratio of the peak area of metformin to that of the internal standard is not more than 1.0%.

Containers and storage Containers—Well-closed containers.

Methamphetamine Hydrochloride

メタンフェタミン塩酸塩

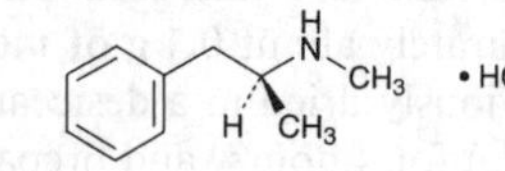

$C_{10}H_{15}N.HCl$: 185.69
(2*S*)-*N*-Methyl-1-phenylpropan-2-amine monohydrochloride
[*51-57-0*]

Methamphetamine Hydrochloride, when dried, contains not less than 98.5% of methamphetamine hydrochloride ($C_{10}H_{15}N.HCl$).

Description Methamphetamine Hydrochloride occurs as colorless crystals or a white crystalline powder. It is odorless.

It is freely soluble in water, in ethanol (95) and in chloroform, and practically insoluble in diethyl ether.

The pH of a solution of 1.0 g of Methamphetamine Hydrochloride in 10 mL of water is between 5.0 and 6.0.

Identification **(1)** To 5 mL of a solution of Methamphetamine Hydrochloride (1 in 100) add 0.5 mL of hydrogen hexachloroplatinate (IV) TS: an orange-yellow, crystalline precipitate is produced.

(2) To 5 mL of a solution of Methamphetamine Hydrochloride (1 in 100) add 0.5 mL of iodine TS: a brown precipitate is produced.

(3) To 5 mL of a solution of Methamphetamine Hydrochloride (1 in 100) add 0.5 mL of 2,4,6-trinitrophenol TS: a yellow, crystalline precipitate is produced.

(4) A solution of Methamphetamine Hydrochloride (1 in 20) responds to Qualitative Tests <*1.09*> for chloride.

Optical rotation <*2.49*> $[\alpha]_D^{20}$: +16 – +19° (after drying, 0.2 g, water, 10 mL, 100 mm).

Melting point <*2.60*> 171 – 175°C

Purity **(1)** Acidity or alkalinity—Dissolve 2.0 g of Methamphetamine Hydrochloride in 40 mL of freshly boiled and cooled water, add 2 drops of methyl red TS, and use this solution as the sample solution.

(i) To 20 mL of the sample solution add 0.20 mL of 0.01 mol/L sulfuric acid VS: a red color develops.

(ii) To 20 mL of the sample solution add 0.20 mL of 0.02 mol/L sodium hydroxide VS: a yellow color develops.

(2) Sulfate <*1.14*>—Dissolve 0.05 g of Methamphetamine Hydrochloride in 40 mL of water, add 1 mL of dilute hydrochloric acid and 1 mL of barium chloride TS, and allow to stand for 10 minutes: the solution remains unchanged.

Loss on drying <*2.41*> Not more than 0.5% (1 g, 105°C, 2 hours).

Residue on ignition <*2.44*> Not more than 0.1% (1 g).

Assay Weigh accurately about 0.4 g of Methamphetamine Hydrochloride, previously dried, and dissolve in 50 mL of a mixture of acetic anhydride and acetic acid (100) (7:3). Titrate <*2.50*> with 0.1 mol/L perchloric acid VS (potentiometric titration). Perform a blank determination in the same manner, and make any necessary correction.

Each mL of 0.1 mol/L perchloric acid VS
= 18.57 mg of $C_{10}H_{15}N.HCl$

Containers and storage Containers—Tight containers.

Storage—Light-resistant.

L-Methionine

L-メチオニン

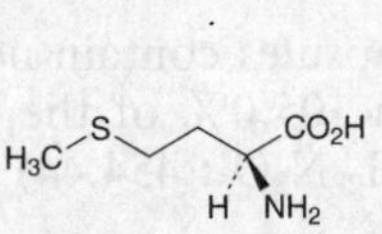

$C_5H_{11}NO_2S$: 149.21
(2*S*)-2-Amino-4-(methylsulfanyl)butanoic acid
[*63-68-3*]

L-Methionine, when dried, contains not less than 98.5% of L-methionine ($C_5H_{11}NO_2S$).

Description L-Methionine occurs as white, crystals or crystalline powder. It has a characteristic odor.

It is freely soluble in formic acid, soluble in water, and very slightly soluble in ethanol (95).

It dissolves in dilute hydrochloric acid.

Identification Determine the infrared absorption spectrum of L-Methionine, previously dried, as directed in the potassium bromide disk method under Infrared Spectrophotometry <*2.25*>, and compare the spectrum with the Reference Spectrum: both spectra exhibit similar intensities of absorption at the same wave numbers.

Optical rotation <*2.49*> $[\alpha]_D^{20}$: +21.0 – +25.0° (after drying, 0.5 g, 6 mol/L hydrochloric acid TS, 25 mL, 100 mm).

pH <*2.54*> Dissolve 0.5 g of L-Methionine in 20 mL of water: the pH of this solution is between 5.2 and 6.2.

Purity (1) Clarity and color of solution—Dissolve 0.5 g of L-Methionine in 20 mL of water: the solution is clear and colorless.

(2) Chloride <*1.03*>—Dissolve 0.5 g of L-Methionine in 20 mL of water, and add 6 mL of dilute nitric acid and water to make 40 mL. Perform the test using this solution as the test solution. Prepare the control solution with 0.30 mL of 0.01 mol/L hydrochloric acid VS, 6 mL of dilute nitric acid and water to make 40 mL. In this test, to the test solution and the control solution add 10 mL each of silver nitrate TS (not more than 0.021%).

(3) Sulfate <*1.14*>—Perform the test with 0.6 g of L-Methionine. Prepare the control solution with 0.35 mL of 0.005 mol/L sulfuric acid VS (not more than 0.028%).

(4) Ammonium <*1.02*>—Perform the test with 0.25 g of L-Methionine. Prepare the control solution with 5.0 mL of Standard Ammonium Solution (not more than 0.02%).

(5) Heavy metals <*1.07*>—Dissolve 1.0 g of L-Methionine in 40 mL of water and 2 mL of dilute acetic acid, dissolve by warming, cool, and add water to make 50 mL. Perform the test using this solution as the test solution. Prepare the control solution as follows: to 2.0 mL of Standard Lead Solution add 2 mL of dilute acetic acid and water to make 50 mL (not more than 20 ppm).

(6) Arsenic <*1.11*>—Transfer 1.0 g of L-Methionine to a 100-mL decomposition flask, add 5 mL of nitric acid and 2 mL of sulfuric acid, put a small funnel on the mouth of the flask, and heat carefully until white fumes are evolved. After cooling, add two 2-mL portions of nitric acid, heat, add 2-mL portions of hydrogen peroxide (30) several times, and heat until the solution becomes colorless or pale yellow. After cooling, add 2 mL of saturated ammonium oxalate monohydrate solution, and heat again until white fumes are evolved. After cooling, add water to make 5 mL, and perform the test with this solution as the test solution (not more than 2 ppm).

(7) Related substances—Dissolve 0.10 g of L-Methionine in 10 mL of water, and use this solution as the sample solution. Pipet 1 mL of the sample solution, and add water to make exactly 50 mL. Pipet 5 mL of this solution, add water to make exactly 20 mL, and use this solution as the standard solution. Perform the test with these solutions as directed under Thin-layer Chromatography <*2.03*>. Spot 5 μL each of the sample solution and standard solution on a plate of silica gel for thin-layer chromatography. After air-drying, immediately develop the plate with a mixture of 1-butanol, water and acetic acid (100) (3:1:1) to a distance of about 10 cm, and dry the plate at 80°C for 30 minutes. Spray evenly a solution of ninhydrin in acetone (1 in 50) on the plate, and heat the plate at 80°C for 5 minutes: the spots other than the principal spot obtained from the sample solution are not more intense than the spot from the standard solution.

Loss on drying <*2.41*> Not more than 0.30% (1 g, 105°C, 3 hours).

Residue on ignition <*2.44*> Not more than 0.1% (1 g).

Assay Weigh accurately about 0.15 g of L-Methionine, previously dried, and dissolve in 3 mL of formic acid, add 50 mL of acetic acid (100), and titrate <*2.50*> with 0.1 mol/L perchloric acid VS (potentiometric titration). Perform a blank determination in the same manner, and make any necessary correction.

Each mL of 0.1 mol/L perchloric acid VS
= 14.92 mg of $C_5H_{11}NO_2S$

Containers and storage Containers—Tight containers.

Methotrexate

メトトレキサート

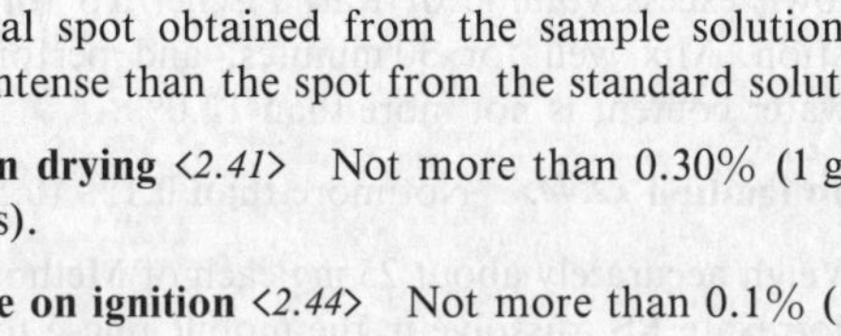

$C_{20}H_{22}N_8O_5$: 454.44
N-{4-[(2,4-Diaminopteridin-6-ylmethyl)(methyl)amino]benzoyl}-L-glutamic acid
[*59-05-2*]

Methotrexate is a mixture of 4-amino-10-methylfolic acid and closely related compounds.

It contains not less than 94.0% and not more than 102.0% of methotrexate ($C_{20}H_{22}N_8O_5$), calculated on the anhydrous basis.

Description Methotrexate occurs as a yellow-brown crystalline powder.

It is slightly soluble in pyridine, and practically insoluble in water, in acetonitrile, in ethanol (95) and in diethyl ether.

It dissolves in dilute sodium hydroxide TS and in dilute sodium carbonate TS.

It is gradually affected by light.

Identification (1) Dissolve 1 mg of Methotrexate in 100 mL of 0.1 mol/L hydrochloric acid TS. Determine the absorption spectrum of this solution as directed under Ultraviolet-visible Spectrophotometry <2.24>, and compare the spectrum with the Reference Spectrum or the spectrum of a solution of Methotrexate RS prepared in the same manner as the sample solution: both spectra exhibit similar intensities of absorption at the same wavelengths.

(2) Determine the infrared absorption spectrum of Methotrexate as directed in the potassium bromide disk method under Infrared Spectrophotometry <2.25>, and compare the spectrum with the Reference Spectrum or the spectrum of Methotrexate RS: both spectra exhibit similar intensities of absorption at the same wave numbers.

Water <2.48> Take 5 mL of pyridine for water determination and 20 mL of methanol for water determination in a dried titration flask, and titrate with Karl Fischer TS until the end point. Weigh accurately about 0.2 g of Methotrexate, immediately place in the titration flask, and add a known excess volume of Karl Fischer TS for water determination. Mix well for 30 minutes, and perform the test: the water content is not more than 12.0%.

Residue on ignition <2.44> Not more than 0.1% (0.5 g).

Assay Weigh accurately about 25 mg each of Methotrexate and Methotrexate RS, dissolve in the mobile phase to make exactly 250 mL, and use these solutions as the sample solution and standard solution. Perform the test with exactly 10 μL each of these solutions as directed under Liquid Chromatography <2.01> according to the following conditions, and determine the peak areas, A_T and A_S, of methotrexate in each solution.

Amount (mg) of methotrexate ($C_{20}H_{22}N_8O_5$) = $M_S \times A_T/A_S$

M_S: Amount (mg) of Methotrexate RS taken, calculated on the anhydrous basis

Operating conditions—

Detector: An ultraviolet absorption photometer (wavelength: 302 nm).

Column: A stainless steel column 4.6 mm in inside diameter and 25 cm in length, packed with octadecylsilanized silica gel for liquid chromatography (10 μm in particle diameter).

Column temperature: A constant temperature of about 25°C.

Mobile phase: A mixture of disodium hydrogen phosphate-citric acid buffer solution (pH 6.0) and acetonitrile (89:11).

Flow rate: Adjust so that the retention time of methotrexate is about 8 minutes.

System suitability—

System performance: Dissolve 10 mg each of Methotrexate and folic acid in 100 mL of the mobile phase. When the procedure is run with 10 μL of this solution under the above operating conditions, folic acid and methotrexate are eluted in this order with the resolution between these peaks being not less than 8.

System repeatability: When the test is repeated 6 times with 10 μL of the standard solution under the above operating conditions, the relative standard deviation of the peak area of methotrexate is not more than 1.0%.

Containers and storage Containers—Tight containers.

Storage—Light-resistant.

Methotrexate Capsules

メトトレキサートカプセル

Methotrexate Capsules contain not less than 95.0% and not more than 105.0% of the labeled amount of methotrexate ($C_{20}H_{22}N_8O_5$: 454.44).

Method of preparation Prepare as directed under Capsules, with Methotrexate.

Identification To an amount of the content of Methotrexate Capsules, equivalent to 2 mg of Methotrexate, add 100 mL of 0.1 mol/L hydrochloric acid TS, shake, and filter. To 10 mL of the filtrate add 0.1 mol/L hydrochloric acid TS to make 20 mL, and determine the absorption spectrum of this solution as directed under Ultraviolet-visible Spectrophotometry <2.24>: it exhibits maxima between 240 nm and 244 nm and between 304 nm and 308 nm.

Uniformity of dosage units <6.02> Perform the test according to the following method: it meets the requirement of the Content uniformity test.

To the content of 1 capsule of Methotrexate Capsules add $3V/5$ mL of the mobile phase, sonicate for 15 minutes, then shake for 25 minutes, and add the mobile phase to make exactly V mL so that each mL contains about 20 μg of methotrexate ($C_{20}H_{22}N_8O_5$). Centrifuge this solution, pipet 2 mL of the supernatant liquid, add exactly 2 mL of the internal standard solution, then add the mobile phase to make 20 mL, and use this solution as the sample solution. Separately, weigh accurately about 10 mg of Methotrexate RS (separately determine the water <2.48> in the same manner as Methotrexate), and dissolve in the mobile phase to make exactly 100 mL. Pipet 10 mL of this solution, and add the mobile phase to make exactly 50 mL. Pipet 2 mL of this solution, add exactly 2 mL of the internal standard solution, then add the mobile phase to make 20 mL, and use this solution as the standard solution. Perform the test with 20 μL each of the sample solution and standard solution as directed under Liquid Chromatography <2.01> according to the following conditions, and calculate the ratios, Q_T and Q_S, of the peak area of methotrexate to that of the internal standard.

Amount (mg) of methotrexate ($C_{20}H_{22}N_8O_5$)
$= M_S \times Q_T/Q_S \times V/500$

M_S: Amount (mg) of Methotrexate RS taken, calculated on the anhydrous basis

*Internal standard solution—*A solution of 4-nitrophenol in methanol (1 in 10,000).

Operating conditions—

Proceed as directed in the operating conditions in the Assay.

System suitability—

System performance: Proceed as directed in the system suitability in the Assay.

System repeatability: When the test is repeated 6 times with 20 μL of the standard solution under the above operating conditions, the relative standard deviation of the ratio of the peak area of methotrexate to that of the internal standard is not more than 1.0%.

Dissolution <6.10> When the test is performed at 50 revolutions per minute according to the Paddle method using the sinker, using 900 mL of water as the dissolution medium, the dissolution rate in 30 minutes of Methotrexate Capsules is not less than 85%.

Start the test with 1 capsule of Methotrexate Capsules, withdraw not less than 20 mL of the medium at the specified minute after starting the test, and filter through a membrane filter with a pore size not exceeding 0.45 µm. Discard not less than 10 mL of the first filtrate, pipet *V* mL of the subsequent filtrate, add water to make exactly *V′* mL so that each mL contains about 2.2 µg of methotrexate ($C_{20}H_{22}N_8O_5$), and use this solution as the sample solution. Separately, weigh accurately about 10 mg of Methotrexate RS (separately determine the water <*2.48*> in the same manner as Methotrexate), and dissolve in the mobile phase to make exactly 100 mL. Pipet 2 mL of this solution, add water to make exactly 100 mL, and use this solution as the standard solution. Perform the test with exactly 50 µL each of the sample solution and standard solution as directed under Liquid Chromatography <*2.01*> according to the following conditions, and determine the peak areas, A_T and A_S, of methotrexate in each solution.

Dissolution rate (%) with respect to the labeled amount of methotrexate ($C_{20}H_{22}N_8O_5$)

$$= M_S \times A_T/A_S \times V'/V \times 1/C \times 18$$

M_S: Amount (mg) of Methotrexate RS taken, calculated on the anhydrous basis

C: Labeled amount (mg) of methotrexate ($C_{20}H_{22}N_8O_5$) in 1 capsule

Operating conditions—

Proceed as directed in the operating conditions in the Assay.

System suitability—

System performance: When the procedure is run with 50 µL of the standard solution under the above operating conditions, the number of theoretical plates and the symmetry factor of the peak of methotrexate are not less than 3500 and not more than 1.5, respectively.

System repeatability: When the test is repeated 6 times with 50 µL of the standard solution under the above operating conditions, the relative standard deviation of the peak area of methotrexate is not more than 1.0%.

Assay Accurately weigh the mass of not less than 20 Methotrexate Capsules, take out all of the content, and accurately weigh the mass of the empty capsules. Powder the content, weigh accurately a portion of the powder, equivalent to about 10 mg of methotrexate ($C_{20}H_{22}N_8O_5$), add 60 mL of the mobile phase, shake for 25 minutes, and add the mobile phase to make exactly 100 mL. Centrifuge this solution, pipet 2 mL of the supernatant liquid, add exactly 2 mL of the internal standard solution, then add the mobile phase to make 20 mL, and use this solution as the sample solution. Separately, weigh accurately about 10 mg of Methotrexate RS (separately determine the water <*2.48*> in the same manner as Methotrexate), and dissolve in the mobile phase to make exactly 100 mL. Pipet 2 mL of this solution, add exactly 2 mL of the internal standard solution, then add the mobile phase to make 20 mL, and use this solution as the standard solution. Perform the test with 20 µL each of the sample solution and standard solution as directed under Liquid Chromatography <*2.01*>, and calculate the ratios, Q_T and Q_S, of the peak area of methotrexate to that of the internal standard.

Amount (mg) of methotrexate ($C_{20}H_{22}N_8O_5$)

$$= M_S \times Q_T/Q_S$$

M_S: Amount (mg) of Methotrexate RS taken, calculated on the anhydrous basis

*Internal standard solution—*A solution of 4-nitrophenol in methanol (1 in 10,000).

Operating conditions—

Detector: An ultraviolet absorption photometer (wavelength: 302 nm).

Column: A stainless steel column 4.6 mm in inside diameter and 25 cm in length, packed with octadecylsilanized silica gel for liquid chromatography (5 µm in particle diameter).

Column temperature: A constant temperature of about 25°C.

Mobile phase: To 250 mL of 0.2 mol/L potassium dihydrogen phosphate TS add 28.5 mL of 0.2 mol/L sodium hydroxide TS and water to make 1000 mL. To 890 mL of this solution add 110 mL of acetonitrile.

Flow rate: Adjust so that the retention time of methotrexate is about 6 minutes.

System suitability—

System performance: Dissolve 10 mg each of methotrexate and folic acid in 100 mL of the mobile phase. To 2 mL of this solution add the mobile phase to make 20 mL. When the procedure is run with 20 µL of this solution under the above operating conditions, folic acid and methotrexate are eluted in this order with the resolution between these peaks being not less than 8.

System repeatability: When the test is repeated 6 times with 20 µL of the standard solution under the above operating conditions, the relative standard deviation of the ratio of the peak area of methotrexate to that of the internal standard is not more than 1.0%.

Containers and storage Containers—Tight containers.

Methotrexate for Injection

注射用メトトレキサート

Methotrexate for Injection is a preparation for injection which is dissolved before use.

It contains not less than 95.0% and not more than 115.0% of the labeled amount of methotrexate ($C_{20}H_{22}N_8O_5$: 454.44).

Method of preparation Prepare as directed under Injections, with Methotrexate.

Description Methotrexate for Injection occurs as a light yellow to reddish yellow crystalline powder or mass.

Identification To 1 mL of a solution of Methotrexate for Injection (1 in 400) add 0.1 mol/L hydrochloric acid TS to make 250 mL. Determine the absorption spectrum of this solution as directed under Ultraviolet-visible Spectrophotometry <*2.24*>: it exhibits maxima between 241 nm and 245 nm, and between 305 nm and 309 nm.

pH Being specified separately when the drug is granted approval based on the Law.

Water Being specified separately when the drug is granted approval based on the Law.

Bacterial endotoxins <*4.01*> Less than 0.1 EU/mg.

Uniformity of dosage units <*6.02*> It meets the requirement of the Mass variation test (*T*: Being specified separately when the drug is granted approval based on the Law.).

Foreign insoluble matter <*6.06*> Perform the test according to Method 2: it meets the requirement.

Insoluble particulate matter <*6.07*> It meets the requirement.

Sterility <*4.06*> Perform the test according to the Membrane filtration method: it meets the requirement.

Assay Dissolve the contents of 20 containers of Methotrexate for Injection in the mobile phase, wash the containers with the mobile phase, combine the solution of the content and washings, and add the mobile phase to make exactly 1000 mL. Pipet V mL of this solution, add the mobile phase to make exactly V' mL so that each mL contains about 0.1 mg of methotrexate ($C_{20}H_{22}N_8O_5$), and use this solution as the sample solution. Separately, weigh accurately about 10 mg of Methotrexate RS (separately determine the water <*2.48*> in the same manner as Methotrexate), add the mobile phase to make exactly 100 mL, and use this solution as the standard solution. Perform the test with exactly 20 μL each of the sample solution and standard solution as directed under Liquid Chromatography <*2.01*> according to the following conditions, and determine the peak areas, A_T and A_S, of methotrexate in each solution.

Amount (mg) of methotrexate ($C_{20}H_{22}N_8O_5$) in 1 container of Methotrexate for Injection
$= M_S \times A_T/A_S \times V'/V \times 1/2$

M_S: Amount (mg) of Methotrexate RS taken, calculated on the anhydrous basis

Operating conditions—

Detector, column temperature, mobile phase, and flow rate: Proceed as directed in the operating conditions in the Assay under Methotrexate.

Column: A stainless steel column of 4.6 mm in inside diameter and 25 cm in length, packed with octadecylsilanized silica gel for liquid chromatography (5 μm in particle diameter).

System suitability—

System performance: Dissolve 10 mg each of methotrexate and folic acid in 100 mL of the mobile phase. When the procedure is run with 20 μL of this solution under the above operating conditions, folic acid and methotrexate are eluted in this order with the resolution between these peaks being not less than 8.

System repeatability: When the test is repeated 6 times with 20 μL of the standard solution under the above operating conditions, the relative standard deviation of the peak area of methotrexate is not more than 1.0%.

Containers and storage Containers—Hermetic containers.
Storage—Light-resistant.

Methotrexate Tablets

メトトレキサート錠

Methotrexate Tablets contain not less than 95.0% and not more than 105.0% of the labeled amount of methotrexate ($C_{20}H_{22}N_8O_5$: 454.44). (This monograph is applied to only 2.5-mg tablets.)

Method of preparation Prepare as directed under Tablets, with Methotrexate.

Identification To a quantity of powdered Methotrexate Tablets, equivalent to 2.5 mg of Methotrexate, add 100 mL of diluted hydrochloric acid (1 in 100), shake, and filter or centrifuge. Determine the absorption spectrum of this solution as directed under Ultraviolet-visible Spectrophotometry <*2.24*>: it exhibits maxima between 241 nm and 245 nm and between 305 nm and 309 nm.

Uniformity of dosage unit <*6.02*> Perform the test according to the following method: it meets the requirement of the Content uniformity test.

To 1 tablet of Methotrexate Tablets add the mobile phase, stir, and add the mobile phase to make exactly V mL so that each mL contains about 0.1 mg of methotrexate ($C_{20}H_{22}N_8O_5$). Centrifuge this solution, and use the supernatant liquid as the sample solution. Then, proceed as directed in the Assay.

Amount (mg) of methotrexate ($C_{20}H_{22}N_8O_5$)
$= M_S \times A_T/A_S \times V/250$

M_S: Amount (mg) of Methotrexate RS taken, calculated on the anhydrous basis

Dissolution <*6.10*> When the test is performed at 50 revolutions per minute according to the Paddle method, using 900 mL of water as the dissolution medium, the dissolution rate in 45 minutes of Methotrexate Tablets is not less than 85%.

Start the test with 1 tablet of Methotrexate Tablets, withdraw not less than 20 mL of the medium at the specified minute after starting the test, and filter through a membrane filter with a pore size not exceeding 0.45 μm. Discard not less than 10 mL of the first filtrate, pipet V mL of the subsequent filtrate, add water to make exactly V' mL so that each mL contains about 2.8 μg of methotrexate ($C_{20}H_{22}N_8O_5$), and use this solution as the sample solution. Separately, weigh accurately about 25 mg of Methotrexate RS (separately determine the water <*2.48*> in the same manner as Methotrexate), and dissolve in the mobile phase to make exactly 100 mL. Pipet 1 mL of this solution, add water to make exactly 100 mL, and use this solution as the standard solution. Perform the test with exactly 50 μL each of the sample solution and standard solution as directed under Liquid Chromatography <*2.01*>, and determine the peak areas, A_T and A_S, of methotrexate in each solution.

Dissolution rate (%) with respect to the labeled amount of methotrexate ($C_{20}H_{22}N_8O_5$)
$= M_S \times A_T/A_S \times V'/V \times 1/C \times 9$

M_S: Amount (mg) of Methotrexate RS taken, calculated on the anhydrous basis
C: Labeled amount (mg) of methotrexate ($C_{20}H_{22}N_8O_5$) in 1 tablet

Operating conditions—

Detector: An ultraviolet absorption photometer (wavelength: 302 nm).

Column: A stainless steel column 4 mm in inside diameter and 15 cm in length, packed with octadecylsilanized silica gel for liquid chromatography (5 μm in particle diameter).

Column temperature: A constant temperature of about 25°C.

Mobile phase: To 250 mL of 0.2 mol/L of potassium dihydrogen phosphate TS add 29 mL of 0.2 mol/L sodium hydroxide TS and water to make 1000 mL. To 890 mL of this solution add 110 mL of acetonitrile.

Flow rate: Adjust so that the retention time of methotrexate is about 4 minutes.

System suitability—

System performance: When the procedure is run with 50 μL of the standard solution under the above operating conditions, the number of theoretical plates and the symmetry factor of the peak of methotrexate are not less than 3000 and

not more than 1.5, respectively.

System repeatability: When the test is repeated 6 times with 50 μL of the standard solution under the above operating conditions, the relative standard deviation of the peak area of methotrexate is not more than 1.0%.

Assay Weigh accurately the mass of not less than 20 Methotrexate Tablets, and powder. Weigh accurately a portion of the powder, equivalent to about 10 mg of methotrexate ($C_{20}H_{22}N_8O_5$), add 50 mL of the mobile phase, shake, and add the mobile phase to make exactly 100 mL. Centrifuge this solution, and use the supernatant liquid as the sample solution. Separately, weigh accurately about 25 mg of Methotrexate RS (separately determine the water <*2.48*> in the same manner as Methotrexate), dissolve in the mobile phase to make exactly 250 mL, and use this solution as the standard solution. Perform the test with exactly 20 μL each of the sample solution and standard solution as directed under Liquid Chromatography <*2.01*> according to the following conditions, and determine the peak areas, A_T and A_S, of methotrexate in each solution.

Amount (mg) of methotrexate ($C_{20}H_{22}N_8O_5$)
$= M_S \times A_T/A_S \times 2/5$

M_S: Amount (mg) of Methotrexate RS taken, calculated on the anhydrous basis

Operating conditions—

Detector: An ultraviolet absorption photometer (wavelength: 302 nm).

Column: A stainless steel column 4.6 mm in inside diameter and 25 cm in length, packed with octadecylsilanized silica gel for liquid chromatography (5 μm in particle diameter).

Column temperature: A constant temperature of about 25°C.

Mobile phase: A mixture of disodium hydrogen phosphate-citric acid buffer solution (pH 6.0) and acetonitrile (89:11).

Flow rate: Adjust so that the retention time of methotrexate is about 8 minutes.

System suitability—

System performance: Dissolve 10 mg each of methotrexate and folic acid in 100 mL of the mobile phase. When the procedure is run with 20 μL of this solution under the above operating conditions, folic acid and methotrexate are eluted in this order with the resolution between these peaks being not less than 8.

System repeatability: When the test is repeated 6 times with 20 μL of the standard solution under the above operating conditions, the relative standard deviation of the peak area of methotrexate is not more than 1.0%.

Containers and storage Containers—Well-closed containers.

Storage—Light-resistant.

Methoxsalen

メトキサレン

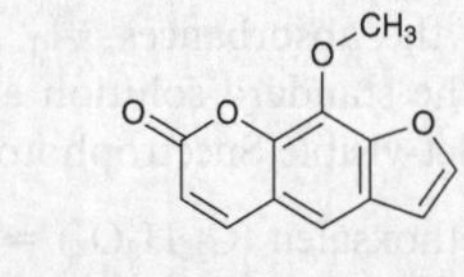

$C_{12}H_8O_4$: 216.19
9-Methoxy-7*H*-furo[3,2-*g*]chromen-7-one
[*298-81-7*]

Methoxsalen contains not less than 98.0% and not more than 102.0% of methoxsalen ($C_{12}H_8O_4$), calculated on the anhydrous basis.

Description Methoxsalen occurs as white to pale yellow, crystals or crystalline powder. It is odorless and tasteless.

It is freely soluble in chloroform, slightly soluble in methanol, in ethanol (95) and in diethyl ether, and practically insoluble in water.

Identification **(1)** To 10 mg of Methoxsalen add 5 mL of dilute nitric acid, and heat: a yellow color develops. Make this solution alkaline with a solution of sodium hydroxide (2 in 5): the color changes to red-brown.

(2) To 10 mg of Methoxsalen add 5 mL of sulfuric acid, and shake: a yellow color develops.

(3) Determine the absorption spectrum of a solution of Methoxsalen in ethanol (95) (1 in 200,000) as directed under Ultraviolet-visible Spectrophotometry <*2.24*>, and compare the spectrum with the Reference Spectrum or the spectrum of a solution of Methoxsalen RS prepared in the same manner as the sample solution: both spectra exhibit similar intensities of absorption at the same wavelengths.

Melting point <*2.60*> 145 – 149°C

Purity **(1)** Heavy metals <*1.07*>—Proceed with 1.0 g of Methoxsalen according to Method 4, and perform the test. Prepare the control solution with 2.0 mL of Standard Lead Solution (not more than 20 ppm).

(2) Arsenic <*1.11*>—Prepare the test solution with 1.0 g of Methoxsalen according to Method 3, and perform the test (not more than 2 ppm).

(3) Related substances—Dissolve 50 mg of Methoxsalen in 10 mL of chloroform, and use this solution as the sample solution. Pipet 2 mL of the sample solution, add chloroform to make exactly 50 mL. Pipet 1 mL of this solution, add chloroform to make exactly 10 mL, and use this solution as the standard solution. Perform the test with these solutions as directed under Thin-layer Chromatography <*2.03*>. Spot 5 μL each of the sample solution and standard solution on a plate of silica gel with fluorescent indicator for thin-layer chromatography. Develop the plate with a mixture of chloroform, hexane and ethyl acetate (40:10:3) to a distance of about 10 cm, and air-dry the plate. Examine under ultraviolet light (main wavelength: 254 nm): the spots other than the principal spot obtained from the sample solution are not more intense than the spot from the standard solution.

Water <*2.48*> Not more than 0.5% (1 g, volumetric titration, direct titration).

Residue on ignition <*2.44*> Not more than 0.1% (1 g).

Assay Weigh accurately about 50 mg each of Methoxsalen and Methoxsalen RS, and dissolve each in ethanol (95) to make exactly 100 mL. Pipet 2 mL each of these solutions, and dilute each with ethanol (95) to make exactly 25 mL. Pipet 10 mL each of these solutions, and dilute each again with ethanol (95) to make exactly 50 mL, and use these solutions as the sample solution and the standard solution, respectively. Determine the absorbances, A_T and A_S, of the sample solution and the standard solution at 300 nm as directed under Ultraviolet-visible Spectrophotometry <*2.24*>.

Amount (mg) of methoxsalen ($C_{12}H_8O_4$) = $M_S \times A_T/A_S$

M_S: Amount (mg) of Methoxsalen RS taken, calculated on the anhydrous basis

Containers and storage Containers—Well-closed containers.

Storage—Light-resistant.

Methylbenactyzium Bromide

メチルベナクチジウム臭化物

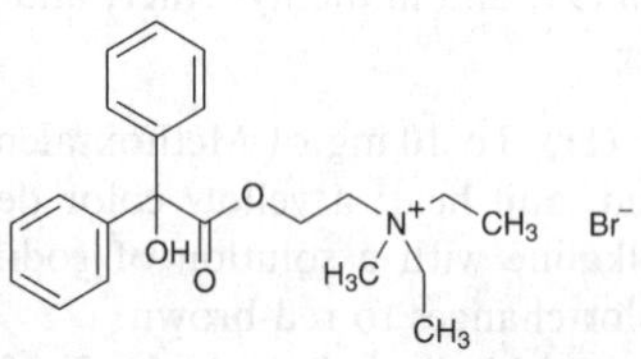

$C_{21}H_{28}BrNO_3$: 422.36

N,*N*-Diethyl-2-[(hydroxyl)(diphenyl)acetoxy]-*N*-methylethylaminium bromide

[*3166-62-9*]

Methylbenactyzium Bromide, when dried, contains not less than 99.0% of methylbenactyzium bromide ($C_{21}H_{28}BrNO_3$).

Description Methylbenactyzium Bromide occurs as white, crystals or crystalline powder. It is odorless, and has an extremely bitter taste.

It is freely soluble in water and in acetic acid (100), soluble in ethanol (95), slightly soluble in acetic anhydride, and practically insoluble in diethyl ether.

The pH of a solution of 1.0 g of Methylbenactyzium Bromide in 50 mL of water is between 5.0 and 6.0.

Identification (1) Shake 0.5 mL of a solution of Methylbenactyzium Bromide (1 in 100) with 5 mL of phosphate buffer solution (pH 7.0), 2 to 3 drops of bromothymol blue TS and 5 mL of chloroform: a yellow color develops in the chloroform layer.

(2) To about 1 g of Methylbenactyzium Bromide add 5 mL of water and 10 mL of sodium hydroxide TS, allow to stand for 5 minutes, add 5 mL of dilute hydrochloric acid, collect the precipitate, wash well with water, recrystallize from a mixture of water and ethanol (95) (10:3), and dry at 105°C for 1 hour: the crystals melt <*2.60*> between 145°C and 150°C. Continue the heating up to about 200°C: a red color develops.

(3) Add 2 mL of dilute nitric acid to 5 mL of a solution of Methylbenactyzium Bromide (1 in 10): the solution responds to Qualitative Tests <*1.09*> (1) for bromide.

Melting point <*2.60*> 168 – 172°C

Purity (1) Clarity and color of solution—Dissolve 1.0 g of Methylbenactyzium Bromide in 10 mL of water: the solution is clear and colorless.

(2) Sulfate <*1.14*>—Perform the test with 0.5 g of Methylbenactyzium Bromide. Prepare the control solution with 0.40 mL of 0.005 mol/L sulfuric acid VS (not more than 0.038%).

(3) Heavy metals <*1.07*>—Proceed with 2.0 g of Methylbenactyzium Bromide according to Method 2, and perform the test. Prepare the control solution with 2.0 mL of Standard Lead Solution (not more than 10 ppm).

Loss on drying <*2.41*> Not more than 0.5% (2 g, 105°C, 2 hours).

Residue on ignition <*2.44*> Not more than 0.1% (1 g).

Assay Weigh accurately about 0.5 g of Methylbenactyzium Bromide, previously dried, and dissolve in 80 mL of a mixture of acetic anhydride and acetic acid (100) (4:1). Titrate <*2.50*> with 0.1 mol/L perchloric acid VS (potentiometric titration). Perform a blank determination in the same manner, and make any necessary correction.

Each mL of 0.1 mol/L perchloric acid VS
= 42.24 mg of $C_{21}H_{28}BrNO_3$

Containers and storage Containers—Tight containers.

Methylcellulose

メチルセルロース

[*9004-67-5*]

This monograph is harmonized with the European Pharmacopoeia and the U.S. Pharmacopeia.

The corresponding part of the attributes/provisions which are agreed as non-harmonized within the scope of the harmonization is marked with symbols (◆ ◆), and the corresponding parts which are agreed as the JP local requirement other than the scope of the harmonization are marked with symbols (◇ ◇).

Information on the harmonization with the European Pharmacopoeia and the U.S. Pharmacopeia is available on the website of the Pharmaceuticals and Medical Devices Agency.

Methylcellulose is a methyl ether of cellulose.

It contains not less than 26.0% and not more than 33.0% of methoxy group (-OCH_3: 31.03), calculated on the dried basis.

The viscosity of Methylcellulose is shown in millipascal second (mPa·s).

◆**Description** Methylcellulose occurs as a white to yellowish white, powder or grains.

It is practically insoluble in ethanol (99.5).

It swells, when water is added, and forms a clear or slightly turbid, viscous liquid.◆

Identification (1) Disperse evenly 1.0 g of Methylcellulose over the surface of 100 mL of water in a beaker, while gently tapping the top of the beaker, if necessary, and allow the beaker to stand: it aggregates on the surface of water.

(2) Add 1.0 g of Methylcellulose to 100 mL of hot water, and stir: it becomes a suspension. Cool the suspension to 5°C, and stir: the resulting liquid is a clear or a slightly cloudy, viscous fluid.

(3) To 0.1 mL of the viscous fluid obtained in (2) add 9 mL of diluted sulfuric acid (9 in 10), shake, heat in a water bath for exactly 3 minutes, and immediately cool in ice water. Add carefully 0.6 mL of ninhydrin TS, shake, and allow to stand at 25°C: the solution shows a red color, and it does not change to purple color within 100 minutes.

(4) Pour and spread out 2 to 3 mL of the viscous fluid obtained in (2) onto a glass plate, and allow the water to evaporate: a transparent film results.

(5) Pipet 50 mL of water, add exactly 50 mL of the viscous fluid obtained in (2), and warm to raise the temperature at a rate of 2 to 5°C per minute while stirring: the temperature, when a white turbidity of the solution starts to increase, is not less than 50°C.

Viscosity <*2.53*> (i) Method I: Apply to Methylcellulose having a labeled viscosity of less than 600 mPa·s. Put an exact amount of Methylcellulose, equivalent to 4.000 g, calculated on the dried basis, in a tared, wide-mouth bottle, add water (between 90°C and 99°C) to make 200 g, stopper the bottle, stir by mechanical means at 350 to 450 revolutions per minute for 10 to 20 minutes to get a homogeneous dispersion. If necessary, take off the sample attached on the walls of the bottle, put them in the dispersed solution, and dissolve by continuing the stirring in a water bath at not exceeding 5°C for 20 to 40 minutes. Add cold water, if necessary, to make 200 g, and use this solution as the sample solution. Centrifuge the solution if necessary to expel any entrapped air bubbles. Perform the test with the sample solution at 20 ± 0.1°C as directed in Method I under Viscosity Determination: not less than 80% and not more than 120% of the labeled viscosity.

(ii) Method II: Apply to Methylcellulose having a labeled viscosity of not less than 600 mPa·s. Put an exact amount of Methylcellulose, equivalent to 10.00 g, calculated on the dried basis, in a tared, wide-mouth bottle, add water (between 90°C and 99°C) to make 500 g, and prepare the sample solution in the same manner as directed in Method I. Perform the test with the sample solution at 20 ± 0.1°C as directed in Method II under Viscosity Determination, using a single cylinder-type rotational viscometer, according to the following operating conditions: not less than 75% and not more than 140% of the labeled viscosity.

Operating conditions—

Apparatus: Brookfield type viscometer LV model or an equivalent apparatus.

Rotor No., rotation frequency, and calculation multiplier: According to the following table, depending on the labeled viscosity.

Labeled viscosity (mPa·s)	Rotor No.	Rotation frequency /min	Calculation multiplier
Not less than 600 and less than 1400	3	60	20
〃 1400 〃 3500	3	12	100
〃 3500 〃 9500	4	60	100
〃 9500 〃 99,500	4	6	1000
〃 99,500	4	3	2000

Procedure of apparatus: Read the value after 2 minutes of rotation, and stop the rotation for at least 2 minutes. Repeat this procedure more two times, and average the three observed values.

pH <*2.54*> The pH of the sample solution obtained in the Viscosity, measured after 5 minutes immersing the electrode in the sample solution, is between 5.0 and 8.0.

◇**Purity** Heavy metals—Put 1.0 g of Methylcellulose in a 100-mL Kjeldahl flask, add a sufficient amount of a mixture of nitric acid and sulfuric acid (5:4) to wet the sample, and heat gently. Repeat this procedure until to use totally 18 mL of the mixture of nitric acid and sulfuric acid (5:4). Then boil gently until the solution changes to black. After cooling, add 2 mL of nitric acid, and heat until the solution changes to black. Repeat this procedure until the solution no longer changes to black, and heat strongly until dense white fumes are evolved. After cooling, add 5 mL of water, boil gently until dense white fumes are evolved, then heat until the volume of the solution becomes to 2 to 3 mL. After cooling, if the solution reveals yellow color by addition of 5 mL of water, add 1 mL of hydrogen peroxide (30), and heat until the volume of the solution becomes to 2 to 3 mL. After cooling, dilute the solution with 2 to 3 mL of water, transfer to a Nessler tube, add water to make 25 mL, and use this solution as the sample solution. Separately, put 2.0 mL of Standard Lead Solution in a 100-mL Kjeldahl flask, add 18 mL of the mixture of nitric acid and sulfuric acid (5:4) and an amount of nitric acid equal to that used for preparation of the sample solution, and heat until dense white fumes are evolved. After cooling, add 10 mL of water. In the case where hydrogen peroxide (30) is added for the preparation of the sample solution, add the same amount of hydrogen peroxide (30), then proceed in the same manner for preparation of the sample solution, and use so obtained solution as the control solution. Adjust the sample solution and the control solution to pH 3.0 to 4.0 with ammonia solution (28), and add water to make 40 mL, respectively. To these solutions add 1.2 mL of thioacetamide-alkaline glycerin TS, 2 mL of acetate buffer solution (pH 3.5) and water to make 50 mL, separately. After allowing to stand for 5 minutes, observe vertically both tubes on a white background: the color obtained with the sample solution is not more intense than that with the control solution (not more than 20 ppm).◇

Loss on drying <*2.41*> Not more than 5.0% (1 g, 105°C, 1 hour).

Residue on ignition <*2.44*> Not more than 1.5% (1 g).

Assay (i) Apparatus—Reaction vial: A 5-mL pressure-tight serum vial, having 20 mm in outside diameter and 50 mm in height, the neck 20 mm in outside diameter and 13 mm in inside diameter, equipped with a septum of butyl-rubber processed the surface with fluoroplastics, which can be fixed tightly to vial with aluminum cap, or equivalent.

Heater: A square-shaped aluminum block, having holes 20 mm in diameter and 32 mm in depth, adopted to the reaction vial. Capable of stirring the content of the reaction vial by means of magnetic stirrer or of reciprocal shaker about 100 times per minute.

(ii) Procedure—Weigh accurately about 65 mg of Methylcellulose, transfer to a reaction vial, add 60 to 100 mg of adipic acid, 2.0 mL of the internal standard solution and 2.0 mL of hydroiodic acid, immediately stopper the vial tightly, and weigh accurately. Using a magnetic stirrer equipped in the heating module, or using a shaker, stir for 60 minutes while heating so that the temperature of the vial content is 130 ± 2°C. In the case when a magnetic stirrer or shaker is not available, heat for 30 minutes with repeated shaking at 5-minute intervals by hand, and continue heating for an additional 30 minutes. Allow the vial to cool, and again weigh accurately. If the mass loss is less than 26 mg and there is no evidence of a leak of the content, use the upper layer of the mixture as the sample solution. Separately, put 60 to 100 mg of adipic acid, 2.0 mL of the internal standard solution and 2.0 mL of hydroiodic acid in a reaction vial, immediately stopper the vial tightly, and weigh accurately. Add 45 μL of iodomethane for assay through the septum using a micro-syringe, weigh accurately, shake, and use the upper layer of the mixture as the standard solution. Perform the test with 1 to 2 μL each of the sample solution and standard solution as directed under Gas Chromatography ⟨*2.02*⟩ according to the following conditions, and calculate the ratios, Q_T and Q_S, of the peak area of iodomethane to that of the internal standard.

Content (%) of methoxy group (CH_3O)
$$= M_S/M \times Q_T/Q_S \times 21.86$$

M_S: Amount (mg) of iodomethane for assay taken
M: Amount (mg) of Methylcellulose taken, calculated on the dried basis

Internal standard solution—A solution of *n*-octane in *o*-xylene (3 in 100).
Operating conditions—
Detector: A thermal conductivity detector or hydrogen flame-ionization detector.
Column: A fused silica column 0.53 mm in inside diameter and 30 m in length, coated with dimethylpolysiloxane for gas chromatography in 3 μm thickness. Use a guard column, if necessary.
Column temperature: Maintain the temperature at 50°C for 3 minutes, raise to 100°C at a rate of 10°C per minute, then raise to 250°C at a rate of 35°C per minute, and maintain at 250°C for 8 minutes.
Injection port temperature: A constant temperature of about 250°C.
Detector temperature: A constant temperature of about 280°C.
Carrier gas: Helium.
Flow rate: 4.3 mL per minute (the retention time of the internal standard is about 10 minutes).
Split ratio: 1:40.
System suitability—
System performance: When the procedure is run with 1 - 2 μL of the standard solution under the above operating conditions, iodomethane and the internal standard are eluted in this order with the resolution between these peaks being not less than 5.
System repeatability: When the test is repeated 6 times with 1 - 2 μL of the standard solution under the above operating conditions, the relative standard deviation of the ratio of the peak area of iodomethane to that of the internal standard is not more than 2.0%.

◆**Containers and storage** Containers—Well-closed containers.◆

Methyldopa Hydrate

メチルドパ水和物

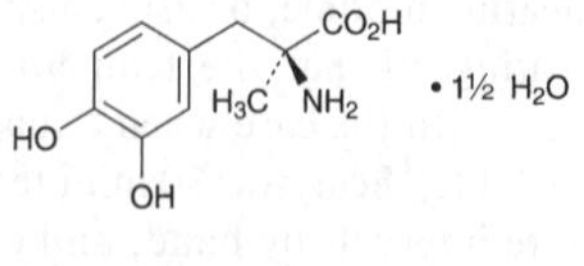

$C_{10}H_{13}NO_4.1\frac{1}{2}H_2O$: 238.24
(2*S*)-2-Amino-3-(3,4-dihydroxyphenyl)-2-methylpropanoic acid sesquihydrate
[*41372-08-1*]

Methyldopa Hydrate contains not less than 98.0% of methyldopa ($C_{10}H_{13}NO_4$: 211.21), calculated on the anhydrous basis.

Description Methyldopa Hydrate occurs as a white to pale grayish white crystalline powder.

It is slightly soluble in water, in methanol and in acetic acid (100), very slightly soluble in ethanol (95), and practically insoluble in diethyl ether.

It dissolves in dilute hydrochloric acid.

Identification **(1)** To 10 mg of Methyldopa Hydrate add 3 drops of ninhydrin TS, and heat in a water bath for 3 minutes: a purple color develops.

(2) Determine the absorption spectrum of a solution of Methyldopa Hydrate in 0.1 mol/L hydrochloric acid TS (1 in 25,000) as directed under Ultraviolet-visible Spectrophotometry ⟨*2.44*⟩, and compare the spectrum with the Reference Spectrum or the spectrum of a solution of Methyldopa RS prepared in the same manner as the sample solution: both spectra exhibit similar intensities of absorption at the same wavelengths.

(3) Determine the infrared absorption spectrum of Methyldopa Hydrate as directed in the potassium bromide disk method under Infrared Spectrophotometry ⟨*2.25*⟩, and compare the spectrum with the Reference Spectrum or the spectrum of Methyldopa RS: both spectra exhibit similar intensities of absorption at the same wave numbers.

Optical rotation ⟨*2.49*⟩ $[\alpha]_D^{20}$: −25 - −28° (1 g calculated on the anhydrous basis, aluminum (III) chloride TS, 20 mL, 100 mm).

Purity **(1)** Acidity—Shake 1.0 g of Methyldopa Hydrate with 100 mL of freshly boiled and cooled water, and add 0.20 mL of 0.1 mol/L sodium hydroxide VS and 2 drops of methyl red TS: a yellow color develops.

(2) Chloride ⟨*1.03*⟩—Perform the test with 0.5 g of Methyldopa Hydrate. Prepare the control solution with 0.40 mL of 0.01 mol/L hydrochloric acid VS (not more than 0.028%).

(3) Heavy metals ⟨*1.07*⟩—Proceed with 2.0 g of Methyldopa Hydrate according to Method 2, and perform the test. Prepare the control solution with 2.0 mL of Standard Lead Solution (not more than 10 ppm).

(4) Arsenic ⟨*1.11*⟩—Prepare the test solution with 1.0 g of Methyldopa Hydrate in 5 mL of dilute hydrochloric acid, and perform the test (not more than 2 ppm).

(5) 3-*O*-Methylmethyldopa—Dissolve 0.10 g of Methyldopa Hydrate in methanol to make exactly 10 mL, and use this solution as the sample solution. Separately, dissolve 5 mg of 3-*O*-methylmethyldopa for thin-layer chromatography in methanol to make exactly 100 mL, and use this solution as the standard solution. Perform the test with these solutions as directed under Thin-layer Chromatography ⟨*2.03*⟩. Spot 20 μL each of the sample solution and standard solution on a plate of cellulose for thin-layer chromatography. Develop the plate with a mixture of 1-butanol, water and acetic acid (100) (13:5:3) to a distance of about 10 cm, and air-dry the plate. Spray evenly 4-nitroaniline-sodium nitrite TS on the plate, and air-dry the plate, then spray evenly a solution of sodium carbonate decahydrate (1 in 4) on the plate: the spot obtained from the sample solution corresponding to that from the standard solution is not more intense than the spot from the standard solution.

Water ⟨*2.48*⟩ 10.0 - 13.0% (0.2 g, volumetric titration, direct titration).

Residue on ignition ⟨*2.44*⟩ Not more than 0.1% (1 g).

Assay Weigh accurately about 0.3 g of Methyldopa Hydrate, dissolve in 80 mL of acetic acid (100), and titrate ⟨*2.50*⟩ with 0.1 mol/L perchloric acid VS until the color of the solution changes from purple through blue to blue-green (indicator: 2 to 3 drops of crystal violet TS). Perform a blank determination in the same manner, and make any necessary correction.

Each mL of 0.1 mol/L perchloric acid VS
$= 21.12$ mg of $C_{10}H_{13}NO_4$

Containers and storage Containers—Well-closed containers.

Storage—Light-resistant.

Methyldopa Tablets

メチルドパ錠

Methyldopa Tablets contain not less than 90.0% and not more than 110.0% of the labeled amount of methyldopa ($C_{10}H_{13}NO_4$: 211.21).

Method of preparation Prepare as directed under Tablets, with Methyldopa Hydrate.

Identification **(1)** To a quantity of powdered Methyldopa Tablets, equivalent to 0.1 g of Methyldopa Hydrate, add 10 mL of water, and heat in a water bath for 5 minutes with occasional shaking. After cooling, centrifuge for 5 minutes at 2000 rotations per minute, apply 1 drop of the supernatant solution to a filter paper, and dry with warm air. Place 1 drop of ninhydrin TS over the spot, and heat for 5 minutes at 100°C: a purple color develops.

(2) To 0.5 mL of the supernatant liquid obtained in (1) add 2 mL of 0.05 mol/L sulfuric acid TS, 2 mL of iron (II) tartrate TS and 4 drops of ammonia TS, and shake well: a deep purple color develops.

(3) To 0.7 mL of the supernatant liquid obtained in (1) add 0.1 mol/L hydrochloric acid TS to make 20 mL. To 10 mL of this solution add 0.1 mol/L hydrochloric acid TS to make 100 mL, and determine the absorption spectrum of the solution as directed under Ultraviolet-visible Spectrophotometry <*2.24*>: it exhibits a maximum between 277 nm and 283 nm.

Uniformity of dosage units <*6.02*> Perform the test according to the following method: it meets the requirement of the Content uniformity test.

To 1 tablet of Methyldopa Tablets add 50 mL of 0.05 mol/L sulfuric acid TS, shake for 15 minutes, then add 0.05 mol/L sulfuric acid TS to make exactly 100 mL, and filter. Discard the first 20 mL of the filtrate, pipet V mL of the subsequent filtrate equivalent to about 5 mg of methyldopa ($C_{10}H_{13}NO_4$), add exactly 5 mL of iron (II) tartrate TS, then add ammonia-ammonium acetate buffer solution (pH 8.5) to make exactly 100 mL, and use this solution as the sample solution. Separately, weigh accurately about 0.11 g of Methyldopa RS (separately determine the loss on drying <*2.41*> at 125°C for 2 hours), and dissolve in 0.05 mol/L sulfuric acid TS to make exactly 100 mL. Pipet 5 mL of this solution, add exactly 5 mL of iron (II) tartrate TS, then add ammonia-ammonium acetate buffer solution (pH 8.5) to make exactly 100 mL, and use this solution as the standard solution. Determine the absorbances at 520 nm, A_T and A_S, of the sample solution and standard solution as directed under Ultraviolet-visible Spectrophotometry <*2.24*>.

Amount (mg) of methyldopa ($C_{10}H_{13}NO_4$)
$= M_S \times A_T/A_S \times 5/V$

M_S: Amount (mg) of Methyldopa RS taken, calculated on the dried basis

Dissolution <*6.10*> When the test is performed at 50 revolutions per minute according to the Paddle method, using 900 mL of water as the dissolution medium, the dissolution rate in 60 minutes of Methyldopa Tablets is not less than 75%.

Start the test with 1 tablet of Methyldopa Tablets, withdraw not less than 30 mL of the medium at the specified minute after starting the test, and filter through a membrane filter with a pore size not exceeding 0.8 μm. Discard not less than 10 mL of the first filtrate, pipet V mL of the subsequent filtrate, add water to make exactly V' mL so that each mL contains about 25 μg of methyldopa ($C_{10}H_{13}NO_4$), and use this solution as the sample solution. Separately, weigh accurately about 56 mg of methyldopa for assay (separately determine the loss on drying <*2.41*> at 125°C for 2 hours), and dissolve in water to make exactly 200 mL. Pipet 10 mL of this solution, add water to make exactly 100 mL, and use this solution as the standard solution. Determine the absorbances, A_T and A_S, of the sample solution and the standard solution at 280 nm as directed under Ultraviolet-visible Spectrophotometry <*2.24*>.

Dissolution rate (%) with respect to the labeled amount of methyldopa ($C_{10}H_{13}NO_4$)
$= M_S \times A_T/A_S \times V'/V \times 1/C \times 45$

M_S: Amount (mg) of methyldopa for assay taken, calculated on the dried basis

C: Labeled amount (mg) of methyldopa ($C_{10}H_{13}NO_4$) in 1 tablet

Assay Weigh accurately and powder not less than 20 Methyldopa Tablets. Weigh accurately a portion of the powder, equivalent to about 0.1 g of methyldopa ($C_{10}H_{13}NO_4$), add 50 mL of 0.05 mol/L sulfuric acid TS, shake thoroughly for 15 minutes, add 0.05 mol/L sulfuric acid TS to make exactly 100 mL, and filter through a dry filter paper. Discard the first 20 mL of the filtrate, and use the subsequent filtrate as the sample solution. Separately, weigh accurately about 0.11 g of Methyldopa RS (separately determine the loss on drying <*2.41*> at 125°C for 2 hours), dissolve in 0.05 mol/L sulfuric acid TS to make exactly 100 mL, and use this solution as the standard solution. Pipet 5 mL each of the sample solution and standard solution, add exactly 5 mL of iron (II) tartrate TS, and add ammonia-ammonium acetate buffer solution (pH 8.5) to make exactly 100 mL. Perform the test with these solutions as directed under Ultraviolet-visible Spectrophotometry <*2.24*>, using a solution prepared with 5 mL of 0.05 mol/L sulfuric acid TS in the same manner, as the blank. Determine the absorbances, A_T and A_S, of the subsequent solutions of the sample solution and the standard solution at 520 nm, respectively.

Amount (mg) of methyldopa ($C_{10}H_{13}NO_4$)
$= M_S \times A_T/A_S$

M_S: amount (mg) of Methyldopa RS taken, calculated on the dried basis

Containers and storage Containers—Well-closed containers.

dl-Methylephedrine Hydrochloride

dl-メチルエフェドリン塩酸塩

and enantiomer

$C_{11}H_{17}NO.HCl$: 215.72
(1*RS*,2*SR*)-2-Dimethylamino-1-phenylpropan-1-ol monohydrochloride
[*18760-80-0*]

dl-Methylephedrine Hydrochloride, when dried, contains not less than 99.0% and not more than 101.0% of *dl*-methylephedrine hydrochloride ($C_{11}H_{17}NO.HCl$).

Description *dl*-Methylephedrine Hydrochloride occurs as colorless crystals or a white crystalline powder.

It is freely soluble in water, sparingly soluble in ethanol (99.5), slightly soluble in acetic acid (100), and practically insoluble in acetic anhydride.

A solution of *dl*-Methylephedrine Hydrochloride (1 in 20) shows no optical rotation.

Identification (1) Determine the absorption spectrum of a solution of *dl*-Methylephedrine Hydrochloride (1 in 2000) as directed under Ultraviolet-visible Spectrophotometry ⟨*2.24*⟩, and compare the spectrum with the Reference Spectrum: both spectra exhibit similar intensities of absorption at the same wavelengths.

(2) Determine the infrared absorption spectrum of *dl*-Methylephedrine Hydrochloride, previously dried, as directed in the potassium chloride disk method under Infrared Spectrophotometry ⟨*2.25*⟩, and compare the spectrum with the Reference Spectrum: both spectra exhibit similar intensities of absorption at the same wave numbers.

(3) A solution of *dl*-Methylephedrine Hydrochloride (1 in 10) responds to Qualitative Tests ⟨*1.09*⟩ for chloride.

pH ⟨*2.54*⟩ The pH of a solution prepared by dissolving 1.0 g of *dl*-Methylephedrine Hydrochloride in 20 mL of water is between 4.5 and 6.0.

Melting point ⟨*2.60*⟩ 207 – 211°C

Purity (1) Clarity and color of solution—Dissolve 1.0 g of *dl*-Methylephedrine Hydrochloride in 10 mL of water: the solution is clear and colorless.

(2) Heavy metals ⟨*1.07*⟩—Proceed with 1.0 g of *dl*-Methylephedrine Hydrochloride according to Method 4, and perform the test. Prepare the control solution with 1.0 mL of Standard Lead Solution (not more than 10 ppm).

(3) Related substances—Dissolve 50 mg of *dl*-Methylephedrine Hydrochloride in 20 mL of water, and use this solution as the sample solution. Pipet 1 mL of the sample solution, add water to make exactly 100 mL, and use this solution as the standard solution. Perform the test with exactly 20 μL each of the sample solution and standard solution as directed under Liquid Chromatography ⟨*2.01*⟩ according to the following conditions, and determine each peak area by the automatic integration method: the total area of the peaks other than the peak of methylephedrine obtained from the sample solution is not larger than the peak area of methylephedrine from the standard solution.

Operating conditions—

Detector: An ultraviolet absorption photometer (wavelength: 257 nm).

Column: A stainless steel column 4.6 mm in inside diameter and 15 cm in length, packed with octadecylsilanized silica gel for liquid chromatography (5 μm in particle diameter).

Column temperature: A constant temperature of about 40°C.

Mobile phase: Dissolve 13.6 g of potassium dihydrogen phosphate and 3 g of sodium 1-heptane sulfonate in 1000 mL of water, and adjust the pH to 2.5 with phosphoric acid. To 900 mL of this solution add 200 mL of acetonitrile.

Flow rate: Adjust so that the retention time of methylephedrine is about 10 minutes.

Time span of measurement: About 2 times as long as the retention time of methylephedrine, beginning after the solvent peak.

System suitability—

Test for required detectability: To exactly 2 mL of the standard solution add water to make exactly 20 mL. Confirm that the peak area of methylephedrine obtained with 20 μL of this solution is equivalent to 7 to 13% of that with 20 μL of the standard solution.

System performance: Dissolve 50 mg of *dl*-Methylephedrine Hydrochloride and 0.4 mg of methyl parahydroxybenzoate in 50 mL of water. When the procedure is run with 20 μL of this solution under the above operating conditions, methylephedrine and methyl parahydroxybenzoate are eluted in this order with the resolution between these peaks being not less than 3.

System repeatability: When the test is repeated 6 times with 20 μL of the standard solution under the above operating conditions, the relative standard deviation of the peak area of methylephedrine is not more than 2.0%.

Loss on drying ⟨*2.41*⟩ Not more than 0.5% (1 g, 105°C, 3 hours).

Residue on ignition ⟨*2.44*⟩ Not more than 0.1% (1 g).

Assay Weigh accurately about 0.4 g of *dl*-Methylephedrine Hydrochloride, previously dried, dissolve in 80 mL of a mixture of acetic anhydride and acetic acid (100) (7:3), and titrate ⟨*2.50*⟩ with 0.1 mol/L perchloric acid VS (potentiometric titration). Perform a blank determination in the same manner, and make any necessary correction.

Each mL of 0.1 mol/L perchloric acid VS
= 21.57 mg of $C_{11}H_{17}NO.HCl$

Containers and storage Containers—Well-closed containers.

Storage—Light-resistant.

10% *dl*-Methylephedrine Hydrochloride Powder

dl-メチルエフェドリン塩酸塩散 10%

10% *dl*-Methylephedrine Hydrochloride Powder contains not less than 9.3% and not more than 10.7% of *dl*-methylephedrine hydrochloride ($C_{11}H_{17}NO.HCl$: 215.72).

Method of preparation

dl-Methylephedrine Hydrochloride	100 g
Starch, Lactose Hydrate or their mixture	a sufficient quantity
To make	1000 g

Prepare as directed under Granules or Powders, with the above ingredients.

Identification To 0.5 g of 10% *dl*-Methylephedrine Hydrochloride Powder add 100 mL of water, shake vigorously for 20 minutes, if necessary, filter the solution. Determine the absorption spectrum of this solution as directed under Ultraviolet-visible Spectrophotometry <2.24>: it exhibits maxima between 250 nm and 253 nm, between 255 nm and 259 nm, and between 261 nm and 264 nm.

Dissolution <6.10> When the test is performed at 50 revolutions per minute according to the Paddle method, using 900 mL of water as the dissolution medium, the dissolution rate in 15 minutes of 10% *dl*-Methylephedrine Hydrochloride Powder is not less than 85%.

Start the test with about 0.5 g of 10% *dl*-Methylephedrine Hydrochloride Powder, accurately weighed, withdraw not less than 20 mL of the medium at the specified minute after starting the test, and filter through a membrane filter with a pore size not exceeding 0.45 μm. Discard not less than 2 mL of the first filtrate, pipet 2 mL of the subsequent filtrate, add exactly 2 mL of the mobile phase, and use this solution as the sample solution. Separately, weigh accurately about 22 mg of *dl*-methylephedrine hydrochloride for assay, previously dried at 105°C for 3 hours, and dissolve in water to make exactly 100 mL. Pipet 25 mL of this solution, and add water to make exactly 100 mL. Pipet 2 mL of this solution, add exactly 2 mL of the mobile phase, and use this solution as the standard solution. Perform the test with exactly 20 μL each of the sample solution and standard solution as directed under Liquid Chromatography <2.01> according to the following conditions, and determine the peak areas, A_T and A_S, of methylephedrine in each solution.

Dissolution rate (%) with respect to the labeled amount of *dl*-methylephedrine hydrochloride ($C_{11}H_{17}NO.HCl$)
$$= M_S/M_T \times A_T/A_S \times 9/4$$

M_S: Amount (mg) of *dl*-methylephedrine hydrochloride for assay taken

M_T: Amount (g) of 10% *dl*-Methylephedrine Hydrochloride Powder taken

Operating conditions—

Column, column temperature, mobile phase, and flow rate: Proceed as directed in the operating conditions in the Assay.

Detector: An ultraviolet absorption photometer (wavelength: 220 nm).

System suitability—

System performance: When the procedure is run with 20 μL of the standard solution under the above operating conditions, the number of theoretical plates and the symmetry factor of the peak of methylephedrine are not less than 5000 and not more than 1.5, respectively.

System repeatability: When the test is repeated 6 times with 20 μL of the standard solution under the above operating conditions, the relative standard deviation of the peak area of methylephedrine is not more than 2.0%.

Assay Weigh accurately about 0.5 g of 10% *dl*-Methylephedrine Hydrochloride Powder, add exactly 4 mL of the internal standard solution and 25 mL of water, shake vigorously for 20 minutes to dissolve, add water to make 50 mL, filter through a membrane filter with a pore size not exceeding 0.45 μm, if necessary, discard the first 10 mL of the filtrate, and use the subsequent filtrate as the sample solution. Separately, weigh accurately about 50 mg of *dl*-methylephedrine hydrochloride for assay, previously dried at 105°C for 3 hours, add exactly 4 mL of the internal standard solution and water to make 50 mL, and use this solution as the standard solution. Perform the test with 20 μL each of the sample solution and standard solution as directed under Liquid Chromatography <2.01> according to the following conditions, and calculate the ratios of the peak area, Q_T and Q_S, of methylephedrine to that of the internal standard.

Amount (mg) of *dl*-methylephedrine hydrochloride ($C_{11}H_{17}NO.HCl$) $= M_S \times Q_T/Q_S$

M_S: Amount (mg) of *dl*-methylephedrine hydrochloride for assay taken

Internal standard solution—A solution of methyl parahydroxybenzoate in acetonitrile (1 in 10,000).

Operating conditions—

Detector: An ultraviolet absorption photometer (wavelength: 257 nm).

Column: A stainless steel column 4.6 mm in inside diameter and 15 cm in length, packed with octadecylsilanized silica gel for liquid chromatography (5 μm in particle diameter).

Column temperature: A constant temperature of about 40°C.

Mobile phase: Dissolve 13.6 g of potassium dihydrogen phosphate and 3 g of sodium 1-heptane sulfonate in 1000 mL of water, and adjust the pH to 2.5 with phosphoric acid. To 900 mL of this solution add 200 mL of acetonitrile.

Flow rate: Adjust so that the retention time of methylephedrine is about 10 minutes.

System suitability—

System performance: When the procedure is run with 20 μL of the standard solution under the above operating conditions, methylephedrine and the internal standard are eluted in this order with the resolution between these peaks being not less than 3.

System repeatability: When the test is repeated 6 times with 20 μL of the standard solution under the above operating conditions, the relative standard deviation of the ratio of the peak area of methylephedrine to that of the internal standard is not more than 1.0%.

Containers and storage Containers—Well-closed containers.

Storage—Light-resistant.

Methylergometrine Maleate

メチルエルゴメトリンマレイン酸塩

$C_{20}H_{25}N_3O_2.C_4H_4O_4$: 455.50
(8*R*)-*N*-[(1*S*)-1-(Hydroxymethyl)propyl]-6-methyl-9,10-didehydroergoline-8-carboxamide monomaleate
[*57432-61-8*]

Methylergometrine Maleate, when dried, contains not less than 95.0% and not more than 105.0% of methylergometrine maleate ($C_{20}H_{25}N_3O_2.C_4H_4O_4$).

Description Methylergometrine Maleate occurs as a white to pale yellow crystalline powder. It is odorless.

It is slightly soluble in water, in methanol and in ethanol (95), and practically insoluble in diethyl ether.

It gradually changes to yellow by light.

Melting point: about 190°C (with decomposition).

Identification **(1)** A solution of Methylergometrine Maleate (1 in 200) shows a blue fluorescence.

(2) The colored solution obtained in the Assay develops a deep blue in color. Determine the absorption spectrum of the colored solution as directed under Ultraviolet-visible Spectrophotometry <*2.24*>, and compare the spectrum with the Reference Spectrum or the spectrum of a solution of Methylergometrine Maleate RS prepared in the same manner as the sample solution: both spectra exhibit similar intensities of absorption at the same wavelengths.

(3) To 5 mL of a solution of Methylergometrine Maleate (1 in 500) add 1 drop of potassium permanganate TS: the red color of the test solution fades immediately.

Optical rotation <*2.49*> $[\alpha]_D^{20}$: +44 – +50° (after drying, 0.1 g, water, 20 mL, 100 mm).

Purity Related substances—Conduct this procedure without exposure to light, using light-resistant vessels. Dissolve 8 mg of Methylergometrine Maleate in 2 mL of a mixture of ethanol (95) and ammonia solution (28) (9:1), and use this solution as the sample solution. Pipet 1 mL of the sample solution, add a mixture of ethanol (95) and ammonia solution (28) (9:1) to make exactly 100 mL, and use this solution as the standard solution. Perform the test immediately with these solutions as directed under Thin-layer Chromatography <*2.03*>. Spot 10 μL each of the sample solution and standard solution on a plate of silica gel with fluorescent indicator for thin-layer chromatography, and immediately develop the plate with a mixture of chloroform, methanol and water (75:25:3) to a distance of about 10 cm, and air-dry the plate. Examine under ultraviolet light (main wavelength: 365 nm): the spots other than the principal spot obtained from the sample solution are not more intense than the spot from the standard solution.

Loss on drying <*2.41*> Not more than 2.0% (0.2 g, in vacuum, phosphorus (V) oxide, 4 hours).

Assay Weigh accurately about 10 mg each of Methylergometrine Maleate and Methylergometrine Maleate RS, previously dried, add water to make exactly 250 mL, and use these solutions as the sample solution and the standard solution. Pipet 2 mL each of the sample solution and the standard solution separately into brown glassstoppered test tubes, add exactly 4 mL each of 4-dimethylaminobenzaldehyde-iron (III) chloride TS while ice cooling, warm for 10 minutes at 45°C, and allow to stand for 20 minutes at room temperature. Perform the test with these solutions as directed under Ultraviolet-visible Spectrophotometry <*2.24*>, using a solution, prepared with 2.0 mL of water in the same manner, as the blank. Determine the absorbances, A_T and A_S, of the subsequent solutions of the sample solution and the standard solution at 545 nm, respectively.

Amount (mg) of methylergometrine maleate ($C_{20}H_{25}N_3O_2.C_4H_4O_4$)
$$= M_S \times A_T/A_S$$

M_S: Amount (mg) of Methylergometrine Maleate RS taken

Containers and storage Containers—Tight containers.
Storage—Light-resistant.

Methylergometrine Maleate Tablets

メチルエルゴメトリンマレイン酸塩錠

Methylergometrine Maleate Tablets contain not less than 90.0% and not more than 110.0% of the labeled amount of methylergometrine maleate ($C_{20}H_{25}N_3O_2.C_4H_4O_4$: 455.50).

Method of preparation Prepare as directed under Tablets, with Methylergometrine maleate.

Identification **(1)** The sample solution obtained in the Assay shows a blue fluorescence.

(2) The colored solution obtained in the Assay shows a deep blue color. Determine the absorption spectrum of the colored solution as directed under Ultraviolet-visible Spectrophotometry <*2.24*>: it exhibits maxima between 543 nm and 547 nm and between 620 nm and 630 nm.

Uniformity of dosage units <*6.02*> Perform the test according to the following method: it meets the requirement of the Content uniformity test.

Transfer 1 tablet of Methylergometrine Maleate Tablets to a brown glass-stoppered centrifuge tube, add 10 mL of water, shake for 10 minutes vigorously, and disintegrate the tablet. Add 3 g of sodium chloride and 2 mL of ammonia solution (28), add exactly 25 mL of chloroform, and after vigorous shaking for 10 minutes, centrifuge for 5 minutes. Discard the water layer, take the chloroform extracts, add chloroform to make exactly *V* mL of a solution containing about 5 μg of methylergometrine maleate ($C_{20}H_{25}N_3O_2.C_4H_4O_4$) per mL, and use this solution as the sample solution. Separately, weigh accurately about 1.25 mg of Methylergometrine Maleate RS, previously dried in a desiccator (in vacuum, phosphorus (V) oxide) for 4 hours, and dissolve in water to make exactly 100 mL. Pipet 10 mL of this solution into a brown glass-stoppered centrifuge tube, and add 3 g of sodium chloride and 2 mL of ammonia solution (28). Add exactly 25 mL of chloroform, shake vigorously for 10 minutes, and centrifuge for 5 minutes. Discard the water layer, and use the chloroform layer as the standard solution. Pipet 20 mL each of the sample solution and the standard solution separately into brown glass-stoppered centrifuge tubes, add immediately exactly 10 mL of dilute 4-dimethylaminobenzaldehyde-iron (III) chloride TS, and shake for 5 minutes vigorously. Centrifuge these solutions for 5 minutes, take the water layers, and allow them to stand for 1 hour. Perform the test with these solutions as directed under Ultraviolet-visible Spectrophotometry <*2.24*>, using dilute 4-dimethylaminobenzaldehyde-iron (III) chloride TS as the blank. Determine the absorbances, A_T and A_S, of the subsequent solutions of the sample solution and standard solution at 545 nm, respectively.

Amount (mg) of methylergometrine maleate ($C_{20}H_{25}N_3O_2.C_4H_4O_4$)
$= M_S \times A_T/A_S \times V/250$

M_S: Amount (mg) of Methylergometrine Maleate RS taken

Dissolution <*6.10*> When the test is performed at 100 revolutions per minute according to the Paddle method, using 900 mL of water as the dissolution medium, the dissolution rate in 30 minutes of Methylergometrine Maleate Tablets is not less than 70%.

Start the test with 1 tablet of Methylergometrine Maleate Tablets, withdraw not less than 20 mL of the medium at the specified minute after starting the test, and filter through a membrane filter with a pore size not exceeding 0.8 μm. Discard not less than 10 mL of the first filtrate, to exactly V mL of the subsequent filtrate add water to make exactly V' mL so that each mL contains about 0.13 μg of methylergometrine maleate ($C_{20}H_{25}N_3O_2.C_4H_4O_4$), and use this solution as the sample solution. Separately, weigh accurately about 25 mg of Methylergometrine Maleate RS, previously dried in a desiccator (in vacuum, phosphorus (V) oxide) for 4 hours, and dissolve in water to make exactly 100 mL. Pipet 5 mL of this solution, add water to make exactly 100 mL, then pipet 1 mL of this solution, add water to make exactly 100 mL, and use this solution as the standard solution. Determine immediately the intensities of the fluorescence, F_T and F_S, of the sample solution and standard solution at 338 nm as the excitation wavelength and at 427 nm as the fluorescence wavelength as directed under Fluorometry <*2.22*>.

Dissolution rate (%) with respect to the labeled amount of methylergometrine maleate ($C_{20}H_{25}N_3O_2.C_4H_4O_4$)
$= M_S \times F_T/F_S \times V'/V \times 1/C \times 9/20$

M_S: Amount (mg) of Methylergometrine Maleate RS taken
C: Labeled amount (mg) of methylergometrine maleate ($C_{20}H_{25}N_3O_2.C_4H_4O_4$) in 1 tablet

Assay Weigh accurately and powder not less than 20 Methylergometrine Maleate Tablets. Weigh accurately a portion of the powder, equivalent to about 0.3 mg of methylergometrine maleate ($C_{20}H_{25}N_3O_2.C_4H_4O_4$), transfer to a brown separator, add 15 mL of sodium hydrogen carbonate solution (1 in 20), and extract with four 20-mL portions of chloroform. Filter each portion of the chloroform extracts through a pledget of absorbent cotton, previously moistened with chloroform, into another dried, brown separator, combine all the extracts, and use this extract as the sample solution. Separately, weigh accurately about 10 mg of Methylergometrine Maleate RS, previously dried in a desiccator (silica gel) for 4 hours, dissolve in water, and add water to make exactly 100 mL. Pipet 3 mL of this solution, and transfer to a brown separator, proceed in the same manner as the preparation of the sample solution, and use this extract as the standard solution. To each total volume of the sample solution and the standard solution add exactly 25 mL each of dilute 4-dimethylaminobenzaldehyde-iron (III) chloride TS, and after vigorous shaking for 5 minutes, allow to stand for 30 minutes. Draw off the water layer, centrifuge, and allow to stand for 1 hour. Perform the test with these solutions as directed under Ultraviolet-visible Spectrophotometry <*2.24*>, using dilute 4-dimethylaminobenzaldehyde-iron (III) chloride TS as the blank. Determine the absorbances, A_T and A_S, of the subsequent solutions of the sample solution and the standard solution at 545 nm, respectively.

Amount (mg) of methylergometrine maleate ($C_{20}H_{25}N_3O_2.C_4H_4O_4$)
$= M_S \times A_T/A_S \times 3/100$

M_S: Amount (mg) of Methylergometrine Maleate RS taken

Containers and storage Containers—Well-closed containers.

Storage—Light-resistant.

Methyl Parahydroxybenzoate

パラオキシ安息香酸メチル

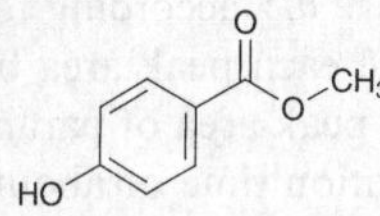

$C_8H_8O_3$: 152.15
Methyl 4-hydroxybenzoate
[*99-76-3*]

This monograph is harmonized with the European Pharmacopoeia and the U.S. Pharmacopeia.

The parts of the text that are not harmonized are marked with symbols (◆ ◆).

Information on the harmonization with the European Pharmacopoeia and the U.S. Pharmacopeia is available on the website of the Pharmaceuticals and Medical Devices Agency.

Methyl Parahydroxybenzoate contains not less than 98.0% and not more than 102.0% of methyl parahydroxybenzoate ($C_8H_8O_3$).

◆**Description** Methyl Parahydroxybenzoate, occurs as colorless crystals or a white crystalline powder.

It is freely soluble in methanol, in ethanol (95) and in acetone, and slightly soluble in water.◆

Identification Determine the infrared absorption spectrum of Methyl Parahydroxybenzoate as directed in the potassium bromide disk method under Infrared Spectrophotometry <*2.25*>, and compare the spectrum with the Reference Spectrum or the spectrum of Methyl Parahydroxybenzoate RS: both spectra exhibit similar intensities of absorption at the same wave numbers.

Melting point <*2.60*> 125 – 128°C

Purity (1) Clarity and color of solution—Dissolve 1.0 g of Methyl Parahydroxybenzoate in ethanol (95) to make 10 mL: the solution is clear and not more intensely colored than the following control solution.

Control solution: To 5.0 mL of Cobalt (II) Chloride CS, 12.0 mL of Iron (III) Chloride CS and 2.0 mL of Copper (II) Sulfate CS add diluted dilute hydrochloric acid (1 in 10) to make 1000 mL.

(2) Acidity—To 2 mL of the solution of Methyl Parahydroxybenzoate obtained in (1) add 3 mL of ethanol (95), add 5 mL of freshly boiled and cooled water and 0.1 mL of bromocresol green-sodium hydroxide-ethanol TS, then add 0.1 mol/L sodium hydroxide VS until the solution shows a blue color: the volume of 0.1 mol/L sodium hydroxide VS used does not exceed 0.1 mL.

◆**(3)** Heavy metals *<1.07>*—Dissolve 1.0 g of Methyl Parahydroxybenzoate in 25 mL of acetone, add 2 mL of dilute acetic acid and water to make 50 mL, and perform the test using this solution as the test solution. Prepare the control solution as follows: to 2.0 mL of Standard Lead Solution add 25 mL of acetone, 2 mL of dilute acetic acid, and water to make 50 mL (not more than 20 ppm).◆

(4) Related substances—Dissolve 50.0 mg of Methyl Parahydroxybenzoate in 2.5 mL of methanol, and add the mobile phase to make exactly 50 mL. Pipet 10 mL of this solution, add the mobile phase to make exactly 100 mL, and use this solution as the sample solution. Pipet 1 mL of the sample solution, and add the mobile phase to make exactly 20 mL. Pipet 1 mL of this solution, add the mobile phase to make exactly 10 mL, and use this solution as the standard solution. Perform the test with exactly 10 μL each of the sample solution and standard solution as directed under Liquid Chromatography *<2.01>* according to the following conditions, and determine each peak area by the automatic integration method: the peak area of parahydroxybenzoic acid having a relative retention time of about 0.6 to methyl parahydroxybenzoate obtained from the sample solution is not larger than the peak area of methyl parahydroxybenzoate from the standard solution (0.5%). For the peak area of parahydroxybenzoic acid, multiply the correction factor, 1.4. Furthermore, the area of the peak other than methyl parahydroxybenzoate and parahydroxybenzoic acid from the sample solution is not larger than the peak area of methyl parahydroxybenzoate from the standard solution (0.5%), and the total area of the peaks other than methyl parahydroxybenzoate from the sample solution is not larger than 2 times the peak area of methyl parahydroxybenzoate from the standard solution (1.0%). For this calculation the peak area not larger than 1/5 times the peak area of methyl parahydroxybenzoate from the standard solution is excluded (0.1%).

Operating conditions—

Detector, column, column temperature, mobile phase, and flow rate: Proceed as directed in the operating conditions in the Assay.

Time span of measurement: About 5 times as long as the retention time of methyl parahydroxybenzoate.

System suitability—

System performance: Proceed as directed in the system suitability in the Assay.

◆Test for required detectability: To exactly 2 mL of the standard solution add the mobile phase to make exactly 10 mL. Confirm that the peak area of methyl parahydroxybenzoate obtained with 10 μL of this solution is equivalent to 14 to 26% of that with 10 μL of the standard solution.◆

◆System repeatability: When the test is repeated 6 times with 10 μL of the standard solution under the above operating conditions, the relative standard deviation of the peak area of methyl parahydroxybenzoate is not more than 2.0%.◆

Residue on ignition *<2.44>* Not more than 0.1% (1 g).

Assay Weigh accurately about 50.0 mg each of Methyl Parahydroxybenzoate and Methyl Parahydroxybenzoate RS, dissolve separately in 2.5 mL each of methanol, and add the mobile phase to make exactly 50 mL. Pipet 10 mL each of these solutions, add the mobile phase to make exactly 100 mL, and use these solutions as the sample solution and the standard solution, respectively. Perform the test with exactly 10 μL each of the sample solution and standard solution as directed under Liquid Chromatography *<2.01>* according to the following conditions, and determine the peak areas, A_T and A_S, of methyl parahydroxybenzoate in each solution.

Amount (mg) of methyl parahydroxybenzoate ($C_8H_8O_3$)
$= M_S \times A_T/A_S$

M_S: Amount (mg) of Methyl Parahydroxybenzoate RS taken

Operating conditions—

Detector: An ultraviolet absorption photometer (wavelength: 272 nm).

Column: A stainless steel column 4.6 mm in inside diameter and 15 cm in length, packed with octadecylsilanized silica gel for liquid chromatography (5 μm in particle diameter).

Column temperature: A constant temperature of about 35°C.

Mobile phase: A mixture of methanol and potassium dihydrogen phosphate solution (17 in 2500) (13:7).

Flow rate: 1.3 mL per minute.

System suitability—

System performance: Dissolve 5 mg each of Methyl Parahydroxybenzoate and parahydroxybenzoic acid in the mobile phase to make exactly 100 mL. Pipet 1 mL of this solution, and add the mobile phase to make exactly 10 mL. When the procedure is run with 10 μL of this solution under the above operating conditions, parahydroxybenzoic acid and methyl parahydroxybenzoate are eluted in this order, the relative retention time of parahydroxybenzoic acid to methyl parahydroxybenzoate is about 0.6, and the resolution between these peaks is not less than 2.0.

System repeatability: When the test is repeated 6 times with 10 μL of the standard solution under the above operating conditions, the relative standard deviation of the peak area of methyl parahydroxybenzoate is not more than 0.85%.

◆**Containers and storage** Containers—Well-closed containers.◆

Methylprednisolone

メチルプレドニゾロン

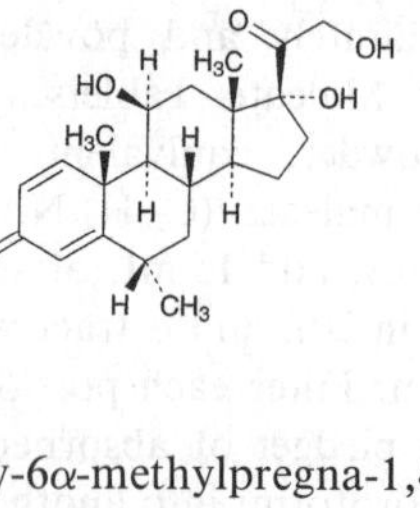

$C_{22}H_{30}O_5$: 374.47
11β,17,21-Trihydroxy-6α-methylpregna-1,4-diene-3,20-dione
[83-43-2]

Methylprednisolone, when dried, contains not less than 96.0% and not more than 104.0% of methylprednisolone ($C_{22}H_{30}O_5$).

Description Methylprednisolone occurs as a white crystalline powder. It is odorless.

It is sparingly soluble in methanol and in ethanol (99.5), and practically insoluble in water.

Melting point: 232 – 240°C (with decomposition).

Identification (1) Add 2 mL of sulfuric acid to 2 mg of Methylprednisolone: a deep red color develops with no fluorescence. Then add 10 mL of water to this solution: the color fades, and a gray, flocculent precipitate is produced.

(2) Dissolve 10 mg of Methylprednisolone in 1 mL of methanol, add 1 mL of Fehling's TS, and heat: a red precipitate is produced.

(3) Determine the absorption spectrum of a solution of Methylprednisolone in methanol (1 in 100,000) as directed under Ultraviolet-visible Spectrophotometry 〈*2.24*〉, and compare the spectrum with the Reference Spectrum: both spectra exhibit similar intensities of absorption at the same wavelengths.

Optical rotation 〈*2.49*〉 $[\alpha]_D^{25}$: +93 – +103° (after drying, 0.1 g, ethanol (99.5), 10 mL, 100 mm).

Purity Related substances—Dissolve 50 mg of Methylprednisolone in 5 mL of a mixture of chloroform and methanol (9:1), and use this solution as the sample solution. Pipet 1 mL of the sample solution, add a mixture of chloroform and methanol (9:1) to make exactly 200 mL, and use this solution as the standard solution. Perform the test with these solutions as directed under Thin-layer Chromatography 〈*2.03*〉. Spot 10 μL each of the sample solution and standard solution on a plate of silica gel for thin-layer chromatography. Develop the plate with a mixture of dichloromethane, diethyl ether, methanol and water (385:75:40:6) to a distance of about 12 cm, and air-dry the plate. Then heat the plate at 105°C for 10 minutes, cool, and spray evenly alkaline blue tetrazolium TS on the plate: the spots other than the principal spot obtained from the sample solution are not more intense than the spot from the standard solution.

Loss on drying 〈*2.41*〉 Not more than 1.0% (0.5 g, 105°C, 3 hours).

Residue on ignition 〈*2.44*〉 Not more than 0.2% (0.2 g).

Assay Weigh accurately about 10 mg of Methylprednisolone, previously dried, and dissolve in methanol to make exactly 100 mL. To exactly 5 mL of this solution add methanol to make exactly 50 mL, and determine the absorbance A at the wavelength of maximum absorption at about 243 nm as directed under Ultraviolet-visible Spectrophotometry 〈*2.24*〉.

$$\text{Amount (mg) of methylprednisolone } (C_{22}H_{30}O_5) = A/400 \times 10{,}000$$

Containers and storage Containers—Tight containers.

Methylprednisolone Succinate

メチルプレドニゾロンコハク酸エステル

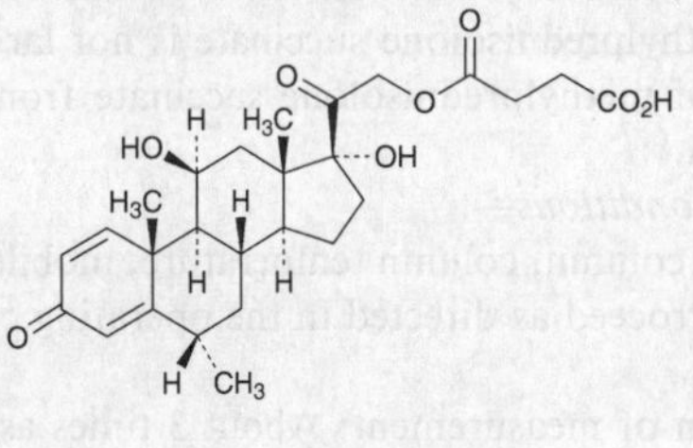

$C_{26}H_{34}O_8$: 474.54

11β,17,21-Trihydroxy-6α-methylpregna-1,4-diene-3,20-dione 21-(hydrogen succinate)

[*2921-57-5*]

Methylprednisolone Succinate, when dried, contains not less than 97.0% and not more than 103.0% of methylprednisolone succinate ($C_{26}H_{34}O_8$).

Description Methylprednisolone Succinate occurs as a white, crystals or crystalline powder.

It is soluble in methanol, sparingly soluble in ethanol (95), and practically insoluble in water.

Melting point: about 235°C (with decomposition).

It shows crystal polymorphism.

Identification (1) Determine the absorption spectrum of a solution of Methylprednisolone Succinate in methanol (1 in 50,000) as directed under Ultraviolet-visible Spectrophotometry 〈*2.24*〉, and compare the spectrum with the Reference Spectrum or the spectrum of a solution of Methylprednisolone Succinate RS prepared in the same manner as the sample solution: both spectra exhibit similar intensities of absorption at the same wavelengths.

(2) Determine the infrared absorption spectrum of Methylprednisolone Succinate, previously dried, as directed in the potassium bromide disk method under Infrared Spectrophotometry 〈*2.25*〉, and compare the spectrum with the Reference Spectrum or the spectrum of previously dried Methylprednisolone Succinate RS: both spectra exhibit similar intensities of absorption at the same wave numbers. In case when some differences are found between the spectra, repeat the test with residues obtained by dissolving these substances in ethanol (95), evaporating to dryness, and drying.

Optical rotation 〈*2.49*〉 $[\alpha]_D^{25}$: +99 – +103° (after drying, 0.2 g, ethanol (95), 20 mL, 100 mm).

Purity (1) Heavy metals 〈*1.07*〉—Proceed with 1.0 g of Methylprednisolone Succinate according to Method 4, and perform the test. Prepare the control solution with 1.0 mL of Standard Lead Solution (not more than 10 ppm).

(2) Arsenic 〈*1.11*〉—Prepare the test solution with 2.0 g of Methylprednisolone Succinate according to Method 3, and perform the test (not more than 1 ppm).

(3) Related substances—Dissolve 15 mg of Methylprednisolone Succinate in 5 mL of methanol, add a mixture of 0.05 mol/L phosphate buffer solution (pH 3.5) and acetonitrile (1:1) to make 50 mL, and use this solution as the sample solution. Pipet 1 mL of the sample solution, add the mixture of 0.05 mol/L phosphate buffer solution (pH 3.5) and acetonitrile (1:1) to make exactly 100 mL, and use this solution as the standard solution. Perform the test with exactly 5 μL each of the sample solution and standard solution as directed under Liquid Chromatography 〈*2.01*〉 according to the following conditions, and determine each peak area by

the automatic integration method: the area of the peaks other than the peak of methylprednisolone succinate obtained from sample solution is not larger than 1/2 times the peak area of methylprednisolone succinate from the standard solution, and the total area of the peaks other than the peak of methylprednisolone succinate is not larger than the peak area of methylprednisolone succinate from the standard solution.

Operating conditions—

Detector, column, column temperature, mobile phase, and flow rate: Proceed as directed in the operating conditions in the Assay.

Time span of measurement: About 3 times as long as the retention time of methylprednisolone succinate.

System suitability—

System performance: Proceed as directed in the System suitability in the Assay.

Test for required detectability: Pipet 1 mL of the standard solution, and add the mixture of 0.05 mol/L phosphate buffer solution (pH 3.5) and acetonitrile (1:1) to make exactly 10 mL. Confirm that the peak area of methylprednisolone succinate obtained with 5 μL of this solution is equivalent to 7 to 13% of that with 5 μL of the standard solution.

System repeatability: When the test is repeated 6 times with 5 μL of the standard solution under the above operating conditions, the relative standard deviation of the peak area of methylprednisolone succinate is not more than 2.5%.

Loss on drying <*2.41*> Not more than 1.0% (1 g, 105°C, 3 hours).

Residue on ignition <*2.44*> Not more than 0.2% (0.5 g).

Assay Weigh accurately about 15 mg each of Methylprednisolone Succinate and Methylprednisolone Succinate RS, previously dried, dissolve separately in 5 mL of methanol, and add the mixture of 0.05 mol/L phosphate buffer solution (pH 3.5) and acetonitrile (1:1) to make exactly 50 mL. Pipet 5 mL each of these solutions, add exactly 5 mL of the internal standard solution, and use these solutions as the sample solution and the standard solution, respectively. Perform the test with 5 μL each of the sample solution and standard solution as directed under Liquid Chromatography <*2.01*> according to the following conditions, and calculate the ratios, Q_T and Q_S, of the peak area of methylprednisolone succinate to that of the internal standard.

Amount (mg) of methylprednisolone succinate ($C_{26}H_{34}O_8$)
$= M_S \times Q_T/Q_S$

M_S: Amount (mg) of Methylprednisolone Succinate RS taken

*Internal standard solution—*A solution of ethyl parahydroxybenzoate in a mixture of 0.05 mol/L phosphate buffer solution (pH 3.5) and acetonitrile (1:1) (3 in 20,000).

Operating conditions—

Detector: An ultraviolet absorption photometer (wavelength: 254 nm).

Column: A stainless steel column 4.6 mm in inside diameter and 25 cm in length, packed with octadecylsilanized silica gel for liquid chromatography (5 μm in particle diameter).

Column temperature: A constant temperature of about 25°C.

Mobile phase: To 1000 mL of 0.05 mol/L potassium dihydrogen phosphate TS add a suitable amount of 0.05 mol/L disodium hydrogen phosphate TS to make a solution having pH 5.5. To 640 mL of this solution add 360 mL of acetonitrile.

Flow rate: Adjust so that the retention time of methylprednisolone succinate is about 6 minutes.

System suitability—

System performance: When the procedure is run with 5 μL of the standard solution under the above operating conditions, methylprednisolone succinate and the internal standard are eluted in this order with the resolution between these peaks being not less than 6.

System repeatability: When the test is repeated 6 times with 5 μL of the standard solution under the above operating conditions, the relative standard deviation of the ratio of the peak area of methylprednisolone succinate to that of the internal standard is not more than 1.0%.

Containers and storage Containers—Tight containers.

Methyl Salicylate

サリチル酸メチル

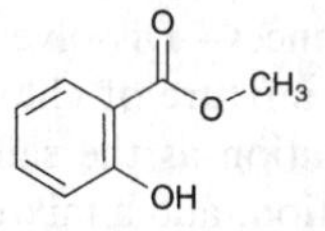

$C_8H_8O_3$: 152.15
Methyl 2-hydroxybenzoate
[*119-36-8*]

Methyl Salicylate contains not less than 98.0% of methyl salicylate ($C_8H_8O_3$).

Description Methyl Salicylate is a colorless to pale yellow liquid. It has a strong, characteristic odor.

It is miscible with ethanol (95) and with diethyl ether.

It is very slightly soluble in water.

Specific gravity d^{20}_{20}: 1.182 – 1.192

Boiling point: 219 – 224°C

Identification Shake 1 drop of Methyl Salicylate thoroughly with 5 mL of water for 1 minute, and add 1 drop of iron (III) chloride TS: a purple color develops.

Purity **(1)** Acidity—Shake 5.0 mL of Methyl Salicylate thoroughly with 25 mL of freshly boiled and cooled water and 1.0 mL of 0.1 mol/L sodium hydroxide VS for 1 minute, add 2 drops of phenol red TS, and titrate <*2.50*> with 0.1 mol/L hydrochloric acid VS until the red color disappears: not more than 0.45 mL of 0.1 mol/L sodium hydroxide VS is consumed.

(2) Heavy metals—Shake 10.0 mL of Methyl Salicylate thoroughly with 10 mL of water, add 1 drop of hydrochloric acid, and saturate with hydrogen sulfide by passing it through the mixture: neither the oily layer nor the aqueous layer shows a dark color.

Assay Weigh accurately about 2 g of Methyl Salicylate, add an exactly measured 50 mL of 0.5 mol/L potassium hydroxide-ethanol VS, and heat on a water bath for 2 hours under a reflux condenser. Cool, and titrate <*2.50*> the excess potassium hydroxide with 0.5 mol/L hydrochloric acid VS (indicator: 3 drops of phenolphthalein TS). Perform a blank determination in the same manner.

Each mL of 0.5 mol/L potassium hydroxide-ethanol VS
$= 76.08$ mg of $C_8H_8O_3$

Containers and storage Containers—Tight containers.

Compound Methyl Salicylate Spirit

複方サリチル酸メチル精

Method of preparation

Methyl Salicylate	40 mL
Capsicum Tincture	100 mL
d- or *dl*-Camphor	50 g
Ethanol	a sufficient quantity
	To make 1000 mL

Prepare as directed under Spirits, with the above ingredients.

Description Compound Methyl Salicylate Spirit is a reddish yellow liquid, having a characteristic odor and a burning taste.

Identification **(1)** Shake 1 mL of Compound Methyl Salicylate Spirit with 5 mL of dilute ethanol, and add 1 drop of iron (III) chloride TS: a purple color is produced (methyl salicylate).

(2) Shake thoroughly 1 mL of Compound Methyl Salicylate Spirit with 10 mL of chloroform, and use this solution as the sample solution. Dissolve 40 mg of methyl salicylate in 10 mL of chloroform, and use this solution as the standard solution. Perform the test with these solutions as directed under Thin-layer Chromatography <*2.03*>. Spot 5 μL each of the sample solution and standard solution on the plate of silica gel with fluorescent indicator for thin-layer chromatography. Develop the plate with a mixture of hexane and chloroform (4:1) to a distance of about 10 cm, air-dry the plate, and examine under ultraviolet light (main wavelength: 254 nm): the spots obtained from the sample solution and the standard solution show the same *R*f value. Spray evenly iron (III) chloride TS upon the plate: the spot from the standard solution and the corresponding spot from the sample solution reveal a purple color.

Containers and storage Containers—Tight containers.

Methyltestosterone

メチルテストステロン

$C_{20}H_{30}O_2$: 302.45
17β-Hydroxy-17α-methylandrost-4-en-3-one
[*58-18-4*]

Methyltestosterone, when dried, contains not less than 98.0% and not more than 102.0% of methyltestosterone ($C_{20}H_{30}O_2$).

Description Methyltestosterone occurs as white to pale yellow, crystals or crystalline powder.

It is freely soluble in methanol and in ethanol (95), and practically insoluble in water.

Identification **(1)** Determine the absorption spectrum of a solution of Methyltestosterone in ethanol (95) (1 in 100,000) as directed under Ultraviolet-visible Spectrophotometry <*2.24*>, and compare the spectrum with the Reference Spectrum or the spectrum of a solution of Methyltestosterone RS prepared in the same manner as the sample solution: both spectra exhibit similar intensities of absorption at the same wavelengths.

(2) Determine the infrared absorption spectrum of Methyltestosterone, previously dried, as directed in the potassium bromide disk method under Infrared Spectrophotometry <*2.25*>, and compare the spectrum with the Reference Spectrum or the spectrum of dried Methyltestosterone RS: both spectra exhibit similar intensities of absorption at the same wave numbers.

Optical rotation <*2.49*> $[\alpha]_D^{20}$: +79 – +85° (after drying, 0.1 g, ethanol (95), 10 mL, 100 mm).

Melting point <*2.60*> 163 – 168°C

Purity Related substances—Dissolve 40 mg of Methyltestosterone in 2 mL of ethanol (95), and use this solution as the sample solution. Pipet 1 mL of the sample solution, add ethanol (95) to make exactly 100 mL, and use this solution as the standard solution. Perform the test with these solutions as directed under Thin-layer Chromatography <*2.03*>. Spot 10 μL each of the sample solution and standard solution on a plate of silica gel with fluorescent indicator for thin-layer chromatography. Develop the plate with a mixture of chloroform and diethylamine (19:1) to a distance of about 15 cm, and air-dry the plate. Examine under ultraviolet light (main wavelength: 254 nm): the spots other than the principal spot obtained from the sample solution are not more intense than the spot from the standard solution.

Loss on drying <*2.41*> Not more than 1.0% (0.5 g, in vacuum, phosphorus (V) oxide, 10 hours).

Residue on ignition <*2.44*> Not more than 0.1% (0.5 g).

Assay Weigh accurately about 20 mg each of Methyltestosterone and Methyltestosterone RS, previously dried in a desiccator (in vacuum, phosphorus (V) oxide) for 10 hours, dissolve each in methanol to make exactly 200 mL. Pipet 5 mL each of these solutions, add exactly 5 mL of the internal standard solution, add methanol to make 50 mL, and use these solutions as the sample solution and standard solution. Perform the test with 10 μL each of the sample solution and standard solution as directed under Liquid Chromatography <*2.01*> according to the following conditions, and calculate the ratios, Q_T and Q_S, of the peak area of methyltestosterone to that of the internal standard.

$$\text{Amount (mg) of methyltestosterone } (C_{20}H_{30}O_2) = M_S \times Q_T/Q_S$$

M_S: Amount (mg) of Methyltestosterone RS taken

Internal standard solution—A solution of propyl parahydroxybenzoate in methanol (1 in 10,000).

Operating conditions—

Detector: An ultraviolet absorption photometer (wavelength: 241 nm).

Column: A stainless steel column 6 mm in inside diameter and 15 cm in length, packed with octadecylsilanized silica gel for liquid chromatography (5 μm in particle diameter).

Column temperature: A constant temperature of about 35°C.

Mobile phase: A mixture of acetonitrile and water (11:9).

Flow rate: Adjust so that the retention time of methyltestosterone is about 10 minutes.

System suitability—

System performance: When the procedure is run with 10 μL of the standard solution under the above operating conditions, the internal standard and methyltestosterone are eluted in this order with the resolution between these peaks being not less than 9.

System repeatability: When the test is repeated 6 times with 10 μL of the standard solution under the above operating conditions, the relative standard deviation of the ratios of the peak area of methyltestosterone to that of the internal standard is not more than 1.0%.

Containers and storage Containers—Tight containers.

Storage—Light-resistant.

Methyltestosterone Tablets

メチルテストステロン錠

Methyltestosterone Tablets contain not less than 90.0% and not more than 110.0% of the labeled amount of methyltestosterone ($C_{20}H_{30}O_2$: 302.45).

Method of preparation Prepare as directed under Tablets, with Methyltestosterone.

Identification To a portion of powdered Methyltestosterone Tablets, equivalent to 10 mg of Methyltestosterone, add 50 mL of acetone, shake for 30 minutes, and filter. Evaporate the filtrate to dryness, dissolve the residue in 10 mL of acetone, and use this solution as the sample solution. Separately, dissolve 10 mg of Methyltestosterone RS in 10 mL of acetone, and use this solution as the standard solution. Perform the test with these solutions as directed under Thin-layer Chromatography <*2.03*>. Spot 10 μL each of the sample solution and standard solution on a plate of silica gel for thin-layer chromatography. Develop the plate with a mixture of chloroform and ethanol (95) (9:1) to a distance of about 12 cm, and air-dry the plate. Spray evenly dilute sulfuric acid on the plate, and heat the plate at 110°C for 10 minutes: the spot obtained from the sample solution and the standard solution show the same *R*f value.

Uniformity of dosage units <*6.02*> Perform the test according to the following method: it meets the requirement of the Content uniformity test.

To 1 tablet of Methyltestosterone Tablets add 5 mL of water to disintegrate, add 50 mL of methanol, and shake for 30 minutes. Add methanol to make exactly 100 mL, and centrifuge. Measure exactly *V* mL of the supernatant liquid, add methanol to make exactly *V′* mL of a solution containing about 10 μg of methyltestosterone ($C_{20}H_{30}O_2$) per ml, and use this solution as the sample solution. Separately, weigh accurately about 10 mg of Methyltestosterone RS, previously dried in a desiccator (in vacuum, phosphorus (V) oxide) for 10 hours, and dissolve in 5 mL of water and 50 mL of methanol, then add methanol to make exactly 100 mL. Pipet 5 mL of this solution, add methanol to make exactly 50 mL, and use this solution as the standard solution. Determine the absorbances, A_T and A_S, of the sample solution and the standard solution at the wavelength of maximum absorption at about 241 nm, respectively, as directed under Ultraviolet-visible Spectrophotometry <*2.25*>.

Amount (mg) of methyltestosterone ($C_{20}H_{30}O_2$)
$= M_S \times A_T/A_S \times V'/V \times 1/10$

M_S: Amount (mg) of Methyltestosterone RS taken

Dissolution <*6.10*> When the test is performed at 100 revolutions per minute according to the Paddle method, using 900 mL of a solution prepared by dissolving 1 g of polysorbate 80 in water to make 5 L as the dissolution medium, the dissolution rate in 30 minutes of a 10-mg tablet is not less than 75% and that in 60 minutes of a 25-mg tablet is not less than 70%.

Start the test with 1 tablet of Methyltestosterone Tablets, withdraw not less than 20 mL of the medium at the specified minute after starting the test, and filter through a membrane filter with a pore size not exceeding 0.45 μm. Discard not less than 10 mL of the first filtrate, pipet *V* mL of the subsequent filtrate, add the dissolution medium to make exactly *V′* mL so that each mL contains about 11 μg of methyltestosterone ($C_{20}H_{30}O_2$), and use this solution as the sample solution. Separately, weigh accurately about 22 mg of Methyltestosterone RS, previously dried in vacuum using phosphorus (V) oxide as a desiccant for 10 hours, and dissolve in ethanol (99.5) to make exactly 100 mL. Pipet 5 mL of this solution, add the dissolution medium to make exactly 100 mL, and use this solution as the standard solution. Determine the absorbances, A_T and A_S, at 249 nm of the sample solution and standard solution as directed under Ultraviolet-visible Spectrophotometry <*2.24*>, using the dissolution medium as the blank.

Dissolution rate (%) with respect to the labeled amount of methyltestosterone ($C_{20}H_{30}O_2$)
$= M_S \times A_T/A_S \times V'/V \times 1/C \times 45$

M_S: Amount (mg) of Methyltestosterone RS taken
C: Labeled amount (mg) of methyltestosterone ($C_{20}H_{30}O_2$) in 1 tablet

Assay Weigh accurately the mass of not less than 20 Methyltestosterone Tablets, and powder. Weigh accurately a portion of the powder, equivalent to about 25 mg of methyltestosterone ($C_{20}H_{30}O_2$), add about 70 mL of methanol, shake for 30 minutes, and add methanol to make exactly 100 mL. Pipet 2 mL of this solution, add exactly 5 mL of the internal standard solution and methanol to make 50 mL, filter through a membrane filter (not exceeding 0.45 μm in pore size), and use the filtrate as the sample solution. Separately, weigh accurately about 20 mg of Methyltestosterone RS, previously dried in a desiccator (in vacuum, phosphorus (V) oxide) for 10 hours, dissolve in methanol to make exactly 200 mL. Pipet 5 mL of this solution, add exactly 5 mL of the internal standard solution, add methanol to make 50 mL, and use this solution as the standard solution. Perform the test with 10 μL each of the sample solution and standard solution as directed under Liquid Chromatography <*2.01*> according to the following conditions, and calculate the ratios, Q_T and Q_S, of the peak area of methyltestosterone to that of the internal standard.

Amount (mg) of methyltestosterone ($C_{20}H_{30}O_2$)
$= M_S \times Q_T/Q_S \times 5/4$

M_S: Amount (mg) of Methyltestosterone RS taken

*Internal standard solution—*A solution of propyl parahydroxybenzoate in methanol (1 in 10,000).

Operating conditions—

Detector: An ultraviolet absorption photometer (wavelength: 241 nm).

Column: A stainless steel column 6 mm in inside diameter and 15 cm in length, packed with octadecylsilanized silica gel for liquid chromatography (5 μm in particle diameter).

Column temperature: A constant temperature of about 35°C.

Mobile phase: A mixture of acetonitrile and water (11:9).

Flow rate: Adjust so that the retention time of methyltestosterone is about 10 minutes.

System suitability—

System performance: When the procedure is run with 10 μL of the standard solution under the above operating conditions, the internal standard and methyltestosterone are eluted in this order with the resolution between these peaks being not less than 9.

System repeatability: When the test is repeated 6 times with 10 μL of the standard solution under the above operating conditions, the relative standard deviation of the ratio of the peak area of methyltestosterone to that of the internal standard is not more than 1.0%.

Containers and storage Containers—Tight containers.

Meticrane

メチクラン

$C_{10}H_{13}NO_4S_2$: 275.34
6-Methylthiochromane-7-sulfonamide 1,1-dioxide
[*1084-65-7*]

Meticrane, when dried, contains not less than 98.0% of meticrane ($C_{10}H_{13}NO_4S_2$).

Description Meticrane occurs as white, crystals or crystalline powder.

It is freely soluble in *N*,*N*-dimethylformamide, slightly soluble in acetonitrile and in methanol, very slightly soluble in ethanol (95), and practically insoluble in water.

Melting point: about 234°C (with decomposition).

Identification **(1)** Determine the absorption spectrum of a solution of Meticrane in methanol (3 in 10,000) as directed under Ultraviolet-visible Spectrophotometry *<2.24>*, and compare the spectrum with the Reference Spectrum: both spectra exhibit similar intensities of absorption at the same wavelengths.

(2) Determine the infrared absorption spectrum of Meticrane, previously dried, as directed in the potassium bromide disk method under Infrared Spectrophotometry *<2.25>*, and compare the spectrum with the Reference Spectrum: both spectra exhibit similar intensities of absorption at the same wave numbers.

Purity **(1)** Ammonium *<1.02>*—Perform the test with 0.10 g of Meticrane. Prepare the control solution with 3.0 mL of Standard Ammonium Solution (not more than 0.03%).

(2) Heavy metals *<1.07>*—Proceed with 1.0 g of Meticrane according to Method 2, and perform the test. Prepare the control solution with 2.0 mL of Standard Lead Solution (not more than 20 ppm).

(3) Arsenic *<1.11>*—Prepare the test solution with 1.0 g of Meticrane according to Method 3, and perform the test (not more than 2 ppm).

(4) Related substances—Dissolve 50 mg of Meticrane in 50 mL of acetonitrile. To 5 mL of this solution add the mobile phase to make 25 mL, and use this solution as the sample solution. Pipet 1 mL of the sample solution, add the mobile phase to make exactly 100 mL, and use this solution as the standard solution. Perform the test with exactly 10 μL each of the sample solution and standard solution as directed under Liquid Chromatography *<2.01>* according to the following conditions, and determine each peak area of both solutions by the automatic integration method: the total area of the peaks other than meticrane obtained from the sample solution is not larger than the peak area of meticrane from the standard solution.

Operating conditions 1—

Detector: An ultraviolet absorption photometer (wavelength: 230 nm).

Column: A stainless steel column 4.6 mm in inside diameter and 15 cm in length, packed with octadecylsilanized silica gel for liquid chromatography (5 μm in particle diameter).

Column temperature: A constant temperature of about 40°C.

Mobile phase: A mixture of water and acetonitrile (17:3).

Flow rate: Adjust so that the retention time of meticrane is about 7 minutes.

Time span of measurement: About 4 times as long as the retention time of meticrane, beginning after the solvent peak.

System suitability 1—

Test for required detectability: To exactly 2 mL of the standard solution add the mobile phase to make exactly 20 mL. Confirm that the peak area of meticrane obtained with 10 μL of this solution is equivalent to 7 to 13% of that with 10 μL of the standard solution.

System performance: Dissolve 10 mg each of Meticrane and caffeine in 100 mL of acetonitrile. To exactly 2 mL of this solution add the mobile phase to make exactly 10 mL. When the procedure is run with 10 μL of this solution under the above operating conditions 1, caffeine and meticrane are eluted in this order with the resolution between these peaks being not less than 10.

System repeatability: When the test is repeated 6 times with 10 μL of the standard solution under the above operating conditions 1, the relative standard deviation of the peak area of meticrane is not more than 2.0%.

Operating conditions 2—

Detector, column, and column temperature: Proceed as directed in the operating conditions 1.

Mobile phase: A mixture of water and acetonitrile (1:1).

Flow rate: Adjust so that the retention time of meticrane is about 2 minutes.

Time span of measurement: About 10 times as long as the retention time of meticrane, beginning after the solvent peak.

System suitability 2—

Test for required detectability: To exactly 2 mL of the standard solution add the mobile phase to make exactly 20 mL. Confirm that the peak area of meticrane obtained with 10 μL of this solution is equivalent to 7 to 13% of that with 10 μL of the standard solution.

System performance: Dissolve 20 mg each of Meticrane and methyl parahydroxybenzoate in 100 mL of acetonitrile. To exactly 2 mL of this solution add the mobile phase to make exactly 10 mL. When the procedure is run with 10 μL of this solution under the above operating conditions 2, meticrane and methyl parahydroxybenzoate are eluted in this order with the resolution between these peaks being not less than 4.

System repeatability: When the test is repeated 6 times with 10 μL of the standard solution under the above operating conditions 2, the relative standard deviation of the peak area of meticrane is not more than 2.0%.

Loss on drying <*2.41*> Not more than 0.5% (1 g, 105°C, 4 hours).

Residue on ignition <*2.44*> Not more than 0.1% (1 g).

Assay Weigh accurately about 0.5 g of Meticrane, previously dried, dissolve in 50 mL of *N*,*N*-dimethylformamide, add 5 mL of water, and titrate <*2.50*> with 0.1 mol/L potassium hydroxide-ethanol VS (potentiometric titration). Perform a blank determination in the same manner, and make any necessary correction.

Each mL of 0.1 mol/L potassium hydroxide-ethanol VS
= 27.54 mg of $C_{10}H_{13}NO_4S_2$

Containers and storage Containers—Well-closed containers.

Metildigoxin

メチルジゴキシン

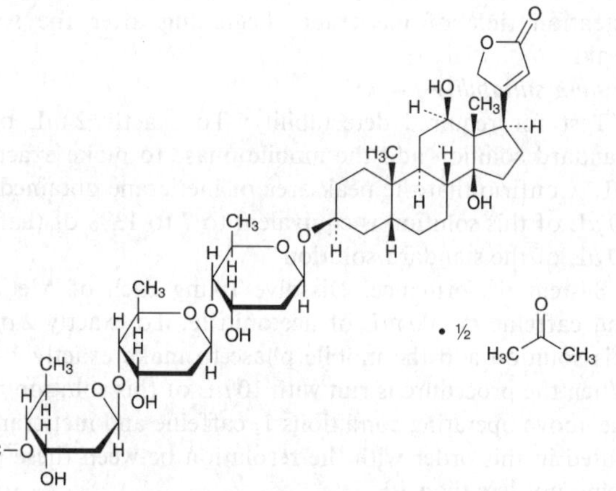

$C_{42}H_{66}O_{14}.\frac{1}{2}C_3H_6O$: 824.00
3*β*-[2,6-Dideoxy-4-*O*-methyl-*β*-D-*ribo*-hexopyranosyl-(1→4)-2,6-dideoxy-*β*-D-*ribo*-hexopyranosyl-(1→4)-2,6-dideoxy-*β*-D-*ribo*-hexopyranosyloxy]-12*β*,14-dihydroxy-5*β*-card-20(22)-enolide—acetone (2/1)
[*30685-43-9*, acetone-free]

Metildigoxin contains not less than 96.0% and not more than 103.0% of metildigoxin ($C_{42}H_{66}O_{14}.\frac{1}{2}C_3H_6O$), calculated on the anhydrous basis.

Description Metildigoxin occurs as a white to light yellow-white crystalline powder.

It is freely soluble in *N*,*N*-dimethylformamide, in pyridine and in acetic acid (100), soluble in chloroform, sparingly soluble in methanol, slightly soluble in ethanol (95) and in acetone, and very slightly soluble in water.

It shows crystal polymorphism.

Identification **(1)** Dissolve 2 mg of Metildigoxin in 2 mL of acetic acid (100), shake well with 1 drop of iron (III) chloride TS, and add gently 2 mL of sulfuric acid to divide into two layers: a brown color develops at the interface, and a deep blue color gradually develops in the acetic acid layer.

(2) Dissolve 2 mg of Metildigoxin in 2 mL of 1,3-dinitrobenzene TS, add 2 mL of a solution of tetramethylammonium hydroxide in ethanol (95) (1 in 200), and shake: a purple color gradually develops, and changes to blue-purple.

(3) Determine the absorption spectrum of a solution of Metildigoxin in methanol (1 in 50,000) as directed under Ultraviolet-visible Spectrophotometry <*2.24*>, and compare the spectrum with the Reference Spectrum or the spectrum of a solution of Metildigoxin RS prepared in the same manner as the sample solution: both spectra exhibit similar intensities of absorption at the same wavelengths.

(4) Determine the infrared absorption spectrum of Metildigoxin as directed in the potassium bromide disk method under Infrared Spectrophotometry <*2.25*>, and compare the spectrum with the Reference Spectrum or the spectrum of Metildigoxin RS: both spectra exhibit similar intensities of absorption at the same wave numbers. If any difference appears between the spectra, dissolve Metildigoxin and Metildigoxin RS in acetone, respectively, then evaporate the acetone to dryness, and repeat the test on the residues.

Optical rotation <*2.49*> $[\alpha]^{20}_{546.1}$: +22.0 – +25.5° (1 g calculated on the anhydrous basis, pyridine, 10 mL, 100 mm).

Purity **(1)** Arsenic <*1.11*>—Prepare the test solution with 0.5 g of Metildigoxin according to Method 3, and perform the test (not more than 4 ppm).

(2) Related substances—Dissolve 10 mg of Metildigoxin in 10 mL of chloroform, and use this solution as the sample solution. Pipet 1 mL of the sample solution, add chloroform to make exactly 50 mL, and use this solution as the standard solution. Perform the test with these solutions as directed under Thin-layer Chromatography <*2.03*>. Spot 20 μL each of the sample solution and standard solution on a plate of silica gel for thin-layer chromatography. Develop the plate with a mixture of 2-butanone and chloroform (3:1) to a distance of about 15 cm, and air-dry the plate. Spray evenly dilute sulfuric acid on the plate, and heat the plate at 110°C for 10 minutes: the spots other than the principal spot obtained from the sample solution are not more intense than the spot from the standard solution.

Acetone Weigh accurately about 0.1 g of Metildigoxin, dissolve in exactly 2 mL of the internal standard solution, add *N*,*N*-dimethylformamide to make 10 mL, and use this solution as the sample solution. Separately, weigh accurately about 0.4 g of acetone in a 50-mL volumetric flask containing about 10 mL of *N*,*N*-dimethylformamide, and add *N*,*N*-dimethylformamide to make 50 mL. Pipet 5 mL of this solution, add exactly 20 mL of the internal standard solution, then add *N*,*N*-dimethylformamide to make 100 mL, and use this solution as the standard solution. Perform the test with 1 μL each of the sample solution and standard solution as directed under Gas Chromatography <*2.02*> according to the following conditions, and calculate the ratios, Q_T and Q_S, of the peak area of acetone to that of the internal standard: the amount of acetone is between 2.0% and 5.0%.

$$\text{Amount (\%) of acetone} = M_S/M_T \times Q_T/Q_S$$

M_S: Amount (g) of acetone taken
M_T: amount (g) of Metildigoxin taken

Internal standard solution—A solution of *t*-butyl alcohol in *N*,*N*-dimethylformamide (1 in 2000).
Operating conditions—

Detector: A hydrogen flame-ionization detector.

Column: A glass column about 2 mm in inside diameter and 1 to 2 m in length, packed with porous ethylvinylbenzene-divinylbenzene copolymer for gas chromatography (150 to 180 μm in particle diameter).

Column temperature: A constant temperature between 170°C and 230°C.

Carrier gas: Nitrogen.

Flow rate: Adjust so that the retention time of acetone is about 2 minutes.

Selection of column: Proceed with 1 μL of the standard

solution under the above operating conditions, and calculate the resolution. Use a column giving elution of acetone and *t*-butyl alcohol in this order with the resolution between these peaks being not less than 2.0.

Water <*2.48*> Not more than 3.0% (0.3 g, volumetric titration, direct titration).

Residue on ignition <*2.44*> Not more than 0.1% (0.5 g).

Assay Weigh accurately 0.1 g each of Metildigoxin and Metildigoxin RS (separately, determine the water <*2.48*> in the same manner as Metildigoxin), and dissolve each in methanol to make exactly 50 mL. Pipet 5 mL each of the solutions, add methanol to each to make exactly 100 mL, and use these solutions as the sample solution and the standard solution, respectively. Pipet 5 mL each of the sample solution and standard solution, add 15 mL of 2,4,6-trinitrophenol-ethanol TS and 2 mL of sodium hydroxide TS to each, shake well, add methanol to make exactly 25 mL, and allow to stand at 20 ± 0.5°C for 20 minutes. Perform the test with these solutions as directed under Ultraviolet-visible Spectrophotometry <*2.24*> using a solution prepared by mixing 15 mL of 2,4,6-trinitrophenol-ethanol TS and 2 mL of sodium hydroxide TS and adding methanol to make exactly 25 mL as the blank. Determine the maximum absorbances, A_T and A_S, of the subsequent solutions obtained from the sample solution and the standard solution, respectively, by measuring every 5 minutes, at 495 nm.

Amount (mg) of metildigoxin ($C_{42}H_{66}O_{14}.{}^{1}\!/_{2}C_3H_6O$)
$= M_S \times A_T/A_S$

M_S: Amount (mg) of Metildigoxin RS taken, calculated on the anhydrous basis

Containers and storage Containers—Tight containers.

Metoclopramide

メトクロプラミド

$C_{14}H_{22}ClN_3O_2$: 299.80
4-Amino-5-chloro-*N*-[2-(diethylamino)ethyl]-2-methoxybenzamide
[*364-62-5*]

Metoclopramide, when dried, contains not less than 99.0% of metoclopramide ($C_{14}H_{22}ClN_3O_2$).

Description Metoclopramide occurs as white, crystals or a crystalline powder, and is odorless.

It is freely soluble in acetic acid (100), soluble in methanol and in chloroform, sparingly soluble in ethanol (95), in acetic anhydride and in acetone, very slightly soluble in diethyl ether, and practically insoluble in water.

It dissolves in dilute hydrochloric acid.

Identification (1) Dissolve 10 mg of Metoclopramide in 1 mL of dilute hydrochloric acid and 4 mL of water: the solution responds to Qualitative Tests <*1.09*> for Primary Aromatic Amines.

(2) Dissolve 10 mg of Metoclopramide in 5 mL of dilute hydrochloric acid and 20 mL of water, and to 5 mL of this solution add 1 mL of Dragendorff's TS: a reddish orange precipitate is produced.

(3) Dissolve 0.1 g of Metoclopramide in 1 mL of 1 mol/L hydrochloric acid TS, and dilute with water to make 100 mL. To 1 mL of the solution add water to make 100 mL, determine the absorption spectrum of the solution as directed under Ultraviolet-visible Spectrophotometry <*2.24*>, and compare the spectrum with the Reference Spectrum: both spectra exhibit similar intensities of absorption at the same wavelengths.

Melting point <*2.60*> 146 – 149°C

Purity (1) Clarity and color of solution—Dissolve 1.0 g of Metoclopramide in 10 mL of 1 mol/L hydrochloric acid TS: the solution is clear and colorless.

(2) Heavy metals <*1.07*>—Proceed with 1.0 g of Metoclopramide as directed under Method 2, and perform the test. Prepare the control solution with 2.0 mL of Standard Lead Solution (not more than 20 ppm).

(3) Arsenic <*1.11*>—Dissolve 1.0 g of Metoclopramide in 5 mL of 1 mol/L hydrochloric acid TS, and use this solution as the sample solution. Perform the test (not more than 2 ppm).

(4) Related substances—Dissolve 0.10 g of Metoclopramide in 10 mL of methanol, and use this solution as the sample solution. Dilute 1 mL of the sample solution, exactly measured, with methanol to make exactly 200 mL, and use this solution as the standard solution. Perform the test with these solutions as directed under Thin-layer Chromatography <*2.03*>. Spot 10 μL each of the sample solution and standard solution on a plate of silica gel with fluorescent indicator for thin-layer chromatography. Develop the plate with a mixture of 1-butanol and ammonia solution (28) (19:1) to a distance of about 10 cm. Dry the plate, first in air and then at 80°C for 30 minutes. Examine under ultraviolet light (main wavelength: 254 nm): the spots other than the principal spot obtained from the sample solution are not more intense than the spot from the standard solution.

Loss on drying <*2.41*> Not more than 0.5% (1 g, 105°C, 3 hours).

Residue on ignition <*2.44*> Not more than 0.1% (1 g).

Assay Dissolve about 0.4 g of Metoclopramide, previously dried and accurately weighed, in 50 mL of acetic acid (100), add 5 mL of acetic anhydride, and warm for 5 minutes. Allow to cool, and titrate <*2.50*> with 0.1 mol/L perchloric acid VS (indicator: 2 drops of crystal violet TS). Perform the blank determination in the same manner, and make any necessary correction.

Each mL of 0.1 mol/L perchloric acid VS
$= 29.98$ mg of $C_{14}H_{22}ClN_3O_2$

Containers and storage Containers—Well-closed containers.

Metoclopramide Tablets

メトクロプラミド錠

Metoclopramide Tablets contain not less than 95.0% and not more than 105.0% of the labeled amount of metoclopramide ($C_{14}H_{22}ClN_3O_2$: 299.80).

Method of preparation Prepare as directed under Tablets, with Metoclopramide.

Identification (1) To a quantity of powdered Metoclopramide Tablets, equivalent to 50 mg of Metoclopramide, add 15 mL of 0.5 mol/L hydrochloric acid TS, and heat in a water bath at 70°C for 15 minutes while frequent shaking. After cooling, centrifuge for 10 minutes, and to 5 mL of the supernatant liquid add 1 mL of 4-dimethylaminobenzaldehyde-hydrochloric acid TS: a yellow color develops.

(2) Determine the absorption spectrum of the sample solution obtained in the Assay as directed under Ultraviolet-visible Spectrophotometry *<2.24>*: it exhibits maxima between 270 nm and 274 nm, and between 306 nm and 310 nm.

Uniformity of dosage units *<6.02>* Perform the test according to the following method: it meets the requirement of the Content uniformity test.

To 1 tablet of Metoclopramide Tablets add 10 mL of 0.1 mol/L hydrochloric acid TS, disperse the particles by sonicating, then add 0.1 mol/L hydrochloric acid TS to make exactly 25 mL, and centrifuge for 10 minutes. Pipet 4 mL of the supernatant liquid, add 0.1 mol/L hydrochloric acid TS to make exactly V mL so that each mL contains about 12 μg of metoclopramide ($C_{14}H_{22}ClN_3O_2$), and use this solution as the sample solution. Separately, weigh accurately about 80 mg of metoclopramide for assay, previously dried at 105°C for 3 hours, and dissolve in 0.1 mol/L hydrochloric acid TS to make exactly 500 mL. Pipet 4 mL of this solution, add 0.1 mol/L hydrochloric acid TS to make exactly 50 mL, and use this solution as the standard solution. Determine the absorbances, A_T and A_S, of the sample solution and standard solution at 308 nm as directed under Ultraviolet-visible Spectrophotometry *<2.24>*.

$$\text{Amount (mg) of metoclopramide } (C_{14}H_{22}ClN_3O_2) = M_S \times A_T/A_S \times V/1000$$

M_S: Amount (mg) of metoclopramide for assay taken

Dissolution Being specified separately when the drug is granted approval based on the Law.

Assay Weigh accurately not less than 20 Metoclopramide Tablets, and powder. Weigh accurately a portion of the powder, equivalent to about 75 mg of metoclopramide ($C_{14}H_{22}ClN_3O_2$), add 300 mL of 0.1 mol/L hydrochloric acid TS, shake for 1 hour, and add 0.1 mol/L hydrochloric acid TS to make exactly 500 mL. Centrifuge for 10 minutes, pipet 4 mL of the supernatant liquid, add 0.1 mol/L hydrochloric acid TS to make exactly 50 mL, and use this solution as the sample solution. Separately, weigh accurately about 80 mg of metoclopramide for assay, previously dried at 105°C for 3 hours, and dissolve in 0.1 mol/L hydrochloric acid TS to make exactly 500 mL. Pipet 4 mL of this solution, add 0.1 mol/L hydrochloric acid TS to make exactly 50 mL, and use this solution as the standard solution. Determine the absorbances, A_T and A_S, of the sample solution and standard solution at 308 nm as directed under Ultraviolet-visible Spectrophotometry *<2.24>*.

$$\text{Amount (mg) of metoclopramide } (C_{14}H_{22}ClN_3O_2) = M_S \times A_T/A_S$$

M_S: Amount (mg) of metoclopramide for assay taken

Containers and storage Containers—Tight containers.

Metoprolol Tartrate

メトプロロール酒石酸塩

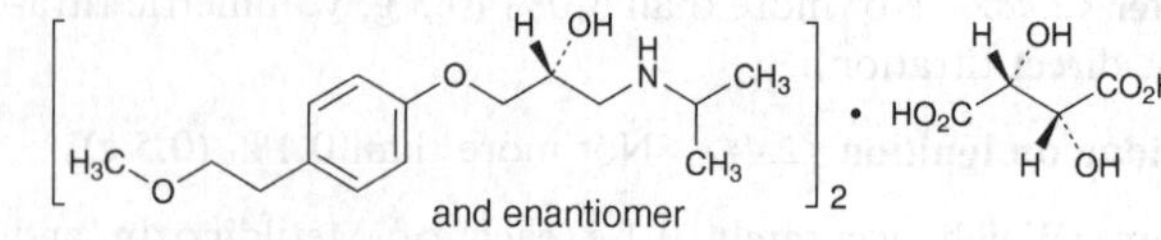

and enantiomer

$(C_{15}H_{25}NO_3)_2.C_4H_6O_6$: 684.81
(2*RS*)-1-[4-(2-Methoxyethyl)phenoxy]-3-[(1-methylethyl)amino]propan-2-ol hemi-(2*R*,3*R*)-tartrate
[*56392-17-7*]

Metoprolol Tartrate, when dried, contains not less than 99.0% and not more than 101.0% of metoprolol tartrate [$(C_{15}H_{25}NO_3)_2.C_4H_6O_6$].

Description Metoprolol Tartrate occurs as a white crystalline powder.

It is very soluble in water, and freely soluble in methanol, in ethanol (95) and in acetic acid (100).

Optical rotation $[\alpha]_D^{20}$: +7.0 – +10.0° (after drying, 1 g, water, 50 mL, 100 mm).

It shows crystal polymorphism.

Identification (1) Determine the absorption spectrum of a solution of Metoprolol Tartrate in ethanol (95) (1 in 10,000) as directed under Ultraviolet-visible Spectrophotometry *<2.24>*, and compare the spectrum with the Reference Spectrum: both spectra exhibit similar intensities of absorption at the same wavelengths.

(2) Determine the infrared absorption spectrum of Metoprolol Tartrate, previously dried, as directed in the paste method under Infrared Spectrophotometry *<2.25>*, and compare the spectrum with the Reference Spectrum: both spectra exhibit similar intensities of absorption at the same wave numbers. If any difference appears between the spectra, recrystallize Metoprolol Tartrate from a solution in acetone (23 in 1000), filter and dry the crystals, and perform the test with the crystals.

(3) A solution of Metoprolol Tartrate (1 in 5) responds to Qualitative Tests *<1.09>* (1) for tartrate.

pH *<2.54>* The pH of a solution obtained by dissolving 1.0 g of Metoprolol Tartrate in 10 mL of water is between 6.0 and 7.0.

Purity (1) Heavy metals *<1.07>*—Proceed with 2.0 g of Metoprolol Tartrate according to Method 1, and perform the test. Prepare the control solution with 2.0 mL of Standard Lead Solution (not more than 10 ppm).

(2) Related substances—Dissolve 0.10 g of Metoprolol Tartrate in 5 mL of methanol, and use this solution as the sample solution. Pipet 1 mL of the sample solution, and add methanol to make exactly 100 mL. Pipet 2 mL of this solution, add methanol to make exactly 10 mL, and use this solution as the standard solution. Perform the test with these solutions as directed under Thin-layer Chromatography *<2.03>*. Spot 10 μL each of the sample solution and standard solution on a plate of silica gel for thin-layer chromatography. After saturating the plate with the atmosphere by allowing to stand in a developing vessel, which contains the developing solvent and a glass vessel containing ammonia water (28), develop with the developing solvent, a mixture of ethyl acetate and methanol (4:1), to a distance of about 12 cm, and air-dry the plate. Allow to stand the plate in an iodine vapors until the spot with the standard solution appears obviously:

the spot other than the principal spot and other than the spot on the original point obtained from the sample solution is not more than three spots, and they are not more intense than the spot from the standard solution.

Loss on drying <*2.41*> Not more than 0.5% (1 g, in vacuum, 60°C, 4 hours).

Residue on ignition <*2.44*> Not more than 0.1% (1 g).

Assay Weigh accurately about 0.5 g of Metoprolol Tartrate, previously dried, dissolve in 50 mL of acetic acid (100), and titrate <*2.50*> with 0.1 mol/L perchloric acid VS (potentiometric titration). Perform a blank determination in the same manner, and make any necessary correction.

Each mL of 0.1 mol/L perchloric acid VS
= 34.24 mg of $(C_{15}H_{25}NO_3)_2.C_4H_6O_6$

Containers and storage Containers—Well-closed containers.

Metoprolol Tartrate Tablets

メトプロロール酒石酸塩錠

Metoprolol Tartrate Tablets contain not less than 93.0% and not more than 107.0% of the labeled amount of metoprolol tartrate [$(C_{15}H_{25}NO_3)_2.C_4H_6O_6$: 684.81].

Method of preparation Prepare as directed under Tablets, with Metoprolol Tartrate.

Identification To an amount of powdered Metoprolol Tartrate Tablets, equivalent to 10 mg of Metoprolol Tartrate, add 100 mL of ethanol (95), shake for 15 minutes, and filter. Determine the absorption spectrum of the filtrate as directed under Ultraviolet-visible Spectrophotometry <*2.24*>: it exhibits maxima between 274 nm and 278 nm and between 281 nm and 285 nm.

Uniformity of dosage units <*6.02*> Perform the Mass variation test, or the Content uniformity test according to the following method: it meets the requirement.

To 1 tablet of Metoprolol Tartrate Tablets add 1 mL of water for every 10 mg of Metoprolol Tartrate, shake for 20 minutes, then add 75 mL of ethanol (95), shake for 15 minutes, add ethanol (95) to make exactly 100 mL, and centrifuge. Pipet V mL of the supernatant liquid, add ethanol (95) to make exactly V' so that each mL contains about 0.1 mg of metoprolol tartrate [$(C_{15}H_{25}NO_3)_2.C_4H_6O_6$], and use this solution as the sample solution. Separately, weigh accurately about 50 mg of metoprolol tartrate for assay, previously dried in vacuum at 60°C for 4 hours, dissolve in 5 mL of water, and add ethanol (95) to make exactly 100 mL. Pipet 10 mL of this solution, add ethanol (95) to make exactly 50 mL, and use this solution as the standard solution. Determine the absorbances, A_T and A_S, of the sample solution and standard solution at 276 nm as directed under Ultraviolet-visible Spectrophotometry <*2.24*>, using ethanol (95) as the blank.

Amount (mg) of metoprolol tartrate [$(C_{15}H_{25}NO_3)_2.C_4H_6O_6$]
$= M_S \times A_T/A_S \times V'/V \times 1/5$

M_S: Amount (mg) of metoprolol tartrate for assay taken

Dissolution <*6.10*> When the test is performed at 50 revolutions per minute according to the Paddle method, using 900 mL of water as the dissolution medium, the dissolution rate in 30 minutes of Metoprolol Tartrate Tablets is not less than 80%.

Start the test with 1 tablet of Metoprolol Tartrate Tablets, withdraw not less than 20 mL of the medium at the specified minute after starting the test, and filter through a membrane filter with a pore size not exceeding 0.5 µm. Discard not less than 10 mL of the first filtrate, pipet V mL of the subsequent filtrate, add water to make exactly V' mL so that each mL contains about 22 µg of metoprolol tartrate [$(C_{15}H_{25}NO_3)_2.C_4H_6O_6$], and use this solution as the sample solution. Separately, weigh accurately about 56 mg of metoprolol tartrate for assay, previously dried in vacuum at 60°C for 4 hours, and dissolve in water to make exactly 200 mL. Pipet 8 mL of this solution, add water to make exactly 100 mL, and use this solution as the standard solution. Perform the test with exactly 50 µL each of the sample solution and standard solution as directed under Liquid Chromatography <*2.01*> according to the following conditions, and determine the peak areas, A_T and A_S, of metoprolol in each solution.

Dissolution rate (%) with respect to the labeled amount of metoprolol tartrate [$(C_{15}H_{25}NO_3)_2.C_4H_6O_6$]
$= M_S \times A_T/A_S \times V'/V \times 1/C \times 36$

M_S: Amount (mg) of metoprolol tartrate for assay taken
C: Labeled amount (mg) of metoprolol tartrate [$(C_{15}H_{25}NO_3)_2.C_4H_6O_6$] in 1 tablet

Operating conditions—

Proceed as directed in the operating conditions in the Assay.

System suitability—

System performance: When the procedure is run with 50 µL of the standard solution under the above operating conditions, the number of theoretical plates and the symmetry factor of the peak of metoprolol are not less than 2000 and not more than 1.5, respectively.

System repeatability: When the test is repeated 6 times with 50 µL of the standard solution under the above operating conditions, the relative standard deviation of the peak area of metoprolol is not more than 2.0%.

Assay Weigh accurately the mass of not less than 20 Metoprolol Tartrate Tablets, and powder. Weigh accurately a portion of the powder, equivalent to about 0.12 g of metoprolol tartrate [$(C_{15}H_{25}NO_3)_2.C_4H_6O_6$], add 60 mL of a mixture of ethanol (99.5) and 1 mol/L hydrochloric acid TS (100:1) and exactly 10 mL of the internal standard solution, shake for 15 minutes, and add the mixture of ethanol (99.5) and 1 mol/L hydrochloric acid TS (100:1) to make 100 mL. Centrifuge, and use the supernatant liquid as the sample solution. Separately, weigh accurately about 0.12 g of metoprolol tartrate for assay, previously dried in vacuum at 60°C for 4 hours, dissolve in 60 mL of the mixture of ethanol (99.5) and 1 mol/L hydrochloric acid TS (100:1), add exactly 10 mL of the internal standard solution, then add the mixture of ethanol (99.5) and 1 mol/L hydrochloric acid TS (100:1) to make 100 mL, and use this solution as the standard solution. Perform the test with 10 µL each of the sample solution and standard solution as directed under Liquid Chromatography <*2.01*> according to the following conditions, and calculate the ratios, Q_T and Q_S, of the peak area of metoprolol to that of the internal standard.

Amount (mg) of metoprolol tartrate [$(C_{15}H_{25}NO_3)_2.C_4H_6O_6$]
$= M_S \times Q_T/Q_S$

M_S: Amount (mg) of metoprolol tartrate for assay taken

Internal standard solution—A solution of ethyl parahydroxybenzoate in the mixture of ethanol (99.5) and 1 mol/L hydrochloric acid TS (100:1) (1 in 500).

Operating conditions—

Detector: An ultraviolet absorption photometer (wavelength: 274 nm).

Column: A stainless steel column 4.6 mm in inside diameter and 15 cm in length, packed with octadecylsilanized silica gel for liquid chromatography (5 μm in particle diameter).

Column temperature: A constant temperature of about 25°C.

Mobile phase: Dissolve 14.0 g of sodium perchlorate monohydrate in 1000 mL of water, and adjust to pH 3.2 with diluted perchloric acid (17 in 2000). To 750 mL of this solution add 250 mL of acetonitrile.

Flow rate: Adjust so that the retention time of metoprolol is about 8 minutes.

System suitability—

System performance: When the procedure is run with 10 μL of the standard solution under the above operating conditions, metoprolol and the internal standard are eluted in this order with the resolution between these peaks being not less than 5.

System repeatability: When the test is repeated 6 times with 10 μL of the standard solution under the above operating conditions, the relative standard deviation of the ratio of the peak area of metoprolol to that of the internal standard is not more than 1.0%.

Containers and storage Containers—Well-closed containers.

Metronidazole

メトロニダゾール

$C_6H_9N_3O_3$: 171.15

2-(2-Methyl-5-nitro-1*H*-imidazol-1-yl)ethanol

[*443-48-1*]

Metronidazole, when dried, contains not less than 99.0% and not more than 101.0% of metronidazole ($C_6H_9N_3O_3$).

Description Metronidazole occurs as white to pale yellow-white, crystals or crystalline powder.

It is freely soluble in acetic acid (100), sparingly soluble in ethanol (99.5) and in acetone, and slightly soluble in water.

It dissolves in dilute hydrochloric acid.

It is colored to yellow-brown by light.

Identification **(1)** Determine the absorption spectrum of a solution of Metronidazole in 0.1 mol/L hydrochloric acid TS (1 in 100,000) as directed under Ultraviolet-visible Spectrophotometry <*2.24*>, and compare the spectrum with the Reference Spectrum: both spectra exhibit similar intensities of absorption at the same wavelengths.

(2) Determine the infrared absorption spectrum of Metronidazole as directed in the potassium bromide disk method under Infrared Spectrophotometry <*2.25*>, and compare the spectrum with the Reference Spectrum: both spectra exhibit similar intensities of absorption at the same wave numbers.

Melting point <*2.60*> 159 – 163°C

Purity **(1)** Heavy metals <*1.07*>—Proceed with 1.0 g of Metronidazole according to Method 2, and perform the test. Prepare the control solution with 2.0 mL of Standard Lead Solution (not more than 20 ppm).

(2) 2-Methyl-5-nitroimidazol—Dissolve 0.10 g of Metronidazole in acetone to make exactly 10 mL, and use this solution as the sample solution. Separately, dissolve 20 mg of 2-methyl-5-nitroimidazole for thin-layer chromatography in acetone to make exactly 20 mL, then pipet 5 mL of this solution, add acetone to make exactly 100 mL, and use this solution as the standard solution. Perform the test with these solutions as directed under Thin-layer Chromatography <*2.03*>. Spot 20 μL each of the sample solution and standard solution on a plate of silica gel with fluorescent indicator for thin-layer chromatography. Immediately develop the plate with a mixture of acetone, water and ethyl acetate (8:1:1) to a distance of about 15 cm, and air-dry the plate. Examine under ultraviolet light (main wavelength: 254 nm): the spot obtained from the sample solution corresponding to the spot from the standard solution is not more intense than the spot from the standard solution.

Loss on drying <*2.41*> Not more than 0.5% (1 g, in vacuum, silica gel, 24 hours).

Residue on ignition <*2.44*> Not more than 0.1% (1 g).

Assay Weigh accurately about 0.2 g of Metronidazole, previously dried, and dissolve in 30 mL of acetic acid (100). Titrate <*2.50*> with 0.1 mol/L perchloric acid VS (indicator: 0.5 mL of *p*-naphtholbenzein TS) until the color of the solution changes from orange-yellow to green. Perform a blank determination in the same manner, and make any necessary correction.

Each mL of 0.1 mol/L perchloric acid VS
= 17.12 mg of $C_6H_9N_3O_3$

Containers and storage Containers—Tight containers.

Storage—Light-resistant.

Metronidazole Tablets

メトロニダゾール錠

Metronidazole Tablets contain not less than 93.0% and not more than 107.0% of the labeled amount of metronidazole ($C_6H_9N_3O_3$: 171.15).

Method of preparation Prepare as directed under Tablets, with Metronidazole.

Identification **(1)** To an amount of powdered Metronidazole Tablets, equivalent to 0.1 g of Metronidazole, add 100 mL of 0.1 mol/L hydrochloric acid TS, and allow to stand for 30 minutes with occasional stirring. Then, shake vigorously, and centrifuge a part of this solution. To 1 mL of the supernatant liquid add 0.1 mol/L hydrochloric acid TS to make 100 mL. Determine the absorption spectrum of this solution as directed under Ultraviolet-visible Spectrophotometry <*2.24*>: it exhibits a maximum between 275 nm and 279 nm.

(2) Shake vigorously a quantity of powdered Metronidazole Tablets, equivalent to 0.20 g of Metronidazole, with 20 mL of acetone for 10 minutes, centrifuge, and use the supernatant liquid as the sample solution. Separately, dissolve 0.10 g of metronidazole in 10 mL of acetone, and use this solution as the standard solution. Perform the test with these solutions as directed under Thin-layer Chromatography <*2.03*>. Spot 5 μL each of the sample solution and standard solution on a plate of silica gel with fluorescent indicator for thin-layer chromatography, develop the plate immediately with a mixture of acetone, water and ethyl acetate (8:1:1) to a distance of about 10 cm, and air-dry the plate. Examine under ultraviolet light (main wavelength: 254 nm): the *R*f value of the principal spots obtained from the sample solution and the standard solution is the same.

Uniformity of dosage units <*6.02*> Perform the test according to the following method: it meets the requirement of the Content uniformity test.

To 1 tablet of Metronidazole Tablets add 25 mL of a mixture of water and methanol (1:1), shake vigorously for 25 minutes, and add the mixture of water and methanol (1:1) to make exactly 50 mL. Pipet 5 mL of this solution, and add a mixture of water and methanol (4:1) to make exactly 100 mL. Filter the solution through a membrane filter with pore size of 0.45 μm, discard the first 3 mL of the filtrate, and use the subsequent filtrate as the sample solution. Hereinafter, proceed as directed in the Assay.

Amount (mg) of metronidazole ($C_6H_9N_3O_3$)
$= M_S \times A_T/A_S \times 10$

M_S: Amount (mg) of metronidazole for assay taken

Dissolution <*6.10*> When the test is performed at 50 revolutions per minute according to the Paddle method, using 900 mL of water as the dissolution medium, the dissolution rate in 90 minutes of Metronidazole Tablets is not less than 70%.

Start the test with 1 tablet of Metronidazole Tablets, withdraw not less than 20 mL of the medium at the specified minute after starting the test, and filter through a membrane filter with a pore size not exceeding 0.45 μm. Discard not less than 10 mL of the first filtrate, pipet V mL of the subsequent filtrate, add water to make exactly V' mL so that each mL contains about 11 μg of metronidazole ($C_6H_9N_3O_3$), and use this solution as the sample solution. Separately, weigh accurately about 22 mg of metronidazole for assay, previously dried in vacuum with silica gel for 24 hours, and dissolve in water to make exactly 100 mL. Pipet 5 mL of this solution, add water to make exactly 100 mL, and use this solution as the standard solution. Determine the absorbances, A_T and A_S, at 320 nm of the sample solution and standard solution as directed under Ultraviolet-visible Spectrophotometry <*2.24*>.

Dissolution rate (%) with respect to the labeled amount of metronidazole ($C_6H_9N_3O_3$)
$= M_S \times A_T/A_S \times V'/V \times 1/C \times 45$

M_S: Amount (mg) of metronidazole for assay taken
C: Labeled amount (mg) of metronidazole ($C_6H_9N_3O_3$) in 1 tablet

Assay Weigh accurately the mass of not less than 20 Metronidazole Tablets, and powder. Weigh accurately a portion of the powder, equivalent to about 0.25 g of metronidazole ($C_6H_9N_3O_3$), add 25 mL of a mixture of water and methanol (1:1), shake vigorously for 10 minutes, and add the mixture of water and methanol (1:1) to make exactly 50 mL. Pipet 5 mL of this solution, and add a mixture of water and methanol (4:1) to make exactly 100 mL. Filter this solution through a membrane filter with pore size of 0.45 μm, discard the first 3 mL of the filtrate, and use the subsequent filtrate as the sample solution. Separately, weigh accurately about 25 mg of metronidazole for assay, previously dried in vacuum on silica gel for 24 hours, dissolve in the mixture of water and methanol (4:1) to make exactly 100 mL, and use this solution as the standard solution. Perform the test with exactly 10 μL each of the sample solution and standard solution as directed under Liquid Chromatography <*2.01*> according to the following conditions, and determine the peak areas, A_T and A_S, of metronidazole in each solution.

Amount (mg) of metronidazole ($C_6H_9N_3O_3$)
$= M_S \times A_T/A_S \times 10$

M_S: Amount (mg) of metronidazole for assay taken

Operating conditions—

Detector: An ultraviolet absorption photometer (wavelength: 320 nm).

Column: A stainless steel column 4.6 mm in inside diameter and 15 cm in length, packed with octadecylsilanized silica gel for liquid chromatography (5 μm in particle diameter).

Column temperature: A constant temperature of about 25°C.

Mobile phase: A mixture of water and methanol (4:1).

Flow rate: Adjust so that the retention time of metronidazole is about 5 minutes.

System suitability—

System performance: When the procedure is run with 10 μL of the standard solution under the above operating conditions, the number of theoretical plates and the symmetry factor of the peak of metronidazole are not less than 3000 and not more than 1.5, respectively.

System repeatability: When the test is repeated 6 times with 10 μL of the standard solution under the above operating conditions, the relative standard deviation of the peak area of metronidazole is not more than 1.0%.

Containers and storage Containers—Tight containers.

Metyrapone

メチラポン

$C_{14}H_{14}N_2O$: 226.27
2-Methyl-1,2-di(pyridin-3-yl)propan-1-one
[54-36-4]

Metyrapone, when dried, contains not less than 98.0% of metyrapone ($C_{14}H_{14}N_2O$).

Description Metyrapone occurs as a white to pale yellow crystalline powder. It has a characteristic odor and a bitter taste.

It is very soluble in methanol, in ethanol (95), in acetic anhydride, in chloroform, in diethyl ether and in nitrobenzene, and sparingly soluble in water.

It dissolves in 0.5 mol/L sulfuric acid TS.

Identification **(1)** Mix 5 mg of Metyrapone with 10 mg of 1-chloro-2,4-dinitrobenzene, melt by gently heating for 5 to 6 seconds, cool, and add 4 mL of potassium hydroxide-ethanol TS: a dark red color develops.

(2) Determine the absorption spectrum of a solution of Metyrapone in 0.5 mol/L sulfuric acid TS (1 in 100,000) as directed under Ultraviolet-visible Spectrophotometry <*2.24*>, and compare the spectrum with the Reference Spectrum:

both spectra exhibit similar intensities of absorption at the same wavelengths.

Melting point ⟨*2.60*⟩ 50 – 54°C

Purity **(1)** Clarity and color of solution—Dissolve 0.5 g of Metyrapone in 5 mL of methanol: the solution is clear and colorless to pale yellow.

(2) Heavy metals ⟨*1.07*⟩—Proceed with 2.0 g of Metyrapone according to Method 2, and perform the test. Prepare the control solution with 2.0 mL of Standard Lead Solution (not more than 10 ppm).

(3) Arsenic ⟨*1.11*⟩—Prepare the test solution with 1.0 g of Metyrapone, according to Method 3, and perform the test (not more than 2 ppm).

(4) Related substances—Dissolve 0.25 g of Metyrapone in 5 mL of methanol, and use this solution as the sample solution. Pipet 1 mL of the sample solution, and add methanol to make exactly 50 mL. Pipet 5 mL of this solution, add methanol to make exactly 50 mL, and use this solution as the standard solution. Perform the test with these solutions as directed under Thin-layer Chromatography ⟨*2.03*⟩. Spot 2 μL each of the sample solution and standard solution on a plate of silica gel with fluorescent indicator for thin-layer chromatography. Develop the plate with a mixture of chloroform and methanol (15:1) to a distance of about 10 cm, and air-dry the plate for about 15 minutes. Examine under ultraviolet light (main wavelength: 254 nm): the spots other than the principal spot obtained from the sample solution is not more intense than the spot from the standard solution.

Loss on drying ⟨*2.41*⟩ Not more than 0.5% (1 g, in vacuum, silica gel, 24 hours).

Residue on ignition ⟨*2.44*⟩ Not more than 0.1% (1 g).

Assay Weigh accurately about 0.2 g of Metyrapone, previously dried, dissolve in 10 mL of nitrobenzene and 40 mL of acetic anhydride, and titrate ⟨*2.50*⟩ with 0.1 mol/L perchloric acid VS (potentiometric titration). Perform a blank determination in the same manner, and make any necessary correction.

Each mL of 0.1 mol/L perchloric acid VS
= 11.31 mg of $C_{14}H_{14}N_2O$

Containers and storage Containers—Tight containers.
Storage—Light-resistant.

Mexiletine Hydrochloride

メキシレチン塩酸塩

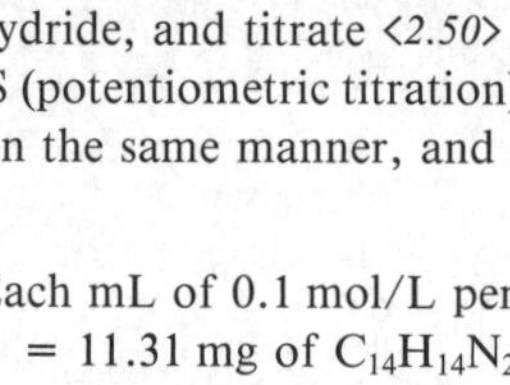

$C_{11}H_{17}NO.HCl$: 215.72
(2*RS*)-1-(2,6-Dimethylphenoxy)propan-2-ylamine monohydrochloride
[*5370-01-4*]

Mexiletine Hydrochloride, when dried, contains not less than 98.0% and not more than 102.0% of mexiletine hydrochloride ($C_{11}H_{17}NO.HCl$).

Description Mexiletine Hydrochloride occurs as a white powder.

It is freely soluble in water and in ethanol (95), and slightly soluble in acetonitrile.

It dissolves in 0.01 mol/L hydrochloric acid TS.

A solution of Mexiletine Hydrochloride (1 in 20) shows no optical rotation.

Mexiletine Hydrochloride shows crystal polymorphism.

Identification **(1)** Determine the absorption spectrum of a solution of Mexiletine Hydrochloride in 0.01 mol/L hydrochloric acid TS (1 in 2000) as directed under Ultraviolet-visible Spectrophotometry ⟨*2.24*⟩, and compare the spectrum with the Reference Spectrum or the spectrum of a solution of Mexiletine Hydrochloride RS prepared in the same manner as the sample solution: both spectra exhibit similar intensities of absorption at the same wavelengths.

(2) Determine the infrared absorption spectrum of Mexiletine Hydrochloride, previously dried, as directed in the potassium chloride disk method under Infrared Spectrophotometry ⟨*2.25*⟩, and compare the spectrum with the Reference Spectrum or the spectrum of dried Mexiletine Hydrochloride RS: both spectra exhibit similar intensities of absorption at the same wave numbers. If any difference appears between the spectra, recrystallize Mexiletine Hydrochloride from ethanol (95), filter, dry the crystals, and perform the test with the crystals.

(3) A solution of Mexiletine Hydrochloride (1 in 100) responds to Qualitative Tests ⟨*1.09*⟩ (2) for chloride.

pH ⟨*2.54*⟩ Dissolve 1.0 g of Mexiletine Hydrochloride in 10 mL of water: the pH of this solution is between 3.8 and 5.8.

Melting point ⟨*2.60*⟩ 200 – 204°C

Purity **(1)** Clarity and color of solution—Dissolve 1.0 g of Mexiletine Hydrochloride in 10 mL of water: the solution is clear and colorless.

(2) Heavy Metals ⟨*1.07*⟩—Proceed with 2.0 g of Mexiletine Hydrochloride according to Method 1, and perform the test. Prepare the control solution with 2.0 mL of Standard Lead Solution (not more than 10 ppm).

(3) Related substances—Dissolve 20 mg of Mexiletine Hydrochloride in 20 mL of the mobile phase, and use this solution as the sample solution. Pipet 1 mL of the sample solution, add the mobile phase to make exactly 250 mL, and use this solution as the standard solution. Perform the test with exactly 20 μL each of the sample solution and standard solution as directed under Liquid Chromatography ⟨*2.01*⟩ according to the following conditions. Determine each peak area of both solutions by the automatic integration method: each peak area other than mexiletine obtained from the sample solution is not larger than the peak area of mexiletine from the standard solution.

Operating conditions—

Detector, column, column temperature, mobile phase, flow rate, and selection of column: Proceed as directed in the operating conditions in the Assay.

Detection sensitivity: Adjust so that the peak height of mexiletine obtained from 20 μL of the standard solution is between 5 mm and 10 mm.

Time span of measurement: About 3 times as long as the retention time of mexiletine, beginning after the solvent peak.

Loss on drying ⟨*2.41*⟩ Not more than 0.5% (1 g, 105°C, 3 hours).

Residue on ignition ⟨*2.44*⟩ Not more than 0.1% (1 g).

Assay Weigh accurately about 20 mg each of Mexiletine Hydrochloride and Mexiletine Hydrochloride RS, each previously dried, and dissolve each in the mobile phase to make exactly 20 mL. Pipet 5 mL each of these solutions, add exactly 5 mL of the internal standard solution, then add the mobile phase to make 100 mL, and use these solutions as the sample solution and the standard solution, respectively. Perform the test with 20 μL each of the sample solution and standard solution as directed under Liquid Chromatography ⟨*2.01*⟩ according to the following conditions, and calculate the ratios, Q_T and Q_S, of the peak area of mexiletine to that of the internal standard, respectively.

Amount (mg) of mexiletine hydrochloride ($C_{11}H_{17}NO.HCl$)
$= M_S \times Q_T/Q_S$

M_S: Amount (mg) of Mexiletine Hydrochloride RS taken

Internal standard solution—A solution of phenetylamine hydrochloride in the mobile phase (3 in 5000).

Operating conditions—

Detector: An ultraviolet absorption photometer (wavelength: 210 nm).

Column: A stainless steel column about 4 mm in inside diameter and about 15 cm in length, packed with octylsilanized silica gel for liquid chromatography (about 7 μm in particle diameter).

Column temperature: A constant temperature of about 30°C.

Mobile phase: Dissolve 2.5 g of sodium lauryl sulfate and 3 g of sodium dihydrogen phosphate dihydrate in 600 mL of water, and add 420 mL of acetonitrile.

Flow rate: Adjust so that the retention time of mexiletine is about 6 minutes.

Selection of column: Proceed with 20 μL of the standard solution under the above conditions, and calculate the resolution. Use a column giving elution of the internal standard and mexiletine in this order with the resolution between these peaks being not less than 9.

Containers and storage Containers—Tight containers.

Storage—Light-resistant.

Miconazole

ミコナゾール

and enantiomer

$C_{18}H_{14}Cl_4N_2O$: 416.13

1-[(2*RS*)-2-(2,4-Dichlorobenzyloxy)-2-(2,4-dichlorophenyl)ethyl]-1*H*-imidazole

[*22916-47-8*]

Miconazole, when dried, contains not less than 98.5% of miconazole ($C_{18}H_{14}Cl_4N_2O$).

Description Miconazole occurs as a white to pale yellow-white crystalline powder.

It is freely soluble in methanol, in ethanol (95) and in acetic acid (100), soluble in diethyl ether, and practically insoluble in water.

A solution of Miconazole in methanol (1 in 20) shows no optical rotation.

Identification **(1)** Determine the absorption spectrum of a solution of Miconazole in methanol (1 in 2500) as directed under Ultraviolet-visible Spectrophotometry ⟨*2.24*⟩, and compare the spectrum with the Reference Spectrum: both spectra exhibit similar intensities of absorption at the same wavelengths.

(2) Determine the infrared absorption spectrum of Miconazole, previously dried, as directed in the potassium bromide disk method under Infrared Spectrophotometry ⟨*2.25*⟩, and compare the spectrum with the Reference Spectrum: both spectra exhibit similar intensities of absorption at the same wave numbers.

Melting point ⟨*2.60*⟩ 84 – 87°C

Purity **(1)** Heavy metals ⟨*1.07*⟩—Proceed with 1.0 g of Miconazole according to Method 2, and perform the test. Prepare the control solution with 1.0 mL of Standard Lead Solution (not more than 10 ppm).

(2) Arsenic ⟨*1.11*⟩—Prepare the test solution with 1.0 g of Miconazole according to Method 3, and perform the test (not more than 2 ppm).

(3) Related substances—Dissolve 0.10 g of Miconazole in 10 mL of methanol, and use this solution as the sample solution. Pipet 1 mL of the sample solution, add methanol to make exactly 20 mL. Pipet 1 mL of this solution, add methanol to make exactly 20 mL, and use this solution as the standard solution. Perform the test with these solutions as directed under Thin-layer Chromatography ⟨*2.03*⟩. Spot 50 μL each of the sample solution and standard solution on a plate of silica gel for thin-layer chromatography. Develop the plate with a mixture of hexane, chloroform, methanol and ammonia solution (28) (60:30:10:1) to a distance of about 12 cm, and air-dry the plate. Allow the plate to stand in iodine vapor for 20 minutes: the spots other than the principal spot obtained from the sample solution are not more intense than the spot from the standard solution.

Loss on drying ⟨*2.41*⟩ Not more than 0.5% (1 g, in vacuum, silica gel, 60%, 3 hours).

Residue on ignition ⟨*2.44*⟩ Not more than 0.1% (1 g).

Assay Weigh accurately about 0.3 g of Miconazole, previously dried, dissolve in 40 mL of acetic acid (100), and titrate ⟨*2.50*⟩ with 0.1 mol/L perchloric acid VS (indicator: 3 drops of *p*-naphtholbenzein TS) until the color of the solution changes from light yellow-brown to light yellow-green. Perform a blank determination in the same manner, and make any necessary correction.

Each mL of 0.1 mol/L perchloric acid VS
$= 41.61$ mg of $C_{18}H_{14}Cl_4N_2O$

Containers and storage Containers—Tight containers.

Miconazole Nitrate

ミコナゾール硝酸塩

and enantiomer

$C_{18}H_{14}Cl_4N_2O.HNO_3$: 479.14
1-[(2*RS*)-2-(2,4-Dichlorobenzyloxy)-2-(2,4-dichlorophenyl)ethyl]-1*H*-imidazole mononitrate
[*22832-87-7*]

Miconazole Nitrate, when dried, contains not less than 98.5% of miconazole nitrate ($C_{18}H_{14}Cl_4N_2O.HNO_3$).

Description Miconazole Nitrate occurs as a white crystalline powder.

It is freely soluble in *N*,*N*-dimethylformamide, sparingly soluble in methanol, slightly soluble in ethanol (95), in acetone and in acetic acid (100), and very slightly soluble in water and in diethyl ether.

Melting point: about 180°C (with decomposition).

Identification **(1)** To 2 mL of a solution of Miconazole Nitrate in methanol (1 in 100) add 2 mL of Reinecke salt TS: a light red precipitate is formed.

(2) Determine the absorption spectrum of a solution of Miconazole Nitrate in methanol (1 in 2500) as directed under Ultraviolet-visible Spectrophotometry <*2.24*>, and compare the spectrum with the Reference Spectrum: both spectra exhibit similar intensities of absorption at the same wavelengths.

(3) Perform the test with a solution of Miconazole Nitrate in methanol (1 in 100) as directed under Flame Coloration Test <*1.04*> (2): a green color appears.

(4) A solution of Miconazole Nitrate in methanol (1 in 100) responds to Qualitative Tests <*1.09*> for nitrate.

Purity **(1)** Clarity and color of solution—Dissolve 1.0 g of Miconazole Nitrate in 100 mL of methanol: the solution is clear and colorless.

(2) Chloride <*1.03*>—Dissolve 0.10 g of Miconazole Nitrate in 6 mL of dilute nitric acid and *N*,*N*-dimethylformamide to make 50 mL. Perform the test using this solution as the test solution. Prepare the control solution as follows: to 0.25 mL of 0.01 mol/L hydrochloric acid VS add 6 mL of dilute nitric acid and *N*,*N*-dimethylformamide to make 50 mL (not more than 0.09%).

(3) Heavy metals <*1.07*>—Proceed with 1.0 g of Miconazole Nitrate according to Method 2, and perform the test. Prepare the control solution with 1.0 mL of Standard Lead Solution (not more than 10 ppm).

(4) Arsenic <*1.11*>—Prepare the test solution with 1.0 g of Miconazole Nitrate according to Method 3, and perform the test (not more than 2 ppm).

(5) Related substances—Dissolve 0.10 g of Miconazole Nitrate in 10 mL of methanol, and use this solution as the sample solution. Pipet 1 mL of the sample solution, add methanol to make exactly 20 mL, pipet 1 mL of this solution, add methanol to make exactly 20 mL, and use this solution as the standard solution. Perform the test with these solutions as directed under Thin-layer Chromatography <*2.03*>. Spot 50 μL each of the sample solution and standard solution on a plate of silica gel for thin-layer chromatography. Develop the plate with a mixture of hexane, chloroform, methanol and ammonia solution (28) (60:30:10:1) to a distance of about 12 cm, and air-dry the plate. Allow the plate in iodine vapor for 20 minutes: the spots other than the principal spot obtained from the sample solution are not more intense than the spot from the standard solution.

Loss on drying <*2.41*> Not more than 0.5% (1 g, in vacuum, silica gel, 60°C, 3 hours).

Residue on ignition <*2.44*> Not more than 0.1% (1 g).

Assay Weigh accurately about 0.35 g of Miconazole Nitrate, previously dried, dissolve in 50 mL of acetic acid (100) by warming, cool, and titrate <*2.50*> with 0.1 mol/L perchloric acid VS (potentiometric titration). Perform a blank determination in the same manner, and make any necessary correction.

Each mL of 0.1 mol/L perchloric acid VS
= 47.91 mg of $C_{18}H_{14}Cl_4N_2O.HNO_3$

Containers and storage Containers—Tight containers.
Storage—Light-resistant.

Micronomicin Sulfate

ミクロノマイシン硫酸塩

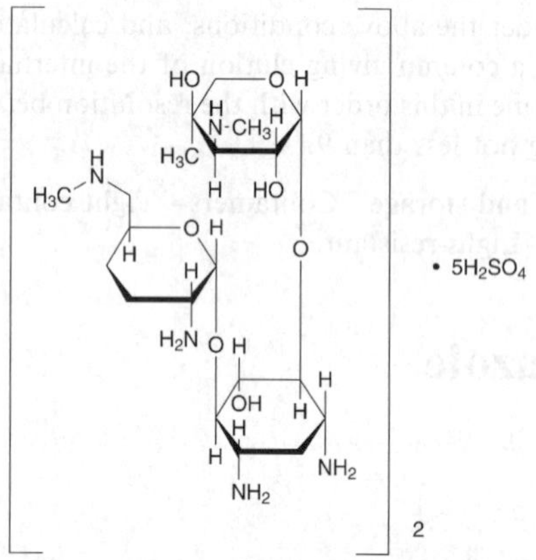

$(C_{20}H_{41}N_5O_7)_2.5H_2SO_4$: 1417.53
2-Amino-2,3,4,6-tetradeoxy-6-methylamino-α-D-*erythro*-hexopyranosyl-(1→4)-[3-deoxy-4-*C*-methyl-3-methylamino-β-L-arabinopyranosyl-(1→6)]-2-deoxy-D-streptamine hemipentasulfate
[*52093-21-7*, Micronomicin]

Micronomicin Sulfate is the sulfate of an aminoglycoside substance having antibacterial activity produced by the growth of *Micromonospora sagamiensis*.

It contains not less than 590 μg (potency) and not more than 660 μg (potency) per mg, calculated on the anhydrous basis. The potency of Micronomicin Sulfate is expressed as mass (potency) of micronomicin ($C_{20}H_{41}N_5O_7$: 463.57).

Description Micronomicin Sulfate occurs as a white to light yellow-white powder.

It is very soluble in water, sparingly soluble in ethylene glycol, and practically insoluble in methanol and in ethanol (99.5).

It is hygroscopic.

Identification **(1)** Dissolve 50 mg each of Micronomicin Sulfate and Micronomicin Sulfate RS in 10 mL of water, and use these solutions as the sample solution and the standard solution. Perform the test with these solutions as directed under Thin-layer Chromatography *<2.03>*. Spot 5 μL of the sample solution and standard solution on a plate of silica gel for thin-layer chromatography. Develop the plate with a mixture of ethanol (99.5), 1-butanol and ammonia solution (28) (10:8:7) to a distance of about 10 cm, and air-dry the plate. Spray evenly a solution of ninhydrin in a mixture of acetone and pyridine (25:1) (1 in 500), and heat the plate at 100°C for 10 minutes: the spots obtained from the sample solution and the standard solution are red-purple to red-brown and their *R*f values are the same.

(2) To 5 mL of a solution of Micronomicin Sulfate (1 in 100) add 1 mL of barium chloride TS: a white precipitate is formed, and it does not dissolve by addition of dilute nitric acid.

Optical rotation *<2.49>* $[\alpha]_D^{20}$: +110 – +130° (0.25 g calculated on the anhydrous basis, water, 25 mL, 100 mm).

pH *<2.54>* The pH of a solution obtained by dissolving 1.0 g of Micronomicin Sulfate in 10 mL of water is between 3.5 and 5.5.

Purity **(1)** Clarity and color of solution—Dissolve 1.5 g of Micronomicin Sulfate in 10 mL of water: the solution is clear and colorless to pale yellow.

(2) Heavy metals *<1.07>*—Proceed with 1.0 g of Micronomicin Sulfate according to Method 2, and perform the test. Prepare the control solution with 2.0 mL of Standard Lead Solution (not more than 20 ppm).

(3) Related substances—Dissolve 0.40 g of Micronomicin Sulfate in 10 mL of water, and use this solution as the sample solution. Pipet 1 mL of the sample solution, add water to make exactly 200 mL, and use this solution as the standard solution. Perform the test with these solutions as directed under Thin-layer Chromatography *<2.03>*. Spot 5 μL of the sample solution and standard solution on a plate of silica gel for thin-layer chromatography. Develop the plate with a mixture of ethanol (99.5), 1-butanol and ammonia solution (28) (10:8:7) to a distance of about 10 cm, and air-dry the plate. Spray evenly a solution of ninhydrin in a mixture of acetone and pyridine (25:1) (1 in 500), and heat the plate at 100°C for 10 minutes: the spot other than the principal spot obtained from the sample solution is not more intense than the spot from the standard solution.

Water *<2.48>* Not more than 10.0% (0.2 g, volumetric titration, back titration). Use a mixture of methanol for water determination and ethylene glycol for water determination (1:1) instead of methanol for water determination.

Assay Perform the test according to the Cylinder-plate method as directed under Microbial Assay for Antibiotics *<4.02>* according to the following conditions.

(i) Test organism—*Bacillus subtilis* ATCC 6633

(ii) Culture medium—Use the medium i in 1) under (1) Agar media for seed and base layer.

(iii) Standard solutions—Weigh accurately an amount of Micronomicin Sulfate RS, equivalent to about 20 mg (potency), dissolve in 0.1 mol/L phosphate buffer solution for antibiotics (pH 8.0) to make exactly 20 mL, and use this solution as the standard stock solution. Keep the standard stock solution at 5 – 15°C, and use within 30 days. Take exactly a suitable amount of the standard stock solution before use, add 0.1 mol/L phosphate buffer solution for antibiotics (pH 8.0) to make solutions so that each mL contains 2 μg (potency) and 0.5 μg (potency), and use these solutions as the high concentration standard solution and the low concentration standard solution, respectively.

(iv) Sample solutions—Weigh accurately an amount of Micronomicin Sulfate, equivalent to about 20 mg (potency), and dissolve in 0.1 mol/L phosphate buffer solution for antibiotics (pH 8.0) to make exactly 20 mL. Take exactly a suitable amount of this solution, add 0.1 mol/L phosphate buffer solution for antibiotics (pH 8.0) to make solutions so that each mL contains 2 μg (potency) and 0.5 μg (potency), and use these solutions as the high concentration sample solution and the low concentration sample solution, respectively.

Containers and storage Containers—Tight containers.

Midecamycin

ミデカマイシン

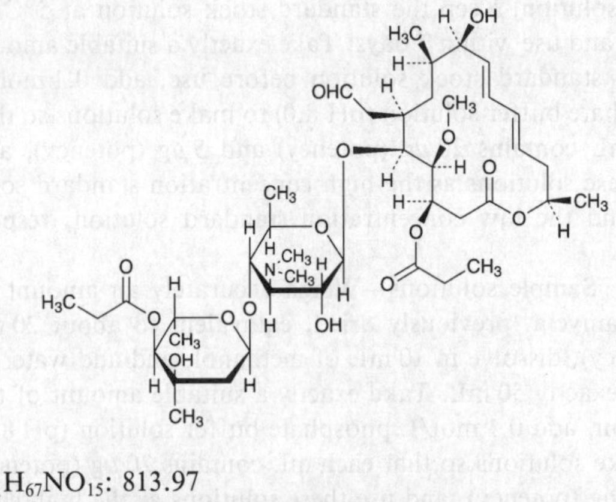

$C_{41}H_{67}NO_{15}$: 813.97
(3*R*,4*R*,5*S*,6*R*,8*R*,9*R*,10*E*,12*E*,15*R*)-
5-[2,6-Dideoxy-3-*C*-methyl-4-*O*-propanoyl-α-L-*ribo*-hexopyranosyl-(1→4)-3,6-dideoxy-3-dimethylamino-β-D-glucopyranosyloxy]-6-formylmethyl-9-hydroxy-4-methoxy-8-methyl-3-propanoyloxyhexadeca-10,12-dien-15-olide
[*35457-80-8*]

Midecamycin is a macrolide substance having antibacterial activity produced by the growth of *Streptomyces mycarofaciens*.

It contains not less than 950 μg (potency) and not more than 1020 μg (potency) per mg, calculated on the dried basis. The potency of Midecamycin is expressed as mass (potency) of midecamycin ($C_{41}H_{67}NO_{15}$).

Description Midecamycin occurs as a white crystalline powder.

It is very soluble in methanol, freely soluble in ethanol (95), and very slightly soluble in water.

Identification **(1)** Determine the absorption spectrum of a solution of Midecamycin in methanol (1 in 50,000) as directed under Ultraviolet-visible Spectrophotometry *<2.24>*, and compare the spectrum with the Reference Spectrum or the spectrum of a solution of Midecamycin RS prepared in the same manner as the sample solution: both spectra exhibit similar intensities of absorption at the same wavelengths.

(2) Determine the infrared absorption spectrum of Midecamycin as directed in the potassium bromide disk method under Infrared Spectrophotometry *<2.25>*, and compare the spectrum with the Reference Spectrum or the spectrum of Midecamycin RS: both spectra exhibit similar intensities of absorption at the same wave numbers.

Melting point <*2.60*> 153 – 158°C

Purity Heavy metals <*1.07*>—Proceed with 1.0 g of Midecamycin according to Method 2, and perform the test. Prepare the control solution with 3.0 mL of Standard Lead Solution (not more than 30 ppm).

Loss on drying <*2.41*> Not more than 2.0% (1.0 g, in vacuum not exceeding 0.67 kPa, 60°C, 3 hours).

Residue on ignition <*2.44*> Not more than 0.2% (1 g).

Assay Perform the test according to the Cylinder-plate method as directed under Microbial Assay for Antibiotics <*4.02*> according to the following conditions.

(i) Test organism—*Bacillus subtilis* ATCC 6633

(ii) Culture medium—Use the medium i in 1) under (1) Agar media for seed and base layer.

(iii) Standard solutions—Weigh accurately an amount of Midecamycin RS, previously dried, equivalent to about 20 mg (potency), dissolve in 10 mL of methanol, add water to make exactly 50 mL, and use this solution as the standard stock solution. Keep the standard stock solution at 5°C or below and use within 7 days. Take exactly a suitable amount of the standard stock solution before use, add 0.1 mol/L phosphate buffer solution (pH 8.0) to make solutions so that each mL contains 20 μg (potency) and 5 μg (potency), and use these solutions as the high concentration standard solution and the low concentration standard solution, respectively.

(iv) Sample solutions—Weigh accurately an amount of Midecamycin, previously dried, equivalent to about 20 mg (potency), dissolve in 10 mL of methanol, and add water to make exactly 50 mL. Take exactly a suitable amount of the solution, add 0.1 mol/L phosphate buffer solution (pH 8.0) to make solutions so that each mL contains 20 μg (potency) and 5 μg (potency), and use these solutions as the high concentration sample solution and the low concentration sample solution, respectively.

Containers and storage Containers—Tight containers.

Midecamycin Acetate

ミデカマイシン酢酸エステル

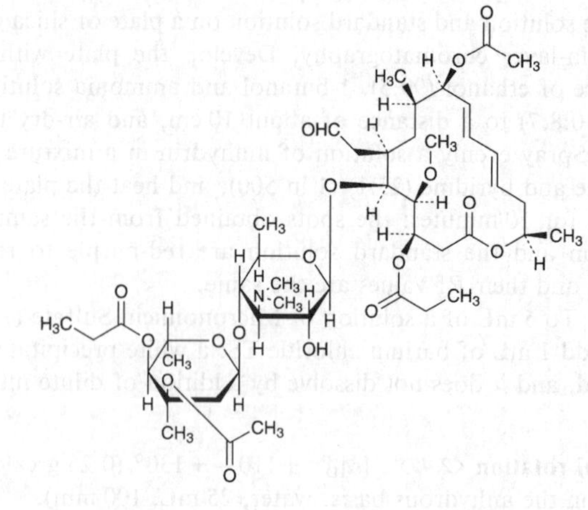

$C_{45}H_{71}NO_{17}$: 898.04

(3*R*,4*S*,5*S*,6*R*,8*R*,9*R*,10*E*,12*E*,15*R*)-9-Acetoxy-5-[3-*O*-acetyl-2,6-dideoxy-3-*C*-methyl-4-*O*-propanoyl-α-L-*ribo*-hexopyranosyl-(1→4)-3,6-dideoxy-3-dimethylamino-β-D-glucopyranosyloxy]-6-formylmethyl-4-methoxy-8-methyl-3-propioyloxyhexadeca-10,12-dien-15-olide

[*55881-07-7*]

Midecamycin Acetate is a derivative of midecamycin.

It contains not less than 950 μg (potency) and not more than 1010 μg (potency) per mg, calculated on the dried basis. The potency of Midecamycin Acetate is expressed as mass (potency) of midecamycin acetate ($C_{45}H_{71}NO_{17}$).

Description Midecamycin Acetate occurs as white, crystals or crystalline powder.

It is sparingly soluble in methanol, slightly soluble in ethanol (95), and practically insoluble in water.

Identification **(1)** Determine the absorption spectrum of a solution of Midecamycin Acetate in methanol (1 in 50,000) as directed under Ultraviolet-visible Spectrophotometry <*2.24*>, and compare the spectrum with the Reference Spectrum or the spectrum of a solution of Midecamycin Acetate RS prepared in the same manner as the sample solution: both spectra exhibit similar intensities of absorption at the same wavelengths.

(2) Determine the infrared absorption spectrum of Midecamycin Acetate, previously dried, as directed in the potassium bromide disk method under Infrared Spectrophotometry <*2.25*>, and compare the spectrum with the Reference Spectrum or spectrum of dried Midecamycin Acetate RS: both spectra exhibit similar intensities of absorption at the same wave numbers.

Purity Heavy metals <*1.07*>—Proceed with 1.0 g of Midecamycin Acetate according to Method 2, and perform the test. Prepare the control solution with 2.0 mL of Standard Lead Solution (not more than 20 ppm).

Loss on drying <*2.41*> Not more than 2.0% (1 g, in vacuum not exceeding 0.67 kPa, 60°C, 3 hours).

Residue on ignition <*2.44*> Not more than 0.2% (1 g).

Assay Perform the test according to the Cylinder-plate method as directed under Microbial Assay for Antibiotics

<*4.02*> according to the following conditions.

(i) Test organism—*Kocuria rhizophila* ATCC 9341

(ii) Culture medium—Use the medium i in 3) under (1) Agar media for seed and base layer.

(iii) Standard solutions—Weigh accurately an amount of Midecamycin Acetate RS, previously dried, equivalent to about 25 mg (potency), and dissolve in methanol to make exactly 50 mL, and use this solution as the standard stock solution. Keep the standard stock solution at 5 - 15°C and use within 7 days. Take exactly a suitable amount of the standard stock solution before use, add 0.1 mol/L phosphate buffer solution (pH 4.5) to make solutions so that each mL contains 20 μg (potency) and 5 μg (potency), and use these solutions as the high concentration standard solution and the low concentration standard solution, respectively.

(iv) Sample solutions—Weigh accurately an amount of Midecamycin Acetate, previously dried, equivalent to about 25 mg (potency), and dissolve in methanol to make exactly 50 mL. Take exactly a suitable amount of the solution, add 0.1 mol/L phosphate buffer solution (pH 4.5) to make solutions so that each mL contains 20 μg (potency) and 5 μg (potency), and use these solutions as the high concentration sample solution and the low concentration sample solution, respectively.

Containers and storage Containers—Tight containers.

Miglitol

ミグリトール

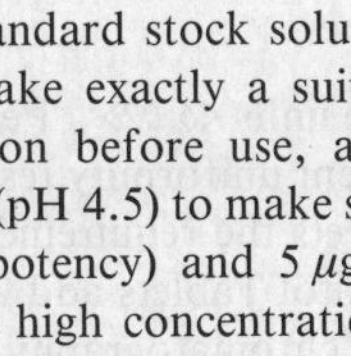

$C_8H_{17}NO_5$: 207.22

(2*R*,3*R*,4*R*,5*S*)-1-(2-Hydroxyethyl)-2-(hydroxymethyl)piperidine-3,4,5-triol

[*72432-03-2*]

Miglitol contains not less than 98.0% and not more than 102.0% of miglitol ($C_8H_{17}NO_5$), calculated on the dried basis.

Description Miglitol is a white to pale yellowish white powder.

It is freely soluble in water, and practically insoluble in ethanol (99.5).

Identification **(1)** Determine the infrared absorption spectrum of Miglitol, previously dried, as directed in the potassium bromide disk method under Infrared Spectrophotometry <*2.25*>, and compare the spectrum with the Reference Spectrum or the spectrum of previously dried Miglitol RS: both spectra exhibit similar intensities of absorption at the same wave numbers.

(2) Dissolve 10 mg each of Miglitol and Miglitol RS in 1 mL of water, and use these solutions as the sample solution and the standard solution. Perform the test with these solutions as directed under Thin-layer Chromatography <*2.03*>. Spot 10 μL each of the sample solution and standard solution on a plate of silica gel for thin-layer chromatography. Develop the plate with a mixture of methanol, ethyl acetate and diluted ammonia solution (28) (9 in 10) (2:2:1) to a distance of about 17 cm, and dry the plate at 105°C. Allow the plate to stand in iodine vapor: the principal spot obtained from the sample solution and the spot from the standard solution show a brown color and the same *Rf* value.

Optical rotation <*2.49*> $[\alpha]_D^{20}$: − 7.3 − − 8.3°(1.2 g calculated on the dried basis, water, 50 mL, 100 mm).

Melting point <*2.60*> 144 - 147°C

Purity **(1)** Clarity and color of solution—Dissolve 2.5 g of Miglitol in 50 mL of water, and use this solution as the test solution. Determine the turbidity of the test solution as directed under Turbidity Measurement <*2.61*>: it exhibits no more turbidity than Reference suspension II, and has no more color than the following control solution.

Control solution: To a mix of 0.3 mL of Cobalt (II) Chloride CS and 1.2 mL of Iron (III) Chloride CS add 38.5 mL of diluted hydrochloric acid (1 in 100).

(2) Heavy metals—Dissolve 2.5 g of Miglitol in 25 mL of water, and use this solution as the sample solution. Separately, to 10 mL of a solution obtained by diluting Standard Lead Stock Solution to 50-fold with water before use, add 2 mL of the sample solution, and use this solution as the control solution. To 12 mL of the sample solution and the control solution add 2 mL of hydrochloric acid-ammonium acetate buffer solution (pH 3.5) and 1.2 mL of thioacetamide TS, mix, allow to stand for 2 minutes, and observe vertically or horizontally both Nessler tubes against a white background: the color obtained with the sample solution is not more intense than that with the control solution (not more than 20 ppm).

(3) Related substances—Dissoble 0.19 g of Miglitol in 50 mL of the mobile phase, and use this solution as the sample solution. Perform the test with 20 μL of the sample solution as directed under Liquid Chromatography <*2.01*> according to the following conditions. Determine each peak area by the automatic integration method, and calculate the amount of them by the area percentage method: the amount of the peaks having the relative retention time of about 0.9 and about 1.5 to miglitol is not more than 0.2%, and the amount of the peaks other than miglitol and the peaks mentioned above is not more than 0.1%. The total amount of the peaks other than miglitol is not more than 0.5%. For the area of the peak, having the relative retention time of about 1.5, multiply the correction factor 4.1.

Operating conditions—

Detector, column, column temperature, mobile phase, and flow rate: Proceed as directed in the operating conditions in the Assay.

Time span of measurement: About 3 times as long as the retention time of miglitol, beginning after the solvent peak.

System suitability—

Test for required detectability: To 1 mL of the sample solution add the mobile phase to make 100 mL, and use this solution as the solution for system suitability test. Pipet 1 mL of the solution for system suitability test, and add the mobile phase to make exactly 10 mL. Confirm that the peak area of miglitol obtained with 20 μL of this solution is equivalent to 7 to 13% of that with 20 μL of the solution for system suitability test.

System performance: When the procedure is run with 20 μL of the solution for system suitability test under the above operating conditions, the number of theoretical plates and the symmetry factor of the peak of miglitol are not less than 5000 and not more than 1.5, respectively.

System repeatability: When the test is repeated 6 times with 20 μL of the solution for system suitability test under the above operating conditions, the relative standard deviation of the peak area of miglitol is not more than 5.0%.

Loss on drying <*2.41*> Not more than 0.5% (0.5 g, in vacuum, 60°C, 6 hours).

Residue on ignition <*2.44*> Not more than 0.1% (1 g).

Assay Weigh accurately about 50 mg each of Miglitol and Miglitol RS (separately determine the loss on drying <*2.41*> under the same conditions as Miglitol), dissolve each in the mobile phase to make exactly 50 mL, and use these solutions as the sample solution and the standard solution, respectively. Perform the test with exactly 20 μL of the sample solution and standard solution as directed under Liquid Chromatography <*2.01*> according to the following conditions, and determine the peak areas, A_T and A_S, of miglitol in each solution.

Amount (mg) of miglitol ($C_8H_{17}NO_5$) = $M_S \times A_T/A_S$

M_S: Amount (mg) of Miglitol RS taken, calculated on the dried basis

Operating conditions—

Detector: An ultraviolet absorption photometer (wavelength: 210 nm).

Column: A stainless steel column 4.6 mm in inside diameter and 25 cm in length, packed with pentaethylenehexaaminated polyvinyl alcohol polymer beads for liquid chromatography (5 μm in particle diameter).

Column temperature: A constant temperature of about 35°C.

Mobile phase: Dissolve 0.6 g of potassium dihydrogen phosphate and 0.28 g of anhydrous disodium hydrogen phosphate in water to make 1000 mL. To 300 mL of this solution add 900 mL of acetonitrile for liquid chromatography.

Flow rate: Adjust so that the retention time of miglitol is about 11 minutes.

System suitability—

System performance: When the procedure is run with 20 μL of the standard solution under the above operating conditions, the number of theoretical plates and the symmetry factor of the peak of miglitol are not less than 5000 and not more than 1.5, respectively.

System repeatability: When the test is repeated 6 times with 20 μL of the standard solution under the above conditions, the relative standard deviation of the peak area of miglitol is not more than 1.0%.

Containers and storage Containers—Tight containers.

Miglitol Tablets

ミグリトール錠

Miglitol Tablets contain not less than 95.0% and not more than 105.0% of the labeled amount of miglitol ($C_8H_{17}NO_5$: 207.22).

Method of preparation Prepare as directed under Tablets, with Miglitol.

Identification To a quantity of powdered Miglitol Tablets, equivalent to 0.1 g of Miglitol, add 50 mL of a mixture of acetonitrile and water (9:1), shake, centrifuge, and use the supernatant liquid as the sample solution. Separately, dissolve 50 mg of miglitol in a mixture of acetonitrile and water (9:1) to make 25 mL, and use this solution as the standard solution. Perform the test with these solutions as directed under Thin-layer Chromatography <*2.03*>. Spot 10 μL each of the sample solution and standard solution on a plate of silica gel for thin-layer chromatography. Develop the plate with a mixture of methanol, ethyl acetate and diluted ammonia solution (28) (9 in 10) (2:2:1) to a distance of about 8 cm, and air-dry the plate. Allow the plate to stand in iodine vapors: the principal spot obtained from the sample solution and the spot from the standard solution show a brown color and the same *R*f value.

Uniformity of dosage units <*6.02*> Perform the Mass variation test, or the Content uniformity test according to the following method: it meets the requirement.

To 1 tablet of Miglitol Tablets add 20 mL of a mixture of acetonitrile for liquid chromatography and water (4:1), sonicate, and add a mixture of acetonitrile for liquid chromatography and water (4:1) to make exactly *V* mL so that each mL contains about 1 mg of miglitol ($C_8H_{17}NO_5$). Centrifuge this solution, and use the supernatant liquid as the sample solution. Then, proceed as directed in the Assay.

Amount (mg) of miglitol ($C_8H_{17}NO_5$)
$= M_S \times A_T/A_S \times V/50$

M_S: Amount (mg) of Miglitol RS taken, calculated on the dried basis

Dissolution <*6.10*> When the test is performed at 75 revolutions per minute according to the Paddle method, using 900 mL of water as the dissolution medium, the dissolution rate in 30 minutes of Miglitol Tablets is not less than 85%.

Start the test with 1 tablet of Miglitol Tablets, withdraw not less than 20 mL of the medium at the specified minute after starting the test, and filter through a membrane filter with a pore size not exceeding 0.45 μm. Discard not less than 10 mL of the first filtrate, pipet *V* mL of the subsequent filtrate, add water to make exactly *V'* mL so that each mL contains about 28 μg of miglitol ($C_8H_{17}NO_5$), and use this solution as the sample solution. Separately, weigh accurately about 56 mg of Miglitol RS (separately determine the loss on drying <*2.41*> under the same conditions as Miglitol), and dissolve in water to make exactly 50 mL. Pipet 5 mL of this solution, add water to make exactly 200 mL and use this solution as the standard solution. Perform the test with exactly 10 μL each of the sample solution and standard solution as directed under Liquid Chromatography <*2.01*> according to the following conditions, and determine the peak areas, A_T and A_S, of miglitol in each solution.

Dissolution rate (%) with respect to the labeled amount of miglitol ($C_8H_{17}NO_5$)
$= M_S \times A_T/A_S \times V'/V \times 1/C \times 45$

M_S: Amount (mg) of Miglitol RS taken, calculated on the dried basis

C: Labeled amount (mg) of miglitol ($C_8H_{17}NO_5$) in 1 tablet

Operating conditions—

Proceed as directed in the operating conditions in the Assay.

System suitability—

System performance: When the procedure is run with 10 μL of the standard solution under the above operating conditions, the number of theoretical plates and the symmetry factor of the peak of miglitol are not less than 1000 and not more than 1.5, respectively.

System repeatability: When the test is repeated 6 times with 10 μL of the standard solution under the above operating conditions, the relative standard deviation of the peak

area of miglitol is not more than 2.0%.

Assay Weigh accurately the mass of not less than 20 Miglitol Tablets, and powder. Weigh accurately a portion of the powder, equivalent to about 0.1 g of miglitol ($C_8H_{17}NO_5$), add 50 mL of a mixture of acetonitrile for liquid chromatography and water (4:1), shake, and add a mixture of acetonitrile for liquid chromatography and water (4:1) to make exactly 100 mL. Centrifuge this solution, and use the supernatant liquid as the sample solution. Separately, weigh accurately about 50 mg of Miglitol RS (separately determine the loss on drying <*2.41*> under the same conditions as Miglitol), and dissolve in a mixture of acetonitrile for liquid chromatography and water (4:1) to make exactly 50 mL, and use this solution as the standard solution. Perform the test with exactly 10 μL each of the sample solution and standard solution as directed under Liquid Chromatography <*2.01*> according to the following conditions, and determine the peak areas, A_T and A_S, of miglitol in each solution.

Amount (mg) of miglitol ($C_8H_{17}NO_5$) = $M_S \times A_T/A_S \times 2$

M_S: Amount (mg) of Miglitol RS taken, calculated on the dried basis

Operating conditions—

Detector: An ultraviolet absorption photometer (wavelength: 210 nm).

Column: A stainless steel column 4.6 mm in inside diameter and 15 cm in length, packed with pentaethylenehexaaminated polyvinyl alcohol polymer beads for liquid chromatography (5 μm in particle diameter).

Column temperature: A constant temperature of about 40°C.

Mobile phase: Dissolve 0.6 g of potassium dihydrogen phosphate and 0.28 g of anhydrous disodium hydrogen phosphate in water to make 1000 mL. To 200 mL of this solution add 800 mL of acetonitrile for liquid chromatography.

Flow rate: Adjust so that the retention time of miglitol is about 8 minutes.

System suitability—

System performance: When the procedure is run with 10 μL of the standard solution under the above operating conditions, the number of theoretical plates and the symmetry factor of the peak of miglitol are not less than 4000 and not more than 1.5, respectively.

System repeatability: When the test is repeated 6 times with 10 μL of the standard solution under the above operating conditions, the relative standard deviation of the peak area of miglitol is not more than 1.0%.

Containers and storage Containers—Tight containers.

Migrenin

ミグレニン

Migrenin is composed of 90 parts of antipyrine, 9 parts of caffeine, and 1 part of citric acid in mass.

Migrenin, when dried, contains not less than 87.0% and not more than 93.0% of antipyrine ($C_{11}H_{12}N_2O$: 188.23) and not less than 8.6% and not more than 9.5% of caffeine ($C_8H_{10}N_4O_2$: 194.19).

Description Migrenin occurs as a white, powder or crystalline powder. It is odorless and has a bitter taste.

It is very soluble in water, freely soluble in ethanol (95) and in chloroform, and slightly soluble in diethyl ether.

The pH of a solution of 1.0 g of Migrenin in 10 mL of water is between 3.0 and 4.0.

It is affected by moisture and light.

Identification **(1)** To 5 mL of a solution of Migrenin (1 in 100) add 2 drops of sodium nitrite TS and 1 mL of dilute sulfuric acid: a deep green color develops.

(2) To 5 mL of a solution of Migrenin (1 in 50) add 1 drop of hydrochloric acid and 0.2 mL of formaldehyde solution, heat in a water bath for 30 minutes, add an excess of ammonia TS, and filter. Acidify the filtrate with hydrochloric acid, shake with 3 mL of chloroform, and separate the chloroform layer. Evaporate the chloroform solution on a water bath, add 10 drops of hydrogen peroxide TS and 1 drop of hydrochloric acid to the residue, and evaporate on a water bath to dryness: the residue shows a yellow-red color. Invert the residue over a vessel containing 2 to 3 drops of ammonia TS: a red-purple color develops, disappearing on the addition of 2 to 3 drops of sodium hydroxide TS.

(3) A solution of Migrenin (1 in 10) responds to Qualitative Tests <*1.09*> for citrate.

Melting point <*2.60*> 104 - 110°C

Purity **(1)** Clarity and color of solution—Dissolve 1.0 g of Migrenin in 40 mL of water: the solution is clear and colorless to pale yellow.

(2) Heavy metals <*1.07*>—Proceed with 1.0 g of Migrenin according to Method 1, and perform the test. Prepare the control solution with 2.0 mL of Standard Lead Solution (not more than 20 ppm).

Loss on drying <*2.41*> Not more than 0.5% (1 g, in vacuum, silica gel, 4 hours).

Residue on ignition <*2.44*> Not more than 0.1% (1 g).

Assay **(1)** Antipyrine—Weigh accurately about 0.25 g of Migrenin, previously dried in an iodine flask, dissolve in 25 mL of sodium acetate TS, add exactly 30 mL of 0.05 mol/L iodine VS, and allow to stand for 20 minutes with occasional shaking. Add 15 mL of chloroform to dissolve the precipitate so obtained, and titrate <*2.50*> the excess iodine with 0.1 mol/L sodium thiosulfate VS (indicator: 3 mL of starch TS). Perform a blank determination in the same manner.

Each mL of 0.05 mol/L iodine VS
= 9.411 mg of $C_{11}H_{12}N_2O$

(2) Caffeine—To about 1 g of Migrenin, previously dried and accurately weighed, add exactly 5 mL of the internal standard solution, dissolve in chloroform to make 10 mL, and use this solution as the sample solution. Separately, weigh accurately about 90 mg of Caffeine RS, previously dried at 80°C for 4 hours, add exactly 5 mL of the internal standard solution, dissolve in chloroform to make 10 mL, and use this solution as the standard solution. Perform the test with 1 μL each of the sample solution and standard solution as directed under Gas Chromatography <*2.02*> according to the following conditions, and calculate the ratios, Q_T and Q_S, of the peak area of caffeine to that of the internal standard.

Amount (mg) of caffeine ($C_8H_{10}N_4O_2$) = $M_S \times Q_T/Q_S$

M_S: Amount (mg) of Caffeine RS taken

Internal standard solution—A solution of ethenzamide in chloroform (1 in 50).

Operating conditions—

Detector: A hydrogen flame-ionization detector.

Column: A glass column 2.6 mm in inside diameter and 210 cm in length, packed with siliceous earth for gas chromatography (180 to 250 μm in particle diameter) coated with 50% phenyl-methyl silicon polymer for gas chromatography at the ratio of 15%.

Column temperature: A constant temperature of about 210°C.

Carrier gas: Nitrogen.

Flow rate: Adjust so that the retention time of ethenzamide is about 4 minutes.

System suitability—

System performance: Dissolve 0.9 g of antipyrine and 0.09 g of caffeine in 10 mL of chloroform. When the procedure is run with 1 μL of this solution under the above operating conditions, caffeine and antipyrine are eluted in this order with the resolution between these peaks being not less than 1.5.

System repeatability: When the test is repeated 6 times with 1 μL of the standard solution under the above operating conditions, the relative standard deviation of the ratios of the peak area of caffeine to that of the internal standard is not more than 1.0%.

Containers and storage Containers—Tight containers.

Storage—Light-resistant.

Minocycline Hydrochloride

ミノサイクリン塩酸塩

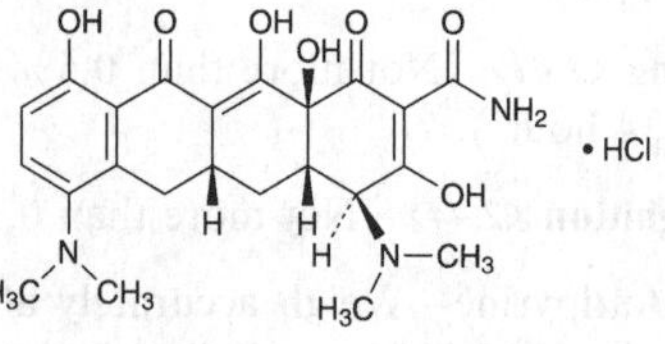

$C_{23}H_{27}N_3O_7.HCl$: 493.94

(4*S*,4a*S*,5a*R*,12a*S*)-4,7-Bis(dimethylamino)-3,10,12,12a-tetrahydroxy-1,11-dioxo-1,4,4a,5,5a,6,11,12a-octahydrotetracene-2-carboxamide monohydrochloride

[*13614-98-7*]

Minocycline Hydrochloride is the hydrochloride of a derivative of tetracycline.

It contains not less than 890 μg (potency) and not more than 950 μg (potency) per mg, calculated on the anhydrous basis. The potency of Minocycline Hydrochloride is expressed as mass (potency) of minocycline ($C_{23}H_{27}N_3O_7$: 457.48).

Description Minocycline Hydrochloride occurs as a yellow crystalline powder.

It is freely soluble in *N*,*N*-dimethylformamide, soluble in methanol, sparingly soluble in water, and slightly soluble in ethanol (95).

Identification **(1)** Determine the absorption spectrum of a solution of Minocycline Hydrochloride in a solution of hydrochloric acid in methanol (19 in 20,000) (1 in 62,500) as directed under Ultraviolet-visible Spectrophotometry <*2.24*>, and compare the spectrum with the Reference Spectrum or the spectrum of a solution of Minocycline Hydrochloride RS prepared in the same manner as the sample solution: both spectra exhibit similar intensities of absorption at the same wavelengths.

(2) Determine the infrared absorption spectrum of Minocycline Hydrochloride as directed in the potassium chloride disk method under Infrared Spectrophotometry <*2.25*>, and compare the spectrum with the Reference Spectrum or the spectrum of Minocycline Hydrochloride RS: both spectra exhibit similar intensities of absorption at the same wave numbers.

(3) A solution of Minocycline Hydrochloride (1 in 100) responds to Qualitative Tests <*1.09*> (2) for chloride.

pH <*2.54*> Dissolve 1.0 g of Minocycline Hydrochloride in 100 mL of water: the pH of the solution is between 3.5 and 4.5.

Purity **(1)** Clarity and color of solution—Dissolve 1.0 g of Minocycline Hydrochloride in 100 mL of water: the solution is clear, and when the test is performed within 1 hour after preparation of this solution, the absorbance of the solution at 560 nm, determined as directed under Ultraviolet-visible Spectrophotometry <*2.24*>, is not more than 0.06.

(2) Heavy metals <*1.07*>—Proceed with 0.5 g of Minocycline Hydrochloride according to Method 2, and perform the test. Prepare the control solution with 2.5 mL of Standard Lead Solution (not more than 50 ppm).

(3) Related substances—Dissolve 50 mg of Minocycline Hydrochloride in 100 mL of the mobile phase, and use this solution as the sample solution. Perform the test, immediately after the preparation of the sample solution, with 20 μL of the sample solution as directed under Liquid Chromatography <*2.01*> according to the following conditions, and determine each peak area by the automatic integration method. Calculate the amount of each peak area by the area percentage method: the amount of epiminocycline is not more than 1.2%, the amount of each peak other than minocycline and epiminocycline is not more than 1.0%, and the total area of the peaks other than minocycline and epiminocycline is not more than 2.0%.

Operating conditions—

Detector, column, column temperature, and mobile phase: Proceed as directed in the operating conditions in the Assay.

Flow rate: Adjust so that the retention time of minocycline is about 12 minutes. The retention time of epiminocycline is about 10 minutes under this condition.

Time span of measurement: About 2.5 times as long as the retention time of minocycline, beginning after the solvent peak.

System suitability—

System performance: Proceed as directed in the system suitability in the Assay.

Test for required detectability: To exactly 2 mL of the sample solution add the mobile phase to make exactly 100 mL, and use this solution as the solution for system suitability test. Pipet 5 mL of the solution for system suitability test, and add the mobile phase to make exactly 100 mL. Confirm that the peak area of minocycline obtained with 20 μL of this solution is equivalent to 3.5 to 6.5% of that with 20 μL of the solution for system suitability test.

System repeatability: When the test is repeated 6 times with 20 μL of the solution for system suitability test under the above operating conditions, the relative standard deviation of the peak area of minocycline is not more than 2.0%.

Water <*2.48*> Not less than 4.3% and not more than 8.0% (0.3 g, volumetric titration, direct titration).

Residue on ignition <*2.44*> Not more than 0.5% (1 g).

Assay Weigh accurately an amount of Minocycline Hydrochloride and Minocycline Hydrochloride RS, equivalent to about 50 mg (potency), dissolve each in the mobile phase to make exactly 100 mL, and use these solutions as the sample solution and the standard solution. Perform the test with exactly 20 μL each of the sample solution and standard solution as directed under Liquid Chromatography <*2.01*> according to the following conditions, and determine the peak areas, A_T and A_S, of minocycline in each solution.

Amount [μg (potency)] of minocycline ($C_{23}H_{27}N_3O_7$)
$= M_S \times A_T/A_S \times 1000$

M_S: Amount [mg (potency)] of Minocycline Hydrochloride RS taken

Operating conditions—

Detector: An ultraviolet absorption photometer (wavelength: 280 nm).

Column: A stainless steel column 4.6 mm in inside diameter and 15 cm in length, packed with octylsilanized silica gel for liquid chromatography (5 μm in particle diameter).

Column temperature: A constant temperature of about 25°C.

Mobile phase: Adjust to pH 6.5 of a mixture of a solution of ammonium oxalate monohydrate (7 in 250), *N,N*-dimethylformamide and 0.1 mol/L disodium dihydrogen ethylenediamine tetraacetate TS (11:5:4) with tetrabutylammonium hydroxide TS.

Flow rate: Adjust so that the retention time of minocycline is about 12 minutes.

System suitability—

System performance: Dissolve 50 mg of Minocycline Hydrochloride in 25 mL of water. Heat 5 mL of this solution on a water bath for 60 minutes, then add water to make 25 mL. When the procedure is run with 20 μL of this solution under the above operating conditions, epiminocycline and minocycline are eluted in this order with the resolution between these peaks being not less than 2.0.

System repeatability: When the test is repeated 6 times with 20 μL of the standard solution under the above operating conditions, the relative standard deviation of peak areas of minocycline is not more than 1.0%.

Containers and storage Containers—Tight containers.

Storage—Light-resistant.

Minocycline Hydrochloride Granules

ミノサイクリン塩酸塩顆粒

Minocycline Hydrochloride Granules contain not less than 90.0% and not more than 110.0% of the labeled potency of minocycline ($C_{23}H_{27}N_3O_7$: 457.48).

Method of preparation Prepare as directed under Granules, with Minocycline Hydrochloride.

Identification To a quantity of Minocycline Hydrochloride Granules, equivalent to 10 mg (potency) of Minocycline Hydrochloride, add 625 mL of a solution of hydrochloric acid in methanol (19 in 20,000), shake thoroughly, and filter. Determine the absorption spectrum of the filtrate as directed under Ultraviolet-visible Spectrophotometry <*2.24*>: it exhibits maxima between 221 nm and 225 nm, between 261 nm and 265 nm, and between 354 nm and 358 nm.

Purity Related substances—Conduct this procedure within 30 minutes after the preparation of the sample solution. To a quantity of Minocycline Hydrochloride Granules, equivalent to 50 mg (potency) of Minocycline Hydrochloride, add 60 mL of the mobile phase, shake vigorously, add the mobile phase to make 100 mL. Centrifuge this solution, and use the supernatant liquid as the sample solution. Perform the test with 20 μL of the sample solution as directed under Liquid Chromatography <*2.01*> according to the following conditions. Determine each peak area by the automatic integration method, and calculate their amounts by the area percentage method: the amount of the peak of epiminocycline, having the relative retention time of about 0.83 to minocycline, is not more than 4.0%.

Operating conditions—

Detector, column, column temperature, mobile phase, and flow rate: Proceed as directed in the operating conditions in the Assay under Minocycline Hydrochloride.

Time span of measurement: About 2.5 times as long as the retention time of minocycline, beginning after the solvent peak.

System suitability—

System performance: Proceed as directed in the system suitability in the Assay under Minocycline Hydrochloride.

Test for required detectability: To 2 mL of the standard solution obtained in the Assay add the mobile phase to make 100 mL, and use this solution as the solution for system suitability test. Pipet 5 mL of the solution for system suitability test, and add the mobile phase to make exactly 100 mL. Confirm that the peak area of minocycline obtained with 20 μL of this solution is equivalent to 3.5 to 6.5% of that with 20 μL of the solution for system suitability test.

System repeatability: When the test is repeated 6 times with 20 μL of the solution for system suitability test under the above operating conditions, the relative standard deviation of the peak area of minocycline is not more than 2.0%.

Water <*2.48*> Not more than 2.0% (4 g of powdered Minocycline Hydrochloride Granules, volumetric titration, back titration).

Uniformity of dosage units <*6.02*> Perform the test according to the following method: Minocycline Hydrochloride Granules in single-dose packages meet the requirement of the Content uniformity test.

To the total content of 1 package of Minocycline Hydrochloride Granules add water to disintegrate, shake thoroughly, add water to make exactly 100 mL, and filter through a membrane filter with a pore size not exceeding 0.45 μm. Discard the first 10 mL of the filtrate, pipet V mL of the subsequent filtrate, add water to make exactly V' mL so that each mL contains about 20 μg (potency) of minocycline ($C_{23}H_{27}N_3O_7$), and use this solution as the sample solution. Separately, weigh accurately an amount of Minocycline Hydrochloride RS, equivalent to about 20 mg (potency), dissolve in water to make exactly 100 mL. Pipet 5 mL of this solution, add water to make exactly 50 mL, and use this solution as the standard solution. Determine the absorbances, A_T and A_S, of the sample solution and standard solution at 348 nm as directed under Ultraviolet-visible Spectrophotometry <*2.24*>.

Amount [mg (potency)] of minocycline ($C_{23}H_{27}N_3O_7$)
$= M_S \times A_T/A_S \times V'/V \times 1/10$

M_S: Amount [mg (potency)] of Minocycline Hydrochloride RS taken

Dissolution <*6.10*> When the test is performed at 50 revolutions per minute according to the Paddle method, using 900 mL of water as the dissolution medium, the dissolution rate in 15 minutes of Minocycline Hydrochloride Granules is not less than 85%.

Start the test with an accurately weighed amount of Minocycline Hydrochloride Granules, equivalent to about 20 mg (potency) of Minocycline Hydrochloride, withdraw not less than 20 mL of the medium at the specified minute after starting the test, and filter through a membrane filter with a pore size not exceeding 0.45 μm. Discard not less than 10 mL of the first filtrate, and use the subsequent filtrate as the sample solution. Separately, weigh accurately an amount of Minocycline Hydrochloride RS, equivalent to about 22 mg (potency), and dissolve in water to make exactly 100 mL. Pipet 5 mL of this solution, add water to make exactly 50 mL, and use this solution as the standard solution. Determine the absorbances, A_T and A_S, of the sample solution and standard solution at 348 nm as directed under Ultraviolet-visible Spectrophotometry <2.24>.

Dissolution rate (%) with respect to the labeled amount of minocycline ($C_{23}H_{27}N_3O_7$)
$= M_S/M_T \times A_T/A_S \times 1/C \times 90$

M_S: Amount [mg (potency)] of Minocycline Hydrochloride RS taken
M_T: Amount (g) of Minocycline Hydrochloride Granules taken
C: Labeled amount [mg (potency)] of minocycline ($C_{23}H_{27}N_3O_7$) in 1 g

Assay Weigh accurately an amount of powdered Minocycline Hydrochloride Granules, equivalent to about 50 mg (potency) of Minocycline Hydrochloride, add the mobile phase, shake vigorously, and add the mobile phase to make exactly 100 mL. Centrifuge this solution, and use the supernatant liquid as the sample solution. Separately, weigh accurately an amount of Minocycline Hydrochloride RS, equivalent to about 25 mg (potency), dissolve in the mobile phase to make exactly 50 mL, and use this solution as the standard solution. Then, proceed as directed in the Assay under Minocycline Hydrochloride.

Amount [mg (potency)] of minocycline ($C_{23}H_{27}N_3O_7$)
$= M_S \times A_T/A_S \times 2$

M_S: Amount [mg (potency)] of Minocycline Hydrochloride RS taken

Containers and storage Containers—Tight containers.
Storage—Light-resistant.

Minocycline Hydrochloride for Injection

注射用ミノサイクリン塩酸塩

Minocycline Hydrochloride for Injection is a preparation for injection, which is dissolved before use.

It contains not less than 90.0% and not more than 110.0% of the labeled potency of minocycline ($C_{23}H_{27}N_3O_7$: 457.48).

Method of preparation Prepare as directed under Injections, with Minocycline Hydrochloride.

Description Minocycline Hydrochloride for Injection occurs as a yellow to yellow-brown, powder or flakes.

Identification Dissolve 4 mg of Minocycline Hydrochloride for Injection in 250 mL of a solution of hydrochloric acid in methanol (19 in 20,000). Determine the absorption spectrum of this solution as directed under Ultraviolet-visible Spectrophotometry <2.24>: it exhibits maxima between 221 nm and 225 nm, between 261 nm and 265 nm, and between 354 nm and 358 nm.

pH <2.54> The pH of a solution, prepared by dissolving an amount of Minocycline Hydrochloride for Injection, equivalent to 0.1 g (potency) of Minocycline Hydrochloride, in 10 mL of water is 2.0 to 3.5.

Purity Related substances—Conduct this procedure rapidly after the preparation of the sample solution. Take an amount of Minocycline Hydrochloride for Injection, equivalent to 0.1 g (potency) of Minocycline Hydrochloride, dissolve in the mobile phase to make 100 mL. To 25 mL of this solution, add the mobile phase to make 50 mL, and use this solution as the sample solution. Perform the test with 20 μL of the sample solution as directed under Liquid Chromatography <2.01> according to the following conditions, and determine each peak area by the automatic integration method. Calculate the amounts of each peak by the area percentage method: the amount of epiminocycline, having the relative retention time of about 0.83 to minocycline, is not more than 6.0%.

Operating conditions—

Detector, column, column temperature, mobile phase and flow rate: Proceed as directed in the operating conditions in the Assay under Minocycline Hydrochloride.

Time span of measurement: About 2.5 times as long as the retention time of minocycline, beginning after the solvent peak.

System suitability—

System performance: Proceed as directed in the system suitability in the Assay under Minocycline Hydrochloride.

Test for required detectability: Pipet 2 mL of the standard solution obtained in the Assay, add the mobile phase to make exactly 100 mL, and use this solution as the solution for system suitability test. Pipet 5 mL of the solution for system suitability test, add the mobile phase to make exactly 100 mL. Confirm that the peak area of minocycline obtained with 20 μL of this solution is equivalent to 3.5 to 6.5% of that with 20 μL of the solution for system suitability test.

System repeatability: When the test is repeated 6 times with 20 μL of the solution for system suitability test under the above operating conditions, the relative standard deviation of the peak area of minocycline is not more than 2.0%.

Water <2.48> Weigh accurately the mass of the content of one container of Minocycline Hydrochloride for Injection, dissolve in exactly 2 mL of methanol for water determination, and perform the test with exactly 1 mL of this solution as directed in the Volumetric titration (back titration): not more than 3.0%.

Bacterial endotoxins <4.01> Less than 1.25 EU/mg (potency).

Uniformity of dosage units <6.02> It meets the requirement of the Mass variation test.

Foreign insoluble matter <6.06> Perform the test according to Method 2: it meets the requirement.

Insoluble particulate matter <6.07> It meets the requirement.

Sterility <4.06> Perform the test according to the Membrane filtration method: it meets the requirement.

Assay Weigh accurately the mass of the contents of not less than 10 containers of Minocycline Hydrochloride for Injection. Weigh accurately an amount of the contents, equivalent to about 0.1 g (potency) of Minocycline Hydrochloride, dissolve in the mobile phase to make exactly 100 mL. Pipet 25 mL of this solution, add the mobile phase to make exactly 50 mL, and use this solution as the sample solution. Separately, weigh accurately an amount of Minocycline Hydrochloride RS, equivalent to about 25 mg (potency), dissolve in the mobile phase to make exactly 50 mL, and use this solution as the standard solution. Then, proceed as directed in the Assay under Minocycline Hydrochloride.

Amount [mg (potency)] of minocycline ($C_{23}H_{27}N_3O_7$)
$= M_S \times A_T/A_S \times 4$

M_S: Amount [mg (potency)] of Minocycline Hydrochloride RS taken

Containers and storage Containers—Hermetic containers.

Minocycline Hydrochloride Tablets

ミノサイクリン塩酸塩錠

Minocycline Hydrochloride Tablets contain not less than 90.0% and not more than 110.0% of the labeled potency of Minocycline ($C_{23}H_{27}N_3O_7$: 457.48).

Method of preparation Prepare as directed under Tablets, with Minocycline Hydrochloride.

Identification To a quantity of powdered Minocycline Hydrochloride Tablets, equivalent to 10 mg (potency) of Minocycline Hydrochloride, add 625 mL of a solution of hydrochloric acid in methanol (19 in 20,000), shake well, and filter. Determine the absorption spectrum of the filtrate as directed under Ultraviolet-visible Spectrophotometry <*2.24*>: it exhibits maxima between 221 nm and 225 nm, between 261 nm and 265 nm, and between 354 nm and 358 nm.

Purity Related substances—Conduct this procedure rapidly after preparation of the sample solution. Powder not less than 5 Minocycline Hydrochloride Tablets. Weigh accurately a portion of the powder, equivalent to 50 mg (potency) of Minocycline Hydrochloride, add 60 mL of the mobile phase, shake vigorously, and add the mobile phase to make 100 mL. Centrifuge this solution, and use the supernatant liquid as the sample solution. Perform the test with 20 μL of the sample solution as directed under Liquid Chromatography <*2.01*> according to the following conditions. Determine each peak area by the automatic integration method. Calculate the amounts of these peaks by the area percentage method: the amount of the peak of epiminocycline, having the relative retention time of about 0.83 to minocycline, is not more than 2.0%.

Operating conditions—

Detector, column, column temperature, mobile phase and flow rate: Proceed as directed in the operating conditions in the Assay under Minocycline Hydrochloride.

Time span of measurement: About 2.5 times as long as the retention time of minocycline, beginning after the solvent peak.

System suitability—

System performance: Proceed as directed in the system suitability in the Assay under Minocycline Hydrochloride.

Test for required detectability: To 2 mL of the sample solution add the mobile phase to make 100 mL, and use this solution as the solution for system suitability test. Pipet 5 mL of the solution for system suitability test, and add the mobile phase to make exactly 100 mL. Confirm that the peak area of minocycline obtained with 20 μL of this solution is equivalent to 3.5 to 6.5% of that with 20 μL of the solution for system suitability test.

System repeatability: When the test is repeated 6 times with 20 μL of the solution for system suitability test under the above operating conditions, the relative standard deviation of the peak area of minocycline is not more than 2.0%.

Water <*2.48*> Not more than 12.0% (0.5 g of powdered Minocycline Hydrochloride Tablets, volumetric titration, back titration).

Uniformity of dosage units <*6.02*> Perform the Mass variation test, or the Content uniformity test according to the following method: it meets the requirement.

To 1 tablet of Minocycline Hydrochloride Tablets add 60 mL of the mobile phase, sonicate for 15 minutes, and add the mobile phase to make exactly *V* mL so that each mL contains about 0.5 mg (potency) of Minocycline Hydrochloride. Centrifuge this solution, and use the supernatant liquid as the sample solution. Then, proceed as directed in the Assay.

Amount [mg (potency)] of minocycline ($C_{23}H_{27}N_3O_7$)
$= M_S \times A_T/A_S \times V/50$

M_S: Amount [mg (potency)] of Minocycline Hydrochloride RS taken

Dissolution <*6.10*> When the test is performed at 50 revolutions per minute according to the Paddle method, using 900 mL of water as the dissolution medium, the dissolution rate in 30 minutes of Minocycline Hydrochloride Tablets is not less than 85%.

Start the test with 1 tablet of Minocycline Hydrochloride Tablets, withdraw not less than 20 mL of the medium at the specified minute after starting the test, and filter through a membrane filter with a pore size not exceeding 0.45 μm. Discard not less than 10 mL of the first filtrate, pipet *V* mL of the subsequent filtrate, add water to make exactly *V′* mL so that each mL contains about 9 μg (potency) of Minocycline Hydrochloride, and use this solution as the sample solution. Separately, weigh accurately an amount of Minocycline Hydrochloride RS, equivalent to about 30 mg (potency), and dissolve in water to make exactly 100 mL. Pipet 4 mL of this solution, add water to make exactly 100 mL, and use this solution as the standard solution. Perform the test with the sample solution and standard solution as directed under Ultraviolet-visible Spectrophotometry <*2.24*>, and determine the absorbances, A_T and A_S, at 348 nm.

Dissolution rate (%) with respect to the labeled amount of minocycline ($C_{23}H_{27}N_3O_7$)
$= M_S \times A_T/A_S \times V'/V \times 1/C \times 36$

M_S: Amount [mg (potency)] of Minocycline Hydrochloride RS taken
C: Labeled amount [mg (potency)] of minocycline ($C_{23}H_{27}N_3O_7$) in 1 tablet

Assay To a number of Minocycline Hydrochloride Tablets, equivalent to about 1 g (potency) of Minocycline Hydrochloride, add 120 mL of the mobile phase, sonicate for 15 minutes, and add the mobile phase to make exactly 200 mL. Centrifuge this solution, pipet 5 mL of the supernatant liquid, add the mobile phase to make exactly 50 mL, and use this solution as the sample solution. Separately, weigh accurately an amount of Minocycline Hydrochloride RS, equivalent to about 25 mg (potency), dissolve in the mobile phase to make exactly 50 mL, and use this solution as the standard solution. Then, proceed as directed in the Assay under

Minocycline Hydrochloride.

Amount [mg (potency)] of minocycline ($C_{23}H_{27}N_3O_7$) $= M_S \times A_T/A_S \times 40$

M_S: Amount [mg (potency)] of Minocycline Hydrochloride RS taken

Containers and storage Containers—Tight containers.
Storage—Light-resistant.

Mitiglinide Calcium Hydrate

ミチグリニドカルシウム水和物

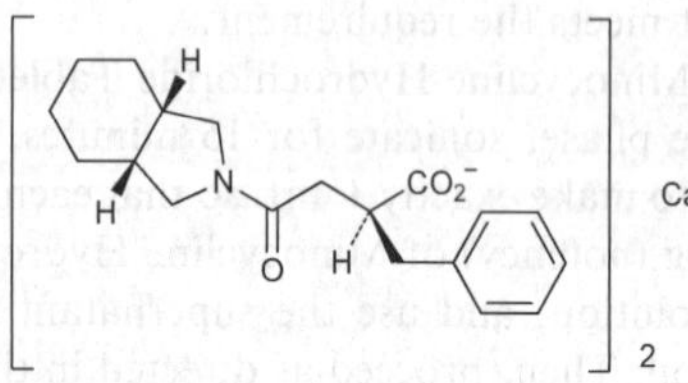

$C_{38}H_{48}CaN_2O_6.2H_2O$: 704.91
Monocalcium bis{(2*S*)-2-benzyl-4-[(3a*R*,7a*S*)-octahydroisoindol-2-yl]-4-oxobutanoate} dihydrate
[207844-01-7]

Mitiglinide Calcium Hydrate contains not less than 98.0% and not more than 102.0% of mitiglinide calcium hydrate ($C_{38}H_{48}CaN_2O_6.2H_2O$).

Description Mitiglinide Calcium Hydrate occurs as a white powder.

It is freely soluble in methanol and in ethanol (99.5), and slightly soluble in water.

It shows crystal polymorphism.

Identification **(1)** Determine the absorption spectrum of a solution of Mitiglinide Calcium Hydrate in methanol (1 in 1000) as directed under Ultraviolet-visible Spectrophotometry *<2.24>*, and compare the spectrum with the Reference Spectrum or the spectrum of a solution of Mitiglinide Calcium RS prepared in the same manner as the sample solution: both spectra exhibit similar intensities of absorption at the same wavelengths.

(2) Determine the infrared absorption spectrum of Mitiglinide Calcium Hydrate as directed in the paste method under Infrared Spectrophotometry *<2.25>*, and compare the spectrum with the Reference Spectrum or the spectrum of Mitiglinide Calcium RS: both spectra exhibit similar intensities of absorption at the same wave numbers.

(3) To 0.5 g of Mitiglinide Calcium Hydrate add 3 mL of 1 mol/L hydrochloric acid TS and 5 mL of diethyl ether, shake, then separate the aqueous layer, and neutralize with ammonia TS: the solution responds to Qualitative Tests *<1.09>* (2) for calcium salt.

Optical rotation *<2.49>* $[\alpha]_D^{20}$: + 8.4 – + 9.0° (0.38 g calculated on the anhydrous basis, methanol, 20 mL, 100 mm).

Purity **(1)** Heavy metals *<1.07>*—Place 1.0 g of Mitiglinide Calcium Hydrate in a crucible, cover the crucible loosely, and ignite at a low temperature until charred. After cooling, add 2 mL of nitric acid and 5 drops of sulfuric acid to the content of the crucible, heat carefully until white fumes are no longer evolved, and ignite between 500 and 600°C. After cooling, moisten the residue with a little amount of sulfuric acid, and incinerate again by ignition. After cooling, add 2 mL of hydrochloric acid, evaporate to dryness on a water bath, moisten the residue with 3 drops of hydrochloric acid, add 10 mL of boiling water, and heat for 2 minutes. Sonicate this solution, add 1 drop of phenolphthalein TS, drop ammonia TS until a slight red color develops, add 2 mL of dilute acetic acid, transfer to a centrifuge tube, centrifuge, and take the supernatant liquid. Wash the residue in the crucible with 15 mL of water, transfer to the former centrifuge tube, sonicate, centrifuge, and take the supernatant liquid. Repeat this operation with 15 mL of water in addition. Combine all the supernatant liquid obtained, put in a Nessler tube, and add water to make 50 mL. Perform the test using this solution as the test solution. Prepare the control solution with 2.0 mL of Standard Lead Solution (not more than 20 ppm).

(2) Related substances—To 0.10 g of Mitiglinide Calcium Hydrate add a mixture of water and acetonitrile (2:1), dissolve by sonicating while occasional shaking, add the mixture of water and acetonitrile (2:1) to make 100 mL, and use this solution as the sample solution. Pipet 2 mL of the sample solution, add the mixture of water and acetonitrile (2:1) to make exactly 50 mL. Pipet 2.5 mL of this solution, add the mixture of water and acetonitrile (2:1) to make exactly 20 mL, and use this solution as the standard solution. Perform the test with exactly 15 μL each of the sample solution and standard solution as directed under Liquid Chromatography *<2.01>* according to the following conditions, and determine each peak area by the automatic integration method: the area of the peak other than mitiglinide obtained from the sample solution is not larger than 1/5 times the peak area of mitiglinide from the standard solution, and the total area of peaks other than mitiglinide from sample solution is not larger than 3/10 times the peak area of mitiglinide from the standard solution.

Operating conditions—

Detector, column, and column temperature: Proceed as directed in the operating conditions in the Assay.

Mobile phase: Adjust to pH 2.0 of a mixture of water, acetonitrile for liquid chromatography and *n*-amyl alcohol (66:33:1) with phosphoric acid.

Flow rate: Adjust so that the retention time of mitiglinide is about 12 minutes.

Time span of measurement: About 2 times as long as the retention time of mitiglinide, beginning after the solvent peak.

System suitability—

Test for required detectability: Pipet 5 mL of the standard solution, add a mixture of water and acetonitrile (2:1) to make exactly 50 mL. Confirm that the peak area of mitiglinide obtained with 15 μL of this solution is equivalent to 7 to 13 % of that with 15 μL of the standard solution.

System performance: When the procedure is run with 15 μL of the standard solution under the above operating conditions, the number of theoretical plates and the symmetry factor of the peak of mitiglinide are not less than 4000 and not more than 1.5, respectively.

System repeatability: When the test is repeated 6 times with 15 μL of the standard solution under the above operating conditions, the relative standard deviation of the peak area of mitiglinide is not more than 2.0%.

Water *<2.48>* 4.5 – 6.0% (50 mg, coulometric titration).

Assay Weigh accurately about 50 mg each of Mitiglinide Calcium Hydrate and Mitiglinide Calcium RS (separately determine the water *<2.48>* in the same manner as Mitiglinide Calcium Hydrate), add a mixture of water and acetonitrile (2:1) to them, dissolve by sonicating while occasional shaking, and add the mixture of water and acetonitrile (2:1) to make exactly 50 mL. Pipet 10 mL each of these solutions, add exactly 10 mL of the internal standard solution, add the mixture of water and acetonitrile (2:1) to make 100 mL, and use these solutions as the sample solution and the standard solution, respectively. Perform the test with 10 μL of the sample solution and standard solution as directed under Liquid Chromatography <*2.01*> according to the following conditions, and calculate the ratios, Q_T and Q_S, of the peak area of mitiglinide to that of the internal standard.

Amount (mg) of mitiglinide calcium hydrate
($C_{38}H_{48}CaN_2O_6.2H_2O$) = $M_S \times Q_T/Q_S \times 1.054$

M_S: Amount (mg) of Mitiglinide Calcium RS taken, calculated on the anhydrous basis

Internal standard solution—A solution of 2-nitrophenol in acetonitrile (1 in 5000).

Operating conditions—

Detector: An ultraviolet absorption photometer (wavelength: 210 nm).

Column: A stainless steel column 4.6 mm in inside diameter and 15 cm in length, packed with palmitamide propylsilanized silica gel for liquid chromatography (5 μm in particle diameter).

Column temperature: A constant temperature of about 35°C.

Mobile phase: Adjust to pH 2.0 of a mixture of water, acetonitrile for liquid chromatography and *n*-amyl alcohol (62:37:1) with phosphoric acid.

Flow rate: Adjust so that the retention time of mitiglinide is about 7.5 minutes.

System suitability—

System performance: When the procedure is run with 10 μL of the standard solution under the above operating conditions, the internal standard and mitiglinide are eluted in this order with the resolution between these peaks being not less than 10.

System repeatability: When the test is repeated 6 times with 10 μL of the standard solution under the above operating conditions, the relative standard deviation of the peak area of mitiglinide is not more than 1.0%.

Containers and storage Containers—Well-closed containers.

Mitiglinide Calcium Tablets

ミチグリニドカルシウム錠

Mitiglinide Calcium Tablets contain not less than 95.0% and not more than 105.0% of the labeled amount of mitiglinide calcium hydrate ($C_{38}H_{48}CaN_2O_6.2H_2O$: 704.91).

Method of preparation Prepare as directed under Tablets, with Mitiglinide Calcium Hydrate.

Identification To 5 mL of the sample solution obtained in the Purity, add a mixture of water and acetonitrile (2:1) to make 10 mL, and use this solution as the sample solution. Separately, to 50 mg of mitiglinide calcium hydrate add the mixture of water and acetonitrile (2:1), dissolve by sonicating while occasional shaking, add the mixture of water and acetonitrile (2:1) to make 100 mL, and use this solution as the standard solution. Perform the test with 15 μL each of the sample solution and standard solution as directed under Liquid Chromatography <*2.01*> according to the following conditions: the principal peaks in the chromatograms obtained from the sample solution and standard solution show the same retention time, and both spectra of these peaks exhibit similar intensities of absorption at the same wavelengths.

Operating conditions—

Column, column temperature, mobile phase, and flow rate: Proceed as directed in the operating conditions in the Purity.

Detector: Photodiode array detector (wavelength: 210 nm, spectrum range of measurement: 200 – 360 nm).

System suitability—

System performance: Proceed as directed in the system suitability in the Purity.

Purity Related substances—Take not less than 10 tablets of Mitiglinide Calcium Tablets, and powder. Weigh a portion of the powder, equivalent to 50 mg of Mitiglinide Calcium Hydrate, add 35 mL of a mixture of water and acetonitrile (2:1), sonicate whiles occasional shaking, add the mixture of water and acetonitrile (2:1) to make 50 mL, and filter through a membrane filter with a pore size not exceeding 0.45 μm. Discard the first 1 mL of the filtrate, and use the subsequent filtrate as the sample solution. Pipet 2 mL of the sample solution, add the mixture of water and acetonitrile (2:1) to make exactly 100 mL, and use this solution as the standard solution. Perform the test with exactly 15 μL each of the sample solution and standard solution as directed under Liquid Chromatography <*2.01*> according to the following conditions. Determine each peak area of both solutions by the automatic integration method: the area of the peak, having the relative retention time of about 0.2 to mitiglinide, obtained from the sample solution is not larger than 1/4 times the peak area of mitiglinide from the standard solution, and the area of peak other than mitiglinide and the peak mentioned above from the sample solution is not larger than 1/8 times the peak area of mitiglinide from the standard solution. In addition, the total area of the peaks other than mitiglinide from the sample solution is not larger than 1/2 times the peak area of mitiglinide from the standard solution.

Operating conditions—

Detector: An ultraviolet absorption photometer (wavelength: 210 nm).

Column: A stainless steel column 4.6 mm in inside diameter and 15 cm in length, packed with palmitamide propylsilanized silica gel for liquid chromatography (5 μm in particle diameter).

Column temperature: A constant temperature of about 35°C.

Mobile phase: Adjust to pH 2.0 of a mixture of water, acetonitrile for liquid chromatography and *n*-amyl alcohol (66:33:1) with phosphoric acid.

Flow rate: Adjust so that the retention time of mitiglinide is about 12 minutes.

Time span of measurement: About 2 times as long as the retention time of mitiglinide, beginning after the solvent peak.

System suitability—

Test for required detectability: Pipet 2.5 mL of the standard solution, add the mixture of water and acetonitrile (2:1) to make exactly 50 mL. Confirm that the peak area of mitiglinide obtained with 15 μL of this solution is equivalent to 3.5 to 6.5% of that with 15 μL of the standard solution.

System performance: When the procedure is run with 15 μL of the standard solution under the above operating conditions, the number of theoretical plates and the symmetry

factor of the peak of mitiglinide are not less than 3000 and not more than 1.5, respectively.

System repeatability: When the test is repeated 6 times with 15 μL of the standard solution under the above operating conditions, the relative standard deviation of the peak area of mitiglinide is not more than 1.5%.

Uniformity of dosage units *<6.02>* Perform the test according to the following method: it meets the requirement of the Content uniformity test.

To 1 tablet of Mitiglinide Calcium Tablets add a mixture of water and acetonitrile (2:1), add exactly *V*/10 mL of the internal standard solution, sonicate while occasional shaking, then add the mixture of water and acetonitrile (2:1) to make *V* mL so that each mL contains about 0.1 mg of mitiglinide calcium hydrate ($C_{38}H_{48}CaN_2O_6.2H_2O$), and filter through a membrane filter with a pore size not exceeding 0.45 μm. Discard the first 1 mL of the filtrate, and use the subsequent filtrate as the sample solution. Separately, weigh accurately about 50 mg of Mitiglinide Calcium RS (separately determine the water *<2.48>* in the same manner as Mitiglinide Calcium Hydrate), add the mixture of water and acetonitrile (2:1), dissolve by sonicating while occasional shaking, and add the mixture of water and acetonitrile (2:1) to make exactly 100 mL. Pipet 20 mL of this solution, add exactly 10 mL of the internal standard solution, add the mixture of water and acetonitrile (2:1) to make 100 mL, and use this solution as the standard solution. Perform the test with 5 μL each of the sample solution and standard solution as directed under Liquid Chromatography *<2.01>* according to the following conditions, and calculate the ratios, Q_T and Q_S, of the peak area of mitiglinide to that of the internal standard.

Amount (mg) of mitiglinide calcium hydrate ($C_{38}H_{48}CaN_2O_6.2H_2O$)
$$= M_S \times Q_T/Q_S \times V/500 \times 1.054$$

M_S: Amount (mg) of Mitiglinide Calcium RS taken, calculated on the anhydrous basis

Internal standard solution—A solution of 2-nitrophenol in acetonitrile (1 in 5000).

Operating conditions—

Proceed as directed in the operating conditions in the Assay under Mitiglinide Calcium Hydrate.

System suitability—

Proceed as directed in the operating conditions in the Assay.

Dissolution *<6.10>* When the test is performed at 50 revolutions per minute according to the Paddle method, using 900 mL of water as the dissolution medium, the dissolution rate in 15 minutes of Mitiglinide Calcium Tablets is not less than 85%.

Start the test with 1 tablet of Mitiglinide Calcium Tablets, withdraw not less than 10 mL of the medium at the specified minute after starting the test, and filter through a membrane filter with a pore size not exceeding 0.45 μm. Discard not less than 1 mL of the first filtrate, pipet *V* mL of the subsequent filtrate, add the mixture of water and acetonitrile (2:1) to make exactly *V′* mL so that each mL contains about 5.6 μg of mitiglinide calcium hydrate ($C_{38}H_{48}CaN_2O_6.2H_2O$), and use this solution as the sample solution. Separately, weigh accurately about 25 mg of Mitiglinide Calcium RS (separately determine the water *<2.48>* in the same manner as Mitiglinide Calcium Hydrate), add the mixture of water and acetonitrile (2:1), dissolve by sonicating while occasional shaking, and add the mixture of water and acetonitrile (2:1) to make exactly 100 mL. Pipet 2 mL of this solution, add water to make exactly 100 mL, and use this solution as the standard solution. Perform the test with exactly 50 μL each of the sample solution and standard solution as directed under Liquid Chromatography *<2.01>* according to the following conditions, and determine the peak areas, A_T and A_S, of mitiglinide in each solution.

Dissolution rate (%) with respect to the labeled amount of mitiglinide calcium hydrate ($C_{38}H_{48}CaN_2O_6.2H_2O$)
$$= M_S \times A_T/A_S \times V'/V \times 1/C \times 18 \times 1.054$$

M_S: Amount (mg) of Mitiglinide Calcium RS taken, calculated on the anhydrous basis

C: Labeled amount (mg) of mitiglinide calcium hydrate ($C_{38}H_{48}CaN_2O_6.2H_2O$) in 1 tablet.

Operating conditions—

Proceed as directed in the operating conditions in the Assay under Mitiglinide Calcium Hydrate.

System suitability—

System performance: When the procedure is run with 50 μL of the standard solution under the above operating conditions, the number of theoretical plates and the symmetry factor of the peak of mitiglinide are not less than 3000 and not more than 2.0, respectively.

System repeatability: When the test is repeated 6 times with 50 μL of the standard solution under the above operating conditions, the relative standard deviation of the peak area of mitiglinide is not more than 1.5%.

Assay Weigh accurately the mass of not less than 20 tablets of Mitiglinide Calcium Tablets, and powder. Weigh accurately a portion of the powder, equivalent to about 10 mg of mitiglinide calcium hydrate ($C_{38}H_{48}CaN_2O_6.2H_2O$), add a mixture of water and acetonitrile (2:1), add exactly 10 mL of the internal standard solution, sonicate while occasional shaking, then add the mixture of water and acetonitrile (2:1) to make 100 mL, and filter through a membrane filter with a pore size not exceeding 0.45 μm. Discard the first 1 mL of the filtrate, and use the subsequent filtrate as the sample solution. Separately, weigh accurately about 50 mg of Mitiglinide Calcium RS (separately determine the water *<2.48>* in the same manner as Mitiglinide Calcium Hydrate), add the mixture of water and acetonitrile (2:1), dissolve by sonicating while occasional shaking, and add the mixture of water and acetonitrile (2:1) to make exactly 100 mL. Pipet 20 mL of this solution, add exactly 10 mL of the internal standard solution, add the mixture of water and acetonitrile (2:1) to make 100 mL, and use this solution as the standard solution. Perform the test with 5 μL each of the sample solution and standard solution as directed under Liquid Chromatography *<2.01>* according to the following conditions, and calculate the ratios, Q_T and Q_S, of the peak area of mitiglinide to that of the internal standard.

Amount (mg) of mitiglinide calcium hydrate ($C_{38}H_{48}CaN_2O_6.2H_2O$)
$$= M_S \times Q_T/Q_S \times 1/5 \times 1.054$$

M_S: Amount (mg) of Mitiglinide Calcium RS taken, calculated on the anhydrous basis

Internal standard solution—A solution of 2-nitrophenol in acetonitrile (1 in 5000).

Operating conditions—

Proceed as directed in the operating conditions in the Assay under Mitiglinide Calcium Hydrate.

System suitability—

System performance: When the procedure is run with 5 μL

of the standard solution under the above operating conditions, the internal standard and mitiglinide are eluted in this order with the resolution between these peaks being not less than 10.

System repeatability: When the test is repeated 6 times with 5 μL of the standard solution under the above operating conditions, the relative standard deviation of the ratio of the peak of mitiglinide to that of the internal standard is not more than 1.0%.

Containers and storage Containers—Well-closed containers.

Mitomycin C

マイトマイシンC

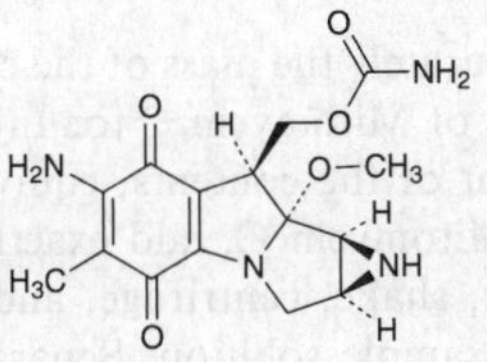

$C_{15}H_{18}N_4O_5$: 334.33
(1a*S*,8*S*,8a*R*,8b*S*)-6-Amino-4,7-dioxo-8a-methoxy-5-methyl-1,1a,2,8,8a,8b-hexahydroazirino[2′,3′:3,4]pyrrolo[1,2-*a*]indol-8-ylmethyl carbamate
[*50-07-7*]

Mitomycin C is a substance having antitumor activity produced by the growth of *Streptomyces caespitosus*.

It contains not less than 970 μg (potency) and not more than 1030 μg (potency) per mg, calculated on the dried basis. The potency of Mitomycin C is expressed as mass (potency) of mitomycin C ($C_{15}H_{18}N_4O_5$).

Description Mitomycin C occurs as blue-purple, crystals or crystalline powder.

It is freely soluble in *N,N*-dimethylacetamide, slightly soluble in water and in methanol, and very slightly soluble in ethanol (99.5).

Identification **(1)** Determine the absorption spectrum of a solution of Mitomycin C (1 in 100,000) as directed under Ultraviolet-visible Spectrophotometry <*2.24*>, and compare the spectrum with the Reference Spectrum or the spectrum of a solution of Mitomycin C RS prepared in the same manner as the sample solution: both spectra exhibit similar intensities of absorption at the same wavelengths.

(2) Determine the infrared absorption spectrum of Mitomycin C as directed in the potassium bromide disk method under Infrared Spectrophotometry <*2.25*>, and compare the spectrum with the Reference Spectrum or the spectrum of Mitomycin C RS: both spectra exhibit similar intensities of absorption at the same wave numbers.

Purity Related substances—Conduct this procedure rapidly after the sample and the standard solutions are prepared. Dissolve 50 mg of Mitomycin C in 10 mL of methanol, and use this solution as the sample solution. Pipet 1 mL of the sample solution, add methanol to make exactly 100 mL, and use this solution as the standard solution. Perform the test with exactly 10 μL each of the sample solution and standard solution as directed under Liquid Chromatography <*2.01*> according to the following conditions, and determine each peak area by the automatic integration method: each area of the peak other than mitomycin C obtained from the sample solution is not larger than the peak area of mitomycin C from the standard solution, and the total area of the peaks other than mitomycin C from the sample solution is not larger than 3 times the peak area of mitomycin C from the standard solution.

Operating conditions—

Detector: An ultraviolet absorption photometer (wavelength: 254 nm).

Column: A stainless steel column 6 mm in inside diameter and 15 cm in length, packed with octadecylsilanized silica gel for liquid chromatography (5 μm in particle diameter).

Column temperature: A constant temperature of about 30°C.

Mobile phase A: To 20 mL of 0.5 mol/L ammonium acetate TS add water to make 1000 mL. To 800 mL of this solution add 200 mL of methanol.

Mobile phase B: To 20 mL of 0.5 mol/L ammonium acetate TS add water to make 1000 mL. To this solution add 1000 mL of methanol.

Flowing of mobile phase: Control the gradient by mixing the mobile phases A and B as directed in the following table.

Time after injection of sample (min)	Mobile phase A (vol%)	Mobile phase B (vol%)
0 – 10	100	0
10 – 30	100 → 0	0 → 100
30 – 45	0	100

Flow rate: About 1.0 mL per minute.

Time span of measurement: About 2 times as long as the retention time of mitomycin C, beginning after the solvent peak.

System suitability—

Test for required detectability: Pipet 10 mL of the standard solution, and add methanol to make exactly 100 mL. Confirm that the peak area of mitomycin C obtained with 10 μL of this solution is equivalent to 7 to 13% of that with 10 μL of the standard solution.

System performance: Dissolve 25 mg of Mitomycin C and 40 mg of 3-ethoxy-4-hydroxybenzaldehyde in 50 mL of methanol. When the procedure is run with 10 μL of this solution under the above operating conditions, mitomycin C and 3-ethoxy-4-hydroxybenzaldehyde are eluted in this order with the resolution between these peaks being not less than 15.

System repeatability: When the test is repeated 3 times with 10 μL of the standard solution under the above operating conditions, the relative standard deviation of the peak area of mitomycin C is not more than 3.0%.

Loss on drying <*2.41*> Not more than 1.0% (0.1 g, reduced pressure not exceeding 0.67 kPa, 60°C, 3 hours).

Assay Weigh accurately an amount of Mitomycin C and Mitomycin C RS, equivalent to about 25 mg (potency), dissolve each in *N,N*-dimethylacetamide to make exactly 50 mL, and use these solutions as the sample solution and standard solution. Perform the test with exactly 10 μL each of the sample solution and standard solution as directed under Liquid Chromatography <*2.01*> according to the following conditions, and determine the peak areas, A_T and A_S, of mitomycin C in each solution.

Amount [μg (potency)] of mitomycin C ($C_{15}H_{18}N_4O_5$)
$= M_S \times A_T/A_S \times 1000$

M_S: Amount [mg (potency)] of Mitomycin C RS taken

Operating conditions—

Detector: An ultraviolet absorption photometer (wavelength: 365 nm).

Column: A stainless steel column 4 mm in inside diameter and 30 cm in length, packed with phenylated silica gel for liquid chromatography (10 μm in particle diameter).

Column temperature: A constant temperature of about 25°C.

Mobile phase: To 40 mL of 0.5 mol/L ammonium acetate TS add 5 mL of diluted acetic acid (100) (1 in 20) and water to make 1000 mL. To 600 mL of this solution add 200 mL of methanol.

Flow rate: Adjust so that the retention time of mitomycin C is about 7 minutes.

System suitability—

System performance: Dissolve about 25 mg of Mitomycin C RS and about 0.375 g of 3-ethoxy-4-hydroxybenzaldehyde in 50 mL of *N,N*-dimethylacetamide. When the procedure is run with 10 μL of this solution under the above operating conditions, mitomycin C and 3-ethoxy-4-hydroxybenzaldehyde are eluted in this order with the resolution between these peaks being not less than 3.

System repeatability: When the test is repeated 6 times with 10 μL of the standard solution under the above operating conditions, the relative standard deviation of the peak area of mitomycin C is not more than 1.0%.

Containers and storage Containers—Tight containers.

Mitomycin C for Injection

注射用マイトマイシンＣ

Mitomycin C for Injection is a preparation for injection, which is dissolved before use.

It contains not less than 90.0% and not more than 110.0% of the labeled potency of mitomycin C ($C_{15}H_{18}N_4O_5$: 334.33).

Method of preparation Prepare as directed under Injections, with Mitomycin C.

Description Mitomycin C for Injection occurs as a blue-purple powder.

Identification Dissolve an amount of Mitomycin C for Injection, equivalent to 2 mg (potency) of Mitomycin C, in 200 mL of water, and determine the absorption spectrum of this solution as directed under Ultraviolet-visible Spectrophotometry <*2.24*>: it exhibits maxima between 216 nm and 220 nm, and between 362 nm and 366 nm.

pH <*2.54*> The pH of a solution, prepared by dissolving 0.25 g of Mitomycin C for Injection in 20 mL of water, is 5.5 to 8.5.

Loss on drying <*2.41*> Not more than 1.0% (0.4 g, in vacuum not exceeding 0.67 kPa, phosphorus (V) oxide, 60°C, 3 hours).

Bacterial endotoxins <*4.01*> Less than 10 EU/mg (potency).

Uniformity of dosage units <*6.02*> Perform the test according to the following method: it meets the requirement of the Content uniformity test.

To the content of 1 container of Mitomycin C for Injection add exactly *V* mL of *N,N*-dimethylacetamide so that each mL contains about 0.5 mg (potency) of Mitomycin C, shake, centrifuge, and use the supernatant liquid as the sample solution. Separately, weigh accurately about 25 mg (potency) of Mitomycin C RS, add *N,N*-dimethylacetamide to make exactly 50 mL, and use this solution as the standard solution. Then, proceed as directed in the Assay under Mitomycin C.

$$\text{Amount [mg (potency)] of mitomycin C } (C_{15}H_{18}N_4O_5) = M_S \times A_T/A_S \times V/50$$

M_S: Amount [mg (potency)] of Mitomycin C RS taken

Foreign insoluble matter <*6.06*> Perform the test according to Method 2: it meets the requirement.

Insoluble particulate matter <*6.07*> It meets the requirement.

Sterility <*4.06*> Perform the test according to the Membrane filtration method: it meets the requirement.

Assay Weigh accurately the mass of the contents of not less than 10 containers of Mitomycin C for Injection. Weigh accurately an amount of the contents, equivalent to about 10 mg (potency) of Mitomycin C, add exactly 20 mL of *N,N*-dimethylacetamide, shake, centrifuge, and use the supernatant liquid as the sample solution. Separately, weigh accurately an amount of Mitomycin C RS, equivalent to about 25 mg (potency), dissolve in *N,N*-dimethylacetamide to make exactly 50 mL, and use this solution as the standard solution. Then, proceed as directed in the Assay under Mitomycin C.

$$\text{Amount [mg (potency)] of mitomycin C } (C_{15}H_{18}N_4O_5) = M_S \times A_T/A_S \times 2/5$$

M_S: Amount [mg (potency)] of Mitomycin C RS taken

Containers and storage Containers—Hermetic containers.

Mizoribine

ミゾリビン

$C_9H_{13}N_3O_6$: 259.22

5-Hydroxy-1-β-D-ribofuranosyl-1*H*-imidazole-4-carboxamide [*50924-49-7*]

Mizoribine contains not less than 98.0% and not more than 102.0% of mizoribine ($C_9H_{13}N_3O_6$), calculated on the anhydrous basis.

Description Mizoribine occurs as a white to yellowish white crystalline powder.

It is freely soluble in water, and practically insoluble in methanol and in ethanol (99.5).

Identification **(1)** Determine the absorption spectrum of a solution of Mizoribine (1 in 100,000) as directed under Ultraviolet-visible Spectrophotometry <*2.24*>, and compare the spectrum with the Reference Spectrum or the spectrum of a solution of Mizoribine RS prepared in the same manner as the sample solution: both spectra exhibit similar intensities of absorption at the same wavelengths.

(2) Determine the infrared absorption spectrum of

Mizoribine as directed in the potassium bromide disk method under Infrared Spectrophotometry <2.25>, and compare the spectrum with the Reference Spectrum or the spectrum of Mizoribine RS: both spectra exhibit similar intensities of absorption at the same wave numbers.

Optical rotation <2.49> $[\alpha]_D^{20}$: −25 – −27° (0.5 g calculated on the anhydrous basis, water, 25 mL, 100 mm).

Purity (1) Heavy metals <1.07>—Proceed with 1.0 g of Mizoribine according to Method 1, and perform the test. Prepare the control solution with 2.0 mL of Standard Lead Solution (not more than 20 ppm).

(2) Related substances—Dissolve 0.10 g of Mizoribine in the mobile phase to make 50 mL, and use this solution as the sample solution. Pipet 5 mL of the sample solution, and add the mobile phase to make exactly 50 mL. Pipet 1 mL of this solution, add the mobile phase to make exactly 100 mL, and use this solution as the standard solution. Perform the test with exactly 5 μL each of the sample solution and standard solution as directed under Liquid Chromatography <2.01> according to the following conditions. Determine each peak area of both solutions by the automatic integration method: the areas of the peaks other than mizoribine obtained from the sample solution are not larger than the peak area of mizoribine from the standard solution.

Operating conditions—

Column, column temperature, mobile phase, and flow rate: Proceed as directed in the operating conditions in the Assay.

Detector: An ultraviolet absorption photometer (wavelength: 220 nm).

Time span of measurement: About 3 times as long as the retention time of mizoribine, beginning after the solvent peak.

System suitability—

Test for required detectability: Pipet 1 mL of the standard solution, and add the mobile phase to make exactly 5 mL. Confirm that the peak area of mizoribine obtained with 5 μL of this solution is equivalent to 14 to 26% of that with 5 μL of the standard solution.

System performance: When the procedure is run with 5 μL of the standard solution under the above operating conditions, the number of theoretical plates and the symmetry factor of the peak of mizoribine are not less than 10,000 and not more than 1.4, respectively.

System repeatability: When the test is repeated 6 times with 5 μL of the standard solution under the above operating conditions, the relative standard deviation of the peak area of mizoribine is not more than 2.0%.

Water <2.48> Not more than 0.5% (0.5 g, volumetric titration, direct titration).

Residue on ignition <2.44> Not more than 0.1% (1 g).

Assay Weigh accurately about 0.1 g of Mizoribine, and dissolve in the mobile phase to make exactly 50 mL. Pipet 5 mL of this solution, add the mobile phase to make exactly 50 mL, and use this solution as the sample solution. Separately, weigh accurately about 10 mg of Mizoribine RS (separately determine the water <2.48> using the same manner as Mizoribine), dissolve in the mobile phase to make exactly 50 mL, and use this solution as the standard solution. Perform the test with exactly 5 μL each of the sample solution and standard solution as directed under Liquid Chromatography <2.01> according to the following conditions, and determine the peak areas, A_T and A_S, of mizoribine in each solution.

$$\text{Amount (mg) of mizoribine } (C_9H_{13}N_3O_6) = M_S \times A_T/A_S \times 10$$

M_S: Amount (mg) of Mizoribine RS taken, calculated on the anhydrous basis

Operating conditions—

Detector: An ultraviolet absorption photometer (wavelength: 279 nm).

Column: A stainless steel column 4.6 mm in inside diameter and 25 cm in length, packed with octadecylsilanized silica gel for liquid chromatography (5 μm in particle diameter).

Column temperature: A constant temperature of about 25°C.

Mobile phase: Diluted phosphoric acid (1 in 1500).

Flow rate: Adjust so that the retention time of mizoribine is about 9 minutes.

System suitability—

System performance: When the procedure is run with 5 μL of the standard solution under the above operating conditions, the number of theoretical plates and the symmetry factor of the peak of mizoribine are not less than 10,000 and not more than 1.4, respectively.

System repeatability: When the test is repeated 6 times with 5 μL of the standard solution under the above operating conditions, the relative standard deviation of the peak area of mizoribine is not more than 1.0%.

Containers and storage Containers—Tight containers.

Storage—At a temperature between 2 and 8°C.

Mizoribine Tablets

ミゾリビン錠

Mizoribine Tablets contain not less than 93.0% and not more than 107.0% of the labeled amount of mizoribine ($C_9H_{13}N_3O_6$: 259.22).

Method of preparation Prepare as directed under Tablets, with Mizoribine.

Identification To a quantity of powdered Mizoribine Tablets, equivalent to 0.1 g of Mizoribine, add 5 mL of water, shake, filter, and use the filtrate as the sample solution. Separately, dissolve 20 mg of Mizoribine RS in 1 mL of water, and use this solution as the standard solution. Perform the test with the sample solution and standard solution as directed under Thin-Layer Chromatography <2.03>. Spot 1 μL each of the sample solution and standard solution on a plate of silica gel for thin-layer chromatography. Then develop the plate with a mixture of methanol, ammonia solution (28) and 1-propanol (2:1:1) to a distance of about 10 cm, and air-dry the plate. Allow the plate to stand in iodine vapor: the principal spot obtained from the sample solution and the spot from the standard solution show a red-brown color and the same *R*f value.

Purity Related substances—To a quantity of powdered Mizoribine Tablets, equivalent to 0.10 g of Mizoribine, add 30 mL of the mobile phase, shake, then add the mobile phase to make 50 mL. Filter the solution through a membrane filter with a pore size not exceeding 0.5 μm and use the filtrate as the sample solution. Pipet 2 mL of the sample solution, add the mobile phase to make exactly 20 mL. Pipet 1 mL of the solution, add the mobile phase to make exactly 20 mL, and use this solution as the standard solution. Perform the test with exactly 5 μL each of the sample solution and standard solution as directed under Liquid Chromatography <*2.01*> according to the following conditions. Determine each peak area by the automatic integration method: the area of the peak, having the relative retention time of about 0.3 to mizoribine, obtained from the sample solution is not larger than the peak area of mizoribine from the standard solution, and the area of the peak other than mizoribine and the peak mentioned above is not larger than 2/5 times the peak area of mizoribine from the standard solution.

Operating conditions—

Column, column temperature, mobile phase, and flow rate: Proceed as directed in the operating conditions in the Assay under Mizoribine.

Detector: An ultraviolet absorption photometer (wavelength: 220 nm).

Time span of measurement: About 3 times as long as the retention time of mizoribine, beginning after the solvent peak.

System suitability—

Test for required detectability: To exactly 1 mL of the standard solution add the mobile phase to make exactly 5 mL. Confirm that the peak area of mizoribine obtained with 5 μL of this solution is equivalent to 14 to 26% of that with 5 μL of the standard solution.

System performance: When the procedure is run with 5 μL of the standard solution under the above operating conditions, the number of theoretical plates and the symmetry factor of the peak of mizoribine are not less than 10,000 and not more than 1.4, respectively.

System repeatability: When the test is repeated 6 times with 5 μL of the standard solution under the above operating conditions, the relative standard deviation of the peak area of mizoribine is not more than 2.0%.

Uniformity of dosage units <*6.02*> Perform the Mass variation test, or the Content uniformity test according to the following method: it meets the requirement.

To 1 tablet of Mizoribine Tablets add 50 mL of water, shake until the tablet is disintegrated, and add water to make exactly 100 mL. Filter the solution, discard not less than 10 mL of the first filtrate, pipet V mL of the subsequent filtrate, add water to make exactly V' mL so that each mL contains about 5 μg of mizoribine ($C_9H_{13}N_3O_6$), and use this solution as the sample solution. Then, proceed as directed in the Assay.

$$\text{Amount of mizoribine } (C_9H_{13}N_3O_6) = M_S \times A_T/A_S \times V'/V \times 1/50$$

M_S: Amount (mg) of Mizoribine RS taken, calculated on the anhydrous basis

Dissolution <*6.10*> When the test is performed at 50 revolutions per minute according to the Paddle method, using 900 mL of water as the dissolution medium, the dissolution rate in 45 minutes of Mizoribine Tablets is not less than 80%.

Start the test with 1 tablet of Mizoribine Tablets, withdraw not less than 20 mL of the medium at the specified minute after starting the test, and filter through a membrane filter with a pore size not exceeding 0.5 μm. Discard not less than 10 mL of the first filtrate, pipet V mL of the subsequent filtrate, add water to make exactly V' mL so that each mL contains about 14 μg of mizoribine ($C_9H_{13}N_3O_6$), and use this solution as the sample solution. Separately, weigh accurately about 28 mg of Mizoribine RS (separately determine the water <*2.48*> in the same manner as Mizoribine), and dissolve in water to make exactly 100 mL. Pipet 1 mL of this solution, add water to make exactly 20 mL, and use this solution as the standard solution. Determine the absorbances, A_T and A_S, at 279 nm of the sample solution and standard solution as directed under Ultraviolet-visible Spectrophotometry <*2.24*>.

$$\text{Dissolution rate (\%) with respect to the labeled amount of mizoribine } (C_9H_{13}N_3O_6) = M_S \times A_T/A_S \times V'/V \times 1/C \times 45$$

M_S: Amount (mg) of Mizoribine RS taken, calculated on the anhydrous basis

C: Labeled amount (mg) of mizoribine ($C_9H_{13}N_3O_6$) in 1 tablet

Assay Weigh accurately not less than 20 Mizoribine Tablets, and powder. Weigh accurately a portion of the powder, equivalent to about 25 mg of mizoribine ($C_9H_{13}N_3O_6$), add 50 mL of water and shake, then add water to make exactly 100 mL. Filter the solution, discard not less than 10 mL of the first filtrate, pipet 2 mL of the subsequent filtrate, add water to make exactly 100 mL, and use this solution as the sample solution. Separately, weigh accurately about 25 mg of Mizoribine RS (separately determine the water <*2.48*> in the same manner as Mizoribine), and dissolve in water to make exactly 100 mL. Pipet 2 mL of the solution, add water to make exactly 100 mL, and use this solution as the standard solution. Determine the absorbances, A_T and A_S, at 279 nm of the sample solution and standard solution as directed under Ultraviolet-visible Spectrophotometry <*2.24*>.

$$\text{Amount (mg) of mizoribine } (C_9H_{13}N_3O_6) = M_S \times A_T/A_S$$

M_S: Amount (mg) of Mizoribine RS taken, calculated on the anhydrous basis

Containers and storage Containers—Tight containers.

Montelukast Sodium

モンテルカストナトリウム

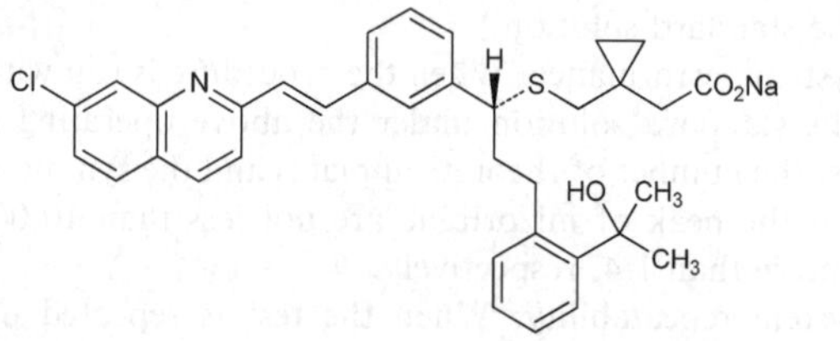

$C_{35}H_{35}ClNNaO_3S$: 608.17

Monosodium {1-[({(1*R*)-1-{3-[(1*E*)-2-(7-chloroquinolin-2-yl)ethenyl]phenyl}-3-[2-(2-hydroxypropan-2-yl)phenyl]propyl}sulfanyl)methyl]cyclopropyl}acetate

[*151767-02-1*]

Montelukast Sodium contains not less than 98.0% and not more than 102.0% of montelukast sodium ($C_{35}H_{35}ClNNaO_3S$), calculated on the anhydrous and residual solvent-free basis.

Description Montelukast Sodium occurs as a white to pale yellow-white powder.

It is very soluble in methanol and in ethanol (99.5), and freely soluble in water.

It is hygroscopic.

It turns yellow on exposure to light.

It shows crystal polymorphism.

Identification **(1)** Place 0.1 g of Montelukast Sodium in a crucible, and ignite until a white residue is formed. To the residue add 2 mL of water, and then filter. To the filtrate add 2 mL of potassium carbonate solution (3 in 20), and heat to boiling: no precipitate is observed. To this solution add 4 mL of potassium hexahydroxoantimonate (V) TS, heat to boiling, and cool immediately in ice water: a white precipitate is formed. Rub the inside wall of the test tube with a glass rod, if necessary.

(2) Determine the absorption spectrum of a solution of Montelukast Sodium in a mixture of methanol and water (3:1) (1 in 100,000) as directed under Ultraviolet-visible Spectrophotometry <*2.24*>, and compare the spectrum with the Reference Spectrum or the spectrum of a solution of Montelukast Sodium for Identification RS prepared in the same manner as the sample solution: both spectra exhibit similar intensities of absorption at the same wavelengths.

(3) Determine the infrared absorption spectrum of Montelukast Sodium as directed in the paste method under Infrared Spectrophotometry <*2.25*>, and compare the spectrum with the Reference Spectrum or the spectrum of Montelukast Sodium for Identification RS: both spectra exhibit similar intensities of absorption at the same wave numbers. Or, perform the test by the potassium bromide disk method or the ATR method, and compare the spectrum with the spectrum of Montelukast Sodium for Identification RS: both spectra exhibit similar intensities of absorption at the same wave numbers. If any difference appears between the spectra, dissolve Montelukast Sodium and Montelukast Sodium for Identification RS in toluene, add heptane, shake, then allow to stand, and remove the supernatant liquid by decantation. Dry the residue at 75°C for 16 hours under reduced pressure, and perform the test by paste method, potassium bromide disk method or the ATR method.

Purity **(1)** Heavy metals—Dissolve 0.5 g of Montelukast Sodium in 20 mL of a mixture of acetone and water (4:1), and use this solution as the sample solution. Separately, take 0.5 mL of Standard Lead Solution, add 20 mL of the mixture of acetone and water (4:1), and use this solution as the standard solution. To the sample solution and the standard solution add 2 mL of acetate buffer solution (pH 3.5), and shake. To these solutions add 1.2 mL of thioacetamide-alkaline glycerin TS, shake immediately, then allow to stand for 2 minutes, and filter through a membrane filter with a pore size 0.45 μm (about 13 mm in diameter). Compare the color on the membrane filters through which each solution is filtered: the color obtained from the sample solution is not darker than that obtained from the standard solution (not more than 10 ppm).

(2) Related substances—Conduct this procedure using light-resistant vessels. Dissolve 50 mg of Montelukast Sodium in 50 mL of a mixture of methanol and water (9:1), and use this solution as the sample solution. Perform the test with 10 μL of the sample solution as directed under Liquid Chromatography <*2.01*> according to the following conditions. Determine each peak area by the automatic integration method, and calculate the amount of them by the area percentage method: the amount of the peak of related substance A, having the relative retention time of about 0.4 to montelukast is not more than 0.2%, the amounts of the peaks, related substance B and related substance E, having respectively the relative retention times of about 0.8 and about 1.2 are not more than 0.15%, the total amount of the two peaks, related substances C and D, both having the relative retention time about 0.9 is not more than 0.15%, the amount of the peak of related substance F having the relative retention time of about 1.9 is not more than 0.3%, and the amount of the peak other than montelukast and other than the peaks mentioned above is not more than 0.10%. Furthermore, the total amount of the peaks other than montelukast is not more than 0.6%.

Operating conditions—

Detector, column, column temperature, mobile phases A and B, flowing of mobile phase, and flow rate: Proceed as directed in the operating conditions in the Assay.

Time span of measurement: For 16 minutes after injection, beginning after the solvent peak.

System suitability—

System performance: Proceed as directed in the system suitability in the Assay.

Test for required detectability: Pipet 1 mL of the sample solution, add the mixture of methanol and water (9:1) to make exactly 100 mL. Pipet 1 mL of this solution, add the mixture of methanol and water (9:1) to make exactly 20 mL, and use this solution as the solution for system suitability test. When the procedure is run with 10 μL of the solution for system suitability test under the above operating conditions, the SN ratio of the peak of montelukast is not less than 10.

For the calculations mentioned above, the peak areas smaller than that of montelukast, founded in the chromatogram obtained with 10 μL of the solution for system suitability test, are excluded.

(3) Enantiomer—Conduct this procedure using light-resistant vessels. Dissolve 50 mg of Montelukast Sodium in 50 mL of a mixture of water and acetonitrile (1:1), and use this solution as the sample solution. Perform the test with 10 μL of the sample solution as directed under Liquid Chromatography <*2.01*> according to the following conditions. Determine each peak area by the automatic integration method, and calculate the amounts of them by the area percentage method: the amount of the peak of the enantiomer having the relative retention time of about 0.7 to montelukast is not more than 0.2%.

Operating conditions—

Detector: An ultraviolet absorption photometer (wavelength: 280 nm).

Column: A stainless steel column 4.0 mm in inside diameter and 15 cm in length, packed with α_1-acid glycoprotein binding silica gel for liquid chromatography (5 μm in particle diameter).

Column temperature: A constant temperature of about 30°C.

Mobile phase A: Dissolve 2.3 g of ammonium acetate in 1000 mL of water, and adjust to pH 5.7 with acetic acid (100).

Mobile phase B: A mixture of methanol and acetonitrile (3:2).

Flowing of mobile phase: Control the gradient by mixing the mobile phases A and B as directed in the following table.

Time after injection of sample (min)	Mobile phase A (vol%)	Mobile phase B (vol%)
0 – 30	70 → 60	30 → 40
30 – 35	60	40

Flow rate: 0.9 mL per minute (the retention time of montelukast is about 25 minutes).

System suitability—

Test for required detectability: Pipet 1 mL of the sample solution, add the mixture of water and acetonitrile (1:1) to make exactly 100 mL. Pipet 1 mL of this solution, add the mixture of water and acetonitrile (1:1) to make exactly 10 mL. When the procedure is run with 10 μL of this solution under the above operating conditions, the SN ratio of the peak of montelukast is not less than 10.

System performance: When the procedure is run with 10 μL of a solution of Montelukast Racemate for System Suitabillity RS in the mixture of water and acetonitrile (1:1) (1 in 10,000) under the above operating conditions, the resolution between the peak of montelukast and the enantiomer is not less than 2.9.

Water <*2.48*> Not more than 4.0% (0.3 g, volumetric titration, direct titration).

Assay Conduct this procedure using light-resistant vessels. Weigh accurately about 50 mg of Montelukast Sodium, and dissolve in a mixture of methanol and water (9:1) to make exactly 50 mL. Pipet 10 mL of this solution, add the mixture of methanol and water (9:1) to make exactly 100 mL, and use this solution as the sample solution. Separately, weigh accurately about 26 mg of Montelukast Dicyclohexylamine RS, dissolve in the mixture of methanol and water (9:1) to make exactly 50 mL. Pipet 5 mL of this solution, add the mixture of methanol and water (9:1) to make exactly 20 mL, and use this solution as the standard solution. Perform the test with exactly 10 μL each of the sample solution and standard solution as directed under Liquid Chromatography <*2.01*> according to the following conditions. Determine the peak areas, A_T and A_S, of montelukast in each solution.

Amount (mg) of montelukast sodium ($C_{35}H_{35}ClNNaO_3S$) $= M_S \times A_T/A_S \times 5/2 \times 0.792$

M_S: Amount (mg) of Montelukast Dicyclohexylamine RS taken

Operating conditions—

Detector: An ultraviolet absorption photometer (wavelength: 238 nm).

Column: A stainless steel column 4.6 mm in inside diameter and 5 cm in length, packed with phenylsilanized silica gel for liquid chromatography (1.8 μm in particle diameter).

Column temperature: A constant temperature of about 30°C.

Mobile phase A: A mixture of water and trifluoroacetic acid (2000:3).

Mobile phase B: A mixture of acetonitrile and trifluoroacetic acid (2000:3).

Flowing of mobile phase: Control the gradient by mixing the mobile phases A and B as directed in the following table.

Time after injection of sample (min)	Mobile phase A (vol%)	Mobile phase B (vol%)
0 – 3	60	40
3 – 16	60 → 49	40 → 51

Flow rate: 1.2 mL per minute (the retention time of montelukast is about 7 minutes).

System suitability—

System performance: Use a solution of Montelukast for System Suitability RS in the mixture of methanol and water (9:1) (1 in 1000) as the solution A for peak identification. Perform the test with 10 μL of the solution A for peak identification under the above operating conditions, and identify the peaks having the relative retention times to montelukast of about 0.4 (related substance A), about 0.9 (related substances C and D), about 1.2 (related substance E), and about 1.9 (related substance F). Place 1 mL of the solution A for peak identification in a clear glass container, allow to stand for about 20 minutes, and use this solution as the solution B for peak identification. When the procedure is run with 10 μL of the solution B for peak identification under the above operating conditions, and identify the peak having the relative retention time of about 0.8 to montelukast (related substance B), the resolution between the peaks of related substance B and montelukast is not less than 2.5, and between the peaks of montelukast and related substance E is not less than 1.5.

System repeatability: When the test is repeated 5 times with 10 μL of the standard solution under the above operating conditions, the relative standard deviation of the peak area of montelukast is not more than 0.73%.

Containers and storage Containers—Tight containers

Storage—Light-resistant.

Others

Related substance A:

(1-{[(1-{3-[(1*E*)-2-(7-Chloroquinolin-2-yl)ethenyl]phenyl}-3-[2-(2-hydroxypropan-2-yl)phenyl]propyl)sulfinyl]methyl}cyclopropyl)acetic acid

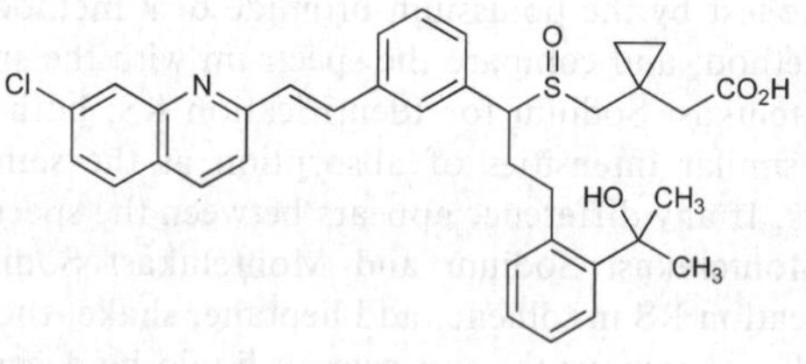

Related substance B:

{1-[({(1*R*)-1-{3-[(1*Z*)-2-(7-Chloroquinolin-2-yl)ethenyl]phenyl}-3-[2-(2-hydroxypropan-2-yl)phenyl]propyl}sulfanyl)methyl]cyclopropyl}acetic acid

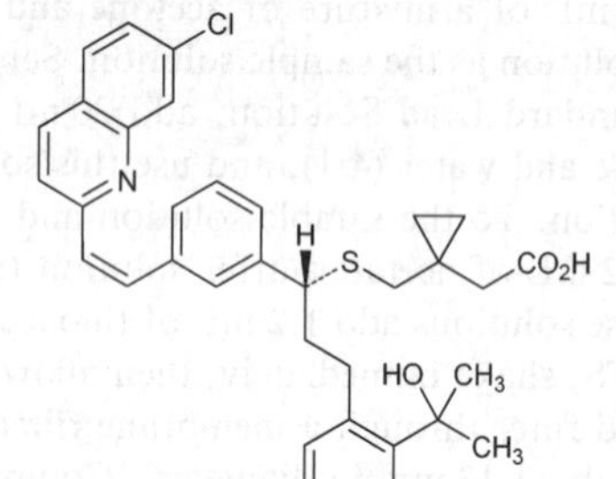

Related substance C:

{1-[({(1*R*)-1-{3-[(1*R*)-1-({[1-(Carboxymethyl)cyclopropyl]methyl}sulfanyl)-2-(7-chloroquinolin-2-yl)ethyl]phenyl}-3-[2-(2-hydroxypropan-2-yl)phenyl]propyl}sulfanyl)methyl]cyclopropyl}acetic acid

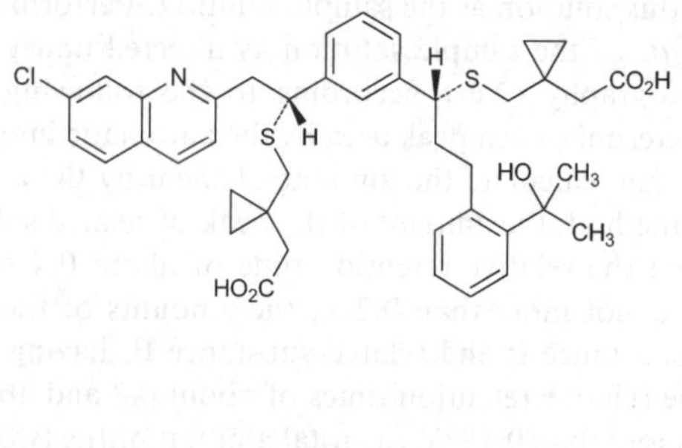

Related substance D:
{1-[({(1*R*)-1-{3-[(1*S*)-1-({[1-(Carboxymethyl)cyclopropyl]methyl}sulfanyl)-2-(7-chloroquinolin-2-yl)ethyl]phenyl}-3-[2-(2-hydroxypropan-2-yl)phenyl]propyl}sulfanyl)methyl]cyclopropyl}acetic acid

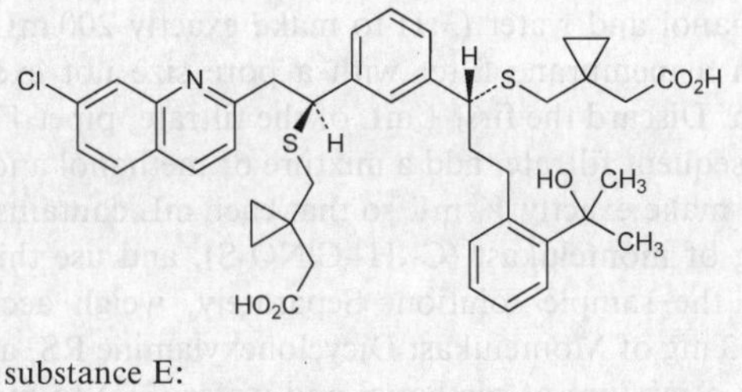

Related substance E:
[1-({[(1*R*)-3-(2-Acetylphenyl)-1-{3-[(1*E*)-2-(7-chloroquinolin-2-yl)ethenyl]phenyl}propyl]sulfanyl}methyl)cyclopropyl]acetic acid

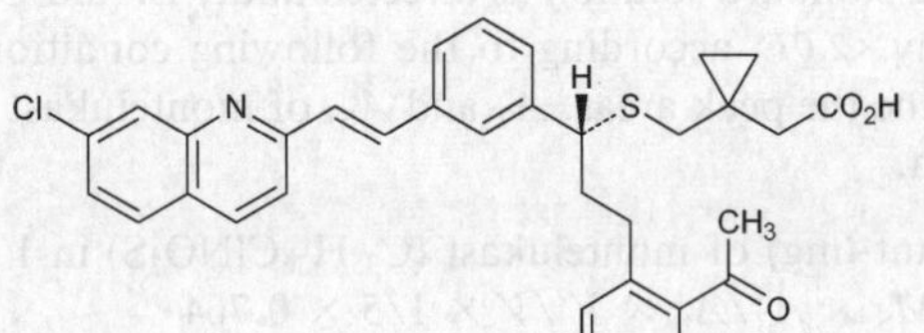

Related substance F:
{1-[({(1*R*)-1-{3-[(1*E*)-2-(7-Chloroquinolin-2-yl)ethenyl]phenyl}-3-[2-(1-methylethenyl)phenyl]propyl}sulfanyl)methyl]cyclopropyl}acetic acid

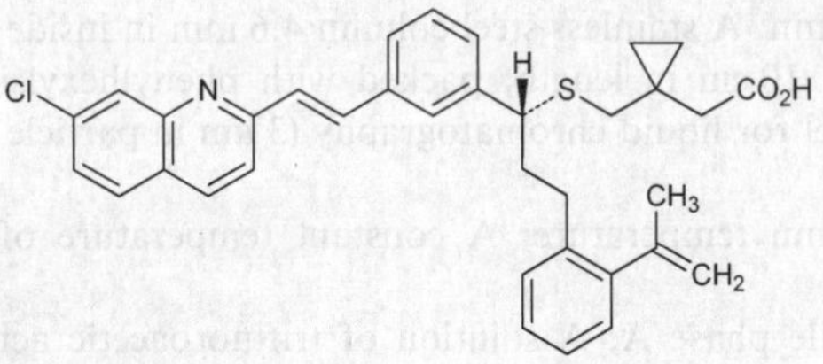

Montelukast Sodium Chewable Tablets

モンテルカストナトリウムチュアブル錠

Montelukast Sodium Chewable Tablets contain not less than 95.0% and not more than 105.0% of the labeled amount of montelukast ($C_{35}H_{36}ClNO_3S$: 586.18).

Method of preparation Prepare as directed under Chewable Tablets, with Montelukast Sodium.

Identification To an amount of powdered Montelukast Sodium Chewable Tablets, equivalent to 5 mg of montelukast ($C_{35}H_{36}ClNO_3S$), add 500 mL of a mixture of methanol and water (3:1), shake, and centrifuge. Determine the absorption spectrum of the supernatant liquid as directed under Ultraviolet-visible Spectrophotometry <2.24>: it exhibits maxima between 281 nm and 285 nm, between 325 nm and 329 nm, between 343 nm and 347 nm and between 357 nm and 361 nm.

Purity Related substances—Use the sample solution obtained in the Assay as the sample solution. Pipet 1 mL of the sample solution, add a mixture of methanol and water (3:1) to make exactly 100 mL, and use this solution as the standard solution. Perform the test with exactly 20 μL each of the sample solution and standard solution as directed under Liquid Chromatography <2.01> according to the following conditions, and determine each peak area by the automatic integration method: the total area of the two peaks of related substance A, having the relative retention time of about 0.45 to montelukast, obtained from the sample solution is not larger than 1.5 times the peak area of montelukast from the standard solution, the area of related substance B having the relative retention time of about 0.92 from the sample solution is not larger than 3/20 times the peak area of montelukast from the standard solution, and the area of the peaks other than montelukast and the peaks mentioned above from the sample solution is not larger than 1/10 times the peak area of montelukast from the standard solution. Furthermore, the total area of the peaks other than montelukast is not larger than 1.8 times the peak area of montelukast from the standard solution. However, the peaks of the related substances derived from Montelukast Sodium [having the relative retention time of about 1.04 (related substance E), about 1.16 (related substance C), about 1.18 (related substance D), about 1.24 and about 1.55 (related substance F)] are excluded. For the area of the peak, having the relative retention time of about 0.71, multiply the correction factor 0.6.

Operating conditions—

Detector, column, column temperature, mobile phase, and flow rate: Proceed as directed in the operating conditions in the Assay.

Time span of measurement: About 1.5 times as long as the retention time of montelukast, beginning after the solvent peak.

System suitability—

System performance: Proceed as directed in the system suitability in the Assay.

Test for required detectability: Pipet 10 mL of the standard solution, and add a mixture of methanol and water (3:1) to make exactly 100 mL. When the procedure is run with 20 μL of this solution under the above operating conditions, the SN ratio of the peak of montelukast is not less than 10.

System repeatability: When the test is repeated 5 times with 20 μL of the standard solution under the above operating conditions, the relative standard deviation of the peak area of montelukast is not more than 2.0%.

Uniformity of dosage units <6.02> Perform the test according to the following method: it meets the requirement of the Content uniformity test.

Conduct this procedure using light-resistant vessels. To 1 tablet of Montelukast Sodium Chewable Tablets add 50 mL of water to disintegrate the tablet, add a suitable amount of methanol, and disperse the fine particles by sonicating. Add methanol to make exactly 200 mL, and centrifuge or filter. Pipet V mL of this solution, add a mixture of methanol and water (3:1) to make exactly V' mL so that each mL contains about 25 μg of montelukast ($C_{35}H_{36}ClNO_3S$) and use this solution as the sample solution. Separately, weigh accurately about 33 mg of Montelukast Dicyclohexylamine RS, and dissolve in a mixture of methanol and water (3:1) to make exactly 200 mL. Pipet 20 mL of this solution, add a mixture of methanol and water (3:1) to make exactly 100 mL, and use this solution as the standard solution. Perform the test with exactly 10 μL each of the sample solution and standard solution as directed under Liquid Chromatography <2.01> according to the following conditions, and determine the peak areas, A_T and A_S, of montelukast in each solution.

$$\text{Amount (mg) of montelukast } (C_{35}H_{36}ClNO_3S) = M_S \times A_T/A_S \times V'/V \times 1/5 \times 0.764$$

M_S: Amount (mg) of Montelukast Dicyclohexylamine RS taken

Operating conditions—

Detector: An ultraviolet absorption photometer (wavelength: 389 nm).

Column: A stainless steel column 3.0 mm in inside diameter and 10 cm in length, packed with phenylated silica gel for liquid chromatography (5 μm in particle diameter).

Column temperature: A constant temperature of about 50°C.

Mobile phase: A solution of trifluoroacetic acid in a mixture of water and acetonitrile for liquid chromatography (1:1) (1 in 500).

Flow rate: Adjust so that the retention time of montelukast is about 2 minutes.

System suitability—

System performance: When the procedure is run with 10 μL of the standard solution under the above operating conditions, the number of theoretical plates and the symmetry factor of the peak of montelukast are not less than 2000 and not more than 1.5, respectively.

System repeatability: When the test is repeated 5 times with 10 μL of the standard solution under the above operating conditions, the relative standard deviation of the peak area of montelukast is not more than 1.0%.

Dissolution <*6.10*> When the test is performed at 50 revolutions per minute according to the Paddle method, using 900 mL of a solution of sodium lauryl sulfate (1 in 200) as the dissolution medium, the dissolution rate in 20 minutes of Montelukast Sodium Chewable Tablets is not less than 85%.

Conduct this procedure using light-resistant vessels. Start the test with 1 tablet of Montelukast Sodium Chewable Tablets, withdraw not less than 15 mL of the medium at the specified minute after starting the test, and centrifuge. Pipet V mL of the supernatant liquid, add the dissolution medium to make exactly V' mL so that each mL contains about 5.6 μg of montelukast ($C_{35}H_{36}ClNO_3S$), and use this solution as the sample solution. Separately, weigh accurately about 35 mg of Montelukast Dicyclohexylamine RS, dissolve in methanol to make exactly 100 mL. Pipet 2 mL of this solution, add the dissolution medium to make exactly 100 mL, and use this solution as the standard solution. Perform the test with exactly 50 μL each of the sample solution and standard solution as directed under Liquid Chromatography <*2.01*> according to the following conditions, and determine the peak areas, A_T and A_S, of montelukast in each solution.

Dissolution rate (%) with respect to the labeled amount of montelukast ($C_{35}H_{36}ClNO_3S$)

$$= M_S \times A_T/A_S \times V'/V \times 1/C \times 18 \times 0.764$$

M_S: Amount (mg) of Montelukast Dicyclohexylamine RS taken

C: Labeled amount (mg) of montelukast ($C_{35}H_{36}ClNO_3S$) in 1 tablet

Operating conditions—

Proceed as directed in the operating conditions in the Uniformity of dosage units.

System suitability—

System performance: When the procedure is run with 50 μL of the standard solution under the above operating conditions, the number of theoretical plates and the symmetry factor of the peak of montelukast are not less than 2000 and not more than 1.5, respectively.

System repeatability: When the test is repeated 5 times with 50 μL of the standard solution under the above operating conditions, the relative standard deviation of the peak area of montelukast is not more than 2.0%.

Assay Conduct this procedure using light-resistant vessels. Disintegrate 10 tablets of Montelukast Sodium Chewable Tablets in 150 mL of a mixture of methanol and water (3:1), disperse the fine particles by sonicating, and add a mixture of methanol and water (3:1) to make exactly 200 mL, filter through a membrane filter with a pore size not exceeding 0.45 μm. Discard the first 1 mL of the filtrate, pipet V mL of the subsequent filtrate, add a mixture of methanol and water (3:1) to make exactly V' mL so that each mL contains about 0.25 mg of montelukast ($C_{35}H_{36}ClNO_3S$), and use this solution as the sample solution. Separately, weigh accurately about 33 mg of Montelukast Dicyclohexylamine RS, and dissolve in a mixture of methanol and water (3:1) to make exactly 100 mL, and use this solution as the standard solution. Perform the test with exactly 20 μL each of the sample solution and standard solution as directed under Liquid Chromatography <*2.01*> according to the following conditions, and determine the peak areas, A_T and A_S, of montelukast in each solution.

Amount (mg) of montelukast ($C_{35}H_{36}ClNO_3S$) in 1 tablet

$$= M_S \times A_T/A_S \times V'/V \times 1/5 \times 0.764$$

M_S: Amount (mg) of Montelukast Dicyclohexylamine RS taken

Operating conditions—

Detector: An ultraviolet absorption photometer (wavelength: 255 nm).

Column: A stainless steel column 4.6 mm in inside diameter and 10 cm in length, packed with phenylhexylsilanized silica gel for liquid chromatography (3 μm in particle diameter).

Column temperature: A constant temperature of about 50°C.

Mobile phase A: A solution of trifluoroacetic acid (1 in 500).

Mobile phase B: A mixture of methanol and acetonitrile for liquid chromatography (3:2).

Flowing of mobile phase: Control the gradient by mixing the mobile phases A and B as directed in the following table.

Time after injection of sample (min)	Mobile phase A (vol%)	Mobile phase B (vol%)
0 – 5	48 → 45	52 → 55
5 – 12	45	55
12 – 22	45 → 25	55 → 75
22 – 23	25	75

Flow rate: 1.5 mL per minute (the retention time of montelukast is about 14 minutes).

System suitability—

System performance: Take 10 mL of the standard solution in a transparent vessel, add 4 μL of hydrogen peroxide (30), and allow to stand under 4000 lx white light for 10 minutes. When the procedure is run with 20 μL of this solution under the above operating conditions, the resolution between the peak of related substance B, having a relative retention time of about 0.92 to montelukast and the peak of montelukast is not less than 1.5. And proceed with 20 μL of the standard solution under the above conditions, the number of theoretical plates and the symmetry factor of the peak of montelukast are not less than 5000 and not more than 2.5, respectively.

System repeatability: When the test is repeated 5 times with 20 μL of the standard solution under the above operating conditions, the relative standard deviation of the peak area of montelukast is not more than 1.0%.

Containers and storage Containers—Tight containers.
Storage—Light-resistant.

Others
Related substances A, B, C, D, E and F: Refer to them described in Montelukast Sodium.

Montelukast Sodium Granules

モンテルカストナトリウム顆粒

Montelukast Sodium Granules contain not less than 95.0% and not more than 105.0% of the labeled amount of montelukast ($C_{35}H_{36}ClNO_3S$: 586.18).

Method of preparation Prepare as directed under Granules, with Montelukast Sodium.

Identification To an amount of Montelukast Sodium Granules, equivalent to 5 mg of montelukast ($C_{35}H_{36}ClNO_3S$), add 500 mL of a mixture of methanol and water (3:1), shake, and centrifuge. Determine the absorption spectrum of the supernatant liquid as directed under Ultraviolet-visible Spectrophotometry <*2.24*>: it exhibits maxima between 281 nm and 285 nm, between 325 nm and 329 nm, between 343 nm and 347 nm, and between 357 nm and 361 nm.

Purity Related substances—Use the sample solution obtained in the Assay as the sample solution. Pipet 1 mL of the sample solution, add a mixture of methanol and water (3:1) to make exactly 100 mL, and use this solution as the standard solution. Perform the test with exactly 20 μL each of the sample solution and standard solution as directed under Liquid Chromatography <*2.01*> according to the following conditions, and determine each peak area by the automatic integration method: the total area of the two peaks of related substance A, having the relative retention time of about 0.45 to montelukast, obtained from the sample solution is not larger than the peak area of montelukast from the standard solution, and the peak area of related substance B, having the relative retention time of about 0.92, from the sample solution is not larger than 3/20 times the peak area of montelukast from the standard solution, and the area of the peak other than montelukast and the peaks mentioned above from the sample solution is not larger than 1/10 times the peak area of montelukast from the standard solution. Furthermore, the total area of the peaks other than montelukast from the sample solution is not larger than 1.2 times the peak area of montelukast from the standard solution. However, the peaks of the related substances derived from Montelukast Sodium [having the relative retention time of about 1.04 (related substance E), about 1.16 (related substance C), about 1.18 (related substance D), about 1.24 and about 1.55 (related substance F)] are excluded. For the area of the peak, having the relative retention time of about 0.71, multiply the correction factor 0.6.

Operating conditions—

Detector, column, column temperature, mobile phase and flow rate: Proceed as directed in the operating conditions in the Assay.

Time span of measurement: About 1.5 times as long as the retention time of montelukast, beginning after the solvent peak.

System suitability—

System performance: Proceed as directed in the system suitability in the Assay.

Test for required detectability: Pipet 10 mL of the standard solution, and add a mixture of methanol and water (3:1) to make exactly 100 mL. When the procedure is run with 20 μL of this solution under the above operating conditions, the SN ratio of the peak of montelukast is not less than 10.

System repeatability: When the test is repeated 5 times with 20 μL of the standard solution under the above operating conditions, the relative standard deviation of the peak area of montelukast is not more than 2.0%.

Uniformity of dosage unit <*6.02*> Perform the test according to the following method: Montelukast Sodium Granules in single-dose packages meet the requirement of the Content uniformity test.

Conduct this procedure using light-resistant vessels. To the total content of 1 package of Montelukast Sodium Granules add 130 mL of methanol, disperse the fine particles by sonicating, and add methanol to make exactly *V* mL so that each mL contains about 20 μg of montelukast ($C_{35}H_{36}ClNO_3S$). Centrifuge, and use the supernatant liquid as the sample solution. Separately, weigh accurately about 33 mg of Montelukast Dicyclohexylamine RS, and dissolve in methanol to make exactly 100 mL. Pipet 8 mL of this solution, add methanol to make exactly 100 mL, and use this solution as the standard solution. Perform the test with exactly 5 μL each of the sample solution and standard solution as directed under Liquid Chromatography <*2.01*> according to the following conditions, and determine the peak areas, A_T and A_S, of montelukast in each solution.

$$\text{Amount (mg) of montelukast } (C_{35}H_{36}ClNO_3S) = M_S \times A_T/A_S \times V/1250 \times 0.764$$

M_S: Amount (mg) of Montelukast Dicyclohexylamine RS taken

Operating conditions—

Detector: An ultraviolet absorption photometer (wavelength: 389 nm).

Column: A stainless steel column 3.0 mm in inside diameter and 10 cm in length, packed with phenylated silica gel for liquid chromatography (5 μm in particle diameter).

Column temperature: A constant temperature of about 50°C.

Mobile phase: A solution of trifluoroacetic acid in a mixture of water and acetonitrile (1:1) (1 in 500).

Flow rate: Adjust so that the retention time of montelukast is about 2 minutes.

System suitability—

System performance: When the procedure is run with 5 μL of the standard solution under the above operating conditions, the number of theoretical plates and the symmetry factor of the peak of montelukast are not less than 1500 and not more than 1.5, respectively.

System repeatability: When the test is repeated 5 times with 5 μL of the standard solution under the above operating conditions, the relative standard deviation of the peak area of montelukast is not more than 1.0%.

Dissolution <*6.10*> When the test is performed at 50 revolutions per minute according to the Paddle method, using 900 mL of a solution of sodium lauryl sulfate (1 in 200) as the dissolution medium, the dissolution rate in 15 minutes of Montelukast Sodium Granules is not less than 85%.

Conduct this procedure using light-resistant vessels. Start the test with an accurately weighed amount of Montelukast

Sodium Granules, equivalent to about 4 mg of montelukast ($C_{35}H_{36}ClNO_3S$), withdraw not less than 15 mL of the medium at the specified minute after starting the test, and filter through a membrane filter with a pore size not exceeding 0.45 μm. Discard not less than 10 mL of the first filtrate, and use the subsequent filtrate as the sample solution. Separately, weigh accurately about 27 mg of Montelukast Dicyclohexylamine RS, and dissolve in methanol to make exactly 100 mL. Pipet 2 mL of this solution, add the dissolution medium to make exactly 100 mL, and use this solution as the standard solution. Perform the test with exactly 25 μL each of the sample solution and standard solution as directed under Liquid Chromatography <*2.01*> according to the following conditions, and determine the peak areas, A_T and A_S, of montelukast in each solution.

Dissolution rate (%) with respect to the labeled amount of montelukast ($C_{35}H_{36}ClNO_3S$)

$$= M_S/M_T \times A_T/A_S \times 1/C \times 18 \times 0.764$$

M_S: Amount (mg) of Montelukast Dicyclohexylamine RS taken

M_T: Amount (g) of Montelukast Sodium Granules taken

C: Labeled amount (mg) of montelukast ($C_{35}H_{36}ClNO_3S$) in 1 g

Operating conditions—

Proceed as directed in the operating conditions in the Uniformity of dosage units.

System suitability—

System performance: When the procedure is run with 25 μL of the standard solution under the above operating conditions, the number of theoretical plates and the symmetry factor of the peak of montelukast are not less than 2000 and not more than 1.5, respectively.

System repeatability: When the test is repeated 6 times with 25 μL of the standard solution under the above operating conditions, the relative standard deviation of the peak area of montelukast is not more than 1.0%.

Assay Conduct this procedure using light-resistant vessels. Weigh accurately an amount of Montelukast Sodium Granules, equivalent to about 48 mg of montelukast ($C_{35}H_{36}ClNO_3S$), and add exactly 200 mL of a mixture of methanol and water (3:1). Disperse the fine particles by sonicating, centrifuge, and use the supernatant liquid as the sample solution. Separately, weigh accurately about 33 mg of Montelukast Dicyclohexylamine RS, and dissolve in a mixture of methanol and water (3:1) to make exactly 100 mL, and use this solution as the standard solution. Perform the test with exactly 20 μL each of the sample solution and standard solution as directed under Liquid Chromatography <*2.01*> according to the following conditions, and determine the peak areas, A_T and A_S, of montelukast in each solution.

Amount (mg) of montelukast ($C_{35}H_{36}ClNO_3S$)

$$= M_S \times A_T/A_S \times 2 \times 0.764$$

M_S: Amount (mg) of Montelukast Dicyclohexylamine RS taken

Operating conditions—

Detector: An ultraviolet absorption photometer (wavelength: 255 nm).

Column: A stainless steel column 4.6 mm in inside diameter and 10 cm in length, packed with phenylhexylsilanized silica gel for liquid chromatography (3 μm in particle diameter).

Column temperature: A constant temperature of about 50°C.

Mobile phase A: A solution of trifluoroacetic acid (1 in 500).

Mobile phase B: A mixture of methanol and acetonitrile (3:2).

Flowing of mobile phase: Control the gradient by mixing the mobile phases A and B as directed in the following table.

Time after injection of sample (min)	Mobile phase A (vol%)	Mobile phase B (vol%)
0 – 5	48 → 45	52 → 55
5 – 12	45	55
12 – 22	45 → 25	55 → 75
22 – 23	25	75

Flow rate: 1.5 mL per minute (the retention time of montelukast is about 14 minutes).

System suitability—

System performance: Take 10 mL of the standard solution in a transparent vessel, add 4 μL of hydrogen peroxide (30), and allow to stand under 4000 lx white light for 10 minutes. When the procedure is run with 20 μL of this solution under the above operating conditions, the resolution between the peak of related substance B, having the relative retention time of about 0.92 to montelukast, and the peak of montelukast is not less than 1.5. And proceed with 20 μL of the standard solution under the above operating conditions, the number of the theoretical plates and the symmetry factor of the peak of montelukast are not less than 5000 and not more than 2.5, respectively.

System repeatability: When the test is repeated 5 times with 20 μL of the standard solution under the above operating conditions, the relative standard deviation of the peak area of montelukast is not more than 1.0%.

Containers and storage Containers—Tight containers.

Storage—Light-resistant.

Others

Related substances A, B, C, D, E and F: Refer to them described in Montelukast Sodium.

Montelukast Sodium Tablets

モンテルカストナトリウム錠

Montelukast Sodium Tablets contain not less than 95.0% and not more than 105.0% of the labeled amount of montelukast ($C_{35}H_{36}ClNO_3S$: 586.18).

Method of preparation Prepare as directed under Tablets, with Montelukast Sodium.

Identification To an amount of powdered Montelukast Sodium Tablets, equivalent to 5 mg of montelukast ($C_{35}H_{36}ClNO_3S$), add 500 mL of a mixture of methanol and water (3:1), shake, and centrifuge. Determine the absorption spectrum of the supernatant liquid as directed under Ultraviolet-visible Spectrophotometry <*2.24*>: it exhibits maxima between 281 nm and 285 nm, between 325 nm and 329 nm, between 343 nm and 347 nm and between 357 nm and 361 nm.

Purity Related substances—Use the sample solution obtained in the Assay as the sample solution. Pipet 1 mL of the sample solution, add a mixture of methanol and water (3:1) to make exactly 100 mL, and use this solution as the standard solution. Perform the test with exactly 20 μL each of the sample solution and standard solution as directed under Liquid Chromatography <2.01> according to the following conditions, and determine each peak area by the automatic integration method: the total area of the two peaks of related substance A, having the relative retention time of about 0.45 to montelukast, obtained from the sample solution is not larger than the peak area of montelukast from the standard solution, the area of related substance B having the relative retention time of about 0.92 from the sample solution is not larger than 3/20 times the peak area of montelukast from the standard solution, and the area of the peaks other than montelukast and the peaks mentioned above from the sample solution is not larger than 1/10 times the peak area of montelukast from the standard solution. Furthermore, the total area of the peaks other than montelukast from the sample solution is not larger than 1.2 times the peak area of montelukast from the standard solution. However, the peaks of the related substances derived from Montelukast Sodium [having the relative retention time of about 1.04 (related substance E), about 1.16 (related substance C), about 1.18 (related substance D), about 1.24 and about 1.55 (related substance F)] are excluded. For the area of the peak, having the relative retention time of about 0.71, multiply the correction factor 0.6.

Operating conditions—

Detector, column, column temperature, mobile phase, and flow rate: Proceed as directed in the operating conditions in the Assay.

Time span of measurement: About 1.5 times as long as the retention time of montelukast, beginning after the solvent peak.

System suitability—

System performance: Proceed as directed in the system suitability in the Assay.

Test for required detectability: Pipet 10 mL of the standard solution, and add a mixture of methanol and water (3:1) to make exactly 100 mL. When the procedure is run with 20 μL of this solution under the above operating conditions, the SN ratio of the peak of montelukast is not less than 10.

System repeatability: When the test is repeated 5 times with 20 μL of the standard solution under the above operating conditions, the relative standard deviation of the peak area of montelukast is not more than 2.0%.

Uniformity of dosage units <*6.02*> Perform the test according to the following method: it meets the requirement of the Content uniformity test.

Conduct this procedure using light-resistant vessels. To 1 tablet of Montelukast Sodium Tablets add 50 mL of water to disintegrate the tablet, add a suitable amount of methanol, and disperse the fine particles by sonicating. Add methanol to make exactly 200 mL, and centrifuge or filter. Pipet V mL of this solution, add a mixture of methanol and water (3:1) to make exactly V' mL so that each mL contains about 25 μg of montelukast ($C_{35}H_{36}ClNO_3S$) and use this solution as the sample solution. Separately, weigh accurately about 33 mg of Montelukast Dicyclohexylamine RS, and dissolve in a mixture of methanol and water (3:1) to make exactly 200 mL. Pipet 20 mL of this solution, add a mixture of methanol and water (3:1) to make exactly 100 mL, and use this solution as the standard solution. Perform the test with exactly 10 μL each of the sample solution and standard solution as directed under Liquid Chromatography <*2.01*> according to the following conditions, and determine the peak areas, A_T and A_S, of montelukast in each solution.

Amount (mg) of montelukast ($C_{35}H_{36}ClNO_3S$)
$= M_S \times A_T/A_S \times V'/V \times 1/5 \times 0.764$

M_S: Amount (mg) of Montelukast Dicyclohexylamine RS taken

Operating conditions—

Detector: An ultraviolet absorption photometer (wavelength: 389 nm).

Column: A stainless steel column 3.0 mm in inside diameter and 10 cm in length, packed with phenylated silica gel for liquid chromatography (5 μm in particle diameter).

Column temperature: A constant temperature of about 50°C.

Mobile phase: A solution of trifluoroacetic acid in a mixture of water and acetonitrile for liquid chromatography (1:1) (1 in 500).

Flow rate: Adjust so that the retention time of montelukast is about 2 minutes.

System suitability—

System performance: When the procedure is run with 10 μL of the standard solution under the above operating conditions, the number of theoretical plates and the symmetry factor of the peak of montelukast are not less than 2000 and not more than 1.5, respectively.

System repeatability: When the test is repeated 5 times with 10 μL of the standard solution under the above operating conditions, the relative standard deviation of the peak area of montelukast is not more than 1.0%.

Dissolution <*6.10*> When the test is performed at 50 revolutions per minute according to the Paddle method, using 900 mL of a solution of sodium lauryl sulfate (1 in 200) as the dissolution medium, the dissolution rate in 20 minutes of Montelukast Sodium Tablets is not less than 85%.

Conduct this procedure using light-resistant vessels. Start the test with 1 tablet of Montelukast Sodium Tablets, withdraw not less than 15 mL of the medium at the specified minute after starting the test, and centrifuge. Pipet V mL of the supernatant liquid, add the dissolution medium to make exactly V' mL so that each mL contains about 5.6 μg of montelukast ($C_{35}H_{36}ClNO_3S$), and use this solution as the sample solution. Separately, weigh accurately about 35 mg of Montelukast Dicyclohexylamine RS, and dissolve in methanol to make exactly 100 mL. Pipet 2 mL of this solution, add the dissolution medium to make exactly 100 mL, and use this solution as the standard solution. Perform the test with exactly 50 μL each of the sample solution and standard solution as directed under Liquid Chromatography <*2.01*> according to the following conditions, and determine the peak areas, A_T and A_S, of montelukast in each solution.

Dissolution rate (%) with respect to the labeled amount of montelukast ($C_{35}H_{36}ClNO_3S$)
$= M_S \times A_T/A_S \times V'/V \times 1/C \times 18 \times 0.764$

M_S: Amount (mg) of Montelukast Dicyclohexylamine RS taken

C: Labeled amount (mg) of montelukast ($C_{35}H_{36}ClNO_3S$) in 1 tablet

Operating conditions—

Proceed as directed in the operating conditions in the Uniformity of dosage units.

System suitability—

System performance: When the procedure is run with 50 μL of the standard solution under the above operating conditions, the number of theoretical plates and the symmetry factor of the peak of montelukast are not less than 2000 and not more than 1.5, respectively.

System repeatability: When the test is repeated 5 times with 50 μL of the standard solution under the above operat-

ing conditions, the relative standard deviation of the peak area of montelukast is not more than 2.0%.

Assay Conduct this procedure using light-resistant vessels. Disintegrate 10 tablets of Montelukast Sodium Tablets in 150 mL of a mixture of methanol and water (3:1), disperse the fine particles by sonicating, and add a mixture of methanol and water (3:1) to make exactly 200 mL, filter through a membrane filter with a pore size not exceeding 0.45 μm. Discard the first 1 mL of the filtrate, pipet *V* mL of the subsequent filtrate, add a mixture of methanol and water (3:1) to make exactly *V′* mL so that each mL contains about 0.25 mg of montelukast ($C_{35}H_{36}ClNO_3S$), and use this solution as the sample solution. Separately, weigh accurately about 33 mg of Montelukast Dicyclohexylamine RS, and dissolve in a mixture of methanol and water (3:1) to make exactly 100 mL, and use this solution as the standard solution. Perform the test with exactly 20 μL each of the sample solution and standard solution as directed under Liquid Chromatography <*2.01*> according to the following conditions, and determine the peak areas, A_T and A_S, of montelukast in each solution.

Amount (mg) of montelukast ($C_{35}H_{36}ClNO_3S$) in 1 tablet
$= M_S \times A_T/A_S \times V/V' \times 1/5 \times 0.764$

M_S: Amount (mg) of Montelukast Dicyclohexylamine RS taken

Operating conditions—

Detector: An ultraviolet absorption photometer (wavelength: 255 nm).

Column: A stainless steel column 4.6 mm in inside diameter and 10 cm in length, packed with phenylhexylsilanized silica gel for liquid chromatography (3 μm in particle diameter).

Column temperature: A constant temperature of about 50°C.

Mobile phase A: A solution of trifluoroacetic acid (1 in 500).

Mobile phase B: A mixture of methanol and acetonitrile for liquid chromatography (3:2).

Flowing of mobile phase: Control the gradient by mixing the mobile phases A and B as directed in the following table.

Time after injection of sample (min)	Mobile phase A (vol%)	Mobile phase B (vol%)
0 - 5	48 → 45	52 → 55
5 - 12	45	55
12 - 22	45 → 25	55 → 75
22 - 23	25	75

Flow rate: 1.5 mL per minute (the retention time of montelukast is about 14 minutes).

System suitability—

System performance: Take 10 mL of the standard solution in a transparent vessel, add 4 μL of hydrogen peroxide (30), and allow to stand under 4000 lx white light for 10 minutes. When the procedure is run with 20 μL of this solution under the above operating conditions, the resolution between the peak of related substance B, having a relative retention time of about 0.92 to montelukast and the peak of montelukast is not less than 1.5. And proceed with 20 μL of the standard solution under the above conditions, the number of theoretical plates and the symmetry factor of the peak of montelukast are not less than 5000 and not more than 2.5, respectively.

System repeatability: When the test is repeated 5 times with 20 μL of the standard solution under the above operating conditions, the relative standard deviation of the peak area of montelukast is not more than 1.0%.

Containers and storage Containers—Tight containers. Storage—Light-resistant.

Others

Related substances A, B, C, D, E and F: Refer to them described in Montelukast Sodium.

Morphine Hydrochloride Hydrate

モルヒネ塩酸塩水和物

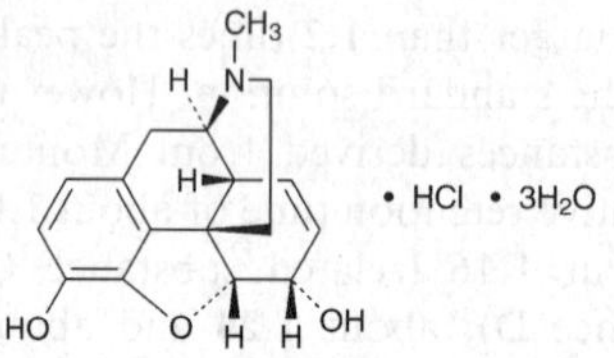

$C_{17}H_{19}NO_3.HCl.3H_2O$: 375.84
(5*R*,6*S*)-4,5-Epoxy-17-methyl-7,8-didehydromorphinan-3,6-diol monohydrochloride trihydrate
[*6055-06-7*]

Morphine Hydrochloride Hydrate contains not less than 98.0% and not more than 102.0% of morphine hydrochloride ($C_{17}H_{19}NO_3.HCl$: 321.80), calculated on the anhydrous basis.

Description Morphine Hydrochloride Hydrate occurs as white, crystals or crystalline powder.

It is freely soluble in formic acid, soluble in water, sparingly soluble in methanol, and slightly soluble in ethanol (95).

It gradually becomes yellow-brown by light.

Identification **(1)** Determine the absorption spectrum of a solution of Morphine Hydrochloride Hydrate (1 in 10,000) as directed under Ultraviolet-visible Spectrophotometry <*2.24*>, and compare the spectrum with the Reference Spectrum 1: both spectra exhibit similar intensities of absorption at the same wavelengths. Separately, determine the absorption spectrum of a solution of Morphine Hydrochloride Hydrate in dilute sodium hydroxide TS (1 in 10,000) as directed under Ultraviolet-visible Spectrophotometry <*2.24*>, and compare the spectrum with the Reference Spectrum 2: both spectra exhibit similar intensities of absorption at the same wavelengths.

(2) Determine the infrared absorption spectrum of Morphine Hydrochloride Hydrate as directed in the potassium bromide disk method under Infrared Spectrophotometry <*2.25*>, and compare the spectrum with the Reference Spectrum: both spectra exhibit similar intensities of absorption at the same wave numbers.

(3) A solution of Morphine Hydrochloride Hydrate (1 in 50) responds to Qualitative Tests <*1.09*> (2) for chloride.

Optical rotation <*2.49*> $[\alpha]_D^{20}$: −111 − −116° (0.5 g calculated on the anhydrous basis, water, 25 mL, 100 mm).

pH <*2.54*> The pH of a solution obtained by dissolving 0.10 g of Morphine Hydrochloride Hydrate in 10 mL of water is between 4.0 and 6.0.

Purity **(1)** Clarity and color of solution—Dissolve 0.40 g of Morphine Hydrochloride Hydrate in 10 mL of water: the solution is clear. When perform the test with this solution as directed under Ultraviolet-visible Spectrophotometry <*2.24*>, the absorbance at 420 nm is not more than 0.12.

(2) Sulfate <*1.14*>—Dissolve 0.20 g of Morphine Hydrochloride Hydrate in 5 mL of water, and add 2 to 3 drops of barium chloride TS: no turbidity is produced.

(3) Meconic acid—Dissolve 0.20 g of Morphine Hydrochloride Hydrate in 5 mL of water, and add 5 mL of dilute hydrochloric acid and 2 drops of iron (III) chloride TS: no red color develops.

(4) Related substances—Dissolve 0.20 g of Morphine Hydrochloride Hydrate in 10 mL of diluted methanol (4 in 5), and use this solution as the sample solution. Pipet 1 mL of the sample solution, add diluted methanol (4 in 5) to make exactly 100 mL, and use this solution as the standard solution (1). Pipet 5 mL of the standard solution (1), add diluted methanol (4 in 5) to make exactly 10 mL, and use this solution as the standard solution (2). Perform the test with these solutions as directed under Thin-layer Chromatography <*2.03*>. Spot 10 μL each of the sample solution and standard solutions (1) and (2) on a plate of silica gel with fluorescent indicator for thin-layer chromatography. Develop the plate with a mixture of acetone, ethanol (99.5) and ammonia solution (28) (21:14:3) to a distance of about 12 cm, and air-dry the plate. Examine under ultraviolet light (main wavelength: 254 nm): the spot having an *Rf* value of about 0.17 obtained from the sample solution is not more intense than the spot from the standard solution (1), and the spots other than the principal spot, the spot mentioned above and the spot of the starting point from the sample solution are not more intense than the spot from the standard solution (2).

Water <*2.48*> 13 – 15% (0.1 g, volumetric titration, direct titration).

Residue on ignition <*2.44*> Not more than 0.1% (0.5 g).

Assay Weigh accurately about 0.5 g of Morphine Hydrochloride Hydrate, dissolve in 3.0 mL of formic acid, add 100 mL of a mixture of acetic anhydride and acetic acid (100) (7:3), mix, and titrate <*2.50*> with 0.1 mol/L perchloric acid VS (potentiometric titration). Perform a blank determination in the same manner, and make any necessary correction.

Each mL of 0.1 mol/L perchloric acid VS
= 32.18 mg of $C_{17}H_{19}NO_3.HCl$

Containers and storage Containers—Tight containers.
Storage—Light-resistant.

Morphine Hydrochloride Injection

モルヒネ塩酸塩注射液

Morphine Hydrochloride Injection is an aqueous injection.

It contains not less than 93.0% and not more than 107.0% of the labeled amount of morphine hydrochloride hydrate ($C_{17}H_{19}NO_3.HCl.3H_2O$: 375.84).

Method of preparation Prepare as directed under Injections, with Morphine Hydrochloride Hydrate.

Description Morphine Hydrochloride Injection is a clear, colorless or pale yellow-brown liquid.

It gradually becomes yellow-brown by light.

pH: 2.5 – 5.0

Identification Take a volume of Morphine Hydrochloride Injection, equivalent to 0.04 g of Morphine Hydrochloride Hydrate, add water to make 20 mL, and use this solution as the sample solution. To 5 mL of the sample solution add water to make 100 mL, and determine the absorption spectrum as directed under Ultraviolet-visible Spectrophotometry <*2.24*>: it exhibits a maximum between 283 nm and 287 nm. And to 5 mL of the sample solution add dilute sodium hydroxide TS to make 100 mL, and determine the absorption spectrum as directed under Ultraviolet-visible Spectrophotometry <*2.24*>: it exhibits a maximum between 296 nm and 300 nm.

Bacterial endotoxins <*4.01*> Less than 1.5 EU/mg.

Extractable volume <*6.05*> It meets the requirement.

Foreign insoluble matter <*6.06*> Perform the test according to Method 1: it meets the requirement.

Insoluble particulate matter <*6.07*> It meets the requirement.

Sterility <*4.06*> Perform the test according to the Membrane filtration method: it meets the requirement.

Assay Take exactly a volume of Morphine Hydrochloride Injection, equivalent to about 80 mg of morphine hydrochloride hydrate ($C_{17}H_{19}NO_3.HCl.3H_2O$), and add water to make exactly 20 mL. Pipet 5 mL of this solution, add exactly 10 mL of the internal standard solution and water to make 50 mL, and use this solution as the sample solution. Separately, weigh accurately about 25 mg of morphine hydrochloride hydrate for assay, dissolve in exactly 10 mL of the internal standard solution, add water to make 50 mL, and use this solution as the standard solution. Perform the test with 20 μL each of the sample solution and standard solution as directed under Liquid Chromatography <*2.01*> according to the following conditions, and calculate the ratios, Q_T and Q_S, of the peak area of morphine to that of the internal standard.

Amount (mg) of morphine hydrochloride hydrate ($C_{17}H_{19}NO_3.HCl.3H_2O$)
$= M_S \times Q_T/Q_S \times 4 \times 1.168$

M_S: Amount (mg) of morphine hydrochloride hydrate for assay taken, calculated on the anhydrous basis

Internal standard solution—A solution of etilefrine hydrochloride (1 in 500).

Operating conditions—

Detector: An ultraviolet absorption photometer (wavelength: 285 nm).

Column: A stainless steel column 4.6 mm in inside diameter and 15 cm in length, packed with octadecylsilanized silica gel for liquid chromatography (5 μm in particle diameter).

Column temperature: A constant temperature of about 40°C.

Mobile phase: Dissolve 1.0 g of sodium lauryl sulfate in 500 mL of diluted phosphoric acid (1 in 1000), and adjust the pH to 3.0 with sodium hydroxide TS. To 240 mL of this solution add 70 mL of tetrahydrofuran, and mix.

Flow rate: Adjust so that retention time of morphine is about 10 minutes.

System suitability—

System performance: When the procedure is run with 20 μL of the standard solution under the above operating conditions, morphine and the internal standard are eluted in this order with the resolution between these peaks being not less than 3.

System repeatability: When the test is repeated 6 times with 20 μL of the standard solution under the above operating conditions, the relative standard deviation of the ratios of the peak area of morphine to that of the internal standard is not more than 1.0%.

Containers and storage Containers—Hermetic containers, and colored containers may be used.

Storage—Light-resistant.

Morphine Hydrochloride Tablets

モルヒネ塩酸塩錠

Morphine Hydrochloride Tablets contain not less than 93.0% and not more than 107.0% of the labeled amount of morphine hydrochloride hydrate ($C_{17}H_{19}NO_3.HCl.3H_2O$: 375.84).

Method of preparation Prepare as directed under Tablets, with Morphine Hydrochloride Hydrate.

Identification Weigh a quantity of powdered Morphine Hydrochloride Tablets equivalent to 0.01 g of Morphine Hydrochloride Hydrate, add 100 mL of water, shake for 10 minutes, and filter. Determine the absorption spectrum of the filtrate as directed under Ultraviolet-visible Spectrophotometry <2.24>: it exhibits a maximum between 283 nm and 287 nm. And weigh a quantity of powdered Morphine Hydrochloride Tablets equivalent to 0.01 g of Morphine Hydrochloride Hydrate, add 100 mL of dilute sodium hydroxide TS, shake for 10 minutes, and filter. Determine the absorption spectrum of the filtrate as directed under Ultraviolet-visible Spectrophotometry <2.24>: it exhibits a maximum between 296 nm and 300 nm.

Uniformity of dosage units <6.02> Perform the test according to the following method: it meets the requirement of the Content uniformity test.

To 1 tablet of Morphine Hydrochloride Tablets add exactly 1 mL of the internal standard solution per 2 mg of morphine hydrochloride hydrate ($C_{17}H_{19}NO_3.HCl.3H_2O$), disperse the tablet into a small particles by sonicating, then sonicate for 15 minutes with occasional stirring, and add water to make V mL so that each mL contains about 0.4 mg of morphine hydrochloride hydrate ($C_{17}H_{19}NO_3.HCl.3H_2O$). Filter the solution, and use the filtrate as the sample solution. Then, proceed as directed in the Assay.

Amount (mg) of morphine hydrochloride hydrate ($C_{17}H_{19}NO_3.HCl.3H_2O$)
$= M_S \times Q_T/Q_S \times V/50 \times 1.168$

M_S: Amount (mg) of morphine hydrochloride hydrate for assay taken, calculated on the anhydrous basis

Internal standard solution—A solution of etilefrine hydrochloride (1 in 500).

Dissolution <6.10> When the test is performed at 50 revolutions per minute according to the Paddle method, using 900 mL of water as the dissolution medium, the dissolution rate in 15 minutes of Morphine Hydrochloride Tablets is not less than 85%.

Start the test with 1 tablet of Morphine Hydrochloride Tablets, withdraw not less than 20 mL of the medium at the specified minute after starting the test, and filter through a membrane filter with a pore size not exceeding 0.45 μm. Discard not less than 10 mL of the first filtrate, and use the subsequent filtrate as the sample solution. Separately, weigh accurately about 28 mg of morphine hydrochloride hydrate for assay (separately, determine the water <2.48> in the same manner as Morphine Hydrochloride Hydrate), and dissolve in water to make exactly 100 mL. Pipet 2 mL of this solution, add water to make exactly 50 mL, and use this solution as the standard solution. Perform the test with exactly 25 μL each of the sample solution and standard solution as directed under Liquid Chromatography <2.01> according to the following conditions, and determine the peak areas, A_T and A_S, of morphine in each solution.

Dissolution rate (%) with respect to the labeled amount of morphine hydrochloride hydrate ($C_{17}H_{19}NO_3.HCl.3H_2O$)
$= M_S \times A_T/A_S \times 1/C \times 36 \times 1.168$

M_S: Amount (mg) of morphine hydrochloride hydrate for assay taken, calculated on the anhydrous basis
C: Labeled amount (mg) of morphine hydrochloride hydrate ($C_{17}H_{19}NO_3.HCl.3H_2O$) in 1 tablet

Operating conditions—

Proceed as directed in the operating conditions in the Assay.

System suitability—

System performance: When the procedure is run with 25 μL of the standard solution under the above operating conditions, the number of theoretical plates and the symmetry factor of the peak of morphine are not less than 5000 and not more than 2.0, respectively.

System repeatability: When the test is repeated 6 times with 25 μL of the standard solution under the above operating conditions, the relative standard deviation of the peak area of morphine is not more than 2.0%.

Assay Take not less than 20 Morphine Hydrochloride Tablets, weigh accurately, and powder. Weigh accurately a quantity of the powder, equivalent to about 20 mg of morphine hydrochloride hydrate ($C_{17}H_{19}NO_3.HCl.3H_2O$), add exactly 10 mL of the internal standard solution, extract the mixture by sonicating for 10 minutes, and add water to make 50 mL. Filter this solution, and use the filtrate as the sample solution. Separately, weigh accurately about 25 mg of morphine hydrochloride hydrate for assay, dissolve in exactly 10 mL of the internal standard solution, add water to make 50 mL, and use this solution as the standard solution. Perform the test with 20 μL each of the sample solution and standard solution as directed under Liquid Chromatography <2.01> according to the following conditions, and calculate the ratios, Q_T and Q_S, of the peak area of morphine to that of the internal standard.

Amount (mg) of morphine hydrochloride hydrate ($C_{17}H_{19}NO_3.HCl.3H_2O$)
$= M_S \times Q_T/Q_S \times 1.168$

M_S: Amount (mg) of morphine hydrochloride hydrate for assay taken, calculated on the anhydrous basis

Internal standard solution—A solution of etilefrine hydrochloride (1 in 500).

Operating conditions—

Detector: An ultraviolet absorption photometer (wavelength: 285 nm).

Column: A stainless steel column 4.6 mm in inside diameter and 15 cm in length, packed with octadecylsilanized silica gel for liquid chromatography (5 μm in particle diameter).

Column temperature: A constant temperature of about 40°C.

Mobile phase: Dissolve 1.0 g of sodium lauryl sulfate in

500 mL of diluted phosphoric acid (1 in 1000), and adjust the pH to 3.0 with sodium hydroxide TS. To 240 mL of this solution add 70 mL of tetrahydrofuran, and mix.

Flow rate: Adjust so that the retention time of morphine is about 10 minutes.

System suitability—

System performance: When the procedure is run with 20 μL of the standard solution under the above operating conditions, morphine and the internal standard are eluted in this order with the resolution between these peaks being not less than 3.

System repeatability: When the test is repeated 6 times with 20 μL of the standard solution under the above operating conditions, the relative standard deviation of the ratios of the peak area of morphine to that of the internal standard is not more than 1.0%.

Containers and storage Containers—Tight containers.

Storage—Light-resistant.

Morphine and Atropine Injection

モルヒネ·アトロピン注射液

Morphine and Atropine Injection is an aqueous injection.

It contains not less than 0.91 w/v% and not more than 1.09 w/v% of morphine hydrochloride hydrate ($C_{17}H_{19}NO_3.HCl.3H_2O$: 375.84), and not less than 0.027 w/v% and not more than 0.033 w/v% of atropine sulfate hydrate [$(C_{17}H_{23}NO_3)_2.H_2SO_4.H_2O$: 694.83].

Method of preparation

Morphine Hydrochloride Hydrate	10 g
Atropine Sulfate Hydrate	0.3 g
Water for Injection or Sterile Water for Injection in Containers	a significant quantity
	To make 1000 mL

Prepare as directed under Injections, with the above ingredients.

Description Morphine and Atropine Injection is a clear, colorless liquid.

It is gradually colored by light.

pH: 2.5 – 5.0

Identification To 2 mL of Morphine and Atropine Injection add 2 mL of ammonia TS, and extract with 10 mL of diethyl ether. Filter the extract with a filter paper, evaporate the filtrate on a water bath to dryness, dissolve the residue in 1 mL of ethanol (99.5), and use this solution as the sample solution. Separately, dissolve 0.1 g of morphine hydrochloride hydrate in 10 mL of water, perform with 2 mL of this solution the same procedure as used for preparation of the sample solution, and use the solution so obtained as the standard solution (1). Separately, dissolve 3 mg of atropine sulfate hydrate in 10 mL of water, perform with 2 mL of this solution the same procedure as used for preparation of the sample solution, and use the solution so obtained as the standard solution (2). Perform the test with these solutions as directed under Thin-layer Chromatography <*2.03*>. Spot 10 μL each of the sample solution and standard solutions (1) and (2) on a plate of silica gel for thin-layer chromatography. Develop the plate with a mixture of methanol and ammonia solution (28) (200:3) to a distance of about 10 cm, and air-dry the plate. Spray evenly Dragendorff's TS on the plate: the two spots obtained from the sample solution show the same color tone and the same *Rf* value with either spot of orange color from the standard solution (1) or the standard solution (2) (morphine and atropine).

Extractable volume <*6.05*> It meets the requirement.

Assay **(1)** Morphine hydrochloride hydrate—Pipet 2 mL of Morphine and Atropine Injection, add exactly 10 mL of the internal standard solution, then add water to make 50 mL, and use this solution as the sample solution. Separately, weigh accurately about 25 mg of morphine hydrochloride hydrate for assay, add exactly 10 mL of the internal standard solution to dissolve, then add water to make 50 mL, and use this solution as the standard solution. Perform the test with 20 μL of the sample solution and standard solution as directed under Liquid Chromatography <*2.01*> according to the following conditions, and calculate the ratios, Q_T and Q_S, of the peak area of morphine to that of the internal standard.

Amount (mg) of morphine hydrochloride hydrate ($C_{17}H_{19}NO_3.HCl.3H_2O$)
$$= M_S \times Q_T/Q_S \times 1.168$$

M_S: Amount (mg) of morphine hydrochloride hydrate for assay taken, calculated on the anhydrous basis

Internal standard solution—A solution of etilefrine hydrochloride (1 in 500).

Operating conditions—

Detector: An ultraviolet absorption photometer (wavelength: 285 nm).

Column: A stainless steel column 4.6 mm in inside diameter and 15 cm in length, packed with octadecylsilanized silica gel for liquid chromatography (5 μm in particle diameter).

Column temperature: A constant temperature of about 40°C.

Mobile phase: Dissolve 1.0 g of sodium lauryl sulfate in 500 mL of diluted phosphoric acid (1 in 1000), and adjust the pH with sodium hydroxide TS to 3.0. To 240 mL of this solution add 70 mL of tetrahydrofuran, and mix.

Flow rate: Adjust so that the retention time of morphine is about 10 minutes.

System suitability—

System performance: When the procedure is run with 20 μL of the standard solution under the above operating conditions, morphine and the internal standard are eluted in this order with the resolution between these peaks being not less than 3.

System repeatability: When the test is repeated 6 times with 20 μL of the standard solution under the above operating conditions, the relative standard deviation of the ratios of the peak area of morphine to that of the internal standard is not more than 1.0%.

(2) Atropine sulfate hydrate—Pipet 2 mL of Morphine and Atropine Injection, add exactly 2 mL of the internal standard solution, and use this solution as the sample solution. Separately, weigh accurately about 15 mg of Atropine Sulfate RS (separately determine the loss on drying <*2.41*> under the same conditions as Atropine Sulfate Hydrate), and dissolve in water to make exactly 50 mL. Pipet 2 mL of this solution, add exactly 2 mL of the internal standard solution, and use this solution as the standard solution. Perform the test with 20 μL each of the sample solution and standard solution as directed under Liquid Chromatography <*2.01*> according to the following conditions, and calculate the ratios, Q_T and Q_S, of the peak areas of atropine to that of the internal standard.

Amount (mg) of atropine sulfate hydrate
$[(C_{17}H_{23}NO_3)_2.H_2SO_4.H_2O]$
$= M_S \times Q_T/Q_S \times 1/25 \times 1.027$

M_S: Amount (mg) of Atropine Sulfate RS taken, calculated on the dried basis

Internal standard solution—A solution of etilefrine hydrochloride (1 in 12,500).

Operating conditions—

Column, column temperature, and mobile phase: Proceed as directed in the operating conditions in the Assay (1).

Detector: An ultraviolet absorption photometer (wavelength: 225 nm).

Flow rate: Adjust so that the retention time of morphine is about 7 minutes.

System suitability—

System performance: When the procedure is run with 20 μL of the sample solution under the above operating conditions, morphine, the internal standard and atropine are eluted in this order, and the resolution between morphine and the internal standard is not less than 3.

System repeatability: When the test is repeated 6 times with 20 μL of the standard solution under the above operating conditions, the relative standard deviation of the ratios of the peak area of atropine to that of the internal standard is not more than 1.0%.

Containers and storage Containers—Hermetic containers, and colored containers may be used.

Storage—Light-resistant.

Morphine Sulfate Hydrate

モルヒネ硫酸塩水和物

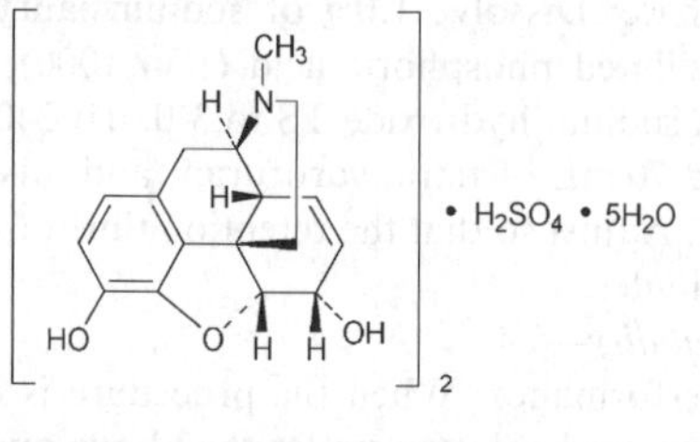

$(C_{17}H_{19}NO_3)_2.H_2SO_4.5H_2O$: 758.83
(5*R*,6*S*)-4,5-Epoxy-17-methyl-7,8-didehydromorphinan-3,6-diol hemisulfate hemipentahydrate
[*6211-15-0*]

Morphine Sulfate Hydrate contains not less than 98.0% and not more than 102.0% of morphine sulfate $[(C_{17}H_{19}NO_3)_2.H_2SO_4$: 668.75], calculated on the anhydrous basis.

Description Morphine Sulfate Hydrate occurs as a white, crystals or crystalline powder.

It is very soluble in formic acid, soluble in water, slightly soluble in methanol, and very slightly soluble in ethanol (99.5).

It dissolves in dilute sodium hydroxide TS.

Identification **(1)** Determine the absorption spectrum of a solution of Morphine Sulfate Hydrate (1 in 10,000) as directed under Ultraviolet-visible Spectrophotometry *<2.24>*, and compare the spectrum with the Reference Spectrum 1: both spectra exhibit similar intensities of absorption at the same wavelengths. Determine the absorption spectrum of a solution of Morphine Sulfate Hydrate in dilute sodium hydroxide TS (1 in 10,000) as directed under Ultraviolet-visible Spectrophotometry *<2.24>*, and compare the spectrum with the Reference Spectrum 2: both spectra exhibit similar intensities of absorption at the same wavelengths.

(2) Determine the infrared absorption spectrum of Morphine Sulfate Hydrate as directed in the paste method under Infrared Spectrophotometry *<2.25>*, and compare the spectrum with the Reference Spectrum: both spectra exhibit similar intensities of absorption at the same wave numbers.

(3) A solution of Morphine Sulfate Hydrate (1 in 25) responds to Qualitative Tests *<1.09>* (1) and (3) for sulfate.

Optical rotation *<2.49>* $[\alpha]_D^{20}$: −107 – −112° (0.2 g calculated on the anhydrous basis, water, 20 mL, 100 mm).

Purity **(1)** Acidity—Dissolve 0.5 g of Morphine Sulfate Hydrate in 15 mL of water, add 2 drops of methyl red TS, and neutralize with 0.02 mol/L sodium hydroxide VS: the necessary volume of 0.02 mol/L sodium hydroxide VS is not more than 0.50 mL.

(2) Ammonium—Being specified separately when the drug is granted approval based on the Law.

(3) Chloride—Dissolve 0.10 g of Morphine Sulfate Hydrate in 10 mL of water, add 1 mL of dilute nitric acid, then add 1 mL of silver nitrate TS: no turbidity is produced.

(4) Meconic acid—Dissolve 0.20 g of Morphine Sulfate Hydrate in 5 mL of water, add 5 mL of dilute hydrochloric acid and 2 drops of iron (III) chloride TS: no red color develops.

(5) Related substances—Dissolve 0.20 g of Morphine Sulfate Hydrate in 10 mL of diluted methanol (4 in 5), and use this solution as the sample solution. Pipet 1 mL of the sample solution, add diluted methanol (4 in 5) to make exactly 100 mL, and use this solution as the standard solution (1). Pipet 5 mL of the standard solution (1), add diluted methanol (4 in 5) to make exactly 10 mL, and use this solution as the standard solution (2). Perform the test with these solutions as directed under Thin-layer Chromatography *<2.03>*. Spot 10 μL each of the sample solution and the standard solutions (1) and (2) on a plate of silica gel with fluorescent indicator for thin-layer chromatography. Develop the plate with a mixture of acetone, ethanol (99.5) and ammonia solution (28) (21:14:3) to a distance of about 12 cm, and air-dry the plate. Examine under ultraviolet light (main wavelength: 254 nm): the spot at an *Rf* value of about 0.17 obtained from the sample solution is not more intense than the spot from the standard solution (1), and the spot other than the principle spot, the spot at an *Rf* value of about 0.17 and the spot at original point from the sample solution is not more intense than the spot from the standard solution (2).

Water *<2.48>* 11.0 – 13.0% (0.1 g, volumetric titration, direct titration).

Residue on ignition *<2.44>* Not more than 0.1% (0.5 g).

Assay Weigh accurately about 0.5 g of Morphine Sulfate Hydrate, dissolve in 3 mL of formic acid, add 100 mL of a mixture of acetic anhydride and acetic acid (100) (7:3), and titrate *<2.50>* with 0.05 mol/L perchloric acid VS (potentiometric titration). Perform a blank determination in the same manner, and make any necessary correction.

Each mL of 0.05 mol/L perchloric acid VS
$= 33.44$ mg of $(C_{17}H_{19}NO_3)_2.H_2SO_4$

Containers and storage Containers—Tight containers.

Storage—Light-resistant.

Mosapride Citrate Hydrate

モサプリドクエン酸塩水和物

and enantiomer

$C_{21}H_{25}ClFN_3O_3.C_6H_8O_7.2H_2O$: 650.05
4-Amino-5-chloro-2-ethoxy-*N*-{[(2*RS*)-4-(4-fluorobenzyl)morpholin-2-yl]methyl}benzamide monocitrate dihydrate
[*636582-62-2*]

Mosapride Citrate Hydrate contains not less than 98.5% and not more than 101.0% of mosapride citrate ($C_{21}H_{25}ClFN_3O_3.C_6H_8O_7$: 614.02), calculated on the anhydrous basis.

Description Mosapride Citrate Hydrate occurs as a white to yellowish white crystalline powder.

It is freely soluble in *N,N*-dimethylformamide and in acetic acid (100), sparingly soluble in methanol, slightly soluble in ethanol (99.5), and practically insoluble in water.

A solution of Mosapride Citrate Hydrate in *N,N*-dimethylformamide (1 in 20) shows no optical rotation.

Identification **(1)** Determine the absorption spectrum of a solution of Mosapride Citrate Hydrate in methanol (1 in 50,000) as directed under Ultraviolet-visible Spectrophotometry <*2.24*>, and compare the spectrum with the Reference Spectrum: both spectra exhibit similar intensities of absorption at the same wavelengths.

(2) Determine the infrared absorption spectrum of Mosapride Citrate Hydrate as directed in the potassium bromide disk method under Infrared Spectrophotometry <*2.25*>, and compare the spectrum with the Reference Spectrum: both spectra exhibit similar intensities of absorption at the same wave numbers.

(3) A solution of Mosapride Citrate Hydrate in *N,N*-dimethylformamide (1 in 10) responds to the Qualitative Tests <*1.09*> (1) for citrate.

Purity **(1)** Heavy metals <*1.07*>—Proceed with 1.0 g of Mosapride Citrate Hydrate in a platinum crucible according to Method 4, and perform the test. Prepare the control solution with 2.0 mL of Standard Lead Solution (not more than 20 ppm).

(2) Related substances—Dissolve 0.10 g of Mosapride Citrate Hydrate in 50 mL of methanol, and use this solution as the sample solution. Pipet 1 mL of the sample solution, and add methanol to make exactly 50 mL. Pipet 1 mL of this solution, add methanol to make exactly 20 mL, and use this solution as the standard solution. Perform the test with exactly 5 μL each of the sample solution and standard solution as directed under Liquid Chromatography <*2.01*> according to the following conditions. Determine each peak area by the automatic integration method: the area of the peak having the relative retention time of about 0.47 to mosapride obtained from the sample solution is not larger than 3 times the peak area of mosapride from the standard solution, and the area of each peak other than mosapride and the peak mentioned above from the sample solution is not larger than the peak area of mosapride from the standard solution. Furthermore, the total area of the peaks other than mosapride from the sample solution is not larger than 5 times the peak area of mosapride from the standard solution.

Operating conditions—

Detector: An ultraviolet absorption photometer (wavelength: 274 nm).

Column: A stainless steel column 4.6 mm in inside diameter and 15 cm in length, packed with octadecylsilanized silica gel for liquid chromatography (5 μm in particle diameter).

Column temperature: A constant temperature of about 40°C.

Mobile phase A: Dissolve 8.82 g of trisodium citrate dihydrate in 800 mL of water, adjust the pH to 4.0 with dilute hydrochloric acid, and add water to make 1000 mL.

Mobile phase B: Acetonitrile.

Flowing of mobile phase: Control the gradient by mixing the mobile phases A and B as directed in the following table.

Time after injection of sample (min)	Mobile phase A (vol%)	Mobile phase B (vol%)
0 – 35	80 → 45	20 → 55

Flow rate: 1.0 mL per minute.

Time span of measurement: For 35 minutes after injection, beginning after the solvent peak.

System suitability—

Test for required detectability: Pipet 4 mL of the standard solution, and add methanol to make exactly 20 mL. Confirm that the peak area of mosapride obtained with 5 μL of this solution is equivalent to 15 to 25% of that with 5 μL of the standard solution.

System performance: When the procedure is run with 5 μL of the standard solution under the above operating conditions, the number of theoretical plates and the symmetry factor of the peak of mosapride are not less than 40,000 and not more than 1.5, respectively.

System repeatability: When the test is repeated 6 times with 5 μL of the standard solution under the above operating conditions, the relative standard deviation of the peak area of mosapride is not more than 5.0%.

Water <*2.48*> 5.0 – 6.5% (0.5 g, volumetric titration, back titration).

Residue on ignition <*2.44*> Not more than 0.1% (1 g, platinum crucible).

Assay Weigh accurately 0.5 g of Mosapride Citrate Hydrate, dissolve in 70 mL of acetic acid (100), and titrate <*2.50*> with 0.1 mol/L perchloric acid VS (potentiometric titration). Perform a blank determination in the same manner, and make any necessary correction.

Each mL of 0.1 mol/L perchloric acid VS
= 61.40 mg of $C_{21}H_{25}ClFN_3O_3.C_6H_8O_7$

Containers and storage Containers—Well-closed containers.

Mosapride Citrate Powder

モサプリドクエン酸塩散

Mosapride Citrate Powder contains not less than 93.0% and not more than 107.0% of the labeled amount of mosapride citrate ($C_{21}H_{25}ClFN_3O_3.C_6H_8O_7$: 614.02).

Method of preparation Prepare as directed under Granules or Powders, with Mosapride Citrate Hydrate.

Identification **(1)** Powder Mosapride Citrate Powder. To a portion of the powder, equivalent to 10 mg of mosapride citrate ($C_{21}H_{25}ClFN_3O_3.C_6H_8O_7$), add 10 mL of dilute acetic acid, shake for 10 minutes, and filter. To 5 mL of the filtrate add 0.3 mL of Dragendorff's TS: an orange precipitate is formed.

(2) Determine the absorption spectrum of the sample solution obtained in the Assay as directed under Ultraviolet-visible Spectrophotometry <*2.24*>: it exhibits maxima between 271 nm and 275 nm and between 306 nm and 310 nm.

Purity Related substances—Powder Mosapride Citrate Powder. To a portion of the powder, equivalent to 10 mg of mosapride citrate ($C_{21}H_{25}ClFN_3O_3.C_6H_8O_7$), moisten with 1 mL of water, then add 9 mL of methanol, shake for 20 minutes, centrifuge, and use the supernatant liquid as the sample solution. Pipet 1 mL of the sample solution, and add methanol to make exactly 20 mL. Pipet 2 mL of this solution, add methanol to make exactly 20 mL, and use this solution as the standard solution. Perform the test with exactly 10 μL each of the sample solution and standard solution as directed under Liquid Chromatography <*2.01*> according to the following conditions, and determine each peak area by the automatic integration method: the area of the two peaks, having the relative retention time of about 0.60 and about 0.85 to mosapride obtained from the sample solution, is not larger than the peak area of mosapride from the standard solution, the area of other than mosapride and the peaks mentioned above from the sample solution is not larger than 2/5 times the peak area of mosapride from the standard solution, and the total area of the peak other than mosapride from the sample solution is not larger than 2 times the peak area of mosapride from the standard solution.

Operating conditions—

Detector, column, column temperature, mobile phases A and B, and flow rate: Proceed as directed in the operating conditions in the Purity (2) under Mosapride Citrate Hydrate.

Flowing of mobile phase: Control the gradient by mixing the mobile phases A and B as directed in the following table.

Time after injection of sample (min)	Mobile phase A (vol%)	Mobile phase B (vol%)
0 – 40	85 – 45	15 – 55

Time span of measurement: For 40 minutes after injection, beginning after the solvent peak.

System suitability—

Test for required detectability: To exactly 1 mL of the standard solution add methanol to make exactly 25 mL. Confirm that the peak area of mosapride obtained with 10 μL of this solution is equivalent to 3.0 to 5.0% of that with 10 μL of the standard solution.

System performance: When the procedure is run with 10 μL of the standard solution under the above operating conditions, the number of theoretical plates and the symmetry factor of the peak of mosapride are not less than 40,000 and not more than 1.5, respectively.

System repeatability: When the test is repeated 6 times with 10 μL of the standard solution under the above operating conditions, the relative standard deviation of the peak area of mosapride is not more than 3.0%.

Uniformity of dosage units <*6.02*> Perform the test according to the following method: the powder in single-dose packages meets the requirement of the Content uniformity test.

To the total amount of the content of 1 package of Mosapride Citrate Powder add 5 mL of water, and shake. Then, add 20 mL of methanol, shake for 20 minutes, and add methanol to make exactly 50 mL. Centrifuge this solution, pipet V mL of the supernatant liquid, add methanol to make exactly V' mL so that each mL contains about 20 μg of mosapride citrate ($C_{21}H_{25}ClFN_3O_3.C_6H_8O_7$), and use this solution as the sample solution. Then, proceed as directed in the Assay.

Amount (mg) of mosapride citrate ($C_{21}H_{25}ClFN_3O_3.C_6H_8O_7$)
$= M_S \times A_T/A_S \times V'/V \times 1/50$

M_S: Amount (mg) of mosapride citrate hydrate for assay taken, calculated on the anhydrous basis

Dissolution <*6.10*> When the test is performed at 50 revolutions per minute according to the Paddle method, using 900 mL of 2nd fluid for dissolution test as the dissolution medium, the dissolution rate in 45 minutes of Mosapride Citrate Powder is not less than 70%.

Start the test with an amount of Mosapride Citrate Powder, equivalent to about 2.5 mg of mosapride citrate ($C_{21}H_{25}ClFN_3O_3.C_6H_8O_7$), withdraw not less than 20 mL of the medium at the specified minute after starting the test, and filter through a membrane filter with a pore size not exceeding 0.45 μm. Discard not less than 10 mL of the first filtrate, and use the subsequent filtrate as the sample solution. Separately, weigh accurately about 30 mg of mosapride citrate hydrate for assay (separately determine the water <*2.48*> in the same manner as Mosapride Citrate Hydrate), and dissolve in the mobile phase to make exactly 100 mL. Pipet 2 mL of this solution, add the mobile phase to make exactly 200 mL, and use this solution as the standard solution. Perform the test with exactly 50 μL each of the sample solution and standard solution as directed under Liquid Chromatography <*2.01*>, and determine the peak areas, A_T and A_S, of mosapride in each solution.

Dissolution rate (%) with respect to the labeled amount of mosapride citrate ($C_{21}H_{25}ClFN_3O_3.C_6H_8O_7$)
$= M_S/M_T \times A_T/A_S \times 1/C \times 9$

M_S: Amount (mg) of mosapride citrate hydrate for assay taken, calculated on the anhydrous basis

M_T: Amount (g) of Mosapride Citrate Powder taken

C: Labeled amount (mg) of mosapride citrate ($C_{21}H_{25}ClFN_3O_3.C_6H_8O_7$) in 1 g

Operating conditions—

Detector: An ultraviolet absorption photometer (wavelength: 274 nm).

Column: A stainless steel column 4.6 mm in inside diameter and 15 cm in length, packed with octadecylsilanized silica gel for liquid chromatography (5 μm in particle diameter).

Column temperature: A constant temperature of about 40°C.

Mobile phase: Dissolve 8.82 g of trisodium citrate dihydrate in 800 mL of water, adjust to pH 3.3 with dilute hydrochloric acid, and add water to make 1000 mL. To 240 mL of this solution add 90 mL of methanol and 70 mL of acetonitrile.

Flow rate: Adjust so that the retention time of mosapride is about 9 minutes.

System suitability—

System performance: When the procedure is run with 50 μL of the standard solution under the above operating conditions, the number of theoretical plates and the symmetry factor of the peak of mosapride are not less than 4000 and not more than 2.0, respectively.

System repeatability: When the test is repeated 6 times with 50 μL of the standard solution under the above operating conditions, the relative standard deviation of the peak area of mosapride is not more than 2.0%.

Assay Powder Mosapride Citrate Powder. Weigh accurately a portion of the powder, equivalent to about 10 mg of mosapride citrate ($C_{21}H_{25}ClFN_3O_3.C_6H_8O_7$), moisten with 2 mL of water, add 70 mL of methanol, shake for 20 minutes, then add methanol to make exactly 100 mL, and centrifuge. Pipet 10 mL of the supernatant liquid, add methanol to make exactly 50 mL, and use this solution as the sample solution. Separately, weigh accurately about 53 mg of mosapride citrate hydrate for assay (separately determine the water <*2.48*> in the same manner as Mosapride Citrate Hydrate), and dissolve in methanol to make exactly 100 mL. To 2 mL of this solution add methanol to make exactly 50 mL, and use this solution as the standard solution. Determine the absorbances, A_T and A_S, of the sample solution and the standard solution at 273 nm as directed under Ultraviolet-visible Spectrophotometry <*2.24*>.

Amount (mg) of mosapride citrate ($C_{21}H_{25}ClFN_3O_3.C_6H_8O_7$)
$= M_S \times A_T/A_S \times 1/5$

M_S: Amount (mg) of mosapride citrate hydrate for assay taken, calculated on the anhydrous basis

Containers and storage Containers—Tight containers.

Mosapride Citrate Tablets

モサプリドクエン酸塩錠

Mosapride Citrate Tablets contain not less than 95.0% and not more than 105.0% of the labeled amount of mosapride citrate ($C_{21}H_{25}ClFN_3O_3.C_6H_8O_7$: 614.02).

Method of preparation Prepare as directed under Tablets, with Mosapride Citrate Hydrate.

Identification **(1)** To an amount of powdered Mosapride Citrate Tablets, equivalent to 10 mg of mosapride citrate ($C_{21}H_{25}ClFN_3O_3.C_6H_8O_7$), add 10 mL of dilute acetic acid, shake for 10 minutes, and filter. To 5 mL of the filtrate add 0.3 mL of Dragendorff's TS: an orange precipitate is formed.

(2) Determine the absorption spectrum of the sample solution obtained in the Assay as directed under Ultraviolet-visible Spectrophotometry <*2.24*>: it exhibits maxima between 271 nm and 275 nm, and between 306 nm and 310 nm.

Purity Related substances—Powder not less than 20 tablets of Mosapride Citrate Tablets. Moisten a portion of the powder, equivalent to 10 mg of mosapride citrate ($C_{21}H_{25}ClFN_3O_3.C_6H_8O_7$), with 1 mL of water. Add 9 mL of methanol, shake for 20 minutes, centrifuge, and use the supernatant liquid as the sample solution. Pipet 1 mL of this solution, add methanol to make exactly 20 mL. Pipet 2 mL of the sample solution, add methanol to make exactly 20 mL, and use this solution as the standard solution. Perform the test with exactly 10 μL each of the sample solution and standard solution as directed under Liquid Chromatography <*2.01*> according to the following conditions. Determine each peak area by the automatic integration method: the area of the peaks having the relative retention times of about 0.60 and about 0.85 to mosapride obtained from the sample solution is not larger than the peak area of mosapride from the standard solution, and the area of each peak other than mosapride and these peaks mentioned above from the sample solution is not larger than 2/5 times the peak area of mosapride from the standard solution. Furthermore, the total area of the peaks other than mosapride from the sample solution is not larger than 2 times the peak area of mosapride from the standard solution.

Operating conditions—

Detector, column, column temperature, mobile phases A and B, and flow rate: Proceed as directed in the operating conditions in the Purity (2) under Mosapride Citrate Hydrate.

Flowing of mobile phase: Control the gradient by mixing the mobile phases A and B as directed in the following table.

Time after injection of sample (min)	Mobile phase A (vol%)	Mobile phase B (vol%)
0 – 40	85 → 45	15 → 55

Time span of measurement: For 40 minutes after injection, beginning after the solvent peak.

System suitability—

Test for required detectability: Pipet 1 mL of the standard solution, and add methanol to make exactly 25 mL. Confirm that the peak area of mosapride obtained with 10 μL of this solution is equivalent to 3.0 to 5.0% of that with 10 μL of the standard solution.

System performance: When the procedure is run with 10 μL of the standard solution under the above operating conditions, the number of theoretical plates and the symmetry factor of the peak of mosapride are not less than 40,000 and not more than 1.5, respectively.

System repeatability: When the test is repeated 6 times with 10 μL of the standard solution under the above operating conditions, the relative standard deviation of the peak area of mosapride is not more than 3.0%.

Uniformity of dosage units <*6.02*> Perform the test according to the following method: it meets the requirement of the Content uniformity test.

To 1 tablet of Mosapride Citrate Tablets add 5 mL of water, and shake well to disintegrate. Add 20 mL of methanol, shake for 20 minutes, and add methanol to make exactly 50 mL. Centrifuge this solution, pipet V mL of the supernatant liquid, add methanol to make exactly V' mL so that each mL contains about 20 μg of mosapride citrate ($C_{21}H_{25}ClFN_3O_3.C_6H_8O_7$), and use this solution as the sample solution. Proceed as directed in the Assay.

Amount (mg) of mosapride citrate ($C_{21}H_{25}ClFN_3O_3.C_6H_8O_7$)
$= M_S \times A_T/A_S \times V'/V \times 1/50$

M_S: Amount (mg) of mosapride citrate hydrate for assay taken, calculated on the anhydrous basis

Dissolution *<6.10>* When the test is performed at 50 revolutions per minute according to the Paddle method, using 900 mL of 2nd fluid for dissolution test as the dissolution medium, the dissolution rate in 45 minutes of Mosapride Citrate Tablets is not less than 80%.

Start the test with 1 tablet of Mosapride Citrate Tablets, withdraw not less than 20 mL of the medium at the specified minute after starting the test, and filter through a membrane filter with a pore size not exceeding 0.45 μm. Discard not less than 10 mL of the first filtrate, pipet V mL of the subsequent filtrate, add the dissolution medium to make exactly V' mL so that each mL contains about 2.8 μg of mosapride citrate ($C_{21}H_{25}ClFN_3O_3.C_6H_8O_7$), and use this solution as the sample solution. Separately, weigh accurately about 30 mg of mosapride citrate hydrate for assay (separately, determine the water *<2.48>* in the same manner as Mosapride Citrate Hydrate), and dissolve in the mobile phase to make exactly 100 mL. Pipet 2 mL of this solution, add the mobile phase to make exactly 200 mL, and use this solution as the standard solution. Perform the test with exactly 50 μL each of the sample solution and standard solution as directed under Liquid Chromatography *<2.01>* according to the following conditions, and determine the peak areas, A_T and A_S, of mosapride in each solution.

Dissolution rate (%) with respect to the labeled amount of mosapride citrate ($C_{21}H_{25}ClFN_3O_3.C_6H_8O_7$)
$= M_S \times A_T/A_S \times V'/V \times 1/C \times 9$

M_S: Amount (mg) of mosapride citrate hydrate for assay taken, calculated on the anhydrous basis
C: Labeled amount (mg) of mosapride citrate ($C_{21}H_{25}ClFN_3O_3.C_6H_8O_7$) in 1 tablet

Operating conditions—

Detector: An ultraviolet absorption photometer (wavelength: 274 nm).

Column: A stainless steel column 4.6 mm in inside diameter and 15 cm in length, packed with octadecylsilanized silica gel for liquid chromatography (5 μm in particle diameter).

Column temperature: A constant temperature of about 40°C.

Mobile phase: Dissolve 8.82 g of trisodium citrate dihydrate in 800 mL of water, adjust the pH to 3.3 with dilute hydrochloric acid, and add water to make 1000 mL. To 240 mL of this solution add 90 mL of methanol and 70 mL of acetonitrile.

Flow rate: Adjust so that the retention time of mosapride is about 9 minutes.

System suitability—

System performance: When the procedure is run with 50 μL of the standard solution under the above operating conditions, the number of theoretical plates and the symmetry factor of the peak of mosapride are not less than 4000 and not more than 2.0, respectively.

System repeatability: When the test is repeated 6 times with 50 μL of the standard solution under the above operating conditions, the relative standard deviation of the peak area of mosapride is not more than 2.0%.

Assay Weigh accurately the mass of not less than 20 Mosapride Citrate Tablets, and powder. Weigh accurately a portion of the powder, equivalent to about 10 mg of mosapride citrate ($C_{21}H_{25}ClFN_3O_3.C_6H_8O_7$), and moisten with 2 mL of water. Add 70 mL of methanol, shake for 20 minutes, add methanol to make exactly 100 mL, and centrifuge. Pipet 10 mL of the supernatant liquid, add methanol to make exactly 50 mL, and use this solution as the sample solution. Separately, weigh accurately about 53 mg of mosapride citrate hydrate for assay (separately, determine the water *<2.48>* in the manner as Mosapride Citrate Hydrate), and dissolve in methanol to make exactly 100 mL. Pipet 2 mL of this solution, add methanol to make exactly 50 mL, and use this solution as the standard solution. Perform the test with the sample solution and standard solution as directed under Ultraviolet-visible Spectrophotometry *<2.24>*, and determine the absorbances, A_T and A_S, at 273 nm.

Amount (mg) of mosapride citrate ($C_{21}H_{25}ClFN_3O_3.C_6H_8O_7$)
$= M_S \times A_T/A_S \times 1/5$

M_S: Amount (mg) of mosapride citrate hydrate for assay taken, calculated on the anhydrous basis

Containers and storage Containers—Tight containers.

Freeze-dried Live Attenuated Mumps Vaccine

乾燥弱毒生おたふくかぜワクチン

Freeze-dried Live Attenuated Mumps Vaccine is a dried preparation containing live attenuated mumps virus.

It conforms to the requirements of Freeze-dried Live Attenuated Mumps Vaccine in the Minimum Requirements of Biologic Products.

Description Freeze-dried Live Attenuated Mumps Vaccine becomes a clear, colorless, yellowish or reddish liquid on addition of solvent.

Mupirocin Calcium Hydrate

ムピロシンカルシウム水和物

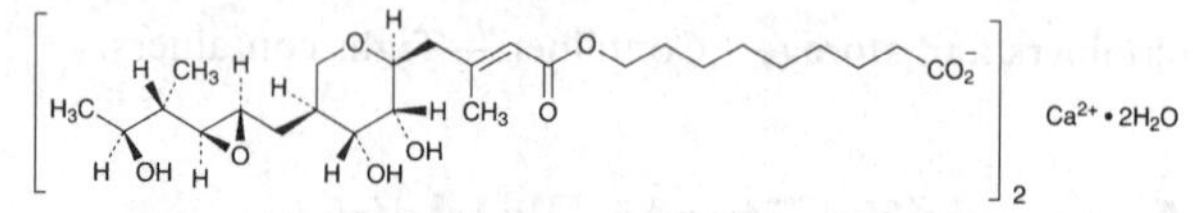

$C_{52}H_{86}CaO_{18}.2H_2O$: 1075.34
Monocalcium bis[9-((2*E*)-4-{(2*S*,3*R*,4*R*,5*S*)-5-[(2*S*,3*S*,4*S*,5*S*)-2,3-epoxy-5-hydroxy-4-methylhexyl]-3,4-dihydroxy-3,4,5,6-tetrahydro-2*H*-pyran-2-yl}-3-methylbut-2-enoyloxy)nonanoate] dihydrate
[*115074-43-6*]

Mupirocin Calcium Hydrate is the calcium salt of a substance having antibacterial activity produced by the growth of *Pseudomonas fluorescens*.

It contains not less than 895 μg (potency) and not more than 970 μg (potency) per mg, calculated on the anhydrous basis. The potency of Mupirocin Calcium Hydrate is expressed as mass (potency) of mupirocin ($C_{26}H_{44}O_9$: 500.62).

Description Mupirocin Calcium Hydrate occurs as a white powder and has a bitter taste.

It is freely soluble in methanol, slightly soluble in water and in ethanol (95), and practically insoluble in diethyl ether.

Identification **(1)** To 1 mL of a solution of Mupirocin Calcium Hydrate in methanol (1 in 200) add 4 mL of hydroxylamine perchlorate-ethanol TS and 1 mL of *N*,*N'*-dicyclohexylcarbodiimide-ethanol TS, shake well, and allow to stand in lukewarm water for 20 minutes. After cooling, add 1 mL of iron (III) perchorate-ethanol TS to the solution, and shake: a dark purple color develops.

(2) Determine the absorption spectrum of a solution of Mupirocin Calcium Hydrate (1 in 50,000) as directed under Ultraviolet-visible Spectrophotometry <*2.24*>: it exhibits a maximum between 219 nm and 224 nm.

(3) Determine the infrared absorption spectrum of Mupirocin Calcium Hydrate as directed in the paste method under Infrared Spectrophotometry <*2.25*>: it exhibits absorption at the wave numbers of about 1708 cm^{-1}, 1648 cm^{-1}, 1558 cm^{-1}, 1231 cm^{-1}, 1151cm^{-1} and 894 cm^{-1}.

(4) A solution of Mupirocin Calcium Hydrate (3 in 1000) responds to Qualitative Tests <*1.09*> (3) for calcium salt.

Optical rotation <*2.49*> $[\alpha]_D^{20}$: $-16 - -20°$ (1 g calculated on the anhydrous basis, methanol, 20 mL, 100 mm).

Purity **(1)** Related substances—Dissolve 50 mg of Mupirocin Calcium Hydrate in a mixture of 0.1 mol/L acetic acid-sodium acetate buffer solution (pH 4.0) and a solution of tetrahydrofuran (3 in 4) (1:1) to make 10 mL, and use this solution as the sample solution (1). Pipet 2 mL of the sample solution (1), add a mixture of 0.1 mol/L acetic acid-sodium acetate buffer solution (pH 4.0) and a solution of tetrahydrofuran (3 in 4) (1:1) to make exactly 100 mL, and use this solution as the sample solution (2). Preserve these sample solutions at a temperature between 4°C and 8°C. Perform the test with exactly 20 μL of the sample solution (1) and the sample solution (2) as directed under Liquid Chromatography <*2.01*> according to the following conditions, and determine the areas of each peak of the sample solution (1) and the sample solution (2) by the automatic integration method. Calculate the amount of the related substances by the following formula: the amount of principal related substance (appeared at about 0.7 of the relative retention time to mupirocin) is not more than 4.0%, and the total amount of related substances (the total area of the peaks other than of the solvent and mupirocin) is not more than 6.0%.

Amount (%) of principal related substance

$$= \frac{A_i}{A + A_m} \times 100 \times \frac{P \times 100}{100 - \dfrac{A \times 100}{A + A_m}}$$

Total amount (%) of related substances

$$= \frac{A}{A + A_m} \times 100 \times \frac{P \times 100}{100 - \dfrac{A \times 100}{A + A_m}}$$

A: Total peak areas other than the solvent and mupirocin from the sample solution (1)

A_i: Peak area of the relative retention time of about 0.7 to mupirocin from the sample solution (1)

A_m: A value of 50 times of peak area of mupirocin from the sample solution (2)

P: Potency per mg obtained from the assay

Operating conditions—

Detector, column, column temperature, mobile phase, and flow rate: Proceed as directed in the operating conditions in the Assay.

Time span of measurement: About 3 times as long as the retention time of mupirocin, beginning after the solvent peak.

System suitability—

System performance: Proceed as directed in the system suitability in the Assay.

Test for required detectability: Pipet 1 mL of the sample solution (2), and add a mixture of 0.1 mol/L acetic acid-sodium acetate buffer solution (pH 4.0) and a solution of tetrahydrofuran (3 in 4) (1:1) to make exactly 20 mL. Confirm that the peak area of mupirocin obtained with 20 μL of this solution is equivalent to 4 to 6% of that with 20 μL of the sample solution (2).

System repeatability: When the test is repeated 6 times with 20 μL of the sample solution (2) under the above operating conditions, the relative standard deviation of the peak areas of mupirocin is not more than 2.0%.

(2) Inorganic salt from manufacturing process—Being specified separately when the drug is granted approval based on the Law.

Water <*2.48*> Not less than 3.0% and not more than 4.5% (0.5 g, volumetric titration, direct titration).

Assay Weigh accurately an amount of Mupirocin Calcium Hydrate and Mupirocin Lithium RS, equivalent to about 20 mg (potency), dissolve in a mixture of 0.1 mol/L acetic acid-sodium acetate buffer solution (pH 4.0) and a solution of tetrahydrofuran (3 in 4) (1:1) to make exactly 200 mL, and use these solutions as the sample solution and the standard solution. Preserve these solutions at a temperature between 4°C and 8°C. Perform the test with exactly 20 μL of the sample solution and standard solution as directed under Liquid Chromatography <*2.01*> according to the following conditions, and determine the peak areas, A_T and A_S, of mupirocin in each solution.

$$\text{Amount [}\mu\text{g (potency)] of mupirocin } (C_{26}H_{44}O_9) = M_S \times A_T/A_S \times 1000$$

M_S: Amount [mg (potency)] of Mupirocin Lithium RS taken

Operating conditions—

Detector: An ultraviolet absorption photometer (wavelength: 240 nm).

Column: A stainless steel column 4.6 mm in inside diameter and 25 cm in length, packed with octadecylsilanized silica gel for liquid chromatography (5 μm in particle diameter).

Column temperature: A constant temperature of about 40°C.

Mobile phase: Dissolve 7.71 g of ammonium acetate in 750 mL of water, adjust the pH to 5.7 with acetic acid (100), and add water to make 1000 mL. To 300 mL of this solution add 100 mL of tetrahydrofuran.

Flow rate: Adjust so that the retention time of mupirocin is about 12.5 minutes.

System suitability—

System performance: Dissolve about 20 mg of Mupirocin Lithium RS and about 5 mg of ethyl parahydroxybenzoate in a mixture of 0.1 mol/L acetic acid-sodium acetate buffer solution (pH 4.0) and a solution of tetrahydrofuran (3 in 4) (1:1) to make 200 mL. When the procedure is run with 20 μL of this solution under the above operating conditions, mupirocin and ethyl parahydroxybenzoate are eluted in this order with the resolution between these peaks being not less than 12.

System repeatability: When the test is repeated 6 times with 20 μL of the standard solution under the above operating conditions, the relative standard deviation of the peak areas of mupirocin is not more than 1.0%.

Containers and storage Containers—Tight containers.

Mupirocin Calcium Ointment

ムピロシンカルシウム軟膏

Mupirocin Calcium Ointment is an oily ointment preparation.

Mupirocin Calcium Ointment contains not less than 95.0% and not more than 105.0% of the labeled potency of mupirocin ($C_{26}H_{44}O_9$: 500.62).

Method of preparation Prepare as directed under Ointments, with Mupirocin Calcium Hydrate.

Identification To an amount of Mupirocin Calcium Ointment, equivalent to 10 mg (potency) of Mupirocin Calcium Hydrate, add 5 mL of water, and warm on a water bath at 60°C for 10 minutes while occasional shaking. After cooling, filter, and to 1 mL of the filtrate add water to make 100 mL. Determine the absorption spectrum of this solution as directed under Ultraviolet-visible Spectrophotometry ⟨*2.24*⟩: it exhibits a maximum between 220 nm and 224 nm.

Purity Related substances—To an amount of Mupirocin Calcium Ointment, equivalent to 50 mg (potency) of Mupirocin Calcium Hydrate, add 5 mL of diluted tetrahydrofuran (3 in 4), and shake vigorously. Then, add 5 mL of 0.1 mol/L acetic acid-sodium acetate buffer solution (pH 4.0), shake vigorously, filter through a glass wool filter, and use the filtrate as the sample solution. Pipet 2 mL of the sample solution, add a mixture of 0.1 mol/L acetic acid-sodium acetate buffer solution (pH 4.0) and diluted tetrahydrofuran (3 in 4) (1:1) to make exactly 100 mL, and use this solution as the standard solution. Perform the test with exactly 20 µL each of the sample solution and standard solution as directed under Liquid Chromatography ⟨*2.01*⟩ according to the following conditions, and determine the area of the peak other than mupirocin obtained from the sample solution and the peak area of mupirocin from the standard solution by the automatic integration method. Calculate the amount of each related substance using the following equation: the amount of the related substance having the relative retention time of about 0.7 to mupirocin is not more than 4.0%, the amount of the related substance other than that is not more than 1.5%, and the total amount of the related substances is not more than 6.0%.

$$\text{Amount (\%) of each related substance} = A/(\Sigma A + A_m) \times 100$$

A: Peak area of each related substance obtained from the sample solution.

ΣA: Total area of the peaks other than mupirocin obtained from the sample solution.

A_m: Amount of 50 times the peak area of mupirocin obtained from the standard solution.

Operating conditions—

Detector, column, column temperature, mobile phase, and flow rate: Proceed as directed in the operating conditions in the Assay under Mupirocin Calcium Hydrate.

Time span of measurement: About 5 times as long as the retention time of mupirocin, beginning after the solvent peak.

System suitability—

System performance: Proceed as directed in the system suitability in the Assay under Mupirocin Calcium Hydrate.

Test for required detectability: To exactly 1 mL of the standard solution add a mixture of 0.1 mol/L acetic acid-sodium acetate buffer solution (pH 4.0) and diluted tetrahydrofuran (3 in 4) (1:1) to make exactly 20 mL. Confirm that the peak area of mupirocin obtained with 20 µL of this solution is equivalent to 4 to 6% of that with 20 µL of the standard solution.

System repeatability: When the test is repeated 6 times with 20 µL of the standard solution under the above operating conditions, the relative standard deviation of the peak area of mupirocin is not more than 2.0%.

Assay Weigh accurately an amount of Mupirocin Calcium Ointment, equivalent to about 2 mg (potency) of Mupirocin Calcium Hydrate, add exactly 10 mL of diluted tetrahydrofuran (3 in 4), and shake vigorously. To this solution add exactly 10 mL of 0.1 mol/L acetic acid-sodium acetate buffer solution (pH 4.0), shake vigorously, filter through a glass wool filter, and use the filtrate as the sample solution. Separately, weigh accurately an amount of Mupirocin Lithium RS, equivalent to about 20 mg (potency), dissolve in a mixture of 0.1 mol/L acetic acid-sodium acetate buffer solution (pH 4.0) and diluted tetrahydrofuran (3 in 4) (1:1) to make exactly 200 mL, and use this solution as the standard solution. Then, proceed as directed in the Assay under Mupirocin Calcium Hydrate.

$$\text{Amount [mg (potency)] of mupirocin } (C_{26}H_{44}O_9) = M_S \times A_T/A_S \times 1/10$$

M_S: Amount [mg (potency)] of Mupirocin Lithium RS taken

Containers and storage Containers—Tight containers.

Nabumetone

ナブメトン

$C_{15}H_{16}O_2$: 228.29

4-(6-Methoxynaphthalen-2-yl)butan-2-one

[*42924-53-8*]

Nabumetone contains not less than 98.0% and not more than 101.0% of nabumetone ($C_{15}H_{16}O_2$), calculated on the anhydrous basis.

Description Nabumetone occurs as white to yellowish white, crystals or a crystalline powder.

It is soluble in acetonitrile, sparingly soluble in methanol and in ethanol (99.5), and practically insoluble in water.

Identification **(1)** Determine the absorption spectrum of a solution of Nabumetone in methanol (1 in 30,000) as directed under Ultraviolet-visible Spectrophotometry ⟨*2.24*⟩, and compare the spectrum with the Reference Spectrum or the spectrum of a solution of Nabumetone RS prepared in the same manner as the sample solution: both spectra exhibit similar intensities of absorption at the same wavelengths.

(2) Determine the infrared absorption spectrum of Nabumetone as directed in the potassium bromide disk method under Infrared Spectrophotometry ⟨*2.25*⟩, and compare the spectrum with the Reference Spectrum or the spectrum of Nabumetone RS: both spectra exhibit similar intensities of absorption at the same wave numbers.

Melting point ⟨*2.60*⟩ 79 – 84°C

Purity **(1)** Heavy metals *<1.07>*—Proceed with 1.0 g of Nabumetone according to Method 2, and perform the test. Prepare the control solution with 1.0 mL of Standard Lead Solution (not more than 10 ppm).

(2) Related substances—Dissolve 20 mg of Nabumetone in 20 mL of acetonitrile, and use this solution as the sample solution. Pipet 5 mL of the sample solution, add acetonitrile to make exactly 50 mL. Pipet 1 mL of this solution, add acetonitrile to make exactly 20 mL, and use this solution as the standard solution. Perform the test with exactly 10 μL each of the sample solution and standard solution as directed under Liquid Chromatography *<2.01>* according to the following conditions. Determine each peak area of both solutions by the automatic integration method: the peak area of the related substance G obtained from the sample solution is not larger than 3/5 times the peak area of nabumetone from the standard solution, and each peak area other than nabumetone and the related substance G is not larger than 1/5 times the peak area of nabumetone from the standard solution. Furthermore, the total area of the peaks other than nabumetone from the sample solution is not larger than 1.6 times the peak area of nabumetone from the standard solution. For each peak area of the related substances A, B, C, D, E, F and G, which are having the relative retention time of about 0.73, 0.85, 0.93, 1.2, 1.9, 2.6 and 2.7 to nabumetone, multiply their correction factors, 0.12, 0.94, 0.25, 0.42, 1.02, 0.91 and 0.1, respectively.

Operating conditions—

Detector, column, and column temperature: Proceed as directed in the operating conditions in the Assay.

Mobile phase A: A mixture of water and acetic acid (100) (999:1).

Mobile phase B: A mixture of acetonitrile and tetrahydrofuran (7:3).

Flowing of mobile phase: Control the gradient by mixing the mobile phases A and B as directed in the following table.

Time after injection of sample (min)	Mobile phase A (vol%)	Mobile phase B (vol%)
0 – 12	60	40
12 – 28	60 → 20	40 → 80

Flow rate: 1.3 mL per minute.

Time span of measurement: About 3 times as long as the retention time of nabumetone, beginning after the solvent peak.

System suitability—

System performance: Proceed as directed in the system suitability in the Assay.

Test for required detectability: Pipet 2 mL of the standard solution, and add acetonitrile to make exactly 10 mL. Confirm that the peak area of nabumetone obtained with 10 μL of this solution is equivalent to 14 to 26% of that with 10 μL of the standard solution.

System repeatability: When the test is repeated 6 times with 10 μL of the standard solution under the above operating conditions, the relative standard deviation of the peak area of nabumetone is not more than 5.0%.

Water *<2.48>* Not more than 0.2% (1 g, volumetric titration, direct titration).

Residue on ignition *<2.44>* Not more than 0.1% (1 g).

Assay Weigh accurately about 20 mg each of Nabumetone and Nabumetone RS (separately determine the water *<2.48>* in the same manner as Nabumetone), dissolve them in acetonitrile to make exactly 20 mL, and use these solutions as the sample solution and the standard solution, respectively. Perform the test with exactly 10 μL each of the sample solution and standard solution as directed under Liquid Chromatography *<2.01>* according to the following conditions, and determine the peak area, A_T and A_S, of nabumetone in each solution.

$$\text{Amount (mg) of nabumetone } (C_{15}H_{16}O_2) = M_S \times A_T/A_S$$

M_S: Amount (mg) of Nabumetone RS taken, calculated on the anhydrous basis

Operating conditions—

Detector: An ultraviolet absorption photometer (wavelength: 254 nm).

Column: A stainless steel column 4.6 mm in inside diameter and 15 cm in length, packed with octadecylsilanized silica gel for liquid chromatography (4 μm in particle diameter).

Column temperature: A constant temperature of about 40°C.

Mobile phase: To 600 mL of a mixture of water and acetic acid (100) (999:1) add 400 mL of a mixture of acetonitrile and tetrahydrofuran (7:3).

Flow rate: Adjust so that the retention time of nabumetone is about 10 minutes.

System suitability—

System performance: When the procedure is run with 10 μL of the standard solution under the above operating conditions, the number of theoretical plates and the symmetry factor of the peak of nabumetone are not less than 6000 and not more than 1.5, respectively.

System repeatability: When the test is repeated 6 times with 10 μL of the standard solution under the above operating conditions, the relative standard deviation of the peak area of nabumetone is not more than 1.0%.

Containers and storage Containers—Tight containers.

Nabumetone Tablets

ナブメトン錠

Nabumetone Tablets contain not less than 95.0% and not more than 105.0% of the labeled amount of nabumetone ($C_{15}H_{16}O_2$: 228.29).

Method of preparation Prepare as directed under Tablets, with Nabumetone.

Identification To a quantity of powdered Nabumetone Tablets, equivalent to 80 mg of Nabumetone, add 50 mL of methanol, shake for 10 minutes and centrifuge the solution. To 1 mL of the supernatant liquid, add methanol to make 50 mL, and determine the absorption spectrum of this solution as directed under Ultraviolet-visible Spectrophotometry *<2.24>*: it exhibits maxima between 259 nm and 263 nm, between 268 nm and 272 nm, between 316 nm and 320 nm, and between 330 nm and 334 nm.

Uniformity of dosage units *<6.02>* It meets the requirement of the Mass variation test.

Dissolution *<6.10>* When the test is performed at 75 revolutions per minute according to the Paddle method, using 900 mL of a solution prepared by dissolving 3 g of polysorbate 80 in water to make 100 mL as the dissolution medium, the dissolution rate in 60 minutes of Nabumetone Tablets is not less than 70%.

Start the test with 1 tablet of Nabumetone Tablets, withdraw not less than 20 mL of the medium at the specified minute after starting the test, and filter through a membrane filter with a pore size not exceeding 0.5 μm. Discard not less than 10 mL of the first filtrate, pipet V mL of the subsequent filtrate, add a solution, prepared by adding to 20 mL of ethanol (99.5) the dissolution medium to make 50 mL, to make exactly V' mL so that each mL contains about 89 μg of nabumetone ($C_{15}H_{16}O_2$), and use this solution as the sample solution. Separately, weigh accurately about 22 mg of Nabumetone RS (separately determine the water *<2.48>* in the same manner as Nabumetone), and dissolve in ethanol (99.5) to make exactly 100 mL. Pipet 10 mL of this solution, add the dissolution medium to make exactly 25 mL, and use this solution as the standard solution. Determine the absorbances, A_T and A_S, at 331 nm of the sample solution and standard solution as directed under Ultraviolet-visible Spectrophotometry *<2.24>*, using a solution prepared by adding to 20 mL of ethanol (99.5) the dissolution medium to make 50 mL as the blank.

Dissolution rate (%) with respect to the labeled amount of nabumetone ($C_{15}H_{16}O_2$)
$= M_S \times A_T/A_S \times V'/V \times 1/C \times 360$

M_S: Amount (mg) of Nabumetone RS taken, calculated on the anhydrous basis
C: Labeled amount (mg) of nabumetone ($C_{15}H_{16}O_2$) in 1 tablet

Assay Weigh accurately the mass of not less than 20 tablets of Nabumetone Tablets, and powder. Weigh accurately a portion of the powder, equivalent to about 0.2 g of nabumetone ($C_{15}H_{16}O_2$), add 10 mL of water and shake, add 40 mL of methanol, shake for 30 minutes, and then add methanol to make exactly 100 mL. Centrifuge this solution, pipet 5 mL of the supernatant liquid, add exactly 5 mL of the internal standard solution, then add methanol to make 50 mL, and use this solution as the sample solution. Separately, weigh accurately about 40 mg of Nabumetone RS (separately determine the water *<2.48>* in the same manner as Nabumetone), dissolve by adding 50 mL of methanol and exactly 20 mL of the internal standard solution, then add methanol to make 200 mL, and use this solution as the standard solution. Perform the test with 10 μL each of the sample solution and standard solution as directed under Liquid Chromatography *<2.01>* according to the following conditions, and calculate the ratios, Q_T and Q_S, of the peak area of nabumetone to that of the internal standard.

Amount (mg) of nabumetone ($C_{15}H_{16}O_2$)
$= M_S \times Q_T/Q_S \times 5$

M_S: Amount (mg) of Nabumetone RS taken, calculated on the anhydrous basis

Internal standard solution—Dissolve 0.12 g of 2-ethylhexyl parahydroxybenzoate in methanol to make 100 mL.
Operating conditions—

Detector: An ultraviolet absorption photometer (wavelength: 254 nm).

Column: A stainless steel column 4 mm in inside diameter and 15 cm in length, packed with octadecylsilanized silica gel for liquid chromatography (5 μm in particle diameter).

Column temperature: A constant temperature of about 25°C.

Mobile phase: A mixture of acetonitrile, water and acetic acid (100) (550:450:1).

Flow rate: Adjust so that the retention time of nabumetone is about 6 minutes.

System suitability—

System performance: When the procedure is run with 10 μL of the standard solution under the above operating conditions, nabumetone and the internal standard are eluted in this order with the resolution between these peaks being not less than 13.

System repeatability: When the test is repeated 6 times with 10 μL of the standard solution under the above operating conditions, the relative standard deviation of the ratio of the peak area of nabumetone to that of the internal standard is not more than 1.0%.

Containers and storage Containers—Well-closed containers.

Nadolol

ナドロール

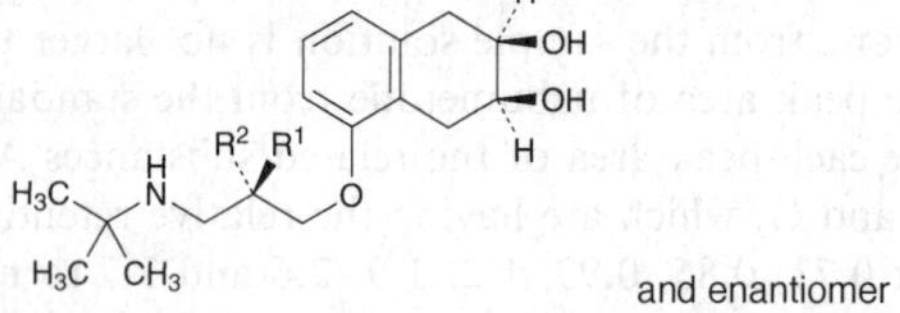

and enantiomer

$C_{17}H_{27}NO_4$: 309.40
$R^1 = OH$, $R^2 = H$
(2*RS*,3*SR*)-5-{(2*SR*)-3-[(1,1-Dimethylethyl)amino]-2-hydroxypropyloxy}-1,2,3,4-tetrahydronaphthalene-2,3-diol

$R^1 = H$, $R^2 = OH$
(2*RS*,3*SR*)-5-{(2*RS*)-3-[(1,1-Dimethylethyl)amino]-2-hydroxypropyloxy}-1,2,3,4-tetrahydronaphthalene-2,3-diol
[42200-33-9]

Nadolol, when dried, contains not less than 98.0% of nadolol ($C_{17}H_{27}NO_4$).

Description Nadolol occurs as a white to yellowish-brown-white crystalline powder.

It is freely soluble in methanol and in acetic acid (100), soluble in ethanol (95), and slightly soluble in water and in chloroform.

A solution of Nadolol in methanol (1 in 100) shows no optical rotation.

Melting point: about 137°C.

Identification **(1)** Determine the absorption spectrum of a solution of Nadolol in methanol (1 in 5000) as directed under Ultraviolet-visible Spectrophotometry *<2.24>*, and compare the spectrum with the Reference Spectrum: both spectra exhibit similar intensities of absorption at the same wavelengths.

(2) Determine the infrared absorption spectrum of Nadolol, previously dried, as directed in the potassium bromide disk method under Infrared Spectrophotometry *<2.25>*: it exhibits absorption at the wave numbers of about 1585 cm^{-1}, 1460 cm^{-1}, 1092 cm^{-1}, 935 cm^{-1} and 770 cm^{-1}.

Purity **(1)** Heavy metals *<1.07>*—Proceed with 1.0 g of Nadolol according to Method 2, and perform the test. Prepare the control solution with 2.0 mL of Standard Lead Solution (not more than 20 ppm).

(2) Related substances—Dissolve 0.5 g of Nadolol in 10 mL of a mixture of methanol and chloroform (1:1), and use this solution as the sample solution. Perform the test with the sample solution as directed under Thin-layer Chromatography <2.03>. Spot 100 μL each of the sample solution and a mixture of methanol and chloroform (1:1) as a control solution with 25 mm each of width at an interval of about 10 mm on the starting line of a plate 0.25 mm in thickness of silica gel with fluorescent indicator for thin-layer chromatography. Develop the plate with a mixture of acetone, chloroform and diluted ammonia TS (1 in 3) (8:1:1) to a distance of about 15 cm, and air-dry the plate. Examine under ultraviolet light (main wavelength: 254 nm), and confirm the positions of the principal spot and the spots other than the principal spot obtained from the sample solution. Scratch and collect the silica gel of the positions of the plate corresponding to the principal spot and the spots other than the principal spot. To the silica gel collected from the principal spot add exactly 30 mL of ethanol (95), and to the silica gel from the spots other than the principal spot add exactly 10 mL of ethanol (95). After shaking them for 60 minutes, centrifuge, and determine the absorbances of these supernatant liquids at 278 nm as directed under Ultraviolet-visible Spectrophotometry <2.24>. Separately, proceed in the same manner with each position of the silica gel from the control solution corresponding to the principal spot and the spots other than the principal spot of the sample solution, and perform a blank determination to make correction. Amount of the related substances calculated by the following equation is not more than 2.0%.

Amount (%) of related substances = $A_b/(A_b + 3A_a) \times 100$

A_a: Corrected absorbance of the principle spot
A_b: Corrected absorbance of the spots other than the principle spot

Loss on drying <2.41> Not more than 1.0% (1 g, in vacuum, 60°C, 3 hours).

Residue on ignition <2.44> Not more than 0.1% (1 g).

Isomer ratio Prepare a paste with 0.01 g of Nadolol as directed in the paste method under Infrared Spectrophotometry <2.25> so that its transmittance at an absorption band at a wave number of about 1585 cm^{-1} is 25 to 30%, and determine the infrared absorption spectrum between 1600 cm^{-1} and 1100 cm^{-1}. Determine the absorbances, A_{1265} and A_{1250}, from the transmittances, T_{1265} and T_{1250}, at wave numbers of about 1265 cm^{-1} (racemic substance A) and 1250 cm^{-1} (racemic substance B), respectively: the ratio A_{1265}/A_{1250} is between 0.72 and 1.08.

Assay Weigh accurately about 0.28 g of Nadolol, previously dried, dissolve in 50 mL of acetic acid (100), and titrate <2.50> with 0.1 mol/L perchloric acid VS until the color of the solution changes from purple through blue to green-blue (indicator: 3 drops of crystal violet TS). Perform a blank determination in the same manner, and make any necessary correction.

Each mL of 0.1 mol/L perchloric acid VS
= 30.94 mg of $C_{17}H_{27}NO_4$

Containers and storage Containers—Tight containers.
Storage—Light-resistant.

Nafamostat Mesilate

ナファモスタットメシル酸塩

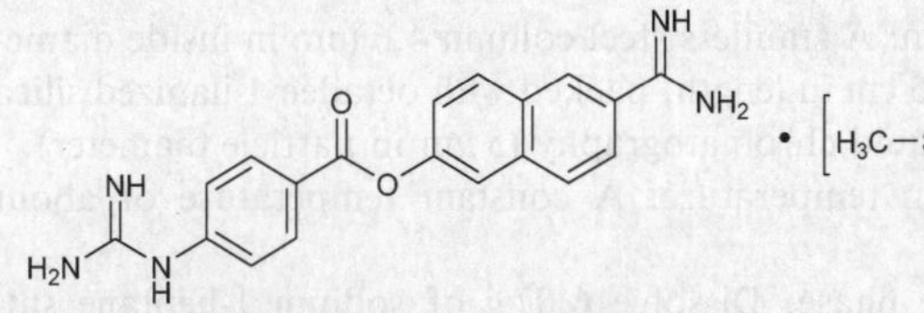

$C_{19}H_{17}N_5O_2.2CH_4O_3S$: 539.58
6-Amidinonaphthalen-2-yl 4-guanidinobenzoate dimethanesulfonate
[82956-11-4]

Nafamostat Mesilate, when dried, contains not less than 99.0% and not more than 101.0% of nafamostat mesilate ($C_{19}H_{17}N_5O_2.2CH_4O_3S$).

Description Nafamostat Mesilate occurs as a white crystalline powder.

It is freely soluble in formic acid, soluble in water, and practically insoluble in ethanol (99.5).

It dissolves in 0.01 mol/L hydrochloric acid TS.

Melting point: about 262°C (with decomposition).

Identification **(1)** Determine the absorption spectrum of a solution of Nafamostat Mesilate in 0.01 mol/L hydrochloric acid TS (1 in 200,000) as directed under Ultraviolet-visible Spectrophotometry <2.24>, and compare the spectrum with the Reference Spectrum: both spectra exhibit similar intensities of absorption at the same wavelengths.

(2) Determine the infrared absorption spectrum of Nafamostat Mesilate as directed in the potassium bromide disk method under Infrared Spectrophotometry <2.25>, and compare the spectrum with the Reference Spectrum: both spectra exhibit similar intensities of absorption at the same wave numbers.

(3) A 0.1-g portion of Nafamostat Mesilate responds to Qualitative Tests <1.09> (1) for mesilate.

pH <2.54> The pH of a solution prepared by dissolving 1.0 g of Nafamostat Mesilate in 50 mL of water is between 4.7 and 5.7.

Purity **(1)** Clarity and color of solution—A solution prepared by dissolving 1.0 g of Nafamostat Mesilate in 50 mL of water is clear and colorless.

(2) Heavy metals <1.07>—Proceed with 2.0 g of Nafamostat Mesilate according to Method 4, and perform the test. Prepare the control solution with 2.0 mL of Standard Lead Solution (not more than 10 ppm).

(3) Related substances—Conduct this procedure using light-resistant vessels. Dissolve 0.10 g of Nafamostat Mesilate in 100 mL of the mobile phase, and use this solution as the sample solution. Pipet 10 mL of the sample solution, add the mobile phase to make exactly 100 mL. Then pipet 5 mL of this solution, add the mobile phase to make exactly 100 mL, and use this solution as the standard solution. Perform the test with exactly 10 μL each of the sample solution and standard solution as directed under Liquid Chromatography <2.01> according to the following conditions. Determine each peak area of each solution by the automatic integration method: the area of each peak other than nafamostat obtained from the sample solution is not larger than 1/5 times the peak area of nafamostat from the standard solution. Furthermore, the total area of the peaks other than nafamostat from the sample solution is not larger than the peak area of nafamostat from the standard solution.

Operating conditions—

Detector: An ultraviolet absorption photometer (wavelength: 260 nm).

Column: A stainless steel column 4.6 mm in inside diameter and 25 cm in length, packed with octadecylsilanized silica gel for liquid chromatography (5 μm in particle diameter).

Column temperature: A constant temperature of about 40°C.

Mobile phase: Dissolve 6.07 g of sodium 1-heptane sulfonate in 1000 mL of diluted acetic acid (100) (3 in 500). To 700 mL of this solution add 300 mL of acetonitrile.

Flow rate: Adjust so that the retention time of nafamostat is about 7 minutes.

Time span of measurement: About 4 times as long as the retention time of nafamostat, beginning after the solvent peak.

System suitability—

Test for required detectability: Pipet 5 mL of the standard solution, and add the mobile phase to make exactly 50 mL. Pipet 15 mL of this solution, and add the mobile phase to make exactly 100 mL. Confirm that the peak area of nafamostat obtained with 10 μL of this solution is equivalent to 1.1 to 1.9% of that with 10 μL of the standard solution.

System performance: Dissolve 0.1 g of nafamostat mesilate in the mobile phase to make 100 mL. To 10 mL of this solution add the mobile phase to make 100 mL. To 5 mL of this solution add 5 mL of a solution of 6-amidino-2-naphthol methanesulfonate in the mobile phase (1 in 20,000). When the procedure is run with 10 μL of this solution under the above operating conditions, 6-amidino-2-naphthol and nafamostat are eluted in this order with the resolution between these peaks being not less than 6.

System repeatability: When the test is repeated 6 times with 10 μL of the standard solution under the above operating conditions, the relative standard deviation of the peak area of nafamostat is not more than 2.0%.

Loss on drying <*2.41*> Not more than 0.5% (1 g, 105°C, 3 hours).

Residue on ignition <*2.44*> Not more than 0.1% (1 g).

Assay Weigh accurately about 0.25 g of Nafamostat Mesilate, previously dried, dissolve in 4 mL of formic acid, add 50 mL of acetic anhydride, and titrate <*2.50*> with 0.1 mol/L perchloric acid VS (potentiometric titration). Perform a blank determination in the same manner, and make any necessary correction.

Each mL of 0.1 mol/L perchloric acid VS
= 26.98 mg of $C_{19}H_{17}N_5O_2.2CH_4O_3S$

Containers and storage Containers—Tight containers.

Naftopidil

ナフトピジル

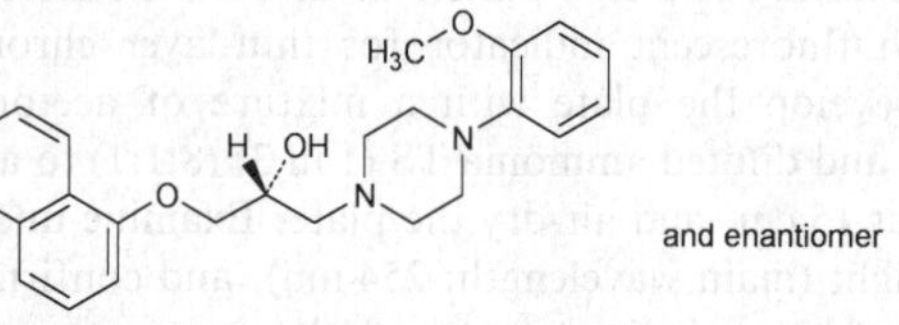

and enantiomer

$C_{24}H_{28}N_2O_3$: 392.49

(2*RS*)-1-[4-(2-Methoxyphenyl)piperazin-1-yl]-3-(naphthalen-1-yloxy)propan-2-ol

[*57149-07-2*]

Naftopidil, when dried, contains not less than 99.0% and not more than 101.0% of naftopidil ($C_{24}H_{28}N_2O_3$).

Description Naftopidil occurs as a white crystalline powder.

It is very soluble in acetic anhydride, freely soluble in *N*,*N*-dimethylformamide and in acetic acid (100), slightly soluble in methanol and in ethanol (99.5), and practically insoluble in water.

It is gradually colored to light brown by light.

A solution of Naftopidil in *N*,*N*-dimethylformamide (1 in 10) shows no optical rotation.

Identification **(1)** Dissolve 50 mg of Naftopidil in 5 mL of acetic acid (100), and add 0.1 mL of Dragendorff's TS: orange colored precipitates are produced.

(2) Determine the absorption spectrum of a solution of Naftopidil in methanol (1 in 100,000) as directed under Ultraviolet-visible Spectrophotometry <*2.24*>, and compare the spectrum with the Reference Spectrum: both spectra exhibit similar intensities of absorption at the same wavelengths.

(3) Determine the infrared absorption spectrum of Naftopidil, previously dried, as directed in the potassium bromide disk method under Infrared Spectrophotometry <*2.25*>, and compare the spectrum with the Reference Spectrum: both spectra exhibit similar intensities of absorption at the same wave numbers.

Melting point <*2.60*> 126 – 129°C

Purity **(1)** Heavy metals <*1.07*>—Proceed with 2.0 g of Naftopidil according to Method 4, and perform the test. Prepare the control solution with 2.0 mL of Standard Lead Solution (not more than 10 ppm).

(2) Related substances—Dissolve 0.10 g of Naftopidil in 60 mL of methanol, add diluted 0.1 mol/L potassium dihydrogen phosphate TS (pH 2.0) (1 in 2) to make 100 mL, and use this solution as the sample solution. Pipet 1 mL of the sample solution, add a mixture of methanol and water (3:2) to make exactly 100 mL. Pipet 4 mL of this solution, add a mixture of methanol and water (3:2) to make exactly 20 mL, and use this solution as the standard solution. Perform the test with exactly 10 μL each of the sample solution and standard solution as directed under Liquid Chromatography <*2.01*> according to the following conditions, and determine each peak area by automatic integration method: each peak area other than naftopidil obtained from the sample solution is not larger than 3/4 times the peak area of naftopidil from the standard solution, and the total area of the peaks other than naftopidil from the sample solution is not larger than 2.5 times the peak area of naftopidil from the standard solution.

Operating conditions—

Detector: An ultraviolet absorption photometer (wavelength: 283 nm).

Column: A stainless steel column 4.0 mm in inside diameter and 15 cm in length, packed with octadecylsilanized silica gel for liquid chromatography (5 μm in particle diameter).

Column temperature: A constant temperature of about 25°C.

Mobile phase: Dissolve 6.80 g of potassium dihydrogen phosphate in 900 mL of water, adjust to pH 4.0 with diluted phosphoric acid (1 in 10), and add water to make 1000 mL. To 450 mL of this solution add 550 mL of methanol.

Flow rate: Adjust so that the retention time of naftopidil is about 10 minutes.

Time span of measurement: About 2 times as long as the retention time of naftopidil, beginning after the solvent peak.

System suitability—

Test for required detectability: Pipet 2.5 mL of the standard solution, add a mixture of methanol and water (3:2) to make exactly 10 mL. Confirm that the peak area of naftopidil obtained with 10 μL of this solution is equivalent to 17.5 to 32.5% of that with 10 μL of the standard solution.

System performance: When the procedure is run with 10 μL of the standard solution under the above operating conditions, the number of theoretical plates and the symmetry factor of the peak of naftopidil are not less than 2500 and not more than 1.5, respectively.

System repeatability: When the test is repeated 6 times with 10 μL of the standard solution under the above operating conditions, the relative standard deviation of the peak area of naftopidil is not more than 3.0%.

Loss on drying *<2.41>* Not more than 0.5% (1 g, 105°C, 3 hours).

Residue on ignition *<2.44>* Not more than 0.1% (1 g).

Assay Weigh accurately about 0.2 g of Naftopidil, previously dried, dissolve in 50 mL of acetic anhydride, and titrate *<2.50>* with 0.1 mol/L perchloric acid VS (potentiometric titration). Perform a blank determination in the same manner, and make any necessary correction.

Each mL of 0.1 mol/L perchloric acid VS
= 39.25 mg of $C_{24}H_{28}N_2O_3$

Containers and storage Containers—Well-closed containers.

Storage—Light-resistant.

Naftopidil Orally Disintegrating Tablets

ナフトピジル口腔内崩壊錠

Naftopidil Orally Disintegrating Tablets contain not less than 95.0% and not more than 105.0% of the labeled amount of naftopidil ($C_{24}H_{28}N_2O_3$: 392.49).

Method of preparation Prepare as directed under Tablets, with Naftopidil.

Identification Powder Naftopidil Orally Disintegrating Tablets. To a portion of the powder, equivalent to 25 mg of Naftopidil add 100 mL of methanol, shake thoroughly, and filter through a membrane filter with a pore size not exceeding 0.45 μm. To 6 mL of the filtrate add methanol to make 50 mL. Determine the absorption spectrum of this solution as directed under Ultraviolet-visible Spectrophotometry *<2.24>*: it exhibits maxima between 281 nm and 285 nm, and between 318 nm and 322 nm.

Uniformity of dosage units *<6.02>* Perform the Mass variation test, or the Content uniformity test according to the following method: it meets the requirement.

To 1 tablet of Naftopidil Orally Disintegrating Tablets add V/10 mL of water, disintegrate and disperse the tablet by sonicating. To this solution add V/2 mL of methanol, shake thoroughly, then add methanol to make exactly V mL so that each mL contains about 0.25 mg of naftopidil ($C_{24}H_{28}N_2O_3$), and filter through a membrane filter with a pore size not exceeding 0.45 μm. Discard the first 10 mL of the filtrate, pipet 6 mL of the subsequent filtrate, add methanol to make exactly 50 mL, and use this solution as the sample solution. Separately, weigh accurately about 50 mg of naftopidil for assay, previously dried at 105°C for 3 hours, dissolve in methanol to make exactly 100 mL. Pipet 3 mL of this solution, add methanol to make exactly 50 mL, and use this solution as the standard solution. Determine the absorbances, A_T and A_S, at 283 nm of the sample solution and standard solution as directed under Ultraviolet-visible Spectrophotometry *<2.24>*.

Amount (mg) of naftopidil ($C_{24}H_{28}N_2O_3$)
$= M_S \times A_T/A_S \times V/200$

M_S: Amount (mg) of naftopidil for assay taken

Disintegration Being specified separately when the drug is granted approval based on the Law.

Dissolution *<6.10>* When the test is performed at 50 revolution per minute according to the Paddle method, using 900 mL of 0.05 mol/L acetic acid-sodium acetate buffer solution (pH 4.0) as the dissolution medium, the dissolution rate in 30 minutes of Naftopidil Orally Disintegrating Tablets is not less than 75%.

Start the test with 1 tablet of Naftopidil Orally Disintegrating Tablets, withdraw not less than 20 mL of the medium at the specified minute after starting the test, and filter through a membrane filter with a pore size not exceeding 0.45 μm. Discard not less than 10 mL of the first filtrate, pipet V mL of the subsequent filtrate, add the dissolution medium to make exactly V' mL so that each mL contains about 28 μg of naftopidil ($C_{24}H_{28}N_2O_3$), and use this solution as the sample solution. Separately, weigh accurately about 28 mg of naftopidil for assay, previously dried at 105°C for 3 hours, dissolve in 50 mL of methanol, then add the dissolution medium to make exactly 100 mL. Pipet 5 mL of this solution, add the dissolution medium to make exactly 50 mL, and use this solution as the standard solution. Determine the absorbances, A_T and A_S, at 283 nm of the sample solution and standard solution as directed under Ultraviolet-visible Spectrophotometry *<2.24>*, using the dissolution medium as the control.

Dissolution rate (%) with respect to the labeled amount of naftopidil ($C_{24}H_{28}N_2O_3$)
$= M_S \times A_T/A_S \times V'/V \times 1/C \times 90$

M_S: Amount (mg) of naftopidil for assay taken
C: Labeled amount (mg) of naftopidil ($C_{24}H_{28}N_2O_3$) in 1 tablet

Assay Weigh accurately the mass of not less than 20 Naftopidil Orally Disintegrating Tablets, and powder. Weigh accurately a portion of the powder, equivalent to about 50 mg of naftopidil ($C_{24}H_{28}N_2O_3$), add 30 mL of methanol, shake thoroughly, add diluted 0.1 mol/L potassium dihydrogen phosphate TS (pH 2.0) (1 in 2) to make exactly 50 mL, and filter through a membrane filter with a pore size not exceeding 0.45 μm. Discard the first 10 mL of the filtrate, pipet 10 mL of the subsequent filtrate, add exactly 10 mL of the internal standard solution, add a mixture of methanol and water (3:2) to make 100 mL, and use this solution as the sample solution. Separately, weigh accurately about 50 mg of naftopidil for assay, previously dried at 105°C for 3 hours, dissolve in 30 mL of methanol, add diluted 0.1 mol/L potassium dihydrogen phosphate TS (pH 2.0) (1 in 2) to make exactly 50 mL. Pipet 10 mL of this solution, add exactly 10 mL of the internal standard solution, add a mixture of methanol and water (3:2) to make 100 mL, and use this solution as the standard solution. Perform the test with 10 μL each of the sample solution and standard solution as directed under Liquid Chromatography <2.01> according to the following conditions, and calculate the ratios, Q_T and Q_S of the peak area of naftopidil to that of the internal standard.

Amount (mg) of naftopidil ($C_{24}H_{28}N_2O_3$) = $M_S \times Q_T/Q_S$

M_S: Amount (mg) of naftopidil for assay taken

Internal standard solution—A solution of butyl parahydroxybenzoate in a mixture of methanol and water (3:2) (3 in 2000).

Operating conditions—

Detector, column, column temperature, mobile phase, and flow rate: Proceed as directed in the operating conditions in the Purity (2) under Naftopidil.

System suitability—

System performance: When the procedure is run with 10 μL of the standard solution under the above operating conditions, naftopidil and the internal standard are eluted in this order with the resolution between these peaks being not less than 4.

System repeatability: When the test is repeated 6 times with 10 μL of the standard solution under the above operating conditions, the relative standard deviation of the ratio of the peak area of naftopidil to that of the internal standard is not more than 1.0%.

Containers and storage Containers—Well-closed containers.

Storage—Light-resistant.

Naftopidil Tablets

ナフトピジル錠

Naftopidil Tablets contain not less than 95.0% and not more than 105.0% of the labeled amount of naftopidil ($C_{24}H_{28}N_2O_3$: 392.49).

Method of preparation Prepare as directed under Tablets, with Naftopidil.

Identification Powder Naftopidil Tablets. To a portion of the powder, equivalent to 25 mg of Naftopidil, add 100 mL of methanol, shake thoroughly, and centrifuge, if necessary. Filter the supernatant liquid through a membrane filter with a pore size not exceeding 0.45 μm. To 6 mL of the filtrate add methanol to make 50 mL. Determine the absorption spectrum of this solution as directed under Ultraviolet-visible Spectrophotometry <2.24>: it exhibits maxima between 281 nm and 285 nm, and between 318 nm and 322 nm.

Uniformity of dosage units <6.02> Perform the test according to the following method: it meets the requirement of the Content uniformity test.

To 1 tablet of Naftopidil Tablets add V/10 mL of water, disintegrate and disperse the tablet with the aid of ultrasonic waves. To this dispersed solution add V/2 mL of methanol, shake thoroughly, add methanol to make exactly V mL so that each mL contains about 0.25 mg of naftopidil ($C_{24}H_{28}N_2O_3$). Centrifuge this solution, if necessary, filter the supernatant liquid through a membrane filter with a pore size not exceeding 0.45 μm. Discard the first 10 mL of the filtrate, pipet 6 mL of the subsequent filtrate, add methanol to make exactly 50 mL, and use this solution as the sample solution. Separately, weigh accurately about 50 mg of naftopidil for assay, previously dried at 105°C for 3 hours, dissolve in methanol to make exactly 100 mL. Pipet 3 mL of this solution, add methanol to make exactly 50 mL, and use this solution as the standard solution. Determine the absorbances, A_T and A_S, at 283 nm of the sample solution and standard solution as directed under Ultraviolet-visible Spectrophotometry <2.24>.

Amount (mg) of naftopidil ($C_{24}H_{28}N_2O_3$)
= $M_S \times A_T/A_S \times V/200$

M_S: Amount (mg) of naftopidil for assay taken

Dissolution <6.10> When the test is performed at 50 revolutions per minute according to the Paddle method, using 900 mL of 0.05 mol/L acetic acid-sodium acetate buffer solution (pH 4.0) as the dissolution medium, the dissolution rate in 15 minutes of 25-mg and 50-mg tablet and in 30 minutes of 75-mg tablet is not less than 75%.

Start the test with 1 tablet of Naftopidil Tablets, withdraw not less than 20 mL of the medium at the specified minute after starting the test, and filter through a membrane filter with a pore size not exceeding 0.45 μm. Discard not less than 10 mL of the first filtrate, pipet V mL of the subsequent filtrate, add the dissolution medium to make exactly V' mL so that each mL contains about 28 μg of naftopidil ($C_{24}H_{28}N_2O_3$), and use this solution as the sample solution. Separately, weigh accurately about 28 mg of naftopidil for assay, previously dried at 105°C for 3 hours, dissolve in 50 mL of methanol, and add the dissolution medium to make exactly 100 mL. Pipet 5 mL of this solution, add the dissolution medium to make exactly 50 mL, and use this solution as the standard solution. Determine the absorbances, A_T and A_S, at 283 nm of the sample solution and standard solution as directed under Ultraviolet-visible Spectrophotometry <2.24>, using the dissolution medium as the control.

Dissolution rate (%) with respect to the labeled amount of naftopidil ($C_{24}H_{28}N_2O_3$)
= $M_S \times A_T/A_S \times V'/V \times 1/C \times 90$

M_S: Amount (mg) of naftopidil for assay taken
C: Labeled amount (mg) of naftopidil ($C_{24}H_{28}N_2O_3$) in 1 tablet

Assay Weigh accurately the mass of not less than 20 Naftopidil Tablets, and powder. Weigh accurately a portion of the powder, equivalent to about 50 mg of naftopidil ($C_{24}H_{28}N_2O_3$), add 30 mL of methanol, shake thoroughly, and add diluted 0.1 mol/L potassium dihydrogen phosphate TS (pH 2.0) (1 in 2) to make exactly 50 mL. Centrifuge this solution, if necessary, filter the supernatant liquid through a membrane filter with a pore size not exceeding 0.45 μm. Discard the first 10 mL of the filtrate, pipet 10 mL of the subsequent filtrate, add exactly 10 mL of the internal standard solution, add a mixture of methanol and water (3:2) to make

100 mL, and use this solution as the sample solution. Separately, weigh accurately about 50 mg of naftopidil for assay, previously dried at 105°C for 3 hours, dissolve in 30 mL of methanol, add diluted 0.1 mol/L potassium dihydrogen phosphate TS (pH 2.0) (1 in 2) to make exactly 50 mL. Pipet 10 mL of this solution, add exactly 10 mL of the internal standard solution, add a mixture of methanol and water (3:2) to make 100 mL, and use this solution as the standard solution. Perform the test with 10 μL each of the sample solution and standard solution as directed under Liquid Chromatography <*2.01*> according to the following conditions, and calculate the ratios, Q_T and Q_S of the peak area of naftopidil to that of the internal standard.

Amount (mg) of naftopidil ($C_{24}H_{28}N_2O_3$) = $M_S \times Q_T/Q_S$

M_S: Amount (mg) of naftopidil for assay taken

Internal standard solution—A solution of butyl parahydroxybenzoate in a mixture of methanol and water (3:2) (3 in 2000).

Operating conditions—

Detector, column, column temperature, mobile phase, and flow rate: Proceed as directed in the operating conditions in the Purity (2) under Naftopidil.

System suitability—

System performance: When the procedure is run with 10 μL of the standard solution under the above operating conditions, naftopidil and the internal standard are eluted in this order with the resolution between these peaks being not less than 4.

System repeatability: When the test is repeated 6 times with 10 μL of the standard solution under the above operating conditions, the relative standard deviation of the ratio of the peak area of naftopidil to that of the internal standard is not more than 1.0%.

Containers and storage Containers—Well-closed containers.

Storage—Light-resistant.

Nalidixic Acid

ナリジクス酸

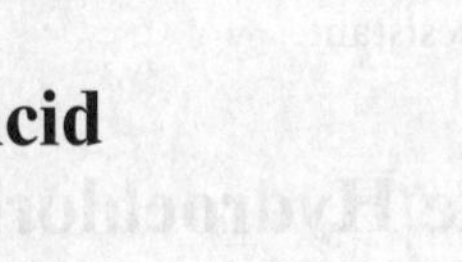

$C_{12}H_{12}N_2O_3$: 232.24

1-Ethyl-7-methyl-4-oxo-1,4-dihydro-1,8-naphthyridine-3-carboxylic acid

[389-08-2]

Nalidixic Acid, when dried, contains not less than 99.0% and not more than 101.0% of nalidixic acid ($C_{12}H_{12}N_2O_3$).

Description Nalidixic Acid occurs as white to light yellow, crystals or crystalline powder.

It is sparingly soluble in *N,N*-dimethylformamide, very slightly soluble in ethanol (99.5), and practically insoluble in water.

It dissolves in sodium hydroxide TS.

Identification **(1)** Determine the absorption spectrum of a solution of Nalidixic Acid in 0.01 mol/L sodium hydroxide TS (1 in 200,000) as directed under Ultraviolet-visible Spectrophotometry <*2.24*>, and compare the spectrum with the Reference Spectrum: both spectra exhibit similar intensities of absorption at the same wavelengths.

(2) Determine the infrared absorption spectrum of Nalidixic Acid, previously dried, as directed in the potassium bromide disk method under Infrared Spectrophotometry <*2.25*>, and compare the spectrum with the Reference Spectrum: both spectra exhibit similar intensities of absorption at the same wave numbers.

Melting point <*2.60*> 225 - 231°C

Purity **(1)** Chloride <*1.03*>—To 2.0 g of Nalidixic Acid add 50 mL of water, warm at 70°C for 5 minutes, cool quickly, and filter. To 25 mL of the filtrate add 6 mL of dilute nitric acid and water to make 50 mL, and perform the test using this solution as the test solution. Prepare the control solution with 0.35 mL of 0.01 mol/L hydrochloric acid VS (not more than 0.012%).

(2) Heavy metals <*1.07*>—Proceed with 1.0 g of Nalidixic Acid according to Method 2, and perform the test. Prepare the control solution with 2.0 mL of Standard Lead Solution (not more than 20 ppm).

(3) Related substances—Dissolve 20 mg of Nalidixic Acid in 20 mL of 0.01 mol/L sodium hydroxide TS. To 5 mL of this solution, add water to make 10 mL, and use this solution as the sample solution. Pipet 2 mL of the sample solution, add water to make exactly 1000 mL, and use this solution as the standard solution. Perform the test with exactly 10 μL each of the sample solution and standard solution as directed under Liquid Chromatography <*2.01*> according to the following conditions, and determine each peak area by the automatic integration method: the area of the peak other than nalidixic acid obtained from the sample solution is not larger than the peak area of nalidixic acid from the standard solution, and the total area of the peaks other than nalidixic acid from the sample solution is not larger than 2.5 times the peak area of nalidixic acid from the standard solution.

Operating conditions—

Detector: An ultraviolet absorption photometer (wavelength: 260 nm).

Column: A stainless steel column 4.6 mm in inside diameter and 15 cm in length, packed with octadecylsilanized silica gel for liquid chromatography (5 μm in particle diameter).

Column temperature: A constant temperature of about 40°C.

Mobile phase: Dissolve 6.24 g of sodium dihydrogen phosphate dihydrate in 950 mL of water, adjust the pH to 2.8 with phosphoric acid, and add water to make 1000 mL. To 300 mL of this solution add 200 mL of methanol.

Flow rate: Adjust so that the retention time of nalidixic acid is about 19 minutes.

Time span of measurement: About 3 times as long as the retention time of nalidixic acid, beginning after the solvent peak.

System suitability—

Test for required detectability: Pipet 5 mL of the standard solution, and add water to make exactly 10 mL. Confirm that the peak area of nalidixic acid obtained with 10 μL of this solution is equivalent to 40 to 60% of that with 10 μL of the standard solution.

System performance: Dissolve 25 mg of methyl parahydroxybenzoate in 100 mL of a mixture of water and methanol (1:1). To 1 mL of this solution add water to make 10 mL. To 5 mL of this solution add 5 mL of the standard solution. When the procedure is run with 10 μL of this solution under the above operating conditions, methyl parahydroxybenzoate and nalidixic acid are eluted in this order with the resolution between these peaks being not less than 13.

System repeatability: When the test is repeated 6 times with 10 μL of the standard solution under the above operating conditions, the relative standard deviation of the peak area of nalidixic acid is not more than 2.0%.

Loss on drying 〈*2.41*〉 Not more than 0.20% (1 g, 105°C, 3 hours).

Residue on ignition 〈*2.44*〉 Not more than 0.2% (1 g).

Assay Weigh accurately about 0.3 g of Nalidixic Acid, previously dried, dissolve in 50 mL of *N,N*-dimethylformamide, and titrate 〈*2.50*〉 with 0.1 mol/L tetramethyl ammonium hydroxide VS (potentiometric titration). Separately, to 50 mL of *N,N*-dimethylformamide add 13 mL of a mixture of water and methanol (89:11), perform a blank determination with the solution in the same manner, and make any necessary correction.

Each mL of 0.1 mol/L tetramethyl ammonium hydroxide VS
= 23.22 mg of $C_{12}H_{12}N_2O_3$

Containers and storage Containers—Tight containers.

Naloxone Hydrochloride

ナロキソン塩酸塩

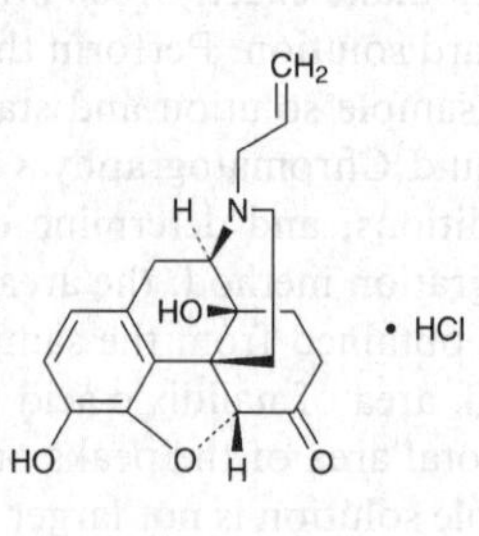

$C_{19}H_{21}NO_4.HCl$: 363.84
(5*R*,14*S*)-17-Allyl-4,5-epoxy-3,14-dihydroxymorphinan-6-one monohydrochloride
[*357-08-4*]

Naloxone Hydrochloride contains not less than 98.5% of naloxone hydrochloride ($C_{19}H_{21}NO_4.HCl$), calculated on the dried basis.

Description Naloxone Hydrochloride occurs as white to yellowish white, crystals or crystalline powder.

It is freely soluble in water, soluble in methanol, slightly soluble in ethanol (99.5) and in acetic acid (100), and very slightly soluble in acetic anhydride.

It is hygroscopic.

It is gradually colored by light.

Identification **(1)** Determine the absorption spectrum of a solution of Naloxone Hydrochloride (1 in 10,000) as directed under Ultraviolet-visible Spectrophotometry 〈*2.24*〉, and compare the spectrum with the Reference Spectrum: both spectra exhibit similar intensities of absorption at the same wavelengths.

(2) Determine the infrared absorption spectrum of Naloxone Hydrochloride, previously dried, as directed in the potassium chloride disk method under Infrared Spectrophotometry 〈*2.25*〉, and compare the spectrum with the Reference Spectrum: both spectra exhibit similar intensities of absorption at the same wave numbers.

(3) A solution of Naloxone Hydrochloride (1 in 50) responds to Qualitative Tests 〈*1.09*〉 (2) for chloride.

Optical rotation 〈*2.49*〉 $[\alpha]_D^{25}$: −170 − −181° (0.25 g calculated on the dried basis, water, 10 mL, 100 mm).

pH 〈*2.54*〉 Dissolve 0.10 g of Naloxone Hydrochloride in 10 mL of freshly boiled and cooled water: the pH of the solution is between 4.5 and 5.5.

Purity Related substances—Conduct this procedure as rapidly as possible without exposure to light, using light-resistant containers. Dissolve 0.08 g of Naloxone Hydrochloride in 10 mL of methanol, and use this solution as the sample solution. Pipet 1 mL of the sample solution, add methanol to make exactly 200 mL, and use this solution as the standard solution. Perform the test with these solutions as directed under Thin-layer Chromatography 〈*2.03*〉. Spot 10 μL each of the sample solution and standard solution on a plate of silica gel for thin-layer chromatography. Develop with a mixture of ammonia-saturated 1-butanol TS and methanol (20:1) to a distance of about 12 cm, and air-dry the plate. Spray evenly iron (III) chloride-potassium hexacyanoferrate (III) TS on the plate: the number of the spot other than the principal spot from the sample solution is not more than 1 and it is not more intense than the spot from the standard solution.

Loss on drying 〈*2.41*〉 Not more than 2.0% [0.1 g, 105°C, 5 hours. Use a desiccator (phosphorus (V) oxide) for cooling].

Residue on ignition 〈*2.44*〉 Not more than 0.2% (0.1 g).

Assay Weigh accurately about 0.3 g of Naloxone Hydrochloride, dissolve in 80 mL of acetic acid (100) by warming. After cooling, add 80 mL of acetic anhydride, and titrate 〈*2.50*〉 with 0.1 mol/L perchloric acid VS (potentiometric titration). Perform a blank determination in the same manner, and make any necessary correction.

Each mL of 0.1 mol/L perchloric acid VS
= 36.38 mg of $C_{19}H_{21}NO_4.HCl$

Containers and storage Containers—Tight containers.
Storage—Light-resistant.

Naphazoline Hydrochloride

ナファゾリン塩酸塩

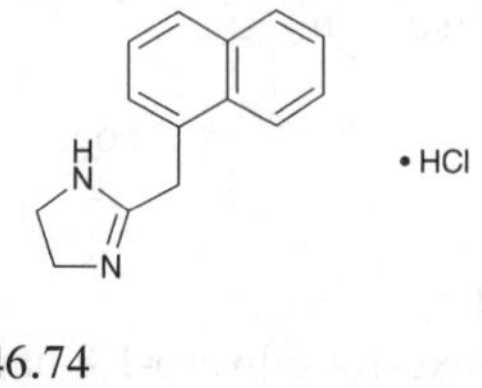

$C_{14}H_{14}N_2.HCl$: 246.74
2-(Naphthalen-1-ylmethyl)-4,5-dihydro-1*H*-imidazole monohydrochloride
[*550-99-2*]

Naphazoline Hydrochloride, when dried, contains not less than 98.5% of naphazoline hydrochloride ($C_{14}H_{14}N_2.HCl$).

Description Naphazoline Hydrochloride occurs as a white crystalline powder. It is odorless, and has a bitter taste.

It is freely soluble in water, soluble in ethanol (95) and in acetic acid (100), very slightly soluble in acetic anhydride, and practically insoluble in diethyl ether.

Melting point: 255 - 260°C (with decomposition).

Identification **(1)** To 10 mL of a solution of Naphazoline

Hydrochloride (1 in 100) add 5 mL of bromine TS, and boil: a deep purple color develops.

(2) To 30 mL of a solution of Naphazoline Hydrochloride (1 in 100) add 2 mL of sodium hydroxide TS, and extract with two 25-mL portions of diethyl ether. Evaporate the combined diethyl ether extracts to dryness with the aid of a current of air. Dry the residue at 80°C for 1 hour: the residue melts ⟨*2.60*⟩ between 117°C and 120°C.

(3) Dissolve 0.02 g of the residue obtained in (2) in 2 to 3 drops of dilute hydrochloric acid and 5 mL of water, and add 2 mL of Reinecke salt TS: a red-purple, crystalline precipitate is formed.

(4) A solution of Naphazoline Hydrochloride (1 in 10) responds to Qualitative Tests ⟨*1.09*⟩ for chloride.

pH ⟨*2.54*⟩ Dissolve 0.10 g of Naphazoline Hydrochloride in 10 mL of freshly boiled and cooled water: the pH of the solution is between 5.0 and 7.0.

Purity **(1)** Clarity and color of solution—Dissolve 1.0 g of Naphazoline Hydrochloride in 10 mL of water: the solution is clear and colorless.

(2) Heavy metals ⟨*1.07*⟩—Proceed with 1.0 g of Naphazoline Hydrochloride according to Method 2, and perform the test. Prepare the control solution with 2.0 mL of Standard Lead Solution (not more than 20 ppm).

Loss on drying ⟨*2.41*⟩ Not more than 0.5% (1 g, 105°C, 2 hours).

Residue on ignition ⟨*2.44*⟩ Not more than 0.1% (1 g).

Assay Weigh accurately about 0.4 g of Naphazoline Hydrochloride, previously dried, dissolve in 50 mL of a mixture of acetic anhydride and acetic acid (100) (7:3), and titrate ⟨*2.50*⟩ with 0.1 mol/L perchloric acid VS (potentiometric titration). Perform a blank determination in the same manner, and make any necessary correction.

Each mL of 0.1 mol/L perchloric acid VS
= 24.67 mg of $C_{14}H_{14}N_2.HCl$

Containers and storage Containers—Tight containers.
Storage—Light-resistant.

Naphazoline Nitrate

ナファゾリン硝酸塩

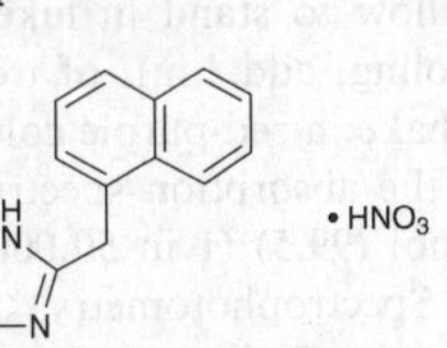

$C_{14}H_{14}N_2.HNO_3$: 273.29
2-(Naphthalen-1-ylmethyl)-4,5-dihydro-1*H*-imidazole mononitrate
[*5144-52-5*]

Naphazoline Nitrate, when dried, contains not less than 98.5% of naphazoline nitrate ($C_{14}H_{14}N_2.HNO_3$).

Description Naphazoline Nitrate occurs as a white crystalline powder. It is odorless, and has a bitter taste.

It is freely soluble in acetic acid (100), soluble in ethanol (95), sparingly soluble in water, slightly soluble in acetic anhydride, and practically insoluble in diethyl ether.

Identification **(1)** To 10 mL of a solution of Naphazoline Nitrate (1 in 100) add 5 mL of bromine TS, and boil: a deep purple color develops.

(2) To 20 mL of a solution of Naphazoline Nitrate (1 in 100) add 5 mL of sodium hydroxide TS, and extract with two 25-mL portions of diethyl ether. Combine the diethyl ether extracts, evaporate to dryness with the aid of a current of air, and dry the residue at 80°C for 1 hour: the residue so obtained melts ⟨*2.60*⟩ between 117°C and 120°C.

(3) A solution of Naphazoline Nitrate (1 in 20) responds to Qualitative Tests ⟨*1.09*⟩ for nitrate.

pH ⟨*2.54*⟩ Dissolve 0.1 g of Naphazoline Nitrate in 10 mL of freshly boiled and cooled water: the pH of the solution is between 5.0 and 7.0.

Melting point ⟨*2.60*⟩ 167 - 170°C

Purity **(1)** Clarity and color of solution—Dissolve 0.5 g of Naphazoline Nitrate in 50 mL of water: the solution is clear and colorless.

(2) Heavy metals ⟨*1.07*⟩—Proceed with 1.0 g of Naphazoline Nitrate according to Method 2, and perform the test. Prepare the control solution with 2.0 mL of Standard Lead Solution (not more than 20 ppm).

Loss on drying ⟨*2.41*⟩ Not more than 0.5% (1 g, 105°C, 2 hours).

Residue on ignition ⟨*2.44*⟩ Not more than 0.1% (1 g).

Assay Weigh accurately about 0.4 g of Naphazoline Nitrate, previously dried, dissolve in 50 mL of a mixture of acetic anhydride and acetic acid (100) (4:1), and titrate ⟨*2.50*⟩ with 0.1 mol/L perchloric acid VS (indicator: 3 drops of crystal violet TS). Perform a blank determination in the same manner, and make any necessary correction.

Each mL of 0.1 mol/L perchloric acid VS
= 27.33 mg of $C_{14}H_{14}N_2.HNO_3$

Containers and storage Containers—Tight containers.
Storage—Light-resistant.

Naphazoline and Chlorpheniramine Solution

ナファゾリン・クロルフェニラミン液

Naphazoline and Chlorpheniramine Solution contains not less than 0.045 w/v% and not more than 0.055 w/v% of naphazoline nitrate ($C_{14}H_{14}N_2.HNO_3$: 273.29), and not less than 0.09 w/v% and not more than 0.11 w/v% of chlorpheniramine maleate ($C_{16}H_{19}ClN_2.C_4H_4O_4$: 390.86).

Method of preparation

Naphazoline Nitrate	0.5 g
Chlorpheniramine Maleate	1 g
Chlorobutanol	2 g
Glycerin	50 mL
Purified Water or Purified Water in Containers	a sufficient quantity
	To make 1000 mL

Dissolve, and mix the above ingredients.

Description Naphazoline and Chlorpheniramine Solution is a clear, colorless liquid.

Identification **(1)** To 20 mL of Naphazoline and Chlorpheniramine Solution add 2 mL of a solution of potassium hydroxide (7 in 10) and 5 mL of pyridine, and heat at 100°C for 5 minutes: a red color is produced (chlorobutanol).

(2) Place 10 mL of Naphazoline and Chlorpheniramine Solution in a glass-stoppered test tube, add 10 mL of ethanol (95), 2 mL of sodium hydroxide TS and 1 mL of a solution of copper (II) chloride dihydrate in ethanol (95) (1 in 10), and shake: a blue color is produced (glycerin).

(3) To 20 mL of Naphazoline and Chlorpheniramine Solution add 5 mL of sodium hydroxide TS, extract with 10 mL of diethyl ether, and separate the diethyl ether layer. Take 5 mL of this solution, distil off the solvent, dissolve the residue in 5 mL of methanol, and use this solution as the sample solution. Separately, dissolve 0.01 g each of naphazoline nitrate and Chlorpheniramine Maleate RS in 10 mL and 5 mL of methanol, respectively, and use these solutions as standard solutions (1) and (2). Perform the test with these solutions as directed under Thin-layer Chromatography *<2.03>*. Spot 5 μL each of the sample solution and standard solutions on a plate of silica gel with fluorescent indicator for thin-layer chromatography. Develop the plate with a mixture of chloroform, methanol, acetone and ammonia solution (28) (73:15:10:2) to a distance of about 10 cm, and air-dry the plate. Examine under ultraviolet light (main wavelength: 254 nm): two spots obtained from the sample solution exhibit the same *Rf* values as the spots from standard solutions (1) and (2). Spray evenly Dragendorff's TS on the plate: the spots from standard solutions (1) and (2) and the corresponding spot from the sample solutions reveal an orange color.

Assay Pipet 4 mL of Naphazoline and Chlorpheniramine Solution, add exactly 4 mL of the internal standard solution, then add water to make 10 mL, and use this solution as the sample solution. Weigh accurately about 50 mg of naphazoline nitrate for assay, dried at 105°C for 2 hours, and about 0.1 g of Chlorpheniramine Maleate RS, dried at 105°C for 3 hours, dissolve in water to make exactly 100 mL. Pipet 4 mL of this solution, add exactly 4 mL of the internal standard solution, then add water to make 10 mL, and use this solution as the standard solution. Perform the test with 10 μL each of the sample solution and standard solutions as directed under Liquid Chromatography *<2.01>* according to the following conditions, and calculate the ratios, Q_{Ta} and Q_{Tb}, of the peak height of naphazoline and chlorpheniramine to that of the internal standard of the sample solution, and the ratios, Q_{Sa} and Q_{Sb}, of the peak height of naphazoline and chlorpheniramine to that of the internal standard of the standard solution.

Amount (mg) of naphazoline nitrate ($C_{14}H_{14}N_2.HNO_3$)
$= M_{Sa} \times Q_{Ta}/Q_{Sa} \times 1/25$

Amount (mg) of chlorpheniramine maleate ($C_{16}H_{19}ClN_2.C_4H_4O_4$)
$= M_{Sb} \times Q_{Tb}/Q_{Sb} \times 1/25$

M_{Sa}: Amount (mg) of naphazoline nitrate for assay taken
M_{Sb}: Amount (mg) of Chlorpheniramine Maleate RS taken

Internal standard solution—A solution of ethenzamide in methanol (1 in 1000).

Operating conditions—

Detector: An ultraviolet absorption photometer (wavelength: 254 nm).

Column: A stainless steel column, about 4 mm in inside diameter and 25 to 30 cm in length, packed with octadecylsilanized silica gel for liquid chromatography (5 μm in particle diameter).

Column temperature: Room temperature.

Mobile phase: A mixture of acetonitrile and a solution of sodium laurylsulfate (1 in 500) in diluted phosphoric acid (1 in 1000) (1:1).

Flow rate: Adjust so that the retention time of chlorpheniramine is about 10 minutes.

Selection of column: Proceed with 10 μL of the standard solution under the above operating conditions. Use a column giving well-resolved peaks of the internal standard, naphazoline and chlorpheniramine in this order.

Containers and storage Containers—Tight containers.
Storage—Light-resistant.

Naproxen

ナプロキセン

$C_{14}H_{14}O_3$: 230.26
(2*S*)-2-(6-Methoxynaphthalen-2-yl)propanoic acid
[22204-53-1]

Naproxen, when dried, contains not less than 98.5% of naproxen ($C_{14}H_{14}O_3$).

Description Naproxen occurs as white, crystals or crystalline powder. It is odorless.

It is freely soluble in acetone, soluble in methanol, in ethanol (99.5) and in chloroform, sparingly soluble in diethyl ether, and practically insoluble in water.

It dissolves in sodium hydroxide TS.

Identification **(1)** Dissolve 0.01 g of Naproxen in 5 mL of methanol, add 5 mL of water, then add 2 mL of potassium iodide TS and 5 mL of a solution of potassium iodate (1 in 100), and shake: a yellow to yellow-brown color develops. To this solution add 5 mL of chloroform, and shake: a light red-purple color develops in the chloroform layer.

(2) To 1 mL of a solution of Naproxen in ethanol (99.5) (1 in 300) add 4 mL of hydroxylamine perchlorate-ethanol TS and 1 mL of *N,N'*-dicyclohexylcarbodiimide-ethanol TS, shake well, and allow to stand in lukewarm water for 20 minutes. After cooling, add 1 mL of iron (III) perchlorate-ethanol TS, and shake: a red-purple color develops.

(3) Determine the absorption spectrum of a solution of Naproxen in ethanol (99.5) (1 in 50,000) as directed under Ultraviolet-visible Spectrophotometry *<2.24>*, and compare the spectrum with the Reference Spectrum: both spectra exhibit similar intensities of absorption at the same wavelengths.

(4) Determine the infrared absorption spectrum of Naproxen, previously dried, as directed in the potassium bromide disk method under Infrared Spectrophotometry *<2.25>*, and compare the spectrum with the Reference Spectrum: both spectra exhibit similar intensities of absorption at the same wave numbers.

Optical rotation *<2.49>* $[\alpha]_D^{25}$: +63.0 – +68.5° (after drying, 0.1 g, chloroform, 10 mL, 100 mm).

Melting point *<2.60>* 154 – 158°C

Purity **(1)** Clarity and color of solution—Dissolve 2.0 g of Naproxen in 20 mL of acetone: the solution is clear. Perform the test with this solution as directed under Ultraviolet-visible Spectrophotometry <*2.24*>: the absorbance at 400 nm is not more than 0.070.

(2) Heavy metals <*1.07*>—Proceed with 2.0 g of Naproxen according to Method 2, and perform the test. Prepare the control solution with 2.0 mL of Standard Lead Solution (not more than 10 ppm).

(3) Arsenic <*1.11*>—Prepare the test solution with 2.0 g of Naproxen according to Method 3, and perform the test (not more than 1 ppm).

(4) Related substances—Conduct this procedure without exposure to light, using light-resistant vessels. Dissolve 0.10 g of Naproxen in 10 mL of a mixture of ethanol (99.5) and chloroform (1:1), and use this solution as the sample solution. Pipet 2 mL of the sample solution, and add a mixture of ethanol (99.5) and chloroform (1:1) to make exactly 100 mL. Pipet 5 mL of this solution, add a mixture of ethanol (99.5) and chloroform (1:1) to make exactly 50 mL, and use this solution as the standard solution. Perform the test with these solutions as directed under Thin-layer Chromatography <*2.03*>. Spot 10 μL each of the sample solution and standard solution on a plate of silica gel with fluorescent indicator for thin-layer chromatography. Develop the plate with a mixture of hexane, dichloromethane, tetrahydrofuran and acetic acid (100) (50:30:17:3) to a distance of about 12 cm, and air-dry the plate. Examine under ultraviolet light (main wavelength: 254 nm): the spots other than the principal spot and the spot of the starting point obtained from the sample solution are not more intense than the spot from the standard solution.

Loss on drying <*2.41*> Not more than 0.5% (1 g, 105°C, 3 hours).

Residue on ignition <*2.44*> Not more than 0.1% (1 g).

Assay Weigh accurately about 0.5g of Naproxen, previously dried, add 100 mL of diluted methanol (4 in 5), dissolve by gentle warming if necessary, and titrate <*2.50*> with 0.1 mol/L sodium hydroxide VS (indicator: 3 drops of phenolphthalein TS). Perform a blank determination in the same manner, and make any necessary correction.

Each mL of 0.1 mol/L sodium hydroxide VS
= 23.03 mg of $C_{14}H_{14}O_3$

Containers and storage Containers—Well-closed containers.

Storage—Light-resistant.

Nartograstim (Genetical Recombination)

ナルトグラスチム(遺伝子組換え)

```
MAPTYRASSL PQSFLLKSLE QVRKIQGDGA ALQEKLCATY KLCHPEELVL
LGHSLGIPWA PLSSCPSQAL QLAGCLSQLH SGLFLYQGLL QALEGISPEL
GPTLDTLQLD VADFATTIWQ QMEELGMAPA LQPTQGAMPA FASAFQRRAG
GVLVASHLQS FLEVSYRVLR HLAQP
```

$C_{850}H_{1344}N_{226}O_{245}S_8$: 18905.65
[*134088-74-7*]

Nartograstim (Genetical Recombination) is an aqueous solution in which a desired product is a recombinant human granulocyte colony-stimulating factor (G-CSF) analog. It is *N*-methionylated, and threonine, leucine, glycine, proline and cysteine residues at the positions, 1, 3, 4, 5 and 17 of G-CSF are substituted by alanine, threonine, tyrosine, arginine and serine, respectively. It is a glycoprotein consisting of 175 amino acid residues.

It contains not less than 0.9 mg and not more than 2.1 mg of protein per mL, and not less than 4.0 × 10^8 units per mg of protein.

Description Nartograstim (Genetical Recombination) occurs as a clear and colorless, liquid.

Identification **(1)** To a suitable amount of Nartograstim (Genetical Recombination) add tris-sodium chloride buffer solution (pH 8.0) so that each mL contains 1 μg of protein, and use this solution as the sample solution. Put 0.1 mL of the sample solution in the well of a 96-well microplate, allow to stand at 5°C for not less than 10 hours, then remove the liquid, and wash the well. Then to the well add 0.25 mL of blocking TS for nartograstim test, and allow to stand at room temperature for 1 hour. Remove the blocking TS, add 0.1 mL of rabbit anti-nartograstim antibody TS to the well, and shake gently at room temperature for 3 hours. Remove the rabbit anti-nartograstim antibody TS, and wash the well. Then, add 0.1 mL of peroxidase labeled anti-rabbit antibody TS, shake gently at room temperature for 2 hours, remove the TS, and wash the well. Then, add 0.1 mL of 2,2′-azinobis(3-ethylbenzothiazoline-6-sulfonic acid) diammonium salt TS, allow to stand at room temperature for 10 minutes, add 0.1 mL of a solution of oxalic acid dihydrate (1 in 50), and name this well as the sample well. Separately, proceed with 0.1 mL of tris-sodium chloride buffer solution (pH 8.0) in the same manner as for the sample solution, and name the well so obtained as the control well. When compare the sample well and the control well, the sample well reveals a green color, while the control well reveals no color.

Washing procedure of well: To the well add 0.25 mL of washing fluid for nartograstim test, allow to stand for 3 minutes, and remove the washing fluid. Repeat this procedure 2 times more.

(2) To a suitable amount of Nartograstim (Genetical Recombination) add water so that each mL contains 1 mg of protein. Replace the solvent of 2 mL of this solution with tris-calcium chloride buffer solution (pH 6.5). To 0.5 mL of the solution so obtained add 0.5 mL of tris-calcium chloride buffer solution (pH 6.5) and 5 μL of thermolysin solution (1 in 1000), allow to stand at 37°C for 21 hours, and use this solution as the sample solution. Separately, proceed with 2 mL of Nartograstim RS in the same manner as for the sample solution, and use the solution so obtained as the standard solution. Perform the test with 20 μL each of the sample solution and standard solution as directed under Liquid Chromatography <*2.01*> according to the following conditions, and compare these chromatograms: the similar peaks appear at the same retention times.

Operating conditions—

Detector: An ultraviolet absorption photometer (wavelength: 220 nm).

Column: A stainless steel column 6 mm in inside diameter and 15 cm in length, packed with octadecylsilanized silica gel for liquid chromatography (5 μm in particle diameter).

Column temperature: A constant temperature of about 35°C.

Mobile phase A: A mixture of water and trifluoroacetic acid (1000:1).

Mobile phase B: A mixture of acetonitrile, water and trifluoroacetic acid (900:100:1).

Flowing of mobile phase: Control the gradient by mixing the mobile phases A and B as directed in the following table.

Time after injection of sample (min)	Mobile phase A (vol%)	Mobile phase B (vol%)
0 – 5	100	0
5 – 90	100 → 40	0 → 60

Flow rate: 1.0 mL per minute.

System suitability—

System performance: When the procedure is run with 20 μL of the standard solution under the above conditions, the number of the peak which shows not less than 1.6 of the resolution between the adjacent peaks is not less than 15.

Molecular mass To a suitable amount of Nartograstim (Genetical Recombination) add reduction buffer solution for nartograstim sample so that each mL contains about 0.5 mg of protein, and use this solution as the sample solution. Separately, to 50 μL of molecular mass marker for nartograstim test add reduction buffer solution for nartograstim sample to make 1.0 mL, and use this solution as the standard solution. Perform the test with 10 μL each of the sample solution and standard solution, both previously warmed at 40°C for 15 minutes, by SDS polyacrylamide gel electrophoresis, using buffer solution for SDS polyacrylamide gel electrophoresis and polyacrylamide gel for nartograstim. After electrophoresis, immerse the gel in a solution of coomassie brilliant blue R-250 in a mixture of water, ethanol (95) and acetic acid (100) (5:4:1) (1 in 1000), and stir gently at room temperature for not less than 12 hours. Then, destain the gel with a mixture of water, ethanol (95) and acetic acid (100) (13:5:2), and dry the gel under reduced pressure. Prepare a calibration curve from the migration distance of the molecular mass markers of the standard solution by plotting the migration distance on the horizontal axis and logarithm of the molecular mass on the vertical axis. Calculate the molecular mass of the sample solution from the calibration curve: the molecular mass of the main band is between 17,000 and 19,000.

Compositions ratio of related substance Being specified separately when the drug is granted approval based on the Law.

pH <*2.54*> 7.0 – 7.5

Purity (1) Related substances—To a suitable amount of Nartograstim (Genetical Recombination) add the buffer solution for nartograstim sample so that each mL contains about 0.5 mg of protein, and use this solution as the sample solution. Pipet 1 mL of the sample solution, add the buffer solution for nartograstim sample to make exactly 100 mL, and use this solution as the standard solution. Perform the test with exactly 10 μL each of the sample solution and standard solution by SDS polyacrylamide gel electrophoresis, using buffer solution for SDS polyacrylamide gel electrophoresis and polyacrylamide gel for nartograstim. After electrophoresis, immerse the gel in a solution of coomassie brilliant blue R-250 in a mixture of water, ethanol (95) and acetic acid (100) (5:4:1) (1 in 1000), and stir gently at room temperature for not less than 12 hours. Then, destain the gel with a mixture of water, ethanol (95) and acetic acid (100) (13:5:2), and dry the gel under reduced pressure. Determine the areas of the colored bands obtained from the sample solution and standard solution by a densitometer at the measure wavelength 560 nm and the control wavelength 400 nm: the total area of the band other than the principal band obtained from the sample solution is not larger than the band area from the standard solution.

(2) Host cell protein—Being specified separately when the drug is granted approval based on the Law.

(3) Host cell DNA—Being specified separately when the drug is granted approval based on the Law.

Bacterial endotoxins <*4.01*> Less than 0.62 EU/μg.

Assay (1) Protein content—To exactly V_1 mL of Nartograstim (Genetical Recombination) add exactly V_2 mL of water so that each mL contains about 0.5 mg of protein, and centrifuge. Determine the absorbance, A, of the supernatant liquid at the absorption maximum at about 280 nm as directed under Ultraviolet-visible Spectrophotometry <*2.24*>.

Amount (mg) of protein in 1 mL of Nartograstim (Genetical Recombination)

$$= A/8.71 \times (V_1 + V_2)/V_1 \times 10$$

8.71: Specific absorbance

(2) Specific activity—To a suitable exact amount of Nartograstim (Genetical Recombination) add potency measuring medium for nartograstim test so that the potency is equivalent to 50% to 150% of the relative potency of the standard solution according to the expected potency, and use this solution as the sample solution. Separately, to a suitable exact amount of Nartograstim RS add an exact amount of the potency measuring medium for nartograstim test so that each mL contains exactly 1.2×10^4 units of nartograstim, and use this solution as the standard solution. Culture NFS-60 cells with subculture medium for nartograstim test, centrifuge the medium, remove the supernatant liquid by suction, and wash the cells with the potency measuring medium for nartograstim test. Repeat the washing procedure twice more, prepare two cell suspensions, containing 8×10^5 cells per mL and 4×10^5 cells per mL in the potency measuring medium for nartograstim test, and use these solutions as the cell suspension (1) and (2), respectively. In 8 wells of the 12th column of a 8 × 12 well-microplate put 50 μL each of the cell suspension (1), and in all wells of the 1st to 11th columns put 50 μL each of the cell suspension (2). Where, the wells of the 1st and 8th lines are not used for the test. To the wells of the 2nd to 4th lines of the 12th column add 50 μL each of the standard solution, and to the wells of 5th to 7th lines of the 12th column add 50 μL each of the sample solution. From the wells of the 12th column take 50 μL each of the content liquid and transfer to the corresponding wells of the 1st column. Then, from the wells of the 1st column take 50 μL each of the content liquid and transfer to the corresponding wells of the 2nd column. Proceed in the same way sequentially to the 10th column to prepare two-fold serial dilution wells. The wells of the 11th column are not performed any process. Incubate the plate under the atmosphere of 5 vol% carbon dioxide at 37°C for about 40 hours. After incubation, add to the all wells 10 μL each of 3-(4,5-dimethylthiazol-2-yl)-2,5-diphenyl-2*H*-tetrazolium bromide TS, and allow to stand under the atmosphere of 5 vol% carbon dioxide at 37°C for 4 – 6 hours. Add 0.125 mL of dimethylsulfoxide, shake for 5 to 10 minutes, then determine the absorbances of all wells at 550 nm and 660 nm, A_1 and A_2, using a spectrophotometer for microplate, and calculate the difference, $(A_1 - A_2)$. Divide by 6 the total of the differences $(A_1 - A_2)$ of six wells of the 11th and the 1st column, which were added the standard solution, and use the value so obtained as the 50% absorbance, A_M. Determine the dilution index numbers (column number) of the two serial wells of the sample solution and standard solution, they are corresponding to just the before and after of the 50% absorbance (A_M), n_{T1}, n_{T2} and n_{S1}, n_{S2}, respectively, where $n_{T1} < n_{T2}$ and

$n_{S1} < n_{S2}$. Differences of the absorbance of the serial wells are named as A_{T1}, A_{T2} and A_{S1}, A_{S2}, respectively. Calculate the relative potencies of each sample solution by the following equation using the mean value of the three standard solutions, and average them. Perform the same procedure by reversing the place of the sample solution and the standard solution. Then, calculate the mean relative potency by averaging both values.

$$\text{Relative potency of the sample solution} = \frac{2^a}{\Sigma 2^b \times \frac{1}{3}}$$

a: $n_{T1} + (A_{T1} - A_M)/(A_{T1} - A_{T2})$
b: $n_{S1} + (A_{S1} - A_M)/(A_{S1} - A_{S2})$

Obtain the potency per mL by the following equation, and calculate the potency per mg of protein using the protein content obtained in (1).

Amount (unit) of nartograstim per mL of Nartograstim (Genetical Recombination)
$= S \times$ mean relative potency of the sample solution $\times d$

S: Concentration (unit/mL) of the standard solution
d: Dilution factor for the sample solution

System suitability—

The absorbance difference of the individual wells of the standard solution of the 3rd column should be not less than A_M, and that of the individual wells of the 8th column should be not more than A_M. If they do not meet the requirements, prepare the standard solution of the range of 1.0×10^3 to 1.6×10^4 units, and perform the test.

Containers and storage Containers—Tight containers.
Storage—Not exceeding −20°C.

Nartograstim for Injection (Genetical Recombination)

注射用ナルトグラスチム(遺伝子組換え)

Nartograstim for Injection (Genetical Recombination) is a preparation for injection which is dissolved before use.

It contains not less than 90.0% and not more than 110.0% of the labeled amount of nartograstim (genetical recombination) ($C_{850}H_{1344}N_{226}O_{245}S_8$: 18905.65).

Method of preparation Prepare as directed under Injections, with Nartograstim (Genetical Recombination).

Description Nartograstim for Injection (Genetical Recombination) occurs as white, masses or powder.

Identification Dissolve the content of 1 package of Nartograstim for Injection (Genetical Recombination) in 1 mL of tris-sodium chloride buffer solution (pH 8.0). To a suitable amount of this solution add tris-sodium chloride buffer solution (pH 8.0) so that each mL contains 1 μg of Nartograstim (Genetical Recombination), and use this solution as the sample solution. Then, proceed with the sample solution as directed in the Identification (1) under Nartograstim (Genetical Recombination).

pH <2.54> Being specified separately when the drug is granted approval based on the Law.

Purity **(1)** Clarity and color of solution—A solution of Nartograstim for Injection (Genetical Recombination) in water, containing 100 μg of Nartograstim (Genetical Recombination) in each mL, is clear and colorless.

(2) Lactose conjugate—Being specified separately when the drug is granted approval based on the Law.

Water <2.48> Not more than 3.0% (50 mg, coulometric titration).

Bacterial endotoxins <4.01> Less than 0.62 EU/μg.

Uniformity of dosage units <6.02> It meets the requirement of the Mass variation test.

Foreign insoluble matter <6.06> Perform the test according to Method 2, using 3 mL of water for injection per 1 Nartograstim for Injection (Genetical Recombination) to dissolve the content: it meets the requirement.

Insoluble particulate matter <6.07> It meets the requirement.

Sterility <4.06> Perform the test according to the Membrane filtration method, using the sample solution prepared by dissolving the sample in water in a concentration to be used for the injection: it meets the requirement.

Specific activity Nartograstim for Injection (Genetical Recombination), when perform the assay and the following test, contains not less than 4.0×10^8 units of nartograstim (genetical recombination) per mg nartograstim (genetical recombination).

Wash out each content of 10 Nartograstim for Injection (Genetical Recombination) with a suitable amount of potency measuring medium for nartograstim test, wash the empty containers with the same medium, combine all washings, and add the same medium to make exactly 50 mL. To an exact amount of this solution add the same medium so that the concentration of nartograstim (genetical recombination) is equivalent to 50% to 150% of that of the standard solution, and use this solution as the sample solution. Separately, weigh accurately a suitable amount of Nartograstim RS, dissolve in the potency measuring medium for nartograstim test so that each mL contains exactly 1.2×10^4 units of nartograstim according to the labeled unit, and use this solution as the standard solution. Then, determine the nartograstim potency (unit) in 1 Nartograstim for Injection (Genetical Recombination) by proceeding as directed in the Assay (2) under Nartograstim (Genetical Recombination), and calculate the ratio against the amount of nartograstim obtained in the Assay.

Nartograstim (genetical recombination) potency (unit) in 1 Nartograstim for Injection (Genetical Recombination)
$= S \times$ mean relative potency of the sample solution $\times d \times 5$

S: Concentration (unit/mL) of the standard solution
d: Dilution factor for the sample solution
5: Amount (mL) of the medium used to dissolve per 1 sample

$$\text{Relative activity of sample solution} = \frac{2^a}{\Sigma 2^b \times \frac{1}{3}}$$

a: $n_{T1} + (A_{T1} - A_M)/(A_{T1} - A_{T2})$
b: $n_{S1} + (A_{S1} - A_M)/(A_{S1} - A_{S2})$

System suitability—

Proceed as directed in the system suitability in the Assay (2) under Nartograstim (Genetical Recombination).

Assay Weigh accurately the mass of each content of not

less than 10 Nartograstim for Injection (Genetical Recombination). Weigh accurately an amount of the content, equivalent to about 0.25 mg of Nartograstim (Genetical Recombination), dissolve in exactly 5 mL of the mobile phase, and use this solution as the sample solution. Separately, dissolve a suitable amount of Nartograstim RS in the mobile phase so that each mL contains about 50 μg of nartograstim, and use this solution as the standard solution. Perform the test with exactly 100 μL each of the sample solution and standard solution as directed under Liquid Chromatography 〈*2.01*〉 according to the following conditions, and determine the peak areas, A_T and A_S, of nartograstim in each solution.

Amount (μg) of nartograstim (genetical recombination) in 1 Nartograstim for Injection (Genetical Recombination)
$= M_S \times A_T/A_S \times M/M_T \times 5$

M_S: Amount (μg) of nartograstim in 1 mL of the standard solution
M: Mean mass (mg) of each content
M_T: Amount (mg) of Nartograstim for Injection (Genetical Recombination) taken

Operating conditions—

Detector: An ultraviolet absorption photometer (wavelength: 280 nm).

Column: A stainless steel column 7.8 mm in inside diameter and 30 cm in length, packed with porous silica gel for liquid chromatography (5 μm in particle diameter).

Column temperature: A constant temperature of about 25°C.

Mobile phase: Dissolve 15.6 g of sodium dihydrogen phosphate dihydrate and 1.0 g of sodium lauryl sulfate in 700 mL of water, adjust to pH 6.5 with sodium hydroxide TS, and add water to make 1000 mL.

Flow rate: Adjust so that the retention time of nartograstim is about 16 minutes.

System suitability—

System performance: When the procedure is run with 100 μL of the standard solution under the above operating conditions, the number of theoretical plates and the symmetry factor of the peak of nartograstim are not less than 3000 and not more than 2.0, respectively.

System repeatability: When the test is repeated 6 times with 100 μL of the standard solution under the above operating conditions, the relative standard deviation of the peak area of nartograstim is not more than 1.5%.

Containers and storage Containers—Hermetic containers.

Storage—Light-resistant, and at a temperature not exceeding 10°C.

Nateglinide

ナテグリニド

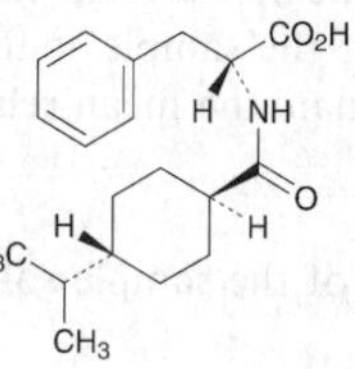

$C_{19}H_{27}NO_3$: 317.42
N-[*trans*-4-(1-Methylethyl)cyclohexanecarbonyl]-D-phenylalanine
[*105816-04-4*]

Nateglinide, when dried, contains not less than 98.0% and not more than 102.0% of nateglinide ($C_{19}H_{27}NO_3$).

Description Nateglinide occurs as a white crystalline powder.

It is freely soluble in methanol and in ethanol (99.5), sparingly soluble in acetonitrile, and practically insoluble in water.

It dissolves in dilute sodium hydroxide TS.

It shows crystal polymorphism.

Identification **(1)** Determine the absorption spectrum of a solution of Nateglinide in methanol (1 in 1000) as directed under Ultraviolet-visible Spectrophotometry 〈*2.24*〉, and compare the spectrum with the Reference Spectrum or the spectrum of a solution of Nateglinide RS prepared in the same manner as the sample solution: both spectra exhibit similar intensities of absorption at the same wavelengths.

(2) Determine the infrared absorption spectrum of Nateglinide as directed in the potassium bromide disk method under Infrared Spectrophotometry 〈*2.25*〉, and compare the spectrum with the Reference Spectrum or the spectrum of Nateglinide RS: both spectra exhibit similar intensities of absorption at the same wave numbers. If any difference appears between the spectra, recrystallize the sample and the reference standard according to the method otherwise specified, filter and dry the crystals, and perform the test with the crystals.

Optical rotation 〈*2.49*〉 $[\alpha]_D^{20}$: -36.5 – $-40.0°$ (after drying, 0.2 g, dilute sodium hydroxide TS, 20 mL, 100 mm).

Purity **(1)** Heavy metals 〈*1.07*〉—Proceed with 2.0 g of Nateglinide according to Method 2, and perform the test. Prepare the control solution with 2.0 mL of Standard Lead Solution (not more than 10 ppm).

(2) Related substances—Dissolve 0.25 g of Nateglinide in 20 mL of acetonitrile. To 4 mL of this solution add the mobile phase to make 25 mL, and use this solution as the sample solution. Pipet 2.5 mL of the sample solution, and add the mobile phase to make exactly 50 mL. Pipet 2 mL of this solution, add the mobile phase to make exactly 100 mL, and use this solution as the standard solution. Perform the test with exactly 10 μL each of the sample solution and standard solution as directed under Liquid Chromatography 〈*2.01*〉 according to the following conditions, and determine each peak area by the automatic integration method: the area of the peak other than nateglinide obtained from the sample solution is not larger than the peak area of nateglinide from the standard solution.

Operating conditions—

Detector, column, column temperature, mobile phase, and

flow rate: Proceed as directed in the operating conditions in the Assay.

Time span of measurement: About 4 times as long as the retention time of nateglinide, beginning after the solvent peak.

System suitability—

System performance: When the procedure is run with 10 μL of the standard solution under the above operating conditions, the number of theoretical plates and the symmetry factor of the peak of nateglinide are not less than 6000 and not more than 1.2, respectively.

System repeatability: When the test is repeated 6 times with 10 μL of the standard solution under the above operating conditions, the relative standard deviation of the peak area of nateglinide is not more than 2.0%.

Loss on drying <*2.41*> Not more than 0.2% (1 g, 105°C, 2 hours).

Residue on ignition <*2.44*> Not more than 0.1% (1 g).

Assay Weigh accurately about 0.1 g of Nateglinide, previously dried, and dissolve in acetonitrile to make exactly 20 mL. Pipet 5 mL of this solution, add exactly 5 mL of the internal standard solution, add the mobile phase to make 50 mL, and use this solution as the sample solution. Separately, weigh accurately about 50 mg of Nateglinide RS, previously dried, and dissolve in acetonitrile to make exactly 20 mL. Pipet 10 mL of this solution, add exactly 5 mL of the internal standard solution, add the mobile phase to make 50 mL, and use this solution as the standard solution. Perform the test with 10 μL each of the sample solution and standard solution as directed under Liquid Chromatography <*2.01*> according to the following conditions, and calculate the ratios, Q_T and Q_S, of the peak area of nateglinide to that of the internal standard.

$$\text{Amount (mg) of nateglinide } (C_{19}H_{27}NO_3) = M_S \times Q_T/Q_S \times 2$$

M_S: Amount (mg) of Nateglinide RS taken

*Internal standard solution—*A solution of propyl parahydroxybenzoate in the mobile phase (1 in 500).

Operating conditions—

Detector: An ultraviolet absorption photometer (wavelength: 210 nm).

Column: A stainless steel column 4.6 mm in inside diameter and 15 cm in length, packed with octadecylsilanized silica gel for liquid chromatography (5 μm in particle diameter).

Column temperature: A constant temperature of about 40°C.

Mobile phase: Adjust 0.05 mol/L sodium dihydrogen phosphate TS to pH 2.5 with phosphoric acid. To 550 mL of this solution add 450 mL of acetonitrile for liquid chromatography.

Flow rate: Adjust so that the retention time of nateglinide is about 10 minutes.

System suitability—

System performance: When the procedure is run with 10 μL of the standard solution under the above operating conditions, the internal standard and nateglinide are eluted in this order with the resolution between these peaks being not less than 19.

System repeatability: When the test is repeated 6 times with 10 μL of the standard solution under the above operating conditions, the relative standard deviation of the ratio of the peak area of nateglinide to that of the internal standard is not more than 1.0%.

Containers and storage Containers—Well-closed containers.

Nateglinide Tablets

ナテグリニド錠

Nateglinide Tablets contain not less than 96.0% and not more than 104.0% of the labeled amount of nateglinide ($C_{19}H_{27}NO_3$: 317.42).

Method of preparation Prepare as directed under Tablets, with Nateglinide.

Identification To an amount of powdered Nateglinide Tablets, equivalent to 20 mg of Nateglinide, add 20 mL of methanol, shake, and filter. Determine the absorption spectrum of the filtrate as directed under Ultraviolet-visible Spectrophotometry <*2.24*>: it exhibits maxima between 246 nm and 250 nm, between 251 nm and 255 nm, between 257 nm and 261 nm and between 262 nm and 266 nm.

Uniformity of dosage units <*6.02*> Perform the Mass variation test, or the Content uniformity test according to the following method: it meets the requirement.

To 1 tablet of Nateglinide Tablets add 10 mL of 0.05 mol/L sodium dihydrogen phosphate TS adjusted to pH 2.5 with phosphoric acid, shake to disintegrate the tablet, and disperse to fine particles by sonicating. Add exactly $3V/50$ mL of the internal standard solution, add $3V/5$ mL of acetonitrile, shake for 10 minutes, and add acetonitrile to make V mL so that each mL contains about 0.6 mg of nateglinide ($C_{19}H_{27}NO_3$). Filter the solution through a membrane filter with a pore size not exceeding 0.45 μm, and discard the first 5 mL of the filtrate. To 8 mL of the subsequent filtrate add the mobile phase to make 10 mL, and use this solution as the sample solution. Separately, weigh accurately about 50 mg of Nateglinide RS, previously dried at 105°C for 2 hours, and dissolve in acetonitrile to make exactly 10 mL. Pipet 6 mL of this solution, add exactly 3 mL of the internal standard solution, and add the mobile phase to make 25 mL. To 8 mL of this solution add the mobile phase to make 20 mL, and use this solution as the standard solution. Perform the test with 10 μL each of the sample solution and standard solution as directed under Liquid Chromatography <*2.01*>, and calculate the ratios, Q_T and Q_S, of the peak area of nateglinide to that of the internal standard.

$$\text{Amount (mg) of nateglinide } (C_{19}H_{27}NO_3) = M_S \times Q_T/Q_S \times 3V/250$$

M_S: Amount (mg) of Nateglinide RS taken

*Internal standard solution—*A solution of propyl parahydroxybenzoate in acetonitrile (1 in 250).

Operating conditions—

Proceed as directed in the operating conditions in the Assay.

System suitability—

System performance: When the procedure is run with 10 μL of the standard solution under the above operating conditions, the internal standard and nateglinide are eluted in this order with the resolution between these peaks being not less than 19.

System repeatability: When the test is repeated 6 times with 10 μL of the standard solution under the above operating conditions, the relative standard deviation of the ratio of the peak area of nateglinide to that of the internal standard is not more than 1.0%.

Dissolution <*6.10*> When the test is performed at 50 revolutions per minute according to the Paddle method, using 900 mL of 2nd fluid for dissolution test as the dissolution medium, the dissolution rate in 45 minutes of a 30-mg tablet and that in 30 minutes of a 90-mg tablet of Nateglinide Tablets is not less than 75%, respectively.

Start the test with 1 tablet of Nateglinide Tablets, withdraw not less than 20 mL of the medium at the specified minute after starting the test, and filter through a membrane filter with a pore size not exceeding 0.45 μm. Discard not less than 5 mL of the first filtrate, pipet V mL of the subsequent filtrate, add the dissolution medium to make exactly V' mL so that each mL contains about 33 μg of nateglinide ($C_{19}H_{27}NO_3$), and use this solution as the sample solution. Separately, weigh accurately about 33 mg of Nateglinide RS, previously dried at 105°C for 2 hours, and dissolve in acetonitrile to make exactly 100 mL. Pipet 5 mL of this solution, add the mobile phase to make exactly 50 mL, and use this solution as the standard solution. Perform the test with exactly 10 μL each of the sample solution and standard solution as directed under Liquid Chromatography <*2.01*> according to the following conditions, and determine the peak areas, A_T and A_S, of nateglinide in each solution.

Dissolution rate (%) with respect to the labeled amount of nateglinide ($C_{19}H_{27}NO_3$)
$= M_S \times A_T/A_S \times V'/V \times 1/C \times 90$

M_S: Amount (mg) of Nateglinide RS taken
C: Labeled amount (mg) of nateglinide ($C_{19}H_{27}NO_3$) in 1 tablet

Operating conditions—

Proceed as directed in the operating conditions in the Assay.

System suitability—

System performance: When the procedure is run with 10 μL of the standard solution under the above operating conditions, the number of theoretical plates and the symmetry factor of the peak of nateglinide are not less than 8000 and not more than 1.5, respectively.

System repeatability: When the test is repeated 6 times with 10 μL of the standard solution under the above operating conditions, the relative standard deviation of the peak area of nateglinide is not more than 2.0%.

Assay To 20 Nateglinide Tablets add $V/5$ mL of 0.05 mol/L sodium dihydrogen phosphate TS adjusted to pH 2.5 with phosphoric acid, shake to disintegrate the tablets, and disperse to fine particles by sonicating. Then, add $V/2$ mL of acetonitrile and exactly $V/10$ mL of the internal standard solution, shake for 10 minutes, and add acetonitrile to make V mL so that each mL contains about 6 mg of nateglinide ($C_{19}H_{27}NO_3$). Filter this solution through a membrane filter with a pore size not exceeding 0.45 μm, discard the first 5 mL of the filtrate, to 4 mL of the subsequent filtrate add the mobile phase to make 50 mL, and use this solution as the sample solution. Separately, weigh accurately about 60 mg of Nateglinide RS, previously dried at 105°C for 2 hours, add exactly 1 mL of the internal standard solution, and add acetonitrile to make 10 mL. To 4 mL of this solution add the mobile phase to make 50 mL, and use this solution as the standard solution. Perform the test with 10 μL each of the sample solution and standard solution as directed under Liquid Chromatography <*2.01*> according to the following conditions, and calculate the ratios, Q_T and Q_S, of the peak area of nateglinide to that of the internal standard.

Amount (mg) of nateglinide ($C_{19}H_{27}NO_3$) in 1 tablet
$= M_S \times Q_T/Q_S \times V/200$

M_S: Amount (mg) of Nateglinide RS taken

*Internal standard solution—*A solution of propyl parahydroxybenzoate in acetonitrile (3 in 125).

Operating conditions—

Detector: An ultraviolet absorption photometer (wavelength: 210 nm).

Column: A stainless steel column 4.6 mm in inside diameter and 15 cm in length, packed with octadecylsilanized silica gel for liquid chromatography (5 μm in particle diameter).

Column temperature: A constant temperature of about 40°C.

Mobile phase: Adjust to pH 2.5 of 0.05 mol/L sodium dihydrogen phosphate TS with phosphoric acid. To 550 mL of this solution add 450 mL of acetonitrile.

Flow rate: Adjust so that the retention time of nateglinide is about 10 minutes.

System suitability—

System performance: When the procedure is run with 10 μL of the standard solution under the above operating conditions, the internal standard and nateglinide are eluted in this order with the resolution between these peaks being not less than 19.

System repeatability: When the test is repeated 6 times with 10 μL of the standard solution under the above operating conditions, the relative standard deviation of the ratio of the peak area of nateglinide to that of the internal standard is not more than 1.0%.

Containers and storage Containers—Tight containers.

Neostigmine Methylsulfate

ネオスチグミンメチル硫酸塩

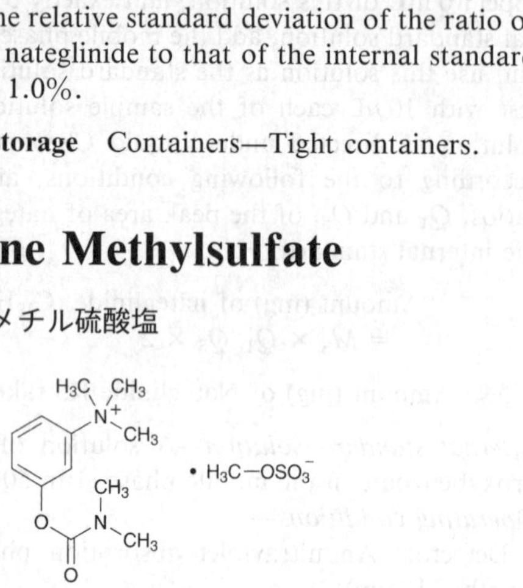

$C_{13}H_{22}N_2O_6S$: 334.39
3-(Dimethylcarbamoyloxy)-*N*,*N*,*N*-trimethylanilinium methyl sulfate
[*51-60-5*]

Neostigmine Methylsulfate, when dried, contains not less than 98.0% and not more than 102.0% of neostigmine methylsulfate ($C_{13}H_{22}N_2O_6S$).

Description Neostigmine Methylsulfate occurs as a white crystalline powder.

It is very soluble in water, and freely soluble in acetonitrile and in ethanol (95).

Identification **(1)** Determine the absorption spectrum of a solution of Neostigmine Methylsulfate (1 in 2000) as directed under Ultraviolet-visible Spectrophotometry <*2.24*>, and compare the spectrum with the Reference Spectrum or the spectrum of a solution of Neostigmine Methylsulfate RS prepared in the same manner as the sample solution: both spectra exhibit similar intensities of absorption at the same wavelengths.

(2) Determine the infrared absorption spectrum of

Neostigmine Methylsulfate as directed in the potassium bromide disk method under Infrared Spectrophotometry <*2.25*>, and compare the spectrum with the Reference Spectrum or the spectrum of dried Neostigmine Methylsulfate RS: both spectra exhibit similar intensities of absorption at the same wave numbers.

pH <*2.54*> Dissolve 1.0 g of Neostigmine Methylsulfate in 10 mL of freshly boiled and cooled water: the pH of the solution is between 3.0 and 5.0.

Melting point <*2.60*> 145 - 149°C

Purity **(1)** Clarity and color of solution—Dissolve 1.0 g of Neostigmine Methylsulfate in 10 mL of water: the solution is clear and colorless.

(2) Sulfate—Dissolve 0.20 g of Neostigmine Methylsulfate in 10 mL of water, add 1 mL of dilute hydrochloric acid and 1 mL of barium chloride TS: no turbidity is produced immediately.

(3) Dimethylaminophenol—Dissolve 0.10 g of Neostigmine Methylsulfate in 5 mL of water, add 1 mL of sodium hydroxide TS, and while cooling with ice, add 1 mL of diazobenzenesulfonic acid TS: no color develops.

Loss on drying <*2.41*> Not more than 1.0% (1 g, 105°C, 3 hours).

Residue on ignition <*2.44*> Not more than 0.1% (1 g).

Assay Weigh accurately about 25 mg each of Neostigmine Methylsulfate and Neostigmine Methylsulfate RS, previously dried, dissolve each in the mobile phase to make exactly 50 mL, and use these solutions as the sample solution and the standard solution, respectively. Perform the test with exactly 10 μL each of the sample solution and standard solution as directed under Liquid Chromatography <*2.01*> according to the following conditions, and determine the peak areas, A_T and A_S, of neostigmine in each solution.

Amount (mg) of neostigmine methylsulfate ($C_{13}H_{22}N_2O_6S$)
$= M_S \times A_T/A_S$

M_S: Amount (mg) of Neostigmine Methylsulfate RS taken

Operating conditions—

Detector: An ultraviolet absorption photometer (wavelength: 259 nm).

Column: A stainless steel column 4.6 mm in inside diameter and 15 cm in length, packed with octadecylsilanized silica gel for liquid chromatography (5 μm in particle diameter).

Column temperature: A constant temperature of about 25°C.

Mobile phase: Dissolve 3.12 g of sodium dihydrogenphosphate dihydrate in 1000 mL of water, adjust to pH 3.0 with phosphoric acid, and add 0.871 g of sodium 1-pentanesulfonate to dissolve. To 890 mL of this solution add 110 mL of acetonitrile.

Flow rate: Adjust so that the retention time of neostigmine is about 9 minutes.

System suitability—

System performance: Dissolve 25 mg of Neostigmine Methylsulfate and 4 mg of dimethylaminophenol in 50 mL of the mobile phase. When the procedure is run with 10 μL of this solution under the above operating conditions, dimethylaminophenol and neostigmine are eluted in this order with the resolution between these peaks being not less than 6.

System repeatability: When the test is repeated 6 times with 10 μL of the standard solution under the above operating conditions, the relative standard deviation of the peak areas of neostigmine methylsulfate is not more than 1.0%.

Containers and storage Containers—Tight containers.

Neostigmine Methylsulfate Injection

ネオスチグミンメチル硫酸塩注射液

Neostigmine Methylsulfate Injection is an aqueous injection.

It contains not less than 93.0% and not more than 107.0% of the labeled amount of neostigmine methylsulfate ($C_{13}H_{22}N_2O_6S$: 334.39).

Method of preparation Prepare as directed under Injections, with Neostigmine Methylsulfate.

Description Neostigmine Methylsulfate Injection is a clear, colorless liquid.

It is slowly affected by light.

pH: 5.0 - 6.5

Identification Take a volume of Neostigmine Methylsulfate Injection, equivalent to 5 mg of neostigmine methylsulfate, add water to make 10 mL if necessary, and determine the absorption spectrum of this solution as directed under Ultraviolet-visible Spectrophotometry <*2.24*>: it exhibits a maximum between 257 nm and 261 nm.

Bacterial endotoxins <*4.01*> Less than 5 EU/mg.

Extractable volume <*6.05*> It meets the requirement.

Foreign insoluble matter <*6.06*> Perform the test according to Method 1: it meets the requirement.

Insoluble particulate matter <*6.07*> It meets the requirement.

Sterility <*4.06*> Perform the test according to the Membrane filtration method: it meets the requirement.

Assay Use Neostigmine Methylsulfate Injection as the sample solution. Separately, weigh accurately about 25 mg of Neostigmine Methylsulfate RS, previously dried at 105°C for 3 hours, dissolve in the mobile phase to make exactly 50 mL, and use this solution as the standard solution. Proceed as directed in the Assay under Neostigmine Methylsulfate.

Amount (mg) of neostigmine methylsulfate ($C_{13}H_{22}N_2O_6S$)
$= M_S \times A_T/A_S$

M_S: Amount (mg) of Neostigmine Methylsulfate RS taken

Containers and storage Containers—Hermetic containers.

Storage—Light-resistant.

Nicardipine Hydrochloride

ニカルジピン塩酸塩

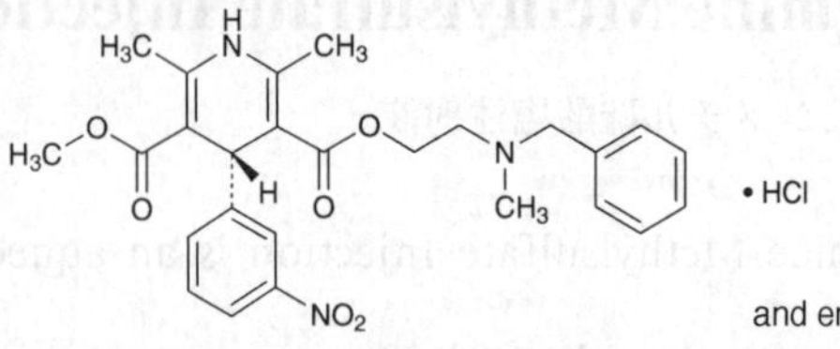

and enantiomer

$C_{26}H_{29}N_3O_6.HCl$: 515.99
2-[Benzyl(methyl)amino]ethyl methyl (4*RS*)-2,6-dimethyl-4-(3-nitrophenyl)-1,4-dihydropyridine-3,5-dicarboxylate monohydrochloride
[*54527-84-3*]

Nicardipine hydrochloride, when dried, contains not less than 98.5% of nicardipine hydrochloride ($C_{26}H_{29}N_3O_6.HCl$).

Description Nicardipine Hydrochloride occurs as a slightly greenish yellow crystalline powder.

It is freely soluble in methanol and in acetic acid (100), sparingly soluble in ethanol (99.5), and slightly soluble in water, in acetonitrile and in acetic anhydride.

A solution of Nicardipine Hydrochloride in methanol (1 in 20) shows no optical rotation.

It is gradually affected by light.

Identification (1) Determine the absorption spectrum of a solution of Nicardipine Hydrochloride in ethanol (99.5) (1 in 100,000) as directed under Ultraviolet-visible Spectrophotometry 〈*2.24*〉, and compare the spectrum with the Reference Spectrum: both spectra exhibit similar intensities of absorption at the same wavelengths.

(2) Determine the infrared absorption spectrum of Nicardipine Hydrochloride, previously dried, as directed in the potassium bromide disk method under Infrared Spectrophotometry 〈*2.25*〉, and compare the spectrum with the Reference Spectrum: both spectra exhibit similar intensities of absorption at the same wave numbers.

(3) Dissolve 0.02 g of Nicardipine Hydrochloride in 10 mL of water and 3 mL of nitric acid: the solution responds to Qualitative Tests 〈*1.09*〉 for chloride.

Melting point 〈*2.60*〉 167 – 171°C

Purity (1) Heavy metals 〈*1.07*〉—Proceed with 1.0 g of Nicardipine Hydrochloride according to Method 4, and perform the test. Prepare the control solution with 2.0 mL of Standard Lead Solution (not more than 20 ppm).

(2) Related substances—Conduct this procedure without exposure to light, using light-resistant vessels. Dissolve 0.10 g of Nicardipine Hydrochloride in 50 mL of the mobile phase, and use this solution as the sample solution. Pipet 1 mL of the sample solution, add the mobile phase to make exactly 50 mL, then take exactly 1 mL of this solution, add the mobile phase to make exactly 10 mL, and use this solution as the standard solution. Perform the test with exactly 10 μL each of the sample solution and standard solution as directed under Liquid Chromatography 〈*2.01*〉 according to the following conditions. Determine each peak area of both solutions by the automatic integration method: the area of each peak other than nicardipine obtained from the sample solution is not larger than the peak area of nicardipine from the standard solution, and the total area of each peak other than nicardipine is not larger than 2 times the peak area of nicardipine from the standard solution.

Operating conditions—

Detector: An ultraviolet absorption photometer (wavelength: 254 nm).

Column: A stainless steel column 4.6 mm in inside diameter and 15 cm in length, packed with octadecylsilanized silica gel for liquid chromatography (5 μm in particle diameter).

Column temperature: A constant temperature of about 30°C.

Mobile phase: A mixture of a solution of perchloric acid (43 in 50,000) and acetonitrile (3:2).

Flow rate: Adjust so that the retention time of nicardipine is about 6 minutes.

Time span of measurement: About 4 times as long as the retention time of nicardipine, beginning after the solvent peak.

System suitability—

Test for required detectability: To exactly 2 mL of the standard solution add the mobile phase to make exactly 20 mL. Confirm that the peak area of nicardipine obtained with 10 μL of this solution is equivalent to 8 to 12% of that with 10 μL of the standard solution.

System performance: Dissolve 2 mg each of Nicardipine Hydrochloride and nifedipine in 50 mL of the mobile phase. When the procedure is run with 10 μL of this solution under the above operating conditions, nicardipine and nifedipine are eluted in this order with the resolution between these peaks being not less than 3.

System repeatability: When the test is repeated 6 times with 10 μL of the standard solution under the above operating conditions, the relative standard deviation of the peak areas of nicardipine is not more than 3%.

Loss on drying 〈*2.41*〉 Not more than 1.0% (1 g, 105°C, 2 hours).

Residue on ignition 〈*2.44*〉 Not more than 0.1% (1 g).

Assay Conduct this procedure without exposure to light, using light-resistant vessels. Weigh accurately about 0.9 g of Nicardipine Hydrochloride, previously dried, dissolve in 100 mL of a mixture of acetic anhydride and acetic acid (100) (7:3), and titrate 〈*2.50*〉 with 0.1 mol/L perchloric acid VS (potentiometric titration). Perform a blank determination in the same manner, and make any necessary correction.

Each mL of 0.1 mol/L perchloric acid VS
= 51.60 mg of $C_{26}H_{29}N_3O_6.HCl$

Containers and storage Containers—Well-closed containers.

Storage—Light-resistant.

Nicardipine Hydrochloride Injection

ニカルジピン塩酸塩注射液

Nicardipine Hydrochloride Injection is an aqueous injection.

It contains not less than 93.0% and not more than 107.0% of the labeled amount of nicardipine hydrochloride ($C_{26}H_{29}N_3O_6.HCl$: 515.99).

Method of preparation Prepare as directed under Injections, with Nicardipine Hydrochloride.

Description Nicardipine Hydrochloride Injection occurs as a clear, pale yellow liquid.

It is gradually changed by light.

Identification To a volume of Nicardipine Hydrochloride Injection, equivalent to 1 mg of Nicardipine Hydrochloride, add ethanol (99.5) to make 100 mL. Determine the absorption spectrum of this solution as directed under Ultraviolet-visible Spectrophotometry 〈*2.24*〉: it exhibits maxima between 235 nm and 239 nm, and between 351 nm and 355 nm.

pH 〈*2.54*〉 3.0 – 4.5

Purity Related substances—Conduct the procedure without exposure to light, using light-resistant vessels. To a volume of Nicardipine Hydrochloride Injection, equivalent to 5 mg of Nicardipine Hydrochloride, add the mobile phase to make 10 mL, and use this solution as the sample solution. To exactly 2 mL of the sample solution add the mobile phase to make exactly 100 mL, and use this solution as the standard solution. Perform the test with exactly 10 μL each of the sample solution and standard solution as directed under Liquid Chromatography 〈*2.01*〉 according to the following conditions, and determine the peak areas of these solutions by the automatic integration method: the areas of the peaks other than nicardipine obtained from the sample solution are not larger than the peak area of nicardipine from the standard solution, and the total of the areas of the peaks other than nicardipine is not larger than 2 times of the peak area of nicardipine from the standard solution.

Operating conditions—

Detector, column, column temperature, mobile phase, and flow rate: Proceed as directed in the operating conditions in the Assay.

Time span of measurement: About 3 times as long as the retention time of nicardipine, beginning after the solvent peak.

System suitability—

System performance: Proceed as directed in the system suitability in the Assay.

Test for required detectability: To exactly 2 mL of the standard solution add the mobile phase to make exactly 20 mL. Confirm that the peak area of nicardipine obtained with 10 μL of this solution is equivalent to 8 to 12% of that with 10 μL of the standard solution.

System repeatability: When the test is repeated 5 times with 10 μL of the standard solution under the above operating conditions, the relative standard deviation of the peak areas of nicardipine is not more than 1.0%.

Bacterial endotoxins 〈*4.01*〉 Less than 8.33 EU/mg.

Extractable volume 〈*6.05*〉 It meets the requirement.

Foreign insoluble matter 〈*6.06*〉 Perform the test according to Method 1: it meets the requirement.

Insoluble particulate matter 〈*6.07*〉 It meets the requirement.

Sterility 〈*4.06*〉 Perform the test according to the Membrane filtration method: it meets the requirement.

Assay Conduct the procedure without exposure to light, using light-resistant vessels. To an exact volume of Nicardipine Hydrochloride Injection, equivalent to about 2 mg of nicardipine hydrochloride ($C_{26}H_{29}N_3O_6.HCl$), add exactly 5 mL of the internal standard solution and methanol to make 50 mL, and use this solution as the sample solution. Separately, weigh accurately about 50 mg of nicardipine hydrochloride for assay, previously dried at 105°C for 2 hours, dissolve in methanol to make exactly 50 mL. Pipet 2 mL of this solution, add exactly 5 mL of the internal standard solution and methanol to make 50 mL, and use this solution as the standard solution. Perform the test with 10 μL each of the sample solution and standard solution as directed under Liquid Chromatography 〈*2.01*〉 according to the following conditions, and calculate the ratios, Q_T and Q_S, of the peak area of nicardipine to that of the internal standard.

Amount (mg) of nicardipine hydrochloride ($C_{26}H_{29}N_3O_6.HCl$)
$= M_S \times Q_T/Q_S \times 1/25$

M_S: Amount (mg) of nicardipine hydrochloride for assay taken

Internal standard solution—A solution of di-*n*-butyl phthalate in methanol (1 in 625).

Operating conditions—

Detector: An ultraviolet absorption photometer (wavelength: 254 nm).

Column: A stainless steel column 4.6 mm in inside diameter and 15 cm in length, packed with octadecylsilanized silica gel for liquid chromatography (5 μm in particle diameter).

Column temperature: A constant temperature of about 40°C.

Mobile phase: Dissolve 1.36 g of potassium dihydrogen phosphate in water to make 1000 mL. To 320 mL of this solution add 680 mL of methanol.

Flow rate: Adjust so that the retention time of nicardipine is about 8 minutes.

System suitability—

System performance: When the procedure is run with 10 μL of the standard solution under the above operating conditions, nicardipine and the internal standard are eluted in this order with the resolution between these peaks being not less than 6.

System repeatability: When the test is repeated 5 times with 10 μL of the standard solution under the above operating conditions, the relative standard deviation of the peak areas of nicardipine is not more than 1.0%.

Containers and storage Containers—Hermetic containers. Colored containers may be used.

Storage—Light-resistant.

Nicergoline

ニセルゴリン

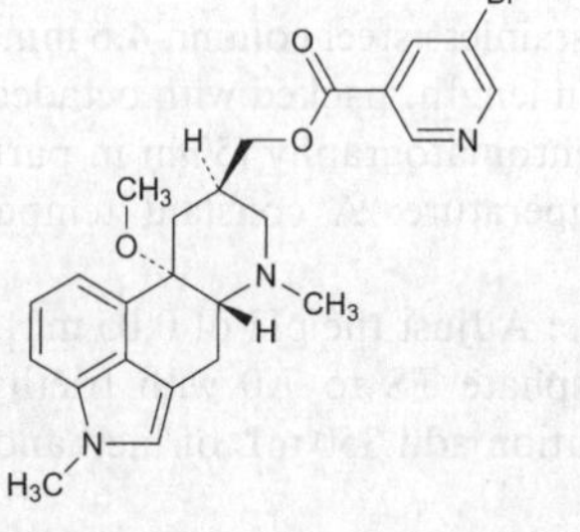

$C_{24}H_{26}BrN_3O_3$: 484.39

[(8*R*,10*S*)-10-Methoxy-1,6-dimethylergolin-8-yl]methyl 5-bromopyridine-3-carboxylate

[*27848-84-6*]

Nicergoline, when dried, contains not less than 98.5% and not more than 101.0% of nicergoline ($C_{24}H_{26}BrN_3O_3$).

Description Nicergoline occurs as white to light yellow, crystals or crystalline powder.

It is soluble in acetonitrile, in ethanol (99.5) and in acetic anhydride, and practically insoluble in water.

It is gradually colored to light brown by light.

Melting point: about 136°C (with decomposition).

Identification **(1)** Determine the absorption spectrum of a solution of Nicergoline in ethanol (99.5) (1 in 100,000) as directed under Ultraviolet-visible Spectrophotometry <*2.24*>, and compare the spectrum with the Reference Spectrum: both spectra exhibit similar intensities of absorption at the same wavelengths.

(2) Determine the infrared absorption spectrum of Nicergoline as directed in the potassium bromide disk method under Infrared Spectrophotometry <*2.25*>, and compare the spectrum with the Reference Spectrum: both spectra exhibit similar intensities of absorption at the same wave numbers.

Optical rotation <*2.49*> $[\alpha]_D^{20}$: +5.2 – +6.2° (after drying, 0.5 g, ethanol (95), 10 mL, 100 mm).

Purity **(1)** Heavy metals <*1.07*>—Proceed with 2.0 g of Nicergoline according to Method 2, and perform the test. Prepare the control solution with 2.0 mL of Standard Lead Solution (not more than 10 ppm).

(2) Related substances—Dissolve 25 mg of Nicergoline in 25 mL of acetonitrile, and use this solution as the sample solution. Pipet 1 mL of the sample solution, and add acetonitrile to make exactly 100 mL. Pipet 10 mL of this solution, add acetonitrile to make exactly 50 mL, and use this solution as the standard solution. Perform the test with exactly 20 μL each of the sample solution and standard solution as directed under Liquid Chromatography <*2.01*> according to the following conditions, and determine each peak area by the automatic integration method: the area of the peak, having the relative retention time of about 0.5 to nicergoline obtained from the sample solution, is not larger than 4 times the peak area of nicergoline from the standard solution, and the area of the peak other than nicergoline and the peak mentioned above from the sample solution is not larger than 2.5 times the peak area of nicergoline from the standard solution. The peak which area is larger than the peak area of nicergoline from the standard solution is not more than two peaks, and the total area of the peaks other than nicergoline from the sample solution is not larger than 7.5 times the peak area of nicergoline from the standard solution.

Operating conditions—

Detector: An ultraviolet absorption photometer (wavelength: 288 nm).

Column: A stainless steel column 4.6 mm in inside diameter and 25 cm in length, packed with octadecylsilanized silica gel for liquid chromatography (5 μm in particle diameter).

Column temperature: A constant temperature of about 25°C.

Mobile phase: Adjust the pH of 0.05 mol/L potassium dihydrogen phosphate TS to 7.0 with triethylamine. To 350 mL of this solution add 350 mL of methanol and 300 mL of acetonitrile.

Flow rate: Adjust so that the retention time of nicergoline is about 25 minutes.

Time span of measurement: About 2 times as long as the retention time of nicergoline, beginning after the solvent peak.

System suitability—

Test for required detectability: To 1 mL of the sample solution add acetonitrile to make exactly 50 mL, and use this solution as the solution for system suitability test. Pipet 5 mL of the solution for system suitability test, and add acetonitrile to make exactly 100 mL. Confirm that the peak area of nicergoline obtained with 20 μL of this solution is equivalent to 3 to 7% of that with 20 μL of the solution for system suitability test.

System performance: When the procedure is run with 20 μL of the sample solution under the above operating conditions, the number of theoretical plates and the symmetry factor of the peak of nicergoline are not less than 8000 and not more than 2.0, respectively.

System repeatability: When the test is repeated 6 times with 20 μL of the standard solution under the above operating conditions, the relative standard deviation of the peak area of nicergoline is not more than 4.0%.

Loss on drying <*2.41*> Not more than 0.5% (2 g, in vacuum, 60°C, 2 hours).

Residue on ignition <*2.44*> Not more than 0.1% (1 g).

Assay Weigh accurately about 0.4 g of Nicergoline, previously dried, add 10 mL of acetic anhydride, and warm to dissolve. After cooling, add 40 mL of nitrobenzene, and titrate <*2.50*> with 0.1 mol/L perchloric acid VS until the color of the solution changes to blue-green from red through a blue-purple (indicator: 10 drops of neutral red TS). Perform a blank determination in the same manner, and make any necessary correction.

Each mL of 0.1 mol/L perchloric acid VS
= 24.22 mg of $C_{24}H_{26}BrN_3O_3$

Containers and storage Containers—Well-closed containers.

Storage—Light-resistant.

Nicergoline Powder

ニセルゴリン散

Nicergoline Powder contains not less than 95.0% and not more than 105.0% of the labeled amount of nicergoline ($C_{24}H_{26}BrN_3O_3$: 484.39).

Method of preparation Prepare as directed under Granules or Powders, with Nicergoline.

Identification Vigorously shake for 10 minutes a quantity of Nicergoline Powder, equivalent to 10 mg of Nicergoline, with 20 mL of diluted ethanol (4 in 5), and centrifuge for 10 minutes. To 2 mL of the supernatant liquid add ethanol (99.5) to make 100 mL. Determine the absorption spectrum of this solution as directed under Ultraviolet-visible Spectrophotometry <*2.24*>: it exhibits maxima between 226 nm and 230 nm, and between 286 nm and 290 nm.

Purity Related substances—Perform the test with 20 μL of the sample solution obtained in the Assay as directed under Liquid Chromatography <*2.01*> according to the following conditions. Determine each peak area by the automatic integration method, and calculate the amount of substances other than nicergoline by the area percentage method: the total amount of them is not more than 2.0%.

Operating conditions—

Detector, column, column temperature, mobile phase, and flow rate: Proceed as directed in the operating conditions in the Assay.

Time span of measurement: About 2 times as long as the retention time of nicergoline, beginning after the solvent peak.

System suitability—

System performance: Proceed as directed in the system suitability in the Assay.

Test for required detectability: To 1 mL of the standard solution obtained in the Assay add a mixture of acetonitrile and water (17:3) to make 50 mL, and use this solution as the solution for system suitability test. Pipet 5 mL of the solution for system suitability test, add the mixture of acetonitrile and water (17:3) to make exactly 100 mL. Confirm that the peak area of nicergoline obtained with 20 μL of this solution is equivalent to 3 to 7% of that with 20 μL of the solution for system suitability test.

System repeatability: When the test is repeated 6 times with 20 μL of the solution for system suitability test under the above operating conditions, the relative standard deviation of the peak area of nicergoline is not more than 1.5%.

Uniformity of dosage units *<6.02>* The Nicergoline Powder in single-dose packages meets the requirement of the Mass variation test.

Dissolution *<6.10>* When the test is performed at 50 revolutions per minute according to the Paddle method, using 900 mL of 2nd fluid for dissolution test as the dissolution medium, the dissolution rate in 15 minutes of Nicergoline Powder is not less than 80%.

Start the test with an accurately weighed amount of Nicergoline Powder, equivalent to about 5 mg of nicergoline ($C_{24}H_{26}BrN_3O_3$), withdraw not less than about 20 mL of the medium at the specified minute after starting the test, and filter through a laminated polyester fiber. Discard not less than 10 mL of the first filtrate, and use the subsequent filtrate as the sample solution. Separately, weigh accurately about 50 mg of nicergoline for assay, previously dried in vacuum at 60°C for 2 hours, and dissolve in 0.1 mol/L hydrochloric acid TS to make exactly 50 mL. Pipet 5 mL of this solution, and add the dissolution medium to make exactly 100 mL. Pipet 10 mL of this solution, add the dissolution medium to make exactly 100 mL, and use this solution as the standard solution. Determine the absorbances at 225 nm, A_{T1} and A_{S1}, and at 250 nm, A_{T2} and A_{S2}, of the sample solution and standard solution as directed under Ultraviolet-visible Spectrophotometry *<2.24>*, using the dissolution medium as the blank.

Dissolution rate (%) with respect to the labeled amount of nicergoline ($C_{24}H_{26}BrN_3O_3$)

$$= M_S/M_T \times (A_{T1} - A_{T2})/(A_{S1} - A_{S2}) \times 1/C \times 9$$

M_S: Amount (mg) of nicergoline for assay taken

M_T: Amount (g) of Nicergoline Powder taken

C: Labeled amount (mg) of nicergoline ($C_{24}H_{26}BrN_3O_3$) in 1 g

Assay Weigh accurately a quantity of Nicergoline Powder, equivalent to about 20 mg of nicergoline ($C_{24}H_{26}BrN_3O_3$), add exactly 20 mL of a mixture of acetonitrile and water (17:3), vigorously shake for 10 minutes, centrifuge for 10 minutes, and use the supernatant liquid as the sample solution. Separately, weigh accurately about 20 mg of nicergoline for assay, previously dried in vacuum at 60°C for 2 hours, dissolve in exactly 20 mL of the mixture of acetonitrile and water (17:3), and use this solution as the standard solution. Perform the test with exactly 20 μL each of the sample solution and standard solution as directed under Liquid Chromatography *<2.01>* according to the following conditions, and determine the peak areas, A_T and A_S, of nicergoline in each solution.

Amount (mg) of nicergoline ($C_{24}H_{26}BrN_3O_3$)

$$= M_S \times A_T/A_S$$

M_S: Amount (mg) of nicergoline for assay taken

Operating conditions—

Detector: An ultraviolet absorption photometer (wavelength: 288 nm).

Column: A stainless steel column 4.6 mm in inside diameter and 25 cm in length, packed with octadecylsilanized silica gel for liquid chromatography (5 μm in particle diameter).

Column temperature: A constant temperature of about 40°C.

Mobile phase: Adjust the pH of 0.05 mol/L potassium dihydrogen phosphate TS to 7.0 with triethylamine. To 350 mL of this solution add 350 mL of methanol and 300 mL of acetonitrile.

Flow rate: Adjust so that the retention time of nicergoline is about 25 minutes.

System suitability—

System performance: When the procedure is run with 20 μL of the standard solution under the above operating conditions, the number of theoretical plates and the symmetry factor of the peak of nicergoline are not less than 8000 and not more than 2.0, respectively.

System repeatability: When the test is repeated 6 times with 20 μL of the standard solution under the above operating conditions, the relative standard deviation of the peak area of nicergoline is not more than 1.0%.

Containers and storage Containers—Tight containers. Storage—Light-resistant.

Nicergoline Tablets

ニセルゴリン錠

Nicergoline Tablets contain not less than 95.0% and not more than 105.0% of the labeled amount of nicergoline ($C_{24}H_{26}BrN_3O_3$: 484.39).

Method of preparation Prepare as directed under Tablets, with Nicergoline.

Identification Take a quantity of powdered Nicergoline Tablets, equivalent to 10 mg of Nicergoline, add 20 mL of ethanol (99.5), shake vigorously for 10 minutes, and filter through a 0.45-μm pore-size membrane filter. To 2 mL of the filtrate add ethanol (99.5) to make 100 mL. Determine the absorption spectrum of this solution as directed under Ultraviolet-visible Spectrophotometry *<2.24>*: it exhibits maxima between 226 nm and 230 nm, and between 286 nm and 290 nm.

Purity Related substances—Perform the test with 20 μL of the sample solution obtained in the Assay as directed under Liquid Chromatography *<2.01>* according to the following conditions. Determine each peak area by the automatic integration method, and calculate the amount of substances other than nicergoline by the area percentage method: the total amount of them is not more than 2.0%.

Operating conditions—

Detector, column, column temperature, mobile phase, and flow rate: Proceed as directed in the operating conditions in the Assay.

Time span of measurement: About 2 times as long as the retention time of nicergoline, beginning after the solvent peak.

System suitability—

System performance: Proceed as directed in the system suitability in the Assay.

Test for required detectability: To 1 mL of the standard solution obtained in the Assay add a mixture of acetonitrile and water (17:3) to make 50 mL, and use this solution as the solution for system suitability test. Pipet 5 mL of the solution for system suitability test, add the mixture of acetonitrile and water (17:3) to make exactly 100 mL. Confirm that the peak area of nicergoline obtained with 20 μL of this solution is equivalent to 3 to 7% of that with 20 μL of the solution for system suitability test.

System repeatability: When the test is repeated 6 times with 20 μL of the solution for system suitability test under the above operating conditions, the relative standard deviation of the peak area of nicergoline is not more than 1.5%.

Uniformity of dosage units <*6.02*> Perform the test according to the following method: it meets the requirement of the Content uniformity test.

To 1 tablet of Nicergoline Tablets add exactly 25 mL of diluted ethanol (4 in 5), disperse to fine particles by sonicating, and shake for 5 minutes. Centrifuge this solution for 10 minutes, pipet 4 mL of the supernatant liquid, add diluted ethanol (4 in 5) to make exactly 25 mL, and use this solution as the sample solution. Separately, weigh accurately about 10 mg of nicergoline for assay, previously dried in vacuum at 60°C for 2 hours, and dissolve in exactly 25 mL of diluted ethanol (4 in 5). Pipet 4 mL of this solution, add diluted ethanol (4 in 5) to make exactly 50 mL, and use this solution as the standard solution. Determine the absorbances at 288 nm, A_{T1} and A_{S1}, and at 340 nm, A_{T2} and A_{S2}, of the sample solution and the standard solution as directed under Ultraviolet-visible Spectrophotometry <*2.24*>.

$$\text{Amount (mg) of nicergoline } (C_{24}H_{26}BrN_3O_3) = M_S \times (A_{T1} - A_{T2})/(A_{S1} - A_{S2}) \times 1/2$$

M_S: Amount (mg) of nicergoline for assay taken

Dissolution Being specified separately when the drug is granted approval based on the Law.

Assay Weigh accurately the mass of not less than 20 Nicergoline Tablets, and powder. Weigh accurately a portion of the powder, equivalent to about 20 mg of nicergoline ($C_{24}H_{26}BrN_3O_3$), add exactly 20 mL of a mixture of acetonitrile and water (17:3), vigorously shake for 10 minutes, centrifuge for 10 minutes, and use the supernatant liquid as the sample solution. Separately, weigh accurately about 20 mg of nicergoline for assay, previously dried in vacuum at 60°C for 2 hours, dissolve in exactly 20 mL of the mixture of acetonitrile and water (17:3), and use this solution as the standard solution. Perform the test with exactly 20 μL each of the sample solution and standard solution as directed under Liquid Chromatography <*2.01*> according to the following conditions, and determine the peak areas, A_T and A_S, of nicergoline in each solution.

$$\text{Amount (mg) of nicergoline } (C_{24}H_{26}BrN_3O_3) = M_S \times A_T/A_S$$

M_S: Amount (mg) of nicergoline for assay taken

Operating conditions—

Detector: An ultraviolet absorption photometer (wavelength: 288 nm).

Column: A stainless steel column 4.6 mm in inside diameter and 25 cm in length, packed with octadecylsilanized silica gel for liquid chromatography (5 μm in particle diameter).

Column temperature: A constant temperature of about 40°C.

Mobile phase: Adjust the pH of 0.05 mol/L potassium dihydrogen phosphate TS to 7.0 with triethylamine. To 350 mL of this solution add 350 mL of methanol and 300 mL of acetonitrile.

Flow rate: Adjust so that the retention time of nicergoline is about 25 minutes.

System suitability—

System performance: When the procedure is run with 20 μL of the standard solution under the above operating conditions, the number of theoretical plates and the symmetry factor of the peak of nicergoline are not less than 8000 and not more than 2.0, respectively.

System repeatability: When the test is repeated 6 times with 20 μL of the standard solution under the above operating conditions, the relative standard deviation of the peak area of nicergoline is not more than 1.0%.

Containers and storage Containers—Tight containers.

Niceritrol

ニセリトロール

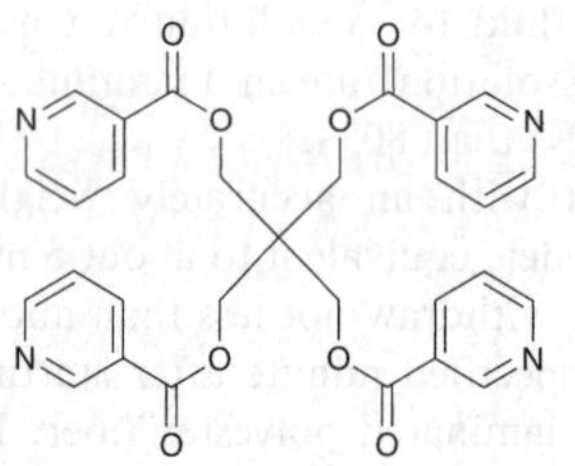

$C_{29}H_{24}N_4O_8$: 556.52

Pentaerythritol tetranicotinate

[*5868-05-3*]

Niceritrol, when dried, contains not less than 99.0% of niceritrol ($C_{29}H_{24}N_4O_8$).

Description Niceritrol occurs as a white to pale yellow-white powder. It is odorless, and has a slightly bitter taste.

It is freely soluble in chloroform, soluble in *N*,*N*-dimethylformamide, very slightly soluble in ethanol (95), and practically insoluble in water and in diethyl ether.

Identification **(1)** Determine the absorption spectrum of a solution of Niceritrol in 0.1 mol/L hydrochloric acid TS (1 in 100,000) as directed under Ultraviolet-visible Spectrophotometry <*2.24*>, and compare the spectrum with the Reference Spectrum: both spectra exhibit similar intensities of absorption at the same wavelengths.

(2) Determine the infrared absorption spectrum of Niceritrol, previously dried, as directed in the potassium bromide disk method under Infrared Spectrophotometry <*2.25*>, and compare the spectrum with the Reference Spectrum: both spectra exhibit similar intensities of absorption at the same wave numbers.

Melting point <*2.60*> 162 – 165°C

Purity **(1)** Chloride <*1.03*>—To 2.0 g of Niceritrol add 50 mL of water, and warm at 70°C for 20 minutes, while shaking occasionally. After cooling, filter, and to 25 mL of the filtrate add 6 mL of dilute nitric acid and water to make 50 mL. Perform the test using this solution as the test solution. Prepare the control solution with 1.0 mL of 0.01 mol/L hydrochloric acid VS (not more than 0.036%).

(2) Heavy metals <*1.07*>—Proceed with 1.0 g of Niceritrol according to Method 2, and perform the test. Prepare the control solution with 2.0 mL of Standard Lead Solution (not more than 20 ppm).

(3) Arsenic 〈*1.11*〉—Prepare the test solution with 1.0 g of Niceritrol according to Method 3, and perform the test. Use 10 mL of a solution of magnesium nitrate hexahydrate in ethanol (95) (1 in 10) (not more than 2 ppm).

(4) Pyridine—Dissolve 0.5 g of Niceritrol in *N,N*-dimethylformamide to make exactly 10 mL, and use this solution as the sample solution. Separately, weigh accurately about 0.1 g of pyridine, and add *N,N*-dimethylformamide to make exactly 100 mL. Pipet 1 mL of this solution, add *N,N*-dimethylformamide to make exactly 100 mL, then pipet 0.5 mL of this solution, add *N,N*-dimethylformamide to make exactly 10 mL, and use this solution as the standard solution. Perform the test with exactly 2 μL each of the sample solution and standard solution as directed under Gas Chromatography 〈*2.02*〉 according to the following conditions. Determine each peak area of pyridine in both solutions: the peak area of pyridine obtained from the sample solution is not larger than the peak area of pyridine from the standard solution.

Operating conditions—

Detector: A hydrogen flame-ionization detector.

Column: A column 3 mm in inside diameter and 3 m in length, packed with polyethylene glycol 20M for gas chromatography coated at the ratio of 10% on acid-treated and silanized siliceous earth for gas chromatography (150 to 180 μm in particle diameter).

Column temperature: A constant temperature of about 160°C.

Carrier gas: Nitrogen.

Flow rate: Adjust so that the retention time of pyridine is about 2 minutes.

System suitability—

System performance: When the procedure is run with 2 μL of the standard solution under the above operating conditions, the number of theoretical plates of the peak of pyridine is not less than 1500.

System repeatability: When the test is repeated 6 times with 2 μL of the standard solution under the above operating conditions, the relative standard deviation of the peak areas of pyridine is not more than 3.0%.

(5) Free acids—Transfer about 1 g of Niceritrol, weighed accurately, to a separator, dissolve in 20 mL of chloroform, and extract with 20 mL and then 10 mL of water while shaking well. Combine the whole extracts, and titrate 〈*2.50*〉 with 0.01 mol/L sodium hydroxide VS (indicator: 3 drops of phenolphthalein TS). Perform a blank determination in the same manner, and make any necessary correction, and calculate the amount of free acid by the following equation: it is not more than 0.1%.

Each mL of 0.01 mol/L sodium hydroxide VS
= 1.231 mg of $C_6H_5NO_2$

(6) Related substances—Dissolve 0.10 g of Niceritrol in 10 mL of chloroform, and use this solution as the sample solution. Pipet 1 mL of the sample solution, and add chloroform to make exactly 20 mL. Pipet 2 mL of this solution, add chloroform to make exactly 20 mL, and use this solution as the standard solution. Perform the test with these solutions as directed under Thin-layer Chromatography 〈*2.03*〉. Spot 10 μL each of the sample solution and standard solution on a plate of silica gel with fluorescent indicator for thin-layer chromatography. Develop the plate with a mixture of chloroform and ethanol (95) (4:1) to a distance of about 10 cm, and air-dry the plate. Examine under ultraviolet light (main wavelength: 254 nm): the spots other than the principal spot obtained from the sample solution are not more intense than the spot from the standard solution.

Loss on drying 〈*2.41*〉 Not more than 0.5% (1 g, 105°C, 3 hours).

Residue on ignition 〈*2.44*〉 Not more than 0.1% (1 g).

Assay Weigh accurately about 1 g of Niceritrol, previously dried, add exactly 25 mL of 0.5 mol/L sodium hydroxide VS, boil gently for 20 minutes under a reflux condenser with a carbon dioxide absorber (soda lime). After cooling, titrate 〈*2.50*〉 immediately the excess sodium hydroxide with 0.5 mol/L hydrochloric acid VS (indicator: 3 drops of phenolphthalein TS). Perform a blank determination in the same manner.

Each mL of 0.5 mol/L sodium hydroxide VS
= 69.57 mg of $C_{29}H_{24}N_4O_8$

Containers and storage Containers—Well-closed containers.

Nicomol

ニコモル

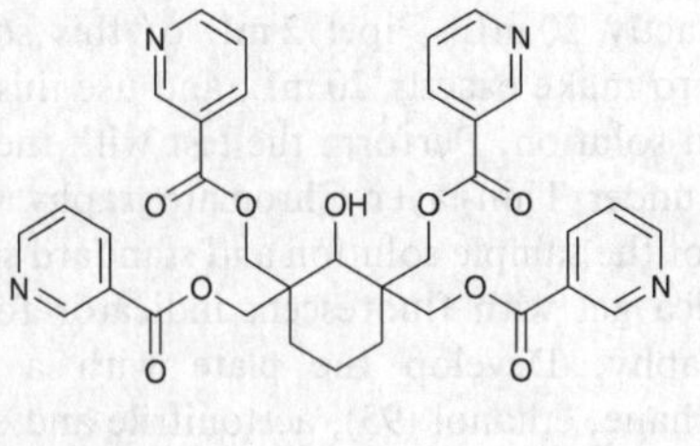

$C_{34}H_{32}N_4O_9$: 640.64
(2-Hydroxycyclohexane-1,1,3,3-tetrayl)tetramethyl tetranicotinate
[*27959-26-8*]

Nicomol, when dried, contains not less than 98.0% of nicomol ($C_{34}H_{32}N_4O_9$).

Description Nicomol occurs as a white crystalline powder. It is odorless and tasteless.

It is soluble in chloroform, and practically insoluble in water, in ethanol (95) and in diethyl ether.

It dissolves in dilute hydrochloric acid and in dilute nitric acid.

Identification **(1)** Mix 0.01 g of Nicomol with 0.02 g of 1-chloro-2,4-dinitrobenzene, add 2 mL of dilute ethanol, heat in a water bath for 5 minutes, cool, and add 4 mL of potassium hydroxide-ethanol TS: a dark red color develops.

(2) Dissolve 0.1 g of Nicomol in 5 mL of dilute hydrochloric acid, and add 5 drops of Reinecke salt TS: a light red precipitate is formed.

(3) Determine the absorption spectrum of a solution of Nicomol in 1 mol/L hydrochloric acid TS (1 in 100,000) as directed under Ultraviolet-visible Spectrophotometry 〈*2.24*〉, and compare the spectrum with the Reference Spectrum: both spectra exhibit similar intensities of absorption at the same wavelengths.

(4) Determine the infrared absorption spectrum of Nicomol, previously dried, as directed in the potassium bromide disk method under Infrared Spectrophotometry 〈*2.25*〉, and compare the spectrum with the Reference Spectrum: both spectra exhibit similar intensities of absorption at the same wave numbers.

Melting point <*2.60*> 181 - 185°C

Purity **(1)** Clarity and color of solution—Dissolve 1.0 g of Nicomol in 10 mL of 1 mol/L hydrochloric acid TS: the solution is clear and colorless.

(2) Acidity—To 1.0 g of Nicomol add 50 mL of freshly boiled and cooled water, shake for 5 minutes, filter, and to 25 mL of the filtrate add 0.60 mL of 0.01 mol/L sodium hydroxide VS and 2 drops of phenolphthalein TS: a red color develops.

(3) Chloride <*1.03*>—Dissolve 0.6 g of Nicomol in 15 mL of dilute nitric acid, and add water to make 50 mL. Perform the test using this solution as the test solution. Prepare the control solution as follows: to 0.40 mL of 0.01 mol/L hydrochloric acid VS add 15 mL of dilute nitric acid and water to make 50 mL (not more than 0.024%).

(4) Heavy metals <*1.07*>—Proceed with 1.0 g of Nicomol according to Method 2, and perform the test. Prepare the control solution with 2.0 mL of Standard Lead Solution (not more than 20 ppm).

(5) Arsenic <*1.11*>—Prepare the test solution with 1.0 g of Nicomol according to Method 3, and perform the test (not more than 2 ppm).

(6) Related substances—Dissolve 0.20 g of Nicomol in 20 mL of chloroform, and use this solution as the sample solution. Pipet 1 mL of the sample solution, and add chloroform to make exactly 20 mL. Pipet 2 mL of this solution, add chloroform to make exactly 20 mL, and use this solution as the standard solution. Perform the test with these solutions as directed under Thin-layer Chromatography <*2.03*>. Spot 10 μL each of the sample solution and standard solution on a plate of silica gel with fluorescent indicator for thin-layer chromatography. Develop the plate with a mixture of dichloromethane, ethanol (95), acetonitrile and ethyl acetate (5:3:1:1) to a distance of about 10 cm, and air-dry the plate. Examine under ultraviolet light (main wavelength: 254 nm): the spots other than the principal spot obtained from the sample solution are not more intense than the spot from the standard solution.

Loss on drying <*2.41*> Not more than 1.0% (1 g, 105°C, 4 hours).

Residue on ignition <*2.44*> Not more than 0.1% (1 g).

Assay Weigh accurately about 1.5 g of Nicomol, previously dried, add exactly 40 mL of 0.5 mol/L sodium hydroxide VS, and boil gently under a reflux condenser connected to a carbon dioxide absorption tube (soda lime) for 10 minutes. After cooling, titrate <*2.50*> immediately the excess sodium hydroxide with 0.25 mol/L sulfuric acid VS (indicator: 3 drops of phenolphthalein TS). Perform a blank determination in the same manner.

Each mL of 0.5 mol/L sodium hydroxide VS
= 80.08 mg of $C_{34}H_{32}N_4O_9$

Containers and storage Containers—Tight containers.

Nicomol Tablets

ニコモール錠

Nicomol Tablets contain not less than 95.0% and not more than 105.0% of the labeled amount of nicomol ($C_{34}H_{32}N_4O_9$: 640.64).

Method of preparation Prepare as directed under Tablets, with Nicomol.

Identification To a portion of powdered Nicomol Tablets, equivalent to 0.5 g of Nicomol, add 20 mL of chloroform, shake, and filter. Evaporate the filtrate on a water bath to dryness. Proceed with the residue as directed in the Identification (1) and (2) under Nicomol.

Uniformity of dosage units <*6.02*> It meets the requirement of the Mass variation test.

Dissolution <*6.10*> When the test is performed at 75 revolutions per minute according to the Paddle method, using 900 mL of 1st fluid for dissolution test as the dissolution medium, the dissolution rate in 60 minutes of Nicomol Tablets is not less than 75%.

Start the test with 1 tablet of Nicomol Tablets, withdraw not less than 20 mL of the medium at the specified minute after starting the test, and filter through a membrane filter with a pore size not exceeding 0.8 μm. Discard not less than 10 mL of the first filtrate, pipet V mL of the subsequent filtrate, add the dissolution medium to make exactly V' mL so that each mL contains about 18 μg of nicomol ($C_{34}H_{32}N_4O_9$), and use this solution as the sample solution. Separately, weigh accurately about 0.1 g of nicomol for assay, previously dried at 105°C for 4 hours, dissolve in the dissolution medium to make exactly 100 mL, then pipet 2 mL of this solution, add the dissolution medium to make exactly 100 mL, and use this solution as the standard solution. Determine the absorbances, A_T and A_S, of the sample solution and standard solution at 262 nm as directed under Ultraviolet-visible Spectrophotometry <*2.24*>.

Dissolution rate (%) with respect to the labeled amount of nicomol ($C_{34}H_{32}N_4O_9$)
$= M_S \times A_T/A_S \times V'/V \times 1/C \times 18$

M_S: Amount (mg) of nicomol for assay taken
C: Labeled amount (mg) of nicomol ($C_{34}H_{32}N_4O_9$) in 1 tablet

Assay Weigh accurately not less than 20 Nicomol Tablets and powder. Weigh accurately a portion of the powder, equivalent to about 1 g of nicomol ($C_{34}H_{32}N_4O_9$), add 100 mL of 1 mol/L hydrochloric acid TS, shake well, add water to make exactly 500 mL, and filter. Discard the first 50 mL of the filtrate, pipet 2 mL of the subsequent filtrate, add 50 mL of 1 mol/L hydrochloric acid TS and water to make exactly 250 mL, and use this solution as the sample solution. Separately, weigh accurately about 80 mg of nicomol for assay, previously dried at 105°C for 4 hours, dissolve in 50 mL of 1 mol/L hydrochloric acid TS, and add water to make exactly 100 mL. Pipet 2 mL of this solution, add 20 mL of 1 mol/L hydrochloric acid TS and water to make exactly 100 mL, and use this solution as the standard solution. Determine the absorbances, A_T and A_S, of the sample solution and standard solution at 262 nm as directed under Ultraviolet-visible Spectrophotometry <*2.24*>.

Amount (mg) of nicomol ($C_{34}H_{32}N_4O_9$)
$= M_S \times A_T/A_S \times 25/2$

M_S: Amount (mg) of nicomol for assay taken

Containers and storage Containers—Tight containers.

Nicorandil

ニコランジル

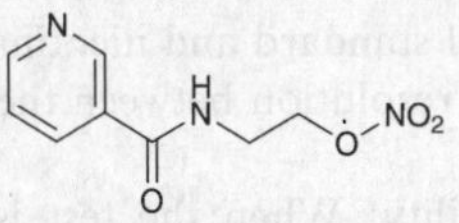

$C_8H_9N_3O_4$: 211.17
N-[2-(Nitrooxy)ethyl]pyridine-3-carboxamide
[65141-46-0]

Nicorandil contains not less than 98.5% and not more than 101.0% of nicorandil ($C_8H_9N_3O_4$), calculated on the anhydrous basis.

Description Nicorandil occurs as white crystals.

It is freely soluble in methanol, in ethanol (99.5) and in acetic acid (100), soluble in acetic anhydride, and sparingly soluble in water.

Melting point: about 92°C (with decomposition).

Identification **(1)** Determine the absorption spectrum of a solution of Nicorandil (1 in 50,000) as directed under Ultraviolet-visible Spectrophotometry <*2.24*>, and compare the spectrum with the Reference Spectrum: both spectra exhibit similar intensities of absorption at the same wavelengths.

(2) Determine the infrared absorption spectrum of Nicorandil as directed in the potassium bromide disk method under Infrared Spectrophotometry <*2.25*>, and compare the spectrum with the Reference Spectrum: both spectra exhibit similar intensities of absorption at the same wave numbers.

Purity **(1)** Sulfate <*1.14*>—Dissolve 2.0 g of Nicorandil in 20 mL of dilute ethanol, add 1 mL of dilute hydrochloric acid and water to make 50 mL, and perform the test using this solution as the test solution. Prepare the control solution with 0.40 mL of 0.005 mol/L sulfuric acid VS, 20 mL of dilute ethanol and 1 mL of dilute hydrochloric acid, and dilute with water to make 50 mL (not more than 0.010%).

(2) Heavy metals <*1.07*>—Proceed with 2.0 g of Nicorandil according to Method 2, and perform the test. Prepare the control solution with 2.0 mL of Standard Lead Solution (not more than 10 ppm).

(3) Related substances—Dissolve 20 mg of Nicorandil in 10 mL of the mobile phase, and use this solution as the sample solution. Perform the test with 10 μL of the sample solution as directed under Liquid Chromatography <*2.01*> according to the following conditions, and determine each peak area by the automatic integration method: the peak area of *N*-(2-hydroxyethyl)isonicotinamide nitric ester, having the relative retention time of about 0.86 to nicorandil, is not more than 0.5% of the peak area of nicorandil, the area of all other peaks is less than 0.1%, and the sum area of the peaks other than nicorandil and *N*-(2-hydroxyethyl)isonicotinamide nitric ester is not more than 0.25% of the total peak area.

Operating conditions—

Detector: An ultraviolet absorption photometer (wavelength: 254 nm).

Column: A stainless steel column 4 mm in inside diameter and 25 cm in length, packed with octadecylsilanized silica gel for liquid chromatography (5 μm in particle diameter).

Column temperature: A constant temperature of about 25°C.

Mobile phase: A mixture of water, tetrahydrofuran, triethylamine and trifluoroacetic acid (982:10:5:3).

Flow rate: Adjust so that the retention time of nicorandil is about 18 minutes.

Time span of measurement: About 3 times as long as the retention time of nicorandil, beginning after the solvent peak.

System suitability—

Test for required detectability: Measure exactly 1 mL of the sample solution, add the mobile phase to make exactly 500 mL, and use this solution as the solution for system suitability test. Pipet 1 mL of the solution for system suitability test, and add the mobile phase to make exactly 20 mL. Confirm that the peak area of nicorandil obtained with 10 μL of this solution is equivalent to 2 to 8% of that with 10 μL of the solution for system suitability test.

System performance: Dissolve 10 mg of *N*-(2-hydroxyethyl)isonicotinamide nitric ester in the mobile phase to make 100 mL. To 1 mL of this solution add 10 mL of the sample solution. When the procedure is run with 10 μL of this solution under the above operating conditions, *N*-(2-hydroxyethyl)isonicotinamide nitric ester and nicorandil are eluted in this order with the resolution between these peaks being not less than 3.0.

System repeatability: When the test is repeated 6 times with 10 μL of the solution for system suitability test under the above operating conditions, the relative standard deviation of the peak area of nicorandil is not more than 1.5%.

Water <*2.48*> Not more than 0.1% (2 g, volumetric titration, direct titration).

Residue on ignition <*2.44*> Not more than 0.1% (1 g).

Assay Weigh accurately about 0.3 g of Nicorandil, dissolve in 30 mL of a mixture of acetic anhydride and acetic acid (100) (7:3), and titrate <*2.50*> with 0.1 mol/L perchloric acid VS (potentiometric titration). Perform a blank determination in the same manner, and make any necessary correction.

Each mL of 0.1 mol/L perchloric acid VS
= 21.12 mg of $C_8H_9N_3O_4$

Containers and storage Containers—Tight containers.

Storage—At a temperature between 2°C and 8°C.

Nicotinamide

ニコチン酸アミド

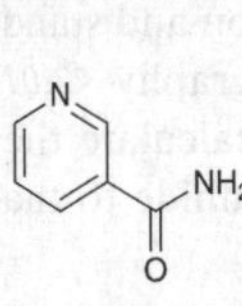

$C_6H_6N_2O$: 122.12
Pyridine-3-carboxamide
[98-92-0]

Nicotinamide, when dried, contains not less than 98.5% and not more than 102.0% of nicotinamide ($C_6H_6N_2O$).

Description Nicotinamide occurs as white, crystals or crystalline powder. It is odorless, and has a bitter taste.

It is freely soluble in water and in ethanol (95), and slightly soluble in diethyl ether.

Identification **(1)** Mix 5 mg of Nicotinamide with 0.01 g of 1-chloro-2,4-dinitrobenzene, heat gently for 5 to 6 seconds, and fuse the mixture. Cool, and add 4 mL of potassium hydroxide-ethanol TS: a red color is produced.

(2) To 0.02 g of Nicotinamide add 5 mL of sodium hydroxide TS, and boil carefully: the gas evolved turns moistened red litmus paper blue.

(3) Dissolve 0.02 g of Nicotinamide in water to make 1000 mL. Determine the absorption spectrum of the solution as directed under Ultraviolet-visible Spectrophotometry <*2.24*>, and compare the spectrum with the Reference Spectrum or the spectrum of a solution of Nicotinamide RS prepared in the same manner as the sample solution: both spectra exhibit similar intensities of absorption at the same wavelengths.

pH <*2.54*> Dissolve 1.0 g of Nicotinamide in 20 mL of water: the pH of this solution is between 6.0 and 7.5.

Melting point <*2.60*> 128 - 131°C

Purity **(1)** Clarity and color of solution—Dissolve 1.0 g of Nicotinamide in 20 mL of water: the solution is clear and colorless.

(2) Chloride <*1.03*>—Take 0.5 g of Nicotinamide, and perform the test. Prepare the control solution with 0.30 mL of 0.01 mol/L hydrochloric acid VS (not more than 0.021%).

(3) Sulfate <*1.14*>—Take 1.0 g of Nicotinamide, and perform the test. Prepare the control solution with 0.40 mL of 0.005 mol/L sulfuric acid VS (not more than 0.019%).

(4) Heavy metals <*1.07*>—Proceed with 1.0 g of Nicotinamide according to Method 1, and perform the test. Prepare the control solution with 3.0 mL of Standard Lead Solution (not more than 30 ppm).

(5) Readily carbonizable substances <*1.15*>—Take 0.20 g of Nicotinamide, and perform the test. The solution has no more color than Matching Fluid A.

Loss on drying <*2.41*> Not more than 0.5% (1 g, in vacuum, silica gel, 4 hours).

Residue on ignition <*2.44*> Not more than 0.1% (1 g).

Assay Weigh accurately about 25 mg each of Nicotinamide and Nicotinamide RS, both previously dried, dissolve separately in 3 mL of water, and add the mobile phase to make exactly 100 mL. Pipet 8 mL each of these solutions, and add the mobile phase to make exactly 50 mL. Pipet 5 mL each of these solutions, add exactly 5 mL of the internal standard solution, and use these solutions as the sample solution and the standard solution, respectively. Perform the test with 20 μL each of the sample solution and standard solution as directed under Liquid Chromatography <*2.01*> according to the following conditions, and calculate the ratios, Q_T and Q_S, of the peak area of nicotinamide to that of the internal standard.

$$\text{Amount (g) of nicotinamide } (C_6H_6N_2O) = M_S \times Q_T/Q_S$$

M_S: Amount (mg) of dried Nicotinamide RS taken

Internal standard solution—A solution of nicotinic acid (1 in 25,000).

Operating conditions—

Detector: An ultraviolet absorption photometer (wavelength: 254 nm).

Column: A stainless steel column 4.6 mm in inside diameter and 25 cm in length, packed with octadecylsilanized silica gel for liquid chromatography (5 μm in particle diameter).

Column temperature: A constant temperature of about 25°C.

Mobile phase: Dissolve 1 g of sodium 1-heptane sulfonate in water to make 1000 mL. To 700 mL of this solution add 300 mL of methanol.

Flow rate: Adjust so that the retention time of nicotinamide is about 7 minutes.

System suitability—

System performance: When the procedure is run with 20 μL of the standard solution under the above operating conditions, the internal standard and nicotinamide are eluted in this order with the resolution between these peaks being not less than 5.

System repeatability: When the test is repeated 6 times with 20 μL of the standard solution under the above operating conditions, the relative standard deviation of the ratio of the peak area of nicotinamide to that of the internal standard is not more than 1.0%.

Containers and storage Containers—Tight containers.

Nicotinic Acid

ニコチン酸

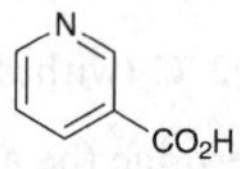

$C_6H_5NO_2$: 123.11

Pyridine-3-carboxylic acid

[59-67-6]

Nicotinic Acid, when dried, contains not less than 99.5% of nicotinic acid ($C_6H_5NO_2$).

Description Nicotinic Acid occurs as white, crystals or crystalline powder. It is odorless, and has a slightly acid taste.

It is sparingly soluble in water, slightly soluble in ethanol (95), and very slightly soluble in diethyl ether.

It dissolves in sodium hydroxide TS and in sodium carbonate TS.

Identification **(1)** Triturate 5 mg of Nicotinic Acid with 0.01 g of 1-chloro-2,4-dinitrobenzene, and fuse the mixture by gentle heating for 5 to 6 seconds. Cool, and add 4 mL of potassium hydroxide-ethanol TS: a dark red color is produced.

(2) Dissolve 0.02 g of Nicotinic Acid in water to make 1000 mL. Determine the absorption spectrum of the solution as directed under Ultraviolet-visible Spectrophotometry <*2.24*>, and compare the spectrum with the Reference Spectrum or the spectrum of a solution of Nicotinic Acid RS prepared in the same manner as the sample solution: both spectra exhibit similar intensities of absorption at the same wavelengths.

pH <*2.54*> Dissolve 0.20 g of Nicotinic Acid in 20 mL of water: the pH of this solution is between 3.0 and 4.0.

Melting point <*2.60*> 234 - 238°C

Purity **(1)** Clarity and color of solution—Dissolve 0.20 g of Nicotinic Acid in 20 mL of water: the solution is clear and colorless.

(2) Chloride <*1.03*>—Perform the test with 0.5 g of Nicotinic Acid. Prepare the control solution with 0.30 mL of 0.01 mol/L hydrochloric acid VS (not more than 0.021%).

(3) Sulfate <*1.14*>—Dissolve 1.0 g of Nicotinic Acid in 3 mL of dilute hydrochloric acid and water to make 50 mL. Perform the test using this solution as the test solution. Prepare the control solution with 0.40 mL of 0.005 mol/L sulfuric acid VS and 3 mL of dilute hydrochloric acid, and dilute with water to make 50 mL (not more than 0.019%).

(4) Nitro compounds—Dissolve 1.0 g of Nicotinic Acid in 8 mL of sodium hydroxide TS, and add water to make 20 mL: the solution has no more color than Matching Fluid A.

(5) Heavy metals *<1.07>*—Proceed with 1.0 g of Nicotinic Acid according to Method 2, and perform the test. Prepare the control solution with 2.0 mL of Standard Lead Solution (not more than 20 ppm).

Loss on drying *<2.41>* Not more than 0.5% (1 g, 105°C, 1 hour).

Residue on ignition *<2.44>* Not more than 0.1% (1 g).

Assay Weigh accurately about 0.3 g of Nicotinic Acid, previously dried, dissolve in 50 mL of water, and titrate *<2.50>* with 0.1 mol/L sodium hydroxide VS (indicator: 5 drops of phenolphthalein TS).

Each mL of 0.1 mol/L sodium hydroxide VS
= 12.31 mg of $C_6H_5NO_2$

Containers and storage Containers—Well-closed containers.

Nicotinic Acid Injection

ニコチン酸注射液

Nicotinic Acid Injection is an aqueous injection.

It contains not less than 95.0% and not more than 110.0% of the labeled amount of nicotinic acid ($C_6H_5NO_2$: 123.11).

Method of preparation Prepare as directed under Injections, with Nicotinic Acid. It may contain Sodium Carbonate or Sodium Hydroxide as a solubilizer.

Description Nicotinic Acid Injection is a clear, colorless liquid.

pH: 5.0 – 7.0

Identification **(1)** To a volume of Nicotinic Acid Injection, equivalent to 0.1 g of Nicotinic Acid, add 0.3 mL of dilute hydrochloric acid, and evaporate on a water bath to 2 mL. After cooling, collect the crystals formed, wash with small portions of ice-cold water until the last washing shows no turbidity on the addition of silver nitrate TS, and dry at 105°C for 1 hour: the crystals melt *<2.60>* between 234°C and 238°C. With the crystals, proceed as directed in the Identification (1) under Nicotinic Acid.

(2) Dissolve 0.02 g of the dried crystals obtained in (1) in water to make 1000 mL, and determine the absorption spectrum as directed under Ultraviolet-visible Spectrophotometry *<2.24>*: it exhibits a maximum between 261 nm and 263 nm, and a minimum between 235 nm and 239 nm. Separately, determine the absorbances of this solution, A_1 and A_2, at each wavelength of maximum and minimum absorption, respectively: the ratio A_2/A_1 is between 0.35 and 0.39.

Bacterial endotoxins *<4.01>* Less than 3.0 EU/mg.

Extractable volume *<6.05>* It meets the requirement.

Foreign insoluble matter *<6.06>* Perform the test according to Method 1: it meets the requirement.

Insoluble particulate matter *<6.07>* It meets the requirement.

Sterility *<4.06>* Perform the test according to the Membrane filtration method: it meets the requirement.

Assay Measure exactly a volume of Nicotinic Acid Injection, equivalent to about 0.1 g of nicotinic acid ($C_6H_5NO_2$), and add the mobile phase to make exactly 100 mL. Pipet 10 mL of this solution, add exactly 10 mL of the internal standard solution, then add the mobile phase to make 100 mL, and use this solution as the sample solution. Separately, weigh accurately about 0.1 g of Nicotinic Acid RS, previously dried at 105°C for 1 hour, and dissolve in the mobile phase to make exactly 100 mL. Pipet 10 mL of this solution, add exactly 10 mL of the internal standard solution, then add the mobile phase to make 100 mL, and use this solution as the standard solution. Perform the test with 10 μL each of the sample solution and standard solution as directed under Liquid Chromatography *<2.01>* according to the following conditions, and calculate the ratios, Q_T and Q_S, of the peak area of nicotinic acid to that of the internal standard.

Amount (mg) of nicotinic acid ($C_6H_5NO_2$)
$= M_S \times Q_T/Q_S$

M_S: Amount (mg) of Nicotinic Acid RS taken

Internal standard solution—A solution of caffeine in the mobile phase (1 in 1000).

Operating conditions—

Detector: An ultraviolet absorption photometer (wavelength: 260 nm).

Column: A stainless steel column 4.6 mm in inside diameter and 15 cm in length, packed with octadecylsilanized silica gel for liquid chromatography (5 μm in particle diameter).

Column temperature: A constant temperature of about 35°C.

Mobile phase: Dissolve 1.1 g of sodium 1-octane sulfonate in a mixture of 0.05 mol/L sodium dihydrogenphosphate TS (pH 3.0) and methanol (4:1) to make 1000 mL.

Flow rate: Adjust so that the retention time of caffeine is about 9 minutes.

System suitability—

System performance: When the procedure is run with 10 μL of the standard solution under the above operating conditions, nicotinic acid and the internal standard are eluted in this order with the resolution between these peaks being not less than 10.

System repeatability: When the test is repeated 6 times with 10 μL of the standard solution under the above operating conditions, the relative standard deviation of the ratios of the peak area of nicotinic acid to that of the internal standard is not more than 1.0%.

Containers and storage Containers—Hermetic containers.

Nifedipine

ニフェジピン

$C_{17}H_{18}N_2O_6$: 346.33
Dimethyl 2,6-dimethyl-4-(2-nitrophenyl)-1,4-dihydropyridine-3,5-dicarboxylate
[21829-25-4]

Nifedipine contains not less than 98.0% and not more than 102.0% of nifedipine ($C_{17}H_{18}N_2O_6$), calculated on the dried basis.

Description Nifedipine occurs as a yellow crystalline powder. It is odorless and tasteless.

It is freely soluble in acetone and in dichloromethane, sparingly soluble in methanol, in ethanol (95) and in acetic acid (100), slightly soluble in diethyl ether, and practically insoluble in water.

It is affected by light.

Identification **(1)** Dissolve 0.05 g of Nifedipine in 5 mL of ethanol (95), and add 5 mL of hydrochloric acid and 2 g of zinc powder. Allow to stand for 5 minutes, and filter: the filtrate responds to Qualitative Tests *<1.09>* for primary aromatic amines, developing a red-purple color.

(2) Determine the absorption spectrum of a solution of Nifedipine in methanol (1 in 100,000) as directed under Ultraviolet-visible Spectrophotometry *<2.24>*, and compare the spectrum with the Reference Spectrum: both spectra exhibit similar intensities of absorption at the same wavelengths.

(3) Determine the infrared absorption spectrum of Nifedipine, previously dried, as directed in the potassium bromide disk method under Infrared Spectrophotometry *<2.25>*, and compare the spectrum with the Reference Spectrum: both spectra exhibit similar intensities of absorption at the same wave numbers.

Melting point *<2.60>* 172 – 175°C

Purity **(1)** Clarity and color of solution—Dissolve 0.5 g of Nifedipine in 5 mL of acetone: the solution is clear and yellow.

(2) Chloride *<1.03>*—To 2.5 g of Nifedipine add 12 mL of dilute acetic acid and 13 mL of water, and heat to boil. After cooling, filter, and discard the first 10 mL of the filtrate. To 5 mL of the subsequent filtrate add 6 mL of dilute nitric acid and water to make 50 mL, and perform the test using this solution as the test solution. Prepare the control solution with 0.30 mL of 0.01 mol/L hydrochloric acid VS (not more than 0.021%).

(3) Sulfate *<1.14>*—To 4 mL of the filtrate obtained in (2) add 1 mL of dilute hydrochloric acid and water to make 50 mL. Perform the test using this solution as the test solution. Prepare the control solution with 0.45 mL of 0.005 mol/L sulfuric acid VS (not more than 0.054%).

(4) Heavy metals *<1.07>*—Proceed with 2.0 g of Nifedipine according to Method 2, and perform the test. Prepare the control solution with 2.0 mL of Standard Lead Solution (not more than 10 ppm).

(5) Arsenic *<1.11>*—Prepare the test solution with 1.0 g of Nifedipine according to Method 3, and perform the test (not more than 2 ppm).

(6) Basic substances—The procedure should be performed under protection from light in light-resistant vessels. Dissolve 5.0 g of Nifedipine in 80 mL of a mixture of acetone and acetic acid (100) (5:3), and titrate *<2.50>* with 0.02 mol/L perchloric acid VS (potentiometric titration). Perform a blank determination in the same manner, and make any necessary correction. Not more than 1.9 mL of 0.02 mol/L perchloric acid VS is consumed.

(7) Dimethyl-2,6-dimethyl-4-(2-nitrosophenyl)-3,5-pyridinedicarboxylate—The procedure should be performed under protection from light in light-resistant vessels. Dissolve 0.15 g of Nifedipine in dichloromethane to make exactly 10 mL, and use this solution as the sample solution. Separately, dissolve 10 mg of dimethyl 2,6-dimethyl-4-(2-nitrosophenyl)-3,5-pyridine-dicarboxylate for thin-layer chromatography in exactly 10 mL of dichloromethane. Measure exactly 1 mL of this solution, add dichloromethane to make exactly 20 mL, and use this solution as the standard solution. Perform the test with these solutions as directed under Thin-layer Chromatography *<2.03>*. Spot 10 μL each of the sample solution and standard solution on a plate of silica gel with fluorescent indicator for thin-layer chromatography. Develop the plate with a mixture of cyclohexane and ethyl acetate (3:2) to a distance of about 10 cm, and air-dry the plate. Examine under ultraviolet light (main wavelength: 254 nm): the spot obtained from the sample solution, corresponding to that from the standard solution, is not more intense than the spot from the standard solution.

Loss on drying *<2.41>* Not more than 0.5% (0.5 g, 105°C, 2 hours).

Residue on ignition *<2.44>* Not more than 0.1% (1 g).

Assay The procedure should be performed under protection from light in light-resistant vessels. Weigh accurately about 0.12 g of Nifedipine, and dissolve in methanol to make exactly 200 mL. Measure exactly 5 mL of this solution, and add methanol to make exactly 100 mL. Determine the absorbance A of this solution at the wavelength of maximum absorption at about 350 nm as directed under Ultraviolet-visible Spectrophotometry *<2.24>*.

$$\text{Amount (mg) of nifedipine } (C_{17}H_{18}N_2O_6) = A/142.3 \times 40{,}000$$

Containers and storage Containers—Tight containers.
Storage—Light-resistant.

Nifedipine Delayed-release Fine Granules

ニフェジピン腸溶細粒

Nifedipine Delayed-release Fine Granules contain not less than 95.0% and not more than 105.0% of the labeled amount of nifedipine ($C_{17}H_{18}N_2O_6$: 346.33).

Method of preparation Prepare as directed under Granules, with Nifedipine.

Identification Conduct this procedure without exposure to light, using light-resistant vessels. Shake for 15 minutes a quantity of powdered Nifedipine Delayed-release Fine Granules, equivalent to 3 mg of Nifedipine, with 100 mL of methanol, and filter. Determine the absorption spectrum of the filtrate so obtained as directed under Ultraviolet-visible Spectrophotometry <2.24>: it exhibits a broad absorption maximum between 335 nm and 356 nm.

Uniformity of dosage units <6.02> Perform the test according to the following method: the Granules in single-dose packages meet the requirement of the Content uniformity test.

Conduct this procedure without exposure to light, using light-resistant vessels. To the total content of 1 package of Nifedipine Delayed-release Fine Granules add 50 mL of a mixture of methanol and water (9:1), sonicate for 15 minutes with occasional shaking, and shake for further 15 minutes. Then, add methanol to make exactly V mL so that each mL contains about 0.1 mg of nifedipine ($C_{17}H_{18}N_2O_6$). Filter this solution through a membrane filter with a pore size not exceeding 0.45 μm. Discard the first 10 mL of the filtrate, pipet 5 mL of the subsequent filtrate, add methanol to make exactly 10 mL, and use this solution as the sample solution. Separately, weigh accurately about 50 mg of nifedipine for assay, previously dried at 105°C for 2 hours, and dissolve in methanol to make exactly 50 mL. Pipet 5 mL of this solution, add methanol to make exactly 100 mL, and use this solution as the standard solution. Then, proceed as directed in the Assay.

Amount (mg) of nifedipine ($C_{17}H_{18}N_2O_6$)
$= M_S \times A_T/A_S \times V/500$

M_S: Amount (mg) of nifedipine for assay taken

Dissolution <6.10> When the tests are performed at 50 revolutions per minute according to the Paddle method, using 900 mL each of 1st and 2nd fluids for dissolution test as the dissolution medium, the dissolution rate in the test using the 1st fluid for dissolution test in 60 minutes is not more than 15%, and that in the test using the 2nd fluid for dissolution test in 30 minutes is not less than 75%.

Conduct this procedure without exposure to light, using light-resistant vessels. Start the test with an accurately weighed amount of Nifedipine Delayed-release Fine Granules, equivalent to about 20 mg of nifedipine ($C_{17}H_{18}N_2O_6$), withdraw not less than 20 mL of the medium at the specified minute after starting the test, and filter through a membrane filter with a pore size not exceeding 0.45 μm. Discard not less than 10 mL of the first filtrate, pipet 5 mL of the subsequent filtrate, add the dissolution medium to make exactly 10 mL, and use this solution as the sample solution. Separately, weigh accurately about 28 mg of nifedipine for assay, previously dried at 105°C for 2 hours, dissolve in 50 mL of methanol, and add the dissolution medium to make exactly 100 mL. Pipet 2 mL of this solution, add the dissolution medium to make exactly 50 mL, and use this solution as the standard solution. Perform the test with exactly 50 μL each of the sample solution and standard solution as directed under Liquid Chromatography <2.01>, and determine the peak areas, A_T and A_S, of nifedipine in each solution.

Dissolution rate (%) with respect to the labeled amount of nifedipine ($C_{17}H_{18}N_2O_6$)
$= M_S/M_T \times A_T/A_S \times 1/C \times 72$

M_S: Amount (mg) of nifedipine for assay taken
M_T: Amount (g) of Nifedipine Delayed-release Fine Granules taken
C: Labeled amount (mg) of nifedipine ($C_{17}H_{18}N_2O_6$) in 1 g

Operating conditions—

Proceed as directed in the operating conditions in the Assay.

System suitability—

System performance: When the procedure is run with 50 μL of the standard solution under the above operating conditions, the number of theoretical plates and the symmetry factor of the peak of nifedipine are not less than 4000 and not more than 1.5, respectively.

System repeatability: When the test is repeated 6 times with 50 μL of the standard solution under the above operating conditions, the relative standard deviation of the peak area of nifedipine is not more than 1.0%.

Assay Conduct this procedure without exposure to light, using light-resistant vessels. Weigh accurately a portion of powdered Nifedipine Delayed-release Fine Granules, equivalent to about 10 mg of nifedipine ($C_{17}H_{18}N_2O_6$), add 50 mL of a mixture of methanol and water (9:1), shake vigorously for 15 minutes, and add methanol to make exactly 100 mL. Filter this solution through a membrane filter with a pore size not exceeding 0.45 μm. Discard the first 10 mL of the filtrate, pipet 5 mL of the subsequent filtrate, add methanol to make exactly 10 mL, and use this solution as the sample solution. Separately, weigh accurately about 50 mg of nifedipine for assay, previously dried at 105°C for 2 hours, and dissolve in methanol to make exactly 50 mL. Pipet 5 mL of this solution, add methanol to make exactly 100 mL, and use this solution as the standard solution. Perform the test with exactly 10 μL each of the sample solution and standard solution as directed under Liquid Chromatography <2.01> according to the following conditions, and determine the peak areas, A_T and A_S, of nifedipine in each solution.

Amount (mg) of nifedipine ($C_{17}H_{18}N_2O_6$)
$= M_S \times A_T/A_S \times 1/5$

M_S: Amount (mg) of nifedipine for assay taken

Operating conditions—

Detector: An ultraviolet absorption photometer (wavelength: 230 nm).

Column: A stainless steel column 4.6 mm in inside diameter and 15 cm in length, packed with octadecylsilanized silica gel for liquid chromatography (5 μm in particle diameter).

Column temperature: A constant temperature of about 40°C.

Mobile phase: Adjust to pH 6.1 of a mixture of methanol and diluted 0.05 mol/L disodium hydrogen phosphate TS (1 in 5) (11:9) with phosphoric acid.

Flow rate: Adjust so that the retention time of nifedipine is about 6 minutes.

System suitability—

System performance: When the procedure is run with 10 μL of the standard solution under the above operating conditions, the number of theoretical plates and the symmetry factor of the peak of nifedipine are not less than 4000 and not more than 1.2, respectively.

System repeatability: When the test is repeated 6 times with 10 μL of the standard solution under the above operating conditions, the relative standard deviation of the peak area of nifedipine is not more than 1.0%.

Containers and storage Containers—Tight containers.

Storage—Light-resistant.

Nifedipine Extended-release Capsules

ニフェジピン徐放カプセル

Nifedipine Extended-release Capsules contain not less than 93.0% and not more than 107.0% of the labeled amount of nifedipine ($C_{17}H_{18}N_2O_6$: 346.33).

Method of preparation Prepare as directed under Capsules, with Nifedipine.

Identification Conduct this procedure without exposure to light, using light-resistant vessels. Take out the content of Nifedipine Extended-release Capsules, and powder. To an amount of the powder, equivalent to 3 mg of Nifedipine, add 100 mL of methanol, shake for 15 minutes, and centrifuge. Determine the absorption spectrum of the supernatant liquid so obtained as directed under Ultraviolet-visible Spectrophotometry <*2.24*>: it exhibits a broad absorption maximum between 335 nm and 356 nm.

Uniformity of dosage units <*6.02*> Perform the test according to the following method: it meets the requirement of the Content uniformity test.

Conduct this procedure without exposure to light, using light-resistant vessels. To the total content of 1 capsule of Nifedipine Extended-release Capsules, add 50 mL of a mixture of methanol and water (9:1), sonicate for 15 minutes with occasional shaking, and shake for further 15 minutes. Then, add methanol to make exactly *V* mL so that each mL contains about 0.1 mg of nifedipine ($C_{17}H_{18}N_2O_6$). Filter this solution through a membrane filter with a pore size not exceeding 0.45 µm. Discard the first 10 mL of the filtrate, pipet 5 mL of the subsequent filtrate, add methanol to make exactly 10 mL, and use this solution as the sample solution. Separately, weigh accurately about 50 mg of nifedipine for assay, previously dried at 105°C for 2 hours, and dissolve in methanol to make exactly 50 mL. Pipet 5 mL of this solution, add methanol to make exactly 100 mL, and use this solution as the standard solution. Then, proceed as directed in the Assay.

$$\text{Amount (mg) of nifedipine } (C_{17}H_{18}N_2O_6) = M_S \times A_T/A_S \times V/500$$

M_S: Amount (mg) of nifedipine for assay taken

Dissolution Being specified separately when the drug is granted approval based on the Law.

Assay Conduct this procedure without exposure to light, using light-resistant vessels. Take out the contents of not less than 20 Nifedipine Extended-release Capsules, weigh accurately the mass of the contents, and powder. Weigh accurately a portion of the powder, equivalent to about 10 mg of nifedipine ($C_{17}H_{18}N_2O_6$), add 50 mL of a mixture of methanol and water (9:1), shake vigorously for 15 minutes, and add methanol to make exactly 100 mL. Filter this solution through a membrane filter with a pore size not exceeding 0.45 µm. Discard the first 10 mL of the filtrate, pipet 5 mL of the subsequent filtrate, add methanol to make exactly 10 mL, and use this solution as the sample solution. Separately, weigh accurately about 50 mg of nifedipine for assay, previously dried at 105°C for 2 hours, and dissolve in methanol to make exactly 50 mL. Pipet 5 mL of this solution, add methanol to make exactly 100 mL, and use this solution as the standard solution. Perform the test with exactly 10 µL each of the sample solution and standard solution as directed under Liquid Chromatography <*2.01*> according to the following conditions, and determine the peak areas, A_T and A_S, of nifedipine in each solution.

$$\text{Amount (mg) of nifedipine } (C_{17}H_{18}N_2O_6) = M_S \times A_T/A_S \times 1/5$$

M_S: Amount (mg) of nifedipine for assay taken

Operating conditions—

Detector: An ultraviolet absorption photometer (wavelength: 230 nm).

Column: A stainless steel column 4.6 mm in inside diameter and 15 cm in length, packed with octadecylsilanized silica gel for liquid chromatography (5 µm in particle diameter).

Column temperature: A constant temperature of about 40°C.

Mobile phase: Adjust to pH 6.1 of a mixture of methanol and diluted 0.05 mol/L disodium hydrogen phosphate TS (1 in 5) (11:9) with phosphoric acid.

Flow rate: Adjust so that the retention time of nifedipine is about 6 minutes.

System suitability—

System performance: When the procedure is run with 10 µL of the standard solution under the above operating conditions, the number of theoretical plates and the symmetry factor of the peak of nifedipine are not less than 4000 and not more than 1.2, respectively.

System repeatability: When the test is repeated 6 times with 10 µL of the standard solution under the above operating conditions, the relative standard deviation of the peak area of nifedipine is not more than 1.0%.

Containers and storage Containers—Tight containers.
Storage—Light-resistant.

Nifedipine Fine Granules

ニフェジピン細粒

Nifedipine Fine Granules contain not less than 95.0% and not more than 105.0% of the labeled amount of nifedipine ($C_{17}H_{18}N_2O_6$: 346.33).

Method of preparation Prepare as directed under Granules, with Nifedipine.

Identification Conduct this procedure without exposure to light, using light-resistant vessels. Shake for 15 minutes a quantity of powdered Nifedipine Fine Granules, equivalent to 6 mg of Nifedipine, with 200 mL of methanol, and centrifuge. Determine the absorption spectrum of the supernatant liquid so obtained as directed under Ultraviolet-visible Spectrophotometry <*2.24*>: it exhibits a broad absorption maximum between 335 nm and 356 nm.

Uniformity of dosage units <*6.02*> Perform the test according to the following method: the Granules in single-dose packages meet the requirement of the Content uniformity test.

Conduct this procedure without exposure to light, using light-resistant vessels. To the total content of 1 package of Nifedipine Fine Granules add 50 mL of a mixture of methanol and water (9:1), sonicate for 15 minutes with occasional shaking, and shake for further 15 minutes. Then, add methanol to make exactly *V* mL so that each mL contains about 0.1 mg of of nifedipine ($C_{17}H_{18}N_2O_6$). Filter this solution through a membrane filter with a pore size not exceeding

0.45 μm. Discard the first 10 mL of the filtrate, pipet 5 mL of the subsequent filtrate, add methanol to make exactly 10 mL, and use this solution as the sample solution. Separately, weigh accurately about 50 mg of nifedipine for assay, previously dried at 105°C for 2 hours, and dissolve in methanol to make exactly 50 mL. Pipet 5 mL of this solution, add methanol to make exactly 100 mL, and use this solution as the standard solution. Then, proceed as directed in the Assay.

Amount (mg) of nifedipine ($C_{17}H_{18}N_2O_6$)
$= M_S \times A_T/A_S \times V/500$

M_S: Amount (mg) of nifedipine for assay taken

Dissolution <*6.10*> When the test is performed at 50 revolutions per minute according to the Paddle method, using 900 mL of water as the dissolution medium, the dissolution rate in 15 minutes of Nifedipine Fine Granules is not less than 85%.

Conduct this procedure without exposure to light, using light-resistant vessels. Start the test with an accurately weighted amount of Nifedipine Fine Granules, equivalent to about 10 mg of nifedipine ($C_{17}H_{18}N_2O_6$), withdraw not less than 20 mL of the medium at the specified minute after starting the test, and filter through a membrane filter with a pore size not exceeding 0.45 μm. Discard not less than 10 mL of the first filtrate, and use the subsequent filtrate as the sample solution. Separately, weigh accurately about 28 mg of nifedipine for assay, previously dried at 105°C for 2 hours, dissolve in 50 mL of methanol, and add water to make exactly 100 mL. Pipet 2 mL of this solution, add water to make exactly 50 mL, and use this solution as the standard solution. Perform the test with exactly 50 μL each of the sample solution and standard solution as directed under Liquid Chromatography <*2.01*> according to the following conditions, and determine the peak areas, A_T and A_S, of nifedipine in each solution.

Dissolution rate (%) with respect to the labeled amount of nifedipine ($C_{17}H_{18}N_2O_6$)
$= M_S/M_T \times A_T/A_S \times 1/C \times 36$

M_S: Amount (mg) of nifedipine for assay taken
M_T: Amount (g) of Nifedipine Fine Granules taken
C: Labeled amount (mg) of nifedipine ($C_{17}H_{18}N_2O_6$) in 1 g

Operating conditions—

Proceed as directed in the operating conditions under the Assay.

System suitability—

System performance: When the procedure is run with 50 μL of the standard solution under the above operating conditions, the number of theoretical plates and the symmetry factor of the peak of nifedipine are not less than 4000 and not more than 1.5, respectively.

System repeatability: When the test is repeated 6 times with 50 μL of the standard solution under the above operating conditions, the relative standard deviation of the peak area of nifedipine is not more than 1.0%.

Assay Conduct this procedure without exposure to light, using light-resistant vessels. Weigh accurately a protein of powdered Nifedipine Fine Granules, equivalent to about 10 mg of nifedipine ($C_{17}H_{18}N_2O_6$), add 50 mL of a mixture of methanol and water (9:1), shake vigorously for 15 minutes, and add methanol to make exactly 100 mL. Filter this solution through a membrane filter with a pore size not exceeding 0.45 μm. Discard the first 10 mL of the filtrate, pipet 5 mL of the subsequent filtrate, add methanol to make exactly 10 mL, and use this solution as the sample solution. Separately, weigh accurately about 50 mg of nifedipine for assay, previously dried at 105°C for 2 hours, and dissolve in methanol to make exactly 50 mL. Pipet 5 mL of this solution, add methanol to make exactly 100 mL, and use this solution as the standard solution. Perform the test with exactly 10 μL each of the sample solution and standard solution as directed under Liquid Chromatography <*2.01*> according to the following conditions, and determine the peak areas, A_T and A_S, of nifedipine in each solution.

Amount (mg) of nifedipine ($C_{17}H_{18}N_2O_6$)
$= M_S \times A_T/A_S \times 1/5$

M_S: Amount (mg) of nifedipine for assay taken

Operating conditions—

Detector: An ultraviolet absorption photometer (wavelength: 230 nm).

Column: A stainless steel column 4.6 mm in inside diameter and 15 cm in length, packed with octadecylsilanized silica gel for liquid chromatography (5 μm in particle diameter).

Column temperature: A constant temperature of about 40°C.

Mobile phase: Adjust to pH 6.1 of a mixture of methanol and diluted 0.05 mol/L disodium hydrogen phosphate TS (1 in 5) (11:9) with phosphoric acid.

Flow rate: Adjust so that the retention time of nifedipine is about 6 minutes.

System suitability—

System performance: When the procedure is run with 10 μL of the standard solution under the above operating conditions, the number of theoretical plates and the symmetry factor of the peak of nifedipine are not less than 4000 and not more than 1.2, respectively.

System repeatability: When the test is repeated 6 times with 10 μL of the standard solution under the above operating conditions, the relative standard deviation of the peak area of nifedipine is not more than 1.0%.

Containers and storage Containers—Tight containers.
Storage—Light-resistant.

Nilvadipine

ニルバジピン

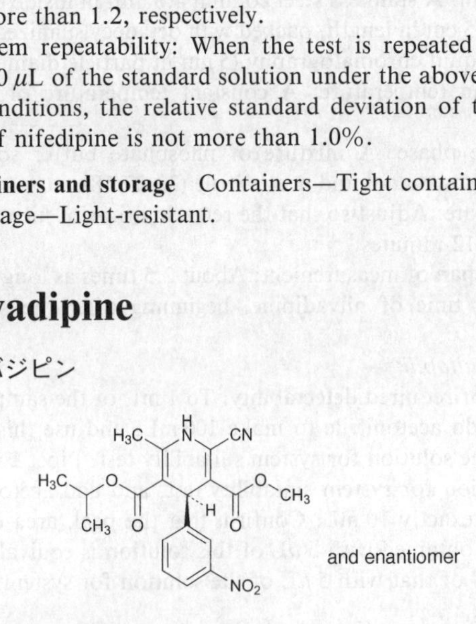

and enantiomer

$C_{19}H_{19}N_3O_6$: 385.37
3-Methyl 5-(1-methylethyl) (4*RS*)-2-cyano-6-methyl-4-(3-nitrophenyl)-1,4-dihydropyridine-3,5-dicarboxylate
[*75530-68-6*]

Nilvadipine contains not less than 98.0% and not more than 102.0% of nilvadipine ($C_{19}H_{19}N_3O_6$).

Description Nilvadipine occurs as a yellow crystalline powder.

It is freely soluble in acetonitrile, soluble in methanol, sparingly soluble in ethanol (99.5), and practically insoluble in water.

A solution of Nilvadipine in acetonitrile (1 in 20) shows no optical rotation.

Identification (1) Determine the absorption spectrum of a solution of Nilvadipine in ethanol (99.5) (1 in 100,000) as directed under Ultraviolet-visible Spectrophotometry <*2.24*>, and compare the spectrum with the Reference Spectrum or the spectrum of a solution of Nilvadipine RS prepared in the same manner as the sample solution: both spectra exhibit similar intensities of absorption at the same wavelengths.

(2) Determine the infrared absorption spectrum of Nilvadipine as directed in the potassium bromide disk method under Infrared Spectrophotometry <*2.25*>, and compare the spectrum with the Reference Spectrum or the spectrum of Nilvadipine RS: both spectra exhibit similar intensities of absorption at the same wave numbers.

Melting point <*2.60*> 167 – 171°C

Purity (1) Heavy metals <*1.07*>—Proceed with 2.0 g of Nilvadipine according to Method 2, and perform the test. Prepare the control solution with 2.0 mL of Standard Lead Solution (not more than 10 ppm).

(2) Related substances—Dissolve 20 mg of Nilvadipine in 20 mL of acetonitrile, and use this solution as the sample solution. Perform the test with 5 μL of the sample solution as directed under Liquid Chromatography <*2.01*> according to the following conditions. Determine each peak area by the automatic integration method, and calculate the amount of them by the area percentage method: the amount of each related substance is not more than 0.3%, and the total of them is not more than 0.5%.

Operating conditions—

Detector: An ultraviolet absorption photometer (wavelength: 240 nm).

Column: A stainless steel column 4.6 mm in inside diameter and 15 cm in length, packed with octadecylsilanized silica gel for liquid chromatography (5 μm in particle diameter).

Column temperature: A constant temperature of about 25°C.

Mobile phase: A mixture of phosphate buffer solution (pH 7.4), methanol and acetonitrile (32:27:18).

Flow rate: Adjust so that the retention time of nilvadipine is about 12 minutes.

Time span of measurement: About 2.5 times as long as the retention time of nilvadipine, beginning after the solvent peak.

System suitability—

Test for required detectability: To 1 mL of the sample solution, add acetonitrile to make 100 mL, and use this solution as the solution for system suitability test. Pipet 1 mL of the solution for system suitability test, and add acetonitrile to make exactly 10 mL. Confirm that the peak area of nilvadipine obtained with 5 μL of this solution is equivalent to 7 to 13% of that with 5 μL of the solution for system suitability test.

System performance: When the procedure is run with 5 μL of the solution for system suitability test under the above operating conditions, the number of theoretical plates and the symmetry factor of the peak of nilvadipine is not less than 3300 and not more than 1.3, respectively.

System repeatability: Pipet 1 mL of the solution for system suitability test, and add acetonitrile to make exactly 10 mL. When the test is repeated 6 times with 5 μL of this solution under the above operating conditions, the relative standard deviation of the peak area of nilvadipine is not more than 1.5%.

Loss on drying <*2.41*> Not more than 0.1% (1 g, 105°C, 2 hours).

Residue on ignition <*2.44*> Not more than 0.1% (1 g).

Assay Weigh accurately about 25 mg each of Nilvadipine and Nilvadipine RS, dissolve in methanol to make exactly 25 mL. Pipet 10 mL each of these solutions, add exactly 20 mL of the internal standard solution, 20 mL of water and methanol to make 100 mL, and use these solutions as the sample solution and the standard solution, respectively. Perform the test with 5 μL each of the sample solution and standard solution as directed under the Liquid Chromatography <*2.01*> according to the following conditions, and calculate the ratios, Q_T and Q_S, of the peak area of nilvadipine to that of the internal standard.

Amount (mg) of nilvadipine ($C_{19}H_{19}N_3O_6$) = $M_S \times Q_T/Q_S$

M_S: Amount (mg) of Nilvadipine RS taken

*Internal standard solution—*A solution of acenaphthene in methanol (1 in 200).

Operating conditions—

Detector: An ultraviolet absorption photometer (wavelength: 254 nm).

Column: A stainless steel column 4 mm in inside diameter and 15 cm in length, packed with octadecylsilanized silica gel for liquid chromatography (5 μm in particle diameter).

Column temperature: A constant temperature of about 25°C.

Mobile phase: Dissolve 2.5 g of diammonium hydrogen phosphate in 1000 mL of water, add 10 mL of tetrabutylammonium hydroxide TS, adjust the pH to 7.0 with diluted phosphoric acid (1 in 10), and add 900 mL of acetonitrile.

Flow rate: Adjust so that the retention time of nilvadipine is about 12 minutes.

System suitability—

System performance: When the procedure is run with 5 μL of the standard solution under the above operating conditions, nilvadipine and the internal standard are eluted in this order with the resolution between these peaks being not less than 8.

System repeatability: When the test is repeated 6 times with 5 μL of the standard solution under the above operating conditions, the relative standard deviation of the ratio of the peak area of nilvadipine to that of the internal standard is not more than 1.0%.

Containers and storage Containers—Well-closed containers.

Nilvadipine Tablets

ニルバジピン錠

Nilvadipine Tablets contain not less than 93.0% and not more than 107.0% of the labeled amount of nilvadipine ($C_{19}H_{19}N_3O_6$: 385.37).

Method of preparation Prepare as directed under Tablets, with Nilvadipine.

Identification To a quantity of powdered Nilvadipine Tablets, equivalent to 1 mg of Nilvadipine, add 100 mL of ethanol (99.5), shake for 10 minutes, centrifuge, and use the supernatant liquid as the sample solution. Determine the absorption spectrum of the sample solution as directed under Ultraviolet-visible Spectrophotometry <*2.24*>: it exhibits a maximum between 239 nm and 243 nm and a maximum having a broad-ranging absorption between 371 nm and 381 nm.

Uniformity of dosage units <*6.02*> Perform the test according to the following method: it meets the requirement of the

Content uniformity test.

To 1 tablet of Nilvadipine Tablets add V mL of a mixture of acetonitrile and water (7:3) so that each mL of the solution contains about 0.2 mg of nilvadipine ($C_{19}H_{19}N_3O_6$), add exactly V mL of the internal standard solution, and disperse the particles by sonicating. Centrifuge for 10 minutes, and use the supernatant liquid as the sample solution. Separately, weigh accurately about 20 mg of Nilvadipine RS, dissolve in the mixture of acetonitrile and water (7:3) to make exactly 20 mL. Pipet 5 mL of this solution, add exactly 25 mL of the internal standard solution and the mixture of acetonitrile and water (7:3) to make 50 mL, and use this solution as the standard solution. Proceed as directed in the Assay.

Amount (mg) of nilvadipine ($C_{19}H_{19}N_3O_6$)
$= M_S \times Q_T/Q_S \times V/100$

M_S: Amount (mg) of Nilvadipine RS taken

Internal standard solution—A solution of acenaphthene in acetonitrile (1 in 500).

Dissolution <*6.10*> When the test is performed at 50 revolutions per minute according to the Paddle method, using 900 mL of water as the dissolution medium, the dissolution rate in 30 minutes of Nilvadipine Tablets is not less than 85%.

Start the test with 1 tablet of Nilvadipine Tablets, withdraw not less than 20 mL of the medium at the specified minute after starting the test, and filter through a membrane filter with a pore size not exceeding 0.5 μm. Discard not less than 10 mL of the first filtrate, pipet 10 mL of the subsequent filtrate, add exactly 1 mL of methanol, and use this solution as the sample solution. Separately, weigh accurately an amount of Nilvadipine RS, equivalent to 10 times the labeled amount of Nilvadipine Tablets, and dissolve in methanol to make exactly 50 mL. Pipet 5 mL of this solution, and add methanol to make exactly 100 mL. Pipet 1 mL of this solution, add exactly 10 mL of water, and use this solution as the standard solution. Perform the test with exactly 20 μL each of the sample solution and standard solution as directed under Liquid Chromatography <*2.01*> according to the following conditions, and determine the peak areas, A_T and A_S, of nilvadipine in each solution.

Dissolution rate (%) with respect to the labeled amount of nilvadipine ($C_{19}H_{19}N_3O_6$)
$= M_S \times A_T/A_S \times 1/C \times 9$

M_S: Amount (mg) of Nilvadipine RS taken
C: Labeled amount (mg) of nilvadipine ($C_{19}H_{19}N_3O_6$) in 1 tablet

Operating conditions—

Detector: An ultraviolet absorption photometer (wavelength: 242 nm).

Column: A stainless steel column 4 mm in inside diameter and 15 cm in length, packed with octadecylsilanized silica gel for liquid chromatography (5 μm in particle diameter).

Column temperature: A constant temperature of about 25°C.

Mobile phase: A mixture of phosphate buffer solution (pH 7.4), methanol and acetonitrile (7:7:6).

Flow rate: Adjust so that the retention time of nilvadipine is about 5 minutes.

System suitability—

System performance: When the procedure is run with 20 μL of the standard solution under the above operating conditions, the number of theoretical plates and the symmetry factor of the peak of nilvadipine are not less than 2000 and not more than 1.5, respectively.

System repeatability: When the test is repeated 6 times with 20 μL of the standard solution under the above operating conditions, the relative standard deviation of the peak area of nilvadipine is not more than 1.5%.

Assay Weigh accurately not less than 20 Nilvadipine Tablets, and powder. Weigh accurately an amount of the powder, equivalent to about 5 mg of nilvadipine ($C_{19}H_{19}N_3O_6$), add 10 mL of a mixture of acetonitrile and water (7:3) and exactly 25 mL of the internal standard solution, shake for 15 minutes, and add the mixture of acetonitrile and water (7:3) to make 50 mL. Centrifuge, and use the supernatant liquid as the sample solution. Separately, weigh accurately about 20 mg of Nilvadipine RS, dissolve in the mixture of acetonitrile and water (7:3) to make exactly 20 mL. Pipet 5 mL of this solution, add exactly 25 mL of the internal standard solution and the mixture of acetonitrile and water (7:3) to make 50 mL, and use this solution as the standard solution. Perform the test with 5 μL each of the sample solution and standard solution as directed under Liquid Chromatography <*2.01*> according to the following conditions, and calculate the ratios, Q_T and Q_S, of the peak area of nilvadipine to that of the internal standard.

Amount (mg) of nilvadipine ($C_{19}H_{19}N_3O_6$)
$= M_S \times Q_T/Q_S \times 1/4$

M_S: Amount (mg) of Nilvadipine RS taken

Internal standard solution—A solution of acenaphthene in acetonitrile (1 in 500).

Operating conditions—

Detector: An ultraviolet absorption photometer (wavelength: 254 nm).

Column: A stainless steel column 4 mm in inside diameter and 15 cm in length, packed with octadecylsilanized silica gel for liquid chromatography (5 μm in particle diameter).

Column temperature: A constant temperature of about 25°C.

Mobile phase: Dissolve 2.5 g of diammonium hydrogen phosphate in 1000 mL of water, add 10 mL of tetrabutylammonium hydroxide TS, adjust the pH to 7.0 with diluted phosphoric acid (1 in 10), and add 900 mL of acetonitrile.

Flow rate: Adjust so that the retention time of nilvadipine is about 12 minutes.

System suitability—

System performance: When the procedure is run with 5 μL of the standard solution under the above operating conditions, nilvadipine and the internal standard are eluted in this order with the resolution between these peaks being not less than 8.

System repeatability: When the test is repeated 6 times with 5 μL of the standard solution under the above operating conditions, the relative standard deviation of the ratio of the peak area of nilvadipine to that of the internal standard is not more than 1.0%.

Containers and storage Containers—Well-closed containers.

Nitrazepam

ニトラゼパム

$C_{15}H_{11}N_3O_3$: 281.27
7-Nitro-5-phenyl-1,3-dihydro-2*H*-1,4-benzodiazepin-2-one
[*146-22-5*]

Nitrazepam, when dried, contains not less than 99.0% of nitrazepam ($C_{15}H_{11}N_3O_3$).

Description Nitrazepam occurs as white to light yellow, crystals or crystalline powder. It is odorless.

It is freely soluble in acetic acid (100), soluble in acetone and in chloroform, slightly soluble in methanol, in ethanol (95) and in ethanol (99.5), very slightly soluble in diethyl ether, and practically insoluble in water.

Melting point: about 227°C (with decomposition).

Identification (1) To 3 mL of a solution of Nitrazepam in methanol (1 in 500) add 0.1 mL of sodium hydroxide TS: a yellow color is produced.

(2) To 0.02 g of Nitrazepam add 15 mL of dilute hydrochloric acid, boil for 5 minutes, cool, and filter: the filtrate responds to Qualitative Tests <*1.09*> for primary aromatic amines.

(3) Neutralize 0.5 mL of the filtrate obtained in (2) with sodium hydroxide TS, add 2 mL of ninhydrin TS, and heat on a water bath: a purple color is produced.

(4) Determine the absorption spectrum of a solution of Nitrazepam in ethanol (99.5) (1 in 100,000) as directed under Ultraviolet-visible Spectrophotometry <*2.24*>, and compare the spectrum with the Reference Spectrum: both spectra exhibit similar intensities of absorption at the same wavelengths.

Purity (1) Clarity and color of solution—Dissolve 0.10 g of Nitrazepam in 20 mL of acetone: the solution is clear and pale yellow to light yellow in color.

(2) Heavy metals <*1.07*>—Proceed with 1.0 g of Nitrazepam according to Method 2, and perform the test. Prepare the control solution with 2.0 mL of Standard Lead Solution (not more than 20 ppm).

(3) Arsenic <*1.11*>—Prepare the test solution with 1.0 g of Nitrazepam according to Method 3, and perform the test (not more than 2 ppm).

(4) Related substances—Dissolve 0.25 g of Nitrazepam in a 10 mL of mixture of methanol and chloroform (1:1), and use this solution as the sample solution. Pipet 1 mL of the sample solution, add a mixture of methanol and chloroform (1:1) to make exactly 20 mL, pipet 2 mL of this solution, add a mixture of methanol and chloroform (1:1) to make exactly 50 mL, and use this solution as the standard solution. Perform the test with these solutions as directed under Thin-layer Chromatography <*2.03*>. Spot 10 μL each of the sample solution and standard solution on a plate of silica gel with fluorescent indicator for thin-layer chromatography. Develop the plate with a mixture of nitromethane and ethyl acetate (17:3) to a distance of about 10 cm, and air-dry the plate. Examine under ultraviolet light (main wavelength: 254 nm): the spots other than the principal spot obtained from the sample solution are not more intense than the spot from the standard solution.

Loss on drying <*2.41*> Not more than 0.5% (1 g, 105°C, 4 hours).

Residue on ignition <*2.44*> Not more than 0.1% (1 g).

Assay Weigh accurately about 0.4 g of Nitrazepam, previously dried, and dissolve in 40 mL of acetic acid (100). Titrate <*2.50*> with 0.1 mol/L perchloric acid VS (potentiometric titration). Perform a blank determination in the same manner, and make any necessary correction.

Each mL of 0.1 mol/L perchloric acid VS
= 28.13 mg of $C_{15}H_{11}N_3O_3$

Containers and storage Containers—Tight containers.
Storage—Light-resistant.

Nitrendipine

ニトレンジピン

and enantiomer

$C_{18}H_{20}N_2O_6$: 360.36
3-Ethyl 5-methyl (4*RS*)-2,6-dimethyl-4-(3-nitrophenyl)-1,4-dihydropyridine-3,5-dicarboxylate
[*39562-70-4*]

Nitrendipine, when dried, contains not less than 98.5% and not more than 101.0% of nitrendipine ($C_{18}H_{20}N_2O_6$).

Description Nitrendipine occurs as a yellow crystalline powder.

It is soluble in acetonitrile, sparingly soluble in methanol and in ethanol (99.5), and practically insoluble in water.

It is gradually colored to brownish yellow by light.

A solution of Nitrendipine in acetonitrile (1 in 50) shows no optical rotation.

Identification (1) Determine the absorption spectrum of a solution of Nitrendipine in methanol (1 in 80,000) as directed under Ultraviolet-visible Spectrophotometry <*2.24*>, and compare the spectrum with the Reference Spectrum: both spectra exhibit similar intensities of absorption at the same wavelengths.

(2) Determine the infrared absorption spectrum of Nitrendipine as directed in the potassium bromide disk method under Infrared Spectrophotometry <*2.25*>, and compare the spectrum with the Reference Spectrum: both spectra exhibit similar intensities of absorption at the same wave numbers.

Melting point <*2.60*> 157 – 161°C

Purity (1) Heavy metals <*1.07*>—Proceed with 2.0 g of Nitrendipine according to Method 4, and perform the test. Prepare the control solution with 2.0 mL of Standard Lead Solution (not more than 10 ppm).

(2) Related substances—Conduct this procedure rapidly using light-resistant vessels. Dissolve 40 mg of Nitrendipine

in 5 mL of acetonitrile, add the mobile phase to make 25 mL, and use this solution as the sample solution. Pipet 1 mL of the sample solution, add the mobile phase to make exactly 100 mL, and use this solution as the standard solution. Perform the test immediately with exactly 10 μL each of the sample solution and standard solution as directed under Liquid Chromatography <*2.01*> according to the following conditions. Determine each peak area by the automatic integration method, and calculate the amount of related substances by the following equation: the amount of the related substance, having the relative retention time of about 0.8 to nitrendipine, is not more than 1.0%, the related substance, having the relative retention time of about 1.3, is not more than 0.25%, and other related substances are not more than 0.2%, respectively. The total amount of the related substances other than nitrendipine is not more than 2.0%.

$$\text{Amount (\%) of related substance} = A_T/A_S$$

A_T: Each peak area other than nitrendipine obtained from the sample solution

A_S: Peak area of nitrendipine obtained from the standard solution

Operating conditions—

Detector: An ultraviolet absorption photometer (wavelength: 254 nm).

Column: A stainless steel column 6 mm in inside diameter and 15 cm in length, packed with octadecylsilanized silica gel for liquid chromatography (5 μm in particle diameter).

Column temperature: A constant temperature of about 25°C.

Mobile phase: A mixture of water, tetrahydrofuran and acetonitrile (14:6:5).

Flow rate: Adjust so that the retention time of nitrendipine is about 12 minutes.

Time span of measurement: About 2.5 times as long as the retention time of nitrendipine, beginning after the solvent peak.

System suitability—

Test for required detectability: To exactly 2 mL of the standard solution add the mobile phase to make exactly 10 mL. Confirm that the peak area of nitrendipine obtained with 10 μL of this solution is equivalent to 14 to 26% of that with 10 μL of the standard solution.

System performance: Dissolve 10 mg of Nitrendipine and 3 mg of propyl parahydroxybenzoate in 5 mL of acetonitrile, and add the mobile phase to make 100 mL. When the procedure is run with 5 μL of this solution under the above operating conditions, propyl parahydroxybenzoate and nitrendipine are eluted in this order with the resolution between these peaks being not less than 6.

System repeatability: When the test is repeated 6 times with 10 μL of the standard solution under the above operating conditions, the relative standard deviation of the peak area of nitrendipine is not more than 2.0%.

Loss on drying <*2.41*> Not more than 0.5% (1 g, 105°C, 2 hours).

Residue on ignition <*2.44*> Not more than 0.1% (1 g).

Assay Weigh accurately about 0.3 g of Nitrendipine, previously dried, dissolve in 60 mL of a solution of sulfuric acid in ethanol (99.5) (3 in 100), add 50 mL of water, and titrate <*2.50*> with 0.1 mol/L serium (IV) tetraammonium sulfate VS until the red-orange color of the solution vanishes (indicator: 3 drops of 1,10-phenanthroline TS). Perform a blank determination in the same manner, and make any necessary correction.

Each mL of 0.1 mol/L serium (IV) tetraammonium sulfate VS
$= 18.02 \text{ mg of } C_{18}H_{20}N_2O_6$

Containers and storage Containers—Tight containers.
Storage—Light-resistant.

Nitrendipine Tablets

ニトレンジピン錠

Nitrendipine Tablets contain not less than 93.0% and not more than 107.0% of the labeled amount of nitrendipine ($C_{18}H_{20}N_2O_6$: 360.36).

Method of preparation Prepare as directed under Tablets, with Nitrendipine.

Identification Shake a quantity of powdered Nitrendipine Tablets, equivalent to 5 mg of Nitrendipine, with 70 mL of methanol, then add methanol to make 100 mL, and centrifuge. To 5 mL of the supernatant liquid add methanol to make 20 mL, and determine the absorption spectrum of this solution as directed under Ultraviolet-visible Spectrophotometry <*2.24*>: it exhibits maxima between 234 nm and 238 nm, and between 350 nm and 354 nm.

Uniformity of dosage units <*6.02*> Perform the test according to the following method: it meets the requirement of the Content uniformity test.

Conduct this procedure using light-resistant vessels. To 1 tablet of Nitrendipine Tablets add 15 mL of diluted acetonitrile (4 in 5), stir until the tablet is completely disintegrated, and further stir for 10 minutes. Add diluted acetonitrile (4 in 5) to make exactly 20 mL, and centrifuge. Pipet V mL of the supernatant liquid, equivalent to about 1 mg of nitrendipine ($C_{18}H_{20}N_2O_6$), add exactly 5 mL of the internal standard solution, then add diluted acetonitrile (4 in 5) to make 25 mL, and use this solution as the sample solution. Proceed as directed in the Assay.

$$\text{Amount (mg) of nitrendipine } (C_{18}H_{20}N_2O_6) = M_S \times Q_T/Q_S \times 1/V \times 1/5$$

M_S: Amount (mg) of nitrendipine for assay taken

Internal standard solution—A solution of propyl parahydroxybenzoate in diluted acetonitrile (4 in 5) (1 in 10,000).

Dissolution <*6.10*> When the test is performed at 100 revolutions per minute according to the Paddle method, using 900 mL of the dissolution medium containing 3 g of polysorbate 80 in 5 L of water for 5-mg tablet and the dissolution medium containing 3 g of polysorbate 80 in 2000 mL of water for 10-mg tablet, the dissolution rate in 45 minutes of Nitrendipine Tablets is not less than 70%.

Conduct this procedure using light-resistant vessels. Start the test with 1 tablet of Nitrendipine Tablets, withdraw not less than 20 mL of the medium at the specified minute after starting the test, and filter through a membrane filter with a pore size not exceeding 0.45 μm. Discard not less than 10 mL of the first filtrate, pipet the subsequent V mL, add the dissolution medium to make exactly V' mL so that each mL contains about 5.6 μg of nitrendipine ($C_{18}H_{20}N_2O_6$), and use this solution as the sample solution. Separately, weigh accurately about 28 mg of nitrendipine for assay, previously dried at 105°C for 2 hours, dissolve in methanol to make exactly 100 mL, then pipet 5 mL of this solution, and add the dissolution medium to make exactly 50 mL. Pipet 5 mL of this solution, add the dissolution medium to make exactly 25 mL, and use this solution as the standard solution. Perform the test with exactly 20 μL each of the sample solution and standard solution as directed under Liquid Chromatography <*2.01*> according to the following conditions, and determine the peak areas, A_T and A_S, of nitrendipine in each solution.

Dissolution rate (%) with respect to the labeled amount of nitrendipine ($C_{18}H_{20}N_2O_6$)
$= M_S \times A_T/A_S \times V'/V \times 1/C \times 18$

M_S: Amount (mg) of nitrendipine for assay taken
C: Labeled amount (mg) of nitrendipine ($C_{18}H_{20}N_2O_6$) in 1 tablet

Operating conditions—

Detector: An ultraviolet absorption photometer (wavelength: 356 nm).

Column: A stainless steel column 4.6 mm in inside diameter and 15 cm in length, packed with octadecylsilanized silica gel for liquid chromatography (5 μm in particle diameter).

Column temperature: A constant temperature of about 25°C.

Mobile phase: A mixture of water, tetrahydrofuran and acetonitrile (14:6:5).

Flow rate: Adjust so that the retention time of nitrendipine is about 9 minutes.

System suitability—

System performance: When the procedure is run with 20 μL of the standard solution under the above operating conditions, the number of theoretical plates and the symmetry factor of the peak of nitrendipine are not less than 5000 and not more than 2.0, respectively.

System repeatability: When the test is repeated 6 times with 20 μL of the standard solution under the above operating conditions, the relative standard deviation of the peak area of nitrendipine is not more than 2.0%.

Assay Conduct this procedure using light-resistant vessels. To 20 tablets of Nitrendipine Tablets add 150 mL of diluted acetonitrile (4 in 5), stir until the tablets completely disintegrate, and stir for further 10 minutes. Add diluted acetonitrile (4 in 5) to make exactly 200 mL, and centrifuge. Pipet a volume of the supernatant liquid, equivalent to about 2 mg of nitrendipine ($C_{18}H_{20}N_2O_6$), add exactly 10 mL of the internal standard solution and diluted acetonitrile (4 in 5) to make 50 mL, and use this solution as the sample solution. Separately, weigh accurately about 0.1 g of nitrendipine for assay, previously dried at 105°C for 2 hours, and dissolve in diluted acetonitrile (4 in 5) to make exactly 200 mL. Pipet 4 mL of this solution, add exactly 10 mL of the internal standard solution and diluted acetonitrile (4 in 5) to make 50 mL, and use this solution as the standard solution. Perform the test with 10 μL each of the sample solution and standard solution as directed under Liquid Chromatography <*2.01*> according to the following conditions, and calculate the ratios, Q_T and Q_S, of the peak area of nitrendipine to that of the internal standard.

Amount (mg) of nitrendipine ($C_{18}H_{20}N_2O_6$)
$= M_S \times Q_T/Q_S \times 1/50$

M_S: Amount (mg) of nitrendipine for assay taken

*Internal standard solution—*A solution of propyl parahydroxybenzoate in diluted acetonitrile (4 in 5) (1 in 10,000).

Operating conditions—

Detector: An ultraviolet absorption photometer (wavelength: 254 nm).

Column: A stainless steel column 6 mm in inside diameter and 15 cm in length, packed with octadecylsilanized silica gel for liquid chromatography (5 μm in particle diameter).

Column temperature: A constant temperature of about 25°C.

Mobile phase: A mixture of water, tetrahydrofuran and acetonitrile (14:6:5).

Flow rate: Adjust so that the retention time of nitrendipine is about 12 minutes.

System suitability—

System performance: When the procedure is run with 10 μL of the standard solution under the above operating conditions, the internal standard and nitrendipine are eluted in this order with the resolution between these peaks being not less than 6.

System repeatability: When the test is repeated 6 times with 10 μL of the standard solution under the above operating conditions, the relative standard deviation of the peak area of nitrendipine is not more than 1.0%.

Containers and storage Containers—Tight containers.

Storage—Light-resistant.

Nitrogen

窒素

N_2: 28.01

Nitrogen is the nitrogen produced by the air liquefaction separation method.

It contains not less than 99.5 vol% of nitrogen (N_2).

Description Nitrogen is a colorless gas at room temperature and under atmospheric pressure, and is odorless.

1 mL of Nitrogen dissolves in 65 mL of water and in 9 mL of ethanol (95) at 20°C and at a pressure of 101.3 kPa.

1000 mL of Nitrogen at 0°C and at a pressure of 101.3 kPa weighs 1.251 g.

Identification Introduce 1 mL each of Nitrogen and nitrogen into a gas-measuring tube or syringe for gas chromatography from a cylinder with a pressure-reducing valve, through a directly connected polyvinyl chloride or stainless steel tube. Perform the test with these gases as directed under Gas Chromatography <*2.02*> according to the following conditions: the principal peak in the chromatogram obtained form Nitrogen has the same retention time as that from nitrogen.

Operating conditions—

Proceed as directed in the operating conditions in the Assay.

Purity Oxygen—The peak area of oxygen obtained from Nitrogen in the Assay is not larger than 1/2 times that from the standard gas mixture.

Assay Introduce 1.0 mL of Nitrogen into a gas-measuring tube or syringe for gas chromatography from a cylinder with a pressure-reducing valve, through a directly connected polyvinyl chloride or stainless steel tube. Perform the test with this gas as directed under Gas Chromatography <*2.02*> according to the following conditions. Measure the peak area A_T of oxygen. Separately, introduce 1.0 mL of oxygen into the gas mixer, add carrier gas to make exactly 100 mL, mix thoroughly, and use this as the standard gas mixture. Proceed with 1.0 mL of this mixture in the same manner under Nitrogen, and measure the peak area A_S of oxygen.

$$\text{Amount (vol\%) of nitrogen } (N_2) = 100 - A_T/A_S$$

Operating conditions—

Detector: A thermal-conductivity detector.

Column: A column 3 mm in inside diameter and 3 m in length, packed with zeolite for gas chromatography (250 to 355 μm in particle diameter; 0.5 nm in pore size).

Column temperature: A constant temperature of about 50°C.

Carrier gas: Hydrogen or helium.

Flow rate: Adjust so that the retention time of oxygen is about 3 minutes.

System suitability—

System performance: Introduce 1.0 mL of oxygen into the gas mixer, add Nitrogen to make 100 mL, and mix thoroughly. When the procedure is run with 1.0 mL of this mixture under the above operating conditions, oxygen and nitrogen are eluted in this order with the resolution between these peaks being not less than 1.5.

System repeatability: When the test is repeated 5 times with 1.0 mL of the standard gas mixture under the above conditions, the relative standard deviation of the peak area of oxygen is not more than 2.0%.

Containers and storage Containers—Pressure-resistant cylinders.

Storage—Not exceeding 40°C.

Nitroglycerin Tablets

ニトログリセリン錠

Nitroglycerin Tablets contain not less than 80.0% and not more than 120.0% of the labeled amount of nitroglycerin ($C_3H_5N_3O_9$: 227.09).

Method of preparation Prepare as directed under Tablets, with nitroglycerin.

Identification (1) Weigh a quantity of powdered Nitroglycerin Tablets, equivalent to 6 mg of nitroglycerin ($C_3H_5N_3O_9$), shake thoroughly with 12 mL of diethyl ether, filter, and use the filtrate as the sample solution. Evaporate 5 mL of the sample solution, dissolve the residue in 1 to 2 drops of sulfuric acid, and add 1 drop of diphenylamine TS: a deep blue color develops.

(2) Evaporate 5 mL of the sample solution obtained in (1), add 5 drops of sodium hydroxide TS, heat over a low flame, and concentrate to about 0.1 mL. Cool, heat the residue with 0.02 g of potassium hydrogen sulfate: the odor of acrolein is perceptible.

Purity Free nitrate ion—Transfer an accurately measured quantity of powdered Nitroglycerin Tablets, equivalent to 20 mg of nitroglycerin ($C_3H_5N_3O_9$), to a separator, add 40 mL of isopropylether and 40 mL of water, shake for 10 minutes, and allow the layers to separate. Collect the aqueous layer, add 40 mL of isopropylether, shake for 10 minutes, collect the aqueous layer, filter, and use the filtrate as the sample solution. Separately, transfer 10 mL of Standard Nitric Acid Solution to a separator, add 30 mL of water and 40 mL of the isopropyl ether layer of the first extraction of the sample solution, shake for 10 minutes, continue the procedure in the same manner as the sample solution, and use the solution so obtained as the standard solution. Transfer 20 mL each of the sample solution and the standard solution to Nessler tubes, respectively, shake well with 30 mL of water and 0.06 g of Griess-Romijin's nitric acid reagent, allow to stand for 30 minutes, and observe the tubes horizontally: the sample solution has no more color than the standard solution.

Uniformity of dosage units <*6.02*> Perform the test according to the following method: it meets the requirement of the Content uniformity test.

Transfer 1 tablet of Nitroglycerin Tablets to a glass-stoppered centrifuge tube, and add exactly V mL of acetic acid (100) to provide a solution containing about 30 μg of nitroglycerin ($C_3H_5N_3O_9$) per ml. Shake vigorously for 1 hour, and after disintegrating the tablet, centrifuge, and use the supernatant liquid as the sample solution. When the tablet does not disintegrate during this procedure, transfer 1 tablet of Nitroglycerin Tablets to a glass-stoppered centrifuge tube, wet the tablet with 0.05 mL of acetic acid (100), and grind down it with a glass rod. While rinsing the glass rod, add acetic acid (100) to make exactly V mL of a solution containing about 30 μg of nitroglycerin ($C_3H_5N_3O_9$) per ml. Shake for 1 hour, centrifuge, and use the supernatant liquid as the sample solution. Separately, weigh accurately about 90 mg of potassium nitrate, previously dried at 105°C for 4 hours, dissolve in 5 mL of water, and add acetic acid (100) to make exactly 100 mL. Pipet 5 mL of the solution, add acetic acid (100) to make exactly 100 mL, and use this solution as the standard solution. Measure exactly 2 mL each of the sample solution and the standard solution, add 2 mL each of salicylic acid TS shake, allow to stand for 15 minutes, and add 10 mL each of water. Render the solution alkaline with about 12 mL of a solution of sodium hydroxide (2 in 5) while cooling in ice, and add water to make exactly 50 mL. Perform the test with these solutions as directed under Ultraviolet-visible Spectrophotometry <*2.24*>, using a solution, prepared with 2 mL of acetic acid (100) in the same manner, as the blank. Determine the absorbances, A_T and A_S, of the subsequent solutions of the sample solution and the standard solution at 410 nm, respectively.

$$\text{Amount (mg) of nitroglycerin } (C_3H_5N_3O_9) = M_S \times A_T/A_S \times V/2000 \times 0.749$$

M_S: Amount (mg) of potassium nitrate taken

Calculate the average content from the contents of 10 tablets: it meets the requirements of the test when each content deviates from the average content by not more than 25%. When there is 1 tablet showing a deviation exceeding 25% and not exceeding 30%, determine the content of an additional 20 tablets in the same manner. Calculate the 30 deviations from the new average of all 30 tablets: it meets the requirements of the test when 1 tablet may deviate from the average content by between 25% and 30%, but no tablet deviates by more than 30%.

Disintegration <*6.09*> It meets the requirement, provided that the time limit of the test is 2 minutes, and the use of the disks is omitted.

Assay Weigh accurately and disintegrate, by soft pressing, not less than 20 Nitroglycerin Tablets. Weigh accurately a portion of the powder, equivalent to about 3.5 mg of nitroglycerin ($C_3H_5N_3O_9$), add exactly 50 mL of acetic acid (100), shake for 1 hour, filter, and use this filtrate as the sample solution. Separately, weigh accurately about 90 mg of potassium nitrate, previously dried at 105°C for 4 hours, dissolve in 5 mL of water, and add acetic acid (100) to make exactly 100 mL. Pipet 10 mL of the solution, add acetic acid (100) to make exactly 100 mL, and use this solution as the standard solution. Measure exactly 2 mL each of the sample solution and the standard solution, to each solution add 2 mL of salicylic acid TS, shake, allow to stand for 15 minutes, and add 10 mL of water. Render the solution alkaline with about 12 mL of a solution of sodium hydroxide (2 in 5) while cooling in ice, and add water to make exactly 50 mL. Perform the test with these solutions as directed under Ultraviolet-visible Spectrophotometry <2.24>, using a solution, prepared with 2 mL of acetic acid (100) in the same manner, as the blank. Determine the absorbances, A_T and A_S, of the subsequent solutions of the sample solution and the standard solution at 410 nm, respectively.

Amount (mg) of nitroglycerin ($C_3H_5N_3O_9$)
$= M_S \times A_T/A_S \times 1/20 \times 0.749$

M_S: Amount (mg) of potassium nitrate taken

Containers and storage Containers—Tight containers.

Storage—Light-resistant, and not exceeding 20°C.

Nitrous Oxide

亜酸化窒素

N_2O: 44.01

Nitrous Oxide contains not less than 97.0 vol% of nitrous oxide (N_2O).

Description Nitrous Oxide is a colorless gas at room temperature and at atmospheric pressure, and is odorless.

1 mL of Nitrous Oxide dissolves in 1.5 mL of water and in 0.4 mL of ethanol (95) at 20°C and at a pressure of 101.3 kPa. It is soluble in diethyl ether and in fatty oils.

1000 mL of Nitrous Oxide at 0°C and at a pressure of 101.3 kPa weighs about 1.96 g.

Identification **(1)** A glowing splinter of wood held in Nitrous Oxide: it bursts into flame immediately.

(2) Transfer 1 mL each of Nitrous Oxide and nitrous oxide directly from metal cylinders with a pressure-reducing valve to gas measuring tubes or syringes for gas chromatography, using a polyvinyl chloride induction tube. Perform the test with these gases as directed under Gas Chromatography <2.02> according to the operating conditions of the Assay: the retention time of the main peak in the chromatogram obtained with Nitrous Oxide coincides with that in the chromatogram obtained with nitrous oxide.

Purity Maintain the containers of Nitrous Oxide between 18°C and 22°C for more than 6 hours before the test, and correct the volume at 20°C and at a pressure of 101.3 kPa.

(1) Acidity or alkalinity—To 400 mL of freshly boiled and cooled water add 0.3 mL of methyl red TS and 0.3 mL of bromothymol blue TS, and boil for 5 minutes. Transfer 50 mL of this solution to each of three Nessler tubes marked A, B and C. Add 0.10 mL of 0.01 mol/L hydrochloric acid VS to tube A, 0.20 mL of 0.01 mol/L hydrochloric acid VS to tube B, stopper each of the tubes, and cool. Pass 1000 mL of Nitrous Oxide through the solution in tube A for 15 minutes, employing delivery tube with an orifice approximately 1 mm in diameter and extending to within 2 mm of the bottom of the Nessler tube: the color of the solution in tube A is not deeper orange-red than that of the solution in tube B and not deeper yellow-green than that of the solution in tube C.

(2) Carbon dioxide—Pass 1000 mL of Nitrous Oxide through 50 mL of barium hydroxide TS in a Nessler tube, in the same manner as directed in (1): any turbidity produced does not exceed that produced in the following control solution.

Control solution: To 50 mL of barium hydroxide TS in a Nessler tube add 1 mL of a solution of 0.1 g of sodium hydrogen carbonate in 100 mL of freshly boiled and cooled water.

(3) Oxidizing substances—Transfer 15 mL of potassium iodide-starch TS to each of two Nessler tubes marked A and B, add 1 drop of acetic acid (100) to each of the tubes, shake, and use these as solution A and solution B, respectively. Pass 2000 mL of Nitrous Oxide through solution A for 30 minutes in the same manner as directed in (1): the color of solution A is the same as that of the stoppered, untreated solution B.

(4) Potassium permanganate-reducing substance—Pour 50 mL of water into each of two Nessler tubes marked A and B, add 0.10 mL of 0.02 mol/L potassium permanganate VS to each of the tubes, and use these as solution A and solution B, respectively. Pass 1000 mL of Nitrous Oxide through solution A in the manner as directed in (1): the color of solution A is the same as that of solution B.

(5) Chloride—Pour 50 mL of water into each of two Nessler tubes marked A and B, add 0.5 mL of silver nitrate TS to each of the tubes, shake, and use these as solution A and solution B, respectively. Pass 1000 mL of Nitrous Oxide through solution A in the same manner as directed in (1): the turbidity of solution A is the same as that of solution B.

(6) Carbon monoxide—Introduce 5.0 mL of Nitrous Oxide into a gas-cylinder or a syringe for gas chromatography from a metal cylinder holding gas under pressure and fitted with a pressure-reducing valve, through a directly connected polyvinyl tube. Perform the test with this under Gas Chromatography <2.02> according to the following conditions: no peak is observed at the same retention time as that of carbon monoxide.

Operating conditions—

Detector: A thermal conductivity detector.

Column: A column about 3 mm in inside diameter and about 3 m in length, packed with 300 to 500 μm zeolite for gas chromatography (0.5 nm in pore size).

Column temperature: A constant temperature of about 50°C.

Carrier gas: Hydrogen or helium.

Flow rate: Adjust so that the retention time of carbon monoxide is about 20 minutes.

Selection of column: To 0.1 mL each of carbon monoxide and air in a gas mixer add carrier gas to make 100 mL, and mix well. Proceed with 5.0 mL of the mixed gas under the above operating conditions. Use a column giving well-resolved peaks of oxygen, nitrogen and carbon monoxide in this order.

Detection sensitivity: Adjust the sensitivity so that the peak height of carbon monoxide obtained from 5.0 mL of the mixed gas used in the selection of column is about 10 cm.

Assay Withdraw Nitrous Oxide as directed in the Purity.

Introduce 1.0 mL of Nitrous Oxide into a gas-measuring tube or syringe for gas chromatography from a metal cylinder under pressure through a pressure-reducing valve and a directly connected polyvinyl tube. Perform the test with this solution as directed under Gas Chromatography <2.02> according to the following conditions, and determine the peak area A_T of air. Separately, introduce 3.0 mL of nitrogen into a gas mixer, add carrier gas to make exactly 100 mL, mix thoroughly, and use this as the standard mixed gas. Proceed with 1.0 mL of this mixture as directed in the case of Nitrous Oxide, and determine the peak area A_S of nitrogen in the same manner.

Amount (vol%) of nitrous oxide (N_2O) = 100 − 3 × A_T/A_S

Operating conditions—

Detector: A thermal conductivity detector.

Column: A column about 3 mm in inside diameter and about 3 m in length, packed with silica gel for gas chromatography (300 to 500 μm in particle diameter).

Column temperature: A constant temperature of about 50°C.

Carrier gas: Hydrogen or helium.

Flow rate: Adjust so that the retention time of nitrogen is about 2 minutes.

Selection of column: To 3.0 mL of nitrogen in a gas mixer add Nitrous Oxide to make 100 mL, and mix well. Proceed with 1.0 mL of the mixed gas under the above operating conditions. Use a column giving well-resolved peaks of nitrogen and nitrous oxide in this order.

System repeatability: Repeat the test five times with the standard mixed gas under the above operating conditions: the relative standard deviation of the peak area of nitrogen is not more than 2.0%.

Containers and storage Containers—Metal cylinders.

Storage—Not exceeding 40°C.

Nizatidine

ニザチジン

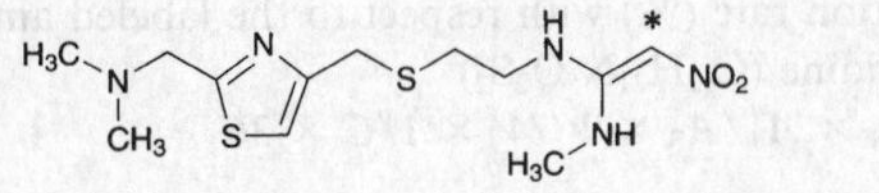

and geometric isomer at C*

$C_{12}H_{21}N_5O_2S_2$: 331.46

(1*EZ*)-*N*-{2-[({2-[(Dimethylamino)methyl]thiazol-4-yl}methyl)sulfanyl]ethyl}-*N'*-methyl-2-nitroethene-1,1-diamine

[*76963-41-2*]

Nizatidine, when dried, contains not less than 98.0% and not more than 101.0% of nizatidine ($C_{12}H_{21}N_5O_2S_2$).

Description Nizatidine occurs as a white to pale yellow-white crystalline powder, and has a characteristic odor.

It is soluble in methanol, sparingly soluble in water, and slightly soluble in ethanol (99.5).

Identification **(1)** Determine the absorption spectrum of a solution of Nizatidine in methanol (1 in 100,000) as directed under Ultraviolet-visible Spectrophotometry *<2.24>*, and compare the spectrum with the Reference Spectrum or the spectrum of a solution of Nizatidine RS prepared in the same manner as the sample solution: both spectra exhibit similar intensities of absorption at the same wavelengths.

(2) Determine the infrared absorption spectrum of Nizatidine, previously dried, as directed in the potassium bromide disk method under Infrared Spectrophotometry *<2.25>*, and compare the spectrum with the Reference Spectrum or the spectrum of dried Nizatidine RS: both spectra exhibit similar intensities of absorption at the same wave numbers.

Melting point *<2.60>* 130 – 135°C (after drying).

Purity **(1)** Heavy metals *<1.07>*—Proceed with 2.0 g of Nizatidine according to Method 4, and perform the test using 3 mL of sulfuric acid. Prepare the control solution with 2.0 mL of Standard Lead Solution (not more than 10 ppm).

(2) Related substances—Dissolve 50 mg of Nizatidine in 10 mL of a mixture of the mobile phase A and mobile phase B (19:6), and use this solution as the sample solution. Pipet 3 mL of the sample solution, add the mixture of the mobile phase A and mobile phase B (19:6) to make exactly 200 mL, and use this solution as the standard solution. Perform the test with exactly 50 μL each of the sample solution and standard solution as directed under Liquid Chromatography *<2.01>* according to the following conditions. Determine each peak area from both solutions by the automatic integration method: the area of the peaks other than nizatidine obtained from the sample solution is not larger than 1/5 times the nizatidine from the standard solution. Furthermore, the total of the areas of peaks other than the nizatidine from the sample solution is not larger than the peak area of nizatidine from the standard solution.

Operating conditions—

Detector: An ultraviolet absorption photometer (wavelength: 254 nm).

Column: A stainless steel column 4.6 mm in inside diameter and 25 cm in length, packed with octadecylsilanized silica gel for liquid chromatography (5 μm in particle diameter).

Column temperature: A constant temperature of about 25°C.

Mobile phase A: Dissolve 5.9 g of ammonium acetate in 760 mL of water, add 1 mL of diethylamine, and adjust to pH 7.5 with acetic acid (100).

Mobile phase B: Methanol.

Flowing of mobile phase: Control the gradient by mixing the mobile phases A and B as directed in the following table.

Time after injection of sample (min)	Mobile phase A (vol%)	Mobile phase B (vol%)
0 – 3	76	24
3 – 20	76 → 50	24 → 50
20 – 45	50	50

Flow rate: 1.0 mL per minute.

Time span of measurement: About 3 times as long as the retention time of nizatidine, beginning after the solvent peak.

System suitability—

Test for required detectability: Pipet 5 mL of the standard solution, and add a mixture of the mobile phase A and mobile phase B (19:6) to make exactly 25 mL. Confirm that the peak area of nizatidine obtained with 50 μL of this solution is equivalent to 15 to 25% of that with 50 μL of the standard solution.

System performance: When the procedure is run with 50 μL of the standard solution under the above operating conditions, the number of theoretical plates and the symmetry factor of the peak of nizatidine are not less than 20,000 and not more than 2.0, respectively.

System repeatability: When the test is repeated 6 times with 50 μL of the standard solution under the above operating conditions, the relative standard deviation of the peak area of nizatidine is not more than 2.0%.

Loss on drying *<2.41>* Not more than 0.5% (2 g, 100°C, 1 hour).

Residue on ignition *<2.44>* Not more than 0.1% (1 g).

Assay Weigh accurately about 15 mg each of Nizatidine and Nizatidine RS, both previously dried, dissolve each in the mobile phase to make exactly 50 mL, and use these solutions as the sample solution and the standard solution, respectively. Perform the test with exactly 10 μL each of the sample solution and standard solution as directed under Liquid Chromatography <*2.01*> according to the following conditions. Determine the peak area, A_T and A_S, of nizatidine in each solution.

Amount (mg) of nizatidine ($C_{12}H_{21}N_5O_2S_2$) = $M_S \times A_T/A_S$

M_S: Amount (mg) of Nizatidine RS taken

Operating conditions—

Detector: An ultraviolet absorption photometer (wavelength: 254 nm).

Column: A stainless steel column 4.6 mm in inside diameter and 15 cm in length, packed with octadecylsilanized silica gel for liquid chromatography (5 μm in particle diameter).

Column temperature: A constant temperature of about 40°C.

Mobile phase: Dissolve 5.9 g of ammonium acetate in 760 mL of water, add 1 mL of diethylamine, and adjust to pH 7.5 with acetic acid (100). To this solution add 240 mL of methanol.

Flow rate: Adjust so that the retention time of nizatidine is about 10 minutes.

System suitability—

System performance: When the procedure is run with 10 μL of the standard solution under the above operating conditions, the number of theoretical plates and the symmetry factor of the peak of nizatidine are not less than 5000 and not more than 1.5, respectively.

System repeatability: When the test is repeated 6 times with 10 μL of the standard solution under the above operating conditions, the relative standard deviation of the peak area of nizatidine is not more than 1.0%.

Containers and storage Containers—Tight containers.

Nizatidine Capsules

ニザチジンカプセル

Nizatidine Capsules contain not less than 95.0% and not more than 105.0% of the labeled amount of nizatidine ($C_{12}H_{21}N_5O_2S_2$: 331.46).

Method of preparation Prepare as directed under Capsules, with Nizatidine.

Identification Take out the contents of Nizatidine Capsules, and powder. To a portion of the powder, equivalent to 50 mg of Nizatidine, add 50 mL of methanol, shake well, and filter. Pipet 1 mL of the filtrate, and add methanol to make 100 mL. Determine the absorption spectrum of the solution as directed under Ultraviolet-visible Spectrophotometry <*2.24*>: it exhibits maxima between 239 nm and 244 nm, and between 323 nm and 327 nm.

Uniformity of dosage units <*6.02*> Perform the Mass variation test, or the Content uniformity test according to the following method: it meets the requirement.

Take out the contents from 1 capsule of Nizatidine Capsules, add the mobile phase to make exactly V mL so that each mL contains about 1.5 mg of nizatidine ($C_{12}H_{21}N_5O_2S_2$). After shaking vigorously for 10 minutes, centrifuge. Pipet 10 mL of the supernatant liquid, add exactly 5 mL of the internal standard solution and add the mobile phase to make 50 mL, and use this solution as the sample solution. Then, proceed as directed in the Assay.

Amount (mg) of nizatidine ($C_{12}H_{21}N_5O_2S_2$)
$= M_S \times Q_T/Q_S \times V/10$

M_S: Amount (mg) of Nizatidine RS taken

Internal standard solution—A solution of phenol in the mobile phase (1 in 100).

Dissolution <*6.10*> When the test is performed at 50 revolutions per minute according to the Paddle method using a sinker, using 900 mL of water as the dissolution medium, the dissolution rate in 15 minutes of Nizatidine Capsules is not less than 80%.

Start the test with 1 capsule of Nizatidine Capsules, withdraw not less than 10 mL of the medium at the specified minute after starting the test, and filter through a membrane filter with a pore size not exceeding 0.45 μm. Discard not less than 2 mL of the first filtrate, pipet V mL of the subsequent filtrate, and add water to make exactly V' mL so that each mL contains about 10 μg of nizatidine ($C_{12}H_{21}N_5O_2S_2$). Use this solution as the sample solution. Separately, weigh accurately about 25 mg of Nizatidine RS, previously dried at 100 °C for 1 hour, and dissolve in water to make exactly 100 mL. Pipet 2 mL of this solution, add water to make exactly 50 mL, and use this solution as the standard solution. Perform the test with the sample solution and standard solution as directed under Ultraviolet-visible Spectrophotometry <*2.24*>, and determine the absorbances, A_T and A_S, at 314 nm.

Dissolution rate (%) with respect to the labeled amount of nizatidine ($C_{12}H_{21}N_5O_2S_2$)
$= M_S \times A_T/A_S \times V'/V \times 1/C \times 36$

M_S: Amount (mg) of Nizatidine RS taken
C: Labeled amount (mg) of nizatidine ($C_{12}H_{21}N_5O_2S_2$) in 1 capsule

Assay Take out the contents of not less than 10 Nizatidine Capsules, weigh accurately the mass of the contents, and powder. Weigh accurately a portion of the powder, equivalent to about 0.15 g of nizatidine ($C_{12}H_{21}N_5O_2S_2$), add exactly 50 mL of the mobile phase, shake vigorously for 10 minutes, and centrifuge. Pipet 5 mL of the supernatant liquid, add exactly 5 mL of the internal standard solution, add the mobile phase to make 50 mL, and use this solution as the sample solution. Separately, weigh accurately about 15 mg of Nizatidine RS, previously dried at 100°C for 1 hour, dissolve in 30 mL of the mobile phase, add exactly 5 mL of the internal standard solution, add the mobile phase to make 50 mL, and use this solution as the standard solution. Perform the test with 10 μL each of the sample solution and standard solution as directed under Liquid Chromatography <*2.01*> according to the following conditions, and calculate the ratios, Q_T and Q_S, of the peak area of nizatidine to that of the internal standard.

Amount (mg) of nizatidine ($C_{12}H_{21}N_5O_2S_2$)
$= M_S \times Q_T/Q_S \times 10$

M_S: Amount (mg) of Nizatidine RS taken

Internal standard solution—A solution of phenol in the mobile phase (1 in 100).

Operating conditions—

Detector: An ultraviolet absorption photometer (wavelength: 254 nm).

Column: A stainless steel column 4.6 mm in inside diameter and 15 cm in length, packed with octadecylsilanized silica gel for liquid chromatography (5 μm in particle diameter).

Column temperature: A constant temperature of about

40°C.

Mobile phase: Dissolve 5.9 g of ammonium acetate in 760 mL of water, add 1 mL of diethylamine, and adjust to pH 7.5 with acetic acid (100). To this solution add 240 mL of methanol.

Flow rate: Adjust so that the retention time of nizatidine is about 10 minutes.

System suitability—

System performance: When the procedure is run with 10 μL of the standard solution under the above operating conditions, the internal standard and nizatidine are eluted in this order with the resolution between these peaks being not less than 3.

System repeatability: When the test is repeated 6 times with 10 μL of the standard solution under the above operating conditions, the relative standard deviation of the ratio of the peak area of nizatidine to that of the internal standard is not more than 1.0%.

Containers and storage Containers—Tight containers.

Noradrenaline

Norepinephrine

ノルアドレナリン

and enantiomer

$C_8H_{11}NO_3$: 169.18

4-[(1*RS*)-2-Amino-1-hydroxyethyl]benzene-1,2-diol

[*51-41-2*]

Noradrenaline, when dried, contains not less than 98.0% of *dl*-noradrenaline ($C_8H_{11}NO_3$).

Description Noradrenaline occurs as a white to light brown or slightly reddish brown crystalline powder.

It is freely soluble in acetic acid (100), very slightly soluble in water, and practically insoluble in ethanol (95).

It dissolves in dilute hydrochloric acid.

It gradually changes to brown by air and by light.

Identification **(1)** Determine the absorption spectrum of a solution of Noradrenaline in 0.1 mol/L hydrochloric acid TS (3 in 100,000) as directed under Ultraviolet-visible Spectrophotometry *<2.24>*, and compare the spectrum with the Reference Spectrum: both spectra exhibit similar intensities of absorption at the same wavelengths.

(2) Determine the infrared absorption spectrum of Noradrenaline, previously dried, as directed in the potassium bromide disk method under Infrared Spectrophotometry *<2.25>*, and compare the spectrum with the Reference Spectrum: both spectra exhibit similar intensities of absorption at the same wave numbers.

Purity **(1)** Clarity and color of solution—Dissolve 0.10 g of Noradrenaline in 10 mL of 0.1 mol/L hydrochloric acid TS, and add water to make 100 mL: the solution is clear and colorless.

(2) Arterenone—Dissolve 50 mg of Noradrenaline in 0.01 mol/L hydrochloric acid TS to make exactly 100 mL. Determine the absorbance of the solution at 310 nm as directed under Ultraviolet-visible Spectrophotometry *<2.24>*: it is not more than 0.1.

(3) Adrenaline—Dissolve 10.0 mg of Noradrenaline in 2.0 mL of diluted acetic acid (100) (1 in 2). Pipet 1 mL of this solution, add water to make 10 mL, then mix with 0.3 mL of a solution of sodium nitrite (1 in 100), and observe after 1 minute: the solution has no more color than the following control solution.

Control solution: Dissolve 2.0 mg of Adrenaline Bitartrate RS for Purity and 90 mg of Noradrenaline Bitartrate RS in water to make exactly 10 mL. Pipet 1 mL of this solution, add 1.0 mL of diluted acetic acid (100) (1 in 2) and water to make 10 mL, and proceed in the same manner.

Loss on drying *<2.41>* Not more than 1.0% (1 g, in vacuum, silica gel, 18 hours).

Residue on ignition *<2.44>* Not more than 0.1% (1 g).

Assay Weigh accurately about 0.3 g of Noradrenaline, previously dried, dissolve in 50 mL of acetic acid for nonaqueous titration by warming, if necessary, and titrate *<2.50>* with 0.1 mol/L perchloric acid VS until the color of the solution changes from blue-purple through blue to blue-green (indicator: 2 drops of crystal violet TS). Perform a blank determination in the same manner, and make any necessary correction.

Each mL of 0.1 mol/L perchloric acid VS
= 16.92 mg of $C_8H_{11}NO_3$

Containers and storage Containers—Tight containers.

Storage—Light-resistant, under nitrogen atmosphere, and in a cold place.

Noradrenaline Injection

Norepinephrine Injection

ノルアドレナリン注射液

Noradrenaline Injection is an aqueous injection.

It contains not less than 90.0% and not more than 110.0% of the labeled amount of *dl*-noradrenaline ($C_8H_{11}NO_3$: 169.18).

Method of preparation Dissolve Noradrenaline in 0.01 mol/L hydrochloric acid TS, and prepare as directed under Injections.

Description Norepinephrine Injection is a clear, colorless liquid.

It gradually becomes a pale red color by light and by air.

pH: 2.3 – 5.0

Identification Transfer a volume of Noradrenaline Injection, equivalent to 1 mg of Noradrenaline, to each of two test tubes A and B, and add 1 mL of water to each tube. Add 10 mL of potassium hydrogen phthalate buffer solution (pH 3.5) to A, and 10 mL of phosphate buffer solution (pH 6.5) to B. To each of these solutions add 1.0 mL of iodine TS, allow to stand for 5 minutes, and add 2.0 mL of sodium thiosulfate TS: no color or a pale red color develops in test tube A, and a deep red-purple color develops in test tube B.

Purity **(1)** Arterenone—Measure a volume of Noradrenaline Injection, equivalent to 10 mg of Noradrenaline, add water to make exactly 20 mL, and determine the absorbance of this solution at 310 nm as directed under Ultraviolet-visible Spectrophotometry *<2.24>*: the absorbance is not more than 0.10.

(2) Adrenaline—Measure a volume of Noradrenaline Injection, equivalent to 5 mg of Noradrenaline, add 1 mL of diluted acetic acid (100) (1 in 2) and water to make exactly 10 mL, and proceed as directed in the Purity (3) under Noradrenaline.

Bacterial endotoxins *<4.01>* Less than 300 EU/mg.

Extractable volume *<6.05>* It meets the requirement.

Foreign insoluble matter *<6.06>* Perform the test according to Method 1: it meets the requirement.

Insoluble particulate matter *<6.07>* It meets the requirement.

Sterility *<4.06>* Perform the test according to the Membrane filtration method: it meets the requirement.

Assay Pipet a volume of Noradrenaline Injection, equivalent to about 5 mg of *dl*-noradrenaline ($C_8H_{11}NO_3$), add water to make exactly 25 mL, and use this solution as the sample solution. Separately, weigh accurately about 10 mg of Noradrenaline Bitartrate RS, previously dried in a desiccator (in vacuum, silica gel) for 24 hours, dissolve in water to make exactly 25 mL, and use this solution as the standard solution. Pipet 5 mL each of the sample solution and standard solution, add 0.2 mL each of starch TS, then add iodine TS dropwise with swirling until a persistent blue color is produced. Add 2 mL of iodine TS, and shake. Adjust the pH of the solution to 6.5 with 0.05 mol/L disodium hydrogenphosphate TS, add 10 mL of phosphate buffer solution (pH 6.5), and shake. Immediately after allowing to stand for 3 minutes, add sodium thiosulfate TS dropwise until a red-purple color develops, then add water to make exactly 50 mL. Determine the absorbances, A_T and A_S, of the subsequent solutions of the sample solution and the standard solution at 515 nm within 5 minutes as directed under Ultraviolet-visible Spectrophotometry *<2.24>*.

Amount (mg) of *dl*-noradrenaline ($C_8H_{11}NO_3$)
$= M_S \times A_T/A_S \times 0.502$

M_S: Amount (mg) of Noradrenaline Bitartrate RS taken

Containers and storage Containers—Hermetic containers, and colored containers may be used.
Storage—Light-resistant.

Norethisterone

ノルエチステロン

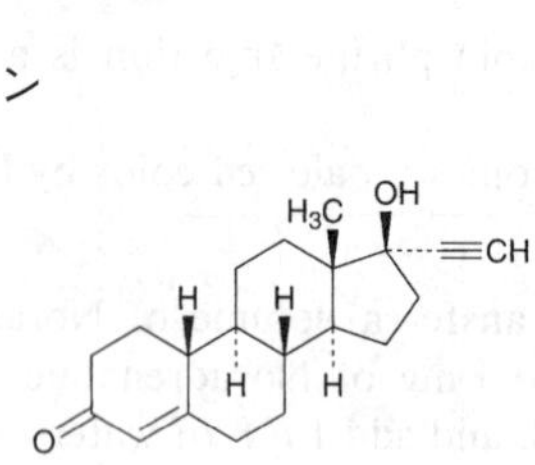

$C_{20}H_{26}O_2$: 298.42
17-Hydroxy-19-nor-17α-pregn-4-en-20-yn-3-one
[68-22-4]

Norethisterone, when dried, contains not less than 97.0% and not more than 103.0% of norethisterone ($C_{20}H_{26}O_2$).

Description Norethisterone occurs as a white to pale yellow-white crystalline powder. It has no odor.

It is sparingly soluble in ethanol (95), in acetone, and in tetrahydrofuran, slightly soluble in diethyl ether, and very slightly soluble in water.

It is affected by light.

Identification **(1)** To 2 mg of Norethisterone add 2 mL of sulfuric acid: the solution shows a red-brown color and a yellow-green fluorescence. Add 10 mL of water to this solution cautiously: a yellow color develops and a yellow-brown precipitate is formed.

(2) Determine the infrared absorption spectrum of Norethisterone as directed in the potassium bromide disk method under Infrared Spectrophotometry *<2.25>*, and compare the spectrum with the Reference Spectrum: both spectra exhibit similar intensities of absorption at the same wave numbers.

Optical rotation *<2.49>* $[\alpha]_D^{20}$: $-32 - -37°$ (after drying, 0.25 g, acetone, 25 mL, 100 mm).

Melting point *<2.60>* 203 - 209°C

Loss on drying *<2.41>* Not more than 0.5% (0.5 g, in vacuum, silica gel, 4 hours).

Residue on ignition *<2.44>* Not more than 0.1% (0.5 g).

Assay Weigh accurately about 0.2 g of Norethisterone, previously dried, dissolve in 40 mL of tetrahydrofuran, add 10 mL of a solution of silver nitrate (1 in 20), and titrate *<2.50>* with 0.1 mol/L sodium hydroxide VS (potentiometric titration). Perform a blank determination in the same manner, and make any necessary correction.

Each mL of 0.1 mol/L sodium hydroxide VS
$= 29.84$ mg of $C_{20}H_{26}O_2$

Containers and storage Containers—Tight containers.
Storage—Light-resistant.

Norfloxacin

ノルフロキサシン

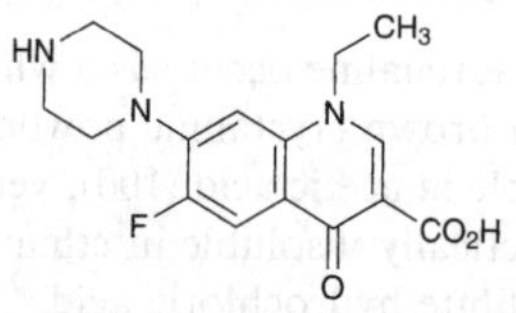

$C_{16}H_{18}FN_3O_3$: 319.33
1-Ethyl-6-fluoro-4-oxo-7-(piperazin-1-yl)-1,4-dihydroquinoline-3-carboxylic acid
[70458-96-7]

Norfloxacin, when dried, contains not less than 99.0% of norfloxacin ($C_{16}H_{18}FN_3O_3$).

Description Norfloxacin occurs as a white to pale yellow crystalline powder.

It is freely soluble in acetic acid (100), slightly soluble in ethanol (99.5) and in acetone, very slightly soluble in methanol, and practically insoluble in water.

It dissolves in dilute hydrochloric acid TS and in sodium hydroxide TS.

It is hygroscopic.

It is gradually colored by light.

Identification **(1)** Dissolve 0.01 g of Norfloxacin in a solution of sodium hydroxide (1 in 250) to make 100 mL. To 5 mL of this solution add a solution of sodium hydroxide (1 in 250) to make 100 mL. Determine the absorption spectrum of this solution as directed under Ultraviolet-visible Spectrophotometry 〈2.24〉, and compare the spectrum with the Reference Spectrum: both spectra exhibit similar intensities of absorption at the same wavelengths.

(2) Dissolve a suitable amount of Norfloxacin in a suitable amount of acetone, evaporate the acetone under reduced pressure, and dry the residue. Determine the infrared absorption spectrum of the residue so obtained as directed in the potassium bromide disk method under Infrared Spectrophotometry 〈2.25〉, and compare the spectrum with the Reference Spectrum: both spectra exhibit similar intensities of absorption at the same wave numbers.

Purity **(1)** Sulfate 〈1.14〉—Dissolve 1.0 g of Norfloxacin in 7 mL of 0.5 mol/L sodium hydroxide TS and 23 mL of water, and add 1 drop of phenolphthalein TS. Add gradually diluted hydrochloric acid (1 in 3) to this solution until the red color disappears, then add 0.5 mL of dilute hydrochloric acid, and cool in ice for 30 minutes. Filter through a glass filter (G4), and wash the residue with 10 mL of water. Combine the filtrate and the washing, and add 1 mL of dilute hydrochloric acid and water to make 50 mL. Perform the test using this solution as the test solution. Prepare the control solution as follows. To 0.50 mL of 0.005 mol/L sulfuric acid VS add 7 mL of 0.5 mol/L sodium hydroxide TS and 1 drop of phenolphthalein TS, add diluted hydrochloric acid (1 in 3) until the red color disappears, then add 1.5 mL of dilute hydrochloric acid, 1 or 2 drops of bromophenol blue TS and water to make 50 mL (not more than 0.024%).

(2) Heavy metals 〈1.07〉—Proceed with 2.0 g of Norfloxacin according to Method 2, and perform the test. Prepare the control solution with 3.0 mL of Standard Lead Solution (not more than 15 ppm).

(3) Arsenic 〈1.11〉—Prepare the test solution with 1.0 g of Norfloxacin according to Method 3, and perform the test (not more than 2 ppm).

(4) Related substances—Conduct this procedure without exposure to light, using light-resistant vessels. Dissolve 0.10 g of Norfloxacin in 50 mL of a mixture of methanol and acetone (1:1), and use this solution as the sample solution. Pipet 1 mL of the sample solution, add a mixture of methanol and acetone (1:1) to make exactly 100 mL. Pipet 2 mL of this solution, add a mixture of methanol and acetone (1:1) to make exactly 10 mL, and use this solution as the standard solution. Perform the test with these solutions as directed under Thin-layer Chromatography 〈2.03〉. Spot 20 μL each of the sample solution and standard solution on a plate of silica gel with fluorescent indicator for thin-layer chromatography (5 to 7 μm in particle diameter). Develop with a mixture of methanol, chloroform, toluene, diethylamine and water (20:20:10:7:4) to a distance of about 9 cm, and air-dry the plate. Examine under ultraviolet light (main wavelength: 254 nm and 366 nm): the number of the spot other than the principal spot obtained from the sample solution is not more than 2 and they are not more intense than the spot from the standard solution.

Loss on drying 〈2.41〉 Not more than 1.0% (1 g, 105°C, 2 hours).

Residue on ignition 〈2.44〉 Not more than 0.1% (1 g).

Assay Weigh accurately about 0.5 g of Norfloxacin, previously dried, dissolve in 50 mL of acetic acid (100), and titrate 〈2.50〉 with 0.1 mol/L perchloric acid VS (potentiometric titration). Perform a blank determination in the same manner, and make any necessary correction.

Each mL of 0.1 mol/L perchloric acid VS
= 31.93 mg of $C_{16}H_{18}FN_3O_3$

Containers and storage Containers—Tight containers.
Storage—Light-resistant.

Norgestrel

ノルゲストレル

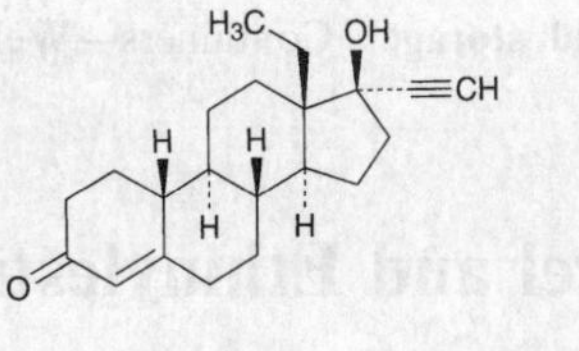

$C_{21}H_{28}O_2$: 312.45
13-Ethyl-17-hydroxy-18,19-dinor-17α-pregn-4-en-20-yn-3-one
[*6533-00-2*]

Norgestrel, when dried, contains not less than 98.0% of norgestrel ($C_{21}H_{28}O_2$).

Description Norgestrel occurs as white, crystals or crystalline powder.

It is soluble in tetrahydrofuran and in chloroform, sparingly soluble in ethanol (95), slightly soluble in diethyl ether, and practically insoluble in water.

Identification **(1)** Dissolve 1 mg of Norgestrel in 2 mL of ethanol (95), and add 1 mL of sulfuric acid: a red-purple color develops. With this solution, examine under ultraviolet light (main wavelength: 365 nm): the solution shows a red-orange fluorescence.

(2) Determine the infrared absorption spectrum of Norgestrel, previously dried, as directed in the potassium bromide disk method under Infrared Spectrophotometry 〈2.25〉, and compare the spectrum with the Reference Spectrum: both spectra exhibit similar intensities of absorption at the same wave numbers.

Melting point 〈2.60〉 206 – 212°C

Purity **(1)** Heavy metals 〈1.07〉—Take 1.0 g of Norgestrel, heat gently to carbonize, cool, add 10 mL of a solution of magnesium nitrate hexahydrate in ethanol (95) (1 in 10), and ignite the ethanol to burn. After cooling, add 1 mL of sulfuric acid, proceed with this solution according to Method 4, and perform the test. Prepare the control solution with 2.0 mL of Standard Lead Solution (not more than 20 ppm).

(2) Related substances—Dissolve 30 mg of Norgestrel in 5 mL of chloroform, and use this solution as the sample solution. Pipet 1 mL of the sample solution, add chloroform to make exactly 100 mL, and use this solution as the standard solution. Perform the test with these solutions as directed under Thin-layer Chromatography 〈2.03〉. Spot 10 μL each of the sample solution and standard solution on a plate of silica gel with fluorescent indicator for thin-layer chromatography. Develop the plate with a mixture of dichloromethane and ethyl acetate (2:1) to a distance of about 10 cm, and air-dry the plate. Examine under ultraviolet light (main wavelength: 254 nm): the spots other than the principal spot obtained from the sample solution are not more intense than the spot from the standard solution.

Loss on drying 〈2.41〉 Not more than 0.5% (1 g, 105°C, 3 hours).

Residue on ignition 〈2.44〉 Not more than 0.2% (0.5 g).

Assay Weigh accurately about 0.2 g of Norgestrel, previously dried, dissolve in 40 mL of tetrahydrofuran, add 10 mL of a solution of silver nitrate (1 in 20), and titrate <*2.50*> with 0.1 mol/L sodium hydroxide VS (potentiometric titration). Perform a blank determination in the same manner, and make any necessary correction.

Each mL of 0.1 mol/L sodium hydroxide VS
= 31.25 mg of $C_{21}H_{28}O_2$

Containers and storage Containers—Well-closed containers.

Norgestrel and Ethinylestradiol Tablets

ノルゲストレル･エチニルエストラジオール錠

Norgestrel and Ethinylestradiol Tablets contain not less than 90.0% and not more than 110.0% of the labeled amount of norgestrel ($C_{21}H_{28}O_2$: 312.45) and ethinylestradiol ($C_{20}H_{24}O_2$: 296.40).

Method of preparation Prepare as directed under Tablets, with Norgestrel and Ethinylestradiol.

Identification **(1)** To a quantity of powdered Norgestrel and Ethinylestradiol Tablets, equivalent to 10 mg of Norgestrel add 10 mL of ethyl acetate, shake for 10 minutes, and filter. To 2 mL of the filtrate add 6 mL of sodium hydroxide TS, shake vigorously, and centrifuge. Take 1 mL of the ethyl acetate layer, evaporate on a water bath to dryness, dissolve the residue in 2 mL of ethanol (95), and add 1 mL of sulfuric acid: a red-purple color develops. Examine under ultraviolet light (main wavelength: 365 nm): this solution shows a red-orange fluorescence (norgestrel).

(2) Take 1 mL of the filtrate obtained in (1), evaporate on a water bath to dryness, add 1 mL of boric acid-methanol buffer solution to the residue, shake, and cool in ice. Add 1 mL of ice-cold diazo TS, shake, add 1 mL of sodium hydroxide TS, and shake: a red-orange color develops (ethinylestradiol).

(3) Use the filtrate obtained in (1) as the sample solution. Separately, dissolve 10 mg of Norgestrel RS and 1 mg of Ethinylestradiol RS, respectively, in 10 mL of ethyl acetate, and use these solutions as the standard solution (1) and the standard solution (2). Perform the test with these solutions as directed under Thin-layer Chromatography <*2.03*>. Spot 20 μL each of the sample solution and standard solutions (1) and (2) on a plate of silica gel for thin-layer chromatography. Develop the plate with a mixture of pentane and ethyl acetate (3:2) to a distance of about 7 cm, and air-dry the plate. Spray evenly a solution of *p*-toluenesulfonic acid monohydrate in ethanol (95) (1 in 5) on the plate, and heat the plate at 105°C for 5 minutes. Examine under ultraviolet light (main wavelength: 365 nm): two spots obtained from the sample solution show the similar color tone and *R*f value to each spot from the standard solutions (1) and (2).

Uniformity of dosage units <*6.02*> Perform the test according to the following method: it meets the requirement of the Content uniformity test.

Add 2 mL of diluted methanol (7 in 10) to 1 tablet of Norgestrel and Ethinylestradiol Tablets, add exactly 2 mL of the internal standard solution, shake for 20 minutes, and centrifuge. Filter the supernatant liquid through a membrane filter with a pore size of not more than 0.2 μm, and use this filtrate as the sample solution. Separately, weigh accurately quantities of Norgestrel RS and of Ethinylestradiol RS, equivalent to 100 times each of the labeled amounts, dissolve in diluted methanol (7 in 10) to make exactly 200 mL. Pipet 2 mL of this solution, add exactly 2 mL of the internal standard solution, and use this solution as the standard solution. Perform the test with 20 μL each of the sample solution and standard solution as directed under Liquid Chromatography <*2.01*> according to the following conditions. Calculate the ratios, Q_{Ta} and Q_{Tb}, of the peak areas of norgestrel and ethinylestradiol to the peak area of the internal standard of the sample solution and also the ratios, Q_{Sa} and Q_{Sb}, of the peak areas of norgestrel and ethinylestradiol to the peak area of the internal standard of the standard solution. Then, proceed as directed in the Assay.

Amount (mg) of norgestrel ($C_{21}H_{28}O_2$)
$= M_{Sa} \times Q_{Ta}/Q_{Sa} \times 1/100$

Amount (mg) of ethinylestradiol ($C_{20}H_{24}O_2$)
$= M_{Sb} \times Q_{Tb}/Q_{Sb} \times 1/100$

M_{Sa}: Amount (mg) of Norgestrel RS taken
M_{Sb}: Amount (mg) of Ethinylestradiol RS taken

Internal standard solution—A solution of diphenyl in diluted methanol (7 in 10) (1 in 50,000).

Operating conditions—

Proceed as directed in the operating conditions in the Assay.

System suitability—

Proceed as directed in the system suitability in the Assay.

Dissolution <*6.10*> When the test is performed at 50 revolutions per minute according to the Paddle method, using 900 mL of water as the dissolution medium, the dissolution rate in 45 minutes of Norgestrel and Ethinylestradiol Tablets is not less than 70%.

Start the test with 1 tablet of Norgestrel and Ethinylestradiol Tablets, withdraw not less than 50 mL of the medium at the specified minute after starting the test, and filter through a membrane filter with a pore size not exceeding 0.8 μm. Discard not less than 10 mL of the first filtrate, pipet exactly *V* mL of the subsequent filtrate, equivalent to about 17 μg of norgestrel ($C_{21}H_{28}O_2$) and about 1.7 μg of ethinylestradiol ($C_{20}H_{24}O_2$), transfer into a chromatography column [prepared by packing 0.36 g of octadecylsilanized silica gel for pretreatment (55 to 105 μm in particle diameter) in a tube about 1 cm in inside diameter]. After washing the column with 15 mL of water, elute with 3 mL of methanol, and evaporate the effluent in a water bath to dryness at about 40°C with the aid of a current air. Dissolve the residue in exactly 2 mL of diluted methanol (7 in 10), and use this solution as the sample solution. Separately, weigh accurately about 25 mg of Norgestrel RS and about 2.5 mg of Ethinylestradiol RS, dissolve in diluted methanol (7 in 10) to make exactly 100 mL, then pipet 3 mL of this solution, add diluted methanol (7 in 10) to make exactly 100 mL, and use this solution as the standard solution. Perform the test with exactly 50 μL each of the sample solution and standard solution as directed under Liquid Chromatography <*2.01*> according to the following conditions. Determine the peak areas, A_{Ta} and A_{Tb}, of norgestrel and ethinylestradiol from the sample solution, and the peak areas, A_{Sa} and A_{Sb}, of norgestrel and ethinylestradiol from the standard solution.

Dissolution rate (%) with respect to the labeled amount of norgestrel ($C_{21}H_{28}O_2$)
$= M_{Sa} \times A_{Ta}/A_{Sa} \times 1/V \times 1/C_a \times 54$

Dissolution rate (%) with respect to the labeled amount of ethinylestradiol ($C_{20}H_{24}O_2$)
$= M_{Sb} \times A_{Tb}/A_{Sb} \times 1/V \times 1/C_b \times 54$

M_{Sa}: Amount (mg) of Norgestrel RS taken
M_{Sb}: Amount (mg) of Ethinylestradiol RS taken
C_a: Labeled amount (mg) of norgestrel ($C_{21}H_{28}O_2$) in 1 tablet
C_b: Labeled amount (mg) of ethinylestradiol ($C_{20}H_{24}O_2$) in 1 tablet

Operating conditions—

Proceed as directed in the operating conditions in the Assay.

System suitability—

Proceed as directed in the system suitability in the Assay.

Assay Weigh accurately not less than 20 Norgestrel and Ethinylestradiol Tablets, and powder. Weigh accurately a portion of the powder, equivalent to about 1 mg of norgestrel ($C_{21}H_{28}O_2$), add 4 mL of diluted methanol (7 in 10), add exactly 4 mL of the internal standard solution, shake for 20 minutes, and centrifuge. Filter the supernatant liquid through a membrane filter with a pore size of not more than 0.2 μm, and use this filtrate as the sample solution. Separately, weigh accurately about 50 mg of Norgestrel RS and about 5 mg of Ethinylestradiol RS, and dissolve in diluted methanol (7 in 10) to make exactly 200 mL. Pipet 4 mL of this solution, add exactly 4 mL of the internal standard solution, and use this solution as the standard solution. Perform the test with 20 μL each of the sample solution and standard solution as directed under Liquid Chromatography <*2.01*> according to the following conditions. Calculate the ratios, Q_{Ta} and Q_{Tb}, of the peak areas of norgestrel and ethinylestradiol to the peak area of the internal standard of the sample solution and also the ratios, Q_{Sa} and Q_{Sb}, of the peak areas of norgestrel and ethinylestradiol to the peak area of the internal standard of the standard solution.

Amount (mg) of norgestrel ($C_{21}H_{28}O_2$)
$= M_{Sa} \times Q_{Ta}/Q_{Sa} \times 1/50$

Amount (mg) of ethinylestradiol ($C_{20}H_{24}O_2$)
$= M_{Sb} \times Q_{Tb}/Q_{Sb} \times 1/50$

M_{Sa}: Amount (mg) of Norgestrel RS taken
M_{Sb}: Amount (mg) of Ethinylestradiol RS taken

Internal standard solution—A solution of diphenyl in diluted methanol (7 in 10) (1 in 50,000).

Operating conditions—

Detector: Norgestrel—An ultraviolet absorption photometer (wavelength: 241 nm).

Ethinylestradiol—A fluorophotometer (excitation wavelength: 281 nm, fluorescence wavelength: 305 nm).

Column: A stainless steel column 4.6 mm in inside diameter and 25 cm in length, packed with octadecylsilanized silica gel for liquid chromatography (10 μm in particle diameter).

Column temperature: A constant temperature of about 25°C.

Mobile phase: A mixture of acetonitrile and water (11:9).

Flow rate: Adjust so that the retention time of norgestrel is about 10 minutes.

System suitability—

System performance: When the procedure is run with 20 μL of the standard solution under the above operating conditions, ethinylestradiol, norgestrel and the internal standard are eluted in this order, and the resolution between the peaks of norgestrel and the internal standard is not less than 8.

System repeatability: When the test is repeated 6 times with 20 μL of the standard solution under the above operating conditions, the relative standard deviation of the ratios of the peak area of ethinylestradiol and norgestrel to that of the internal standard are not more than 1.0%, respectively.

Containers and storage Containers—Tight containers.

Nortriptyline Hydrochloride

ノルトリプチリン塩酸塩

• HCl

$C_{19}H_{21}N.HCl$: 299.84
3-(10,11-Dihydro-5*H*-dibenzo[*a,d*]cyclohepten-5-ylidene)-*N*-methylpropylamine monohydrochloride
[*894-71-3*]

Nortriptyline Hydrochloride, when dried, contains not less than 98.5% of nortriptyline hydrochloride ($C_{19}H_{21}N.HCl$).

Description Nortriptyline Hydrochloride occurs as a white to yellowish white crystalline powder. It is odorless, or has a faint, characteristic odor.

It is freely soluble in acetic acid (100) and in chloroform, soluble in ethanol (95), sparingly soluble in water, and practically insoluble in diethyl ether.

The pH of a solution of 1.0 g of Nortriptyline Hydrochloride in 100 mL of water is about 5.5.

Melting point: 215 - 220°C

Identification **(1)** To 5 mL of a solution of Nortriptyline Hydrochloride (1 in 100) add 1 mL of bromine TS: the color of the test solution disappears.

(2) To 5 mL of a solution of Nortriptyline Hydrochloride (1 in 100) add 1 to 2 drops of a solution of quinhydrone in methanol (1 in 40): a red color gradually develops.

(3) Determine the absorption spectrum of a solution of Nortriptyline Hydrochloride (1 in 100,000) as directed under Ultraviolet-visible Spectrophotometry <*2.24*>, and compare the spectrum with the Reference Spectrum: both spectra exhibit similar intensities of absorption at the same wavelengths.

(4) Determine the infrared absorption spectrum of Nortriptyline Hydrochloride, previously dried, as directed in the potassium chloride disk method under Infrared Spectrophotometry <*2.25*>, and compare the spectrum with the Reference Spectrum: both spectra exhibit similar intensities of absorption at the same wave numbers.

(5) A solution of Nortriptyline Hydrochloride (1 in 100) responds to Qualitative Tests <*1.09*> for chloride.

Purity **(1)** Clarity and color of solution—Dissolve 0.10 g of Nortriptyline Hydrochloride in 10 mL of water: the solution is clear and colorless to very light yellow.

(2) Heavy metals <*1.07*>—Proceed with 1.0 g of Nortriptyline Hydrochloride according to Method 2, and perform the test. Prepare the control solution with 2.0 mL of Standard Lead Solution (not more than 20 ppm).

(3) Arsenic <*1.11*>—Prepare the test solution with 1.0 g of Nortriptyline Hydrochloride according to Method 3, and perform the test (not more than 2 ppm).

(4) Related substances—Dissolve 0.50 g of Nortriptyline

Hydrochloride in 20 mL of chloroform, and use this solution as the sample solution. Pipet 2 mL of the sample solution, and add chloroform to make exactly 100 mL. Pipet 5 mL of this solution, add chloroform to make exactly 50 mL, and use this solution as the standard solution. Perform the test with these solutions as directed under Thin-layer Chromatography *<2.03>*. Spot 4 μL each of the sample solution and standard solution on a plate of silica gel with fluorescent indicator for thin-layer chromatography. Develop the plate with a mixture of cyclohexane, methanol and diethylamine (8:1:1) to a distance of about 15 cm, and air-dry the plate. Examine under ultraviolet light (main wavelength: 254 nm): the spots other than the principal spot obtained from the sample solution are not more intense than the spot from the standard solution.

Loss on drying *<2.41>* Not more than 0.5% (1 g, 105°C, 2 hours).

Residue on ignition *<2.44>* Not more than 0.1% (1 g).

Assay Weigh accurately about 0.5 g of Nortriptyline Hydrochloride, previously dried, dissolve in 5 mL of acetic acid (100), add 50 mL of acetic anhydride, and titrate *<2.50>* with 0.1 mol/L perchloric acid VS (potentiometric titration). Perform a blank determination in the same manner, and make any necessary correction.

Each mL of 0.1 mol/L perchloric acid VS
= 29.98 mg of $C_{19}H_{21}N.HCl$

Containers and storage Containers—Well-closed containers.

Storage—Light-resistant.

Nortriptyline Hydrochloride Tablets

ノルトリプチリン塩酸塩錠

Nortriptyline Hydrochloride Tablets contain not less than 95.0% and not more than 105.0% of the labeled amount of nortriptyline ($C_{19}H_{21}N$: 263.38).

Method of preparation Prepare as directed under Tablets, with Nortriptyline Hydrochloride.

Identification **(1)** Determine the absorption spectrum of the sample solution obtained in the Assay as directed under Ultraviolet-visible Spectrophotometry *<2.24>*, using diluted 0.1 mol/L hydrochloric acid TS (1 in 50) as the blank: it exhibits a maximum between 237 nm and 241 nm.

(2) To a quantity of powdered Nortriptyline Hydrochloride Tablets, equivalent to 10 mg of nortriptyline ($C_{19}H_{21}N$), add 10 mL of ethanol (99.5), shake thoroughly, centrifuge, and use the supernatant liquid as the sample solution. Separately, dissolve 11 mg of nortriptyline hydrochloride in 10 mL of ethanol (99.5), and use this solution as the standard solution. Perform the test with these solutions as directed under Thin-layer Chromatography *<2.03>*. Spot 10 μL each of the sample solution and standard solution on a plate of silica gel with fluorescent indicator for thin-layer chromatography. Develop the plate with a mixture of 1-butanol, water and acetic acid (100) (4:1:1) to a distance of about 10 cm, and air-dry the plate. Examine under ultraviolet light (main wavelength: 254 nm): the principal spot obtained from the sample solution and the spot from the standard solution show the same *Rf* value.

Uniformity of dosage units *<6.02>* Perform the test according to the following method: it meets the requirement of the Content uniformity test.

To 1 tablet of Nortriptyline Hydrochloride Tablets add a suitable volume of 0.1 mol/L hydrochloric acid TS, disperse the fine particles by sonicating, add a suitable volume of 0.1 mol/L hydrochloric acid TS, sonicate, and extract for 15 minutes while occasional shaking. Shake for 15 minutes, and add 0.1 mol/L hydrochloric acid TS to make exactly V mL so that each mL contains about 0.5 mg of nortriptyline ($C_{19}H_{21}N$). Centrifuge this solution, pipet 2 mL of the supernatant liquid, add water to make exactly 100 mL, and use this solution as the sample solution. Then, proceed as directed in the Assay.

Amount (mg) of nortriptyline ($C_{19}H_{21}N$)
$= M_S \times A_T/A_S \times V/50 \times 0.878$

M_S: Amount (mg) of nortriptyline hydrochloride for assay taken

Dissolution *<6.10>* When the test is performed at 50 revolutions per minute according to the Paddle method, using 900 mL of water as the dissolution medium, the dissolution rates in 30 minutes of a 10-mg tablet and a 25-mg tablet are not less than 70% and not less than 80%, respectively.

Start the test with 1 tablet of Nortriptyline Hydrochloride Tablets, withdraw not less than 20 mL of the medium at the specified minute after starting the test, and filter through a membrane filter with a pore size not exceeding 0.45 μm. Discard not less than 10 mL of the first filtrate, pipet V mL of the subsequent filtrate, add water to make exactly V' mL so that each mL contains about 11 μg of nortriptyline ($C_{19}H_{21}N$), and use this solution as the sample solution. Separately, weigh accurately about 25 mg of nortriptyline hydrochloride for assay, previously dried at 105°C for 2 hours, and dissolve in water to make exactly 100 mL. Pipet 5 mL of this solution, add water to make exactly 100 mL, and use this solution as the standard solution. Determine the absorbances, A_T and A_S, of the sample solution and standard solution at 239 nm as directed under Ultraviolet-visible Spectrophotometry *<2.24>*.

Dissolution rate (%) with respect to the labeled amount of nortriptyline ($C_{19}H_{21}N$)
$= M_S \times A_T/A_S \times V'/V \times 1/C \times 45 \times 0.878$

M_S: Amount (mg) of nortriptyline hydrochloride for assay taken

C: Labeled amount (mg) of nortriptyline ($C_{19}H_{21}N$) in 1 tablet

Assay Weigh accurately the mass of not less than 20 tablets of Nortriptyline Hydrochloride Tablets, and powder. Weigh accurately a portion of the powder, equivalent to about 50 mg of nortriptyline ($C_{19}H_{21}N$), add 50 mL of 0.1 mol/L hydrochloric acid TS, sonicate, and extract for 15 minutes while occasional shaking. Shake for 15 minutes, and add 0.1 mol/L hydrochloric acid TS to make exactly 100 mL. Centrifuge this solution, pipet 2 mL of the supernatant liquid, add water to make exactly 100 mL, and use this solution as the sample solution. Separately, weigh accurately about 28 mg of nortriptyline hydrochloride for assay, previously dried at 105°C for 2 hours, and dissolve in 0.1 mol/L hydrochloric acid TS to make exactly 50 mL. Pipet 2 mL of this solution, add water to make exactly 100 mL, and use this solution as the standard solution. Determine the absorbances, A_T and A_S, of the sample solution and standard solution at 239 nm as directed under Ultraviolet-visible Spectrophotometry *<2.24>*, using diluted 0.1 mol/L hydrochloric acid TS (1 in 50) as the blank.

Amount (mg) of nortriptyline ($C_{19}H_{21}N$)
$= M_S \times A_T/A_S \times 2 \times 0.878$

M_S: Amount (mg) of nortriptyline hydrochloride for assay taken

Containers and storage Containers—Tight containers.

Noscapine

ノスカピン

$C_{22}H_{23}NO_7$: 413.42
(3*S*)-6,7-Dimethoxy-3-[(5*R*)-4-methoxy-6-methyl-5,6,7,8-tetrahydro[1,3]dioxolo[4,5-*g*]isoquinolin-5-yl]isobenzofuran-1(3*H*)-one
[*128-62-1*]

Noscapine, when dried, contains not less than 98.5% of noscapine ($C_{22}H_{23}NO_7$).

Description Noscapine occurs as white, crystals or crystalline powder. It is odorless and tasteless.

It is very soluble in acetic acid (100), slightly soluble in ethanol (95) and in diethyl ether, and practically insoluble in water.

Identification **(1)** Determine the absorption spectrum of a solution of Noscapine in methanol (1 in 20,000) as directed under Ultraviolet-visible Spectrophotometry <*2.24*>, and compare the spectrum with the Reference Spectrum: both spectra exhibit similar intensities of absorption at the same wavelengths.

(2) Determine the infrared absorption spectrum of Noscapine, previously dried, as directed in the potassium bromide disk method under the Infrared Spectrophotometry <*2.25*>, and compare the spectrum with the Reference Spectrum: both spectra exhibit similar intensities of absorption at the same wave numbers.

Optical rotation <*2.49*> $[\alpha]_D^{20}$: +42 – +48° (after drying, 0.5 g, 0.1 mol/L hydrochloric acid TS, 25 mL, 100 nm).

Melting point <*2.60*> 174 – 177°C

Purity **(1)** Chloride <*1.03*>—Dissolve 0.7 g of Noscapine in 20 mL of acetone, add 6 mL of dilute nitric acid and water to make 50 mL, and perform the test with this solution. Prepare the control solution as follows: To 0.4 mL of 0.01 mol/L hydrochloric acid VS add 20 mL of acetone, 6 mL of dilute nitric acid and water to make 50 mL (not more than 0.02%).

(2) Heavy metals <*1.07*>—Proceed with 2.0 g of Noscapine according to Method 2, and perform the test. Prepare the control solution with 2.0 mL of Standard Lead Solution (not more than 10 ppm).

(3) Morphine—Dissolve 10 mg of Noscapine in 1 mL of water and 5 mL of 1-nitroso-2-naphthol TS with shaking, add 2 mL of a solution of potassium nitrate (1 in 10), and warm at 40°C for 2 minutes. Add 1 mL of a solution of sodium nitrite (1 in 5000), and warm at 40°C for 5 minutes. After cooling, shake the solution with 10 mL of chloroform, centrifuge, and collect the aqueous layer: the solution so obtained has no more color than a pale red.

(4) Related substances—Dissolve 0.7 g of Noscapine in 50 mL of acetone, and use this solution as the sample solution. Pipet 5 mL of the sample solution, add acetone to make exactly 50 mL. Pipet 5 mL of this solution, add acetone to make exactly 100 mL, and use this solution as the standard solution. Perform the test with these solutions as directed under Thin-layer Chromatography <*2.03*>. Spot 10 μL each of the sample solution and standard solution on a plate of silica gel for thin-layer chromatography. Develop the plate with a mixture of acetone, toluene, ethanol (99.5) and ammonia solution (28) (60:60:9:2) to a distance of about 10 cm, and air-dry the plate. Spray evenly dilute bismuth subnitrate-potassium iodide TS for spraying on the plate: the spots other than the principal spot obtained from the sample solution are not more intense than the spot from the standard solution.

Loss on drying <*2.41*> Not more than 0.5% (2 g, 105°C, 4 hours).

Residue on ignition <*2.44*> Not more than 0.1% (1 g).

Assay Weigh accurately about 0.8 g of Noscapine, previously dried, dissolve in 30 mL of acetic acid (100) and titrate <*2.50*> with 0.1 mol/L perchloric acid VS (indicator: 3 drops of crystal violet TS). Perform a blank determination in the same manner, and make any necessary correction.

Each mL of 0.1 mol/L perchloric acid VS
$= 41.34$ mg of $C_{22}H_{23}NO_7$

Containers and storage Containers—Well-closed containers.

Storage—Light-resistant.

Noscapine Hydrochloride Hydrate

ノスカピン塩酸塩水和物

$C_{22}H_{23}NO_7.HCl.xH_2O$
(3*S*)-6,7-Dimethoxy-3-[(5*R*)-4-methoxy-6-methyl-5,6,7,8-tetrahydro[1,3]dioxolo[4,5-*g*]isoquinolin-5-yl]isobenzofuran-1(3*H*)-one monohydrochloride hydrate
[*912-60-7*, anhydride]

Noscapine Hydrochloride Hydrate, when dried, contains not less than 98.0% of noscapine hydrochloride ($C_{22}H_{23}NO_7.HCl$: 449.88).

Description Noscapine Hydrochloride Hydrate occurs as colorless or white, crystals or crystalline powder. It is odorless, and has a bitter taste.

It is freely soluble in water, in acetic anhydride, and in acetic acid (100), soluble in ethanol (95), and practically insoluble in diethyl ether.

Identification **(1)** To 1 mg of Noscapine Hydrochloride Hydrate add 1 drop of formaldehyde-sulfuric acid TS: a purple color, changing to yellow-brown, is produced.

(2) To 1 mg of Noscapine Hydrochloride Hydrate add 1 drop of a solution of ammonium vanadate (V) in sulfuric acid (1 in 200): an orange color is produced.

(3) Dissolve 0.02 g of Noscapine Hydrochloride Hydrate in 1 mL of water, and add 3 drops of sodium acetate TS: a white, flocculent precipitate is produced.

(4) Dissolve 1 mg of Noscapine Hydrochloride Hydrate in 1 mL of diluted sulfuric acid (1 in 35), shake with 5 drops of a solution of disodium chromotropate dihydrate (1 in 50), and add 2 mL of sulfuric acid dropwise: a purple color is produced.

(5) Dissolve 0.1 g of Noscapine Hydrochloride Hydrate in 10 mL of water, make the solution alkaline with ammonia TS, and shake with 10 mL of chloroform. Separate the chloroform layer, wash with 5 mL of water, and filter. Distil most of the filtrate on a water bath, add 1 mL of ethanol (99.5), and evaporate to dryness. Dry the residue at 105°C for 4 hours: the residue so obtained melts <*2.60*> between 174°C and 177°C.

(6) Make a solution of Noscapine Hydrochloride Hydrate (1 in 50) alkaline with ammonia TS, and filter the precipitate. Acidify the filtrate with dilute nitric acid: the solution responds to Qualitative Tests <*1.09*> (2) for chloride.

Purity Morphine—Dissolve 10 mg of Noscapine Hydrochloride Hydrate in 1 mL of water, add 5 mL of 1-nitroso-2-naphthol TS and 2 mL of a solution of potassium nitrate (1 in 10), and warm at 40°C for 2 minutes. Add 1 mL of a solution of sodium nitrite (1 in 5000), and warm at 40°C for 5 minutes. After cooling, shake the mixture with 10 mL of chloroform, centrifuge, and separate the aqueous layer: the solution so obtained has no more color than a pale red color.

Loss on drying <*2.41*> Not more than 9.0% (0.5 g, 120°C, 4 hours).

Residue on ignition <*2.44*> Not more than 0.5% (1 g).

Assay Weigh accurately about 0.5 g of Noscapine Hydrochloride Hydrate, previously dried, dissolve in 50 mL of a mixture of acetic anhydride and acetic acid (100) (7:3), and titrate <*2.50*> with 0.1 mol/L perchloric acid VS (potentiometric titration). Perform a blank determination in the same manner, and make any necessary correction.

Each mL of 0.1 mol/L perchloric acid VS
= 44.99 mg of $C_{22}H_{23}NO_7.HCl$

Containers and storage Containers—Well-closed containers.

Storage—Light-resistant.

Nystatin

ナイスタチン

Nystatin is a mixture of polyene macrolide substances having antifungal activity produced by the growth of *Streptomyces noursei*.

It contains not less than 4600 units (potency) per mg, calculated on the dried basis. The potency of Nystatin is expressed as the unit of nystatin ($C_{47}H_{75}NO_{17}$: 926.09), and one unit corresponds to 0.27 μg of nystatin ($C_{47}H_{75}NO_{17}$).

Description Nystatin occurs as a white to light yellow-brown powder.

It is soluble in formamide, sparingly soluble in methanol, slightly soluble in ethanol (95), and very slightly soluble in water.

It dissolves in sodium hydroxide TS.

Identification **(1)** Dissolve 1 mg of Nystatin in 5 mL of water and 1 mL of sodium hydroxide TS, heat for 2 minutes, and cool. To this solution add 3 mL of a solution of 4-aminoacetophenone in methanol (1 in 200) and 1 mL of hydrochloric acid: a red-purple color develops.

(2) To 10 mg of Nystatin add 50.25 mL of a mixture of diluted methanol (4 in 5) and sodium hydroxide TS (200:1), heat at not exceeding 50°C to dissolve, then add diluted methanol (4 in 5) to make 500 mL. Determine the absorption spectrum of this solution as directed under Ultraviolet-visible Spectrophotometry <*2.24*>, and compare the spectrum with the Reference Spectrum or the spectrum of a solution of Nystatin RS prepared in the same manner as the sample solution: both spectra exhibit similar intensities of absorption at the same wavelengths.

Purity Heavy metals <*1.07*>—Proceed with 1.0 g of Nystatin according to Method 4, and perform the test. Prepare the control solution with 2.0 mL of Standard Lead Solution (not more than 20 ppm).

Loss on drying <*2.41*> Not more than 5.0% (0.3 g, in vacuum, 60°C, 3 hours).

Assay Perform the test according to the Cylinder-plate method as directed under Microbial Assay for Antibiotics <*4.02*> according to the following conditions.

(i) Test organism—*Saccharomyces cerevisiae* ATCC 9763

(ii) Culture medium—Use the medium 2) under (1) Agar media for seed and base layer.

(iii) Standard solutions—Use a light-resistant container. Weigh accurately an amount of Nystatin RS equivalent to about 60,000 units, previously dried at 40°C for 2 hours in vacuum (not more than 0.67 kPa), dissolve in formamide to make a solution of 3000 units per mL, and use this solution as the standard stock solution. Keep the standard stock solution at 5°C or below and use within 3 days. Take exactly a suitable amount of the standard stock solution before use, add phosphate buffer solution (pH 6.0) to make solutions so that each mL contains 300 units and 150 units, and use these solutions as the high concentration standard solution and the low concentration standard solution, respectively.

(iv) Sample solutions—Use a light-resistant container. Weigh accurately an amount of Nystatin equivalent to about 60,000 units, dissolve in formamide to make a solution of 3000 units per mL, and use this solution as the sample stock solution. Take exactly a suitable amount of the sample stock solution, add phosphate buffer solution (pH 6.0) to make solutions so that each mL contains 300 units and 150 units, and use these solutions as the high concentration sample solution and the low concentration sample solution, respectively.

Containers and storage Containers—Tight containers.

Storage—Light-resistant, and in a cold place.

Ofloxacin

オフロキサシン

and enantiomer

$C_{18}H_{20}FN_3O_4$: 361.37
(3*RS*)-9-Fluoro-3-methyl-10-(4-methylpiperazin-1-yl)-7-oxo-2,3-dihydro-7*H*-pyrido[1,2,3-*de*][1,4]benzoxazine-6-carboxylic acid
[*82419-36-1*]

Ofloxacin, when dried, contains not less than 99.0% and not more than 101.0% of ofloxacin ($C_{18}H_{20}FN_3O_4$).

Description Ofloxacin occurs as pale yellowish white to light yellow-white, crystals or crystalline powder.

It is freely soluble in acetic acid (100), slightly soluble in water, and very slightly soluble in acetonitrile and in ethanol (99.5).

A soluton of Ofloxacin in sodium hydroxide TS (1 in 20) does not show optical rotation.

It is changed in color by light.

Melting point: about 265°C (with decomposition).

Identification **(1)** Determine the absorption spectrum of a solution of Ofloxacin in 0.1 mol/L hydrochloric acid TS (1 in 150,000) as directed under Ultraviolet-visible Spectrophotometry <*2.24*>, and compare the spectrum with the Reference Spectrum: both spectra exhibit similar intensities of absorption at the same wavelengths.

(2) Determine the infrared absorption spectrum of Ofloxacin as directed in the potassium bromide disk method under Infrared Spectrophotometry <*2.25*>, and compare the spectrum with the Reference Spectrum: both spectra exhibit similar intensities of absorption at the same wave numbers.

Purity **(1)** Heavy metals <*1.07*>—Proceed with 2.0 g of Ofloxacin according to Method 4, and perform the test. Prepare the control solution with 2.0 mL of Standard Lead Solution (not more than 10 ppm).

(2) Related substances—Conduct this procedure without exposure to light. Dissolve 10 mg of Ofloxacin in 50 mL of a mixture of water and acetonitrile (6:1), and use this solution as the sample solution. Pipet 1 mL of the sample solution, and add a mixture of water and acetonitrile (6:1) to make exactly 20 mL. Pipet 1 mL of this solution, add a mixture of water and acetonitrile (6:1) to make exactly 10 mL, and use this solution as the standard solution. Perform the test with exactly 10 μL each of the sample solution and standard solution as directed under Liquid Chromatography <*2.01*> according to the following conditions, and determine each peak area by the automatic integration method: the area of the peak other than ofloxacin obtained from the sample solution is not larger than 2/5 times the peak area of ofloxacin from the standard solution, and the total area of the peaks other than ofloxacin is not larger than the peak area from the standard solution.

Operating conditions—

Detector: An ultraviolet absorption photometer (wavelength: 294 nm).

Column: A stainless steel column 4.6 mm in inside diameter and 25 cm in length, packed with octadecylsilanized silica gel for liquid chromatography (5 μm in particle diameter).

Column temperature: A constant temperature of about 45°C.

Mobile phase: Dissolve 7.0 g of sodium perchlorate monohydrate and 4.0 g of ammonium acetate in 1300 mL of water, adjust the pH to 2.2 with phosphoric acid, and add 240 mL of acetonitrile.

Flow rate: Adjust so that the retention time of ofloxacin is about 20 minutes.

Time span of measurement: About 1.8 times as long as the retention time of ofloxacin, beginning after the solvent peak.

System suitability—

Test for required detectability: Pipet 1 mL of the standard solution, and add a mixture of water and acetonitrile (6:1) to make exactly 20 mL. Confirm that the peak area of ofloxacin obtained with 10 μL of this solution is equivalent to 4 to 6% of that with 10 μL of the standard solution.

System performance: To 0.5 mL of the sample solution add 1 mL of a solution of ofloxacin demethyl substance in a mixture of water and acetonitrile (6:1) (1 in 20,000) and a mixture of water and acetonitrile (6:1) to make 100 mL. When the procedure is run with 10 μL of this solution under the above operating conditions, ofloxacin demethyl substance and ofloxacin are eluted in this order with the resolution between these peaks being not less than 2.5.

System repeatability: When the test is repeated 6 times with 10 μL of the standard solution under the above operating conditions, the relative standard deviation of the peak area of ofloxacin is not more than 2.0%.

Loss on drying <*2.41*> Not more than 0.2% (1 g, 105°C, 4 hours).

Residue on ignition <*2.44*> Not more than 0.1% (1 g).

Assay Weigh accurately about 0.3 g of Ofloxacin, previously dried, dissolve in 100 mL of acetic acid (100), and titrate <*2.50*> with 0.1 mol/L perchloric acid VS (potentiometric titration). Perform a blank determination in the same manner, and make any necessary correction.

Each mL of 0.1 mol/L perchloric acid VS
= 36.14 mg of $C_{18}H_{20}FN_3O_4$

Containers and storage Containers—Tight containers.

Storage—Light-resistant.

Olmesartan Medoxomil

オルメサルタン　メドキソミル

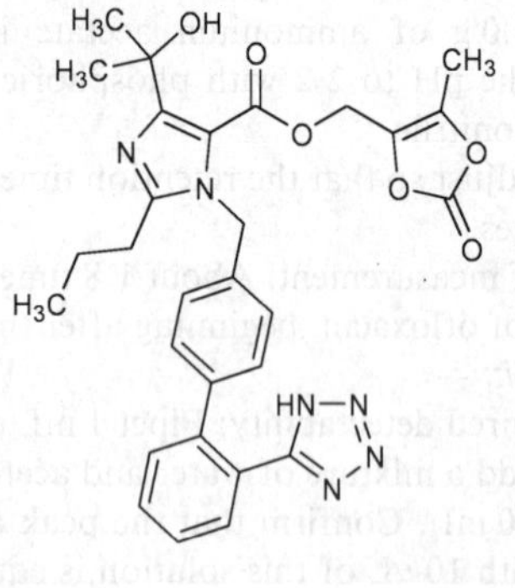

$C_{29}H_{30}N_6O_6$: 558.59

(5-Methyl-2-oxo-1,3-dioxol-4-yl)methyl 4-(2-hydroxypropan-2-yl)-2-propyl-1-{[2′-(1*H*-tetrazol-5-yl)biphenyl-4-yl]methyl}-1*H*-imidazole-5-carboxylate

[*144689-63-4*]

Olmesartan Medoxomil contains not less than 98.5% and not more than 101.5% of olmesartan medoxomil ($C_{29}H_{30}N_6O_6$), calculated on the anhydrous and residual solvent-free basis.

Description Olmesartan Medoxomil occurs as a white to pale yellow-white crystalline powder.

It is slightly soluble in acetonitrile and in ethanol (99.5), and practically insoluble in water.

Identification **(1)** Determine the absorption spectrum of a solution of Olmesartan Medoxomil in acetonitrile (1 in 100,000) as directed under Ultraviolet-visible Spectrophotometry ⟨*2.24*⟩, and compare the spectrum with the Reference Spectrum or the spectrum of a solution of Olmesartan Medoxomil RS prepared in the same manner as the sample solution: both spectra exhibit similar intensities of absorption at the same wavelengths.

(2) Determine the infrared absorption spectrum of Olmesartan Medoxomil as directed in the potassium bromide disk method under Infrared Spectrophotometry ⟨*2.25*⟩, and compare the spectrum with the Reference Spectrum or the spectrum of Olmesartan Medoxomil RS: both spectra exhibit similar intensities of absorption at the same wave numbers.

Purity **(1)** Heavy metals ⟨*1.07*⟩—Proceed with 2.0 g of Olmesartan Medoxomil according to Method 4, and perform the test. Prepare the control solution with 2.0 mL of Standard Lead Solution (not more than 10 ppm).

(2) Related substances—Dissolve 20 mg of Olmesartan Medoxomil in 20 mL of acetonitrile, and use this solution as the sample solution. Pipet 1 mL of the sample solution, add acetonitrile to make exactly 100 mL, and use this solution as the standard solution. Perform the test with exactly 10 μL each of the sample solution and standard solution as directed under Liquid Chromatography ⟨*2.01*⟩ according to the following conditions, and determine each peak area by the automatic integration method: the areas of the peaks, having the relative retention times of about 0.2 and about 1.6 to olmesartan medoxomil, obtained from the sample solution are not larger than 2/5 times and 3/10 times the peak area of olmesartan medoxomil from the standard solution, respectively, the area of the peaks other than olmesartan medoxomil and the peaks mentioned above from the sample solution is not larger than 1/10 times the peak area of olmesartan medoxomil from the standard solution, and the total area of these peaks is not larger than 3/10 times the peak area of olmesartan medoxomil from the standard solution. In addition, the total area of the peaks other than olmesartan medoxomil from the sample solution is not larger than 4/5 times the peak area of olmesartan medoxomil from the standard solution. For the areas of the peaks, having the relative retention times of about 0.7 and about 3.4 to olmesartan medoxomil, multiply their correction factors 0.65 and 1.39, respectively.

Operating conditions—

Detector: An ultraviolet absorption photometer (wavelength: 250 nm).

Column: A stainless steel column 4.6 mm in inside diameter and 10 cm in length, packed with octylsilanized silica gel for liquid chromatography (3.5 μm in particle diameter).

Column temperature: A constant temperature of about 40°C.

Mobile phase A: Dissolve 2.04 g of potassium dihydrogen phosphate in water to make 1000 mL, and adjust to pH 3.5 with a solution prepared by dissolving 1.73 g of phosphoric acid in water to make 1000 mL. To 400 mL of this solution add 100 mL of acetonitrile.

Mobile phase B: Dissolve 2.04 g of potassium dihydrogen phosphate in water to make 1000 mL, and adjust to pH 3.5 with a solution prepared by dissolving 1.73 g of phosphoric acid in water to make 1000 mL. To 100 mL of this solution add 400 mL of acetonitrile.

Flowing of mobile phase: Control the gradient by mixing the mobile phases A and B as directed in the following table.

Time after injection of sample (min)	Mobile phase A (vol%)	Mobile phase B (vol%)
0 – 10	75	25
10 – 35	75 → 0	25 → 100
35 – 45	0	100

Flow rate: 1.0 mL per minute.

Time span of measurement: For 45 minutes after injection, beginning after the solvent peak.

System suitability—

Test for required detectability: Pipet 1 mL of the standard solution, add acetonitrile to make exactly 20 mL. Confirm that the peak area of olmesartan medoxomil obtained with 10 μL of this solution is equivalent to 3.5 to 6.5% of that with 10 μL of the standard solution.

System performance: When the procedure is run with 10 μL of the standard solution under the above operating conditions, the number of theoretical plates and the symmetry factor of the peak of olmesartan medoxomil are not less than 5000 and not more than 1.5, respectively.

System repeatability: When the test is repeated 6 times with 10 μL of the standard solution under the above operating conditions, the relative standard deviation of the peak area of olmesartan medoxomil is not more than 2.0%.

Water ⟨*2.48*⟩ Not more than 0.5% (0.5 g, coulometric titration).

Residue on ignition ⟨*2.44*⟩ Not more than 0.1% (1 g).

Assay Weigh accurately about 50 mg each of Olmesartan Medoxomil and Olmesartan Medoxomil RS (separately determine the water ⟨*2.48*⟩ and the residual solvent in the same manners as Olmesartan Medoxomil), dissolve them separately in a mixture of acetonitrile and water (4:1) to make exactly 50 mL. Pipet 5 mL each of these solutions, add exactly

5 mL of the internal standard solution, add a mixture of water and acetonitrile (3:2) to make 100 mL, and use these solutions as the sample solution and the standard solution, respectively. Perform the test with 10 μL each of the sample solution and standard solution as directed under Liquid Chromatography <*2.01*> according to the following conditions, and calculate the ratios, Q_T and Q_S, of the peak area of olmesartan medoxomil to that of the internal standard.

Amount (mg) of olmesartan medoxomil ($C_{29}H_{30}N_6O_6$)
$= M_S \times Q_T/Q_S$

M_S: Amount (mg) of Olmesartan Medoxomil RS taken, calculated on the anhydrous and residual solvent-free basis

Internal standard solution—A solution of isobutyl parahydroxybenzoate in a mixture of water and acetonitrile (3:2) (1 in 2000).

Operating conditions—

Detector: An ultraviolet absorption photometer (wavelength: 250 nm).

Column: A stainless steel column 4.6 mm in inside diameter and 15 cm in length, packed with octadecylsilanized silica gel for liquid chromatography (5 μm in particle diameter).

Column temperature: A constant temperature of about 40°C.

Mobile phase: Dissolve 2.04 g of potassium dihydrogen phosphate in water to make 1000 mL, and adjust to pH 3.4 with a solution prepared by dissolving 1.73 g of phosphoric acid in water to make 1000 mL. To 330 mL of this solution add 170 mL of acetonitrile.

Flow rate: Adjust so that the retention time of olmesartan medoxomil is about 16 minutes.

System suitability—

System performance: When the procedure is run with 10 μL of the standard solution under the above operating conditions, olmesartan medoxomil and the internal standard are eluted in this order with the resolution between these peaks being not less than 4.

System repeatability: When the test is repeated 6 times with 10 μL of the standard solution under the above operating conditions, the relative standard deviation of the ratio of the peak area of olmesartan medoxomil to that of the internal standard is not more than 0.5%.

Containers and storage Containers—Well-closed containers.

Olmesartan Medoxomil Tablets

オルメサルタン　メドキソミル錠

Olmesartan Medoxomil Tablets contain not less than 95.0% and not more than 105.0% of the labeled amount of olmesartan medoxomil ($C_{29}H_{30}N_6O_6$: 558.59).

Method of preparation Prepare as directed under Tablets, with Olmesartan Medoxomil.

Identification To a quantity of powdered Olmesartan Medoxomil Tablets, equivalent to 20 mg of Olmesartan Medoxomil, add 60 mL of a mixture of acetonitrile and water (3:2), sonicate for 10 minutes, and add a mixture of acetonitrile and water (3:2) to make 100 mL. Centrifuge this solution, to 5 mL of the supernatant liquid add a mixture of acetonitrile and water (3:2) to make 100 mL, and determine the absorption spectrum of this solution as directed under Ultraviolet-visible Spectrophotometry <*2.24*>: it exhibits a maximum between 255 nm and 259 nm.

Purity Related substances—To a quantity of powdered Olmesartan Medoxomil Tablets, equivalent to 20 mg of Olmesartan Medoxomil, add 20 mL of a mixture of acetonitrile and water (9:1), sonicate for 15 minutes, centrifuge, and filter the supernatant liquid through a membrane filter with a pore size not exceeding 0.5 μm. Discard the first 5 mL of the filtrate, and use the subsequent filtrate as the sample solution. Pipet 1 mL of the sample solution, add a mixture of acetonitrile and water (9:1) to make exactly 100 mL, and use this solution as the standard solution. Perform the test with exactly 10 μL each of the sample solution and standard solution as directed under Liquid Chromatography <*2.01*> according to the following conditions. Determine each peak area by the automatic integration method: the areas of the peaks, having the relative retention time of about 0.2 and about 1.6 to olmesartan medoxomil, obtained from the sample solution are not larger than 3/5 times the peak area of olmesartan medoxomil from the standard solution, and the area of the peak other than olmesartan medoxomil and the peaks mentioned above from the sample solution is not larger than 1/5 times the peak area of olmesartan medoxomil from the standard solution. Furthermore, the total area of the peaks other than olmesartan medoxomil from the sample solution is not larger than 1.4 times the peak area of olmesartan medoxomil from the standard solution. For the areas of the peaks, having the relative retention time of about 0.7 and about 3.4 to olmesartan medoxomil, multiply their collection factors, 0.65 and 1.39, respectively.

Operating conditions—

Detector, column, column temperature, mobile phase, flowing of mobile phase, and flow rate: Proceed as directed in the operating conditions in the Purity (2) under Olmesartan Medoxomil.

Time span of measurement: For 45 minutes after injection, beginning after the solvent peak.

System suitability—

Test for required detectability: To exactly 1 mL of the standard solution add a mixture of acetonitrile and water (9:1) to make exactly 20 mL. Confirm that the peak area of olmesartan medoxomil obtained with 10 μL of this solution is equivalent to 3.5 to 6.5% of that with 10 μL of the standard solution.

System performance: When the procedure is run with 10 μL of the standard solution under the above operating conditions, the number of theoretical plates and the symmetry factor of the peak of olmesartan medoxomil are not less than 5500 and not more than 1.5, respectively.

System repeatability: When the test is repeated 6 times with 10 μL of the standard solution under the above operating conditions, the relative standard deviation of the peak area of olmesartan medoxomil is not more than 2.0%.

Uniformity of dosage units <*6.02*> Perform the test according to the following method: it meets the requirement of the Content uniformity test.

To 1 tablet of Olmesartan Medoxomil Tablets add $5V/7$ mL of a mixture of acetonitrile and water (3:2) and exactly $V/10$ mL of the internal standard solution. Sonicate for 10 minutes with occasional stirring, and add a mixture of acetonitrile and water (3:2) to make V mL so that each mL contains about 0.2 mg of olmesartan medoxomil ($C_{29}H_{30}N_6O_6$). Centrifuge this solution, to 5 mL of the supernatant liquid add a mixture of acetonitrile and water (3:2) to make 25 mL, and use this solution as the sample solution. Then, proceed as directed in the Assay.

Amount (mg) of olmesartan medoxomil ($C_{29}H_{30}N_6O_6$)
$= M_S \times Q_T/Q_S \times V/200$

M_S: Amount (mg) of Olmesartan Medoxomil RS taken, calculated on the anhydrous and residual solvent-free basis

Internal standard solution—A solution of isobutyl parahydroxybenzoate in a mixture of acetonitrile and water (3:2) (1 in 1000).

Dissolution <*6.10*> When the test is performed at 50 revolutions per minute according to the Paddle method, using 900 mL of 2nd fluid for dissolution test as the dissolution medium, the dissolution rates in 30 minutes of 5-mg, 10-mg and 20-mg tablets are not less than 80%, and that in 30 minutes of 40-mg tablet is not less than 75%.

Start the test with 1 tablet of Olmesartan Medoxomil Tablets, withdraw not less than 20 mL of the medium at the specified minute after starting the test, and filter through a membrane filter with a pore size not exceeding 0.45 μm. Discard not less than 10 mL of the first filtrate, pipet V mL of the subsequent filtrate, add the dissolution medium to make exactly V' mL so that each mL contains about 6 μg of olmesartan medoxomil ($C_{29}H_{30}N_6O_6$), and use this solution as the sample solution. Separately, weigh accurately about 40 mg of Olmesartan Medoxomil RS (separately, determine the water <*2.48*> and the residual solvent in the same manner as Olmesartan Medoxomil), dissolve in 15 mL of ethanol (99.5) by warming at 50 - 60°C, and after cooling add ethanol (99.5) to make exactly 20 mL. Pipet 5 mL of this solution, add ethanol (99.5) to make exactly 50 mL. Then, pipet 5 mL of this solution, add the dissolution medium to make exactly 200 mL, and use this solution as the standard solution. Determine the absorbances, A_T and A_S, at 257 nm of the sample solution and standard solution as directed under Ultraviolet-visible Spectrophotometry <*2.24*> using the dissolution medium as the control.

Dissolution rate (%) with respect to the labeled amount of olmesartan medoxomil ($C_{29}H_{30}N_6O_6$)
$= M_S \times A_T/A_S \times V'/V \times 1/C \times 45/4$

M_S: Amount (mg) of Olmesartan Medoxomil RS taken, calculated on the anhydrous and residual solvent-free basis

C: Labeled amount (mg) of olmesartan medoxomil ($C_{29}H_{30}N_6O_6$) in 1 tablet

Assay Weigh accurately the mass of not less than 20 Olmesartan Medoxomil Tablets, and powder. Weigh accurately a portion of the powder, equivalent to about 20 mg of olmesartan medoxomil ($C_{29}H_{30}N_6O_6$), add 70 mL of a mixture of acetonitrile and water (3:2) and exactly 10 mL of the internal standard solution. Sonicate for 15 minutes with occasional stirring, and add a mixture of acetonitrile and water (3:2) to make 100 mL. Centrifuge this solution, to 5 mL of the supernatant liquid add a mixture of acetonitrile and water (3:2) to make 25 mL, and use this solution as the sample solution. Separately, weigh accurately about 40 mg of Olmesartan Medoxomil RS (separately determine the water <*2.48*> and the residual solvent in the same manner as Olmesartan Medoxomil), dissolve in 60 mL of a mixture of acetonitrile and water (3:2), add exactly 20 mL of the internal standard solution, then add a mixture of acetonitrile and water (3:2) to make 100 mL. To 5 mL of this solution add a mixture of acetonitrile and water (3:2) to make 50 mL, and use this solution as the standard solution. Perform the test with 10 μL each of the sample solution and standard solution as directed under Liquid Chromatography <*2.01*> according to the following conditions, and calculate the ratios, Q_T and Q_S, of the peak area of olmesartan medoxomil to that of the internal standard.

Amount (mg) of olmesartan medoxomil ($C_{29}H_{30}N_6O_6$)
$= M_S \times Q_T/Q_S \times 1/2$

M_S: Amount (mg) of Olmesartan Medoxomil RS taken, calculated on the anhydrous and residual solvent-free basis

Internal standard solution—A solution of isobutyl parahydroxybenzoate in a mixture of acetonitrile and water (3:2) (1 in 1000).

Operating conditions—

Detector: An ultraviolet absorption photometer (wavelength: 250 nm).

Column: A stainless steel column 4.6 mm in inside diameter and 15 cm in length, packed with octadecylsilanized silica gel for liquid chromatography (5 μm in particle diameter).

Column temperature: A constant temperature of about 40°C.

Mobile phase: Dissolve 2.04 g of potassium dihydrogen phosphate in water to make 1000 mL, and adjust to pH 3.4 with a solution prepared by dissolving 1.73 g of phosphoric acid in water to make 1000 mL. To 330 mL of this solution add 170 mL of acetonitrile.

Flow rate: Adjust so that the retention time of olmesartan medoxomil is about 16 minutes.

System suitability—

System performance: When the procedure is run with 10 μL of the standard solution under the above operating conditions, olmesartan medoxomil and the internal standard are eluted in this order with the resolution between these peaks being not less than 4.

System repeatability: When the test is repeated 6 times with 10 μL of the standard solution under the above operating conditions, the relative standard deviations of the ratio of the peak area of olmesartan medoxomil to that of the internal standard is not more than 1.0%.

Containers and storage Containers—Tight containers.

Olopatadine Hydrochloride

オロパタジン塩酸塩

$C_{21}H_{23}NO_3.HCl$: 373.87

{11-[(1*Z*)-3-(Dimethylamino)propylidene]-6,11-dihydrodibenzo[*b*,*e*]oxepin-2-yl}acetic acid monohydrochloride

[*140462-76-6*]

Olopatadine Hydrochloride, when dried, contains not less than 99.0% and not more than 101.0% of olopatadine hydrochloride ($C_{21}H_{23}NO_3.HCl$).

Description Olopatadine Hydrochloride occurs as white,

crystals or crystalline powder.

It is very soluble in formic acid, sparingly soluble in water, and very slightly soluble in ethanol (99.5).

It dissolves in 0.01 mol/L hydrochloric acid TS.

The pH of a solution obtained by dissolving 1.0 g of Olopatadine Hydrochloride in 100 mL of water is 2.3 to 3.3.

Melting point: about 250°C (with decomposition).

Identification **(1)** Determine the absorption spectrum of a solution of Olopatadine Hydrochloride in 0.01 mol/L hydrochloric acid TS (1 in 40,000) as directed under Ultraviolet-visible Spectrophotometry <*2.24*>, and compare the spectrum with the Reference Spectrum: both spectra exhibit similar intensities of absorption at the same wavelengths.

(2) Determine the infrared absorption spectrum of Olopatadine Hydrochloride as directed in the potassium chloride disk method under Infrared Spectrophotometry <*2.25*>, and compare the spectrum with the Reference Spectrum: both spectra exhibit similar intensities of absorption at the same wave numbers.

(3) To 5 mL of a solution of Olopatadine Hydrochloride (1 in 100) add 1 mL of dilute nitric acid: this solution responds to Qualitative Tests <*1.09*> (2) for chloride.

Purity **(1)** Heavy metals <*1.07*>—Proceed with 2.0 g of Olopatadine Hydrochloride according to Method 2, and perform the test. Prepare the control solution with 2.0 mL of Standard Lead Solution (not more than 10 ppm).

(2) Related substances—Dissolve 50 mg of Olopatadine Hydrochloride in 100 mL of a mixture of 0.05 mol/L phosphate buffer solution (pH 3.5) and acetonitrile (3:2), and use this solution as the sample solution. Pipet 1 mL of the sample solution, add a mixture of 0.05 mol/L phosphate buffer solution (pH 3.5) and acetonitrile (3:2) to make exactly 100 mL, and use this solution as the standard solution. Perform the test with exactly 20 μL each of the sample solution and standard solution as directed under Liquid Chromatography <*2.01*> according to the following conditions, and determine each peak area by the automatic integration method: the area of the peak other than olopatadine obtained from the sample solution is not larger than 1/10 times the peak area of olopatadine from the standard solution.

Operating conditions—

Detector: An ultraviolet absorption photometer (wavelength: 299 nm).

Column: A stainless steel column 4.6 mm in inside diameter and 25 cm in length, packed with octylsilanized silica gel for liquid chromatography (5 μm in particle diameter).

Column temperature: A constant temperature of about 40°C.

Mobile phase: Dissolve 2.3 g of sodium lauryl sulfate in a mixture of 0.05 mol/L phosphate buffer solution (pH 3.5) and acetonitrile (11:9) to make 1000 mL.

Flow rate: Adjust so that the retention time of olopatadine is about 11 minutes.

Time span of measurement: About 2 times as long as the retention time of olopatadine, beginning after the solvent peak.

System suitability—

Test for required detectability: Pipet 1 mL of the standard solution, add a mixture of 0.05 mol/L phosphate buffer solution (pH 3.5) and acetonitrile (3:2) to make exactly 20 mL. Confirm that the peak area of olopatadine obtained with 20 μL of this solution is equivalent to 3.5 to 6.5% of that with 20 μL of the standard solution.

System performance: When the procedure is run with 20 μL of the standard solution under the above operating conditions, the number of theoretical plates and the symmetry factor of the peak of olopatadine are not less than 8000 and not more than 2.0, respectively.

System repeatability: When the test is repeated 6 times with 20 μL of the standard solution under the above operating conditions, the relative standard deviation of the peak area of olopatadine is not more than 2.0%.

Loss on drying <*2.41*> Not more than 0.3% (1 g, 105°C, 3 hours).

Residue on ignition <*2.44*> Not more than 0.1% (1 g).

Assay Weigh accurately about 0.5 g of Olopatadine Hydrochloride, previously dried, dissolve in 3 mL of formic acid, add 50 mL of a mixture of acetic anhydride and acetic acid (100) (7:3), and titrate <*2.50*> with 0.1 mol/L perchloric acid VS (potentiometric titration). Perform a blank determination in the same manner, and make any necessary correction.

Each mL of 0.1 mol/L perchloric acid VS
= 37.39 mg of $C_{21}H_{23}NO_3.HCl$

Containers and storage Containers—Well-closed containers.

Olopatadine Hydrochloride Tablets

オロパタジン塩酸塩錠

Olopatadine Hydrochloride Tablets contain not less than 95.0% and not more than 105.0% of the labeled amount of olopatadine hydrochloride ($C_{21}H_{23}NO_3$.HCl: 373.87).

Method of preparation Prepare as directed under Tablets, with Olopatadine Hydrochloride.

Identification Shake well a quantity of powdered Olopatadine Hydrochloride Tablets, equivalent to 5 mg of Olopatadine Hydrochloride, with 100 mL of 0.01 mol/L hydrochloric acid TS, and filter through a membrane filter with a pore size not exceeding 0.45 μm. Determine the absorption spectrum of the filtrate as directed under Ultraviolet-visible Spectrophotometry <*2.24*>: it exhibits a maximum between 295 nm and 299 nm.

Uniformity of dosage units <*6.02*> Perform the test according to the following method: it meets the requirement of the Content uniformity test.

To 1 tablet of Olopatadine Hydrochloride Tablets add $4V/5$ mL of a mixture of 0.05 mol/L phosphate buffer solution (pH 3.5) and acetonitrile (3:2). To this solution add exactly $V/10$ mL of the internal standard solution, shake well, and add a mixture of 0.05 mol/L phosphate buffer solution (pH 3.5) and acetonitrile (3:2) to make V mL so that each mL contains about 50 μg of olopatadine hydrochloride ($C_{21}H_{23}NO_3$.HCl). Filter this solution through a membrane filter with a pore size not exceeding 0.45 μm, and use this filtrate as the sample solution. Then, proceed as directed in the Assay.

Amount (mg) of olopatadine hydrochloride
($C_{21}H_{23}NO_3$.HCl)
$= M_S \times Q_T/Q_S \times V/1000$

M_S: Amount (mg) of olopatadine hydrochloride for assay taken

Internal standard solution—A solution of doxepin hydrochloride in a mixture of 0.05 mol/L phosphate buffer solu tion (pH 3.5) and acetonitrile (3:2) (7 in 20,000).

Dissolution <*6.10*> When the test is performed at 50 revolutions per minute according to the Paddle method using the sinker, using 900 mL of water as the dissolution medium, the dissolution rate in 15 minutes of Olopatadine Hydrochloride Tablets is not less than 85%.

Start the test with 1 tablet of Olopatadine Hydrochloride Tablets, withdraw not less than 10 mL of the medium at the specified minute after starting the test, and filter through a membrane filter with a pore size not exceeding 0.45 μm. Discard not less than 5 mL of the first filtrate, pipet V mL of the subsequent filtrate, add water to make exactly V' mL so that each mL contains about 2.8 μg of olopatadine hydrochloride ($C_{21}H_{23}NO_3.HCl$), and use this solution as the sample solution. Separately, weigh accurately about 28 mg of olopatadine hydrochloride for assay, previously dried at 105 °C for 3 hours, dissolve in water to make exactly 100 mL. Pipet 10 mL of this solution, add water to make exactly 100 mL. Then pipet 10 mL of this solution, add water to make exactly 100 mL, and use this solution as the standard solution. Perform the test with exactly 50 μL each of the sample solution and standard solution as directed under Liquid Chromatography <*2.01*> according to the following conditions, and determine the peak areas, A_T and A_S, of olopatadine in each solution.

Dissolution rate (%) with respect to the labeled amount of olopatadine hydrochloride ($C_{21}H_{23}NO_3.HCl$)
$= M_S \times A_T/A_S \times V'/V \times 1/C \times 9$

M_S: Amount (mg) of olopatadine hydrochloride for assay taken

C: Labeled amount (mg) of olopatadine hydrochloride ($C_{21}H_{23}NO_3.HCl$) in 1 tablet

Operating conditions—

Proceed as directed in the operating conditions in the Assay.

System suitability—

System performance: When the procedure is run with 50 μL of the standard solution under the above operating conditions, the number of theoretical plates and the symmetry factor of the peak of olopatadine are not less than 10,000 and not more than 2.0, respectively.

System repeatability: When the test is repeated 6 times with 50 μL of the standard solution under the above operating conditions, the relative standard deviation of the peak area of olopatadine is not more than 1.5%.

Assay Weigh accurately the mass of not less than 20 Olopatadine Hydrochloride Tablets, and powder. Weigh accurately a portion of the powder, equivalent to about 5 mg of olopatadine hydrochloride ($C_{21}H_{23}NO_3.HCl$), add 80 mL of a mixture of 0.05 mol/L phosphate buffer solution (pH 3.5) and acetonitrile (3:2), and add exactly 10 mL of the internal standard solution. Shake well for 10 minutes, add a mixture of 0.05 mol/L phosphate buffer solution (pH 3.5) and acetonitrile (3:2) to make 100 mL. Filter this solution through a membrane filter with a pore size not exceeding 0.45 μm, and use this filtrate as the sample solution. Separately, weigh accurately about 50 mg of olopatadine hydrochloride for assay, previously dried at 105°C for 3 hours, and dissolve in a mixture of 0.05 mol/L phosphate buffer solution (pH 3.5) and acetonitrile (3:2) to make exactly 100 mL. Pipet 10 mL of this solution, add exactly 10 mL of the internal standard solution, then add a mixture of 0.05 mol/L phosphate buffer solution (pH 3.5) and acetonitrile (3:2) to make 100 mL, and use this solution as the standard solution. Perform the test with 20 μL each of the sample solution and standard solution as directed under Liquid Chromatography <*2.01*> according to the following conditions, and calculate the ratios, Q_T and Q_S, of the peak area of olopatadine to that of the internal standard.

Amount (mg) of olopatadine hydrochloride ($C_{21}H_{23}NO_3.HCl$)
$= M_S \times Q_T/Q_S \times 1/10$

M_S: Amount (mg) of olopatadine hydrochloride for assay taken

Internal standard solution—A solution of doxepin hydrochloride in a mixture of 0.05 mol/L phosphate buffer solution (pH 3.5) and acetonitrile (3:2) (7 in 20,000).

Operating conditions—

Detector: An ultraviolet absorption photometer (wavelength: 299 nm).

Column: A stainless steel column 4.6 mm in inside diameter and 25 cm in length, packed with octylsilanized silica gel for liquid chromatography (5 μm in particle diameter).

Column temperature: A constant temperature of about 40°C.

Mobile phase: Dissolve 2.3 g of sodium lauryl sulfate in a mixture of 0.05 mol/L phosphate buffer solution (pH 3.5) and acetonitrile (11:9) to make 1000 mL.

Flow rate: Adjust so that the retention time of olopatadine is about 11 minutes.

System suitability—

System performance: When the procedure is run with 20 μL of the standard solution under the above operating conditions, olopatadine and the internal standard are eluted in this order with the resolution between these peaks being not less than 13.

System repeatability: When the test is repeated 6 times with 20 μL of the standard solution under the above operating conditions, the relative standard deviation of the peak area of olopatadine is not more than 1.0%.

Containers and storage Containers—Well-closed containers.

Omeprazole

オメプラゾール

$C_{17}H_{19}N_3O_3S$: 345.42

(*RS*)-5-Methoxy-2-{[(4-methoxy-3,5-dimethylpyridin-2-yl)methyl]sulfinyl}-1*H*-benzimidazole

[*73590-58-6*]

Omeprazole, when dried, contains not less than 99.0% and not more than 101.0% of omeprazole ($C_{17}H_{19}N_3O_3S$).

Description Omeprazole occurs as a white to yellowish white crystalline powder.

It is freely soluble in *N*,*N*-dimethylformamide, sparingly soluble in ethanol (99.5), and practically insoluble in water.

A solution of Omeprazole in *N*,*N*-dimethylformamide (1 in 25) shows no optical rotation.

It gradually turns yellowish white on exposure to light.

Melting point: about 150°C (with decomposition).

Identification (1) Add phosphate buffer solution (pH 7.4) to 1 mL of a solution of Omeprazole in ethanol (99.5) (1 in 1000) to make 50 mL. Determine the absorption spectrum of this solution as directed under Ultraviolet-visible Spectrophotometry <*2.24*>, and compare the spectrum with the Reference Spectrum: both spectra exhibit similar intensities of absorption at the same wavelengths.

(2) Determine the infrared absorption spectrum of Omeprazole as directed in the potassium bromide disk method under Infrared Spectrophotometry <*2.25*>, and compare the spectrum with the Reference Spectrum: both spectra exhibit similar intensities of absorption at the same wave numbers.

Purity (1) Clarity and color of solution—Dissolve 0.5 g of Omeprazole in 25 mL of *N,N*-dimethylformamide: the solution is clear and colorless or light yellow. Perform the test with this solution as directed under Ultraviolet-visible Spectrophotometry <*2.24*>: the absorbance at 420 nm is not more than 0.3.

(2) Heavy metals <*1.07*>—Proceed with 2.0 g of Omeprazole according to Method 2, and perform the test. Prepare the control solution with 2.0 mL of Standard Lead Solution (not more than 10 ppm).

(3) Related substances—Conduct the procedure soon after preparation of the sample solution. Dissolve 50 mg of Omeprazole in 50 mL of the mobile phase, and use this solution as the sample solution. Perform the test with 10 μL of the sample solution as directed under Liquid Chromatography <*2.01*> according to the following conditions. Determine each of the peak areas of the sample solution by the automatic integration method, and calculate the amounts of them by the area percentage method: the amount of the peaks other than omeprazole is not more than 0.1%, and the total amount of the peaks other than omeprazole is not more than 0.5%.

Operating conditions—

Detector: An ultraviolet absorption photometer (wavelength: 280 nm).

Column: A stainless steel column 4.6 mm in inside diameter and 15 cm in length, packed with octylsilanized silica gel for liquid chromatography (5 μm in particle diameter).

Column temperature: A constant temperature of about 25°C.

Mobile phase: Dissolve 2.83 g of disodium hydrogen phosphate dodecahydrate and 0.21 g of sodium dihydrogen phosphate dihydrate in water to make 1000 mL. If necessary, adjust the pH to 7.6 with diluted phosphoric acid (1 in 100). Add 11 volumes of acetonitrile to 29 volumes of this solution.

Flow rate: Adjust so that the retention time of omeprazole is about 8 minutes.

Time span of measurement: About 10 times as long as the retention time of omeprazole, beginning after the solvent peak.

System suitability—

Test for required detectability: Pipet 5 mL of the sample solution, and add the mobile phase to make exactly 100 mL. Pipet 5 mL of this solution, add the mobile phase to make exactly 50 mL, and use this solution as the solution for system suitability test. Pipet 5 mL of the solution for system suitability test, and add the mobile phase to make exactly 25 mL. Confirm that the peak area of omeprazole obtained with 10 μL of this solution is equivalent to 15 to 25% of that with 10 μL of the solution for system suitability test.

System performance: Dissolve 10 mg of Omeprazole and 25 mg of 1,2-dinitrobenzene in 5 mL of sodium borate solution (19 in 5000) and 95 mL of ethanol (99.5). When the procedure is run with 10 μL of this solution under the above conditions, omeprazole and 1,2-dinitrobenzene are eluted in this order with the resolution between these peaks being not less than 10.

System repeatability: When the test is repeated 6 times with 10 μL of the solution for system suitability test under the above operating conditions, the relative standard deviation of the peak area of omeprazole is not more than 2.0%.

Loss on drying <*2.41*> Not more than 0.2% (1 g, in vacuum, phosphorus (V) oxide, 50°C, 2 hours).

Residue on ignition <*2.44*> Not more than 0.1% (1 g).

Assay Weigh accurately about 0.4 g of Omeprazole, previously dried, dissolve in 70 mL of *N,N*-dimethylformamide, and titrate <*2.50*> with 0.1 mol/L tetramethylammonium hydroxide VS (potentiometric titration). Separately, perform a blank determination in the same manner on a solution consisting of 70 mL of *N,N*-dimethylformamide and 12 mL of water, and make any necessary correction.

Each mL of 0.1 mol/L tetramethylammonium hydroxide VS
= 34.54 mg of $C_{17}H_{19}N_3O_3S$

Containers and storage Containers—Tight containers.

Storage—Light-resistant, in a cold place.

Omeprazole Delayed-release Tablets

オメプラゾール腸溶錠

Omeprazole Delayed-release Tablets contain not less than 95.0% and not more than 105.0% of the labeled amount of omeprazole ($C_{17}H_{19}N_3O_3S$: 345.42).

Method of preparation Prepare as directed under Tablets, with Omeprazole.

Identification Powder Omeprazole Delayed-release Tablets. To a portion of the powder, equivalent to 10 mg of Omeprazole, add 10 mL of ethanol (95), shake for 10 minutes, and centrifuge. To 1 mL of the supernatant liquid add phosphate buffer solution (pH 7.4) to make 50 mL. Determine the absorption spectrum of this solution as directed under Ultraviolet-visible Spectrophotometry <*2.24*>: it exhibits maxima between 273 nm and 277 nm, and between 299 nm and 303 nm.

Uniformity of dosage units <*6.02*> Perform the test according to the following method: it meets the requirement of the Content uniformity test.

To 1 tablet of Omeprazole Delayed-release Tablets add V/20 mL of a solution of sodium tetraborate decahydrate (19 in 5000), and shake thoroughly to disintegrate the tablet. Then, proceed as directed in the Assay.

$$\text{Amount (mg) of omeprazole } (C_{17}H_{19}N_3O_3S) = M_S \times Q_T/Q_S \times V/50$$

M_S: Amount (mg) of omeprazole for assay taken

Internal standard solution—A solution of 1,2-dinitrobenzene in ethanol (95) (1 in 400).

Dissolution <*6.10*> When the tests are performed at 50 revolutions per minute according to the Paddle method, using 900 mL each of 1st fluid for dissolution test and 2nd fluid for dissolution test as the dissolution medium, the dissolution rates of 10-mg tablet and 20-mg tablet in 120 minutes of the test using the 1st fluid for dissolution test are not more than 5%, respectively, and those of 10-mg tablet in 20 minutes and 20-mg tablet in 15 minutes of the test using the 2nd fluid for dissolution test are not less than 85%, respectively.

Start the test with 1 tablet of Omeprazole Delayed-release Tablets, withdraw not less than 20 mL of the medium at the specified minute after starting the test, and filter through a membrane filter with a pore size not exceeding 0.45 μm. Discard not less than 10 mL of the first filtrate, pipet V mL of the subsequent filtrate, add the dissolution medium to make exactly V' mL so that each mL contains about 11 μg of omeprazole ($C_{17}H_{19}N_3O_3S$), and use this solution as the sample solution. Separately, weigh accurately about 22 mg of omeprazole for assay, previously dried in vacuum at 50°C using phosphorus (V) oxide as desiccant for 2 hours, and dissolve in ethanol (95) to make exactly 100 mL. Pipet 5 mL of this solution, add the dissolution medium to make exactly 100 mL, and use this solution as the standard solution. Determine the absorbances, A_T and A_S, of the sample solution and standard solution as directed under Ultraviolet-visible Spectrophotometry <2.24> at 323 nm when the test is performed using the 1st fluid as the dissolution medium and at 293 nm when the test is performed using the 2nd fluid as the dissolution medium, using the dissolution medium as the blank.

Dissolution rate (%) with respect to the labeled amount of omeprazole ($C_{17}H_{19}N_3O_3S$)
$= M_S \times A_T/A_S \times V'/V \times 1/C \times 45$

M_S: Amount (mg) of omeprazole for assay taken
C: Labeled amount (mg) of omeprazole ($C_{17}H_{19}N_3O_3S$) in 1 tablet

Assay To 20 Omeprazole Delayed-release Tablets add $V/20$ mL of a solution of sodium tetraborate decahydrate (19 in 5000), shake to disintegrate. To this solution add $3V/5$ mL of ethanol (95), shake for 15 minutes, then add ethanol (95) to make exactly V mL so that each mL contains about 0.4 mg of omeprazole ($C_{17}H_{19}N_3O_3S$), and centrifuge. Pipet 10 mL of the supernatant liquid, add exactly 4 mL of the internal standard solution, add a mixture of ethanol (95) and a solution of sodium tetraborate decahydrate (19 in 5000) (19:1) to make 20 mL, and use this solution as the sample solution. Separately, weigh accurately about 20 mg of omeprazole for assay, previously dried in vacuum at 50°C with phosphorus (V) oxide as the desiccant for 2 hours, dissolve in a mixture of ethanol (95) and a solution of sodium tetraborate decahydrate (19 in 5000) (19:1), add exactly 20 mL of the internal standard solution, add a mixture of ethanol (95) and a solution of sodium tetraborate decahydrate (19 in 5000) (19:1) to make 100 mL, and use this solution as the standard solution. Perform the test with 5 μL each of the sample solution and standard solution as directed under Liquid Chromatography <2.01> according to the following conditions, and calculate the ratios, Q_T and Q_S, of the peak area of omeprazole to that of the internal standard.

Amount (mg) of omeprazole ($C_{17}H_{19}N_3O_3S$) in tablet
$= M_S \times Q_T/Q_S \times V/1000$

M_S: Amount (mg) of omeprazole for assay taken

Internal standard solution—A solution of 1,2-dinitrobenzene in ethanol (95) (1 in 400).
Operating conditions—

Detector: An ultraviolet absorption photometer (wavelength: 280 nm).

Column: A stainless steel column 4.6 mm in inside diameter and 15 cm in length, packed with octylsilanized silica gel for liquid chromatography (5 μm in particle diameter).

Column temperature: A constant temperature of about 25°C.

Mobile phase: Dissolve 2.83 g of disodium hydrogen phosphate dodecahydrate and 0.21 g of sodium dihydrogen phosphate dihydrate in water to make 1000 mL, and adjust to pH 7.6 with diluted phosphoric acid (1 in 100). To 290 mL of this solution add 110 mL of acetonitrile.

Flow rate: Adjust so that the retention time of omeprazole is about 8 minutes.
System suitability—

System performance: When the procedure is run with 5 μL of the standard solution under the above operating conditions, omeprazole and the internal standard are eluted in this order with the resolution between these peaks being not less than 10.

System repeatability: When the test is repeated 6 times with 5 μL of the standard solution under the above operating conditions, the relative standard deviation of the ratio of the peak area of omeprazole to that of the internal standard is not more than 1.0%.

Containers and storage Containers—Tight containers.

Opium Alkaloids Hydrochlorides

アヘンアルカロイド塩酸塩

Opium Alkaloids Hydrochlorides consist of the hydrochlorides of some of the main alkaloids obtained from opium.

It contains not less than 47.0% and not more than 52.0% of morphine ($C_{17}H_{19}NO_3$: 285.34), and not less than 35.0% and not more than 41.0% of other opium alkaloids.

Description Opium Alkaloids Hydrochlorides occur as a white to light brown powder.

It is soluble in water, and slightly soluble in ethanol (99.5).

It is colored by light.

Identification **(1)** Dissolve 0.1 g of Opium Alkaloids Hydrochlorides in 10 mL of diluted ethanol (1 in 2), and use this solution as the sample solution. Separately, dissolve 60 mg of Morphine Hydrochloride Hydrate, 40 mg of Noscapine Hydrochloride Hydrate, 10 mg of Codein Phosphate Hydrate and 10 mg of Papaverine Hydrochloride in 10 mL each of diluted ethanol (1 in 2), and use these solutions as the standard solutions (1), (2), (3) and (4), respectively. Perform the test with these solutions as directed under Thin-layer Chromatography <2.03>. Spot 20 μL each of the sample solution and standard solutions on a plate of silica gel with fluorescent indicator for thin-layer chromatography. Develop the plate with a mixture of acetone, toluene, ethanol (99.5) and ammonia solution (28) (20:20:3:1) to a distance of about 10 cm, and air-dry the plate. Examine under ultraviolet light (main wavelength: 254 nm): each spot obtained from the sample solution is the same in color tone and Rf value with the corresponding spot from the standard solutions (1), (2), (3) and (4) (morphine, noscapine, codeine and papaverine).

(2) A solution of Opium Alkaloids Hydrochlorides (1 in 50) responds to Qualitative Tests <1.09> (2) for chloride.

pH <2.54> Dissolve 1.0 g of Opium Alkaloids Hydrochlorides in 50 mL of water: the pH of the solution is between

3.0 and 4.0.

Purity (1) Clarity and color of solution—Dissolve 0.5 g of Opium Alkaloids Hydrochlorides in 10 mL of water: the solution is clear, and its absorbance <*2.24*> at 420 nm is not more than 0.20.

(2) Meconic acid—Dissolve 0.1 g of Opium Alkaloids Hydrochlorides in 2 mL of water, and pour into a polyethylene column 1 cm in inside diameter, packed with about 0.36 g of aminopropylsilanized silica gel for pretreatment (55 - 105 μm in particle diameter) and previously washed through with 5 mL of water. Then, wash the column with 5 mL of water, 5 mL of methanol and 10 mL of 0.1 mol/L hydrochloric acid in this order, then elute with 2 mL of 1 mol/L hydrochloric acid, and use the eluate as the test solution. To the test solution add 2 mL of dilute sodium hydroxide TS and 1 drop of iron (III) chloride TS: no red color develops.

Loss on drying <*2.41*> Not more than 6.0% (0.5 g, 120°C, 8 hours).

Residue on ignition <*2.44*> Not more than 0.5% (0.5 g).

Assay Weigh accurately about 0.1 g of Opium Alkaloids Hydrochlorides, and dissolve in water to make exactly 50 mL, and use this solution as the sample solution. Separately, weigh accurately about 60 mg of morphine hydrochloride hydrate for assay, dissolve in water to make exactly 50 mL, and use this solution as the standard solution. Perform the test with exactly 20 μL each of the sample solution and standard solution as directed under Liquid Chromatography <*2.01*> according to the following conditions, and determine the peak areas of morphine, codeine, papaverine, thebaine, narceine and noscapine, A_{T1}, A_{T2}, A_{T3}, A_{T4}, A_{T5} and A_{T6}, from the sample solution, and the peak area of morphine, A_S, from the standard solution.

$$\text{Amount (mg) of morphine } (C_{17}H_{19}NO_3) = M_S \times A_{T1}/A_S \times 0.887$$

$$\text{Amount (mg) of other opium alkaloids} = M_S \times \{(A_{T2} + 0.29A_{T3} + 0.20A_{T4} + 0.19A_{T5} + A_{T6})/A_S\} \times 0.887$$

M_S: Amount (mg) of morphine hydrochloride hydrate for assay taken, calculated on the anhydrous basis

The relative retention time of codine, papaverine, thebaine, narceine and noscapine to morphine obtained under the following operating conditions are as follows.

Component	Relative retention time
codeine	1.1
papaverine	1.9
thebaine	2.5
narceine	2.8
noscapine	3.6

Operating conditions—

Detector: An ultraviolet absorption photometer (wavelength: 285 nm).

Column: A stainless steel column 4.6 mm in inside diameter and 15 cm in length, packed with octadecylsilanized silica gel for liquid chromatography (5 μm in particle diameter).

Column temperature: A constant temperature of about 40°C.

Mobile phase: Dissolve 1.0 g of sodium lauryl sulfate in 500 mL of diluted phosphoric acid (1 in 1000), and adjust the pH to 3.0 with sodium hydroxide TS. To 240 mL of this solution add 70 mL of tetrahydrofuran, and mix.

Flow rate: Adjust so that the retention time of morphine is about 10 minutes.

System suitability—

System performance: Dissolve 60 mg of Morphine Hydrochloride Hydrate, 10 mg of Codeine Phosphate Hydrate, 10 mg of Papaverine Hydrochloride and 40 mg of Noscapine Hydrochloride Hydrate in water to make 50 mL. When the procedure is run with 20 μL of this solution under the above operating conditions, morphine, codeine, papaverine and noscapine are eluted in this order with the complete separation between these peaks and with the resolution between the peaks of morphine and codeine being not less than 1.5.

System repeatability: When the test is repeated 6 times with 20 μL of the standard solution under the above operating conditions, the relative standard deviation of the peak area of morphine is not more than 1.0%.

Containers and storage Containers—Tight containers.

Storage—Light-resistant.

Opium Alkaloids Hydrochlorides Injection

アヘンアルカロイド塩酸塩注射液

Opium Alkaloids Hydrochlorides Injection is an aqueous injection.

It contains not less than 0.90 w/v% and not more than 1.10 w/v% of morphine ($C_{17}H_{19}NO_3$: 285.34).

Method of preparation

Opium Alkaloids Hydrochlorides	20 g
Water for Injection or Sterile Water for Injection in Containers	a sufficient quantity
To make	1000 mL

Prepare as directed under Injections, with the above ingredients.

Description Opium Alkaloids Hydrochlorides Injection is a clear, colorless or light brown liquid.

It is affected by light.

pH: 2.5 - 3.5

Identification To 1 mL of Opium Alkaloids Hydrochlorides Injection add 1 mL of ethanol (99.5), mix, and use this solution as the sample solution, and proceed as directed in the Identification (1) under Opium Alkaloids Hydrochlorides.

Extractable volume <*6.05*> It meets the requirement.

Assay Pipet 2 mL of Opium Alkaloids Hydrochlorides Injection, add exactly 10 mL of the internal standard solution and water to make 50 mL, and use this solution as the sample solution. Separately, weigh accurately about 25 mg of morphine hydrochloride hydrate for assay, and dissolve in exactly 10 mL of the internal standard solution, add water to make 50 mL, and use this solution as the standard solution. Perform the test with 20 μL each of the sample solution and standard solution as directed under Liquid Chromatography <*2.01*> according to the following conditions, and calculate the ratios, Q_T and Q_S, of the peak area of morphine to that of the internal standard.

$$\text{Amount (mg) of morphine } (C_{17}H_{19}NO_3) = M_S \times Q_T/Q_S \times 0.887$$

M_S: Amount (mg) of morphine hydrochloride hydrate for assay taken, calculated on the anhydrous basis

Internal standard solution—A solution of etilefrine hydrochloride (1 in 500).

Operating conditions—

Detector: An ultraviolet absorption photometer (wavelength: 285 nm).

Column: A stainless steel column 4.6 mm in inside diameter and 15 cm in length, packed with octadecylsilanized silica gel for liquid chromatography (5 μm in particle diameter).

Column temperature: A constant temperature of about 40°C.

Mobile phase: Dissolve 1.0 g of sodium lauryl sulfate in 500 mL of diluted phosphoric acid (1 in 1000), and adjust the pH to 3.0 with sodium hydroxide TS. To 240 mL of this solution add 70 mL of tetrahydrofuran, and mix.

Flow rate: Adjust so that the retention time of morphine is about 10 minutes.

System suitability—

System performance: When the procedure is run with 20 μL of the standard solution under the above operating conditions, morphine and the internal standard are eluted in this order with the resolution between these peaks being not less than 3.

System repeatability: When the test is repeated 6 times with 20 μL of the standard solution under the above operating conditions, the relative standard deviation of the ratios of the peak area of morphine to that of the internal standard is not more than 1.0%.

Containers and storage Containers—Hermetic containers, and colored containers may be used.

Storage—Light-resistant.

Opium Alkaloids and Atropine Injection

アヘンアルカロイド・アトロピン注射液

Opium Alkaloids and Atropine Injection is an aqueous injection.

It contains not less than 0.90 w/v% and not more than 1.10 w/v% of morphine ($C_{17}H_{19}NO_3$: 285.34), and not less than 0.027 w/v% and not more than 0.033 w/v% of atropine sulfate hydrate [$(C_{17}H_{23}NO_3)_2.H_2SO_4.H_2O$: 694.84].

Method of preparation

Opium Alkaloids Hydrochlorides	20 g
Atropine Sulfate Hydrate	0.3 g
Water for Injection or Sterile Water for Injection in Containers	a sufficient quantity
	To make 1000 mL

Prepare as directed under Injections, with the above ingredients.

Description Opium Alkaloids and Atropine Injection is a colorless or light brown, clear liquid.

It is affected by light.

pH: 2.5 – 3.5

Identification **(1)** To 1 mL of Opium Alkaloids and Atropine Injection add 1 mL of ethanol (99.5), mix, and use this solution as the sample solution. Proceed with the sample solution as directed in the Identification (1) under Opium Alkaloids Hydrochlorides.

(2) To 2 mL of Opium Alkaloids and Atropine Injection add 2 mL of ammonia TS, extract with 10 mL of diethyl ether, and filter the diethyl ether layer. Evaporate the filtrate on a water bath to dryness, add 1 mL of ethanol (99.5) to the residue, and heat to dissolve. Allow to stand this solution in an ice water for 30 minutes with occasional shaking. After crystals are formed, use the supernatant liquid as the sample solution. Separately, dissolve 0.03 g of Atropine Sulfate RS in 100 mL of water, proceed with 2 mL of this solution in the same manner as for the sample solution, and use a solution so obtained as the standard solution. Perform the test with these solutions as directed under Thin-layer Chromatography <2.03>. Spot 10 μL each of the sample solution and standard solution on a plate of silica gel for thin-layer chromatography. Develop the plate with a mixture of methanol and ammonia water (28) (200:3) to a distance of about 10 cm, and air-dry the plate. Spray evenly Dragendorff's TS for spraying on the plate: a spot of about 0.2 *R*f value among the several spots obtained from the sample solution and an orange colored spot from the standard solution show the same color tone, and have the same *R*f value (atropine).

Extractable volume <6.05> It meets the requirements.

Assay **(1)** Morphine—Pipet 2 mL of Opium Alkaloids and Atropine Injection, add exactly 10 mL of the internal standard solution, then add water to make 50 mL, and use this solution as the sample solution. Separately, weigh accurately about 25 mg of morphine hydrochloride hydrate for assay, dissolve in exactly 10 mL of the internal standard solution, then add water to make 50 mL, and use this solution as the standard solution. Perform the test with 20 μL each of the sample solution and standard solution as directed under Liquid Chromatography <2.01> according to the following conditions, and calculate the ratios, Q_T and Q_S, of the peak area of morphine to that of the internal standard.

$$\text{Amount (mg) of morphine } (C_{17}H_{19}NO_3) = M_S \times Q_T/Q_S \times 0.887$$

M_S: Amount (mg) of morphine hydrochloride hydrate for assay taken, calculated on the anhydrous basis

Internal standard solution—A solution of etilefrine hydrochloride (1 in 500).

Operating conditions—

Detector: An ultraviolet absorption photometer (wavelength: 285 nm).

Column: A stainless steel column 4.6 mm in inside diameter and 15 cm in length, packed with octadecylsilanized silica gel for liquid chromatography (5 μm in particle diameter).

Column temperature: A constant temperature of about 40°C.

Mobile phase: Dissolve 1.0 g of sodium lauryl sulfate in 500 mL of diluted phosphoric acid (1 in 1000), and adjust the pH to 3.0 with sodium hydroxide TS. To 240 mL of this solution add 70 mL of tetrahydrofuran, and mix.

Flow rate: Adjust so that the retention time of morphine is about 10 minutes.

System suitability—

System performance: When the procedure is run with 20 μL of the standard solution under the above operating conditions, morphine and the internal standard are eluted in this order with the resolution between these peaks being not less than 3.

System repeatability: When the test is repeated 6 times with 20 μL of the standard solution under the above operating conditions, the relative standard deviation of the ratios of the peak area of morphine to that of the internal standard is not more than 2.0%.

(2) Atropine sulfate hydrate—Pipet 2 mL of Opium Alkaloids and Atropine Injection, add exactly 2 mL of the internal standard solution, and add 10 mL of diluted dilute hydrochloric acid (1 in 10). Shake this solution with two 10-mL portions of dichloromethane. Remove the dichloromethane layer, to the water layer add 2 mL of ammonia TS, immediately add 20 mL of dichloromethane, shake vigorously, filter the dichloromethane extract through filter paper on which 5 g of anhydrous sodium sulfate is placed, and evaporate the filtrate to dryness under reduced pressure. To the residue add 0.5 mL of 1,2-dichloroethane and 0.5 mL of bis-trimethyl silyl acetamide, stopper tightly, warm in a water bath at 60°C for 15 minutes, and use this solution as the sample solution. Separately, weigh accurately about 30 mg of Atropine Sulfate RS (determine separately the loss on drying <*2.41*> under the same conditions as Atropine Sulfate Hydrate), and dissolve in water to make exactly 100 mL. Pipet 2 mL of this solution, and add exactly 2 mL of the internal standard solution. Proceed with this solution in the same manner as directed for the sample solution, and use this solution as the standard solution. Perform the test with 2 μL each of the sample solution and standard solution as directed under Gas Chromatography <*2.02*> according to the following conditions, and calculate the ratios, Q_T and Q_S, of the peak area of atropine to that of the internal standard.

Amount (mg) of atropine sulfate hydrate
$[(C_{17}H_{23}NO_3)_2.H_2SO_4.H_2O]$
$= M_S \times Q_T/Q_S \times 1/50 \times 1.027$

M_S: Amount (mg) of Atropine Sulfate RS taken, calculated on the dried basis

Internal standard solution—A solution of homatropine hydrobromide (1 in 4000).

Operating conditions—

Detector: A hydrogen flame-ionization detector.

Column: A glass column 3 mm in inside diameter and 1.5 m in length, packed with 180 to 250 μm siliceous earth for gas chromatography coated in 1 to 3% with 50% phenyl-methyl silicone polymer for gas chromatography.

Column temperature: A constant temperature of about 210°C.

Carrier gas: Nitrogen or helium.

Flow rate: Adjust so that the retention time of atropine is about 5 minutes.

System suitability—

System performance: When the procedure is run with 2 μL of the standard solution under the above operating conditions, the internal standard and atropine are eluted in this order with the resolution between these peaks being not less than 3.

System repeatability: When the test is repeated 5 times with 2 μL of the standard solution under the above operating conditions, the relative standard deviation of the ratios of the peak area of atropine to that of the internal standard is not more than 2.0%.

Containers and storage Containers—Hermetic containers, and colored containers may be used.

Storage—Light-resistant.

Opium Alkaloids and Scopolamine Injection

アヘンアルカロイド·スコポラミン注射液

Opium Alkaloids and Scopolamine Injection is an aqueous injection.

It contains not less than 1.80 w/v% and not more than 2.20 w/v% of morphine ($C_{17}H_{19}NO_3$: 285.34) and not less than 0.054 w/v% and not more than 0.066 w/v% of scopolamine hydrobromide hydrate ($C_{17}H_{21}NO_4.HBr.3H_2O$: 438.31).

Method of preparation

Opium Alkaloids Hydrochlorides	40 g
Scopolamine Hydrobromide Hydrate	0.6 g
Water for Injection or Sterile Water for Injection in Containers	a sufficient quantity
To make	1000 mL

Prepare as directed under Injections, with the above ingredients.

Description Opium Alkaloids and Scopolamine Injection is a clear, colorless to light brown liquid.

It is affected by light.

pH: 2.5 – 3.5

Identification **(1)** To 1 mL of Opium Alkaloids and Scopolamine Injection add 1 mL of water and 2 mL of ethanol (99.5), mix, and use this solution as the sample solution. Proceed with the sample solution as directed in the Identification (1) under Opium Alkaloids Hydrochlorides.

(2) To 1 mL of Opium Alkaloids and Scopolamine Injection add 1 mL of water and 2 mL of ammonia TS, extract with 10 mL of diethyl ether, and filter the diethyl ether layer. Evaporate the filtrate on a water bath to dryness, add 1 mL of ethanol (99.5) to the residue, and heat to dissolve. Allow to stand this solution in an ice water for 30 minutes with occasional shaking. After crystals are formed, use the supernatant liquid as the sample solution. Separately, dissolve 0.03 g of Scopolamine Hydrobromide RS in 100 mL of water. To 2 mL of this solution add 2 mL of ammonia TS, proceed with this solution in the same manner as for the sample solution, and use a solution so obtained as the standard solution. Perform the test with these solutions as directed under Thin-layer Chromatography <*2.03*>. Spot 10 μL each of the sample solution and standard solution on a plate of silica gel for thin-layer chromatography. Develop the plate with a mixture of methanol and ammonia water (28) (200:3) to a distance of about 10 cm, and air-dry the plate. Spray evenly Dragendorff's TS for spraying on the plate: a spot with an *R*f value of about 0.7 among the several spots obtained from the sample solution and an orange colored spot from the standard solution show the same color tone, and have the same *R*f value (scopolamine).

Extractable volume <*6.05*> It meets the requirements.

Assay **(1)** Morphine—Pipet 1 mL of Opium Alkaloids and Scopolamine Injection, add 10 mL of the internal standard solution and water to make 50 mL, and use this solution as the sample solution. Separately, weigh accurately about 25 mg of morphine hydrochloride hydrate for assay, dissolve in exactly 10 mL of the internal standard solution, add water to make 50 mL, and use this solution as the standard solution. Perform the test with 20 μL each of the sample solution and standard solution as directed under Liquid Chromatography <*2.01*> according to the following conditions, and calculate the ratios, Q_T and Q_S, of the peak area of morphine to that of the internal standard.

$$\text{Amount (mg) of morphine } (C_{17}H_{19}NO_3) = M_S \times Q_T/Q_S \times 0.887$$

M_S: Amount (mg) of morphine hydrochloride hydrate for assay taken, calculated on the anhydrous basis

Internal standard solution—A solution of etilefrin hydrochloride (1 in 500).

Operating conditions—

Detector: An ultraviolet absorption photometer (wavelength: 285 nm).

Column: A stainless steel column 4.6 mm in inside diameter and 15 cm in length, packed with octadecylsilanized silica gel for liquid chromatography (5 μm in particle diameter).

Column temperature: A constant temperature of about 40°C.

Mobile phase: Dissolve 1.0 g of sodium lauryl sulfate in 500 mL of diluted phosphoric acid (1 in 1000), and adjust the pH to 3.0 with sodium hydroxide TS. To 240 mL of this solution add 70 mL of tetrahydrofuran, and mix.

Flow rate: Adjust so that the retention time of morphine is about 10 minutes.

System suitability—

System performance: When the procedure is run with 20 μL of the standard solution under the above operating conditions, morphine and the internal standard are eluted in this order with the resolution between these peaks being not less than 3.

System repeatability: When the test is repeated 6 times with 20 μL of the standard solution under the above operating conditions, the relative standard deviation of the ratios of the peak area of morphine to that of the internal standard is not more than 2.0%.

(2) Scopolamine hydrobromide hydrate—Pipet 2 mL of Opium Alkaloids and Scopolamine Injection, and add exactly 2 mL of the internal standard solution. To this solution add 10 mL of diluted dilute hydrochloric acid (1 in 10), and shake with two 10-mL portions of dichloromethane. Remove the dichloromethane layer, to the water layer add 2 mL of ammonia TS, add immediately 20 mL of dichloromethane, shake vigorously, filter the dichloromethane extract through a filter paper on which 5 g of anhydrous sodium sulfate is placed, and evaporate the filtrate to dryness under reduced pressure. To the residue add 0.5 mL of 1,2-dichloroethane and 0.5 mL of bis-trimethyl silyl acetamide, stopper tightly, warm in a water bath at 60°C for 15 minutes, and use this solution as the sample solution. Separately, weigh accurately about 60 mg of Scoporamine Hydrobromide RS (determine separately the loss on drying <*2.41*> under the same conditions as Scopolamine Hydrobromide Hydrate), and dissolve in water to make exactly 100 mL. Pipet 2 mL of this solution, add exactly 2 mL of the internal standard solution. Proceed with this solution in the same manner as for the sample solution, and use thus obtained solution as the standard solution. Perform the test with 2 μL each of the sample solution and standard solution as directed under Gas Chromatography <*2.02*> according to the following conditions, and calculate the ratios, Q_T and Q_S, of the peak area of scopolamine to that of the internal standard.

$$\text{Amount (mg) of scopolamine hydrobromide hydrate } (C_{17}H_{21}NO_4.HBr.3H_2O) = M_S \times Q_T/Q_S \times 1/50 \times 1.141$$

M_S: Amount (mg) of Scopolamine Hydrobromide RS taken, calculated on the dried basis

Internal standard solution—A solution of homatropine hydrobromide (1 in 4000).

Operating conditions—

Detector: A hydrogen flame-ionization detector.

Column: A glass column 3 mm in inside diameter and 1.5 m in length, packed with 180 to 250 μm siliceous earth for gas chromatography coated in 1 to 3% with 50% phenyl-methyl silicone polymer for gas chromatography.

Column temperature: A constant temperature of about 210°C.

Carrier gas: Nitrogen or helium.

Flow rate: Adjust so that the retention time of scopolamine is about 8 minutes.

System suitability—

System performance: When the procedure is run with 2 μL of the standard solution under the above operating conditions, the internal standard and scopolamine are eluted in this order with the resolution between these peaks being not less than 6.

System repeatability: When the test is repeated 5 times with 2 μL of the standard solution under the above operating conditions, the relative standard deviation of the ratios of the peak area of scopolamine to that of the internal standard is not more than 2.0%.

Containers and storage Containers—Hermetic containers, and colored containers may be used.

Storage—Light-resistant.

Weak Opium Alkaloids and Scopolamine Injection

弱アヘンアルカロイド·スコポラミン注射液

Weak Opium Alkaloids and Scopolamine Injection is an aqueous injection.

It contains not less than 0.90 w/v% and not more than 1.10 w/v% of morphine ($C_{17}H_{19}NO_3$: 285.34) and not less than 0.027 w/v% and not more than 0.033 w/v% of scopolamine hydrobromide hydrate ($C_{17}H_{21}NO_4.HBr.3H_2O$: 438.31).

Method of preparation

Opium Alkaloids Hydrochlorides	20 g
Scopolamine Hydrobromide Hydrate	0.3 g
Water for Injection or Sterile Water for Injection in Containers	a sufficient quantity
To make	1000 mL

Prepare as directed under Injections, with the above ingredients.

Description Weak Opium Alkaloids and Scopolamine Injection is a clear, colorless or light brown liquid.

It is affected by light.

pH: 2.5 – 3.5

Identification **(1)** To 1 mL of Weak Opium Alkaloids and Scopolamine Injection add 1 mL of ethanol (99.5), mix, and use this solution as the sample solution. Proceed with the sample solution as directed in the Identification (1) under Opium Alkaloids Hydrochlorides.

(2) To 2 mL of Weak Opium Alkaloids and Scopolamine

Injection add 2 mL of ammonia TS, extract with 10 mL of diethyl ether, and filter the diethyl ether layer. Evaporate the filtrate on a water bath to dryness, add 1 mL of ethanol (99.5) to the residue, and heat to dissolve. Allow to stand this solution in an ice water for 30 minutes with occasional shaking. After crystals are formed, use the supernatant liquid as the sample solution. Separately, dissolve 0.03 g of Scopolamine Hydrobromide RS in 100 mL of water, proceed with 2 mL of this solution in the same manner as for the sample solution, and use a solution so obtained as the standard solution. Perform the test with these solutions as directed under Thin-layer Chromatography <*2.03*>. Spot 10 μL each of the sample solution and standard solution on a plate of silica gel for thin-layer chromatography. Develop the plate with a mixture of methanol and ammonia water (28) (200:3) to a distance of about 10 cm, and air-dry the plate. Spray evenly Dragendorff's TS for spraying on the plate: a spot with an *R*f value of about 0.7 among the several spots from the sample solution and an orange colored spot from the standard solution show the same color tone, and have the same *R*f value (scopolamine).

Extractable volume <*6.05*> It meets the requirements.

Assay **(1)** Morphine—Pipet 2 mL of Weak Opium Alkaloids and Scopolamine Injection, add exactly 10 mL of the internal standard solution and water to make 50 mL, and use this solution as the sample solution. Separately, weigh accurately about 25 mg of morphine hydrochloride hydrate for assay, dissolve in exactly 10 mL of the internal standard solution, add water to make 50 mL, and use this solution as the standard solution. Perform the test with 20 μL each of the sample solution and standard solution as directed under Liquid Chromatography <*2.01*> according to the following conditions, and calculate the ratios, Q_T and Q_S, of the peak area of morphine to that of the internal standard.

$$\text{Amount (mg) of morphine } (C_{17}H_{19}NO_3) = M_S \times Q_T \times Q_S \times 0.887$$

M_S: Amount (mg) of morphine hydrochloride hydrate for assay taken, calculated on the anhydrous basis

Internal standard solution—A solution of etilefrin hydrochloride (1 in 500).

Operating conditions—

Detector: An ultraviolet absorption photometer (wavelength: 285 nm).

Column: A stainless steel column 4.6 mm in inside diameter and 15 cm in length, packed with octadecylsilanized silica gel for liquid chromatography (5 μm in particle diameter).

Column temperature: A constant temperature of about 40°C.

Mobile phase: Dissolve 1.0 g of sodium lauryl sulfate in 500 mL of diluted phosphoric acid (1 in 1000), and adjust the pH to 3.0 with sodium hydroxide TS. To 240 mL of this solution add 70 mL of tetrahydrofuran, and mix.

Flow rate: Adjust so that the retention time of morphine is about 10 minutes.

System suitability—

System performance: When the procedure is run with 20 μL of the standard solution under the above operating conditions, morphine and the internal standard are eluted in this order with the resolution between these peaks being not less than 3.

System repeatability: When the test is repeated 6 times with 20 μL of the standard solution under the above operating conditions, the relative standard deviation of the ratios of the peak area of morphine to that of the internal standard is not more than 2.0%.

(2) Scopolamine hydrobromide hydrate—Pipet 4 mL of Weak Opium Alkaloids and Scopolamine Injection, and add exactly 2 mL of the internal standard solution. To this solution add 10 mL of diluted dilute hydrochloric acid (1 in 10), and shake with two 10-mL portions of dichloromethane. Remove the dichloromethane layer, to the water layer add 2 mL of ammonia TS, add immediately 20 mL of dichloromethane, shake vigorously, filter the dichloromethane extract through a filter paper on which 5 g of anhydrous sodium sulfate is placed, and evaporate the filtrate to dryness under reduced pressure. To the residue add 0.5 mL of 1,2-dichloroethane and 0.5 mL of bis-trimethyl silyl acetamide, stopper tightly, warm in a water bath at 60°C for 15 minutes, and use this solution as the sample solution. Separately, weigh accurately about 60 mg of Scoporamine Hydrobromide RS (separately determine the loss on drying <*2.41*> under the same conditions as Scopolamine Hydrobromide Hydrate), and dissolve in water to make exactly 100 mL. Pipet 2 mL of this solution, add exactly 2 mL of the internal standard solution. Proceed with this solution in the same manner as for the sample solution, and use so obtained solution as the standard solution. Perform the test with 2 μL each of the sample solution and standard solution as directed under Gas Chromatography <*2.02*> according to the following conditions, and calculate the ratios, Q_T and Q_S, of the peak area of scopolamine to that of the internal standard.

$$\text{Amount (mg) of scopolamine hydrobromide hydrate } (C_{17}H_{21}NO_4.HBr.3H_2O) = M_S \times Q_T/Q_S \times 1/50 \times 1.141$$

M_S: Amount (mg) of Scopolamine Hydrobromide RS taken, calculated on the dried basis

Internal standard solution—A solution of homatropine hydrobromide (1 in 4000).

Operating conditions—

Detector: A hydrogen flame-ionization detector.

Column: A glass column 3 mm in inside diameter and 1.5 m in length, packed with 180 to 250 μm siliceous earth for gas chromatography coated in 1 to 3% with 50% phenyl-methyl silicone polymer for gas chromatography.

Column temperature: A constant temperature of about 210°C.

Carrier gas: Nitrogen or helium.

Flow rate: Adjust so that the retention time of scopolamine is about 8 minutes.

System suitability—

System performance: When the procedure is run with 2 μL of the standard solution under the above operating conditions, the internal standard and scopolamine are eluted in this order with the resolution between these peaks being not less than 6.

System repeatability: When the test is repeated 5 times with 2 μL of the standard solution under the above operating conditions, the relative standard deviation of the ratios of the peak area of scopolamine to that of the internal standard is not more than 2.0%.

Containers and storage Containers—Hermetic containers, and colored containers may be used.

Storage—Light-resistant.

Orciprenaline Sulfate

オルシプレナリン硫酸塩

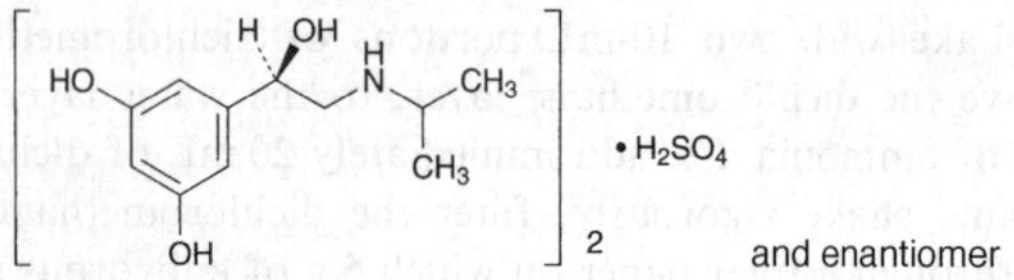

$(C_{11}H_{17}NO_3)_2.H_2SO_4$: 520.59
5-{(1*RS*)-1-Hydroxy-
2-[(1-methylethyl)amino]ethyl}benzene-1,3-diol
hemisulfate
[*5874-97-5*]

Orciprenaline Sulfate contains not less than 98.5% of orciprenaline sulfate [$(C_{11}H_{17}NO_3)_2.H_2SO_4$], calculated on the dried basis.

Description Orciprenaline Sulfate occurs as white, crystals or crystalline powder.

It is freely soluble in water, slightly soluble in ethanol (95) and in acetic acid (100), and practically insoluble in diethyl ether.

A solution of Orciprenaline Sulfate (1 in 20) shows no optical rotation.

Melting point: about 220°C (with decomposition).

Identification **(1)** Determine the absorption spectrum of a solution of Orciprenaline Sulfate in 0.01 mol/L hydrochloric acid TS (1 in 10,000) as directed under Ultraviolet-visible Spectrophotometry <*2.24*>, and compare the spectrum with the Reference Spectrum: both spectra exhibit similar intensities of absorption at the same wavelengths.

(2) Determine the infrared absorption spectrum of Orciprenaline Sulfate, previously dried, as directed in the potassium bromide disk method under Infrared Spectrophotometry <*2.25*>: it exhibits absorption at the wave numbers of about 1607 cm^{-1}, 1153 cm^{-1}, 1131 cm^{-1} and 1110 cm^{-1}.

(3) A solution of Orciprenaline Sulfate (1 in 100) responds to Qualitative Tests <*1.09*> for sulfate.

pH <*2.54*> Dissolve 1.0 g of Orciprenaline Sulfate in 10 mL of water: the pH of this solution is between 4.0 and 5.5.

Purity **(1)** Clarity and color of solution—Dissolve 1.0 g of Orciprenaline Sulfate in 10 mL of water: the solution is clear, and has no more color than the following control solution.

Control solution: To 3 mL of Matching Fluid T add 1 mL of diluted hydrochloric acid (1 in 40).

(2) Heavy metals <*1.07*>—Proceed with 2.0 g of Orciprenaline Sulfate according to Method 2, and perform the test. Prepare the control solution with 2.0 mL of Standard Lead Solution (not more than 10 ppm).

(3) Orciprenalone—Dissolve 0.200 g of Orciprenaline Sulfate in 0.01 mol/L hydrochloric acid TS to make exactly 20 mL. Perform the test with this solution as directed under Ultraviolet-visible Spectrophotometry <*2.24*>: the absorbance at 328 nm is not more than 0.075.

Loss on drying <*2.41*> Not more than 1.5% (1 g, in vacuum, 105°C, 4 hours).

Residue on ignition <*2.44*> Not more than 0.1% (1 g).

Assay Weigh accurately about 0.7 g of Orciprenaline Sulfate, dissolve in 100 mL of acetic acid (100) by warming on a water bath, and titrate <*2.50*> with 0.1 mol/L perchloric acid VS (potentiometric titration). Perform a blank determination in the same manner, and make any necessary correction.

Each mL of 0.1 mol/L perchloric acid VS
= 52.06 mg of $(C_{11}H_{17}NO_3)_2.H_2SO_4$

Containers and storage Containers—Tight containers.
Storage—Light-resistant.

Oxapium Iodide

オキサピウムヨウ化物

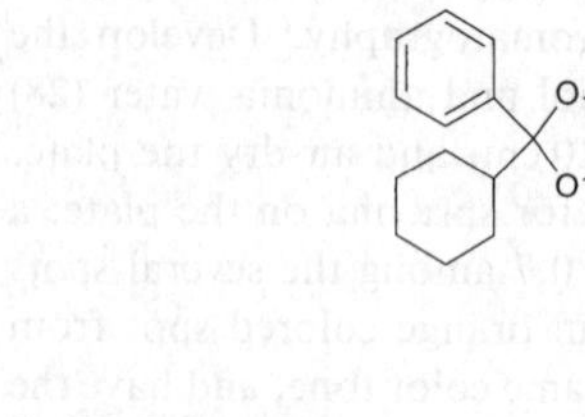

$C_{22}H_{34}INO_2$: 471.42
1-(2-Cyclohexyl-2-phenyl-1,3-dioxolan-4-ylmethyl)-1-methylpiperidinium iodide
[*6577-41-9*]

Oxapium Iodide, when dried, contains not less than 98.5% of oxapium iodide ($C_{22}H_{34}INO_2$).

Description Oxapium Iodide occurs as a white crystalline powder.

It is soluble in acetonitrile, in methanol and in ethanol (95), slightly soluble in water, in acetic anhydride and in acetic acid (100), and practically insoluble in diethyl ether.

A solution of Oxapium Iodide in methanol (1 in 100) does not show optical rotation.

Identification **(1)** Determine the infrared absorption spectrum of Oxapium Iodide, previously dried, as directed in the paste method under Infrared Spectrophotometry <*2.25*>, and compare the spectrum with the Reference Spectrum: both spectra exhibit similar intensities of absorption at the same wave numbers.

(2) Dissolve 0.1 g of Oxapium Iodide in 10 mL of methanol, and add 2 mL of dilute nitric acid and 2 mL of silver nitrate TS: a greenish yellow precipitate is formed.

Melting point <*2.60*> 198 – 203°C

Purity **(1)** Heavy metals <*1.07*>—Proceed with 1.0 g of Oxapium Iodide according to Method 2, and perform the test. Prepare the control solution with 2.0 mL of Standard Lead Solution (not more than 20 ppm).

(2) Related substances—Dissolve 0.05 g of Oxapium Iodide in 100 mL of a mixture of water and acetonitrile (1:1), and use this solution as the sample solution. Pipet 1 mL of the sample solution, add a mixture of water and acetonitrile (1:1) to make exactly 50 mL, and use this solution as the standard solution. Perform the test with exactly 50 μL each of the sample solution and standard solution as directed under Liquid Chromatography <*2.01*> according to the following conditions. Determine each peak area of each solution by the automatic integration method: the total area of the peaks other than oxapium obtained from the sample solution is not larger than the area of the peak of oxapium from the standard solution.

Operating conditions—

Detector: An ultraviolet absorption photometer (wavelength: 254 nm).

Column: A stainless steel column about 4 mm in inside diameter and about 15 cm in length, packed with octadecylsilanized silica gel for liquid chromatography (5 μm in particle diameter).

Column temperature: A constant temperature of 20°C to 30°C.

Mobile phase: To 57 mL of acetic acid (100) and 139 mL of triethylamine add water to make 1000 mL. To 50 mL of this solution add 500 mL of acetonitril, 10 mL of dilute acetic acid and 440 mL of water.

Flow rate: Adjust so that the retention time of oxapium is about 4 minutes.

Selection of column: Dissolve 0.05 g of Oxapium Iodide and 3 mg of benzophenone in 100 mL of the mobile phase. Proceed with 20 μL of this solution under the above operating conditions, and calculate the resolution. Use a column giving elution of oxapium and benzophenone in this order with the resolution between these peaks being not less than 5.

Detection sensitivity: Adjust the detection sensitivity so that the peak height of oxapium obtained from 50 μL of the standard solution composes 5 to 15% of the full scale.

Time span of measurement: About 6 times as long as the retention time of oxapium, beginning after the peak of iodide ion.

Loss on drying <*2.41*> Not more than 0.5% (1 g, 105°C, 4 hours).

Residue on ignition <*2.44*> Not more than 0.1% (1 g).

Assay Weigh accurately about 0.7 g of Oxapium Iodide, previously dried, dissolve in 50 mL of a mixture of acetic anhydride and acetic acid (100) (9:1), and titrate <*2.50*> with 0.1 mol/L perchloric acid VS (potentiometric titration, platinum electrode). Perform a blank determination in the same manner, and make any necessary correction.

Each mL of 0.1 mol/L perchloric acid VS
= 47.14 mg of $C_{22}H_{34}INO_2$

Containers and storage Containers—Tight containers.
Storage—Light-resistant.

Oxaprozin

オキサプロジン

$C_{18}H_{15}NO_3$: 293.32
3-(4,5-Diphenyloxazol-2-yl)propanoic acid
[*21256-18-8*]

Oxaprozin, when dried, contains not less than 98.5% of oxaprozin ($C_{18}H_{15}NO_3$).

Description Oxaprozin occurs as a white to yellowish white crystalline powder.

It is sparingly soluble in methanol and in ethanol (95), slightly soluble in diethyl ether, and practically insoluble in water.

It is gradually affected by light.

Identification Determine the infrared absorption spectrum of Oxaprozin, previously dried, as directed in the potassium bromide disk method under Infrared Spectrophotometry <*2.25*>, and compare the spectrum with the Reference Spectrum: both spectra exhibit similar intensities of absorption at the same wave numbers.

Absorbance <*2.24*> $E^{1\%}_{1\,cm}$ (285 nm): 455 – 495 (after drying, 10 mg, methanol, 1000 mL).

Melting point <*2.60*> 161 – 165°C

Purity (1) Heavy metals <*1.07*>—Proceed with 2.0 g of Oxaprozin according to Method 4, and perform the test. Prepare the control solution with 2.0 mL of Standard Lead Solution (not more than 10 ppm).

(2) Arsenic <*1.11*>—Prepare the test solution with 2.0 g of Oxaprozin according to Method 3, and perform the test (not more than 1 ppm).

(3) Related substances—Dissolve 0.10 g of Oxaprozin in 10 mL of methanol, and use this solution as the sample solution. Pipet 1 mL of the sample solution, add methanol to make exactly 100 mL, and use this solution as the standard solution (1). Pipet 5 mL, 3 mL and 1 mL of the standard solution (1), add methanol to each to make exactly 10 mL, and use these solutions as the standard solutions (2), (3) and (4), respectively. Perform the test with these solutions as directed under Thin-layer Chromatography <*2.03*>. Spot 10 μL each of the sample solution and standard solutions (1), (2), (3) and (4) on a plate of silica gel with fluorescent indicator for thin-layer chromatography. Develop the plate with a mixture of ethyl acetate and acetic acid (100) (99:1) to a distance of about 15 cm, and air-dry the plate. Examine under ultraviolet light (main wavelength: 254 nm): the total intensity of the spots other than the principal spot obtained from the sample solution is not more than 1.0% calculated on the basis of intensities of the spots from the standard solutions (1), (2), (3) and (4).

Loss on drying <*2.41*> Not more than 0.3% (1 g, 105°C, 2 hours).

Residue on ignition <*2.44*> Not more than 0.3% (1 g).

Assay Weigh accurately about 0.5 g of Oxaprozin, previously dried, dissolve in 50 mL of ethanol (95), and titrate <*2.50*> with 0.1 mol/L sodium hydroxide VS (potentiometric titration). Perform a blank determination in the same manner, and make any necessary correction.

Each mL of 0.1 mol/L sodium hydroxide VS
= 29.33 mg of $C_{18}H_{15}NO_3$

Containers and storage Containers—Tight containers.
Storage—Light-resistant.

Oxazolam

オキサゾラム

$C_{18}H_{17}ClN_2O_2$: 328.79
10-Chloro-2-methyl-11b-phenyl-2,3,7,11b-tetrahydro[1,3]oxazolo[3,2-*d*][1,4]benzodiazepin-6(5*H*)-one
[*24143-17-7*]

Oxazolam, when dried, contains not less than 99.0% of oxazolam ($C_{18}H_{17}ClN_2O_2$).

Description Oxazolam occurs as white, crystals or crystalline powder. It is odorless and tasteless.

It is freely soluble in acetic acid (100), soluble in 1,4-dioxane and in dichloromethane, slightly soluble in ethanol (95) and in diethyl ether, and practically insoluble in water.

It dissolves in dilute hydrochloric acid.

It gradually changes in color by light.

Melting point: about 187°C (with decomposition).

Identification **(1)** Dissolve 0.01 g of Oxazolam in 10 mL of ethanol (95) by heating, and add 1 drop of hydrochloric acid: a light yellow color develops, and the solution shows a yellow-green fluorescence under ultraviolet light (main wavelength: 365 nm). Add 1 mL of sodium hydroxide TS to this solution: the color and fluorescence of this solution disappear immediately.

(2) Dissolve 0.01 g of Oxazolam in 5 mL of dilute hydrochloric acid by heating in a water bath for 10 minutes. After cooling, 1 mL of this solution responds to Qualitative Tests <*1.09*> for primary aromatic amines.

(3) Place 2 g of Oxazolam in a 200-mL flask, add 50 mL of ethanol (95) and 25 mL of 6 mol/L hydrochloric acid TS, and boil under a reflux condenser for 5 hours. After cooling, neutralize with a solution of sodium hydroxide (1 in 4), and extract with 30 mL of dichloromethane. Dehydrate with 3 g of anhydrous sodium sulfate, filter, and evaporate the dichloromethane of the filtrate. Dissolve the residue in 20 mL of methanol by heating on a water bath, and cool immediately in an ice bath. Collect the crystals, and dry in vacuum at 60°C for 1 hour: the crystals melt <*2.60*> between 96°C and 100°C.

(4) Determine the absorption spectrum of a solution of Oxazolam in ethanol (95) (1 in 100,000) as directed under Ultraviolet-visible Spectrophotometry <*2.24*>, and compare the spectrum with the Reference Spectrum: both spectra exhibit similar intensities of absorption at the same wavelengths.

(5) Proceed with Oxazolam as directed under Flame Coloration Test <*1.04*> (2), and perform the test: a green color appears.

Absorbance <*2.24*> $E^{1\%}_{1\,cm}$ (246 nm): 410 – 430 (after drying, 1 mg, ethanol (95), 100 mL).

Purity **(1)** Chloride <*1.03*>—To 1.0 g of Oxazolam add 50 mL of water, allow to stand for 1 hour with occasional shaking, and filter. To 25 mL of this filtrate add 6 mL of dilute nitric acid and water to make 50 mL, and perform the test using this solution as the test solution. Prepare the control solution with 0.20 mL of 0.01 mol/L hydrochloric acid VS (not more than 0.014%).

(2) Heavy metals <*1.07*>—Proceed with 1.0 g of Oxazolam according to Method 2, and perform the test. Prepare the control solution with 2.0 mL of Standard Lead Solution (not more than 20 ppm).

(3) Arsenic <*1.11*>—Place 1.0 g of Oxazolam in a Kjeldahl flask, add 5 mL of sulfuric acid and 5 mL of nitric acid, and heat gently. Repeat the addition of 2 to 3 mL of nitric acid at times, and continue to heat until a colorless to light yellow solution is obtained. After cooling, add 15 mL of saturated ammonium oxalate monohydrate solution, heat the solution until dense white fumes are evolved, and evaporate to a volume of 2 to 3 mL. After cooling, dilute with water to 10 mL, and perform the test with this solution as the test solution (not more than 2 ppm).

(4) Related substances—Dissolve 0.05 g of Oxazolam in 10 mL of dichloromethane, and use this solution as the sample solution. Pipet 1 mL of the sample solution, add dichloromethane to make exactly 200 mL, and use this solution as the standard solution. Perform the test with these solutions as directed under Thin-layer Chromatography <*2.03*>. Spot 10 μL each of the sample solution and standard solution on a plate of silica gel with fluorescent indicator for thin-layer chromatography. Immediately air-dry, develop the plate with a mixture of toluene and acetone (8:1) to a distance of about 10 cm, and air-dry the plate. Examine under ultraviolet light (main wavelength: 254 nm): the spots other than the principal spot obtained from the sample solution are not more intense than the spot from the standard solution.

Loss on drying <*2.41*> Not more than 0.5% (1 g, 105°C, 3 hours).

Residue on ignition <*2.44*> Not more than 0.1% (1 g).

Assay Weigh accurately about 0.65 g of Oxazolam, previously dried, dissolve in 100 mL of a mixture of acetic acid (100) and 1,4-dioxane (1:1). Titrate <*2.50*> with 0.1 mol/L perchloric acid VS until the color of the solution changes from purple through blue to blue-green (indicator: 2 drops of crystal violet TS). Perform a blank determination in the same manner, and make any necessary correction.

Each mL of 0.1 mol/L perchloric acid VS
= 32.88 mg of $C_{18}H_{17}ClN_2O_2$

Containers and storage Containers—Tight containers.
Storage—Light-resistant.

Oxethazaine

Oxetacaine

オキセサゼイン

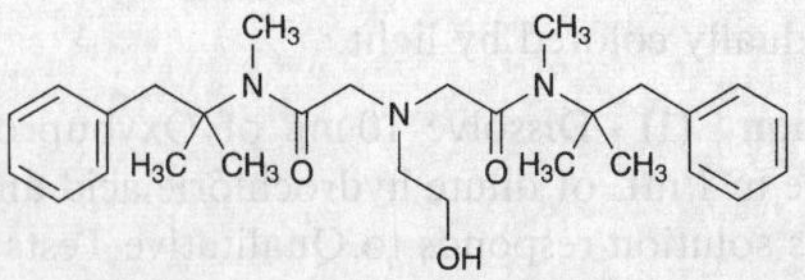

$C_{28}H_{41}N_3O_3$: 467.64
2,2′-(2-Hydroxyethylimino)bis[*N*-(1,1-dimethyl-2-phenylethyl)-*N*-methylacetamide]
[126-27-2]

Oxethazaine, when dried, contains not less than 98.5% of oxethazaine ($C_{28}H_{41}N_3O_3$).

Description Oxethazaine occurs as a white to pale yellow-white crystalline powder.

It is very soluble in acetic acid (100), freely soluble in methanol and in ethanol (95), sparingly soluble in diethyl ether, and practically insoluble in water.

Identification **(1)** Determine the absorption spectrum of a solution of Oxethazaine in ethanol (95) (1 in 2500) as directed under Ultraviolet-visible Spectrophotometry *<2.24>*, and compare the spectrum with the Reference Spectrum: both spectra exhibit similar intensities of absorption at the same wavelengths.

(2) Determine the infrared absorption spectrum of Oxethazaine as directed in the potassium bromide disk method under Infrared Spectrophotometry *<2.25>*, and compare the spectrum with the Reference Spectrum: both spectra exhibits similar intensities of absorption at the same wave numbers.

Melting point *<2.60>* 101 - 104°C

Purity **(1)** Chloride *<1.03>*—Dissolve 1.0 g of Oxethazaine in 20 mL of ethanol (95), add 6 mL of dilute nitric acid and water to make 50 mL. Perform the test using this solution as the test solution. Prepare the control solution with 0.30 mL of 0.01 mol/L hydrochloric acid VS, 20 mL of ethanol (95), 6 mL of dilute nitric acid and water to make 50 mL (not more than 0.011%).

(2) Heavy metals *<1.07>*—Proceed with 2.0 g of Oxethazaine according to Method 2, and perform the test. Prepare the control solution with 2.0 mL of Standard Lead Solution (not more than 10 ppm).

(3) Related substances—Dissolve 0.40 g of Oxethazaine in 10 mL of ethanol (95), and use this solution as the sample solution. Pipet 1 mL of the sample solution, add ethanol (95) to make exactly 100 mL, and use this solution as the standard solution. Perform the test with these solutions as directed under Thin-layer Chromatography *<2.03>*. Spot 10 μL each of the sample solution and standard solution on a plate of silica gel with fluorescent indicator for thin-layer chromatography. Develop the plate with a mixture of isopropylether, tetrahydrofuran, methanol and ammonia solution (28) (24:10:5:1) to a distance of about 10 cm, and air-dry the plate. Examine under ultraviolet light (main wavelength: 254 nm): the spots other than the principal spot obtained from the sample solution are not more intense than the spot from the standard solution.

(4) 2-Aminoethanol—To 1.0 g of Oxethazaine add methanol to make exactly 10 mL, then add 0.1 mL of a solution of 1-fluoro-2,4-dinitrobenzene in methanol (1 in 25), shake well, and heat at 60°C for 20 minutes: the solution has no more color than the following control solution.

Control solution: To 0.10 g of 2-aminoethanol add methanol to make exactly 200 mL, pipet 1 mL of this solution, and add methanol to make exactly 10 mL. Proceed as directed above.

Loss on drying *<2.41>* Not more than 0.5% (1 g, in vacuum, 60°C, 3 hours).

Residue on ignition *<2.44>* Not more than 0.1% (1 g).

Assay Weigh accurately about 0.9 g of Oxethazaine, previously dried, dissolve in 50 mL of acetic acid (100), and titrate *<2.50>* with 0.1 mol/L perchloric acid VS (indicator: 2 drops of crystal violet TS). Perform a blank determination in the same manner, and make any necessary correction.

Each mL of 0.1 mol/L perchloric acid VS
= 46.76 mg of $C_{28}H_{41}N_3O_3$

Containers and storage Containers—Tight containers.

Oxprenolol Hydrochloride

オクスプレノロール塩酸塩

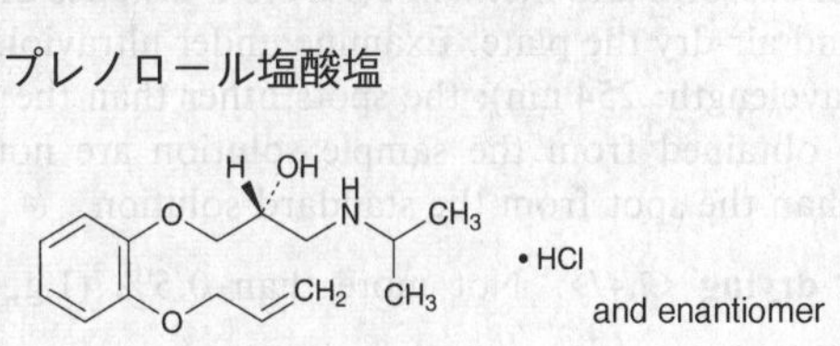

and enantiomer

$C_{15}H_{23}NO_3.HCl$: 301.81
(2*RS*)-1-[2-(Allyloxy)phenoxy]-3-(1-methylethyl)aminopropan-2-ol monohydrochloride
[6452-73-9]

Oxprenolol Hydrochloride, when dried, contains not less than 98.5% of oxprenolol hydrochloride ($C_{15}H_{23}NO_3.HCl$).

Description Oxprenolol Hydrochloride occurs as a white crystalline powder.

It is very soluble in water, freely soluble in ethanol (95) and in acetic acid (100), slightly soluble in acetic anhydride, and practically insoluble in diethyl ether.

Identification **(1)** To 2 mL of a solution of Oxprenolol Hydrochloride (1 in 100) add 1 drop of copper (II) sulfate TS and 2 mL of sodium hydroxide TS: a blue-purple color develops. To this solution add 1 mL of diethyl ether, shake well, and allow to stand: a red-purple color develops in the diethyl ether layer, and a blue-purple color develops in the water layer.

(2) To 3 mL of a solution of Oxprenolol Hydrochloride (1 in 150) add 3 drops of Reinecke salt TS: a light red precipitate is formed.

(3) Determine the infrared absorption spectrum of Oxprenolol Hydrochloride, previously dried, as directed in the potassium chloride disk method under Infrared Spectrophotometry *<2.25>*, and compare the spectrum with the Reference Spectrum: both spectra exhibit similar intensities of absorption at the same wave numbers.

(4) A solution of Oxprenolol Hydrochloride (1 in 50) responds to Qualitative Tests *<1.09>* for chloride.

pH *<2.54>* Dissolve 1.0 g of Oxprenolol Hydrochloride in 10 mL of water: the pH of this solution is between 4.5 and

6.0.

Melting point <*2.60*> 107 – 110°C

Purity **(1)** Clarity and color of solution—Dissolve 1.0 g of Oxprenolol Hydrochloride in 10 mL of water: the solution is clear and colorless.

(2) Heavy metals <*1.07*>—Proceed with 2.0 g of Oxprenolol Hydrochloride according to Method 4, and perform the test. Prepare the control solution with 2.0 mL of Standard Lead Solution (not more than 10 ppm).

(3) Arsenic <*1.11*>—Prepare the test solution with 1.0 g of Oxprenolol Hydrochloride according to Method 3, and perform the test (not more than 2 ppm).

(4) Related substances—Dissolve 0.25 g of Oxprenolol Hydrochloride in 10 mL of water, and use this solution as the sample solution. Pipet 4 mL of the sample solution, and add water to make exactly 100 mL. Pipet 5 mL of this solution, add water to make exactly 100 mL, and use this solution as the standard solution. Perform the test with these solutions as directed under Thin-layer Chromatography <*2.03*>. Spot 10 μL each of the sample solution and standard solution on a plate of silica gel with fluorescent indicator for thin-layer chromatography. Develop the plate in a developing chamber saturated with ammonia vapor with a mixture of chloroform and methanol (9:1) to a distance of about 10 cm, and air-dry the plate. Examine under ultraviolet light (main wavelength: 254 nm): the spots other than the principal spot obtained from the sample solution are not more intense than the spot from the standard solution.

Loss on drying <*2.41*> Not more than 0.5% (1 g, 80°C, 3 hours).

Residue on ignition <*2.44*> Not more than 0.1% (1 g).

Assay Weigh accurately about 0.6 g of Oxprenolol Hydrochloride, previously dried, dissolve in 50 mL of a mixture of acetic anhydride and acetic acid (100) (7:3), and titrate <*2.50*> with 0.1 mol/L perchloric acid VS (potentiometric titration). Perform a blank determination in the same manner, and make any necessary correction.

Each mL of 0.1 mol/L perchloric acid VS
= 30.18 mg of $C_{15}H_{23}NO_3.HCl$

Containers and storage Containers—Tight containers.

Oxybuprocaine Hydrochloride

Benoxinate Hydrochloride

オキシブプロカイン塩酸塩

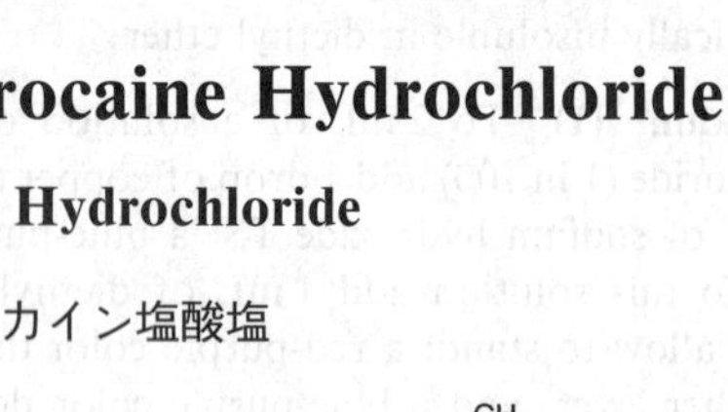

$C_{17}H_{28}N_2O_3.HCl$: 344.88
2-(Diethylamino)ethyl 4-amino-3-butyloxybenzoate monohydrochloride
[*5987-82-6*]

Oxybuprocaine Hydrochloride, when dried, contains not less than 99.0% of oxybuprocaine hydrochloride ($C_{17}H_{28}N_2O_3.HCl$).

Description Oxybuprocaine Hydrochloride occurs as white, crystals or crystalline powder. It is odorless, and has a saline taste. It exhibits anesthetic properties when placed on the tongue.

It is very soluble in water, freely soluble in ethanol (95) and in chloroform, and practically insoluble in diethyl ether.

The pH of a solution of 1.0 g of Oxybuprocaine Hydrochloride in 10 mL of water is between 5.0 and 6.0.

It is gradually colored by light.

Identification **(1)** Dissolve 10 mg of Oxybuprocaine Hydrochloride in 1 mL of dilute hydrochloric acid and 4 mL of water. This solution responds to Qualitative Tests <*1.09*> for primary aromatic amines.

(2) Dissolve 0.1 g of Oxybuprocaine Hydrochloride in 8 mL of water, and add 3 mL of ammonium thiocyanate TS: an oily substance is produced. Rub the inner surface of the container with a glass rod: white crystals are formed. Collect the crystals so obtained, recrystallize from water, and dry in a desiccator (in vacuum, phosphorus (V) oxide) for 5 hours: the crystals melt <*2.60*> between 103°C and 106°C.

(3) Determine the absorption spectrum of a solution of Oxybuprocaine Hydrochloride (1 in 100,000) as directed under Ultraviolet-visible Spectrophotometry <*2.24*>, and compare the spectrum with the Reference Spectrum: both spectra exhibit similar intensities of absorption at the same wavelengths.

(4) A solution of Oxybuprocaine Hydrochloride (1 in 10) responds to Qualitative Tests <*1.09*> for chloride.

Melting point <*2.60*> 158 – 162°C

Purity **(1)** Clarity and color of solution—Dissolve 1.0 g of Oxybuprocaine Hydrochloride in 10 mL of water: the solution is clear and colorless.

(2) Heavy metals <*1.07*>—Proceed with 1.0 g of Oxybuprocaine Hydrochloride according to Method 1, and perform the test. Prepare the control solution with 2.0 mL of Standard Lead Solution (not more than 20 ppm).

(3) Related substances—Dissolve 0.25 g of Oxybuprocaine Hydrochloride in 10 mL of chloroform, and use this solution as the sample solution. Pipet 1 mL of the sample solution, and add chloroform to make exactly 20 mL. Pipet 1 mL of this solution, add chloroform to make exactly 50 mL, and use this solution as the standard solution. Perform the test with these solutions as directed under Thin-layer Chromatography <*2.03*>. Spot 10 μL each of the sample solution and standard solution on a plate of silica gel for thin-layer chromatography. Develop the plate with a mixture of chloroform, ethanol (95) and formic acid (7:2:1) to a distance of about 10 cm, and air-dry the plate. Spray evenly 4-dimethylaminobenzaldehyde TS for spraying on the plate: the spots other than the principal spot obtained from the sample solution are not more intense than the spot from the standard solution.

Loss on drying <*2.41*> Not more than 0.5% (1 g, 105°C, 2 hours).

Residue on ignition <*2.44*> Not more than 0.1% (1 g).

Assay Weigh accurately about 0.6 g of Oxybuprocaine Hydrochloride, previously dried, dissolve in 50 mL of a mixture of acetic anhydride and acetic acid (100) (7:3), and titrate <*2.50*> with 0.1 mol/L perchloric acid VS (potentiometric titration). Perform a blank determination in the same manner, and make any necessary correction.

Each mL of 0.1 mol/L perchloric acid VS
= 34.49 mg of $C_{17}H_{28}N_2O_3.HCl$

Containers and storage Containers—Well-closed contain-

ers.

Storage—Light-resistant.

Oxycodone Hydrochloride Hydrate

オキシコドン塩酸塩水和物

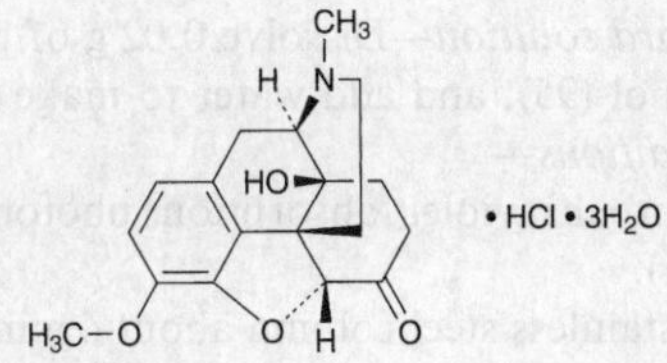

$C_{18}H_{21}NO_4.HCl.3H_2O$: 405.87
(5*R*)-4,5-Epoxy-14-hydroxy-3-methoxy-17-methylmorphinan-6-one monohydrochloride trihydrate
[*124-90-3*, anhydride]

Oxycodone Hydrochloride Hydrate contains not less than 98.0% and not more than 101.0% of oxycodone hydrochloride ($C_{18}H_{21}NO_4.HCl$: 351.83), calculated on the anhydrous basis.

Description Oxycodone Hydrochloride Hydrate occurs as a white crystalline powder.

It is freely soluble in water, in methanol and in acetic acid (100), sparingly soluble in ethanol (95), slightly soluble in acetic anhydride.

The pH of a solution dissolved 1.0 g of Oxycodone Hydrochloride Hydrate in 10 mL of water is between 3.8 and 5.8.

It is affected by light.

Identification **(1)** Determine the absorption spectrum of a solution of Oxycodone Hydrochloride Hydrate (1 in 10,000) as directed under Ultraviolet-visible Spectrophotometry <*2.24*>, and compare the spectrum with the Reference Spectrum: both spectra exhibit similar intensities of absorption at the same wavelengths.

(2) Determine the infrared absorption spectrum of Oxycodone Hydrochloride Hydrate as directed in the potassium bromide disk method under Infrared Spectrophotometry <*2.25*>, and compare the spectrum with the Reference Spectrum: both spectra exhibit similar intensities of absorption at the same wave numbers.

(3) A solution of Oxycodone Hydrochloride Hydrate (1 in 50) responds to Qualitative Tests <*1.09*> (2) for chloride.

Optical rotation <*2.49*> $[\alpha]_D^{20}$: −140 – −149° (0.5 g calculated on the anhydrous basis, water, 25 mL, 100 mm).

Purity **(1)** Clarity and color of solution—Dissolve 0.5 g of Oxycodone Hydrochloride Hydrate in 10 mL of water: the solution is clear and colorless.

(2) Related substances—Dissolve 26 mg of Oxycodone Hydrochloride Hydrate in 20 mL of the mobile phase A, and use this solution as the sample solution. Pipet 1 mL of the sample solution, add the mobile phase A to make exactly 100 mL, and use this solution as the standard solution. Perform the test with exactly 50 μL each of the sample solution and standard solution as directed under Liquid Chromatography <*2.01*> according to the following conditions. Determine each peak area by the automatic integration method: the area of the peak other than oxycodone obtained from the sample solution is not larger than 1/5 times the peak area of oxycodone from the standard solution, and the total area of the peaks other than oxycodone from the sample solution is not larger than 3/5 times the peak area of oxycodone from the standard solution. For the area of the peak, having the relative retention time of about 1.8 to oxycodone, multiply the correction factor 0.17.

Operating conditions—

Detector: An ultraviolet absorption photometer (wavelength: 280 nm).

Column: A stainless steel column 4.6 mm in inside diameter and 10 cm in length, packed with octadecylsilanized silica gel for liquid chromatography (3 μm in particle diameter).

Column temperature: A constant temperature of about 40°C.

Mobile phase A: Dissolve 1.0 g of sodium lauryl sulfate in 500 mL of diluted phosphoric acid (1 in 1000), and adjust to pH 3.0 with sodium hydroxide TS. To 4 volumes of this solution add 1 volume of tetrahydrofuran for liquid chromatography.

Mobile phase B: Dissolve 1.0 g of sodium lauryl sulfate in 500 mL of diluted phosphoric acid (1 in 1000), and adjust to pH 3.0 with sodium hydroxide TS. To 1 volume of this solution add 1 volume of tetrahydrofuran for liquid chromatography.

Flowing of mobile phase: Control the gradient by mixing the mobile phases A and B as directed in the following table.

Time after injection of sample (min)	Mobile phase A (vol%)	Mobile phase B (vol%)
0 – 30	100	0
30 – 70	100 → 0	0 → 100

Flow rate: 1.0 mL per minute.

Time span of measurement: About 5 times as long as the retention time of oxycodone, beginning after the solvent peak.

System suitability—

Test for required detectability: Pipet 2.5 mL of the standard solution, add the mobile phase A to make exactly 50 mL. Confirm that the peak area of oxycodone obtained with 50 μL of this solution is equivalent to 3.5 to 6.5% of that with 50 μL of the standard solution.

System performance: When the procedure is run with 50 μL of the standard solution under the above operating conditions, the number of theoretical plates and the symmetry factor of the peak of oxycodone are not less than 3000 and between 0.7 and 1.3, respectively.

System repeatability: When the test is repeated 6 times with 50 μL of the standard solution under the above operating conditions, the relative standard deviation of the peak area of oxycodone is not more than 2.0%.

Water <*2.48*> 12 – 15% (0.2 g, volumetric titration, direct titration).

Residue on ignition <*2.44*> Not more than 0.1% (0.5 g).

Assay Weigh accurately about 0.5 g of Oxycodone Hydrochloride Hydrate, dissolve in 50 mL of a mixture of acetic anhydride and acetic acid (100) (7:3), and titrate <*2.50*> with 0.1 mol/L perchloric acid VS (potentiometric titration). Perform a blank determination in the same manner, and make any necessary correction.

Each mL of 0.1 mol/L perchloric acid VS
= 35.18 mg of $C_{18}H_{21}NO_4.HCl$

Containers and storage Containers—Tight containers.

Storage—Light-resistant.

Compound Oxycodone Injection

複方オキシコドン注射液

Compound Oxycodone Injection is an aqueous injection.

It contains not less than 0.74 w/v% and not more than 0.86 w/v% of oxycodone hydrochloride hydrate ($C_{18}H_{21}NO_4.HCl.3H_2O$: 405.87), and not less than 0.18 w/v% and not more than 0.22 w/v% of hydrocotarnine hydrochloride hydrate ($C_{12}H_{15}NO_3.HCl.H_2O$: 275.73).

Method of preparation

Oxycodone Hydrochloride Hydrate	8 g
Hydrocotarnine Hydrochloride Hydrate	2 g
Water for Injection or Sterile Water for Injection in Containers	a sufficient quantity
To make	1000 mL

Prepare as directed under Injections, with the above ingredients.

Description Compound Oxycodone Injection is a clear, colorless to pale yellow liquid.

It is affected by light.

pH: 2.5 – 4.0

Identification **(1)** To 1 mL of Compound Oxycodone Injection add 1 mL of 2,4-dinitrophenylhydrazine-ethanol TS: a yellow precipitate is formed (oxycodone).

(2) Evaporate 1 mL of Compound Oxycodone Injection on a water bath. Dissolve the residue in 2 mL of sulfuric acid: a yellow color is produced. Heat the solution: it changes to red, and then to deep orange-red (hydrocotarnine).

(3) Evaporate 1 mL of Compound Oxycodone Injection on a water bath. Dissolve the residue in 3 mL of sulfuric acid, add 2 drops of a solution of tannic acid in ethanol (95) (1 in 20), and allow to stand: a deep green color is produced (hydrocotarnine).

Extractable volume *<6.05>* It meets the requirement.

Assay Pipet 2 mL of Compound Oxycodone Injection, add exactly 10 mL of the internal standard solution, and use this solution as the sample solution. Separately, weigh accurately about 0.4 g of oxycodone hydrochloride hydrate for assay (separately determine the water *<2.48>* in the same manner as Oxycodone Hydrochloride Hydrate) and about 0.1 g of hydrocotarnine hydrochloride hydrate for assay previously dried at 105°C for 3 hours, and dissolve in water to make exactly 50 mL. Pipet 2 mL of this solution, add exactly 10 mL of the internal standard solution, and use this solution as the standard solution. Perform the test with 10 μL each of the sample solution and standard solution as directed under Liquid Chromatography *<2.01>* according to the following conditions. Calculate the ratios, Q_{Ta} and Q_{Tb}, of the peak area of oxycodone and hydrocotarnine to that of the internal standard obtained from the sample solution, and the ratios, Q_{Sa} and Q_{Sb}, of the peak area of oxycodone and hydrocotarnine to that of the internal standard from the standard solution.

Amount (mg) of oxycodone hydrochloride hydrate ($C_{18}H_{21}NO_4.HCl.3H_2O$)
$= M_{Sa} \times Q_{Ta}/Q_{Sa} \times 1/25 \times 1.154$

Amount (mg) of hydrocotarnine hydrochloride hydrate ($C_{12}H_{15}NO_3.HCl.H_2O$)
$= M_{Sb} \times Q_{Tb}/Q_{Sb} \times 1/25 \times 1.070$

M_{Sa}: Amount (mg) of oxycodone hydrochloride hydrate for assay taken, calculated on the anhydrous basis

M_{Sb}: Amount (mg) of hydrocotarnine hydrochloride hydrate for assay taken

Internal standard solution—Dissolve 0.02 g of phenacetin in 10 mL of ethanol (95), and add water to make 100 mL.

Operating conditions—

Detector: An ultraviolet absorption photometer (wavelength: 285 nm).

Column: A stainless steel column about 4 mm in inside diameter and about 15 cm in length, packed with octadecylsilanized polyvinyl alcohol gel polymer for liquid chromatography (5 μm in particle diameter).

Column temperature: A constant temperature of about 25°C.

Mobile phase: To 500 mL of 0.05 mol/L disodium hydrogen phosphate TS add 0.05 mol/L sodium dihydrogen phosphate TS, and adjust the pH to 8.0. To 300 mL of this solution add 200 mL of acetonitrile, and mix.

Flow rate: Adjust so that the retention time of oxycodone is about 8 minutes.

Selection of column: Proceed with 10 μL of the standard solution under the above operating conditions, and use a column giving elution of the internal standard, oxycodone and hydrocotarnine in this order, with complete separation of these peaks.

Containers and storage Containers—Hermetic containers, and colored containers may be used.

Storage—Light-resistant.

Compound Oxycodone and Atropine Injection

複方オキシコドン・アトロピン注射液

Compound Oxycodone and Atropine Injection is an aqueous injection.

It contains not less than 0.74 w/v% and not more than 0.86 w/v% of oxycodone hydrochloride hydrate ($C_{18}H_{21}NO_4.HCl.3H_2O$: 405.87), not less than 0.18 w/v% and not more than 0.22 w/v% of hydrocotarnine hydrochloride hydrate ($C_{12}H_{15}NO_3.HCl.H_2O$: 275.73), and not less than 0.027 w/v% and not more than 0.033 w/v% of atropine sulfate hydrate [$(C_{17}H_{23}NO_3)_2.H_2SO_4.H_2O$: 694.83].

Method of preparation

Oxycodone Hydrochloride Hydrate	8 g
Hydrocotarnine Hydrochloride Hydrate	2 g
Atropine Sulfate Hydrate	0.3 g
Water for Injection or Sterile Water for Injection in Containers	a sufficient quantity
To make	1000 mL

Prepare as directed under Injections, with the above ingredients.

Description Compound Oxycodone and Atropine Injection is a colorless or pale yellow, clear liquid.

It is affected by light.

pH: 2.5 – 4.0

Identification (1) To 1 mL of Compound Oxycodone and Atropin Injection add 1 mL of 2,4-dinitrophenylhydrazine-ethanol TS: a yellow precipitate is formed (oxycodone).

(2) Evaporate 1 mL of Compound Oxycodone and Atropin Injection on a water bath, and dissolve the residue in 2 mL of sulfuric acid: a yellow color is produced. Heat the solution: it changes to red, and then to deep orange-red (hydrocotarnine).

(3) Evaporate 1 mL of Compound Oxycodone and Atropin Injection on a water bath. Dissolve the residue in 3 mL of sulfuric acid, add 2 drops of a solution of tannic acid in ethanol (95) (1 in 20), and allow to stand: a deep green color is produced (hydrocotarnine).

(4) To 1 mL of Compound Oxycodone and Atropine Injection add 0.5 mL of 2,4-dinitrophenylhydrazine-ethanol TS, and allow to stand for 1 hour. Centrifuge, and add acetone to the supernatant liquid until no more precipitate is produced. Allow to stand for 20 minutes, and centrifuge. To the supernatant liquid add potassium hydroxide TS until the liquid is light purple. Shake the liquid with 5 mL of dichloromethane, and separate the dichloromethane layer. Take 0.5 mL of the dichloromethane layer, and evaporate to dryness on a water bath. Add 5 drops of fuming nitric acid to the residue, and evaporate to dryness on a water bath. Cool, dissolve the residue in 1 mL of *N,N*-dimethylformamide, and add 6 drops of tetraethylammonium hydroxide TS: a red-purple color is produced (atropine).

Extractable volume <*6.05*> It meets the requirement.

Assay (1) Oxycodone hydrochloride hydrate and hydrocotarnine hydrochloride hydrate—Pipet 2 mL of Compound Oxycodone and Atropine Injection, add exactly 10 mL of the internal standard solution, and use this solution as the sample solution. Separately, weigh accurately about 0.4 g of oxycodone hydrochloride hydrate for assay (separately determine the water <*2.48*> in the same manner as Oxycodone Hydrochloride Hydrate) and about 0.1 g of hydrocotarnine hydrochloride hydrate for assay previously dried at 105°C for 3 hours, and dissolve in water to make exactly 50 mL. Pipet 2 mL of this solution, add exactly 10 mL of the internal standard solution, and use this solution as the standard solution. Perform the test with 10 μL each of the sample solution and standard solution as directed under Liquid Chromatography <*2.01*> according to the following conditions. Calculate the ratios, Q_{Ta} and Q_{Tb}, of the peak area of oxycodone and hydrocotarnine to that of the internal standard obtained from the sample solution, and the ratios, Q_{Sa} and Q_{Sb}, of the peak area of oxycodone and hydrocotarnine to that of the internal standard from the standard solution.

Amount (mg) of oxycodone hydrochloride hydrate ($C_{18}H_{21}NO_4.HCl.3H_2O$)
$= M_{Sa} \times Q_{Ta}/Q_{Sa} \times 1/25 \times 1.154$

Amount (mg) of hydrocotarnine hydrochloride hydrate ($C_{12}H_{15}NO_3.HCl.H_2O$)
$= M_{Sb} \times Q_{Tb}/Q_{Sb} \times 1/25 \times 1.070$

M_{Sa}: Amount (mg) of oxycodone hydrochloride hydrate for assay taken, calculated on the anhydrous basis

M_{Sb}: Amount (mg) of hydrocotarnine hydrochloride hydrate for assay taken

Internal standard solution—Dissolve 0.02 g of phenacetin in 10 mL of ethanol (95), and add water to make 100 mL.

Operating conditions—

Detector: An ultraviolet absorption photometer (wavelength: 285 nm).

Column: A stainless steel column about 4 mm in inside diameter and about 15 cm in length, packed with octadecylsilanized polyvinyl alcohol gel polymer for liquid chromatography (5 μm in particle diameter).

Column temperature: A constant temperature of about 25°C.

Mobile phase: To 500 mL of 0.05 mol/L disodium hydrogenphosphate TS add 0.05 mol/L sodium dihydrogenphosphate TS, and adjust the pH to 8.0. To 300 mL of this solution add 200 mL of acetonitrile, and mix.

Flow rate: Adjust so that the retention time of oxycodone hydrochloride is about 8 minutes.

Selection of column: Proceed with 10 μL of the standard solution under the above operating conditions, and use a column giving elution of the internal standard, oxycodone and hydrocotarine in this order with complete separation of these peaks.

(2) Atropine sulfate hydrate—Pipet 2 mL of Compound Oxycodone and Atropine Injection, and add exactly 2 mL of the internal standard solution. To this solution add 10 mL of diluted dilute hydrochloric acid (1 in 10) and 2 mL of ammonia TS, immediately add 20 mL of dichloromethane, shake vigorously, filter the dichloromethane layer through filter paper on which 5 g of anhydrous sodium sulfate is placed, and evaporate the filtrate to dryness under reduced pressure. To the residue add 0.5 mL of 1,2-dichloroethane and 0.5 mL of bis-trimethyl silyl acetamide, stopper tightly, warm in a water bath at 60°C for 15 minutes, and use this solution as the sample solution. Separately, weigh accurately about 30 mg of Atropine Sulfate RS (separately determine the loss on drying <*2.41*> under the same conditions as Atropine Sulfate Hydrate), and dissolve in water to make exactly 100 mL. Pipet 2 mL of this solution, and add exactly 2 mL of the internal standard solution. Proceed with this solution in the same manner as directed for the sample solution, and use so obtained solution as the standard solution. Perform the test with 2 μL each of the sample solution and standard solution as directed under Gas Chromatography <*2.02*> according to the following conditions, and calculate the ratios, Q_T and Q_S, of the peak area of atropine to that of the internal standards.

Amount (mg) of atropine sulfate hydrate
$[(C_{17}H_{23}NO_3)_2.H_2SO_4.H_2O]$
$= M_S \times Q_T/Q_S \times 1/50 \times 1.027$

M_S: Amount (mg) of Atropine Sulfate RS taken, calculated on the dried basis

Internal standard solution—A solution of homatropine hydrobromide (1 in 4000).

Operating conditions—

Detector: A hydrogen flame-ionization detector.

Column: A glass column about 3 mm in inside diameter and about 1.5 m in length, packed with 180- to 250-μm siliceous earth for gas chromatography coated with 1 to 3% of 50% phenyl-methylsilicone polymer.

Column temperature: A constant temperature of about 210°C.

Carrier gas: Nitrogen or helium.

Flow rate: Adjust so that the retention time of atropine is about 5 minutes.

Selection of column: Proceed with 2 μL of the standard solution under the above operating conditions, and calculate the resolution. Use a column giving elution of the internal standard and atropine in this order with the resolution between these peaks being not less than 3.

Containers and storage Containers—Hermetic containers,

and colored containers may be used.

Storage—Light-resistant.

Oxydol

オキシドール

Oxydol contains not less than 2.5 w/v% and not more than 3.5 w/v% of hydrogen peroxide (H_2O_2: 34.01). It contains suitable stabilizers.

Description Oxydol occurs as a clear, colorless liquid. It is odorless or has an odor resembling that of ozone.

It gradually decomposes upon standing or upon vigorous agitation.

It rapidly decomposes when in contact with oxidizing substances as well as reducing substances.

It, when alkalized, decomposes with effervescence.

It is affected by light.

pH: 3.0 – 5.0

Specific gravity d^{20}_{20}: about 1.01

Identification 1 mL of Oxydol responds to Qualitative Tests <*1.09*> for peroxide.

Purity **(1)** Acidity—To 25.0 mL of Oxydol add 2 drops of phenolphthalein TS and 2.5 mL of 0.1 mol/L sodium hydroxide VS: a red color develops.

(2) Heavy metals <*1.07*>—To 5.0 mL of Oxydol add 20 mL of water and 2 mL of ammonia TS, evaporate on a water bath to dryness, dissolve the residue in 2 mL of dilute acetic acid by heating, add water to make 50 mL, and perform the test using this solution as the test solution. Prepare the control solution with 2.5 mL of Standard Lead Solution, 2 mL of dilute acetic acid and water to make 50 mL (not more than 5 ppm).

(3) Arsenic <*1.11*>—To 1.0 mL of Oxydol add 1 mL of ammonia TS, evaporate on a water bath to dryness, take the residue, prepare the test solution according to Method 1, and perform the test (not more than 2 ppm).

(4) Organic stabilizer—Extract 100 mL of Oxydol with 50-mL, 25-mL and 25-mL portions of a mixture of chloroform and diethyl ether (3:2) successively, combine the extracts in a tared vessel, and evaporate the combined extract on a water bath. Dry the residue over silica gel to constant mass: the mass of the residue is not more than 50 mg.

(5) Nonvolatile residue—Evaporate 20.0 mL of Oxydol on a water bath to dryness, and dry the residue at 105°C for 1 hour: the mass of the residue is not more than 20 mg.

Assay Pipet 1.0 mL of Oxydol, transfer it to a flask containing 10 mL of water and 10 mL of dilute sulfuric acid, and titrate <*2.50*> with 0.02 mol/L potassium permanganate VS.

Each mL of 0.02 mol/L potassium permanganate VS
= 1.701 mg of H_2O_2

Containers and storage Containers—Tight containers.

Storage—Light-resistant, and not exceeding 30°C.

Oxygen

酸素

O_2: 32.00

Oxygen is oxygen produced by the air liquification separation method.

It contains not less than 99.5 v/v% of oxygen (O_2).

Description Oxygen is a colorless gas under atmospheric pressure, and is odorless.

1 mL of Oxygen dissolves in 32 mL of water, and in 7 mL of ethanol (95) at 20°C and at a pressure of 101.3 kPa.

1000 mL of Oxygen at 0°C and at a pressure of 101.3 kPa weighs 1.429 g.

Identification Transfer 1 mL each of Oxygen and oxygen directly from cylinders with a pressure-reducing valve to gas-measuring tubes or syringes for gas chromatography, using a polyvinyl chloride induction tube. Perform the test with these gases as directed under Gas Chromatography <*2.02*> according to the following conditions: the retention time of principal peak in the chromatogram obtained from Oxygen is the same as that of the peak in the chromatogram from oxygen.

Operating conditions—

Proceed as directed in the operating conditions in the Purity.

Purity Nitrogen—Transfer 1.0 mL of Oxygen directly from cylinder with a pressure-reducing valve to gas-measuring tube or syringe for gas chromatography, using a polyvinyl chloride induction tube. Perform the test with this gas as directed under Gas Chromatography <*2.02*> according to the following conditions, and determine the peak area A_T of nitrogen. Introduce 0.50 mL of nitrogen into the gas mixer, draw carrier gas into the mixer to make exactly 100 mL, allow to mix thoroughly and use this gas as the standard mixed gas. Perform the test in the same manner with 1.0 mL of this mixture as directed above, and determine the peak area A_S of nitrogen: A_T is not larger than A_S.

Operating conditions—

Detector: A thermal conductivity detector.

Column: A column 3 mm in inside diameter and 3 m in length, packed with zeolite for gas chromatography 250- to 355-μm in particle diameter (a porosity of 0.5 nm).

Column temperature: A constant temperature of about 50°C.

Carrier gas: Hydrogen or helium.

Flow rate: Adjust so that the retention time of nitrogen is about 5 minutes.

System suitability—

System performance: Introduce 0.5 mL of nitrogen into a gas mixer, add Oxygen to make 100 mL, and mix thoroughly. When the test is run with 1.0 mL of the mixture under the above operating conditions, oxygen and nitrogen are eluted in this order with the resolution between these peaks being not less than 1.5.

System repeatability: When the test is repeated 5 times with 1.0 mL of the standard mixed gas under the above operating conditions, the relative standard deviation of the peak area of nitrogen is not more than 2.0%.

Assay Perform the assay by using the magnetic analysis.

(i) Apparatus—Oxygen zero gas for assay and oxygen span gas for assay are delivered individually into an apparatus via a sample gas-introducing system and a switching valve. An apparatus with a pressure detector of magnetic force method has an introducing system not only for the above gases but also for oxygen reference gas for assay. Each gas is delivered at the flow rate specified for the apparatus under control of a flow meter and a manometer.

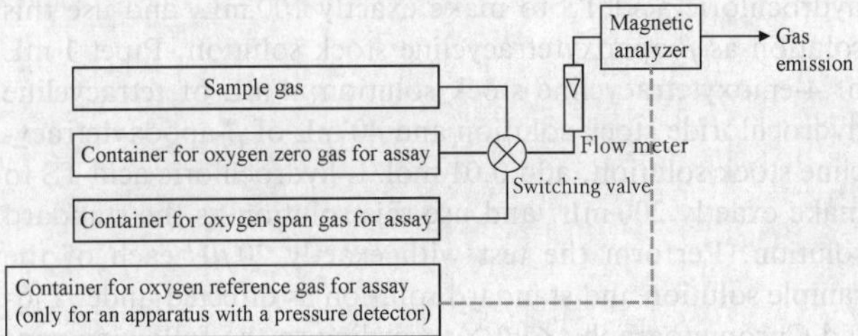

(ii) Procedure—Inject oxygen zero gas for assay into the apparatus at the set flow rate, and set the zero after reaching a stable indication. Then inject oxygen span gas for assay at the specified flow rate, and set the span after reaching a stable indication. Confirm that both these indicated values after the settings are within the specification of the apparatus to confirm the suitability of the apparatus. Stop injecting each calibration gas, inject the sample gas at the specified flow rate, and read the indication V (vol%).

$$\text{Volume (vol\%) of oxygen} = V \text{ (vol\%)}$$

When the apparatus is controlled by periodic calibration, determine appropriately the frequency of calibration according to the apparatus manufacturer's recommendations, past control records, or statistical methods, and maintain the environment for use and the conditions of injection of the sample gas within the range recommended by the apparatus manufacturer.

Containers and storage Containers—Cylinders.

Storage—Not exceeding 40°C.

Oxymetholone

オキシメトロン

$C_{21}H_{32}O_3$: 332.48

17*β*-Hydroxy-2-hydroxymethylene-17*α*-methyl-5*α*-androstan-3-one

[434-07-1]

Oxymetholone, when dried, contains not less than 97.0% and not more than 103.0% of oxymetholone ($C_{21}H_{32}O_3$).

Description Oxymetholone occurs as a white to pale yellow-white crystalline powder. It is odorless.

It is freely soluble in chloroform, soluble in 1,4-dioxane, sparingly soluble in methanol, in ethanol (95) and in acetone, slightly soluble in diethyl ether, and practically insoluble in water.

It is gradually colored and decomposed by light.

Identification **(1)** Dissolve 2 mg of Oxymetholone in 1 mL of ethanol (95), and add 1 drop of iron (III) chloride TS: a purple color develops.

(2) Dissolve 0.01 g of Oxymetholone in methanol to make 50 mL. To 5 mL of the solution add 5 mL of sodium hydroxide-methanol TS and methanol to make 50 mL. Determine the absorption spectrum of the solution as directed under Ultraviolet-visible Spectrophotometry 〈*2.24*〉, and compare the spectrum with the Reference Spectrum: both spectra exhibit similar intensities of absorption at the same wavelengths.

(3) Determine the infrared absorption spectrum of Oxymetholone as directed in the potassium bromide disk method under Infrared Spectrophotometry 〈*2.25*〉, and compare the spectrum with the Reference Spectrum: both spectra exhibit similar intensities of absorption at the same wave numbers.

Optical rotation 〈*2.49*〉 $[\alpha]_D^{20}$: +34 – +38° (after drying, 0.2 g, 1,4-dioxane, 10 mL, 100 mm).

Melting point 〈*2.60*〉 175 – 182°C

Purity **(1)** Clarity and color of solution—Dissolve 0.5 g of Oxymetholone in 25 mL of 1,4-dioxane: the solution is clear, and shows a colorless to pale yellow color.

(2) Related substances—Dissolve 50 mg of Oxymetholone in 5 mL of chloroform, and use this solution as the sample solution. Pipet 1 mL of the sample solution, add chloroform to make exactly 200 mL, and use this solution as the standard solution. Perform the test with these solutions as directed under Thin-layer Chromatography 〈*2.03*〉. Spot 10 *μ*L each of the sample solution and standard solution on a plate of silica gel for thin-layer chromatography, and air-dry the spot. Develop immediately the plate with a mixture of toluene and ethanol (99.5) (49:1) to a distance of about 12 cm, and air-dry the plate. Spray evenly vanillin-sulfuric acid TS on the plate, and heat the plate at 100°C for 3 to 5 minutes: any spot other than the principal spot and starting point obtained from the sample solution is not more intense than the spot from the standard solution.

Loss on drying 〈*2.41*〉 Not more than 1.0% (0.5 g, in vacuum, phosphorus (V) oxide, 4 hours).

Residue on ignition 〈*2.44*〉 Not more than 0.1% (0.5 g).

Assay Weigh accurately about 40 mg of Oxymetholone, previously dried, and dissolve in methanol to make exactly 50 mL. Pipet 5 mL of this solution, and add methanol to make exactly 50 mL. To exactly measured 5 mL of this solution add 5 mL of sodium hydroxide-methanol TS and methanol to make exactly 50 mL. Determine the absorbance A of this solution at the wavelength of maximum absorption at about 315 nm as directed under Ultraviolet-visible Spectrophotometry 〈*2.24*〉, using a solution, prepared by adding methanol to 5 mL of sodium hydroxide-methanol TS to make 50 mL, as the blank.

$$\text{Amount (mg) of oxymetholone } (C_{21}H_{32}O_3) = A/541 \times 50{,}000$$

Containers and storage Containers—Tight containers.

Storage—Light-resistant.

Oxytetracycline Hydrochloride

オキシテトラサイクリン塩酸塩

$C_{22}H_{24}N_2O_9.HCl$: 496.89
(4*S*,4a*R*,5*S*,5a*R*,6*S*,12a*S*)-4-Dimethylamino-3,5,6,10,12,12a-hexahydroxy-6-methyl-1,11-dioxo-1,4,4a,5,5a,6,11,12a-octahydrotetracene-2-carboxamide monohydrochloride
[*2058-46-0*]

Oxytetracycline Hydrochloride is the hydrochloride of a tetracycline substance having antibacterial activity produced by the growth of *Streptomyces rimosus*.

It contains not less than 880 μg (potency) and not more than 945 μg (potency) per mg, calculated on the dried basis. The potency of Oxytetracycline Hydrochloride is expressed as mass (potency) of oxytetracycline ($C_{22}H_{24}N_2O_9$: 460.43).

Description Oxytetracycline Hydrochloride occurs as yellow, crystals or crystalline powder.

It is freely soluble in water, and slightly soluble in ethanol (99.5).

It shows crystal polymorphism.

Identification **(1)** Determine the absorption spectrum of a solution of Oxytetracycline Hydrochloride in 0.1 mol/L hydrochloric acid TS (1 in 50,000) as directed under Ultraviolet-visible Spectrophotometry <*2.24*>, and compare the spectrum with the Reference Spectrum or the spectrum of a solution of Oxytetracycline Hydrochloride RS prepared in the same manner as the sample solution: both spectra exhibit similar intensities of absorption at the same wavelengths.

(2) Determine the infrared absorption spectrum of Oxytetracycline Hydrochloride, previously dried, as directed in the potassium chloride disk method under Infrared Spectrophotometry <*2.25*>, and compare the spectrum with the Reference Spectrum or the spectrum of Oxytetracycline Hydrochloride RS: both spectra exhibit similar intensities of absorption at the same wave numbers. If any difference appears between the spectra, dissolve the sample and the Reference Standard separately in methanol, evaporate the solvent, and perform the test with the residues.

(3) Dissolve 20 mg of Oxytetracycline Hydrochloride in 3 mL of water, and add 1 drop of silver nitrate TS: a white turbidity is produced.

Optical rotation <*2.49*> $[\alpha]_D^{20}$: −188 – −200° (0.25 g calculated on the dried basis, 0.1 mol/L hydrochloric acid, 25 mL, 100 mm).

Purity **(1)** Heavy metals <*1.07*>—Proceed with 0.5 g of Oxytetracycline Hydrochloride according to Method 2, and perform the test. Prepare the control solution with 2.5 mL of Standard Lead Solution (not more than 50 ppm).

(2) Related substances—Dissolve 20 mg of Oxytetracycline Hydrochloride in 0.01 mol/L hydrochloric acid TS to make exactly 25 mL, and use this solution as the sample solution. Separately, dissolve 20 mg of 4-epioxytetracycline in 0.01 mol/L hydrochloric acid TS to make exactly 25 mL, and use this solution as 4-epioxytetracycline stock solution. Separately, dissolve 20 mg of tetracycline hydrochloride in 0.01 mol/L hydrochloric acid TS to make exactly 25 mL, and use this solution as tetracycline hydrochloride stock solution. Separately, dissolve 8 mg of β-apooxytetracycline in 5 mL of 0.01 mol/L sodium hydroxide TS, add 0.01 mol/L hydrochloric acid TS to make exactly 100 mL, and use this solution as β-apooxytetracycline stock solution. Pipet 1 mL of 4-epioxytetracycline stock solution, 4 mL of tetracycline hydrochloride stock solution and 40 mL of β-apooxytetracycline stock solution, add 0.01 mol/L hydrochloric acid TS to make exactly 200 mL, and use this solution as the standard solution. Perform the test with exactly 20 μL each of the sample solution and standard solution as directed under Liquid Chromatography <*2.01*> according to the following conditions, and determine each peak area by the automatic integration method: the peak areas of 4-epioxytetracycline and tetracycline obtained from the sample solution are not larger than each of the peak area from the standard solution, and the total area of the peaks, α-apooxytetracycline having the relative retention time of about 2.1 to oxytetracycline, β-apooxytetracycline and the peaks, which appear between α-apooxytetracycline and β-apooxytetracycline, is not larger than the peak area of β-apooxytetracycline from the standard solution. The peak area of 2-acetyl-2-decarboxamide oxytetracycline, which appears after the principal peak, from the sample solution is not larger than 4 times the peak area of 4-epioxytetracycline from the standard solution.

Operating conditions—

Detector: An ultraviolet absorption photometer (wavelength: 254 nm).

Column: A stainless steel column 4.6 mm in inside diameter and 25 cm in length, packed with styrene-divinylbenzene copolymer for liquid chromatography (8 μm in particle diameter).

Column temperature: A constant temperature of about 60°C.

Mobile phase A: Mix 60 mL of 0.33 mol/L potassium dihydrogen phosphate TS, 100 mL of a solution of tetrabutylammonium hydrogensulfate (1 in 100), 10 mL of a solution of disodium dihydrogen ethylenediamine tetraacetate dihydrate (1 in 2500) and 200 mL of water, and adjust the pH to 7.5 with 2 mol/L sodium hydroxide TS. To this solution add 30 g of *t*-butyl alcohol and water to make 1000 mL.

Mobile phase B: Mix 60 mL of 0.33 mol/L potassium dihydrogen phosphate TS, 50 mL of a solution of tetrabutylammonium hydrogensulfate (1 in 100), 10 mL of a solution of disodium dihydrogen ethylenediamine tetraacetate dihydrate (1 in 2500) and 200 mL of water, and adjust the pH to 7.5 with 2 mol/L sodium hydroxide TS. To this solution add 100 g of *t*-butyl alcohol and water to make 1000 mL.

Flowing of mobile phase: Control the gradient by mixing the mobile phases A and B as directed in the following table.

Time after injection of sample (min)	Mobile phase A (vol%)	Mobile phase B (vol%)
0 – 20	70 → 10	30 → 90
20 – 35	10 → 20	90 → 80

Flow rate: 1.0 mL per minute.

Time span of measurement: About 3.5 times as long as the retention time of oxytetracycline, beginning after the solvent peak.

System suitability—

Test for required detectability: Pipet 1 mL of 4-epioxytetracycline stock solution, and add 0.01 mol/L hydrochloric acid TS to make exactly 200 mL. Pipet 4 mL of this solution, and add 0.01 mol/L hydrochloric acid TS to make exactly 20 mL. Confirm that the peak area of 4-epioxytetracycline obtained with 20 μL of this solution is equivalent to 14 to 26% of that with 20 μL of the standard solution.

System performance: Dissolve 8 mg of α-apooxytetracycline in 5 mL of 0.01 mol/L sodium hydroxide TS, add 0.01 mol/L hydrochloric acid TS to make 100 mL, and use this solution as α-apooxytetracycline stock solution. Mix 3 mL of the sample solution, 2 mL of 4-epioxytetracycline stock solution, 6 mL of tetracycline hydrochloride stock solution, 6 mL of β-apooxytetracycline stock solution and 6 mL of α-apooxytetracycline stock solution, and add 0.01 mol/L hydrochloric acid TS to make 50 mL. When the procedure is run with 20 μL of this solution under the above operating conditions, 4-epioxytetracycline, oxytetracycline, tetracycline, α-apooxytetracycline and β-apooxytetracycline are eluted in this order with the resolutions between the peaks, 4-epioxytetracycline and oxytetracycline, oxytetracycline and tetracycline, and α-apooxytetracycline and β-apooxytetracycline being not less than 4, not less than 5 and not less than 4, respectively, and the symmetry factor of the peak of oxytetracycline is not more than 1.3.

System repeatability: Pipet 1 mL of 4-epioxytetracycline stock solution, and add 0.01 mol/L hydrochloric acid TS to make exactly 200 mL. When the test is repeated 6 times with 20 μL of this solution under the above operating conditions, the relative standard deviation of the peak area of 4-epioxytetracycline is not more than 2.0%.

Loss on drying *<2.41>* Not more than 2.0% (1 g, in vacuum, 60°C, 3 hours).

Residue on ignition *<2.44>* Not more than 0.5% (1 g).

Assay Weigh accurately an amount of Oxytetracycline Hydrochloride and Oxytetracycline Hydrochloride RS, equivalent to about 50 mg (potency), and dissolve each in diluted hydrochloric acid (1 in 100) to make exactly 50 mL. Pipet 5 mL each of these solutions, add diluted methanol (3 in 20) to make exactly 50 mL, and use these solutions as the sample solution and the standard solution. Perform the test with exactly 20 μL each of the sample solution and standard solution as directed under Liquid Chromatography *<2.01>* according to the following conditions, and determine the peak areas, A_T and A_S, of oxytetracycline in each solution.

Amount [μg (potency)] of oxytetracycline ($C_{22}H_{24}N_2O_9$)
$= M_S \times A_T/A_S \times 1000$

M_S: Amount [mg (potency)] of Oxytetracycline Hydrochloride RS taken

Operating conditions—

Detector: An ultraviolet absorption photometer (wavelength: 263 nm).

Column: A stainless steel column 4.6 mm in inside diameter and 25 cm in length, packed with strongly acidic ion exchange resin for liquid chromatography (5 μm in particle diameter).

Column temperature: A constant temperature of about 30°C.

Mobile phase: Dissolve 3.402 g of potassium dihydrogen phosphate and 9.306 g of disodium dihydrogen ethylenediamine tetraacetate dihydrate in 700 mL of water, add 300 mL of methanol, and adjust the pH to 4.5 with dilute hydrochloric acid.

Flow rate: Adjust so that the retention time of oxytetracycline is about 7 minutes.

System suitability—

System performance: When the procedure is run with 20 μL of the standard solution under the above operating conditions, the number of the theoretical plates and the symmetry factor of the peak of oxytetracycline are not less than 1000 and not more than 2.0, respectively.

System repeatability: When the test is repeated 6 times with 20 μL of the standard solution under the above operating conditions, the relative standard deviation of the peak area of oxytetracycline is not more than 1.0%.

Containers and storage Containers—Tight containers.

Storage—Light-resistant.

Oxytocin

オキシトシン

Cys-Tyr-Ile-Gln-Asn-Cys-Pro-Leu-Gly-NH_2

$C_{43}H_{66}N_{12}O_{12}S_2$: 1007.19
[50-56-6]

Oxytocin is synthetic human oxytocin, and is a peptide consisting of 9 amino acid residues.

It contains not less than 540 oxytocin Units and not more than 600 oxytocin Units per mg, calculated on the anhydrous and residual acetic acid-free basis.

Description Oxytocin occurs as a white powder.

It is very soluble in water, and freely soluble in ethanol (99.5).

It dissolves in hydrochloric acid TS.

The pH of a solution prepared by dissolving 0.10 g of Oxytocin in 10 mL of freshly boiled and cooled water is between 4.0 and 6.0.

It is hygroscopic.

Identification Determine the absorption spectrum of a solution of Oxytocin (1 in 2000) as directed under Ultraviolet-visible Spectrophotometry *<2.24>*, and compare the spectrum with the Reference Spectrum: both spectra exhibit similar intensities of absorption at the same wavelengths.

Constituent amino acids Put about 1 mg of Oxytocin in a test tube for hydrolysis, add 6 mol/L hydrochloric acid TS to dissolve, replace the air in the tube with Nitrogen, seal the tube under reduced pressure, and heat at 110 to 115°C for 16 hours. After cooling, open the tube, evaporate the hydrolyzate to dryness under reduced pressure, add 2 mL of 0.02 mol/L hydrochloric acid TS to dissolve the residue, and use this solution as the sample solution. Separately, weigh accurately about 27 mg of L-aspartic acid, about 24 mg of L-threonine, about 21 mg of L-serine, about 29 mg of L-glutamic acid, about 23 mg of L-proline, about 15 mg of glycine, about 18 mg of L-alanine, about 23 mg of L-valine, about 48 mg of L-cystine, about 30 mg of methionine, about 26 mg of L-isoleucine, about 26 mg of L-leucine, about 36 mg of L-tyrosine, about 33 mg of phenylalanine, about 37 mg of L-lysine hydrochloride, about 42 mg of L-histidine hydrochloride monohydrate and about 42 mg of L-arginine hydrochloride, dissolve them in 10 mL of 1 mol/L hydrochloric acid TS, and add water to make exactly 100 mL. Pipet 5 mL of this solution, add water to make exactly 20 mL, and use this solution as the standard solution. Perform the test with exactly 20 μL each of the sample solution and standard solution as directed under Liquid Chromatography *<2.01>*

according to the following conditions, and calculate the respective molar ratios with respect to leucine: 0.95 – 1.05 for aspartic acid, 0.95 – 1.05 for glutamic acid, 0.95 – 1.05 for proline, 0.95 – 1.05 for glycine, 0.80 – 1.10 for isoleucine, 0.80 – 1.05 for tyrosine and 0.80 – 1.05 for cystine, and not more than 0.01 each for others.

Operating conditions—

Detector: A visible spectrophotometer (wavelength: 440 nm and 570 nm).

Column: A stainless steel column 4.6 mm in inside diameter and 8 cm in length, packed with strongly acidic ion-exchange resin for liquid chromatography (Na type) composed with a sulfonated polystyrene copolymer (3 μm in particle diameter).

Column temperature: A constant temperature of about 57°C.

Chemical reaction bath temperature: A constant temperature of about 130°C.

Color developing time: About 1 minute.

Mobile phase: Prepare mobile phases A, B and C according to the following table.

Mobile phase	A	B	C
Citric acid monohydrate	19.80 g	22.00 g	6.10 g
Trisodium citrate dihydrate	6.19 g	7.74 g	26.67 g
Sodium chloride	5.66 g	7.07 g	54.35 g
Ethanol (99.5)	260.0 mL	20.0 mL	—
Benzyl alcohol	—	—	5.0 mL
Thiodiglycol	5.0 mL	5.0 mL	—
Lauromacrogol solution (1 in 4)	4.0 mL	4.0 mL	4.0 mL
Caprylic acid	0.1 mL	0.1 mL	0.1 mL
Water	a sufficient amount	a sufficient amount	a sufficient amount
Total amount	2000 mL	1000 mL	1000 mL

Flowing of mobile phase: Control the gradient by mixing the mobile phases A, B and C as directed in the following table.

Time after injection of sample (min)	Mobile phase A (vol%)	Mobile phase B (vol%)	Mobile phase C (vol%)
0 – 9	100	0	0
9 – 25	0	100	0
25 – 61	0	100 → 0	0 → 100
61 – 80	0	0	100

Reaction reagent: Mix 407 g of lithium acetate dihydrate, 245 mL of acetic acid (100) and 801 mL of 1-methoxy-2-propanol, add water to make 2000 mL, stir for more than 10 minutes while passing Nitrogen, and use this solution as Solution A. Separately, to 1957 mL of 1-methoxy-2-propanol add 77 g of ninhydrin and 0.134 g of sodium borohydride, stir for more than 30 minutes while passing Nitrogen, and use this solution as Solution B. Mix Solution A and Solution B before use.

Flow rate of mobile phase: About 0.26 mL per minute.

Flow rate of reaction reagent: About 0.3 mL per minute.

System suitability—

System performance: When the procedure is run with 20 μL of the standard solution under the above operating conditions, aspartic acid, threonine, serine, glutamic acid, proline, glycine, alanine, valine, cystine, methionine, isoleucine, leucine, tyrosine, phenylalanine, lysine, histidine and arginine are eluted in this order with the resolutions between the peaks of threonine and serine, glycine and alanine, and isoleucine and leucine being not less than 1.5, 1.4 and 1.2, respectively.

System repeatability: When the test is repeated 3 times with 20 μL of the standard solution under the above operating conditions, the relative standard deviations of the peak area of aspartic acid, proline, valine and arginine are not more than 2.0%, respectively.

Purity **(1)** Acetic acid—Weigh accurately about 15 mg of Oxytocin, dissolve in the internal standard solution to make exactly 10 mL, and use this solution as the sample solution. Separately, weigh accurately about 1 g of acetic acid (100), add the internal standard solution to make exactly 100 mL. Pipet 2 mL of this solution, add the internal standard solution to make exactly 200 mL, and use this solution as the standard solution. Perform the test with 10 μL each of the sample solution and standard solution as directed under Liquid Chromatography <2.01> according to the following conditions, and calculate the ratios, Q_T and Q_S, of the peak area of acetic acid to that of the internal standard: the amount of acetic acid is not less than 6.0% and not more than 10.0%.

$$\text{Amount (\%) of acetic acid } (C_2H_4O_2) = M_S/M_T \times Q_T/Q_S \times 1/10$$

M_S: Amount (mg) of acetic acid (100) taken
M_T: Amount (mg) of Oxytocin taken

*Internal standard solution—*A solution of propionic acid in the mobile phase (1 in 10,000).

Operating conditions—

Detector: An ultraviolet absorption photometer (wavelength: 210 nm).

Column: A stainless steel column 4.6 mm in inside diameter and 15 cm in length, packed with octadecylsilanized silica gel for liquid chromatography (5 μm in particle diameter).

Column temperature: A constant temperature of about 40°C.

Mobile phase: To 0.7 mL of phosphoric acid add 900 mL of water, adjust the pH to 3.0 with 8 mol/L sodium hydroxide TS, and add water to make 1000 mL. To 950 mL of this solution add 50 mL of methanol.

Flow rate: Adjust so that the retention time of acetic acid is about 3 minutes.

System suitability—

System performance: When the procedure is run with 10 μL of the standard solution under the above operating conditions, acetic acid and propionic acid are eluted in this order with the resolution between these peaks being not less than 14.

System repeatability: When the test is repeated 6 times with 10 μL of the standard solution under the above operating conditions, the relative standard deviation of the ratio of the peak area of acetic acid to that of the internal standard is not more than 2.0%.

(2) Related substances—Dissolve 25 mg of Oxytocin in 100 mL of the mobile phase A, and use this solution as the sample solution. Perform the test with 50 μL of the sample solution as directed under Liquid Chromatography <2.01> according to the following conditions, determine each peak area by the automatic integration method, and calculate the amount of them by the area percentage method: the amount of each peak other than Oxytocin is not more than 1.5%, and the total of them is not more than 5.0%.

Operating conditions—

Detector, column, column temperature, mobile phase, flowing of mobile phase, and flow rate: Proceed as directed in the operating conditions in the Assay.

Time span of measurement: About 2.5 times as long as the retention time of oxytocin.

System suitability—

Test for required detectability: Measure exactly 1 mL of the sample solution, add the mobile phase A to make exactly 100 mL, and use this solution as the solution for system suitability test. Pipet 1 mL of the solution for system suitability test, and add the mobile phase A to make exactly 10 mL. Confirm that the peak area of oxytocin obtained with 50 μL of this solution is equivalent to 5 to 15% of that with 50 μL of the solution for system suitability test.

System performance: Dissolve an adequate amount of oxytocin and vasopressin in the mobile phase A, so that each mL contains about 0.1 mg each of them. When the procedure is run with 50 μL of this solution under the above operating conditions, vasopressin and oxytocin are eluted in this order with the resolution between these peaks being not less than 14, and the symmetry factor of the peak of oxytocin is not more than 1.5.

System repeatability: When the test is repeated 6 times with 50 μL of the solution for system suitability test under the above operating conditions, the relative standard deviation of the peak area of oxytocin is not more than 2.0%.

Water <*2.48*> Not more than 5.0% (50 mg, coulometric titration).

Assay Weigh accurately an amount of Oxytocin, equivalent to about 13,000 Units, dissolve in the mobile phase A to make exactly 100 mL, and use this solution as the sample solution. Separately, dissolve 1 bottle of the Oxytocin RS in the mobile phase A to make a known concentration solution containing each mL contains about 130 Units, and use this solution as the standard solution. Perform the test with exactly 25 μL each of the sample solution and standard solution as directed under Liquid Chromatography <*2.01*> according to the following conditions, and determine the peak areas, A_T and A_S, of oxytocin in each solution.

Units per mg of Oxytocin, calculated on the anhydrous and residual acetic acid-free basis
$$= M_S/M_T \times A_T/A_S \times 100$$

M_S: Units per mL of the standard solution

M_T: Amount (mg) of Oxytocin taken, calculated on the anhydrous and residual acetic acid-free basis

Operating conditions—

Detector: An ultraviolet absorption photometer (wavelength: 220 nm).

Column: A stainless steel column 4.6 mm in inside diameter and 15 cm in length, packed with octadecylsilanized silica gel for liquid chromatography (5 μm in particle diameter).

Column temperature: A constant temperature of about 25°C.

Mobile phase A: Dissolve 15.6 g of sodium dihydrogen phosphate dihydrate in 1000 mL of water.

Mobile phase B: A mixture of water and acetonitrile (1:1).

Flowing of mobile phase: Control the gradient by mixing the mobile phases A and B as directed in the following table.

Time after injection of sample (min)	Mobile phase A (vol%)	Mobile phase B (vol%)
0 – 30	70 → 40	30 → 60
30 – 30.1	40 → 70	60 → 30
30.1 – 45	70	30

Flow rate: 1.0 mL per minute.

System suitability—

System performance: Dissolve an adequate amount of oxytocin and vasopressin in the mobile phase A, so that each mL contains about 0.1 mg each of them. When the procedure is run with 25 μL of this solution under the above operating conditions, vasopressin and oxytocin are eluted in this order with the resolution between these peaks being not less than 14, and the symmetry factor of the peak of oxytocin is not more than 1.5.

System repeatability: When the test is repeated 6 times with 25 μL of the standard solution under the above operating conditions, the relative standard deviation of the peak area of oxytocin is not more than 1.0%.

Containers and storage Containers—Tight containers.

Storage—At 2 to 8°C.

Oxytocin Injection

オキシトシン注射液

Oxytocin Injection is an aqueous injection.

It contains not less than 90.0% and not more than 110.0% of the labeled oxytocin Units.

Method of preparation Prepare as directed under Injections, with Oxytocin.

Description Oxytocin Injection is a colorless, clear liquid.

pH <*2.54*> 2.5 – 4.5

Bacterial endotoxins <*4.01*> Less than 10 EU/oxytocin Unit.

Extractable volume <*6.05*> It meets the requirement.

Foreign insoluble matter <*6.06*> Perform the test according to the Method 1: it meets the requirement.

Insoluble particulate matter <*6.07*> It meets the requirement.

Sterility <*4.06*> Perform the test according to the Membrane filtration method: it meets the requirement.

Assay Measure exactly a portion of Oxytocin Injection according to the labeled Units, dilute with the diluent so that each mL contains about 1 Unit, and use this solution as the sample solution. Separately, dissolve 1 bottle of Oxytocin RS in the mobile phase A to make exactly 20 mL. Pipet a suitable volume of this solution, dilute with the diluent to make a known concentration solution so that each mL contains about 1 Unit, and use this solution as the standard solution. Perform the test with exactly 100 μL each of the sample solution and standard solution as directed under Liquid Chromatography <*2.01*> according to the following conditions, and determine the peak areas, A_T and A_S, of oxytocin in each solution.

Units per mL of Oxytocin Injection
$$= M_S \times A_T/A_S \times b/a$$

M_S: Units per mL of the standard solution
a: Volume (mL) of Oxytocin Injection taken
b: Total volume of the sample solution prepared by diluting with the diluent

Diluent: Dissolve 5 g of chlorobutanol, 1.1 g of sodium acetate trihydrate, 5 g of acetic acid (100) and 6 mL of ethanol (99.5) in water to make 1000 mL.

Operating conditions—

Detector: An ultraviolet absorption photometer (wavelength: 220 nm).

Column: A stainless steel column 4.6 mm in inside diameter and 15 cm in length, packed with octadecylsilanized silica gel for liquid chromatography (5 μm in particle diameter).

Column temperature: A constant temperature of about 25°C.

Mobile phase A: Dissolve 15.6 g of sodium dihydrogen phosphate dihydrate in 1000 mL of water.

Mobile phase B: A mixture of water and acetonitrile (1:1).

Flowing of mobile phase: Control the gradient by mixing the mobile phases A and B as directed in the following table.

Time after injection of sample (min)	Mobile phase A (vol%)	Mobile phase B (vol%)
0 - 30	70 → 40	30 → 60
30 - 30.1	40 → 70	60 → 30
30.1 - 45	70	30

Flow rate: 1.0 mL per minute.

System suitability—

System performance: Dissolve an adequate amount of oxytocin and vasopressin in the mobile phase A, so that each mL contains about 0.02 mg each of them. When the procedure is run with 100 μL of this solution under the above operating conditions, vasopressin and oxytocin are eluted in this order with the resolution between these peaks being not less than 14, and the symmetry factor of the peak of oxytocin is not more than 1.5.

System repeatability: When the test is repeated 6 times with 100 μL of the standard solution under the above operating conditions, the relative standard deviation of the peak area of oxytocin is not more than 2.0%.

Containers and storage Containers—Hermetic containers.
Storage—In a cold place, and avoid freezing.

Ozagrel Sodium

オザグレルナトリウム

$C_{13}H_{11}N_2NaO_2$: 250.23
Monosodium (2*E*)-3-[4-(1*H*-imidazol-1-ylmethyl)phenyl]prop-2-enoate
[*189224-26-8*]

Ozagrel Sodium, when dried, contains not less than 98.0% and not more than 102.0% of ozagrel sodium ($C_{13}H_{11}N_2NaO_2$).

Description Ozagrel Sodium occurs as white, crystals or crystalline powder.

It is freely soluble in water, soluble in methanol, and practically insoluble in ethanol (99.5).

Identification (1) Determine the absorption spectrum of a solution of Ozagrel Sodium (1 in 200,000) as directed under Ultraviolet-visible Spectrophotometry <*2.24*>, and compare the spectrum with the Reference Spectrum or the spectrum of a solution of Ozagrel Sodium RS prepared in the same manner as the sample solution: both spectra exhibit similar intensities of absorption at the same wavelengths.

(2) Determine the infrared absorption spectrum of Ozagrel Sodium as directed in the potassium bromide disk method under Infrared Spectrophotometry <*2.25*>, and compare the spectrum with the Reference Spectrum or the spectrum of Ozagrel Sodium RS: both spectra exhibit similar intensities of absorption at the same wave numbers.

(3) A solution of Ozagrel Sodium (1 in 20) responds to Qualitative Tests <*1.09*> for sodium salt.

pH <*2.54*> The pH of a solution prepared by dissolving 0.5 g of Ozagrel Sodium in 10 mL of water is between 9.5 and 10.5.

Purity (1) Clarity and color of solution—Dissolve 0.5 g of Ozagrel Sodium in 10 mL of water: the solution is clear and colorless.

(2) Chloride <*1.03*>—Dissolve 2.0 g of Ozagrel Sodium in 30 mL of water, add 1 mL of acetic acid (100) and water to make 50 mL, shake, and allow to stand for 30 minutes. Filter the solution, discard the first 5 mL of the filtrate, and to 25 mL of the subsequent filtrate add 6 mL of dilute nitric acid and water to make 50 mL. Perform the test with this solution as the test solution. Prepare the control solution as follows: To 0.35 mL of 0.01 mol/L hydrochloric acid VS add 0.5 mL of acetic acid (100), 6 mL of dilute nitric acid and water to make 50 mL (not more than 0.012%).

(3) Heavy metals <*1.07*>—Proceed with 2.0 g of Ozagrel Sodium according to Method 2, and perform the test. Prepare the control solution with 2.0 mL of Standard Lead Solution (not more than 10 ppm).

(4) Related substances—Dissolve 50 mg of Ozagrel Sodium in 100 mL of the mobile phase, and use this solution as the sample solution. Perform the test with 5 μL of the sample solution as directed under Liquid Chromatography <*2.01*> according to the following conditions. Determine each peak area by the automatic integration method, and calculate the amount of them by the area percentage method: each of the amount other than ozagrel is not more than 0.2%, and the total amount other than ozagrel is not more than 0.5%.

Operating conditions—

Column, column temperature, mobile phase, and flow rate: Proceed as directed in the operating conditions in the Assay.

Detector: An ultraviolet absorption photometer (wavelength: 220 nm).

Time span of measurement: About 2 times as long as the retention time of ozagrel, beginning after the solvent peak.

System suitability—

Test for required detectability: Pipet 1 mL of the sample solution, and add the mobile phase to make exactly 200 mL, and use this solution as the solution for system suitability test. Pipet 2 mL of the solution for system suitability test, and add the mobile phase to make exactly 10 mL. Confirm that the peak area of ozagrel obtained with 5 μL of this solution is equivalent to 15 to 25% of that with 5 μL of the solution for system suitability test.

System performance: When the procedure is run with 5 μL of the solution for system suitability test under the above operating conditions, the number of theoretical plates and the symmetry factor of the peak of ozagrel are not less than 6000 and not more than 2.0, respectively.

System repeatability: When the test is repeated 6 times with 5 μL of the solution for system suitability test under the above operating conditions, the relative standard deviation of the peak area of ozagrel is not more than 2.0%.

Loss on drying *<2.41>* Not more than 0.5% (1 g, 105°C, 4 hours).

Assay Weigh accurately about 25 mg each of Ozagrel Sodium and Ozagrel Sodium RS, both previously dried, and dissolve each in methanol to make exactly 25 mL. Pipet 5 mL each of these solutions, add exactly 5 mL of the internal standard solution, and use these solutions as the sample solution and the standard solution, respectively. Perform the test with 1 μL each of the sample solution and standard solution as directed under Liquid Chromatography *<2.01>* according to the following conditions, and calculate the ratios, Q_T and Q_S, of the peak area of ozagrel to that of the internal standard.

Amount (mg) of ozagrel sodium ($C_{13}H_{11}N_2NaO_2$)
$= M_S \times Q_T/Q_S$

M_S: Amount (mg) of Ozagrel Sodium RS taken

Internal standard solution—A solution of benzoic acid in methanol (1 in 100).

Operating conditions—

Detector: An ultraviolet absorption photometer (wavelength: 272 nm).

Column: A stainless steel column 4.6 mm in inside diameter and 15 cm in length, packed with octadecylsilanized silica gel for liquid chromatography (5 μm in particle diameter).

Column temperature: A constant temperature of about 25°C.

Mobile phase: A mixture of a solution of ammonium acetate (3 in 1000) and methanol (4:1).

Flow rate: Adjust so that the retention time of ozagrel is about 10 minutes.

System suitability—

System performance: When the procedure is run with 1 μL of the standard solution under the above operating conditions, the internal standard and ozagrel are eluted in this order with the resolution between these peaks being not less than 2.0, and the symmetry factor of the peak of ozagrel is not more than 2.0.

System repeatability: When the test is repeated 6 times with 1 μL of the standard solution under the above operating conditions, the relative standard deviation of the ratio of the peak area of ozagrel to that of the internal standard is not more than 1.0%.

Containers and storage Containers—Tight containers.

Storage—Light-resistant.

Ozagrel Sodium Injection

オザグレルナトリウム注射液

Ozagrel Sodium Injection is an aqueous injection.

It contains not less than 95.0% and not more than 105.0% of the labeled amount of ozagrel sodium ($C_{13}H_{11}N_2NaO_2$: 250.23).

Method of preparation Prepare as directed under Injections, with Ozagrel Sodium.

Description Ozagrel Sodium Injection occurs as a clear and colorless liquid.

Identification To a suitable volume of Ozagrel Sodium Injection add water so that each mL contains 5 μg of Ozagrel Sodium. Determine the absorption spectrum of this solution as directed under Ultraviolet-visible Spectrophotometry *<2.24>*: it exhibits a maximum between 269 nm and 273 nm.

pH Being specified separately when the drug is granted approval based on the Law.

Purity Related substance—To a suitable volume of Ozagrel Sodium Injection add the mobile phase so that each mL contains 0.4 mg of Ozagrel Sodium, and use this solution as the sample solution. Then, proceed as directed in the Purity (4) under Ozagrel Sodium.

Bacterial endotoxins *<4.01>* Less than 3.7 EU/mg.

Extractable volume *<6.05>* It meets the requirement.

Foreign insoluble matter *<6.06>* Perform the test according to Method 1: it meets the requirement.

Insoluble particulate matter *<6.07>* It meets the requirement.

Sterility *<4.06>* Perform the test according to the Membrane filtration method: it meets the requirement.

Assay Perform the test following the test 1). The test 2) may be performed instead of 1), if possible.

1) To exactly a volume of Ozagrel Sodium Injection, equivalent to about 4 mg of ozagrel sodium ($C_{13}H_{11}N_2NaO_2$), add exactly 5 mL of the internal standard solution and methanol to make 100 mL, and use this solution as the sample solution. Separately, weigh accurately about 40 mg of Ozagrel Sodium RS, previously dried at 105°C for 4 hours, and dissolve in methanol to make exactly 50 mL. Pipet 5 mL of this solution, add exactly 5 mL of the internal standard solution, add 10 mL of water, then add methanol to make 100 mL, and use this solution as the standard solution. Then, proceed as directed in the Assay under Ozagrel Sodium.

Amount (mg) of ozagrel sodium ($C_{13}H_{11}N_2NaO_2$)
$= M_S \times Q_T/Q_S \times 1/10$

M_S: Amount (mg) of Ozagrel Sodium RS taken

Internal standard solution—A solution of benzoic acid in methanol (1 in 100).

2) To exactly a volume of Ozagrel Sodium Injection, equivalent to about 20 mg of ozagrel sodium ($C_{13}H_{11}N_2NaO_2$) add water to make exactly 10 mL. Pipet 1 mL of this solution, add exactly 2 mL of the internal standard solution, add 1 mL of water, and use this solution as the sample solution. Separately, weigh accurately about 25 mg of Ozagrel Sodium RS, previously dried at 105°C for 4 hours, and dissolve in methanol to make exactly 25 mL. Pipet 1 mL of this solution, add exactly 1 mL of the internal standard solution, and use this solution as the standard solution. Then, proceed as directed in the Assay under Ozagrel Sodium.

Amount (mg) of ozagrel sodium ($C_{13}H_{11}N_2NaO_2$)
$= M_S \times Q_T/Q_S \times 4/5$

M_S: Amount (mg) of Ozagrel Sodium RS taken

Internal standard solution—A solution of benzoic acid in methanol (1 in 100).

Containers and storage Containers—Hermetic containers.

Plastic containers for aqueous injections may be used.
Storage—Light-resistant.

Ozagrel Sodium for Injection

注射用オザグレルナトリウム

Ozagrel Sodium for Injection is a preparation for injection, which is dissolved before use.

It contains not less than 95.0% and not more than 105.0% of the labeled amount of ozagrel sodium ($C_{13}H_{11}N_2NaO_2$: 250.23).

Method of preparation Prepare as directed under Injections, with Ozagrel Sodium.

Description Ozagrel Sodium for Injection occurs as white, masses or powder.

Identification Dissolve an amount of Ozagrel Sodium for Injection, equivalent to 40 mg of Ozagrel Sodium, in water to make 40 mL. To 1 mL of this solution add water to make 200 mL, and determine the absorption spectrum of this solution as directed under Ultraviolet-visible Spectrophotometry <*2.24*>: it exhibits a maximum between 269 nm and 273 nm.

pH Being specified separately when the drug is granted approval based on the Law.

Purity Related substances—Dissolve an amount of Ozagrel Sodium for Injection, equivalent to 0.20 g of Ozagrel Sodium, in the mobile phase to make 100 mL. To 5 mL of this solution add the mobile phase to make 20 mL, and use this solution as the sample solution. Then, proceed as directed in the Purity (4) under Ozagrel Sodium.

Bacterial endotoxins <*4.01*> Less than 3.7 EU/mg.

Uniformity of dosage units <*6.02*> It meets the requirement of the Mass variation test.

Foreign insoluble matter <*6.06*> Perform the test according to Method 2: it meets the requirement.

Insoluble particulate matter <*6.07*> It meets the requirement.

Sterility <*4.06*> Perform the test according to the Membrane filtration method: it meets the requirement.

Assay Take a number of Ozagrel Sodium for Injection, equivalent to about 0.4 g of ozagrel sodium ($C_{13}H_{11}N_2NaO_2$), and dissolve all the contents in water to make exactly 200 mL. Pipet 5 mL of this solution, add exactly 10 mL of the internal standard solution and 5 mL of water, mix, and use this solution as the sample solution. Separately, weigh accurately about 25 mg of Ozagrel Sodium RS, previously dried at 105°C for 4 hours, and dissolve in methanol to make exactly 25 mL. Pipet 5 mL of this solution, add exactly 5 mL of the internal standard solution, and use this solution as the standard solution. Then, proceed as directed in the Assay under Ozagrel Sodium.

$$\text{Amount (mg) of ozagrel sodium } (C_{13}H_{11}N_2NaO_2) = M_S \times Q_T/Q_S \times 16$$

M_S: Amount (mg) of Ozagrel Sodium RS taken

Internal standard solution—A solution of benzoic acid in methanol (1 in 100).

Containers and storage Containers—Hermetic containers.

Pancreatin

パンクレアチン

Pancreatin is a substance containing enzymes prepared from the pancreas of edible animals, mostly the hog, and has amylolytic, proteolytic and lipolytic activities.

It contains not less than 2800 starch saccharifying activity units, not less than 28,000 proteolytic activity units, and not less than 960 lipolytic activity units per g.

It is usually diluted with suitable excipients.

Description Pancreatin occurs as a white to light yellow powder. It has a characteristic odor.

Purity (1) Rancidity—Pancreatin has no unpleasant or rancid odor and is tasteless.

(2) Fat—Add 20 mL of diethyl ether to 1.0 g of Pancreatin, extract with occasional shaking for 30 minutes, and filter. Wash the residue with 10 mL of diethyl ether, combine the washing with the filtrate, evaporate the diethyl ether, and dry the residue at 105°C for 2 hours: the mass of the residue does not exceed 20 mg.

Loss on drying <*2.41*> Not more than 4.0% (1 g, in vacuum, phosphorus (V) oxide, 24 hours).

Residue on ignition <*2.44*> Not more than 5% (1 g).

Assay (1) Starch digestive activity <*4.03*>

(i) Substrate solution—Use potato starch TS for amylolytic activity test, prepared by adding 10 mL of phosphate buffer solution for pancreatin instead of 10 mL of 1 mol/L acetic acid-sodium acetate buffer solution (pH 5.0).

(ii) Sample solution—Weigh accurately about 0.1 g of Pancreatin, add a suitable amount of ice-cold water, stir, and add ice-cold water to make exactly 100 mL. Pipet 10 mL of this solution, and add ice-cold water to make exactly 100 mL.

(iii) Procedure—Proceed as directed in 1.1. Measurement of starch saccharifying activity of 1. Assay for starch digestive activity under Digestion Test.

(2) Protein digestive activity <*4.03*>

(i) Substrate solution—Use the substrate solution 2 described in 2.3. (ii) of 2. Assay for protein digestive activity under Digestion Test after adjusting the pH to 8.5.

(ii) Sample solution—Weigh accurately about 0.1 g of Pancreatin, add a suitable amount of ice-cold water, stir, and add ice-cold water to make exactly 200 mL.

(iii) Procedure—Proceed as directed in 2. Assay for protein digestive activity under Digestion Test, using trichloroacetic acid TS B as the precipitation reagent.

(3) Fat digestive activity <*4.03*>

(i) Emulsifier—Prepare with 18 g of polyvinyl alcohol I and 2 g of polyvinyl alcohol II as directed in 3. Assay for fat digestive activity under Digestion Test.

(ii) Substrate solution—Use the substrate solution described in 3. Assay for fat digestive activity under the Digestion Test.

(iii) Sample solution—Weigh accurately about 0.1 g of Pancreatin, add a suitable amount of ice-cold water, stir, and add ice-cold water to make exactly 100 mL.

(iv) Procedure—Proceed as directed in 3. Assay for fat digestive activity under Digestion Test, using phosphate buffer solution (pH 8.0) as the buffer solution.

Containers and storage Containers—Tight containers.
Storage—Not exceeding 30°C.

Pancuronium Bromide

パンクロニウム臭化物

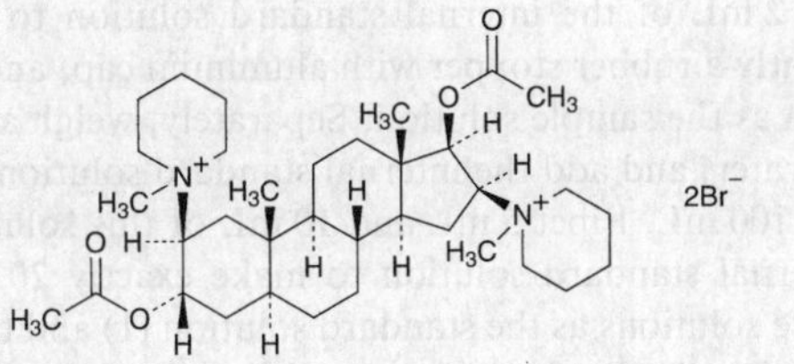

$C_{35}H_{60}Br_2N_2O_4$: 732.67
1,1′-(3α,17β-Diacetoxy-5α-androstan-2β,16β-diyl)bis(1-methylpiperidinium) dibromide
[*15500-66-0*]

Pancuronium Bromide contains not less than 98.0% and not more than 102.0% of pancuronium bromide ($C_{35}H_{60}Br_2N_2O_4$), calculated on the anhydrous basis.

Description Pancuronium Bromide occurs as a white crystalline powder.

It is very soluble in water, and freely soluble in ethanol (95) and in acetic anhydride.

It is hygroscopic.

Identification **(1)** Determine the infrared absorption spectrum of Pancuronium Bromide as directed in the potassium bromide disk method under Infrared Spectrophotometry <*2.25*>, and compare the spectrum with the Reference Spectrum: both spectra exhibit similar intensities of absorption at the same wave numbers.

(2) A solution of Pancuronium Bromide (1 in 100) responds to Qualitative Tests <*1.09*> (1) for bromide.

Optical rotation <*2.49*> $[\alpha]_D^{20}$: +38 – +42° (0.75 g calculated on the anhydrous basis, water, 25 mL, 100 mm).

pH <*2.54*> The pH of a solution of Pancuronium Bromide (1 in 100) is between 4.5 and 6.5.

Purity **(1)** Clarity and color of solution—Dissolve 1.0 g of Pancuronium Bromide in 10 mL of water: the solution is clear and colorless.

(2) Related substances—Dissolve 50 mg of Pancuronium Bromide in 5 mL of ethanol (95), and use this solution as the sample solution. Pipet 1 mL of the sample solution, add ethanol (95) to make exactly 100 mL, and use this solution as the standard solution (1). Separately, weigh exactly 5 mg of dacuronium bromide for thin-layer chromatography, add ethanol (95) to make exactly 25 mL, and use this solution as the standard solution (2). Perform the test with these solutions as directed under Thin-layer Chromatography <*2.03*>. Spot 2 μL each of the sample solution and standard solutions (1) and (2) on a plate of silica gel for thin-layer chromatography. Develop the plate with a mixture of 2-propanol, acetonitrile and a solution of sodium iodide (1 in 5) (17:2:1) to a distance of about 12 cm, and air-dry the plate. Spray evenly a solution of sodium nitrite in methanol (1 in 100) on the plate, allow to stand for 2 minutes, and spray evenly potassium bismuth iodide TS on the plate: a spot obtained from the sample solution, corresponding to that from the standard solution (2), has no more color than that from the standard solution (2), and the spots other than the principal spot and the above mentioned spot from the sample solution have no more color than the spot from the standard solution (1).

Water <*2.48*> Not more than 8.0% (0.3 g, volumetric titration, direct titration).

Residue on ignition <*2.44*> Not more than 0.1% (1 g).

Assay Weigh accurately about 0.2 g of Pancuronium Bromide, dissolve in 50 mL of acetic anhydride by warming, and titrate <*2.50*> with 0.1 mol/L perchloric acid VS (potentiometric titration). Perform a blank determination in the same manner, and make any necessary correction.

Each mL of 0.1 mol/L perchloric acid VS
= 36.63 mg of $C_{35}H_{60}Br_2N_2O_4$

Containers and storage Containers—Tight containers.
Storage—Light-resistant.

Panipenem

パニペネム

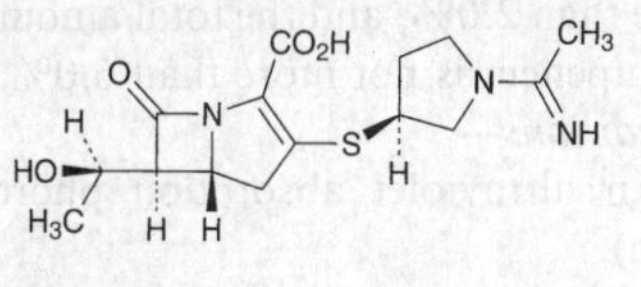

$C_{15}H_{21}N_3O_4S$: 339.41
(5*R*,6*S*)-6-[(1*R*)-1-Hydroxyethyl]-3-[(3*S*)-1-(1-iminoethyl)pyrrolidin-3-ylsulfanyl]-7-oxo-1-azabicyclo[3.2.0]hept-2-ene-2-carboxylic acid
[*87726-17-8*]

Panipenem contains not less than 900 μg (potency) and not more than 1010 μg (potency) per mg, calculated on the anhydrous and residual solvent-free basis. The potency of Panipenem is expressed as mass (potency) of panipenem ($C_{15}H_{21}N_3O_4S$).

Description Panipenem occurs as a white to light yellow, crystalline powder or mass.

It is very soluble in water, freely soluble in methanol, slightly soluble in ethanol (99.5), and practically insoluble in diethyl ether.

It is hygroscopic.

It deliquesces in the presence of moisture.

Identification **(1)** Dissolve 20 mg of Panipenem in 2 mL of water, add 1 mL of hydroxylammonium chloride-ethanol TS, allow to stand for 3 minutes, add 1 mL of acidic ammonium iron (III) sulfate TS, and shake: a red-brown color develops.

(2) Determine the absorption spectrum of a solution of Panipenem in 0.02 mol/L 3-(*N*-morpholino)propanesulfonic acid buffer solution (pH 7.0) (1 in 50,000) as directed under Ultraviolet-visible Spectrophotometry <*2.24*>, and compare the spectrum with the Reference Spectrum: both spectra exhibit similar intensities of absorption at the same wavelengths.

(3) Determine the infrared absorption spectrum of Panipenem as directed in the potassium bromide disk method under Infrared Spectrophotometry <*2.25*>, and compare the spectrum with the Reference Spectrum: both spectra exhibit similar intensities of absorption at the same wave numbers.

Optical rotation <*2.49*> $[\alpha]_D^{20}$: +55 – +65° (0.1 g calculated on the anhydrous and residual solvent-free basis, 0.1 mol/L

3-(*N*-morpholino)propanesulfonic acid buffer solution (pH 7.0), 10 mL, 100 mm).

pH <*2.54*> Dissolve 0.5 g of Panipenem in 10 mL of water: the pH of the solution is between 4.5 and 6.5.

Purity **(1)** Clarity and color of solution—Dissolve 0.30 g of Panipenem in 40 mL of water, and observe immediately: the solution is clear and its absorbance at 400 nm determined as directed under Ultraviolet-visible Spectrophotometry <*2.24*> is not more than 0.4.

(2) Heavy metals <*1.07*>—Proceed with 1.0 g of Panipenem according to Method 4, and perform the test. Prepare the control solution with 2.0 mL of Standard Lead Solution (not more than 20 ppm).

(3) Related substances—Keep the sample solution at 5°C or below. Dissolve 50 mg of Panipenem in 50 mL of water, and use this solution as the sample solution. Perform the test with 10 μL of the sample solution as directed under Liquid Chromatography <*2.01*> according to the following conditions. Determine each peak area by the automatic integration method, and calculate the amount of them by the area percentage method: the amount of the peak other than panipenem is not more than 2.0%, and the total amount of the peaks other than panipenem is not more than 6.0%.

Operating conditions—

Detector: An ultraviolet absorption photometer (wavelength: 220 nm).

Column: A stainless steel column 4 mm in inside diameter and 25 cm in length, packed with octadecylsilanized porous glass for liquid chromatography (7 μm in particle diameter).

Column temperature: A constant temperature of about 40°C.

Mobile phase A: Dissolve 3.12 g of sodium dihydrogen phosphate dihydrate in 700 mL of water, adjust to pH 8.0 with dilute sodium hydroxide TS, then add water to make 1000 mL, and add 20 mL of acetonitrile.

Mobile phase B: Dissolve 3.12 g of sodium dihydrogen phosphate dihydrate in 700 mL of water, adjust to pH 8.0 with dilute sodium hydroxide TS, then add water to make 1000 mL. To 750 mL of this solution add 250 mL of acetonitrile.

Flowing of mobile phase: Control the gradient by mixing the mobile phases A and B as directed in the following table.

Time after injection of sample (min)	Mobile phase A (vol%)	Mobile phase B (vol%)
0 – 15	100	0
15 – 50	100 → 0	0 → 100

Flow rate: 1.0 mL per minute (the retention time of panipenem is about 16 minutes).

Time span of measurement: For 50 minutes after injection, beginning after the solvent peak.

System suitability—

Test for required detectability: Use a solution of Panipenem (1 in 100,000) as the solution for system suitability test. Pipet 1 mL of the solution for system suitability test, add water to make exactly 10 mL. Confirm that the peak area of panipenem obtained with 10 μL of this solution is equivalent to 7 to 13% of that with 10 μL of the solution for system suitability test.

System performance: When the procedure is run with 10 μL of the solution for system suitability test under the above conditions, the number of theoretical plates and the symmetry factor of the peak of panipenem are not less than 3000 and not more than 1.5, respectively.

System repeatability: When the test is repeated 6 times with 10 μL of the solution for system suitability test under the above conditions, the relative standard deviation of the peak area of panipenem is not more than 2.0%.

Water Weigh accurately about 0.5 g of Panipenem, transfer to a 15-mL narrow-mouthed cylindrical glass bottle, add exactly 2 mL of the internal standard solution to dissolve, seal tightly a rubber stopper with aluminum cap, and use this solution as the sample solution. Separately, weigh accurately 2 g of water, and add the internal standard solution to make exactly 100 mL. Pipet 5 mL and 10 mL of this solution, add the internal standard solution to make exactly 20 mL, and use these solutions as the standard solution (1) and the standard solution (2). Perform the test with 1 μL of the sample solution and standard solutions (1) and (2) as directed under Gas Chromatography <*2.02*> according to the following condition, and calculate the ratios, Q_T, Q_{S1} and Q_{S2} of the peak area of water to that of the internal standard. Calculate the amount of water by the following formula: water is not more than 5.0%.

$$\text{Amount of water (\%)} = M_S/M_T \times (Q_T + Q_{S2} - 2Q_{S1})/2(Q_{S2} - Q_{S1}) \times 1/100 \times 100$$

M_S: Amount (g) of water taken

M_T: Amount (g) of Panipenem taken

Internal standard solution—A solution of acetonitrile in methanol (1 in 100).

Operating conditions—

Detector: A thermal conductivity detector.

Column: A glass column 3 mm in inside diameter and 2 m in length, packed with porous ethyl vinylbenzene-divinylbenzene copolymer for gas chromatography (150 to 180 μm in particle diameter).

Column temperature: A constant temperature of about 125°C.

Carrier gas: Helium.

Flow rate: Adjust so that the retention time of acetonitrile is about 8 minutes.

System suitability—

System performance: When the procedure is run with 1 μL of the standard solution (2) under the above operating conditions, water, methanol, and the internal standard are eluted in this order with the resolution between the peaks of water and internal standard being not less than 10.

System repeatability: When the test is repeated 6 times with 1 μL of the standard solution (2) under the above operating conditions, the relative standard deviation of the ratios of the peak area of water to that of the internal standard is not more than 5.0%.

Residue on ignition <*2.44*> Not more than 0.5% (1 g).

Assay Conduct this procedure within 30 minutes after preparation of the sample and standard solutions. Weigh accurately an amount of Panipenem and Panipenem RS, equivalent to about 0.1 g (potency), dissolve them separately in 0.02 mol/L 3-(*N*-morpholino)propanesulfonic acid buffer solution (pH 7.0) to make exactly 100 mL. Pipet 5 mL each of these solutions, add exactly 5 mL of the internal standard solution, add 0.02 mol/L 3-(*N*-morpholino)propanesulfonic acid buffer solution (pH 7.0) to make 20 mL, and use these solutions as the sample solution and the standard solution, respectively. Perform the test with 10 μL of the sample solution and standard solution as directed under Liquid Chromatography <*2.01*> according to the following conditions, and calculate the ratios, Q_T and Q_S, of the peak area of panipenem to that of the internal standard.

$$\text{Amount } [\mu g \text{ (potency)}] \text{ of panipenem } (C_{15}H_{21}N_3O_4S) = M_S \times Q_T/Q_S \times 1000$$

M_S: Amount [mg (potency)] of Panipenem RS taken

Internal standard solution—A solution of sodium *p*-styrenesulfonate in 0.02 mol/L 3-(*N*-morpholino)propanesulfonic acid buffer solution (pH 7.0) (1 in 1000).

Operating conditions—

Detector: An ultraviolet absorption photometer (wavelength: 280 nm).

Column: A stainless steel column 4.6 mm in inside diameter and 25 cm in length, packed with octadecylsilanized silicone polymer coated silica gel for liquid chromatography (5 μm in particle diameter).

Column temperature: A constant temperature of about 40°C.

Mobile phase: A mixture of 0.02 mol/L 3-(*N*-morpholino)propanesulfonic acid buffer solution (pH 8.0) and acetonitrile (50:1).

Flow rate: Adjust so that the retention time of the internal standard is about 12 minutes.

System suitability—

System performance: When the procedure is run with 10 μL of the standard solution under the above operating conditions, panipenem and the internal standard are eluted in this order with the resolution between these peaks being not less than 3.

System repeatability: When the test is repeated 6 times with 10 μL of the standard solution under the above operating conditions, the relative standard deviation of the ratios of the peak area of panipenem to that of the internal standard is not more than 2.0%.

Containers and storage Containers—Tight containers.

Storage—At a temperature not exceeding −10°C.

Panipenem and Betamipron for Injection

注射用パニペネム・ベタミプロン

Panipenem and Betamipron for Injection is a preparation for injection which is dissolved before use.

It contains not less than 90.0% and not more than 105.0% of the labeled potency of panipenem ($C_{15}H_{21}N_3O_4S$: 339.41), and not less than 95.0% and not more than 105.0% of labeled amount of betamipron ($C_{10}H_{11}NO_3$: 193.20).

Method of preparation Prepare as directed under Injections, with Panipenem and Betamipron.

Description Panipenem and Betamipron for Injection occurs as two layers of upper and lower. The former occurs pale yellowish white to light yellow, masses or masses containing powder, and the latter white, masses or masses containing powder.

It is deliquescent.

Identification **(1)** Powder Panipenem and Betamipron for Injection, weigh a portion of the powder, equivalent to 40 mg (potency) of Panipenem, dissolve in 4 mL of water, add 1 mL of hydroxylammonium chloride-ethanol TS, allow to stand for 3 minutes, add 1 mL of acidic ammonium iron (III) sulfate TS, and shake: a red-brown color develops (panipenem).

(2) Powder Panipenem and Betamipron for Injection. Dissolve a portion of the powder, equivalent to 50 mg of Betamipron, in 4 mL of diluted methanol (1 in 2), and use this solution as the sample solution. Separately, dissolve 12 mg of betamipron in 1 mL of diluted methanol (1 in 2), and use this solution as the standard solution. Perform the test with these solutions as directed under Thin-layer Chromatography <*2.03*>. Spot 1 μL each of the sample solution and standard solution on a plate of silica gel with fluorescent indicator for thin-layer chromatography. Develop the plate with a mixture of ethanol (99.5) and triethylamine (19:1) to a distance of about 8 cm, and air-dry the plate. Examine under ultraviolet light (main wavelength: 254 nm): the principal spot obtained from the sample solution and the spot from the standard solution show the same *R*f value (betamipron).

pH <*2.54*> The pH of a solution of an amount of Panipenem and Betamipron for Injection, equivalent to 0.5 mg (potency) of Panipenem, in 100 mL of isotonic sodium chloride solution is 5.8 to 7.8.

Purity **(1)** Clarity and color of solution—A solution of an amount of Panipenem and Betamipron for Injection, equivalent to 0.5 g (potency) of Panipenem, in 10 mL of water is clear, and has no more color than Matching Fluid J.

(2) Related substances—After preparation of the sample solution, keep it at not exceeding 5°C and use within 60 minutes. Take 1 container of Panipenem and Betamipron for Injection, dissolve in water so that each mL contains 1 mg (potency) of panipenem, and use this solution as the sample solution. Perform the test with 10 μL of the sample solution as directed under Liquid Chromatography <*2.01*> according to the following conditions, and determine each peak area by the automatic integration method, and calculate the amount of them by the area percentage method: the amount of each peak other than panipenem and betamipron is not more than 8.0%, and the total amount of peaks other than panipenem and betamipron is not more than 13.0%.

Operating conditions—

Detector: An ultraviolet absorption photometer (wavelength: 220 nm).

Column: A stainless steel column 4.6 mm in inside diameter, 15 cm in length, packed with octadecylsilanized silica gel for liquid chromatography (3 μm in particle diameter).

Column temperature: A constant temperature of about 40°C.

Mobile phase A: A mixture of 0.02 mol/L phosphate buffer (pH 8.0) and acetonitrile (100:1).

Mobile phase B: A mixture of 0.02 mol/L phosphate buffer (pH 8.0) and acetonitrile (3:1).

Flowing of mobile phase: Control the gradient by mixing the mobile phase A and B as directed in the following table.

Time after injection of sample (min)	Mobile phase A (vol%)	Mobile phase B (vol%)
0 – 22	100	0
22 – 25	100 → 90	0 → 10
25 – 30	90	10
30 – 35	90 → 85	10 → 15
35 – 40	85 → 77	15 → 23
40 – 50	77 → 0	23 → 100
50 – 55	0	100

Flow rate: 1.0 mL per minute.

Time span of measurement: About 3 times as long as the retention time of panipenem.

System suitability—

Test for required detectability: Use the diluted sample solution (1 in 100) as the solution for system suitability test. Pipet 1 mL of the solution for system suitability test, add water to make exactly 10 mL. Confirm that the peak area of panipenem obtained with 10 μL of this solution is equivalent to 7 to 13% of that with 10 μL of the solution for system suitability test.

System performance: When the procedure is run with 10 μL of the solution for system suitability test under the above operating conditions, the number of theoretical plates and the symmetry factor of the peak of panipenem are not less than 4000 and 0.8 to 1.2, respectively.

System repeatability: When the test is repeated 3 times with 10 μL of the solution for system suitability test under the above operating conditions, the relative standard deviation of the peak area of panipenem is not more than 0.95%.

Bacterial endotoxins <*4.01*> Less than 0.15 EU/mg (potency).

Uniformity of dosage units <*6.02*> Perform the test according to the following method: it meets the requirement of Content uniformity test.

After preparation of the sample solution and standard solution, keep them at not exceeding 5°C. Dissolve the content of 1 container of Panipenem and Betamipron for Injection in 0.02 mol/L 3-(*N*-morpholino)propanesulfonic acid buffer solution (pH 7.0) to make exactly 500 mL. Take exactly *V* mL of this solution, equivalent to 5 mg (potency) of Panipenem, add exactly 5 mL of the internal standard solution, add 0.02 mol/L 3-(*N*-morpholino)propanesulfonic acid buffer solution (pH 7.0) to make 20 mL, and use this solution as the sample solution. Then, proceed as directed in the Assay.

Amount [mg (potency)] of panipenem ($C_{15}H_{21}N_3O_4S$)
$= M_{S1} \times Q_{T1}/Q_{S1} \times 25/V$

Amount (mg) of betamipron ($C_{10}H_{11}NO_3$)
$= M_{S2} \times Q_{T2}/Q_{S2} \times 25/V$

M_{S1}: Amount [mg (potency)] of Panipenem RS taken
M_{S2}: Amount (mg) of betamipron for assay taken, calculated on the anhydrous basis

*Internal standard solution—*A solution of sodium *p*-styrenesulfonate in 0.02 mol/L 3-(*N*-morpholino)propanesulfonic acid buffer solution (pH 7.0) (1 in 10,000).

Foreign insoluble matter <*6.06*> Perform the test according to Method 2: it meets the requirement.

Insoluble particulate matter <*6.07*> It meets the requirement.

Sterility <*4.06*> Perform the test according to the Membrane filtration method: it meets the requirement.

Assay After preparation of the sample solution and standard solution, keep them at not exceeding 5°C. Dissolve the total amount of the contents of 10 containers of Panipenem and Betamipron for Injection in 0.02 mol/L 3-(*N*-morpholino)propanesulfonic acid buffer solution (pH 7.0) to make exactly 500 mL. Take exactly *V* mL of this solution, equivalent to about 50 mg (potency) of Panipenem, add 0.02 mol/L 3-(*N*-morpholino)-propanesulfonic acid buffer solution (pH 7.0) to make exactly 50 mL. Pipet 5 mL of this solution, add exactly 5 mL of the internal standard solution, add 0.02 mol/L 3-(*N*-morpholino)propanesulfonic acid buffer solution (pH 7.0) to make 20 mL, and use this solution as the sample solution. Separately, weigh accurately about 50 mg (potency) of Panipenem RS and about 50 mg of betamipron for assay (separately determine the water <*2.48*> in the same manner as Betamipron), dissolve in 0.02 mol/L 3-(*N*-morpholino)propanesulfonic acid buffer solution (pH 7.0) to make exactly 50 mL. Pipet 5 mL of this solution, add exactly 5 mL of the internal standard solution, add 0.02 mol/L 3-(*N*-morpholino)propanesulfonic acid buffer solution (pH 7.0) to make 20 mL, and use this solution as the standard solution. Perform the test with 10 μL each of the sample solution and standard solution as directed under Liquid Chromatography <*2.01*> according to the following conditions, and calculate the ratios, Q_{T1} and Q_{T2}, of the peak areas of panipenem and betamipron to that of the internal standard obtained from the sample solution, and the ratios, Q_{S1}, and Q_{S2}, of the peak areas of panipenem and betamipron to that of the internal standard obtained from the standard solution.

Amount [mg (potency)] of panipenem ($C_{15}H_{21}N_3O_4S$)
$= M_{S1} \times Q_{T1}/Q_{S1} \times 25/V$

Amount (mg) of betamipron ($C_{10}H_{11}NO_3$)
$= M_{S2} \times Q_{T2}/Q_{S2} \times 25/V$

M_{S1}: Amount [mg (potency)] of Panipenem RS taken
M_{S2}: Amount (mg) of betamipron for assay taken, calculated on the anhydrous basis

*Internal standard solution—*A solution of sodium *p*-styrenesulfonate in 0.02 mol/L 3-(*N*-morpholino)propanesulfonic acid buffer solution (pH 7.0) (1 in 10,000).

Operating conditions—

Column, column temperature, and mobile phase: Proceed as directed in the operating conditions in the Assay under Panipenem.

Detector: An ultraviolet absorption photometer (wavelength: 260 nm).

Flow rate: Adjust so that the retention time of panipenem is about 9 minutes.

System suitability—

System performance: When the procedure is run with 10 μL of the standard solution under the above operating conditions, betamipron, panipenem and the internal standard are eluted in this order, and the resolutions between the peaks of betamipron and panipenem, and panipenem and the internal standard are not less than 3, respectively.

System repeatability: When the test is repeated 6 times with 10 μL of the standard solution under the above operating conditions, the relative standard deviation of the ratios of the peak area of betamipron and panipenem to that of the internal standard are not more than 1.0%, respectively.

Containers and storage Containers—Hermetic containers.

Shelf life 24 months after preparation.

Pantethine

パンテチン

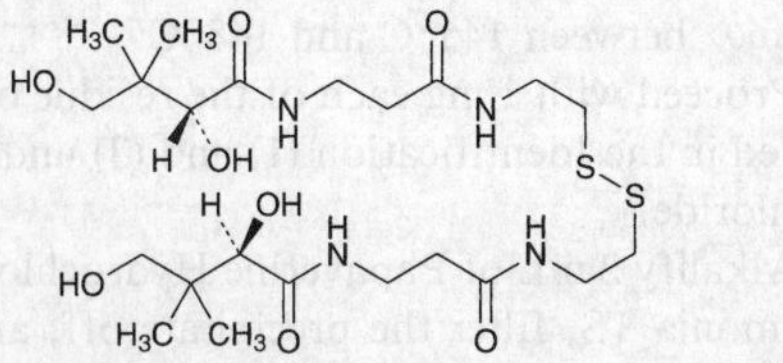

$C_{22}H_{42}N_4O_8S_2$: 554.72
Bis(2-{3-[(2*R*)-2,4-dihydroxy-3,3-dimethylbutanoylamino]propanoylamino}ethyl) disulfide
[*16816-67-4*]

Pantethine is an aqueous solution containing 80% of pantethine.

Pantethine contains not less than 98.0% of pantethine ($C_{22}H_{42}N_4O_8S_2$), calculated on the anhydrous basis.

Description Pantethine is a clear, colorless to pale yellow viscous liquid.

It is miscible with water, with methanol and with ethanol (95).

It is decomposed by light.

Identification **(1)** To 0.7 g of Pantethine add 5 mL of sodium hydroxide TS, shake, and add 1 to 2 drops of copper (II) sulfate TS: a blue-purple color develops.

(2) To 0.7 g of Pantethine add 3 mL of water, shake, add 0.1 g of zinc powder and 2 mL of acetic acid (100), and boil for 2 to 3 minutes. After cooling, add 1 to 2 drops of sodium pentacyanonitrosylferrate (III) TS: a red-purple color develops.

(3) To 1.0 g of Pantethine add 500 mL of water, and shake. To 5 mL of this solution add 3 mL of 1 mol/L hydrochloric acid TS, and heat on a water bath for 30 minutes. After cooling, add 7 mL of a solution of hydroxylammonium chloride in sodium hydroxide TS (3 in 140), and allow to stand for 5 minutes. Add 3 drops of 2,4-dinitrophenol TS, and add 1 mol/L hydrochloric acid TS dropwise until the solution has no color, and then add 1 mL of iron (III) chloride TS: a red-purple color develops.

Optical rotation <*2.49*> $[\alpha]_D^{20}$: +15.0 – +18.0° (1 g calculated on the anhydrous basis, water, 25 mL, 100 mm).

Purity **(1)** Heavy metals <*1.07*>—Proceed with 2.0 g of Pantethine according to Method 1, and perform the test. Prepare the control solution with 2.0 mL of Standard Lead Solution (not more than 10 ppm).

(2) Arsenic <*1.11*>—Prepare the test solution with 2.0 g of Pantethine according to Method 3, and perform the test (not more than 1 ppm).

(3) Related substances—Dissolve 0.6 g of Pantethine in 10 mL of water, and use this solution as the sample solution. Pipet 2 mL of the sample solution, add water to make exactly 100 mL, and use this solution as the standard solution. Perform the test with these solutions as directed under Thin-layer Chromatography <*2.03*>. Spot 2 μL each of the sample solution and standard solution on a plate of silica gel for thin-layer chromatography. Develop the plate with 2-butanone saturated with water to a distance of about 10 cm, and air-dry the plate. Allow the plate to stand for about 10 minutes in iodide vapor: the spots other than the principal spot obtained from the sample solution are not more intense than the spot from the standard solution.

(4) Mercapto compounds—To 1.5 g of Pantethine add 20 mL of water, shake, add 1 drop of ammonia TS and 1 to 2 drops of sodium pentacyanonitrosylferrate (III) TS: a red color is not developed.

Water <*2.48*> 18 – 22% (0.2 g, volumetric titration, direct titration).

Residue on Ignition <*2.44*> Not more than 0.1% (2 g).

Assay Weigh accurately about 0.3 g of Pantethine, add water to make exactly 20 mL. Transfer exactly 5 mL of this solution in an iodine bottle, and add exactly 25 mL of 0.05 mol/L bromine VS and 100 mL of water. Add 5 mL of diluted sulfuric acid (1 in 5) rapidly, stopper tightly immediately, and warm at 40 to 50°C for 15 minutes with occasional shaking. After cooling, carefully add 5 mL of a solution of potassium iodide (2 in 5), then immediately stopper tightly, shake, add 100 mL of water and titrate <*2.50*> the liberated iodine with 0.1 mol/L sodium thiosulfate VS (indicator: 2 mL of starch TS). Perform a blank determination in the same manner.

Each mL of 0.05 mol/L bromine VS
= 5.547 mg of $C_{22}H_{42}N_4O_8S_2$

Containers and storage Containers—Tight containers.

Storage—Light-resistant, at a temperature not exceeding 10°C.

Papaverine Hydrochloride

パパベリン塩酸塩

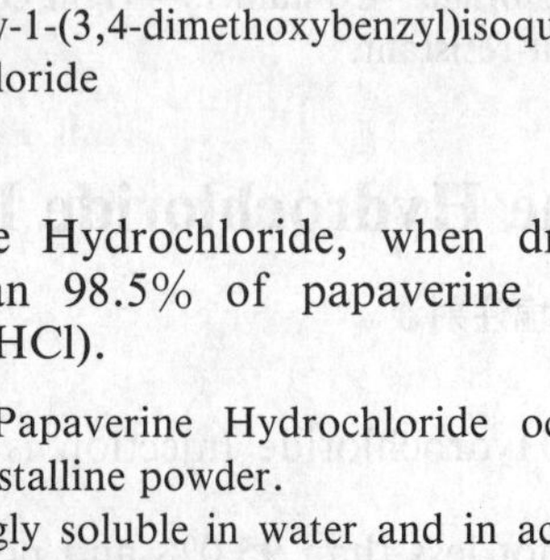

$C_{20}H_{21}NO_4.HCl$: 375.85
6,7-Dimethoxy-1-(3,4-dimethoxybenzyl)isoquinoline monohydrochloride
[*61-25-6*]

Papaverine Hydrochloride, when dried, contains not less than 98.5% of papaverine hydrochloride ($C_{20}H_{21}NO_4.HCl$).

Description Papaverine Hydrochloride occurs as white crystals or crystalline powder.

It is sparingly soluble in water and in acetic acid (100), slightly soluble in ethanol (95), and practically insoluble in acetic anhydride and in diethyl ether.

The pH of a solution of 1.0 g of Papaverine Hydrochloride in 50 mL of water is between 3.0 and 4.0.

Identification **(1)** To 1 mg of Papaverine Hydrochloride add 1 drops of formaldehyde-sulfuric acid TS: a colorless to light yellow-green color is produced, and it gradually changes to deep red, then to brown.

(2) Dissolve 0.02 g of Papaverine Hydrochloride in 1 mL of water, and add 3 drops of sodium acetate TS: a white precipitate is produced.

(3) Dissolve 1 mg of Papaverine Hydrochloride in 3 mL of acetic anhydride and 5 drops of sulfuric acid, heat in a water bath for 1 minute, and examine under ultraviolet light (main wavelength: 365 nm): the solution shows a yellow-green fluorescence.

(4) Dissolve 0.1 g of Papaverine Hydrochloride in 10 mL of water, make alkaline with ammonia TS, and shake with 10 mL of diethyl ether. Draw off the diethyl ether layer, wash with 5 mL of water, and filter. Evaporate the filtrate on a water bath, and dry the residue at 105°C for 3 hours: the residue so obtained melts <*2.60*> between 145°C and 148°C.

(5) Alkalify a solution of Papaverine Hydrochloride (1 in 50) with ammonia TS, and filter the precipitate. Acidify the filtrate with dilute nitric acid: the solution responds to Qualitative Tests <*1.09*> (2) for chloride.

Purity **(1)** Clarity and color of solution—Dissolve 0.10 g of Papaverine Hydrochloride in 10 mL of water: the solution is clear and colorless.

(2) Morphine—Dissolve 10 mg of Papaverine Hydrochloride in 1 mL of water, add 5 mL of 1-nitroso-2-naphthol TS and 2 mL of a solution of potassium nitrate (1 in 10), and warm at 40°C for 2 minutes. Add 1 mL of a solution of sodium nitrate (1 in 5000), and warm at 40°C for 5 minutes. After cooling, shake the mixture with 10 mL of chloroform, centrifuge, and separate the aqueous layer: the solution so obtained has no more color than a pale red color.

(3) Readily carbonizable substances <*1.15*>—Perform the test with 0.12 g of Papaverine Hydrochloride: the solution has no more color than Matching Fluid S or P.

Loss on drying <*2.41*> Not more than 1.0% (1 g, 105°C, 4 hours).

Residue on ignition <*2.44*> Not more than 0.2% (1 g).

Assay Weigh accurately about 0.5 g of Papaverine Hydrochloride, previously dried, dissolve in 100 mL of a mixture of acetic anhydride and acetic acid (100) (7:3) by warming, cool, and titrate <*2.50*> with 0.1 mol/L perchloric acid VS (potentiometric titration). Perform a blank determination in the same manner, and make any necessary correction.

Each mL of 0.1 mol/L perchloric acid VS
= 37.59 mg of $C_{20}H_{21}NO_4.HCl$

Containers and storage Containers—Tight containers.
Storage—Light-resistant.

Papaverine Hydrochloride Injection

パパベリン塩酸塩注射液

Papaverine Hydrochloride Injection is an aqueous injection.

It contains not less than 95.0% and not more than 105.0% of the labeled amount of papaverine hydrochloride ($C_{20}H_{21}NO_4.HCl$: 375.85).

Method of preparation Prepare as directed under Injections, with Papaverine Hydrochloride.

Description Papaverine Hydrochloride Injection is a clear, colorless liquid.

pH: 3.0 – 5.0

Identification **(1)** To 1 mL of Papaverine Hydrochloride Injection add 3 drops of sodium acetate TS: a white precipitate is produced.

(2) Dilute a volume of Papaverine Hydrochloride Injection, equivalent to 0.1 g of Papaverine Hydrochloride, with water to 10 mL, render the solution alkaline with ammonia TS, and shake with 10 mL of diethyl ether. Draw off the diethyl ether layer, wash with 5 mL of water, and filter. Evaporate the filtrate on a water bath to dryness, and dry the residue at 105°C for 3 hours: the residue so obtained melts <*2.60*> between 145°C and 148°C.

(3) Proceed with 1 mg each of the residue obtained in (2) as directed in the Identification (1) and (3) under Papaverine Hydrochloride.

(4) Alkalify 2 mL of Papaverine Hydrochloride Injection with ammonia TS, filter the precipitate off, and acidity the filtrate with dilute nitric acid: the solution responds to Qualitative Tests <*1.09*> (2) for chloride.

Bacterial endotoxins <*4.01*> Less than 6.0 EU/mg.

Extractable volume <*6.05*> It meets the requirement.

Foreign insoluble matter <*6.06*> Perform the test according to Method 1: it meets the requirement.

Insoluble particulate matter <*6.07*> It meets the requirement.

Sterility <*4.06*> Perform the test according to the Membrane filtration method: it meets the requirement.

Assay Dilute an exactly measured volume of Papaverine Hydrochloride Injection, equivalent to about 0.2 g of papaverine hydrochloride ($C_{20}H_{21}NO_4.HCl$), with water to 10 mL, render the solution alkaline with ammonia TS, and extract with 20-mL, 15-mL, 10-mL and 10-mL portions of chloroform. Combine the extracts, wash with 10 mL of water, and re-extract the washings with two 5-mL portions of chloroform. Combine all the chloroform extracts, and distil the chloroform on a water bath. Dissolve the residue in 30 mL of acetic acid (100), and titrate <*2.50*> with 0.05 mol/L perchloric acid VS (indicator: 2 drops of crystal violet TS). Perform a blank determination in the same manner, and make any necessary correction.

Each mL of 0.05 mol/L perchloric acid VS
= 18.79 mg of $C_{20}H_{21}NO_4.HCl$

Containers and storage Containers—Hermetic containers.
Storage—Light-resistant.

Paraffin

パラフィン

Paraffin is a mixture of solid hydrocarbons obtained from petroleum.

Description Paraffin occurs as a colorless or white, more or less transparent, crystalline mass. It is odorless and tasteless.

It is sparingly soluble in diethyl ether and practically insoluble in water, in ethanol (95) and in ethanol (99.5).

Specific gravity d^{20}_{20}: about 0.92 (proceed as directed in 4.2. in 4. Specific gravity under Fats and Fatty Oils Test <*1.13*>).

Identification **(1)** Heat Paraffin strongly in a porcelain dish, and ignite: it burns with a bright flame and the odor of paraffin vapor is perceptible.

(2) Heat 0.5 g of Paraffin with 0.5 g of sulfur with shaking carefully: the odor of hydrogen sulfide is perceptible.

Melting point <*2.60*> 50 – 75°C (Method 2).

Purity **(1)** Acidity or alkalinity—Boil 10.0 g of Paraffin with 10 mL of hot water and 1 drop of phenolphthalein TS in a water bath for 5 minutes, and shake vigorously: a red color is not produced. Add 0.20 mL of 0.02 mol/L sodium hydroxide VS to this solution, and shake: a red color is produced.

(2) Heavy metals *<1.07>*—Ignite 2.0 g of Paraffin in a crucible, first moderately until charred, then between 450°C and 550°C to ash. Cool, add 2 mL of hydrochloric acid, and evaporate on a water bath to dryness. To the residue add 2 mL of dilute acetic acid and water to make 50 mL, and perform the test using this solution as the test solution. Prepare the control solution as follows: to 2.0 mL of Standard Lead Solution add 2 mL of dilute acetic acid and water to make 50 mL (not more than 10 ppm).

(3) Arsenic *<1.11>*—Prepare the test solution with 1.0 g of Paraffin according to Method 3, and perform the test (not more than 2 ppm).

(4) Sulfur compounds—To 4.0 g of Paraffin add 2 mL of ethanol (99.5), further add 2 drops of a clear saturated solution of lead (II) oxide in a solution of sodium hydroxide (1 in 5), and heat for 10 minutes at 70°C with occasional shaking: no dark brown color develops in the aqueous layer.

(5) Readily carbonizable substances—Melt 5.0 g of Paraffin placed in a Nessler tube at a temperature near the melting point. Add 5 mL of sulfuric acid for readily carbonizable substances, and warm at 70°C for 5 minutes in a water bath. Remove the tube from the water bath, immediately shake vigorously and vertically for 3 seconds, and warm for 1 minute in a water bath at 70°C. Repeat this procedure 5 times: the color of the sulfuric acid layer is not darker than that of the following control solution.

Control solution: Add 1.5 mL of Cobalt (II) Chloride CS, 0.5 mL of Copper (II) Sulfate CS and 5 mL of liquid paraffin to 3.0 mL of Iron (III) Chloride CS, and shake vigorously.

Containers and storage Containers—Well-closed containers.

Liquid Paraffin

流動パラフィン

Liquid Paraffin is a mixture of liquid hydrocarbons obtained from petrolatum.

Tocopherols of a suitable form may by added at a concentration not exceeding 0.001% as a stabilizer.

Description Liquid Paraffin is a colorless, transparent, oily liquid, nearly free from fluorescence. It is odorless and tasteless.

It is freely soluble in diethyl ether, very slightly soluble in ethanol (99.5), and practically insoluble in water and in ethanol (95).

Boiling point: above 300°C.

Identification **(1)** Heat Liquid Paraffin strongly in a porcelain dish, and fire: it burns with a bright flame and the odor of paraffin vapor is perceptible.

(2) Heat 0.5 of Liquid Paraffin with 0.5 g of sulfur with shaking carefully: the odor of hydrogen sulfide is perceptible.

Specific gravity *<2.56>* d_{20}^{20}: 0.860 – 0.890

Viscosity *<2.53>* Not less than 37 mm^2/s (Method 1, 37.8°C).

Purity **(1)** Odor—Transfer a suitable amount of Liquid Paraffin to a small beaker, and heat on a water bath: a foreign odor is not perceptible.

(2) Acidity or alkalinity—Shake vigorously 10 mL of Liquid Paraffin with 10 mL of hot water and 1 drop of phenolphthalein TS: no red color develops. Shake this solution with 0.20 mL of 0.02 mol/L sodium hydroxide VS: a red color develops.

(3) Heavy metals *<1.07>*—Ignite 2.0 g of Liquid Paraffin in a crucible, first moderately until charred, then between 450°C and 550°C to ash. Cool, add 2 mL of hydrochloric acid, and evaporate on a water bath to dryness. To the residue add 2 mL of dilute acetic acid and water to make 50 mL, and perform the test using this solution as the test solution. Prepare the control solution as follows: to 2.0 mL of Standard Lead Solution add 2 mL of dilute acetic acid and water to make 50 mL (not more than 10 ppm).

(4) Arsenic *<1.11>*—Prepare the test solution with 1.0 g of Liquid Paraffin, according to Method 3 except that after addition of 10 mL of a solution of magnesium nitrate hexahydrate in ethanol (95) (1 in 50), add 1.5 mL of hydrogen peroxide (30), fire to burn, and perform the test (not more than 2 ppm).

(5) Solid paraffin—Transfer 50 mL of Liquid Paraffin, previously dried at 105°C for 2 hours, to a Nessler tube, and cool in ice water for 4 hours: the turbidity produced, if any, is not deeper than that of the following control solution.

Control solution: To 1.5 mL of 0.01 mol/L hydrochloric acid VS add 6 mL of dilute nitric acid and water to make 50 mL, add 1 mL of silver nitrate TS, and allow to stand for 5 minutes.

(6) Sulfur compounds—Prepare a saturated solution of lead (II) oxide in a solution of sodium hydroxide (1 in 5), and mix 2 drops of this clear solution with 4.0 mL of Liquid Paraffin and 2 mL of ethanol (99.5). Heat at 70°C for 10 minutes with frequent shaking, and cool: no dark brown color develops.

(7) Polycyclic aromatic hydrocarbons—Take 25 mL of Liquid Paraffin by a 25-mL measuring cylinder, transfer to a 100-mL separator, and wash out the cylinder with 25 mL of hexane for ultraviolet-visible spectrophotometry. Combine the washings with the liquid in the separator, and shake vigorously. Shake this solution vigorously for 2 minutes with 5.0 mL of dimethylsulfoxide for ultraviolet-visible spectrophotometry, and allow to stand for 15 minutes. Transfer the lower layer to a 50-mL separator, add 2 mL of hexane for ultraviolet-visible spectrophotometry, shake vigorously for 2 minutes, and allow to stand for 2 minutes. Transfer the lower layer to a 10-mL glass-stoppered centrifuge tube, and centrifuge between 2500 revolutions per minute and 3000 revolutions per minute for about 10 minutes, and use the clear solution obtained as the sample solution. Transfer 25 mL of hexane for ultraviolet-visible spectrophotometry to another 50-mL separator, shake vigorously for 2 minutes with 5.0 mL of dimethylsulfoxide for ultraviolet-visible spectrophotometry, and allow to stand for 2 minutes. Transfer the lower layer to a 10-mL glass-stoppered centrifuge tube, centrifuge between 2500 revolutions per minute and 3000 revolutions per minute for about 10 minutes, and use the clear solution thus obtained as a control solution. Immediately determine the absorbance of the sample solution using the control solution as the blank as directed under Ultraviolet-visible Spectrophotometry *<2.24>*: not more than 0.10 at the wavelength region between 260 nm and 350 nm.

(8) Readily carbonizable substances—Transfer 5 mL of Liquid Paraffin to a Nessler tube, and add 5 mL of sulfuric acid for readily carbonizable substances. After heating in a water bath for 2 minutes, remove the tube from the water bath, and immediately shake vigorously and vertically for 5 seconds. Repeat this procedure 4 times: the Liquid Paraffin layer remains unchanged in color, and the sulfuric acid layer has no more color than the following control solution.

Control solution: Mix 3.0 mL of Iron (III) Chloride CS with 1.5 mL of Cobalt (II) Chloride CS and 0.50 mL of Copper (II) Sulfate CS.

Containers and storage Containers—Tight containers.

Light Liquid Paraffin

軽質流動パラフィン

Light Liquid Paraffin is a mixture of liquid hydrocarbons obtained from petroleum.

Tocopherols of a suitable form may be added at a concentration not exceeding 0.001% as a stabilizer.

Description Light Liquid Paraffin is a clear, colorless oily liquid, nearly free from fluorescence. It is odorless and tasteless.

It is freely soluble in diethyl ether, and practically insoluble in water and in ethanol (95).

Boiling point: above 300°C.

Identification **(1)** Heat Light Liquid Paraffin strongly in a porcelain dish, and fire: it burns with a bright flame and the odor of paraffin vapor is perceptible.

(2) Heat 0.5 of Light Liquid Paraffin with 0.5 g of sulfur with shaking carefully: the odor of hydrogen sulfide is perceptible.

Specific gravity <*2.56*> d^{20}_{20}: 0.830 – 0.870

Viscosity <*2.53*> Less than 37 mm²/s (Method 1, 37.8°C).

Purity **(1)** Odor—Transfer a suitable amount of Light Liquid Paraffin to a small beaker, and heat on a water bath: no foreign odor is perceptible.

(2) Acidity or alkalinity—Shake vigorously 10 mL of Light Liquid Paraffin with 10 mL of hot water and 1 drop of phenolphthalein TS: no red color develops. Shake this solution with 0.20 mL of 0.02 mol/L sodium hydroxide VS: a red color develops.

(3) Heavy metals <*1.07*>—Ignite 2.0 g of Light Liquid Paraffin in a crucible, first moderately until charred, then between 450°C and 550°C to ash. Cool, add 2 mL of hydrochloric acid, and evaporate on a water bath to dryness. To the residue add 2 mL of dilute acetic acid and water to make 50 mL, and perform the test using this solution as the test solution. Prepare the control solution as follows: to 2.0 mL of Standard Lead Solution add 2 mL of dilute acetic acid and water to make 50 mL (not more than 10 ppm).

(4) Arsenic <*1.11*>—Prepare the test solution with 1.0 g of Light Liquid Paraffin according to Method 3, and perform the test (not more than 2 ppm).

(5) Solid paraffin—Transfer 50 mL of Light Liquid Paraffin, previously dried at 105°C for 2 hours, to a Nessler tube, and cool in ice water for 4 hours: the turbidity produced, if any, is not deeper than that of the following control solution.

Control solution: To 1.5 mL of 0.01 mol/L hydrochloric acid VS add 6 mL of dilute nitric acid and water to make 50 mL, add 1 mL of silver nitrate TS, and allow to stand for 5 minutes.

(6) Sulfur compounds—Prepare a saturated solution of lead (II) oxide in a solution of sodium hydroxide (1 in 5), and mix 2 drops of this clear solution with 4.0 mL of Light Liquid Paraffin and 2 mL of ethanol (99.5). Heat at 70°C for 10 minutes with frequent shaking, and cool: no dark brown color develops.

(7) Polycyclic aromatic hydrocarbons—Take 25 mL of Light Liquid Paraffin by a 25-mL measuring cylinder, transfer to a 100-mL separator, and wash out the cylinder with 25 mL of hexane for ultraviolet-visible spectrophotometry. Combine the washings with the liquid in the separator, and shake vigorously. Shake this solution vigorously for 2 minutes with 5.0 mL of dimethylsulfoxide for ultraviolet-visible spectrophotometry, and allow to stand for 15 minutes. Transfer the lower layer to a 50-mL separator, add 2 mL of hexane for ultraviolet-visible spectrophotometry, shake vigorously for 2 minutes, and allow to stand for 2 minutes. Transfer the lower layer to a glass-stoppered 10-mL centrifuge tube, and centrifuge between 2500 revolutions per minute and 3000 revolutions per minute for about 10 minutes, and use the clear solution so obtained as the sample solution. Separately, transfer 25 mL of hexane for ultraviolet-visible spectrophotometry to a 50-mL separator, add 5.0 mL of dimethylsulfoxide for ultraviolet-visible spectrophotometry, shake vigorously for 2 minutes, and allow to stand for 2 minutes. Transfer the lower layer to a glass-stoppered 10-mL centrifuge tube, centrifuge between 2500 revolutions per minute and 3000 revolutions per minute for about 10 minutes, and use the clear solution so obtained as a control solution. Immediately determine the absorbance of the sample solution using the control solution as the blank as directed under Ultraviolet-visible Spectrophotometry <*2.24*>: not more than 0.10 at the wavelength region between 260 nm and 350 nm.

(8) Readily carbonizable substances—Transfer 5 mL of Light Liquid Paraffin to a Nessler tube, and add 5 mL of sulfuric acid for readily carbonizable substances. After heating in a water bath for 2 minutes, remove the tube from the water bath, and immediately shake vigorously and vertically for 5 seconds. Repeat this procedure four times: the liquid paraffin layer remains unchanged in color, and sulfuric acid layer has no more color than the following control solution.

Control solution: Mix 3.0 mL of Iron (III) Chloride CS with 1.5 mL of Cobalt (II) Chloride CS and 0.50 mL of Copper (II) Sulfate CS.

Containers and storage Containers—Tight containers.

Paraformaldehyde

パラホルムアルデヒド

$(CH_2O)_n$
Poly(oxymethylene)
[*30525-89-4*]

Paraformaldehyde contains not less than 95.0% of formaldehyde (CH_2O: 30.03).

Description Paraformaldehyde occurs as a white powder. It has a slight odor of formaldehyde, but a very strong irritating odor is perceptible when it is heated.

It is practically insoluble in water, in ethanol (95) and in diethyl ether.

It dissolves in hot water, in hot dilute hydrochloric acid, in sodium hydroxide TS and in ammonia TS.

It sublimes at about 100°C.

Identification (1) Dissolve 0.1 g of Paraformaldehyde in 5 mL of ammonia TS, add 5 mL of silver nitrate TS, shake, and add 3 mL of a solution of sodium hydroxide (1 in 10): a mirror of metallic silver is immediately formed on the sides of the container.

(2) Add a solution of 0.04 g of salicylic acid in 5 mL of sulfuric acid to 0.02 g of Paraformaldehyde, and warm slowly: a persistent, dark red color is produced.

Purity (1) Clarity and color of solution—Dissolve 0.20 g of Paraformaldehyde in 10 mL of ammonia TS: the solution is clear and colorless.

(2) Acidity or alkalinity—To 0.5 g of Paraformaldehyde add 10 mL of water, shake vigorously for 1 minute, and filter: the filtrate is neutral.

(3) Chloride <*1.03*>—Dissolve 1.5 g of Paraformaldehyde in 75 mL of water and 7.5 mL of sodium carbonate TS, evaporate on a water bath to dryness, and ignite at about 500°C. Dissolve the residue in 15 mL of water, filter, if necessary, neutralize with diluted nitric acid (3 in 10), and add 6 mL of dilute nitric acid and water to make 50 mL. Perform the test using this solution as the test solution. Prepare the control solution as follows: to 0.25 mL of 0.01 mol/L hydrochloric acid VS add 7.5 mL of sodium carbonate TS, a volume of diluted nitric acid (3 in 10) required for neutralization of the sample, 6 mL of dilute nitric acid and water to make 50 mL (not more than 0.006%).

(4) Sulfate <*1.14*>—Dissolve 1.5 g of Paraformaldehyde in 45 mL of water and 4.5 mL of sodium carbonate TS, evaporate on a water bath to dryness, and ignite at about 500°C. Dissolve the residue in 15 mL of water, filter, if necessary, neutralize the diluted hydrochloric acid (3 in 5), and boil for 5 minutes. After cooling, add 1 mL of dilute hydrochloric acid and water to make 50 mL. Perform the test using this solution as the test solution. Prepare the control solution as follows: to 4.5 mL of sodium carbonate TS add an equal volume of diluted hydrochloric acid (3 in 5) for the neutralization of the sample and 15 mL of water, and boil for 5 minutes. After cooling, add 0.35 mL of 0.005 mol/L sulfuric acid VS, 1 mL of dilute hydrochloric acid and water to make 50 mL (not more than 0.011%).

Residue on ignition <*2.44*> Not more than 0.1% (1 g).

Assay Dissolve about 50 mg of Paraformaldehyde, accurately weighed, in 10 mL of potassium hydroxide TS in an iodine flask. Add 40 mL of water and an exactly measured 50 mL of 0.05 mol/L iodine VS, stopper, and allow to stand for 5 minutes. Then add 5 mL of dilute hydrochloric acid, stopper immediately, allow to stand for 15 minutes, and titrate <*2.50*> the excess iodine with 0.1 mol/L sodium thiosulfate VS (indicator: 1 mL of starch TS). Perform a blank determination in the same manner.

Each mL of 0.05 mol/L iodine VS = 1.501 mg of CH_2O

Containers and storage Containers—Tight containers.

Dental Paraformaldehyde Paste

歯科用パラホルムパスタ

Method of preparation

Paraformaldehyde, finely powdered	35 g
Procaine Hydrochloride, finely powdered	35 g
Hydrous Lanolin	a sufficient quantity
To make	100 g

Prepare as directed under Ointments, with the above ingredients.

Description Dental Paraformaldehyde Paste is yellowish white in color. It has a characteristic odor.

Identification (1) To 0.15 g of Dental Paraformaldehyde Paste add 20 mL of diethyl ether and 20 mL of 0.5 mol/L sodium hydroxide TS, shake well, separate the water layer, and dilute with water to make 100 mL. To 1 mL of this solution add 10 mL of acetylacetone TS, and heat on a water bath for 10 minutes: a yellow color is produced (paraformaldehyde).

(2) To the diethyl ether layer obtained in (1) add 5 mL of dilute hydrochloric acid and 20 mL of water, shake well, and separate the water layer: the solution responds to Qualitative Tests <*1.09*> for primary aromatic amines (procaine hydrochloride).

(3) To 0.15 g of Dental Paraformaldehyde Paste add 25 mL of diethyl ether and 25 mL of water, shake, separate the water layer, filter, and use the filtrate as the sample solution. Separately, dissolve 0.01 g of procaine hydrochloride in 5 mL of water, and use this solution as standard solution. Perform the test with these solutions as directed under Thin-layer Chromatography <*2.03*>. Spot 5 μL each of the sample solution and standard solution on a plate of silica gel with fluorescent indicator for thin-layer chromatography. Develop the plate with a mixture of ethyl acetate, ethanol (99.5) and ammonia solution (28) (50:5:1) to a distance of about 10 cm, and air-dry the plate. Examine under ultraviolet light (main wavelength: 254 nm): spots obtained from the sample solution and standard solution show the same *R*f value.

Containers and storage Containers—Tight containers.

Parnaparin Sodium

パルナパリンナトリウム

$R^1, R^3, R^4 = SO_3Na$ or H

$R^2 = SO_3Na$ or $COCH_3$

$R^5 = CO_2Na$, $R^6 = H$
or
$R^5 = H$, $R^6 = CO_2Na$

n = 4−21

Parnaparin Sodium is a low-molecular heparin sodium obtained by depolymerization, with hydrogen peroxide and copper (II) acetate or with sodium hypochlorite, of heparins sodium from the healthy edible porcine intestinal mucosa. The mass-average molecular mass ranges between 4500 and 6500.

The potency is not less than 70 low-molecular-mass-heparin units and not more than 95 low-molecular-mass-heparin units of anti-factor Xa activity per mg, calculated on the dried basis.

Description Parnaparin Sodium occurs as a white or light yellow powder.

It is freely soluble in water, and practically insoluble in ethanol (99.5).

It is hygroscopic.

Identification **(1)** Mix 0.1 mL of a solution of Parnaparin Sodium (1 in 20) and 10 mL of a solution of tritoluidine blue O (1 in 100,000), and shake the mixture: the blue color of solution immediately changes to purple.

(2) A solution of Parnaparin Sodium (1 in 20) responds to Qualitative Tests *<1.09>* for sodium salt.

pH *<2.54>* Dissolve 0.1 g of Parnaparin Sodium in 10 mL of water: the pH of this solution is between 6.0 and 8.0.

Purity **(1)** Clarity and color of solution—Dissolve 1.0 g of Parnaparin Sodium in 10 mL of water: the solution is clear and colorless or pale yellow.

(2) Heavy metals *<1.07>*—Proceed with 1.0 g of Parnaparin Sodium according to Method 2, and perform the test. Prepare the control solution with 2.0 mL of Standard Lead Solution (not more than 20 ppm).

Loss on drying *<2.41>* Not more than 8.0% (0.2 g, in vacuum, phosphorus (V) oxide, 60°C, 3 hours).

Molecular mass Calculate the molecular mass of Parnaparin Sodium by the following methods: The mass-average molecular mass ranges between 4500 and 6500.

(i) Creation of calibration curve—Weigh 20 mg of low-molecular mass heparin for calibration of molecular mass, and dissolve it in 2.0 mL of the mobile phase as the standard solution. Perform the test with 50 μL of the standard solution as directed under Liquid Chromatography *<2.01>* according to the following conditions. Determine the peak height, H_{UV}, in chromatogram obtained by the ultraviolet absorption photometer, and determine the peak height, H_{RI}, in chromatogram obtained by the differential refractometer. Calculate the ratio of H_{UV} to H_{RI}, H_{RI}/H_{UV}, at each peak. Assume the molecular mass in the 4th peak from the low molecular mass in chromatogram obtained by the ultraviolet absorption photometer as 2400, and make the calculation of the standard coefficient from dividing 2400 by the H_{RI}/H_{UV} at the corresponding peak. Make the calculation to multiply the H_{RI}/H_{UV} at each peak by the standard coefficient, and determine the molecular mass of each peak by the calculation. Prepare the calculation curve by plotting the logarithm of molecular masses at each peak on the vertical axis and the retention time on the chromatogram obtained by the differential refractometer on the horizontal axis.

Operating conditions—

Detector: An ultraviolet absorption photometer (wavelength: 234 nm) and a differential refractometer.

Column: Connect 2 stainless steel columns which are 7.5 mm in inside diameter and 30 cm in length, and are packed with porous silica gel for liquid chromatography; one column, the molecular mass of limited size exclusion is about 500,000; the other, the molecular mass of limited size exclusion is about 100,000. Connect a pump, the about 500,000-molecular mass of limited size exclusion column, the about 100,000-molecular mass of limited size exclusion column, the ultraviolet absorption photometer and the differential refractometer in this order.

Column temperature; A constant temperature of about 40°C.

Mobile phase: Dissolve 28.4 g of sodium sulfate anhydride in 1000 mL of water, and 5.0 with 0.05 mol/L sulfuric acid TS.

Flow rate: 0.5 mL per minute.

System suitability—

System performance: When the procedure is run with 50 μL of the standard solution under the above operating conditions, confirm that more than 10 peaks in chromatogram obtained as directed under either the Ultraviolet-visible Spectrophotometry, or the Differential Refractometry are observed.

System repeatability: When the tests repeated 6 times with 50 μL of the standard solution under the above operating conditions, relative standard deviation of the 4th peak height in chromatogram (H_{UV} and H_{RI}) is not more than 3.0%.

(ii) Determination of molecular mass—Dissolve the 20 mg of Parnaparin Sodium with 2.0 mL of mobile phase, and use this solution as the sample solution. Perform the test with 50 μL of the sample solution as directed under Liquid Chromatography *<2.01>* according to the following conditions. Divide the main peak observed between 30 minutes and 45 minutes to 30 sec-interval fractions, and determine the strength of differential refractometer of each 30 sec-interval fraction. Determine the molecular mass of each fraction using the calibration curve and the retention time of each fraction. Determine the mean of molecular mass in the entire peak using the strength of differential refractometer and the molecular mass in every fractions.

$$\text{Mean molecular mass of parnaparin sodium} = \Sigma(n_i \cdot M_i)/\Sigma n_i$$

n_i: The differential refractometer strength of fraction i in the main peak of chromatogram

M_i: Molecular mass of fraction i in main peak

Operating conditions—

Detector: A differential refractometer.

Column, column temperature, mobile phase, and flow

rate: Proceed as directed in the operating conditions in (i) Creation of calibration curve.

System suitability—

Proceed as directed in (i) Creation of calibration curve.

Distribution of molecular mass The molecular mass of Parnaparin Sodium is calculated as directed in the determination of molecular mass and the distribution of molecular mass is calculated by the following equation: the molecular mass of not less than 80% parnaparin sodium is between 1500 and 10,000.

Distribution of molecular mass (%)
$= (\Sigma n_j / \Sigma n_i) \times 100$

n_i: The differential refractometer strength of fraction i in the main peak of chromatogram

Σn_j: Sum of differential refractometer strength in the each fraction between 1500 and 10,000 molecular mass in the main peak

The degree of sulfate ester Dissolve 0.5 g of Parnaparin Sodium with 10 mL water. Treat the solution with 5 mL of a strongly basic ion exchange resin, and subsequently with 10 mL of a strongly acidic ion exchange resin. Dilute the solution with water to 50 mL, and titrate <*2.50*> with 0.1 mol/L Sodium hydroxide VS (potentiometric titration). Calculate the degree of sulfate ester of Parnaparin Sodium from the equivalence point by the following equation; it is between 2.0 and 2.4.

The degree of sulfate ester
= the first equivalence point (mL)/[the second equivalence point (mL) − first equivalence point (mL)]

Total nitrogen Weigh accurately about 0.10 g of Parnaparin Sodium which is dried, and perform the test as directed under Nitrogen Determination <*1.08*>: it contains not less than 1.9% and not more than 2.3% of nitrogen (N:14.01).

Anti-factor IIa activity Determine the potency of anti-factor IIa activity of Parnaparin Sodium according to the following method, it contains not less than 35 and not more than 60 low-molecular-mass-heparin unit per mg, calculated on the dried basis.

(i) Standard solution—Dissolve Low-molecular Mass Heparin RS with isotonic sodium chloride solution to make solutions which contain 0.1, 0.2 and 0.3 low-molecular-mass-heparin unit (anti-factor IIa activity) in 1 mL, respectively.

(ii) Sample solution—Weigh accurately about 50 mg of Parnaparin Sodium, and dissolve it with isotonic sodium chloride solution to adjust the solution which contains 4 μg parnaparin sodium in 1 mL.

(iii) Procedure—To each plastic tube add 0.10 mL of the sample solution and the standard solution, separately. To each tube add 0.10 mL of human normal plasma and mix, and incubate at 37 ± 1°C accurately for 1 minute. Next, to each test tube add 0.10 mL of activated thromboplastin-time assay solution, which is pre-warmed at 37 ± 1°C, and after the mixing incubate accurately for 5 minutes at 37 ± 1°C. Then, to each tube add 0.10 mL of calcium chloride solution (277 in 100,000) which is pre-warmed at 37 ± 1°C, mix, start a stop watch simultaneously, and permit to stand at the same temperature. Determine the time for the first appearance of fibrin clot.

(iv) Calculation—Determine the low-molecular-mass-heparin unit (anti-factor IIa activity) of the sample solution from calibration curve obtained plots of clotting times for each standard solution; calculate the low-molecular-mass-heparin unit (anti-factor IIa activity) for 1 mg of parnaparin sodium as following equation.

The low-molecular-mass-heparin unit (anti-factor IIa activity) for 1 mg of parnaparin sodium
= the low-molecular-mass-heparin unit (anti-factor IIa activity) in 1 mL of sample solution × b/a

a: Amount (mg) of Parnaparin Sodium

b: The total volume (mL) in which Parnaparin Sodium has been dissolved with isotonic sodium chloride solution for the preparation of sample solution

The ratio of anti-factor Xa activity to anti-factor IIa activity Divide the anti-factor Xa activity, obtained in the Assay, by the anti-factor IIa activity which has been obtained from the test according to the method of anti-factor IIa activity; the ratio of anti-factor Xa activity to anti-factor IIa activity is between 1.5 and 2.5.

Assay

(i) Standard solution—Dissolve Low-molecular Mass-Heparin RS in isotonic sodium chloride solution to make solutions which contain 0.4, 0.6 and 0.8 low-molecular-mass-heparin units (anti-factor Xa activity) in 1 mL, respectively.

(ii) Sample solution—Weigh accurately about 50 mg of Parnaparin Sodium, and dissolve it in isotonic sodium chloride solution to make a solution which contains 7 μg parnaparin sodium in 1 mL.

(iii) Procedure—To each plastic tube add 0.10 mL of either the sample solution or the standard solution, separately. Subsequently to the every tubes add 0.70 mL of Tris-buffered solution (pH 8.4), 0.10 mL of anti-thrombin III TS, and 0.10 mL of normal human plasma, and mix them. To another plastic tube transfer 0.20 mL of these solutions, separately, and incubate for accurate 3 minutes at 37 ± 1°C. Next, to each tube add 0.10 mL of facter Xa TS and mix it, permit to stand 37 ± 1°C accurately for 30 seconds, and immediately add 0.20 mL of chromogenic synthetic substrate solution (3 in 4000) and mix it, and subsequently incubate accurately for 3 min at 37 ± 1°C. To each test tube add 0.30 mL of diluted acetic acid (100) solution (1 in 2) to stop the reaction. Separately, to plastic tube add 0.10 mL of isotonic sodium chloride solution, 0.70 mL of Tris-buffered solution (pH 8.4), 0.10 mL of anti-thrombin III TS, and 0.10 mL of normal human plasma to every tubes, and mix well. To another plastic tube transfer 0.20 mL of the solution, separately, and add both 0.30 mL of water and 0.30 mL of diluted acetic acid (100) (1 in 2). Determine the absorbance of both the sample solution and the standard solution at 405 nm as directed under Ultraviolet-visible Spectrophotometry <*2.24*> using a solution obtained from this solution as the blank.

(iv) Calculation method—Determine the low-molecular-mass unit (anti-factor Xa activity) of the sample solution using the calibration curve prepared from the absorbance of the standard solutions and their logarithmic concentrations, and calculate the low-molecular-mass unit (anti-factor Xa activity) in 1 mg of Parnaparin Sodium.

Low-molecular-mass-heparin unit (anti-factor Xa activity) in 1 mg of Parnaparin Sodium
= the low-molecular-mass-heparin unit (anti-factor Xa activity) in 1 mL of the sample solution × b/a

a: Amount (mg) of Parnaparin Sodium taken

b: The total volume (mL) in which Parnaparin Sodium has been dissolved with isotonic sodium chloride solution for the preparation of sample solution

Containers and storage Containers—Well-closed containers.

Paroxetine Hydrochloride Hydrate

パロキセチン塩酸塩水和物

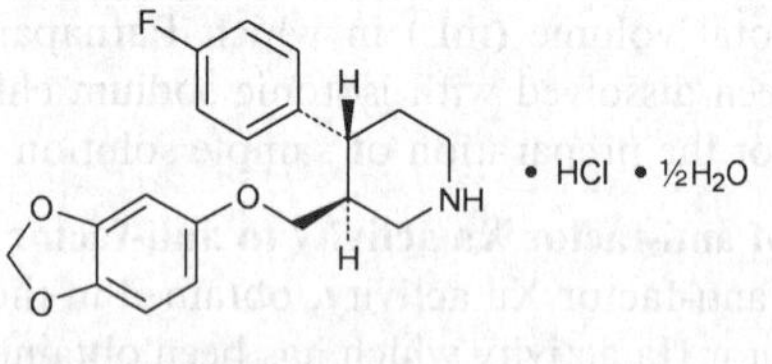

$C_{19}H_{20}FNO_3.HCl.{}^1\!/_2H_2O$: 374.83
(3*S*,4*R*)-3-[(1,3-Benzodioxol-5-yloxy)methyl]-4-(4-fluorophenyl)piperidine monohydrochloride hemihydrate
[*110429-35-1*]

Paroxetine Hydrochloride Hydrate contains not less than 98.5% and not more than 101.5% of paroxetine hydrochloride ($C_{19}H_{20}FNO_3.HCl$: 365.83), calculated on the anhydrous basis.

Description Paroxetine Hydrochloride Hydrate occurs as a white crystalline powder.

It is freely soluble in methanol, soluble in ethanol (99.5), and slightly soluble in water.

Optical rotation $[\alpha]_D^{20}$: −83 – −93°(0.1 g calculated on the anhydrous basis, ethanol (99.5), 20 mL, 100 mm).

Melting point: about 140°C (with decomposition).

Identification **(1)** Determine the absorption spectrum of a solution of Paroxetine Hydrochloride Hydrate in ethanol (99.5) (1 in 20,000) as directed under Ultraviolet-visible Spectrophotometry *<2.24>*, and compare the spectrum with the Reference Spectrum or the spectrum of a solution of Paroxetine Hydrochloride RS prepared in the same manner as the sample solution: both spectra exhibit similar intensities of absorption at the same wavelengths.

(2) Determine the infrared absorption spectrum of Paroxetine Hydrochloride Hydrate as directed in the potassium chloride disk method under Infrared Spectrophotometry *<2.25>*, and compare the spectrum with the Reference Spectrum or the spectrum of Paroxetine Hydrochloride RS: both spectra exhibit similar intensities of absorption at the same wave numbers.

(3) A solution of Paroxetine Hydrochloride Hydrate (1 in 500) responds to Qualitative Tests *<1.09>* for chloride.

Purity **(1)** Heavy metals *<1.07>*—Proceed with 1.0 g of Paroxetine Hydrochloride Hydrate according to Method 4, and perform the test. Use a solution of magnesium nitrate hexahydrate in ethanol (95) (1 in 30). Prepare the control solution with 1.0 mL of Standard Lead Solution (not more than 10 ppm).

(2) 4-(4-Fluorophenyl)-1-methyl-1,2,3,6-tetrahydropyridine—Dissolve 0.42 g of Paroxetine Hydrochloride Hydrate in 10 mL of a mixture of water and acetonitrile (4:1), and use this solution as the sample solution. Pipet 1 mL of the sample solution, and add a mixture of water and acetonitrile (4:1) to make exactly 100 mL. Pipet 1 mL of this solution, and add a mixture of water and acetonitrile (4:1) to make exactly 100 mL. Pipet 2 mL of this solution, add a mixture of water and acetonitrile (4:1) to make exactly 20 mL, and use this solution as the standard solution. Perform the test with exactly 75 μL each of the sample solution and standard solution as directed under Liquid Chromatography *<2.01>* according to the following conditions. Determine each peak area by the automatic integration method: the area of the peak, having the relative retention time of about 0.8 to paroxetine, obtained from the sample solution is not larger than the peak area of paroxetine from the standard solution. For the area of the peak, having the relative retention time of about 0.8 to paroxetine, multiply the correction factor 0.86.

Operating conditions—

Detector: An ultraviolet absorption photometer (wavelength: 242 nm).

Column: A stainless steel column 4.0 mm in inside diameter and 25 cm in length, packed with octadecylsilanized silica gel for liquid chromatography (5 μm in particle diameter).

Column temperature: A constant temperature of about 30°C.

Mobile phase A: Dissolve 30 g of sodium perchlorate monohydrate in 900 mL of water, add 3.5 mL of phosphoric acid, 2.4 mL of triethylamine and water to make 1000 mL, and then adjust to pH 2.0 with phosphoric acid or triethylamine.

Mobile phase B: Acetonitrile.

Flowing of mobile phase: Control the gradient by mixing the mobile phases A and B as directed in the following table.

Time after injection of sample (min)	Mobile phase A (vol%)	Mobile phase B (vol%)
0 – 20	85 → 80	15 → 20
20 – 27	80 → 55	20 → 45
27 – 36	55	45

Flow rate: 1.5 mL per minute.

System suitability—

System performance: When the procedure is run with 75 μL of the standard solution under the above operating conditions, the number of theoretical plates and the symmetry factor of the peak of paroxetine are not less than 100,000 and not more than 2.0, respectively.

System repeatability: When the test is repeated 6 times with 75 μL of the standard solution under the above operating conditions, the relative standard deviation of the peak area of paroxetine is not more than 5.0%.

(3) Related substances—Dissolve 20 mg of Paroxetine Hydrochloride Hydrate in 20 mL of a mixture of water and tetrahydrofuran (9:1), and use this solution as the sample solution. Pipet 1 mL of the sample solution, and add a mixture of water and tetrahydrofuran (9:1) to make exactly 100 mL. Pipet 1 mL of this solution, and add a mixture of water and tetrahydrofuran (9:1) to make exactly 10 mL, and use this solution as the standard solution. Perform the test with exactly 20 μL each of the sample solution and standard solution as directed under Liquid Chromatography *<2.01>* according to the following conditions. Determine each peak area by the automatic integration method: the area of the peak other than paroxetine obtained from the sample solution is not larger than the peak area of paroxetine from the standard solution. For the areas of the peaks, having the relative retention time of about 0.29, about 0.66, about 0.73, about 0.85, about 0.91, about 1.14, about 1.51, and about 1.84 to paroxetine, multiply their correction factors 0.46, 0.82, 1.10, 0.95, 0.93, 0.82, 1.55, and 1.54, respectively.

Operating conditions—

Detector: An ultraviolet absorption photometer (wavelength: 285 nm).

Column: A stainless steel column 4.6 mm in inside diameter and 25 cm in length, packed with octylsilanized silica gel for liquid chromatography (5 μm in particle diameter).

Column temperature: A constant temperature of about 40°C.

Mobile phase A: A mixture of water, tetrahydrofuran and trifluoroacetic acid (180:20:1).

Mobile phase B: A mixture of acetonitrile, tetrahyrofuran and trifluoroacetic acid (180:20:1).

Flowing of mobile phase: Control the gradient by mixing the mobile phases A and B as directed in the following table.

Time after injection of sample (min)	Mobile phase A (vol%)	Mobile phase B (vol%)
0 – 30	80	20
30 – 50	80 → 20	20 → 80
50 – 60	20	80

Flow rate: 1.0 mL per minute.

Time span of measurement: For 60 minutes after injection, beginning after the solvent peak.

System suitability—

System performance: When the procedure is run with 20 μL of the standard solution under the above operating conditions, the number of theoretical plates and the symmetry factor of the peak of paroxetine are not less than 5000 and not more than 2.0, respectively.

System repeatability: When the test is repeated 6 times with 20 μL of the standard solution under the above operating conditions, the relative standard deviation of the peak area of paroxetine is not more than 2.0%.

(4) Enantiomer—Dissolve 0.10 g of Paroxetine Hydrochloride Hydrate in 20 mL of methanol, add a solution of sodium chloride (29 in 1000) to make 100 mL, and use this solution as the sample solution. Pipet 1 mL of the sample solution, add 10 mL of methanol, and add a solution of sodium chloride (29 in 1000) to make exactly 50 mL. Pipet 2 mL of this solution, add 4 mL of methanol, add a solution of sodium chloride (29 in 1000) to make exactly 20 mL, and use this solution as the standard solution. Perform the test with exactly 10 μL each of the sample solution and standard solution as directed under Liquid Chromatography <2.01> according to the following conditions, and determine each peak area by the automatic integration method: the area of the peak of the enantiomer, having the relative retention time of about 0.4 to paroxetine, obtained from the sample solution is not larger than the peak area of paroxetine from the standard solution.

Operating conditions—

Detector: An ultraviolet absorption photometer (wavelength: 295 nm).

Column: A stainless steel column 4 mm in inside diameter and 10 cm in length, packed with α_1-acid glycoprotein-binding silica gel for liquid chromatography (5 μm in particle diameter).

Column temperature: A constant temperature of about 18°C.

Mobile phase: A mixture of sodium chloride solution (29 in 1000) and methanol (4:1).

Flow rate: Adjust so that the retention time of paroxetine is about 22 minutes.

System suitability—

System performance: When the procedure is run with 10 μL of the standard solution under the above operating conditions, the number of theoretical plates and the symmetry factor of the peak of paroxetine are not less than 500 and not more than 2.0, respectively.

System repeatability: When the test is repeated 6 times with 10 μL of the standard solution under the above operating conditions, the relative standard deviation of the peak area of paroxetine is not more than 2.0%.

Water *<2.48>* 2.0 – 3.0% (0.2 g, volumetric titration, direct titration).

Residue on ignition *<2.44>* Not more than 0.1% (1 g, platinum crucible).

Assay Weigh accurately about 50 mg each of Paroxetine Hydrochloride Hydrate and Paroxetine Hydrochloride RS (separately determine the water *<2.48>* in the same manner as Paroxetine Hydrochloride Hydrate), dissolve them separately in water to make exactly 100 mL, and use these solutions as the sample solution and the standard solution, respectively. Perform the test with exactly 10 μL each of the sample solution and standard solution as directed under Liquid Chromatography *<2.01>* according to the following conditions, and determine the peak areas, A_T and A_S, of paroxetine in each solution.

Amount (mg) of paroxetine hydrochloride ($C_{19}H_{20}FNO_3.HCl$)
$$= M_S \times A_T/A_S$$

M_S: Amount (mg) of Paroxetine Hydrochloride RS taken, calculated on the anhydrous basis

Operating conditions—

Detector: An ultraviolet absorption photometer (wavelength: 295 nm).

Column: A stainless steel column 4.6 mm in inside diameter and 25 cm in length, packed with trimethylsilanized silica gel for liquid chromatography (5 μm in particle diameter).

Column temperature: A constant temperature of about 30°C.

Mobile phase: Dissolve 3.85 g of ammonium acetate in 1000 mL of water, and adjust to pH 4.5 with acetic acid (100). To 600 mL of this solution, add 400 mL of acetonitrile and 10 mL of triethylamine, then adjust to pH5.5 with acetic acid (100).

Flow rate: Adjust so that the retention time of paroxetine is about 9 minutes.

System suitability—

System performance: When the procedure is run with 10 μL of the standard solution under the above operating conditions, the number of theoretical plates and the symmetry factor of the peak of paroxetine are not less than 5000 and not more than 2.0, respectively.

System repeatability: When the test is repeated 6 times with 10 μL of the standard solution under the above operating conditions, the relative standard deviation of the peak area of paroxetine is not more than 1.0%.

Containers and storage Containers—Tight containers.

Paroxetine Hydrochloride Tablets

パロキセチン塩酸塩錠

Paroxetine Hydrochloride Tablets contain not less than 95.0% and not more than 105.0% of the labeled amount of paroxetine ($C_{19}H_{20}FNO_3$: 329.37).

Method of preparation Prepare as directed under Tablets, with Paroxetine Hydrochloride Hydrate.

Identification Powder Paroxetine Hydrochloride Tablets. To a portion of the powder, equivalent to 10 mg of paroxetine ($C_{19}H_{20}FNO_3$), add 140 mL of ethanol (99.5), sonicate for 5 minutes, add ethanol (99.5) to make 200 mL, and filter. Determine the absorption spectrum of the filtrate as directed under Ultraviolet-visible Spectrophotometry <*2.24*>: it exhibits maxima between 233 nm and 237 nm, between 263 nm and 267 nm, between 269 nm and 273 nm, and between 293 nm and 297 nm.

Uniformity of dosage units <*6.02*> Perform the test according to the following method: it meets the requirement of the Content uniformity test.

To 1 tablet of Paroxetine Hydrochloride Tablets add $V/5$ mL of 0.1 mol/L hydrochloric acid TS, disintegrate by sonicating for 10 minutes, add $3V/5$ mL of a mixture of water and 2-propanol (1:1), and sonicate for 20 minutes. To this solution add a mixture of water and 2-propanol (1:1) to make exactly V mL so that each mL contains about 0.2 mg of paroxetine ($C_{19}H_{20}FNO_3$), filter through a membrane filter with a pore size not exceeding 0.45 μm, and use the filtrate as the sample solution. Then, proceed as directed in the Assay.

Amount (mg) of paroxetine ($C_{19}H_{20}FNO_3$)
$= M_S \times A_T/A_S \times V/100 \times 0.900$

M_S: Amount (mg) of Paroxetine Hydrochloride RS taken, calculated on the anhydrous basis

Dissolution <*6.10*> When the test is performed at 50 revolutions per minute according to the Paddle method, using 900 mL of 1st fluid for dissolution test as the dissolution medium, the dissolution rate in 45 minutes of 5-mg and 10-mg tablet is not less than 80%, and of 20-mg tablet is not less than 75%.

Start the test with 1 tablet of Paroxetine Hydrochloride Tablets, withdraw not less than 20 mL of the medium at the specified minute after starting the test, and filter through a membrane filter with a pore size not exceeding 0.45 μm. Discard not less than 10 mL of the first filtrate, pipet V mL of the subsequent filtrate, add the dissolution medium to make exactly V' mL so that each mL contains about 5.6 μg of paroxetine ($C_{19}H_{20}FNO_3$), and use this solution as the sample solution. Separately, weigh accurately about 11 mg of Paroxetine Hydrochloride RS (separately determine the water <*2.48*> in the same manner as Paroxetine Hydrochloride Hydrate), and dissolve in the dissolution medium to make exactly 100 mL. Pipet 3 mL of this solution, add the dissolution medium to make exactly 50 mL, and use this solution as the standard solution. Perform the test with exactly 25 μL each of the sample solution and standard solution as directed under Liquid Chromatography <*2.01*> according to the following conditions, and determine the peak areas, A_T and A_S, of paroxetine in each solution.

Dissolution rate (%) with respect to the labeled amount of paroxetine ($C_{19}H_{20}FNO_3$)
$= M_S \times A_T/A_S \times V'/V \times 1/C \times 54 \times 0.900$

M_S: Amount (mg) of Paroxetine Hydrochloride RS taken, calculated on the anhydrous basis
C: Labeled amount (mg) of paroxetine ($C_{19}H_{20}FNO_3$) in 1 tablet

Operating conditions—

Proceed as directed in the operating conditions in the Assay.

System suitability—

System performance: When the procedure is run with 25 μL of the standard solution under the above operating conditions, the number of theoretical plates and the symmetry factor of the peak of paroxetine are not less than 5000 and not more than 2.0, respectively.

System repeatability: When the test is repeated 6 times with 25 μL of the standard solution under the above operating conditions, the relative standard deviation of the peak area of paroxetine is not more than 2.0%.

Assay Weigh accurately the mass of not less than 20 Paroxetine Hydrochloride Tablets, and powder. Weigh accurately a portion of the powder, equivalent to about 20 mg of paroxetine ($C_{19}H_{20}FNO_3$), add 20 mL of 0.1 mol/L hydrochloric acid TS, sonicate for 10 minutes. To this solution add 60 mL of a mixture of water and 2-propanol (1:1), and sonicate for 20 minutes. Then add a mixture of water and 2-propanol (1:1) to make exactly 100 mL, filter through a membrane filter with a pore size not exceeding 0.45 μm, and use the filtrate as the sample solution. Separately, weigh accurately about 23 mg of Paroxetine Hydrochloride RS (separately determine the water <*2.48*> in the same manner as Paroxetine Hydrochloride Hydrate), and dissolve in 20 mL of 0.1 mol/L hydrochloric acid TS, add a mixture of water and 2-propanol (1:1) to make exactly 100 mL, and use this solution as the standard solution. Perform the test with exactly 25 μL each of the sample solution and standard solution as directed under Liquid Chromatography <*2.01*> according to the following conditions, and determine the peak areas, A_T and A_S, of paroxetine in each solution.

Amount (mg) of paroxetine ($C_{19}H_{20}FNO_3$)
$= M_S \times A_T/A_S \times 0.900$

M_S: Amount (mg) of Paroxetine Hydrochloride RS taken, calculated on the anhydrous basis

Operating conditions—

Detector: An ultraviolet absorption photometer (wavelength: 295 nm).

Column: A stainless steel column 4.6 mm in inside diameter and 25 cm in length, packed with trimethylsilanized silica gel for liquid chromatography (5 μm in particle diameter).

Column temperature: A constant temperature of about 30°C.

Mobile phase: Dissolve 3.85 g of ammonium acetate in 1000 mL of water, and adjust to pH 4.5 with acetic acid (100). To 600 mL of this solution, add 400 mL of acetonitrile and 10 mL of triethylamine, then adjust to pH 5.5 with acetic acid (100).

Flow rate: Adjust so that the retention time of paroxetine is about 9 minutes.

System suitability—

System performance: When the procedure is run with 25 μL of the standard solution under the above operating conditions, the number of theoretical plates and the symmetry factor of the peak of paroxetine are not less than 5000 and not more than 3.0, respectively.

System repeatability: When the test is repeated 6 times with 25 μL of the standard solution under the above operating conditions, the relative standard deviation of the peak area of paroxetine is not more than 1.0%.

Containers and storage Containers—Well-closed containers.

Pazufloxacin Mesilate

パズフロキサシンメシル酸塩

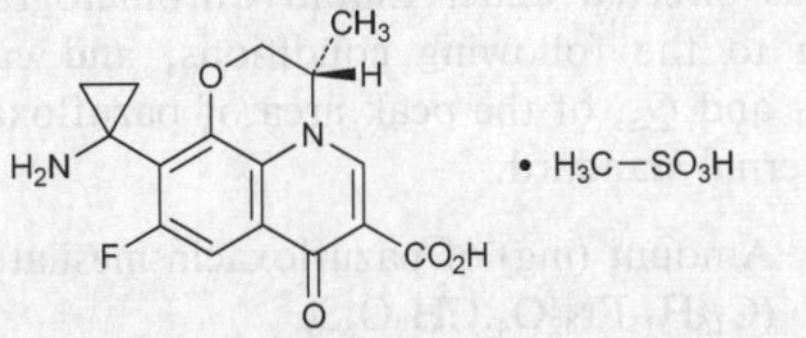

$C_{16}H_{15}FN_2O_4.CH_4O_3S$: 414.41
(3*S*)-10-(1-Aminocyclopropyl)-9-fluoro-3-methyl-7-oxo-2,3-dihydro-7*H*-pyrido[1,2,3-*de*][1,4]benzoxazine-6-carboxylic acid monomethanesulfonate
[*163680-77-1*]

Pazufloxacin Mesilate, when dried, contains not less than 98.0% and not more than 102.0% of pazufloxacin mesilate ($C_{16}H_{15}FN_2O_4.CH_4O_3S$).

Description Pazufloxacin Mesilate occurs as a white to light yellow crystalline powder.

It is freely soluble in water, and slightly soluble in ethanol (99.5).

It dissolves in sodium hydroxide TS.

The pH of a solution prepared by dissolving 0.4 g of Pazufloxacin Mesilate in 10 mL of water is between 3.0 and 4.0.

Melting point: about 258°C (with decomposition).

It shows crystal polymorphism.

Identification (1) Determine the absorption spectrum of a solution of Pazufloxacin Mesilate in a mixture of methanol and 1 mol/L hydrochloric acid TS (49:1) (1 in 100,000) as directed under Ultraviolet-visible Spectrophotometry <*2.24*>, and compare the spectrum with the Reference Spectrum or the spectrum of a solution of Pazufloxacin Mesilate RS prepared in the same manner as the sample solution: both spectra exhibit similar intensities of absorption at the same wavelengths.

(2) Determine the infrared absorption spectrum of Pazufloxacin Mesilate, previously dried, as directed in the paste method under Infrared Spectrophotometry <*2.25*>, and compare the spectrum with the Reference Spectrum or the spectrum of dried Pazufloxacin Mesilate RS: both spectra exhibit similar intensities of absorption at the same wave numbers.

(3) Pazufloxacin Mesilate responds to Qualitative Tests <*1.09*> for mesilate.

Optical rotation <*2.49*> $[\alpha]_D^{20}$: −61 − −65° (after drying, 0.2 g, sodium hydroxide TS, 20 mL, 100 mm).

Purity (1) Heavy metals <*1.07*>—Proceed with 1.0 g of Pazufloxacin Mesilate according to Method 2, and perform the test. Prepare the control solution with 2.0 mL of Standard Lead Solution (not more than 20 ppm).

(2) Related substances—Dissolve 26 mg of Pazufloxacin Mesilate in 100 mL of the mobile phase, and use this solution as the sample solution. Perform the test with 20 μL of the sample solution as directed under Liquid Chromatography <*2.01*> according to the following conditions. Determine each peak area by the automatic integration method, and calculate the amounts of them by the area percentage method: the amount of the peak other than pazufloxacin is not more than 0.10%. For the area of the peak, having the relative retention time of about 2.7 to pazufloxacin, multiply the correction factor, 1.6.

Operating conditions—

Detector: An ultraviolet absorption photometer (wavelength: 254 nm).

Column: A stainless steel column 4.6 mm in inside diameter and 15 cm in length, packed with octadecylsilanized silica gel for liquid chromatography (5 μm in particle diameter).

Column temperature: A constant temperature of about 40°C.

Mobile phase: Dissolve 1.08 g of sodium 1-octanesulfonate in 1000 mL of a mixture of diluted phosphoric acid (1 in 1000) and acetonitrile (39:11).

Flow rate: Adjust so that the retention time of pazufloxacin is about 8 minutes.

Time span of measurement: About 6 times as long as the retention time of pazufloxacin, beginning after the solvent peak.

System suitability—

Test for required detectability: To 1 mL of the sample solution add the mobile phase to make 100 mL, and use this solution as the solution for system suitability test. Pipet 1 mL of the solution for system suitability test, and add the mobile phase to make exactly 10 mL. Confirm that the peak area of pazufloxacin obtained with 20 μL of this solution is equivalent to 7 to 13% of that with 20 μL of the solution for system suitability test.

System performance: When the procedure is run with 20 μL of the solution for system suitability test under the above operating conditions, the number of theoretical plates and the symmetry factor of the peak of pazufloxacin are not less than 2500 and not more than 2.0, respectively.

System repeatability: When the test is repeated 6 times with 20 μL of the solution for system suitability test under the above operating conditions, the relative standard deviation of the peak area of pazufloxacin is not more than 2.0%.

Loss on drying <*2.41*> Not more than 0.5% (1 g, 105°C, 3 hours).

Residue on ignition <*2.44*> Not more than 0.1% (0.2 g, platinum crucible).

Assay Weigh accurately about 26 mg each of Pazufloxacin Mesilate and Pazufloxacin Mesilate RS, both previously dried, dissolve each in water to make exactly 100 mL. Pipet 5 mL each of these solutions, add exactly 5 mL of the internal standard solution, and use these solutions as the sample solution and the standard solution, respectively. Perform the test with 10 μL each of the sample solution and standard solution as directed under Liquid Chromatography <*2.01*> according to the following conditions, and calculate the ratios, Q_T and Q_S, of the peak area of pazufloxacin to that of the internal standard.

$$\text{Amount (mg) of pazufloxacin mesilate } (C_{16}H_{15}FN_2O_4.CH_4O_3S) = M_S \times Q_T/Q_S$$

M_S: Amount (mg) of Pazufloxacin Mesilate RS taken

Internal standard solution—A solution of acetanilide in the mobile phase (3 in 10,000).

Operating conditions—

Detector: An ultraviolet absorption photometer (wavelength: 254 nm).

Column: A stainless steel column 4 mm in inside diameter and 25 cm in length, packed with octadecylsilanized silica gel for liquid chromatography (10 μm in particle diameter).

Column temperature: A constant temperature of about 25°C.

Mobile phase: To 200 mL of water add gradually 30 mL

of methanesulfonic acid while ice-cooling, then add 30 mL of triethylamine in the same manner, and add water to make 300 mL. To 50 mL of this solution add 150 mL of acetonitrile, 35 mL of 1 mol/L dipotassium hydrogen phosphate TS for buffer solution and water to make 1000 mL.

Flow rate: Adjust so that the retention time of pazufloxacin is about 5 minutes.

System suitability—

System performance: When the procedure is run with 10 μL of the standard solution under the above operating conditions, pazufloxacin and the internal standard are eluted in this order with the resolution between these peaks being not less than 3.

System repeatability: When the test is repeated 6 times with 10 μL of the standard solution under the above operating conditions, the relative standard deviation of the ratio of the peak area of pazufloxacin to that of the internal standard is not more than 1.0%.

Containers and storage Containers—Tight containers.

Pazufloxacin Mesilate Injection

パズフロキサシンメシル酸塩注射液

Pazufloxacin Mesilate Injection is an aqueous injection.

It contains not less than 95.0% and not more than 105.0% of the labeled amount of pazufloxacin mesilate ($C_{16}H_{15}FN_2O_4.CH_4O_3S$: 414.41).

Method of preparation Prepare as directed under Injections, with Pazufloxacin Mesilate.

Description Pazufloxacin Mesilate Injection is a clear, colorless liquid.

Identification To a volume of Pazufloxacin Mesilate Injection, equivalent to 20 mg of Pazufloxacin Mesilate, add a mixture of methanol and 1 mol/L hydrochloric acid TS (49:1) to make 100 mL. To 5 mL of this solution add a mixture of methanol and 1 mol/L hydrochloric acid TS (49:1) to make 100 mL. Determine the absorption spectrum of this solution as directed under Ultraviolet-visible Spectrophotometry <*2.24*>: it exhibits maxima between 237 nm and 241 nm, between 314 nm and 324 nm, between 328 nm and 332 nm, and between 343 nm and 347 nm.

pH Being specified separately when the drug is granted approval based on the Law.

Bacterial endotoxins <*4.01*> Less than 0.30 EU/mg.

Extractable volume <*6.05*> It meets the requirement.

Foreign insoluble matter <*6.06*> Perform the test according to Method 1: it meets the requirement.

Insoluble particulate matter <*6.07*> It meets the requirement.

Sterility <*4.06*> Perform the test according to the Membrane filtration method: it meets the requirement.

Assay Pipet a volume of Pazufloxacin Mesilate Injection, equivalent to about 12 mg of pazufloxacin mesilate ($C_{16}H_{15}FN_2O_4.CH_4O_3S$), and add water to make exactly 50 mL. Pipet 5 mL of this solution, add exactly 5 mL of the internal standard solution, and use this solution as the sample solution. Separately, weigh accurately about 23 mg of Pazufloxacin Mesilate RS, previously dried at 105°C for 3 hours, and add water to make exactly 100 mL. Pipet 5 mL of this solution, add exactly 5 mL of the internal standard solution, and use this solution as the standard solution. Perform the test with 10 μL each of the sample solution and standard solution as directed under Liquid Chromatography <*2.01*> according to the following conditions, and calculate the ratios, Q_T and Q_S, of the peak area of pazufloxacin to that of the internal standard.

Amount (mg) of pazufloxacin mesilate ($C_{16}H_{15}FN_2O_4.CH_4O_3S$)

$$= M_S \times Q_T/Q_S \times 1/2$$

M_S: Amount (mg) of Pazufloxacin Mesilate RS taken

*Internal standard solution—*A solution of acetanilide in the mobile phase (3 in 10,000).

Operating conditions—

Proceed as directed in the operating conditions in the Assay under Pazufloxacin Mesilate.

System suitability—

System performance: When the procedure is run with 10 μL of the standard solution under the above operating conditions, pazufloxacin and acetanilide are eluted in this order with the resolution between these peaks being not less than 3.

System repeatability: When the test is repeated 6 times with 10 μL of the standard solution under the above operating conditions, the relative standard deviation of the ratio of the peak area of pazufloxacin to that of the internal standard is not more than 1.0%.

Containers and storage Containers—Hermetic containers. Plastic containers for aqueous injections may be used.

Storage—Light-resistant.

Pemirolast Potassium

ペミロラストカリウム

$C_{10}H_7KN_6O$: 266.30

Monopotassium 5-(9-methyl-4-oxo-4*H*-pyrido[1,2-*a*]pyrimidin-3-yl)-1*H*-tetrazol-1-ide

[*100299-08-9*]

Pemirolast Potassium contains not less than 98.5% and not more than 101.0% of pemirolast potassium ($C_{10}H_7KN_6O$), calculated on the anhydrous basis.

Description Pemirolast Potassium occurs as a light yellow crystalline powder.

It is freely soluble in water, slightly soluble in methanol, and very slightly soluble in ethanol (99.5).

It dissolves in potassium hydroxide TS.

Melting point: about 322°C (with decomposition).

Identification **(1)** Determine the absorption spectrum of a solution of Pemirolast Potassium in diluted potassium hydroxide TS (1 in 10,000) (1 in 100,000) as directed under Ultraviolet-visible Spectrophotometry <*2.24*>, and compare the spectrum with the Reference Spectrum or the spectrum of a solution of Pemirolast Potassium RS prepared in the same manner as the sample solution: both spectra exhibit similar intensities of absorption at the same wavelengths.

(2) Determine the infrared absorption spectrum of Pemirolast Potassium as directed in the potassium bromide disk method under Infrared Spectrophotometry *<2.25>*, and compare the spectrum with the Reference Spectrum or the spectrum of Pemirolast Potassium RS: both spectra exhibit similar intensities of absorption at the same wave numbers.

(3) Pemirolast Potassium responds to Qualitative Tests *<1.09>* (1) for potassium salt.

Purity **(1)** Clarity of solution—A solution obtained by dissolving 0.5 g of Pemirolast Potassium in 10 mL of water is clear.

(2) Heavy metals *<1.07>*—Proceed with 0.5 g of Pemirolast Potassium according to Method 2, and perform the test. Prepare the control solution with 1.0 mL of Standard Lead Solution (not more than 20 ppm).

(3) Related substances—Dissolve 50 mg of Pemirolast Potassium in 50 mL of a mixture of phosphate buffer solution (pH 8.0) and methanol (3:2), and use this solution as the sample solution. Pipet 2 mL of the sample solution, and add a mixture of phosphate buffer solution (pH 8.0) and methanol (3:2) to make exactly 100 mL. To exactly 2.5 mL of this solution add a mixture of phosphate buffer solution (pH 8.0) and methanol (3:2) to make exactly 50 mL, and use this solution as the standard solution. Perform the test with exactly 10 μL each of the sample solution and standard solution as directed under Liquid Chromatography *<2.01>* according to the following conditions. Determine each peak area by the automatic integration method: the area of the peak other than pemirolast obtained from the sample solution is not larger than the peak area of pemirolast from the standard solution.

Operating conditions—

Detector, column, column temperature, mobile phase, and flow rate: Proceed as directed in the operating conditions in the Assay.

Time span of measurement: About 9 times as long as the retention time of pemirolast.

System suitability—

Test for required detectability: To exactly 5 mL of the standard solution add a mixture of phosphate buffer solution (pH 8.0) and methanol (3:2) to make exactly 25 mL. Confirm that the peak area of pemirolast obtained with 10 μL of this solution is equivalent to 15 to 25% of that with 10 μL of the standard solution.

System performance: When the procedure is run with 10 μL of the standard solution under the above operating conditions, the number of theoretical plates and the symmetry factor of the peak of pemirolast are not less than 3000 and not more than 1.7, respectively.

System repeatability: When the test is repeated 6 times with 10 μL of the standard solution under the above operating conditions, the relative standard deviation of the peak area of pemirolast is not more than 2.0%.

Water *<2.48>* Not more than 0.5% (0.1 g, coulometric titration).

Assay Weigh accurately about 50 mg each of Pemirolast Potassium and Pemirolast Potassium RS (separately determine the water *<2.48>* in the same manner as Pemirolast Potassium), dissolve in a mixture of phosphate buffer solution (pH 8.0) and methanol (3:2) to make them exactly 50 mL. Pipet 5 mL each of these solutions, add exactly 5 mL of the internal standard solution, then add a mixture of phosphate buffer solution (pH 8.0) and methanol (3:2) to make 50 mL, and use these solutions as the sample solution and the standard solution, respectively. Perform the test with 10 μL each of the sample solution and standard solution as directed under Liquid Chromatography *<2.01>* according to the following conditions, and calculate the ratios, Q_T and Q_S, of the peak area of pemirolast to that of the internal standard.

$$\text{Amount (mg) of pemirolast potassium } (C_{10}H_7KN_6O) = M_S \times Q_T/Q_S$$

M_S: Amount (mg) of Pemirolast Potassium RS taken, calculated on the anhydrous basis

Internal standard solution—A solution of ethyl aminobenzoate in methanol (1 in 1000).

Operating conditions—

Detector: An ultraviolet absorption photometer (wavelength: 260 nm).

Column: A stainless steel column 4.6 mm in inside diameter and 15 cm in length, packed with octadecylsilanized silica gel for liquid chromatography (5 μm in particle diameter).

Column temperature: A constant temperature of about 25°C.

Mobile phase: A mixture of water, methanol and acetic acid (100) (30:20:1).

Flow rate: Adjust so that the retention time of pemirolast is about 5 minutes.

System suitability—

System performance: When the procedure is run with 10 μL of the standard solution under the above operating conditions, pemirolast and the internal standard are eluted in this order with the resolution between these peaks being not less than 5.

System repeatability: When the test is repeated 6 times with 10 μL of the standard solution under the above operating conditions, the relative standard deviation of the ratio of the peak area of pemirolast to that of the internal standard is not more than 1.0%.

Containers and storage Containers—Tight containers.

Storage—Light-resistant.

Pemirolast Potassium Ophthalmic Solution

ペミロラストカリウム点眼液

Pemirolast Potassium Ophthalmic Solution is an aqueous ophthalmic preparation.

It contains not less than 95.0% and not more than 105.0% of the labeled amount of pemirolast potassium ($C_{10}H_7KN_6O$: 266.30).

Method of preparation Prepare as directed under Ophthalmic Liquids and Solutions, with Pemirolast Potassium.

Description Pemirolast Potassium Ophthalmic Solution is a clear, colorless liquid.

Identification To a volume of Pemirolast Potassium Ophthalmic Solution, equivalent to 1 mg of Pemirolast Potassium, add diluted 0.1 mol/L phosphate buffer solution for antibiotics (pH 8.0) (1 in 10) to make 100 mL. Determine the absorption spectrum of this solution as directed under Ultraviolet-visible Spectrophotometry *<2.24>*: it exhibits maxima between 255 nm and 259 nm, and between 355 nm and 359 nm.

Osmotic pressure ratio Being specified separately when the drug is granted approval based on the Law.

pH Being specified separately when the drug is granted approval based on the Law.

Purity Related substances—To a volume of Pemirolast Potassium Ophthalmic Solution, equivalent to 2 mg of Pemirolast Potassium, add 1 mL of methanol and diluted 0.1 mol/L phosphate buffer solution for antibiotics (pH 8.0) (1 in 10) to make 5 mL, and use this solution as the sample solution. Pipet 1 mL of the sample solution, add 20 mL of methanol and diluted 0.1 mol/L phosphate buffer solution for antibiotics (pH 8.0) (1 in 10) to make exactly 100 mL, and use this solution as the standard solution. Perform the test with exactly 10 μL each of the sample solution and standard solution as directed under Liquid Chromatography <*2.01*> according to the following conditions. Determine each peak area by the automatic integration method: the area of the peak other than pemirolast obtained from the sample solution is not larger than 3/10 times the peak area of pemirolast from the standard solution, and the total area of the peaks other than pemirolast from the sample solution is not larger than the peak area of pemirolast from the standard solution.

Operating conditions—

Detector: An ultraviolet spectrophotometer (wavelength: 260 nm).

Column: A stainless steel column 4.6 mm in inside diameter and 15 cm in length, packed with octadecylsilanized silica gel for liquid chromatography (5 μm in particle diameter).

Column temperature: A constant temperature of about 40°C.

Mobile phase A: A mixture of trifluoroacetic acid TS and methanol (4:1).

Mobile phase B: A mixture of methanol and trifluoroacetic acid TS (3:2).

Flowing of mobile phase: Control the gradient by mixing the mobile phases A and B as directed in the following table.

Time after injection of sample (min)	Mobile phase A (vol%)	Mobile phase B (vol%)
0 - 60	100 → 0	0 → 100

Flow rate: Adjust so that the retention time of pemirolast is about 19 minutes.

Time span of measurement: About 3 times as long as the retention time of pemirolast, beginning after the solvent peak.

System suitability—

Test for required detectability: Pipet 2 mL of the standard solution, and add diluted 0.1 mol/L phosphate buffer solution for antibiotics (pH 8.0) (1 in 10) to make exactly 20 mL. Confirm that the peak area of pemirolast obtained with 10 μL of this solution is equivalent to 7 to 13% of that with 10 μL of the standard solution.

System performance: Dissolve 10 mg of pemirolast potassium in 10 mL of diluted 0.1 mol/L phosphate buffer solution for antibiotics (pH 8.0) (1 in 10), transfer this solution to a colorless test tube, and illuminate with a D_{65} fluorescent lamp (3000 lx) for 72 hours. To 2 mL of this solution add 1 mL of methanol and diluted 0.1 mol/L phosphate buffer solution for antibiotics (pH 8.0) (1 in 10) to make 5 mL. When the procedure is run with 10 μL of this solution under the above operating conditions, the resolution between the peak, having the relative retention time about 0.9 to pemirolast, and the peak of pemirolast is not less than 3.

System repeatability: When the test is repeated 6 times with 10 μL of the standard solution under the above operating conditions, the relative standard deviation of the peak area of pemirolast is not more than 2.0%.

Foreign insoluble matter <*6.11*> It meets the requirement.

Insoluble particulate matter <*6.08*> It meets the requirement.

Sterility <*4.06*> Perform the test according to the Membrane filtration method: it meets the requirement.

Assay Pipet a volume of Pemirolast Potassium Ophthalmic Solution, equivalent to 2 mg of pemirolast potassium ($C_{10}H_7KN_6O$), add exactly 2 mL of the internal standard solution, then add a mixture of diluted 0.1 mol/L phosphate buffer solution for antibiotics (pH 8.0) (1 in 10) and methanol (3:2) to make 20 mL, and use this solution as the sample solution. Separately, weigh accurately about 50 mg of Pemirolast Potassium RS (separately determine the water <*2.48*> in the same manner as Pemirolast Potassium), and dissolve in water to make exactly 50 mL. Pipet 2 mL of this solution, add exactly 2 mL of the internal standard solution, then add a mixture of diluted 0.1 mol/L phosphate buffer solution for antibiotics (pH 8.0) (1 in 10) and methanol (3:2) to make 20 mL, and use this solution as the standard solution. Perform the test with 10 μL each of the sample solution and standard solution as directed under Liquid Chromatography <*2.01*> according to the following conditions. Calculate the ratios, Q_T and Q_S of the peak area of pemirolast to that of the internal standard.

Amount (mg) of pemirolast potassium ($C_{10}H_7KN_6O$)
$= M_S \times Q_T/Q_S \times 1/25$

M_S: Amount (mg) of Pemirolast Potassium RS taken, calculated on the anhydrous basis

Internal standard solution—A solution of ethyl aminobenzoate in methanol (1 in 1000).

Operating conditions—

Detector: An ultraviolet spectrophotometer (wavelength: 260 nm).

Column: A stainless steel column 3.9 mm in inside diameter and 15 cm in length, packed with octadecylsilanized silica gel for liquid chromatography (4 μm in particle diameter).

Column temperature: A constant temperature of about 40°C.

Mobile phase: A mixture of water, methanol and acetic acid (100) (30:20:1).

Flow rate: Adjust so that the retention time of pemirolast is about 4 minutes.

System suitability—

System performance: When the procedure is run with 10 μL of the standard solution under the above operating conditions, pemirolast and the internal standard are eluted in this order with the resolution between these peaks being not less than 6.

System repeatability: When the test is repeated 6 times with 10 μL of the standard solution under the above operating conditions, the relative standard deviation of the ratio of the peak area of pemirolast to that of the internal standard is not more than 1.0%.

Containers and storage Containers—Tight containers.

Pemirolast Potassium for Syrup

シロップ用ペミロラストカリウム

Pemirolast Potassium for Syrup is a preparation for syrup, which is dissolved before use.

It contains not less than 95.0% and not more than 105.0% of the labeled amount of pemirolast potassium ($C_{10}H_7KN_6O$: 266.30).

Method of preparation Prepare as directed under Preparations for Syrups, with Pemirolast Potassium.

Identification Determine the absorption spectrum of the sample solution obtained in the Assay as directed under Ultraviolet-visible Spectrophotometry <*2.24*>: it exhibits maxima between 255 nm and 259 nm and between 355 nm and 359 nm.

pH Being specified separately when the drug is granted approval based on the Law.

Uniformity of dosage units <*6.02*> Perform the test according to the following method: Pemirolast Potassium for Syrup in single-dose packages meet the requirement of the Content uniformity test.

Dissolve the total amount of the content of 1 package of Pemirolast Potassium for Syrup in water to make exactly V mL so that each mL contains about 50 μg of pemirolast potassium ($C_{10}H_7KN_6O$). Pipet 10 mL of this solution, add water to make exactly 50 mL, and use this solution as the sample solution. Then, proceed as directed in the Assay.

Amount (mg) of pemirolast potassium ($C_{10}H_7KN_6O$)
$= M_S \times A_T/A_S \times V/400$

M_S: Amount (mg) of Pemirolast Potassium RS taken, calculated on the anhydrous basis

Assay Powder Pemirolast Potassium for Syrup. Weigh accurately a portion of the powder, equivalent to about 5 mg of pemirolast potassium ($C_{10}H_7KN_6O$), and dissolve in water to make exactly 100 mL. Pipet 10 mL of this solution, add water to make exactly 50 mL, and use this solution as the sample solution. Separately, weigh accurately about 20 mg of Pemirolast Potassium RS (separately determine the water <*2.48*> in the same manner as Pemirolast Potassium), and dissolve in water to make exactly 100 mL. Pipet 5 mL of this solution, add water to make exactly 100 mL, and use this solution as the standard solution. Determine the absorbances, A_T and A_S, at 357 nm of the sample solution and standard solution as directed under Ultraviolet-visible Spectrophotometry <*2.24*>.

Amount (mg) of pemirolast potassium ($C_{10}H_7KN_6O$)
$= M_S \times A_T/A_S \times 1/4$

M_S: Amount (mg) of Pemirolast Potassium RS taken, calculated on the anhydrous basis

Containers and storage Containers—Tight containers.
Storage—Light-resistant.

Pemirolast Potassium Tablets

ペミロラストカリウム錠

Pemirolast Potassium Tablets contain not less than 95.0% and not more than 105.0% of the labeled amount of pemirolast potassium ($C_{10}H_7KN_6O$: 266.30).

Method of preparation Prepare as directed under Tablets, with Pemirolast Potassium.

Identification Determine the absorption spectrum of the sample solution obtained in the Assay as directed under Ultraviolet-visible Spectrophotometry <*2.24*>: it exhibits maxima between 255 nm and 259 nm, and between 355 nm and 359 nm.

Uniformity of dosage units <*6.02*> Perform the test according to the following method: it meets the requirement of the Content uniformity test.

To 1 tablet of Pemirolast Potassium Tablets add 50 mL of water for 5 mg of pemirolast potassium ($C_{10}H_7KN_6O$), and shake to disintegrate the tablet completely. Then, add water to make exactly V mL so that each mL contains about 50 μg of pemirolast potassium ($C_{10}H_7KN_6O$), and filter. Discard the first 10 mL of the filtrate, pipet 10 mL of the subsequent filtrate, add 1 mL of diluted potassium hydroxide TS (1 in 100), add water to make exactly 50 mL, and use this solution as the sample solution. Then, proceed as directed in the Assay.

Amount (mg) of pemirolast potassium ($C_{10}H_7KN_6O$)
$= M_S \times A_T/A_S \times V/400$

M_S: Amount (mg) of Pemirolast Potassium RS taken, calculated on the anhydrous basis

Dissolution <*6.10*> When the test is performed at 50 revolutions per minute according to the Paddle method, using 900 mL of disodium hydrogen phosphate-citric acid buffer solution (pH 5.0) as the dissolution medium, the dissolution rate in 45 minutes of a 5-mg tablet is not less than 75%, and that in 60 minutes of a 10-mg tablet is not less than 70%.

Start the test with 1 tablet of Pemirolast Potassium Tablets, withdraw not less than 20 mL of the medium at the specified minute after starting the test, and filter through a membrane filter with a pore size not exceeding 0.45 μm. Discard not less than 10 mL of the first filtrate, pipet V mL of the subsequent filtrate, and add the dissolution medium to make exactly V' mL so that each mL contains about 5.6 μg of pemirolast potassium ($C_{10}H_7KN_6O$). Pipet 4 mL of this solution, add exactly 2 mL of diluted potassium hydroxide TS (1 in 10), and use this solution as the sample solution. Separately, weigh accurately about 28 mg of Pemirolast Potassium RS (separately determine the water <*2.48*> in the same manner as Pemirolast Potassium), dissolve in water to make exactly 100 mL. Pipet 5 mL of this solution, add water to make exactly 50 mL. Pipet 5 mL of this solution, add water to make exactly 25 mL. Pipet 4 mL of this solution, add exactly 2 mL of diluted potassium hydroxide TS (1 in 10), and use this solution as the standard solution. Then, proceed as directed in the Assay.

Dissolution rate (%) with respect to the labeled amount of pemirolast potassium ($C_{10}H_7KN_6O$)
$= M_S \times A_T/A_S \times V'/V \times 1/C \times 18$

M_S: Amount (mg) of Pemirolast Potassium RS taken, calculated on the anhydrous basis

C: Labeled amount (mg) of pemirolast potassium ($C_{10}H_7KN_6O$) in 1 tablet

Assay Accurately weigh the mass of not less than 20 Pemirolast Potassium Tablets, and powder. Weigh accurately a portion of the powder, equivalent to about 5 mg of pemirolast potassium ($C_{10}H_7KN_6O$), add 50 mL of water, shake thoroughly for 20 minutes, then add water to make exactly 100 mL. Filter, discard the first 10 mL of the filtrate, pipet 10 mL of the subsequent filtrate, add 1 mL of diluted potassium hydroxide TS (1 in 100), add water to make exactly 50 mL, and use this solution as the sample solution. Separately, weigh accurately about 20 mg of Pemirolast Potassium RS (separately determine the water <*2.48*> in the same manner as Pemirolast Potassium), and dissolve in water to make exactly 100 mL. Pipet 5 mL of this solution, add 1 mL of diluted potassium hydroxide TS (1 in 100), add water to make exactly 100 mL, and use this solution as the standard solution. Determine the absorbances, A_T sand A_S, at 357 nm of the sample solution and standard solution as directed under Ultraviolet-visible Spectrophotometry <*2.24*>, using water as the blank.

Amount (mg) of pemirolast potassium ($C_{10}H_7KN_6O$)
$= M_S \times A_T/A_S \times 1/4$

M_S: Amount (mg) of Pemirolast Potassium RS taken, calculated on the anhydrous basis

Containers and storage Containers—Tight containers.
Storage—Light-resistant.

Penbutolol Sulfate

ペンブトロール硫酸塩

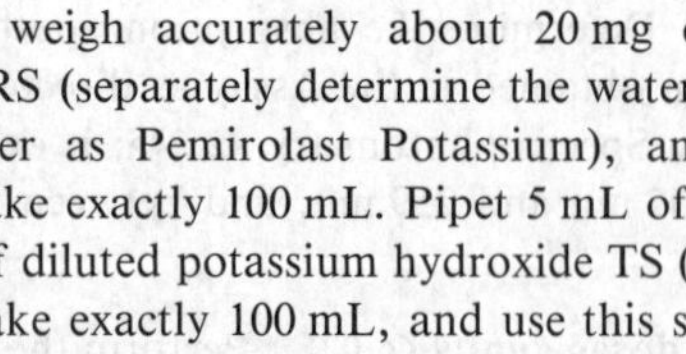

$(C_{18}H_{29}NO_2)_2.H_2SO_4$: 680.94
(2*S*)-3-(2-Cyclopentylphenoxy)-1-(1,1-dimethylethyl)aminopropan-2-ol hemisulfate
[*38363-32-5*]

Penbutolol Sulfate, when dried, contains not less than 98.5% of penbutolol sulfate [$(C_{18}H_{29}NO_2)_2.H_2SO_4$].

Description Penbutolol Sulfate occurs as a white crystalline powder.

It is very soluble in acetic acid (100), freely soluble in methanol, sparingly soluble in ethanol (95), slightly soluble in water, and practically insoluble in acetic anhydride and in diethyl ether.

Identification **(1)** Determine the absorption spectrum of a solution of Penbutolol Sulfate in methanol (1 in 10,000) as directed under Ultraviolet-visible Spectrophotometry <*2.24*>, and compare the spectrum with the Reference Spectrum: both spectra exhibit similar intensities of absorption at the same wavelengths.

(2) Determine the infrared absorption spectrum of Penbutolol Sulfate, previously dried, as directed in the paste method under Infrared Spectrophotometry <*2.25*>, and compare the spectrum with the Reference Spectrum: both spectra exhibit similar intensities of absorption at the same wave numbers.

(3) Dissolve 0.1 g of Penbutolol Sulfate in 25 mL of water by warming, and cool: this solution responds to Qualitative Tests <*1.09*> for sulfate.

Optical rotation <*2.49*> $[\alpha]_D^{20}$: −23 – −25° (after drying, 0.2 g, methanol, 20 mL, 100 mm).

Melting point <*2.60*> 213 – 217°C

Purity **(1)** Heavy metals <*1.07*>—Proceed with 2.0 g of Penbutolol Sulfate according to Method 2, and perform the test. Prepare the control solution with 2.0 mL of Standard Lead Solution (not more than 10 ppm).

(2) Arsenic <*1.11*>—Prepare the test solution with 1.0 g of Penbutolol Sulfate according to Method 4, and perform the test (not more than 2 ppm).

(3) Related substances—Dissolve 0.8 g of Penbutolol Sulfate in 10 mL of methanol, and use this solution as the sample solution. Pipet 1 mL of the sample solution, add methanol to make exactly 200 mL, and use this solution as the standard solution. Perform the test with these solutions as directed under Thin-layer Chromatography <*2.03*>. Spot 10 μL each of the sample solution and standard solution on a plate of silica gel with fluorescent indicator for thin-layer chromatography. Develop the plate with a mixture of 2-propanol, ethanol (95) and ammonia solution (28) (85:12:3) to a distance of about 10 cm, and air-dry the plate. Examine under ultraviolet light (main wavelength: 254 nm): the spots other than the principal spot obtained from the sample solution are not more intense than the spot from the standard solution.

Loss on drying <*2.41*> Not more than 0.5% (0.5 g, 105°C, 3 hours).

Residue on ignition <*2.44*> Not more than 0.2% (1 g).

Assay Weigh accurately about 0.8 g of Penbutolol Sulfate, previously dried, dissolve in 50 mL of a mixture of acetic anhydride and acetic acid (100) (7:3), and titrate <*2.50*> with 0.1 mol/L perchloric acid VS (potentiometric titration). Perform a blank determination in the same manner, and make any necessary correction.

Each mL of 0.1 mol/L perchloric acid VS
= 68.09 mg of $(C_{18}H_{29}NO_2)_2.H_2SO_4$

Containers and storage Containers—Well-closed containers.

Pentazocine

ペンタゾシン

and enantiomer

$C_{19}H_{27}NO$: 285.42
(2*RS*,6*RS*,11*RS*)-6,11-Dimethyl-3-(3-methylbut-2-en-1-yl)-1,2,3,4,5,6-hexahydro-2,6-methano-3-benzoazocin-8-ol
[*359-83-1*]

Pentazocine, when dried, contains not less than 99.0% of pentazocine ($C_{19}H_{27}NO$).

Description Pentazocine occurs as a white to pale yellowish-white, crystalline powder. It is odorless.

It is freely soluble in acetic acid (100) and in chloroform, soluble in ethanol (95), sparingly soluble in diethyl ether and practically insoluble in water.

Identification **(1)** To 1 mg of Pentazocine add 0.5 mL of formaldehyde-sulfuric acid TS: a deep red color is produced, and it changes to grayish brown immediately.

(2) Dissolve 5 mg of Pentazocine in 5 mL of sulfuric acid, add 1 drop of iron (III) chloride TS, and heat in a water bath for 2 minutes: the color of the solution changes from light yellow to deep yellow. Shake the solution with 1 drop of nitric acid: the solution remains yellow in color.

(3) Determine the absorption spectrum of a solution of Pentazocine in 0.01 mol/L hydrochloric acid TS (1 in 10,000) as directed under Ultraviolet-visible Spectrophotometry <*2.24*>, and compare the spectrum with the Reference Spectrum: both spectra exhibit similar intensities of absorption at the same wavelengths.

Absorbance <*2.24*> $E^{1\%}_{1\,\mathrm{cm}}$ (278 nm): 67.5 – 71.5 (after drying, 0.1 g, 0.01 mol/L hydrochloric acid TS, 1000 mL).

Melting point <*2.60*> 150 – 158°C

Purity **(1)** Clarity and color of solution—Dissolve 0.10 g of Pentazocine in 20 mL of 0.1 mol/L hydrochloric acid TS: the solution is clear and colorless.

(2) Heavy metals <*1.07*>—Proceed with 1.0 g of Pentazocine according to Method 2, and perform the test. Prepare the control solution with 2.0 mL of Standard Lead Solution (not more than 20 ppm).

(3) Arsenic <*1.11*>—Prepare the test solution with 1.0 g of Pentazocine according to Method 3, and perform the test with a solution of magnesium nitrate hexahydrate in ethanol (95) (1 in 10) (not more than 2 ppm).

(4) Related substances—Dissolve 0.20 g of Pentazocine in 10 mL of chloroform, and use this solution as the sample solution. Pipet 1 mL of the sample solution, add chloroform to make exactly 100 mL, and use this solution as the standard solution. Perform the test with these solutions as directed under Thin-layer Chromatography <*2.03*>. Spot 10 μL each of the sample solution and standard solution on a plate of silica gel for thin-layer chromatography. Develop the plate with a mixture of chloroform, methanol and isopropylamine (94:3:3) to a distance of about 13 cm, and air-dry the plate. Allow to stand for 5 minutes in iodine vapor: any spot other than the principal spot obtained from the sample solution is not more intense than the spot from the standard solution.

Loss on drying <*2.41*> Not more than 0.5% (1 g, in vacuum, phosphorus (V) oxide, 60°C, 5 hours).

Residue on ignition <*2.44*> Not more than 0.2% (1 g).

Assay Weigh accurately about 0.5 g of Pentazocine, previously dried, dissolve in 50 mL of acetic acid (100), and titrate <*2.50*> with 0.1 mol/L perchloric acid VS (indicator: 2 drops of crystal violet TS). Perform a blank determination in the same manner, and make any necessary correction.

Each mL of 0.1 mol/L perchloric acid VS
= 28.54 mg of $C_{19}H_{27}NO$

Containers and storage Containers—Well-closed containers.

Pentobarbital Calcium

ペントバルビタールカルシウム

and enantiomer

$C_{22}H_{34}CaN_4O_6$: 490.61
Monocalcium bis[5-ethyl-5-[(1*RS*)-1-methylbutyl]-4,6-dioxo-1,4,5,6-tetrahydropyrimidin-2-olate]
[*76-74-4*, Pentobarbital]

Pentobarbital Calcium contains not less than 98.0% and not more than 102.0% of pentobarbital calcium ($C_{22}H_{34}CaN_4O_6$), calculated on the dried basis.

Description Pentobarbital Calcium occurs as a white powder.

It is sparingly soluble in water, slightly soluble in ethanol (95), and practically insoluble in acetonitrile.

A solution of Pentobarbital Calcium (1 in 100) shows no optical rotation.

Identification **(1)** Determine the infrared absorption spectrum of Pentobarbital Calcium as directed in the potassium bromide disk method under Infrared Spectrophotometry <*2.25*>, and compare the spectrum with the Reference Spectrum: both spectra exhibit similar intensities of absorption at the same wave numbers.

(2) To 1 g of Pentobarbital Calcium add 5 mL of ethanol (95) and 5 mL of dilute hydrochloric acid, dissolve by warming with shaking, shake with 5 mL of dilute hydrochloric acid and 10 mL of water, allow to cool, and filter. To the filtrate add 1 drop of methyl red TS, and add ammonia TS until a slight yellow color develops: the solution responds to Qualitative Tests <*1.09*> (1), (2) and (3) for calcium salt.

Purity **(1)** Chloride <*1.03*>—To 1.0 g of Pentobarbital Calcium add 5 mL of ethanol (95) and 2.5 mL of dilute nitric acid, dissolve by warming with shaking, cool, add water to make 50 mL, shake well, and filter. Discard the first 10 mL of the filtrate, and to 15 mL of the subsequent filtrate add 6 mL of dilute nitric acid and water to make 50 mL. Perform the test using this solution as the test solution. Prepare the control solution as follows: To 0.30 mL of 0.01 mol/L hydrochloric acid VS add 1.5 mL of ethanol (95), 6 mL of dilute nitric acid and water to make 50 mL (not more than 0.035%).

(2) Heavy metals <*1.07*>—To 2.0 g of Pentobarbital Calcium add 5 mL of ethanol (95) and 5 mL of dilute hydrochloric acid, dissolve by warming with shaking, cool, add water to make 80 mL, shake well, and filter. Discard the first 10 mL of the filtrate, to 40 mL of the subsequent filtrate add 1 drop of phenolphthalein TS, add dropwise ammonia TS until a pale red color develops, and add 2 mL of dilute acetic acid and water to make 50 mL. Perform the test using this solution as the test solution. Prepare the control solution as follows: To 2.5 mL of ethanol (95) add 2.5 mL of dilute hydrochloric acid and water to make 30 mL. Add 1 drop of phenolphthalein TS, add dropwise ammonia TS until a pale red color develops, then add 2.0 mL of Standard Lead Solution, 2 mL of dilute acetic acid and water to make 50 mL (not more than 20 ppm).

(3) Related substances—Dissolve 10 mg of Pentobarbital Calcium in 100 mL of water, and use this solution as the sample solution. Pipet 1 mL of the sample solution, add water to make exactly 100 mL, and use this solution as the standard solution. Perform the test with exactly 20 μL each of the sample solution and standard solution as directed under Liquid Chromatography <*2.01*> according to the following conditions, and determine the areas of each peak by the automatic integration method: the area of any peak other than the peak of pentobarbital obtained from the sample solution is not larger than 3/10 times the peak area of pentobarbital from the standard solution, and the total of these peak area is not larger than the peak area of pentobarbital from the standard solution.

Operating conditions—

Detector, column, column temperature, mobile phase, and flow rate: Proceed as directed in the operating conditions in the Assay.

Time span of measurement: About 3 times as long as the retention time of pentobarbital, beginning after the solvent peak.

System suitability—

System performance: Proceed as directed in the system performance in the Assay.

Test for required detectability: Pipet 2 mL of the standard solution, add water to make exactly 20 mL, and confirm that the peak area of pentobarbital obtained with 20 μL of this solution is equivalent to 5 to 15% of that with 20 μL of the standard solution.

System repeatability: When the test is repeated 6 times with 20 μL of the standard solution under the above operating conditions, the relative standard deviation of the peak areas of pentobarbital is not more than 5%.

Loss on drying <*2.41*> Not more than 7.0% (1 g, 105°C, 5 hours).

Assay Weigh accurately about 20 mg of Pentobarbital Calcium, dissolve in 5 mL of water, add exactly 5 mL of the internal standard solution and water to make 50 mL. To 5 mL of this solution add water to make 20 mL. To 2 mL of this solution add water to make 20 mL, and use this solution as the sample solution. Separately, weigh accurately about 18 mg of Pentobarbital RS, previously dried at 105°C for 2 hours, dissolve in 10 mL of acetonitrile for liquid chromatography, add exactly 5 mL of the internal standard solution, and add water to make 50 mL. To 5 mL of this solution add water to make 20 mL. To 2 mL of this solution add water to make 20 mL, and use this solution as the standard solution. Perform the test with 20 μL each of the sample solution and standard solution as directed under Liquid Chromatography <*2.01*> according to the following conditions, and calculate the ratios, Q_T and Q_S, of the peak area of pentobarbital to that of the internal standard.

Amount (mg) of pentobarbital calcium ($C_{22}H_{34}CaN_4O_6$)
$= M_S \times Q_T/Q_S \times 1.084$

M_S: Amount (mg) of Pentobarbital RS taken

*Internal standard solution—*Dissolve 0.2 g of isopropyl parahydroxybenzoate in 20 mL of acetonitrile for liquid chromatography, and add water to make 100 mL.

Operating conditions—

Detector: An ultraviolet absorption photometer (wavelength: 210 nm).

Column: A stainless steel column 4.6 mm in inside diameter and 15 cm in length, packed with octadecylsilanized silica gel for liquid chromatography (5 μm in particle diameter).

Column temperature: A constant temperature of about 40°C.

Mobile phase: Dissolve 1.36 g of potassium dihydrogen phosphate in 1000 mL of water, and adjust to pH 4.0 with diluted phosphoric acid (1 in 10). To 650 mL of this solution add 350 mL of acetonitrile for liquid chromatography.

Flow rate: Adjust so that the retention time of pentobarbital is about 7 minutes.

System suitability—

System performance: When the procedure is run with 20 μL of the standard solution under the above operating conditions, pentobarbital and the internal standard are eluted in this order with the resolution between these peaks being not less than 5.

System repeatability: When the test is repeated 6 times with 20 μL of the standard solution under the above operating conditions, the relative standard deviation of the ratios of the peak area of pentobarbital to that of the internal standard is not more than 1.0%.

Containers and storage Containers—Well-closed containers.

Pentobarbital Calcium Tablets

ペントバルビタールカルシウム錠

Pentobarbital Calcium Tablets contain not less than 95.0% and not more than 105.0% of the labeled amount of pentobarbital calcium ($C_{22}H_{34}CaN_4O_6$: 490.61).

Method of preparation Prepare as directed under Tablets, with Pentobarbital Calcium.

Identification To a quantity of powdered Pentobarbital Calcium Tablets, equivalent to 5.6 mg of Pentobarbital Calcium, add 60 mL of water, shake thoroughly, then add water to make 100 mL, and filter. To 6 mL of the filtrate add dilute sodium hydroxide TS to make 20 mL, and determine the absorption spectrum of this solution as directed under Ultraviolet-visible Spectrophotometry <*2.24*>: it exhibits a maximum between 240 nm and 244 nm.

Uniformity of dosage unit <*6.02*> Perform the Mass variation test, or the Content uniformity test according to the following method: it meets the requirement.

To 1 tablet of Pentobarbital Calcium Tablets add exactly V/10 mL of the internal standard solution, add 60 mL of water, shake vigorously until the tablet is completely disintegrated, then add water to make 100 mL, and filter through a membrane filter with a pore size not exceeding 0.45 μm. Discard the first 10 mL of the filtrate, to 2 mL of the subsequent filtrate add water to make *V* mL so that each mL contains about 10 μg of pentobarbital calcium ($C_{22}H_{34}CaN_4O_6$), and use this solution as the sample solution. Then, proceed as directed in the Assay.

Amount (mg) of pentobarbital calcium ($C_{22}H_{34}CaN_4O_6$)
$= M_S \times Q_T/Q_S \times V/50 \times 1.084$

M_S: Amount (mg) of Pentobarbital Calcium RS taken

Internal standard solution—Dissolve 0.5 g of isopropyl parahydroxybenzoate in 20 mL of acetonitrile for liquid chromatography, and add water to make 200 mL.

Dissolution <*6.10*> When the test is performed at 50 revolutions per minute according to the Paddle method, using 900 mL of 2nd fluid for dissolution test as the dissolution medium, the dissolution rate in 15 minutes of Pentobarbital Calcium Tablets is not less than 80%.

Start the test with 1 tablet of Pentobarbital Calcium Tablets, withdraw not less than 20 mL of the medium at the specified minute after starting the test, and filter through a membrane filter with a pore size not exceeding 0.45 μm. Discard not less than 10 mL of the first filtrate, pipet *V* mL of the subsequent filtrate, add the dissolution medium to make exactly *V′* mL so that each mL contains about 56 μg of pentobarbital calcium ($C_{22}H_{34}CaN_4O_6$). Pipet 3 mL of this solution, add dilute sodium hydroxide TS to make exactly 10 mL, and use this solution as the sample solution. Separately, weigh accurately about 26 mg of Pentobarbital RS, previously dried at 105°C for 2 hours, dissolve in 2 mL of ethanol (99.5), and add water to make exactly 100 mL. Pipet 4 mL of this solution, and add the dissolution medium to make exactly 20 mL. Pipet 3 mL of this solution, add dilute sodium hydroxide TS to make exactly 10 mL, and use this solution as the standard solution. Determine the absorbances, A_T and A_S, of the sample solution and standard solution at 241 nm as directed under Ultraviolet-visible Spectrophotometry <*2.24*>, using a solution, prepared by adding dilute sodium hydroxide TS to 3 mL of the dissolution medium to make 10 mL, as the blank.

Dissolution rate (%) with respect to the labeled amount of pentobarbital calcium ($C_{22}H_{34}CaN_4O_6$)
$= M_S \times A_T/A_S \times V'/V \times 1/C \times 180 \times 1.084$

M_S: Amount (mg) of Pentobarbital RS taken
C: Labeled amount (mg) of pentobarbital calcium ($C_{22}H_{34}CaN_4O_6$) in 1 tablet

Assay To 20 Pentobarbital Calcium Tablets add 120 mL of water, shake vigorously for 10 minutes, then add water to make exactly 200 mL, and filter through a membrane filter with a pore size not exceeding 0.45 μm. Discard the first 10 mL of the filtrate, pipet 5 mL of the subsequent filtrate, add exactly *V*/10 mL of the internal standard solution, and add water to make *V* mL so that each mL contains about 0.5 mg of pentobarbital calcium ($C_{22}H_{34}CaN_4O_6$). To 2 mL of this solution, add water to make 100 mL, and use this solution as the sample solution. Separately, weigh accurately about 23 mg of Pentobarbital RS, previously dried at 105°C for 2 hours, dissolve in 10 mL of acetonitrile for liquid chromatography, add exactly 5 mL of the internal standard solution, and add water to make 50 mL. To 2 mL of this solution add water to make 100 mL, and use this solution as the standard solution. Perform the test with 20 μL each of the sample solution and standard solution as directed under Liquid Chromatography <*2.01*> according to the following conditions, and calculate the ratios, Q_T and Q_S, of the peak area of pentobarbital to that of the internal standard.

Amount (mg) of pentobarbital calcium ($C_{22}H_{34}CaN_4O_6$) in 1 tablet
$= M_S \times Q_T/Q_S \times V/25 \times 1.084$

M_S: Amount (mg) of Pentobarbital RS taken

Internal standard solution—Dissolve 0.5 g of isopropyl parahydroxybenzoate in 20 mL of acetonitrile for liquid chromatography, and add water to make 200 mL.

Operating conditions—

Detector: An ultraviolet absorption photometer (wavelength: 210 nm).

Column: A stainless steel column 4.6 mm in inside diameter and 15 cm in length, packed with octadecylsilanized silica gel for liquid chromatography (5 μm in particle diameter).

Column temperature: A constant temperature of about 40°C.

Mobile phase: Dissolve 1.36 g of potassium dihydrogen phosphate in 1000 mL of water, and adjust to pH 4.0 with diluted phosphoric acid (1 in 10). To 650 mL of this solution add 350 mL of acetonitrile for liquid chromatography.

Flow rate: Adjust so that the retention time of pentobarbital is about 7 minutes.

System suitability—

System performance: When the procedure is run with 20 μL of the standard solution under the above operating conditions, pentobarbital and the internal standard are eluted in this order with the resolution between these peaks being not less than 5.

System repeatability: When the test is repeated 6 times with 20 μL of the standard solution under the above operating conditions, the relative standard deviation of the ratio of the peak area of pentobarbital to that of the internal standard is not more than 1.0%.

Containers and storage Containers—Tight containers.

Pentoxyverine Citrate

ペントキシベリンクエン酸塩

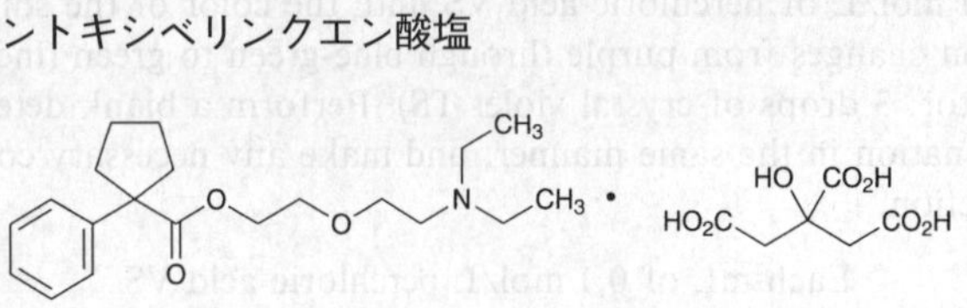

$C_{20}H_{31}NO_3.C_6H_8O_7$: 525.59
2-[2-(Diethylamino)ethoxy]ethyl 1-phenylcyclopentanecarboxylate monocitrate
[23142-01-0]

Pentoxyverine Citrate, when dried, contains not less than 98.5% of pentoxyverine citrate ($C_{20}H_{31}NO_3.C_6H_8O_7$).

Description Pentoxyverine Citrate occurs as a white crystalline powder.

It is very soluble in acetic acid (100), freely soluble in water and in ethanol (95), and practically insoluble in diethyl ether.

Identification **(1)** Dissolve 0.1 g of Pentoxyverine Citrate in 10 mL of water, and add 10 mL of Reinecke salt TS: a light red precipitate is formed.

(2) Determine the infrared absorption spectrum of Pentoxyverine Citrate, previously dried, as directed in the paste method under Infrared Spectrophotometry <2.25>, and compare the spectrum with the Reference Spectrum: both spectra exhibit similar intensities of absorption at the same wave numbers.

(3) A solution of Pentoxyverine Citrate (1 in 10) responds to Qualitative Tests <1.09> (1) and (2) for citrate.

Melting point <2.60> 92 - 95°C

Purity **(1)** Clarity and color of solution—Dissolve 1.0 g of Pentoxyverine Citrate in 10 mL of water: the solution is clear and colorless.

(2) Heavy metals <1.07>—Proceed with 2.0 g of Pentoxyverine Citrate according to Method 2, and perform the test. Prepare the control solution with 2.0 mL of Standard Lead Solution (not more than 10 ppm).

(3) Arsenic <1.11>—Prepare the test solution with 1.0 g of Pentoxyverine Citrate according to Method 3, and perform the test (not more than 2 ppm).

(4) Related substances—Dissolve 0.20 g of Pentoxyverine Citrate in 10 mL of ethanol (95), and use this solution as the sample solution. Pipet 1 mL of the sample solution, add ethanol (95) to make exactly 200 mL, and use this solution as the standard solution. Perform the test with these solutions as directed under Thin-layer Chromatography <2.03>. Spot 15 μL each of the sample solution and standard solution on a plate of silica gel for thin-layer chromatography. Immediately after air-drying, develop the plate with a mixture of chloroform, methanol, ethyl acetate and ammonia solution (28) (25:10:10:1) to a distance of about 10 cm, and air-dry the plate. Allow to stand in iodine vapor for 10 minutes: the spots other than the principal spot obtained from the sample solution are not more intense than the spot from the standard solution.

Loss on drying <2.41> Not more than 0.5% (1 g, in vacuum, phosphorus (V) oxide, 60°C, 4 hours).

Residue on ignition <2.44> Not more than 0.1% (1 g).

Assay Weigh accurately about 0.5 g of Pentoxyverine Citrate, previously dried, dissolve in 30 mL of acetic acid (100), add 30 mL of acetic anhydride, and titrate <2.50> with 0.1 mol/L of perchloric acid VS until the color of the solution changes from purple through blue-green to green (indicator: 3 drops of crystal violet TS). Perform a blank determination in the same manner, and make any necessary correction.

Each mL of 0.1 mol/L perchloric acid VS
= 52.56 mg of $C_{20}H_{31}NO_3.C_6H_8O_7$

Containers and storage Containers—Well-closed containers.

Peplomycin Sulfate

ペプロマイシン硫酸塩

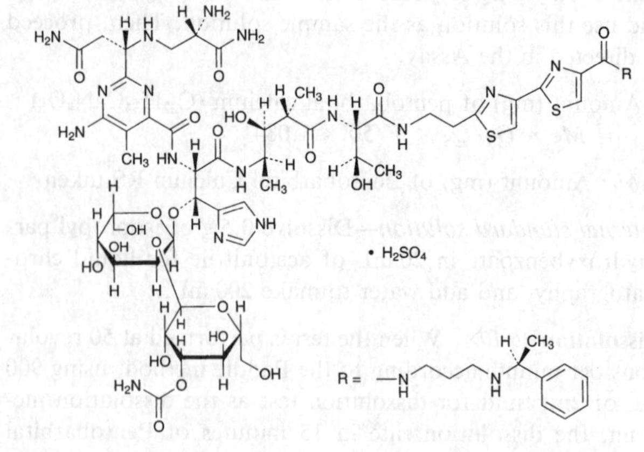

$C_{61}H_{88}N_{18}O_{21}S_2.H_2SO_4$: 1571.67
N[1]-{3-[(1*S*)-(1-Phenylethyl)amino]propyl}bleomycinamide monosulfate
[*70384-29-1*]

Peplomycin Sulfate is the sulfate of a substance having antitumor activity produced by the growth of *Streptomyces verticillus*.

It contains not less than 865 μg (potency) and not more than 1010 μg (potency) per mg, calculated on the dried basis. The potency of Peplomycin Sulfate is expressed as mass (potency) of peplomycin ($C_{61}H_{88}N_{18}O_{21}S_2$: 1473.59).

Description Peplomycin Sulfate occurs as a white to light yellow-white powder.

It is freely soluble in water, and practically insoluble in ethanol (95).

It is hygroscopic.

Identification **(1)** To 4 mg of Peplomycin Sulfate add 5 μL of copper (II) sulfate TS, and dissolve in water to make 100 mL. Determine the absorption spectrum of this solution as directed under Ultraviolet-visible Spectrophotometry <2.24>, and compare the spectrum with the Reference Spectrum or the spectrum of a solution of Peplomycin Sulfate RS prepared in the same manner as the sample solution: both spectra exhibit similar intensities of absorption at the same wavelengths.

(2) Determine the infrared absorption spectrum of Peplomycin Sulfate as directed in the paste method under Infrared Spectrophotometry <2.25>, and compare the spectrum with the Reference Spectrum or the spectrum of Peplomycin Sulfate RS: both spectra exhibit similar intensities of absorption at the same wave numbers.

(3) Dissolve 10 mg each of Peplomycin Sulfate and Peplomycin Sulfate RS in 6 mL of water, add 0.5 mL of a solution of copper (II) sulfate pentahydrate (1 in 125), and use these solutions as the sample solution and the standard solution, respectively. Perform the test with 10 μL each of the sample solution and standard solution as directed under Liquid Chromatography <2.01> according to the following conditions: the retention time of the principal peak in the chromatogram obtained from the sample solution is the same as that in the chromatogram from the standard solution.

Operating conditions—

Detector, column, column temperature, mobile phase

stock solution, mobile phase A, mobile phase B, flowing of mobile phase, and flow rate: Proceed as directed in the operating conditions in the Purity (3).

(4) A solution of Peplomycin Sulfate (1 in 200) responds to Qualitative Tests <*1.09*> (1) and (2) for sulfate.

Optical rotation <*2.49*> $[\alpha]_D^{20}$: −2 – −5° (0.1 g calculated on the dried basis, 0.1 mol/L phosphate buffer solution (pH 5.3), 10 mL, 100 mm).

pH <*2.54*> The pH of a solution obtained by dissolving 0.10 g of Peplomycin Sulfate in 20 mL of water is between 4.5 and 6.0.

Purity (1) Clarity and color of solution—Dissolve 80 mg of Peplomycin Sulfate in 4 mL of water: the solution is clear and colorless.

(2) Copper—Dissolve exactly 75 mg of Peplomycin Sulfate in 10 mL of diluted nitric acid (1 in 100), and use this solution as the sample solution. Separately, to 5.0 mL of Standard Copper Stock Solution add diluted nitric acid (1 in 100) to make exactly 100 mL. To 3.0 mL of this solution add diluted nitric acid (1 in 100) to make exactly 100 mL, and use this solution as the standard solution. Perform the test with the sample solution and standard solution as directed under Atomic Absorption Spectrophotometry <*2.23*> according to the following conditions: the absorbance of the sample solution is not more than that of the standard solution (not more than 200 ppm).

Gas: Combustible gas—Acetylene.
Supporting gas—Air.

Lamp: Copper hollow cathode lamp.

Wavelength: 324.8 nm.

(3) Related substances—Dissolve about 10 mg of Peplomycin Sulfate in 6 mL of water, add 0.5 mL of a solution of copper (II) sulfate pentahydrate (1 in 125), and use this solution as the sample solution. Perform the test with 10 μL of the sample solution as directed under Liquid Chromatography <*2.01*> according to the following conditions. Determine the areas of the peaks, appeared after the peak of copper sulfate, by the automatic integration method, and calculate the amounts of them by the area percentage method: the total amount of the peaks other than peplomycin is not more than 7.0%.

Operating conditions—

Detector: An ultraviolet absorption photometer (wavelength: 254 nm).

Column: A stainless steel column 4.6 mm in inside diameter and 25 cm in length, packed with octadecylsilanized silica gel for liquid chromatography (7 μm in particle diameter).

Column temperature: A constant temperature of about 40°C.

Mobile phase stock solution: Dissolve 0.96 g of sodium 1-pentanesulfonate and 1.86 g of disodium dihydrogen ethylenediamine tetraacetate dihydrate in 1000 mL of water and 5 mL of acetic acid (100), and adjust the pH to 4.3 with ammonia TS.

Mobile phase A: A mixture of mobile phase stock solution and methanol (9:1).

Mobile phase B: A mixture of mobile phase stock solution and methanol (3:2).

Flowing of mobile phase: Control the gradient by mixing the mobile phases A and B as directed in the following table.

Time after injection of sample (min)	Mobile phase A (vol%)	Mobile phase B (vol%)
0 – 60	100 → 0	0 → 100
60 – 75	0	100

Flow rate: 1.2 mL per minute.

Time span of measurement: As long as 20 minutes after elution of peplomycin, beginning after the peak of copper sulfate.

System suitability—

Test for required detectability: Measure exactly 1 mL of the sample solution, add water to make exactly 10 mL, and use this solution as the solution for system suitability test. Pipet 1 mL of the solution for system suitability test, and add water to make exactly 10 mL. Confirm that the peak area of peplomycin obtained with 10 μL of this solution is equivalent to 7 to 13% of that with 10 μL of the solution for system suitability test.

System performance: When the procedure is run with 10 μL of the sample solution under the above operating conditions, the number of theoretical plates and the symmetry factor of the peak of peplomycin are not less than 30,000 and not more than 2.0, respectively.

System repeatability: When the test is repeated 6 times with 10 μL of the sample solution under the above operating conditions, the relative standard deviation of the peak area of peplomycin is not more than 2.0%.

Loss on drying <*2.41*> Not more than 3.0% (60 mg, in vacuum, phosphorus (V) oxide, 60°C, 3 hours). Handle the sample avoiding absorption of moisture.

Assay Weigh accurately an amount of Peplomycin Sulfate and Peplomycin Sulfate RS, both previously dried, equivalent to about 50 mg (potency), dissolve them separately in the mobile phase to make exactly 100 mL. Pipet 4 mL each of these solutions, add exactly 10 mL of the internal standard solution, then add the mobile phase to make 50 mL, and use these solutions as the sample solution and the standard solution, respectively. Perform the test with 1 μL each of the sample solution and standard solution as directed under Liquid Chromatography <*2.01*> according to the following conditions, and calculate the ratios, Q_T and Q_S, of the peak area of peplomycin to that of the internal standard.

Amount [μg (potency)] of peplomycin sulfate ($C_{61}H_{88}N_{18}O_{21}S_2.H_2SO_4$)
$= M_S \times Q_T/Q_S \times 1000$

M_S: Amount [mg (potency)] of Peplomycin Sulfate RS taken

*Internal standard solution—*A solution of 1-aminonaphthalene in mobile phase (1 in 20,000).

Operating conditions—

Detector: An ultraviolet absorption photometer (wavelength: 254 nm).

Column: A stainless steel column 3.0 mm in inside diameter and 5 cm in length, packed with octadecylsilanized silica gel for liquid chromatography (2.2 μm in particle diameter).

Column temperature: A constant temperature of about 40°C.

Mobile phase: Dissolve 0.96 g of sodium 1-pentane sulfonate and 1.86 g of disodium dihydrogen ethylenediamine tetraacetate dihydrate in 1000 mL of water, add 5 mL of acetic acid (100), and adjust to pH 4.3 with ammonia TS. To 650 mL of this solution add 350 mL of methanol.

Flow rate: Adjust so that the retention time of peplomycin is about 3 minutes.

System suitability—

System performance: When the procedure is run with 1 μL of the standard solution under the above operating conditions, peplomycin and the internal standard are eluted in this order with the resolution between these peaks being not less than 7.

System repeatability: When the test is repeated 6 times with 1 μL of the standard solution under the above operating conditions, the relative standard deviation of the ratio of the peak area of peplomycin to that of the internal standard is not more than 1.0%.

Containers and storage Containers—Tight containers.

Peplomycin Sulfate for Injection

注射用ペプロマイシン硫酸塩

Peplomycin Sulfate for Injection is a preparation for injection which is dissolved before use.

It contains not less than 90.0% and not more than 115.0% of the labeled potency of peplomycin ($C_{61}H_{88}N_{18}O_{21}S_2$: 1473.59).

Method of preparation Prepare as directed under Injections, with Peplomycin Sulfate.

Description Peplomycin Sulfate for Injection occurs as white light masses or powder.

Identification Take an amount of Peplomycin Sulfate for Injection, equivalent to 10 mg (potency) of Peplomycin Sulfate, and dissolve in 15 μL of Copper (II) sulfate TS and water to make 2 mL. Apply this solution to the column (prepared by filling a 15 mm inside diameter and 15 cm long chromatography tube with 15 mL of strongly basic ion exchange resin (Cl type) for column chromatography (75 - 150 μm in particle diameter) and run off. Then wash the column using water at 2.5 mL per minute, collect about 30 mL of the effluent. Add water to the effluent to make 250 mL, and determine the absorption spectrum of this solution as directed under Ultraviolet-visible Spectrophotometry <2.24>: it exhibits maxima between 242 nm and 246 nm, and between 291 nm and 295 nm. Further determine the absorbances A_1 and A_2, at 243 nm and 293 nm, respectively: the ratio A_1/A_2 is 1.20 to 1.30.

Osmotic pressure ratio Being specified separately when the drug is granted approval based on the Law.

pH <2.54> The pH of a solution prepared by dissolving an amount of Peplomycin Sulfate for Injection, equivalent to 50 mg (potency) of Peplomycin Sulfate, in 10 mL of water is 4.5 to 6.0.

Purity Clarity and color of solution—A solution prepared by dissolving an amount of Peplomycin Sulfate for Injection, equivalent to 10 mg (potency) of Peplomycin Sulfate, in 10 mL of water is clear and colorless.

Loss on drying <2.41> Not more than 4.0% (60 mg, in vacuum, phosphorus (V) oxide, 60°C, 3 hours). Perform the sampling preventing from moisture absorption.

Bacterial endotoxins <4.01> Less than 1.5 EU/mg (potency).

Uniformity of dosage units <6.02> It meets the requirement of the Mass variation test.

Foreign insoluble matter <6.06> Perform the test according to Method 2: it meets the requirement.

Insoluble particulate matter <6.07> It meets the requirement.

Sterility <4.06> Perform the test according to the Membrane filtration method: it meets the requirement.

Assay Perform the test according to the Cylinder-plate method as directed under Microbial Assay for Antibiotics <4.02> according to the following conditions.

(i) Test organism—*Mycobacterium smegmatis* ATCC 607

(ii) Agar media for base layer, seed and transferring test organisms—

Glycerin 10.0 g
Peptone 10.0 g
Meat extract 10.0 g
Sodium chloride 3.0 g
Agar 15.0 g
Water 1000 mL

Mix all the ingredients, and sterilize. Adjust to pH 6.9 to 7.1 with sodium hydroxide TS after sterilization.

(iii) Liquid media for suspending the test organism

Glycerin 10.0 g
Peptone 10.0 g
Meat extract 10.0 g
Sodium chloride 3.0 g
Water 1000 mL

Mix all the components, and sterilize. Adjust to pH 6.9 to 7.1 with sodium hydroxide TS after sterilization.

(iv) Preparation of seeded agar layer—Cultivate the test organism on the slant of the agar medium for transferring the test organism at 27°C for 40 to 48 hours, then inoculate the test organism thus obtained in 100 mL of the liquid media for suspending the test organism, cultivate with shaking at between 25°C and 27°C for 5 days, and use this as the suspension of test organism. Store the suspension of test organism at a temperature not exceeding 5°C, and use within 14 days. Add 0.5 mL of the suspension of test organism in 100 mL of the agar medium for seed previously kept at 48°C, mix thoroughly, and use as the seeded agar layer.

(v) Preparation of cylinder-agar plate—Proceed as directed in 1.7. Preparation of cylinder-agar plates under the Microbial Assay for Antibiotics, dispensing 5.0 mL of agar medium for base layer and 8.0 mL of the agar medium for seed into the Petri dish.

(vi) Standard solutions—Weigh accurately an amount of Peplomycin Sulfate RS, equivalent to about 20 mg (potency), dissolve in 0.1 mol/L phosphate buffer solution (pH 6.8) to make exactly 100 mL, and use this solution as the standard stock solution. Keep the standard stock solution at 5°C or below, and use within 15 days. Measure exactly a suitable amount of the standard stock solution before use, add 0.1 mol/L phosphate buffer solution (pH 6.8) to make solutions so that each mL contains 4 μg (potency) and 2 μg (potency), and use these solutions as the high concentration standard solution and low concentration standard solution, respectively.

(vii) Sample solutions—Weigh accurately the mass of the contents of not less than 10 containers of Peplomycin Sulfate for Injection. Weigh accurately an amount of the contents, equivalent to about 10 mg (potency) of Peplomycin Sulfate, dissolve in 0.1 mol/L phosphate buffer solution (pH 6.8) to make exactly 100 mL. Measure exactly a suitable amount of this solution, add 0.1 mol/L phosphate buffer solution (pH 6.8) to make solutions so that each mL contains 4 μg (potency) and 2 μg (potency), and use these solutions as the high concentration sample solution and low concentration sample solution, respectively.

Containers and storage Containers—Hermetic containers.

Perphenazine

ペルフェナジン

$C_{21}H_{26}ClN_3OS$: 403.97
2-{4-[3-(2-Chloro-10*H*-phenothiazin-10-yl)propyl]piperazin-1-yl}ethanol
[58-39-9]

Perphenazine, when dried, contains not less than 98.5% of perphenazine ($C_{21}H_{26}ClN_3OS$).

Description Perphenazine occurs as white to light yellow, crystals or crystalline powder. It is odorless, and has a bitter taste.

It is freely soluble in methanol and in ethanol (95), soluble in acetic acid (100), sparingly soluble in diethyl ether, and practically insoluble in water.

It dissolves in dilute hydrochloric acid.

It is gradually colored by light.

Identification **(1)** Dissolve 5 mg of Perphenazine in 5 mL of sulfuric acid: a red color, changing to deep red-purple upon warming, is produced.

(2) Dissolve 0.2 g of Perphenazine in 2 mL of methanol, add this solution to 10 mL of a warm solution of 2,4,6-trinitrophenol in methanol (1 in 25), and allow to stand for 4 hours. Collect the crystals, wash with a small volume of methanol, and dry at 105°C for 1 hour: the crystals so obtained melt *⟨2.60⟩* between 237°C and 244°C (with decomposition).

(3) Determine the absorption spectrum of a solution of Perphenazine in 0.1 mol/L hydrochloric acid TS (1 in 200,000) as directed under Ultraviolet-visible Spectrophotometry *⟨2.24⟩*, and compare the spectrum with the Reference Spectrum 1 or the spectrum of a solution of Perphenazine RS prepared in the same manner as the sample solution: both spectra exhibit similar intensities of absorption at the same wavelengths. Separately, to 10 mL of the solution add 10 mL of water. Determine the absorption spectrum of the solution as directed under Ultraviolet-visible Spectrophotometry *⟨2.24⟩*, and compare the spectrum with the Reference Spectrum 2 or the spectrum of a solution of Perphenazine RS prepared in the same manner as the sample solution: both spectra exhibit similar intensities of absorption at the same wavelengths.

(4) Perform the test with Perphenazine as directed under Flame Coloration Test *⟨1.04⟩* (2): a green color appears.

Melting point *⟨2.60⟩* 95 - 100°C

Purity **(1)** Heavy metals *⟨1.07⟩*—Proceed with 1.0 g of Perphenazine according to Method 2, and perform the test. Prepare the control solution with 2.0 mL of Standard Lead Solution (not more than 20 ppm).

(2) Related substances—Perform the test in the current of nitrogen in light-resistant containers under the protection from light. Dissolve 0.10 g of Perphenazine in 10 mL of ethanol (95), and use this solution as the sample solution. Pipet 1 mL of the sample solution, and add ethanol (95) to make exactly 10 mL. Pipet 1 mL of this solution, add ethanol (95) to make exactly 20 mL, and use this solution as the standard solution. Perform the test with these solutions as directed under Thin-layer Chromatography *⟨2.03⟩*. Spot 10 μL each of the sample solution and standard solution on a plate of silica gel with fluorescent indicator for thin-layer chromatography. Develop the plate with a mixture of 1-butanol and 1 mol/L ammonia TS (5:1) to a distance of about 12 cm, and air-dry the plate. Examine under ultraviolet light (main wavelength: 254 nm): any spot other than the principal spot obtained from the sample solution is not more intense than that from the standard solution.

Loss on drying *⟨2.41⟩* Not more than 0.5% (1 g, in vacuum, phosphorus (V) oxide, 65°C, 4 hours).

Residue on ignition *⟨2.44⟩* Not more than 0.1% (1 g).

Assay Weigh accurately about 0.4 g of Perphenazine, previously dried, dissolve in 50 mL of acetic acid (100), and titrate *⟨2.50⟩* with 0.1 mol/L perchloric acid VS until the color of the solution changes from purple through blue-purple to blue-green (indicator: 3 drops of crystal violet TS). Perform a blank determination in the same manner, and make any necessary correction.

Each mL of 0.1 mol/L perchloric acid VS
= 20.20 mg of $C_{21}H_{26}ClN_3OS$

Containers and storage Containers—Tight containers.
Storage—Light-resistant.

Perphenazine Tablets

ペルフェナジン錠

Perphenazine Tablets contain not less than 90.0% and not more than 110.0% of the labeled amount of perphenazine ($C_{21}H_{26}ClN_3OS$: 403.97).

Method of preparation Prepare as directed under Tablets, with Perphenazine.

Identification **(1)** Shake well a quantity of powdered Perphenazine Tablets, equivalent to 25 mg of Perphenazine, with 10 mL of methanol, and filter. Evaporate 2 mL of the filtrate on a water bath to dryness. With the residue, proceed as directed in the Identification (1) under Perphenazine.

(2) Add 5 mL of the filtrate obtained in (1) to 10 mL of a warm solution of 2,4,6-trinitrophenol in methanol (1 in 25), and proceed as directed in the Identification (2) under Perphenazine.

(3) Determine the absorption spectrum of the filtrate obtained in the Assay as directed under Ultraviolet-visible Spectrophotometry *⟨2.24⟩*: it exhibits a maximum between 309 nm and 313 nm. Add 30 mL of methanol to another 10 mL of the filtrate, and determine the absorption spectrum: it exhibits a maximum between 256 nm and 260 nm.

Uniformity of dosage units *⟨6.02⟩* Perform the test according to the following method: it meets the requirement of the Content uniformity test.

Disintegrate 1 tablet of Perphenazine Tablets by shaking with 5 mL of water, shake well with 70 mL of methanol, and add methanol to make exactly 100 mL. Centrifuge this solution, pipet V mL of the supernatant liquid, add methanol to make exactly V' mL of a solution containing about 4 μg of perphenazine ($C_{21}H_{26}ClN_3OS$) in each ml, and use this solution as the sample solution. Separately, weigh accurately about 10 mg of Perphenazine RS, previously dried in vacuum over phosphorus (V) oxide at 65°C for 4 hours, dissolve in methanol to make exactly 250 mL. Pipet 5 mL of this solution, add methanol to make exactly 50 mL, and use this solution as the standard solution. Determine the absorbances, A_T and A_S, of the sample solution and standard solution at 258 nm as directed under Ultraviolet-visible Spectrophotometry <*2.24*>.

Amount (mg) of perphenazine ($C_{21}H_{26}ClN_3OS$)
$= M_S \times A_T/A_S \times V'/V \times 1/25$

M_S: Amount (mg) of Perphenazine RS taken

Dissolution <*6.10*> When the test is performed at 100 revolutions per minute according to the Paddle method, using 900 mL of 2nd fluid for dissolution test as the dissolution medium, the dissolution rate in 90 minutes of Perphenazine Tablets is not less than 70%.

Start the test with 1 tablet of Perphenazine Tablets, withdraw not less than 20 mL of the medium at the specified minute after starting the test, and filter through a membrane filter with a pore size not exceeding 0.8 μm. Discard not less than 10 mL of the first filtrate, and use the subsequent filtrate as the sample solution. Separately, weigh accurately about 10 mg of Perphenazine RS, previously dried in vacuum with phosphorus (V) oxide at 65°C for 4 hours, dissolve in 5 mL of 0.1 mol/L hydrochloric acid TS, and add the dissolution medium to make exactly 250 mL. Pipet 5 mL of this solution, add the dissolution medium to make exactly 100 mL, and use this solution as the standard solution. Determine the absorbances, A_T and A_S, of the sample solution and standard solution at 255 nm as directed under Ultraviolet-visible Spectrophotometry <*2.24*>.

Dissolution rate (%) with respect to the labeled amount of perphenazine ($C_{21}H_{26}ClN_3OS$)
$= M_S \times A_T/A_S \times 1/C \times 18$

M_S: Amount (mg) of Perphenazine RS taken
C: Labeled amount (mg) of perphenazine ($C_{21}H_{26}ClN_3OS$) in 1 tablet

Assay Weigh accurately and powder not less than 20 Perphenazine Tablets. Weigh accurately a portion of the powder, equivalent to about 4 mg of perphenazine ($C_{21}H_{26}ClN_3OS$), add 70 mL of methanol, shake well, and add methanol to make exactly 100 mL. Filter the solution, and discard the first 20 mL of the filtrate. Pipet 5 mL of the subsequent filtrate, add methanol to make exactly 50 mL, and use this solution as the sample solution. Weigh accurately about 10 mg of Perphenazine RS, previously dried in vacuum over phosphorus (V) oxide at 65°C for 4 hours, and dissolve in methanol to make exactly 250 mL. Pipet 5 mL of this solution, add methanol to make exactly 50 mL, and use this solution as the standard solution. Determine the absorbances, A_T and A_S, of the sample solution and the standard solution at 258 nm as directed under Ultraviolet-visible Spectrophotometry <*2.24*>.

Amount (mg) of perphenazine ($C_{21}H_{26}ClN_3OS$)
$= M_S \times A_T/A_S \times 2/5$

M_S: Amount (mg) of Perphenazine RS taken

Containers and storage Containers—Tight containers.
Storage—Light-resistant.

Perphenazine Maleate

ペルフェナジンマレイン酸塩

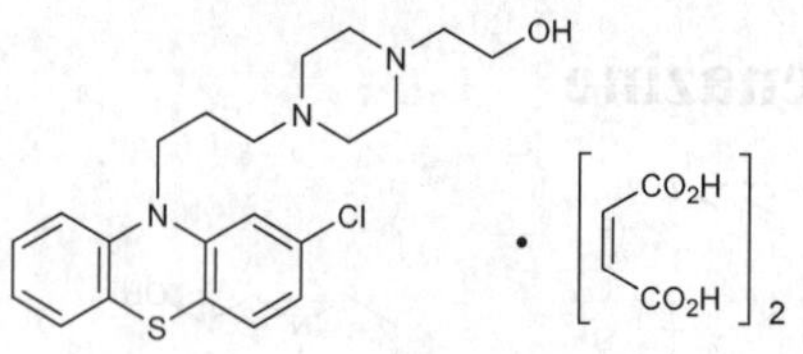

$C_{21}H_{26}ClN_3OS.2C_4H_4O_4$: 636.11
2-{4-[3-(2-Chloro-10*H*-phenothiazin-10-yl)propyl]piperazin-1-yl}ethanol dimaleate
[*58-39-9*, Perphenazine]

Perphenazine Maleate, when dried, contains not less than 98.0% of perphenazine maleate ($C_{21}H_{26}ClN_3OS.2C_4H_4O_4$).

Description Perphenazine Maleate occurs as a white to light yellow powder. It is odorless.

It is sparingly soluble in acetic acid (100), slightly soluble in water and in ethanol (95), and practically insoluble in chloroform.

It dissolves in dilute hydrochloric acid.

It is gradually colored by light.

Melting point: about 175°C (with decomposition).

Identification **(1)** Dissolve 8 mg of Perphenazine Maleate in 5 mL of sulfuric acid: a red color is produced, which becomes deep red-purple on warming.

(2) Dissolve 0.3 g of Perphenazine Maleate in 3 mL of dilute hydrochloric acid, add 2 mL of water and 3 mL of ammonia solution (28), shake, and extract with three 10-mL portions of chloroform. [Reserve the aqueous layer, and use for test (5)]. Evaporate the combined chloroform extracts on a water bath to dryness, dissolve the residue in 20 mL of methanol, and pour into 10 mL of a warm solution of 2,4,6-trinitrophenol in methanol (1 in 25). Allow to stand for 4 hours, collect the crystals, wash with a small amount of methanol, and dry at 105°C for 1 hour: the crystals melt <*2.60*> between 237°C and 244°C (with decomposition).

(3) Determine the absorption spectrum of a solution of Perphenazine Maleate (1 in 20,000) as directed under Ultraviolet-visible Spectrophotometry <*2.24*>, and compare the spectrum with the Reference Spectrum 1: both spectra exhibit similar intensities of absorption at the same wavelengths. Separately, to 10 mL of the solution add 30 mL of water. Determine the absorption spectrum of the solution as directed under Ultraviolet-visible Spectrophotometry <*2.24*>, and compare the spectrum with the Reference Spectrum 2: both spectra exhibit similar intensities of absorption at the same wavelengths.

(4) Perform the test with Perphenazine Maleate as directed under Flame Coloration Test <*1.04*> (2): a green color appears.

(5) Evaporate the aqueous layer reserved in (2) to dryness. To the residue add 1 mL of dilute sulfuric acid and 5 mL of water, and extract with four 25-mL portions of diethyl ether. Combine the diethyl ether extracts, and evaporate in a water bath at about 35°C with the aid of a current of air: the residue melts <*2.60*> between 128°C and 136°C.

Purity **(1)** Heavy metals <*1.07*>—Proceed with 2.0 g of perphenazine maleate according to Method 2, and perform the test. Prepare the control solution with 2.0 mL of Standard Lead Solution (not more than 10 ppm).

(2) Arsenic <*1.11*>—Prepare the test solution with 1.0 g of Perphenazine Maleate according to Method 3, and perform the test (not more than 2 ppm).

Loss on drying <*2.41*> Not more than 0.5% (1 g, 105°C, 3 hours).

Residue on ignition <*2.44*> Not more than 0.1% (1 g).

Assay Weigh accurately about 0.5 g of Perphenazine Maleate, previously dried, dissolve in 70 mL of acetic acid (100), and titrate <*2.50*> with 0.1 mol/L perchloric acid VS until the color of the solution changes from purple through blue to blue-green (indicator: 3 drops of crystal violet TS). Perform a blank determination in the same manner, and make any necessary correction.

Each mL of 0.1 mol/L perchloric acid VS
= 31.81 mg of $C_{21}H_{26}ClN_3OS.2C_4H_4O_4$

Containers and storage Containers—Well-closed containers.

Storage—Light-resistant.

Perphenazine Maleate Tablets

ペルフェナジンマレイン酸塩錠

Perphenazine Maleate Tablets contain not less than 93.0% and not more than 107.0% of the labeled amount of perphenazine maleate ($C_{21}H_{26}ClN_3OS.2C_4H_4O_4$: 636.11).

Method of preparation Prepare as directed under Tablets, with Perphenazine Maleate.

Identification **(1)** Shake a quantity of powdered Perphenazine Maleate Tablets, equivalent to 0.04 g of Perphenazine Maleate, with 3 mL of dilute hydrochloric acid and 30 mL of water, centrifuge. Filter the supernatant liquid, add 3 mL of ammonia solution (28) to the filtrate, and extract with three 10-mL portions of chloroform. [Reserve the aqueous layer, and use for test (4).] Wash the combined chloroform extracts with two 5-mL portions of water, and separate the chloroform layer. Evaporate 6 mL of the chloroform solution on a water bath to dryness. Proceed with the residue as directed in the Identification (1) under Perphenazine Maleate.

(2) Evaporate 20 mL of the chloroform solution obtained in (1) on a water bath to dryness, dissolve the residue in 20 mL of methanol, and filter, if necessary. Warm the filtrate, add 5 mL of a warm solution of 2,4,6-trinitrophenol in methanol (1 in 25), allow to stand for 4 hours, and proceed as directed in the Identification (2) under Perphenazine Maleate.

(3) To 2 mL of the filtrate obtained in the Assay add water to make 50 mL. Determine the absorption spectrum of the solution as directed under Ultraviolet-visible Spectrophotometry <*2.24*>: it exhibits maxima between 253 nm and 257 nm and between 303 nm and 313 nm.

(4) Filter, if necessary, the aqueous layer reserved in (1), evaporate the filtrate to make about 5 mL, add 2 mL of dilute sulfuric acid, and extract with two 10-mL portions of diethyl ether. Combine the diethyl ether extracts, evaporate on a water bath to dryness, dissolve the residue in 5 mL of sulfuric acid TS, and add 1 to 2 drops of potassium permanganate TS: the red color of potassium permanganate TS fades immediately.

Uniformity of dosage units <*6.02*> Perform the test according to the following method: it meets the requirement of the Content uniformity test.

Disintegrate 1 tablet of Perphenazine Maleate Tablets by shaking with 15 mL of 0.1 mol/L hydrochloric acid TS, shake vigorously with 50 mL of methanol, add water to make exactly 100 mL, and centrifuge. Pipet V mL of the supernatant liquid, add water to make exactly V' mL of a solution containing about 6 μg of perphenazine maleate ($C_{21}H_{26}ClN_3OS.2C_4H_4O_4$) in each ml, and use this solution as the sample solution. Separately, weigh accurately 30 mg of perphenazine maleate for assay, previously dried at 105°C for 3 hours, dissolve in 15 mL of 0.1 mol/L hydrochloric acid TS and 50 mL of methanol, and add water to make exactly 100 mL. Pipet 5 mL of this solution, add 3 mL of 0.1 mol/L hydrochloric acid TS, 10 mL of methanol and water to make exactly 250 mL, and use this solution as the standard solution. Determine the absorbances, A_T and A_S, of the sample solution and standard solution at 255 nm as directed under Ultraviolet-visible Spectrophotometry <*2.24*>, using water as the blank.

Amount (mg) of perphenazine maleate ($C_{21}H_{26}ClN_3OS.2C_4H_4O_4$)
$= M_S \times A_T/A_S \times V'/V \times 1/50$

M_S: Amount (mg) of perphenazine maleate for assay taken

Dissolution <*6.10*> When the test is performed at 75 revolutions per minute according to the Paddle method, using 900 mL of 2nd fluid for dissolution test as the dissolution medium, the dissolution rate in 30 minutes of Perphenazine Maleate Tablets is not less than 70%.

Conduct this procedure without exposure to light. Start the test with 1 tablet of Perphenazine Maleate Tablets, withdraw not less than 20 mL of the medium at the specified minute after starting the test, and filter through a membrane filter with a pore size not exceeding 0.45 μm. Discard not less than 10 mL of the first filtrate, pipet V mL of the subsequent filtrate, add the dissolution medium to make exactly V' mL so that each mL contains about 3.5 μg of perphenazine maleate ($C_{21}H_{26}ClN_3OS.2C_4H_4O_4$), and use this solution as the sample solution. Separately, weigh accurately about 28 mg of perphenazine maleate for assay, previously dried at 105°C for 3 hours, dissolve in 10 mL of 0.1 mol/L hydrochloric acid TS, and add the dissolution medium to make exactly 200 mL. Pipet 5 mL of this solution, add the dissolution medium to make exactly 200 mL, and use this solution as the standard solution. Determine the absorbances, A_T and A_S, at 255 nm of the sample solution and standard solution as directed under Ultraviolet-visible Spectrophotometry <*2.24*>.

Dissolution rate (%) with respect to the labeled amount of perphenazine maleate ($C_{21}H_{26}ClN_3OS.2C_4H_4O_4$)
$= M_S \times A_T/A_S \times V'/V \times 1/C \times 45/4$

M_S: Amount (mg) of perphenazine maleate for assay taken

C: Labeled amount (mg) of perphenazine maleate ($C_{21}H_{26}ClN_3OS.2C_4H_4O_4$) in 1 tablet

Assay Weigh accurately and powder not less than 20 Perphenazine Maleate Tablets. Weigh accurately a portion of the powder, equivalent to about 40 mg of perphenazine maleate ($C_{21}H_{26}ClN_3OS.2C_4H_4O_4$), shake well with 15 mL of 1 mol/L hydrochloric acid TS and 50 mL of methanol, add water to make exactly 100 mL, and filter. Discard the first 20 mL of the filtrate, measure exactly 5 mL of the subsequent filtrate, add water to make exactly 250 mL, and use this solution as the sample solution. Separately, weigh accurately about 40 mg of perphenazine maleate for assay, previously dried at 105°C for 3 hours, dissolve in 15 mL of 1 mol/L hydrochloric acid TS and 50 mL of methanol, and add water to make exactly 100 mL. Pipet 5 mL of this solution, add water to make exactly 250 mL, and use this solution as the standard solution. Determine the absorbances, A_T and A_S, of the sample solution and the standard solution at 255 nm as directed under Ultraviolet-visible Spectrophotometry <*2.24*>, using water as the blank.

Amount (mg) of perphenazine maleate ($C_{21}H_{26}ClN_3OS.2C_4H_4O_4$)
$= M_S \times A_T/A_S$

M_S: Amount (mg) of perphenazine maleate for assay taken

Containers and storage Containers—Tight containers.
Storage—Light-resistant.

Adsorbed Purified Pertussis Vaccine

沈降精製百日せきワクチン

Adsorbed Purified Pertussis Vaccine is a liquid for injection prepared by adding an aluminum salt to a liquid containing the protective antigen of *Bordetella pertussis* to make the antigen insoluble.

It conforms to the requirements of Adsorbed Purified Pertussis Vaccine in the Minimum Requirements for Biological Products.

Description Adsorbed Purified Pertussis Vaccine forms a homogeneous, white turbidity on shaking.

Pethidine Hydrochloride

ペチジン塩酸塩

$C_{15}H_{21}NO_2.HCl$: 283.79
Ethyl 1-methyl-4-phenylpiperidine-4-carboxylate monohydrochloride
[*50-13-5*]

Pethidine Hydrochloride, when dried, contains not less than 98.0% of pethidine hydrochloride ($C_{15}H_{21}NO_2.HCl$).

Description Pethidine Hydrochloride occurs as a white crystalline powder.

It is very soluble in water and in acetic acid (100), freely soluble in ethanol (95), sparingly soluble in acetic anhydride, and practically insoluble in diethyl ether.

The pH of a solution dissolved 1.0 g of Pethidine Hydrochloride in 20 mL of water is between 3.8 and 5.8.

Identification **(1)** Determine the absorption spectrum of a solution of Pethidine Hydrochloride (1 in 2000) as directed under Ultraviolet-visible Spectrophotometry <*2.24*>, and compare the spectrum with the Reference Spectrum: both spectra exhibit similar intensities of absorption at the same wavelengths.

(2) Determine the infrared absorption spectrum of Pethidine Hydrochloride, previously dried, as directed in the potassium bromide disk method under Infrared Spectrophotometry <*2.25*>, and compare the spectrum with the Reference Spectrum: both spectra exhibit similar intensities of absorption at the same wave numbers.

(3) A solution of Pethidine Hydrochloride (1 in 50) responds to Qualitative Tests <*1.09*> (2) for chloride.

Melting point <*2.60*> 187 – 189°C

Purity **(1)** Clarity and color of solution—Dissolve 1.0 g of Pethidine Hydrochloride in 10 mL of water: the solution is clear and colorless.

(2) Sulfate <*1.14*>—Perform the test with 0.20 g of Pethidine Hydrochloride. Prepare the control solution with 1.0 mL of 0.005 mol/L sulfuric acid VS (not more than 0.240%).

(3) Related substances—Dissolve 0.05 g of Pethidine Hydrochloride in 20 mL of the mobile phase, and use this solution as the sample solution. Pipet 1 mL of the sample solution, add the mobile phase to make exactly 100 mL, and use this solution as the standard solution. Perform the test with exactly 20 μL each of the sample solution and standard solution as directed under Liquid Chromatography <*2.01*> according to the following conditions. Determine each peak area obtained from both solutions by the automatic integration method: the total area of the peaks other than pethidine obtained from the sample solution is not larger than the peak area of pethidine from the standard solution.

Operating conditions—

Detector: An ultraviolet absorption photometer (wavelength: 257 nm).

Column: A stainless steel column 4.6 mm in inside diameter and 15 cm in length, packed with octadecylsilanized silica gel for liquid chromatography (5 μm in particle diameter).

Column temperature: A constant temperature of about 40°C.

Mobile phase: Dissolve 2.0 g of sodium lauryl sulfate in 1000 mL of diluted phosphoric acid (1 in 1000), adjust the pH to 3.0 with sodium hydroxide TS, and to 550 mL of this solution add 450 mL of acetonitrile.

Flow rate: Adjust so that the retention time of pethidine is about 7 minutes.

Time span of measurement: About 2 times as long as the retention time of pethidine, beginning after the solvent peak.

System suitability—

Test for required detectability: To exactly 2 mL of the standard solution add the mobile phase to make exactly 20 mL. Confirm that the peak area of pethidine obtained with 20 μL of this solution is equivalent to 5 to 15% of that with 20 μL of the standard solution.

System performance: To 2 mL each of the sample solution and a solution of isoamyl parahydroxybenzoate in the mobile phase (1 in 50,000) add the mobile phase to make 10 mL. When the procedure is run with 20 μL of this solution according to the above operating conditions, pethidine and isoamyl parahydroxybenzoate are eluted in this order with the resolution between these peaks being not less than 2.0.

System repeatability: When the test is repeated 6 times with 20 μL of the standard solution under the above operating conditions, the relative standard deviation of the peak

area of pethidine is not more than 2.0%.

Loss on drying <2.41>　Not more than 0.5% (1 g, 105°C, 3 hours).

Residue on ignition <2.44>　Not more than 0.1% (0.5 g).

Assay　Weigh accurately about 0.5 g of Pethidine Hydrochloride, previously dried, dissolve in 50 mL of a mixture of acetic anhydride and acetic acid (100) (7:3), and titrate <2.50> with 0.1 mol/L perchloric acid VS (potentiometric titration). Perform a blank determination in the same manner, and make any necessary correction.

Each mL of 0.1 mol/L perchloric acid VS
= 28.38 mg of $C_{15}H_{21}NO_2.HCl$

Containers and storage　Containers—Tight containers.
Storage—Light-resistant.

Pethidine Hydrochloride Injection

ペチジン塩酸塩注射液

Pethidine Hydrochloride Injection is an aqueous injection.

It contains not less than 95.0% and not more than 105.0% of the labeled amount of pethidine hydrochloride ($C_{15}H_{21}NO_2.HCl$: 283.79).

Method of preparation　Prepare as directed under Injections, with Pethidine Hydrochloride.

Description　Pethidine Hydrochloride Injection is a clear, colorless liquid.

It is affected by light.

pH 4.0 – 6.0

Identification　Take a volume of Pethidine Hydrochloride Injection equivalent to 0.1 g of Pethidine Hydrochloride, and add water to make 200 mL. Determine the absorption spectrum of this solution as directed under Ultraviolet-visible Spectrophotometry <2.24>: it exhibits maxima between 250 nm and 254 nm, between 255 nm and 259 nm, and between 261 nm and 265 nm.

Bacterial endotoxins <4.01>　Less than 6.0 EU/mg.

Extractable volume <6.05>　It meets the requirement.

Foreign insoluble matter <6.06>　Perform the test according to Method 1: it meets the requirement.

Insoluble particulate matter <6.07>　It meets the requirement.

Sterility <4.06>　Perform the test according to the Membrane filtration method: it meets the requirement.

Assay　Measure exactly a volume of Pethidine Hydrochloride Injection, equivalent to about 0.1 g of pethidine hydrochloride ($C_{15}H_{21}NO_2.HCl$), add exactly 10 mL of the internal standard solution, and add the mobile phase to make 50 mL. To 5 mL of this solution add the mobile phase to make 20 mL, and use this solution as the sample solution. Separately, weigh accurately about 0.1 g of pethidine hydrochloride for assay, previously dried at 105°C for 3 hours, add exactly 10 mL of the internal standard solution, and add the mobile phase to make 50 mL. To 5 mL of this solution add the mobile phase to make 20 mL, and use this solution as the standard solution. Perform the test with 20 μL of the sample solution and standard solution as directed under Liquid Chromatography <2.01> according to the following conditions, and calculate the ratios, Q_T and Q_S, of the peak area of pethidine to that of the internal standard.

Amount (mg) of pethidine hydrochloride ($C_{15}H_{21}NO_2.HCl$)
$= M_S \times Q_T/Q_S$

M_S: Amount (mg) of pethidine hydrochloride for assay taken

Internal standard solution—A solution of isoamyl parahydroxybenzoate in the mobile phase (1 in 12,500).

Operating conditions—

Detector: An ultraviolet absorption photometer (wavelength: 257 nm).

Column: A stainless steel column 4.6 mm in inside diameter and 15 cm in length, packed with octadecylsilanized silica gel for liquid chromatography (5 μm in particle diameter).

Column temperature: A constant temperature of about 40°C.

Mobile phase: Dissolve 2.0 g of sodium lauryl sulfate in 1000 mL of diluted phosphoric acid (1 in 1000), adjust the pH to 3.0 with sodium hydroxide TS, and to 550 mL of this solution add 450 mL of acetonitrile.

Flow rate: Adjust so that the retention time of pethidine is about 7 minutes.

System suitability—

System performance: When the procedure is run with 20 μL of the standard solution under the above operating conditions, pethidine and the internal standard are eluted in this order with the resolution between these peaks being not less than 2.0.

System repeatability: When the test is repeated 6 times with 20 μL of the standard solution under the above operating conditions, the relative standard deviation of the ratios of the peak area of pethidine to that of the internal standard is not more than 1.0%.

Containers and storage　Containers—Hermetic containers, and colored containers may be used.
Storage—Light-resistant.

White Petrolatum

白色ワセリン

White Petrolatum is a decolorized and purified mixture of hydrocarbons obtained from petroleum.

Description　White Petrolatum is a white to pale yellow, homogeneous, unctuous mass. It is odorless and tasteless.

It is practically insoluble in water, in ethanol (95) and in ethanol (99.5).

It dissolves in diethyl ether making a clear liquid or producing slight insoluble substances.

It becomes a clear liquid when warmed.

Melting point <2.60>　38 – 60°C (Method 3).

Purity　**(1)**　Color—Melt White Petrolatum by warming, and pour 5 mL of it into a test tube, and keep the content in a liquid condition: the liquid has no more color than the following control solution, when observed transversely from side against a white background.

Control solution: Add 3.4 mL of water to 1.6 mL of Iron (III) Chloride CS.

(2)　Acidity or alkalinity—To 35.0 g of White Petrolatum add 100 mL of hot water, shake vigorously for 5 minutes, and then draw off the aqueous layer. Treat the White

Petrolatum layer in the same manner using two 50-mL portions of hot water. To the combined aqueous layer add 1 drop of phenolphthalein TS, and boil: no red color is produced. Further add 2 drops of methyl orange TS: no red color is produced.

(3) Heavy metals *<1.07>*—Proceed with 1.0 g of White Petrolatum according to Method 2, and perform the test. Prepare the control solution with 3.0 mL of Standard Lead Solution (not more than 30 ppm).

(4) Arsenic *<1.11>*—Prepare the test solution with 1.0 g of White Petrolatum, according to Method 3, and perform the test. Add 10 mL of a solution of magnesium nitrate hexahydrate in ethanol (95) (1 in 50), then add 1.5 mL of hydrogen peroxide (30), and fire to burn (not more than 2 ppm).

(5) Sulfur compound—To 4.0 g of White Petrolatum add 2 mL of ethanol (99.5) and 2 drops of sodium hydroxide solution (1 in 5) saturated with lead (II) oxide, warm the mixture for 10 minutes at about 70°C with frequent shaking, and allow to cool: no dark color is produced.

(6) Organic acids—To 100 mL of dilute ethanol add 1 drop of phenolphthalein TS, and titrate with 0.01 mol/L sodium hydroxide VS, until the color of the solution changes to light red. Mix this solution with 20.0 g of White Petrolatum, and boil for 10 minutes under a reflux condenser. Add 2 to 3 drops of phenolphthalein TS to the mixture and 0.40 mL of 0.1 mol/L sodium hydroxide VS with vigorous shaking: the color of the solution remains red.

(7) Fats and fatty oils or resins—To 10.0 g of White Petrolatum add 50 mL of sodium hydroxide solution (1 in 5), and boil for 30 minutes under a reflux condenser. Cool the mixture, separate the aqueous layer, and filter, if necessary. To the aqueous layer add 200 mL of dilute sulfuric acid: neither oily matter nor precipitate is produced.

Residue on ignition *<2.44>* Not more than 0.05% (2 g).

Containers and storage Containers—Tight containers.

Hydrophilic Petrolatum

親水ワセリン

Method of preparation

White Beeswax	80 g
Stearyl Alcohol or Cetanol	30 g
Cholesterol	30 g
White Petrolatum	a sufficient quantity
To make	1000 g

Melt and mix Stearyl Alcohol or Cetanol, White Beeswax and White Petrolatum on a water bath. Add Cholesterol, and melt completely by stirring. Stop warming, and stir until the mixture congeals.

Description Hydrophilic Petrolatum is white in color. It has a slight, characteristic odor.

When mixed with an equal volume of water, it retains the consistency of ointment.

Containers and storage Containers—Tight containers.

Yellow Petrolatum

黄色ワセリン

Yellow Petrolatum is a purified mixture of hydrocarbons obtained from petroleum.

Description Yellow Petrolatum occurs as a yellow, homogeneous, unctuous mass, It is odorless and tasteless.

It is slightly soluble in ethanol (95), and practically insoluble in water.

It dissolves in diethyl ether, in petroleum benzine and in turpentine oil, making a clear liquid or producing slight insoluble substances.

It becomes a yellow, clear liquid with slight fluorescence when warmed.

Melting point *<2.60>* 38 – 60°C (Method 3).

Purity **(1)** Color—Melt Yellow Petrolatum by warming, and pour 5 mL of it into a test tube, and keep the content in a liquid condition: the liquid has no more color than the following control solution, when observed transversely from side against a white background.

Control solution: To 3.8 mL of Iron (III) Chloride CS add 1.2 mL of Cobalt (II) Chloride CS.

(2) Acidity or alkalinity—To 35.0 g of Yellow Petrolatum add 100 mL of hot water, shake vigorously for 5 minutes, and then draw off the aqueous layer. Treat the Yellow Petrolatum layer in the same manner using two 50-mL portions of hot water. To the combined aqueous layer add 1 drop of phenolphthalein TS, and boil: no red color is produced. Further add 2 drops of methyl orange TS: no red color is produced.

(3) Heavy metals *<1.07>*—Proceed with 1.0 g of Yellow Petrolatum according to Method 2, and perform the test. Prepare the control solution with 3.0 mL of Standard Lead Solution (not more than 30 ppm).

(4) Arsenic *<1.11>*—Prepare the test solution with 1.0 g of Yellow Petrolatum, according to Method 3, and perform the test. Add 10 mL of a solution of magnesium nitrate hexahydrate in ethanol (95) (1 in 50), then add 1.5 mL of hydrogen peroxide (30), and fire to burn (not more than 2 ppm).

(5) Sulfur compound—To 4.0 g of Yellow Petrolatum add 2 mL of ethanol (99.5) and 2 drops of sodium hydroxide solution (1 in 5) saturated with lead (II) oxide, warm the mixture for 10 minutes at about 70°C with frequent shaking, and allow to cool: no dark color is produced.

(6) Organic acids—To 100 mL of dilute ethanol add 1 drop of phenolphthalein TS, and titrate with 0.01 mol/L sodium hydroxide VS, until the color of the solution changes to light red. Mix this solution with 20.0 g of Yellow Petrolatum, and boil for 10 minutes under a reflux condenser. Add 2 to 3 drops of phenolphthalein TS to the mixture and 0.40 mL of 0.1 mol/L sodium hydroxide VS with vigorous shaking: the color of the solution remains red.

(7) Fats and fatty oils or resins—To 10.0 g of Yellow Petrolatum add 50 mL of sodium hydroxide solution (1 in 5), and boil for 30 minutes under a reflux condenser. Cool the mixture, separate the aqueous layer, and filter, if necessary. To the aqueous layer add 200 mL of dilute sulfuric acid: neither oily matter nor precipitate is produced.

Residue on ignition *<2.44>* Not more than 0.05% (2 g).

Containers and storage Containers—Tight containers.

Petroleum Benzin

石油ベンジン

Petroleum Benzin is a mixture of low-boiling point hydrocarbons from petroleum.

Description Petroleum Benzin occurs as a colorless, clear, volatile liquid. It shows no fluorescence. It has a chracteristic odor.

It is miscible with ethanol (99.5) and with diethyl ether.

It is practically insoluble in water.

It is very flammable.

Specific gravity d_{20}^{20}: 0.65 – 0.71

Purity **(1)** Acid—Shake vigorously 10 mL of Petroleum Benzin with 5 mL of water for 2 minutes, and allow to stand: the separated aqueous layer does not change moistened blue litmus paper to red.

(2) Sulfur compounds and reducing substances—To 10 mL of Petroleum Benzin add 2.5 mL of ammonia-ethanol TS and 2 to 3 drops of silver nitrate TS, and warm the mixture at about 50°C for 5 minutes, protected from light: no brown color develops.

(3) Fatty oil and sulfur compounds—Drop and evaporate 10 mL of Petroleum Benzin in small portions on odorless filter paper spread on a previously warmed glass plate: no spot or no foreign odor is perceptible.

(4) Benzene—Warm 5 drops of Petroleum Benzin with 2 mL of sulfuric acid and 0.5 mL of nitric acid for about 10 minutes, allow to stand for 30 minutes, transfer the mixture to a porcelain dish, and dilute with water: no odor of nitrobenzene is perceptible.

(5) Residue on evaporation—Evaporate 140 mL of Petroleum Benzin on a water bath to dryness, and heat the residue at 105°C to constant mass: the mass is not more than 1 mg.

(6) Readily carbonizable substances—Shake vigorously 5 mL of Petroleum Benzin with 5 mL of sulfuric acid for readily carbonizable substances for 5 minutes in a Nessler tube, and allow to stand: the sulfuric acid layer has no more color than Matching Fluid A.

Distilling range *<2.57>* 50 – 80°C, not less than 90 vol%.

Containers and storage Containers—Tight containers.

Storage—Remote from fire, and not exceeding 30°C.

Phenethicillin Potassium

フェネチシリンカリウム

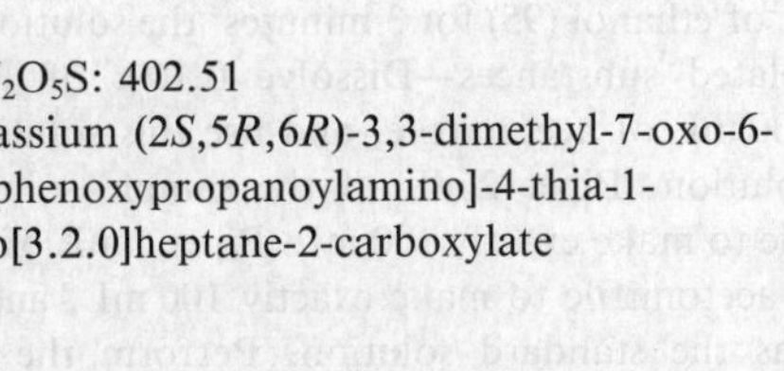

and epimer at C*

$C_{17}H_{19}KN_2O_5S$: 402.51

Monopotassium (2*S*,5*R*,6*R*)-3,3-dimethyl-7-oxo-6-[(2*RS*)-2-phenoxypropanoylamino]-4-thia-1-azabicyclo[3.2.0]heptane-2-carboxylate

[132-93-4]

Phenethicillin Potassium contains not less than 1400 units and not more than 1480 units per mg, calculated on the dried basis. The potency of Phenethicillin Potassium is expressed as unit based on the amount of phenethicillin potassium ($C_{17}H_{19}KN_2O_5S$). One unit of Phenethicillin Potassium is equivalent to 0.68 μg of phenethicillin potassium ($C_{17}H_{19}KN_2O_5S$).

Description Phenethicillin Potassium occurs as a white to light yellow-white crystalline powder.

It is freely soluble in water, and slightly soluble in ethanol (99.5).

Identification **(1)** Determine the absorption spectrum of a solution of Phenethicillin Potassium (1 in 5000) as directed under Ultraviolet-visible Spectrophotometry *<2.24>*, and compare the spectrum with the Reference Spectrum: both spectra exhibit similar intensities of absorption at the same wavelengths.

(2) Determine the infrared absorption spectrum of Phenethicillin Potassium as directed in the potassium bromide disk method under Infrared Spectrophotometry *<2.25>*, and compare the spectrum with the Reference Spectrum: both spectra exhibit similar intensities of absorption at the same wave numbers.

(3) Phenethicillin Potassium responds to Qualitative Tests *<1.09>* (1) for potassium salt.

Optical rotation *<2.49>* $[\alpha]_D^{20}$: +217 – +244° (1 g calculated on the dried basis, phosphate TS, 100 mL, 100 mm).

L-α-Phenethicillin potassium Dissolve about 50 mg of Phenethicillin Potassium in the mobile phase to make 50 mL, and use this solution as the sample solution. Perform the test with 10 μL of the sample solution as directed under Liquid Chromatography *<2.01>* according to the following conditions, and determine the peak areas, A_D and A_L, of D-α-phenethicillin and L-α-phenethicillin by the automatic integration method: $A_L/(A_D + A_L)$ is between 0.50 and 0.70.

Operating conditions—

Detector: An ultraviolet absorption photometer (wavelength: 254 nm).

Column: A stainless steel column 6 mm in inside diameter and 15 cm in length, packed with octadecylsilanized silica gel for liquid chromatography (5 μm in particle diameter).

Column temperature: A constant temperature of about 30°C.

Mobile phase: Adjust the pH of a mixture of a solution of diammonium hydrogen phosphate (1 in 150) and acetonitrile (41:10) to 7.0 with phosphoric acid.

Flow rate: Adjust so that the retention time of L-α-phenethicillin is about 25 minutes.

System suitability—

System performance: When the procedure is run with 10 μL of the sample solution under the above operating conditions, D-α-phenethicillin and L-α-phenethicillin are eluted in this order with the resolution between these peaks being not less than 1.5.

System repeatability: When the test is repeated 6 times with 10 μL of the sample solution under the above operating conditions, the relative standard deviation of the peak area of L-α-phenethicillin is not more than 2.0%.

Purity **(1)** Heavy metals *<1.07>*—Proceed with 1.0 g of Phenethicillin Potassium according to Method 2, and perform the test. Prepare the control solution with 1.0 mL of Standard Lead Solution (not more than 10 ppm).

(2) Arsenic *<1.11>*—Prepare the test solution with 1.0 g of Phenethicillin Potassium according to Method 4 and, perform the test (not more than 2 ppm).

(3) Related substances—Dissolve 50 mg of Phenethicillin Potassium in 50 mL of the mobile, and use this solution as the sample solution. Pipet 1 mL of the sample solution, add the mobile phase to make exactly 100 mL, and use this solution as the standard solution. Perform the test with exactly 10 μL each of the sample solution and standard solution as directed under Liquid Chromatography <*2.01*> according to the following conditions, and determine each peak area by the automatic integration method: the total of the peak areas other than D-α-phenethicillin and L-α-phenethicillin obtained from the sample solution is not larger than 5 times the total of the peak areas of D-α-phenethicillin and L-α-phenethicillin from the standard solution.

Operating conditions—

Detector, column, column temperature, mobile phase, and flow rate: Proceed as directed in the operating conditions in the L-α-Phenethicillin potassium.

Time span of measurement: About 1.5 times as long as the retention time of L-α-phenethicillin.

System suitability—

System performance, and system repeatability: Proceed as directed in the system suitability in the L-α-Phenethicillin potassium.

Test for required detectability: Measure exactly 2 mL of the standard solution, and add the mobile phase to make exactly 10 mL. Confirm that the peak area of L-α-phenethicillin obtained with 10 μL of this solution is equivalent to 14 to 26% of that with 10 μL of the standard solution.

Loss on drying <*2.41*> Not more than 1.0% (0.1 g, in vacuum, 60°C, 3 hours).

Assay Weigh accurately an amount of Phenethicillin Potassium and dried Phenethicillin Potassium RS, equivalent to about 40,000 units, dissolve each in phosphate buffer solution (pH 6.0) to make exactly 20 mL, and use these solutions as the sample solution and the standard solution, respectively. Pipet 2 mL each of these solutions in 100-mL glass-stoppered flasks, add 2.0 mL of sodium hydroxide TS to them, and allow to stand for exactly 15 minutes. To them add 2.0 mL of diluted hydrochloric acid (1 in 10) and exactly 10 mL of 0.005 mol/L iodine VS, and allow them to stand for exactly 15 minutes. Add 0.2 - 0.5 mL of starch TS, and titrate <*2.50*> with 0.01 mol/L sodium thiosulfate VS until the color of the solution disappears. Separately, to exactly 2 mL each of the sample solution and standard solution add exactly 10 mL of 0.005 mol/L iodine VS, then proceed in the same manner as above without allowing to stand for 15 minutes as a blank determination, and make any necessary correction. Determine the volumes, V_T and V_S, of 0.005 mol/L iodine VS consumed in the sample solution and standard solution.

Amount (unit) of phenethicillin potassium ($C_{17}H_{19}KN_2O_5S$)
$= M_S \times V_T/V_S$

M_S: Amount (unit) of Phenethicillin Potassium RS taken

Containers and storage Containers—Well-closed containers.

Phenobarbital

フェノバルビタール

$C_{12}H_{12}N_2O_3$: 232.24
5-Ethyl-5-phenylpyrimidine-2,4,6(1*H*,3*H*,5*H*)-trione
[*50-06-6*]

Phenobarbital, when dried, contains not less than 99.0% and not more than 101.0% of phenobarbital ($C_{12}H_{12}N_2O_3$).

Description Phenobarbital occurs as white, crystals or crystalline powder.

It is very soluble in *N*,*N*-dimethylformamide, freely soluble in ethanol (95) and in acetone, sparingly soluble in acetonitrile, and very slightly soluble in water.

It dissolves in sodium hydroxide TS.

The pH of a saturated solution of Phenobarbital is between 5.0 and 6.0.

Identification **(1)** Determine the absorption spectrum of a solution of Phenobarbital in boric acid-potassium chloride-sodium hydroxide buffer solution (pH 9.6) (1 in 100,000) as directed under Ultraviolet-visible Spectrophotometry <*2.24*>, and compare the spectrum with the Reference Spectrum: both spectra exhibit similar intensities of absorption at the same wavelengths.

(2) Determine the infrared absorption spectrum of Phenobarbital as directed in the potassium bromide disk method under Infrared Spectrophotometry <*2.25*>, and compare the spectrum with the Reference Spectrum: both spectra exhibit similar intensities of absorption at the same wave numbers.

Melting point <*2.60*> 175 - 179°C

Purity **(1)** Clarity and color of solution—Dissolve 0.5 g of Phenobarbital in 5 mL of sodium hydroxide TS: the solution is clear and colorless.

(2) Chloride <*1.03*>—Dissolve 0.30 g of Phenobarbital in 20 mL of acetone, and add 6 mL of dilute nitric acid and water to make 50 mL. Perform the test using this solution as the test solution. Prepare the control solution as follows: take 0.30 mL of 0.01 mol/L hydrochloric acid VS, 20 mL of acetone and 6 mL of dilute nitric acid, and add water to make 50 mL (not more than 0.035%).

(3) Heavy metals <*1.07*>—Proceed with 1.0 g of Phenobarbital according to Method 2, and perform the test. Prepare the control solution with 2.0 mL of Standard Lead solution (not more than 20 ppm).

(4) Phenylbarbituric acid—Boil 1.0 g of Phenobarbital with 5 mL of ethanol (95) for 3 minutes: the solution is clear.

(5) Related substances—Dissolve 0.10 g of Phenobarbital in 100 mL of acetonitrile, and use this solution as the sample solution. Pipet 2 mL of the sample solution, add acetonitrile to make exactly 100 mL. Pipet 5 mL of this solution, add acetonitrile to make exactly 100 mL, and use this solution as the standard solution. Perform the test with exactly 10 μL each of the sample solution and standard solution as directed under Liquid Chromatography <*2.01*> according to the following conditions, and determine each peak area of both solutions by the automatic integration method: the area of the peak other than phenobarbital obtained from the sample solution is not larger than the peak area of phenobarbital from the standard solution.

Operating conditions—

Detector: An ultraviolet absorption photometer (wavelength: 210 nm).

Column: A stainless steel column 4.6 mm in inside diameter and 15 cm in length, packed with octadecylsilanized silica gel for liquid chromatography (5 μm in particle diameter).

Column temperature: A constant temperature of about 45°C.

Mobile phase: A mixture of water and acetonitrile (11:9).

Flow rate: Adjust so that the retention time of phenobarbital is about 5 minutes.

Time span of measurement: About 12 times as long as the retention time of phenobarbital, beginning after the solvent peak.

System suitability—

Test for required detectability: Pipet 5 mL of the standard solution, and add acetonitrile to make exactly 20 mL. Confirm that the peak area of phenobarbital obtained with 10 μL of this solution is equivalent to 20 to 30% of that with 10 μL of the standard solution.

System performance: When the procedure is run with 10 μL of the standard solution under the above operating conditions, the number of theoretical plates and the symmetry factor of the peak of phenobarbital are not less than 3000 and not more than 2.0, respectively.

System repeatability: When the test is repeated 6 times with 10 μL of the standard solution under the above operating conditions, the relative standard deviation of the peak area of phenobarbital is not more than 3.0%.

Loss on drying <*2.41*> Not more than 1.0% (1 g, 105°C, 2 hours).

Residue on ignition <*2.44*> Not more than 0.1% (1 g).

Assay Weigh accurately about 0.5 g of Phenobarbital, previously dried, dissolve in 50 mL of *N,N*-dimethylformamide, and titrate <*2.50*> with 0.1 mol/L potassium hydroxide-ethanol VS until the color of the solution change from yellow to yellow-green (indicator: 1 mL of alizarin yellow GG-thymolphthalein TS). Perform a blank determination using a mixture of 50 mL of *N,N*-dimethylformamide and 22 mL of ethanol (95) in the same manner, and make any necessary correction.

Each mL of 0.1 mol/L potassium hydroxide-ethanol VS
= 23.22 mg of $C_{12}H_{12}N_2O_3$

Containers and storage Containers—Well-closed containers.

10% Phenobarbital Powder

フェノバルビタール散10%

10% Phenobarbital Powder contains not less than 9.3% and not more than 10.7% of phenobarbital ($C_{12}H_{12}N_2O_3$: 232.24).

Method of preparation

Phenobarbital	100 g
Starch, Lactose Hydrate or their mixture	a sufficient quantity
To make	1000 g

Prepare as directed under Granules or Powders, with the above ingredients.

Identification (1) Determine the absorption spectrum of the sample solution obtained in the Assay as directed under Ultraviolet-visible Spectrophotometry <*2.24*>: it exhibits a maximum between 238 nm and 242 nm.

(2) To 6 g of 10% Phenobarbital Powder add 150 mL of ethanol, shake well, and filter. Condense the filtrate on a water bath to about 5 mL, add about 50 mL of water, filter to collect the formed crystals, and dry them at 105°C for 2 hours. Determine the infrared absorption spectrum of the crystals as directed in the potassium bromide disk method under Infrared Spectrophotometry <*2.25*>, and compare the spectrum with the Reference Spectrum: both spectra exhibit similar intensities of absorption at the same wave numbers.

Dissolution <*6.10*> When the test is performed at 50 revolutions per minute according to the Paddle method, using 900 mL of water as the dissolution medium, the dissolution rate in 30 minutes of 10% Phenobarbital Powder is not less than 80%.

Start the test with an accurately weighted about 0.3 g of 10% Phenobarbital Powder, withdraw not less than 20 mL of the medium at the specified minute after starting the test, and filter through a membrane filter with a pore size not exceeding 0.45 μm. Discard not less than 10 mL of the first filtrate, pipet 5 mL of the subsequent filtrate, add exactly 10 mL of boric acid-potassium chloride-sodium hydroxide buffer solution (pH 9.6) and use this solution as the sample solution. Separately, weigh accurately about 17 mg of phenobarbital for assay, previously dried at 105°C for 2 hours, and dissolve in water to make exactly 100 mL. Pipet 5 mL of this solution, and add water to make exactly 25 mL. Pipet 5 mL of this solution, add exactly 10 mL of boric acid-potassium chloride-sodium hydroxide buffer solution (pH 9.6) and use this solution as the standard solution. Perform the test with the sample solution and standard solution as directed under Ultraviolet-visible Spectrophotometry <*2.24*>, using a mixture of boric acid-potassium chloride-sodium hydroxide buffer solution (pH 9.6) and water (2:1) as the blank, and determine the absorbances, A_T and A_S, at 240 nm.

Dissolution rate (%) with respect to the labeled amount of phenobarbital ($C_{12}H_{12}N_2O_3$)
$= M_S/M_T \times A_T/A_S \times 1/C \times 180$

M_S: Amount (mg) of phenobarbital for assay taken
M_T: Amount (g) of 10% Phenobarbital Powder taken
C: Labeled amount (mg) of phenobarbital ($C_{12}H_{12}N_2O_3$) in 1 g

Assay Weigh accurately about 0.2 g of 10% Phenobarbital

Powder, dissolve in a boric acid-potassium chloride-sodium hydroxide buffer solution (pH 9.6) to make exactly 100 mL. Pipet 5 mL of this solution, add a boric acid-potassium chloride-sodium hydroxide buffer solution (pH 9.6) to make exactly 100 mL, and use this solution as the sample solution. Separately, weigh accurately about 20 mg of phenobarbital for assay, previously dried at 105°C for 2 hours, and add a boric acid-potassium chloride-sodium hydroxide buffer solution (pH 9.6) to make exactly 100 mL. Pipet 5 mL of this solution, add a boric acid-potassium chloride-sodium hydroxide buffer solution (pH 9.6) to make exactly 100 mL, and use this solution as the standard solution. Perform the test with the sample solution and standard solution as directed under Ultraviolet-visible Spectrophotometry <*2.24*>, using a boric acid-potassium chloride-sodium hydroxide buffer solution (pH 9.6) as the blank, and determine the absorbances, A_T and A_S, at 240 nm.

Amount (mg) of phenobarbital ($C_{12}H_{12}N_2O_3$)
$= M_S \times A_T/A_S$

M_S: Amount (mg) of phenobarbital for assay taken

Containers and storage Containers—Well-closed containers.

Phenobarbital Tablets

フェノバルビタール錠

Phenobarbital Tablets contain not less than 95.0% and not more than 105.0% of the labeled amount of phenobarbital ($C_{12}H_{12}N_2O_3$: 232.24).

Method of preparation Prepare as directed under Tablets, with Phenobarbital.

Identification To a quantity of powdered Phenobarbital Tablets, equivalent to 20 mg of Phenobarbital, add 20 mL of boric acid-potassium chloride-sodium hydroxide buffer solution (pH 9.6), shake, and centrifuge. To 1 mL of the supernatant liquid add boric acid-potassium chloride-sodium hydroxide buffer solution (pH 9.6) to make 100 mL. Determine the absorption spectrum of this solution as directed under Ultraviolet-visible Spectrophotometry <*2.24*>: it exhibits a maximum between 238 nm and 242 nm.

Uniformity of dosage units <*6.02*> Perform the Mass variation test, or the Content uniformity test according to the following method: it meets the requirement.

To 1 tablet of Phenobarbital Tablets add exactly V mL of a mixture of water and acetonitrile (1:1) so that each mL contains about 1 mg of phenobarbital ($C_{12}H_{12}N_2O_3$), sonicate to disintegrate, shake for 10 minutes, and centrifuge. Pipet 1 mL of the supernatant liquid, add a mixture of water and acetonitrile (1:1) to make exactly 20 mL, and use this solution as the sample solution. Then, proceed as directed in the Assay.

Amount (mg) of phenobarbital ($C_{12}H_{12}N_2O_3$)
$= M_S \times A_T/A_S \times V/30$

M_S: Amount (mg) of phenobarbital for assay taken

Dissolution <*6.10*> When the test is performed at 50 revolutions per minute according to the Paddle method, using 900 mL of water as the dissolution medium, the dissolution rate in 30 minutes of Phenobarbital Tablets is not less than 75%.

Start the test with 1 tablet of Phenobarbital Tablets, withdraw not less than 20 mL of the medium at the specified minute after starting the test, and filter through a membrane filter with a pore size not exceeding 0.45 μm. Discard not less than 10 mL of the first filtrate, pipet V mL of the subsequent filtrate, and add water to make exactly V' mL so that each mL contains about 33 μg of phenobarbital ($C_{12}H_{12}N_2O_3$). Pipet 5 mL of this solution, add exactly 10 mL of boric acid-potassium chloride-sodium hydroxide buffer solution (pH 9.6), and use this solution as the sample solution. Separately, weigh accurately about 17 mg of phenobarbital for assay, previously dried at 105°C for 2 hours, and dissolve in water to make exactly 100 mL. Pipet 5 mL of this solution, and add water to make exactly 25 mL. Pipet 5 mL of this solution, add exactly 10 mL of boric acid-potassium chloride-sodium hydroxide buffer solution (pH 9.6), and use this solution as the standard solution. Determine the absorbances, A_T and A_S, at 240 nm of the sample solution and standard solution as directed under Ultraviolet-visible Spectrophotometry <*2.24*>, using a mixture of boric acid-potassium chloride-sodium hydroxide buffer solution (pH 9.6) and water (2:1) as the blank.

Dissolution rate (%) with respect to the labeled amount of phenobarbital ($C_{12}H_{12}N_2O_3$)
$= M_S \times A_T/A_S \times V'/V \times 1/C \times 180$

M_S: Amount (mg) of phenobarbital for assay taken
C: Labeled amount (mg) of phenobarbital ($C_{12}H_{12}N_2O_3$) in 1 tablet

Assay Weigh accurately the mass of not less than 20 tablets of Phenobarbital Tablets, and powder. Weigh accurately a portion of the powder, equivalent to about 30 mg of phenobarbital ($C_{12}H_{12}N_2O_3$), add exactly 30 mL a mixture of water and acetonitrile (1:1), shake for 10 minutes, and centrifuge. Pipet 1 mL of the supernatant liquid, add a mixture of water and acetonitrile (1:1) to make exactly 20 mL, and use this solution as the sample solution. Separately, weigh accurately about 30 mg of phenobarbital for assay, previously dried at 105°C for 2 hours, and dissolve in exactly 30 mL of a mixture of water and acetonitrile (1:1). Pipet 1 mL of this solution, add a mixture of water and acetonitrile (1:1) to make exactly 20 mL, and use this solution as the standard solution. Perform the test with exactly 10 μL each of the sample solution and standard solution as directed under Liquid Chromatography <*2.01*> according to the following conditions, and determine the peak areas, A_T and A_S, of phenobarbital in each solution.

Amount (mg) of phenobarbital ($C_{12}H_{12}N_2O_3$)
$= M_S \times A_T/A_S$

M_S: Amount (mg) of phenobarbital for assay taken

Operating conditions—

Detector: An ultraviolet absorption photometer (wavelength: 210 nm).

Column: A stainless steel column 4.6 mm in inside diameter and 15 cm in length, packed with octadecylsilanized silica gel for liquid chromatography (5 μm in particle diameter).

Column temperature: A constant temperature of about 45°C.

Mobile phase: A mixture of water and acetonitrile for liquid chromatography (11:9).

Flow rate: Adjust so that the retention time of phenobarbital is about 3 minutes.

System suitability—

System performance: When the procedure is run with 10 μL of the standard solution under the above operating conditions, the number of theoretical plates and the symmetry factor of the peak of phenobarbital are not less than 3000

and not more than 1.5, respectively.

System repeatability: When the test is repeated 6 times with 10 μL of the standard solution under the above operating conditions, the relative standard deviation of the peak area of phenobarbital is not more than 1.0%.

Containers and storage Containers—Well-closed containers.

Phenol

フェノール

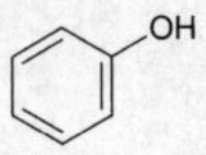

C_6H_6O: 94.11
Phenol
[*108-95-2*]

Phenol contains not less than 98.0% of phenol (C_6H_6O).

Description Phenol occurs as colorless to slightly red, crystals or crystalline masses. It has a characteristic odor.

It is very soluble in ethanol (95) and in diethyl ether, and soluble in water.

Phenol (10 g) is liquefied by addition of 1 mL of water.

The color changes gradually through red to dark red by light or air.

It cauterizes the skin, turning it white.

Congealing point: about 40°C

Identification **(1)** Add 1 drop of iron (III) chloride TS to 10 mL of a solution of Phenol (1 in 100): a blue-purple color develops.

(2) Add bromine TS dropwise to 5 mL of a solution of Phenol (1 in 10,000): a white precipitate is produced, which at first dissolves with shaking, but becomes permanent as excess of the reagent is added.

Purity **(1)** Clarity and color of solution and acidity or alkalinity—Dissolve 1.0 g of Phenol in 15 mL of water: the solution is clear, and neutral or only faintly acid. Add 2 drops of methyl orange TS: no red color develops.

(2) Residue on evaporation—Weigh accurately about 5 g of Phenol, evaporate on a water bath, and dry the residue at 105°C for 1 hour: the mass is not more than 0.05% of the mass of the sample.

Assay Dissolve about 1.5 g of Phenol, accurately weighed, in water to make exactly 1000 mL. Transfer exactly 25 mL of this solution to an iodine flask, add exactly 30 mL of 0.05 mol/L bromine VS, then 5 mL of hydrochloric acid, and immediately stopper the flask. Shake the flask repeatedly for 30 minutes, allow to stand for 15 minutes, then add 7 mL of potassium iodide TS, at once stopper the flask, and shake well. Add 1 mL of chloroform, stopper the flask, and shake thoroughly. Titrate *<2.50>* the liberated iodine with 0.1 mol/L sodium thiosulfate VS (indicator: 1 mL of starch TS). Perform a blank determination in the same manner.

Each mL of 0.05 mol/L bromine VS
= 1.569 mg of C_6H_6O

Containers and storage Containers—Tight containers.

Storage—Light-resistant.

Liquefied Phenol

液状フェノール

Liquefied Phenol is Phenol maintained in a liquid condition by the presence of 10% of Water, Purified Water or Purified Water in Containers.

It contains not less than 88.0% of phenol (C_6H_6O: 94.11).

Description Liquefied Phenol is a colorless or slightly reddish liquid. It has a characteristic odor.

It is miscible with ethanol (95), with diethyl ether and with glycerin.

A mixture of equal volumes of Liquefied Phenol and glycerin is miscible with water.

The color changes gradually to dark red on exposure to light or air.

It cauterizes the skin, turning it white.

Specific gravity d_{20}^{20}: about 1.065

Identification **(1)** Add 1 drop of iron (III) chloride TS to 10 mL of a solution of Liquefied Phenol (1 in 100): a blue-purple color develops.

(2) Add bromine TS dropwise to 5 mL of a solution of Liquefied Phenol (1 in 10,000): a white precipitate is produced, which at first dissolves with shaking, but becomes permanent as excess of the reagent is added.

Boiling point *<2.57>* Not more than 182°C.

Purity **(1)** Clarity and color of solution and acidity or alkalinity—Dissolve 1.0 g of Liquefied Phenol in 15 mL of water: the solution is clear, and neutral or only faintly acid. Add 2 drops of methyl orange TS: no red color develops.

(2) Residue on evaporation—Weigh accurately about 5 g of Liquefied Phenol, evaporate on a water bath, and dry the residue at 105°C for 1 hour: the mass is not more than 0.05% of the mass of the sample.

Assay Dissolve about 1.7 g of Liquefied Phenol, accurately weighed, in a water to make exactly 1000 mL. Transfer exactly 25 mL of this solution to an iodine flask, add exactly 30 mL of 0.05 mol/L bromine VS, then 5 mL of hydrochloric acid, and immediately stopper the flask. Shake the flask repeatedly for 30 minutes, allow to stand for 15 minutes, then add 7 mL of potassium iodide TS, at one stopper the flask tightly, and shake well. Add 1 mL of chloroform, stopper the flask, and shake thoroughly. Titrate *<2.50>* the liberated iodine with 0.1 mol/L sodium thiosulfate VS (indicator: 1 mL of starch TS). Perform a blank determination in the same manner.

Each mL of 0.05 mol/L bromine VS
= 1.569 mg of C_6H_6O

Containers and storage Containers—Tight containers.

Storage—Light-resistant.

Phenol for Disinfection

消毒用フェノール

Phenol for Disinfection contains not less than 95.0% of phenol (C_6H_6O: 94.11).

Description Phenol for Disinfection occurs as colorless to slightly, red crystals, crystalline masses, or liquid containing these crystals. It has a characteristic odor.

It is very soluble in ethanol (95) and in diethyl ether, and freely soluble in water.

Phenol for Disinfection (10 g) is liquefied by addition of 1 mL of water.

It cauterizes the skin, turning it white.

Congealing point: about 30°C.

Identification (1) To 10 mL of a solution of Phenol for Disinfection (1 in 100) add 1 drop of iron (III) chloride TS: a blue-purple color is produced.

(2) To 5 mL of a solution of Phenol for Disinfection (1 in 10,000) add bromine TS dropwise: a white precipitate is formed, and it dissolves at first upon shaking but becomes permanent as excess of the reagent is added.

Purity (1) Clarity of solution—Dissolve 1.0 g of Phenol for Disinfection in 15 mL of water: the solution is clear.

(2) Residue on evaporation—Weigh accurately about 5 g of Phenol for Disinfection, evaporate on a water bath, and dry the residue at 105°C for 1 hour: the mass is not more than 0.10% of the mass of the sample.

Assay Dissolve about 1 g of Phenol for Disinfection, accurately weighed, in water to make exactly 1000 mL. Pipet 25 mL of the solution into an iodine flask, add exactly 30 mL of 0.05 mol/L bromine VS and 5 mL of hydrochloric acid, stopper immediately, shake for 30 minutes and allow to stand for 15 minutes. Add 7 mL of potassium iodide TS, stopper immediately, shake well, and titrate *<2.50>* the liberated iodine with 0.1 mol/L sodium thiosulfate VS (indicator: 1 mL of starch TS). Perform a blank determination in the same manner.

Each mL of 0.05 mol/L bromine VS
= 1.569 mg of C_6H_6O

Containers and storage Containers—Tight containers.
Storage—Light-resistant.

Phenolated Water

フェノール水

Phenolated Water contains not less than 1.8 w/v% and not more than 2.3 w/v% of phenol (C_6H_6O: 94.11).

Method of preparation

Liquefied Phenol	22 mL
Water, Purified Water or Purified Water in Containers	a sufficient quantity
To make	1000 mL

Mix the above ingredients.

Description Phenolated Water is a colorless, clear liquid, having the odor of phenol.

Identification (1) Add 1 drop of iron (III) chloride TS to 10 mL of Phenolated Water: blue-purple color develops.

(2) To 5 mL of a solution of Phenolated Water (1 in 200) add bromine TS dropwise: a white precipitate is formed, and it dissolves at first upon shaking but becomes permanent as excess of the reagent is added.

Assay Take exactly 2 mL of Phenolated Water into an iodine flask, add 25 mL of water, then add exactly 40 mL of 0.05 mol/L bromine VS and 5 mL of hydrochloric acid, stopper immediately, shake for 30 minutes, and allow to stand for 15 minutes. Add 7 mL of potassium iodide TS, stopper tightly at once, shake well, and titrate *<2.50>* the liberated iodine with 0.1 mol/L sodium thiosulfate VS (indicator: 1 mL of starch TS). Perform a blank determination in the same manner.

Each mL of 0.05 mol/L bromine VS
= 1.569 mg of C_6H_6O

Containers and storage Containers—Tight containers.

Phenolated Water for Disinfection

消毒用フェノール水

Phenolated Water for Disinfection contains not less than 2.8 w/v% and not more than 3.3 w/v% of phenol (C_6H_6O: 94.11).

Method of preparation

Phenol for Disinfection	31 g
Water, Purified Water or Purified Water in Containers	a sufficient quantity
To make	1000 mL

Mix the above ingredients.

Description Phenolated Water for Disinfection is a clear, colorless liquid, having the odor of phenol.

Identification (1) Add 1 drop of iron (III) chloride TS to 10 mL of Phenolated Water for Disinfection: a blue-purple color develops.

(2) Proceed with 5 mL of a solution of Phenolated Water for Disinfection (1 in 200) as directed in the Identification (2) under Phenol for Disinfection.

Assay Take exactly 5 mL of Phenolated Water for Disinfection, add water to make exactly 100 mL, then pipet 25 mL of the solution into an iodine flask, and proceed as directed in the Assay under Phenol for Disinfection.

Each mL of 0.05 mol/L bromine VS
= 1.569 mg of C_6H_6O

Containers and storage Containers—Tight containers.

Dental Phenol with Camphor

歯科用フェノール・カンフル

Method of preparation

Phenol	35 g
d- or *dl*-Camphor	65 g
To make	100 g

Melt Phenol by warming, add *d*-Camphor or *dl*- Camphor, and mix.

Description Dental Phenol with Camphor is a colorless or light red liquid. It has a characteristic odor.

Containers and storage Containers—Tight containers.
Storage—Light-resistant.

Phenol and Zinc Oxide Liniment

フェノール·亜鉛華リニメント

Method of preparation

Liquefied Phenol	22 mL
Powdered Tragacanth	20 g
Carmellose Sodium	30 g
Glycerin	30 mL
Zinc Oxide	100 g
Purified Water or Purified Water in Containers	a sufficient quantity
To make	1000 g

Mix Liquefied Phenol, Glycerin and Purified Water or Purified Water in Containers, add Powdered Tragacanth in small portions by stirring, and allow the mixture to stand overnight. To the mixture add Carmellose Sodium in small portions by stirring to make a pasty mass, add Zinc Oxide in small portions, and mix. Less than 5 g of Powdered Tragacanth or Carmellose Sodium can be replaced by each other to make 50 g in total.

Description Phenol and Zinc Oxide Liniment is a white pasty mass. It has a slight odor of phenol.

Identification **(1)** Shake well 1 g of Phenol and Zinc Oxide Liniment with 10 mL of diethyl ether, and filter. To the filtrate add 10 mL of dilute sodium hydroxide TS, shake well, and separate the water layer. To 1 mL of the water layer add 1 mL of sodium nitrite TS and 1 mL of dilute hydrochloric acid, shake, and add 3 mL of sodium hydroxide TS: a yellow color develops (phenol).

(2) Place 1 g of Phenol and Zinc Oxide Liniment in a porcelain crucible, heat gradually raising the temperature until the content is charred, and then ignite it strongly: a yellow color develops, and disappears on cooling. To the residue add 10 mL of water and 5 mL of dilute hydrochloric acid, shake well, and filter. To the filtrate add 2 to 3 drops of potassium hexacyanoferrate (II) TS: a white precipitate is produced (zinc oxide).

(3) Shake 0.5 g of Phenol and Zinc Oxide Liniment with 1 mL of water and 5 mL of chloroform, separate the chloroform layer, and use this solution as the sample solution. Separately, dissolve 0.01 g of phenol in 5 mL of chloroform, and use this solution as the standard solution. Perform the test with these solutions as directed under Thin-layer Chromatography <*2.03*>. Spot 5 μL each of the sample solution and standard solution on a plate of silica gel for thin-layer chromatography. Develop the plate with a mixture of ethyl acetate, ethanol (99.5) and ammonia solution (28) (50:5:1) to a distance of about 10 cm, and air-dry the plate. Allow the plate to stand in iodine vapor: the spots obtained from the sample solution and the standard solution show the same *R*f value.

Containers and storage Containers—Tight containers.

Phenolsulfonphthalein

フェノールスルホンフタレイン

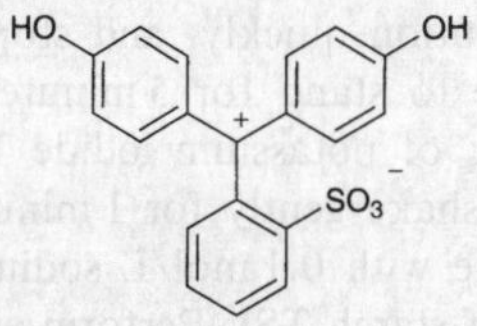

$C_{19}H_{14}O_5S$: 354.38

2-[Bis(4-hydroxyphenyl)methyliumyl]benzenesulfonate

[*143-74-8*]

Phenolsulfonphthalein, when dried, contains not less than 98.0% of phenolsulfonphthalein ($C_{19}H_{14}O_5S$).

Description Phenolsulfonphthalein occurs as a vivid red to dark red crystalline powder.

It is very slightly soluble in water and in ethanol (95).

It dissolves in sodium hydroxide TS.

Identification **(1)** Dissolve 5 mg of Phenolsulfonphthalein in 2 to 3 drops of sodium hydroxide TS, add 2 mL of 0.05 mol/L bromine VS and 1 mL of dilute sulfuric acid, shake well, and allow to stand for 5 minutes. Render the solution alkaline with sodium hydroxide TS: a deep blue-purple color develops.

(2) Dissolve 0.01 g of Phenolsulfonphthalein in diluted sodium carbonate TS (1 in 10) to make 200 mL. To 5 mL of this solution add diluted sodium carbonate TS (1 in 10) to make 100 mL. Perform the test with this solution as directed under Ultraviolet-visible Spectrophotometry <*2.24*>, and compare the spectrum with the Reference Spectrum: both spectra exhibit similar intensities of absorption at the same wavelengths.

Purity **(1)** Insoluble substances—To about 1 g of Phenolsulfonphthalein, accurately weighed, add 20 mL of a solution of sodium hydrogen carbonate (1 in 40). Allow the mixture to stand for 1 hour with frequent shaking, dilute with water to 100 mL, and allow to stand for 24 hours. Collect the insoluble substances using a tared glass filter (G4), wash with 25 mL of a solution of sodium hydrogen carbonate (1 in 100) and with five 5-mL portions of water, and dry at 105°C for 1 hour: the mass of the residue is not more than 0.2%.

(2) Related substances—Dissolve 0.10 g of Phenolsulfonphthalein in 5 mL of dilute sodium hydroxide TS, and use this solution as the sample solution. Pipet 0.5 mL of the sample solution, add dilute sodium hydroxide TS to make exactly 100 mL, and use this solution as the standard solution. Perform the test with these solutions as directed under Thin-layer Chromatography <*2.03*>. Spot 10 μL each of the sample solution and standard solution on a plate of silica gel with fluorescent indicator for thin-layer chromatography. Develop the plate with a mixture of *t*-amyl alcohol, acetic acid (100) and water (4:1:1) to a distance of about 15 cm, and air-dry the plate. After allowing the plate to stand in an ammonia vapor, examine under ultraviolet light (main wavelength: 254 nm): the spots other than the principal spot obtained from the sample solution are not more intense than the spot from the standard solution.

Loss on drying <*2.41*> Not more than 1.0% (1 g, silica gel, 4 hours).

Residue on ignition <*2.44*> Not more than 0.2% (1 g).

Assay Weigh accurately about 0.15 g of Phenolsulfonphthalein, previously dried, transfer to an iodine flask, dissolve in 30 mL of a solution of sodium hydroxide (1 in 250), and add water to make 200 mL. Add exactly measured 50 mL of 0.05 mol/L bromine VS, add 10 mL of hydrochloric acid to the solution quickly, and stopper immediately. Allow the mixture to stand for 5 minutes with occasional shaking, add 7 mL of potassium iodide TS, stopper again immediately, and shake gently for 1 minute. Titrate <*2.50*> the liberated iodine with 0.1 mol/L sodium thiosulfate VS (indicator: 1 mL of starch TS). Perform a blank determination in the same manner.

Each mL of 0.05 mol/L bromine VS
= 4.430 mg of $C_{19}H_{14}O_5S$

Containers and storage Containers—Well-closed containers.

Phenolsulfonphthalein Injection

フェノールスルホンフタレイン注射液

Phenolsulfonphthalein Injection is an aqueous injection.

It contains not less than 0.54 w/v% and not more than 0.63 w/v% of phenolsulfonphthalein ($C_{19}H_{14}O_5S$: 354.38).

Method of preparation

Phenolsulfonphthalein	6 g
Sodium Chloride	9 g
Sodium Bicarbonate	1.43 g
(or Sodium Hydroxide	0.68 g)
Water for Injection or Sterile Water for Injection in Containers	a sufficient quantity
To make	1000 mL

Prepare as directed under Injections, with the above ingredients.

Description Phenolsulfonphthalein Injection is a clear, orange-yellow to red liquid.

Identification To 1 mL of Phenolsulfonphthalein Injection add 2 to 3 drops of sodium hydroxide TS, and proceed as directed in the Identification (1) under Phenolsulfonphthalein.

pH <*2.54*> 6.0 – 7.6

Bacterial endotoxins <*4.01*> Less than 7.5 EU/mg.

Extractable volume <*6.05*> It meets the requirement.

Foreign insoluble matter <*6.06*> Perform the test according to Method 1: it meets the requirement.

Insoluble particulate matter <*6.07*> Perform the test according to Method 2: it meets the requirement.

Sterility <*4.06*> Perform the test according to the Membrane filtration method: it meets the requirement.

Sensitivity To 1.0 mL of Phenolsulfonphthalein Injection add 5 mL of water. To 0.20 mL of this solution add 50 mL of freshly boiled and cooled water and 0.40 mL of 0.01 mol/L sodium hydroxide VS: a deep red-purple color develops, and it changes to light yellow on the addition of 0.40 mL of 0.005 mol/L sulfuric acid VS.

Assay Pipet 5 mL of Phenolsulfonphthalein Injection, and add a solution of anhydrous sodium carbonate (1 in 100) to make exactly 250 mL. Pipet 5 mL of this solution, add a solution of anhydrous sodium carbonate (1 in 100) to make exactly 200 mL, and use this solution as the sample solution. Separately, weigh accurately about 30 mg of phenolsulfonphthalein for assay, previously dried in a desiccator (silica gel) for 4 hours, and dissolve in a solution of anhydrous sodium carbonate (1 in 100) to make exactly 250 mL. Pipet 5 mL of this solution, add a solution of anhydrous sodium carbonate (1 in 100) to make exactly 200 mL, and use this solution as the standard solution. Determine the absorbances, A_T and A_S, of the sample solution and standard solution at 559 nm as directed under Ultraviolet-visible Spectrophotometry <*2.24*>.

Amount (mg) of phenolsulfonphthalein ($C_{19}H_{14}O_5S$)
$= M_S \times A_T/A_S$

M_S: Amount (mg) of phenolsulfonphthalein for assay taken

Containers and storage Containers—Hermetic containers.

L-Phenylalanine

L-フェニルアラニン

$C_9H_{11}NO_2$: 165.19
(2*S*)-2-Amino-3-phenylpropanoic acid
[*63-91-2*]

L-Phenylalanine, when dried, contains not less than 98.5% of L-phenylalanine ($C_9H_{11}NO_2$).

Description L-Phenylalanine occurs as white, crystals or crystalline powder. It is odorless or has a faint characteristic odor, and has a slightly bitter taste.

It is freely soluble in formic acid, sparingly soluble in water, and practically insoluble in ethanol (95).

It dissolves in dilute hydrochloric acid.

Identification Determine the infrared absorption spectrum of L-Phenylalanine, previously dried, as directed in the potassium bromide disk method under Infrared Spectrophotometry <*2.25*>, and compare the spectrum with the Reference Spectrum: both spectra exhibit similar intensities of absorption at the same wave numbers.

Optical rotation <*2.49*> $[\alpha]_D^{20}$: −33.0 – −35.5° (after drying, 0.5 g, water, 25 mL, 100 mm).

pH <*2.54*> Dissolve 0.20 g of L-Phenylalanine in 20 mL of water: the pH of this solution is between 5.3 and 6.3.

Purity **(1)** Clarity and color of solution—Dissolve 0.5 g of L-Phenylalanine in 10 mL of 1 mol/L hydrochloric acid TS: the solution is clear and colorless.

(2) Chloride <*1.03*>—Perform the test with 0.5 g of L-Phenylalanine. Prepare the control solution with 0.30 mL of 0.01 mol/L hydrochloric acid VS (not more than 0.021%).

(3) Sulfate <*1.14*>—Perform the test with 0.6 g of L-Phenylalanine. Prepare the control solution with 0.35 mL of 0.005 mol/L sulfuric acid VS (not more than 0.028%).

(4) Ammonium <*1.02*>—Perform the test with 0.25 g of L-Phenylalanine. Prepare the control solution with 5.0 mL of Standard Ammonium Solution (not more than 0.02%).

(5) Heavy metals <1.07>—Dissolve 1.0 g of L-Phenylalanine in 40 mL of water and 2 mL of dilute acetic acid by warming, cool, and add water to make 50 mL. Perform the test using this solution as the test solution. Prepare the control solution as follows: to 2.0 mL of Standard Lead Solution add 2 mL of dilute acetic acid and water to make 50 mL (not more than 20 ppm).

(6) Arsenic <1.11>—Dissolve 1.0 g of L-Phenylalanine in 5 mL of dilute hydrochloric acid and 15 mL of water, and perform the test with this solution as the test solution (not more than 2 ppm).

(7) Related substances—Dissolve 0.10 g of L-Phenylalanine in 25 mL of water, and use this solution as the sample solution. Pipet 1 mL of the sample solution, and add water to make exactly 50 mL. Pipet 5 mL of this solution, add water to make exactly 20 mL, and use this solution as the standard solution. Perform the test with these solutions as directed under Thin-layer Chromatography <2.03>. Spot 5 μL each of the sample solution and standard solution on a plate of silica gel for thin-layer chromatography. Develop the plate with a mixture of 1-butanol, water and acetic acid (100) (3:1:1) to a distance of about 10 cm, and dry the plate at 80°C for 30 minutes. Spray evenly a solution of ninhydrin in acetone (1 in 50) on the plate, and heat the plate at 80°C for 5 minutes: the spots other than the principal spot obtained from the sample solution are not more intense than the spot from the standard solution.

Loss on drying <2.41> Not more than 0.30% (1 g, 105°C, 3 hours).

Residue on ignition <2.44> Not more than 0.1% (1 g).

Assay Weigh accurately about 0.17 g of L-Phenylalanine, previously dried, and dissolve in 3 mL of formic acid, add 50 mL of acetic acid (100), and titrate <2.50> with 0.1 mol/L perchloric acid VS (potentiometric titration). Perform a blank determination in the same manner, and make any necessary correction.

Each mL of 0.1 mol/L perchloric acid VS
= 16.52 mg of $C_9H_{11}NO_2$

Containers and storage Containers—Tight containers.

Phenylbutazone

フェニルブタゾン

$C_{19}H_{20}N_2O_2$: 308.37
4-Butyl-1,2-diphenylpyrazolidine-3,5-dione
[50-33-9]

Phenylbutazone, when dried, contains not less than 99.0% of phenylbutazone ($C_{19}H_{20}N_2O_2$).

Description Phenylbutazone occurs as a white to pale yellow-white crystalline powder. It is odorless, and is at first tasteless but leaves a slightly bitter aftertaste.

It is freely soluble in acetone, soluble in ethanol (95) and in diethyl ether, and practically insoluble in water.

It dissolves in sodium hydroxide TS.

Identification (1) To 0.1 g of Phenylbutazone add 1 mL of acetic acid (100) and 1 mL of hydrochloric acid, and heat on a water bath under a reflux condenser for 30 minutes. Add 10 mL of water, and cool with ice water. Filter, and to the filtrate add 3 to 4 drops of sodium nitrite TS. To 1 mL of this solution add 1 mL of 2-naphthol TS and 3 mL of chloroform, and shake: a deep red color develops in the chloroform layer.

(2) Dissolve 1 mg of Phenylbutazone in 10 mL of dilute sodium hydroxide TS, and dilute with water to make 100 mL. Determine the absorption spectrum of the solution as directed under Ultraviolet-visible Spectrophotometry <2.24>, and compare the spectrum with the Reference Spectrum: both spectra exhibit similar intensities of absorption at the same wavelengths.

Melting point <2.60> 104 - 107°C

Purity (1) Clarity of solution—Dissolve 1.0 g of Phenylbutazone in 20 mL of sodium hydroxide solution (2 in 25), and allow to stand at 25 ± 1°C for 3 hours: the solution is clear. Determine the absorbance of this solution at 420 nm as directed under Ultraviolet-visible Spectrophotometry <2.24>: it is not more than 0.05.

(2) Heavy metals <1.07>—Proceed with 2.0 g of Phenylbutazone according to Method 2, and perform the test. Prepare the control solution with 2.0 mL of Standard Lead Solution (not more than 10 ppm).

(3) Arsenic <1.11>—Prepare the test solution with 1.0 g of phenylbutazone, according to Method 3, and perform the test (not more than 2 ppm).

(4) Readily carbonizable substances—Dissolve 1.0 g of Phenylbutazone in 20 mL of sulfuric acid, and allow to stand at 25 ± 1°C for exactly 30 minutes: the solution is clear. Determine the absorbance of this solution at 420 nm as directed under Ultraviolet-visible Spectrophotometry <2.24>: it is not more than 0.10.

Loss on drying <2.41> Not more than 0.5% (1 g, in vacuum, silica gel, 4 hours).

Residue on ignition <2.44> Not more than 0.1% (1 g).

Assay Weigh accurately about 0.5 g of Phenylbutazone, previously dried, dissolve in 25 mL of acetone, and titrate <2.50> with 0.1 mol/L sodium hydroxide VS until the solution shows a blue color which persists for 15 seconds (indicator: 5 drops of bromothymol blue TS). Perform a blank determination with a mixture of 25 mL of acetone and 16 mL of water in the same manner, and make any necessary correction.

Each mL of 0.1 mol/L sodium hydroxide VS
= 30.84 mg of $C_{19}H_{20}N_2O_2$

Containers and storage Containers—Tight containers.

Phenylephrine Hydrochloride

フェニレフリン塩酸塩

$C_9H_{13}NO_2.HCl$: 203.67
(1*R*)-1-(3-Hydroxyphenyl)-2-methylaminoethanol monohydrochloride
[*61-76-7*]

Phenylephrine Hydrochloride, when dried, contains not less than 98.0% and not more than 102.0% of phenylephrine hydrochloride ($C_9H_{13}NO_2.HCl$).

Description Phenylephrine Hydrochloride occurs as white crystals or crystalline powder. It is odorless, and has a bitter taste.

It is very soluble in water, freely soluble in ethanol (95), and practically insoluble in diethyl ether.

The pH of a solution of 1.0 g of Phenylephrine Hydrochloride in 100 mL of water is 4.5 to 5.5.

Identification **(1)** To 1 mL of a solution of Phenylephrine Hydrochloride (1 in 100) add 1 drop of copper (II) sulfate TS and 1 mL of a solution of sodium hydroxide (1 in 5): a blue color is produced. To the solution so obtained add 1 mL of diethyl ether, and shake vigorously: no blue color develops in the diethyl ether layer.

(2) To 1 mL of a solution of Phenylephrine Hydrochloride (1 in 100) add 1 drop of iron (III) chloride TS: a persistent purple color is produced.

(3) Dissolve 0.3 g of Phenylephrine Hydrochloride in 3 mL of water, add 1 mL of ammonia TS, and rub the inner side of the test tube with a glass rod: a precipitate is produced. Collect the precipitate, wash with a few drops of ice-cold water, and dry at 105°C for 2 hours: it melts <*2.60*> between 170°C and 177°C.

(4) A solution of Phenylephrine Hydrochloride (1 in 100) responds to Qualitative Tests <*1.09*> (2) for chloride.

Optical rotation <*2.49*> $[\alpha]_D^{20}$: −42.0 – −47.5° (after drying, 0.5 g, water, 10 mL, 100 mm).

Melting point <*2.60*> 140 – 145°C

Purity **(1)** Clarity and color of solution—Dissolve 1.0 g of Phenylephrine Hydrochloride in 10 mL of water: the solution is clear and colorless.

(2) Sulfate <*1.14*>—Take 0.5 g of Phenylephrine Hydrochloride, and perform the test. Prepare the control solution with 0.50 mL of 0.005 mol/L sulfuric acid VS (not more than 0.048%).

(3) Ketone—Dissolve 0.20 g of Phenylephrine Hydrochloride in 1 mL of water, and add 2 drops of sodium pentacyanonitrosylferrate (III) TS, 1 mL of sodium hydroxide TS and then 0.6 mL of acetic acid (100): the solution has no more color than the following control solution.

Control solution: Prepare as directed above without Phenylephrine Hydrochloride.

Loss on drying <*2.41*> Not more than 0.5% (1 g, 105°C, 2 hours).

Residue on ignition <*2.44*> Not more than 0.2% (1 g).

Assay Weigh accurately about 0.1 g of Phenylephrine Hydrochloride, previously dried, dissolve in 40 mL of water contained in an iodine flask, add exactly measured 50 mL of 0.05 mol/L bromine VS, then add 5 mL of hydrochloric acid, and immediately stopper tightly. Shake the mixture, and allow to stand for 15 minutes. To this solution add 10 mL of potassium iodide TS carefully, stopper tightly immediately, shake thoroughly, allow to stand for 5 minutes, and titrate <*2.50*> with 0.1 mol/L sodium thiosulfate VS (indicator: 1 mL of starch TS). Perform a blank determination in the same manner.

Each mL of 0.05 mol/L bromine VS
= 3.395 mg of $C_9H_{13}NO_2.HCl$

Containers and storage Containers—Tight containers.
Storage—Light-resistant.

Phenytoin

フェニトイン

$C_{15}H_{12}N_2O_2$: 252.27
5,5-Diphenylimidazolidine-2,4-dione
[*57-41-0*]

Phenytoin, when dried, contains not less than 99.0% of phenytoin ($C_{15}H_{12}N_2O_2$).

Description Phenytoin occurs as a white, crystalline powder or granules. It is odorless and tasteless.

It is sparingly soluble in ethanol (95) and in acetone, slightly soluble in diethyl ether, and practically insoluble in water.

It dissolves in sodium hydroxide TS.

Melting point: about 296°C (with decomposition).

Identification **(1)** Dissolve 0.02 g of Phenytoin in 2 mL of ammonia TS, and add 5 mL of silver nitrate TS: a white precipitate is produced.

(2) Boil a mixture of 0.01 g of Phenytoin, 1 mL of ammonia TS and 1 mL of water, and add dropwise 2 mL of a mixture prepared from 50 mL of a solution of copper (II) sulfate pentahydrate (1 in 20) and 10 mL of ammonia TS: a red, crystalline precipitate is produced.

(3) Heat 0.1 g of Phenytoin with 0.2 g of sodium hydroxide, and fuse: the gas evolved turns moistened red litmus paper blue.

(4) Add 3 mL of chlorinated lime TS to 0.1 g of Phenytoin, shake for 5 minutes, and dissolve the oily precipitate in 15 mL of hot water. After cooling, add 1 mL of dilute hydrochloric acid dropwise, then add 4 mL of water. Filter the white precipitate thus obtained, wash with water, and press it with dry filter paper to remove the accompanying water. Dissolve the precipitate with 1 mL of chloroform, add 5 mL of diluted ethanol (9 in 10), and rub the inner surface of the flask to produce a white, crystalline precipitate. Collect the precipitate, wash with ethanol (95), and dry: the melting point <*2.60*> is between 165°C and 169°C.

Purity **(1)** Clarity and color of solution—Dissolve 0.20 g of Phenytoin in 10 mL of 0.2 mol/L sodium hydroxide VS: the solution is clear and colorless. Then heat the solution: no turbidity is produced. Cool, and mix the solution with 5 mL of acetone: the solution is clear and colorless.

(2) Acidity or alkalinity—Shake 2.0 g of Phenytoin with 40 mL of water for 1 minute, filter, and perform the following tests using this filtrate as the sample solution.

(i) To 10 mL of the sample solution add 2 drops of phenolphthalein TS: no color develops. Then add 0.15 mL of 0.01 mol/L sodium hydroxide VS: a red color develops.

(ii) To 10 mL of the sample solution add 0.30 mL of 0.01 mol/L hydrochloric acid VS and 5 drops of methyl red TS: a red to orange color develops.

(3) Chloride *<1.03>*—Dissolve 0.30 g of Phenytoin in 30 mL of acetone, and add 6 mL of dilute nitric acid and water to make 50 mL. Perform the test using this solution as the test solution. Prepare the control solution from 0.60 mL of 0.01 mol/L hydrochloric acid VS, 30 mL of acetone and 6 mL of dilute nitric acid, and add water to 50 mL (not more than 0.071%).

(4) Heavy metals *<1.07>*—Proceed with 1.0 g of Phenytoin according to Method 2, and perform the test. Prepare the control solution with 2.0 mL of Standard Lead Solution (not more than 20 ppm).

Loss on drying *<2.41>* Not more than 0.5% (2 g, 105°C, 2 hours).

Residue on ignition *<2.44>* Not more than 0.1% (1 g).

Assay Weigh accurately about 0.5 g of Phenytoin, previously dried, dissolve in 40 mL of ethanol (95) with the aid of gentle heating, add 0.5 mL of thymolphthalein TS immediately, and titrate with 0.1 mol/L sodium hydroxide VS until a light blue color develops. Then add 1 mL of pyridine, 5 drops of phenolphthalein TS and 25 mL of silver nitrate TS, and titrate *<2.50>* with 0.1 mol/L sodium hydroxide VS until a light red color, which persists for 1 minute, develops.

Each mL of 0.1 mol/L sodium hydroxide VS
= 25.23 mg of $C_{15}H_{12}N_2O_2$

Containers and storage Containers—Well-closed containers.

Phenytoin Powder

フェニトイン散

Phenytoin Powder contains not less than 95.0% and not more than 105.0% of the labeled amount of phenytoin ($C_{15}H_{12}N_2O_2$: 252.27).

Method of preparation Prepare as directed under Granules or Powders, with Phenytoin.

Identification Weigh a portion of Phenytoin Powder, equivalent to 0.3 g of Phenytoin, stir well with two 100-mL portions of diethyl ether, and extract. Combine the diethyl ether extracts, and filter. Evaporate the filtrate on a water bath to dryness, and proceed with the residue as directed in the Identification under Phenytoin.

Dissolution Being specified separately when the drug is granted approval based on the Law.

Assay Weigh accurately an amount of Phenytoin Powder, equivalent to about 50 mg of phenytoin ($C_{15}H_{12}N_2O_2$), add 30 mL of methanol, sonicate for 15 minutes with occasional shaking, shake for another 10 minutes, and add methanol to make exactly 50 mL. Centrifuge this solution, pipet 5 mL of the supernatant liquid, add exactly 5 mL of the internal standard solution, and use this solution as the sample solution. Separately, weigh accurately about 25 mg of phenytoin for assay, previously dried at 105°C for 2 hours, and dissolve in methanol to make exactly 25 mL. Pipet 5 mL of this solution, add exactly 5 mL of the internal standard solution, and use this solution as the standard solution. Perform the test with 10 μL each of the sample solution and standard solution as directed under Liquid Chromatography *<2.01>* according to the following conditions, and calculate the ratios, Q_T and Q_S, of the peak area of phenytoin to that of the internal standard.

Amount (mg) of phenytoin ($C_{15}H_{12}N_2O_2$)
$= M_S \times Q_T/Q_S \times 2$

M_S: Amount (mg) of phenytoin for assay taken

Internal standard solution—A solution of propyl parahydroxybenzoate in the mobile phase (1 in 25,000).

Operating conditions—

Detector: An ultraviolet absorption photometer (wavelength: 258 nm).

Column: A stainless steel column 4.6 mm in inside diameter and 15 cm in length, packed with octadecylsilanized silica gel for liquid chromatography (5 μm in particle diameter).

Column temperature: A constant temperature of about 40°C.

Mobile phase: A mixture of methanol and 0.02 mol/L phosphate buffer solution (pH 3.5) (11:9).

Flow rate: Adjust so that the retention time of phenytoin is about 5 minutes.

System suitability—

System performance: When the procedure is run with 10 μL of the standard solution under the above operating conditions, phenytoin and the internal standard are eluted in this order with the resolution between these peaks being not less than 8.

System repeatability: When the test is repeated 6 times with 10 μL of the standard solution under the above operating conditions, the relative standard deviation of the ratio of the peak area of phenytoin to that of the internal standard is not more than 1.0%.

Containers and storage Containers—Well-closed containers.

Phenytoin Tablets

フェニトイン錠

Phenytoin Tablets contain not less than 95.0% and not more than 105.0% of the labeled amount of phenytoin ($C_{15}H_{12}N_2O_2$: 252.27).

Method of preparation Prepare as directed under Tablets, with Phenytoin.

Identification Weigh a portion of powdered Phenytoin Tablets, equivalent to about 0.3 g of Phenytoin, transfer to a separator, and add 1 mL of dilute hydrochloric acid and 10 mL of water. Extract with 100 mL of diethyl ether, then with four 25-mL potions of diethyl ether. Combine the extracts, evaporate the diethyl ether on a water bath, and dry the residue at 105°C for 2 hours. Proceed with the residue as directed in the Identification under Phenytoin.

Uniformity of dosage units *<6.02>* Perform the Mass variation test, or the Content uniformity test according to the following method: it meets the requirement.

To 1 tablet of Phenytoin Tablets add $3V/5$ mL of a mixture of water and acetonitrile (1:1), sonicate for 15 minutes with occasional shaking, shake for another 10 minutes, and add a mixture of water and acetonitrile (1:1) to make exactly V mL so that each mL contains about 1 mg of phenytoin ($C_{15}H_{12}N_2O_2$). Centrifuge this solution, pipet 5 mL of the supernatant liquid, add exactly 5 mL of the internal standard solution, and use this solution as the sample solution. Proceed as directed in the Assay.

$$\text{Amount (mg) of phenytoin } (C_{15}H_{12}N_2O_2) = M_S \times Q_T/Q_S \times V/25$$

M_S: Amount (mg) of phenytoin for assay taken

Internal standard solution—A solution of propyl parahydroxybenzoate in the mobile phase (1 in 25,000).

Dissolution Being specified separately when the drug is granted approval based on the Law.

Assay Weigh accurately the mass of not less than 20 Phenytoin Tablets, and powder in an agate mortar. Weigh accurately a portion of the powder, equivalent to about 50 mg of phenytoin ($C_{15}H_{12}N_2O_2$), add 30 mL of a mixture of water and acetonitrile (1:1), sonicate for 15 minutes with occasional shaking, shake for another 10 minutes, and add a mixture of water and acetonitrile (1:1) to make exactly 50 mL. Centrifuge this solution, pipet 5 mL of the supernatant liquid, add exactly 5 mL of the internal standard solution, and use this solution as the sample solution. Separately, weigh accurately about 25 mg of phenytoin for assay, previously dried at 105°C for 2 hours, and dissolve in a mixture of water and acetonitrile (1:1) to make exactly 25 mL. Pipet 5 mL of this solution, add exactly 5 mL of the internal standard solution, and use this solution as the standard solution. Perform the test with 10 μL each of the sample solution and standard solution as directed under Liquid Chromatography <*2.01*> according to the following conditions, and calculate the ratios, Q_T and Q_S, of the peak area of phenytoin to that of the internal standard.

$$\text{Amount (mg) of phenytoin } (C_{15}H_{12}N_2O_2) = M_S \times Q_T/Q_S \times 2$$

M_S: Amount (mg) of phenytoin for assay taken

Internal standard solution—A solution of propyl parahydroxybenzoate in the mobile phase (1 in 25,000).
Operating conditions—

Detector: An ultraviolet absorption photometer (wavelength: 258 nm).

Column: A stainless steel column 4.6 mm in inside diameter and 15 cm in length, packed with octadecylsilanized silica gel for liquid chromatography (5 μm in particle diameter).

Column temperature: A constant temperature of about 40°C.

Mobile phase: A mixture of methanol and 0.02 mol/L phosphate buffer solution (pH 3.5) (11:9).

Flow rate: Adjust so that the retention time of phenytoin is about 5 minutes.
System suitability—

System performance: When the procedure is run with 10 μL of the standard solution under the above operating conditions, phenytoin and the internal standard are eluted in this order with the resolution between these peaks being not less than 8.

System repeatability: When the test is repeated 6 times with 10 μL of the standard solution under the above operating conditions, the relative standard deviation of the ratio of the peak area of phenytoin to that of the internal standard is not more than 1.0%.

Containers and storage Containers—Well-closed containers.

Phenytoin Sodium for Injection

注射用フェニトインナトリウム

$C_{15}H_{11}N_2NaO_2$: 274.25
Monosodium 5,5-diphenyl-4-oxoimidazolidin-2-olate
[*630-93-3*]

Phenytoin Sodium for Injection is a preparation for injection which is dissolved before use.

When dried, it contains not less than 98.5% of phenytoin sodium ($C_{15}H_{11}N_2NaO_2$), and contains not less than 92.5% and not more than 107.5% of the labeled amount of phenytoin sodium ($C_{15}H_{11}N_2NaO_2$).

Method of preparation Prepare as directed under Injections.

Description Phenytoin Sodium for Injection occurs as white, crystals or crystalline powder. It is odorless.

It is soluble in water and in ethanol (95), and practically insoluble in chloroform and in diethyl ether.

The pH of a solution of 1.0 g of Phenytoin Sodium for Injection in 20 mL of water is about 12.

It is hygroscopic.

A solution of Phenytoin Sodium for Injection absorbs carbon dioxide gradually when exposed to air, and a crystalline precipitate of phenytoin is produced.

Identification **(1)** With the residue obtained in the Assay, proceed as directed in the Identification under Phenytoin.

(2) Ignite 0.5 g of Phenytoin Sodium for Injection, cool, and dissolve the residue in 10 mL of water: the solution changes red litmus paper to blue, and responds to Qualitative Tests <*1.09*> (1) for sodium salt.

Purity **(1)** Clarity and color of solution—Dissolve 1.0 g of Phenytoin Sodium for Injection in 20 mL of freshly boiled and cooled water in a glass-stoppered test tube: the solution is clear and colorless. If any turbidity is produced, add 4.0 mL of 0.1 mol/L sodium hydroxide VS: the solution becomes clear and colorless.

(2) Heavy metals <*1.07*>—Proceed with 1.0 g of Phenytoin Sodium for Injection according to Method 2, and perform the test. Prepare the control solution with 2.0 mL of Standard Lead Solution (not more than 20 ppm).

Loss on drying <*2.41*> Not more than 2.5% (1 g, 105°C, 4 hours).

Assay Weigh accurately the content of not less than 10 containers of Phenytoin Sodium for Injection, transfer about 0.3 g of the content, previously dried and accurately weighed, to a separator, dissolve in 50 mL of water, add 10 mL of dilute hydrochloric acid, and extract with 100 mL of diethyl ether, then with four 25-mL portions of diethyl ether. Combine the diethyl ether extracts, and evaporate on a water bath. Dry the residue at 105°C for 2 hours, and weigh it as the mass of phenytoin ($C_{15}H_{12}N_2O_2$: 252.27).

Amount (mg) of phenytoin sodium ($C_{15}H_{11}N_2NaO_2$)
= amount (mg) of phenytoin ($C_{15}H_{12}N_2O_2$) × 1.087

Containers and storage Containers—Hermetic containers.

Phytonadione

Vitamin K_1

フィトナジオン

$C_{31}H_{46}O_2$: 450.70
2-Methyl-3-[(2*E*,7*R*,11*R*)-3,7,11,15-tetramethylhexadec-2-en-1-yl]-1,4-naphthoquinone
[84-80-0]

Phytonadione contains not less than 97.0% and not more than 102.0% of phytonadione ($C_{31}H_{46}O_2$).

Description Phytonadione is a clear yellow to orange-yellow viscous liquid.

It is miscible with isooctane.

It is soluble in ethanol (99.5), and practically insoluble in water.

It decomposes gradually and changes to a red-brown by light.

Specific gravity d^{20}_{20}: about 0.967

Identification (1) Determine the absorption spectrum of a solution of Phytonadione in isooctane (1 in 100,000) as directed under Ultraviolet-visible Spectrophotometry <*2.24*>, and compare the spectrum with the Reference Spectrum 1: both spectra exhibit similar intensities of absorption at the same wavelengths. Separately, determine the absorption spectrum of a solution of Phytonadione in isooctane (1 in 10,000) as directed under Ultraviolet-visible Spectrophotometry <*2.24*>, and compare the spectrum with the Reference Spectrum 2: both spectra exhibit similar intensities of absorption at the same wavelengths.

(2) Determine the infrared absorption spectrum of Phytonadione as directed in the liquid film method under Infrared Spectrophotometry <*2.25*>, and compare the spectrum with the Reference Spectrum: both spectra exhibit similar intensities of absorption at the same wave numbers.

Refractive index <*2.45*> n^{20}_{D}: 1.525 – 1.529

Purity (1) Ratio of absorbances—Determine the absorbances, A_1, A_2 and A_3, of a solution of Phytonadione in isooctane (1 in 100,000) at 248.5 nm, 253.5 nm and 269.5 nm, respectively, as directed under Ultraviolet-visible Spectrophotometry <*2.24*>: the ratio A_2/A_1 is between 0.69 and 0.73, and the ratio A_2/A_3 is between 0.74 and 0.78. Determine the absorbances, A_4 and A_5, of a solution of Phytonadione in isooctane (1 in 10,000) at 284.5 nm and 326 nm, respectively: the ratio A_4/A_5 is between 0.28 and 0.34.

(2) Heavy metals <*1.07*>—Carbonize 1.0 g of Phytonadione by gentle heating. Cool, add 10 mL of a solution of magnesium nitrate hexahydrate in ethanol (95) (1 in 10), and ignite the ethanol to burn. Cool, add 1 mL of sulfuric acid, proceed according to Method 4, and perform the test. Prepare the control solution with 2.0 mL of Standard Lead Solution (not more than 20 ppm).

(3) Menadione—Dissolve 20 mg of Phytonadione in 0.5 mL of a mixture of water and ethanol (95) (1:1), add 1 drop of a solution of 3-methyl-1-phenyl-5-pyrazolone in ethanol (95) (1 in 20) and 1 drop of ammonia solution (28), and allow to stand for 2 hours: no blue-purple color develops.

Isomer ratio Conduct this procedure rapidly and without exposure to light. Dissolve 30 mg of Phytonadione in 50 mL of the mobile phase. To 4 mL of this solution add the mobile phase to make 25 mL. To 10 mL of this solution add the mobile phase to make 25 mL, and use this solution as the sample solution. Perform the test with 50 μL of the sample solution as directed under Liquid Chromatography <*2.01*> according to the following conditions, and determine the peak areas of *Z*-isomer and *E*-isomer, A_{TZ} and A_{TE}: $A_{TZ}/(A_{TZ} + A_{TE})$ is between 0.05 and 0.18.

Operating conditions—

Proceed as directed in the operating conditions in the Assay.

System suitability—

System performance: When the procedure is run with 50 μL of the sample solution under the above operating conditions, *Z*-isomer and *E*-isomer are eluted in this order with the resolution between these peaks being not less than 1.5.

System repeatability: When the test is repeated 6 times with 50 μL of the sample solution under the above operating conditions, the relative standard deviation of the total area of the peaks of *Z*-isomer and *E*-isomer is not more than 2.0%.

Assay Conduct this procedure rapidly and without exposure to light. Weigh accurately about 30 mg each of Phytonadione and Phytonadione RS, and dissolve each in the mobile phase to make exactly 50 mL. Pipet 4 mL each of these solutions, and add the mobile phase to make exactly 25 mL. To exactly 10 mL each of these solutions add exactly 7 mL of the internal standard solution and the mobile phase to make 25 mL, and use these as the sample solution and the standard solution, respectively. Perform the test with 50 μL each of the sample solution and standard solution as directed under Liquid Chromatography <*2.01*> according to the following conditions, and calculate the ratios, Q_T and Q_S, of the total area of the peaks of *Z*-isomer and *E*-isomer to the peak area of the internal standard.

Amount (mg) of phytonadione ($C_{31}H_{46}O_2$) = $M_S \times Q_T/Q_S$

M_S: Amount (mg) of Phytonadione RS taken

Internal standard solution—A solution of cholesterol benzoate in the mobile phase (1 in 400).

Operating conditions—

Detector: An ultraviolet absorption photometer (wavelength: 254 nm).

Column: A stainless steel column 4.6 mm in inside diameter and 25 cm in length, packed with porous silica gel for liquid chromatography (5 μm in particle diameter).

Column temperature: A constant temperature of about 30°C.

Mobile phase: A mixture of hexane and *n*-amyl alcohol (4000 : 3).

Flow rate: Adjust so that the retention time of the peak of *E*-isomer of phytonadione is about 25 minutes.

System suitability—

System performance: When the procedure is run with 50 μL of the standard solution under the above operating conditions, the internal standard, *Z*-isomer and *E*-isomer are eluted in this order with the resolution between the peaks of *Z*-isomer and *E*-isomer being not less than 1.5.

System repeatability: When the test is repeated 6 times with 50 μL of the standard solution under the above operating conditions, the relative standard deviation of the ratio of the total area of the peaks of *Z*-isomer and *E*-isomer to the peak area of the internal standard is not more than 1.0%.

Containers and storage Containers—Tight containers.

Storage—Light-resistant, at a cold place or in containers in which air has been displaced by Nitrogen.

Pilocarpine Hydrochloride

ピロカルピン塩酸塩

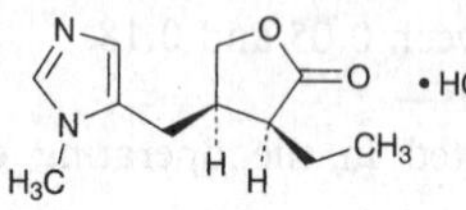

$C_{11}H_{16}N_2O_2.HCl$: 244.72
(3*S*,4*R*)-3-Ethyl-4-(1-methyl-1*H*-imidazol-5-ylmethyl)-4,5-dihydrofuran-2(3*H*)-one monohydrochloride
[*54-71-7*]

Pilocarpine Hydrochloride, when dried, contains not less than 99.0% of pilocarpine hydrochloride ($C_{11}H_{16}N_2O_2.HCl$).

Description Pilocarpine Hydrochloride occurs as colorless crystals or white powder. It is odorless, and has a slightly bitter taste.

It is very soluble in acetic acid (100), freely soluble in water, in methanol and in ethanol (95), soluble in acetic anhydride, and practically insoluble in diethyl ether.

The pH of a solution of 1.0 g of Pilocarpine Hydrochloride in 10 mL of water is between 3.5 and 4.5.

It is hygroscopic.

It is affected by light.

Identification **(1)** Dissolve 0.1 g of Pilocarpine Hydrochloride in 5 mL of water, add 1 drop of dilute nitric acid, 1 mL of hydrogen peroxide TS, 1 mL of chloroform and 1 drop of a potassium dichromate solution (1 in 300), and shake the mixture vigorously: a violet color develops in the chloroform layer while no color or a light yellow color is produced in the aqueous layer.

(2) To 1 mL of a solution of Pilocarpine Hydrochloride (1 in 20) add 1 mL of dilute nitric acid and 2 to 3 drops of silver nitrate TS: a white precipitate or opalescence is produced.

Melting point 〈*2.60*〉 200 – 203°C

Purity **(1)** Sulfate—Dissolve 0.5 g of Pilocarpine Hydrochloride in 20 mL of water, and use this solution as the sample solution. To 5.0 mL of the sample solution add 1 mL of dilute hydrochloric acid and 0.5 mL of barium chloride TS: no turbidity is produced.

(2) Nitrate—To 2.0 mL of the sample solution obtained in (1) add 2 mL of iron (II) sulfate TS, and superimpose the mixture upon 4 mL of sulfuric acid: no dark brown color develops at the zone of contact.

(3) Related substances—Dissolve 0.3 g of Pilocarpine Hydrochloride in 10 mL of methanol, and use this solution as the sample solution. Pipet 1 mL of the sample solution, add methanol to make exactly 100 mL, and use this solution as the standard solution. Perform the test with these solutions as directed under Thin-layer Chromatography 〈*2.03*〉. Spot 10 μL each of the sample solution and standard solution on a plate of silica gel for thin-layer chromatography. Develop the plate with a mixture of chloroform, methanol and ammonia TS (85:14:2) to a distance of about 13 cm, and dry the plate at 105°C for 10 minutes. Cool, and spray evenly bismuth potassium iodide TS on the plate: the spots other than the principal spot obtained from the sample solution are not more intense than the spot from the standard solution.

(4) Readily carbonizable substances 〈*1.15*〉—Take 0.25 g of Pilocarpine Hydrochloride, and perform the test: the solution has no more color than Matching Fluid B.

Loss on drying 〈*2.41*〉 Not more than 3.0% (1 g, 105°C, 2 hours).

Residue on ignition 〈*2.44*〉 Not more than 0.5% (0.1 g).

Assay Weigh accurately about 0.5 g of Pilocarpine Hydrochloride, previously dried, dissolve in 50 mL of a mixture of acetic anhydride and acetic acid (100) (7:3), and titrate 〈*2.50*〉 with 0.1 mol/L perchloric acid VS (potentiometric titration). Perform a blank determination in the same manner, and make any necessary correction.

Each mL of 0.1 mol/L perchloric acid VS
= 24.47 mg of $C_{11}H_{16}N_2O_2.HCl$

Containers and storage Containers—Tight containers.

Storage—Light-resistant.

Pilocarpine Hydrochloride Tablets

ピロカルピン塩酸塩錠

Pilocarpine Hydrochloride Tablets contain not less than 95.0% and not more than 105.0% of the labeled amount of pilocarpine hydrochloride ($C_{11}H_{16}N_2O_2$.HCl: 244.72).

Method of preparation Prepare as directed under Tablets, with Pilocarpine Hydrochloride.

Identification Perform the test with 10 μL each of the sample solution and the standard solution, both obtained in the assay, as directed under Liquid Chromatography 〈*2.01*〉 according to the following conditions: the principal peaks in the chromatograms obtained from the sample solution and standard solution show the same retention time, and both spectra of these peaks in the chromatograms exhibit similar intensities of absorption at the same wavelengths.

Operating conditions—

Column, column temperature, mobile phase, and flow rate: Proceed as directed in the operating conditions in the Assay.

Detector: Photodiode array detector (wavelength: 215 nm; spectrum range of measurement: 200 – 370 nm).

System suitability—

System performance: Proceed as directed in the system suitability in the Assay.

Purity Related substances—Use the sample solution obtained in the Assay as the sample solution. Pipet 1 mL of the sample solution, add phosphate buffer solution (pH 4.0) to make exactly 100 mL, and use this solution as the standard solution. Perform the test with exactly 10 μL each of the sample solution and standard solution as directed under Liquid Chromatography 〈*2.01*〉 according to the following conditions, and determine each peak area by the automatic integration method: the area of the two peaks, having the relative retention time of about 0.78 and about 0.92 to pilocarpine, obtained from the sample solution is not larger than the peak area of pilocarpine from the standard solution, the area of the peak other than pilocarpine and the peaks mentioned above from the sample solution is not larger than 1/5 times the peak area of pilocarpine from the standard solution, and the total area of the peaks other than pilocarpine from the sample solution is not larger than 2 times the peak area of pilocarpine from the standard solution.

Operating conditions—

Detector, column, column temperature, mobile phase, and flow rate: Proceed as directed in the operating conditions in the Assay.

Time span of measurement: About 1.3 times as long as the retention time of pilocarpine, beginning after the solvent peak.

System suitability—

Test for required detectability: To exactly 2 mL of the standard solution add phosphate buffer solution (pH 4.0) to make exactly 20 mL. Confirm that the peak area of pilocarpine obtained with 10 μL of this solution is equivalent to 7 – 13% of that with 10 μL of the standard solution.

System performance: When the procedure is run with 10 μL of the standard solution under the above operating conditions, the number of theoretical plates and the symmetry factor of the peak of pilocarpine are not less than 3000 and not more than 2.0, respectively.

System repeatability: When the test is repeated 6 times with 10 μL of the standard solution under the above operating conditions, the relative standard deviation of the peak area of pilocarpine is not more than 2.0%.

Uniformity of dosage units <*6.02*> Perform the test according to the following method: it meets the requirement of the Content uniformity test.

To 1 tablet of Pilocarpine Hydrochloride Tablets add a suitable amount of phosphate buffer solution (pH 4.0), shake until the tablet is completely disintegrated, then add phosphate buffer solution (pH 4.0) to make exactly *V* mL so that each mL contains about 0.2 mg of pilocarpine hydrochloride ($C_{11}H_{16}N_2O_2.HCl$), and filter through a membrane filter with a pore size not exceeding 0.45 μm. Discard the first 3 mL of the filtrate, and use the subsequent filtrate as the sample solution. Separately, weigh accurately about 40 mg of pilocarpine hydrochloride for assay, previously dried at 105°C for 2 hours, and dissolve in phosphate buffer solution (pH 4.0) to make exactly 100 mL. Pipet 5 mL of this solution, add phosphate buffer solution (pH 4.0) to make exactly 10 mL, and use this solution as the standard solution. Perform the test with exactly 20 μL each of the sample solution and standard solution as directed under Liquid Chromatography <*2.01*> according to the following conditions, and determine the peak areas, A_T and A_S, of pilocarpine in each solution.

Amount (mg) of pilocarpine hydrochloride ($C_{11}H_{16}N_2O_2.HCl$)
$= M_S \times A_T/A_S \times V/200$

M_S: Amount (mg) of pilocarpine hydrochloride for assay taken

Operating conditions—

Proceed as directed in the operating conditions in the Assay.

System suitability—

System performance: When the procedure is run with 20 μL of the standard solution under the above operating conditions, the number of theoretical plates and the symmetry factor of the peak of pilocarpine are not less than 3000 and not more than 2.0, respectively.

System repeatability: When the test is repeated 6 times with 20 μL of the standard solution under the above operating conditions, the relative standard deviation of the peak area of pilocarpine is not more than 1.0%.

Dissolution <*6.10*> When the test is performed at 50 revolutions per minute according to the Paddle method, using 900 mL of 2nd fluid for dissolution test as the dissolution medium, the dissolution rate in 30 minutes of Pilocarpine Hydrochloride Tablets is not less than 80%.

Start the test with 1 tablet of Pilocarpine Hydrochloride Tablets, withdraw not less than 10 mL of the medium at the specified minute after starting the test, and filter through a membrane filter with a pore size not exceeding 0.45 μm. Discard not less than 3 mL of the first filtrate, pipet *V* mL of the subsequent filtrate, add the dissolution medium to make exactly *V′* mL so that each mL contains about 5.6 μg of pilocarpine hydrochloride ($C_{11}H_{16}N_2O_2.HCl$), and use this solution as the sample solution. Separately, weigh accurately about 50 mg of pilocarpine hydrochloride for assay, previously dried at 105°C for 2 hours, and dissolve in the dissolution medium to make exactly 100 mL. Pipet 2 mL of this solution, add the dissolution medium to make exactly 200 mL, and use this solution as the standard solution. Perform the test with exactly 50 μL each of the sample solution and standard solution as directed under Liquid Chromatography <*2.01*> according to the following conditions, and determine the peak areas, A_T and A_S, of pilocarpine in each solution.

Dissolution rate (%) with respect to the labeled amount of pilocarpine hydrochloride ($C_{11}H_{16}N_2O_2.HCl$)
$= M_S \times A_T/A_S \times V'/V \times 1/C \times 9$

M_S: Amount (mg) of pilocarpine hydrochloride for assay taken

C: Labeled amount (mg) of pilocarpine hydrochloride ($C_{11}H_{16}N_2O_2.HCl$) in 1 tablet

Operating conditions—

Proceed as directed in the operating conditions in the Assay.

System suitability—

System performance: When the procedure is run with 50 μL of the standard solution under the above operating conditions, the number of theoretical plates and the symmetry factor of the peak of pilocarpine are not less than 3000 and not more than 2.0, respectively.

System repeatability: When the test is repeated 6 times with 50 μL of the standard solution under the above operating conditions, the relative standard deviation of the peak area of pilocarpine is not more than 1.0%.

Assay To 20 Pilocarpine Hydrochloride Tablets add a suitable amount of phosphate buffer solution (pH 4.0), shake until the tablets are completely disintegrated, then add phosphate buffer solution (pH 4.0) to make exactly *V* mL so that each mL contains about 0.4 mg of pilocarpine hydrochloride ($C_{11}H_{16}N_2O_2.HCl$), and filter through a membrane filter with a pore size not exceeding 0.45 μm. Discard the first 3 mL of the filtrate, and use the subsequent filtrate as the sample solution. Separately, weigh accurately about 40 mg of pilocarpine hydrochloride for assay, previously dried at 105°C for 2 hours, dissolve in phosphate buffer solution (pH 4.0) to make exactly 100 mL, and use this solution as the standard solution. Perform the test with exactly 10 μL each of the sample solution and standard solution as directed under Liquid Chromatography 〈*2.01*〉 according to the following conditions, and determine the peak areas, A_T and A_S, of pilocarpine in each solution.

Amount (mg) of pilocarpine hydrochloride ($C_{11}H_{16}N_2O_2.HCl$) in 1 tablet
$$= M_S \times A_T/A_S \times V/2000$$

M_S: Amount (mg) of pilocarpine hydrochloride for assay taken

Operating conditions—

Detector: An ultraviolet absorption photometer (wavelength: 215 nm).

Column: A stainless steel column 3.9 mm in inside diameter and 30 cm in length, packed with phenylated silica gel for liquid chromatography (10 μm in particle diameter).

Column temperature: A constant temperature of about 25°C.

Mobile phase: To 1000 mL of 0.05 mol/L potassium dihydrogen phosphate TS add phosphoric acid to adjust to pH 2.5. To this solution add 5.0 mL of triethylamine, and adjust to pH 2.5 with phosphoric acid.

Flow rate: Adjust so that the retention time of pilocarpine is about 12 minutes.

System suitability—

System performance: When the procedure is run with 10 μL of the standard solution under the above operating conditions, the number of theoretical plates and the symmetry factor of the peak of pilocarpine are not less than 3000 and not more than 2.0, respectively.

System repeatability: When the test is repeated 6 times with 10 μL of the standard solution under the above operating conditions, the relative standard deviation of the peak area of pilocarpine is not more than 1.0%.

Containers and storage Containers—Tight containers.

Pilsicainide Hydrochloride Hydrate

ピルシカイニド塩酸塩水和物

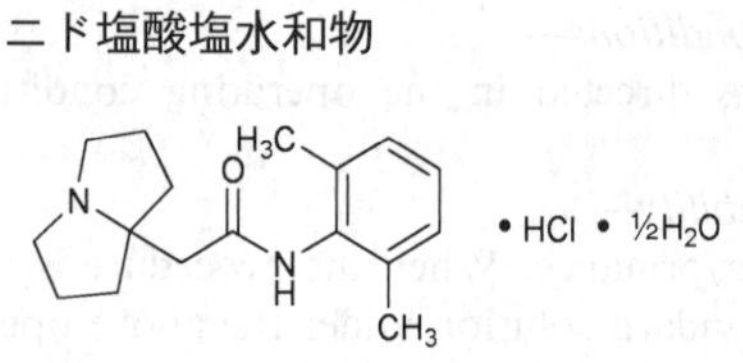

$C_{17}H_{24}N_2O.HCl.\frac{1}{2}H_2O$: 317.85
N-(2,6-Dimethylphenyl)tetrahydro-1*H*-pyrrolizin-7a(5*H*)-ylacetamide monohydrochloride hemihydrate
[*88069-49-2*, anhydride]

Pilsicainide Hydrochloride Hydrate contains not less than 99.0% and not more than 101.0% of pilsicainide hydrochloride hydrate ($C_{17}H_{24}N_2O.HCl.\frac{1}{2}H_2O$).

Description Pilsicainide Hydrochloride Hydrate occurs as white, crystals or crystalline powder.

It is very soluble in acetic acid (100), and freely soluble in water, in methanol and in ethanol (99.5).

It dissolves in 0.1 mol/L hydrochloric acid TS.

Identification (1) Determine the absorption spectrum of a solution of Pilsicainide Hydrochloride Hydrate in 0.1 mol/L hydrochloric acid TS (1 in 2000) as directed under Ultraviolet-visible Spectrophotometry 〈*2.24*〉, and compare the spectrum with the Reference Spectrum: both spectra exhibit similar intensities of absorption at the same wavelengths.

(2) Determine the infrared absorption spectrum of Pilsicainide Hydrochloride Hydrate as directed in the potassium chloride disk method under Infrared Spectrophotometry 〈*2.25*〉, and compare the spectrum with the Reference Spectrum: both spectra exhibit similar intensities of absorption at the same wave numbers.

(3) A solution of Pilsicainide Hydrochloride Hydrate (1 in 100) responds to Qualitative Tests 〈*1.09*〉 (2) for chloride.

pH 〈*2.54*〉 Dissolve 1.0 g of Pilsicainide Hydrochloride Hydrate in 50 mL of water: the pH of this solution is between 5.3 and 6.1.

Melting point 〈*2.60*〉 210.5 – 213.5°C (Heat the bath to 160°C in advance).

Purity (1) Heavy metals 〈*1.07*〉—Proceed with 2.0 g of Pilsicainide Hydrochloride Hydrate according to Method 1, and perform the test. Prepare the control solution with 2.0 mL of Standard Lead Solution (not more than 10 ppm).

(2) Related substances—Dissolve 40 mg of Pilsicainide Hydrochloride Hydrate in 20 mL of water, and use this solution as the sample solution. Pipet 1 mL of the sample solution, and add water to make exactly 20 mL. Pipet 1 mL of this solution, add water to make exactly 50 mL, and use this solution as the standard solution. Perform the test with exactly 20 μL each of the sample solution and standard solution as directed under Liquid Chromatography 〈*2.01*〉 according to the following conditions, and determine each peak area by the automatic integration method: the area of the peaks other than pilsicainide obtained from the sample solution is not larger than the peak area of pilsicainide from the standard solution.

Operating conditions—

Detector: An ultraviolet absorption photometer (wavelength: 210 nm).

Column: A stainless steel column 4.6 mm in inside diameter and 15 cm in length, packed with octadecylsilanized silica gel for liquid chromatography (5 μm in particle diameter).

Column temperature: A constant temperature of about 40°C.

Mobile phase: To 750 mL of water add 5 mL of triethylamine, adjust to pH 4.0 with phosphoric acid, and add water to make 1000 mL. To this solution add 200 mL of acetonitrile for liquid chromatography.

Flow rate: Adjust so that the retention time of pilsicainide is about 5 minutes.

Time span of measurement: About 5 times as long as the retention time of pilsicainide, beginning after the solvent peak.

System suitability—

System performance: When the procedure is run with 20 μL of the standard solution under the above operating conditions, the number of theoretical plates and the symmetry factor of the peak of pilsicainide are not less than 5000 and not more than 1.5, respectively.

System repeatability: When the test is repeated 6 times with 20 μL of the standard solution under the above operating conditions, the relative standard deviation of the peak area of pilsicainide is not more than 2.0%.

Water 〈*2.48*〉 2.5 – 3.3% (50 mg, coulometric titration).

Residue on ignition 〈*2.44*〉 Not more than 0.1% (1 g).

Assay Weigh accurately about 0.3 g of Pilsicainide Hydrochloride Hydrate, dissolve it in 10 mL of acetic acid (100), add 40 mL of acetic anhydride, and titrate <2.50> with 0.1 mol/L perchloric acid VS (potentiometric titration). Perform a blank determination in the same manner, and make any necessary correction.

Each mL of 0.1 mol/L perchloric acid VS
= 31.79 mg of $C_{17}H_{24}N_2O.HCl.\frac{1}{2}H_2O$

Containers and storage Containers—Tight containers.

Pilsicainide Hydrochloride Capsules

ピルシカイニド塩酸塩カプセル

Pilsicainide Hydrochloride Capsules contain not less than 95.0% and not more than 105.0% of the labeled amount of pilsicainide hydrochloride hydrate ($C_{17}H_{24}N_2O.HCl.\frac{1}{2}H_2O$: 317.85).

Method of preparation Prepare as directed under Capsules, with Pilsicainide Hydrochloride Hydrate.

Identification Take out the contents of Pilsicainide Hydrochloride Capsules, to a quantity of the content, equivalent to 50 mg of Pilsicainide Hydrochloride Hydrate, add 10 mL of water, and shake well. Centrifuge this solution, and filter the supernatant liquid through a membrane filter with a pore size not exceeding 0.45 μm. To 1 mL of the filtrate, add 1 mL of 1 mol/L hydrochloric acid TS and 8 mL of water. Determine the absorption spectrum of this solution as directed under Ultraviolet-visible Spectrophotometry <2.24>: it exhibits maxima between 261 nm and 265 nm, and between 268 nm and 272 nm.

Uniformity of dosage units <6.02> Perform the Mass variation test, or the Content uniformity test according to the following method: it meets the requirement.

To 1 capsule of Pilsicainide Hydrochloride Capsules, add water, and shake to disperse the content of the capsule uniformly while warming in a water bath. After cooling, add exactly V mL of the internal standard solution so that 0.2 mL of the internal standard solution is added for each mg of pilsicainide hydrochloride hydrate ($C_{17}H_{24}N_2O.HCl.\frac{1}{2}H_2O$), then, add water so that each mL contains about 0.5 mg of pilsicainide hydrochloride hydrate ($C_{17}H_{24}N_2O.HCl.\frac{1}{2}H_2O$). To 5 mL of this solution, add water to make 50 mL, and filter. Discard the first 10 mL of the filtrate, and use the subsequent filtrate as the sample solution. Then, proceed as directed in the Assay.

Amount (mg) of pilsicainide hydrochloride hydrate ($C_{17}H_{24}N_2O.HCl.\frac{1}{2}H_2O$)
$= M_S \times Q_T/Q_S \times V/10$

M_S: Amount (mg) of pilsicainide hydrochloride hydrate for assay taken

Internal Standard Solution—Dissolve 2.5 g of lidocaine for assay in 20 mL of 0.5 mol/L hydrochloric acid TS, and add water to make 1000 mL.

Dissolution <6.10> When the test is performed at 50 revolutions per minute according to the Paddle method using the sinker, using 900 mL of water as the dissolution medium, the dissolution rate in 30 minutes of Pilsicainide Hydrochloride Capsules is not less than 85%.

Start the test with 1 capsule of Pilsicainide Hydrochloride Capsules, withdraw not less than 20 mL of the medium at the specified minute after starting the test, and filter through a membrane filter with a pore size not exceeding 0.45 μm. Discard not less than 10 mL of the first filtrate, pipet V mL of the subsequent filtrate, add water to make exactly V' mL so that each mL contains about 28 μg of pilsicainide hydrochloride hydrate ($C_{17}H_{24}N_2O.HCl.\frac{1}{2}H_2O$), and use this solution as the sample solution. Separately, weigh accurately about 28 mg of pilsicainide hydrochloride hydrate for assay, dissolve in water to make exactly 100 mL. Pipet 5 mL of this solution, add water to make exactly 50 mL, and use this solution as the standard solution. Perform the test with exactly 20 μL each of the sample solution and standard solution as directed under Liquid Chromatography <2.01> according to the following conditions, and determine the peak areas, A_T and A_S, of pilsicainide in each solution.

Dissolution rate (%) with respect to the labeled amount of pilsicainide hydrochloride hydrate ($C_{17}H_{24}N_2O.HCl.\frac{1}{2}H_2O$)
$= M_S \times A_T/A_S \times V'/V \times 1/C \times 90$

M_S: Amount (mg) of pilsicainide hydrochloride hydrate for assay taken

C: Labeled amount (mg) of pilsicainide hydrochloride hydrate ($C_{17}H_{24}N_2O.HCl.\frac{1}{2}H_2O$) in 1 capsule

Operating conditions—

Proceed as directed in the operating conditions in the Assay.

System suitability—

System performance: When the procedure is run with 20 μL of the standard solution under the above operating conditions, the number of theoretical plates and the symmetry factor of the peak of pilsicainide are not less than 4000 and not more than 1.5, respectively.

System repeatability: When the test is repeated 6 times with 20 μL of the standard solution under the above operating conditions, the relative standard deviation of the peak area of pilsicainide is not more than 1.0%.

Assay Take out the contents of not less than 20 Pilsicainide Hydrochloride Capsules, weigh accurately the mass of the contents, and powder. Weigh accurately a portion of the powder, equivalent to about 50 mg of pilsicainide hydrochloride hydrate ($C_{17}H_{24}N_2O.HCl.\frac{1}{2}H_2O$), add 50 mL of water and shake well. After adding exactly 10 mL of the internal standard solution, add water to make 100 mL. To 5 mL of this solution add water to make 50 mL, and filter the solution. Discard the first 10 mL of the filtrate, and use the subsequent filtrate as the sample solution. Separately, weigh accurately about 50 mg of pilsicainide hydrochloride hydrate for assay, dissolve in exactly 10 mL of the internal standard solution, and add water to make 100 mL. To 5 mL of this solution add water to make 50 mL, and use this solution as the standard solution. Perform the test with 20 μL each of the sample solution and standard solution as directed under Liquid Chromatography <2.01> according to the following conditions, and calculate the ratios, Q_T and Q_S, of the peak area of pilsicainide to that of the internal standard.

Amount (mg) of pilsicainide hydrochloride hydrate ($C_{17}H_{24}N_2O.HCl.\frac{1}{2}H_2O$)
$= M_S \times Q_T/Q_S$

M_S: Amount (mg) of pilsicainide hydrochloride hydrate for assay taken

Internal Standard Solution—Dissolve 2.5 g of lidocaine for assay in 20 mL of 0.5 mol/L hydrochloric acid TS, and add water to make 1000 mL.

Operating conditions—

Detector: An ultraviolet absorption photometer (wavelength: 210 nm).

Column: A stainless steel column 4.6 mm in inside diameter and 15 cm in length, packed with octadecylsilanized silica gel for liquid chromatography (5 μm in particle diameter).

Column temperature: A constant temperature of around 40°C.

Mobile phase: To 750 mL of water add 5 mL of triethylamine, adjust the pH to 4.0 with phosphoric acid, and add water to make 1000 mL. To this solution, add 200 mL of acetonitrile for liquid chromatography.

Flow rate: Adjust so that the retention time of pilsicainide is about 5 minutes.

System suitability—

System performance: When the procedure is run with 20 μL of the standard solution under the above operating conditions, the internal standard and pilsicainide are eluted in this order with the resolution between these peaks being not less than 2.0.

System repeatability: When the test is repeated 6 times with 20 μL of the standard solution under the above operating conditions, the relative standard deviation of the ratio of the peak area of pilsicainide to that of the internal standard is not more than 1.0%.

Containers and storage Containers—Tight containers.

Pimaricin

Natamycin

ピマリシン

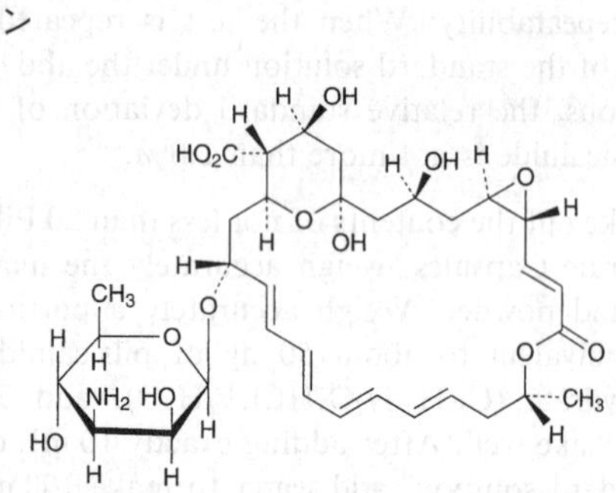

$C_{33}H_{47}NO_{13}$: 665.73
(1*R**,3*S**,5*R**,7*R**,8*E*,12*R**,14*E*,16*E*,18*E*,20*E*,22*R**,
24*S**,25*R**,26*S**)-22-(3-Amino-3,6-dideoxy-β-D-mannopyranosyloxy)-1,3,26-trihydroxy-12-methyl-10-oxo-6,11,28-trioxatricyclo[22.3.1.0^{5,7}]octacosa-8,14,16,18,20-pentaene-25-carboxylic acid
[*7681-93-8*]

Pimaricin is a polyene macrolide substance having antifungal activity produced by the growth of *Streptomyces natalensis*.

It contains not less than 900 μg (potency) and not more than 1020 μg (potency) per mg, calculated on the anhydrous basis. The potency of Pimaricin is expressed as mass (potency) of pimaricin ($C_{33}H_{47}NO_{13}$).

Description Pimaricin occurs as white to yellow-white crystalline powder.

It is slightly soluble in methanol and in acetic acid (100), and practically insoluble in water and in ethanol (99.5).

Identification (1) To 3 mg of Pimaricin add 1 mL of hydrochloric acid, and mix: a blue-purple color appears.

(2) Dissolve 5 mg of Pimaricin in a solution of acetic acid (100) in methanol (1 in 100) to make 1000 mL. Determine the absorption spectrum of this solution as directed under Ultraviolet-visible Spectrophotometry <*2.24*>, and compare the spectrum with the Reference Spectrum or the spectrum of a solution of Pimaricin RS prepared in the same manner as the sample solution: both spectra exhibit similar intensities of absorption at the same wavelengths.

Optical rotation <*2.49*> $[\alpha]_D^{20}$: +243 – +259° (0.1 g, acetic acid (100), 25 mL, 100 mm).

Purity (1) Heavy metals <*1.07*>—Proceed with 1.0 g of Pimaricin according to Method 4, and perform the test. Prepare the control solution with 3.0 mL of Standard Lead Solution (not more than 30 ppm).

(2) Related substances—Dissolve 20 mg of Pimaricin in methanol to make 100 mL, and use this solution as the sample solution. Perform the test with 10 μL of the sample solution as directed under Liquid Chromatography <*2.01*> according to the following conditions, and determine the total area of the peaks other than pimaricin by the automatic integration method. Calculate the amount of the peaks by the area percentage method: not more than 4.0%.

Operating conditions—

Detector: An ultraviolet absorption photometer (wavelength: 303 nm).

Column: A stainless steel column 3.9 mm in inside diameter and 30 cm in length, packed with octadecylsilanized silica gel for liquid chromatography (10 μm in particle diameter).

Column temperature: A constant temperature of about 40°C.

Mobile phase: Dissolve 1.0 g of ammonium acetate in 1000 mL of a mixture of water, methanol and tetrahydrofuran (47:44:2).

Flow rate: Adjust so that the retention time of pimaricin is about 10 minutes.

Time span of measurement: About 3 times as long as the retention time of pimaricin.

System suitability—

Test for required detectability: Measure exactly 1 mL of the sample solution, add methanol to make exactly 100 mL, and use this solution as the solution for system suitability test. Pipet 1 mL of the solution for system suitability test, and add methanol to make exactly 10 mL. Confirm that the peak area of pimaricin obtained with 10 μL of this solution is equivalent to 7 to 13% of that with 10 μL of the solution for system suitability test.

System performance: When the procedure is run with 10 μL of the solution for system suitability test under the above operating conditions, the number of theoretical plates and the symmetry factor of the peak of pimaricin are not less than 1500 and not more than 2.0, respectively.

System repeatability: When the test is repeated 6 times with 10 μL of the solution for system suitability test under the above operating conditions, the relative standard deviation of the peak area of pimaricin is not more than 2.0%.

Water <*2.48*> Between 6.0% and 9.0% (0.2 g, volumetric titration, direct titration).

Assay Weigh accurately an amount of Pimaricin and Pimaricin RS, equivalent to about 25 mg (potency), and dissolve each in methanol to make exactly 100 mL. Pipet 2 mL each of these solutions, add a solution of acetic acid (100) in methanol (1 in 100) to make exactly 100 mL, and use these solutions as the sample solution and standard solution. Determine the absorbances at 295.5 nm, A_{T1} and A_{S1}, at 303 nm, A_{T2} and A_{S2}, and at 311 nm, A_{T3} and A_{S3}, of the sample solution and standard solution as directed under Ultraviolet-visible Spectrophotometry ⟨*2.24*⟩.

Amount [μg (potency)] of pimaricin ($C_{33}H_{47}NO_{13}$)

$$= M_S \times \frac{A_{T2} - \frac{A_{T1} + A_{T3}}{2}}{A_{S2} - \frac{A_{S1} + A_{S3}}{2}} \times 1000$$

M_S: Amount [mg (potency)] of Pimaricin RS taken

Containers and storage Containers—Tight containers.
Storage—Light resistant.

Pimozide

ピモジド

$C_{28}H_{29}F_2N_3O$: 461.55
1-{1-[4,4-Bis(4-fluorophenyl)butyl]piperidin-4-yl}-1,3-dihydro-2*H*-benzimidazol-2-one
[*2062-78-4*]

Pimozide contains not less than 98.5% and not more than 101.0% of pimozide ($C_{28}H_{29}F_2N_3O$).

Description Pimozide occurs as a white to pale yellow-white powder.

It is freely soluble in acetic acid (100), slightly soluble in methanol and in ethanol (99.5), and practically insoluble in water.

Identification **(1)** Determine the absorption spectrum of a solution of Pimozide in methanol (1 in 25,000) as directed under Ultraviolet-visible Spectrophotometry ⟨*2.24*⟩, and compare the spectrum with the Reference Spectrum: both spectra exhibit similar intensities of absorption at the same wavelengths.

(2) Determine the infrared absorption spectrum of Pimozide as directed in the potassium bromide disk method under Infrared Spectrophotometry ⟨*2.25*⟩, and compare the spectrum with the Reference Spectrum: both spectra exhibit similar intensities of absorption at the same wave numbers.

Melting point ⟨*2.60*⟩ 216 – 220°C

Purity **(1)** Heavy metals ⟨*1.07*⟩—Proceed with 2.0 g of Pimozide according to Method 2, and perform the test. Prepare the control solution with 2.0 mL of Standard Lead Solution by using 5 mL of sulfuric acid (not more than 10 ppm).

(2) Arsenic ⟨*1.11*⟩—Prepare the test solution with 1.0 g of Pimozide according to Method 3, and perform the test (not more than 2 ppm).

(3) Related substances—Dissolve 0.10 g of Pimozide in 10 mL of methanol, and use this solution as the sample solution. Pipet 1 mL of the sample solution, add methanol to make exactly 200 mL, and use this solution as the standard solution. Perform the test with exactly 10 μL each of the sample solution and standard solution as directed under Liquid Chromatography ⟨*2.01*⟩ according to the following conditions. Determine each peak area of both solutions by the automatic integration method: the area of the peak other than the peak of pimozide obtained from the sample solution is not larger than the peak area of pimozide from the standard solution, and the total area of the peaks other than the peak of pimozide from the sample solution is not larger than 1.5 times of the peak area of pimozide from the standard solution.

Operating conditions—

Detector: An ultraviolet absorption photometer (wavelength: 280 nm).

Column: A stainless steel column 4.6 mm in inside diameter and 10 cm in length, packed with octadecylsilanized silica gel for liquid chromatography (3 μm in particle diameter).

Column temperature: A constant temperature of about 25°C.

Mobile phase A: Dissolve 2.5 g of ammonium acetate and 8.5 g of tetrabutylammonium hydrogensulfate in water to make 1000 mL.

Mobile phase B: Acetonitrile.

Flowing of mobile phase: Control the gradient by mixing the mobile phases A and B as directed in the following table.

Time after injection of sample (min)	Mobile phase A (vol%)	Mobile phase B (vol%)
0 – 10	80 → 70	20 → 30
10 – 15	70	30

Flow rate: 2.0 mL per minute.

Time span of measurement: 1.5 times as long as the retention time of pimozide.

System suitability—

Test for required detectability: Pipet 1 mL of the standard solution, and add methanol to make exactly 10 mL. Confirm that the peak area of pimozide obtained with 10 μL of this solution is equivalent to 8 to 12% of that with 10 μL of the standard solution.

System performance: Dissolve 5 mg of Pimozide and 2 mg of mebendazole in methanol to make 100 mL. When the procedure is run with 10 μL of this solution under the above operating conditions, mebendazole and pimozide are eluted in this order with the resolution between these peaks being not less than 5.

System repeatability: When the test is repeated 6 times with 10 μL of the standard solution under the above operating conditions, the relative standard deviation of the peak area of pimozide is not more than 2.0%.

Loss on drying ⟨*2.41*⟩ Not more than 0.5% (1 g, 105°C, 3 hours).

Residue on ignition ⟨*2.44*⟩ Not more than 0.1% (1 g).

Assay Weigh accurately about 70 mg of Pimozide, previously dried, dissolve in 25 mL of acetic acid for nonaqueous titration, and titrate ⟨*2.50*⟩ with 0.02 mol/L perchloric acid VS (indicator: 2 drops of crystal violet TS). Perform a blank determination in the same manner, and make any necessary correction.

Each mL of 0.02 mol/L perchloric acid VS
= 9.231 mg of $C_{28}H_{29}F_2N_3O$

Containers and storage Containers—Well-closed containers.

Pindolol

ピンドロール

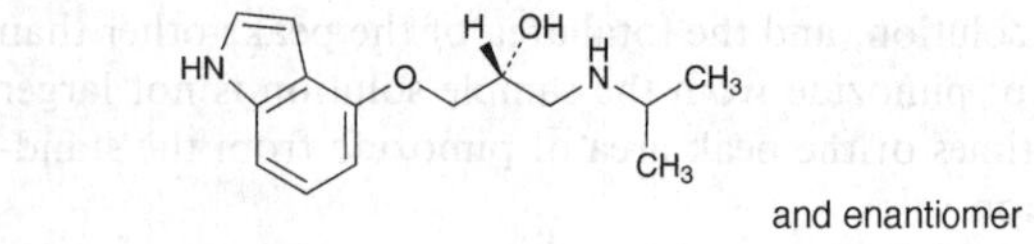

and enantiomer

$C_{14}H_{20}N_2O_2$: 248.32
(2*RS*)-1-(1*H*-Indol-4-yloxy)-
3-(1-methylethyl)aminopropan-2-ol
[*13523-86-9*]

Pindolol, when dried, contains not less than 98.5% of pindolol ($C_{14}H_{20}N_2O_2$).

Description Pindolol occurs as a white crystalline powder. It has a slight, characteristic odor.

It is sparingly soluble in methanol, slightly soluble in ethanol (95), and practically insoluble in water and in diethyl ether.

It dissolves in dilute sulfuric acid and in acetic acid (100).

Identification (1) To 1 mL of a solution of Pindolol in methanol (1 in 10,000) add 1 mL of a solution of 1-(4-pyridyl)-pyridinium chloride hydrochloride (1 in 1000) and 1 mL of sodium hydroxide TS, then add 1 mL of hydrochloric acid: a blue to blue-purple color, changing to red-purple, is produced.

(2) Dissolve 0.05 g of Pindolol in 1 mL of dilute sulfuric acid, and add 1 mL of Reinecke salt TS: a light red precipitate is produced.

(3) Determine the absorption spectrum of a solution of Pindolol in methanol (1 in 50,000) as directed under Ultraviolet-visible Spectrophotometry <*2.24*>, and compare the spectrum with the Reference Spectrum: both spectra exhibit similar intensities of absorption at the same wavelengths.

(4) Determine the infrared absorption spectrum of Pindolol, previously dried, as directed in the potassium bromide disk method under Infrared Spectrophotometry <*2.25*>, and compare the spectrum with the Reference Spectrum: both spectra exhibit similar intensities of absorption at the same wave numbers.

Absorbance <*2.24*> $E^{1\%}_{1\,\mathrm{cm}}$ (264 nm): 333 – 350 (10 mg, methanol, 500 mL).

Melting point <*2.60*> 169 – 173°C

Purity (1) Clarity and color of solution—Dissolve 0.5 g of Pindolol in 10 mL of acetic acid (100), and observe immediately: the solution is clear, and has no more color than the following control solution.

Control solution: Measure accurately 4 mL of Matching Fluid A, add exactly 6 mL of water, and mix.

(2) Heavy metals <*1.07*>—Proceed with 1.0 g of Pindolol according to Method 2, and perform the test. Prepare the control solution with 2.0 mL of Standard Lead Solution (not more than 20 ppm).

(3) Arsenic <*1.11*>—Prepare the test solution with 1.0 g of Pindolol according to Method 3, and perform the test (not more than 2 ppm).

(4) Related substances—Dissolve 0.10 g of Pindolol in 10 mL of methanol, and use this solution as the sample solution. Pipet 2 mL of the sample solution, and add methanol to make exactly 100 mL. Pipet 5 mL of this solution, add methanol to make exactly 20 mL, and use this solution as the standard solution. Perform the test with these solutions as directed under Thin-layer Chromatography <*2.03*>. Spot 5 μL each of the sample solution and standard solution on a plate of silica gel for thin-layer chromatography. Develop the plate with a mixture of chloroform, acetone and isopropylamine (5:4:1) to a distance of about 12 cm, and air-dry the plate. Spray evenly diluted sulfuric acid (3 in 5) and a sodium nitrite solution (1 in 50) on the plate: the spots other than the principal spot obtained from the sample solution are not more intense than the spot from the standard solution.

Loss on drying <*2.41*> Not more than 0.5% (1 g, 105°C, 4 hours).

Residue on ignition <*2.44*> Not more than 0.1% (1 g).

Assay Weigh accurately about 0.5 g of Pindolol, previously dried, dissolve in 80 mL of methanol, and titrate <*2.50*> with 0.1 mol/L hydrochloric acid VS (potentiometric titration). Perform a blank determination in the same manner, and make any necessary correction.

Each mL of 0.1 mol/L hydrochloric acid VS
= 24.83 mg of $C_{14}H_{20}N_2O_2$

Containers and storage Containers—Tight containers.
Storage—Light-resistant.

Pioglitazone Hydrochloride

ピオグリタゾン塩酸塩

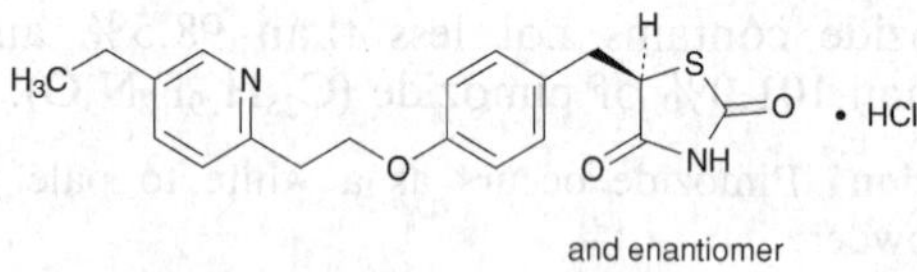

and enantiomer

$C_{19}H_{20}N_2O_3S.HCl$: 392.90
(5*RS*)-5-{4-[2-(5-Ethylpyridin-
2-yl)ethoxy]benzyl}thiazolidine-2,4-dione
monohydrochloride
[*112529-15-4*]

Pioglitazone Hydrochloride contains not less than 99.0% and not more than 101.0% of pioglitazone hydrochloride ($C_{19}H_{20}N_2O_3S.HCl$), calculated on the anhydrous basis.

Description Pioglitazone Hydrochloride occurs as white, crystals or crystalline powder.

It is soluble in *N*,*N*-dimethylformamide and in methanol, slightly soluble in ethanol (99.5), and practically insoluble in water.

It dissolves in 0.1 mol/L hydrochloric acid TS.

A solution of Pioglitazone Hydrochloride in *N*,*N*-dimethylformamide (1 in 20) shows no optical rotation.

Identification (1) Determine the absorption spectrum of a solution of Pioglitazone Hydrochloride in 0.1 mol/L hydrochloric acid TS (1 in 50,000) as directed under Ultraviolet-visible Spectrophotometry <*2.24*>, and compare the spectrum with the Reference Spectrum or the spectrum of a solution of Pioglitazone Hydrochloride RS prepared in the same manner as the sample solution: both spectra exhibit similar intensities of absorption at the same wavelengths.

(2) Determine the infrared absorption spectrum of Pioglitazone Hydrochloride as directed in the potassium bromide disk method under Infrared Spectrophotometry <*2.25*>,

and compare the spectrum with the Reference Spectrum or the spectrum of Pioglitazone Hydrochloride RS: both spectra exhibit similar intensities of absorption at the same wave numbers.

(3) Dissolve 50 mg of Pioglitazone Hydrochloride in 1 mL of nitric acid, and add 4 mL of dilute nitric acid: the solution responds to Qualitative Tests 〈*1.09*〉 (2) for chloride.

Purity **(1)** Heavy metals 〈*1.07*〉—Proceed with 1.0 g of Pioglitazone Hydrochloride according to Method 4, and perform the test. After incineration, use 3 mL of hydrobromic acid instead of 3 mL of hydrochloric acid. Prepare the control solution with 1.0 mL of Standard Lead Solution (not more than 10 ppm).

(2) Related substances—Dissolve 20 mg of Pioglitazone Hydrochloride in 20 mL of methanol, add the mobile phase to make 100 mL, and use this solution as the sample solution. Pipet 1 mL of the sample solution, add the mobile phase to make exactly 200 mL, and use this solution as the standard solution. Perform the test with exactly 40 μL each of the sample solution and standard solution as directed under Liquid Chromatography 〈*2.01*〉 according to the following conditions. Determine each peak area of both solutions by the automatic integration method: the area of the peaks, having the relative retention times of about 0.7, about 1.4 and about 3.0 to pioglitazone obtained from the sample solution, is not larger than 2/5 times the peak area of pioglitazone from the standard solution, and the area of each peak other than pioglitazone and those peaks mentioned above from the sample solution is smaller than 1/5 times the peak area of pioglitazone from the standard solution. Furthermore, the total area of the peaks other than pioglitazone from the sample solution is not larger than the peak area of pioglitazone from the standard solution.

Operating conditions—

Detector, column, column temperature, mobile phase and flow rate: Proceed as directed in the operating conditions in the Assay.

Time span of measurement: About 4 times as long as the retention time of pioglitazone, beginning after the solvent peak.

System suitability—

Test for required detectability: Pipet 1 mL of the standard solution, and add the mobile phase to make exactly 10 mL. Confirm that the peak area of pioglitazone obtained with 40 μL of this solution is equivalent to 7 to 13% of that with 40 μL of the standard solution.

System performance: Dissolve 50 mg of Pioglitazone Hydrochloride in 10 mL of a solution of benzophenone in methanol (1 in 750), and add methanol to make 100 mL. To 1 mL of this solution add the mobile phase to make 20 mL. When the procedure is run with 40 μL of this solution under the above operating conditions, pioglitazone and benzophenone are eluted in this order with the resolution between these peaks being not less than 10.

System repeatability: When the test is repeated 6 times with 40 μL of the standard solution under the above operating conditions, the relative standard deviation of the peak area of pioglitazone is not more than 2.0%.

Water 〈*2.48*〉 Not more than 0.2% (0.5 g, coulometric titration). For anolyte solution, use anode solution A for water determination.

Residue on ignition 〈*2.44*〉 Not more than 0.1% (1 g).

Assay Weigh accurately about 50 mg each of Pioglitazone Hydrochloride and Pioglitazone Hydrochloride RS (separately, determine the water 〈*2.48*〉 in the same manner as Pioglitazone Hydrochloride), add exactly 10 mL of the internal standard solution and methanol to make 100 mL. Pipet 2 mL each of these solutions, add the mobile phase to make 20 mL, and use these solutions as the sample solution and the standard solution, respectively. Perform the test with 20 μL each of the sample solution and standard solution as directed under Liquid Chromatography 〈*2.01*〉 according to the following conditions, and calculate the ratios, Q_T and Q_S, of the peak area of pioglitazone to that of the internal standard.

Amount (mg) of pioglitazone hydrochloride ($C_{19}H_{20}N_2O_3S.HCl$)
$$= M_S \times Q_T/Q_S$$

M_S: Amount (mg) of Pioglitazone Hydrochloride RS taken, calculated on the anhydrous basis

*Internal standard solution—*A solution of benzophenone in methanol (1 in 750).

Operating conditions—

Detector: An ultraviolet absorption photometer (wavelength: 269 nm).

Column: A stainless steel column 4.6 mm in inside diameter and 15 cm in length, packed with octadecylsilanized silica gel for liquid chromatography (5 μm in particle diameter).

Column temperature: A constant temperature of about 25°C.

Mobile phase: A mixture of ammonium acetate solution (77 in 10,000), acetonitrile and acetic acid (100) (25:25:1).

Flow rate: Adjust so that the retention time of pioglitazone is about 7 minutes.

System suitability—

System performance: When the procedure is run with 20 μL of the standard solution under the above operating conditions, pioglitazone and the internal standard are eluted in this order with the resolution between these peaks being not less than 10.

System repeatability: When the test is repeated 6 times with 20 μL of the standard solution under the above operating conditions, the relative standard deviation of the peak area of pioglitazone is not more than 1.0%.

Containers and storage Containers—Well-closed containers.

Pioglitazone Hydrochloride Tablets

ピオグリタゾン塩酸塩錠

Pioglitazone Hydrochloride Tablets contain not less than 95.0% and not more than 105.0% of the labeled amount of pioglitazone hydrochloride ($C_{19}H_{20}N_2O_3S.HCl$: 392.90).

Method of preparation Prepare as directed under Tablets, with Pioglitazone Hydrochloride.

Identification To an amount of powdered Pioglitazone Hydrochloride Tablets, equivalent to 2.8 mg of Pioglitazone Hydrochloride, add 100 mL of 0.1 mol/L hydrochloric acid TS, shake, and filter through a membrane filter with a pore size not exceeding 0.45 μm. Determine the absorption spectrum of the filtrate as directed under Ultraviolet-visible Spectrophotometry 〈*2.24*〉: it exhibits a maximum between 267 nm and 271 nm.

Uniformity of dosage units 〈*6.02*〉 Perform the Mass variation test, or the Content uniformity test according to the following method: it meets the requirement.

Disintegrate 1 tablet of Pioglitazone Hydrochloride Tablets with 10 mL of 0.1 mol/L hydrochloric acid TS, add 70 mL of methanol, shake vigorously for 10 minutes, then add methanol to make exactly 100 mL, and centrifuge. Take exactly V mL of the supernatant liquid, add a mixture of methanol and 0.1 mol/L hydrochloric acid TS (9:1) to make exactly V' mL so that each mL contains about 26 μg of pioglitazone hydrochloride ($C_{19}H_{20}N_2O_3S.HCl$), and use this solution as the sample solution. Separately, weigh accurately about 33 mg of Pioglitazone Hydrochloride RS (separately, determine the water <2.48> in the same manner as Pioglitazone Hydrochloride), dissolve in 10 mL of 0.1 mol/L hydrochloric acid TS, and add methanol to make exactly 100 mL. Pipet 4 mL of this solution, add a mixture of methanol and 0.1 mol/L hydrochloric acid TS (9:1) to make exactly 50 mL, and use this solution as the standard solution. Determine the absorbances, A_T and A_S, of the sample solution and standard solution at 269 nm as directed under Ultraviolet-visible Spectrophotometry <2.24> using a mixture of methanol and 0.1 mol/L hydrochloric acid TS (9:1) as the blank.

Amount (mg) of pioglitazone hydrochloride ($C_{19}H_{20}N_2O_3S.HCl$)
$= M_S \times A_T/A_S \times V'/V \times 2/25$

M_S: Amount (mg) of Pioglitazone Hydrochloride RS taken, calculated on the anhydrous basis

Dissolution <6.10> When the test is performed at 50 revolutions per minute according to the Paddle method, using 900 mL of a solution, which is prepared by mixing 50 mL of 0.2 mol/L hydrochloric acid TS and 150 mL of potassium chloride solution (3 in 20), adding water to make 1000 mL and adjusting to pH 2.0 with 5 mol/L hydrochloric acid TS, as the dissolution medium, the dissolution rate in 45 minutes of Pioglitazone Hydrochloride Tablets is not less than 80%.

Start the test with 1 tablet of Pioglitazone Hydrochloride Tablets, withdraw 10 mL of the medium at the specified minute after starting the test, and filter through a membrane filter with a pore size not exceeding 0.45 μm. Discard not less than 5 mL of the first filtrate, pipet V mL of the subsequent filtrate, add the dissolution medium to make exactly V' mL so that each mL contains about 18 μg of pioglitazone hydrochloride ($C_{19}H_{20}N_2O_3S.HCl$), and use this solution as the sample solution. Separately, weigh accurately about 23 mg of Pioglitazone Hydrochloride RS (separately determine the water <2.48> in the same manner as Pioglitazone Hydrochloride), dissolve in 10 mL of methanol, and add the dissolution medium to make exactly 50 mL. Pipet 2 mL of this solution, add the dissolution medium to make exactly 50 mL, and use this solution as the standard solution. Determine the absorbances, A_T and A_S, of the sample solution and standard solution at 269 nm as directed under Ultraviolet-visible Spectrophotometry <2.24> using the dissolution medium as the blank.

Dissolution rate (%) with respect to the labeled amount of pioglitazone hydrochloride ($C_{19}H_{20}N_2O_3S.HCl$)
$= M_S \times A_T/A_S \times V'/V \times 1/C \times 72$

M_S: Amount (mg) of Pioglitazone Hydrochloride RS taken, calculated on the anhydrous basis

C Labeled amount (mg) of pioglitazone hydrochloride ($C_{19}H_{20}N_2O_3S.HCl$) in 1 tablet

Assay Accurately weigh the mass of not less than 20 Pioglitazone Hydrochloride Tablets, and powder. Weigh accurately a portion of the powder, equivalent to about 25 mg of pioglitazone hydrochloride ($C_{19}H_{20}N_2O_3S.HCl$), add 45 mL of methanol and exactly 5 mL of the internal standard solution, sonicate, and centrifuge. To 2 mL of the supernatant liquid add the mobile phase to make 20 mL, and use this solution as the sample solution. Separately, weigh accurately about 25 mg of Pioglitazone Hydrochloride RS (separately, determine the water <2.48> in the same manner as Pioglitazone Hydrochloride), dissolve in 45 mL of methanol, and add exactly 5 mL of the internal standard solution. Pipet 2 mL of this solution, add the mobile phase to make 20 mL, and use this solution as the standard solution. Perform the test with 20 μL each of the sample solution and standard solution as directed under Liquid Chromatography <2.01> according to the following conditions, and calculate the ratios, Q_T and Q_S, of the peak area of pioglitazone to that of the internal standard.

Amount (mg) of pioglitazone hydrochloride ($C_{19}H_{20}N_2O_3S.HCl$)
$= M_S \times Q_T/Q_S$

M_S: Amount (mg) of Pioglitazone Hydrochloride RS taken, calculated on the anhydrous basis

Internal standard solution—A solution of benzophenone in methanol (1 in 750).

Operating conditions—

Detector: An ultraviolet absorption photometer (wavelength: 269 nm).

Column: A stainless steel column 4.6 mm in inside diameter and 15 cm in length, packed with octadecylsilanized silica gel for liquid chromatography (5 μm in particle diameter).

Column temperature: A constant temperature of about 25°C.

Mobile phase: A mixture of ammonium acetate solution (77 in 10,000), acetonitrile and acetic acid (100) (25:25:1).

Flow rate: Adjust so that the retention time of pioglitazone is about 7 minutes.

System suitability—

System performance: When the procedure is run with 20 μL of the standard solution under the above operating conditions, pioglitazone and the internal standard are eluted in this order with the resolution between these peaks being not less than 10.

System repeatability: When the test is repeated 6 times with 20 μL of the standard solution under the above operating conditions, the relative standard deviation of the ratio of the peak area of pioglitazone to that of the internal standard is not more than 1.0%.

Containers and storage Containers—Tight containers.

Pioglitazone Hydrochloride and Glimepiride Tablets

ピオグリタゾン塩酸塩・グリメピリド錠

Pioglitazone Hydrochloride and Glimepiride Tablets contain not less than 95.0% and not more than 105.0% of the labeled amount of pioglitazone hydrochloride ($C_{19}H_{20}N_2O_3S.HCl$: 392.90), and not less than 93.0% and not more than 107.0% of the labeled amount of glimepiride ($C_{24}H_{34}N_4O_5S$: 490.62).

Method of Preparation Prepare as directed under Tablets, with Pioglitazone Hydrochloride and Glimepiride.

Identification **(1)** Powder Pioglitazone Hydrochloride and Glimepiride Tablets, weigh a portion of the powder, equivalent to 33 mg of Pioglitazone Hydrochloride, add 20 mL of 0.1 mol/L hydrochloric acid TS, and disintegrate completely by vigorous shaking for several minutes. Filter 2 mL of this solution through a membrane filter with a pore size not exceeding 0.45 μm. To 1 mL of the filtrate add 0.1 mol/L hydrochloric acid TS to make 50 mL. Determine the absorption spectrum of this solution as directed under Ultraviolet-visible Spectrophotometry <*2.24*>: it exhibits a maximum between 267 nm and 271 nm.

(2) Wash the membrane filter obtained in (1) with 100 mL of 0.1 mol/L hydrochloric acid TS, and extract with methanol so that each mL contains about 10 μg of glimepiride ($C_{24}H_{34}N_4O_5S$). Determine the absorption spectrum of this solution as directed under Ultraviolet-visible Spectrophotometry <*2.24*>: it exhibits a maximum between 227 nm and 231 nm.

Purity Related substances—Powder Pioglitazone Hydrochloride and Glimepiride Tablets, weigh a portion of the powder, equivalent to 10 mg of Glimepiride, add 30 mL of a mixture of acetonitrile and 0.1 mol/L hydrochloric acid TS (9:1), shake vigorously for 20 minutes, and add the mobile phase A to make 50 mL. Filter this solution through a membrane filter with a pore size not exceeding 0.2 μm, discard the first 4 mL of the filtrate, and use the subsequent filtrate as the sample solution. Pipet 1 mL of the sample solution, add the mobile phase A to make exactly 100 mL, and use this solution as the standard solution. Perform the test with exactly 40 μL each of the sample solution and standard solution as directed under Liquid Chromatography <*2.01*> according to the following conditions. Determine each peak area by the automatic integration method: the area of the peak, having a relative retention time of about 0.23 to glimepiride obtained from the sample solution is not larger than 2.5 times the peak area of glimepiride from the standard solution. The area of the peak other than glimepiride and other than the peak mentioned above from the sample solution is not larger than 1/2 times the peak area of glimepiride from the standard solution, and the total area of these peaks is not larger than the peak area of glimepiride from the standard solution. The total area of the peaks other than glimepiride from the sample solution is not larger than 3 times the peak area of glimepiride from the standard solution.

Operating conditions—

Detector: An ultraviolet absorption photometer (wavelength: 228 nm).

Column: A stainless steel column 4.6 mm in inside diameter and 25 cm in length, packed with octadecylsilanized silica gel for liquid chromatography (5 μm in particle diameter).

Column temperature: A constant temperature of about 25°C.

Mobile phase A: Dissolve 1.1 g of sodium dihydrogen phosphate dihydrate in water to make 1000 mL, and adjust to pH 1.6 with diluted phosphoric acid (1 in 10). To 650 mL of this solution add 600 mL of acetonitrile.

Mobile phase B: Dissolve 1.1 g of sodium dihydrogen phosphate dihydrate in water to make 1000 mL, and adjust to pH 1.6 with diluted phosphoric acid (1 in 10). To 300 mL of this solution add 700 mL of acetonitrile.

Flowing of mobile phase: Control the gradient by mixing the mobile phases A and B as directed in the following table.

Time after injection of sample (min)	Mobile phase A (vol%)	Mobile phase B (vol%)
0 – 15	100	0
15 – 60	100 → 0	0 → 100

Flow rate: 1.0 mL per minute.

Time span of measurement: For 60 minutes after injection, beginning after the peak having a relative retention time of about 0.23 to glimepiride.

System suitability—

Test for required detectability: Pipet 2 mL of the standard solution, and add the mobile phase A to make exactly 20 mL. Confirm that the peak area of glimepiride obtained with 40 μL of this solution is equivalent to 7 to 13% of that with 40 μL of the standard solution.

System performance: When the procedure is run with 40 μL of the standard solution under the above operating conditions, the number of theoretical plates and the symmetry factor of the peak of glimepiride are not less than 20,000 and not more than 1.5, respectively.

System repeatability: When the test is repeated 6 times with 40 μL of the standard solution under the above operating conditions, the relative standard deviation of the peak area of glimepiride is not more than 2.0%.

Uniformity of dosage units <*6.02*> Perform the test according to the following method: it meets the requirement of the Content uniformity test.

(1) Pioglitazone hydrochloride—To 1 tablet of Pioglitazone Hydrochloride and Glimepiride Tablets add 30 mL of a mixture of acetonitrile and 0.1 mol/L hydrochloric acid TS (9:1), shake vigorously for 20 minutes, and add the mixture of acetonitrile and 0.1 mol/L hydrochloric acid TS (9:1) to make exactly 50 mL. Filter this solution through a membrane filter with a pore size not exceeding 0.2 μm. Discard the first 5 mL of the filtrate, pipet V mL of the subsequent filtrate, add exactly $V'/10$ mL of the internal standard solution, add the mobile phase to make V' mL so that each mL contains about 66 μg of pioglitazone hydrochloride ($C_{19}H_{20}N_2O_3S.HCl$), and use this solution as the sample solution. Then, proceed as directed in the Assay (1).

$$\text{Amount (mg) of pioglitazone hydrochloride } (C_{19}H_{20}N_2O_3S.HCl) = M_S \times Q_T/Q_S \times V'/V \times 1/10$$

M_S: Amount (mg) of Pioglitazone Hydrochloride RS taken, calculated on the anhydrous basis

Internal standard solution—A solution of ethyl benzoate in the mobile phase (1 in 10,000).

(2) Glimepiride—To 1 tablet of Pioglitazone Hydrochloride and Glimepiride Tablets add 30 mL of a mixture of acetonitrile and 0.1 mol/L hydrochloric acid TS (9:1), shake vigorously for 20 minutes, and add the mixture of acetonitrile and 0.1 mol/L hydrochloric acid TS (9:1) to make exactly 50 mL. Filter this solution through a membrane filter with a pore size not exceeding 0.2 μm. Discard the first 5 mL of the filtrate, pipet V mL of the subsequent filtrate, add exactly $V'/10$ mL of the internal standard solution, add the mobile phase to make V' mL so that each mL contains about 6 μg of glimepiride ($C_{24}H_{34}N_4O_5S$), and use this solution as the sample solution. Then, proceed as directed in the Assay (2).

$$\text{Amount (mg) of glimepiride } (C_{24}H_{34}N_4O_5S) = M_S \times Q_T/Q_S \times V'/V \times 1/100$$

M_S: Amount (mg) of Glimepiride RS taken, calculated on the anhydrous basis

Internal standard solution—A solution of ethyl benzoate in the mobile phase (1 in 10,000).

Dissolution ⟨*6.10*⟩ **(1)** Pioglitazone hydrochloride—When the test is performed at 50 revolutions per minute according to the Paddle method, using 900 mL of a solution, which is prepared by mixing 50 mL of 0.2 mol/L hydrochloric acid TS and 150 mL of potassium chloride solution (3 in 20), adding water to make 1000 mL and adjusting to pH 2.0 with 5 mol/L hydrochloric acid TS, as the dissolution medium, the dissolution rate in 45 minutes of Pioglitazone Hydrochloride and Glimepiride Tablets is not less than 80%.

Start the test with 1 tablet of Pioglitazone Hydrochloride and Glimepiride Tablets, withdraw not less than 10 mL of the medium at the specified minute after starting the test, and filter through a membrane filter with a pore size not exceeding 0.45 μm. Discard not less than 5 mL of the first filtrate, pipet V mL of the subsequent filtrate, add the dissolution medium to make exactly V' mL so that each mL contains about 18 μg of pioglitazone hydrochloride ($C_{19}H_{20}N_2O_3S.HCl$), and use this solution as the sample solution. Separately, weigh accurately about 37 mg of Pioglitazone Hydrochloride RS (separately determine the water ⟨*2.48*⟩ in the same manner as Pioglitazone Hydrochloride), dissolve in 20 mL of methanol, and add the dissolution medium to make exactly 100 mL. Pipet 5 mL of this solution, add the dissolution medium to make exactly 100 mL, and use this solution as the standard solution. Perform the test with exactly 20 μL each of the sample solution and standard solution as directed under Liquid Chromatography ⟨*2.01*⟩ according to the following conditions, and determine the peak areas, A_T and A_S, of pioglitazone in each solution.

Dissolution rate (%) with respect to the labeled amount of pioglitazone hydrochloride ($C_{19}H_{20}N_2O_3S.HCl$)
$= M_S \times A_T/A_S \times V'/V \times 1/C \times 45$

M_S: Amount (mg) of Pioglitazone Hydrochloride RS taken, calculated on the anhydrous basis
C: Labeled amount (mg) of pioglitazone hydrochloride ($C_{19}H_{20}N_2O_3S.HCl$) in 1 tablet

Operating conditions—

Proceed as directed in the operating conditions in the Assay (1) (Pioglitazone Hydrochloride).

System suitability—

System performance: When the procedure is run with 20 μL of the standard solution under the above operating conditions, the number of theoretical plates and the symmetry factor of the peak of pioglitazone are not less than 1500 and not more than 2.0, respectively.

System repeatability: When the test is repeated 6 times with 20 μL of the standard solution under the above conditions, the relative standard deviation of the peak area of pioglitazone is not more than 1.0 %.

(2) Glimepiride—When the test is performed at 50 revolutions per minute according to the Paddle method, using 900 mL of disodium hydrogen phosphate-citrate buffer solution (pH 7.5) as the dissolution medium, the dissolution rate in 30 minutes of Pioglitazone Hydrochloride and Glimepiride Tablets is not less than 80%.

Start the test with 1 tablet of Pioglitazone Hydrochloride and Glimepiride Tablets, withdraw not less than 10 mL of the medium at the specified minute after starting the test, and filter through a membrane filter with a pore size not exceeding 0.45 μm. Discard not less than 5 mL of the first filtrate, pipet V mL of the subsequent filtrate, add the dissolution medium to make exactly V' mL so that each mL contains about 1.1 μg of glimepiride ($C_{24}H_{34}N_4O_5S$), and use this solution as the sample solution. Separately, weigh accurately about 55 mg of Glimepiride RS (separately determine the water ⟨*2.48*⟩ in the same manner as Glimepiride), dissolve in acetonitrile to make exactly 250 mL. Pipet 10 mL of this solution, and add acetonitrile to make exactly 100 mL. Pipet 5 mL of this solution, add the dissolution medium to make exactly 100 mL, and use this solution as the standard solution. Perform the test with exactly 20 μL each of the sample solution and standard solution as directed under Liquid Chromatography ⟨*2.01*⟩ according to the following conditions, and determine the peak areas, A_T and A_S, of glimepiride in each solution.

Dissolution rate (%) with respect to the labeled amount of glimepiride ($C_{24}H_{34}N_4O_5S$)
$= M_S \times A_T/A_S \times V'/V \times 1/C \times 9/5$

M_S: Amount (mg) of Glimepiride RS taken, calculated on the anhydrous basis
C: Labeled amount (mg) of glimepiride ($C_{24}H_{34}N_4O_5S$) in 1 tablet

Operating conditions—

Detector, column, column temperature and mobile phase: Proceed as directed in the operating conditions in the Assay (1) (Pioglitazone Hydrochloride).

Flow rate: Adjust so that the retention time of glimepiride is about 5.4 minutes.

System suitability—

System performance: When the procedure is run with 20 μL of the standard solution under the above operating conditions, the number of theoretical plates and the symmetry factor of the peak of glimepiride are not less than 5000 and not more than 1.5, respectively.

System repeatability: When the test is repeated 6 times with 20 μL of the standard solution under the above conditions, the relative standard deviation of the peak area of glimepiride is not more than 2.0%.

Assay **(1)** Pioglitazone hydrochloride—Weigh accurately the mass of not less than 20 Pioglitazone Hydrochloride and Glimepiride Tablets, and powder. Weigh accurately a portion of the powder, equivalent to about 33 mg of pioglitazone hydrochloride ($C_{19}H_{20}N_2O_3S.HCl$), add 30 mL of a mixture of acetonitrile and 0.1 mol/L hydrochloric acid TS (9:1), shake vigorously for 20 minutes, and add a mixture of acetonitrile and 0.1 mol/L hydrochloric acid TS (9:1) to make exactly 50 mL. Filter this solution through a membrane filter with a pore size not exceeding 0.2 μm. Discard the first 5 mL of the filtrate, pipet 5 mL of the subsequent filtrate, add exactly 5 mL of the internal standard solution, add the mobile phase to make 50 mL, and use this solution as the sample solution. Separately, weigh accurately about 33 mg of Pioglitazone Hydrochloride RS (separately determine the water ⟨*2.48*⟩ in the same manner as Pioglitazone Hydrochloride), dissolve in a mixture of acetonitrile and 0.1 mol/L hydrochloric acid TS (9:1) to make exactly 50 mL. Pipet 5 mL of this solution, add exactly 5 mL of the internal standard solution, add the mobile phase to make 50 mL, and use this solution as the standard solution. Perform the test with 20 μL each of the sample solution and standard solution as directed under Liquid Chromatography ⟨*2.01*⟩ according to the following conditions, and calculate the ratios, Q_T and Q_S, of the peak area of pioglitazone to that of the internal standard.

Amount (mg) of pioglitazone hydrochloride ($C_{19}H_{20}N_2O_3S.HCl$)
$= M_S \times Q_T/Q_S$

M_S: Amount (mg) of Pioglitazone Hydrochloride RS taken, calculated on the anhydrous basis

Internal standard solution—A solution of ethyl benzoate in the mobile phase (1 in 10,000).

Operating conditions—

Detector: An ultraviolet absorption photometer (wavelength: 228 nm).

Column: A stainless steel column 4.6 mm in inside diameter and 5 cm in length, packed with octadecylsilanized silica gel for liquid chromatography (3 μm in particle diameter).

Column temperature: A constant temperature of about 25°C.

Mobile phase: Dissolve 7.80 g of sodium dihydrogen phosphate dihydrate in water to make 1000 mL, and adjust to pH 4.0 with diluted phosphoric acid (1 in 10). To 500 mL of this solution add 500 mL of acetonitrile.

Flow rate: Adjust so that the retention time of pioglitazone is about 2.3 minutes.

System suitability—

System performance: To 33 mg of Pioglitazone Hydrochloride RS add 5 mL of the glimepiride standard stock solution obtained in (2), and add a mixture of acetonitrile and 0.1 mol/L hydrochloric acid TS (9:1) to make 50 mL. To 5 mL of this solution add 5 mL of the internal standard solution, and add the mobile phase to make 50 mL. When the procedure is run with 20 μL of this solution under the above operating conditions, pioglitazone, the internal standard, and glimepiride are eluted in this order, and the resolutions between the peaks of pioglitazone and the internal standard and between the peaks of the internal standard and glimepiride are not less than 4 and not less than 3, respectively.

System repeatability: When the test is repeated 6 times with 20 μL of the standard solution under the above conditions, the relative standard deviation of the ratio of the peak area of pioglitazone to that of the internal standard is not more than 1.0%.

(2) Glimepiride—Weigh accurately the mass of not less than 20 Pioglitazone Hydrochloride and Glimepiride Tablets, and powder. Weigh accurately a portion of the powder, equivalent to about 3 mg of glimepiride ($C_{24}H_{34}N_4O_5S$), add 30 mL of a mixture of acetonitrile and 0.1 mol/L hydrochloric acid TS (9:1), shake vigorously for 20 minutes, and add a mixture of acetonitrile and 0.1 mol/L hydrochloric acid TS (9:1) to make exactly 50 mL. Filter this solution through a membrane filter with a pore size not exceeding 0.2 μm. Discard the first 5 mL of the filtrate, pipet 5 mL of the subsequent filtrate, add exactly 5 mL of the internal standard solution, add the mobile phase to make 50 mL, and use this solution as the sample solution. Separately, weigh accurately about 30 mg of Glimepiride RS (separately determine the water *<2.48>* in the same manner as Glimepiride), dissolve in the mixture of acetonitrile and 0.1 mol/L hydrochloric acid TS (9:1) to make exactly 50 mL, and use this solution as the glimepiride standard stock solution. Pipet 10 mL of the glimepiride standard stock solution, and add the mixture of acetonitrile and 0.1 mol/L hydrochloric acid TS (9:1) to make exactly 100 mL. Pipet 5 mL of this solution, add exactly 5 mL of the internal standard solution, add the mobile phase to make 50 mL, and use this solution as the standard solution. Perform the test with 20 μL each of the sample solution and standard solution as directed under Liquid Chromatography *<2.01>* according to the following conditions, and calculate the ratios, Q_T and Q_S, of the peak area of glimepiride to that of the internal standard.

Amount (mg) of glimepiride ($C_{24}H_{34}N_4O_5S$)
$= M_S \times Q_T/Q_S \times 1/10$

M_S: Amount (mg) of Glimepiride RS taken, calculated on the anhydrous basis

Internal standard solution—A solution of ethyl benzoate in the mobile phase (1 in 10,000).

Operating conditions—

Proceed as directed in the operating conditions in the Assay (1).

System suitability—

System performance: To 33 mg of Pioglitazone Hydrochloride RS add 5 mL of the glimepiride standard stock solution, and add a mixture of acetonitrile and 0.1 mol/L hydrochloric acid TS (9:1) to make 50 mL. To 5 mL of this solution add 5 mL of the internal standard solution, and add the mobile phase to make 50 mL. When the procedure is run with 20 μL of this solution under the above operating conditions, pioglitazone, the internal standard and glimepiride are eluted in this order, and the resolutions between the peaks of pioglitazone and the internal standard and between the peaks of the internal standard and glimepiride are not less than 4 and not less than 3, respectively.

System repeatability: When the test is repeated 6 times with 20 μL of the standard solution under the above conditions, the relative standard deviation of the ratio of the peak area of glimepiride to that of the internal standard is not more than 1.0%.

Containers and storage Containers—Tight containers.

Pioglitazone Hydrochloride and Metformin Hydrochloride Tablets

ピオグリタゾン塩酸塩・メトホルミン塩酸塩錠

Pioglitazone Hydrochloride and Metformin Hydrochloride Tablets contain not less than 95.0% and not more than 105.0% of the labeled amount of pioglitazone hydrochloride ($C_{19}H_{20}N_2O_3S.HCl$: 392.90) and metformin hydrochloride ($C_4H_{11}N_5.HCl$: 165.62).

Method of preparation Prepare as directed under Tablets, with Pioglitazone Hydrochloride and Metformin Hydrochloride.

Identification **(1)** Shake vigorously a quantity of powdered Pioglitazone Hydrochloride and Metformin Hydrochloride Tablets, equivalent to 0.33 mg of Pioglitazone Hydrochloride, with 10 mL of water, and filter through a membrane filter with a pore size not exceeding 0.45 μm. After washing the membrane filter with 10 mL of water, dissolve the retained substance on the filter by running through 10 mL of 0.1 mol/L hydrochloric acid TS, and determine the absorption spectrum of the filtrate so obtained as directed under Ultraviolet-visible Spectrophotometry *<2.24>*: it exhibits a maximum between 267 nm and 271 nm.

(2) Shake vigorously a quantity of powdered Pioglitazone Hydrochloride and Metformin Hydrochloride Tablets, equivalent to 20 mg of Metformin Hydrochloride, with 50 mL of water, and filter through a membrane filter with a pore size not exceeding 0.45 μm. To 1 mL of the filtrate add water to make 50 mL, and determine the absorption spectrum of this solution as directed under Ultraviolet-visible Spectrophotometry *<2.24>*: it exhibits a maximum between

230 nm and 234 nm.

Uniformity of dosage units <*6.02*> Perform the test according to the following method: it meets the requirement of the Content uniformity test.

(1) Pioglitazone hydrochloride—To 1 tablet of Pioglitazone Hydrochloride and Metformin Hydrochloride Tablets add 40 mL of 0.1 mol/L hydrochloric acid TS, shake vigorously for 10 minutes, add 40 mL of methanol, and shake. To this solution add a mixture of 0.1 mol/L hydrochloric acid TS and methanol (1:1) to make exactly 100 mL, and filter through a membrane filter with a pore size not exceeding 0.45 μm. Discard the first 5 mL of the filtrate, pipet *V* mL of the subsequent filtrate, add exactly *V'*/20 mL of the internal standard solution, then add a mixture of 0.1 mol/L hydrochloric acid TS and methanol (1:1) to make *V'* mL so that each mL contains about 16.5 μg of pioglitazone hydrochloride ($C_{19}H_{20}N_2O_3S.HCl$), and use this solution as the sample solution. Then, proceed as directed in the Assay (1).

Amount (mg) of pioglitazone hydrochloride ($C_{19}H_{20}N_2O_3S.HCl$)
$= M_S \times Q_T/Q_S \times V'/V \times 1/20$

M_S: Amount (mg) of Pioglitazone Hydrochloride RS taken, calculated on the anhydrous basis

Internal standard solution—A solution of butyl parahydroxybenzoate in a mixture of 0.1 mol/L hydrochloric acid TS and methanol (1:1) (1 in 2500).

(2) Metformin hydrochloride—To 1 tablet of Pioglitazone Hydrochloride and Metformin Hydrochloride Tablets add 40 mL of 0.1 mol/L hydrochloric acid TS, shake vigorously for 10 minutes, add 40 mL of methanol, and shake. To this solution add a mixture of 0.1 mol/L hydrochloric acid TS and methanol (1:1) to make exactly 100 mL, and filter through a membrane filter with a pore size not exceeding 0.45 μm. Discard the first 5 mL of the filtrate, pipet *V* mL of the subsequent filtrate, add exactly *V'*/20 mL of the internal standard solution, then add a mixture of 0.1 mol/L hydrochloric acid TS and methanol (1:1) to make *V'* mL so that each mL contains about 0.25 mg of metformin hydrochloride ($C_4H_{11}N_5.HCl$), and use this solution as the sample solution. Then, proceed as directed in the Assay (2).

Amount (mg) of metformin hydrochloride ($C_4H_{11}N_5.HCl$)
$= M_S \times Q_T/Q_S \times V'/V \times 1/2$

M_S: Amount (mg) of metformin hydrochloride for assay taken

Internal standard solution—A solution of 4′-methoxyacetophenone in a mixture of 0.1 mol/L hydrochloric acid TS and methanol (1:1) (1 in 2000).

Dissolution <*6.10*> **(1)** Pioglitazone hydrochloride—When the test is performed at 50 revolutions per minute according to the Paddle method, using 900 mL of a solution, which is prepared by mixing 50 mL of 0.2 mol/L hydrochloric acid TS and 150 mL of potassium chloride solution (3 in 20), adding water to make 1000 mL and adjusting to pH 2.0 with 5 mol/L hydrochloric acid TS, as the dissolution medium, the dissolution rate in 30 minutes of Pioglitazone Hydrochloride and Metformin Hydrochloride Tablets is not less than 80%.

Start the test with 1 tablet of Pioglitazone Hydrochloride and Metformin Hydrochloride Tablets, withdraw not less than 10 mL of the medium at the specified minute after starting the test, and filter through a membrane filter with a pore size not exceeding 0.45 μm. Discard not less than 5 mL of the first filtrate, pipet *V* mL of the subsequent filtrate, add the dissolution medium to make exactly *V'* mL so that each mL contains about 18.4 μg of pioglitazone hydrochloride ($C_{19}H_{20}N_2O_3S.HCl$), and use this solution as the sample solution. Separately, weigh accurately about 37 mg of Pioglitazone Hydrochloride RS (separately, determine the water <*2.48*> in the same manner as Pioglitazone Hydrochloride), and dissolve in a mixture of 0.1 mol/L hydrochloric acid TS and methanol (1:1) to make exactly 100 mL. Pipet 5 mL of this solution, add the dissolution medium to make exactly 100 mL, and use this solution as the standard solution. Perform the test with exactly 5 μL each of the sample solution and standard solution as directed under Liquid Chromatography <*2.01*> according to the following conditions, and determine the peak areas, A_T and A_S, of pioglitazone in each solution.

Dissolution rate (%) with respect to the labeled amount of pioglitazone hydrochloride ($C_{19}H_{20}N_2O_3S.HCl$)
$= M_S \times A_T/A_S \times V'/V \times 1/C \times 45$

M_S: Amount (mg) of Pioglitazone Hydrochloride RS taken, calculated on the anhydrous basis

C: Labeled amount (mg) of pioglitazone hydrochloride ($C_{19}H_{20}N_2O_3S.HCl$) in 1 tablet

Operating conditions—

Proceed as directed in the operating conditions in the Assay (1).

System suitability—

System performance: When the procedure is run with 5 μL of the standard solution under the above operating conditions, the number of theoretical plates and the symmetry factor of the peak of pioglitazone are not less than 8000 and not more than 2.0, respectively.

System repeatability: When the test is repeated 6 times with 5 μL of the standard solution under the above operating conditions, the relative standard deviation of the peak area of pioglitazone is not more than 1.0%.

(2) Metformin hydrochloride—When the test is performed at 50 revolutions per minute according to the Paddle method, using 900 mL of the dissolution medium used in (1), the dissolution rate in 30 minutes of Pioglitazone Hydrochloride and Metformin Hydrochloride Tablets is not less than 80%.

Start the test with 1 tablet of Pioglitazone Hydrochloride and Metformin Hydrochloride Tablets, withdraw not less than 10 mL of the medium at the specified minute after starting the test, and filter through a membrane filter with a pore size not exceeding 0.45 μm. Discard not less than 5 mL of the first filtrate, pipet *V* mL of the subsequent filtrate, add the dissolution medium to make exactly *V'* mL so that each mL contains about 0.56 mg of metformin hydrochloride ($C_4H_{11}N_5.HCl$), and use this solution as the sample solution. Separately, weigh accurately about 28 mg of metformin hydrochloride for assay, previously dried at 105°C for 3 hours, and dissolve in the dissolution medium to make exactly 50 mL, use this solution as the standard solution. Perform the test with exactly 5 μL each of the sample solution and standard solution as directed under Liquid Chromatography <*2.01*> according to the following conditions, and determine the peak areas, A_T and A_S, of metformin in each solution.

Dissolution rate (%) with respect to the labeled amount of metformin hydrochloride ($C_4H_{11}N_5.HCl$)
$= M_S \times A_T/A_S \times V'/V \times 1/C \times 1800$

M_S: Amount (mg) of metformin hydrochloride for assay taken

C: Labeled amount (mg) of metformin hydrochloride ($C_4H_{11}N_5.HCl$) in 1 tablet

Operating conditions—

Proceed as directed in the operating conditions in the Assay (2).

System suitability—

System performance: When the procedure is run with 5 μL of the standard solution under the above operating conditions, the number of theoretical plates and the symmetry factor of the peak of metformin are not less than 6000 and not more than 2.5, respectively.

System repeatability: When the test is repeated 6 times with 5 μL of the standard solution under the above operating conditions, the relative standard deviation of the peak area of metformin is not more than 1.0%.

Assay (1) Pioglitazone hydrochloride—Weigh accurately the mass of not less than 20 Pioglitazone Hydrochloride and Metformin Hydrochloride Tablets, and powder. Weigh accurately a portion of the powder, equivalent to about 33 mg of pioglitazone hydrochloride ($C_{19}H_{20}N_2O_3S.HCl$), add 40 mL of 0.1 mol/L hydrochloric acid TS, shake vigorously for 10 minutes, add 40 mL of methanol, and shake. Add a mixture of 0.1 mol/L hydrochloric acid TS and methanol (1:1) to make exactly 100 mL, and filter through a membrane filter with a pore size not exceeding 0.45 μm. Discard the first 5 mL of the filtrate, pipet 5 mL of the subsequent filtrate, add exactly 5 mL of the internal standard solution, then add a mixture of 0.1 mol/L hydrochloric acid TS and methanol (1:1) to make 100 mL, and use this solution as the sample solution. Separately, weigh accurately about 33 mg of Pioglitazone Hydrochloride RS (separately determine the water <*2.48*> in the same manner as Pioglitazone Hydrochloride), and dissolve in a mixture of 0.1 mol/L hydrochloric acid TS and methanol (1:1) to make exactly 100 mL. Pipet 5 mL of this solution, add exactly 5 mL of the internal standard solution, then add a mixture of 0.1 mol/L hydrochloric acid TS and methanol (1:1) to make 100 mL, and use this solution as the standard solution. Perform the test with 10 μL each of the sample solution and standard solution as directed under Liquid Chromatography <*2.01*> according to the following conditions, and calculate the ratios, Q_T and Q_S, of the peak area of pioglitazone to that of the internal standard.

Amount (mg) of pioglitazone hydrochloride ($C_{19}H_{20}N_2O_3S.HCl$)
$= M_S \times Q_T/Q_S$

M_S: Amount (mg) of Pioglitazone Hydrochloride RS taken, calculated on the anhydrous basis

Internal standard solution—A solution of butyl parahydroxybenzoate in a mixture of 0.1 mol/L hydrochloric acid TS and methanol (1:1) (1 in 2500).

Operating conditions—

Detector: An ultraviolet absorption photometer (wavelength: 225 nm).

Column: A stainless steel column 6 mm in inside diameter and 15 cm in length, packed with octylsilanized silica gel for liquid chromatography (5 μm in particle diameter).

Column temperature: A constant temperature of about 25°C.

Mobile phase: Dissolve 7.2 g of sodium lauryl sulfate in 1000 mL of a mixture of a solution of ammonium dihydrogen phosphate (23 in 4000) and acetonitrile (1:1).

Flow rate: Adjust so that the retention time of pioglitazone is about 9 minutes.

System suitability—

System performance: When the procedure is run with 10 μL of the standard solution under the above operating conditions, pioglitazone and the internal standard are eluted in this order with the resolution between these peaks being not less than 2.5.

System repeatability: When the test is repeated 6 times with 10 μL of the standard solution under the above operating conditions, the relative standard deviation of the ratio of the peak area of pioglitazone to that of the internal standard is not more than 1.0%.

(2) Metformin hydrochloride—Weigh accurately the mass of not less than 20 Pioglitazone Hydrochloride and Metformin Hydrochloride Tablets, and powder. Weigh accurately a portion of the powder, equivalent to about 0.5 g of metformin hydrochloride ($C_4H_{11}N_5.HCl$), add 40 mL of 0.1 mol/L hydrochloric acid TS, shake vigorously for 10 minutes, add 40 mL of methanol, and shake. Add a mixture of 0.1 mol/L hydrochloric acid TS and methanol (1:1) to make exactly 100 mL, and filter through a membrane filter with a pore size not exceeding 0.45 μm. Discard the first 5 mL of the filtrate, pipet 5 mL of the subsequent filtrate, add exactly 5 mL of the internal standard solution, then add a mixture of 0.1 mol/L hydrochloric acid TS and methanol (1:1) to make 100 mL, and use this solution as the sample solution. Separately, weigh accurately about 50 mg of metformin hydrochloride for assay, previously dried at 105°C for 3 hours, and dissolve in a mixture of 0.1 mol/L hydrochloric acid TS and methanol (1:1) to make exactly 10 mL. Pipet 5 mL of this solution, add exactly 5 mL of the internal standard solution, then add a mixture of 0.1 mol/L hydrochloric acid TS and methanol (1:1) to make 100 mL, and use this solution as the standard solution. Perform the test with 10 μL each of the sample solution and standard solution as directed under Liquid Chromatography <*2.01*> according to the following conditions, and calculate the ratios, Q_T and Q_S, of the peak area of metformin to that of the internal standard.

Amount (mg) of metformin hydrochloride ($C_4H_{11}N_5.HCl$)
$= M_S \times Q_T/Q_S \times 10$

M_S: Amount (mg) of metformin hydrochloride for assay taken

Internal standard solution—A solution of 4′-methoxyacetophenone in a mixture of 0.1 mol/L hydrochloric acid TS and methanol (1:1) (1 in 2000).

Operating conditions—

Detector: An ultraviolet absorption photometer (wavelength: 255 nm).

Column: A stainless steel column 6 mm in inside diameter and 15 cm in length, packed with octylsilanized silica gel for liquid chromatography (5 μm in particle diameter).

Column temperature: A constant temperature of about 25°C.

Mobile phase: Dissolve 7.2 g of sodium lauryl sulfate in 1000 mL of a mixture of a solution of ammonium dihydrogen phosphate (23 in 4000) and acetonitrile (1:1).

Flow rate: Adjust so that the retention time of metformin is about 5 minutes.

System suitability—

System performance: When the procedure is run with 10 μL of the standard solution under the above operating conditions, metformin and the internal standard are eluted in this order with the resolution between these peaks being not less than 2.5.

System repeatability: When the test is repeated 6 times with 10 μL of the standard solution under the above operat-

ing conditions, the relative standard deviation of the ratio of the peak area of metformin to that of the internal standard is not more than 1.0%.

Containers and storage Containers—Tight containers.

Pipemidic Acid Hydrate

ピペミド酸水和物

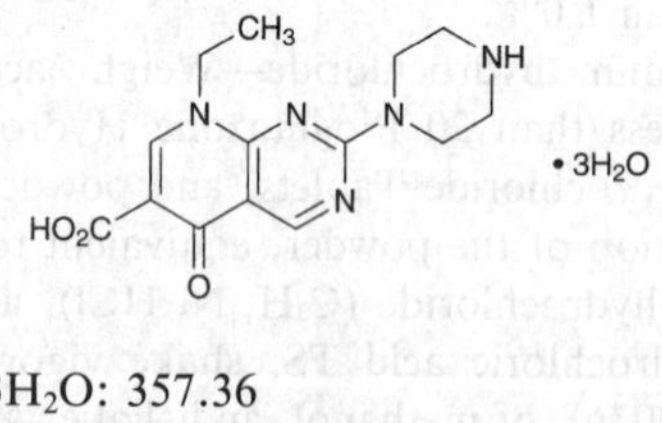

$C_{14}H_{17}N_5O_3.3H_2O$: 357.36
8-Ethyl-5-oxo-2-(piperazin-1-yl)-
5,8-dihydropyrido[2,3-*d*]pyrimidine-
6-carboxylic acid trihydrate
[*51940-44-4*, anhydride]

Pipemidic Acid Hydrate contains not less than 98.5% and not more than 101.0% of pipemidic acid ($C_{14}H_{17}N_5O_3$: 303.32), calculated on the anhydrous basis.

Description Pipemidic Acid Hydrate occurs as a pale yellow crystalline powder.

It is freely soluble in acetic acid (100), very slightly soluble in water, and practically insoluble in methanol and in ethanol (99.5).

It dissolves in sodium hydroxide TS.

It is gradually colored on exposure to light.

Melting point: about 250°C (with decomposition).

Identification (1) Dissolve 0.1 g of Pipemidic Acid Hydrate in 20 mL of sodium hydroxide TS, and dilute with water to make 200 mL. To 1 mL of the solution add water to make 100 mL. Determine the absorption spectrum of the solution as directed under Ultraviolet-visible Spectrophotometry <*2.24*>, and compare the spectrum with the Reference Spectrum: both spectra exhibit similar intensities of absorption at the same wavelengths.

(2) Determine the infrared absorption spectrum of Pipemidic Acid Hydrate as directed in the potassium bromide disk method under Infrared Spectrophotometry <*2.25*>, and compare the spectrum with the Reference Spectrum: both spectra exhibit similar intensities of absorption at the same wave numbers.

Purity (1) Chloride <*1.03*>—Dissolve 1.0 g of Pipemidic Acid Hydrate in 35 mL of water and 10 mL of sodium hydroxide TS, then add 15 mL of dilute nitric acid, shake well, and filter through a glass filter (G3). To 30 mL of the filtrate add 6 mL of dilute nitric acid and water to make 50 mL. Perform the test using this solution as the test solution. Prepare the control solution as follows: to 0.30 mL of 0.01 mol/L hydrochloric acid VS add 5 mL of sodium hydroxide TS, 13.5 mL of dilute nitric acid and water to make 50 mL (not more than 0.021%).

(2) Sulfate <*1.14*>—Dissolve 1.0 g of Pipemidic Acid Hydrate in 35 mL of water and 10 mL of sodium hydroxide TS, then add 15 mL of dilute hydrochloric acid, shake well, and filter through a glass filter (G3). To 30 mL of the filtrate add water to make 50 mL. Perform the test using this solution as the test solution. Prepare the control solution as follows: to 0.50 mL of 0.005 mol/L sulfuric acid VS add 5 mL of sodium hydroxide TS, 7.5 mL of dilute hydrochloric acid and water to make 50 mL (not more than 0.048%).

(3) Heavy metals <*1.07*>—Proceed with 2.0 g of Pipemidic Acid Hydrate according to Method 2, and perform the test. Prepare the control solution with 2.0 mL of Standard Lead Solution (not more than 10 ppm).

(4) Arsenic <*1.11*>—Prepare the test solution with 1.0 g of Pipemidic Acid Hydrate according to Method 3, and perform the test (not more than 2 ppm).

(5) Related substances—Dissolve 0.10 g of Pipemidic Acid Hydrate in 10 mL of diluted acetic acid (100) (1 in 20), and use this solution as the sample solution. Pipet 1 mL of the sample solution, add diluted acetic acid (100) (1 in 20) to make exactly 200 mL, and use this solution as the standard solution. Perform the test with these solutions as directed under Thin-layer Chromatography <*2.03*>. Spot 5 μL each of the sample solution and standard solution on a plate of silica gel with fluorescent indicator for thin-layer chromatography. Develop the plate with a mixture of chloroform, methanol, formic acid and triethylamine (25:15:5:1) to a distance of about 10 cm, and air-dry the plate. Examine under ultraviolet light (main wavelength: 254 nm): the spots other than the principal spot obtained from the sample solution are not more intense than the spot from the standard solution.

Water <*2.48*> 14.5 – 16.0% (20 mg, coulometric titration).

Residue on ignition <*2.44*> Not more than 0.1% (1 g).

Assay Weigh accurately about 0.35 g of Pipemidic Acid Hydrate, dissolve in 40 mL of acetic acid (100), and titrate <*2.50*> with 0.1 mol/L perchloric acid VS (potentiometric titration). Perform a blank determination in the same manner, and make any necessary correction.

Each mL of 0.1 mol/L perchloric acid VS
= 30.33 mg of $C_{14}H_{17}N_5O_3$

Containers and storage Containers—Well-closed containers.

Storage—Light-resistant.

Piperacillin Hydrate

ピペラシリン水和物

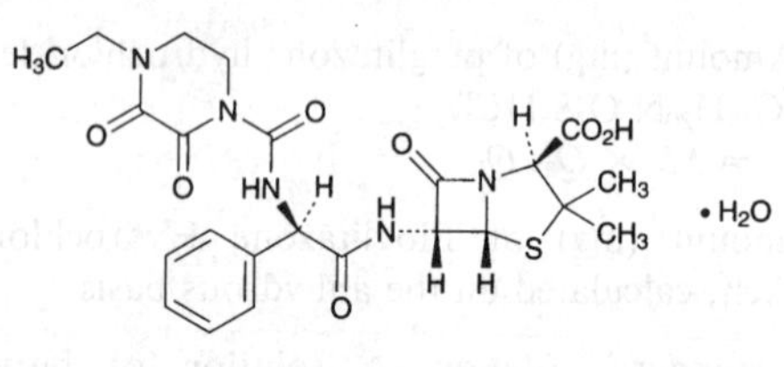

$C_{23}H_{27}N_5O_7S.H_2O$: 535.57
(2*S*,5*R*,6*R*)-6-{(2*R*)-2-[(4-Ethyl-2,3-dioxopiperazine-1-carbonyl)amino]-2-phenylacetylamino}-3,3-dimethyl-7-oxo-4-thia-1-azabicyclo[3.2.0]heptane-2-carboxylic acid monohydrate
[*66258-76-2*]

Piperacillin Hydrate contains not less than 970 μg (potency) and not more than 1020 μg (potency) per mg, calculated on the anhydrous basis. The potency of Piperacillin Hydrate is expressed as mass (potency) of piperacillin ($C_{23}H_{27}N_5O_7S$: 517.55).

Description Piperacillin Hydrate occurs as a white crystalline powder.

It is freely soluble in methanol, soluble in ethanol (99.5)

and in dimethylsulfoxide, and very slightly soluble in water.

Identification **(1)** Determine the infrared absorption spectrum of Piperacillin Hydrate as directed in the potassium bromide disk method under Infrared Spectrophotometry <*2.25*>, and compare the spectrum with the Reference Spectrum or the spectrum of Piperacillin RS: both spectra exhibit similar intensities of absorption at the same wave numbers.

(2) Determine the ^{1}H spectrum of a solution of Piperacillin Hydrate in deuterated dimethylsulfoxide for nuclear magnetic resonance spectroscopy (1 in 3) as directed under Nuclear Magnetic Resonance Spectroscopy <*2.21*>, using tetramethylsilane for nuclear magnetic resonance spectroscopy as an internal reference compound: it exhibits a triplet signal A at about δ 1.1 ppm, a singlet signal B at about δ 4.2 ppm, and a multiplet signal C at about δ 7.4 ppm, and the ratio of the integrated intensity of each signal, A:B:C, is about 3:1:5.

Optical rotation <*2.49*> $[\alpha]_D^{20}$: +162 – +172° (0.2 g, methanol, 20 mL, 100 mm).

Purity **(1)** Heavy metals <*1.07*>—Proceed with 2.0 g of Piperacillin Hydrate according to Method 2, and perform the test. Prepare the control solution with 2.0 mL of Standard Lead Solution (not more than 10 ppm).

(2) Related substances 1—Conduct this procedure rapidly after the preparation of the sample solution and standard solution. Dissolve 20 mg of Piperacillin Hydrate in 20 mL of the mobile phase, and use this solution as the sample solution. Pipet 1 mL of the sample solution, add the mobile phase to make exactly 200 mL, and use this solution as the standard solution (1). Pipet 2 mL of the standard solution (1), add the mobile phase to make exactly 10 mL, and use this solution as the standard solution (2). Perform the test with exactly 20 μL each of the sample solution and the standard solutions (1) and (2) as directed under Liquid Chromatography <*2.01*> according to the following conditions, and determine each peak area by the automatic integration method: the total area of the peaks, having the relative retention time of about 0.38 and about 0.50 to piperacillin, obtained from the sample solution is not larger than 2 times the peak area of piperacillin from the standard solution (2), the total area of the peaks, having the relative retention time of about 0.82 and about 0.86, from the sample solution is not larger than the peak area of piperacillin from the standard solution (2), and the area of the peak other than piperacillin and the peaks having the relative retention time of about 0.38, about 0.50, about 0.82 and about 0.86, from the sample solution, is not larger than the peak area of piperacillin from the standard solution (2). Furthermore, the total area of the peaks other than piperacillin from the sample solution is not larger than the peak area of piperacillin from the standard solution (1).

Operating conditions—

Detector, column, column temperature, mobile phase, and flow rate: Proceed as directed in the operating conditions in the Assay.

Time span of measurement: About 3 times as long as the retention time of piperacillin, beginning after the solvent peak.

System suitability—

Test for required detectability: Confirm that the peak area of piperacillin obtained with 20 μL of the standard solution (2) is equivalent to 15 to 25% of that with 20 μL of the standard solution (1).

System performance: When the procedure is run with 20 μL of the standard solution (1) under the above operating conditions, the number of theoretical plates and the symmetry factor of the peak of piperacillin are not less than 3000 and not more than 1.5, respectively.

System repeatability: When the test is repeated 6 times with 20 μL of the standard solution (2) under the above operating conditions, the relative standard deviation of the peak area of piperacillin is not more than 3.0%.

(3) Related substances 2—Dissolve 20 mg of Piperacillin Hydrate in 20 mL of the mobile phase, and use this solution as the sample solution. Pipet 1 mL of the sample solution, add the mobile phase to make exactly 200 mL, and use this solution as the standard solution (1). Pipet 2 mL of the standard solution (1), add the mobile phase to make exactly 10 mL, and use this solution as the standard solution (2). Perform the test with exactly 20 μL each of the sample solution, and the standard solutions (1) and (2) as directed under Liquid Chromatography <*2.01*> according to the following conditions, and determine each peak area by the automatic integration method: the area of the peak, having the relative retention time of about 6.6 to piperacillin, obtained from the sample solution is not larger than 3 times the peak area of piperacillin from the standard solution (2), and the area of the peaks other than piperacillin and the peak mentioned above from the sample solution are not larger than 1.4 times the peak area of piperacillin from the standard solution (2). Furthermore, the total area of the peaks other than the peak of piperacillin from the sample solution is not larger than the area of the peak of piperacillin from the standard solution (1). For the area of the peak, having the relative retention time of about 6.6, multiply the correction factor, 2.0.

Operating conditions—

Detector, column and column temperature: Proceed as directed in the operating conditions in the Assay.

Mobile phase: Take 60.1 g of acetic acid (100) and 101.0 g of triethylamine, add water to make 1000 mL. To 25 mL of this solution add 300 mL of acetonitrile and 25 mL of dilute acetic acid, and add water to make 1000 mL.

Flow rate: Adjust so that the retention time of piperacillin is about 1.2 minutes.

Time span of measurement: About 8 times as long as the retention time of piperacillin, beginning after the piperacillin peak.

System suitability—

Test for required detectability: Confirm that the peak area of piperacillin obtained with 20 μL of the standard solution (2) is equivalent to 15 to 25% of that with 20 μL of the standard solution (1).

System performance: When the procedure is run with 20 μL of the standard solution (1) under the above operating conditions, the number of theoretical plates and the symmetry factor of the peak of piperacillin are not less than 1500 and not more than 2.0, respectively.

System repeatability: When the test is repeated 6 times with 20 μL of the standard solution (2) under the above operating conditions, the relative standard deviation of the peak area of piperacillin is not more than 4.0%.

(4) Residual solvents <*2.46*>—Transfer exactly 10 mg of Piperacillin Hydrate to an about 3 mL-vial, add exactly 1 mL of saturated sodium hydrogen carbonate solution to dissolve and stop the vial tightly. After heating this at 90°C for 10 minutes, use the gas inside the container as the sample gas. Separately, measure exactly 1 mL of ethyl acetate, dissolve in water to make exactly 200 mL. Pipet 10 mL of this solution, add water to make exactly 20 mL. Pipet 2 μL of this solution in an about 3-mL vial containing exactly 1 mL of saturated sodium hydrogen carbonate solution, and stop the vial tightly. Run the procedure similarly to the sample, and use the gas as the standard gas. Perform the test with exactly 0.5 mL each of the sample gas and standard gas as directed under Gas Chromatography <*2.02*> according to the following conditions, and determine the peak area of ethyl acetate by the automatic integration method: the peak area of ethyl acetate obtained from the sample gas is not larger than that from the standard gas.

Operating conditions—

Detector: A hydrogen flame-ionization detector.

Column: A glass column 3 mm in inside diameter and 1 m in length, packed with porous stylene-divinyl benzene copolymer for gas chromatography (average pore diameter of 0.0085 μm, 300 – 400 m^2/g) with the particle size of 125 to 150 μm.

Column temperature: A constant temperature of about 145°C.

Carrier gas: Nitrogen.

Flow rate: Adjust so that the retention time of ethyl acetate is about 4 minutes.

System suitability—

System performance: Take 1 mL of saturated sodium hydrogen carbonate solution in an about 3 mL-vial, add 2 μL each of ethyl acetate solution (1 in 400) and acetone solution (1 in 400), and stop the vial tightly. When the procedure is run under the above operating conditions, acetone and ethyl acetate are eluted in this order with the resolution between these peaks being not less than 2.0.

System repeatability: Take 1 mL of saturated sodium hydrogen carbonate solution in an about 3 mL-vial, add 2 μL of ethyl acetate solution (1 in 400), stop the vial tightly, and perform the test under the above operating conditions. When the procedure is repeated 6 times, the relative standard deviation of the peak area of ethyl acetate is not more than 10%.

Water <*2.48*> Not less than 3.2% and not more than 3.8% (0.5 g, volumetric titration, direct titration).

Residue on ignition <*2.44*> Not more than 0.1% (1 g).

Bacterial endotoxins <*4.01*> Less than 0.07 EU/mg (potency).

Assay Weigh accurately an amount of Piperacillin Hydrate and Piperacillin RS, equivalent to about 50 mg (potency), dissolve each in the mobile phase to make exactly 50 mL. Pipet 5 mL each of these solutions, add exactly 5 mL of the internal standard solution, and use these solutions as the sample solution and the standard solution, respectively. Perform the test with 5 μL each of the sample solution and standard solution as directed under Liquid Chromatography <*2.01*> according to the following conditions, and calculate the ratios, H_T and H_S, of the peak height of piperacillin to that of the internal standard.

Amount [μg (potency)] of piperacillin ($C_{23}H_{27}N_5O_7S$)
$= M_S \times H_T/H_S \times 1000$

M_S: Amount [mg (potency)] of Piperacillin RS taken

*Internal standard solution—*A solution of acetanilide in the mobile phase (1 in 5000).

Operating conditions—

Detector: An ultraviolet absorption photometer (wavelength: 254 nm).

Column: A stainless steel column 4 mm in inside diameter and 15 cm in length, packed with octadecylsilanized silica gel for liquid chromatography (5 μm in particle diameter).

Column temperature: A constant temperature of about 25°C.

Mobile phase: Take 60.1 g of acetic acid (100) and 101.0 g of triethylamine, add water to make 1000 mL. To 25 mL of this solution add 210 mL of acetonitrile and 25 mL of dilute acetic acid, and add water to make 1000 mL.

Flow rate: Adjust so that the retention time of piperacillin is about 5 minutes.

System suitability—

System performance: When the procedure is run with 5 μL of the standard solution under the above operating conditions, the internal standard and piperacillin are eluted in this order with the resolution between these peaks being not less than 3.

System repeatability: When the test is repeated 6 times with 5 μL of the standard solution under the above operating conditions, the relative standard deviation of the ratio of the peak height of piperacillin to that of the internal standard is not more than 1.0%.

Containers and storage Containers—Tight containers.

Piperacillin Sodium

ピペラシリンナトリウム

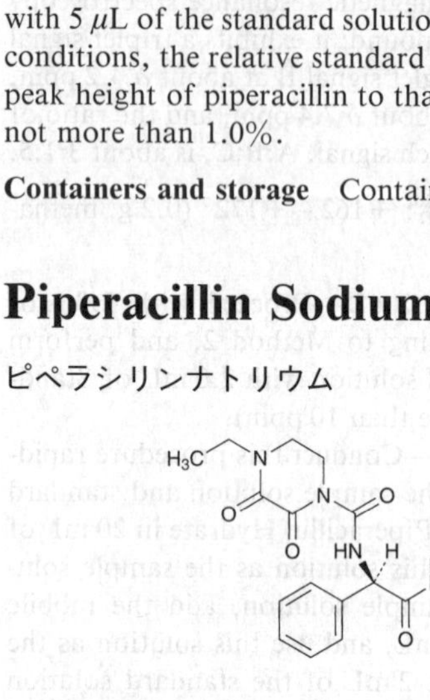

$C_{23}H_{26}N_5NaO_7S$: 539.54

Monosodium (2*S*,5*R*,6*R*)-6-{(2*R*)-2-[(4-ethyl-2,3-dioxopiperazine-1-carbonyl)amino]-2-phenylacetylamino}-3,3-dimethyl-7-oxo-4-thia-1-azabicyclo[3.2.0]heptane-2-carboxylate

[59703-84-3]

Piperacillin Sodium contains not less than 863 μg (potency) and not more than 978 μg (potency) per mg, calculated on the anhydrous basis. The potency of Piperacillin Sodium is expressed as mass (potency) of piperacillin ($C_{23}H_{27}N_5O_7S$: 517.55).

Description Piperacillin Sodium occurs as a white, powder or mass.

It is very soluble in water, freely soluble in methanol and in ethanol (95), and practically insoluble in acetonitrile.

Identification **(1)** Determine the infrared absorption spectrum of Piperacillin Sodium as directed in the potassium bromide disk method under Infrared Spectrophotometry <*2.25*>, and compare the spectrum with the Reference Spectrum: both spectra exhibit similar intensities of absorption at the same wave numbers.

(2) Piperacillin Sodium responds to Qualitative Tests <*1.09*> (1) for sodium salt.

Optical rotation <*2.49*> $[\alpha]_D^{20}$: +175 – +190° (0.8 g calculated on the anhydrous basis, water, 20 mL, 100 mm).

pH <*2.54*> Dissolve 1.0 g of Piperacillin Sodium in 4 mL of water: the pH of the solution is between 5.0 and 7.0.

Purity **(1)** Clarity and color of solution—Dissolve 1.0 g of Piperacillin Sodium in 10 mL of water: the solution is clear and colorless.

(2) Heavy metals <*1.07*>—Proceed with 2.0 g of Piperacillin Sodium according to Method 4, and perform the test. Prepare the control solution with 2.0 mL of Standard Lead

Solution (not more than 10 ppm).

(3) Arsenic <*1.11*>—Prepare the test solution with 2.0 g of Piperacillin Sodium according to Method 4, and perform the test (not more than 1 ppm).

(4) Related substances—Dissolve 0.10 g of Piperacillin Sodium in 50 mL of the mobile phase A, and use this solution as the sample solution. Pipet 1 mL of the sample solution, add the mobile phase A to make exactly 100 mL, and use this solution as the standard solution. Perform the test with exactly 20 μL each of the sample solution and standard solution as directed under Liquid Chromatography <*2.01*> according to the following conditions, and determine the areas of each peak by the automatic integration method: the area of the peak of ampicillin appeared at the retention time of about 7 minutes obtained from the sample solution is not larger than 1/2 times that of piperacillin from the standard solution, the total area of related compounds 1 appeared at the retention times of about 17 minutes and about 21 minutes is not larger than 2 times of the peak area of piperacillin from the standard solution, the peak area of related compound 2 appeared at the retention time of about 56 minutes is not larger than that of piperacillin from the standard solution, and the total area of the peaks other than piperacillin is not larger than 5 times of the peak area of piperacillin from the standard solution. For the peak areas of ampicillin, related compound 1 and related compound 2, multiply their correction factors, 1.39, 1.32 and 1.11, respectively.

Operating conditions—

Detector: An ultraviolet absorption photometer (wavelength: 220 nm).

Column: A stainless steel column 4.6 mm in inside diameter and 15 cm in length, packed with octadecylsilanized silica gel for liquid chromatography (5 μm in particle diameter).

Column temperature: A constant temperature of about 25°C.

Mobile phase A: A mixture of water, acetonitrile and 0.2 mol/L potassium dihydrogen phosphate (45:4:1).

Mobile phase B: A mixture of acetonitrile, water and 0.2 mol/L potassium dihydrogen phosphate (25:24:1).

Flowing of mobile phase: Control the gradient by mixing the mobile phases A and B as directed in the following table.

Time after injection of sample (min)	Mobile phase A (vol%)	Mobile phase B (vol%)
0 – 7	100	0
7 – 13	100 → 83	0 → 17
13 – 41	83	17
41 – 56	83 → 20	17 → 80
56 – 60	20	80

Flow rate: 1.0 mL per minute (the retention time of piperacillin is about 33 minutes).

Time span of measurement: About 1.8 times as long as the retention time of piperacillin, beginning after the solvent peak.

System suitability—

Test for required detectability: To exactly 2 mL of the standard solution add the mobile phase A to make exactly 20 mL. Confirm that the peak area of piperacillin obtained with 20 μL of this solution is equivalent to 7 to 13% of that with 20 μL of the standard solution.

System performance: When the procedure is run with 20 μL of the standard solution under the above operating conditions, the number of theoretical plates and the symmetry factor of the peak of piperacillin are not less than 15,000 and not more than 1.5, respectively.

System repeatability:When the test is repeated 3 times with 20 μL of the standard solution under the above operating conditions, the relative standard deviation of the peak area of piperacillin is not more than 2.0%.

Water <*2.48*> Not more than 1.0% (3 g, volumetric titration, direct titration).

Assay Weigh accurately an amount of Piperacillin Sodium, equivalent to about 0.1 g (potency), and dissolve in water to make exactly 100 mL. To exactly 5 mL of this solution add exactly 5 mL of the internal standard solution, and use this solution as the sample solution. Separately, weigh accurately an amount of Piperacillin RS, equivalent to about 0.1 g (potency), and dissolve in the mobile phase to make exactly 100 mL. Pipet 5 mL of this solution, add exactly 5 mL of the internal standard solution, and use this solution as the standard solution. Perform the test with 5 μL each of the sample solution and standard solution as directed under Liquid Chromatography <*2.01*> according to the following conditions, and calculate the ratios, Q_T and Q_S, of the peak height of piperacillin to that of the internal standard.

Amount [μg (potency)] of piperacillin ($C_{23}H_{27}N_5O_7S$)
$= M_S \times Q_T/Q_S \times 1000$

M_S: Amount [mg (potency)] of Piperacillin RS taken

Internal standard solution—A solution of acetanilide in the mobile phase (1 in 5000).

Operating conditions—

Detector: An ultraviolet absorption photometer (wavelength: 254 nm).

Column: A stainless steel column 4.6 mm in inside diameter and 15 cm in length, packed with octadecylsilanized silica gel for liquid chromatography (5 μm in particle diameter).

Column temperature: A constant temperature of about 25°C.

Mobile phase: To 60.1 g of acetic acid (100) and 101.0 g of triethylamine add water to make exactly 1000 mL. To 25 mL of this solution add 25 mL of dilute acetic acid and 210 mL of acetonitrile, and add water to make exactly 1000 mL.

Flow rate: Adjust so that the retention time of piperacillin is about 5 minutes.

System suitability—

System performance: When the procedure is run with 5 μL of the standard solution under the above operating conditions, the internal standard and piperacillin are eluted in this order with the resolution between these peaks being not less than 3.

System repeatability: When the test is repeated 6 times with 5 μL of the standard solution under the above operating conditions, the relative standard deviation of the ratios of the peak height of piperacillin to that of the internal standard is not more than 1.0%.

Containers and storage Containers—Hermetic containers.

Piperacillin Sodium for Injection

注射用ピペラシリンナトリウム

Piperacillin Sodium for Injection is a preparation for injection which is dissolved before use.

It contains not less than 93.0% and not more than 107.0% of the labeled potency of piperacillin ($C_{23}H_{27}N_5O_7S$: 517.55).

Method of preparation Prepare as directed under Injections, with Piperacillin Sodium.

Description Piperacillin Sodium for Injection is a white, powder or masses.

Identification Proceed as directed in the Identification under Piperacillin Sodium.

pH *<2.54>* The pH of a solution prepared by dissolving an amount of Piperacillin Sodium for Injection, equivalent to 1.0 g (potency) of Piperacillin Sodium, in 4 mL of water is 5.0 – 7.0.

Purity (1) Clarity and color of solution—Dissolve an amount of Piperacillin Sodium for Injection, equivalent to 4.0 g (potency) of Piperacillin Sodium, in 17 mL of water: the solution is clear and colorless.

(2) Related substances—Proceed as directed in the Purity (4) under Piperacillin Sodium.

Water *<2.48>* Not more than 1.0% (3 g, volumetric titration, direct titration).

Bacterial endotoxins *<4.01>* Less than 0.04 EU/mg (potency).

Uniformity of dosage units *<6.02>* It meets the requirement of the Mass variation test.

Foreign insoluble matter *<6.06>* Perform the test according to Method 2: it meets the requirement.

Insoluble particulate matter *<6.07>* It meets the requirement.

Sterility *<4.06>* Perform the test according to the Membrane filtration method: it meets the requirement.

Assay Weigh accurately the mass of the contents of not less than 10 Piperacillin Sodium for Injection. Weigh accurately an amount of the contents, equivalent to about 20 mg (potency) of Piperacillin Sodium, dissolve in water to make exactly 20 mL. Pipet 5 mL of this solution, add exactly 5 mL of the internal standard solution, and use this solution as the sample solution. Separately, weigh accurately about 20 mg (potency) of Piperacillin RS, and dissolve in the mobile phase to make exactly 20 mL. Pipet 5 mL of this solution, add exactly 5 mL of the internal standard solution, and use this solution as the standard solution. Proceed as directed in the Assay under Piperacillin Sodium.

Amount [mg (potency)] of piperacillin ($C_{23}H_{27}N_5O_7S$)
$= M_S \times Q_T/Q_S$

M_S: Amount [mg (potency)] of Piperacillin RS taken

Internal standard solution—A solution of acetanilide in the mobile phase (1 in 5000).

Containers and storage Containers—Hermetic containers. Plastic containers for aqueous injections may be used.

Piperazine Adipate

ピペラジンアジピン酸塩

$C_4H_{10}N_2.C_6H_{10}O_4$: 232.28
Piperazine hexanedioate
[*142-88-1*]

Piperazine Adipate, when dried, contains not less than 98.5% of piperazine adipate ($C_4H_{10}N_2.C_6H_{10}O_4$).

Description Piperazine Adipate occurs as a white crystalline powder. It is odorless, and has a slightly acid taste.

It is soluble in water and in acetic acid (100), and practically insoluble in ethanol (95), in acetone and in diethyl ether.

Melting point: about 250°C (with decomposition).

Identification (1) Dissolve 0.5 g of Piperazine Adipate in 10 mL of water, add 1 mL of hydrochloric acid, and extract with two 20-mL portions of diethyl ether. Combine the diethyl ether extracts, evaporate to dryness on a water bath, and dry the residue at 105°C for 1 hour: the melting point *<2.60>* is between 152°C and 155°C.

(2) To 3 mL of a solution of Piperazine Adipate (1 in 100) add 3 drops of Reinecke salt TS: a light red precipitate is formed.

(3) Determine the infrared absorption spectrum of Piperazine Adipate, previously dried, as directed in the potassium bromide disk method under Infrared Spectrophotometry *<2.25>*, and compare the spectrum with the Reference Spectrum: both spectra exhibit similar intensities of absorption at the same wave numbers.

pH *<2.54>* The pH of a solution of 1.0 g of Piperazine Adipate in 20 mL of water is between 5.0 and 6.0.

Purity (1) Clarity and color of solution—Dissolve 1.0 g of Piperazine Adipate in 30 mL of water: the solution is clear and colorless.

(2) Heavy metals *<1.07>*—Proceed with 2.0 g of Piperazine Adipate according to Method 2, and perform the test. Prepare the control solution with 2.0 mL of Standard Lead Solution (not more than 10 ppm).

Loss on drying *<2.41>* Not more than 0.5% (1 g, 105°C, 4 hours).

Residue on ignition *<2.44>* Not more than 0.1% (1 g).

Assay Weigh accurately about 0.2 g of Piperazine Adipate, previously dried, dissolve in a mixture of 20 mL of acetic acid for nonaqueous titration and 40 mL of acetone for nonaqueous titration, and titrate *<2.50>* with 0.1 mol/L perchloric acid VS until the red-purple color of the solution changes to blue-purple (indicator: 6 drops of bromocresol green-methylrosaniline chloride TS). Perform a blank determination, and make any necessary correction in the same manner.

Each mL of 0.1 mol/L perchloric acid VS
$= 11.61$ mg of $C_4H_{10}N_2.C_6H_{10}O_4$

Containers and storage Containers—Well-closed containers.

Piperazine Phosphate Hydrate

ピペラジンリン酸塩水和物

$\cdot H_3PO_4 \cdot H_2O$

$C_4H_{10}N_2.H_3PO_4.H_2O$: 202.15
Piperazine monophosphate monohydrate
[18534-18-4]

Piperazine Phosphate Hydrate contains not less than 98.5% of piperazine phosphate ($C_4H_{10}N_2.H_3PO_4$: 184.13), calculated on the anhydrous basis.

Description Piperazine Phosphate Hydrate occurs as white, crystals or crystalline powder. It is odorless, and has a slightly acid taste.

It is soluble in formic acid, sparingly soluble in water, very slightly soluble in acetic acid (100), and practically insoluble in methanol, in ethanol (95) and in diethyl ether.

It dissolves in dilute hydrochloric acid.

Melting point: about 222°C (with decomposition).

Identification **(1)** To 3 mL of a solution of Piperazine Phosphate Hydrate (1 in 100) add 3 drops of Reinecke salt TS:a light red precipitate is formed.

(2) Determine the infrared absorption spectrum of Piperazine Phosphate Hydrate as directed in the potassium bromide disk method under Infrared Spectrophotometry *<2.25>*, and compare the spectrum with the Reference Spectrum: both spectra exhibit similar intensities of absorption at the same wave numbers.

(3) A solution of Piperazine Phosphate Hydrate (1 in 100) responds to Qualitative Tests *<1.09>* (1) and (3) for phosphate.

pH *<2.54>* Dissolve 1.0 g of Piperazine Phosphate Hydrate in 100 mL of water: the pH of the solution is between 6.0 and 6.5.

Purity **(1)** Chloride *<1.03>*—To 0.5 g of Piperazine Phosphate Hydrate add 6 mL of dilute nitric acid and water to make 50 mL. Use this solution as the test solution, and perform the test. Prepare the control solution with 0.25 mL of 0.01 mol/L hydrochloric acid VS (not more than 0.018%).

(2) Heavy metals *<1.07>*—To 2.0 g of Piperazine Phosphate Hydrate add 5 mL of dilute hydrochloric acid, 30 mL of water and 2 mL of dilute acetic acid, and dissolve. Add sodium hydroxide TS, adjust the pH of the solution to 3.3, and add water to make 50 mL. Perform the test using this solution as the test solution. Prepare the control solution with 2.0 mL of Standard Lead Solution (not more than 10 ppm).

(3) Arsenic *<1.11>*—Dissolve 2.0 g of Piperazine Phosphate Hydrate in 5 mL of dilute hydrochloric acid, and use this solution as the test solution. Perform the test (not more than 1 ppm).

(4) Related substances—Dissolve 50 mg of Piperazine Phosphate Hydrate in 10 mL of water, and use this solution as the sample solution. Pipet 1 mL of the sample solution, add water to make exactly 100 mL, and use this solution as the standard solution. Perform the test with these solutions as directed under Thin-layer Chromatography *<2.03>*. Spot 5 μL each of the sample solution and standard solution on a plate of cellulose for thin-layer chromatography. Develop the plate with a mixture of ethyl acetate, ammonia solution (28), acetone and ethanol (99.5) (8:3:3:2) to a distance of about 13 cm, and air-dry the plate. Spray evenly 4-dimethylaminocinnamaldehyde TS, and allow to stand for 15 minutes: the spots other than the principal spot and the spot on the starting line obtained from the sample solution are not more intense than the spot from the standard solution.

Water *<2.48>* 8.0 – 9.5% (0.3 g, volumetric titration, direct titration).

Assay Weigh accurately about 0.15 g of Piperazine Phosphate Hydrate, dissolve in 10 mL of formic acid, add 60 mL of acetic acid (100), and titrate *<2.50>* with 0.1 mol/L perchloric acid VS (potentiometric titration). Perform a blank determination in the same manner, and make any necessary correction.

Each mL of 0.1 mol/L perchloric acid VS
= 9.207 mg of $C_4H_{10}N_2.H_3PO_4$

Containers and storage Containers—Well-closed containers.

Piperazine Phosphate Tablets

ピペラジンリン酸塩錠

Piperazine Phosphate Tablets contain not less than 95.0% and not more than 105.0% of the labeled amount of piperazine phosphate hydrate ($C_4H_{10}N_2.H_3PO_4.H_2O$: 202.15).

Method of preparation Prepare as directed under Tablets, with Piperazine Phosphate Hydrate.

Identification Take a quantity of Piperazine Phosphate Tablets equivalent to 0.1 g of Piperazine Phosphate Hydrate, previously powdered, add 10 mL of water, shake while warming for 10 minutes, allow to cool, and filter. To 3 mL of the filtrate add 3 drops of Reinecke salt TS: a light red precipitate is formed.

Disintegration *<6.09>* It meets the requirement. The time limit of the test is 10 minutes.

Assay Weigh accurately not less than 20 Piperazine Phosphate Tablets, and powder. Weigh accurately a quantity of the powder, equivalent to about 0.15 g of piperazine phosphate hydrate ($C_4H_{10}N_2.H_3PO_4.H_2O$). Add 5 mL of formic acid, shake for 5 minutes, centrifuge, and collect the supernatant liquid. To the residue add 5 mL of formic acid, shake for 5 minutes, centrifuge, and collect the supernatant liquid. Repeat twice the same procedure with 5 mL each of acetic acid (100), combine all the supernatant liquids, add 50 mL of acetic acid (100), and titrate *<2.50>* with 0.1 mol/L perchloric acid VS (potentiometric titration). Perform a blank determination, and make any necessary correction.

Each mL of 0.1 mol/L perchloric acid VS
= 10.11 mg of $C_4H_{10}N_2.H_3PO_4.H_2O$

Containers and storage Containers—Tight containers.

Pirarubicin

ピラルビシン

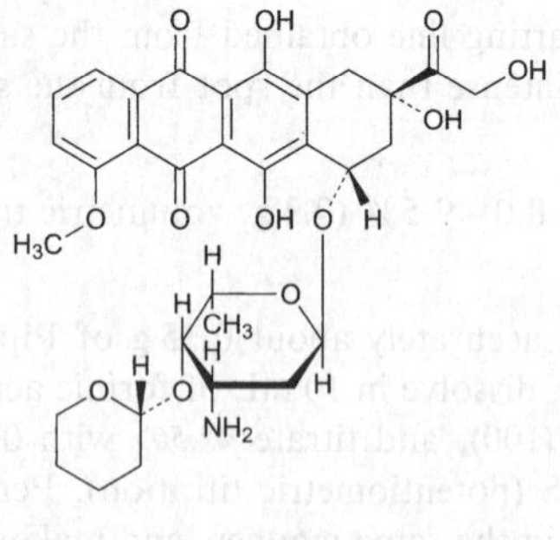

$C_{32}H_{37}NO_{12}$: 627.64
(2*S*,4*S*)-4-{3-Amino-2,3,6-trideoxy-4-*O*-[(2*R*)-3,4,5,6-tetrahydro-2*H*-pyran-2-yl]-α-L-*lyxo*-hexopyranosyloxy}-2,5,12-trihydroxy-2-hydroxyacetyl-7-methoxy-1,2,3,4-tetrahydrotetracene-6,11-dione
[*72496-41-4*]

Pirarubicin is a derivative of daunorubicin.

It contains not less than 950 μg (potency) per mg, calculated on the anhydrous basis. The potency of Pirarubicin is expressed as mass (potency) of pirarubicin ($C_{32}H_{37}NO_{12}$).

Description Pirarubicin occurs as a red-orange crystalline powder.

It is soluble in chloroform, very slightly soluble in acetonitrile, in methanol and in ethanol (99.5), and practically insoluble in water.

Identification (1) Dissolve 10 mg of Pirarubicin in 80 mL of methanol and 6 mL of diluted hydrochloric acid (1 in 5000), and add water to make 100 mL. To 10 mL of this solution add diluted methanol (4 in 5) to make 100 mL. Determine the absorption spectrum of this solution as directed under Ultraviolet-visible Spectrophotometry *<2.24>*, and compare the spectrum with the Reference Spectrum or the spectrum of a solution of Pirarubicin RS prepared in the same manner as the sample solution: both spectra exhibit similar intensities of absorption at the same wavelengths.

(2) Dissolve 5 mg each of Pirarubicin and Pirarubicin RS in 5 mL of chloroform, and use these solutions as the sample solution and standard solution. Perform the test with these solutions as directed under Thin-layer Chromatography *<2.03>*. Spot 5 μL each of the sample solution and standard solution on a plate of silica gel for thin-layer chromatography. Develop the plate with a mixture of chloroform and methanol (5:1) to a distance of about 10 cm, and air-dry the plate. Examine the spots: the principal spot obtained from the sample solution and the spot from the standard solution show a red-orange color and the same *R*f value.

Optical rotation *<2.49>* $[\alpha]_D^{20}$: +195 – +215° (10 mg, chloroform, 10 mL, 100 mm).

Purity (1) Clarity and color of solution—Dissolve 10 mg of Pirarubicin in 10 mL of 0.01 mol/L hydrochloric acid TS: the solution is clear and red.

(2) Heavy metals *<1.07>*—Proceed with 1.0 g of Pirarubicin according to Method 2, and perform the test. Prepare the control solution with 2.0 mL of Standard Lead Solution (not more than 20 ppm).

(3) Related substances—Dissolve 10 mg of Pirarubicin in 20 mL of the mobile phase, and use this solution as the sample solution. Pipet 1 mL of the sample solution, add the mobile phase to make exactly 200 mL, and use this solution as the standard solution. Perform the test with exactly 20 μL each of the sample solution and standard solution as directed under Liquid Chromatography *<2.01>* according to the following conditions, and determine each peak area by the automatic integration method: the peak area of doxorubicin, having the relative retention time of about 0.45 to pirarubicin, and the area of the peak, having the relative retention time of about 1.2, obtained from the sample solution are not larger than the peak area of pirarubicin from the standard solution, respectively, and the sum of the areas of the peaks, having the relative retention times of about 1.9 and about 2.0, from the sample solution is not larger than 5 times the peak area of pirarubicin from the standard solution. For the peak area for doxorubicin, multiply the correction factor 0.94 and the area for the two peaks, having the relative retention times of about 1.9 and about 2.0, multiply their correction factors, 1.09, respectively.

Operating conditions—

Detector, column, column temperature, mobile phase, and flow rate: Proceed as directed in the operating conditions in the Assay.

Time span of measurement: About 4 times as long as the retention time of pirarubicin.

System suitability—

System performance, and system repeatability: Proceed as directed in the system suitability in the Assay.

Test for required detectability: Measure exactly 2 mL of the standard solution, and add the mobile phase to make exactly 10 mL. Confirm that the peak area of pirarubicin obtained with 20 μL of this solution is equivalent to 14 to 26% of that with 20 μL of the standard solution.

Water *<2.48>* Not more than 2.0% (0.1 g, volumetric titration, direct titration).

Assay Weigh accurately an amount of Pirarubicin and Pirarubicin RS, equivalent to about 10 mg (potency), and dissolve in the mobile phase to make exactly 10 mL. Pipet 5 mL of these solutions, add exactly 5 mL of the internal standard solution, and use these solutions as the sample solution and standard solution. Perform the test with 20 μL each of the sample solution and standard solution as directed under Liquid Chromatography *<2.01>* according to the following conditions, and calculate the ratios, Q_T and Q_S, of the peak area of pirarubicin to that of the internal standard.

Amount [μg (potency)] of pirarubicin ($C_{32}H_{37}NO_{12}$)
$$= M_S \times Q_T/Q_S \times 1000$$

M_S: Amount [mg (potency)] of Pirarubicin RS taken

Internal standard solution—A solution of 2-naphthol in the mobile phase (1 in 1000).

Operating conditions—

Detector: An ultraviolet absorption photometer (wavelength: 254 nm).

Column: A stainless steel column 6 mm in inside diameter and 15 cm in length, packed with octadecylsilanized silica gel for liquid chromatography (5 μm in particle diameter).

Column temperature: A constant temperature of about 25°C.

Mobile phase: A mixture of 0.05 mol/L ammonium formate buffer solution (pH 4.0) and acetonitrile (3:2).

Flow rate: Adjust so that the retention time of pirarubicin is about 7 minutes.

System suitability—

System performance: When the procedure is run with 20

μL of the standard solution under the above operating conditions, pirarubicin and the internal standard are eluted in this order with the resolution between these peaks being not less than 9.

System repeatability: When the test is repeated 6 times with 20 μL of the standard solution under the above operating conditions, the relative standard deviation of the ratios of the peak area of pirarubicin to that of the internal standard is not more than 1.0%.

Containers and storage Containers—Hermetic containers.

Pirenoxine

ピレノキシン

$C_{16}H_8N_2O_5$: 308.25
1-Hydroxy-5-oxo-5*H*-pyrido[3,2-*a*]phenoxazine-3-carboxylic acid
[*1043-21-6*]

Pirenoxine, when dried, contains not less than 98.0% of pirenoxine ($C_{16}H_8N_2O_5$).

Description Pirenoxine occurs as a yellow-brown powder. It is odorless, and has a slightly bitter taste.

It is very slightly soluble in dimethylsulfoxide, and practically insoluble in water, in acetonitrile, in ethanol (95), in tetrahydrofuran and in diethyl ether.

Melting point: about 250°C (with decomposition).

Identification **(1)** Dissolve 2 mg of Pirenoxine in 10 mL of phosphate buffer solution (pH 6.5), add 5 mL of a solution of L-ascorbic acid (1 in 50), and shake vigorously: a dark purple precipitate is formed.

(2) Determine the absorption spectrum of a solution of Pirenoxine in phosphate buffer solution (pH 6.5) (1 in 200,000) as directed under Ultraviolet-visible Spectrophotometry 〈*2.24*〉, and compare the spectrum with the Reference Spectrum: both spectra exhibit similar intensities of absorption at the same wavelengths.

(3) Determine the infrared absorption spectrum of Pirenoxine, previously dried, as directed in the potassium bromide disk method under Infrared Spectrophotometry 〈*2.25*〉, and compare the spectrum with the Reference Spectrum: both spectra exhibit similar intensities of absorption at the same wave numbers.

Purity **(1)** Heavy metals 〈*1.07*〉—Proceed with 1.0 g of Pirenoxine according to Method 2, and perform the test. Prepare the control solution with 2.0 mL of Standard Lead Solution (not more than 20 ppm).

(2) Related substances—Dissolve 10 mg of Pirenoxine in 50 mL of the mobile phase, and use this solution as the sample solution. Pipet 3 mL of the sample solution, add the mobile phase to make exactly 200 mL, and use this solution as the standard solution. Perform the test with exactly 5 μL each of the sample solution and standard solution as directed under Liquid Chromatography 〈*2.01*〉 according to the following conditions. Determine each peak area of both solutions by the automatic integration method: the total area of the peaks other than pirenoxine obtained from the sample solution is not larger than the peak area of pirenoxine from the standard solution.

Operating conditions—

Detector: An ultraviolet absorption photometer (wavelength: 230 nm).

Column: A stainless steel column 4 mm in inside diameter and 15 cm in length, packed with octadecylsilanized silica gel for liquid chromatography (5 μm in particle diameter).

Column temperature: A constant temperature of about 35°C.

Mobile phase: Dissolve 1.39 g of tetra *n*-butylammonium chloride and 4.5 g of disodium hydrogen phosphate dodecahydrate in 1000 mL of water, and adjust the pH to 6.5 with phosphoric acid. To 700 mL of this solution add 200 mL of acetonitrile and 30 mL of tetrahydrofuran, and mix.

Flow rate: Adjust so that the retention time of pirenoxine is about 10 minutes.

Time span of measurement: About 3 times as long as the retention time of pirenoxine.

System suitability—

Test for required detectability: To exactly 2 mL of the standard solution add the mobile phase to make exactly 30 mL. Confirm that the peak area of pirenoxine obtained with 5 μL of this solution is equivalent to 5 to 8% of that with 5 μL of the standard solution.

System performance: Dissolve 3 mg of Pirenoxine and 16 mg of methyl parahydroxybenzoate in 100 mL of the mobile phase. When the procedure is run with 5 μL of this solution under the above operating conditions, pirenoxine and methyl parahydroxybenzoate are eluted in this order with the resolution between these peaks being not less than 2.0.

System repeatability: When the test is repeated 6 times with 5 μL of the standard solution under the above operating conditions, the relative standard deviation of the peak area of pirenoxine is not more than 1.0%.

Loss on drying 〈*2.41*〉 Not more than 1.5% (0.5 g, in vacuum, 80°C, 3 hours).

Residue on ignition 〈*2.44*〉 Not more than 0.1% (1 g).

Assay Weigh accurately about 0.1 g of Pirenoxine, previously dried, dissolve in 140 mL of dimethylsulfoxide by heating on a water bath. After cooling, add 30 mL of water, and titrate 〈*2.50*〉 immediately with 0.02 mol/L sodium hydroxide VS (potentiometric titration). Perform a blank determination in the same manner, and make any necessary correction.

Each mL of 0.02 mol/L sodium hydroxide VS
= 6.165 mg of $C_{16}H_8N_2O_5$

Containers and storage Containers—Tight containers.

Pirenzepine Hydrochloride Hydrate

ピレンゼピン塩酸塩水和物

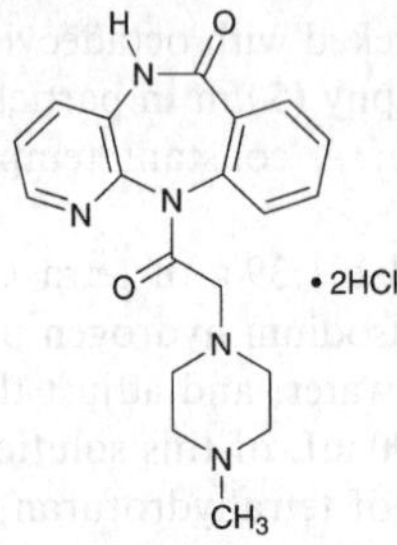

$C_{19}H_{21}N_5O_2.2HCl.H_2O$: 442.34

11-[(4-Methylpiperazin-1-yl)acetyl]-5,11-dihydro-6*H*-pyrido[2,3-*b*][1,4]benzodiazepin-6-one dihydrochloride monohydrate

[*29868-97-1*, anhydride]

Pirenzepine Hydrochloride Hydrate contains not less than 98.5% and not more than 101.0% of pirenzepine hydrochloride ($C_{19}H_{21}N_5O_2.2HCl$: 424.32), calculated on the anhydrous basis.

Description Pirenzepine Hydrochloride Hydrate occurs as a white to pale yellow crystalline powder.

It is freely soluble in water and in formic acid, slightly soluble in methanol, and very slightly soluble in ethanol (99.5).

The pH of a solution obtained by dissolving 1 g of Pirenzepine Hydrochloride Hydrate in 10 mL of water is between 1.0 and 2.0.

Melting point: about 245°C (with decomposition).

It is gradually colored by light.

Identification **(1)** Determine the absorption spectrum of a solution of Pirenzepine Hydrochloride Hydrate (1 in 40,000) as directed under Ultraviolet-visible Spectrophotometry <*2.24*>, and compare the spectrum with the Reference Spectrum: both spectra exhibit similar intensities of absorption at the same wavelengths.

(2) Determine the infrared absorption spectrum of Pirenzepine Hydrochloride Hydrate as directed in the potassium chloride disk method under Infrared Spectrophotometry <*2.25*>, and compare the spectrum with the Reference Spectrum: both spectra exhibit similar intensities of absorption at the same wave numbers.

(3) A solution of Pirenzepine Hydrochloride Hydrate (1 in 50) responds to Qualitative Tests <*1.09*> for chloride.

Purity **(1)** Clarity and color of solution—A solution obtained by dissolving 1.0 g of Pirenzepine Hydrochloride Hydrate in 10 mL of water is clear and not more color than that of the following control solution.

Control solution: To 1.2 mL of Matching Fluid F add 8.8 mL of diluted hydrochloric acid (1 in 40).

(2) Heavy metals <*1.07*>—Proceed with 2.0 g of Pirenzepine Hydrochloride Hydrate according to Method 2, and perform the test. Prepare the control solution with 2.0 mL of Standard Lead Solution (not more than 10 ppm).

(3) Related substances—Dissolve 0.3 g of Pirenzepine Hydrochloride Hydrate in 10 mL of water. To 1 mL of this solution add 5 mL of methanol and the mobile phase A to make 10 mL, and use this solution as the sample solution. Pipet 1 mL of the sample solution, and add 5 mL of methanol and the mobile phase A to make exactly 10 mL. Pipet 1 mL of this solution, add 5 mL of methanol and the mobile phase A to make exactly 10 mL, and use this solution as the standard solution. Perform the test with exactly 10 μL each of the sample solution and standard solution as directed under Liquid Chromatography <*2.01*> according to the following conditions, and determine each peak area by the automatic integration method: the area of the peak other than pirenzepine obtained from the sample solution is not larger than 3/10 times the peak area of pirenzepine from the standard solution, and the total area of the peaks other than pirenzepine from the sample solution is not larger than 3/5 times the peak area of pirenzepine from the standard solution.

Operating conditions—

Detector: An ultraviolet absorption photometer (wavelength: 283 nm).

Column: A stainless steel column 4.6 mm in inside diameter and 15 cm in length, packed with octadecylsilanized silica gel for liquid chromatography (5 μm in particle diameter).

Column temperature: A constant temperature of about 40°C.

Mobile phase A: Dissolve 2 g of sodium lauryl sulfate in 900 mL of water, adjust the pH to 3.2 with acetic acid (100), and add water to make 1000 mL.

Mobile phase B: Methanol.

Mobile phase C: Acetonitrile.

Flowing of mobile phase: Control the gradient by mixing the mobile phases A, B and C as directed in the following table.

Time after injection of sample (min)	Mobile phase A (vol%)	Mobile phase B (vol%)	Mobile phase C (vol%)
0 – 15	55 → 25	30	15 → 45
15 –	25	30	45

Flow rate: Adjust so that the retention time of pirenzepine is about 8 minutes.

Time span of measurement: About 2 times as long as the retention time of pirenzepine, beginning after the solvent peak.

System suitability—

Test for required detectability: Pipet 1 mL of the standard solution, and add 5 mL of methanol and the mobile phase A to make exactly 10 mL. Confirm that the peak area of pirenzepine obtained with 10 μL of this solution is equivalent to 7 to 13% of that with 10 μL of the standard solution.

System performance: Dissolve 0.1 g of 1-phenylpiperazine hydrochloride in 10 mL of methanol. Mix 1 mL of this solution and 1 mL of the sample solution, and add 5 mL of methanol and the mobile phase A to make 10 mL. When the procedure is run with 10 μL of this solution under the above operating conditions, pirenzepine and phenylpiperazine are eluted in this order with the resolution between these peaks being not less than 5.

System repeatability: When the test is repeated 6 times with 10 μL of the standard solution under the above operating conditions, the relative standard deviation of the peak area of pirenzepine is not more than 2.0%.

Water <*2.48*> Not less than 3.5% and not more than 5.0% (0.3 g, volumetric titration, direct titration).

Residue on ignition <*2.44*> Not more than 0.1% (1 g).

Assay Weigh accurately about 0.2 g of Pirenzepine Hydrochloride Hydrate, dissolve in 2 mL of formic acid, add 60 mL of acetic anhydride, and titrate <*2.50*> with 0.1 mol/L perchloric acid VS (potentiometric titration). Perform a blank determination in the same manner, and make any necessary correction.

Each mL of 0.1 mol/L perchloric acid VS
= 14.14 mg of $C_{19}H_{21}N_5O_2.2HCl$

Containers and storage Containers—Well-closed containers.

Storage—Light-resistant.

Piroxicam

ピロキシカム

$C_{15}H_{13}N_3O_4S$: 331.35
4-Hydroxy-2-methyl-*N*-(pyridin-2-yl)-2*H*-1,2-benzothiazine-3-carboxamide 1,1-dioxide
[*36322-90-4*]

Piroxicam contains not less than 98.5% and not more than 101.0% of piroxicam ($C_{15}H_{13}N_3O_4S$), calculated on the dried basis.

Description Piroxicam occurs as a white to light yellow crystalline powder.

It is slightly soluble in acetonitrile and in ethanol (99.5), and practically insoluble in water.

Melting point: about 200°C (with decomposition).

It shows crystal polymorphism.

Identification **(1)** Dissolve 0.1 g of Piroxicam in a mixture of methanol and 0.5 mol/L hydrochloric acid TS (490:1) to make 200 mL. To 1 mL of this solution add the mixture of methanol and 0.5 mol/L hydrochloric acid TS (490:1) to make 100 mL. Determine the absorption spectrum of this solution as directed under Ultraviolet-visible Spectrophotometry 〈*2.24*〉, and compare the spectrum with the Reference Spectrum: both spectra exhibit similar intensities of absorption at the same wavelengths.

(2) Determine the infrared absorption spectrum of Piroxicam as directed in the potassium bromide disk method under Infrared Spectrophotometry 〈*2.25*〉, and compare the spectrum with the Reference Spectrum: both spectra exhibit similar intensities of absorption at the same wave numbers. If any difference appears between the spectra, dissolve the Piroxicam with dichloromethane, evaporate the solvent, dry the residue on a water bath, and perform the test.

Purity **(1)** Heavy metals 〈*1.07*〉—Proceed with 1.0 g of Piroxicam according to Method 2, and perform the test. Prepare the control solution with 2.0 mL of Standard Lead Solution (not more than 20 ppm).

(2) Related substances—Dissolve 75 mg of Piroxicam in 50 mL of acetonitrile for liquid chromatography, and use this solution as the sample solution. Pipet 1 mL of the sample solution, add acetonitrile for liquid chromatography to make exactly 10 mL. Pipet 1 mL of this solution, add acetonitrile for liquid chromatography to make exactly 50 mL, and use this solution as the standard solution. Perform the test with exactly 20 μL each of the sample solution and standard solution as directed under Liquid Chromatography 〈*2.01*〉 according to the following conditions, and determine each peak area by the automatic integration method: the area of the peak other than piroxicam obtained from the sample solution is not larger than the peak area of piroxicam from the standard solution, and the total area of the peaks other than piroxicam from the sample solution is not larger than 2 times the peak area of piroxicam from the standard solution.

Operating conditions—

Detector: An ultraviolet absorption photometer (wavelength: 230 nm).

Column: A stainless steel column 4.6 mm in inside diameter and 25 cm in length, packed with octadecylsilanized silica gel for liquid chromatography (5 μm in particle diameter).

Column temperature: A constant temperature of about 40°C.

Mobile phase: A mixture of 0.05 mol/L potassium dihydrogen phosphate TS (pH 3.0) and acetonitrile for liquid chromatography (3:2).

Flow rate: Adjust so that the retention time of piroxicam is about 10 minutes.

Time span of measurement: About 5 times as long as the retention time of piroxicam, beginning after the solvent peak.

System suitability—

Test for required detectability: To exactly 5 mL of the standard solution add acetonitrile for liquid chromatography to make exactly 20 mL. Confirm that the peak area of piroxicam obtained with 20 μL of this solution is equivalent to 17.5 to 32.5% of that with 20 μL of the standard solution.

System performance: When the procedure is run with 20 μL of the standard solution under the above operating conditions, the number of theoretical plates and the symmetry factor of the peak of piroxicam are not less than 6000 and not more than 1.5, respectively.

System repeatability: When the test is repeated 6 times with 20 μL of the standard solution under the above operating conditions, the relative standard deviation of the peak area of piroxicam is not more than 2.0%.

Loss on drying 〈*2.41*〉 Not more than 0.5% (1 g, 105°C, 3 hours).

Residue on ignition 〈*2.44*〉 Not more than 0.2% (1 g).

Assay Weigh accurately about 0.25 g of Piroxicam, dissolve in 60 mL of a mixture of acetic anhydride and acetic acid (100) (1:1), and titrate 〈*2.50*〉 with 0.1 mol/L perchloric acid VS (potentiometric titration). Perform a blank determination in the same manner, and make any necessary correction.

Each mL of 0.1 mol/L perchloric acid VS
= 33.14 mg of $C_{15}H_{13}N_3O_4S$

Containers and storage Containers—Tight containers.

Pitavastatin Calcium Hydrate

ピタバスタチンカルシウム水和物

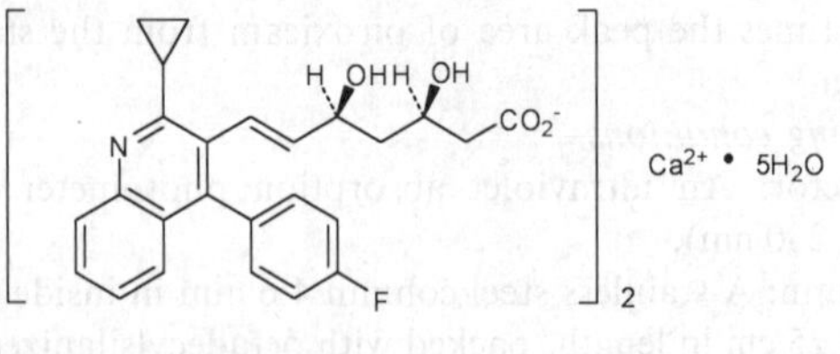

$C_{50}H_{46}CaF_2N_2O_8.5H_2O$: 971.06
Monocalcium bis{(3*R*,5*S*,6*E*)-7-[2-cyclopropyl-4-(4-fluorophenyl)quinolin-3-yl]-3,5-dihydroxyhept-6-enoate} pentahydrate
[*147526-32-7*, anhydride]

Pitavastatin Calcium Hydrate contains not less than 98.0% and not more than 102.0% of pitavastatin calcium ($C_{50}H_{46}CaF_2N_2O_8$: 880.98), calculated on the anhydrous basis.

Description Pitavastatin Calcium Hydrate occurs as a white to pale yellow powder.

It is slightly soluble in methanol, very slightly soluble in water and in ethanol (99.5).

It dissolves in dilute hydrochloric acid.

It shows crystal polymorphism.

Identification (1) Determine the absorption spectrum of a solution of Pitavastatin Calcium Hydrate in methanol (1 in 125,000) as directed under Ultraviolet-visible Spectrophotometry <*2.24*>, and compare the spectrum with the Reference Spectrum: both spectra exhibit similar intensities of absorption at the same wavelengths.

(2) Determine the infrared absorption spectrum of Pitavastatin Calcium Hydrate as directed in the potassium bromide disk method under Infrared Spectrophotometry <*2.25*>: it exhibits absorption at the wave numbers of 3400 – 3300 cm^{-1}, about 1560 cm^{-1}, 1490 cm^{-1}, 1219 cm^{-1}, 1066 cm^{-1} and 766 cm^{-1}.

(3) Dissolve 0.25 g of Pitavastatin Calcium Hydrate in 5 mL of dilute hydrochloric acid, neutralize with ammonia TS, and filter: the filtrate responds to Qualitative Tests <*1.09*> (1), (2), and (3) for calcium.

Optical rotation <*2.49*> $[\alpha]_D^{20}$: +22.0 – +24.5° (0.1 g calculated on the anhydrous basis, a mixture of water and acetonitrile (1:1), 10 mL, 100 mm).

Purity (1) Heavy metals <*1.07*>—To 1.0 g of Pitavastatin Calcium Hydrate in a quartz crucible add 10 mL of a solution of magnesium nitrate hexahydrate in ethanol (95) (1 in 10) and mix well, then fire the ethanol to burn, and heat gradually to carbonize. After cooling, moisten the residue with 1.5 mL of sulfuric acid, heat carefully, then ignite at 550°C until the residue is incinerated. After cooling, moisten the residue with 1.5 mL of nitric acid, heat carefully, then ignite at 550°C until the residue is completely incinerated. After cooling, dissolve the residue in 3 mL of hydrochloric acid, and evaporate the solvent to dryness on a water bath. Moisten the residue with 3 drops of hydrochloric acid, dissolve in 10 mL of hot water with the aid of gentle heat, and filter. Wash the residue with 20 mL of water, and pour the filtrates and washings into a Nessler tube. Add 1 drop of phenolphthalein TS, add ammonia TS dropwise until the solution develops a pale red color, then add 2 mL of dilute acetic acid, add water to make 50 mL, and use this solution as the test solution. The control solution is prepared as follows: Take 10 mL of a solution of magnesium nitrate hexahydrate in ethanol (95) (1 in 10), and fire the ethanol to burn. Hereafter, proceed as for the test solution, then add 2.0 mL of Standard Lead Solution, 2 mL of acetic acid and water to make 50 mL (not more than 20 ppm).

(2) Related substances—Conduct this procedure using light-resistant vessels. Dissolve 0.10 g of Pitavastatin Calcium Hydrate in 100 mL of a mixture of acetonitrile and water (3:2), and use this solution as the sample solution. Pipet 1 mL of the sample solution, add a mixture of acetonitrile and water (3:2) to make exactly 100 mL, and use this solution as the standard solution. Perform the test with exactly 10 μL each of the sample solution and standard solution as directed under Liquid Chromatography <*2.01*> according to the following conditions, and determine each peak area by the automatic integration method: the area of the peak of related substance A, having the relative retention time of about 1.1 to pitavastatin, obtained from the sample solution is not more than 1/2 times the peak area of pitavastatin from the standard solution, and the area of the peak other than pitavastatin and the peak mentioned above from the sample solution is not more than 1/10 times the peak area of pitavastatin from the standard solution. Furthermore, the total area of the peaks other than pitavastatin from the sample solution is not larger than the peak area of pitavastatin from the standard solution. For the area of the peak of related substance B, having the relative retention time of about 1.4, multiply the correction factor, 1.8.

Operating conditions—

Detector, column, and column temperature: Proceed as directed in the operating conditions in the Assay.

Mobile phase A: To 10 mL of dilute acetic acid add water to make 1000 mL. To 800 mL of this solution add diluted sodium acetate TS (1 in 100) to adjust to pH 3.8.

Mobile phase B: Acetonitrile for liquid chromatography.

Flowing of mobile phase: Control the gradient by mixing the mobile phases A and B as directed in the following table.

Time after injection of sample (min)	Mobile phase A (vol%)	Mobile phase B (vol%)
0 – 20	60	40
20 – 40	60 → 10	40 → 90
40 – 60	10	90

Flow rate: Adjust so that the retention time of pitavastatin is about 23 minutes.

Time span of measurement: About 2.5 times as long as the retention time of pitavastatin, beginning after the solvent peak.

System suitability—

Test for required detectability: Pipet 1 mL of the standard solution, add a mixture of acetonitrile and water (3:2) to make exactly 20 mL. Confirm that the peak area of pitavastatin obtained with 10 μL of this solution is equivalent to 4 to 6% of that with 10 μL of the standard solution.

System performance: When the procedure is run with 10 μL of the standard solution under the above operating conditions, the number of theoretical plates and the symmetry factor of the peak of pitavastatin are not less than 17,000 and not more than 1.3, respectively.

System repeatability: When the test is repeated 6 times with 10 μL of the standard solution under the above operating conditions, the relative standard deviation of the peak area of pitavastatin is not more than 2.0%.

Water <*2.48*> 9.0 – 13.0% (0.2 g, volumetric titration, direct titration. Use a mixture of pyridine for water determination and ethylene glycol for water determination (83:17) instead of methanol for water determination).

Assay Conduct this procedure using light-resistant vessels. Weigh accurately about 0.1 g of Pitavastatin Calcium Hydrate, dissolve in a mixture of acetonitrile and water (3:2) to make exactly 100 mL. Pipet 5 mL of this solution, add exactly 5 mL of the internal standard solution, then add a mixture of acetonitrile and water (3:2) to make 50 mL, and use this solution as the sample solution. Separately, weigh accurately about 30 mg of Pitavastatin Methylbenzylamine RS (separately determine the water <*2.48*> by coulometric titration using 0.1 g), dissolve in a mixture of acetonitrile and water (3:2) to make exactly 25 mL. Pipet 5 mL of this solution, add exactly 5 mL of the internal standard solution, then add a mixture of acetonitrile and water (3:2) to make 50 mL, and use this solution as the standard solution. Perform the test with 10 μL each of the sample solution and standard solution as directed under Liquid Chromatography <*2.01*> according to the following conditions, and calculate the ratios, Q_T and Q_S, of the peak area of pitavastatin to that of the internal standard.

Amount (mg) of pitavastatin calcium ($C_{50}H_{46}CaF_2N_2O_8$)
$= M_S \times Q_T/Q_S \times 4 \times 0.812$

M_S: Amount (mg) of Pitavastatin Methylbenzylamine RS taken, calculated on the anhydrous basis

Internal standard solution—Butyl parahydroxybenzoate in a mixture of acetonitrile and water (3:2) (3 in 2000).

Operating conditions—

Detector: An ultraviolet absorption photometer (wavelength: 245 nm).

Column: A stainless steel column 4.6 mm in inside diameter and 25 cm in length, packed with octadecylsilanized silica gel for liquid chromatography (5 μm in particle diameter).

Column temperature: A constant temperature of about 40°C.

Mobile phase: To 10 mL of dilute acetic acid add water to make 1000 mL. To 350 mL of this solution add 650 mL of methanol, and dissolve 0.29 g of sodium chloride in this solution.

Flow rate: Adjust so that the retention time of pitavastatin is about 17 minutes.

System suitability—

System performance: When the procedure is run with 10 μL of the standard solution under the above operating conditions, the internal standard and pitavastatin are eluted in this order with the resolution between these peaks being not less than 8.

System repeatability: When the test is repeated 6 times with 10 μL of the standard solution under the above operating conditions, the relative standard deviation of the ratio of the peak area of pitavastatin to that of the internal standard is not more than 1.0%.

Containers and storage Containers—Tight containers.

Storage—Light-resistant.

Others

Related substance A:
(3*RS*,5*RS*)-7-[2-Cyclopropyl-4-(4-fluorophenyl)quinolin-3-yl]-3,5-dihydroxyhept-6-enoic acid

and enantiomer

Related substance B:
7-[2-Cyclopropyl-4-(4-fluorophenyl)quinolin-3-yl]-3-hydroxy-5-oxohept-6-enoic acid

Pitavastatin Calcium Orally Disintegrating Tablets

ピタバスタチンカルシウム口腔内崩壊錠

Pitavastatin Calcium Orally Disintegrating Tablets contain not less than 95.0% and not more than 105.0% of the labeled amount of pitavastatin calcium ($C_{50}H_{46}CaF_2N_2O_8$: 880.98).

Method of preparation Prepare as directed under Tablets, with Pitavastatin Calcium Hydrate.

Identification To a quantity of Pitavastatin Calcium Orally Disintegrating Tablets, equivalent to 4 mg of pitavastatin calcium ($C_{50}H_{46}CaF_2N_2O_8$), add 10 mL of methanol, shake thoroughly, and centrifuge. To 1 mL of the supernatant liquid add methanol to make 50 mL. Determine the absorption spectrum of this solution as directed under Ultraviolet-visible Spectrophotometry <*2.24*>: it exhibits a maximum between 243 nm and 247 nm.

Purity Related substances—Conduct this procedure using light-resistant vessels. To a quantity of Pitavastatin Calcium Orally Disintegrating Tablets, equivalent to 20 mg of pitavastatin calcium ($C_{50}H_{46}CaF_2N_2O_8$), add 60 mL of a mixture of acetonitrile and water (3:2), sonicate to disintegrate, add a mixture of acetonitrile and water (3:2) to make 100 mL. Filter this solution through a membrane filter with a pore size not exceeding 0.45 μm, and use the filtrate as the sample solution. Perform the test with 10 μL of the sample solution as directed under Liquid Chromatography <*2.01*> according to the following conditions. Determine each peak area by the automatic integration method, and calculate the amounts of them by the area percentage method: the amount of related substance A having the relative retention times of about 1.1 to pitavastatin is not more than 0.5%, the amount of related substance B having the relative retention times of about 1.5 is not more than 0.2%, the amount of related substance TA having the relative retention times of about 1.7 is not more than 0.5%, and the amount of the peak other than pitavastatin and the peaks mentioned above is not more than 0.1%. Furthermore, the total amount of the peaks other than pitavastatin is not more than 2.0%.

Operating conditions—

Detector: An ultraviolet absorption photometer (wavelength: 245 nm).

Column: A stainless steel column 4.6 mm in inside diameter and 25 cm in length, packed with octadecylsilanized silica gel for liquid chromatography (5 μm in particle diameter).

Column temperature: A constant temperature of about 40°C.

Mobile phase A: To 10 mL of dilute acetic acid add water to make 1000 mL. To 800 mL of this solution add diluted sodium acetate TS (1 in 100) to adjust to pH 3.8.

Mobile phase B: Acetonitrile for liquid chromatography.

Flowing of mobile phase: Control the gradient by mixing the mobile phases A and B as directed in the following table.

Time after injection of sample (min)	Mobile phase A (vol%)	Mobile phase B (vol%)
0 – 20	60	40
20 – 40	60 → 30	40 → 70
40 – 65	30	70

Flow rate: Adjust so that the retention time of pitavastatin is about 23 minutes.

Time span of measurement: About 2.7 times as long as the retention time of pitavastatin, beginning after the solvent peak.

System suitability—

Test for required detectability: To 1 mL of the sample solution, add a mixture of acetonitrile and water (3:2) to make 100 mL, and use this solution as the solution for system suitability test. Pipet 5 mL of the solution for system suitability test, add a mixture of acetonitrile and water (3:2) to make exactly 50 mL. Confirm that the peak area of pitavastatin obtained with 10 μL of this solution is equivalent to 7 to 13% of that with 10 μL of the solution for system suitability test.

System performance: When the procedure is run with 10 μL of the solution for system suitability test under the above operating conditions, the number of theoretical plates and the symmetry factor of the peak of pitavastatin are not less than 7500 and not more than 2.0, respectively.

System repeatability: When the test is repeated 6 times with 10 μL of the solution for system suitability test under the above operating conditions, the relative standard deviation of the peak area of pitavastatin is not more than 2.0%.

Uniformity of dosage units <*6.02*> Perform the test according to the following method: it meets the requirement of the Content uniformity test.

Conduct this procedure using light-resistant vessels. To 1 tablet of Pitavastatin Calcium Orally Disintegrating Tablets add exactly *V* mL of the internal standard solution so that each mL contains about 0.2 mg of pitavastatin calcium ($C_{50}H_{46}CaF_2N_2O_8$), and add *V* mL of a mixture of acetonitrile and water (3:2), and sonicate to disintegrate. Filter this solution through a membrane filter with a pore size not exceeding 0.45 μm, and use the filtrate as the sample solution. Then, proceed as directed in the Assay.

Amount (mg) of pitavastatin calcium ($C_{50}H_{46}CaF_2N_2O_8$)
$= M_S \times Q_T/Q_S \times V/100 \times 0.812$

M_S: Amount (mg) of Pitavastatin Methylbenzylamine RS taken, calculated on the anhydrous basis

*Internal standard solution—*A solution of butyl parahydroxybenzoate in a mixture of acetonitrile and water (3:2) (3 in 10,000).

Disintegration Being specified separately when the drug is granted approval based on the Law.

Dissolution <*6.10*> When the test is performed at 50 revolutions per minute according to the Paddle method, using 900 mL of 2nd fluid for dissolution test as the dissolution medium, the dissolution rate in 15 minutes of Pitavastatin Calcium Orally Disintegrating Tablets is not less than 75%.

Conduct this procedure using light-resistant vessels. Start the test with 1 tablet of Pitavastatin Calcium Orally Disintegrating Tablets, withdraw not less than 20 mL of the medium at the specified minute after starting the test, and filter through a membrane filter with a pore size not exceeding 0.45 μm. Discard not less than 5 mL of the first filtrate, pipet *V* mL of the subsequent filtrate, add the dissolution medium to make exactly *V′* mL so that each mL contains about 1.1 μg of pitavastatin calcium ($C_{50}H_{46}CaF_2N_2O_8$), and use this solution as the sample solution. Separately, weigh accurately about 24 mg of Pitavastatin Methylbenzylamine RS (separately determine the water <*2.48*> by coulometric titration using 0.1 g) and dissolve in a mixture of acetonitrile and water (3:2) to make exactly 200 mL. Pipet 1 mL of this solution, add the dissolution medium to make exactly 100 mL, and use this solution as the standard solution. Perform the test with exactly 50 μL each of the sample solution and standard solution as directed under Liquid Chromatography <*2.01*> according to the following conditions, and determine the peak areas, A_T and A_S, of pitavastatin in each solution.

Dissolution rate (%) with respect to the labeled amount of pitavastatin calcium ($C_{50}H_{46}CaF_2N_2O_8$)
$= M_S \times A_T/A_S \times V'/V \times 1/C \times 9/2 \times 0.812$

M_S: Amount (mg) of Pitavastatin Methylbenzylamine RS taken, calculated on the anhydrous basis

C: Labeled amount (mg) of pitavastatin calcium ($C_{50}H_{46}CaF_2N_2O_8$) in 1 tablet

Operating conditions—

Proceed as directed in the operating conditions in the Assay.

System suitability—

System performance: When the procedure is run with 50 μL of the standard solution under the above operating conditions, the number of theoretical plates and the symmetry factor of the peak of pitavastatin are not less than 4500 and not more than 2.0, respectively.

System repeatability: When the test is repeated 6 times with 50 μL of the standard solution under the above operating conditions, the relative standard deviation of the peak area of pitavastatin is not more than 1.0%.

Assay Conduct this procedure using light-resistant vessels. To not less than 20 tablets of Pitavastatin Calcium Orally Disintegrating Tablets add exactly *V* mL of a mixture of acetonitrile and water (3:2) so that each mL contains about 0.2 mg of pitavastatin calcium ($C_{50}H_{46}CaF_2N_2O_8$), and sonicate to disintegrate the tablets. Pipet 5 mL of this solution, add exactly 5 mL of the internal standard solution, shake, then filter through a membrane filter with a pore size not exceeding 0.45 μm, and use the filtrate as the sample solution. Separately weigh accurately about 24 mg of Pitavastatin Methylbenzylamine RS (separately determine the water <*2.48*> by coulometric titration using 0.1 g), dissolve in a mixture of acetonitrile and water (3:2) to make exactly 100 mL. Pipet 5 mL of this solution, add exactly 5 mL of the internal standard solution, and use this solution as the standard solution. Perform the test with 10 μL each of the sample solution and standard solution as directed under Liquid Chromatography *<2.01>* according to the following conditions, and calculate the ratios, Q_T and Q_S, of the peak area of pitavastatin to that of the internal standard.

Amount (mg) of pitavastatin calcium ($C_{50}H_{46}CaF_2N_2O_8$) in 1 tablet
$= M_S \times Q_T/Q_S \times V/N \times 1/100 \times 0.812$

M_S: Amount (mg) of Pitavastatin Methylbenzylamine RS taken, calculated on the anhydrous basis
N: Number of tablets taken

Internal standard solution—A solution of butyl parahydroxybenzoate in a mixture of acetonitrile and water (3:2) (3 in 10,000).
Operating conditions—

Proceed as directed in the operating conditions in the Assay under Pitavastatin Calcium Hydrate.
System suitability—

System performance: When the procedure is run with 10 μL of the standard solution under the above operating conditions, the internal standard and pitavastatin are eluted in this order with the resolution between these peaks being not less than 2.0.

System repeatability: When the test is repeated 6 times with 10 μL of the standard solution under the above operating conditions, the relative standard deviation of the ratio of the peak area of pitavastatin to that of the internal standard is not more than 1.0%.

Containers and storage Containers—Tight containers.
Storage—Light-resistant.

Others
Related substances A and B: Refer to them described in Pitavastatin Calcium Hydrate.
Related substances TA:
6-{2-[2-Cyclopropyl-4-(4-fluorophenyl)quinolin-3-yl]ethenyl}-4-hydroxyoxan-2-one

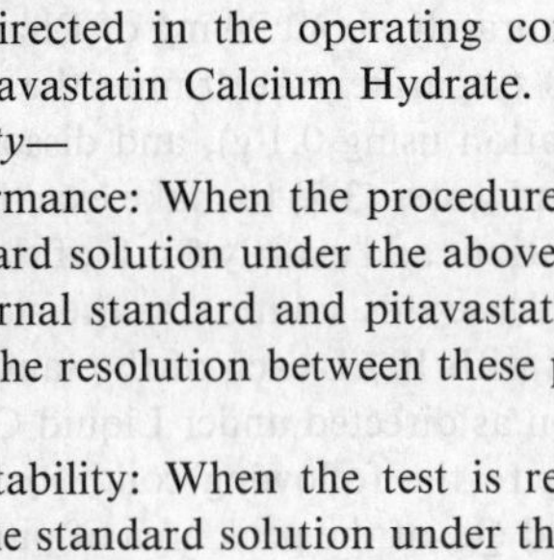

Pitavastatin Calcium Tablets

ピタバスタチンカルシウム錠

Pitavastatin Calcium Tablets contain not less than 95.0% and not more than 105.0% of the labeled amount of pitavastatin calcium ($C_{50}H_{46}CaF_2N_2O_8$: 880.98).

Method of preparation Prepare as directed under Tablets, with Pitavastatin Calcium Hydrate.

Identification Powder Pitavastatin Calcium Tablets. Weigh a portion of the powder, equivalent to 4 mg of pitavastatin calcium ($C_{50}H_{46}CaF_2N_2O_8$), add 10 mL of methanol and shake well, and centrifuge. To 1 mL of the supernatant liquid, add methanol to make 50 mL. Determine the absorption spectrum of this solution as directed under Ultraviolet-visible Spectrophotometry *<2.24>*: it exhibits a maximum between 242 nm and 246 nm.

Purity Related substances—Conduct this procedure using light-resistant vessels. Take a quantity of Pitavastatin Calcium Tablets, equivalent to 20 mg of pitavastatin calcium ($C_{50}H_{46}CaF_2N_2O_8$), add 60 mL of a mixture of acetonitrile and water (3:2), sonicate to disintegrate, and add a mixture of acetonitrile and water (3:2) to make 100 mL. Filter this solution through a membrane filter with a pore size not exceeding 0.45 μm, and use the filtrate as the sample solution. Perform the test with 50 μL of the sample solution as directed under Liquid Chromatography *<2.01>* according to the following conditions, and determine each peak area by the automatic integration method. Calculate the amount of the peaks by the area percentage method: the amounts of the peak of related substance A and related substance TA, having the relative retention times of about 1.1 and about 1.7 to pitavastatin, respectively, obtained from sample solution is not more than 0.5%, the amount of the peak other than pitavastatin and the peaks mentioned above is not more than 0.1%, and the total amount of the peaks other than pitavastatin is not more than 1.5%.
Operating conditions—

Detector: An ultraviolet absorption photometer (wavelength: 245 nm).

Column: A stainless steel column 4.6 mm in inside diameter and 25 cm in length, packed with octadecylsilanized silica gel for liquid chromatography (5 μm in particle diameter).

Column temperature: A constant temperature of about 40°C.

Mobile phase A: To 10 mL of dilute acetic acid add water to make 1000 mL. To 800 mL of this solution add diluted sodium acetate TS (1 in 100) to adjust to pH 3.8.

Mobile phase B: Acetonitrile for liquid chromatography.

Flowing of mobile phase: Control the gradient by mixing the mobile phases A and B as directed in the following table.

Time after injection of sample (min)	Mobile phase A (vol%)	Mobile phase B (vol%)
0 – 20	60	40
20 – 40	60 → 30	40 → 70
40 – 65	30	70

Flow rate: Adjust so that the retention time of pitavastatin is about 23 minutes.

Time span of measurement: About 2.7 times as long as the retention time of pitavastatin, beginning after the solvent peak.
System suitability—

Test for required detectability: To 1 mL of the sample solution add a mixture of acetonitrile and water (3:2) to make 100 mL, and use this solution as the solution for system suitability test. Pipet 5 mL of the solution for system suitability test, add a mixture of acetonitrile and water (3:2) to make exactly 50 mL. Confirm that the peak area of pitavastatin obtained with 50 μL of this solution is equivalent to 7 to 13% of that with 50 μL of the solution for system suitability test.

System performance: When the procedure is run with 50 μL of the solution for system suitability test under the above operating conditions, the number of theoretical plates and the symmetry factor of the peak of pitavastatin are not less than 7500 and not more than 2.0, respectively.

System repeatability: When the test is repeated 6 times with 50 μL of the solution for system suitability test under the above operating conditions, the relative standard deviation of the peak area of pitavastatin is not more than 2.0%.

Uniformity of dosage units <*6.02*> Perform the test according to the following method: it meets the requirement of the Content uniformity test.

Conduct this procedure using light-resistant vessels. To 1 tablet of Pitavastatin Calcium Tablets add exactly V mL of the internal standard solution so that each mL contains about 0.2 mg of pitavastatin calcium ($C_{50}H_{46}CaF_2N_2O_8$), and add V mL of a mixture of acetonitrile and water (3:2), shake well until the tablet is disintegrated completely. Filter this solution through a membrane filter with a pore size not exceeding 0.45 μm, and use the filtrate as the sample solution. Then, proceed as directed in the Assay.

Amount (mg) of pitavastatin calcium ($C_{50}H_{46}CaF_2N_2O_8$)
$= M_S \times Q_T/Q_S \times V/100 \times 0.812$

M_S: Amount (mg) of Pitavastatin Methylbenzylamine RS taken, calculated on the anhydrous basis

Internal standard solution—A solution of butyl parahydroxybenzoate in a mixture of acetonitrile and water (3:2) (3 in 10,000).

Dissolution <*6.10*> When the test is performed at 50 revolutions per minute according to the Paddle method, using 900 mL of water as the dissolution medium, the dissolution rates in 15 minutes of Pitavastatin Calcium Tablets is not less than 85%.

Conduct this procedure using light-resistant vessels. Start the test with 1 tablet of Pitavastatin Calcium Tablets, withdraw not less than 10 mL of the medium at the specified minute after starting the test, and filter through a membrane filter with a pore size not exceeding 0.45 μm. Discard not less than 5 mL of the first filtrate, pipet V mL of the subsequent filtrate, add water to make exactly V' mL so that each mL contains about 1.1 μg of pitavastatin calcium ($C_{50}H_{46}CaF_2N_2O_8$), and use this solution as the sample solution. Separately, weigh accurately about 24 mg of Pitavastatin Methylbenzylamine RS (separately determine the water <*2.48*> by coulometric titration using 0.1 g), and dissolve in a mixture of acetonitrile and water (3:2) to make exactly 200 mL. Pipet 1 mL of this solution, add water to make exactly 100 mL, and use this solution as the standard solution. Perform the test with exactly 50 μL each of the sample solution and standard solution as directed under Liquid Chromatography <*2.01*> according to the following conditions, and determine the peak areas, A_T and A_S, of pitavastatin in each solution.

Dissolution rate (%) with respect to the labeled amount of pitavastatin calcium ($C_{50}H_{46}CaF_2N_2O_8$)
$= M_S \times A_T/A_S \times V'/V \times 1/C \times 9/2 \times 0.812$

M_S: Amount (mg) of Pitavastatin Methylbenzylamine RS taken, calculated on the anhydrous basis
C: Labeled amount (mg) of pitavastatin calcium ($C_{50}H_{46}CaF_2N_2O_8$) in 1 tablet

Operating conditions—

Proceed as directed in the operating conditions in the Assay.

System suitability—

System performance: When the procedure is run with 50 μL of the standard solution under the above operating conditions, the number of theoretical plates and the symmetry factor of the peak of pitavastatin are not less than 4500 and not more than 2.0, respectively.

System repeatability: When the test is repeated 6 times with 50 μL of the standard solution under the above operating conditions, the relative standard deviation of the peak area of pitavastatin is not more than 2.0%.

Assay Conduct this procedure using light-resistant vessels. Weigh accurately the mass of not less than 20 Pitavastatin Calcium Tablets, and powder. Weigh accurately a portion of the powder, equivalent to about 10 mg of pitavastatin calcium ($C_{50}H_{46}CaF_2N_2O_8$), add 30 mL of a mixture of acetonitrile and water (3:2), and sonicate for 10 minutes. To this solution, add a mixture of acetonitrile and water (3:2) to make exactly 50 mL. Filter this solution through a membrane filter with a pore size not exceeding 0.45 μm. Pipet 5 mL of this filtrate, add exactly 5 mL of the internal standard solution, and use this solution as the sample solution. Separately, weigh accurately about 24 mg of Pitavastatin Methylbenzylamine RS (separately determine the water <*2.48*> by coulometric titration using 0.1 g), and dissolve in a mixture of acetonitrile and water (3:2) to make exactly 100 mL. Pipet 5 mL of this solution, add exactly 5 mL of the internal standard solution, and use this solution as the standard solution. Perform the test with 10 μL each of the sample solution and standard solution as directed under Liquid Chromatography <*2.01*> according to the following conditions, and calculate the ratios, Q_T and Q_S, of the peak area of pitavastatin to that of the internal standard.

Amount (mg) of pitavastatin calcium ($C_{50}H_{46}CaF_2N_2O_8$)
$= M_S \times Q_T/Q_S \times 1/2 \times 0.812$

M_S: Amount (mg) of Pitavastatin Methylbenzylamine RS taken, calculated on the anhydrous basis

Internal standard solution—A solution of butyl parahydroxybenzoate in a mixture of acetonitrile and water (3:2) (3 in 10,000).

Operating conditions—

Detector: An ultraviolet absorption photometer (wavelength: 245 nm).

Column: A stainless steel column 4.6 mm in inside diameter and 15 cm in length, packed with octadecylsilanized silica gel for liquid chromatography (3 μm in particle diameter).

Column temperature: A constant temperature of about 40°C.

Mobile phase: To 10 mL of dilute acetic acid add water to make 1000 mL. To 350 mL of this solution add 650 mL of methanol, and dissolve 0.29 g of sodium chloride in this solution.

Flow rate: Adjust so that the retention time of pitavastatin is about 5 minutes.

System suitability—

System performance: When the procedure is run with 10 μL of the standard solution under the above operating conditions, the internal standard and pitavastatin are eluted in this order with the resolution between these peaks being not less than 2.0.

System repeatability: When the test is repeated 6 times with 10 μL of the standard solution under the above operating conditions, the relative standard deviation of the ratio of the peak area of pitavastatin to that of the internal standard is not more than 1.0%.

Containers and storage Containers—Tight containers.

Storage—Light-resistant.

Others

Related substance A: Refer to it described in Pitavastatin Calcium Hydrate.

Related substance TA:

6-{2-[2-cyclopropyl-4-(4-fluorophenyl)quinolin-3-yl]ethenyl}-4-hydroxyoxane-2-one

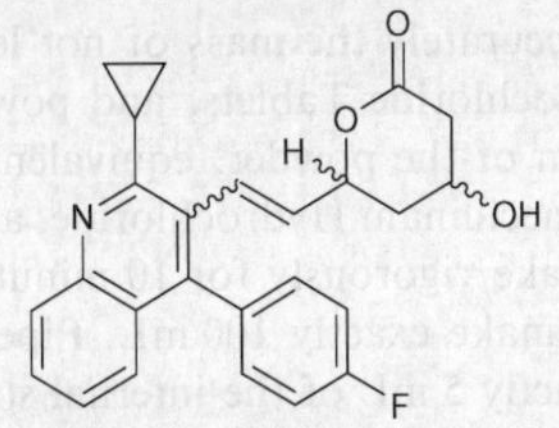

Pivmecillinam Hydrochloride

ピブメシリナム塩酸塩

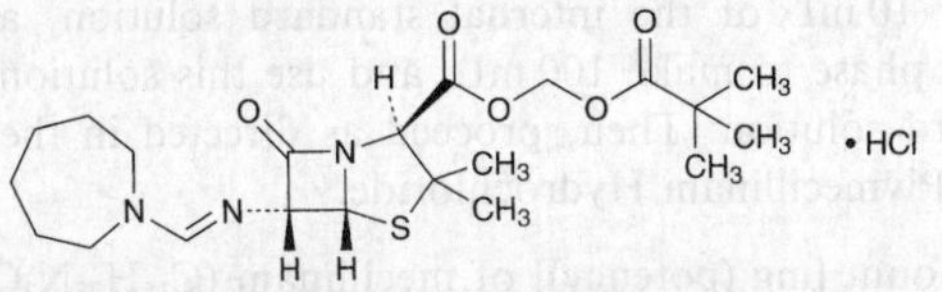

$C_{21}H_{33}N_3O_5S.HCl$: 476.03

2,2-Dimethylpropanoyloxymethyl (2*S*,5*R*,6*R*)-6-[(azepan-1-ylmethylene)amino]-3,3-dimethyl-7-oxo-4-thia-1-azabicyclo[3.2.0]heptane-2-carboxylate monohydrochloride
[*32887-03-9*]

Pivmecillinam Hydrochloride contains not less than 630 μg (potency) and not more than 710 μg (potency) per mg, calculated on the anhydrous basis. The potency of Pivmecillinam Hydrochloride is expressed as mass (potency) of mecillinam ($C_{15}H_{23}N_3O_3S$: 325.43).

Description Pivmecillinam Hydrochloride occurs as a white to yellowish white crystalline powder.

It is very soluble in methanol and in acetic acid (100), freely soluble in water and in ethanol (99.5), and soluble in acetonitrile.

Identification **(1)** Determine the infrared absorption spectrum of Pivmecillinam Hydrochloride as directed in the potassium bromide disk method under Infrared Spectrophotometry *<2.25>*, and compare the spectrum with the Reference Spectrum or the spectrum of Pivmecillinam Hydrochloride RS: both spectra exhibit similar intensities of absorption at the same wave numbers.

(2) Dissolve 0.5 g of Pivmecillinam Hydrochloride in 10 mL of water, and add 1 mL of dilute nitric acid and 1 drop of silver nitrate TS: a white precipitate is formed.

Optical rotation *<2.49>* $[\alpha]_D^{20}$: +200 – +220° (1 g calculated on the anhydrous basis, water, 100 mL, 100 mm).

Purity **(1)** Heavy metals *<1.07>*—To 1.0 g of Pivmecillinam Hydrochloride in a crucible add 10 mL of a solution of magnesium nitrate hexahydrate in ethanol (95) (1 in 10), fire the ethanol to burn, and heat gradually to incinerate. If a carbonized substance remains, moisten with a small amount of nitric acid, and ignite to incinerate. Cool, add 3 mL of hydrochloric acid to the residue, dissolve by warming on a water bath, and heat to dryness. To the residue add 10 mL of water, and dissolve by warming on a water bath. After cooling, adjust the pH to 3 to 4 with ammonia TS, add 2 mL of dilute acetic acid, filter if necessary, and wash the crucible and the filter with 10 mL of water. Put the filtrate and the washings to a Nessler tube, add water to make 50 mL, and use this solution as the test solution. Prepare the control solution in the same manner as the test solution with 2.0 mL of Standard Lead Solution (not more than 20 ppm).

(2) Arsenic *<1.11>*—Prepare the test solution with 1.0 g of Pivmecillinam Hydrochloride according to Method 4, and perform the test (not more than 2 ppm).

(3) Related substances—Dissolve 50 mg of Pivmecillinam Hydrochloride in 4.0 mL of a mixture of acetonitrile and acetic acid (100) (97:3), and use this solution as the sample solution. Separately, dissolve 2.0 mg of Pivmecillinam Hydrochloride RS in 4.0 mL of water, and use this solution as the standard solution. Perform the test with these solutions as directed under Thin-layer Chromatography *<2.03>*. Spot 2 μL of the standard solution on a plate of silica gel for thin-layer chromatography, allow to stand for 30 minutes, then spot 2 μL of the sample solution on the plate. Immediately, develop the plate with a mixture of acetone, water and acetic acid (100) (10:1:1) to a distance of about 12 cm, and air-dry the plate. Allow the plate to stand for 10 minutes in iodine vapor: the spot obtained from the sample solution appeared at the position corresponding to the spot from the standard solution is not larger and not more intense than the spot from the standard solution, and any spot other than the principal spot and the above spot from the sample solution is not observable.

Water *<2.48>* Not more than 1.0% (0.25 g, coulometric titration).

Assay Weigh accurately an amount of Pivmecillinam Hydrochloride and Pivmecillinam Hydrochloride RS, equivalent to about 20 mg (potency), dissolve in a suitable amount of the mobile phase, add exactly 10 mL of the internal standard solution and the mobile phase to make 100 mL, and use these solutions as the sample solution and the standard solution, respectively. Perform the test with 10 μL each of the sample solution and standard solution as directed under Liquid Chromatography *<2.01>* according to the following conditions, and calculate the ratios, Q_T and Q_S, of the peak area of pivmecillinam to that of the internal standard.

$$\text{Amount [}\mu\text{g (potency)] of mecillinam } (C_{15}H_{23}N_3O_3S) = M_S \times Q_T/Q_S \times 1000$$

M_S: Amount [mg (potency)] of Pivmecillinam Hydrochloride RS taken

Internal standard solution—A solution of diphenyl in the mobile phase (1 in 12,500).

Operating conditions—

Detector: An ultraviolet absorption photometer (wavelength: 254 nm).

Column: A stainless steel column 4 mm in inside diameter and 30 cm in length, packed with octadecylsilanized silica gel for liquid chromatography (10 μm in particle diameter).

Column temperature: A constant temperature of about 25°C.

Mobile phase: Dissolve 0.771 g of ammonium acetate in about 900 mL of water, adjust the pH to 3.5 with acetic acid (100), and add water to make 1000 mL. To 400 mL of this solution add 600 mL of acetonitrile.

Flow rate: Adjust so that the retention time of pivmecillinam is about 6.5 minutes.

System suitability—

System performance: When the procedure is run with 10 μL of the standard solution under the above operating conditions, pivmecillinam and the internal standard are eluted in this order with the resolution between these peaks being not less than 4.

System repeatability: When the test is repeated 6 times with 10 μL of the standard solution under the above operat-

ing conditions, the relative standard deviation of the ratios of the peak area of pivmecillinam to that of the internal standard is not more than 1.0%.

Containers and storage Containers—Tight containers.

Pivmecillinam Hydrochloride Tablets

ピブメシリナム塩酸塩錠

Pivmecillinam Hydrochloride Tablets contain not less than 93.0% and not more than 107.0% of the labeled potency of mecillinam ($C_{15}H_{23}N_3O_3S$: 325.43).

Method of preparation Prepare as directed under Tablets, with Pivmecillinam Hydrochloride.

Identification Powder Pivmecillinam Hydrochloride Tablets, dissolve a portion of the powder, equivalent to 35 mg (potency) of Pivmecillinam Hydrochloride, in 4 mL of a mixture of acetonitrile and acetic acid (100) (97:3), and filter through a membrane filter with a pore size not exceeding 0.45 μm. Discard the first 2 mL of the filtrate, and use the subsequent filtrate as the sample solution. Separately dissolve 25 mg of Pivmecillinam Hydrochloride RS in 2 mL of a mixture of acetonitrile and acetic acid (100) (97:3), and use this solution as the standard solution. Perform the test with these solutions as directed under Thin-layer Chromatography <2.03>. Spot 2 μL each of the sample solution and standard solution on a plate of silica gel for thin-layer chromatography, and immediately develop the plate with a mixture of acetone, water and acetic acid (100) (10:1:1) to a distance of about 12 cm, and air-dry the plate. Allow the plate to stand in iodine vapor for 10 minutes: the principal spot obtained from the sample solution has the same *Rf* value as the spot from the standard solution.

Water <2.48> Not more than 3.0% (1 g of powdered Pivmecillinam Hydrochloride Tablets, volumetric titration, direct titration).

Uniformity of dosage units <6.02> Perform the test according to the following method: it meets the requirement of the Content uniformity test.

To 1 tablet of Pivmecillinam Hydrochloride Tablets add 40 mL of the mobile phase, shake vigorously for 10 minutes, and add the mobile phase to make exactly 50 mL. Pipet *V* mL, equivalent to about 10 mg (potency) of Pivmecillinam Hydrochloride, add exactly 5 mL of the internal standard solution and the mobile phase to make 50 mL, filter through a membrane filter with a pore size not exceeding 0.45 μm, discard the first 10 mL of the filtrate, and use the subsequent filtrate as the sample solution. Separately, weigh accurately an amount of Pivmecillinam Hydrochloride RS, equivalent to about 20 mg (potency), dissolve in the mobile phase, add exactly 10 mL of the internal standard solution, add the mobile phase to make 100 mL, and use this solution as the standard solution. Then, proceed as directed in the Assay under Pivmecillinam Hydrochloride.

Amount [mg (potency)] of mecillinam ($C_{15}H_{23}N_3O_3S$)
$= M_S \times Q_T/Q_S \times 25/V$

M_S: Amount [mg (potency)] of Pivmecillinam Hydrochloride RS taken

Internal standard solution—A solution of diphenyl in the mobile phase (1 in 12,500).

Disintegration <6.09> Perform the test using the disk: it meets the requirement.

Assay Weigh accurately the mass of not less than 20 Pivmecillinam Hydrochloride Tablets, and powder. Weigh accurately a portion of the powder, equivalent to about 0.1 g (potency) of Pivmecillinam Hydrochloride, add 50 mL of the mobile phase, shake vigorously for 10 minutes, and add the mobile phase to make exactly 100 mL. Pipet 10 mL of this solution, add exactly 5 mL of the internal standard solution and the mobile phase to make 50 mL, filter through a membrane filter with a pore size not exceeding 0.45 μm, discard the first 10 mL of the filtrate, and use the subsequent filtrate as the sample solution. Separately, weigh accurately an amount of Pivmecillinam Hydrochloride RS, equivalent to about 20 mg (potency), dissolve in the mobile phase, add exactly 10 mL of the internal standard solution, add the mobile phase to make 100 mL, and use this solution as the standard solution. Then, proceed as directed in the Assay under Pivmecillinam Hydrochloride.

Amount [mg (potency)] of mecillinam ($C_{15}H_{23}N_3O_3S$)
$= M_S \times Q_T/Q_S \times 5$

M_S: Amount [mg (potency)] of Pivmecillinam Hydrochloride RS taken

Internal standard solution—A solution of diphenyl in the mobile phase (1 in 12,500).

Containers and storage Containers—Tight containers.

Polaprezinc

ポラプレジンク

$(C_9H_{12}N_4O_3Zn)_n$
catena-Poly{zinc-μ-[β-alanyl-L-histidinato(2-)-$N,N^N,O:N^\tau$]}
[*107667-60-7*]

Polaprezinc contains not less than 98.0% and not more than 102.0% of polaprezinc ($C_9H_{12}N_4O_3Zn$: 289.60), and contains not less than 21.5% and not more than 23.0% of zinc (Zn: 65.38), calculated on the anhydrous basis.

Description Polaprezinc occurs as a white to pale yellowwhite crystalline powder.

It is practically insoluble in water, in methanol and in ethanol (99.5).

It dissolves in dilute hydrochloric acid.

Identification **(1)** To 2 mL of a solution of Polaprezinc in 0.2 mol/L hydrochloric acid TS (1 in 1000) add 0.5 mL of a solution of sulfanilic acid in 1 mol/L hydrochloric acid TS (1 in 200), 0.5 mL of a solution of sodium nitrite (1 in 20) and 3 mL of sodium carbonate TS: a red color is produced.

(2) A solution of Polaprezinc in 0.2 mol/L hydrochloric acid TS (1 in 1000) responds to Qualitative Tests <1.09> for zinc salt.

(3) Determine the infrared absorption spectrum of Polaprezinc as directed in the potassium bromide disk method under Infrared Spectrophotometry <2.25>, and compare the spectrum with the Reference Spectrum: both spectra exhibit similar intensities of absorption at the same wave numbers.

Optical rotation *<2.49>* $[\alpha]_D^{20}$: +8 – +9° (1 g calculated on the anhydrous basis, 3 mol/L hydrochloric acid TS, 50 mL, 100 mm).

Purity **(1)** Lead—Weigh accurately about 0.5 g of Polaprezinc, dissolve in 3 mL of dilute nitric acid, add water to make exactly 10 mL, and use this solution as the sample solution. Separately, pipet 0.5 mL, 1.0 mL, 1.5 mL and 2.0 mL of Standard Lead Solution, to each solution add 3 mL of dilute nitric acid and water to make exactly 10 mL, and use these solutions as the standard solutions. Perform the test with the sample solution and standard solutions as directed under Atomic Absorption Spectrophotometry *<2.23>* according to the following conditions, and calculate the amount of lead in the sample solution using a calibration curve obtained from the absorbances of the standard solutions: not more than 10 ppm.

Gas: Combustible gas—Acetylene.
Supporting gas—Air.
Lamp: Lead hollow-cathode lamp.
Wavelength: 283.3 nm.

(2) Related substances—Dissolve 50 mg of Polaprezinc in 10 mL of 0.1 mol/L hydrochloric acid TS, add the mobile phase to make 100 mL, and use this solution as the sample solution. Pipet 1 mL of the sample solution, add the mobile phase to make exactly 100 mL, and use this solution as the standard solution. Perform the test with exactly 10 μL each of the sample solution and standard solution as directed under Liquid Chromatography *<2.01>* according to the following conditions. Determine each peak area by the automatic integration method: the peak area of L-histidine, having the relative retention time of about 0.38 to L-carnosine, obtained from the sample solution is not larger than 1/5 times of the peak area of L-carnosine from the standard solution, the area of the peak other than L-carnosine and the peak mentioned above from the sample solution is not larger than 1/10 times of the peak area of L-carnosine from the standard solution. Furthermore, the total area of the peaks other than L-carnosine from the sample solution is not larger than the peak area of L-carnosine from the standard solution.

Operating conditions—

Detector, column, column temperature, mobile phase, and flow rate: Proceed as directed in the operating conditions in the Assay.

Time span of measurement: About 4 times as long as the retention time of L-carnosine, beginning after the solvent peak.

System suitability—

Test for required detectability: Pipet 2 mL of the standard solution, add the mobile phase to make exactly 20 mL. Confirm that the peak area of L-carnosine obtained with 10 μL of this solution is equivalent to 7 to 13% of that with 10 μL of the standard solution.

System performance: Dissolve 50 mg each of Polaprezinc and L-histidine in 10 mL of 0.1 mol/L hydrochloric acid TS, and add the mobile phase to make 100 mL. When the procedure is run with 10 μL of this solution under the above operating conditions, L-histidine and L-carnosine are eluted in this order with the resolution between these peaks being not less than 12.

System repeatability: When the test is repeated 6 times with 10 μL of the standard solution under the above operating conditions, the relative standard deviation of the peak area of L-carnosine is not more than 2.0%.

Water *<2.48>* Not more than 5.0% (0.2 g, volumetric titration, direct titration, stir for 30 minutes).

Assay **(1)** Polaprezinc—Weigh accurately about 25 mg of Polaprezinc, dissolve in 5 mL of 0.1 mol/L hydrochloric acid TS, add the mobile phase to make exactly 100 mL, and use this solution as the sample solution. Separately, weigh accurately about 20 mg of L-Carnosine RS, previously dried at 105°C for 3 hours, dissolve in 5 mL of 0.1 mol/L hydrochloric acid TS, add the mobile phase to make exactly 100 mL, and use this solution as the standard solution. Perform the test with exactly 10 μL each of the sample solution and standard solution as directed under Liquid Chromatography *<2.01>* according to the following conditions. Determine the peak areas, A_T and A_S, of L-carnosine in each solution.

$$\text{Amount (mg) of polaprezinc } (C_9H_{12}N_4O_3Zn) = M_S \times A_T/A_S \times 1.292$$

M_S: Amount (mg) of L-Carnosine RS taken

Operating conditions—

Detector: An ultraviolet absorption photometer (wavelength: 210 nm).

Column: A stainless steel column 4.6 mm in inside diameter and 15 cm in length, packed with octadecylsilanized silica gel for liquid chromatography (5 μm in particle diameter).

Column temperature: A constant temperature of about 45°C.

Mobile phase: Dissolve 1.4 g of potassium dihydrogen phosphate in 1000 mL of water, adjust to pH 3.5 with diluted phosphoric acid (1 in 100). Dissolve 2 g of sodium 1-octane sulfonate in 900 mL of this solution, and add 100 mL of acetonitrile for liquid chromatography.

Flow rate: Adjust so that the retention time of L-carnosine is about 15 minutes.

System suitability—

System performance: Dissolve 5 mg of L-histidine in 20 mL of the standard solution. When the procedure is run with 10 μL of this solution under the above operating conditions, L-histidine and L-carnosine are eluted in this order with the resolution between these peaks being not less than 12.

System repeatability: When the test is repeated 6 times with 10 μL of the standard solution under the above operating conditions, the relative standard deviation of the peak area of L-carnosine is not more than 1.0%.

(2) Zinc—Weigh accurately about 0.2 g of Polaprezinc, dissolve in 3 mL of dilute hydrochloric acid, and add water to make exactly 100 mL. Pipet 25 mL of this solution, add 10 mL of ammonia-ammonium chloride buffer solution (pH 10.7), and titrate *<2.50>* with 0.01 mol/L disodium dihydrogen ethylenediamine tetraacetate VS (indicator: 40 mg of eriochrome black T-sodium chloride indicator).

Each mL of 0.01 mol/L disodium dihydrogen ethylenediamine tetraacetate VS
= 0.6538 mg Zn

Containers and storage Containers—Tight containers.

Polaprezinc Granules

ポラプレジンク顆粒

Polaprezinc Granules contain not less than 95.0% and not more than 105.0% of the labeled amount of polaprezinc [$(C_9H_{12}N_4O_3Zn)_n$].

Method of preparation Prepare as directed under Granules, with Polaprezinc.

Identification **(1)** To a quantity of Polaprezinc Granules, equivalent to 20 mg of Polaprezinc, add 20 mL of 0.2 mol/L hydrochloric acid TS, shake for 10 minutes, centrifuge, and use the supernatant liquid as the sample solution. To 2 mL of the sample solution add 0.5 mL of a solution of sulfanilic acid in 1 mol/L hydrochloric acid TS (1 in 200), 0.5 mL of a solution of sodium nitrite (1 in 20) and 3 mL of sodium carbonate TS: a red color develops.

(2) The sample solution obtained in (1) responds to Qualitative Tests <*1.09*> for zinc salt.

Uniformity of dosage units <*6.02*> Perform the test according to the following method: Polaprezinc Granules in single-dose packages meet the requirement of the Content uniformity test.

To the total content of 1 package of Polaprezinc Granules add exactly *V* mL of 0.2 mol/L hydrochloric acid TS so that each mL contains about 5 mg of polaprezinc [$(C_9H_{12}N_4O_3Zn)_n$], shake vigorously for 10 minutes, and centrifuge. Pipet 5 mL of the supernatant liquid, add exactly 5 mL of the internal standard solution, add the mobile phase to make 50 mL, and use this solution as the sample solution. Then, proceed as directed in the Assay.

Amount (mg) of polaprezinc [$(C_9H_{12}N_4O_3Zn)_n$]
$= M_S \times Q_T/Q_S \times V/5 \times 1.292$

M_S: Amount (mg) of L-Carnosine RS taken

Dissolution <*6.10*> When the test is performed at 50 revolutions per minute according to the Paddle method, using 900 mL of 0.05 mol/L acetic acid-sodium acetate buffer solution (pH 4.0) as the dissolution medium, the dissolution rate in 15 minutes of Polaprezinc Granules is not less than 80%.

Start the test with an accurately weighed amount of Polaprezinc Granules, equivalent to about 75 mg of polaprezinc [$(C_9H_{12}N_4O_3Zn)_n$], withdraw not less than 20 mL of the medium at the specified minute after starting the test, and filter through a membrane filter with a pore size not exceeding 0.45 μm. Discard not less than 10 mL of the first filtrate, pipet 1 mL of the subsequent filtrate, add diluted nitric acid (77 in 10,000) to make exactly 25 mL, and use this solution as the sample solution. Separately, pipet suitable volumes of Standard Zinc Stock Solution, to each solution add diluted nitric acid (77 in 10,000) so that each mL contains 0.4 to 0.8 μg of zinc (Zn: 65.38), and use these solutions as the standard solutions. Perform the test with the sample solution and standard solutions as directed under Atomic Absorption Spectrophotometry <*2.23*> according to the following conditions, and calculate the amount of zinc in the sample solution using a calibration curve obtained from the absorbances of the standard solutions.

Dissolution rate (%) with respect to the labeled amount of polaprezinc [$(C_9H_{12}N_4O_3Zn)_n$]
= Content (μg/mL) of zinc in the sample solution/M_T $\times 1/C \times 2250 \times 4.429$

M_T: Amount (g) of Polaprezinc Granules taken
C: Labeled amount (mg) of polaprezinc [$(C_9H_{12}N_4O_3Zn)_n$] in 1 g

Gas: Combustible gas—Acetylene.
Supporting gas—Air.
Lamp: Zinc hollow-cathode lamp.
Wavelength: 213.9 nm.

Assay Weigh accurately an amount of Polaprezinc Granules, equivalent to about 0.1 g of polaprezinc [$(C_9H_{12}N_4O_3Zn)_n$], add exactly 20 mL of 0.2 mol/L hydrochloric acid TS, shake vigorously for 10 minutes, and centrifuge. Pipet 5 mL of the supernatant liquid, add exactly 5 mL of the internal standard solution, add the mobile phase to make 50 mL, and use this solution as the sample solution. Separately, weigh accurately about 20 mg of L-Carnosine RS, previously dried at 105°C for 3 hours, dissolve in 5 mL of 0.2 mol/L hydrochloric acid TS, add exactly 5 mL of the internal standard solution, add the mobile phase to make 50 mL, and use this solution as the standard solution. Perform the test with 5 μL each of the sample solution and standard solution as directed under Liquid Chromatography <*2.01*> according to the following conditions, and calculate the ratios, Q_T and Q_S, of the peak area of L-carnosine to that of the internal standard.

Amount (mg) of polaprezinc [$(C_9H_{12}N_4O_3Zn)_n$]
$= M_S \times Q_T/Q_S \times 4 \times 1.292$

M_S: Amount (mg) of L-Carnosine RS taken

Internal standard solution—Dissolve 0.25 g of 4-aminoacetophenone in 5 mL of acetonitrile, and add the mobile phase to make 100 mL.

Operating conditions—

Proceed as directed in the operating conditions in the Assay (1) under Polaprezinc.

System suitability—

System performance: When the procedure is run with 5 μL of the standard solution under the above operating conditions, 4-aminoacetophenone and L-carnosine are eluted in this order with the resolution between these peaks being not less than 6.

System repeatability: When the test is repeated 6 times with 5 μL of the standard solution under the above operating conditions, the relative standard deviation of the ratio of the peak area of L-carnosine to that of the internal standard is not more than 1.0%.

Containers and storage Containers—Tight containers.

Polymixin B Sulfate

ポリミキシンB硫酸塩

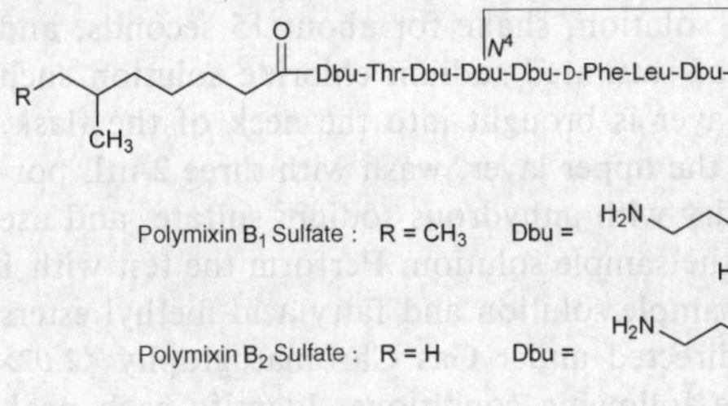

Polymixin B_1 Sulfate $C_{56}H_{98}N_{16}O_{13}.xH_2SO_4$
Polymixin B_2 Sulfate $C_{55}H_{96}N_{16}O_{13}.xH_2SO_4$

Polymixin B Sulfate is the sulfate of a mixture of peptide substances having antibacterial activity produced by the growth of *Bacillus polymyxa*.

It contains not less than 6500 units and not more than 10,500 units per mg, calculated on the dried basis. The potency of Polymixin B Sulfate is expressed as mass unit of polymixin B ($C_{55-56}H_{96-98}N_{16}O_{13}$). One unit of Polymixin B Sulfate is equivalent to 0.129 μg of polymixin B sulfate ($C_{55-56}H_{96-98}N_{16}O_{13}.1-2H_2SO_4$).

Description Polymixin B Sulfate occurs as a white powder.

It is freely soluble in water, and practically insoluble in ethanol (99.5).

Identification **(1)** To 5 mL of a solution of Polymixin B Sulfate (1 in 10) add 5 mL of a solution of sodium hydroxide (1 in 10), add 5 drops of a solution of copper (II) sulfate pentahydrate (1 in 100) while shaking: a purple color develops.

(2) Transfer 5 mg each of Polymixin B Sulfate and Polymixin B Sulfate RS separately into two glass stoppered test tubes, add 1 mL of diluted hydrochloric acid (1 in 2), stopper the tube, heat at 135°C for 5 hours, then heat to dryness on a water bath, and keep the heating until no more hydrochloric acid odor is evolved. Dissolve the residue in 0.5 mL of water, and use these solutions as the sample solution and standard solution (1). Separately, dissolve 20 mg each of L-leucine, L-threonine, phenylalanine and L-serine separately in 10 mL of water, and use these solutions as the standard solutions (2), (3), (4) and (5), respectively. Perform the test with these solutions as directed under Thin-layer Chromatography <*2.03*>. Spot 3 μL each of the sample solution, the standard solutions (1), (2), (3), (4) and (5) on a plate of silica gel for thin-layer chromatography, and expose the plate to a saturated vapor of the developing solvent for 15 hours. Develop the plate with a mixture of phenol and water (3:1) to a distance of about 13 cm while without exposure to light, and dry the plate at 110°C for 5 minutes. Spray evenly ninhydrin-acetic acid TS on the plate, and heat at 110°C for 5 minutes: *R*f value of each spot obtained from the sample solution is the same with *R*f value of the corresponding spots from the standard solution (1). Each of the spots from the sample solution appears at the position corresponding to each of the spots from the standard solutions (2), (3) and (4), but not appears at the position corresponding to the spot from the standard solution (5).

(3) A solution of Polymixin B Sulfate (1 in 20) responds to Qualitative Tests <*1.09*> for sulfate.

Optical rotation <*2.49*> $[\alpha]_D^{20}$: −78 – −90° (0.5 g calculated on the dried basis, water, 25 mL, 100 mm).

pH <*2.54*> The pH of a solution obtained by dissolving 1.0 g of Polymixin B Sulfate in 50 mL of water is between 5.0 and 7.0.

Phenylalanine Weigh accurately about 0.375 g of Polymixin B Sulfate, dissolve in 0.1 mol/L hydrochloric acid VS to make exactly 100 mL. Determine absorbances, A_1, A_2, A_3, A_4 and A_5, of this solution at 252 nm, at 258 nm, at 264 nm, at 280 nm and at 300 nm, respectively, as directed under Ultraviolet-visible Spectrophotometry <*2.24*>, and calculate the amount of phenylalanine by the following equation: the amount of phenylalanine is not less than 9.0% and not more than 12.0%.

Amount (%) of phenylalanine

$$= (A_2 - 0.5A_1 + 0.5A_3 - 1.8A_4 + 0.8A_5)/M_T \times 9.4787$$

M_T: Amount (g) of Polymixin B Sulfate taken, calculated on the dried basis

Purity Heavy metals <*1.07*>—Proceed with 1.0 g of Polymixin B Sulfate according to Method 2, and perform the test. Prepare the control solution with 2.0 mL of Standard Lead Solution (not more than 20 ppm).

Loss on drying <*2.41*> Not more than 6.0% (1 g, in vacuum, 60°C, 3 hours).

Residue on ignition <*2.44*> Not more than 0.75% (1 g).

Assay Perform the test according to the Cylinder-plate method as directed under Microbial Assay for Antibiotics <*4.02*> according to the following conditions.

(i) Test organism—*Escherichia coli* NIHJ

(ii) Agar media for seed and base layer

Peptone	10.0 g
Meat extract	3.0 g
Sodium chloride	30.0 g
Agar	20.0 g
Water	1000 mL

Mix all the ingredients, and sterilize. Adjust the pH <*2.54*> of the solution so that it will be 6.5 to 6.6 after sterilization.

(iii) Standard solutions—Weigh accurately an amount of Polymixin B Sulfate RS, equivalent to about 200,000 units, dissolve in phosphate buffer solution (pH 6.0) to make exactly 20 mL, and use this solution as the standard stock solution. Keep the standard stock solution at not exceeding 5°C and use within 14 days. Take exactly a suitable amount of the standard stock solution before use, add phosphate buffer solution (pH 6.0) to make solutions so that each mL contains 4000 units and 1000 units, and use these solutions as the high concentration standard solution and the low concentration standard solution, respectively.

(iv) Sample solutions—Weigh accurately an amount of Polymixin B Sulfate, equivalent to about 200,000 units, and dissolve in phosphate buffer solution (pH 6.0) to make exactly 20 mL. Take exactly a suitable amount of this solution, add phosphate buffer solution (pH 6.0) to make solutions so that each mL contains 4000 units and 1000 units, and use these solutions as the high concentration sample solution and the low concentration sample solution, respectively.

Containers and storage Containers—Tight containers.

Storage—Light-resistant.

Polyoxyl 40 Stearate

ステアリン酸ポリオキシル 40

Polyoxyl 40 Stearate is the monostearate of condensation polymers of ethylene oxide represented by the formula $H(OCH_2CH_2)_nOCOC_{17}H_{35}$, in which n is approximately 40.

Description Polyoxyl 40 Stearate occurs as a white to light yellow, waxy solid or powder. It is odorless or has a faint fat-like odor.

It is soluble in water, in ethanol (95) and in diethyl ether.

Congealing point <*2.42*> 39.0 – 44.0°C

Congealing point of the fatty acid <*1.13*> Not below 53°C.

Acid value <*1.13*> Not more than 1.

Saponification value <*1.13*> 25 – 35

Purity **(1)** Clarity and color of solution—Dissolve 1.0 g of Polyoxyl 40 Stearate in 20 mL of water: the solution is clear and colorless.

(2) Heavy metals <*1.07*>—Proceed with 2.0 g of Polyoxyl 40 Stearate according to Method 2, and perform the test. Prepare the control solution with 2.0 mL of Standard Lead Solution (not more than 10 ppm).

(3) Arsenic <*1.11*>—Prepare the test solution with 0.67 g of Polyoxyl 40 Stearate, according to Method 3, and perform the test (not more than 3 ppm).

Residue on ignition <*2.44*> Not more than 0.1% (1 g).

Containers and storage Containers—Tight containers.

Polysorbate 80

ポリソルベート 80

This monograph is harmonized with the European Pharmacopoeia and the U.S. Pharmacopeia.

The parts of the text that are not harmonized are marked with symbols (◆ ◆).

Information on the harmonization with the European Pharmacopoeia and the U.S. Pharmacopeia is available on the website of the Pharmaceuticals and Medical Devices Agency.

Polysorbate 80 is a mixture of partial esters of fatty acids, mainly oleic acid, with sorbitol and its anhydrides ethoxylated with approximately 20 moles of ethylene oxide for each mole of sorbitol and sorbitol anhydrides.

◆**Description** Polysorbate 80 is a colorless or brownish yellow, clear or slightly opalescent, oily liquid.

It is miscible with water, with methanol, with ethanol (99.5) and with ethyl acetate.

It is practically insoluble in fatty oils and in liquid paraffin.

Viscosity: about 400 mPa·s (25°C).

Specific gravity d^{20}_{20}: about 1.10◆

Identification It meets the requirements of the Composition of fatty acids.

Composition of fatty acids Dissolve 0.10 g of Polysorbate 80 in 2 mL of a solution of sodium hydroxide in methanol (1 in 50) in a 25-mL conical flask, and boil under a reflux condenser for 30 minutes. Add 2.0 mL of boron trifluoride-methanol TS through the condenser, and boil for 30 minutes. Add 4 mL of heptane through the condenser, and boil for 5 minutes. After cooling, add 10.0 mL of saturated sodium chloride solution, shake for about 15 seconds, and add a quantity of saturated sodium chloride solution such that the upper layer is brought into the neck of the flask. Collect 2 mL of the upper layer, wash with three 2-mL portions of water, dry with anhydrous sodium sulfate, and use this solution as the sample solution. Perform the test with 1 μL each of the sample solution and fatty acid methyl esters mixture TS as directed under Gas Chromatography <*2.02*> according to the following conditions. Identify each peak obtained with the sample solution using the chromatogram with fatty acid methyl esters mixture TS. Determine each peak area with the sample solution by the automatic integration method, and calculate the composition of fatty acids by the area percentage method: myristic acid is not more than 5.0%, palmitic acid is not more than 16.0%, palmitoleic acid is not more than 8.0%, stearic acid is not more than 6.0%, oleic acid is not less than 58.0%, linoleic acid is not more than 18.0% and linolenic acid is not more than 4.0%.

Operating conditions—

Detector: A hydrogen flame-ionization detector.

Column: A fused silica column 0.32 mm in inside diameter and 30 m in length, coated with polyethylene glycol 20 M for gas chromatography 0.5 μm in thickness.

Column temperature: Inject at a constant temperature of about 80°C, raise the temperature to 220°C at a rate of 10°C per minute, and maintain at 220°C for 40 minutes.

Injection port temperature: A constant temperature of about 250°C.

Detector temperature: A constant temperature of about 250°C.

Carrier gas: Helium.

Flow rate: 50 cm per second.

Split ratio: 1: 50.

System suitability—

Test for required detectability: Dissolve 0.50 g of the mixture of fatty acid methyl esters described in the following table in heptane to make exactly 50 mL, and use this solution as the solution for system suitability test. Pipet 1 mL of the solution for system suitability test add heptane to make exactly 10 mL. When the procedure is run with 1 μL of this solution under the above operating conditions, the SN ratio of methyl myristate is not less than 5.

Mixture of fatty acid methyl esters	Composition (%)
Methyl myristate for gas chromatography	5
Methyl palmitate for gas chromatography	10
Methyl stearate for gas chromatography	15
Methyl arachidate for gas chromatography	20
Methyl oleate for gas chromatography	20
Methyl eicosenoate for gas chromatography	10
Methyl behenate	10
Methyl lignocerate for gas chromatography	10

System performance: When the procedure is run with 1 μL of the solution for system suitability test under the above operating conditions, ◆methyl stearate and methyl oleate are eluted in this order,◆ the resolution between these peaks is not less than 1.8, and the number of theoretical plates of the peak of methyl stearate is not less than 30,000.

◆**Acid value** ⟨*1.13*⟩ Not more than 2.0 (using ethanol (95) instead).◆

Saponification value Introduce about 4 g of Polysorbate 80, accurately weighed, into a 250-mL borosilicate glass flask. Add exactly 30 mL of 0.5 mol/L potassium hydroxide-ethanol VS and a few glass beads. Attach a reflux condenser, and heat for 60 minutes. Add 1 mL of phenolphthalein TS and 50 mL of ethanol (99.5), and titrate ⟨*2.50*⟩ immediately with 0.5 mol/L hydrochloric acid VS. Perform a blank determination in the same manner. Calculate the saponification value by the following equation: 45 – 55.

$$\text{Saponification value} = (a - b) \times 28.05/M$$

M: Amount (g) of Polysorbate 80 taken
a: Volume (mL) of 0.5 mol/L hydrochloric acid VS required for blank determination
b: Volume (mL) of 0.5 mol/L hydrochloric acid VS required for sample determination

Hydroxyl value Introduce about 2 g of Polysorbate 80, accurately weighed, into a 150-mL round bottom flask, add exactly 5 mL of acetic anhydride-pyridine TS, and attach an air condenser. Heat the flask in a water bath for 1 hour keeping the level of the water about 2.5 cm above the level of the liquid in the flask. Withdraw the flask and allow to cool. Add 5 mL of water through the condenser. If a cloudiness appears add sufficient pyridine to clear it, noting the volume added. Shake the flask, and heat in the water bath for 10 minutes. Withdraw the flask and allow to cool. Rinse the condenser and the walls of the flask with 5 mL of neutralized ethanol, and titrate ⟨*2.50*⟩ with 0.5 mol/L potassium hydroxide-ethanol VS (indicator: 0.2 mL of phenolphthalein TS). Perform a blank determination in the same manner. Calculate the hydroxyl value by the following equation: 65 – 80.

$$\text{Hydroxyl value} = (a - b) \times 28.05/M + \text{acid value}$$

M: Amount (g) of Polysorbate 80 taken
a: Volume (mL) of 0.5 mol/L potassium hydroxide-ethanol VS required for blank determination
b: Volume (mL) of 0.5 mol/L potassium hydroxide-ethanol VS required for sample determination

Purity ◆**(1)** Heavy metals ⟨*1.07*⟩—Proceed with 1.0 g of Polysorbate 80 according to Method 2, and perform the test. Prepare the control solution with 2.0 mL of Standard Lead Solution (not more than 20 ppm).◆

(2) Ethylene oxide and 1,4-dioxane—Transfer exactly 1.00 g of Polysorbate 80 into a 10-mL headspace vial, add exactly 2 mL of water, seal the vial immediately with a septum of silicon rubber coated the surface with fluororesin and an aluminum cap. Mix carefully, and use the content as the sample solution. Separately, pipet 0.5 mL of a solution, prepared by dissolving ethylene oxide in dichloromethane so that each mL contains 50 mg, and add water to make exactly 50 mL. Allow to stand to reach room temperature. Pipet 1 mL of this solution, add water to make exactly 250 mL, and use this solution as ethylene oxide stock solution. Separately, pipet 1 mL of 1,4-dioxane, add water to make exactly 200 mL. Pipet 1 mL of this solution, add water to make exactly 100 mL, and use this solution as 1,4-dioxane stock solution. To exact 6 mL of ethylene oxide stock solution and exact 2.5 mL of 1,4-dioxane stock solution add water to make exactly 25 mL, and use this solution as ethylene oxide-1,4-dioxane standard stock solution. Separately, transfer exactly 1.00 g of Polysorbate 80 into a 10-mL headspace vial, add exactly 2 mL of ethylene oxide-1,4-dioxane standard stock solution, seal the vial immediately with a septum of silicon rubber coated the surface with fluororesin and an aluminum cap. Mix carefully, and use the content as the standard solution. Perform the test with the sample solution and standard solution as directed in the head-space method under Gas Chromatography ⟨*2.02*⟩ according to the following conditions. The amounts of ethylene oxide and 1,4-dioxane, calculated by the following equations, are not more than 1 ppm and not more than 10 ppm, respectively.

$$\text{Amount (ppm) of ethylene oxide} = 2 \times C_{EO} \times A_a/(A_b - A_a)$$

C_{EO}: Concentration (μg/mL) of added ethylene oxide in the standard solution
A_a: Peak area of ethylene oxide obtained with the sample solution
A_b: Peak area of ethylene oxide obtained with the standard solution

$$\text{Amount (ppm) of 1,4-dioxane} = 2 \times 1.03 \times C_D \times A'_a \times 1000/(A'_b - A'_a)$$

C_D: Concentration (μL/mL) of added 1,4-dioxane in the standard solution
1.03: Density (g/mL) of 1,4-dioxane
A'_a: Peak area of 1,4-dioxane obtained with the sample solution
A'_b: Peak area of 1,4-dioxane obtained with the standard solution

Head-space injection conditions—

Equilibration temperature in vial: A constant temperature of about 80°C.

Equilibration time in vial: 30 minutes.

Carrier gas: Helium.

Injection volume of sample: 1.0 mL.

Operating conditions—

Detector: A hydrogen flame-ionization detector.

Column: A fused silica column 0.53 mm in inside diameter and 50 m in length, coated the inside surface with 5% diphenyl-95% dimethylpolysiloxane for gas chromatography 5 μm in thickness.

Column temperature: Inject at a constant temperature of about 70°C, raise the temperature to 250°C at a rate of 10°C per minute, and maintain at 250°C for 5 minutes.

Injection port temperature: A constant temperature of about 85°C.

Detector temperature: A constant temperature of about 250°C.

Carrier gas: Helium.

Flow rate: 4.0 mL per minute.

Split ratio: 1:3.5.

System suitability—

System performance: Introduce 0.100 g of acetaldehyde in a 100-mL volumetric flask, and add water to make 100 mL. To exact 1 mL of this solution add water to make exactly 100 mL. Transfer exactly 2 mL of this solution and exactly 2 mL of ethylene oxide stock solution into a 10-mL headspace vial, seal the vial immediately with a fluororesin coated silicon septum and an aluminum cap. Mix carefully, and use the content as the solution for system suitability test. When perform the test with ◆the standard solution and◆ the solution for system suitability test under the above conditions, acetaldehyde, ethylene oxide and 1,4-dioxane are eluted in this order, and the resolution between the peaks of acetaldehyde and ethylene oxide is not less than 2.0.

(3) Peroxide value—Introduce about 10 g of Polysorbate 80, accurately weighed, into a 100-mL beaker, dissolve in 20 mL of acetic acid (100). Add 1 mL of saturated potassium iodide solution and allow to stand for 1 minute. Add 50 mL of fleshly boiled and cooled water, and titrate <*2.50*> with 0.01 mol/L sodium thiosulfate VS, while stirring with a magnetic stirrer (potentiometric titration). Perform a blank determination in the same manner, and make any necessary correction. Calculate peroxide value by the following equation: not more than 10.0.

$$\text{Peroxide value} = (a - b) \times 10/M$$

M: Amount (g) of Polysorbate 80 taken
a: Volume (mL) of 0.01 mol/L sodium thiosulfate VS required for sample determination
b: Volume (mL) of 0.01 mol/L sodium thiosulfate VS required for blank determination

Water <*2.48*> Not more than 3.0% (1 g, volumetric titration, direct titration).

Residue on ignition Heat a quartz or platinum crucible to redness for 30 minutes, allow to cool in a desiccator (silica gel or other appropriate desiccants), and weigh accurately. Evenly distribute 2.00 g of Polysorbate 80 in the crucible, dry at 100 - 105°C for 1 hour, ◆and gradually heat with as lower temperature as possible to carbonize completely.◆ Then after igniting to constant mass in an electric furnace at 600 ± 25°C, allow the crucible to cool in a desiccator, and weigh the mass accurately. Flames should not be produced at any time during the procedure. If after prolonged ignition the ash still contains black particles, take up the ash with hot water, filter through a filter paper for quantitative analysis, and ignite the residue and the filter paper. Combine the filtrate with the ash, carefully evaporate to dryness, and ignite to constant mass: not more than 0.25%.

Containers and storage Containers—Tight containers.
Storage—Light-resistant.

Potash Soap

カリ石ケン

Potash Soap contains not less than 40.0% as fatty acids.

Method of preparation

Fixed oil	470 mL
Potassium Hydroxide	a sufficient quantity
Water, Purified Water or Purified Water in Containers	a sufficient quantity
To make	1000 g

Dissolve Potassium Hydroxide, in required quantity for saponification, in Water, Purified Water or Purified Water in Containers, add this solution to fixed oil, previously warmed, add a sufficient quantity of Ethanol if necessary, stir thoroughly, heat in a water bath, and continue the saponification. After complete saponification, add Water, Purified Water or Purified Water in Containers to make 1000 g.

Description Potash Soap occurs as a yellow-brown, transparent, unctuous, soft mass, having a characteristic odor.

It is freely soluble in water and in ethanol (95).

Purity Silicic acid and alkalinity—Dissolve 10 g of Potash Soap in 30 mL of ethanol (95), and add 0.50 mL of 1 mol/L hydrochloric acid VS: no turbidity is produced. Add 1 drop of phenolphthalein TS to this solution: no red color develops.

Assay Weigh accurately about 5 g of Potash Soap, dissolve in 100 mL of hot water, and transfer to a separator. Acidify the mixture with dilute sulfuric acid, and cool. Extract the solution with 50-mL, 40-mL, and 30-mL portions of diethyl ether. Wash the combined diethyl ether extracts with 10-mL portions of water until the washing contains no acid. Transfer the diethyl ether solution to a tared flask, evaporate diethyl ether on a water bath at a temperature as low as possible. Dry the residue at 80°C to constant mass, and weigh as fatty acids.

Containers and storage Containers—Tight containers.

Potassium Bromide

臭化カリウム

KBr: 119.00

Potassium Bromide, when dried, contains not less than 99.0% of potassium bromide (KBr).

Description Potassium Bromide occurs as colorless or white crystals, granules or crystalline powder. It is odorless.

It is freely soluble in water and in glycerin, soluble in hot ethanol (95), and slightly soluble in ethanol (95).

Identification A solution of Potassium Bromide (1 in 10) responds to Qualitative Tests <*1.09*> for potassium salt and for bromide.

Purity (1) Clarity and color of solution—Dissolve 1.0 g of Potassium Bromide in 3 mL of water: the solution is clear and colorless.

(2) Alkalinity—Dissolve 1.0 g of Potassium Bromide in 10 mL of water, add 0.10 mL of 0.05 mol/L sulfuric acid VS and 1 drop of phenolphthalein TS, heat to boiling, and cool: no color develops.

(3) Chloride—Make a calculation from the result obtained in the Assay: not more than 84.5 mL of 0.1 mol/L silver nitrate VS is consumed for 1 g of Potassium Bromide.

(4) Sulfate <*1.14*>—Proceed with 2.0 g of Potassium Bromide, and perform the test. Prepare the control solution with 1.0 mL of 0.005 mol/L sulfuric acid VS (not more than 0.024%).

(5) Iodide—Dissolve 0.5 g of Potassium Bromide in 10 mL of water, add 2 to 3 drops of iron (III) chloride TS and 1 mL of chloroform, and shake: no red-purple to purple color develops in the chloroform layer.

(6) Bromate—Dissolve 1.0 g of Potassium Bromide in 10 mL of freshly boiled and cooled water, and add 0.1 mL of potassium iodide TS, 1 mL of starch TS and 3 drops of dilute sulfuric acid. Shake the mixture gently, and allow to stand for 5 minutes: no blue color develops.

(7) Heavy metals <*1.07*>—Proceed with 2.0 g of Potassium Bromide according to Method 1, and perform the test. Prepare the control solution with 2.0 mL of Standard Lead Solution (not more than 10 ppm).

(8) Barium—Dissolve 0.5 g of Potassium Bromide in 10 mL of water, add 0.5 mL of dilute hydrochloric acid and 1 mL of potassium sulfate TS, and allow to stand for 10 minutes: no turbidity is produced.

(9) Arsenic <*1.11*>—Prepare the test solution with 1.0 g of Potassium Bromide according to Method 1, and perform the test (not more than 2 ppm).

Loss on drying *<2.41>* Not more than 1.0% (1 g, 110°C, 4 hours).

Assay Weigh accurately about 0.4 g of Potassium Bromide, previously dried, and dissolve in 50 mL of water. Add 10 mL of dilute nitric acid and exactly measured 50 mL of 0.1 mol/L silver nitrate VS, and titrate *<2.50>* the excess silver nitrate with 0.1 mol/L ammonium thiocyanate VS (indicator: 2 mL of ammonium iron (III) sulfate TS). Perform a blank determination in the same manner.

Each mL of 0.1 mol/L silver nitrate VS
= 11.90 mg of KBr

Containers and storage Containers—Tight containers.

Potassium Canrenoate

カンレノ酸カリウム

$C_{22}H_{29}KO_4$: 396.56
Monopotassium 17-hydroxy-3-oxo-17α-pregna-4,6-diene-21-carboxylate
[*2181-04-6*]

Potassium Canrenoate, when dried, contains not less than 98.0% and not more than 102.0% of potassium canrenoate ($C_{22}H_{29}KO_4$).

Description Potassium Canrenoate occurs as a pale yellow-white to pale yellow-brown, crystalline powder.

It is freely soluble in water, soluble in methanol, sparingly soluble in ethanol (95), and practically insoluble in chloroform and in diethyl ether.

Identification **(1)** Dissolve 2 mg of Potassium Canrenoate in 2 drops of sulfuric acid: an orange color develops. Observe under ultraviolet light (main wavelength: 365 nm): the solution shows a yellow-green fluorescence. Add 1 drop of acetic anhydride to this solution: the color of the solution changes to red.

(2) Determine the absorption spectrum of a solution of Potassium Canrenoate in methanol (1 in 100,000) as directed under Ultraviolet-visible Spectrophotometry *<2.24>*, and compare the spectrum with the Reference Spectrum: both spectra exhibit similar intensities of absorption at the same wavelengths.

(3) Determine the infrared absorption spectrum of Potassium Canrenoate, previously dried, as directed in the potassium bromide disk method under Infrared Spectrophotometry *<2.25>*, and compare the spectrum with the Reference Spectrum: both spectra exhibit similar intensities of absorption at the same wave numbers.

(4) The solution of Potassium Canrenoate (1 in 10) responds to Qualitative Tests *<1.09>* (1) for potassium salt.

Optical rotation *<2.49>* $[\alpha]_D^{20}$: −71 – −76° (after drying, 0.2 g, methanol, 20 mL, 100 mm).

pH *<2.54>* Dissolve 1.0 g of Potassium Canrenoate in 20 mL of water: the pH of this solution is between 8.4 and 9.4.

Purity **(1)** Clarity and color of solution—Dissolve 0.5 g of Potassium Canrenoate in 5 mL of water: the solution is clear, and shows a pale yellow to light yellow color.

(2) Heavy metals *<1.07>*—Proceed with 2.0 g of Potassium Canrenoate according to Method 2, and perform the test. Prepare the control solution with 2.0 mL of Standard Lead Solution (not more than 10 ppm).

(3) Arsenic *<1.11>*—Prepare the test solution with 1.0 g of Potassium Canrenoate according to Method 3, and perform the test (not more than 2 ppm).

(4) Canrenone—Place 0.40 g of Potassium Canrenoate in a glass-stoppered centrifuge tube, cool in ice-water to a temperature not higher than 5°C, add 6 mL of boric acid-potassium chloride-sodium hydroxide buffer solution (pH 10.0) being cooled to a temperature not higher than 5°C to dissolve, and add 8 mL of water being cooled to a temperature not higher than 5°C. Add exactly 10 mL of chloroform, allow to stand for 3 minutes at a temperature not higher than 5°C, shake vigorously for 2 minutes, and centrifuge. Drain off the water layer, collect 5 mL of the chloroform layer, transfer to a glass-stoppered centrifuge tube containing 3 mL of boric acid-potassium chloride-sodium hydroxide buffer solution (pH 10.0) cooled to a temperature not higher than 5°C, and 4 mL of water cooled to a temperature not higher than 5°C, shake for 1 minute, and centrifuge. Drain off the water layer, pipet 2 mL of the chloroform layer, and add chloroform to make exactly 10 mL. Determine the absorbance of this solution at 283 nm as directed under Ultraviolet-visible Spectrophotometry *<2.24>*: it is not more than 0.67.

Loss on drying *<2.41>* Not more than 0.5% (1 g, 105°C, 4 hours).

Assay Weigh accurately about 0.2 g of Potassium Canrenoate, previously dried, dissolve in 75 mL of acetic acid (100), and titrate *<2.50>* with 0.1 mol/L perchloric acid VS (potentiometric titration). Use a solution of saturated potassium chloride-acetic acid (100) as the internal liquid.). Perform a blank determination in the same manner, and make any necessary correction.

Each mL of 0.1 mol/L perchloric acid VS
= 39.66 mg of $C_{22}H_{29}KO_4$

Containers and storage Containers—Tight containers.

Potassium Carbonate

炭酸カリウム

K_2CO_3: 138.21

Potassium Carbonate, when dried, contains not less than 99.0% of potassium carbonate (K_2CO_3).

Description Potassium Carbonate occurs as white granules or powder. It is odorless.

It is very soluble in water, and practically insoluble in ethanol (95).

A solution of Potassium Carbonate (1 in 10) is alkaline.

It is hygroscopic.

Identification A solution of Potassium Carbonate (1 in 10) responds to Qualitative Tests *<1.09>* for potassium salt and for carbonate.

Purity **(1)** Clarity and color of solution—Dissolve 1.0 g of Potassium Carbonate in 20 mL of water: the solution is clear and colorless.

(2) Heavy metals *<1.07>*—Dissolve 1.0 g of Potassium

Carbonate in 2 mL of water and 6 mL of dilute hydrochloric acid, and evaporate to dryness on a water bath. Dissolve the residue in 35 mL of water and 2 mL of dilute acetic acid, dilute with water to 50 mL, and perform the test using this solution as the test solution. Prepare the control solution as follows: evaporate 6 mL of dilute hydrochloric acid on a water bath to dryness, add 2 mL of dilute acetic acid and 2.0 mL of Standard Lead Solution, and dilute with water to 50 mL (not more than 20 ppm).

(3) Sodium—Dissolve 1.0 g of Potassium Carbonate in 20 mL of water, and perform the test as directed under Flame Coloration Test <*1.04*> (1): no persisting yellow color is produced.

(4) Arsenic <*1.11*>—Prepare the test solution with 0.5 g of Potassium Carbonate, according to Method 1, and perform the test (not more than 4 ppm).

Loss on drying <*2.41*> Not more than 1.0% (3 g, 180°C, 4 hours).

Assay Dissolve about 1.5 g of Potassium Carbonate, previously dried and accurately weighed, in 25 mL of water, titrate with 0.5 mol/L sulfuric acid VS until the blue color of the solution changes to yellow-green, boil cautiously, then cool, and titrate <*2.50*> until a greenish yellow color develops (indicator: 2 drops of bromocresol green TS).

Each mL of 0.5 mol/L sulfuric acid VS
= 69.11 mg of K_2CO_3

Containers and storage Containers—Tight containers.

Potassium Chloride

塩化カリウム

KCl: 74.55

Potassium Chloride, when dried, contains not less than 99.0% of potassium chloride (KCl).

Description Potassium Chloride occurs as colorless or white crystals or crystalline powder. It is odorless, and has a saline taste.

It is freely soluble in water, and practically insoluble in ethanol (95) and in diethyl ether.

A solution of Potassium Chloride (1 in 10) is neutral.

Identification A solution of Potassium Chloride (1 in 50) responds to Qualitative Tests <*1.09*> for potassium salt and for chloride.

Purity (1) Clarity and color of solution—Dissolve 1.0 g of Potassium Chloride in 5 mL of water: the solution is clear and colorless.

(2) Acidity and alkalinity—Dissolve 5.0 g of Potassium Chloride in 50 mL of freshly boiled and cooled water, and add 3 drops of phenolphthalein TS: no red color develops. Then add 0.50 mL of 0.01 mol/L sodium hydroxide VS: a red color develops.

(3) Bromide—Dissolve 1.0 g of Potassium Chloride in water to make 100 mL. To 5 mL of the solution add 3 drops of dilute hydrochloric acid and 1 mL of chloroform, and add 3 drops of sodium toluensulfonchloramide TS dropwise while shaking: no yellow to yellow-red color develops in the chloroform layer.

(4) Iodide—Dissolve 0.5 g of Potassium Chloride in 10 mL of water, add 3 drops of iron (III) chloride TS and 1 mL of chloroform, shake, allow to stand for 30 minutes, and shake again: no red-purple to purple color develops in the chloroform layer.

(5) Heavy metals <*1.07*>—Proceed with 4.0 g of Potassium Chloride according to Method 1, and perform the test. Prepare the control solution with 2.0 mL of Standard Lead Solution (not more than 5 ppm).

(6) Calcium and magnesium—Dissolve 0.20 g of Potassium Chloride in 20 mL of water, add 2 mL of ammonia TS, 2 mL of ammonium oxalate TS and 2 mL of disodium hydrogenphosphate TS, and then allow to stand for 5 minutes: no turbidity is produced.

(7) Sodium—Dissolve 1.0 g of Potassium Chloride in 20 mL of water, and perform Flame Coloration Test <*1.04*> (1): no persistent, yellow color develops.

(8) Arsenic <*1.11*>—Prepare the test solution with 1.0 g of Potassium Chloride according to Method 1, and perform the test (not more than 2 ppm).

Loss on drying <*2.41*> Not more than 0.5% (1 g, 130°C, 2 hours).

Assay Weigh accurately about 0.2 g of Potassium Chloride, previously dried, dissolve in 50 mL of water, and titrate <*2.50*> with 0.1 mol/L silver nitrate VS while shaking vigorously (indicator: 3 drops of fluorescein sodium TS).

Each mL of 0.1 mol/L silver nitrate VS = 7.455 mg of KCl

Containers and storage Containers—Tight containers.

Potassium Clavulanate

クラブラン酸カリウム

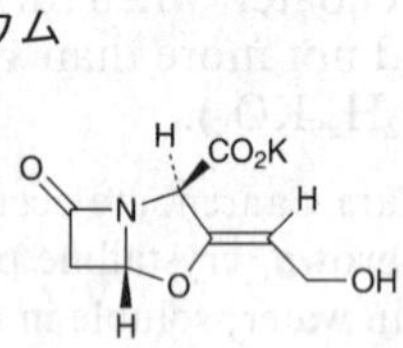

$C_8H_8KNO_5$: 237.25
Monopotassium (2*R*,5*R*)-3-[(1*Z*)-2-hydroxyethylidene]-7-oxo-4-oxa-1-azabicyclo[3.2.0]heptane-2-carboxylate
[*61177-45-5*]

Potassium Clavulanate is the potassium salt of a substance having *β*-lactamase inhibiting activity produced by the growth of *Streptomyces clavuligerus*.

It contains not less than 810 *μ*g (potency) and not more than 860 *μ*g (potency) per mg, calculated on the anhydrous basis. The potency of Potassium Clavulanate is expressed as mass (potency) of clavularic acid ($C_8H_9NO_5$: 199.16).

Description Potassium Clavulanate occurs as a white to light yellow-white, crystalline powder.

It is very soluble in water, soluble in methanol, and slightly soluble in ethanol (95).

It is hygroscopic.

Identification (1) To 1 mL of a solution of Potassium Clavulanate (1 in 50,000) add 5 mL of imidazole TS, and warm in a water bath at 30°C for 12 minutes. After cooling, determine the absorption spectrum of this solution as directed under Ultraviolet-visible Spectrophotometry <*2.24*>, and compare the spectrum with the Reference Spectrum: both spectra exhibit similar intensities of absorption at the same wavelengths.

(2) Determine the infrared absorption spectrum of Potassium Clavulanate as directed in the potassium bromide disk method under Infrared Spectrophotometry <2.25>, and compare the spectrum with the Reference Spectrum: both spectra exhibit similar intensities of absorption at the same wave numbers.

(3) Potassium Clavulanate responds to Qualitative Tests <1.09> (1) for potassium salt.

Optical rotation <2.49> $[\alpha]_D^{20}$: +53 – +63° (0.5 g calculated on the anhydrous basis, water, 50 mL, 100 mm).

Purity **(1)** Heavy metals <1.07>—Proceed with 2.0 g of Potassium Clavulanate according to Method 2, and perform the test. Prepare the control solution with 4.0 mL of Standard Lead Solution (not more than 20 ppm).

(2) Arsenic <1.11>—Prepare the test solution with 1.0 g of Potassium Clavulanate according to Method 3, and perform the test (not more than 2 ppm).

(3) Related substances—Dissolve 0.10 g of Potassium Clavulanate in 10 mL of the mobile phase A, and use this solution as the sample solution. Pipet 1 mL of the sample solution, add the mobile phase A to make exactly 100 mL, and use this solution as the standard solution. Perform the test with exactly 20 μL each of the sample solution and standard solution as directed under Liquid Chromatography <2.01> according to the following conditions, and determine each peak area by the automatic integration method: the area of each peak other than clavulanic acid obtained from the sample solution is not larger than the peak area of clavulanic acid from the standard solution, and the total area of the peaks other than clavulanic acid from the sample solution is not larger than 2 times of the peak area of clavulanic acid from the standard solution.

Operating conditions—

Detector: An ultraviolet absorption photometer (wavelength: 230 nm).

Column: A stainless steel column 4.6 mm in inside diameter and 10 cm in length, packed with octadecylsilanized silica gel for liquid chromatography (5 μm in particle diameter).

Column temperature: A constant temperature of about 40°C.

Mobile phase A: Adjust the pH of 0.05 mol/L sodium dihydrogen phosphate TS to 4.0 with phosphoric acid.

Mobile phase B: A mixture of the mobile phase A and methanol (1:1).

Flowing of mobile phase: Control the gradient by mixing the mobile phases A and B as directed in the following table.

Time after injection of sample (min)	Mobile phase A (vol%)	Mobile phase B (vol%)
0 – 4	100	0
4 – 15	100 → 0	0 → 100
15 – 25	0	100

Flow rate: 1.0 mL per minute.

Time span of measurement: About 6 times as long as the retention time of clavulanic acid.

System suitability—

Test for required detectability: Pipet 1 mL of the standard solution, and add the mobile phase A to make exactly 10 mL. Confirm that the peak area of clavulanic acid obtained with 20 μL of this solution is equivalent to 7 to 13% of that with 20 μL of the standard solution.

System performance: Dissolve 10 mg each of Potassium Clavulanate and amoxycillin hydrate in 100 mL of the mobile phase A. When the procedure is run with 20 μL of this solution under the above operating conditions, clavulanic acid and amoxycillin are eluted in this order with the resolution between these peaks being not less than 8 and the number of theoretical plates of the peak of clavulanic acid is not less than 2500.

System repeatability: When the test is repeated 3 times with 20 μL of the standard solution under the above operating conditions, the relative standard deviation of the peak area of clavulanic acid is not more than 2.0%.

Water <2.48> Not more than 1.5% (5 g, volumetric titration, direct titration).

Assay Weigh accurately an amount of Potassium Clavulanate and Lithium Clavulanate RS, equivalent to about 12.5 mg (potency), dissolve each in 30 mL of water, add exactly 5 mL of the internal standard solution and water to make 50 mL, and use these solutions as the sample solution and the standard solution, respectively. Perform the test with 5 μL each of the sample solution and standard solution as directed under Liquid Chromatography <2.01> according to the following conditions, and calculate the ratios, Q_T and Q_S, of the peak area of clavularic acid to that of the internal standard.

Amount [μg (potency)] of clavularic acid ($C_8H_9NO_5$)
$= M_S \times Q_T/Q_S \times 1000$

M_S: Amount [mg (potency)] of Lithium Clavulanate RS taken

Internal standard solution—Dissolve 0.3 g of sulfanilamide in 30 mL of methanol, and add water to make 100 mL.

Operating conditions—

Detector: An ultraviolet absorption photometer (wavelength: 230 nm).

Column: A stainless steel column 4.6 mm in inside diameter and 25 cm in length, packed with octadecylsilanized silica gel for liquid chromatography (5 μm in particle diameter).

Column temperature: A constant temperature of about 25°C.

Mobile phase: Dissolve 1.36 g of sodium acetate trihydrate in 900 mL of water, adjust to pH 4.5 with diluted acetic acid (31) (2 in 5), and add 30 mL of methanol and water to make 1000 mL.

Flow rate: Adjust so that the retention time of clavularic acid is about 6 minutes.

System suitability—

System performance: When the procedure is run with 5 μL of the standard solution under the above operating conditions, clavularic acid and the internal standard are eluted in this order with the resolution between these peaks being not less than 4.

System repeatability: When the test is repeated 6 times with 5 μL of the standard solution under the above operating conditions, the relative standard deviation of the ratios of the peak area of clavularic acid to that of the internal standard is not more than 1.0%.

Containers and storage Containers—Tight containers.

Potassium Guaiacolsulfonate

グアヤコールスルホン酸カリウム

$C_7H_7KO_5S$: 242.29

Monopotassium 4-hydroxy-3-methoxybenzenesulfonate

[*16241-25-1*]

Potassium Guaiacolsulfonate contains not less than 98.5% of potassium guaiacolsulfonate ($C_7H_7KO_5S$), calculated on the anhydrous basis.

Description Potassium Guaiacolsulfonate occurs as white crystals or crystalline powder. It is odorless or has a slight, characteristic odor and a slightly bitter taste.

It is freely soluble in water and in formic acid, soluble in methanol, and practically insoluble in ethanol (95), in acetic anhydride and in diethyl ether.

Identification **(1)** To 10 mL of a solution of Potassium Guaiacolsulfonate (1 in 100) add 2 drops of iron (III) chloride TS: a blue-purple color develops.

(2) Dissolve 0.25 g of Potassium Guaiacolsulfonate in water to make 500 mL, and to 10 mL of this solution add phosphate buffer solution (pH 7.0) to make 100 mL. Determine the absorption spectrum of this solution as directed under Ultraviolet-visible Spectrophotometry 〈*2.24*〉, and compare the spectrum with the Reference Spectrum: both spectra exhibit similar intensities of absorption at the same wavelengths.

(3) A solution of Potassium Guaiacolsulfonate (1 in 10) responds to Qualitative Tests 〈*1.09*〉 for potassium salt.

pH 〈*2.54*〉 Dissolve 1.0 g of Potassium Guaiacolsulfonate in 20 mL of water: the pH of the solution is between 4.0 and 5.5.

Purity **(1)** Clarity and color of solution—Dissolve 1.0 g of Potassium Guaiacolsulfonate in 20 mL of water: the solution is clear and colorless.

(2) Sulfate 〈*1.14*〉—Perform the test with 0.8 g of Potassium Guaiacolsulfonate. Prepare the control solution with 0.50 mL of 0.005 mol/L sulfuric acid VS (not more than 0.030%).

(3) Heavy metals 〈*1.07*〉—Proceed with 1.0 g of Potassium Guaiacolsulfonate according to Method 1, and perform the test. Prepare the control solution with 2.0 mL of Standard Lead Solution (not more than 20 ppm).

(4) Arsenic 〈*1.11*〉—Prepare the test solution with 1.0 g of Potassium Guaiacolsulfonate according to Method 1, and perform the test (not more than 2 ppm).

(5) Related substances—Dissolve 0.20 g of Potassium Guaiacolsulfonate in 200 mL of mobile phase, and use this solution as the sample solution. Pipet 1 mL of the sample solution, add the mobile phase to make exactly 100 mL, and use this solution as the standard solution. Perform the test with exactly 5 μL each of the sample solution and standard solution as directed under Liquid Chromatography 〈*2.01*〉 according to the following conditions. Determine each peak area by the automatic integration method: the total area of peaks other than potassium guaiacolsulfonate obtained from the sample solution is not larger than the peak area of potassium guaiacolsulfonate from the standard solution.

Operating conditions—

Detector: An ultraviolet absorption photometer (wavelength: 279 nm).

Column: A stainless steel column 4 mm in inside diameter and 20 to 25 cm in length, packed with dimethylaminopropylsilanized silica gel for liquid chromatography (5 to 10 μm in particle diameter).

Column temperature: A constant temperature of about 30°C.

Mobile phase: A mixture of 0.05 mol/L potassium dihydrogenphosphate TS and methanol (20:1).

Flow rate: Adjust so that the retention time of potassium guaiacolsulfonate is about 10 minutes.

Selection of column: Weigh 50 mg each of potassium guaiacolsulfonate and guaiacol, and dissolve in 50 mL of the mobile phase. Proceed with 5 μL of this solution under the above operating conditions, and calculate the resolution. Use a column giving elution of guaiacol and potassium guaiacolsulfonate in this order with the resolution of these peaks being not less than 4.

Detection sensitivity: Adjust the sensitivity so that the peak height of potassium guaiacolsulfonate from 5 μL of the standard solution is not less than 10 mm.

Time span of measurement: About twice as long as the retention time of potassium guaiacolsulfonate.

Water 〈*2.48*〉 3.0 – 4.5% (0.3 g, volumetric titration, direct titration).

Assay Weigh accurately about 0.3 g of Potassium Guaiacolsulfonate, dissolve in 2.0 mL of formic acid, add 50 mL of acetic anhydride, and titrate 〈*2.50*〉 with 0.1 mol/L perchloric acid VS (potentiometric titration). Perform a blank determination in the same manner, and make any necessary correction.

Each mL of 0.1 mol/L perchloric acid VS
= 24.23 mg of $C_7H_7KO_5S$

Containers and storage Containers—Well-closed containers.

Storage—Light-resistant.

Potassium Hydroxide

水酸化カリウム

KOH: 56.11

Potassium Hydroxide contains not less than 85.0% of potassium hydroxide (KOH).

Description Potassium Hydroxide occurs as white fused masses, in small pellets, in flakes, in sticks and in other forms. It is hard and brittle, and shows a crystalline fracture.

It is freely soluble in water and in ethanol (95), and practically insoluble in diethyl ether.

It rapidly absorbs carbon dioxide in air.

It deliquesces in the presence of moisture.

Identification **(1)** A solution of Potassium Hydroxide (1 in 500) is alkaline.

(2) A solution of Potassium Hydroxide (1 in 25) responds to Qualitative Tests 〈*1.09*〉 for potassium salt.

Purity **(1)** Clarity and color of solution—Dissolve 1.0 g of Potassium Hydroxide in 20 mL of water: the solution is clear and colorless.

(2) Chloride 〈*1.03*〉—Dissolve 2.0 g of Potassium Hydroxide in water to make 100 mL. To 25 mL of the solution add 8 mL of dilute nitric acid and water to make 50 mL. Perform the test using this solution as the test solution. Prepare the control solution with 0.7 mL of 0.01 mol/L hydrochloric acid VS (not more than 0.050%).

(3) Heavy metals <*1.07*>—Dissolve 1.0 g of Potassium Hydroxide in 5 mL of water, add 7 mL of dilute hydrochloric acid, and evaporate on a water bath to dryness. Dissolve the residue in 35 mL of water, 2 mL of dilute acetic acid and 1 drop of ammonia TS, add water to make 50 mL, and perform the test using this solution as the test solution. Prepare the control solution as follows: evaporate 7 mL of dilute hydrochloric acid on a water bath to dryness, dissolve the residue in 2 mL of dilute acetic acid and 3.0 mL of Standard Lead Solution, and add water to make 50 mL (not more than 30 ppm).

(4) Sodium—Dissolve 0.10 g of Potassium Hydroxide in 10 mL of dilute hydrochloric acid, and perform the test as directed under Flame Coloration Test <*1.04*> (1): no persistent yellow color develops.

(5) Potassium carbonate—The amount of potassium carbonate (K_2CO_3: 138.21) is not more than 2.0% when calculated by the following equation using *B* (mL) obtained in the Assay.

Amount of potassium carbonate (mg) = 138.21 × *B*

Assay Weigh accurately about 1.5 g of Potassium Hydroxide, and dissolve in 40 mL of freshly boiled and cooled water. Cool the solution to 15°C, add 2 drops of phenolphthalein TS, and titrate <*2.50*> with 0.5 mol/L sulfuric acid VS until the red color of the solution disappears. Record the amount *A* (mL) of 0.5 mol/L sulfuric acid VS consumed, then add 2 drops of methyl orange TS, and titrate <*2.50*> again with 0.5 mol/L sulfuric acid VS until the solution changes to a persistent light red color. Record the amount *B* (mL) of 0.5 mol/L sulfuric acid VS consumed.

Calculate the amount potassium hydroxide (KOH) from the amount, *A* (mL) − *B* (mL).

Each mL of 0.5 mol/L sulfuric acid VS
= 56.11 mg of KOH

Containers and storage Containers—Tight containers.

Potassium Iodide

ヨウ化カリウム

KI: 166.00

Potassium Iodide, when dried, contains not less than 99.0% of potassium iodide (KI).

Description Potassium Iodide occurs as colorless or white crystals, or a white crystalline powder.

It is very soluble in water, soluble in ethanol (95), and practically insoluble in diethyl ether.

It is slightly deliquescent in moist air.

Identification A solution of Potassium Iodide (1 in 20) responds to Qualitative Tests <*1.09*> for potassium salt and for iodide.

Purity **(1)** Clarity and color of solution—Dissolve 1.0 g of Potassium Iodide in 2 mL of water: the solution is clear and colorless.

(2) Alkalinity—Dissolve 1.0 g of Potassium Iodide in 10 mL of freshly boiled and cooled water, and add 0.50 mL of 0.005 mol/L sulfuric acid VS and 1 drop of phenolphthalein TS: no color develops.

(3) Chloride, bromide and thiosulfate—Dissolve 0.20 g of Potassium Iodide in 5 mL of ammonia TS, add 15.0 mL of 0.1 mol/L silver nitrate VS, shake for 2 to 3 minutes, and filter. To 10 mL of the filtrate, add 15 mL of dilute nitric acid: no brown color develops. The solution has no more turbidity than that of the following control solution.

Control solution: To 0.30 mL of 0.01 mol/L hydrochloric acid VS add 2.5 mL of ammonia TS, and 7.5 mL of 0.1 mol/L silver nitrate VS and 15 mL of dilute nitric acid.

(4) Nitrate, nitrite and ammonium—Place 1.0 g of Potassium Iodide in a 40-mL test tube, and add 5 mL of water, 5 mL of sodium hydroxide TS and 0.2 g of aluminum wire. Insert the absorbent cotton in the mouth of the test tube, and place a piece of moistened red litmus paper on it. Heat the test tube carefully on a water bath for 15 minutes: the gas evolved does not turn red litmus paper to blue.

(5) Cyanide—Dissolve 0.5 g of Potassium Iodide in 10 mL of water. To 5 mL of this solution add 1 drop of iron (II) sulfate TS and 2 mL of sodium hydroxide TS, warm, then add 4 mL of hydrochloric acid: no green color develops.

(6) Iodate—Dissolve 0.5 g of Potassium Iodide in 10 mL of freshly boiled and cooled water, and add 2 drops of dilute sulfuric acid and 1 drop of starch TS: no blue color develops immediately.

(7) Heavy metals <*1.07*>—Proceed with 2.0 g of Potassium Iodide according to Method 1, and perform the test. Prepare the control solution with 2.0 mL of Standard Lead Solution (not more than 10 ppm).

(8) Barium—Dissolve 0.5 g of Potassium Iodide in 10 mL of water, add 1 mL of dilute sulfuric acid, and allow to stand for 5 minutes: no turbidity is produced.

(9) Sodium—Dissolve 1.0 g of Potassium Iodide in 10 mL of water, and perform Flame Coloration Test <*1.04*> (1): a yellow color develops, but does not persist.

(10) Arsenic <*1.11*>—Prepare the test solution with 0.40 g of Potassium Iodide according to Method 1, and perform the test (not more than 5 ppm).

Loss on drying <*2.41*> Not more than 1.0% (2 g, 105°C, 4 hours).

Assay Weigh accurately about 0.5 g of Potassium Iodide, previously dried, in an iodine flask, dissolve in 10 mL of water, add 35 mL of hydrochloric acid and 5 mL of chloroform, and titrate <*2.50*> with 0.05 mol/L potassium iodate VS with shaking until the red-purple color of the chloroform layer disappears. The end point is reached when the red-purple color does not reappear in the chloroform layer within 5 minutes after the layer has been decolorized.

Each mL of 0.05 mol/L potassium iodate VS
= 16.60 mg of KI

Containers and storage Containers—Tight containers.
Storage—Light-resistant.

Potassium Permanganate

過マンガン酸カリウム

$KMnO_4$: 158.03

Potassium Permanganate, when dried, contains not less than 99.0% of potassium permanganate ($KMnO_4$).

Description Potassium Permanganate occurs as dark purple crystals and has a metallic luster.

It is soluble in water.

A solution of Potassium Permanganate (1 in 1000) has a slightly sweet, astringent taste.

Identification A solution of Potassium Permanganate (1 in 100) responds to Qualitative Tests *<1.09>* for permanganate.

Purity **(1)** Water-insoluble substances—Dissolve 2.0 g of Potassium Permanganate, previously powdered, in 200 mL of water. Filter the insoluble substances through a tared glass filter (G4), wash with water until the last washing shows no color, and dry at 105°C for 2 hours: the mass of the residue is not more than 4 mg.

(2) Arsenic *<1.11>*—Dissolve 0.40 g of Potassium Permanganate in 10 mL of water, add 1 mL of sulfuric acid, add hydrogen peroxide (30) dropwise until the solution remains colorless, and evaporate on a sand bath nearly to dryness. Dissolve the residue in 5 mL of water, and perform the test with this solution as the test solution: the color produced is not more intense than the following color standard.

Color standard: To 10 mL of water add 1 mL of sulfuric acid and the same volume of hydrogen peroxide (30) as used for the preparation of the test solution. Evaporate the solution on a sand bath nearly to dryness, add 2.0 mL of Standard Arsenic Solution and water to make 5 mL, and carry out the test with this solution in the same manner as the test solution (not more than 5 ppm).

Loss on drying *<2.41>* Not more than 0.5% (1 g, silica gel, 18 hours).

Assay Weigh accurately about 0.6 g of Potassium Permanganate, previously dried, dissolve in water to make exactly 200 mL, and use this solution as the sample solution. Pipet 25 mL of 0.05 mol/L oxalic acid VS into a 500-mL conical flask, add 200 mL of diluted sulfuric acid (1 in 20), and keep at a temperature between 30°C and 35°C. Transfer the sample solution to a buret. Add quickly 23 mL of the sample solution from the buret to the flask while shaking gently, and then allow the flask to stand until the red color disappears. Warm the mixture to a temperature between 55°C and 60°C, and continue the titration *<2.50>* slowly until the red color persists for 30 seconds.

Each mL of 0.05 mol/L oxalic acid VS
= 3.161 mg of $KMnO_4$

Containers and storage Containers—Tight containers.

Potassium Sulfate

硫酸カリウム

K_2SO_4: 174.26

Potassium Sulfate, when dried, contains not less than 99.0% of potassium sulfate (K_2SO_4).

Description Potassium Sulfate occurs as colorless crystals or a white, crystalline powder. It has a slightly saline, somewhat bitter taste.

It is soluble in water and practically insoluble in ethanol (95).

Identification A solution of Potassium Sulfate (1 in 20) responds to Qualitative Tests *<1.09>* for potassium salt and for sulfate.

Purity **(1)** Clarity and color of solution, and acid or alkali—Dissolve 1.0 g of Potassium Sulfate in 20 mL of water: the solution is clear, colorless and neutral.

(2) Chloride *<1.03>*—Perform the test with 0.5 g of Potassium Sulfate. Prepare the control solution with 0.40 mL of 0.01 mol/L hydrochloric acid VS (not more than 0.028%).

(3) Heavy metals *<1.07>*—Proceed with 2.0 g of Potassium Sulfate according to Method 1, and perform the test. Prepare the control solution with 2.0 mL of Standard Lead Solution (not more than 10 ppm).

(4) Sodium—Dissolve 1.0 g of Potassium Sulfate in 20 mL of water, and perform the test as directed under Flame Coloration Test *<1.04>* (1): no persistent yellow color develops.

(5) Arsenic *<1.11>*—Prepare the test solution with 0.40 g of Potassium Sulfate according to Method 1, and perform the test (not more than 5 ppm).

Loss on drying *<2.41>* Not more than 1.0% (1 g, 110°C, 4 hours).

Assay Weigh accurately about 0.5 g of Potassium Sulfate, previously dried, boil with 200 mL of water and 1.0 mL of hydrochloric acid, and add gradually 8 mL of boiling barium chloride TS. Heat the mixture on a water bath for 1 hour, collect the precipitate, and wash the precipitate with water until the last washing shows no opalescence on the addition of silver nitrate TS. Dry, heat strongly to constant mass between 500°C and 600°C by raising the temperature gradually, and weigh as barium sulfate ($BaSO_4$: 233.39).

Amount (mg) of potassium sulfate (K_2SO_4)
= amount (mg) of barium sulfate ($BaSO_4$) × 0.747

Containers and storage Containers—Well-closed containers.

Povidone

ポビドン

$(C_6H_9NO)_n$
Poly[1-(2-oxopyrrolidin-1-yl)ethylene]
[*9003-39-8*]

This monograph is harmonized with the European Pharmacopoeia and the U.S. Pharmacopeia.

The parts of the text that are not harmonized are marked with symbols (◆ ◆).

Information on the harmonization with the European Pharmacopoeia and the U.S. Pharmacopeia is available on the website of the Pharmaceuticals and Medical Devices Agency.

Povidone is a chain polymer of 1-vinyl-2-pyrrolidone.

It contains not less than 11.5% and not more than 12.8% of nitrogen (N: 14.01), calculated on the anhydrous basis.

It has a nominal K-value of not less than 10 and not more than 120.

The nominal K-value is shown on the label.

◆**Description** Povidone occurs as a white to slightly yellowish fine powder. It is odorless or has a faint, characteristic odor.

It is freely soluble in water, in methanol and in ethanol (99.5).

It is hygroscopic.◆

Identification **(1)** To 0.5 g of Povidone add 10 mL of water, and shake: it dissolves.

(2) Determine the infrared absorption spectrum of Povidone, previously dried at 105°C for 6 hours, as directed in the potassium bromide disk method under Infrared Spectrophotometry *<2.25>*, and compare the spectrum with the Reference Spectrum or the spectrum of Povidone for Identification RS (previously dried at 105°C for 6 hours): both spectra exhibit similar intensities of absorption at the same wave numbers.

pH *<2.54>* Dissolve 1.0 g of Povidone in 20 mL of water: the pH of this solution is between 3.0 and 5.0 for Povidone having the nominal K-value of 30 or less, and between 4.0 and 7.0 for Povidone having the nominal K-value exceeding 30.

Purity ◆**(1)** Clarity and color of solution—Dissolve 1.0 g of Povidone in 20 mL of water: the solution is clear and colorless to pale yellow, or pale red.◆

◆**(2)** Heavy metals *<1.07>*—Proceed with 2.0 g of Povidone according to Method 2, and perform the test. Prepare the control solution with 2.0 mL of Standard Lead Solution (not more than 10 ppm).◆

(3) Aldehydes—Weigh accurately about 1 g of Povidone and dissolve in 0.05 mol/L pyrophosphate buffer solution (pH 9.0) to make exactly 100 mL. Stopper, heat at 60°C for 60 minutes, allow to cool to room temperature, and use this solution as the sample solution. Separately, dissolve 0.140 g of acetaldehyde ammonia trimer trihydrate in water to make exactly 200 mL. Pipet 1 mL of this solution, add 0.05 mol/L pyrophosphate buffer solution (pH 9.0) to make exactly 100 mL, and use this solution as the standard solution. Measure exactly 0.5 mL each of the sample solution, standard solution and water, transfer to separate 1-cm cells, add 2.5 mL of 0.05 mol/L pyrophosphate buffer solution (pH 9.0) and 0.2 mL of β-nicotinamide adenine dinucleotide TS to each of these cells, mix and stopper tightly. Allow to stand for 2 to 3 minutes at 22 ± 2°C, and perform the test with these solutions as directed under Ultraviolet-visible Spectrophotometry *<2.24>* using water as the control solution. Determine the absorbances, A_{T1}, A_{S1} and A_{B1} of the subsequent solutions of the sample solution, the standard solution and water at 340 nm. Add 0.05 mL of aldehyde dehydrogenase TS to each of the cells, mix and stopper tightly. Allow to stand for 5 minutes at 22 ± 2°C. Determine the absorbances, A_{T2}, A_{S2} and A_{B2} of these solutions in the same manner as above, and calculate the content of aldehydes by the follwing equation: the content of aldehydes is not more than 500 ppm.

Content (ppm) of aldehydes [as acetaldehyde (CH_3CHO)]
$$= C/M \times \{(A_{T2} - A_{T1}) - (A_{B2} - A_{B1})\}/\{(A_{S2} - A_{S1}) - (A_{B2} - A_{B1})\} \times 100{,}000$$

M: Amount (g) of Povidone taken, calculated on the anhydrous basis

C: Concentration (mg/mL) of acetaldehyde in the standard solution, using 0.72 as conversion factor for acetaldehyde ammonia trimer trihydrate to acetaldehyde

(4) 1-Vinyl-2-pyrrolidone—Weigh accurately about 0.25 g of Povidone, dissolve in a mixture of water and acetonitrile (9:1) to make exactly 10 mL, and use this solution as the sample solution. Separately, dissolve 50 mg of 1-vinyl-2-pyrrolidone in a mixture of water and acetonitrile (9:1) to make exactly 100 mL. Pipet 1 mL of this solution and add a mixture of water and acetonitrile (9:1) to make exactly 100 mL. Pipet 5 mL of this solution, add a mixture of water and acetonitrile (9:1) to make exactly 100 mL, and use this solution as the standard solution. Perform the test with exactly 20 μL each of the sample solution and standard solution as directed under Liquid Chromatography *<2.01>* according to the following conditions, determine the peak areas, A_T and A_S, of 1-vinyl-2-pyrrolidone in each solution, and calculate the content of 1-vinyl-2-pyrrolidone by the following equation: it is not more than 10 ppm.

Content (ppm) of 1-vinyl-2-pyrrolidone
$$= 1/M \times A_T/A_S \times 2.5$$

M: Amount (g) of Povidone taken, calculated on the anhydrous basis

Operating conditions—

Detector: An ultraviolet spectrophotometer (detection wavelength: 235 nm).

Column: Stainless steel columns 4.0 mm in inside diameter and 10 mm in length, and 4.6 mm in inside diameter and 150 mm in length, packed with octadecylsilanized silica gel for liquid chromatography (5 μm in particle diameter), and use them as a guard column and a separation column, respectively.

Column temperature: A constant temperature of about 40°C.

Mobile phase: A mixture of water and acetonitrile (9:1).

Flow rate: 1.0 mL per minutes.

System suitability—

System performance: Dissolve 10 mg of 1-vinyl-2-pyrrolidone and 0.5 g of vinyl acetate in 100 mL of methanol. To 1 mL of this solution add a mixture of water and acetonitrile

(9:1) to make 100 mL. When the procedure is run with 20 μL of this solution under the above operating conditions, 1-vinyl-2-pyrrolidone and vinyl acetate are eluted in this order with the resolution between these peaks being not less than 2.0.

System repeatability: When the test is repeated 6 times with 20 μL of the standard solution under the above operating conditions, the relative standard deviation of the peak area of 1-vinyl-2-pyrrolidone is not more than 2.0%.

(5) Peroxides—Weigh exactly an amount of Povidone, equivalent to 4.0 g calculated on the anhydrous basis, dissolve in water to make exactly 100 mL, and use this solution as the sample solution. To 25 mL of the sample solution add 2 mL of titanium (III) chloride-sulfuric acid TS, and mix. Allow to stand for 30 minutes, and perform the test with this solution as directed under Ultraviolet-visible Spectrophotometry <*2.24*>, using a solution prepared by adding 2 mL of diluted sulfuric acid (13 in 100) to 25 mL of the sample solution as a blank: the absorbance of the solution at 405 nm is not more than 0.35 (not more than 400 ppm, expressed as hydrogen peroxide).

(6) Hydrazine—Weigh exactly an amount of Povidone equivalent to 2.5 g calculated on the anhydrous basis, transfer to a 50-mL centrifuge tube, add 25 mL of water, and stir to dissolve. Add 500 μL of a solution of salicylaldehyde in methanol (1 in 20), stir and warm at 60°C for 15 minutes in a water bath. Allow to cool, add 2.0 mL of toluene, stopper tightly, shake vigorously for 2 minutes, centrifuge, and use the upper layer of the mixture as the sample solution. Separately, dissolve 90 mg of salicylaldazine in toluene to make exactly 100 mL. Pipet 1 mL of this solution, add toluene to make exactly 100 mL, and use this solution as the standard solution. Perform the test with these solutions as directed under Thin-layer Chromatography <*2.03*>. Spot 10 μL each of the sample solution and standard solution on a plate of dimethylsilanized silica gel with fluorescent indicator for thin-layer chromatography. Develop the plate with a mixture of methanol and water (2:1) to a distance of about three-fourths of the length of the plate, and air-dry the plate. Examine under ultraviolet light (main wavelength: 365 nm): the fluorescence of the spot obtained from the sample solution corresponding to the spot having a *R*f value of about 0.3 from the standard solution is not more intense than that of the spot from the standard solution (not more than 1 ppm).

(7) Formic acid—Weigh accurately about 2 g of Pivodone, dissolve in water to make exactly 100 mL, and use this solution as the sample stock solution. Transfer a strongly acidic ion exchange resin (H type) for column chromatography previously suspended in water to a column of about 8 mm in inside diameter to give a packing depth of about 20 mm in length, and keep the resin layer constantly immersed in water. Pour 5 mL of water to the column, and adjust the flow rate about 1 mL per minute. When the level of the water comes down to near the top of the resin layer, put the sample stock solution into the column, discard the first 2 mL of the eluent, take 1.5 mL of the subsequent eluent, and use this solution as the sample solution. Separately, weigh accurately about 0.1 g of formic acid, dissolve in water to make exactly 100 mL. Pipet 1 mL of this solution, add water to make exactly 100 mL, and use this solution as the standard solution. Perform the test with exactly 50 μL each of the sample solution and standard solution as directed under Liquid Chromatography <*2.01*> according to the following conditions, and determine the peak areas, A_T and A_S, of formic acid in each solution. Calculate the content of formic acid by the following equation: it is not more than 0.5%.

$$\text{Content of formic acid(\%)} = M_S/M_T \times A_T/A_S$$

M_S: Amount (g) of formic acid taken

M_T: Amount (g) of Povidone taken, calculated on the anhydrous basis

Operating conditions—

Detector: An ultraviolet absorption photometer (wavelength: 210 nm).

Column: A stainless steel column 7.8 mm in inside diameter and 300 mm in length, packed with strongly acidic ion exchange resin for liquid chromatography (9 μm in particle diameter).

Column temperature: A constant temperature of about 35°C.

Mobile phase: Diluted perchloric acid (1 in 700).

Flow rate: 1.0 mL per minute.

System suitability—

System performance: When the procedure is run with 50 μL of the standard solution under the above operating conditions, the number of theoretical plates and the symmetry factor of the peak of formic acid are not less han 1000 and 0.5 to 1.5, respectively.

System repeatability: When the test is repeated 6 times with 50 μL of the standard solution under the above operating conditions, the relative standard deviation of the peak area of formic acid is not more than 2.0%.

(8) 2-Pyrrolidone—Weigh accurately about 0.5 g of Povidone, dissolve in a mixture of water and methanol for liquid chromatography (19:1) to make exactly 100 mL, and use this solution as the sample solution. Separately, dissolve 0.150 g of 2-pyrrolidone in a mixture of water and methanol for liquid chromatography (19:1) to make exactly 100 mL. Pipet 2 mL of this solution, add a mixture of water and methanol for liquid chromatography (19:1) to make exactly 100 mL, and use this solution as the standard solution. Perform the test with exactly 50 μL each of the sample solution and standard solution as directed under Liquid Chromatography <*2.01*> according to the following conditions, and determine the peak areas, A_T and A_S, of 2-pyrrolidone in each solution. Calculate the content of 2-pyrrolidone by the following equation: not more than 3.0%.

$$\text{Content (\%) of 2-pyrrolidone} = 1/M \times A_T/A_S \times 0.3$$

M: The amount (g) of Povidone taken, calculated on the anhydrous basis

Operating conditions—

Detector: An ultraviolet absorption photometer (wavelength: 205 nm).

Column: Stainless steel columns 4.0 mm in inside diameter and 10 mm in length, and 4.6 mm in inside diameter and 150 mm in length, packed with octadecylsilanized silica gel for liquid chromatography (5 μm in particle diameter), and use them as a guard column and a separation column, respectively.

Column temperature: A constant temperature of about 40°C.

Mobile phase: A mixture of water and methanol for liquid chromatography (19 : 1).

Flow rate: 0.8 mL per min.

System suitability—

System performance: When the procedure is run with 50 μL of the standard solution under the above operating conditions, the number of theoretical plates and the symmetry factor of the peak of 2-pyrrolidone are not less than 5000 and not more than 1.5, respectively.

System repeatability: When the test is repeated 6 times

with 50 μL of the standard solution under the above operating conditions, the relative standard deviation of the peak area of 2-pyrrolidone is not more than 2.0%.

Water *<2.48>* Not more than 5.0% (0.5 g, volumetric titration, direct titration).

Residue on ignition *<2.44>* Not more than 0.1% (1 g).

K-value Weigh accurately an amount of Povidone, calculated on the anhydrous basis, specified in the table below according to the nominal K-value, dissolve in water to make exactly 100 mL, allow to stand for 60 minutes, and use this solution as the sample solution. Perform the test with the sample solution and with water at 25°C as directed in Method 1 under Viscosity Determination *<2.53>*, and calculate the K-value by the following formula.

$$K = \frac{1.5 \log \nu_{rel.} - 1}{0.15 + 0.003\,c} + \frac{\sqrt{300\,c \log \nu_{rel.} + (c + 1.5\,c \log \nu_{rel.})^2}}{0.15\,c + 0.003\,c^2}$$

c: Mass (g) of Povidone in 100 mL of the solution, calculated on the anhydrous basis

$\nu_{rel.}$: Kinematic viscosity of the sample solution relative to that of water

Nominal K-value	Amount (g) calculated on anhydrous basis
Not more than 18	5.00
More than 18 and not more than 95	1.00
More than 95	0.10

The K-value is not less than 85% and not more than 115.0% of the nominal K-value when the nominal K-value is not more than 15, and the K-value is not less than 90.0% and not more than 108.0% of the nominal K-value when the nominal K-value is more than 15.

Assay Weigh accurately about 0.1 g of Povidone, and place in a Kjeldahl flask. Add 5 g of a decomposition accelerator (a powdered mixture of 33 g of potassium sulfate, 1 g of copper (II) sulfate pentahydrate and 1 g of titanium (IV) oxide), and wash down any adhering sample from the neck of the flask with a small amount of water. Add 7 mL of sulfuric acid allowing to flow down the inside wall of the flask. Heat the flask gradually over a free flame until the solution has a clear, yellow-green color and the inside wall of the flask is free from a carbonaceous material, and then heat for further 45 minutes. After cooling, add cautiously 20 mL of water, and connect the flask to the distillation apparatus previously washed by passing steam through it. To the absorption flask add 30 mL of a solution of boric acid (1 in 25), 3 drops of bromocresol green-methyl red TS and sufficient water to immerse the lower end of the condenser tube. Add 30 mL of a solution of sodium hydroxide (2 in 5) through the funnel, rinse cautiously the funnel with 10 ml of water, immediately close the clamp attached to the rubber tube, then start the distillation with steam to get 80 to 100 mL of the distillate. Remove the absorption flask from the lower end of the condenser tube, rinsing the end part with a small quantity of water, and titrate *<2.50>* the distillate with 0.025 mol/L sulfuric acid VS until the color of the solution changes from green through pale grayish blue to pale grayish red-purple. Perform a blank determination in the same manner, and make any necessary correction.

Each mL of 0.025 mol/L sulfuric acid VS
= 0.700 mg of N

◆**Containers and storage** Containers—Tight containers.◆

Povidone-Iodine

ポビドンヨード

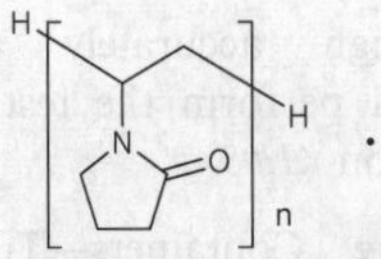

$(C_6H_9NO)_n.xI$

Poly[1-(2-oxopyrrolidin-1-yl)ethylene] iodine

[25655-41-8]

Povidone-Iodine is a complex of iodine with 1-vinyl-2-pyrrolidone polymer.

It contains not less than 9.0% and not more than 12.0% of available iodine (I: 126.90), and not less than 9.5% and not more than 11.5% of nitrogen (N: 14.01), calculated on the dried basis.

Description Povidone-Iodine occurs as a dark red-brown powder. It has a faint, characteristic odor.

It is freely soluble in water and in ethanol (99.5).

The pH of a solution obtained by dissolving 1.0 g of Povidone-Iodine in 100 mL of water is between 1.5 and 3.5.

Identification **(1)** To 10 mL of diluted starch TS (1 in 10) add 1 drop of a solution of Povidone-Iodine (1 in 10): a deep blue color develops.

(2) To 1 mL of a solution of Povidone-Iodine (1 in 100) add 1 mL of sodium thiosulfate TS, and add 1 mL of ammonium thiocyanate-cobalt (II) nitrate TS and 2 drops of mol/L hydrochloric acid TS: a blue color develops, and a blue precipitate is gradually formed.

Purity **(1)** Clarity and color of solution—Dissolve 0.30 g of Povidone-Iodine in 100 mL of water: the solution is clear and brown.

(2) Heavy metals *<1.07>*—Proceed with 1.0 g of Povidone-Iodine according to Method 2, and perform the test. Prepare the control solution with 2.0 mL of Standard Lead Solution (not more than 20 ppm).

(3) Arsenic *<1.11>*—Prepare the test solution with 1.0 g of Povidone-Iodine according to Method 4, and perform the test (not more than 2 ppm).

(4) Iodide ion—Weigh accurately about 0.5 g of Povidone-Iodine, dissolve in 100 mL of water, and add sodium hydrogensulfite TS until the color of iodine completely disappears. To this solution add exactly 25 mL of 0.1 mol/L silver nitrate VS, shake thoroughly with 10 mL of nitric acid, titrate *<2.50>* the excess silver nitrate with 0.1 mol/L ammonium thiocyanate VS until the solution develops a red-brown color, and calculate the total amount of iodine (indicator: 1 mL of ammonium iron (III) sulfate TS). Perform a blank determination in the same manner.

Each mL of 0.1 mol/L ammonium thiocyanate VS
= 12.69 mg of I

Obtain the amount of iodide ion, calculated on the dried basis, by deducting the amount (%) of available iodine from the total amount (%) of iodine: not more than 6.6%.

Loss on drying *<2.41>* Not more than 8.0% (1 g, 100°C, 3 hours).

Residue on ignition *<2.44>* Not more than 0.05% (5 g).

Assay **(1)** Available iodine—Weigh accurately about 0.5 g of Povidone-Iodine, dissolve in 30 mL of water, and titrate <*2.50*> with 0.02 mol/L sodium thiosulfate VS (indicator: 2 mL of starch TS).

Each mL of 0.02 mol/L sodium thiosulfate VS
= 2.538 mg of I

(2) Nitrogen—Weigh accurately about 20 mg of Povidone-Iodine, and perform the test as directed under Nitrogen Determination <*1.08*>.

Containers and storage Containers—Tight containers.

Pranlukast Hydrate

プランルカスト水和物

$C_{27}H_{23}N_5O_4 \cdot \frac{1}{2}H_2O$: 490.51
N-[4-Oxo-2-(1*H*-tetrazol-5-yl)-4*H*-chromen-8-yl]-4-(4-phenylbutyloxy)benzamide hemihydrate
[*150821-03-7*]

Pranlukast Hydrate contains not less than 98.0% and not more than 101.0% of pranlukast ($C_{27}H_{23}N_5O_4$: 481.50), calculated on the anhydrous basis.

Description Pranlukast Hydrate occurs as a white to light yellow crystalline powder.

It is very slightly soluble in ethanol (99.5), and practically insoluble in water.

Melting point: about 233°C (with decomposition).

Identification **(1)** Determine the absorption spectrum of a solution of Pranlukast Hydrate in ethanol (99.5) (1 in 100,000) as directed under Ultraviolet-visible Spectrophotometry <*2.24*>, and compare the spectrum with the Reference Spectrum or the spectrum of a solution of Pranlukast RS prepared in the same manner as the sample solution: both spectra exhibit similar intensities of absorption at the same wavelengths.

(2) Determine the infrared absorption spectrum of Pranlukast Hydrate as directed in the potassium bromide disk method under Infrared Spectrophotometry <*2.25*>, and compare the spectrum with the Reference Spectrum or the spectrum of Pranlukast RS: both spectra exhibit similar intensities of absorption at the same wave numbers.

Purity **(1)** Heavy metals <*1.07*>—Suspend 1.0 g of Pranlukast Hydrate in 10 mL of *N*,*N*-dimethylformamide, proceed according to Method 4, and perform the test. Prepare the control solution with 10 mL of *N*,*N*-dimethylformamide in the same manner as preparation of the test solution, and add 2.0 mL of Standard Lead Solution (not more than 20 ppm).

(2) Arsenic <*1.11*>—Suspend 1.0 g of Pranlukast Hydrate in 10 mL of *N*,*N*-dimethylformamide, then proceed according to Method 4, and perform the test (not more than 2 ppm).

(3) Related substances—Dissolve 20 mg of Pranlukast Hydrate in 50 mL of a mixture of acetonitrile and dimethylsulfoxide (3:1), and use this solution as the sample solution. Pipet 1 mL of the sample solution, add a mixture of acetonitrile and dimethylsulfoxide (3:1) to make exactly 100 mL, and use this solution as the standard solution. Perform the test with exactly 10 μL each of the sample solution and standard solution as directed under Liquid Chromatography <*2.01*> according to the following conditions. Determine each peak area by the automatic integration method: the area of the peak, having the relative retention time about 1.5 to pranlukast, obtained from the sample solution is not larger than 1/2 times that of pranlukast from the standard solution, the area of the peak other than pranlukast and the peak mentioned above from the sample solution is not larger than 1/5 times that of pranlukast from the standard solution, and the total area of the peaks other than pranlukast from the sample solution is not larger than the peak area of pranlukast from the standard solution.

Operating conditions—

Detector, column, column temperature, mobile phase, and flow rate: Proceed as directed in the operating conditions in the Assay.

Time span of measurement: About 5 times as long as the retention time of pranlukast, beginning after the solvent peak.

System suitability—

Test for required detectability: Pipet 5 mL of the standard solution, add a mixture of acetonitrile and dimethylsulfoxide (3:1) to make exactly 50 mL. Confirm that the peak area of pranlukast obtained with 10 μL of this solution is equivalent to 7 to 13% of that with 10 μL of the standard solution.

System performance: When the procedure is run with 10 μL of the standard solution under the above operating conditions, the number of theoretical plates and the symmetry factor of the peak of pranlukast are not less than 6000 and not more than 1.5, respectively.

System repeatability: When the test is repeated 6 times with 10 μL of the standard solution under the above operating conditions, the relative standard deviation of the peak area of pranlukast is not more than 2.0%.

Water <*2.48*> 1.5 - 2.2% (50 mg, coulometric titration).

Residue on ignition <*2.44*> Not more than 0.2% (1 g).

Assay Weigh accurately about 20 mg each of Pranlukast Hydrate and Pranlukast RS (separately determine the water <*2.48*> in the same manner as Pranlukast Hydrate), dissolve them separately in a mixture of acetonitrile and dimethylsulfoxide (3:1) to make exactly 50 mL. To exactly 5 mL each of these solutions add exactly 5 mL of the internal standard solution, and use these solutions as the sample solution and the standard solution, respectively. Perform the test with 4 μL each of the sample solution and standard solution as directed under Liquid Chromatography <*2.01*> according to the following conditions, and calculate the ratios, Q_T and Q_S, of the peak area of pranlukast to that of the internal standard.

Amount (mg) of pranlukast ($C_{27}H_{23}N_5O_4$)
$= M_S \times Q_T/Q_S$

M_S: Amount (mg) of Pranlukast RS taken, calculated on the anhydrous basis

Internal standard solution—A solution of isoamyl parahydroxybenzoate in a mixture of acetonitrile and dimethylsulfoxide (3:1) (1 in 2500).

Operating conditions—

Detector: An ultraviolet absorption photometer (wavelength: 260 nm).

Column: A stainless steel column 6 mm in inside diameter and 15 cm in length, packed with octylsilanized silica gel for liquid chromatography (5 μm in particle diameter).

Column temperature: A constant temperature of about 25°C.

Mobile phase: A mixture of 0.02 mol/L potassium dihydrogen phosphate TS, acetonitrile and methanol (5:5:1).

Flow rate: Adjust so that the retention time of pranlukast is about 10 minutes.

System suitability—

System performance: When the procedure is run with 4 μL of the standard solution under the above operating conditions, pranlukast and the internal standard are eluted in this order with the resolution between these peaks being not less than 3.

System repeatability: When the test is repeated 6 times with 4 μL of the standard solution under the above operating conditions, the relative standard deviation of the ratio of the peak area of pranlukast to that of the internal standard is not more than 1.0%.

Containers and storage Containers—Tight containers.

Pranoprofen

プラノプロフェン

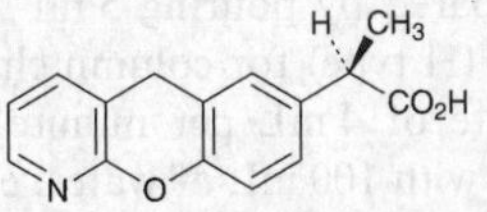

and enantiomer

$C_{15}H_{13}NO_3$: 255.27
(2*RS*)-2-(10*H*-9-Oxa-1-azaanthracen-6-yl)propanoic acid
[*52549-17-4*]

Pranoprofen, when dried, contains not less than 98.5% of pranoprofen ($C_{15}H_{13}NO_3$).

Description Pranoprofen occurs as a white to pale yellow-white crystalline powder.

It is freely soluble in *N,N*-dimethylformamide, soluble in acetic acid (100), sparingly soluble in methanol, slightly soluble in acetonitrile, in ethanol (95) and in acetic anhydride, very slightly soluble in diethyl ether, and practically insoluble in water.

A solution of Pranoprofen in *N,N*-dimethylformamide (1 in 30) shows no optical rotation.

Identification **(1)** Dissolve 0.02 g of Pranoprofen in 1 mol/L hydrochloric acid TS to make 100 mL, and dilute 10 mL of the solution with water to make 100 mL. Determine the absorption spectrum of the solution as directed under Ultraviolet-visible Spectrophotometry ⟨*2.24*⟩, and compare the spectrum with the Reference Spectrum: both spectra exhibit similar intensities of absorption at the same wavelengths.

(2) Determine the infrared absorption spectrum of Pranoprofen as directed in the potassium bromide disk method under Infrared Spectrophotometry ⟨*2.25*⟩, and compare the spectrum with the Reference Spectrum: both spectra exhibit similar intensities of absorption at the same wave numbers.

Melting point ⟨*2.60*⟩ 186 – 190°C

Purity **(1)** Chloride ⟨*1.03*⟩—Dissolve 0.5 g of Pranoprofen in 40 mL of methanol, and 6 mL of dilute nitric acid, and add water to make 50 mL. Perform the test using this solution as the test solution. Prepare the control solution as follows. To 0.30 mL of 0.01 mol/L hydrochloric acid VS add 40 mL of methanol, 6 mL of dilute nitric acid and water to make 50 mL (not more than 0.021%).

(2) Heavy metals ⟨*1.07*⟩—Proceed with 2.0 g of Pranoprofen according to Method 4, and perform the test. Prepare the control solution with 2.0 mL of the Standard Lead Solution (not more than 10 ppm).

(3) Related Substances—Dissolve 50 mg of Pranoprofen in 50 mL of the mobile phase, and use this solution as the sample solution. Pipet 1 mL of the sample solution, add the mobile phase to make exactly 200 mL, and use this solution as the standard solution. Perform the test with exactly 10 μL each of the sample solution and standard solution as directed under Liquid Chromatography ⟨*2.01*⟩ according to the following conditions. Determine each peak area from both solutions by the automatic integration method: the each area of the peaks other than pranoprofen obtained from the sample solution is not larger than the peak area of pranoprofen from the standard solution, and the total peak area of them is not larger than 2 times the peak area of pranoprofen from the standard solution.

Operating conditions—

Detector: An ultraviolet absorption photometer (wavelength: 275 nm).

Column: A stainless steel column about 6 mm in inside diameter and about 15 cm in length, packed with octadecylsilanized silica gel for liquid chromatography (5 μm in particle diameter).

Column temperature: A constant temperature of about 25°C.

Mobile phase: Dissolve 7.02 g of sodium perchlorate monohydrate in 1000 mL of water, and adjust the pH to 2.5 with perchloric acid. To 2 volumes of this solution add 1 volume of acetonitrile.

Flow rate: Adjust so that the retention time of pranoprofen is about 10 minutes.

Selection of column: Dissolve 4 mg each of Pranoprofen and ethyl parahydroxybenzoate in 200 mL of the mobile phase. Proceed with 10 μL of this solution under the above operating conditions, and calculate the resolution. Use a column giving elution of pranoprofen and ethyl parahydroxybenzoate in this order with the resolution between these peaks being not less than 2.1.

Detection sensitivity: Adjust the detection sensitivity so that the peak height of pranoprofen obtained from 10 μL of the standard solution is between 10 mm and 20 mm.

Time span of measurement: About three times as long as the retention time of pranoprofen.

Loss on drying ⟨*2.41*⟩ Not more than 0.5% (1 g, in vacuum, phosphorus (V) oxide, 4 hours).

Residue on ignition ⟨*2.44*⟩ Not more than 0.1% (1 g).

Assay Weigh accurately about 0.4 g of Pranoprofen, previously dried, dissolve in 70 mL of a mixture of acetic anhydride and acetic acid (100) (7:3), and titrate ⟨*2.50*⟩ with 0.1 mol/L perchloric acid VS (potentiometric titration). Perform a blank determination in the same manner, and make any necessary correction.

Each mL of 0.1 mol/L perchloric acid VS
= 25.53 mg of $C_{15}H_{13}NO_3$

Containers and storage Containers—Tight containers.

Storage—Light-resistant.

Prasterone Sodium Sulfate Hydrate

プラステロン硫酸エステルナトリウム水和物

$C_{19}H_{27}NaO_5S.2H_2O$: 426.50
Monosodium 17-oxoandrost-5-en-3β-yl sulfate dihydrate
[*1099-87-2*, anhydride]

Sodium Prasterone Sulfate Hydrate contains not less than 98.0% of prasterone sodium sulfate ($C_{19}H_{27}NaO_5S$: 390.47), calculated on the dried basis.

Description Prasterone Sodium Sulfate Hydrate occurs as white crystals or crystalline powder. It is odorless.

It is soluble in methanol, sparingly soluble in water and in ethanol (95), and practically insoluble in acetone and in diethyl ether.

The pH of a solution of 1.0 g of Prasterone Sodium Sulfate Hydrate in 200 mL of water is between 4.5 and 6.5.

Melting point: about 160°C (with decomposition, after drying).

Identification **(1)** Dissolve 0.01 g of Prasterone Sodium Sulfate Hydrate in 4 mL of ethanol (95), add 2 mL of 1,3-dinitrobenzene TS and 2 mL of a solution of sodium hydroxide (1 in 8): a red-purple color develops, and gradually changes to brown.

(2) To 10 mL of a solution of Prasterone Sodium Sulfate Hydrate (1 in 200) add 0.5 mL of bromine TS: the color of bromine TS immediately disappears.

(3) Determine the infrared absorption spectrum of Prasterone Sodium Sulfate Hydrate as directed in the potassium bromide disk method under the Infrared Spectrophotometry <*2.25*>, and compare the spectrum with the Reference Spectrum: both spectra exhibit similar intensities of absorption at the same wave numbers.

(4) A solution of Prasterone Sodium Sulfate Hydrate (1 in 200) responds to Qualitative Tests <*1.09*> for sodium salt.

Optical rotation <*2.49*> $[\alpha]_D^{20}$: +10.7 – +12.1° (0.73 g calculated on the dried basis, methanol, 20 mL, 100 mm).

Purity **(1)** Clarity and color of solution—Dissolve 0.25 g of Prasterone Sodium Sulfate Hydrate in 50 mL of water: the solution is clear and colorless.

(2) Chloride <*1.03*>—Dissolve 1.0 g of Prasterone Sodium Sulfate Hydrate in 20 mL of acetone and 20 mL of water, and add 6 mL of dilute nitric acid and water to make 50 mL. Perform the test using this solution as the test solution. Prepare the control solution as follows: to 0.30 mL of 0.01 mol/L hydrochloric acid VS add 20 mL of acetone, 6 mL of dilute nitric acid and water to make 50 mL (not more than 0.011%).

(3) Sulfate <*1.14*>—To 1.2 g of Prasterone Sodium Sulfate Hydrate add 20 mL of water, shake vigorously for 5 minutes, and filter. To 10 mL of the filtrate add 20 mL of acetone, 1 mL of dilute hydrochloric acid and water to make 50 mL. Perform the test using this solution as the test solution. Prepare the control solution as follows: to 0.40 mL of 0.005 mol/L sulfuric acid VS add 20 mL of acetone, 1 mL of dilute hydrochloric acid and water to make 50 mL (not more than 0.032%).

(4) Heavy metals <*1.07*>—Proceed with 2.0 g of Prasterone Sodium Sulfate Hydrate according to Method 2, and perform the test. Prepare the control solution with 2.0 mL of Standard Lead Solution (not more than 10 ppm).

(5) Related substances—Dissolve 0.10 g of Prasterone Sodium Sulfate Hydrate in 10 mL of methanol, and use this solution as the sample solution. Pipet 1 mL of the sample solution, add methanol to make exactly 200 mL, and use this solution as the standard solution. Perform the test with these solutions as directed under Thin-layer Chromatography <*2.03*>. Spot 5 μL each of the sample solution and standard solution on a plate of silica gel with fluorescent indicator for thin-layer chromatography. Develop the plate with a mixture of chloroform, methanol and water (75:22:3) to a distance of about 10 cm, and air-dry the plate. Spray evenly a mixture of sulfuric acid and ethanol (95) (1:1) on the plate, and heat the plate at 80°C for 5 minutes: the spots other than the principal spot obtained from the sample solution are not more intense than the spot from the standard solution.

Loss on drying <*2.41*> 8.0 – 9.0% (0.5 g, in vacuum, phosphorus (V) oxide, 60°C, 3 hours).

Assay Weigh accurately about 0.25 g of Prasterone Sodium Sulfate Hydrate, dissolve in 30 mL of water. Apply this solution to a chromatographic column 10 mm in inside diameter, previously prepared by pouring 5 mL of strongly acidic ion-exchange resin (H type) for column chromatography, and elute at the rate of 4 mL per minute. Wash the chromatographic column with 100 mL of water, combine the washings with above effluent solution, and titrate <*2.50*> with 0.05 mol/L sodium hydroxide VS (potentiometric titration). Perform a blank determination in the same manner, and make any necessary correction.

Each mL of 0.05 mol/L sodium hydroxide VS
= 19.52 mg of $C_{19}H_{27}NaO_5S$

Containers and storage Containers—Tight containers.

Pravastatin Sodium

プラバスタチンナトリウム

$C_{23}H_{35}NaO_7$: 446.51
Monosodium (3*R*,5*R*)-3,5-dihydroxy-
7-{(1*S*,2*S*,6*S*,8*S*,8a*R*)-6-hydroxy-2-methyl-
8-[(2*S*)-2-methylbutanoyloxy]-
1,2,6,7,8,8a-hexahydronaphthalen-1-yl}heptanoate
[*81131-70-6*]

Pravastatin Sodium contains not less than 98.5% and not more than 101.0% of pravastatin sodium ($C_{23}H_{35}NaO_7$), calculated on the anhydrous and residual solvent-free basis.

Description Pravastatin Sodium occurs as a white to yellowish white, powder or crystalline powder.

It is freely soluble in water and in methanol, and soluble in ethanol (99.5).

It is hygroscopic.

Identification **(1)** Determine the absorption spectrum of a solution of Pravastatin Sodium (1 in 100,000) as directed under Ultraviolet-visible Spectrophotometry *<2.24>*, and compare the spectrum with the Reference Spectrum: both spectra exhibit similar intensities of absorption at the same wavelengths.

(2) Determine the infrared absorption spectrum of Pravastatin Sodium as directed in the potassium bromide disk method under Infrared Spectrophotometry *<2.25>*: it exhibits absorption at the wave numbers of about 2970 cm^{-1}, 2880 cm^{-1}, 1727 cm^{-1} and 1578 cm^{-1}.

(3) Dissolve 50 mg of Pravastatin Sodium in 5 mL of methanol, and use this solution as the sample solution. Separately, dissolve 24 mg of Pravastatin 1,1,3,3-Tetramethylbutylammonium RS in 2 mL of methanol, and use this solution as the standard solution. Perform the test with these solutions as directed under Thin-layer Chromatography *<2.03>*. Spot 2 μL each of the sample solution and standard solution on a plate of silica gel with fluorescent indicator for thin-layer chromatography. Develop the plate with a mixture of ethyl acetate, ethanol (99.5) and acetic acid (100) (80:16:1) to a distance of about 8 cm, and air-dry the plate. Examine under ultraviolet light (main wavelength: 254 nm): the color tone and the *R*f value of the principal spot obtained from the sample solution are not different with them of the spot from the standard solution.

(4) A solution of Pravastatin Sodium (1 in 10) responds to Qualitative Tests *<1.09>* (1) for sodium salt.

Optical rotation *<2.49>* $[\alpha]_D^{20}$: +153 – +159° (0.1 g calculated on the anhydrous and residual solvent-free basis, water, 20 mL, 100 mm).

pH *<2.54>* The pH of a solution obtained by dissolving 1.0 g of Pravastatin Sodium in 20 mL of freshly boiled and cooled water is between 7.2 and 8.2.

Purity **(1)** Heavy metals *<1.07>*—Proceed with 1.0 g of Pravastatin Sodium according to Method 2, and perform the test. Prepare the control solution with 1.0 mL of Standard Lead Solution (not more than 10 ppm).

(2) Related substances—Dissolve 0.10 g of Pravastatin Sodium in 100 mL of a mixture of water and methanol (11:9), and use this solution as the sample solution. Pipet 10 mL of the sample solution, add the mixture of water and methanol (11:9) to make exactly 100 mL. Pipet 5 mL of this solution, add the mixture of water and methanol (11:9) to make exactly 100 mL, and use this solution as the standard solution. Perform the test with exactly 10 μL each of the sample solution and standard solution as directed under Liquid Chromatography *<2.01>* according to the following conditions, and determine each peak area by the automatic integration method: the area of the peak other than pravastatin from the sample solution is not larger than 1/5 times the peak area of pravastatin from the standard solution, and the total area of the peaks other than pravastatin from the sample solution is not larger than the peak area of pravastatin from the standard solution. Keep the sample solution and standard solution at not over than15°C.

Operating conditions—

Detector, column, column temperature, mobile phase, and flow rate: Proceed as directed in the operating conditions in the Assay.

Time span of measurement: About 2.5 times as long as the retention time of pravastatin, beginning after the solvent peak.

System suitability—

Test for required detectability: To exactly 5 mL of the standard solution add a mixture of water and methanol (11:9) to make exactly 50 mL. Confirm that the peak area of pravastatin obtained with 10 μL of this solution is equivalent to 7 to 13% of that obtained with 10 μL of the standard solution.

System performance: Dissolve 5 mg of pravastatin sodium in 50 mL of the mixture of water and methanol (11:9). When the procedure is run with 10 μL of this solution under the above operating conditions, the number of theoretical plates and the symmetry factor of the peak of pravastatin are not less than 3500 and not more than 1.6, respectively.

System repeatability: When the test is repeated 6 times with 10 μL of the standard solution under the above operating conditions, the relative standard deviation of the peak area of pravastatin is not more than 2.0%.

Water *<2.48>* Not more than 4.0% (0.5 g, volumetric titration, direct titration).

Assay Weigh accurately about 0.1 g of Pravastatin Sodium, and dissolve in a mixture of water and methanol (11:9) to make exactly 100 mL. Pipet 10 mL of this solution, add exactly 10 mL of the internal standard solution and the mixture of water and methanol (11:9) to make 100 mL, and use this solution as the sample solution. Separately, weigh accurately about 30 mg of Pravastatin 1,1,3,3-Tetramethylbutylammonium RS (previously determine the water *<2.48>* with 0.5 g by direct titration in volumetric titration) dissolve in the mixture of water and methanol (11:9) to make exactly 25 mL. Pipet 10 mL of this solution, add exactly 10 mL of the internal standard solution, add a mixture of water and methanol (11:9) to make 100 mL, and use this solution as the standard solution. Perform the test with 10 μL each of the sample solution and standard solution as directed under Liquid Chromatography *<2.01>* according to the following conditions, and calculate the ratios, Q_T and Q_S, of the peak area of pravastatin to that of the internal standard.

$$\text{Amount (mg) of pravastatin sodium } (C_{23}H_{35}NaO_7) = M_S \times Q_T/Q_S \times 4 \times 1.052$$

M_S: Amount (mg) of pravastatin in taken Pravastatin 1,1,3,3-Tetramethylbutylammonium RS, calculated on the anhydrous basis

*Internal standard solution—*A solution of ethyl parahydroxybenzoate in the mixture of water and methanol (11:9) (3 in 4000).

Operating conditions—

Detector: An ultraviolet absorption photometer (wavelength: 238 nm).

Column: A stainless steel column 4.6 mm in inside diameter and 15 cm in length, packed with octadecylsilanized silica gel for liquid chromatography (5 μm in particle diameter).

Column temperature: A constant temperature of about 25°C.

Mobile phase: A mixture of water, methanol, acetic acid (100) and triethylamine (550:450:1:1).

Flow rate: Adjust so that the retention time of pravastatin is about 21 minutes.

System suitability—

System performance: When the procedure is run with 10 μL of the standard solution under the above operating conditions, the internal standard and pravastatin are eluted in this order with the resolution between these peaks being not less than 10.

System repeatability: When the test is repeated 6 times with 10 μL of the standard solution under the above operating conditions, the relative standard deviation of the ratio of the peak area of pravastatin to that of the internal standard is not more than 1.0%.

Containers and storage Containers—Tight containers.

Pravastatin Sodium Fine Granules

プラバスタチンナトリウム細粒

Pravastatin Sodium Fine Granules contain not less than 95.0% and not more than 105.0% of the labeled amount of pravastatin sodium ($C_{23}H_{35}NaO_7$: 446.51).

Method of preparation Prepare as directed under Granules, with Pravastatin Sodium.

Identification To an amount of Pravastatin Sodium Fine Granules, equivalent to 10 mg of Pravastatin Sodium, add 20 mL of water, sonicate for 15 minutes, and centrifuge. Filter the supernatant liquid, discard the first 5 mL of the filtrate, and add water to 1 mL of the subsequent filtrate to make 50 mL. Determine the absorption spectrum of this solution as directed under Ultraviolet-visible Spectrophotometry <*2.24*>: it exhibits a maximum between 237 nm and 241 nm.

Purity Related substances—The sample solution and the standard solution are stored at not exceeding 5°C after preparation. To an amount of Pravastatin Sodium Fine Granules, equivalent to 25 mg of Pravastatin Sodium, add 25 mL of a mixture of water and methanol (1:1), sonicate for 15 minutes, and centrifuge. Filter the supernatant liquid, discard the first 5 mL of the filtrate, and use the subsequent filtrate as the sample solution. Pipet 1 mL of the sample solution, add a mixture of water and methanol (1:1) to make exactly 100 mL, and use this solution as the standard solution. Perform the test with exactly 20 μL each of the sample solution and standard solution as directed under Liquid Chromatography <*2.01*> according to the following conditions. Determine each peak area by the automatic integration method: the area of the peaks, having the relative retention time of about 0.36 and about 1.9 to pravastatin, obtained from the sample solution is not larger than 1/2 times and 3 times the peak area of pravastatin from the standard solution, respectively, the area of the peak other than pravastatin and the peaks mentioned above from the sample solution is not larger than 1/5 times the peak area of pravastatin from the standard solution, and the total area of the peaks other than pravastatin from the sample solution is not larger than 4.5 times the peak area of pravastatin from the standard solution. For the area of the peaks, having the relative retention time of about 0.28, about 0.36 and about 0.88, multiply their correction factors, 1.16, 1.72 and 1.22, respectively.

Operating conditions—

Detector: An ultraviolet spectrophotometer (wavelength: 238 nm).

Column: A stainless steel column 4.6 mm in inside diameter and 15 cm in length, packed with octadecylsilanized silica gel for liquid chromatography (5 μm in particle diameter).

Column temperature: A constant temperature of about 25°C.

Mobile phase A: A mixture of water, methanol, acetic acid (100) and triethylamine (750:250:1:1).

Mobile phase B: A mixture of methanol, water, acetic acid (100) and triethylamine (650:350:1:1).

Flowing of mobile phase: Control the gradient by mixing the mobile phases A and B as directed in the following table.

Time after injection of sample (min)	Mobile phase A (vol%)	Mobile phase B (vol%)
0 – 50	50	50
50 – 75	50 → 0	50 → 100

Flow rate: 1.3 mL per minute.

Time span of measurement: For 75 minutes after injection, beginning after the solvent peak.

System suitability—

Test for required detectability: To exactly 1 mL of the standard solution add a mixture of water and methanol (1:1) to make exactly 10 mL. Confirm that the peak area of pravastatin obtained with 20 μL of this solution is equivalent to 7 to 13% of that with 20 μL of the standard solution.

System performance: When the procedure is run with 20 μL of the standard solution under the above operating conditions, the number of theoretical plates and the symmetry factor of the peak of pravastatin are not less than 3500 and not more than 1.6, respectively.

System repeatability: When the test is repeated 6 times with 20 μL of the standard solution under the above operating conditions, the relative standard deviation of the peak area of pravastatin is not more than 1.5%.

Uniformity of dosage units <*6.02*> Perform the test according to the following method: the Pravastatin Sodium Fine Granules in single-dose packages meet the requirement of the Content uniformity test.

To the total amount of the content of 1 package of Pravastatin Sodium Fine Granules add exactly V mL of the internal standard solution so that each mL contains 0.25 mg of pravastatin sodium ($C_{23}H_{35}NaO_7$), sonicate for 15 minutes, and centrifuge. Filter the supernatant liquid, discard the first 5 mL of the filtrate, pipet 2 mL of the subsequent filtrate add a mixture of water and methanol (1 in 1) to make 20 mL, and use this solution as the sample solution. Then, proceed as directed in the Assay.

$$\text{Amount (mg) of pravastatin sodium } (C_{23}H_{35}NaO_7) = M_S \times Q_T/Q_S \times V/100 \times 1.052$$

M_S: Amount (mg) of pravastatin in taken Pravastatin 1,1,3,3-Tetramethylbutylammonium RS, calculated on the anhydrous basis

Internal standard solution—A solution of propyl parahydroxybenzoate in a mixture of water and methanol (1:1) (3 in 10,000).

Dissolution <*6.10*> When the test is performed at 50 revolutions per minute according to the Paddle method, using 900 mL of water as the dissolution medium, the dissolution rate in 15 minutes of Pravastatin Sodium Fine Granules is not less than 80%.

Start the test with an accurately weighed amount of Pravastatin Sodium Fine Granules, equivalent to about 5 mg of pravastatin sodium ($C_{23}H_{35}NaO_7$), withdraw not less than 20 mL of the medium at the specified minute after starting the test, and filter through a membrane filter with a pore size not exceeding 0.45 μm. Discard not less than 10 mL of the first filtrate, and use the subsequent filtrate as the sample solution. Separately, weigh accurately about 23 mg of Pravastatin 1,1,3,3-Tetramethylbutylammonium RS (separately determine the water <*2.48*> in the same manner as Pravastatin Sodium), and dissolve in water to make exactly 100 mL. Pipet 3 mL of this solution, add water to make exactly 100 mL, and use this solution as the standard solution.

Determine the absorbances, A_{T1} and A_{S1}, at 238 nm and A_{T2} and A_{S2} at 265 nm of the sample solution and standard solution as directed under Ultraviolet-visible Spectrophotometry <2.24>.

Dissolution rate (%) with respect to the labeled amount of pravastatin sodium ($C_{23}H_{35}NaO_7$)

$$= M_S/M_T \times (A_{T1} - A_{T2})/(A_{S1} - A_{S2}) \times 1/C \times 27 \times 0.806$$

M_S: Amount (mg) of Pravastatin 1,1,3,3-Tetramethylbutylammonium RS taken, calculated on the anhydrous basis
M_T: Amount (g) of Pravastatin Sodium Fine Granules taken
C: Labeled amount (mg) of pravastatin sodium ($C_{23}H_{35}NaO_7$) in 1 g

Assay Weigh accurately an amount of Pravastatin Sodium Fine Granules, equivalent to about 5 mg of pravastatin sodium ($C_{23}H_{35}NaO_7$), add exactly 20 mL of the internal standard solution, sonicate for 15 minute, and centrifuge. Filter the supernatant liquid, discard the first 5 mL of the filtrate, to 2 mL of the subsequent filtrate add a mixture of water and methanol (1:1) to make 20 mL, and use this solution as the sample solution. Separately, weigh accurately about 32 mg of Pravastatin 1,1,3,3-Tetramethylbutylammonium RS (separately determine the water <2.48> in the same manner as Pravastatin Sodium), and dissolve in a mixture of water and methanol (1:1) to make exactly 100 mL. Pipet 5 mL of this solution, add exactly 5 mL of the internal standard solution, then add a mixture of water and methanol (1:1) to make 50 mL, and use this solution as the standard solution. Perform the test with 10 μL each of the sample solution and standard solution as directed under Liquid Chromatography <2.01> according to the following conditions, and calculate the ratios, Q_T and Q_S, of the peak area of pravastatin to that of the internal standard.

Amount (mg) of pravastatin sodium ($C_{23}H_{35}NaO_7$)

$$= M_S \times Q_T/Q_S \times 1/5 \times 1.052$$

M_S: Amount (mg) of pravastatin in taken Pravastatin 1,1,3,3-Tetramethylbutylammonium RS, calculated on the anhydrous basis

Internal standard solution—A solution of propyl parahydroxybenzoate in a mixture of water and methanol (1:1) (3 in 10,000).

Operating conditions—

Proceed as directed in the operating conditions in the Assay under Pravastatin Sodium.

System suitability—

System performance: When the procedure is run with 10 μL of the standard solution under the above operating conditions, the internal standard and pravastatin are eluted in this order with the resolution between these peaks being not less than 4.

System repeatability: When the test is repeated 6 times with 10 μL of the standard solution under the above operating conditions, the relative standard deviation of the ratio of the peak area of pravastatin to that of the internal standard is not more than 1.0%.

Containers and storage Containers—Well-closed containers.

Pravastatin Sodium Solution

プラバスタチンナトリウム液

Pravastatin Sodium Solution contains not less than 95.0% and not more than 105.0% of the labeled amount of pravastatin sodium ($C_{23}H_{35}NaO_7$: 446.51).

Method of preparation Prepare as directed under Liquids and Solutions for Oral Administration, with Pravastatin Sodium.

Identification Pass a volume of Pravastatin Sodium Solution, equivalent to 1 mg of Pravastatin Sodium, through a column [5.5 mm in inside diameter, packed with 30 mg of divinylbenzene-*N*-vinyl pyrrolidone copolymer for column chromatography (30 μm in particle size), and washed with 1 mL of methanol and 1 mL of water]. Then wash with 1 mL of water, and elute with 1 mL of methanol. To 0.1 mL of the eluate add water to make 10 mL, and determine the absorption spectrum of this solution as directed under Ultraviolet-visible Spectrophotometry <2.24>: it exhibits a maximum between 237 nm and 241 nm.

pH Being specified separately when the drug is granted approval based on the Law.

Purity Related substances—The sample solution and the standard solution are stored at not exceeding 15°C after preparation. To a volume of Pravastatin Sodium Solution, equivalent to 2 mg of Pravastatin Sodium, add a mixture of methanol and water (5:3) to make 10 mL, and use this solution as the sample solution. Pipet 1 mL of the sample solution, add a mixture of water and methanol (1:1) to make exactly 100 mL, and use this solution as the standard solution. Perform the test with exactly 10 μL each of the sample solution and standard solution as directed under Liquid Chromatography <2.01> according to the following conditions. Determine each peak area of both solutions by the automatic integration method: the area of the peaks, having the relative retention time about 0.24 and about 0.85 to pravastatin, obtained from the sample solution is not larger than 2 times the peak area of pravastatin from the standard solution, the area of the peak other than pravastatin and the peaks mentioned above from the sample solution is not larger than 3/10 times the peak area of pravastatin from the standard solution, and the total area of the peaks other than pravastatin from the sample solution is not larger than 3.5 times the peak area of pravastatin from the standard solution.

Operating conditions—

Detector, column, column temperature, mobile phase, and flow rate: Proceed as directed in the operating conditions in the Assay.

Time span of measurement: About 2 times as long as the retention time of pravasatin, beginning after the solvent peak.

System suitability—

Test for required detectability: Pipet 2 mL of the standard solution, and add a mixture of water and methanol (1:1) to make exactly 10 mL. Confirm that the peak area of pravastatin obtained with 10 μL of this solution is equivalent to 15 to 25% of that with 10 μL of the standard solution.

System performance: When the procedure is run with 10 μL of the standard solution under the above operating conditions, the number of theoretical plates and the symmetry factor of the peak of pravastatin are not less than 3400 and not more than 1.6, respectively.

System repeatability: When the test is repeated 6 times with 10 μL of the standard solution under the above operating conditions, the relative standard deviation of the peak area of pravastatin is not more than 2.5%.

Uniformity of dosage units <*6.02*> The solution in single-dose packages meet the requirement of the Mass variation test.

Microbial limit <*4.05*> The acceptance criteria of TAMC and TYMC are 10^2 CFU/mL and 10^1 CFU/mL, respectively. *Escherichia coli* is not observed.

Assay To an exact volume of Pravastatin Sodium Solution, equivalent to 2 mg of pravastatin sodium ($C_{23}H_{35}NaO_7$), add exactly 5 mL of the internal standard solution, add water to make 100 mL, and use this solution as the sample solution. Separately, weigh accurately about 20 mg of Pravastatin 1,1,3,3-Tetramethylbutylammonium RS (separately determine the water <*2.48*> in the same manner as Pravastatin Sodium), and dissolve in a solution of disodium hydrogen phosphate dodecahydrate (1 in 200) to make exactly 50 mL. Pipet 6 mL of this solution, add exactly 5 mL of the internal standard solution, add water to make 100 mL, and use this solution as the standard solution. Perform the test with 10 μL each of the sample solution and standard solution as directed under Liquid Chromatography <*2.01*> according to the following conditions. Calculate the ratios, Q_T and Q_S, of the peak area of pravastatin to that of the internal standard.

$$\text{Amount (mg) of pravastatin sodium} = M_S \times Q_T/Q_S \times 3/25 \times 1.052$$

M_S: Amount (mg) of pravastatin in taken Pravastatin 1,1,3,3-Tetramethylbutylammonium RS, calculated on the anhydrous basis

Internal standard solution—A solution of ethyl parahydroxybenzoate in methanol (3 in 10,000).

Operating conditions—

Detector: An ultraviolet spectrophotometer (wavelength: 238 nm).

Column: A stainless steel column 3.9 mm in inside diameter and 30 cm in length, packed with octadecylsilanized silica gel for liquid chromatography (10 μm in particle diameter).

Column temperature: A constant temperature of about 30°C.

Mobile phase: A mixture of water, methanol, acetic acid (100) and triethylamine (500:500:1:1).

Flow rate: Adjust so that the retention time of pravastatin is about 20 minutes.

System suitability—

System performance: When the procedure is run with 10 μL of the standard solution under the above operating conditions, the internal standard and pravastatin are eluted in this order with the resolution between these peaks being not less than 8.

System repeatability: When the test is repeated 6 times with 10 μL of the standard solution under the above operating conditions, the relative standard deviation of the ratio of the peak area of pravastatin to that of the internal standard is not more than 1.0%.

Containers and storage Containers—Tight containers.

Pravastatin Sodium Tablets

プラバスタチンナトリウム錠

Pravastatin Sodium Tablets contain not less than 95.0% and not more than 105.0% of the labeled amount of pravastatin sodium ($C_{23}H_{35}NaO_7$: 446.51).

Method of preparation Prepare as directed under Tablets, with Pravastatin Sodium.

Identification To a quantity of powdered Pravastatin Sodium Tablets, equivalent to 10 mg of Pravastatin Sodium, add 20 mL of water, sonicate for 15 minutes, and centrifuge. Filter the supernatant liquid, discard the first 5 mL of the filtrate, and add water to 1 mL of the subsequent filtrate to make 50 mL. Determine the absorption spectrum of this solution as directed under Ultraviolet-visible Spectrophotometry <*2.24*>: it exhibits a maximum between 237 nm and 241 nm.

Purity Related substances—The sample solution and the standard solution are stored at not exceeding 15°C after preparation. To an amount of powdered Pravastatin Sodium Tablets, equivalent to 50 mg of Pravastatin Sodium, add 40 mL of a mixture of water and methanol (1:1), sonicate, then add a mixture of water and methanol (1:1) to make 50 mL, centrifuge, and use the supernatant liquid as the sample solution. Pipet 1 mL of the sample solution, add a mixture of water and methanol (1:1) to make exactly 100 mL, and use this solution as the standard solution. Perform the test with exactly 20 μL each of the sample solution and standard solution as directed under Liquid Chromatography <*2.01*> according to the following conditions. Determine each peak area by the automatic integration method: the area of the peaks, having the relative retention time about 0.36 and about 1.9 to pravastatin obtained from the sample solution is not larger than 3/10 times and 2 times the peak area of pravastatin from the standard solution, respectively, the area of the peak other than pravastatin and the peak mentioned above from the sample solution is not larger than 1/5 times the peak area of pravastatin from the standard solution, and the total area of the peaks other than pravastatin from the sample solution is not larger than 3 times the peak area of pravastatin from the standard solution. For the area of the peaks, having the relative retention time about 0.28, about 0.36 and about 0.88, multiply their correction factors, 1.16, 1.72 and 1.22, respectively.

Operating conditions—

Detector: An ultraviolet spectrophotometer (wavelength: 238 nm).

Column: A stainless steel column 4.6 mm in inside diameter and 15 cm in length, packed with octadecylsilanized silica gel for liquid chromatography (5 μm in particle diameter).

Column temperature: A constant temperature of about 25°C.

Mobile phase A: A mixture of water, methanol, acetic acid (100) and triethylamine (750:250:1:1).

Mobile phase B: A mixture of methanol, water, acetic acid (100) and triethylamine (650:350:1:1).

Flowing of mobile phase: Control the gradient by mixing the mobile phases A and B as directed in the following table.

Time after injection of sample (min)	Mobile phase A (vol%)	Mobile phase B (vol%)
0 – 50	50	50
50 – 75	50 → 0	50 → 100

Flow rate: 1.3 mL per minute.

Time span of measurement: For 75 minutes after injection, beginning after the solvent peak.

System suitability—

Test for required detectability: Pipet 1 mL of the standard solution, and add a mixture of water and methanol (1:1) to make exactly 10 mL. Confirm that the peak area of pravastatin obtained with 20 μL of this solution is equivalent to 7 to 13% of that with 20 μL of the standard solution.

System performance: When the procedure is run with 20 μL of the standard solution under the above operating conditions, the number of theoretical plates and the symmetry factor of the peak of pravastatin are not less than 3500 and not more than 1.6, respectively.

System repeatability: When the test is repeated 6 times with 20 μL of the standard solution under the above operating conditions, the relative standard deviation of the peak area of pravastatin is not more than 1.5%.

Uniformity of dosage units <6.02> Perform the test according to the following method: it meets the requirement of the Content uniformity test.

To 1 tablet of Pravastatin Sodium Tablets add exactly V mL of the internal standard solution so that each mL contains 0.25 mg of pravastatin sodium ($C_{23}H_{35}NaO_7$), sonicate for 15 minutes, and centrifuge. To 2 mL of the supernatant liquid add a mixture of water and methanol (1:1) to make 20 mL, and use this solution as the sample solution. Then, proceed as directed in the Assay.

Amount (mg) of pravastatin sodium ($C_{23}H_{35}NaO_7$)
$= M_S \times Q_T/Q_S \times V/100 \times 1.052$

M_S: Amount (mg) of pravastatin in taken Pravastatin 1,1,3,3-Tetramethylbutylammonium RS, calculated on the anhydrous basis

*Internal standard solution—*A solution of propyl parahydroxybenzoate in a mixture of water and methanol (1:1) (3 in 10,000).

Dissolution <6.10> When the test is performed at 50 revolutions per minute according to the Paddle method, using 900 mL of water as the dissolution medium, the dissolution rate in 30 minutes of Pravastatin Sodium Tablets is not less than 85%.

Start the test with 1 tablet of Pravastatin Sodium Tablets, withdraw not less than 20 mL of the medium at the specified minute after starting the test, and filter through a membrane filter with a pore size not exceeding 0.45 μm. Discard not less than 10 mL of the first filtrate, pipet V mL of the subsequent filtrate, add water to make exactly V' mL so that each mL contains about 5.5 μg of pravastatin ($C_{23}H_{36}O_7$), and use this solution as the sample solution. Separately, weigh accurately about 23 mg of Pravastatin 1,1,3,3-Tetramethylbutylammonium RS (separately determine the water <2.48> in the same manner as Pravastatin Sodium), and dissolve in water to make exactly 100 mL. Pipet 3 mL of this solution, add water to make exactly 100 mL, and use this solution as the standard solution. Determine the absorbances, A_{T1} and A_{S1}, at 238 nm and A_{T2} and A_{S2} at 256 nm of the sample solution and standard solution as directed under Ultraviolet-visible Spectrophotometry <2.24>.

Dissolution rate (%) with respect to the labeled amount of pravastatin sodium ($C_{23}H_{35}NaO_7$)
$= M_S \times (A_{T1} - A_{T2})/(A_{S1} - A_{S2})$
$\times V'/V \times 1/C \times 27 \times 0.806$

M_S: Amount (mg) of Pravastatin 1,1,3,3-Tetramethylbutylammonium RS taken, calculated on the anhydrous basis

C: Labeled amount (mg) of pravastatin sodium ($C_{23}H_{35}NaO_7$) in 1 tablet

Assay Weigh accurately and powder not less than 20 Pravastatin Sodium Tablets. Weigh accurately a portion of the powder, equivalent to about 10 mg of pravastatin sodium ($C_{23}H_{35}NaO_7$), add exactly 40 mL of the internal standard solution, sonicate for 15 minutes, and centrifuge. Filter the supernatant liquid, discard the first 5 mL of the filtrate, to 2 mL of the subsequent filtrate add a mixture of water and methanol (1:1) to make 20 mL, and use this solution as the sample solution. Separately, weigh accurately about 32 mg of Pravastatin 1,1,3,3-Tetramethylbutylammonium RS (separately determine the water <2.48> in the same manner as Pravastatin Sodium), and dissolve in a mixture of water and methanol (1:1) to make exactly 100 mL. Pipet 5 mL of this solution, add exactly 5 mL of the internal standard solution, then add a mixture of water and methanol (1:1) to make 50 mL, and use this solution as the standard solution. Perform the test with 10 μL each of the sample solution and standard solution as directed under Liquid Chromatography <2.01> according to the following conditions. Calculate the ratios, Q_T and Q_S, of the peak area of pravastatin to that of the internal standard.

Amount (mg) of pravastatin sodium ($C_{23}H_{35}NaO_7$)
$= M_S \times Q_T/Q_S \times 2/5 \times 1.052$

M_S: Amount (mg) of pravastatin in taken Pravastatin 1,1,3,3-Tetramethylbutylammonium RS, calculated on the anhydrous basis

*Internal standard solution—*A solution of propyl parahydroxybenzoate in a mixture of water and methanol (1:1) (3 in 10,000).

Operating conditions—

Proceed as directed in the operating conditions in the Assay under Pravastatin Sodium.

System suitability—

System performance: When the procedure is run with 10 μL of the standard solution under the above operating conditions, the internal standard and pravastatin are eluted in this order with the resolution between these peaks being not less than 4.

System repeatability: When the test is repeated 6 times with 10 μL of the standard solution under the above operating conditions, the relative standard deviation of the ratio of the peak area of pravastatin to that of the internal standard is not more than 1.0%.

Containers and storage Containers—Well-closed containers.

Prazepam

プラゼパム

$C_{19}H_{17}ClN_2O$: 324.80
7-Chloro-1-(cyclopropylmethyl)-5-phenyl-1,3-dihydro-2*H*-1,4-benzodiazepin-2-one
[*2955-38-6*]

Prazepam, when dried, contains not less than 98.5% of prazepam ($C_{19}H_{17}ClN_2O$).

Description Prazepam occurs as white to light yellow crystals or crystalline powder. It is odorless.

It is freely soluble in acetone, soluble in acetic anhydride, sparingly soluble in ethanol (99.5) and in diethyl ether, and practically insoluble in water.

Identification **(1)** Dissolve 0.01 g of Prazepam in 3 mL of sulfuric acid, and observe under ultraviolet light (main wavelength: 365 nm): the solution shows a grayish blue fluorescence.

(2) Dissolve 0.01 g of Prazepam in 1000 mL of a solution of sulfuric acid in ethanol (99.5) (3 in 1000). Determine the absorption spectrum of the solution as directed under Ultraviolet-visible Spectrophotometry *<2.24>*, and compare the spectrum with the Reference Spectrum: both spectra exhibit similar intensities of absorption at the same wavelengths.

(3) Determine the infrared absorption spectrum of Prazepam, previously dried, as directed in the potassium bromide disk method under Infrared Spectrophotometry *<2.25>*, and compare the spectrum with the Reference Spectrum: both spectra exhibit similar intensities of absorption at the same wave numbers.

(4) Perform Flame Coloration Tests *<1.04>* (2) with Prazepam: a green color appears.

Melting point *<2.60>* 145 – 148°C

Purity **(1)** Chloride *<1.03>*—To 1.0 g of Prazepam add 50 mL of water, allow to stand for 1 hour with occasional shaking, and filter. To 20 mL of the filtrate add 6 mL of dilute nitric acid and water to make 50 mL. Perform the test using this solution as the test solution. Prepare the control solution with 0.40 mL of 0.01 mol/L hydrochloric acid VS (not more than 0.036%).

(2) Sulfate *<1.14>*—To 20 mL of the filtrate obtained in (1) add 1 mL of dilute hydrochloric acid and water to make 50 mL. Perform the test using this solution as the test solution. Prepare the control solution with 0.40 mL of 0.005 mol/L sulfuric acid VS (not more than 0.048%).

(3) Heavy metals *<1.07>*—Proceed with 2.0 g of Prazepam according to Method 2, and perform the test. Prepare the control solution with 2.0 mL of Standard Lead Solution (not more than 10 ppm).

(4) Arsenic *<1.11>*—Prepare the test solution with 1.0 g of Prazepam according to Method 3, and perform the test (not more than 2 ppm).

(5) Related substances—Dissolve 0.40 g of Prazepam in 10 mL of acetone, and use this solution as the sample solution. Pipet 1 mL of the sample solution, and add acetone to make exactly 20 mL. Pipet 1 mL of this solution, add acetone to make exactly 25 mL, and use this solution as the standard solution. Perform the test with these solutions as directed under Thin-layer Chromatography *<2.03>*. Spot 5 μL each of the sample solution and standard solution on a plate of silica gel with fluorescent indicator for thin-layer chromatography. Develop the plate with a mixture of chloroform and acetone (9:1) to a distance of about 10 cm, and air-dry the plate. Examine under ultraviolet light (main wavelength: 254 nm): the spots other than the principal spot obtained from the sample solution are not more intense than the spot from the standard solution.

Loss on drying *<2.41>* Not more than 0.20% (1 g, 105°C, 2 hours).

Residue on ignition *<2.44>* Not more than 0.1% (1 g).

Assay Weigh accurately about 0.4 g of Prazepam, previously dried, dissolve in 60 mL of acetic anhydride, and titrate *<2.50>* with 0.1 mol/L perchloric acid VS (potentiometric titration). Perform a blank determination in the same manner, and make any necessary correction.

Each mL of 0.1 mol/L perchloric acid VS
= 32.48 mg of $C_{19}H_{17}ClN_2O$

Containers and storage Containers—Tight containers.

Prazepam Tablets

プラゼパム錠

Prazepam Tablets contain not less than 93.0% and not more than 107.0% of the labeled amount of prazepam ($C_{19}H_{17}ClN_2O$: 324.80).

Method of preparation Prepare as directed under Tablets, with Prazepam.

Identification **(1)** To a quantity of powdered Prazepam Tablets, equivalent to 0.05 g of Prazepam, add 25 mL of acetone, shake well, and filter. Take 5 mL of the filtrate, evaporate on a water bath to dryness, and dissolve the residue in 3 mL of sulfuric acid. With this solution, proceed as directed in the Identification (1) under Prazepam.

(2) To a quantity of powdered Prazepam Tablets, equivalent to 0.02 g of Prazepam, add 200 mL of a solution of sulfuric acid in ethanol (99.5) (3 in 1000), shake well, and filter. To 5 mL of the filtrate add a solution of sulfuric acid in ethanol (99.5) (3 in 1000) to make 50 mL, and determine the absorption spectrum as directed under Ultraviolet-visible Spectrophotometry *<2.24>*: it exhibits maxima between 241 nm and 245 nm, between 283 nm and 287 nm and between 363 nm and 367 nm, and minima between 263 nm and 267 nm and between 334 nm and 338 nm.

Dissolution *<6.10>* When the test is performed at 100 revolutions per minute according to the Basket method, using 900 mL of 0.1 mol/L hydrochloric acid TS as the dissolution medium, the dissolution rate in 30 minutes of Prazepam Tablets is not less than 80%.

Start the test with 1 tablet of Prazepam Tablets, withdraw not less than 20 mL of the medium at the specified minute after starting the test, and filter through a membrane filter with a pore size not exceeding 0.8 μm. Discard not less than 10 mL of the first filtrate, measure exactly the subsequent *V* mL of the filtrate, add the dissolution medium to make exactly V' mL so that each mL contains about 5 μg of prazepam ($C_{19}H_{17}ClN_2O$), and use this solution as the sample solution. Separately, weigh accurately about 5 mg of prazepam for assay, previously dried at 105°C for 2 hours, add 200 mL of the dissolution medium and dissolve with shaking, or by sonicating if necessary, add the dissolution medium to make exactly 1000 mL, and use this solution as the standard solution. Determine the absorbances, A_T and A_S, of the sample solution and standard solution at 240 nm as directed under Ultraviolet-visible Spectrophotometry *<2.24>*.

Dissolution rate (%) with respect to the labeled amount of prazepam ($C_{19}H_{17}ClN_2O$)

$$= M_S \times A_T/A_S \times V'/V \times 1/C \times 90$$

M_S: Amount (mg) of prazepam for assay taken

C: Labeled amount (mg) of prazepam ($C_{19}H_{17}ClN_2O$) in 1 tablet

Assay Weigh accurately not less than 20 Prazepam Tablets, and powder. Weigh accurately a quantity of the powder, equivalent to about 50 mg of prazepam ($C_{19}H_{17}ClN_2O$), add 30 mL of acetone, shake well, centrifuge, and separate the supernatant liquid. Repeat the same procedure twice with 30 mL each of acetone, combine all the supernatants liquid, and evaporate on a water bath to dryness. Dissolve the residue in 50 mL of a mixture of acetic anhydride and acetic acid (100) (7:3), and titrate *<2.50>* with 0.02 mol/L perchloric acid VS (potentiometric titration). Perform a blank determination in the same manner, and make any necessary correction.

Each mL of 0.02 mol/L perchloric acid VS
$= 6.496$ mg of $C_{19}H_{17}ClN_2O$

Containers and storage Containers—Tight containers.

Prazosin Hydrochloride

プラゾシン塩酸塩

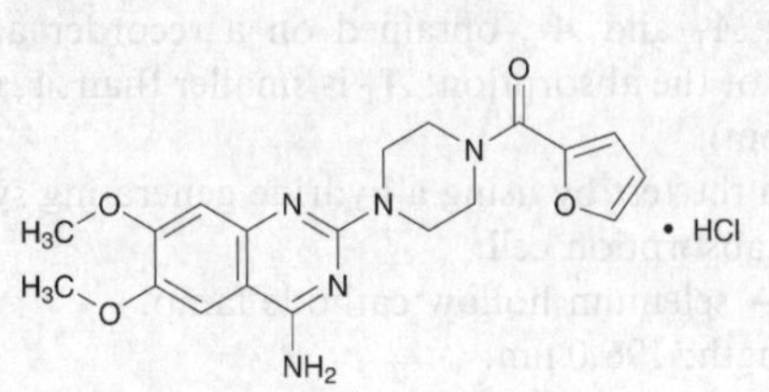

$C_{19}H_{21}N_5O_4.HCl$: 419.86

1-(4-Amino-6,7-dimethoxy-quinazolin-2-yl)-
4-(2-furoyl)piperazine monohydrochloride
[*19237-84-4*]

Prazosin Hydrochloride, when dried, contains not less than 97.0% and not more than 103.0% of prazosin hydrochloride ($C_{19}H_{21}N_5O_4.HCl$).

Description Prazosin Hydrochloride occurs as a white crystalline powder.

It is slightly soluble in methanol, very slightly soluble in ethanol (99.5) and practically insoluble in water.

It gradually turns pale yellow-white on exposure to light.

Melting point: about 270°C (with decomposition).

Identification **(1)** Determine the absorption spectrum of a solution of Prazosin Hydrochloride in 0.01 mol/L hydrochloric acid-methanol TS (1 in 200,000) as directed under Ultraviolet-visible Spectrophotometry *<2.24>*, and compare the spectrum with the Reference Spectrum or the spectrum of a solution of Prazosin Hydrochloride RS prepared in the same manner as the sample solution: both spectra exhibit similar intensities of absorption at the same wavelengths.

(2) Determine the infrared absorption spectrum of Prazosin Hydrochloride as directed in the potassium chloride disk method under Infrared Spectrophotometry *<2.25>*, and compare the spectrum with the Reference Spectrum or the spectrum of Prazosin Hydrochloride RS: both spectra exhibit similar intensities of absorption at the same wave numbers.

(3) To 0.1 g of Prazosin Hydrochloride add 5 mL of water and 1 mL of ammonia TS, shake, allow to stand for 5 minutes, and filter. Render the filtrate acid with acetic acid (100): the solution responds to Qualitative Tests *<1.09>* for chloride.

Purity **(1)** Heavy metals *<1.07>*—Proceed with 1.0 g of Prazosin Hydrochloride according to Method 4, and perform the test. Prepare the control solution with 1.0 mL of Standard Lead Solution (not more than 10 ppm).

(2) Related substances—Dissolve 20 mg of Prazosin Hydrochloride in 20 mL of the mobile phase, and use this solution as the sample solution. Pipet 1 mL of the sample solution, and add the mobile phase to make exactly 100 mL. Pipet 1 mL of this solution, add the mobile phase to make exactly 10 mL, and use this solution as the standard solution. Perform the test with exactly 20 μL each of the sample solution and standard solution as directed under Liquid Chromatography *<2.01>* according to the following conditions. Determine each peak area of both solutions by the automatic integration method: the area of each peak other than prazosin obtained from the sample solution is not larger than 2 times the peak area of prazosin from the standard solution, and the total area of the peaks other than prazosin from the sample solution is not larger than 5 times the peak area of prazosin from the standard solution.

Operating conditions—

Detector: An ultraviolet absorption photometer (wavelength: 254 nm).

Column: A stainless steel column 4.6 mm in inside diameter and 25 cm in length, packed with octadecylsilanized silica gel for liquid chromatography (5 μm in particle diameter).

Column temperature: A constant temperature of about 25°C.

Mobile phase: Dissolve 3.484 g of sodium 1-pentane sulfonate and 18 mL of tetramethylammonium hydroxide in 900 mL of water, adjust the pH to 5.0 with acetic acid (100), and add water to make 1000 mL. To this solution add 1000 mL of methanol.

Flow rate: Adjust so that the retention time of prazosin is about 9 minutes.

Time span of measurement: About 6 times as long as the retention time of prazosin.

System suitability—

Test for required detectability: Pipet 5 mL of the standard solution, and add the mobile phase to make exactly 10 mL. Confirm that the peak area of prazosin obtained with 20 μL of this solution is equivalent to 35 to 65% of that with 20 μL of the standard solution.

System performance: When the procedure is run with 20 μL of the standard solution under the above operating conditions, the number of theoretical plates and the symmetry factor of the peak of prazosin are not less than 4000 and not more than 2.0, respectively.

System repeatability: When the test is repeated 6 times with 20 μL of the standard solution under the above operating conditions, the relative standard deviation of the peak

area of prazosin is not more than 2.0%.

Loss on drying <*2.41*> Not more than 1.0% (1 g, 105°C, 2 hours).

Residue on ignition <*2.44*> Not more than 0.2% (1 g).

Assay Weigh accurately about 25 mg each of Prazosin Hydrochloride and Prazosin Hydrochloride RS, previously dried, and dissolve each in methanol to make exactly 50 mL. Pipet 3 mL each of these solutions, and add a mixture of methanol and water (7:3) to make exactly 100 mL, and use these solutions as the sample solution and the standard solution, respectively. Perform the test with exactly 10 μL each of the sample solution and standard solution as directed under Liquid Chromatography <*2.01*> according to the following conditions, and determine the peak areas, A_T and A_S, of prazosin in each solution.

Amount (mg) of prazosin hydrochloride ($C_{19}H_{21}N_5O_4.HCl$) $= M_S \times A_T/A_S$

M_S: Amount (mg) of Prazosin Hydrochloride RS taken

Operating conditions—

Detector: An ultraviolet absorption photometer (wavelength: 254 nm).

Column: A stainless steel column 4.6 mm in inside diameter and 25 cm in length, packed with silica gel for liquid chromatography (5 μm in particle diameter).

Column temperature: A constant temperature of about 25°C.

Mobile phase: A mixture of methanol, water, acetic acid (100) and diethylamine (3500:1500:50:1).

Flow rate: Adjust so that the retention time of prazosin is about 8 minutes.

System suitability—

System performance: When the procedure is run with 10 μL of the standard solution under the above operating conditions, the number of theoretical plates and the symmetry factor of the peak of prazosin are not less than 5000 and not more than 2.0, respectively.

System repeatability: When the test is repeated 6 times with 10 μL of the standard solution under the above operating conditions, the relative standard deviation of the peak area of prazosin is not more than 1.0%.

Containers and storage Containers—Well-closed containers.

Storage—Light-resistant.

Prednisolone

プレドニゾロン

$C_{21}H_{28}O_5$: 360.44
11*β*,17,21-Trihydroxypregna-1,4-diene-3,20-dione
[50-24-8]

Prednisolone, when dried, contains not less than 97.0% and not more than 102.0% of prednisolone ($C_{21}H_{28}O_5$).

Description Prednisolone occurs as a white crystalline powder.

It is soluble in methanol and in ethanol (95), slightly soluble in ethyl acetate, and very slightly soluble in water.

Melting point: about 235°C (with decomposition).

It shows crystal polymorphism.

Identification **(1)** To 2 mg of Prednisolone add 2 mL of sulfuric acid, and allow to stand for 2 to 3 minutes: a deep red color, without fluorescence, develops. To this solution add 10 mL of water cautiously: the color disappears and a gray, flocculent precipitate is formed.

(2) Determine the infrared absorption spectrum of Prednisolone, previously dried, as directed in the potassium bromide disk method under Infrared Spectrophotometry <*2.25*>, and compare the spectrum with the Reference Spectrum or the spectrum of previously dried Prednisolone RS: both spectra exhibit similar intensities of absorption at the same wave numbers. If any difference appears between the spectra, dissolve Prednisolone and Prednisolone RS in ethyl acetate, respectively, then evaporate the ethyl acetate to dryness, and repeat the test on the residues.

Optical rotation <*2.49*> $[\alpha]_D^{20}$: +113 – +119° (after drying, 0.2 g, ethanol (95), 20 mL, 100 mm).

Purity **(1)** Selenium—To 0.10 g of Prednisolone add 0.5 mL of a mixture of perchloric acid and sulfuric acid (1:1) and 2 mL of nitric acid, and heat on a water bath until no more brown gas evolves and the solution becomes to be a light yellow clear solution. After cooling, add 4 mL of nitric acid to this solution, then add water to make exactly 50 mL, and use this solution as the sample solution. Separately, pipet 3 mL of Standard Selenium Solution, add 0.5 mL of a mixture of perchloric acid and sulfuric acid (1:1) and 6 mL of nitric acid, then add water to make exactly 50 mL, and use this solution as the standard solution. Perform the test with the sample solution and standard solution as directed under Atomic Absorption Spectrophotometry <*2.23*> according to the following conditions, and determine constant absorbances, A_T and A_S, obtained on a recorder after rapid increasing of the absorption: A_T is smaller than A_S (not more than 30 ppm).

Perform the test by using a hydride generating system and a thermal absorption cell.

Lamp: A selenium hollow cathode lamp.

Wavelength: 196.0 nm.

Temperature of sample atomizer: When an electric furnace is used, about 1000°C.

Carrier gas: Nitrogen or argon.

(2) Related substances—Dissolve 20 mg of Prednisolone in exactly 2 mL of a mixture of methanol and chloroform (1:1), and use this solution as the sample solution. Separately, dissolve 20 mg of hydrocortisone and 10 mg of prednisolone acetate each in a mixture of methanol and chloroform (1:1) to make exactly 100 mL, and use these solutions as the standard solution (1) and standard solution (2). Perform the test with these solutions as directed under Thin-layer Chromatography <*2.03*>. Spot 5 μL each of the sample solution and standard solutions (1) and (2) on a plate of silica gel for thin-layer chromatography. Develop the plate with a mixture of acetone, toluene and diethylamine (55:45:2) to a distance of about 15 cm, and air-dry the plate (do not dip the filter paper in the developing vessel). Spray evenly alkaline blue tetrazolium TS on the plate: the spots obtained from the sample solution corresponding to those from the standard solutions (1) and (2) are not more intense than the spots from the standard solutions (1) and (2), and no spots other than the principal spot, hydrocortisone and prednisolone acetate appear from the sample solution.

Loss on drying *<2.41>* Not more than 1.0% (0.5 g, 105°C, 3 hours).

Residue on ignition *<2.44>* Not more than 0.1% (0.5 g).

Assay Dissolve about 25 mg each of Prednisolone and Prednisolone RS, previously dried, and accurately weighed, in 50 mL of methanol, add exactly 25 mL of the internal standard solution to each, and add methanol to make 100 mL. To 1 mL each of these solutions add the mobile phase to make 10 mL, and use these solutions as the sample solution and standard solution. Perform the test with 20 μL each of these solutions as directed under Liquid Chromatography *<2.01>* according to the following conditions, and calculate the ratios, Q_T and Q_S, of the peak area of prednisolone to that of the internal standard.

Amount (mg) of prednisolone ($C_{21}H_{28}O_5$) = $M_S \times Q_T/Q_S$

M_S: Amount (mg) of Prednisolne RS taken

Internal standard solution—A solution of methyl parahydroxybenzoate in methanol (1 in 2000).

Operating conditions—

Detector: An ultraviolet absorption photometer (wavelength: 247 nm).

Column: A stainless steel column 4.6 mm in inside diameter and 15 cm in length, packed with fluorosilanized silica gel for liquid chromatography (5 μm in particle diameter).

Column temperature: A constant temperature of about 40°C.

Mobile phase: A mixture of water and methanol (13:7).

Flow rate: Adjust so that the retention time of prednisolone is about 15 minutes.

System suitability—

System performance: Dissolve 25 mg of Prednisolone and 25 mg of hydrocortisone in 100 mL of methanol. To 1 mL of this solution add the mobile phase to make 10 mL. When the procedure is run with 20 μL of this solution under the above operating conditions, hydrocortisone and prednisolone are eluted in this order with the resolution between these peaks being not less than 1.5.

System repeatability: When the test is repeated 6 times with 20 μL of the standard solution under the above operating conditions, the relative standard deviation of the ratios of the peak area of prednisolone to that of the internal standard is not more than 1.0%.

Containers and storage Containers—Tight containers.

Prednisolone Tablets

プレドニゾロン錠

Prednisolone Tablets contain not less than 90.0% and not more than 110.0% of the labeled amount of prednisolone ($C_{21}H_{28}O_5$: 360.44).

Method of preparation Prepare as directed under Tablets, with Prednisolone.

Identification (1) Weigh a quantity of powdered Prednisolone Tablets, equivalent to 0.05 g of Prednisolone, add 10 mL of chloroform, shake for 15 minutes, and filter. Evaporate the filtrate on a water bath to dryness. Dry the residue at 105°C for 1 hour, and proceed as directed in the Identification (1) under Prednisolone.

(2) Determine the infrared absorption spectra of the residue obtained in (1) and Prednisolone RS, previously dried, as directed in the potassium bromide disk method under Infrared Spectrophotometry *<2.25>*: both spectra exhibit similar intensities of absorption at the same wave numbers. If any difference appears, dissolve the sample and the RS in ethyl acetate, evaporate to dryness, and repeat the test on the residues.

Uniformity of dosage units *<6.02>* Perform the test according to the following method: it meets the requirement of the Content uniformity test.

Transfer 1 tablet of Prednisolone Tablets to a volumetric flask, and shake with 10 mL of water until the tablet is disintegrated. Add 50 mL of methanol, shake for 30 minutes, and add methanol to make exactly 100 mL. Centrifuge this solution, pipet *V* mL of the supernatant liquid, and add methanol to make exactly *V′* mL to provide a solution that contains about 10 μg of prednisolone ($C_{21}H_{28}O_5$) per ml, and use this solution as the sample solution. Separately, weigh accurately about 10 mg of Prednisolone RS, previously dried at 105°C for 3 hours, dissolve in 10 mL of water and 50 mL of methanol, and add methanol to make exactly 100 mL. Pipet 5 mL of this solution, add methanol to make exactly 50 mL, and use this solution as the standard solution. Determine the absorbances, A_T and A_S, of the sample solution and standard solution at 242 nm as directed under Ultraviolet-visible Spectrophotometry *<2.24>*.

Amount (mg) of prednisolone ($C_{21}H_{28}O_5$)
$= M_S \times A_T/A_S \times V'/V \times 1/10$

M_S: Amount (mg) of Prednisolone RS taken

Dissolution *<6.10>* When the test is performed at 100 revolutions per minute according to the Paddle method, using 900 mL of water as the dissolution medium, the dissolution rate in 20 minutes of Prednisolone Tablets is not less than 70%.

Start the test with 1 tablet of Prednisolone Tablets, withdraw not less than 20 mL of the medium at the specified minute after starting the test, and filter through a membrane filter with a pore size not exceeding 0.8 μm. Discard not less than 10 mL of the first filtrate, and use the subsequent filtrate as the sample solution. Separately, weigh accurately about 10 mg of Prednisolone RS, previously dried at 105°C for 3 hours, and dissolve in ethanol (95) to make exactly 100 mL. Pipet 5 mL of this solution, add water to make exactly 100 mL, and use this solution as the standard solution. Determine the absorbances, A_T and A_S, of the sample solution and standard solution at the maximum wavelength at about 242 nm as directed under Ultraviolet-visible Spectrophotometry *<2.24>*, using water as the blank.

Dissolution rate (%) with respect to the labeled amount of prednisolone ($C_{21}H_{28}O_5$)
$= M_S \times A_T/A_S \times 1/C \times 45$

M_S: Amount (mg) of Prednisolone RS taken
C: Labeled amount (mg) of prednisolone ($C_{21}H_{28}O_5$) in 1 tablet

Assay Weigh accurately and powder not less than 20 Prednisolone Tablets using an agate mortar. Weigh accurately a portion of the powder, equivalent to about 5 mg of prednisolone ($C_{21}H_{28}O_5$), add 1 mL of water, and shake gently. Add exactly 5 mL of the internal standard solution and 15 mL of methanol, and shake vigorously for 20 minutes. To 1 mL of this solution add the mobile phase to make 10 mL, and filter through a membrane filter with pore size of 0.45 μm. Discard the first 3 mL of the filtrate, and use the subsequent filtrate as the sample solution. Separately, weigh accurately about 25 mg of Prednisolone RS, previously dried at 105°C for 3 hours, dissolve in 50 mL of methanol, add exactly 25 mL of the internal standard solution, and add methanol to make 100 mL. To 1 mL of this solution add the mobile phase to make 10 mL, and use this solution as the standard solution. Proceed as directed in the Assay under Prednisolone with these solutions.

$$\text{Amount (mg) of prednisolone } (C_{21}H_{28}O_5) = M_S \times Q_T/Q_S \times 1/5$$

M_S: Amount (mg) of Prednisolone RS taken

Internal standard solution—A solution of methyl parahydroxybenzoate in methanol (1 in 2000).

Containers and storage Containers—Tight containers.

Prednisolone Acetate

プレドニゾロン酢酸エステル

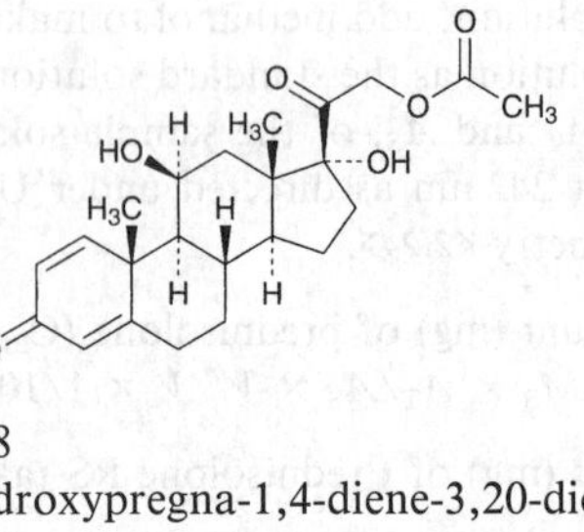

$C_{23}H_{30}O_6$: 402.48
11*β*,17,21-Trihydroxypregna-1,4-diene-3,20-dione
21-acetate
[52-21-1]

Prednisolone Acetate, when dried, contains not less than 96.0% and not more than 102.0% of prednisolone acetate ($C_{23}H_{30}O_6$).

Description Prednisolone Acetate occurs as a white crystalline powder.

It is slightly soluble in methanol and in ethanol (99.5), and practically insoluble in water.

Melting point: about 235°C (with decomposition).

It shows crystal polymorphism.

Identification **(1)** To 2 mg of Prednisolone Acetate add 2 mL of sulfuric acid, and allow to stand for 2 to 3 minutes: a deep red color, without fluorescence, develops. To this solution add 10 mL of water cautiously: the color disappears and a gray, flocculent precipitate is formed.

(2) Determine the infrared absorption spectra of Prednisolone Acetate, previously dried, as directed in the potassium bromide disk method under Infrared Spectrophotometry ⟨*2.25*⟩, and compare the spectrum in a range between 4000 cm^{-1} and 650 cm^{-1} with the Infrared Reference Spectrum or the spectrum of previously dried Prednisolone Acetate RS: both spectra exhibit similar intensities of absorption at the same wave numbers. If any difference appears, dissolve the sample and the RS in ethanol (99.5), respectively, evaporate to dryness, and repeat the test on the residues.

Optical rotation ⟨*2.49*⟩ $[\alpha]_D^{20}$: +128 – +137° (after drying, 70 mg, methanol, 20 mL, 100 mm).

Purity Related substances—Dissolve 0.20 g of Prednisolone Acetate in exactly 10 mL of a mixture of chloroform and methanol (9:1), and use this solution as the sample solution. Separately, dissolve 20 mg each of prednisolone, cortisone acetate and hydrocortisone acetate in exactly 10 mL of a mixture of chloroform and methanol (9:1). Pipet 1 mL of this solution, add a mixture of chloroform and methanol (9:1) to make exactly 10 mL, and use this solution as the standard solution. Perform the test with these solutions as directed under Thin-layer Chromatography ⟨*2.03*⟩. Spot 5 µL each of the sample solution and standard solution on a plate of silica gel with fluorescent indicator for thin-layer chromatography. Develop the plate with a mixture of dichloromethane, diethyl ether, methanol and water (385:75:40:6) to a distance of about 15 cm, and air-dry the plate. Examine under ultraviolet light (wavelength: 254 mm): the spots obtained from the sample solution corresponding to those from the standard solution are not more intense than the spots from the standard solution, and any spot from the sample solution other than the principal spot and the spots from prednisolone, cortisone acetate and hydrocortisone acetate does not appear.

Loss on drying ⟨*2.41*⟩ Not more than 1.0% (0.5 g, 105°C, 3 hours).

Residue on ignition ⟨*2.44*⟩ Not more than 0.1% (0.5 g).

Assay Dissolve about 10 mg each of Prednisolone Acetate and Prednisolone Acetate RS, previously dried and accurately weighed, in 60 mL each of methanol, add exactly 2 mL each of the internal standard solution, then add methanol to make 100 mL, and use these solutions as the sample solution and standard solution. Perform the test with 10 µL each of the sample solution and standard solution as directed under Liquid Chromatography ⟨*2.01*⟩ according to the following conditions, and calculate the ratios, Q_T and Q_S, of the peak height of prednisolone acetate to that of the internal standard.

$$\text{Amount (mg) of prednisolone acetate } (C_{23}H_{30}O_6) = M_S \times Q_T/Q_S$$

M_S: Amount (mg) of Prednisolone Acetate RS taken

Internal standard solution—A solution of butyl parahydroxybenzoate in methanol (3 in 1000).

Operating conditions—

Detector: An ultraviolet absorption photometer (wavelength: 254 nm).

Column: A stainless steel column 4.0 mm in inside diameter and 15 cm in length, packed with octadecylsilanized silica gel for liquid chromatography (5 µm in particle diameter).

Column temperature: A constant temperature of about 25°C.

Mobile phase: A mixture of water and acetonitrile (3:2).

Flow rate: Adjust so that the retention time of prednisolone acetate is about 10 minutes.

System suitability—

System performance: When the procedure is run with 10 µL of the standard solution under the above operating conditions, prednisolone acetate and the internal standard are eluted in this order with the resolution between these peaks being not less than 10.

System repeatability: When the test is repeated 6 times with 10 µL of the standard solution under the above operating conditions, the relative standard deviation of the ratios of the peak height of prednisolone acetate to that of the internal standard is not more than 1.0%.

Containers and storage Containers—Tight containers.

Prednisolone Sodium Phosphate

プレドニゾロンリン酸エステルナトリウム

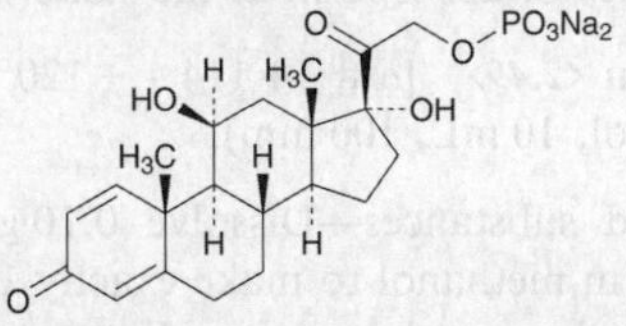

$C_{21}H_{27}Na_2O_8P$: 484.39
11β,17,21-Trihydroxypregna-1,4-diene 3,20-dione 21-(disodium phosphate)
[125-02-0]

Prednisolone Sodium Phosphate contains not less than 97.0% and not more than 103.0% of prednisolone sodium phosphate ($C_{21}H_{27}Na_2O_8P$), calculated on the anhydrous basis.

Description Prednisolone Sodium Phosphate occurs as a white to pale yellow powder.

It is freely soluble in water, soluble in methanol, and practically insoluble in ethanol (99.5).

It is hygroscopic.

Identification (1) Moisten 1.0 g of Prednisolone Sodium Phosphate with a small amount of sulfuric acid, and gradually heat to incinerate. After cooling, dissolve the residue in 10 mL of dilute nitric acid, and heat in a water bath for 30 minutes. After cooling, filter if necessary. This solution responds to Qualitative Tests *<1.09>* for phosphate.

(2) Dissolve 2 mg of Prednisolone Sodium Phosphate in 2 mL of sulfuric acid, and allow to stand for 2 minutes: a deep red color, without fluorescence, develops.

(3) Determine the absorption spectrum of a solution of Prednisolone Sodium Phosphate (1 in 50,000) as directed under Ultraviolet-visible Spectrophotometry *<2.24>*, and compare the spectrum with the Reference Spectrum: both spectra exhibit similar intensities of absorption at the same wavelengths.

(4) Determine the infrared absorption spectrum of Prednisolone Sodium Phosphate as directed in the potassium bromide disk method under Infrared Spectrophotometry *<2.25>*, and compare the spectrum with the Reference Spectrum: both spectra exhibit similar intensities of absorption at the same wave numbers.

(5) The solution obtained in (1) responds to Qualitative Tests *<1.09>* for sodium salt.

Optical rotation *<2.49>* $[\alpha]_D^{20}$: +96 – +103° (1 g calculated on the anhydrous basis, phosphate buffer solution (pH 7.0), 100 mL, 100 mm).

pH *<2.54>* Dissolve 1.0 g of Prednisolone Sodium Phosphate in 100 mL of water: the pH of the solution is between 7.5 and 9.0.

Purity (1) Clarity and color of solution—Dissolve 1.0 g of Prednisolone Sodium Phosphate in 10 mL of water: the solution is clear and not more colored than the following control solution.

Control solution: To a mixture of 3.0 mL of Cobalt (II) Chloride CS, 3.0 mL of Iron (III) Chloride CS and 2.4 mL of Copper (II) Sulfate CS add diluted hydrochloric acid (1 in 40) to make 10 mL. To 2.5 mL of this solution add diluted hydrochloric acid (1 in 40) to make 100 mL.

(2) Heavy metals *<1.07>*—Proceed with 0.5 g of Prednisolone Sodium Phosphate according to Method 3, and perform the test. Prepare the control solution with 2.0 mL of Standard Lead Solution (not more than 40 ppm).

(3) Free phosphoric acid—Weigh accurately about 0.25 g of Prednisolone Sodium Phosphate, dissolve in water to make exactly 100 mL, and use this solution as the sample solution. Pipet 5 mL each of the sample solution and Phosphoric Acid Standard Solution, add 2.5 mL of hexaammonium heptamolybdate-sulfuric acid TS and 1 mL of 1-amino-2-naphtol-4-sulfonic acid TS, shake, add water to make exactly 25 mL, and allow to stand at 20 ± 1°C for 30 minutes. Perform the test with these solutions as directed under Ultraviolet-visible Spectrophotometry *<2.24>*, using a solution prepared with 5 mL of water in the same manner as the blank. Determine the absorbances, A_T and A_S, of each solution from the sample solution and standard solution at 740 nm: the content of free phosphoric acid is not more than 1.0%.

Content (%) of free phosphoric acid (H_3PO_4)
$= 1/M \times A_T/A_S \times 258.0$

M: Amount (mg) of Prednisolone Sodium Phosphate taken, calculated on the anhydrous basis

(4) Related substances—Dissolve 10 mg of Prednisolone Sodium Phosphate in 100 mL of the mobile phase, and use this solution as the sample solution. Pipet 2 mL of the sample solution, add the mobile phase to make exactly 100 mL, and use this solution as the standard solution. Perform the test with exactly 20 μL each of the sample solution and standard solution as directed under Liquid Chromatography *<2.01>* according to the following conditions. Determine each peak area of both solutions by the automatic integration method: the area of each peak other than prednisolone phosphate obtained from the sample solution is not larger than 1.5 times the peak area of prednisolone phosphate from the standard solution, and the total area of the peaks other than prednisolone phosphate from the sample solution is not larger than 2.5 times the peak area of prednisolone phosphate from the standard solution.

Operating conditions—

Detector: An ultraviolet absorption photometer (wavelength: 245 nm).

Column: A stainless steel column 4.6 mm in inside diameter and 10 cm in length, packed with octadecylsilanized silica gel for liquid chromatography (3 μm in particle diameter).

Column temperature: A constant temperature of about 40°C.

Mobile phase: Dissolve 6.80 g of potassium dihydrogen phosphate in water to make 1000 mL, and adjust the pH to 2.5 with phosphoric acid. To 1000 mL of this solution add 250 mL of acetonitrile.

Flow rate: Adjust so that the retention time of prednisolone phosphate is about 7 minutes.

Time span of measurement: About 4 times as long as the retention time of prednisolone phosphate.

System suitability—

Test for required detectability: Pipet 5 mL of the standard solution, and add the mobile phase to make exactly 50 mL. Confirm that the peak area of prednisolone phosphate obtained with 20 μL of this solution is equivalent to 7 to 13% of that with 20 μL of the standard solution.

System performance: When the procedure is run with 20 μL of the standard solution under the above operating conditions, the number of theoretical plates and the symmetry factor of the peak of prednisolone phosphate are not less than 3000 and not more than 2.0, respectively.

System repeatability: When the test is repeated 6 times with 20 μL of the standard solution under the above operating conditions, the relative standard deviation of the peak area of prednisolone phosphate is not more than 2.0%.

Water ⟨*2.48*⟩ Not more than 8.0% (0.1 g, volumetric titration, direct titration).

Assay Weigh accurately about 0.1 g of Prednisolone Sodium Phosphate, and dissolve in water to make exactly 100 mL. Pipet 2 mL of this solution, add 1 mL of alkaline phosphatase TS, and allow to stand for 2 hours with occasional shaking. To this solution add exactly 20 mL of 1-octanol, and shake vigorously. Centrifuge this solution, pipet 10 mL of the 1-octanol layer, add 1-octanol to make exactly 50 mL, and use this solution as the sample solution. Separately, weigh accurately about 25 mg of Prednisolone RS, previously dried at 105°C for 3 hours, and dissolve in 1-octanol to make exactly 100 mL. Pipet 6 mL of this solution, add a solution prepared by adding 1 mL of alkaline phosphatase TS to 2 mL water and being allowed to stand for 2 hours with occasional gentle shaking, add exactly 14 mL of 1-octanol, and shake vigorously. Proceed in the same manner as the sample solution to make the standard solution. Perform the test with the sample solution and standard solution as directed under Ultraviolet-visible Spectrophotometry ⟨*2.24*⟩, using 1-octanol as the blank, and determine the absorbances, A_T and A_S, at 245 nm.

Amount (mg) of prednisolone sodium phosphate ($C_{21}H_{27}Na_2O_8P$)
$= M_S \times A_T/A_S \times 3 \times 1.344$

M_S: Amount (mg) of Prednisolone RS taken

Containers and storage Containers—Tight containers.

Prednisolone Succinate

プレドニゾロンコハク酸エステル

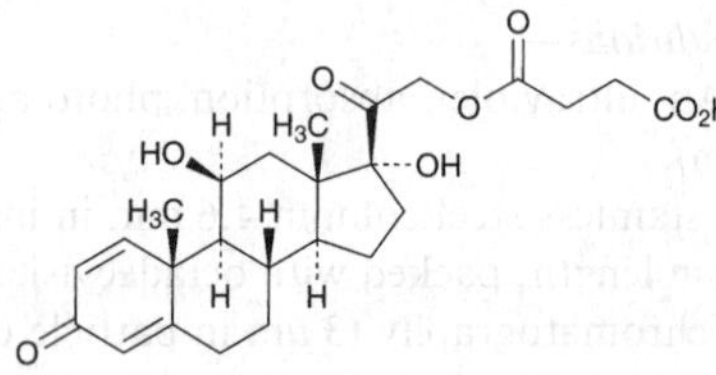

$C_{25}H_{32}O_8$: 460.52
11β,17,21-Trihydroxypregna-1,4-diene-3,20-dione 21-(hydrogen succinate)
[*2920-86-7*]

Prednisolone Succinate, when dried, contains not less than 97.0% and not more than 103.0% of prednisolone succinate ($C_{25}H_{32}O_8$).

Description Prednisolone Succinate occurs as a white, fine, crystalline powder. It is odorless.

It is freely soluble in methanol, soluble in ethanol (95), and very slightly soluble in water and in diethyl ether.

Melting point: about 205°C (with decomposition).

Identification **(1)** To 2 mg of Prednisolone Succinate add 2 mL of sulfuric acid, and allow to stand for 2 to 3 minutes: a deep red color, without fluorescence, develops. To this solution add 10 mL of water cautiously: the color disappears and a gray, flocculent precipitate is formed.

(2) Determine the infrared absorption spectrum of Prednisolone Succinate as directed in the potassium bromide disk method under Infrared Spectrophotometry ⟨*2.25*⟩, and compare the spectrum with the Reference Spectrum or the spectrum of Prednisolone Succinate RS: both spectra exhibit similar intensities of absorption at the same wave numbers.

Optical rotation ⟨*2.49*⟩ $[\alpha]_D^{20}$: +114 – +120° (after drying, 67 mg, methanol, 10 mL, 100 mm).

Purity Related substances—Dissolve 0.10 g of Prednisolone Succinate in methanol to make exactly 10 mL, and use this solution as the sample solution. Separately, dissolve 30 mg of prednisolone in methanol to make exactly 10 mL. Pipet 1 mL of the solution, add methanol to make exactly 10 mL, and use this solution as the standard solution. Perform the test with these solutions as directed under Thin-layer Chromatography ⟨*2.03*⟩. Spot 5 μL of the sample solution and standard solution on a plate of silica gel with fluorescent indicator for thin-layer chromatography. Develop the plate with a mixture of ethyl acetate and ethanol (95) (2:1) to a distance of about 10 cm, and air-dry the plate. Examine the plate under ultraviolet light (main wavelength: 254 nm): the spots other than the principal spot obtained from the sample solution are not more intense than the spot from the standard solution.

Loss on drying ⟨*2.41*⟩ Not more than 0.5% (1 g, in vacuum, phosphorus (V) oxide, 60°C, 6 hours).

Residue on ignition ⟨*2.44*⟩ Not more than 0.1% (1 g).

Assay Weigh accurately about 10 mg each of Prednisolone Succinate and Prednisolone Succinate RS, previously dried, and dissolve each in methanol to make exactly 100 mL. Pipet 5 mL each of these solutions, add methanol to make exactly 50 mL, and use these solutions as the sample solution and standard solution. Determine the absorbances, A_T and A_S, of the sample solution and standard solution at 242 nm as directed under Ultraviolet-visible Spectrophotometry ⟨*2.24*⟩.

Amount (mg) of prednisolone succinate ($C_{25}H_{32}O_8$)
$= M_S \times A_T/A_S$

M_S: Amount (mg) of Prednisolone Succinate RS taken

Containers and storage Containers—Tight containers.

Prednisolone Sodium Succinate for Injection

注射用プレドニゾロンコハク酸エステルナトリウム

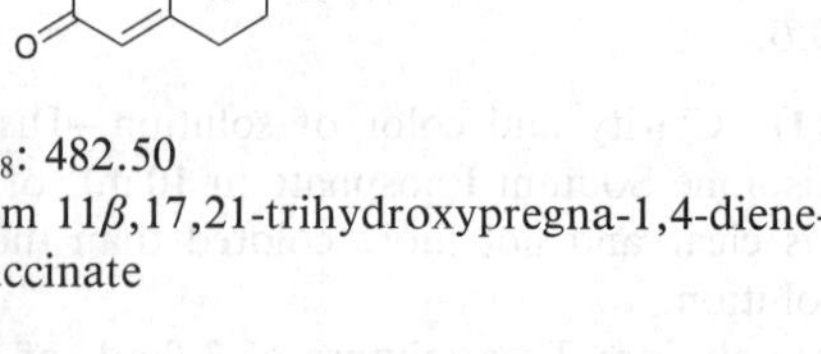

$C_{25}H_{31}NaO_8$: 482.50
Monosodium 11β,17,21-trihydroxypregna-1,4-diene-3,20-dione 21-succinate
[*1715-33-9*]

Prednisolone Sodium Succinate for Injection is a preparation for injection which is dissolved before use.

It contains not less than 72.4% and not more than 83.2% of prednisolone sodium succinate

($C_{25}H_{31}NaO_8$), and the equivalent of not less than 90.0% and not more than 110.0% of the labeled amount of prednisolone ($C_{21}H_{28}O_5$: 360.44).

The amount should be stated as the amount of prednisolone ($C_{21}H_{28}O_5$).

Method of preparation Prepare as directed under Injections, with Prednisolone Succinate and Dried Sodium Carbonate or Sodium Hydroxide.

It contains a suitable buffer agent.

Description Prednisolone Sodium Succinate for Injection occurs as a white, powder or porous, friable mass.

It is freely soluble in water.

It is hygroscopic.

Identification **(1)** To 2 mg of Prednisolone Sodium Succinate for Injection add 2 mL of sulfuric acid, and allow to stand for 2 to 3 minutes: a deep red color, without fluorescence, develops. To this solution add 10 mL of water cautiously: the color disappears and a gray, flocculent precipitate is formed.

(2) Dissolve 0.01 g of Prednisolone Sodium Succinate for Injection in 1 mL of methanol, add 1 mL of Fehling's TS, and heat: an orange to red precipitate is formed.

(3) Dissolve 0.1 g of Prednisolone Sodium Succinate for Injection in 2 mL of sodium hydroxide TS, allow to stand for 10 minutes, and filter. Add 1 mL of dilute hydrochloric acid to the filtrate, shake, and filter if necessary. Adjust the solution with diluted ammonia TS (1 in 10) to a pH of about 6, and add 2 to 3 drops of iron (III) chloride TS: a brown precipitate is formed.

(4) Prednisolone Sodium Succinate for Injection responds to Qualitative Tests *<1.09>* (1) for sodium salt.

pH *<2.54>* Dissolve 1.0 g of Prednisolone Sodium Succinate for Injection in 40 mL of water: the pH of the solution is between 6.5 and 7.2.

Purity Clarity and color of solution—Dissolve 0.25 g of Prednisolone Sodium Succinate for Injection in 10 mL of water: the solution is clear and colorless.

Loss on drying *<2.41>* Not more than 2.0% (0.15 g, in vacuum, phosphorus (V) oxide, 60°C, 3 hours).

Bacterial endotoxins *<4.01>* Less than 2.4 EU/mg of prednisolone ($C_{21}H_{28}O_5$).

Uniformity of dosage units *<6.02>* It meets the requirement of the Mass variation test.

Foreign insoluble matter *<6.06>* Perform the test according to Method 2: it meets the requirement.

Insoluble particulate matter *<6.07>* It meets the requirement.

Sterility *<4.06>* Perform the test according to the Membrane filtration method: it meets the requirement.

Assay Take a quantity of sealed containers of Prednisolone Sodium Succinate for Injection, equivalent to about 0.1 g of prednisolone ($C_{21}H_{28}O_5$), and dissolve the contents in a suitable amount of diluted methanol (1 in 2), and transfer to a 100-mL volumetric flask. Wash each container with diluted methanol (1 in 2), collect the washings in the volumetric flask, and add diluted methanol (1 in 2) to make volume. Pipet 4 mL of this solution, add diluted methanol (1 in 2) to make exactly 50 mL. Pipet 5 mL of this solution, add exactly 5 mL of the internal standard solution, mix, and use this solution as the sample solution. Separately, weigh accurately about 25 mg of Prednisolone Succinate RS, previously dried in a desiccator for 6 hours (in vacuum, phosphorus (V) oxide, 60°C), dissolve in methanol to make exactly 25 mL. Pipet 5 mL of this solution, add diluted methanol (1 in 2) to make exactly 50 mL. Pipet 5 mL of this solution, add exactly 5 mL of the internal standard solution, mix, and use this solution as the standard solution. Perform the test with 10 μL of the sample solution and standard solution as directed under Liquid Chromatography according *<2.01>* to the following conditions, and calculate the ratios, Q_T and Q_S, of the peak area of prednisolone succinate to that of the internal standard.

Amount (mg) of prednisolone sodium succinate ($C_{25}H_{31}NaO_8$)
$= M_S \times Q_T/Q_S \times 5 \times 1.048$

Amount (mg) of prednisolone ($C_{21}H_{28}O_5$)
$= M_S \times Q_T/Q_S \times 5 \times 0.783$

M_S: Amount (mg) of Prednisolone Succinate RS taken

Internal standard solution—A solution of propyl parahydroxybenzoate in diluted methanol (1 in 2) (1 in 25,000).

Operating conditions—

Detector: An ultraviolet absorption photometer (wavelength: 254 nm).

Column: A stainless steel column 4.6 mm in inside diameter and 25 cm in length, packed with octadecylsilanized silica gel for liquid chromatography (5 μm in particle diameter).

Column temperature: A constant temperature of about 25°C.

Mobile phase: Dissolve 0.32 g of tetra *n*-butylammonium bromide, 3.22 g of disodium hydrogen phosphate dodecahydrate and 6.94 g of potassium dihydrogen phosphate in 1000 mL of water. To 840 mL of this solution add 1160 mL of methanol.

Flow rate: Adjust so that the retention time of prednisolone succinate is about 15 minutes.

System suitability—

System performance: When the procedure is run with 10 μL of the standard solution under the above operating conditions, prednisolone succinate and the internal standard are eluted in this order with the resolution between these peaks being not less than 6.

System repeatability: When the test is repeated 6 times with 10 μL of the standard solution under the above operating conditions, the relative standard deviation of the ratios of the peak area of prednisolone succinate to that of the internal standard is not more than 1.0%.

Containers and storage Containers—Hermetic containers.

Primidone

プリミドン

$C_{12}H_{14}N_2O_2$: 218.25
5-Ethyl-5-phenyl-2,3-dihyropyrimidine-4,6(1*H*,5*H*)-dione
[*125-33-7*]

Primidone, when dried, contains not less than 98.5% of primidone ($C_{12}H_{14}N_2O_2$).

Description Primidone occurs as a white, crystalline powder or granules. It is odorless and has a slightly bitter taste.

It is soluble in *N*,*N*-dimethylformamide, sparingly soluble in pyridine, slightly soluble in ethanol (95), very slightly soluble in water, and practically insoluble in diethyl ether.

Identification **(1)** Heat 0.5 g of Primidone with 5 mL of diluted sulfuric acid (1 in 2): the odor of formaldehyde is perceptible.

(2) Mix 0.2 g of Primidone with 0.2 g of anhydrous sodium carbonate, and heat: the gas evolved changes moistened red litmus paper to blue.

Melting point ⟨*2.60*⟩ 279 – 284°C

Purity **(1)** Clarity and color of solution—Dissolve 0.10 g of Primidone in 10 mL of *N*,*N*-dimethylformamide: the solution is clear and colorless.

(2) Heavy metals ⟨*1.07*⟩—Proceed with 2.0 g of Primidone according to Method 2, and perform the test. Prepare the control solution with 2.0 mL of Standard Lead Solution (not more than 10 ppm).

(3) 2-Ethyl-2-phenylmalonediamide—Dissolve 0.10 g of Primidone in 2 mL of pyridine, add exactly 2 mL of the internal standard solution, then add 1 mL of bis-trimethyl silyl acetamide, shake well, and heat at 100°C for 5 minutes. Cool, add pyridine to make 10 mL, and use this solution as the sample solution. Separately, dissolve 50 mg of 2-ethyl-2-phenylmalonediamide in pyridine to make exactly 100 mL. Pipet 2 mL of this solution, add exactly 2 mL of the internal standard solution, proceed in the same manner as Primidone, and use this solution as the standard solution. Perform the test with 2 μL of the sample solution and standard solution as directed under Gas Chromatography ⟨*2.02*⟩ according to the following conditions, and calculate the ratios, Q_T and Q_S, of the peak area of 2-ethyl-2-phenylmalonediamide to that of the internal standard: Q_T is not more than Q_S.

Internal standard solution—A solution of stearylalcohol in pyridine (1 in 2000).

Operating conditions—

Detector: A hydrogen flame-ionization detector.

Column: A glass column 3 mm in inside diameter and 150 cm in length, packed with siliceous earth for gas chromatography (125 to 150 μm in particle diameter) coated with 50% phenyl-methyl silicon polymer for gas chromatography at the ratio of 3%.

Column temperature: A constant temperature of about 195°C.

Carrier gas: Nitrogen.

Flow rate: Adjust so that the retention time of stearylalcohol is about 10 minutes.

System suitability—

System performance: When the procedure is run with 2 μL of the standard solution under the above operating conditions, 2-ethyl-2-phenylmalonediamide and the internal standard are eluted in this order with the resolution between these peaks being not less than 3.

System repeatability: When the test is repeated 5 times with 2 μL of the standard solution under the above operating conditions, the relative standard deviation of the ratios of the peak area of 2-ethyl-2-phenylmalonediamide to that of the internal standard is not more than 1.5%.

Loss on drying ⟨*2.41*⟩ Not more than 0.5% (1 g, 105°C, 2 hours).

Residue on ignition ⟨*2.44*⟩ Not more than 0.2% (1 g).

Assay Weigh accurately about 20 mg each of Primidone and Primidone RS, previously dried, dissolve each in 20 mL of ethanol (95) by warming, and after cooling, add ethanol (95) to make exactly 25 mL, and use these solutions as the sample solution and the standard solution, respectively. Determine the absorbance, A_1, of the sample solution and standard solution at the wavelength of maximum absorption at about 257 nm, and the absorbances, A_2 and A_3, at the wavelength of minimum absorption at about 254 nm and at about 261 nm, as directed under Ultraviolet-visible Spectrophotometry ⟨*2.24*⟩, using ethanol (95) as the blank.

$$\text{Amount (mg) of primidone } (C_{12}H_{14}N_2O_2) = M_S \times (2A_1 - A_2 - A_3)_T/(2A_1 - A_2 - A_3)_S$$

M_S: Amount (mg) of Primidone RS taken

where, $(2A_1 - A_2 - A_3)_T$ is the value from the sample solution, and $(2A_1 - A_2 - A_3)_S$ is from the standard solution.

Containers and storage Containers—Tight containers.

Probenecid

プロベネシド

$C_{13}H_{19}NO_4S$: 285.36
4-(Dipropylaminosulfonyl)benzoic acid
[*57-66-9*]

Probenecid, when dried, contains not less than 98.0% of probenecid ($C_{13}H_{19}NO_4S$).

Description Probenecid occurs as white, crystals or crystalline powder. It is odorless, and has a slightly bitter taste, followed by unpleasant bitter.

It is sparingly soluble in ethanol (99.5), and practically insoluble in water.

It dissolves in sodium hydroxide TS and in ammonia TS.

Melting point: 198 – 200°C

Identification **(1)** Heat Probenecid strongly: the odor of sulfur dioxide is perceptible.

(2) Determine the absorption spectrum of a solution of Probenecid in ethanol (99.5) (1 in 50,000) as directed under Ultraviolet-visible Spectrophotometry ⟨*2.24*⟩, and compare the spectrum with the Reference Spectrum or the spectrum of a solution of Probenecid RS prepared in the same manner as the sample solution: both spectra exhibit similar intensities of absorption at the same wavelengths.

Purity **(1)** Acidity—To 2.0 g of Probenecid add 100 mL of water, heat on a water bath with occasional shaking for 30 minutes, cool, and filter. To the filtrate add 1 drop of phenolphthalein TS and 0.50 mL of 0.1 mol/L sodium hydroxide VS: a red color develops.

(2) Chloride *<1.03>*—To 1.0 g of Probenecid add 100 mL of water and 1 mL of nitric acid, and heat on a water bath with occasional shaking for 30 minutes. After cooling, add, if necessary, water to make 100 mL, and filter. Perform the test using 50 mL of the filtrate as the test solution. Prepare the control solution with 0.30 mL of 0.01 mol/L hydrochloric acid VS (not more than 0.021%).

(3) Sulfate *<1.14>*—To 1.0 g of Probenecid add 100 mL of water and 1 mL of hydrochloric acid, and heat on a water bath with occasional shaking for 30 minutes. After cooling, add, if necessary, water to make 100 mL, and filter. Perform the test using 50 mL of the filtrate as the test solution. Prepare the control solution with 0.40 mL of 0.005 mol/L sulfuric acid VS (not more than 0.038%).

(4) Heavy metals *<1.07>*—Proceed with 2.0 g of Probenecid according to Method 2, and perform the test. Prepare the control solution with 2.0 mL of Standard Lead Solution (not more than 10 ppm).

(5) Arsenic *<1.11>*—Prepare the test solution with 1.0 g of Probenecid according to Method 3, and perform the test (not more than 2 ppm).

Loss on drying *<2.41>* Not more than 0.5% (1 g, 105°C, 4 hours).

Residue on ignition *<2.44>* Not more than 0.1% (1 g).

Assay Weigh accurately about 0.5 g of Probenecid, previously dried, and dissolve in 50 mL of neutralized ethanol. Titrate *<2.50>* with 0.1 mol/L sodium hydroxide VS (indicator: 3 drops of phenolphthalein TS).

Each mL of 0.1 mol/L sodium hydroxide VS
= 28.54 mg of $C_{13}H_{19}NO_4S$

Containers and storage Containers—Well-closed containers.

Probenecid Tablets

プロベネシド錠

Probenecid Tablets contain not less than 95.0% and not more than 105.0% of the labeled amount of probenecid ($C_{13}H_{19}NO_4S$: 285.36).

Method of preparation Prepare as directed under Tablets, with Probenecid.

Identification **(1)** Weigh a quantity of powdered Probenecid Tablets, equivalent to 0.5 g of Probenecid, add 50 mL of ethanol (95) and 1 mL of 1 mol/L hydrochloric acid TS, shake, and filter. Evaporate the filtrate on a water bath to about 20 mL. After cooling, collect produced crystals, recrystallize with 50 mL of dilute ethanol, and dry at 105°C for 4 hours: it melts *<2.60>* between 196°C and 200°C. With the crystals so obtained, proceed as directed in the Identification (1) under Probenecid.

(2) Determine the absorption spectrum of a solution of the dried crystals obtained in (1) in ethanol (99.5) (1 in 50,000) as directed under Ultraviolet-visible Spectrophotometry *<2.24>*, and compare the spectrum with the Reference Spectrum or the spectrum of a solution of Probenecid RS prepared in the same manner as the sample solution: both spectra exhibit similar intensities of absorption at the same wavelengths.

Uniformity of dosage units *<6.02>* Perform the test according to the following method: it meets the requirement of the Content uniformity test.

To 1 tablet of Probenecid Tablets add 30 mL of water and 2 mL of 1 mol/L hydrochloric acid TS, sonicate with occasional shaking to disintegrate the tablet completely, and add ethanol (99.5) to make exactly 100 mL. Centrifuge this solution, pipet 3 mL of the supernatant liquid, and add 1 mL of 1 mol/L hydrochloric acid TS and ethanol (99.5) to make exactly 50 mL. Pipet 5 mL of this solution, and add ethanol (99.5) to make exactly V mL so that each mL contains about 15 μg of probenecid ($C_{13}H_{19}NO_4S$), and use this solution as the sample solution. Separately, weigh accurately about 0.125 g of Probenecid RS, previously dried at 105°C for 4 hours, dissolve in 15 mL of water, 1 mL of 1 mol/L hydrochloric acid TS and ethanol (99.5) to make exactly 50 mL. Pipet 3 mL of this solution, and add 1 mL of 1 mol/L hydrochloric acid TS and ethanol (99.5) to make exactly 50 mL. Pipet 5 mL of this solution, add ethanol (99.5) to make exactly 50 mL, and use this solution as the standard solution. Perform the test with the sample solution and standard solution as directed under Ultraviolet-visible Spectrophotometry *<2.24>*, using a solution, prepared by adding ethanol (99.5) to 1 mL of 0.1 mol/L hydrochloric acid TS to make exactly 50 mL, as the blank, and determine the absorbances, A_T and A_S, at 248 nm.

Amount (mg) of probenecid ($C_{13}H_{19}NO_4S$)
$= M_S \times A_T/A_S \times V/25$

M_S: Amount (mg) of Probenecid RS taken

Dissolution *<6.10>* When the test is performed at 50 revolutions per minute according to the Paddle method, using 900 mL of the 2nd fluid for dissolution test as the dissolution medium, the dissolution rate in 30 minutes of Probenecid Tablets is not less than 80%.

Start the test with 1 tablet of Probenecid Tablets, withdraw not less than 20 mL of the medium at the specified minute after starting the test, and filter through a membrane filter with a pore size not exceeding 0.8 μm. Discard not less than 10 mL of the first filtrate, pipet V mL of the subsequent filtrate, add the dissolution medium to make exactly V' mL so that each mL contains about 14 μg of probenecid ($C_{13}H_{19}NO_4S$), and use this solution as the sample solution. Separately, weigh accurately about 70 mg of Probenecid RS, previously dried at 105°C for 4 hours, and dissolve in the dissolution medium to make exactly 100 mL. Pipet 1 mL of this solution, add the dissolution medium to make exactly 50 mL, and use this solution as the standard solution. Determine the absorbances, A_T and A_S, at 244 nm of the sample solution and standard solution as directed under Ultraviolet-visible Spectrophotometry *<2.24>*.

Dissolution rate (%) with respect to the labeled amount of probenecid ($C_{13}H_{19}NO_4S$)
$= M_S \times A_T/A_S \times V'/V \times 1/C \times 18$

M_S: Amount (mg) of Probenecid RS taken
C: Labeled amount (mg) of probenecid ($C_{13}H_{19}NO_4S$) in 1 tablet

Assay Weigh accurately, and powder not less than 20 Probenecid Tablets. Weigh accurately a portion of the powder, equivalent to about 0.25 g of probenecid ($C_{13}H_{19}NO_4S$), add 30 mL of water and 2 mL of 1 mol/L hydrochloric acid TS, shake, add 30 mL of ethanol (99.5), disperse the particles by sonicating, and add ethanol (99.5) to make exactly 100 mL. Centrifuge the solution, pipet 3 mL of the supernatant liquid, add 1 mL of 1 mol/L hydrochloric acid TS, and add ethanol (99.5) to make exactly 50 mL. Pipet 5 mL of the solution, add ethanol (99.5) to make exactly 50 mL, and use this solution as the sample solution. Separately, weigh accurately about 0.125 g of Probenecid RS, previously dried at 105°C for 4 hours, add 15 mL of water and 1 mL of 1 mol/L hydrochloric acid TS, then add ethanol (99.5) to make exactly 50 mL. Pipet 3 mL of this solution, add 1 mL of 1 mol/L hydrochloric acid TS, and add ethanol (99.5) to make exactly 50 mL. Pipet 5 mL of the solution, add ethanol (99.5) to make exactly 50 mL, and use this solution as the standard solution. Determine the absorbances, A_T and A_S, of the sample solution and standard solution at 248 nm as directed under Ultraviolet-visible Spectrophotometry <*2.24*>, using a solution, prepared by mixing 1 mL of 0.1 mol/L hydrochloric acid TS and sufficient ethanol (99.5) to make exactly 50 mL, as the blank.

Amount (mg) of probenecid ($C_{13}H_{19}NO_4S$)
$= M_S \times A_T/A_S \times 2$

M_S: Amount (mg) of Probenecid RS taken

Containers and storage Containers—Well-closed containers.

Probucol

プロブコール

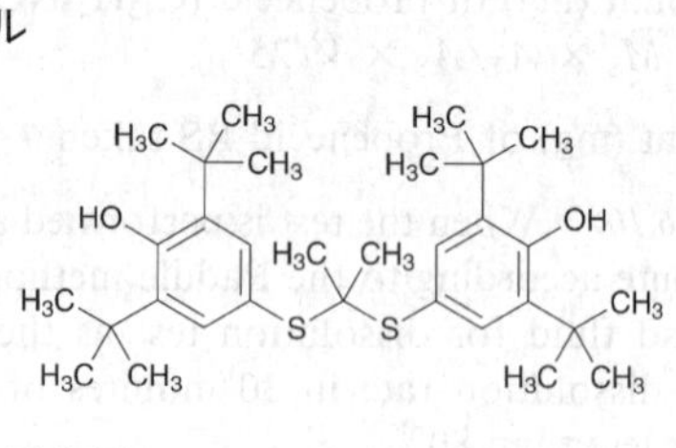

$C_{31}H_{48}O_2S_2$: 516.84
4,4′-[Propan-2,2-diylbis(sulfandiyl)]bis[2,6-bis(1,1-dimethylethyl)phenol]
[23288-49-5]

Probucol, when dried, contains not less than 98.5% and not more than 101.0% of probucol ($C_{31}H_{48}O_2S_2$).

Description Probucol occurs as a white crystalline powder.

It is very soluble in tetrahydrofuran, freely soluble in ethanol (99.5), soluble in methanol, and practically insoluble in water.

It gradually turns light yellow on exposure to light.

Identification **(1)** Determine the absorption spectrum of a solution of Probucol in methanol (1 in 100,000) as directed under Ultraviolet-visible Spectrophotometry <*2.24*>, and compare the spectrum with the Reference Spectrum or the spectrum of a solution of Probucol RS prepared in the same manner as the sample solution: both spectra exhibit similar intensities of absorption at the same wavelengths.

(2) Determine the infrared absorption spectrum of Probucol as directed in the potassium bromide disk method under Infrared Spectrophotometry <*2.25*>, and compare the spectrum with the Reference Spectrum or the spectrum of Probucol RS: both spectra exhibit similar intensities of absorption at the same wave numbers.

Melting point <*2.60*> 125 – 128°C

Purity **(1)** Heavy metals <*1.07*>—Proceed with 2.0 g of Probucol according to Method 2, and perform the test. Prepare the control solution with 2.0 mL of Standard Lead Solution (not more than 10 ppm).

(2) Related substances—Conduct this procedure using light-resistant vessels. Dissolve 0.40 g of Probucol in 5 mL of ethanol (99.5), add the mobile phase to make 20 mL, and use this solution as the sample solution. Pipet 1 mL of the sample solution, and add the mobile phase to make exactly 50 mL. Pipet 1 mL of this solution, add the mobile phase to make exactly 100 mL, and use this solution as the standard solution. Perform the test with exactly 5 μL each of the sample solution and standard solution as directed under Liquid Chromatography <*2.01*> according to the following conditions. Determine each peak area of both solutions by the automatic integration method: the area of the peak having the relative retention time of about 0.9 to probucol obtained from the sample solution is not larger than the peak area of probucol from the standard solution, and the area of peak having the relative retention time of about 1.9 from the sample solution is not larger than 25 times the peak area of probucol from the standard solution, and the area of each peak other than probucol and the peaks mentioned above from the sample solution is not larger than 5 times the peak area of probucol from the standard solution. Furthermore, the total area of the peaks other than probucol from the sample solution is not larger than 50 times the peak area of probucol from the standard solution. For the areas of the peaks, having the relative retention times of about 0.9 and about 1.9 to probucol, multiply their correction factors, 1.2 and 1.4, respectively.

Operating conditions—

Detector, column, column temperature, mobile phase and flow rate: Proceed as directed in the operating conditions in the Assay.

Time span of measurement: About 3 times as long as the retention time of probucol, beginning after the solvent peak, excluding the peak having the relative retention time of about 0.5 to probucol.

System suitability—

Test for required detectability: Pipet 2 mL of the standard solution, and add the mobile phase to make exactly 10 mL. Confirm that the peak area of probucol obtained with 5 μL of this solution is equivalent to 14 to 26% of that with 5 μL of the standard solution.

System performance: To 1 mL of the sample solution add the mobile phase to make 50 mL. To 1 mL of this solution add 1 mL of a solution of phthalic acid bis(cis-3,3,5-trimethylcyclohexyl) in the mobile phase (1 in 1000), 5 mL of ethanol (99.5), and the mobile phase to make 20 mL. When the procedure is run with 5 μL of this solution under the above operating conditions, phthalic acid bis(cis-3,3,5-trimethylcyclohexyl) and probucol are eluted in this order with the resolution between these peaks being not less than 6.

System repeatability: When the test is repeated 6 times with 5 μL of the standard solution under the above operating conditions, the relative standard deviation of the peak area of probucol is not more than 5%.

Loss on drying <*2.41*> Not more than 0.5% (1 g, in vacuum, 80°C, 1 hour).

Residue on ignition <*2.44*> Not more than 0.1% (1 g).

Assay Weigh accurately about 60 mg each of Probucol and Probucol RS, previously dried, dissolve each in 5 mL of tetrahydrofuran, and add the mobile phase to make exactly

50 mL. Pipet 5 mL each of these solutions, add exactly 5 mL of the internal standard solution and the mobile phase to make 100 mL, and use these solutions as the sample solution and standard solution. Perform the test with 10 μL each of the sample solution and standard solution as directed under Liquid Chromatography <*2.01*> according to the following conditions, and calculate the ratios, Q_T and Q_S, of the peak area of probucol to that of the internal standard.

$$\text{Amount (mg) of probucol } (C_{31}H_{48}O_2S_2) = M_S \times Q_T/Q_S$$

M_S: Amount (mg) of Probucol RS taken

Internal standard solution—Dissolve 0.2 g of bis(cis-3,3,5-trimethylcyclohexyl) phthalate in 1 mL of tetrahydrofuran, and add the mobile phase to make 50 mL.

Operating conditions—

Detector: An ultraviolet absorption photometer (wavelength: 242 nm).

Column: A stainless steel column 4.6 mm in inside diameter and 25 cm in length, packed with octadecylsilanized silica gel for liquid chromatography (5 μm in particle diameter).

Column temperature: A constant temperature of about 40°C.

Mobile phase: A mixture of acetonitrile and water (93:7).

Flow rate: Adjust so that the retention time of probucol is about 13 minutes.

System suitability—

System performance: When the procedure is run with 10 μL of the standard solution under the above operating conditions, the internal standard and probucol are eluted in this order with the resolution between these peaks being not less than 6.

System repeatability: When the test is repeated 6 times with 10 μL of the standard solution under the above operating conditions, the relative standard deviation of the ratio of the peak area of probucol to that of the internal standard is not more than 1.0%.

Containers and storage Containers—Tight containers.

Storage—Light-resistant.

Probucol Fine Granules

プロブコール細粒

Probucol Fine Granules contain not less than 95.0% and not more than 105.0% of the labeled amount of probucol ($C_{31}H_{48}O_2S_2$: 516.84).

Method of preparation Prepare as directed under Granules, with Probucol.

Identification To an amount of powdered Probucol Fine Granules, equivalent to 50 mg of Probucol, add 100 mL of methanol, shake, and filter. To 2 mL of the filtrate add methanol to make 100 mL. Determine the absorption spectrum of this solution as directed under Ultraviolet-visible Spectrophotometry <*2.24*>: it exhibits a maximum between 240 nm and 244 nm.

Uniformity of dosage units <*6.02*> Perform the test according to the following method: the granules in single-dose packages meet the requirement of the Content uniformity test.

To the total amount of the content of 1 package of Probucol Fine Granules add 70 mL of methanol, shake thoroughly, and add methanol to make exactly 100 mL. Centrifuge, pipet V mL of the supernatant liquid, equivalent to about 5 mg of probucol ($C_{31}H_{48}O_2S_2$), add exactly 5 mL of the internal standard solution, add methanol to make 100 mL, and use this solution as the sample solution. Then, proceed as directed in the Assay.

$$\text{Amount (mg) of probucol } (C_{31}H_{48}O_2S_2) = M_S \times Q_T/Q_S \times 10/V$$

M_S: Amount (mg) of Probucol RS taken

Internal standard solution—A solution of bis(*cis*-3,3,5-trimethylcyclohexyl) phthalate in methanol (1 in 250).

Assay Weigh accurately an amount of powdered Probucol Fine Granules, equivalent to about 0.25 g of probucol ($C_{31}H_{48}O_2S_2$), add 70 mL of methanol, shake thoroughly, and add methanol to make exactly 100 mL. Centrifuge, pipet 2 mL of the supernatant liquid, add exactly 5 mL of the internal standard solution, add methanol to make 100 mL, and use this solution as the sample solution. Separately, weigh accurately about 50 mg of Probucol RS, previously dried under reduced pressure at 80°C for 1 hour, and dissolve in methanol to make exactly 20 mL. Pipet 2 mL of this solution, add exactly 5 mL of the internal standard solution, add methanol to make 100 mL, and use this solution as the standard solution. Perform the test with 10 μL each of the sample solution and standard solution as directed under Liquid Chromatography <*2.01*> according to the following conditions, and calculate the ratios, Q_T and Q_S, of the peak area of probucol to that of the internal standard.

$$\text{Amount (mg) of probucol } (C_{31}H_{48}O_2S_2) = M_S \times Q_T/Q_S \times 5$$

M_S: Amount (mg) of Probucol RS taken

Internal standard solution—A solution of bis(*cis*-3,3,5-trimethylcyclohexyl) phthalate in methanol (1 in 250).

Operating conditions—

Detector, column temperature, mobile phase, and flow rate: Proceed as directed in the operating conditions in the Assay under Probucol.

Column: A stainless steel column 4.6 mm in inside diameter and 15 cm in length, packed with octadecylsilanized silica gel for liquid chromatography (5 μm in particle diameter).

System suitability—

System performance: When the procedure is run with 10 μL of the standard solution under the above operating conditions, the internal standard and probucol are eluted in this order with the resolution between these peaks being not less than 3.

System repeatability: When the test is repeated 6 times with 10 μL of the standard solution under the above operating conditions, the relative standard deviation of the ratio of the peak area of probucol to that of the internal standard is not more than 1.0%.

Containers and storage Containers—Well-closed containers.

Probucol Tablets

プロブコール錠

Probucol Tablets contain not less than 95.0% and not more than 105.0% of probucol ($C_{31}H_{48}O_2S_2$: 516.84).

Method of preparation Prepare as directed under Tablets, with Probucol.

Identification To an amount of powdered Probucol Tablets, equivalent to 50 mg of Probucol, add 100 mL of methanol, shake, and filter. To 2 mL of the filtrate add methanol to make 100 mL. Determine the absorption spectrum of this solution as directed under Ultraviolet-visible Spectrophotometry *<2.24>*: it exhibits a maximum between 240 nm and 244 nm.

Uniformity of dosage units *<6.02>* Perform the test according to the following method: it meets the requirement of the Content uniformity test.

Shake 1 tablet of Probucol Tablets with a suitable amount of methanol until the tablet is disintegrated, and add methanol to make exactly *V* mL so that each mL of the solution contains about 2.5 mg of probucol ($C_{31}H_{48}O_2S_2$). Centrifuge the solution, pipet 2 mL of the supernatant liquid, add exactly 5 mL of the internal standard solution, then add methanol to make 100 mL, and use this solution as the sample solution. Then, proceed as directed in the Assay.

$$\text{Amount (mg) of probucol } (C_{31}H_{48}O_2S_2) = M_S \times Q_T/Q_S \times V/20$$

M_S: Amount (mg) of Probucol RS taken

Internal standard solution—A solution of bis(*cis*-3,3,5-trimethylcyclohexyl) phthalate in methanol (1 in 250).

Disintegration *<6.09>* It meets the requirement.

Assay Weigh accurately the mass of 20 Probucol Tablets, and powder the tablets. Weigh accurately a portion of the powder, equivalent to about 0.25 g of probucol ($C_{31}H_{48}O_2S_2$), add 70 mL of methanol, shake thoroughly, and add methanol to make exactly 100 mL. Centrifuge, pipet 2 mL of the supernatant liquid, add exactly 5 mL of the internal standard solution, add methanol to make 100 mL, and use this solution as the sample solution. Separately, weigh accurately about 50 mg of Probucol RS, previously dried under reduced pressure at 80°C for 1 hour, and dissolve in methanol to make exactly 20 mL. Pipet 2 mL of this solution, add exactly 5 mL of the internal standard solution, add methanol to make 100 mL, and use this solution as the standard solution. Perform the test with 10 μL each of the sample solution and standard solution as directed under Liquid Chromatography *<2.01>* according to the following conditions, and calculate the ratios, Q_T and Q_S, of the peak area of probucol to that of the internal standard.

$$\text{Amount (mg) of probucol } (C_{31}H_{48}O_2S_2) = M_S \times Q_T/Q_S \times 5$$

M_S: Amount (mg) of Probucol RS taken

Internal standard solution—A solution of bis(*cis*-3,3,5-trimethylcyclohexyl) phthalate in methanol (1 in 250).

Operating conditions—

Detector, column temperature, mobile phase, and flow rate: Proceed as directed in the operating conditions in the Assay under Probucol.

Column: A stainless steel column 4.6 mm in inside diameter and 15 cm in length, packed with octadecylsilanized silica gel for liquid chromatography (5 μm in particle diameter).

System suitability—

System performance: When the procedure is run with 10 μL of the standard solution under the above operating conditions, the internal standard and probucol are eluted in this order with the resolution between these peaks being not less than 3.

System repeatability: When the test is repeated 6 times with 10 μL of the standard solution under the above operating conditions, the relative standard deviation of the ratio of the peak area of probucol to that of the internal standard is not more than 1.0%.

Containers and storage Containers—Well-closed containers.

Procainamide Hydrochloride

プロカインアミド塩酸塩

$C_{13}H_{21}N_3O.HCl$: 271.79

4-Amino-*N*-(2-diethylaminoethyl)benzamide monohydrochloride

[614-39-1]

Procainamide Hydrochloride, when dried, contains not less than 98.0% and not more than 101.0% of procainamide hydrochloride ($C_{13}H_{21}N_3O.HCl$).

Description Procainamide Hydrochloride occurs as a white to light yellow crystalline powder.

It is very soluble in water and soluble in ethanol (99.5).

It is hygroscopic.

Identification **(1)** Determine the infrared absorption spectrum of Procainamide Hydrochloride, previously dried, as directed in the potassium chloride disk method under Infrared Spectrophotometry *<2.25>*, and compare the spectrum with the Reference Spectrum: both spectra exhibit similar intensities of absorption at the same wave numbers.

(2) A solution of Procainamide Hydrochloride (1 in 20) responds to Qualitative Tests *<1.09>* for chloride.

pH *<2.54>* Dissolve 1.0 g of Procainamide Hydrochloride in 10 mL of water: the pH of this solution is between 5.0 and 6.5.

Melting point *<2.60>* 165 - 169°C

Purity **(1)** Clarity and color of solution—Dissolve 1.0 g of Procainamide Hydrochloride in 10 mL of water: the solution is clear and colorless.

(2) Heavy metals *<1.07>*—Proceed with 2.0 g of Procainamide Hydrochloride according to Method 2, and perform the test. Prepare the control solution with 2.0 mL of Standard Lead Solution (not more than 10 ppm).

(3) Arsenic *<1.11>*—Prepare the test solution with 1.0 g of Procainamide Hydrochloride according to Method 1, and perform the test (not more than 2 ppm).

(4) Related substances—Dissolve 50 mg of Procainamide Hydrochloride in 100 mL of the mobile phase, and use this solution as the sample solution. Pipet 1 mL of the sample solution, and add the mobile phase to make exactly 50 mL. Pipet 2 mL of this solution, add the mobile phase to make exactly 20 mL, and use this solution as the standard solution. Perform the test with exactly 10 μL each of the sample solution and standard solution as directed under Liquid Chromatography <2.01> according to the following conditions. Determine each peak area of both solutions by the automatic integration method: the total area of the peaks other than procainamide obtained from the sample solution is not larger than the peak area of procainamide from the standard solution.

Operating conditions—

Detector: An ultraviolet absorption photometer (wavelength: 270 nm).

Column: A stainless steel column 4.6 mm in inside diameter and 25 cm in length, packed with octadecylsilanized silica gel for liquid chromatography (5 μm in particle diameter).

Column temperature: A constant temperature of about 40°C.

Mobile phase: A mixture of 0.02 mol/L phosphate buffer solution (pH 3.0) and methanol (9:1).

Flow rate: Adjust so that the retention time of procainamide is about 9 minutes.

Time span of measurement: About 2 times as long as the retention time of procainamide.

System suitability—

Test for required detectability: Pipet 10 mL of the standard solution, and add the mobile phase to make exactly 20 mL. Confirm that the peak area of procainamide obtained with 10 μL of this solution is equivalent to 40 to 60% of that with 10 μL of the standard solution.

System performance: When the procedure is run with 10 μL of the standard solution under the above operating conditions, the number of theoretical plates and the symmetry factor of the peak of procainamide are not less than 10,000 and not more than 1.5, respectively.

System repeatability: When the test is repeated 6 times with 10 μL of the standard solution under the above operating conditions, the relative standard deviation of the peak area of procainamide is not more than 2.0%.

Loss on drying *<2.41>* Not more than 0.3% (2 g, 105°C, 4 hours).

Residue on ignition *<2.44>* Not more than 0.1% (2 g).

Assay Weigh accurately about 0.5 g of Procainamide Hydrochloride, previously dried, dissolve in 50 mL of a mixture of acetic anhydride and acetic acid (100) (7:3), and titrate *<2.50>* with 0.1 mol/L perchloric acid VS (potentiometric titration). Perform a blank determination in the same manner, and make any necessary correction.

Each mL of 0.1 mol/L perchloric acid VS
= 27.18 mg of $C_{13}H_{21}N_3O.HCl$

Containers and storage Containers—Tight containers.

Procainamide Hydrochloride Injection

プロカインアミド塩酸塩注射液

Procainamide Hydrochloride Injection is an aqueous injection.

It contains not less than 95.0% and not more than 105.0% of the labeled amount of procainamide hydrochloride ($C_{13}H_{21}N_3O.HCl$: 271.79).

Method of preparation Prepare as directed under Injections, with Procainamide Hydrochloride.

Description Procainamide Hydrochloride Injection is a clear, colorless or light yellow liquid.

pH: 4.0 – 6.0

Identification **(1)** To a volume of Procainamide Hydrochloride Injection, equivalent to 10 mg of Procainamide Hydrochloride, add 1 mL of dilute hydrochloric acid and water to make 5 mL: the solution responds to Qualitative Tests *<1.09>* (1) for primary aromatic amines.

(2) To a volume of Procainamide Hydrochloride Injection, equivalent to 0.1 g of Procainamide Hydrochloride, add water to make 100 mL. To 1 mL of this solution add water to make 100 mL. Determine the absorption spectrum of this solution as directed under Ultraviolet-visible Spectrophotometry *<2.24>*: it exhibits a maximum between 277 nm and 281 nm.

(3) Procainamide Hydrochloride Injection responds to Qualitative Tests *<1.09>* (2) for chloride.

Bacterial endotoxins *<4.01>* Less than 0.30 EU/mg.

Extractable volume *<6.05>* It meets the requirement.

Foreign insoluble matter *<6.06>* Perform the test according to Method 1: it meets the requirement.

Insoluble particulate matter *<6.07>* It meets the requirement.

Sterility *<4.06>* Perform the test according to the Membrane filtration method: it meets the requirement.

Assay Dilute an accurately measured volume of Procainamide Hydrochloride Injection, equivalent to about 0.5 g of procainamide hydrochloride ($C_{13}H_{21}N_3O.HCl$), with 5 mL of hydrochloric acid and water to 50 mL, add 10 mL of potassium bromide solution (3 → 10), cool to 15°C or lower, and titrate *<2.50>* with 0.1 mol/L sodium nitrite VS (potentiometric titration method or amperometric titration).

Each mL of 0.1 mol/L sodium nitrite VS
= 27.18 mg of $C_{13}H_{21}N_3O.HCl$

Containers and storage Containers—Hermetic containers.

Procainamide Hydrochloride Tablets

プロカインアミド塩酸塩錠

Procainamide Hydrochloride Tablets contain not less than 95.0% and not more than 105.0% of the labeled amount of procainamide hydrochloride ($C_{13}H_{21}N_3O.HCl$: 271.79).

Method of preparation Prepare as directed under Tablets, with Procainamide Hydrochloride.

Identification To a quantity of powdered Procainamide Hydrochloride Tablets, equivalent to 1.5 g of Procainamide Hydrochloride, add 30 mL of water, shake well, filter, and use the filtrate as the sample solution. To 0.2 mL of the sample solution add 1 mL of dilute hydrochloric acid and 4 mL of water: the solution responds to Qualitative Tests <*1.09*> for primary aromatic amines.

Uniformity of dosage units <*6.02*> Perform the test according to the following method: it meets the requirement of the Content uniformity test.

To 1 tablet of Procainamide Hydrochloride Tablets add $3V/5$ mL of 0.02 mol/L phosphate buffer solution (pH 3.0), sonicate to disintegrate the tablet completely, add 0.02 mol/L phosphate buffer solution (pH 3.0) to make exactly V mL so that each mL contains about 2.5 mg of procainamide hydrochloride ($C_{13}H_{21}N_3O.HCl$), and shake for 5 minutes. Centrifuge this solution, pipet 1 mL of the supernatant liquid, add 0.02 mol/L phosphate buffer solution (pH 3.0) to make exactly 250 mL, and use this solution as the sample solution. Proceed as directed in the Assay.

Amount (mg) of procainamide hydrochloride ($C_{13}H_{21}N_3O.HCl$)
$= M_S \times A_T/A_S \times V/20$

M_S: Amount (mg) of procainamide hydrochloride for assay taken

Dissolution <*6.10*> When the test is performed at 50 revolutions per minute according to the Paddle method, using 900 mL of water as the dissolution medium, the dissolution rate in 30 minutes of Procainamide Hydrochloride Tablets is not less than 80%.

Start the test with 1 tablet of Procainamide Hydrochloride Tablets, withdraw not less than 30 mL of the medium at the specified minute after starting the test, and filter through a membrane filter with a pore size not exceeding 0.8 μm. Discard not less than 10 mL of the first filtrate, pipet V mL of the subsequent filtrate, add 2nd fluid for dissolution test to make exactly V' mL so that each mL contains about 7 μg of procainamide hydrochloride ($C_{13}H_{21}N_3O.HCl$), and use this solution as the sample solution. Separately, weigh accurately about 0.125 g of procainamide hydrochloride for assay, previously dried at 105°C for 4 hours, and dissolve in water to make exactly 1000 mL. Pipet 5 mL of this solution, add 2nd fluid for dissolution test to make exactly 100 mL, and use this solution as the standard solution. Perform the test with the sample solution and standard solution as directed under Ultraviolet-visible Spectrophotometry <*2.24*>, and determine the absorbances, A_T and A_S, at 278 nm.

Dissolution rate (%) with respect to the labeled amount of procainamide hydrochloride ($C_{13}H_{21}N_3O.HCl$)
$= M_S \times A_T/A_S \times V'/V \times 1/C \times 9/2$

M_S: Amount (mg) of procainamide hydrochloride for assay taken
C: Labeled amount (mg) of procainamide hydrochloride ($C_{13}H_{21}N_3O.HCl$) in 1 tablet

Assay To 10 Procainamide Hydrochloride Tablets add about 300 mL of 0.02 mol/L phosphate buffer solution (pH 3.0) and sonicate to disintegrate the tablets completely. To this solution add 0.02 mol/L phosphate buffer solution (pH 3.0) to make exactly 500 mL, and stir for 5 minutes. Centrifuge this solution, pipet V mL of the supernatant liquid, and add 0.02 mol/L phosphate buffer solution (pH 3.0) to make exactly V' mL so that each mL contains about 10 μg of procainamide hydrochloride ($C_{13}H_{21}N_3O.HCl$). Filter this solution through a membrane filter with a pore size not exceeding 0.45 μm, discard the first 10 mL of the filtrate, and use the subsequent filtrate as the sample solution. Separately, weigh accurately about 50 mg of procainamide hydrochloride for assay, previously dried at 105°C for 4 hours, dissolve in 0.02 mol/L phosphate buffer solution (pH 3.0) to make exactly 100 mL. Pipet 2 mL of this solution, add 0.02 mol/L phosphate buffer solution (pH 3.0) to make exactly 100 mL, and use this solution as the standard solution. Perform the test with exactly 10 μL each of the sample solution and standard solution as directed under Liquid Chromatography <*2.01*> according to the following conditions, and determine the peak areas, A_T and A_S, of procainamide in each solution.

Amount (mg) of procainamide hydrochloride ($C_{13}H_{21}N_3O.HCl$)
$= M_S \times A_T/A_S \times V'/V \times 1/10$

M_S: Amount (mg) of procainamide hydrochloride for assay taken

Operating conditions—

Detector: An ultraviolet absorption photometer (wavelength: 270 nm).

Column: A stainless steel column 4.6 mm in inside diameter and 25 cm in length, packed with octadecylsilanized silica gel for liquid chromatography (5 μm in particle diameter).

Column temperature: A constant temperature of about 40°C.

Mobile phase: A mixture of 0.02 mol/L phosphate buffer solution (pH 3.0) and methanol (9:1).

Flow rate: Adjust so that the retention time of procainamide is about 9 minutes.

System suitability—

System performance: When the procedure is run with 10 μL of the standard solution under the above operating conditions, the number of theoretical plates and the symmetry factor of the peak of procainamide are not less than 10,000 and not more than 1.5, respectively.

System repeatability: When the test is repeated 6 times with 10 μL of the standard solution under the above operating conditions, the relative standard deviation of the peak area of procainamide is not more than 1.0%.

Containers and storage Containers—Tight containers.

Procaine Hydrochloride

プロカイン塩酸塩

$C_{13}H_{20}N_2O_2.HCl$: 272.77
2-(Diethylamino)ethyl 4-aminobenzoate monohydrochloride
[*51-05-8*]

Procaine Hydrochloride, when dried, contains not less than 99.0% of procaine hydrochloride ($C_{13}H_{20}N_2O_2.HCl$).

Description Procaine Hydrochloride occurs as white, crystals or crystalline powder.

It is very soluble in water, soluble in ethanol (95), and practically insoluble in diethyl ether.

Identification **(1)** Determine the absorption spectrum of a solution of Procaine Hydrochloride (1 in 100,000) as directed under Ultraviolet-visible Spectrophotometry 〈*2.24*〉, and compare the spectrum with the Reference Spectrum: both spectra exhibit similar intensities of absorption at the same wavelengths.

(2) Determine the infrared absorption spectrum of Procaine Hydrochloride, previously dried, as directed in the potassium chloride disk method under Infrared Spectrophotometry 〈*2.25*〉, and compare the spectrum with the Reference Spectrum: both spectra exhibit similar intensities of absorption at the same wave numbers.

(3) A solution of Procaine Hydrochloride (1 in 10) responds to Qualitative Tests 〈*1.09*〉 for chloride.

pH 〈*2.54*〉 The pH of a solution prepared by dissoluing 1.0 g of Procaine Hydrochloride in 20 mL of water is between 5.0 and 6.0.

Melting point 〈*2.60*〉 155 – 158°C

Purity **(1)** Clarity and color of solution—Dissolve 1.0 g of Procaine Hydrochloride in 10 mL of water: the solution is clear and colorless.

(2) Heavy metals 〈*1.07*〉—Proceed with 1.0 g of Procaine Hydrochloride according to Method 1, and perform the test. Prepare the control solution with 2.0 mL of Standard Lead Solution (not more than 20 ppm).

(3) Related substances—To 1.0 g of Procaine Hydrochloride add 5 mL of ethanol (95), dissolve by mixing well, add water to make exactly 10 mL, and use this solution as the sample solution. Separately, dissolve 10 mg of 4-aminobenzoic acid in ethanol (95) to make exactly 20 mL, then pipet 1 mL of this solution, add 4 mL of ethanol (95) and water to make exactly 10 mL, and use this solution as the standard solution. Perform the test with these solutions as directed under Thin-layer Chromatography 〈*2.03*〉. Spot 5 μL each of the sample solution and standard solution on a plate of silica gel with fluorescent indicator for thin-layer chromatography. Develop the plate with a mixture of dibutyl ether, *n*-hexane and acetic acid (100) (20:4:1) to a distance of about 10 cm, and air-dry the plate. After drying the plate more at 105°C for 10 minutes, examine under ultraviolet light (main wavelength: 254 nm): the spots other than the principal spot obtained from the sample solution are not more intense than the spot from the standard solution. The principal spot from the sample solution stays at the origin.

Loss on drying 〈*2.41*〉 Not more than 0.5% (1 g, silica gel, 4 hours).

Residue on ignition 〈*2.44*〉 Not more than 0.1% (1 g).

Assay Weigh accurately about 0.4 g of Procaine Hydrochloride, previously dried, dissolve in 5 mL of hydrochloric acid and 60 mL of water, add 10 mL of a solution of potassium bromide (3 in 10), cool to below 15°C, and titrate 〈*2.50*〉 with 0.1 mol/L sodium nitrite VS (potentiometric titration or amperometric titration).

Each mL of 0.1 mol/L sodium nitrite VS
= 27.28 mg of $C_{13}H_{20}N_2O_2.HCl$

Containers and storage Containers—Well-closed containers.

Procaine Hydrochloride Injection

プロカイン塩酸塩注射液

Procaine Hydrochloride Injection is an aqueous injection.

It contains not less than 95.0% and not more than 105.0% of the labeled amount of procaine hydrochloride ($C_{13}H_{20}N_2O_2.HCl$: 272.77).

Method of preparation Prepare as directed under Injections, with Procaine Hydrochloride.

Description Procaine Hydrochloride Injection is a clear, colorless liquid.

Identification **(1)** To a volume of Procaine Hydrochloride Injection, equivalent to 0.01 g of Procaine Hydrochloride, add water to make 1000 mL. Determine the absorption spectrum of this solution as directed under Ultraviolet-visible Spectrophotometry 〈*2.24*〉: it exhibits maxima between 219 nm and 223 nm, and between 289 nm and 293 nm.

(2) Procaine Hydrochloride Injection responds to Qualitative Tests 〈*1.09*〉 (2) for chloride.

pH 〈*2.54*〉 3.3 – 6.0

Bacterial endotoxins 〈*4.01*〉 Less than 0.02 EU/unit. Apply to the preparations intended for intraspinal administration.

Extractable volume 〈*6.05*〉 It meets the requirement.

Foreign insoluble matter 〈*6.06*〉 Perform the test according to Method 1: it meets the requirement.

Insoluble particulate matter 〈*6.07*〉 It meets the requirement.

Sterility 〈*4.06*〉 Perform the test according to the Membrane filtration method: it meets the requirement.

Assay To an exactly measured volume of Procaine Hydrochloride Injection, equivalent to about 20 mg of procaine hydrochloride ($C_{13}H_{20}N_2O_2.HCl$), add the mobile phase to make exactly 20 mL. Pipet 5 mL of this solution, add exactly 5 mL of the internal standard solution and the mobile phase to make 20 mL, and use this solution as the sample solution. Separately, weigh accurately about 50 mg of procaine hydrochloride for assay, previously dried in a desiccator (silica gel) for 4 hours, dissolve in the mobile phase to make exactly 50 mL. Pipet 5 mL of this solution, add exactly 5 mL of the internal standard solution and the mobile phase to make 20 mL, and use this solution as the standard solution. Perform the test with 5 μL each of the sample solution and standard solution as directed under Liquid Chromatography <*2.01*> according to the following conditions, and calculate the ratios, Q_T and Q_S, of the peak area of procaine hydrochloride to that of the internal standard.

Amount (mg) of procaine hydrochloride ($C_{13}H_{20}N_2O_2.HCl$)
$= M_S \times Q_T/Q_S \times 2/5$

M_S: Amount (mg) of procaine hydrochloride for assay taken

Internal standard solution—A solution of caffeine in the mobile phase (1 in 1000).

Operating conditions—

Detector: An ultraviolet absorption photometer (wavelength: 254 nm).

Column: A stainless steel column about 6 mm in inside diameter and about 15 cm in length, packed with octadecylsilanized silica gel for liquid chromatography (5 μm in particle diameter).

Column temperature: A constant temperature of about 40°C.

Mobile phase: Adjust the pH of 0.05 mol/L potassium dihydrogen phosphate TS to 3.0 with phosphoric acid, and add an amount of sodium 1-pentane sulfonate to make a solution so that containing 0.1%. To 800 mL of this solution add 200 mL of methanol.

Flow rate: Adjust so that the retention time of procaine is about 10 minutes.

System suitability—

System performance: When the procedure is run with 5 μL of the standard solution under the above operating conditions, procaine and the internal standard are eluted in this order with the resolution between these peaks being not less than 8.

System repeatability: When the test is repeated 6 times with 5 μL of the standard solution under the above operating conditions, the relative standard deviation of the ratios of the peak area of procaine to that of the internal standard is not more than 1.0%.

Containers and storage Containers—Hermetic containers.

Procarbazine Hydrochloride

プロカルバジン塩酸塩

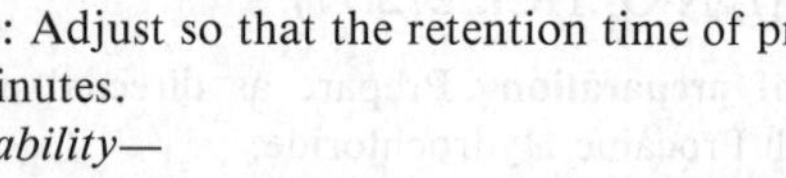

$C_{12}H_{19}N_3O.HCl$: 257.76
N-(1-Methylethyl)-
4-[(2-methylhydrazino)methyl]benzamide
monohydrochloride
[366-70-1]

Procarbazine Hydrochloride, when dried, contains not less than 98.5% and not more than 101.0% of procarbazine hydrochloride ($C_{12}H_{19}N_3O.HCl$).

Description Procarbazine Hydrochloride occurs as white to light yellowish white, crystals or crystalline powder.

It is freely soluble in water, and slightly soluble in ethanol (99.5).

It dissolves in dilute hydrochloric acid.

Melting point: about 223°C (with decomposition).

Identification **(1)** Dissolve 0.01 g of Procarbazine Hydrochloride in 1 mL of diluted copper (II) sulfate TS (1 in 10), and add 4 drops of sodium hydroxide TS: a green precipitate is formed immediately, and the color changes from green through yellow to orange.

(2) Determine the absorption spectrum of a solution of Procarbazine Hydrochloride in 0.1 mol/L hydrochloric acid TS (1 in 100,000) as directed under Ultraviolet-visible Spectrophotometry <*2.24*>, and compare the spectrum with the Reference Spectrum: both spectra exhibit similar intensities of absorption at the same wavelengths.

(3) Determine the infrared absorption spectrum of Procarbazine Hydrochloride, previously dried, as directed in the potassium chloride disk method under Infrared Spectrophotometry <*2.25*>, and compare the spectrum with the Reference Spectrum: both spectra exhibit similar intensities of absorption at the same wave numbers.

(4) A solution of Procarbazine Hydrochloride (1 in 20) responds to Qualitative Tests <*1.09*> for chloride.

pH <*2.54*> Dissolve 0.10 g of Procarbazine Hydrochloride in 10 mL of water: the pH of this solution is between 3.0 and 5.0.

Purity **(1)** Heavy metals <*1.07*>—Proceed with 1.0 g of Procarbazine Hydrochloride according to Method 4, and perform the test. Prepare the control solution with 2.0 mL of Standard Lead Solution (not more than 20 ppm).

(2) Related substances—Dissolve 50 mg of Procarbazine Hydrochloride in 5.0 mL of a solution of L-cysteine hydrochloride monohydrate in diluted methanol (7 in 10) (1 in 200), and use this solution as the sample solution. Pipet 1 mL of the sample solution, add a solution of L-cysteine hydrochloride monohydrate in diluted methanol (7 in 10) (1 in 200) to make exactly 50 mL, and use this solution as the standard solution. Perform the test with these solutions as directed under Thin-layer Chromatography <*2.03*>. Immerse slowly, by inclining, a plate of silica gel with fluorescent indicator for thin-layer chromatography in a solution of L-cysteine hydrochloride monohydrate in diluted methanol (7 in 10) (1 in 200), allow to stand for 1 minute, lift the plate from the solution, dry it in cold wind for 10 minutes, then dry in warm wind for 5 minutes, and then dry at 60°C for 5 minutes. After cooling, spot 5 μL each of the sample solution and standard solution on the plate. Develop the plate with a mixture of methanol and ethyl acetate (1:1) to a distance of about 12 cm, and air-dry the plate. Examine under ultraviolet light (main wavelength: 254 nm): not more than 1 spot other than the principal spot and the spot of the starting point obtained from the sample solution appears, and is not more intense than the spot from the standard solution.

Loss on drying <*2.41*> Not more than 0.5% (1 g, 105°C, 2 hours).

Residue on ignition <*2.44*> Not more than 0.1% (1 g).

Assay Weigh accurately about 0.15 g of Procarbazine Hydrochloride, previously dried, place in a glass-stoppered flask, dissolve in 25 mL of water, add 25 mL of hydrochloric acid, and cool to room temperature. To this solution add 5 mL of chloroform, and titrate <*2.50*>, while shaking, with 0.05 mol/L potassium iodate VS until the purple color of the chloroform layer disappears. The end point is reached when the red-purple color of the chloroform layer no more reappears within 5 minutes after the purple color disappeared.

Each mL of 0.05 mol/L potassium iodate VS
= 8.592 mg of $C_{12}H_{19}N_3O.HCl$

Containers and storage Containers—Tight containers.

Procaterol Hydrochloride Hydrate

プロカテロール塩酸塩水和物

and enantiomer

$C_{16}H_{22}N_2O_3.HCl.\frac{1}{2}H_2O$: 335.83
8-Hydroxy-5-{(1*RS*,2*SR*)-1-hydroxy-2-[(1-methylethyl)amino]butyl]}quinolin-2(1*H*)-one monohydrochloride hemihydrate
[*62929-91-3*, anhydride]

Procaterol Hydrochloride Hydrate contains not less than 98.5% of procaterol hydrochloride ($C_{16}H_{22}N_2O_3.HCl$: 326.82), calculated on the anhydrous basis.

Description Procaterol Hydrochloride Hydrate occurs as white to pale yellow-white, crystals or crystalline powder.

It is soluble in water, in formic acid and in methanol, slightly soluble in ethanol (95), and practically insoluble in diethyl ether.

The pH of a solution of 1.0 g of Procaterol Hydrochloride Hydrate in 100 mL of water is between 4.0 and 5.0.

It is gradually colored by light.

The solution of Procaterol Hydrochloride Hydrate (1 in 20) shows no optical rotation.

Melting point: about 195°C (with decomposition).

Identification (1) Determine the absorption spectrum of a solution of Procaterol Hydrochloride Hydrate (7 in 1,000,000) as directed under Ultraviolet-visible Spectrophotometry *<2.24>*, and compare the spectrum with the Reference Spectrum: both spectra exhibit similar intensities of absorption at the same wavelengths.

(2) Determine the infrared absorption spectrum of Procaterol Hydrochloride Hydrate as directed in the potassium bromide disk method under Infrared Spectrophotometry *<2.25>*, and compare the spectrum with the Reference Spectrum: both spectra exhibit similar intensities of absorption at the same wave numbers.

(3) A solution of Procaterol Hydrochloride Hydrate (1 in 50) responds to Qualitative Tests *<1.09>* for chloride.

Purity (1) Clarity and color of solution—Dissolve 1.0 g of Procaterol Hydrochloride Hydrate in 30 mL of water: the solution is clear, and has no more color than the following control solution.

Control solution: To 3.0 mL of Iron (III) Chloride CS add water to make 50 mL.

(2) Heavy metals *<1.07>*—Proceed with 2.0 g of Procaterol Hydrochloride Hydrate according to Method 2, and perform the test. Prepare the control solution with 2.0 mL of Standard Lead Solution (not more than 10 ppm).

(3) Related substances—Dissolve 0.10 g of Procaterol Hydrochloride Hydrate in 100 mL of diluted methanol (1 in 2), and use this solution as the sample solution. Pipet 1 mL of the sample solution, add diluted methanol (1 in 2) to make exactly 100 mL, and use this solution as the standard solution. Perform the test with exactly 2 μL each of the sample solution and standard solution as directed under Liquid Chromatography *<2.01>* according to the following conditions. Determine each peak area of these solutions by the automatic integration method: the total area of the peaks other than procaterol obtained from the sample solution is not larger than the peak area of procaterol from the standard solution.

Operating conditions—

Detector: An ultraviolet absorption photometer (wavelength: 254 nm).

Column: A stainless steel column about 4 mm in inside diameter and about 25 cm in length, packed with octadecylsilanized silica gel for liquid chromatography (5 μm in particle diameter).

Column temperature: A constant temperature of about 40°C.

Mobile phase: Dissolve 0.87 g of sodium 1-pentanesulfonate in 1000 mL of water. To 760 mL of this solution add 230 mL of methanol and 10 mL of acetic acid (100).

Flow rate: Adjust so that the retention time of procaterol is about 15 minutes.

Selection of column: Dissolve 20 mg each of Procaterol Hydrochloride Hydrate and threoprocaterol hydrochloride in 100 mL of diluted methanol (1 in 2). To 15 mL of this solution add diluted methanol (1 in 2) to make 100 mL. Proceed with 2 μL of this solution under the above operating conditions, and calculate the resolution. Use a column giving elution of procaterol and threoprocaterol in this order with the resolution of these peaks being not less than 3.

Detection sensitivity: Adjust the detection sensitivity so that the peak height of procaterol obtained from 2 μL of the standard solution is not less than 10 mm.

Time span of measurement: 2.5 times as long as the retention time of procaterol, beginning after the solvent peak.

Water *<2.48>* 2.5 – 3.3% (0.5 g, volumetric titration, direct titration).

Residue on ignition *<2.44>* Not more than 0.1% (1 g).

Assay Weigh accurately about 0.25 g of Procaterol Hydrochloride Hydrate, add 2 mL of formic acid, dissolve by warming, and add exactly 15 mL of 0.1 mol/L perchloric acid VS. Add 1 mL of acetic anhydride, heat on a water bath for 30 minutes, cool, add 60 mL of acetic anhydride, and titrate *<2.50>* the excess perchloric acid with 0.1 mol/L sodium acetate VS (potentiometric titration). Perform a blank determination in the same manner.

Each mL of 0.1 mol/L perchloric acid VS
= 32.68 mg of $C_{16}H_{22}N_2O_3.HCl$

Containers and storage Containers—Well-closed containers.

Storage—Light-resistant.

Prochlorperazine Maleate

プロクロルペラジンマレイン酸塩

$C_{20}H_{24}ClN_3S.2C_4H_4O_4$: 606.09
2-Chloro-10-[3-(4-methylpiperazin-1-yl)propyl]-10*H*-phenothiazine dimaleate
[*84-02-6*]

Prochlorperazine Maleate, when dried, contains not less than 98.0% of prochlorperazine maleate ($C_{20}H_{24}ClN_3S.2C_4H_4O_4$).

Description Prochlorperazine Maleate occurs as a white to light yellow powder. It is odorless, and has a slightly bitter taste.

It is slightly soluble in acetic acid (100), very slightly soluble in water and in ethanol (95), and practically insoluble in diethyl ether.

It gradually acquires a red tint by light.

Melting point: 195 – 203°C (with decomposition).

Identification **(1)** Dissolve 5 mg of Prochlorperazine Maleate in 5 mL of sulfuric acid: a red color develops, which darkens slowly on standing. Warm a half of the solution: the color changes to red-purple. To the remainder add 1 drop of potassium dichromate TS: a green-brown color develops, which changes to brown on standing.

(2) Boil 0.5 g of Prochlorperazine Maleate with 10 mL of hydrobromic acid under a reflux condenser for 10 minutes. After cooling, add 100 mL of water, and filter through glass filter (G4). Wash the residue with three 10-mL portions of water, and dry at 105°C for 1 hour: it melts <*2.60*> between 195°C and 198°C (with decomposition).

(3) Dissolve 0.2 g of Prochlorperazine Maleate in 5 mL of a solution of sodium hydroxide (1 in 10), and extract with three 3-mL portions of diethyl ether [reserve the aqueous layer, and use for test (4)]. Evaporate the combined diethyl ether extracts on a water bath to dryness, dissolve the residue in 10 mL of methanol by warming, and pour into 30 mL of a solution of 2,4,6-trinitrophenol in methanol (1 in 75), previously warmed to 50°C. Allow to stand for 1 hour, collect the crystals, wash with a small amount of methanol, and dry at 105°C for 1 hour: the crystals melt <*2.60*> between 252°C and 258°C (with decomposition).

(4) To the aqueous layer reserved in (3) add boiling chips, and heat on a water bath for 10 minutes. Cool, add 2 mL of bromine TS, heat on a water bath for 10 minutes, and heat the solution to boil. After cooling, add 2 drops of this solution to 3 mL of a solution of resorcinol in sulfuric acid (1 in 300), and heat on a water bath for 15 minutes: a red-purple color is produced.

Purity Heavy metals <*1.07*>—Proceed with 1.0 g of Prochlorperazine Maleate according to Method 2, and perform the test. Prepare the control solution with 1.0 mL of Standard Lead Solution (not more than 10 ppm).

Loss on drying <*2.41*> Not more than 1.0% (1 g, 105°C, 3 hours).

Residue on ignition <*2.44*> Not more than 0.1% (1 g).

Assay Weigh accurately about 0.3 g of Prochlorperazine Maleate, previously dried, dissolve in 60 mL of acetic acid (100) while stirring and warming. Cool, and titrate <*2.50*> with 0.05 mol/L perchloric acid VS until the color of the solution changes from orange to green (indicator: 0.5 mL of *p*-naphtholbenzein TS). Perform a blank determination in the same manner, and make any necessary correction.

Each mL of 0.05 mol/L perchloric acid VS
= 15.15 mg of $C_{20}H_{24}ClN_3S.2C_4H_4O_4$

Containers and storage Containers—Tight containers.
Storage—Light-resistant.

Prochlorperazine Maleate Tablets

プロクロルペラジンマレイン酸塩錠

Prochlorperazine Maleate Tablets contain not less than 95.0% and not more than 105.0% of the labeled amount of prochlorperazine maleate ($C_{20}H_{24}ClN_3S.2C_4H_4O_4$: 606.09).

Method of preparation Prepare as directed under Tablets, with Prochlorperazine Maleate.

Identification **(1)** Weigh a quantity of powdered Prochlorperazine Maleate Tablets, equivalent to 5 mg of Prochlorperazine Maleate, add 15 mL of acetic acid (100), shake, and filter. To 5 mL of the filtrate add 3 mL of sulfuric acid, and shake: a light red color develops. To this solution add 1 drop of potassium dichromate TS: a green-brown color is produced and changes to brown on standing.

(2) Weigh a quantity of powdered Prochlorperazine Maleate Tablets, equivalent to 0.08 g of Prochlorperazine Maleate, add 15 mL of methanol and 1 mL of dimethylamine, shake, centrifuge, and use the supernatant liquid as the sample solution. Separately, dissolve 0.08 g of Prochlorperazine Maleate RS in 15 mL of methanol and 1 mL of dimethylamine, and use this solution as the standard solution. Perform the test with these solutions as directed under Thin-layer Chromatography <*2.03*>. Spot 10 μL each of the sample solution and standard solution on a plate of silica gel for thin-layer chromatography. Develop the plate with a mixture of 1-butanol and ammonia TS (15:2) to a distance of about 10 cm, and air-dry the plate. Spray evenly palladium (II) chloride TS on the plate: the spots obtained from the sample solution and standard solution show a red-purple color, and has the same *R*f value.

(3) To a quantity of powdered Prochlorperazine Maleate Tablets, equivalent to 0.04 g of Prochlorperazine Maleate, add 10 mL of 1 mol/L hydrochloric acid TS and 20 mL of diethyl ether, shake, and centrifuge. Transfer the diethyl ether layer to a separator, wash with 5 mL of 0.05 mol/L sulfuric acid TS, and evaporate on a water bath to dryness. Dissolve the residue in 5 mL of sulfuric acid TS, filter, if necessary, and add 1 to 2 drops of potassium permanganate TS: the red color of the test solution is discharged immediately.

Uniformity of dosage units <*6.02*> Perform the test according to the following method: it meets the requirement of the Content uniformity test.

Conduct this procedure using light-resistant vessels. To 1 tablet of Prochlorperazine Maleate Tablets add 3*V*/5 mL of a mixture of dilute phosphoric acid (1 in 500) and ethanol (99.5) (1:1), sonicate until the tablet is disintegrated, and shake vigorously for 10 minutes. Add exactly *V*/20 mL of the internal standard solution, and a mixture of dilute phosphoric acid (1 in 500) and ethanol (99.5) (1:1) to make V mL so that each mL contains about 80 μg of prochlorperazine maleate ($C_{20}H_{24}ClN_3S.2C_4H_4O_4$). Centrifuge this solution, and use the supernatant liquid as the sample solution. Proceed as directed in the Assay.

Amount (mg) of prochlorperazine maleate ($C_{20}H_{24}ClN_3S.2C_4H_4O_4$)
$= M_S \times Q_T/Q_S \times V/250$

M_S: Amount (mg) of Prochlorperazine Maleate RS taken

Internal standard solution—A solution of butyl parahydroxybenzoate in a mixture of diluted phosphoric acid (1 in 500) and ethanol (99.5) (1:1) (1 in 1000).

Dissolution <*6.10*> When the test is performed at 50 revolutions per minute according to the Paddle method, using 900 mL of 2nd fluid for dissolution test as the dissolution medium, the dissolution rate in 45 minutes of Prochlorperazine Maleate Tablets is not less than 75%.

Start the test with 1 tablet of Prochlorperazine Maleate Tablets, withdraw not less than 20 mL of the medium at the specified minute after starting the test, and filter through a membrane filter with a pore size not exceeding 0.45 μm. Discard not less than 10 mL of the first filtrate, pipet V mL of the subsequent filtrate, add the dissolution medium to make exactly V' mL so that each mL contains about 9 μg of prochlorperazine maleate ($C_{20}H_{24}ClN_3S.2C_4H_4O_4$), and use this solution as the sample solution. Separately, weigh accurately about 18 mg of Prochlorperazine Maleate RS, previously dried at 105°C for 3 hours, and dissolve in methanol to make exactly 100 mL. Pipet 5 mL of this solution, add the dissolution medium to make exactly 100 mL, and use this solution as the standard solution. Perform the test with the sample solution and standard solution as directed under Ultraviolet-visible Spectrophotometry <*2.24*>, using the dissolution medium as the blank, and determine the absorbances, A_T and A_S, at 255 nm.

Dissolution rate (%) with respect to the labeled amount of prochlorperazine maleate ($C_{20}H_{24}ClN_3S.2C_4H_4O_4$)
$= M_S \times A_T/A_S \times V'/V \times 1/C \times 45$

M_S: Amount (mg) of Prochlorperazine Maleate RS taken
C: Labeled amount (mg) of prochlorperazine maleate ($C_{20}H_{24}ClN_3S.2C_4H_4O_4$) in 1 tablet

Assay Conduct this procedure using light-resistant vessels. Weigh accurately the mass of not less than 20 Prochlorperazine Maleate Tablets, and powder in an agate mortar. Weigh accurately a portion of the powder, equivalent to about 8 mg of prochlorperazine maleate ($C_{20}H_{24}ClN_3S.2C_4H_4O_4$), add 60 mL of a mixture of diluted phosphoric acid (1 in 500) and ethanol (99.5) (1:1), and shake vigorously for 10 minutes. Add exactly 5 mL of the internal standard solution, and add a mixture of diluted phosphoric acid (1 in 500) and ethanol (99.5) (1:1) to make 100 mL. Centrifuge this solution, and use the supernatant liquid as the sample solution. Separately, weigh accurately about 20 mg of Prochlorperazine Maleate RS, previously dried at 105°C for 3 hours, and dissolve in a mixture of diluted phosphoric acid (1 in 500) and ethanol (99.5) (1:1) to make exactly 25 mL. Pipet 10 mL of this solution, add exactly 5 mL of the internal standard solution and a mixture of diluted phosphoric acid (1 in 500) and ethanol (99.5) (1:1) to make 100 mL, and use this solution as the standard solution. Perform the test with 5 μL each of the sample solution and standard solution as directed under Liquid Chromatography <*2.01*> according to the following conditions, and calculate the ratios, Q_T and Q_S, of the peak area of prochlorperazine to that of the internal standard.

Amount (mg) of prochlorperazine maleate ($C_{20}H_{24}ClN_3S.2C_4H_4O_4$)
$= M_S \times Q_T/Q_S \times 2/5$

M_S: Amount (mg) of Prochlorperazine Maleate RS taken

Internal standard solution—A solution of butyl parahydroxybenzoate in a mixture of diluted phosphoric acid (1 in 500) and ethanol (99.5) (1:1) (1 in 1000).

Operating conditions—

Detector: An ultraviolet absorption photometer (wavelength: 257 nm).

Column: A stainless steel column 4.6 mm in inside diameter and 15 cm in length, packed with octadecylsilanized silica gel for liquid chromatography (5 μm in particle diameter).

Column temperature: A constant temperature of about 25°C.

Mobile phase: A mixture of diluted 0.05 mol/L sodium dihydrogen phosphate TS (1 in 2) and acetonitrile (11:9).

Flow rate: Adjust so that the retention time of prochlorperazine is about 5 minutes.

System suitability—

System performance: When the procedure is run with 5 μL of the standard solution under the above operating conditions, prochlorperazine and the internal standard are eluted in this order with the resolution between these peaks being not less than 10.

System repeatability: When the test is repeated 6 times with 5 μL of the standard solution under the above operating conditions, the relative standard deviation of the ratio of the peak area of prochlorperazine to that of the internal standard is not more than 1.0%.

Containers and storage Containers—Tight containers.

Storage—Light-resistant.

Progesterone

プロゲステロン

$C_{21}H_{30}O_2$: 314.46
Pregn-4-ene-3,20-dione
[*57-83-0*]

Progesterone, when dried, contains not less than 97.0% and not more than 103.0% of progesterone ($C_{21}H_{30}O_2$).

Description Progesterone occurs as white, crystals or crystalline powder.

It is soluble in methanol and in ethanol (99.5), and practically insoluble in water.

It shows crystal polymorphism.

Identification **(1)** Determine the absorption spectrum of a solution of Progesterone in ethanol (99.5) (1 in 100,000) as directed under Ultraviolet-visible Spectrophotometry <*2.24*>, and compare the spectrum with the Reference Spectrum or the spectrum of a solution of Progesterone RS prepared in the same manner as the sample solution: both spectra exhibit similar intensities of absorption at the same wavelengths.

(2) Determine the infrared absorption spectrum of Progesterone, as directed in the potassium bromide disk method under Infrared Spectrophotometry <*2.25*>, and compare the spectrum with the Reference Spectrum or the spectrum of Progesterone RS: both spectra exhibit similar intensities of absorption at the same wave numbers. If any difference appears between the spectra, dissolve Progesterone and Progesterone RS in ethanol (95), respectively, then evaporate the ethanol to dryness, and repeat the test on the residues.

Optical rotation <*2.49*> $[\alpha]_D^{20}$: +184 – +194° (after drying, 0.2 g, ethanol (99.5), 10 mL, 100 mm).

Melting point <*2.60*> 128 – 133°C or 120 – 122°C

Purity Related substances—Dissolve 80 mg of Progesterone in 2 mL of methanol, and use this solution as the sample solution. Pipet 1 mL of the sample solution, add methanol to make exactly 100 mL, and use this solution as the standard solution. Perform the test with these solutions as directed under Thin-layer Chromatography <*2.03*>. Spot 5 μL each of the sample solution and standard solution on a plate of silica gel with fluorescent indicator for thin-layer chromatography. Develop the plate with a mixture of diethyl ether and diethylamine (19:1) to a distance of about 15 cm, and air-dry the plate. Examine under ultraviolet light (main wavelength: 254 nm): the spot other than the principal spot obtained from the sample solution is not more intense than the spot from the standard solution.

Loss on drying <*2.41*> Not more than 0.5% (0.5 g, in vacuum, phosphorus (V) oxide, 4 hours).

Residue on ignition <*2.44*> Not more than 0.1% (0.5 g).

Assay Weigh accurately about 10 mg each of Progesterone and Progesterone RS, previously dried, and dissolve each in ethanol (99.5) to make exactly 100 mL. Pipet 5 mL each of these solutions, add ethanol (99.5) to make exactly 50 mL, and use these solution as the sample solution and the standard solution, respectively. Determine the absorbances, A_T and A_S, of the sample solution and standard solution at the wavelength of maximum absorption at about 241 nm as directed under Ultraviolet-visible Spectrophotometry <*2.24*>.

$$\text{Amount (mg) of progesterone } (C_{21}H_{30}O_2) = M_S \times A_T/A_S$$

M_S: Amount (mg) of Progesterone RS taken

Containers and storage Containers—Tight containers.
Storage—Light-resistant.

Progesterone Injection

プロゲステロン注射液

Progesterone Injection is an oily solution for injection.

It contains not less than 95.0% and not more than 105.0% of the labeled amount of progesterone ($C_{21}H_{30}O_2$: 314.46).

Method of preparation Prepare as directed under Injections, with Progesterone.

Description Progesterone Injection is a clear, colorless to pale yellow, oily liquid.

Identification To 1 mL of Progesterone Injection add 1 mL of diluted ethanol (9 in 10), shake well, take the ethanol layer, shake well with 1 mL of petroleum benzin, and use the ethanol layer as the sample solution. Separately, dissolve about 5 mg of Progesterone RS in 1 mL of ethanol (99.5), and use this solution as the standard solution. Perform the test with these solutions as directed under Thin-layer Chromatography <*2.03*>. Spot 2 μL each of the sample solution and standard solution on a plate of silica gel for thin-layer chromatography. Develop the plate with a mixture of diethyl ether and diethylamine (19:1) to a distance of about 10 cm, and air-dry the plate. Spray evenly sulfuric acid on the plate, and heat the plate at 105°C for 10 minutes: the principal spot obtained from the sample solution has the same *R*f value as the spot from the standard solution.

Extractable volume <*6.05*> It meets the requirement.

Foreign insoluble matter <*6.06*> Perform the test according to Method 1: it meets the requirement.

Insoluble particulate matter <*6.07*> It meets the requirement.

Sterility <*4.06*> Perform the test according to the Membrane filtration method: it meets the requirement.

Assay Measure the specific gravity of Progesterone Injection. Weigh accurately the mass of Progesterone Injection, equivalent to about 1 mL, mix with 2 mL of tetrahydrofuran, and add ethanol (99.5) to make exactly *V* mL so that each mL contains about 0.5 mg of progesterone ($C_{21}H_{30}O_2$). Pipet 2 mL of this solution, add exactly 10 mL of the internal standard solution and ethanol (99.5) to make 20 mL, and use this solution as the sample solution. Separately, weigh accurately about 10 mg of Progesterone RS, previously dried in vacuum for 4 hours using phosphorus (V) oxide as the desiccant, dissolve in 2 mL of tetrahydrofuran, and add ethanol (99.5) to make exactly 20 mL. Pipet 2 mL of this solution, add exactly 10 mL of the internal standard solution and ethanol (99.5) to make 20 mL, and use this solution as the standard solution. Perform the test with 5 μL each of the sample solution and standard solution as directed under Liquid Chromatography <*2.01*> according to the following conditions, and calculate the ratios, Q_T and Q_S, of the peak area of progesterone to that of the internal standard.

$$\text{Amount (mg) of progesterone } (C_{21}H_{30}O_2) = M_S \times Q_T/Q_S \times V/20$$

M_S: Amount (mg) of Progesterone RS taken

Internal standard solution—A solution of testosterone propionate in ethanol (99.5) (1 in 4000).

Operating conditions—

Detector: An ultraviolet absorption photometer (wavelength: 241 nm).

Column: A stainless steel column 4.6 mm in inside diameter and 15 cm in length, packed with octadecylsilanized silica gel for liquid chromatography (5 μm in particle diameter).

Column temperature: A constant temperature of about 35°C.

Mobile phase: A mixture of acetonitrile and water (7:3).

Flow rate: Adjust so that the retention time of progesterone is about 6 minutes.

System suitability—

System performance: When the procedure is run with 5 μL of the standard solution under the above operating conditions, progesterone and the internal standard are eluted in this order with the resolution between these peaks being not less than 9.

System repeatability: When the test is repeated 6 times with 5 μL of the standard solution under the above operating conditions, the relative standard deviation of the ratio of the peak area of progesterone to that of the internal standard is not more than 1.0%.

Containers and storage Containers—Hermetic containers.

Storage—Light-resistant.

Proglumide

プログルミド

and enantiomer

$C_{18}H_{26}N_2O_4$: 334.41
(4*RS*)-4-Benzoylamino-*N*,*N*-dipropylglutaramic acid
[*6620-60-6*]

Proglumide, when dried, contains not less than 98.5% of proglumide ($C_{18}H_{26}N_2O_4$).

Description Proglumide occurs as white, crystals or crystalline powder.

It is freely soluble in methanol, soluble in ethanol (95), sparingly soluble in diethyl ether, and very slightly soluble in water.

A solution of Proglumide in methanol (1 in 10) shows no optical rotation.

Identification **(1)** Put 0.5 g of Proglumide in a round bottom tube, add 5 mL of hydrochloric acid, seal the tube, and heat the tube carefully at 120°C for 3 hours. After cooling, open the tube, filter the content to collect crystals separated out, wash the crystals with 50 mL of cold water, and dry at 100°C for 1 hour: the melting point <*2.60*> of the crystals is between 121°C and 124°C.

(2) Determine the infrared absorption spectrum of Proglumide, previously dried, as directed in the potassium bromide disk method under Infrared Spectrophotometry <*2.25*>, and compare the spectrum with the Reference Spectrum: both spectra exhibit similar intensities of absorption at the same wave numbers.

Absorbance <*2.24*> $E^{1\%}_{1\,\mathrm{cm}}$ (225 nm): 384 – 414 (after drying, 4 mg, methanol, 250 mL).

Melting point <*2.60*> 148 – 150°C

Purity **(1)** Heavy metals <*1.07*>—Proceed with 1.0 g of Proglumide according to Method 2, and perform the test. Prepare the control solution with 2.0 mL of Standard Lead Solution (not more than 20 ppm).

(2) Arsenic <*1.11*>—To 1.0 g of Proglumide add 10 mL of a solution of magnesium nitrate hexahydrate in ethanol (95) (1 in 10) and 1.5 mL of hydrogen peroxide (30), burn the ethanol, and prepare the test solution according to Method 3, and perform the test (not more than 2 ppm).

(3) Related substances—Dissolve 0.10 g of Proglumide in 5 mL of methanol, and use this solution as the sample solution. Pipet 1 mL of the sample solution, add methanol to make exactly 200 mL, and use this solution as the standard solution. Perform the test with these solutions as directed under Thin-layer Chromatography <*2.03*>. Spot 10 μL each of the sample solution and standard solution on a plate of silica gel with fluorescent indicator for thin-layer chromatography. Develop the plate with a mixture of cyclohexane, ethyl acetate, acetic acid (100) and methanol (50:18:5:4) to a distance of about 10 cm, and air-dry the plate. Examine under ultraviolet light (main wavelength: 254 nm): the spots other than the principal spot obtained from the sample solution are not more intense than the spot from the standard solution.

Loss on drying <*2.41*> Not more than 0.10% (1 g, reduced pressure, phosphorus (V) oxide, 60°C, 3 hours).

Residue on ignition <*2.44*> Not more than 0.1% (1 g).

Assay Weigh accurately about 0.16 g of Proglumide, previously dried, dissolve in 40 mL of methanol, add 10 mL of water, and titrate <*2.50*> with 0.1 mol/L sodium hydroxide VS (potentiometric titration). Perform a blank determination in the same manner, and make any necessary correction.

Each mL of 0.1 mol/L sodium hydroxide VS
= 33.44 mg of $C_{18}H_{26}N_2O_4$

Containers and storage Containers—Well-closed containers.

L-Proline

L-プロリン

$C_5H_9NO_2$: 115.13
(2*S*)-Pyrrolidine-2-carboxylic acid
[*147-85-3*]

L-Proline contains not less than 99.0% and not more than 101.0% of L-proline ($C_5H_9NO_2$), calculated on the dried basis.

Description L-Proline occurs as white, crystals or crystalline powder. It has a slightly sweet taste.

It is very soluble in water and in formic acid, and slightly soluble in ethanol (99.5).

It is deliquescent.

Identification Determine the infrared absorption spectrum of L-Proline as directed in the potassium bromide disk method under Infrared Spectrophotometry <*2.25*>, and compare the spectrum with the Reference Spectrum: both spectra exhibit similar intensities of absorption at the same wave numbers.

Optical rotation <*2.49*> $[\alpha]^{20}_{D}$: −84.0 – −86.0° (1 g calculated on the dried basis, water, 25 mL, 100 mm).

pH <*2.54*> The pH of a solution of 1.0 g of L-Proline in 10 mL of water is 5.9 to 6.9.

Purity **(1)** Clarity and color of solution—Dissolve 1.0 g of L-Proline in 10 mL of water: the solution is clear and colorless.

(2) Chloride <*1.03*>—Perform the test with 0.5 g of L-Proline. Prepare the control solution with 0.30 mL of 0.01 mol/L hydrochloric acid VS (not more than 0.021%).

(3) Sulfate <*1.14*>—Perform the test with 0.6 g of L-Proline. Prepare the control solution with 0.35 mL of 0.005 mol/L sulfuric acid VS (not more than 0.028%).

(4) Ammonium <*1.02*>—Perform the test with 0.25 g of L-Proline. Prepare the control solution with 5.0 mL of Standard Ammonium Solution (not more than 0.02%).

(5) Heavy metals <*1.07*>—Proceed with 1.0 g of L-Proline according to Method 1, and perform the test. Prepare the control solution with 1.0 mL of Standard Lead Solution (not more than 10 ppm).

(6) Iron <*1.10*>—Prepare the test solution with 1.0 g of L-Proline according to Method 1, and perform the test according to Method A. Prepare the control solution with 1.0 mL of Standard Iron Solution (not more than 10 ppm).

(7) Related substances—Weigh accurately about 0.5 g of L-Proline, and dissolve in 0.5 mL of hydrochloric acid and water to make exactly 100 mL. Pipet 10 mL of this solution, add 0.02 mol/L hydrochloric acid TS to make exactly 50 mL, and use this solution as the sample solution. Separately, weigh accurately an amount, equivalent to 2.5 mmol, of L-aspartic acid, L-threonine, L-serine, L-glutamic acid, L-proline, glycine, L-alanine, L-cystine, L-valine, L-methionine, L-isoleucine, L-leucine, L-tyrosine, L-phenylalanine, L-lysine hydrochloride, ammonium chloride, L-histidine and L-arginine, dissolve them in 0.1 mol/L hydrochloric acid TS to make exactly 1000 mL, and use this solution as the standard stock solution. Pipet 5 mL of the standard stock solution, and add 0.02 mol/L hydrochloric acid TS to make exactly 100 mL. Pipet 4 mL of this solution, add 0.02 mol/L hydrochloric acid TS to make exactly 50 mL, and use this solution as the standard solution. Perform the test with exactly 20 μL each of the sample solution and standard solution as directed under Liquid Chromatography <*2.01*> according to the following conditions, and calculate the mass percentage of each amino acid, using the mass of amino acid other than proline in 1 mL of the sample solution from the height of the peaks obtained from the sample and standard solution: the amount of each amino acid other than proline is not more than 0.1 %.

Operating conditions—

Detector: A visible absorption photometer (wavelength: 570 nm).

Column: A stainless steel column 4.6 mm in inside diameter and 8 cm in length, packed with strongly acidic ion-exchange resin for liquid chromatography composed with a sulfonated polystyrene (3 μm in particle diameter) (Na type).

Column temperature: A constant temperature of about 57°C.

Chemical reaction vessel temperature: A constant temperature of about 130°C.

Reaction time: About 1 minute.

Mobile phase: Prepare the mobile phases A, B, C, D and E according to the following table, and add 0.1 mL each of caprylic acid.

Mobile phase	A	B	C	D	E
Citric acid monohydrate	19.80 g	22.00 g	12.80 g	6.10 g	—
Trisodium citrate dihydrate	6.19 g	7.74 g	13.31 g	26.67 g	—
Sodium chloride	5.66 g	7.07 g	3.74 g	54.35 g	—
Sodium hydroxide	—	—	—	—	8.00 g
Ethanol (99.5)	130 mL	20 mL	4 mL	—	100 mL
Thiodiglycol	5 mL	5 mL	5 mL	—	—
Benzyl alcohol	—	—	—	5 mL	—
Lauromacrogol solution (1 in 4)	4 mL	4 mL	4 mL	4 mL	4 mL
Water	a sufficient amount	a sufficient amount	a sufficient amount	a sufficient amount	a sufficient amount
Total amount	1000 mL	1000 mL	1000 mL	1000 mL	1000 mL

Switching of mobile phase: Switch the mobile phases A, B, C, D and E sequentially so that when proceed with 20 μL of the standard solution under the above conditions, aspartic acid, threonine, serine, glutamic acid, proline, glycine, alanine, cystine, valine, methionine, isoleucine, leucine, tyrosine, phenylalanine, lysine, ammonia, histidine and arginine are eluted in this order with the resolution between the peaks of isoleucine and leucine being not less than 1.2.

Reaction reagent: Dissolve 204 g of lithium acetate dihydrate in an appropriate amount of water, add 123 mL of acetic acid (100), 401 mL of 1-methoxy-2-propanol and water to make 1000 mL, pass nitrogen for 10 minutes, and use this solution as Solution (I). Separately, to 979 mL of 1-methoxy-2-propanol add 39 g of ninhydrin, pass nitrogen for 5 minutes, add 81 mg of sodium borohydride, pass nitrogen for 30 minutes, and use this solution as Solution (II). Prepare a mixture with an equal volume of the Solution (I) and (II). (Prepare before use).

Flow rate of mobile phase: 0.20 mL per minute.

Flow rate of reaction regent: 0.24 mL per minute.

System suitability—

System performance: When the test is run with 20 μL of the standard solution under the above operating conditions, the resolution between the peaks of glycine and alanine is not less than 1.2.

System repeatability: When the test is repeated 6 times with 20 μL of the standard solution under the above operating conditions, the relative standard deviations of the peak height of each amino acid other than proline in the standard solution is not more than 5.0%, and the relative standard deviation of the retention time is not more than 1.0%.

Loss on drying <*2.41*> Not more than 0.3% (1 g, 105°C, 3 hours).

Residue on ignition <*2.44*> Not more than 0.1% (1 g).

Assay Weigh accurately about 0.12 g of L-Proline, dissolve in 3 mL of formic acid, add 50 mL of acetic acid (100), and titrate <*2.50*> with 0.1 mol/L perchloric acid VS (potentiometric titration). Perform a blank determination in the same manner, and make any necessary correction.

Each mL of 0.1 mol/L perchloric acid VS
= 11.51 mg of $C_5H_9NO_2$

Containers and storage Containers—Tight containers.

Promethazine Hydrochloride

プロメタジン塩酸塩

• HCl

and enantiomer

$C_{17}H_{20}N_2S.HCl$: 320.88
(2*RS*)-*N*,*N*-Dimethyl-1-(10*H*-phenothiazin-10-yl)propan-2-ylamine monohydrochloride
[*58-33-3*]

Promethazine Hydrochloride, when dried, contains not less than 98.0% of promethazine hydrochloride ($C_{17}H_{20}N_2S.HCl$).

Description Promethazine Hydrochloride occurs as a white to light yellow powder.

It is very soluble in water, freely soluble in ethanol (95) and in acetic acid (100), sparingly soluble in acetic anhydride, and practically insoluble in diethyl ether.

It is gradually colored by light.

A solution of Promethazine Hydrochloride (1 in 25) shows no optical rotation.

Melting point: about 223°C (with decomposition).

Identification **(1)** Determine the absorption spectrum of a solution of Promethazine Hydrochloride (1 in 100,000) as directed under Ultraviolet-visible Spectrophotometry <*2.24*>, and compare the spectrum with the Reference Spectrum: both spectra exhibit similar intensities of absorption at the same wavelengths.

(2) Determine the infrared absorption spectrum of Promethazine Hydrochloride, previously dried, as directed in the potassium bromide disk method under Infrared Spectrophotometry <*2.25*>, and compare the spectrum with the Reference Spectrum: both spectra exhibit similar intensities of absorption at the same wave numbers.

(3) Dissolve 0.5 g of Promethazine Hydrochloride in 5 mL of water, add 2 mL of ammonia TS, and filter. To 5 mL of the filtrate add dilute nitric acid to make acidic: the solution responds to Qualitative Tests <*1.09*> (2) for chloride.

pH <*2.54*> The pH of a solution of Promethazine Hydrochloride (1 in 10) is between 4.0 and 5.5.

Purity **(1)** Clarity and color of solution—Dissolve 1.0 g of Promethazine Hydrochloride in 10 mL of water, protecting from light: the solution is clear and colorless.

(2) Heavy metals <*1.07*>—Proceed with 1.0 g of Promethazine Hydrochloride according to Method 2, and perform the test. Prepare the control solution with 2.0 mL of Standard Lead Solution (not more than 20 ppm).

(3) Related substances—Perform the test under the protection from sunlight. Dissolve 0.10 g of Promethazine Hydrochloride in exactly 5 mL of ethanol (95), and use this solution as the sample solution. Pipet 1 mL of the sample solution, add ethanol (95) to make exactly 200 mL, and use this solution as the standard solution (1). Separately, dissolve 20 mg of isopromethazine hydrochloride for thin-layer chromatography in ethanol (95) to make exactly 100 mL, and use this solution as the standard solution (2). Perform the test with these solutions as directed under Thin-layer Chromatography <*2.03*>. Spot 10 μL each of the sample solution and standard solutions (1) and (2) on a plate of silica gel with fluorescent indicator for thin-layer chromatography. Develop the plate with a mixture of methanol and diethylamine (19:1) to a distance of about 12 cm, and air-dry the plate. Examine under ultraviolet light (main wavelength: 254 nm): the spots obtained from the sample solution corresponding to the spots from the standard solution (2) are not more intense than the spot from the standard solution (2), and any spot other than the principal spot from the sample solution is not more intense than the spot from the standard solution (1).

Loss on drying <*2.41*> Not more than 0.5% (1 g, 105°C, 3 hours).

Residue on ignition <*2.44*> Not more than 0.1% (1 g).

Assay Weigh accurately about 0.5 g of Promethazine Hydrochloride, previously dried, dissolve in 50 mL of a mixture of acetic anhydride and acetic acid (100) (7:3), and titrate <*2.50*> with 0.1 mol/L perchloric acid VS (potentiometric titration). Perform a blank determination in the same manner, and make any necessary correction.

Each mL of 0.1 mol/L perchloric acid VS
= 32.09 mg of $C_{17}H_{20}N_2S.HCl$

Containers and storage Containers—Tight containers.
Storage—Light-resistant.

Propafenone Hydrochloride

プロパフェノン塩酸塩

• HCl

and enantiomer

$C_{21}H_{27}NO_3.HCl$: 377.90
1-{2-[(2*RS*)-2-Hydroxy-3-(propylamino)propyloxy]phenyl}-3-phenylpropan-1-one monohydrochloride
[*34183-22-7*]

Propafenone Hydrochloride, when dried, contains not less than 98.5% and not more than 101.0% of propafenone hydrochloride ($C_{21}H_{27}NO_3.HCl$).

Description Propafenone Hydrochloride occurs as white crystals or a white crystalline powder.

It is freely soluble in formic acid, sparingly soluble in methanol, and slightly soluble in water and in ethanol (99.5).

A solution of Propafenone Hydrochloride in methanol (1 in 100) shows no optical rotation.

Identification **(1)** Dissolve 0.1 g of Propafenone Hydrochloride in 20 mL of water by warming. After cooling, to 3 mL of this solution add water to make 500 mL. Determine the absorption spectrum of this solution as directed under Ultraviolet-visible Spectrophotometry <*2.24*>, and compare the spectrum with the Reference Spectrum: both spectra exhibit similar intensities of absorption at the same wavelengths.

(2) Determine the infrared absorption spectrum of Propafenone Hydrochloride as directed in the potassium chloride disk method under Infrared Spectrophotometry <*2.25*>, and compare the spectrum with the Reference Spectrum: both spectra exhibit similar intensities of absorption at the same wave numbers.

(3) Dissolve 0.1 g of Propafenone Hydrochloride in 20 mL of water by warming. After cooling, to 10 mL of this solution add 1 mL of dilute nitric acid, and filter to separate formed precipitate: the filtrate responds to Qualitative Tests <*1.09*> (2) for chloride.

Melting point <*2.60*> 172 – 175°C

Purity **(1)** Heavy metals <*1.07*>—Proceed with 1.0 g of Propafenone Hydrochloride according to Method 4, and perform the test. Prepare the control solution with 2.0 mL of Standard Lead Solution (not more than 20 ppm).

(2) Related substances—Dissolve 0.10 g of Propafenone Hydrochloride in 20 mL of the mobile phase in the operating conditions 1, and use this solution as the sample solution. Pipet 2 mL of the sample solution, and add the mobile phase in the operating conditions 1 to make exactly 50 mL. Pipet 2.5 mL of this solution, add 2.5 mL of a solution of diphenyl phthalate in methanol (1 in 2000), add the mobile phase in the operating conditions 1 to make exactly 100 mL, and use this solution as the standard solution. Perform the test with exactly 10 μL each of the sample solution and standard solution as directed under Liquid Chromatography <*2.01*> according to the following conditions 1 and 2. Determine each peak area of both solutions by the automatic integration method: the area of each peak other than the peak of propafenone obtained from the sample solution is not larger than the peak area of propafenone from the standard solution.

Operating conditions 1—

Detector: An ultraviolet absorption photometer (wavelength: 254 nm).

Column: A stainless steel column 4.6 mm in inside diameter and 15 cm in length, packed with octadecylsilanized silica gel for liquid chromatography (5 μm in particle diameter).

Column temperature: A constant temperature of about 40°C.

Mobile phase: Dissolve 4.6 g of sodium 1-nonanesulfonate and 2.3 g of phosphoric acid in water to make 1000 mL, and filter through a membrane filter with a pore size not exceeding 0.45 μm. To 900 mL of the filtrate add 600 mL of acetonitrile.

Flow rate: Adjust so that the retention time of diphenyl phthalate is about 39 minutes.

Time span of measurement: Beginning after the solvent peak to the retention time of diphenyl phthalate.

System suitability 1—

System performance: Dissolve 12 mg of Propafenone Hydrochloride and 50 mg of isopropyl benzoate in 100 mL of methanol. When the procedure is run with 10 μL of this solution under the above operating conditions 1, propafenone and isopropyl benzoate are eluted in this order with the resolution between these peaks being not less than 5.

System repeatability: When the test is repeated 6 times with 10 μL of the standard solution under the above operating conditions 1, the relative standard deviation of the peak area of propafenone is not more than 2.0%.

Operating conditions 2—

Detector, column and column temperature: Proceed as directed in the operating conditions 1.

Mobile phase: Dissolve 7.33 g of sodium 1-decanesulfonate and 2.3 g of phosphoric acid in water to make 1000 mL, and filter through a membrane filter with a pore size not exceeding 0.45 μm. To 700 mL of the filtrate add 700 mL of acetonitrile.

Flow rate: Adjust so that the retention time of diphenyl phthalate is about 11 minutes.

Time span of measurement: About 2.5 times as long as the retention time of diphenyl phthalate, beginning after the retention time of diphenyl phthalate.

System suitability 2—

System performance: When the procedure is run with 10 μL of the standard solution under the above operating conditions 2, propafenone and diphenyl phthalate are eluted in this order with the resolution between these peaks being not less than 21.

System repeatability: When the test is repeated 6 times with 10 μL of the standard solution under the above operating conditions 2, the relative standard deviation of the peak area of propafenone is not more than 2.0%.

Loss on drying <*2.41*> Not more than 0.5% (1 g, 105°C, 2 hours).

Residue on ignition <*2.44*> Not more than 0.1% (1 g).

Assay Weigh accurately about 0.3 g of Propafenone Hydrochloride, previously dried, dissolve in 2 mL of formic acid, add 50 mL of acetic anhydride, and titrate <*2.50*> with 0.05 mol/L perchloric acid VS (potentiometric titration). Perform a blank determination in the same manner, and make any necessary correction.

Each mL of 0.05 mol/L perchloric acid VS
= 18.90 mg of $C_{21}H_{27}NO_3.HCl$

Containers and storage Containers—Well-closed containers.

Propafenone Hydrochloride Tablets

プロパフェノン塩酸塩錠

Propafenone Hydrochloride Tablets contain not less than 96.0% and not more than 104.0% of the labeled amount of propafenone hydrochloride ($C_{21}H_{27}NO_3.HCl$: 377.90).

Method of preparation Prepare as directed under Tablets, with Propafenone Hydrochloride.

Identification To a quantity of Propafenone Hydrochloride Tablets, equivalent to 0.3 g of Propafenone Hydrochloride, add 60 mL of water, and disintegrate by warming. After cooling, centrifuge, and to 3 mL of the supernatant liquid add water to make 500 mL. Determine the absorption spectrum of this solution as directed under Ultraviolet-visible Spectrophotometry <*2.24*>: it exhibits maxima between 247 nm and 251 nm, and between 302 nm and 306 nm. Separately, determine the both maximal absorbances, A_1 and A_2, of the solution, the ratio of A_1/A_2 is between 2.30 and 2.55.

Uniformity of dosage units <*6.02*> Perform the Mass variation test, or the Content uniformity test according to the following method: it meets the requirement.

To 1 tablet of Propafenone Hydrochloride Tablets add 30 mL of a mixture of water and acetonitrile (1:1), shake well to disintegrate, add a mixture of water and acetonitrile (1:1) to make exactly 50 mL, and centrifuge. Pipet V mL of the supernatant liquid, equivalent to about 6 mg of propafenone hydrochloride ($C_{21}H_{27}NO_3.HCl$), add exactly 5 mL of the internal standard solution, add methanol to make 50 mL, and use this solution as the sample solution. Proceed as directed in the Assay.

Amount (mg) of propafenone hydrochloride ($C_{21}H_{27}NO_3.HCl$)
$= M_S \times Q_T/Q_S \times 10/V$

M_S: Amount (mg) of propafenone hydrochloride for assay taken

Internal standard solution—A solution of isopropyl benzoate in methanol (1 in 200).

Dissolution <*6.10*> When the test is performed at 50 revolutions per minute according to the Paddle method, using 900 mL of water as the dissolution medium, the dissolution rate in 30 minutes of Propafenone Hydrochloride Tables is not less than 75%.

Start the test with 1 tablet of Propafenone Hydrochloride Tablets, withdraw not less than 20 mL of the medium at the specified minute after starting the test, and filter through a membrane filter with a pore size not exceeding 0.5 μm. Discard not less than 10 mL of the first filtrate, pipet V mL of the subsequent filtrate, add water to make exactly V' mL so that each mL contains about 67 μg of propafenone hydrochloride ($C_{21}H_{27}NO_3.HCl$), and use this solution as the sample solution. Separately, weigh accurately about 13 mg of propafenone hydrochloride for assay, previously dried at 105°C for 2 hours, dissolve in water to make exactly 200 mL, and use this solution as the standard solution. Determine the absorbances, A_T and A_S, of the sample solution and standard solution at 305 nm as directed under Ultraviolet-visible Spectrophotometry <*2.24*>.

Dissolution rate (%) with respect to the labeled amount of propafenone hydrochloride ($C_{21}H_{27}NO_3.HCl$)
$= M_S \times A_T/A_S \times V'/V \times 1/C \times 450$

M_S: Amount (mg) of propafenone hydrochloride for assay taken

C: Labeled amount (mg) of propafenone hydrochloride ($C_{21}H_{27}NO_3.HCl$) in 1 tablet

Assay To a quantity of Propafenone Hydrochloride Tablets, equivalent to 1.5 g of propafenone hydrochloride ($C_{21}H_{27}NO_3.HCl$), add 70 mL of a mixture of water and acetonitrile (1:1), shake well to disintegrate, shake well for another 5 minutes, add a mixture of water and acetonitrile (1:1) to make exactly 100 mL, and centrifuge. Pipet 4 mL of the supernatant liquid, and add methanol to make exactly 50 mL. Pipet 5 mL of the solution, add exactly 5 mL of the internal standard solution, add methanol to make 50 mL, and use this solution as the sample solution. Separately, weigh accurately about 30 mg of propafenone hydrochloride for assay, previously dried at 105°C for 2 hours, and dissolve in methanol to make exactly 50 mL. Pipet 10 mL of this solution, add exactly 5 mL of the internal standard solution, add methanol to make 50 mL, and use this solution as the standard solution. Perform the test with 10 μL each of the sample solution and standard solution as directed under Liquid Chromatography <*2.01*> according to the following conditions, and calculate the ratios, Q_T and Q_S, of the peak area of propafenone to that of the internal standard.

Amount (mg) of propafenone hydrochloride ($C_{21}H_{27}NO_3.HCl$)
$= M_S \times Q_T/Q_S \times 50$

M_S: Amount (mg) of propafenone hydrochloride for assay taken

Internal standard solution—A solution of isopropyl benzoate in methanol (1 in 200).

Operating conditions—

Detector: An ultraviolet absorption photometer (wavelength: 254 nm).

Column: A stainless steel column 4.6 mm in inside diameter and 15 cm in length, packed with octadecylsilanized silica gel for liquid chromatography (5 μm in particle diameter).

Column temperature: A constant temperature of about 40°C.

Mobile phase: Dissolve 4.6 g of sodium 1-nonanesulfonate and 2.3 g of phosphoric acid in water to make 1000 mL, and filter through a membrane filter with a pore size not exceeding 0.45 μm. To 900 mL of the filtrate add 600 mL of acetonitrile.

Flow rate: Adjust so that the retention time of propafenone is about 8 minutes.

System suitability—

System performance: When the procedure is run with 10 μL of the standard solution under the above operating conditions, propafenone and the internal standard are eluted in this order with the resolution between these peaks being not less than 5.

System repeatability: When the test is repeated 6 times with 10 μL of the standard solution under the above operating conditions, the relative standard deviation of the ratio of the peak area of propafenone to that of the internal standard is not more than 1.0%.

Containers and storage Containers—Tight containers.

Propantheline Bromide

プロパンテリン臭化物

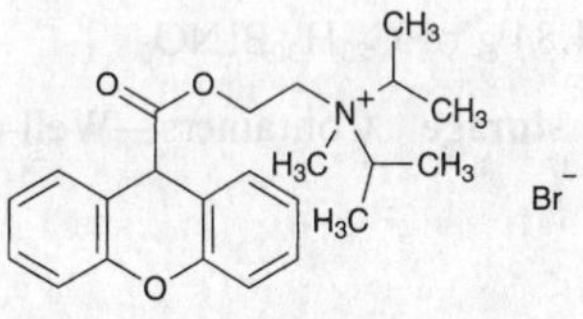

$C_{23}H_{30}BrNO_3$: 448.39
N-Methyl-*N*,*N*-bis(1-methylethyl)-2-[(9*H*-xanthen-9-ylcarbonyl)oxy]ethylaminium bromide
[*50-34-0*]

Propantheline Bromide, when dried, contains not less than 98.0% and not more than 102.0% of propantheline bromide ($C_{23}H_{30}BrNO_3$).

Description Propantheline Bromide occurs as a white to yellowish white crystalline powder. It is odorless and has a very bitter taste.

It is very soluble in water, in ethanol (95), in acetic acid (100) and in chloroform, soluble in acetic anhydride, and practically insoluble in diethyl ether.

The pH of a solution of 1.0 g of Propantheline Bromide in 50 mL of water is between 5.0 and 6.0.

Melting point: about 161°C (with decomposition, after drying).

Identification **(1)** To 5 mL of a solution of Propantheline Bromide (1 in 20) add 10 mL of sodium hydroxide TS, heat to boil for 2 minutes. Cool to 60°C, and add 5 mL of dilute hydrochloric acid. After cooling, collect the precipitates, and wash with water. Recrystallize from dilute ethanol, and dry at 105°C for 1 hour: the crystals melt <*2.60*> between 217°C and 222°C.

(2) Dissolve 0.01 g of the crystals obtained in (1) in 5 mL of sulfuric acid: a vivid yellow to yellow-red color develops.

(3) To 5 mL of a solution of Propantheline Bromide (1 in 10) add 2 mL of dilute nitric acid: this solution responds to Qualitative Tests <*1.09*> (1) for bromide.

Purity Xanthene-9-carboxylic acid and xanthone—Dissolve 10 mg of Propantheline Bromide in exactly 2 mL of chloroform, and use this solution as the sample solution. Separately, dissolve 1.0 mg of xanthene-9-carboxylic acid and 1.0 mg of xanthone in exactly 40 mL of chloroform, and use this solution as the standard solution. Perform the test immediately with these solutions as directed under Thin-layer Chromatography <*2.03*>. Spot 25 μL each of the sample solution and standard solution on a plate of silica gel with fluorescent indicator for thin-layer chromatography, and air-dry the plate for 10 minutes. Develop the plate with a mixture of 1,2-dichloroethane, methanol, water and formic acid (56:24:1:1) to a distance of about 12 cm, and air-dry the plate. Examine under ultraviolet light: the spots obtained from the sample solution corresponding to the spots from the standard solution are not more intense than those from the standard solution.

Loss on drying <*2.41*> Not more than 0.5% (2 g, 105°C, 4 hours).

Residue on ignition <*2.44*> Not more than 0.1% (1 g).

Assay Weigh accurately about 1 g of Propantheline Bromide, previously dried, dissolve in 50 mL of a mixture of acetic anhydride and acetic acid (100) (7:3), and titrate <*2.50*> with 0.1 mol/L perchloric acid VS (potentiometric titration). Perform a blank determination in the same manner, and make any necessary correction.

Each mL of 0.1 mol/L perchloric acid VS
= 44.84 g of $C_{23}H_{30}BrNO_3$

Containers and storage Containers—Well-closed containers.

Propiverine Hydrochloride

プロピベリン塩酸塩

$C_{23}H_{29}NO_3.HCl$: 403.94
1-Methylpiperidin-4-yl 2,2-diphenyl-2-propoxyacetate monohydrochloride
[*54556-98-8*]

Propiverine Hydrochloride, when dried, contains not less than 98.5% and not more than 101.5% of propiverine hydrochloride ($C_{23}H_{29}NO_3.HCl$).

Description Propiverine Hydrochloride occurs as white, crystals or crystalline powder.

It is soluble in water and in ethanol (99.5).

Identification **(1)** Dissolve 50 mg of Propiverine Hydrochloride in 20 mL of water, and add acetonitrile to make 100 mL. Determine the absorption spectrum of this solution as directed under Ultraviolet-visible Spectrophotometry <*2.24*>, and compare the spectrum with the Reference Spectrum or the spectrum of a solution of Propiverine Hydrochroride RS prepared in the same manner as the sample solution: both spectra exhibit similar intensities of absorption at the same wavelengths.

(2) Determine the infrared absorption spectrum of Propiverine Hydrochloride, previously dried, as directed in the potassium chloride disk method under Infrared Spectrophotometry <*2.25*>, and compare the spectrum with the Reference Spectrum or the spectrum of dried Propiverine Hydrochloride RS: both spectra exhibit similar intensities of absorption at the same wave numbers.

(3) To 5 mL of a solution of Propiverine Hydrochloride (1 in 100) add 6 mL of ethyl acetate, and add 3 drops of silver nitrate TS: a white precipitate is formed, which does not dissolve on the addition of 0.5 mL of dilute nitric acid and shaking. The precipitate dissolves on the addition of 2 mL of ammonia TS and shaking.

Melting point <*2.60*> 213 - 218°C

Purity **(1)** Sulfate <*1.14*>—Perform the test with 0.40 g of Propiverine Hydrochloride. Prepare the control solution with 0.40 mL of 0.005 mol/L sulfuric acid VS (not more than 0.048%).

(2) Heavy metals <*1.07*>—Proceed with 1.0 g of Propiverine Hydrochloride according to Method 2, and perform the test. Prepare the control solution with 2.0 mL of Standard Lead Solution (not more than 20 ppm).

(3) Related substances—Dissolve 50 mg of Propiverine Hydrochloride in 100 mL of the mobile phase, and use this solution as the sample solution. Pipet 1 mL of the sample solution, add the mobile phase to make exactly 100 mL, and use this solution as the standard solution. Perform the test with exactly 15 μL each of the sample solution and standard solution as directed under Liquid Chromatography <*2.01*> according to the following conditions. Determine each peak area by the automatic integration method: the area of the peak, having the relative retention time about 0.28 to propiverine, obtained from the sample solution is not larger than 3/10 times the peak area of propiverine from the standard solution, the area of the peak other than propiverine and the peak mentioned above from the sample solution is not larger than 1/10 times the peak area of propiverine from the standard solution, and the total area of the peaks other than propiverine from the sample solution is not larger than 1/2 times the peak area of propiverine from the standard solution.

Operating conditions—

Detector, column, column temperature, mobile phase, and flow rate: Proceed as directed in the operating conditions in the Assay.

Time span of measurement: About 2.5 times as long as the retention time of propiverine, beginning after the solvent peak.

System suitability—

Test for required detectability: Pipet 1 mL of the standard solution, and add the mobile phase to make exactly 20 mL. Confirm that the peak area of propiverine obtained with 15 μL of this solution is equivalent to 3.5 to 6.5% of that with 15 μL of the standard solution.

System performance: When the procedure is run with 15 μL of the standard solution under the above operating conditions, the number of theoretical plates and the symmetry factor of the peak of propiverine are not less than 7000 and not more than 1.5, respectively.

System repeatability: When the test is repeated 6 times with 15 μL of the standard solution under the above operating conditions, the relative standard deviation of the peak area of propiverine is not more than 2.0%.

Loss on drying <*2.41*> Not more than 1.0% (1 g, 105°C, 1 hour).

Residue on ignition <*2.44*> Not more than 0.1% (1 g).

Assay Weigh accurately about 50 mg each of Propiverine Hydrochloride and Propiverine Hydrachloride RS, both previously dried, and dissolve each in the mobile phase to make exactly 100 mL. Pipet 10 mL each of these solutions, add the mobile phase to make exactly 50 mL, and use these solutions as the sample solution and the standard solution, respectively. Perform the test with exactly 15 μL each of the sample solution and standard solution as directed under Liquid Chromatography <*2.01*> according to the following conditions, and determine the peak areas, A_T and A_S, of propiverine in each solution.

Amount (mg) of propiverine hydrochloride ($C_{23}H_{29}NO_3.HCl$)
$$= M_S \times A_T/A_S$$

M_S: Amount (mg) of Propiverine Hydrochloride RS taken

System suitability—

Detector: An ultraviolet absorption photometer (wavelength: 210 nm).

Column: A stainless steel column 4.6 mm in inside diameter and 15 cm in length, packed with phenylated silica gel for liquid chromatography (5 μm in particle diameter).

Column temperature: A constant temperature of about 40°C.

Mobile phase: Dissolve 2.21 g of potassium dihydrogen phosphate and 1.51 g of sodium 1-octane sulfonate in 650 mL of water, adjust to pH 3.2 with phosphoric acid, and add 350 mL of acetonitrile.

Flow rate: Adjust so that the retention time of propiverine is about 17 minutes.

System suitability—

System performance: When the procedure is run with 15 μL of the standard solution under the above operating conditions, the number of theoretical plates and the symmetry factor of the peak of propiverine are not less than 6000 and not more than 2.0, respectively.

System repeatability: When the test is repeated 6 times with 15 μL of the standard solution under the above operating conditions, the relative standard deviation of the peak area of propiverine is not more than 1.0%.

Containers and storage Containers—Tight containers.

Propiverine Hydrochloride Tablets

プロピベリン塩酸塩錠

Propiverine Hydrochloride Tablets contain not less than 95.0% and not more than 105.0% of propiverine hydrochloride ($C_{23}H_{29}NO_3.HCl$: 403.94).

Method of preparation Prepare as directed under Tablets, with Propiverine Hydrochloride.

Identification Shake vigorously a quantity of powdered Propiverine Hydrochloride Tablets, equivalent to 50 mg of Propiverine Hydrochloride, with 20 mL of water. Add acetonitrile to make 100 mL, centrifuge, and filter the supernatant liquid, if necessary. Determine the absorption spectrum of the supernatant liquid or the filtrate under Ultraviolet-visible Spectrophotometry <*2.24*>: it exhibits a maximum between 257 nm and 261 nm.

Purity Related substances—Shake vigorously a quantity of powdered Propiverine Hydrochloride Tablets, equivalent to 50 mg of Propiverine Hydrochloride, with the mobile phase, add the mobile phase to make 100 mL, centrifuge, and use the supernatant liquid as the sample solution. Pipet 1 mL of the sample solution, add the mobile phase to make exactly 100 mL, and use this solution as the standard solution. Perform the test with exactly 15 μL each of the sample solution and standard solution as directed under Liquid Chromatography <*2.01*> according to the following conditions. Determine each peak area by the automatic integration method: the area of the peak, having the relative retention time about 0.28 to propiverine, obtained from the sample solution is not larger than 3/10 times the peak area of propiverine from the standard solution, the area of the peak other than propiverine and the peak mentioned above from the sample solution is not larger than 1/5 times the peak area of propiverine from the standard solution, and the total area of the peaks other than propiverine from the sample solution is not larger than 7/10 times the peak area of propiverine from the standard solution.

Operating conditions—

Detector, column, column temperature, mobile phase, and flow rate: Proceed as directed in the operating conditions in the Assay under Propiverine Hydrochloride.

Time span of measurement: About 2.5 times as long as the retention time of propiverine, beginning after the solvent peak.

System suitability—

Test for required detectability: Pipet 1 mL of the standard solution, and add the mobile phase to make exactly 20 mL. Confirm that the peak area of propiverine obtained with 15 μL of this solution is equivalent to 3.5 to 6.5% of that with 15 μL of the standard solution.

System performance: When the procedure is run with 15 μL of the standard solution under the above operating conditions, the number of theoretical plates and the symmetry factor of the peak of propiverine are not less than 7000 and not more than 1.5, respectively.

System repeatability: When the test is repeated 6 times with 15 μL of the standard solution under the above operating conditions, the relative standard deviation of the peak area of propiverine is not more than 2.0%.

Uniformity of dosage units <*6.02*> Perform the test according to the following method: it meets the requirement of the Content uniformity test.

To 1 tablet of Propiverine Hydrochloride Tablets add the mobile phase, shake vigorously, add the mobile phase to make exactly V mL so that each mL contains about 0.1 mg of propiverine hydrochloride ($C_{23}H_{29}NO_3.HCl$), centrifuge, and use the supernatant liquid as the sample solution. Separately, weigh accurately about 50 mg of Propirevine Hydrochloride RS, previously dried at 105°C for 1 hour, and dissolve in the mobile phase to make exactly 100 mL. Pipet 10 mL of this solution, add the mobile phase to make exactly 50 mL, and use this solution as the standard solution. Then, proceed as directed in the Assay under Propiverine Hydrochloride.

Amount (mg) of propiverine hydrochloride ($C_{23}H_{29}NO_3.HCl$)
$$= M_S \times A_T/A_S \times V/500$$

M_S: Amount (mg) of Propiverine Hydrochloride RS taken

Dissolution <*6.10*> When the test is performed at 50 revolutions per minute according to Paddle method, using 900 mL of 2nd fluid for dissolution test as the dissolution medium, the dissolution rate in 20 minutes of Propiverine Hydrochloride Tablets is not less than 85%.

Start the test with 1 tablet of Propiverine Hydrochloride Tablets, withdraw not less than 25 mL of the medium at the specified minute after starting the test, and filter through a membrane filter with a pore size not exceeding 0.45 μm. Discard not less than 10 mL of the first filtrate, pipet V mL of the subsequent filtrate, add the dissolution medium to make exactly V' mL so that each mL contains about 11 μg of propiverine hydrochloride ($C_{23}H_{29}NO_3.HCl$). Pipet 15 mL of this solution, add exactly 2 mL of 0.1 mol/L hydrochloric acid TS, and use this solution as the sample solution. Separately, weigh accurately about 28 mg of Propiverine Hydrochloride RS, previously dried at 105°C for 1 hour, and dissolve in the dissolution medium to make exactly 100 mL. Pipet 4 mL of this solution, and add the dissolution medium to make exactly 100 mL. Further, pipet 15 mL of this solution, add exactly 2 mL of 0.1 mol/L hydrochloric acid TS, and use this solution as the standard solution. Perform the test with exactly 20 μL each of the sample solution and standard solution as directed under Liquid Chromatography *<2.01>* according to the following conditions, and determine the peak areas, A_T and A_S, of propiverine in each solution.

Dissolution rate (%) with respect to the labeled amount of propiverine hydrochloride ($C_{23}H_{29}NO_3.HCl$)
$= M_S \times A_T/A_S \times V'/V \times 1/C \times 36$

M_S: Amount (mg) of Propiverine Hydrochloride RS taken
C: Labeled amount (mg) of propiverine hydrochloride ($C_{23}H_{29}NO_3.HCl$) in 1 tablet

Operating conditions—

Detector: An ultraviolet absorption photometer (wavelength: 220 nm).

Column: A stainless steel column 4.6 mm in inside diameter and 15 cm in length, packed with octadecylsilanized silica gel for liquid chromatography (5 μm in particle diameter).

Column temperature: A constant temperature of about 25°C.

Mobile phase: To diluted 0.02 mol/L potassium dihydrogen phosphate TS (1 → 2) add phosphoric acid, and adjust to pH 2.0. To 560 mL of this solution add 440 mL of acetonitrile.

Flow rate: Adjust so that the retention time of propirevine is about 6 minutes.

System suitability—

System performance: When the procedure is run with 20 μL of the standard solution under the above operating conditions, the number of theoretical plates and the symmetry factor of the peak of propiverine are not less than 4000 and not more than 2.0, respectively.

System repeatability: When the test is repeated 6 times with 20 μL of the standard solution under the above operations conditions, the relative standard deviation of the peak area of propiverine is not more than 2.0%.

Assay Weigh accurately and powder not less than 20 Propiverine Hydrochloride Tablets. Weigh accurately a portion of the powder, equivalent to about 50 mg of propiverine hydrochloride ($C_{23}H_{29}NO_3.HCl$), add the mobile phase, shake vigorously, and add the mobile phase to make exactly 100 mL. Centrifuge this solution, pipet 10 mL of the supernatant liquid, add the mobile phase to make exactly 50 mL, and use this solution as the sample solution. Separately, weigh accurately about 50 mg of Propiverine Hydrochloride RS, previously dried at 105°C for 1 hour, and dissolve in the mobile phase to make exactly 100 mL. Pipet 10 mL of this solution, add the mobile phase to make exactly 50 mL, and use this solution as the standard solution. Then, proceed as directed in the Assay under Propiverine Hydrochloride.

Amount (mg) of propiverine hydrochloride ($C_{23}H_{29}NO_3.HCl$)
$= M_S \times A_T/A_S$

M_S: Amount (mg) of Propiverine Hydrochloride RS taken

Containers and storage Containers—Tight containers.

Propranolol Hydrochloride

プロプラノロール塩酸塩

and enantiomer

$C_{16}H_{21}NO_2.HCl$: 295.80
(2*RS*)-1-(1-Methylethyl)amino-3-(naphthalen-1-yloxy)propan-2-ol monohydrochloride
[318-98-9]

Propranolol Hydrochloride, when dried, contains not less than 99.0% and not more than 101.0% of propranolol hydrochloride ($C_{16}H_{21}NO_2.HCl$).

Description Propranolol Hydrochloride occurs as a white crystalline powder.

It is freely soluble in methanol, soluble in water and in acetic acid (100), and sparingly soluble in ethanol (99.5).

A solution of Propranolol Hydrochloride in methanol (1 in 40) shows no optical rotation.

It is graduauly colored to yellowish white to light brown by light.

Identification **(1)** Determine the absorption spectrum of a solution of Propranolol Hydrochloride in methanol (1 in 50,000) as directed under Ultraviolet-visible Spectrophotometry *<2.24>*, and compare the spectrum with the Reference Spectrum: both spectra exhibit similar intensities of absorption at the same wavelengths.

(2) Determine the infrared absorption spectrum of Propranolol Hydrochloride, previously dried, as directed in the potassium chloride disk method under Infrared Spectrophotometry *<2.25>*, and compare the spectrum with the Reference Spectrum: both spectra exhibit similar intensities of absorption at the same wave numbers.

(3) A solution of Propranolol Hydrochloride (1 in 50) responds to Qualitative Tests *<1.09>* (2) for chloride.

pH *<2.54>* The pH of a solution prepared by dissolving 0.5 g of Propranolol Hydrochloride in 50 mL of water is 5.0 – 6.0.

Melting point *<2.60>* 163 – 166°C

Purity **(1)** Clarity and color of solution—Dissolve 1.0 g of Propranolol Hydrochloride in 20 mL of water: the solution is clear and colorless.

(2) Heavy metals *<1.07>*—Proceed with 1.0 g of Propranolol Hydrochloride according to Method 4, and perform the test. Prepare the control solution with 2.0 mL of Standard Lead Solution (not more than 20 ppm).

(3) Related substances—Dissolve 20 mg of Propranolol Hydrochloride in 10 mL of the mobile phase, and use this solution as the sample solution. Pipet 2 mL of the sample solution, and add the mobile phase to make exactly 100 mL.

Pipet 1 mL of this solution, add the mobile phase to make exactly 10 mL, and use this solution as the standard solution. Perform the test with exactly 20 μL each of the sample solution and standard solution as directed under Liquid Chromatography <*2.01*> according to the following conditions, and determine each peak area by the automatic integration method: the area of the peak other than propranolol obtained from the sample solution is not larger than 1/2 times the peak area of propranolol from the standard solution, and the total area of the peaks other than the peak of propranolol from the sample solution is not larger than 2 times the peak area of propranolol from the standard solution.

Operating conditions—

Detector: An ultraviolet absorption photometer (wavelength: 292 nm).

Column: A stainless steel column 4.6 mm in inside diameter and 25 cm in length, packed with octadecylsilanized silica gel for liquid chromatography (5 μm in particle diameter).

Column temperature: A constant temperature of about 25°C.

Mobile phase: Dissolve 1.6 g of sodium lauryl sulfate and 0.31 g of tetrabutylammonium dihydrogen phosphate in 450 mL of water, add 1 mL of sulfuric acid and 550 mL of acetonitrile for liquid chromatography, and adjust to pH 3.3 with 2 mol/L sodium hydroxide TS.

Flow rate: Adjust so that the retention time of propranolol is about 4 minutes.

Time span of measurement: About 5 times as long as the retention time of propranolol.

System suitability—

Test for required detectability: Measure exactly 5 mL of the standard solution, and add the mobile phase to make exactly 20 mL. Confirm that the peak area of propranolol obtained with 20 μL of this solution is equivalent to 17 to 33% of that with 20 μL of the standard solution.

System performance: When the procedure is run with 20 μL of the standard solution under the above operating conditions, the number of theoretical plates and the symmetry factor of the peak of propranolol is not less than 3000 and not more than 2.0, respectively.

System repeatability: When the test is repeated 6 times with 20 μL of the standard solution under the above operating conditions, the relative standard deviation of the peak area of propranolol is not more than 2.0%.

Loss on drying <*2.41*> Not more than 0.5% (1 g, 105°C, 4 hours).

Residue on ignition <*2.44*> Not more than 0.1% (1 g).

Assay Weigh accurately about 0.5 g of Propranolol Hydrochloride, previously dried, dissolve in 50 mL of a mixture of acetic anhydride and acetic acid (100) (7:3), and titrate <*2.50*> with 0.1 mol/L perchloric acid VS (potentiometric titration). Perform a blank determination in the same manner, and make any necessary correction.

Each mL of 0.1 mol/L perchloric acid VS
= 29.58 mg of $C_{16}H_{21}NO_2.HCl$

Containers and storage Containers—Well-closed containers.

Storage—Light-resistant.

Propranolol Hydrochloride Tablets

プロプラノロール塩酸塩錠

Propranolol Hydrochloride Tablets contain not less than 95.0% and not more than 105.0% of the labeled amount of propranolol hydrochloride ($C_{16}H_{21}NO_2.HCl$: 295.80).

Method of preparation Prepare as directed under Tablets, with Propranolol Hydrochloride.

Identification Determine the absorption spectrum of the sample solution obtained in the Assay as directed under Ultraviolet-visible Spectrophotometry <*2.24*>: it exhibits maxima between 288 nm and 292 nm, and between 317 nm and 321 nm.

Uniformity of dosage units <*6.02*> Perform the test according to the following method: it meets the requirement of the Content uniformity test.

To 1 tablet of Propranolol Hydrochloride Tablets add 20 mL of water, and shake until the tablet is completely disintegrated. Add 50 mL of methanol, shake vigorously for 10 minutes, then add methanol to make exactly 100 mL, and filter. Discard the first 20 mL of the filtrate, pipet V mL of the subsequent filtrate, add methanol to make exactly V' mL so that each mL contains about 20 μg of propranolol hydrochloride ($C_{16}H_{21}NO_2.HCl$), and use this solution as the sample solution. Separately, weigh accurately about 50 mg of propranolol hydrochloride for assay, previously dried at 105°C for 4 hours, and dissolve in methanol to make exactly 50 mL. Pipet 2 mL of this solution, add methanol to make exactly 100 mL, and use this solution as the standard solution. Determine the absorbances, A_T and A_S, of the sample solution and standard solution at 290 nm as directed under Ultraviolet-visible Spectrophotometry <*2.24*>.

Amount (mg) of propranolol hydrochloride ($C_{16}H_{21}NO_2.HCl$)
$= M_S \times A_T/A_S \times V'/V \times 1/25$

M_S: Amount (mg) of propranolol hydrochloride for assay taken

Dissolution <*6.10*> When the test is performed at 50 revolutions per minute according to the Paddle method, using 900 mL of water as the dissolution medium, the dissolution rate in 15 minutes of Propranolol Hydrochloride Tablets is not less than 80%.

Start the test with 1 tablet of Propranolol Hydrochloride Tablets, withdraw not less than 20 mL of the medium at the specified minute after starting the test, and filter through a membrane filter with a pore size not exceeding 0.45 μm. Discard not less than 10 mL of the first filtrate, pipet V mL of the subsequent filtrate, add water to make exactly V' mL so that each mL contains about 10 μg of propranolol hydrochloride ($C_{16}H_{21}NO_2.HCl$), and use this solution as the sample solution. Separately, weigh accurately about 50 mg of propranolol hydrochloride for assay, previously dried at 105°C for 4 hours, and dissolve in water to make exactly 50 mL. Pipet 1 mL of this solution, add water to make exactly 100 mL, and use this solution as the standard solution. Determine the absorbances, A_T and A_S, of the sample solution and standard solution at 290 nm as directed under Ultraviolet-visible Spectrophotometry <*2.24*>.

Dissolution rate (%) with respect to the labeled amount of propranolol hydrochloride ($C_{16}H_{21}NO_2.HCl$)
$= M_S \times A_T/A_S \times V'/V \times 1/C \times 18$

M_S: Amount (mg) of propranolol hydrochloride for assay taken

C: Labeled amount (mg) of propranolol hydrochloride ($C_{16}H_{21}NO_2.HCl$) in 1 tablet

Assay Weigh accurately the mass of not less than 20 Propranolol Hydrochloride Tablets, and powder. Weigh accurately a portion of the powder, equivalent to about 20 mg of propranolol hydrochloride ($C_{16}H_{21}NO_2.HCl$), add 60 mL of methanol, shake for 10 minutes, and add methanol to make exactly 100 mL. Filter, discard the first 20 mL of the filtrate, pipet 10 mL of the subsequent filtrate, add methanol to make exactly 100 mL, and use this solution as the sample solution. Separately, weigh accurately about 50 mg of propranolol hydrochloride for assay, previously dried at 105°C for 4 hours, and dissolve in methanol to make exactly 50 mL. Pipet 2 mL of this solution, add methanol to make exactly 100 mL, and use this solution as the standard solution. Determine the absorbances, A_T and A_S, of the sample solution and standard solution at 290 nm as directed under Ultraviolet-visible Spectrophotometry <*2.24*>.

Amount (mg) of propranolol hydrochloride ($C_{16}H_{21}NO_2.HCl$)
$= M_S \times A_T/A_S \times 2/5$

M_S: Amount (mg) of propranolol hydrochloride for assay taken

Containers and storage Containers—Well-closed containers.

Storage—Light-resistant.

Propylene Glycol

プロピレングリコール

H OH
H₃C OH and enantiomer

$C_3H_8O_2$: 76.09
(2*RS*)-Propane-1,2-diol
[*57-55-6*]

Description Propylene Glycol is a clear, colorless, viscous liquid. It is odorless, and has a slightly bitter taste.

It is miscible with water, with methanol, with ethanol (95) and with pyridine.

It is freely soluble in diethyl ether.

It is hygroscopic.

Identification (1) Mix 2 to 3 drops of Propylene Glycol with 0.7 g of triphenylchloromethane, add 1 mL of pyridine, and heat under a reflux condenser on a water bath for 1 hour. After cooling, dissolve the mixture in 20 mL of acetone by warming, shake with 0.02 g of activated charcoal, and filter. Concentrate the filtrate to about 10 mL, and cool. Collect the separated crystals, and dry in a desiccator (silica gel) for 4 hours: the crystals melt <*2.60*> between 174°C and 178°C.

(2) Heat gently 1 mL of Propylene Glycol with 0.5 g of potassium hydrogen sulfate: a characteristic odor is evolved.

Specific gravity <*2.56*> d_{20}^{20}: 1.035 – 1.040

Purity (1) Acidity—Mix 10.0 mL of Propylene Glycol with 50 mL of freshly boiled and cooled water, and add 5 drops of phenolphthalein TS and 0.30 mL of 0.1 mol/L sodium hydroxide VS: the solution has a red color.

(2) Chloride <*1.03*>—Perform the test with 2.0 g of Propylene Glycol. Prepare the control solution with 0.40 mL of 0.01 mol/L hydrochloric acid VS (not more than 0.007%).

(3) Sulfate <*1.14*>—Perform the test with 10.0 g of Propylene Glycol. Prepare the control solution with 0.40 mL of 0.005 mol/L sulfuric acid VS (not more than 0.002%).

(4) Heavy metals <*1.07*>—Perform the test with 5.0 g of Propylene Glycol according to Method 1. Prepare the control solution with 2.5 mL of Standard Lead Solution (not more than 5 ppm).

(5) Arsenic <*1.11*>—Prepare the test solution with 1.0 g of Propylene Glycol according to Method 1, and perform the test (not more than 2 ppm).

(6) Glycerin—Heat 1.0 g of Propylene Glycol with 0.5 g of potassium hydrogen sulfate and evaporate to dryness: no odor of acrolein is perceptible.

(7) Ethylene glycol, diethylene glycol and related substances—Weigh accurately about 5 g of Propylene Glycol, mix with methanol to make exactly 100 mL, and use this solution as the sample solution. Separately, weigh accurately about 0.1 g each of ethylene glycol and diethylene glycol, and mix with methanol to make exactly 100 mL. Pipet 5 mL of this solution, and transfer to a 100-mL volumetric flask. Separately, weigh 5.0 g of propylene glycol for gas chromatography, mix with a suitable amount of methanol and put in the 100-mL volumetric flask, dilute with methanol to volume, and use this solution as the standard solution. Perform the test with exactly 1 μL each of the sample solution and standard solution as directed under Gas Chromatography <*2.02*> according to the following conditions, and determine the peak areas, A_{T1} and A_{S1}, of ethylene glycol and, A_{T2} and A_{S2}, of diethylene glycol by the automatic integration method. The amounts of ethylene glycol and diethylene glycol calculated by the following equations are not more than 0.1%, respectively. The amount of the peak other than propylene glycol, ethylene glycol and diethylene glycol obtained from the sample solution, calculated by the area percentage method, is not more than 0.1%, and the total amount of the peaks other than propylene glycol is not more than 1.0%.

Amount (%) of ethylene glycol
$= M_{S1}/M_T \times A_{T1}/A_{S1} \times 5$

Amount (%) of diethylene glycol
$= M_{S2}/M_T \times A_{T2}/A_{S2} \times 5$

M_{S1}: Amount (g) of ethylene glycol taken
M_{S2}: Amount (g) of diethylene glycol taken
M_T: Amount (g) of Propylene Glycol taken

Operating conditions—

Detector: A hydrogen flame-ionization detector.

Column: A fused silica tube 0.32 mm in inside diameter and 30 m in length, coated the inside surface 1 μm in thickness with 14% cyanopropylphenyl-86% dimethyl silicone polymer for gas chromatography.

Column temperature: Inject at a constant temperature of about 100°C, rise the temperature at the rate of 7.5°C per minute to 220°C, and maintain at a constant temperature of about 220°C.

Injection port temperature: A constant temperature of about 220°C.

Detector temperature: A constant temperature of about 250°C.

Carrier gas: Helium.
Flow rate: about 38 cm per second.
Split ratio: 1:20.

Time span of measurement: About 3 times as long as the retention time of propylene glycol, beginning after the solvent peak.

System suitability—

System performance: Mix 50 mg each of ethylene glycol, diethylene glycol and propylene glycol for gas chromatography with 100 mL of methanol. When the procedure is run with 1 μL of this mixture under the above operating conditions, ethylene glycol, propylene glycol and diethylene glycol are eluted in this order, and the resolution between the peaks of ethylene glycol and propylene glycol is not less than 5, and that between the peaks of propylene glycol and diethylene glycol is not less than 50.

System repeatability: When the test is repeated 6 times with 1 μL of the standard solution under the above operating conditions, the relative standard deviation of the peak area of ethylene glycol and diethylene glycol is not more than 10%.

Water *<2.48>* Not more than 0.5% (2 g, volumetric titration, direct titration).

Residue on ignition *<2.44>* Weigh accurately about 20 g of Propylene Glycol in a tared crucible, and heat to boiling. Stop heating, and immediately ignite to burn. Cool, moisten the residue with 0.2 mL of sulfuric acid, and heat strongly with care to constant mass: the mass of the residue is not more than 0.005%.

Distilling range *<2.57>* 184 – 189°C, not less than 95 vol%.

Containers and storage Containers—Tight containers.

Propyl Parahydroxybenzoate

パラオキシ安息香酸プロピル

$C_{10}H_{12}O_3$: 180.20
Propyl 4-hydroxybenzoate
[94-13-3]

This monograph is harmonized with the European Pharmacopoeia and the U.S. Pharmacopeia.

The parts of the text that are not harmonized are marked with symbols (◆ ◆).

Information on the harmonization with the European Pharmacopoeia and the U.S. Pharmacopeia is available on the website of the Pharmaceuticals and Medical Devices Agency.

Propyl Parahydroxybenzoate contains not less than 98.0% and not more than 102.0% of propyl parahydroxybenzoate ($C_{10}H_{12}O_3$).

◆**Description** Propyl Parahydroxybenzoate occurs as colorless crystals or a white crystalline powder.

It is freely soluble in methanol, in ethanol (95) and in acetone, and very slightly soluble in water.◆

Identification Determine the infrared absorption spectrum of Propyl Parahydroxybenzoate as directed in the potassium bromide disk method under Infrared Spectrophotometry *<2.25>*, and compare the spectrum with the Reference Spectrum or the spectrum of Propyl Parahydroxybenzoate RS: both spectra exhibit similar intensities of absorption at the same wave numbers.

Melting point *<2.60>* 96 – 99°C

Purity (1) Clarity and color of solution—Dissolve 1.0 g of Propyl Parahydroxybenzoate in ethanol (95) to make 10 mL: the solution is clear and not more intensely colored than the following control solution.

Control solution: To 5.0 mL of Cobalt (II) Chloride CS, 12.0 mL of Iron (III) Chloride CS and 2.0 mL of Copper (II) Sulfate CS add diluted dilute hydrochloric acid (1 in 10) to make 1000 mL.

(2) Acidity—To 2 mL of the solution of Propyl Parahydroxybenzoate obtained in (1) add 3 mL of ethanol (95), add 5 mL of freshly boiled and cooled water and 0.1 mL of bromocresol green-sodium hydroxide-ethanol TS, then add 0.1 mol/L sodium hydroxide VS until the solution shows a blue color: the volume of 0.1 mol/L sodium hydroxide VS used does not exceed 0.1 mL.

◆(3) Heavy metals *<1.07>*—Dissolve 1.0 g of Propyl Parahydroxybenzoate in 25 mL of acetone, add 2 mL of dilute acetic acid and water to make 50 mL, and perform the test using this solution as the test solution. Prepare the control solution as follows: to 2.0 mL of Standard Lead Solution add 25 mL of acetone, 2 mL of dilute acetic acid, and water to make 50 mL (not more than 20 ppm).◆

(4) Related substances—Dissolve 50.0 mg of Propyl Parahydroxybenzoate in 2.5 mL of methanol, and add the mobile phase to make exactly 50 mL. Pipet 10 mL of this solution, add the mobile phase to make exactly 100 mL, and use this solution as the sample solution. Pipet 1 mL of the sample solution, and add the mobile phase to make exactly 20 mL. Pipet 1 mL of this solution, add the mobile phase to make exactly 10 mL, and use this solution as the standard solution. Perform the test with exactly 10 μL each of the sample solution and standard solution as directed under Liquid Chromatography *<2.01>* according to the following conditions, and determine each peak area by the automatic integration method: the peak area of parahydroxybenzoic acid having a relative retention time of about 0.3 to propyl parahydroxybenzoate obtained from the sample solution is not larger than the peak area of propyl parahydroxybenzoate from the standard solution (0.5%). For the peak area of parahydroxybenzoic acid, multiply the correction factor, 1.4. Furthermore, the area of the peak other than propyl parahydroxybenzoate and parahydroxybenzoic acid from the sample solution is not larger than the peak area of propyl parahydroxybenzoate from the standard solution (0.5%), and the total area of the peaks other than propyl parahydroxybenzoate from the sample solution is not larger than 2 times the peak area of propyl parahydroxybenzoate from the standard solution (1.0%). For this calculation the peak area not larger than 1/5 times the peak area of propyl parahydroxybenzoate from the standard solution is excluded (0.1%).

Operating conditions—

Detector, column, column temperature, mobile phase, and flow rate: Proceed as directed in the operating conditions in the Assay.

Time span of measurement: About 2.5 times as long as the retention time of propyl parahydroxybenzoate.

System suitability—

System performance: Proceed as directed in the system suitability in the Assay.

◆Test for required detectability: To exactly 2 mL of the standard solution add the mobile phase to make exactly 10 mL. Confirm that the peak area of propyl parahydroxybenzoate obtained with 10 μL of this solution is equivalent to 14 to 26% of that with 10 μL of the standard solution.◆

◆System repeatability: When the test is repeated 6 times with 10 μL of the standard solution under the above operating conditions, the relative standard deviation of the peak area of propyl parahydroxybenzoate is not more than 2.0%.◆

Residue on ignition <*2.44*> Not more than 0.1% (1 g).

Assay Weigh accurately about 50.0 mg each of Propyl Parahydroxybenzoate and Propyl Parahydroxybenzoate RS, dissolve separately in 2.5 mL each of methanol, and add the mobile phase to make exactly 50 mL. Pipet 10 mL each of these solutions, add the mobile phase to make exactly 100 mL, and use these solutions as the sample solution and the standard solution, respectively. Perform the test with exactly 10 μL each of the sample solution and standard solution as directed under Liquid Chromatography <*2.01*> according to the following conditions, and determine the peak areas, A_T and A_S, of propyl parahydroxybenzoate in each solution.

Amount (mg) of propyl parahydroxybenzoate ($C_{10}H_{12}O_3$)
$= M_S \times A_T/A_S$

M_S: Amount (mg) of Propyl Parahydroxybenzoate RS taken

Operating conditions—

Detector: An ultraviolet absorption photometer (wavelength: 272 nm).

Column: A stainless steel column 4.6 mm in inside diameter and 15 cm in length, packed with octadecylsilanized silica gel for liquid chromatography (5 μm in particle diameter).

Column temperature: A constant temperature of about 35°C.

Mobile phase: A mixture of methanol and potassium dihydrogen phosphate solution (17 in 2500) (13:7).

Flow rate: 1.3 mL per minute.

System suitability—

System performance: Dissolve 5 mg each of Propyl Parahydroxybenzoate, ethyl parahydroxybenzoate and parahydroxybenzoic acid in the mobile phase to make exactly 100 mL. Pipet 1 mL of this solution, and add the mobile phase to make exactly 10 mL. When the procedure is run with 10 μL of this solution under the above operating conditions, parahydroxybenzoic acid, ethyl parahydroxybenzoate and propyl parahydroxybenzoate are eluted in this order, the relative retention times of parahydroxybenzoic acid and ethyl parahydroxybenzoate to propyl parahydroxybenzoate are about 0.3 and about 0.7, respectively, and the resolution between the peaks of ethyl parahydroxybenzoate and propyl parahydroxybenzoate is not less than 3.0.

System repeatability: When the test is repeated 6 times with 10 μL of the standard solution under the above operating conditions, the relative standard deviation of the peak area of propyl parahydroxybenzoate is not more than 0.85%.

◆**Containers and storage** Containers—Well-closed containers.◆

Propylthiouracil

プロピルチオウラシル

$C_7H_{10}N_2OS$: 170.23
6-Propyl-2-thiouracil
[*51-52-5*]

Propylthiouracil, when dried, contains not less than 98.0% of propylthiouracil ($C_7H_{10}N_2OS$).

Description Propylthiouracil occurs as a white powder. It is odorless, and has a bitter taste.

It is sparingly soluble in ethanol (95), and very slightly soluble in water and in diethyl ether.

It dissolves in sodium hydroxide TS and in ammonia TS.

Identification **(1)** Shake well 0.02 g of Propylthiouracil with 7 mL of bromine TS for 1 minute, and heat until the color of bromine TS disappears. Cool, filter, and add 10 mL of barium hydroxide TS to the filtrate: a white precipitate is produced. The color of the precipitate does not turn purple within 1 minute.

(2) To 5 mL of a hot saturated solution of Propylthiouracil add 2 mL of a solution of sodium pentacyanoammine ferroate (II) *n*-hydrate (1 in 100): a green color develops.

Melting point <*2.60*> 218 – 221°C

Purity **(1)** Sulfate <*1.14*>—Triturate Propylthiouracil finely in a mortar. To 0.75 g of the powder add 25 mL of water, heat for 10 minutes on a water bath, cool, filter, and wash the residue with water until the volume of the filtrate becomes 30 mL. To 10 mL of the filtrate add 1 mL of dilute hydrochloric acid and water to make 50 mL, and perform the test using this solution as the test solution. Prepare the control solution with 0.40 mL of 0.005 mol/L sulfuric acid VS (not more than 0.077%).

(2) Thiourea—Dissolve 0.30 g of Propylthiouracil in 50 mL of water by heating under a reflux condenser for 5 minutes, cool, and filter. To 10 mL of the filtrate add 3 mL of ammonia TS, shake well, and add 2 mL of silver nitrate TS: the solution has no more color than the following control solution.

Control solution: Weigh exactly 60 mg of thiourea, and dissolve in water to make exactly 100 mL. Pipet 1 mL of this solution, add water to make exactly 100 mL, and proceed with 10 mL of this solution in the same manner.

Loss on drying <*2.41*> Not more than 0.5% (1 g, 105°C, 2 hours).

Residue on ignition <*2.44*> Not more than 0.1% (1 g).

Assay Weigh accurately about 0.3 g of Propylthiouracil, previously dried, and add 30 mL of water. Add 30 mL of 0.1 mol/L sodium hydroxide VS from a burette, heat to boil, and dissolve by stirring. Wash down the solid adhering to the wall of the flask with a small amount of water, and add 50 mL of 0.1 mol/L silver nitrate VS with stirring. Boil gently for 5 minutes, add 1 to 2 mL of bromothymol blue TS, and titrate <*2.50*> with 0.1 mol/L sodium hydroxide VS until a persistent blue-green color develops. Determine the total volume of 0.1 mol/L sodium hydroxide VS consumed.

Each mL of 0.1 mol/L sodium hydroxide VS
= 8.512 mg of $C_7H_{10}N_2OS$

Containers and storage Containers—Well-closed containers.

Storage—Light-resistant.

Propylthiouracil Tablets

プロピルチオウラシル錠

Propylthiouracil Tablets contain not less than 93.0% and not more than 107.0% of the labeled amount of propylthiouracil ($C_7H_{10}N_2OS$: 170.23).

Method of preparation Prepare as directed under Tablets, with Propylthiouracil.

Identification To a quantity of powdered Propylthiouracil Tablets, equivalent to 0.3 g of Propylthiouracil, add 5 mL of ammonia TS, allow to stand for 5 minutes with occasional shaking, add 10 mL of water, and centrifuge. To the supernatant liquid add acetic acid (31), collect the precipitate produced, recrystallize from water, and dry at 105°C for 1 hour: it melts <*2.60*> between 218°C and 221°C. Proceed with the residue as directed in the Identification under Propylthiouracil.

Uniformity of dosage units <*6.02*> Perform the Mass variation test, or the Content uniformity test according to the following method: it meets the requirement.

To 1 tablet of Propylthiouracil Tablets add $3V/4$ mL of 2nd fluid for dissolution test, sonicate until the tablet is disintegrated, and add 2nd fluid for dissolution test to make exactly V mL so that each mL contains about 0.25 mg of propylthiouracil ($C_7H_{10}N_2OS$). Filter this solution through a membrane filter with a pore size not exceeding 0.45 μm, discard the first 5 mL of the filtrate, pipet 2 mL of the subsequent filtrate, add 2nd fluid for dissolution test to make exactly 100 mL, and use this solution as the sample solution. Proceed as directed in the Assay.

Amount (mg) of propylthiouracil ($C_7H_{10}N_2OS$)
$= M_S \times A_T/A_S \times V/200$

M_S: Amount (mg) of propylthiouracil for assay taken

Dissolution <*6.10*> When the test is performed at 75 revolutions per minute according to the Paddle method, using 900 mL of 2nd fluid for dissolution test as the dissolution medium, the dissolution rate in 30 minutes of Propylthiouracil Tablets is not less than 80%.

Start the test with 1 tablet of Propylthiouracil Tablets, withdraw not less than 20 mL of the medium at the specified minute after starting the test, and filter through a membrane filter with a pore size not exceeding 0.8 μm. Discard not less than 10 mL of the first filtrate, pipet V mL of the subsequent filtrate, add the dissolution medium to make exactly V' mL so that each mL contains about 5.6 μg of propylthiouracil ($C_7H_{10}N_2OS$), and use this solution as the sample solution. Separately, weigh about 50 mg of propylthiouracil for assay, previously dried at 105°C for 3 hours, and dissolve in the dissolution medium to make exactly 1000 mL. Pipet 5 mL of this solution, add the dissolution medium to make exactly 50 mL, and use this solution as the standard solution. Determine the absorbance at 274 mm, A_T and A_S, of the sample solution and standard solution as directed under Ultraviolet-visible Spectrophotometry <*2.24*>.

Dissolution rate (%) with respect to the labeled amount of propylthiouracil ($C_7H_{10}N_2OS$)
$= M_S \times A_T/A_S \times V'/V \times 1/C \times 9$

M_S: Amount (mg) of propylthiouracil for assay taken
C: Labeled amount (mg) of propylthiouracil ($C_7H_{10}N_2OS$) in 1 tablet

Assay Weigh accurately the mass of not less than 20 Propylthiouracil Tablets, and powder. Weigh accurately a portion of the powder, equivalent to about 50 mg of propylthiouracil ($C_7H_{10}N_2OS$), add 150 mL of 2nd fluid for dissolution test, disperse finely the particles by sonicating, and add 2nd fluid for dissolution test to make exactly 200 mL. Filter this solution through a membrane filter with a pore size not exceeding 0.45 μm, discard the first 5 mL of the filtrate, pipet 2 mL of the subsequent filtrate, add 2nd fluid for dissolution test to make exactly 100 mL, and use this solution as the sample solution. Separately, weigh accurately about 50 mg of propylthiouracil for assay, previously dried at 105°C for 2 hours, and dissolve in 2nd fluid for dissolution test to make exactly 200 mL. Pipet 2 mL of this solution, add 2nd fluid for dissolution test to make exactly 100 mL, and use this solution as the standard solution. Determine the absorbance at 274 nm, A_T and A_S, of the sample solution and standard solution as directed under Ultraviolet-visible Spectrophotometry <*2.24*>.

Amount (mg) of propylthiouracil ($C_7H_{10}N_2OS$)
$= M_S \times A_T/A_S$

M_S: Amount (mg) of propylthiouracil for assay taken

Containers and storage Containers—Well-closed containers.

Storage—Light-resistant.

Protamine Sulfate

プロタミン硫酸塩

Protamine Sulfate is the sulfate of protamine prepared from the mature spermary of fish belonging to the family *Salmonidae*.

It has a property to bind with heparin.

It binds with not less than 100 Units of heparin per mg, calculated on the dried basis.

Description Protamine Sulfate occurs as a white powder.

It is sparingly soluble in water.

Identification **(1)** Dissolve 1 mg of Protamine Sulfate in 2 mL of water, add 0.4 mL of sodium hydroxide TS, and immediately add 5 drops of a solution prepared by dissolving 0.1 g of 1-naphthol in 100 mL of diluted ethanol (7 in 10) and 5 drops of sodium hypochlorite TS: a vivid red color develops.

(2) Dissolve 5 mg of Protamine Sulfate in 1 mL of water by warming, add 1 drop of a solution of sodium hydroxide (1 in 10) and 2 drops of copper (II) sulfate TS: a red-purple color develops.

(3) An aqueous solution of Protamine Sulfate (1 in 20) responds to Qualitative Tests <*1.09*> for sulfate.

pH <*2.54*> Dissolve 1.0 g of Protamine Sulfate in 100 mL of water: the pH of this solution is between 6.5 and 7.5.

Purity **(1)** Clarity and color of solution—Dissolve 0.10 g of Protamine Sulfate in 10 mL of water: the solution is clear and colorless.

(2) Absorbance—Dissolve 0.10 g of Protamine Sulfate in 10 mL of water, and determine the absorption spectrum as directed under Ultraviolet-visible Spectrophotometry *<2.24>*: the absorbance between 260 nm and 280 nm is not more than 0.1.

Loss on drying *<2.41>* Not more than 5.0% (1 g, 105°C, 3 hours).

Nitrogen content Weigh accurately about 10 mg of Protamine Sulfate, and perform the test as directed under Nitrogen Determination *<1.08>*: the amount of nitrogen (N:14.01) is 22.5 – 25.5%, calculated on the dried basis.

Heparin-binding capacity

(i) Sample solution (a)—Weigh accurately about 15 mg of Protamine Sulfate, and dissolve in water to make exactly 100 mL. Repeat this procedure 3 times, and use the solutions so obtained as the sample solutions (a_1), (a_2) and (a_3).

(ii) Sample solution (b)—Pipet 10 mL each of the sample solutions (a_1), (a_2) and (a_3), add exactly 5 mL of water to them, and use these solutions as the sample solutions (b_1), (b_2) and (b_3).

(iii) Sample solution (c)—Pipet 10 mL each of the sample solutions (a_1), (a_2) and (a_3), add exactly 20 mL of water to them, and use these solutions as the sample solutions (c_1), (c_2) and (c_3).

(iv) Standard solution—Dissolve Heparin Sodium RS in water to make a solution containing exactly about 20 Units per mL.

(v) Procedure—Transfer exactly 2 mL of the sample solution to a cell for spectrophotometer, add the standard solution dropwise while mixing, and determine the transmittance at 500 nm as directed under Ultraviolet-visible Spectrophotometry *<2.24>*. Continue the addition until a sharp change in the transmittance is observed, and note the volume, *V* mL, of the standard solution added. Repeat this procedure 2 times for each sample solution.

(vi) Calculation—Calculate the amount of heparin bound with 1 mg of the sample by the following formula from the volume of titrant on each sample solution, and calculate the average of 18 results obtained. The assay is not valid unless each relative standard deviation of 6 results obtained from the sample solution (a), sample solution (b) and sample solution (c) is not more than 5%, respectively, and also unless each relative standard deviation of 6 results obtained from 3 sets, (a_1, b_1, c_1), (a_2, b_2, c_2) and (a_3, b_3, c_3) is not more than 5%, respectively.

Amount (heparin Unit) of heparin bound to 1 mg of Protamine Sulfate

$$= S \times V \times 50/M_T \times d$$

S: Amount (heparin Unit) of heparin sodium in 1 mL of the standard solution

M_T: Amount (mg) of Protamine Sulfate taken, calculated on the dried basis

d: Dilution factor for each sample solution from the sample solution (a)

Sulfate content Weigh accurately about 0.15 g of Protamine Sulfate, dissolve in 75 mL of water, add 5 mL of 3 mol/L hydrochloric acid TS, and heat to boil. Add gradually 10 mL of barium chloride TS while boiling, and allow to stand for 1 hour while heating. Filter the precipitate formed, wash the precipitate with warm water several times, and transfer the precipitate into a tared crucible. Dry the precipitate, and incinerate by ignition to constant mass: the amount of sulfate (SO_4) is 16 – 22%, calculated on the dried basis, where 1 g of the residue is equivalent to 0.4117 g of SO_4.

Containers and storage Containers—Tight containers.

Protamine Sulfate Injection

プロタミン硫酸塩注射液

Protamine Sulfate Injection is an aqueous injection.

It contains not less than 92.0% and not more than 108.0% of the labeled amount of Protamine Sulfate. It binds with not less than 100 Units of heparin per mg of the labeled amount.

Method of preparation Prepare as directed under Injections, with Protamine Sulfate.

Description Protamine Sulfate Injection is a colorless liquid. It is odorless or has the odor of preservatives.

Identification **(1)** Dilute a volume of Protamine Sulfate Injection, equivalent to 1 mg of Protamine Sulfate, with water to make 2 mL, and proceed as directed in the Identification (1) under Protamine Sulfate.

(2) Dilute a volume of Protamine Sulfate Injection, equivalent to 5 mg of Protamine Sulfate, with water to make 1 mL, and proceed as directed in the Identification (2) under Protamine Sulfate.

pH *<2.54>* 5.0 – 7.0

Bacterial endotoxins *<4.01>* Less than 6.0 EU/mg.

Extractable volume *<6.05>* It meets the requirement.

Foreign insoluble matter *<6.06>* Perform the test according to Method 1: it meets the requirement.

Insoluble particulate matter *<6.07>* It meets the requirement.

Sterility *<4.06>* Perform the test according to the Membrane filtration method: it meets the requirement.

Assay **(1)** Protein—Pipet a volume of Protamine Sulfate Injection, equivalent to about 10 mg of Protamine Sulfate, transfer to a Kjeldahl flask, evaporate on a water bath to dryness with the aid of a current of air, determine the nitrogen as directed under Nitrogen Determination *<1.08>*, and calculate the amount of protein by converting 0.24 mg of nitrogen (N: 14.01) to 1 mg of protein.

(2) Heparin-binding activity—Proceed the test as directed in the Heparin-binding capacity under Protamine Sulfate, changing the sample solution (a) as below, and determine the amount of heparin bound to 1 mg of protein by dividing by the amount of protein.

(i) Sample solution (a)—Pipet a volume of Protamine Sulfate Injection, equivalent to 15.0 mg of Protamine Sulfate, and add water to make exactly 100 mL. Repeat this procedure two more times, and designate the solutions so obtained as the sample solutions (a_1), (a_2) and (a_3).

Containers and storage Containers—Hermetic containers.

Prothionamide

プロチオナミド

$C_9H_{12}N_2S$: 180.27
2-Propylpyridine-4-carbothioamide
[*14222-60-7*]

Prothionamide, when dried, contains not less than 98.0% of prothionamide ($C_9H_{12}N_2S$).

Description Prothionamide occurs as yellow, crystals or crystalline powder. It has a slight, characteristic odor.

It is freely soluble in methanol and in acetic acid (100), soluble in ethanol (95), slightly soluble in diethyl ether, and practically insoluble in water.

It dissolves in dilute hydrochloric acid and in dilute sulfuric acid.

Identification **(1)** Mix 0.05 g of Prothionamide with 0.1 g of 1-chloro-2,4-dinitrobenzene, transfer about 10 mg of this mixture to a test tube, and heat for several seconds over a small flame until the mixture is fused. Cool, and add 3 mL of potassium hydroxide-ethanol TS: a red to orange-red color develops.

(2) Place 0.5 g of Prothionamide in a 100-mL beaker, and dissolve in 20 mL of sodium hydroxide TS by heating while shaking occasionally: the gas evolved turns a moistened red litmus paper to blue. Boil gently, and evaporate the solution to 3 to 5 mL. After cooling, add gradually 20 mL of acetic acid (100), and heat on a water bath: the gas evolved darkens moistened lead (II) acetate paper. Evaporate the solution on a water bath to 3 to 5 mL with the aid of a current of air, cool, add 10 mL of water, and mix well. Filter the crystals by suction, recrystallize from water immediately, and dry in a desiccator (in vacuum, silica gel) for 6 hours: the crystals melt 〈*2.60*〉 between 198°C and 203°C (with decomposition).

Melting point 〈*2.60*〉 142 – 145°C

Purity **(1)** Clarity and color of solution—Dissolve 0.5 g of Prothionamide in 20 mL of ethanol (95): the solution is clear, and shows a yellow color.

(2) Acidity—Dissolve 3.0 g of Prothionamide in 20 mL of methanol with warming. Add 100 mL of water to the solution, cool in an ice water bath with agitation, and remove any precipitate by filtration. Allow 80 mL of the filtrate to cool to room temperature, and add 0.8 mL of cresol red TS and 0.20 mL of 0.1 mol/L sodium hydroxide VS: a red color develops.

(3) Heavy metals 〈*1.07*〉—Proceed with 1.0 g of Prothionamide according to Method 2, and perform the test. Prepare the control solution with 2.0 mL of Standard Lead Solution (not more than 20 ppm).

(4) Arsenic 〈*1.11*〉—Prepare the test solution with 0.6 g of Prothionamide according to Method 3, and perform the test. To the test solution add 10 mL of a solution of magnesium nitrate hexahydrate in ethanol (95) (1 in 50), then add 1.5 mL of hydrogen peroxide (30), and ignite to burn (not more than 3.3 ppm).

Loss on drying 〈*2.41*〉 Not more than 0.5% (1 g, 80°C, 3 hours).

Residue on ignition 〈*2.44*〉 Not more than 0.1% (1 g).

Assay Weigh accurately about 0.3 g of Prothionamide, previously dried, dissolve in 50 mL of acetic acid (100), and titrate 〈*2.50*〉 with 0.1 mol/L perchloric acid VS until the color of the solution changes from orange-red to dark orange-brown (indicator: 2 mL of *p*-naphtholbenzein TS). Perform a blank determination in the same manner, and make any necessary correction.

Each mL of 0.1 mol/L perchloric acid VS
= 18.03 mg of $C_9H_{12}N_2S$

Containers and storage Containers—Well-closed containers.

Storage—Light-resistant.

Protirelin

プロチレリン

$C_{16}H_{22}N_6O_4$: 362.38
5-Oxo-L-prolyl-L-histidyl-L-prolinamide
[*24305-27-9*]

Protirelin contains not less than 98.5% of protirelin ($C_{16}H_{22}N_6O_4$), calculated on the anhydrous basis.

Description Protirelin occurs as a white powder.

It is freely soluble in water, in methanol, in ethanol (95) and in acetic acid (100).

It is hygroscopic.

Identification **(1)** Take 0.01 g of Protirelin in a test tube made of hard glass, add 0.5 mL of 6 mol/L hydrochloric acid TS, seal the upper part of the tube, and heat carefully at 110°C for 5 hours. After cooling, open the seal, transfer the contents into a beaker, and evaporate on a water bath to dryness. Dissolve the residue in 1 mL of water, and use this solution as the sample solution. Separately, dissolve 0.08 g of L-glutamic acid, 0.12 g of L-histidine hydrochloride monohydrate and 0.06 g of L-proline in 20 mL of water, and use this solution as the standard solution. Perform the test with these solutions as directed under Thin-layer Chromatography 〈*2.03*〉. Spot 5 μL each of the sample solution and standard solution on a plate of silica gel for thin-layer chromatography. Develop the plate with a mixture of 1-butanol, water, acetic acid (100) and pyridine (4:1:1:1) to a distance of about 12 cm, and dry the plate at 100°C for 30 minutes. Spray evenly a solution of ninhydrin in acetone (1 in 50) on the plate, and heat the plate at 80°C for 5 minutes: the three spots obtained from the sample solution show the same color and the same *R*f value as each corresponding spots from the standard solution.

(2) Determine the infrared absorption spectrum of Protirelin, as directed in the potassium bromide disk method under Infrared Spectrophotometry 〈*2.25*〉, and compare the spectrum with the Reference Spectrum: both spectra exhibit similar intensities of absorption at the same wave numbers.

Optical rotation 〈*2.49*〉 $[\alpha]_D^{20}$: −66.0 – −69.0° (0.1 g, calculated on the anhydrous basis, water, 20 mL, 100 mm).

pH *<2.54>* Dissolve 0.20 g of Protirelin in 10 mL of water: the pH of this solution is between 7.5 and 8.5.

Purity **(1)** Clarity and color of solution—Dissolve 0.10 g of Protirelin in 10 mL of water: the solution is clear and colorless.

(2) Heavy metals *<1.07>*—Proceed with 1.0 g of Protirelin according to Method 2, and perform the test. Prepare the control solution with 2.0 mL of Standard Lead Solution (not more than 20 ppm).

(3) Related substances—Dissolve 0.20 g of Protirelin in 10 mL of water, and use this solution as the sample solution. Pipet 1 mL of the sample solution, add water to make exactly 200 mL, and use this solution as the standard solution. Perform the test with these solutions as directed under Thin-layer Chromatography *<2.03>*. Spot 5 μL each of the sample solution and standard solution on a plate (1) of silica gel for thin-layer chromatography, and spot 5 μL of the sample solution on a plate (2) of silica gel for thin-layer chromatography. Develop the plates with a mixture of 1-butanol, water, pyridine and acetic acid (100) (4:2:1:1) to a distance of about 12 cm, and dry the plates at 100°C for 30 minutes. Spray evenly a mixture of a solution of sulfanilic acid in 1 mol/L hydrochloric acid TS (1 in 200) and a solution of sodium nitrite (1 in 20) (1:1) on the plate (1), and air-dry the plates. Successively spray evenly a solution of sodium carbonate decahydrate (1 in 10) on it: the spots other than the principal spot obtained from the sample solution are not more intense than the spot from the standard solution. Spray evenly a solution of ninhydrin in acetone (1 in 50) on the plate (2), and heat the plate at 80°C for 5 minutes: no colored spot appears.

Water *<2.48>* Not more than 5.0% (0.1 g, volumetric titration, direct titration).

Residue on ignition *<2.44>* Not more than 0.3% (0.2 g).

Assay Weigh accurately about 70 mg of Protirelin dissolve in 50 mL of acetic acid (100), and titrate *<2.50>* with 0.02 mol/L perchloric acid VS (potentiometric titration). Perform a blank determination in the same manner, and make any necessary correction.

Each mL of 0.02 mol/L perchloric acid VS
= 7.248 mg of $C_{16}H_{22}N_6O_4$

Containers and storage Containers—Tight containers.

Protirelin Tartrate Hydrate

プロチレリン酒石酸塩水和物

$C_{16}H_{22}N_6O_4.C_4H_6O_6.H_2O$: 530.49
5-Oxo-L-prolyl-L-histidyl-L-prolinamide monotartrate monohydrate
[*24305-27-9*, Protirelin]

Protirelin Tartrate Hydrate, calculated on the anhydrous basis, contains not less than 98.5% of protirelin tartrate ($C_{16}H_{22}N_6O_4.C_4H_6O_6$: 512.48).

Description Protirelin Tartrate Hydrate occurs as white to pale yellowish white, crystals or crystalline powder.

It is freely soluble in water, sparingly soluble in acetic acid (100), and practically insoluble in ethanol (95) and in diethyl ether.

Melting point: about 187°C (with decomposition).

Identification **(1)** To 1 mL of a solution of Protirelin Tartrate Hydrate (1 in 1000) add 2 mL of a solution of 4-nitrobenzene diazonium fluoroborate (1 in 2000) and 2 mL of boric acid-potassium chloride-sodium hydroxide buffer solution (pH 9.0): a red color develops.

(2) Dissolve 0.03 g of Protirelin Tartrate Hydrate in 5 mL of sodium hydroxide TS, add 1 drop of copper (II) sulfate TS: a purple color develops.

(3) To 0.20 g of Protirelin Tartrate Hydrate add 5.0 mL of 6 mol/L hydrochloric acid TS, and boil for 7 hours under a reflux condenser. After cooling, evaporate 2.0 mL of this solution on a water bath to dryness, dissolve the residue in 2.0 mL of water and use this solution as the sample solution. Separately, dissolve 22 mg of L-glutamic acid, 32 mg of L-histidine hydrochloride monohydrate and 17 mg of L-proline in 2.0 mL of 0.1 mol/L hydrochloric acid TS by heating, and use this solution as the standard solution. Perform the test with these solutions as directed under Thin-layer Chromatography *<2.03>*. Spot 2 μL each of the sample solution and standard solution on a plate of silica gel for thin-layer chromatography. Develop the plate with a mixture of 1-butanol, water, acetic acid (100) and pyridine (4:1:1:1) to a distance of about 12 cm, and dry at 100°C for 30 minutes. Spray evenly a solution of ninhydrin in acetone (1 in 50) on the plate, and heat the plate at 80°C for 5 minutes: the three spots obtained from the sample solution show, respectively, the same color and the same Rf value as the corresponding spot from the standard solution.

(4) A solution of Protirelin Tartrate Hydrate (1 in 40) responds to Qualitative Tests *<1.09>* for tartrate.

Optical rotation *<2.49>* $[\alpha]_D^{20}$: −50.0 – −53.0° (0.5 g calculated on the anhydrous basis, water, 25 mL, 100 mm).

pH *<2.54>* Dissolve 1.0 g of Protirelin Tartrate Hydrate in 100 mL of water: the pH of this solution is between 3.0 and 4.0.

Purity **(1)** Clarity and color of solution—Dissolve 0.10 g of Protirelin Tartrate Hydrate in 10 mL of water: the solution is clear and colorless.

(2) Heavy metals *<1.07>*—Proceed with 1.0 g of Protirelin Tartrate Hydrate according to Method 2, and perform the test. Prepare the control solution with 2.0 mL of Standard Lead Solution (not more than 20 ppm).

(3) Arsenic *<1.11>*—Take 1.0 g of Protirelin Tartrate Hydrate in a porcelain crucible. Add 10 mL of a solution of magnesium nitrate hexahydrate in ethanol (95) (1 in 10), ignite the ethanol, and heat gradually to incinerate. If a carbonized material still remains in this method, moisten with a small quantity of nitric acid, and ignite to incinerate. After cooling, add 10 mL of dilute hydrochloric acid, heat on a water bath to dissolve the residue, use this solution as the test solution, and perform the test (not more than 2 ppm).

(4) Related substances—Dissolve 0.60 g of Protirelin Tartrate Hydrate in 10 mL of water, and use this solution as the sample solution. Pipet 1 mL of the sample solution, add water to make exactly 200 mL, and use this solution as the standard solution. Perform the test with these solutions as directed under Thin-layer Chromatography *<2.03>*. Spot 5 μL each of the sample solution and standard solution on a plate (1) of silica gel for thin-layer chromatography. Spot 5 μL of the sample solution on a plate (2) of silica gel for thin-layer chromatography. Develop the plates with a mixture of chloroform, methanol and ammonia solution (28) (6:4:1) to a distance of about 10 cm, and dry at 100°C for 30 minutes. Spray evenly a mixture of a solution of sulfanilic acid in 1 mol/L hydrochloric acid TS (1 in 200) and a solution of sodium nitrite (1 in 20) (1:1) on the plate (1), and air-dry the plate. Then, spray evenly a solution of sodium carbonate decahydrate (1 in 10) on the plate: the spots other than the principal spot obtained from the sample solution are not more intense than those from the standard solution in color. On the other hand, spray evenly a solution of ninhydrin in acetone (1 in 50) on the plate (2), and heat the plate at 80°C for 5 minutes: no colored spot is obtained.

Water *<2.48>* Not more than 4.5% (0.2 g, volumetric titration, direct titration).

Residue on ignition *<2.44>* Not more than 0.2% (0.5 g).

Assay Weigh accurately about 0.5 g of Protirelin Tartrate Hydrate, dissolve in 80 mL of acetic acid (100) by warming, cool, and titrate *<2.50>* with 0.1 mol/L perchloric acid VS (potentiometric titration). Perform a blank determination in the same manner, and make any necessary correction.

Each mL of 0.1 mol/L perchloric acid VS
= 51.25 mg of $C_{16}H_{22}N_6O_4.C_4H_6O_6$

Containers and storage Containers—Well-closed containers.

Pullulan

プルラン

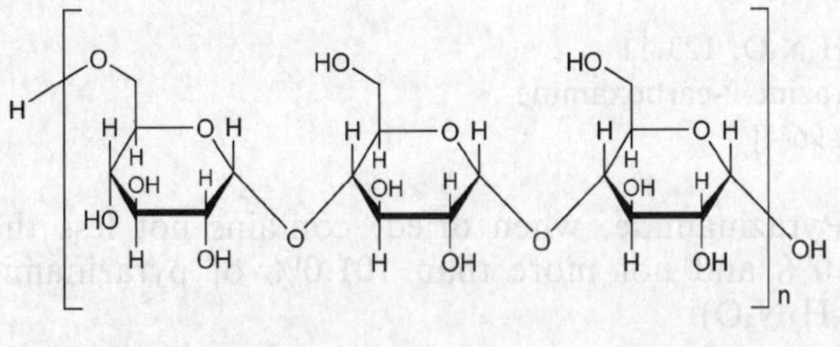

$(C_{18}H_{30}O_{15})_n$
Poly[6)-α-D-glucopyranosyl-(1→4)-α-D-glucopyranosyl-(1→4)-α-D-glucopyranosyl-(1→]
[9057-02-7]

Pullulan is a neutral simple polysaccharide produced by the growth of *Aureobasidium pullulans*. It has a chain structure of repeated α-1,6 binding of maltotriose composed of three glucoses in α-1,4 binding.

Description Pullulan occurs as a white powder.

It is freely soluble in water, and practically insoluble in ethanol (99.5).

Identification **(1)** Dissolve 10 g of Pullulan in 100 mL of water with stirring by adding in small portions: a viscous solution is produced.

(2) Mix 10 mL of the viscous solution obtained in (1) with 0.1 mL of pullulanase TS, and allow to stand: the solution loses its viscosity.

(3) To 10 mL of a solution of Pullulan (1 in 50) add 2 mL of macrogol 600: a white precipitate is formed immediately.

Viscosity *<2.53>* Weigh exactly 10.0 g of Pullulan, previously dried, dissolve in water to make exactly 100 g, and perform the test at 30 ± 0.1°C as directed in Method 1: the kinematic viscosity is between 100 mm^2/s and 180 mm^2/s.

pH *<2.54>* Dissolve 1.0 g of Pullulan in 10 mL of freshly boiled and cooled water: the pH is between 4.5 and 6.5.

Purity **(1)** Heavy metals *<1.07>*—Proceed with 4.0 g of Pullulan according to Method 2, and perform the test. Prepare the control solution with 2.0 mL of Standard Lead Solution (not more than 5 ppm).

(2) Nitrogen—Weigh accurately about 3 g of Pullulan, previously dried, and perform the test as directed under Nitrogen Determination *<1.08>*: the amount of nitrogen (N: 14.01) is not more than 0.05%. Use 12 mL of sulfuric acid for the decomposition, and add 40 mL of a solution of sodium hydroxide (2 in 5).

(3) Monosaccharide and oligosaccharides—Dissolve 0.8 g of Pullulan, previously dried, in 100 mL of water, and designate this solution as the sample stock solution. To 1 mL of the sample stock solution add 0.1 mL of potassium chloride saturated solution, and shake vigorously with 3 mL of methanol. Centrifuge, and use the supernatant liquid as the sample solution. Separately, pipet 1 mL of the sample stock solution, add water to make exactly 50 mL, and use this solution as the standard solution. Pipet 0.2 mL each of the sample solution, the standard solution and water, transfer them gently to each test tube containing 5 mL of a solution of anthrone in diluted sulfuric acid (3 in 4) (1 in 500) cooled in ice water, stir immediately, then heat at 90°C for 10 minutes, and cool immediately. Perform the test with these solutions so obtained as directed under Ultraviolet-visible Spectrophtometry *<2.24>* using water as a blank, and determine the absorbances at 620 nm, A_T, A_S and A_B: the amount of monosaccharide and oligosaccharides is not more than 10.0%.

Amount (%) of monosaccharide and oligosaccharides
$= (A_T - A_B)/(A_S - A_B) \times 8.2$

Loss on drying *<2.41>* Not more than 6.0% (1 g, in vacuum, 90°C, 6 hours).

Residue on ignition *<2.44>* Not more than 0.3% (2 g).

Containers and storage Containers—Well-closed containers.

Pyrantel Pamoate

ピランテルパモ酸塩

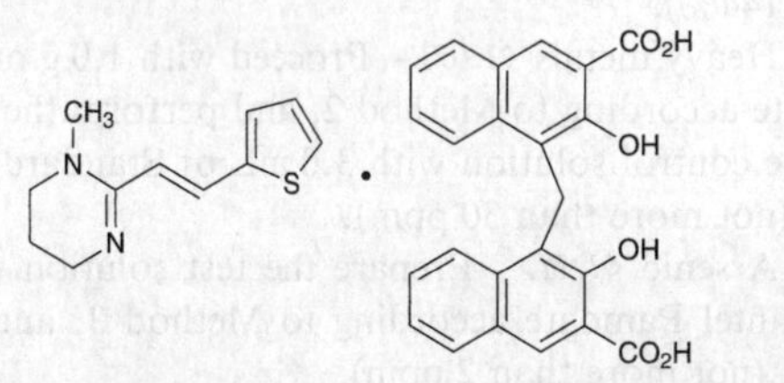

$C_{11}H_{14}N_2S.C_{23}H_{16}O_6$: 594.68
1-Methyl-2-[(1*E*)-2-(thien-2-yl)vinyl]-1,4,5,6-tetrahydropyrimidine mono[4,4′-methylenebis(3-hydroxy-2-naphthoate)]
[22204-24-6]

Pyrantel Pamoate, when dried, contains not less than 98.0% of pyrantel pamoate ($C_{11}H_{14}N_2S.C_{23}H_{16}O_6$).

Description Pyrantel Pamoate occurs as a light yellow to yellow crystalline powder. It is odorless and tasteless.

It is sparingly soluble in *N*,*N*-dimethylformamide, very slightly soluble in methanol and in ethanol (95), and practically insoluble in water, in ethyl acetate and in diethyl ether.

Melting point: 256 – 264°C (with decomposition).

Identification **(1)** To 0.05 g of Pyrantel Pamoate add 10 mL of methanol and 1 mL of a mixture of hydrochloric acid and methanol (1:1), and shake vigorously: a yellow precipitate is produced. Filter the solution, and use the filtrate as the sample solution. Use the precipitate for the test (2). To 0.5 mL of the sample solution add 1 mL of a solution of 2,3-indolinedione in sulfuric acid (1 in 1000): a red color develops.

(2) Collect the precipitate obtained in the test (1), wash with methanol, and dry at 105°C for 1 hour. To 0.01 g of the dried precipitate add 10 mL of methanol, shake well, and filter. To 5 mL of the filtrate add 1 drop of iron (III) chloride TS: a green color develops.

(3) Dissolve 0.1 g of Pyrantel Pamoate in 50 mL of *N*,*N*-dimethylformamide, and add methanol to make 200 mL. To 2 mL of the solution add a solution of hydrochloric acid in methanol (9 in 1000) to make 100 mL. Determine the absorption spectrum of the solution as directed under Ultraviolet-visible Spectrophotometry <*2.24*>, and compare the spectrum with the Reference Spectrum: both spectra exhibit similar intensities of absorption at the same wavelengths.

(4) Determine the infrared absorption spectrum of Pyrantel Pamoate, previously dried, as directed in the potassium bromide disk method under Infrared Spectrophotometry <*2.25*>, and compare the spectrum with the Reference Spectrum: both spectra exhibit similar intensities of absorption at the same wave numbers.

Purity **(1)** Chloride <*1.03*>—To 1.0 g of Pyrantel Pamoate add 10 mL of dilute nitric acid and 40 mL of water, and heat on a water bath with shaking for 5 minutes. After cooling, add water to make 50 mL, and filter. To 20 mL of the filtrate add 2 mL of dilute nitric acid and water to make 50 mL. Proceed the test using this solution as the test solution. Prepare the control solution with 0.40 mL of 0.01 mol/L hydrochloric acid VS (not more than 0.036%).

(2) Sulfate <*1.14*>—To 0.75 g of Pyrantel Pamoate add 5 mL of dilute hydrochloric acid and water to make 100 mL, and heat on a water bath for 5 minutes with shaking. After cooling, add water to make 100 mL, and filter. To 20 mL of the filtrate add water to make 50 mL. Proceed the test using this solution as the test solution. Prepare the control solution with 0.45 mL of 0.005 mol/L sulfuric acid VS (not more than 0.144%).

(3) Heavy metals <*1.07*>—Proceed with 1.0 g of Pyrantel Pamoate according to Method 2, and perform the test. Prepare the control solution with 3.0 mL of Standard Lead Solution (not more than 30 ppm).

(4) Arsenic <*1.11*>—Prepare the test solution with 1.0 g of Pyrantel Pamoate according to Method 3, and perform the test (not more than 2 ppm).

(5) Related substances—The procedure should be performed under protection from light in light-resistant vessels. Dissolve 0.10 g of Pyrantel Pamoate in 10 mL of *N*,*N*-dimethylformamide, and use this solution as the sample solution. Pipet 1 mL of the sample solution, add *N*,*N*-dimethylformamide to make exactly 100 mL, and use this solution as the standard solution. Perform the test with these solutions as directed under Thin-layer Chromatography <*2.03*>. Spot 5 μL each of the sample solution and standard solution on a plate of silica gel with fluorescent indicator for thin-layer chromatography. Develop the plate with a mixture of ethyl acetate, water and acetic acid (100) (3:1:1) to a distance of about 10 cm, and air-dry the plate. Examine under ultraviolet light (main wavelength: 254 nm): the spots other than the spot of pyrantel and the spot of pamoic acid obtained from the sample solution are not more intense than the spot of pyrantel (*R*f value: about 0.3) from the standard solution.

Loss on drying <*2.41*> Not more than 1.0% (1 g, 105°C, 2 hours).

Residue on ignition <*2.44*> Not more than 0.3% (1 g).

Assay Weigh accurately about 0.5 g of Pyrantel Pamoate, previously dried, add 25 mL of chloroform and 25 mL of sodium hydroxide TS, shake for 15 minutes, and extract. Extract further with two 25-mL portions of chloroform. Filter each extract through 5 g of anhydrous sodium sulfate on a pledget of absorbent cotton. Combine the chloroform extracts, add 30 mL of acetic acid (100), and titrate <*2.50*> with 0.1 mol/L perchloric acid VS (indicator: 2 drops of crystal violet TS). Perform a blank determination in the same manner, and make any necessary correction.

Each mL of 0.1 mol/L perchloric acid VS
= 59.47 mg of $C_{11}H_{14}N_2S.C_{23}H_{16}O_6$

Containers and storage Containers—Tight containers.

Pyrazinamide

ピラジナミド

$C_5H_5N_3O$: 123.11
Pyrazine-2-carboxamide
[*98-96-4*]

Pyrazinamide, when dried, contains not less than 99.0% and not more than 101.0% of pyrazinamide ($C_5H_5N_3O$).

Description Pyrazinamide occurs as white, crystals or crystalline powder.

It is sparingly soluble in water and in methanol, and slightly soluble in ethanol (99.5) and in acetic anhydride.

Identification **(1)** Determine the absorption spectrum of a solution of Pyrazinamide in 0.1 mol/L hydrochloric acid TS (1 in 100,000) as directed under Ultraviolet-visible Spectrophotometry <*2.24*>, and compare the spectrum with the Reference Spectrum: both spectra exhibit similar intensities of absorption at the same wavelengths.

(2) Determine the infrared absorption spectrum of Pyrazinamide, previously dried, as directed in the potassium bromide disk method under Infrared Spectrophotometry <*2.25*>, and compare the spectrum with the Reference Spectrum: both spectra exhibit similar intensities of absorption at the same wave numbers.

Melting point <*2.60*> 188 – 193°C

Purity **(1)** Heavy metals <*1.07*>—Proceed with 1.0 g of Pyrazinamide according to Method 2, and perform the test. Prepare the control solution with 2.0 mL of Standard Lead Solution (not more than 20 ppm).

(2) Related substances—Dissolve 0.10 g of Pyrazinamide in 10 mL of methanol, and use this solution as the sample solution. Pipet 1 mL of the sample solution, add methanol to make exactly 200 mL, and use this solution as the standard solution. Perform the test with these solutions as directed under Thin-layer Chromatography <*2.03*>. Spot 20 μL each of the sample solution and standard solution on a plate of silica gel with fluorescent indicator for thin-layer chromatography. Develop the plate with a mixture of 1-butanol, water and acetic acid (100) (3:1:1) to a distance of about 10 cm, and air-dry the plate. Examine under ultraviolet light (main wavelength: 254 nm): the spot other than the principal spot obtained from the sample solution is not more intense than the spot from the standard solution.

Loss on drying <*2.41*> Not more than 0.5% (1 g, in vacuum, silica gel, 4 hours).

Residue on ignition <*2.44*> Not more than 0.1% (1 g).

Assay Weigh accurately about 0.1 g of Pyrazinamide, previously dried, dissolve in 50 mL of acetic anhydride, and titrate <*2.50*> with 0.1 mol/L perchloric acid VS (potentiometric titration). Perform a blank determination in the same manner, and make any necessary correction.

Each mL of 0.1 mol/L perchloric acid VS
= 12.31 mg of $C_5H_5N_3O$

Containers and storage Containers—Well-closed containers.

Pyridostigmine Bromide

ピリドスチグミン臭化物

$C_9H_{13}BrN_2O_2$: 261.12
3-Dimethylcarbamoyloxy-1-methylpyridinium bromide
[*101-26-8*]

Pyridostigmine Bromide, when dried, contains not less than 98.5% of pyridostigmine bromide ($C_9H_{13}BrN_2O_2$).

Description Pyridostigmine Bromide occurs as a white crystalline powder. It is odorless or has a slightly characteristic odor.

It is very soluble in water, freely soluble in ethanol (95) and in acetic acid (100), and practically insoluble in diethyl ether.

The pH of a solution of 1.0 g of Pyridostigmine Bromide in 10 mL of water is between 4.0 and 6.0.

It is deliquescent.

Identification **(1)** Dissolve 0.02 g of Pyridostigmine Bromide in 10 mL of water, add 5 mL of Reinecke salt TS: a light red precipitate is produced.

(2) To 0.1 g of Pyridostigmine Bromide add 0.6 mL of sodium hydroxide TS: the unpleasant odor of dimethylamine is perceptible.

(3) Determine the absorption spectrum of a solution of Pyridostigmine Bromide in 0.1 mol/L hydrochloric acid TS (1 in 30,000) as directed under Ultraviolet-visible Spectrophotometry <*2.24*>, and compare the spectrum with the Reference Spectrum: both spectra exhibit similar intensities of absorption at the same wavelengths.

(4) A solution of Pyridostigmine Bromide (1 in 50) responds to Qualitative Tests <*1.09*> for Bromide.

Melting point <*2.60*> 153 – 157°C

Purity **(1)** Clarity and color of solution—Dissolve 1.0 g of Pyridostigmine Bromide in 10 mL of water: the solution is clear and colorless.

(2) Heavy metals <*1.07*>—Proceed with 1.0 g of Pyridostigmine Bromide according to Method 1, and perform the test. Prepare the control solution with 2.0 mL of Standard Lead Solution (not more than 20 ppm).

(3) Arsenic <*1.11*>—Prepare the test solution with 1.0 g of Pyridostigmine Bromide according to Method 1, and perform the test (not more than 2 ppm).

(4) Related substances—Dissolve 0.10 g of Pyridostigmine Bromide in 10 mL of ethanol (95), and use this solution as the sample solution. Pipet 2 mL of the sample solution, and add ethanol (95) to make exactly 10 mL. Pipet 1 mL of this solution, add ethanol (95) to make exactly 25 mL, and use this solution as the standard solution. Perform the test with these solutions as directed under Thin-layer Chromatography <*2.03*>. Spot 10 μL each of the sample solution and standard solution on a plate of silica gel with fluorescent indicator for thin-layer chromatography. Develop the plate with a mixture of methanol, chloroform and ammonium chloride TS (5:4:1) to a distance of about 12 cm, and air-dry the plate. Examine under ultraviolet light (main wavelength: 254 nm): the spots other than the principal spot obtained from the sample solution are not more intense than the spot from the standard solution in color.

Loss on drying <*2.41*> Not more than 2.0% (1 g, in vacuum, phosphorus (V) oxide, 100°C, 5 hours).

Residue on ignition <*2.44*> Not more than 0.1% (1 g).

Assay Weigh accurately about 0.3 g of Pyridostigmine Bromide, previously dried, dissolve in 10 mL of acetic acid (100), add 40 mL of acetic anhydride, and titrate <*2.50*> with 0.1 mol/L perchloric acid VS (potentiometric titration). Perform a blank determination in the same manner, and make any necessary correction.

Each mL of 0.1 mol/L perchloric acid VS
= 26.11 mg of $C_9H_{13}BrN_2O_2$

Containers and storage Containers—Hermetic containers.

Pyridoxal Phosphate Hydrate

ピリドキサールリン酸エステル水和物

$C_8H_{10}NO_6P.H_2O$: 265.16
(4-Formyl-5-hydroxy-6-methylpyridin-
3-yl)methyl dihydrogenphosphate monohydrate
[*41468-25-1*]

Pyridoxal Phosphate Hydrate contains not less than 98.0% and not more than 101.0% of pyridoxal phosphate ($C_8H_{10}NO_6P$: 247.14), calculated on the anhydrous basis.

Description Pyridoxal Phosphate Hydrate occurs as a pale yellow-white to light yellow crystalline powder.

It is slightly soluble in water, and practically insoluble in ethanol (99.5).

It dissolves in dilute hydrochloric acid and in sodium hydroxide TS.

The pH of a solution prepared by dissolving 0.1 g of Pyridoxal Phosphate Hydrate in 200 mL of water is between 3.0 and 3.5.

Pyridoxal Phosphate Hydrate is colored to light red by light.

Identification (1) Determine the absorption spectrum of a solution of Pyridoxal Phosphate Hydrate in phosphate buffer solution (pH 6.8) (1 in 50,000) as directed under Ultraviolet-visible Spectrophotometry *<2.24>*, and compare the spectrum with the Reference Spectrum or the spectrum of a solution of Pyridoxal Phosphate RS prepared in the same manner as the sample solution: both spectra exhibit similar intensities of absorption at the same wavelengths.

(2) Determine the infrared absorption spectrum of Pyridoxal Phosphate Hydrate as directed in the potassium bromide disk method under Infrared Spectrophotometry *<2.25>*, and compare the spectrum with the Reference Spectrum or the spectrum of Pyridoxal Phosphate RS: both spectra exhibit similar intensities of absorption at the same wave numbers.

Purity (1) Heavy metals *<1.07>*—Proceed with 4.0 g of Pyridoxal Phosphate Hydrate according to Method 2, and perform the test. Prepare the control solution with 2.0 mL of Standard Lead Solution (not more than 5 ppm).

(2) Arsenic *<1.11>*—Dissolve 1.0 g of Pyridoxal Phosphate Hydrate in 5 mL of dilute hydrochloric acid. Use this solution as the test solution, and perform the test (not more than 2 ppm).

(3) Free phosphoric acid—Weigh accurately about 0.1 g of Pyridoxal Phosphate Hydrate, dissolve in water to make exactly 100 mL, and use this solution as the sample solution. Pipet 5 mL each of the sample solution and Standard Phosphoric Acid Solution, to each add 2.5 mL of hexaammonium heptamolybdate-sulfuric acid TS and 1 mL of 1-amino-2-naphthol-4-sulfonic acid TS, and shake. Add water to make exactly 25 mL, and allow to stand at 20 ± 1°C for 30 minutes. Perform the test with these solutions as directed under Ultraviolet-visible Spectrophotometry *<2.24>*, using a solution prepared with 5 mL of water in the same manner as the blank. Determine the absorbances, A_T and A_S, of each solution from the sample solution and Standard Phosphoric Acid Solution at 740 nm: the amount of free phosphoric acid is not more than 0.5%.

$$\text{Content (\%) of free phosphoric acid } (H_3PO_4) = 1/M \times A_T/A_S \times 258.0$$

M: Amount (mg) of Pyridoxal Phosphate Hydrate taken, calculated on the anhydrous basis

(4) Related substances—Dissolve 50 mg of Pyridoxal Phosphate Hydrate in 20 mL of the mobile phase, and use this solution as the sample solution. Pipet 1 mL of the sample solution, add the mobile phase to make exactly 100 mL, and use this solution as the standard solution. Perform the test with exactly 5 µL each of the sample solution and standard solution as directed under Liquid Chromatography *<2.01>* according to the following conditions. Determine each peak area by the automatic integration method: the area of the peak other than pyridoxal phosphate obtained from the sample solution is not larger than the peak area of pyridoxal phosphate from the standard solution, and the total area of the peaks other than pyridoxal phosphate from the sample solution is not larger than 2 times the peak area of pyridoxal phosphate from the standard solution.

Operating conditions—

Detector: An ultraviolet absorption photometer (wavelength: 254 nm).

Column: A stainless steel column 4.6 mm in inside diameter and 25 cm in length, packed with octadecylsilanized silica gel for liquid chromatography (5 µm in particle diameter).

Column temperature: A constant temperature of about 30°C.

Mobile phase: Dissolve 3.63 g of potassium dihydrogen phosphate and 5.68 g of anhydrous disodium hydrogen phosphate in water to make 1000 mL.

Flow rate: Adjust so that the retention time of pyridoxal phosphate is about 6 minutes.

Time span of measurement: About 2.5 times as long as the retention time of pyridoxal phosphate, beginning after the solvent peak.

System suitability—

Test for required detectability: Pipet 2 mL of the standard solution, and add the mobile phase to make exactly 20 mL. Confirm that the peak area of pyridoxal phosphate obtained with 5 µL of this solution is equivalent to 7 to 13% of that with 5 µL of the standard solution.

System performance: When the procedure is run with 5 µL of the standard solution under the above operating conditions, the number of theoretical plates and the symmetry factor of the peak of pyridoxal phosphate are not less than 3000 and not more than 1.5, respectively.

System repeatability: When the test is repeated 6 times with 5 µL of the standard solution under the above operating conditions, the relative standard deviation of the peak area of pyridoxal phosphate is not more than 2.0%.

Water *<2.48>* 6.0 - 9.0% (0.1 g, volumetric titration, direct titration. Use a solution prepared by dissolving 50 g of imidazole for water determination in 100 mL of the dissolving solution instead of methanol for water determination).

Dissolving solution: A solution containing 80% of 1-methoxy-2-propanol, 18% of ethanol (99.5), 1% of imidazole and 1% of imidazole hydrobromide.

Assay Weigh accurately about 45 mg each of Pyridoxal Phosphate Hydrate and Pyridoxal Phosphate RS (separately determine the water *<2.48>* in the same manner as Pyridoxal Phosphate Hydrate), and dissolve each in phosphate buffer solution (pH 6.8) to make exactly 250 mL. Pipet 10 mL each of these solutions, add phosphate buffer solution (pH 6.8) to make exactly 100 mL, and use these solutions as the sample solution and the standard solution. Determine the absorbances, A_T and A_S, of the sample solution and standard solution at 388 nm as directed under Ultraviolet-visible Spectrophotometry *<2.24>* using phosphate buffer solution (pH 6.8) as the blank.

$$\text{Amount (mg) of pyridoxal phosphate } (C_8H_{10}NO_6P) = M_S \times A_T/A_S$$

M_S: Amount (mg) of Pyridoxal Phosphate RS taken, calculated on the anhydrous basis

Containers and storage Containers—Well-closed containers.

Storage—Light-resistant.

Pyridoxine Hydrochloride

Vitamin B_6

ピリドキシン塩酸塩

$C_8H_{11}NO_3.HCl$: 205.64
4,5-Bis(hydroxymethyl)-2-methylpyridin-3-ol monohydrochloride
[58-56-0]

Pyridoxine Hydrochloride, when dried, contains not less than 98.0% and not more than 101.0% of pyridoxine hydrochloride ($C_8H_{11}NO_3.HCl$).

Description Pyridoxine Hydrochloride occurs as a white to pale yellow crystalline powder.

It is freely soluble in water, slightly soluble in ethanol (99.5), and practically insoluble in acetic anhydride and in acetic acid (100).

It is gradually affected by light.

Melting point: about 206°C (with decomposition).

Identification **(1)** Determine the absorption spectrum of a solution of Pyridoxine Hydrochloride in 0.1 mol/L hydrochloric acid TS (1 in 100,000) as directed under Ultraviolet-visible Spectrophotometry 〈*2.24*〉, and compare the spectrum with the Reference Spectrum or the spectrum of a solution of Pyridoxine Hydrochloride RS prepared in the same manner as the sample solution: both spectra exhibit similar intensities of absorption at the same wavelengths.

(2) Determine the infrared absorption spectrum of Pyridoxine Hydrochloride, previously dried, as directed in the potassium chloride disk method under Infrared Spectrophotometry 〈*2.25*〉, and compare the spectrum with the Reference Spectrum or the spectrum of Pyridoxine Hydrochloride RS: both spectra exhibit similar intensities of absorption at the same wave numbers.

(3) A solution of Pyridoxine Hydrochloride (1 in 10) responds to Qualitative Tests 〈*1.09*〉 for chloride.

pH 〈*2.54*〉 The pH of a solution prepared by dissolving 1.0 g of Pyridoxine Hydrochloride in 50 mL of water is between 2.5 and 3.5.

Purity **(1)** Clarity and color of solution—Dissolve 1.0 g of Pyridoxine hydrochloride in 20 mL of water: the solution is clear and colorless.

(2) Heavy metals 〈*1.07*〉—Proceed with 1.0 g of Pyridoxine Hydrochloride according to Method 1, and perform the test. Prepare the control solution with 3.0 mL of Standard Lead Solution (not more than 30 ppm).

(3) Related substances—Dissolve 1.0 g of Pyridoxine Hydrochloride in 10 mL of water, and use this solution as the sample solution. Pipet 2.5 mL of the sample solution, and add water to make exactly 100 mL. Pipet 1 mL of this solution, add water to make exactly 10 mL, and use this solution as the standard solution. Perform the test with these solutions as directed under Thin-layer Chromatography 〈*2.03*〉. Spot 2 μL each of the sample solution and standard solution on a plate of silica gel for thin-layer chromatography, and air-dry the plate. Develop the plate with a mixture of acetone, tetrahydrofuran, hexane and ammonia solution (28) (65:13:13:9) to a distance of about 10 cm, and air-dry the plate. Spray evenly a solution of sodium carbonate in diluted ethanol (3 in 10) (1 in 20) on the plate. After air-drying, spray evenly a solution of 2,6-dibromo-*N*-chloro-1,4-benzoquinone monoimine in ethanol (99.5) (1 in 1000) on the plate, and air-dry: the spot other than the principal spot obtained from the sample solution is not more intense than the spot from the standard solution.

Loss on drying 〈*2.41*〉 Not more than 0.30% (1 g, in vacuum, silica gel, 4 hours).

Residue on ignition 〈*2.44*〉 Not more than 0.1% (1 g).

Assay Weigh accurately about 0.2 g of Pyridoxine Hydrochloride, previously dried, add 5 mL of acetic acid (100) and 5 mL of acetic anhydride, dissolve by gentle boiling, cool, add 30 mL of acetic anhydride, and titrate 〈*2.50*〉 with 0.1 mol/L perchloric acid VS (potentiometric titration). Perform a blank determination in the same manner, and make any necessary correction.

Each mL of 0.1 mol/L perchloric acid VS
= 20.56 mg of $C_8H_{11}NO_3.HCl$

Containers and storage Containers—Tight containers.
Storage—Light-resistant.

Pyridoxine Hydrochloride Injection

Vitamin B_6 Injection

ピリドキシン塩酸塩注射液

Pyridoxine Hydrochloride Injection is an aqueous injection.

It contains not less than 95.0% and not more than 105.0% of the labeled amount of pyridoxine hydrochloride ($C_8H_{11}NO_3.HCl$: 205.64).

Method of preparation Prepare as directed under Injections, with Pyridoxine Hydrochloride.

Description Pyridoxine Hydrochloride Injection is a colorless or pale yellow, clear liquid.

It is gradually affected by light.

pH: 3.0 – 6.0

Identification **(1)** To a volume of Pyridoxine Hydrochloride Injection, equivalent to 0.05 g of Pyridoxine Hydrochloride, add 0.1 mol/L hydrochloric acid TS to make 100 mL. To 2 mL of this solution add 0.1 mol/L hydrochloric acid TS to make 100 mL, and determine the absorption spectrum of this solution as directed under Ultraviolet-visible spectrophotometry 〈*2.24*〉: it exhibits a maximum between 288 nm and 292 nm.

(2) To a volume of Pyridoxine Hydrochloride Injection, equivalent to 0.01 g of Pyridoxine Hydrochloride, add water to make 10 mL, and use this solution as the sample solution. Separately, dissolve 0.01 g of Pyridoxine Hydrochloride RS in 10 mL of water, and use this solution as the standard solution. Perform the test with these solutions as directed under Thin-layer Chromatography 〈*2.03*〉. Spot 2 μL each of the sample solution and standard solution on a plate of silica gel for thin-layer chromatography, and air-dry the plate. Develop the plate with a mixture of acetone, tetrahydrofuran, hexane and ammonia solution (28) (65:13:13:9) to a distance of about 10 cm, and air-dry the plate. Spray evenly a solution of sodium carbonate in diluted ethanol (3 in 10) (1 in 20) on the plate. After air-drying, spray evenly a solution of 2,6-dibromo-*N*-chloro-1,4-benzoquinone monoimine in ethanol (99.5) (1 in 1000) on the plate: the spots obtained from the sample solution and the standard solution are blue in color and have the same *Rf* value.

Bacterial endotoxins *<4.01>* Less than 3.0 EU/mg.

Extractable volume *<6.05>* It meets the requirement.

Foreign insoluble matter *<6.06>* Perform the test according to Method 1: it meets the requirement.

Insoluble particulate matter *<6.07>* It meets the requirement.

Sterility *<4.06>* Perform the test according to the Membrane filtration method: it meets the requirement.

Assay Measure exactly a volume of Pyridoxine Hydrochloride Injection, equivalent to about 20 mg of pyridoxine hydrochloride ($C_8H_{11}NO_3.HCl$), dilute with water, if necessary, and add water to make exactly 100 mL. Pipet 25 mL of this solution, add water to make exactly 200 mL, and use this solution as the sample solution. Separately, weigh accurately about 0.1 g of Pyridoxine Hydrochloride RS, previously dried in a desiccator (in vacuum, silica gel) for 4 hours, and dissolve in water to make exactly 100 mL. Pipet 5 mL of this solution, add water to make exactly 200 mL, and use this solution as the standard solution. Pipet 1 mL each of the sample solution and standard solution, add 2.0 mL of barbital buffer solution, 9.0 mL of 2-propanol and 2.0 mL of a freshly prepared solution of 2,6-dibromo-*N*-chloro-1,4-benzoquinone monoimine in ethanol (95) (1 in 4000), shake well, add 2-propanol to make exactly 25 mL, and allow to stand for 90 minutes. Determine the absorbances, A_T and A_S, of the subsequent sample solution and subsequent standard solution, respectively, at 650 nm as directed under Ultraviolet-visible Spectrophotometry *<2.24>*, using a solution, prepared in the same manner with 1 mL of water, as the blank.

$$\text{Amount (mg) of pyridoxine hydrochloride } (C_8H_{11}NO_3.HCl) = M_S \times A_T/A_S \times 1/5$$

M_S: Amount (mg) of Pyridoxine Hydrochloride RS taken

Containers and storage Containers—Hermetic containers, and colored containers may be used.

Storage—Light-resistant.

Pyroxylin

ピロキシリン

Pyroxylin is a nitric acid ester of cellulose. It is usually moistened with 2-propanol or some other solvent.

Description Pyroxylin occurs as a white cotton-like substance or white flakes.

It is freely soluble in acetone, and very slightly soluble in diethyl ether.

Upon heating or exposure to light, it is decomposed with the evolution of nitrous acid vapors.

Identification Ignite Pyroxylin: it burns very rapidly with a luminous flame.

Purity (1) Clarity of solution—Dissolve 1.0 g of Pyroxylin, previously dried at 80°C for 2 hours, in 25 mL of a mixture of diethyl ether and ethanol (95) (3:1): the solution is clear.

(2) Acidity—Shake 1.0 g of Pyroxylin, previously dried at 80°C for 2 hours, with 20 mL of water for 10 minutes: the filtrate is neutral.

(3) Water-soluble substances—Evaporate 10 mL of the filtrate obtained in (2) on a water bath to dryness, and dry at 105°C for 1 hour: the mass of the residue is not more than 1.5 mg.

(4) Residue on ignition—Weigh accurately about 2 g of Pyroxylin, previously dried at 80°C for 2 hours, and moisten with 10 mL of a solution of castor oil in acetone (1 in 20) to gelatinize the sample. Ignite the contents to carbonize the sample, heat strongly at about 500°C for 2 hours, and allow to cool in a desicator (silica gel): the amount of the residue is not more than 0.30%.

Containers and storage Containers—Tight containers.

Storage—Light-resistant, packed loosely, remote from fire, and preferably in a cold place.

Pyrrolnitrin

ピロールニトリン

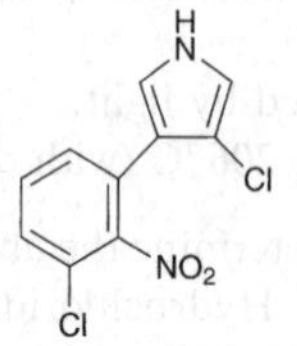

$C_{10}H_6Cl_2N_2O_2$: 257.07
3-Chloro-4-(3-chloro-2-nitrophenyl)pyrrole
[*1018-71-9*]

Pyrrolnitrin contains not less than 970 μg (potency) and not more than 1020 μg (potency) per mg, calculated on the dried basis. The potency of Pyrrolnitrin is expressed as mass (potency) of pyrrolnitrin ($C_{10}H_6Cl_2N_2O_2$).

Description Pyrrolnitrin occurs as yellow to yellow-brown, crystals or crystalline powder.

It is freely soluble in methanol and in ethanol (95), and practically insoluble in water.

Identification (1) Determine the absorption spectrum of a solution of Pyrrolnitrin in ethanol (95) (1 in 100,000) as directed under Ultraviolet-visible Spectrophotometry *<2.24>*, and compare the spectrum with the Reference Spectrum or the spectrum of a solution of Pyrrolnitrin RS prepared in the same manner as the sample solution: both spectra exhibit similar intensities of absorption at the same wavelengths.

(2) Determine the infrared absorption spectrum of Pyrrolnitrin as directed in the potassium bromide disk method under Infrared Spectrophotometry *<2.25>*, and compare the spectrum with the Reference Spectrum or the spectrum of Pyrrolnitrin RS: both spectra exhibit similar intensities of absorption at the same wave numbers.

Melting point *<2.60>* 124 – 128°C

Purity Related substances—Dissolve 0.10 g of Pyrrolnitrin in 10 mL of methanol, and use this solution as the sample solution. Pipet 1 mL of the sample solution, and add methanol to make exactly 100 mL. Pipet 3 mL of this solution, add methanol to make exactly 10 mL, and use this solution as the standard solution. Perform the test with these solutions as directed under Thin-layer Chromatography *<2.03>*. Spot 10

μL each of the sample solution and standard solution on a plate of silica gel for thin-layer chromatography. Develop the plate with a mixture of xylene, ethyl acetate and formic acid (18:2:1) to a distance of about 10 cm, and dry the plate at 80°C for 30 minutes. Spray evenly diluted sulfuric acid (1 in 3) on the plate, and heat the plate at 100°C for 30 minutes: the spot other than the principal spot obtained from the sample solution is not more intense than the spot from the standard solution.

Loss on drying <2.41> Not more than 0.5% (1 g, reduced pressure not exceeding 0.67 kPa, 60°C, 3 hours).

Residue on ignition <2.44> Not more than 0.1% (1 g).

Assay Conduct this procedure using light-resistant vessels. Weigh accurately an amount of Pyrrolnitrin and Pyrrolnitrin RS, equivalent to about 50 mg (potency) each, and dissolve separetely in diluted acetonitrile (3 in 5) to make exactly 50 mL. Pipet 10 mL each of these solutions, add exactly 10 mL of the internal standard solution, add diluted acetonitrile (3 in 5) to make 100 mL, and use these solutions as the sample solution and standard solution. Perform the test with 5 μL each of the sample solution and standard solution as directed under Liquid Chromatography <2.01> according to the following conditions, and calculate the ratios, Q_T and Q_S, of the peak area of pyrrolnitrin to that of the internal standard.

Amount [μg (potency)] of pyrrolnitrin ($C_{10}H_6Cl_2N_2O_2$)
$= M_S \times Q_T/Q_S \times 1000$

M_S: Amount [mg (potency)] of Pyrrolnitrin RS taken

Internal standard solution—A solution of benzyl benzoate in diluted acetonitrile (3 in 5) (3 in 500).

Operating conditions—

Detector: An ultraviolet absorption photometer (wavelength: 254 nm).

Column: A stainless steel column 4 mm in inside diameter and 15 cm in length, packed with octylsilanized silica gel for liquid chromatography (5 μm in particle diameter).

Column temperature: A constant temperature of about 25°C.

Mobile phase: A mixture of water and acetonitrile (11:9).

Flow rate: Adjust so that the retention time of pyrrolnitrin is about 9 minutes.

System suitability—

System performance: When the procedure is run with 5 μL of the standard solution under the above operating conditions, pyrrolnitrin and the internal standard are eluted in this order with the resolution between these peaks being not less than 3.

System repeatability: When the test is repeated 6 times with 5 μL of the standard solution under the above operating conditions, the relative standard deviation of the ratios of the peak area of pyrrolnitrin to that of the internal standard is not more than 1.0%.

Containers and storage Containers—Tight containers.

Storage—Light-resistant.

Quetiapine Fumarate

クエチアピンフマル酸塩

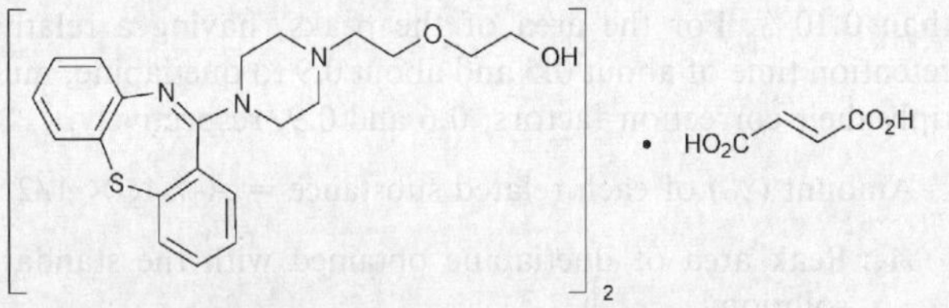

$(C_{21}H_{25}N_3O_2S)_2.C_4H_4O_4$: 883.09

2-[2-(4-Dibenzo[*b,f*][1,4]thiazepin-11-ylpiperazin-1-yl)ethoxy]ethanol hemifumarate

[111974-72-2]

Quetiapine Fumarate contains not less than 98.0% and not more than 102.0% of quetiapine fumarate [$(C_{21}H_{25}N_3O_2S)_2.C_4H_4O_4$], calculated on the anhydrous basis.

Description Quetiapine Fumarate occurs as a white powder.

It is sparingly soluble in methanol, and slightly soluble in water and in ethanol (99.5).

Identification (1) Determine the absorption spectrum of a solution of Quetiapine Fumarate in a mixture of water and acetonitrile (1:1) (3 in 200,000) as directed under Ultraviolet-visible Spectrophotometry <2.24>, and compare the spectrum with the Reference Spectrum or the spectrum of a solution of Quetiapine Fumarate RS prepared in the same manner as the sample solution: both spectra exhibit similar intensities of absorption at the same wavelengths.

(2) Determine the infrared absorption spectrum of Quetiapine Fumarate as directed in the potassium bromide disk method under Infrared Spectrophotometry <2.25>, and compare the spectrum with the Reference Spectrum or the spectrum of Quetiapine Fumarate RS: both spectra exhibit similar intensities of absorption at the same wave numbers.

(3) Dissolve 40 mg of Quetiapine Fumarate and 10 mg of fumaric acid for thin-layer chromatography in separate 10 mL of methanol, and use these solutions as the sample solution and the standard solution, respectively. Perform the test with these solutions as directed under Thin-layer Chromatography <2.03>. Spot 10 μL each of the sample solution and standard solution on a plate of silica gel with fluorescent indicator for thin-layer chromatography. Develop the plate with a mixture of isopropyl ether, formic acid and water (90:7:3) to a distance of about 10 cm, and air-dry the plate. Examine under ultraviolet light (main wavelength: 254 nm): the spot having a larger *R*f value among the spots obtained from the sample solution and the spot from the standard solution show the same *R*f value.

Purity (1) Heavy metals <1.07>—Proceed with 2.0 g of Quetiapine Fumarate according to Method 2, and perform the test. Prepare the control solution with 2.0 mL of Standard Lead Solution (not more than 10 ppm).

(2) Related substances (i)—To 20 mg of Quetiapine Fumarate add 30 mL of the mobile phase, dissolve by sonicating, add the mobile phase to make 50 mL, and use this solution as the sample solution. Pipet 5 mL of the sample solution, add the mobile phase to make exactly 100 mL. Pipet 5 mL of this solution, and add the mobile phase to make exactly 50 mL, and use this solution as the standard solution. Perform the test with exactly 50 μL each of the

sample solution and standard solution as directed under Liquid Chromatography <*2.01*> according to the following conditions. Determine each peak area by the automatic integration method, and calculate the amount of each related substance by the following equation: the amount is not more than 0.10%. For the area of the peaks, having a relative retention time of about 0.5 and about 0.9 to quetiapine, multiply their correction factors, 0.6 and 0.9, respectively.

Amount (%) of each related substance = $A_T/A_S \times 1/2$

A_S: Peak area of quetiapine obtained with the standard solution

A_T: Each peak area other than quetiapine obtained with the sample solution

Operating conditions—

Detector, column, column temperature, mobile phase, and flow rate: Proceed as directed in the operating conditions in the Assay.

Time span of measurement: About 1.8 times as long as the retention time of quetiapine, beginning after the solvent peak.

System suitability—

Test for required detectability: Pipet 5 mL of the standard solution, and add the mobile phase to make exactly 50 mL. Confirm that the peak area of quetiapine obtained with 50 μL of this solution is equivalent to 7 to 13% of that with 50 μL of the standard solution.

System performance: When the procedure is run with 50 μL of the standard solution under the above operating conditions, the number of theoretical plates and the symmetry factor of the peak of quetiapine are not less than 6000 and not more than 2.0, respectively.

System repeatability: When the test is repeated 6 times with 50 μL of the standard solution under the above operating conditions, the relative standard deviation of the peak area of quetiapine is not more than 2.0%.

(ii)—To 20 mg of Quetiapine Fumarate add 30 mL of a mixture of acetonitrile, water and the mobile phase (2:1:1), dissolve by sonicating, add the same mixture to make 50 mL, and use this solution as the sample solution. Pipet 5 mL of the sample solution, and add the same mixture to make exactly 100 mL. Pipet 5 mL of this solution, add the same mixture to make exactly 50 mL, and use this solution as the standard solution. Perform the test with exactly 50 μL each of the sample solution and standard solution as directed under Liquid Chromatography <*2.01*> according to the following conditions. Determine each peak area by the automatic integration method, and calculate the amount of each related substance by the following equation: the amount is not more than 0.10%. For the area of the peak, having a relative retention time of about 1.9 to quetiapine, multiply its correction factor, 0.8.

Amount (%) of each related substance = $A_T/A_S \times 1/2$

A_S: Peak area of quetiapine obtained from the standard solution

A_T: Each peak area other than quetiapine obtained from the sample solution

Operating conditions—

Detector: An ultraviolet absorption photometer (wavelength: 250 nm).

Column: A stainless steel column 4.6 mm in inside diameter and 25 cm in length, packed with octylsilanized silica gel for liquid chromatography (5 μm in particle diameter).

Column temperature: A constant temperature of about 25°C.

Mobile phase: A mixture of methanol, diammonium hydrogen phosphate solution (33 in 12,500) and acetonitrile (70:21:9).

Flow rate: Adjust so that the retention time of quetiapine is about 3.5 minutes.

Time span of measurement: About 8 times as long as the retention time of quetiapine, beginning from about 1.2 times the retention time of quetiapine.

System suitability—

Test for required detectability: Pipet 5 mL of the standard solution, and add a mixture of acetonitrile, water and the mobile phase (2:1:1) to make exactly 50 mL. Confirm that the peak area of quetiapine obtained with 50 μL of this solution is equivalent to 7 to 13% of that with 50 μL of the standard solution.

System performance: When the procedure is run with 50 μL of the standard solution under the above operating conditions, the number of theoretical plates and the symmetry factor of the peak of quetiapine are not less than 3000 and not more than 2.0, respectively.

System repeatability: When the test is repeated 6 times with 50 μL of the standard solution under the above operating conditions, the relative standard deviation of the peak area of quetiapine is not more than 2.0%.

(iii)—The total amount of the related substances obtained in (i) and (ii) is not more than 0.5%.

Water <*2.48*> Not more than 0.5% (Weigh accurately about 0.1 g of Quetiapine Fumarate, transfer to a centrifuge tube, add exactly 4 mL of methanol for water determination, shake vigorously for 1 minute, and centrifuge at 2000 round per minute for 5 minutes. Pipet 1 mL of the supernatant liquid and perform the test. Perform a blank determination in the same manner, and make any necessary correction. Coulometric titration).

Residue on ignition <*2.44*> Not more than 0.1% (1 g).

Assay Weigh accurately about 20 mg each of Quetiapine Fumarate and Quetiapine Fumarate RS (separately determine the water <*2.48*> in the same manner as Quetiapine Fumarate), add 60 mL of the mobile phase to them, dissolve by sonicating, and add the mobile phase to make exactly 100 mL. Pipet 10 mL each of these solutions, add the mobile phase to make exactly 25 mL, and use these solutions as the sample solution and the standard solution, respectively. Perform the test with exactly 50 μL each of the sample solution and standard solution as directed under Liquid Chromatography <*2.01*> according to the following conditions, and determine the peak areas, A_T and A_S, of quetiapine in each solution.

$$\text{Amount (mg) of quetiapine fumarate } [(C_{21}H_{25}N_3O_2S)_2.C_4H_4O_4] = M_S \times A_T/A_S$$

M_S: Amount (mg) of Quetiapine Fumarate RS taken, calculated on the anhydrous basis

Operating conditions—

Detector: An ultraviolet absorption photometer (wavelength: 230 nm).

Column: A stainless steel column 4.6 mm in inside diameter and 25 cm in length, packed with octylsilanized silica gel for liquid chromatography (5 μm in particle diameter).

Column temperature: A constant temperature of about 25°C.

Mobile phase: Dissolve 2.6 g of diammonium hydrogen phosphate in 1000 mL of water, and adjust to pH 6.5 with phosphoric acid. To 39 volumes of this solution add 54 volumes of methanol and 7 volumes of acetonitrile.

Flow rate: Adjust so that the retention time of quetiapine is about 15 minutes.

System suitability—

System performance: When the procedure is run with 50 μL of the standard solution under the above operating conditions, the number of theoretical plates and the symmetry factor of the peak of quetiapine are not less than 6000 and not more than 2.0, respectively.

System repeatability: When the test is repeated 6 times with 50 μL of the standard solution under the above operating conditions, the relative standard deviation of the peak area of quetiapine is not more than 1.0%.

Containers and storage Containers—Tight containers.

Quetiapine Fumarate Fine Granules

クエチアピンフマル酸塩細粒

Quetiapine Fumarate Fine Granules contain not less than 95.0% and not more than 105.0% of the labeled amount of quetiapine ($C_{21}H_{25}N_3O_2S$: 383.51).

Method of preparation Prepare as directed under Granules, with Quetiapine Fumarate.

Identification Powder Quetiapine Fumarate Fine Granules. To a portion of the powder, equivalent to 12.5 mg of quetiapine ($C_{21}H_{25}N_3O_2S$), add 60 mL of a mixture of water and acetonitrile (1:1), shake, then add the same mixture to make 100 mL, and filter. To 3 mL of the filtrate add the same mixture to make 25 mL. Determine the absorption spectrum of this solution as directed under Ultraviolet-visible Spectrophotometry <2.24>: it exhibits a maximum between 290 nm and 296 nm.

Dissolution <6.10> When the test is performed at 50 revolutions per minute according to the Paddle method, using 900 mL of water as the dissolution medium, the dissolution rate in 30 minutes of Quetiapine Fumarate Fine Granules is not less than 80%.

Start the test with an accurately weighed amount of Quetiapine Fumarate Fine Granules, equivalent to about 0.1 g of quetiapine ($C_{21}H_{25}N_3O_2S$), withdraw not less than 10 mL of the medium at the specified minute after starting the test, and filter through a membrane filter with a pore size not exceeding 1.0 μm. Discard not less than 5 mL of the first filtrate, pipet 4 mL of the subsequent filtrate, add water to make exactly 20 mL, and use this solution as the sample solution. Separately, weigh accurately about 32 mg of Quetiapine Fumarate RS (separately determine the water <2.48> in the same manner as Quetiapine Fumarate), and dissolve in water to make exactly 50 mL. Pipet 4 mL of this solution, add water to make exactly 100 mL, and use this solution as the standard solution. Determine the absorbances, A_T and A_S, at 289 nm of the sample solution and standard solution as directed under Ultraviolet-visible Spectrophotometry <2.24>.

Dissolution rate (%) with respect to the labeled amount of quetiapine ($C_{21}H_{25}N_3O_2S$)

$$= M_S/M_T \times A_T/A_S \times 1/C \times 360 \times 0.869$$

M_S: Amount (mg) of Quetiapine Fumarate RS taken, calculated on the anhydrous basis

M_T: Amount (g) of Quetiapine Fumarate Fine Granules taken

C: Labeled amount (mg) of quetiapine ($C_{21}H_{25}N_3O_2S$) in 1 g

Assay To an accurately weighed amount of Quetiapine Fumarate Fine Granules, equivalent to about 0.25 g of quetiapine ($C_{21}H_{25}N_3O_2S$), add 10 mL of water, and allow to stand for 15 minutes. Add 100 mL of the mobile, shake for 15 minutes, then add the mobile phase to make exactly 200 mL, and stir the solution thoroughly. After standing for 15 minutes, pipet 6 mL of the supernatant liquid, add the mobile phase to make exactly 50 mL, and filter through a membrane filter with a pore size not exceeding 0.45 μm. Discard the first 5 mL of the filtrate, and use the subsequent filtrate as the sample solution. Separately, weigh accurately about 17 mg of Quetiapine Fumarate RS (separately determine the water <2.48> in the same manner as Quetiapine Fumarate), add 60 mL of the mobile phase, dissolve by sonicating, then add the mobile phase to make exactly 100 mL, and use this solution as the standard solution. Perform the test with exactly 50 μL each of the sample solution and standard solution as directed under Liquid Chromatography <2.01> according to the following conditions, and determine the peak areas, A_T and A_S, of quetiapine in each solution.

Amount (mg) of quetiapine ($C_{21}H_{25}N_3O_2S$)

$$= M_S \times A_T/A_S \times 50/3 \times 0.869$$

M_S: Amount (mg) of Quetiapine Fumarate RS taken, calculated on the anhydrous basis

Operating conditions—

Detector: An ultraviolet absorption photometer (wavelength: 230 nm).

Column: A stainless steel column 4.6 mm in inside diameter and 25 cm in length, packed with octylsilanized silica gel for liquid chromatography (5 μm in particle diameter).

Column temperature: A constant temperature of about 25°C.

Mobile phase: A mixture of methanol, diammonium hydrogen phosphate solution (33 in 12,500) and acetonitrile (54:39:7).

Flow rate: Adjust so that the retention time of quetiapine is about 15 minutes.

System suitability—

System performance: When the procedure is run with 50 μL of the standard solution under the above operating conditions, the number of theoretical plates and the symmetry factor of the peak of quetiapine are not less than 7000 and not more than 1.5, respectively.

System repeatability: When the test is repeated 6 times with 50 μL of the standard solution under the above operating conditions, the relative standard deviation of the peak area of quetiapine is not more than 1.0%.

Containers and storage Containers—Tight containers.

Quetiapine Fumarate Tablets

クエチアピンフマル酸塩錠

Quetiapine Fumarate Tablets contain not less than 95.0% and not more than 105.0% of the labeled amount of quetiapine ($C_{21}H_{25}N_3O_2S$: 383.51).

Method of preparation Prepare as directed under Tablets, with Quetiapine Fumarate.

Identification Powder Quetiapine Fumarate Tablets. To a portion of the powder, equivalent to about 12.5 mg of quetiapine ($C_{21}H_{25}N_3O_2S$), add 5 mL of water, shake, add 60

mL of a mixture of water and acetonitrile (1:1), shake, then add the same mixture to make 100 mL, and filter. To 3 mL of the filtrate add the same mixture to make 25 mL. Determine the absorption spectrum of this solution as directed under Ultraviolet-visible Spectrophotometry <*2.24*>: it exhibits a maximum between 290 nm and 296 nm.

Purity Related substances—To 10 Quetiapine Fumarate Tablets add 10 mL of water, allow to stand for 15 minutes, then shake for 25 minutes, and add a mixture of water and acetonitrile (1:1) to make exactly 200 mL. Stir this solution for 4 hours, and allow to stand for 15 minutes. Pipet 3 mL of this solution, add the mobile phase so that each mL contains about 0.15 mg of quetiapine ($C_{21}H_{25}N_3O_2S$), and filter through a membrane filter with a pore size not exceeding 0.45 μm. Discard the first 5 mL of the filtrate, and use the subsequent filtrate as the sample solution. Pipet 1 mL of the sample solution, add the mobile phase to make exactly 100 mL, and use this solution as the standard solution. Perform the test with exactly 50 μL each of the sample solution and standard solution as directed under Liquid Chromatography <*2.01*> according to the following conditions. Determine each peak area by the automatic integration method: the area of the peak with the relative retention time of about 0.6 to quetiapine obtained from the sample solution is not larger than 1/5 times the peak area of quetiapine from the standard solution, the area of the peak other than quetiapine and the peak mentioned above from the sample solution is not larger than 1/10 times the peak area of quetiapine from the standard solution, and the total area of the peaks other than quetiapine and the peak with the relative retention time of about 0.6 is not larger than 1/5 times the peak area of quetiapine from the standard solution.

Operating conditions—

Detector, column, column temperature, mobile phase, and flow rate: Proceed as directed in the operating conditions in the Assay.

Time span of measurement: About 2.3 times as long as the retention time of quetiapine, beginning after the peak of fumaric acid.

System suitability—

Test for required detectability: Pipet 5 mL of the standard solution, and add the mobile phase to make exactly 50 mL. Confirm that the peak area of quetiapine obtained with 50 μL of this solution is equivalent to 7 to 13% of that with 50 μL of the standard solution.

System performance: When the procedure is run with 50 μL of the standard solution under the above operating conditions, the number of theoretical plates and the symmetry factor of the peak of quetiapine are not less than 7000 and not more than 1.5, respectively.

System repeatability: When the test is repeated 6 times with 50 μL of the standard solution under the above operating conditions, the relative standard deviation of the peak area of quetiapine is not more than 2.0%.

Uniformity of dosage units <*6.02*> Perform the Mass variation test, or the Content uniformity test according to the following method: it meets the requirement.

To 1 tablet of Quetiapine Fumarate Tablets add 5 mL of water, allow to stand for 15 minutes, then shake for 25 minutes, add 30 mL of a mixture of water and acetonitrile (1:1), shake, and add the same mixture to make exactly 50 mL. Stir this solution for 4 hours, and allow to stand for 15 minutes. To exactly 8 mL of this solution, add the mobile phase to make exactly *V* mL so that each mL contains about 0.16 mg of quetiapine ($C_{21}H_{25}N_3O_2S$), and filter through a membrane filter with a pore size not exceeding 0.45 μm. Discard the first 5 mL of the filtrate, and use the subsequent filtrate as the sample solution. Separately, weigh accurately about 18 mg of Quetiapine Fumarate RS (separately determine the water <*2.48*> in the same manner as Quetiapine Fumarate), add 60 mL of the mobile phase, dissolve by sonicating, then add the mobile phase to make exactly 100 mL, and use this solution as the standard solution. Then, proceed as directed in the Assay.

$$\text{Amount (mg) of quetiapine } (C_{21}H_{25}N_3O_2S) = M_S \times A_T/A_S \times V/16 \times 0.869$$

M_S: Amount (mg) of Quetiapine Fumarate RS taken, calculated on the anhydrous basis

Dissolution <*6.10*> When the test is performed at 50 revolutions per minute according to the Paddle method, using 900 mL of water as the dissolution medium, the dissolution rate in 30 minutes of Quetiapine Fumarate Tablets is not less than 75%.

Start the test with 1 tablet of Quetiapine Fumarate Tablets, withdraw not less than 20 mL of the medium at the specified minute after starting the test, and filter through a membrane filter with a pore size not exceeding 0.45 μm. Discard not less than 5 mL of the first filtrate, pipet *V* mL of the subsequent filtrate, add the mobile phase to make exactly *V′* mL so that each mL contains about 14 μg of quetiapine ($C_{21}H_{25}N_3O_2S$), and use this solution as the sample solution. Separately, weigh accurately about 20 mg of Quetiapine Fumarate RS (separately determine the water <*2.48*> in the same manner as Quetiapine Fumarate), add 60 mL of the mobile phase, sonicate to dissolve, and add the mobile phase to make exactly 100 mL. Pipet 8 mL of this solution, add the mobile phase to make exactly 100 mL, and use this solution as the standard solution. Perform the test with exactly 50 μL each of the sample solution and standard solution as directed under Liquid Chromatography <*2.01*> according to the following conditions, and determine the peak areas, A_T and A_S, of quetiapine in each solution.

$$\text{Dissolution rate (\%) with respect to the labeled amount of quetiapine } (C_{21}H_{25}N_3O_2S) = M_S \times A_T/A_S \times V'/V \times 1/C \times 72 \times 0.869$$

M_S: Amount (mg) of Quetiapine Fumarate RS taken, calculated on the anhydrous basis

C: Labeled amount (mg) of quetiapine ($C_{21}H_{25}N_3O_2S$) in 1 tablet

Operating conditions—

Detector: An ultraviolet absorption photometer (wavelength: 230 nm).

Column: A stainless steel column 4 mm in inside diameter and 8 cm in length, packed with octylsilanized silica gel for liquid chromatography (5 μm in particle diameter).

Column temperature: A constant temperature of about 25°C.

Mobile phase: A mixture of methanol, a solution of diammonium hydrogen phosphate (33 in 12,500) and acetonitrile (54:39:7).

Flow rate: Adjust so that the retention time of quetiapine is about 4 minutes.

System suitability—

System performance: When the procedure is run with 50 μL of the standard solution under the above operating conditions, the number of theoretical plates and the symmetry factor of the peak of quetiapine are not less than 1400 and not more than 1.5, respectively.

System repeatability: When the test is repeated 6 times with 50 μL of the standard solution under the above operat-

ing conditions, the relative standard deviation of the peak area of quetiapine is not more than 2.0%.

Assay To 20 Quetiapine Fumarate Tablets add 20 mL of water, allow to stand for 15 minutes, shake for 25 minutes, and add a mixture of water and acetonitrile (1:1) to make exactly 500 mL. Stir the solution for 4 hours. After standing for 15 minutes, pipet 4 mL of this solution, and add the mobile phase to make exactly *V* mL so that each mL contains about 0.16 mg of quetiapine ($C_{21}H_{25}N_3O_2S$). Filter this solution through a membrane filter with a pore size not exceeding 0.45 μm. Discard the first 5 mL of the filtrate, and use the subsequent filtrate as the sample solution. Separately, weigh accurately about 18 mg of Quetiapine Fumarate RS (separately determine the water <*2.48*> in the same manner as Quetiapine Fumarate), add 60 mL of the mobile phase, dissolve by sonicating, then add the mobile phase to make exactly 100 mL, and use this solution as the standard solution. Perform the test with exactly 50 μL each of the sample solution and standard solution as directed under Liquid Chromatography <*2.01*> according to the following conditions, and determine the peak areas, A_T and A_S, of quetiapine in each solution.

Amount (mg) of quetiapine ($C_{21}H_{25}N_3O_2S$) in 1 tablet of Quetiapine Fumarate Tablets
$= M_S \times A_T/A_S \times V/16 \times 0.869$

M_S: Amount (mg) of Quetiapine Fumarate RS taken, calculated on the anhydrous basis

Operating conditions—

Detector: An ultraviolet absorption photometer (wavelength: 230 nm).

Column: A stainless steel column 4.6 mm in inside diameter and 25 cm in length, packed with octylsilanized silica gel for liquid chromatography (5 μm in particle diameter).

Column temperature: A constant temperature of about 25°C.

Mobile phase: A mixture of methanol, diammonium hydrogen phosphate solution (33 in 12,500) and acetonitrile (54:39:7).

Flow rate: Adjust so that the retention time of quetiapine is about 15 minutes.

System suitability—

System performance: When the procedure is run with 50 μL of the standard solution under the above operating conditions, the number of theoretical plates and the symmetry factor of the peak of quetiapine are not less than 7000 and not more than 1.5, respectively.

System repeatability: When the test is repeated 6 times with 50 μL of the standard solution under the above operating conditions, the relative standard deviation of the peak area of quetiapine is not more than 1.0%.

Containers and storage Containers—Tight containers.

Quinapril Hydrochloride

キナプリル塩酸塩

$C_{25}H_{30}N_2O_5.HCl$: 474.98
(3*S*)-2-((2*S*)-2-{[(1*S*)-1-Ethoxycarbonyl-3-phenylpropyl]amino}propanoyl)-1,2,3,4-tetrahydroisoquinoline-3-carboxylic acid monohydrochloride
[*82586-55-8*]

Quinapril Hydrochloride contains not less than 99.0% and not more than 101.0% of quinapril hydrochloride ($C_{25}H_{30}N_2O_5.HCl$), calculated on the anhydrous basis.

Description Quinapril Hydrochloride occurs as a white powder.

It is very soluble in methanol, freely soluble in water and in ethanol (99.5), and soluble in acetic acid (100).

It is deliquescent.

Identification (1) Determine the absorption spectrum of a solution of Quinapril Hydrochloride in methanol (1 in 2000) as directed under Ultraviolet-visible Spectrophotometry <*2.24*>, and compare the spectrum with the Reference Spectrum: both spectra exhibit similar intensities of absorption at the same wavelengths.

(2) Determine the infrared absorption spectrum of Quinapril Hydrochloride as directed in the potassium chloride disk method under Infrared Spectrophotometry <*2.25*>, and compare the spectrum with the Reference Spectrum: both spectra exhibit similar intensities of absorption at the same wave numbers.

(3) A solution of Quinapril Hydrochloride (1 in 20) responds to Qualitative Tests <*1.09*> for chloride.

Optical rotation <*2.49*> $[\alpha]_D^{20}$: +14.4 – +16.0° (0.5 g calculated on the anhydrous basis, methanol, 25 mL, 100 mm).

Purity (1) Heavy metals <*1.07*>—Proceed with 1.0 g of Quinapril Hydrochloride according to Method 2, and perform the test. Prepare the control solution with 2.0 mL of Standard Lead Solution (not more than 20 ppm).

(2) Related substances—Dissolve 50 mg of Quinapril Hydrochloride in 50 mL of a mixture of phosphate buffer solution (pH 7.0) and acetonitrile for liquid chromatography (1:1), and use this solution as the sample solution. Pipet 1 mL of the sample solution, add a mixture of phosphate buffer solution (pH 7.0) and acetonitrile for liquid chromatography (1:1) to make exactly 200 mL, and use this solution as the standard solution. Perform the test with exactly 10 μL each of the sample solution and standard solution as directed under Liquid Chromatography <*2.01*> according to the following conditions. Determine each peak area by the automatic integration method: the area of the peaks, having the relative retention time of about 0.5 and about 2.0 to quinapril, obtained from the sample solution are not larger than the peak area of quinapril from the standard solution, respectively, the area of peak other than quinapril and the peak mentioned above from the sample solution are not larger than 2/5 times the peak area of quinapril from the standard solution, and the total area of the peaks other than

quinapril from the sample solution is not larger than 3 times the peak area of quinapril from the standard solution.

Operating conditions—

Detector: An ultraviolet absorption photometer (wavelength: 214 nm).

Column: A stainless steel column 6 mm in inside diameter and 15 cm in length, packed with octadecylsilanized silica gel for liquid chromatography (5 μm in particle diameter).

Column temperature: A constant temperature of about 25°C.

Mobile phase: While keeping the temperature not below 25°C, adjust to pH 2.0 of 0.2 mol/L potassium dihydrogen phosphate TS with perchloric acid. To 1000 mL of this solution add 1000 mL of acetonitrile for liquid chromatography.

Flow rate: Adjust so that the retention time of quinapril is about 7 minutes.

Time span of measurement: About 4 times as long as the retention time of quinapril, beginning after the solvent peak.

System suitability—

Test for required detectability: Pipet 10 mL of the standard solution, and add a mixture of phosphate buffer solution (pH 7.0) and acetonitrile for liquid chromatography (1:1) to make exactly 100 mL. Confirm that the peak area of quinapril obtained with 10 μL of this solution is equivalent to 7 to 13% of that with 10 μL of the standard solution.

System performance: When the procedure is run with 10 μL of the standard solution under the above operating conditions, the number of theoretical plates and the symmetry factor of the peak of quinapril are not less than 5000 and not more than 1.5, respectively.

System repeatability: When the test is repeated 6 times with 10 μL of the standard solution under the above operating conditions, the relative standard deviation of the peak area of quinapril is not more than 2.0%.

Water 〈*2.48*〉 Not more than 1.0% (0.2 g, coulometric titration).

Residue on ignition 〈*2.44*〉 Not more than 0.1% (1 g).

Assay Start to titrate within 3 minutes after dissolving Quinapril Hydrochloride. Weigh accurately about 0.5 g of Quinapril Hydrochloride, dissolve in 70 mL of acetic acid (100), add 4 mL of bismuth nitrate TS, and titrate 〈*2.50*〉 with 0.1 mol/L perchloric acid VS (potentiometric titration). Perform a blank determination in the same manner, and make any necessary correction.

Each mL of 0.1 mol/L perchloric acid VS
= 47.50 mg of $C_{25}H_{30}N_2O_5.HCl$

Containers and storage Containers—Tight containers.

Storage—In a cold place.

Quinapril Hydrochloride Tablets

キナプリル塩酸塩錠

Quinapril Hydrochloride Tablets contain not less than 93.0% and not more than 107.0% of the labeled amount of quinapril hydrochloride ($C_{25}H_{30}N_2O_5.HCl$: 474.98).

Method of preparation Prepare as directed under Tablets, with Quinapril Hydrochloride.

Identification To a quantity of powdered Quinapril Hydrochloride Tablets, equivalent to 20 mg of Quinapril Hydrochloride, add 10 mL of methanol, shake for 5 minutes, and centrifuge. To 5 mL of the supernatant liquid add 0.5 mL of dilute hydrochloric acid, and add methanol to make 20 mL. Determine the absorption spectrum of this solution as directed under Ultraviolet-visible Spectrophotometry 〈*2.24*〉: it exhibits maxima between 256 nm and 260 nm, between 262 nm and 266 nm, and between 269 nm and 273 nm.

Purity To an amount of the supernatant liquid obtained in the Assay add a mixture of phosphate buffer solution (pH 7.0) and acetonitrile for liquid chromatography (1:1) so that each mL contains 0.2 mg of Quinapril Hydrochloride, and use this solution as the sample solution. Pipet 3 mL of the sample solution, add a mixture of phosphate buffer solution (pH 7.0) and acetonitrile for liquid chromatography (1:1) to make exactly 200 mL, and use this solution as the standard solution. Perform the test with exactly 10 μL each of the sample solution and standard solution as directed under Liquid Chromatography 〈*2.01*〉 according to the following conditions. Determine each peak area by the automatic integration method: the area of the peak having the relative retention time of about 0.5 to quinapril obtained from the sample solution is not larger than 2 times the peak area of quinapril from the standard solution, and the area of the peak, having the relative retention time of about 2.0 from the sample solution is not larger than the peak area of quinapril from the standard solution.

Operating conditions—

Proceed as directed in the operating conditions in the Purity (2) under Quinapril Hydrochloride.

System suitability—

System performance: When the procedure is run with 10 μL of the standard solution under the above operating conditions, the number of theoretical plates and the symmetry factor of the peak of quinapril are not less than 5000 and not more than 1.5, respectively.

System repeatability: When the test is repeated 6 times with 10 μL of the standard solution under the above operating conditions, the relative standard deviation of the peak area of quinapril is not more than 2.0%.

Uniformity of dosage units 〈*6.02*〉 Perform the test according to the following method: it meets the requirement of the Content uniformity test.

To 1 tablet of Quinapril Hydrochloride Tablets add $3V/5$ mL of a mixture of phosphate buffer solution (pH 7.0) and acetonitrile for liquid chromatography (1:1), shake vigorously to disintegrate the tablet, shake again for 10 minutes, add a mixture of phosphate buffer solution (pH 7.0) and acetonitrile for liquid chromatography (1:1) to make exactly V mL so that each mL contains about 0.22 mg of quinapril hydrochloride ($C_{25}H_{30}N_2O_5.HCl$), and centrifuge. Pipet 15 mL of the supernatant liquid, add exactly 2 mL of the internal standard solution, add a mixture of phosphate buffer solution (pH 7.0) and acetonitrile for liquid chromatography (1:1) to make 50 mL, and use this solution as the sample solution. Then, proceed as directed in the Assay.

Amount (mg) of quinapril hydrochloride ($C_{25}H_{30}N_2O_5.HCl$)
$= M_S \times Q_T/Q_S \times V/120$

M_S: Amount (mg) of quinapril hydrochloride for assay taken, calculated on the anhydrous basis

Internal standard solution—A solution of butyl parahydroxybenzoate in a mixture of phosphate buffer solution (pH 7.0) and acetonitrile for liquid chromatography (1:1) (1 in 800).

Dissolution 〈*6.10*〉 When the test is performed at 75 revolutions per minute according to the Paddle method, using 900 mL of water as the dissolution medium, the dissolution rate in 15 minutes of Quinapril Hydrochloride Tablets is not less than 80%.

Start the test with 1 tablet of Quinapril Hydrochloride Tablets, withdraw not less than 20 mL of the medium at the specified minute after starting the test, and filter through a membrane filter with a pore size not exceeding 0.45 μm. Discard not less than 10 mL of the first filtrate, pipet *V* mL of the subsequent filtrate, add a mixture of phosphate buffer solution (pH 7.0) and acetonitrile for liquid chromatography (1:1) to make exactly *V′* mL so that each mL contains about 1.2 μg of quinapril hydrochloride ($C_{25}H_{30}N_2O_5.HCl$), and use this solution as the sample solution. Separately, weigh accurately about 24 mg of quinapril hydrochloride for assay (separately, determine the water *<2.48>* in the same manner as Quinapril Hydrochloride), and dissolve in a mixture of phosphate buffer solution (pH 7.0) and acetonitrile for liquid chromatography (1:1) to make exactly 200 mL. Pipet 2 mL of this solution, add a mixture of phosphate buffer solution (pH 7.0) and acetonitrile for liquid chromatography (1:1) to make exactly 200 mL, and use this solution as the standard solution. Perform the test with exactly 10 μL each of the sample solution and standard solution as directed under Liquid Chromatography *<2.01>* according to the following conditions, and determine the peak areas, A_T and A_S, of quinapril in each solution.

Dissolution rate (%) with respect to the labeled amount of quinapril hydrochloride ($C_{25}H_{30}N_2O_5.HCl$)
$= M_S \times A_T/A_S \times V'/V \times 1/C \times 9/2$

M_S: Amount (mg) of quinapril hydrochloride for assay taken, calculated on the anhydrous basis
C: Labeled amount (mg) of quinapril hydrochloride ($C_{25}H_{30}N_2O_5.HCl$) in 1 tablet

Operating conditions—

Detector: An ultraviolet absorption photometer (wavelength: 214 nm).

Column: A stainless steel column 4.6 mm in inside diameter and 15 cm in length, packed with octadecylsilanized silica gel for liquid chromatography (5 μm in particle diameter).

Column temperature: A constant temperature of about 25°C.

Mobile phase: While keeping the temperature not below 25°C, adjust to pH 2.0 of 0.1 mol/L potassium dihydrogen phosphate TS with perchloric acid. To 1000 mL of this solution add 1500 mL of acetonitrile for liquid chromatography.

Flow rate: Adjust so that the retention time of quinapril is about 7 minutes.

System suitability—

System performance: When the procedure is run with 10 μL of the standard solution under the above operating conditions, the number of theoretical plates and the symmetry factor of the peak of quinapril are not less than 2000 and not more than 2.0, respectively.

System repeatability: When the test is repeated 6 times with 10 μL of the standard solution under the above operating conditions, the relative standard deviation of the peak area of quinapril is not more than 2.0%.

Assay To 20 Quinapril Hydrochloride Tablets add 300 mL of a mixture of phosphate buffer solution (pH 7.0) and acetonitrile for liquid chromatography (1:1), shake vigorously to disintegrate the tablets, shake again for 10 minutes, and add a mixture of phosphate buffer solution (pH 7.0) and acetonitrile for liquid chromatography (1:1) to make exactly 500 mL. Centrifuge this solution, pipet *V* mL of the supernatant liquid, equivalent to about 6.5 mg of quinapril hydrochloride ($C_{25}H_{30}N_2O_5.HCl$), add exactly 4 mL of the internal standard solution, add a mixture of phosphate buffer solution (pH 7.0) and acetonitrile for liquid chromatography (1:1) to make 100 mL, and use this solution as the sample solution. Separately, weigh accurately about 25 mg of quinapril hydrochloride for assay (separately, determine the water *<2.48>* in the same manner as Quinapril Hydrochloride), and dissolve in a mixture of phosphate buffer solution (pH 7.0) and acetonitrile for liquid chromatography (1:1) to make exactly 100 mL. Pipet 25 mL of this solution, add exactly 4 mL of the internal standard solution, add a mixture of phosphate buffer solution (pH 7.0) and acetonitrile for liquid chromatography (1:1) to make 100 mL, and use this solution as the standard solution. Perform the test with 10 μL each of the sample solution and standard solution as directed under Liquid Chromatography *<2.01>* according to the following conditions. Calculate the ratios, Q_T and Q_S, of the peak area of quinapril to that of the internal standard.

Amount (mg) of quinapril hydrochloride ($C_{25}H_{30}N_2O_5.HCl$) in 1 tablet
$= M_S \times Q_T/Q_S \times 1/V \times 25/4$

M_S: Amount (mg) of quinapril hydrochloride for assay taken, calculated on the anhydrous basis

*Internal standard solution—*A solution of butyl parahydroxybenzoate in a mixture of phosphate buffer solution (pH 7.0) and acetonitrile for liquid chromatography (1:1) (1 in 800).

Operating conditions—

Detector: An ultraviolet spectrophotometer (wavelength: 214 nm).

Column: A stainless steel column 6 mm in inside diameter and 15 cm in length, packed with octadecylsilanized silica gel for liquid chromatography (5 μm in particle diameter).

Column temperature: A constant temperature of about 25°C.

Mobile phase: While keeping the temperature not below 25°C, adjust to pH 2.0 of 0.2 mol/L potassium dihydrogen phosphate TS with perchloric acid. To 1000 mL of this solution add 1000 mL of acetonitrile for liquid chromatography.

Flow rate: Adjust so that the retention time of quinapril is about 7 minutes.

System suitability—

System performance: When the procedure is run with 10 μL of the standard solution under the above operating conditions, quinapril and the internal standard are eluted in this order with the resolution between these peaks being not less than 6.

System repeatability: When the test is repeated 6 times with 10 μL of the standard solution under the above operating conditions, the relative standard deviation of the ratio of the peak area of quinapril to that of the internal standard is not more than 1.0%.

Containers and storage Containers—Tight containers.

Quinidine Sulfate Hydrate

キニジン硫酸塩水和物

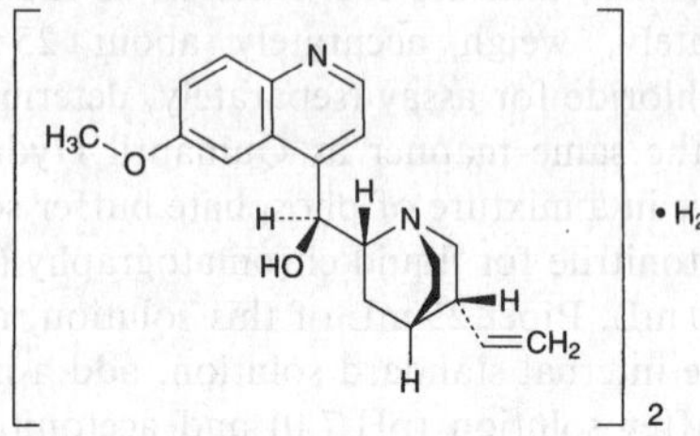

$(C_{20}H_{24}N_2O_2)_2.H_2SO_4.2H_2O$: 782.94

(9*S*)-6′-Methoxycinchonan-9-ol hemisulfate monohydrate

[6591-63-5]

Quinidine Sulfate Hydrate, when dried, contains not less than 98.5% of quinidine sulfate [$(C_{20}H_{24}N_2O_2)_2.H_2SO_4$: 746.91].

Description Quinidine Sulfate Hydrate occurs as white crystals. It is odorless, and has a very bitter taste.

It is freely soluble in ethanol (95) and in boiling water, sparingly soluble in water, and practically insoluble in diethyl ether. It, previously dried, is freely soluble in chloroform.

It darkens gradually by light.

Optical rotation $[\alpha]_D^{20}$: +275 – +287° (after drying, 0.5 g, 0.1 mol/L hydrochloric acid VS, 25 mL, 100 mm).

Identification **(1)** Dissolve 0.01 g of Quinidine Sulfate Hydrate in 10 mL of water and 2 to 3 drops of dilute sulfuric acid: a blue fluorescence is produced.

(2) To 5 mL of a solution of Quinidine Sulfate Hydrate (1 in 1000) add 1 to 2 drops of bromine TS, then add 1 mL of ammonia TS: a green color develops.

(3) To 5 mL of a solution of Quinidine Sulfate Hydrate (1 in 100) add 1 mL of silver nitrate TS, stir with a glass rod, and allow to stand for a short interval: a white precipitate is produced, and it dissolves on addition of nitric acid.

(4) Dissolve 0.4 g of Quinidine Sulfate Hydrate in 20 mL of water and 1 mL of dilute hydrochloric acid: the solution responds to Qualitative Tests <*1.09*> for sulfate.

pH <*2.54*> Dissolve 1.0 g of Quinidine Sulfate Hydrate in 100 mL of freshly boiled and cooled water: the pH of this solution is between 6.0 and 7.0.

Purity **(1)** Chloroform-ethanol-insoluble substances—Warm 2.0 g of Quinidine Sulfate Hydrate with 15 mL of a mixture of chloroform and ethanol (99.5) (2:1) at about 50°C for 10 minutes. After cooling, filter through a tared glass filter (G4) by gentle suction. Wash the residue with five 10-mL portions of a mixture of chloroform and ethanol (99.5) (2:1), and dry at 105°C for 1 hour: the mass of the residue is not more than 2.0 mg.

(2) Related substances—Dissolve 20 mg of Quinidine Sulfate Hydrate in the mobile phase to make exactly 100 mL, and use this solution as the sample solution. Separately, dissolve 25 mg of cinchonine in the mobile phase to make exactly 100 mL. Pipet 2 mL of this solution, add the mobile phase to make exactly 100 mL, and use this solution as the standard solution. Perform the test with exactly 50 μL each of the sample solution and standard solution as directed under Liquid Chromatography <*2.01*> according to the following conditions. Determine each peak area of the sample solution by the automatic integration method, and calculate their amounts by the area percentage method: the amount of dihydroquinidine sulfate is not more than 15.0%, and those of quinine sulfate and dihydroquinine sulfate are not more than 1.0%. The total area of the peaks other than the principal peak and the peaks mentioned above obtained from the sample solution is not larger than the peak area of cinchonine from the standard solution.

Operating conditions—

Detector: An ultraviolet absorption photometer (wavelength: 235 nm).

Column: A column about 4 mm in inside diameter and about 25 cm in length, packed with octadecylsilanized silica gel (10 μm in particle diameter).

Temperature: Room temperature.

Mobile phase: A mixture of water, acetonitrile, methanesulfonic acid TS and a solution of diethylamine (1 in 10) (43:5:1:1).

Flow rate: Adjust so that the retention time of quinidine is about 10 minutes.

Selection of column: Dissolve 0.01 g each of Quinidine Sulfate Hydrate and quinine sulfate hydrate in 5 mL of methanol, and add the mobile phase to make 50 mL. Proceed with 50 μL of this solution under the above operating conditions, and calculate the resolution. Use a column giving elution of quinidine, quinine, dihydroquinidine and dihydroquinine in this order with a resolution between quinidine and quinine and that between quinine and dihydroquinidine being not less than 1.2, respectively.

Detection sensitivity: Adjust the detection sensitivity so that the peak height of cinchonine obtained with 50 μL of the standard solution is between 5 mm and 10 mm.

Time span of measurement: About 2 times as long as the retention time of quinidine, beginning after the solvent peak.

(3) Readily carbonizable substances <*1.15*>—Take 0.20 g of Quinidine Sulfate Hydrate and perform the test: the solution has no more color than Matching Fluid M.

Loss on drying <*2.41*> Not more than 5.0% (1 g, 130 °C, 3 hours).

Residue on ignition <*2.44*> Not more than 0.1% (1 g).

Assay Weigh accurately about 0.5 g of Quinidine Sulfate Hydrate, previously dried, dissolve in 20 mL of acetic acid (100), and add 80 mL of acetic anhydride, and titrate <*2.50*> with 0.1 mol/L perchloric acid VS until the color of the solution changes from purple through blue to blue-green (indicator: 3 drops of crystal violet TS). Perform a blank determination in the same manner, and make any necessary correction.

Each mL of 0.1 mol/L perchloric acid VS
= 24.90 mg of $(C_{20}H_{24}N_2O_2)_2.H_2SO_4$

Containers and storage Containers—Well-closed containers.

Storage—Light-resistant.

Quinine Ethyl Carbonate

キニーネエチル炭酸エステル

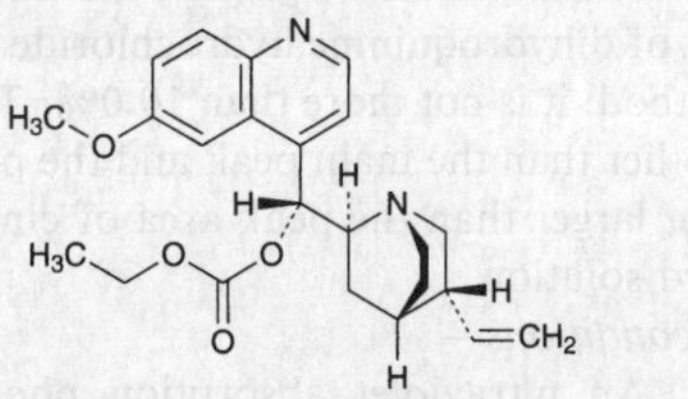

$C_{23}H_{28}N_2O_4$: 396.48
Ethyl (8*S*,9*R*)-6′-methoxycinchonan-9-yl carbonate
[*83-75-0*]

Quinine Ethyl Carbonate contains not less than 98.5% of quinine ethyl carbonate ($C_{23}H_{28}N_2O_4$), calculated on the anhydrous basis.

Description Quinine Ethyl Carbonate occurs as white crystals. It is odorless, and tasteless at first but slowly develops a bitter taste.

It is very soluble in methanol, freely soluble in ethanol (95) and in ethanol (99.5), soluble in diethyl ether, and practically insoluble in water.

It dissolves in dilute hydrochloric acid.

Identification **(1)** Determine the absorption spectrum of a solution of Quinine Ethyl Carbonate in methanol (1 in 20,000) as directed under Ultraviolet-visible Spectrophotometry 〈*2.24*〉, and compare the spectrum with the Reference Spectrum: both spectra exhibit similar intensities of absorption at the same wavelengths.

(2) Determine the infrared absorption spectrum of Quinine Ethyl Carbonate as directed in the potassium bromide disk method under Infrared Spectrophotometry 〈*2.25*〉, and compare the spectrum with the Reference Spectrum: both spectra exhibit similar intensities of absorption at the same wave numbers.

Optical rotation 〈*2.49*〉 $[\alpha]_D^{20}$: −42.2 – −44.0° (0.5 g calculated on the anhydrous basis, methanol, 50 mL, 100 mm).

Melting point 〈*2.60*〉 91 – 95°C

Purity **(1)** Chloride—Dissolve 0.30 g of Quinine Ethyl Carbonate in 10 mL of dilute nitric acid and 20 mL of water. To 5 mL of the solution add 2 to 3 drops of silver nitrate TS: no color develops.

(2) Sulfate 〈*1.14*〉—Dissolve 1.0 g of Quinine Ethyl Carbonate in 5 mL of dilute hydrochloric acid and water to make 50 mL, and perform the test using this solution as the test solution. Prepare the control solution with 1.0 mL of 0.005 mol/L sulfuric acid VS, 5 mL of dilute hydrochloric acid and water to make 50 mL (not more than 0.048%).

(3) Heavy metals 〈*1.07*〉—Proceed with 2.0 g of Quinine Ethyl Carbonate according to Method 2, and perform the test. Prepare the control solution with 2.0 mL of Standard Lead Solution (not more than 10 ppm).

(4) Related substances—Dissolve 20 mg of Quinine Ethyl Carbonate in the mobile phase to make exactly 100 mL, and use this solution as the sample solution. Separately, dissolve 25 mg of quinine sulfate hydrate in the mobile phase to make exactly 100 mL. Pipet 2 mL of this solution, add mobile phase to make exactly 100 mL, and use this solution as the standard solution. Perform the test with exactly 10 μL each of the sample solution and standard solution as directed under Liquid Chromatography 〈*2.01*〉 according to the following conditions. Determine each peak area of these solutions by the automatic integration method, and calculate the amount of a main impurity in the sample solution which appears at about 1.2 times of the retention time of quinine ethyl carbonate by the area percentage method: it is not more than 10.0%. The total area of the peaks other than the principal peak and the peak mentioned above obtained from the sample solution is not larger than the peak area of quinine from the standard solution.

Operating conditions—

Detector: An ultraviolet absorption photometer (wavelength: 235 nm).

Column: A stainless steel column about 4 mm in inside diameter and about 15 cm in length, packed with octadecylsilanized silica gel for liquid chromatography (5 μm in particle diameter).

Column temperature: A constant temperature of about 40°C.

Mobile phase: Dissolve 1.2 g of sodium 1-octanesulfonate in 1000 mL of a mixture of water and methanol (1:1), and adjust to pH 3.5 with diluted phosphoric acid (1 in 20).

Flow rate: Adjust so that the retention time of the peak of quinine ethyl carbonate is about 20 minutes.

Selection of column: Dissolve 5 mg each of Quinine Ethyl Carbonate and quinine sulfate hydrate in the mobile phase to make 50 mL. Proceed with 10 μL of this solution under the above operating conditions, and calculate the resolution. Use a column giving elution of quinine, dihydroquinine, quinine ethyl carbonate and the main impurity of quinine ethyl carbonate in this order with the resolution between the peaks of quinine and dihydroquinine being not less than 2.7, and between the peaks of quinine and quinine ethyl carbonate being not less than 5.

Detection sensitivity: Adjust the detection sensitivity so that the peak height of quinine obtained from 10 μL of the standard solution is between 5 mm and 10 mm.

Time span of measurement: About 2 times as long as the retention time of quinine ethyl carbonate.

Water 〈*2.48*〉 Not more than 3.0% (0.5 g, volumetric titration, direct titration).

Residue on ignition 〈*2.44*〉 Not more than 0.1% (1 g).

Assay Weigh accurately about 0.3 g of Quinine Ethyl Carbonate, dissolve in 60 mL of acetic acid (100), add 2 mL of acetic anhydride, and titrate 〈*2.50*〉 with 0.1 mol/L perchloric acid VS (potentiometric titration). Perform a blank determination in the same manner, and make any necessary correction.

Each mL of 0.1 mol/L perchloric acid VS
= 19.82 mg of $C_{23}H_{28}N_2O_4$

Containers and storage Containers—Well-closed containers.

Quinine Hydrochloride Hydrate

キニーネ塩酸塩水和物

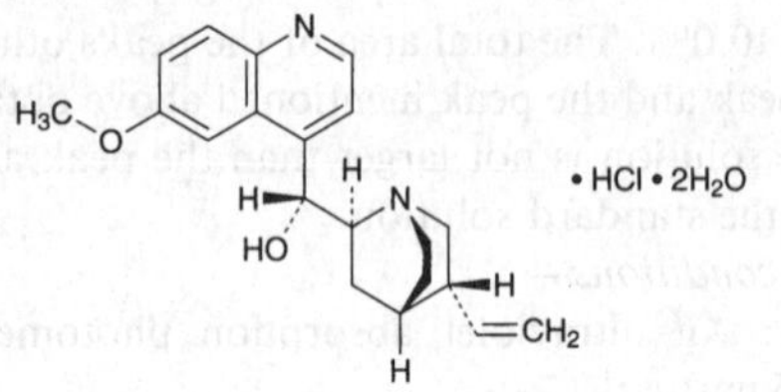

$C_{20}H_{24}N_2O_2.HCl.2H_2O$: 396.91
(8*S*,9*R*)-6′-Methoxycinchonan-9-ol monohydrochloride dihydrate
[*6119-47-7*]

Quinine Hydrochloride Hydrate, when dried, contains not less than 98.5% of quinine hydrochloride ($C_{20}H_{24}N_2O_2.HCl$: 360.88).

Description Quinine Hydrochloride Hydrate occurs as white crystals. It is odorless, and has a very bitter taste.

It is very soluble in ethanol (99.5), freely soluble in acetic acid (100), in acetic anhydride and in ethanol (95), soluble in water, and practically insoluble in diethyl ether.

It, previously dried, is freely soluble in chloroform.

It gradually changes to brown by light.

Identification (1) A solution of Quinine Hydrochloride Hydrate (1 in 50) shows no fluorescence. To 1 mL of the solution add 100 mL of water and 1 drop of dilute sulfuric acid: a blue fluorescence is produced.

(2) To 5 mL of a solution of Quinine Hydrochloride Hydrate (1 in 1000) add 1 to 2 drops of bromine TS and 1 mL of ammonia TS: a green color develops.

(3) To 5 mL of a solution of Quinine Hydrochloride Hydrate (1 in 50) add 1 mL of dilute nitric acid and 1 mL of silver nitrate TS: a white precipitate is produced. Collect the precipitate, and add an excess of ammonia TS: it dissolves.

Optical rotation <*2.49*> $[\alpha]_D^{20}$: −245 – −255° (after drying, 0.5 g, 0.1 mol/L hydrochloric acid VS, 25 mL, 100 mm).

pH <*2.54*> Dissolve 1.0 g of Quinine Hydrochloride Hydrate in 100 mL of freshly boiled and cooled water: the pH of this solution is between 6.0 and 7.0.

Purity (1) Sulfate <*1.14*>—Perform the test with 1.0 g of Quinine Hydrochloride Hydrate. Prepare the control solution with 1.0 mL of 0.005 mol/L sulfuric acid VS (not more than 0.048%).

(2) Barium—Dissolve 0.5 g of Quinine hydrochloride Hydrate in 10 mL of water by warming, and add 1 mL of dilute sulfuric acid: no turbidity is produced.

(3) Chloroform-ethanol-insoluble substances—Warm 2.0 g of Quinine Hydrochloride Hydrate with 15 mL of a mixture of chloroform and ethanol (99.5) (2:1) at 50°C for 10 minutes. After cooling, filter through a tared glass filter (G4) by gentle suction. Wash the residue with five 10-mL portions of a mixture of chloroform and ethanol (99.5) (2:1), dry at 105°C for 1 hour, and weigh: the mass of the residue so obtained is not more than 2.0 mg.

(4) Related substances—Dissolve 20 mg of Quinine Hydrochloride Hydrate in the mobile phase to make exactly 100 mL, and use this solution as the sample solution. Separately, dissolve 25 mg of cinchonidine in the mobile phase to make exactly 100 mL. Pipet 2 mL of this solution, add the mobile phase to make exactly 100 mL, and use this solution as the standard solution. Perform the test with exactly 50 μL each of the sample solution and standard solution as directed under Liquid Chromatography <*2.01*> according to the following conditions. Determine each peak area of the sample solution by the automatic integration method, and calculate the amount of dihydroquinine hydrochloride by the area percentage method: it is not more than 10.0%. The total area of the peaks other than the main peak and the peaks mentioned above is not larger than the peak area of cinchonidine from the standard solution.

Operating conditions—

Detector: An ultraviolet absorption photometer (wavelength: 235 nm).

Column: A stainless steel column about 4 mm in inside diameter and about 25 cm in length, packed with octadecylsilanized silica gel (10 μm in particle diameter).

Column temperature: Room temperature.

Mobile phase: A mixture of water, acetonitrile, methanesulfonic acid TS and a solution of diethylamine (1 in 10) (43:5:1:1).

Flow rate: Adjust so that the retention time of quinine is about 10 minutes.

Selection of column: Dissolve 10 mg each of Quinine Hydrochloride Hydrate and quinidine sulfate hydrate in 5 mL of methanol, and add the mobile phase to make 50 mL. Proceed with 50 μL of this solution under the above operating conditions. Use a column giving elution of quinidine, quinine, dihydroquinidine and dihydroquinine in this order with the resolution between quinidine and quinine, and that between quinine and dihydroquinidine being not less than 1.2, respectively.

Detection sensitivity: Adjust the detection sensitivity so that the peak height of cinchonidine from 50 μL of the standard solution is between 5 mm and 10 mm.

Time span of measurement: About 2 times as long as the retention time of quinine, beginning after the solvent peak.

(5) Readily carbonizable substances <*1.15*>—Perform the test with 0.25 g of Quinine Hydrochloride Hydrate. The solution has no more color than Matching Fluid M.

Loss on drying <*2.41*> Not more than 10.0% (1 g, 105°C, 5 hours).

Residue on ignition <*2.44*> Not more than 0.1% (1 g).

Assay Weigh accurately about 0.4 g of Quinine Hydrochloride Hydrate, previously dried, dissolve in 100 mL of a mixture of acetic anhydride and acetic acid (100) (7:3) by warming, cool, and titrate <*2.50*> with 0.1 mol/L perchloric acid VS (potentiometric titration). Perform a blank determination in the same manner, and make any necessary correction.

Each mL of 0.1 mol/L perchloric acid VS
= 18.04 mg of $C_{20}H_{24}N_2O_2.HCl$

Containers and storage Containers—Well-closed containers.

Storage—Light-resistant.

Quinine Sulfate Hydrate

キニーネ硫酸塩水和物

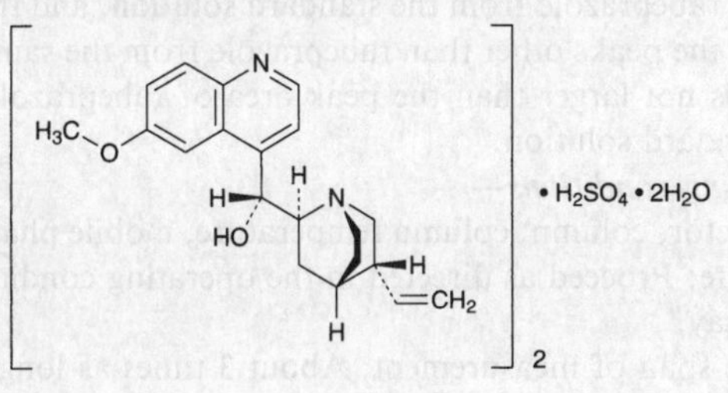

$(C_{20}H_{24}N_2O_2)_2.H_2SO_4.2H_2O$: 782.94
(8*S*,9*R*)-6′-Methoxycinchonan-9-ol hemisulfate monohydrate
[*6119-70-6*]

Quinine Sulfate Hydrate contains not less than 98.5% of quinine sulfate [$(C_{20}H_{24}N_2O_2)_2.H_2SO_4$: 746.91], calculated on the dried basis.

Description Quinine Sulfate Hydrate occurs as white, crystals or crystalline powder. It is odorless, and has a very bitter taste.

It is freely soluble in acetic acid (100), slightly soluble in water, in ethanol (95), in ethanol (99.5) and in chloroform, and practically insoluble in diethyl ether.

It gradually changes to brown by light.

Identification **(1)** Determine the absorption spectrum of a solution of Quinine Sulfate Hydrate (1 in 20,000) as directed under Ultraviolet-visible Spectrophotometry <*2.24*>, and compare the spectrum with the Reference Spectrum: both spectra exhibit similar intensities of absorption at the same wavelengths.

(2) Determine the infrared absorption spectrum of Quinine Sulfate Hydrate, previously dried, as directed in the potassium bromide disk method under Infrared Spectrophotometry <*2.25*>, and compare the spectrum with the Reference Spectrum: both spectra exhibit similar intensities of absorption at the same wave numbers.

(3) To 0.4 g of Quinine Sulfate Hydrate add 20 mL of water and 1 mL of dilute hydrochloric acid: the solution responds to Qualitative Tests <*1.09*> for sulfate.

Optical rotation <*2.49*> $[\alpha]_D^{20}$: −235 − −245°(after drying, 0.5 g, 0.1 mol/L hydrochloric acid VS, 25 mL, 100 mm).

pH <*2.54*> Shake 2.0 g of Quinine Sulfate Hydrate in 20 mL of freshly boiled and cooled water, and filter: the pH of this filtrate is between 5.5 and 7.0.

Purity **(1)** Heavy metals <*1.07*>—Proceed with 2.0 g of Quinine Sulfate Hydrate according to Method 2, and perform the test. Prepare the control solution with 2.0 mL of Standard Lead Solution (not more than 10 ppm).

(2) Chloroform-ethanol-insoluble substances—Warm 2.0 g of Quinine Sulfate Hydrate with 15 mL of a mixture of chloroform and ethanol (99.5) (2:1) at 50°C for 10 minutes. After cooling, filter through a tared glass filter (G4) by gentle suction. Wash the residue with five 10-mL portions of a mixture of chloroform and ethanol (99.5) (2:1), dry at 105°C for 1 hour, and weigh: the mass of the residue is not more than 2.0 mg.

(3) Related substances—Dissolve 20 mg of Quinine Sulfate Hydrate in the mobile phase to make exactly 100 mL, and use this solution as the sample solution. Separately, dissolve 25 mg of cinchonidine in the mobile phase to make exactly 100 mL. Pipet 2 mL of this solution, add the mobile phase to make exactly 100 mL, and use this solution as the standard solution. Perform the test with exactly 50 μL each of the sample solution and standard solution as directed under Liquid Chromatography <*2.01*> according to the following conditions. Determine each peak area from the sample solution by the automatic integration method, and calculate the amount of dihydroquinine sulfate by the area percentage method: it is not more than 5%. The total area of the peaks other than the main peak and the peaks mentioned above is not larger than the peak area of cinchonidine from the standard solution.

Operating conditions—

Detector: An ultraviolet absorption photometer (wavelength: 235 nm).

Column: A column about 4 mm in inside diameter and about 25 cm in length, packed with octadecylsilanized silica gel (10 μm in particle diameter).

Temperature: Room temperature.

Mobile phase: A mixture of water, acetonitrile, methane sulfonic acid TS and a solution of diethylamine (1 in 10) (43:5:1:1).

Flow rate: Adjust so that the retention time of quinine is about 10 minutes.

Selection of column: Dissolve 0.01 g each of Quinine Sulfate Hydrate and quinidine sulfate hydrate in 5 mL of methanol, and add the mobile phase to make 50 mL. Proceed with 50 μL of this solution under the above operating conditions, and calculate the resolution. Use a column giving elution of quinidine, quinine, dihydroquinidine and dihydroquinine in this order with the resolution between quinidine and quinine and that between quinine and dihydroquinidine being not less than 1.2, respectively.

Detection sensitivity: Adjust the detection sensitivity so that the peak height of cinchonidine obtained from 50 μL of the standard solution is between 5 mm and 10 mm.

Time span of measurement: About 2 times as long as the retention time of quinine, beginning after the solvent peak.

Loss on drying <*2.41*> 3.0% − 5.0% (1 g, 105°C, 3 hours).

Residue on ignition <*2.44*> Not more than 0.1% (1 g).

Assay Weigh accurately about 0.5 g of Quinine Sulfate Hydrate, dissolve in 20 mL of acetic acid (100), add 80 mL of acetic anhydride, and titrate <*2.50*> with 0.1 mol/L perchloric acid VS until the color of the solution changes from purple through blue to blue-green (indicator: 2 drops of crystal violet TS). Perform a blank determination in the same manner, and make any necessary correction.

Each mL of 0.1 mol/L perchloric acid VS
= 24.90 mg of $(C_{20}H_{24}N_2O_2)_2.H_2SO_4$

Containers and storage Containers—Well-closed containers.

Storage—Light-resistant.

Rabeprazole Sodium

ラベプラゾールナトリウム

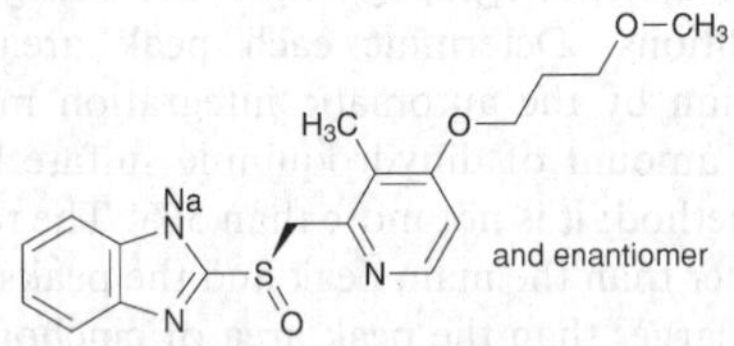

$C_{18}H_{20}N_3NaO_3S$: 381.42

Monosodium (*RS*)-2-({[4-(3-methoxypropoxy)-3-methylpyridin-2-yl]methyl}sulfinyl)-1*H*-benzimidazolide

[*117976-90-6*]

Rabeprazole Sodium contains not less than 98.0% and not more than 101.0% of rabeprazole sodium ($C_{18}H_{20}N_3NaO_3S$), calculated on the dried basis.

Description Rabeprazole Sodium occurs as a white to pale yellow-white powder.

It is very soluble in water, and freely soluble in ethanol (99.5).

It dissolves in 0.01 mol/L sodium hydroxide TS.

It is hygroscopic.

A solution of Rabeprazole Sodium (1 in 20) shows no optical rotation.

Rabeprazole Sodium shows crystal polymorphism.

Identification **(1)** Determine the absorption spectrum of a solution of Rabeprazole Sodium in 0.01 mol/L sodium hydroxide TS (1 in 100,000) as directed under Ultraviolet-visible Spectrophotometry <*2.24*>, and compare the spectrum with the Reference Spectrum or the spectrum of a solution of Rabeprazole Sodium RS prepared in the same manner as the sample solution: both spectra exhibit similar intensities of absorption at the same wavelengths.

(2) Determine the infrared absorption spectrum of Rabeprazole Sodium as directed in the potassium bromide disk method under Infrared Spectrophotometry <*2.25*>, and compare the spectrum with the Reference Spectrum or the spectrum of Rabeprazole Sodium RS: both spectra exhibit similar intensities of absorption at the same wave numbers. If any difference appears between the spectra, dissolve the sample, or the sample and the RS separately in ethanol (99.5), evaporate the ethanol at 40°C, dry the residues in vacuum at 55°C for 24 hours, and perform the test with the residues.

(3) A solution of Rabeprazole Sodium (1 in 10) responds to Qualitative Tests <*1.09*> for sodium salt.

Purity **(1)** Heavy metals <*1.07*>—Proceed with 2.0 g of Rabeprazole Sodium according to Method 2, and perform the test. Prepare the control solution with 2.0 mL of Standard Lead Solution (not more than 10 ppm).

(2) Related substances—Dissolve 50 mg of Rabeprazole Sodium in 50 mL of a mixture of methanol and 0.01 mol/L sodium hydroxide TS (3:2), and use this solution as the sample solution. Pipet 1 mL of the sample solution, add a mixture of methanol and 0.01 mol/L sodium hydroxide TS (3:2) to make exactly 100 mL, and use this solution as the standard solution. Perform the test with exactly 10 μL each of the sample solution and standard solution as directed under Liquid Chromatography <*2.01*> according to the following conditions, and determine each peak area by the automatic integration method: the area of the peak having the relative retention time of about 0.7 to rabeprazole obtained from the sample solution is not larger than 4/5 times the peak area of rabeprazole from the standard solution, the area of the peak other than rabeprazole and the peak mentioned above from the sample solution is not larger than 1/10 times the peak area of rabeprazole from the standard solution, and the total area of the peaks other than rabeprazole from the sample solution is not larger than the peak area of rabeprazole from the standard solution.

Operating conditions—

Detector, column, column temperature, mobile phase, and flow rate: Proceed as directed in the operating conditions in the Assay.

Time span of measurement: About 3 times as long as the retention time of rabeprazole, beginning after the solvent peak.

System suitability—

Test for required detectability: Pipet 5 mL of the standard solution, and add a mixture of methanol and 0.01 mol/L sodium hydroxide TS (3:2) to make exactly 100 mL. Confirm that the peak area of rabeprazole obtained with 10 μL of this solution is equivalent to 3.5 to 6.5% of that with 10 μL of the standard solution.

System performance: When the procedure is run with 10 μL of the standard solution under the above operating conditions, the number of theoretical plates and the symmetry factor of the peak of rabeprazole are not less than 3000 and not more than 1.5, respectively.

System repeatability: When the test is repeated 6 times with 10 μL of the standard solution under the above operating conditions, the relative standard deviation of the peak area of rabeprazole is not more than 2.0%.

Loss on drying <*2.41*> Not more than 1.0% (1 g, in vacuum, phosphorus (V) oxide, 24 hours. Take the sample to be tested while avoiding moisture absorption.).

Assay Take the sample to be tested while avoiding moisture absorption. Weigh accurately about 0.1 g each of Rabeprazole Sodium and Rabeprazole Sodium RS (separately determine the loss on drying <*2.41*> under the same conditions as Rabeprazole Sodium), dissolve each in a mixture of methanol and 0.01 mol/L sodium hydroxide TS (3:2) to make exactly 25 mL. Pipet 5 mL each of these solutions, add exactly 10 mL of the internal standard solution to each, then add a mixture of methanol and 0.01 mol/L sodium hydroxide TS (3:2) to make 100 mL, and use these solutions as the sample solution and the standard solution, respectively. Perform the test with 10 μL each of the sample solution and standard solution as directed under Liquid Chromatography <*2.01*> according to the following conditions, and calculate the ratios, Q_T and Q_S, of the peak area of rabeprazole to that of the internal standard.

Amount (mg) of sodium rabeprazole ($C_{18}H_{20}N_3NaO_3S$)
$= M_S \times Q_T/Q_S$

M_S: Amount (mg) of Rabeprazole Sodium RS taken, calculated on the dried basis

Internal standard solution—A solution of 1-amino-2-methylnaphthalene in a mixture of methanol and 0.01 mol/L sodium hydroxide TS (3:2) (1 in 250).

Operating conditions—

Detector: An ultraviolet absorption photometer (wavelength: 290 nm).

Column: A stainless steel column 4.6 mm in inside diameter and 15 cm in length, packed with octadecylsilanized silica gel for liquid chromatography (5 μm in particle diameter).

Column temperature: A constant temperature of about

30°C.

Mobile phase: A mixture of methanol and 0.05 mol/L phosphate buffer solution (pH 7.0) (3:2).

Flow rate: Adjust so that the retention time of rabeprazole is about 5 minutes.

System suitability—

System performance: When the procedure is run with 10 μL of the standard solution under the above operating conditions, rabeprazole and the internal standard are eluted in this order with the resolution between these peaks being not less than 4, and the symmetry factor of the peak of rabeprazole is not more than 2.0.

System repeatability: When the test is repeated 6 times with 10 μL of the standard solution under the above operating conditions, the relative standard deviation of the ratio of the peak area of rabeprazole to that of the internal standard is not more than 1.0%.

Containers and storage Containers—Tight containers.

Freeze-dried Inactivated Tissue Culture Rabies Vaccine

乾燥組織培養不活化狂犬病ワクチン

Freeze-dried Inactivated Tissue Culture Rabies Vaccine is a dried preparation containing inactivated rabies virus.

It conforms to the requirements of Freeze-dried Inactivated Tissue Culture Rabies Vaccine in the Minimum Requirements of Biologic Products.

Description Freeze-dried Inactivated Tissue Culture Rabies Vaccine becomes a colorless or light yellow-red clear liquid on addition of solvent.

Ranitidine Hydrochloride

ラニチジン塩酸塩

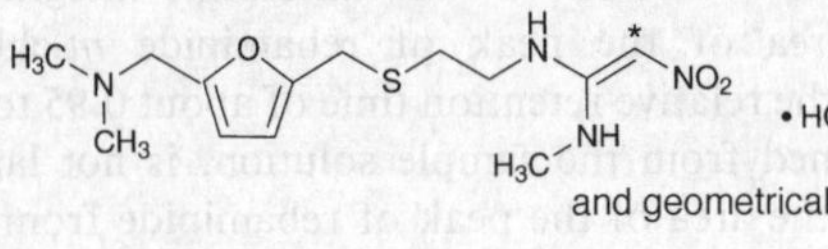

and geometrical isomer at C*

$C_{13}H_{22}N_4O_3S.HCl$: 350.86
(1*EZ*)-*N*-{2-[({5-[(Dimethylamino)methyl]furan-2-yl}methyl)sulfanyl]ethyl}-*N′*-methyl-2-nitroethene-1,1-diamine monohydrochloride
[66357-59-3]

Ranitidine Hydrochloride, when dried, contains not less than 97.5% and not more than 102.0% of ranitidine hydrochloride ($C_{13}H_{22}N_4O_3S.HCl$).

Description Ranitidine Hydrochloride occurs as a white to pale yellow, crystalline or fine granular powder.

It is very soluble in water, freely soluble in methanol, and slightly soluble in ethanol (99.5).

It is hygroscopic.

It is gradually colored by light.

Melting point: about 140°C (with decomposition).

Identification (1) Determine the absorption spectrum of a solution of Ranitidine Hydrochloride (1 in 100,000) as directed under Ultraviolet-visible Spectrophotometry 〈*2.24*〉, and compare the spectrum with the Reference Spectrum or the spectrum of a solution of Ranitidine Hydrochloride RS prepared in the same manner as the sample solution: both spectra exhibit similar intensities of absorption at the same wavelengths.

(2) Determine the infrared absorption spectrum of Ranitidine Hydrochloride as directed in the paste method under Infrared Spectrophotometry 〈*2.25*〉, and compare the spectrum with the Reference Spectrum or the spectrum of previously dried Ranitidine Hydrochloride RS: both spectra exhibit similar intensities of absorption at the same wave numbers.

(3) A solution of Ranitidine Hydrochloride (1 in 50) responds to Qualitative Tests 〈*1.09*〉 for chloride.

pH 〈*2.54*〉 The pH of a solution obtained by dissolving 1.0 g of Ranitidine Hydrochloride in 100 mL of water is between 4.5 and 6.0.

Purity (1) Clarity and color of solution—A solution of Ranitidine Hydrochloride (1 in 10) is clear and pale yellow to light yellow.

(2) Heavy metals 〈*1.07*〉—Proceed with 2.0 g of Ranitidine Hydrochloride according to Method 2, and perform the test. Prepare the control solution with 2.0 mL of Standard Lead Solution (not more than 10 ppm).

(3) Arsenic 〈*1.11*〉—Prepare the test solution with 1.0 g of Ranitidine Hydrochloride according to Method 4, and perform the test (not more than 2 ppm).

(4) Related substances—Conduct this procedure without exposure to light, using light-resistant vessels. Dissolve 0.22 g of Ranitidine Hydrochloride in methanol to make exactly 10 mL, and use this solution as the sample solution. Pipet 0.5 mL of the sample solution, add methanol to make exactly 100 mL, and use this solution as the standard solution (1). Pipet 6 mL, 4 mL, 2 mL and 1 mL of the standard solution (1), add to each methanol to make exactly 10 mL, and use these solutions as the standard solution (2), the standard solution (3), the standard solution (4) and the standard solution (5), respectively. Separately, dissolve 12.7 mg of ranitidinediamine in methanol to make exactly 10 mL, and use this solution as the standard solution (6). Perform the test with these solutions as directed under Thin-layer Chromatography 〈*2.03*〉. Spot 10 μL each of the sample solution and standard solutions (1), (2), (3), (4) and (5) on a plate of silica gel for thin-layer chromatography. Separately, spot 10 μL of the sample solution on the plate, then spot 10 μL of the standard solution (6) on the spotted position of the sample solution. Immediately develop the plate with a mixture of ethyl acetate, 2-propanol, ammonia solution (28) and water (25:15:5:1) to a distance of about 15 cm, and air-dry the plate. Allow the plate to stand in iodine vapor until the spot from the standard solution (5) appears: the spot obtained from the standard solution (6) is completely separated from the principal spot from the sample solution. The spot having *R*f value of about 0.7 from the sample solution is not more intense than the spot from the standard solution (1), the spots other than the principal spot and the spot of *R*f value of about 0.7 from the sample solution are not more intense than the spot from the standard solution (2), and the total amount of these related substances, calculated by comparison with the spots from the standard solutions (1), (2), (3), (4) and (5), is not more than 1.0%.

Loss on drying 〈*2.41*〉 Not more than 0.75% (1 g, in vacuum, 60°C, 3 hours).

Residue on ignition 〈*2.44*〉 Not more than 0.1% (1 g).

Assay Weigh accurately about 20 mg of Ranitidine Hydrochloride and Ranitidine Hydrochloride RS, previously dried, dissolve each in the mobile phase to make exactly 200 mL, and use these solutions as the sample solution and standard solution. Perform the test with exactly 10 μL each of the sample solution and standard solution as directed under Liquid Chromatography *<2.01>* according to the following conditions, and determine the peak areas, A_T and A_S, of ranitidine in each solution.

Amount (mg) of ranitidine hydrochloride ($C_{13}H_{22}N_4O_3S.HCl$)
$= M_S \times A_T/A_S$

M_S: Amount (mg) of Ranitidine Hydrochloride RS taken

Operating conditions—

Detector: An ultraviolet absorption photometer (wavelength: 322 nm).

Column: A stainless steel column 4.6 mm in inside diameter and 20 cm in length, packed with octadecylsilanized silica gel for liquid chromatography (10 μm in particle diameter).

Column temperature: A constant temperature of about 25°C.

Mobile phase: A mixture of methanol and diluted 0.5 mol/L ammonium acetate TS (1 in 5) (17:3).

Flow rate: Adjust so that the retention time of ranitidine is about 5 minutes.

System suitability—

System performance: Dissolve 20 mg of Ranitidine Hydrochloride and 5 mg of benzalphthalide in 200 mL of the mobile phase. When the procedure is run with 10 μL of this solution under the above operating conditions, benzalphthalide and ranitidine are eluted in this order with the resolution between these peaks being not less than 2.0.

System repeatability: When the test is repeated 6 times with 10 μL of the standard solution under the above operating conditions, the relative standard deviation of the peak area of ranitidine is not more than 1.0%.

Containers and storage Containers—Tight containers.

Storage—Light-resistant.

Rebamipide

レバミピド

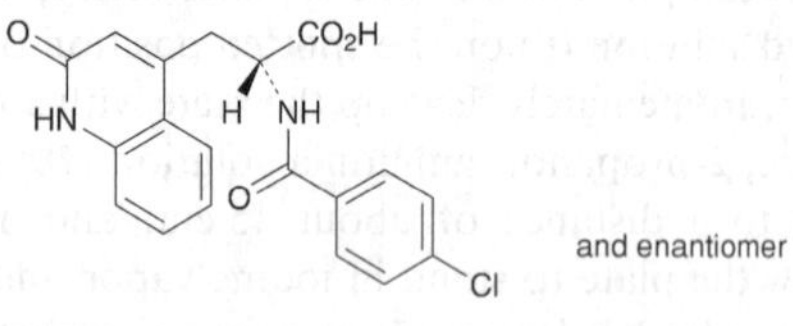

$C_{19}H_{15}ClN_2O_4$: 370.79

(2*RS*)-2-(4-Chlorobenzoylamino)-3-(2-oxo-1,2-dihydroquinolin-4-yl)propanoic acid

[*90098-04-7*]

Rebamipide, when dried, contains not less than 99.0% and not more than 101.0% of rebamipide ($C_{19}H_{15}ClN_2O_4$).

Description Rebamipide occurs as a white crystalline powder. It has a bitter taste.

It is soluble in *N,N*-dimethylformamide, very slightly soluble in methanol and in ethanol (99.5), and practically insoluble in water.

A solution of Rebamipide in *N,N*-dimethylformamide (1 in 20) shows no optical rotation.

Melting point: about 291°C (with decomposition).

Identification **(1)** Determine the absorption spectrum of a solution of Rebamipide in methanol (7 in 1,000,000) as directed under Ultraviolet-visible Spectrophotometry *<2.24>*, and compare the spectrum with the Reference Spectrum: both spectra exhibit similar intensities of absorption at the same wavelengths.

(2) Determine the infrared absorption spectrum of Rebamipide as directed in the potassium bromide disk method under Infrared Spectrophotometry *<2.25>*, and compare the spectrum with the Reference Spectrum: both spectra exhibit similar intensities of absorption at the same wave numbers.

(3) Perform the test with Rebamipide as directed under Flame Coloration Test *<1.04>* (2): a green color appears.

Purity **(1)** Chloride *<1.03>*—Dissolve 0.5 g of Rebamipide in 40 mL of *N,N*-dimethylformamide, and add 6 mL of dilute nitric acid and water to make 50 mL. Perform the test using this solution as the test solution. Prepare the control solution as follows: To 0.40 mL of 0.01 mol/L hydrochloric acid VS add 40 mL of *N,N*-dimethylformamide, 6 mL of dilute nitric acid and water to make 50 mL (not more than 0.028%).

(2) Heavy metals *<1.07>*—Proceed with 2.0 g of Rebamipide according to Method 2, and perform the test. Prepare the control solution with 2.0 mL of Standard Lead Solution (not more than 10 ppm).

(3) Rebamipide *m*-chloro isomer—Dissolve 40 mg of Rebamipide in a mixture of water, 0.05 mol/L phosphate buffer solution (pH 6.0) and methanol (7:7:6) to make 100 mL, and use this solution as the sample solution. Pipet 2 mL of the sample solution, and add a mixture of water, 0.05 mol/L phosphate buffer solution (pH 6.0) and methanol (7:7:6) to make exactly 20 mL. Pipet 2 mL of this solution, add a mixture of water, 0.05 mol/L phosphate buffer solution (pH 6.0) and methanol (7:7:6) to make exactly 50 mL, and use this solution as the standard solution. Perform the test with exactly 10 μL each of the sample solution and standard solution as directed under Liquid Chromatography *<2.01>* according to the following conditions. Determine each peak area of both solutions by the automatic integration method: the area of the peak of rebamipide *m*-chloro isomer, having the relative retention time of about 0.95 to rebamipide obtained from the sample solution, is not larger than 3/8 times the area of the peak of rebamipide from the standard solution.

Operating conditions—

Detector: An ultraviolet absorption photometer (wavelength: 222 nm).

Column: A stainless steel column 4.6 mm in inside diameter and 15 cm in length, packed with octadecylsilanized silica gel for liquid chromatography (5 μm in particle diameter).

Column temperature: A constant temperature of about 25°C.

Mobile phase: To 300 mL of phosphate buffer solution (pH 6.2) add 750 mL of water. To 830 mL of this solution add 170 mL of acetonitrile.

Flow rate: Adjust so that the retention time of rebamipide is about 20 minutes.

System suitability—

Test for required detectability: Pipet 5 mL of the standard solution, and add a mixture of water, 0.05 mol/L phosphate buffer solution (pH 6.0) and methanol (7:7:6) to make exactly 25 mL. Confirm that the peak area of rebamipide obtained with 10 μL of this solution is equivalent to 15 to 25% of that with 10 μL of the standard solution.

System performance: To 1 mL of the sample solution add a mixture of water, 0.05 mol/L phosphate buffer solution (pH 6.0) and methanol (7:7:6) to make 100 mL. When the procedure is run with 10 μL of this solution under the above operating conditions, the number of theoretical plates and the symmetry factor of the peak of rebamipide are not less than 11,000 and not more than 1.2, respectively.

System repeatability: When the test is repeated 6 times with 10 μL of the standard solution under the above operating conditions, the relative standard deviation of the peak area of rebamipide is not more than 2.0%.

(4) Related substances—Perform the test with exactly 10 μL each of the sample solution and standard solution obtained in (3) as directed under Liquid Chromatography <*2.01*> according to the following conditions. Determine each peak area of both solutions by the automatic integration method: each area of the peaks of rebamipide *o*-chloro isomer and debenzoylated isomer, having the relative retention times of about 0.5 and about 0.7, respectively, to rebamipide obtained from the sample solution, is not larger than 3/8 times the peak area of rebamipide from the standard solution, the area of each peak other than rebamipide and the peak mentioned above from the sample solution is not larger than 1/4 times the peak area of rebamipide from the standard solution, and the total area of the peaks other than rebamipide from the sample solution is not larger than the peak area of rebamipide from the standard solution. For the peak area of rebamipide *o*-chloro isomer, multiply the correction factor, 1.4.

Operating conditions—

Detector: An ultraviolet absorption photometer (wavelength: 232 nm).

Column: A stainless steel column 4.6 mm in inside diameter and 25 cm in length, packed with octadecylsilanized silica gel for liquid chromatography (5 μm in particle diameter).

Column temperature: A constant temperature of about 40°C.

Mobile phase: Dissolve 2.44 g of sodium 1-decanesulfonate in 1000 mL of water and to this solution add 1000 mL of methanol and 10 mL of phosphoric acid.

Flow rate: Adjust so that the retention time of rebamipide is about 12 minutes.

Time span of measurement: About 3 times as long as the retention time of rebamipide, beginning after the solvent peak.

System suitability—

Test for required detectability: Pipet 5 mL of the standard solution, and add a mixture of water, 0.05 mol/L phosphate buffer solution (pH 6.0) and methanol (7:7:6) to make exactly 50 mL. Confirm that the peak area of rebamipide obtained with 10 μL of this solution is equivalent to 7 to 13% of that with 10 μL of the standard solution.

System performance: Dissolve 20 mg of 4-chlorobenzoate in methanol to make 50 mL. To 5 mL of this solution add 5 mL of the sample solution and a mixture of water, 0.05 mol/L phosphate buffer solution (pH 6.0) and methanol (7:7:6) to make 50 mL. When the procedure is run with 10 μL of this solution under the above operating conditions, rebamipide and 4-chlorobenzoate are eluted in this order with the resolution between these peaks being not less than 8.

System repeatability: When the test is repeated 6 times with 10 μL of the standard solution under the above operating conditions, the relative standard deviation of the peak area of rebamipide is not more than 2.0%.

Loss on drying <*2.41*> Not more than 3.0% (1 g, 105°C, 2 hours).

Residue on ignition <*2.44*> Not more than 0.1% (1 g).

Assay Weigh accurately about 0.6 g of Rebamipide, previously dried, dissolve in 60 mL of *N*,*N*-dimethylformamide, and titrate <*2.50*> with 0.1 mol/L potassium hydroxide VS until the color of the solution changes from pale yellow to colorless (indicator: 2 drops of phenol red TS). Perform a blank determination in the same manner, and make any necessary correction.

Each mL of 0.1 mol/L potassium hydroxide VS
= 37.08 mg of $C_{19}H_{15}ClN_2O_4$

Containers and storage Containers—Well-closed containers.

Storage—Light-resistant.

Rebamipide Tablets

レバミピド錠

Rebamipide Tablets contain not less than 95.0% and not more than 105.0% of the labeled amount of rebamipide ($C_{19}H_{15}ClN_2O_4$: 370.79).

Method of preparation Prepare as directed under Tablets, with Rebamipide.

Identification To a quantity of powdered Rebamipide Tablets, equivalent to 30 mg of Rebamipide, add 5 mL of a mixture of methanol and ammonia solution (28) (9:1), shake for 10 minutes, centrifuge, and use the supernatant liquid as the sample solution. Separately, dissolve 30 mg of rebamipide for assay in 5 mL of a mixture of methanol and ammonia solution (28) (9:1), and use this solution as the standard solution. Perform the test with these solutions as directed under Thin-layer Chromatography <*2.03*>. Spot 5 μL each of the sample solution and standard solution on a plate of silica gel with fluorescent indicator for thin-layer chromatography. Develop the plate with a mixture of ethyl acetate, methanol and formic acid (75:25:2) to a distance of about 10 cm, and air-dry the plate. Examine under ultraviolet light (main wavelength: 254 nm): the principal spot obtained from the sample solution has the same *R*f value as the spot from the standard solution.

Uniformity of dosage units <*6.02*> Perform the Mass variation test, or the Content uniformity test according to the following method: it meets the requirement.

To 1 tablet of Rebamipide Tablets add 10 mL of water, shake well for 10 minutes, add exactly 10 mL of the internal standard solution, add 10 mL of *N*,*N*-dimethylformamide, shake well for 5 minutes, and add *N*,*N*-dimethylformamide to make 50 mL. Centrifuge this solution, pipet *V* mL of the supernatant liquid, equivalent to 3 mg of rebamipide ($C_{19}H_{15}ClN_2O_4$), and add 20 mL of *N*,*N*-dimethylformamide and water to make 50 mL. Filter this solution through a membrane filter with a pore size not exceeding 0.5 μm, discard the first 1 mL of the filtrate, and use the subsequent filtrate as the sample solution. Separately, weigh accurately about 0.1 g of rebamipide for assay, previously dried at 105°C for 2 hours, dissolve in *N*,*N*-dimethylformamide, and add exactly 10 mL of the internal standard solution and *N*,*N*-dimethylformamide to make 50 mL. Pipet 1.5 mL of this solution, add 20 mL of *N*,*N*-dimethylformamide, add water to make 50 mL, and use this solution as the standard solution. Proceed as directed in the Assay.

Amount (mg) of rebamipide ($C_{19}H_{15}ClN_2O_4$)
$= M_S \times Q_T/Q_S \times 3/2V$

M_S: Amount (mg) of rebamipide for assay taken

Internal standard solution—A solution of acetanilide in *N,N*-dimethylformamide (1 in 150).

Dissolution ⟨*6.10*⟩ When the test is performed at 50 revolutions per minute according to the Paddle method, using 900 mL of diluted disodium hydrogen phosphate-citric acid buffer solution (pH 6.0) (1 in 4), as the dissolution medium, the dissolution rate in 60 minutes of Rebamipide Tablets is not less than 75%.

Start the test with 1 tablet of Rebamipide Tablets, withdraw not less than 20 mL of the medium at the specified minute after starting the test, and filter through a membrane filter with a pore size not exceeding 0.45 μm. Discard not less than 10 mL of the first filtrate, pipet V mL of the subsequent filtrate, add the dissolution medium to make exactly V' mL so that each mL contains about 22 μg of rebamipide ($C_{19}H_{15}ClN_2O_4$), and use this solution as the sample solution. Separately, weigh accurately about 50 mg of rebamipide for assay, previously dried at 105°C for 2 hours, and dissolve in *N,N*-dimethylformamide to make exactly 25 mL. Pipet 2 mL of this solution, add the dissolution medium to make exactly 200 mL, and use this solution as the standard solution. Perform the test with the sample solution and standard solution as directed under Ultraviolet-visible Spectrophotometry ⟨*2.24*⟩, using the dissolution medium as the blank, and determine the absorbances, A_T and A_S, at 326 nm.

Dissolution rate (%) with respect to the labeled amount of rebamipide ($C_{19}H_{15}ClN_2O_4$)
$= M_S \times A_T/A_S \times V'/V \times 1/C \times 36$

M_S: Amount (mg) of rebamipide for assay taken
C: Labeled amount (mg) of rebamipide ($C_{19}H_{15}ClN_2O_4$) in 1 tablet

Assay To 10 Rebamipide Tablets add exactly V/5 mL of the internal standard solution and 50 mL of *N,N*-dimethylformamide, and disintegrate the tablets by sonicating. Shake this solution for 5 minutes, add *N,N*-dimethylformamide to make V mL so that each mL contains about 10 mg of rebamipide ($C_{19}H_{15}ClN_2O_4$). Centrifuge this solution, and to 5 mL of the supernatant liquid add *N,N*-dimethylformamide to make 50 mL. To 2 mL of this solution add 20 mL of *N,N*-dimethylformamide and water to make 50 mL. Filter, if necessary, through a membrane filter with a pore size not exceeding 0.5 μm, and use the filtrate as the sample solution. Separately, weigh accurately about 0.1 g of rebamipide for assay, previously dried at 105°C for 2 hours, dissolve in *N,N*-dimethylformamide, and add exactly 2 mL of the internal standard solution and *N,N*-dimethylformamide to make 100 mL. To 2 mL of this solution, add 20 mL of *N,N*-dimethylformamide and water to make 50 mL, and use this solution as the standard solution. Perform the test with 20 μL each of the sample solution and standard solution as directed under Liquid Chromatography ⟨*2.01*⟩ according to the following conditions, and calculate the ratios, Q_T and Q_S, of the peak area of rebamipide to that of the internal standard.

Amount (mg) of rebamipide ($C_{19}H_{15}ClN_2O_4$)
$= M_S \times Q_T/Q_S \times V/100$

M_S: Amount (mg) of rebamipide for assay taken

Internal standard solution—A solution of acetanilide in *N,N*-dimethylformamide (1 in 20).

Operating conditions—

Detector: An ultraviolet absorption photometer (wavelength: 254 nm).

Column: A stainless steel column 4.6 mm in inside diameter and 15 cm in length, packed with octadecylsilanized silica gel for liquid chromatography (5 μm in particle diameter).

Column temperature: A constant temperature of about 25°C.

Mobile phase: To 300 mL of phosphate buffer solution (pH 6.2) add 750 mL of water. To 830 mL of this solution add 170 mL of acetonitrile.

Flow rate: Adjust so that the retention time of rebamipide is about 20 minutes.

System suitability—

System performance: When the procedure is run with 20 μL of the standard solution under the above operating conditions, the internal standard and rebamipide are eluted in this order with the resolution between these peaks being not less than 8.

System repeatability: When the test is repeated 6 times with 20 μL of the standard solution under the above operating conditions, the relative standard deviation of the ratio of the peak area of rebamipide to that of the internal standard is not more than 1.0%.

Containers and storage Containers—Well-closed containers.

Reserpine

レセルピン

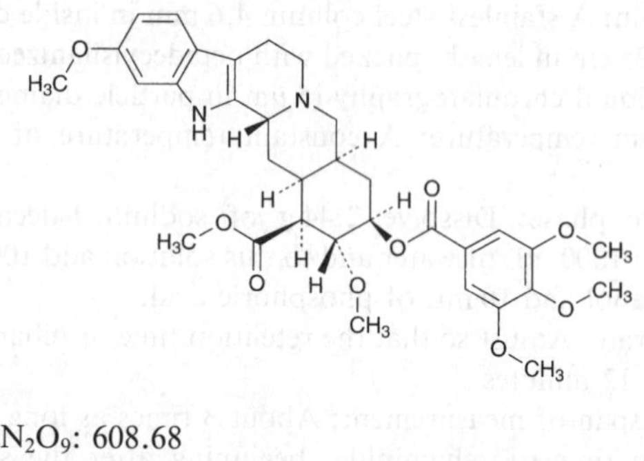

$C_{33}H_{40}N_2O_9$: 608.68
Methyl (3*R*,16*S*,17*R*,18*R*,20*S*)-11,17-dimethoxy-18-(3,4,5-trimethoxybenzoyloxy)yohimban-16-carboxylate
[*50-55-5*]

Reserpine, when dried, contains not less than 96.0% of reserpine ($C_{33}H_{40}N_2O_9$).

Description Reserpine occurs as white to light yellow, crystals or crystalline powder.

It is freely soluble in acetic acid (100) and in chloroform, slightly soluble in acetonitrile, very slightly soluble in ethanol (95), and practically insoluble in water and in diethyl ether.

It is affected by light.

Identification **(1)** To 1 mg of Reserpine add 1 mL of vanillin-hydrochloric acid TS, and warm: a vivid red-purple color develops.

(2) Determine the absorption spectrum of a solution of Reserpine in acetonitrile (1 in 50,000) as directed under Ultraviolet-visible Spectrophotometry ⟨*2.24*⟩, and compare the spectrum with the Reference Spectrum or the spectrum of a solution of Reserpine RS prepared in the same manner as the sample solution: both spectra exhibit similar intensities of absorption at the same wavelengths.

(3) Determine the infrared absorption spectrum of Reserpine, previously dried, as directed in the potassium bromide disk method under Infrared Spectrophotometry <*2.25*>, and compare the spectrum with the Reference Spectrum or the spectrum of previously dried Reserpine RS: both spectra exhibit similar intensities of absorption at the same wave numbers.

Optical rotation <*2.49*> $[\alpha]_D^{20}$: −114 – −127° (after drying, 0.25 g, chloroform, 25 mL, 100 mm).

Purity Related substances—Conduct this procedure without exposure to light, using light-resistant vessels. Dissolve 50 mg of Reserpine in 50 mL of acetonitrile, and use this solution as the sample solution. Pipet 3 mL of the sample solution, add acetonitrile to make exactly 100 mL, and use this solution as the standard solution. Perform the test with exactly 10 μL each of the sample solution and standard solution as directed under Liquid Chromatography <*2.01*> according to the following conditions. Determine each peak area from these solutions by the automatic integration method: the total area of the peaks other than reserpine obtained from the sample solution is not larger than the peak area of reserpine from the standard solution.

Operating conditions—

Detector, column, and column temperature: Proceed as directed in the operating conditions in the Assay.

Mobile phase: A mixture of 0.05 mol/L potassium dihydrogen phosphate (pH 3.0) and acetonitrile (13:7).

Flow rate: Adjust so that the retention time of reserpine is about 20 minutes.

Time span of measurement: About 2 times as long as the retention time of reserpine.

System suitability—

Test for required detectability: To exactly 2 mL of the standard solution add acetonitorile to make exactly 50 mL. Confirm that the peak area of reserpine obtained with 10 μL of this solution is equivalent to 3 to 5% of that with 10 μL of the standard solution.

System performance: Dissolve 0.01 g of Reserpine and 4 mg of butyl parahydroxybenzoate in 100 mL of acetonitrile. To 5 mL of this solution add acetonitrile to make 50 mL. When the procedure is run with 20 μL of this solution according to the operating conditions in the Assay, reserpine and butyl parahydroxybenzoate are eluted in this order with the resolution between these peaks being not less than 2.0.

System repeatability: When the test is repeated 6 times with 10 μL of the standard solution under the above operating conditions, the relative standard deviation of the peak area of reserpine is not more than 2.0%.

Loss on drying <*2.41*> Not more than 0.5% (0.2 g, in vacuum, 60°C, 3 hours).

Residue on ignition <*2.44*> Not more than 0.2% (0.2 g).

Assay Conduct this procedure without exposure to light, using light-resistant vessels. Weigh accurately about 10 mg each of Reserpine and Reserpine RS, previously dried, and dissolve each in acetonitrile to make exactly 100 mL. Pipet 5 mL each of these solutions, add exactly 10 mL of the internal standard solution, 5 mL of acetonitrile and water to make 50 mL, and use these solutions as the sample solution and the standard solution, respectively. Perform the test with 20 μL each of the sample solution and standard solution as directed under Liquid Chromatography <*2.01*> according to the following conditions, and calculate the ratios, Q_T and Q_S, of the peak area of reserpine to that of the internal standard.

Amount (mg) of reserpine ($C_{33}H_{40}N_2O_9$) = $M_S \times Q_T/Q_S$

M_S: Amount (mg) of Reserpine RS taken

Internal standard solution—A solution of butyl parahydroxybenzoate in acetonitrile (1 in 50,000).

Operating conditions—

Detector: An ultraviolet absorption photometer (wavelength: 268 nm).

Column: A stainless steel column 4 mm in inside diameter and 25 cm in length, packed with octadecylsilanized silica gel for liquid chromatography (5 μm in particle diameter).

Column temperature: A constant temperature of about 40°C.

Mobile phase: A mixture of 0.05 mol/L potassium dihydrogen phosphate (pH 3.0) and acetonitrile (11:9).

Flow rate: Adjust so that the retention time of reserpine is about 10 minutes.

System suitability—

System performance: When the procedure is run with 20 μL of the standard solution under the above operating conditions, reserpine and the internal standard are eluted in this order with the resolution between these peaks being not less than 2.0.

System repeatability: When the test is repeated 6 times with 20 μL of the standard solution under the above operating conditions, the relative standard deviation of the ratios of the peak area of reserpine to that of the internal standard is not more than 2.0%.

Containers and Storage Containers—Well-closed containers.

Storage—Light-resistant.

Reserpine Injection

レセルピン注射液

Reserpine Injection is an aqueous injection.

It contains not less than 90.0% and not more than 110.0% of the labeled amount of reserpine ($C_{33}H_{40}N_2O_9$: 608.68).

Method of preparation Prepare as directed under Injections, with Reserpine.

Description Reserpine Injection is a clear, colorless or pale yellow liquid.

pH: 2.5 – 4.0

Identification Measure a volume of Reserpine Injection, equivalent to 1.5 mg of Reserpine, add 10 mL of diethyl ether, shake for 10 minutes, and take the aqueous layer. If necessary, add 10 mL of diethyl ether to the aqueous layer, and shake for 10 minutes to repeat the process. To the aqueous layer add water to make 50 mL, and determine the absorption spectrum of this solution as directed under Ultraviolet-visible Spectrophotometry <*2.24*>: it exhibits a maximum between 265 nm and 269 nm.

Extractable volume <*6.05*> It meets the requirement.

Foreign insoluble matter <*6.06*> Perform the test according to Method 1: it meets the requirement.

Insoluble particulate matter <*6.07*> It meets the requirement.

Sterility <*4.06*> Perform the test according to the Membrane filtration method: it meets the requirement.

Assay Measure exactly a volume of Reserpine Injection, equivalent to about 4 mg of reserpine ($C_{33}H_{40}N_2O_9$). Separately, weigh accurately about 4 mg of Reserpine RS, previously dried in vacuum at 60°C for 3 hours. Transfer them to separate separator, add 10 mL each of water and 5 mL each of ammonia TS, and extract with one 20-mL portion of chloroform, then with three 10-mL portions of chloroform with shaking vigorously. Combine the chloroform extracts, wash with two 50-mL portions of diluted hydrochloric acid (1 in 1000), and combine the washings. Then wash the chloroform extract with two 50-mL portions of a solution of sodium hydrogen carbonate (1 in 100), and combine the all washings. Extract the combined washing with two 10-mL portions of chloroform, and combine the washings with the former chloroform extract. Transfer the chloroform solution to a 100-mL volumetric flask through a pledget of absorbent cotton previously wetted with chloroform, wash with a small amount of chloroform, dilute with chloroform to make 100 mL, and use these solutions as the sample solution and the standard solution, respectively. Determine the absorbances, A_T and A_S, of the sample solution and the standard solution, respectively, at 295 nm as directed under Ultraviolet-visible Spectrophotometry <*2.24*>.

$$\text{Amount (mg) of reserpine } (C_{33}H_{40}N_2O_9) = M_S \times A_T/A_S$$

M_S: Amount (mg) of Reserpine RS taken

Containers and storage Containers—Hermetic containers, and colored containers may be used.

Storage—Light-resistant.

0.1% Reserpine Powder

レセルピン散 **0.1%**

0.1% Reserpine Powder contains not less than 0.09% and not more than 0.11% of reserpine ($C_{33}H_{40}N_2O_9$: 608.68).

Method of preparation

Reserpine	1 g
Lactose Hydrate	a sufficient quantity
To make	1000 g

Prepare as directed under Powders, with the above ingredients.

Identification To 0.4 g of 0.1% Reserpine Powder add 20 mL of acetonitrile, shake for 30 minutes, and centrifuge. Determine the absorption spectrum of the supernatant liquid as directed under Ultraviolet-visible Spectrophotometry <*2.24*>: it exhibits maxima between 265 nm and 269 nm, and between 294 nm and 298 nm.

Dissolution Being specified separately when the drug is granted approval based on the Law.

Assay Conduct this procedure without exposure to light, using light-resistant vessels. Weigh accurately a quantity of 0.1% Reserpine Powder, equivalent to about 0.5 mg of reserpine ($C_{33}H_{40}N_2O_9$), disperse in 12 mL of water, add exactly 10 mL of the internal standard solution and 10 mL of acetonitrile, and dissolve by warming at 50°C for 15 minutes, then add water to make 50 mL, and use this solution as the sample solution. Separately, weigh accurately about 10 mg of Reserpine RS, previously dried at 60°C in vacuum for 3 hours, dissolve in acetonitrile to make exactly 100 mL. Pipet 5 mL of this solution, add exactly 10 mL of the internal standard solution, 5 mL of acetonitrile and water to make 50 mL, and use this solution as the standard solution. Then, proceed as directed in the Assay under Reserpine.

$$\text{Amount (mg) of reserpine } (C_{33}H_{40}N_2O_9) = M_S \times Q_T/Q_S \times 1/20$$

M_S: Amount (mg) of Reserpine RS taken

Internal standard solution—A solution of butyl parahydroxybenzoate in acetonitrile (1 in 50,000).

Containers and storage Containers—Well-closed containers.

Storage—Light-resistant.

Reserpine Tablets

レセルピン錠

Reserpine Tablets contain not less than 90.0% and not more than 110.0% of the labeled amount of reserpine ($C_{33}H_{40}N_2O_9$: 608.68).

Method of preparation Prepare as directed under Tablets, with Reserpine.

Identification Take a portion of powdered Reserpine Tablets, equivalent to 0.4 mg of Reserpine, add 20 mL of acetonitrile, shake for 30 minutes, and centrifuge. Determine the absorption spectrum of the supernatant liquid as directed under Ultraviolet-visible Spectrophotometry <*2.24*>: it exhibits maxima between 265 nm and 269 nm, and between 294 nm and 298 nm.

Uniformity of dosage units <*6.02*> Perform the test according to the following method: it meets the requirement of the Content uniformity test.

Conduct this procedure without exposure to light, using light-resistant vessels. To 1 tablet of Reserpine Tablets add 2 mL of water, disintegrate by warming at 50°C for 15 minutes while shaking. After cooling, add exactly 2 mL of the internal standard solution per 0.1 mg of reserpine ($C_{33}H_{40}N_2O_9$), add 2 mL of acetonitrile, warm at 50°C for 15 minutes while shaking, and after cooling, add water to make 10 mL. Centrifuge the solution, and use the supernatant liquid as the sample solution. Separately, weigh accurately about 10 mg of Reserpine RS, previously dried at 60°C in vacuum for 3 hours, dissolve in acetonitrile to make exactly 100 mL. Pipet 5 mL of this solution add exactly 10 mL of the internal standard solution, 5 mL of acetonitrile and water to make 50 mL, and use this solution as the standard solution. Then, proceed as directed in the Assay under Reserpine.

$$\text{Amount (mg) of reserpine } (C_{33}H_{40}N_2O_9) = M_S \times Q_T/Q_S \times C/10$$

M_S: Amount (mg) of Reserpine RS taken

C: Labeled amount (mg) of reserpine ($C_{33}H_{40}N_2O_9$) in 1 tablet

Internal standard solution—A solution of butyl parahydroxybenzoate in acetonitrile (1 in 50,000).

Dissolution <*6.10*> When the test is performed at 100 revolutions per minute according to the Paddle method, using 500 mL of a solution prepared by dissolving 1 g of polysorbate 80 in diluted dilute acetic acid (1 in 200) to make 20 L as the dissolution medium, the dissolution rate in 30 minutes of Reserpine Tablets is not less than 70%.

Start the test with 1 tablet of Reserpine Tablets, withdraw not less than 20 mL of the medium at the specified minute after starting the test, filter through a filter laminated with polyester fibers, discard not less than 10 mL of the first filtrate, and use the subsequent filtrate as the sample solution. Separately, dry Reserpine RS at 60°C in vacuum for 3 hours, weigh accurately an amount 100 times the labeled amount of Reserpine Tablets, dissolve in 1 mL of chloroform and 80 mL of ethanol (95), and add the dissolution medium to make exactly 200 mL. Pipet 1 mL of this solution, add the dissolution medium to make exactly 250 mL, and use this solution as the standard solution. Pipet 5 mL each of the sample solution and standard solution, transfer to glass-stoppered brown test tubes T and S, respectively, add exactly 5 mL each of ethanol (99.5), shake well, add exactly 1 mL each of diluted vanadium (V) oxide TS (1 in 2), shake vigorously, and allow to stand for 30 minutes. Perform the test with these solutions as directed under Fluorometry 〈*2.22*〉, and determine the intensity of fluorescence, F_T and F_S, at the wavelength of excitation at 400 nm and at the wavelength of fluorescence at 500 nm.

Dissolution rate (%) with respect to the labeled amount of reserpine ($C_{33}H_{40}N_2O_9$)

$$= M_S \times F_T/F_S \times 1/C$$

M_S: Amount (mg) of Reserpine RS taken
C: Labeled amount (mg) of reserpine ($C_{33}H_{40}N_2O_9$) in 1 tablet

Assay Conduct this procedure without exposure to light, using light-resistant vessels. Weigh accurately and powder not less than 20 Reserpine Tablets. Weigh accurately a quantity of the powder, equivalent to about 0.5 mg of reserpine ($C_{33}H_{40}N_2O_9$), add 3 mL of water, and warm at 50°C for 15 minutes while shaking. After cooling, add exactly 10 mL of the internal standard solution, 10 mL of acetonitrile and warm at 50°C for 15 minutes while shaking. After cooling, add water to make 50 mL, centrifuge, and use the supernatant liquid as the sample solution. Separately, weigh accurately about 10 mg of Reserpine RS, previously dried at 60°C in vacuum for 3 hours, and dissolve in acetonitrile to make exactly 100 mL. Pipet 5 mL of this solution, add exactly 10 mL of the internal standard solution, 5 mL of acetonitrile and water to make 50 mL, and use this solution as the standard solution. Then, proceed as directed in the Assay under Reserpine.

$$\text{Amount (mg) of reserpine } (C_{33}H_{40}N_2O_9) = M_S \times Q_T/Q_S \times 1/20$$

M_S: Amount (mg) of Reserpine RS taken

Internal standard solution—A solution of butyl parahydroxybenzoate in acetonitrile (1 in 50,000).

Containers and storage Containers—Well-closed containers.

Storage—Light-resistant.

Retinol Acetate

Vitamin A Acetate

レチノール酢酸エステル

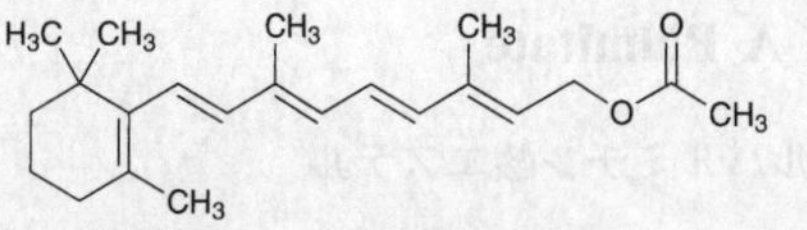

$C_{22}H_{32}O_2$: 328.49
(2*E*,4*E*,6*E*,8*E*)-3,7-Dimethyl-9-(2,6,6-trimethylcyclohex-1-en-1-yl)nona-2,4,6,8-tetraen-1-yl acetate
[*127-47-9*]

Retinol Acetate is synthetic retinol acetate or synthetic retinol acetate diluted with fixed oil.

It contains not less than 2,500,000 Vitamin A Units per gram.

A suitable antioxidant may be added.

It contains not less than 95.0% and not more than 105.0% of the labeled Units.

Description Retinol Acetate occurs as pale yellow to yellow-red, crystals or an ointment-like substance, and has a faint, characteristic odor, but has no rancid odor.

It is freely soluble in petroleum ether, soluble in ethanol (95), and practically insoluble in water.

It is decomposed by air and by light.

Identification Dissolve Retinol Acetate and Retinol Acetate RS, equivalent to 15,000 Units each, in 5 mL of petroleum ether, and use these solutions as the sample solution and standard solution. Perform the test with these solutions as directed under Thin-layer Chromatography 〈*2.03*〉. Spot 5 μL each of the sample solution and standard solution on a plate of silica gel for thin-layer chromatography. Develop with a mixture of cyclohexane and diethyl ether (12:1) to a distance of about 10 cm, and air-dry the plate. Spray evenly antimony (III) chloride TS: the principal spot obtained from the sample solution is the same in color tone and *R*f value with the blue spot from the standard solution.

Purity **(1)** Acid value 〈*1.13*〉—Take exactly 5.0 g of Retinol Acetate, and perform the test: not more than 2.0.

(2) Peroxide—Weigh accurately about 5 g of Retinol Acetate, transfer in a 250-mL glass-stoppered conical flask, add 50 mL of a mixture of acetic acid (100) and isooctane (3:2), and gently mix to dissolve completely. Replace the air of the inside gradually with about 600 mL of Nitrogen, then add 0.1 mL of saturated potassium iodide TS under a current of Nitrogen. Immediately stopper tightly, and mix with a swirling motion for 1 minute. Add 30 mL of water, stopper tightly, and shake vigorously for 5 to 10 seconds. Titrate 〈*2.50*〉 this solution with 0.01 mol/L sodium thiosulfate VS until the blue color of the solution disappears after addition of 0.5 mL of starch TS near the end point where the solution is a pale yellow color. Calculate the amount of peroxide by the following formula: not more than 10 mEq/kg.

$$\text{Amount (mEq/kg) of peroxide} = V/M \times 10$$

V: Volume (mL) of 0.01 mol/L sodium thiosulfate VS consumed
M: Amount (g) of Retinol Acetate taken

Assay Proceed as directed in Method 1-1 under Vitamin A Assay 〈*2.55*〉.

Containers and storage Containers—Tight containers.

Storage—Light-resistant, and almost well-filled, or under Nitrogen atmosphere, and in a cold place.

Retinol Palmitate

Vitamin A Palmitate

レチノールパルミチン酸エステル

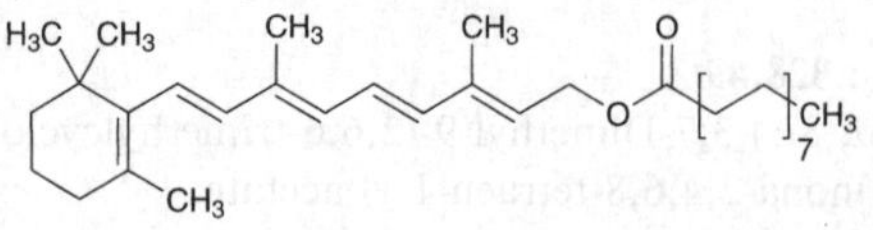

$C_{36}H_{60}O_2$: 524.86
(2*E*,4*E*,6*E*,8*E*)-3,7-Dimethyl-9-(2,6,6-trimethylcyclohex-1-en-1-yl)nona-2,4,6,8-tetraen-1-yl palmitate
[*79-81-2*]

Retinol Palmitate is a synthetic retinol palmitate or a synthetic retinol palmitate diluted with fixed oil.

It contains not less than 1,500,000 Vitamin A Units per gram.

A suitable antioxidant may be added.

It contains not less than 95.0% and not more than 105.0% of the labeled Units.

Description Retinol Palmitate occurs as a light yellow to yellow-red, ointment-like or an oily substance. It has a faint, characteristic odor, but has no rancid odor.

It is very soluble in petroleum ether, slightly soluble in ethanol (95), and practically insoluble in water.

It is decomposed by air and by light.

Identification Dissolve Retinol Palmitate and Retinol Palmitate RS, equivalent to 15,000 Units each, in 5 mL of petroleum ether, and use these solutions as the sample solution and standard solution. Perform the test with these solutions as directed under Thin-layer Chromatography <*2.03*>. Spot 5 μL each of the sample solution and standard solution on a plate of silica gel for thin-layer chromatography. Develop with a mixture of cyclohexane and diethyl ether (12:1) to a distance of about 10 cm, and air-dry the plate. Spray evenly antimony (III) chloride TS: the principal spot obtained from the sample solution is the same in color tone and *R*f value with the blue spot from the standard solution.

Purity **(1)** Acid value <*1.13*>—Take exactly 5.0 g of Retinol Palmitate, and perform the test: not more than 2.0.

(2) Peroxide—Weigh accurately about 5 g of Retinol Palmitate, transfer in a 250-mL glass-stoppered conical flask, add 50 mL of a mixture of acetic acid (100) and isooctane (3:2), and gently mix to dissolve completely. Replace the air of the inside gradually with about 600 mL of Nitrogen, then add 0.1 mL of saturated potassium iodide TS under a current of Nitrogen. Immediately stopper tightly, and mix with a swirling motion for 1 minute. Add 30 mL of water, stopper tightly, and shake vigorously for 5 to 10 seconds. Titrate <*2.50*> this solution with 0.01 mol/L sodium thiosulfate VS until the blue color of the solution disappears after addition of 0.5 mL of starch TS near the end point where the solution is a pale yellow color. Calculate the amount of peroxide by the following formula: not more than 10 mEq/kg.

$$\text{Amount (mEq/kg) of peroxide} = V/M \times 10$$

V: Volume (mL) of 0.01 mol/L sodium thiosulfate VS
M: Amount (g) of Retinol Palmitate taken

Assay Proceed as directed in Method 1-1 under the Vitamin A Assay <*2.55*>.

Containers and storage Containers—Tight containers.

Storage—Light-resistant, and almost well-filled, or under Nitrogen atmosphere, and in a cold place.

Ribavirin

リバビリン

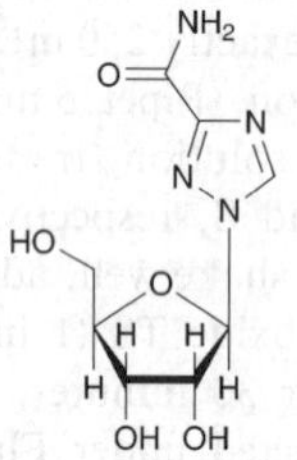

$C_8H_{12}N_4O_5$: 244.20
1-*β*-D-Ribofuranosyl-1*H*-1,2,4-triazole-3-carboxamide
[*36791-04-5*]

Ribavirin, when dried, contains not less than 98.0% and not more than 102.0% of ribavirin ($C_8H_{12}N_4O_5$).

Description Ribavirin occurs as a white crystalline powder.

It is freely soluble in water and in *N*, *N*-dimethylformamide, slightly soluble in methanol, and practically insoluble in ethanol (99.5).

Melting point: 167 – 171°C

Ribavirin shows crystal polymorphism.

Identification **(1)** Determine the absorption spectrum of a solution of Ribavirin (1 in 100,000) as directed under Ultraviolet-visible Spectrophotometry <*2.24*>, and compare the spectrum with the Reference Spectrum or the spectrum of a solution of Ribavirin RS prepared in the same manner as the sample solution: both spectra exhibit similar intensities of absorption at the same wavelengths.

(2) Determine the infrared absorption spectrum of previously dried Ribavirin as directed in the potassium bromide disk method under Infrared Spectrophotometry <*2.25*>, and compare the spectrum with the Reference Spectrum or the spectrum of previously dried Ribavirin RS: both spectra exhibit similar intensities of absorption at the same wave numbers.

Optical rotation <*2.49*> $[\alpha]_D^{20}$: − 33.0 – − 37.0°(after drying, 0.1 g, water, 10 mL, 100 mm).

Purity **(1)** Heavy metals <*1.07*>—Proceed with 1.0 g of Ribavirin according to Method 1, and perform the test. Prepare the control solution with 1.0 mL of Standard Lead Solution (not more than 10 ppm).

(2) Arsenic <*1.11*>—Prepare the test solution with 1.0 g of Ribavirin according to Method 5, and perform the test (not more than 2 ppm).

(3) Related substances—Use the sample solution obtained in the Assay as the sample solution. Pipet 1 mL of the sample solution, add water to make exactly 200 mL, and use this solution as the standard solution. Perform the test with exactly 5 μL each of the sample solution and standard solution as directed under Liquid Chromatography <*2.01*> according to the following conditions, and determine each peak area by the automatic integration method: the area of the peak, having the relative retention time of about 0.85 to ribavirin, obtained from the sample solution, is not larger than 2/5 times the peak area of ribavirin from the standard solution, and the area of the peak other than ribavirin and other than the peak mentioned above from the sample solution is not larger than 1/5 times the peak area of ribavirin from the standard solution. Furthermore, the total area of the peaks other than ribavirin and other than the peak mentioned above from the sample solution is not larger than 2/5 times the peak area of ribavirin from the standard solution, and the total area of the peaks other than ribavirin from the sample solution is not larger than the peak area of ribavirin from the standard solution. For the area of the peaks, having the relative retention time of about 0.59 and about 0.85 to ribavirin, multiply their correction factors 0.6 and 1.7, respectively.

Operating conditions—

Detector, column, column temperature, mobile phases A and B, flowing of mobile phase, and flow rate: Proceed as directed in the operating conditions in the Assay.

Time span of measurement: For 35 minutes after the injection, beginning after the solvent peak.

System suitability—

Test for required detectability: To exactly 1 mL of the standard solution add water to make exactly 10 mL. Confirm that the peak area of ribavirin obtained with 5 μL of this solution is equivalent to 7 to 13% of that with 5 μL of the standard solution.

System performance: To 5 mL of the sample solution add 1 mL of sodium hydroxide TS, allow to stand for 30 minutes, and add 1 mL of 1 mol/L hydrochloric acid TS. To 1 mL of this solution add water to make 200 mL. When the procedure is run with 5 μL of this solution under the above operating conditions, the resolution between the peak having the relative retention time of about 0.85 to ribavirin and the peak of ribavirin is not less than 4.0, and when the procedure is run with 5 μL of the standard solution under the above operating conditions, the symmetry factor of the peak of ribavirin is not more than 1,5.

System repeatability: When the test is repeated 6 times with 5 μL of the standard solution under the above operating conditions, the relative standard deviation of the peak area of ribavirin is not more than 2.0%.

Loss on drying <*2.41*> Not more than 0.5% (1 g, 105°C, 5 hours).

Residue on ignition <*2.44*> Not more than 0.1% (1 g).

Assay Weigh accurately an amount of Ribavirin and Ribavirin RS, both previously dried, equivalent to about 25 mg each, dissolve in water to make exactly 50 mL, and use these solutions as the sample solution and the standard solution, respectively. Perform the test with exactly 5 μL each of the sample solution and standard solution as directed under Liquid Chromatography <*2.01*> according to the following conditions, and determine the peak areas, A_T and A_S, of ribavirin in each solution.

Amount (mg) of ribavirin ($C_8H_{12}N_4O_5$) = $M_S \times A_T/A_S$

M_S: Amount (mg) of Ribavirin RS taken

Operating conditions—

Detector: An ultraviolet absorption photometer (wavelength: 220 nm).

Column: A stainless steel column 4.6 mm in inside diameter and 15 cm in length, packed with octadecylsilanized silica gel for liquid chromatography (3 μm in particle diameter).

Column temperature: A constant temperature of about 25°C.

Mobile phase A: Dissolve 2.0 g of anhydrous sodium sulfate in 300 mL of water, add 8 mL of phosphoric acid solution (1 in 20) and water to make 2000 mL.

Mobile phase B: A mixture of mobile phase A and acetonitrile for liquid chromatography (19:1).

Flowing of mobile phase: Control the gradient by mixing the mobile phases A and B as directed in the following table.

Time after injection of sample (min)	Mobile phase A (vol%)	Mobile phase B (vol%)
0 – 15	100	0
15 – 25	100 → 0	0 → 100
25 – 35	0	100

Flow rate: 1.0 mL per minute.

System suitability—

System performance: To 5 mL of the standard solution add 1 mL of sodium hydroxide TS, allow to stand for 30 minutes, and add 1 mL of 1 mol/L hydrochloric acid TS. When the procedure is run with 5 μL of this solution under the above operating conditions, the resolution between the peak having the relative retention time of about 0.85 to ribavirin and the peak of ribavirin is not less than 4.0, and when the procedure is run with 5 μL of the standard solution under the above operating conditions, the symmetry factor of the peak of ribavirin is not more than 1.5.

System repeatability: When the test is repeated 6 times with 5 μL of the standard solution under the above operating conditions, the relative standard deviation of the peak area of ribavirin is not more than 1.0%.

Containers and storage Containers—Well-closed containers.

Ribavirin Capsules

リバビリンカプセル

Ribavirin Capsules contain not less than 95.0% and not more than 105.0% of the labeled amount of ribavirin ($C_8H_{12}N_4O_5$: 244.20).

Method of preparation Prepare as directed under Capsules, with Ribavirin.

Identification Take out the content of Ribavirin Capsules. Shake thoroughly an amount of the content, equivalent to 0.1 g of Ribavirin, with 10 mL of water, allow to stand for 1 minute, filter, and use the filtrate as the sample solution. Separately, dissolve 50 mg of ribavirin in 5 mL of water, and use this solution as the standard solution. Perform the test with these solutions as directed under Thin-layer Chromatography <*2.03*>. Spot 10 μL each of the sample solution and standard solution on a plate of silica gel with fluorescent indicator for thin-layer chromatography. Develop the plate with a mixture of acetonitrile and diluted ammonium chloride TS (1 in 20) (9:2) to a distance of about 15 cm, and air-dry the plate. Examine under ultraviolet light (main wavelength: 254 nm): the principal spot obtained from the sample solution and the spot from the standard solution have the same *Rf* value.

Uniformity of dosage units <*6.02*> Perform the Mass variation test, or the Content uniformity test according to the following method: it meets the requirement.

To 1 capsule of Ribavirin Capsules add 250 mL of water previously warmed to 37°C, shake in a water bath of 37°C for 15 minutes, then allow standing to cool to room temperature, add water to make exactly 500 mL, and filter. Discard the first 3 mL of the filtrate, pipet *V* mL of the subsequent filtrate, add water to make exactly *V′* mL so that each mL contains about 20 μg of ribavirin ($C_8H_{12}N_4O_5$), and use this solution as the sample solution. Separately, weigh accurately about 20 mg of Ribavirin RS, previously dried at 105°C for 5 hours, dissolve in water to make exactly 100 mL. Pipet 5 mL of this solution, add water to make exactly 50 mL, and use this solution as the standard solution. Perform the test with exactly 20 μL each of the sample solution and standard solution as directed under Liquid Chromatography <*2.01*> according to the following conditions, and determine the peak areas, A_T and A_S, of ribavirin in each solution.

Amount (mg) of ribavirin ($C_8H_{12}N_4O_5$)
$= M_S \times A_T/A_S \times V'/V \times 1/2$

M_S: Amount (mg) of Ribavirin RS taken

Operating conditions—

Proceed as directed in the operating conditions in the Dissolution.

System suitability—

Proceed as directed in the system suitability in the Dissolution.

Dissolution <*6.10*> When the test is performed at 50 revolutions per minute according to the Paddle method using the sinker, using 900 mL of water as the dissolution medium, the dissolution rate in 30 minutes of Ribavirin Capsules is not less than 85%.

Start the test with 1 capsule of Ribavirin Capsules, withdraw not less than 10 mL of the medium at the specified minute after starting the test, and filter through a membrane filter with a pore size not exceeding 0.8 μm. Discard not less than 3 mL of the first filtrate, pipet *V* mL of the subsequent filtrate, add water to make exactly *V′* mL so that each mL contains about 22 μg of ribavirin ($C_8H_{12}N_4O_5$), and use this solution as the sample solution. Separately, weigh accurately about 20 mg of Ribavirin RS, previously dried at 105°C for 5 hours, and dissolve in water to make exactly 100 mL. Pipet 5 mL of this solution, add water to make exactly 50 mL, and use this solution as the standard solution. Perform the test with exactly 20 μL each of the sample solution and standard solution as directed under Liquid Chromatography <*2.01*> according to the following conditions, and determine the peak areas, A_T and A_S, of ribavirin in each solution.

Dissolution rate (%) with respect to the labeled amount of ribavirin ($C_8H_{12}N_4O_5$)
$= M_S \times A_T/A_S \times V'/V \times 1/C \times 90$

M_S: Amount (mg) of Ribavirin RS taken
C: Labeled amount (mg) of ribavirin ($C_8H_{12}N_4O_5$) in 1 capsule

Operating conditions—

Detector: An ultraviolet absorption photometer (wavelength: 207 nm).

Column: A stainless steel column 7.8 mm in inside diameter and 10 cm in length, packed with strongly acidic ion-exchange resin for liquid chromatography composed with sulfonic acid group bound styrene-divinylbenzene copolymer (9 μm in particle diameter).

Column temperature: A constant temperature of about 40°C.

Mobile phase: Adjust to pH 2.5 of water with 0.5 mol/L sulfuric acid TS.

Flow rate: Adjust so that the retention time of ribavirin is about 4 minutes.

System suitability—

System performance: When the procedure is run with 20 μL of the standard solution under the above operating conditions, the number of theoretical plates and the symmetry factor of the peak of ribavirin are not less than 500 and not more than 1.5, respectively.

System repeatability: When the test is repeated 6 times with 20 μL of the standard solution under the above operating conditions, the relative standard deviation of the peak area of ribavirin is not more than 2.0%.

Assay Cut and open the capsules of not less than 20 Ribavirin Capsules, take out the contents and weigh the mass accurately, and mix uniformly. Weigh accurately an amount of the content, equivalent to about 0.1 g of ribavirin ($C_8H_{12}N_4O_5$), add 100 mL of water, shake for 30 minutes, then add water to make exactly 200 mL, and use this solution as the sample solution. Separately, weigh accurately about 25 mg of Ribavirin RS, previously dried at 105°C for 5 hours, dissolve in water to make exactly 50 mL, and use this solution as the standard solution. Perform the test with exactly 5 μL each of the sample solution and standard solution as directed under Liquid Chromatography <*2.01*> according to the following conditions, and determine the peak areas, A_T and A_S, of ribavirin in each solution.

Amount (mg) of ribavirin ($C_8H_{12}N_4O_5$)
$= M_S \times A_T/A_S \times 4$

M_S: Amount (mg) of Ribavirin RS taken

Operating conditions—

Detector, column, column temperature, mobile phase A, and flow rate: Proceed as directed in the operating conditions in the Assay under Ribavirin.

Mobile phase B: A mixture of mobile phase A and acetonitrile for liquid chromatography (9:1).

Flowing of mobile phase: Control the gradient by mixing the mobile phases A and B as directed in the following table.

Time after injection of sample (min)	Mobile phase A (vol%)	Mobile phase B (vol%)
0 – 15	100	0
15 – 20	100 → 0	0 → 100

System suitability—

System performance: To 5 mL of the standard solution add 1 mL of sodium hydroxide TS, allow to stand for 30 minutes, and add 1 mL of 1 mol/L hydrochloric acid TS. When the procedure is run with 5 μL of this solution under the above operating conditions, the resolution between the peak having the relative retention time of about 0.85 to ribavirin and the peak of ribavirin is not less than 4.0. Furthermore, when the procedure is run with 5 μL of the standard solution under the above operating conditions, the symmetry factor of the peak of ribavirin is not more than 1.5.

System repeatability: When the test is repeated 6 times with 5 μL of the standard solution under the above operating conditions, the relative standard deviation of the peak area of ribavirin is not more than 1.0%.

Containers and storage Containers—Tight containers.

Riboflavin

Vitamin B_2

リボフラビン

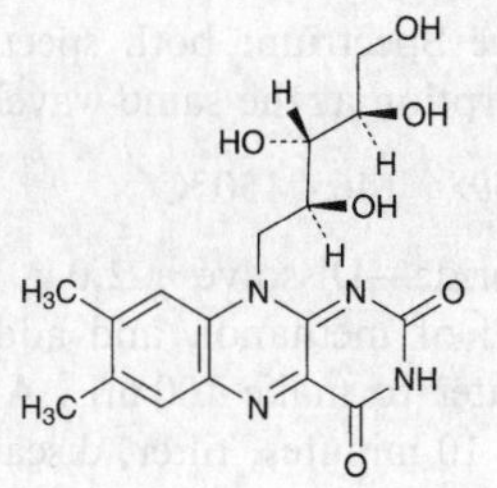

$C_{17}H_{20}N_4O_6$: 376.36
7,8-Dimethyl-10-[(2*S*,3*S*,4*R*)-2,3,4,5-tetrahydroxypentyl]benzo[*g*]pteridine-2,4(3*H*,10*H*)-dione
[*83-88-5*]

Riboflavin, when dried, contains not less than 98.0% of riboflavin ($C_{17}H_{20}N_4O_6$).

Description Riboflavin occurs as yellow to orange-yellow crystals. It has a slight odor.

It is very slightly soluble in water, practically insoluble in ethanol (95), in acetic acid (100), and in diethyl ether.

It dissolves in sodium hydroxide TS.

A saturated solution of Riboflavin is neutral.

It is decomposed by light.

Melting point: about 290°C (with decomposition).

Identification **(1)** A solution of Riboflavin (1 in 100,000) is light yellow-green in color and has an intense yellow-green fluorescence. The color and fluorescence of the solution disappear upon the addition of 0.02 g of sodium hydrosulfite to 5 mL of the solution, and reappear on shaking the mixture in air. This fluorescence disappears upon the addition of dilute hydrochloric acid or sodium hydroxide TS.

(2) To 10 mL of a solution of Riboflavin (1 in 100,000) placed in a glass-stoppered test tube add 1 mL of sodium hydroxide TS, and after illumination with a fluorescence lamp of 10 to 30 watts at 20-cm distance for 30 minutes between 20°C and 40°C, acidify with 0.5 mL of acetic acid (31), and shake with 5 mL of chloroform: the chloroform layer shows a yellow-green fluorescence.

(3) Determine the absorption spectrum of a solution of Riboflavin in phosphate buffer solution (pH 7.0) (1 in 100,000) as directed under Ultraviolet-visible Spectrophotometry <*2.24*>, and compare the spectrum with the Reference Spectrum or the spectrum of a solution of Rivoflavin RS prepared in the same manner as the sample solution: both spectra exhibit similar intensities of absorption at the same wavelengths.

Optical rotation <*2.49*> $[\alpha]_D^{20}$: −128 – −142° Weigh accurately about 0.1 g of dried Riboflavin, dissolve in exactly 4 mL of dilute sodium hydroxide TS, add 10 mL of freshly boiled and cooled water, add exactly 4 mL of aldehyde-free ethanol while shaking, add freshly boiled and cooled water to make exactly 20 mL, and determine the rotation in a 100-mm cell within 30 minutes after preparing the solution.

Purity Lumiflavin—Shake 25 mg of Riboflavin with 10 mL of ethanol-free chloroform for 5 minutes, and filter: the filtrate has no more color than the following control solution.

Control solution: To 2.0 mL of 1/60 mol/L potassium dichromate VS add water to make 1000 mL.

Loss on drying <*2.41*> Not more than 1.5% (0.5 g, 105°C, 2 hours).

Residue on ignition <*2.44*> Not more than 0.2% (1 g).

Assay Conduct this procedure without exposure to light, using light-resistant vessels. Weigh accurately about 15 mg of Riboflavin, previously dried, dissolve in 800 mL of diluted acetic acid (100) (1 in 400) by warming, cool, add water to make exactly 1000 mL, and use this solution as the sample solution. Dry Riboflavin RS at 105°C for 2 hours, weigh accurately about 15 mg, dissolve in 800 mL of diluted acetic acid (100) (1 in 400) by warming, cool, add water to make exactly 1000 mL, and use this solution as the standard solution. Perform the test with the sample solution and standard solution as directed under Ultraviolet-visible Spectrophotometry <*2.24*>, using water as the blank, and determine the absorbances, A_T and A_S, at 445 nm. Add 0.02 g of sodium hydrosulfite to 5 mL of each solution, shake until decolorized, and immediately measure the absorbances, $A_T{}'$ and $A_S{}'$, of the solutions.

$$\text{Amount (mg) of riboflavin } (C_{17}H_{20}N_4O_6) = M_S \times (A_T - A_T{}')/(A_S - A_S{}')$$

M_S: Amount (mg) of Riboflavin RS taken

Containers and storage Containers—Tight containers.
Storage—Light-resistant.

Riboflavin Powder

Vitamin B_2 Powder

リボフラビン散

Riboflavin Powder contains not less than 95.0% and not more than 115.0% of the labeled amount of riboflavin ($C_{17}H_{20}N_4O_6$: 376.36).

Method of preparation Prepare as directed under Granules or Powders, with Riboflavin.

Identification Shake a portion of Riboflavin Powder, equivalent to 1 mg of Riboflavin, with 100 mL of water, filter, and proceed with the filtrate as directed in the Identification (1) and (2) under Riboflavin.

Purity Rancidity—Riboflavin Powder is free from any unpleasant or rancid odor or taste.

Dissolution <*6.10*> When the test is performed at 75 revolutions per minute according to the Paddle method, using 900 mL of water as the dissolution medium, the dissolution rate in 60 minutes of Riboflavin Powder is not less than 80%.

Conduct this procedure without exposure to light. Start the test with an accurately weighed amount of Riboflavin Powder, equivalent to about 5 mg of riboflavin ($C_{17}H_{20}N_4O_6$), withdraw not less than 20 mL of the medium at the specified minute after starting the test, and filter through a membrane filter with a pore size not exceeding 0.45 μm. Discard not less than 10 mL of the first filtrate, and use the subsequent filtrate as the sample solution. Separately, weigh accurately about 22 mg of Riboflavin RS, previously dried at 105°C for 2 hours, dissolve in water by warming and add water to make exactly 200 mL after cooling. Pipet 5 mL of this solution, add water to make exactly 100 mL, and use this solution as the standard solution. Determine the absorbances, A_T and A_S, at 445 nm of the sample solution and standard solution as directed under Ultraviolet-visible Spectrophotometry <2.24>.

Dissolution rate (%) with respect to the labeled amount of riboflavin ($C_{17}H_{20}N_4O_6$)

$$= M_S/M_T \times A_T/A_S \times 1/C \times 45/2$$

M_S: Amount (mg) of Riboflavin RS taken
M_T: Amount (g) of Riboflavin Powder taken
C: Labeled amount (mg) of riboflavin ($C_{17}H_{20}N_4O_6$) in 1 g

Assay Conduct this procedure without exposure to light, using light-resistant vessels. Weigh accurately Riboflavin Powder equivalent to about 15 mg of riboflavin ($C_{17}H_{20}N_4O_6$), add 800 mL of diluted acetic acid (100) (1 in 400), and extract by warming for 30 minutes with occasional shaking. Cool, dilute with water to make exactly 1000 mL, and filter through a glass filter (G4). Use this filtrate as the sample solution, and proceed as directed in the Assay under Riboflavin.

Amount (mg) of riboflavin ($C_{17}H_{20}N_4O_6$)

$$= M_S \times (A_T - A_T')/(A_S - A_S')$$

M_S: Amount (mg) of Riboflavin RS taken

Containers and storage Containers—Tight containers.
Storage—Light-resistant.

Riboflavin Butyrate

Vitamin B_2 Butyrate

リボフラビン酪酸エステル

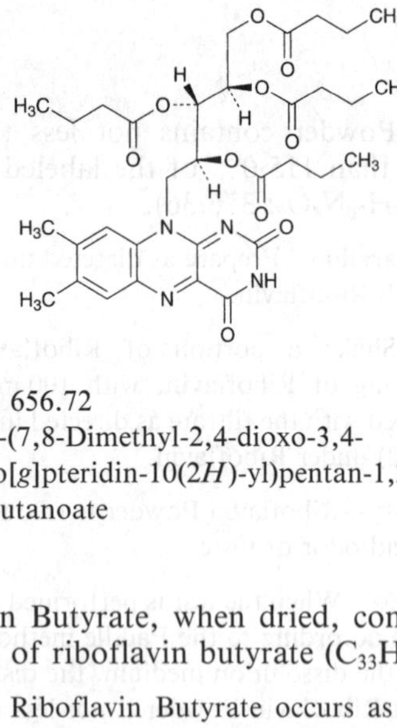

$C_{33}H_{44}N_4O_{10}$: 656.72
(2*R*,3*S*,4*S*)-5-(7,8-Dimethyl-2,4-dioxo-3,4-dihydrobenzo[*g*]pteridin-10(2*H*)-yl)pentan-1,2,3,4-tetrayl tetrabutanoate
[*752-56-7*]

Riboflavin Butyrate, when dried, contains not less than 98.5% of riboflavin butyrate ($C_{33}H_{44}N_4O_{10}$).

Description Riboflavin Butyrate occurs as orange-yellow, crystals or crystalline powder. It has a slight, characteristic odor and a slightly bitter taste.

It is freely soluble in methanol, in ethanol (95) and in chloroform, slightly soluble in diethyl ether, and practically insoluble in water.

It is decomposed by light.

Identification **(1)** A solution of Riboflavin Butyrate in ethanol (95) (1 in 100,000) shows a light yellow-green color with a strong yellowish green fluorescence. To the solution add dilute hydrochloric acid or sodium hydroxide TS: the fluorescence disappears.

(2) Dissolve 0.01 g of Riboflavin Butyrate in 5 mL of ethanol (95), add 2 mL of a mixture of a solution of sodium hydroxide (3 in 20) and a solution of hydroxylammonium chloride (3 in 20) (1:1), and shake well. To this solution add 0.8 mL of hydrochloric acid and 0.5 mL of iron (III) chloride TS, and add 8 mL of ethanol (95): a deep red-brown color develops.

(3) Determine the absorption spectrum of the sample solution obtained in the Assay as directed under Ultraviolet-visible Spectrophotometry <2.24>, and compare the spectrum with the Reference Spectrum: both spectra exhibit similar intensities of absorption at the same wavelengths.

Melting point <2.60> 146 - 150°C

Purity **(1)** Chloride—Dissolve 2.0 g of Riboflavin Butyrate in 10 mL of methanol, and add 24 mL of dilute nitric acid and water to make 100 mL. After shaking well, allow to stand for 10 minutes, filter, discard the first 10 mL of the filtrate, and use the subsequent filtrate as the sample solution. To 25 mL of the sample solution add water to make 50 mL, then add 1 mL of silver nitrate TS, and allow to stand for 5 minutes: the turbidity of the solution is no more than that of the following control solution.

Control solution: To 25 mL of the sample solution add 1 mL of silver nitrate TS, allow to stand for 10 minutes, and filter. Wash the precipitate with four 5-mL portions of water, and combine the washings with the filtrate. To this solution add 0.30 mL of 0.01 mol/L hydrochloric acid VS and water to make 50 mL, add 1 mL of water, and mix (not more than 0.021%).

(2) Heavy metals <1.07>—Proceed with 2.0 g of Riboflavin Butyrate according to Method 2, and perform the test. Prepare the control solution with 2.0 mL of Standard Lead Solution (not more than 10 ppm).

(3) Free acid—To 1.0 g of Riboflavin Butyrate add 50 mL of freshly boiled and cooled water, shake, and filter. To 25 mL of the filtrate add 0.50 mL of 0.01 mol/L sodium hydroxide VS and 2 drops of phenolphthalein TS: the solution shows a red color.

(4) Related substances—Dissolve 0.10 g of Riboflavin Butyrate in 10 mL of chloroform, and use this solution as the sample solution. Pipet 1 mL of the sample solution, and add chloroform to make exactly 50 mL. Pipet 5 mL of this solution, add chloroform to make exactly 20 mL, and use this solution as the standard solution. Perform the test with these solutions as directed under Thin-layer Chromatography <2.03>. Spot 10 μL each of the sample solution and standard solution on a plate of silica gel with fluorescent indicator for thin-layer chromatography. Develop the plate with a mixture of chloroform and 2-propanol (9:1) to a distance of about 10 cm, and air-dry the plate. Examine under ultraviolet light (main wavelength: 254 nm): the spots other than the principal spot obtained from the sample solution are not more intense than the spot from the standard solution.

Loss on drying <2.41> Not more than 0.5% (1 g, in vacuum, silica gel, 4 hours).

Residue on ignition <2.44> Not more than 0.1% (1 g).

Assay Conduct this procedure without exposure to light, using light-resistant vessels. Weigh accurately about 40 mg of Riboflavin Butyrate, previously dried, dissolve in ethanol (95) to make exactly 500 mL, and pipet 10 mL of this solution, add ethanol (95) to make exactly 50 mL, and use this solution as the sample solution. Separately, weigh accurately about 50 mg of Riboflavin RS, previously dried at 105°C for 2 hours, dissolve in 150 mL of diluted acetic acid (100) (2 in 75) by warming, and after cooling, add water to make exactly 500 mL. Pipet 5 mL of this solution, add ethanol (95) to make exactly 50 mL, and use this solution as the standard solution. Determine the absorbances, A_T and A_S, of the sample solution and standard solution at 445 nm as directed under Ultraviolet-visible Spectrophotometry ⟨*2.24*⟩.

Amount (mg) of riboflavin butyrate ($C_{33}H_{44}N_4O_{10}$)
$= M_S \times A_T/A_S \times 1/2 \times 1.745$

M_S: Amount (mg) of Riboflavin RS taken

Containers and storage Containers—Tight containers.
Storage—Light-resistant.

Riboflavin Sodium Phosphate

Vitamin B_2 Phosphate Ester

リボフラビンリン酸エステルナトリウム

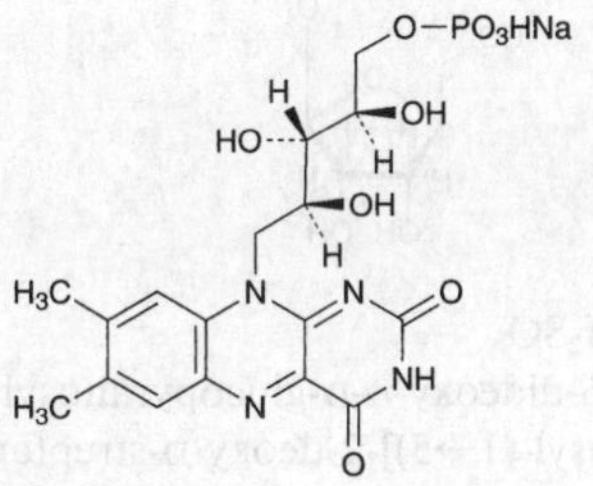

$C_{17}H_{20}N_4NaO_9P$: 478.33
Monosodium (2*R*,3*S*,4*S*)-5-(7,8-dimethyl-2,4-dioxo-3,4-dihydrobenzo[*g*]pteridin-10(2*H*)-yl)-2,3,4-trihydroxypentyl monohydrogen phosphate
[*130-40-5*]

Riboflavin Sodium Phosphate contains not less than 92% of riboflavin sodium phosphate ($C_{17}H_{20}N_4NaO_9P$), calculated on the anhydrous basis.

Description Riboflavin Sodium Phosphate is a yellow to orange-yellow crystalline powder. It is odorless, and has a slightly bitter taste.

It is soluble in water, and practically insoluble in ethanol (95), in chloroform and in diethyl ether.

It is decomposed on exposure to light.

It is very hygroscopic.

Identification **(1)** A solution of Riboflavin Sodium Phosphate (1 in 100,000) is light yellow-green in color and has an intense yellow-green fluorescence. The color and fluorescence of the solution disappear upon the addition of 0.02 g of sodium hydrosulfite to 5 mL of the solution, and reappear on shaking the mixture in air. This fluorescence disappears upon the addition of dilute hydrochloric acid or sodium hydroxide TS.

(2) To 10 mL of a solution of Riboflavin Sodium Phosphate (1 in 100,000) placed in a glass-stoppered test tube add 1 mL of sodium hydroxide TS, and after illumination with a fluorescence lamp of 10 to 30 watts at 20-cm distance for 30 minutes between 20°C and 40°C, acidify with 0.5 mL of acetic acid (31), and shake with 5 mL of chloroform: the chloroform layer shows a yellow-green fluorescence.

(3) Determine the absorption spectrum of a solution of Riboflavin Sodium Phosphate in phosphate buffer solution (pH 7.0) (1 in 100,000) as directed under Ultraviolet-visible Spectrophotometry ⟨*2.24*⟩, and compare the spectrum with the Reference Spectrum: both spectra exhibit similar intensities of absorption at the same wavelengths.

(4) To 0.05 g of Riboflavin Sodium Phosphate add 10 mL of nitric acid, evaporate on a water bath to dryness, and ignite. Boil the residue with 10 mL of diluted nitric acid (1 in 50) for 5 minutes, after cooling, neutralize this solution with ammonia TS, and filter, if necessary: the solution responds to Qualitative Tests ⟨*1.09*⟩ for sodium salt and phosphate.

Optical rotation ⟨*2.49*⟩ $[\alpha]_D^{20}$: +38 – +43° (0.3 g calculated on the anhydrous basis, 5 mol/L hydrochloric acid TS, 20 mL, 100 mm).

pH ⟨*2.54*⟩ Dissolve 0.20 g of Riboflavin Sodium Phosphate in 20 mL of water: the pH of the solution is between 5.0 and 6.5.

Purity **(1)** Clarity and color of solution—Dissolve 0.20 g of Riboflavin Sodium Phosphate in 10 mL of water: the solution is clear and yellow to orange-yellow in color.

(2) Lumiflavin—To 35 mg of Riboflavin Sodium Phosphate add 10 mL of ethanol-free chloroform, and shake for 5 minutes, then filter: the filtrate has no more color than the control solution.

Control solution: To 3.0 mL of 1/60 mol/L potassium dichromate VS add water to make 1000 mL.

(3) Free phosphoric acid—Weigh accurately about 0.4 g of Riboflavin Sodium Phosphate, dissolve in water to make exactly 100 mL, and use this solution as the sample solution. Measure exactly 5 mL each of the sample solution and Standard Phosphoric Acid Solution, transfer to separate 25-mL volumetric flasks, add 2.5 mL of hexaammonium heptamolybdate-sulfuric acid TS and 1 mL of 1-amino-2-naphthol-4-sulfonic acid TS to each of these flasks, mix, and add water to make 25 mL. Allow to stand for 30 minutes at 20 ± 1°C, and perform the test with these solutions as directed under Ultraviolet-visible Spectrophotometry ⟨*2.24*⟩, using a solution prepared with 5 mL of water in the same manner as a blank. Determine the absorbances, A_T and A_S, of the subsequent solutions of the sample solution and Standard Phosphoric Acid Solution at 740 nm: the free phosphoric acid content is not more than 1.5%.

Content (%) of free phosphoric acid (H_3PO_4)
$= 1/M \times A_T/A_S \times 258.0$

M: Amount (mg) of Riboflavin Sodium Phosphate taken, calculated on the anhydrous basis

Water ⟨*2.48*⟩ Place 25 mL of a mixture of methanol for water determination and ethylene glycol for water determination (1:1) in a dry flask for titration, and titrate with Karl Fischer TS for water determination to the end point. Weigh accurately about 0.1 g of Riboflavin Sodium Phosphate, place quickly into the flask, add a known excess volume of Karl Fischer TS for water determination, mix for 10 minutes, and perform the test: the water content is not more than 10.0%.

Assay Conduct this procedure without exposure to light, using light-resistant vessels. To about 0.1 g of Riboflavin Sodium Phosphate, accurately weighed, dissolve in diluted acetic acid (100) (1 in 500) to make exactly 1000 mL, then pipet 10 mL of this solution, and add diluted acetic acid (100) (1 in 500) to make exactly 50 mL. Use this solution as the sample solution. Separately, dry Riboflavin RS at 105°C for 2 hours, weigh accurately about 15 mg, dissolve in 800 mL of diluted acetic acid (100) (1 in 400) by warming, cool, add water to make exactly 1000 mL, and use this solution as the standard solution. Perform the test with the sample solution and standard solution as directed under Ultraviolet-visible Spectrophotometry ⟨*2.24*⟩, using water as the blank, and determine the absorbances, A_T and A_S, at 445 nm. Add 0.02 g of sodium hydrosulfite to 5 mL of each solution, shake until decolorized, and immediately measure the absorbances, A_T' and A_S', of the solutions.

Amount (mg) of riboflavin sodium phosphate ($C_{17}H_{20}N_4NaO_9P$)
$= M_S \times (A_T - A_T')/(A_S - A_S') \times 5 \times 1.271$

M_S: Amount (mg) of Riboflavin RS taken

Containers and storage Containers—Tight containers.
Storage—Light-resistant.

Riboflavin Sodium Phosphate Injection

Vitamin B$_2$ Phosphate Ester Injection

リボフラビンリン酸エステルナトリウム注射液

Riboflavin Sodium Phosphate Injection is an aqueous injection.

It contains not less than 95.0% and not more than 120.0% of the labeled amount of riboflavin ($C_{17}H_{20}N_4O_6$: 376.36).

The concentration of Riboflavin Sodium Phosphate Injection should be stated as the amount of riboflavin ($C_{17}H_{20}N_4O_6$).

Method of preparation Prepare as directed under Injections, with Riboflavin Sodium Phosphate.

Description Riboflavin Sodium Phosphate Injection is a clear, yellow to orange-yellow liquid.

pH: 5.0 – 7.0

Identification **(1)** To a measured volume of Riboflavin Sodium Phosphate Injection, equivalent to 1 mg of Riboflavin, add water to make 100 mL, and proceed with this solution as directed in the Identification (1) and (2) under Riboflavin Sodium Phosphate.

(2) To a measured volume of Riboflavin Sodium Phosphate Injection, equivalent to 0.05 g of Riboflavin, and evaporate on a water bath to dryness. Proceed with this residue as directed in the Identification (4) under Riboflavin Sodium Phosphate.

Bacterial endotoxins <*4.01*> Less than 10 EU/mg.

Extractable volume <*6.05*> It meets the requirement.

Foreign insoluble matter <*6.06*> Perform the test according to Method 1: it meets the requirement.

Insoluble particulate matter <*6.07*> It meets the requirement.

Sterility <*4.06*> Perform the test according to the Membrane filtration method: it meets the requirement.

Assay Conduct this procedure without exposure to light, using light-resistant vessels. To an accurately measured volume of Riboflavin Sodium Phosphate Injection, equivalent to about 15 mg of riboflavin ($C_{17}H_{20}N_4O_6$), add diluted acetic acid (100) (1 in 500) to make exactly 1000 mL, and use this solution as the sample solution. Proceed as directed in the Assay under Riboflavin Sodium Phosphate.

Amount (mg) of Riboflavin ($C_{17}H_{20}N_4O_6$)
$= M_S \times (A_T - A_T')/(A_S - A_S')$

M_S: Amount (mg) of Riboflavin RS taken

Containers and storage Containers—Hermetic containers.
Storage—Light-resistant.

Ribostamycin Sulfate

リボスタマイシン硫酸塩

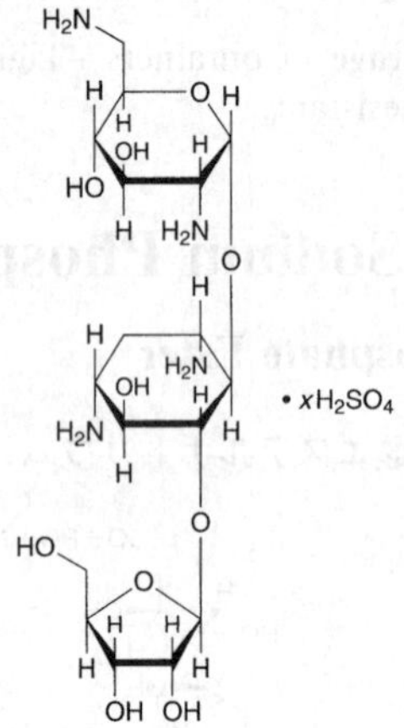

$C_{17}H_{34}N_4O_{10}.xH_2SO_4$
2,6-Diamino-2,6-dideoxy-α-D-glucopyranosyl-(1→4)-[β-D-ribofuranosyl-(1→5)]-2-deoxy-D-streptamine sulfate
[*53797-35-6*]

Ribostamycin Sulfate is the sulfate of an aminoglycoside substance having antibacterial activity produced by the growth of *Streptomyces ribosidificus*.

It contains not less than 680 μg (potency) and not more than 780 μg (potency) per mg, calculated on the dried basis. The potency of Ribostamycin Sulfate is expressed as mass (potency) of ribostamycin ($C_{17}H_{34}N_4O_{10}$: 454.47).

Description Ribostamycin Sulfate occurs as a white to yellow-white powder.

It is freely soluble in water, and practically insoluble in ethanol (95).

Identification **(1)** Dissolve 20 mg of Ribostamycin Sulfate in 2 mL of phosphate buffer solution (pH 6.0), add 1 mL of ninhydrin TS, and boil: a blue-purple color develops.

(2) Dissolve 0.12 g each of Ribostamycin Sulfate and Ribostamycin Sulfate RS in 20 mL of water, and use these solutions as the sample solution and standard solution. Perform the test with these solutions as directed under Thin-layer Chromatography <*2.03*>. Spot 5 μL each of the sample solution and standard solution on a plate of silica gel for thin-layer chromatography. Develop the plate with a solution of potassium dihydrogen phosphate (3 in 40) to a distance of about 10 cm, and air-dry the plate. Spray evenly 0.2% ninhydrin-water saturated 1-butanol TS, and heat at 100°C for 10 minutes: the principal spots obtained from the sample solution and standard solution show a purple-brown color and the same *R*f value.

(3) To 2 mL of a solution of Ribostamycin Sulfate (1 in 5) add 1 drop of barium chloride TS: a white turbidity is produced.

Optical rotation <*2.49*> $[\alpha]_D^{20}$: +42 – +49° (after drying, 0.25 g, water, 25 mL, 100 mm).

pH <*2.54*> The pH of a solution obtained by dissolving 1.0 g of Ribostamycin Sulfate in 20 mL of water is between 6.0 and 8.0.

Purity (1) Clarity and color of solution—Dissolve 2.9 g of Ribostamycin Sulfate in 10 mL of water: the solution is clear. Determine the absorbance of this solution at 400 nm as directed under Ultraviolet-visible Spectrophotometry <*2.24*>: not more than 0.10.

(2) Heavy metals <*1.07*>—Proceed with 1.0 g of Ribostamycin Sulfate according to Method 1, and perform the test. Prepare the control solution with 3.0 mL of Standard Lead Solution (not more than 30 ppm).

(3) Arsenic <*1.11*>—Prepare the test solution with 1.0 g of Ribostamycin Sulfate according to Method 1, and perform the test (not more than 2 ppm).

(4) Related substances—Dissolve 0.12 g of Ribostamycin Sulfate in water to make exactly 20 mL, and use this solution as the sample solution. Pipet 5 mL of the sample solution, add water to make exactly 100 mL, and use this solution as the standard solution. Perform the test with these solutions as directed under Thin-layer Chromatography <*2.03*>. Spot 5 μL each of the sample solution and standard solution on a plate of silica gel for thin-layer chromatography. Develop the plate with a solution of potassium dihydrogen phosphate (3 in 40) to a distance of about 10 cm, and air-dry the plate. Spray evenly 0.2% ninhydrin-water saturated 1-butanol TS on the plate, and heat the plate at 100°C for 10 minutes: the spot other than the principal spot obtained from the sample solution is not more intense than the spot from the standard solution.

Loss on drying <*2.41*> Not more than 5.0% (0.5 g, reduced pressure not exceeding 0.67 kPa, 60°C, 3 hours).

Residue on ignition <*2.44*> Not more than 1.0% (1 g).

Assay Perform the test according to the Cylinder-plate method as directed under Microbial Assay for Antibiotics <*4.02*> according to the following conditions.

(i) Test organism—*Bacillus subtilis* ATCC 6633

(ii) Culture medium—Use the medium i in 1) Medium under (1) Agar media for seed and base layer.

(iii) Standard solutions—Weigh accurately an amount of Ribostamycin Sulfate RS, previously dried, equivalent to about 20 mg (potency), dissolve in diluted phosphate buffer solution (pH 6.0) (1 in 2) to make exactly 50 mL, and use this solution as the standard stock solution. Keep the standard stock solution at 5 to 15°C and use within 20 days. Take exactly a suitable amount of the standard stock solution before use, add 0.1 mol/L phosphate buffer solution (pH 8.0) to make solutions so that each mL contains 20 μg (potency) and 5 μg (potency), and use these solutions as the high concentration standard solution and the low concentration standard solution, respectively.

(iv) Sample solutions—Weigh accurately an amount of Ribostamycin Sulfate, equivalent to about 20 mg (potency), and dissolve in water to make exactly 50 mL. Take exactly a suitable amount of this solution, add 0.1 mol/L phosphate buffer solution (pH 8.0) to make solutions so that each mL contains 20 μg (potency) and 5 μg (potency), and use these solutions as the high concentration sample solution and the low concentration sample solution, respectively.

Containers and storage Containers—Tight containers.

Rifampicin

リファンピシン

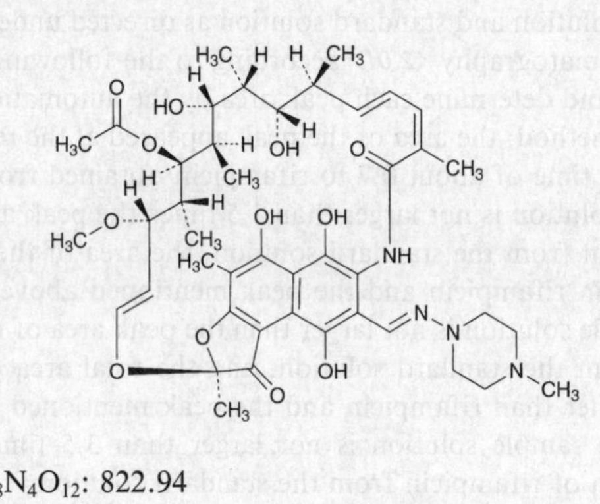

$C_{43}H_{58}N_4O_{12}$: 822.94

(2*S*,12*Z*,14*E*,16*S*,17*S*,18*R*,19*R*,20*R*,21*S*,22*R*,23*S*,24*E*)-5,6,9,17,19-Pentahydroxy-23-methoxy-2,4,12,16,18,20,22-heptamethyl-8-(4-methylpiperazin-1-yliminomethyl)-1,11-dioxo-1,2-dihydro-2,7-(epoxypentadeca[1,11,13]trienimino)naphtho[2,1-*b*]furan-21-yl acetate

[*13292-46-1*]

Rifampicin is a derivative of a substance having antibacterial activity produced by the growth of *Streptomyces mediterranei*.

It contains not less than 970 μg (potency) and not more than 1020 μg (potency) per mg, calculated on the dried basis. The potency of Rifampicin is expressed as mass (potency) of rifampicin ($C_{43}H_{58}N_4O_{12}$).

Description Rifampicin occurs as orange-red to red-brown, crystals or crystalline powder.

It is slightly soluble in water, in acetonitrile, in methanol and in ethanol (95).

Identification (1) To 5 mL of a solution of Rifampicin in methanol (1 in 5000) add 0.05 mol/L phosphate buffer solution (pH 7.0) to make 100 mL. Determine the absorption spectrum of this solution as directed under Ultraviolet-visible Spectrophotometry <*2.24*>, and compare the spectrum with the Reference Spectrum or the spectrum of a solution of Rifampicin RS prepared in the same manner as the sample solution: both spectra exhibit similar intensities of absorption at the same wavelengths.

(2) Determine the infrared absorption spectrum of Rifampicin as directed in the potassium bromide disk method under the Infrared Spectrophotometry <*2.25*>, and compare the spectrum with the Reference Spectrum or the spectrum of Rifampicin RS: both spectra exhibit similar intensities of absorption at the same wave numbers.

Purity (1) Heavy metals <*1.07*>—Proceed with 1.0 g of Rifampicin according to Method 2, and perform the test. Prepare the control solution with 2.0 mL of Standard Lead Solution (not more than 20 ppm).

(2) Arsenic <*1.11*>—Prepare the test solution with 1.0 g of Rifampicin according to Method 3, and perform the test (not more than 2 ppm).

(3) Related substances—Perform the test immediately after preparing of the sample and standard solutions. Dissolve 0.10 g of Rifampicin in 50 mL of acetonitrile, and use this solution as the sample stock solution. Pipet 5 mL of the sample stock solution, add citric acid-phosphate-acetonitrile TS to make exactly 50 mL, and use this solution as the sample solution. Separately, pipet 1 mL of the sample stock so-

lution, and add acetonitrile to make exactly 100 mL. Pipet 5 mL of this solution, add citric acid-phosphate-acetonitrile TS to make exactly 50 mL, and use this solution as the standard solution. Perform the test with exactly 50 μL each of the sample solution and standard solution as directed under Liquid Chromatography <*2.01*> according to the following conditions, and determine each peak area by the automatic integration method: the area of the peak appeared at the relative retention time of about 0.7 to rifampicin obtained from the sample solution is not larger than 1.5 times the peak area of rifampicin from the standard solution, the area of the peak other than rifampicin and the peak mentioned above from the sample solution is not larger than the peak area of rifampicin from the standard solution, and the total area of the peaks other than rifampicin and the peak mentioned above from the sample solution is not larger than 3.5 times the peak area of rifampicin from the standard solution.

Operating conditions—

Detector, column, column temperature, mobile phase, and flow rate: Proceed as directed in the operating conditions in the Assay.

Time span of measurement: About 3 times as long as the retention time of rifampicin, beginning after the peak of the solvent.

System suitability—

System performance: Proceed as directed in the system suitability in the Assay.

Test for required detectability: Measure exactly 2 mL of the standard solution, and add citric acid-phosphate-acetonitrile TS to make exactly 20 mL. Confirm that the peak area of rifampicin obtained with 50 μL of this solution is equivalent to 7 to 13% of that with 50 μL of the standard solution.

System repeatability: When the test is repeated 6 times with 50 μL of the standard solution under the above operating conditions, the relative standard deviation of the peak area of rifampicin is not more than 2.0%.

Loss on drying <*2.41*> Not more than 2.0% (1 g, reduced pressure not exceeding 0.67 kPa, 60°C, 3 hours).

Residue on ignition <*2.44*> Not more than 0.1% (1 g).

Assay Weigh accurately an amount of Rifampicin and Rifampicin RS, equivalent to about 40 mg (potency), and dissolve each in acetonitrile to make exactly 200 mL. Pipet 10 mL each of these solutions, add citric acid-phosphate-acetonitrile TS to make exactly 100 mL, and use these solutions as the sample solution and standard solution. Perform the test with exactly 50 μL each of the sample solution and standard solution as directed under Liquid Chromatography <*2.01*> according to the following conditions, and determine the peak areas, A_T and A_S, of rifampicin in each solution.

Amount [μg (potency)] of rifampicin ($C_{43}H_{58}N_4O_{12}$)
$= M_S \times A_T/A_S \times 1000$

M_S: Amount [mg (potency)] of Rifampicin RS taken

Operating conditions—

Detector: An ultraviolet absorption photometer (wavelength: 254 nm).

Column: A stainless steel column 4.6 mm in inside diameter and 10 cm in length, packed with octylsilanized silica gel for liquid chromatography (5 μm in particle diameter).

Column temperature: A constant temperature of about 25°C.

Mobile phase: Dissolve 4.2 g of citric acid monohydrate and 1.4 g of sodium perchlorate in 1000 mL of a mixture of water, acetonitrile and phosphate buffer solution (pH 3.1) (11:7:2).

Flow rate: Adjust so that the retention time of rifampicin is about 8 minutes.

System suitability—

System performance: To 5 mL of a solution of Rifampicin in acetonitrile (1 in 5000) add 1 mL of a solution of butyl parahydroxybenzoate in acetonitrile (1 in 5000) and citric acid-phosphate-acetonitrile TS to make 50 mL. When the procedure is run with 50 μL of this solution under the above operating conditions, butyl parahydroxybenzoate and rifampicin are eluted in this order with the resolution between these peaks being not less than 1.5.

System repeatability: When the test is repeated 5 times with 50 μL of the standard solution under the above operating conditions, the relative standard deviation of the peak area of rifampicin is not more than 1.0%.

Containers and storage Containers—Tight containers.

Rifampicin Capsules

リファンピシンカプセル

Rifampicin Capsules contain not less than 93.0% and not more than 105.0% of the labeled potency of rifampicin ($C_{43}H_{58}N_4O_{12}$: 822.94).

Method of preparation Prepare as directed under Capsules, with Rifampicin.

Identification Take out the content of Rifampicin Capsules, mix well, and powder, if necessary. Dissolve an amount of the content, equivalent to 20 mg (potency) of Rifampicin, in methanol to make 100 mL, and filter. To 5 mL of the filtrate add 0.05 mol/L phosphate buffer solution (pH 7.0) to make 100 mL. Determine the absorption spectrum of this solution as directed under Ultraviolet-visible Spectrophotometry <*2.24*>: it exhibits maxima between 234 nm and 238 nm, between 252 nm and 256 nm, between 331 nm and 335 nm, and between 472 nm and 476 nm.

Purity Related substances—Perform the test quickly after the sample solution and standard solution are prepared. Open the capsules of not less than 20 Rifampicin Capsules, carefully take out the content, weigh accurately, and powder. Weigh accurately a portion of the powder, equivalent to about 20 mg (potency) of Rifampicin, and dissolve in acetonitrile to make exactly 10 mL. Pipet 2 mL of this solution, add a mixture of acetonitrile and methanol (1:1) to make exactly 20 mL, and use this solution as the sample solution. Separately, weigh accurately an amount of Rifampicin RS, equivalent to about 20 mg (potency), and dissolve in acetonitrile to make exactly 10 mL. Pipet 2 mL of this solution, and add the mixture of acetonitrile and methanol (1:1) to make exactly 20 mL. Pipet 1 mL of this solution, add the mixture of acetonitrile and methanol (1:1) to make exactly 50 mL, and use this solution as the standard solution. Perform the test with exactly 20 μL each of the sample solution and standard solution as directed under Liquid Chromatography <*2.01*> according to the following conditions, and determine each peak area by the automatic integration method: the amount of the peaks of quinone substance and *N*-oxide substance, having the relative retention time of about 0.5 and about 1.2 to rifampicin, obtained from the sample solution are not more than 4.0% and not more than 1.5%, respectively. The amount of the peak other than the peaks mentioned above is not more than 1.0%, and the total amount of these related substances is not more than 2.0%.

For the areas of the peaks of the quinone substance and *N*-oxide substance, multiply their correction factors, 1.24 and 1.16, respectively.

$$\text{Amount (mg) of quinone substance} = M_S/M_T \times A_{Ta}/A_S \times 2.48$$

$$\text{Amount (mg) of } N\text{-oxide substance} = M_S/M_T \times A_{Tb}/A_S \times 2.32$$

Each amount (mg) of related substances other than quinone and *N*-oxide substances = $M_S/M_T \times A_{Ti}/A_S \times 2$

M_S: Amount [mg (potency)] of Rifampicin RS taken
M_T: Amount [mg (potency)] of sample taken
A_S: Peak area of the standard solution
A_{Ta}: Peak area of quinone substance
A_{Tb}: Peak area of *N*-oxide substance
A_{Ti}: Each peak area of related substances other than quinone and *N*-oxide substances

Operating conditions—

Detector: An ultraviolet absorption photometer (wavelength: 254 nm).

Column: A stainless steel column 4.6 mm in inside diameter and 25 cm in length, packed with octylsilanized silica gel for liquid chromatography (5 μm in particle diameter).

Column temperature: A constant temperature of about 25°C.

Mobile phase: Dissolve 2.1 g of sodium perchlorate, 6.5 g of citric acid monohydrate and 2.3 g of potassium dihydrogen phosphate in 1100 mL of water, and add 900 mL of acetonitrile.

Flow rate: Adjust so that the retention time of rifampicin is about 12 minutes.

Time span of measurement: About 2.5 times as long as the retention time of rifampicin.

System suitability—

Test for required detectability: To exactly 1 mL of the standard solution add a mixture of acetonitrile and methanol (1:1) to make exactly 20 mL. Confirm that the peak area of rifampicin obtained with 20 μL of this solution is equivalent to 3.5 to 6.5% of that with 20 μL of the standard solution.

System performance: When the procedure is run with 20 μL of the standard solution under the above operating conditions, the number of theoretical plates and the symmetry factor of the peak of rifampicin is not less than 2500 and not more than 4.0, respectively.

System repeatability: When the test is repeated 6 times with 20 μL of the standard solution under the above operating conditions, the relative standard deviation of the peak area of rifampicin is not more than 2.0%.

Uniformity of dosage units <*6.02*> It meets the requirement of the Mass variation test.

Dissolution <*6.10*> When the test is performed at 75 revolutions per minute according to the Paddle method using a sinker, using 900 mL of water as the dissolution medium, the dissolution rate in 45 minutes of Rifampicin Capsules is not less than 80%.

Start the test with 1 capsule of Rifampicin Capsules, withdraw not less than 20 mL of the medium at the specified minute after starting the test, and filter through a membrane filter with a pore size not exceeding 0.45 μm. Discard not less than 10 mL of the first filtrate, pipet *V* mL of the subsequent filtrate, add water to make exactly *V′* mL so that each mL contains about 17 μg (potency) of rifampicin ($C_{43}H_{58}N_4O_{12}$), and use this solution as the sample solution. Separately, weigh accurately about 17 mg (potency) of Rifampicin RS, dissolve in 5 mL of methanol, and add water to make exactly 100 mL. Pipet 2 mL of this solution, add water to make exactly 20 mL, and use this solution as the standard solution. Determine the absorbances, A_T and A_S, at 334 nm of the sample solution and standard solution as directed under Ultraviolet-visible Spectrophotometry <*2.24*>, using water as the blank.

Dissolution rate (%) with respect to the labeled amount of rifampicin ($C_{43}H_{58}N_4O_{12}$)
$$= M_S \times A_T/A_S \times V'/V \times 1/C \times 90$$

M_S: Amount [mg (potency)] of Rifampicin RS taken
C: Labeled amount [mg (potency)] of rifampicin ($C_{43}H_{58}N_4O_{12}$) in 1 capsule

Assay Open the capsules of not less than 20 Rifampicin Capsules, take out the content, weigh accurately the mass of the content, and powder. Weigh accurately a portion of the powder, equivalent to about 75 mg (potency) of Rifampicin, dissolve in a mixture of acetonitrile and methanol (1:1) to make exactly 50 mL. Pipet 10 mL of this solution, and add acetonitrile to make exactly 50 mL. Pipet 5 mL of this solution, add a solution prepared by dissolving 2.1 g of citric acid monohydrate, 27.6 g of disodium hydrogen phosphate dodecahydrate and 3.1 g of potassium dihydrogen phosphate in 1000 mL of a mixture of water and acetonitrile (3:1) to make exactly 50 mL, and use this solution as the sample solution. Separately, weigh accurately an amount of Rifampicin RS, equivalent to about 30 mg (potency), dissolve in 20 mL of a mixture of acetonitrile and methanol (1:1), and add acetonitrile to make exactly 100 mL. Pipet 5 mL of this solution, add the solution prepared by dissolving 2.1 g of citric acid monohydrate, 27.6 g of disodium hydrogen phosphate dodecahydrate and 3.1 g of potassium dihydrogen phosphate in 1000 mL of the mixture of water and acetonitrile (3:1) to make exactly 50 mL, and use this solution as the standard solution. Perform the test with exactly 50 μL each of the sample solution and standard solution as directed under Liquid Chromatography <*2.01*> according to the following conditions, and determine the peak areas, A_T and A_S, of rifampicin in each solution.

$$\text{Amount [mg (potency)] of rifampicin } (C_{43}H_{58}N_4O_{12}) = M_S \times A_T/A_S \times 5/2$$

M_S: Amount [mg (potency)] of Rifampicin RS taken

Operating conditions—

Proceed as directed in the operating conditions in the Assay under Rifampicin.

System suitability—

System performance: Dissolve 30 mg (potency) of Rifampicin RS in 20 mL of the mixture of acetonitrile and methanol (1:1), and add acetonitrile to make 100 mL. To 5 mL of this solution add 2 mL of a solution of butyl parahydroxybenzoate in the mixture of acetonitrile and methanol (1:1) (1 in 5000), then add the solution prepared by dissolving 2.1 g of citric acid monohydrate, 27.6 g of disodium hydrogen phosphate dodecahydrate and 3.1 g of potassium dihydrogen phosphate in 1000 mL of a mixture of water and acetonitrile (3:1) to make exactly 50 mL. When the procedure is run with 50 μL of this solution under the above operating conditions, butyl parahydroxybenzoate and rifampicin are eluted in this order with the resolution between these peaks being not less than 1.5.

System repeatability: When the test is repeated 5 times with 50 μL of the standard solution under the above operating conditions, the relative standard deviation of the peak area of rifampicin is not more than 1.0%.

Containers and storage Containers—Tight containers.

Rilmazafone Hydrochloride Hydrate

リルマザホン塩酸塩水和物

$C_{21}H_{20}Cl_2N_6O_3.HCl.2H_2O$: 547.82
5-[(2-Aminoacetamido)methyl]-1-[4-chloro-2-(2-chlorobenzoyl)phenyl]-*N*,*N*-dimethyl-1*H*-1,2,4-triazole-3-carboxamide monohydrochloride dihydrate
[*85815-37-8*, anhydride]

Rilmazafone Hydrochloride Hydrate contains not less than 98.0% and not more than 102.0% of rilmazafone hydrochloride ($C_{21}H_{20}Cl_2N_6O_3.HCl$: 511.79), calculated on the anhydrous basis.

Description Rilmazafone Hydrochloride Hydrate occurs as a white to pale yellow-white crystalline powder.

It is very soluble in methanol, soluble in water, and slightly soluble in ethanol (99.5).

Identification **(1)** Determine the absorption spectrum of a solution of Rilmazafone Hydrochloride Hydrate (1 in 100,000) as directed under Ultraviolet-visible Spectrophotometry *<2.24>*, and compare the spectrum with the Reference Spectrum or the spectrum of a solution of Rilmazafone Hydrochloride RS prepared in the same manner as the sample solution: both spectra exhibit similar intensities of absorption at the same wavelengths.

(2) Determine the infrared absorption spectrum of Rilmazafone Hydrochloride Hydrate as directed in the potassium chloride disk method under Infrared Spectrophotometry *<2.25>*, and compare the spectrum with the Reference Spectrum or the spectrum of Rilmazafone Hydrochloride RS: both spectra exhibit similar intensities of absorption at the same wave numbers.

(3) A solution of Rilmazafone Hydrochloride Hydrate (1 in 200) responds to Qualitative Tests *<1.09>* (2) for chloride.

Purity **(1)** Heavy metals *<1.07>*—Proceed with 1.0 g of Rilmazafone Hydrochloride Hydrate according to Method 2, and perform the test. Prepare the control solution with 1.0 mL of Standard Lead Solution (not more than 10 ppm).

(2) Related substances—Dissolve 25 mg of Rilmazafone Hydrochloride Hydrate in 50 mL of a mixture of water and acetonitrile (1:1), and use this solution as the sample solution. Pipet 1 mL of the sample solution, add a mixture of water and acetonitrile (1:1) to make exactly 200 mL, and use this solution as the standard solution. Perform the test with exactly 10 μL each of the sample solution and standard solution as directed under Liquid Chromatography *<2.01>* according to the following conditions, and determine each peak area by the automatic integration method: the area of the peak, having the relative retention time of about 0.87 to rilmazafone, obtained from the sample solution is not larger than the peak area of rilmazafone from the standard solution, and the area of the peak other than rilmazafone and the peak mentioned above from the sample solution is not larger than 1/5 times the peak area of rilmazafone from the standard solution. Furthermore, the total area of the peaks other than rilmazafone from the sample solution is not larger than 2 times the peak area of rilmazafone from the standard solution.

Operating conditions—

Detector: An ultraviolet absorption photometer (wavelength: 254 nm).

Column: A stainless steel column 4.6 mm in inside diameter and 25 cm in length, packed with octadecylsilanized silica gel for liquid chromatography (5 μm in particle diameter).

Column temperature: A constant temperature of about 25°C.

Mobile phase A: 0.02 mol/L phosphate buffer solution (pH 3.0).

Mobile phase B: Acetonitrile.

Flowing of mobile phase: Control the gradient by mixing the mobile phases A and B as directed in the following table.

Time after injection of sample (min)	Mobile phase A (vol%)	Mobile phase B (vol%)
0 – 3	75	25
3 – 20	75 → 70	25 → 30
20 – 30	70 → 50	30 → 50
30 – 45	50	50

Flow rate: 1.0 mL per minute.

Time span of measurement: For 45 minutes after injection, beginning after the solvent peak.

System suitability—

Test for required detectability: Pipet 2 mL of the standard solution, and add a mixture of water and acetonitrile (1:1) to make exactly 20 mL. Confirm that the peak area of rilmazafone obtained with 10 μL of this solution is equivalent to 7 to 13% of that with 10 μL of the standard solution.

System performance: When the procedure is run with 10 μL of the standard solution under the above operating conditions, the number of theoretical plates and the symmetry factor of the peak of rilmazafone are not less than 20,000 and not more than 1.3, respectively.

System repeatability: When the test is repeated 6 times with 10 μL of the standard solution under the above operating conditions, the relative standard deviation of the peak area of rilmazafone is not more than 2.0%.

Water *<2.48>* 5.5 – 7.5% (0.2 g, volumetric titration, direct titration).

Residue on ignition *<2.44>* Not more than 0.1% (1 g).

Assay Weigh accurately about 40 mg each of Rilmazafone Hydrochloride Hydrate and Rilmazafone Hydrochloride RS (separately determine the water *<2.48>* in the same manner as Rilmazafone Hydrochloride Hydrate), dissolve each in water to make exactly 200 mL. Pipet 10 mL each of these solutions, add exactly 20 mL of the internal standard solution to each solution, and use these solutions as the sample solution and the standard solution, respectively. Perform the test with 15 μL each of the sample solution and standard solution as directed under Liquid Chromatography *<2.01>* according to the following conditions, and calculate the ratios, Q_T and Q_S, of the peak area of rilmazafone to that of the internal standard.

Amount (mg) of rilmazafone hydrochloride
($C_{21}H_{20}Cl_2N_6O_3.HCl$)
$= M_S \times Q_T/Q_S$

M_S: Amount (mg) of Rilmazafone Hydrochloride RS taken, calculated on the anhydrous basis

Internal standard solution—A solution of propyl parahydroxybenzoate in a mixture of water and acetonitrile (1:1) (3 in 100,000).

Operating conditions—

Detector: An ultraviolet absorption photometer (wavelength: 254 nm).

Column: A stainless steel column 4.6 mm in inside diameter and 15 cm in length, packed with octadecylsilanized silica gel for liquid chromatography (5 μm in particle diameter).

Column temperature: A constant temperature of about 25°C.

Mobile phase: Dissolve 1.1 g of sodium 1-heptanesulfonate in 1000 mL of water, and adjust to pH 3.0 with acetic acid (100). To 500 mL of this solution add 300 mL of acetonitrile.

Flow rate: Adjust so that the retention time of rilmazafone is about 5 minutes.

System suitability—

System performance: When the procedure is run with 15 μL of the standard solution under the above operating conditions, rilmazafone and the internal standard are eluted in this order with the resolution between these peaks being not less than 13.

System repeatability: When the test is repeated 6 times with 15 μL of the standard solution under the above operating conditions, the relative standard deviation of the ratios of the peak area of rilmazafone to that of the internal standard is not more than 1.0%.

Containers and storage Containers—Well-closed containers.

Rilmazafone Hydrochloride Tablets

リルマザホン塩酸塩錠

Rilmazafone Hydrochloride Tablets contain not less than 93.0% and not more than 107.0% of the labeled amount of rilmazafone hydrochloride hydrate ($C_{21}H_{20}Cl_2N_6O_3.HCl.2H_2O$: 547.82).

Method of preparation Prepare as directed under Tablets, with Rilmazafone Hydrochloride Hydrate.

Identification To a quantity of powdered Rilmazafone Hydrochloride Tablets, equivalent to 10 mg of Rilmazafone Hydrochloride Hydrate, add 5 mL of methanol, shake for 10 minutes, and centrifuge. Filter the supernatant liquid with a membrane filter with a pore size not exceeding 0.45 μm, and use the filtrate as the sample solution. Separately, dissolve 2 mg of rilmazafone hydrochloride hydrate in 1 mL of methanol, and use this solution as the standard solution. Perform the test with these solutions as directed under Thin-layer Chromatography <*2.03*>. Spot 10 μL each of the sample solution and standard solution on a plate of silica gel with fluorescent indicator for thin-layer chromatography. Develop the plate with a mixture of ethyl acetate, acetonitrile, water and acetic acid (100) (8:4:3:3) to a distance of about 10 cm, and air-dry the plate. Examine under ultraviolet light (main wavelength: 254 nm): the principal spot obtained from the sample solution and the spot from the standard solution show the same *R*f value.

Uniformity of dosage units <*6.02*> Perform the test according to the following method: it meets the requirement of the Content uniformity test.

To 1 tablet of Rilmazafone Hydrochloride Tablets add *V* mL of water so that each mL contains about 0.2 mg of rilmazafone hydrochloride hydrate ($C_{21}H_{20}Cl_2N_6O_3.HCl.2H_2O$). Add exactly 2*V* mL of the internal standard solution, shake vigorously for 10 minutes, and filter with a membrane filter with a pore size not exceeding 0.45 μm. Discard the first 5 mL of the filtrate, and use the subsequent filtrate as the sample solution. Separately, weigh accurately about 20 mg of Rilmazafone Hydrochloride RS (separately determine the water <*2.48*> in the same manner as Rilmazafone Hydrochloride Hydrate), and dissolve in water to make exactly 100 mL. Pipet 10 mL of this solution, add exactly 20 mL of the internal standard solution, and use this solution as the standard solution. Then, proceed as directed in the Assay under Rilmazafone Hydrochloride Hydrate.

Amount (mg) of rilmazafone hydrochloride hydrate
($C_{21}H_{20}Cl_2N_6O_3.HCl.2H_2O$)
$= M_S \times Q_T/Q_S \times V/100 \times 1.070$

M_S: Amount (mg) of Rilmazafone Hydrochloride RS taken, calculated on the anhydrous basis

Internal standard solution—A solution of propyl parahydroxybenzoate in a mixture of water and acetonitrile (1:1) (3 in 100,000).

Dissolution <*6.10*> When the test is performed at 50 revolutions per minute according to the Paddle method, using 900 mL of water as the dissolution medium, the dissolution rate in 15 minutes of Rilmazafone Hydrochloride Tablets is not less than 85%.

Start the test with 1 tablet of Rilmazafone Hydrochloride Tablets, withdraw not less than 20 mL of the medium at the specified minute after starting the test, and filter through a membrane filter with a pore size not exceeding 0.45 μm. Discard not less than 10 mL of the first filtrate, pipet *V* mL of the subsequent filtrate, add water to make exactly *V′* mL so that each mL contains about 1.1 μg of rilmazafone hydrochloride hydrate ($C_{21}H_{20}Cl_2N_6O_3.HCl.2H_2O$), and use this solution as the sample solution. Separately, weigh accurately about 22 mg of Rilmazafone Hydrochloride RS (separately determine the water <*2.48*> in the same manner as Rilmazafone Hydrochloride Hydrate), and dissolve in water to make exactly 100 mL. Pipet 5 mL of this solution, add water to make exactly 100 mL. Then, pipet 5 mL of this solution, add water to make exactly 50 mL, and use this solution as the standard solution. Perform the test with exactly 50 μL each of the sample solution and standard solution as directed under Liquid Chromatography <*2.01*> according to the following conditions, and determine the peak areas, A_T and A_S, of rilmazafone in each solution.

Dissolution rate (%) with respect to the labeled amount of rilmazafone hydrochloride hydrate
($C_{21}H_{20}Cl_2N_6O_3.HCl.2H_2O$)
$= M_S \times A_T/A_S \times V'/V \times 1/C \times 9/2 \times 1.070$

M_S: Amount (mg) of Rilmazafone Hydrochloride RS taken, calculated on the anhydrous basis

C: Labeled amount (mg) of rilmazafone hydrochloride hydrate ($C_{21}H_{20}Cl_2N_6O_3.HCl.2H_2O$) in 1 tablet

Operating conditions—

Proceed as directed in the operating conditions in the

Assay under Rilmazafone Hydrochloride Hydrate.

System suitability—

System performance: When the procedure is run with 50 μL of the standard solution under the above operating conditions, the number of theoretical plates and the symmetry factor of the peak of rilmazafone are not less than 5000 and not more than 1.5, respectively.

System repeatability: When the test is repeated 6 times with 50 μL of the standard solution under the above operating conditions, the relative standard deviation of the peak area of rilmazafone is not more than 2.0%.

Assay Weigh accurately the mass of not less than 20 tablets of Rilmazafone Hydrochloride Tablets, and powder. Weigh accurately a portion of the powder, equivalent to about 2 mg of rilmazafone hydrochloride hydrate ($C_{21}H_{20}Cl_2N_6O_3.HCl.2H_2O$), add 10 mL of water and exactly 20 mL of the internal standard solution, shake vigorously for 10 minutes, and filter through a membrane filter with a pore size not exceeding 0.45 μm. Discard the first 5 mL of the filtrate, and use the subsequent filtrate as the sample solution. Separately, weigh accurately about 20 mg of Rilmazafone Hydrochloride RS (separately determine the water <2.48> in the same manner as Rilmazafone Hydrochloride Hydrate), and dissolve in water to make exactly 100 mL. Pipet 10 mL of this solution, add exactly 20 mL of the internal standard, and use this solution as the standard solution. Then, proceed as directed in the Assay under Rilmazafone Hydrochloride Hydrate.

Amount (mg) of rilmazafone hydrochloride hydrate ($C_{21}H_{20}Cl_2N_6O_3.HCl.2H_2O$)
$= M_S \times Q_T/Q_S \times 1/10 \times 1.070$

M_S: Amount (mg) of Rilmazafone Hydrochloride RS taken, calculated on the anhydrous basis

Internal standard solution—A solution of propyl parahydroxybenzoate in a mixture of water and acetonitrile (1:1) (3 in 100,000).

Containers and storage Containers—Well-closed containers.

Ringer's Solution

リンゲル液

Ringer's Solution is an aqueous injection.

It contains not less than 0.53 w/v% and not more than 0.58 w/v% of chlorine [as (Cl: 35.45)], and not less than 0.030 w/v% and not more than 0.036 w/v% of calcium chloride hydrate ($CaCl_2.2H_2O$: 147.01).

Method of preparation

Sodium Chloride	8.6 g
Potassium Chloride	0.3 g
Calcium Chloride Hydrate	0.33 g
Water for Injection or Sterile Water for Injection in Containers	a sufficient quantity
To make	1000 mL

Prepare as directed under Injections, with the above ingredients.

No preservative may be added.

Description Ringer's Solution is a clear and colorless liquid. It has a slightly saline taste.

Identification (1) Evaporate 10 mL of Ringer's Solution to 5 mL: the solution responds to Qualitative Tests <1.09> for potassium salt.

(2) Evaporate 10 mL of Ringer's Solution to 5 mL: the solution responds to Qualitative Test <1.09> for calcium salt.

(3) Ringer's Solution responds to Qualitative Tests <1.09> for sodium salt.

(4) Ringer's Solution responds to Qualitative Tests <1.09> for chloride.

pH <2.54> 5.0 – 7.5

Purity (1) Heavy metals <1.07>—Evaporate 100 mL of Ringer's Solution to about 40 mL on a water bath. Add 2 mL of dilute acetic acid and water to make 50 mL, and perform the test using this solution as the test solution.

Control solution: To 3.0 mL of Standard Lead Solution add 2 mL of dilute acetic acid and water to make 50 mL (not more than 0.3 ppm).

(2) Arsenic <1.11>—Perform the test with 20 mL of Ringer's Solution as the test solution (not more than 0.1 ppm).

Bacterial endotoxins <4.01> Less than 0.50 EU/mL.

Extractable volume <6.05> It meets the requirement.

Foreign insoluble matter <6.06> Perform the test according to Method 1: it meets the requirement.

Insoluble particulate matter <6.07> It meets the requirement.

Sterility <4.06> Perform the test according to the Membrane filtration method: it meets the requirement.

Assay (1) Chlorine—To 20 mL of Ringer's Solution, accurately measured, add 30 mL of water. Titrate <2.50> with 0.1 mol/L silver nitrate VS while shaking vigorously (indicator: 3 drops of fluorescein sodium TS).

Each mL of 0.1 mol/L silver nitrate VS
= 3.545 mg of Cl

(2) Calcium chloride Hydrate—To 50 mL of Ringer's Solution, exactly measured, add 2 mL of 8 mol/L potassium hydroxide TS and 50 mg of NN indicator, and titrate <2.50> immediately with 0.01 mol/L disodium dihydrogen ethylenediamine tetraacetate VS, until the color of the solution changes from red-purple to blue.

Each mL of 0.01 mol/L disodium dihydrogen ethylenediamine tetraacetate VS
= 1.470 mg of $CaCl_2.2H_2O$

Containers and storage Containers—Hermetic containers. Plastic containers for aqueous infusions may be used.

Risperidone

リスペリドン

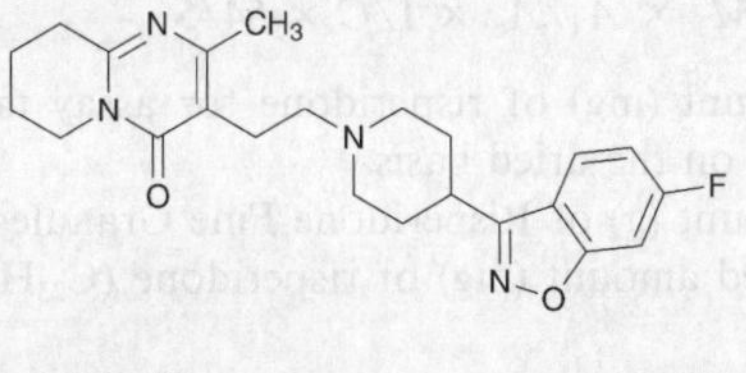

$C_{23}H_{27}FN_4O_2$: 410.48
3-{2-[4-(6-Fluoro-1,2-benzisoxazol-3-yl)piperidin-1-yl]ethyl}-2-methyl-6,7,8,9-tetrahydro-4*H*-pyrido[1,2-*a*]pyrimidin-4-one
[*106266-06-2*]

Risperidone contains not less than 98.5% and not more than 101.0% of risperidone ($C_{23}H_{27}FN_4O_2$), calculated on the dried basis.

Description Risperidone occurs as a white to pale yellowwhite crystalline powder.

It is sparingly soluble in methanol and in ethanol (99.5), very slightly soluble in 2-propanol, and practically insoluble in water.

Identification **(1)** Determine the absorption spectrum of a solution of Risperidone in 2-propanol (1 in 40,000) as directed under Ultraviolet-visible Spectrophotometry <*2.24*>, and compare the spectrum with the Reference Spectrum: both spectra exhibit similar intensities of absorption at the same wavelengths.

(2) Determine the infrared absorption spectrum of Risperidone, previously dried, as directed in the potassium bromide disk method under Infrared Spectrophotometry <*2.25*>, and compare the spectrum with the Reference Spectrum: both spectra exhibit similar intensities of absorption at the same wave numbers.

Melting point <*2.60*> 169 – 173°C

Purity **(1)** Heavy metals <*1.07*>—Proceed with 1.0 g of Risperidone according to Method 4, and perform the test. Prepare the control solution with 1.0 mL of Standard Lead Solution (not more than 10 ppm).

(2) Related substances—Dissolve 0.10 g of Risperidone in 10 mL of methanol, and use this solution as the sample solution. Pipet 1 mL of the sample solution, and add methanol to make exactly 100 mL. Pipet 5 mL of this solution, add methanol to make exactly 25 mL, and use this solution as the standard solution. Perform the test with exactly 10 μL each of the sample solution and standard solution as directed under Liquid Chromatography <*2.01*> according to the following conditions, and determine each peak area by the automatic integration method: the area of the peak other than risperidone obtained from the sample solution is not larger than the peak area of risperidone from the standard solution, and the total area of the peaks other than risperidone from the sample solution is not larger than 1.5 times the peak area of risperidone from the standard solution.

Operating conditions—

Detector: An ultraviolet absorption photometer (wavelength: 260 nm).

Column: A stainless steel column 4.6 mm in inside diameter and 10 cm in length, packed with octadecylsilanized silica gel for liquid chromatography (3 μm in particle diameter).

Column temperature: A constant temperature of about 30°C.

Mobile phase A: A solution of ammonium acetate (1 in 200).

Mobile phase B: Methanol.

Flowing of mobile phase: Control the gradient by mixing the mobile phases A and B as directed in the following table.

Time after injection of sample (min)	Mobile phase A (vol%)	Mobile phase B (vol%)
0 – 2	70	30
2 – 17	70 → 30	30 → 70
17 – 22	30	70

Flow rate: 1.5 mL per minute.

Time span of measurement: About 1.6 times as long as the retention time of risperidone.

System suitability—

Test for required detectability: Pipet 2 mL of the standard solution, and add methanol to make exactly 20 mL. Confirm that the peak area of risperidone obtained with 10 μL of this solution is equivalent to 7 to 13% of that with 10 μL of the standard solution.

System performance: When the procedure is run with 10 μL of the standard solution under the above operating conditions, the number of theoretical plates and the symmetry factor of the peak of risperidone are not less than 10,000 and not more than 2.0, respectively.

System repeatability: When the test is repeated 6 times with 10 μL of the standard solution under the above operating conditions, the relative standard deviation of the peak area of risperidone is not more than 2.0%.

Loss on drying <*2.41*> Not more than 0.5% (1 g, in vacuum, 80°C, 4 hours).

Residue on ignition <*2.44*> Not more than 0.1% (1 g, platinum crucible).

Assay Weigh accurately about 0.16 g of Risperidone, dissolve in 70 mL of a mixture of 2-butanone and acetic acid (100) (7:1), and titrate <*2.50*> with 0.1 mol/L perchloric acid VS (potentiometric titration). Perform a blank determination in the same manner, and make any necessary correction.

Each mL of 0.1 mol/L perchloric acid VS
= 20.52 mg of $C_{23}H_{27}FN_4O_2$

Containers and storage Containers—Tight containers.

Risperidone Fine Granules

リスペリドン細粒

Risperidone Fine Granules contain not less than 95.0% and not more than 105.0% of the labeled amount of risperidone ($C_{23}H_{27}FN_4O_2$: 410.48).

Method of preparation Prepare as directed under Granules, with Risperidone.

Identification To an amount of Risperidone Fine Granules, equivalent to 2 mg of Risperidone, add 100 mL of 2-propanol, shake thoroughly, and filter. Determine the absorption spectrum of the filtrate as directed under Ultraviolet-visible Spectrophotometry <*2.24*>: it exhibits maxima between 277 nm and 281 nm and between 283 nm and 287 nm.

Purity Related substances—To an amount of Risperidone Fine Granules, equivalent to 2 mg of Risperidone, add 20 mL of a mixture of 0.1 mol/L hydrochloric acid TS and methanol (3:2), shake, and filter through a membrane filter with a pore size not exceeding 0.45 μm. Discard the first 1 mL of the filtrate, and use the subsequent filtrate as the sample solution. Pipet 1 mL of the sample solution, add a mixture of 0.1 mol/L hydrochloric acid TS and methanol (3:2) to make exactly 100 mL, and use this solution as the standard solution. Perform the test with exactly 10 μL each of the sample solution and standard solution as directed under Liquid Chromatography <*2.01*> according to the following conditions, and determine each peak area by the automatic integration method: the area of the peak other than risperidone obtained from the sample solution is not larger than 1/2 times the peak area of risperidone from the standard solution, and the total area of the peaks other than risperidone from the sample solution is not larger than the peak area of risperidone from the standard solution. For the area of the peaks, having the relative retention time of about 0.4 and about 1.6 to risperidone, multiply their correction factors, 1.9 and 1.5, respectively.

Operating conditions—

Detector, column, column temperature, mobile phase, and flow rate: Proceed as directed in the operating conditions in the Assay.

Time span of measurement: About 2.5 times as long as the retention time of risperidone, beginning after the solvent peak.

System suitability—

Test for required detectability: To exactly 5 mL of the standard solution add a mixture of 0.1 mol/L hydrochloric acid TS and methanol (3:2) to make exactly 50 mL. Confirm that the peak area of risperidone obtained with 10 μL of this solution is equivalent to 7.5 to 12.5% of that with 10 μL of the standard solution.

System performance: When the procedure is run with 10 μL of the standard solution under the above operating conditions, the number of theoretical plates and the symmetry factor of the peak of risperidone are not less than 4000 and not more than 2.5, respectively.

System repeatability: When the test is repeated 6 times with 10 μL of the standard solution under the above operating conditions, the relative standard deviation of the peak area of risperidone is not more than 2.5%.

Dissolution <*6.10*> When the test is performed at 50 revolutions per minute according to the Paddle method, using 900 mL of water as the dissolution medium, the dissolution rate in 30 minutes of Risperidone Fine Granules is not less than 75%.

Start the test with an accurately weighed amount of Risperidone Fine Granules, equivalent to about 3 mg of risperidone ($C_{23}H_{27}FN_4O_2$), withdraw not less than 20 mL of the medium at the specified minute after starting the test, and filter through a membrane filter with a pore size not exceeding 0.45 μm. Discard not less than 10 mL of the first filtrate, pipet 5 mL of the subsequent filtrate, add diluted hydrochloric acid (1 in 137) to make exactly 10 mL, and use this solution as the sample solution. Separately, weigh accurately about 28 mg of risperidone for assay (separately determine the loss on drying <*2.41*> under the same conditions as Risperidone), and dissolve in methanol to make exactly 50 mL. Pipet 15 mL of this solution, add methanol to make exactly 25 mL. Pipet 2 mL of this solution, and add water to make exactly 200 mL. Pipet 3 mL of this solution, add exactly 3 mL of diluted hydrochloric acid (1 in 137), and use this solution as the standard solution. Perform the test with exactly 100 μL each of the sample solution and standard solution as directed under Liquid Chromatography <*2.01*> according to the following conditions, and determine the peak areas, A_T and A_S, of risperidone in each solution.

Dissolution rate (%) with respect to the labeled amount of risperidone ($C_{23}H_{27}FN_4O_2$)
$= M_S/M_T \times A_T/A_S \times 1/C \times 54/5$

M_S: Amount (mg) of risperidone for assay taken, calculated on the dried basis
M_T: Amount (g) of Risperidone Fine Granules taken
C: Labeled amount (mg) of risperidone ($C_{23}H_{27}FN_4O_2$) in 1 g

Operating conditions—

Detector: An ultraviolet absorption photometer (wavelength: 237 nm).

Column: A stainless steel column 4.6 mm in inside diameter and 15 cm in length, packed with octadecylsilanized silica gel for liquid chromatography (5 μm in particle diameter).

Column temperature: A constant temperature of about 25°C.

Mobile phase: To 1000 mL of a mixture of water and acetonitrile (13:7) add 1 mL of trifluoroacetic acid, and adjust to pH 3.0 with ammonia solution (28).

Flow rate: Adjust so that the retention time of risperidone is about 3 minutes.

System suitability—

System performance: When the procedure is run with 100 μL of the standard solution under the above operating conditions, the number of theoretical plates and the symmetry factor of the peak of risperidone are not less than 3500 and not more than 2.5, respectively.

System repeatability: When the test is repeated 6 times with 100 μL of the standard solution under the above operating conditions, the relative standard deviation of the peak area of risperidone is not more than 2.0%.

Assay If necessary powder Risperidone Fine Granules, and weigh accurately an amount, equivalent to about 2 mg of risperidone ($C_{23}H_{27}FN_4O_2$), add 8 mL of a mixture of 0.1 mol/L hydrochloric acid TS and methanol (3:2), shake, and add a mixture of 0.1 mol/L hydrochloric acid TS and methanol (3:2) to make exactly 20 mL. Filter the solution through a membrane filter with a pore size not exceeding 0.45 μm. Discard the first 1 mL of the filtrate, and use the subsequent filtrate as the sample solution. Separately, weigh accurately about 50 mg of risperidone for assay (separately determine the loss on drying <*2.41*> under the same conditions as Risperidone), and dissolve in a mixture of 0.1 mol/L hydrochloric acid TS and methanol (3:2) to make exactly 50 mL. Pipet 10 mL of this solution, add a mixture of 0.1 mol/L hydrochloric acid TS and methanol (3:2) to make exactly 100 mL, and use this solution as the standard solution. Perform the test with exactly 10 μL each of the sample solution and standard solution as directed under Liquid Chromatography <*2.01*> according to the following conditions, and determine the peak areas, A_T and A_S, of risperidone in each solution.

Amount (mg) of risperidone ($C_{23}H_{27}FN_4O_2$)
$= M_S \times A_T/A_S \times 1/25$

M_S: Amount (mg) of risperidone for assay taken, calculated on the dried basis

Operating conditions—

Detector: An ultraviolet absorption photometer (wavelength: 275 nm).

Column: A stainless steel column 3.0 mm in inside diameter and 15 cm in length, packed with octadecylsilanized silica gel for liquid chromatography (3.5 μm in particle diameter).

Column temperature: A constant temperature of about 25°C.

Mobile phase: To 1000 mL of a mixture of water and acetonitrile (4:1) add 1.5 mL of trifluoroacetic acid, and adjust to pH 3.0 with ammonia solution (28).

Flow rate: Adjust so that the retention time of risperidone is about 13 minutes.

System suitability—

System performance: When the procedure is run with 10 μL of the standard solution under the above operating conditions, the number of theoretical plates and the symmetry factor of the peak of risperidone are not less than 4000 and not more than 2.5, respectively.

System repeatability: When the test is repeated 6 times with 10 μL of the standard solution under the above operating conditions, the relative standard deviation of the peak area of risperidone is not more than 1.0%.

Containers and storage Containers—Tight containers.

Risperidone Oral Solution

リスペリドン内服液

Risperidone Oral Solution contains not less than 95.0% and not more than 105.0% of the labeled amount of risperidone ($C_{23}H_{27}FN_4O_2$: 410.48).

Method of preparation Prepare as directed under Liquids and Solutions for Oral Administration, with Risperidone.

Description Risperidone Oral Solution occurs as a clear and colorless liquid.

Identification To a volume of Risperidone Oral Solution, equivalent to 2 mg of Risperidone, add 50 mg of sodium hydrogen carbonate and 10 mL of diethyl ether, shake, centrifuge, and evaporate the supernatant liquid to dryness in lukewarm water. Determine the absorption spectrum of a solution of the residue in 100 mL of 2-propanol as directed under Ultraviolet-visible Spectrophotometry <*2.24*>: it exhibits maxima between 277 nm and 281 nm and between 283 nm and 287 nm.

pH Being specified separately when the drug is granted approval based on the Law.

Purity Related substances—To a volume of Risperidone Oral Solution, equivalent to 2 mg of Risperidone, add methanol to make 20 mL, and use this solution as the sample solution. Pipet 1 mL of the sample solution, add a mixture of methanol and water (9:1) to make exactly 100 mL, and use this solution as the standard solution. Perform the test with exactly 10 μL each of the sample solution and standard solution as directed under Liquid Chromatography <*2.01*> according to the following conditions, and determine each peak area by the automatic integration method: the area of the peak other than risperidone obtained from the sample solution is not larger than 1/2 times the peak area of risperidone from the standard solution, and the total area of the peaks other than risperidone from the sample solution is not larger than the peak area of risperidone from the standard solution. For the area of the peaks, having the relative retention time of about 0.4 and about 1.6 to risperidone, multiply their correction factors, 1.9 and 1.5, respectively.

Operating conditions—

Detector, column, column temperature, mobile phase, and flow rate: Proceed as directed in the operating conditions in the Assay.

Time span of measurement: About 2.5 times as long as the retention time of risperidone, beginning after the solvent peak.

System suitability—

Test for required detectability: To exactly 5 mL of the standard solution add a mixture of methanol and water (9:1) to make exactly 50 mL. Confirm that the peak area of risperidone obtained with 10 μL of this solution is equivalent to 7.5 to 12.5% of that with 10 μL of the standard solution.

System performance: When the procedure is run with 10 μL of the standard solution under the above operating conditions, the number of theoretical plates and the symmetry factor of the peak of risperidone are not less than 4000 and not more than 2.5, respectively.

System repeatability: When the test is repeated 6 times with 10 μL of the standard solution under the above operating conditions, the relative standard deviation of the peak area of risperidone is not more than 2.5%.

Uniformity of dosage units <*6.02*> Risperidone Oral Solution in single-dose packages meet the requirement of the Mass variation test.

Microbial limit <*4.05*> The acceptance criteria of TAMC and TYMC are 10^2 CFU/mL and 10^1 CFU/mL, respectively. *Escherichia coli* is not observed.

Assay To an exact volume of Risperidone Oral Solution, equivalent to about 2 mg of risperidone ($C_{23}H_{27}FN_4O_2$), add methanol to make exactly 20 mL, and use this solution as the sample solution. Separately, weigh accurately about 50 mg of risperidone for assay (separately determine the loss on drying <*2.41*> under the same conditions as Risperidone), and dissolve in methanol to make exactly 50 mL. Pipet 10 mL of this solution, add 10 mL of water, then add methanol to make exactly 100 mL, and use this solution as the standard solution. Perform the test with exactly 10 μL each of the sample solution and standard solution as directed under Liquid Chromatography <*2.01*> according to the following conditions, and determine the peak areas, A_T and A_S, of risperidone in each solution.

$$\text{Amount (mg) of risperidone } (C_{23}H_{27}FN_4O_2) = M_S \times A_T/A_S \times 1/25$$

M_S: Amount (mg) of risperidone for assay taken, calculated on the dried basis

Operating conditions—

Detector: An ultraviolet absorption photometer (wavelength: 275 nm).

Column: A stainless steel column 3.0 mm in inside diameter and 15 cm in length, packed with octadecylsilanized silica gel for liquid chromatography (3.5 μm in particle diameter).

Column temperature: A constant temperature of about 25°C.

Mobile phase: To 1000 mL of a mixture of water and acetonitrile (4:1) add 1.5 mL of trifluoroacetic acid, and adjust to pH 3.0 with ammonia solution (28).

Flow rate: Adjust so that the retention time of risperidone is about 13 minutes.

System suitability—

System performance: When the procedure is run with 10 μL of the standard solution under the above operating conditions, the number of theoretical plates and the symmetry factor of the peak of risperidone are not less than 4000 and not more than 2.5, respectively.

System repeatability: When the test is repeated 6 times with 10 μL of the standard solution under the above operat-

ing conditions, the relative standard deviation of the peak area of risperidone is not more than 1.0%.

Containers and storage Containers—Tight containers.

Risperidone Tablets

リスペリドン錠

Risperidone Tablets contain not less than 95.0% and not more than 105.0% of the labeled amount of risperidone ($C_{23}H_{27}FN_4O_2$: 410.48).

Method of preparation Prepare as directed under Tablets, with Risperidone.

Identification Powder Risperidone Tablets. To a portion of the powder, equivalent to 2 mg of Risperidone, add 100 mL of 2-propanol, shake thoroughly, and filter. Determine the absorption spectrum of the filtrate as directed under Ultraviolet-visible Spectrophotometry <*2.24*>: it exhibits maxima between 277 nm and 281 nm and between 283 nm and 287 nm.

Purity Related substances—Powder Risperidone Tablets. To a portion of the powder, equivalent to 2 mg of Risperidone, add 20 mL of a mixture of 0.1 mol/L hydrochloric acid TS and methanol (3:2), shake, and filter through a membrane filter with a pore size not exceeding 0.45 μm. Discard the first 1 mL of the filtrate, and use the subsequent filtrate as the sample solution. Pipet 1 mL of the sample solution, add a mixture of 0.1 mol/L hydrochloric acid TS and methanol (3:2) to make exactly 100 mL, and use this solution as the standard solution. Perform the test with exactly 10 μL each of the sample solution and standard solution as directed under Liquid Chromatography <*2.01*> according to the following conditions, and determine each peak area by the automatic integration method: the area of the peak other than risperidone obtained from the sample solution is not larger than 1/2 times the peak area of risperidone from the standard solution, and the total area of the peaks other than risperidone from the sample solution is not larger than the peak area of risperidone from the standard solution. For the area of the peaks, having the relative retention time of about 0.4 and about 1.6 to risperidone, multiply their correction factors, 1.9 and 1.5, respectively.

Operating conditions—

Detector, column, column temperature, mobile phase, and flow rate: Proceed as directed in the operating conditions in the Assay.

Time span of measurement: About 2.5 times as long as the retention time of risperidone, beginning after the solvent peak.

System suitability—

Test for required detectability: To exactly 5 mL of the standard solution add a mixture of 0.1 mol/L hydrochloric acid TS and methanol (3:2) to make exactly 50 mL. Confirm that the peak area of risperidone obtained with 10 μL of this solution is equivalent to 7.5 to 12.5% of that with 10 μL of the standard solution.

System performance: When the procedure is run with 10 μL of the standard solution under the above operating conditions, the number of theoretical plates and the symmetry factor of the peak of risperidone are not less than 4000 and not more than 2.5, respectively.

System repeatability: When the test is repeated 6 times with 10 μL of the standard solution under the above operating conditions, the relative standard deviation of the peak area of risperidone is not more than 2.5%.

Uniformity of dosage units <*6.02*> Perform the test according to the following method: it meets the requirement of the Content uniformity test.

To 1 tablet of Risperidone Tablets add $3V/5$ mL of a mixture of 0.1 mol/L hydrochloric acid TS and methanol (3:2), shake, and add a mixture of 0.1 mol/L hydrochloric acid TS and methanol (3:2) to make exactly V mL so that each mL contains 0.1 mg of risperidone ($C_{23}H_{27}FN_4O_2$). Filter this solution through a membrane filter with a pore size not exceeding 0.45 μm, discard the first 1 mL of the filtrate, and use the subsequent filtrate as the sample solution. Then, proceed as directed in the Assay.

$$\text{Amount (mg) of risperidone } (C_{23}H_{27}FN_4O_2) = M_S \times A_T/A_S \times V/500$$

M_S: Amount (mg) of risperidone for assay taken, calculated on the dried basis

Dissolution <*6.10*> When the test is performed at 50 revolutions per minute according to the Paddle method, using 900 mL of water as the dissolution medium, the dissolution rate in 30 minutes of Risperidone Tablets is not less than 75%.

Start the test with 1 tablet of Risperidone Tablets, withdraw not less than 20 mL of the medium at the specified minute after starting the test, and filter through a membrane filter with a pore size not exceeding 0.45 μm. Discard not less than 10 mL of the first filtrate, pipet V mL of the subsequent filtrate, add diluted hydrochloric acid (1 in 137) to make exactly V' mL so that each mL contains about 0.56 μg of risperidone ($C_{23}H_{27}FN_4O_2$), and use this solution as the sample solution. Separately, weigh accurately about 28 mg of risperidone for assay (separately determine the loss on drying <*2.41*> under the same conditions as Risperidone), and dissolve in methanol to make exactly 50 mL. Pipet 5 mL of this solution, add methanol to make exactly 25 mL. Pipet 2 mL of this solution, and add water to make exactly 200 mL. Pipet 3 mL of this solution, add exactly 3 mL of diluted hydrochloric acid (1 in 137), and use this solution as the standard solution. Perform the test with exactly 100 μL each of the sample solution and standard solution as directed under Liquid Chromatography <*2.01*> according to the following conditions, and determine the peak areas, A_T and A_S, of risperidone in each solution.

$$\text{Dissolution rate (\%) with respect to the labeled amount of risperidone } (C_{23}H_{27}FN_4O_2) = M_S \times A_T/A_S \times V'/V \times 1/C \times 9/5$$

M_S: Amount (mg) of risperidone for assay taken, calculated on the dried basis

C: Labeled amount (mg) of risperidone ($C_{23}H_{27}FN_4O_2$) in 1 tablet

Operating conditions—

Detector: An ultraviolet absorption photometer (wavelength: 237 nm).

Column: A stainless steel column 4.6 mm in inside diameter and 15 cm in length, packed with octadecylsilanized silica gel for liquid chromatography (5 μm in particle diameter).

Column temperature: A constant temperature of about 25°C.

Mobile phase: To 1000 mL of a mixture of water and acetonitrile (13:7) add 1 mL of trifluoroacetic acid, and adjust to pH 3.0 with ammonia solution (28).

Flow rate: Adjust so that the retention time of risperidone is about 3 minutes.

System suitability—

System performance: When the procedure is run with 100 μL of the standard solution under the above operating conditions, the number of theoretical plates and the symmetry factor of the peak of risperidone are not less than 3500 and not more than 2.5, respectively.

System repeatability: When the test is repeated 6 times with 100 μL of the standard solution under the above operating conditions, the relative standard deviation of the peak area of risperidone is not more than 2.0%.

Assay Weigh accurately the mass of not less than 20 Risperidone Tablets, and powder. Weigh accurately a portion of the powder, equivalent to about 2 mg of risperidone ($C_{23}H_{27}FN_4O_2$), add 8 mL of a mixture of 0.1 mol/L hydrochloric acid TS and methanol (3:2), shake, and add a mixture of 0.1 mol/L hydrochloric acid TS and methanol (3:2) to make exactly 20 mL. Filter the solution through a membrane filter with a pore size not exceeding 0.45 μm. Discard the first 1 mL of the filtrate, and use the subsequent filtrate as the sample solution. Separately, weigh accurately about 50 mg of risperidone for assay (separately determine the loss on drying <*2.41*> under the same conditions as Risperidone), and dissolve in a mixture of 0.1 mol/L hydrochloric acid TS and methanol (3:2) to make exactly 50 mL. Pipet 10 mL of this solution, add a mixture of 0.1 mol/L hydrochloric acid TS and methanol (3:2) to make exactly 100 mL, and use this solution as the standard solution. Perform the test with exactly 10 μL each of the sample solution and standard solution as directed under Liquid Chromatography <*2.01*> according to the following conditions, and determine the peak areas, A_T and A_S, of risperidone in each solution.

$$\text{Amount (mg) of risperidone } (C_{23}H_{27}FN_4O_2) = M_S \times A_T/A_S \times 1/25$$

M_S: Amount (mg) of risperidone for assay taken, calculated on the dried basis

Operating conditions—

Detector: An ultraviolet absorption photometer (wavelength: 275 nm).

Column: A stainless steel column 3.0 mm in inside diameter and 15 cm in length, packed with octadecylsilanized silica gel for liquid chromatography (3.5 μm in particle diameter).

Column temperature: A constant temperature of about 25°C.

Mobile phase: To 1000 mL of a mixture of water and acetonitrile (4:1) add 1.5 mL of trifluoroacetic acid, and adjust to pH 3.0 with ammonia solution (28).

Flow rate: Adjust so that the retention time of risperidone is about 13 minutes.

System suitability—

System performance: When the procedure is run with 10 μL of the standard solution under the above operating conditions, the number of theoretical plates and the symmetry factor of the peak of risperidone are not less than 4000 and not more than 2.5, respectively.

System repeatability: When the test is repeated 6 times with 10 μL of the standard solution under the above operating conditions, the relative standard deviation of the peak area of risperidone is not more than 1.0%.

Containers and storage Containers—Tight containers.

Ritodrine Hydrochloride

リトドリン塩酸塩

and enantiomer

$C_{17}H_{21}NO_3 \cdot HCl$: 323.81

(1*RS*,2*SR*)-1-(4-Hydroxyphenyl)-2-{[2-(4-hydroxyphenyl)ethyl]amino}propan-1-ol monohydrochloride

[*23239-51-2*]

Ritodrine Hydrochloride, when dried, contains not less than 98.0% and not more than 102.0% of ritodrine hydrochloride ($C_{17}H_{21}NO_3.HCl$).

Description Ritodrine Hydrochloride occurs as a white crystalline powder.

It is freely soluble in water, in methanol and in ethanol (99.5).

It dissolves in 0.01 mol/L hydrochloric acid TS.

A solution of Ritodrine Hydrochloride (1 in 10) shows no optical rotation.

It is gradually colored to light yellow by light.

Melting point: about 196°C (with decomposition).

Identification **(1)** Determine the absorption spectrum of a solution of Ritodrine Hydrochloride in 0.01 mol/L hydrochloric acid TS (1 in 20,000) as directed under Ultraviolet-visible Spectrophotometry <*2.24*>, and compare the spectrum with the Reference Spectrum or the spectrum of a solution of Ritodrine Hydrochloride RS prepared in the same manner as the sample solution: both spectra exhibit similar intensities of absorption at the same wavelengths.

(2) Determine the infrared absorption spectrum of Ritodrine Hydrochloride as directed in the potassium chloride disk method under Infrared Spectrophotometry <*2.25*>, and compare the spectrum with the Reference Spectrum or the spectrum of Ritodrine Hydrochloride RS: both spectra exhibit similar intensities of absorption at the same wave numbers.

(3) A solution of Ritodrine Hydrochloride (1 in 50) responds to the Qualitative Tests <*1.09*> (2) for chloride.

pH <*2.54*> The pH of a solution obtained by dissolving 1.0 g of Ritodrine Hydrochloride in 50 mL of water is between 4.5 and 5.5.

Purity **(1)** Clarity and color of solution—A solution obtained by dissolving 1.0 g of Ritodrine Hydrochloride in 10 mL of water is clear and colorless.

(2) Heavy metals <*1.07*>—Proceed with 2.0 g of Ritodrine Hydrochloride according to Method 4, and perform the test. Prepare the control solution with 2.0 mL of Standard Lead Solution (not more than 10 ppm).

(3) Related substances—Dissolve 20 mg of Ritodrine Hydrochloride in 20 mL of the mobile phase, and use this solution as the sample solution. Pipet 1 mL of the sample solution, add the mobile phase to make exactly 200 mL, and use this solution as the standard solution. Perform the test with exactly 10 μL each of the sample solution and standard solution as directed under Liquid Chromatography <*2.01*> according to the following conditions, and determine each peak area by the automatic integration method: the area of the peak of ritodrine threo-isomer, having the relative retention time of about 1.2 to ritodrine, obtained from the sample solution is not larger than 4/5 times the peak area of ritodrine from the standard solution, the area of the peak other than ritodrine and ritodrine threo-isomer from the sample solution is not larger than 3/10 times the peak area of ritodrine from the standard solution, and the total area of the peaks other than ritodrine and ritodrine threo-isomer from the sample solution is not larger than 4 times the peak area of ritodrine from the standard solution.

Operating conditions—

Column, column temperature, and mobile phase: Proceed as directed in the operating conditions in the Assay.

Detector: An ultraviolet absorption photometer (wavelength: 220 nm).

Flow rate: Adjust so that the retention time of ritodrine is about 10 minutes.

Time span of measurement: About 3 times as long as the retention time of ritodrine, beginning after the solvent peak.

System suitability—

Test for required detectability: To exactly 5 mL of the standard solution add the mobile phase to make exactly 50 mL. Confirm that the peak area of ritodrine obtained with 10 μL of this solution is equivalent to 7 to 13% of that with 10 μL of the standard solution.

System performance: To 20 mg of Ritodrine Hydrochloride add 50 mL of the mobile phase and 5.6 mL of sulfuric acid, and add the mobile phase to make 100 mL. Heat a portion of this solution at about 85°C for about 2 hours, and allow to cool. Pipet 10 mL of this solution, and add exactly 10 mL of 2 mol/L sodium hydroxide TS. When the procedure is run with 10 μL of this solution under the above operating conditions, ritodrine and the threo-isomer are eluted in this order with the resolution between these peaks being not less than 3.

System repeatability: When the test is repeated 6 times with 10 μL of the standard solution under the above operating conditions, the relative standard deviation of the peak area of ritodrine is not more than 2.0%.

Loss on drying <*2.41*> Not more than 1.0% (1 g, 105°C, 2 hours).

Residue on ignition <*2.44*> Not more than 0.2% (1 g).

Assay Weigh accurately about 30 mg each of Ritodrine Hydrochloride and Ritodrine Hydrochloride RS, previously dried, and dissolve in methanol to make exactly 50 mL. Pipet 25 mL of these solutions, add exactly 5 mL of the internal standard solution, then add water to make 50 mL, and use these solutions as the sample solution and standard solution. Perform the test with 10 μL of the sample solution and standard solution as directed under Liquid Chromatography <*2.01*> according to the following conditions, and calculate the ratios, Q_T and Q_S, of the peak area of ritodrine to that of the internal standard.

Amount (mg) of ritodrine hydrochloride ($C_{17}H_{21}NO_3.HCl$)
$= M_S \times Q_T/Q_S$

M_S: Amount (mg) of Ritodrine Hydrochloride RS taken

Internal standard solution—A solution of methyl parahydroxybenzoate in methanol (3 in 5000).

Operating conditions—

Detector: An ultraviolet absorption photometer (wavelength: 274 nm).

Column: A stainless steel column 4.6 mm in inside diameter and 15 cm in length, packed with octadecylsilanized silica gel for liquid chromatography (5 μm in particle diameter).

Column temperature: A constant temperature of about 25°C.

Mobile phase: Dissolve 6.6 g of diammonium hydrogen phosphate and 1.1 g of sodium 1-heptanesulfonate in 700 mL of water, and add 300 mL of methanol. Adjust to pH 3.0 with phosphoric acid.

Flow rate: Adjust so that the retention time of ritodrine is about 6 minutes.

System suitability—

System performance: When the procedure is run with 10 μL of the standard solution under the above operating conditions, ritodrine and the internal standard are eluted in this order with the resolution between these peaks being not less then 3.

System repeatability: When the test is repeated 6 times with 10 μL of the standard solution under the above operating conditions, the relative standard deviation of the ratio of the peak area of ritodrine to that of the internal standard is not more than 1.0%.

Containers and storage Containers—Tight containers.

Storage—Light-resistant.

Ritodrine Hydrochloride Injection

リトドリン塩酸塩注射液

Ritodrine Hydrochloride Injection is an aqueous injection.

It contains not less than 95.0% and not more than 105.0% of the labeled amount of ritodrine hydrochloride ($C_{17}H_{21}NO_3.HCl$: 323.81).

Method of preparation Prepare as directed under Injections, with Ritodrine Hydrochloride.

Manufacture Ritodrine Hydrochloride Injection is produced by the formulation and the manufacturing method to ensure that the amounts of related substances do not exceed the limit values of related substances under Ritodrine Hydrochloride.

Description Ritodrine Hydrochloride Injection is a clear and colorless liquid.

Identification To a volume of Ritodrine Hydrochloride Injection, equivalent to 50 mg of Ritodrine Hydrochloride, add 0.01 mol/L hydrochloric acid TS to make 100 mL. To 10 mL of this solution add 0.01 mol/L hydrochloric acid TS to make 100 mL. Determine the absorption spectrum of this solution as directed under Ultraviolet-visible Spectrophotometry <*2.24*>: it exhibits a maximum between 272 nm and 276 nm.

pH Being specified separately when the drug is granted approval based on the Law.

Bacterial endotoxins <*4.01*> Less than 25 EU/mg.

Extractable volume <*6.05*> It meets the requirement.

Foreign insoluble matter <*6.06*> Perform the test according to Method 1: it meets the requirement.

Insoluble particulate matter <*6.07*> It meets the requirement.

Sterility <*4.06*> Perform the test according to the Membrane filtration method: it meets the requirement.

Assay Pipet a volume of Ritodrine Hydrochloride Injection, equivalent to about 20 mg of ritodrine hydrochloride

($C_{17}H_{21}NO_3.HCl$), and add a mixture of 0.02 mol/L sodium dihydrogen phosphate dihydrate solution and methanol (7:3) to make exactly 250 mL, and use this solution as the sample solution. Separately, weigh accurately about 20 mg of Ritodrine Hydrochloride RS, previously dried at 105°C for 2 hours, dissolve in a mixture of 0.02 mol/L sodium dihydrogen phosphate dihydrate solution and methanol (7:3) to make exactly 250 mL, and use this solution as the standard solution. Perform the test with exactly 10 μL each of the sample solution and standard solution as directed under Liquid Chromatography <*2.01*> according to the following conditions. Determine the peak areas, A_T and A_S, of ritodrine in each solution.

Amount (mg) of ritodrine hydrochloride ($C_{17}H_{21}NO_3.HCl$)
$= M_S \times A_T/A_S$

M_S: Amount (mg) of Ritodrine Hydrochloride RS taken

Operating conditions—

Detector: An ultraviolet absorption photometer (wavelength: 220 nm).

Column: A stainless steel column 6 mm in inside diameter and 15 cm in length, packed with octylsilanized silica gel for liquid chromatography (5 μm in particle diameter).

Column temperature: A constant temperature of about 25°C.

Mobile phase: Dissolve 6.6 g of diammonium hydrogen phosphate and 1.1 g of sodium 1-heptansulfonate in 840 mL of water, add 160 mL of acetonitrile for liquid chromatography, and adjust to pH 3.0 with phosphoric acid.

Flow rate: Adjust so that the retention time of ritodrine is about 19 minutes.

System Suitability—

System performance: Dissolve 10 mg of ritodrine hydrochloride in 50 mL of dilute sulfuric acid. Heat a portion of this solution in a water bath for about 30 minutes, and allow to cool. Measure a portion of this solution, and add the same volume of 2 mol/L sodium hydroxide TS. Dissolve 2 mg of ritodrine hydrochloride in 10 mL of this solution, and add a mixture of 0.02 mol/L sodium dihydrogen phosphate dihydrate solution and methanol (7:3) to make 25 mL. When the procedure is run with 10 μL of this solution under the above operating conditions, ritodrine and ritodrine threo-isomer are eluted in this order with the resolution between these peaks being not less than 3.

System repeatability: When the test is repeated 6 times with 10 μL of the standard solution under the above operating conditions, the relative standard deviation of the peak area of ritodrine is not more than 1.0%.

Containers and storage Containers—Hermetic containers.
Storage—At a temperature between 2°C and 8°C.

Ritodrine Hydrochloride Tablets

リトドリン塩酸塩錠

Ritodrine Hydrochloride Tablets contain not less than 93.0% and not more than 107.0% of the labeled amount of ritodrine hydrochloride ($C_{17}H_{21}NO_3.HCl$: 323.81).

Method of preparation Prepare as directed under Tablets, with Ritodrine Hydrochloride.

Identification To 10 mL of the filtrate obtained in the Assay add 0.01 mol/L hydrochloric acid TS to make 100 mL. Determine the absorption spectrum of this solution as directed under Ultraviolet-visible Spectrophotometry <*2.24*>: it exhibits a maximum between 272 nm and 276 nm.

Uniformity of dosage units <*6.02*> Perform the test according to the following method: it meets the requirement of the Content uniformity test.

To 1 tablet of Ritodrine Hydrochloride Tablets add 9 mL of 0.01 mol/L hydrochloric acid TS, shake until the tablet is completely disintegrated, add 0.01 mol/L hydrochloric acid TS to make exactly 10 mL, and filter through a membrane filter having pore size of 0.45 μm. Pipet 3 mL of the filtrate, add exactly 1 mL of the internal standard solution, and use this solution as the sample solution. Separately, weigh accurately about 25 mg of Ritodrine Hydrochloride RS, previously dried at 105°C for 2 hours, and dissolve in 0.01 mol/L hydrochloric acid TS to make exactly 50 mL. Pipet 3 mL of this solution, add exactly 1 mL of the internal standard solution, and use this solution as the standard solution. Perform the test with 10 μL each of the sample solution and standard solution as directed under Liquid Chromatography <*2.01*> according to the following conditions, and calculate the ratios, Q_T and Q_S, of the peak area of ritodrine to that of the internal standard.

Amount (mg) of ritodrine hydrochloride ($C_{17}H_{21}NO_3.HCl$)
$= M_S \times Q_T/Q_S \times 1/5$

M_S: Amount (mg) of Ritodrine Hydrochloride RS taken

*Internal standard solution—*A solution of methyl parahydroxybenzoate in methanol (3 in 10,000).

Operating conditions—

Proceed as directed in the operating conditions in the Assay.

System suitability—

System performance: When the procedure is run with 10 μL of the standard solution under the above operating conditions, ritodrine and the internal standard are eluted in this order with the resolution between these peaks being not less than 3.

System repeatability: When the test is repeated 6 times with 10 μL of the standard solution under the above operating conditions, the relative standard deviation of the ratio of the peak area of ritodrine to that of the internal standard is not more than 1.0%.

Dissolution <*6.10*> When the test is performed at 50 revolutions per minute according to the Paddle method, using 900 mL of water as the dissolution medium, the dissolution rate in 15 minutes of Ritodrine Hydrochloride Tablets is not less than 80%.

Start the test with 1 tablet of Ritodrine Hydrochloride Tablets, withdraw not less than 20 mL of the medium at the specified minute after starting the test, and filter through a membrane filter with a pore size not exceeding 0.45 μm. Discard not less than 10 mL of the first filtrate, pipet V mL of the subsequent filtrate, add water to make exactly V' mL so that each mL contains about 5.6 μg of ritodrine hydrochloride ($C_{17}H_{21}NO_3.HCl$), and use this solution as the sample solution. Separately, weigh accurately about 28 mg of Ritodrine Hydrochloride RS, previously dried at 105°C for 2 hours, and dissolve in water to make exactly 100 mL. Pipet 2 mL of this solution, add water to make exactly 100 mL, and use this solution as the standard solution. Perform the test with exactly 80 μL each of the sample solution and standard solution as directed under Liquid Chromatography <*2.01*> according to the following conditions, and determine the peak areas, A_T and A_S, of ritodrine in each solution.

Dissolution rate (%) with respect to the labeled amount of ritodrine hydrochloride ($C_{17}H_{21}NO_3.HCl$)

$$= M_S \times A_T/A_S \times V'/V \times 1/C \times 18$$

M_S: Amount (mg) of Ritodrine Hydrochloride RS taken
C: Labeled amount (mg) of ritodrine hydrochloride ($C_{17}H_{21}NO_3.HCl$) in 1 tablet

Operating conditions—

Proceed as directed in the operating conditions in the Assay.

System suitability—

System performance: When the procedure is run with 80 μL of the standard solution under the above operating conditions, the number of theoretical plates and the symmetry factor of the peak of ritodrine are not less than 3000 and not more than 1.5, respectively.

System repeatability: When the test is repeated 6 times with 80 μL of the standard solution under the above operating conditions, the relative standard deviation of the peak area of ritodrine is not more than 1.5%.

Assay To 20 Ritodrine Hydrochloride Tablets add 150 mL of 0.01 mol/L hydrochloric acid TS, shake for 20 minutes, and add 0.01 mol/L hydrochloric acid TS to make exactly 200 mL. Filter through a glass filter (G4), and discard the first 20 mL of the filtrate. Pipet 30 mL of the subsequent filtrate, add exactly 5 mL of the internal standard solution and 0.01 mol/L hydrochloric acid TS to make 50 mL, and use this solution as the sample solution. Separately, weigh accurately about 25 mg of Ritodrine Hydrochloride RS, previously dried at 105°C for 2 hours, and dissolve in 0.01 mol/L hydrochloric acid TS to make exactly 50 mL. Pipet 30 mL of this solution, add exactly 5 mL of the internal standard solution and 0.01 mol/L hydrochloric acid TS to make 50 mL, and use this solution as the standard solution. Perform the test with 10 μL each of the sample solution and standard solution as directed under Liquid Chromatography <*2.01*> according to the following conditions, and calculate the ratios, Q_T and Q_S, of the peak area of ritodrine to that of the internal standard.

Amount (mg) of ritodrine hydrochloride ($C_{17}H_{21}NO_3.HCl$)

$$= M_S \times Q_T/Q_S \times 4$$

M_S: Amount (mg) of Ritodrine Hydrochloride RS taken

Internal standard solution—A solution of methyl parahydroxybenzoate in methanol (3 in 5000).

Operating conditions—

Detector: An ultraviolet absorption photometer (wavelength: 274 nm).

Column: A stainless steel column 4.6 mm in inside diameter and 15 cm in length, packed with octadecylsilanized silica gel for liquid chromatography (5 μm in particle diameter).

Column temperature: A constant temperature of about 25°C.

Mobile phase: Dissolve 6.6 g of diammonium hydrogen phosphate and 1.1 g of sodium 1-heptanesulfonate in 700 mL of water, and add 300 mL of methanol. Adjust to pH 3.0 with phosphoric acid.

Flow rate: Adjust so that the retention time of ritodrine is about 6 minutes.

System suitability—

System performance: When the procedure is run with 10 μL of the standard solution under the above operating conditions, ritodrine and the internal standard are eluted in this order with the resolution between these peaks being not less than 3.

System repeatability: When the test is repeated 6 times with 10 μL of the standard solution under the above operating conditions, the relative standard deviation of the ratio of the peak area of ritodrine to that of the internal standard is not more than 1.0%.

Containers and storage Containers—Tight containers.
Storage—Light-resistant.

Rosuvastatin Calcium

ロスバスタチンカルシウム

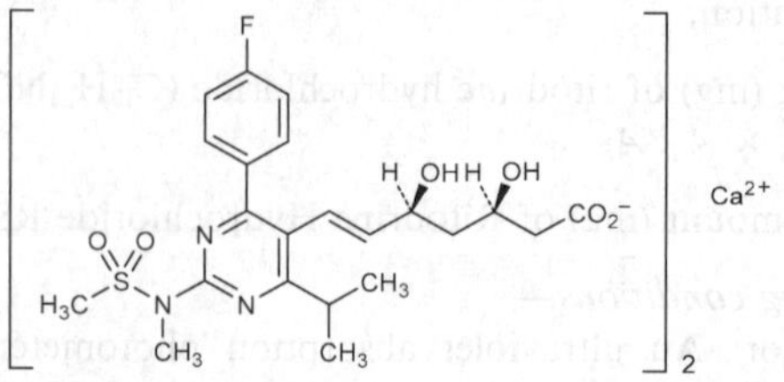

$(C_{22}H_{27}FN_3O_6S)_2Ca$: 1001.14
Monocalcium bis[(3*R*,5*S*,6*E*)-7-{4-(4-fluorophenyl)-6-(1-methylethyl)-2-[methyl(methylsulfonyl)amino]pyrimidin-5-yl}-3,5-dihydroxyhept-6-enoate]
[*147098-20-2*]

Rosuvastatin Calcium contains not less than 97.0% and not more than 102.0% of rosuvastatin calcium [$(C_{22}H_{27}FN_3O_6S)_2Ca$], calculated on the anhydrous basis.

Description Rosuvastatin Calcium occurs as a white powder.

It is freely soluble in acetonitrile, soluble in methanol, and slightly soluble in water and in ethanol (99.5).

It is hygroscopic.

Identification **(1)** Determine the absorption spectrum of a solution of Rosuvastatin Calcium in methanol (1 in 100,000) as directed under Ultraviolet-visible Spectrophotometry <*2.24*>, and compare the spectrum with the Reference Spectrum or the spectrum of a solution of Rosuvastatin Calcium RS prepared in the same manner as the sample solution: both spectra exhibit similar intensities of absorption at the same wavelengths.

(2) Determine the infrared absorption spectrum of Rosuvastatin Calcium as directed in the potassium bromide disk method under Infrared Spectrophotometry <*2.25*>, and compare the spectrum with the Reference Spectrum or the spectrum of Rosuvastatin Calcium RS: both spectra exhibit similar intensities of absorption at the same wave numbers.

(3) A solution of Rosuvastatin Calcium in a mixture of water and methanol (1:1) (1 in 125) responds to Qualitative Tests <*1.09*> (3) for calcium salt.

Purity **(1)** Inorganic impurities (chloride)—Being specified separately when the drug is granted approval based on the Law.

(2) Heavy metals <*1.07*>—Proceed with 1.0 g of Rosuvastatin Calcium according to Method 2, and perform the test. Prepare the control solution with 2.0 mL of Standard Lead Solution (not more than 20 ppm).

(3) Related substances—Conduct this procedure using light-resistant vessels. Use the sample solution obtained in the Assay as the sample solution. Separately, pipet 1 mL of the standard solution obtained in the Assay, add a mixture of water and acetonitrile (3:1) to make exactly 10 mL. Pipet 1 mL of this solution, add a mixture of water and acetonitrile (3:1) to make exactly 50 mL, and use this solution as the standard solution. Perform the test with exactly 10 μL each of the sample solution and standard solution as directed under Liquid Chromatography <*2.01*> according to the following conditions. Determine each peak area of related substances, A_T, in the sample solution and the peak area of rosuvastatin, A_S, in the standard solution by the automatic integration method, and calculate the amount of the related substances by the following equation: the amount of related substance A having the relative retention time of about 0.90 to rosuvastatin is not more than 0.2%, the amount of related substance B (diastereomer) having the relative retention time of about 1.1 is not more than 0.5%, the amount of related substance C having the relative retention time of about 1.5 is not more than 0.7%, the amount of related substance D having the relative retention time of about 1.7 is not more than 0.15%, and each amount of other related substance is not more than 0.1%. Furthermore the total amount of the related substances is not more than 1.1%. For the area of the peak of related substance C, multiply the correction factor 1.4.

Amount (%) of related substance
$= M_S/M_T \times A_T/A_S \times 1/5$

M_S: Amount (mg) of Rosuvastatin Calcium RS taken, calculated on the anhydrous basis

M_T: Amount (mg) of Rosuvastatin Calcium taken, calculated on the anhydrous basis

Operating conditions—

Detector, column, column temperature, mobile phase, and flow rate: Proceed as directed in the operating conditions in the Assay.

Time span of measurement: About 2.8 times as long as the retention time of rosuvastatin, beginning after the solvent peak.

System suitability—

System performance: Proceed as directed in the system suitability in the Assay.

Test for required detectability: Pipet 5 mL of the standard solution obtained in the Assay, add 24 mL of acetonitrile, and add water to make exactly 100 mL. Pipet 1 mL of this solution, add 24 mL of acetonitrile, and add water to make exactly 100 mL. Confirm that the peak area of rosuvastatin obtained with 10 μL of this solution is equivalent to 0.035 to 0.065% of that with 10 μL of the standard solution in the Assay.

System repeatability: When the test is repeated 5 times with 10 μL of the standard solution in the Assay under the above operating conditions, the relative standard deviation of the peak area of rosuvastatin is not more than 2.0%.

(4) Enantiomer—Dissolve 25 mg of Rosuvastatin Calcium in 6 mL of acetonitrile, add water to make exactly 25 mL, and use this solution as the sample solution. Pipet 1 mL of this solution, add a mixture of water and acetonitrile (3:1) to make exactly 200 mL, and use this solution as the standard solution. Perform the test with exactly 10 μL each of the sample solution and standard solution as directed under Liquid Chromatography <*2.01*> according to the following conditions, and determine each peak area by the automatic integration method: the area of related substance E (enantiomer) having the relative retention time of about 0.92 to rosuvastatin obtained from the sample solution is not larger than 1/5 times the peak area of rosuvastatin from the standard solution.

Operating conditions—

Detector: An ultraviolet absorption photometer (wavelength: 242 nm).

Column: A stainless steel column 4.6 mm in inside diameter and 15 cm in length, packed with silica gel coated with cellulose tris(4-methylbenzoate) for liquid chromatography (5 μm in particle diameter).

Column temperature: A constant temperature of about 35°C.

Mobile phase: A mixture of diluted trifluoroacetic acid (1 in 1000) and acetonitrile (3:1).

Flow rate: Adjust so that the retention time of rosuvastatin is about 26.5 minutes.

System suitability—

Test for required detectability: Pipet 5 mL of the standard solution, add a mixture of water and acetonitrile (3:1) to make exactly 50 mL. Confirm that the peak area of rosuvastatin obtained with 10 μL of this solution is equivalent to 7 to 13% of that with the standard solution.

System performance: To 5 mg of rosuvastatin calcium enantiomer add 12 mL of acetonitrile and 10 mL of water, sonicate to dissolve, and add water to make 50 mL. To 1 mL of this solution and 6 mL of acetonitrile add 25 mg of Rosuvastatin Calcium, sonicate to dissolve, and add water to make 25 mL. When the procedure is run with 10 μL of this solution under the above operating conditions, rosuvastatin enantiomer and rosuvastatin are eluted in this order with the resolution between these peaks being not less than 1.5, and the symmetry factor of the peak of rosuvastatin is 1.0 – 1.5.

System repeatability: When the test is repeated 6 times with 10 μL of the standard solution under the above operating conditions, the relative standard deviation of the peak area of rosuvastatin is not more than 2.0%.

Water <*2.48*> Not more than 6.1% (20 mg, coulometric titration).

Assay Conduct this procedure using light-resistant vessels. Weigh accurately about 35 mg each of Rosuvastatin Calcium and Rosuvastatin Calcium RS (separately determine the water <*2.48*> in the same manner as Rosuvastatin Calcium), dissolve each in 12 mL of acetonitrile, add water to make exactly 50 mL, and use these solutions as the sample solution and the standard solution, respectively. Perform the test with exactly 10 μL each of the sample solution and standard solution as directed under Liquid Chromatography <*2.01*> according to the following conditions, and determine the peak areas, A_T and A_S, of rosuvastatin in each solution.

Amount (mg) of rosuvastatin calcium [$(C_{22}H_{27}FN_3O_6S)_2Ca$]
$= M_S \times A_T/A_S$

M_S: Amount (mg) of Rosuvastatin Calcium RS taken, calculated on the anhydrous basis

Operating conditions—

Detector: An ultraviolet absorption photometer (wavelength: 242 nm).

Column: A stainless steel column 3 mm in inside diameter and 15 cm in length, packed with octadecylsilanized silica gel for liquid chromatography (3 μm in particle diameter).

Column temperature: A constant temperature of about 40°C.

Mobile phase A: A mixture of water, acetonitrile and diluted trifluoroacetic acid (1 in 100) (70:29:1).

Mobile phase B: A mixture of acetonitrile, water, and diluted trifluoroacetic acid (1 in 100) (75:24:1).

Flowing of mobile phase: Control the gradient by mixing the mobile phases A and B as directed in the following table.

Time after injection of sample (min)	Mobile phase A (vol%)	Mobile phase B (vol%)
0 – 30	100	0
30 – 50	100 → 60	0 → 40
50 – 60	60 → 0	40 → 100
60 – 70	0	100

Flow rate: 0.75 mL per minute.

System suitability—

System performance: Dissolve 10 mg of Rosuvastatin Calcium in 10 mL of a solution of trifluoroacetic acid in acetonitrile (1 in 100), and allow to stand at 40°C for 1 hour. After cooling, add 20 mL of water, adjust to pH 6 – 8 with sodium hydroxide TS, and add water to make 50 mL. To 3 mL of this solution, add water to make 50 mL. When the procedure is run with 10 μL of this solution under the above operating conditions, rosuvastatin and the related substance B (diastereomer) are eluted in this order with the resolution between these peaks being not less than 2.5, and the symmetry factor of the peak of rosuvastatin is not more than 1.5.

System repeatability: When the test is repeated 5 times with 10 μL of the standard solution under the above operating conditions, the relative standard deviation of the peak area of rosuvastatin is not more than 2.0%.

Containers and storage Containers—Tight containers.

Storage—Light-resistant, at a temperature between 2°C and 8°C.

Others

Rosuvastatin enantiomer:
(3*S*,5*R*,6*E*)-7-{4-(4-Fluorophenyl)-6-(1-methylethyl)-2-[methyl(methylsulfonyl)amino]pyrimidin-5-yl}-3,5-dihydroxyhept-6-enoic acid

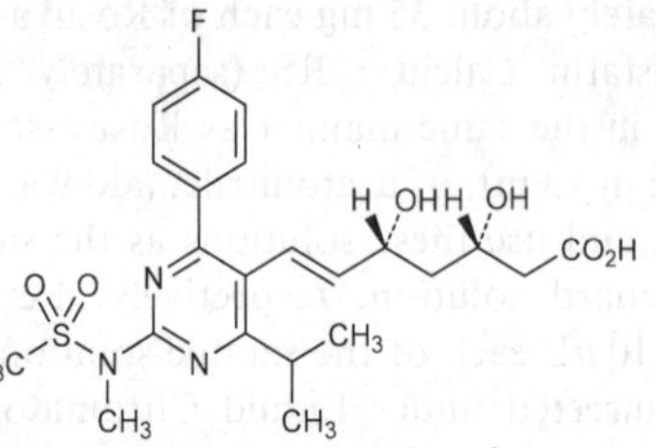

Related substance A:
(3*R*,5*S*,6*E*)-7-[4-(4-Fluorophenyl)-2-{[(2-hydroxy-2-methylpropyl)sulfonyl]methylamino}-6-(1-methylethyl)pyrimidin-5-yl]-3,5-dihydroxyhept-6-enoic acid

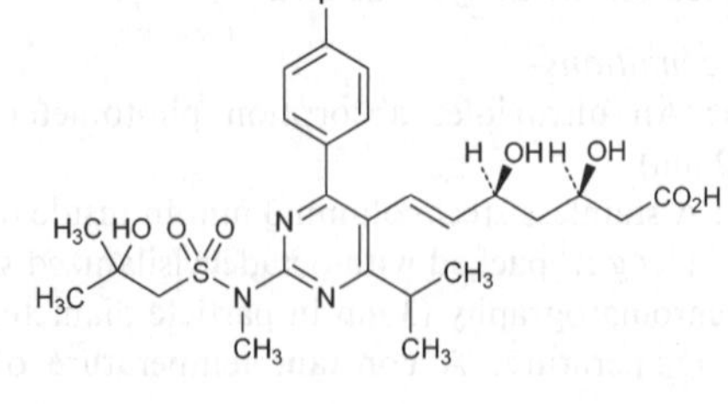

Related substance B (diastereomer):
(3*RS*,5*RS*,6*E*)-7-{4-(4-Fluorophenyl)-6-(1-methylethyl)-2-[methyl(methylsulfonyl)amino]pyrimidin-5-yl}-3,5-dihydroxyhept-6-enoic acid

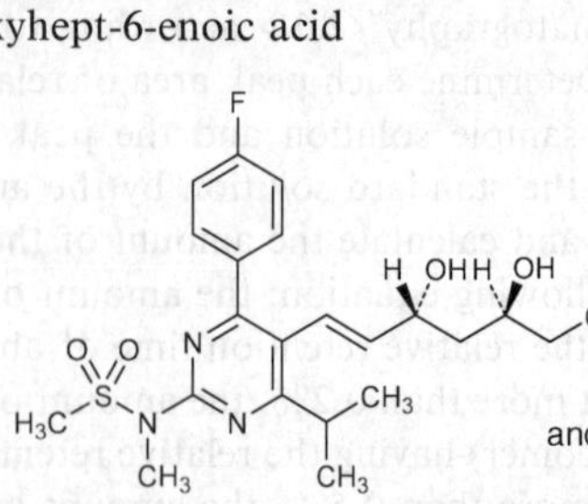

and enantiomer

Related substance C:
(3*R*,6*E*)-7-{4-(4-Fluorophenyl)-6-(1-methylethyl)-2-[methyl(methylsulfonyl)amino]pyrimidin-5-yl}-3-hydroxy-5-oxohept-6-enoic acid

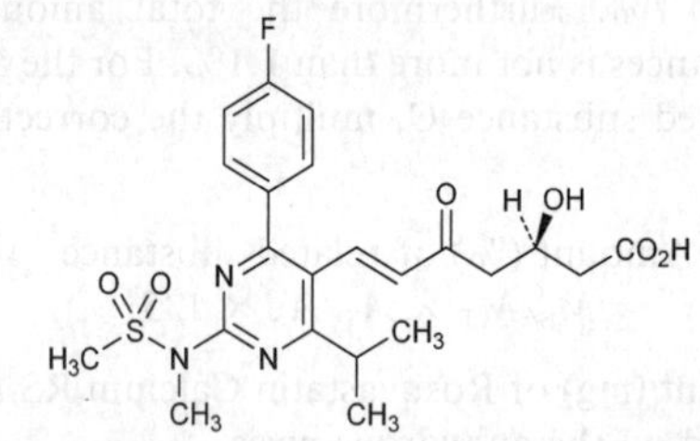

Related substance D:
N-[4-(4-Fluorophenyl)-5-{(1*E*)-2-[(2*S*,4*R*)-4-hydroxy-6-oxotetrahydro-2*H*-pyran-2-yl]ethenyl}-6-(1-methylethyl)pyrimidin-2-yl]-*N*-methylmethanesulfonamide

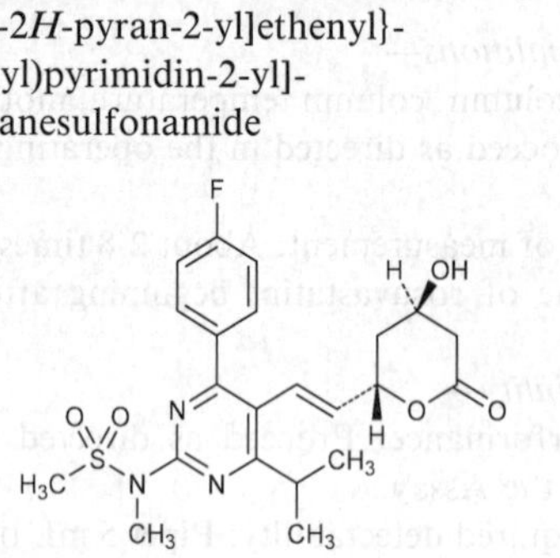

Related substance E (enantiomer):
(3*S*,5*R*,6*E*)-7-{4-(4-Fluorophenyl)-6-(1-methylethyl)-2-[methyl(methylsulfonyl)amino]pyrimidin-5-yl}-3,5-dihydroxyhept-6-enoic acid

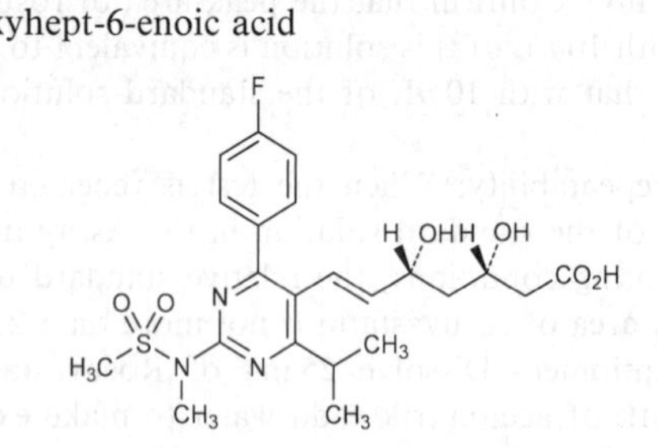

Rosuvastatin Calcium Tablets

ロスバスタチンカルシウム錠

Rosuvastatin Calcium Tablets contain not less than 95.0% and not more than 105.0% of the labeled amount of rosuvastatin ($C_{22}H_{28}FN_3O_6S$: 481.54).

Method of preparation Prepare as directed under Tablets, with Rosuvastatin Calcium.

Identification Perform the test with 10 μL each of the sample solution and standard solution obtained in the Assay, as directed under Liquid Chromatography <2.01> according to the following conditions: the principal peaks in the chromatograms obtained from the sample solution and the standard solution show the same retention time, and both spectra of these peaks in the chromatograms exhibit similar intensities of absorption at the same wavelengths.

Operating conditions—

Column, column temperature, mobile phase, and flow rate: Proceed as directed in the operating conditions in the Assay.

Detector: A photodiode array detector (wavelength: 242 nm; spectrum range of measurement: 220 – 400 nm).

System suitability—

System performance: Proceed as directed in the system suitability in the Assay.

Purity Related substances—To an amount of Rosuvastatin Calcium Tablets, equivalent to 0.1 g of rosuvastatin ($C_{22}H_{28}FN_3O_6S$), add 50 mL of water, shake for 30 minutes, then add 25 mL of acetonitrile, and shake for 30 minutes. To this solution add water to make 100 mL, and filter through a membrane filter with a pore size not exceeding 0.45 μm. Discard the first 5 mL of the filtrate, and use the subsequent filtrate as the sample solution. Pipet 1 mL of the sample solution, add a mixture of water and acetonitrile (3:1) to make exactly 100 mL, and use this solution as the standard solution. Perform the test with exactly 10 μL each of the sample solution and standard solution as directed under Liquid Chromatography <2.01> according to the following conditions, and determine each peak area by the automatic integration method: the peak area of related substance C, having the relative retention time of about 1.6 to rosuvastatin, obtained from the sample solution is not larger than 1.4 times the peak area of rosuvastatin from the standard solution, the peak area of related substance D, having the relative retention time of about 2.3, from the sample solution is not larger than 7/10 times the peak area of rosuvastatin from the standard solution, and the area of the peak other than the peaks of rosuvastatin and related substance B (diastereomer) having a relative retention time of about 1.1 and the peaks mentioned above from the sample solution is not larger than 1/5 times the peak area of rosuvastatin from the standard solution. Furthermore, the total area of the peaks other than rosuvastatin from the sample solution is not larger than 2.1 times the peak area of rosuvastatin from the standard solution. For the area of the peak of related substance C, multiply the correction factor 1.4.

Operating conditions—

Detector, column, column temperature, mobile phase, and flow rate: Proceed as directed in the operating conditions in the Assay.

Time span of measurement: About 2.5 times as long as the retention time of rosuvastatin, beginning after the solvent peak.

System suitability—

System performance: Proceed as directed in the system suitability in the Assay.

Test for required detectability: Pipet 5 mL of the standard solution, add a mixture of water and acetonitrile (3:1) to make exactly 100 mL. Confirm that the peak area of rosuvastatin obtained with 10 μL of this solution is equivalent to 3.5 to 6.5% of that with 10 μL of the standard solution.

System repeatability: When the test is repeated 6 times with 10 μL of the standard solution under the above operating conditions, the relative standard deviation of the peak area of rosuvastatin is not more than 2.0%.

Uniformity of dosage units <6.02> Perform the test according to the following method: it meets the requirement of the Content uniformity test.

To 1 tablet of Rosuvastatin Calcium Tablets add 3V/4 mL of 0.1 mol/L phosphate buffer solution (pH 7), and shake for 45 minutes. To this solution add 0.1 mol/L phosphate buffer solution (pH 7) to make exactly V mL so that each mL contains about 25 μg of rosuvastatin ($C_{22}H_{28}FN_3O_6S$), and filter through a membrane filter with a pore size not exceeding 0.2 μm. Discard the first 5 mL of the filtrate, and use the subsequent filtrate as the sample solution. Separately, weigh accurately about 0.1 g of Rosuvastatin Calcium RS (separately determine the water <2.48> in the same manner as Rosuvastatin Calcium), add 0.1 mol/L phosphate buffer solution (pH 7) to make exactly 250 mL. Pipet 15 mL of this solution, add 0.1 mol/L phosphate buffer solution (pH 7) to make exactly 250 mL, and use this solution as the standard solution. Determine the absorbances, A_T and A_S, of the sample solution and standard solution at 241 nm as directed under Ultraviolet-visible Spectrophotometry <2.24>.

Amount (mg) of rosuvastatin ($C_{22}H_{28}FN_3O_6S$)
$= M_S \times A_T/A_S \times 3V/12{,}500 \times 0.962$

M_S: Amount (mg) of Rosuvastatin Calcium RS taken, calculated on the anhydrous basis

Dissolution <6.10> When the test is performed at 50 revolutions per minute according to the Paddle method, using 900 mL of 0.05 mol/L citrate buffer solution (pH 6.6) as the dissolution medium, the dissolution rate in 30 minutes of Rosuvastatin Calcium Tablets is not less than 80%.

Start the test with 1 tablet of Rosuvastatin Calcium Tablets, withdraw not less than 20 mL of the medium at the specified minute after starting the test, and filter through a membrane filter with a pore size not exceeding 0.45 μm. Discard not less than 5 mL of the first filtrate, pipet V mL of the subsequent filtrate, add the dissolution medium to make exactly V' mL so that each mL contains about 2.8 μg of rosuvastatin ($C_{22}H_{28}FN_3O_6S$), and use this solution as the sample solution. Separately, weigh accurately about 0.1 g of Rosuvastatin Calcium RS (separately determine the water <2.48> in the same manner as Rosuvastatin Calcium), add 50 mL of water, sonicate, add 25 mL of acetonitrile to dissolve, and add water to make exactly 100 mL. Pipet 10 mL of this solution, add the dissolution medium to make exactly 200 mL. Pipet 10 mL of this solution, and add the dissolution medium to make exactly 200 mL, and use this solution as the standard solution. Perform the test with exactly 20 μL each of the sample solution and standard solution as directed under Liquid Chromatography <2.01> according to the following conditions, and determine the peak areas, A_T and A_S, of rosuvastatin in each solution.

Dissolution rate (%) with respect to the labeled amount of rosuvastatin ($C_{22}H_{28}FN_3O_6S$)
$= M_S \times A_T/A_S \times V'/V \times 1/C \times 9/4 \times 0.962$

M_S: Amount (mg) of Rosuvastatin Calcium RS taken, calculated on the anhydrous basis
C: Labeled amount (mg) of rosuvastatin ($C_{22}H_{28}FN_3O_6S$) in 1 tablet

Operating conditions—

Detector: An ultraviolet absorption photometer (wavelength: 242 nm).

Column: A stainless steel column 4.6 mm in inside diameter and 5 cm in length, packed with octadecylsilanized silica gel for liquid chromatography (5 μm in particle diameter).

Column temperature: A constant temperature of about

25°C.

Mobile phase: A mixture of water, acetonitrile and phosphoric acid (600:400:1).

Flow rate: Adjust so that the retention time of rosuvastatin is about 2 minutes.

System suitability—

System performance: When the procedure is run with 20 μL of the standard solution under the above operating conditions, the number of theoretical plates and the symmetry factor of the peak of rosuvastatin are not less than 1900 and not more than 1.4, respectively.

System repeatability: When the test is repeated 6 times with 20 μL of the standard solution under the above operating conditions, the relative standard deviation of the peak area of rosuvastatin is not more than 1.5%.

Assay To 10 tablets of Rosuvastatin Calcium Tablets add exactly 300 mL of water, and shake for 30 minutes. To this solution add 125 mL of acetonitrile, shake for 15 minutes, and add water to make exactly 500 mL. Pipet 5 mL of this solution, add a mixture of water and acetonitrile (3:1) to make exactly V mL so that each mL contains about 25 μg of rosuvastatin ($C_{22}H_{28}FN_3O_6S$), and filter this solution through a membrane filter with a pore size not exceeding 0.45 μm. Discard the first 5 mL of the filtrate, and use the subsequent filtrate as the sample solution. Separately, weigh accurately about 0.1 g of Rosuvastatin Calcium RS (separately determine the water <*2.48*> in the same manner as Rosuvastatin Calcium), add 50 mL of water, sonicate, add 25 mL of acetonitrile, and add water to make exactly 100 mL. Pipet 5 mL of this solution, add a mixture of water and acetonitrile (3:1) to make exactly 200 mL, and use this solution as the standard solution. Perform the test with exactly 10 μL each of the sample solution and standard solution as directed under Liquid Chromatography <*2.01*> according to the following conditions, and determine the peak areas, A_T and A_S, of rosuvastatin in each solution.

Amount (mg) of rosuvastatin ($C_{22}H_{28}FN_3O_6S$) in 1 tablet of Rosuvastatin Calcium Tablets
$= M_S \times A_T/A_S \times V/400 \times 0.962$

M_S: Amount (mg) of Rosuvastatin Calcium RS taken, calculated on the anhydrous basis

Operating conditions—

Detector: An ultraviolet absorption photometer (wavelength: 242 nm).

Column: A stainless steel column 3.2 mm in inside diameter and 25 cm in length, packed with octadecylsilanized silica gel for liquid chromatography (5 μm in particle diameter).

Column temperature: A constant temperature of about 40°C.

Mobile phase: A mixture of water, acetonitrile and diluted trifluoroacetic acid (1 in 100) (62:37:1).

Flow rate: Adjust so that the retention time of rosuvastatin is about 13 minutes.

System suitability—

System performance: To 10 mg of rosuvastatin calcium add 100 mL of water and 20 mL of 1 mol/L hydrochloric acid TS, heat on a water bath of 60°C for 2 hours, and neutralize with sodium hydroxide TS. After cooling, add 50 mL of acetonitrile and water to make 200 mL. To 10 mL of this solution add 10 mL of a mixture of water and acetonitrile (3:1). When the procedure is run with 10 μL of this solution under the above operating conditions, the resolution between rosuvastatin and related substance B (diastereomer) is not less than 1.5.

System repeatability: When the test is repeated 6 times with 10 μL of the standard solution under the above operating conditions, the relative standard deviation of the peak area of rosuvastatin is not more than 1.5%.

Containers and storage Containers—Tight containers.

Others

Related substances B (diastereomer), C and D: Refer to them described in Rosuvastatin Calcium.

Roxatidine Acetate Hydrochloride

ロキサチジン酢酸エステル塩酸塩

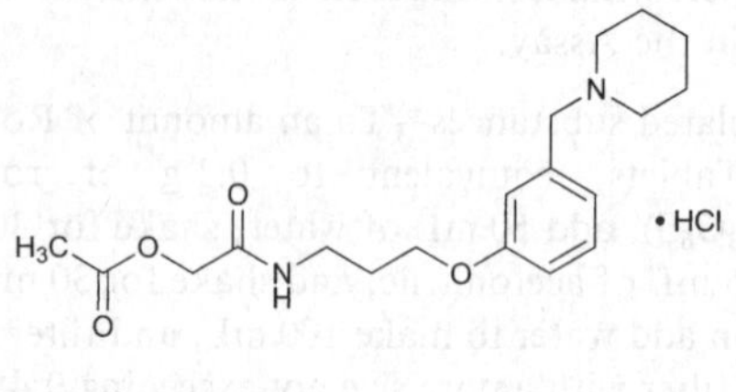

$C_{19}H_{28}N_2O_4 \cdot HCl$: 384.90
(3-{3-[(Piperidin-1-yl)methyl]phenoxy}propylcarbamoyl)methyl acetate monohydrochloride
[93793-83-0]

Roxatidine Acetate Hydrochloride, when dried, contains not less than 99.0% and not more than 101.0% of roxatidine acetate hydrochloride ($C_{19}H_{28}N_2O_4.HCl$).

Description Roxatidine Acetate Hydrochloride occurs as white, crystals or crystalline powder.

It is very soluble in water, freely soluble in acetic acid (100), and sparingly soluble in ethanol (99.5).

Identification **(1)** Determine the absorption spectrum of a solution of Roxatidine Acetate Hydrochloride in ethanol (99.5) (1 in 10,000) as directed under Ultraviolet-visible Spectrophotometry <*2.24*>, and compare the spectrum with the Reference Spectrum or the spectrum of a solution of Roxatidine Acetate Hydrochloride RS prepared in the same manner as the sample solution: both spectra exhibit similar intensities of absorption at the same wavelengths.

(2) Determine the infrared absorption spectrum of Roxatidine Acetate Hydrochloride as directed in the potassium chloride disk method under Infrared Spectrophotometry <*2.25*>, and compare the spectrum with the Reference Spectrum or the spectrum of Roxatidine Acetate Hydrochloride RS: both spectra exhibit similar intensities of absorption at the same wave numbers.

(3) A solution of Roxatidine Acetate Hydrochloride (1 in 50) responds to Qualitative Tests <*1.09*> (2) for chloride.

pH <*2.54*> Dissolve 1.0 g of Roxatidine Acetate Hydrochloride in 20 mL of water: the pH of this solution is between 4.0 and 6.0.

Melting point <*2.60*> 147 – 151°C (after drying).

Purity **(1)** Clarity and color of solution—Dissolve 1.0 g of Roxatidine Acetate Hydrochloride in 10 mL of water: the solution is clear and colorless.

(2) Heavy metals <*1.07*>—Proceed with 2.0 g of Roxatidine Acetate Hydrochloride according to Method 1, and perform the test. Prepare the control solution with 2.0 mL of Standard Lead Solution (not more than 10 ppm).

(3) Related substances—Dissolve 50 mg of Roxatidine

Acetate Hydrochloride in 10 mL of ethanol (99.5), and use this solution as the sample solution. Pipet 1 mL of the sample solution, add ethanol (99.5) to make exactly 100 mL, and use this solution as the standard solution. Perform the test with exactly 10 μL each of the sample solution and standard solution as directed under Liquid Chromatography <2.01> according to the following conditions, and determine each peak area by the automatic integration method: the area of the peak other than roxatidine acetate obtained from sample solution is not larger than 1/5 times the peak area of roxatidine acetate from the standard solution, and the total area of the peaks other than roxatidine acetate from the sample solution is not larger than 1/2 times the peak area of roxatidine acetate from the standard solution.

Operating conditions—

Detector: An ultraviolet absorption photometer (wavelength: 274 nm).

Column: A stainless steel column 4 mm in inside diameter and 25 cm in length, packed with cyanopropylsilanized silica gel for liquid chromatography (5 μm in particle diameter).

Column temperature: A constant temperature of about 35°C.

Mobile phase: A mixture of hexane, ethanol (99.5), triethylamine and acetic acid (100) (384:16:2:1).

Flow rate: Adjust so that the retention time of roxatidine acetate is about 10 minutes.

Time span of measurement: About 1.5 times as long as the retention time of roxatidine acetate, beginning after the solvent peak.

System suitability—

Test for required detectability: To 5 mL of the standard solution add ethanol (99.5) to make 10 mL, and use this solution as the solution for system suitability test. Pipet 1 mL of the solution for system suitability test, and add ethanol (99.5) to make exactly 10 mL. Confirm that the peak area of roxatidine acetate obtained with 10 μL of this solution is equivalent to 7 to 13% of that with 10 μL of the solution for system suitability test.

System performance: Dissolve 50 mg of roxatidine acetate hydrochloride and 10 mg of benzoic acid in 25 mL of ethanol (99.5). When the procedure is run with 10 μL of this solution under the above operating conditions, benzoic acid and roxatidine acetate are eluted in this order with the resolution between these peaks being not less than 10.

System repeatability: When the test is repeated 6 times with 10 μL of the standard solution under the above operating conditions, the relative standard deviation of the peak area of roxatidine acetate is not more than 1.0%.

Loss on drying <2.41> Not more than 0.3% (1 g, in vacuum, phosphorus (V) oxide, 4 hours).

Residue on ignition <2.44> Not more than 0.1% (1 g).

Assay Weigh accurately about 0.3 g of Roxatidine Acetate Hydrochloride, previously dried, dissolve in 5 mL of acetic acid (100), add 50 mL of acetic anhydride, and titrate <2.50> with 0.1 mol/L perchloric acid VS (potentiometric titration). Perform a blank determination in the same manner, and make any necessary correction.

Each mL of 0.1 mol/L perchloric acid VS
= 38.49 mg of $C_{19}H_{28}N_2O_4.HCl$

Containers and storage Containers—Tight containers.

Roxatidine Acetate Hydrochloride Extended-release Capsules

ロキサチジン酢酸エステル塩酸塩徐放カプセル

Roxatidine Acetate Hydrochloride Extended-release Capsules contain not less than 93.0% and not more than 107.0% of the labeled amount of roxatidine acetate hydrochloride ($C_{19}H_{28}N_2O_4.HCl$: 384.90).

Method of preparation Prepare as directed under Capsules, with Roxatidine Acetate Hydrochloride.

Identification To 1 mL of the filtrate obtained in the Assay add ethanol (99.5) to make 20 mL, and determine the absorption spectrum as directed under Ultraviolet-visible Spectrophotometry <2.24>: it exhibits maxima between 275 nm and 278 nm, and between 282 nm and 285 nm.

Uniformity of dosage units <6.02> Perform the Mass variation test, or the Content uniformity test according to the following method: it meets the requirement.

Take out the contents of 1 capsule of Roxatidine Acetate Hydrochloride Extended-release Capsules, add exactly V mL of ethanol (99.5) so that each mL contains about 2.5 mg of roxatidine acetate hydrochloride ($C_{19}H_{28}N_2O_4.HCl$), disperse the particles by sonicating, and filter through a membrane filter with a pore size of not more than 1.0 μm. To exactly 8 mL of the filtrate add exactly 2 mL of the internal standard solution, mix, and use this solution as the sample solution. Proceed as directed in the Assay.

Amount (mg) of roxatidine acetate hydrochloride
($C_{19}H_{28}N_2O_4.HCl$) = $M_S \times Q_T/Q_S \times V/20$

M_S: Amount (mg) of Roxatidine Acetate Hydrochloride RS taken

*Internal standard solution—*A solution of benzoic acid in ethanol (99.5) (1 in 500).

Dissolution <6.10> When the test is performed at 50 revolutions per minute according to the Paddle method using the sinker, using 900 mL of water as the dissolution medium, the dissolution rates of a 37.5-mg capsule in 45 minutes, in 90 minutes and in 8 hours are 10 – 40%, 35 – 65%, and not less than 70%, respectively, and of a 75-mg capsule in 60 minutes, in 90 minutes and in 8 hours are 20 – 50%, 35 – 65%, and not less than 70%, respectively.

Start the test with 1 capsule of Roxatidine Acetate Hydrochloride Extended-release Capsules, withdraw exactly 20 mL of the medium at the specified minute after starting the test, and supply exactly 20 mL of warmed water to 37 ± 0.5°C immediately after withdrawing of the medium every time, and filter the media withdrawn through a membrane filter with a pore size not exceeding 0.45 μm. Discard not less than 10 mL of the first filtrate, pipet V mL of the subsequent filtrate, add water to make exactly V' mL so that each mL contains about 42 μg of roxatidine acetate hydrochloride ($C_{19}H_{28}N_2O_4.HCl$), and use this solution as the sample solution. Separately, weigh accurately about 21 mg of Roxatidine Acetate Hydrochloride RS, previously dried in a desiccator (in vacuum, phosphorus (V) oxide) for 4 hours, and dissolve in water to make exactly 50 mL. Pipet 2 mL of this solution, add water to make exactly 20 mL, and use this solution as the standard solution. Perform the test with exactly 100 μL each of the sample solutions and standard solution as directed under Liquid Chromatography <2.01> according to the following conditions, and determine the peak areas, $A_{T(n)}$ and A_S, of roxatidine acetate in each solution.

Dissolution rate (%) with respect to the labeled amount of roxatidine acetate hydrochloride ($C_{19}H_{28}N_2O_4.HCl$) on the nth medium withdrawing (n = 1,2,3)

$$= M_S \times \left[\frac{A_{T(n)}}{A_S} + \sum_{i=1}^{n-1}\left(\frac{A_{T(i)}}{A_S} \times \frac{1}{45}\right)\right] \times \frac{V'}{V} \times \frac{1}{C} \times 180$$

M_S: Amount (mg) of Roxatidine Acetate Hydrochloride RS taken

C: Labeled amount (mg) of roxatidine acetate hydrochloride ($C_{19}H_{28}N_2O_4.HCl$) in 1 capsule

Operating conditions—

Detector: An ultraviolet absorption photometer (wavelength: 274 nm).

Column: A stainless steel column 4.6 mm in inside diameter and 15 cm in length, packed with octadecylsilanized silica gel for liquid chromatography (5 μm in particle diameter).

Column temperature: A constant temperature of about 40°C.

Mobile phase: A mixture of water, acetonitrile, triethylamine and acetic acid (100) (340:60:2:1).

Flow rate: Adjust so that the retention time of roxatidine acetate is about 5 minutes.

System suitability—

System performance: When the procedure is run with 100 μL of the standard solution under the above operating conditions, the number of theoretical plates and the symmetry factor of the peak of roxatidine acetate are not less than 3000 and not more than 2.0, respectively.

System repeatability: When the test is repeated 6 times with 100 μL of the standard solution under the above operating conditions, the relative standard deviation of the peak area of roxatidine acetate is not more than 1.0%.

Assay Take out the contents of not less than 20 Roxatidine Acetate Hydrochloride Extended-release Capsules, weigh accurately the mass of the contents, and powder. Weigh accurately a portion of the powder, equivalent to about 75 mg of roxatidine acetate hydrochloride ($C_{19}H_{28}N_2O_4.HCl$), add exactly 30 mL of ethanol (99.5), shake, and filter through a membrane filter with a pore size of not more than 1.0 μm. To exactly 8 mL of the filtrate add exactly 2 mL of the internal standard solution, mix, and use this solution as the sample solution. Separately, weigh accurately about 50 mg of Roxatidine Acetate Hydrochloride RS, previously dried in a desiccator (in vacuum, phosphorus (V) oxide) for 4 hours, and dissolve in ethanol (99.5) to make exactly 20 mL. To exactly 8 mL of this solution add exactly 2 mL of the internal standard solution, mix, and use this solution as the standard solution. Perform the test with 10 μL each of the sample solution and standard solution as directed under Liquid Chromatography *<2.01>* according to the following conditions, and calculate the ratios, Q_T and Q_S, of the peak area of roxatidine acetate to that of the internal standard.

Amount (mg) of roxatidine acetate hydrochloride ($C_{19}H_{28}N_2O_4.HCl$)
$= M_S \times Q_T/Q_S \times 3/2$

M_S: Amount (mg) of Roxatidine Acetate Hydrochloride RS taken

*Internal standard solution—*A solution of benzoic acid in ethanol (99.5) (1 in 500).

Operating conditions—

Detector: An ultraviolet absorption photometer (wavelength: 274 nm).

Column: A stainless steel column 4.0 mm in inside diameter and 25 cm in length, packed with cyanopropylsilanized silica gel for liquid chromatography (5 μm in particle diameter).

Column temperature: A constant temperature of about 35°C.

Mobile phase: A mixture of hexane, ethanol (99.5), triethylamine and acetic acid (100) (384:16:2:1).

Flow rate: Adjust so that the retention time of roxatidine acetate is about 10 minutes.

System suitability—

System performance: When the procedure is run with 10 μL of the standard solution under the above operating conditions, the internal standard and roxatidine acetate are elute in this order with the resolution between these peaks being not less than 10.

System repeatability: When the test is repeated 6 times with 10 μL of the standard solution under the above operating conditions, the relative standard deviation of the ratio of the peak area of roxatidine acetate to that of the internal standard is not more than 1.0%.

Containers and storage Containers—Tight containers.

Roxatidine Acetate Hydrochloride Extended-release Tablets

ロキサチジン酢酸エステル塩酸塩徐放錠

Roxatidine Acetate Hydrochloride Extended-release Tablets contain not less than 93.0% and not more than 107.0% of the labeled amount of roxatidine acetate hydrochloride ($C_{19}H_{28}N_2O_4.HCl$: 384.90).

Method of preparation Prepare as directed under Tablets, with Roxatidine Acetate Hydrochloride.

Identification Powder Roxatidine Acetate Hydrochloride Extended-release Tablets. To a portion of the powder, equivalent to 37.5 mg of Roxatidine Acetate Hydrochloride, add 40 mL of ethanol (99.5), and disperse the particles by sonicating for 10 minutes with occasional shaking. After shaking thoroughly, add ethanol (99.5) to make 50 mL. Filter the solution, and to 4 mL of the filtrate add ethanol (99.5) to make 25 mL. Determine the absorption spectrum of this solution as directed under Ultraviolet-visible Spectrophotometry *<2.24>*: it exhibits maxima between 274 nm and 278 nm and between 281 nm and 285 nm.

Uniformity of dosage units *<6.02>* Perform the test according to the following method: it meets the requirement of the Content uniformity test.

To 1 tablet of Roxatidine Acetate Hydrochloride Extended-release Tablets add 5 mL of a mixture of water, triethylamine and acetic acid (100) (340:2:1), sonicate for 5 minutes with occasional shaking, then add 7.5 mL of acetonitrile, then sonicate again for 5 minutes. Add 5 mL of a mixture of water, triethylamine and acetic acid (100) (340:2:1), sonicate for 5 minutes, shake thoroughly, add a mixture of water, triethylamine and acetic acid (100) (340:2:1) to make exactly 50 mL, centrifuge, and filter the supernatant liquid. Discard the first 10 mL of the filtrate, pipet V mL of the subsequent filtrate, equivalent to 6 mg of roxatidine acetate hydrochloride ($C_{19}H_{28}N_2O_4.HCl$), add exactly 3 mL of the internal standard solution, then add the mobile phase to make 20 mL, and use this solution as the sample solution. Then, proceed as directed in the Assay.

Amount (mg) of roxatidine acetate hydrochloride
($C_{19}H_{28}N_2O_4.HCl$)
$= M_S \times Q_T/Q_S \times 8/V$

M_S: Amount (mg) of Roxatidine Acetate Hydrochloride RS taken

Internal standard solution—A solution of sodium benzoate in the mobile phase (3 in 2000).

Dissolution Being specified separately when the drug is granted approval based on the Law.

Assay Weigh accurately the mass of not less than 20 Roxatidine Acetate Hydrochloride Extended-release Tablets, and powder. Weigh accurately a portion of the powder, equivalent to about 37.5 mg of roxatidine acetate hydrochloride ($C_{19}H_{28}N_2O_4.HCl$), add 40 mL of the mobile phase, and sonicate for 10 minutes with occasional shaking. Further shake thoroughly, add the mobile phase to make exactly 50 mL, centrifuge, and filter the supernatant liquid. Discard the first 10 mL of the filtrate, pipet 8 mL of the subsequent filtrate, add exactly 3 mL of the internal standard solution, add the mobile phase to make 20 mL, and use this solution as the sample solution. Separately, weigh accurately about 38 mg of Roxatidine Acetate Hydrochloride RS, previously dried in a desiccator (in vacuum, phosphorous (V) oxide) for 4 hours, dissolve in the mobile phase to make exactly 50 mL. Pipet 8 mL of this solution, add exactly 3 mL of the internal standard solution, then add the mobile phase to make 20 mL, and use this solution as the standard solution. Perform the test with 20 μL each of the sample solution and standard solution as directed under Liquid Chromatography <*2.01*> under the following conditions, and calculate the ratios, Q_T and Q_S, of the peak area of roxatidine acetate to that of the internal standard.

Amount (mg) of roxatidine acetate hydrochloride
($C_{19}H_{28}N_2O_4.HCl$)
$= M_S \times Q_T/Q_S$

M_S: Amount (mg) of Roxatidine Acetate Hydrochloride RS taken

Internal standard solution—A solution of sodium benzoate in the mobile phase (3 in 2000).
Operating conditions—

Detector: An ultraviolet absorption photometer (wavelength: 274 nm).

Column: A stainless steel column 4 mm in inside diameter and 15 cm in length, packed with octadecylsilanized silica gel for liquid chromatography (5 μm in particle diameter).

Column temperature: A constant temperature of about 40°C.

Mobile phase: A mixture of water, acetonitrile, triethylamine and acetic acid (100) (340:60:2:1).

Flow rate: Adjust so that the retention time of roxatidine acetate is about 8 minutes.
System suitability—

System performance: When the procedure is run with 20 μL of the standard solution under the above operating conditions, the internal standard and roxatidine acetate are eluted in this order with the resolution between these peaks being not less than 10.

System repeatability: When the test is repeated 6 times with 20 μL of the standard solution under the above operating conditions, the relative standard deviation of the ratio of the peak area of roxatidine acetate to that of the internal standard is not more than 1.0%.

Containers and storage Containers—Well-closed containers.

Roxatidine Acetate Hydrochloride for Injection

注射用ロキサチジン酢酸エステル塩酸塩

Roxatidine Acetate Hydrochloride for Injection is a preparation for injection which is dissolved before use.

It contains not less than 95.0% and not more than 105.0% of the labeled amount of roxatidine acetate hydrochloride ($C_{19}H_{28}N_2O_4.HCl$: 384.90).

Method of preparation Prepare as directed under Injections, with Roxatidine Acetate Hydrochloride.

Description It occurs as white, masses or powder.

Identification To an amount of Roxatidine Acetate Hydrochloride for Injection, equivalent to 75 mg of Roxatidine Acetate Hydrochloride, add 30 mL of ethanol (99.5), shake, and filter through a membrane filter with a pore size not exceeding 0.45 μm. To 1 mL of the filtrate add ethanol (99.5) to make 20 mL. Determine the absorption spectrum of this solution as directed under Ultraviolet-visible Spectrophotometry <*2.24*>: it exhibits maxima between 275 nm and 279 nm and between 282 nm and 286 nm.

pH Being specified separately when the drug is granted approval based on the Law.

Purity Clarity and color of solution Dissolve an amount of Roxatidine Acetate Hydrochloride for Injection, equivalent to 75 mg of Roxatidine Acetate Hydrochloride, in 20 mL of isotonic sodium chloride solution: the solution is clear and colorless.

Bacterial endotoxins <*4.01*> Less than 4.0 EU/mg.

Uniformity of dosage units <*6.02*> It meets the requirements of the Mass variation test.

Foreign insoluble matter <*6.06*> Perform the test according to Method 2: it meets the requirement.

Insoluble particulate matter <*6.07*> It meets the requirement.

Sterility <*4.06*> Perform the test according to the Membrane filtration method: it meets the requirement.

Assay Dissolve with water each content of 10 Roxatidine Acetate Hydrochloride for Injection, wash the containers with water, combine the solution of the content and washings, and add water to make exactly V mL so that each mL contains about 3.75 mg of roxatidine acetate hydrochloride ($C_{19}H_{28}N_2O_4.HCl$). Pipet 5 mL of this solution, add water to make exactly 50 mL. Pipet 5 mL of this solution, add exactly 5 mL of the internal standard solution, and use this solution as the sample solution. Separately, weigh accurately about 20 mg of Roxatidine Acetate Hydrochloride RS, previously dried in a desiccator (in vacuum, phosphorous (V) oxide) for 4 hours, dissolve in water to make exactly 50 mL. Pipet 5 mL of this solution, add exactly 5 mL of the internal standard solution, and use this solution as the standard solution. Perform the test with 10 μL each of the sample solution and standard solution as directed under Liquid Chromatography <*2.01*> according to the following conditions, and calculate the ratios, Q_T and Q_S, of the peak area of roxatidine acetate to that of the internal standard.

Amount (mg) of roxatidine acetate hydrochloride ($C_{19}H_{28}N_2O_4.HCl$) in 1 Roxatidine Acetate Hydrochloride for Injection
$= M_S \times Q_T/Q_S \times V/50$

M_S: Amount (mg) of Roxatidine Acetate Hydrochloride RS taken

Internal standard solution—Dissolve 20 mg of guanine in 10 mL of 2 mol/L hydrochloric acid TS, add 50 mL of water, then add 20 mL of a solution of sodium hydroxide (1 in 25) and water to make 100 mL. To 10 mL of this solution add water to make 100 mL.

Operating conditions—

Detector: An ultraviolet absorption photometer (wavelength: 274 nm).

Column: A stainless steel column 4.6 mm in inside diameter and 15 cm in length, packed with octadecylsilanized silica gel for liquid chromatography (5 μm in particle diameter).

Column temperature: A constant temperature of about 40°C.

Mobile phase: A mixture of water, acetonitrile, triethylamine and acetic acid (100) (340:60:2:1).

Flow rate: Adjust so that the retention time of roxatidine acetate is about 14 minutes.

System suitability—

System performance: When the procedure is run with 10 μL of the standard solution under the above operating conditions, the internal standard and roxatidine acetate are eluted in this order with the resolution between these peaks being not less than 10.

System repeatability: When the test is repeated 6 times with 10 μL of the standard solution under the above operating conditions, the relative standard deviation of the ratio of the peak area of roxatidine acetate to that of the internal standard is not more than 1.0%.

Containers and storage Containers—Hermetic containers.

Roxithromycin

ロキシスロマイシン

$C_{41}H_{76}N_2O_{15}$: 837.05
(2*R*,3*S*,4*S*,5*R*,6*R*,8*R*,9*E*,10*R*,11*R*,12*S*,13*R*)-5-(3,4,6-Trideoxy-3-dimethylamino-β-D-*xylo*-hexopyranosyloxy)-3-(2,6-dideoxy-3-*C*-methyl-3-*O*-methyl-α-L-*ribo*-hexopyranosyloxy)-6,11,12-trihydroxy-9-(2-methoxyethoxy)methoxyimino-2,4,6,8,10,12-hexamethylpentadecan-13-olide
[*80214-83-1*]

Roxithromycin is a derivative of erythromycin.

It contains not less than 970 μg (potency) and not more than 1020 μg (potency) per mg, calculated on the anhydrous basis. The potency of Roxithromycin is expressed as mass (potency) of roxithromycin ($C_{41}H_{76}N_2O_{15}$).

Description Roxithromycin occurs as a white crystalline powder.

It is freely soluble in ethanol (95) and in acetone, soluble in methanol, and practically insoluble in water.

Identification Determine the infrared absorption spectrum of Roxithromycin as directed in the potassium bromide disk method under Infrared Spectrophotometry <*2.25*>, and compare the spectrum with the Reference Spectrum or the spectrum of Roxithromycin RS: both spectra exhibit similar intensities of absorption at the same wave numbers.

Optical rotation <*2.49*> $[\alpha]_D^{20}$: −93 – −96° (0.5 g calculated on the anhydrous basis, acetone, 50 mL, 100 mm).

Purity **(1)** Heavy metals <*1.07*>—Proceed with 2.0 g of Roxithromycin according to Method 2, and perform the test. Prepare the control solution with 2.0 mL of Standard Lead Solution (not more than 10 ppm).

(2) Related substances—Dissolve exactly 40 mg of Roxithromycin in the mobile phase A to make exactly 10 mL, and use this solution as the sample solution. Separately, dissolve exactly 20 mg of Roxithromycin RS in the mobile phase A to make exactly 10 mL. Pipet 1 mL of this solution, add the mobile phase A to make exactly 100 mL, and use this solution as the standard solution. Perform the test with exactly 20 μL each of the sample solution and standard solution as directed under Liquid Chromatography <*2.01*> according to the following conditions, and determine each peak area by the automatic integration method: the area of the peak having a relative retention time of about 1.05 to roxithromycin obtained from the sample solution is not larger than 2 times the peak area of roxithromycin from the standard solution. The area of the peak other than roxithromycin and the peak mentioned above from the sample solution is not larger than the peak area of roxithromycin from the standard solution, and the total area of the peaks other than roxithromycin from the sample solution is not larger than 6 times the peak area of roxithromycin from the standard solution.

Operating conditions—

Detector: An ultraviolet absorption photometer (wavelength: 205 nm).

Column: A stainless steel column 4.6 mm in inside diameter and 25 cm in length, packed with octadecylsilanized silica gel for liquid chromatography (5 μm in particle diameter).

Column temperature: A constant temperature of about 25°C.

Mobile phase A: To 200 mL of a solution of ammonium dihydrogenphosphate (17 in 100) add 510 mL of water, and adjust to pH 5.3 with 2 mol/L sodium hydroxide TS. To this solution add 315 mL of acetonitrile for liquid chromatography.

Mobile phase B: A mixture of acetonitrile for liquid chromatography and water (7:3).

Flowing of mobile phase: Control the gradient by mixing the mobile phases A and B as directed in the following table.

Time after injection of sample (min)	Mobile phase A (vol%)	Mobile phase B (vol%)
0 – 38	100	0
38 – 39	100 → 90	0 → 10
39 – 80	90	10

Flow rate: Adjust so that the retention time of roxithromycin is about 21 minutes.

Time span of measurement: For 80 minutes after injection of the sample solution.

System suitability—

Test for required detectability: To exactly 2 mL of the standard solution add the mobile phase A to make exactly 10 mL. Confirm that the peak area of roxithromycin obtained with 20 μL of this solution is equivalent to 15 to 25% of that with 20 μL of the standard solution.

System performance: When the procedure is run with 20 μL of the standard solution under the above operating conditions, the number of theoretical plates and the symmetry factor of the peak of roxithromycin are not less than 9000 and not more than 1.5, respectively.

System repeatability: When the test is repeated 5 times with 20 μL of the standard solution under the above operating conditions, the relative standard deviation of the peak areas of roxithromycin is not more than 2.0%.

Water <*2.48*> Not more than 3.0% (0.3 g, volumetric titration, direct titration).

Residue on ignition <*2.44*> Not more than 0.1% (1 g).

Assay Weigh accurately an amount of Roxithromycin and Roxithromycin RS, equivalent to about 38 mg (potency), dissolve them separately in a suitable amount of the mobile phase, then add exactly 1 mL of the internal standard, add the mobile phase to make 25 mL, and use these solutions as the sample solution and the standard solution, respectively. Perform the test with 10 μL each of the sample solution and standard solution as directed under Liquid Chromatography <*2.01*> according to the following conditions, and calculate the ratios, Q_T and Q_S, of the peak area of roxithromycin to that of the internal standard.

Amount [μg (potency)] of roxithromycin ($C_{41}H_{76}N_2O_{15}$)
$= M_S \times Q_T/Q_S \times 1000$

M_S: Amount [mg (potency)] of Roxithromycin RS taken

Internal standard solution—A solution of isopropyl parahydroxybenzoate in the mobile phase (1 in 800).

Operating conditions—

Detector: An ultraviolet absorption photometer (wavelength: 230 nm).

Column: A stainless steel column 4.6 mm in inside diameter and 25 cm in length, packed with octadecylsilanized silica gel for liquid chromatography (5 μm in particle diameter).

Column temperature: A constant temperature of about 25°C.

Mobile phase: Dissolve 49.1 g of ammonium dihydrogen phosphate in water to make 1000 mL, and adjust to pH 5.3 with 2 mol/L sodium hydroxide TS. To 690 mL of this solution add 310 mL of acetonitrile.

Flow rate: Adjust so that the retention time of roxithromycin is about 12 minutes.

System suitability—

System performance: When the procedure is run with 10 μL of the standard solution under the above operating conditions, roxithromycin and the internal standard are eluted in this order with the resolution between these peaks being not less than 10.

System repeatability: When the test is repeated 6 times with 10 μL of the standard solution under the above operating conditions, the relative standard deviation of the ratio of the peak area of roxithromycin to that of the internal standard is not more than 1.0%.

Containers and storage Containers—Tight containers.

Roxithromycin Tablets

ロキシスロマイシン錠

Roxithromycin Tablets contain not less than 95.0% and not more than 110.0% of the labeled potency of roxithromycin ($C_{41}H_{76}N_2O_{15}$: 837.05).

Method of preparation Prepare as directed under Tablets, with Roxithromycin.

Identification To a quantity of powdered Roxithromycin Tablets, equivalent to 0.3 g (potency) of Roxithromycin, add 10 mL of acetonitrile, shake, and centrifuge. Evaporate the supernatant liquid on a water bath under reduced pressure, dry the residue at 60°C under reduced pressure for 1 hour, and determine the infrared absorption spectrum of the residue as directed in the potassium bromide disk method under Infrared Spectrophotometry <*2.25*>: it exhibits absorption at the wave numbers of about 3460 cm^{-1}, 2940 cm^{-1}, 1728 cm^{-1}, 1633 cm^{-1} and 1464 cm^{-1}.

Uniformity of dosage unit <*6.02*> Perform the Mass variation test, or the Content uniformity test according to the following method: it meets the requirement.

To 1 tablet of Roxithromycin Tablets add 7*V*/10 mL of the mobile phase, sonicate to disintegrate the tablet, shake, add exactly *V*/25 mL of the internal standard solution, and add the mobile phase to make *V* mL so that each mL contains about 1.5 mg (potency) of roxithromycin ($C_{41}H_{76}N_2O_{15}$). Filter this solution through a membrane filter with a pore size not exceeding 0.45 μm, discard the first 5 mL of the filtrate, and use the subsequent filtrate as the sample solution. Then, proceed as directed in the Assay.

Amount [mg (potency)] of roxithromycin ($C_{41}H_{76}N_2O_{15}$)
$= M_S \times Q_T/Q_S \times V/25$

M_S: Amount [mg (potency)] of Roxithromycin RS taken

Internal standard solution—A solution of isopropyl parahydroxybenzoate in the mobile phase (1 in 800).

Dissolution <*6.10*> When the test is performed at 50 revolutions per minute according to the Paddle method, using 900 mL of 2nd fluid for dissolution test as the dissolution medium, the dissolution rate in 30 minutes of Roxithromycin Tablets is not less than 80%.

Start the test with 1 tablet of Roxithromycin Tablets, withdraw not less than 20 mL of the medium at the specified minute after starting the test, and filter through a membrane filter with a pore size not exceeding 0.45 μm. Discard not less than 10 mL of the first filtrate, pipet V mL of the subsequent filtrate, add the dissolution medium to make exactly V' mL so that each mL contains about 0.17 mg (potency) of roxithromycin ($C_{41}H_{76}N_2O_{15}$), and use this solution as the sample solution. Separately, weigh accurately about 33 mg (potency) of Roxithromycin RS, dissolve in the dissolution medium to make exactly 200 mL, and use this solution as the standard solution. Perform the test with exactly 50 μL each of the sample solution and standard solution as directed under Liquid Chromatography <*2.01*> according to the following conditions, and determine the peak areas, A_T and A_S, of roxithromycin in each solution.

Dissolution rate (%) with respect to the labeled amount [mg (potency)] of roxithromycin ($C_{41}H_{76}N_2O_{15}$)
$= M_S \times A_T/A_S \times V'/V \times 1/C \times 450$

M_S: Amount [mg (potency)] of Roxithromycin RS taken
C: Labeled amount [mg (potency)] of roxithromycin ($C_{41}H_{76}N_2O_{15}$) in 1 tablet

Operating conditions—

Detector, column temperature and mobile phase: Proceed as directed in the operating conditions in the Assay.

Column: A stainless steel column 4.6 mm in inside diameter and 15 cm in length, packed with octadecylsilanized silica gel for liquid chromatography (5 μm in particle diameter).

Flow rate: Adjust so that the retention time of roxithromycin is about 5 minutes.

System suitability—

System performance: When the procedure is run with 50 μL of the standard solution under the above operating conditions, the number of theoretical plates and the symmetry factor of the peak of roxithromycin are not less than 2300 and not more than 2.0, respectively.

System repeatability: When the test is repeated 6 times with 50 μL of the standard solution under the above operating conditions, the relative standard deviation of the peak area of roxithromycin is not more than 1.0%.

Assay Weigh accurately the mass of not less than 20 Roxithromycin Tablets, and powder. Weigh accurately a portion of the powder, equivalent to about 38 mg (potency) of roxithromycin ($C_{41}H_{76}N_2O_{15}$), add 20 mL of the mobile phase, shake vigorously, add exactly 1 mL of the internal standard solution, and then add the mobile phase to make 25 mL. Filter the solution through a membrane filter with a pore size not exceeding 0.45 μm, discard the first 5 mL of the filtrate, and use the subsequent filtrate as the sample solution. Separately, weigh accurately about 38 mg (potency) of Roxithromycin RS, dissolve in the mobile phase, add exactly 1 mL of the internal standard solution, then add the mobile phase to make 25 mL, and use this solution as the standard solution. Perform the test with 10 μL each of the sample solution and standard solution as directed under Liquid Chromatography <*2.01*> according to the following conditions, and calculate the ratios, Q_T and Q_S, of the peak area of roxithromycin to that of the internal standard.

Amount [mg (potency)] of roxithromycin ($C_{41}H_{76}N_2O_{15}$)
$= M_S \times Q_T/Q_S$

M_S: Amount [mg (potency)] of Roxithromycin RS taken

Internal standard solution—A solution of isopropyl parahydroxybenzoate in the mobile phase (1 in 800).

Operating conditions—

Detector: An ultraviolet absorption photometer (wavelength: 230 nm).

Column: A stainless steel column 4.6 mm in inside diameter and 25 cm in length, packed with octadecylsilanized silica gel for liquid chromatography (5 μm in particle diameter).

Column temperature: A constant temperature of about 25°C.

Mobile phase: Dissolve 49.1 g of ammonium dihydrogen phosphate in water to make 1000 mL, and adjust to pH 5.3 with 2 mol/L sodium hydroxide TS. To 690 mL of this solution add 310 mL of acetonitrile.

Flow rate: Adjust so that the retention time of roxithromycin is about 12 minutes.

System suitability—

System performance: When the procedure is run with 10 μL of the standard solution under the above operating conditions, roxithromycin and the internal standard are eluted in this order with the resolution between these peaks being not less than 10.

System repeatability: When the test is repeated 6 times with 10 μL of the standard solution under the above operating conditions, the relative standard deviation of the ratio of the peak area of roxithromycin to that of the internal standard is not more than 1.0%.

Containers and storage Containers—Tight containers.

Freeze-dried Live Attenuated Rubella Vaccine

乾燥弱毒生風しんワクチン

Freeze-dried Live Attenuated Rubella Vaccine is a preparation for injection which is dissolved before use.

It contains live attenuated rubella virus.

It conforms to the requirements of Freeze-dried Live Attenuated Rubella Vaccine in the Minimum Requirements for Biological Products.

Description Freeze-dried Live Attenuated Rubella Vaccine becomes a colorless, yellowish or reddish, clear liquid on addition of solvent.

Saccharated Pepsin

含糖ペプシン

Saccharated Pepsin is a mixture of pepsin obtained from the gastric mucosa of hog or cattle and Lactose Hydrate, and it is an enzyme drug having a proteolytic activity.

It contains not less than 3800 units and not more

than 6000 units per g.

Description Saccharated Pepsin occurs as a white powder. It has a characteristic odor, and has a slightly sweet taste.

It dissolves in water to give a slightly turbid liquid, and does not dissolve in ethanol (95) and in diethyl ether.

It is slightly hygroscopic.

Purity (1) Rancidity—Saccharated Pepsin has no unpleasant or rancid odor.

(2) Acidity—Dissolve 0.5 g of Saccharated Pepsin in 50 mL of water, and add 0.50 mL of 0.1 mol/L sodium hydroxide VS and 2 drops of phenolphthalein TS: the solution is red in color.

Loss on drying <*2.41*> Not more than 1.0% (1 g, 80°C, 4 hours).

Residue on ignition <*2.44*> Not more than 0.5% (1 g).

Assay (i) Substrate solution—Use the substrate solution 1 described in Assay for protein digestive activity under Digestion Test <*4.03*> after adjusting the pH to 2.0.

(ii) Sample solution—Weigh accurately an amount of Saccharated Pepsin equivalent to about 1250 units, dissolve in ice-cold 0.01 mol/L hydrochloric acid TS to make exactly 50 ml.

(iii) Standard solution—Weigh accurately a suitable amount of Saccharated Pepsin RS, and dissolve in ice-cold 0.01 mol/L hydrochloric acid TS to make a solution containing about 25 units per mL.

(iv) Procedure—Proceed as directed in Assay for protein digestive activity under Digestion Test <*4.03*>, and determine the absorbances, A_T and A_{TB}, of the sample solution, using trichloroacetic acid TS A as the precipitation reagent. Separately, determine the absorbances, A_S and A_{SB}, of the standard solution in the same manner as the sample solution.

Units in 1 g of Saccharated Pepsin

$$= U_S \times (A_T - A_{TB})/(A_S - A_{SB}) \times 1/M$$

U_S: Units per mL of the standard solution

M: Amount (g) of Saccharated Pepsin per mL of the sample solution taken

Containers and storage Containers—Tight containers.

Storage—Not exceeding 30°C.

Saccharin

サッカリン

$C_7H_5NO_3S$: 183.18

1,2-Benzo[*d*]isothiazol-3(2*H*)-one 1,1-dioxide

[*81-07-2*]

Saccharin contains not less than 98.0% and not more than 102.0% of saccharin ($C_7H_5NO_3S$), calculated on the dried basis.

Description Saccharin occurs as colorless to white crystals or a white crystalline powder.

It is sparingly soluble in ethanol (95), and slightly soluble in water.

It dissolves in sodium hydroxide TS.

Identification Determine the infrared absorption spectrum of Saccharin as directed in the potassium bromide disk method under Infrared Spectrophotometry <*2.25*>, and compare the spectrum with the Reference Spectrum: both spectra exhibit similar intensities of absorption at the same wave numbers.

Melting point <*2.60*> 226 – 230°C

Purity (1) Clarity and color of solution—Dissolve 5.0 g of Saccharin in 25 mL of a solution of sodium acetate trihydrate (1 in 5): the clarity of the solution is equivalent to that of water or a solution of sodium acetate trihydrate (1 in 5), or its degree of opalescence is not more than Reference suspension I, and it has the appearance of water in color or is not more intensely colored than a solution of sodium acetate trihydrate (1 in 5) or the following control solution.

Control solution: Mix 3.0 mL of Cobalt (II) Chloride CS, 3.0 mL of Iron (III) Chloride CS and 2.4 mL of Copper (II) Sulfate CS, and add diluted dilute hydrochloric acid (1 in 10) to make 1000 mL.

(2) Heavy metals <*1.07*>—Proceed with 2.0 g of Saccharin according to Method 2, and perform the test. Prepare the control solution with 2.0 mL of Standard Lead Solution (not more than 10 ppm).

(3) Benzoate and salicylate—To 10 mL of a saturated solution of Saccharin in hot water add 3 drops of iron (III) chloride TS: no precipitate is formed, and no red-purple to purple color develops.

(4) *o*-Toluene sulfonamide—Dissolve 10 g of Saccharin in 70 mL of sodium hydroxide TS, and extract with three 30-mL portions of ethyl acetate. Combine all the ethyl acetate extracts, wash with 30 mL of a solution of sodium chloride (1 in 4), dehydrate with 5 g of anhydrous sodium sulfate, then evaporate the solvent. To the residue add exactly 5 mL of the internal standard solution to dissolve, and use this solution as the sample solution. Separately, dissolve 0.10 g of *o*-toluene sulfonamide in ethyl acetate to make exactly 100 mL. Pipet 1 mL of this solution, evaporate to dryness on a water bath, dissolve the residue in exactly 5 mL of the internal standard solution, and use this solution as the standard solution. Perform the test with 1 μL each of the sample solution and standard solution as directed under Gas Chromatography <*2.02*> according to the following conditions, and calculate the ratios, Q_T and Q_S, of the peak height of *o*-toluene sulfonamide to that of the internal standard: Q_T is not more than Q_S.

Internal standard solution—A solution of caffeine in ethyl acetate (1 in 500).

Operating conditions—

Detector: A hydrogen flame-ionization detector.

Column: A glass column 3 mm in inside diameter and 1 m in length, packed with siliceous earth for gas chromatography coated 3% with diethylene glycol succinate polyester for gas chromatography (180 – 250 μm in particle diameter).

Column temperature: A constant temperature of about 200°C.

Temperature of injection port: A constant temperature of about 225°C.

Temperature of detector: A constant temperature of about 250°C.

Carrier gas: Nitrogen.

Flow rate: Adjust so that the retention time of caffeine is about 6 minutes.

System suitability—

System performance: When the procedure is run with 1 μL of the standard solution under the above operating conditions, the internal standard and *o*-toluene sulfonamide are eluted in this order with the resolution between these peaks being not less than 2.0.

System repeatability: When the test is repeated 6 times with 1 μL of the standard solution under the above operating conditions, the relative standard deviation of the ratio of the peak height of *o*-toluene sulfonamide to that of the internal standard is not more than 2.0%.

(5) Readily carbonizable substances—Transfer 0.20 g of Saccharin to a Nessler tube, add 5 mL of sulfuric acid, mix to dissolve, and warm at 48 to 50°C for 10 minutes: the solution is not more intensely colored than Matching Fluid A, when compared both solutions against a white background by viewing transversely.

Loss on drying <*2.41*> Not more than 1.0% (1 g, 105°C, 2 hours).

Residue on ignition <*2.44*> Not more than 0.2% (1 g).

Assay Weigh accurately about 50 mg of Saccharin, and dissolve in a mixture of water and methanol (1:1) to make exactly 50 mL. Pipet 5 mL of this solution, add a mixture of water and methanol (1:1) to make exactly 50 mL, and use this solution as the sample solution. Separately, weigh accurately about 25 mg of Saccharin RS (separately determine the loss on drying <*2.41*> in the same conditions as Saccharin), dissolve in a mixture of water and methanol (1:1) to make exactly 25 mL, and use this solution as the standard stock solution. Pipet 5 mL of the standard stock solution, add a mixture of water and methanol (1:1) to make exactly 50 mL, and use this solution as the standard solution. Perform the test with exactly 10 μL each of the sample solution and standard solution as directed under Liquid Chromatography <*2.01*> according to the following conditions, and determine the peak areas, A_T and A_S, of saccharin in each solution.

$$\text{Amount (mg) of saccharin } (C_7H_5NO_3S) = M_S \times A_T/A_S \times 2$$

M_S: Amount (mg) of Saccharin RS taken, calculated on the dried basis

Operating conditions—

Detector: An ultraviolet spectrophotometer (wavelength: 230 nm).

Column: A stainless steel column 4.6 mm in inside diameter and 15 cm in length, packed with octadecylsilanized silica gel for liquid chromatography (3.5 μm in particle diameter).

Column temperature: A constant temperature of about 20°C.

Mobile phase A: Dissolve 8.7 g of dipotassium hydrogen phosphate in diluted phosphoric acid (1 in 1000) to make 1000 mL.

Mobile phase B: Methanol.

Flowing of mobile phase: Control the gradient by mixing the mobile phases A and B as directed in the following table.

Time after injection of sample (min)	Mobile phase A (vol%)	Mobile phase B (vol%)
0 – 7.0	90	10
7.0 – 8.0	90 → 5	10 → 95
8.0 – 10.0	5	95
10.0 – 10.1	5 → 90	95 → 10
10.1 – 10.5	90	10

Flow rate: 1.0 mL per minute (the retention time of saccharin is about 7.3 minutes).

System suitability—

System performance: Dissolve 25 mg of phthalic anhydride in a mixture of water and methanol (1:1) to make 25 mL. To 5 mL of this solution add 5 mL of the standard stock solution and a mixture of water and methanol (1:1) to make 50 mL. When the procedure is run with 10 μL of this solution under the above operating conditions, phthalic anhydride and saccharin are eluted in this order with the resolution between these peaks being not less than 1.5. When the procedure is run with 10 μL of the standard solution under the above operating conditions, the symmetry factor of the peak of saccharin is not more than 1.5.

System repeatability: When the test is repeated 5 times with 10 μL of the standard solution under the above operating conditions, the relative standard deviation of the peak area of saccharin is not more than 0.73%.

Containers and storage Containers—Well-closed containers.

Saccharin Sodium Hydrate

サッカリンナトリウム水和物

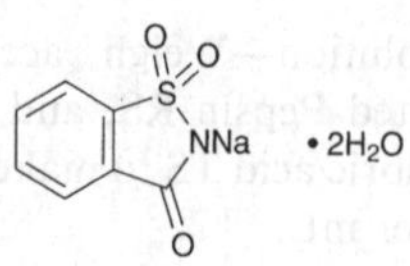

$C_7H_4NNaO_3S.2H_2O$: 241.20

2-Sodio-1,2-benzo[*d*]isothiazol-3(2*H*)-one 1,1-dioxide dihydrate

[*6155-57-3*]

Saccharin Sodium Hydrate contains not less than 98.0% and not more than 102.0% of saccharin sodium ($C_7H_4NNaO_3S$: 205.17), calculated on the anhydrous basis.

Description Saccharin Sodium Hydrate occurs as colorless crystals or a white crystalline powder.

It is freely soluble in water and in methanol, and sparingly soluble in ethanol (95).

It effloresces slowly and loses about half the amount of water of crystallization in air.

Identification **(1)** Determine the infrared absorption spectrum of Saccharin Sodium Hydrate, previously dried at 105°C to constant mass, as directed in the potassium bromide disk method under Infrared Spectrophotometry <*2.25*>, and compare the spectrum with the spectrum of Saccharin Sodium RS dried in the same manner as Saccharin Sodium Hydrate: both spectra exhibit similar intensities of absorption at the same wave numbers.

(2) A solution of Saccharin Sodium Hydrate (1 in 10) responds to Qualitative Tests <*1.09*> for sodium salt.

Purity **(1)** Clarity and color of solution—Dissolve 2.0 g of Saccharin Sodium Hydrate in water to make 10 mL, and use this solution as the test solution. Perform the test with the test solution as directed under Turbidity Measurement <*2.61*>: the solution is clear. Perform the test with the test solution according to Method 2 under Methods for Color Matching <*2.65*>: the solution is colorless.

(2) Acidity or alkalinity—Dissolve 1.0 g of Saccharin Sodium Hydrate in 10 mL of water, and add 1 drop of phenolphthalein TS: the solution is colorless. Add 1 drop of 0.1 mol/L sodium hydroxide VS to the solution: the color changes to red.

(3) Heavy metals <*1.07*>—Dissolve 2.0 g of Saccharin Sodium Hydrate in 40 mL of water, add 0.7 mL of dilute hydrochloric acid, dilute with water to make 50 mL, and rub the inner wall of the vessel with a glass rod until crystallization begins. Allow the solution to stand for 1 hour after the beginning of crystallization, and then filter through dry filter paper. Reject the first 10 mL of the filtrate, and take 25 mL of the subsequent filtrate. Add 2 mL of dilute acetic acid and water to make 50 mL, and perform the test, using this solution as the test solution. To 1.0 mL of Standard Lead Solution add 2 mL of dilute acetic acid and water to make 50 mL, and use this solution as the control solution (not more than 10 ppm).

(4) Benzoate and salicylate—Dissolve 0.5 g of Saccharin Sodium Hydrate in 10 mL of water, add 5 drops of acetic acid (31) and 3 drops of iron (III) chloride TS: no turbidity is produced, and no red-purple to purple color develops.

(5) *o*-Toluene sulfonamide—Dissolve 10 g of Saccharin Sodium Hydrate in 50 mL of water, and extract with three 30-mL portions of ethyl acetate. Combine all the ethyl acetate extracts, wash with 30 mL of a solution of sodium chloride (1 in 4), dehydrate with 5 g of anhydrous sodium sulfate, and evaporate ethyl acetate. To the residue add exactly 5 mL of the internal standard solution to dissolve, and use this solution as the sample solution. Separately, dissolve 0.10 g of *o*-toluene sulfonamide in ethyl acetate to make exactly 100 mL. Pipet 1 mL of this solution, evaporate on a water bath to dryness, dissolve the residue in exactly 5 mL of the internal standard solution, and use this solution as the standard solution. Perform the test with 1 μL each of the sample solution and standard solution as directed under Gas Chromatography <*2.02*> according to the following conditions, and calculate the ratios, Q_T and Q_S, of the peak height of *o*-toluene sulfonamide to that of the internal standard: Q_T is not more than Q_S.

Internal standard solution—A solution of caffeine in ethyl acetate (1 in 500).

Operating conditions—

Detector: A hydrogen flame-ionization detector.

Column: A glass column 3 mm in inside diameter and 1 m in length, packed with siliceous earth for gas chromatography (180 to 250 μm in diameter), coated with diethylene glycol succinate polyester for gas chromatography at the ratio of 3%.

Column temperature: A constant temperature of about 200°C.

Injection port temperature: A constant temperature of about 225°C.

Detector temperature: A constant temperature of about 250°C.

Carrier gas: Nitrogen.

Flow rate: Adjust so that the retention time of caffeine is about 6 minutes.

System suitability—

System performance: When the procedure is run with 1 μL of the standard solution under the above operating conditions, the internal standard and *o*-toluene sulfonamide are eluted in this order with the resolution between these peaks being not less than 2.0.

System repeatability: When the test is repeated 6 times with 1 μL of the standard solution under the above operating conditions, the relative standard deviation of the ratio of the peak height of *o*-toluene sulfonamide to that of the internal standard is not more than 2.0%.

(6) Readily carbonizable substances <*1.15*>—Perform the test with 0.20 g of Saccharin Sodium Hydrate. Allow the solution to stand between 48°C and 50°C for 10 minutes: the solution has no more color than Matching Fluid A.

Water <*2.48*> Not more than 15.0% (0.1 g, volumetric titration, direct titration).

Assay Weigh accurately about 50 mg of Saccharin Sodium Hydrate, and dissolve in a mixture of water and methanol (1:1) to make exactly 50 mL. Pipet 5 mL of this solution, add a mixture of water and methanol (1:1) to make exactly 50 mL, and use this solution as the sample solution. Separately, weigh accurately about 25 mg of Saccharin Sodium RS (separately determine the water <*2.48*> in the same manner as Saccharin Sodium Hydrate), dissolve in a mixture of water and methanol (1:1) to make exactly 25 mL, and use this solution as the standard stock solution. Pipet 5 mL of the standard stock solution, add a mixture of water and methanol (1:1) to make exactly 50 mL, and use this solution as the standard solution. Perform the test with exactly 10 μL each of the sample solution and standard solution as directed under Liquid Chromatography <*2.01*> according to the following conditions, and determine the peak areas, A_T and A_S, of saccharin in each solution.

Amount (mg) of saccharin sodium ($C_7H_4NNaO_3S$)
$= M_S \times A_T/A_S \times 2$

M_S: Amount (mg) of Saccharin Sodium RS taken, calculated on the anhydrous basis

Operating conditions—

Detector: An ultraviolet spectrophotometer (wavelength: 230 nm).

Column: A stainless steel column 4.6 mm in inside diameter and 15 cm in length, packed with octadecylsilanized silica gel for liquid chromatography (3.5 μm in particle diameter).

Column temperature: A constant temperature of about 20°C.

Mobile phase A: Dissolve 8.7 g of dipotassium hydrogen phosphate in diluted phosphoric acid (1 in 1000) to make 1000 mL.

Mobile phase B: Methanol.

Flowing of mobile phase: Control the gradient by mixing the mobile phases A and B as directed in the following table.

Time after injection of sample (min)	Mobile phase A (vol%)	Mobile phase B (vol%)
0 – 7.0	90	10
7.0 – 8.0	90 → 5	10 → 95
8.0 – 10.0	5	95
10.0 – 10.1	5 → 90	95 → 10
10.1 – 10.5	90	10

Flow rate: 1.0 mL per minute (the retention time of saccharin is about 7.3 minutes).

System suitability—

System performance: Dissolve 25 mg of phthalic anhydride in a mixture of water and methanol (1:1) to make 25 mL. To 5 mL of this solution add 5 mL of the standard stock solution and a mixture of water and methanol (1:1) to make 50 mL. When the procedure is run with 10 μL of this solution under the above operating conditions, phthalic anhydride and saccharin are eluted in this order with the resolution between these peaks being not less than 1.5. When the procedure is run with 10 μL of the standard solution under the above operating conditions, the symmetry factor of the peak of saccharin is not more than 1.5.

System repeatability: When the test is repeated 5 times

with 10 μL of the standard solution under the above operating conditions, the relative standard deviation of the peak area of saccharin is not more than 0.73%.

Containers and storage Containers—Well-closed containers.

Salazosulfapyridine

Sulfasalazine

サラゾスルファピリジン

$C_{18}H_{14}N_4O_5S$: 398.39
2-Hydroxy-5-[4-(pyridin-2-ylsulfamoyl)phenylazo]benzoic acid
[599-79-1]

Salazosulfapyridine, when dried, contains not less than 96.0% of salazosulfapyridine ($C_{18}H_{14}N_4O_5S$).

Description Salazosulfapyridine occurs as a yellow to yellow-brown fine powder. It is odorless and tasteless.

It is sparingly soluble in pyridine, slightly soluble in ethanol (95), practically insoluble in water, in chloroform and in diethyl ether.

It dissolves in sodium hydroxide TS.

Melting point: 240 – 249°C (with decomposition).

Identification **(1)** Dissolve 0.1 g of Salazosulfapyridine in 20 mL of dilute sodium hydroxide TS: a red-brown color develops. This color gradually fades upon gradual addition of 0.5 g of sodium hydrosulfite with shaking. Use this solution in the following tests (2) to (4).

(2) To 1 mL of the solution obtained in (1) add 40 mL of water, neutralize with 0.1 mol/L hydrochloric acid TS, and add water to make 50 mL. To 5 mL of this solution add 2 to 3 drops of dilute iron (III) chloride TS: a red color develops and changes to purple, then fades when dilute hydrochloric acid is added dropwise.

(3) The solution obtained in (1) responds to Qualitative Tests <*1.09*> for primary aromatic amines.

(4) To 1 mL of the solution obtained in (1) add 1 mL of pyridine and 2 drops of copper (II) sulfate TS, and shake. Add 3 mL of water and 5 mL of chloroform, shake, and allow to stand: a green color develops in the chloroform layer.

(5) Determine the absorption spectrum of a solution of Salazosulfapyridine in dilute sodium hydroxide TS (1 in 100,000) as directed under Ultraviolet-visible Spectrophotometry <*2.24*>, and compare the spectrum with the Reference Spectrum: both spectra exhibit similar intensities of absorption at the same wavelengths.

Purity **(1)** Chloride <*1.03*>—Dissolve 2.0 g of Salazosulfapyridine in 12 mL of sodium hydroxide TS and 36 mL of water, add 2 mL of nitric acid, shake, and filter. To 25 mL of the filtrate add 6 mL of dilute nitric acid and water to make 50 mL, and perform the test using this solution as the test solution. Prepare the control solution with 0.40 mL of 0.01 mol/L hydrochloric acid VS (not more than 0.014%).

(2) Sulfate <*1.14*>—Dissolve 2.0 g of Salazosulfapyridine in 12 mL of sodium hydroxide TS and 36 mL of water, add 2 mL of hydrochloric acid, shake, and filter. To 25 mL of the filtrate add 1 mL of dilute hydrochloric acid and water to make 50 mL, and perform the test using this solution as the test solution. Prepare the control solution with 1.0 mL of 0.005 mol/L sulfuric acid VS (not more than 0.048%).

(3) Heavy metals <*1.07*>—Proceed with 1.0 g of Salazosulfapyridine according to Method 2, and perform the test. Prepare the control solution with 2.0 mL of Standard Lead Solution (not more than 20 ppm).

(4) Arsenic <*1.11*>—Take 1.0 g of Salazosulfapyridine in a decomposition flask, add 20 mL of nitric acid, and heat gently until it becomes fluid. After cooling, add 5 mL of sulfuric acid, and heat until white fumes are evolved. Add, if necessary, 5 mL of nitric acid after cooling, and heat again. Repeat this operation until the solution becomes colorless to slightly yellow. After cooling, add 15 mL of a saturated solution of ammonium oxalate monohydrate, and heat until white fumes are evolved again. After cooling, add water to make 25 mL. Perform the test with 5 mL of this solution as the test solution: the color of the test solution is not deeper than that of the following color standard.

Color standard: Proceed in the same manner without Salazosulfapyridine, transfer 5 mL of the obtained solution to a generator bottle, add exactly 2 mL of Standard Arsenic Solution, and proceed in the same manner as the test solution with this solution (not more than 10 ppm).

(5) Related substances—Dissolve 0.20 g of Salazosulfapyridine in 20 mL of pyridine, and use this solution as the sample solution. Pipet 1 mL of the sample solution, add pyridine to make exactly 100 mL, and use this solution as the standard solution. Perform the test with these solutions as directed under Thin-layer Chromatography <*2.03*>. Spot 10 μL each of the sample solution and standard solution on a plate of silica gel with fluorescent indicator for thin-layer chromatography. Develop the plate with diluted methanol (9 in 10) to a distance of about 10 cm, and air-dry the plate. Examine the plate under ultraviolet light (main wavelength: 254 nm): the spots other than the principal spot obtained from the sample solution are not more intense than the spot from the standard solution.

(6) Salicylic acid—To 0.10 g of Salazosulfapyridine add 15 mL of diethyl ether, and shake vigorously. Add 5 mL of dilute hydrochloric acid, shake vigorously for 3 minutes, collect the diethyl ether layer, and filter. To the water layer add 15 mL of diethyl ether, shake vigorously for 3 minutes, collect the diethyl ether layer, filter, and combine the filtrates. Wash the residue on the filter paper with a small quantity of diethyl ether, and combine the washings and the filtrate. Evaporate the diethyl ether with the aid of air-stream at room temperature. To the residue add dilute ammonium iron (III) sulfate TS, shake, and filter, if necessary. Wash the residue on the filter paper with a small quantity of dilute ammonium iron (III) sulfate TS, combine the washings and the filtrate, add dilute ammonium iron (III) sulfate TS to make exactly 20 mL, and use this solution as the sample solution. Separately, weigh accurately about 10 mg of salicylic acid for assay, previously dried in a desiccator (silica gel) for 3 hours, dissolve in dilute ammonium iron (III) sulfate TS to make exactly 400 mL, and use this solution as the standard solution. Determine the absorbances, A_T and A_S, at 535 nm of the sample solution and standard solution as directed under Ultraviolet-visible Spectrophotometry <*2.24*>: salicylic acid content is not more than 0.5%.

$$\text{Content (\%) of salicylic acid } (C_7H_6O_3) = M_S \times A_T/A_S \times 1/20$$

M_S: Amount (mg) of salicylic acid for assay taken

Loss on drying <2.41> Not more than 2.0% (1 g, 105°C, 4 hours).

Residue on ignition <2.44> Not more than 0.2% (1 g).

Assay Weigh accurately about 20 mg of Salazosulfapyridine, previously dried, and perform the test as directed in the procedure of determination for sulfur under Oxygen Flask Combustion Method <1.06>, using 10 mL of diluted hydrogen peroxide (30) (1 in 40) as an absorbing liquid.

Each mL of 0.005 mol/L barium perchlorate VS
= 1.992 mg of $C_{18}H_{14}N_4O_5S$

Containers and storage Containers—Tight containers.

Storage—Light-resistant.

Salbutamol Sulfate

サルブタモール硫酸塩

$(C_{13}H_{21}NO_3)_2.H_2SO_4$: 576.70
(1*RS*)-2-(1,1-Dimethylethyl)amino-1-(4-hydroxy-3-hydroxymethylphenyl)ethanol hemisulfate
[*51022-70-9*]

Salbutamol Sulfate, when dried, contains not less than 98.0% of salbutamol sulfate [$(C_{13}H_{21}NO_3)_2.H_2SO_4$].

Description Salbutamol Sulfate occurs as a white powder.

It is freely soluble in water, slightly soluble in ethanol (95), and in acetic acid (100) and practically insoluble in diethyl ether.

A solution of Salbutamol Sulfate (1 in 20) shows no optical rotation.

Identification **(1)** Determine the absorption spectrum of a solution of Salbutamol Sulfate in 0.1 mol/L hydrochloric acid TS (1 in 12,500) as directed under Ultraviolet-visible Spectrophotometry <2.24>, and compare the spectrum with the Reference Spectrum: both spectra exhibit similar intensities of absorption at the same wavelengths.

(2) Determine the infrared absorption spectrum of Salbutamol Sulfate, previously dried, as directed in the potassium bromide disk method under Infrared Spectrophotometry <2.25>, and compare the spectrum with the Reference Spectrum: both spectra exhibit similar intensities of absorption at the same wave numbers.

(3) A solution of Salbutamol Sulfate (1 in 20) responds to Qualitative Tests <1.09> for sulfate.

Purity **(1)** Clarity and color of solution—Dissolve 1.0 g of Salbutamol Sulfate in 20 mL of water: the solution is clear and colorless.

(2) Heavy metals <1.07>—Proceed with 1.0 g of Salbutamol Sulfate according to Method 1, and perform the test. Prepare the control solution with 2.0 mL of Standard Lead Solution (not more than 20 ppm).

(3) Related substances—Dissolve 20 mg of Salbutamol Sulfate in 10 mL of water, and use this solution as the sample solution. Pipet 1 mL of the sample solution, add water to make exactly 100 mL, and use this solution as the standard solution. Perform the test with these solutions as directed under Thin-layer Chromatography <2.03>. Spot 5 μL each of the sample solution and standard solution on a plate of silica gel for thin-layer chromatography. Develop the plate with a mixture of ethyl acetate, 2-propanol, water and ammonia solution (28) (25:15:8:2) to a distance of about 15 cm, and air-dry the plate. Leave the plate in a well-closed vessel saturated with diethylamine vapor for 5 minutes, and spray evenly 4-nitrobenzenediazonium chloride TS: the spots other than the principal spot obtained from the sample solution are not more intense than the spot from the standard solution in color.

(4) Boron—Take 50 mg of Salbutamol Sulfate and 5.0 mL of the Standard Boron Solution, and transfer to a platinum crucible. Add 5 mL of potassium carbonate-sodium carbonate TS, evaporate on a water bath to dryness, and dry at 120°C for 1 hour. Ignite the residue immediately. After cooling, add 0.5 mL of water and 3 mL of curcumin TS to the residue, warm gently in a water bath for 5 minutes. After cooling, add 3 mL of acetic acid-sulfuric acid TS, mix, and allow to stand for 30 minutes. Add ethanol (95) to make exactly 100 mL, and filter. Discard the first 10 mL of the filtrate, and use the subsequent filtrate as the sample solution and standard solution. Perform the test with these solutions as directed under Ultraviolet-visible Spectrophotometry <2.24>, using ethanol (95) as the blank: the absorbance of the sample solution at 555 nm is not larger than that of the standard solution.

Loss on drying <2.41> Not more than 0.5% (1 g, in vacuum at a pressure not exceeding 0.67 kPa, 100°C, 3 hours).

Residue on ignition <2.44> Not more than 0.1% (1 g).

Assay Weigh accurately about 0.9 g of Salbutamol Sulfate, previously dried, and dissolve in 50 mL of acetic acid (100) by warming. After cooling, titrate <2.50> with 0.1 mol/L perchloric acid VS until the color of the solution changes from purple through blue to blue-green (indicator: 3 drops of crystal violet TS). Perform a blank determination in the same manner, and make any necessary correction.

Each mL of 0.1 mol/L perchloric acid VS
= 57.67 mg of $(C_{13}H_{21}NO_3)_2.H_2SO_4$

Containers and storage Containers—Tight containers.

Salicylic Acid

サリチル酸

$C_7H_6O_3$: 138.12
2-Hydroxybenzoic acid
[*69-72-7*]

Salicylic Acid, when dried, contains not less than 99.5% and not more than 101.0% of salicylic acid ($C_7H_6O_3$).

Description Salicylic Acid occurs as white, crystals or crystalline powder. It has a slightly acid, followed by an acrid taste.

It is freely soluble in ethanol (95) and in acetone, and slightly soluble in water.

Identification **(1)** A solution of Salicylic Acid (1 in 500) responds to Qualitative Tests <*1.09*> (1) and (3) for salicylate.

(2) Determine the absorption spectrum of a solution of Salicylic Acid in ethanol (95) (3 in 200,000) as directed under Ultraviolet-visible Spectrophotometry <*2.24*>, and compare the spectrum with the Reference Spectrum: both spectra exhibit similar intensities of absorption at the same wavelengths.

(3) Determine the infrared absorption spectrum of Salicylic Acid as directed in the potassium bromide disk method under Infrared Spectrophotometry <*2.25*>, and compare the spectrum with the Reference Spectrum: both spectra exhibit similar intensities of absorption at the same wave numbers.

Melting point <*2.60*> 158 – 161°C

Purity **(1)** Chloride <*1.03*>—Dissolve 5.0 g of Salicylic Acid in 90 mL of water by heating, cool, dilute with water to 100 mL, and filter. Discard the first 20 mL of the filtrate, take 30 mL of the subsequent filtrate, add 6 mL of dilute nitric acid and water to make 50 mL, and perform the test using this solution as the test solution. Prepare the control solution with 0.35 mL of 0.01 mol/L hydrochloric acid VS (not more than 0.008%).

(2) Sulfate <*1.14*>—To 20 mL of the filtrate obtained in (1) add 1 mL of dilute hydrochloric acid and water to make 50 mL, and perform the test using this solution as the test solution. Prepare the control solution with 0.40 mL of 0.005 mol/L sulfuric acid VS (not more than 0.019%).

(3) Heavy metals <*1.07*>—Dissolve 2.0 g of Salicylic Acid in 25 mL of acetone, add 4 mL of sodium hydroxide TS, 2 mL of dilute acetic acid and water to make 50 mL, and perform the test using this solution as the test solution. Prepare the control solution as follows: to 2.0 mL of Standard Lead Solution add 25 mL of acetone, 2 mL of dilute acetic acid and water to make 50 mL (not more than 10 ppm).

(4) Related substances—Dissolve 0.50 g of Salicylic Acid in the mobile phase to make exactly 100 mL, and use this solution as the sample solution. Separately, dissolve exactly 10 mg of phenol, exactly 25 mg of 4-hydroxyisophthalic acid and exactly 50 mg of parahydroxybenzoic acid in the mobile phase to make exactly 100 mL. Pipet 1 mL of this solution, add the mobile phase to make exactly 100 mL, and use this solution as the standard solution. Perform the test with exactly 10 μL each of the sample solution and standard solution as directed under Liquid Chromatography <*2.01*> according to the following conditions, and determine each peak area by the automatic integration method: the peak areas of parahydroxybenzoic acid, 4-hydroxyisophthalic acid and phenol obtained from the sample solution are not larger than the area of each respective peak from the standard solution, the area of the peak other than salicylic acid and the substances mentioned above is not larger than the peak area of 4-hydroxisophthalic acid from the standard solution, and the total area of peaks other than salicylic acid is not larger than 2 times the peak area of parahydroxybenzoic acid from the standard solution.

Operating conditions—

Detector: An ultraviolet absorption photometer (wavelength: 270 nm).

Column: A stainless steel column 4.6 mm in inside diameter and 15 cm in length, packed with octadecylsilanized silica gel for liquid chromatography (5 μm in particle diameter).

Column temperature: A constant temperature of about 35°C.

Mobile phase: A mixture of water, methanol and acetic acid (100) (60:40:1).

Flow rate: Adjust so that the retention time of salicylic acid is about 17 minutes.

Time span of measurement: About 2 times as long as the retention time of salicylic acid, beginning after the solvent peak.

System suitability—

Test for required detectability: Pipet 2 mL of the standard solution, and add the mobile phase to make exactly 10 mL. Confirm that the peak areas of parahydroxybenzoic acid, 4-hydroxyisophthalic acid and phenol obtained with 10 μL of this solution are equivalent to 14 to 26% of the area of each respective peak with 10 μL of the standard solution.

System performance: Dissolve 10 mg of phenol, 25 mg of 4-hydroxyisophthalic acid and 50 mg of parahydroxybenzoic acid in 100 mL of the mobile phase. To 1 mL of this solution add the mobile phase to make 10 mL. When the procedure is run with 10 μL of this solution under the above operating conditions, parahydroxybenzoic acid, 4-hydroxyisophthalic acid and phenol are eluted in this order with the resolution between the peaks of 4-hydroxyisophthalic acid and phenol being not less than 4.

System repeatability: When the test is repeated 6 times with 10 μL of the standard solution under the above operating conditions, the relative standard deviation of the peak areas of parahydroxybenzoic acid, 4-hydroxyisophthalic acid and phenol is not more than 2.0%, respectively.

Loss on drying <*2.41*> Not more than 0.5% (2 g, silica gel, 3 hours).

Residue on ignition <*2.44*> Not more than 0.1% (1 g).

Assay Weigh accurately about 0.5 g of Salicylic Acid, previously dried, dissolve in 25 mL of neutralized ethanol, and titrate <*2.50*> with 0.1 mol/L sodium hydroxide VS (indicator: 3 drops of phenolphthalein TS).

Each mL of 0.1 mol/L sodium hydroxide VS
= 13.81 mg of $C_7H_6O_3$

Containers and storage Containers—Well-closed containers.

Salicylic Acid Adhesive Plaster

サリチル酸絆創膏

Method of preparation

Salicylic Acid, finely powdered	500 g
Adhesive plaster base	a sufficient quantity
To make	1000 g

Adhesive Plaster consists of a mixture of the above ingredients with carefully selected rubber, resins, zinc oxide and other substances. It has adhesive properties. It spreads evenly on a fabric.

Description The surface of Salicylic Acid Adhesive Plaster is whitish in color and adheres well to the skin.

Containers and storage Containers—Well-closed containers.

Storage—Light-resistant.

Salicylic Acid Spirit

サリチル酸精

Salicylic Acid Spirit contains not less than 2.7 w/v% and not more than 3.3 w/v% of salicylic acid ($C_7H_6O_3$: 138.12).

Method of preparation

Salicylic Acid	30 g
Glycerin	50 mL
Ethanol	a sufficient quantity
To make	1000 mL

Prepare as directed under Spirits, with the above ingredients.

Description Salicylic Acid Spirit is a clear, colorless liquid.

Specific gravity d_{20}^{20}: about 0.86

Identification The solution obtained in the Assay has a red-purple color. Determine the absorption spectrum of the solution as directed under Ultraviolet-visible Spectrophotometry <*2.24*>: it exhibits a maximum between 520 nm and 535 nm (salicylic acid).

Alcohol number <*1.01*> Not less than 8.8 (Method 2).

Assay Measure exactly 10 mL of Salicylic Acid Spirit, add 10 mL of ethanol (95) and water to make exactly 100 mL. Pipet 3 mL of this solution, and dilute with hydrochloric acid-potassium chloride buffer solution (pH 2.0) to make exactly 100 mL. Use this solution as the sample solution. Dissolve about 0.3 g of salicylic acid for assay, previously dried in a desiccator (silica gel) for 3 hours and accurately weighed, in 10 mL of ethanol (95) and water to make exactly 100 mL. Pipet 3 mL of this solution, dilute with hydrochloric acid-potassium chloride buffer solution (pH 2.0) to make exactly 100 mL, and use this solution as the standard solution. Pipet 10 mL each of the sample solution and standard solution, to each add exactly 5 mL of a solution of iron (III) nitrate enneahydrate (1 in 200), dilute with hydrochloric acid-potassium chloride buffer solution (pH 2.0) to exactly 25 mL. Determine the absorbances, A_T and A_S, of both solutions at 530 nm as directed under Ultraviolet-visible Spectrophotometry <*2.24*>, using a blank solution prepared in the same manner with water.

$$\text{Amount (mg) of salicylic acid } (C_7H_6O_3) = M_S \times A_T/A_S$$

M_S: Amount (mg) of salicylic acid for assay taken

Containers and storage Containers—Tight containers.

Compound Salicylic Acid Spirit

複方サリチル酸精

Compound Salicylic Acid Spirit contains not less than 1.8 w/v% and not more than 2.2 w/v% of salicylic acid ($C_7H_6O_3$: 138.12), and not less than 0.43 w/v% and not more than 0.53 w/v% of phenol (C_6H_6O: 94.11).

Method of preparation

Salicylic Acid	20 g
Liquefied Phenol	5 mL
Glycerin	40 mL
Ethanol	800 mL
Water, Purified Water or Purified Water in Containers	a sufficient quantity
To make	1000 mL

Prepare as directed under Spirits, with the above ingredients.

Description Compound Salicylic Acid Spirit is a clear, colorless to light red liquid.

Specific gravity d_{20}^{20}: about 0.88

Identification **(1)** To 1 mL of Compound Salicylic Acid Spirit add hydrochloric acid-potassium chloride buffer solution (pH 2.0) to make 200 mL, and to 5 mL of this solution add 5 mL of a solution of iron (III) nitrate enneahydrate (1 in 200): a red-purple color is produced (salicylic acid).

(2) To 1 mL of Compound Salicylic Acid Spirit add 20 mL of water and 5 mL of dilute hydrochloric acid, and extract with 20 mL of diethyl ether. Wash the diethyl ether extract with two 5-mL portions of sodium hydrogen carbonate TS, and extract with 10 mL of dilute sodium hydroxide TS. Shake 1 mL of the extract with 1 mL of sodium nitrite TS and 1 mL of dilute hydrochloric acid, allow to stand for 10 minutes, and add 3 mL of sodium hydroxide TS: a yellow color is produced (phenol).

(3) To 0.5 mL of Compound Salicylic Acid Spirit add 5 mL of dilute hydrochloric acid, extract with 5 mL of chloroform, and use the extract as the sample solution (1). To 2 mL of Compound Salicylic Acid Spirit add 5 mL of dilute hydrochloric acid, extract with 5 mL of chloroform, wash the extract with two 5-mL portions of sodium hydrogen carbonate TS, and use the chloroform extract as the sample solution (2). Separately, dissolve 0.01 g each of salicylic acid and phenol in 5 mL each of chloroform, and use both solutions as the standard solutions (1) and (2). Perform the test with these solutions as directed under Thin-layer Chromatography <*2.03*>. Spot 5 μL each of the sample solutions (1) and (2) and the standard solutions (1) and (2) on a plate of silica gel with fluorescent indicator for thin-layer chromatography. Develop the plate with a mixture of chloroform, acetone and acetic acid (100) (45:5:1) to a distance of about 10 cm, and air-dry the plate. Examine under ultraviolet light (main wavelength: 254 nm): the spots obtained from the sample solution (1) and standard solution (1) show the same *R*f value, and the spots from the sample solution (2) and the standard solution (2) show the same *R*f value. Spray evenly iron (III) chloride TS upon the plate: the spot from the standard solution (1) and the corresponding spot from the sample solution (1) reveal a purple color.

Alcohol number <*1.01*> Not less than 7.5 (Method 2).

Assay Measure accurately 2 mL of Compound Salicylic Acid Spirit, add exactly 5 mL of the internal standard solution and diluted methanol (1 in 2) to make 100 mL, and use this solution as the sample solution. Weigh accurately about 0.2 g of salicylic acid for assay, previously dried in a desiccator (silica gel) for 3 hours, and about 50 mg of phenol for assay, dissolve in diluted methanol (1 in 2) to make exactly 100 mL. Pipet 20 mL of this solution, add exactly 5 mL of the internal standard solution and diluted methanol (1 in 2) to make 100 mL, and use this solution as the standard solution. Perform the test with 15 μL each of the sample solution and standard solution as directed under Liquid Chromatography <*2.01*> according to the following conditions, and calculate the ratios, Q_{Ta} and Q_{Tb}, of the peak area of salicylic acid and phenol to that of the internal standard in the sample solution, and the ratios, Q_{Sa} and Q_{Sb}, of the peak area of salicylic acid and phenol to that of the internal standard in the standard solution.

Amount (mg) of salicylic acid ($C_7H_6O_3$)
$= M_{Sa} \times Q_{Ta}/Q_{Sa} \times 1/5$

Amount (mg) of phenol (C_6H_6O)
$= M_{Sb} \times Q_{Tb}/Q_{Sb} \times 1/5$

M_{Sa}: Amount (mg) of salicylic acid for assay taken
M_{Sb}: Amount (mg) of phenol for assay taken

Internal standard solution—A solution of theophylline in methanol (1 in 1250).

Operating conditions—

Detector: An ultraviolet absorption photometer (wavelength: 270 nm).

Column: A stainless steel column about 4 mm in inside diameter and 25 to 30 cm in length, packed with octadecylsilanized silica gel for liquid chromatography (5 μm in particle diameter).

Column temperature: Room temperature.

Mobile phase: A mixture of 0.1 mol/L phosphate buffer solution (pH 7.0) and methanol (3:1).

Flow rate: Adjust so that the retention time of salicylic acid is about 6 minutes.

Selection of column: Dissolve 0.2 g of benzoic acid, 0.2 g of salicylic acid and 0.05 g of theophylline in 100 mL of diluted methanol (1 in 2). To 10 mL of this solution add 90 mL of diluted methanol (1 in 2). Proceed with 10 μL of this solution under the above operating conditions. Use a column giving elution of benzoic acid, salicylic acid and theophylline in this order, and clearly dividing each peak.

Containers and storage Containers—Tight containers.

Salicylated Alum Powder

サリチル・ミョウバン散

Salicylated Alum Powder contains not less than 2.7% and not more than 3.3% of salicylic acid ($C_7H_6O_3$: 138.12).

Method of preparation

Salicylic Acid, finely powdered	30 g
Dried Aluminum Potassium Sulfate, very finely powdered	640 g
Talc, very finely powdered	a sufficient quantity
To make	1000 g

Prepare as directed under Powders, with the above ingredients.

Description Salicylated Alum Powder occurs as a white powder.

Identification **(1)** The colored solution obtained in the Assay has a red-purple color. Determine the absorption spectrum of the solution as directed under Ultraviolet-visible Spectrophotometry <*2.24*>: it exhibits a maximum between 520 nm and 535 nm (salicylic acid).

(2) Shake 0.3 g of Salicylated Alum Powder with 5 mL of methanol, filter, and use the filtrate as the sample solution. Separately, dissolve 0.01 g of salicylic acid in 5 mL of methanol, and use this solution as the standard solution. Perform the test with these solutions as directed under Thin-layer Chromatography <*2.03*>. Spot 5 μL each of the sample solution and standard solution on the plate of silica gel with fluorescent indicator for thin-layer chromatography. Develop the plate with a mixture of chloroform, acetone and acetic acid (100) (45:5:1) to a distance of about 10 cm, and air-dry the plate. Examine the plate under ultraviolet light (main wavelength: 254 nm): the spot obtained from the sample solution and that from the standard solution show the same *R*f value. Spray evenly iron (III) chloride TS upon the plate: the spot from the standard solution and the corresponding spot from the sample solution reveal a purple color.

Assay Weigh accurately about 0.33 g of Salicylated Alum Powder, add 80 mL of ethanol (95), and shake vigorously. Dilute with ethanol (95) to make exactly 100 mL, filter, and discard the first 10 mL of the filtrate. Use the subsequent filtrate as the sample solution. Dissolve about 0.1 g of salicylic acid for assay, previously dried in a desiccator (silica gel) for 3 hours and accurately weighed, in sufficient ethanol (95) to make exactly 100 mL. Pipet 10 mL of this solution, dilute with ethanol (95) to make exactly 100 mL, and use the solution as the standard solution. Pipet 10 mL each of the sample solution and standard solution, to each add exactly 5 mL of a solution of iron (III) nitrate enneahydrate (1 in 200), and dilute with hydrochloric acid-potassium chloride buffer solution (pH 2.0) to make exactly 25 mL. Determine the absorbances, A_T and A_S, of both solutions at 530 nm as directed under Ultraviolet-visible Spectrophotometry <*2.24*>, using a solution prepared in the same manner with 10 mL of ethanol (95) as the blank.

Amount (mg) of salicylic acid ($C_7H_6O_3$)
$= M_S \times A_T/A_S \times 1/10$

M_S: Amount (mg) of salicylic acid for assay taken

Containers and storage Containers—Well-closed contain-

ers.

Santonin

サントニン

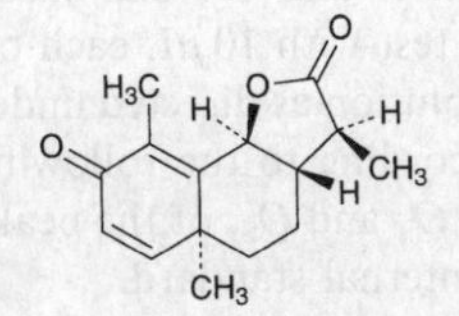

$C_{15}H_{18}O_3$: 246.30
(3*S*,3a*S*,5a*S*,9b*S*)-3,5a,9-Trimethyl-3a,5,5a,9b-tetrahydronaphtho[1,2-*b*]furan-2,8(3*H*,4*H*)-dione
[*481-06-1*]

Santonin, when dried, contains not less than 98.5% and not more than 101.0% of santonin ($C_{15}H_{18}O_3$).

Description Santonin occurs as colorless crystals, or a white crystalline powder.

It is freely soluble in chloroform, sparingly soluble in ethanol (95), and practically insoluble in water.

It becomes yellow by light.

Identification **(1)** Determine the absorption spectrum of a solution of Santonin in ethanol (95) (3 in 250,000) as directed under Ultraviolet-visible Spectrophotometry *<2.24>*, and compare the spectrum with the Reference Spectrum: both spectra exhibit similar intensities of absorption at the same wavelengths.

(2) Determine the infrared absorption spectrum of Santonin as directed in the potassium bromide disk method under Infrared Spectrophotometry *<2.25>*, and compare the spectrum with the Reference Spectrum: both spectra exhibit similar intensities of absorption at the same wave numbers.

Optical rotation *<2.49>* $[\alpha]_D^{20}$: −170 – −175° (0.2 g, chloroform, 10 mL, 100 mm).

Melting point *<2.60>* 172 – 175°C

Purity **(1)** Heavy metals *<1.07>*—Proceed with 1.0 g of Santonin according to Method 4, and perform the test. Prepare the control solution with 2.0 mL of Standard Lead Solution (not more than 20 ppm).

(2) Alkaloids—Boil 0.5 g of Santonin with 20 mL of diluted sulfuric acid (1 in 100), cool, and filter. Dilute 10 mL of the filtrate with water to 30 mL, add 3 drops of iodine TS, and allow to stand for 3 hours: no turbidity is produced.

(3) Artemisin—Dissolve 1.0 g of powdered Santonin in 2 mL of chloroform by slight warming: the solution is clear and colorless, or any yellow color produced is not darker than Matching Fluid A.

(4) Phenols—Boil 0.20 g of Santonin with 10 mL of water, cool, and filter. To the filtrate add bromine TS until the color of the solution becomes yellow: no turbidity is produced.

(5) Acid-coloring substances—Moisten 10 mg of Santonin with nitric acid: no color develops immediately. Moisten Santonin with sulfuric acid, previously cooled to 0°C: no color is produced immediately.

Loss on drying *<2.41>* Not more than 0.5% (1 g, 105°C, 3 hours).

Residue on ignition *<2.44>* Not more than 0.2% (1 g).

Assay Weigh accurately about 0.25 g of Santonin, previously dried, dissolve in 10 mL of ethanol (95) by warming, add exactly 20 mL of 0.1 mol/L sodium hydroxide VS, and heat on a water bath under a reflux condenser for 5 minutes. Cool quickly, and titrate *<2.50>* the excess sodium hydroxide with 0.05 mol/L hydrochloric acid VS (indicator: 3 drops of phenolphthalein TS). Perform a blank determination in the same manner.

Each mL of 0.1 mol/L sodium hydroxide VS
= 24.63 mg of $C_{15}H_{18}O_3$

Containers and storage Containers—Tight containers.
Storage—Light-resistant.

Sarpogrelate Hydrochloride

サルポグレラート塩酸塩

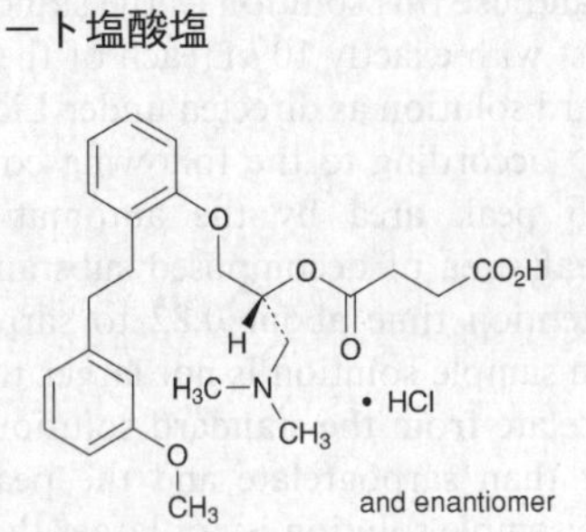

$C_{24}H_{31}NO_6.HCl$: 465.97
(2*RS*)-1-Dimethylamino-3-{2-[2-(3-methoxyphenyl)ethyl]phenoxy}propan-2-yl hydrogen succinate monohydrochloride
[*135159-51-2*]

Sarpogrelate Hydrochloride contains not less than 98.5% and not more than 101.0% of sarpogrelate hydrochloride ($C_{24}H_{31}NO_6.HCl$), calculated on the anhydrous basis.

Description Sarpogrelate Hydrochloride occurs as a white crystalline powder.

It is slightly soluble in water and in ethanol (99.5).

It dissolves in 0.01 mol/L hydrochloric acid TS.

A solution of Sarpogrelate Hydrochloride (1 in 100) shows no optical rotation.

Sarpogrelate Hydrochloride shows crystal polymorphism.

Identification **(1)** Determine the absorption spectrum of a solution of Sarpogrelate Hydrochloride in 0.01 mol/L hydrochloric acid TS (1 in 20,000) as directed under Ultraviolet-visible Spectrophotometry *<2.24>*, and compare the spectrum with the Reference Spectrum or the spectrum of a solution of Sarpogrelate Hydrochloride RS prepared in the same manner as the sample solution: both spectra exhibit similar intensities of absorption at the same wavelengths.

(2) Determine the infrared absorption spectrum of Sarpogrelate Hydrochloride as directed in the potassium chloride disk method under Infrared Spectrophotometry *<2.25>*, and compare the spectrum with the Reference Spectrum or the spectrum of Sarpogrelate Hydrochloride RS: both spectra exhibit similar intensities of absorption at the same wave numbers. If any difference appears between the spectra, recrystallize the Sarpogrelate Hydrochloride, or the Sarpogrelate Hydrochloride and the Sarpogrelate Hydrochloride RS separately with acetone by heating and suspending, filter and dry the crystals at 50°C for 1 hour, and perform the test with the crystals.

(3) Dissolve 0.3 g of Sarpogrelate Hydrochloride in 6 mL of sodium hydroxide TS, shake well, allow to stand for 10 minutes, and filter. To 1 mL of the filtrate add 1 mL of dilute nitric acid. This solution responds to Qualitative Tests <*1.09*> for chloride.

Purity **(1)** Heavy metals <*1.07*>—Proceed with 2.0 g of Sarpogrelate Hydrochloride according to Method 4, and perform the test. Prepare the control solution with 2.0 mL of Standard Lead Solution (not more than 10 ppm).

(2) Arsenic <*1.11*>—Prepare the test solution with 2.0 g of Sarpogrelate Hydrochloride according to Method 4, and perform the test (not more than 1 ppm).

(3) Related substances—Conduct this procedure within 3 hours after preparation of the sample solution. Dissolve 20 mg of Sarpogrelate Hydrochloride in 10 mL of the mobile phase, and use this solution as the sample solution. Pipet 2 mL of the sample solution, add the mobile phase to make exactly 200 mL, and use this solution as the standard solution. Perform the test with exactly 10 μL each of the sample solution and standard solution as directed under Liquid Chromatography <*2.01*> according to the following conditions, and determine each peak area by the automatic integration method: the peak area of decomposed substance A, having the relative retention time about 0.82 to sarpogrelate, obtained from the sample solution is not larger than 1/5 times that of sarpogrelate from the standard solution, the area of the peak other than sarpogrelate and the peak mentioned above from the sample solution is not larger than 1/10 times the peak area of sarpogrelate from the standard solution, and the total area of the peaks other than sarpogrelate from the sample solution is not larger than 1/2 times the peak area of sarpogrelate from the standard solution. For the peak area of the decomposed substance A, multiply the correction factor, 0.78.

Operating conditions—

Detector, column, column temperature, mobile phase, and flow rate: Proceed as directed in the operating conditions in the Assay.

Time span of measurement: About 2.5 times as long as the retention time of sarpogrelate, beginning after the solvent peak.

System suitability—

Test for required detectability: Pipet 5 mL of the standard solution, add the mobile phase to make exactly 50 mL. Confirm that the peak area of sarpogrelate obtained with 10 μL of this solution is equivalent to 7 to 13% of that with 10 μL of the standard solution.

System performance: Dissolve 50 mg of Sarpogrelate Hydrochloride in 20 mL of water, and use as the sarpogrelate hydrochloride stock solution. To 1 mL of the sarpogrelate hydrochloride stock solution add 2 mL of sodium hydroxide TS, shake thoroughly, allow to stand for 10 minutes, and add 3 mL of 1 mol/L hydrochloric acid TS. To this solution add 1 mL of the sarpogrelate hydrochloride stock solution, and add the mobile phase to make 50 mL. When the procedure is run with 10 μL of this solution under the above operating conditions, the decomposed substance A and sarpogrelate are eluted in this order with the resolution between these peaks being not less than 3.

System repeatability: When the test is repeated 6 times with 10 μL of the standard solution under the above operating conditions, the relative standard deviation of the peak area of sarpogrelate is not more than 2.0%.

Water <*2.48*> Not more than 0.5% (1 g, coulometric titration).

Residue on ignition <*2.44*> Not more than 0.1% (1 g).

Assay Weigh accurately about 50 mg each of Sarpogrelate Hydrochloride and Sarpogrelate Hydrochloride RS (separately determine the water <*2.48*> in the same manner as Sarpogrelate Hydrochloride), add to them exactly 2.5 mL of the internal standard solution, and dissolve them in the mobile phase to make 50 mL. To 5 mL each of these solutions add the mobile phase to make 50 mL, and use these solutions as the sample solution and the standard solution, respectively. Perform the test with 10 μL each of the sample solution and standard solution as directed under Liquid Chromatography <*2.01*> according to the following conditions, and calculate the ratios, Q_T and Q_S, of the peak area of sarpogrelate to that of the internal standard.

Amount (mg) of sarpogrelate hydrochloride ($C_{24}H_{31}NO_6.HCl$)
$= M_S \times Q_T/Q_S$

M_S: Amount (mg) of Sarpogrelate Hydrochloride RS taken, calculated on the anhydrous basis

Internal standard solution—A solution of isopropyl parahydroxybenzoate in the mobile phase (3 in 1000).

Operating conditions—

Detector: An ultraviolet absorption photometer (wavelength: 272 nm).

Column: A stainless steel column 4.6 mm in inside diameter and 15 cm in length, packed with octadecylsilanized silica gel for liquid chromatography (5 μm in particle diameter).

Column temperature: A constant temperature of about 40°C.

Mobile phase: A mixture of water, acetonitrile and trifluoroacetic acid (1300:700:1).

Flow rate: Adjust so that the retention time of sarpogrelate is about 8 minutes.

System suitability—

System performance: When the procedure is run with 10 μL of the standard solution under the above operating conditions, sarpogrelate and the internal standard are eluted in this order with the resolution between these peaks being not less than 3.

System repeatability: When the test is repeated 6 times with 10 μL of the standard solution under the above operating conditions, the relative standard deviation of the ratio of the peak area of sarpogrelate to that of the internal standard is not more than 1.0%.

Containers and storage Containers—Tight containers.

Sarpogrelate Hydrochloride Fine Granules

サルポグレラート塩酸塩細粒

Sarpogrelate Hydrochloride Fine Granules contain not less than 95.0% and not more than 105.0% of the labeled amount of sarpogrelate hydrochloride ($C_{24}H_{31}NO_6.HCl$: 465.97).

Method of preparation Prepare as directed under Granules, with Sarpogrelate Hydrochloride.

Identification To an amount of Sarpogrelate Hydrochloride Fine Granules, equivalent to 50 mg of Sarpogrelate Hydrochloride, add 10 mL of 0.01 mol/L hydrochloric acid TS, allow to stand at room temperature for 10 minutes, then add 0.01 mol/L hydrochloric acid TS to make 100 mL, and disperse the particles by sonicating. Centrifuge this solution, and to 5 mL of the supernatant liquid add 0.01 mol/L hydrochloric acid TS to make 50 mL. Determine the absorption spectrum of this solution as directed under Ultraviolet-visible Spectrophotometry <*2.24*>: it exhibits maxima between 269 nm and 273 nm and between 274 nm and 278 nm.

Purity Related substances—Conduct this procedure within 3 hours after preparation of the sample solution. Powder Sarpogrelate Hydrochloride Fine Granules. To a portion of the powder, equivalent to 0.10 g of Sarpogrelate Hydrochloride, add 50 mL of the mobile phase, and disperse the particles by sonicating. Filter thorough a membrane filter with a pore size not exceeding 0.45 μm, discard the first 3 mL of the filtrate, and use the subsequent filtrate as the sample solution. Pipet 2 mL of the sample solution, add the mobile phase to make exactly 200 mL, and use this solution as the standard solution. Perform the test with exactly 10 μL each of the sample solution and standard solution as directed under Liquid Chromatography <*2.01*> according to the following conditions, and determine each peak area by the automatic integration method: the peak area of decomposed substance A, having the relative retention time about 0.82 to sarpogrelate, obtained from the sample solution is not larger than 2.5 times that of sarpogrelate from the standard solution, and the area of the peak other than sarpogrelate and the peak mentioned above from the sample solution is not larger than 1/10 times the peak area of sarpogrelate from the standard solution. For the peak area of the decomposed substance A, multiply the correction factor, 0.78.

Operating conditions—

Detector, column, column temperature, mobile phase, and flow rate: Proceed as directed in the operating conditions in the Assay under Sarpogrelate Hydrochloride.

Time span of measurement: About 2.5 times as long as the retention time of sarpogrelate, beginning after the solvent peak.

System suitability—

Test for required detectability: Pipet 5 mL of the standard solution, and add the mobile phase to make exactly 50 mL. Confirm that the peak area of sarpogrelate obtained with 10 μL of this solution is equivalent to 7 to 13% of that with 10 μL of the standard solution.

System performance: Dissolve 50 mg of sarpogrelate hydrochloride in 20 mL of water, and use this solution as the sarpogrelate hydrochloride stock solution. To 1 mL of the sarpogrelate hydrochloride stock solution add 2 mL of sodium hydroxide TS, shake thoroughly, allow to stand for 10 minutes, and add 3 mL of 1 mol/L hydrochloric acid TS. To this solution add 1 mL of the sarpogrelate hydrochloride stock solution, and add the mobile phase to make 50 mL. When the procedure is run with 10 μL of this solution under the above operating conditions, the decomposed substance A and sarpogrelate are eluted in this order with the resolution between these peaks being not less than 3.

System repeatability: When the test is repeated 6 times with 10 μL of the standard solution under the above operating conditions, the relative standard deviation of the peak area of sarpogrelate is not more than 2.0%.

Uniformity of dosage units <*6.02*> Perform the test according to the following method: Sarpogrelate Hydrochloride Fine Granules in single-dose packages meet the requirement of the Content uniformity test.

To the total amount of the content of 1 package of Sarpogrelate Hydrochloride Fine Granules add exactly V/10 mL of the internal standard solution, and add 4V/5 mL of the mobile phase, disperse the particles by sonicating, then add the mobile phase to make V mL so that each mL contains about 1 mg of sarpogrelate hydrochloride ($C_{24}H_{31}NO_6$.HCl), and centrifuge. To 5 mL of the supernatant liquid add the mobile phase to make 50 mL, and use this solution as the sample solution. Then, proceed as directed in the Assay.

Amount (mg) of sarpogrelate hydrochloride ($C_{24}H_{31}NO_6$.HCl)
$= M_S \times Q_T/Q_S \times V/50$

M_S: Amount (mg) of Sarpogrelate Hydrochloride RS taken, calculated on the anhydrous basis

Internal standard solution—A solution of isopropyl parahydroxybenzoate in the mobile phase (1 in 1000).

Dissolution <*6.10*> When the test is performed at 50 revolutions per minute according to the Paddle method, using 900 mL of water as the dissolution medium, the dissolution rate in 15 minutes of Sarpogrelate Hydrochloride Fine Granules is not less than 85%.

Start the test with an accuretely weighed amount of Sarpogrelate Hydrochloride Fine Granules, equivalent to about 50 mg of sarpogrelate hydrochloride ($C_{24}H_{31}NO_6$.HCl), withdraw not less than 20 mL of the medium at the specified minute after starting the test, and filter through a membrane filter with a pore size not exceeding 0.45 μm. Discard not less than 10 mL of the first filtrate, and use the subsequent filtrate as the sample solution. Separately, weigh accurately about 25 mg of Sarpogrelate Hydrochloride RS (separately determine the water <*2.48*> in the same manner as Sarpogrelate Hydrochloride), and dissolve in water to make exactly 50 mL. Pipet 5 mL of this solution, add water to make exactly 50 mL, and use this solution as the standard solution. Determine the absorbances, A_T and A_S, of the sample solution and standard solution at 270 nm as directed under Ultraviolet-visible Spectrophotometry <*2.24*>.

Dissolution rate (%) with respect to the labeled amount of sarpogrelate hydrochloride ($C_{24}H_{31}NO_6$.HCl)
$= M_S/M_T \times A_T/A_S \times 1/C \times 180$

M_S: Amount (mg) of Sarpogrelate Hydrochloride RS taken, calculated on the anhydrous basis
M_T: Amount (g) of Sarpogrelate Hydrochloride Fine Granules taken
C: Labeled amount (mg) of sarpogrelate hydrochloride ($C_{24}H_{31}NO_6$.HCl) in 1 g

Assay Powder Sarpogrelate Hydrochloride Fine Granules. Weigh accurately a portion of the powder, equivalent to about 0.25 g of sarpogrelate hydrochloride ($C_{24}H_{31}NO_6$.HCl), add exactly 25 mL of the internal standard solution, add 200 mL of the mobile phase, and disperse the particles by sonicating. To this solution add the mobile phase to make 250 mL, and centrifuge. To 5 mL of the supernatant liquid add the mobile phase to make 50 mL, and use this solution as the sample solution. Separately, weigh accurately about 50 mg of Sarpogrelate Hydrochloride RS (separately determine the water <*2.48*> in the same manner as Sarpogrelate Hydroxide), add exactly 5 mL of the internal standard solution, and add the mobile phase to make 50 mL. To 5 mL of this solution add the mobile phase to make 50 mL, and use this solution as the standard solution. Perform the test with 10 μL each of the sample solution and standard solution as directed under Liquid Chromatography <*2.01*> according to the following conditions, and calculate the ratios, Q_T and Q_S, of the peak area of sarpogrelate to that of the internal standard.

Amount (mg) of sarpogrelate hydrochloride ($C_{24}H_{31}NO_6$.HCl)
$= M_S \times Q_T/Q_S \times 5$

M_S: Amount (mg) of Sarpogrelate Hydrochloride RS taken, calculated on the anhydrous basis

Internal standard solution—A solution of isopropyl parahydroxybenzoate in the mobile phase (1 in 1000).

Operating conditions—

Proceed as directed in the operating conditions in the Assay under Sarpogrelate Hydrochloride.

System suitability—

System performance: When the procedure is run with 10 μL of the standard solution under the above operating conditions, sarpogrelate and the internal standard are eluted in this order with the resolution between these peaks being not less than 3.

System repeatability: When the test is repeated 6 times with 10 μL of the standard solution under the above operating conditions, the relative standard deviation of the ratio of the peak area of sarpogrelate to that of the internal standard is not more than 1.0%.

Containers and storage Containers—Tight containers.

Sarpogrelate Hydrochloride Tablets

サルポグレラート塩酸塩錠

Sarpogrelate Hydrochloride Tablets contain not less than 95.0% and not more than 105.0% of the labeled amount of sarpogrelate hydrochloride ($C_{24}H_{31}NO_6$.HCl: 465.97).

Method of preparation Prepare as directed under Tablets, with Sarpogrelate Hydrochloride.

Identification Powder Sarpogrelate Hydrochloride Tablets. To a portion of the powder, equivalent to 50 mg of Sarpogrelate Hydrochloride, add 10 mL of 0.01 mol/L hydrochloric acid TS, allow to stand at room temperature for 10 minutes, then add 0.01 mol/L hydrochloric acid TS to make 100 mL, and disperse the particles by sonicating. Centrifuge this solution, and to 5 mL of the supernatant liquid add 0.01 mol/L hydrochloric acid TS to make 50 mL. Determine the absorption spectrum of this solution as directed under Ultraviolet-visible Spectrophotometry *<2.24>*: it exhibits maxima between 269 nm and 273 nm, and between 274 nm and 278 nm.

Purity Related substances—Conduct this procedure within 12 hours after preparation of the sample solution. Powder Sarpogrelate Hydrochloride Tablets. To a portion of the powder, equivalent to 0.10 g of Sarpogrelate Hydrochloride, add 50 mL of the mobile phase, and disperse the particles by sonicating. Filter the solution through a membrane filter with a pore size not exceeding 0.45 μm, discard the first 3 mL of the filtrate, and use the subsequent filtrate as the sample solution. Pipet 2 mL of the sample solution, add the mobile phase to make exactly 200 mL, and use this solution as the standard solution. Perform the test with exactly 10 μL each of the sample solution and standard solution as directed under Liquid Chromatography *<2.01>* according to the following conditions, and determine each peak area by the automatic integration method: the peak area of decomposed substance A, having the relative retention time about 0.82 to sarpogrelate, obtained from the sample solution is not larger than 1.5 times that of sarpogrelate from the standard solution, and the area of the peak other than sarpogrelate and the peak mentioned above from the sample solution is not larger than 1/10 times the peak area of sarpogrelate from the standard solution. For the peak area of the decomposed substance A, multiply the correction factor, 0.78.

Operating conditions—

Detector, column, column temperature, mobile phase, and flow rate: Proceed as directed in the operating conditions in the Assay under Sarpogrelate Hydrochloride.

Time span of measurement: About 2.5 times as long as the retention time of sarpogrelate, beginning after the solvent peak.

System suitability—

Test for required detectability: To exactly 5 mL of the standard solution add the mobile phase to make exactly 50 mL. Confirm that the peak area of sarpogrelate obtained with 10 μL of this solution is equivalent to 7 to 13% of that with 10 μL of the standard solution.

System performance: Dissolve 50 mg of sarpogrelate hydrochloride in 20 mL of water, and use this solution as the sarpogrelate hydrochloride stock solution. To 1 mL of the sarpogrelate hydrochloride stock solution add 2 mL of sodium hydroxide TS, shake thoroughly, allow to stand for 10 minutes, and add 3 mL of 1 mol/L hydrochloric acid TS. To this solution add 1 mL of the sarpogrelate hydrochloride stock solution, and add the mobile phase to make 50 mL. When the procedure is run with 10 μL of this solution under the above operating conditions, the decomposed substance A and sarpogrelate are eluted in this order with the resolution between these peaks being not less than 3.

System repeatability: When the test is repeated 6 times with 10 μL of the standard solution under the above operating conditions, the relative standard deviation of the peak area of sarpogrelate is not more than 2.0%.

Uniformity of dosage units *<6.02>* Perform the Mass variation test, or the Content uniformity test according to the following method: it meets the requirement.

To 1 tablet of Sarpogrelate Hydrochloride Tablets add exactly V/10 mL of the internal standard solution, and disintegrate the tablet. Add 4V/5 mL of the mobile phase, disperse the particles by sonicating, then add the mobile phase to make V mL so that each mL contains about 1 mg of sarpogrelate hydrochloride ($C_{24}H_{31}NO_6$.HCl), and centrifuge. To 5 mL of the supernatant liquid add the mobile phase to make 50 mL, and use this solution as the sample solution. Then, proceed as directed in the Assay.

Amount (mg) of sarpogrelate hydrochloride ($C_{24}H_{31}NO_6$.HCl)

$$= M_S \times Q_T/Q_S \times V/50$$

M_S: Amount (mg) of Sarpogrelate Hydrochloride RS taken, calculated on the anhydrous basis

Internal standard solution—A solution of isopropyl parahydroxybenzoate in the mobile phase (1 in 1000).

Dissolution *<6.10>* When the test is performed at 50 revolutions per minute according to the Paddle method, using 900 mL of water as the dissolution medium, the dissolution rate in 30 minutes of Sarpogrelate Hydrochloride Tablets is not less than 80%.

Start the test with 1 tablet of Sarpogrelate Hydrochloride Tablets, withdraw not less than 20 mL of the medium at the specified minute after starting the test, and filter through a membrane filter with a pore size not exceeding 0.45 μm. Discard not less than 10 mL of the first filtrate, pipet V mL of the subsequent filtrate, add water to make exactly V' mL so that each mL contains about 55.6 μg of sarpogrelate hydrochloride ($C_{24}H_{31}NO_6$.HCl), and use this solution as the sample solution. Separately, weigh accurately about 25 mg of

Sarpogrelate Hydrochloride RS (separately determine the water <*2.48*> in the same manner as Sarpogrelate Hydrochloride), and dissolve in water to make exactly 50 mL. Pipet 5 mL of this solution, add water to make exactly 50 mL, and use this solution as the standard solution. Determine the absorbances, A_T and A_S, of the sample solution and standard solution at 270 nm as directed under Ultraviolet-visible Spectrophotometry <*2.24*>.

Dissolution rate (%) with respect to the labeled amount of sarpogrelate hydrochloride ($C_{24}H_{31}NO_6.HCl$)

$$= M_S \times A_T/A_S \times V'/V \times 1/C \times 180$$

M_S: Amount (mg) of Sarpogrelate Hydrochloride RS taken, calculated on the anhydrous basis

C: Labeled amount (mg) of sarpogrelate hydrochloride ($C_{24}H_{31}NO_6.HCl$) in 1 tablet

Assay Weigh accurately the mass of not less than 20 Sarpogrelate Hydrochloride Tablets, and powder. Weigh accurately a portion of the powder, equivalent to about 0.25 g of sarpogrelate hydrochloride ($C_{24}H_{31}NO_6.HCl$), add exactly 25 mL of the internal standard solution, add about 200 mL of the mobile phase, and disperse the particles by sonicating. To this solution add the mobile phase to make 250 mL, and centrifuge. To 5 mL of the supernatant liquid add the mobile phase to make 50 mL, and use this solution as the sample solution. Separately, weigh accurately about 50 mg of Sarpogrelate Hydrochloride RS (separately determine the water <*2.48*> in the same manner as Sarpogrelate Hydroxide), add exactly 5 mL of the internal standard solution, and add the mobile phase to make 50 mL. To 5 mL of this solution add the mobile phase to make 50 mL, and use this solution as the standard solution. Perform the test with 10 μL each of the sample solution and standard solution as directed under Liquid Chromatography <*2.01*> under the following conditions, and calculate the ratios, Q_T and Q_S, of the peak area of sarpogrelate to that of the internal standard.

Amount (mg) of sarpogrelate hydrochloride ($C_{24}H_{31}NO_6.HCl$)

$$= M_S \times Q_T/Q_S \times 5$$

M_S: Amount (mg) of Sarpogrelate Hydrochloride RS taken, calculated on the anhydrous basis

Internal standard solution—A solution of isopropyl parahydroxybenzoate in the mobile phase (1 in 1000).

Operating conditions—

Proceed as directed in the operating conditions in the Assay under Sarpogrelate Hydrochloride.

System suitability—

System performance: When the procedure is run with 10 μL of the standard solution under the above operating conditions, sarpogrelate and the internal standard are eluted in this order with the resolution between these peaks being not less than 3.

System repeatability: When the test is repeated 6 times with 10 μL of the standard solution under the above operating conditions, the relative standard deviation of the ratio of the peak area of sarpogrelate to that of the internal standard is not more than 1.0%.

Containers and storage Containers—Tight containers.

Scopolamine Butylbromide

ブチルスコポラミン臭化物

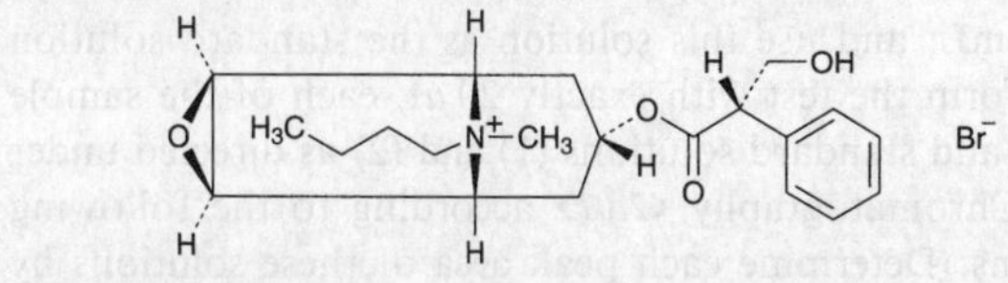

$C_{21}H_{30}BrNO_4$: 440.37

(1*R*,2*R*,4*S*,5*S*,7*s*,9*r*)-9-Butyl-7-[(2*S*)-3-hydroxy-2-phenylpropanoyloxy]-9-methyl-3-oxa-9-azoniatricyclo[3.3.1.0^{2,4}]nonane bromide

[*149-64-4*]

Scopolamine Butylbromide, when dried, contains not less than 98.5% of scopolamine butylbromide ($C_{21}H_{30}BrNO_4$).

Description Scopolamine Butylbromide occurs as white, crystals or crystalline powder.

It is very soluble in water, freely soluble in acetic acid (100), soluble in ethanol (95), sparingly soluble in methanol, slightly soluble in acetic anhydride, and practically insoluble in diethyl ether.

Melting point: about 140°C (with decomposition).

Identification **(1)** To 1 mg of Scopolamine Butylbromide add 3 to 4 drops of fuming nitric acid, and evaporate on a water bath to dryness. After cooling, dissolve the residue in 1 mL of *N*,*N*-dimethylformamide, and add 6 drops of tetraethylammonium hydroxide TS: a red-purple color develops.

(2) Determine the absorption spectrum of a solution of Scopolamine Butylbromide (1 in 1000) as directed under Ultraviolet-visible Spectrophotometry <*2.24*>, and compare the spectrum with the Reference Spectrum: both spectra exhibit similar intensities of absorption at the same wavelengths.

(3) Determine the infrared absorption spectrum of Scopolamine Butylbromide, previously dried, as directed in the potassium bromide disk method under Infrared Spectrophotometry <*2.25*>, and compare the spectrum with the Reference Spectrum: both spectra exhibit similar intensities of absorption at the same wave numbers.

(4) A solution of Scopolamine Butylbromide (1 in 20) responds to Qualitative Tests <*1.09*> for bromide.

Optical rotation <*2.49*> $[\alpha]_D^{20}$: −18.0 – −20.0° (after drying, 1 g, water, 10 mL, 100 mm).

pH <*2.54*> Dissolve 1.0 g of Scopolamine Butylbromide in 10 mL of water: the pH of this solution is between 5.5 and 6.5.

Purity **(1)** Clarity and color of solution—Dissolve 1.0 g of Scopolamine Butylbromide in 10 mL of water: the solution is clear, and has no more color than the following control solution.

Control solution: To 0.5 mL of Matching Fluid F add diluted hydrochloric acid (1 in 40) to make 20 mL.

(2) Heavy metals <*1.07*>—Proceed with 2.0 g of Scopolamine Butylbromide according to Method 1, and perform the test. Prepare the control solution with 2.0 mL of Standard Lead Solution (not more than 10 ppm).

(3) Related substances—Dissolve 0.10 g of Scopolamine Butylbromide in the mobile phase to make exactly 10 mL, and use this solution as the sample solution. Separately, dissolve 10 mg of scopolamine hydrobromide hydrate in the mobile phase to make exactly 100 mL. Pipet 10 mL of this solution, add the mobile phase to make exactly 50 mL, and use this solution as the standard solution (1). Pipet 5 mL of the standard solution (1), add the mobile phase to make exactly 10 mL, and use this solution as the standard solution (2). Perform the test with exactly 20 μL each of the sample solution and standard solutions (1) and (2) as directed under Liquid Chromatography <*2.01*> according to the following conditions. Determine each peak area of these solutions by the automatic integration method: the peak area of scopolamine obtained from the sample solution is not larger than that from the standard solution (2), and each area of the peaks other than the peak appearing in the first elution and the peak of scopolamine and butylscopolamine from the sample solution are not larger than the peak area from the standard solution (1).

Operating conditions—

Detector: An ultraviolet absorption photometer (wavelength: 210 nm).

Column: A stainless steel column 4.6 mm in inside diameter and 15 cm in length, packed with octylsilanized silica gel for liquid chromatography (10 μm in particle diameter).

Column temperature: A constant temperature of about 30°C.

Mobile phase: Dissolve 2 g of sodium lauryl sulfate in 370 mL of water and 680 mL of methanol, and adjust the pH to 3.6 with diluted phosphoric acid (1 in 10).

Flow rate: Adjust so that the retention time of butylscopolamine is about 7 minutes.

Time span of measurement: About 2 times as long as the retention time of butylscopolamine.

System suitability—

System performance: Dissolve 5 mg each of Scopolamine Butylbromide and scopolamine hydrobromide hydrate in 50 mL of the mobile phase. When the procedure is run with 20 μL of this solution under the above operating conditions, scopolamine and butylscopolamine are eluted in this order with the resolution between these peaks being not less than 5.

System repeatability: When the test is repeated 6 times with 20 μL of the standard solution (2) under the above operating conditions, the relative standard deviation of the peak area of scopolamine is not more than 2.0%.

Loss on drying <*2.41*> Not more than 1.0% (1 g, 105°C, 4 hours).

Residue on ignition <*2.44*> Not more than 0.1% (1 g).

Assay Weigh accurately about 0.8 g of Scopolamine Butylbromide, previously dried, dissolve in 40 mL of acetic acid (100) and 30 mL of acetic anhydride, and titrate <*2.50*> with 0.1 mol/L perchloric acid VS (potentiometric titration). Perform a blank determination in the same manner, and make any necessary correction.

Each mL of 0.1 mol/L perchloric acid VS
= 44.04 mg of $C_{21}H_{30}BrNO_4$

Containers and storage Containers—Tight containers.

Scopolamine Hydrobromide Hydrate

スコポラミン臭化水素酸塩水和物

$C_{17}H_{21}NO_4.HBr.3H_2O$: 438.31
(1*R*,2*R*,4*S*,5*S*,7*s*)-9-Methyl-3-oxa-9-azatricyclo[3.3.1.$0^{2,4}$]non-7-yl (2*S*)-3-hydroxy-2-phenylpropanoate monohydrobromide trihydrate
[*6533-68-2*]

Scopolamine Hydrobromide Hydrate, when dried, contains not less than 98.5% of scopolamine hydrobromide ($C_{17}H_{21}NO_4.HBr$: 384.26).

Description Scopolamine Hydrobromide Hydrate occurs as colorless or white crystals, or white granules or powder. It is odorless.

It is freely soluble in water, sparingly soluble in ethanol (95) and in acetic acid (100), and practically insoluble in diethyl ether.

Identification **(1)** To 1 mg of Scopolamine Hydrobromide Hydrate add 3 to 4 drops of fuming nitric acid, evaporate on a water bath to dryness, and cool. Dissolve the residue in 1 mL of *N*,*N*-dimethylformamide, and add 6 drops of tetraethylammonium hydroxide TS: a red-purple color is produced.

(2) A solution of Scopolamine Hydrobromide Hydrate (1 in 20) responds to Qualitative Tests <*1.09*> for bromide.

Optical rotation <*2.49*> $[\alpha]_D^{20}$: −24.0 – −26.0° (after drying, 0.5 g, water, 10 mL, 100 mm).

Melting point <*2.60*> 195 – 199°C (after drying, previously heat the bath to 180°C).

Purity **(1)** Clarity and color of solution—Dissolve 0.5 g of Scopolamine Hydrobromide Hydrate in 10 mL of water: the solution is clear and colorless.

(2) Acidity—Dissolve 0.50 g of Scopolamine Hydrobromide Hydrate in 15 mL of water, and add 0.50 mL of 0.02 mol/L sodium hydroxide VS and 1 drop of methyl red-methylene blue TS: a green color develops.

(3) Apoatropine—Dissolve 0.20 g of Scopolamine Hydrobromide Hydrate in 20 mL of water, add 0.60 mL of 0.002 mol/L potassium permanganate VS, and allow to stand for 5 minutes: the red color in the solution does not disappear.

(4) Related substances—Dissolve 0.15 g of Scopolamine Hydrobromide Hydrate in 3 mL of water, and use this solution as the sample solution.

(i) To 1 mL of the sample solution add 2 to 3 drops of ammonia TS: no turbidity is produced.

(ii) To 1 mL of the sample solution add 2 to 3 drops of potassium hydroxide TS: a transient white turbidity might be produced, and disappears clearly in a little while.

Loss on drying <*2.41*> Not more than 13.0% [1.5 g, first dry in a desiccator (silica gel) for 24 hours, then dry at 105°C for 3 hours].

Residue on ignition <*2.44*> Not more than 0.1% (1 g).

Assay Weigh accurately about 0.5 g of Scopolamine Hydrobromide Hydrate, previously dried, in 10 mL of acetic acid (100) by warming. After cooling, add 40 mL of acetic anhydride, and titrate <*2.50*> with 0.1 mol/L perchloric acid VS (potentiometric titration). Perform a blank determination in the same manner, and make any necessary correction.

Each mL of 0.1 mol/L perchloric acid VS
= 38.43 mg of $C_{17}H_{21}NO_4.HBr$

Containers and storage Containers—Tight containers.
Storage—Light-resistant.

L-Serine

L-セリン

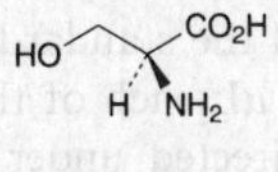

$C_3H_7NO_3$: 105.09
(2*S*)-2-Amino-3-hydroxypropanoic acid
[*56-45-1*]

L-Serine, when dried, contains not less than 98.5% and not more than 101.0% of L-serine ($C_3H_7NO_3$).

Description L-Serine occurs as white, crystals or a crystalline powder. It has a slight sweet taste.

It is freely soluble in water and in formic acid, and practically insoluble in ethanol (99.5).

It dissolves in 2 mol/L hydrochloric acid TS.

Identification Determine the infrared absorption spectrum of L-Serine as directed in the potassium bromide disk method under Infrared Spectrophotometry <*2.25*>, and compare the spectrum with the Reference Spectrum: both spectra exhibit similar intensities of absorption at the same wave numbers.

Optical rotation <*2.49*> $[\alpha]_D^{20}$: +14.0 – +16.0° (After drying, 2.5 g, 2 mol/L hydrochloric acid TS, 25 mL, 100 mm).

pH <*2.54*> The pH of a solution prepared by dissolving 1.0 g of L-Serine in 10 mL of water is between 5.2 and 6.2.

Purity **(1)** Clarity and color of solution—Dissolve 1.0 g of L-Serine in 10 mL of water: the solution is clear and colorless.

(2) Chloride <*1.03*>—Perform the test with 0.5 g of L-Serine. Prepare the control solution with 0.30 mL of 0.01 mol/L hydrochloric acid VS (not more than 0.021%).

(3) Sulfate <*1.14*>—Perform the test with 0.6 g of L-Serine. Prepare the control solution with 0.35 mL of 0.005 mol/L sulfuric acid VS (not more than 0.028%).

(4) Ammonium <*1.02*>—Perform the test with 0.25 g of L-Serine. Prepare the control solution with 5.0 mL of Standard Ammonium Solution (not more than 0.02%).

(5) Heavy metals <*1.07*>—Proceed with 2.0 g of L-Serine according to Method 1, and perform the test. Prepare the control solution with 2.0 mL of Standard Lead Solution (not more than 10 ppm).

(6) Iron <*1.10*>—Prepare the test solution with 1.0 g of L-Serine according to Method 1, and perform the test according to Method A. Prepare the control solution with 1.0 mL of Standard Iron Solution (not more than 10 ppm).

(7) Related substances—Dissolve 0.10 g of L-Serine in 10 mL of water, and use this solution as the sample solution. Pipet 1 mL of the sample solution, add water to make exactly 10 mL. Pipet 1 mL of this solution, add water to make exactly 50 mL, and use this solution as the standard solution. Perform the test with these solutions as directed under Thin-layer Chromatography <*2.03*>. Spot 5 μL each of the sample solution and standard solution on a plate of silica gel for thin-layer chromatography. Then develop with a mixture of 1-butanol, water and acetic acid (100) (3:1:1) to a distance of about 10 cm, and dry the plate at 80°C for 30 minutes. Spray evenly a solution of ninhydrin in a mixture of methanol and acetic acid (100) (97:3) (1 in 100) on the plate, and heat the plate at 80°C for 10 minutes: the spot other than the principal spot obtained from the sample solution is not more intense than the spot from the standard solution.

Loss on drying <*2.41*> Not more than 0.3% (1 g, 105°C, 3 hours).

Residue on Ignition <*2.44*> Not more than 0.1% (1 g).

Assay Weigh accurately about 0.11 g of L-Serine, previously dried, dissolve in 3 mL of formic acid, add 50 mL of acetic acid (100), and titrate <*2.50*> with 0.1 mol/L perchloric acid VS (potentiometric titration). Perform a blank determination in the same manner, and make any necessary correction.

Each mL of 0.1 mol/L perchloric acid VS
= 10.51 mg of $C_3H_7NO_3$

Containers and storage Containers—Tight containers.

Sevoflurane

セボフルラン

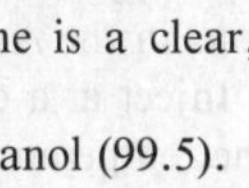

$C_4H_3F_7O$: 200.05
1,1,1,3,3,3-Hexafluoro-2-(fluoromethoxy)propane
[*28523-86-6*]

Sevoflurane contains not less than 99.0% and not more than 101.0% of sevoflurane ($C_4H_3F_7O$), calculated on the anhydrous basis.

Description Sevoflurane is a clear, colorless, and mobile liquid.

It is miscible with ethanol (99.5).

It is very slightly soluble in water.

It is volatile and not inflammable.

Refractive index n_D^{20}: 1.2745 – 1.2760

Boiling point: about 58.6°C

Identification Transfer about 1 μL of Sevoflurane to a gas cell having light path 10 cm in length, and determine the infrared absorption spectrum as directed in the gas sampling method under Infrared Spectrophotometry <*2.25*>, and compare the spectrum with the Reference Spectrum or the spectrum of Sevoflurane RS: both spectra exhibit similar intensities of absorption at the same wave numbers.

Specific gravity <*2.56*> d_{20}^{20}: 1.510 – 1.530

Purity **(1)** Acidity or alkalinity—To 50 mL of Sevoflurane with 50 mL of freshly boiled and cooled water vigorously for 3 minutes. Separate the water layer and use this solution as the sample solution. To 20 mL of the sample solution add 1 drop of bromocresol purple TS and 0.10 mL of 0.01 mol/L sodium hydroxide VS: a red-purple color develops. To 20 mL of the sample solution add 1 drop of bromocresol purple TS and 0.6 mL of 0.01 mol/L hydrochloric acid VS: a yellow color is produced.

(2) Soluble fluoride—To 6 g of Sevoflurane add 12 mL of diluted 0.01 mol/L sodium hydroxide TS (1 in 20), and shake for 10 minutes. Transfer 4.0 mL of diluted 0.01 mol/L sodium hydroxide solution (1 in 20) layer into a Nessler tube. Add 30 mL of a mixture of alizarin complexone TS, acetic acid-potassium acetate buffer solution (pH 4.3) and cerium (III) nitrate TS (1:1:1), add water to make 50 mL, allow to stand for 60 minutes, and use this solution as the sample solution. Separately, transfer 0.2 mL of the fluorine standard solution and 4.0 mL of diluted 0.01 mol/L sodium hydroxide TS (1 in 20) into a Nessler tube, and add 30 mL of a mixture of alizarin complexone TS, acetic acid-potassium acetate buffer solution (pH 4.3) and cerium (III) nitrate TS (1:1:1). Proceed in the same manner as directed for the preparation of the sample solution, and use this solution as the standard solution. Determine the absorbances of the sample solution and standard solution at 600 nm as directed under Ultraviolet-visible Spectrophotometry <*2.24*>, using a solution, prepared with 4.0 mL of diluted 0.01 mol/L sodium hydroxide TS (1 in 20) in the same manner, as the blank: the absorbance of the sample solution is not more than that of the standard solution (not more than 1 ppm).

Fluorine standard solution: Dissolve exactly 2.21 g of sodium fluoride in water to make exactly 1000 mL. Pipet 10 mL of this solution and add water to make exactly 1000 mL. Each mL of this solution contains 0.01 mg of fluorine (F).

(3) Related substances—Perform the test with 2 μL of Sevoflurane as directed under Gas Chromatography <*2.02*> according to the following conditions. Determine each peak area by the automatic integration method and calculate the amount of them by the area percentage method: the amount of the peak of hexafluoroisopropyl methyl ether, having the relative retention time of about 0.84 to sevoflurane, is not more than 0.005%, the amount of each peak other than the peaks of sevoflurane and hexafluoroisopropyl methyl ether is not more than 0.0025%, and the total amount of the peaks other than the peaks of sevoflurane and hexafluoroisopropyl methyl ether is not more than 0.005%.

Operating conditions—

Detector, column, injection port temperature, detector temperature, carrier gas and split ratio: Proceed as directed in the operating conditions in the Assay.

Column temperature: Inject at a constant temperature of about 40°C, maintain the temperature for 10 minutes, raise at a rate of 10°C per minute to 200°C, and maintain at a constant temperature of about 200°C.

Flow rate: Adjust so that the retention time of sevoflurane is about 7 minutes.

Time span of measurement: About 6 times as long as the retention time of sevoflurane.

System suitability—

Test for required detectability: To 20 μL of Sevoflurane add *o*-xylene to make 20 mL. To 1 mL of this solution add *o*-xylene to make 20 mL, and use this solution as the solution for system suitability test. Pipet 1 mL of the solution for system suitability test and add *o*-xylene to make exactly 10 mL. Confirm that the peak area of sevoflurane obtained with 2 μL of this solution is equivalent to 7 to 13% of the peak area of sevoflurane with 2 μL of the solution for system suitability test.

System performance: When the procedure is run with 2 μL of the solution for system suitability test under the above operating conditions, the number of theoretical plates and symmetry factor of the peak of sevoflurane are not less than 6000 and not more than 1.5, respectively.

System repeatability: When the test is repeated 6 times with 2 μL of the solution for system suitability test under the above operating conditions, the relative standard deviation of the peak area of Sevoflurane is not more than 5.0%.

(4) Residue on evaporation—Evaporate 10 mL of Sevoflurane, exactly measured, on a water bath to dryness, and dry at 105°C for 2 hours: the mass of the residue is not more than 1.0 mg.

Water <*2.48*> Not more than 0.2 w/v% (5 mL, volumetric titration, direct titration).

Assay Pipet 5 mL each of Sevoflurane and Sevoflurane RS (separately determine the water <*2.48*> in the same manner as Sevoflurane), to each add exactly 5 mL of dimethoxymethane as an internal standard, and use these solutions as the sample solution and the standard solution, respectively. Perform the test with 1 μL each of the sample solution and standard solution as directed under Gas Chromatography <*2.02*> according to the following conditions, and calculate the ratios, Q_T and Q_S, of the peak area of sevoflurane to that of the internal standard.

$$\text{Amount (mg) of sevoflurane } (C_4H_3F_7O) = V_S \times Q_T/Q_S \times 1000 \times 1.521$$

V_S: Amount (mL) of Sevoflurane RS taken, calculated on the anhydrous basis

1.521: Specific gravity of Sevoflurane (d^{20}_{20})

Operating conditions—

Detector: A hydrogen flame-ionization detector.

Column: A fused silica column 0.32 mm in inside diameter and 30 m in length, coated inside with cyanopropyl methylphenyl silicone for gas chromatography in 1.8 μm thickness.

Column temperature: 40°C.

Injection port temperature: A constant temperature of about 200°C.

Detector temperature: A constant temperature of about 225°C.

Carrier gas: Helium.

Flow rate: Adjust so that the retention time of Sevoflurane is about 3 minutes.

Split ratio: 1:20.

System suitability—

System performance: When the procedure is run with 1 μL of the standard solution under the above operating conditions, sevoflurane and the internal standard are eluted in this order with the resolution between these peaks being not less than 3.

System repeatability: When the test is repeated 6 times with 1 μL of the standard solution under the above operating conditions, the relative standard deviation of the ratio of the peak area of sevoflurane to that of the internal standard is not more than 1.0 %.

Containers and storage Containers—Tight containers.

Purified Shellac

精製セラック

Purified Shellac is a resin-like substance obtained from a purified secretion of *Laccifer lacca* Kerr (*Coccidae*).

Description Purified Shellac occurs as light yellow-brown to brown, lustrous, hard, brittle scutella. It is odorless or has a faint, characteristic odor.

It is freely soluble in ethanol (95) and in ethanol (99.5), and practically insoluble in water and in diethyl ether.

It dissolves in sodium hydroxide TS.

Acid value *<1.13>* 60 – 80 Weigh accurately about 1 g of Purified Shellac, add 40 mL of neutralized ethanol, and dissolve by warming. After cooling, titrate *<2.50>* with 0.1 mol/L potassium hydroxide VS (potentiometric titration).

Purity **(1)** Heavy metals *<1.07>*—Proceed with 2.0 g of Purified Shellac according to Method 2, and perform the test. Prepare the control solution with 2.0 mL of Standard Lead Solution (not more than 10 ppm).

(2) Arsenic *<1.11>*—Prepare the test solution with 0.40 g of Purified Shellac according to Method 3, and perform the test. Add 10 mL of a solution of magnesium nitrate hexahydrate in ethanol (95) (1 in 50), then add 1.5 mL of hydrogen peroxide (30), and fire to burn (not more than 5 ppm).

(3) Ethanol-insoluble substances—Dissolve about 5 g of Purified Shellac, accurately weighed, in 50 mL of ethanol (95) on a water bath while shaking. Pour the ethanol solution into a tared extraction thimble, previously dried at 105°C for 2 hours, in a Soxhlet extractor, and extract with ethanol (95) for 3 hours. Dry the extraction thimble at 105°C for 3 hours: the mass of the residue is not more than 2.0%. Use a cylindrical weighing bottle for taring the extraction thimble.

(4) Rosin—To 2.0 g of Purified Shellac add 10 mL of ethanol (99.5), shake thoroughly to dissolve, and add gradually 50 mL of hexane while shaking. Transfer the solution to a separator, wash with two 50-mL portions of water, filter the upper layer, and evaporate the filtrate on a water bath to dryness. To the residue add 5 mL of acetic anhydride, and heat on a water bath to dissolve, if necessary. Transfer this solution to a Nessler tube, and add 1 drop of sulfuric acid: the color of the solution does not change from red-purple through purple to reddish yellow.

(5) Wax—Dissolve 10.0 g of Purified Shellac in 150 mL of a solution of sodium carbonate decahydrate (9 in 200) with shaking on a water bath, and continue the heating for 2 hours. After cooling, collect the floating wax by filtration, wash the wax and the filter paper with water, transfer to a beaker, and dry at 65°C until the water is almost evaporated. Transfer the wax together with the filter paper to an extraction thimble in a Soxhlet extractor. Dissolve the wax remaining in the beaker with a suitable quantity of chloroform by warming. Pour the solution into the thimble, and extract with chloroform for 2 hours. Evaporate the chloroform solution to dryness, and dry the residue at 105°C for 3 hours: the mass of the residue is not more than 20 mg.

Loss on drying Not more than 2.0%. Weigh accurately about 1 g of moderately fine powder of Purified Shellac, and dry at 40°C for 4 hours, then for 15 hours in a desiccator (calcium chloride for drying).

Total ash *<5.01>* Not more than 1.0% (1 g).

Containers and storage Containers—Well-closed containers.

White Shellac

白色セラック

White Shellac is a resin-like substance obtained from a bleached secretion of *Laccifer lacca* Kerr (*Coccidae*).

Description White Shellac occurs as yellow-white to light yellow, hard, brittle granules. It is odorless or has a faint, characteristic odor.

It is sparingly soluble in ethanol (95), and practically insoluble in water.

It dissolves in sodium hydroxide TS.

Acid value *<1.13>* 65 – 90 Weigh accurately about 0.5 g of White Shellac, add 50 mL of neutralized ethanol, and dissolve by warming. After cooling, perform the test as directed in the Acid value under Purified Shellac.

Purity **(1)** Chloride *<1.03>*—Shake and dissolve 0.40 g of White Shellac in 5 mL of ethanol (95) while warming, add 40 mL of water, and cool. Add 12 mL of dilute nitric acid and water to make 100 mL, and filter. Perform the test using 50 mL of the filtrate as the test solution. Prepare the control solution as follows: to 0.80 mL of 0.01 mol/L hydrochloric acid VS add 2.5 mL of ethanol (95), 6 mL of dilute nitric acid and water to make 50 mL (not more than 0.140%).

(2) Sulfate *<1.14>*—Shake and dissolve 0.40 g of White Shellac in 5 mL of ethanol (95) by warming, add 40 mL of water, and cool. Add 2 mL of dilute hydrochloric acid and water to make 100 mL, and filter. Perform the test using 50 mL of the filtrate as the test solution. Prepare the control solution as follows: to 0.45 mL of 0.005 mol/L sulfuric acid VS add 2.5 mL of ethanol (95), 1 mL of dilute hydrochloric acid and water to make 50 mL (not more than 0.110%).

(3) Heavy metals *<1.07>*—Proceed with 2.0 g of White Shellac according to Method 2, and perform the test. Prepare the control solution with 2.0 mL of Standard Lead Solution (not more than 10 ppm.)

(4) Arsenic *<1.11>*—Prepare the test solution with 0.40 g of White Shellac according to Method 3, and perform the test. Add 10 mL of a solution of magnesium nitrate hexahydrate in ethanol (95) (1 in 50), then add 1.5 mL of hydrogen peroxide (30), and fire to burn (not more than 5 ppm).

(5) Ethanol-insoluble substances—Dissolve about 5 g of White Shellac, accurately weighed, in 50 mL of ethanol (95) on a water bath while shaking. Pour the ethanol solution into a tared extraction thimble, previously dried at 105°C for 2 hours, in a Soxhlet extractor, and extract with ethanol (95) for 3 hours. Dry the extraction thimble at 105°C for 3 hours: the mass of the residue is not more than 2.0%. Use a cylindrical weighing bottle for taring the extraction thimble.

(6) Rosin—To 2.0 g of White Shellac add 10 mL of ethanol (99.5), shake thoroughly to dissolve, and add gradually 50 mL of hexane while shaking. Transfer the solution to a separator, wash with two 50-mL portions of water, filter the upper layer, and evaporate the filtrate on a water bath to dryness. To the residue add 5 mL of acetic anhydride, and heat on a water bath to dissolve, if necessary. Transfer this solution to a Nessler tube, and add 1 drop of sulfuric acid: the color of the solution does not change from red-purple through purple to reddish yellow.

(7) Wax—Dissolve 10.0 g of White Shellac in 150 mL of

a solution of sodium carbonate decahydrate (9 in 200) with shaking on a water bath, and continue the heating for 2 hours. After cooling, collect the floating wax by filtration, wash the wax and the filter paper with water, transfer to a beaker, and dry at 65°C until the water is almost evaporated. Transfer the wax together with the filter paper to an extraction thimble in a Soxhlet extractor. Dissolve the wax remaining in the beaker with a suitable quantity of chloroform by warming. Pour the solution into the thimble, and extract with chloroform for 2 hours. Evaporate the chloroform solution to dryness, and dry the residue at 105°C for 3 hours: the mass of the residue is not more than 20 mg.

Loss on drying Not more than 6.0%. Weigh accurately about 1 g of moderately fine powder of White Shellac, and dry at 40°C for 4 hours, then for 15 hours in a desiccator (calcium chloride for drying).

Total ash <*5.01*> Not more than 1.0% (1 g).

Containers and storage Containers—Well-closed containers.

Storage—In a cold place.

Light Anhydrous Silicic Acid

軽質無水ケイ酸

Light Anhydrous Silicic Acid contains not less than 98.0% of silicon dioxide (SiO_2: 60.08), calculated on the incinerated basis.

Description Light Anhydrous Silicic Acid occurs as a white to bluish white, light, fine power. It is odorless and tasteless, and smooth to the touch.

It is practically insoluble in water, in ethanol (95), and in diethyl ether.

It dissolves in hydrofluoric acid, in hot potassium hydroxide TS and in hot sodium hydroxide TS, and does not dissolve in dilute hydrochloric acid.

Identification **(1)** Dissolve 0.1 g of Light Anhydrous Silicic Acid in 20 mL of sodium hydroxide TS by boiling, and add 12 mL of ammonium chloride TS: a white, gelatinous precipitate is produced. The precipitate does not dissolve in dilute hydrochloric acid.

(2) To the precipitate obtained in (1) add 10 mL of a solution of methylene blue trihydrate (1 in 10,000), and wash with water: the precipitate has a blue color.

(3) Prepare a bead by fusing ammonium sodium hydrogenphosphate tetrahydrate on a platinum loop. Bring the hot, transparent bead into contact with Light Anhydrous Silicic Acid, and fuse again: an insoluble matter is perceptible in the bead. The resulting bead, upon cooling, becomes opaque and acquires a reticulated appearance.

Purity **(1)** Chloride <*1.03*>—Dissolve 0.5 g of Light Anhydrous Silicic Acid in 20 mL of sodium hydroxide TS by boiling, cool, filter if necessary, and wash with 10 mL of water. Combine the filtrate and washings, add 18 mL of dilute nitric acid, shake, and add water to make 50 mL. Perform the test using this solution as the test solution. To 0.15 mL of 0.01 mol/L hydrochloric acid VS add 20 mL of sodium hydroxide TS, 18 mL of dilute nitric acid and water to make 50 mL, and use this solution as the control solution (not more than 0.011%).

(2) Heavy metals <*1.07*>—Dissolve 0.5 g of Light Anhydrous Silicic Acid in 20 mL of sodium hydroxide TS by boiling, cool, add 15 mL of acetic acid (31), shake, filter if necessary, wash with 10 mL of water, combine the filtrate and washings, and add water to make 50 mL. Perform the test using this solution as the test solution. Add acetic acid (31) to 20 mL of sodium hydroxide TS and 1 drop of phenolphthalein TS until the color of this solution disappears, add 2.0 mL of Standard Lead Solution, 2 mL of dilute acetic acid and water to make 50 mL, and use this solution as the control solution (not more than 40 ppm).

(3) Iron <*1.10*>—To 0.040 g of Light Anhydrous Silicic Acid add 10 mL of dilute hydrochloric acid, and heat for 10 minutes in a water bath while shaking. After cooling, add 0.5 g of L-tartaric acid to dissolve by shaking. Prepare the test solution with this solution according to Method 2, and perform the test according to Method B. Prepare the control solution with 2.0 mL of Standard Iron Solution (not more than 500 ppm).

(4) Aluminum—Dissolve 0.5 g of Light Anhydrous Silicic Acid in 40 mL of sodium hydroxide TS by boiling, cool, add sodium hydroxide TS to make 50 mL, and filter. Measure 10 mL of the filtrate, add 17 mL of acetic acid (31), shake, add 2 mL of aluminon TS and water to make 50 mL, and allow to stand for 30 minutes: the color of this solution is not deeper than that of the following control solution.

Control solution: Dissolve 0.176 g of aluminum potassium sulfate dodecahydrate in water, and add water to make 1000 mL. To 15.5 mL of this solution add 10 mL of sodium hydroxide TS, 17 mL of acetic acid (31), 2 mL of aluminon TS and water to make 50 mL.

(5) Calcium—Dissolve 1.0 g of Light Anhydrous Silicic Acid in 30 mL of sodium hydroxide TS by boiling, cool, add 20 mL of water, 1 drop of phenolphthalein TS and dilute nitric acid until the color of this solution disappears, immediately add 5 mL of dilute acetic acid, shake, add water to make 100 mL, and obtain a clear liquid by centrifugation or filtration. To 25 mL of this liquid add 1 mL of oxalic acid TS and ethanol (95) to make 50 mL, immediately shake, and allow to stand for 10 minutes: the turbidity of this solution is not deeper than that of the following control solution.

Control solution: Dissolve 0.250 g of calcium carbonate, previously dried at 180°C for 4 hours, in 3 mL of dilute hydrochloric acid, and add water to make 100 mL. To 4 mL of this solution add 5 mL of dilute acetic acid and water to make 100 mL. To 25 mL of this solution add 1 mL of oxalic acid TS and ethanol (95) to make 50 mL, and shake.

(6) Arsenic <*1.11*>—Dissolve 0.40 g of Light Anhydrous Silicic Acid in 10 mL of sodium hydroxide TS by boiling in a porcelain crucible, cool, add 5 mL of water and 5 mL of dilute hydrochloric acid, shake, and perform the test with this solution as the test solution (not more than 5 ppm).

Loss on drying <*2.41*> Not more than 7.0% (1 g, 105°C, 4 hours).

Loss on ignition <*2.43*> Not more than 12.0% (1 g, 850 – 900°C, constant mass).

Assay Weigh accurately about 1 g of Light Anhydrous Silicic Acid, add 20 mL of hydrochloric acid, and evaporate to dryness on a sand bath. Moisten the residue with hydrochloric acid, evaporate to dryness, and heat between 110°C and 120°C for 2 hours. Cool, add 5 mL of dilute hydrochloric acid, and heat. Allow to cool to room temperature, add 20 to 25 mL of hot water, filter rapidly, and wash the residue with warm water until the last washing becomes negative to Qualitative Tests <*1.09*> (2) for chloride. Transfer the residue together with the filter paper to a platinum crucible, ignite to ash, and continue the ignition for 30 minutes. Cool, weigh the crucible, and designate the mass as *a* (g). Moisten the residue in the crucible with water, add 6 mL of hydrofluoric acid and 3 drops of sulfuric acid, and evaporate to dryness. Heat strongly for 5 minutes, cool, weigh the crucible, and designate the mass as *b* (g).

$$\text{Amount (g) of silicon dioxide } (SiO_2) = a - b$$

Containers and storage Containers—Tight containers.

Silodosin

シロドシン

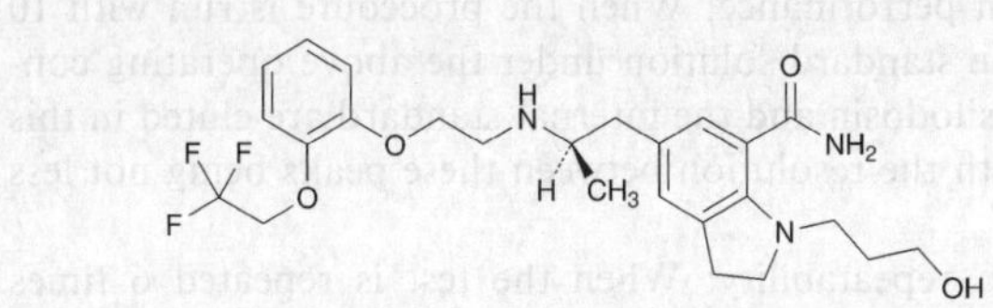

$C_{25}H_{32}F_3N_3O_4$: 495.53
1-(3-Hydroxypropyl)-5-[(2*R*)-2-({2-[2-(2,2,2-trifluoroethoxy)phenoxy]ethyl}amino)propyl]-2,3-dihydro-1*H*-indole-7-carboxamide
[*160970-54-7*]

Silodosin contains not less than 98.0% and not more than 102.0% of silodosin ($C_{25}H_{32}F_3N_3O_4$), calculated on the anhydrous basis.

Description Silodosin occurs as a white to pale yellow-white powder.

It is freely soluble in methanol and in ethanol (99.5), and very slightly soluble in water.

It gradually becomes yellow-white on exposure to light.

Optical rotation $[\alpha]_D^{20}$: $-13 - -17°$ (0.2 g calculated on the anhydrous basis, methanol, 20 mL, 100 mm).

Melting point: 105 – 109°C

Silodosin shows crystal polymorphism.

Identification **(1)** Prepare the test solution with 10 mg of Silodosin as directed under Oxygen Flask Combustion Method <*1.06*>, using a mixture of 0.5 mL of 0.01 mol/L sodium hydroxide TS and 20 mL of water as the absorbing liquid: the solution responds to Qualitative Tests <*1.09*> (2) for fluoride.

(2) Determine the absorption spectrum of a solution of Silodosin in methanol (1 in 20,000) as directed under Ultraviolet-visible Spectrophotometry <*2.24*>, and compare the spectrum with the Reference Spectrum or the spectrum of a solution of Silodosin RS prepared in the same manner as the sample solution: both spectra exhibit similar intensities of absorption at the same wavelengths.

(3) Determine the infrared absorption spectrum of Silodosin as directed in the paste method under Infrared Spectrophotometry <*2.25*>, and compare the spectrum with the Reference Spectrum or the spectrum of Silodosin RS: both spectra exhibit similar intensities of absorption at the same wave numbers. If any difference appears between the spectra, recrystallize the sample and the Reference Standard according to the method otherwise specified, filter and dry the crystals, and perform the test using the crystals.

Purity **(1)** Heavy metals <*1.07*>—Proceed with 2.0 g of Silodosin in a platinum crucible according to Method 2, and perform the test. Prepare the control solution with 2.0 mL of Standard Lead Solution (not more than 10 ppm).

(2) Related substances—Conduct this procedure using light-resistant vessels. Dissolve 50 mg of Silodosin in 100 mL of methanol, and use this solution as the sample solution. Pipet 1 mL of the sample solution, add methanol to make exactly 100 mL, and use this solution as the standard solution. Perform the test with exactly 10 μL each of the sample solution and standard solution as directed under Liquid Chromatography <*2.01*> according to the following conditions, and determine each peak area by the automatic integration method: the area of the peak of related substance A, having the relative retention time of about 1.3 to silodosin, obtained from the sample solution is not larger than 3/20 times the peak area of silodosin from the standard solution, the peak areas of related substance B and related substance C, having the relative retention time of about 1.6 and about 2.0, respectively, is not larger than 1/16 times the peak area of silodosin from the standard solution, and the area of the peak other than silodosin and the peaks mentioned above from the sample solution is not larger than 1/10 times the peak area of silodosin from the standard solution. In addition, the total area of the peaks other than silodosin from the sample solution is not larger than 7/20 times the peak area of silodosin from the standard solution. For the areas of the peaks of related substance A, related substance B, and related substance C, multiply the correction factor 0.6, respectively.

Operating conditions—

Detector: An ultraviolet absorption photometer (wavelength: 225 nm).

Column: A stainless steel column 4.6 mm in inside diameter and 25 cm in length, packed with octadecylsilanized silica gel for liquid chromatography (5 μm in particle diameter).

Column temperature: A constant temperature of about 40°C.

Mobile phase A: Dissolve 3.9 g of sodium dihydrogen phosphate dihydrate in 1000 mL of water, and adjust to pH 3.4 with diluted phosphoric acid (1 in 10).

Mobile phase B: Acetonitrile for liquid chromatography.

Flowing of mobile phase: Control the gradient by mixing the mobile phases A and B as directed in the following table.

Time after injection of sample (min)	Mobile phase A (vol%)	Mobile phase B (vol%)
0 – 15	75	25
15 – 35	75 → 50	25 → 50
35 – 45	50	50

Flow rate: Adjust so that the retention time of silodosin is about 13 minutes.

Time span of measurement: About 3 times as long as the retention time of silodosin, beginning after the solvent peak.

System suitability—

Test for required detectability: Pipet 1 mL of the standard solution, and add methanol to make exactly 20 mL. Confirm that the peak area of silodosin obtained with 10 μL of this solution is equivalent to 3.5 to 6.5% of that with 10 μL of the standard solution.

System performance: Thinly spread out an amount of Silodosin in a petri dish, exposure to a 4000 lx light for not less than 24 hours using a D_{65} fluorescent lamp, and dissolve 4 mg of this sample in 8 mL of methanol. When the procedure is run with 10 μL of this solution under the above operating conditions, the resolution between the peaks of silodosin and related substance A is not less than 6.

System repeatability: When the test is repeated 6 times with 10 μL of the standard solution under the above operat-

ing conditions, the relative standard deviation of the peak area of silodosin is not more than 2.5%.

(3) Enantiomer—Conduct this procedure using light-resistant vessels. Dissolve 0.1 g of Silodosin in 10 mL of ethanol (99.5), and use this solution as the sample solution. Pipet 1 mL of the sample solution, add ethanol (99.5) to make exactly 200 mL. Pipet 3 mL of this solution, add ethanol (99.5) to make exactly 10 mL, and use this solution as the standard solution. Perform the test with exactly 5 μL each of the sample solution and standard solution as directed under Liquid Chromatography <*2.01*> according to the following conditions, and determine each peak area by the automatic integration method: the area of the peak of the enantiomer, having the relative retention time of about 0.8 to silodosin, obtained from the sample solution is not larger than the peak area of silodosin from the standard solution.

Operating conditions—

Detector: An ultraviolet absorption photometer (wavelength: 270 nm).

Column: A stainless steel column 4.6 mm in inside diameter and 25 cm in length, packed with silica gel coated with cellulose tris(4-methylbenzoate) for liquid chromatography (10 μm in particle diameter).

Column temperature: A constant temperature of about 40°C.

Mobile phase: A mixture of hexane, diethylamine and ethanol (99.5) (93:10:7).

Flow rate: Adjust so that the retention time of silodosin is about 29 minutes.

System suitability—

System performance: When the procedure is run with 5 μL of the standard solution under the above operating conditions, the number of theoretical plates and the symmetry factor of the peak of silodosin are not less than 1000 and not more than 1.5, respectively.

System repeatability: When the test is repeated 6 times with 5 μL of the standard solution under the above operating conditions, the relative standard deviation of the peak area of silodosin is not more than 5%.

Water <*2.48*> Not more than 0.1%, using a water vaporization device (heating temperature: 150°C; heating time: 2 minutes) (1.5 g, coulometric titration).

Residue on ignition <*2.44*> Not more than 0.1% (1 g, platinum crucible).

Assay Conduct this procedure using light-resistant vessels. Weigh accurately about 50 mg each of Silodosin and Silodosin RS (separately determine the water <*2.48*> in the same manner as Silodosin), dissolve each in methanol to make exactly 100 mL. Pipet 5 mL of both solutions, add exactly 5 mL of the internal standard solution to them, add methanol to make 25 mL, and use these solutions as the sample solution and the standard solution, respectively. Perform the test with 10 μL each of the sample solution and standard solution as directed under Liquid Chromatography <*2.01*> according to the following conditions, and calculate the ratios, Q_T and Q_S, of the peak area of silodosin to that of the internal standard.

Amount (mg) of silodosin ($C_{25}H_{32}F_3N_3O_4$) = $M_S \times Q_T/Q_S$

M_S: Amount (mg) of Silodosin RS taken, calculated on the anhydrous basis

Internal standard solution—A solution of ethyl parahydroxybenzoate in methanol (1 in 8000).

Operating conditions—

Detector: An ultraviolet absorption photometer (wavelength: 270 nm).

Column: A stainless steel column 4.6 mm in inside diameter and 15 cm in length, packed with octadecylsilanized silica gel for liquid chromatography (5 μm in particle diameter).

Column temperature: A constant temperature of about 40°C.

Mobile phase: Dissolve 3.9 g of sodium dihydrogen phosphate dihydrate in 1000 mL of water, and adjust to pH 3.4 with diluted phosphoric acid (1 in 10). To 730 mL of this solution add 270 mL of acetonitrile.

Flow rate: Adjust so that the retention time of silodosin is about 6 minutes.

System suitability—

System performance: When the procedure is run with 10 μL of the standard solution under the above operating conditions, silodosin and the internal standard are eluted in this order with the resolution between these peaks being not less than 10.

System repeatability: When the test is repeated 6 times with 10 μL of the standard solution under the above operating conditions, the relative standard deviation of the ratio of the peak area of silodosin to that of the internal standard is not more than 1.0%.

Containers and storage Containers—Well-closed containers.

Storage—Light-resistant.

Others

Related substance A:
1-(3-Hydroxylpropyl)-5-[2-({2-[2-(2,2,2-trifluoroethoxy)phenoxy]ethyl}amino)propyl]-1*H*-indole-7-carboxamide

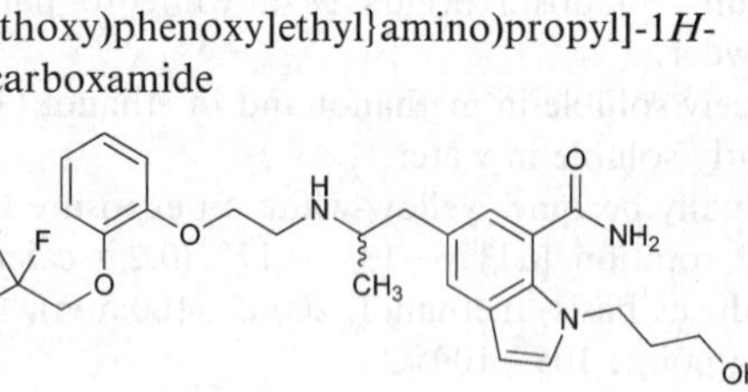

Related substance B:
5-[2-({2-[2-(2,2,2-Trifluoroethoxy)phenoxy]ethyl}amino)propyl]-2,3-dihydro-1*H*-indole-7-carboxamide

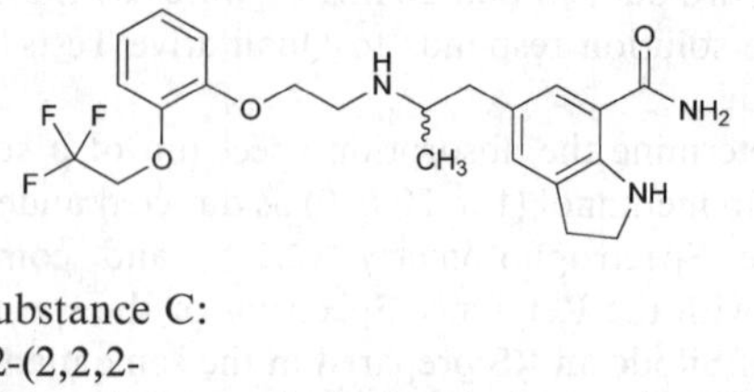

Related substance C:
5-[2-({2-[2-(2,2,2-Trifluoroethoxy)phenoxy]ethyl}amino)propyl]-1*H*-indole-7-carboxamide

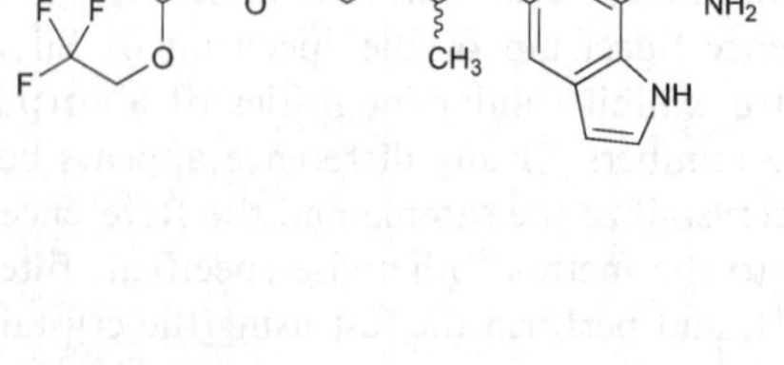

Silodosin Orally Disintegrating Tablets

シロドシン口腔内崩壊錠

Silodosin Orally Disintegrating Tablets contain not less than 95.0% and not more than 105.0% of the labeled amount of silodosin ($C_{25}H_{32}F_3N_3O_4$: 495.53).

Method of preparation Prepare as directed under Tablets, with Silodosin.

Identification Conduct this procedure using light-resistant vessels. To 1 tablet of Silodosin Orally Disintegrating Tablets add 15 mL of a mixture of methanol and a solution of sodium chloride (1 in 200) (7:3) per 1 mg of Silodosin, and sonicate until the tablet is completely disintegrated while occasional shaking. Add a mixture of methanol and a solution of sodium chloride (1 in 200) (7:3) so that each mL contains about 40 μg of Silodosin, and filter through a membrane filter with a pore size not exceeding 0.45 μm. Discard the first 3 mL of the filtrate, and use the subsequent filtrate as the sample solution. Separately, dissolve 20 mg of Silodosin RS in a mixture of methanol and a solution of sodium chloride (1 in 200) (7:3) to make 50 mL. To 5 mL of this solution add a mixture of methanol and a solution of sodium chloride (1 in 200) (7:3) to make 50 mL, and use this solution as the standard solution. Perform the test with 10 μL each of the sample solution and standard solution as directed under Liquid Chromatography <*2.01*> according to the following conditions: the retention times of the principal peaks in the chromatograms obtained from the sample solution and standard solution are the same, and both absorption spectra of these peaks exhibit similar intensities of absorption at the same wavelengths.

Operating conditions—

Column, column temperature, mobile phase, and flow rate: Proceed as directed in the operating conditions in the Assay.

Detector: A photodiode array detector (wavelength: 270 nm, spectrum range of measurement: 200 – 370 nm).

System suitability—

System performance: Proceed as directed in the system suitability in the Assay.

Purity Related substances—Conduct this procedure using light-resistant vessels. To a number of Silodosin Orally Disintegrating Tablets, equivalent to 20 mg of Silodosin, add 60 mL of a mixture of methanol and a solution of sodium chloride (1 in 200) (7:3), sonicate until the tablet is completely disintegrated while occasional shaking, and add a mixture of methanol and a solution of sodium chloride (1 in 200) (7:3) to make 100 mL. Centrifuge this solution, and filter the supernatant liquid through a membrane filter with a pore size not exceeding 0.45 μm. Discard the first 3 mL of the filtrate, and use the subsequent filtrate as the sample solution. Pipet 1 mL of the sample solution, add a mixture of methanol and a solution of sodium chloride (1 in 200) (7:3) to make exactly 100 mL, and use this solution as the standard solution. Perform the test with exactly 25 μL each of the sample solution and standard solution as directed under Liquid Chromatography <*2.01*> according to the following conditions, and determine each peak area by the automatic integration method: the peak area of related substance A, having the relative retention time of about 1.3 to silodosin, obtained from the sample solution is not lager than the peak area of silodosin from the standard solution, the area of the peak other than silodosin and the peak mentioned above from the sample solution is not larger than 1/4 times the peak area of silodosin from the standard solution. Furthermore, the total area of the peaks other than silodosin from the sample solution is not larger than 2 times the peak area of silodosin from the standard solution. For the peak area of related substance A, multiply the correction factor 0.6.

Operating conditions—

Detector, column, column temperature, and mobile phases A and B: Proceed as directed in the Purity (2) under Silodosin.

Flowing of the mobile phase: Control the gradient by mixing the mobile phases A and B as directed in the following table.

Time after injection of sample (min)	Mobile phase A (vol%)	Mobile phase B (vol%)
0 – 15	75	25
15 – 47	75 → 35	25 → 65
47 – 53	35	65

Flow rate: Adjust so that the retention time of silodosin is about 13 minutes.

Time span of measurement: About 3.5 times as long as the retention time of silodosin, beginning after the solvent peak.

System suitability—

Test for required detectability: Pipet 1 mL of the standard solution, and add a mixture of methanol and a solution of sodium chloride (1 in 200) (7:3) to make exactly 20 mL. Confirm that the peak area of silodosin obtained with 25 μL of this solution is equivalent to 3.5 to 6.5% of that with 25 μL of the standard solution.

System performance: Thinly spread out an amount of silodosin in a petri dish, exposure to a 4000 lx light for not less than 24 hours using a D_{65} fluorescent lamp, and dissolve 4 mg of this sample in a mixture of methanol and a solution of sodium chloride (1 in 200) (7:3) to make 20 mL. When the procedure is run with 25 μL of this solution under the above operating conditions, the resolution between the peaks of silodosin and related substance A is not less than 6.

System repeatability: When the test is repeated 6 times with 25 μL of the standard solution under the above operating conditions, the relative standard deviation of the peak area of silodosin is not more than 2.0%.

Uniformity of dosage units <*6.02*> Perform the test according to the following method: it meets the requirement of the Content uniformity test.

Conduct this procedure using light-resistant vessels. To 1 tablet of Silodosin Orally Disintegrating Tablets add $3V/5$ mL of a mixture of methanol and a solution of sodium chloride (1 in 200) (7:3), sonicate until the tablet is completely disintegrated while occasional shaking. Add a mixture of methanol and a solution of sodium chloride (1 in 200) (7:3) to make exactly V mL so that each mL contains about 40 μg of silodosin ($C_{25}H_{32}F_3N_3O_4$), and filter through a membrane filter with a pore size not exceeding 0.45 μm. Discard the first 3 mL of the filtrate, and use the subsequent filtrate as the sample solution. Then, proceed as directed in the Assay.

$$\text{Amount (mg) of silodosin } (C_{25}H_{32}F_3N_3O_4) = M_S \times A_T/A_S \times V/500$$

M_S: Amount (mg) of Silodosin RS taken, calculated on the anhydrous basis

Disintegration Being specified separately when the drug is granted approval based on the Law.

Dissolution ⟨*6.10*⟩ When the test is performed at 50 revolutions per minute according to the Paddle method, using 900 mL of 2nd fluid for dissolution test as the dissolution medium, the dissolution rate in 15 minutes of Silodosin Orally Disintegrating Tablets is not less than 80%.

Start the test with 1 tablet of Silodosin Orally Disintegrating Tablets, withdraw not less than 9 mL of the medium at the specified minute after starting the test, and filter through a membrane filter with a pore size not exceeding 0.45 μm. Discard not less than 5 mL of the first filtrate, pipet V mL of the subsequent filtrate, add 0.2 mol/L hydrochloric acid TS to make exactly V' mL so that each mL contains about 1.1 μg of silodosin ($C_{25}H_{32}F_3N_3O_4$), and use this solution as the sample solution. Separately, weigh accurately about 22 mg of Silodosin RS (separately determine the water ⟨*2.48*⟩ in the same manner as Silodosin), and dissolve in 0.1 mol/L hydrochloric acid TS to make exactly 100 mL. Pipet 5 mL of this solution, add 0.1 mol/L hydrochloric acid TS to make exactly 50 mL. Pipet 5 mL of this solution, add 0.1 mol/L hydrochloric acid TS to make exactly 100 mL, and use this solution as the standard solution. Perform the test with exactly 100 μL each of the sample solution and standard solution as directed under Liquid Chromatography ⟨*2.01*⟩ according to the following conditions, and determine the peak areas, A_T and A_S, of silodosin in each solution.

Dissolution rate (%) with respect to the labeled amount of silodosin ($C_{25}H_{32}F_3N_3O_4$)
$= M_S \times A_T/A_S \times V'/V \times 1/C \times 9/2$

M_S: Amount (mg) of Silodosin RS taken, calculated on the anhydrous basis

C: Labeled amount (mg) of silodosin ($C_{25}H_{32}F_3N_3O_4$) in 1 tablet

Operating conditions—

Proceed as directed in the Assay.

System suitability—

System performance: When the procedure is run with 100 μL of the standard solution under the above operating conditions, the number of theoretical plates and the symmetry factor of the peak of silodosin are not less than 3000 and not more than 1.6, respectively.

System repeatability: When the test is repeated 6 times with 100 μL of the standard solution under the above operating conditions, the relative standard deviation of the peak area of silodosin is not more than 2.0%.

Assay Conduct this procedure using light-resistant vessels. To 20 tablets of Silodosin Orally Disintegrating Tablets add $3V/5$ mL of a mixture of methanol and a solution of sodium chloride (1 in 200) (7:3), and sonicate until the tablet is completely disintegrated while occasional shaking. Add a mixture of methanol and a solution of sodium chloride (1 in 200) (7:3) to make exactly V mL so that each mL contains about 160 μg of silodosin ($C_{25}H_{32}F_3N_3O_4$). Pipet 5 mL of this solution, add a mixture of methanol and a solution of sodium chloride (1 in 200) (7:3) to make exactly 20 mL, and filter through a membrane filter with a pore size not exceeding 0.45 μm. Discard the first 3 mL of the filtrate, and use the subsequent filtrate as the sample solution. Separately, weigh accurately about 20 mg of Silodosin RS (separately determine the water ⟨*2.48*⟩ in the same manner as Silodosin), and dissolve in a mixture of methanol and a solution of sodium chloride (1 in 200) (7:3) to make exactly 50 mL. Pipet 5 mL of this solution, add a mixture of methanol and a solution of sodium chloride (1 in 200) (7:3) to make exactly 50 mL, and use this solution as the standard solution. Perform the test with exactly 10 μL each of the sample solution and standard solution as directed under Liquid Chromatography ⟨*2.01*⟩ according to the following conditions, and determine the peak areas, A_T and A_S, of silodosin in each solution.

Amount (mg) of silodosin ($C_{25}H_{32}F_3N_3O_4$) in 1 tablet
$= M_S \times A_T/A_S \times V/2500$

M_S: Amount (mg) of Silodosin RS taken, calculated on the anhydrous basis

Operating conditions—

Detector: An ultraviolet absorption photometer (wavelength: 270 nm).

Column: A stainless steel column 4.6 mm in inside diameter and 15 cm in length, packed with octadecylsilanized silica gel for liquid chromatography (5 μm in particle diameter).

Column temperature: A constant temperature of about 40°C.

Mobile phase: Dissolve 3.9 g of sodium dihydrogen phosphate dihydrate in 1000 mL of water, and adjust to pH 3.4 with diluted phosphoric acid (1 in 10). To 730 mL of this solution add 270 mL of acetonitrile.

Flow rate: Adjust so that the retention time of silodosin is about 6 minutes.

System suitability—

System performance: When the procedure is run with 10 μL of the standard solution under the above operating conditions, the number of theoretical plates and the symmetry factor of the peak of silodosin are not less than 3000 and not more than 1.6, respectively.

System repeatability: When the test is repeated 6 times with 10 μL of the standard solution under the above operating conditions, the relative standard deviation of the peak area of silodosin is not more than 1.0%.

Containers and storage Containers—Tight containers.

Storage—Light-resistant.

Others

Related substance A: Refer to it described in Silodosin.

Silodosin Tablets

シロドシン錠

Silodosin Tablets contain not less than 95.0% and not more than 105.0% of the labeled amount of silodosin ($C_{25}H_{32}F_3N_3O_4$: 495.53).

Method of preparation Prepare as directed under Tablets, with Silodosin.

Identification Conduct this procedure using light-resistant vessels. To an amount of powdered Silodosin Tablets, equivalent to 2 mg of Silodosin, add a mixture of methanol and a solution of sodium chloride (1 in 200) (7:3), sonicate with occasional shaking, then add a mixture of methanol and a solution of sodium chloride (1 in 200) (7:3) to make 50 mL, and filter through a membrane filter with a pore size not exceeding 0.45 μm. Discard the first 3 mL of the filtrate, and use the subsequent filtrate as the sample solution. Separately, dissolve 20 mg of Silodosin RS in a mixture of methanol and a solution of sodium chloride (1 in 200) (7:3) to make 50 mL. To 5 mL of this solution add a mixture of methanol and a solution of sodium chloride (1 in 200) (7:3) to make 50 mL, and use this solution as the standard solution. Perform the test with 25 μL each of the sample solution and standard solution as directed under Liquid Chromatography <*2.01*> according to the following conditions: the retention times of the principal peaks in the chromatograms obtained from these solutions are the same, and the absorption spectra of these peaks exhibit similar intensities of absorption at the same wavelengths.

Operating conditions—

Column, column temperature, mobile phase, and flow rate: Proceed as directed in the operating conditions in the Assay under Silodosin.

Detector: A photodiode array detector (wavelength: 270 nm, spectrum measuring range: 220 – 370 nm).

System suitability—

System performance: When the procedure is run with 25 μL of the standard solution under the above operating conditions, the number of theoretical plates and the symmetry factor of the peak of silodosin are not less than 3000 and not more than 1.6, respectively.

Purity Related substances—Conduct this procedure using light-resistant vessels. Powder not less than 10 Silodosin Tablets. To a portion of the powder, equivalent to 20 mg of Silodosin, add a mixture of methanol and a solution of sodium chloride (1 in 200) (7:3), sonicate with occasional shaking, and add a mixture of methanol and a solution of sodium chloride (1 in 200) (7:3) to make 100 mL. Centrifuge this solution, and filter the supernatant liquid through a membrane filter with a pore size not exceeding 0.45 μm. Discard the first 3 mL of the filtrate, and use the subsequent filtrate as the sample solution. Pipet 1 mL of the sample solution, add a mixture of methanol and a solution of sodium chloride (1 in 200) (7:3) to make exactly 100 mL, and use this solution as the standard solution. Perform the test with exactly 25 μL each of the sample solution and standard solution as directed under Liquid Chromatography <*2.01*> according to the following conditions, and determine each peak area by the automatic integration method: the peak area of related substance A, having the relative retention time of about 1.3 to silodosin, obtained from the sample solution is not larger than the peak area of silodosin from the standard solution, the area of the peak other than silodosin and the peak mentioned above from the sample solution is not larger than 1/4 times the peak area of silodosin from the standard solution. Furthermore, the total area of the peaks other than silodosin from the sample solution is not larger than 2 times the peak area of silodosin from the standard solution. For the peak area of related substance A, multiply the correction factor 0.6.

Operating conditions—

Detector, column, column temperature, mobile phase A and mobile phase B: Proceed as directed in the operating conditions in the Purity (2) under Silodosin.

Flowing of mobile phase: Control the gradient by mixing the mobile phases A and B as directed in the following table.

Time after injection of sample (min)	Mobile phase A (vol%)	Mobile phase B (vol%)
0 – 15	75	25
15 – 47	75 → 35	25 → 65
47 – 53	35	65

Flow rate: Adjust so that the retention time of silodosin is about 13 minutes.

Time span of measurement: About 3.5 times as long as the retention time of silodosin, beginning after the solvent peak.

System suitability—

Test for required detectability: Pipet 1 mL of the standard solution, and add a mixture of methanol and a solution of sodium chloride (1 in 200) (7:3) to make exactly 20 mL. Confirm that the peak area of silodosin obtained with 25 μL of this solution is equivalent to 3.5 to 6.5% of that with 25 μL of the standard solution.

System performance: Thinly spread out an amount of silodosin in a petri dish, exposure it to a 4000 lx light for not less than 24 hours using a D_{65} lamp, and dissolve 4 mg of this sample in a mixture of methanol and a solution of sodium chloride (1 in 200) (7:3) to make 20 mL. When the procedure is run with 25 μL of this solution under the above operating conditions, the resolution between the peak of silodosin and related substance A is not less than 6.

System repeatability: When the test is repeated 6 times with 25 μL of the standard solution under the above operating conditions, the relative standard deviation of the peak area of silodosin is not more than 2.5%.

Uniformity of dosage units <*6.02*> Perform the test according to the following method: it meets the requirement of the Content uniformity test.

Conduct this procedure using light-resistant vessels. To 1 tablet of Silodosin Tablets add exactly $2V/25$ mL of the internal standard solution, then add a suitable amount of a mixture of methanol and a solution of sodium chloride (1 in 200) (7:3), sonicate until the tablet is completely disintegrated with occasional stirring, and add a mixture of methanol and a solution of sodium chloride (1 in 200) (7:3) to make V mL so that each mL contains about 40 μg of silodosin ($C_{25}H_{32}F_3N_3O_4$), and filter through a membrane filter with a pore size not exceeding 0.45 μm. Discard the first 3 mL of the filtrate, and use the subsequent filtrate as the sample solution. Separately, weigh accurately about 20 mg of Silodosin RS (separately determine the water <*2.48*> in the same manner as Silodosin), and dissolve in a mixture of methanol and a solution of sodium chloride (1 in 200) (7:3) to make exactly 50 mL. Pipet 5 mL of this solution, add exactly 4 mL of the internal standard solution, then add a mixture of methanol and a solution of sodium chloride (1 in 200) (7:3) to make 50 mL, and use this solution as the standard solution. Perform the test with 25 μL each of the sample solution and standard solution as directed under Liquid Chromatography <*2.01*> according to the following conditions, and calculate the ratios, Q_T and Q_S, of the peak area of silodosin to that of the internal standard.

$$\text{Amount (mg) of silodosin } (C_{25}H_{32}F_3N_3O_4) = M_S \times Q_T/Q_S \times V/500$$

M_S: Amount (mg) of Silodosin RS taken, calculated on the anhydrous basis

Internal standard solution—A solution of ethyl parahydroxybenzoate in a mixture of methanol and a solution of sodium chloride (1 in 200) (7:3) (1 in 8000).

Operating conditions—

Proceed as directed in the operating conditions in the Assay under Silodosin.

System suitability—

Proceed as directed in the system suitability in the Assay.

Dissolution <*6.10*> When the test is performed at 50 revolutions per minute according to the Paddle method, using 900 mL of water as the dissolution medium, the dissolution rate in 15 minutes of Silodosin Tablets is not less than 80%.

Start the test with 1 tablet of Silodosin Tablets, withdraw not less than 9 mL of the medium at the specified minute after starting the test, and filter through a membrane filter with a pore size not exceeding 0.45 μm. Discard not less than 5 mL of the first filtrate, pipet V mL of the subsequent filtrate, add 0.2 mol/L hydrochloric acid TS to make exactly V' mL so that each mL contains about 1.1 μg of silodosin ($C_{25}H_{32}F_3N_3O_4$), and use this solution as the sample solution. Separately, weigh accurately about 22 mg of Silodosin RS (separately determine the water *<2.48>* in the same manner as Silodosin), and dissolve in 0.1 mol/L hydrochloric acid TS to make exactly 100 mL. Pipet 5 mL of this solution, add 0.1 mol/L hydrochloric acid TS to make exactly 50 mL. Pipet 5 mL of this solution, add 0.1 mol/L hydrochloric acid TS to make exactly 100 mL, and use this solution as the standard solution. Perform the test with exactly 100 μL each of the sample solution and standard solution as directed under Liquid Chromatography *<2.01>* according to the following conditions, and determine the peak areas, A_T and A_S, of silodosin in each solution.

Dissolution rate (%) with respect to the labeled amount of silodosin ($C_{25}H_{32}F_3N_3O_4$)
$= M_S \times A_T/A_S \times V'/V \times 1/C \times 9/2$

M_S: Amount (mg) of Silodosin RS taken, calculated on the anhydrous basis
C: Labeled amount (mg) of silodosin ($C_{25}H_{32}F_3N_3O_4$) in 1 tablet

Operating conditions—

Proceed as directed in the operating conditions in the Assay under Silodosin.

System suitability—

System performance: When the procedure is run with 100 μL of the standard solution under the above operating conditions, the number of theoretical plates and the symmetry factor of the peak of silodosin are not less than 3000 and not more than 1.6, respectively.

System repeatability: When the test is repeated 6 times with 100 μL of the standard solution under the above operating conditions, the relative standard deviation of the peak area of silodosin is not more than 2.0%.

Assay Conduct this procedure using light-resistant vessels. Weigh accurately the mass of not less than 20 Silodosin Tablets, and powder. Weigh accurately a portion of the powder, equivalent to about 40 mg of silodosin ($C_{25}H_{32}F_3N_3O_4$), add exactly 8 mL of the internal standard solution, then add a suitable amount of a mixture of methanol and a solution of sodium chloride (1 in 200) (7:3), sonicate with occasional shaking, and add a mixture of methanol and a solution of sodium chloride (1 in 200) (7:3) to make 100 mL. To 5 mL of this solution add a mixture of methanol and a solution of sodium chloride (1 in 200) (7:3) to make 50 mL, and filter through a membrane filter with a pore size not exceeding 0.45 μm. Discard the first 3 mL of the filtrate, and use the subsequent filtrate as the sample solution. Separately, weigh accurately about 20 mg of Silodosin RS (separately determine the water *<2.48>* in the same manner as Silodosin), add exactly 4 mL of the internal standard solution and a mixture of methanol and a solution of sodium chloride (1 in 200) (7:3) to make 50 mL. To 5 mL of this solution add a mixture of methanol and a solution of sodium chloride (1 in 200) (7:3) to make 50 mL, and use this solution as the standard solution. Perform the test with 25 μL each of the sample solution and standard solution as directed under Liquid Chromatography *<2.01>* according to the following conditions, and calculate the ratios, Q_T and Q_S, of the peak area of silodosin to that of the internal standard.

Amount (mg) of silodosin ($C_{25}H_{32}F_3N_3O_4$)
$= M_S \times Q_T/Q_S \times 2$

M_S: Amount (mg) of Silodosin RS taken, calculated on the anhydrous basis

Internal standard solution—A solution of ethyl parahydroxybenzoate in a mixture of methanol and a sodium chloride solution (1 in 200) (7:3) (1 in 800).

Operating conditions—

Proceed as directed in the operating conditions the Assay under Silodosin.

System suitability—

System performance: When the procedure is run with 25 μL of the standard solution under the above operating conditions, silodosin and the internal standard are eluted in this order with the resolution between these peaks being not less than 10.

System repeatability: When the test is repeated 6 times with 25 μL of the standard solution under the above operating conditions, the relative standard deviation of the ratio of the peak area of silodosin to that of the internal standard is not more than 1.0%.

Containers and storage Containers—Tight containers.
Storage—Light-resistant.

Others

Related substance A: Refer to it described in Silodosin.

Silver Nitrate

硝酸銀

$AgNO_3$: 169.87

Silver Nitrate, when dried, contains not less than 99.8% of silver nitrate ($AgNO_3$).

Description Silver Nitrate occurs as lustrous, colorless or white crystals.

It is very soluble in water, soluble in ethanol (95), and practically insoluble in diethyl ether.

It gradually turns grayish black by light.

Identification A solution of Silver Nitrate (1 in 50) responds to Qualitative Tests *<1.09>* for silver salt and for nitrate.

Purity **(1)** Clarity and color of solution, and acidity or alkalinity—Dissolve 1.0 g of Silver Nitrate in 10 mL of freshly boiled and cooled water: the solution is clear and colorless. It is neutral.

(2) Bismuth, copper and lead—To 5 mL of a solution of Silver Nitrate (1 in 10) add 3 mL of ammonia TS: the solution is clear and colorless.

Loss on drying *<2.41>* Not more than 0.20% (2 g, silica gel, light resistant, 4 hours).

Assay Weigh accurately about 0.7 g of Silver Nitrate, previously powdered and dried, dissolve in 50 mL of water, add 2 mL of nitric acid, and titrate *<2.50>* with 0.1 mol/L ammonium thiocyanate VS (indicator: 2 mL of ammonium iron (III) sulfate TS).

Each mL of 0.1 mol/L ammonium thiocyanate VS
$= 16.99$ mg of $AgNO_3$

Containers and storage Containers—Tight containers.
Storage—Light-resistant.

Silver Nitrate Ophthalmic Solution

硝酸銀点眼液

Silver Nitrate Ophthalmic Solution is an aqueous ophthalmic preparation.

It contains not less than 0.95 w/v% and not more than 1.05 w/v% of silver nitrate ($AgNO_3$: 169.87).

Method of preparation

Silver Nitrate	10 g
Purified Water or Purified Water in Containers	a sufficient quantity
To make	1000 mL

Prepare as directed under Ophthalmic Liquids and Solutions, with the above ingredients.

Description Silver Nitrate Ophthalmic Solution is a clear, colorless liquid.

Identification Silver Nitrate Ophthalmic Solution responds to Qualitative Tests *<1.09>* for silver salt and for nitrate.

Assay Measure accurately 20 mL of Silver Nitrate Ophthalmic Solution, add 30 mL of water and 2 mL of nitric acid, and titrate *<2.50>* with 0.1 mol/L ammonium thiocyanate VS (indicator: 2 mL of ammonium iron (III) sulfate TS).

Each mL of 0.1 mol/L ammonium thiocyanate VS
= 16.99 mg of $AgNO_3$

Containers and storage Containers—Tight containers.
Storage—Light-resistant.

Silver Protein

プロテイン銀

Silver Protein is a compound of silver and proteins.

It contains not less than 7.5% and not more than 8.5% of silver (Ag: 107.87).

Description Silver Protein occurs as a light yellow-brown to brown powder. It is odorless.

It (1 g) dissolves slowly in 2 mL of water. It is practically insoluble in ethanol (95), in diethyl ether and in chloroform.

The pH of a solution of 1.0 g of Silver Protein in 10 mL of water is between 7.0 and 8.5.

It is slightly hygroscopic.

It is affected by light.

Identification **(1)** To 10 mL of a solution of Silver Protein (1 in 100) add 2 mL of dilute hydrochloric acid, shake frequently for 5 minutes, and filter. To the filtrate add 5 mL of a solution of sodium hydroxide (1 in 10), and add 2 mL of diluted copper (II) sulfate TS (2 in 25): a purple color develops.

(2) To 5 mL of a solution of Silver Protein (1 in 100) add dropwise iron (III) chloride TS: the color of the solution fades and a precipitate is gradually formed.

(3) Incinerate 0.2 g of Silver Protein by strong heating, dissolve the residue in 1 mL of nitric acid by warming, and add 10 mL of water: this solution responds to Qualitative Tests *<1.09>* (1) for silver salt.

Purity Silver salt—Dissolve 0.10 g of Silver Protein in 10 mL of water, and filter. To the filtrate add 1 mL of potassium chromate TS: no turbidity is produced.

Assay Transfer about 1 g of Silver Protein, accurately weighed, to a 100-mL decomposition flask, add 10 mL of sulfuric acid, cover the flask with a funnel, and boil for 5 minutes. Cool, add dropwise 3 mL of nitric acid with caution, and heat for 30 minutes without boiling. Cool, add 1 mL of nitric acid, boil, and, if necessary, repeat this operation until the solution becomes colorless. After cooling, transfer the solution to a 250-mL conical flask with 100 mL of water, and titrate *<2.50>* with 0.1 mol/L ammonium thiocyanate VS (indicator: 3 mL of ammonium iron (III) sulfate TS).

Each mL of 0.1 mol/L ammonium thiocyanate VS
= 10.79 mg of Ag

Containers and storage Containers—Tight containers.
Storage—Light-resistant.

Silver Protein Solution

プロテイン銀液

Silver Protein Solution contains not less than 0.22 w/v% and not more than 0.26 w/v% of silver (Ag: 107.87).

Method of preparation

Silver Protein	30 g
Glycerin	100 mL
Mentha Water	a sufficient quantity
To make	1000 mL

Dissolve and mix the above ingredients.

Description Silver Protein Solution is a clear, brown liquid, having the odor of mentha oil.

Identification **(1)** To 1 mL of Silver Protein Solution add 10 mL of ethanol (95), mix, and add 2 mL of sodium hydroxide TS. Add immediately 1 mL of a solution of copper (II) chloride dihydrate in ethanol (95) (1 in 10), shake, and filter: the filtrate is blue in color (glycerin).

(2) To 3 mL of Silver Protein Solution add water to make 10 mL, add 2 mL of dilute hydrochloric acid, shake frequently for 5 minutes, and filter. Add 5 mL of a solution of sodium hydroxide (1 in 10) to the filtrate, and add 2 mL of diluted copper (II) sulfate TS (2 in 25): a purple color develops (silver protein).

(3) To 5 mL of the sample solution obtained in (2) add iron (III) chloride TS dropwise: a brown precipitate is formed (silver protein).

(4) Place 3 mL of Silver Protein Solution in a crucible, heat cautiously, and evaporate almost to dryness. Then incinerate gradually by strong heating, dissolve the residue in 1 mL of nitric acid by warming, and add 10 mL of water: the solution responds to Qualitative Tests *<1.09>* (1) for silver salt.

Assay Pipet 25 mL of Silver Protein Solution into a 250-mL Kjeldahl flask, and heat cautiously until a white gas of glycerin is evolved. After cooling, add 25 mL of sulfuric acid, cover the flask with a funnel, and heat gently for 5 minutes. After cooling, drop gradually 5 mL of nitric acid, heat with occasional shaking in a water bath for 45 minutes, and cool. Add 2 mL of nitric acid, boil gently, and repeat this operation until the solution becomes colorless upon cooling. Transfer cautiously the cooled content in the flask into a 500-mL conical flask with 250 mL of water. Boil gently for 5 minutes, cool, and titrate <*2.50*> with 0.1 mol/L ammonium thiocyanate VS (indicator: 3 mL of ammonium iron (III) sulfate TS).

Each mL of 0.1 mol/L ammonium thiocyanate VS
= 10.79 mg of Ag

Containers and storage Containers—Tight containers.
Storage—Light-resistant.

Simple Syrup

単シロップ

Simple Syrup is an aqueous solution of Sucrose.

Method of preparation

Sucrose	850 g
Purified Water or Purified Water in Containers	a sufficient quantity
	To make 1000 mL

Prepare as directed under Syrups, with the above materials.

Description Simple Syrup is a clear, colorless to pale yellow, viscous liquid. It is odorless and has a sweet taste.

Identification (1) Evaporate Simple Syrup on a water bath to dryness. 1 g of the residue so obtained, when ignited, melts to swell, and decomposes, emitting an odor of caramel, to bulky charcoal.

(2) To 0.1 g of the residue obtained in (1) add 2 mL of dilute sulfuric acid, boil, add 4 mL of sodium hydroxide TS and 3 mL of Fehling's TS, and heat to boiling: a red to dark red precipitate is produced.

Specific gravity <*2.56*> d_{20}^{20}: 1.310 – 1.325

Purity (1) Artificial sweetening agents—To 100 mL of Simple Syrup add 100 mL of water, shake, acidify a 50-mL portion of the solution with dilute sulfuric acid, and make another 50-mL portion alkaline with sodium hydroxide TS. To each portion add 100 mL of diethyl ether, shake, separate the diethyl ether layer, and evaporate the combined diethyl ether extract on a water bath to dryness: the residue has no sweet taste.

(2) Salicylic acid—To the residue obtained in (1) add 2 to 3 drops of dilute iron (III) chloride TS: no purple color develops.

Containers and storage Containers—Tight containers.

Simvastatin

シンバスタチン

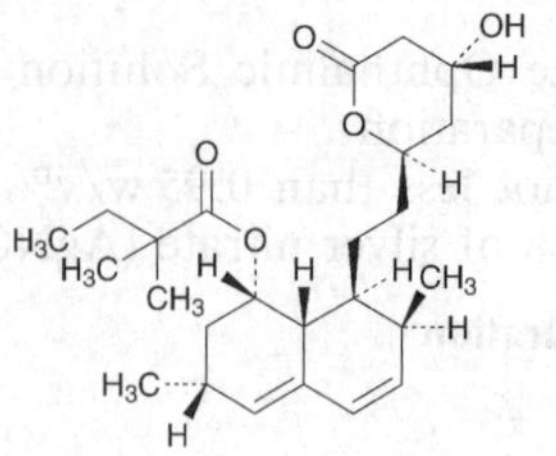

$C_{25}H_{38}O_5$: 418.57
(1*S*,3*R*,7*S*,8*S*,8a*R*)-8-{2-[(2*R*,4*R*)-4-Hydroxy-6-oxotetrahydro-2*H*-pyran-2-yl]ethyl}-3,7-dimethyl-1,2,3,7,8,8a-hexahydronaphthalen-1-yl 2,2-dimethylbutanoate
[*79902-63-9*]

Simvastatin contains not less than 98.0% and not more than 101.0% of simvastatin ($C_{25}H_{38}O_5$), calculated on the dried basis.

It may contain a suitable antioxidant.

Description Simvastatin occurs as a white crystalline powder.

It is freely soluble in acetonitrile, in methanol and in ethanol (99.5), and practically insoluble in water.

Identification (1) Determine the absorption spectrum of a solution of Simvastatin in acetonitrile (1 in 100,000) as directed under Ultraviolet-visible Spectrophotometry <*2.24*> and compare the spectrum with the Reference Spectrum or the spectrum of a solution of Simvastatin RS prepared in the same manner as the sample solution: both spectra exhibit similar intensities of absorption at the same wavelengths.

(2) Determine the infrared absorption spectrum of Simvastatin as directed in the potassium bromide disk method under Infrared Spectrophotometry <*2.25*>, and compare the spectrum with the Reference Spectrum or the spectrum of Simvastatin RS: both spectra exhibit similar intensities of absorption at the same wave numbers.

Optical rotation <*2.49*> $[\alpha]_D^{20}$: +285 – +300° (50 mg calculated on the dried basis, acetonitrile, 10 mL, 100 mm).

Purity (1) Clarity and color of solution—Dissolve 1 g of Simvastatin in 10 mL of methanol: the solution is clear. Perform the test with this solution as directed under Ultraviolet-visible Spectrophotometry <*2.24*>: the absorbance at 440 nm is not more than 0.10.

(2) Heavy metals <*1.07*>—To 1.0 g of Simvastatin add 2 mL of sulfuric acid, and heat gently to carbonize. After cooling, add 2 mL of nitric acid and 1 mL of sulfuric acid, heat gently until the white fumes no more evolve, and heat to incinerate at 500 to 600°C. If the incineration is not accomplished, add 0.5 mL of nitric acid, heat in the same manner as above, and ignite at 500 to 600°C to incinerate completely. After cooling, add 2 mL of hydrochloric acid, proceed with this solution according to Method 2, and perform the test. Prepare the control solution by using the same quantities of the same reagents as directed for the preparation of the test solution, and add 2.0 mL of Standard Lead solution and water to make 50 mL (not more than 20 ppm).

(3) Related substances—Dissolve 30 mg of Simvastatin in 20 mL of a mixture of acetonitrile and 0.01 mol/L potassium dihydrogen phosphate TS (pH 4.0) (3:2), and use this solution as the sample solution. Perform the test with 5 μL of the sample solution as directed under Liquid Chromatography <*2.01*> according to the following conditions. Determine each peak area from the sample solution by the automatic integration method, and calculate the amount of them by the area percentage method: the amounts of the peaks, having the relative retention times of about 0.45, about 0.80, about 2.42, and about 3.80 to simvastatin are not more than 0.2%, respectively; the amount of the peak, having a relative retention time of about 2.38 is not more than 0.3%; the amount of the peak, having a relative retention time of about 0.60 is not more than 0.4%; and the amount of each peak other than simvastatin and the peaks mentioned above is not more than 0.1%. Furthermore, the total amount of the peaks other than simvastatin and the peak with relative retention time of about 0.60 is not more than 1.0%.

Operating conditions—

Detector, column, and column temperature: Proceed as directed in the operating conditions in the Assay.

Mobile phase A: A mixture of diluted phosphoric acid (1 in 1000) and acetonitrile for liquid chromatography (1:1).

Mobile phase B: A solution of phosphoric acid in acetonitrile for liquid chromatography (1 in 1000).

Flowing of mobile phase: Control the gradient by mixing the mobile phases A and B as directed in the following table.

Time after injection of sample (min)	Mobile phase A (vol%)	Mobile phase B (vol%)
0 – 4.5	100	0
4.5 – 4.6	100 → 95	0 → 5
4.6 – 8.0	95 → 25	5 → 75
8.0 – 11.5	25	75

Flow rate: 3.0 mL per minute.

Time span of measurement: About 5 times as long as the retention time of simvastatin.

System suitability—

System performance: Proceed as directed in the system suitability in the Assay.

Test for required detectability: To 0.5 mL of the sample solution, add a mixture of acetonitrile and 0.01 mol/L potassium dihydrogen phosphate TS (pH 4.0) (3:2), to make 100 mL, and use this solution as the solution for system suitability test. Pipet 2 mL of the solution for system suitability test, add a mixture of acetonitrile and 0.01 mol/L potassium dihydrogen phosphate TS (pH 4.0) (3:2), to make exactly 10 mL. Confirm that the peak area of simvastatin obtained with 5 μL of this solution is equivalent to 16 to 24% of that with 5 μL of the solution for system suitability test.

System repeatability: When the test is repeated 6 times with 5 μL of the solution for system suitability test under the above conditions, the relative standard deviation of the peak area of simvastatin is not more than 1.0%.

Loss on drying <*2.41*> Not more than 0.5% (1 g, in vacuum not exceeding 0.67 kPa, 60°C, 3 hours).

Residue on ignition <*2.44*> Not more than 0.1% (1 g).

Assay Weigh accurately about 30 mg each of Simvastatin and Simvastatin RS (previously determine the loss on drying <*2.41*> under the same conditions as Simvastatin), dissolve each in a mixture of acetonitrile and 0.01 mol/L potassium dihydrogen phosphate TS (pH 4.0) (3:2), to make exactly 20 mL, and use these solutions as the sample solution and the standard solution, respectively. Perform the test with exactly 5 μL each of the sample solution and standard solution as directed under Liquid Chromatography <*2.01*> according to the following conditions, and determine the peak areas, A_T and A_S, of simvastatin in each solution.

$$\text{Amount (mg) of simvastatin } (C_{25}H_{38}O_5) = M_S \times A_T/A_S$$

M_S: Amount (mg) of Simvastatin RS taken, calculated on the dried basis

Operating conditions—

Detector: An ultraviolet absorption photometer (wavelength: 238 nm).

Column: A stainless steel column 4.6 mm in inside diameter and 33 mm in length, packed with octadecylsilanized silica gel for liquid chromatography (3 μm in particle diameter).

Column temperature: A constant temperature of about 25°C.

Mobile phase: A mixture of diluted phosphoric acid (1 in 1000) and acetonitrile for liquid chromatography (1:1).

Flow rate: Adjust so that the retention time of simvastatin is about 3 minutes.

System suitability—

System performance: Dissolve 3 mg of lovastatin in 2 mL of the standard solution. When the procedure is run with 5 μL of this solution under the above operating conditions, lovastatin and simvastatin are eluted in this order with the resolution between these peaks being not less than 3.

System repeatability: When the test is repeated 6 times with 5 μL of the standard solution under the above operating conditions, the relative standard deviation of the peak area of simvastatin is not more than 1.0%.

Containers and storage Containers—Tight containers.

Storage—Under nitrogen atmosphere.

Simvastatin Tablets

シンバスタチン錠

Simvastatin Tablets contain not less than 93.0% and not more than 107.0% of the labeled amount of simvastatin ($C_{25}H_{38}O_5$: 418.57).

Method of preparation Prepare as directed under Tablets, with Simvastatin.

Identification To an amount of powdered Simvastatin Tablets, equivalent to about 2.5 mg of Simvastatin, add 25 mL of acetonitrile, sonicate for 15 minutes, and centrifuge. To 2 mL of the supernatant liquid add acetonitrile to make 20 mL. Determine the absorption spectrum of this solution as directed under Ultraviolet-visible Spectrophotometry <*2.24*>: it exhibits maxima between 229 nm and 233 nm, between 236 nm and 240 nm, and between 245 nm and 249 nm.

Purity Related substances—Powder not less than 20 Simvastatin Tablets. To a portion of the powder, equivalent to about 50 mg of Simvastatin, add 200 mL of a mixture of acetonitrile and 0.05 mol/L acetate buffer solution (pH 4.0) (4:1), and sonicate for 15 minutes. After cooling, add the same mixture to make 250 mL, and centrifuge. To 5 mL of the supernatant liquid add the same mixture to make 10 mL, and use this solution as the sample solution. Pipet 1 mL of the sample solution, add a mixture of acetonitrile and 0.05 mol/L acetate buffer solution (pH 4.0) (4:1) to make exactly 200 mL, and use this solution as the standard solution. Perform the test with exactly 10 μL each of the sample solution and standard solution as directed under Liquid Chromatography <2.01> according to the following conditions. Determine each peak area by the automatic integration method: the area of the peak, having the relative retention time of about 0.5 to simvastatin obtained from the sample solution is not larger than 1.6 times the peak area of simvastatin from the standard solution, the area of the peak having the relative retention time of about 2.0 from the sample solution is not larger than the peak area of simvastatin from the standard solution, and the total area of the peaks other than simvastatin is not larger than 4 times the peak area of simvastatin from the standard solution.

Operating conditions—

Detector, column, column temperature, mobile phase, and flow rate: Proceed as directed in the operating conditions in the Assay.

Time span of measurement: About 2.5 times as long as the retention time of simvastatin, beginning after the solvent peak.

System suitability—

Test for required detectability: Pipet 2 mL of the standard solution, and add the mobile phase to make exactly 10 mL. Confirm that the peak area of simvastatin obtained with 10 μL of this solution is equivalent to 14 to 26% of that with 10 μL of the standard solution.

System performance: When the procedure is run with 10 μL of the standard solution under the above operating conditions, the number of theoretical plates and the symmetry factor of the peak of simvastatin are not less than 6000 and 0.9 – 1.1, respectively.

System repeatability: When the test is repeated 6 times with 10 μL of the standard solution under the above operating conditions, the relative standard deviation of the peak area of simvastatin is not more than 2.0%.

Uniformity of dosage units <6.02> Perform the test according to the following method: it meets the requirement of the Content uniformity test.

To 1 tablet of Simvastatin Tablets add $V/20$ mL of water, and disintegrate the tablet by sonicating. Add a mixture of acetonitrile and 0.05 mol/L acetate buffer solution (pH 4.0) (4:1) to make $3V/4$ mL, and sonicate for 15 minutes. After cooling, add the same mixture to make exactly V mL so that each mL contains about 0.1 mg of simvastatin ($C_{25}H_{38}O_5$), centrifuge, and use the supernatant liquid as the sample solution. Then, proceed as directed in the Assay.

$$\text{Amount (mg) of simvastatin } (C_{25}H_{38}O_5) = M_S \times A_T/A_S \times V/200$$

M_S: Amount (mg) of Simvastatin RS taken, calculated on the dried basis

Dissolution <6.10> When the test is performed at 50 revolutions per minute according to the Paddle method, using 900 mL of a solution of polysorbate 80, prepared by dissolving 3 g in water to make 1000 mL, as the dissolution medium, the dissolution rate in 45 minutes of Simvastatin Tablets is not less than 70%.

Start the test with 1 tablet of Simvastatin Tablets, withdraw not less than 10 mL of the medium at the specified minute after starting the test, and filter through a membrane filter with a pore size not exceeding 0.45 μm. Discard not less than 5 mL of the first filtrate, pipet V mL of the subsequent filtrate, add water to make exactly V' mL so that each mL contains about 5.6 μg of simvastatin ($C_{25}H_{38}O_5$), and use this solution as the sample solution. Separately, weigh accurately about 22 mg of Simvastatin RS (separately determine the loss on drying <2.41> under the same conditions as Simvastatin), and dissolve in acetonitrile to make exactly 100 mL. Pipet 5 mL of this solution, add the mobile phase to make exactly 200 mL, and use this solution as the standard solution. Perform the test with exactly 20 μL each of the sample solution and standard solution as directed under Liquid Chromatography <2.01>, according to the following conditions, and determine the peak areas, A_T and A_S, of simvastatin in each solution.

$$\text{Dissolution rate (\%) with respect to the labeled amount of simvastatin } (C_{25}H_{38}O_5) = M_S \times A_T/A_S \times V'/V \times 1/C \times 45/2$$

M_S: Amount (mg) of Simvastatin RS taken, calculated on the dried basis

C: Labeled amount (mg) of simvastatin ($C_{25}H_{38}O_5$) in 1 tablet

Operating conditions—

Detector: An ultraviolet absorption photometer (wavelength: 238 nm).

Column: A stainless steel column 3.9 mm in inside diameter and 15 cm in length, packed with octadecylsilanized silica gel for liquid chromatography (5 μm in particle diameter).

Column temperature: A constant temperature of about 50°C.

Mobile phase: A mixture of methanol and 0.02 mol/L potassium dihydrogen phosphate TS (4:1).

Flow rate: Adjust so that the retention time of simvastatin is about 4 minutes.

System suitability—

System performance: When the procedure is run with 20 μL of the standard solution under the above operating conditions, the number of theoretical plates and the symmetry factor of the peak of simvastatin are not less than 3000 and not more than 2.0, respectively.

System repeatability: When the test is repeated 6 times with 20 μL of the standard solution under the above operating conditions, the relative standard deviation of the peak area of simvastatin is not more than 1.0%.

Assay Weigh accurately the mass of not less than 20 Simvastatin Tablets, and powder. Weigh accurately a portion of the powder, equivalent to about 50 mg of simvastatin ($C_{25}H_{38}O_5$), add 200 mL of a mixture of acetonitrile and 0.05 mol/L acetate buffer solution (pH 4.0) (4:1), and sonicate for 15 minutes. After cooling, add the same mixture to make exactly 250 mL, and centrifuge. Pipet 5 mL of the supernatant liquid, add the same mixture to make exactly 10 mL, and use this solution as the sample solution. Separately, weigh accurately about 20 mg of Simvastatin RS (separately determine the loss on drying <2.41> under the same conditions as Simvastatin), dissolve in a mixture of acetonitrile and 0.05 mol/L acetate buffer solution (pH 4.0) (4:1) to make exactly 200 mL, and use this solution as the standard solution. Perform the test as directed under Liquid Chromatography <2.01> according to the following conditions, and determine the peak areas, A_T and A_S, of simvastatin in each solution.

$$\text{Amount (mg) of simvastatin } (C_{25}H_{38}O_5) = M_S \times A_T/A_S \times 5/2$$

M_S: Amount (mg) of Simvastatin RS taken, calculated on the dried basis

Operating conditions—

Detector: An ultraviolet absorption photometer (wavelength: 238 nm).

Column: A stainless steel column 4.6 mm in inside diame-

ter and 25 cm in length, packed with octadecylsilanized silica gel for liquid chromatography (5 μm in particle diameter).

Column temperature: A constant temperature of about 45°C.

Mobile phase: Dissolve 3.90 g of sodium dihydrogen phosphate dihydrate in 900 mL of water, adjust to pH 4.5 with sodium hydroxide TS or phosphoric acid, and add water to make 1000 mL. To 700 mL of this solution add 1300 mL of acetonitrile.

Flow rate: Adjust so that the retention time of simvastatin is about 9 minutes.

System suitability—

System performance: When the procedure is run with 10 μL of the standard solution under the above operating conditions, the number of theoretical plates and the symmetry factor of the peak of simvastatin are not less than 6000 and 0.9 – 1.1, respectively.

System repeatability: When the test is repeated 6 times with 10 μL of the standard solution under the above operating conditions, the relative standard deviation of the peak area of simvastatin is not more than 1.0%.

Containers and storage Containers—Tight containers.

Sitagliptin Phosphate Hydrate

シタグリプチンリン酸塩水和物

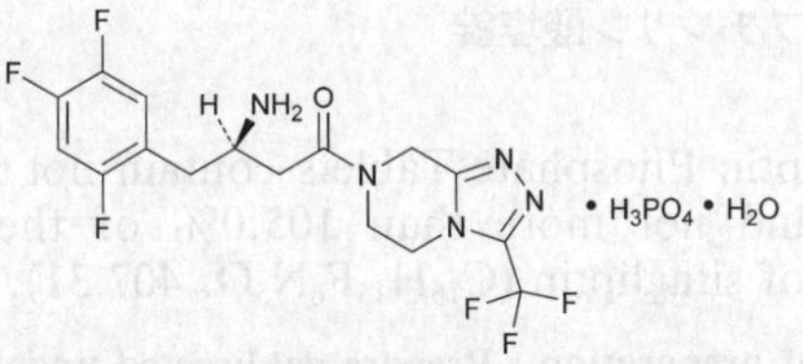

$C_{16}H_{15}F_6N_5O.H_3PO_4.H_2O$: 523.32
(3*R*)-3-Amino-1-[3-(trifluoromethyl)-5,6-dihydro[1,2,4]triazolo[4,3-*a*]pyrazin-7(8*H*)-yl]-4-(2,4,5-trifluorophenyl)butan-1-one monophosphate monohydrate
[*654671-77-9*]

Sitagliptin Phosphate Hydrate contains not less than 98.0% and not more than 102.0% of sitagliptin phosphate ($C_{16}H_{15}F_6N_5O.H_3PO_4$: 505.31), calculated on the anhydrous basis.

Description Sitagliptin Phosphate Hydrate occurs as a white powder.

It is soluble in water, sparingly soluble in methanol, very slightly soluble in acetonitrile and in ethanol (99.5).

Identification **(1)** Determine the absorption spectrum of a solution of Sitagliptin Phosphate Hydrate (1 in 10,000) as directed under Ultraviolet-visible Spectrophotometry *<2.24>*, and compare the spectrum with the Reference Spectrum or the spectrum of a solution of Sitagliptin Phosphate RS prepared in the same manner as the sample solution: both spectra exhibit similar intensities of absorption at the same wavelengths.

(2) Determine the infrared absorption spectrum of Sitagliptin Phosphate Hydrate as directed in the paste method under Infrared Spectrophotometry *<2.25>*, and compare the spectrum with the Reference Spectrum or the spectrum of Sitagliptin Phosphate RS: both spectra exhibit similar intensities of absorption at the same wave numbers. Alternatively, perform the test by the potassium bromide disk method or the ATR method, and compare the spectrum with the spectrum of Sitagliptin Phosphate RS: both spectra exhibit similar intensities of absorption at the same wave numbers.

(3) A solution of Sitagliptin Phosphate Hydrate (1 in 25) responds to Qualitative Tests *<1.09>* (1) for phosphate.

Purity **(1)** Heavy metals—Being specified separately when the drug is granted approval based on the Law.

(2) Related substances—Use the sample solution obtained in the Assay as the sample solution. Pipet 1 mL of the sample solution, add a mixture of diluted phosphoric acid (1 in 1000) and acetonitrile for liquid chromatography (19:1) to make exactly 1000 mL, and use this solution as the standard solution. Perform the test with exactly 20 μL each of the sample solution and standard solution as directed under Liquid Chromatography *<2.01>* according to the following conditions. Determine each peak area by the automatic integration method: the area of the peak other than sitagliptin obtained from the sample solution is not larger than the peak area of sitagliptin from the standard solution, and the total area of the peaks other than sitagliptin from the sample solution is not larger than 5 times the peak area of sitagliptin from the standard solution. For this calculation the peak area not larger than 1/2 times the peak area of sitagliptin from the standard solution is excluded.

Operating conditions—

Detector, column, column temperature, mobile phase and flow rate: Proceed as directed in the operating conditions in the Assay.

Time span of measurement: About 5.5 times as long as the retention time of sitagliptin, beginning after the solvent peak.

System suitability—

System performance: Proceed as directed in the system suitability in the Assay.

Test for required detectability: Pipet 5 mL of the standard solution, and add a mixture of diluted phosphoric acid (1 in 1000) and acetonitrile for liquid chromatography (19:1) to make exactly 10 mL. When the procedure is run with 20 μL of this solution under the above operating conditions, the SN ratio of the peak of sitagliptin is not less than 10.

System repeatability: When the test is repeated 6 times with 20 μL of the standard solution under the above operating conditions, the relative standard deviation of the peak area of sitagliptin is not more than 2.0%.

(3) Enantiomer—Dissolve 80 mg of Sitagliptin Phosphate Hydrate in a mixture of methanol and water (9:1) to make 10 mL, and use this solution as the sample solution. Perform the test with 10 μL of the sample solution as directed under Liquid Chromatography *<2.01>* according to the following conditions. Determine the total peak area, A_T, of sitagliptin and related substance A (enantiomer), having the relative retention time of about 0.9 to sitagliptin and the peak area, A_S, of related substance A (enantiomer), and calculate the amount of the enantiomer by the following equation: not more than 0.5%.

$$\text{Amount (\%) of enantiomer} = A_S/A_T \times 100$$

Operating conditions—

Detector: An ultraviolet absorption photometer (wavelength: 268 nm).

Column: A stainless steel column 4.6 mm in inside diameter and 25 cm in length, packed with silica gel coated with amylose tris-(3,5-dimethylphenylcarbamate) coated silica gel for liquid chromatography (5 μm in particle diameter).

Column temperature: A constant temperature of about 35°C.

The JP Drugs are to be tested according to the provisions given in the pertinent monographs, General Notices, General Rules for Crude Drugs, General Rules for Preparations, and General Tests for their conformity to the Japanese Pharmacopoeia. (See the General Notices 5.)

Mobile phase: A mixture of ethanol (99.5), heptane, water and diethylamine (600:400:1:1).

Flow rate: 0.8 mL per minute.

System suitability—

Test for required detectability: Pipet 1 mL of the sample solution, and dissolve in a mixture of methanol and water (9:1) to make exactly 100 mL. Pipet 1 mL of this solution, add a mixture of methanol and water (9:1) to make exactly 10 mL. When the procedure is run with 10 μL of this solution under the above operating conditions, the SN ratio of the peak of sitagliptin is not less than 10.

System performance: Dissolve 8 mg of Sitagliptin Phosphate for System Suitability RS in 1 mL of a mixture of methanol and water (9:1). When the procedure is run with 10 μL of this solution under the above operating conditions, the resolution between the peaks of related substance A (enantiomer) and sitagliptin is not less than 1.5.

Water 〈*2.48*〉 3.3 – 3.7% (0.3 g, volumetric titration, direct titration).

Residue on ignition 〈*2.44*〉 Not more than 0.2% (1 g, platinum crucible).

Assay Weigh accurately about 20 mg each of Sitagliptin Phosphate Hydrate and Sitagliptin Phosphate RS (separately determine the water 〈*2.48*〉 in the same manner as Sitagliptin Phosphate Hydrate), dissolve each in a mixture of diluted phosphoric acid (1 in 1000) and acetonitrile for liquid chromatography (19:1) to make exactly 200 mL, and use these solutions as the sample solution and the standard solution, respectively. Perform the test with exactly 20 μL each of the sample solution and standard solution as directed under Liquid Chromatography 〈*2.01*〉 according to the following conditions, and determine the peak areas, A_T and A_S, of sitagliptin in each solution.

Amount (mg) of sitagliptin phosphate ($C_{16}H_{15}F_6N_5O.H_3PO_4$)
$$= M_S \times A_T/A_S$$

M_S: Amount (mg) of Sitagliptin Phosphate RS taken, calculated on the anhydrous basis

Operating conditions—

Detector: An ultraviolet absorption photometer (wavelength: 205 nm).

Column: A stainless steel column 4.6 mm in inside diameter and 15 cm in length, packed with cyanopropylsilanized silica gel for liquid chromatography (5 μm in particle diameter).

Column temperature: A constant temperature of about 30°C.

Mobile phase: Dissolve 1.36 g of potassium dihydrogen phosphate in 900 mL of water, adjust to pH 2.0 with phosphoric acid, and add water to make 1000 mL. To 850 mL of this solution add 150 mL of acetonitrile for liquid chromatography.

Flow rate: 1.0 mL per minute.

System suitability—

System performance: Place 10 mg of Sitagliptin Phosphate RS and 1 mg of sodium stearyl fumarate in a vial, and add 1 mL of water. Stopper the vial tightly, and heat at 80°C for 20 to 48 hours. Take out the contents of the vial, wash the vial 3 times with a mixture of diluted phosphoric acid (1 in 1000) and acetonitrile for liquid chromatography (19:1), combine the washings and the content, and add a mixture of diluted phosphoric acid (1 in 1000) and acetonitrile for liquid chromatography (19:1) to make 100 mL. Stir this solution for 1 hour, and centrifuge for 10 minutes or until the solution becomes clear. Use the supernatant liquid as the solution for system suitability test. When the procedure is run with 20 μL of the solution for system suitability test under the above operating conditions, the resolution between sitagliptin and the peak having the relative retention time of about 1.2 to sitagliptin is not less than 1.5.

System repeatability: When the test is repeated 6 times with 20 μL of the standard solution under the above operating conditions, the relative standard deviation of the peak area of sitagliptin is not more than 1.0%.

Containers and storage Containers—Tight containers.

Others

Related substance A (enantiomer):
(3*S*)-3-Amino-1-[3-(trifluoromethyl)-5,6-dihydro[1,2,4]triazolo[4,3-*a*]pyrazin-7(8*H*)-yl]-4-(2,4,5-trifuluorophenyl)butan-1-one

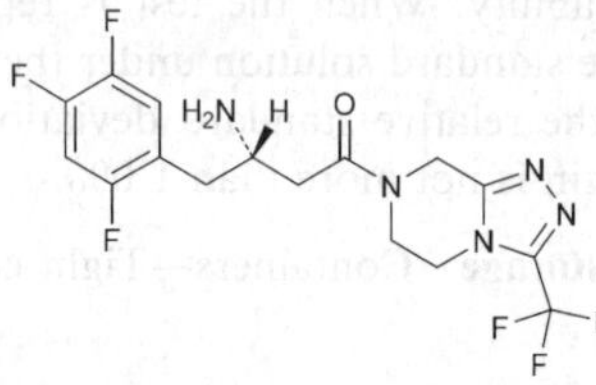

Sitagliptin Phosphate Tablets

シタグリプチンリン酸塩錠

Sitagliptin Phosphate Tablets contain not less than 95.0% and not more than 105.0% of the labeled amount of sitagliptin ($C_{16}H_{15}F_6N_5O$: 407.31).

Method of preparation Prepare as directed under Tablets, with Sitagliptin Phosphate Hydrate.

Manufacture The management strategy of Sitagliptin Phosphate Tablets is based on systematic development methods, which put emphasis on prior setting targets, understanding of products and processes, and process control, and which is based on quality risk management and proven science. In addition when it can be scientifically possible to explain that a disintegration test ensure quality with distinguishability equal or better than a dissolution test, the following disintegration is alternative for the estimation of dissolution.

Disintegration 〈*6.09*〉 Perform the test for 5 minutes: it meets the requirement.

Identification **(1)** To 1 tablet of Sitagliptin Phosphate Tablets add water so that each mL contains about 0.2 mg of sitagliptin ($C_{16}H_{15}F_6N_5O$), and shake thoroughly to disintegrate. Centrifuge this solution. Determine the absorption spectrum of the supernatant liquid as directed under Ultraviolet-visible Spectrophotometry 〈*2.24*〉: it exhibits a maximum between 265 nm and 269 nm.

(2) Perform the test with 20 μL of the sample solution and standard solution obtained in the Assay as directed under Liquid Chromatography 〈*2.01*〉 according to the operating conditions in the Assay: the retention times of the principal peaks in the chromatograms obtained from the sample solution and the standard solution are the same.

Purity Related substances—Use the sample solution obtained in the Assay as the sample solution. Separately, pipet 1 mL of the standard solution obtained in the Assay, add a mixture of diluted phosphoric acid (1 in 1000) and acetonitrile for liquid chromatography (19:1) to make exactly 500 mL, and use this solution as the standard solution. Perform the test with exactly 20 μL each of the sample solution and standard solution as directed under Liquid Chromatography <2.01> according to the following conditions. Determine the peak area, A_T, of related substance obtained from the sample solution and the peak area, A_S, of sitagliptin from the standard solution, and calculate the amount of related substances by the following equation: the total amount of related substances is not more than 0.2%. For this calculation the peak area of the related substance not more than 0.1 % is excluded.

Amount (%) of related substance
$= M_S \times A_T/A_S \times V'/V \times 1/C \times 1/50 \times 0.806$

M_S: Amount (mg) of Sitagliptin Phosphate RS taken, calculated on the anhydrous basis
V'/V: Dilution factor for the sample solution in the Assay
C: Labeled amount (mg) of sitagliptin ($C_{16}H_{15}F_6N_5O$) in 1 tablet

Operating conditions—

Detector, column, column temperature, mobile phase and flow rate: Proceed as directed in the operating conditions in the Assay.

Time span of measurement: About 5.5 times as long as the retention time of sitagliptin, beginning after the solvent peak.

System suitability—

System performance and system repeatability: Proceed as directed in the system suitability in the Assay.

Test for required detectability: To 5 mL of the standard solution add a mixture of diluted phosphoric acid (1 in 1000) and acetonitrile for liquid chromatography (19:1) to make exactly 10 mL. When the procedure is run with 20 μL of this solution under the above operating conditions, the SN ratio of the peak of sitagliptin is not less than 10.

Uniformity of dosage units <6.02> Perform the Mass variation test, or the Content uniformity test according to the following method: it meets the requirement.

To 1 tablet of Sitagliptin Phosphate Tablets add a mixture of diluted phosphoric acid (1 in 1000) and acetonitrile for liquid chromatography (19:1) to make exactly 25 mL, and stir thoroughly. Pipet V mL of this solution, and add a mixture of diluted phosphoric acid (1 in 1000) and acetonitrile for liquid chromatography (19:1) to make exactly V' mL so that each mL contains about 80 μg of sitagliptin ($C_{16}H_{15}F_6N_5O$). Centrifuge this solution, and use the supernatant liquid as the sample solution. Then, proceed as directed in the Assay.

Amount (mg) of sitagliptin ($C_{16}H_{15}F_6N_5O$)
$= M_S \times A_T/A_S \times V'/V \times 1/10 \times 0.806$

M_S: Amount (mg) of Sitagliptin Phosphate RS taken, calculated on the anhydrous basis

Dissolution <6.10> When the test is performed at 100 revolutions per minute according to the Basket method, using 900 mL of water as the dissolution medium, the dissolution rate in 15 minutes of Sitagliptin Phosphate Tablets is not less than 85%.

Start the test with 1 tablet of Sitagliptin Phosphate Tablets, withdraw not less than 4 mL of the medium at the specified minute after starting the test, and filter through a membrane filter with a pore size of 0.45 μm. Discard not less than 2 mL of the first filtrate, pipet V mL of the subsequent filtrate, add water to make exactly V' mL so that each mL contains about 14 μg of sitagliptin ($C_{16}H_{15}F_6N_5O$), and use this solution as the sample solution. Separately, weigh accurately about 29 mg of Sitagliptin Phosphate RS (separately determine the water <2.48> in the same manner as Sitagliptin Phosphate Hydrate), and dissolve in a solution of sodium chloride (37 in 25,000) to make exactly 100 mL. Pipet 6 mL of this solution, and add a solution of sodium chloride (37 in 25,000) to make exactly 100 mL, and use this solution as the standard solution. Perform the test with exactly 20 μL each of the sample solution and standard solution as directed under Liquid Chromatography <2.01> according to the following conditions, and determine the peak areas, A_T and A_S, of sitagliptin in each solution.

Dissolution rate (%) with respect to the labeled amount of sitagliptin ($C_{16}H_{15}F_6N_5O$)
$= M_S \times A_T/A_S \times V'/V \times 1/C \times 54 \times 0.806$

M_S: Amount (mg) of Sitagliptin Phosphate RS taken, calculated on the anhydrous basis
C: Labeled amount (mg) of sitagliptin ($C_{16}H_{15}F_6N_5O$) in 1 tablet

Operating conditions—

Column, column temperature and flow rate: Proceed as directed in the operating conditions in the Assay.

Detector: An ultraviolet absorption photometer (wavelength: 267 nm).

Mobile phase: Dissolve 1.36 g of potassium dihydrogen phosphate in 900 mL of water, adjust to pH 2.0 with phosphoric acid, and add water to make 1000 mL. To 750 mL of this solution add 250 mL of acetonitrile for liquid chromatography.

System suitability—

System performance: When the procedure is run with 20 μL of the standard solution under the above operating conditions, the number of theoretical plates and the symmetry factor of the peak of sitagliptin are not less than 5000 and not more than 1.5, respectively.

System repeatability: When the test is repeated 6 times with 20 μL of the standard solution under the above operating conditions, the relative standard deviation of the peak area of sitagliptin is not more than 1.0%.

Assay To 10 Sitagliptin Phosphate Tablets add a mixture of diluted phosphoric acid (1 in 1000) and acetonitrile for liquid chromatography (19:1) to make exactly 250 mL, and stir thoroughly. Pipet V mL of this solution, and add a mixture of diluted phosphoric acid (1 in 1000) and acetonitrile for liquid chromatography (19:1) to make exactly V' mL so that each mL contains about 80 μg of sitagliptin ($C_{16}H_{15}F_6N_5O$). Centrifuge this solution, and use the supernatant liquid as the sample solution. Separately, weigh accurately about 26 mg of Sitagliptin Phosphate RS (separately determine the water <2.48> in the same manner as Sitagliptin Phosphate Hydrate), dissolve in a mixture of diluted phosphoric acid (1 in 1000) and acetonitrile for liquid chromatography (19:1) to make exactly 250 mL, and use this solution as the standard solution. Perform the test with exactly 20 μL each of the sample solution and standard solution as directed under Liquid Chromatography <2.01> according to the following conditions, and determine the peak areas, A_T and A_S, of sitagliptin in each solution.

Amount (mg) of sitagliptin ($C_{16}H_{15}F_6N_5O$) in 1 tablet of Sitagliptin Phosphate Tablets
$= M_S \times A_T/A_S \times V'/V \times 1/10 \times 0.806$

M_S: Amount (mg) of Sitagliptin Phosphate RS taken, calculated on the anhydrous basis

Operating conditions—

Detector: An ultraviolet absorption photometer (wavelength: 205 nm).

Column: A stainless steel column 4.6 mm in inside diameter and 15 cm in length, packed with cyanopropylsilanized silica gel for liquid chromatography (5 μm in particle diameter).

Column temperature: A constant temperature of about 30°C.

Mobile phase: Dissolve 1.36 g of potassium dihydrogen phosphate in 900 mL of water, adjust to pH 2.0 with phosphoric acid, and add water to make 1000 mL. To 850 mL of this solution add 150 mL of acetonitrile for liquid chromatography.

Flow rate: 1.0 mL per minute.

System suitability—

System performance: Proceed as directed in the system suitability in the Assay under Sitagliptin Phosphate Hydrate. The following method can be applied when sodium stearyl fumarate is contained in the additive of the tablet.

Crush 1 tablet of Sitagliptin Phosphate Tablets, transfer to a vial, and add 1 mL of water. Stopper the vial tightly, and heat at 80°C for 20 to 48 hours. Take out the contents of the vial, wash the vial 3 times with a mixture of diluted phosphoric acid (1 in 1000) and acetonitrile for liquid chromatography (19:1), combine the washings and the content, and add a mixture of diluted phosphoric acid (1 in 1000) and acetonitrile for liquid chromatography (19:1) to make 100 mL. Stir this solution for 1 hour, and centrifuge for 10 minutes or until the solution becomes clear. When the procedure is run with 20 μL of the supernatant liquid under the above operating conditions, the resolution between sitagliptin and the peak having the relative retention time of about 1.2 to sitagliptin is not less than 1.5.

System repeatability: When the test is repeated 6 times with 20 μL of the standard solution under the above operating conditions, the relative standard deviation of the peak area of sitagliptin is not more than 1.0%.

Containers and storage Containers—Tight containers.

Sivelestat Sodium Hydrate

シベレスタットナトリウム水和物

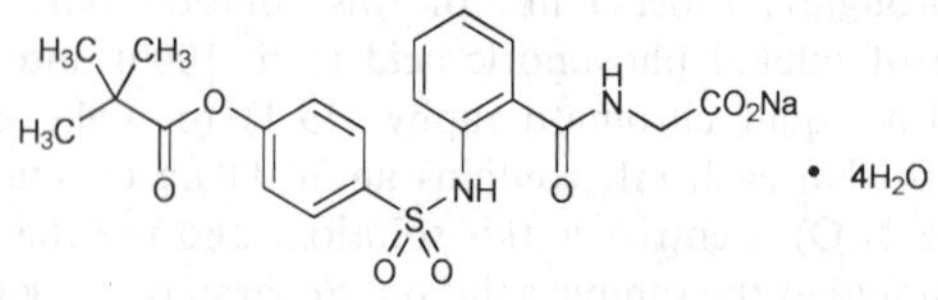

$C_{20}H_{21}N_2NaO_7S.4H_2O$: 528.51
Monosodium *N*-{2-[4-(2,2-dimethylpropanoyloxy)phenylsulfonylamino]benzoyl}aminoacetate tetrahydrate
[*201677-61-4*]

Sivelestat Sodium Hydrate contains not less than 98.0% and not more than 102.0% of sivelestat sodium ($C_{20}H_{21}N_2NaO_7S$: 456.44), calculated on the anhydrous basis.

Description Sivelestat Sodium Hydrate occurs as a white crystalline powder.

It is freely soluble in methanol, slightly soluble in ethanol (99.5), and practically insoluble in water.

It dissolves in sodium hydroxide TS.

Melting point: about 190°C (with decomposition, after drying in vacuum, 60°C, 2 hours).

Identification **(1)** Determine the absorption spectrum of a solution of Sivelestat Sodium Hydrate in boric acid-potassium chloride-sodium hydroxide buffer solution (pH 9.0) (1 in 40,000) as directed under Ultraviolet-visible Spectrophotometry <*2.24*>, and compare the spectrum with the Reference Spectrum: both spectra exhibit similar intensities of absorption at the same wavelengths.

(2) Determine the infrared absorption spectrum of Sivelestat Sodium Hydrate as directed in the paste method under Infrared Spectrophotometry <*2.25*>, and compare the spectrum with the Reference Spectrum: both spectra exhibit similar intensities of absorption at the same wave numbers.

(3) Dissolve 50 mg of Sivelestat Sodium Hydrate in 5 mL of water with one drop of ammonia TS: the solution responds to Qualitative Tests <*1.09*> for sodium salt.

Purity **(1)** Heavy metals <*1.07*>—Proceed with 2.0 g of Sivelestat Sodium Hydrate according to Method 4, and perform the test. Prepare the control solution with 2.0 mL of Standard Lead Solution (not more than 10 ppm).

(2) Related substances—Dissolve 10 mg of Sivelestat Sodium Hydrate in 10 mL of a mixture of water and acetonitrile (1:1), and use this solution as the sample solution. Pipet 1 mL of the sample solution, add a mixture of water and acetonitrile (1:1) to make exactly 100 mL, and use this solution as the standard solution. Perform the test with exactly 10 μL each of the sample solution and standard solution as directed under Liquid Chromatography <*2.01*> according to the following conditions, and determine each peak area by the automatic integration method: the area of the peak, having the relative retention time of about 1.2 to sivelestat, obtained from the sample solution is not larger than 1/2 times the peak area of sivelestat from the standard solution, the areas of the peaks, having the relative retention time of about 0.25, about 0.60, and about 2.7, from the sample solution is not larger than 3/10 times the peak area of sivelestat from the standard solution, the area of the peaks other than sivelestat and peaks mentioned above from the sample solution is not larger than 1/10 times the peak area of sivelestat from the standard solution, and the total area of the peaks other than sivelestat from the sample solution is not larger than the peak area of sivelestat from the standard solution.

Operating conditions—

Column, column temperature, mobile phase and flow rate: Proceed as directed in the operating conditions in the Assay.

Detector: An ultraviolet absorption photometer (wavelength: 220 nm).

Time span of measurement: About 4 times as long as the retention time of sivelestat, beginning after the solvent peak.

System suitability—

Test for required detectability: Pipet 1 mL of the standard solution, and add a mixture of water and acetonitrile (1:1) to make exactly 20 mL. Confirm that the peak area of sivelestat obtained with 10 μL of this solution is equivalent to 4 to 6% of that with 10 μL of the standard solution.

System performance: When the procedure is run with 10 μL of the standard solution under the above operating conditions, the number of theoretical plates and the symmetry factor of the peak of sivelestat are not less than 5000 and not more than 1.5, respectively.

System repeatability: When the test is repeated 6 times with 10 μL of the standard solution under the above operating conditions, the relative standard deviation of the peak

area of sivelestat is not more than 2.0%.

Water <*2.48*> 12.0 – 14.0% (0.2 g, volumetric titration, direct titration).

Assay Weigh accurately about 50 mg of Sivelestat Sodium Hydrate, dissolve in a mixture of water and acetonitrile (1:1) to make exactly 50 mL. Pipet 5 mL of this solution, and add exactly 5 mL of the internal standard solution. To 4 mL of this solution, add 7 mL of acetonitrile and 9 mL of water, and use this solution as the sample solution. Separately, weigh accurately about 40 mg of Sivelestat RS, previously dried (in vacuum, 60°C, 2 hours), and dissolve in acetonitrile to make exactly 50 mL. Pipet 5 mL of this solution, and add exactly 5 mL of the internal standard solution. To 2 mL of this solution, add 3 mL of acetonitrile and 5 mL of water, and use this solution as the standard solution. Perform the test with 10 μL each of the sample solution and standard solution as directed under Liquid Chromatography <*2.01*> according to the following conditions, and calculate the ratios, Q_T and Q_S, of the peak area of sivelestat to that of the internal standard.

Amount (mg) of sivelestat sodium ($C_{20}H_{21}N_2NaO_7S$)
$= M_S \times Q_T/Q_S \times 1.051$

M_S: Amount (mg) of Sivelestat RS taken

Internal standard solution—A solution of propyl parahydroxybenzoate in acetonitrile (1 in 2500).

Operating conditions—

Detector: An ultraviolet absorption photometer (wavelength: 240 nm).

Column: A stainless steel column 4.6 mm in inside diameter and 15 cm in length, packed with octadecylsilanized silica gel for liquid chromatography (5 μm in particle diameter).

Column temperature: A constant temperature of about 25°C.

Mobile phase: Dissolve 5.44 g of potassium dihydrogen phosphate in water to make 1000 mL, then adjust to pH 3.5 with phosphoric acid. To 5 volumes of this solution, add 4 volumes of acetonitrile.

Flow rate: Adjust so that the retention time of sivelestat is about 10 minutes.

System suitability—

System performance: When the procedure is run with 10 μL of the standard solution under the above operating conditions, the internal standard and sivelestat are eluted in this order with the resolution between these peaks being not less than 5.

System repeatability: When the test is repeated 6 times with 10 μL of the standard solution under the above operating conditions, the relative standard deviation of the ratio of the peak area of sivelestat to that of the internal standard is not more than 1.0%.

Containers and storage Containers—Tight containers.

Sivelestat Sodium for Injection

注射用シベレスタットナトリウム

Sivelestat Sodium for Injection is a preparation for injection which is dissolved before use.

It contains not less than 95.0% and not more than 105.0% of the labeled amount of sivelestat sodium hydrate ($C_{20}H_{21}N_2NaO_7S.4H_2O$: 528.51).

Method of preparation Prepare as directed under Injections, with Sivelestat Sodium Hydrate.

Description Sivelestat Sodium for Injection occurs as white, masses or powder.

Identification **(1)** Dissolve an amount of Sivelestat Sodium for Injection, equivalent to 0.1 g of Sivelestat Sodium Hydrate, in 10 mL of water. To 1 mL of this solution add boric acid-potassium chloride-sodium hydroxide buffer solution (pH 9.0) to make 100 mL. Determine the absorption spectrum of this solution as directed under Ultraviolet-visible Spectrophotometry <*2.24*>: it exhibits a maximum between 311 nm and 315 nm.

(2) Take an amount of Sivelestat Sodium for Injection, equivalent to 0.1 g of Sivelestat Sodium Hydrate, add 10 mL of methanol, and shake. Take 1 mL of the supernatant liquid, add methanol to make 10 mL, and use this solution as the sample solution. Separately, dissolve 10 mg of sivelestat sodium hydrate in 10 mL of methanol, and use this solution as the standard solution. Perform the test with these solutions as directed under Thin-layer Chromatography <*2.03*>. Spot 5 μL each of the sample solution and standard solution on a plate of silica gel with fluorescent indicator for thin-layer chromatography. Develop the plate with a mixture of ethyl acetate and acetic acid (100) (20:1) to a distance of about 10 cm, and air-dry the plate. Examine under ultraviolet light (main wavelength: 254 nm): the principal spot obtained from the sample solution and the spot from the standard solution show the same *R*f value.

pH Being specified separately when the drug is granted approval based on the Law.

Purity Related substances—Dissolve an amount of Sivelestat Sodium for Injection, equivalent to 1.0 g of Sivelestat Sodium Hydrate, in water to make 100 mL. To 1 mL of this solution add 9 mL of a mixture of acetonitrile and water (5:4), and use the solution as the sample solution. Pipet 1 mL of the sample solution, add a mixture of water and acetonitrile (1:1) to make exactly 100 mL, and use this solution as the standard solution. Perform the test with exactly 10 μL each of the sample solution and standard solution as directed under Liquid Chromatography <*2.01*> according to the following conditions, and determine each peak area by the automatic integration method: the area of the peak, having the relative retention time of about 0.25 to sivelestat, obtained from the sample solution is not larger than 3 times the peak area of sivelestat from the standard solution.

Operating conditions—

Column, column temperature, mobile phase and flow rate: Proceed as directed in the operating conditions in the Assay under Sivelestat Sodium Hydrate.

Detector: An ultraviolet absorption photometer (wavelength: 220 nm).

System suitability—

Proceed as directed in the system suitability in the Purity (2) under Sivelestat Sodium Hydrate.

Bacterial endotoxins <*4.01*> Less than 25 EU/mg.

Uniformity of dosage units <*6.02*> It meets the requirement of the Mass variation test.

Foreign insoluble matter <*6.06*> Perform the test according to Method 2: it meets the requirement.

Insoluble particulate matter <*6.07*> It meets the requirement.

Sterility <*4.06*> Perform the test according to the Mem-

brane filtration method: it meets the requirement.

Assay Take a number of Sivelestat Sodium for Injection, equivalent to about 1 g of sivelestat sodium hydrate ($C_{20}H_{21}N_2NaO_7S.4H_2O$), and dissolve all the contents in water to make exactly 100 mL. Pipet 5 mL of this solution, add water to make exactly 100 mL. Pipet 10 mL of this solution, add exactly 5 mL of the internal standard solution and 5 mL of acetonitrile. To 2 mL of this solution add 3 mL of a mixture of water and acetonitrile (1:1), and use the solution as the sample solution. Then, proceed as directed in the Assay under Sivelestat Sodium Hydrate.

Amount (mg) of sivelestat sodium hydrate ($C_{20}H_{21}N_2NaO_7S.4H_2O$)
$= M_S \times Q_T/Q_S \times 20 \times 1.216$

M_S: Amount (mg) of Sivelestat RS taken

Internal standard solution—A solution of propyl parahydroxybenzoate in acetonitrile (1 in 2500).

Containers and storage Containers—Hermetic containers.
Storage—Light-resistant.

Freeze-dried Smallpox Vaccine

乾燥痘そうワクチン

Freeze-dried Smallpox Vaccine is a preparation for injection which is dissolved before use. It contains live vaccinia virus.

It conforms to the requirements of Freeze-dried Smallpox Vaccine in the Minimum Requirements for Biological Products.

Description Freeze-dried Smallpox Vaccine becomes a white to gray, turbid liquid on addition of solvent.

Freeze-dried Smallpox Vaccine Prepared in Cell Culture

乾燥細胞培養痘そうワクチン

Freeze-dried Smallpox Vaccine Prepared in Cell Culture is a preparation for injection which is dissolved before use. It contains live vaccinia virus.

It conforms to the requirements of Freeze-dried Smallpox Vaccine Prepared in Cell Culture in the Minimum Requirements for Biological Products.

Description Freeze-dried Smallpox Vaccine Prepared in Cell Culture becomes a reddish clear liquid on addition of solvent.

Sodium Acetate Hydrate

酢酸ナトリウム水和物

$H_3C—CO_2Na \cdot 3H_2O$

$C_2H_3NaO_2.3H_2O$: 136.08
Monosodium acetate trihydrate
[6131-90-4]

Sodium Acetate Hydrate, when dried, contains not less than 99.5% of sodium acetate ($C_2H_3NaO_2$: 82.03).

Description Sodium Acetate Hydrate occurs as colorless crystals or a white crystalline powder. It is odorless or has a slight, acetous odor. It has a cool, saline and slightly bitter taste.

It is very soluble in water, freely soluble in acetic acid (100), soluble in ethanol (95), and practically insoluble in diethyl ether.

It is efflorescent in warm, dry air.

Identification A solution of Sodium Acetate Hydrate (1 in 10) responds to Qualitative Tests <*1.09*> for acetate and for sodium salt.

Purity **(1)** Clarity and color of solution—Dissolve 2.0 g of Sodium Acetate Hydrate in 20 mL of water: the solution is clear and colorless.

(2) Acidity or alkalinity—Dissolve 1.0 g of Sodium Acetate Hydrate in 20 mL of freshly boiled and cooled water, and add 3 drops of phenolphthalein TS: a red color develops. When cooled to 10°C, or 1.0 mL of 0.01 mol/L hydrochloric acid VS is added after cooling to 10°C, the red color disappears.

(3) Chloride <*1.03*>—Perform the test with 1.0 g of Sodium Acetate Hydrate. Prepare the control solution with 0.30 mL of 0.01 mol/L hydrochloric acid VS (not more than 0.011%).

(4) Sulfate <*1.14*>—Perform the test with 1.0 g of Sodium Acetate Hydrate. Prepare the control solution with 0.35 mL of 0.005 mol/L sulfuric acid VS (not more than 0.017%).

(5) Heavy metals <*1.07*>—Proceed with 2.0 g of Sodium Acetate Hydrate according to Method 1, and perform the test. Prepare the control solution with 2.0 mL of Standard Lead Solution (not more than 10 ppm).

(6) Calcium and magnesium—Dissolve 4.0 g of Sodium Acetate Hydrate in 25 mL of water, add 6 g of ammonium chloride, 20 mL of ammonia solution (28) and 0.25 mL of a solution of sodium sulfite heptahydrate (1 in 10), and titrate <*2.50*> with 0.01 mol/L disodium dihydrogen ethylenediamine tetraacetate VS until the blue color changes to grayish blue (indicator: 0.1 g of methylthymol blue-potassium nitrate indicator): the amount of 0.01 mol/L disodium dihydrogen ethylenediamine tetraacetate VS consumed is not more than 0.5 mL.

(7) Arsenic <*1.11*>—Prepare the test solution with 1.0 g of Sodium Acetate Hydrate, according to Method 1, and perform the test (not more than 2 ppm).

(8) Potassium permanganate-reducing substance—Dissolve 1.0 g of Sodium Acetate Hydrate in 100 mL of water, add 5 mL of dilute sulfuric acid, boil, add 0.50 mL of 0.002 mol/L potassium permanganate VS, and further boil for 5 minutes: the red color of the solution does not disappear.

Loss on drying <*2.41*> 39.0 – 40.5% (1 g, first at 80°C for 2 hours, and then at 130°C for 2 hours).

Assay Weigh accurately about 0.2 g of Sodium Acetate Hydrate, previously dried, dissolve in 50 mL of acetic acid (100), and titrate <*2.50*> with 0.1 mol/L perchloric acid VS until the color of the solution changes from yellow to green (indicator: 1 mL of *p*-naphtholbenzein TS). Perform a blank determination in the same manner, and make any necessary correction.

Each mL of 0.1 mol/L perchloric acid VS
= 8.203 mg of $C_2H_3NaO_2$

Containers and storage Containers—Tight containers.

Sodium Aurothiomalate

金チオリンゴ酸ナトリウム

H S–Au
R^1O_2C CO_2R^2 and enantiomer

Mixture of $C_4H_3AuNa_2O_4S$: 390.08 and
$C_4H_4AuNaO_4S$: 368.09
R^1, R^2 = Na, H
Monogold monosodium monohydrogen (2*RS*)-2-sulfidobutane-1,4-dioate
R^1, R^2 = Na
Monogold disodium (2*RS*)-2-sulfidobutane-1,4-dioate
[*12244-57-4*, Sodium Aurothiomalate]

Sodium Aurothiomalate contains not less than 49.0% and not more than 52.5% of gold (Au: 196.97), calculated on the anhydrous and ethanol-free basis.

Description Sodium Aurothiomalate occurs as a white to light yellow, powder or granules.

It is very soluble in water, and practically insoluble in ethanol (99.5).

It is hygroscopic.

It changes in color by light to greenish pale yellow.

Identification **(1)** To 2 mL of a solution of Sodium Aurothiomalate (1 in 10) add 1 mL of a solution of calcium nitrate tetrahydrate (1 in 10): a white precipitate is produced, and it dissolves in dilute nitric acid and reappears on the addition of ammonium acetate TS.

(2) To 2 mL of a solution of Sodium Aurothiomalate (1 in 10) add 3 mL of silver nitrate TS: a yellow precipitate is produced, and it dissolves in an excess of ammonia TS.

(3) Place 2 mL of a solution of Sodium Aurothiomalate (1 in 10) in a porcelain crucible, add 1 mL of ammonia TS and 1 mL of hydrogen peroxide (30), evaporate to dryness, and ignite. Add 20 mL of water to the residue, and filter: the residue on the filter paper occurs as a yellow or dark yellow, powder or granules.

(4) The filtrate obtained in (3) responds to Qualitative Tests <*1.09*> for sodium salt.

(5) The filtrate obtained in (3) responds to Qualitative Tests <*1.09*> for sulfate.

pH <*2.54*> Dissolve 1.0 g of Sodium Aurothiomalate in 10 mL of water: the pH of this solution is between 5.8 and 6.5.

Purity **(1)** Clarity and color of solution—Dissolve 1.0 g of Sodium Aurothiomalate in 10 mL of water: the solution is clear and light yellow.

(2) Heavy metals <*1.07*>—Proceed with 1.0 g of Sodium Aurothiomalate according to Method 2, and perform the test. Prepare the control solution with 3.0 mL of Standard Lead Solution (not more than 30 ppm).

(3) Arsenic <*1.11*>—Prepare the test solution with 1.0 g of Sodium Aurothiomalate according to Method 3, and perform the test (not more than 2 ppm).

(4) Ethanol—Weigh accurately about 0.2 g of Sodium Aurothiomalate, add exactly 3 mL of the internal standard solution and 2 mL of water to dissolve, and use this solution as the sample solution. Separately, pipet 3 mL of ethanol (99.5), and add water to make exactly 1000 mL. Pipet 2 mL of this solution, add exactly 3 mL of the internal standard solution, and use this solution as the standard solution. Perform the test with 2 μL each of the sample solution and standard solution as directed under Gas Chromatography <*2.02*> according to the following conditions, and calculate the ratios of the peak area of ethanol to that of the internal standard, Q_T and Q_S: the amount of ethanol is not more than 3.0%.

Amount (mg) of ethanol = $Q_T/Q_S \times 6 \times 0.793$

0.793: Density (g/mL) of ethanol (99.5) at 20°C

Internal standard solution—A solution of 2-propanol (1 in 500).
Operating conditions—
Detector: A hydrogen flame-ionization detector.
Column: A column 3 mm in inside diameter and 3 m in length, packed with porous styrene-divinylbenzene copolymer for gas chromatography (particle diameter: 150 – 180 μm) (average pore size: 0.0085 μm; 300 – 400 m^2/g).
Column temperature: A constant temperature of about 180°C.
Carrier gas: Nitrogen.
Flow rate: Adjust so that the retention time of the internal standard is about 7 minutes.
System suitability—
System performance: When the procedure is run with 2 μL of the standard solution under the above operating conditions, ethanol and the internal standard are eluted in this order with the resolution between these peaks being not less than 4.
System repeatability: When the test is repeated 6 times with 2 μL of the standard solution under the above operating conditions, the relative standard deviation of the ratio of the peak area of ethanol to that of the internal standard is not more than 2.0%.

Water <*2.48*> Not more than 5.0% (0.1 g, coulometric titration). Use a water vaporizer (heating temperature: 105°C; heating time: 30 minutes).

Assay Weigh accurately about 25 mg of Sodium Aurothiomalate, and dissolve in 2 mL of aqua regia by heating. After cooling, add water to make exactly 100 mL. Pipet 2 mL of the solution, add water to make exactly 25 mL, and use this solution as the sample solution. Separately, pipet 5 mL, 10 mL and 15 mL of Standard Gold Solution for atomic absorption spectrophotometry, add water to make exactly 25 mL, and use these solutions as the standard solutions (1), (2) and (3), respectively. Perform the test with the sample solution and standard solutions (1), (2) and (3) as directed under Atomic Absorption Spectrophotometry <*2.23*> under the following conditions. Determine the amount of gold in the sample solution using the calibration curve obtained from the absorbances of the standard solutions.

Gas: Combustible gas—Acetylene.
Supporting gas—Air.
Lamp: Gold hollow-cathode lamp.
Wavelength: 242.8 nm.

Containers and storage Containers—Tight containers.

Storage—Light-resistant.

Sodium Benzoate

安息香酸ナトリウム

$C_7H_5NaO_2$: 144.10
Monosodium benzoate
[532-32-1]

Sodium Benzoate, when dried, contains not less than 99.0% of sodium benzoate ($C_7H_5NaO_2$).

Description Sodium Benzoate occurs as white, granules, crystals or crystalline powder. It is odorless, and has a sweet and saline taste.

It is freely soluble in water, slightly soluble in ethanol (95), and practically insoluble in diethyl ether.

Identification A solution of Sodium Benzoate (1 in 100) responds to Qualitative Tests 〈*1.09*〉 for benzoate and Qualitative Tests 〈*1.09*〉 (1) and (2) for sodium salt.

Purity **(1)** Clarity and color of solution—Dissolve 1.0 g of Sodium Benzoate in 5 mL of water: the solution is clear and colorless.

(2) Acidity or alkalinity—Dissolve 2.0 g of Sodium Benzoate in 20 mL of freshly boiled and cooled water, and add 2 drops of phenolphthalein TS and 0.20 mL of 0.05 mol/L sulfuric acid VS: the solution remains colorless. To this solution add 0.40 mL of 0.1 mol/L sodium hydroxide VS: a red color develops.

(3) Sulfate 〈*1.14*〉—Dissolve 0.40 g of Sodium Benzoate in 40 mL of water, add slowly 3.5 mL of dilute hydrochloric acid with thorough stirring, allow to stand for 5 minutes, and filter. Discard the first 5 mL of the filtrate, take the subsequent 20 mL of the filtrate, add water to make 50 mL, and perform the test using this solution as the test solution. Prepare the control solution with 0.40 mL of 0.005 mol/L sulfuric acid VS (not more than 0.120%).

(4) Heavy metals 〈*1.07*〉—Dissolve 2.0 g of Sodium Benzoate in 44 mL of water, add gradually 6 mL of dilute hydrochloric acid with thorough stirring, and filter. Discard the first 5 mL of the filtrate, take the subsequent 25 mL of the filtrate, neutralize with ammonia TS, add 2 mL of dilute acetic acid and water to make 50 mL, and perform the test using this solution as the test solution. Prepare the control solution as follows: to 2.0 mL of Standard Lead Solution add 2 mL of dilute acetic acid and water to make 50 mL (not more than 20 ppm).

(5) Arsenic 〈*1.11*〉—Mix well 1.0 g of Sodium Benzoate with 0.40 g of calcium hydroxide, ignite, dissolve the residue in 10 mL of dilute hydrochloric acid, and perform the test using this solution as the test solution (not more than 2 ppm).

(6) Chlorinated compounds—Dissolve 1.0 g of Sodium Benzoate in 10 mL of water, add 10 mL of dilute sulfuric acid, and extract with two 20-mL portions of diethyl ether. Combine the diethyl ether extracts, and evaporate the diethyl ether on a water bath. Place 0.5 g of the residue and 0.7 g of calcium carbonate in a crucible, mix with a small amount of water, and dry. Ignite it at about 600°C, dissolve in 20 mL of dilute nitric acid, and filter. Wash the residue with 15 mL of water, combine the filtrate and the washing, add water to make 50 mL, and add 0.5 mL of silver nitrate TS: this solution has no more turbidity than the following control solution.

Control solution: Dissolve 0.7 g of calcium carbonate in 20 mL of dilute nitric acid, and filter. Wash the residue with 15 mL of water, combine the filtrate and the washings, add 1.2 mL of 0.01 mol/L Hydrochloric acid VS and water to make 50 mL, and add 0.5 mL of silver nitrate TS.

(7) Phthalic acid—To 0.10 g of Sodium Benzoate add 1 mL of water and 1 mL of resorcinol-sulfuric acid TS, and heat the mixture in an oil bath heated at a temperature between 120°C and 125°C to evaporate the water, then heat the residue for further 90 minutes, cool, and dissolve in 5 mL of water. To 1 mL of the solution add 10 mL of a solution of sodium hydroxide (43 in 500), shake, then examine under light at a wavelength between 470 nm and 490 nm: the green fluorescence of the solution is not more intense than that of the following control solution.

Control solution: Dissolve 61 mg of potassium hydrogen phthalate in water to make exactly 1000 mL. Pipet exactly 1 mL of the solution, add 1 mL of resorcinol-sulfuric acid TS, and proceed as directed above.

Loss on drying 〈*2.41*〉 Not more than 1.5% (2 g, 110°C, 4 hours).

Assay Weigh accurately about 1.5 g of Sodium Benzoate, previously dried, and transfer to a 300-mL glass-stoppered flask. Dissolve in 25 mL of water, add 75 mL of diethyl ether and 10 drops of bromophenol blue TS, and titrate 〈*2.50*〉 with 0.5 mol/L hydrochloric acid VS, while mixing the aqueous and diethyl ether layers by vigorous shaking, until a persistent, light green color is produced in the aqueous layer.

Each mL of 0.5 mol/L hydrochloric acid VS
= 72.05 mg of $C_7H_5NaO_2$

Containers and storage Containers—Well-closed containers.

Sodium Bicarbonate

Sodium Hydrogen Carbonate

炭酸水素ナトリウム

$NaHCO_3$: 84.01

Sodium Bicarbonate contains not less than 99.0% of sodium bicarbonate ($NaHCO_3$).

Description Sodium Bicarbonate occurs as white, crystals or crystalline powder. It is odorless, and has a characteristic, saline taste.

It is soluble in water, and practically insoluble in ethanol (95) and in diethyl ether.

It slowly decomposes in moist air.

Identification A solution of Sodium Bicarbonate (1 in 30) responds to Qualitative Tests 〈*1.09*〉 for sodium salt and for bicarbonate.

pH 〈*2.54*〉 Dissolve 1.0 g of Sodium Bicarbonate in 20 mL of water: the pH of this solution is between 7.9 and 8.4.

Purity **(1)** Clarity and color of solution—Dissolve 1.0 g of Sodium Bicarbonate in 20 mL of water: the solution is clear and colorless.

(2) Chloride 〈*1.03*〉—To 0.40 g of Sodium Bicarbonate

add 4 mL of dilute nitric acid, heat to boil, cool, and add 6 mL of dilute nitric acid and water to make 50 mL. Perform the test using this solution as the test solution. Prepare the control solution with 0.45 mL of 0.01 mol/L hydrochloric acid VS (not more than 0.040%).

(3) Carbonate—Dissolve 1.0 g of Sodium Bicarbonate in 20 mL of freshly boiled and cooled water with very gentle swirling at a temperature not exceeding 15°C. Add 2.0 mL of 0.1 mol/L hydrochloric acid VS and 2 drops of phenolphthalein TS: no red color develops immediately.

(4) Ammonium—Heat 1.0 g of Sodium Bicarbonate: the gas evolved does not change moistened red litmus paper to blue.

(5) Heavy metals <*1.07*>—Dissolve 4.0 g of Sodium Bicarbonate in 5 mL of water and 4.5 mL of hydrochloric acid, and evaporate on a water bath to dryness. Dissolve the residue in 2 mL of dilute acetic acid, 35 mL of water and 1 drop of ammonia TS, dilute with water to 50 mL, and perform the test using this solution as the test solution. Prepare the control solution as follows: evaporate 4.5 mL of hydrochloric acid to dryness, and add 2 mL of dilute acetic acid, 2.0 mL of Standard Lead Solution and water to make 50 mL (not more than 5 ppm).

(6) Arsenic <*1.11*>—Dissolve 1.0 g of Sodium Bicarbonate in 3 mL of water and 2 mL of hydrochloric acid, and perform the test using this solution as the test solution (not more than 2 ppm).

Assay Weigh accurately about 2 g of Sodium Bicarbonate, dissolve in 25 mL of water, and titrate with 0.5 mol/L sulfuric acid VS. When the color of the solution changes from blue to yellow-green, boil with caution, cool, and continue the titration <*2.50*> until a greenish yellow color develops (indicator: 2 drops of bromocresol green TS).

Each mL of 0.5 mol/L sulfuric acid VS
= 84.01 mg of $NaHCO_3$

Containers and storage Containers—Tight containers.

Sodium Bicarbonate Injection

炭酸水素ナトリウム注射液

Sodium Bicarbonate Injection is an aqueous injection.

It contains not less than 95.0% and not more than 105.0% of the labeled amount of sodium hydrogen carbonate ($NaHCO_3$: 84.01).

Method of preparation Prepare as directed under Injections, with Sodium Bicarbonate.

Description Sodium Bicarbonate Injection is a clear, colorless liquid.

Identification To a volume of Sodium Bicarbonate Injection, equivalent to 1 g of Sodium Bicarbonate, add water to make 30 mL: the solution responds to Qualitative Tests <*1.09*> for sodium salt and for bicarbonate.

pH <*2.54*> 7.0 – 8.5

Bacterial endotoxins <*4.01*> Less than 5.0 EU/mEq.

Extractable volume <*6.05*> It meets the requirement.

Foreign insoluble matter <*6.06*> Perform the test according to Method 1: it meets the requirement.

Insoluble particulate matter <*6.07*> It meets the requirement.

Sterility <*4.06*> Perform the test according to the Membrane filtration method: it meets the requirement.

Assay Measure exactly a volume of Sodium Bicarbonate Injection, equivalent to about 2 g of sodium hydrogen carbonate ($NaHCO_3$), titrate with 0.5 mol/L sulfuric acid VS, and proceed as directed in the Assay under Sodium Bicarbonate.

Each mL of 0.5 mol/L sulfuric acid VS
= 84.01 mg of $NaHCO_3$

Containers and storage Containers—Hermetic containers.
Plastic containers for aqueous injections may be used.

Sodium Bisulfite

亜硫酸水素ナトリウム

$NaHSO_3$: 104.06

Sodium Bisulfite is a mixture of sodium hydrogensulfite and sodium pyrosulfite.

It contains not less than 64.0% and not more than 67.4% of sulfur dioxide (SO_2: 64.06).

Description Sodium Bisulfite occurs as white, granules or powder, having the odor of sulfur dioxide.

It is freely soluble in water, and practically insoluble in ethanol (95) and in diethyl ether.

A solution of Sodium Bisulfite (1 in 20) is acid.

Sodium Bisulfite is slowly affected by air or by light.

Identification A solution of Sodium Bisulfite (1 in 20) responds to Qualitative Tests <*1.09*> for sodium salt and for bisulfite.

Purity **(1)** Clarity and color of solution—Dissolve 1.0 g of Sodium Bisulfite in 10 mL of water: the solution is clear and colorless.

(2) Thiosulfate—Dissolve 1.0 g of Sodium Bisulfite in 15 mL of water, add slowly 5 mL of dilute hydrochloric acid, shake, and allow to stand for 5 minutes: no turbidity is produced.

(3) Heavy metals <*1.07*>—Dissolve 1.0 g of Sodium Bisulfite in 10 mL of water, add 5 mL of hydrochloric acid, and evaporate on a water bath to dryness. To the residue add 2 mL of dilute acetic acid and water to make 50 mL, and perform the test using this solution as the test solution. Prepare the control solution as follows: evaporate 5 mL of hydrochloric acid on a water bath to dryness, and add 2 mL of dilute acetic acid and 2.0 mL of Standard Lead Solution, and dilute with water to make 50 mL (not more than 20 ppm).

(4) Iron <*1.10*>—Prepare the test solution with 1.0 g of Sodium Bisulfite according to Method 1, and perform the test according to Method A. Prepare the control solution with 2.0 mL of Standard Iron Solution (not more than 20 ppm).

(5) Arsenic <*1.11*>—Dissolve 0.5 g of Sodium Bisulfite in 10 mL of water. Add 1 mL of sulfuric acid, heat on a sand bath until white fumes are evolved, add water to make 5 mL, and perform the test with this solution as the test solution (not more than 4 ppm).

Assay Weigh accurately about 0.15 g of Sodium Bisulfite, and transfer immediately into an iodine flask containing exactly 50 mL of 0.05 mol/L iodine VS, stopper, shake, and allow to stand for 5 minutes in a dark place. Add 1 mL of hydrochloric acid, and titrate <*2.50*> the excess iodine with 0.1 mol/L sodium thiosulfate VS (indicator: 1 mL of starch TS). Perform a blank determination in the same manner.

Each mL of 0.05 mol/L iodine VS = 3.203 mg of SO_2

Containers and storage Containers—Tight containers.

Storage—Light-resistant, preferably well-filled, and not exceeding 30°C.

Sodium Borate

ホウ砂

$Na_2B_4O_7.10H_2O$: 381.37

Sodium Borate contains not less than 99.0% and not more than 103.0% of sodium borate ($Na_2B_4O_7.10H_2O$).

Description Sodium Borate occurs as colorless or white crystals or a white crystalline powder. It is odorless, and has a slightly characteristic, saline taste.

It is freely soluble in glycerin, soluble in water, and practically insoluble in ethanol (95), in ethanol (99.5) and in diethyl ether.

When placed in dry air, Sodium Borate effloresces and is coated with a white powder.

Identification A solution of Sodium Borate (1 in 20) responds to Qualitative Tests <*1.09*> for sodium salt and for borate.

pH <*2.54*> Dissolve 1.0 g of Sodium Borate in 20 mL of water: the pH of this solution is between 9.1 and 9.6.

Purity **(1)** Clarity and color of solution—Dissolve 1.0 g of Sodium Borate in 20 mL of water by warming slightly: the solution is clear and colorless.

(2) Carbonate or bicarbonate—Dissolve 1.0 g of powdered Sodium Borate in 20 mL of freshly boiled and cooled water, and add 3 mL of dilute hydrochloric acid: the solution does not effervesce.

(3) Heavy metals <*1.07*>—Dissolve 1.5 g of Sodium Borate in 25 mL of water and 7 mL of 1 mol/L hydrochloric acid TS, add 1 drop of phenolphthalein TS, and add ammonia TS until a pale red color develops. Then add dilute acetic acid until the solution becomes colorless again, add 2 mL of dilute acetic acid, and add water to make 50 mL. Perform the test using this solution as the test solution. Prepare the control solution as follows: to 3.0 mL of Standard Lead Solution add 2 mL of dilute acetic acid and water to make 50 mL (not more than 20 ppm).

(4) Arsenic <*1.11*>—Prepare the test solution with 0.40 g of Sodium Borate according to Method 1, and perform the test (not more than 5 ppm).

Assay Weigh accurately about 2 g of Sodium Borate, dissolve in 50 mL of water, and titrate <*2.50*> with 0.5 mol/L hydrochloric acid VS (indicator: 3 drops of methyl red TS).

Each mL of 0.5 mol/L hydrochloric acid VS
= 95.34 mg of $Na_2B_4O_7.10H_2O$

Containers and storage Containers—Tight containers.

Sodium Bromide

臭化ナトリウム

NaBr: 102.89

Sodium Bromide, when dried, contains not less than 99.0% of sodium bromide (NaBr).

Description Sodium Bromide occurs as colorless or white, crystals or crystalline powder. It is odorless.

It is freely soluble in water, and soluble in ethanol (95).

It is hygroscopic, but not deliquescent.

Identification A solution of Sodium Bromide (1 in 10) responds to Qualitative Tests <*1.09*> for sodium salt and for bromide.

Purity **(1)** Clarity and color of solution—Dissolve 1.0 g of Sodium Bromide in 3 mL of water: the solution is clear and colorless.

(2) Alkalinity—Dissolve 1.0 g of Sodium Bromide in 10 mL of water, add 0.10 mL of 0.005 mol/L sulfuric acid VS and 1 drop of phenolphthalein TS, heat to boil, and cool: the solution is colorless.

(3) Chloride—Make a calculation from the result obtained in the Assay. Not more than 97.9 mL of 0.1 mol/L silver nitrate VS is consumed for 1 g of Sodium Bromide.

(4) Sulfate <*1.14*>—Perform the test with 2.0 g of Sodium Bromide. Prepare the control solution with 1.0 mL of 0.005 mol/L sulfuric acid VS (not more than 0.024%).

(5) Iodide—Dissolve 0.5 g of Sodium Bromide in 10 mL of water, add 2 to 3 drops of iron (III) chloride TS and 1 mL of chloroform, and shake: no red-purple color develops in the chloroform layer.

(6) Bromate—Dissolve 1.0 g of Sodium Bromide in 10 mL of freshly boiled and cooled water, and add 2 drops of potassium iodide TS, 1 mL of starch TS and 3 drops of dilute sulfuric acid. Shake the mixture gently, and allow to stand for 5 minutes: no blue color develops.

(7) Heavy metals <*1.07*>—Proceed with 2.0 g of Sodium Bromide according to Method 1, and perform the test. Prepare the control solution with 2.0 mL of Standard Lead Solution (not more than 10 ppm).

(8) Barium—Dissolve 0.5 g of Sodium Bromide in 10 mL of water, add 0.5 mL of dilute hydrochloric acid and 1 mL of potassium sulfate TS, and allow to stand for 10 minutes: no turbidity is produced.

(9) Arsenic <*1.11*>—Prepare the test solution with 1.0 g of Sodium Bromide according to Method 1, and perform the test (not more than 2 ppm).

Loss on drying <*2.41*> Not more than 5.0% (1 g, 110°C, 4 hours).

Assay Weigh accurately about 0.4 g of Sodium Bromide, previously dried, and dissolve in 50 mL of water. Add 10 mL of dilute nitric acid and 50 mL of 0.1 mol/L silver nitrate VS, exactly measured, and titrate <*2.50*> the excess silver nitrate with 0.1 mol/L ammonium thiocyanate VS (indicator: 2 mL of ammonium iron (III) sulfate TS). Perform a blank determination in the same manner.

Each mL of 0.1 mol/L silver nitrate VS
= 10.29 mg of NaBr

Containers and storage Containers—Tight containers.

Dried Sodium Carbonate

乾燥炭酸ナトリウム

Na_2CO_3: 105.99

Dried Sodium Carbonate, when dried, contains not less than 99.0% of sodium carbonate (Na_2CO_3).

Description Dried Sodium Carbonate occurs as white crystals or crystalline powder.

It is freely soluble in water, and practically insoluble in ethanol (95) and in diethyl ether.

A solution of Dried Sodium Carbonate (1 in 10) is alkaline.

Dried Sodium Carbonate is hygroscopic.

Identification A solution of Dried Sodium Carbonate (1 in 20) responds to Qualitative Tests <*1.09*> for sodium salt and for carbonate.

Purity **(1)** Clarity and color of solution—Dissolve 1.0 g of Dried Sodium Carbonate in 10 mL of water: the solution is clear and colorless.

(2) Chloride <*1.03*>—Dissolve 0.5 g of Dried Sodium Carbonate in 10 mL of water, add 12 mL of dilute nitric acid, dilute with water to make 50 mL, and perform the test using this solution as the test solution. Prepare the control solution with 1.0 mL of 0.01 mol/L hydrochloric acid VS (not more than 0.071%).

(3) Heavy metals <*1.07*>—Dissolve 1.0 g of Dried Sodium Carbonate in 10 mL of water, add 7.5 mL of dilute hydrochloric acid, and evaporate on a water bath to dryness. Dissolve the residue in 35 mL of water and 2 mL of dilute acetic acid, dilute with water to make 50 mL, and perform the test using this solution as the test solution. Prepare the control solution as follows: evaporate 7.5 mL of dilute hydrochloric acid on a water bath to dryness, add 2 mL of dilute acetic acid and 2.0 mL of Standard Lead Solution, and dilute with water to make 50 mL (not more than 20 ppm).

(4) Arsenic <*1.11*>—Prepare the test solution with 0.65 g of Dried Sodium Carbonate according to Method 1, and perform the test (not more than 3.1 ppm).

Loss on drying <*2.41*> Not more than 2.0% (2 g, 106°C, 4 hours).

Assay Dissolve about 1.2 g of Dried Sodium Carbonate, weighed accurately, in 25 mL of water, and titrate with 0.5 mol/L sulfuric acid VS until the color of the solution changes from blue to yellow-green. Then boil cautiously, cool, and further titrate <*2.50*> until a greenish yellow color develops (indicator: 2 drops of bromocresol green TS).

Each mL of 0.5 mol/L sulfuric acid VS
= 53.00 mg of Na_2CO_3

Containers and storage Containers—Tight containers.

Sodium Carbonate Hydrate

炭酸ナトリウム水和物

$Na_2CO_3.10H_2O$: 286.14

Sodium Carbonate Hydrate contains not less than 99.0% and not more than 103.0% of sodium carbonate hydrate ($Na_2CO_3.10H_2O$).

Description Sodium Carbonate Hydrate occurs as colorless or white crystals.

It is freely soluble in water, and practically insoluble in ethanol (95) and in diethyl ether.

A solution of Sodium Carbonate Hydrate (1 in 10) is alkaline.

Sodium Carbonate Hydrate is efflorescent in air.

It liquefies in its water of crystallization at 34°C, and becomes anhydrous at above 100°C.

Identification A solution of Sodium Carbonate Hydrate (1 in 20) responds to Qualitative Tests <*1.09*> for sodium salt and for carbonate.

Purity **(1)** Clarity and color of solution—Dissolve 1.0 g of Sodium Carbonate Hydrate in 5 mL of water: the solution is clear and colorless.

(2) Chloride <*1.03*>—Dissolve 0.5 g of Sodium Carbonate Hydrate in 10 mL of water, add 7 mL of dilute nitric acid, dilute with water to make 50 mL, and perform the test using this solution as the test solution. Prepare the control solution with 1.0 mL of 0.01 mol/L hydrochloric acid VS (not more than 0.071%).

(3) Heavy metals <*1.07*>—Dissolve 2.0 g of Sodium Carbonate Hydrate in 10 mL of water, add 8 mL of dilute hydrochloric acid, and evaporate to dryness on a water bath. Dissolve the residue in 35 mL of water and 2 mL of dilute acetic acid, dilute with water to make 50 mL, and perform the test using this solution as the test solution. Prepare the control solution as follows: evaporate 8 mL of dilute hydrochloric acid on a water bath to dryness, add 2 mL of dilute acetic acid and 2.0 mL of Standard Lead Solution, and dilute with water to make 50 mL (not more than 10 ppm).

(4) Arsenic <*1.11*>—Prepare the test solution with 0.65 of Sodium Carbonate Hydrate according to Method 1, and perform the test (not more than 3.1 ppm).

Loss on drying <*2.41*> 61.0 – 63.0% (1 g, 105°C, 4 hours).

Assay Dissolve about 3 g of Sodium Carbonate Hydrate, weighed accurately, in 25 mL of water, and titrate with 0.5 mol/L sulfuric acid VS until the color of the solution changes from blue to yellow-green. Boil cautiously, cool, and further titrate <*2.50*> until a greenish yellow color appears (indicator: 2 drops of bromocresol green TS).

Each mL of 0.5 mol/L sulfuric acid VS
= 143.1 mg of $Na_2CO_3.10H_2O$

Containers and storage Containers—Tight containers.

Sodium Chloride

塩化ナトリウム

NaCl: 58.44

This monograph is harmonized with the European Pharmacopoeia and the U.S. Pharmacopeia.

The parts of the text that are not harmonized are marked with symbols (◆ ◆).

Information on the harmonization with the European Pharmacopoeia and the U.S. Pharmacopeia is available on the website of the Pharmaceuticals and Medical Devices Agency.

Sodium Chloride contains not less than 99.0% and not more than 100.5% of sodium chloride (NaCl), calculated on the dried basis.

◆**Description** Sodium Chloride occurs as colorless or white, crystals or crystalline powder.

It is freely soluble in water, and practically insoluble in ethanol (99.5).◆

Identification **(1)** A solution of Sodium Chloride (1 in 20) responds to Qualitative Tests <*1.09*> for sodium salt.

(2) A solution of Sodium Chloride (1 in 20) responds to Qualitative Tests <*1.09*> for chloride.

Purity ◆**(1)** Clarity and color of solution—Dissolve 1.0 g of Sodium Chloride in 5 mL of water: the solution is clear and colorless.◆

(2) Acidity or alkalinity—Dissolve 20.0 g of Sodium Chloride in freshly boiled and cooled water to make exactly 100 mL, and use this solution as the sample solution. To 20 mL of the sample solution add 0.1 mL of bromothymol blue-sodium hydroxide-ethanol TS and 0.5 mL of 0.01 mol/L hydrochloric acid VS: the color of the solution is yellow. Separately, to 20 mL of the sample solution add 0.1 mL of bromothymol blue-sodium hydroxide-ethanol TS and 0.5 mL of 0.01 mol/L sodium hydroxide VS: the color of the solution is blue.

(3) Sulfates—To 7.5 mL of the sample solution obtained in (2) add water to make 30 mL, and use this solution as the sample solution. Separately, dissolve 0.181 g of potassium sulfate in diluted ethanol (3 in 10) to make exactly 500 mL. Pipet 5 mL of this solution, and add diluted ethanol (3 in 10) to make exactly 100 mL. To 4.5 mL of this solution add 3 mL of a solution of barium chloride dihydrate (1 in 4), shake, and allow to stand for 1 minutes. To 2.5 mL of this solution add 15 mL of the sample solution and 0.5 mL of acetic acid (31), and allow to stand for 5 minutes: any turbidity produced does not more than that produced in the following control solution.

Control solution: Dissolve 0.181 g of potassium sulfate in water to make exactly 500 mL. Pipet 5 mL of this solution, add water to make exactly 100 mL, and proceed in the same manner as directed above using this solution instead of the sample solution.

(4) Phosphates—To 2.0 mL of the sample solution obtained in (2) add water to make exactly 100 mL, then add 4 mL of molybdenium-sulfuric acid TS, mix, add 0.1 mL of tin (II) chloride-hydrochloric acid TS, and allow to stand for 10 minutes: the color of the solution is not darker than the following control solution.

Control solution: To 1.0 mL of Standard Phosphoric Acid Solution add 12.5 mL of 2 mol/L sulfuric acid TS and water to make exactly 250 mL. Then, proceed in the same manner as above with 100 mL of this solution.

(5) Bromides—To 0.50 mL of the sample solution obtained in (2) add 4.0 mL of water, 2.0 mL of dilute phenol red TS and 1.0 mL of a freshly prepared solution of sodium toluenesulfonchloramide trihydrate (1 in 10,000), and mix immediately. After allowing to stand for 2 minutes, add 0.15 mL of 0.1 mol/L sodium thiosulfate VS, mix, add water to make exactly 10 mL, and use this solution as the sample solution. Separately, to 5.0 mL of a solution of potassium bromide (3 in 1,000,000) add 2.0 mL of dilute phenol red TS and 1.0 mL of a solution of sodium toluenesulfonchloramide trihydrate (1 in 10,000), and mix immediately. Proceed in the same manner as the preparation of the sample solution, and use the solution so obtained as the standard solution. Perform the test with the sample solution and standard solution as directed under Ultraviolet-visible Spectrophotometry <*2.24*> using water as the control: the absorbance at 590 nm of the sample solution is not more than that of the standard solution.

(6) Iodides—Wet 5 g of Sodium Chloride by adding dropwise a freshly prepared mixture of soluble starch TS, 0.5 mol/L sulfuric acid TS and sodium nitrite TS (1000:40:3), allow to stand for 5 minutes, and examine: a blue color does not appear.

(7) Ferrocyanides—Dissolve 2.0 g of Sodium Chloride in 6 mL of water, and add 0.5 mL of a mixture of a solution of iron (II) sulfate heptahydrate (1 in 100) and a solution of ammonium iron (III) sulfate dodecahydrate in diluted sulfuric acid (1 in 400) (1 in 100) (19:1): a blue color does not develop within 10 minutes.

◆**(8)** Heavy metals <*1.07*>—Proceed with 5.0 g of Sodium Chloride according to Method 1, and perform the test. Prepare the control solution with 1.5 mL of Standard Lead Solution (not more than 3 ppm).◆

(9) Iron—To 10 mL of the sample solution obtained in (2) add 2 mL of a solution of citric acid monohydrate (1 in 5) and 0.1 mL of mercapto acetic acid, alkalize with ammonia TS, add water to make exactly 20 mL, and allow to stand for 5 minutes: the solution has not more color than the following control solution.

Control solution: Pipet 1 mL of Standard Iron Solution, and add water to make exactly 25 mL. To 10 mL of this solution add 2 mL of a solution of citric acid monohydrate (1 in 5) and 0.1 mL of mercapto acetic acid, and proceed in the same manner as directed for the sample solution.

(10) Barium—To 5.0 mL of the sample solution obtained in (2) add 5.0 mL of water and 2.0 mL of dilute sulfuric acid, and allow to stand for 2 hours: the solution has not more turbidity than the following control solution.

Control solution: To 5.0 mL of the sample solution obtained in (2) add 7.0 mL of water, and allow to stand for 2 hours.

(11) Magnesium and alkaline-earth materials—To 200 mL of water add 0.1 g of hydroxylammonium chloride, 10 mL of ammonium chloride buffer solution (pH 10), 1 mL of 0.1 mol/L zinc sulfate VS and 0.15 g of eriochrome black T-sodium chloride indicator, and warm to 40°C. Add 0.01 mol/L disodium dihydrogen ethylenediamine tetraacetate VS dropwise until the purple color of the solution changes to blue. To this solution add a solution prepared by dissolving 10.0 g of Sodium Chloride in 100 mL of water, and add 2.5 mL of 0.01 mol/L disodium dihydrogen ethylenediamine tetraacetate VS: the color of the solution is a blue.

◆**(12)** Arsenic <*1.11*>—Prepare the test solution with 1.0 g of Sodium Chloride according to Method 1, and perform the test (not more than 2 ppm).◆

Loss on drying <2.41> Not more than 0.5% (1 g, 105°C, 2 hours).

Assay Weigh accurately about 50 mg of Sodium Chloride, dissolve in 50 mL of water, and titrate <2.50> with 0.1 mol/L silver nitrate VS (potentiometric titration).

Each mL of 0.1 mol/L silver nitrate VS
= 5.844 mg of NaCl

◆**Containers and storage** Containers—Tight containers.◆

10% Sodium Chloride Injection

10% 塩化ナトリウム注射液

10% Sodium Chloride Injection is an aqueous injection.

It contains not less than 9.5 w/v% and not more than 10.5 w/v% of sodium chloride (NaCl: 58.44).

Method of preparation

Sodium Chloride	100 g
Water for Injection or Sterile Water for Injection in Containers	a sufficient quantity
To make	1000 mL

Prepare as directed under Injections, with the above ingredients.

Description 10% Sodium Chloride Injection is a clear, colorless liquid. It has a saline taste.

It is neutral.

Identification 10% Sodium Chloride Injection responds to Qualitative Tests <1.09> for sodium salt and for chloride.

Bacterial endotoxins <4.01> Less than 3.6 EU/mL.

Extractable volume <6.05> It meets the requirement.

Foreign insoluble matter <6.06> Perform the test according to Method 1: it meets the requirement.

Insoluble particulate matter <6.07> It meets the requirement.

Sterility <4.06> Perform the test according to the Membrane filtration method: it meets the requirement.

Assay Pipet 10 mL of 10% Sodium Chloride Injection, and add water to make exactly 100 mL. Pipet 20 mL of this solution, add 30 mL of water, and titrate <2.50>, with vigorous shaking, with 0.1 mol/L silver nitrate VS (indicator: 3 drops of fluorescein sodium TS).

Each mL 0.1 mol/L silver nitrate VS
= 5.844 mg of NaCl

Containers and storage Containers—Hermetic containers.

Plastic containers for aqueous injections may be used.

Isotonic Sodium Chloride Solution

0.9% Sodium Chloride Injection

生理食塩液

Isotonic Sodium Chloride Solution is an aqueous injection.

It contains not less than 0.85 w/v% and not more than 0.95 w/v% of sodium chloride (NaCl: 58.44).

Method of preparation

Sodium Chloride	9 g
Water for Injection or Sterile Water for Injection in Containers	a sufficient quantity
To make	1000 mL

Prepare as directed under Injections, with the above ingredients.

No preservative is added.

Description Isotonic Sodium Chloride Solution is a clear, colorless liquid. It has a slightly saline taste.

Identification Isotonic Sodium Chloride Solution responds to Qualitative Tests <1.09> for sodium salt and for chloride.

pH <2.54> 4.5 – 8.0

Purity **(1)** Heavy metals <1.07>—Concentrate 100 mL of Isotonic Sodium Chloride Solution to about 40 mL on a water bath, and add 2 mL of dilute acetic acid and water to make 50 mL. Perform the test using this solution as the test solution. Prepare the control solution with 3.0 mL of Standard Lead Solution and 2 mL of dilute acetic acid, and add water to make 50 mL (not more than 0.3 ppm).

(2) Arsenic <1.11>—Prepare the test solution with 20 mL of Isotonic Sodium Chloride Solution, and perform the test (not more than 0.1 ppm).

Bacterial endotoxins <4.01> Less than 0.50 EU/mL.

Extractable volume <6.05> It meets the requirement.

Foreign insoluble matter <6.06> Perform the test according to Method 1: it meets the requirement.

Insoluble particulate matter <6.07> It meets the requirement.

Sterility <4.06> Perform the test according to the Membrane filtration method: it meets the requirement.

Assay Measure exactly 20 mL of Isotonic Sodium Chloride Solution, add 30 mL of water, and titrate <2.50> with 0.1 mol/L silver nitrate VS with vigorous shaking (indicator: 3 drops of fluorescein sodium TS).

Each mL of 0.1 mol/L silver nitrate VS
= 5.844 mg of NaCl

Containers and storage Containers—Hermetic containers.

Plastic containers for aqueous injections may be used.

Sodium Chromate (^{51}Cr) Injection

クロム酸ナトリウム(^{51}Cr)注射液

Sodium Chromate (^{51}Cr) Injection is an aqueous injection.

It contains a chromium-51 (^{51}Cr) in the form of sodium chromate.

It conforms to the requirements of Sodium Chromate (^{51}Cr) Injection in the Minimum Requirements for Radiopharmaceuticals.

Test for Extractable Volume of Parenteral Preparations and Insoluble Particulate Matter Test for Injections are not applied to this injection.

Description Sodium Chromate (^{51}Cr) Injection is a clear, light yellow liquid. It is odorless or has an odor of the preservatives.

Sodium Citrate Hydrate

クエン酸ナトリウム水和物

HO CO2Na / NaO2C CO2Na •2H2O

$C_6H_5Na_3O_7.2H_2O$: 294.10
Trisodium 2-hydroxypropane-1,2,3-tricarboxylate dihydrate
[*6132-04-3*]

Sodium Citrate Hydrate, when dried, contains not less than 99.0% and not more than 101.0% of sodium citrate ($C_6H_5Na_3O_7$: 258.07).

Description Sodium Citrate Hydrate occurs as colorless crystals, or a white crystalline powder. It is odorless, and has a cooling, saline taste.

It is freely soluble in water, and practically insoluble in ethanol (95) and in diethyl ether.

Identification A solution of Sodium Citrate Hydrate (1 in 20) responds to Qualitative Tests ⟨*1.09*⟩ for citrate and for sodium salt.

pH ⟨*2.54*⟩ Dissolve 1.0 g of Sodium Citrate Hydrate in 20 mL of water: the pH of this solution is between 7.5 and 8.5.

Purity **(1)** Clarity and color of solution—A solution of 1.0 g of Sodium Citrate Hydrate in 10 mL of water is clear and colorless.

(2) Chloride ⟨*1.03*⟩—Take 0.6 g of Sodium Citrate Hydrate, and perform the test. Prepare the control solution with 0.25 mL of 0.01 mol/L hydrochloric acid VS (not more than 0.015%).

(3) Sulfate ⟨*1.14*⟩—To 0.5 g of Sodium Citrate Hydrate add water to make 40 mL, then add 3.0 mL of dilute hydrochloric acid and water to make 50 mL, and perform the test. Prepare the control solution with 0.50 mL of 0.005 mol/L sulfuric acid VS (not more than 0.048%).

(4) Heavy metals ⟨*1.07*⟩—Proceed with 2.5 g of Sodium Citrate Hydrate according to Method 2, and perform the test. Prepare the control solution with 2.5 mL of Standard Lead Solution (not more than 10 ppm).

(5) Arsenic ⟨*1.11*⟩—Prepare the test solution with 1.0 g of Sodium Citrate Hydrate according to Method 1, and perform the test (not more than 2 ppm).

(6) Tartrate—To a solution of 1.0 g of Sodium Citrate Hydrate in 2 mL of water add 1 mL of potassium acetate TS and 1 mL of acetic acid (31): no crystalline precipitate is formed after the sides of the tube have been rubbed with a glass rod.

(7) Oxalate—Dissolve 1.0 g of Sodium Citrate Hydrate in a mixture of 1 mL of water and 3 mL of dilute hydrochloric acid, add 4 mL of ethanol (95) and 0.2 mL of calcium chloride TS, and allow to stand for 1 hour: the solution is clear.

(8) Readily carbonizable substances ⟨*1.15*⟩—Take 0.5 g of Sodium Citrate Hydrate, and perform the test by heating at 90°C for 1 hour: the solution has no more color than Matching Fluid K.

Loss on drying ⟨*2.41*⟩ 10.0 – 13.0% (1 g, 180°C, 2 hours).

Assay Weigh accurately about 0.2 g of Sodium Citrate Hydrate, previously dried, add 30 mL of acetic acid for nonaqueous titration, warm to dissolve, and titrate ⟨*2.50*⟩ with 0.1 mol/L perchloric acid VS (potentiometric titration). Perform a blank determination in the same manner, and make any necessary correction.

Each mL of 0.1 mol/L perchloric acid VS
= 8.602 mg of $C_6H_5Na_3O_7$

Containers and storage Containers—Tight containers.

Sodium Citrate Injection for Transfusion

輸血用クエン酸ナトリウム注射液

Sodium Citrate Injection for Transfusion is an aqueous injection.

It contains not less than 9.5 w/v% and not more than 10.5 w/v% of sodium citrate hydrate ($C_6H_5Na_3O_7.2H_2O$: 294.10).

Method of preparation

Sodium Citrate Hydrate	100 g
Water for Injection or Sterile Water for Injection in Containers	a sufficient quantity
To make	1000 mL

Prepare as directed under Injections, with the above ingredients.

No preservatives may be added.

Description Sodium Citrate Injection for Transfusion is a clear, colorless liquid.

Identification Sodium Citrate Injection for Transfusion responds to Qualitative Tests ⟨*1.09*⟩ for sodium salt and for citrate.

pH ⟨*2.54*⟩ 7.0 – 8.5

Bacterial endotoxins ⟨*4.01*⟩ Less than 5.6 EU/mL.

Extractable volume ⟨*6.05*⟩ It meets the requirement.

Foreign insoluble matter ⟨*6.06*⟩ Perform the test according to Method 1: it meets the requirement.

Insoluble particulate matter ⟨*6.07*⟩ It meets the requirement.

Sterility ⟨*4.06*⟩ Perform the test according to the Membrane filtration method: it meets the requirement.

Assay Pipet 5 mL of Sodium Citrate Injection for Transfusion, and add water to make exactly 25 mL. Evaporate 10 mL of this solution, exactly measured, on a water bath to dryness, dry the residue at 180°C for 2 hours, and dissolve in 30 mL of acetic acid (100) by warming. Cool, titrate <*2.50*> with 0.1 mol/L perchloric acid VS (indicator: 3 drops of crystal violet TS). Perform a blank determination in the same manner, and make any necessary correction.

Each mL of 0.1 mol/L perchloric acid VS
= 9.803 mg of $C_6H_5Na_3O_7.2H_2O$

Containers and storage Containers—Hermetic containers.

Diagnostic Sodium Citrate Solution

診断用クエン酸ナトリウム液

Diagnostic Sodium Citrate Solution contains not less than 3.3 w/v% and not more than 4.3 w/v% of sodium citrate hydrate ($C_6H_5Na_3O_7.2H_2O$: 294.10).

The requirements as described for aqueous injections under Injections are applicable.

Method of preparation

Sodium Citrate Hydrate	38 g
Water for Injection or Sterile Water for Injection in Containers	a sufficient quantity
To make	1000 mL

Prepare as directed under Injections, with the above ingredients.

No preservative may be added.

Description Diagnostic Sodium Citrate Solution is a clear, colorless liquid.

Identification Diagnostic Sodium Citrate Solution responds to Qualitative Tests <*1.09*> for sodium salt and for citrate.

pH <*2.54*> 7.0 – 8.5

Assay Pipet 5 mL of Diagnostic Sodium Citrate Solution, evaporate on a water bath to dryness, dry the residue at 180°C for 2 hours, and dissolve in 30 mL of acetic acid (100) by warming. Cool, and titrate <*2.50*> with 0.1 mol/L perchloric acid VS (indicator: 3 drops of crystal violet TS). Perform a blank determination in the same manner, and make any necessary correction.

Each mL of 0.1 mol/L perchloric acid VS
= 9.803 mg of $C_6H_5Na_3O_7.2H_2O$

Containers and storage Containers—Hermetic containers.

Sodium Cromoglicate

クロモグリク酸ナトリウム

$C_{23}H_{14}Na_2O_{11}$: 512.33
Disodium 5,5′-(2-hydroxypropane-1,3-diyl)bis(oxy)bis(4-oxo-4*H*-chromene-2-carboxylate)
[*15826-37-6*]

Sodium Cromoglicate contains not less than 98.0% of sodium cromoglicate ($C_{23}H_{14}Na_2O_{11}$), calculated on the dried basis.

Description Sodium Cromoglicate occurs as a white crystalline powder. It is odorless and tasteless at first, and later develops a slightly bitter taste.

It is freely soluble in water, sparingly soluble in propylene glycol, very slightly soluble in ethanol (95), and practically insoluble in 2-propanol and in diethyl ether.

It is hygroscopic.

It gradually acquires a yellow color by light.

Identification **(1)** Dissolve 0.1 g of Sodium Cromoglicate in 2 mL of water, add 2 mL of sodium hydroxide TS, and boil for 1 minute: a yellow color is produced. After cooling, add 0.5 mL of concentrated diazobenzene sulfonic acid TS: a dark red color is produced.

(2) Determine the absorption spectrum of a solution of Sodium Cromoglicate in phosphate buffer solution (pH 7.4) (1 in 100,000) as directed under Ultraviolet-visible Spectrophotometry <*2.24*>, and compare the spectrum with the Reference Spectrum: both spectra exhibit similar intensities of absorption at the same wavelengths.

(3) Sodium Cromoglicate responds to Qualitative Tests <*1.09*> for sodium salt.

Purity **(1)** Clarity and color of solution—Dissolve 0.50 g of Sodium Cromoglicate in 10 mL of water: the solution is clear and colorless to pale yellow.

(2) Acidity or alkalinity—Dissolve 2.0 g of Sodium Cromoglicate in 40 mL of freshly boiled and cooled water, add 6 drops of bromothymol blue TS, and use this solution as the sample solution. To 20 mL of the sample solution add 0.25 mL of 0.1 mol/L sodium hydroxide VS: a blue color is produced. To another 20 mL of the sample solution add 0.25 mL of 0.1 mol/L hydrochloric acid VS: a yellow color is produced.

(3) Heavy metals <*1.07*>—Proceed with 1.0 g of Sodium Cromoglicate according to Method 2, and perform the test. Prepare the control solution with 2.0 mL of Standard Lead Solution (not more than 20 ppm).

(4) Oxalate—Dissolve 0.25 g of Sodium Cromoglicate in water to make exactly 50 mL, and use this solution as the sample solution. Separately, dissolve 49 mg of oxalic acid dihydrate, exactly weighed, in water to make exactly 100 mL. Pipet 5 mL of this solution, add water to make exactly 100 mL, and use this solution as the standard solution. Pipet 20 mL each of the sample solution and standard solution, add exactly 5 mL of iron salicylate TS to each solution, and add water to make 50 mL. Determine the absorbances of these solutions as directed under Ultraviolet-visible Spectrophotometry <*2.24*> using water as the blank: the absorbance of the sample solution at 480 nm is not smaller than that of the standard solution.

(5) Related substances—Dissolve 0.20 g of Sodium Cromoglicate in 10 mL of water, and use this solution as the sample solution. Pipet 1 mL of the sample solution, add water to make exactly 10 mL, pipet 1 mL of this solution, add water to make exactly 20 mL, and use this solution as the standard solution. Perform the test with these solutions as directed under Thin-layer Chromatography *<2.03>*. Spot 10 μL each of the sample solution and standard solution on a plate of silica gel with fluorescent indicator for thin-layer chromatography. Develop the plate with a mixture of methanol, chloroform and acetic acid (100) (9:9:2) to a distance of about 10 cm, and air-dry the plate. Examine under ultraviolet light (main wavelength: 254 nm): spots other than the principal spot obtained from the sample solution is not more intense than the spot from the standard solution.

Loss on drying *<2.41>* Not more than 10.0% (1 g, in vacuum, 105°C, 4 hours).

Assay Weigh accurately about 0.18 g of Sodium Cromoglicate, and dissolve in a mixture of 25 mL of propylene glycol and 5 mL of 2-propanol by warming. After cooling, add 30 mL of 1,4-dioxane, and titrate *<2.50>* with 0.1 mol/L perchloric acid-1,4-ioxane VS (potentiometric titration). Perform a blank determination in the same manner, and make any necessary correction.

Each mL of 0.1 mol/L perchloric acid-1,4-dioxane VS
= 25.62 mg of $C_{23}H_{14}Na_2O_{11}$

Containers and storage Containers—Tight containers.
Storage—Light-resistant.

Disodium Edetate Hydrate

エデト酸ナトリウム水和物

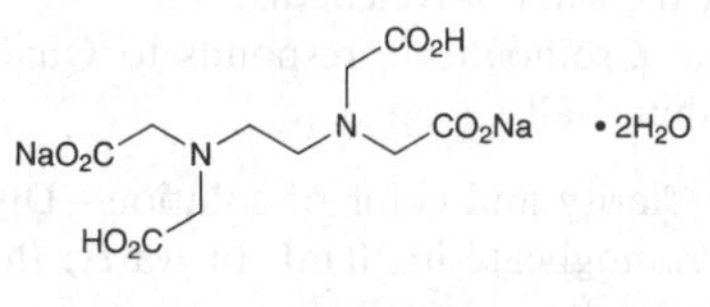

$C_{10}H_{14}N_2Na_2O_8.2H_2O$: 372.24
Disodium dihydrogen ethylenediaminetetraacetate dihydrate
[6381-92-6]

Disodium Edetate Hydrate contains not less than 99.0% of disodium edetate hydrate ($C_{10}H_{14}N_2Na_2O_8.2H_2O$).

Description Disodium Edetate Hydrate occurs as white, crystals or crystalline powder. It is odorless and has a slight, acid taste.

It is soluble in water, and practically insoluble in ethanol (95) and in diethyl ether.

Identification **(1)** Dissolve 0.01 g of Disodium Edetate Hydrate in 5 mL of water, add 2 mL of a solution of potassium chromate (1 in 200) and 2 mL of arsenic trioxide TS, and heat in a water bath for 2 minutes: a purple color develops.

(2) Dissolve 0.5 g of Disodium Edetate Hydrate in 20 mL of water, and add 1 mL of dilute hydrochloric acid: a white precipitate is produced. Collect the precipitate, wash with 50 mL of water, and dry at 105°C for 1 hour: the precipitate melts *<2.60>* between 240°C and 244°C (with decomposition).

(3) A solution of Disodium Edetate Hydrate (1 in 20) responds to Qualitative Tests *<1.09>* (1) for sodium salt.

pH *<2.54>* Dissolve 1.0 g of Disodium Edetate Hydrate in 100 mL of water: the pH of this solution is between 4.3 and 4.7.

Purity **(1)** Clarity and color of solution—Dissolve 1.0 g of Disodium Edetate Hydrate in 50 mL of water: the solution is clear and colorless.

(2) Cyanide—Transfer 1.0 g of Disodium Edetate Hydrate to a round-bottomed flask, dissolve in 100 mL of water, add 10 mL of phosphoric acid, and distil. Place 15 mL of 0.5 mol/L sodium hydroxide VS in a 100-mL measuring cylinder, which is used as a receiver, and immerse the bottom end of the condenser into the solution. Distil the mixture until the distillate measures 100 mL, and use this solution as the sample solution. Transfer 20 mL of the sample solution to a glass-stoppered test tube, add 1 drop of phenolphthalein TS, neutralize with dilute acetic acid, and add 5 mL of phosphate buffer solution (pH 6.8) and 1.0 mL of diluted sodium toluenesulfonchloramide TS (1 in 5). Immediately stopper the tube, mix gently, and allow to stand for a few minutes. Mix well with 5 mL of pyridine-pyrazolone TS, and allow to stand between 20°C and 30°C for 50 minutes: the solution has no more color than the following control solution.

Control solution: Pipet 1.0 mL of Standard Cyanide Solution, add 15 mL of 0.5 mol/L sodium hydroxide VS and water to make exactly 1000 mL, transfer 20 mL of this solution to a glass-stoppered test tube, and proceed as directed for the sample solution.

(3) Heavy metals *<1.07>*—Proceed with 2.0 g of Disodium Edetate Hydrate according to Method 2, and perform the test. Prepare the control solution with 2.0 mL of Standard Lead Solution (not more than 10 ppm).

(4) Arsenic *<1.11>*—Prepare the test solution with 1.0 g of Disodium Edetate Hydrate according to Method 1, and perform the test (not more than 2 ppm).

Residue on ignition *<2.44>* 37.0 – 39.0% (1 g).

Assay Weigh accurately about 1 g of Disodium Edetate Hydrate, dissolve in 50 mL of water, add 2 mL of ammonia-ammonium chloride buffer solution (pH 10.7) and 0.04 g of eriochrome black T-sodium chloride indicator, and titrate *<2.50>* with 0.1 mol/L zinc VS until the color of the solution changes from blue to red.

Each mL of 0.1 mol/L zinc VS
= 37.22 mg of $C_{10}H_{14}N_2Na_2O_8.2H_2O$

Containers and storage Containers—Well-closed containers.

Sodium Fusidate

フシジン酸ナトリウム

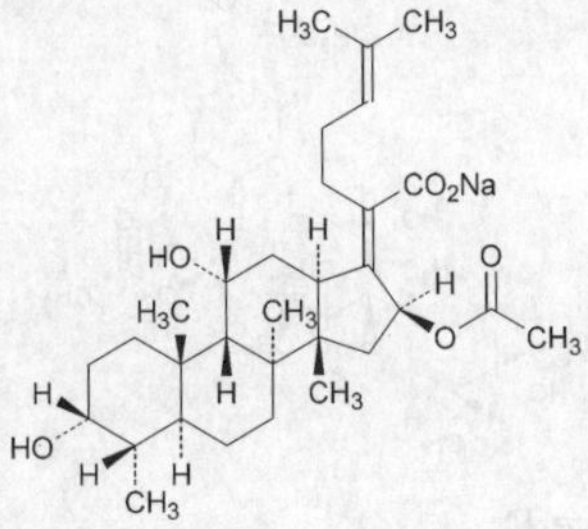

$C_{31}H_{47}NaO_6$: 538.69
Monosodium (17Z)-*ent*-16α-acetoxy-3β,11β-dihydroxy-4β,8β,14α-trimethyl-18-nor-5β,10α-cholesta-17(20),24-dien-21-oate
[*751-94-0*]

Sodium Fusidate is the sodium salt of a substance having antibacterial activity produced by the growth of *Fusidium coccineum*.

It contains not less than 935 μg (potency) and not more than 969 μg (potency) per mg, calculated on the anhydrous basis. The potency of Sodium Fusidate is expressed as mass (potency) of fusidic acid ($C_{31}H_{48}O_6$: 516.71).

Description Sodium Fusidate occurs as white, crystals or crystalline powder.

It is freely soluble in water, in methanol and in ethanol (99.5).

Identification (1) Determine the infrared absorption spectra of Sodium Fusidate as directed in the potassium bromide disk method under Infrared Spectrophotometry <*2.25*>, and compare the spectrum with the Reference Spectrum: both spectra exhibit similar intensities of absorption at the same wave numbers.

(2) Sodium Fusidate responds to Qualitative Tests <*1.09*> (1) for sodium salt.

Purity (1) Heavy metals <*1.07*>—Proceed with 2.0 g of Sodium Fusidate according to Method 4, and perform the test. Prepare the control solution with 2.0 mL of Standard Lead Solution (not more than 10 ppm).

(2) Related substances—Dissolve 25 mg of Sodium Fusidate in a mixture of acetonitrile for liquid chromatography, diluted phosphoric acid (3 in 1000) and methanol (5:4:1) to make 10 mL, and use this solution as the sample solution. Pipet 1 mL of the sample solution, add water to make exactly 100 mL, and use this solution as the standard solution. Perform the test with exactly 20 μL each of the sample solution and standard solution as directed under Liquid Chromatography <*2.01*> according to the following conditions. Determine each peak area by the automatic integration method: the peak area of the related substance A, having the relative retention time of about 0.4 to fusidic acid, obtained from the sample solution is not larger than 3/10 times the peak area of fusidic acid from the standard solution, the peak area of the related substance B, having the relative retention time of about 0.5, from the sample solution is not larger than 2/5 times the peak area of fusidic acid from the standard solution, the peak areas of the related substance C having the relative retention time of about 0.6, the related substance D having the relative retention time of about 0.63, the unknown substance having the relative retention time of about 0.65, the related substance E having the relative retention time of about 0.7, the related substance G having the relative retention time of about 0.96 and the related substance H having the relative retention time of about 1.18, from the sample solution are not larger than 1/5 times the peak area of fusidic acid from the standard solution, the peak area of the related substance F, having the relative retention time of about 0.82, from the sample solution is not larger than 7/10 times the peak area of fusidic acid from the standard solution, the peak area of the related substance I, having the relative retention time of about 1.23, from the sample solution is not larger than 1/2 times the peak area of fusidic acid from the standard solution, the peak area of the related substance J, having the relative retention time of about 1.4, from the sample solution is not larger than the peak area of fusidic acid from the standard solution, the area of the peak other than fusidic acid and the peaks mentioned above from the sample solution is not larger than 1/10 times the peak area of fusidic acid from the standard solution. Furthermore, the total area of the peaks other than fusidic acid from the sample solution is not larger than 2 times the peak area of fusidic acid from the standard solution. For the areas of the peaks, the related substances C, D, E, G and H, multiply their correction factors, 0.7, 0.7, 0.3, 0.6 and 0.6, respectively.

Operating conditions—

Detector: An ultraviolet absorption photometer (wavelength: 235 nm).

Column: A stainless steel column 4.6 mm in inside diameter and 15 cm in length, packed with octadecylsilanized silica gel for liquid chromatography (3.5 μm in particle diameter).

Column temperature: A constant temperature of about 30°C.

Mobile phase A: A mixture of diluted phosphoric acid (3 in 1000), acetonitrile for liquid chromatography and methanol (2:2:1).

Mobile phase B: A mixture of acetonitrile for liquid chromatography, methanol and diluted phosphoric acid (3 in 1000) (7:2:1).

Flowing of mobile phase: Control the gradient by mixing the mobile phases A and B as directed in the following table.

Time after injection of sample (min)	Mobile phase A (vol%)	Mobile phase B (vol%)
0 – 3	100	0
3 – 28	100 → 0	0 → 100
28 – 33	0	100

Flow rate: 1.0 mL per minute.

Time span of measurement: For 33 minutes after injection, beginning after the solvent peak.

System suitability—

Test for required detectability: Pipet 1 mL of the standard solution, and add a mixture of acetonitrile for liquid chromatography, diluted phosphoric acid (3 in 1000) and methanol (5:4:1) to make exactly 20 mL. Confirm that the peak area of fusidic acid obtained with 20 μL of this solution is equivalent to 3.5 to 6.5% of that with 20 μL of the standard solution.

System performance: When the procedure is run with 20 μL of the standard solution under the above operating conditions, the number of theoretical plates and the symmetry factor of the peak of fusidic acid are not less than 43,000 and not more than 1.5, respectively.

System repeatability: When the test is repeated 6 times with 20 μL of the standard solution under the above operating conditions, the relative standard deviation of the peak area of fusidic acid is not more than 2.0%.

Water <*2.48*> Not more than 2.0% (1 g, volumetric titration, direct titration).

Assay Perform the test according to the Cylinder-plate method as directed under Microbial Assay for Antibiotics <*4.02*> according to the following conditions.

(i) Test organism—*Staphylococcus aureus* ATCC 6538 P

(ii) Culture medium—Use the medium ii in 3) under (1) Agar media for seed and base layer.

(iii) Standard solutions—Weigh accurately an amount of Diethanolamine Fusidate RS, equivalent to about 20 mg (potency), dissolve in 2 mL of ethanol (95), add water to make exactly 20 mL, and use this solution as the standard stock solution. Keep the standard stock solution at a temperature not exceeding 5°C and use within 7 days. Take exactly a suitable amount of the standard stock solution before use, add phosphate buffer solution (pH 6.0) to make solutions so that each mL contains 4 μg (potency) and 1 μg (potency), and use these solutions as the high concentration standard solution and the low concentration standard solution, respectively.

(iv) Sample solutions—Weigh accurately an amount of Sodium Fusidate, equivalent to about 20 mg (potency), and dissolve in water to make exactly 20 mL. Take exactly a suitable amount of this solution, add phosphate buffer solution (pH 6.0) to make solutions so that each mL contains 4 μg (potency) and 1 μg (potency), and use these solutions as the high concentration sample solution and the low concentration sample solution, respectively.

Containers and storage Containers—Tight containers.

Storage—Light-resistant, and at a temperature 2 to 8°C.

Others

Related substance A:
(24*RS*,17*Z*)-*ent*-16α-Acetoxy-3β,11β,24,25-tetrahydroxy-4β,8β,14α-trimethyl-18-nor-5β,10α-cholest-17(20)-en-21-oic acid

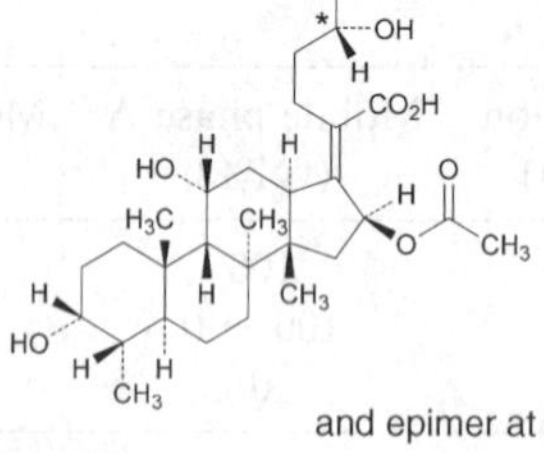

and epimer at C*

Related substance B:
(17*Z*)-*ent*-3β,11β-Dihydroxy-17-[(6*SR*)-6-hydroxy-7,7-dimethyl-2-oxooxepan-3-ylidene]-4β,8β,14α-trimethyl-18-nor-5β,10α-androstan-16α-yl acetate

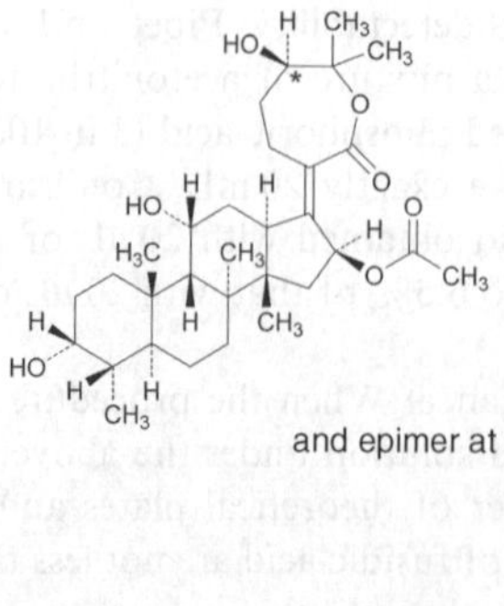

and epimer at C*

Related substance C:
(17*Z*)-*ent*-3β,11β-Dihydroxy-17-[(6*S*)-6-(2-hydroxypropan-2-yl)-2-oxodihydro-2*H*-pyran-3(4*H*)-ylidene]-4β,8β,14α-trimethyl-18-nor-5β,10α-androstan-16α-yl acetate

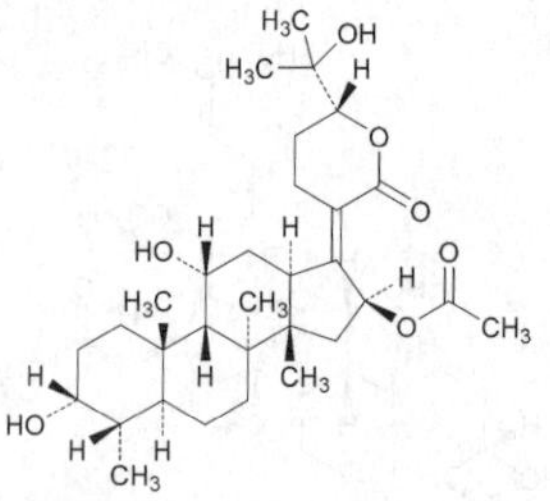

Related substance D:
(17*Z*)-*ent*-3β,11β-Dihydroxy-17-[(6*R*)-6-(2-hydroxypropan-2-yl)-2-oxodihydro-2*H*-pyran-3(4*H*)-ylidene]-4β,8β,14α-trimethyl-18-nor-5β,10α-androstan-16α-yl acetate

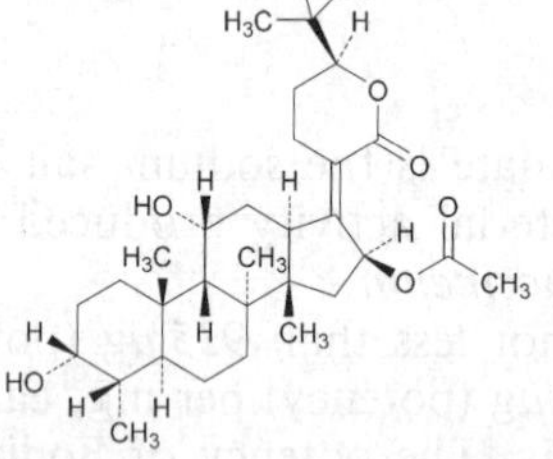

Related substance E:
(17*Z*,24*EZ*)-*ent*-16α-Acetoxy-3β,11β-dihydroxy-4β,8β,14α-trimethyl-26-oxo-18-nor-5β,10α-cholesta-17(20),24-dien-21-oic acid

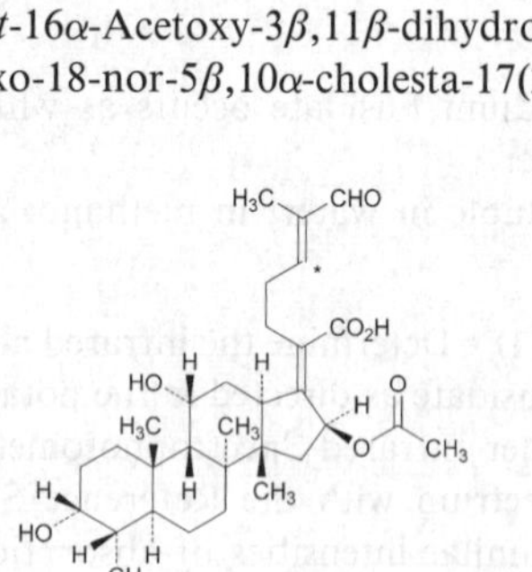

and epimer at C*

Related substance F:
(17*Z*)-*ent*-16α-Acetoxy-11β-hydroxy-4β,8β,14α-trimethyl-3-oxo-18-nor-5β,10α-cholesta-17(20),24-dien-21-oic acid

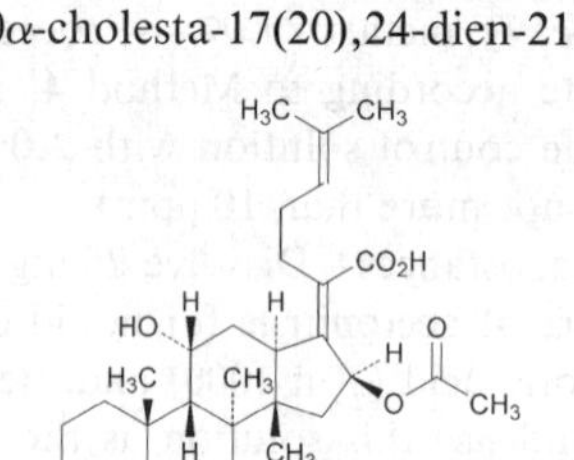

Related substance G:
(17*Z*)-*ent*-3β,11β,16β-Trihydroxy-4β,8β,14α-trimethyl-18-nor-5β,10α-cholesta-17(20),24-dien-21-oic acid

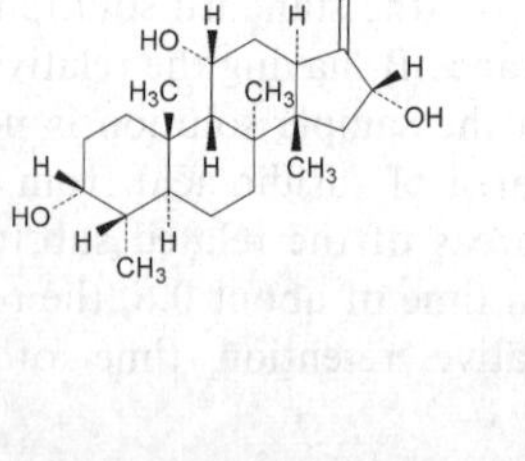

Related substance H:
(17*Z*)-*ent*-3β,11β-Dihydroxy-4β,8β,14α-trimethyl-18-nor-5β,10α-cholesta-17(20),24-dieno-21,16α-lactone

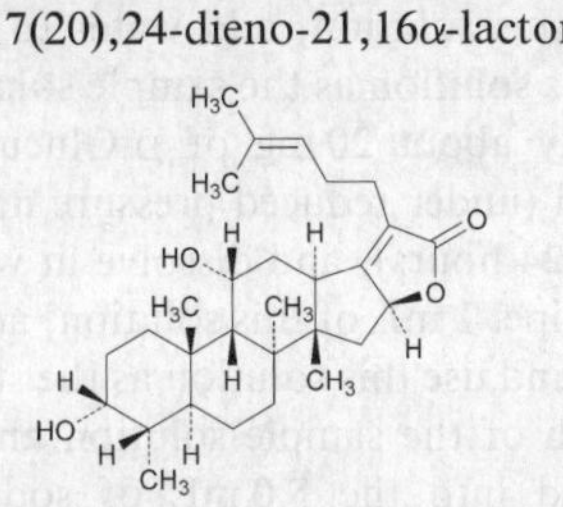

Related substance I:
(17*Z*)-*ent*-16α-Acetoxy-3β-hydroxy-4β,8β,14α-trimethyl-18-nor-5β,10α-cholesta-9(11),17(20),24-trien-21-oic acid

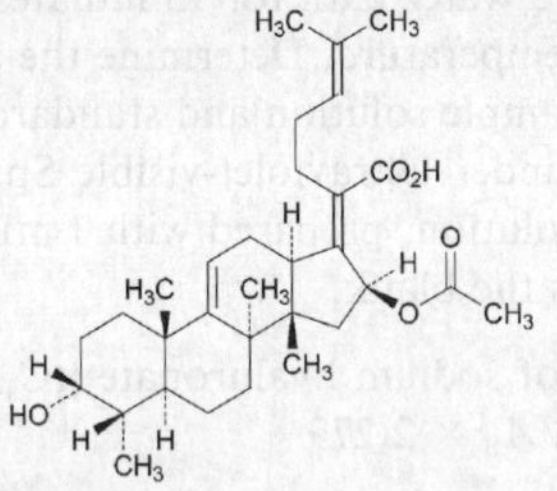

Related substance J:
(17*Z*)-*ent*-16α-Acetoxy-3β-hydroxy-4β,8β,14α-trimethyl-18-nor-5β,10α-cholesta-17(20),24-dien-21-oic acid

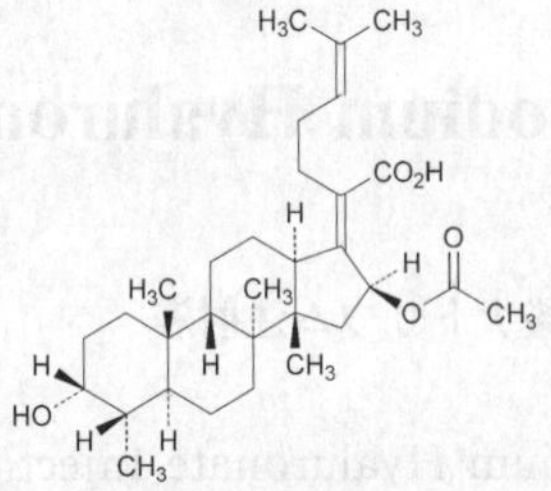

Purified Sodium Hyaluronate

精製ヒアルロン酸ナトリウム

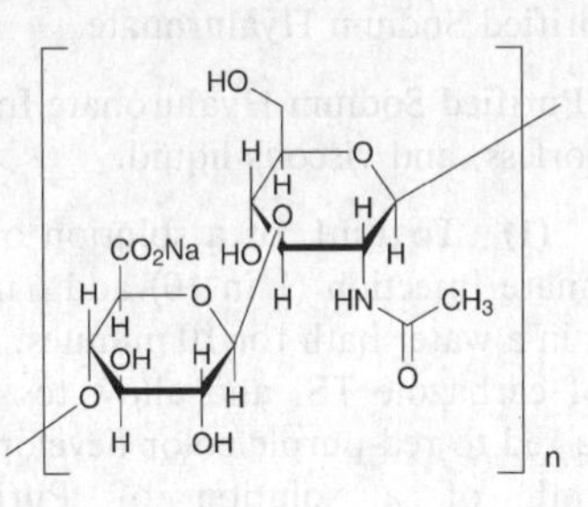

$(C_{14}H_{20}NNaO_{11})_n$
[9067-32-7]

Purified Sodium Hyaluronate is the sodium salt of glycosaminoglycans composed of disaccharide units of D-glucuronic acid and *N*-acetyl-D-glucosamine obtained from cockscomb or microorganisms.

It contains not less than 90.0% and not more than 105.5% of sodium hyaluronate [$(C_{14}H_{20}NNaO_{11})_n$], calculated on the dried basis.

It is composed of an average molecular mass of the sodium salt of hyaluronic acid between 500,000 and 1,490,000 or between 1,500,000 and 3,900,000.

The average molecular mass of Purified Sodium Hyaluronate should be labeled.

Description Purified Sodium Hyaluronate occurs as white, powder, granules or fibrous masses.

It is sparingly soluble in water, and practically insoluble in ethanol (99.5).

It is hygroscopic.

Identification (1) Determine the infrared absorption spectrum of Purified Sodium Hyaluronate, previously dried, as directed in the potassium bromide disk method under Infrared Spectrophotometry <*2.25*>, and compare the spectrum with the Reference Spectrum: both spectra exhibit similar intensities of absorption at the same wave numbers.

(2) A solution of Purified Sodium Hyaluronate (1 in 1000) responds to Qualitative Tests <*1.09*> (1) for sodium salt.

Viscosity <*2.53*> Weigh accurately an amount of Purified Sodium Hyaluronate so that the downflowing time of its solution in 100 mL of 0.2 mol/L sodium chloride TS is 2.0 to 2.4 times longer than that of 0.2 mol/L sodium chloride TS, dissolve in 0.2 mol/L sodium chloride TS to make exactly 100 mL, and use this solution as the sample solution (1). Pipet 16 mL, 12 mL and 8 mL of the sample solution (1), to each add 0.2 mol/L sodium chloride TS to make exactly 20 mL, and use these solutions as the sample solutions (2), (3) and (4), respectively. Perform the test with the sample solutions (1), (2), (3) and (4) as directed under Method 1 at 30 ± 0.1°C using an Ubbelohde-type viscometer in which the downflowing time for 0.2 mol/L sodium chloride TS is 200 to 300 seconds: the intrinsic viscosity calculated on the dried basis is between 10.0 dL/g and 24.9 dL/g or between 25.0 dL/g and 55.0 dL/g.

Purity (1) Clarity and color of solution—Dissolve 0.10 g of Purified Sodium Hyaluronate in 10 mL of water: the solution is clear and colorless.

(2) Chloride <*1.03*>—Dissolve 0.20 g of Purified Sodium Hyaluronate in 15 mL of water, add 6 mL of dilute nitric acid, and heat on a water bath for 30 minutes. After cooling, add water to make 50 mL. Perform the test using this solution as the test solution. Prepare the control solution with 0.70 mL of 0.01 mol/L hydrochloric acid VS (not more than 0.124%).

(3) Heavy metals <*1.07*>—Proceed with 1.0 g of Purified Sodium Hyaluronate according to Method 2, and perform the test. Prepare the control solution with 2.0 mL of Standard Lead Solution (not more than 20 ppm).

(4) Protein—Weigh accurately about 20 mg of Purified Sodium Hyaluronate, calculated on the dried basis, dissolve in 1.0 mL of dilute sodium hydroxide TS, and use this solution as the sample solution. Separately, weigh accurately about 10 mg of bovine serum albumin, dissolve in dilute sodium hydroxide TS to make exactly 1000 mL, and use this solution as the standard solution. To 1.0 mL each of the sample solution and standard solution add 5.0 mL of alkaline copper TS (2), immediately stir, allow to stand at room temperature for 10 minutes, add 0.5 mL of diluted Folin's TS (1 in 2), immediately stir, and allow to stand at room temperature for 30 minutes. Perform the test with these solutions as directed under Ultraviolet-visible Spectrophotometry <*2.24*>, using a solution, prepared with 1.0 mL of dilute sodium hydrochloride in the same manner, as the blank: the absorbance of the sample solution at 750 nm does not exceed the absorbance of the standard solution (not more than 0.05%).

(5) Nucleic acid—Determine the absorbance of a solution of 0.10 g Purified Sodium Hyaluronate in 50 mL of water as directed under Ultraviolet-visible Spectrophotometry <*2.24*>, using water as the blank: the absorbance at 260 nm is not more than 0.02.

(6) Other acidic mucopolysaccharides—(In the case of chicken-derived samples) Dissolve 0.25 g of Purified Sodium Hyaluronate in 100 mL of water, and use this solution as the sample solution. Immerse a cellulose acetate membrane 6 cm in length in 0.2 mol/L pyridine-formic acid buffer solution (pH 3.0). Take out the membrane and remove excessive buffer solution using a filter paper. Place the membrane in an electrophoresis vessel saturated with 0.2 mol/L pyridine-formic acid buffer solution (pH 3.0) and run at 0.5 mA/cm for 1 minute. Apply 2 μL of the sample solution to the membrane in an area 1 cm in width at 1.5 cm from the anode. Carry out electrophoresis at 0.5 mA/cm for 1 hour. After the electrophoresis, stain the membrane by immersing it in alcian blue staining solution for 10 to 20 minutes. After staining, decolorize sufficiently with diluted acetic acid (100) (3 in 100): no bands other than the principal band appears.

(7) Hemolytic streptococci—(In the case of microorganism-derived samples) Dissolve 0.5 g of Purified Sodium Hyaluronate in sterile isotonic sodium chloride solution to make exactly 100 mL. Take 0.5 mL of this solution, apply to 2 blood agar plates, respectively, using a Conradi stick, and incubate at 37°C for 48 hours: no hemolytic colonies appear, or if any, no streptococci are observed in the colony under a microscope.

(8) Hemolysis—(In the case of microorganism-derived samples) Dissolve 0.40 g of Purified Sodium Hyaluronate in sterile isotonic sodium chloride solution to make exactly 100 mL. To 0.5 mL of this solution add 0.5 mL of 1% blood suspension, mix, allow to stand at 37°C for 2 hours, and, if necessary, centrifuge at 3000 revolutions per minute for 10 minutes: the erythrocytes precipitate and the supernatant liquid is clear as in a blank determination performed in the same manner using 0.5 mL of sterile isotonic sodium chloride solution as the blank and 0.5 mL of sterile purified water as the positive control.

Loss on drying <*2.41*> Not more than 15.0% (0.1 g, reduced pressure not exceeding 0.67 kPa, phosphorus (V) oxide, 60°C, 5 hours).

Microbial limit <*4.05*> The acceptance criteria of TAMC and TYMC are 10^2 CFU/g and 10^1 CFU/g, respectively. In the case of the sample of the labeled average molecular mass between 500,000 and 1,490,000, perform the test with 1 g, and of the labeled average molecular mass between 1,500,000 and 3,900,000, perform the test with 0.3 g.

Average molecular mass

1) In the case of the labeled average molecular mass of between 500,000 and 1,490,000.

Calculate the average molecular mass of Purified Sodium Hyaluronate according to the following equation: it is between 500,000 and 1,490,000. For $[\eta]$, use the maximum viscosity under Viscosity.

$$\text{Average molecular mass} = \left(\frac{[\eta] \times 10^5}{36}\right)^{\frac{1}{0.78}}$$

2) In the case of the labeled average molecular mass of between 1,500,000 and 3,900,000.

Calculate the average molecular mass of Purified Sodium Hyaluronate according to the following equation: it is between 1,500,000 and 3,900,000. For $[\eta]$, use the maximum viscosity under Viscosity.

$$\text{Average molecular mass} = \left(\frac{[\eta] \times 10^5}{22.8}\right)^{\frac{1}{0.816}}$$

Assay Weigh accurately about 50 mg of Purified Sodium Hyaluronate, and dissolve in water to make exactly 50 mL. Pipet 1 mL of this solution, add water to make exactly 20 mL, and use this solution as the sample solution. Separately, weigh accurately about 20 mg of D-Glucuronolactone RS, previously dried (under reduced pressure not exceeding 0.67 kPa, silica gel, 24 hours), and dissolve in water to make exactly 100 mL. Pipet 1 mL of this solution, add water to make exactly 10 mL, and use this solution as the standard solution. Pipet 1 mL each of the sample solution and standard solution, gently add into the 5.0 mL of sodium tetraborate-sulfuric acid TS, previously cooled in ice water, stir while cooling, heat in a water bath for 10 minutes, and cool in ice water. To each solution add exactly 0.2 mL of carbazole TS, stir well, heat in a water bath for 15 minutes, and cool in ice water to room temperature. Determine the absorbances, A_T and A_S, of the sample solution and standard solution at 530 nm as directed under Ultraviolet-visible Spectrophotometry <*2.24*>, using a solution, prepared with 1 mL of water in the same manner, as the blank.

Amount (mg) of sodium hyaluronate $[(C_{14}H_{20}NNaO_{11})_n]$
$= M_S \times A_T/A_S \times 2.279$

M_S: Amount (mg) of D-Glucuronolactone RS taken

Containers and storage Containers—Tight containers.
Storage—Light-resistant, at not exceeding 15°C.

Purified Sodium Hyaluronate Injection

精製ヒアルロン酸ナトリウム注射液

Purified Sodium Hyaluronate Injection is an aqueous injection.

It contains not less than 90.0% and not more than 110.0% of the labeled amount of sodium hyaluronate $[(C_{14}H_{20}NNaO_{11})_n]$.

Method of preparation Prepare as directed under Injections, with Purified Sodium Hyaluronate.

Description Purified Sodium Hyaluronate Injection occurs as a clear, colorless, and viscous liquid.

Identification **(1)** To 1 mL of a solution of Purified Sodium Hyaluronate Injection (1 in 10) add 6 mL of sulfuric acid, and heat in a water bath for 10 minutes. After cooling, add 0.2 mL of carbazole TS, and allow to stand at room temperature: a red to red-purple color develops.

(2) To 1 mL of a solution of Purified Sodium Hyaluronate Injection (1 in 10) add 0.2 mL of 1 mol/L acetic acid-sodium acetate buffer solution (pH 6.0) and 5 units of hyaluronidase, and allow to stand at 50°C for 1 hour. To this solution add 1 mL of a solution of dipotassium tetraborate tetrahydrate (1 in 20), heat in a water bath for 7 minutes. After cooling, add 6 mL of acetic acid (100) and 2.4 mL of 4-dimethylaminobenzaldehyde-hydrochloric acid-acetic acid TS, and allow to stand at room temperature: a yellowish red to red color develops.

(3) To 1 mL of a solution of Purified Sodium Hyaluronate Injection (1 in 10) add 2 to 3 drops of a solution of cetylpyridinium chloride monohydrate (1 in 20): a white precipitate is formed.

Viscosity <*2.53*>

1) Apply to the preparation which labeled average mo-

lecular mass of sodium hyaluronate is 600,000 to 1,200,000. Weigh accurately an amount of Purified Sodium Hyaluronate Injection, equivalent to about 10 mg of Purified Sodium Hyaluronate, add 0.2 mol/L sodium chloride TS to make exactly 20 mL, and use this solution as the sample solution. Perform the test with the sample solution at 30 ± 0.1°C according to Method 1, using an Ubbelohde-type viscometer showing the downflowing time of 0.2 mol/L sodium chloride TS is between 200 and 300 seconds. Calculate the intrinsic viscosity $[\eta]$ according to the following equation, where c is the content obtained in the Assay expressed as the concentration (g/dL): 11.8 – 19.5 dL/g.

$$[\eta] = \sqrt{2(\eta_{sp} - \ln \eta_{rel})}/c \times 0.87 + 1.33$$

η_{sp} (specific viscosity) $= \eta_{rel} - 1$

η_{rel} (relative viscosity) $= t/t_0$

2) Apply to the preparation which labeled average molecular mass of sodium hyaluronate is 1,500,000 to 2,000,000. Weigh accurately an amount of Purified Sodium Hyaluronate Injection, equivalent to about 4 mg of Purified Sodium Hyaluronate, add 0.2 mol/L sodium chloride TS to make exactly 20 mL, and use this solution as the sample solution. Perform the test with the sample solution at 30 ± 0.1°C according to Method 1, using an Ubbelohde-type viscometer showing the downflowing time of 0.2 mol/L sodium chloride TS is between 200 and 300 seconds. Calculate the intrinsic viscosity $[\eta]$ according to the following equation: 24.5 – 31.5 dL/g.

$$[\eta] = (1 - \sqrt{1 - 0.432 \cdot \ln \eta_{rel}})/(0.0108 \times M)$$

η_{rel} (relative viscosity) $= t/t_0$

M: Amount (g) of Purified Sodium Hyaluronate Injection taken

Osmotic pressure ratio Being specified separately when the drug is granted approval based on the Law.

pH Being specified separately when the drug is granted approval based on the Law.

Bacterial endotoxins <4.01> Less than 0.003 EU/mg.

Extractable volume <6.05> It meets the requirements.

Foreign insoluble matter <6.06> Perform the test according to Method 1: it meets the requirement.

Insoluble particulate matter <6.07> It meets the requirement.

Sterility <4.06> Perform the test according to the Direct inoculation method: it meets the requirement.

Average molecular mass

1) Apply to the preparation which labeled average molecular mass of sodium hyaluronate is 600,000 to 1,200,000. Calculate the average molecular mass by the following equation, where $[\eta]$ is the intrinsic viscosity obtained in the Viscosity: it is 600,000 to 1,200,000.

$$\text{Average molecular mass} = \left(\frac{[\eta] \times 10^5}{36}\right)^{\frac{1}{0.78}}$$

2) Apply to the preparation which labeled average molecular mass of sodium hyaluronate is 1,500,000 to 2,000,000.
Calculate the average molecular mass by the following equation, where $[\eta]$ is the intrinsic viscosity obtained in the Viscosity: it is 1,500,000 to 2,000,000.

$$\text{Average molecular mass} = \left(\frac{[\eta] \times 10^5}{22.8}\right)^{\frac{1}{0.816}}$$

Assay Weigh accurately an amount of Purified Sodium Hyaluronate Injection, equivalent to about 10 mg of Purified Sodium Hyaluronate, and add 0.2 mol/L sodium chloride TS to make exactly 20 mL. Pipet 1 mL of this solution, add water to make exactly 10 mL, and use this solution as the sample solution. Then, proceed as directed in the Assay under Purified Sodium Hyaluronate.

Content (mg) of sodium hyaluronate $[(C_{14}H_{20}NNaO_{11})_n]$ per mL of Purified Sodium Hyaluronate Injection
$= M_S/M_T \times A_T/A_S \times 1/5 \times \rho \times 2.279$

M_S: Amount (mg) of D-Glucuronolactone RS taken

M_T: Amount (g) of Purified Sodium Hyaluronate Injection taken

ρ: Density (g/mL) of Purified Sodium Hyaluronate Injection measured as directed under Determination of Specific Gravity and Density <2.56>

Containers and storage Containers—Hermetic containers. Plastic containers for aqueous injections may be used.

Purified Sodium Hyaluronate Ophthalmic Solution

精製ヒアルロン酸ナトリウム点眼液

Purified Sodium Hyaluronate Ophthalmic Solution is an aqueous ophthalmic preparation.

It contains not less than 90.0% and not more than 110.0% of the labeled amount of purified sodium hyaluronate $[(C_{14}H_{20}NNaO_{11})_n]$.

Method of preparation Prepare as directed under Ophthalmic Liquids and Solutions, with Purified Sodium Hyaluronate.

Description Purified Sodium Hyaluronate Ophthalmic Solution occurs as a clear, colorless, and viscous liquid.

Identification **(1)** To 1 mL of Purified Sodium Hyaluronate Ophthalmic Solution add 0.2 mL of 1 mol/L acetic acid-sodium acetate buffer solution (pH 6.0) and 5 units of hyaluronidase, and allow to stand at 50°C for 1 hour. Add 1 mL of a solution of dipotassium tetraborate tetrahydrate (1 in 20), and heat in a water bath for 7 minutes. After cooling, add 6 mL of acetic acid (100) and 2.4 mL of 4-dimethylaminobenzaldehyde-hydrochloric acid-acetic acid TS, and allow to stand at room temperature: a yellowish red to red color develops.

(2) To 1 volume of Purified Sodium Hyaluronate Ophthalmic Solution, equivalent to 7.5 mg of purified sodium hyaluronate $[(C_{14}H_{20}NNaO_{11})_n]$, add 2 volumes of acetone, shake well, and centrifuge at 3000 rpm for 10 minutes. Remove the acetone, wash the precipitate with a mixture of acetone and water (5:1), dry the precipitate under reduced pressure (not exceeding 0.67 kPa) at 60°C for 5 hours using phosphorus (V) oxide as a desiccant, and determine the infrared absorption spectrum as directed in ATR method under Infrared Spectrophotometry <2.25>: it exhibits absorption at the wave numbers of about 1605 cm^{-1}, 1404 cm^{-1}, 1375 cm^{-1}, 1150 cm^{-1}, 1025 cm^{-1} and 945 cm^{-1}.

Osmotic pressure ratio Being specified separately when the drug is granted approval based on the Law.

pH Being specified separately when the drug is granted approval based on the Law.

Viscosity <*2.53*> Perform the test according to Method 1 at 30 ± 0.1°C: the kinematic viscosity is 3.0 to 4.0 mm^2/s or 17 to 30 mm^2/s.

Foreign insoluble matter <*6.11*> It meets the requirement.

Insoluble particulate matter <*6.08*> It meets the requirement.

Sterility <*4.06*> Perform the test according to the Membrane filtration method: it meets the requirement.

Average molecular mass When determined by the following method it is between 600,000 and 1,200,000.

(i) Determination of viscosity <*2.53*>

Weigh accurately an amount of Purified Sodium Hyaluronate Ophthalmic Solution, equivalent to about 15 mg of purified sodium hyaluronate [$(C_{14}H_{20}NNaO_{11})_n$], add 0.2 mol/L sodium chloride TS to make exactly 30 mL, and use this solution as the sample solution. Perform the test with the sample solution according to Method 1 at 30 ± 0.1°C, using an Ubbelohde-type viscometer with the down-flowing time of 0.2 mol/L sodium chloride TS is between 200 and 300 seconds. Calculate the intrinsic viscosity [η] according to the following equation, where c is the content obtained in the Assay expressed as the concentration (g/dL): 11.8 - 19.5 dL/g.

$$[\eta] = \sqrt{2(\eta_{sp} - \ln \eta_{rel})}/c \times 0.87 + 1.33$$

η_{sp} (specific viscosity) = $\eta_{rel} - 1$
η_{rel} (relative e viscosity) = t/t_0

(ii) Calculation of average molecular mass

Calculate by the following equation, using the intrinsic viscosity obtained in (i) for [η].

$$\text{Average molecular mass} = \left(\frac{[\eta] \times 10^5}{36}\right)^{\frac{1}{0.78}}$$

Assay To exactly V mL of Purified Sodium Hyaluronate Ophthalmic Solution, equivalent to about 1.5 mg of purified sodium hyaluronate [$(C_{14}H_{20}NNaO_{11})_n$], add the mobile phase to make exactly 30 mL, and use this solution as the sample solution. Separately, weigh accurately about 50 mg of sodium hyaluronate for assay, previously dried under reduced pressure (not exceeding 0.67 kPa) at 60°C for 5 hours using phosphorus (V) oxide as a desiccant, and dissolve in a solution of sodium chloride (9 in 1000) to make exactly 50 mL. Pipet 1 mL of this solution, add the mobile phase to make exactly 20 mL, and use this solution as the standard solution. Perform the test with exactly 20 μL each of the sample solution and standard solution as directed under Liquid Chromatography <*2.01*> according to the following conditions, and determine the peak areas, A_T and A_S, of hyaluronic acid in each solution.

Amount (mg) of purified sodium hyaluronate [$(C_{14}H_{20}NNaO_{11})_n$]
$= M_S \times A_T/A_S \times 1/V \times 3/100$

M_S: Amount (mg) of sodium hyaluronate for assay taken

Operating conditions—

Detector: An ultraviolet absorption photometer (wavelength: 210 nm).

Column: A stainless steel column 7.8 mm in inside diameter and 30 cm in length, packed with porous polymethacrylate for liquid chromatography (7 μm in particle diameter).

Column temperature: A constant temperature of about 40°C.

Mobile phase: Dissolve 32.2 g of sodium sulfate decahydrate in water to make 1000 mL.

Flow rate: Adjust so that the retention time of hyaluronic acid is about 5 minutes.

System suitability—

System performance: Dissolve 50 mg of purified sodium hyaluronate in 50 mL of sodium chloride solution (9 in 1000). To 1 mL of this solution and 2 mL of a solution of ε-aminocaproic acid (1 in 500) add the mobile phase to make 20 mL, and use this solution as the solution for system suitability test. When the procedure is run with 20 μL of the solution for system suitability test under the above operating conditions, hyaluronic acid and ε-aminocaproic acid are eluted in this order with the resolution between these peaks being not less than 5.

System repeatability: When the test is repeated 6 times with 20 μL of the standard solution under the above operating conditions, the relative standard deviation of the peak area of hyaluronic acid is not more than 2.0%.

Containers and storage Containers—Tight containers.

Sodium Hydroxide

水酸化ナトリウム

NaOH: 40.00

Sodium Hydroxide contains not less than 95.0% of sodium hydroxide (NaOH).

Description Sodium Hydroxide occurs as white, fused masses, in small pellets, in flakes, in sticks, and in other forms. It is hard and brittle, and shows a crystalline fracture.

It is freely soluble in water and in ethanol (95), and practically insoluble in diethyl ether.

It rapidly absorbs carbon dioxide in air.

It deliquesces in moist air.

Identification **(1)** A solution of Sodium Hydroxide (1 in 500) is alkaline.

(2) A solution of Sodium Hydroxide (1 in 25) responds to Qualitative Tests <*1.09*> for sodium salt.

Purity **(1)** Clarity and color of solution—Dissolve 1.0 g of Sodium Hydroxide in 20 mL of water: the solution is clear and colorless.

(2) Chloride <*1.03*>—Dissolve 2.0 g of Sodium Hydroxide in water, and add water to make 100 mL. To 25 mL of the solution add 10 mL of dilute nitric acid and water to make 50 mL, and perform the test using this solution as the test solution. Prepare the control solution with 0.7 mL of 0.01 mol/L hydrochloric acid VS (not more than 0.050%).

(3) Heavy metals <*1.07*>—Dissolve 1.0 g of Sodium Hydroxide in 5 mL of water, add 11 mL of dilute hydrochloric acid, and evaporate on a water bath to dryness. Dissolve the residue in 35 mL of water, add 2 mL of dilute acetic acid and 1 drop of ammonia TS, add water to make 50 mL, and perform the test using this solution as the test solution. Evaporate 11 mL of dilute hydrochloric acid on a water bath to dryness, dissolve the residue in 2 mL of dilute acetic acid and 3.0 mL of Standard Lead Solution, add water to make 50 mL, and use this solution as the control solution (not more than 30 ppm).

(4) Potassium—Dissolve 0.10 g of Sodium Hydroxide in water and dilute with water to make 40 mL. Add 1.0 mL of dilute acetic acid to 4.0 mL of this solution, and shake. Add 5.0 mL of a solution of sodium tetraphenylboron (1 in 30), shake immediately, and allow to stand for 10 minutes: the solution has no more turbidity than the following control solution.

Control solution: Dissolve 9.5 mg of potassium chloride in water, and dilute with water to make 1000 mL. Add 1.0 mL of dilute acetic acid to 4.0 mL of this solution, shake, and proceed as directed above.

(5) Sodium carbonate—The amount of sodium carbonate (Na_2CO_3: 105.99) is not more than 2.0%, when calculated by the following equation using *B* (mL) which is obtained in the Assay.

$$\text{Amount (mg) of sodium carbonate} = 105.99 \times B$$

(6) Mercury—Dissolve 2.0 g of Sodium Hydroxide in 1 mL of a solution of potassium permanganate (3 in 50) and 30 mL of water, neutralize gradually with purified hydrochloric acid, and add 5 mL of diluted sulfuric acid (1 in 2). To this solution add a solution of hydroxylammonium chloride (1 in 5) until the precipitate of manganese dioxide disappears, add water to make exactly 100 mL, and use this solution as the sample solution. Perform the tests according to Atomic Absorption Spectrophotometry *<2.23>* (Cold vapor type) with the sample solution. Place the sample solution in the sample bottle of an atomic absorption spectrophotometer, add 10 mL of tin (II) chloride-sulfuric acid TS, connect the bottle immediately to the atomic absorption spectrophotometer, and circulate air. Read the absorbance A_T of the sample solution when the indication of the recorder rises rapidly and becomes constant at the wavelength of 253.7 nm. On the other hand, to 2.0 mL of Standard Mercury Solution add 1 mL of a solution of potassium permanganate (3 in 50), 30 mL of water and a volume of purified hydrochloric acid equal to that used in the preparation of the sample solution, and read the absorbance A_S of the solution obtained by the same procedure as used for the sample solution: A_T is smaller than A_S.

Assay Weigh accurately about 1.5 g of Sodium Hydroxide, and dissolve in 40 mL of freshly boiled and cooled water. Cool the solution to 15°C, add 2 drops of phenolphthalein TS, and titrate *<2.50>* with 0.5 mol/L sulfuric acid VS until the red color of the solution disappears. Record the amount, *A* (mL), of 0.5 mol/L sulfuric acid VS consumed. Then add 2 drops of methyl orange TS to the solution, and further titrate *<2.50>* with 0.5 mol/L sulfuric acid VS until the solution shows a persistent light red color. Record the amount, *B* (mL), of 0.5 mol/L sulfuric acid VS consumed. Calculate the amount of NaOH from the difference, *A* (mL) − *B* (mL).

Each mL of 0.5 mol/L sulfuric acid VS
= 40.00 mg of NaOH

Containers and storage Containers—Tight containers.

Sodium Iodide

ヨウ化ナトリウム

NaI: 149.89

Sodium Iodide, when dried, contains not less than 99.0% of sodium iodide (NaI).

Description Sodium Iodide occurs as colorless crystals or a white crystalline powder. It is odorless.

It is very soluble in water, and freely soluble in glycerin and in ethanol (95).

It deliquesces in moist air.

Identification A solution of Sodium Iodide (1 in 20) responds to Qualitative Tests *<1.09>* for sodium salt and for iodide.

Purity **(1)** Clarity and color of solution—Dissolve 1.0 g of Sodium Iodide in 2 mL of water: the solution is clear and colorless.

(2) Alkalinity—Dissolve 1.0 g of Sodium Iodide in 10 mL of freshly boiled and cooled water, and add 1.0 mL of 0.005 mol/L sulfuric acid VS and 1 drop of phenolphthalein TS: no color is produced.

(3) Chloride, bromide and thiosulfate—Dissolve 0.20 g of Sodium Iodide in 5 mL of ammonia TS, add 15.0 mL of 0.1 mol/L silver nitrate VS, shake for a few minutes, and filter. To 10 mL of the filtrate add 15 mL of dilute nitric acid: no brown color appears. The solution has no more turbidity than the following control solution.

Control solution: To 0.30 mL of 0.01 mol/L hydrochloric acid VS add 2.5 mL of ammonia TS, 7.5 mL of 0.1 mol/L silver nitrate VS and 15 mL of dilute nitric acid.

(4) Nitrate, nitrite and ammonium—Place 1.0 g of Sodium Iodide in a 40-mL test tube, and add 5 mL of water, 5 mL of sodium hydroxide TS and 0.2 g of aluminum wire. Insert a pledget of absorbent cotton in the mouth of the test tube, and place a piece of moistened red litmus paper on the cotton. Heat the test tube on a water bath for 15 minutes: the evolved gas does not turn moistened red litmus paper to blue.

(5) Cyanide—Dissolve 0.5 g of Sodium Iodide in 10 mL of water. To 5 mL of this solution add 1 drop of iron (II) sulfate TS and 2 mL of sodium hydroxide TS, warm, and add 4 mL of hydrochloric acid: no green color develops.

(6) Iodate—Dissolve 0.5 g of Sodium Iodide in 10 mL of freshly boiled and cooled water, and add 2 drops of dilute sulfuric acid and 1 drop of starch TS: no blue color develops immediately.

(7) Heavy metals *<1.07>*—Proceed with 2.0 g of Sodium Iodide according to Method 1, and perform the test. Prepare the control solution with 2.0 mL of Standard Lead Solution (not more than 10 ppm).

(8) Barium—Dissolve 0.5 g of Sodium Iodide in 10 mL of water, add 1 mL of dilute sulfuric acid, and allow to stand for 5 minutes: no turbidity is produced.

(9) Potassium—Dissolve 1.0 g of Sodium Iodide in water, and add water to make 100 mL. To 4.0 mL of this solution add 1.0 mL of dilute acetic acid, shake, add 5.0 mL of a solution of sodium tetraphenylboron (1 in 30), immediately shake, and allow to stand for 10 minutes: the solution has no more turbidity than the following control solution.

Control solution: Dissolve 9.5 mg of potassium chloride in water, and add water to make 1000 mL. To 4.0 mL of this solution add 1.0 mL of dilute acetic acid, shake, and then proceed as directed above.

(10) Arsenic *<1.11>*—Prepare the test solution with 0.40 g of Sodium Iodide according to Method 1, and perform the test (not more than 5 ppm).

Loss on drying *<2.41>* Not more than 5.0% (2 g, 120°C, 2 hours).

Assay Weigh accurately about 0.4 g of Sodium Iodide, previously dried, in an iodine flask, dissolve in 10 mL of water, add 35 mL of hydrochloric acid and 5 mL of chloroform, and titrate *<2.50>* with 0.05 mol/L potassium iodate VS while shaking vigorously until the red-purple color of the chloroform layer disappears. The end point is attained when the red-purple color does not reappear in the chloroform layer within 5 minutes after the layer has been decolorized.

Each mL of 0.05 mol/L potassium iodate VS
= 14.99 mg of NaI

Containers and storage Containers—Tight containers.
Storage—Light-resistant.

Sodium Iodide (^{123}I) Capsules

ヨウ化ナトリウム (^{123}I) カプセル

Sodium Iodide (^{123}I) Capsules contain iodine-123 in the form of sodium iodide.

It conforms to the requirements of Sodium Iodide (^{123}I) Capsules in the Minimum Requirements for Radiopharmaceuticals.

Sodium Iodide (^{131}I) Capsules

ヨウ化ナトリウム (^{131}I) カプセル

Sodium Iodide (^{131}I) Capsules contain iodine-131 in the form of sodium iodide.

It conforms to the requirements of Sodium Iodide (^{131}I) Capsules in the Minimum Requirements for Radiopharmaceuticals.

Sodium Iodide (^{131}I) Solution

ヨウ化ナトリウム (^{131}I) 液

Sodium Iodide (^{131}I) Solution contains iodine-131 (^{131}I) in the form of sodium iodide.

It conforms to the requirements of Sodium Iodide (^{131}I) Solution in the Minimum Requirements for Radiopharmaceuticals.

Description Sodium Iodide (^{131}I) Solution is a clear, colorless liquid. It is odorless, or has an odor due to the preservatives or stabilizers.

Sodium Iodohippurate (^{131}I) Injection

ヨウ化ヒプル酸ナトリウム (^{131}I) 注射液

Sodium Iodohippurate (^{131}I) Injection is an aqueous injection containing iodine-131 (^{131}I) in the form of sodium *o*-iodohippurate.

It conforms to the requirements of Sodium Iodohippurate (^{131}I) Injection in the Minimum Requirements for Radiopharmaceuticals.

Test for Extractable Volume of Parenteral Preparations and Insoluble Particulate Matter Test for Injections are not applied to this injection.

Description Sodium Iodohippurate (^{131}I) Injection is a clear, colorless liquid. It is odorless or has an odor of the preservatives or stabilizers.

Sodium Iotalamate Injection

イオタラム酸ナトリウム注射液

Sodium Iotalamate Injection is an aqueous injection.

It contains not less than 95.0% and not more than 105.0% of the labeled amount of iotalamic acid ($C_{11}H_9I_3N_2O_4$: 613.91).

Method of preparation

(1)

Iotalamic Acid	645 g
Sodium Hydroxide	42 g
Water for Injection or Sterile Water for Injection in Containers	a sufficient quantity
To make	1000 mL

(2)

Iotalamic Acid	772.5 g
Sodium Hydroxide	50.5 g
Water for Injection or Sterile Water for Injection in Containers	a sufficient quantity
To make	1000 mL

Prepare as directed under Injections, with the above ingredients (1) or (2).

Description Sodium Iotalamate Injection is a clear, colorless or pale yellow, slightly viscous liquid.

It is gradually colored by light.

Identification **(1)** To a volume of Sodium Iotalamate Injection, equivalent to 1 g of Iotalamic Acid, add 25 mL of water, and add 2.5 mL of dilute hydrochloric acid with thorough stirring: a white precipitate is produced. Filter the precipitate by suction through a glass filter (G4), wash the precipitate with two 10-mL portions of water, and dry at 105°C for 1 hour. Proceed with the precipitate as directed in the Identification (2) under Iotalamic Acid.

(2) Sodium Iotalamate Injection responds to Qualitative Tests <*1.09*> (1) for sodium salt.

pH <*2.54*> 6.5 – 7.7

Purity **(1)** Primary aromatic amines—To a volume of Sodium Iotalamate Injection, equivalent to 0.20 g of Iotalamic Acid, add 15 mL of water, shake, add 4 mL of a solution of sodium nitrite (1 in 100) under ice-cooling, and proceed as directed in the Purity (2) under Iotalamic Acid: the absorbance is not more than 0.17.

(2) Iodine and iodide—To a volume of Sodium Iotalamate Injection, equivalent to 1.5 g of Iotalamic Acid, add 20 mL of water and 5 mL of dilute sulfuric acid, shake well, and filter the precipitate by suction through a glass filter (G4). To the filtrate add 5 mL of toluene, and shake vigorously: the toluene layer is colorless. Then add 2 mL of a solution of sodium nitrite (1 in 100), and shake vigorously: the toluene layer has no more color than the following control solution.

Control solution: Dissolve 0.25 g of potassium iodide in water to make 1000 mL. To 2.0 mL of this solution add 20 mL of water, 5 mL of dilute sulfuric acid, 5 mL of toluene and 2 mL of a solution of sodium nitrite (1 in 100), and shake vigorously.

Bacterial endotoxins <*4.01*> Less than 3.4 EU/mL.

Extractable volume <*6.05*> It meets the requirement.

Foreign insoluble matter <*6.06*> Perform the test according to Method 1: it meets the requirement.

Insoluble particulate matter <*6.07*> It meets the requirement.

Sterility <*4.06*> Perform the test according to the Direct inoculation method: it meets the requirement.

Assay Pipet a volume of Sodium Iotalamate Injection, equivalent to about 4 g of iotalamic acid ($C_{11}H_9I_3N_2O_4$), add water to make exactly 200 mL. Pipet 2 mL of this solution, add water to make exactly 200 mL. To exactly 5 mL of this solution add exactly 5 mL of the internal standard solution, add the mobile phase to make 100 mL, and use this solution as the sample solution. Separately, weigh accurately about 0.4 g of iotalamic acid for assay, previously dried at 105°C for 4 hours, dissolve in 100 mL of water and 1 mL of sodium hydroxide TS, and add water to make exactly 200 mL. Pipet 5 mL of this solution, add water to make exactly 50 mL. To exactly 5 mL of this solution add exactly 5 mL of the internal standard solution, add the mobile phase to make 100 mL, and use this solution as the standard solution. Perform the test with 10 μL each of the sample solution and standard solution as directed under Liquid Chromatography <*2.01*> according to the following conditions, and calculate the ratios, Q_T and Q_S, of the peak area of iotalamic acid to that of the internal standard.

$$\text{Amount (mg) of iotalamic acid } (C_{11}H_9I_3N_2O_4) = M_S \times Q_T/Q_S$$

M_S: Amount (mg) of iotalamic acid for assay taken

Internal standard solution—A solution of L-tryptophan in the mobile phase (3 in 2500).

Operating conditions—

Detector: An ultraviolet absorption photometer (wavelength: 240 nm).

Column: A stainless steel column 4.6 mm in inside diameter and 15 cm in length, packed with octadecylsilanized silica gel for liquid chromatography (5 μm in particle diameter).

Column temperature: A constant temperature of about 20°C.

Mobile phase: To 3.9 g of phosphoric acid and 2.8 mL of triethylamine add water to make 2000 mL. To this solution add 100 mL of acetonitrile.

Flow rate: Adjust so that the retention time of iotalamic acid is about 6 minutes.

System suitability—

System performance: When the procedure is run with 10 μL of the standard solution under the above operating conditions, iotalamic acid and the internal standard are eluted in this order with the resolution between these peaks being not less than 5.

System repeatability: When the test is repeated 6 times with 10 μL of the standard solution under the above operating conditions, the relative standard deviation of the ratios of the peak area of iotalamic acid to that of the internal standard is not more than 1.0%.

Containers and storage Containers—Hermetic containers, and colored containers may be used.

Storage—Light-resistant.

Sodium L-Lactate Solution

L-乳酸ナトリウム液

Sodium L-Lactate Solution is an aqueous solution of sodium salt of L-lactic acid.

It contains not less than 95.0% and not more than 105.0% of the labeled amount of sodium L-lactate ($C_3H_5NaO_3$).

The label states the content amount of sodium L-lactate.

Description Sodium L-Lactate Solution occurs as a clear and colorless viscous liquid. It has no odor or has a slight characteristic odor, and has a slight saline taste.

It is miscible with water or with ethanol (99.5).

Identification To an amount of Sodium L-Lactate Solution, equivalent to 1 g of sodium L-lactate ($C_3H_5NaO_3$), add water to make 50 mL. This solution responds to Qualitative Tests <*1.09*> for sodium salt and for lactate.

Optical rotation <*2.49*> $[\alpha]_D^{20}$: −38 − −44° To an exact amount of Sodium L-Lactate Solution, equivalent to 2.5 g of sodium L-lactate ($C_3H_5NaO_3$), add 30 mL of water and 5.0 g of hexaammonium heptamolybdate tetrahydrate, then add water to make exactly 50 mL, and determine using a 100-mm cell.

pH <*2.54*> To an amount of Sodium L-Lactate Solution, equivalent to 5 g of sodium L-lactate ($C_3H_5NaO_3$), add water to make 50 mL: the pH of this solution is between 6.5 and 7.5.

Purity (1) Chloride <*1.03*>—Perform the test with an amount of Sodium L-Lactate Solution, equivalent to 1.0 g of sodium L-lactate ($C_3H_5NaO_3$). Prepare the control solution with 0.40 mL of 0.01 mol/L hydrochloric acid VS (not more than 0.014%).

(2) Sulfate <*1.14*>—To an amount of Sodium L-Lactate Solution, equivalent to 2.0 g of sodium L-lactate ($C_3H_5NaO_3$), add 7 mL of dilute hydrochloric acid and water to make 50 mL. Perform the test using this solution as the test solution. Prepare the control solution with 0.40 mL of 0.005 mol/L sulfuric acid VS (not more than 0.010%).

(3) Heavy metals <*1.07*>—To an amount of Sodium L-Lactate Solution, equivalent to 2.0 g of sodium L-lactate ($C_3H_5NaO_3$), add 5 mL of dilute hydrochloric acid, 2 mL of dilute acetic acid and water to make 50 mL. Perform the test using this solution as the test solution. Prepare the control solution as follows: To 2.0 mL of Standard Lead Solution add 2 mL of dilute acetic acid and water to make 50 mL (not more than 10 ppm).

(4) Iron <*1.10*>—Prepare the test solution with an amount of Sodium L-Lactate Solution, equivalent to 2.0 g of sodium L-lactate ($C_3H_5NaO_3$), according to Method 1, and perform the test according to Method A. Prepare the control solution with 1.0 mL of Standard Iron Solution (not more than 5 ppm).

(5) Arsenic <*1.11*>—To an amount of Sodium L-Lactate Solution, equivalent to 2.5 g of sodium L-lactate ($C_3H_5NaO_3$), and add water to make 10 mL. Perform the test using 2 mL of this solution as the test solution (not more than 4 ppm).

(6) Sugars—To an amount of Sodium L-Lactate Solution, equivalent to 1.0 g of sodium L-lactate ($C_3H_5NaO_3$), add 10 mL of water and 10 mL of Fehling's TS, and boil for 5 minutes: no red precipitate is produced.

(7) Citric, oxalic, phosphoric and L-tartaric acids—To an amount of Sodium L-Lactate Solution, equivalent to 1.0 g of sodium L-lactate ($C_3H_5NaO_3$), add 1 mL of water and 1 mL of dilute hydrochloric acid, then add 40 mL of calcium hydroxide TS, and boil for 2 minutes: the solution is not changed.

(8) Volatile fatty acids—To an amount of Sodium L-Lactate Solution, equivalent to 3.0 g of sodium L-lactate ($C_3H_5NaO_3$), add 2 mL of dilute sulfuric acid, and heat on a water bath: no acetic acid like nor lactic acid like odor is produced.

(9) Cyanide—Transfer an amount of Sodium L-Lactate Solution, equivalent to 1.0 g of sodium L-lactate ($C_3H_5NaO_3$), to a Nessler tube, add 10 mL of water and 1 drop of phenolphthalein TS, then add dropwise a solution of sodium hydroxide (1 in 10) while shaking until a pale red color appears. Add further 1.5 mL of a solution of sodium hydroxide (1 in 10) and water to make 20 mL, and heat in a water bath for 10 minutes. After cooling, add dropwise dilute hydrochloric acid until a red color of the solution disappears, then add 1 drop of acetic acid (31), 10 mL of phosphate buffer solution (pH 6.8) and 0.25 mL of sodium toluenesulfonchloramide TS, stopper immediately, mix gently, and allow to stand for 5 minutes. Add 15 mL of pyridine-pyrazolone TS and water to make 50 mL, and allow to stand at 25°C for 30 minutes: the color of the solution is not more intense than that of the following control solution.

Control solution: To 1.0 mL of Standard Cyanide Solution add water to make 20 mL. Transfer 1.0 mL of this solution to a Nessler tube, add 10 mL of water and 1 drop of phenolphthalein TS, then proceed in the same manner as descried above.

(10) Methanol—Transfer an amount of Sodium L-Lactate Solution, equivalent to 5.0 g of sodium L-lactate ($C_3H_5NaO_3$), to a distilling flask of the apparatus for alcohol number determination *<1.01>*, add 10 mL of water, and distill. Pipet 5 mL of the distillate, add water to make exactly 10 mL, and use this solution as the sample solution. Separately, to exactly 1.0 mL of methanol add water to make exactly 100 mL. Pipe 5 mL of this solution, add water to make exactly 200 mL. Pipet 5 mL of this solution, add water to make exactly 10 mL, and use this solution as the standard solution. Perform the test with exactly 10 μL each of the sample solution and standard solution as directed under Gas Chromatography *<2.02>* according to the following conditions: the peak area of methanol obtained from the sample solution is not larger than that from the standard solution (not more than 0.025%).

Operating conditions—

Detector: A hydrogen flame-ionization detector.

Column: A glass column 3 mm in inside diameter and 1.5 m in length, packed with porous ethyl vinylbenzene-divinylbenzene copolymer for gas chromatography (149 - 177 μm in particle diameter).

Column temperature: A constant temperature of about 120°C.

Injection port and detector temperature: A constant temperature of about 125°C.

Carrier gas: Nitrogen.

Flow rate: Adjust so that the retention time of methanol is about 2 minutes.

System suitability—

System performance: To 1 mL of methanol and 1 mL of ethanol (99.5) add water to make 100 mL. To 5 mL of this solution add water to make 200 mL. To 5 mL of this solution add water to make 10 mL. When the procedure is run with 10 μL of this solution under the above operating conditions, methanol and ethanol are eluted in this order with the resolution between these peaks being not less than 2.0.

System repeatability: When the test is repeated 6 times with 10 μL of the standard solution under the above operating conditions, the relative standard deviation of the peak area of methanol is not more than 5%.

Assay Weigh accurately an amount of Sodium L-Lactate Solution, equivalent to about 0.25 g of sodium L-lactate ($C_3H_5NaO_3$), dry at 105°C for 4 hours, add 50 mL of acetic acid (100), and titrate *<2.50>* with 0.1 mol/L perchloric acid VS until the color of solution changes from purple to yellow-green through blue-green (indicator: 2 drops of crystal violet TS). Perform a blank determination in the same manner, and make any necessary correction.

Each mL of 0.1 mol/L perchloric acid VS
= 11.21 mg of $C_3H_5NaO_3$

Containers and storage Containers—Tight containers.

Sodium L-Lactate Ringer's Solution

L-乳酸ナトリウムリンゲル液

Sodium L-Lactate Ringer's Solution is an aqueous injection.

It contains not less than 0.285 w/v% and not more than 0.330 w/v% of sodium (as Na: 22.99), not less than 0.0149 w/v% and not more than 0.0173 w/v% of potassium (as K: 39.10), not less than 0.00518 w/v% and not more than 0.00600 w/v% of calcium (as Ca: 40.08), not less than 0.369 w/v% and not more than 0.427 w/v% of chlorine (as Cl: 35.45), and not less than 0.234 w/v% and not more than 0.271 w/v% of L-lactic acid (as $C_3H_5O_3$: 89.07).

Method of preparation

Sodium Chloride	6.0 g
Potassium Chloride	0.30 g
Calcium Chloride Hydrate	0.20 g
Sodium L-Lactate Solution (as sodium L-lactate)	3.1 g
Water for Injection or Sterile Water for Injection in Containers	a sufficient amount
Total amount	1000 mL

Prepare as directed under Injections, with the components above. Any preservatives are not added.

Description Sodium L-Lactate Ringer's Solution occurs as a clear and colorless liquid.

Identification **(1)** Sodium L-Lactate Ringer's Solution responds to Qualitative Tests *<1.09>* (1) for sodium salt.

(2) A solution, obtained by concentrating 10 mL of Sodium L-Lactate Ringer's Solution to 5 mL by heating on a water bath, responds to Qualitative Tests *<1.09>* (1) for potassium salt.

(3) A solution, obtained by concentrating 10 mL of Sodium L-Lactate Ringer's Solution to 5 mL by heating on a water bath, responds to Qualitative Tests *<1.09>* (3) for calcium salt.

(4) Sodium L-Lactate Ringer's Solution responds to Qualitative Tests *<1.09>* (2) for chloride.

(5) Sodium L-Lactate Ringer's Solution responds to Qualitative Tests *<1.09>* for lactate.

pH *<2.54>* 6.0 - 7.5

Purity Heavy metals *<1.07>*—Concentrate 100 mL of Sodium L-Lactate Ringer's Solution on a water bath to about 40 mL, and add 2 mL of dilute acetic acid and water to make 50 mL. Perform the test with this solution as the test solution. Prepare the control solution with 3.0 mL of Standard Lead Solution by adding 2 mL of dilute acetic acid and water to make 50 mL (not more than 0.3 ppm).

Bacterial endotoxins *<4.01>* Less than 0.25 EU/mL.

Extractable volume *<6.05>* It meets the requirement.

Foreign insoluble matter *<6.06>* Perform the test according to Method 1: it meets the requirement.

Insoluble particulate matter *<6.07>* It meets the requirement.

Sterility *<4.06>* Perform the test according to the Membrane filtration method: it meets the requirement.

Assay **(1)** Sodium, potassium, and calcium—Pipet 10 mL of Sodium L-Lactate Ringer's Solution, add exactly 5 mL of the internal standard solution and water to make 50 mL, and use this solution as the sample solution. Separately, pipet 10 mL of standard stock solution, add exactly 5 mL of the internal standard solution and water to make 50 mL, and use this solution as the standard solution. Perform the test with 20 μL each of the sample solution and standard solution as directed under Liquid Chromatography *<2.01>* according to the following conditions, and calculate the ratios, Q_{Ta}, Q_{Tb} and Q_{Tc}, of respective peak area of sodium, potassium and calcium to that of the internal standard in the sample solution, and the ratios, Q_{Sa}, Q_{Sb} and Q_{Sc}, of respective peak area of sodium, potassium and calcium to that of the internal standard in the standard solution.

Amount (w/v%) of sodium (Na)
$$= (M_{Sa1} \times f/100 \times 0.205 + M_{Sa2} \times 0.393) \times Q_{Ta}/Q_{Sa} \times 1/10$$

Amount (w/v%) of potassium (K)
$$= M_{Sb} \times Q_{Tb}/Q_{Sb} \times 1/10 \times 0.524$$

Amount (w/v%) of calcium (Ca)
$$= M_{Sc} \times Q_{Tc}/Q_{Sc} \times 1/10 \times 0.273$$

M_{Sa1}: Amount (g) of sodium L-lactate solution for assay taken
f: Content (%) of sodium L-lactate solution for assay
M_{Sa2}: Amount (g) of sodium chloride for assay taken
M_{Sb}: Amount (g) of potassium chloride for assay taken
M_{Sc}: Amount (g) of calcium chloride hydrate for assay taken

Standard stock solution: Weigh accurately an amount of sodium L-lactate solution for assay equivalent to about 3.1 g of sodium L-lactate ($C_3H_5NaO_3$), about 6 g of dried sodium chloride for assay, about 0.3 g of dried potassium chloride for assay and about 0.2 g of calcium chloride hydrate for assay, respectively, and dissolve in water to make exactly 1000 mL.

Internal standard solution—A solution of rubidium chloride (1 in 200).

Operating conditions—

Detector: A conductivity detector.

Column: A plastic column 4 mm in inside diameter and 25 cm in length, packed with a weakly acidic ion-exchange resin for liquid chromatography composed with carboxylic acid and phosphonic acid groups combining ethylvinylbenzene-divinylbenzene copolymer (8.5 μm in particle diameter).

Column temperature: A constant temperature of about 25°C.

Mobile phase: To 4 mL of methanesulfonic acid add water to make 3000 mL.

Flow rate of mobile phase: Adjust so that the retention time of potassium is about 6 minutes.

Suppressor: An anion elimination device with anion-exchange membrane.

Refreshing liquid: Diluted 40% tetrabutylammonium hydroxide TS (1 in 40).

Flow rate of refreshing liquid: 2 mL per minute.

System suitability—

System performance: When the procedure is run with 20 μL of the standard solution under the above operating conditions, sodium, potassium, the internal standard and calcium are eluted in this order with the resolution between these peaks being not less than 1.5.

System repeatability: When the test is repeated 6 times with 20 μL of the standard solution under the above operating conditions, the relative standard deviation of the ratio of the peak area of sodium, potassium and calcium to that of the internal standard is not more than 1.0%.

(2) Chlorine—Pipet 1 mL of Sodium L-Lactate Ringer's Solution, add exactly 5 mL of the internal standard solution and water to make 100 mL, and use this solution as the sample solution. Separately, pipet 10 mL of standard stock solution obtained in (1), and add water to make exactly 50 mL. Take exactly 4 mL and 6 mL of this solution, add exactly 5 mL of the internal standard solution to them and water to make 100 mL, and use these solutions as the low concentration standard solution and the high concentration standard solution, respectively. Perform the test with 20 μL each of the sample solution, the low concentration standard solution and the high concentration standard solution as directed under Liquid Chromatography *<2.01>* according to the following conditions, and calculate the ratios, Q_T, Q_{SL} and Q_{SH}, of the peak area of chlorine to that of the internal standard.

Amount (w/v%) of chlorine (Cl)
$$= (M_{Sa} \times 0.607 + M_{Sb} \times 0.476 + M_{Sc} \times 0.482) \times (Q_T - 3Q_{SL} + 2Q_{SH})/(Q_{SH} - Q_{SL}) \times 1/25$$

M_{Sa}: Amount (g) of sodium chloride for assay taken
M_{Sb}: Amount (g) of potassium chloride for assay taken
M_{Sc}: Amount (g) of calcium chloride hydrate for assay taken

Internal standard solution—A solution of sodium bromide (1 in 500).

Operating conditions—

Detector: A conductivity detector.

Column: A plastic column 4 mm in inside diameter and 25 cm in length, packed with a strongly basic ion-exchange resin for liquid chromatography composed with quaternary ammonium group combining ethylvinylbenzene-divinylbenzene copolymer (9 μm in particle diameter).

Column temperature: A constant temperature of about 25°C.

Mobile phase: Dissolve 0.25 g of sodium hydrogen carbonate and 0.64 g of anhydrous sodium carbonate in 2000 mL of water.

Flow rate of mobile phase: Adjust so that the retention time of chlorine is about 4 minutes.

Suppressor: A cation elimination device with cation-exchange membrane.

Refreshing liquid: Diluted sulfuric acid (3 in 4000).

Flow rate of refreshing liquid: 2 mL per minute.

System suitability—

System performance: When the procedure is run with 20 μL of the low concentration standard solution under the above operating conditions, lactic acid, chlorine and the internal standard are eluted in this order and the resolution between the peaks of lactic acid and chlorine is not less than 1.5.

System repeatability: When the test is repeated 6 times with 20 μL of the low concentration standard solution under the above operating conditions, the relative standard deviation of the ratio of the peak area of chlorine to that of the internal standard is not more than 1.0%.

(3) L-Lactic acid—Pipet 20 mL of Sodium L-Lactate Ringer's Solution, add exactly 5 mL of the internal standard solution and water to make 50 mL, and use this solution as the sample solution. Separately, pipet 20 mL of standard stock solution obtained in (1), add exactly 5 mL of the internal standard solution and water to make 50 mL, and use this solution as the standard solution. Perform the test with 20 μL each of the sample solution and standard solution as directed under Liquid Chromatography <*2.01*> according to the following conditions, and calculate the ratios, Q_T and Q_S, of the peak area of lactic acid to that of the internal standard.

$$\text{Amount (w/v\%) of L-lactic acid } (C_3H_5O_3) = M_S \times f/100 \times Q_T/Q_S \times 1/10 \times 0.795$$

M_S: Amount (g) of sodium L-lactate solution for assay taken

f: Content (%) of sodium L-lactate solution for assay

Internal standard solution—A solution of sodium acetate trihydrate (1 in 50).

Operating conditions—

Detector: A conductivity detector.

Column: A stainless steel column 7.8 mm in inside diameter and 30 cm in length, packed with a strongly acidic ion-exchange resin for liquid chromatography composed with sulfonic acid group combining styrene-divinylbenzene copolymer (5 μm in particle diameter).

Column temperature: A constant temperature of about 25°C.

Mobile phase: To 3000 mL of water add 0.5 mL of heptafluorobutylic acid.

Flow rate of mobile phase: Adjust so that the retention time of lactic acid is about 9 minutes.

Suppressor: A cation elimination device with cation-exchange membrane.

Refreshing liquid: Diluted 40% tetrabutylammonium hydroxide TS (13 in 2000).

Flow rate of refreshing liquid: 2 mL per minute.

System suitability—

System performance: When the procedure is run with 20 μL of the standard solution under the above operating conditions, lactic acid and the internal standard are eluted in this order with the resolution between these peaks being not less than 2.0.

System repeatability: When the test is repeated 6 times with 20 μL of the standard solution under the above operating conditions, the relative standard deviation of the ratio of the peak area of lactic acid to that of the internal standard is not more than 1.0%.

Containers and storage Containers—Hermetic containers. Plastic containers for aqueous injections may be used.

Sodium Lauryl Sulfate

ラウリル硫酸ナトリウム

$C_{12}H_{25}NaO_4S$: 288.38

Monosodium monododecyl sulfate

[151-21-3]

This monograph is harmonized with the European Pharmacopoeia and the U.S. Pharmacopeia.

The corresponding part of the attributes/provisions which are agreed as non-harmonized within the scope of the harmonization is marked with symbols (◆ ◆), and the corresponding parts which are agreed as the JP local requirement other than the scope of the harmonization are marked with symbols (◇ ◇).

Information on the harmonization with the European Pharmacopoeia and the U.S. Pharmacopeia is available on the website of the Pharmaceuticals and Medical Devices Agency.

Sodium Lauryl Sulfate is a mixture of sodium alkyl sulfate consisting chiefly of sodium lauryl sulfate.

It contains not less than 85.0% of sodium alkyl sulfate [as sodium lauryl sulfate ($C_{12}H_{25}NaO_4S$)].

◆**Description** Sodium Lauryl Sulfate occurs as white to light yellow, crystals or powder. It has a slightly characteristic odor.

It is sparingly soluble in ethanol (95).

A solution of 1 g of Sodium Lauryl Sulfate in 10 mL of water is a clear or an opalescent solution.◆

Identification **(1)** Determine the infrared absorption spectrum of Sodium Lauryl Sulfate as directed in the potassium bromide disk method under Infrared Spectrophotometry <*2.25*>, and compare the spectrum with the Reference Spectrum: both spectra exhibit similar intensities of absorption at the same wave numbers.

(2) Put 2.5 g of Sodium Lauryl Sulfate in a platinum or quartz crucible, and add 2 mL of 5 mol/L sulfuric acid TS. Heat on a water bath, cautiously raise the temperature gradually with a burner, and ignite. Ignite, preferably in an electric furnace, at 600 ± 25°C and incinerate the residue completely. After cooling, add a few drops of 1 mol/L sulfuric acid TS, and heat and ignite as above. After cooling, add a few drops of ammonium carbonate TS, evaporate to dryness, and further ignite as above. After cooling, dissolve the residue in 50 mL of water, and stir. To 2 mL of this solution add 4 mL of potassium hexahydroxoantimonate (V) TS. If necessary, rub the inside wall of the vessel with a glass rod: a white crystalline precipitate is formed.

(3) Acidify a solution of Sodium Lauryl Sulfate (1 in 10) with hydrochloric acid, and boil for 20 minutes: no precipitate is formed. To this solution add barium chloride TS: a white precipitate is formed.

Purity **(1)** Alkalinity—Dissolve 1.0 g of Sodium Lauryl Sulfate in 100 mL of water, add 0.1 mL of phenol red TS, and titrate <*2.50*> with 0.1 mol/L hydrochloric acid VS: the consumed volume is not more than 0.5 mL.

(2) Sodium chloride—Dissolve about 5 g of Sodium Lauryl Sulfate, accurately weighed, in 50 mL of water, neutralize the solution with dilute nitric acid, if necessary, add exactly 5 mL of 0.1 mol/L sodium chloride TS, and titrate <*2.50*> with 0.1 mol/L silver nitrate VS until the color of the solution changes from yellow-green through yellow to orange (indicator: 2 drops of fluorescein sodium TS). Perform a blank determination in the same manner, and make any necessary correction.

Each mL of 0.1 mol/L silver nitrate VS
= 5.844 mg of NaCl

The combined content of sodium chloride (NaCl: 58.44) and sodium sulfate (Na_2SO_4: 142.04) obtained in (3) is not more than 8.0%.

(3) Sodium sulfate—Dissolve about 1 g of Sodium Lauryl Sulfate, accurately weighed, in 10 mL of water, add 100 mL of ethanol (95), and heat at a temperature just below the boiling point for 2 hours. Filter through a glass filter (G4) while hot, and wash with 100 mL of boiling ethanol (95). Dissolve the residue on the glass filter by washing with 150 mL of water, collecting the washings in a beaker. Add 10 mL of dilute hydrochloric acid, heat to boiling, add 25 mL of barium chloride TS, and allow to stand overnight. Collect the precipitate, and wash with water until the last washing produces no opalescence with silver nitrate TS. Dry the precipitate together with the filter paper, ignite to a constant mass between 500°C and 600°C by raising the temperature gradually, and weigh as barium sulfate ($BaSO_4$: 233.39).

Amount (mg) of sodium sulfate (Na_2SO_4)
= amount (mg) of barium sulfate ($BaSO_4$) × 0.6086

(4) Unsulfated alcohols—Dissolve about 10 g of Sodium Lauryl Sulfate, accurately weighed, in 100 mL of water, add 100 mL of ethanol (95), and transfer to a separator. Extract the solution with three 50-mL portions of pentane. If an emulsion forms, sodium chloride may be added to promote separation of the two layers. Combine the pentane extracts, wash with three 50-mL portions of water, dehydrate with anhydrous sodium sulfate, and filter. Put the filtrate to a tared beaker, and evaporate the pentane on a water bath. Dry the residue at 105°C for 30 minutes, cool, and weigh: the mass of the residue is not more than 4.0%.

◇**Water** *<2.48>* Not more than 5.0% (0.5 g, volumetric titration, direct titration).◇

◇**Total alcohol content** Dissolve about 5 g of Sodium Lauryl Sulfate, accurately weighed, in 150 mL of water and 50 mL of hydrochloric acid, and boil under a reflux condenser for 4 hours. Cool, extract with two 75-mL portions of diethyl ether, and evaporate the combined diethyl ether extracts on a water bath. Dry the residue at 105°C for 30 minutes, and weigh: the mass of the residue is not less than 59.0%.◇

Assay Weigh accurately about 1.15 g of Sodium Lauryl Sulfate, and dissolve in water to make exactly 1000 mL, by warming if necessary. Transfer exactly 20 mL of this solution to a 100-mL stoppered graduated cylinder, add 15 mL of dichloromethane and 10 mL of dimidium bromide-patent blue TS, and shake. Titrate *<2.50>* with 0.004 mol/L benzethonium chloride VS until the color of the dichloromethane layer changes from light red to grayish blue, while shaking vigorously. Allow the layers to separate before each titration.

Each mL of 0.004 mol/L benzethonium chloride VS
= 1.154 mg of $C_{12}H_{25}NaO_4S$

◆**Containers and storage** Containers—Well-closed containers.◆

Sodium Pertechnetate (^{99m}Tc) Injection

過テクネチウム酸ナトリウム (^{99m}Tc) 注射液

Sodium Pertechnetate (^{99m}Tc) Injection is an aqueous injection. It contains technetium-99*m* (^{99m}Tc) in the form of sodium pertechnetate.

It conforms to the requirements of Sodium Pertechnetate (^{99m}Tc) Injection in the Minimum Requirements for Radiopharmaceuticals.

Test for Extractable Volume of Parenteral Preparations and Insoluble Particulate Matter Test for Injections are not applied to this injection.

Description Sodium Pertechnetate (^{99m}Tc) Injection is a clear, colorless liquid.

Dibasic Sodium Phosphate Hydrate

リン酸水素ナトリウム水和物

$Na_2HPO_4.12H_2O$: 358.14

Dibasic Sodium Phosphate Hydrate contains not less than 98.0% of disodium hydrogen phosphate (Na_2HPO_4: 141.96), calculated on the dried basis.

Description Dibasic Sodium Phosphate Hydrate occurs as colorless or white crystals. It is odorless.

It is freely soluble in water, and practically insoluble in ethanol (95) and in diethyl ether.

It effloresces in warm, dry air.

Identification (1) A solution of Dibasic Sodium Phosphate Hydrate (1 in 10) responds to Qualitative Tests *<1.09>* (1) and (2) for sodium salt.

(2) A solution of Dibasic Sodium Phosphate Hydrate (1 in 10) responds to Qualitative Tests *<1.09>* (1) and (3) for phosphate.

(3) Dissolve 0.1 g of Dibasic Sodium Phosphate Hydrate in 5 mL of dilute nitric acid, warm at 70°C for 1 to 2 minutes, and add 2 mL of hexaammonium heptamolybdate TS: a yellow precipitate is formed.

pH *<2.54>* Dissolve 1.0 g of Dibasic Sodium Phosphate Hydrate in 50 mL of water: the pH of this solution is between 9.0 and 9.4.

Purity (1) Clarity and color of solution—Dissolve 1.0 g of Dibasic Sodium Phosphate Hydrate in 20 mL of water: the solution is clear and colorless.

(2) Chloride *<1.03>*—Dissolve 1.0 g of Dibasic Sodium Phosphate Hydrate in 7 mL of dilute nitric acid and water to make 50 mL. Perform the test using this solution as the test solution. Prepare the control solution with 0.40 mL of 0.01 mol/L hydrochloric acid VS (not more than 0.014%).

(3) Sulfate *<1.14>*—Dissolve 0.5 g of Dibasic Sodium Phosphate Hydrate in 2 mL of dilute hydrochloric acid and water to make 50 mL. Perform the test using this solution as the test solution. Prepare the control solution with 0.40 mL of 0.005 mol/L sulfuric acid VS (not more than 0.038%).

(4) Carbonate—To 2.0 g of Dibasic Sodium Phosphate Hydrate add 5 mL of water, boil, and add 2 mL of hydrochloric acid after cooling: the solution does not effervesce.

(5) Heavy metals *<1.07>*—Dissolve 2.0 g of Dibasic Sodium Phosphate Hydrate in 4 mL of acetic acid (31) and water to make 50 mL. Perform the test using this solution as the test solution. Prepare the control solution with 2.0 mL of Standard Lead Solution by adding 2 mL of dilute acetic acid and water to make 50 mL (not more than 10 ppm).

(6) Arsenic <*1.11*>—Prepare the test solution with 1.0 g of Dibasic Sodium Phosphate Hydrate according to Method 1, and perform the test (not more than 2 ppm).

Loss on drying <*2.41*> 57.0 - 61.0% (1 g, at 40°C for 3 hours and then at 105°C for 5 hours, not exceeding 2 mm in sample layer).

Assay Weigh accurately about 6 g of Dibasic Sodium Phosphate Hydrate, dissolve in 50 mL of water, and then titrate <*2.50*> with 0.5 mol/L sulfuric acid VS at 15°C until the green color of the solution changes to dark-greenish red-purple (indicator: 3 to 4 drops of methyl orange-xylenecyanol FF TS).

Each mL of 0.5 mol/L sulfuric acid VS
= 142.0 mg of Na_2HPO_4

Containers and storage Containers—Tight containers.

Sodium Picosulfate Hydrate

ピコスルファートナトリウム水和物

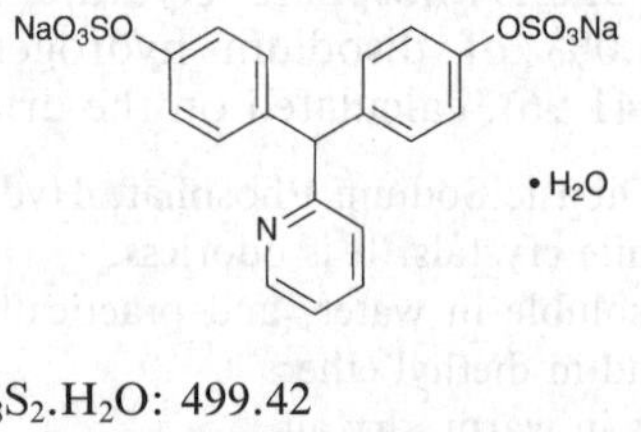

$C_{18}H_{13}NNa_2O_8S_2.H_2O$: 499.42
Disodium 4,4′-(pyridin-2-ylmethylene)bis(phenyl sulfate) monohydrate
[*10040-45-6*, anhydride]

Sodium Picosulfate Hydrate contains not less than 98.5% of sodium picosulfate ($C_{18}H_{13}NNa_2O_8S_2$: 481.41), calculated on the anhydrous basis.

Description Sodium Picosulfate Hydrate occurs as a white crystalline powder. It is odorless and tasteless.

It is very soluble in water, soluble in methanol, slightly soluble in ethanol (99.5), and practically insoluble in diethyl ether.

It is gradually colored by light.

The pH of a solution of 1.0 g of Sodium Picosulfate Hydrate in 20 mL of water is between 7.4 and 9.4.

Identification **(1)** Mix 5 mg of Sodium Picosulfate Hydrate with 0.01 g of 1-chloro-2,4-dinitrobenzene, and melt by gentle heating for 5 to 6 seconds. After cooling, add 4 mL of potassium hydroxide-ethanol TS: an orange-red color develops.

(2) To 0.2 g of Sodium Picosulfate Hydrate add 5 mL of dilute hydrochloric acid, boil for 5 minutes, cool, and add 1 mL of barium chloride TS: a white precipitate is formed.

(3) Determine the absorption spectrum of a solution of Sodium Picosulfate Hydrate (1 in 25,000) as directed under Ultraviolet-visible Spectrophotometry <*2.24*>, and compare the spectrum with the Reference Spectrum: both spectra exhibit similar intensities of absorption at the same wavelengths.

(4) Determine the infrared absorption spectrum of Sodium Picosulfate Hydrate, previously dried at 105° C in vacuum for 4 hours, as directed in the potassium bromide disk method under Infrared Spectrophotometry <*2.25*>, and compare the spectrum with the Reference Spectrum: both spectra exhibit similar intensities of absorption at the same wave numbers.

(5) A solution of Sodium Picosulfate Hydrate (1 in 10) responds to Qualitative Tests <*1.09*> for sodium salt.

Absorbance <*2.24*> $E^{1\%}_{1\,cm}$ (263 nm): 120 - 130 (4 mg calculated on the anhydrous basis, water, 100 mL).

Purity **(1)** Clarity and color of solution—Dissolve 1.0 g of Sodium Picosulfate Hydrate in 10 mL of water: the solution is clear and colorless to pale yellow.

(2) Chloride <*1.03*>—Perform the test with 0.5 g of Sodium Picosulfate Hydrate. Prepare the control solution with 0.40 mL of 0.01 mol/L hydrochloric acid VS (not more than 0.028%).

(3) Sulfate <*1.14*>—Perform the test with 0.40 g of Sodium Picosulfate Hydrate. Prepare the control solution with 0.35 mL of 0.005 mol/L sulfuric acid VS (not more than 0.042%).

(4) Heavy metals <*1.07*>—Proceed with 2.0 g of Sodium Picosulfate Hydrate according to Method 2, and perform the test. Prepare the control solution with 2.0 mL of Standard Lead Solution (not more than 10 ppm).

(5) Arsenic <*1.11*>—Prepare the test solution with 2.0 g of Sodium Picosulfate Hydrate according to Method 3, and perform the test (not more than 1 ppm).

(6) Related substances—Dissolve 0.25 g of Sodium Picosulfate Hydrate in 5 mL of methanol, and use this solution as the sample solution. Pipet 1 mL of the sample solution, add methanol to make exactly 500 mL, and use this solution as the standard solution. Perform the test with these solutions as directed under Thin-layer Chromatography <*2.03*>. Spot 5 μL each of the sample solution and standard solution on a plate of silica gel with fluorescent indicator for thin-layer chromatography. Develop the plate with a mixture of 1-butanol, water and acetic acid (100) (74:20:19) to a distance of about 10 cm, and air-dry the plate. Examine under ultraviolet light (main wavelength: 254 nm): the spots other than the principal spot obtained from the sample solution are not more intense than the spot from the standard solution.

Water <*2.48*> 3.0 - 4.5% (0.5 g, volumetric titration, direct titration).

Assay Weigh accurately about 0.4 g of Sodium Picosulfate Hydrate, dissolve in 50 mL of methanol, add 7 mL of acetic acid (100), and titrate <*2.50*> with 0.1 mol/L perchloric acid VS (potentiometric titration). Perform a blank determination in the same manner, and make any necessary correction.

Each mL of 0.1 mol/L perchloric acid VS
= 48.14 mg of $C_{18}H_{13}NNa_2O_8S_2$

Containers and storage Containers—Tight containers.
Storage—Light-resistant.

Sodium Polystyrene Sulfonate

ポリスチレンスルホン酸ナトリウム

Sodium Polystyrene Sulfonate is a cation exchange resin prepared as the sodium form of the sulfonated styrene divinylbenzene copolymer.

It contains not less than 9.4% and not more than 11.0% of sodium (Na: 22.99), calculated on the anhydrous basis.

Each g of Sodium Polystyrene Sulfonate, calculated on the anhydrous basis, exchanges with not less than 0.110 g and not more than 0.135 g of potassium (K: 39.10).

Description Sodium Polystyrene Sulfonate occurs as a yellow-brown powder. It is odorless and tasteless.

It is practically insoluble in water, in ethanol (95), in acetone and in diethyl ether.

Identification **(1)** Determine the infrared absorption spectrum of Sodium Polystyrene Sulfonate as directed in the potassium bromide disk method under Infrared Spectrophotometry <*2.25*>, and compare the spectrum with the Reference Spectrum: both spectra exhibit similar intensities of absorption at the same wave numbers.

(2) To 1 g of Sodium Polystyrene Sulfonate add 10 mL of dilute hydrochloric acid, stir, and filter. Add ammonia TS to the filtrate to neutralize: the solution responds to Qualitative Tests <*1.09*> for sodium salt.

Purity **(1)** Ammonium—Place 1.0 g of Sodium Polystyrene Sulfonate in a flask, add 5 mL of sodium hydroxide TS, cover the flask with a watch glass having a moistened strip of red litmus paper on the underside, and boil for 15 minutes: the gas evolved does not change the red litmus paper to blue.

(2) Heavy metals <*1.07*>—Proceed with 2.0 g of Sodium Polystyrene Sulfonate according to Method 2, and perform the test. Prepare the control solution with 2.0 mL of Standard Lead Solution (not more than 10 ppm).

(3) Arsenic <*1.11*>—Prepare the test solution with 2.0 g of Sodium Polystyrene Sulfonate according to Method 3, and perform the test (not more than 1 ppm).

(4) Styrene—To 10.0 g of Sodium Polystyrene Sulfonate add 10 mL of acetone, shake for 30 minutes, centrifuge, and use the supernatant liquid as the sample solution. Separately, dissolve 10 mg of styrene in acetone to make exactly 100 mL. Pipet 1 mL of this solution, add acetone to make exactly 100 mL, and use this solution as the standard solution. Perform the test with exactly 20 μL each of the sample solution and standard solution as directed under Liquid Chromatography <*2.01*> according to the following conditions, and determine peak areas, A_T and A_S, of styrene in each solution: A_T is not larger than A_S.

Operating conditions—

Detector: An ultraviolet absorption photometer (wavelength: 254 nm).

Column: A stainless steel column 4 mm in inside diameter and 15 cm in length, packed with octadecylsilanized silica gel for liquid chromatography (5 μm in particle diameter).

Column temperature: A constant temperature of about 25°C.

Mobile phase: A mixture of water and acetonitrile (1:1).

Flow rate: Adjust so that the retention time of styrene is about 8 minutes.

System suitability—

System performance: Dissolve 20 mg each of styrene and butyl parahydroxybenzoate in 100 mL of acetone. To 5 mL of this solution add acetone to make 100 mL. When the procedure is run with 20 μL of this solution under the above operating conditions, butyl parahydroxybenzoate and styrene are eluted in this order with the resolution between these peaks being not less than 5.

System repeatability: When the test is repeated 6 times with 20 μL of the standard solution under the above operating conditions, the relative standard deviation of the peak area of styrene is not more than 2.0%.

Water <*2.48*> Not more than 10.0% (0.2 g, volumetric titration, direct titration).

Assay **(1)** Sodium—Weigh accurately about 1 g of Sodium Polystyrene Sulfonate, calculated on the anhydrous basis, in a glass-stoppered flask, add exactly 50 mL of 3 mol/L hydrochloric acid TS, shake for 60 minutes, and filter. Discard the first 20 mL of the filtrate, pipet 5 mL of the subsequent filtrate, and add water to make exactly 100 mL. Pipet 20 mL of this solution, add water to make exactly 1000 mL, and use this solution as the sample solution. Separately, pipet a suitable quantity of Standard Sodium Stock Solution, dilute exactly with water so that each ml of the solution contains 1 to 3 μg of sodium (Na: 22.99), and use these solutions as the standard solutions. Perform the test with the sample solution and the standard solutions as directed under Atomic Absorption Spectrophotometry <*2.23*> according to the following conditions, and calculate the amount of sodium in the sample solution using the calibration curve obtained from the standard solutions.

Gas: Combustible gas—Acetylene.

Supporting gas—Air.

Lamp: A sodium hollow-cathode lamp.

Wavelength: 589.0 nm.

(2) Potassium exchange capacity—Weigh accurately about 1.5 g of Sodium Polystyrene Sulfonate, calculated on the anhydrous basis, in a glass-stoppered flask, add exactly 100 mL of Standard Potassium Stock Solution, shake for 15 minutes, and filter. Discard the first 20 mL of the filtrate, pipet 10 mL of the subsequent filtrate, and add water to make exactly 100 mL. Pipet 10 mL of this solution, add water to make exactly 1000 mL, and use this solution as the sample solution. Separately, pipet a suitable quantity of Standard Potassium Stock Solution, dilute exactly with water so that each mL of the solution contains 1 to 5 μg of potassium (K: 39.10), and use these solutions as the standard solutions. Perform the test with these solutions as directed under Atomic Absorption Spectrophotometry <*2.23*> according to the following conditions, and calculate the amount Y (mg) of potassium in 1000 mL of the sample solution using the calibration curve obtained from the standard solution. The quantity of potassium absorbed on each g of Sodium Polystyrene Sulfonate, calculated on the anhydrous basis, is calculated from the following equation: it is between 0.110 g and 0.135 g.

Quantity (mg) of potassium (K) absorbed on 1 g of Sodium Polystyrene Sulfonate, calculated on the anhydrous basis
$= (X - 100Y)/M$

X: Amount (mg) of potassium in 100 mL of the Standard Potassium Stock Solution before exchange

M: Mass (g) of Sodium Polystyrene Sulfonate taken, calculated on the anhydrous basis

Gas: Combustible gas—Acetylene.

Supporting gas—Air.

Lamp: A potassium hollow-cathode lamp.

Wavelength: 766.5 nm.

Containers and storage Containers—Tight containers.

Sodium Pyrosulfite

Sodium Metabisulfite

ピロ亜硫酸ナトリウム

$Na_2S_2O_5$: 190.11

Sodium Pyrosulfite contains not less than 95.0% of sodium pyrosulfite ($Na_2S_2O_5$).

Description Sodium Pyrosulfite occurs as white, crystals or crystalline powder. It has the odor of sulfur dioxide.

It is freely soluble in water, very slightly soluble in ethanol (95), and practically insoluble in diethyl ether.

A solution of Sodium Pyrosulfite (1 in 20) is acid.

It is hygroscopic.

It decomposes slowly on exposure to air.

Identification A solution of Sodium Pyrosulfite (1 in 20) responds to Qualitative Tests *<1.09>* for sodium salt and for bisulfite.

Purity (1) Clarity and color of solution—Dissolve 1.0 g of Sodium Pyrosulfite in 10 mL of water: the solution is clear and colorless.

(2) Thiosulfate—Dissolve 1.0 g of Sodium Pyrosulfite in 15 mL of water, add slowly 5 mL of dilute hydrochloric acid, shake, and allow to stand for 5 minutes: no turbidity is produced.

(3) Heavy metals *<1.07>*—Dissolve 1.0 g of Sodium Pyrosulfite in 10 mL of water, and evaporate with 5 mL of hydrochloric acid on a water bath to dryness. Dissolve the residue in 10 mL of water, add 1 drop of phenolphthalein TS, and add ammonia TS until the solution becomes slightly red. Add 2 mL of dilute acetic acid and water to make 50 mL. Perform the test using this solution as the test solution. Prepare the control solution as follows: evaporate 5 mL of hydrochloric acid on a water bath to dryness, and to the residue add 2 mL of dilute acetic acid, 2.0 mL of Standard Lead Solution and water to make 50 mL (not more than 20 ppm).

(4) Iron *<1.10>*—Prepare the test solution with 1.0 g of Sodium Pyrosulfite according to Method 1, and perform the test according to Method A. Prepare the control solution with 2.0 mL of Standard Iron Solution (not more than 20 ppm).

(5) Arsenic *<1.11>*—Dissolve 0.5 g of Sodium Pyrosulfite in 10 mL of water, heat with 1 mL of sulfuric acid on a sand bath until white fumes are evolved, and add water to make 5 mL. Perform the test with this solution as the test solution (not more than 4 ppm).

Assay Weigh accurately about 0.15 g of Sodium Pyrosulfite, and transfer to an iodine flask containing an exactly measured 50 mL of 0.05 mol/L iodine VS. Stopper tightly, shake well, and allow to stand for 5 minutes in a dark place. Add 1 mL of hydrochloric acid, and titrate *<2.50>* the excess of iodine with 0.1 mol/L sodium thiosulfate VS (indicator: 1 mL of starch TS). Perform a blank determination in the same manner.

Each mL of 0.05 mol/L iodine VS = 4.753 mg of $Na_2S_2O_5$

Containers and storage Containers—Tight containers.

Storage—Light-resistant, preferably well-filled, and not exceeding 30°C.

Sodium Risedronate Hydrate

リセドロン酸ナトリウム水和物

$C_7H_{10}NNaO_7P_2.2\frac{1}{2}H_2O$: 350.13

Monosodium trihydrogen 1-hydroxy-2-(pyridin-3-yl)ethane-1,1-diyldiphosphonate hemipentahydrate

[329003-65-8]

Sodium Risedronate Hydrate contains not less than 98.0% and not more than 102.0% of sodium risedronate ($C_7H_{10}NNaO_7P_2$: 305.09), calculated on the anhydrous basis.

Description Sodium Risedronate Hydrate occurs as a white crystalline powder.

It is soluble in water, and practically insoluble in ethanol (99.5).

It dissolves in diluted dilute sodium hydroxide TS (1 in 20).

Identification (1) Determine the absorption spectrum of a solution of Sodium Risedronate Hydrate in diluted dilute sodium hydroxide TS (1 in 20) (1 in 20,000) as directed under Ultraviolet-visible Spectrophotometry *<2.24>*, and compare the spectrum with the Reference Spectrum: both spectra exhibit similar intensities of absorption at the same wavelengths.

(2) Determine the infrared absorption spectrum of Sodium Risedronate Hydrate as directed in the potassium bromide disk method under Infrared Spectrophotometry *<2.25>*, and compare the spectrum with the Reference Spectrum: both spectra exhibit similar intensities of absorption at the same wave numbers.

(3) Sodium Risedronate Hydrate responds to Qualitative Tests *<1.09>* (1) for sodium salt.

Purity (1) Heavy metals—To 0.50 g of Sodium Risedronate Hydrate in a quartz crucible add 0.50 g of magnesium oxide, mix, heat until the content becomes a light gray while mixing occasionally with a glass rod, then incinerate at 800°C. After cooling, dissolve the residue with 3 mL of hydrochloric acid, and add 3 mL of water. Adjust this solution to pH 8.5 with ammonia TS, then adjust to pH 4 with acetic acid (100), and adjust the pH to 3.4 with dilute hydrochloric acid. Filter the solution into a Nessler tube using a filter paper, rinse the crucible and filter with water, add the rinsings to the Nessler tube, then add water to make 50 mL, and use this solution as the test solution. Separately, to 1.0 mL of Standard Lead Solution add 0.50 g of magnesium oxide, dryness at 110°C, and proceed with the residue in the same manner as for the test solution, and use the solution so obtained as the control solution. To the test and control solutions add 1 drop each of sodium sulfide TS, mix, and allow to stand for 5 minutes, and compare the colors of both solutions against a white background: the color of the test solution is not more intense than that of the control solution (not more than 20 ppm).

(2) Arsenic *<1.11>*—Prepare the test solution by dissolving 1.0 g of Sodium Risedronate Hydrate in 5 mL of a solution of sodium hydroxide (1 in 5), and perform the test (not more than 2 ppm).

(3) Related substance 1—Dissolve 50 mg of Sodium Risedronate Hydrate in 1.5 mL of 0.2 mol/L sodium hydroxide TS, add the mobile phase to make 25 mL, and use this solution as the sample solution. Pipet 2.5 mL of the sample solution, and add the mobile phase to make exactly 50 mL. Pipet 2 mL of this solution, add the mobile phase to make exactly 100 mL, and use this solution as the standard solution. Perform the test with exactly 20 μL each of the sample solution and standard solution as directed under Liquid Chromatography <*2.01*> according to the following conditions, and determine each peak area by the automatic integration method: the area of the peak other than risedronic acid obtained from the sample solution is not larger than the peak area of risedronic acid from the standard solution.

Operating conditions—

Detector, column, column temperature, mobile phase, and flow rate: Proceed as directed in the operating conditions in the Assay.

Time span of measurement: About 2 times as long as the retention time of risedronic acid, beginning after the solvent peak.

System suitability—

System performance: When the procedure is run with 20 μL of the standard solution under the above operating conditions, the number of theoretical plates and the symmetry factor of the peak of risedronic acid are not less than 4500 and not more than 1.5, respectively.

System repeatability: When the test is repeated 6 times with 20 μL of the standard solution under the above operating conditions, the relative standard deviation of the peak area of risedronic acid is not more than 5.0%.

(4) Related substance 2—Dissolve 0.10 g of Sodium Risedronate Hydrate in 3 mL of 0.2 mol/L sodium hydroxide TS, add the diluting solution below to make 50 mL, and use this solution as the sample solution. Pipet 2.5 mL of the sample solution, and add the diluting solution to make exactly 50 mL. Pipet 2 mL of this solution, add the diluting solution to make exactly 100 mL, and use this solution as the standard solution. Perform the test with exactly 50 μL each of the sample solution and standard solution as directed under Liquid Chromatography <*2.01*> according to the following conditions, and determine each peak area by the automatic integration method: the area of the peak other than risedronic acid obtained from the sample solution is not larger than the peak area of risedronic acid from the standard solution.

Diluting solution: Dissolve 0.11 g of disodium dihydrogen ethylenediamine tetraacetate dihydrate and 2.47 g of tetradecyl trimethylammonium bromide in 1000 mL of water, and adjust to pH 6.5 with 0.2 mol/L sodium hydroxide TS. To 700 mL of this solution add 300 mL of acetonitrile.

Operating conditions—

Detector: An ultraviolet absorption photometer (wavelength: 263 nm).

Column: A stainless steel column 4.6 mm in inside diameter and 15 cm in length, packed with octadecylsilanized silica gel for liquid chromatography (5 μm in particle diameter).

Column temperature: A constant temperature of about 25°C.

Mobile phase: Dissolve 0.14 g of disodium dihydrogen ethylenediamine tetraacetate dihydrate, 3.16 g of tetradecyl trimethylammonium bromide, 4.81 g of ammonium dihydrogen phosphate and 2.93 g of diammonium hydrogen phosphate in 1280 mL of water, and add 720 mL of acetonitrile.

Flow rate: Adjust so that the retention time of risedronic acid is about 5 minutes.

Time span of measurement: About 10 times as long as the retention time of risedronic acid, beginning after the solvent peak.

System suitability—

System performance: When the procedure is run with 50 μL of the standard solution under the above operating conditions, the number of theoretical plates and the symmetry factor of the peak of risedronic acid are not less than 5000 and not more than 1.4, respectively.

System repeatability: When the test is repeated 6 times with 50 μL of the standard solution under the above operating conditions, the relative standard deviation of the peak area of risedronic acid is not more than 2.0%.

Water <*2.48*> 11.9 – 13.9% (40 mg, volumetric titration, direct titration. Use a mixture of formamide for water determination and methanol for water determination (1:1) instead of methanol for water determination).

Assay Weigh accurately about 50 mg of Sodium Risedronate Hydrate, dissolve in 1.5 mL of 0.2 mol/L sodium hydroxide TS, and add the mobile phase to make exactly 25 mL. Pipet 10 mL of this solution, add exactly 5 mL of the internal standard solution, then add the mobile phase to make 25 mL, and use this solution as the sample solution. Separately, weigh accurately about 50 mg of Risedronic Acid RS (separately determine the water <*2.48*> using 80 mg, in the same manner as Sodium Risedronate Hydrate), dissolve in 3 mL of 0.2 mol/L sodium hydroxide TS, and add the mobile phase to make exactly 25 mL. Pipet 10 mL of this solution, add exactly 5 mL of the internal standard solution, then add the mobile phase to make 25 mL, and use this solution as the standard solution. Perform the test with 20 μL each of the sample solution and standard solution as directed under Liquid Chromatography <*2.01*> according to the following conditions, and calculate the ratios, Q_T and Q_S, of the peak area of risedronic acid to that of the internal standard.

Amount (mg) of sodium risedronate ($C_7H_{10}NNaO_7P_2$)
$= M_S \times Q_T/Q_S \times 1.078$

M_S: Amount (mg) of Risedronic Acid RS taken, calculated on the anhydrous basis

Internal standard solution—A solution of sodium benzoate in the mobile phase (1 in 125).

Operating conditions—

Detector: An ultraviolet absorption photometer (wavelength: 263 nm).

Column: A polyether ether ketone column 4 mm in inside diameter and 25 cm in length, packed with quaternary alkylaminated styrene-divinylbenzene copolymer for liquid chromatography (10 μm in particle diameter).

Column temperature: A constant temperature of about 25°C.

Mobile phase: Dissolve 1.8 g of disodium dihydrogen ethylenediamine tetraacetate dihydrate in 1000 mL of water, and adjust to pH 9.5 with 0.2 mol/L sodium hydroxide TS.

Flow rate: Adjust so that the retention time of risedronic acid is about 14 minutes.

System suitability—

System performance: When the procedure is run with 20 μL of the standard solution under the above operating conditions, the internal standard and risedronic acid are eluted in this order with the resolution between these peaks being not less than 6.

System repeatability: When the test is repeated 6 times with 20 μL of the standard solution under the above operat-

ing conditions, the relative standard deviation of the peak area of risedronic acid is not more than 1.0%.

Containers and storage Containers—Well-closed containers.

Sodium Risedronate Tablets

リセドロン酸ナトリウム錠

Sodium Risedronate Tablets contain not less than 95.0% and not more than 105.0% of the labeled amount of sodium risedronate ($C_7H_{10}NNaO_7P_2$: 305.09).

Method of preparation Prepare as directed under Tablets, with Sodium Risedronate Hydrate.

Identification Powder Sodium Risedronate Tablets. To a portion of the powder, equivalent to 2.5 mg of sodium risedronate ($C_7H_{10}NNaO_7P_2$), add 50 mL of diluted dilute sodium hydroxide TS (1 in 20), shake, and centrifuge. Filter the supernatant liquid through a membrane filter with a pore size not exceeding 0.2 μm. Discard the first 2 mL of the filtrate, and determine the absorption spectrum of the subsequent filtrate as directed under Ultraviolet-visible Spectrophotometry <*2.24*>: it exhibits a maximum between 260 nm and 264 nm.

Uniformity of dosage units <*6.02*> Perform the Mass variation test, or the Content uniformity test according to the following method: it meets the requirement.

To 1 tablet of Sodium Risedronate Tablets add exactly 10 mL of the mobile phase, shake, and allow to stand for 10 minutes. Disperse the particles by sonicating for 10 minutes with occasional shaking, then centrifuge, and filter the supernatant liquid through a membrane filter with a pore size not exceeding 0.2 μm. Discard the first 1 mL of the filtrate, pipet exactly V mL of the subsequent filtrate, equivalent to about 1.75 mg of sodium risedronate ($C_7H_{10}NNaO_7P_2$), add exactly 1 mL of the internal standard solution and the mobile phase to make 10 mL, and use this solution as the sample solution. Separately, weigh accurately about 70 mg of Risedronic Acid RS (separately determine the water <*2.48*> using 80 mg, in the same manner as Sodium Risedronate Hydrate), dissolve in 3 mL of 0.2 mol/L sodium hydroxide TS, and add the mobile phase to make exactly 100 mL. Pipet 5 mL of this solution, add exactly 2 mL of the internal standard solution, then add the mobile phase to make 20 mL, and use this solution as the standard solution. Perform the test with 20 μL each of the sample solution and standard solution as directed under Liquid Chromatography <*2.01*> according to the following conditions, and calculate the ratios, Q_T and Q_S, of the peak area of risedronic acid to that of the internal standard.

Amount (mg) of sodium risedronate ($C_7H_{10}NNaO_7P_2$)
$= M_S \times Q_T/Q_S \times 1/V \times 1/4 \times 1.078$

M_S: Amount (mg) of Risedronic Acid RS taken, calculated on the anhydrous basis

Internal standard solution—A solution of sodium benzoate in the mobile phase (7 in 2000).

Operating conditions—

Proceed as directed in the operating conditions in the Assay under Sodium Risedronate Hydrate.

System suitability—

System performance: When the procedure is run with 20 μL of the standard solution under the above operating conditions, the internal standard and risedronic acid are eluted in this order with the resolution between these peaks being not less than 6.

System repeatability: When the test is repeated 6 times with 20 μL of the standard solution under the above operating conditions, the relative standard deviation of the ratio of the peak area of risedronic acid to that of the internal standard is not more than 1.0%.

Dissolution <*6.10*> When the test is performed at 50 revolutions per minute according to the Paddle method, using 900 mL of water as the dissolution medium, the dissolution rate in 20 minutes of Sodium Risedronate Tablets is not less than 80%.

Start the test with 1 tablet of Sodium Risedronate Tablets, withdraw 10 mL of the medium at the specified minute after starting the test, and filter through a membrane filter with a pore size not exceeding 0.45 μm. Discard not less than 2 mL of the first filtrate, pipet V mL of the subsequent filtrate, add water to make exactly V' mL so that each mL contains about 2.8 μg of sodium risedronate ($C_7H_{10}NNaO_7P_2$), and use this solution as the sample solution. Separately, weigh accurately about 50 mg of Risedronic Acid RS (separately determine the water <*2.48*> using 80 mg, in the same manner as Sodium Risedronate Hydrate), dissolve in 3 mL of 0.2 mol/L sodium hydroxide TS, and add water to make exactly 50 mL. Pipet 5 mL of this solution, and add water to make exactly 100 mL. Pipet 5 mL of this solution, add water to make exactly 100 mL, and use this solution as the standard solution. Perform the test with exactly 200 μL each of the sample solution and standard solution as directed under Liquid Chromatography <*2.01*> according to the following conditions, and determine the peak areas, A_T and A_S, of risedronic acid in each solution.

Dissolution rate (%) with respect to the labeled amount of sodium risedronate ($C_7H_{10}NNaO_7P_2$)
$= M_S \times A_T/A_S \times V'/V \times 1/C \times 9/2 \times 1.078$

M_S: Amount (mg) of Risedronic Acid RS taken, calculated on the anhydrous basis

C: Labeled amount (mg) of sodium risedronate ($C_7H_{10}NNaO_7P_2$) in 1 tablet

Operating conditions—

Detector: An ultraviolet absorption photometer (wavelength: 263 nm).

Column: A stainless steel column 4.6 mm in inside diameter and 15 cm in length, packed with octadecylsilanized silica gel for liquid chromatography (5 μm in particle diameter).

Column temperature: A constant temperature of about 25°C.

Mobile phase: Dissolve 0.15 g of disodium dihydrogen ethylenediamine tetraacetate dihydrate, 3.36 g of tetradecyl trimethylammonium bromide, 5.11 g of ammonium dihydrogen phosphate and 3.11 g of diammonium hydrogen phosphate in 1360 mL of water, and add 640 mL of acetonitrile.

Flow rate: Adjust so that the retention time of risedronic acid is about 12 minutes.

System suitability—

System performance: When the procedure is run with 200 μL of the standard solution under the above operating conditions, the number of theoretical plates and the symmetry factor of the peak of risedronic acid are not less than 5000 and not more than 1.5, respectively.

System repeatability: When the test is repeated 6 times with 200 μL of the standard solution under the above operat-

ing conditions, the relative standard deviation of the peak area of risedronic acid is not more than 2.0%.

Assay Weigh accurately the mass of not less than 20 Sodium Risedronate Tablets, and powder. Weigh accurately a portion of the powder, equivalent to about 50 mg of sodium risedronate ($C_7H_{10}NNaO_7P_2$), add exactly 10 mL of the internal standard solution, add 190 mL of the mobile phase, shake, and allow to stand for 10 minutes. Disperse the particles by sonicating with occasional shaking, then centrifuge, and filter through a membrane filter with a pore size not exceeding 0.2 μm. Discard the first 2 mL of the filtrate, and use the subsequent filtrate as the sample solution. Separately, weigh accurately about 50 mg of Risedronic Acid RS (separately determine the water *<2.48>* using 80 mg, in the same manner as Sodium Risedronate Hydrate), dissolve in 3 mL of 0.2 mol/L sodium hydroxide TS, add exactly 10 mL of the internal standard solution, then add the mobile phase to make 200 mL, and use this solution as the standard solution. Then, proceed as directed in the Assay under Sodium Risedronate Hydrate.

Amount (mg) of sodium risedronate ($C_7H_{10}NNaO_7P_2$)
$= M_S \times Q_T/Q_S \times 1.078$

M_S: Amount (mg) of Risedronic Acid RS taken, calculated on the anhydrous basis

Internal standard solution—A solution of sodium benzoate in the mobile phase (1 in 100).

Containers and storage Containers—Well-closed containers.

Sodium Salicylate

サリチル酸ナトリウム

$C_7H_5NaO_3$: 160.10
Monosodium 2-hydroxybenzoate
[*54-21-7*]

Sodium Salicylate, when dried, contains not less than 99.5% of sodium salicylate ($C_7H_5NaO_3$).

Description Sodium Salicylate occurs as white, crystals or crystalline powder.

It is very soluble in water, freely soluble in acetic acid (100), and soluble in ethanol (95).

It is gradually colored by light.

Identification **(1)** Determine the infrared absorption spectrum of Sodium Salicylate, previously dried, as directed in the potassium bromide disk method under Infrared Spectrophotometry *<2.25>*, and compare the spectrum with the Reference Spectrum: both spectra exhibit similar intensities of absorption at the same wave numbers.

(2) A solution of Sodium Salicylate (1 in 20) responds to Qualitative Tests *<1.09>* for sodium salt.

pH *<2.54>* The pH of a solution of 2.0 g of Sodium Salicylate in 20 mL of water is between 6.0 and 8.0.

Purity **(1)** Clarity and color of solution—Dissolve 1.0 g of Sodium Salicylate in 10 mL of water: the solution is clear, and its absorbance at 420 nm determined as directed under Ultraviolet-visible Spectrophotometry *<2.24>* is not more than 0.02.

(2) Chloride *<1.03>*—Dissolve 0.5 g of Sodium Salicylate in 15 mL of water, add 6 mL of dilute nitric acid and ethanol (95) to make 50 mL, and perform the test using this solution as the test solution. Prepare the control solution with 0.30 mL of 0.01 mol/L hydrochloric acid VS, 28 mL of ethanol (95), 6 mL of dilute nitric acid and water to make 50 mL (not more than 0.021%).

(3) Sulfate—Dissolve 0.25 g of Sodium Salicylate in 5 mL of water, and add 0.5 mL of barium chloride TS: the solution shows no change.

(4) Sulfite and thiosulfate—Dissolve 1.0 g of Sodium Salicylate in 20 mL of water, add 1 mL of hydrochloric acid, and filter. Add 0.15 mL of 0.05 mol/L iodine VS to the filtrate: a yellow color develops.

(5) Heavy metals *<1.07>*—Proceed with 1.0 g of Sodium Salicylate according to Method 2, and perform the test. Prepare the control solution with 2.0 mL of Standard Lead Solution (not more than 20 ppm).

(6) Arsenic *<1.11>*—To 1.0 g of Sodium Salicylate in a decomposition flask add 5 mL of nitric acid and 2 mL of sulfuric acid, and heat carefully until white fumes are evolved. After cooling, add 2 mL of nitric acid, and heat. After cooling, add several 2-mL portions of hydrogen peroxide (30), and heat until the solution is colorless to pale yellow. Repeat the procedure of adding nitric acid and hydrogen peroxide (30) and heating, if necessary. After cooling, add 2 mL of a saturated solution of ammonium oxalate monohydrate, and heat until white fumes are evolved. After cooling, add water to make 5 mL, and perform the test with this solution (not more than 2 ppm).

Loss on drying *<2.41>* Not more than 0.5% (1 g, 105°C, 2 hours).

Assay Weigh accurately about 0.3 g of Sodium Salicylate, previously dried, dissolve in 50 mL of acetic acid (100), and titrate *<2.50>* with 0.1 mol/L perchloric acid VS (potentiometric titration). Perform a blank determination in the same manner, and make any necessary correction.

Each mL of 0.1 mol/L perchloric acid VS
= 16.01 mg of $C_7H_5NaO_3$

Containers and storage Containers—Tight containers.

Storage—Light-resistant.

Sodium Starch Glycolate

デンプングリコール酸ナトリウム

[*9063-38-1*]

This monograph is harmonized with the European Pharmacopoeia and the U.S. Pharmacopeia.

The parts of the text that are not harmonized are marked with symbols (◆ ◆).

Information on the harmonization with the European Pharmacopoeia and the U.S. Pharmacopeia is available on the website of the Pharmaceuticals and Medical Devices Agency.

Sodium Starch Glycolate is the sodium salt of a carboxymethyl ether of starch or of a cross-linked carboxymethyl ether of starch.

There are two neutralization types of Sodium Starch Glycolate, Type A and Type B, and their insoluble matter in a mixture of ethanol (99.5) and water (8:2), when dried, contains not less than 2.8% and not more than 4.2%, and not less than 2.0% and not more than 3.4% of sodium (Na: 22.99), respectively.

◆The label states the type of neutralization.◆

◆**Description** Sodium Starch Glycolate occurs as a white powder, and has a characteristic salty taste.

It practically insoluble in ethanol (99.5).

It swells with water, and becomes viscous, pasty liquid.

It is hygroscopic.◆

Identification **(1)** Acidify 5 mL of a solution of Sodium Starch Glycolate (1 in 500) with dilute hydrochloric acid, then add one drop of iodine TS, and stir: a blue to violet color is produced.

◆**(2)** Determine the infrared absorption spectrum of Sodium Starch Glycolate as directed in the potassium bromide disk method under Infrared Spectrophotometry <*2.25*>, and compare the spectrum with the Reference Spectrum: both spectra exhibit similar intensities of absorption at the same wave numbers.◆

(3) The sample solution obtained in the Purity (2) responds to Qualitative Tests <*1.09*> (2) for sodium salt. Perform the test using 2 mL of the sample solution and 4 mL of potassium hexahydroxoantimonate (V) TS.

pH <*2.54*> To 1 g of Sodium Starch Glycolate add 30 mL of water and stir: the pH of the resulting suspension of Type A is 5.5 – 7.5, and that of Type B is 3.0 – 5.0.

Purity ◆**(1)** Heavy metals <*1.07*>—Proceed with 1.0 g of Sodium Starch Glycolate according to Method 2, and perform the test. Prepare the control solution with 2.0 mL of Standard Lead Solution (not more than 20 ppm).◆

(2) Iron

(i) Sample solution Take 2.5 g of Sodium Starch Glycolate in a silica or platinum crucible, add 2 mL of 5 mol/L sulfuric acid TS. Heat on a water bath, then ignite cautiously with a gas burner or preferably in an electric furnace at 600 ± 25°C, and incinerate the residue completely. Allow to cool, add a few drops of 1 mol/L sulfuric acid TS, and heat and ignite as above. Allow to cool, add a few drops of ammonium carbonate TS, evaporate to dryness on a water bath, and heat and ignite as above. After cooling, dissolve the residue by adding 50 mL of water.

(ii) Standard solution Weigh accurately 863.4 mg of ammonium iron (III) sulfate dodecahydrate, dissolve in water, add 25 mL of 1 mol/L sulfuric acid TS, and add water to make exactly 500 mL. Pipet 10 mL of this solution, and add water to make exactly 100 mL. Pipet 5 mL of this solution, and add water to make exactly 100 mL. Each mL of this solution contains 1.0 μg of iron (Fe).

(iii) Procedure Pipet 10 mL each of the sample solution and standard solution, and to each solution add 2 mL of citric acid solution (1 in 5) and 0.1 mL of thioglycolic acid. Then add ammonia solution (28) dropwise to render the solution alkaline, using litmus paper as an indicator. Add water to make 20 mL, and use these solutions as the test solution and the control solution, respectively. Allow these solutions to stand for 5 minutes, and compare the color of the solutions using white background: the color of the test solution is not deeper than that of the control solution (not more than 20 ppm).

(3) Sodium glycolate—Conduct this procedure without exposure to light, using light-resistant vessels.

(i) Sample solution Weigh accurately 0.200 g of Sodium Starch Glycolate in a beaker, add 4 mL of 6 mol/L acetic acid TS and 5 mL of water, and stir to dissolve. Add 50 mL of acetone and 1 g of sodium chloride, stir, and filter through a filter paper previously soaked with acetone. Rinse the beaker and the filter paper with acetone, combine the filtrate and washings, and add acetone to make exactly 100 mL. Allow to stand for 24 hours, and use the supernatant liquid as the sample solution.

(ii) Standard solution To exactly 0.310 g of glycolic acid, previously dried in a desiccator (silica gel) for 18 hours, add water to dissolve to make exactly 500 mL. Pipet 5 mL of this solution, add 4 mL of 6 mol/L acetic acid TS, and allow to stand for 30 minutes. Add 50 mL of acetone and 1 g of sodium chloride, proceed as (i) above, and use the supernatant liquid as the standard solution.

(iii) Procedure Pipet 2.0 mL each of the sample solution and standard solution into 25-mL stoppered test tubes, and heat on a water bath for 20 minutes to remove acetone. After cooling, add 20.0 mL of 2,7-dihydroxynaphthalene TS to the residue, stopper the test tube, and heat on a water bath for 20 minutes. Cool under running water, and transfer whole quantity of the content to a 25-mL volumetric flask. Maintain the flask under running water, and add sulfuric acid to make 25 mL. Within 10 minutes, determine the absorbance of these solutions at 540 nm using water as the blank as directed under Ultraviolet-visible Spectrophotometry <*2.24*>; the absorbance of the sample solution is not larger than that of the standard solution (not more than 2.0%).

(4) Sodium chloride—Weigh accurately about 0.5 g of Sodium Starch Glycolate in a beaker, disperse in 100 mL of water, and add 1 ml of nitric acid. Titrate <*2.50*> with 0.1 mol/L silver nitrate VS (potentiometric titration): the amount of sodium chloride (NaCl: 58.44) is not more than 7.0%.

Each mL of 0.1 mol/L silver nitrate VS = 5.844 mg of NaCl

Loss on drying <*2.41*> Not more than 10.0% (1 g, 130°C, 90 minutes).

Microbial limits <*4.05*> *Salmonella* and *Escherichia coli* are not observed.

Assay To about 1 g of Sodium Starch Glycolate add 20 mL of a mixture of ethanol (99.5) and water (8:2), stir for 10 minutes, and filter. Repeat this procedure until no more turbidity is produced by adding silver nitrate TS, and dry the residue on the filter paper at 105°C to constant mass. Weigh accurately 0.7 g of the mass, add 80 mL of acetic acid (100), and heat the mixture under a reflux condenser on a water bath for 2 hours. After cooling, titrate <*2.50*> with 0.1 mol/L perchloric acid VS (potentiometric titration).

$$\text{Content (\%) of sodium (Na)} = V \times 2.299 \times 100/M$$

V: Consumed amount (mL) of 0.1 mol/L perchloric acid VS

M: Mass (mg) of the dried residue

◆**Containers and storage** Containers—Tight containers.◆

Dried Sodium Sulfite

乾燥亜硫酸ナトリウム

Na_2SO_3: 126.04

Dried Sodium Sulfite contains not less than 97.0% of sodium sulfite (Na_2SO_3).

Description Dried Sodium Sulfite is white, crystals or powder. It is odorless.

It is freely soluble in water, and practically insoluble in ethanol (95) and in diethyl ether.

The pH of a solution of 1.0 g of Dried Sodium Sulfite in 10 mL of water is about 10.

It gradually changes in moist air.

Identification An aqueous solution of Dried Sodium Sulfite (1 in 20) responds to Qualitative Tests *<1.09>* for sodium salt and sulfite.

Purity (1) Thiosulfate—Dissolve 1.0 g of Dried Sodium Sulfite in 15 mL of water, add gradually 5 mL of hydrochloric acid, shake, and allow to stand for 5 minutes: no turbidity is produced.

(2) Heavy metals *<1.07>*—Dissolve 1.0 g of Dried Sodium Sulfite in 5 mL of water, add 2 mL of hydrochloric acid gradually, and evaporate the mixture on a water bath to dryness. Add 3 mL of boiling water and 1 mL of hydrochloric acid to the residue, and again evaporate to dryness on a water bath. Dissolve the residue in 2 mL of dilute acetic acid and water to make 50 mL, and perform the test using this solution as the test solution. Prepare the control solution as follows: evaporate 3 mL of hydrochloric acid to dryness, and add 2 mL of dilute acetic acid, 2.0 mL of Standard Lead Solution and water to make 50 mL (not more than 20 ppm).

(3) Arsenic *<1.11>*—Dissolve 0.5 g of Dried Sodium Sulfite in 5 mL of water, add 1 mL of sulfuric acid, and evaporate on a sand bath until white fumes are evolved. Add water to make 5 mL, take this solution as the sample solution, and perform the test (not more than 4 ppm).

Assay Weigh accurately about 0.2 g of Dried Sodium Sulfite, transfer immediately to an iodine flask containing exactly 50 mL of 0.05 mol/L iodine VS, stopper, shake, and allow to stand for 5 minutes in a dark place. Add 1 mL of hydrochloric acid, and titrate *<2.50>* the excess iodine with 0.1 mol/L sodium thiosulfate VS (indicator: 1 mL of starch TS). Perform a blank determination in the same manner.

Each mL of 0.05 mol/L iodine VS = 6.302 mg of Na_2SO_3

Containers and storage Containers—Tight containers.

Sodium Thiosulfate Hydrate

チオ硫酸ナトリウム水和物

$Na_2S_2O_3.5H_2O$: 248.18

Sodium Thiosulfate Hydrate, when dried, contains not less than 99.0% and not more than 101.0% of sodium thiosulfate ($Na_2S_2O_3$: 158.11).

Description Sodium Thiosulfate Hydrate occurs as colorless, crystals or crystalline powder. It is odorless.

It is very soluble in water, and practically insoluble in ethanol (99.5).

It effloresces in dry air, and is deliquescent in moist air.

Identification (1) A solution of Sodium Thiosulfate Hydrate (1 in 10) responds to Qualitative Tests *<1.09>* for thiosulfate.

(2) A solution of Sodium Thiosulfate Hydrate (1 in 10) responds to Qualitative Tests *<1.09>* for sodium salt.

pH *<2.54>* Dissolve 1.0 g of Sodium Thiosulfate Hydrate in 10 mL of water: the pH of the solution is between 6.0 and 8.0.

Purity (1) Clarity and color of solution—Dissolve 1.0 g of Sodium Thiosulfate Hydrate in 10 mL of water: the solution is clear and colorless.

(2) Heavy metals *<1.07>*—Dissolve 1.0 g of Sodium Thiosulfate Hydrate in 10 mL of water, add slowly 5 mL of dilute hydrochloric acid, and evaporate on a water bath to dryness. Add 15 mL of water to the residue, boil gently for 2 minutes, and filter. Heat the filtrate to boil, and add bromine TS to the hot filtrate to produce a clear solution and provide a slight excess of bromine. Boil the solution to expel the bromine. Cool, add 1 drop of phenolphthalein TS, and add dropwise sodium hydroxide TS until a slight red color is produced. Add 2 mL of dilute acetic acid and water to make 50 mL. Perform the test using this solution as the test solution. Prepare the control solution as follows: to 2.0 mL of Standard Lead Solution add 2 mL of dilute acetic acid and water to make 50 mL (not more than 20 ppm).

(3) Calcium—Dissolve 1.0 g of Sodium Thiosulfate in 10 mL of water, add 2 mL of ammonium oxalate TS, and allow to stand for 4 minutes: no turbidity is produced.

(4) Arsenic *<1.11>*—To 0.40 g of Sodium Thiosulfate add 3 mL of nitric acid and 5 mL of water, evaporate on a water bath to dryness, and perform the test with the residue. Prepare the test solution according to Method 2, and perform the test (not more than 5 ppm).

Loss on drying *<2.41>* 32.0 – 37.0% (1 g, in vacuum, 40 – 45°C, 16 hours).

Assay Weigh accurately about 0.4 g of Sodium Thiosulfate, previously dried, dissolve in 30 mL of water, and titrate *<2.50>* with 0.05 mol/L iodine VS (indicator: 1 mL of starch TS).

Each mL of 0.05 mol/L iodine VS
= 15.81 mg of $Na_2S_2O_3$

Containers and storage Containers—Tight containers.

Sodium Thiosulfate Injection

チオ硫酸ナトリウム注射液

Sodium Thiosulfate Injection is an aqueous injection.

It contains not less than 95.0% and not more than 105.0% of the labeled amount of sodium thiosulfate hydrate ($Na_2S_2O_3.5H_2O$: 248.18).

Method of preparation Prepare as directed under Injections, with Sodium Thiosulfate Hydrate.

Description Sodium Thiosulfate Injection is a clear, colorless liquid.

Identification Sodium Thiosulfate Injection responds to Qualitative Tests *<1.09>* for sodium salt and for thiosulfate.

Bacterial endotoxins <*4.01*> Less than 0.01 EU/mg.

Extractable volume <*6.05*> It meets the requirement.

Foreign insoluble matter <*6.06*> Perform the test according to Method 1: it meets the requirement.

Insoluble particulate matter <*6.07*> It meets the requirement.

Sterility <*4.06*> Perform the test according to the Membrane filtration method: it meets the requirement.

Assay Measure exactly a volume of Sodium Thiosulfate Injection, equivalent to about 0.5 g of sodium thiosulfate hydrate ($Na_2S_2O_3.5H_2O$), add water to make 30 mL, and titrate <*2.50*> with 0.05 mol/L iodine VS (indicator: 1 mL of starch TS).

Each mL of 0.05 mol/L iodine VS
= 24.82 mg of $Na_2S_2O_3.5H_2O$

Containers and storage Containers—Hermetic containers.

Sodium Valproate

バルプロ酸ナトリウム

$C_8H_{15}NaO_2$: 166.19
Monosodium 2-propylpentanoate
[*1069-66-5*]

Sodium Valproate, when dried, contains not less than 98.5% and not more than 101.0% of sodium valproate ($C_8H_{15}NaO_2$).

Description Sodium Valproate occurs as a white crystalline powder.

It is very soluble in water, freely soluble in ethanol (99.5) and in acetic acid (100).

It is hygroscopic.

Identification **(1)** To 5 mL of a solution of Sodium Valproate (1 in 20) add 1 mL of a solution of cobalt (II) nitrate hexahydrate (1 in 20) and warm on a water bath: a purple precipitate is formed.

(2) Dissolve 0.5 g of Sodium Valproate in 5 mL of water, add 5 mL of diethyl ether and 1 mL of 2 mol/L hydrochloric acid TS, and shake vigorously for 1 minute. Separate the diethyl ether layer, dehydrate with anhydrous sodium sulfate, and filter. Evaporate the solvent of the filtrate, determine the infrared spectrum of the residue as directed in the liquid film method under Infrared Spectrophotometry <*2.25*>, and compare the spectrum with the Reference Spectrum: both spectra exhibit similar intensities of absorption at the same wave numbers.

(3) A solution of Sodium Valproate (1 in 10) responds to Qualitative Tests <*1.09*> for sodium salt.

pH <*2.54*> Dissolve 1.0 g of Sodium Valproate in 20 mL of water: the pH of this solution is between 7.0 and 8.5.

Purity **(1)** Heavy metals <*1.07*>—Dissolve 2.0 g of Sodium Valproate in 44 mL of water, shake with 6 mL of dilute hydrochloric acid, allow to stand for 5 minutes, and filter. Discard the first 5 mL of the filtrate, neutralize 25 mL of the subsequent filtrate with ammonia TS, and add 2 mL of dilute acetic acid and water to make 50 mL. Perform the test using this solution as the test solution. Prepare the control solution as follows: to 2.0 mL of Standard Lead Solution add 2 mL of dilute acetic acid and water to make 50 mL (not more than 20 ppm).

(2) Related substances—Dissolve 0.10 g of Sodium Valproate in 10 mL of a mixture of formic acid and methyl acetate (1:1), and use this solution as the sample solution. Pipet 1 mL of the sample solution, add a mixture of formic acid and methyl acetate (1:1) to make exactly 200 mL, and use this solution as the standard solution. Perform the test with exactly 2 μL each of the sample solution and standard solution as directed under Gas Chromatography <*2.02*> according to the following conditions. Determine each peak area of both solutions by automatic integration method: the total area of the peaks other than valproic acid obtained from the sample solution is not larger than the peak area of valproic acid from the standard solution.

Operating conditions—

Detector: A hydrogen flame-ionization detector.

Column: A glass column 3 mm in inside diameter and 2 m in length, packed with siliceous earth for gas chromatography (150 to 180 μm in particle diameter) coated with diethylene glycol adipate ester for gas chromatography and phosphoric acid at the ratios of 5% and 1%, respectively.

Column temperature: A constant temperature of about 145°C.

Carrier gas: Nitrogen.

Flow rate: Adjust so that the retention time of valproic acid is about 7 minutes.

Time span of measurement: About 2 times as long as the retention time of valproic acid, beginning after the solvent peak.

System suitability—

System performance: To 2 mL of the sample solution and 8 μL of *n*-valerianic acid, add a mixture of formic acid and methyl acetate (1:1) to make 10 mL. When the procedure is run with 2 μL of this solution under the above operating conditions, *n*-valerianic acid and valproic acid are eluted in this order with the resolution between these peaks being not less than 5.

System repeatability: Pipet 2 mL of the standard solution and add a mixture of formic acid and methyl acetate (1:1) to make exactly 10 mL. When the test is repeated 6 times with 2 μL of this solution under the above operating conditions, the relative standard deviation of the peak area of valproic acid is not more than 5.0%.

Loss on drying <*2.41*> Not more than 1.0% (1 g, 105°C, 3 hours).

Assay Weigh accurately about 0.2 g of Sodium Valproate, previously dried, dissolve in 80 mL of acetic acid (100), and titrate <*2.50*> with 0.1 mol/L perchloric acid VS (potentiometric titration). Perform a blank determination in the same manner, and make any necessary correction.

Each mL of 0.1 mol/L perchloric acid VS
= 16.62 mg of $C_8H_{15}NaO_2$

Containers and storage Containers—Tight containers.

Sodium Valproate Extended-release Tablets A

バルプロ酸ナトリウム徐放錠A

Sodium Valproate Extended-release Tablets A contain not less than 95.0% and not more than 105.0% of the labeled amount of sodium valproate ($C_8H_{15}NaO_2$: 166.19).

Method of preparation Prepare as directed under Tablets, with Sodium Valproate.

Identification To a quantity of powdered Sodium Valproate Extended-release Tablets A, equivalent to 0.2 g of Sodium Valproate, add 20 mL of water, shake thoroughly, and centrifuge. To 2 mL of the supernatant liquid add 1 mL of a solution of cobalt (II) nitrate hexahydrate (1 in 20), and heat on a water bath: a purple precipitate is formed.

Uniformity of dosage units <*6.02*> Perform the test according to the following method: it meets the requirement of the Content uniformity test.

Crush 1 tablet of Sodium Valproate Extended-release Tablets A, add exactly $V/40$ mL of the internal standard solution, add $4V/5$ mL of a mixture of methanol and water (3:2), shake vigorously, add a mixture of methanol and water (3:2) to make V mL so that each mL contains about 1 mg of sodium valproate ($C_8H_{15}NaO_2$), and filter through a membrane filter with a pore size not exceeding 0.45 μm. Discard the first 5 mL of the filtrate, and use the subsequent filtrate as the sample solution. Separately, weigh accurately about 0.1 g of sodium valproate for assay, previously dried at 105°C for 3 hours, add exactly 2.5 mL of the internal standard solution, add a mixture of methanol and water (3:2) to make 100 mL, and use this solution as the standard solution. Then, proceed as directed in the Assay.

$$\text{Amount (mg) of sodium valproate } (C_8H_{15}NaO_2) = M_S \times Q_T/Q_S \times V/100$$

M_S: Amount (mg) of sodium valproate for assay taken

Internal standard solution—A solution of ethyl parahydroxybenzoate in a mixture of methanol and water (3:2) (1 in 5000).

Dissolution <*6.10*> When the test is performed at 50 revolutions per minute according to the Paddle method, using 900 mL of water as the dissolution medium, the dissolution rates of a 100-mg tablet in 4 hours, in 6 hours and in 12 hours are 15 to 45%, 40 to 70%, and not less than 75%, respectively, and those of a 200-mg tablet in 4 hours, in 6 hours and in 12 hours are 15 to 45%, 35 to 65%, and not less than 75%, respectively.

Start the test with 1 tablet of Sodium Valproate Extended-release Tablets A, withdraw exactly 20 mL of the medium at the specified minutes after starting the test and supply exactly 20 mL of water warmed to 37 ± 0.5°C immediately after withdrawing of the medium every time. Filter the media through a membrane filter with a pore size not exceeding 0.45 μm. Discard not less than 10 mL of the first filtrate, pipet V mL of the subsequent filtrate, add water to make exactly V' mL so that each mL contains about 0.11 mg of sodium valproate ($C_8H_{15}NaO_2$), and use these solutions as the sample solutions. Separately, weigh accurately about 56 mg of sodium valproate for assay, previously dried at 105°C for 3 hours, and dissolve in water to make exactly 50 mL. Pipet 5 mL of this solution, add water to make exactly 50 mL, and use this solution as the standard solution. Perform the test with exactly 50 μL each of the sample solutions and standard solution as directed under Liquid Chromatography <*2.01*> according to the following conditions, and determine the peak areas, $A_{T(n)}$ and A_S, of valproic acid in each solution.

Dissolution rate (%) with respect to the labeled amount of sodium valproate ($C_8H_{15}NaO_2$) on the nth medium withdrawing (n = 1, 2, 3)

$$= M_S \times \left\{\frac{A_{T(n)}}{A_S} + \sum_{i=1}^{n-1}\left(\frac{A_{T(i)}}{A_S} \times \frac{1}{45}\right)\right\} \times \frac{V'}{V} \times \frac{1}{C} \times 180$$

M_S: Amount (mg) of sodium valproate for assay taken

C: Labeled amount (mg) of sodium valproate ($C_8H_{15}NaO_2$) in 1 tablet

Operating conditions—

Proceed as directed in the operating conditions in the Assay.

System suitability—

System performance: When the procedure is run with 50 μL of the standard solution under the above operating conditions, the number of theoretical plates and the symmetry factor of the peak of valproic acid are not less than 3000 and not more than 2.0, respectively.

System repeatability: When the test is repeated 6 times with 50 μL of the standard solution under the above operating conditions, the relative standard deviation of the peak area of valproic acid is not more than 1.5%.

Assay Weigh accurately the mass of not less than 20 Sodium Valproate Extended-release Tablets A, and powder. Weigh accurately a portion of the powder, equivalent to about 0.1 g of sodium valproate ($C_8H_{15}NaO_2$), add about 80 mL of the mobile phase, shake thoroughly, add the mobile phase to make exactly 100 mL, and centrifuge. Pipet 20 mL of the supernatant liquid, add exactly 5 mL of the internal standard solution, and use this solution as the sample solution. Separately, weigh accurately about 0.1 g of sodium valproate for assay, previously dried at 105°C for 3 hours, dissolve in the mobile phase to make exactly 100 mL. Pipet 20 mL of this solution, add exactly 5 mL of the internal standard solution, and use this solution as the standard solution. Perform the test with 10 μL each of the sample solution and standard solution as directed under Liquid Chromatography <*2.01*> according to the following conditions, and calculate the ratios, Q_T and Q_S, of the peak area of valproic acid to that of the internal standard.

$$\text{Amount (mg) of sodium valproate } (C_8H_{15}NaO_2) = M_S \times Q_T/Q_S$$

M_S: Amount (mg) of sodium valproate for assay taken

Internal standard solution—A solution of ethyl parahydroxybenzoate in the mobile phase (1 in 50,000).

Operating conditions—

Detector: An ultraviolet absorption photometer (wavelength: 210 nm).

Column: A stainless steel column 4.6 mm in inside diameter and 15 cm in length, packed with octadecylsilanized silica gel for liquid chromatography (5 μm in particle diameter).

Column temperature: A constant temperature of about 25°C.

Mobile phase: A mixture of 0.05 mol/L sodium dihydrogen phosphate TS (pH 3.0) and acetonitrile for liquid chromatography (1:1).

Flow rate: Adjust so that the retention time of valproic acid is about 6 minutes.

System suitability—

System performance: When the procedure is run with 10 μL of the standard solution under the above operating conditions, the internal standard and valproic acid are eluted in this order with the resolution between these peaks being not less than 7.

System repeatability: When the test is repeated 6 times with 10 μL of the standard solution under the above operating conditions, the relative standard deviation of the ratio of the peak area of valproic acid to that of the internal standard is not more than 1.0%.

Containers and storage Containers—Tight containers.

Sodium Valproate Extended-release Tablets B

バルプロ酸ナトリウム徐放錠 B

Sodium Valproate Extended-release Tablets B contain not less than 95.0% and not more than 105.0% of the labeled amount of sodium valproate ($C_8H_{15}NaO_2$: 166.19).

Method of preparation Prepare as directed under Tablets, with Sodium Valproate.

Identification To a quantity of the powdered Sodium Valproate Extended-release Tablets B, equivalent to 1.0 g of Sodium Valproate, add 10 mL of water, heat on a water bath for 30 minutes, and filter. To 2.5 mL of the filtrate add 2.5 mL of water and 1 mL of a solution of cobalt (II) nitrate hexahydrate (1 in 20), and heat on a water bath: a purple precipitate is formed.

Uniformity of dosage units <*6.02*> Perform the Mass variation test, or the Content uniformity test according to the following method: it meets the requirement.

To 1 tablet of Sodium Valproate Extended-release Tablets B add 150 mL of the mobile phase, allow to stand for not less than 16 hours, shake until the film is disintegrated, and add the mobile phase to make exactly 200 mL. Pipet V mL of this solution, and add the mobile phase to make exactly V' mL so that each mL contains about 1 mg of sodium valproate ($C_8H_{15}NaO_2$). Centrifuge this solution, and filter the supernatant liquid through a membrane filter with a pore size not exceeding 0.45 μm. Discard the first 5 mL of the filtrate, pipet 20 mL of the subsequent filtrate, add exactly 5 mL of the internal standard solution, and use this solution as the sample solution. Then, proceed as directed in the Assay.

$$\text{Amount (mg) of sodium valproate } (C_8H_{15}NaO_2) = M_S \times Q_T/Q_S \times V'/V \times 2$$

M_S: Amount (mg) of sodium valproate for assay taken

Internal standard solution—A solution of methyl parahydroxybenzoate in the mobile phase (1 in 50,000).

Dissolution <*6.10*> When the test is performed at 50 revolutions per minute according to the Paddle method, using 900 mL of water as the dissolution medium, the dissolution rates of a 200-mg tablet in 8 hours, in 11 hours and in 20 hours are 15 to 45%, 35 to 65%, and not less than 70%, respectively, and those of a 400-mg tablet in 9 hours, in 12 hours and in 21 hours are 15 to 45%, 35 to 65%, and not less than 70%, respectively.

Start the test with 1 tablet of Sodium Valproate Extended-release Tablets B, withdraw exactly 20 mL of the medium at the specified minutes after starting the test and supply exactly 20 mL of water warmed to 37 ± 0.5°C immediately after withdrawing of the medium every time. Filter the media through a membrane filter with a pore size not exceeding 0.45 μm. Discard not less than 2 mL of the first filtrate, pipet V mL of the subsequent filtrate, add water to make exactly V' mL so that each mL contains about 0.22 mg of sodium valproate ($C_8H_{15}NaO_2$), and use these solutions as the sample solutions. Separately, weigh accurately about 55 mg of sodium valproate for assay, previously dried at 105°C for 3 hours, dissolve in water to make exactly 250 mL, and use this solution as the standard solution. Perform the test with exactly 20 μL each of the sample solutions and standard solution as directed under Liquid Chromatography <*2.01*> according to the following conditions, and determine the peak areas, $A_{T(n)}$ and A_S, of valproic acid in each solution.

Dissolution rate (%) with respect to the labeled amount of sodium valproate ($C_8H_{15}NaO_2$) on the nth medium withdrawing (n = 1, 2, 3)

$$= M_S \times \left\{ \frac{A_{T(n)}}{A_S} + \sum_{i=1}^{n-1} \left(\frac{A_{T(i)}}{A_S} \times \frac{1}{45} \right) \right\} \times \frac{V'}{V} \times \frac{1}{C} \times 360$$

M_S: Amount (mg) of sodium valproate for assay taken
C: Labeled amount (mg) of sodium valproate ($C_8H_{15}NaO_2$) in 1 tablet

Operating conditions—

Proceed as directed in the operating conditions in the Assay.

System suitability—

System performance: When the procedure is run with 20 μL of the standard solution under the above operating conditions, the number of theoretical plates and the symmetry factor of the peak of valproic acid are not less than 3000 and not more than 2.0, respectively.

System repeatability: When the test is repeated 6 times with 20 μL of the standard solution under the above operating conditions, the relative standard deviation of the peak area of valproic acid is not more than 1.0%.

Assay To 20 Sodium Valproate Extended-release Tablets B add 150 mL of the mobile phase, allow to stand for not less than 16 hours, shake until the film is disintegrated, and add the mobile phase to make exactly 200 mL. Pipet 5 mL of this solution, add the mobile phase to make exactly V mL so that each mL contains about 1 mg of sodium valproate ($C_8H_{15}NaO_2$). Centrifuge this solution, and filter the supernatant liquid through a membrane filter with a pore size not exceeding 0.45 μm. Discard the first 5 mL of the filtrate, pipet 20 mL of the subsequent filtrate, add exactly 5 mL of the internal standard solution, and use this solution as the sample solution. Separately, weigh accurately about 0.1 g of sodium valproate for assay, previously dried at 105°C for 3 hours, dissolve in the mobile phase to make exactly 100 mL. Pipet 20 mL of this solution, add exactly 5 mL of the internal standard solution, and use this solution as the standard solution. Perform the test with 10 μL each of the sample solution and standard solution as directed under Liquid Chromatography <*2.01*> according to the following conditions, and calculate the ratios, Q_T and Q_S, of the peak area of valproic acid to that of the internal standard.

$$\text{Amount (mg) of sodium valproate } (C_8H_{15}NaO_2) \text{ in 1 tablet} = M_S \times Q_T/Q_S \times V/50$$

M_S: Amount (mg) of sodium valproate for assay taken

Internal standard solution—A solution of methyl parahydroxybenzoate in the mobile phase (1 in 50,000).

Operating conditions—

Detector: An ultraviolet absorption photometer (wavelength: 210 nm).

Column: A stainless steel column 4.6 mm in inside diameter and 15 cm in length, packed with octadecylsilanized silica gel for liquid chromatography (5 μm in particle diameter).

Column temperature: A constant temperature of about 25°C.

Mobile phase: A mixture of 0.05 mol/L sodium dihydrogen phosphate TS (pH 3.0) and acetonitrile for liquid chromatography (1:1).

Flow rate: Adjust so that the retention time of valproic acid is about 6 minutes.

System suitability—

System performance: When the procedure is run with 10 μL of the standard solution under the above operating conditions, the internal standard and valproic acid are eluted in this order with the resolution between these peaks being not less than 7.

System repeatability: When the test is repeated 6 times with 10 μL of the standard solution under the above operating conditions, the relative standard deviation of the ratio of the peak area of valproic acid to that of the internal standard is not more than 1.0%.

Containers and storage Containers—Tight containers.

Sodium Valproate Syrup

バルプロ酸ナトリウムシロップ

Sodium Valproate Syrup contains not less than 95.0% and not more than 105.0% of the labeled amount of sodium valproate ($C_8H_{15}NaO_2$: 166.19).

Method of preparation Prepare as directed under Syrups, with Sodium Valproate.

Identification To a volume of Sodium Valproate Syrup, equivalent to 50 mg of Sodium Valproate, add water to make 10 mL. To 5 mL of this solution add 1 mL of a solution of cobalt (II) nitrate hexahydrate (1 in 20) and warm on a water bath: a purple precipitate is formed.

Microbial limit <*4.05*> The acceptance criteria of TAMC and TYMC are 10^2 CFU/mL and 10^1 CFU/mL, respectively. *Escherichia coli* is not observed.

Assay Pipet a volume of Sodium Valproate Syrup, equivalent to about 0.1 g of sodium valproate ($C_8H_{15}NaO_2$) and add water to make exactly 100 mL. Pipet 20 mL of this solution, add exactly 5 mL of internal standard solution, and use this solution as the sample solution. Separately, weigh accurately about 50 mg of sodium valproate for assay, previously dried at 105°C for 3 hours, dissolve in water to make exactly 50 mL. Pipet 20 mL of this solution, add exactly 5 mL of the internal standard solution, and use this solution as the standard solution. Perform the test with 10 μL each of the sample solution and standard solution as directed under Liquid Chromatography <*2.01*> according to the following conditions, and calculate the ratios, Q_T and Q_S, of the peak area of valproic acid to that of the internal standard.

$$\text{Amount (mg) of sodium valproate } (C_8H_{15}NaO_2) = M_S \times Q_T/Q_S \times 2$$

M_S: Amount (mg) of sodium valproate for assay taken

*Internal standard solution—*A solution of ethyl parahydroxybenzoate in the mobile phase (1 in 50,000).

Operating conditions—

Detector: An ultraviolet absorption photometer (wavelength: 210 nm).

Column: A stainless steel column 4.6 mm in inside diameter and 15 cm in length packed with octadecylsilanized silica gel for liquid chromatography (5 μm in particle diameter).

Column temperature: A constant temperature of about 25°C.

Mobile phase: A mixture of 0.05 mol/L sodium dihydrogenphosphate TS (pH 3.0) and acetonitrile (1:1).

Flow rate: Adjust so that the retention time of valproic acid is about 6 minutes.

System suitability—

System performance: When the procedure is run with 10 μL of the standard solution under the above operating conditions, the internal standard and valproic acid are eluted in this order with the resolution between these peaks being not less than 7.

System repeatability: When the test is repeated 6 times with 10 μL of the standard solution under the above operating conditions, the relative standard deviation of the ratio of the peak area of valproic acid to that of the internal standard is not more than 1.0%.

Containers and storage Containers—Tight containers.

Sodium Valproate Tablets

バルプロ酸ナトリウム錠

Sodium Valproate Tablets contain not less than 95.0% and not more than 105.0% of the labeled amount of sodium valproate ($C_8H_{15}NaO_2$: 166.19).

Method of preparation Prepare as directed under Tablets, with Sodium Valproate.

Identification To a quantity of powdered Sodium Valproate Tablets, equivalent to 0.5 g of Sodium Valproate, add 10 mL of water, shake well, and centrifuge. To 5 mL of the supernatant liquid add 1 mL of a solution of cobalt (II) nitrate hexahydrate (1 in 20) and warm on a water bath: a purple precipitate is formed.

Uniformity of dosage units <*6.02*> Perform the Mass variation test, or the Content uniformity test according to the following method: it meets the requirement.

To 1 tablet of Sodium Valproate Tablets add $7V/10$ mL of the mobile phase, shake vigorously, add the mobile phase to make exactly V mL so that each mL contains about 1 mg of sodium valproate ($C_8H_{15}NaO_2$), and centrifuge. Filter the supernatant liquid, pipet 20 mL of the filtrate, add exactly 5 mL of the internal standard solution, shake vigorously, and use this solution as the sample solution. Then, proceed as directed in the Assay.

$$\text{Amount (mg) of sodium valproate } (C_8H_{15}NaO_2) = M_S \times Q_T/Q_S \times V/100$$

M_S: Amount (mg) of sodium valproate for assay taken

*Internal standard solution—*A solution of ethyl parahydroxybenzoate in the mobile phase (1 in 50,000).

Dissolution <*6.10*> When the test is performed at 50 revolutions per minute according to the Paddle method using the sinker, using 900 mL of water as the dissolution medium, the dissolution rate in 30 minutes of Sodium Valproate Tablets is not less than 85%.

Start the test with 1 tablet of Sodium Valproate Tablets, withdraw not less than 20 mL of the medium at the specified minute after starting the test, and filter through a membrane filter with a pore size not exceeding 0.45 μm. Discard not less than 10 mL of the first filtrate, pipet V mL of the subsequent filtrate, add water to make exactly V' mL so that each mL contains about 0.11 mg of sodium valproate ($C_8H_{15}NaO_2$), and use this solution as the sample solution. Separately, weigh accurately about 56 mg of sodium valproate for assay, previously dried at 105°C for 3 hours, and dissolve in water to make exactly 50 mL. Pipet 5 mL of this solution, add water to make exactly 50 mL of the solution, and use this solution as the standard solution. Perform the test with exactly 50 μL each of the sample solution and standard solution as directed under Liquid Chromatography *<2.01>* according to the following conditions, and determine the peak areas, A_T and A_S, of valproic acid in each solution.

Dissolution rate (%) with respect to the labeled amount of sodium valproate ($C_8H_{15}NaO_2$)

$$= M_S \times A_T/A_S \times V'/V \times 1/C \times 180$$

M_S: Amount (mg) of sodium valproate for assay taken

C: Labeled amount (mg) of sodium valproate ($C_8H_{15}NaO_2$) in 1 tablet

Operating conditions—

Proceed as directed in the operating conditions in the Assay.

System suitability—

System performance: When the procedure is run with 50 μL of the standard solution under the above operating conditions, the number of theoretical plates and symmetry factor of the peak of valproic acid are not less than 3000 and not more than 2.0, respectively.

System repeatability: When the test is repeated 6 times with 50 μL of the standard solution under the above operating conditions, the relative standard deviation of the peak area of valproic acid is not more than 1.5%.

Assay Weigh accurately the mass of not less than 20 Sodium Valproate Tablets, and powder. Weigh accurately a portion of the powder, equivalent to about 0.2 g of sodium valproate ($C_8H_{15}NaO_2$), add about 160 mL of the mobile phase, shake well, add the mobile phase to make exactly 200 mL, and centrifuge. Filter the supernatant liquid, pipet 20 mL of the filtrate, add exactly 5 mL of the internal standard solution, and use this solution as the sample solution. Separately, weigh accurately about 0.1 g of sodium valproate for assay, previously dried at 105°C for 3 hours, and dissolve in the mobile phase to make exactly 100 mL. Pipet 20 mL of this solution, add exactly 5 mL of the internal standard solution, and use this solution as the standard solution. Perform the test with 10 μL each of the sample solution and standard solution as directed under Liquid Chromatography *<2.01>* according to the following conditions, and calculate the ratios, Q_T and Q_S, of the peak area of valproic acid to that of the internal standard.

Amount (mg) of sodium valproate ($C_8H_{15}NaO_2$)

$$= M_S \times Q_T/Q_S \times 2$$

M_S: Amount (mg) of sodium valproate for assay taken

Internal standard solution—A solution of ethyl parahydroxybenzoate in the mobile phase (1 in 50,000).

Operating conditions—

Detector: An ultraviolet absorption photometer (wavelength: 210 nm).

Column: A stainless steel column 4.6 mm in inside diameter and 15 cm in length, packed with octadecylsilanized silica gel for liquid chromatography (5 μm in particle diameter).

Column temperature: A constant temperature of about 25°C.

Mobile phase: A mixture of 0.05 mol/L sodium dihydrogen phosphate TS (pH 3.0) and acetonitrile (1:1).

Flow rate: Adjust so that the retention time of valproic acid is about 6 minutes.

System suitability—

System performance: When the procedure is run with 10 μL of the standard solution under the above operating conditions, the internal standard and valproic acid are eluted in this order with the resolution between these peaks being not less than 7.

System repeatability: When the test is repeated 6 times with 10 μL of the standard solution under the above operating conditions, the relative standard deviation of the ratio of the peak area of valproic acid to that of the internal standard is not more than 1.0%.

Containers and storage Containers—Tight containers.

Sorbitan Sesquioleate

ソルビタンセスキオレイン酸エステル

Sorbitan Sesquioleate is a mixture of monoester and diester of sorbitol anhydride, partially esterified with oleic acid.

Description Sorbitan Sesquioleate is a pale yellow to light yellow-brown, viscous oily liquid. It has a faint, characteristic odor and a slightly bitter taste.

It is freely soluble in diethyl ether, slightly soluble in ethanol (95), and very slightly soluble in methanol.

It is dispersed as fine oily drops in water.

Identification **(1)** To 0.5 g of Sorbitan Sesquioleate add 5 mL of ethanol (95) and 5 mL of dilute sulfuric acid, and heat on a water bath for 30 minutes. Cool, shake with 5 mL of petroleum ether, and allow to stand, and separate the upper layer and the lower layer. Shake 2 mL of the lower layer with 2 mL of freshly prepared catechol solution (1 in 10), then with 5 mL of sulfuric acid: a red to red-brown color develops.

(2) Heat the upper layer obtained in (1) on a water bath, and evaporate petroleum ether. To the residue add 2 mL of diluted nitric acid (1 in 2), and then add 0.5 g of potassium nitrite between 30°C and 35°C with stirring: the solution develops an opalescence, and, when cooled, crystals are formed.

Specific gravity *<1.13>* d_{25}^{25}: 0.960 – 1.020

Saponification value *<1.13>* 150 – 168

Purity **(1)** Acidity—To 2.0 g of Sorbitan Sesquioleate add 50 mL of neutralized ethanol, and heat on a water bath nearly to boiling with stirring once or twice. Cool, add 4.3 mL of 0.1 mol/L sodium hydroxide VS and 5 drops of phenolphthalein TS: a red color develops.

(2) Heavy metals *<1.07>*—Proceed with 1.0 g of Sorbitan Sesquioleate according to Method 2, and perform the test. Prepare the control solution with 2.0 mL of Standard Lead Solution (not more than 20 ppm).

(3) Arsenic *<1.11>*—Prepare the test solution with 1.0 g of Sorbitan Sesquioleate according to Method 2, and perform the test (not more than 2 ppm).

Water *<2.48>* Not more than 3.0% (1 g, volumetric titration, direct titration, stir for 30 minutes).

Residue on ignition *<2.44>* Not more than 1.0% (1 g).

Containers and storage Containers—Tight containers.

D-Sorbitol

D-ソルビトール

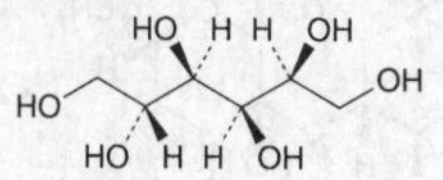

$C_6H_{14}O_6$: 182.17
D-Glucitol
[50-70-4]

D-Sorbitol, when dried, contains not less than 97.0% of D-sorbitol ($C_6H_{14}O_6$).

Description D-Sorbitol occurs as white, granules, powder, or crystalline masses. It is odorless, and has a sweet taste with a cold sensation.

It is very soluble in water, sparingly soluble in ethanol (95), and practically insoluble in diethyl ether.

It is hygroscopic.

Identification **(1)** To 1 mL of a solution of D-Sorbitol (7 in 10) add 2 mL of iron (II) sulfate TS and 1 mL of a solution of sodium hydroxide (1 in 5): a blue-green color develops, but no turbidity is produced.

(2) Shake thoroughly 1 mL of a solution of D-Sorbitol (1 in 20) with 1 mL of a freshly prepared solution of catechol (1 in 10), add rapidly 2 mL of sulfuric acid, and shake: a reddish purple to red-purple color immediately develops.

(3) Boil 0.5 g of D-Sorbitol with 10 mL of acetic anhydride and 1 mL of pyridine under a reflux condenser for 10 minutes, cool, shake with 25 mL of water, and allow to stand in a cold place. Transfer the solution to a separator, extract with 30 mL of chloroform, and evaporate the extract on a water bath. Add 80 mL of water to the oily residue, heat for 10 minutes on a water bath, then filter the hot mixture. After cooling, collect the produced precipitate through a glass filter (G3), wash with water, recrystallize once from ethanol (95), and dry in a desiccator (in vacuum, silica gel) for 4 hours: the precipitate melts *<2.60>* between 97°C and 101°C.

Purity **(1)** Clarity and color of solution, and acidity or alkalinity—Dissolve 5 g of D-Sorbitol in 20 mL of water by warming with shaking: the solution is clear, colorless, and neutral.

(2) Chloride *<1.03>*—Perform the test with 2.0 g of D-Sorbitol. Prepare the control solution with 0.30 mL of 0.01 mol/L hydrochloric acid VS (not more than 0.005%).

(3) Sulfate *<1.14>*—Perform the test with 4.0 g of D-Sorbitol. Prepare the control solution with 0.50 mL of 0.005 mol/L sulfuric acid VS (not more than 0.006%).

(4) Heavy metals *<1.07>*—Proceed with 5.0 g of D-Sorbitol according to Method 1, and perform the test. Prepare the control solution with 2.5 mL of Standard Lead Solution (not more than 5 ppm).

(5) Nickel—Dissolve 0.5 g of D-Sorbitol in 5 mL of water, add 3 drops of dimethylglyoxime TS and 3 drops of ammonia TS, and allow to stand for 5 minutes: no red color develops.

(6) Arsenic *<1.11>*—Prepare the test solution with 1.5 g of D-Sorbitol according to Method 1, and perform the test (not more than 1.3 ppm).

(7) Glucose—Dissolve 20.0 g of D-Sorbitol in 25 mL of water, and boil gently with 40 mL of Fehling's TS for 3 minutes. After cooling, filter the supernatant liquid cautiously through a glass filter (G4), leaving the precipitate in the flask as much as possible, wash the precipitate with hot water until the last washings no longer show an alkali reaction, and filter the washings through the glass filter. Dissolve the precipitate in the flask in 20 mL of iron (III) sulfate TS, filter through the glass filter, and wash with water. Combine the filtrate and the washings, heat at 80°C, and titrate *<2.50>* with 0.02 mol/L potassium permanganate VS: not more than 6.3 mL of volume for titration consumed or consumption is required.

(8) Sugars—Dissolve 20.0 g of D-Sorbitol in 25 mL of water, and heat with 8 mL of dilute hydrochloric acid under a reflux condenser in a water bath for 3 hours. After cooling, add 2 drops of methyl orange TS, followed by sodium hydroxide TS until an orange color develops, and add water to make 100 mL. Boil gently 10 mL of this solution with 10 mL of water and 40 mL of Fehling's TS for 3 minutes and proceed as directed in (7).

Loss on drying *<2.41>* Not more than 2.0% (0.5 g, in vacuum, phosphorus (V) oxide, 80°C, 3 hours).

Residue on ignition *<2.44>* Not more than 0.02% (5 g).

Assay Weigh accurately about 0.2 g of D-Sorbitol, previously dried, dissolve in water and add water to make exactly 100 mL. Pipet 10 mL of the solution into an iodine flask, add exactly 50 mL of potassium periodate TS, and heat for 15 minutes in a water bath. Cool, add 2.5 g of potassium iodide, immediately stopper tightly, and shake well. Allow to stand for 5 minutes in a dark place, and titrate *<2.50>* with 0.1 mol/L sodium thiosulfate VS (indicator: 3 mL of starch TS). Perform a blank determination in the same manner.

Each mL of 0.1 mol/L sodium thiosulfate VS
= 1.822 mg of $C_6H_{14}O_6$

Containers and storage Containers—Tight containers.

D-Sorbitol Solution

D-ソルビトール液

D-Sorbitol Solution contains not less than 97.0% and not more than 103.0% of the labeled amount of D-sorbitol ($C_6H_{14}O_6$: 182.17).

Description D-Sorbitol Solution is a clear, colorless liquid. It is odorless, and has a sweet taste.

It is miscible with water, with ethanol (95), with glycerin and with propylene glycol.

It sometimes separates crystalline masses.

Identification **(1)** To a volume of D-Sorbitol Solution, equivalent to 0.7 g of D-Sorbitol, add 2 mL of iron (II) sulfate TS and 1 mL of a solution of sodium hydroxide (1 in 5): a blue-green color develops, but no turbidity is produced.

(2) To a volume of D-Sorbitol Solution, equivalent to 1 g of D-Sorbitol, add water to make 20 mL. To 1 mL of this solution add 1 mL of a freshly prepared solution of catechol (1 in 10), mix well, then add rapidly 2 mL of sulfuric acid, and mix: a reddish purple to red-purple color immediately develops.

Purity **(1)** Acidity or alkalinity—D-Sorbitol Solution is neutral.

(2) Chloride <*1.03*>—Proceed with a volume of D-Sorbitol Solution, equivalent to 2.0 g of D-Sorbitol, and perform the test. Prepare the control solution with 0.30 mL of 0.01 mol/L hydrochloric acid VS (not more than 0.005%).

(3) Sulfate <*1.14*>—To a volume of D-Sorbitol Solution, equivalent to 4.0 g of D-Sorbitol, and perform the test. Prepare the control solution with 0.50 mL of 0.005 mol/L sulfuric acid VS (not more than 0.006%).

(4) Heavy metals <*1.07*>—Proceed with a volume of D-Sorbitol Solution, equivalent to 5.0 g of D-Sorbitol, and according to Method 1, perform the test. Prepare the control solution with 2.5 mL of Standard Lead Solution (not more than 5 ppm).

(5) Nickel—Take a volume of D-Sorbitol Solution, equivalent to 0.5 g of D-Sorbitol, add 3 drops of dimethylglyoxime TS and 3 drops of ammonia TS, and allow to stand for 5 minutes: no red color develops.

(6) Arsenic <*1.11*>—Take a volume of D-Sorbitol Solution, equivalent to 1.5 g of D-Sorbitol, dilute with water or concentrate to 5 mL on a water bath, if necessary, cool, and perform the test using this solution as the test solution (not more than 1.3 ppm).

(7) Glucose—Take a volume of D-Sorbitol Solution, equivalent to 20.0 g of D-Sorbitol, dilute with water or concentrate to 40 mL on a water bath, if necessary, add 40 mL of Fehling's TS, and boil gently for 3 minutes. After cooling, filter the supernatant liquid cautiously through a glass filter (G4), leaving the precipitate in the flask as much as possible, wash the precipitate with hot water until the last washings no longer show alkalinity, and filter the washings through the glass filter. Dissolve the precipitate in the flask in 20 mL of iron (III) sulfate TS, filter through the glass filter, and wash the filter with water. Combine the filtrate and the washings, heat at 80°C, and titrate <*2.50*> with 0.02 mol/L potassium permanganate VS: not more than 6.3 mL of 0.02 mol/L potassium permanganate VS is required.

(8) Sugars—Take a volume of D-Sorbitol Solution, equivalent to 20.0 g of D-Sorbitol, dilute with water or concentrate to 40 mL of a water bath, if necessary, add 8 mL of dilute hydrochloric acid, and heat under a reflux condenser in a water bath for 3 hours. After cooling, add 2 drops of methyl orange TS, followed by sodium hydroxide TS until an orange color develops, and add water to make 100 mL. Boil gently 10 mL of this solution with 10 mL of water and 40 mL of Fehling's TS for 3 minutes and proceed as directed in (7).

Residue on ignition <*2.44*> Measure exactly a volume of D-Sorbitol Solution, equivalent to 5 g of D-Sorbitol, add 3 to 4 drops of sulfuric acid, and heat gently to evaporate. Ignite to burn, cool, and perform the test with the residue: not more than 1 mg.

Assay Measure exactly a volume of D-Sorbitol Solution, equivalent to about 5 g of D-sorbitol ($C_6H_{14}O_6$), and add water to make exactly 250 mL. Pipet 10 mL of this solution, add water to make exactly 100 mL. Pipet 10 mL of the solution into an iodine flask, add exactly 50 mL of potassium periodate TS, and heat for 15 minutes in a water bath. Cool, add 2.5 g of potassium iodide, immediately stopper tightly, and shake well. Allow to stand for 5 minutes in a dark place, and titrate <*2.50*> with 0.1 mol/L sodium thiosulfate VS (indicator: 3 mL of starch TS). Perform a blank determination in the same manner.

Each mL of 0.1 mol/L sodium thiosulfate VS
= 1.822 mg of $C_6H_{14}O_6$

Containers and storage Containers—Tight containers.

Spectinomycin Hydrochloride Hydrate

スペクチノマイシン塩酸塩水和物

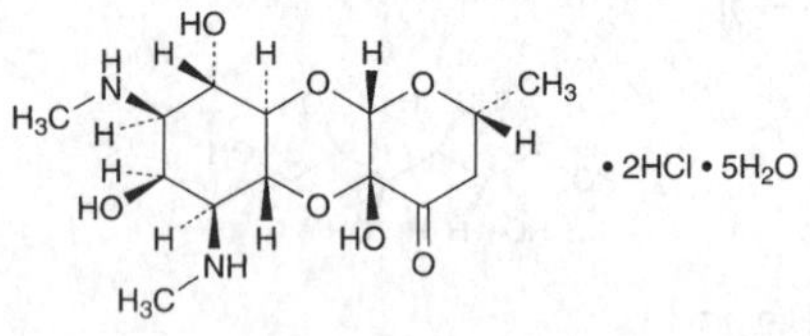

$C_{14}H_{24}N_2O_7.2HCl.5H_2O$: 495.35
(2*R*,4a*R*,5a*R*,6*S*,7*S*,8*R*,9*S*,9a*R*,10a*S*)-
4a,7,9-Trihydroxy-2-methyl-6,8-bis(methylamino)-
2,3,4a,5a,6,7,8,9,9a,10a-decahydro-
4*H*-pyrano[2,3-*b*][1,4]benzodioxin-4-one
dihydrochloride pentahydrate
[*22189-32-8*]

Spectinomycin Hydrochloride Hydrate is the hydrochloride of a substance having antibacterial activity produced by the growth of *Streptomyces spectabilis*.

It contains not less than 763 μg (potency) and not more than 831 μg (potency) per mg, calculated on the anhydrous basis. The potency of Spectinomycin Hydrochloride Hydrate is expressed as mass (potency) of spectinomycin ($C_{14}H_{24}N_2O_7$: 332.35).

Description Spectinomycin Hydrochloride Hydrate occurs as a white to light yellow-white crystalline powder.

It is freely soluble in water, and practically insoluble in ethanol (95).

Identification **(1)** To 5 mL of a solution of Spectinomycin Hydrochloride Hydrate (1 in 100) add gently anthrone TS: a blue to blue-green color is produced at the zone of contact.

(2) Determine the infrared absorption spectra of Spectinomycin Hydrochloride Hydrate and Spectinomycin Hydrochloride RS as directed in the paste method under Infrared Spectrophotometry <*2.25*>, and compare these spectra: both spectra exhibit similar intensities of absorption at the same wave numbers.

(3) To 3 mL of a solution of Spectinomycin Hydrochloride Hydrate (1 in 150) add 1 drop of silver nitrate TS: a white turbidity is produced.

Optical rotation <*2.49*> $[\alpha]_D^{20}$: +15 – +21° (2.1 g calculated on the anhydrous basis, water, 25 mL, 200 mm).

pH <*2.54*> Dissolve 0.10 g of Spectinomycin Hydrochloride Hydrate in 10 mL of water: the pH of the solution is between 4.0 and 5.6.

Purity Related substances—Dissolve 0.20 g of Spectinomycin Hydrochloride Hydrate in 5 mL of water, and use this solution as the sample solution. Pipet 1 mL of the sample solution, add water to make exactly 100 mL, and use this solution as the standard solution. Perform the test with these solutions as directed under Thin-layer Chromatography <*2.03*>. Spot 5 μL each of the sample solution and standard solution on a plate of silica gel for thin-layer chromatography. Develop the plate with a mixture of 1-propanol, water, pyridine and acetic acid (100) (10:8:1:1) to a distance of about 12 cm, and air-dry the plate. Spray evenly alkaline 1.6% potassium periodate-0.2% potassium permanganate TS: the spot other than the principal spot obtained from the sample solution is not more intense than the spot from the standard solution.

Water <2.48> Not less than 16.0% and not more than 20.0% (0.3 g, volumetric titration, direct titration).

Residue on ignition <2.44> Not more than 1.0% (1 g).

Assay Weigh accurately an amount of both Spectinomycin Hydrochloride Hydrate and Spectinomycin Hydrochloride RS, equivalent to about 20 mg (potency), add exactly 10 mL of the internal standard solution to them, add 1 mL of 1,1,1,3,3,3-hexamethyldisilazan, allow to stand at room temperature for 1 hour, and use these solutions as the sample solution and the standard solution, respectively. Perform the test with 1 μL each of the sample solution and standard solution as directed under Gas Chromatography <2.02> according to the following conditions, and calculate the ratios, Q_T and Q_S, of the peak area of spectinomycin to that of the internal standard.

Amount [μg (potency)] of spectinomycin ($C_{14}H_{24}N_2O_7$)
$= M_S \times Q_T/Q_S \times 1000$

M_S: Amount [mg (potency)] of Spectinomycin Hydrochloride RS taken

Internal standard solution—A solution of triphenylantimony in *N,N*-dimethylformamide (1 in 500).

Operating conditions—

Detector: A hydrogen flame-ionization detector.

Column: A glass column 3 mm in inside diameter and 60 cm in length, packed with 150 to 180 μm siliceous earth for gas chromatography coated in 5% with 5% phenyl-methyl silicone polymer for gas chromatography.

Column temperature: A constant temperature of about 190°C.

Injection port temperature: A constant temperature of about 215°C.

Detector temperature: A constant temperature of about 220°C.

Carrier gas: Helium.

Flow rate: Adjust so that the retention time of spectinomycin is about 10 minutes.

System suitability—

System performance: When the procedure is run with 1 μL of the standard solution under the above operating conditions, the internal standard and spectinomycin are eluted in this order with the resolution between these peaks being not less than 2.0.

System repeatability: When the test is repeated 6 times with 1 μL of the standard solution under the above operating conditions, the relative standard deviation of the ratio of the peak area of spectinomycin to that of the internal standard is not more than 1.5%.

Containers and storage Containers—Tight containers.

Spectinomycin Hydrochloride for Injection

注射用スペクチノマイシン塩酸塩

Spectinomycin Hydrochloride for Injection is a preparation for injection which is suspended before use.

It contains not less than 97.5% and not more than 117.5% of the labeled potency of spectinomycin ($C_{14}H_{24}N_2O_7$: 332.35).

Method of preparation Prepare as directed under Injections, with Spectinomycin Hydrochloride Hydrate.

Description Spectinomycin Hydrochloride for Injection occurs as a white to light yellow-white crystalline powder.

Identification Proceed as directed in the Identification (2) under Spectinomycin Hydrochloride Hydrate.

pH <2.54> Dissolve an amount of Spectinomycin Hydrochloride for Injection, equivalent to 70 mg (potency) of Spectinomycin Hydrochloride Hydrate, in 10 mL of water: the pH of the solution is between 4.0 and 5.6.

Purity Clarity and color of solution—A solution dissolved an amount of Spectinomycin Hydrochloride for Injection, equivalent to 0.70 g (potency) of Spectinomycin Hydrochloride Hydrate, in 10 mL of water is clear, and its absorbance at 425 nm, determined as directed under Ultraviolet-visible Spectrophotometry <2.24>, is not more than 0.10.

Water <2.48> 16.0 - 20.0% (0.3 g, volumetric titration, direct titration).

Uniformity of dosage units <6.02> It meets the requirement of the Mass variation test (*T*: 107.5%).

Sterility <4.06> Perform the test according to the Membrane filtration method: it meets the requirement.

Assay Weigh accurately the mass of the contents of not less than 10 Spectinomycin Hydrochloride for Injection. Weigh accurately a portion of the content, equivalent to about 20 mg (potency) of Spectinomycin Hydrochloride Hydrate, dissolve in exactly 10 mL of the internal standard solution, add 1 mL of 1,1,1,3,3,3-hexamethyldisilazan, allow to stand at room temperature for 1 hour, and use this solution as the sample solution. Separately, weigh accurately an amount of Spectinomycin Hydrochloride RS, equivalent to about 20 mg (potency), dissolve in exactly 10 mL of the internal standard solution, add 1 mL of 1,1,1,3,3,3-hexamethyldisilazan, allow to stand at room temperature for 1 hour, and use this solution as the standard solution. Then, proceed as directed in the Assay under Spectinomycin Hydrochloride Hydrate.

Amount [mg (potency)] of spectinomycin ($C_{14}H_{24}N_2O_7$)
$= M_S \times Q_T/Q_S$

M_S: Amount [mg (potency)] of Spectinomycin Hydrochloride RS taken

Internal standard solution—A solution of triphenylantimony in *N, N*-dimethylformamide (1 in 500).

Containers and storage Containers—Hermetic containers.

Spiramycin Acetate

スピラマイシン酢酸エステル

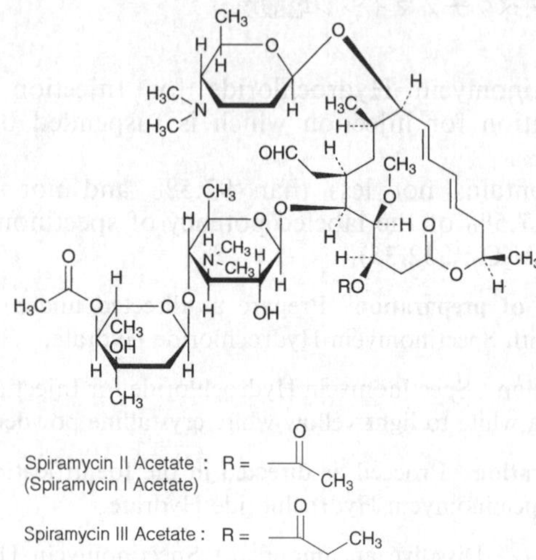

Spiramycin II Acetate : R =
(Spiramycin I Acetate)

Spiramycin III Acetate : R =

(Spiramycin II Acetate (Spiramycin I Acetate))
(3*R*,4*S*,5*S*,6*R*,8*R*,9*R*,10*E*,12*E*,15*R*)-3-Acetoxy-5-[4-*O*-acetyl-2,6-dideoxy-3-*C*-methyl-*α*-L-*ribo*-hexopyranosyl-(1→4)-3,6-dideoxy-3-dimethylamino-*β*-D-glucopyranosyloxy]-9-(2,3,4,6-tetradeoxy-4-dimethylamino-*β*-D-*erythro*-hexopyranosyloxy)-6-formylmethyl-4-methoxy-8-methylhexadeca-10,12-dien-15-olide
[*87111-42-0*]
(Spiramycin III Acetate)
(3*R*,4*S*,5*S*,6*R*,8*R*,9*R*,10*E*,12*E*,15*R*)-5-[4-*O*-Acetyl-2,6-dideoxy-3-*C*-methyl-*α*-L-*ribo*-hexopyranosyl-(1→4)-3,6-dideoxy-3-dimethylamino-*β*-D-glucopyranosyloxy]-9-(2,3,4,6-tetradeoxy-4-dimethylamino-*β*-D-*erythro*-hexopyranosyloxy)-6-formylmethyl-4-methoxy-8-methyl-3-propanoyloxyhexadeca-10,12-dien-15-olide
[*112501-15-2*]

Spiramycin Acetate is a derivative of a mixture of macrolide substances having antibacterial activity produced by the growth of *Streptomyces ambofaciens*.

It contains not less than 900 μg (potency) and not more than 1450 μg (potency) per mg, calculated on the dried basis. The potency of Spiramycin Acetate is expressed as mass (potency) of spiramycin II acetate ($C_{47}H_{78}N_2O_{16}$: 927.13). One mg (potency) of Spiramycin Acetate is equivalent to 0.7225 mg of spiramycin II acetate ($C_{47}H_{78}N_2O_{16}$).

Description Spiramycin Acetate occurs as a white to light yellow-white powder.

It is very soluble in acetonitrile and in methanol, freely soluble in ethanol (99.5), and practically insoluble in water.

Identification **(1)** Determine the absorption spectrum of a solution of Spiramycin Acetate in methanol (1 in 50,000) as directed under Ultraviolet-visible Spectrophotometry *<2.24>*, and compare the spectrum with the Reference Spectrum: both spectra exhibit similar intensities of absorption at the same wavelengths.

(2) Determine the infrared absorption spectrum of Spiramycin Acetate as directed in the potassium bromide disk method under Infrared Spectrophotometry *<2.25>*, and compare the spectrum with the Reference Spectrum: both spectra exhibit similar intensities of absorption at the same wave numbers.

Content ratio of the active principle Dissolve 25 mg of Spiramycin Acetate in 25 mL of the mobile phase, and use this solution as the sample solution. Perform the test with 5 μL of the sample solution as directed under Liquid Chromatography *<2.01>* according to the following conditions, and determine the areas, A_{II}, A_{III}, A_{IV}, A_V, A_{VI} and A_{VII}, of the peaks of spiramycin II acetate, spiramycin III acetate, spiramycin IV acetate, spiramycin V acetate, spiramycin VI acetate and spiramycin VII acetate, respectively, by the automatic integration method, and calculate the ratios of the amounts of A_{II}, A_{IV} and the total of A_{III} and A_V to the total amount of all these peaks: the amount of A_{II} is 30 – 45%, A_{IV} is 30 – 45%, and the total of A_{III} and A_V is not more than 25%. The relative retention times of spiramycin III acetate, spiramycin IV acetate, spiramycin V acetate, spiramycin VI acetate and spiramycin VII acetate to spiramycin II acetate are about 1.3, about 1.7, about 2.3, about 0.85 and about 1.4, respectively.

Operating conditions—

Detector: An ultraviolet absorption photometer (wavelength: 231 nm).

Column: A stainless steel column 6 mm in inside diameter and 15 cm in length, packed with octadecylsilanized silica gel for liquid chromatography (3 μm in particle diameter).

Column temperature: A constant temperature of about 35°C.

Mobile phase: A mixture of acetonitrile, 0.02 mol/L potassium dihydrogen phosphate TS and a solution of dipotassium hydrogen phosphate (87 in 25,000) (26:7:7).

Flow rate: Adjust so that the retention time of spiramycin II acetate is about 10 minutes.

System suitability—

System performance: Dissolve 25 mg of Spiramycin II Acetate RS in the mobile phase to make 100 mL. When the procedure is run with 5 μL of this solution under the above operating conditions, the number of theoretical plates and the symmetry factor of the peak of spiramycin II acetate are not less than 14,500 and not more than 2.0, respectively.

System repeatability: When the test is repeated 6 times with 5 μL of the sample solution under the above operating conditions, the relative standard deviation of the peak area of spiramycin II acetate is not more than 2.0%.

Purity Heavy metals *<1.07>*—Proceed with 1.0 g of Spiramycin Acetate according to Method 2, and perform the test. Prepare the control solution with 1.0 mL of Standard Lead Solution (not more than 10 ppm).

Loss on drying *<2.41>* Not more than 3.0% (1 g, in vacuum, phosphorus (V) oxide, 60°C, 3 hours).

Residue on ignition *<2.44>* Not more than 0.5% (1 g).

Assay Perform the test according to the Cylinder-plate method as directed under Microbial Assay for Antibiotics *<4.02>* according to the following conditions.

(i) Test organism—*Bacillus subtilis* ATCC 6633

(ii) Culture medium—Use the medium i in 1) under (1) Agar media for seed and base layer.

(iii) Standard solutions—Weigh accurately an amount of Spiramycin II Acetate RS, equivalent to about 50 mg (potency), dissolve in 20 mL of methanol, add 0.1 mol/L phosphate buffer solution for antibiotics (pH 8.0) to make exactly 50 mL, and use this solution as the standard stock solution. Keep the standard stock solution at not exceeding 5°C, and use within 3 days. Take exactly a suitable amount of the standard stock solution before use, add 0.1 mol/L phosphate buffer solution for antibiotics (pH 8.0) to make solutions so that each mL contains 80 μg (potency) and 20 μg (potency), and use these solutions as the high concentration standard solution and the low concentration standard solution, respectively.

(iv) Sample solutions—Weigh accurately an amount of Spiramycin Acetate, equivalent to about 50 mg (potency), dissolve in 20 mL of methanol, and add 0.1 mol/L phosphate buffer solution for antibiotics (pH 8.0) to make exactly 50 mL. Take exactly a suitable amount of this solution, add 0.1 mol/L phosphate buffer solution for antibiotics (pH 8.0) to make solutions so that each mL contains 80 μg (potency) and 20 μg (potency), and use these solutions as the high concentration sample solution and the low concentration sample solution, respectively.

Containers and storage Containers—Tight containers.

Spironolactone

スピロノラクトン

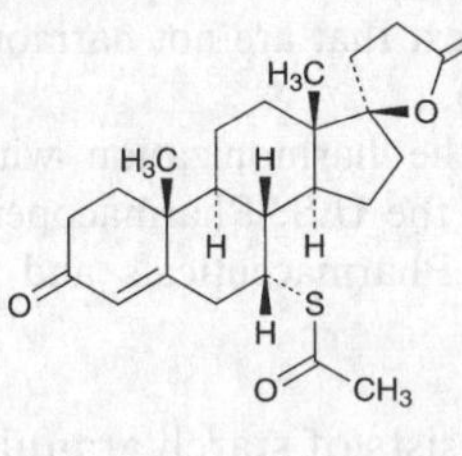

$C_{24}H_{32}O_4S$: 416.57
7α-Acetylsulfanyl-3-oxo-17α-pregn-4-ene-21,17-carbolactone
[52-01-7]

Spironolactone, when dried, contains not less than 97.0% and not more than 103.0% of spironolactone ($C_{24}H_{32}O_4S$).

Description Spironolactone occurs as a white to light yellow-brown fine powder.

It is freely soluble in chloroform, soluble in ethanol (95), slightly soluble in methanol, and practically insoluble in water.

Melting point: 198 – 207°C (Insert the capillary tube into a bath at about 125°C, and continue the heating so that the temperature rises at a rate of about 10°C per minute in the range between 140°C and 185°C, and when the temperature is near the expected melting range, reduce the heating so that the temperature rises at a rate of about 3°C per minute.)

It shows crystal polymorphism.

Identification **(1)** Determine the absorption spectrum of a solution of Spironolactone in methanol (1 in 100,000) as directed under Ultraviolet-visible Spectrophotometry *<2.24>*, and compare the spectrum with the Reference Spectrum or the spectrum of a solution of Spironolactone RS prepared in the same manner as the sample solution: both spectra exhibit similar intensities of absorption at the same wavelengths.

(2) Determine the infrared absorption spectrum of Spironolactone, previously dried, as directed in the potassium bromide disk method under Infrared Spectrophotometry *<2.25>*, and compare the spectrum with the Reference Spectrum or the spectrum of Spironolactone RS: both spectra exhibit similar intensities of absorption at the same wave numbers. If any difference appears between the spectra, dissolve Spironolactone and Spironolactone RS in methanol, respectively, then evaporate methanol to dryness, and repeat the test on the residues.

Optical rotation *<2.49>* $[\alpha]_D^{20}$: −33 – −37° (after drying, 0.25 g, chloroform, 25 mL, 200 mm).

Purity **(1)** Mercapto compounds—Shake 2.0 g of Spironolactone with 20 mL of water, and filter. To 10 mL of the filtrate add 1 mL of starch TS and 0.05 mL of 0.01 mol/L iodine VS, and mix: a blue color develops.

(2) Related substances—Dissolve 0.20 g of Spironolactone in 10 mL of ethanol (95), and use this solution as the sample solution. Pipet 1 mL of the sample solution, add ethanol (95) to make exactly 100 mL, and use this solution as the standard solution. Perform the test with these solutions as directed under Thin-layer Chromatography *<2.03>*. Spot 5 μL each of the sample solution and standard solution on a plate of silica gel for thin-layer chromatography. Develop the plate with *n*-butyl acetate to a distance of about 15 cm, and air-dry the plate. Spray evenly a solution of sulfuric acid in methanol (1 in 10) on the plate, and heat the plate at 105°C for 10 minutes: the spots other than the principal spot obtained from the sample solution are not more intense than the spot from the standard solution.

Loss on drying *<2.41>* Not more than 0.5% (1 g, 105°C, 2 hours).

Residue on ignition *<2.44>* Not more than 0.1% (1 g).

Assay Weigh accurately about 50 mg each of Spironolactone and Spironolactone RS, previously dried at 105°C for 2 hours, dissolve in methanol to make exactly 250 mL. Pipet 5 mL each of these solutions, add methanol to make exactly 100 mL, and use these solutions as the sample solution and the standard solution, respectively. Perform the test with these solutions as directed under Ultraviolet-visible Spectrophotometry *<2.24>*, and determine the absorbances, A_T and A_S, of the sample solution and standard solution at 238 nm.

$$\text{Amount (mg) of spironolactone } (C_{24}H_{32}O_4S) = M_S \times A_T/A_S$$

M_S: amount (mg) of Spironolactone RS taken

Containers and storage Containers—Tight containers.

Spironolactone Tablets

スピロノラクトン錠

Spironolactone Tablets contain not less than 95.0% and not more than 105.0% of the labeled amount of spironolactone ($C_{24}H_{32}O_4S$: 416.57).

Method of preparation Prepare as directed under Tablets, with Spironolactone.

Identification To an amount of powdered Spironolactone Tablets, equivalent to 10 mg of Spironolactone, add 100 mL of methanol, shake vigorously, and centrifuge. To 5 mL of the supernatant liquid add methanol to make 50 mL, and determine the absorption spectrum of this solution as directed under Ultraviolet-visible Spectrophotometry *<2.24>*: it exhibits a maximum between 236 nm and 240 nm.

Uniformity of dosage units *<6.02>* Perform the Mass variation test, or the Content uniformity test according to the following method: it meets the requirement.

To 1 tablet of Spironolactone Tablets add a mixture of water and acetonitrile (1:1) to make exactly *V* mL so that each mL contains about 0.5 mg of spironolactone ($C_{24}H_{32}O_4S$). After stirring for 30 minutes, centrifuge, and use the supernatant liquid as the sample solution. Then, proceed as directed in the Assay.

Amount (mg) of spironolactone ($C_{24}H_{32}O_4S$)
$= M_S \times A_T/A_S \times V/50$

M_S: Amount (mg) of Spironolactone RS taken

Dissolution <*6.10*> When the test is performed at 50 revolutions per minute according to the Paddle method, using 900 mL of a solution prepared by dissolving 1 g of polysorbate 80 in water to make 500 mL as the dissolution medium, the dissolution rate in 30 minutes of a 25-mg tablet and a 50-mg tablet are not less than 80% and not less than 70%, respectively.

Start the test with 1 tablet of Spironolactone Tablets, withdraw not less than 20 mL of the medium at the specified minute after starting the test, and filter through a membrane filter with a pore size not exceeding 0.45 μm. Discard not less than 10 mL of the first filtrate, pipet V mL of the subsequent filtrate, add the dissolution medium to make exactly V' mL so that each mL contains about 14 μg of spironolactone ($C_{24}H_{32}O_4S$), and use this solution as the sample solution. Separately, weigh accurately about 28 mg of Spironolactone RS, previously dried at 105°C for 2 hours, dissolve in 20 mL of ethanol (95), and add the dissolution medium to make exactly 100 mL. Pipet 5 mL of this solution, add the dissolution medium to make exactly 100 mL, and use this solution as the standard solution. Determine the absorbances, A_T and A_S, at 243 nm of the sample solution and standard solution as directed under Ultraviolet-visible Spectrophotometry <*2.24*>, using the dissolution medium as the blank.

Dissolution rate (%) with respect to the labeled amount of spironolactone ($C_{24}H_{32}O_4S$)
$= M_S \times A_T/A_S \times V'/V \times 1/C \times 45$

M_S: Amount (mg) of Spironolactone RS taken
C: Labeled amount (mg) of spironolactone ($C_{24}H_{32}O_4S$) in 1 tablet

Assay Weigh accurately the mass of not less than 10 Spironolactone Tablets, and powder. Weigh accurately a portion of the powder, equivalent to about 50 mg of spironolactone ($C_{24}H_{32}O_4S$), add a mixture of water and acetonitrile (1:1) to make exactly 100 mL. After stirring this solution for 30 minutes, centrifuge, and use the supernatant liquid as the sample solution. Separately, weigh accurately about 25 mg of Spironolactone RS, previously dried at 105°C for 2 hours, dissolve in a mixture of water and acetonitrile (1:1) to make exactly 50 mL, and use this solution as the standard solution. Perform the test with exactly 10 μL each of the sample solution and standard solution as directed under Liquid Chromatography <*2.01*> according to the following conditions, and determine the peak areas, A_T and A_S, of spironolactone in each solution.

Amount (mg) of spironolactone ($C_{24}H_{32}O_4S$)
$= M_S \times A_T/A_S \times 2$

M_S: Amount (mg) of Spironolactone RS taken

Operating conditions—

Detector: An ultraviolet absorption photometer (wavelength: 230 nm).

Column: A stainless steel column 4.6 mm in inside diameter and 15 cm in length, packed with octadecylsilanized silica gel for liquid chromatography (5 μm in particle diameter).

Column temperature: A constant temperature of about 25°C.

Mobile phase: A mixture of methanol and water (3:2).

Flow rate: Adjust so that the retention time of spironolactone is about 11 minutes.

System suitability—

System performance: When the procedure is run with 10 μL of the standard solution under the above operating conditions, the number of theoretical plates and the symmetry factor of the peak of spironolactone are not less than 4000 and not more than 1.5, respectively.

System repeatability: When the test is repeated 6 times with 10 μL of the standard solution under the above operating conditions, the relative standard deviation of the peak area of spironolactone is not more than 1.0%.

Containers and storage Containers—Tight containers.

Corn Starch

トウモロコシデンプン

This monograph is harmonized with the European Pharmacopoeia and the U.S. Pharmacopeia.

The parts of the text that are not harmonized are marked with symbols (◆ ◆).

Information on the harmonization with the European Pharmacopoeia and the U.S. Pharmacopeia is available on the website of the Pharmaceuticals and Medical Devices Agency.

Corn Starch consists of starch granules derived from the ripen seeds of *Zea mays* Linné (*Gramineae*).

◆**Description** Corn Starch occurs as white to pale yellow-white, masses or powder.

It is practically insoluble in water and in ethanol (99.5).◆

Identification **(1)** Examined under a microscope <*5.01*>, using mixture of water and glycerin (1:1), Corn Starch appears as either angular polyhedral granules of irregular sizes with diameters of 2 – 23 μm or as rounded or spheroidal granules of irregular sizes with diameters of 25 – 35 μm. The central hilum consists of a distinct cavity or two- to five-rayed cleft, and there are no concentric striations. Between orthogonally oriented polarizing plates or prisms, the starch granules show a distinct black cross intersecting at the hilum.

(2) To 1 g of Corn Starch add 50 mL of water, boil for 1 minute, and allow to cool: a thin, cloudy mucilage is formed.

(3) To 1 mL of the mucilage obtained in (2) add 0.05 mL of diluted iodine TS (1 in 10): an orange-red to deep blue color is formed and the color disappears by heating.

pH <*2.54*> Put 5.0 g of Corn Starch in a non-metal vessel, add 25.0 mL of freshly boiled and cooled water, mix gently for 1 minute, and allow to stand for 15 minutes: the pH of the solution is between 4.0 and 7.0.

Purity **(1)** Iron—To 1.5 g of Corn Starch add 15 mL of 2 mol/L hydrochloric acid TS, mix, filter, and use the filtrate as the test solution. To 2.0 mL of Standard Iron Solution add water to make 20 mL, and use this solution as the control solution. Put 10 mL each of the test solution and the control solution in test tubes, add 2 mL of a solution of citric acid (1 in 5) and 0.1 mL of mercapto acetic acid, and mix. Alkalize with ammonia solution (28) to litmus paper, add water to make 20 mL, and mix. Transfer 10 mL each of these solutions into test tubes, allow to stand for 5 minutes, and compare the color of these solutions against a white background: the color of the test solution is not more intense than that of the control solution (not more than 10 ppm).

(2) Oxidizing substances—To 4.0 g of Corn Starch add 50.0 mL of water, shake for 5 minutes, and centrifuge. To 30.0 mL of the supernatant liquid add 1 mL of acetic acid (100) and 0.5 to 1.0 g of potassium iodide, shake, and allow to stand for 25 to 30 minutes at a dark place. Add 1 mL of starch TS, and titrate *<2.50>* with 0.002 mol/L sodium thiosulfate VS until the color of the solution disappears. Perform a blank determination in the same manner, and make any necessary correction: the volume of 0.002 mol/L sodium thiosulfate VS consumed is not more than 1.4 mL (not more than 20 ppm, calculated as hydrogen peroxide).

(3) Sulfur dioxide—

(i) Apparatus Use as shown in the following figure.

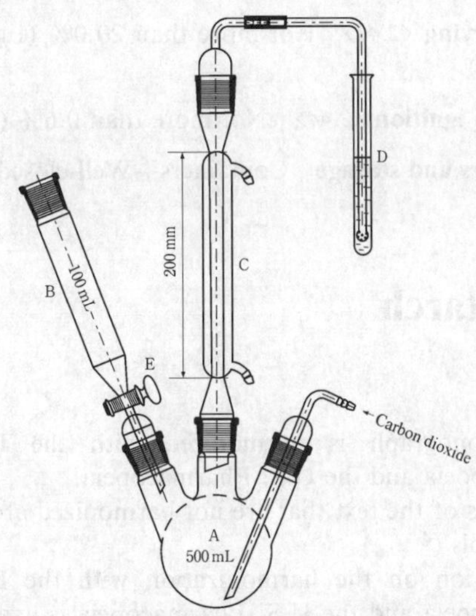

A: Three-necked round-bottom flask (500 mL)
B: Cylindrical dropping funnel (100 mL)
C: Condenser
D: Test tube
E: Tap

(ii) Procedure Introduce 150 mL of water into the three-necked round-bottom flask, close the tap of the cylindrical dropping funnel, and pass carbon dioxide through the whole system at a rate of 100 ± 5 mL per minute. Pass cooling water through the condenser, and place 10 mL of hydrogen peroxide-sodium hydroxide TS in the test tube. After 15 minutes, remove the funnel without interrupting the stream of carbon dioxide, and introduce through the opening into the flask about 25 g of Corn Starch, accurately weighed, with the aid of 100 mL of water. Apply tap grease to the outside of the connection part of the funnel, and load the funnel. Close the tap of the funnel, pour 80 mL of 2 mol/L hydrochloric acid TS into the funnel, open the tap to introduce the hydrochloric acid into the flask, and close the tap while several mL of the hydrochloric acid remains, in order to avoid losing sulfur dioxide. Place the flask in a water bath, and heat the mixture for 1 hour. Transfer the contents of the test tube with the aid of a little water to a wide-necked conical flask. Heat in a water bath for 15 minutes, and cool. Add 0.1 mL of bromophenol blue TS, and titrate *<2.50>* with 0.1 mol/L sodium hydroxide VS until the color changes from yellow to violet-blue lasting for at least 20 seconds. Perform a blank determination in the same manner, and make any necessary correction. Calculate the amount of sulfur dioxide by applying the following formula: it is not more than 50 ppm.

$$\text{Amount (ppm) of sulfur dioxide} = V/M \times 1000 \times 3.203$$

M: Amount (g) of Corn Starch taken
V: Amount (mL) of 0.1 mol/L sodium hydroxide VS consumed

◆**(4)** Foreign matter—Under a microscope *<5.01>*, Corn Starch does not contain starch granules of any other origin. It may contain a minute quantity, if any, of fragments of the tissue of the original plant.◆

Loss on drying *<2.41>* Not more than 15.0% (1 g, 130°C, 90 minutes).

Residue on ignition *<2.44>* Not more than 0.6% (1 g).

◆**Containers and storage** Containers—Well-closed containers.◆

Potato Starch

バレイショデンプン

This monograph is harmonized with the European Pharmacopoeia and the U.S. Pharmacopeia.

The parts of the text that are not harmonized are marked with symbols (◆ ◆).

Information on the harmonization with the European Pharmacopoeia and the U.S. Pharmacopeia is available on the website of the Pharmaceuticals and Medical Devices Agency.

Potato Starch consists of starch granules derived from the tuber of *Solanum tuberosum* Linné (*Solanaceae*).

◆**Description** Potato Starch occurs as a white powder.

It is practically insoluble in water and in ethanol (99.5).◆

Identification **(1)** Examined under a microscope *<5.01>* using a mixture of water and glycerin (1:1), Potato Starch presents granules, either irregularly shaped, ovoid or pear-shaped, usually 30 - 100 μm in size but occasionally exceeding 100 μm, or rounded, 10 - 35 μm in size. There are occasional compound granules having two to four components. The ovoid and pear-shaped granules have an eccentric hilum and the rounded granules acentric or slightly eccentric hilum. All granules show clearly visible concentric striations. Between orthogonally oriented polarizing plates or prisms, the granules show a distinct black cross intersecting at the hilum.

(2) To 1 g of Potato Starch add 50 mL of water, boil for 1 minute, and allow to cool: a thick, opalescent mucilage is formed.

(3) To 1 mL of the mucilage obtained in (2) add 0.05 mL of diluted iodine TS (1 in 10): an orange-red to deep blue color is formed, and the color disappears by heating.

pH *<2.54>* Put 5.0 g of Potato Starch in a non-metal vessel, add 25.0 mL of freshly boiled and cooled water, mix gently for 1 minute, and allow to stand for 15 minutes: the pH of the solution is between 5.0 and 8.0.

Purity **(1)** Iron—To 1.5 g of Potato Starch add 15 mL of 2 mol/L hydrochloric acid TS, mix, filter, and use the filtrate as the test solution. To 2.0 mL of Standard Iron Solution add water to make 20 mL, and use this solution as the control solution. Put 10 mL each of the test solution and the control solution in test tubes, add 2 mL of a solution of citric acid (1 in 5) and 0.1 mL of mercapto acetic acid, and mix. Alkalize with ammonia solution (28) to litmus paper, add water to make 20 mL, and mix. Transfer 10 mL each of these solutions into test tubes, allow to stand for 5 minutes, and compare the color of these solutions against a white background: the color of the test solution is not more intense than that of the control solution (not more than 10 ppm).

(2) Oxidizing substances—To 4.0 g of Potato Starch add 50.0 mL of water, shake for 5 minutes, and centrifuge. To 30.0 mL of the supernatant liquid add 1 mL of acetic acid (100) and 0.5 to 1.0 g of potassium iodide, shake, and allow to stand for 25 to 30 minutes at a dark place. Add 1 mL of starch TS, and titrate *<2.50>* with 0.002 mol/L sodium thiosulfate VS until the color of the solution disappears. Perform a blank determination in the same manner, and make any necessary correction: the volume of 0.002 mol/L sodium thiosulfate VS consumed is not more than 1.4 mL (not more than 20 ppm, calculated as hydrogen peroxide).

(3) Sulfur dioxide—

(i) Apparatus Use as shown in the figure.

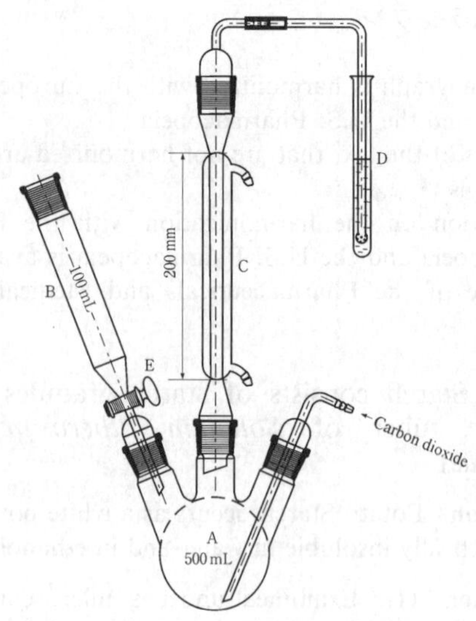

A: Three-necked round-bottom flask (500 mL)
B: Cylindrical dropping funnel (100 mL)
C: Condenser
D: Test tube
E: Tap

(ii) Procedure Introduce 150 mL of water into the three-necked round-bottom flask, close the tap of the cylindrical dropping funnel, and pass carbon dioxide through the whole system at a rate of 100 ± 5 mL per minute. Pass cooling water through the condenser, and place 10 mL of hydrogen peroxide-sodium hydroxide TS in the test tube. After 15 minutes, remove the funnel without interrupting the stream of carbon dioxide, and introduce through the opening into the flask about 25 g of Potato Starch, accurately weighed, with the aid of 100 mL of water. Apply tap grease to the outside of the connection part of the funnel, and load the funnel. Close the tap of the funnel, pour 80 mL of 2 mol/L hydrochloric acid TS into the funnel, open the tap to introduce the hydrochloric acid into the flask, and close the tap while several mL of the hydrochloric acid remains, in order to avoid losing sulfur dioxide. Place the flask in a water bath, and heat the mixture for 1 hour. Transfer the contents of the test tube with the aid of a little water to a wide-necked conical flask. Heat in a water bath for 15 minutes, and cool. Add 0.1 mL of bromophenol blue TS, and titrate *<2.50>* with 0.1 mol/L sodium hydroxide VS until the color changes from yellow to violet-blue lasting for at least 20 seconds. Perform a blank determination in the same manner, and make any necessary correction. Calculate the amount of sulfur dioxide by applying the following formula: it is not more than 50 ppm.

Amount (ppm) of sulfur dioxide
$= V/M \times 1000 \times 3.203$

M: Amount (g) of Potato Starch taken
V: Amount (mL) of 0.1 mol/L sodium hydroxide VS consumed

◆**(4)** Foreign matter—Under a microscope *<5.01>*, Potato Starch does not contain starch granules of any other origin. It may contain a minute quantity, if any, of fragments of the tissue of the original plant.◆

Loss on drying *<2.41>* Not more than 20.0% (1 g, 130°C, 90 minutes).

Residue on ignition *<2.44>* Not more than 0.6% (1 g).

◆**Containers and storage** Containers—Well-closed containers.◆

Rice Starch

コメデンプン

This monograph is harmonized with the European Pharmacopoeia and the U.S. Pharmacopeia.

The parts of the text that are not harmonized are marked with symbols (◆ ◆).

Information on the harmonization with the European Pharmacopoeia and the U.S. Pharmacopeia is available on the website of the Pharmaceuticals and Medical Devices Agency.

Rice Starch consists of the starch granules obtained from the caryopsis of *Oryza sativa* Linné (*Gramineae*).

◆**Description** Rice Starch occurs as a white mass or powder.

It is practically insoluble in water and in ethanol (99.5).◆

Identification **(1)** Examined under a microscope *<5.01>* using a mixture of water and glycerin (1:1), Rice Starch presents polyhedral, simple grains 1 - 10 μm, mostly 4 - 6 μm, in size. These simple grains often gather in ellipsoidal, compound grains 50 - 100 μm in diameter. The granules have a poorly visible central hilum and there are no concentric striations. Between orthogonally orientated polarizing plates or prisms, the starch granules show a distinct black cross intersecting at the hilum.

(2) To 1 g of Rice Starch add 50 mL of water, boil for 1 minute, and allow to cool: a thin, cloudy mucilage is formed.

(3) To 1 mL of the mucilage obtained in (2) add 0.05 mL of diluted iodine TS (1 in 10): an orange-red to dark-blue color is produced which disappears on heating.

pH *<2.54>* To 5.0 g of Rice Starch add 25 mL of freshly boiled and cooled water, and mix gently for 1 minute to achieve suspension. Allow to stand for 15 minutes: the pH of the solution is between 5.0 and 8.0.

Purity **(1)** Iron—To 1.5 g of Rice Starch add 15 mL of 2 mol/L hydrochloric acid TS, mix, filter, and use the filtrate as the test solution. To 2.0 mL of Standard Iron Solution add water to make 20 mL, and use this solution as the control solution. Put 10 mL each of the test solution and the control solution in test tubes, add 2 mL of a solution of citric acid (1 in 5) and 0.1 mL of mercapto acetic acid, and mix. Add ammonia solution (28) to these solutions until the color of a litmus paper to change from red to blue, add water to make 20 mL, and mix. Transfer 10 mL each of these solutions into test tubes, allow to stand for 5 minutes, and compare the color of these solutions against a white background: the color of the test solution is not more intense than that of the control solution (not more than 10 ppm).

(2) Oxidizing substances—To 4.0 g of Rice Starch add 50 mL of water, shake for 5 minutes, and centrifuge. To 30 mL of the supernatant liquid add 1 mL of acetic acid (100) and 0.5 to 1.0 g of potassium iodide, shake, and allow to stand for 25 to 30 minutes in the dark. Add 1 mL of starch TS, and titrate *⟨2.50⟩* with 0.002 mol/L sodium thiosulfate VS until the starch-iodine color disappears. Perform a blank determination in the same manner, and make any necessary correction. Not more than 1.4 mL of 0.002 mol/L sodium thiosulfate VS is required (not more than 20 ppm, calculated as hydrogen peroxide).

(3) Sulfur dioxide—

(i) Apparatus Use as shown in the figure.

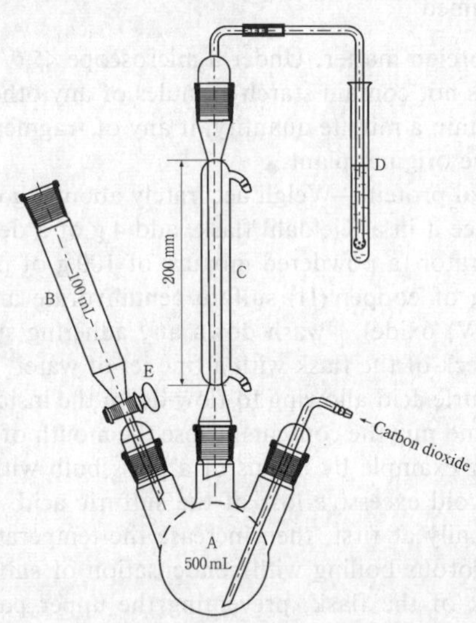

A: Three-necked round-bottom flask (500 mL)
B: Cylindrical dropping funnel (100 mL)
C: Condenser
D: Test tube
E: Tap

(ii) Procedure Introduce 150 mL of water into the three-necked round-bottom flask, close the tap of the cylindrical dropping funnel, and pass carbon dioxide through the whole system at a rate of 100 ± 5 mL per minute. Pass cooling water through the condenser, and place 10 mL of hydrogen peroxide-sodium hydroxide TS in the test tube. After 15 minutes, remove the funnel without interrupting the stream of carbon dioxide, and introduce through the opening into the flask about 25 g of Rice Starch, accurately weighed, with the aid of 100 mL of water. Apply tap grease to the outside of the connection part of the funnel, and load the funnel. Close the tap of the funnel, pour 80 mL of 2 mol/L hydrochloric acid TS into the funnel, open the tap to introduce the hydrochloric acid into the flask, and close the tap while several mL of the hydrochloric acid remains, in order to avoid losing sulfur dioxide. Place the flask in a water bath, and heat the mixture for 1 hour. Transfer the contents of the test tube with the aid of a little water to a wide-necked conical flask. Heat on a water bath for 15 minutes and allow to cool. Add 0.1 mL of bromophenol blue TS, and titrate *⟨2.50⟩* with 0.1 mol/L sodium hydroxide VS until the color changes from yellow to violet-blue lasting for at least 20 seconds. Perform a blank determination in the same manner, and make any necessary correction. Calculate the amount of sulfur dioxide by applying the following formula: it is not more than 50 ppm.

$$\text{Amount (ppm) of sulfur dioxide} = V/M \times 1000 \times 3.203$$

M: Amount (g) of Rice Starch taken
V: Amount (mL) of 0.1 mol/L sodium hydroxide VS consumed

◆**(4)** Foreign matter—Under a microscope *⟨5.01⟩*, Rice Starch does not contain starch granules of any other origin. It may contain a minute quantity, if any, of fragments of the tissue of the original plant.◆

Loss on drying *⟨2.41⟩* Not more than 15.0% (1 g, 130°C, 90 minutes).

Residue on ignition *⟨2.44⟩* Not more than 0.6% (1 g).

◆**Containers and storage** Containers—Well-closed containers.◆

Wheat Starch

コムギデンプン

This monograph is harmonized with the European Pharmacopoeia and the U.S. Pharmacopeia.

The corresponding part of the attributes/provisions which are agreed as non-harmonized within the scope of the harmonization is marked with symbols (◆ ◆), and the corresponding parts which are agreed as the JP local requirement other than the scope of the harmonization are marked with symbols (◇ ◇).

Information on the harmonization with the European Pharmacopoeia and the U.S. Pharmacopeia is available on the website of the Pharmaceuticals and Medical Devices Agency.

Wheat Starch consists of the starch granules obtained from caryopsis of wheat, *Triticum aestivum* Linné (*Gramineae*).

◆**Description** Wheat Starch occurs as white masses or powder.

It is practically insoluble in water and in ethanol (99.5).◆

Identification **(1)** Examine under a microscope *⟨5.01⟩* using a mixture of water and glycerin (1:1), Wheat Starch presents large and small granules, and, very rarely, intermediate sizes. The large granules, usually 10 – 60 μm in diameter, are discoid or, more rarely, reniform when seen face-on. The central hilum and striations are invisible or barely visible and the granules sometimes show cracks on the edges. Seen in profile, the granules are elliptical and fusiform and the hilum appears as a slit along the main axis. The small granules, rounded or polyhedral, are 2 – 10 μm in diameter. Between orthogonally oriented polarizing plates or prisms, the granules show a distinct black cross intersecting at the hilum.

(2) To 1 g of Wheat Starch add 50 mL of water, boil for 1 minute, and allow to cool: a thin, cloudy mucilage is formed.

(3) To 1 mL of the mucilage obtained in (2) add 0.05 mL of diluted iodine TS (1 in 10): a deep blue color is formed, and the color disappears by heating.

pH <*2.54*> Put 5.0 g of Wheat Starch in a non-metal vessel, add 25.0 mL of freshly boiled and cooled water, mix gently for 1 minute, and allow to stand for 15 minutes: the pH of the solution is between 4.5 and 7.0.

Purity **(1)** Iron—To 1.5 g of Wheat Starch add 15 mL of 2 mol/L hydrochloric acid TS, mix, filter, and use the filtrate as the test solution. To 2.0 mL of Standard Iron Solution add water to make 20 mL, and use this solution as the control solution. Put 10 mL each of the test solution and the control solution in test tubes, add 2 mL of a solution of citric acid (2 in 10) and 0.1 mL of mercapto acetic acid, and mix. Alkalize with ammonia solution (28) to litmus paper, add water to make 20 mL, and mix. Transfer 10 mL each of these solutions into test tubes, allow to stand for 5 minutes, and compare the color of these solutions against a white background: the color of the test solution is not more intense than that of the control solution (not more than 10 ppm).

(2) Oxidizing substances—To 4.0 g of Wheat Starch add 50 mL of water, shake for 5 minutes, and centrifuge. To 30 mL of the supernatant liquid add 1 mL of acetic acid (100) and 0.5 to 1.0 g of potassium iodide, shake, and allow to stand for 25 to 30 minutes at a dark place. Add 1 mL of starch TS, and titrate <*2.50*> with 0.002 mol/L sodium thiosulfate VS until the color of the solution disappears. Perform a blank determination in the same manner, and make any necessary correction: the volume of 0.002 mol/L sodium thiosulfate VS consumed is not more than 1.4 mL (not more than 20 ppm, calculated as hydrogen peroxide).

(3) Sulfur dioxide—

(i) Apparatus Use as shown in the figure.

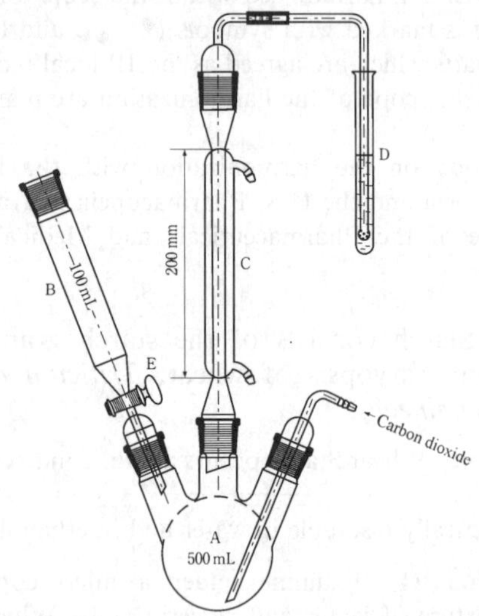

A: Three-necked round-bottom flask (500 mL)
B: Cylindrical dropping funnel (100 mL)
C: Condenser
D: Test tube
E: Tap

(ii) Procedure Introduce 150 mL of water into the three-necked round-bottom flask, close the tap of the cylindrical dropping funnel, and pass carbon dioxide through the whole system at a rate of 100 ± 5 mL per minute. Pass cooling water through the condenser, and place 10 mL of hydrogen peroxide-sodium hydroxide TS in the test tube. After 15 minutes, remove the funnel without interrupting the stream of carbon dioxide, and introduce through the opening into the flask about 25 g of Wheat Starch, accurately weighed, with the aid of 100 mL of water. Apply tap grease to the outside of the connection part of the funnel, and load the funnel. Close the tap of the funnel, pour 80 mL of 2 mol/L hydrochloric acid TS into the funnel, open the tap to introduce the hydrochloric acid into the flask, and close the tap while several mL of the hydrochloric acid remains, in order to avoid losing sulfur dioxide. Place the flask in a water bath, and heat the mixture for 1 hour. Transfer the contents of the test tube with the aid of a little water to a wide-necked conical flask. Heat in a water bath for 15 minutes, and cool. Add 0.1 mL of bromophenol blue TS, and titrate <*2.50*> with 0.1 mol/L sodium hydroxide VS until the color changes from yellow to violet-blue lasting for at least 20 seconds. Perform a blank determination in the same manner, and make any necessary correction. Calculate the amount of sulfur dioxide by applying the following formula: it is not more than 50 ppm.

$$\text{Amount (ppm) of sulfur dioxide} = V/M \times 1000 \times 3.203$$

M: Amount (g) of Wheat Starch taken
V: Amount (mL) of 0.1 mol/L sodium hydroxide VS consumed

◆**(4)** Foreign matter. Under a microscope <*5.01*>, Wheat Starch does not contain starch granules of any other origin. It may contain a minute quantity, if any of fragments of the tissue of the original plant.◆

(5) Total protein—Weigh accurately about 3 g of Wheat Starch, place it in a Kjeldahl flask, add 4 g of a decomposition accelerator (a powdered mixture of 100 g of potassium sulfate, 3 g of copper (II) sulfate pentahydrate and 3 g of titanium (IV) oxide), ◇wash down any adhering substances from the neck of the flask with a fine jet of water.◇ Add 25 mL of sulfuric acid allowing to flow down the inside wall of the flask, and mix the contents. Close the mouth of the flask loosely, for example by means of a glass bulb with a short stem, to avoid excessive loss of the sulfuric acid. Heat the flask gradually at first, then increase the temperature until there is vigorous boiling with condensation of sulfuric acid in the neck of the flask, preventing the upper part of the flask from becoming overheated. Continue the heating until the solution become clear, ◇and the inside wall of the flask is free from a carbonaceous material.◇ After cooling, dissolve the solid material by adding cautiously 25 mL of water, cool again, and place in a steam-distillation apparatus previously washed by passing steam. Add exactly 25 mL of 0.01 mol/L hydrochloric acid VS and a suitable amount of water into the receiver, and immerse the tip of the condenser in this acid solution. Add the same quantity of a solution of sodium hydroxide (21 in 50) as used for a blank determination through the funnel, and distill immediately by passing steam through the mixture. Collect about 40 mL of distillate, lower the receiver so that the tip of the condenser is above the surface of the acid solution, ◇then continue the distillation for a while, and rinse the end part of the condenser with a small amount of water.◇ Titrate <*2.50*> the excessive hydrochloric acid with 0.025 mol/L sodium hydroxide VS until the color of the solution changes from red-purple through grayish blue to green (indicator: 3 drops of methyl red-methylene blue TS). Perform a blank determination in the same manner. The amount of a solution of sodium hydroxide (21 in 50) to be added from the funnel is sufficient to change the color of the solution in the flask from bluish green to dark brown or black.

Amount (%) of nitrogen = $(a - b) \times 0.035/M$

M: Amount (g) of Wheat Starch taken
a: Volume (mL) of 0.025 mol/L sodium hydroxide VS consumed in a blank determination
b: Volume (mL) of 0.025 mol/L sodium hydroxide VS consumed in the sample determination

The amount of total protein is not more than 0.3% [0.048% as nitrogen (N:14.01) (using conversion factor of nitrogen to protein, 6.25)].

Loss on drying <*2.41*> Not more than 15.0% (1 g, 130°C, 90 minutes).

Residue on ignition <*2.44*> Not more than 0.6% (1 g).

◆**Containers and storage** Containers—Well-closed containers.◆

Stearic Acid

ステアリン酸

This monograph is harmonized with the European Pharmacopoeia and the U.S. Pharmacopeia.

The parts of the text that are not harmonized are marked with symbols (◆ ◆).

Information on the harmonization with the European Pharmacopoeia and the U.S. Pharmacopeia is available on the website of the Pharmaceuticals and Medical Devices Agency.

Stearic Acid is a mixture consisting mainly of stearic acid ($C_{18}H_{36}O_2$: 284.48) and palmitic acid ($C_{16}H_{32}O_2$: 256.42) obtained from fats or oils of vegetable or animal origin.

It occurs as three types, stearic acid 50, stearic acid 70 and stearic acid 95, composed with different fatty acid composition. Each type contains respectively the amount of stearic acid and the sum of stearic acid and palmitic acid as shown in the following table.

Type	Fatty acid composition	
	Stearic acid (%)	Sum of stearic acid and palmitic acid (%)
Stearic acid 50	40.0 – 60.0	not less than 90.0
Stearic acid 70	60.0 – 80.0	not less than 90.0
Stearic acid 95	not less than 90.0	not less than 96.0

The label states the type of Stearic Acid.

◆**Description** Stearic acid occurs as white, unctuous masses, crystalline masses or powder. It has a faint, fatty odor.

It is soluble in ethanol (99.5), and practically insoluble in water.◆

Congealing point The apparatus consists of a test tube about 25 mm in diameter and 150 mm long placed inside a test tube about 40 mm in diameter and 160 mm long. The inner tube is closed by a stopper which carries a thermometer about 175 mm long and graduated in 0.2°C fixed so that ◆the upper end of◆ the bulb is about 15 mm above the bottom of the tube. The stopper has a hole allowing the passage of the stem of a stirrer made from a glass rod or other suitable material formed at one end into a loop of about 18 mm overall diameter at right angles to the rod. The inner tube with its jacket is supported centrally in a 1-L beaker containing a suitable cooling liquid to within 20 mm of the top. A thermometer is supported in the cooling bath.

Place in the inner tube sufficient quantity of the liquid or previously melted substance to be examined, to cover the thermometer bulb and determine the approximate congealing point by cooling rapidly. Place the inner tube in a bath about 5°C above the approximate congealing point until all but the last traces of crystals are melted. Fill the beaker with water or a saturated solution of sodium chloride, at a temperature about 5°C lower than the expected congealing point, insert the inner tube into the outer tube, ensuring that some seed crystals are present, and stir thoroughly until solidification takes place. Note the highest temperature observed during solidification.

◆The apparatus directed under Congealing Point Determination <*2.42*> is also can be used. Transfer the melted sample into sample container B up to the marked line C. Adjust the immersion line H of thermometer F to the same level of the meniscus of the sample, and then determine the approximate congealing point by cooling rapidly. Place the sample container B in a bath at a temperature about 5°C above the approximate congealing point until all but the last traces of crystals are melted. Fill bath D with water or a saturated solution of sodium chloride, at a temperature about 5°C lower than the expected congealing point, and set the sample container B in A. Ensuring that some seed crystals are present, stir thoroughly until solidification takes place. Note the highest temperature observed during solidification.◆

The congealing point of stearic acid 50 is 53 – 59°C, of stearic acid 70 is 57 – 64°C, and of stearic acid 95 is 64 – 69°C.

Acid value <*1.13*> 194 – 212

Iodine value Introduce about 1 g of Stearic Acid, weighed accurately, into a 250-mL flask fitted with a ground-glass stopper and previously dried or rinsed with acetic acid (100), and dissolve it in 15 mL of chloroform unless otherwise prescribed. Add very slowly exactly 25 mL of iodine bromide (II) TS. Close the flask and keep it in the dark for 30 minutes unless otherwise prescribed, shaking frequently. Add 10 mL of a solution of potassium iodine (1 in 10) and 100 mL of water. Titrate <*2.50*> with 0.1 mol/L sodium thiosulfate VS, shaking vigorously until the yellow color is almost discharged. Add 5 mL of starch TS and continue the titration adding the 0.1 mol/L sodium thiosulfate VS dropwise until the color is discharged. Perform a blank determination in the same manner. When the iodine value is calculated by the following equation, that of stearic acid 50 and 70 is not more than 4.0, and of stearic acid 95 is not more than 1.5.

Iodine value = $(a - b) \times 1.269/M$

M: Amount (g) of Stearic Acid taken
a: Volume (mL) of 0.1 mol/L sodium thiosulfate VS consumed in the blank determination
b: Volume (mL) of 0.1 mol/L sodium thiosulfate VS consumed in the test

Purity **(1)** Acidity—Melt 5.0 g, shake for 2 minutes with 10 mL of hot carbon dioxide-free water, cool slowly and filter. To the filtrate add 0.05 mL of methyl orange TS: no red color develops.

◆**(2)** Heavy metals <*1.07*>—Proceed with 1.0 g of Stearic Acid according to Method 2, and perform the test. Prepare the control solution with 2.0 mL of Standard Lead Solution (not more than 20 ppm).◆

◆**Residue on ignition** <2.44> Not more than 0.1% (1 g).◆

Assay Place 0.100 g of Stearic Acid in a ◆small◆ conical flask fitted with a reflux condenser. Add 5.0 mL of boron trifluoride-methanol TS, ◆shake, and◆ boil under reflux for about 10 minutes ◆to dissolve.◆ Add 4 mL of heptane through the condenser, and boil again under reflux for 10 minutes. Allow to cool, add 20 mL of a saturated solution of sodium chloride, shake and allow the layers to separate. Remove 2 mL of the separated heptane layer, and dry it over about 0.2 g of anhydrous sodium sulphate, ◆previously washed with heptane.◆ Take 1.0 mL of the dried heptane layer in a 10-mL volumetric flask, add heptane to make up to 10 mL, and use this solution as the sample solution. Perform the test with 1 µL of the sample solution as directed under Gas Chromatography <2.02> according to the following conditions, and determine the peak area of methyl stearate, A, and the area of all of fatty acid ester peaks, B, and calculate the content (%) of stearic acid in the fatty acid fraction by the following equation.

$$\text{Content (\%) of stearic acid} = A/B \times 100$$

In the same way, calculate the content (%) of palmitic acid, and calculate the sum (%) of stearic acid and palmitic acid.

Operating conditions—

Detector: A hydrogen flame-ionization detector.

Column: A fused silica column 0.32 mm in inside diameter and 30 m in length, coated the inside surface with a layer about 0.5 µm thick of polyethylene glycol 20 M for gas chromatography.

Column temperature: Maintain at 70°C for 2 minutes after injection, raise the temperature at a rate of 5°C per minute to 240°C, and maintain at 240°C for 5 minutes.

Injection port temperature: A constant temperature of about 220°C.

Detector temperature: A constant temperature of about 260°C.

Carrier gas: Helium.

Flow rate: 2.4 mL per minute.

◆Splitless.◆

◆Time span of measurement: For 41 minutes after sample injection, beginning after the solvent peak.◆

System suitability—

◆Test for required detectability: Put 50 mg each of stearic acid for gas chromatography and palmitic acid for gas chromatography in a small conical flask fitted with a reflux condenser. Add 5.0 mL of boron trifluoride-methanol TS, mix, then proceed as the same manner for the sample solution, and use the solution so obtained as the solution for system suitability test. Pipet 1 mL of the solution for system suitability test, add heptane to make exactly 10 mL. Pipet 1 mL of this solution, add heptane to make exactly 10 mL. Again, pipet 1 mL of this solution, and add heptane to make exactly 10 mL. Confirm that the peak area of methyl stearate obtained with 1 µL of this solution is equivalent to 0.05 to 0.15% of that with 1 µL of the solution for system suitability test.◆

System performance: When the procedure is run with 1 µL of the solution for system suitability test under the above operating conditions, the relative retention time of methyl palmitate to methyl stearate is about 0.9, and the resolution between these peaks is not less than 5.0.

System repeatability: When the test is repeated 6 times with 1 µL of the solution for system suitability test under the above operating conditions, the relative standard deviation of the peak areas of methyl palmitate and methyl stearate is not more than 3.0%. Furthermore, the relative standard deviation of the ratio of the peak area of methyl palmitate to the peak area of methyl stearate obtained from the 6-time repetition is not more than 1.0%.

◆**Containers and storage** Containers—Well-closed containers.◆

Stearyl Alcohol

ステアリルアルコール

Stearyl Alcohol is a mixture of solid alcohols, and consists chiefly of stearyl alcohol ($C_{18}H_{38}O$: 270.49).

Description Stearyl Alcohol occurs as a white unctuous matter. It has a faint, characteristic odor. It is tasteless.

It is freely soluble in ethanol (95), in ethanol (99.5) and in diethyl ether, and practically insoluble in water.

Melting point <1.13> 56 - 62°C Prepare the sample according to Method 2 under Melting Point Determination, then attach tightly a capillary tube to the bottom of the thermometer by means of a rubber band or by any suitable means, and make the bottom of the capillary tube equal in position to the lower end of the thermometer. Insert this thermometer into a test tube about 17 mm in inside diameter and about 170 mm in height, fasten the thermometer with cork stopper so that the lower end of the thermometer is about 25 mm distant from the bottom of the test tube. Suspend the test tube in a beaker containing water, and heat the beaker with constant stirring until the temperature rises to 5°C below the expected melting point. Then regulate the rate of increase to 1°C per minute. The temperature at which the sample is transparent and no turbidity is produced is taken as the melting point.

Acid value <1.13> Not more than 1.0.

Ester value <1.13> Not more than 3.0.

Hydroxyl value <1.13> 200 - 220

Iodine value <1.13> Not more than 2.0.

Purity **(1)** Clarity of solution—Dissolve 3.0 g of Stearyl Alcohol in 25 mL of ethanol (99.5) by warming: the solution is clear.

(2) Alkalinity—To the solution obtained in (1) add 2 drops of phenolphthalein TS: no red color develops.

Residue on ignition <2.44> Not more than 0.05% (2 g).

Containers and storage Containers—Well-closed containers.

Streptomycin Sulfate

ストレプトマイシン硫酸塩

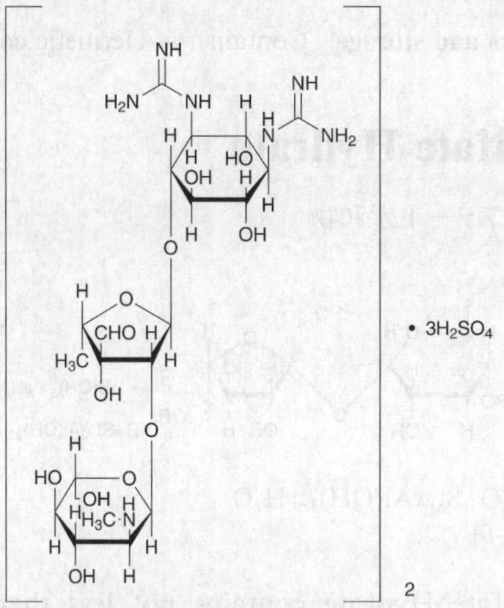

$(C_{21}H_{39}N_7O_{12})_2.3H_2SO_4$: 1457.38
2-Deoxy-2-methylamino-α-L-glucopyranosyl-(1→2)-5-deoxy-3-*C*-formyl-α-L-lyxofuranosyl-(1→4)-*N*,*N′*-diamidino-D-streptamine sesquisulfate
[*3810-74-0*]

Streptomycin Sulfate is the sulfate of an aminoglycoside substance having antibacterial activity produced by the growth of *Streptomyces griseus*.

It contains not less than 740 μg (potency) and not more than 820 μg (potency) per mg, calculated on the dried basis. The potency of Streptomycin Sulfate is expressed as mass (potency) of streptomycin ($C_{21}H_{39}N_7O_{12}$: 581.57).

Description Streptomycin Sulfate occurs as a white to light yellow-white powder.

It is freely soluble in water, and very slightly soluble in ethanol (95).

Identification (1) Dissolve 50 mg of Streptomycin Sulfate in 5 mL of water, add 1 mL of ninhydrin TS and 0.5 mL of pyridine, and heat for 10 minutes: a purple color is developed.

(2) Dissolve 10 mg each of Streptomycin Sulfate and Streptomycin Sulfate RS in 10 mL of water, and use these solutions as the sample solution and standard solution. Perform the test with these solutions as directed under Thin-layer Chromatography ⟨*2.03*⟩. Spot 10 μL each of the sample solution and standard solution on a plate of silica gel for thin-layer chromatography. Develop the plate with a solution of potassium dihydrogen phosphate (7 in 100) to a distance of about 12 cm, and air-dry the plate. Spray evenly a mixture of a solution of 1,3-dihydroxynaphthalene in ethanol (95) (1 in 500) and diluted sulfuric acid (1 in 5) (1:1) on the plate, and heat the plate at about 150°C for about 5 minutes: the principal spots obtained from the sample solution and the standard solution show the same in color tone and *R*f value.

(3) A solution of Streptomycin Sulfate (1 in 5) responds to Qualitative Tests ⟨*1.09*⟩ for sulfate.

Optical rotation ⟨*2.49*⟩ $[\alpha]_D^{20}$: −79 – −88° (0.5 g calculated on the dried basis, water, 50 mL, 100 mm).

pH ⟨*2.54*⟩ The pH of a solution obtained by dissolving 2.0 g of Streptomycin Sulfate in 10 mL of water is between 4.5 and 7.0.

Purity (1) Clarity and color of solution—Dissolve 1.0 g of Streptomycin Sulfate in 5 mL of water: the solution is clear, and its absorbance at 400 nm determined as directed under Ultraviolet-visible Spectrophotometry ⟨*2.24*⟩ is not more than 0.17.

(2) Heavy metals ⟨*1.07*⟩—Proceed with 2.0 g of Streptomycin Sulfate according to Method 4, and perform the test. Prepare the control solution with 2.0 mL of Standard Lead Solution (not more than 10 ppm).

(3) Arsenic ⟨*1.11*⟩—Prepare the test solution with 2.0 g of Streptomycin Sulfate according to Method 3 and perform the test (not more than 1 ppm).

(4) Related substances—Dissolve exactly 0.20 g of Streptomycin Sulfate in a mixture of methanol and sulfuric acid (97:3) to make 5 mL, and heat under a reflux condenser for 1 hour. After cooling, wash the inside of the condenser with a suitable amount of a mixture of methanol and sulfuric acid (97:3), add a mixture of methanol and sulfuric acid (97:3) to make exactly 20 mL, and use this solution as the sample solution. Separately, dissolve exactly 36 mg of D-mannose in a mixture of methanol and sulfuric acid (97:3) to make 5 mL, and heat under a reflux condenser for 1 hour. After cooling, wash the inside of the condenser with a suitable amount of a mixture of methanol and sulfuric acid (97:3), and add a mixture of methanol and sulfuric acid (97:3) to make exactly 50 mL. Pipet 5 mL of this solution, add a mixture of methanol and sulfuric acid (97:3) to make exactly 50 mL, and use this solution as the standard solution. Perform the test with these solutions as directed under Thin-layer Chromatography ⟨*2.03*⟩. Spot 10 μL each of the sample solution and standard solution on a plate of silica gel for thin-layer chromatography, develop with a mixture of toluene, methanol and acetic acid (100) (2:1:1) to a distance of 13 to 15 cm, and air-dry the plate. Spray evenly a mixture of a solution of 1,3-dihydroxynaphthalene in ethanol (95) (1 in 500) and diluted sulfuric acid (1 in 5) (1:1) on the plate, and heat the plate at 110°C for 5 minutes: the spot obtained from the sample solution corresponding to the spot from the standard solution is not more intense than the spot from the standard solution.

Loss on drying ⟨*2.41*⟩ Not more than 5.0% (0.5 g, reduced pressure not exceeding 0.67 kPa, 60°C, 3 hours).

Residue on ignition ⟨*2.44*⟩ Not more than 1.0% (1 g).

Assay Perform the test according to the Cylinder-plate method as directed under Microbial Assay for Antibiotics ⟨*4.02*⟩ according to the following conditions.

(i) Test organism—*Bacillus subtilis* ATCC 6633

(ii) Culture medium—Use the medium i in 1) under (1) Agar media for seed and base layer, having pH 7.8 – 8.0 after sterilization.

(iii) Standard solutions—Weigh accurately an amount of Streptomycin Sulfate RS, previously dried, equivalent to about 20 mg (potency), dissolve in diluted phosphate buffer solution (pH 6.0) (1 in 2) to make exactly 50 mL, and use this solution as the standard stock solution. Keep the standard stock solution between 5°C and 15°C, and use within 30 days. Take exactly a suitable amount of the standard stock solution before use, add 0.1 mol/L phosphate buffer solution (pH 8.0) to make solutions so that each mL contains 8 μg (potency) and 2 μg (potency), and use these solutions as the high concentration standard solution and the low concentration standard solution, respectively.

(iv) Sample solutions—Weigh accurately an amount of Streptomycin Sulfate, equivalent to about 20 mg (potency), dissolve in water to make exactly 50 mL. Take exactly a suitable amount of this solution, add 0.1 mol/L phosphate buffer solution (pH 8.0) to make solutions so that each mL contains 8 μg (potency) and 2 μg (potency), and use these solutions as the high concentration sample solution and the low concentration sample solution, respectively.

Containers and storage Containers—Tight containers.

Streptomycin Sulfate for Injection

注射用ストレプトマイシン硫酸塩

Streptomycin Sulfate for Injection is a preparation for injection, which is dissolved before use.

It contains not less than 90.0% and not more than 110.0% of the labeled potency of streptomycin ($C_{21}H_{39}N_7O_{12}$: 581.57).

Method of preparation Prepare as directed under Injections, with Streptomycin Sulfate.

Description Streptomycin Sulfate for Injection occurs as a white or light yellow-white, masses or powder.

Identification Perform the test as directed in the Identification (2) under Streptomycin Sulfate.

Osmotic pressure ratio Being specified separately when the drug is granted approval based on the Law.

pH *<2.54>* The pH of a solution prepared by dissolving an amount of Streptomycin Sulfate for Injection, equivalent to 2.0 g (potency) of Streptomycin Sulfate, in 10 mL of water is 4.5 to 7.0.

Purity Clarity and color of solution—Dissolve an amount of Streptomycin Sulfate for Injection, equivalent to 1.0 g (potency) of Streptomycin Sulfate, in 3 mL of water: The solution is clear, and the absorbance of this solution at 400 nm, determined as directed under Ultraviolet-visible Spectrophotometry *<2.24>*, is not more than 0.50.

Loss on drying *<2.41>* Not more than 4.0% (0.5 g, reduced pressure not exceeding 0.67 kPa, 60°C, 3 hours).

Bacterial endotoxins *<4.01>* Less than 0.10 EU/mg (potency).

Uniformity of dosage units *<6.02>* It meets the requirement of the Mass variation test.

Foreign insoluble matter *<6.06>* Perform the test according to Method 2: it meets the requirement.

Insoluble particulate matter *<6.07>* It meets the requirement.

Sterility *<4.06>* Perform the test according to the Membrane filtration method: it meets the requirement.

Assay Perform the test according to the Cylinder-plate method as directed under Microbial Assay for Antibiotics *<4.02>* according to the following conditions.

(i) Test organisms, culture medium and standard solutions—Proceed as directed in the Assay under Streptomycin Sulfate.

(ii) Sample solution—Weigh accurately the contents of not less than 10 Streptomycin Sulfate for Injection. Weigh accurately an amount of the contents, equivalent to 1 g (potency) of Streptomycin Sulfate, and dissolve in water to make exactly 200 mL. Take exactly a suitable amount of this solution, add 0.1 mol/L phosphate buffer solution (pH 8.0) to make a solutions so that each mL contains 8 μg (potency) and 2 μg (potency), and use these solutions as the high concentration sample solution and the low concentration sample solution, respectively.

Containers and storage Containers—Hermetic containers.

Sucralfate Hydrate

スクラルファート水和物

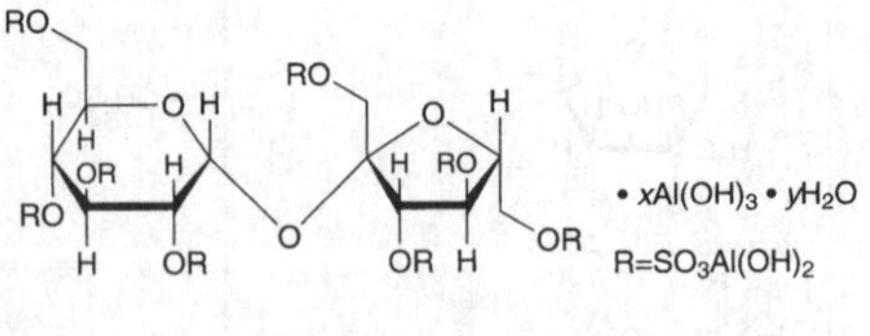

$C_{12}H_{30}Al_8O_{51}S_8.xAl(OH)_3.yH_2O$
[54182-58-0]

Sucralfate Hydrate contains not less than 17.0% and not more than 21.0% of aluminum (Al: 26.98) and not less than 34.0% and not more than 43.0% of sucrose octasulfate ester ($C_{12}H_{22}O_{35}S_8$: 982.80), calculated on the dried basis.

Description Sucralfate Hydrate occurs as a white powder. It is odorless and tasteless.

It is practically insoluble in water, in hot water, in ethanol (95) and in diethyl ether.

It dissolves in dilute hydrochloric acid and in sulfuric acid-sodium hydroxide TS.

Identification **(1)** To 0.05 g of Sucralfate Hydrate in a small test tube add 0.05 g of fresh pieces of sodium, and melt by careful heating. Immerse the test tube immediately in 100 mL of water, break the test tube, shake well, and filter. To 5 mL of the filtrate add 1 drop of sodium pentacyanonitrosylferrate (III) TS: a red-purple color develops.

(2) Dissolve 40 mg of Sucralfate Hydrate in 2 mL of dilute sulfuric acid, and add gently 2 mL of anthrone TS to make 2 layers: a blue color develops at the zone of contact, and gradually changes to blue-green.

(3) Dissolve 0.5 g of Sucralfate Hydrate in 10 mL of dilute hydrochloric acid: the solution responds to Qualitative Tests *<1.09>* for aluminum.

Purity **(1)** Clarity and color of solution—Dissolve 1.0 g of Sucralfate Hydrate in 10 mL of dilute sulfuric acid: the solution is clear and colorless.

(2) Chloride *<1.03>*—Dissolve 0.5 g of Sucralfate Hydrate in 30 mL of dilute nitric acid, and heat gently to boiling. After cooling, add water to make 100 mL, and to 10 mL of this solution add 3 mL of dilute nitric acid and water to make 50 mL. Perform the test using this solution as the test solution. Prepare the control solution with 0.70 mL of 0.01 mol/L hydrochloric acid VS (not more than 0.50%).

(3) Heavy metals *<1.07>*—Dissolve 1.0 g of Sucralfate Hydrate in 20 mL of a solution of sodium chloride (1 in 5) and 1 mL of dilute hydrochloric acid, and to this solution add 2 mL of dilute acetic acid and water to make 50 mL. Perform the test using this solution as the test solution. Prepare the control solution as follows: evaporate 1 mL of dilute hydrochloric acid on a water bath to dryness, and add 20 mL of a solution of sodium chloride (1 in 5), 2 mL of dilute acetic acid, 2.0 mL of Standard Lead Solution and water to make 50 mL (not more than 20 ppm).

(4) Arsenic <*1.11*>—Dissolve 1.0 g of Sucralfate Hydrate in 5 mL of dilute hydrochloric acid, use this solution as the test solution, and perform the test (not more than 2 ppm).

(5) Free aluminum—To 3.0 g of Sucralfate Hydrate add 50 mL of water, heat in a water bath for 5 minutes, cool, and filter. Wash the residue with four 5-mL portions of water, combine the filtrate with the washings, add 2 mL of dilute hydrochloric acid, and heat in a water bath for 30 minutes. After cooling, neutralize the solution with sodium hydroxide TS, add water to make exactly 100 mL, and use this solution as the sample solution. Pipet 50 mL of the sample solution, add exactly 25 mL of 0.05 mol/L disodium dihydrogen ethylenediamine tetraacetate VS and 20 mL of acetic acid-ammonium acetate buffer solution (pH 4.5) and boil for 5 minutes. After cooling, add 50 mL of ethanol (95), and titrate <*2.50*> the excess disodium dihydrogen ethylenediamine tetraacetate with 0.05 mol/L zinc acetate VS until the color of the solution changes from green-purple through purple to red (indicator: 3 mL of dithizone TS). Perform a blank determination in the same manner (not more than 0.2 %).

Each mL of 0.05 mol/L disodium dihydrogen ethylenediamine tetraacetate VS
= 1.349 mg of Al

(6) Related substances—Proceed with 50 μL of the sample solution obtained in the Assay (2) Sucrose octasulfate ester as directed in the Assay (2) Sucrose octasulfate ester, and perform the test as directed under Liquid Chromatography <*2.01*>. Determine the peak area of sucrose octasulfate ester obtained from the sample solution and that of a related substance with the relative retention time about 0.7 to sucrose octasulfate ester by the automatic integration method, and calculate the ratio of the peak area of the related substance to that of sucrose octasulfate ester: it is not more than 0.1.

Detection sensitivity: Adjust so that the peak height of sucrose octasulfate ester from 50 μL of the standard solution obtained in the Assay (2) Sucrose octasulfate ester composes 60 to 100% of the full scale.

Loss on drying <*2.41*> Not more than 14.0% (1 g, 105°C, 3 hours).

Acid-consuming capacity Weigh accurately about 0.25 g of Sucralfate Hydrate, previously dried, place in a 200-mL glass-stoppered conical flask, add exactly 100 mL of 0.1 mol/L hydrochloric acid VS, stopper the flask tightly, and shake at 37 ± 2°C for exactly 1 hour (150 shakings per minute, amplitude: 20 mm). After cooling in water for 5 minutes, pipet 10 mL of the supernatant liquid, and titrate <*2.50*> the excess acid with 0.1 mol/L sodium hydroxide VS until the pH becomes 3.5. Perform a blank determination in the same manner. The amount of 0.1 mol/L hydrochloric acid VS consumed per g of Sucralfate Hydrate is not less than 130 mL.

Assay **(1)** Aluminum—Weigh accurately about 1 g of Sucralfate Hydrate, dissolve in 10 mL of dilute hydrochloric acid by warming on a water bath, cool, and add water to make exactly 250 mL. Pipet 25 mL of this solution, add exactly 25 mL of 0.05 mol/L disodium dihydrogen ethylenediamine tetraacetate VS and 20 mL of acetic acid-ammonium acetate buffer solution (pH 4.5) and boil for 5 minutes. After cooling, add 50 mL of ethanol (95), and titrate <*2.50*> the excess disodium dihydrogen ethylenediamine tetraacetate with 0.05 mol/L zinc acetate VS until the color of the solution changes from green-purple through purple to red (indicator: 3 mL of dithizone TS). Perform a blank determination in the same manner.

Each mL of 0.05 mol/L disodium dihydrogen ethylenediamine tetraacetate VS
= 1.349 mg of Al

(2) Sucrose octasulfate ester—Weigh accurately about 0.55 g of Sucralfate Hydrate, add exactly 10 mL of sulfuric acid-sodium hydroxide TS, shake vigorously, and dissolve by sonicating at below 30°C for 5 minutes. To this solution add 0.1 mol/L sodium hydroxide VS to make exactly 25 mL, and use this solution as the sample solution. Separately, weigh accurately about 0.25 g of Potassium Sucrose Octasulfate RS, add the mobile phase to make exactly 25 mL, and use this solution as the standard solution. Prepare rapidly the sample solution and the standard solution, and perform the test immediately. Pipet 50 μL each of the sample solution and standard solution, and perform the test as directed under Liquid Chromatography <*2.01*> according to the following conditions. Determine the peak areas, A_T and A_S, of sucrose octasulfate ester in each solution.

Amount (mg) of sucrose octasulfate ester ($C_{12}H_{22}O_{35}S_8$)
$= M_S \times A_T/A_S \times 0.763$

M_S: Amount (mg) of Potassium Sucrose Octasulfate RS taken, calculated on the anhydrous basis

Operating conditions—

Detector: A differential refractometer.

Column: A stainless steel column about 4 mm in inside diameter and about 30 cm in length, packed with aminopropylsilanized silica gel for liquid chromatography (about 8 μm in particle diameter).

Column temperature: Room temperature.

Mobile phase: Dissolve a suitable amount (26 to 132 g) of ammonium sulfate in 1000 mL of water, and adjust with phosphoric acid to pH 3.5. Allow a solution of Potassium Sucrose Octasulfate RS in dilute hydrochloric acid (1 in 100) to stand at 60°C for 10 minutes, cool, and perform the test immediately. Adjust the amount of ammonium sulfate in the mobile phase so that the peak of a related substance with the relative retention time about 0.7 to sucrose octasulfate ester almost returns to the base line, and the peak of sucrose octasulfate ester elutes most rapidly.

Flow rate: Adjust so that the retention time of sucrose octasulfate ester is between 6 and 11 minutes.

Selection of column: Allow a solution of Potassium Sucrose Octasulfate RS in dilute hydrochloric acid (1 in 100) to stand at 60°C for 10 minutes, cool, and proceed immediately with 50 μL of this solution under the above operating conditions. Use a column with a resolution being not less than 1.5 between sucrose octasulfate ester and a related substance with the relative retention time about 0.7 to sucrose octasulfate ester.

System repeatability: Repeat the test 6 times with the standard solution under the above operating conditions: the relative standard deviation of the peak area of sucrose octasulfate ester is not more than 2.0%.

Containers and storage Containers—Tight containers.

White Soft Sugar

白糖

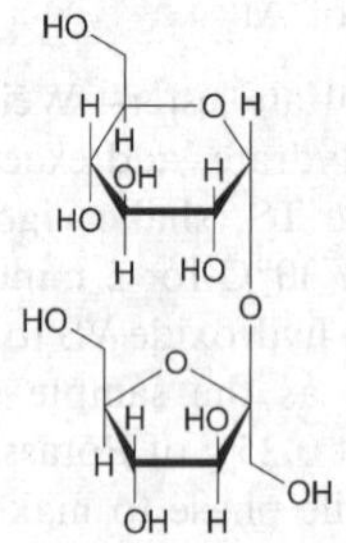

$C_{12}H_{22}O_{11}$: 342.30
β-D-Fructofuranosyl *α*-D-glucopyranoside
[57-50-1]

Description White Soft Sugar is colorless or white, crystals or crystalline powder. It is odorless and has a sweet taste.

It is very soluble in water, very slightly soluble in ethanol (95), and practically insoluble in diethyl ether.

A solution of White Soft Sugar (1 in 10) is neutral.

Identification **(1)** When 1 g of White Soft Sugar is ignited, it melts and swells, and decomposes, emitting an odor of caramel, to bulky charcoal.

(2) To 0.1 g of White Soft Sugar add 2 mL of dilute sulfuric acid, boil, add 4 mL of sodium hydroxide TS and 3 mL of Fehling's TS, and heat to boiling: a red to dark red precipitate is produced.

Optical rotation ⟨*2.49*⟩ $[\alpha]_D^{20}$: +65.0 – +67.0° (after drying, 13 g, water, 50 mL, 100 mm).

Purity **(1)** Clarity and color of solution—Dissolve 100 g of White Soft Sugar in 100 mL of water, take 50 mL of this solution in a Nessler tube, and view transversely the Nessler tube against a white background: the solution is colorless or only slightly yellow and has no blue color. Fill the solution in the Nessler tube, stopper, and allow to stand for 2 days: no precipitate is produced.

(2) Chloride ⟨*1.03*⟩—To 10.0 g of White Soft Sugar add water to make 100 mL, and use this solution as the sample solution. To 20 mL of the sample solution add 6 mL of dilute nitric acid and water to make 50 mL. Perform the test using this solution as the test solution. Prepare the control solution with 0.30 mL of 0.01 mol/L hydrochloric acid VS (not more than 0.005%).

(3) Sulfate ⟨*1.14*⟩—To 40 mL of the sample solution obtained in (2) add 1 mL of dilute hydrochloric acid and water to make 50 mL. Perform the test using this solution as the test solution. Prepare the control solution with 0.50 mL of 0.005 mol/L sulfuric acid VS (not more than 0.006%).

(4) Calcium—To 10 mL of the sample solution obtained in (2) add 1 mL of ammonium oxalate TS: this solution shows immediately no change.

(5) Heavy metals ⟨*1.07*⟩—Proceed with 5.0 g of White Soft Sugar according to Method 1, and perform the test. Prepare the control solution with 2.5 mL of Standard Lead Solution (not more than 5 ppm).

(6) Arsenic ⟨*1.11*⟩—Prepare the test solution with 1.0 g of White Soft Sugar according to Method 1, and perform the test (not more than 2 ppm).

(7) Invert sugar—Dissolve 5.0 g of White Soft Sugar in water to make 100 mL, filter if necessary, and use this solution as the sample solution. Separately place 100 mL of alkaline copper (II) sulfate TS in a 300-mL beaker, cover the beaker with a watch glass, and boil. Immediately add 50.0 mL of the sample solution, boil the mixture exactly for 5 minutes, add at once 50 mL of freshly boiled and cooled water, dip it in a water bath of a temperature below 10°C for 5 minutes, and collect the precipitate in a tared glass filter (G4). Wash the residue on the filter with water until the last washing is neutral, then wash with 10 mL of ethanol (95) and 10 mL of diethyl ether, and dry at 105°C for 30 minutes: the mass of the residual precipitate is not more than 0.120 g.

Loss on drying ⟨*2.41*⟩ Not more than 1.30% (15 g, 105°C, 2 hours).

Residue on ignition ⟨*2.44*⟩ Not more than 0.1% (2 g).

Containers and storage Containers—Well-closed containers.

Sucrose

精製白糖

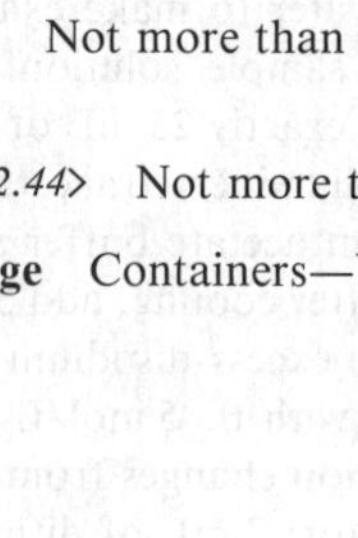

$C_{12}H_{22}O_{11}$: 342.30
β-D-Fructofuranosyl *α*-D-glucopyranoside
[57-50-1]

This monograph is harmonized with the European Pharmacopoeia and the U.S.Pharmacopeia.

The parts of the text that are not harmonized are marked with symbols (◆ ◆).

Information on the harmonization with the European Pharmacopoeia and the U.S. Pharmacopeia is available on the website of the Pharmaceuticals and Medical Devices Agency.

Sucrose contains no additives.

For Sucrose used for preparation of the parenteral infusions, the label states the purpose.

◆**Description** Sucrose is a white crystalline powder, or lustrous colorless or white crystals.

It is very soluble in water, and practically insoluble in ethanol (99.5).◆

◆**Identification** Determine the infrared absorption spectrum of Sucrose as directed in the potassium bromide disk method under Infrared Spectrophotometry ⟨*2.25*⟩, and compare the spectrum with the Reference Spectrum: both spectra exhibit similar intensities of absorption at the same wave numbers.◆

Optical rotation ⟨*2.49*⟩ $[\alpha]_D^{20}$: +66.3 – +67.0° (26 g, water, 100 mL, ◆100 mm◆).

Purity ◆**(1)** Color value—Dissolve 50.0 g of Sucrose in 50.0 mL of water, filter through a membrane filter with 0.45 *μ*m in pore size, degas, and use this solution as the sample solution. Measure the absorbance of the sample solution at 420 nm as directed under Ultraviolet-visible Spectrophotometry ⟨*2.24*⟩, using a cell of at least 4 cm (a cell length of

10 cm or more is preferred), and calculate the color value by the following equation: not more than 45.

$$\text{Color value} = A \times 1000/b/c$$

A: Absorbance measured at 420 nm
b: Path length (cm)
c: Concentration (g/mL) of Sucrose in the sample solution, calculated from the refractive index (n_D^{20}) obtained as directed under Refractive Index Determination <2.45>. Use the following table and interpolate the value, if necessary.

n_D^{20}	c (g/mL)
1.4138	0.570
1.4159	0.585
1.4179	0.600
1.4200	0.615
1.4221	0.630
1.4243	0.645
1.4264	0.661

System suitability—

System repeatability: When the test is repeated 2 times with the sample solution, the difference between 2 results is not larger than 3.◆

(2) Clarity of solution—Dissolve 50.0 g of Sucrose in water to make 100 mL, and use this solution as the sample solution: the sample solution is clear, and its clarity is not different from water, or its opalescence is not more than that of reference suspension 1.

(3) Sulfite

(i) Enzyme reaction: Sulfite is oxidized by sulfite oxidase to sulfuric acid and hydrogen peroxide which in turn is reduced by nicotinamide adenine dinucleotide peroxidase in the presence of nicotinamide adenine dinucleotide reduced form (NADH). The amount of NADH oxidized is proportional to the amount of sulfite. Calculate the amount of oxidized NADH from the degree of reduction of the absorbance at 340 nm. A suitable kit may be used.

(ii) Procedure: Dissolve 4.0 g of Sucrose in freshly prepared distilled water to make exactly 10 mL, and use this solution as the sample solution. Separately, dissolve 4.0 g of Sucrose in freshly prepared distilled water, add exactly 0.5 mL of Standard Sulfite Solution, then add freshly prepared distilled water to make exactly 10 mL, and use this solution as the standard solution. Use freshly prepared distilled water as a blank. Separately, introduce 2.0 mL each of the sample solution, the standard solution and the blank in 10-mm cells, add 1.00 mL of β-nicotinamide adenine dinucleotide reduced form TS and 10 μL of NADH peroxidase TS, stir with a plastic stirring rod, and allow to stand at 20 - 25°C for 5 minutes. Measure the absorbance of these solutions at 340 nm, A_{T1}, A_{S1} and A_{B1}, as directed under Ultraviolet-visible Spectrophotometry <2.24>, using water as the blank. Then, to these solutions add 50 μL each of sulfite oxidase TS, stir, allow to stand at 20 - 25°C for 30 minutes, then measure the absorbance of these solutions in the same manner as above, A_{T2}, A_{S2} and A_{B2}: the result of $(A_{T1} - A_{T2}) - (A_{B1} - A_{B2})$ is not larger than half the result of $(A_{S1} - A_{S2}) - (A_{B1} - A_{B2})$ (not more than 10 ppm expressed as SO_2).

(4) Reducing sugars—Transfer 5 mL of the sample solution obtained in (2) to a test-tube about 150 mm long and about 16 mm in diameter, add 5 mL of water, 1.0 mL of 1 mol/L sodium hydroxide VS and 1.0 mL of methylene blue TS, mix, and heat in a water bath. After exactly 2 minutes, take the tube out of the bath, and examine the solution immediately: the blue color does not disappear completely. Ignore any blue color at the air and solution interface.

Conductivity *<2.51>* Dissolve 31.3 g of Sucrose in freshly prepared distilled water to make 100 mL, and use this solution as the sample solution. Measure the conductivity of the sample solution (κ_1 (μS·cm^{-1})) while gently stirring with a magnetic stirrer at 20 ± 0.1°C. Measure the conductivity of the water used for preparing the sample solution (κ_2 (μS·cm^{-1})) in the same manner as above. The measured conductivity must be stable within 1% in the rate of change per 30 seconds. Calculate the corrected conductivity of the sample solution (κ_C) by the following expression: κ_C is not more than 35 μS·cm^{-1}.

$$\kappa_C\ (\mu\text{S}\cdot\text{cm}^{-1}) = \kappa_1 - 0.35\kappa_2$$

Loss on drying *<2.41>* Not more than 0.1% (2 g, 105°C, 3 hours).

Dextrins For Sucrose used to prepare parenteral infusions, to 2 mL of the sample solution obtained in the Purity (2) add 8 mL of water, 0.05 mL of 2 mol/L hydrochloric acid and 0.05 mL of iodine TS: the solution remains yellow.

Bacterial endotoxins *<4.01>* Less than 0.25 EU/mg, for Sucrose used to prepare parenteral infusions.

◆**Containers and storage** Containers—Well-closed containers.◆

Sulbactam Sodium

スルバクタムナトリウム

$C_8H_{10}NNaO_5S$: 255.22
Monosodium (2*S*,5*R*)-3,3-dimethyl-7-oxo-4-thia-1-azabicyclo[3.2.0]heptane-2-carboxylate 4,4-dioxide
[*69388-84-7*]

Sulbactam Sodium contains not less than 875 μg (potency) and not more than 941 μg (potency) per mg, calculated on the anhydrous basis. The potency of Sulbactam Sodium is expressed as mass (potency) of sulbactam ($C_8H_{11}NO_5S$: 233.24).

Description Sulbactam Sodium occurs as a white to yellowish white crystalline powder.

It is freely soluble in water, sparingly soluble in methanol, very slightly soluble in ethanol (99.5), and practically insoluble in acetonitrile.

Identification **(1)** Determine the infrared absorption spectrum of Sulbactam Sodium as directed in the potassium bromide disk method under Infrared Spectrophotometry *<2.25>*, and compare the spectrum with the Reference Spectrum: both spectra exhibit similar intensities of absorption at the same wave numbers.

(2) Sulbactam Sodium responds to Qualitative Tests *<1.09>* (1) for sodium salt.

Optical rotation *<2.49>* $[\alpha]_D^{20}$: +219 – +233° (1 g, water, 100 mL, 100 mm).

pH <*2.54*> Dissolve 1.0 g of Sulbactam Sodium in 20 mL of water: the pH of the solution is between 5.2 and 7.2.

Purity **(1)** Clarity and color of solution—Dissolve 1.0 g of Sulbactam Sodium in 20 mL of water: the solution is clear, and its absorbance at 430 nm determined as directed under Ultraviolet-visible Spectrophotometry <*2.24*> is not more than 0.10.

(2) Heavy metals <*1.07*>—Proceed with 1.0 g of Sulbactam Sodium according to Method 2, and perform the test. Prepare the control solution with 2.0 mL of Standard Lead Solution (not more than 20 ppm).

(3) Sulbactam penicillamine—Weigh accurately about 0.2 g of Sulbactam Sodium, dissolve in the mobile phase to make exactly 50 mL, and use this solution as the sample solution. Separately, weigh accurately about 40 mg of sulbactam sodium for sulbactam penicillamine, dissolve in 2 mL of water, and add 0.5 mL of sodium hydroxide TS. Allow to stand at room temperature for 10 minutes, add 0.5 mL of 1 mol/L hydrochloric acid TS, and then add the mobile phase to make exactly 100 mL. Pipet 5 mL of this solution, add the mobile phase to make exactly 50 mL, and use this solution as the standard solution. Perform the test with exactly 10 μL each of the sample solution and standard solution as directed under Liquid Chromatography <*2.01*> according to the following conditions, and determine the peak areas, A_T and A_S, of sulbactam penicillamine by the automatic integration method: the amount of sulbactam penicillamine is not more than 1.0%.

Amount (%) of sulbactam penicillamine
$= M_S/M_T \times A_T/A_S \times 5$

M_S: Amount (mg) of sulbactam sodium for sulbactam penicillamine taken
M_T: Amount (mg) of Sulbactam Sodium taken

Operating conditions—

Column, column temperature, mobile phase, and flow rate: Proceed as directed in the operating conditions in the Assay.

Detector: An ultraviolet absorption photometer (wavelength: 230 nm).

System suitability—

System performance: Proceed as directed in the system suitability in the Assay.

System repeatability: When the test is repeated 6 times with 10 μL of the standard solution under the above operating conditions, the relative standard deviation of the peak area of sulbactam penicillamine is not more than 2.0%.

Water <*2.48*> Not more than 1.0% (0.5 g, volumetric titration, direct titration).

Assay Weigh accurately amounts of Sulbactam Sodium and Sulbactam RS, equivalent to about 50 mg (potency), dissolve each in a suitable amount of the mobile phase, add exactly 5 mL of the internal standard solution, then add the mobile phase to make 50 mL, and use these solutions as the sample solution and the standard solution, respectively. Perform the test with 10 μL each of the sample solution and standard solution as directed under Liquid Chromatography <*2.01*> according to the following conditions, and calculate the ratios, Q_T and Q_S, of the peak area of sulbactam to that of the internal standard.

Amount [μg (potency)] of sulbactam ($C_8H_{11}NO_5S$)
$= M_S \times Q_T/Q_S \times 1000$

M_S: Amount [mg (potency)] of Sulbactam RS taken

Internal standard solution—A solution of ethyl parahydroxybenzoate in the mobile phase (7 in 1000).

Operating conditions—

Detector: An ultraviolet absorption photometer (wavelength: 220 nm).

Column: A stainless steel column 3.9 mm in inside diameter and 30 cm in length, packed with octadecylsilanized silica gel for liquid chromatography (10 μm in particle diameter).

Column temperature: A constant temperature of about 35°C.

Mobile phase: To 750 mL of 0.005 mol/L tetrabutylammonium hydroxide TS add 250 mL of acetonitrile for liquid chromatography.

Flow rate: Adjust so that the retention time of sulbactam is about 6 minutes.

System suitability—

System performance: When the procedure is run with 10 μL of the standard solution under the above operating conditions, sulbactam and the internal standard are eluted in this order with the resolution between these peaks being not less than 1.5.

System repeatability: When the test is repeated 6 times with 10 μL of the standard solution under the above operating conditions, the relative standard deviation of the peak area of sulbactam is not more than 1.0%.

Containers and storage Containers—Tight containers.

Sulbenicillin Sodium

スルベニシリンナトリウム

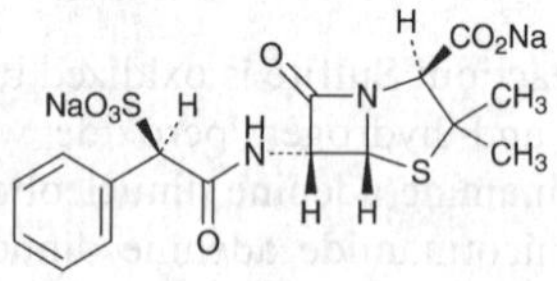

$C_{16}H_{16}N_2Na_2O_7S_2$: 458.42
Disodium (2*S*,5*R*,6*R*)-3,3-dimethyl-7-oxo-6-[(2*R*)-2-phenyl-2-sulfonatoacetylamino]-4-thia-1-azabicyclo[3.2.0]heptane-2-carboxylate
[*28002-18-8*]

Sulbenicillin Sodium contains not less than 900 μg (potency) and not more than 970 μg (potency) per mg, calculated on the anhydrous basis. The potency of Sulbenicillin Sodium is expressed as mass (potency) of sulbenicillin ($C_{16}H_{18}N_2O_7S_2$: 414.45).

Description Sulbenicillin Sodium occurs as white to light yellow-white powder.

It is very soluble in water, freely soluble in methanol, and slightly soluble in ethanol (99.5).

It is hygroscopic.

Identification **(1)** Determine the infrared absorption spectrum of Sulbenicillin Sodium as directed in the potassium bromide disk method under Infrared Spectrophotometry <*2.25*>, and compare the spectrum with the Reference Spectrum or the spectrum of Sulbenicillin Sodium RS: both spectra exhibit similar intensities of absorption at the same wave numbers.

(2) Sulbenicillin Sodium responds to Qualitative Tests <*1.09*> (1) for sodium salt.

Optical rotation <*2.49*> $[\alpha]_D^{20}$: +167 – +182° (1 g calculated on the anhydrous basis, water, 20 mL, 100 mm).

pH *<2.54>* The pH of a solution obtained by dissolving 0.20 g of Sulbenicillin Sodium in 10 mL of water is between 4.5 and 7.0.

Purity (1) Clarity and color of solution—Dissolve 2.5 g of Sulbenicillin Sodium in 5 mL of water: the solution is clear and colorless to pale yellow.

(2) Heavy metals *<1.07>*—Proceed with 1.0 g of Sulbenicillin Sodium according to Method 1, and perform the test. Prepare the control solution with 2.0 mL of Standard Lead Solution (not more than 20 ppm).

(3) Arsenic *<1.11>*—Prepare the test solution with 1.0 g of Sulbenicillin Sodium according to Method 1, and perform the test (not more than 2 ppm).

(4) Related substances—Dissolve 0.10 g of Sulbenicillin Sodium in 15 mL of the mobile phase, and use this solution as the sample solution. Perform the test with 10 μL of the sample solution as directed under Liquid Chromatography *<2.01>* according to the following conditions, determine each peak area by the automatic integration method, and calculate the amount of these peaks by the area percentage method: the amount of the each peak other than the two peaks of sulbenicillin is not more than 2.0%, and the total amount of the peaks other than the two peaks of sulbenicillin is not more than 5.0%.

Operating conditions—

Detector: An ultraviolet absorption photometer (wavelength: 254 nm).

Column: A stainless steel column 3.9 mm in inside diameter and 30 cm in length, packed with octadecylsilanized silica gel for liquid chromatography (5 μm in particle diameter).

Column temperature: A constant temperature of about 25°C.

Mobile phase: Dissolve 10 g of potassium dihydrogen phosphate in 750 mL of water, adjust the pH to 6.0 ± 0.1 with sodium hydroxide TS, and add water to make 1000 mL. To 940 mL of this solution add 60 mL of acetonitrile.

Flow rate: Adjust so that the retention time of the lately eluted peak of sulbenicillin is about 18 minutes.

Time span of measurement: About 1.5 times as long as the retention time of the lately eluted peak of sulbenicillin, beginning after the solvent peak.

System suitability—

Test for required detectability: Measure exactly 1 mL of the sample solution, add the mobile phase to make exactly 100 mL, and use this solution as the solution for system suitability test. Pipet 1 mL of the solution for system suitability test, and add the mobile phase to make exactly 10 mL. Confirm that the total area of the two peaks of sulbenicillin obtained with 10 μL of this solution is equivalent to 7 to 13% of that with 10 μL of the solution for system suitability test.

System performance: When the procedure is run with 10 μL of the sample solution under the above operating conditions, the resolution between the two peaks of sulbenicillin is not less than 2.0.

System repeatability: When the test is repeated 6 times with 10 μL of the solution for system suitability test under the above operating conditions, the relative standard deviation of the total areas of the two peaks of sulbenicillin is not more than 5.0%.

Water *<2.48>* Not more than 6.0% (0.5 g, volumetric titration, direct titration).

Assay Perform the test according to the Cylinder-plate method as directed under Microbial Assay for Antibiotics *<4.02>* according to the following conditions.

(i) Test organism—*Bacillus subtilis* ATCC 6633

(ii) Culture medium—Use the medium i in 1) under (1) Agar media for seed and base layer. Adjust the pH of the medium so that it will be 6.4 to 6.6 after sterilization.

(iii) Standard solutions—Weigh accurately an amount of Sulbenicillin Sodium RS, equivalent to about 50 mg (potency), dissolve in phosphate buffer solution (pH 6.0) to make exactly 50 mL, and use this solution as the standard stock solution. Keep the standard stock solution in a freezer, and use within 4 days. Take exactly a suitable amount of the standard stock solution before use, add phosphate buffer solution (pH 6.0) to make solutions so that each mL contains 40 μg (potency) and 10 μg (potency), and use these solutions as the high concentration standard solution and the low concentration standard solution, respectively.

(iv) Sample solutions—Weigh accurately an amount of Sulbenicillin Sodium, equivalent to about 50 mg (potency), and dissolve in phosphate buffer solution (pH 6.0) to make exactly 50 mL. Take exactly a suitable amount of this solution, add phosphate buffer solution (pH 6.0) to make solutions so that each mL contains 40 μg (potency) and 10 μg (potency), and use these solutions as the high concentration sample solution and the low concentration sample solution, respectively.

Containers and storage Containers—Hermetic containers.

Sulfadiazine Silver

スルファジアジン銀

$C_{10}H_9AgN_4O_2S$: 357.14

Monosilver 4-amino-*N*-(pyrimidin-2-yl)-benzenesulfonamidate

[*22199-08-2*]

Sulfadiazine Silver, when dried, contains not less than 99.0% and not more than 102.0% of sulfadiazine silver ($C_{10}H_9AgN_4O_2S$).

Description Sulfadiazine Silver occurs as a white to pale yellow crystalline powder. It is odorless.

It is practically insoluble in water, in ethanol (95) and in diethyl ether.

It dissolves in ammonia TS.

It is gradually colored by light.

Melting point: about 275°C (with decomposition).

Identification Determine the infrared absorption spectrum of Sulfadiazine Silver, previously dried, as directed in the paste method under Infrared Spectrophotometry *<2.25>*, and compare the spectrum with the Reference Spectrum or the spectrum of previously dried Sulfadiazine Silver RS: both spectra exhibit similar intensities of absorption at the same wave numbers.

Purity (1) Nitrate—To 250 mL of water add 1.0 g of Sulfadiazine Silver, shake well for 50 minutes, filter, and use this filtrate as the sample solution. Separately, weigh accurately 0.25 g of potassium nitrate, and dissolve in water to make exactly 2000 mL. Pipet 5 mL of this solution and add water to make exactly 200 mL, and use this solution as the standard solution. Pipet 2.0 mL each of the sample solution and standard solution, and add 5 mL of a solution of disodium chromotropate dihydrate in sulfuric acid (1 in 10,000) and sulfuric acid to make exactly 10 mL. Determine the absorbances, A_T and A_S, of the sample solution and standard solution at 408 nm as directed under Ultraviolet-visible Spectrophotometry <*2.24*>, using a solution, prepared with exactly 2.0 mL of water in the same manner, as the blank: A_T is not larger than A_S (not more than 0.05%).

(2) Related substances—Dissolve 50 mg of Sulfadiazine Silver in 5 mL of a mixture of ethanol (95) and ammonia solution (28) (3:2), and use this solution as the sample solution. Pipet 2 mL of the sample solution, and add a mixture of ethanol (95) and ammonia solution (28) (3:2) to make exactly 20 mL. Pipet 2 mL of this solution, add a mixture of ethanol (95) and ammonia solution (28) (3:2) to make exactly 20 mL, and use this solution as the standard solution. Perform the test with these solutions as directed under Thin-layer Chromatography <*2.03*>. Spot 5 μL each of the sample solution and standard solution on a plate of silica gel with fluorescent indicator for thin-layer chromatography. Develop the plate with a mixture of chloroform, methanol and ammonia solution (28) (10:5:2) to a distance of about 15 cm, and air-dry the plate. Examine under ultraviolet light (main wavelength: 254 nm): the spots other than the principal spot and spot of the starting point obtained from the sample solution are not more intense than the spot from the standard solution.

Loss on drying <*2.41*> Not more than 0.5% (1 g, in vacuum, phosphorus (V) oxide, 80°C, 4 hours).

Residue on ignition <*2.44*> 41 - 45% (1 g).

Silver content Weigh accurately about 50 mg of Sulfadiazine Silver, previously dried, dissolve in 2 mL of nitric acid, and add water to make exactly 100 mL. Pipet 1 mL of this solution, add water to make exactly 100 mL, and use this solution as the sample solution. Measure accurately a suitable quantity of Standard Silver Solution for Atomic Absorption Spectrophotometry, dilute with water to make solutions containing 1.0 to 2.0 μg of silver (Ag:107.87) per mL, and use these solutions as the standard solutions. Perform the test with the sample solution and standard solutions as directed under Atomic Absorption Spectrophotometry <*2.23*> according to the following conditions, and calculate the silver content of the sample solution from the calibration curve obtained from the absorbances of the standard solutions: it contains not less than 28.7% and not more than 30.8% of silver.

Gas: Combustible gas—Acetylene.
Supporting gas—Air.
Lamp: A silver hollow cathode lamp.
Wavelength: 328.1 nm.

Assay Weigh accurately about 0.1 g each of Sulfadiazine Silver and Sulfadiazine Silver RS, each previously dried, and add ammonia TS to make exactly 100 mL, respectively. Pipet 1 mL each of these solutions, add water to make exactly 100 mL, and use these solutions as the sample solution and the standard solution, respectively. Determine the absorbances, A_T and A_S, of the sample solution and standard solution at 255 nm, as directed under Ultraviolet-visible Spectrophotometry <*2.24*>, using a solution, prepared with exactly 1 mL of ammonia TS and a sufficient water to make exactly 100 mL, as the blank.

Amount (mg) of sulfadiazine silver ($C_{10}H_9AgN_4O_2S$)
$= M_S \times A_T/A_S$

M_S: Amount (mg) of Sulfadiazine Silver RS taken

Containers and storage Containers—Well-closed containers.
Storage—Light-resistant.

Sulfamethizole

スルファメチゾール

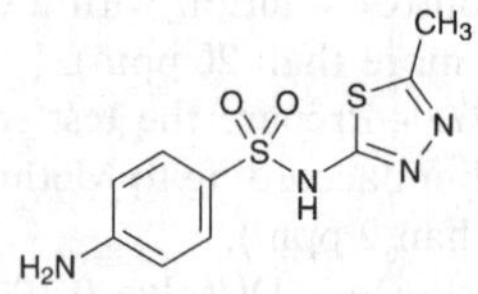

$C_9H_{10}N_4O_2S_2$: 270.33
4-Amino-*N*-(5-methyl-1,3,4-thiadiazol-2-yl)-benzenesulfonamide
[*144-82-1*]

Sulfamethizole, when dried, contains not less than 99.0% of sulfamethizole ($C_9H_{10}N_4O_2S_2$).

Description Sulfamethizole occurs as white to yellowish white, crystals or crystalline powder. It is odorless.

It is slightly soluble in ethanol (95), and in acetic acid (100) and practical insoluble in water and in diethyl ether.

It dissolves in dilute hydrochloric acid and in sodium hydroxide TS.

It is gradually colored by light.

Identification Determine the infrared absorption spectrum of Sulfamethizole, previously dried, as directed in the potassium bromide disk method under Infrared Spectrophotometry <*2.25*>, and compare the spectrum with the Reference Spectrum: both spectra exhibit similar intensities of absorption at the same wave numbers.

Melting point <*2.60*> 208 - 211°C

Purity **(1)** Clarity and color of solution—Dissolve 0.5 g of Sulfamethizole in 3 mL of sodium hydroxide TS and 20 mL of water: the solution is clear and colorless.

(2) Acidity—To 1.0 g of Sulfamethizole add 50 mL of water, warm at 70°C for 5 minutes, allow to stand for 1 hour in an ice bath, and filter. To 25 mL of the filtrate add 2 drops of methyl red TS and 0.60 mL of 0.1 mol/L sodium hydroxide VS: a yellow color develops.

(3) Heavy metals <*1.07*>—Proceed with 1.0 g of Sulfamethizole according to Method 2, and perform the test. Prepare the control solution with 2.0 mL of Standard Lead Solution (not more than 20 ppm).

(4) Arsenic <*1.11*>—Prepare the test solution with 1.0 g of Sulfamethizole according to Method 3, and perform the test (not more than 2 ppm).

(5) Related substances—Dissolve 0.10 g of Sulfamethizole in 10 mL of acetone, and use this solution as the sample solution. Pipet 1 mL of the sample solution, add acetone to make exactly 50 mL, then pipet 5 mL of this solution, add acetone to make exactly 20 mL, and use this solution as the standard solution. Perform the test with these solutions as directed under Thin-layer Chromatography <*2.03*>. Spot 5 μL each of the sample solution and standard solution on a plate of silica gel with fluorescent indicator for thin-layer chromatography. Develop the plate with a mixture of ethyl acetate and acetic acid (100) (20:1) to a distance of about 10 cm, and air-dry the plate. Examine under ultraviolet light (main wavelength: 254 nm): the spots other than the principal spot obtained from the sample solution are not more intense than the spot from the standard solution.

Loss on drying 〈*2.41*〉 Not more than 0.5% (1 g, 105°C, 4 hours).

Residue on ignition 〈*2.44*〉 Not more than 0.1% (1 g).

Assay Weigh accurately about 0.4 g of Sulfamethizole, previously dried, dissolve in 5 mL of hydrochloric acid and 50 mL of water, add 10 mL of a solution of potassium bromide (3 in 10), cool below 15°C, and titrate 〈*2.50*〉 with 0.1 mol/L sodium nitrite VS according to the potentiometric titration method or the amperometric titration method.

Each mL of 0.1 mol/L sodium nitrite VS
= 27.03 mg of $C_9H_{10}N_4O_2S_2$

Containers and storage Containers—Well-closed containers.

Storage—Light-resistant.

Sulfamethoxazole

スルファメトキサゾール

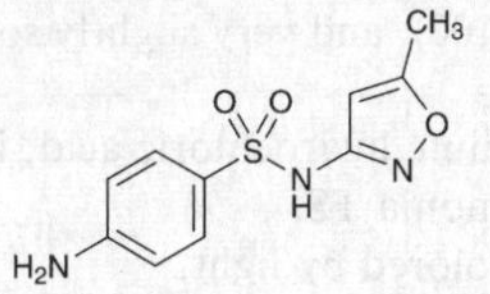

$C_{10}H_{11}N_3O_3S$: 253.28
4-Amino-*N*-(5-methylisoxazol-3-yl)benzenesulfonamide
[*723-46-6*]

Sulfamethoxazole, when dried, contains not less than 99.0% of sulfamethoxazole ($C_{10}H_{11}N_3O_3S$).

Description Sulfamethoxazole occurs as white, crystals or crystalline powder. It is odorless, and has a slightly bitter taste.

It is very soluble in *N,N*-dimethylformamide, sparingly soluble in ethanol (95), slightly soluble in diethyl ether, and very slightly soluble in water.

It dissolves in sodium hydroxide TS.

It is gradually colored by light.

Identification Determine the infrared absorption spectrum of Sulfamethoxazole, previously dried, as directed in the potassium bromide disk method under Infrared Spectrophotometry 〈*2.25*〉, and compare the spectrum with the Reference Spectrum: both spectra exhibit similar intensities of absorption at the same wave numbers.

Melting point 〈*2.60*〉 169 – 172°C

Purity **(1)** Clarity and color of solution—Dissolve 1.0 g of Sulfamethoxazole in 5 mL of sodium hydroxide TS, and add 20 mL of water: the solution is clear and colorless.

(2) Acidity—To 1.0 g of Sulfamethoxazole add 50 mL of water, heat at 70°C for 5 minutes, allow to stand in ice water for 1 hour, and filter. To 25 mL of the filtrate add 2 drops of methyl red TS and 0.60 mL of 0.1 mol/L sodium hydroxide VS: a yellow color develops.

(3) Heavy metals 〈*1.07*〉—Proceed with 1.0 g of Sulfamethoxazole according to Method 2, and perform the test. Prepare the control solution with 2.0 mL of Standard Lead Solution (not more than 20 ppm).

(4) Arsenic 〈*1.11*〉—Prepare the test solution with 1.0 g of Sulfamethoxazole according to Method 3, and perform the test (not more than 2 ppm).

(5) Related substances—Dissolve 0.20 g of Sulfamethoxazole in 10 mL of a solution of ammonia solution (28) in methanol (1 in 50), and use this solution as the sample solution. Pipet 1 mL of the sample solution, add a solution of ammonia solution (28) in methanol (1 in 50) to make exactly 10 mL. Pipet 1 mL of this solution, add a solution of ammonia solution (28) in methanol (1 in 50) to make exactly 20 mL, and use this solution as the standard solution. Perform the test with these solutions as directed under Thin-layer Chromatography 〈*2.03*〉. Spot 5 μL each of the sample solution and standard solution on a plate of silica gel with fluorescent indicator for thin-layer chromatography. Develop the plate with a mixture of ethyl acetate, acetonitrile and diluted ammonia solution (28) (7 in 100) (10:8:1) to a distance of about 10 cm, and air-dry the plate. Examine under ultraviolet light (main wavelength: 254 nm): the spots other than the principal spot obtained from the sample solution are not more intense than the spot from the standard solution.

Loss on drying 〈*2.41*〉 Not more than 0.5% (1 g, 105°C, 4 hours).

Residue on ignition 〈*2.44*〉 Not more than 0.1% (1 g).

Assay Weigh accurately about 0.4 g of Sulfamethoxazole, previously dried, dissolve in 30 mL of *N,N*-dimethylformamide, add 10 mL of water, and titrate 〈*2.50*〉 with 0.1 mol/L sodium hydroxide VS until a light blue color is produced (indicator: 0.5 mL of thymolphthalein TS). Separately, perform a blank determination in the same manner with a mixture of 30 mL of *N,N*-dimethylformamide and 26 mL of water, and make any necessary correction.

Each mL of 0.1 mol/L sodium hydroxide VS
= 25.33 mg of $C_{10}H_{11}N_3O_3S$

Containers and storage Containers—Well-closed containers.

Storage—Light-resistant.

Sulfamonomethoxine Hydrate

スルファモノメトキシン水和物

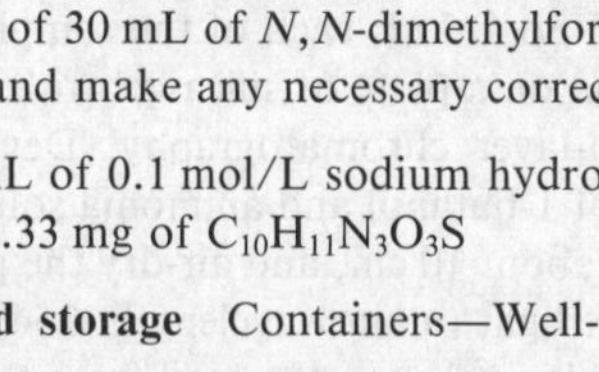

$C_{11}H_{12}N_4O_3S.H_2O$: 298.32
4-Amino-*N*-(6-methoxypyrimidin-4-yl)benzenesulfonamide monohydrate
[*1220-83-3*, anhydride]

Sulfamonomethoxine Hydrate, when dried, contains not less than 99.0% of sulfamonomethoxine ($C_{11}H_{12}N_4O_3S$: 280.31).

Description Sulfamonomethoxine Hydrate occurs as white to pale yellow, crystals, granules or crystalline powder. It is odorless.

It is soluble in acetone, slightly soluble in ethanol (95), very slightly soluble in diethyl ether, and practically insoluble in water.

It dissolves in dilute hydrochloric acid and in sodium hydroxide TS.

It is gradually colored by light.

Identification Determine the infrared absorption spectrum of Sulfamonomethoxine Hydrate as directed in the potassium bromide disk method under Infrared Spectrophotometry <*2.25*>, and compare the spectrum with the Reference Spectrum: both spectra exhibit similar intensities of absorption at the same wave numbers.

Melting point <*2.60*> 204 - 206°C

Purity **(1)** Clarity and color of solution—Dissolve 1.0 g of Sulfamonomethoxine Hydrate in 5 mL of sodium hydroxide TS and 20 mL of water: the solution is clear and colorless to pale yellow. Dissolve 0.5 g of Sulfamonomethoxine Hydrate in 5 mL of sodium hydroxide TS, and heat: no turbidity is produced. After cooling, add 5 mL of acetone: the solution is clear.

(2) Heavy metals <*1.07*>—Proceed with 1.0 g of Sulfamonomethoxine Hydrate according to Method 2, and perform the test. Prepare the control solution with 2.0 mL of Standard Lead Solution (not more than 20 ppm).

(3) Arsenic <*1.11*>—Prepare the test solution with 1.0 g of Sulfamonomethoxine Hydrate according to Method 3, and perform the test (not more than 2 ppm).

(4) Related substances—Dissolve 0.02 g of Sulfamonomethoxine Hydrate in 10 mL of ethanol (95), and use this solution as the sample solution. Pipet 1 mL of the sample solution, add ethanol (95) to make exactly 200 mL, and use this solution as the standard solution. Perform the test with these solutions as directed under Thin-layer Chromatography <*2.03*>. Spot 5 μL each of the sample solution and standard solution on a plate of silica gel with fluorescent indicator for thin-layer chromatography. Develop the plate with a mixture of 1-butanol and ammonia solution (28) (4:1) to a distance of about 10 cm, and air-dry the plate. Examine under ultraviolet light (main wavelength: 254 nm): the spots other than the principal spot obtained from the sample solution are not larger and not more intense than the spot from the standard solution.

Loss on drying <*2.41*> 4.5 - 6.5% (1 g, 105°C, 4 hours).

Residue on ignition <*2.44*> Not more than 0.10% (1 g).

Assay Weigh accurately about 0.5 g of Sulfamonomethoxine Hydrate, previously dried, dissolve in 5 mL of hydrochloric acid and 50 mL of water, add 10 mL of a solution of potassium bromide (3 in 10), cool below 15°C, and titrate <*2.50*> with 0.1 mol/L sodium nitrite VS (potentiometric titration or amperometric titration).

Each mL of 0.1 mol/L sodium nitrite VS
= 28.03 mg of $C_{11}H_{12}N_4O_3S$

Containers and storage Containers—Well-closed containers.

Storage—Light-resistant.

Sulfisoxazole

Sulfafurazole

スルフイソキサゾール

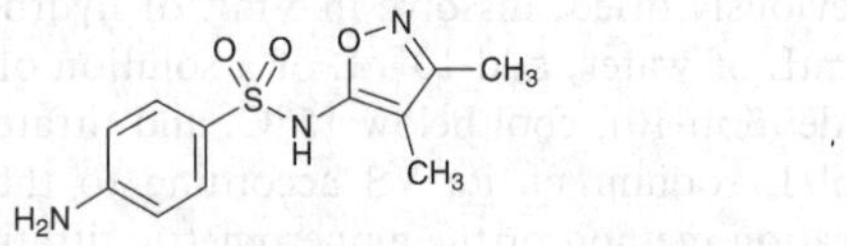

$C_{11}H_{13}N_3O_3S$: 267.30
4-Amino-*N*-(3,4-dimethylisoxazol-5-yl)benzenesulfonamide
[*127-69-5*]

Sulfisoxazole, when dried, contains not less than 99.0% of sulfisoxazole ($C_{11}H_{13}N_3O_3S$).

Description Sulfisoxazole occurs as white, crystals or crystalline powder. It is odorless, and has a slightly bitter taste.

It is freely soluble in pyridine and in *n*-butylamine, soluble in methanol, sparingly soluble in ethanol (95), slightly soluble in acetic acid (100), and very slightly soluble in water and in diethyl ether.

It dissolves in dilute hydrochloric acid, in sodium hydroxide TS and in ammonia TS.

It is gradually colored by light.

Identification **(1)** Dissolve 0.01 g of Sulfisoxazole in 1 mL of dilute hydrochloric acid and 4 mL of water: the solution responds to Qualitative Tests <*1.09*> for primary aromatic amines.

(2) Dissolve 0.02 g of Sulfisoxazole in 5 mL of water and 1 mL of *n*-butylamine, add 2 to 3 drops of copper (II) sulfate TS, and shake well. Add 5 mL of chloroform, shake, and allow to stand: a blue-green color develops in the chloroform layer.

(3) Dissolve 0.01 g of Sulfisoxazole in 1 mL of pyridine, add 2 drops of copper (II) sulfate TS, and shake. Add 3 mL of water and 5 mL of chloroform, shake, and allow to stand: a light yellow-brown color develops in the chloroform layer.

(4) To 0.5 g of Sulfisoxazole add 2 mL of acetic acid (100), dissolve by heating under a reflux condenser, add 1 mL of acetic anhydride, and boil for 10 minutes. Add 10 mL of water, cool, and alkalize with about 7 mL of a solution of sodium hydroxide (3 in 10). Filter, if necessary, immediately acidify by adding acetic acid (100) dropwise, collect the produced precipitate, recrystallize from methanol, and dry at 105°C for 1 hour: the crystals melt <*2.60*> between 208°C and 210°C.

Melting point <*2.60*> 192 - 196°C (with decomposition).

Purity **(1)** Clarity and color of solution—Dissolve 1.0 g of Sulfisoxazole in 5 mL of sodium hydroxide TS and 20 mL of water: the solution is clear and colorless to pale yellow.

(2) Acidity—To 1.0 g of Sulfisoxazole add 50 mL of water, warm at 70°C for 5 minutes, allow to stand in an ice bath for 1 hour, and filter. To 25 mL of the filtrate add 2 drops of methyl red TS and 0.20 mL of 0.1 mol/L sodium hydroxide VS: a yellow color develops.

(3) Heavy metals <*1.07*>—Proceed with 1.0 g of Sulfisoxazole according to Method 2, and perform the test. Prepare the control solution with 2.0 mL of Standard Lead Solution (not more than 20 ppm).

Loss on drying <*2.41*> Not more than 0.5% (2 g, 105°C,

4 hours).

Residue on ignition ⟨*2.44*⟩ Not more than 0.1% (1 g).

Assay Weigh accurately about 1 g of Sulfisoxazole, previously dried, dissolve in 50 mL of methanol by warming, cool and titrate ⟨*2.50*⟩ with 0.2 mol/L sodium hydroxide VS (indicator: 3 drops of phenolphthalein TS). Perform a blank determination in the same manner using a mixture of 50 mL of methanol and 18 mL of water, and make any necessary correction.

Each mL of 0.2 mol/L sodium hydroxide VS
= 53.46 mg of $C_{11}H_{13}N_3O_3S$

Containers and storage Containers—Well-closed containers.

Storage—Light-resistant.

Sulfobromophthalein Sodium

スルホブロモフタレインナトリウム

$C_{20}H_8Br_4Na_2O_{10}S_2$: 838.00
Disodium 5,5′-(4,5,6,7-tetrabromo-3-oxo-1,3-dihydroisobenzofuran-1,1-diyl)bis(2-hydroxybenzenesulfonate)
[*71-67-0*]

Sulfobromophthalein Sodium, when dried, contains not less than 96.0% and not more than 104.0% of sulfobromophthalein sodium ($C_{20}H_8Br_4Na_2O_{10}S_2$).

Description Sulfobromophthalein Sodium occurs as a white crystalline powder. It is odorless.

It is soluble in water, and practically insoluble in ethanol (95) and in diethyl ether.

It is hygroscopic.

Identification **(1)** Dissolve 0.02 g of Sulfobromophthalein Sodium in 10 mL of water, and add 1 mL of sodium carbonate TS: a blue-purple color is produced. Add 1 mL of dilute hydrochloric acid to the solution: the color of the solution disappears.

(2) Transfer 0.2 g of Sulfobromophthalein Sodium to a porcelain crucible, mix well with 0.5 g of anhydrous sodium carbonate, and ignite until the mixture is charred. After cooling, add 15 mL of hot water to the residue, heat for 5 minutes on a water bath, filter, and render the filtrate slightly acid with hydrochloric acid: the solution responds to Qualitative Tests ⟨*1.09*⟩ for bromide, and (1) and (2) for sulfate.

(3) Sulfobromophthalein Sodium responds to Qualitative Tests ⟨*1.09*⟩ (1) for sodium salt.

pH ⟨*2.54*⟩ The pH of a solution of 1.0 g of Sulfobromophthalein Sodium in 20 mL of water is between 4.0 and 5.5.

Purity **(1)** Clarity and color of solution—Dissolve 0.5 g of Sulfobromophthalein Sodium in 10 mL of water: the solution is clear and colorless to pale yellow.

(2) Chloride ⟨*1.03*⟩—Perform the test with 2.0 g of Sulfobromophthalein Sodium. Prepare the control solution with 0.10 mL of 0.01 mol/L hydrochloric acid VS (not more than 0.002%).

(3) Sulfate—To 10 mL of a solution of Sulfobromophthalein Sodium (1 in 500) add 5 drops of dilute hydrochloric acid, heat to boil, and add 1 mL of hot barium chloride TS: the solution is clear when observed 1 minute after the addition of the barium chloride TS.

(4) Calcium—Weigh accurately about 5 g of Sulfobromophthalein Sodium, transfer to a porcelain dish, heat gently to char, and heat strongly between 700°C and 750°C until the residue is incinerated. After cooling, add 10 mL of dilute hydrochloric acid, and heat for 5 minutes on a water bath. Transfer the contents to a flask with 50 mL of water, and add 5 mL of 8 mol/L potassium hydroxide TS and 0.1 g of NN indicator. Titrate ⟨*2.50*⟩ with 0.01 mol/L disodium dihydrogen ethylenediamine tetraacetate VS until the red-purple color of the solution changes to blue.

Each mL of 0.01 mol/L disodium dihydrogen
ethylenediamine tetraacetate VS
= 0.4008 mg of Ca

The content of calcium (Ca: 40.08) is not more than 0.05%.

(5) Heavy metals ⟨*1.07*⟩—Proceed with 1.0 g of Sulfobromophthalein Sodium according to Method 2, and perform the test. Prepare the control solution with 2.0 mL of Standard Lead Solution (not more than 20 ppm).

(6) Arsenic ⟨*1.11*⟩—Transfer 0.65 g of Sulfobromophthalein Sodium to a crucible, add 10 mL of a solution of magnesium nitrate hexahydrate in ethanol (95) (1 in 50), fire to burn, then heat gently until the residue is incinerated. If any carbon remains, moisten the residue with a small amount of nitric acid, and incinerate again by ignition. After cooling, add 10 mL of dilute sulfuric acid, and heat until white fumes are evolved. After cooling, add 5 mL of water to the residue, and perform the test with this solution as the test solution (not more than 3.1 ppm).

Loss on drying ⟨*2.41*⟩ Not more than 5.0% (0.5 g, 105°C, 3 hours).

Residue on ignition ⟨*2.44*⟩ 14 – 19% (after drying, 0.5 g, 700 – 750°C).

Assay Dissolve about 0.1 g of Sulfobromophthalein Sodium, previously dried and accurately weighed, in water to make exactly 500 mL. Pipet 5 mL of this solution, and add a solution of anhydrous sodium carbonate (1 in 100) to make exactly 200 mL. Perform the test with this solution as directed under Ultraviolet-visible Spectrophotometry ⟨*2.24*⟩. Determine the absorbance A of this solution at the wavelength of maximum absorption at about 580 nm, using water as the blank.

Amount (mg) of sulfobromophthalein sodium
($C_{20}H_8Br_4Na_2O_{10}S_2$)
$= A/881 \times 200{,}000$

Containers and storage Containers—Tight containers.

Storage—Light-resistant.

Sulfobromophthalein Sodium Injection

スルホブロモフタレインナトリウム注射液

Sulfobromophthalein Sodium Injection is an aqueous Injection.

It contains not less than 94.0% and not more than 106.0% of the labeled amount of sulfobromophthalein sodium ($C_{20}H_8Br_4Na_2O_{10}S_2$: 838.00).

Method of preparation Prepare as directed under Injections, with Sulfobromophthalein Sodium.

Description Sulfobromophthalein Sodium Injection is a clear and colorless or pale yellow liquid.

pH: 5.0 – 6.0

Identification **(1)** Measure a volume of Sulfobromophthalein Sodium Injection, equivalent to 0.02 g of Sulfobromophthalein Sodium, and proceed as directed in the Identification (1) under Sulfobromophthalein Sodium.

(2) Measure a volume of Sulfobromophthalein Sodium Injection, equivalent to 0.1 g of Sulfobromophthalein Sodium, add 0.5 g of anhydrous sodium carbonate, and evaporate on a water bath to dryness. Ignite the residue until it is charred. Proceed as directed in the Identification (2) under Sulfobromophthalein Sodium.

Extractable volume <*6.05*> It meets the requirement.

Pyrogen <*4.04*> Add isotonic sodium chloride solution to Sulfobromophthalein Sodium Injection to make a 0.5 w/v% solution of Sulfobromophthalein Sodium. Inject into each of the rabbits 5 mL of this solution per kg of body mass: it meets the requirement.

Assay Measure exactly a volume of Sulfobromophthalein Sodium Injection, equivalent to about 0.1 g of sulfobromophthalein sodium ($C_{20}H_8Br_4Na_2O_{10}S_2$), add water to make exactly 500 mL, and proceed as directed in the Assay under Sulfobromophthalein Sodium.

Amount (mg) of sulfobromophthalein sodium ($C_{20}H_8Br_4Na_2O_{10}S_2$)
$= A/881 \times 200{,}000$

Containers and storage Containers—Hermetic containers.
Storage—Light-resistant.

Sulfur

イオウ

S: 32.07

Sulfur, when dried, contains not less than 99.5% of sulfur (S).

Description Sulfur occurs as a light yellow to yellow powder. It is odorless and tasteless.

It is freely soluble in carbon disulfide, and practically insoluble in water, in ethanol (95) and in diethyl ether.

Identification **(1)** Ignite Sulfur: it burns with a blue flame and gives a pungent odor of sulfur dioxide.

(2) Dissolve 5 mg of Sulfur in 5 mL of sodium hydroxide TS by heating in a water bath, cool, and add 1 drop of sodium pentacyanonitrosylferrate (III) TS: a blue-purple color develops.

(3) Boil 1 mg of Sulfur with 2 mL of pyridine and 0.2 mL of sodium hydrogen carbonate TS: a blue color develops.

Purity **(1)** Clarity of solution—Dissolve 1.0 g of Sulfur in a mixture of 20 mL of a solution of sodium hydroxide (1 in 6) and 2 mL of ethanol (95) by boiling: the solution is clear. Dissolve 2.0 g of Sulfur in 10 mL of carbon disulfide: the solution is almost clear or slightly opalescent.

(2) Acidity or alkalinity—Shake 2.0 g of Sulfur with 50 mL of freshly boiled and cooled water, and add 2 drops of phenolphthalein TS: no red color develops. Further add 1.0 mL of 0.1 mol/L sodium hydroxide VS: a red color develops.

(3) Arsenic <*1.11*>—Prepare the test solution with 0.20 g of Sulfur according to Method 3, and perform the test (not more than 10 ppm).

Loss on drying <*2.41*> Not more than 1.0% (1 g, in vacuum, not more than 0.67 kPa, silica gel, 4 hours).

Residue on ignition <*2.44*> Not more than 0.2% (1 g).

Assay Weigh accurately about 0.4 g of Sulfur, previously dried, dissolve in 20 mL of potassium hydroxide-ethanol TS and 10 mL of water by boiling, cool, and add water to make exactly 100 mL. Transfer exactly 25 mL of the solution to a 400-mL beaker, add 50 mL of hydrogen peroxide TS, and heat on a water bath for 1 hour. Acidify the solution with dilute hydrochloric acid, add 200 mL of water, heat to boil, add hot barium chloride TS dropwise until no more precipitate is formed, and heat on a water bath for 1 hour. Collect the precipitate, and wash with water until the last washing shows no opalescence with silver nitrate TS. Dry the precipitate, heat strongly to constant mass, and weigh as barium sulfate ($BaSO_4$: 233.39). Perform a blank determination in the same manner, and make any necessary correction.

Amount (mg) of sulfur (S)
= amount (mg) of barium sulfate ($BaSO_4$) $\times$ 0.13739

Containers and storage Containers—Well-closed containers.

Sulfur and Camphor Lotion

イオウ・カンフルローション

Method of preparation

Sulfur	60 g
d-Camphor or *dl*-Camphor	5 g
Hydroxypropylcellulose	4 g
Calcium Hydroxide	1 g
Ethanol	4 mL
Water, Purified Water or Purified Water in Containers	a sufficient quantity
To make	1000 mL

Dissolve Hydroxypropylcellulose in 200 mL of Water, Purified Water or Purified Water in Containers. Add this solution in small portions to the triturate of Sulfur with the Ethanol solution of *d*-Camphor or *dl*-Camphor, and triturate again the mixture. Separately, dissolve Calcium Hydroxide in 500 mL of Water, Purified Water or Purified Water in Containers, stopper tightly, shake, and allow to stand. Add 300 mL of this supernatant liquid to the above mixture, then add Water, Purified Water or Purified Water in Containers to make 1000 mL, and shake thoroughly.

Description Sulfur and Camphor Lotion is a light yellow suspension.

A part of the components separates out on standing.

Identification **(1)** To 5 mL of well shaken Sulfur and Camphor Lotion add 25 mL of water, and centrifuge [use this supernatant liquid for test (3)]. To 0.02 g of the precipitate add 2 mL of pyridine and 0.2 mL of sodium hydrogen carbonate TS, and boil: a blue color develops (sulfur).

(2) To 10 mL of well shaken Sulfur and Camphor Lotion add 5 mL of diethyl ether, and mix. Separate the diethyl ether layer, and filter through a pledget of cotton. Wash the cotton with a small portion of diethyl ether, combine the washings with the filtrate, and distil cautiously on a water bath to remove the diethyl ether. Dissolve the residue in 1 mL of methanol, add 1 mL of 2,4-dinitrophenylhydrazine TS, and heat for about 2 minutes on a water bath. Cool, dilute with water to make about 5 mL, and allow to stand. Filter the produced precipitate through a glass filter (G4), and wash the residue on the filter with water until the last washing is colorless. Dissolve the residue in 10 mL of ethanol (95), add 5 mL of sodium hydroxide TS, and allow to stand for 2 minutes: a red color develops (*d*-camphor or *dl*-camphor).

(3) The supernatant liquid obtained in (1) responds to Qualitative Tests <*1.09*> (2) and (3) for calcium salt.

Containers and storage Containers—Tight containers.

Sulfur, Salicylic Acid and Thianthol Ointment

イオウ·サリチル酸·チアントール軟膏

Method of preparation

Sulfur	100 g
Salicylic Acid, finely powdered	30 g
Thianthol	100 mL
Zinc Oxide, very finely powdered	100 g
Simple Ointment or a suitable ointment base	a sufficient quantity
To make	1000 g

Prepare as directed under Ointments, with above ingredients.

Description Sulfur, Salicylic Acid and Thianthol Ointment is light yellow in color.

Identification **(1)** Stir well 0.5 g of Sulfur, Salicylic Acid and Thianthol Ointment with 10 mL of water while heating, cool, and filter. To 1 mL of the filtrate add 5 mL of iron (III) nitrate TS: a purple color is produced (salicylic acid).

(2) Shake 1 g of Sulfur, Salicylic Acid and Thianthol Ointment with 20 mL of diethyl ether, remove the supernatant liquid and floating materials. Wash the residue with 10 mL of diethyl ether, and remove the diethyl ether by suction. To the residue add 2 mL of pyridine and 0.2 mL of sodium hydrogen carbonate TS, and boil: a light blue to blue color is produced (sulfur).

(3) To 1 g of Sulfur, Salicylic Acid and Thianthol Ointment add 15 mL of ethanol (95), stir well while warming on a water bath, cool, and filter. Use the filtrate as the sample solution. Dissolve 0.01 g each of salicylic acid and thianthol in 5 mL of ethanol (95), and use these solutions as the standard solution (1) and standard solution (2). Perform the test with these solutions as directed under Thin-layer Chromatography <*2.03*>. Spot 5 μL each of the sample solution and standard solutions (1) and (2) on a plate of silica gel with fluorescent indicator for thin-layer chromatography. Develop the plate with a mixture of chloroform, acetone and acetic acid (100) (45:5:1) to a distance of about 10 cm, and air-dry the plate. Examine under ultraviolet light (main wavelength: 254 nm): the spots of each component obtained from the sample solution and standard solutions (1) and (2) show the same *R*f value. Spray iron (III) chloride TS upon the plate evenly: the spot from the standard solution (1) and that from the corresponding sample solution reveal a purple color.

Containers and storage Containers—Tight containers.

Sulindac

スリンダク

$C_{20}H_{17}FO_3S$: 356.41

(1*Z*)-(5-Fluoro-2-methyl-1-{4-[(*RS*)-methylsulfinyl]benzylidene}-1*H*-inden-3-yl)acetic acid

[*38194-50-2*]

Sulindac, when dried, contains not less than 99.0% and not more than 101.0% of sulindac ($C_{20}H_{17}FO_3S$).

Description Sulindac occurs as a yellow crystalline powder.

It is sparingly soluble in methanol and in ethanol (99.5), and practically insoluble in water.

A solution of Sulindac in methanol (1 in 100) shows no optical rotation.

Melting point: about 184°C (with decomposition).

Identification **(1)** Dissolve 15 mg of Sulindac in 1000 mL of a solution of hydrochloric acid in methanol (1 in 120). Determine the absorption spectrum of this solution as directed under Ultraviolet-visible Spectrophotometry <*2.24*> and compare the spectrum with the Reference Spectrum: both spectra exhibit similar intensities of absorption at the same wavelengths.

(2) Determine the infrared absorption spectrum of Sulindac as directed in the potassium bromide disc method under Infrared Spectrophotometry <*2.25*>, and compare the spectrum with the Reference Spectrum: both spectra exhibit similar intensities of absorption at the same wave numbers.

Purity **(1)** Heavy metals <*1.07*>—Proceed with 2.0 g of Sulindac according to Method 2 and perform the test. Prepare the control solution with 2.0 mL of Standard Lead Solution (not more than 10 ppm).

(2) Arsenic <*1.11*>—Prepare the test solution with 1.0 g of Sulindac according to Method 3 and perform the test (not more than 2 ppm).

(3) Related substances—Dissolve 0.25 g of Sulindac in 10 mL of methanol and use this solution as the sample solution. Pipet 1 mL of the sample solution and add methanol to make exactly 100 mL. Pipet 5 mL, 4 mL and 2 mL of this solution, to each add methanol to make exactly 10 mL, and use these solutions as the standard solutions (1), (2) and (3). Perform the test with these solutions as directed under Thin-layer Chromatography 〈*2.03*〉. Spot 4 μL each of the sample solution, standard solution (1), (2) and (3) on a plate of silica gel for thin-layer chromatography. Develop the plate with a mixture of ethyl acetate and acetic acid (100) (97:3) to a distance of about 17 cm, and air-dry the plate. Examine under ultraviolet light (main wavelength: 254 nm): the spots other than the principal spot obtained from the sample solution are not more intense than the spot from the standard solution (1), and the total intensity of spots other than the principal spot from the sample solution is not more than 1.0% calculated on the basis of intensities of the spots from the standard solution (1), (2) and (3).

Loss on drying 〈*2.41*〉 Not more than 0.5% (1 g, in vacuum not exceeding 0.7 kPa, 100°C, 2 hours).

Residue on ignition 〈*2.44*〉 Not more than 0.1% (1 g, platinum crucible).

Assay Weigh accurately about 0.3 g of Sulindac, previously dried, dissolve in 50 mL of methanol and titrate 〈*2.50*〉 with 0.1 mol/L sodium hydroxide VS (potentiometric titration). Perform a blank determination in the same manner, and make any necessary correction.

Each mL of 0.1 mol/L sodium hydroxide VS
= 35.64 mg of $C_{20}H_{17}FO_3S$

Containers and storage Containers—Tight containers.

Sulpiride

スルピリド

$C_{15}H_{23}N_3O_4S$: 341.43
N-(1-Ethylpyrolidin-2-ylmethyl)-2-methoxy-5-sulfamoylbenzamide
[*15676-16-1*]

Sulpiride, when dried, contains not less than 98.5% and not more than 101.0% of sulpiride ($C_{15}H_{23}N_3O_4S$).

Description Sulpiride is a white crystalline powder.

It is freely soluble in acetic acid (100) and in dilute acetic acid, sparingly soluble in methanol, slightly soluble in ethanol (99.5), and practically insoluble in water.

It is soluble in 0.05 mol/L sulfuric acid TS.

A solution of Sulpiride in methanol (1 in 100) shows no optical rotation.

Melting point: about 178°C (with decomposition).

Identification **(1)** Dissolve 0.1 g of Sulpiride in 0.05 mol/L sulfuric acid TS to make 100 mL. Dilute 5 mL of the solution with water to make 100 mL. Determine the absorption spectrum of the solution as directed under Ultraviolet-visible Spectrophotometry 〈*2.24*〉, using water as the blank, and compare the spectrum with the Reference Spectrum: both spectra exhibit similar intensities of absorption at the same wavelengths.

(2) Determine the infrared absorption spectrum of Sulpiride as directed in the potassium bromide disk method under Infrared Spectrophotometry 〈*2.25*〉, and compare the spectrum with the Reference Spectrum: both spectra exhibit similar intensities of absorption at the same wave numbers.

Purity **(1)** Clarity and color of solution—Dissolve 2.0 g of Sulpiride in 7 mL of dilute acetic acid, and add water to make 20 mL: the solution is clear. Perform the test with the solution as directed under Ultraviolet-visible Spectrophotometry 〈*2.24*〉, using water as the blank: the absorbance at a wavelength of 450 nm does not exceed 0.020.

(2) Heavy metals 〈*1.07*〉—Proceed with 2.0 g of Sulpiride as directed under Method 2, and perform the test. Prepare the control solution with 2.0 mL of Standard Lead Solution (not more than 10 ppm).

(3) Related substances—Dissolve 50 mg of Sulpiride in 10 mL of methanol, and use this solution as the sample solution. Dilute 1 mL of the sample solution, accurately measured, with methanol to make exactly 100 mL. Dilute 2 mL of this solution, accurately measured, with methanol to make exactly 10 mL, and use this solution as the standard solution. Perform the test with these solutions as directed under Thin-layer Chromatography 〈*2.03*〉. Spot 20 μL each of the sample solution and standard solution on a plate of silica gel with fluorescent indicator for thin-layer chromatography. Develop the plate with a mixture of 1-butanol, water and acetic acid (100) (4:2:1) to a distance of about 10 cm, and air-dry the plate. Examine under ultraviolet light (main wavelength: 254 nm): the number of the spots other than the principal spot obtained from the sample solution is not more than 2, and they have no more intense than the spot from the standard solution. When the plate is exposed to iodine vapor for 30 minutes, the number of the spots other than the principal spot from the sample solution is not more than 2, and they have no more intense than the spot from the standard solution.

Loss on drying 〈*2.41*〉 Not more than 0.5% (1 g, 105°C, 3 hours).

Residue on ignition 〈*2.44*〉 Not more than 0.1% (1 g).

Assay Dissolve about 0.4 g of Sulpiride, previously dried and accurately weighed, in 80 mL of acetic acid (100), and titrate 〈*2.50*〉 with 0.1 mol/L perchloric acid VS (indicator: 2 drops of crystal violet TS) until the color of the solution changes from violet through blue to bluish green. Perform a blank determination in the same manner, and make any necessary correction.

Each mL of 0.1 mol/L perchloric acid VS
= 34.14 mg of $C_{15}H_{23}N_3O_4S$

Containers and storage Containers—Well-closed containers.

Sulpiride Capsules

スルピリドカプセル

Sulpiride Capsules contain not less than 95.0% and not more than 105.0% of the labeled amount of sulpiride ($C_{15}H_{23}N_3O_4S$: 341.43).

Method of preparation Prepare as directed under Capsules, with Sulpiride.

Identification Determine the absorption spectrum of the sample solution obtained in the Assay as directed under Ultraviolet-visible Spectrophotometry 〈*2.24*〉, using water as the blank: it exhibits a maximum between 289 nm and 293 nm.

Uniformity of dosage units <6.02> Perform the Mass variation test, or the Content uniformity test according to the following method: it meets the requirement.

To 1 capsule of Sulpiride Capsules add 30 mL of 0.05 mol/L sulfuric acid TS, shake for 30 minutes, add 0.05 mol/L sulfuric acid TS to make exactly V mL so that each mL contains about 1 mg of sulpiride ($C_{15}H_{23}N_3O_4S$), and filter the solution. Discard the first 20 mL of the filtrate, pipet 5 mL of the subsequent filtrate, add water to make exactly 100 mL, and use this solution as the sample solution. Proceed as directed in the Assay.

Amount (mg) of sulpiride ($C_{15}H_{23}N_3O_4S$)
$= M_S \times A_T/A_S \times V/50$

M_S: Amount (mg) of sulpiride for assay taken

Dissolution Being specified separately when the drug is granted approval based on the Law.

Assay Cut the capsule of not less than 20 Sulpiride Capsules, weigh accurately the mass of the contents, and powder. Weigh accurately a portion of the powder, equivalent to about 0.1 g of sulpiride ($C_{15}H_{23}N_3O_4S$), add 70 mL of 0.05 mol/L sulfuric acid TS, shake for 30 minutes, and add 0.05 mol/L sulfuric acid TS to make exactly 100 mL, and filter. Discard the first 20 mL of the filtrate, pipet 5 mL of the subsequent filtrate, add water to make exactly 100 mL, and use this solution as the sample solution. Separately, weigh accurately about 50 mg of sulpiride for assay, previously dried at 105°C for 3 hours, and dissolve in 0.05 m/L sulfuric acid TS to make exactly 50 mL. Pipet 5 mL of this solution, add water to make exactly 100 mL, and use this solution as the standard solution. Determine the absorbances, A_T and A_S, of the sample solution and standard solution at 291 nm as directed under Ultraviolet-visible Spectrophotometry <2.24>, using water as the blank.

Amount (mg) of sulpiride ($C_{15}H_{23}N_3O_4S$)
$= M_S \times A_T/A_S \times 2$

M_S: Amount (mg) of sulpiride for assay taken

Containers and storage Containers—Tight containers.

Sulpiride Tablets

スルピリド錠

Sulpiride Tablets contain not less than 95.0% and not more than 105.0% of the labeled amount of sulpiride ($C_{15}H_{23}N_3O_4S$: 341.43).

Method of preparation Prepare as directed under Tablets, with Sulpiride.

Identification Determine the absorption spectrum of the sample solution obtained in the Assay as directed under Ultraviolet-visible Spectrophotometry <2.24>, using water as the blank: it exhibits a maximum between 289 nm and 293 nm.

Uniformity of dosage units <6.02> Perform the Mass variation test, or the Content uniformity test according to the following method: it meets the requirement.

To 1 tablet of Sulpiride Tablets add 30 mL of 0.05 mol/L sulfuric acid TS, shake for 30 minutes, add 0.05 mol/L sulfuric acid TS to make exactly V mL so that each mL contains about 1 mg of sulpiride ($C_{15}H_{23}N_3O_4S$), and filter the solution. Discard the first 20 mL of the filtrate, pipet 5 mL of the subsequent filtrate, add water to make exactly 100 mL, and use this solution as the sample solution. Proceed as directed in the Assay.

Amount (mg) of sulpiride ($C_{15}H_{23}N_3O_4S$)
$= M_S \times A_T/A_S \times V/50$

M_S: Amount (mg) of sulpiride for assay taken

Dissolution <6.10> When the test is performed at 50 revolutions per minute according to the Paddle method, using 900 mL of 2nd fluid for dissolution test as the dissolution medium, the dissolution rate of a 50-mg tablet in 30 minutes is not less than 80%, that of a 100-mg tablet in 45 minutes is not less than 75%, and that of a 200-mg tablet in 45 minutes is not less than 70%.

Start the test with 1 tablet of Sulpiride Tablets, withdraw not less than 20 mL of the medium at the specified minute after starting the test, and filter through a membrane filter with a pore size not exceeding 0.5 μm. Discard not less than 10 mL of the first filtrate, pipet V mL of the subsequent filtrate, add the dissolution medium to make exactly V' mL so that each mL contains about 56 μg of sulpiride ($C_{15}H_{23}N_3O_4S$), and use this solution as the sample solution. Separately, weigh accurately about 28 mg of sulpiride for assay, previously dried at 105°C for 3 hours, and dissolve in the dissolution medium to make exactly 100 mL. Pipet 5 mL of this solution, add the dissolution medium to make exactly 25 mL, and use this solution as the standard solution. Determine the absorbances, A_T and A_S, at 291 nm of the sample solution and standard solution as directed under Ultraviolet-visible Spectrophotometry <2.24>.

Dissolution rate (%) with respect to the labeled amount of sulpiride ($C_{15}H_{23}N_3O_4S$)
$= M_S \times A_T/A_S \times V'/V \times 1/C \times 180$

M_S: Amount (mg) of sulpiride for assay taken
C: Labeled amount (mg) of sulpiride ($C_{15}H_{23}N_3O_4S$) in 1 tablet

Assay Weigh accurately, and powder not less than 20 Sulpiride Tablets. Weigh accurately a portion of the powder, equivalent to about 0.1 g of sulpiride ($C_{15}H_{23}N_3O_4S$), add 70 mL of 0.05 mol/L sulfuric acid TS, shake for 30 minutes, and add 0.05 mol/L sulfuric acid TS to make exactly 100 mL, and filter. Discard the first 20 mL of the filtrate, pipet 5 mL of the subsequent filtrate, add water to make exactly 100 mL, and use this solution as the sample solution. Separately, weigh accurately about 50 mg of sulpiride for assay, previously dried at 105°C for 3 hours, and dissolve in 0.05 mol/L sulfuric acid TS to make exactly 50 mL. Pipet 5 mL of this solution, add water to make exactly 100 mL, and use this solution as the standard solution. Determine the absorbances, A_T and A_S, of the sample solution and standard solution at 291 nm as directed under Ultraviolet-visible Spectrophotometry <2.24>, using water as the blank.

Amount (mg) of sulpiride ($C_{15}H_{23}N_3O_4S$)
$= M_S \times A_T/A_S \times 2$

M_S: Amount (mg) of sulpiride for assay taken

Containers and storage Containers—Tight containers.

Sulpyrine Hydrate

スルピリン水和物

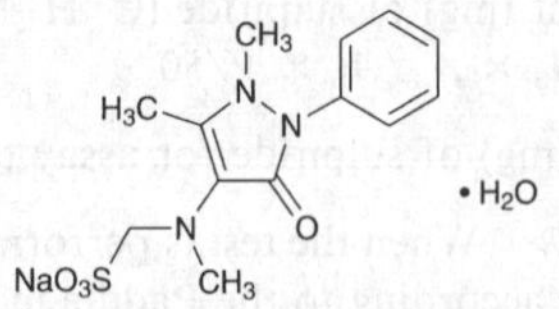

$C_{13}H_{16}N_3NaO_4S.H_2O$: 351.35
Monosodium [(1,5-dimethyl-3-oxo-2-phenyl-2,3-dihydro-1*H*-pyrazol-4-yl)(methyl)amino]methanesulfonate monohydrate
[*5907-38-0*]

Sulpyrine Hydrate contains not less than 98.5% of sulpyrine ($C_{13}H_{16}N_3NaO_4S$: 333.34), calculated on the dried basis.

Description Sulpyrine Hydrate occurs as white to light yellow, crystals or crystalline powder. It is odorless, and has a bitter taste.

It is very soluble in water, slightly soluble in ethanol (95), and practically insoluble in diethyl ether.

It is colored by light.

Identification **(1)** Add 2 drops of dilute sulfuric acid and 1 mL of chlorinated lime TS to 3 mL of a solution of Sulpyrine Hydrate (1 in 15): a deep blue color develops at first, but the color immediately turns red, then gradually changes to yellow.

(2) Boil 5 mL of a solution of Sulpyrine Hydrate (1 in 25) with 3 mL of dilute hydrochloric acid: the odor of sulfur dioxide is perceptible at first, and on further boiling, the odor of formaldehyde is perceptible.

(3) A solution of Sulpyrine Hydrate (1 in 10) responds to Qualitative Tests <*1.09*> for sodium salt.

Purity **(1)** Clarity of solution, and acidity or alkalinity—Dissolve 1.0 g of Sulpyrine Hydrate in 10 mL of water: the solution is clear and neutral.

(2) Sulfate <*1.14*>—Dissolve 0.20 g of Sulpyrine Hydrate in 0.05 mol/L hydrochloric acid VS to make 50 mL, and perform the test using this solution as the test solution. Prepare the control solution with 0.50 mL of 0.005 mol/L sulfuric acid VS and 0.05 mol/L hydrochloric acid VS to make 50 mL (not more than 0.120%).

(3) Heavy metals <*1.07*>—Proceed with 1.0 g of Sulpyrine Hydrate according to Method 2, and perform the test. Prepare the control solution with 2.0 mL of Standard Lead Solution (not more than 20 ppm).

(4) Merbuline—Transfer 0.10 g of Sulpyrine Hydrate with 2 mL of water and 1 mL of dilute sulfuric acid into a flask, cover with a funnel, and boil gently for 15 minutes. Cool, add 2 mL of a solution of sodium acetate trihydrate (1 in 2) and water to make 5 mL, shake this solution with 5 mL of benzaldehyde-saturated solution, and allow to stand for 5 minutes: the solution is clear.

(5) Chloroform-soluble substances—Mix, by frequent shaking, 1.0 g of Sulpyrine Hydrate and 10 mL of chloroform for 30 minutes. Collect the precipitate, wash with two 5-mL portions of chloroform, combine the washings with the filtrate, and evaporate on a water bath to dryness. Dry the residue at 105°C for 4 hours: the mass of the residue is not more than 5.0 mg.

Loss on drying <*2.41*> Not more than 6.0% (1 g, 105°C, 4 hours).

Assay Weigh accurately about 0.25 g of Sulpyrine Hydrate, dissolve in 100 mL of diluted hydrochloric acid (1 in 20), previously cooled below 10°C. Titrate <*2.50*> immediately with 0.05 mol/L iodine VS while keeping the temperature between 5°C and 10°C, until the color of the solution remains blue upon shaking vigorously for 1 minute after the addition of 0.05 mol/L iodine VS (indicator: 1 mL of starch TS).

Each mL of 0.05 mol/L iodine VS
= 16.67 mg of $C_{13}H_{16}N_3NaO_4S$

Containers and storage Containers—Tight containers.
Storage—Light-resistant.

Sulpyrine Injection

スルピリン注射液

Sulpyrine Injection is an aqueous injection.

It contains not less than 95.0% and not more than 105.0% of the labeled amount of sulpyrine hydrate ($C_{13}H_{16}N_3NaO_4S.H_2O$: 351.35).

Method of preparation Prepare as directed under Injections, with Sulpyrine Hydrate.

Description Sulpyrine Injection is a clear, colorless or pale yellow liquid.

pH: 5.0 – 8.5

Identification **(1)** To a volume of Sulpyrine Injection, equivalent to 0.2 g of Sulpyrine Hydrate, add water to make 3 mL, then add 2 drops of dilute sulfuric acid and 1 mL of chlorinated lime TS: a deep blue color develops at first, and the color immediately turns red and gradually changes to yellow.

(2) To a volume of Sulpyrine Injection, equivalent to 0.2 g of Sulpyrine Hydrate, add water to make 5 mL, and boil this solution with 3 mL of dilute hydrochloric acid: the odor of sulfur dioxide is perceptible at first, and on further boiling the odor of formaldehyde is perceptible.

Extractable volume <*6.05*> It meets the requirement.

Foreign insoluble matter <*6.06*> Perform the test according to Method 1: it meets the requirement.

Insoluble particulate matter <*6.07*> It meets the requirement.

Sterility <*4.06*> Perform the test according to the Membrane filtration method: it meets the requirement.

Assay Pipet 2 mL of Sulpyrine Injection, dilute with water to exactly 100 mL. Measure exactly a volume (*V* mL) of this solution, equivalent to about 50 mg of sulpyrine hydrate ($C_{13}H_{16}N_3NaO_4S.H_2O$), and add water to make exactly 100 mL. Pipet 5 mL of this solution, add water to exactly 100 mL, and use this solution as the sample solution. Weigh accurately about 50 mg of sulpyrine for assay (previously determine the loss on drying <*2.41*> under the same conditions as Sulpyrine Hydrate), and dissolve in water to make exactly 100 mL. Pipet 5 mL of this solution, add water to exactly 100 mL, and use this solution as the standard solution. Pipet 2 mL each of the sample solution and standard solution into separate 25-mL volumetric flasks, add 5 mL of ethanol (95), 2 mL of a solution of 4-dimethylaminocinnamaldehyde in ethanol (95) (1 in 250) and 2 mL of acetic acid (100) to each of these solutions, shake well, allow to stand for 15 minutes, and add water to make 25 mL. Perform the test with these solutions as directed under Ultraviolet-visible Spectrophotometry <2.24>, using a solution prepared with 2 mL of water in the same manner as the blank. Determine the absorbances, A_T and A_S, of the subsequent solutions of the sample solution and the standard solution at 510 nm.

Amount (mg) of sulpyrine hydrate ($C_{13}H_{16}N_3NaO_4S.H_2O$) in 1 mL of Sulpyrine Injection

$$= M_S \times A_T/A_S \times 50/V \times 1.054$$

M_S: Amount (mg) of sulpyrine for assay taken, calculated on the dried basis

Containers and storage Containers—Hermetic containers, and colored containers may be used.

Storage—Light-resistant, and under nitrogen atmosphere.

Sultamicillin Tosilate Hydrate

スルタミシリントシル酸塩水和物

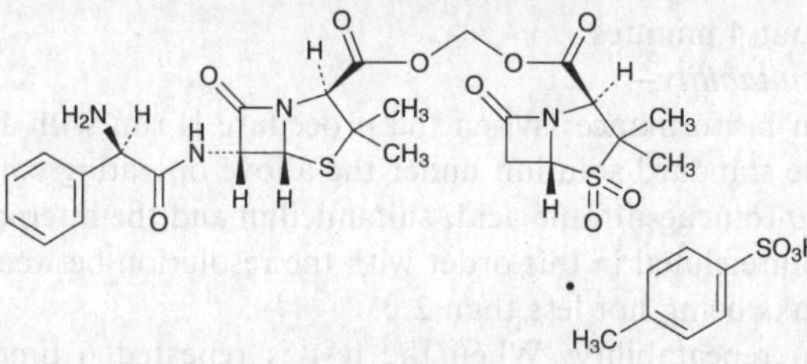

$C_{25}H_{30}N_4O_9S_2.C_7H_8O_3S.2H_2O$: 802.89
(2*S*,5*R*)-(3,3-Dimethyl-4,4,7-trioxo-4-thia-1-azabicyclo[3.2.0]hept-2-ylcarbonyloxy)methyl (2*S*,5*R*,6*R*)-6-[(2*R*)-2-amino-2-phenylacetylamino]-3,3-dimethyl-7-oxo-4-thia-1-azabicyclo[3.2.0]heptane-2-carboxylate mono-4-toluenesulfonate dihydrate
[*83105-70-8*, anhydride]

Sultamicillin Tosilate Hydrate contains not less than 698 μg (potency) and not more than 800 μg (potency) per mg, calculated on the anhydrous and residual solvent-free basis. The potency of Sultamicillin Tosilate Hydrate is expressed as mass (potency) of sultamicillin ($C_{25}H_{30}N_4O_9S_2$: 594.66).

Description Sultamicillin Tosilate Hydrate occurs as a white to yellowish white crystalline powder.

It is freely soluble in acetonitrile, in methanol and in ethanol (99.5), and very slightly soluble in water.

Identification (1) Determine the absorption spectrum of a solution of Sultamicillin Tosilate Hydrate in methanol (1 in 1000) as directed under Ultraviolet-visible Spectrophotometry <2.24>, and compare the spectrum with the Reference Spectrum or the spectrum of a solution of Sultamicillin Tosilate RS prepared in the same manner as the sample solution: both spectra exhibit similar intensities of absorption at the same wavelengths.

(2) Determine the infrared absorption spectrum of Sultamicillin Tosilate Hydrate as directed in the paste method under Infrared Spectrophotometry <2.25>, and compare the spectrum with the Reference Spectrum or the spectrum of Sultamicillin Tosilate RS: both spectra exhibit similar intensities of absorption at the same wave numbers.

Optical rotation <2.49> $[\alpha]_D^{20}$: +173 – +187° (0.5 g calculated on the anhydrous bases, a mixture of water and acetonitrile (3:2), 25 mL, 100 mm).

Purity (1) Heavy metals <1.07>—Proceed with 1.0 g of Sultamicillin Tosilate Hydrate according to Method 2, and perform the test. Prepare the control solution with 2.0 mL Standard Lead Solution (not more than 20 ppm).

(2) Ampicillin—Perform the procedure rapidly. Weigh accurately about 20 mg of Sultamicillin Tosilate Hydrate, dissolve in the mobile phase to make exactly 50 mL, and use this solution as the sample solution. Separately, weigh accurately an amount of Ampicillin RS, equivalent to about 20 mg (potency), dissolve in the mobile phase to make exactly 100 mL. Pipet 6 mL of this solution, add the mobile phase to make exactly 100 mL, and use this solution as the standard solution. Perform the test with exactly 25 μL each of the sample solution and standard solution as directed under Liquid Chromatography <2.01> according to the following conditions, and determine the peak area of ampicillin by the automatic integration method: the peak area obtained from the sample solution is not larger than that from the standard solution.

Operating conditions—

Detector, column, and column temperature: Proceed as directed in the operating conditions in the Assay.

Mobile phase: Dissolve 3.12 g of sodium dihydrogen phosphate dihydrate in about 750 mL of water, adjust to pH 3.0 with diluted phosphoric acid (1 in 10), and add water to make 1000 mL. To 80 mL of acetonitrile for liquid chromatography add this solution to make 1000 mL.

Flow rate: Adjust so that the retention time of ampicillin is about 14 minutes.

System suitability—

System performance: Dissolve 12 mg of Ampicillin RS, 4 mg of Sulbactam RS and 4 mg of *p*-toluenesulfonic acid monohydrate in 1000 mL of the mobile phase. When the procedure is run with 25 μL of this solution under the above operating conditions, sulbactam, *p*-toluenesulfonic acid and ampicillin are eluted in this order, and the resolutions between these peaks are not less than 2.0, respectively.

System repeatability: When the test is repeated 6 times with 25 μL of the standard solution under the above operating conditions, the relative standard deviation of the peak area of ampicillin is not more than 2.0%.

(3) Sulbactam—Perform the procedure rapidly. Weigh accurately about 20 mg of Sultamicillin Tosilate Hydrate, dissolve in the mobile phase to make exactly 50 mL, and use this solution as the sample solution. Separately, weigh accurately an amount of Sulbactam RS, equivalent to about 20 mg (potency), dissolve in the mobile phase to make exactly 100 mL. Pipet 2 mL of this solution, add the mobile phase to make exactly 100 mL, and use this solution as the standard solution. Perform the test with exactly 25 μL each of the sample solution and standard solution as directed under Liquid Chromatography <2.01> according to the following conditions, and determine the peak area of sulbactam of each solution by the automatic integration method: the peak area obtained from the sample solution is not larger than that from the standard solution.

Operating conditions—

Proceed as directed in the operating conditions in the Purity (2).

System suitability—

Proceed as directed in the system suitability in the Purity (2).

(4) Penicilloic acids—Weigh accurately about 25 mg of Sultamicillin Tosilate Hydrate, dissolve in 1 mL of acetonitrile, and add 25 mL of 0.02 mol/L phosphate buffer solu-

tion (pH 3.0) in a 100-mL glass-stoppered flask. Add exactly 5 mL of 0.005 mol/L iodine VS, and allow to stand the stoppered flask for 5 minutes. Titrate <2.50> with 0.005 mol/L sodium thiosulfate VS (indicator: 1.0 mL of starch TS). Perform a blank determination in the same manner, and make any necessary correction. Calculate the amount of penicilloic acid ($C_{25}H_{34}N_4O_{11}S_2$: 630.69) by using the following equation: it is not more than 3.0%.

Each mL of 0.005 mol/L sodium thiosulfate VS
= 0.2585 mg of $C_{25}H_{34}N_4O_{11}S_2$

(5) Residual solvent *<2.46>*—Weigh accurately about 0.1 g of Sultamicillin Tosilate Hydrate, dissolve in 2 mL of methanol, add water to make exactly 20 mL, and use this solution as the sample solution. Separately, weigh accurately about 1 g of ethyl acetate, and mix with water to make exactly 200 mL. Pipet 2 mL of this solution, add 10 mL of methanol, then add water to make exactly 100 mL, and use this solution as the standard solution. Perform the test with exactly 5 μL each of the sample solution and standard solution as directed under Gas Chromatography *<2.02>* according to the following conditions, and determine the peak areas, A_T and A_S, of ethyl acetate in each solution. Calculate the amount of ethyl acetate by the following equation: not more than 2.0%.

Amount (%) of ethyl acetate $= M_S/M_T \times A_T/A_S \times 1/5$

M_S: Amount (mg) of ethyl acetate taken

M_T: Amount (mg) of the Sultamicillin Tosilate Hydrate taken

Operating conditions—

Detector: A hydrogen flame-ionization detector.

Column: A column 3 mm in inside diameter and 1 m in length, packed with porous styrene-divinylbenzene copolymer for gas chromatography (average pore diameter: 0.0085 μm, 300 – 400 m^2/g) (150 to 180 μm in particle diameter).

Column temperature: A constant temperature of about 155°C.

Carrier gas: Nitrogen.

Flow rate: Adjust so that the retention time of ethyl acetate is about 6 minutes.

System suitability—

System performance: When the procedure is run with 5 μL of the standard solution under the above operating conditions, the number of theoretical plates and the symmetry factor of the peak of ethyl acetate are not less than 500 and not more than 1.5, respectively.

System repeatability: When the test is repeated 6 times with 5 μL of the standard solution under the above operating conditions, the relative standard deviation of the peak area of ethyl acetate is not more than 5%.

Water *<2.48>* 4.0 – 6.0% (0.5 g, volumetric titration, direct titration).

Residue on ignition *<2.44>* Not more than 0.2% (1 g).

Assay Perform the procedure rapidly. Weigh accurately an amount of Sultamicillin Tosilate Hydrate and Sultamicillin Tosilate RS, equivalent to about 50 mg (potency), dissolve each in the mobile phase to make exactly 50 mL. Pipet 5 mL each of these solutions, add exactly 5 mL of the internal standard solution, add the mobile phase to make 25 mL, and use these solutions as the sample solution and the standard solution, respectively. Perform the test with 10 μL each of these solutions as directed under Liquid Chromatography *<2.01>* according to the following conditions, and calculate the ratios, Q_T and Q_S, of the peak area of sultamicillin to that of the internal standard in each solution.

Amount [μg (potency)] of sultamicillin ($C_{25}H_{30}N_4O_9S_2$)
$= M_S \times Q_T/Q_S \times 1000$

M_S: Amount [mg (potency)] of Sultamicillin Tosilate RS taken

Internal standard solution—A solution of isopropyl-4-aminobenzoate in the mobile phase (1 in 2500).

Operating conditions—

Detector: An ultraviolet absorption photometer (wavelength: 215 nm).

Column: A stainless steel column 3.9 mm in inside diameter and 30 cm in length, packed with octadecylsilanized silica gel for liquid chromatography (10 μm in particle diameter).

Column temperature: A constant temperature of about 35°C.

Mobile phase: Dissolve 3.12 g of sodium dihydrogenphosphate in about 750 mL of water, adjust to pH 3.0 with diluted phosphoric acid (1 in 10), and add water to make 1000 mL. To 400 mL of acetonitrile for liquid chromatography add this solution to make 1000 mL.

Flow rate: Adjust so that the retention time of sultamicillin is about 4 minutes.

System suitability—

System performance: When the procedure is run with 10 μL of the standard solution under the above operating conditions, *p*-toluenesulfonic acid, sultamicillin and the internal standard are eluted in this order with the resolution between these peaks being not less than 2.0.

System repeatability: When the test is repeated 6 times with 10 μL of the standard solution under the above operating conditions, the relative standard deviation of the peak area of sultamicillin is not more than 2.0%.

Containers and storage Containers—Tight containers.

Sultamicillin Tosilate Tablets

スルタミシリントシル酸塩錠

Sultamicillin Tosilate Tablets contains not less than 90.0% and not more than 105.0% of the labeled potency of sultamicillin ($C_{25}H_{30}N_4O_9S_2$: 594.66).

Method of preparation Prepare as directed under Tablets, with Sultamicillin Tosilate Hydrate.

Identification Powder Sultamicillin Tosilate Tablets, take a portion of the powder, equivalent to 7 mg (potency) of Sultamicillin Tosilate Hydrate, add 2 mL of methanol and shake well, then centrifuge this solution. To 1 mL of the supernatant liquid add 1 mL of hydroxylammonium chloride-ethanol TS, allow to stand for 3 minutes, then add 1 mL of acidic ammonium iron (III) sulfate TS: a red-brown color is produced.

Purity Penicilloic acid—Weigh accurately the mass of not less than 5 Sultamicillin Tosilate Tablets, and powder. Weigh accurately a portion of the powder, equivalent to about 30 mg (potency) of Sultamicillin Tosilate Hydrate, add 0.02 mol/L phosphate buffer (pH 3.0) and sonicate for 5 minutes with occasional shaking, then add 0.02 mol/L phosphate buffer (pH 3.0) to make exactly 50 mL. Filter this solution through a membrane filter with a pore size not exceeding 0.45 μm, and discard the first 5 mL of the filtrate. Pipet 10 mL of the subsequent filtrate into a glass-stoppered flask, add exactly 5 mL of 0.005 mol/L iodine VS, and stopper tightly. After standing for 5 minutes, titrate <*2.50*> this solution with 0.005 mol/L sodium thiosulfate VS (indicator: 1.0 mL of starch TS). Perform a blank determination in the same manner, and make any necessary correction: the amount of penicilloic acid ($C_{25}H_{34}N_4O_{11}S_2$: 630.69) is not more than 5.5%.

Each mL of 0.005 mol/L sodium thiosulfate VS
= 0.2585 mg of $C_{25}H_{34}N_4O_{11}S_2$

Uniformity of dosage units <*6.02*> Perform the Mass variation test, or the Content uniformity test according to the following method: it meets the requirement.

Perform the procedure within 2 hours after preparation of the sample solution and standard solution. To 1 tablet of Sultamicillin Tosilate Tablets add a suitable amount of the mobile phase, disperse the tablet by sonicating, and add the mobile phase to make exactly 200 mL. If it is necessary, filter or centrifuge. Pipet *V* mL of this solution, equivalent to about 5.6 mg (potency) of Sultamicillin Tosilate Hydrate, add exactly 5 mL of the internal standard solution, then add the mobile phase to make 25 mL, and use this solution as the sample solution. Separately, weigh accurately about 47 mg (potency) of Sultamicillin Tosilate RS, dissolve in the mobile phase to make exactly 25 mL. Pipet 3 mL of this solution, add exactly 5 mL of the internal standard solution, add the mobile phase to make 25 mL, and use this solution as the standard solution. Then, proceed as directed in the Assay under Sultamicillin Tosilate Hydrate.

Amount [mg (potency)] of Sultamicillin ($C_{25}H_{30}N_4O_9S_2$)
$= M_S \times Q_T/Q_S \times 24/V$

M_S: Amount [mg (potency)] of Sultamicillin Tosilate RS taken

Internal standard solution: A solution of isopropyl-4-aminobenzoate in the mobile phase (1 in 2500).

Dissolution <*6.10*> When the test is performed at 50 revolutions per minute according to the Paddle method, using 900 mL of water as the dissolution medium, the dissolution rate in 15 minutes of Sultamicillin Tosilate Tablets is not less than 75%.

Start the test with 1 tablet of Sultamicillin Tosilate Tablets, withdraw not less than 20 mL of the medium at the specified minute after starting the test, and filter through a membrane filter with a pore size not exceeding 0.45 μm. Discard not less than 10 mL of the first filtrate, pipet *V* mL of the subsequent filtrate, add water to make exactly *V′* mL so that each mL contains about 0.42 mg (potency) of sultamicillin ($C_{25}H_{30}N_4O_9S_2$), and use this solution as the sample solution. Separately, weigh accurately about 27 mg of *p*-toluenesulfonic acid monohydrate, previously dried in a desiccator using sulfuric acid as desiccant for 18 hours, dissolve in water to make exactly 200 mL, and use this solution as the standard solution. Perform the test with exactly 10 μL each of the sample solution and standard solution as directed under Liquid Chromatography <*2.01*> according to the following conditions, and determine the peak areas, A_T and A_S, of *p*-toluenesulfonic acid in each solution.

Dissolution rate (%) with respect to the labeled amount of sultamicillin ($C_{25}H_{30}N_4O_9S_2$)
$= M_S \times A_T/A_S \times V'/V \times 1/C \times 450 \times 3.126$

M_S: Amount (mg) of *p*-toluenesulfonic acid monohydrate taken

C: Labeled amount [mg (potency)] of sultamicillin ($C_{25}H_{30}N_4O_9S_2$) in 1 tablet

Operating conditions—

Detector: An ultraviolet absorption photometer (wavelength: 222 nm).

Column: A stainless steel column 4.6 mm in inside diameter and 15 cm in length, packed with octadecylsilanized silica gel for liquid chromatography (5 μm in particle diameter).

Column temperature: A constant temperature of about 35°C.

Mobile phase: Dissolve 13.6 g of potassium dihydrogen phosphate in water to make 1000 mL, and adjust to pH 5.5 with potassium hydroxide TS. To 950 mL of this solution add 50 mL of acetonitrile.

Flow rate: Adjust so that the retention time of *p*-toluenesulfonic acid is about 8 minutes.

System suitability—

System performance: When the procedure is run with 10 μL of the standard solution under the above operating conditions, the number of theoretical plates and the symmetry factor of the peak of *p*-toluenesulfonic acid are not less than 4000 and not more than 2.0, respectively.

System repeatability: When the test is repeated 6 times with 10 μL of the standard solution under the above operating conditions, the relative standard deviation of the peak area of *p*-toluenesulfonic acid is not more than 1.5%.

Assay Perform the procedure within 2 hours after the preparation of the sample solution and standard solution. Weigh accurately the mass of not less than 20 tablets of Sultamicillin Tosilate Tablets, and powder. Weigh accurately a portion of the powder, equivalent to about 50 mg (potency) of Sultamicillin Tosilate Hydrate, add 40 mL of the mobile phase, sonicate, and add the mobile phase to make exactly 50 mL. If it is necessary, filter or centrifuge. Pipet 5 mL of this solution, add exactly 5 mL of the internal standard solution, add the mobile phase to make 25 mL, and use this solution as the sample solution. Separately, weigh accurately about 50 mg (potency) of Sultamicillin Tosilate RS, dissolve in the mobile phase to make exactly 50 mL. Pipet 5 mL of this solution, add exactly 5 mL of the internal standard solution, add the mobile phase to make 25 mL, and use this solution as the standard solution. Then, proceed as directed in the Assay under Sultamicillin Tosilate Hydrate.

Amount [mg (potency)] of sultamicillin ($C_{25}H_{30}N_4O_9S_2$)
$= M_S \times Q_T/Q_S$

M_S: Amount [mg (potency)] of Sultamicillin Tosilate RS taken

Internal standard solution: A solution of isopropyl-4-aminobenzoate in the mobile phase (1 in 2500).

Containers and storage Containers—Tight containers.

Sultiame

スルチアム

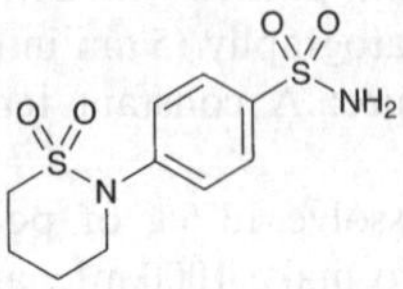

$C_{10}H_{14}N_2O_4S_2$: 290.36
4-(3,4,5,6-Tetrahydro-2*H*-1,2-thiazin-2-yl)benzenesulfonamide *S*,*S*-dioxide
[*61-56-3*]

Sultiame, when dried, contains not less than 98.5% of sultiame ($C_{10}H_{14}N_2O_4S_2$).

Description Sultiame occurs as white, crystals or crystalline powder. It is odorless, and has a slightly bitter taste.

It is very soluble in *N*,*N*-dimethylformamide, freely soluble in *n*-butylamine, slightly soluble in methanol and in ethanol (95), very slightly soluble in water, and practically insoluble in diethyl ether.

It dissolves in sodium hydroxide TS.

Identification **(1)** Dissolve 0.02 g of Sultiame in 5 mL of water and 1 mL of *n*-butylamine, add 2 to 3 drops of copper (II) sulfate TS, and shake well. To this solution add 5 mL of chloroform, shake, and allow to stand: a green color develops in the chloroform layer.

(2) Mix 0.1 g of Sultiame with 0.5 g of sodium carbonate decahydrate, and melt carefully: the gas evolved changes moistened red litmus paper to blue. After cooling, crush the fused substance with a glass rod, stir with 10 mL of water, and filter. To 4 mL of the filtrate add 2 drops of hydrogen peroxide (30), 5 mL of diluted hydrochloric acid (1 in 5) and 2 to 3 drops of barium chloride TS: a white precipitate is formed.

(3) Determine the absorption spectrum of a solution of Sultiame in methanol (1 in 100,000) as directed under Ultraviolet-visible Spectrophotometry *<2.24>*, and compare the spectrum with the Reference Spectrum: both spectra exhibit similar intensities of absorption at the same wavelengths.

Melting point *<2.60>* 185 – 188°C

Purity **(1)** Chloride *<1.03>*—Dissolve 1.0 g of Sultiame in 20 mL of sodium hydroxide TS by warming, cool, and add 2 mL of acetic acid (100) and water to make 100 mL. After shaking, filter, and discard the first 10 mL of the filtrate. To 40 mL of the subsequent filtrate add 6 mL of dilute nitric acid and water to make 50 mL, and perform the test using this solution as the test solution. Prepare the control solution as follows: to 0.25 mL of 0.01 mol/L hydrochloric acid VS add 8 mL of sodium hydroxide TS, 0.8 mL of acetic acid (100), 6 mL of dilute nitric acid and water to make 50 mL (not more than 0.022%).

(2) Sulfate *<1.14>*—Dissolve 1.0 g of Sultiame in 20 mL of sodium hydroxide TS by warming, cool, and add 8 mL of dilute hydrochloric acid and water to make 100 mL. After shaking, filter, and discard the first 10 mL of the filtrate. To 40 mL of the subsequent filtrate add 1 mL of dilute hydrochloric acid and water to make 50 mL, and perform the test using this solution as the test solution. Prepare the control solution as follows: to 0.40 mL of 0.005 mol/L sulfuric acid VS add 8 mL of sodium hydroxide TS, 4.2 mL of dilute hydrochloric acid and water to make 50 mL (not more than 0.048%).

(3) Heavy metals *<1.07>*—Proceed with 2.0 g of Sultiame according to Method 2, and perform the test. Prepare the control solution with 2.0 mL of Standard Lead Solution (not more than 10 ppm).

(4) Arsenic *<1.11>*—Prepare the test solution with 1.0 g of Sultiame according to Method 3, and perform the test (not more than 2 ppm).

(5) Related substances—Dissolve 0.10 g of Sultiame in methanol to make exactly 20 mL, and use this solution as the sample solution. Separately, dissolve 10 mg of sulfanilamide in methanol to make exactly 100 mL. Pipet 10 mL of this solution, add methanol to make exactly 100 mL, and use this solution as the standard solution. Perform the test with these solutions as directed under Thin-layer Chromatography *<2.03>*. Spot 20 μL each of the sample solution and standard solution on a plate of silica gel with fluorescent indicator for thin-layer chromatography. Develop the plate with a mixture of chloroform, methanol and ammonia solution (28) (30:8:1) to a distance of about 12 cm, and air-dry the plate. Examine under ultraviolet light (main wavelength: 254 nm): the spots other than the principal spot obtained from the sample solution are not more intense than the spot from the standard solution.

Loss on drying *<2.41>* Not more than 0.5% (1 g, 105°C, 3 hours).

Residue on ignition *<2.44>* Not more than 0.1% (1 g).

Assay Weigh accurately about 0.8 g of Sultiame, previously dried, dissolve in 70 mL of *N*,*N*-dimethylformamide, and titrate *<2.50>* with 0.2 mol/L tetramethylammonium hydroxide VS (potentiometric titration). Perform a blank determination in the same manner, and make any necessary correction.

Each mL of 0.2 mol/L tetramethylammonium hydroxide VS
= 58.07 mg of $C_{10}H_{14}N_2O_4S_2$

Containers and storage Containers—Well-closed containers.

Suxamethonium Chloride Hydrate

スキサメトニウム塩化物水和物

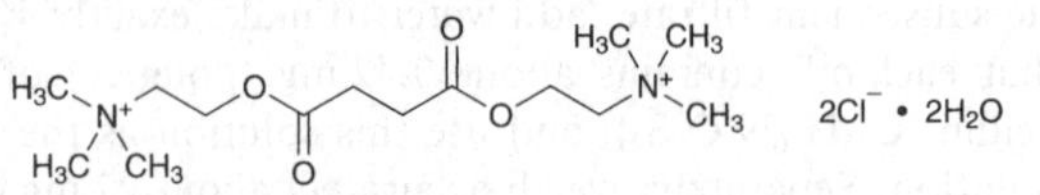

$C_{14}H_{30}Cl_2N_2O_4.2H_2O$: 397.34
2,2′-Succinyldioxybis(*N*,*N*,*N*-trimethylethylaminium) dichloride dihydrate
[*6101-15-1*]

Suxamethonium Chloride Hydrate contains not less than 98.0% of suxamethonium chloride ($C_{14}H_{30}Cl_2N_2O_4$: 361.31), calculated on the anhydrous basis.

Description Suxamethonium Chloride Hydrate occurs as a white crystalline powder.

It is freely soluble in water, in methanol and in acetic acid (100), slightly soluble in ethanol (95), very slightly soluble in acetic anhydride, and practically insoluble in diethyl ether.

Identification **(1)** Determine the infrared absorption spec-

trum of Suxamethonium Chloride Hydrate as directed in the potassium bromide disk method under Infrared Spectrophotometry <*2.25*>, and compare the spectrum with the Reference Spectrum: both spectra exhibit similar intensities of absorption at the same wave numbers.

(2) A solution of Suxamethonium Chloride Hydrate (1 in 20) responds to Qualitative Tests <*1.09*> for chloride.

pH <*2.54*> The pH of a solution of 0.1 g of Suxamethonium Chloride Hydrate in 10 mL of water is between 4.0 and 5.0.

Melting point <*2.60*> 159 - 164°C (hydrate form).

Purity **(1)** Clarity and color of solution—Dissolve 1.0 g of Suxamethonium Chloride Hydrate in 10 mL of water: the solution is clear and colorless.

(2) Related substances—Dissolve 0.25 g of Suxamethonium Chloride Hydrate in 5 mL of water, and use this solution as the sample solution. Pipet 1 mL of the sample solution, add water to make exactly 200 mL, and use this solution as the standard solution. Perform the test with these solutions as directed under Thin-layer Chromatography <*2.03*>. Spot 1 μL each of the sample solution and standard solution on a plate of cellulose for thin-layer chromatography. Develop the plate with a mixture of a solution of ammonium acetate (1 in 100), acetone, 1-butanol and formic acid (20:20:20:1) to a distance of about 10 cm, and dry the plate at 105°C for 15 minutes. Spray evenly hydrogen hexachloroplatinate (IV)-potassium iodide TS on the plate, and allow to stand for 15 minutes: the spots other than the principal spot from the sample solution are not more intense than the spot from the standard solution.

Water <*2.48*> 8.0 - 10.0% (0.4 g, volumetric titration, direct titration).

Residue on ignition <*2.44*> Not more than 0.1% (1 g).

Assay Weigh accurately about 0.4 g of Suxamethonium Chloride Hydrate, dissolve in 80 mL of a mixture of acetic anhydride and acetic acid (100) (7:3), and titrate <*2.50*> with 0.1 mol/L perchloric acid VS (potentiometric titration).

Each mL of 0.1 mol/L perchloric acid VS
= 18.07 mg of $C_{14}H_{30}Cl_2N_2O_4$

Containers and storage Containers—Tight containers.

Suxamethonium Chloride Injection

スキサメトニウム塩化物注射液

Suxamethonium Chloride Injection is an aqueous injection.

It contains not less than 93.0% and not more than 107.0% of the labeled amount of suxamethonium chloride ($C_{14}H_{30}Cl_2N_2O_4$: 361.31).

The concentration of Suxamethonium Chloride Injection should be stated as the amount of suxamethonium chloride ($C_{14}H_{30}Cl_2N_2O_4$).

Method of preparation Prepare as directed under Injections, with Suxamethonium Chloride Hydrate.

Description Suxamethonium Chloride Injection is a clear, colorless liquid.

Identification Take a volume of Suxamethonium Chloride Injection, equivalent to 0.05 g of Suxamethonium Chloride Hydrate, add water to make 10 mL, and use this solution as the sample solution. Separately, dissolve 0.05 g of suxamethonium chloride for thin-later chromatography in 10 mL of water, and use this solution as the standard solution. Perform the test with these solutions as directed under Thin-layer Chromatography <*2.03*>. Spot 1 μL each of the sample solution and standard solution on a plate of cellulose for thin-layer chromatography. Develop the plate with a mixture of a solution of ammonium acetate (1 in 100), acetone, 1-butanol and formic acid (20:20:20:1) to a distance of about 10 cm, and dry the plate at 105°C for 15 minutes. Spray evenly hydrogen hexachloroplatinate (IV)-potassium iodide TS on the plate: the spots obtained from the sample solution and standard solution are blue-purple in color and have similar *Rf* value.

pH <*2.54*> 3.0 - 5.0

Purity Hydrolysis products—Perform the preliminary neutralization with 0.1 mol/L sodium hydroxide VS in the Assay: not more than 0.7 mL of 0.1 mol/L sodium hydroxide VS is required for each 200 mg of Suxamethonium Chloride ($C_{14}H_{30}Cl_2N_2O_4$) taken.

Bacterial endotoxins <*4.01*> Less than 2.0 EU/mg.

Extractable volume <*6.05*> It meets the requirement.

Foreign insoluble matter <*6.06*> Perform the test according to Method 1: it meets the requirement.

Insoluble particulate matter <*6.07*> It meets the requirement.

Sterility <*4.06*> Perform the test according to the Membrane filtration method: it meets the requirement.

Assay Transfer to a separator an accurately measured volume of Suxamethonium Chloride Injection, equivalent to about 0.2 g of suxamethonium chloride ($C_{14}H_{30}Cl_2N_2O_4$), add 30 mL of freshly boiled and cooled water, and wash the solution with five 20-mL portions of diethyl ether. Combine the diethyl ether washings, and extract the combined diethyl ether layer with two 10-mL portions of freshly boiled and cooled water. Wash the combined water extracts with two 10-mL portions of diethyl ether. Combine the solution and the water extracts, add 2 drops of bromothymol blue TS, and neutralize with 0.1 mol/L sodium hydroxide VS. Add accurately measured 25 mL of 0.1 mol/L sodium hydroxide VS, and boil for 40 minutes under a reflux condenser, and cool. Titrate <*2.50*> the excess sodium hydroxide with 0.1 mol/L hydrochloric acid VS. Transfer 50 mL of the freshly boiled and cooled water to a flask, add 2 drops of bromothymol blue TS, neutralize the solution with 0.1 mol/L sodium hydroxide VS, and perform a blank determination in the same manner.

Each mL of 0.1 mol/L sodium hydroxide VS
= 18.07 mg of $C_{14}H_{30}Cl_2N_2O_4$

Containers and storage Containers—Hermetic containers.

Storage—Not exceeding 5°C, and avoid freezing.

Shelf life 12 months after preparation.

Suxamethonium Chloride for Injection

注射用スキサメトニウム塩化物

Suxamethonium Chloride for Injection is a preparation for injection which is dissolved before use.

It contains not less than 93.0% and not more than 107.0% of the labeled amount of suxamethonium chloride ($C_{14}H_{30}Cl_2N_2O_4$: 361.31).

The concentration of Suxamethonium Chloride for Injection should be stated as the amount of suxamethonium chloride ($C_{14}H_{30}Cl_2N_2O_4$).

Method of preparation Prepare as directed under Injections, with Suxamethonium Chloride Hydrate.

Description Suxamethonium Chloride for Injection occurs as a white, crystalline powder or mass.

Identification Take an amount of Suxamethonium Chloride for Injection, equivalent to 0.05 g of Suxamethonium Chloride Hydrate, dissolve in water to make 10 mL, and use this solution as the sample solution. Separately, dissolve 0.05 g of suxamethonium chloride for thin-layer chromatography in 10 mL of water, and use this solution as the standard solution. Perform the test with these solutions as directed under Thin-layer Chromatography *<2.03>*. Spot 1 μL each of the sample solution and standard solution on a plate of cellulose for thin-layer chromatography. Develop the plate with a mixture of a solution of ammonium acetate (1 in 100), acetone, 1-butanol and formic acid (20:20:20:1) to a distance of about 10 cm, and dry the plate at 105°C for 15 minutes. Spray evenly hydrogen hexachloroplatinate (IV)-potassium iodide TS on the plate: the spots obtained from the sample solution and standard solution are blue-purple in color and have similar *R*f value.

pH *<2.54>* The pH of a solution of 0.1 g of Suxamethonium Chloride for Injection in 10 mL of water is between 4.0 and 5.0.

Purity Related substances—Take an amount of Suxamethonium Chloride for Injection, equivalent to 0.25 g of Suxamethonium Chloride Hydrate, and proceed as directed in the Purity (2) under Suxamethonium Chloride Hydrate.

Bacterial endotoxins *<4.01>* Less than 1.5 EU/mg.

Uniformity of dosage units *<6.02>* It meets the requirement of the Mass variation test.

Foreign insoluble matter *<6.06>* Perform the test according to Method 2: it meets the requirement.

Insoluble particulate matter *<6.07>* It meets the requirement.

Sterility *<4.06>* Perform the test according to the Membrane filtration method: it meets the requirement.

Assay Weigh accurately the contents of not less than 10 preparations of Suxamethonium Chloride for Injection. Weigh accurately about 0.5 g of the contents, and proceed as directed in the Assay under Suxamethonium Chloride Hydrate.

Each mL of 0.1 mol/L perchloric acid VS
= 18.07 mg of $C_{14}H_{30}Cl_2N_2O_4$

Containers and storage Containers—Hermetic containers.

Tacalcitol Hydrate

タカルシトール水和物

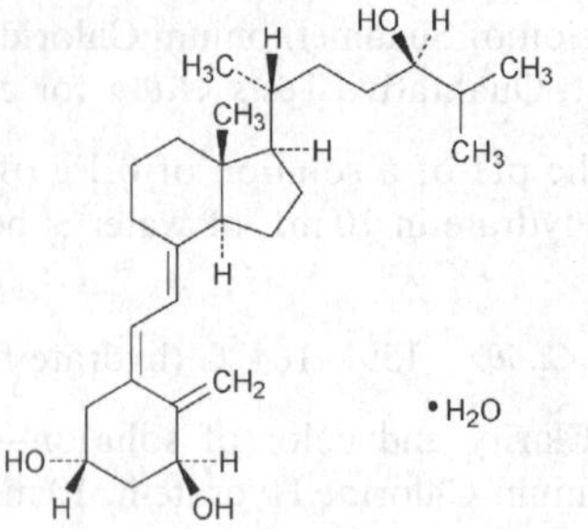

$C_{27}H_{44}O_3.H_2O$: 434.65
(1*S*,3*R*,5*Z*,7*E*,24*R*)-9,10-Secocholesta-5,7,10(19)-triene-1,3,24-triol monohydrate
[*93129-94-3*]

Tacalcitol Hydrate contains not less than 97.0% and not more than 103.0% of tacalcitol ($C_{27}H_{44}O_3$: 416.64), calculated on the anhydrous basis.

Description Tacalcitol Hydrate occurs as white, crystals or crystalline powder.

It is very soluble in methanol and in ethanol (99.5), and practically insoluble in water.

It decomposes on exposure to light.

Melting point: about 100°C. Place Tacalcitol Hydrate in a capillary tube and immediately flame-seal, put the tube in a bath heated at a temperature of about 10°C below the predicted melting point, then start the determination by rising the temperature at the rate of 1°C per minute.

Identification **(1)** Determine the absorption spectrum of a solution of Tacalcitol Hydrate in ethanol (99.5) (1 in 100,000) as directed under Ultraviolet-visible Spectrophotometry *<2.24>*, and compare the spectrum with the Reference Spectrum or the spectrum of a solution of Tacalcitol RS prepared in the same manner as the sample solution: both spectra exhibit similar intensities of absorption at the same wavelengths.

(2) Determine the infrared absorption spectrum of Tacalcitol Hydrate as directed in the potassium bromide disk method under Infrared Spectrophotometry *<2.25>*, and compare the spectrum with the Reference Spectrum or the spectrum of Tacalcitol RS: both spectra exhibit similar intensities of absorption at the same wave numbers.

Optical rotation *<2.49>* $[\alpha]_D^{20}$: +58 – +63° (25 mg calculated on the anhydrous basis, ethanol (99.5), 5 mL, 100 mm).

Purity **(1)** 1α,24(*S*)-Dihydroxycolecalciferol — Conduct this procedure avoiding contact to the air as possible and using light-resistant vessels. Dissolve 1 mg of Tacalcitol Hydrate in 20 mL of methanol, and use this solution as the sample solution. Perform the test with 30 μL of the sample solution as directed under Liquid Chromatography *<2.01>* according to the following conditions. Determine the peak area of tacalcitol, A_a, and the area of a peak, having the relative retention time of about 1.1 to tacalcitol, A_b, by the automatic integration method: $A_b/(A_a + A_b)$ is not more than 0.02.

Operating conditions—

Detector: An ultraviolet absorption photometer (wavelength: 265 nm).

Column: A stainless steel column 4.6 mm in inside diameter and 15 cm in length, packed with triacontylsilanized silica gel for liquid chromatography (3 μm in particle diameter).

Column temperature: A constant temperature of about 15°C.

Mobile phase: A mixture of acetonitrile and water (3:2).

Flow rate: Adjust so that the retention time of tacalcitol is about 26 minutes.

System suitability—

Test for required detectability: To 2 mL of the sample solution add methanol to make 20 mL, and use this solution as the solution for system suitability test. Pipet 4 mL of the solution for system suitability test, and add methanol to make exactly 20 mL. Confirm that the peak area of tacalcitol obtained with 30 μL of this solution is equivalent to 15 to 25% of that with 30 μL of the solution for system suitability test.

System performance: Dissolve 1 mg of Tacalcitol Hydrate in ethanol (99.5) to make 20 mL. Put 1 mL of this solution in a glass ampoule, flame-seal, heat at 100°C for 1 hour, and cool quickly to room temperature. Open the ampoule, evaporate to dryness the content under the nitrogen stream. Dissolve the residue with 1 mL of methanol. When the procedure is run with 30 μL of this solution under the above operating conditions, the resolution between the peaks corresponding to pre-tacalcitol, having the relative retention time of about 0.85 to tacalcitol and tacalcitol is not less than 4.

System repeatability: When the test is repeated 6 times with 30 μL of the solution for system suitability test under the above operating conditions, the relative standard deviation of the peak area of tacalcitol is not more than 2.0%.

(2) Related substances—Dissolve 1 mg of Tacalcitol Hydrate in 0.2 mL of ethanol (99.5), and use this solution as the sample solution. Pipet 50 μL of the sample solution, add ethanol (99.5) to make exactly 5 mL, and use this solution as the standard solution. Perform the test with these solutions as directed under Thin-layer Chromatography *<2.03>*. Spot 20 μL each of the sample solution and standard solution on a plate of silica gel for thin-layer chromatography. Develop the plate with a mixture of toluene and acetone (4:3) to a distance of about 15 cm, and air-dry the plate. Spray evenly a mixture of sulfuric acid and methanol (1:1) on the plate, and heat the plate at 105°C for 5 minutes: the spot other than the principal spot obtained from the sample solution is not more than one, and not more intense than the spot from the standard solution.

Water *<2.48>* 3.7 - 4.6% (10 mg, coulometric titration).

Assay Conduct this procedure avoiding contact to the air as possible and using light-resistant vessels. Weigh accurately about 1 mg each of Tacalcitol Hydrate and Tacalcitol RS (separately determine the water *<2.48>* in the same manner as Tacalcitol Hydrate), and dissolve each in methanol to make exactly 50 mL. Pipet 5 mL each of these solutions, add methanol to make exactly 20 mL, and use these solutions as the sample solution and the standard solution, respectively. Perform the test with exactly 40 μL each of the sample solution and standard solution as directed under Liquid Chromatography *<2.01>* according to the following conditions, and determine the peak area, A_T and A_S, of tacalcitol in each solution.

$$\text{Amount (mg) of tacalcitol } (C_{27}H_{44}O_3) = M_S \times A_T/A_S$$

M_S: Amount (mg) of Tacalcitol RS taken, calculated on the anhydrous basis

Operating conditions—

Detector: An ultraviolet absorption photometer (wavelength: 265 nm).

Column: A stainless steel column 4.6 mm in inside diameter and 25 cm in length, packed with octadecylsilanized silica gel for liquid chromatography (5 μm in particle diameter).

Column temperature: A constant temperature of about 35°C.

Mobile phase: A mixture of acetonitrile and water (3:1).

Flow rate: Adjust so that the retention time of tacalcitol is about 10 minutes.

System suitability—

System performance: When the procedure is run with 40 μL of the standard solution under the above operating conditions, the number of theoretical plates and the symmetry factor of the peak of tacalcitol are not less than 1500 and not more than 1.5, respectively.

System repeatability: When the test is repeated 6 times with 40 μL of the standard solution under the above operating conditions, the relative standard deviation of the peak area of tacalcitol is not more than 1.0%.

Containers and storage Containers—Tight containers.

Storage—Light-resistant, and at a temperature of 2 - 8°C.

Tacalcitol Lotion

タカルシトールローション

Tacalcitol Lotion contains not less than 90.0% and not more than 110.0% of tacalcitol ($C_{27}H_{44}O_3$: 416.64).

Method of preparation Prepare as directed under Lotions, with Tacalcitol Hydrate.

Identification Perform the test with 30 μL each of the sample solution and standard solution, both are obtained in the Assay, as directed under Liquid Chromatography *<2.01>* according to the following conditions: the retention time of the principal peaks in the chromatograms obtained from the sample solution and standard solution is the same, and both adsorption spectra of these peaks exhibit similar intensities of absorption at the same wavelengths.

Operating conditions—

Column, column temperature, mobile phase, and flow rate: Proceed as directed in the operating conditions in the Assay.

Detector: A photodiode array detector (wavelength: 265 nm; spectrum range of measurement: 210 - 400 nm).

System suitability—

System performance: Proceed as directed in the system suitability in the Assay.

Assay Weigh accurately an amount of Tacalcitol Lotion, equivalent to about 2 μg of tacalcitol ($C_{27}H_{44}O_3$), add exactly 4 mL of methanol and exactly 1 mL of the internal standard solution, and shake. Add 5 mL of hexane, shake thoroughly for 30 minutes, centrifuge at 4°C, filter the lower layer through a membrane filter with a pore size not exceeding 0.2 μm, and use the filtrate as the sample solution. Separately, weigh accurately about 1 mg of Tacalcitol RS (separately determine the water *<2.48>* in the same manner as Tacalcitol Hydrate), and dissolve in methanol to make exactly 20 mL. Pipet 1 mL of this solution, and add methanol to make exactly 100 mL. Pipet 4 mL of this solution, add exactly 1 mL of the internal standard solution, shake, add 5 mL of hexane and shake well for 30 minutes, then centrifuge at 4°C, filter the lower layer through a membrane filter with a pore size not exceeding 0.2 μm, and use the filtrate as the standard solution. Perform the test with 30 μL each of the sample solution and standard solution as directed under Liquid Chromatography <*2.01*> according to the following conditions, and calculate the ratios, Q_T and Q_S, of the peak area of tacalcitol to that of the internal standard.

$$\text{Amount } (\mu g) \text{ of tacalcitol } (C_{27}H_{44}O_3) = M_S \times Q_T/Q_S \times 2$$

M_S: Amount (mg) of Tacalcitol RS taken, calculated on the anhydrous basis

Internal standard solution—A solution of hexyl parahydroxybenzoate in methanol (3 in 2,500,000).

Operating conditions—

Detector: An ultraviolet absorption photometer (wavelength: 265 nm).

Column: A stainless steel column 4.6 mm in inside diameter and 25 cm in length, packed with octadecylsilanized silica gel for liquid chromatography (5 μm in particle diameter).

Column temperature: A constant temperature of about 30°C.

Mobile phase: A mixture of acetonitrile for liquid chromatography and diluted 0.25 mol/L acetic acid TS (1 in 10) (13:7).

Flow rate: Adjust so that the retention time of tacalcitol is about 18 minutes.

System suitability—

System performance: When the procedure is run with 30 μL of the standard solution under the above operating conditions, the internal standard and tacalcitol are eluted in this order with the resolution between these peaks being not less than 14.

System repeatability: When the test is repeated 6 times with 30 μL of the standard solution under the above operating conditions, the relative standard deviation of the ratio of the peak area of tacalcitol to that of the internal standard is not more than 2.0%.

Containers and storage Containers—Tight containers.

Storage—Light-resistant.

Tacalcitol Ointment

タカルシトール軟膏

Tacalcitol Ointment contains not less than 90.0% and not more than 115.0% of the labeled amount of tacalcitol ($C_{27}H_{44}O_3$: 416.64).

Method of preparation Prepare as directed under Ointments, with Tacalcitol Hydrate.

Identification Perform the test with 30 μL each of the sample solution and standard solution, both are obtained in the Assay, as directed under Liquid Chromatography <*2.01*> according to the following conditions: the retention time of the principal peaks in the chromatograms obtained from the sample solution and standard solution is the same, and both adsorption spectra of these peaks exhibit similar intensities of absorption at the same wavelengths.

Operating conditions—

Column, column temperature, mobile phase and flow rate: Proceed as directed in the operating conditions in the Assay.

Detector: A photodiode array detector (wavelength: 265 nm, spectrum range of measurement: 210 – 400 nm).

System suitability—

System performance: Proceed as directed in the system suitability in the Assay.

Purity Related substances—This test is only applied to the preparations of 20 μg/g.

Conduct this procedure using light-resistant vessels. To an amount of Tacalcitol Ointment, equivalent to about 20 μg of tacalcitol ($C_{27}H_{44}O_3$), add 5 mL of hexane and 5 mL of methanol, shake thoroughly for 15 minutes, and centrifuge. Discard the upper layer, pipet 5 mL of the lower layer, and evaporate the solvents in vacuum. Dissolve the residue in 1 mL of methanol, filter this solution through a membrane filter with a pore size not exceeding 0.2 μm, and use the filtrate as the sample solution. Perform the test with 30 μL of the sample solution as directed under Liquid Chromatography <*2.01*> according to the following conditions. Determine each peak area by the automatic integration method, and calculate their amounts by the area percentage method: the amount of the peak other than tacalcitol and pre-tacalcitol, having a relative retention time of about 0.83 to tacalcitol, is not more than 0.8%, and the total amount of the peaks other than tacalcitol and pre-tacalcitol is not more than 2.0%.

Operating conditions—

Detector, column and column temperature: Proceed as directed in the operating conditions in the Assay.

Mobile phase A: Water.

Mobile phase B: Acetonitrile for liquid chromatography.

Flowing of mobile phase: Control the gradient by mixing the mobile phases A and B as directed in the following table.

Time after injection of sample (min)	Mobile phase A (vol%)	Mobile phase B (vol%)
0 – 30	40	60
30 – 50	40 → 0	60 → 100
50 – 60	0	100

Flow rate: Adjust so that the retention time of tacalcitol is about 24 minutes.

Time span of measurement: For 60 minutes after injection, beginning after the solvent peak.

System suitability—

Test for required detectability: To 0.5 mL of the sample solution add methanol to make 50 mL, and use this solution as the solution for system suitability test. Pipet 4 mL of the solution for system suitability test, and add methanol to make exactly 10 mL. Confirm that the peak area of tacalcitol obtained with 30 μL of this solution is equivalent to 28 to 52% of that with 30 μL of the solution for system suitability test.

System performance: When the procedure is run with 30 μL of the sample solution under the above operating conditions, pre-tacalcitol and tacalcitol are eluted in this order with the resolution between these peaks being not less than 5.

System repeatability: When the test is repeated 6 times with 30 μL of the solution for system suitability test under the above operating conditions, the relative standard deviation of the peak area of tacalcitol is not more than 10%.

Assay Weigh accurately an amount of Tacalcitol Ointment, equivalent to about 2 μg of tacalcitol ($C_{27}H_{44}O_3$), add exactly 5 mL of hexane, exactly 4 mL of methanol, and exactly 1 mL of the internal standard solution, shake thoroughly for 15 minutes, and centrifuge. Filter the lower layer through a membrane filter with a pore size not exceeding 0.2

μm, and use the filtrate as the sample solution. Separately, weigh accurately about 1 mg of Tacalcitol RS (separately determine the water ⟨2.48⟩ in the same manner as Tacalcitol Hydrate), and dissolve in methanol to make exactly 20 mL. Pipet 1 mL of this solution, and add methanol to make exactly 100 mL. Pipet 4 mL of this solution, add exactly 1 mL of the internal standard solution and exactly 5 mL of hexane, shake thoroughly for 15 minutes, and centrifuge. Filter the lower layer through a membrane filter with a pore size not exceeding 0.2 μm, and use the filtrate as the standard solution. Perform the test with 30 μL each of the sample solution and standard solution as directed under Liquid Chromatography ⟨2.01⟩ according to the following conditions, and calculate the ratios, Q_T and Q_S, of the peak area of tacalcitol to that of the internal standard.

$$\text{Amount } (\mu g) \text{ of tacalcitol } (C_{27}H_{44}O_3) = M_S \times Q_T/Q_S \times 2$$

M_S: Amount (mg) of Tacalcitol RS taken, calculated on the anhydrous basis

Internal standard solution—A solution of hexyl parahydroxybenzoate in methanol (3 in 2,500,000).

Operating conditions—

Detector: An ultraviolet absorption photometer (wavelength: 265 nm).

Column: A stainless steel column 4.6 mm in inside diameter and 25 cm in length, packed with octadecylsilanized silica gel for liquid chromatography (5 μm in particle diameter).

Column temperature: A constant temperature of about 30°C.

Mobile phase: A mixture of acetonitrile for liquid chromatography and diluted 0.25 mol/L acetic acid TS (1 in 10) (13:7).

Flow rate: Adjust so that the retention time of tacalcitol is about 18 minutes.

System suitability—

System performance: When the procedure is run with 30 μL of the standard solution under the above operating conditions, the internal standard and tacalcitol are eluted in this order with the resolution between these peaks being not less than 14.

System repeatability: When the test is repeated 6 times with 30 μL of the standard solution under the above operating conditions, the relative standard deviation of the ratio of the peak area of tacalcitol to that of the internal standard is not more than 2.0%.

Containers and storage Containers—Tight containers.

Storage—Light-resistant.

Tacrolimus Hydrate

タクロリムス水和物

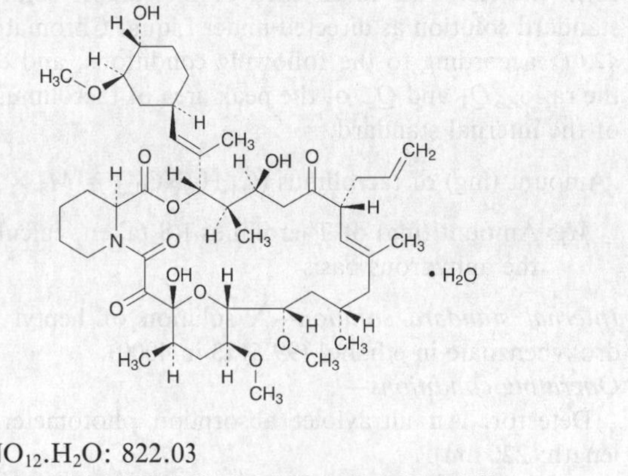

$C_{44}H_{69}NO_{12}.H_2O$: 822.03

(3*S*,4*R*,5*S*,8*R*,9*E*,12*S*,14*S*,15*R*,16*S*,18*R*,19*R*,26a*S*)-5,19-Dihydroxy-3-{(1*E*)-2-[(1*R*,3*R*,4*R*)-4-hydroxy-3-methoxycyclohexyl]-1-methylethenyl}-14,16-dimethoxy-4,10,12,18-tetramethyl-8-(prop-2-en-1-yl)-15,19-epoxy-5,6,8,11,12,13,14,15,16,17,18,19,24,25,26,26a-hexadecahydro-3*H*-pyrido[2,1-*c*][1,4]oxaazacyclotricosine-1,7,20,21(4*H*,23*H*)-tetrone monohydrate

[*109581-93-3*]

Tacrolimus Hydrate contains not less than 98.0% and not more than 102.0% of tacrolimus ($C_{44}H_{69}NO_{12}$: 804.02), calculated on the anhydrous basis.

Description Tacrolimus Hydrate occurs as white, crystals or crystalline powder.

It is very soluble in methanol and in ethanol (99.5), freely soluble in *N*,*N*-dimethylformamide and in ethanol (95), and practically insoluble in water.

Identification (1) Dissolve 5 mg of Tacrolimus Hydrate in 1 mL of ethanol (95), add 1 mL of 1,3-dinitrobenzene TS and 1 mL of sodium hydroxide TS, and shake: a red-purple color develops.

(2) Determine the infrared absorption spectrum of Tacrolimus Hydrate as directed in the paste method under Infrared Spectrophotometry ⟨2.25⟩, and compare the spectrum with the Reference Spectrum or the spectrum of Tacrolimus RS: both spectra exhibit similar intensities of absorption at the same wave numbers.

Optical rotation ⟨2.49⟩ $[\alpha]_D^{25}$: −112 – −117° (0.2 g calculated on the anhydrous basis, *N*,*N*-dimethylformamide, 20 mL, 100 mm).

Purity (1) Heavy metals ⟨1.07⟩—Proceed with 2.0 g of Tacrolimus Hydrate according to Method 2, and perform the test. Prepare the control solution with 2.0 mL of Standard Lead Solution (not more than 10 ppm).

(2) Related substances—Being specified separately when the drug is granted approval based on the Law.

Water ⟨2.48⟩ 1.9 – 2.5% (0.5 g, volumetric titration, direct titration).

Residue on ignition ⟨2.44⟩ Not more than 0.1% (1 g).

Isomer Being specified separately when the drug is granted approval based on the Law.

Assay Weigh accurately about 25 mg each of Tacrolimus Hydrate and Tacrolimus RS (separately determine the water ⟨2.48⟩ in the same manner as Tacrolimus Hydrate) and dissolve each in 15 mL of ethanol (99.5), to each add exactly 10 mL of the internal standard solution, add 25 mL of water, allow to stand for 6 hours, and use these solutions as the sample solution and the standard solution, respectively. Perform the test with 10 μL each of the sample solution and standard solution as directed under Liquid Chromatography <*2.01*> according to the following conditions, and calculate the ratios, Q_T and Q_S, of the peak area of tacrolimus to that of the internal standard.

$$\text{Amount (mg) of tacrolimus } (C_{44}H_{69}NO_{12}) = M_S \times Q_T/Q_S$$

M_S: Amount (mg) of Tacrolimus RS taken, calculated on the anhydrous basis

Internal standard solution—A solution of heptyl parahydroxybenzoate in ethanol (99.5) (3 in 4000).
Operating conditions—

Detector: An ultraviolet absorption photometer (wavelength: 220 nm).

Column: A stainless steel column 4.6 mm in inside diameter and 15 cm in length, packed with octadecylsilanized silica gel for liquid chromatography (5 μm in particle diameter).

Column temperature: A constant temperature of about 50°C.

Mobile phase: A mixture of water, 2-propanol for liquid chromatography and tetrahydrofuran for liquid chromatography (5:2:2).

Flow rate: Adjust so that the retention time of tacrolimus is about 10 minutes.

System suitability—

System performance: When the procedure is run with 10 μL of the standard solution under the above operating conditions, tacrolimus and the internal standard are eluted in this order with the resolution between these peaks being not less than 6.

System repeatability: When the test is repeated 6 times with 10 μL of the standard solution under the above operating conditions, the relative standard deviation of the ratio of the peak area of tacrolimus to that of internal standard is not more than 1.0%.

Containers and storage Containers—Well-closed containers.

Tacrolimus Capsules

タクロリムスカプセル

Tacrolimus Capsules contain not less than 93.0% and not more than 107.0% of the labeled amount of tacrolimus ($C_{44}H_{69}NO_{12}$: 804.02).

Method of preparation Prepare as directed under Capsules, with Tacrolimus Hydrate.

Identification Take out the contents of Tacrolimus Capsules, to a quantity of the contents, equivalent to 5 mg of tacrolimus ($C_{44}H_{69}NO_{12}$), add 2 mL of ethanol (95), shake for 10 minutes, and centrifuge. To 1 mL of the supernatant liquid add 0.5 mL of 1,3-dinitrobenzene TS and 0.5 mL of sodium hydroxide TS, shake, and allow to stand for 3 minutes: a light red-purple develops.

Purity Related substances—Being specified separately when the drug is granted approval based on the Law.

Isomer Being specified separately when the drug is granted approval based on the Law.

Uniformity of dosage units <*6.02*> Perform the test according to the following method: it meets the requirement of the Content uniformity test.

To 1 capsule of Tacrolimus Capsules add exactly 3*V*/5 mL of the internal standard solution, then add ethanol (99.5) to make *V* mL so that each mL contains about 0.1 mg of tacrolimus ($C_{44}H_{69}NO_{12}$), and sonicate for 10 minutes with occasional shaking. Centrifuge this solution, take 2 mL of the supernatant liquid, add 2 mL of water, allow to stand 6 hours, and use this solution as the sample solution. Separately, weigh accurately about 25 mg of Tacrolimus RS (separately determine the water <*2.48*> in the same manner as Tacrolimus Hydrate), and dissolve in ethanol (99.5) to make exactly 100 mL. Pipet 2 mL of this solution, add exactly 3 mL of the internal standard solution, add 5 mL of water, allow to stand for 6 hours, and use this solution as the standard solution. Then, proceed as directed in the Assay.

$$\text{Amount (mg) of tacrolimus } (C_{44}H_{69}NO_{12}) = M_S \times Q_T/Q_S \times V/250$$

M_S: Amount (mg) of Tacrolimus RS taken, calculated on the anhydrous basis

Internal standard solution—A solution of heptyl parahydroxybenzoate in ethanol (99.5) (1 in 20,000).

Dissolution Being specified separately when the drug is granted approval based on the Law.

Assay Take out the contents of not less than 20 Tacrolimus Capsules, weigh accurately the mass of the contents, and powder. Weigh accurately a portion of the powder, equivalent to about 25 mg of tacrolimus ($C_{44}H_{69}NO_{12}$), add 15 mL of ethanol (99.5) and exactly 10 mL of the internal standard solution, and sonicate for 10 minutes with occasional shaking. Centrifuge this solution, to 5 mL of the supernatant liquid add 5 mL of water, allow to stand for 6 hours, and use this solution as the sample solution. Separately, weigh accurately about 25 mg of Tacrolimus RS (separately determine the water <*2.48*> in the same manner as Tacrolimus Hydrate), dissolve in 15 mL of ethanol (99.5), add exactly 10 mL of the internal standard solution, add 25 mL of water, allow to stand for 6 hours, and use this solution as the standard solution. Perform the test with 10 μL each of the sample solution and standard solution as directed under Liquid Chromatography <*2.01*> according to the following conditions, and calculate the ratios, Q_T and Q_S, of the peak area of tacrolimus to that of the internal standard.

$$\text{Amount (mg) of tacrolimus } (C_{44}H_{69}NO_{12}) = M_S \times Q_T/Q_S$$

M_S: Amount (mg) of Tacrolimus RS taken, calculated on the anhydrous basis

Internal standard solution—A solution of heptyl parahydroxybenzoate in ethanol (99.5) (3 in 4000).
Operating conditions—

Detector: An ultraviolet absorption photometer (wavelength: 220 nm).

Column: A stainless steel column 4.6 mm in inside diameter and 15 cm in length, packed with octadecylsilanized silica gel for liquid chromatography (5 μm in particle diameter).

Column temperature: A constant temperature of about 50°C.

Mobile phase: A mixture of water, 2-propanol for liquid chromatography and tetrahydrofuran for liquid chromatography (5:2:2).

Flow rate: Adjust so that the retention time of tacrolimus is about 10 minutes.

System suitability—

System performance: When the procedure is run with 10 μL of the standard solution under the above operating conditions, tacrolimus and the internal standard are eluted in this order with the resolution between these peaks being not less than 6, and the number of theoretical plates and the symmetry factor of the peak of tacrolimus are not less than 3000 and not more than 1.5, respectively.

System repeatability: When the test is repeated 5 times with 10 μL of the standard solution under the above operating conditions, the relative standard deviation of the ratio of the peak area of tacrolimus to that of the internal standard is not more than 1.0%.

Containers and storage Containers—Tight containers.

Talampicillin Hydrochloride

タランピシリン塩酸塩

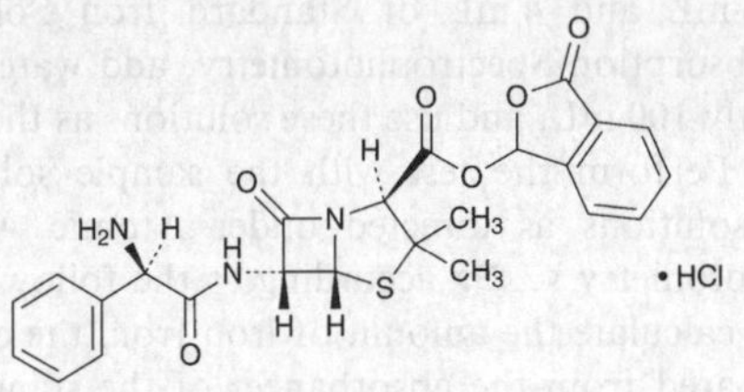

$C_{24}H_{23}N_3O_6S.HCl$: 517.98
3-Oxo-1,3-dihydroisobenzofuran-1-yl (2*S*,5*R*,6*R*)-6-[(2*R*)-2-amino-2-phenylacetylamino]-3,3-dimethyl-7-oxo-4-thia-1-azabicyclo[3.2.0]heptane-2-carboxylate monohydrochloride
[47747-56-8]

Talampicillin Hydrochloride is the hydrochloride of ampicillin phthalidyl ester.

It contains not less than 600 μg (potency) and not more than 700 μg (potency) per mg, calculated on the anhydrous basis. The potency of Talampicillin Hydrochloride is expressed as mass (potency) of ampicillin ($C_{16}H_{19}N_3O_4S$: 349.40).

Description Talampicillin Hydrochloride occurs as a white to light yellow-white powder.

It is very soluble in methanol, and freely soluble in water and in ethanol (99.5).

Identification (1) To 1 mL of a solution of Talampicillin Hydrochloride (1 in 30) add 1 mL of sodium hydroxide TS, mix, allow to stand for 5 minutes, and add 2 mL of dilute sulfuric acid and 2 to 3 drops of 2,4-dinitrophenylhydrazine TS: an orange-yellow precipitate is formed.

(2) Determine the infrared absorption spectrum of Talampicillin Hydrochloride as directed in the potassium bromide disk method under Infrared Spectrophotometry <*2.25*>, and compare the spectrum with the Reference Spectrum or the spectrum of Talampicillin Hydrochloride RS: both spectra exhibit similar intensities of absorption at the same wave numbers.

(3) To 10 mL of a solution of Talampicillin Hydrochloride (1 in 300) add 1 mL of dilute nitric acid, and add silver nitrate TS: a white precipitate is formed.

Optical rotation <*2.49*> $[\alpha]_D^{20}$: +151 – +171° (0.2 g calculated on the anhydrous basis, ethanol (99.5), 20 mL, 100 mm).

Purity (1) Heavy metals <*1.07*>—Proceed with 1.0 g of Talampicillin Hydrochloride according to Method 2, and perform the test. Prepare the control solution with 2.0 mL of Standard Lead Solution (not more than 20 ppm).

(2) Arsenic <*1.11*>—Prepare the test solution with 1.0 g of Talampicillin Hydrochloride according to Method 4, and perform the test (not more than 2 ppm).

(3) Related substances—Dissolve 50 mg of Talampicillin Hydrochloride in ethanol (99.5) to make exactly 10 mL, and use this solution as the sample solution. Pipet 1 mL, 2 mL and 3 mL of the sample solution, add ethanol (99.5) to each to make exactly 100 mL, and use these solutions as the standard solution (1), the standard solution (2) and the standard solution (3), respectively. Perform the test with these solutions as directed under Thin-layer Chromatography <*2.03*>. Spot 10 μL each of the sample solution and standard solutions (1), (2) and (3) on a plate of silica gel for thin-layer chromatography. Develop the plate with a mixture of tetrahydrofuran, ethyl acetate, water and ethanol (95) (4:4:2:1) to a distance of about 13 cm, and air-dry the plate. Spray evenly a solution of ninhydrin in ethanol (99.5) (1 in 500) on the plate, and heat the plate at 110°C for 5 minutes: the spots other than the principal spot obtained from the sample solution is not more intense than the spot from the standard solution (3), and the total of the amount of each spot other than the principal spot from the sample solution, which is calculated by the comparison with the spots from the standard solutions (1), (2) and (3), is not more than 5%.

(4) 2-Formylbenzoic acid—Dissolve 50 mg of Talampicillin Hydrochloride in ethanol (99.5) to make exactly 10 mL, and use this solution as the sample solution. Separately, dissolve 10 mg of 2-formylbenzoic acid in ethanol (99.5) to make exactly 100 mL. Pipet 5 mL of this solution, add ethanol (99.5) to make exactly 10 mL, and use this solution as the standard solution. Perform the test with these solutions as directed under Thin-layer Chromatography <*2.03*>. Spot 10 μL each of the sample solution and standard solution on a plate of silica gel for thin-layer chromatography, develop the plate with a mixture of chloroform and acetic acid (100) (4:1) to a distance of about 13 cm, and air-dry the plate. Spray evenly a solution of 2,4-dinitrophenylhydrazine in diluted sulfuric acid (6 in 25) (1 in 500): the spot of 2-formylbenzoic acid obtained from the sample solution is not more intense than that from the standard solution.

Water <*2.48*> Not more than 3.0% (0.5 g, volumetric titration, direct titration).

Assay Weigh accurately an amount of Talampicillin Hydrochloride and Talampicillin Hydrochloride RS, equivalent to about 20 mg (potency), dissolve in water to make exactly 20 mL each, and use these solutions as the sample solution and the standard solution. The standard solution should be prepared before use. Pipet 2 mL each of the sample solution and standard solution in separate 100-mL glass-stoppered flasks, add 2.0 mL of sodium hydroxide TS, and allow them to stand for exactly 15 minutes. Add 2.0 mL of diluted hydrochloric acid (1 in 10) and exactly 10 mL of 0.005 mol/L iodine VS, allow them to stand for exactly 15 minutes, and titrate <*2.50*> with 0.01 mol/L sodium thiosulfate VS until the color of the solution is disappeared. If necessary, add 0.2 to 0.5 mL of starch TS. Separately, pipet 2 mL each of the sample solution and the standard solution in separate 100-mL glass-stoppered flasks, add exactly 10 mL of 0.005 mol/L iodine VS, titrate <*2.50*> with 0.01 mol/L sodium thiosulfate VS until the color of the solution is disappeared, and make any necessary correction. For this titration, add 0.2 to 0.5 mL of starch TS, if necessary. Calculate the amount (mL) of 0.005 mol/L iodine VS, V_T and V_S, consumed by the sample solution and the standard solution, respectively.

Amount [μg (potency)] of ampicillin ($C_{16}H_{19}N_3O_4S$)
$= M_S \times V_T/V_S \times 1000$

M_S: Amount [mg (potency)] of Talampicillin Hydrochloride RS taken

Containers and storage Containers—Tight containers.

Talc

タルク

This monograph is harmonized with the European Pharmacopoeia and the U.S. Pharmacopeia.

The parts of the text that are not harmonized are marked with symbols (◆ ◆).

Information on the harmonization with the European Pharmacopoeia and the U.S. Pharmacopeia is available on the website of the Pharmaceuticals and Medical Devices Agency.

Talc is a powdered, selected, natural, hydrated magnesium silicate. Pure talc is $Mg_3Si_4O_{10}(OH)_2$: 379.27. It may contain related mineral substances consisting chiefly of chlorite (hydrous magnesium aluminum silicate), magnesite (magnesium carbonate), calcite (calcium carbonate) and dolomite (calcium magnesium carbonate).

It contains no asbestos.

It contains not less than 17.0% and not more than 19.5% of magnesium (Mg: 24.31).

◆**Description** Talc occurs as a white to grayish white, fine, crystalline powder.

It is unctuous, and adheres readily to the skin.

It is practically insoluble in water and in ethanol (99.5).◆

Identification Determine the infrared absorption spectrum of Talc as directed in the potassium bromide disk method under Infrared Spectrophotometry <*2.25*>: it exhibits absorption at the wave numbers of about 3680 cm^{-1}, 1018 cm^{-1} and 669 cm^{-1}.

Purity **(1)** Acidity or alkalinity—To 2.5 g of Talc add 50 mL of freshly boiled and cooled water, and heat under a reflux condenser. Filter the liquid by suction, add 0.1 mL of bromothymol blue-sodium hydroxide-ethanol TS to 10 mL of the filtrate, and add 0.01 mol/L hydrochloric acid VS until the color of the solution changes: the necessary volume of the VS is not more than 0.4 mL. Separately, to 10 mL of the filtrate add 0.1 mL of phenolphthalein TS, and add 0.01 mol/L sodium hydroxide VS until the color of the solution changes to light red: the necessary volume of the VS is not more than 0.3 mL.

◆**(2)** Acid-soluble substances—Weigh accurately about 1 g of Talc, heat with 20 mL of dilute hydrochloric acid at 50°C for 15 minutes with stirring. Cool, add water to make exactly 50 mL, and filter. Centrifuge, if necessary, until the filtrate becomes clear. To 25 mL of the filtrate add 1 mL of dilute sulfuric acid, evaporate to dryness, and ignite to constant mass at 800 ± 25°C: the amount of the residue is not more than 2.0%.◆

◆**(3)** Water-soluble substances—To 10.0 g of Talc add 50 mL of water, weigh the mass, and boil for 30 minutes, supplying water lost by evaporation. Cool, add water to restore the original mass, and filter. Centrifuge, if necessary, until the filtrate becomes clear. Evaporate 20 mL of the filtrate to dryness, and dry the residue at 105°C for 1 hour: the mass of the residue is not more than 4.0 mg.◆

(4) Iron—Weigh accurately about 10 g of Talc, add 50 mL of 0.5 mol/L hydrochloric acid TS gently while stirring, and heat under a reflux condenser on a water bath for 30 minutes. After cooling, transfer the content to a beaker, and allow to settle the insoluble matter. Filter the supernatant liquid through a filter paper for quantitative analysis (No. 5B), leaving the precipitate in the beaker as much as possible, wash the remaining precipitate in the beaker with three 10-mL portions of hot water, and also wash the filter paper with 15 mL of hot water, and combine the washings and the filtrate. After cooling, add water to make exactly 100 mL, and use this solution as the sample stock solution. Pipet 2.5 mL of the stock solution, add 50 mL of 0.5 mol/L hydrochloric acid TS, then add water to make exactly 100 mL, and use this solution as the sample solution. Separately, to 50 mL each of 0.5 mol/L hydrochloric acid TS add exactly 2 mL, 2.5 mL, 3 mL and 4 mL of Standard Iron Solution for Atomic Absorption Spectrophotometry, add water to make them exactly 100 mL, and use these solutions as the standard solutions. Perform the test with the sample solution and standard solutions as directed under Atomic Absorption Spectrophotometry <*2.23*> according to the following conditions, and calculate the amount of iron from the calibration curve prepared from the absorbances of the standard solutions: not more than 0.25%.

Gas: Combustible gas—Acetylene.
Supporting gas—Air.
Lamp: Iron hollow-cathode lamp.
Wavelength: 248.3 nm.

(5) Aluminum—Pipet 5 mL of the sample stock solution obtained in the Assay, add 10 mL of cesium chloride TS and 10 mL of hydrochloric acid, then add water to make exactly 100 mL, and use this solution as the sample solution. Separately, to 10 mL of hydrochloric acid and 10 mL of cesium chloride TS add exactly 5 mL, 10 mL, 15 mL and 20 mL of Standard Aluminum Solution for Atomic Absorption Spectrophotometry, add water to make them exactly 100 mL, and use these solutions as the standard solutions. Perform the test with the sample solution and standard solutions as directed under Atomic Absorption Spectrophotometry <*2.23*> according to the following conditions, and calculate the amount of aluminum from the calibration curve prepared from the absorbances of the standard solutions: not more than 2.0%.

Gas: Combustible gas—Acetylene.
Supporting gas—Nitrous oxide.
Lamp: Aluminum hollow-cathode lamp.
Wavelength: 309.3 nm.

(6) Lead—Use the sample stock solution obtained in (4) as the sample solution. Separately, to 50 mL of 0.5 mol/L hydrochloric acid TS add exactly 5 mL, 7.5 mL, 10 mL and 12.5 mL of Standard Lead Solution, add water to make them exactly 100 mL, and use these solutions as the standard solutions. Perform the test with the sample solution and standard solutions as directed under Atomic Absorption Spectrophotometry <*2.23*> according to the following conditions, and calculate the amount of lead from the calibration curve prepared from the absorbances of the standard solutions: not more than 10 ppm.

Gas: Combustible gas—Acetylene.
Supporting gas—Air.
Lamp: Lead hollow-cathode lamp.
Wavelength: 217.0 nm.

(7) Calcium—Pipet 5 mL of the sample stock solution obtained in the Assay, add 10 mL of hydrochloric acid and 10 mL of lanthanum chloride TS, then add water to make exactly 100 mL, and use this solution as the sample solution. Separately, to 10 mL of hydrochloric acid and 10 mL of lanthanum chloride TS add exactly 1 mL, 2 mL, 3 mL and 5 mL of Standard Calcium Solution, add water to make them exactly 100 mL, and use these solutions as the standard solutions. Perform the test with the sample solution and standard solutions as directed under Atomic Absorption Spectrophotometry *<2.23>* according to the following conditions, and calculate the amount of calcium from the calibration curve prepared from the absorbances of the standard solutions: not more than 0.9%.

Gas: Combustible gas—Acetylene.

Supporting gas—Nitrous oxide.

Lamp: Calcium hollow-cathode lamp.

Wavelength: 422.7 nm.

◆**(8)** Arsenic *<1.11>*—To 0.5 g of Talc add 5 mL of dilute sulfuric acid, and heat gently to boiling with shaking. Cool immediately, filter, and wash the residue with 5 mL of dilute sulfuric acid, then with 10 mL of water. Combine the filtrate and the washings, evaporate to 5 mL on a water bath, and perform the test with this solution as the test solution (not more than 4 ppm).◆

Loss on ignition *<2.43>* Not more than 7.0% (1 g, 1050 – 1100°C, constant mass).

Assay Weigh accurately about 0.5 g of Talc in a polytetrafluoroethylene dish, add 5 mL of hydrochloric acid, 5 mL of nitric acid and 5 mL of perchloric acid, then add 35 mL of hydrofluoric acid while mixing gently, and evaporate to dryness on a hot plate by heating gradually. Add 5 mL of hydrochloric acid to the residue, cover the dish with a watch glass, and heat to boil. After cooling, transfer the content to a volumetric flask while washing the watch glass and dish with water, further wash the dish with water, transfer the washings to the flask, then add water to make exactly 50 mL, and use this solution as the sample stock solution. Pipet 0.5 mL of the sample stock solution, and add water to make exactly 100 mL. Pipet 4 mL of this solution, add 10 mL of hydrochloric acid and 10 mL of lanthanum chloride TS, then add water to make exactly 100 mL, and use this solution as the sample solution. Separately, to 10 mL of hydrochloric acid and 10 mL of lanthanum chloride TS add exactly 2.5 mL, 3 mL, 4 mL and 5 mL of Standard Magnesium Solution for Atomic Absorption Spectrophotometry, add water to make them exactly 100 mL, and use these solutions as the standard solutions. Perform the test with the sample solution and standard solutions as directed under Atomic Absorption Spectrophotometry *<2.23>* according to the following conditions, and calculate the amount of magnesium from the calibration curve prepared from the absorbances of the standard solutions.

Gas: Combustible gas—Acetylene.

Supporting gas—Air.

Lamp: Magnesium hollow-cathode lamp.

Wavelength: 285.2 nm.

◆**Containers and storage** Containers—Well-closed containers.◆

Taltirelin Hydrate

タルチレリン水和物

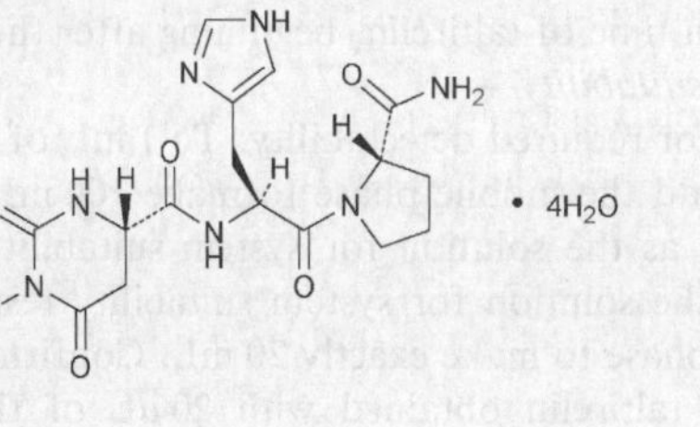

$C_{17}H_{23}N_7O_5.4H_2O$: 477.47

N-[(4*S*)-1-Methyl-2,6-dioxohexahydropyrimidine-4-carbonyl]-L-histidyl-L-prolinamide tetrahydrate

[201677-75-0]

Taltirelin Hydrate contains not less than 98.5% and not more than 101.0% of taltirelin ($C_{17}H_{23}N_7O_5$: 405.41), calculated on the anhydrous basis.

Description Taltirelin Hydrate occurs as white, crystals or crystalline powder.

It is freely soluble in water, in ethanol (99.5) and in acetic acid (100), and soluble in methanol.

It dissolves in 1 mol/L hydrochloric acid TS.

It shows crystal polymorphism.

Identification **(1)** Dissolve 30 mg of Taltirelin Hydrate in 10 mL of water. To 0.5 mL of this solution add 2 mL of a solution of 4-nitrobenzenediazonium fluoroborate (1 in 2000) and 3 mL of boric acid-potassium chloride-sodium hydroxide buffer solution (pH 9.0): a red color is produced.

(2) Determine the infrared absorption spectrum of Taltirelin Hydrate as directed in the potassium bromide disk method under Infrared Spectrophotometry *<2.25>*, and compare the spectrum with the Reference Spectrum: both spectra exhibit similar intensities of absorption at the same wave numbers.

Optical rotation *<2.49>* $[\alpha]_D^{20}$: −22.5 – −24.5° (1 g calculated on the anhydrous basis, 1 mol/L hydrochloric acid TS, 50 mL, 100 mm).

Purity **(1)** Heavy metals *<1.07>*—Proceed with 2.0 g of Taltirelin Hydrate according to Method 4, and perform the test. Prepare the control solution with 2.0 mL of Standard Lead Solution (not more than 10 ppm).

(2) Related substances—Dissolve 10 mg of Taltirelin Hydrate in 20 mL of the mobile phase, and use this solution as the sample solution. Perform the test with 20 μL of the sample solution as directed under Liquid Chromatography *<2.01>* according to the following conditions, determine each peak area by the automatic integration method, and calculate their amounts by the area percentage method: the amount of the peak other than taltirelin is not more than 0.1 %, and the total amount of the peaks other than taltirelin is not more than 0.5%.

Operating conditions—

Detector: An ultraviolet absorption photometer (wavelength: 210 nm).

Column: A stainless steel column 4.6 mm in inside diameter and 15 cm in length, packed with octadecylsilanized silica gel for liquid chromatography (5 μm in particle diameter).

Column temperature: A constant temperature of about 40°C.

Mobile phase: Dissolve 3.4 g of potassium dihydrogen phosphate in 1000 mL of water, adjust to pH 2.5 with phosphoric acid, and add 1.7 g of sodium 1-octanesulfonate. To 900 mL of this solution add 100 mL of acetonitrile.

Flow rate: Adjust so that the retention time of taltirelin is about 15 minutes.

Time span of measurement: About 1.5 times as long as the retention time of taltirelin, beginning after the solvent peak.

System suitability—

Test for required detectability: To 1 mL of the sample solution add the mobile phase to make 100 mL, and use this solution as the solution for system suitability test. Pipet 1 mL of the solution for system suitability test, and add the mobile phase to make exactly 20 mL. Confirm that the peak area of taltirelin obtained with 20 μL of this solution is equivalent to 3.5 to 6.5% of that with 20 μL of the solution for system suitability test.

System performance: When the procedure is run with 20 μL of the solution for system suitability test under the above operating conditions, the number of theoretical plates and the symmetry factor of the peak of taltirelin are not less than 7000 and not more than 1.5, respectively.

System repeatability: When the test is repeated 6 times with 20 μL of the solution for system suitability test under the above operating conditions, the relative standard deviation of the peak area of taltirelin is not more than 2.0%.

Water <*2.48*> 14.0 - 15.5% (0.2 g, volumetric titration, direct titration).

Residue on ignition <*2.44*> Not more than 0.1% (1 g).

Assay Weigh accurately about 0.7 g of Taltirelin Hydrate, dissolve in 70 mL of acetic acid (100), and titrate <*2.50*> with 0.1 mol/L perchloric acid VS until the color of solution changes from violet through blue to blue-green (indicator: 3 drops of crystal violet TS). Perform a blank determination in the same manner, and make any necessary correction.

Each mL of 0.1 mol/L perchloric acid VS
= 40.54 mg of $C_{17}H_{23}N_7O_5$

Containers and storage Containers—Well-closed containers.

Taltirelin Orally Disintegrating Tablets

タルチレリン口腔内崩壊錠

Taltirelin Orally Disintegrating Tablets contain not less than 95.0% and not more than 105.0% of the labeled amount of taltirelin hydrate ($C_{17}H_{23}N_7O_5.4H_2O$: 477.47).

Method of preparation Prepare as directed under Tablets, with Taltirelin Hydrate.

Identification Powder Taltirelin Orally Disintegrating Tablets. To a portion of the powder, equivalent to 30 mg of Taltirelin Hydrate, add 10 mL of water, shake for 5 minutes, and filter. To 0.5 mL of the filtrate add 2 mL of a solution of 4-nitrobenzenediazonium fluoroborate (1 in 2000) and 3 mL of boric acid-potassium chloride-sodium hydroxide buffer solution (pH 9.0): a red color is produced.

Purity Related substances—Powder Taltirelin Orally Disintegrating Tablets. To a portion of the powder, equivalent to 5 mg of Taltirelin Hydrate, add 20 mL of the mobile phase, shake for 5 minutes, and filter through a membrane filter with a pore size not exceeding 0.45 μm. Discard the first 2 mL of the filtrate, and use the subsequent filtrate as the sample solution. Perform the test with 20 μL of the sample solution as directed under Liquid Chromatography <*2.01*> according to the following conditions. Determine each peak area by the automatic integration method, and calculate their amounts by the area percentage method: the amount of the peak with the relative retention time of about 0.7 to taltirelin is not more than 0.7% and the peaks with the relative retention time of about 0.8 and about 0.9, respectively, are not more than 0.3%, and the peak other than taltirelin and the peaks mentioned above is not more than 0.1%. And the total amount of the peaks other than taltirelin is not more than 1.0%.

Operating conditions—

Detector, column, and column temperature: Proceed as directed in the operating conditions in the Assay.

Mobile phase: Dissolve 3.4 g of potassium dihydrogen phosphate in 1000 mL of water, adjust to pH 2.5 with phosphoric acid, and add 1.7 g of sodium 1-octanesulfonate. To 900 mL of this solution add 100 mL of acetonitrile.

Flow rate: Adjust so that the retention time of taltirelin is about 15 minutes.

Time span of measurement: About 1.5 times as long as the retention time of taltirelin, beginning from 1/3 times the retention time of taltirelin.

System suitability—

Test for required detectability: To 1 mL of the sample solution add the mobile phase to make 100 mL, and use this solution as the solution for system suitability test. Pipet 1 mL of the solution for system suitability test, and add the mobile phase to make exactly 20 mL. Confirm that the peak area of taltirelin obtained with 20 μL of this solution is equivalent to 3.5 to 6.5% of that with 20 μL of the solution for system suitability test.

System performance: When the procedure is run with 20 μL of the solution for system suitability test under the above operating conditions, the number of theoretical plates and the symmetry factor of the peak of taltirelin are not less than 7000 and not more than 1.5, respectively.

System repeatability: When the test is repeated 6 times with 20 μL of the solution for system suitability test under the above operating conditions, the relative standard deviation of the peak area of taltirelin is not more than 2.0%.

Uniformity of dosage units <*6.02*> Perform the test according to the following method: it meets the requirement of the Content uniformity test.

To 1 tablet of Taltirelin Orally Disintegrating Tablets add $V/2$ mL of the mobile phase and exactly $V/10$ mL of the internal standard solution, and shake vigorously for 5 minutes. Then, add the mobile phase to make V mL so that each mL contains about 0.1 mg of taltirelin hydrate ($C_{17}H_{23}N_7O_5.4H_2O$), and filter through a membrane filter with a pore size not exceeding 0.45 μm. Discard the first 2 mL of the filtrate, and use the subsequent filtrate as the sample solution. Then, proceed as directed in the Assay.

Amount (mg) of taltirelin hydrate ($C_{17}H_{23}N_7O_5.4H_2O$)
$= M_S \times Q_T/Q_S \times V/500 \times 1.178$

M_S: Amount (mg) of taltirelin hydrate for assay taken, calculated on the anhydrous basis

*Internal standard solution—*A solution of *o*-acetanisidide (1 in 2500).

Disintegration Being specified separately when the drug is granted approval based on the Law.

Dissolution <*6.10*> When the test is performed at 50 revolutions per minute according to the Paddle method, using 900 mL of water as the dissolution medium, the dissolution rate in 15 minutes of Taltirelin Orally Disintegrating Tablets is not less than 85%.

Start the test with 1 tablet of Taltirelin Orally Disintegrating Tablets, withdraw not less than 20 mL of the medium at the specified minute after starting the test, and filter through a membrane filter with a pore size not exceeding 0.45 μm. Discard not less than 10 mL of the first filtrate, pipet V mL of the subsequent filtrate, add water to make exactly V' mL so that each mL contains about 5.6 μg of taltirelin hydrate ($C_{17}H_{23}N_7O_5.4H_2O$), and use this solution as the sample solution. Separately, weigh accurately about 28 mg of taltirelin hydrate for assay (separately determine the water <*2.48*> in the same manner as Taltirelin Hydrate), and dissolve in water to make exactly 100 mL. Pipet 2 mL of this solution, add water to make exactly 100 mL, and use this solution as the standard solution. Perform the test with exactly 20 μL each of the sample solution and standard solution as directed under Liquid Chromatography <*2.01*>, according to the following conditions, and determine the peak areas, A_T and A_S, of taltirelin in each solution.

Dissolution rate (%) with respect to the labeled amount of taltirelin hydrate ($C_{17}H_{23}N_7O_5.4H_2O$)
$= M_S \times A_T/A_S \times V'/V \times 1/C \times 18 \times 1.178$

M_S: Amount (mg) of taltirelin hydrate for assay taken, calculated on the anhydrous basis
C: Labeled amount (mg) of taltirelin hydrate ($C_{17}H_{23}N_7O_5.4H_2O$) in 1 tablet

Operating conditions—

Proceed as directed in the operating conditions in the Assay.

System suitability—

System performance: When the procedure is run with 20 μL of the standard solution under the above operating conditions, the number of theoretical plates and the symmetry factor of the peak of taltirelin are not less than 3000 and not more than 2.0, respectively.

System repeatability: When the test is repeated 6 times with 20 μL of the standard solution under the above operating conditions, the relative standard deviation of the peak area of taltirelin is not more than 2.0%.

Assay Weigh accurately, and powder not less than 20 Taltirelin Orally Disintegrating Tablets. Weigh accurately a portion of the powder, equivalent to about 5 mg of taltirelin hydrate ($C_{17}H_{23}N_7O_5.4H_2O$), add 25 mL of the mobile phase and exactly 5 mL of the internal standard solution, shake for 5 minutes, add the mobile phase to make 50 mL, and filter through a membrane filter with a pore size not exceeding 0.45 μm. Discard the first 2 mL of the filtrate, and use the subsequent filtrate as the sample solution. Separately, weigh accurately about 50 mg of taltirelin hydrate for assay (separately determine the water <*2.48*> in the same manner as Taltirelin Hydrate), and dissolve in the mobile phase to make exactly 50 mL. Pipet 5 mL of this solution, add exactly 5 mL of the internal standard solution, add the mobile phase to make 50 mL, and use this solution as the standard solution. Perform the test with 20 μL each of the sample solution and standard solution as directed under Liquid Chromatography <*2.01*>, according to the following conditions, and calculate the ratios, Q_T and Q_S, of the peak area of taltirelin to that of the internal standard.

Amount (mg) of taltirelin hydrate ($C_{17}H_{23}N_7O_5.4H_2O$)
$= M_S \times Q_T/Q_S \times 1/10 \times 1.178$

M_S: Amount (mg) of taltirelin hydrate for assay taken, calculated on the anhydrous basis

Internal standard solution—A solution of *o*-acetanisidide (1 in 2500).

Operating conditions—

Detector: An ultraviolet absorption photometer (wavelength: 210 nm).

Column: A stainless steel column 4.6 mm in inside diameter and 15 cm in length, packed with octadecylsilanized silica gel for liquid chromatography (5 μm in particle diameter).

Column temperature: A constant temperature of about 40°C.

Mobile phase: Dissolve 3.4 g of potassium dihydrogen phosphate in 1000 mL of water, adjust to pH 2.5 with phosphoric acid, and add 1.7 g of sodium 1-octanesulfonate. To 850 mL of this solution add 150 mL of acetonitrile.

Flow rate: Adjust so that the retention time of taltirelin is about 5 minutes.

System suitability—

System performance: When the procedure is run with 20 μL of the standard solution under the above operating conditions, taltirelin and the internal standard are eluted in this order with the resolution between these peaks being not less than 10.

System repeatability: When the test is repeated 6 times with 20 μL of the standard solution under the above operating conditions, the relative standard deviation of the ratio of the peak area of taltirelin to that of the internal standard is not more than 1.0%.

Containers and storage Containers—Tight containers.

Taltirelin Tablets

タルチレリン錠

Taltirelin Tablets contain not less than 95.0% and not more than 105.0% of the labeled amount of taltirelin hydrate ($C_{17}H_{23}N_7O_5.4H_2O$: 477.47).

Method of preparation Prepare as directed under Tablets, with Taltirelin Hydrate.

Identification Powder Taltirelin Tablets. To a portion of the powder, equivalent to 30 mg of Taltirelin Hydrate, add 10 mL of water, shake for 15 minutes, and filter. To 0.5 mL of the filtrate add 2 mL of a solution of 4-nitrobenzendiazonium fluoroborate (1 in 2000) and 3 mL of boric acid-potassium chloride-sodium hydroxide buffer solution (pH 9.0): a red color is produced.

Purity Related substances—Powder Taltirelin Tablets. To a portion of the powder, equivalent to 5 mg of Taltirelin Hydrate, add 20 mL of the mobile phase, shake for 20 minutes, and filter through a membrane filter with a pore size not exceeding 0.45 μm. Discard the first 2 mL of the filtrate, and use the subsequent filtrate as the sample solution. Perform the test with 20 μL of the sample solution as directed under Liquid Chromatography <*2.01*> according to the following conditions. Determine each peak area by the automatic integration method, and calculate these amounts by the area percentage method: the amount of the peak with the relative retention time of about 0.7 to taltirelin is not more than 0.7% and the peaks with the relative retention time of about 0.8 and about 0.9, respectively, are not more than 0.3%, and the peak other than taltirelin and the peaks mentioned above is not more than 0.1%. And the total amount of the peaks other than taltirelin is not more than 1.0%.

Operating conditions—

Detector, column, and column temperature: Proceed as directed in the operating conditions in the Assay.

Mobile phase: Dissolve 3.4 g of potassium dihydrogen phosphate in 1000 mL of water, adjust to pH 2.5 with phosphoric acid, and add 1.7 g of sodium 1-octanesulfonate. To 900 mL of this solution add 100 mL of acetonitrile.

Flow rate: Adjust so that the retention time of taltirelin is about 15 minutes.

Time span of measurement: About 1.5 times as long as the retention time of taltirelin, beginning from 1/3 times the retention time of taltirelin.

System suitability—

Test for required detectability: To 1 mL of the sample solution add the mobile phase to make 100 mL, and use this solution as the solution for system suitability test. Pipet 1 mL of the solution for system suitability test, and add the mobile phase to make exactly 20 mL. Confirm that the peak area of taltirelin obtained with 20 μL of this solution is equivalent to 3.5 to 6.5% of that with 20 μL of the solution for system suitability test.

System performance: When the procedure is run with 20 μL of the solution for system suitability test under the above operating conditions, the number of theoretical plates and the symmetry factor of the peak of taltirelin are not less than 7000 and not more than 1.5, respectively.

System repeatability: When the test is repeated 6 times with 20 μL of the solution for system suitability test under the above operating conditions, the relative standard deviation of the peak area of taltirelin is not more than 2.0%.

Uniformity of dosage units <*6.02*> Perform the test according to the following method: it meets the requirement of the Content uniformity test.

To 1 tablet of Taltirelin Tablets add $V/2$ mL of the mobile phase and exactly $V/10$ mL of the internal standard solution, and sonicate for 10 minutes while occasional shaking. Then, add the mobile phase to make V mL so that each mL contains about 0.1 mg of taltirelin hydrate ($C_{17}H_{23}N_7O_5.4H_2O$), and filter through a membrane filter with a pore size not exceeding 0.45 μm. Discard the first 2 mL of the filtrate, and use the subsequent filtrate as the sample solution. Then, proceed as directed in the Assay.

Amount (mg) of taltirelin hydrate ($C_{17}H_{23}N_7O_5.4H_2O$)
$= M_S \times Q_T/Q_S \times V/500 \times 1.178$

M_S: Amount (mg) of taltirelin hydrate for assay taken, calculated on the anhydrous basis

Internal standard solution—A solution of *o*-acetanisidide (1 in 2500).

Dissolution <*6.10*> When the test is performed at 50 revolutions per minute according to the Paddle method, using 900 mL of water as the dissolution medium, the dissolution rate in 30 minutes of Taltirelin Tablets is not less than 85%.

Start the test with 1 tablet of Taltirelin Tablets, withdraw not less than 20 mL of the medium at the specified minute after starting the test, and filter through a membrane filter with a pore size not exceeding 0.45 μm. Discard not less than 10 mL of the first filtrate, pipet V mL of the subsequent filtrate, add water to make exactly V' mL so that each mL contains about 5.6 μg of taltirelin hydrate ($C_{17}H_{23}N_7O_5.4H_2O$), and use this solution as the sample solution. Separately, weigh accurately about 28 mg of taltirelin hydrate for assay (separately determine the water <*2.48*> in the same manner as Taltirelin Hydrate), and dissolve in water to make exactly 100 mL. Pipet 2 mL of this solution, add water to make exactly 100 mL, and use this solution as the standard solution. Perform the test with 20 μL each of the sample solution and standard solution as directed under Liquid Chromatography <*2.01*>, according to the following conditions, and determine the peak areas, A_T and A_S, of taltirelin in each solution.

Dissolution rate (%) with respect to the labeled amount of taltirelin hydrate ($C_{17}H_{23}N_7O_5.4H_2O$)
$= M_S \times A_T/A_S \times V'/V \times 1/C \times 18 \times 1.178$

M_S: Amount (mg) of taltirelin hydrate for assay taken, calculated on the anhydrous basis

C: Labeled amount (mg) of taltirelin hydrate ($C_{17}H_{23}N_7O_5.4H_2O$) in 1 tablet

Operating conditions—

Proceed as directed in the operating conditions in the Assay.

System suitability—

System performance: When the procedure is run with 20 μL of the standard solution under the above operating conditions, the number of theoretical plates and the symmetry factor of the peak of taltirelin are not less than 3000 and not more than 2.0, respectively.

System repeatability: When the test is repeated 6 times with 20 μL of the standard solution under the above operating conditions, the relative standard deviation of the peak area of taltirelin is not more than 2.0%.

Assay Weigh accurately, and powder not less than 20 Taltirelin Tablets. Weigh accurately a portion of the powder, equivalent to about 5 mg of taltirelin hydrate ($C_{17}H_{23}N_7O_5.4H_2O$), add 25 mL of the mobile phase and exactly 5 mL of the internal standard solution, shake for 20 minutes, add the mobile phase to make 50 mL, and filter through a membrane filter with a pore size not exceeding 0.45 μm. Discard the first 2 mL of the filtrate, and use the subsequent filtrate as the sample solution. Separately, weigh accurately about 50 mg of taltirelin hydrate for assay (separately determine the water <*2.48*> in the same manner as Taltirelin Hydrate), and dissolve in the mobile phase to make exactly 50 mL. Pipet 5 mL of this solution, add exactly 5 mL of the internal standard solution, add the mobile phase to make 50 mL, and use this solution as the standard solution. Perform the test with 20 μL each of the sample solution and standard solution as directed under Liquid Chromatography <*2.01*>, according to the following conditions, and calculate the ratios, Q_T and Q_S, of the peak area of taltirelin to that of the internal standard.

Amount (mg) of taltirelin hydrate ($C_{17}H_{23}N_7O_5.4H_2O$)
$= M_S \times Q_T/Q_S \times 1/10 \times 1.178$

M_S: Amount (mg) of taltirelin hydrate for assay taken, calculated on the anhydrous basis

Internal standard solution—A solution of *o*-acetanisidide (1 in 2500).

Operating conditions—

Detector: An ultraviolet absorption photometer (wavelength: 210 nm).

Column: A stainless steel column 4.6 mm in inside diameter and 15 cm in length, packed with octadecylsilanized silica gel for liquid chromatography (5 μm in particle diameter).

Column temperature: A constant temperature of about 40°C.

Mobile phase: Dissolve 3.4 g of potassium dihydrogen phosphate in 1000 mL of water, adjust to pH 2.5 with phosphoric acid, and add 1.7 g of sodium 1-octanesulfonate. To

850 mL of this solution add 150 mL of acetonitrile.

Flow rate: Adjust so that the retention time of taltirelin is about 5 minutes.

System suitability—

System performance: When the procedure is run with 20 μL of the standard solution under the above operating conditions, taltirelin and the internal standard are eluted in this order with the resolution between these peaks being not less than 10.

System repeatability: When the test is repeated 6 times with 20 μL of the standard solution under the above operating conditions, the relative standard deviation of the ratio of the peak area of taltirelin to that of the internal standard is not more than 1.0%.

Containers and storage Containers—Tight containers.

Tamoxifen Citrate

タモキシフェンクエン酸塩

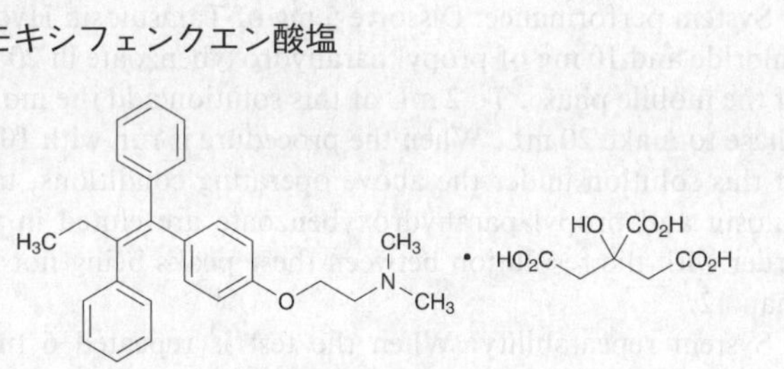

$C_{26}H_{29}NO.C_6H_8O_7$: 563.64
2-{4-[(1*Z*)-1,2-Diphenylbut-1-en-1-yl]phenoxy}-*N*,*N*-dimethylethylamine monocitrate
[*54965-24-1*]

Tamoxifen Citrate, when dried, contains not less than 99.0% and not more than 101.0% of tamoxifen citrate ($C_{26}H_{29}NO.C_6H_8O_7$).

Description Tamoxifen Citrate occurs as a white crystalline powder.

It is freely soluble in acetic acid (100), sparingly soluble in methanol, and slightly soluble in water and in ethanol (99.5).

Identification **(1)** Determine the absorption spectrum of a solution of Tamoxifen Citrate in methanol (1 in 50,000) as directed under Ultraviolet-visible Spectrophotometry <*2.24*>, and compare the spectrum with the Reference Spectrum: both spectra exhibit similar intensities of absorption at the same wavelengths.

(2) Determine the infrared absorption spectrum of Tamoxifen Citrate as directed in the potassium bromide disk method under Infrared Spectrophotometry <*2.25*>, and compare the spectrum with the Reference Spectrum: both spectra exhibit similar intensities of absorption at the same wave numbers.

(3) A solution of Tamoxifen Citrate (1 in 100) responds to Qualitative Tests <*1.09*> (1) for citrate.

Purity **(1)** Heavy metals <*1.07*>—Proceed with 2.0 g of Tamoxifen Citrate according to Method 2, and perform the test. Prepare the control solution with 2.0 mL of Standard Lead Solution (not more than 10 ppm).

(2) Related substances—Conduct this procedure rapidly, using light-resistant vessels. Dissolve 15 mg of Tamoxifen Citrate in 10 mL of the mobile phase, and use this solution as the sample solution. Pipet 1 mL of the sample solution, add the mobile phase to make exactly 100 mL, and use this solution as the standard solution. Perform the test with 10 μL each of the sample solution and standard solution as directed under Liquid Chromatography <*2.01*> according to the following conditions. Determine each peak area by the automatic integration method: the area of the peak other than tamoxifen obtained from the sample solution is not larger than 3/10 times the peak area of tamoxifen from the standard solution, and the total area of the peaks other than tamoxifen from the sample solution is not larger than 4/5 times the peak area of tamoxifen from the standard solution.

Operating conditions—

Detector: An ultraviolet absorption photometer (wavelength: 240 nm).

Column: A stainless steel column 4.6 mm in inside diameter and 25 cm in length, packed with octadecylsilanized silica gel for liquid chromatography (5 μm in particle diameter).

Column temperature: A constant temperature of about 25°C.

Mobile phase: Dissolve 4.8 g of *N*,*N*-dimethyl-*n*-octylamine in 1000 mL of water. Separately, dissolve 0.9 g of sodium dihydrogen phosphate dihydrate in 1000 mL of water. Mix these solutions, and adjust to pH 3.0 with phosphoric acid. To 600 mL of this solution add 400 mL of acetonitrile.

Flow rate: Adjust so that the retention time of tamoxifen is about 21 minutes.

Time span of measurement: About 2.5 times as long as the retention time of tamoxifen, beginning after the solvent peak.

System suitability—

Test for required detectability: Pipet 1 mL of the standard solution, and add the mobile phase to make exactly 10 mL. Confirm that the peak area of tamoxifen obtained with 10 μL of this solution is equivalent to 8 to 12% of that with 10 μL of the standard solution.

System performance: When the procedure is run with 10 μL of the standard solution under the above operating conditions, the number of theoretical plates and the symmetry factor of the peak of tamoxifen are not less than 5000 and not more than 1.5, respectively.

System repeatability: When the test is repeated 6 times with 10 μL of the standard solution under the above operating conditions, the relative standard deviation of the peak area of tamoxifen is not more than 1.5%.

Loss on drying <*2.41*> Not more than 0.5% (1 g, 105°C, 4 hours).

Residue on ignition <*2.44*> Not more than 0.1% (1 g).

Assay Weigh accurately about 1 g of Tamoxifen Citrate, previously dried, dissolve in 150 mL of acetic acid (100), and titrate <*2.50*> with 0.1 mol/L perchloric acid VS (potentiometric titration). Perform the blank determination in the same manner, and make any necessary correction.

Each mL of 0.1 mol/L perchloric acid VS
= 56.36 mg of $C_{26}H_{29}NO.C_6H_8O_7$

Containers and storage Containers—Well-closed containers.

Storage—Light-resistant.

Tamsulosin Hydrochloride

タムスロシン塩酸塩

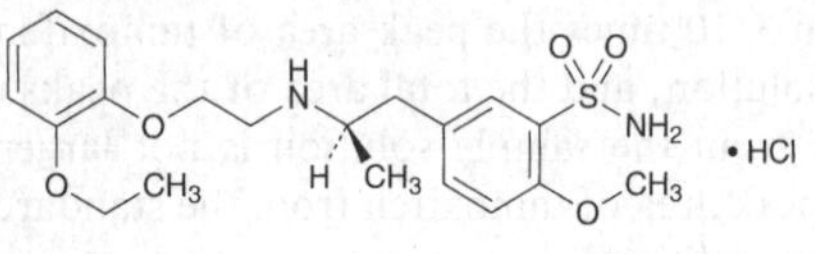

$C_{20}H_{28}N_2O_5S.HCl$: 444.97
5-{(2*R*)-2-[2-(2-Ethoxyphenoxy)ethylamino]propyl}-2-methoxybenzenesulfonamide monohydrochloride
[*106463-17-6*]

Tamsulosin Hydrochloride, when dried, contains not less than 98.5% and not more than 101.0% of tamsulosin hydrochloride ($C_{20}H_{28}N_2O_5S.HCl$).

Description Tamsulosin Hydrochloride occurs as white crystals.

It is freely soluble in formic acid, sparingly soluble in water, slightly soluble in acetic acid (100), and very slightly soluble in ethanol (99.5).

Melting point: about 230°C (with decomposition).

Identification **(1)** Determine the absorption spectrum of a solution of Tamsulosin Hydrochloride (3 in 160,000) as directed under Ultraviolet-visible Spectrophotometry <*2.24*>, and compare the spectrum with the Reference Spectrum: both spectra exhibit similar intensities of absorption at the same wavelengths.

(2) Determine the infrared absorption spectrum of Tamsulosin Hydrochloride as directed in the potassium chloride disk method under Infrared Spectrophotometry <*2.25*>, and compare the spectrum with the Reference Spectrum: both spectra exhibit similar intensities of absorption at the same wave numbers.

(3) To 5 mL of an ice cooled solution of Tamsulosin Hydrochloride (3 in 400) add 3 mL of dilute nitric acid, shake well, allow to stand at room temperature for 30 minutes, and filter: the filtrate responds to Qualitative Tests <*1.09*> for chloride.

Optical rotation <*2.49*> $[\alpha]_D^{20}$: −17.5 − −20.5° (after drying, 0.15 g, water, warming, after cooling, 20 mL, 100 mm).

Purity **(1)** Heavy metals <*1.07*>—Proceed with 1.0 g of Tamsulosin Hydrochloride according to Method 4, and perform the test. Prepare the control solution with 2.0 mL of Standard Lead Solution (not more than 20 ppm).

(2) Related substances—

(i) Dissolve 50 mg of Tamsulosin Hydrochloride in 10 mL of the mobile phase, and use this solution as the sample solution. Pipet 2 mL of the sample solution, and add the mobile phase to make exactly 50 mL. Pipet 2.5 mL of this solution, add the mobile phase to make exactly 50 mL, and use this solution as the standard solution. Perform the test with exactly 10 μL each of the sample solution and standard solution as directed under Liquid Chromatography <*2.01*> according to the following conditions, and determine each peak area by the automatic integration method: the area of the peak other than tamsulosin obtained from the sample solution is not larger than 1/2 times the peak area of tamsulosin from the standard solution.

Operating conditions—

Detector: An ultraviolet absorption photometer (wavelength: 225 nm).

Column: A stainless steel column 4 mm in inside diameter and 15 cm in length, packed with octadecylsilanized silica gel for liquid chromatography (5 μm in particle diameter).

Column temperature: A constant temperature of about 40°C.

Mobile phase: Dissolve 4.4 mL of perchloric acid and 1.5 g of sodium hydroxide in 950 mL of water, adjust the pH to 2.0 with sodium hydroxide TS, and add water to make 1000 mL. To 700 mL of this solution add 300 mL of acetonitrile for liquid chromatography.

Flow rate: Adjust so that the retention time of tamsulosin is about 6 minutes.

Time span of measurement: Until tamsulosin is eluted, beginning after the solvent peak.

System suitability—

Test for required detectability: Measure exactly 1 mL of the standard solution, and add the mobile phase to make exactly 50 mL. Confirm that the peak area of tamsulosin obtained with 10 μL of this solution is equivalent to 1.4 to 2.6% of that with 10 μL of the standard solution.

System performance: Dissolve 5 mg of Tamsulosin Hydrochloride and 10 mg of propyl parahydroxybenzoate in 20 mL of the mobile phase. To 2 mL of this solution add the mobile phase to make 20 mL. When the procedure is run with 10 μL of this solution under the above operating conditions, tamsulosin and propyl parahydroxybenzoate are eluted in this order with the resolution between these peaks being not less than 12.

System repeatability: When the test is repeated 6 times with 10 μL of the standard solution under the above operating conditions, the relative standard deviation of the peak area of tamsulosin is not more than 4.0%.

(ii) Perform the test with exactly 10 μL each of the sample solution and standard solution which are obtained in above (i) as directed under Liquid Chromatography <*2.01*> according to the following conditions, and determine each peak area by the automatic integration method: the area of the peak other than tamsulosin obtained from the sample solution is not larger than 1/2 times the peak area of tamsulosin from the standard solution.

Operating conditions—

Detector, column, and column temperature: Proceed as directed in the operating conditions in the Purity (2) (i).

Mobile phase: Dissolve 4.4 mL of perchloric acid and 1.5 g of sodium hydroxide in 950 mL of water, adjust the pH to 2.0 with sodium hydroxide TS, and add water to make 1000 mL. To this solution add 1000 mL of acetonitrile for liquid chromatography.

Flow rate: Adjust so that the retention time of tamsulosin is about 2.5 minutes.

Time span of measurement: About 5 times as long as the retention time of tamsulosin, beginning after the peak of tamsulosin.

System suitability—

System performance: Proceed as directed in the system suitability in the Purity (2) (i).

Test for required detectability: Measure exactly 1 mL of the standard solution, and add the mobile phase used in the Purity (2) (i) to make exactly 50 mL. Confirm that the peak area of tamsulosin obtained with 10 μL of this solution is equivalent to 1.4 to 2.6% of that with 10 μL of the standard solution.

System repeatability: When the test is repeated 6 times with 10 μL of the standard solution under the above operating conditions, the relative standard deviation of the peak area of tamsulosin is not more than 4.0%.

Loss on drying <*2.41*> Not more than 0.5% (1 g, 105°C,

2 hours).

Residue on ignition <2.44> Not more than 0.1% (1 g).

Assay Weigh accurately about 0.7 g of Tamsulosin Hydrochloride, previously dried, dissolve in 5 mL of formic acid, add 75 mL of a mixture of acetic acid (100) and acetic anhydride (3:2), and immediately titrate <2.50> with 0.1 mol/L perchloric acid VS (potentiometric titration). Perform a blank determination in the same manner, and make any necessary correction.

Each mL of 0.1 mol/L perchloric acid VS
= 44.50 mg of $C_{20}H_{28}N_2O_5S.HCl$

Containers and storage Containers—Well-closed containers.

Tamsulosin Hydrochloride Extended-release Tablets

タムスロシン塩酸塩徐放錠

Tamsulosin Hydrochloride Extended-release Tablets contain not less than 94.0% and not more than 106.0% of the labeled amount of tamsulosin hydrochloride ($C_{20}H_{28}N_2O_5S.HCl$: 444.97).

Method of preparation Prepare as directed under Tablets, with Tamsulosin Hydrochloride.

Identification To an amount of powdered Tamsulosin Hydrochloride Extended-release Tablets, equivalent to 1 mg of Tamsulosin Hydrochloride, add about 5 g of porcelain balls with about 5 mm in diameter, add 20 mL of 0.2 mol/L sodium hydroxide TS, warm at 50°C for 10 minutes, and shake vigorously for 15 minutes. Then, add 7 mL of acetonitrile, shake slightly, and centrifuge. Take the supernatant liquid, add 2.5 g of sodium chloride and 5 mL of ethyl acetate, shake vigorously for 5 minutes, and centrifuge. Take the supernatant liquid, evaporate to dryness at 50°C in a water bath under reduced pressure, dissolve the residue with 20 mL of water, and filter through a membrane filter with a pore size not exceeding 0.45 μm. Determine the absorption spectrum of the filtrate as directed under Ultraviolet-visible Spectrophotometry <2.24>: it exhibits maxima between 222 nm and 226 nm, and between 278 nm and 282 nm.

Uniformity of dosage units <6.02> Perform the test according to the following method: it meets the requirement of the Content uniformity test.

To 1 tablet of Tamsulosin Hydrochloride Extended-release Tablets add about 5 g of porcelain balls with about 5 mm in diameter and 5 mL of water, and shake to disintegrate the tablet. Add 20 mL of a solution of sodium hydroxide (1 in 500), warm at 50°C for 10 minutes, shake vigorously for 30 minutes, and add 10 mL of acetonitrile and 5 mL of 0.2 mol/L hydrochloric acid TS. To this solution add exactly 5 mL of the internal standard solution for every 0.1 mg of tamsulosin hydrochloride, add the mobile phase to make 50 mL, shake slightly, and centrifuge. Filter the supernatant liquid through a membrane filter with a pore size not exceeding 0.45 μm. To V mL of the filtrate add the mobile phase to make V' mL so that each mL contains about 2 μg of tamsulosin hydrochloride ($C_{20}H_{28}N_2O_5S.HCl$), and use this solution as the sample solution. Then, proceed as directed in the Assay.

Amount (mg) of tamsulosin hydrochloride
($C_{20}H_{28}N_2O_5S.HCl$)
$= M_S \times Q_T/Q_S \times V'/V \times 1/100$

M_S: Amount (mg) of tamsulosin hydrochloride for assay taken

Internal standard solution—A solution of methyl parahydroxybenzoate in the mobile phase (1 in 25,000).

Dissolution Being specified separately when the drug is granted approval based on the Law.

Assay Weigh accurately the mass of not less than 20 Tamsulosin Hydrochloride Extended-release Tablets, and powder. Weigh accurately a portion of the powder, equivalent to about 0.1 mg of tamsulosin hydrochloride ($C_{20}H_{28}N_2O_5S.HCl$), add about 5 g of porcelain balls with about 5 mm in diameter and 5 mL of water, shake, then add 20 mL of a solution of sodium hydroxide (1 in 500), warm at 50°C for 10 minutes, and shake vigorously for 30 minutes. To this solution add 10 mL of acetonitrile, 5 mL of 0.2 mol/L hydrochloric acid TS and exactly 5 mL of the internal standard solution, then add 5 mL of the mobile phase, shake slightly, and centrifuge. Filter the supernatant liquid through a membrane filter with a pore size not exceeding 0.45 μm, and use the filtrate as the sample solution. Separately, weigh accurately about 10 mg of tamsulosin hydrochloride for assay, previously dried at 105°C for 2 hours, and dissolve in the mobile phase to make exactly 100 mL. Pipet 2 mL of this solution, add exactly 10 mL of the internal standard solution, add the mobile phase to make 100 mL, and use this solution as the standard solution. Perform the test with 20 μL each of the sample solution and standard solution as directed under Liquid Chromatography <2.01> according to the following conditions, and calculate the ratios, Q_T and Q_S, of the peak area of tamsulosin to that of the internal standard.

Amount (mg) of tamsulosin hydrochloride
($C_{20}H_{28}N_2O_5S.HCl$)
$= M_S \times Q_T/Q_S \times 1/100$

M_S: Amount (mg) of tamsulosin hydrochloride for assay taken

Internal standard solution—A solution of methyl parahydroxybenzoate in the mobile phase (1 in 25,000).
Operating conditions—

Detector: An ultraviolet absorption photometer (wavelength: 225 nm).

Column: A stainless steel column 4.6 mm in inside diameter and 15 cm in length, packed with octadecylsilanized silica gel for liquid chromatography (5 μm in particle diameter).

Column temperature: A constant temperature of about 40°C.

Mobile phase: Dissolve 4.4 mL of perchloric acid and 1.5 g of sodium hydroxide in 950 mL of water, adjust to pH 2.0 with sodium hydroxide TS, and add water to make 1000 mL. To 700 mL of this solution add 300 mL of acetonitrile for liquid chromatography.

Flow rate: Adjust so that the retention time of tamsulosin is about 6 minutes.

System suitability—

System performance: When the procedure is run with 20 μL of the standard solution under the above operating conditions, the internal standard and tamsulosin are eluted in this order with the resolution between these peaks being not less than 6.

System repeatability: When the test is repeated 6 times with 20 μL of the standard solution under the above operat-

ing conditions, the relative standard deviation of the ratio of the peak area of tamsulosin to that of the internal standard is not more than 1.0%.

Containers and storage Containers—Well-closed containers.

Tannic Acid

タンニン酸

Tannic Acid is the tannin usually obtained from nutgalls or rhusgalls.

Description Tannic Acid occurs as a yellow-white to light brown amorphous powder, glistening leaflets, or spongy masses. It is odorless or has a faint, characteristic odor, and has a strongly astringent taste.

It is very soluble in water and in ethanol (95), and practically insoluble in diethyl ether.

Identification **(1)** To 5 mL of a solution of Tannic Acid (1 in 400) add 2 drops of iron (III) chloride TS: a blue-black color develops. Allow the solution to stand: a blue-black precipitate is produced.

(2) To 5 mL of a solution of Tannic Acid (1 in 20) add 1 drop each of albumin TS, gelatin TS, or 1 mL of starch TS: a precipitate is produced in each solution.

Purity **(1)** Gum, dextrin and sucrose—Dissolve 3.0 g of Tannic Acid in 15 mL of boiling water: the solution is clear or slightly turbid. Cool, and filter the solution. To 5 mL of the filtrate add 5 mL of ethanol (95): no turbidity is produced. Add further 3 mL of diethyl ether to this solution: no turbidity is produced.

(2) Resinous substances—To 5 mL of the filtrate obtained in (1) add 10 mL of water: no turbidity is produced.

Loss on drying <*2.41*> Not more than 12.0% (1 g, 105°C, 2 hours).

Residue on ignition <*2.44*> Not more than 1.0% (0.5 g).

Containers and storage Containers—Tight containers.
Storage—Light-resistant.

Tartaric Acid

酒石酸

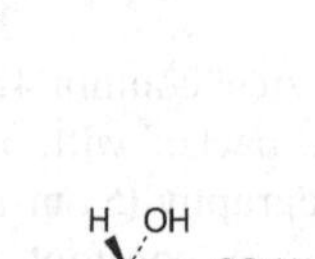

$C_4H_6O_6$: 150.09
(2*R*,3*R*)-2,3-Dihydroxybutanedioic acid
[*87-69-4*]

Tartaric Acid, when dried, contains not less than 99.7% of tartaric acid ($C_4H_6O_6$).

Description Tartaric Acid occurs as colorless crystals or a white crystalline powder. It is odorless, and has a strong acid taste.

It is very soluble in water, freely soluble in ethanol (95), and slightly soluble in diethyl ether.

A solution of Tartaric Acid (1 in 10) is dextrorotatory.

Identification **(1)** Ignite Tartaric Acid gradually: it decomposes and an odor of burning sugar is perceptible.

(2) A solution of Tartaric Acid (1 in 10) changes blue litmus paper to red, and responds to Qualitative Tests <*1.09*> for tartrate.

Purity **(1)** Sulfate <*1.14*>—Perform the test with 0.5 g of Tartaric Acid. Prepare the control solution with 0.50 mL of 0.005 mol/L sulfuric acid VS (not more than 0.048%).

(2) Oxalate—Dissolve 1.0 g of Tartaric Acid in 10 mL of water, and add 2 mL of calcium chloride TS: no turbidity is produced.

(3) Heavy metals <*1.07*>—Proceed with 2.0 g of Tartaric Acid according to Method 4, and perform the test. Prepare the control solution with 2.0 mL of Standard Lead Solution (not more than 10 ppm).

(4) Calcium—Neutralize a solution of 1.0 g of Tartaric Acid in 10 mL of water with ammonia TS, and add 1 mL of ammonium oxalate TS: no turbidity is produced.

(5) Arsenic <*1.11*>—Prepare the test solution with 2.0 g of Tartaric Acid according to Method 1, and perform the test (not more than 1 ppm).

Loss on drying <*2.41*> Not more than 0.5% (3 g, silica gel, 3 hours).

Residue on ignition <*2.44*> Not more than 0.05% (1 g).

Assay Weigh accurately about 1.5 g of Tartaric Acid, previously dried, dissolve in 40 mL of water, and titrate <*2.50*> with 1 mol/L sodium hydroxide VS (indicator: 2 drops of phenolphthalein TS).

Each mL of 1 mol/L sodium hydroxide VS
= 75.05 mg of $C_4H_6O_6$

Containers and storage Containers—Well-closed containers.

Taurine

タウリン

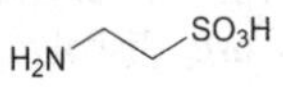

$C_2H_7NO_3S$: 125.15
2-Aminoethanesulfonic acid
[*107-35-7*]

Taurine, when dried, contains not less than 99.0% and not more than 101.0% of taurine ($C_2H_7NO_3S$).

Description Taurine occurs as colorless or white crystals, or a white crystalline powder.

It is soluble in water, and practically insoluble in ethanol (99.5).

The pH of a solution prepared by dissolving 1.0 g of Taurine in 20 mL of freshly boiled and cooled water is between 4.1 and 5.6.

Identification Determine the infrared absorption spectrum of Taurine as directed in the potassium bromide disk method under Infrared Spectrophotometry <*2.25*>, and compare the spectrum with the Reference Spectrum: both spectra exhibit similar intensities of absorption at the same wave numbers.

Purity **(1)** Clarity and color of solution—A solution obtained by dissolving 1.0 g of Taurine in 20 mL of water is clear and colorless.

(2) Chloride <*1.03*>—Perform the test with 1.0 g of Taurine. Prepare the control solution with 0.30 mL of 0.01

mol/L hydrochloric acid VS (not more than 0.011%).

(3) Sulfate <*1.14*>—Perform the test with 2.0 g of Taurine. Prepare the control solution with 0.40 mL of 0.005 mol/L sulfuric acid VS (not more than 0.010%).

(4) Ammonium <*1.02*>—Perform the test with 0.25 g of Taurine. Prepare the control solution with 5.0 mL of Standard Ammonium Solution (not more than 0.02%).

(5) Heavy metals <*1.07*>—Proceed with 2.0 g of Taurine according to Method 1, and perform the test. Prepare the control solution with 2.0 mL of Standard Lead Solution (not more than 10 ppm).

(6) Iron <*1.10*>—Prepare the test solution with 2.0 g of Taurine according to Method 1, and perform the test according to Method A. Prepare the control solution with 2.0 mL of Standard Iron Solution (not more than 10 ppm).

(7) Related substances—Dissolve 1.0 g of Taurine in 50 mL of water, and use this solution as the sample solution. Pipet 1 mL of the sample solution, and add water to make exactly 50 mL. Pipet 1 mL of this solution, add water to make exactly 10 mL, and use this solution as the standard solution. Perform the test with these solutions as directed under Thin-layer Chromatography <*2.03*>. Spot 5 μL each of the sample solution and standard solution on a plate of silica gel for thin-layer chromatography. Develop the plate with a mixture of water, ethanol (99.5), 1-butanol and acetic acid (100) (150:150:100:1) to a distance of about 10 cm, and air-dry the plate. Spray evenly ninhydrin-butanol TS on the plate, and heat the plate at 105°C for 5 minutes: the spot other than the principle spot obtained from the sample solution is not more than one spot, and it is not more intense than the spot from the standard solution.

Loss on drying <*2.41*> Not more than 0.20% (1 g, 105°C, 2 hours).

Residue on ignition <*2.44*> Not more than 0.1% (1 g).

Assay Weigh accurately about 0.2 g of Taurine, previously dried, dissolve in 50 mL of water, add 5 mL of formaldehyde solution, and titrate <*2.50*> with 0.1 mol/L sodium hydroxide VS (potentiometric titration). Perform a blank determination in the same manner, and make any necessary correction.

Each mL of 0.1 mol/L sodium hydroxide VS
= 12.52 mg of $C_2H_7NO_3S$

Containers and storage Containers—Well-closed containers.

Tazobactam

タゾバクタム

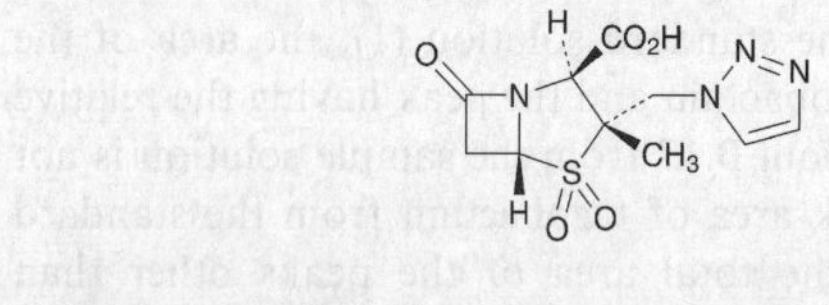

$C_{10}H_{12}N_4O_5S$: 300.29
(2*S*,3*S*,5*R*)-3-Methyl-7-oxo-3-(1*H*-1,2,3-triazol-1-ylmethyl)-4-thia-1-azabicyclo[3.2.0]heptane-2-carboxylic acid 4,4-dioxide
[*89786-04-9*]

Tazobactam contains not less than 980 μg (potency) and not more than 1020 μg (potency) per 1 mg, calculated on the anhydrous basis. The potency of Tazobactam is expressed as mass (potency) of tazobactam ($C_{10}H_{12}N_4O_5S$).

Description Tazobactam occurs as a white to pale yellowish white crystalline powder.

It is freely soluble in dimethylsulfoxide and in *N*,*N*-dimethylformamide, and slightly soluble in water, in methanol and in ethanol (99.5).

It dissolves in a solution of sodium hydrogen carbonate (3 in 100).

Identification **(1)** Determine the infrared absorption spectrum of Tazobactam as directed in the potassium bromide disk method under Infrared Spectrophotometry <*2.25*>, and compare the spectrum with the Reference Spectrum or the spectrum of Tazobactam RS: both spectra exhibit similar intensities of absorption at the same wave numbers.

(2) Determine the ^{1}H spectrum of a solution of Tazobactam in deuterated dimethylsulfoxide for nuclear magnetic resonance spectroscopy (1 in 35) as directed under Nuclear Magnetic Resonance Spectroscopy <*2.21*>, using tetramethylsilane for nuclear magnetic resonance spectroscopy as an internal reference compound: it exhibits a singlet signal A at around δ 1.3 ppm, and doublet signals, B and C, at around δ 7.8 ppm and at around δ 8.1 ppm. The ratio of the integrated intensity of each signal, A:B:C, is about 3:1:1.

Optical rotation <*2.49*> $[\alpha]_D^{20}$: +162 – +167° (1 g calculated on the anhydrous basis, *N*,*N*-dimethylformamide, 100 mL, 100 mm).

Purity **(1)** Clarity and color of solution—Dissolve 1.0 g of Tazobactam in 10 mL of sodium hydrogen carbonate (3 in 100): the solution is clear. Perform the test with the solution as directed under Ultraviolet-visible Spectrophotometry <*2.24*>: the absorbance at 420 nm is not more than 0.14.

(2) Heavy metals <*1.07*>—Proceed with 1.0 g of Tazobactam according to Method 2, and perform the test. Prepare the control solution with 1.0 mL of Standard Lead Solution (not more than 10 ppm).

(3) Related substances—This operation must be performed quickly. Dissolve 50 mg of Tazobactam in 20 mL of the mobile phase, and use this solution as the sample solution. Pipet 1 mL of the sample solution, add the mobile phase to make exactly 100 mL, and use this solution as the standard solution (1). Pipet 1 mL of the standard solution (1), add the mobile phase to make exactly 10 mL, and use this solution as the standard solution (2). Perform the test with exactly 50 μL each of the sample solution, the standard solutions (1) and (2) as directed under Liquid Chromatography <*2.01*> according to the following conditions. Determine each peak area of these solutions by the automatic integration method: the area of the peak, having the relative retention time of about 0.17 to tazobactam, obtained from the sample solution is not larger than 4/5 times the peak area of tazobactam from the standard solution (1), the area of the peak other than tazobactam and the peak having the relative retention time of about 0.17 from the sample solution is not larger than the peak area of tazobactam from the standard solution (2), and the total area of the peaks other than tazobactam and the peak having the relative retention time of about 0.17 from the sample solution is not larger than 2 times the peak area of tazobactam from the standard solution (2).

Operating conditions—

Detector, column, column temperature, mobile phase, and flow rate: Proceed as directed in the operating conditions in the Assay.

Time span of measurement: About 3 times as long as the retention time of tazobactam.

System suitability—

Test for required detectability: Pipet 1 mL of the standard solution (1), and add the mobile phase to make exactly 20 mL. Confirm that the peak area of tazobactam obtained with 50 μL of this solution is equivalent to 3 to 7% of that of tazobactam with 50 μL of the standard (1).

System performance: When the procedure is run with 50 μL of the standard solution (1) under the above operating conditions, the number of theoretical plates and the symmetry factor of the peak of tazobactam are not less than 2000 and 0.8 - 1.2, respectively.

System repeatability: When the test is repeated 6 times with 50 μL of the standard solution (1) under the above operating conditions, the relative standard deviations of the peak area of tazobactam is not more than 1.0%.

Water <*2.48*> Not more than 0.5% (1 g, volumetric titration, direct titration. Use a mixture of formamide for water determination and methanol for water determination (3:1) instead of methanol for water determination).

Residue on ignition <*2.44*> Not more than 0.1% (1 g).

Bacterial endotoxins <*4.01*> Less than 0.04 EU/mg (potency).

Assay Weigh accurately an amount of Tazobactam and Tazobactam RS, equivalent to about 50 mg (potency), dissolve each in exactly 10 mL of the internal standard solution, add water to make 100 mL, and use these solutions as the sample solution and the standard solution, respectively. Perform the test with 10 μL each of the sample solution and standard solution as directed under the Liquid Chromatography <*2.01*> according to the following conditions, and calculate the ratios, Q_T and Q_S, of the peak areas of tazobactam to that of the internal standard.

$$\text{Amount [}\mu\text{g (potency)] of tazobactam } (C_{10}H_{12}N_4O_5S) = M_S \times (Q_T/Q_S) \times 1000$$

M_S: Amount [mg (potency)] of Tazobactam RS taken

*Internal standard solution—*A solution of phenylalanine (1 in 400).

Operating conditions—

Detector: An ultraviolet absorption photometer (wavelength: 210 nm).

Column: A stainless steel column 4.6 mm in inside diameter and 25 cm in length, packed with octadecylsilanized silica gel for liquid chromatography (10 μm in particle diameter).

Column temperature: A constant temperature of about 25°C.

Mobile phase: Dissolve 1.32 g of diammonium hydrogen phosphate in 750 mL of water, adjust the pH to 2.5 with phosphoric acid, add water to make 1000 mL, and add 25 mL of acetonitrile.

Flow rate: Adjust so that the retention time of tazobactam is about 10 minutes.

System suitability—

System performance: When the procedure is run with 10 μL of the standard solution under the above operating conditions, the internal standard and tazobactam are eluted in this order with the resolution between these peaks being not less than 4.

System repeatability: When the test is repeated 6 times with 10 μL of the standard solution under the above operating conditions, the relative standard deviation of the ratios of the peak area of tazobactam to that of the internal standard is not more than 1.0%.

Containers and storage Containers—Tight containers.

Shelf life 24 months after preparation.

Tazobactam and Piperacillin for Injection

注射用タゾバクタム·ピペラシリン

Tazobactam and Piperacillin for Injection is a preparation for injection which is dissolved before use.

It contains not less than 93.0% and not more than 107.0% of the labeled potency of tazobactam ($C_{10}H_{12}N_4O_5S$: 300.29) and not less than 95.0% and not more than 105.0% of the labeled potency of piperacillin ($C_{23}H_{27}N_5O_7S$: 517.55).

Method of preparation Prepare as directed under Injections, with Tazobactam, Piperacillin Hydrate and Sodium Hydrogen Carbonate.

Description Tazobactam and Piperacillin for Injection occurs as white to pale yellowish white, masses or powder.

Identification **(1)** Determine ^1H spectrum of a solution of Tazobactam and Piperacillin for Injection in heavy water for nuclear magnetic resonance spectroscopy (1 in 10) as directed under Nuclear Magnetic Resonance Spectroscopy <*2.21*>, using sodium 3-trimethylsilylpropionate-d_4 for nuclear magnetic resonance spectroscopy as an internal reference compound: it exhibits a singlet signal A at around δ 4.2 ppm, a multiplet signal B at δ 7.3 - 7.5 ppm, a doublet signal C at around δ 7.8 ppm and a doublet signal D at around δ 8.1 ppm. The ratio of integrated intensity of these signals, A:B and C:D, is about 1:5 and about 1:1, respectively.

(2) Tazobactam and Piperacillin for Injection responds to Qualitative Tests <*1.09*> (1) for sodium salt.

pH <*2.54*> The pH of a solution of an amount of Tazobactam and Piperacillin for Injection, equivalent to 4.0 g (potency) of Piperacillin Hydrate, in 40 mL of water is 5.1 to 6.3.

Purity **(1)** Clarity and color of solution—A solution of an amount of Tazobactam and Piperacillin for Injection, equivalent to 4.0 g (potency) of Piperacillin Hydrate, in 40 mL of water is clear and colorless.

(2) Related substances—Keep the sample solution at

5°C. Dissolve an amount of Tazobactam and Piperacillin for Injection, equivalent to 0.1 g (potency) of Piperacillin Hydrate, in 100 mL of dissolving solution, and use this solution as the sample solution. Pipet 1 mL of the sample solution, add dissolving solution to make exactly 100 mL, and use this solution as the standard solution. Perform the test with exactly 20 μL each of the sample solution and standard solution as directed under Liquid Chromatography <*2.01*> according to the following conditions, and determine each peak area by the automatic integration method: the area of the peak, having the relative retention time of about 0.06 to piperacillin, obtained from the sample solution is not larger than 1.3 times the peak area of tazobactam from the standard solution, the area of the peak, having the relative retention time of about 0.05, about 0.07, about 0.19, about 0.45 and about 0.53, from the sample solution is not larger than 1/10 times the peak area of tazobactam from the standard solution, and the total area of the peaks, having the relative retention time of about 0.05, about 0.06, about 0.07, about 0.19, about 0.45 and about 0.53, from the sample solution is not larger than 1.5 times the peak area of tazobactam from the standard solution. Furthermore, the area of the peak, having the relative retention time of about 1.20 and about 1.36, from the sample solution is not larger than 1/5 times the peak area of piperacillin from the standard solution, the area of the peak, having the relative retention time of about 0.15 and about 0.63, from the sample solution is not larger than 3/10 times the peak area of piperacillin from the standard solution, the area of the peak, having the relative retention time of about 0.91 and about 1.53, from the sample solution is not larger than 2/5 times the peak area of piperacillin from the standard solution, the total area of the peaks eluted between the relative retention time of about 0.85 and about 0.87, from the sample solution is not larger than 1/2 times the peak area of piperacillin from the standard solution, the total area of the peaks, having the relative retention time of about 0.85 and about 0.87, from the sample solution is not larger than 1.5 times the peak area of piperacillin from the standard solution, and the area of the peak other than tazobactam, piperacillin and the peaks mentioned above from the sample solution is not larger than 1/10 times the peak area of piperacillin from the standard solution. The total area of the peaks other than tazobactam, piperacillin and the peaks, having the relative retention time of about 0.05, about 0.06, about 0.07, about 0.19, about 0.45 and about 0.53, from the sample solution is not larger than 4.0 times the peak area of piperacillin from the standard solution. For the area of the peaks, having the relative retention time of about 0.05, about 0.06, about 0.07, about 0.15, about 0.19, about 0.45, about 0.53, about 0.63, about 0.68, about 0.79, about 0.91 and about 1.53, multiply their correction factors 2.09, 0.70, 0.92, 0.42, 0.69, 0.56, 0.19, 1.37, 1,93, 1.64, 1.73 and 1.29, respectively, and for the total area of the peaks having the relative retention time of about 0.85 and about 0.87 and the total area of the peaks that are eluted between the peaks having the relative retention time of about 0.85 and about 0.87, multiply their correction factors, 1.79 and 2.50, respectively.

Dissolving solution: To 950 mL of diluted 1 mol/L dipotassium hydrogen phosphate TS for buffer solution (1 in 100) adjusted to pH 6.5 with phosphoric acid, add 50 mL of acetonitrile.

Operating conditions—

Detector, column, column temperature, mobile phase A, mobile phase B, flowing of mobile phase and flow rate: Proceed as directed in the operating conditions in the Assay (1).

Time span of measurement: For 36 minutes after injection, beginning after the solvent peak.

System suitability—

Test for required detectability: To exactly 1 mL of the standard solution add dissolving solution to make exactly 20 mL. Confirm that the peak area of tazobactam obtained with 20 μL of this solution is equivalent to 3.5 to 6.5% of that with 20 μL of the standard solution.

System performance: When the procedure is run with 20 μL of the standard solution under the above operating conditions, tazobactam and piperacillin are eluted in this order with the resolution between these peaks being not less than 50, and the number of theoretical plates and the symmetry factor of the peak of tazobactam are not less than 40,000 and not more than 1.5, respectively, and those of piperacillin are not less than 150,000 and not more than 1.5, respectively. Furthermore, when warm the sample solution at 40°C for 60 minutes and proceed with 20 μL of this solution under the above conditions, the resolution between the two peaks, having the relative retention time of about 0.85 and about 0.87 to piperacillin, is not less than 2.9.

System repeatability: When the test is repeated 6 times with 20 μL of the standard solution under the above conditions, the relative standard deviations of the peak area of tazobactam and piperacillin are not more than 2.0%, respectively.

Water <*2.48*> Weigh accurately the mass of the content of 1 container of Tazobactam and Piperacillin for Injection, dissolve in 20 mL of methanol for water determination, and perform the test with this solution according to the direct titration of Volumetric titration: not more than 0.6%. Perform a blank determination in the same manner, and make any necessary correction.

Bacterial endotoxins <*4.01*> Less than 0.07 EU/mg (potency) of Piperacillin Hydrate.

Uniformity of dosage units <*6.02*> It meets the requirement of the Mass variation test.

Foreign insoluble matter <*6.06*> Perform the test according to Method 2: it meets the requirement.

Insoluble particulate matter <*6.07*> It meets the requirement.

Sterility <*4.06*> Perform the test according to the Membrane filtration method: it meets the requirement.

Assay (1) Tazobactam—Dissolve the contents of 10 containers of Tazobactam and Piperacillin for Injection in a suitable amount of dissolving solution. Washout these empty containers with dissolving solution, combine the washings and the former solution, and add dissolving solution to make exactly V mL so that each mL contains about 5 mg (potency) of Tazobactam. Pipet 5 mL of this solution, add dissolving solution to make exactly 200 mL, and use this solution as the sample solution. Separately, weigh accurately about 25 mg (potency) of Tazobactam RS, dissolve in 10 mL of acetonitrile, dilute with an amount of diluted 1 mol/L dipotassium hydrogen phosphate TS for buffer solution (1 in 100) adjusted to pH 6.5 with phosphoric acid to make exactly 200 mL, and use this solution as the standard solution. Perform the test with exactly 20 μL each of the sample solution and standard solution as directed under Liquid Chromatography <*2.01*> according to the following conditions and determine the peak areas, A_T and A_S, of tazobactam in each solution.

Amount [g (potency)] of tazobactam ($C_{10}H_{12}N_4O_5S$) in 1 container of Tazobactam and Piperacillin for Injection
$= M_S \times A_T/A_S \times V/50{,}000$

M_S: Amount [mg (potency)] of Tazobactam RS taken

Dissolving solution: To 950 mL of diluted 1 mol/L dipotassium hydrogen phosphate TS for buffer solution (1 in 100) adjusted to pH 6.5 with phosphoric acid, add 50 mL of acetonitrile.

Operating conditions—

Detector: An ultraviolet absorption photometer (wavelength: 220 nm).

Column: A stainless steel column 3.9 mm in inside diameter and 10 cm in length, packed with octadecylsilanized silica gel for liquid chromatography (3 μm in particle diameter).

Column temperature: A constant temperature of about 35°C.

Mobile phase A: Dissolve 1.74 g of dipotassium hydrogen phosphate in 1000 mL of water, and adjust to pH 2.6 with phosphoric acid.

Mobile phase B: Acetonitrile.

Flowing of mobile phase: Control the gradient by mixing the mobile phases A and B as directed in the following table.

Time after injection of sample (min)	Mobile phase A (vol%)	Mobile phase B (vol%)
0 – 5	100	0
5 – 15	100 → 76	0 → 24
15 – 25	76 → 65	24 → 35
25 – 36	65	35

Flow rate: 1.5 mL per minute.

System suitability—

System performance: Dissolve 50 mg (potency) of piperacillin hydrate in the standard solution to make 50 mL, and use this solution as the solution for system suitability test. When the procedure is run with 20 μL of the solution for system suitability test under the above operating conditions, tazobactam and piperacillin are eluted in this order with the resolution between these peaks being not less than 50, and the number of theoretical plates and the symmetry factor of the peak of tazobactam are not less than 25,000 and not more than 2.0, respectively.

System repeatability: When the test is repeated 6 times with 20 μL of the standard solution under the above conditions, the relative standard deviations of the peak area of tazobactam is not more than 1.0%.

(2) Piperacillin—Dissolve the contents of 10 containers of Tazobactam and Piperacillin for Injection in a suitable amount of dissolving solution. Washout these empty containers with dissolving solution, combine the washings and the former solution, and add dissolving solution to make exactly V mL so that each mL contains about 40 mg (potency) of Piperacillin Hydrate. Pipet 5 mL of this solution, add dissolving solution to make exactly 200 mL, and use this solution as the sample solution. Separately, weigh accurately about 50 mg (potency) of Piperacillin RS, dissolve in 2.5 mL of acetonitrile, dilute with an amount of diluted 1 mol/L dipotassium hydrogen phosphate TS for buffer solution (1 in 100) adjusted to pH 6.5 with phosphoric acid to make exactly 50 mL, and use this solution as the standard solution. Perform the test with exactly 20 μL each of the sample solution and standard solution as directed under Liquid Chromatography <*2.01*> according to the following conditions, and determine the peak areas, A_T and A_S, of piperacillin in each solution.

Amount [g (potency)] of piperacillin ($C_{23}H_{27}N_5O_7S$) in 1 container of Tazobactam and Piperacillin for Injection
$= M_S \times A_T/A_S \times V/12{,}500$

M_S: Amount [mg (potency)] of Piperacillin RS taken

Dissolving solution: To 950 mL of diluted 1 mol/L dipotassium hydrogen phosphate TS for buffer solution (1 in 100) adjusted to pH 6.5 with phosphoric acid, add 50 mL of acetonitrile.

Operating conditions—

Proceed as directed in the operating conditions in the Assay (1).

System suitability—

System performance: When the procedure is run with 20 μL of the solution for system suitability test obtained in the Assay (1) under the above operating conditions, tazobactam and piperacillin are eluted in this order with the resolution between these peaks being not less than 50, and the number of theoretical plates and the symmetry factor of the peak of piperacillin are not less than 100,000 and not more than 2.0, respectively.

System repeatability: When the test is repeated 6 times with 20 μL of the standard solution under the above conditions, the relative standard deviations of the peak area of piperacillin is not more than 1.0%.

Containers and storage Containers—Hermetic containers.

Teceleukin (Genetical Recombination)

テセロイキン(遺伝子組換え)

```
MAPTSSSTKK TQLQLEHLLL DLQMILNGIN NYKNPKLTRM LTFKFYMPKK
ATELKHLQCL EEELKPLEEV LNLAQSKNFH LRPRDLISNI NVIVLELKGS
ETTFMCEYAD ETATIVEFLN RWITFCQSII STLT
```

$C_{698}H_{1127}N_{179}O_{204}S_8$: 15547.01
[136279-32-8]

Teceleukin (Genetical Recombination) is a recombinant human interleukin-2, and is a protein consisting of 134 amino acid residues with methionine at the N-terminus. It is a solution.

It contains potency between 7.7×10^6 and 1.54×10^7 units per mL, and not less than 7.7×10^6 units per mg of protein.

Description Teceleukin (Genetical Recombination) occurs as a clear and colorless liquid.

Identification **(1)** Pipet an appropriate amount of Teceleukin (Genetical Recombination), add an accurate amount of potency measuring medium for teceleukin so that each mL contains about 200 units, and use this solution as the sample stock solution. Dilute reference anti-interleukin-2 antibody for teceleukin with potency measuring medium for teceleukin to a concentration of approximately 200 neutral units per mL and use this solution as the interleukin-2 neutral antibody solution. Accurately add an equivalent volume of the interleukin-2 neutral antibody solution to the sample stock solution, shake, and then leave for 1 hour in a 37°C incubator in air containing 5% carbon dioxide. This solution is used as the sample solution. Prepare a standard solution by accurately adding an equivalent volume of potency measuring medium for teceleukin to the sample stock solution, mixing, and then processing in the same way. Process the sample and standard solutions according to the assay method, determine their respective dilution coefficients, D_N and D_T, and then calculate the neutralization rate, which should be at least 90%, using the following formula.

$$\text{Neutralization rate (\%)} = (D_T - D_N)/D_T \times 100$$

If the mean values of the absorbance of the maximum uptake control solution and absorbance of the minimum uptake control solution do not fit the standard curve, the neutralization coefficient is to be determined within the following range.

$$\text{Neutralization coefficient (\%)} > (D_T - 2)/D_T \times 100$$

(2) When hydrolyzed according to modified Method 2 and Method 4 as directed in 1. Hydrolysis of Protein and Peptide, and performed the test according to Method 1 in 2. Methodologies of Amino Acid Analysis under Amino Acid Analysis of Proteins <*2.04*>, the molar ratios of the respective amino acids are as follows: aspartic acid is 11.4 to 12.6, glutamic acid is 17.1 to 18.9, proline is 4.5 to 5.5, glycine is 1.8 to 2.2, cysteine 2.7 to 3.3, methionine is 4.5 to 5.5, leucine is 20.9 to 23.1, tyrosine is 2.7 to 3.3, phenylalanine is 5.4 to 6.6, lysine is 10.5 to 11.6, histidine is 2.7 to 3.3, tryptophan is 0.7 to 1.2, and arginine is 3.6 to 4.4. Furthermore, the peaks of the constituent 18 amino acids are observed in the chromatogram obtained from the sample solution (1).

(i) Hydrolysis—Place a volume of Teceleukin (Genetical Recombination) corresponding to approximately 50 μg of protein in 2 test tubes for hydrolysis, evaporate to dryness under vacuum, and use one as the sample (1). To the other, add 50 μL of a mixture of formic acid and hydrogen peroxide (30) (9:1) that has been left at room temperature for 1 hour, cool for 4 hours in ice, add 0.5 mL of water, and then evaporate to dryness under vacuum to give the sample (2). To 1.3 mL of methanesulfonic acid add 3.7 mL of water, mix well, and dissolve 10 mg of 3-(2-aminoethyl)indole, to make a 4 mol/L methanesulfonic acid solution. Dissolve 39.2 g of trisodium citrate dihydrate, 33 mL of hydrochloric acid, 40 mL of thiodiglycol, and 4 mL of lauromacrogol solution (1 in 4) in 700 mL of water, adjust the pH to 2.2, add water to make 1000 mL, add 100 μL of capric acid, and mix to make a sodium citrate solution for dilution. Add 50 μL of freshly prepared 4 mol/L methanesulfonic acid to the sample (1) and sample (2), cool to −70°C, and then deaerate under vacuum. Heat to 115°C ± 2°C for 24 hours after sealing these test tubes under reduced pressure. After cooling, unseal, add 50 μL of 4 mol/L sodium hydroxide TS followed by 0.4 mL of sodium citrate solution for dilution to make the sample solution (1) and sample solution (2). Separately, weigh accurately 0.25 mmol amounts of L-aspartic acid, L-threonine, L-serine, L-glutamic acid, L-proline, glycine, L-alanine, L-valine, L-methionine, L-isoleucine, L-leucine, L-tyrosine, L-phenylalanine, L-lysine hydrochloride, ammonium chloride, L-histidine hydrochloride monohydrate, and L-arginine hydrochloride as well as 0.125 mmol of L-cysteine, and then dissolve in 0.1 mol/L hydrochloric acid TS to make exactly 100 mL. This solution is used as the amino acid standard stock solution. Pipet 1 mL of the amino acid standard stock solution, and add sodium citrate solution for dilution to make exactly 25 mL. This solution is used as solution A. Weigh accurately about 20 mg of L-tryptophan and dissolve in water to make exactly 1000 mL. This solution is used as solution B. Pipet 10 mL of both solution A and solution B, combine together, and add sodium citrate solution for dilution to make exactly 50 mL. This solution is used as the amino acid standard solution. Separately, weigh accurately about 17 mg of L-cysteic acid and dissolve in sodium citrate solution for dilution to make exactly 50 mL. Pipet 1 mL of this solution and add sodium citrate solution for dilution to make exactly 100 mL. This solution is used as the cysteic acid standard solution.

(ii) Amino acid analysis—Accurately measure 0.25 mL each of the sample solution (1), the sample solution (2), the amino acid standard solution, and the cysteic acid standard solution, perform the test by Liquid Chromatography <*2.01*> under the following conditions, and confirm the peaks of amino acids appeared on the chromatogram obtained from the sample solution (1). Also, measure the peak area of each amino acid in the sample solution (1) and the amino acid standard solution, and taking the molar number of alanine in the sample solution (1) as 5.0, determine the concentrations of aspartic acid, glutamic acid, proline, glycine, methionine, leucine, tyrosine, phenylalanine, lysine, histidine, tryptophan, and arginine and then calculate the molar ratio for each amino acid. Also, measure the cysteic acid peak areas of the sample solution (2) and the cysteic acid standard solution, determine the concentration of the cysteine, and calculate the molar ratio of cysteine taking the molar number of alanine in the sample solution (2) as 5.0.

Operating conditions—

Detector: Visible absorption photometer [wavelengths: 440 nm (proline) and 570 nm (amino acids other than proline)].

Column: A stainless steel column 4 mm in inside diameter and 25 cm in length, packed with a strongly acidic ion exchange resin for liquid chromatography consisting of polystyrene to which sulfonate group binds (5 μm in particle diameter).

Column temperature: A constant temperature of about 50°C when the sample is injected. After a certain time, increase the temperature to a constant temperature of about 62°C.

Reaction temperature: A constant temperature of about 98°C.

Time for color formation: Approximately 2 minutes.

Mobile phase: After preparing mobile phases A, B, and C according to the following table, add 0.1 mL of capric acid to each.

	Mobile phase A	Mobile phase B	Mobile phase C
Citric acid monohydrate	18.70 g	10.50 g	7.10 g
Trisodium citrate dihydrate	7.74 g	14.71 g	26.67 g
Sodium chloride	7.07 g	2.92 g	54.35 g
Ethanol (99.5)	60 mL	—	—
Benzyl alcohol	—	—	10 mL
Thiodiglycol	5 mL	5 mL	—
Lauromacrogol solution (1 in 4)	4 mL	4 mL	4 mL
Water	Appropriate amount	Appropriate amount	Appropriate amount
pH	3.2	4.3	4.7
Total volume	1000 mL	1000 mL	1000 mL

Changing mobile phases and column temperature: When operating under the above conditions using 0.25 mL of the amino acid standard solution, the amino acids will elute in the following order; aspartic acid, threonine, serine, glutamic acid, proline, glycine, alanine, cystine, valine, methionine, isoleucine, leucine, tyrosine, phenylalanine, lysine, ammonia, histidine, tryptophan, and arginine. Switchover to the mobile phases A, B, and C, in sequence so that the resolution between the peaks of cystine and valine is 2.0 or more and that between ammonia and histidine is 1.5 or more. Also, increase the temperature after a constant length of time so that the resolution between the peaks of glutamic acid and proline is at least 2.0.

Reaction reagents: Dissolve 408 g of lithium acetate dihydrate in water, and add 100 mL of acetic acid (100) and water to make 1000 mL. To this solution add 1200 mL of dimethylsulfoxide and 800 mL of 2-methoxyethanol. This solution is used as solution (I). Separately, mix together 600 mL of dimethylsulfoxide and 400 mL of 2-methoxyethanol and then add 80 g of ninhydrin and 0.15 g of sodium borohydride. This solution is used as solution (II). After gassing 3000 mL of the solution (I) for 20 minutes with nitrogen, rapidly add 1000 mL of the solution (II) and then mix by gassing for 10 minutes with nitrogen.

Mobile phase flow rate: About 0.275 mL per minute.

Reaction reagent flow rate: About 0.3 mL per minute.

System suitability—

System performance: When the procedure is run with 0.25 mL of the amino acid standard solution under the above operating conditions, the resolution between the peaks of threonine and serine is at least 1.5.

Molecular mass Dissolve 0.242 g of 2-amino-2-hydroxymethyl-1,3-propanediol, 5.0 g of sodium lauryl sulfate, and 74 mg of disodium dihydrogen ethylenediamine tetraacetate dihydrate in 60 mL of water. After adjusting the pH to 8.0 with 1 mol/L hydrochloric acid TS, add water to make 100 mL. This solution is used as the molecular mass determination buffer solution. Pipet 20 μL of Teceleukin (Genetical Recombination), add exactly 20 μL of the molecular mass determination buffer solution and exactly 2 μL of 2-mercaptoethanol, and then heat at 90 to 100°C for 5 minutes on a water bath without allowing any water evaporation from the mixture. After cooling, add exactly 1 μL of bromophenol blue solution (1 in 2000) and then shake. This solution is used as the sample solution. Separately, pipet 5 μL of molecular mass marker for teceleukin, and add exactly 50 μL of water, exactly 55 μL of the molecular mass determination buffer solution, and exactly 5 μL of 2-mercaptoethanol, and then heat at 90 to 100°C for 5 minutes on a water bath without allowing any water evaporation from the mixture. After cooling, add exactly 1 μL of bromophenol blue solution (1 in 2000), and shake well. This solution is used as the molecular mass standard solution. When conducting a test using SDS-polyacrylamide gel electrophoresis with 1 μL each of the sample solution and the molecular mass standard solution, the molecular mass of the main band is between 14,000 and 16,000.

Operating conditions—

Equipment: Horizontal electrophoresis vessel with a cooling unit, a device that accumulates load voltage over time, and a direct current power source device that controls the amperage, voltage, wattage.

Spotting of solutions: Solutions are spotted on concentrating gel of polyacrylamide gel sheets.

Electrophoresis conditions

Polyacrylamide gel sheet: Polyester sheet to which a polyacrylamide gel (width, about 43 mm, length, about 50 mm, and thickness, about 0.5 mm) is closely adhered. The polyacrylamide gel consists of a concentrating gel with a gel support concentration of 7.5% and a 3% degree of crosslinking and a separating gel with corresponding values of 20% and 2%. The gel contains tris-acetate buffer (pH 6.5).

Buffer solution for electrode: Prepared by dissolving 35.83 g of tricine, 24.23 g of 2-amino-2-hydroxymethyl-1,3-propanediol, and 5.5 g of sodium lauryl sulfate in water to make 1000 mL.

Cooling temperature of gel support plate: 15°C.

Running conditions

Pre-electrophoresis and electrophoresis: The voltage, amperage, and wattage should not exceed 250 V, 10 mA, and 3 W, respectively. The amperage and wattage should be proportional to the number of polyacrylamide sheets.

Immediately after adding sample: The voltage, amperage, and wattage should not exceed 250 V, 1 mA, and 3 W, respectively. The amperage and wattage should be proportional to the number of polyacrylamide sheets.

Electrophoresis time

Before adding sample: Until value of load voltage integrated to time reaches 60 V·h.

Immediately after adding sample: Until value of load voltage integrated to time reaches 1 V·h.

Main electrophoresis: Until value of load voltage integrated to time reaches 140 V·h.

Fixation and staining

Dissolve 25 g of anhydrous sodium carbonate and 0.8 mL of formaldehyde solution in water to make 1000 mL. This solution is used as the developing solution. After immersing the polyacrylamide gel sheet in a mixture of ethanol (99.5), water and acetic acid (100) (5:4:1) for 2 minutes, immerse for 2 minutes in a mixture of water, ethanol (99.5) and acetic acid (100) (17:2:1). Change the mixture, immerse for another 4 minutes, immerse in water for 2 minutes to rinse the polyacrylamide gel sheet, and change the water to immerse for 2 minutes. This procedure is carried out with warming to 50°C. Next, while warming at 40°C, immerse for 10 to 15 minutes in diluted silver nitrate TS (1 in 7), warm to 30°C, and gently rinse the polyacrylamide gel sheet with water. While warming at 30°C, immerse the polyacrylamide gel sheet in freshly prepared developing solution. After obtaining adequate color formation, immerse the polyacrylamide gel sheet in diluted acetic acid (100) (1 in 20) to terminate the color formation.

Estimation of molecular mass

Plot graphs for each band obtained from the molecular mass standard solution, distance from the border of the concentrating gel and separating gel, and the logarithm of the molecular mass of proteins in each band. Calculate the molecular mass by reading the corresponding position of the major band obtained from the sample solution on the graph.

Isoelectric point The isoelectric point determined from the electrophoresis position is 7.4 to 7.9 when 3 μL of Teceleukin (Genetical Recombination) and 8 μL of isoelectric marker for teceleukin are tested by the polyacrylamide gel isoelectric method.

Operating conditions—

Equipment: Horizontal electrophoretic vessel with a cooling unit and direct current power source that can perform constant wattage control.

Preparation of polyacrylamide gel: Dissolve 1.62 g of acrylamide and 50 mg of *N*,*N*′-methylenebisacrylamide in water to make 25 mL. Accurately measure 7.5 mL of this solution, 2 mL of a 10 mL solution prepared by adding water to 5 g of glycerin, and 0.64 mL of a pH 3 to pH 10 amphoteric electrolyte solution, and degas under reduced pressure while stirring thoroughly. Next, accurately measure 74 μL of freshly prepared ammonium peroxodisulfate solution (1 in

50), 3 μL of *N,N,N',N'*-tetramethylethylenediamine, and 50 μL of freshly prepared riboflavin sodium phosphate solution (1 in 1000), stir well, immediately pour on a gel preparation plate (10 cm wide, 11 cm long, and 0.8 mm thick), and then expose to a fluorescent light source for 60 minutes to gelate.

Spotting

Add Teceleukin (Genetical Recombination) or isoelectric marker for teceleukin 30 minutes after starting electrophoresis to wells in gel plates to which plastic tape (3.5 mm wide, 3.5 mm long, 0.4 mm thick) has been applied in advance and that have undergone gelation.

Electrophoresis conditions

Cathode solution: Sodium hydroxide TS.

Anode solution: DL-Aspartic acid solution (133 in 25,000).

Cooling temperature of gel support plate: 2 ± 1°C.

Running conditions: After starting the electrophoresis, a constant wattage of 10 W for 20 minutes and 20 W thereafter. However, the voltage should be 3000 V or less.

Running time: 120 to 140 minutes while blowing Nitrogen into the electrophoresis vessel.

Fixation and washing

Dissolve 28.75 g of trichloroacetic acid and 8.65 g of 5-sulfosalicylic acid dihydrate in 75 mL of methanol and 175 mL of water. Immerse the gel in this solution for 60 minutes to fix the protein to the gel. After fixation, immerse for 10 minutes in a mixture of water, ethanol (99.5) and acetic acid (100) (67:25:8).

Staining and decolorization

Dissolve 0.11 g of Coomassie brilliant blue G-250 in 25 mL of ethanol (99.5), and add 8 mL of acetic acid (100) and water to make 100 mL. This solution is used as the staining solution. Immerse the gel for 10 minutes while warming at 60°C in freshly filtered staining solution. After staining, decolorize by immersing in a mixture of water, ethanol (99.5) and acetic acid (100) (67:25:8).

Determination of isoelectric point

Plot the protein isoelectric points and the distance from the cathode of each band obtained from the isoelectric markers for teceleukin. Calculate the isoelectric point from the corresponding position of the major bands obtained from the sample solution.

pH <*2.54*> 2.7 – 3.5

Purity (1) Desmethionyl form—To Teceleukin (Genetical Recombination) add water so that each mL contains about 0.17 mg of protein, and use this solution as the sample solution. Perform the test with 1.2 mL of the sample solution as directed under Liquid Chromatography <*2.01*> according to the following conditions. Determine the peak area, A_2, of teceleukin and the peak area of the desmethionyl form having the relative retention time of about 0.8 to teceleukin, A_1, by the automatic integration method. The amount of the desmethionyl form is not more than 1.0% when determined using the following formula.

$$\text{Amount (\%) of desmethionyl form} = A_1/(A_1 + A_2) \times 100$$

Operating conditions—

Detector: Ultraviolet absorption photometer (wavelength: 280 nm).

Columns: Two stainless steel columns with inside diameters of 7.5 mm and lengths of 7.5 cm connected in sequence and packed with 10 μm synthetic polymer bound to diethylaminoethyl base for liquid chromatography.

Column temperature: A constant temperature of about 25°C.

Mobile phase A: Mix 0.658 g of diethanolamine in 400 mL of water, adjust the pH to 9.0 with 1 mol/L hydrochloric acid TS, and then add water to make 500 mL.

Mobile phase B: Add 300 mL of water to 2.6 mL of a pH 6 to 9 amphoteric electrolyte solution and 0.5 mL of a pH 8 to 10.5 amphoteric electrolyte solution, adjust to pH 7 with diluted hydrochloric acid (9 in 100), and then add water to make 400 mL.

Switching mobile phases and sample injection: Inject the sample solution while running the mobile phase A. Repeatedly inject 10 times a sample solution volume of 0.11 mL followed by a single injection of 100 μL. After injecting the entire volume and running mobile phase A for 60 minutes, switch to mobile phase B. After measuring the sample solution and after running 1 mol/L sodium chloride TS for 10 minutes for postreatment and cleaning of the columns, inject 100 μL of sodium hydroxide TS while running the mobile phase A and then 55 minutes later start injection of the next sample solution.

Flow rate: Adjust the flow of the mobile phase B so that the retention time for teceleukin is 45 to 65 minutes. Measure the retention time from the point at which the mobile phase is switched to the mobile phase B.

System suitability—

System performance: Dissolve in water a mixture of two kinds of equine heart-derived myoglobin whose isoelectric points are 6.76 and 7.16 to make a concentration of approximately 0.5 mg/mL. Mix together 50 μL of this solution, 50 μL of Teceleukin (Genetical Recombination), and 1.47 mL of water. When the procedure is run with 1.2 mL of this solution under the above operating conditions, myoglobin and teceleukin are eluted in this order, and their respective peaks are completely separated.

(2) Dimer—Prepare a sample solution by adding 20 μL of 0.2% sodium laurylsulfate TS to 20 μL of Teceleukin (Genetical Recombination). Perform the test as directed under Liquid Chromatography <*2.01*> with 20 μL of the sample solution according to the following conditions. Determine the teceleukin peak area, A_2, and the peak area, A_1, of the dimer with the relative retention time of 0.8 to 0.9 in relation to teceleukin, by the automatic integration method. The amount of the dimer is not more than 1.0% by the following formula.

$$\text{Amount (\%) of dimer} = A_1/(A_1 + A_2) \times 100$$

Operating conditions—

Detector: Ultraviolet absorption photometer (wavelength: 220 nm).

Column: A stainless steel column 7.5 mm in inside diameter and 60 cm in length, packed with glycol etherifized silica gel for liquid chromatography (10 μm in particle diameter).

Column temperature: A constant temperature of about 25°C.

Mobile phase: Dissolve 1.0 g of sodium lauryl sulfate in 0.1 mol/L sodium phosphate buffer (pH 7.0) to make 1000 mL.

Flow rate: Adjust so that the retention time of teceleukin is 30 – 40 minutes.

System suitability—

System performance: Add 20 μL of 0.2% sodium lauryl sulfate TS to 20 μL of a solution consisting of 5 mg of carbonic anhydrase and 5 mg of α-lactoalbumin dissolved in 100 mL of water. When the procedure is run with 20 μL of this solution under the above operating conditions, carbonic anhydrase and α-lactoalbumin are eluted in this order with the resolution between these peaks being not less than 1.5.

System repeatability: To exactly 1 mL of the sample solution add the mobile phase to make exactly 20 mL. To exactly

1 mL of this solution add the mobile phase to make exactly 10 mL. When the test is repeated 3 times with 20 μL of this solution under the above operating conditions, the relative standard deviation of the teceleukin peak area is not more than 7%.

(3) Tetracycline hydrochloride—Serially subculture through 2 passages at 35 to 37°C the test bacteria *Kocuria rhizophila* ATCC9341 in a slant culture of test bacteria inoculation media for teceleukin and then dilute this 100-fold by adding sterilized purified water. This solution is used as the test bacteria solution. Store the test bacteria solution at 5°C or less and use the solution within 5 days. Dilute the test bacteria solution serially by adding sterilized purified water, add an appropriate amount to 100 mL of normal agar medium for teceleukin, conduct a preliminary test, and determine the amount of tetracycline hydrochloride that shows an inhibition zone corresponding to standard solution containing 0.5 μg (potency) of tetracycline hydrochloride ($C_{22}H_{24}N_2O_8$.HCl) in 1 mL. Add this amount to 100 mL of normal agar medium for teceleukin dissolved and then cooled to 45 to 50°C and mix. Pipet 25 mL of this solution into square Petri dishes (135 × 95 mm) and spread horizontally to solidify. Prepare plates for testing by making an appropriate number of wells in this agar medium. The volume of the test bacteria solution to which 100 mL of normal agar medium for teceleukin has been added is 0.25 to 1.0 mL. Pipet an appropriate amount of Tetracycline Hydrochloride RS and dilute accurately with water to make a clear solution with a concentration of 1 mg (potency) of tetracycline hydrochloride ($C_{22}H_{24}N_2O_8$.HCl) per mL. Pipet an appropriate amount of this solution and dilute precisely with water to make standard solutions with concentrations of 4, 2, 1 and 0.5 μg (potency)/mL. Separately, dilute Teceleukin (Genetical Recombination) with diluted acetic acid (100) (3 in 1000), if necessary, or alternatively concentrate under reduced pressure, to make a sample solution with a protein concentration of 0.8 to 1.2 mg/mL. Pipet 25 μL of the sample solution and each standard solution, and add each to the wells in the same test plate. Repeat the same procedure for at least 3 more test plates. Leave the test plates at room temperature for 30 to 60 minutes and then incubate at 35 to 37°C for 16 to 18 hours. Measure the inhibitions zones to a diameter of 0.25 mm. Determine the mean among the test plates for each of the solutions.

Prepare a standard curve by plotting a graph with the concentration of each standard solution in logarithmic scale on the horizontal axis and the diameter of the inhibition zone on the vertical axis. Match the diameter of the inhibition zone of teceleukin from the standard curve and determine A, the concentration of tetracycline hydrochloride. When the amount of tetracycline hydrochloride per mg of protein is determined by the following formula, the amount is not more than 0.7 μg. However, if an inhibition zone is not seen, or is seen but the diameter is smaller than 0.5 μg/mL on the standard curve, A is taken as being 0.5 μg/mL or less.

Amount [μg (potency)] of tetracycline hydrochloride ($C_{22}H_{24}N_2O_8$.HCl) per mg of protein
$= A/P$

P: The protein concentration (mg/mL) of the sample solution.

(4) Other related proteins—Perform the test with 5 μL of Teceleukin (Genetical Recombination) as directed under Liquid Chromatography <2.01> according to the following conditions, and measure the area of each peak by the automatic integration method. When the amounts of the peak are calculated by the area percent method, the total amount of peaks other than the teceleukin and solvent peaks is not more than 1.0%.

Operating conditions—

Detector: Ultraviolet absorption photometer (wavelength: 220 nm).

Column: A stainless steel column with an inside diameter of 4.6 mm and 15 cm in length, packed with octadecylsilanized silica gel for liquid chromatography (5 μm in particle diameter).

Column temperature: A constant temperature of about 30°C.

Mobile phase A: A solution of trifluoroacetic acid in a mixture of water and acetonitrile (19:1) (1 in 1000).

Mobile phase B: A solution of trifluoroacetic acid in acetonitrile (7 in 10,000).

Flowing of mobile phase: Control the gradient by mixing the mobile phases A and B as follows.

Time after injection of sample (min)	Mobile phase A (vol%)	Mobile phase B (vol%)
0 – 12	60 → 50	40 → 50
12 – 25	50	50
25 – 45	50 → 0	50 → 100
45 – 50	0	100

Flow rate: 1.0 mL per minute.

Time span of measurement: About 1.2 times as long as the retention time of teceleukin.

System suitability—

System performance: Add 3.8 μL of water and 16.6 μL of polysorbate 80 solution (1 in 100) to 83.6 μL of Teceleukin (Genetical Recombination) and let stand for at least 1 hour. When the procedure is run with 5 μL of this solution under the above operating conditions, there is complete separation between the teceleukin peak and the peak with the relative retention time of about 0.98 to the teceleukin.

(5) Host cell proteins—Being specified separately when the drug is granted approval based on the Law.

(6) Host cell DNA—Being specified separately when the drug is granted approval based on the Law.

Bacterial endotoxins <4.01> Less than 5EU per mg of protein.

Acetic acid Pipet 0.25 mL of Teceleukin (Genetical Recombination) and add exactly 0.25 mL of the internal standard solution to make the sample solution. Separately, pipet 3 mL of acetic acid (100) and add water to make exactly 100 mL. Pipet 10 mL of this solution and add water to make exactly 100 mL. Pipet 2 mL of this solution and add exactly 2 mL of the internal standard solution to make the standard solution. Perform the test with 1 μL each of the sample solution and standard solution as directed under Gas Chromatography <2.02> according to the following conditions. Calculate the ratios of the peak area of acetic acid to that of the internal standard, Q_T and Q_S, and the amount of acetic acid ($C_2H_4O_2$) in 1 mL of Teceleukin (Genetical Recombination) calculated by the following formula is between 2.85 mg and 3.15 mg.

Amount (mg) of acetic acid ($C_2H_4O_2$) in 1 mL of Teceleukin (Genetical Recombination)
$= Q_T/Q_S \times 1.5 \times 1.049 \times 2$

1.5: Concentration (μL/mL) of acetic acid (100) in the standard solution

1.049: Density (mg/μL) of acetic acid (100) at 25°C
2: Dilution factor

Internal standard solution—Diluted propionic acid (1 in 500).
Operating conditions—
Detector: A hydrogen flame-ionization detector.
Column: A glass column with an inside diameter of 1.2 mm and 40 m in length, whose inside is covered with chemically-bound polyethylene glycol for gas chromatography 1.0 μm in thickness.
Column temperature: A constant temperature of about 110°C.
Carrier gas: Helium.
Flow rate: Adjust so that the retention time of acetic acid is about 8 minutes.
System suitability—
System performance: When the procedure is run with 1 μL of the standard solution under the above operating conditions, acetic acid and the internal standard are eluted in this order with the resolution between these peaks being not less than 3.
System repeatability: When the test is repeated 6 times with 1 μL of standard solution under the above operating conditions, the relative standard deviation of the ratio of the peak area of acetic acid to that of the internal standard is not more than 5%.

Specific activity Pipet an appropriate amount of Teceleukin (Genetical Recombination), and add water accurately so that each mL contains about 0.1 mg. This solution is used as the sample solution. Separately, pipet about 25 mg of human serum albumin for assay, dissolve in water to make exactly 50 mL. Pipet an appropriate amount of this solution, and accurately dilute with water to make standard solutions with concentrations of 0.05, 0.10, and 0.15 mg per mL. Pipet 1 mL each of the sample solution, the standard solutions, and water, add 2.5 mL of alkaline copper solution, mix, leave for at least 10 minutes to dissolve, add exactly 2.5 mL of water and 0.5 mL of diluted Folin TS (1 in 2), immediately shake vigorously, and then leave at 37°C for 30 minutes. Perform the test with these solutions, with water as a control, as directed under Ultraviolet-visible Spectrophotometry <*2.24*>, and measure the absorbance at 750 nm. With the concentration of the standard solution as the *x*-axis and the absorbance as the *y*-axis, perform linear regression using their respective reciprocals, and calculate the protein content.
Calculate the ratio of the potency determined by Assay and the protein content.

Assay Pipet an appropriate amount of Teceleukin (Genetical Recombination) and, depending on the cell sensitivity, dilute precisely by adding potency measuring medium for teceleukin to a constant concentration of 10 to 50 units/mL (estimated value). This solution is used as the sample solution. Separately, dissolve Interleukin-2 RS in 1 mL of sterilized purified water, and, depending on the cell sensitivity, dilute precisely by adding potency measuring medium for teceleukin to a constant concentration of 10 to 50 units/mL. This solution is used as the standard solution. Add exactly 50 μL of potency measuring medium for teceleukin to all but 8 wells in a 96-well microplate. Add exactly 50 μL of the sample solution and standard solution to 2 wells each containing potency measuring medium for teceleukin. From these 4 wells, remove exactly 50 μL and add to 4 other wells containing potency measuring medium for teceleukin. From these 4 wells, remove exactly 50 μL and add to 4 other wells containing potency measuring medium for teceleukin and repeat this procedure to prepare 2 wells that contain each of 1/2, 1/4, 1/8, 1/16, 1/32, 1/64, 1/128, and 1/256 dilutions of the sample solution and standard solution. Add 50 μL of the standard solution to each of the 8 empty wells to make maximum uptake controls. The 8 wells containing only potency measuring medium for teceleukin serve as the minimum uptake controls. After adding exactly 50 μL of cell suspension solution for teceleukin to each well in the microplate, leave for 15 to 17 hours in an incubator at 37°C filled with air containing 5% carbon dioxide. After adding exactly 25 μL of MTT TS to each of the wells in the microplate, leave for 4 hours in an incubator at 37°C filled with air containing 5% carbon dioxide. Transfer the culture medium in all of the wells to empty wells into another microplate. To each of the empty wells from which the culture medium was removed, add 100 μL of hydrochloric acid-2-propanol TS, and then shake the plates horizontally for 5 minutes to elute the pigment. After returning the transferred culture medium to each original well, perform the test with the solution in each well, determine the difference in absorption at wavelengths of 560 nm and 690 nm, and calculate the mean values of the identical respective solutions in the two wells (dilution solutions of the sample solution and standard solutions) as well as the 8 wells containing the maximum or minimum uptake controls. Prepare standard curves by plotting the values obtained from each dilution solution of the sample solution, with the dilution coefficient of the sample solution on the microplate in logarithmic scale on the horizontal axis and the absorbance on the vertical axis. Determine the mean absorbance values of the maximum and minimum uptake controls, find the values on the standard curve, and then calculate the dilution coefficient, D_T. Perform the same plot for the dilution solution of the standard solution, calculate the dilution coefficient, D_S, and then calculate the potency in 1 mL by the following formula.

Teceleukin potency (unit) in 1 mL of Teceleukin (Genetical Recombination)
$$= S \times D_T/D_S \times d$$

S: Concentration of standard solution (unit/mL)
d: Dilution coefficient when sample solution prepared

Containers and storage Containers—Tight containers
Storage—Store at −70°C or lower.

Teceleukin for Injection (Genetical Recombination)

注射用テセロイキン(遺伝子組換え)

Teceleukin for Injection (Genetical Recombination) is a preparation for injection which is dissolved before use.

It contains not less than 70.0% and not more than 150.0% of the labeled amount of teceleukin (genetical recombination) ($C_{698}H_{1127}N_{179}O_{204}S_8$: 15547.01).

Method of preparation Prepare as directed under Injection, with Teceleukin (Genetical Recombination).

Description Teceleukin for Injection (Genetical Recombination) occurs as a white, light mass or powder.

Identification Dissolve the content of 1 container of Teceleukin for Injection (Genetical Recombination) in 1 mL of sterilized purified water, dilute exactly with potency measuring medium for teceleukin to make the sample stock solution containing about 200 units of Teceleukin (Genetical Recombination) per mL. Proceed as directed in the Identification (1) under Teceleukin (Genetical Recombination).

pH <*2.54*> Being specified separately when the drug is granted approval based on the Law.

Purity Clarity and color of solution—Dissolve the content of 1 container of Teceleukin for Injection (Genetical Recombination) in 1 mL of water: the solution is clear and colorless.

Loss on drying Transfer the content of the container of Teceleukin for Injection (Genetical Recombination) to a weighing bottle under the atmosphere not exceeding 10% relative humidity, and perform the test as directed in the Water content determination described in the Minimum Requirements for Biological Products: not more than 5%.

Bacterial endotoxins <*4.01*> Less than 5 EU/350,000 units.

Uniformity of dosage units <*6.02*> It meets the requirement of the Mass variation test. Calculate as $|M - A| = 0$.

Foreign insoluble matter <*6.06*> Perform the test according to Method 2: it meets the requirement.

Insoluble particulate matter <*6.07*> It meets the requirement.

Sterility <*4.06*> Perform the test according to the Membrane filtration method: it meets the requirement.

Assay Dissolve the content of 1 container of Teceleukin for Injection (Genetical Recombination) in exactly 1 mL of sterilized purified water, dilute exactly with culture medium for assay of teceleukin to make the sample solution containing a definite concentration of 10 to 50 units/mL (estimate). Proceed as directed in the Assay under Teceleukin (Genetical Recombination), and calculate the amount (unit) of teceleukin in 1 container by the following formula.

$$\text{Amount (unit) of teceleukin in 1 container} = S \times D_T/D_S \times d \times 1$$

S: Concentration of the standard solution (unit/mL)
d: Dilution coefficient when sample solution prepared
1: Volume (mL) of the sample solution

Containers and storage Containers—Hermetic containers.
Storage—Light-resistant, not exceeding 10°C, avoiding freezing.

Tegafur

テガフール

and enantiomer

$C_8H_9FN_2O_3$: 200.17
5-Fluoro-1-[(2*RS*)-tetrahydrofuran-2-yl]uracil
[*17902-23-7*]

Tegafur, when dried, contains not less than 98.0% of tegafur ($C_8H_9FN_2O_3$).

Description Tegafur occurs as a white crystalline powder.
It is soluble in methanol, and sparingly soluble in water and in ethanol (95).
It dissolves in dilute sodium hydroxide TS.
A solution of Tegafur in methanol (1 in 50) shows no optical rotation.
It shows crystal polymorphism.

Identification **(1)** Prepare the test solution with 0.01 g of Tegafur as directed under Oxygen Flask Combustion Method <*1.06*>, using a mixture of 0.5 mL of 0.01 mol/L sodium hydroxide TS and 20 mL of water as an absorbing liquid: the test solution responds to Qualitative Tests <*1.09*> (2) for fluoride.

(2) Determine the absorption spectrum of a solution of Tegafur in 0.01 mol/L sodium hydroxide TS (1 in 100,000) as directed under Ultraviolet-visible Spectrophotometry <*2.24*>, and compare the spectrum with the Reference Spectrum: both spectra exhibit similar intensities of absorption at the same wavelengths.

(3) Determine the infrared absorption spectrum of Tegafur, previously dried, as directed in the potassium bromide disk method under Infrared Spectrophotometry <*2.25*>, and compare the spectrum with the Reference Spectrum: both spectra exhibit similar intensities of absorption at the same wave numbers. If any difference appears between the spectra, recrystallize the sample with a mixture of methanol and acetone (1:1), filter and dry the crystals, and perform the test with the crystals.

pH <*2.54*> Dissolve 0.5 g of Tegafur in 50 mL of water: the pH of this solution is between 4.2 and 5.2.

Melting point <*2.60*> 166 - 171°C

Purity **(1)** Clarity and color of solution—Dissolve 0.2 g of Tegafur in 10 mL of dilute sodium hydroxide TS: the solution is clear and colorless.

(2) Chloride <*1.03*>—Dissolve 0.8 g of Tegafur in 40 mL of water by warming, cool, filter if necessary, and add 6 mL of dilute nitric acid and water to make 50 mL. Perform the test using this solution as the test solution. Prepare the control solution with 0.25 mL of 0.01 mol/L hydrochloric acid VS (not more than 0.011%).

(3) Heavy metals <*1.07*>—Dissolve 1.0 g of Tegafur in 40 mL of water by warming, cool, filter if necessary, and add 2 mL of dilute acetic acid and water to make 50 mL. Perform the test using this solution as the test solution. Prepare the control solution with 1.0 mL of Standard Lead Solution (not more than 10 ppm).

(4) Arsenic <*1.11*>—Prepare the test solution in a platinum crucible with 1.0 g of Tegafur according to Method 4, incinerating by ignition between 750°C and 850°C, and perform the test (not more than 2 ppm).

(5) Related substances—Dissolve 0.10 g of Tegafur in 10 mL of methanol, and use this solution as the sample solution. Pipet 1 mL of the sample solution, add methanol to make exactly 200 mL, and use this solution as the standard solution. Perform the test with these solutions as directed under Thin-layer Chromatography <*2.03*>. Spot 5 μL each of the sample solution and standard solution on a plate of silica gel with fluorescent indicator for thin-layer chromatography. Develop the plate with a mixture of chloroform and ethanol (95) (5:1) to a distance of about 10 cm, and air-dry the plate. Examine under ultraviolet light (main wavelength: 254 nm): the spots other than the principal spot obtained from the sample solution are not more intense than the spot from the standard solution.

Loss on drying <*2.41*> Not more than 0.5% (1 g, 105°C, 4 hours).

Residue on ignition <*2.44*> Not more than 0.1% (1 g, platinum crucible).

Assay Weigh accurately about 0.15 g of Tegafur, previously dried, place in an iodine bottle, dissolve in 75 mL of water, and add exactly 25 mL of 1/60 mol/L potassium bromate VS. Add rapidly 1.0 g of potassium bromide and 12 mL of hydrochloric acid, stopper the bottle tightly at once, and allow to stand for 30 minutes with occasional shaking. To this solution add 1.6 g of potassium iodide, shake gently, allow to stand for exactly 5 minutes, and titrate <*2.50*> the liberated iodine with 0.1 mol/L sodium thiosulfate VS (indicator: 2 mL of starch TS). Perform a blank determination in the same manner.

Each mL of 1/60 mol/L potassium bromate VS
= 10.01 mg of $C_8H_9FN_2O_3$

Containers and storage Containers—Tight containers.

Teicoplanin

テイコプラニン

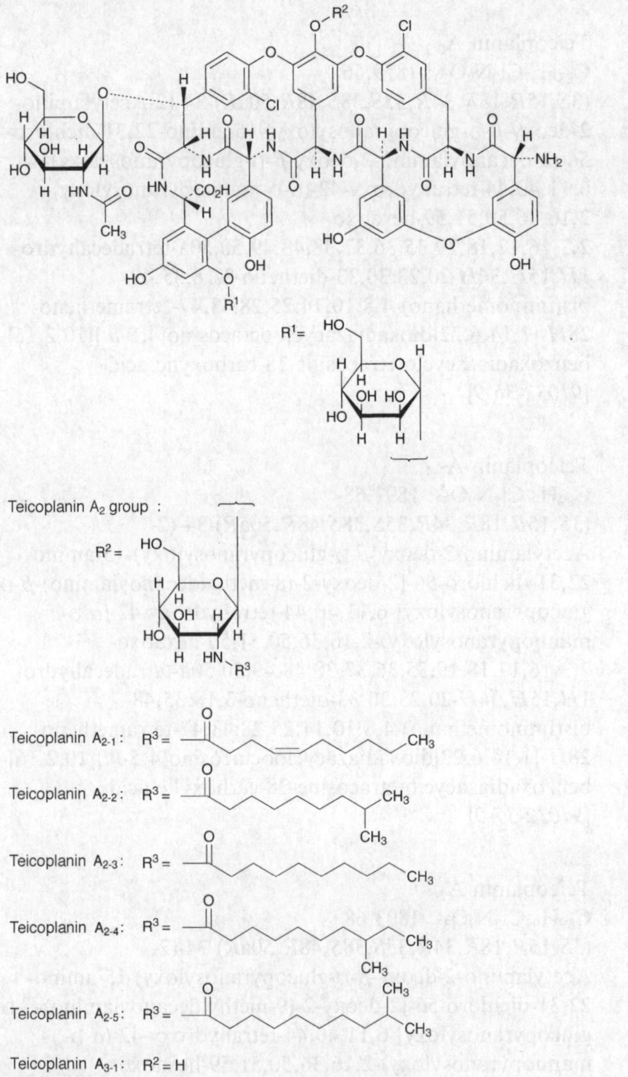

Teicoplanin A_2 group :

Teicoplanin $A_{2\text{-}1}$: R^3 =

Teicoplanin $A_{2\text{-}2}$: R^3 =

Teicoplanin $A_{2\text{-}3}$: R^3 =

Teicoplanin $A_{2\text{-}4}$: R^3 =

Teicoplanin $A_{2\text{-}5}$: R^3 =

Teicoplanin $A_{3\text{-}1}$: R^2 = H

Teicoplanin $A_{2\text{-}1}$
$C_{88}H_{95}Cl_2N_9O_{33}$: 1877.64
(3*S*,15*R*,18*R*,34*R*,35*S*,38*S*,48*R*,50a*R*)-34-(2-Acetylamino-2-deoxy-β-D-glucopyranosyloxy)-15-amino-22,31-dichloro-56-[2-(4*Z*)-dec-4-enoylamino-2-deoxy-β-D-glucopyranosyloxy]-6,11,40,44-tetrahydroxy-42-(α-D-mannopyranosyloxy)-2,16,36,50,51,59-hexaoxo-2,3,16,17,18,19,35,36,37,38,48,49,50,50a-tetradecahydro-1*H*,15*H*,34*H*-20,23:30,33-dietheno-3,18:35,48-bis(iminomethano)-4,8:10,14:25,28:43,47-tetrametheno-28*H*-[1,14,6,22]dioxadiazacyclooctacosino[4,5-*m*][10,2,16]-benzoxadiazacyclotetracosine-38-carboxylic acid
[*91032-34-7*]

Teicoplanin $A_{2\text{-}2}$
$C_{88}H_{97}Cl_2N_9O_{33}$: 1879.66
(3*S*,15*R*,18*R*,34*R*,35*S*,38*S*,48*R*,50a*R*)-34-(2-Acetylamino-2-deoxy-β-D-glucopyranosyloxy)-15-amino-22,31-dichloro-56-[2-deoxy-2-(8-methylnonanoylamino)-β-D-glucopyranosyloxy]-6,11,40,44-tetrahydroxy-42-(α-D-mannopyranosyloxy)-2,16,36,50,51,59-hexaoxo-2,3,16,17,18,19,35,36,37,38,48,49,50,50a-tetradecahydro-1*H*,15*H*,34*H*-20,23:30,33-dietheno-3,18:35,48-

bis(iminomethano)-4,8:10,14:25,28:43,47-tetrametheno-28*H*-[1,14,6,22]dioxadiazacyclooctacosino[4,5-*m*][10,2,16]-benzoxadiazacyclotetracosine-38-carboxylic acid
[*91032-26-7*]

Teicoplanin $A_{2\text{-}3}$
$C_{88}H_{97}Cl_2N_9O_{33}$: 1879.66
(3*S*,15*R*,18*R*,34*R*,35*S*,38*S*,48*R*,50a*R*)-34-(2-Acetylamino-2-deoxy-*β*-D-glucopyranosyloxy)-15-amino-22,31-dichloro-56-(2-decanoylamino-2-deoxy-*β*-D-glucopyranosyloxy)-6,11,40,44-tetrahydroxy-42-(*α*-D-mannopyranosyloxy)-2,16,36,50,51,59-hexaoxo-2,3,16,17,18,19,35,36,37,38,48,49,50,50a-tetradecahydro-1*H*,15*H*,34*H*-20,23:30,33-dietheno-3,18:35,48-bis(iminomethano)-4,8:10,14:25,28:43,47-tetrametheno-28*H*-[1,14,6,22]dioxadiazacyclooctacosino[4,5-*m*][10,2,16]-benzoxadiazacyclotetracosine-38-carboxylic acid
[*91032-36-9*]

Teicoplanin $A_{2\text{-}4}$
$C_{89}H_{99}Cl_2N_9O_{33}$: 1893.68
(3*S*,15*R*,18*R*,34*R*,35*S*,38*S*,48*R*,50a*R*)-34-(2-Acetylamino-2-deoxy-*β*-D-glucopyranosyloxy)-15-amino-22,31-dichloro-56-[2-deoxy-2-(8-methyldecanoylamino)-*β*-D-glucopyranosyloxy]-6,11,40,44-tetrahydroxy-42-(*α*-D-mannopyranosyloxy)-2,16,36,50,51,59-hexaoxo-2,3,16,17,18,19,35,36,37,38,48,49,50,50a-tetradecahydro-1*H*,15*H*,34*H*-20,23:30,33-dietheno-3,18:35,48-bis(iminomethano)-4,8:10,14:25,28:43,47-tetrametheno-28*H*-[1,14,6,22]dioxadiazacyclooctacosino[4,5-*m*][10,2,16]-benzoxadiazacyclotetracosine-38-carboxylic acid
[*91032-37-0*]

Teicoplanin $A_{2\text{-}5}$
$C_{89}H_{99}Cl_2N_9O_{33}$: 1893.68
(3*S*,15*R*,18*R*,34*R*,35*S*,38*S*,48*R*,50a*R*)-34-(2-Acetylamino-2-deoxy-*β*-D-glucopyranosyloxy)-15-amino-22,31-dichloro-56-[2-deoxy-2-(9-methyldecanoylamino)-*β*-D-glucopyranosyloxy]-6,11,40,44-tetrahydroxy-42-(*α*-D-mannopyranosyloxy)-2,16,36,50,51,59-hexaoxo-2,3,16,17,18,19,35,36,37,38,48,49,50,50a-tetradecahydro-1*H*,15*H*,34*H*-20,23:30,33-dietheno-3,18:35,48-bis(iminomethano)-4,8:10,14:25,28:43,47-tetrametheno-28*H*-[1,14,6,22]dioxadiazacyclooctacosino[4,5-*m*][10,2,16]-benzoxadiazacyclotetracosine-38-carboxylic acid
[*91032-38-1*]

Teicoplanin $A_{3\text{-}1}$
$C_{72}H_{68}Cl_2N_8O_{28}$: 1564.25
(3*S*,15*R*,18*R*,34*R*,35*S*,38*S*,48*R*,50a*R*)-34-(2-Acetylamino-2-deoxy-*β*-D-glucopyranosyloxy)-15-amino-22,31-dichloro-6,11,40,44,56-pentahydroxy-42-(*α*-D-mannopyranosyloxy)-2,16,36,50,51,59-hexaoxo-2,3,16,17,18,19,35,36,37,38,48,49,50,50a-tetradecahydro-1*H*,15*H*,34*H*-20,23:30,33-dietheno-3,18:35,48-bis(iminomethano)-4,8:10,14:25,28:43,47-tetrametheno-28*H*-[1,14,6,22]dioxadiazacyclooctacosino[4,5-*m*][10,2,16]-benzoxadiazacyclotetracosine-38-carboxylic acid
[*93616-27-4*]

[*61036-62-2*, Teicoplanin]

Teicoplanin is a mixture of glycopeptide substances having antibacterial activity produced by the growth of *Actinoplanes teichomyceticus*.

It contains not less than 900 *μ*g (potency) and not more than 1120 *μ*g (potency) per 1 mg, calculated on the anhydrous, sodium chloride-free and residual solvent-free basis. The potency of Teicoplanin is expressed as mass (potency) of teicoplanin ($C_{72\text{-}89}H_{68\text{-}99}Cl_2N_{8\text{-}9}O_{28\text{-}33}$).

Description Teicoplanin occurs as a white to light yellowish white powder.

It is freely soluble in water, sparingly soluble in *N,N*-dimethylformamide, and practically insoluble in acetonitrile, in methanol, in ethanol (95), in acetone, in acetic acid (100) and in diethyl ether.

Identification **(1)** To 1 mL of a solution of Teicoplanin (1 in 100) add 2 mL of ninhydrin TS, and warm for 5 minutes: a blue-purple color develops.

(2) To 1 mL of a solution of Teicoplanin (3 in 100) add slowly 2 mL of anthrone TS, and shake gently: a dark brown color develops.

(3) Determine the infrared absorption spectra of Teicoplanin and Teicoplanin RS as directed in the potassium bromide disk method under Infrared Spectrophotometry <*2.25*>, and compare the spectrum with the spectrum of Teicoplanin RS: both spectra exhibit similar intensities of absorption at the same wave numbers.

pH <*2.54*> Dissolve 0.5 g of Teicoplanin in 10 mL of water: the pH of the solution is between 6.3 and 7.7.

Content ratio of the active principle Dissolve about 20 mg of Teicoplanin in water to make 10 mL, and use this solution as the sample solution. Perform the test with 20 *μ*L of the sample solution as directed under Liquid Chromatography <*2.01*> according to the following conditions, and determine the sum of peak areas of teicoplanin A_2 group, S_a, the sum of peak areas of teicoplanin A_3 group, S_b, and the sum of peak areas of other contents, S_c from the sample solution by the automatic integration method. Calculate the content ratio of them by the formula given below: teicoplanin A_2 group, teicoplanin A_3 group, and the other are not less than 80.0%, not more than 15.0% and not more than 5.0%, respectively.

The elution order of each content and the relative retention time of each content to teicoplanin $A_{2\text{-}2}$ are shown in the following table.

Name of content	Elution order	Relative retention time
teicoplanin A_3 group		≦0.42
teicoplanin $A_{3\text{-}1}$	1	0.29
teicoplanin A_2 group		0.42<, ≦1.25
teicoplanin $A_{2\text{-}1}$	2	0.91
teicoplanin $A_{2\text{-}2}$	3	1.00
teicoplanin $A_{2\text{-}3}$	4	1.04
teicoplanin $A_{2\text{-}4}$	5	1.17
teicoplanin $A_{2\text{-}5}$	6	1.20
others		1.25<

Content ratio (%) of teicoplanin A_2 group
$= S_a/(S_a + 0.83S_b + S_c) \times 100$

Content ratio (%) of teicoplanin A_3 group
$= 0.83S_b/(S_a + 0.83S_b + S_c) \times 100$

Content ratio (%) of others
$= S_c/(S_a + 0.83S_b + S_c) \times 100$

Operating conditions—

Detector: An ultraviolet absorption photometer (wavelength: 254 nm).

Column: A stainless steel column 4.6 mm in inside diameter and 25 cm in length, packed with octadecylsilanized silica gel for liquid chromatography (5 μm in particle diameter).

Column temperature: A constant temperature of about 25°C.

Mobile phase A: Dissolve 7.80 g of sodium dihydrogen phosphate dihydrate in 1650 mL of water, add 300 mL of acetonitrile, adjust pH to 6.0 with sodium hydroxide TS, and add water to make 2000 mL.

Mobile phase B: Dissolve 7.80 g of sodium dihydrogen phosphate dihydrate in 550 mL of water, add 1400 mL of acetonitrile, adjust the pH to 6.0 with sodium hydroxide TS, and add water to make 2000 mL.

Flowing of mobile phase: Flow mobile phase A for 10 minutes before injection. After injection, control the gradient by mixing the mobile phases A and B as directed in the following table.

Time after injection of sample (min)	Mobile phase A (vol%)	Mobile phase B (vol%)
0 – 32	100 → 70	0 → 30
32 – 40	70 → 50	30 → 50
40 – 42	50 → 100	50 → 0

Flow rate: About 1.8 mL per minute.

Time span of measurement: About 1.7 times as long as the retention time of teicoplanin $A_{2\text{-}2}$, beginning after the solvent peak.

System suitability—

Test for required detectability: Confirm that peak height of teicoplanin $A_{2\text{-}2}$ obtained with the sample solution is equivalent to 90% of the full scale.

System performance: When the procedure is run with 20 μL of the sample solution under the above operating conditions, the symmetry factor of the peak of teicoplanin $A_{3\text{-}1}$ is not more than 2.2.

System repeatability: When the test is repeated 3 times with 20 μL of the sample solution under the above operating conditions, the relative standard deviation of the peak area of teicoplanin $A_{2\text{-}2}$ is not more than 2.0%.

Purity **(1)** Clarity and color of solution—Dissolve 0.8 g of Teicoplanin in 10 mL of water: the solution is clear. Perform the test with this solution according to Method 1 under Methods for Color Matching <*2.65*>: the color is not more colored than Matching Fluids BY3 and B4.

(2) Sodium chloride—Weigh accurately about 0.5 g of Teicoplanin, dissolve in 50 mL of water, titrate <*2.50*> with 0.1 mol/L silver nitrate VS (indicator: 1 mL of potassium chromate TS), and calculate an amount of sodium chloride: not more than 5.0%.

Each mL of 0.1 mol/L silver nitrate VS
= 5.844 mg of NaCl

(3) Heavy metals <*1.07*>—Place 2.0 g of Teicoplanin in a quartz or porcelain crucible, cover loosely with a lid, and heat gently to carbonize. After cooling, add 2 mL of nitric acid and 5 drops of sulfuric acid, heat cautiously until white fumes are no longer evolved, and incinerate by ignition between 500°C and 600°C. If a carbonized substance remains, add 2 mL of nitric acid and 5 drops of sulfuric acid, heat in the same manner as above, and incinerate by ignition between 500°C and 600°C. Cool, then proceed according to Method 2, and perform the test. The control solution is prepared as follows: Evaporate a mixture of 4 mL of nitric acid, 10 drops of sulfuric acid and 2 mL of hydrochloric acid on a water bath, further evaporate to dryness on a sand bath, and moisten the residue with 3 drops of hydrochloric acid. Then proceed in the same manner as the test solution, and add 1.0 mL of Standard Lead Solution and water to make 50 mL (not more than 5 ppm).

(4) Arsenic <*1.11*>—Prepare the test solution with 1.0 g of Teicoplanin according to Method 3, and perform the test (not more than 2 ppm).

(5) Residual solvents <*2.46*>—Weigh accurately about 0.1 g of Teicoplanin, dissolve in *N*,*N*-dimethylformamide to make exactly 10 mL, and use this solution as the sample solution. Separately, weigh accurately about 1 g each of methanol and acetone, and add *N*,*N*-dimethylformamide to make exactly 100 mL. Pipet 1 mL of this solution, add *N*,*N*-dimethylformamide to make exactly 100 mL, and use this solution as the standard solution. Perform the test with exactly 4 μL each of the sample solution and standard solution as directed under Gas Chromatography <*2.02*> according to the following conditions. Determine the peak area of methanol, A_1, and the peak area of acetone, A_2, obtained from the sample solution, and the peak area of methanol, A_{S1}, and the peak area of acetone, A_{S2}, from the standard solution by the automatic integration method, and calculate the amounts of methanol and acetone by the following formula: not more than 0.5% and not more than 1.0%, respectively.

$$\text{Amount (\%) of methanol} = M_{S1} \times A_1/A_{S1} \times 0.001 \times 1/M_T \times 100$$

$$\text{Amount (\%) of acetone} = M_{S2} \times A_2/A_{S2} \times 0.001 \times 1/M_T \times 100$$

M_{S1}: Amount (g) of methanol taken
M_{S2}: Amount (g) of acetone taken
M_T: Amount (g) of Teicoplanin taken

Operating conditions—

Detector: A Hydrogen flame-ionization detector.

Column: A glass column 2 mm in inside diameter and 3 m in length, packed with graphite carbon for gas chromatography, 150 to 180 μm in particle diameter, coated with 0.1% of polyethylene glycol esterified.

Column temperature: Inject the sample at a constant temperature of about 70°C, maintain the temperature for 4 minutes, then program to raise the temperature to 210°C at the rate of 8°C per minute.

Detector temperature: A constant temperature of about 240°C.

Carrier gas: Nitrogen.

Flow rate: Adjust so that the retention times of methanol and acetone are about 2 minutes and 5 minutes, respectively.

System suitability—

Test for required detectability: Confirm that the peak height of acetone obtained from 4 μL of the standard solution is equivalent to about the full scale.

System performance: When the procedure is run with 4 μL of the standard solution under the above operating conditions, methanol and acetone are eluted in this order with the resolution between these peaks being not less than 2.0.

System repeatability: When the test is repeated 3 times with 4 μL of the standard solution under the above operating conditions, the relative standard deviation of the peak areas of acetone is not more than 3%.

Water <*2.48*> Not more than 15.0% (0.2 g, volumetric titration, direct titration).

Assay Perform the test according to the Cylinder-plate method as directed under Microbial Assay for Antibiotics *<4.02>* according to the following conditions.

(i) Test organism—*Bacillus subtilis* ATCC 6633

(ii) Culture medium—Use the medium i in 1) under (1) Agar media for seed and base layer.

(iii) Standard solutions—Weigh accurately an amount of Teicoplanin RS equivalent to about 50 mg (potency), dissolve in phosphate buffer solution (pH 6.0) to make exactly 50 mL, and use this solution as the standard stock solution. Keep the standard stock solution at not exceeding 5°C and use within 14 days. Take exactly a suitable amount of this solution before use, add phosphate buffer solution (pH 6.0) to make solutions so that each mL contains 160 μg (potency) and 40 μg (potency), and use these solutions as the high concentration standard solution and the low concentration standard solution, respectively.

(iv) Sample solutions—Weigh accurately an amount of Teicoplanin equivalent to about 50 mg (potency), dissolve in phosphate buffer solution (pH 6.0) to make exactly 50 mL. Take exactly a suitable amount of this solution, add phosphate buffer solution (pH 6.0) to make solutions so that each mL contains 160 μg (potency) and 40 μg (potency), and use these solutions as the high concentration sample solution and the low concentration sample solution, respectively.

Containers and storage Containers—Tight containers.

Storage—Light-resistant, and at a temperature between 2°C and 8°C.

Telmisartan

テルミサルタン

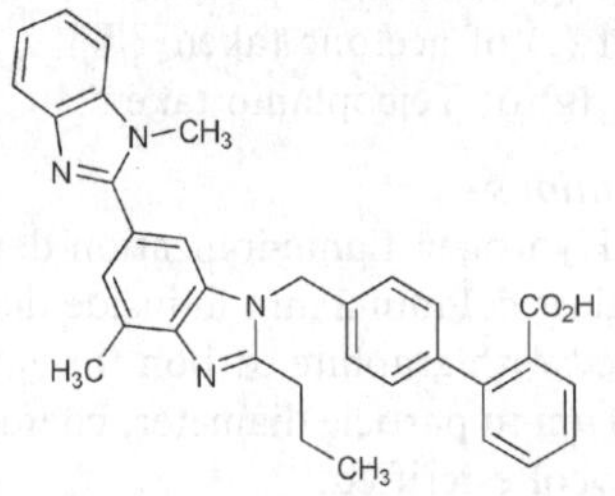

$C_{33}H_{30}N_4O_2$: 514.62

4′-{[4-Methyl-6-(1-methyl-1*H*-benzimidazol-2-yl)-2-propyl-1*H*-benzimidazol-1-yl]methyl}biphenyl-2-carboxylic acid

[*144701-48-4*]

Telmisartan, when dried, contains not less than 99.0% and not more than 101.0% of telmisartan ($C_{33}H_{30}N_4O_2$).

Description Telmisartan occurs as a white to pale yellow crystalline powder.

It is freely soluble in formic acid, slightly soluble in methanol, very slightly soluble in ethanol (99.5), and practically insoluble in water.

It shows crystal polymorphism.

Identification **(1)** Determine the absorption spectrum of a solution of Telmisartan in methanol (7 in 1,000,000) as directed under Ultraviolet-visible Spectrophotometry *<2.24>*, and compare the spectrum with the Reference Spectrum: both spectra exhibit similar intensities of absorption at the same wavelengths.

(2) Determine the infrared absorption spectrum of Telmisartan as directed in the potassium bromide disk method under Infrared Spectrophotometry *<2.25>*, and compare the spectrum with the Reference Spectrum: both spectra exhibit similar intensities of absorption at the same wave numbers. If any difference appears between the spectra, dissolve Telmisartan in ethanol (95) by warming, and cool in ice. Collect the crystals formed, dry, and perform the test with the crystals.

Purity **(1)** Heavy metals *<1.07>*—Proceed with 2.0 g of Telmisartan according to Method 2, and perform the test. Prepare the control solution with 2.0 mL of Standard Lead solution (not more than 10 ppm).

(2) Related substances—To 25 mg of Telmisartan add 5 mL of methanol and 0.1 mL of sodium hydroxide TS, and dissolve by sonicating. To this solution add methanol to make 10 mL, and use this solution as the sample solution. Pipet 1 mL of the sample solution, add methanol to make exactly 100 mL, and use this solution as the standard solution. Perform the test with exactly 2 μL each of the sample solution and standard solution as directed under Liquid Chromatography *<2.01>* according to the following conditions, and determine each peak area by the automatic integration method: the area of the peak, having the relative retention time of about 1.7 to telmisartan, obtained from the sample solution is not larger than 1/5 times the peak area of telmisartan from the standard solution, the area of the peak other than telmisartan and the peak mentioned above from the sample solution is not larger than 1/10 times the peak area of telmisartan from the standard solution, and the total area of the peaks other than telmisartan from the sample solution is not larger than the peak area of telmisartan from the standard solution. For the area of the peak, having the relative retention time of about 0.7, multiply its correction factor 1.2.

Operating conditions—

Detector: An ultraviolet absorption photometer (wavelength: 230 nm).

Column: A stainless steel column 4.0 mm in inside diameter and 12.5 cm in length, packed with octadecylsilanized silica gel for liquid chromatography (5 μm in particle diameter).

Column temperature: A constant temperature of about 40°C.

Mobile phase A: Dissolve 2.0 g of potassium dihydrogen phosphate and 3.4 g of sodium 1-pentanesulfonate in 1000 mL of water, and adjust to pH 3.0 with diluted phosphoric acid (1 in 10).

Mobile phase B: A mixture of acetonitrile and methanol (4:1).

Flowing of mobile phase: Control the gradient by mixing the mobile phases A and B as directed in the following table.

Time after injection of sample (min)	Mobile phase A (vol%)	Mobile phase B (vol%)
0 - 25	70 → 20	30 → 80

Flow rate: 1.0 mL per minute.

Time span of measurement: About 2 times as long as the retention time of telmisartan, beginning after the solvent peak.

System suitability—

Test for required detectability: Pipet 5 mL of the standard solution, add methanol to make exactly 100 mL. Confirm that the peak area of telmisartan obtained with 2 μL of this solution is equivalent to 3.5 to 6.5% of that with 2 μL of the standard solution.

System performance: When the procedure is run with 2 μL of the standard solution under the above operating conditions, the number of theoretical plates and the symmetry factor of the peak of telmisartan are not less than 45,000 and not more than 1.2, respectively.

System repeatability: When the test is repeated 6 times with 2 μL of the standard solution under the above operating conditions, the relative standard deviation of the peak area of telmisartan is not more than 5%.

Loss on drying <*2.41*> Not more than 0.5% (1 g, 105°C, 4 hours).

Residue on ignition <*2.44*> Not more than 0.1% (1 g).

Assay Weigh accurately about 0.19 g of Telmisartan, previously dried, dissolve in 5 mL of formic acid, add 75 mL of acetic anhydride, and titrate <*2.50*> with 0.1 mol/L perchloric acid VS (potentiometric titration). Perform a blank determination in the same manner, and make any necessary correction.

Each mL of 0.1 mol/L perchloric acid VS
= 25.73 mg of $C_{33}H_{30}N_4O_2$

Containers and storage Containers—Tight containers.

Telmisartan and Amlodipine Besilate Tablets

テルミサルタン・アムロジピンベシル酸塩錠

Telmisartan and Amlodipine Besilate Tablets contain not less than 95.0% and not more than 105.0% of the labeled amount of telmisartan ($C_{33}H_{30}N_4O_2$: 514.62) and amlodipine besilate ($C_{20}H_{25}ClN_2O_5.C_6H_6O_3S$: 567.05)

Method of preparation Prepare as directed under Tablets, with Telmisartan and Amlodipine Besilate.

Identification **(1)** Perform the test with 5 μL each of the sample solution and standard solution obtained in the Assay (1) as directed under Liquid Chromatography <*2.01*> according to the following conditions: the retention times of the peaks of telmisartan in the chromatograms obtained from the sample solution and the standard solution are the same, and both absorption spectra of these peaks exhibit similar intensities of absorption at the same wavelengths.

Operating conditions—

Column, column temperature, mobile phase A, mobile phase B, flowing of mobile phase, and flow rate: Proceed as directed in the operating conditions in the Assay (1).

Detector: A photodiode array detector (wavelength: 270 nm; spectrum range of measurement: 210 – 400 nm).

System suitability -

System performance: Proceed as directed in the system suitability in the Assay (1).

(2) Perform the test with 5 μL each of the sample solution and standard solution obtained in the Assay (2) as directed under Liquid Chromatography <*2.01*> according to the following conditions: the retention times of the peaks of amlodipine besilate in the chromatograms obtained from the sample solution and the standard solution are the same, and both spectra of these peaks in the chromatograms exhibit similar intensities of absorption at the same wavelengths.

Operating conditions—

Column, column temperature, mobile phase A, mobile phase B, flowing of mobile phase, and flow rate: Proceed as directed in the operating conditions in the Assay (2).

Detector: A photodiode array detector (wavelength: 237 nm; spectrum range of measurement: 210 – 400 nm).

System suitability—

System performance: Proceed as directed in the system suitability in the Assay (2).

Uniformity of dosage unit <*6.02*> Perform the test according to the following method: it meets the requirement of the Content uniformity test.

(1) Telmisartan—To 1 tablet of Telmisartan and Amlodipine Besilate Tablets add $4V/5$ mL of the dissolving solution, disintegrate by sonicating, and add the dissolving solution to make exactly V mL so that each mL contains about 1.6 mg of telmisartan ($C_{33}H_{30}N_4O_2$). Centrifuge this solution, pipet 5 mL of the supernatant liquid, add the buffer solution to make exactly 25 mL, and use this solution as the sample solution. Then, proceed as directed in the Assay (1).

Amount (mg) of telmisartan ($C_{33}H_{30}N_4O_2$)
$= M_S \times A_T/A_S \times V/50$

M_S: Amount (mg) of telmisartan for assay taken

Dissolving solution: Dissolve 2 g of ammonium dihydrogen phosphate in 1000 mL of water, and adjust to pH 1.8 with phosphoric acid. To 1000 mL of this solution add 1000 mL of acetonitrile.

Buffer solution: Dissolve 2 g of ammonium dihydrogen phosphate in 1000 mL of water, and adjust to pH 1.8 with phosphoric acid.

(2) Amlodipine Besilate—To 1 tablet of Telmisartan and Amlodipine Besilate Tablets add $4V/5$ mL of the dissolving solution, disintegrate by sonicating, and add the dissolving solution to make exactly V mL so that each mL contains about 0.138 mg of amlodipine besilate ($C_{20}H_{25}ClN_2O_5.C_6H_6O_3S$). Centrifuge this solution, pipet 5 mL of the supernatant liquid, add the buffer solution to make exactly 25 mL, and use this solution as the sample solution. Then, proceed as directed in the Assay (2).

Amount (mg) of amlodipine besilate
($C_{20}H_{25}ClN_2O_5.C_6H_6O_3S$)
$= M_S \times A_T/A_S \times V/250$

M_S: Amount (mg) of Amlodipine Besilate RS taken, calculated on the anhydrous basis

Dissolving solution: Dissolve 2 g of ammonium dihydrogen phosphate in 1000 mL of water, and adjust to pH 1.8 with phosphoric acid. To 1000 mL of this solution add 1000 mL of acetonitrile.

Buffer solution: Dissolve 2 g of ammonium dihydrogen phosphate in 1000 mL of water, and adjust to pH 1.8 with phosphoric acid.

Dissolution <*6.10*> **(1)** Telmisartan—Being specified separately when the drug is granted approval based on the Law.

(2) Amlodipine Besilate—Being specified separately when the drug is granted approval based on the Law.

Assay **(1)** Telmisartan—Weigh accurately the mass of not less than 20 Telmisartan and Amlodipine Besilate Tablets, and powder. Weigh accurately a portion of the powder, equivalent to about 80 mg of telmisartan ($C_{33}H_{30}N_4O_2$), add 40 mL of the dissolving solution, disintegrate by sonicating, and add the dissolving solution to make exactly 50 mL. Centrifuge this solution, pipet 5 mL of the supernatant liquid, add the buffer solution to make exactly 25 mL, and use this solution as the sample solution. Separately, weigh accurately about 80 mg of telmisartan for assay, previously dried at 105°C for 4 hours, add the dissolving solution to make exactly 50 mL, and use this solution as the telmisartan standard stock solution. Pipet 5 mL of the telmisartan standard stock solution, add the buffer solution to make exactly 25 mL, and use this solution as the standard solution. Perform the test with exactly 5 μL each of the sample solution and standard solution as directed under Liquid Chromatography <*2.01*> according to the following conditions, and determine the peak areas, A_T and A_S, of telmisartan in each solution.

Amount (mg) of telmisartan ($C_{33}H_{30}N_4O_2$)
$$= M_S \times A_T/A_S$$

M_S: Amount (mg) of telmisartan for assay taken

Dissolving solution: Dissolve 2 g of ammonium dihydrogen phosphate in 1000 mL of water, and adjust to pH 1.8 with phosphoric acid. To 1000 mL of this solution add 1000 mL of acetonitrile.

Buffer solution: Dissolve 2 g of ammonium dihydrogen phosphate in 1000 mL of water, and adjust to pH 1.8 with phosphoric acid.

Operating conditions—

Detector: An ultraviolet absorption photometer (wavelength: 270 nm).

Column: A stainless steel column 3.0 mm in inside diameter and 7.5 cm in length, packed with octylsilanized silica gel for liquid chromatography (5 μm in particle diameter).

Column temperature: A constant temperature of about 40°C.

Mobile phase A: Dissolve 2 g of ammonium dihydrogen phosphate in 1000 mL of water, and adjust to pH 3.5 with phosphoric acid.

Mobile phase B: Acetonitrile.

Flowing of mobile phase: Control the gradient by mixing the mobile phases A and B as directed in the following table.

Time after injection of sample (min)	Mobile phase A (vol%)	Mobile phase B (vol%)
0 – 2.0	90	10
2.0 – 7.0	90 → 20	10 → 80
7.0 – 8.0	20	80

Flow rate: 0.8 mL per minute.

System suitability—

System performance: To each 5 mL of the telmisartan standard stock solution and the amlodipine besilate standard stock solution obtained in (2) add the buffer solution to make 25 mL. When the procedure is run with 5 μL of this solution under the above operating conditions, amlodipine and telmisartan are eluted in this order with the resolution between these peaks being not less than 5.

System repeatability: When the test is repeated 6 times with 5 μL of the standard solution under the above operating conditions, the relative standard deviation of the peak area of telmisartan is not more than 1.0%.

(2) Amlodipine Besilate—Weigh accurately the mass of not less than 20 Telmisartan and Amlodipine Besilate Tablets, and powder. Weigh accurately a portion of the powder, equivalent to about 6.9 mg of amlodipine besilate ($C_{20}H_{25}ClN_2O_5.C_6H_6O_3S$), add 40 mL of the dissolving solution, disintegrate by sonicating, and add the dissolving solution to make exactly 50 mL. Centrifuge this solution, pipet 5 mL of the supernatant liquid, add the buffer solution to make exactly 25 mL, and use this solution as the sample solution. Separately, weigh accurately about 35 mg of Amlodipine Besilate RS (separately determine the water <*2.48*> in the same manner as Amlodipine Besilate) and add the dissolving solution to make exactly 100 mL. Pipet 20 mL of this solution, add the dissolving solution to make exactly 50 mL, and use this solution as the amlodipine besilate standard stock solution. Pipet 5 mL of the amlodipine besilate standard stock solution, add the buffer solution to make exactly 25 mL, and use this solution as the standard solution. Perform the test with exactly 5 μL each of the sample solution and standard solution as directed under Liquid Chromatography <*2.01*> according to the following conditions, and determine the peak areas, A_T and A_S, of amlodipine in each solution.

Amount (mg) of amlodipine besilate
($C_{20}H_{25}ClN_2O_5.C_6H_6O_3S$)
$$= M_S \times A_T/A_S \times 1/5$$

M_S: Amount (mg) of Amlodipine Besilate RS taken, calculated on the anhydrous basis

Dissolving solution: Dissolve 2 g of ammonium dihydrogen phosphate in 1000 mL of water, and adjust to pH 1.8 with phosphoric acid. To 1000 mL of this solution add 1000 mL of acetonitrile.

Buffer solution: Dissolve 2 g of ammonium dihydrogen phosphate in 1000 mL of water, and adjust to pH 1.8 with phosphoric acid.

Operating conditions—

Detector: An ultraviolet absorption photometer (wavelength: 237 nm).

Column: A stainless steel column 3.0 mm in inside diameter and 7.5 cm in length, packed with octylsilanized silica gel for liquid chromatography (5 μm in particle diameter).

Column temperature: A constant temperature of about 40°C.

Mobile phase A: Dissolve 2 g of ammonium dihydrogen phosphate in 1000 mL of water, and adjust to pH 3.5 with phosphoric acid.

Mobile phase B: Acetonitrile.

Flowing of mobile phase: Control the gradient by mixing the mobile phases A and B as directed in the following table.

Time after injection of sample (min)	Mobile phase A (vol%)	Mobile phase B (vol%)
0 – 2.0	90	10
2.0 – 7.0	90 → 20	10 → 80
7.0 – 8.0	20	80

Flow rate: 0.8 mL per minute.

System suitability—

System performance: To 5 mL each of the telmisartan standard stock solution obtained in (1) and the amlodipine besilate standard stock solution add the buffer solution to make 25 mL. When the procedure is run with 5 μL of this solution under the above operating conditions, amlodipine and telmisartan are eluted in this order with the resolution between these peaks being not less than 5.

System repeatability: When the test is repeated 6 times with 5 μL of the standard solution under the above operating conditions, the relative standard deviation of the peak area of amlodipine is not more than 1.0%.

Containers and storage Containers—Tight containers.

Telmisartan Tablets

テルミサルタン錠

Telmisartan Tablets contain not less than 95.0% and not more than 105.0% of the labeled amount of telmisartan ($C_{33}H_{30}N_4O_2$: 514.62).

Method of preparation Prepare as directed under Tablets, with Telmisartan.

Identification Powder Telmisartan Tablets. To a portion of the powder, equivalent to 0.7 mg of Telmisartan, add 100 mL of methanol, shake well, and filter through a membrane filter with a pore size not exceeding 0.45 μm. Determine the absorption spectrum of the filtrate as directed under Ultraviolet-visible Spectrophotometry <*2.24*>: it exhibits maxima between 226 nm and 230 nm and between 295 nm and 299 nm.

Uniformity of dosage units <*6.02*> Perform the test according to the following method: it meets the requirement of the Content uniformity test.

To 1 tablet of Telmisartan Tablets add $4V/5$ mL of a mixture of water and methanol (1:1), disintegrate the tablet by sonicating, and add a mixture of water and methanol (1:1) to make exactly V mL so that each mL contains about 0.8 mg of telmisartan ($C_{33}H_{30}N_4O_2$). Filter this solution through a membrane filter with a pore size not exceeding 0.45 μm, discard 10 mL of the first filtrate, pipet 5 mL of the subsequent filtrate, add a mixture of water and methanol (1:1) to make exactly 50 mL, and use this solution as the sample solution. Then, proceed as directed in the Assay.

Amount (mg) of telmisartan ($C_{33}H_{30}N_4O_2$)
$= M_S \times A_T/A_S \times V/25$

M_S: Amount (mg) of telmisartan for assay taken

Dissolution <*6.10*> When the test is performed at 50 revolutions per minute according to the Paddle method, using 900 mL of 2nd fluid for dissolution test as the dissolution medium, the dissolution rate in 30 minutes of Telmisartan Tablets is not less than 85%.

Start the test with 1 tablet of Telmisartan Tablets, withdraw not less than 20 mL of the medium at the specified minute after starting the test, and filter through a membrane filter with a pore size not exceeding 0.45 μm. Discard not less than 5 mL of the first filtrate, pipet V mL of the subsequent filtrate, add the dissolution medium to make exactly V' mL so that each mL contains about 11 μg of telmisartan ($C_{33}H_{30}N_4O_2$), and use this solution as the sample solution. Separately, weigh accurately about 22 mg of telmisartan for assay, previously dried at 105°C for 4 hours, add 10 mL of a solution of meglumine in methanol (1 in 500), dissolve by sonicating, and add methanol to make exactly 50 mL. Pipet 5 mL of this solution, add the dissolution medium to make exactly 200 mL, and use this solution as the standard solution. Determine the absorbances, A_T and A_S, at 296 nm of the sample solution and standard solution as directed under Ultraviolet-visible Spectrophotometry <*2.24*>, using the dissolution medium as the control.

Dissolution rate (%) with respect to the labeled amount of telmisartan ($C_{33}H_{30}N_4O_2$)
$= M_S \times A_T/A_S \times V'/V \times 1/C \times 45$

M_S: Amount (mg) of telmisartan for assay taken
C: Labeled amount (mg) of telmisartan ($C_{33}H_{30}N_4O_2$) in 1 tablet

Assay Weigh accurately the mass of not less than 20 Telmisartan Tablets, and powder. Weigh accurately a portion of the powder, equivalent to about 80 mg of telmisartan ($C_{33}H_{30}N_4O_2$), add 80 mL of a mixture of water and methanol (1:1), shake thoroughly, and add a mixture of water and methanol (1:1) to make exactly 100 mL. Filter this solution through a membrane filter with a pore size not exceeding 0.45 μm. Discard the first 10 mL of the filtrate, pipet 5 mL of the subsequent filtrate, add a mixture of water and methanol (1:1) to make exactly 50 mL, and use this solution as the sample solution. Separately, weigh accurately about 20 mg of telmisartan for assay, previously dried at 105°C for 4 hours, add 10 mL of a solution of meglumine in a mixture of water and methanol (1:1) (1 in 500), dissolve by shaking well, and add a mixture of water and methanol (1:1) to make exactly 25 mL. Pipet 5 mL of this solution, add a mixture of water and methanol (1:1) to make exactly 50 mL, and use this solution as the standard solution. Perform the test with exactly 10 μL each of the sample solution and standard solution as directed under Liquid Chromatography <*2.01*> according to the following conditions, and determine the peak areas, A_T and A_S, of telmisartan in each solution.

Amount (mg) of telmisartan ($C_{33}H_{30}N_4O_2$)
$= M_S \times A_T/A_S \times 4$

M_S: Amount (mg) of telmisartan for assay taken

Operating conditions—

Detector: An ultraviolet absorption photometer (wavelength: 295 nm).

Column: A stainless steel column 4.6 mm in inside diameter and 15 cm in length, packed with octadecylsilanized silica gel for liquid chromatography (5 μm in particle diameter).

Column temperature: A constant temperature of about 40°C.

Mobile phase: Dissolve 2 g of diammonium hydrogenphosphate in 1000 mL of water, and adjust to pH 3.0 with diluted phosphoric acid (1 in 10). To 300 mL of this solution add 700 mL of methanol.

Flow rate: Adjust so that the retention time of telmisartan is about 6 minutes.

System suitability—

System performance: When the procedure is run with 10 μL of the standard solution under the above operating conditions, the number of theoretical plates and the symmetry factor of the peak of telmisartan are not less than 3000 and not more than 2.0, respectively.

System repeatability: When the test is repeated 6 times with 10 μL of the standard solution under the above operating conditions, the relative standard deviation of the peak area of telmisartan is not more than 1.0%.

Containers and storage Containers—Tight containers.

Telmisartan and Hydrochlorothiazide Tablets

テルミサルタン・ヒドロクロロチアジド錠

Telmisartan and Hydrochlorothiazide Tablets contain not less than 95.0% and not more than 105.0% of the labeled amount of telmisartan ($C_{33}H_{30}N_4O_2$: 514.62) and hydrochlorothiazide ($C_7H_8ClN_3O_4S_2$: 297.74).

Method of preparation Prepare as directed under Tablets, with Telmisartan and Hydrochlorothiazide.

Identification (1) Perform the test with 5 μL each of the sample solution and standard solution obtained in the Assay (1) as directed under Liquid Chromatography <*2.01*> according to the following conditions: the retention times of the peaks of telmisartan in the chromatograms obtained from the sample solution and standard solution are the same, and absorption spectra of these peaks exhibit similar intensities of absorption at the same wavelengths.

Operating conditions—

Column, column temperature, mobile phase, and flow rate: Proceed as directed in the operating conditions in the Assay (1).

Detector: A photodiode array detector (wavelength: 270 nm, spectrum range of measurement: 210 – 400 nm).

System suitability—

System performance: Proceed as directed in the system suitability in the Assay (1).

(2) Perform the test with 5 μL each of the sample solution and standard solution obtained in the Assay (2) as directed under Liquid Chromatography <*2.01*> according to the following conditions: the retention times of the peaks of hydrochlorothiazide in the chromatograms obtained from the sample solution and standard solution are the same, and absorption spectra of these peaks exhibit similar intensities of absorption at the same wavelengths.

Operating conditions—

Column, column temperature, mobile phase, and flow rate: Proceed as directed in the operating conditions in the Assay (1).

Detector: A photodiode array detector (wavelength: 270 nm, spectrum range of measurement: 210 – 400 nm).

System suitability—

System performance: Proceed as directed in the system suitability in the Assay (2).

Purity Related substances—To a quantity of powdered Telmisartan and Hydrochlorothiazide Tablets, equivalent to 12.5 mg of Hydrochlorothiazide, add 40 mL of the dissolving solution, disperse by sonicating, add the dissolving solution to make exactly 50 mL. Centrifuge this solution, and use the supernatant liquid as the sample solution. Pipet 1 mL of the sample solution, add the dissolving solution to make exactly 100 mL, and use this solution as the standard solution. Perform the test with exactly 20 μL each of the sample solution and standard solution as directed under Liquid Chromatography <*2.01*> according to the following conditions, and determine each peak area by the automatic integration method: the area of the peak having the relative retention time of about 0.9 to hydrochlorothiazide, obtained from the sample solution is not larger than the peak area of hydrochlorothiazide from the standard solution.

Dissolving solution: Dissolve 2 g of ammonium dihydrogen phosphate in 1000 mL of water, and adjust to pH 1.8 with phosphoric acid. To 1000 mL of this solution add 1000 mL of acetonitrile.

Operating conditions—

Detector: An ultraviolet absorption photometer (wavelength: 270 nm).

Column: A stainless steel column 4.0 mm in inside diameter and 15 cm in length, packed with octylsilanized silica gel for liquid chromatography (3 μm in particle diameter).

Column temperature: A constant temperature of about 40°C.

Mobile phase A: Dissolve 2 g of ammonium dihydrogen phosphate in 1000 mL of water, and adjust to pH 3.5 with phosphoric acid.

Mobile phase B: Acetonitrile.

Flowing of mobile phase: Control the gradient by mixing the mobile phases A and B as directed in the following table.

Time after injection of sample (min)	Mobile phase A (vol%)	Mobile phase B (vol%)
0 – 8	90 → 50	10 → 50
8 – 12	50	50
12 – 18	50 → 20	50 → 80
18 – 20	20	80

Flow rate: 1.0 mL per minute.

System suitability—

Test for required detectability: Pipet 5 mL of the standard solution and add the dissolving solution to make exactly 50 mL. Confirm that the peak area of hydrochlorothiazide obtained with 20 μL of this solution is equivalent to 7 to 13% of that with 20 μL of the standard solution.

System performance: When the procedure is run with 20 μL of the standard solution under the above operating conditions, the number of theoretical plates and the symmetry factor of the peak of hydrochlorothiazide are not less than 6000 and not more than 2.0, respectively.

System repeatability: When the test is repeated 6 times with 20 μL of the standard solution under the above operating conditions, the relative standard deviation of the peak area of hydrochlorothiazide is not more than 2.0%.

Uniformity of dosage units <*6.02*> Perform the test according to the following method: it meets the requirement of the Content uniformity test.

(1) Telmisartan—To 1 tablet of Telmisartan and Hydrochlorothiazide Tablets add $4V/5$ mL of the dissolving solution, disintegrate by sonicating, add the dissolving solution to make exactly V mL so that each mL contains about 1.6 mg of telmisartan ($C_{33}H_{30}N_4O_2$). Centrifuge this solution, pipet 5 mL of the supernatant liquid, add the buffer solution to make exactly 25 mL, and use this solution as the sample solution. Proceed as directed in the Assay (1).

$$\text{Amount (mg) of telmisartan } (C_{33}H_{30}N_4O_2) = M_S \times A_T/A_S \times V/50$$

M_S: Amount (mg) of telmisartan for assay taken

Dissolving solution: Dissolve 2 g of ammonium dihydrogen phosphate in 1000 mL of water, and adjust to pH 1.8 with phosphoric acid. To 1000 mL of this solution add 1000 mL of acetonitrile.

Buffer solution: Dissolve 2 g of ammonium dihydrogen phosphate in 1000 mL of water, and adjust to pH 1.8 with phosphoric acid.

(2) Hydrochlorothiazide—To 1 tablet of Telmisartan

and Hydrochlorothiazide Tablets add $4V/5$ mL of the dissolving solution, disintegrate by sonicating, add the dissolving solution to make exactly V mL so that each mL contains about 0.25 mg of hydrochlorothiazide ($C_7H_8ClN_3O_4S_2$). Centrifuge this solution, pipet 5 mL of the supernatant liquid, add the buffer solution to make exactly 25 mL, and use this solution as the sample solution. Proceed as directed in the Assay (2).

Amount (mg) of hydrochlorothiazide ($C_7H_8ClN_3O_4S_2$)
$= M_S \times A_T/A_S \times V/50$

M_S: Amount (mg) of Hydrochlorothiazide RS taken

Dissolving solution: Dissolve 2 g of ammonium dihydrogen phosphate in 1000 mL of water, and adjust to pH 1.8 with phosphoric acid. To 1000 mL of this solution add 1000 mL of acetonitrile.

Buffer solution: Dissolve 2 g of ammonium dihydrogen phosphate in 1000 mL of water, and adjust to pH 1.8 with phosphoric acid.

Dissolution <*6.10*> (1) Telmisartan—When the test is performed at 50 revolutions per minute according to the Paddle method, using 900 mL of 2nd fluid for dissolution test as the dissolution medium, the dissolution rates in 45 minutes of a telmisartan 40-mg and hydrochlorothiazide 12.5-mg tablet and a telmisartan 80-mg and hydrochlorothiazide 12.5-mg tablet are not less than 85% and not less than 80%, respectively.

Start the test with 1 tablet of Telmisartan and Hydrochlorothiazide Tablets, withdraw not less than 20 mL of the medium at the specified minute after starting the test, and filter through a membrane filter with a pore size not exceeding 0.45 μm. Discard not less than 15 mL of the first filtrate, pipet V mL of the subsequent filtrate, add the dissolution medium to make exactly V' mL so that each mL contains about 44 μg of telmisartan ($C_{33}H_{30}N_4O_2$), and use this solution as the sample solution. Separately, weigh accurately about 44 mg of telmisartan for assay, previously dried at 105°C for 4 hours, dissolve in 10 mL of a solution of meglumine in methanol (1 in 250), and add methanol to make exactly 50 mL. Pipet 5 mL of this solution, add water to make exactly 100 mL, and use this solution as the standard solution. Perform the test with exactly 25 μL each of the sample solution and standard solution as directed under Liquid Chromatography <*2.01*> according to the following conditions, and determine the peak areas, A_T and A_S, of telmisartan in each solution.

Dissolution rate (%) with respect to the labeled amount of telmisartan ($C_{33}H_{30}N_4O_2$)
$= M_S \times A_T/A_S \times V'/V \times 1/C \times 90$

M_S: Amount (mg) of telmisartan for assay taken
C: Labeled amount (mg) of telmisartan ($C_{33}H_{30}N_4O_2$) in 1 tablet

Operating conditions—

Proceed as directed in the operating conditions in the Assay (1).

System suitability—

System performance: When the procedure is run with 25 μL of the standard solution under the above operating conditions, the number of theoretical plates and the symmetry factor of the peak of telmisartan are not less than 25,000 and not more than 2.0, respectively.

System repeatability: When the test is repeated 6 times with 25 μL of the standard solution under the above operating conditions, the relative standard deviation of the peak area of telmisartan is not more than 2.0%.

(2) Hydrochlorothiazide—When the test is performed at 75 revolutions per minute according to the Paddle method, using 900 mL of 2nd fluid for dissolution test as the dissolution medium, the dissolution rate in 45 minutes of Telmisartan and Hydrochlorothiazide Tablets is not less than 80%.

Start the test with 1 tablet of Telmisartan and Hydrochlorothiazide Tablets, withdraw not less than 20 mL of the medium at the specified minute after starting the test, and filter through a membrane filter with a pore size not exceeding 0.45 μm. Discard not less than 15 mL of the first filtrate, pipet V mL of the subsequent filtrate, add the dissolution medium to make exactly V' mL so that each mL contains about 14 μg of hydrochlorothiazide ($C_7H_8ClN_3O_4S_2$), and use this solution as the sample solution. Separately, weigh accurately about 14 mg of Hydrochlorothiazide RS, previously dried at 105°C for 2 hours, and dissolve in methanol to make exactly 50 mL. Pipet 5 mL of this solution, add water to make exactly 100 mL, and use this solution as the standard solution. Perform the test with exactly 25 μL each of the sample solution and standard solution as directed under Liquid Chromatography <*2.01*> according to the following conditions, and determine the peak areas, A_T and A_S, of hydrochlorothiazide in each solution.

Dissolution rate (%) with respect to the labeled amount of hydrochlorothiazide ($C_7H_8ClN_3O_4S_2$)
$= M_S \times A_T/A_S \times V'/V \times 1/C \times 90$

M_S: Amount (mg) of Hydrochlorothiazide RS taken
C: Labeled amount (mg) of hydrochlorothiazide ($C_7H_8ClN_3O_4S_2$) in 1 tablet

Operating conditions—

Proceed as directed in the operating conditions in the Assay (1).

System suitability—

System performance: When the procedure is run with 25 μL of the standard solution under the above operating conditions, the number of theoretical plates and the symmetry factor of the peak of hydrochlorothiazide are not less than 1000 and not more than 2.0, respectively.

System repeatability: When the test is repeated 6 times with 25 μL of the standard solution under the above operating conditions, the relative standard deviation of the peak area of hydrochlorothiazide is not more than 2.0%.

Assay (1) Telmisartan—Weigh accurately the mass of not less than 20 Telmisartan and Hydrochlorothiazide Tablets, and powder. Weigh accurately a portion of the powder, equivalent to about 80 mg of telmisartan ($C_{33}H_{30}N_4O_2$), add 40 mL of the dissolving solution, sonicate, and add the dissolving solution to make exactly 50 mL. Centrifuge this solution, pipet 5 mL of the supernatant liquid, add the buffer solution to make exactly 25 mL, and use this solution as the sample solution. Separately, weigh accurately about 80 mg of telmisartan for assay, previously dried at 105°C for 4 hours, and dissolve in the dissolving solution to make exactly 50 mL. Pipet 5 mL of this solution, add the buffer solution to make exactly 25 mL, and use this solution as the standard solution. Perform the test with exactly 5 μL each of the sample solution and standard solution as directed under Liquid Chromatography <*2.01*> according to the following conditions, and determine the peak areas, A_T and A_S, of telmisartan in each solution.

Amount (mg) of telmisartan ($C_{33}H_{30}N_4O_2$)
$= M_S \times A_T/A_S$

M_S: Amount (mg) of telmisartan for assay taken

Dissolving solution: Dissolve 2 g of ammonium dihydrogen phosphate in 1000 mL of water, and adjust to pH 1.8 with phosphoric acid. To 1000 mL of this solution add 1000 mL of acetonitrile.

Buffer solution: Dissolve 2 g of ammonium dihydrogen phosphate in 1000 mL of water, and adjust to pH 1.8 with phosphoric acid.

Operating conditions—

Detector: An ultraviolet absorption photometer (wavelength: 270 nm).

Column: A stainless steel column 3.0 mm in inside diameter and 7.5 cm in length, packed with octylsilanized silica gel for liquid chromatography (5 μm in particle diameter).

Column temperature: A constant temperature of about 40°C.

Mobile phase A: Dissolve 2 g of ammonium dihydrogen phosphate in 1000 mL of water, and adjust to pH 3.5 with phosphoric acid.

Mobile phase B: Acetonitrile.

Flowing of mobile phase: Control the gradient by mixing the mobile phases A and B as directed in the following table.

Time after injection of sample (min)	Mobile phase A (vol%)	Mobile phase B (vol%)
0 - 2	90	10
2 - 7	90 → 20	10 → 80
7 - 8	20	80

Flow rate: 0.8 mL per minute.

System suitability—

System performance: When the procedure is run with 5 μL of the standard solution under the above operating conditions, the number of theoretical plates and the symmetry factor of the peak of telmisartan are not less than 15,000 and not more than 2.0, respectively.

System repeatability: When the test is repeated 6 times with 5 μL of the standard solution under the above operating conditions, the relative standard deviation of the peak area of telmisartan is not more than 1.0%.

(2) Hydrochlorothiazide—Weigh accurately the mass of not less than 20 Telmisartan and Hydrochlorothiazide Tablets, and powder. Weigh accurately a portion of the powder, equivalent to about 12.5 mg of hydrochlorothiazide ($C_7H_8ClN_3O_4S_2$), add 40 mL of the dissolving solution, sonicate, and add the dissolving solution to make exactly 50 mL. Centrifuge this solution, pipet 5 mL of the supernatant liquid, add the buffer solution to make exactly 25 mL, and use this solution as the sample solution. Separately, weigh accurately about 12.5 mg of Hydrochlorothiazide RS, previously dried at 105°C for 2 hours, and dissolve in the dissolving solution to make exactly 50 mL. Pipet 5 mL of this solution, add the buffer solution to make exactly 25 mL, and use this solution as the standard solution. Perform the test with exactly 5 μL each of the sample solution and standard solution as directed under Liquid Chromatography *<2.01>* according to the following conditions, and determine the peak areas, A_T and A_S, of hydrochlorothiazide in each solution.

Amount (mg) of hydrochlorothiazide ($C_7H_8ClN_3O_4S_2$)
$= M_S \times A_T/A_S$

M_S: Amount (mg) of Hydrochlorothiazide RS taken

Dissolving solution: Dissolve 2 g of ammonium dihydrogen phosphate in 1000 mL of water, and adjust to pH 1.8 with phosphoric acid. To 1000 mL of this solution add 1000 mL of acetonitrile.

Buffer solution: Dissolve 2 g of ammonium dihydrogen phosphate in 1000 mL of water, and adjust to pH 1.8 with phosphoric acid.

Operating conditions—

Proceed as directed in the operating conditions in (1).

System suitability—

System performance: When the procedure is run with 5 μL of the standard solution under the above operating conditions, the number of theoretical plates and the symmetry factor of the peak of hydrochlorothiazide are not less than 1500 and not more than 2.0, respectively.

System repeatability: When the test is repeated 6 times with 5 μL of the standard solution under the above operating conditions, the relative standard deviation of the peak area of hydrochlorothiazide is not more than 1.0%.

Containers and storage Containers—Tight containers.

Temocapril Hydrochloride

テモカプリル塩酸塩

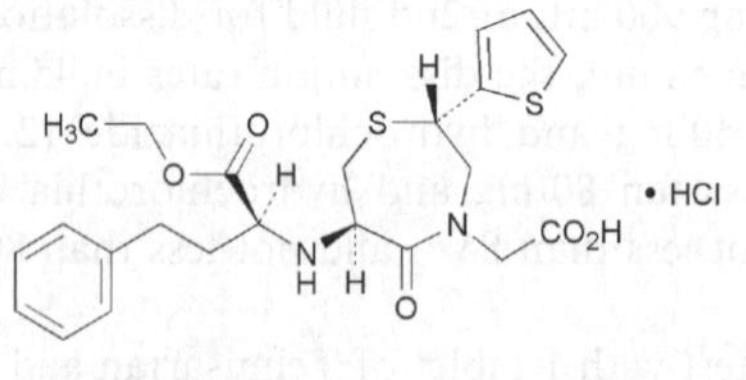

$C_{23}H_{28}N_2O_5S_2.HCl$: 513.07

2-[(2*S*,6*R*)-6-{[(1*S*)-1-(Ethoxycarbonyl)-3-phenylpropyl]amino}-5-oxo-2-(thiophen-2-yl)-2,3,6,7-tetrahydro-1,4-thiazepin-4(5*H*)-yl] acetic acid monohydrochloride

[*110221-44-8*]

Temocapril Hydrochloride contains not less than 99.0% and not more than 101.0% of temocapril hydrochloride ($C_{23}H_{28}N_2O_5S_2.HCl$), calculated on the anhydrous basis.

Description Temocapril Hydrochloride occurs as a white crystalline powder.

It is freely soluble in ethanol (99.5), and vey slightly soluble in water.

Identification **(1)** Determine the absorption spectrum of a solution of Temocapril Hydrochloride in ethanol (99.5) (1 in 50,000) as directed under Ultraviolet-visible Spectrophotometry *<2.24>*, and compare the spectrum with the Reference Spectrum: both spectra exhibit similar intensities of absorption at the same wavelengths.

(2) Determine the infrared absorption spectrum of Temocapril Hydrochloride as directed in the paste method under Infrared Spectrophotometry *<2.25>*, and compare the spectrum with the Reference Spectrum: both spectra exhibit similar intensities of absorption at the same wave numbers.

(3) A solution of Temocapril Hydrochloride in ethanol (99.5) (1 in 100) responds to Qualitative Tests *<1.09>* (2) for chloride.

Optical rotation *<2.49>* $[\alpha]_D^{20}$: +60 - +64° (0.2 g calculated on the anhydrous basis, ethanol (99.5), 20 mL, 100 mm).

Purity **(1)** Heavy metals *<1.07>*—Proceed with 1.0 g of Temocapril Hydrochloride according to Method 4, and perform the test. Prepare the control solution with 2.0 mL of Standard Lead Solution (not more than 20 ppm).

(2) Related substances—Dissolve 50 mg of Temocapril Hydrochloride in 100 mL of diluted acetonitrile (1 in 2), and use this solution as the sample solution. Pipet 1 mL of the sample solution, add diluted acetonitrile (1 in 2) to make exactly 100 mL, and use this solution as the standard solution. Perform the test with exactly 10 μL each of the sample solution and standard solution as directed under Liquid Chromatography ⟨*2.01*⟩ according to the following conditions. Determine each peak area by the automatic integration method: the area of the peak other than temocapril obtained from the sample solution is not larger than 1/5 times the peak area of temocapril from the standard solution, and the total area of the peaks other than temocapril from the sample solution is not larger than 1/2 times the peak area of temocapril from the standard solution.

Operating conditions—

Detector: An ultraviolet absorption photometer (wavelength: 234 nm).

Column: A stainless steel column 6.0 mm in inside diameter and 15 cm in length, packed with octadecylsilanized silica gel for liquid chromatography (5 μm in particle diameter).

Column temperature: A constant temperature of about 40°C.

Mobile phase: A mixture of diluted phosphoric acid (1 in 500) and acetonitrile (63:37).

Flow rate: Adjust so that the retention time of temocapril is about 11 minutes.

Time span of measurement: About 4 times as long as the retention time of temocapril, beginning after the solvent peak.

System suitability—

Test for required detectability: Pipet 1 mL of the standard solution, and add diluted acetonitrile (1 in 2) to make exactly 10 mL. Confirm that the peak area of temocapril obtained with 10 μL of this solution is equivalent to 7 to 13% of that with 10 μL of the standard solution.

System performance: When the procedure is run with 10 μL of the standard solution under the above operating conditions, the number of theoretical plates and the symmetry factor of the peak of temocapril are not less than 7000 and not more than 1.5, respectively.

System repeatability: When the test is repeated 6 times with 10 μL of the standard solution under the above operating conditions, the relative standard deviation of the peak area of temocapril is not more than 2.0%.

Water ⟨*2.48*⟩ Not more than 1.0% (0.3 g, coulometric titration).

Residue on ignition ⟨*2.44*⟩ Not more than 0.1% (1 g).

Assay Weigh accurately about 0.8 g of Temocapril Hydrochloride, dissolve in 80 mL of a mixture of acetic anhydrate and acetic acid (100) (7:3), and titrate ⟨*2.50*⟩ with 0.1 mol/L perchloric acid VS (potentiometric titration). Perform a blank determination in the same manner, and make any necessary correction.

Each mL of 0.1 mol/L perchloric acid VS
= 51.31 mg of $C_{23}H_{28}N_2O_5S_2$.HCl

Containers and storage Containers—Well-closed containers.

Temocapril Hydrochloride Tablets

テモカプリル塩酸塩錠

Temocapril Hydrochloride Tablets contain not less than 95.0% and not more than 105.0% of the labeled amount of temocapril hydrochloride ($C_{23}H_{28}N_2O_5S_2$.HCl: 513.07).

Method of preparation Prepare as directed under Tablets, with Temocapril Hydrochloride.

Identification To an amount of powdered Temocapril Hydrochloride Tablets, equivalent to 2.5 mg of Temocapril Hydrochloride, add 25 mL of diluted acetonitrile (1 in 2), shake vigorously for 10 minutes, and centrifuge. To 5 mL of the supernatant liquid add diluted acetonitrile (1 in 2) to make 25 mL, and determine the absorption spectrum of this solution as directed under Ultraviolet-visible Spectrophotometry ⟨*2.24*⟩: it exhibits a maximum between 232 nm and 236 nm.

Uniformity of dosage units ⟨*6.02*⟩ Perform the test according to the following method: it meets the requirement of the Content uniformity test.

To 1 tablet of Temocapril Hydrochloride Tablets add exactly 20 mL of diluted acetonitrile (1 in 2), and sonicate for 10 minutes. Furthermore, shake for 10 minutes, and centrifuge. Pipet V mL of the supernatant liquid equivalent to about 0.8 mg of temocapril hydrochloride ($C_{23}H_{28}N_2O_5S_2$.HCl), add exactly 2 mL of the internal standard solution, then add diluted acetonitrile (1 in 2) to make 20 mL, and use this solution as the sample solution. Separately, weigh accurately about 40 mg of temocapril hydrochloride for assay (separately determine the water ⟨*2.48*⟩ in the same manner as Temocapril Hydrochloride), dissolve in diluted acetonitrile (1 in 2) to make exactly 200 mL. Pipet 4 mL of this solution, add exactly 2 mL of the internal standard solution, then add diluted acetonitrile (1 in 2) to make 20 mL, and use this solution as the standard solution. Perform the test with 10 μL each of the sample solution and standard solution as directed under Liquid Chromatography ⟨*2.01*⟩ according to the following conditions, and calculate the ratios, Q_T and Q_S, of the peak area of temocapril to that of the internal standard.

Amount (mg) of temocapril hydrochloride ($C_{23}H_{28}N_2O_5S_2$.HCl)
$= M_S \times Q_T/Q_S \times 1/V \times 2/5$

M_S: Amount (mg) of temocapril hydrochloride for assay taken, calculated on the anhydrous basis

*Internal standard solution—*A solution of propyl parahydroxybenzoate in diluted acetonitrile (1 in 2) (1 in 3000).

Operating conditions—

Proceed as directed in the operating conditions in the Assay.

System suitability—

System performance: When the procedure is run with 10 μL of the standard solution under the above operating conditions, temocapril and the internal standard are eluted in this order with the resolution between these peaks being not less than 7.

System repeatability: When the test is repeated 6 times with 10 μL of the standard solution under the above operating conditions, the relative standard deviation of the ratio of the peak area of temocapril to that of the internal standard is not more than 1.0%.

Dissolution ⟨*6.10*⟩ When the test is performed at 50 revolutions per minute according to the Paddle method, using 900 mL of water as the dissolution medium, the dissolution rate in 30 minutes of Temocapril Hydrochloride Tablets is not less than 85%.

Start the test with 1 tablet of Temocapril Hydrochloride Tablets, withdraw not less than 20 mL of the medium at the specified minute after starting the test, and filter through a membrane filter with a pore size not exceeding 0.45 μm. Discard not less than 10 mL of the first filtrate, pipet *V* mL of the subsequent filtrate, add water to make exactly *V′* mL so that each mL contains about 1.1 μg of temocapril hydrochloride ($C_{23}H_{28}N_2O_5S_2.HCl$), and use this solution as the sample solution. Separately, weigh accurately about 22 mg of temocapril hydrochloride for assay (separately determine the water *<2.48>* in the same manner as Temocapril Hydrochloride), and dissolve in diluted acetonitrile (1 in 2) to make exactly 50 mL. Pipet 5 mL of this solution, and add water to make exactly 100 mL. Pipet 5 mL of this solution, add water to make exactly 100 mL, and use this solution as the standard solution. Perform the test with exactly 50 μL each of the sample solution and standard solution as directed under Liquid Chromatography *<2.01>* according to the following conditions, and determine the peak areas, A_T and A_S, of temocapril in each solution.

Dissolution rate (%) with respect to the labeled amount of temocapril hydrochloride ($C_{23}H_{28}N_2O_5S_2.HCl$)
$= M_S \times A_T/A_S \times V'/V \times 1/C \times 9/2$

M_S: Amount (mg) of temocapril hydrochloride for assay taken, calculated on the anhydrous basis
C: Labeled amount (mg) of temocapril hydrochloride ($C_{23}H_{28}N_2O_5S_2.HCl$) in 1 tablet

Operating conditions—

Detector, column, and column temperature: Proceed as directed in the operating conditions in the Assay.

Mobile phase: A mixture of diluted phosphoric acid (1 in 500) and acetonitrile (43:32).

Flow rate: Adjust so that the retention time of temocapril is about 7 minutes.

System suitability—

System performance: When the procedure is run with 50 μL of the standard solution under the above operating conditions, the number of theoretical plates and the symmetry factor of the peak of temocapril are not less than 9000 and not more than 2.0, respectively.

System repeatability: When the test is repeated 6 times with 50 μL of the standard solution under the above operating conditions, the relative standard deviation of the peak area of temocapril is not more than 2.0%.

Assay Weigh accurately the mass of not less than 20 Temocapril Hydrochloride Tablets, and powder. Weigh accurately a portion of the powder, equivalent to about 10 mg of temocapril hydrochloride ($C_{23}H_{28}N_2O_5S_2.HCl$), add exactly 20 mL of the internal standard solution, and sonicate for 10 minutes. Furthermore, shake for 10 minutes, and centrifuge. To 2 mL of the supernatant liquid add diluted acetonitrile (1 in 2) to make 20 mL, and use this solution as the sample solution. Separately, weigh accurately about 50 mg of temocapril hydrochloride for assay (separately determine the water *<2.48>* in the same manner as Temocapril Hydrochloride), and dissolve in diluted acetonitrile (1 in 2) to make exactly 50 mL. Pipet 5 mL of this solution, add exactly 10 mL of the internal standard solution, then add diluted acetonitrile (1 in 2) to make 100 mL, and use this solution as the standard solution. Perform the test with 10 μL each of the sample solution and standard solution as directed under Liquid Chromatography *<2.01>* according to the following conditions, and calculate the ratios, Q_T and Q_S, of the peak area of temocapril to that of the internal standard.

Amount (mg) of temocapril hydrochloride ($C_{23}H_{28}N_2O_5S_2.HCl$)
$= M_S \times Q_T/Q_S \times 1/5$

M_S: Amount (mg) of temocapril hydrochloride for assay taken, calculated on the anhydrous basis

Internal standard solution—A solution of propyl parahydroxybenzoate in diluted acetonitrile (1 in 2) (1 in 3000).

Operating conditions—

Detector: An ultraviolet absorption photometer (wavelength: 234 nm).

Column: A stainless steel column 6.0 mm in inside diameter and 15 cm in length, packed with octadecylsilanized silica gel for liquid chromatography (5 μm in particle diameter).

Column temperature: A constant temperature of about 40°C.

Mobile phase: A mixture of diluted phosphoric acid (1 in 500) and acetonitrile (63:37).

Flow rate: Adjust so that the retention time of temocapril is about 10 minutes.

System suitability—

System performance: When the procedure is run with 10 μL of the standard solution under the above operating conditions, temocapril and the internal standard are eluted in this order with the resolution between these peaks being not less than 7.

System repeatability: When the test is repeated 6 times with 10 μL of the standard solution under the above operating conditions, the relative standard deviation of the ratio of the peak area of temocapril to that of the internal standard is not more than 1.0%.

Containers and storage Containers—Well-closed containers.

Teprenone

テプレノン

$C_{23}H_{38}O$: 330.55
(5*E*,9*E*,13*E*)-6,10,14,18-Tetramethylnonadeca-5,9,13,17-tetraen-2-one
(5*Z*,9*E*,13*E*)-6,10,14,18-Tetramethylnonadeca-5,9,13,17-tetraen-2-one
[6809-52-5]

Teprenone contains not less than 97.0% and not more than 101.0% of teprenone ($C_{23}H_{38}O$).

Teprenone is comprised of mono-cis and all-trans isomers, with their ratio being about 2:3.

Description Teprenone occurs as a colorless to pale yellow clear oily liquid, with slight, characteristic odor.

It is miscible with ethanol (99.5), with ethyl acetate and with hexane.

It is practically insoluble in water.

It is oxidized by air, and gradually turns yellow.

Identification **(1)** To 2 mL of a solution of Teprenone in ethanol (99.5) (1 in 100) add 1 mL of a solution of phosphomolybdic acid *n*-hydrate in acetic acid (100) (1 in 100), heat in a water bath for 5 minutes, and continue heating with addition of 5 to 6 drops of sulfuric acid: blue to bluish green color develops.

(2) To 2 mL of a solution of Teprenone in ethanol (99.5) (1 in 100) add 2 mL of 2,4-dinitrophenylhydrazine TS, and shake: a yellow to orange-yellow precipitate is formed.

(3) Determine the infrared absorption spectrum of Teprenone as directed in the liquid film method under Infrared Spectrophotometry <*2.25*>, and compare the spectrum with the Reference Spectrum or the spectrum of Teprenone RS: both spectra exhibit similar intensities of absorption at the same wave numbers.

Refractive index <*2.45*> n_D^{20}: 1.485 – 1.491

Specific gravity <*2.56*> d_{20}^{20}: 0.882 – 0.890

Purity **(1)** Clarity and color of solution—To 1.0 mL of Teprenone add 9 mL of ethanol (99.5) and shake: the solution is clear, and its absorbance at 400 nm determined as directed under Ultraviolet-visible Spectrophotometry <*2.24*> is not more than 0.02.

(2) Heavy metals <*1.07*>—Proceed with 1.0 g of Teprenone according to Method 2 and perform the test. Prepare the control solution with 2.0 mL of Standard Lead Solution (not more than 20 ppm).

(3) Related substances—Dissolve 30 mg of Teprenone in 6 mL of hexane, and use this solution as the sample solution. Perform the test with 3 μL of the sample solution as directed under Gas Chromatography <*2.02*> according to the following conditions. Determine each peak area from the sample solution by the automatic integration method and calculate the amounts of them by the area percentage method: the peak area of the di-cis isomer of teprenone, having the relative retention time of about 0.8 to the all-trans isomer of teprenone, is not more than 0.5%, and each area of the peaks other than the mono-cis and all-trans isomers of the teprenone and the other than mentioned above is not more than 0.2%. Furthermore, the total area of the peaks other than the mono-cis, all-trans and di-cis isomers of teprenone is not more than 1.0%.

Operating conditions—

Detector, column, column temperature, carrier gas and flow rate: Proceed as directed in the operating conditions in the Assay.

Time span of measurement: About 2 times as long as the retention time for the all-trans isomer of teprenone, beginning after the solvent peak.

System suitability—

Test for required detectability: To 1 mL of the sample solution add hexane to make 100 mL, and use this solution as the solution for system suitability test. Pipet 1 mL of the solution for system suitability test, and add hexane to make exactly 10 mL. Confirm that the sum of the peak areas of the mono-cis and all-trans isomers of teprenone obtained with 3 μL of this solution is 7 to 13% of the peak areas of the mono-cis and all-trans isomers of teprenone with 3 μL of the solution for system suitability test.

System performance: When the procedure is run with 3 μL of the solution for system suitability test under the above operating conditions, the mono-cis and all-trans isomers of teprenone are eluted in this order with the resolution between these peaks being not less than 1.1.

System repeatability: When the test is repeated 6 times with 3 μL of the solution for system suitability test under the above operating conditions, the relative standard deviation of the sum of the peak areas of the mono-cis and all-trans isomers of teprenone is not more than 3.0%.

Residue on ignition <*2.44*> Not more than 0.1% (1 g).

Isomer ratio Dissolve 30 mg of Teprenone in 6 mL of hexane, and use this solution as the sample solution. Perform the test with 3 μL of the sample solution as directed under Gas Chromatography <*2.02*> according to the following conditions. Determine the areas of two adjacent peaks, A_a and A_b, having retention times of about 18 minutes, where A_a is the peak area of the mono-cis isomer, having the shorter retention time, and A_b is the peak area of the all-trans isomer, having the longer retention time: A_a/A_b is 0.60 to 0.70.

Operating conditions—

Proceed as directed in the operating conditions in the Assay.

System suitability—

System performance, and system repeatability: Proceed as directed in the system suitability in the Purity (3).

Assay Weigh accurately about 50 mg each of Teprenone and Teprenone RS, dissolve each in exactly 5 mL of the internal standard solution, add ethyl acetate to make 50 mL, and use these solutions as the sample solution and the standard solution, respectively. Perform the test with 3 μL each of the sample solution and standard solution as directed under Gas Chromatography <*2.02*> according to the following conditions, and calculate the ratios, Q_T and Q_S, of the peak area of teprenone (sum of the peak areas of mono-cis and all-trans isomers) to that of the internal standard.

$$\text{Amount (mg) of teprenone } (C_{23}H_{38}O) = M_S \times Q_T/Q_S$$

M_S: Amount (mg) of Teprenone RS taken

Internal standard solution—A solution of di-*n*-butyl phthalate in ethyl acetate (1 in 200).

Operating conditions—

Detector: A hydrogen flame-ionization detector.

Column: A glass column 3 mm in inside diameter and 2 m in length, packed with 149 to 177 μm silica-gel for gas chromatography coated in 5% with polyethylene glycol 2-nitroterephthalate for gas chromatography.

Column temperature: A constant temperature of about 235°C.

Carrier gas: Nitrogen or helium.

Flow rate: Adjust so that the retention time of the peak of all-trans isomer of teprenone, having the larger retention time among the adjacent two main peaks appearing at a retention time of about 18 minutes, is about 19 minutes.

System suitability—

System performance: When the procedure is run with 3 μL of the standard solution under the above operating conditions, the internal standard and the mono-cis and all-trans isomers of teprenone are eluted in this order with the resolution between the mono-cis and all-trans isomers being not less than 1.1.

System repeatability: When the test is repeated 6 times with 3 μL of the standard solution under the above operating conditions, the relative standard deviation of the ratio of the sum of the peak areas of the mono-cis and all-trans isomers of teprenone to that of the internal standard is not more than 1.0%.

Containers and storage Containers—Tight Containers.

Storage—Under Nitrogen atmosphere at 2 to 8°C.

Teprenone Capsules

テプレノンカプセル

Teprenone Capsules contain not less than 95.0% and not more than 105.0% of the labeled amount of teprenone ($C_{23}H_{38}O$: 330.55).

Method of preparation Prepare as directed under Capsules, with Teprenone.

Identification **(1)** Take out the contents of Teprenone Capsules, to a quantity of the content, equivalent to 0.1 g of Teprenone, add 10 mL of ethanol (99.5), shake well, and centrifuge. To 2 mL of the supernatant liquid add 1 mL of a solution of phosphomolybdic acid *n*-hydrate in acetic acid (100) (1 in 100), heat in a water bath for 5 minutes, add 5-6 drops of sulfuric acid, and continue heating: a blue to bluish green color develops.

(2) Take out the contents of Teprenone Capsules, to a quantity of the content, equivalent to 0.1 g of Teprenone, add 10 mL of ethanol (99.5), shake well, and centrifuge. To 2 mL of the supernatant liquid add 2 mL of 2,4-dinitrophenyl hydrazine TS, and shake: a yellow to orange-yellow precipitate is formed.

Uniformity of dosage units *<6.02>* Perform the Mass variation test, or the Content uniformity test according to the following method: it meets the requirement of the Content uniformity test.

Take out the contents of 1 capsule of Teprenone Capsules, add exactly 1 mL of the internal standard solution for each 10 mg of teprenone ($C_{23}H_{38}O$), and add ethyl acetate to make *V* mL so that each mL contains 1 mg of teprenone ($C_{23}H_{38}O$). Stand for 30 minutes with shaking occasionally, and filter. Discard the first 10 mL of the filtrate, and use the subsequent filtrate as the sample solution. Separately, weigh accurately about 50 mg of Teprenone RS, add exactly 5 mL of the internal standard solution, then add ethyl acetate to make 50 mL, and use this solution as the standard solution. Then, proceed as directed in the Assay.

$$\text{Amount (mg) of teprenone } (C_{23}H_{38}O) = M_S \times Q_T/Q_S \times V/50$$

M_S: Amount (mg) of Teprenone RS taken

Internal standard solution—A solution of di-*n*-butyl phthalate in ethyl acetate (1 in 200).

Dissolution *<6.10>* When the test is performed at 100 revolutions per minute according to the Paddle method using the sinker, using 900 mL of a solution of sodium lauryl sulfate in disodium hydrogen phosphate-citric acid buffer solution (pH 6.8) (1 in 20) as the dissolution medium, the dissolution rate in 60 minutes of Teprenone Capsules is not less than 70%.

Start the test with 1 capsule of Teprenone Capsules, withdraw not less than 20 mL of the medium at the specified minute after starting the test, and filter through a membrane filter with a pore size not exceeding 0.45 μm. Discard not less than 10 mL of the first filtrate, pipet *V* mL of the subsequent filtrate, add the dissolution medium to make exactly *V′* mL so that each mL contains about 56 μg of teprenone ($C_{23}H_{38}O$), and use this solution as the sample solution. Separately, weigh accurately about 28 mg of Teprenone RS, and dissolve in ethanol (99.5) to make exactly 50 mL. Pipet 5 mL of this solution, add the dissolution medium to make exactly 50 mL, and use this solution as the standard solution. Perform the test with exactly 10 μL each of the sample solution and standard solution as directed under Liquid Chromatography *<2.01>* according to the following conditions, and determine the sum of the peak areas of mono-cis and all-trans isomer of teprenone, A_T and A_S, in each solution.

Dissolution rate (%) with respect to the labeled amount of teprenone ($C_{23}H_{38}O$)

$$= M_S \times A_T/A_S \times V'/V \times 1/C \times 180$$

M_S: Amount (mg) of Teprenone RS taken

C: Labeled amount (mg) of teprenone ($C_{23}H_{38}O$) in 1 capsule

Operating conditions—

Detector: An ultraviolet absorption photometer (wavelength: 210 nm).

Column: A stainless steel column 4.6 mm in inside diameter and 15 cm in length, packed with octadecylsilanized silica gel for liquid chromatography (5 μm in particle diameter).

Column temperature: A constant temperature of about 40°C.

Mobile phase: A mixture of acetonitrile and water (87:13).

Flow rate: Adjust so that the retention time of all-trans isomer of teprenone is about 8 minutes.

System suitability—

System performance: When the procedure is run with 10 μL of the standard solution under the above operating conditions, the mono-cis and the all-trans isomer of teprenone are eluted in this order with the resolution between these peaks being not less than 1.0.

System repeatability: When the test is repeated 6 times with 10 μL of the standard solution under the above operating conditions, the relative standard deviation of the sum of the peak areas of the mono-cis and all-trans isomer of teprenone is not more than 1.5%.

Assay Take out the contents of not less than 20 Teprenone Capsules. Weigh accurately the total mass of the contents, and powder. Weigh accurately a portion of the powder, equivalent to about 50 mg of teprenone ($C_{23}H_{38}O$), add exactly 5 mL of the internal standard solution, add ethyl acetate to make 50 mL. Stand for 30 minutes with shaking occasionally, and filter. Discard the first 10 mL of the filtrate, and use the subsequent filtrate as the sample solution. Separately, weigh accurately about 50 mg of Teprenone RS, add exactly 5 mL of the internal standard solution, add ethyl acetate to make 50 mL, and use this solution as the standard solution. Then, proceed as directed in the Assay under Teprenone.

$$\text{Amount (mg) of teprenone } (C_{23}H_{38}O) = M_S \times Q_T/Q_S$$

M_S: Amount (mg) of Teprenone RS taken

Internal standard solution—A solution of di-*n*-butyl phthalate in ethyl acetate (1 in 200).

Containers and storage Containers—Tight containers.

Terbinafine Hydrochloride

テルビナフィン塩酸塩

$C_{21}H_{25}N.HCl$: 327.89

(2*E*)-*N*,6,6-Trimethyl-*N*-(naphthalen-1-ylmethyl)hept-2-en-4-yn-1-amine monohydrochloride

[*78628-80-5*]

Terbinafine Hydrochloride, when dried, contains not less than 99.0% and not more than 101.0% of terbinafine hydrochloride ($C_{21}H_{25}N.HCl$).

Description Terbinafine Hydrochloride occurs as a white to pale yellow-white crystalline powder.

It is freely soluble in methanol, in ethanol (99.5) and in acetic acid (100), and slightly soluble in water.

The pH of a solution of 1.0 g of Terbinafine Hydrochloride in 1000 mL of water is 3.5 to 4.5.

Melting point: about 205°C (with decomposition).

Identification **(1)** Determine the absorption spectrum of a solution of Terbinafine Hydrochloride in methanol (1 in 40,000) as directed under Ultraviolet-visible Spectrophotometry 〈*2.24*〉, and compare the spectrum with the Reference Spectrum: both spectra exhibit similar intensities of absorption at the same wavelengths.

(2) Determine the infrared absorption spectrum of Terbinafine Hydrochloride, previously dried, as directed in the potassium chloride disk method under Infrared Spectrophotometry 〈*2.25*〉, and compare the spectrum with the Reference Spectrum: both spectra exhibit similar intensities of absorption at the same wave numbers.

(3) A solution of Terbinafine Hydrochloride in ethanol (99.5) (1 in 100) responds to Qualitative Tests 〈*1.09*〉 (2) for chloride.

Purity **(1)** Heavy metals 〈*1.07*〉—Proceed with 1.0 g of Terbinafine Hydrochloride according to Method 4, and perform the test. Prepare the control solution with 2.0 mL of Standard Lead Solution (not more than 20 ppm).

(2) Related substances—Conduct this procedure using light-resistant vessels. Dissolve 50 mg of Terbinafine Hydrochloride in 100 mL of a mixture of water and acetonitrile (1:1), and use this solution as the sample solution. Pipet 1 mL of the sample solution, and add a mixture of water and acetonitrile (1:1) to make exactly 100 mL. Pipet 5 mL of this solution, add a mixture of water and acetonitrile (1:1) to make exactly 50 mL, and use this solution as the standard solution. Perform the test with exactly 20 μL each of the sample solution and standard solution as directed under Liquid Chromatography 〈*2.01*〉 according to the following conditions, and determine each peak area by the automatic integration method: the peak area of a dimer, having the relative retention time of about 1.7 to terbinafine obtained from the sample solution is not larger than 1/2 times the peak area of terbinafine from the standard solution, the area of the peaks other than terbinafine and the dimer from the sample solution is not larger than the peak area of terbinafine from the standard solution, and the total area of the peaks other than terbinafine is not larger than 3 times the peak area of terbinafine from the standard solution.

Operating conditions—

Detector: An ultraviolet absorption photometer (wavelength: 280 nm).

Column: A stainless steel column 3 mm in inside diameter and 15 cm in length, packed with octadecylsilanized silica gel for liquid chromatography (5 μm in particle diameter).

Column temperature: A constant temperature of about 40°C.

Mobile phase A: To 700 mL of a mixture of methanol and acetonitrile (3:2) add 300 mL of a solution of triethylamine (1 in 500) adjusted to pH 7.5 with dilute acetic acid.

Mobile phase B: To 950 mL of a mixture of methanol and acetonitrile (3:2) add 50 mL of a solution of triethylamine (1 in 500) adjusted to pH 7.5 with dilute acetic acid.

Flowing of mobile phase: Control the gradient by mixing the mobile phases A and B as directed in the following table.

Time after injection of sample (min)	Mobile phase A (vol%)	Mobile phase B (vol%)
0 – 4	100	0
4 – 25	100 → 0	0 → 100
25 – 30	0	100

Flow rate: Adjust so that the retention time of terbinafine is about 15 minutes.

Time span of measurement: About 2 times as long as the retention time of terbinafine, beginning after the solvent peak.

System suitability—

Test for required detectability: Pipet 5 mL of the standard solution, and add a mixture of water and acetonitrile (1:1) to make exactly 20 mL. Confirm that the peak area of terbinafine obtained with 20 μL of this solution is equivalent to 18 to 32% of that with 20 μL of the standard solution.

System performance: Dissolve 20 mg of Terbinafine Hydrochloride in 20 mL of a mixture of water and acetonitrile (1:1), and irradiate under a short-wave lamp (main wavelength: 254 nm) for 1 hour. When the procedure is run with 20 μL of this solution under the above operating conditions, the resolution between the peak of cis-terbinafine, having the relative retention time of about 0.94 to terbinafine, and the peak of terbinafine is not less than 2.0.

System repeatability: When the test is repeated 6 times with 20 μL of the standard solution under the above operating conditions, the relative standard deviation of the peak area of terbinafine is not more than 2.0%.

Loss on drying 〈*2.41*〉 Not more than 0.5% (1 g, 105°C, 4 hours).

Residue on ignition 〈*2.44*〉 Not more than 0.1% (1 g).

Assay Weigh accurately about 0.26 g of Terbinafine Hydrochloride, previously dried, dissolve in 5 mL of acetic acid (100), add 50 mL of acetic anhydride, and titrate 〈*2.50*〉 with 0.1 mol/L perchloric acid VS (potentiometric titration). Perform a blank determination in the same manner, and make any necessary correction.

Each mL of 0.1 mol/L perchloric acid VS
= 32.79 mg of $C_{21}H_{25}N.HCl$

Containers and storage Containers—Tight containers.

Storage—Light-resistant.

Terbinafine Hydrochloride Cream

テルビナフィン塩酸塩クリーム

Terbinafine Hydrochloride Cream contains not less than 95.0% and not more than 105.0% of the labeled amount of terbinafine hydrochloride ($C_{21}H_{25}N.HCl$: 327.89).

Method of preparation Prepare as directed under Creams, with Terbinafine Hydrochloride.

Identification To quantity of Terbinafine Hydrochloride Cream, equivalent to 10 mg of Terbinafine Hydrochloride, dissolve in 20 mL of 2-propanol, and use this solution as the sample solution. Separately, dissolve 10 mg of terbinafine hydrochloride for assay in 20 mL of 2-propanol, and use this solution as the standard solution. Perform the test with these solutions as directed under Thin-layer Chromatography <*2.03*>. Spot 10 μL each of the sample solution and standard solution on a plate of silica gel with fluorescent indicator for thin-layer chromatography. Develop the plate with the upper layer of a mixture of 80 volumes of hexane, 20 volumes of ethyl acetate and 1 volume of ammonia solution (28) to a distance of about 15 cm, and air-dry the plate. Examine the plate under ultraviolet light (main wavelength: 254 nm): the principal spot obtained from the sample solution shows the same *Rf* value with the spot from the standard solution.

Assay Weigh accurately an amount of Terbinafine Hydrochloride Cream, equivalent to about 10 mg of terbinafine hydrochloride ($C_{21}H_{25}N.HCl$), dissolve in 2-propanol to make exactly 50 mL, and use this solution as the sample solution. Separately, weigh accurately about 40 mg of terbinafine hydrochloride for assay, previously dried at 105°C for 4 hours, and dissolve in 2-propanol to make exactly 200 mL, and use this solution as the standard solution. Perform the test with exactly 10 μL each of the sample solution and standard solution as directed under Liquid Chromatography <*2.01*> according to the following conditions, and determine the peak areas, A_T and A_S, of terbinafine in each solution.

Amount (mg) of terbinafine hydrochloride ($C_{21}H_{25}N.HCl$)
$= M_S \times A_T/A_S \times 1/4$

M_S: Amount (mg) of terbinafine hydrochloride for assay taken

Operating conditions—

Detector: An ultraviolet absorption photometer (wavelength: 282 nm).

Column: A stainless steel column 4.0 mm in inside diameter and 125 mm in length, packed with octadecylsilanized silica gel for liquid chromatography (5 μm in particle diameter).

Column temperature: A constant temperature of about 25°C.

Mobile phase: A mixture of a solution of tetramethylammonium hydroxide (9 in 2000) adjusted to pH 8.0 with diluted phosphoric acid (1 in 25), acetonitrile and tetrahydrofuran (2:2:1).

Flow rate: Adjust so that the retention time of terbinafine is about 8.5 minutes.

System suitability—

System performance: Dissolve 40 mg of terbinafine hydrochloride for assay and 3.5 mg of terphenyl in 200 mL of methanol. When the procedure is run with 10 μL of this solution under the above operating conditions, terphenyl and terbinafine are eluted in this order with the resolution between these peaks being not less than 6.

System repeatability: When the test is repeated 6 times with 10 μL of the standard solution under the above operating conditions, the relative standard deviation of the peak area of terbinafine is not more than 1.0%.

Containers and storage Containers—Tight containers.

Terbinafine Hydrochloride Solution

テルビナフィン塩酸塩液

Terbinafine Hydrochloride Solution is a liquid for external use.

It contains not less than 95.0% and not more than 105.0% of the labeled amount of terbinafine hydrochloride ($C_{21}H_{25}N.HCl$: 327.89).

Method of preparation Prepare as directed under Liquids and Solutions for Cutaneous Application, with Terbinafine Hydrochloride.

Identification To a volume of Terbinafine Hydrochloride Solution, equivalent to 10 mg of Terbinafine Hydrochloride, add methanol to make 10 mL, and use this solution as the sample solution. Separately, dissolve 10 mg of terbinafine hydrochloride for assay in 10 mL of methanol, and use this solution as the standard solution. Perform the test with these solutions as directed under Thin-layer Chromatography <*2.03*>. Spot 5 μL each of the sample solution and standard solution on a plate of silica gel with fluorescent indicator for thin-layer chromatography. Develop the plate with the upper layer of a mixture of 80 volumes of hexane, 20 volumes of ethyl acetate and 1 volume of ammonia solution (28) to a distance of about 15 cm, and air-dry the plate. Examine under ultraviolet light (main wavelength: 254 nm): the principal spot obtained from the sample solution shows the same *Rf* value with the spot from the standard solution.

pH Being specified separately when the drug is granted approval based on the Law.

Assay Weigh accurately an amount of Terbinafine Hydrochloride Solution, equivalent to about 10 mg of terbinafine hydrochloride ($C_{21}H_{25}N.HCl$), add methanol to make exactly 50 mL, and use this solution as the sample solution. Separately, weigh accurately about 40 mg of terbinafine hydrochloride for assay, previously dried at 105°C for 4 hours, dissolve in methanol to make exactly 200 mL, and use this solution as the standard solution. Perform the test with exactly 10 μL each of the sample solution and standard solution as directed under Liquid Chromatography <*2.01*> according to the following conditions, and determine the peak areas, A_T and A_S, of terbinafine in each solution.

Amount (mg) of terbinafine hydrochloride ($C_{21}H_{25}N.HCl$)
$= M_S \times A_T/A_S \times 1/4$

M_S: Amount (mg) of terbinafine hydrochloride for assay taken

Operating conditions—

Detector: An ultraviolet absorption photometer (wavelength: 282 nm).

Column: A stainless steel column 4.0 mm in inside diameter and 125 mm in length, packed with octadecylsilanized silica gel for liquid chromatography (5 μm in particle diameter).

Column temperature: A constant temperature of about 25°C.

Mobile phase: A mixture of a solution of tetramethylammonium hydroxide (9 in 2000) adjusted to pH 8.0 with diluted phosphoric acid (1 in 25), acetonitrile and tetrahydrofuran (2:2:1).

Flow rate: Adjust so that the retention time of terbinafine is about 8.5 minutes.

System suitability—

System performance: Dissolve 40 mg of terbinafine hydrochloride for assay and 3.5 mg of terphenyl in 200 mL of methanol. When the procedure is run with 10 μL of this solution under the above operating conditions, terphenyl and terbinafine are eluted in this order with the resolution between these peaks being not less than 6.

System repeatability: When the test is repeated 6 times with 10 μL of the standard solution under the above operating conditions, the relative standard deviation of the peak area of terbinafine is not more than 1.0%.

Containers and storage Containers—Tight containers.

Terbinafine Hydrochloride Spray

テルビナフィン塩酸塩スプレー

Terbinafine Hydrochloride Spray contains not less than 95.0% and not more than 105.0% of the labeled amount of terbinafine hydrochloride ($C_{21}H_{25}N.HCl$: 327.89).

Method of preparation Prepare as directed under Pump Sprays for Cutaneous Application, with Terbinafine Hydrochloride.

Identification To an amount of Terbinafine Hydrochloride Spray, equivalent to 10 mg of Terbinafine Hydrochloride, add methanol to make 10 mL, and use this solution as the sample solution. Separately, dissolve 10 mg of terbinafine hydrochloride for assay in 10 mL of methanol, and use this solution as the standard solution. Perform the test with these solutions as directed under Thin-layer Chromatography <*2.03*>. Spot 5 μL each of the sample solution and standard solution on a plate of silica gel with fluorescent indicator for thin-layer chromatography. Develop the plate with the upper layer of a mixture of 80 volumes of hexane, 20 volumes of ethyl acetate and 1 volume of ammonia solution (28) to a distance of about 15 cm, and air-dry the plate. Examine the plate under ultraviolet light (main wavelength: 254 nm): the principal spot obtained from the sample solution shows the same *R*f value with the spot from the standard solution.

pH Being specified separately when the drug is granted approval based on the Law.

Assay Weigh accurately an amount of Terbinafine Hydrochloride Spray, equivalent to about 10 mg of terbinafine hydrochloride ($C_{21}H_{25}N.HCl$), dissolve in methanol to make exactly 50 mL, and use this solution as the sample solution. Separately, weigh accurately about 40 mg of terbinafine hydrochloride for assay, previously dried at 105°C for 4 hours, dissolve in methanol to make exactly 200 mL, and use this solution as the standard solution. Perform the test with exactly 10 μL each of the sample solution and standard solution as directed under Liquid Chromatography <*2.01*> according to the following conditions, and determine the peak areas, A_T and A_S, of terbinafine in each solution.

Amount (mg) of terbinafine hydrochloride ($C_{21}H_{25}N.HCl$)
$= M_S \times A_T/A_S \times 1/4$

M_S: Amount (mg) of terbinafine hydrochloride for assay taken

Operating conditions—

Detector: An ultraviolet absorption photometer (wavelength: 282 nm).

Column: A stainless steel column 4.0 mm in inside diameter and 125 mm in length, packed with octadecylsilanized silica gel for liquid chromatography (5 μm in particle diameter).

Column temperature: A constant temperature of about 25°C.

Mobile phase: A mixture of a solution of tetramethylammonium hydroxide (9 in 2000) adjusted to pH 8.0 with diluted phosphoric acid (1 in 25), acetonitrile and tetrahydrofuran (2:2:1).

Flow rate: Adjust so that the retention time of terbinafine is about 8.5 minutes.

System suitability—

System performance: Dissolve 40 mg of terbinafine hydrochloride for assay and 3.5 mg of terphenyl in 200 mL of methanol. When the procedure is run with 10 μL of this solution under the above operating conditions, terphenyl and terbinafine are eluted in this order with the resolution between these peaks being not less than 6.

System repeatability: When the test is repeated 6 times with 10 μL of the standard solution under the above operating conditions, the relative standard deviation of the peak area of terbinafine is not more than 1.0%.

Containers and storage Containers—Tight containers.

Terbinafine Hydrochloride Tablets

テルビナフィン塩酸塩錠

Terbinafine Hydrochloride Tablets contain not less than 95.0% and not more than 105.0% of the labeled amount of terbinafine hydrochloride ($C_{21}H_{25}N.HCl$: 327.89).

Method of preparation Prepare as directed under Tablets, with Terbinafine Hydrochloride.

Identification To an amount of powdered Terbinafine Hydrochloride Tablets, equivalent to 10 mg of Terbinafine Hydrochloride, add 10 mL of methanol, shake thoroughly, centrifuge, and use the supernatant liquid as the sample solution. Separately, dissolve 10 mg of terbinafine hydrochloride for assay in 10 mL of methanol, and use this solution as the standard solution. Perform the test with these solutions as directed under Thin-layer Chromatography <*2.03*>. Spot 5 μL each of the sample solution and standard solution on a plate of silica gel with fluorescent indicator for thin-layer chromatography. Develop the plate with the upper layer of a mixture of 80 volumes of hexane, 20 volumes of ethyl acetate and 1 volume of ammonia solution (28) to a distance of about 15 cm, and air-dry the plate. Examine under ultraviolet light (main wavelength: 254 nm): the principal spot obtained from the sample solution and the spot from the standard solution show the same *R*f value.

Uniformity of dosage units <*6.02*> Perform the Mass variation test, or the Content uniformity test according to the following method: it meets the requirement.

To 1 tablet of Terbinafine Hydrochloride Tablets add 40 mL of methanol, shake thoroughly until completely integrated, and add methanol to make exactly 50 mL. Centrifuge this solution, pipet V mL of the supernatant liquid, add methanol to make exactly V' mL so that each mL contains about 0.28 mg of terbinafine hydrochloride ($C_{21}H_{25}N.HCl$), and use this solution as the sample solution. Then, proceed as directed in the Assay.

Amount (mg) of terbinafine hydrochloride ($C_{21}H_{25}N.HCl$)
$= M_S \times A_T/A_S \times V'/V \times 1/2$

M_S: Amount (mg) of terbinafine hydrochloride for assay taken

Dissolution <*6.10*> When the test is performed at 50 revolutions per minute according to the Paddle method, using 900 mL of 0.05 mol/L acetic acid-sodium acetate buffer solution (pH 4.0) as the dissolution medium, the dissolution rate in 30 minutes of Terbinafine Hydrochloride Tablets is not less than 75%.

Start the test with 1 tablet of Terbinafine Hydrochloride Tablets, withdraw not less than 20 mL of the medium at the specified minute after starting the test, and filter through a membrane filter with a pore size not exceeding 0.5 μm. Discard not less than 10 mL of the first filtrate, pipet V mL of the subsequent filtrate, add the dissolution medium to make exactly V' mL so that each mL contains about 0.16 mg of terbinafine hydrochloride ($C_{21}H_{25}N.HCl$). Pipet 2 mL of this solution, add diluted acetic acid (100) (1 in 100) to make exactly 20 mL, and use this solution as the sample solution. Separately, weigh accurately about 16 mg of terbinafine hydrochloride for assay, previously dried at 105°C for 4 hours, dissolve in diluted acetic acid (100) (1 in 100) to make exactly 100 mL. Pipet 5 mL of this solution, add 5 mL of the dissolution medium, add diluted acetic acid (100) (1 in 100) to make exactly 50 mL, and use this solution as the standard solution. Determine the absorbances, A_T and A_S, at 283 nm of the sample solution and standard solution as directed under Ultraviolet-visible Spectrophotometry <*2.24*>, using a solution, prepared by adding diluted acetic acid (100) (1 in 100) to 5 mL of the dissolution medium to make 50 mL, as the blank.

Dissolution rate (%) with respect to the labeled amount of terbinafine hydrochloride ($C_{21}H_{25}N.HCl$)
$= M_S \times A_T/A_S \times V'/V \times 1/C \times 900$

M_S: Amount (mg) of terbinafine hydrochloride for assay taken
C: Labeled amount (mg) of terbinafine hydrochloride ($C_{21}H_{25}N.HCl$) in 1 tablet

Assay Weigh accurately the mass of not less than 20 Terbinafine Hydrochloride Tablets, and powder. Weigh accurately a portion of the powder, equivalent to about 0.14 g of terbinafine hydrochloride ($C_{21}H_{25}N.HCl$), add 40 mL of methanol, shake thoroughly, then add methanol to make exactly 50 mL. Centrifuge, pipet 5 mL of the supernatant liquid, add methanol to make exactly 50 mL, and use this solution as the sample solution. Separately, weigh accurately about 28 mg of terbinafine hydrochloride for assay, previously dried at 105°C for 4 hours, dissolve in methanol to make exactly 100 mL, and use this solution as the standard solution. Perform the test with exactly 10 μL each of the sample solution and standard solution as directed under Liquid Chromatography <*2.01*> according to the following conditions, and determine the peak areas, A_T and A_S, of terbinafine in each solution.

Amount (mg) of terbinafine hydrochloride ($C_{21}H_{25}N.HCl$)
$= M_S \times A_T/A_S \times 5$

M_S: Amount (mg) of terbinafine hydrochloride for assay taken

Operating conditions—

Detector: An ultraviolet absorption photometer (wavelength: 282 nm).

Column: A stainless steel column 4.0 mm in inside diameter and 125 mm in length, packed with octadecylsilanized silica gel for liquid chromatography (5 μm in particle diameter).

Column temperature: A constant temperature of about 25°C.

Mobile phase: A mixture of a solution of tetramethylammonium hydroxide (9 in 2000) adjusted to pH 8.0 with diluted phosphoric acid (1 in 25), acetonitrile and tetrahydrofuran (2:2:1).

Flow rate: Adjust so that the retention time of terbinafine is about 8.5 minutes.

System suitability—

System performance: Dissolve 40 mg of terbinafine hydrochloride for assay and 3.5 mg of telphenyl in 200 mL of methanol. When the procedure is run with 10 μL of this solution under the above operating conditions, telphenyl and terbinafine are eluted in this order with the resolution between these peaks being not less than 6.

System repeatability: When the test is repeated 6 times with 10 μL of the standard solution under the above operating conditions, the relative standard deviation of the peak area of terbinafine is not more than 1.0%.

Containers and storage Containers—Tight containers.

Terbutaline Sulfate

テルブタリン硫酸塩

$(C_{12}H_{19}NO_3)_2.H_2SO_4$: 548.65
5-[(1*RS*)-2-(1,1-Dimethylethylamino)-1-hydroxyethyl]benzene-1,3-diol hemisulfate
[*23031-32-5*]

Terbutaline Sulfate contains not less than 98.5% of terbutaline sulfate [$(C_{12}H_{19}NO_3)_2.H_2SO_4$], calculated on the anhydrous basis.

Description Terbutaline Sulfate is white to brownish white, crystals or crystalline powder. It is odorless or has a faint odor of acetic acid.

It is freely soluble in water, and practically insoluble in acetonitrile, in ethanol (95), in acetic acid (100), in chloroform, and in diethyl ether.

It is gradually colored by light and by air.

Melting point: about 255°C (with decomposition).

Identification **(1)** Dissolve 1 mg of Terbutaline Sulfate in 1 mL of water, and add 5 mL of Tris buffer solution (pH 9.5), 0.5 mL of 4-aminoantipyrine solution (1 in 50) and 2 drops of potassium hexacyanoferrate (III) solution (2 in 25): a reddish purple color is produced.

(2) Determine the absorption spectrum of a solution of Terbutaline Sulfate in 0.01 mol/L hydrochloric acid TS (1 in 10,000) as directed under Ultraviolet-visible Spectrophotometry *<2.24>*, and compare the spectrum with the Reference Spectrum: both spectra exhibit similar intensities of absorption at the same wavelengths. This maximum can be biphasic.

(3) A solution of Terbutaline Sulfate (1 in 50) responds to Qualitative Tests *<1.09>* for sulfate.

pH *<2.54>* Dissolve 0.10 g of Terbutaline Sulfate in 10 mL of water: the pH of this solution is between 4.0 and 4.8.

Purity **(1)** Clarity and color of solution—Dissolve 0.10 g of Terbutaline Sulfate in 10 mL of water: the solution is clear and colorless or pale yellow.

(2) Chloride *<1.03>*—Perform the test with 2.0 g of Terbutaline Sulfate. Prepare the control solution with 0.25 mL of 0.01 mol/L hydrochloric acid VS (not more than 0.004%).

(3) Acetic acid—Dissolve 0.50 g of Terbutaline Sulfate in a solution of phosphoric acid (59 in 1000) to make exactly 10 mL, and use this solution as the sample solution. Separately, dissolve 1.50 g of acetic acid (100) in a solution of phosphoric acid (59 in 1000) to make exactly 100 mL. Dilute 2 mL of this solution, accurately measured, with a solution of phosphoric acid (59 in 1000) to make exactly 200 mL, and use this solution as the standard solution. Perform the test with exactly 2 μL each of the sample solution and standard solution as directed under Gas Chromatography *<2.02>* according to the following conditions. Determine the peak areas, A_T and A_S, of acetic acid in each solution: A_T is not larger than A_S.

Operating conditions—

Detector: A hydrogen flame-ionization detector.

Column: A glass column 3 mm in inside diameter and 1 m in length, packed with 10% of macrogol 6000 on 180- to 250-μm terephthalic acid for gas chromatography.

Column temperature: A constant temperature at about 120°C.

Carrier gas: Nitrogen.

Flow rate: Adjust so that the retention time of acetic acid is about 5 minutes.

System suitability—

System performance: Mix 0.05 g each of acetic acid (100) and propionic acid in 100 mL of diluted phosphoric acid (59 in 1000). When the procedure is run with 2 μL of this solution under the above conditions, acetic acid and propionic acid are eluted in this order with the resolution between these peaks being not less than 2.0.

System repeatability: When the test is repeated 6 times with 2 μL of the standard solution under the above operating conditions, the relative standard deviation of the peak areas of acetic acid is not more than 3.0%.

(4) 3,5-Dihydroxy-ω-*tert*-butylaminoacetophenone sulfate—Dissolve 0.50 g of Terbutaline Sulfate in 0.01 mol/L hydrochloric acid TS to make exactly 25 mL, and perform the test as directed under Ultraviolet-visible Spectrophotometry *<2.24>*: the absorbance at a wavelength of 330 nm does not exceed 0.47.

(5) Heavy metals *<1.07>*—Proceed with 2.0 g of Terbutaline Sulfate as directed under Method 2, and perform the test. Prepare the control solution with 2.0 mL of Standard Lead Solution (not more than 10 ppm).

(6) Arsenic *<1.11>*—Prepare the test solution with 1.0 g of Terbutaline Sulfate according to method 3, and perform the test (not more than 2 ppm).

Water *<2.48>* Not more than 0.5% (1 g, volumetric titration, direct titration).

Residue on ignition *<2.44>* Not more than 0.2% (1 g).

Assay Weigh accurately about 0.5 g of Terbutaline Sulfate, dissolve in 50 mL of a mixture of acetonitrile and acetic acid (100) (1:1) by stirring and warming. Allow to cool, and titrate *<2.50>* with 0.1 mol/L perchloric acid VS (potentiometric titration, substituting a saturated solution of potassium chloride in methanol for the internal fluid).

Each mL of 0.1 mol/L perchloric acid VS
= 54.87 mg of $(C_{12}H_{19}NO_3)_2.H_2SO_4$

Containers and storage Containers—Tight containers.
Storage—Light-resistant.

Testosterone Enanthate

テストステロンエナント酸エステル

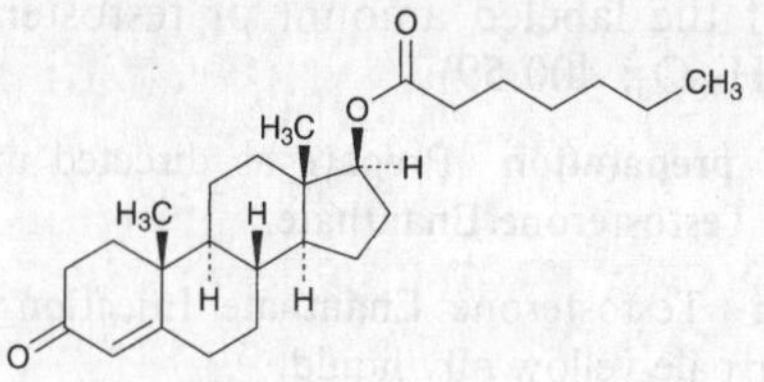

$C_{26}H_{40}O_3$: 400.59
3-Oxoandrost-4-en-17β-yl heptanoate
[315-37-7]

Testosterone Enanthate, when dried, contains not less than 95.0% and not more than 105.0% of testosterone enanthate ($C_{26}H_{40}O_3$).

Description Testosterone Enanthate occurs as white to pale yellow, crystals or crystalline powder, or a pale yellow-brown viscous liquid. It is odorless or has a slight, characteristic odor.

It is freely soluble in ethanol (99.5), and practically insoluble in water.

Melting point: about 36°C

Identification Heat 25 mg of Testosterone Enanthate with 2 mL of a solution of potassium hydroxide in methanol (1 in 100) under a reflux condenser on a water bath for 1 hour, cool, and add 10 mL of water. Collect the produced precipitate by suction, wash with water until the last washing is neutral, and dry the precipitate in a desiccator (in vacuum, phosphorus (V) oxide) for 4 hours: the precipitate melts *<2.60>* between 151°C and 157°C.

Optical rotation *<2.49>* $[\alpha]_D^{25}$: +76 – +86° (after drying, 0.1 g, ethanol (99.5), 10 mL, 100 mm).

Purity Acidity—Dissolve 0.5 g of Testosterone Enanthate in 10 mL of ethanol (95) which has previously been rendered neutral to bromothymol blue TS, and add 2 drops of bromothymol blue TS and 0.50 mL of 0.01 mol/L sodium hydroxide VS: the color of the solution is light blue.

Loss on drying *<2.41>* Not more than 0.5% (0.5 g, in vacuum, phosphorus (V) oxide, 4 hours).

Residue on ignition *<2.44>* Not more than 0.1% (0.5 g).

Assay Weigh accurately about 0.1 g of Testosterone Enanthate, previously dried, and dissolve in ethanol (95) to make exactly 100 mL. Measure exactly 10 mL of this solution, and dilute with ethanol (95) to make exactly 100 mL. Measure exactly 10 mL of this solution, and dilute with ethanol (95) to make exactly 100 mL. Perform the test as directed under Ultraviolet-visible Spectrophotometry <*2.24*> with this solution. Determine the absorbance A of this solution at the wavelength of maximum absorption at about 241 nm.

Amount (mg) of testosterone enanthate ($C_{26}H_{40}O_3$)
$= A/426 \times 100{,}000$

Containers and storage Containers—Tight containers.
Storage—Light-resistant, and not exceeding 30°C.

Testosterone Enanthate Injection

テストステロンエナント酸エステル注射液

Testosterone Enanthate Injection is an oily solution for injection.

It contains not less than 90.0% and not more than 110.0% of the labeled amount of testosterone enanthate ($C_{26}H_{40}O_3$: 400.59).

Method of preparation Prepare as directed under Injections, with Testosterone Enanthate.

Description Testosterone Enanthate Injection is a clear, colorless or pale yellow oily liquid.

Identification Measure a volume of Testosterone Enanthate Injection, equivalent to 0.05 g of Testosterone Enanthate, add 8 mL of petroleum ether, and extract with three 10-mL portions of diluted acetic acid (100) (7 in 10). Combine the extracts, wash with 10 mL of petroleum ether, add 0.5 mL of diluted sulfuric acid (7 in 10) to 0.1 mL of the extract, and heat on a water bath for 5 minutes. Cool, and add 0.5 mL of iron (III) chloride-acetic acid TS: the color of the solution is blue.

Extractable volume <*6.05*> It meets the requirement.

Foreign insoluble matter <*6.06*> Perform the test according to Method 1: it meets the requirement.

Insoluble particulate matter <*6.07*> Perform the test according to Method 2: it meets the requirement.

Sterility <*4.06*> Perform the test according to the Membrane filtration method: it meets the requirement.

Assay Measure accurately a volume of Testosterone Enanthate Injection, equivalent to about 25 mg of testosterone enanthate ($C_{26}H_{40}O_3$), and dissolve in chloroform to make exactly 25 mL. Pipet 3 mL of this solution, add chloroform to make exactly 50 mL, and use this solution as the sample solution. Separately, weigh accurately about 25 mg of Testosterone Propionate RS, proceed in the same manner as for the sample solution, and use this solution as the standard solution. Pipet 5 mL each of the sample solution and standard solution, add exactly 10 mL of isoniazid TS, add methanol to make exactly 20 mL, and allow to stand for 45 minutes. Determine the absorbances, A_T and A_S, of these solutions at 380 nm, respectively, as directed under Ultraviolet-visible Spectrophotometry <*2.24*>, using a solution obtained by proceeding with 5 mL of chloroform as the blank.

Amount (mg) of testosterone enanthate ($C_{26}H_{40}O_3$)
$= M_S \times A_T/A_S \times 1.163$

M_S: Amount (mg) of Testosterone Propionate RS taken

Containers and storage Containers—Hermetic containers.
Storage—Light-resistant.

Testosterone Propionate

テストステロンプロピオン酸エステル

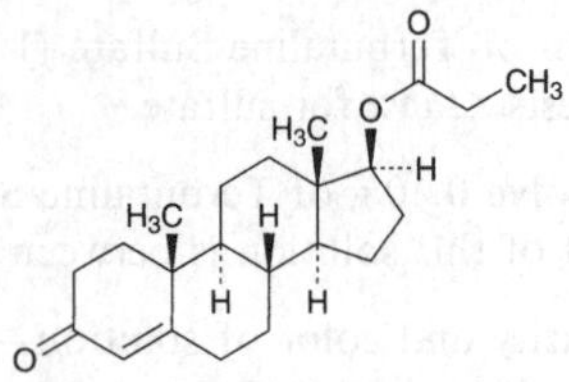

$C_{22}H_{32}O_3$: 344.49
3-Oxoandrost-4-en-17β-yl propanoate
[*57-85-2*]

Testosterone Propionate, when dried, contains not less than 97.0% and not more than 103.0% of testosterone propionate ($C_{22}H_{32}O_3$).

Description Testosterone Propionate occurs as white to pale yellow, crystals or crystalline powder.

It is freely soluble in methanol and in ethanol (95), and practically insoluble in water.

Identification **(1)** Determine the absorption spectrum of a solution of Testosterone Propionate in ethanol (95) (1 in 100,000) as directed under Ultraviolet-visible Spectrophotometry <*2.24*>, and compare the spectrum with the Reference Spectrum or the spectrum of a solution of Testosterone Propionate RS prepared in the same manner as the sample solution: both spectra exhibit similar intensities of absorption at the same wavelengths.

(2) Determine the infrared absorption spectrum of Testosterone Propionate, previously dried, as directed in the potassium bromide disk method under Infrared Spectrophotometry <*2.25*>, and compare the spectrum with the Reference Spectrum or the spectrum of Testosterone Propionate RS: both spectra exhibit similar intensities of absorption at the same wave numbers.

Optical rotation <*2.49*> $[\alpha]_D^{20}$: +83 – +90° (after drying, 0.1 g, ethanol (95), 10 mL, 100 mm).

Melting point <*2.60*> 118 – 123°C

Purity Related substances—Dissolve 40 mg of Testosterone Propionate in 2 mL of ethanol (95), and use this solution as the sample solution. Pipet 1 mL of the sample solution, add ethanol (95) to make exactly 100 mL, and use this solution as the standard solution. Perform the test with these solutions as directed under Thin-layer Chromatography <*2.03*>. Spot 10 μL each of the sample solution and standard solution on a plate of silica gel with fluorescent indicator for thin-layer chromatography. Develop the plate with a mixture of chloroform and diethylamine (19:1) to a distance of about 15 cm, and air-dry the plate. Examine under ultraviolet light (main wavelength: 254 nm): the spots other than the principal spot obtained from the sample solution are not more intense than the spot from the standard solution.

Loss on drying <*2.41*> Not more than 0.5% (0.5 g, in vacuum, phosphorus (V) oxide, 4 hours).

Residue on ignition <*2.44*> Not more than 0.1% (0.5 g).

Assay Weigh accurately each about 10 mg of Testosterone Propionate and Testosterone Propionate RS, previously dried, and dissolve in methanol to make exactly 100 mL. To exactly 5 mL of these solutions add exactly 5 mL of the internal standard solution and methanol to make 20 mL, and use these solutions as the sample solution and standard solution. Perform the test with 5 μL each of the sample solution and standard solution as directed under Liquid Chromatography <*2.01*> according to the following conditions, and calculate the ratios, Q_T and Q_S, of the peak area of testosterone propionate to that of the internal standard.

Amount (mg) of testosterone propionate ($C_{22}H_{32}O_3$)
$= M_S \times Q_T/Q_S$

M_S: Amount (mg) of Testosterone Propionate RS taken

Internal standard solution—A solution of progesterone in methanol (9 in 100,000).
Operating conditions—

Detector: An ultraviolet absorption photometer (wavelength: 241 nm).

Column: A stainless steel column 4.6 mm in inside diameter and 15 cm in length, packed with octadecylsilanized silica gel for liquid chromatography (5 μm in particle diameter).

Column temperature: A constant temperature of about 35°C.

Mobile phase: A mixture of acetonitrile and water (7:3).

Flow rate: Adjust so that the retention time of testosterone propionate is about 10 minutes.
System suitability—

System performance: When the procedure is run with 5 μL of the standard solution under the above operating conditions, the internal standard and testosterone propionate are eluted in this order with the resolution between these peaks being not less than 9.

System repeatability: When the test is repeated 6 times with 5 μL of the standard solution under the above operating conditions, the relative standard deviation of the ratio of the peak area of testosterone propionate to that of the internal standard is not more than 1.0%.

Containers and storage Containers—Tight containers.

Storage—Light-resistant.

Testosterone Propionate Injection

テストステロンプロピオン酸エステル注射液

Testosterone Propionate Injection is an oily solution for injection.

It contains not less than 92.5% and not more than 107.5% of the labeled amount of testosterone propionate ($C_{22}H_{32}O_3$: 344.49).

Method of preparation Prepare as directed under Injections, with Testosterone Propionate.

Description Testosterone Propionate Injection is a clear, colorless or pale yellow oily liquid.

Identification Dissolve the residue obtained as directed in the procedure in the Assay in exactly 20 mL of methanol, and use this solution as the sample solution. Separately, dissolve 1 mg of Testosterone Propionate RS in 10 mL of methanol, and use this solution as the standard solution. Perform the test with these solutions as directed under Thin-layer Chromatography <*2.03*>. Spot 10 μL each of the sample solution and standard solution on a plate of silica gel with fluorescent indicator for thin-layer chromatography. Develop the plate with a mixture of chloroform and diethylamine (19:1) to a distance of about 15 cm, and air-dry the plate. Examine under ultraviolet light (main wavelength: 254 nm): the *R*f values of the principal spot obtained from the sample solution and of the spot from the standard solution are not different each other.

Extractable volume <*6.05*> It meets the requirement.

Foreign insoluble matter <*6.06*> Perform the test according to Method 1: it meets the requirement.

Insoluble particulate matter <*6.07*> Perform the test according to Method 2: it meets the requirement.

Sterility <*4.06*> Perform the test according to the Membrane filtration method: it meets the requirement.

Assay (i) Chromatographic tube A glass tube about 1 cm in inside diameter and about 18 cm in length, with a glass filter (G3) at the lower end.

(ii) Chromatographic column To about 2 g of silica gel for liquid chromatography add 5 mL of dichloromethane, and mix gently. Transfer and wash into the chromatographic tube with the aid of dichloromethane, allow to elute the dichloromethane through the column, and put a filter paper on the upper end of the silica gel.

(iii) Standard solution Weigh accurately about 10 mg of Testosterone Propionate RS, previously dried at 105°C for 4 hours, and dissolve in methanol to make exactly 100 mL. Pipet 5 mL of this solution, add exactly 5 mL of the internal standard solution and methanol to make 20 mL.

(iv) Sample stock solution To exactly a volume of Testosterone Propionate Injection, equivalent to about 20 mg of testosterone propionate ($C_{22}H_{32}O_3$), add dichloromethane to make exactly 20 mL.

(v) Procedure Transfer exactly 2 mL of the sample stock solution into the chromatographic column, and elute to the upper surface of the silica gel. Wash the inner surface of the chromatographic tube with 15 mL of dichloromethane, elute to the upper surface of the silica gel, and discard the effluent. Elute 15 mL of a mixture of dichloromethane and methanol (39:1), discard the first 5 mL of the effluent, and collect the subsequent effluent. Wash the lower part of the column with a few amount of dichloromethane, combine the washings and the effluent, and evaporate the solvent under reduced pressure. Dissolve the residue so obtained with methanol to make exactly 20 mL. Pipet 5 mL of this solution, add exactly 5 mL of the internal standard solution and methanol to make 20 mL, and use this solution as the sample solution. Perform the test with 5 μL each of the sample solution and standard solution as directed in the Assay under Testosterone Propionate.

Amount (mg) of testosterone propionate ($C_{22}H_{32}O_3$)
$= M_S \times Q_T/Q_S \times 2$

M_S: Amount (mg) of Testosterone Propionate RS taken

Internal standard solution—A solution of progesterone in methanol (9 in 100,000).

Containers and storage Containers—Hermetic containers.

Adsorbed Tetanus Toxoid

沈降破傷風トキソイド

Adsorbed Tetanus Toxoid is a liquid for injection containing tetanus toxoid prepared by treating tetanus toxin with formaldehyde by a method involving no appreciable loss of the immunogenicity and rendered insoluble by the addition of aluminum salt.

It conforms to the requirements of Adsorbed Tetanus Toxoid in the Minimum Requirements for Biological Products.

Description Adsorbed Tetanus Toxoid becomes a uniform white-turbid liquid on shaking.

Tetracaine Hydrochloride

テトラカイン塩酸塩

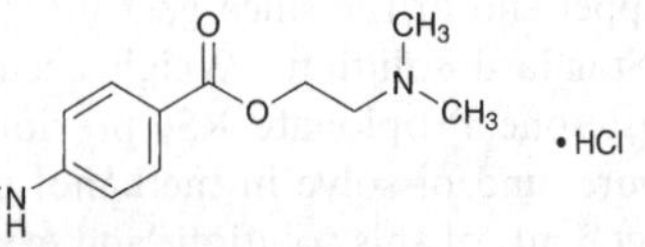

$C_{15}H_{24}N_2O_2.HCl$: 300.82
2-(Dimethylamino)ethyl 4-(butylamino)benzoate monohydrochloride
[136-47-0]

Tetracaine Hydrochloride, when dried, contains not less than 98.5% of tetracaine hydrochloride ($C_{15}H_{25}N_2O_2.HCl$).

Description Tetracaine Hydrochloride occurs as white, crystals or crystalline powder. It is odorless, and has a slightly bitter taste followed by a sense of numbness on the tongue.

It is very soluble in formic acid, freely soluble in water, soluble in ethanol (95), sparingly soluble in ethanol (99.5), slightly soluble in acetic anhydride, and practically insoluble in diethyl ether.

A solution of Tetracaine Hydrochloride (1 in 10) is neutral.

Melting point: about 148°C.

Identification **(1)** Dissolve 0.5 g of Tetracaine Hydrochloride in 50 mL of water, add 5 mL of ammonia TS, shake, and allow to stand in a cold place. Collect the precipitate, wash with water until the washings become neutral, and dry in a desiccator (silica gel) for 24 hours: it melts *<2.60>* between 42°C and 44°C.

(2) Dissolve 0.1 g of Tetracaine Hydrochloride in 8 mL of water, and add 3 mL of ammonium thiocyanate TS: a crystalline precipitate is produced. Collect the precipitate, recrystallize from water, and dry at 80°C for 2 hours: it melts *<2.60>* between 130°C and 132°C.

(3) Determine the absorption spectrum of a solution of Tetracaine Hydrochloride in ethanol (99.5) (1 in 200,000) as directed under Ultraviolet-visible Spectrophotometry *<2.24>*, and compare the spectrum with the Reference Spectrum: both spectra exhibit similar intensities of absorption at the same wavelengths.

(4) A solution of Tetracaine Hydrochloride (1 in 10) responds to Qualitative Tests *<1.09>* for chloride.

Purity Heavy metals *<1.07>*—Proceed with 1.0 g of Tetracaine Hydrochloride according to Method 1, and perform the test. Prepare the control solution with 2.0 mL of Standard Lead Solution (not more than 20 ppm).

Loss on drying *<2.41>* Not more than 1.0% (1 g, 105°C, 4 hours).

Residue on ignition *<2.44>* Not more than 0.1% (1 g).

Assay Weigh accurately about 0.5 g of Tetracaine Hydrochloride, previously dried, dissolve in 2 mL of formic acid, add 80 mL of acetic anhydride, allow to stand at 30°C on a water bath for 15 minutes, cool, and titrate *<2.50>* with 0.1 mol/L perchloric acid VS (potentiometric titration). Perform a blank determination in the same manner, and make any necessary correction.

Each mL of 0.1 mol/L perchloric acid VS
= 30.08 mg of $C_{15}H_{24}N_2O_2.HCl$

Containers and storage Containers—Tight containers.

Tetracycline Hydrochloride

テトラサイクリン塩酸塩

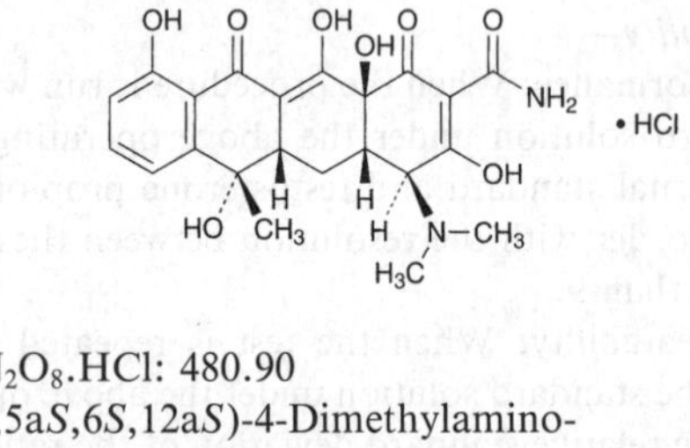

$C_{22}H_{24}N_2O_8.HCl$: 480.90
(4*S*,4a*S*,5a*S*,6*S*,12a*S*)-4-Dimethylamino-3,6,10,12,12a-pentahydroxy-6-methyl-1,11-dioxo-1,4,4a,5,5a,6,11,12a-octahydrotetracene-2-carboxamide monohydrochloride
[64-75-5]

Tetracycline Hydrochloride is the hydrochloride of a tetracycline substance having antibacterial activity produced by the growth of *Streptomyces aureofaciens*.

It contains not less than 950 μg (potency) and not more than 1010 μg (potency) per mg, calculated on the dried basis. The potency of Tetracycline Hydrochloride is expressed as mass (potency) of tetracycline hydrochloride ($C_{22}H_{24}N_2O_8.HCl$).

Description Tetracycline Hydrochloride occurs as a yellow to pale brownish yellow crystalline powder.

It is freely soluble in water, and sparingly soluble in ethanol (95).

Identification **(1)** Determine the absorption spectrum of a solution of Tetracycline Hydrochloride (1 in 62,500) as directed under Ultraviolet-visible Spectrophotometry *<2.24>*, and compare the spectrum with the Reference Spectrum or the spectrum of a solution of Tetracycline Hydrochloride RS prepared in the same manner as the sample solution: both spectra exhibit similar intensities of absorption at the same wavelengths.

(2) Determine the infrared absorption spectrum of Tetracycline Hydrochloride as directed in the potassium chloride disk method under Infrared Spectrophotometry *<2.25>*, and compare the spectrum with the Reference Spectrum or the spectrum of Tetracycline Hydrochloride RS: both spectra exhibit similar intensities of absorption at the same wave numbers.

(3) A solution of Tetracycline Hydrochloride (1 in 100) responds to Qualitative Tests 〈*1.09*〉 (2) for chloride.

pH 〈*2.54*〉 Dissolve 1.0 g of Tetracycline Hydrochloride in 100 mL of water: the pH of the solution is between 1.8 and 2.8.

Purity **(1)** Heavy metals 〈*1.07*〉—Proceed with 1.0 g of Tetracycline Hydrochloride according to Method 2, and perform the test. Prepare the control solution with 1.0 mL of Standard Lead Solution (not more than 10 ppm).

(2) Related substances—Dissolve 25 mg of Tetracycline Hydrochloride in 50 mL of 0.01 mol/L hydrochloric acid TS, and use this solution as the sample solution. Pipet 3 mL of the sample solution, add 0.01 mol/L hydrochloric acid TS to make exactly 100 mL, and use this solution as the standard solution. Perform the test with exactly 20 μL each of the sample solution and standard solution as directed under Liquid Chromatography 〈*2.01*〉 according to the following conditions, and determine each peak area by the automatic integration method: the area of the peak other than tetracycline obtained from the sample solution is not larger than the peak area of tetracycline from the standard solution, and the total area of the peaks other than tetracycline from the sample solution is not larger than 3 times the peak area of tetracycline from the standard solution.

Operating conditions—

Detector, column, column temperature, mobile phase, and flow rate: Proceed as directed in the operating conditions in the Assay.

Time span of measurement: About 7 times as long as the retention time of tetracycline, beginning after the solvent peak.

System suitability—

System performance: Proceed as directed in the system suitability in the Assay.

Test for required detectability: Pipet 3 mL of the standard solution, add 0.1 mol/L hydrochloric acid TS to make exactly 100 mL, and confirm that the peak area of tetracycline obtained with 20 μL of this solution is equivalent to 1 to 5% of that with 20 μL of the standard solution.

System repeatability: When the test is repeated 6 times with 20 μL of the standard solution under the above operating conditions, the relative standard deviation of the peak area of tetracycline is not more than 1.0%.

Loss on drying 〈*2.41*〉 Not more than 2.0% (1 g, in vacuum, 60°C, 3 hours).

Residue on ignition 〈*2.44*〉 Not more than 0.3% (1.0 g).

Assay Weigh accurately an amount of Tetracycline Hydrochloride and Tetracycline Hydrochloride RS, equivalent to about 25 mg (potency), and dissolve each in 0.1 mol/L hydrochloric acid TS to make exactly 50 mL, and use these solutions as the sample solution and the standard solution, respectively. Perform the test with exactly 20 μL each of these solutions as directed under Liquid Chromatography 〈*2.01*〉 according to the following conditions, and determine the peak areas, A_T and A_S, of tetracycline in each solution.

Amount [μg (potency)] of tetracycline hydrochloride ($C_{22}H_{24}N_2O_8.HCl$)
$= M_S \times A_T/A_S \times 1000$

M_S: Amount [mg (potency)] of Tetracycline Hydrochloride RS taken

Operating conditions—

Detector: An ultraviolet absorption photometer (wavelength: 254 nm).

Column: A stainless steel column 4.6 mm in inside diameter and 25 cm in length, packed with stylene-divinylbenzene copolymer for liquid chromatography (0.01 μm in pore diameter).

Column temperature: A constant temperature of about 60°C.

Mobile phase: Dissolve 3.5 g of dipotassium hydrogenphosphate, 2.0 g of tetrabutylammonium hydrogensulfate and 0.4 g of disodium dihydrogen ethylenediamine tetraacetate dihydrate in 300 mL of water, adjust to pH 9.0 with sodium hydroxide TS, add 90.0 g of *t*-butyl alcohol, and add water to make 1000 mL.

Flow rate: Adjust so that the retention time of tetracycline is about 5 minutes.

System suitability—

System performance: Dissolve 0.05 g of Tetracycline Hydrochloride RS in water to make 25 mL. Heat 5 mL of this solution on a water bath for 60 minutes, then add water to make 25 mL. When the procedure is run with 20 μL of this solution under the above operating conditions, the retention time of 4-epitetracycline is about 3 minutes, and 4-epitetracycline and tetracycline are eluted in this order with the resolution between these peaks being not less than 2.5.

System repeatability: When the test is repeated 6 times with 20 μL of the standard solution under the above operating conditions, the relative standard deviation of the peak areas of tetracycline is not more than 1.0%.

Containers and storage Containers—Tight containers.
Storage—Light-resistant.

Thallium (^{201}Tl) Chloride Injection

塩化タリウム (^{201}Tl) 注射液

Thallium (^{201}Tl) Chloride Injection is an aqueous injection

It contains thallium-201 (^{201}Tl) in the form of thallous chloride.

It conforms to the requirements of Thallium (^{201}Tl) Chloride Injection in the Minimum Requirements for Radiopharmaceuticals.

Test for Extractable Volume of Parenteral Preparations and Insoluble Particulate Matter Test for Injections are not applied to this injection.

Description Thallium (^{201}Tl) Chloride Injection is a clear, colorless liquid.

Theophylline

テオフィリン

$C_7H_8N_4O_2$: 180.16
1,3-Dimethyl-1*H*-purine-2,6(3*H*,7*H*)-dione
[*58-55-9*]

Theophylline, when dried, contains not less than 99.0% of theophylline ($C_7H_8N_4O_2$).

Description Theophylline occurs as white, crystals or crystalline powder.

It is soluble in *N,N*-dimethylformamide, and slightly soluble in water and in ethanol (99.5).

It dissolves in 0.1 mol/L hydrochloric acid TS.

Identification **(1)** Determine the absorption spectrum of a solution of Theophylline in 0.1 mol/L hydrochloric acid TS (1 in 200,000) as directed under Ultraviolet-visible Spectrophotometry <*2.24*>, and compare the spectrum with the Reference Spectrum: both spectra exhibit similar intensities of absorption at the same wavelengths.

(2) Determine the infrared absorption spectrum of Theophylline, previously dried, as directed in the potassium bromide disk method under Infrared Spectrophotometry <*2.25*>, and compare the spectrum with the Reference Spectrum: both spectra exhibit similar intensities of absorption at the same wave numbers.

Melting point <*2.60*> 271 – 275°C

Purity **(1)** Acidity—To 0.5 g of Theophylline add 75 mL of water, 2.0 mL of 0.01 mol/L sodium hydroxide VS and 1 drop of methyl red TS: a yellow color develops.

(2) Heavy metals <*1.07*>—Proceed with 1.0 g of Theophylline according to Method 4, and perform the test. Prepare the control solution with 2.0 mL of Standard Lead Solution (not more than 20 ppm).

(3) Arsenic <*1.11*>—Prepare the test solution with 1.0 g of Theophylline according to Method 3, and perform the test (not more than 2 ppm).

(4) Related substances—Dissolve 0.10 g of Theophylline in 3 mL of *N,N*-dimethylformamide, add 10 mL of methanol, and use this solution as the sample solution. Pipet 1 mL of the sample solution, add methanol to make exactly 200 mL, and use this solution as the standard solution. Perform the test with these solutions as directed under Thin-layer Chromatography <*2.03*>. Spot 10 μL each of the sample solution and standard solution on a plate of silica gel with fluorescent indicator for thin-layer chromatography. Develop the plate with a mixture of acetone, chloroform, methanol, 1-butanol and ammonia solution (28) (3:3:2:2:1) to a distance of about 10 cm, and air-dry the plate. Examine under ultraviolet light (main wavelength: 254 nm): the spots other than the principal spot obtained from the sample solution are not more intense than the spot from the standard solution.

Loss on drying <*2.41*> Not more than 0.5% (1 g, 105°C, 4 hours).

Residue on ignition <*2.44*> Not more than 0.1% (1 g).

Assay Weigh accurately about 0.25 g of Theophylline, previously dried, and dissolve in 100 mL of water, add exactly 20 mL of 0.1 mol/L silver nitrate VS, shake the mixture, and titrate <*2.50*> with 0.1 mol/L sodium hydroxide VS (potentiometric titration). Perform a blank determination in the same manner, and make any necessary correction.

Each mL of 0.1 mol/L sodium hydroxide VS
= 18.02 mg of $C_7H_8N_4O_2$

Containers and storage Containers—Well-closed containers.

Thiamazole

チアマゾール

$C_4H_6N_2S$: 114.17
1-Methyl-1*H*-imidazole-2-thiol
[*60-56-0*]

Thiamazole, when dried, contains not less than 98.0% of thiamazole ($C_4H_6N_2S$).

Description Thiamazole occurs as white to pale yellowwhite, crystals or crystalline powder. It has a faint, characteristic odor, and has a bitter taste.

It is freely soluble in water and in ethanol (95), and slightly soluble in diethyl ether.

The pH of a solution of 1.0 g of Thiamazole in 50 mL of water is between 5.0 and 7.0.

Identification **(1)** Dissolve 5 mg of Thiamazole in 1 mL of water, shake with 1 mL of sodium hydroxide TS, and add 3 drops of sodium pentacyanonitrosylferrate (III) TS: a yellow color develops, and it gradually changes to yellow-green to green. To this solution add 1 mL of acetic acid (31): it changes to blue.

(2) To 2 mL of a solution of Thiamazole (1 in 200) add 1 mL of sodium carbonate TS and 1 mL of diluted Folin's TS (1 in 5): a deep blue color develops.

Melting point <*2.60*> 144 – 147°C

Purity **(1)** Selenium—Proceed with 0.10 g of Thiamazole as directed under Oxygen Flask Combustion Method <*1.06*>, using 25 mL of diluted nitric acid (1 in 30) as the absorbing liquid, and prepare the test solution. Apply a small amount of water to the upper part of apparatus A, pull out C carefully, and transfer the test solution to a beaker. Wash C, B and the inner side of A with 25 mL of water, and combine the washings with the test solution. Boil gently for 10 minutes, cool to room temperature, add water to make exactly 50 mL, and use this solution as the sample solution. Separately, weigh exactly 40 mg of selenium, dissolve in 100 mL of diluted nitric acid (1 in 2), heat to dissolve on a water bath if necessary, and add water to make exactly 1000 mL. Pipet 5 mL of this solution, and add water to make exactly 200 mL. To 2 mL of this solution, exactly measured, add diluted nitric acid (1 in 60) to make exactly 50 mL, and use this solution as the standard solution. Pipet 40 mL each of the sample solution and standard solution into separate beakers, and adjust each solution with ammonia solution (28) to a pH of 1.8 to 2.2. To each solution add 0.2 g of hydroxylammonium chloride, shake gently to dissolve. To these solutions add 5 mL of a solution prepared by dissolving 0.10 g of 2,3-diaminonaphthalene and 0.5 g of hydroxylammonium chloride in 0.1 mol/L hydrochloric acid TS to make 100 mL, shake, and allow to stand for 100 minutes. Transfer these solutions to corresponding separators, rinse the beakers with 10 mL of water, combine the rinsings in the respective separators, shake well with 5.0 mL of cyclohexane for 2 minutes, and extract. Centrifuge the cyclohexane extracts to remove any water remaining in these solutions. Perform the test with these solutions as directed under Ultraviolet-visible Spectrophotometry <*2.24*>, using a solution prepared with 40 mL of diluted nitric acid (1 in 60) in the same manner as the blank.

The absorbance of of the sample solution at the wavelength of maximum absorbance at about 378 nm does not exceed the absorbance of the standard solution.

(2) Heavy metals *<1.07>*—Proceed with 1.0 g of Thiamazole according to Method 2, and perform the test. Prepare the control solution with 2.0 mL of Standard Lead Solution (not more than 20 ppm).

(3) Arsenic *<1.11>*—Prepare the test solution with 1.0 g of Thiamazole according to Method 1, and perform the test (not more than 2 ppm).

Loss on drying *<2.41>* Not more than 0.5% (1 g, 105°C, 2 hours).

Residue on ignition *<2.44>* Not more than 0.1% (1 g).

Assay Weigh accurately about 0.25 g of Thiamazole, previously dried, dissolve in 75 mL of water, add 15 mL of 0.1 mol/L sodium hydroxide VS from a burette, and add 30 mL of 0.1 mol/L silver nitrate VS with stirring. Add 1 mL of bromothymol blue TS, and titrate *<2.50>* with 0.1 mol/L sodium hydroxide VS, until a persistent blue-green color is produced. Determine the total volume of 0.1 mol/L sodium hydroxide VS consumed.

Each mL of 0.1 mol/L sodium hydroxide VS
= 11.42 mg of $C_4H_6N_2S$

Containers and storage Containers—Well-closed containers.

Storage—Light-resistant.

Thiamazole Tablets

チアマゾール錠

Thiamazole Tablets contain not less than 94.0% and not more than 106.0% of the labeled amount of thiamazole ($C_4H_6N_2S$: 114.17).

Method of preparation Prepare as directed under Tablets, with Thiamazole.

Identification **(1)** To a quantity of powdered Thiamazole Tablets, equivalent to 0.05 g of Thiamazole, add 20 mL of hot ethanol (95), shake for 15 minutes, filter, and evaporate the filtrate on a water bath to dryness. Dissolve the residue in 10 mL of water, filter if necessary, and use this solution as the sample solution. To 1 mL of the sample solution add 1 mL of sodium hydroxide TS, shake, and add 3 drops of sodium pentacyanonitrosylferrate (III) TS: a yellow color develops, and it gradually changes to yellow-green to green. To this solution add 1 mL of acetic acid (31): it changes to blue.

(2) With 2 mL of the sample solution obtained in (1), proceed as directed in the Identification (2) under Thiamazole.

Assay Weigh accurately and powder not less than 20 Thiamazole Tablets. Weigh accurately a quantity of the powder, equivalent to about 0.15 g of thiamazole ($C_4H_6N_2S$), add 80 mL of water, shake for 15 minutes, add water to make exactly 100 mL, and centrifuge. Filter, discard the first 20 mL of the filtrate, pipet 50 mL of the subsequent filtrate, add 1 mL of bromothymol blue TS, and if a blue color develops, neutralize with 0.1 mol/L hydrochloric acid VS until the color of the solution changes to green. To this solution add 4.5 mL of 0.1 mol/L sodium hydroxide VS from a burette, add 15 mL of 0.1 mol/L silver nitrate VS while stirring, and titrate *<2.50>* with 0.1 mol/L sodium hydroxide VS. Continue the titration until a persistent blue-green color is produced, and determine the total volume of 0.1 mol/L sodium hydroxide VS consumed.

Each mL of 0.1 mol/L sodium hydroxide VS
= 11.42 mg of $C_4H_6N_2S$

Containers and storage Containers—Well-closed containers.

Storage—Light-resistant.

Thiamine Chloride Hydrochloride

Vitamin B_1 Hydrochloride

チアミン塩化物塩酸塩

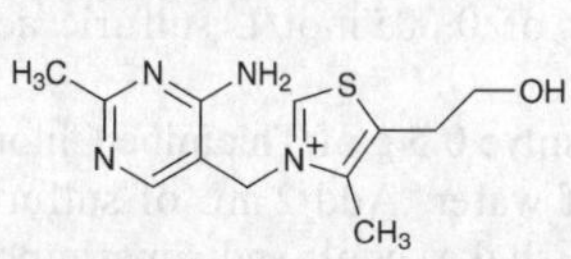

$C_{12}H_{17}ClN_4OS.HCl$: 337.27
3-(4-Amino-2-methylpyrimidin-5-ylmethyl)-5-(2-hydroxyethyl)-4-methylthiazolium chloride monohydrochloride
[67-03-8]

Thiamine Chloride Hydrochloride contains not less than 98.5% and not more than 101.0% of thiamine chloride hydrochloride ($C_{12}H_{17}ClN_4OS.HCl$), calculated on the anhydrous basis.

Description Thiamine Chloride Hydrochloride occurs as white, crystals or crystalline powder. It is odorless or has a slight, characteristic odor.

It is freely soluble in water, sparingly soluble in methanol, and slightly soluble in ethanol (95).

Melting point: about 245°C (with decomposition).

It shows crystal polymorphism.

Identification **(1)** To 5 mL of a solution of Thiamine Chloride Hydrochloride (1 in 500) add 2.5 mL of sodium hydroxide TS and 0.5 mL of potassium hexacyanoferrate (III) TS. Then add 5 mL of 2-methyl-1-propanol, shake the mixture vigorously for 2 minutes, allow to stand, and examine under ultraviolet light (main wavelength: 365 nm): the 2-methyl-1-propanol layer shows a blue-purple fluorescence. This fluorescence disappears when the mixture is acidified, but reappears when it is again made alkaline.

(2) Determine the absorption spectrum of a solution of Thiamine Chloride Hydrochloride (1 in 100,000) as directed under Ultraviolet-visible Spectrophotometry *<2.24>*, and compare the spectrum with the Reference Spectrum or the spectrum of a solution of Thiamine Chloride Hydrochloride RS prepared in the same manner as the sample solution: both spectra exhibit similar intensities of absorption at the same wavelengths.

(3) Determine the infrared absorption spectrum of Thiamine Chloride Hydrochloride, previously dried at 105°C for 2 hours, as directed in the potassium chloride disk method under the Infrared Spectrophotometry *<2.25>*, and compare the spectrum with the Reference Spectrum, or the spectrum of Thiamine Chloride Hydrochloride RS previously dried at 105°C for 2 hours: both spectra exhibit similar intensities of absorption at the same wave numbers. In case when some differences are found between the spectra, repeat the test with residues obtained by dissolving these substances in water, evaporating to dryness, and drying at 105°C for 2 hours.

(4) A solution of Thiamine Chloride Hydrochloride (1 in 500) responds to Qualitative Tests <*1.09*> for chloride.

pH <*2.54*> Dissolve 1.0 g of Thiamine Chloride Hydrochloride in 100 mL of water: the pH of this solution is between 2.7 and 3.4.

Purity (1) Clarity and color of solution—Dissolve 1.0 g of Thiamine Chloride Hydrochloride in 10 mL of water: the solution is clear, and has no more color than the following control solution.

Control solution: To 1.5 mL of 1/60 mol/L potassium dichromate VS add water to make 1000 mL.

(2) Sulfate <*1.14*>—Weigh 1.5 g of Thiamine Chloride Hydrochloride, and perform the test. Prepare the control solution with 0.35 mL of 0.005 mol/L sulfuric acid VS (not more than 0.011%).

(3) Nitrate—Dissolve 0.5 g of Thiamine Chloride Hydrochloride in 25 mL of water. Add 2 mL of sulfuric acid to 2 mL of this solution, shake, cool, and superimpose iron (II) sulfate TS: no dark brown ring is produced at the junction of the two layers.

(4) Heavy metals <*1.07*>—Proceed with 1.0 g of Thiamine Chloride Hydrochloride according to Method 1, and perform the test. Prepare the control solution with 2.0 mL of Standard Lead Solution (not more than 20 ppm).

(5) Related substances—Dissolve 0.10 g of Thiamine Chloride Hydrochloride in 100 mL of the mobile phase, and use this solution as the sample solution. Pipet 1 mL of the sample solution, add the mobile phase to make exactly 100 mL, and use this solution as the standard solution. Perform the test with exactly 10 μL each of the sample solution and standard solution as directed under Liquid Chromatography <*2.01*> according to the following conditions, and determine the area of each peak by the automatic integration method: the total area of the peaks other than thiamine obtained from the sample solution is not larger than the peak area of thiamine from the standard solution.

Operating conditions—

Detector, column, column temperature, mobile phase, and flow rate: Proceed as directed in the operating conditions in the Assay.

Time span of measurement: About 3 times as long as the retention time of thiamine.

System suitability—

System performance: Proceed as directed in the system suitability in the Assay.

Test for required detectability: To exactly 5 mL of the standard solution add water to make exactly 50 mL. Confirm that the peak area of thiamine obtained with 10 μL of this solution is equivalent to 7 to 13% of that with 10 μL of the standard solution.

System repeatability: When the test is repeated 6 times with 10 μL of the standard solution under the above operating conditions, the relative standard deviation of the peak area of thiamine is not more than 1.0%.

Water <*2.48*> Not more than 5.0% (30 mg, coulometric titration).

Residue on ignition <*2.44*> Not more than 0.2% (1 g).

Assay Weigh accurately about 0.1 g each of Thiamine Chloride Hydrochloride and Thiamine Chloride Hydrochloride RS (separately determine the water <*2.48*> in the same manner as Thiamine Chloride Hydrochloride), and dissolve them in the mobile phase to make exactly 50 mL. To 10 mL each of the solutions, accurately measured, add exactly 5 mL each of the internal standard solution, add the mobile phase to make 50 mL, and use these solutions as the sample solution and standard solution. Perform the test with 10 μL each of the sample solution and standard solution as directed under Liquid Chromatography <*2.01*> according to the following conditions, and calculate the ratios, Q_T and Q_S, of the peak area of thiamine to that of the internal standard.

Amount (mg) of thiamine chloride hydrochloride ($C_{12}H_{17}ClN_4OS.HCl$)

$$= M_S \times Q_T/Q_S$$

M_S: Amount (mg) of Thiamine Chloride Hydrochloride RS taken, calculated on the anhydrous basis

*Internal standard solution—*A solution methyl benzoate in methanol (1 in 50).

Operating conditions—

Detector: An ultraviolet absorption photometer (wavelength: 254 nm).

Column: A stainless steel column 4.6 mm in inside diameter and 15 cm in length, packed with octadecylsilanized silica gel for liquid chromatography (5 μm in particle diameter).

Column temperature: A constant temperature of about 25°C.

Mobile phase: Dissolve 1.1 g of sodium 1-octanesulfonate in 1000 mL of diluted acetic acid (100) (1 in 100). To 600 mL of this solution add 400 mL of a mixture of methanol and acetonitrile (3:2).

Flow rate: Adjust so that the retention time of thiamine is about 12 minutes.

System suitability—

System performance: When the procedure is run with 10 μL of the standard solution under the above operating conditions, thiamine and the internal standard are eluted in this order with the resolution between these peaks being not less than 6.

System repeatability: When the test is repeated 6 times with 10 μL of the standard solution under the above operating conditions, the relative standard deviation of the ratio of the peak area of thiamine to that of the internal standard is not more than 1.0%.

Containers and storage Containers—Tight containers.
Storage—Light-resistant.

Thiamine Chloride Hydrochloride Injection

Vitamin B$_1$ Hydrochloride Injection

チアミン塩化物塩酸塩注射液

Thiamine Chloride Hydrochloride Injection is an aqueous injection.

It contains not less than 95.0% and not more than 115.0% of the labeled amount of thiamine Chloride hydrochloride ($C_{12}H_{17}ClN_4OS.HCl$: 337.27).

Method of preparation Prepare as directed under Injections, with Thiamine Chloride Hydrochloride.

Description Thiamine Chloride Hydrochloride Injection is a clear, colorless liquid.

pH: 2.5 – 4.5

Identification To a volume of Thiamine Chloride Hydrochloride Injection, equivalent to 0.05 g of Thiamine Chloride Hydrochloride, add water to make 25 mL. Proceed with 5 mL of this solution as directed in the Identification (1) under Thiamine Chloride Hydrochloride.

Bacterial endotoxins ⟨*4.01*⟩ Less than 6.0 EU/mg.

Extractable volume ⟨*6.05*⟩ It meets the requirement.

Foreign insoluble matter ⟨*6.06*⟩ Perform the test according to Method 1: it meets the requirement.

Insoluble particulate matter ⟨*6.07*⟩ It meets the requirement.

Sterility ⟨*4.06*⟩ Perform the test according to the Membrane filtration method: it meets the requirement.

Assay Dilute with 0.001 mol/L hydrochloric acid TS if necessary, then measure exactly a volume of Thiamine Chloride Hydrochloride Injection, equivalent to about 20 mg of thiamine chloride hydrochloride ($C_{12}H_{17}ClN_4OS.HCl$), and add 20 mL of methanol and 0.001 mol/L hydrochloric acid TS to make exactly 100 mL. To 25 mL of this solution, exactly measured, add exactly 5 mL of the internal standard solution, add 0.001 mol/L hydrochloric acid TS to make 50 mL, and use this solution as the sample solution. Separately, weigh accurately about 0.1 g of Thiamine Chloride Hydrochloride RS (separately determine the water ⟨*2.48*⟩ in the same manner as Thiamine Chloride Hydrochloride), and dissolve in 0.001 mol/L hydrochloric acid TS to make exactly 50 mL. To 10 mL of this solution, exactly measured, add 20 mL of methanol and 0.001 mol/L hydrochloric acid TS to make exactly 100 mL. To 25 mL of this solution, exactly measured, add exactly 5 mL of the internal standard solution, add 0.001 mol/L hydrochloric acid TS to make 50 mL, and use this solution as the standard solution. Proceed as directed in the Assay under Thiamine Chloride Hydrochloride.

Amount (mg) of thiamine chloride hydrochloride ($C_{12}H_{17}ClN_4OS.HCl$)
$= M_S \times Q_T/Q_S \times 1/5$

M_S: Amount (mg) of Thiamine Chloride Hydrochloride RS taken, calculated on the anhydrous basis

Internal standard solution—A solution of methyl benzoate in methanol (1 in 200).

Containers and storage Containers—Hermetic containers.
Storage—Light-resistant.

Thiamine Chloride Hydrochloride Powder

Vitamin B$_1$ Hydrochloride Powder

チアミン塩化物塩酸塩散

Thiamine Chloride Hydrochloride Powder contains not less than 95.0% and not more than 115.0% of the labeled amount of thiamine chloride hydrochloride ($C_{12}H_{17}ClN_4OS.HCl$: 337.27).

Method of preparation Prepare as directed under Powders, with Thiamine Chloride Hydrochloride.

Identification To a portion of Thiamine Chloride Hydrochloride Powder, equivalent to 0.02 g of Thiamine Chloride Hydrochloride, add 50 mL of water and 10 mL of dilute acetic acid, shake, and filter. Proceed with 5 mL of the filtrate as directed in the Identification (1) under Thiamine Chloride Hydrochloride.

Purity Rancidity—Thiamine Chloride Hydrochloride Powder has no unpleasant or rancid odor. It is tasteless.

Assay Weigh accurately a quantity of Thiamine Chloride Hydrochloride Powder, equivalent to about 20 mg of thiamine chloride hydrochloride ($C_{12}H_{17}ClN_4OS.HCl$), add 60 mL of 0.01 mol/L hydrochloric acid TS, and heat on a water bath for 30 minutes. Shake vigorously for 10 minutes, cool, add methanol to make exactly 100 mL, and centrifuge. Pipet 25 mL of the supernatant liquid, add exactly 5 mL of the internal standard solution, add water to make 50 mL, and use this solution as the sample solution. Separately, weigh accurately about 0.1 g of Thiamine Chloride Hydrochloride RS (separately determine the water ⟨*2.48*⟩ in the same manner as Thiamine Chloride Hydrochloride), and dissolve in 0.01 mol/L hydrochloric acid TS to make exactly 50 mL. To 10 mL of this solution, exactly measured, add 50 mL of 0.01 mol/L hydrochloric acid TS, and add methanol to make exactly 100 mL. To 25 mL of this solution, exactly measured, add exactly 5 mL of the internal standard solution, add water to make 50 mL, and use this solution as the standard solution. Proceed as directed in the Assay under Thiamine Chloride Hydrochloride.

Amount (mg) of thiamine chloride hydrochloride ($C_{12}H_{17}ClN_4OS.HCl$)
$= M_S \times Q_T/Q_S \times 1/5$

M_S: Amount (mg) of Thiamine Chloride Hydrochloride RS taken, calculated on the anhydrous basis

Internal standard solution—A solution of methyl benzoate in methanol (1 in 200).

Containers and storage Containers—Tight containers.
Storage—Light-resistant.

Thiamine Nitrate

Vitamin B$_1$ Nitrate

チアミン硝化物

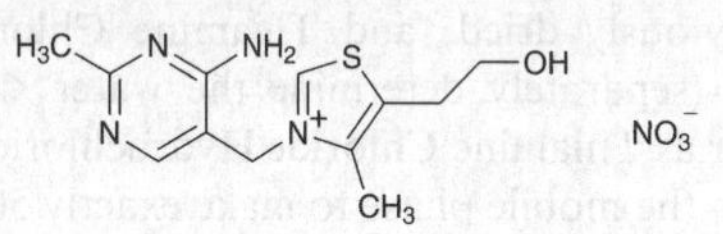

$C_{12}H_{17}N_5O_4S$: 327.36
3-(4-Amino-2-methylpyrimidin-5-ylmethyl)-5-(2-hydroxyethyl)-4-methylthiazolium nitrate
[*532-43-4*]

Thiamine Nitrate, when dried, contains not less than 98.0% and not more than 102.0% of thiamine nitrate ($C_{12}H_{17}N_5O_4S$).

Description Thiamine Nitrate occurs as white, crystals or crystalline powder. It is odorless or a slight, characteristic odor.

It is sparingly soluble in water, and very slightly soluble in ethanol (95), and practically insoluble in diethyl ether.

Melting point: about 193°C (with decomposition).

Identification **(1)** Take 2-mL portions of a solution of Thiamine Nitrate (1 in 500), and add 2 to 3 drops of iodine TS: a red-brown precipitate or turbidity is produced. Upon further addition of 1 mL of 2,4,6-trinitrophenol TS, a yellow precipitate or turbidity is produced.

(2) To 1 mL of a solution of Thiamine Nitrate (1 in 500) add 1 mL of lead (II) acetate TS and 1 mL of a solution of sodium hydroxide (1 in 10), and warm: the color of the solution changes through yellow to brown, and on standing, a black-brown precipitate is produced.

(3) To 5 mL of a solution of Thiamine Nitrate (1 in 500) add 2.5 mL of sodium hydroxide TS and 0.5 mL of potassium hexacyanoferrate (III) TS. Then add 5 mL of 2-methyl-1-propanol, shake the mixture vigorously for 2 minutes, allow to stand, and examine under ultraviolet light (main wavelength: 365 nm): the 2-methyl-1-propanol layer shows a blue-purple fluorescence. This fluorescence disappears when the mixture is acidified, but reappears when it is again made alkaline.

(4) A solution of Thiamine Nitrate (1 in 50) responds to Qualitative Tests <*1.09*> (1) and (2) for nitrate.

pH <*2.54*> Dissolve 1.0 g of Thiamine Nitrate in 100 mL of water: the pH of this solution is between 6.5 and 8.0.

Purity **(1)** Chloride <*1.03*>—Perform the test with 0.20 g of Thiamine Nitrate. Prepare the control solution with 0.30 mL of 0.01 mol/L hydrochloric acid VS (not more than 0.053%).

(2) Sulfate <*1.14*>—Dissolve 1.5 g of Thiamine Nitrate in 30 mL of water and 2 mL of dilute hydrochloric acid, and add water to make 50 mL. Perform the test using this solution as the test solution. Prepare the control solution with 0.35 mL of 0.005 mol/L sulfuric acid VS and 2 mL of dilute hydrochloric acid, and add water to make 50 mL (not more than 0.011%).

(3) Heavy metals <*1.07*>—Dissolve 1.0 g of Thiamine Nitrate in 30 mL of water by warming, cool, and add 12 mL of 6 mol/L acetic acid TS and water to make 50 mL. Perform the test with this solution as the test solution. Prepare the control solution with 2.0 mL of Standard Lead Solution (not more than 20 ppm).

Loss on drying <*2.41*> Not more than 1.0% (0.5 g, 105°C, 2 hours).

Residue on ignition <*2.44*> Not more than 0.2% (1 g).

Assay Weigh accurately about 0.1 g each of Thiamine Nitrate, previously dried, and Thiamine Chloride Hydrochloride RS (separately determine the water <*2.48*> in the same manner as Thiamine Chloride Hydrochloride), and dissolve them in the mobile phase to make exactly 50 mL. To 10 mL each of the solutions, accurately measured, add exactly 5 mL each of the internal standard solution, add the mobile phase to make 50 mL, and use these solutions as the sample solution and standard solution. Perform the test with 10 μL each of the sample solution and standard solution as directed under Liquid Chromatography <*2.01*> according to the following conditions and calculate the ratios, Q_T and Q_S, of the peak area of thiamine to that of the internal standard.

$$\text{Amount (mg) of thiamine nitrate } (C_{12}H_{17}N_5O_4S) = M_S \times Q_T/Q_S \times 0.971$$

M_S: Amount (mg) of Thiamine Chloride Hydrochloride RS taken, calculated on the anhydrous basis

Internal standard solution—A solution of methyl benzoate in methanol (1 in 50).

Operating conditions—

Detector: An ultraviolet spectrophotometer (wavelength: 254 nm).

Column: A stainless steel column 4.6 mm in inside diameter and 15 cm in length, packed with octadecylsilanized silica gel for liquid chromatography (5 μm in particle diameter).

Column temperature: A constant temperature of about 30°C.

Mobile phase: Dissolve 1.1 g of sodium 1-octanesulfonate in 1000 mL of diluted acetic acid (100) (1 in 100). To 600 mL of this solution add 400 mL of a mixture of methanol and acetonitrile (3:2).

Flow rate: Adjust so that the retention time of thiamine is about 12 minutes.

System suitability—

System performance: When the procedure is run with 10 μL of the standard solution under the above operating conditions, thiamine and the internal standard are eluted in this order with the resolution between these peaks being not less than 6.

System repeatability: When the test is repeated 6 times with 10 μL of the standard solution under the above operating conditions, the relative standard deviation of the ratios of the peak area of thiamine to that of the internal standard is not more than 1.0%.

Containers and storage Containers—Tight containers.
Storage—Light-resistant.

Thiamylal Sodium

チアミラールナトリウム

and enantiomer

$C_{12}H_{17}N_2NaO_2S$: 276.33
Monosodium 5-allyl-5-[(1*RS*)-1-methylbutyl]-4,6-dioxo-1,4,5,6-tetrahydropyrimidine-2-thiolate
[*337-47-3*]

Thiamylal Sodium contains not less than 97.5% and not more than 101.0% of thiamylal sodium ($C_{12}H_{17}N_2NaO_2S$), calculated on the dried basis.

Description Thiamylal Sodium occurs as light yellow, crystals or powder.

It is very soluble in water, and freely soluble in ethanol (95).

The pH of a solution of 1.0 g of Thiamylal Sodium in 10 mL of water is between 10.0 and 11.0.

It is hygroscopic.

It is gradually decomposed by light.

Its solution in ethanol (95) (1 in 10) shows no optical rotation.

Identification **(1)** Determine the absorption spectrum of a solution of Thiamylal Sodium in ethanol (95) (7 in 1,000,000) as directed under Ultraviolet-visible Spectrophotometry <*2.24*>, and compare spectrum with the Reference Spectrum: both spectra exhibit similar intensities of absorption at the same wavelengths.

(2) Determine the infrared absorption spectrum of Thiamylal Sodium, previously dried, as directed in the potassium bromide disk method under Infrared Spectrophotometry <*2.25*>, and compare the spectrum with the Reference Spectrum: both spectra exhibit similar intensities of absorption at the same wave numbers.

(3) A solution of Thiamylal Sodium (1 in 10) responds to Qualitative Tests <*1.09*> for sodium salt.

Purity **(1)** Clarity and color of solution—To 1.0 g of Thiamylal Sodium in a 11- to 13-mL glass-stoppered test tube add 10 mL of freshly boiled and cooled water, stopper tightly, allow to stand, and dissolve by occasional gentle shaking: the solution is clear and light yellow.

(2) Heavy metals <*1.07*>—Proceed with 1.0 g of Thiamylal Sodium according to Method 2, and perform the test. Prepare the control solution with 2.0 mL of Standard Lead Solution (not more than 20 ppm).

(3) Related substances—Dissolve 0.10 g of Thiamylal Sodium in 10 mL of ethanol (95), and use this solution as the sample solution. Pipet 1 mL and 3 mL of the sample solution, add ethanol (95) to make exactly 200 mL, and use these solutions as the standard solution (1) and the standard solution (2). Perform the test with these solutions as directed under Thin-layer Chromatography <*2.03*>. Spot 10 μL each of the sample solution and standard solutions (1) and (2) on a plate of silica gel for thin-layer chromatography, develop with a mixture of toluene, methanol and ethyl acetate (40:7:3) to a distance of about 12 cm, and air-dry the plate. Allow the plate to stand in iodine vapor for a night: the spot at an *R*f value of about 0.1 obtained from the sample solution is not more intense than the spot from the standard solution (2), and the spot other than the principal spot, the spot at origin and the spot mentioned above from the sample solution is not more intense than the spot from the standard solution (1).

Loss on drying <*2.41*> Not more than 2.0% (1 g, 105°C, 1 hour).

Assay Weigh accurately about 0.25 g of Thiamylal Sodium, dissolve in 50 mL of methanol and 5 mL of dilute hydrochloric acid, and add methanol to make exactly 100 mL. Pipet 10 mL of this solution, and add methanol to make exactly 100 mL. Pipet 5 mL of this solution, add exactly 10 mL of the internal standard solution and the mobile phase to make 200 mL, and use this solution as the sample solution. Separately, weigh accurately about 23 mg of Thiamylal RS, previously dried at 105°C for 1 hour, dissolve in 50 mL of methanol and 0.5 mL of dilute hydrochloric acid, and add methanol to make exactly 100 mL. Pipet 5 mL of this solution, add exactly 10 mL of the internal standard solution and the mobile phase to make 200 mL, and use this solution as the standard solution. Perform the test with 20 μL each of the sample solution and standard solution as directed under Liquid Chromatography <*2.01*> according to the following conditions, and calculate the ratios, Q_T and Q_S, of the peak area of thiamylal to that of the internal standard.

$$\text{Amount (mg) of thiamylal sodium } (C_{12}H_{17}N_2NaO_2S) = M_S \times Q_T/Q_S \times 10 \times 1.086$$

M_S: Amount (mg) of Thiamylal RS taken

Internal standard solution—A solution of phenyl benzoate in methanol (3 in 500).

Operating conditions—

Detector: An ultraviolet absorption photometer (wavelength: 289 nm).

Column: A stainless steel column about 4 mm in inside diameter and about 15 cm in length, packed with octadecylsilanized silica gel for liquid chromatography (5 μm in particle diameter).

Column temperature: A constant temperature of about 25°C.

Mobile phase: A mixture of methanol and 0.05 mol/L acetic acid-sodium acetate buffer solution (pH 4.6) (13:7).

Flow rate: Adjust so that the retention time of thiamylal is about 6 minutes.

System suitability—

System performance: When the procedure is run with 20 μL of the standard solution under the above operating conditions, thiamylal and the internal standard are eluted in this order with the resolution between these peaks being not less than 12.

System repeatability: When the test is repeated 6 times with 20 μL of the standard solution under the above operating conditions, the relative standard deviation of the ratio of the peak area of thiamylal to that of the internal standard is not more than 1.0%.

Containers and storage Containers—Tight containers.

Storage—Light-resistant.

Thiamylal Sodium for Injection

注射用チアミラールナトリウム

Thiamylal Sodium for Injection is a preparation for injection which is dissolved before use.

It contains not less than 93.0% and not more than 107.0% of the labeled amount of thiamylal sodium ($C_{12}H_{17}N_2NaO_2S$: 276.33).

Method of preparation Prepare as directed under Injections, with 100 parts of Thiamylal Sodium and 7 parts of Dried Sodium Carbonate in mass.

Description Thiamylal Sodium for Injection occurs as light yellow, crystals, powder or masses.

It is hygroscopic.

It is gradually decomposed by light.

Identification **(1)** To 1.0 g of Thiamylal Sodium for Injection add 20 mL of ethanol (95), shake vigorously, and filter. Dissolve the precipitate so obtained in 1 mL of water, and add 1 mL of barium chloride TS: a white precipitate is produced. Centrifuge this solution, take off the supernatant liquid, and to the precipitate add dilute hydrochloric acid dropwise: the precipitate dissolves with effervescence.

(2) To 50 mg of Thiamylal Sodium for Injection add 100 mL of ethanol (95), shake vigorously, and filter. To 3 mL of the filtrate add ethanol (95) to make 200 mL. Determine the absorption spectrum of this solution as directed under Ultraviolet-visible Spectrophotometry <*2.24*>: it exhibits maxima between 236 nm and 240 nm, and between 287 nm and 291 nm.

pH <*2.54*> The pH of a solution obtained by dissolving 1.0 g of Thiamylal Sodium for Injection in 40 mL of water is between 10.5 and 11.5.

Purity Related substances—To 0.10 g of Thiamylal Sodium for Injection add 10 mL of ethanol (95), shake vigorously, filter, and use the filtrate as the sample solution. Proceed as directed in the Purity (3) under Thiamylal Sodium.

Bacterial endotoxins <*4.01*> Less than 1.0 EU/mg.

Uniformity of dosage units <*6.02*> It meets the requirement of the Mass variation test.

Foreign insoluble matter <*6.06*> Perform the test according to Method 2: it meets the requirement.

Insoluble particulate matter <*6.07*> It meets the requirement.

Sterility ‹*4.06*› Perform the test according to the Membrane filtration method: it meets the requirement.

Assay Open carefully 10 containers of Thiamylal Sodium for Injection, dissolve the contents with water, wash out the inside of each container with water, combine them, and add water to make exactly V mL so that each mL contains about 5 mg of thiamylal sodium ($C_{12}H_{17}N_2NaO_2S$). Pipet 5 mL of this solution, and add 0.5 mL of dilute hydrochloric acid and methanol to make exactly 100 mL. Pipet 5 mL of this solution, add exactly 10 mL of the internal standard solution and the mobile phase to make 200 mL, and use this solution as the sample solution. Proceed the test with the sample solution as directed in the Assay under Thiamylal Sodium.

Amount (mg) of thiamylal sodium ($C_{12}H_{17}N_2NaO_2S$) in 1 container

$$= M_S \times Q_T/Q_S \times V/50 \times 1.086$$

M_S: Amount (mg) of Thiamylal RS taken

Internal standard solution—A solution of phenyl benzoate in methanol (3 in 500).

Containers and storage Containers—Hermetic containers. Storage—Light-resistant.

Thianthol

チアントール

Thianthol consists of dimethylthianthrene and ditoluene disulfide.

It contains not less than 23.5% and not more than 26.5% of sulfur (S: 32.07).

Description Thianthol is a yellowish, viscous liquid. It has a faint, agreeable odor.

It is freely soluble in diethyl ether, slightly soluble in ethanol (95), and practically insoluble in water.

It, when cold, may separate crystals, which melt on warming.

Specific gravity d^{20}_{20}: 1.19 – 1.23

Identification To 0.1 g of Thianthol add cautiously 5 mL of sulfuric acid: a blue-purple color develops. Add 5 to 6 drops of nitric acid to the solution: the color of the solution changes to yellow-red with evolution of gas.

Purity **(1)** Acidity or alkalinity—Shake 10 g of Thianthol with 20 mL of water, allow to stand, and separate the water layer. The solution is neutral.

(2) Sulfate—To 10 mL of the water layer obtained in (1) add 2 to 3 drops of barium chloride TS: no opalescence is produced.

Residue on ignition ‹*2.44*› Not more than 0.1% (1 g).

Assay Weigh accurately about 10 mg of Thianthol, and proceed as directed in the sulfur determination of Oxygen Flask Combustion Method ‹*1.06*›, using a mixture of 5 mL of diluted sodium hydroxide TS (1 in 10) and 1.0 mL of hydrogen peroxide TS as an absorbing liquid.

Containers and storage Containers—Tight containers.

Compound Thianthol and Salicylic Acid Solution

複方チアントール・サリチル酸液

Compound Thianthol and Salicylic Acid Solution contains not less than 1.8 w/v% and not more than 2.2 w/v% of salicylic acid ($C_7H_6O_3$: 138.12), and not less than 1.8 w/v% and not more than 2.2 w/v% of phenol (C_6H_6O: 94.11).

Method of preparation

Thianthol	200 mL
Salicylic Acid	20 g
Phenol	20 g
Olive Oil	50 mL
Ether	100 mL
Petroleum Benzin	a sufficient quantity
To make	1000 mL

Dissolve Salicylic Acid and Phenol in Ether, add Thianthol, Olive Oil and Petroleum Benzin to this solution, mix and dissolve to make 1000 mL.

Description Compound Thianthol and Salicylic Acid Solution is a light yellow liquid, having a characteristic odor.

Identification **(1)** Place 1 mL of Compound Thianthol and Salicylic Acid Solution to a porcelain dish, and evaporate on a water bath to dryness. To the residue add cautiously 5 mL of sulfuric acid: a blue-purple color develops. Add 5 to 6 drops of nitric acid to the solution: the color of the solution changes to yellow-red with evolution of gas (thianthol).

(2) Shake 10 mL of Compound Thianthol and Salicylic Acid Solution with 10 mL of sodium hydrogen carbonate TS, and separate the water layer. To 0.5 mL of the water layer add hydrochloric acid-potassium chloride buffer solution (pH 2.0) to make 50 mL, and to 5 mL of this solution add 5 mL of a solution of iron (III) nitrate enneahydrate (1 in 200): a red-purple color is produced (salicylic acid).

(3) Wash the upper phase obtained in (2) with 10 mL of sodium hydrogen carbonate TS, and extract with 10 mL of dilute sodium hydroxide TS. Shake 1 mL of the extract with 1 mL of sodium nitrate TS and 1 mL of dilute hydrochloric acid, and add 3 mL of sodium hydroxide TS: a yellow color is produced (phenol).

(4) To 1 mL of Compound Thianthol and Salicylic Acid Solution add 10 mL of ethanol (95), mix, and use this solution as the sample solution. Dissolve 0.01 g each of salicylic acid, phenol and thianthol in 5 mL each of ethanol (95), and use each solution as standard solutions (1), (2) and (3). Perform the test with these solutions as directed under Thin-layer Chromatography ‹*2.03*›. Spot 5 μL each of the sample solution and standard solutions on a plate of silica gel with fluorescent indicator for thin-layer chromatography. Develop the plate with a mixture of chloroform, acetone and acetic acid (100) (45:5:1) to a distance of about 10 cm, and air-dry the plate. Examine under ultraviolet light (main wavelength: 254 nm): three spots obtained from the sample solution and the corresponding spots from the standard solutions (1), (2) and (3) show the same Rf value. Spray evenly iron (III) chloride TS on the plate: the spot from standard solution (1) and the corresponding spot from the sample solution reveal a purple color.

Assay Pipet 2 mL of Compound Thianthol and Salicylic Acid Solution, add exactly 10 mL of the internal standard solution, then add 70 mL of diluted methanol (1 in 2), mix well, and add diluted methanol (1 in 2) to make 100 mL. Filter, discard the first 10 mL of the filtrate, and use the subsequent filtrate as the sample solution. Weigh accurately about 0.2 g of salicylic acid for assay, previously dried in a desiccator (silica gel) for 3 hours, and about 0.2 g of phenol for assay, dissolve in diluted methanol (1 in 2) to make exactly 50 mL. Pipet 10 mL of this solution, add exactly 10 mL of the internal standard solution and diluted methanol (1 in 2) to make 100 mL, and use this solution as the standard solution. With 5 μL each of the sample solution and standard solution, perform the test as directed under Liquid Chromatography <*2.01*> according to the following conditions, and calculate the ratios, Q_{Ta} and Q_{Tb}, of the peak area of salicylic acid and phenol to that of the internal standard in the sample solution, and the ratios, Q_{Sa} and Q_{Sb}, of the peak area of salicylic acid and phenol to that of the internal standard in the standard solution.

Amount (mg) of salicylic acid ($C_7H_6O_3$)
$= M_{Sa} \times Q_{Ta}/Q_{Sa} \times 1/5$

Amount (mg) of phenol (C_6H_6O)
$= M_{Sb} \times Q_{Tb}/Q_{Sb} \times 1/5$

M_{Sa}: Amount (mg) of salicylic acid for assay taken
M_{Sb}: Amount (mg) of phenol for assay taken

Internal standard solution—A solution of theophylline in methanol (1 in 10,000).
Operating conditions—

Detector: An ultraviolet absorption photometer (wavelength: 270 nm).

Column: A stainless steel column about 4 mm in inside diameter and 25 to 30 cm in length, packed with octadecylsilanized silica gel for liquid chromatography (5 μm in particle diameter).

Column temperature: Room temperature.

Mobile phase: A mixture of 0.1 mol/L phosphate buffer solution (pH 7.0) and methanol (3:1).

Flow rate: Adjust so that the retention time of salicylic acid is about 6 minutes.

Selection of column: Dissolve 0.2 g of benzoic acid, 0.2 g of salicylic acid and 0.05 g of theophylline in 100 mL of diluted methanol (1 in 2). To 10 mL of this solution add 90 mL of diluted methanol (1 in 2). Proceed with 10 μL of this solution under the above operating conditions. Use a column giving elution of benzoic acid, salicylic acid and theophylline in this order, and clearly dividing each peak.

Containers and storage Containers—Tight containers.

Storage—Light-resistant, and not exceeding 25°C.

Thiopental Sodium

チオペンタールナトリウム

and enantiomer

$C_{11}H_{17}N_2NaO_2S$: 264.32
Monosodium 5-ethyl-5-[(1*RS*)-1-methylbutyl]-4,6-dioxo-1,4,5,6-tetrahydropyrimidine-2-thiolate
[*71-73-8*]

Thiopental Sodium, when dried, contains not less than 97.0% of thiopental sodium ($C_{11}H_{17}N_2NaO_2S$).

Description Thiopental Sodium occurs as a light yellow powder. It has a faint, characteristic odor.

It is very soluble in water, freely soluble in ethanol (95), and practically insoluble in diethyl ether.

A solution of Thiopental Sodium (1 in 10) is alkaline.

It is hygroscopic.

Its solution gradually decomposes on standing.

Identification (1) Dissolve 0.2 g of Thiopental Sodium in 5 mL of sodium hydroxide TS, and add 2 mL of lead (II) acetate TS: a white precipitate, which dissolves upon heating, is produced. Boil the solution thus obtained: a black precipitate forms gradually, and the precipitate responds to Qualitative Tests <*1.09*> for sulfide.

(2) Dissolve 0.5 g of Thiopental Sodium in 15 mL of water, add 10 mL of dilute hydrochloric acid to produce white precipitate, and extract with four 25-mL portions of chloroform. Combine the chloroform extracts, evaporate on a water bath, and dry at 105°C for 2 hours: the residue melts <*2.60*> between 157°C and 162°C.

(3) A solution of Thiopental Sodium (1 in 10) responds to Qualitative Tests <*1.09*> (1) and (2) for sodium salt.

Purity (1) Clarity and color of solution—Dissolve 1.0 g of Thiopental Sodium in 10 mL of freshly boiled and cooled water: the solution is clear and light yellow.

(2) Heavy metals <*1.07*>—Dissolve 2.0 g of Thiopental Sodium in 76 mL of water, add 4 mL of dilute hydrochloric acid, shake, and filter through a glass filter (G4). To 40 mL of the filtrate add 2 mL of ammonium acetate TS, dilute with water to 50 mL, and perform the test using this solution as the test solution. Prepare a control solution as follows: to 2.0 mL of Standard Lead Solution add 2 mL of dilute acetic acid, 2 mL of ammonium acetate TS and water to make 50 mL (not more than 20 ppm).

(3) Neutral and basic substances—Weigh accurately about 1 g of Thiopental Sodium, dissolve in 10 mL of water and 5 mL of sodium hydroxide TS, and shake vigorously with 40 mL of chloroform. Separate the chloroform layer, wash with two 5-mL portions of water, filter, and evaporate the filtrate on a water bath to dryness. Dry the residue at 105°C for 1 hour: the amount of the residue is not more than 0.50%.

(4) Related substances—Dissolve 50 mg of Thiopental Sodium in 50 mL of the mobile phase, and use this solution as the sample solution. Pipet 1 mL of the sample solution, add the mobile phase to make exactly 200 mL, and use this solution as the standard solution. Perform the test with exactly 20 μL each of the sample solution and the standard solution as directed under Liquid Chromatography <*2.01*> ac-

cording to the following conditions. Determine each peak area by the automatic integration method: the total area of peaks other than thiopental obtained from the sample solution is not larger than the peak area of thiopental from the standard solution.

Operating conditions—

Detector: An ultraviolet absorption photometer (wavelength: 254 nm).

Column: A stainless steel column 4.6 mm in inside diameter and 15 cm in length, packed with octadecylsilanized silica gel (5 μm in particle diameter).

Column temperature: A constant temperature of about 40°C.

Mobile phase: Dissolve 1 g of potassium dihydrogen phosphate in 1000 mL of water, and adjust the pH to 3.0 with phosphoric acid. To 700 mL of this solution add 300 mL of acetonitrile.

Flow rate: Adjust so that the retention time of thiopental is about 15 minutes.

Time span of measurement: About 1.5 times as long as the retention time of thiopental.

System suitability—

Test for required detectability: To exactly 2 mL of the standard solution add the mobile phase to make exactly 10 mL. Confirm that the peak area of thiopental obtained with 20 μL of this solution is equivalent to 15 to 25% of that with 20 μL of the standard solution.

System performance: Dissolve 5 mg each of isopropyl parahydroxybenzoate and propyl parahydroxybenzoate in 50 mL of acetonitrile, and add water to make 100 mL. When the procedure is run with 20 μL of this solution under the above operating conditions, isopropyl parahydroxybenzoate and propyl parahydroxybenzoate are eluted in this order with the resolution between these peaks being not less than 1.9.

System repeatability: When the test is repeated 6 times with 20 μL of the standard solution under the above operating conditions, the relative standard deviation of the peak area of thiopental is not more than 2.0%.

Loss on drying <*2.41*> Not more than 2.0% (1 g, in vacuum, 80°C, 4 hours).

Assay Weigh accurately about 0.5 g of Thiopental Sodium, previously dried, transfer to a separator, dissolve in 20 mL of water, add 5 mL of ethanol (95) and 10 mL of dilute hydrochloric acid, and extract with 50 mL of chloroform, then with three 25-mL portions of chloroform. Combine the chloroform extracts, wash with two 5-mL portions of water, and extract the washings with two 10-mL portions of chloroform. Filter the combined chloroform extracts into a conical flask, and wash the filter paper with three 5-mL portions of chloroform. Combine the filtrate and the washings, and add 10 mL of ethanol (95). Titrate <*2.50*> with 0.1 mol/L potassium hydroxide-ethanol VS until the color of the solution changes from yellow through light blue to purple (indicator: 2 mL of alizarin yellow GG-thymolphthalein TS). Perform a blank determination in the same manner with a mixture of 160 mL of chloroform and 30 mL of ethanol (95), and make any necessary correction.

Each mL of 0.1 mol/L potassium hydroxide-ethanol VS
= 26.43 mg of $C_{11}H_{17}N_2NaO_2S$

Containers and storage Containers—Tight containers.

Storage—Light-resistant.

Thiopental Sodium for Injection

注射用チオペンタールナトリウム

Thiopental Sodium for Injection is a preparation for injection which is dissolved before use.

It contains not less than 93.0% and not more than 107.0% of the labeled amount of thiopental sodium ($C_{11}H_{17}N_2NaO_2S$: 264.32).

Method of preparation Prepare as directed under Injections, with 100 parts of Thiopental Sodium and 6 parts of Dried Sodium Carbonate in mass.

Description Thiopental Sodium for Injection is a light yellow, powder or mass, and has a slight, characteristic odor.

It is very soluble in water, and practically insoluble in dehydrated diethyl ether.

It is hygroscopic.

Identification **(1)** Dissolve 0.1 g of Thiopental Sodium for Injection in 10 mL of water, and add 0.5 mL of barium chloride TS: a white precipitate is formed. Collect the precipitate, and add dilute hydrochloric acid dropwise: the precipitate dissolves with effervescence.

(2) Proceed as directed in the Identification under Thiopental Sodium.

pH <*2.54*> Dissolve 1.0 g of Thiopental Sodium for Injection in 40 mL of water: the pH of this solution is between 10.2 and 11.2.

Purity Proceed as directed in the Purity under Thiopental Sodium.

Loss on drying <*2.41*> Not more than 2.0% (1 g, in vacuum, 80°C, 4 hours).

Bacterial endotoxins <*4.01*> Less than 0.30 EU/mg.

Uniformity of dosage units <*6.02*> It meets the requirement of the Mass variation test.

Foreign insoluble matter <*6.06*> Perform the test according to Method 2: it meets the requirement.

Insoluble particulate matter <*6.07*> It meets the requirement.

Sterility <*4.06*> Perform the test according to the Membrane filtration method: it meets the requirement.

Assay Open carefully 10 containers of Thiopental Sodium for Injection, dissolve each content with water, wash each container with water, combine the washings with the former solution, and add water to make exactly 1000 mL. Pipet 10 mL of this solution, and add water to make exactly 100 mL. Measure exactly a volume (V mL) of this solution, equivalent to about 15 mg of thiopental sodium ($C_{11}H_{17}N_2NaO_2S$), and add water to make exactly 1000 mL. Pipet 10 mL of this solution, add 15 mL of diluted dilute sodium hydroxide TS (1 in 100), add water to make exactly 30 mL, and use this solution as the sample solution. Separately, weigh accurately about 46 mg of thiopental for assay, previously dried at 105° C for 3 hours, dissolve in 50 mL of dilute sodium hydroxide TS, and add water to make exactly 200 mL. Pipet 2 mL of this solution, add water to make exactly 100 mL, and use this solution as the standard solution. Perform the test with the sample solution and standard solution as directed under Ultraviolet-visible Spectrophotometry <*2.24*>, and determine the absorbances, A_T and A_S, at 304 nm.

Amount (mg) of thiopental sodium ($C_{11}H_{17}N_2NaO_2S$) in each sample of Thiopental Sodium for Injection
$= M_S \times A_T/A_S \times 300/V \times 1.091$

M_S: Amount (mg) of thiopental sodium for assay taken

Containers and storage Containers—Hermetic containers. Storage—Light-resistant.

Thioridazine Hydrochloride

チオリダジン塩酸塩

and enantiomer

$C_{21}H_{26}N_2S_2.HCl$: 407.04
10-{2-[(2*RS*)-1-Methylpiperidin-2-yl]ethyl}-2-methylsulfanyl-10*H*-phenothiazine monohydrochloride
[*130-61-0*]

Thioridazine Hydrochloride, when dried, contains not less than 99.0% of thioridazine hydrochloride ($C_{21}H_{26}N_2S_2.HCl$).

Description Thioridazine Hydrochloride occurs as a white to pale yellow crystalline powder. It is odorless, and has a bitter taste.

It is freely soluble in water, in methanol, in ethanol (95) and in acetic acid (100), sparingly soluble in acetic anhydride, and practically insoluble in diethyl ether.

The pH of a solution of 1.0 g of Thioridazine Hydrochloride in 100 mL of water is between 4.2 and 5.2.

It is gradually colored by light.

Identification **(1)** Dissolve 0.01 g of Thioridazine Hydrochloride in 2 mL of sulfuric acid: a deep blue color develops.

(2) Dissolve 0.01 g of Thioridazine Hydrochloride in 2 mL of water, and add 1 drop of cerium (IV) tetraammonium sulfate TS: a blue color develops, and the color disappears on the addition of excess of the reagent.

(3) Determine the infrared absorption spectrum of Thioridazine Hydrochloride, previously dried, as directed in the potassium chloride disk method under Infrared Spectrophotometry <*2.25*>, and compare the spectrum with the Reference Spectrum: both spectra exhibit similar intensities of absorption at the same wave numbers.

(4) To 5 mL of a solution of Thioridazine Hydrochloride (1 in 100) add 2 mL of ammonia TS, and heat on a water bath for 5 minutes. After cooling, filter, and acidify the filtrate with dilute nitric acid: the solution responds to Qualitative Tests <*1.09*> (2) for chloride.

Melting point <*2.60*> 159 – 164°C

Purity **(1)** Heavy metals <*1.07*>—Proceed with 1.0 g of Thioridazine Hydrochloride according to Method 2, and perform the test. Prepare the control solution with 2.0 mL of Standard Lead Solution (not more than 20 ppm).

(2) Arsenic <*1.11*>—Prepare the test solution with 1.0 g of Thioridazine Hydrochloride, according to Method 3, and perform the test (not more than 2 ppm).

(3) Related substances—Conduct this procedure without exposure to light. Dissolve 0.10 g of Thioridazine Hydrochloride in 10 mL of methanol, and use this solution as the sample solution. Pipet 1 mL of the sample solution, and add methanol to make exactly 20 mL. Pipet 2 mL of this solution, add methanol to make exactly 10 mL, and use this solution as the standard solution. Perform the test with these solutions as directed under Thin-layer Chromatography <*2.03*>. Spot 5 μL each of the sample solution and standard solution on a plate of silica gel with fluorescent indicator for thin-layer chromatography. Develop the plate with a mixture of chloroform, 2-propanol and ammonia solution (28) (74:25:1) to a distance of about 10 cm, and air-dry the plate. Examine the plate under ultraviolet light (main wavelength: 254 nm): the spots other than the principal spot obtained from the sample solution are not more intense than the spot from the standard solution.

Loss on drying <*2.41*> Not more than 0.5% (1 g, 105°C, 4 hours).

Residue on ignition <*2.44*> Not more than 0.1% (1 g).

Assay Weigh accurately about 0.35 g of Thioridazine Hydrochloride, previously dried, dissolve in 80 mL of a mixture of acetic anhydride and acetic acid (100) (1:1), and titrate <*2.50*> with 0.1 mol/L perchloric acid VS (potentiometric titration). Perform a blank determination in the same manner, and make any necessary correction.

Each mL of 0.1 mol/L perchloric acid VS
= 40.70 mg of $C_{21}H_{26}N_2S_2.HCl$

Containers and storage Containers—Tight containers. Storage—Light-resistant.

L-Threonine

L-トレオニン

$C_4H_9NO_3$: 119.12
(2*S*,3*R*)-2-Amino-3-hydroxybutanoic acid
[*72-19-5*]

L-Threonine, when dried, contains not less than 98.5% of L-threonine ($C_4H_9NO_3$).

Description L-Threonine occurs as white, crystals or crystalline powder. It is odorless or has a slight, characteristic odor, and has a slightly sweet taste.

It is freely soluble in formic acid, soluble in water, and practically insoluble in ethanol (95).

Identification Determine the infrared absorption spectrum of L-Threonine, previously dried, as directed in the potassium bromide disk method under the Infrared Spectrophotometry <*2.25*>, and compare the spectrum with the Reference Spectrum: both spectra exhibit similar intensities of absorption at the same wave numbers.

Optical rotation <*2.49*> $[\alpha]_D^{20}$: $-26.0 - -29.0°$ (after drying, 1.5 g, water, 25 mL, 100 mm).

pH <*2.54*> Dissolve 0.20 g of L-Threonine in 20 mL of water: the pH of this solution is between 5.2 and 6.2.

Purity **(1)** Clarity and color of solution—Dissolve 1.0 g of L-Threonine in 20 mL of water: the solution is clear and colorless.

(2) Chloride <*1.03*>—Perform the test with 0.5 g of L-Threonine. Prepare the control solution with 0.30 mL of 0.01 mol/L hydrochloric acid VS (not more than 0.021%).

(3) Sulfate <*1.14*>—Perform the test with 0.6 g of L-Threonine. Prepare the control solution with 0.35 mL of 0.005 mol/L sulfuric acid VS (not more than 0.028%).

(4) Ammonium <*1.02*>—Perform the test with 0.25 g of L-Threonine. Prepare the control solution with 5.0 mL of Standard Ammonium Solution (not more than 0.02%).

(5) Heavy metals <*1.07*>—Proceed with 1.0 g of L-Threonine according to Method 1, and perform the test. Prepare the control solution with 2.0 mL of Standard Lead Solution (not more than 20 ppm).

(6) Arsenic <*1.11*>—Dissolve 1.0 g of L-Threonine in 5 mL of dilute hydrochloric acid, and perform the test with this solution as the test solution (not more than 2 ppm).

(7) Related substances—Dissolve 0.30 g of L-Threonine in 50 mL of water, and use this solution as the sample solution. Pipet 1 mL of the sample solution, and add water to make exactly 50 mL. Pipet 5 mL of this solution, add water to make exactly 20 mL, and use this solution as the standard solution. Perform the test with these solutions as directed under Thin-layer Chromatography <*2.03*>. Spot 5 μL each of the sample solution and standard solution on a plate of silica gel for thin-layer chromatography. Develop the plate with a mixture of 1-butanol, water and acetic acid (100) (3:1:1) to a distance of about 10 cm, and dry the plate at 80°C for 30 minutes. Spray evenly the plate with a solution of ninhydrin in acetone (1 in 50), and heat the plate at 80°C for 5 minutes: the spots other than the principal spot obtained from the sample solution are not more intense than the spot from the standard solution.

Loss on drying <*2.41*> Not more than 0.20% (1 g, 105°C, 3 hours).

Residue on ignition <*2.44*> Not more than 0.1% (1 g).

Assay Weigh accurately about 0.12 g of L-Threonine, previously dried, dissolve in 3 mL of formic acid, add 50 mL of acetic acid (100), and titrate <*2.50*> with 0.1 mol/L perchloric acid VS (potentiometric titration). Perform a blank determination in the same manner, and make any necessary correction.

Each mL of 0.1 mol/L perchloric acid VS
= 11.91 mg of $C_4H_9NO_3$

Containers and storage Containers—Tight containers.

Thrombin

トロンビン

Thrombin is prepared from prothrombin obtained from blood of man or bull, through interaction with added thromboplastin in the presence of calcium ions, sterilized and lyophilized.

It contains not less than 80% and not more than 150% of the labeled Units of thrombin.

Each mg contains not less than 10 Units of thrombin.

Description Thrombin is a white to light yellow, amorphous substance.

Thrombin (500 Units) dissolves in 1.0 mL of isotonic sodium chloride solution clearly or with slight turbidity within 1 minute.

Loss on drying <*2.41*> Not more than 3% (50 mg, in vacuum, phosphorus (V) oxide, 4 hours).

Sterility <*4.06*> It meets the requirement.

Assay (i) Fibrinogen solution—Weigh accurately about 30 mg of fibrinogen, and dissolve in 3 mL of isotonic sodium chloride solution. Allow the solution to clot sufficiently with frequent shaking after the addition of about 3 Units of thrombin. Wash the precipitated clot thoroughly until the washings yield no turbidity on addition of silver nitrate TS, weigh the clot after drying at 105°C for 3 hours, and calculate the percentage of the clot in the fibrinogen. Dissolve the fibrinogen in isotonic sodium chloride solution so that the clot should be 0.20%, adjust the pH of the solution between 7.0 and 7.4 by addition of 0.05 mol/L dibasic sodium phosphate TS (or if necessary, use 0.5 mol/L disodium hydrogenphosphate TS), and dilute with isotonic sodium chloride solution to make a 0.10% solution.

(ii) Procedure—Dissolve Thrombin RS in isotonic sodium chloride solution, and prepare four kinds of standard solutions which contain 4.0, 5.0, 6.2, and 7.5 Units in 1 mL. Transfer accurately 0.10 mL each of the standard solutions maintained at a given degree ± 1°C between 20°C and 30°C to a small test tube, 10 mm in inside diameter, 100 mm in length, blow out 0.90 mL of the fibrinogen solution at the same temperature into the test tube from a pipet, start a stop watch simultaneously, shake the tube constantly, and determine the time for the first appearance of clot. Calculate the average values of five determinations for the four kinds of standard solutions, respectively. If the deviation between the maximum and the minimum values of five determinations is more than 10% of the average value, reject the whole run, and try the experiment again. The concentration of the standard solution may be changed appropriately within the range between 14 and 60 seconds of the clotting time. The determination proceeds at the same temperature described above. Next, weigh accurately the whole contents of a single container of Thrombin, dissolve it in isotonic sodium chloride solution to provide a solution which is presumed to contain about 5 Units in each mL, treat 0.10 mL of the solution with the same reagents in the same manner five times, determine the clotting times, and calculate the average value. Plot the average values of the clotting times of the four kinds of the standard solutions on a logarithmic graph, using Units as the abscissa and clotting times as the ordinate, and draw a calibration line which best fits the four plotted points. Using this line, read the Units U from the average value of the clotting times of the sample solution.

$$\text{Units of 1 container of Thrombin} = U \times 10 \times V$$

V: The number of mL of the volume in which the contents of 1 container of Thrombin has been dissolved

Calculate the units for 1 mg of the contents.

Containers and storage Containers—Hermetic containers.
Storage—Not exceeding 10°C.

Shelf life 36 months after preparation.

Thymol

チモール

$C_{10}H_{14}O$: 150.22
5-Methyl-2-(1-methylethyl)phenol
[89-83-8]

Thymol contains not less than 98.0% of thymol ($C_{10}H_{14}O$).

Description Thymol occurs as colorless crystals or white crystalline masses. It has an aromatic odor, and has a burning taste.

It is very soluble in acetic acid (100), freely soluble in ethanol (95) and in diethyl ether, and slightly soluble in water.

It sinks in water, but when warmed, it melts and rises to the surface of water.

Identification **(1)** To 1 mL of a solution of Thymol in acetic acid (100) (1 in 300) add 6 drops of sulfuric acid and 1 drop of nitric acid: a blue-green color develops by reflected light and a red-purple color develops by transmitted light.

(2) Dissolve 1 g of Thymol in 5 mL of a solution of sodium hydroxide (1 in 10) by heating in a water bath, and continue heating for several minutes: a light yellow-red color slowly develops. Allow this solution to stand at room temperature: the color changes to dark yellow-brown. Shake this solution with 2 to 3 drops of chloroform: a purple color gradually develops.

(3) Triturate Thymol with an equal mass of camphor or menthol: the mixture liquefies.

Melting point <*2.60*> 49 – 51°C

Purity **(1)** Non-volatile residue—Volatilize 2.0 g of Thymol by heating on a water bath, and dry the residue at 105°C for 2 hours: the mass is not more than 1.0 mg.

(2) Other phenols—Shake vigorously 1.0 g of Thymol with 20 mL of warm water for 1 minute, and filter. To 5 mL of the filtrate add 1 drop of iron (III) chloride TS: a green color may develop, but no blue to purple color develops.

Assay Weigh accurately about 0.5 g of Thymol, dissolve in 10 mL of sodium hydroxide TS, and add water to make exactly 100 mL. Measure exactly 10 mL of the solution into an iodine flask, add 50 mL of water and 20 mL of dilute sulfuric acid, and cool in ice water for 30 minutes. Add exactly 20 mL of 0.05 mol/L bromine VS, stopper tightly immediately, allow to stand for 30 minutes in ice water with occasional shaking in a dark place, add 14 mL of potassium iodide TS and 5 mL of chloroform, stopper tightly, shake vigorously, and titrate <*2.50*> the liberated iodine with 0.1 mol/L sodium thiosulfate VS (indicator: 3 mL of starch TS). Stopper tightly, shake vigorously near the end point, and continue the titration until the blue color in the chloroform layer disappears. Perform a blank determination in the same manner.

Each mL of 0.05 mol/L bromine VS
= 3.756 mg of $C_{10}H_{14}O$

Containers and storage Containers—Tight containers.
Storage—Light-resistant.

Dried Thyroid

乾燥甲状腺

Dried Thyroid is the fresh thyroid gland, previously deprived of connective tissue and fat, minced, dried rapidly at a temperature not above 50°C, and powdered, or diluted with suitable diluents. It is obtained from domesticated animals that are used for food by man.

It contains not less than 0.30% and not more than 0.35% of iodine (I: 126.90) in the form of organic compounds peculiar to the thyroid gland.

Description Dried Thyroid occurs as a light yellow to grayish brown powder. It has a slight, characteristic, meat-like odor.

Identification Mount Dried Thyroid in diluted formaldehyde solution (1 in 10), stain in hematoxylin TS for 10 to 30 minutes, wash with water, soak in a mixture of 1 mL of hydrochloric acid and 99 mL of diluted ethanol (7 in 10) for 5 to 10 seconds, and again wash with water for about 1 hour. Stain in a solution of eosin Y (1 in 100) for 1 to 5 minutes, wash with water, dehydrate, and soak successively in diluted ethanol (7 in 10) for 5 to 10 seconds, in diluted ethanol (4 in 5) for 5 to 10 seconds, in diluted ethanol (9 in 10) for 1 to 2 minutes, in ethanol (95) for 1 to 5 minutes then in ethanol (99.5) for 1 to 5 minutes. Interpenetrate in xylene, seal with balsam, and examine under a microscope: epithelial nuclei forming follicles peculiar to the thyroid gland are observed.

Purity **(1)** Inorganic iodides—Mix 1.0 g of Dried Thyroid with 10 mL of a saturated solution of zinc sulfate, shake for 5 minutes, and filter. To 5 mL of the filtrate add 0.5 mL of starch TS, 4 drops of sodium nitrite TS and 4 drops of dilute sulfuric acid with thorough shaking: no blue color is produced.

(2) Fat—Extract 1.0 g of Dried Thyroid with diethyl ether for 2 hours using a Soxhlet extractor. Evaporate the diethyl ether extract, and dry the residue at 105°C to constant mass: the mass of the residue is not more than 30 mg.

Loss on drying <*2.41*> Not more than 6.0% (1 g, 105°C, constant mass).

Total ash <*5.01*> Not more than 5.0% (0.5 g).

Assay Transfer about 1 g of Dried Thyroid, accurately weighed, to a crucible, add 7 g of potassium carbonate, mix carefully, and gently tap the crucible on the table to compact the mixture. Overlay with 10 g of potassium carbonate, and compact again thoroughly by tapping. Place the crucible in a muffle furnace preheated to a temperature between 600°C and 700°C, and ignite the mixture for 25 minutes. Cool, add 20 mL of water, heat gently to boiling, and filter into a flask. To the residue add 20 mL of water, boil, and filter into the same flask. Rinse the crucible and the char on the funnel with boiling water until the filtrate measures 200 mL. Add slowly 7 mL of freshly prepared bromine TS, 40 mL of diluted phosphoric acid (1 in 2), and boil until starch iodide paper is no longer colored blue by the evolved gas. Wash down inside of the flask with water, and continue boiling for 5 minutes. During the boiling add water from time to time to maintain a volume at not less than 200 mL. Cool, add 5 mL of a solution of phenol (1 in 20), again rinse inside of the flask with water, and allow to stand for 5 minutes. Add 2 mL of diluted phosphoric acid (1 in 2) and 5 mL of potassium iodide TS, and titrate <*2.50*> immediately the liberated iodine with 0.01 mol/L sodium thiosulfate VS (indicator: 3 mL of starch TS). Perform a blank determination in the same manner, and make any necessary correction.

Each mL of 0.01 mol/L sodium thiosulfate VS
= 0.2115 mg of I

Containers and storage Containers—Tight containers.

Tiapride Hydrochloride

チアプリド塩酸塩

$C_{15}H_{24}N_2O_4S.HCl$: 364.89
N-[2-(Diethylamino)ethyl]-2-methoxy-5-(methylsulfonyl)benzamide monohydrochloride
[*51012-33-0*]

Tiapride Hydrochloride, when dried, contains not less than 99.0% and not more than 101.0% of tiapride hydrochloride ($C_{15}H_{24}N_2O_4S.HCl$).

Description Tiapride Hydrochloride occurs as a white to pale yellow-white, crystal or crystalline powder.

It is very soluble in water, freely soluble in acetic acid (100), soluble in methanol, slightly soluble in ethanol (99.5) and very slightly soluble in acetic anhydride.

It dissolves in 0.1 mol/L hydrochloric acid TS.

Identification **(1)** Determine the absorption spectrum of a solution of Tiapride Hydrochloride in 0.1 mol/L hydrochloric acid TS (1 in 10,000) as directed under Ultraviolet-visible Spectrophotometry <*2.24*>, and compare the spectrum with the Reference Spectrum: both spectra exhibit similar intensities of absorption at the same wavelengths.

(2) Determine the infrared absorption spectrum of Tiapride Hydrochloride as directed in the potassium chloride disk method under Infrared Spectrophotometry <*2.25*>: both spectra exhibit similar intensities of absorption at the same wave numbers.

(3) A solution of Tiapride Hydrochloride (1 in 20) responds to Qualitative Tests <*1.09*> for chloride.

Purity **(1)** Heavy metals <*1.07*>—Proceed with 1.0 g of Tiapride Hydrochloride according to Method 1 and perform the test. Prepare the control solution with 2.0 mL of Standard Lead Solution (not more than 20 ppm).

(2) Related substances—Dissolve 0.20 g of Tiapride Hydrochloride in 10 mL of methanol and use this solution as the sample solution. Pipet 1 mL of the sample solution, and add methanol to make exactly 100 mL. Pipet 1 mL of this solution, add methanol to make exactly 10 mL, and use this solution as the standard solution. Perform the test with these solutions as directed under Thin-layer Chromatography <*2.03*>. Spot rapidly 10 μL each of the sample solution and standard solution on a plate of silica gel with fluorescent indicator for thin-layer chromatography under a stream of nitrogen. Develop the plate with a mixture of water, 1-butanol and acetic acid (100) (2:2:1) to a distance of about 10 cm, and air-dry, and then dry the plate at 80°C for 30 minutes. Examine under ultraviolet light (main wavelength: 254 nm): the spots other than the principal spot obtained from the sample solution are not more intense than the spot from the standard solution.

Loss on drying <*2.41*> Not more than 0.5% (1 g, 105°C, 2 hours).

Residue on ignition <*2.44*> Not more than 0.1% (1 g).

Assay Weigh accurately about 0.4 g of Tiapride Hydrochloride, previously dried, dissolve in 50 mL of a mixture of acetic anhydride and acetic acid (100) (7:3), and titrate <*2.50*> with 0.1 mol/L perchloric acid VS (potentiometric titration). Perform a blank determination in the same manner, and make any necessary correction.

Each mL of 0.1 mol/L perchloric acid VS
= 36.49 mg of $C_{15}H_{24}N_2O_4S.HCl$

Containers and storage Containers—Well-closed containers.

Tiapride Hydrochloride Tablets

チアプリド塩酸塩錠

Tiapride Hydrochloride Tablets contain not less than 95.0% and not more than 105.0% of the labeled amount of tiapride ($C_{15}H_{24}N_2O_4S$: 328.43).

Method of preparation Prepare as directed under Tablets, with Tiapride Hydrochloride.

Identification To a quantity of powdered Tiapride Hydrochloride Tablets, equivalent to 10 mg of tiapride ($C_{15}H_{24}N_2O_4S$), add 100 mL of 0.1 mol/L hydrochloric acid TS, shake well, and filter. Determine the absorption spectrum of the filtrate as directed under Ultraviolet-visible Spectrophotometry <*2.24*>: it exhibits a maximum between 286 nm and 290 nm.

Uniformity of dosage units <*6.02*> Perform the Mass variation test, or the Content uniformity test according to the following method: it meets the requirement.

To 1 tablet of Tiapride Hydrochloride Tablets add V/10 mL of 0.1 mol/L hydrochloric acid TS, sonicate until the tablet is disintegrated, and add 4V/10 mL of methanol. To this solution add exactly V/10 mL of the internal standard solution, shake for 30 minutes, and add methanol to make V mL so that each mL contains about 1 mg of tiapride ($C_{15}H_{24}N_2O_4S$). Centrifuge this solution for 10 minutes, and use the supernatant liquid as the sample solution. Proceed as directed in the Assay.

Amount (mg) of tiapride ($C_{15}H_{24}N_2O_4S$)
$= M_S \times Q_T/Q_S \times V/100 \times 0.900$

M_S: Amount (mg) of tiapride hydrochloride for assay taken

Internal standard solution—A solution of methyl parahydroxybenzoate in methanol (1 in 500).

Dissolution Being specified separately when the drug is granted approval based on the Law.

Assay Weigh accurately the mass of not less than 20 Tiapride Hydrochloride Tablets and powder. Weigh accurately a portion of the powder, equivalent to about 0.1 g of tiapride ($C_{15}H_{24}N_2O_4S$), add about 10 mL of 0.1 mol/L hydrochloric acid TS and 40 mL of methanol, add exactly 10 mL of the internal standard solution, shake for 30 minutes, and add methanol to make 100 mL. Centrifuge this solution and use the supernatant liquid as the sample solution. Separately, weigh accurately about 0.11 g of tiapride chloride for assay, previously dried at 105°C for 2 hours, dissolve in 10 mL of 0.1 mol/L hydrochloric acid TS, add exactly 10 mL of the internal standard solution, add methanol to make 100 mL, and use this solution as the standard solution. Perform the test with 5 μL each of the sample solution and standard solution as directed under Liquid Chromatography <*2.01*> according to the following conditions, and calculate the ratios, Q_T and Q_S, of the peak area of Tiapride to that of the internal standard.

$$\text{Amount (mg) of tiapride } (C_{15}H_{24}N_2O_4S) = M_S \times Q_T/Q_S \times 0.900$$

M_S: Amount (mg) of tiapride chloride for assay taken

Internal standard solution—A solution of methyl parahydroxybenzoate in methanol (1 in 500).

Operating conditions—

Detector: An ultraviolet absorption photometer (wavelength: 254 nm).

Column: A stainless steel column 4 mm in inside diameter and 15 cm in length, packed with octadecylsilanized silica gel for liquid chromatography (5 μm in particle diameter).

Column temperature: A constant temperature of about 25°C.

Mobile phase: Dissolve 11.2 g of sodium perchlorate in 800 mL of water, add 5 mL of diluted perchloric acid (17 in 2000). To 800 mL of this solution add 200 mL of acetonitrile.

Flow rate: Adjust so that the retention time of tiapride is about 8 minutes.

System suitability—

System performance: When the procedure is run with 5 μL of the standard solution under the above operating conditions, tiapride and the internal standard are eluted in this order with the resolution between these peaks being not less than 8.

System repeatability: When the test is repeated 6 times with 5 μL of the standard solution under the above operating conditions, the relative standard deviation of the ratio of the peak area of tiapride to that of the internal standard is not more than 1.0%.

Containers and storage Containers—Well-closed containers.

Tiaramide Hydrochloride

チアラミド塩酸塩

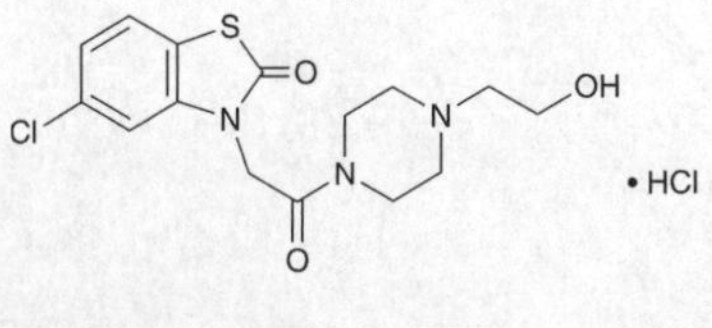

$C_{15}H_{18}ClN_3O_3S.HCl$: 392.30
5-Chloro-3-{2-[4-(2-hydroxyethyl)piperazin-1-yl]-2-oxoethyl}-1,3-benzothiazol-2(3*H*)-one monohydrochloride
[*35941-71-0*]

Tiaramide Hydrochloride, when dried, contains not less than 98.5% of tiaramide hydrochloride ($C_{15}H_{18}ClN_3O_3S.HCl$).

Description Tiaramide Hydrochloride occurs as a white crystalline powder. It is odorless.

It is freely soluble in water, slightly soluble in ethanol (95) and in acetic acid (100), and practically insoluble in acetic anhydride and in diethyl ether.

The pH of a solution of 1.0 g of Tiaramide Hydrochloride in 20 mL of water is between 3.0 and 4.5.

Melting point: about 265°C (with decomposition).

Identification (1) Dissolve 5 mg of Tiaramide Hydrochloride in 5 mL of 0.1 mol/L hydrochloric acid TS, and add 3 drops of Dragendorff's TS: an orange precipitate is formed.

(2) Determine the infrared absorption spectrum of Tiaramide Hydrochloride, previously dried, as directed in the potassium chloride disk method under the Infrared Spectrophotometry <*2.25*>, and compare the spectrum with the Reference Spectrum: both spectra exhibit similar intensities of absorption at the same wave numbers.

(3) A solution of Tiaramide Hydrochloride (1 in 50) responds to Qualitative Tests <*1.09*> for chloride.

Purity (1) Clarity and color of solution—Dissolve 0.5 g of Tiaramide Hydrochloride in 10 mL of water: the solution is clear and colorless.

(2) Heavy metals <*1.07*>—Proceed with 2.0 g of Tiaramide Hydrochloride according to Method 2, and perform the test. Prepare the control solution with 2.0 mL of Standard Lead Solution (not more than 10 ppm).

(3) Arsenic <*1.11*>—Prepare the test solution with 1.0 g of Tiaramide Hydrochloride according to Method 1, and perform the test. In the procedure, add 20 mL of diluted hydrochloric acid (1 in 2) (not more than 2 ppm).

(4) Related substances—Dissolve 0.20 g of Tiaramide Hydrochloride in 10 mL of diluted ethanol (7 in 10), and use this solution as the sample solution. Pipet 1 mL of the sample solution, and add diluted ethanol (7 in 10) to make exactly 100 mL. Pipet 2 mL of this solution, add diluted ethanol (7 in 10) to make exactly 10 mL, and use this solution as the standard solution. Perform the test with these solutions as directed under Thin-layer Chromatography <*2.03*>. Spot 5 μL each of the sample solution and standard solution on a plate of silica gel with fluorescent indicator for thin-layer chromatography. After air-drying, immediately develop the plate with a mixture of 1-butanol, water and acetic acid (100) (4:2:1) to a distance of about 10 cm, air-dry the plate, and then dry at 100°C for 30 minutes. After cooling, examine under ultraviolet light (main wavelength: 254 nm): the spots other than the principal spot and the spot of the starting point obtained from the sample solution are not more intense than the spot from the standard solution. Allow the plate to stand in iodine vapor for 30 minutes: the spots other than the principal spot and the spot of the starting point from the sample solution are not more intense than the spot from the standard solution.

Loss on drying <*2.41*> Not more than 0.5% (1 g, 105°C, 3 hours).

Residue on ignition <*2.44*> Not more than 0.1% (1 g).

Assay Weigh accurately about 0.5 g of Tiaramide Hydrochloride, previously dried, dissolve in 50 mL of a mixture of acetic anhydride and acetic acid (100) (7:3) by warming, cool, and titrate <*2.50*> with 0.1 mol/L perchloric acid VS until the color of the solution changes from red through purple to blue-purple (indicator: 3 drops of neutral red TS). Perform a blank determination in the same manner, and make any necessary correction.

$$\text{Each mL of 0.1 mol/L perchloric acid VS} = 39.23 \text{ mg of } C_{15}H_{18}ClN_3O_3S.HCl$$

Containers and storage Containers—Well-closed containers.

Tiaramide Hydrochloride Tablets

チアラミド塩酸塩錠

Tiaramide Hydrochloride Tablets contain not less than 95.0% and not more than 105.0% of the labeled amount of tiaramide ($C_{15}H_{18}ClN_3O_3S$: 355.84).

Method of preparation Prepare as directed under Tablets, with Tiaramide Hydrochloride.

Identification **(1)** Determine the absorption spectrum of the sample solution obtained in the Assay as directed under Ultraviolet-visible Spectrophotometry ⟨*2.24*⟩: it exhibits maxima between 285 nm and 289 nm, and between 292 nm and 296 nm.

(2) To a quantity of powdered Tiaramide Hydrochloride Tablets, equivalent to 0.1 g of tiaramide ($C_{15}H_{18}ClN_3O_3S$), add 10 mL of diluted ethanol (7 in 10), shake well, filter, and use the filtrate as the sample solution. Separately, dissolve 0.11 g of tiaramide hydrochloride for assay in 10 mL of diluted ethanol (7 in 10), and use this solution as the standard solution. Perform the test with these solutions as directed under Thin-layer Chromatography ⟨*2.03*⟩. Spot 20 μL each of the sample solution and standard solution on a plate of silica gel for thin-layer chromatography, develop with a mixture of 1-butamol, water and acetic acid (100) (4:2:1) to a distance of about 10 cm, and dry the plate at 100°C for 30 minutes. Spray evenly Dragendorff's TS for spraying followed by diluted nitric acid (1 in 50) on the plate: the principal spot obtained from the sample solution and the spot from the standard solution are yellow-red in color and have the same *R*f value.

Uniformity of dosage units ⟨*6.02*⟩ Perform the test according to the following method: it meets the requirement of the Content uniformity test.

To 1 tablet of Tiaramide Hydrochloride Tablets add $3V/5$ mL of 0.1 mol/L hydrochloric acid TS, shake for 60 minutes. Add 0.1 mol/L hydrochloric acid TS to make exactly V mL so that each mL contains about 1 mg of tiaramide ($C_{15}H_{18}ClN_3O_3S$), and filter. Discard the first 20 mL of the filtrate, pipet 5 mL of the subsequent filtrate, add water to make exactly 100 mL, and use this solution as the sample solution. Separately, weigh accurately about 55 mg of tiaramide hydrochloride for assay, previously dried at 105°C for 3 hours, and dissolve in 0.1 mol/L hydrochloric acid TS to make exactly 50 mL. Pipet 5 mL of this solution, add water to make exactly 100 mL, and use this solution as the standard solution. Determine the absorbances, A_T and A_S, of the sample solution and standard solution at 294 nm as directed under Ultraviolet-visible Spectrophotometry ⟨*2.24*⟩.

$$\text{Amount (mg) of tiaramide } (C_{15}H_{18}ClN_3O_3S) = M_S \times A_T/A_S \times V/50 \times 0.907$$

M_S: Amount (mg) of tiaramide hydrochloride for assay taken

Dissolution ⟨*6.10*⟩ When the test is performed at 50 revolutions per minute according to the Paddle method, using 900 mL of water as the dissolution medium, the dissolution rates of a 50-mg tablet in 15 minutes and of a 100-mg tablet in 30 minutes are not less than 80%.

Start the test with 1 tablet of Tiaramide Hydrochloride Tablets, withdraw not less than 20 mL of the medium at the specified minute after starting the test, and filter through a membrane filter with a pore size not exceeding 0.5 μm. Discard not less than 10 mL of the first filtrate, pipet V mL of the subsequent filtrate, add water to make exactly V' mL so that each mL contains about 56 μg of tiaramide ($C_{15}H_{18}ClN_3O_3S$), and use this solution as the sample solution. Separately, weigh accurately about 15 mg of tiaramide hydrochloride for assay, previously dried at 105°C for 3 hours, and dissolve in water to make exactly 50 mL. Pipet 5 mL of this solution, add water to make exactly 25 mL, and use this solution as the standard solution. Determine the absorbances, A_T and A_S, at 294 nm of the sample solution and standard solution as directed under Ultraviolet-visible Spectrophotometry ⟨*2.24*⟩.

$$\text{Dissolution rate (\%) with respect to the labeled amount of tiaramide } (C_{15}H_{18}ClN_3O_3S) = M_S \times A_T/A_S \times V'/V \times 1/C \times 360 \times 0.907$$

M_S: Amount (mg) of tiaramide hydrochloride for assay taken
C: Labeled amount (mg) of tiaramide ($C_{15}H_{18}ClN_3O_3S$) in 1 tablet

Assay Weigh accurately the mass of more than 20 Tiaramide Hydrochloride Tablets, and powder. Weigh accurately an amount of the powder, equivalent to about 0.1 g of tiaramide ($C_{15}H_{18}ClN_3O_3S$), add 60 mL of 0.1 mol/L hydrochloric acid TS, shake for 30 minutes, add 0.1 mol/L hydrochloric acid TS to make exactly 100 mL, and filter. Discard the first 20 mL of the filtrate, pipet 5 mL of the subsequent filtrate, add water to make exactly 100 mL, and use this solution as the sample solution. Separately, weigh accurately about 0.11 g of tiaramide hydrochloride for assay, previously dried at 105°C for 3 hours, and dissolve in 0.1 mol/L hydrochloric acid TS to make exactly 100 mL. Pipet 5 mL of this solution, add water to make exactly 100 mL, and use this solution as the standard solution. Determine the absorbances, A_T and A_S, of the sample solution and standard solution at 294 nm as directed under Ultraviolet-visible Spectrophotometry ⟨*2.24*⟩.

$$\text{Amount (mg) of tiaramide } (C_{15}H_{18}ClN_3O_3S) = M_S \times A_T/A_S \times 0.907$$

M_S: Amount (mg) of tiaramide hydrochloride for assay taken

Containers and storage Containers—Tight containers.

Ticlopidine Hydrochloride

チクロピジン塩酸塩

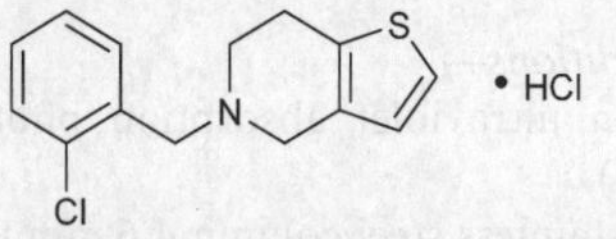

$C_{14}H_{14}ClNS.HCl$: 300.25
5-(2-Chlorobenzyl)-4,5,6,7-tetrahydrothieno[3,2-*c*]pyridine monohydrochloride
[53885-35-1]

Ticlopidine Hydrochloride contains not less than 99.0% of ticlopidine hydrochloride ($C_{14}H_{14}ClNS.HCl$), calculated on the anhydrous basis.

Description Ticlopidine Hydrochloride occurs as a white to pale yellow-white crystalline powder.

It is freely soluble in acetic acid (100), soluble in water and in methanol, sparingly soluble in ethanol (95), and practically insoluble in diethyl ether.

Identification **(1)** Determine the infrared absorption spectrum of Ticlopidine Hydrochloride as directed in the potassium bromide disk method under Infrared Spectrophotometry <*2.25*>, and compare the spectrum with the Reference Spectrum: both spectra exhibit similar intensities of absorption at the same wave numbers.

(2) A solution of Ticlopidine Hydrochloride (1 in 20) responds to Qualitative Tests <*1.09*> (2) for chloride.

Purity **(1)** Heavy metals <*1.07*>—Proceed with 2.0 g of Ticlopidine Hydrochloride according to Method 3, and perform the test. Prepare the control solution with 2.0 mL of Standard Lead Solution (not more than 10 ppm).

(2) Arsenic <*1.11*>—Prepare the test solution with 1.0 g of Ticlopidine Hydrochloride according to Method 4, and perform the test (not more than 2 ppm).

(3) Related substances—Dissolve 0.5 g of Ticlopidine Hydrochloride in 20 mL of a solution of hydrochloric acid in methanol (1 in 20,000), and use this solution as the sample solution. To exactly 5 mL of the sample solution add a solution of hydrochloric acid in methanol (1 in 20,000) to make exactly 200 mL, and use this solution as the standard solution (1). Separately, pipet 1 mL of the sample solution, add a solution of hydrochloric acid in methanol (1 in 20,000) to make exactly 50 mL, and use this solution as the standard solution (2). Perform the test with these solutions as directed under Thin-layer Chromatography <*2.03*>. Spot 10 μL each of the sample solution and standard solution (1) on a plate of silica gel for thin-layer chromatography (Plate 1), and spot 10 μL each of the sample solution and standard solution (2) on another plate of silica gel for thin-layer chromatography (Plate 2). Develop the plates with an upper layer of a mixture of water, 1-butanol and acetic acid (100) (5:4:1) to a distance of about 15 cm, and air-dry the plates. Spray evenly a solution of ninhydrin in acetone (1 in 50) on Plate 1, and heat the plate at 100°C for 20 minutes: the spots other than the principal spot obtained from the sample solution are not more intense than the spot from the standard solution (1). Allow Plate 2 to stand in an iodine vapor for 30 minutes: the spots other than the principal spot obtained from the sample solution are not more intense than the spot from the standard solution (2).

(4) Formaldehyde—Dissolve 0.80 g of Ticlopidine Hydrochloride in 19.0 mL of water, add 1.0 mL of 4 mol/L sodium hydroxide TS, shake well, centrifuge, and filter the supernatant liquid. To 5.0 mL of the filtrate add 5.0 mL of acetylacetone TS, mix, and warm at 40°C for 40 minutes: the solution has no more color than the following control solution.

Control solution: Weigh exactly 0.54 g of formaldehyde solution, and add water to make exactly 1000 mL. To exactly 10 mL of this solution add water to make exactly 1000 mL. Prepare before use. To 8.0 mL of this solution add water to make 20.0 mL, and filter. To 5.0 mL of the filtrate add 5.0 mL of acetylacetone TS, and proceed in the same manner.

Water <*2.48*> Not more than 1.0% (0.3 g, volumetric titration, direct titration).

Residue on ignition <*2.44*> Not more than 0.1% (1 g).

Assay Weigh accurately about 0.4 g of Ticlopidine Hydrochloride, dissolve in 20 mL of acetic acid (100), add 40 mL of acetic anhydride, and titrate <*2.50*> with 0.1 mol/L perchloric acid VS (potentiometric titration). Perform a blank determination in the same manner, and make any necessary correction.

Each mL of 0.1 mol/L perchloric acid VS
= 30.03 mg of $C_{14}H_{14}ClNS.HCl$

Containers and storage Containers—Well-closed containers.

Ticlopidine Hydrochloride Tablets

チクロピジン塩酸塩錠

Ticlopidine Hydrochloride Tablets contain not less than 95.0% and not more than 105.0% of the labeled amount of ticlopidine hydrochloride ($C_{14}H_{14}ClNS.HCl$: 300.25).

Method of preparation Prepare as directed under Tablets, with Ticlopidine Hydrochloride.

Identification Determine the absorption spectrum of the sample solution obtained in the Uniformity of dosage units as directed under Ultraviolet-visible Spectrophotometry <*2.24*>: it exhibits maxima between 212 nm and 216 nm, and between 231 nm and 235 nm.

Uniformity of dosage units <*6.02*> Perform the Mass variation test, or the Content uniformity test according to the following method: it meets the requirement.

To 1 tablet of Ticlopidine Hydrochloride Tablets add 70 mL of water, thoroughly shake until the tablet is completely disintegrated, then add water to make exactly 100 mL, and filter through a membrane filter with a pore size not exceeding 0.45 μm. Discard the first 10 mL of the filtrate, pipet *V* mL of the subsequent filtrate, add water to make exactly *V′* mL so that each mL contains about 20 μg of ticlopidine hydrochloride ($C_{14}H_{14}ClNS.HCl$), and use this solution as the sample solution. Separately, weigh accurately about 25 mg of ticlopidine hydrochloride for assay (separately determine the water <*2.48*> in the same manner as Ticlopidine Hydrochloride), and dissolve in water to make exactly 50 mL. Pipet 2 mL of this solution, add water to make exactly 50 mL, and use this solution as the standard solution. Determine the absorbances, A_T and A_S, at 233 nm of the sample solution and standard solution as directed under Ultraviolet-visible Spectrophotometry <*2.24*>.

Amount (mg) of ticlopidine hydrochloride ($C_{14}H_{14}ClNS.HCl$)
$= M_S \times A_T/A_S \times V'/V \times 2/25$

M_S: Amount (mg) of ticlopidine hydrochloride for assay taken, calculated on the anhydrous basis

Dissolution *<6.10>* When the test is performed at 50 revolutions per minute according to the Paddle method, using 900 mL of water as the dissolution medium, the dissolution rate in 35 minutes of Ticlopidine Hydrochloride Tablets is not less than 85%.

Start the test with 1 tablet of Ticlopidine Hydrochloride Tablets, withdraw not less than 20 mL of the medium at the specified minute after starting the test, and filter through a membrane filter with a pore size not exceeding 0.45 μm. Discard not less than 10 mL of the first filtrate, pipet *V* mL of the subsequent filtrate, add water to make exactly *V′* mL so that each mL contains about 11 μg of ticlopidine hydrochloride ($C_{14}H_{14}ClNS.HCl$), and use this solution as the sample solution. Separately, weigh accurately about 22 mg of ticlopidine hydrochloride for assay (separately determine the water *<2.48>* in the same manner as Ticlopidine Hydrochloride), and dissolve in water to make exactly 200 mL. Pipet 2 mL of this solution, add water to make exactly 20 mL, and use this solution as the standard solution. Determine the absorbances, A_T and A_S, at 233 nm of the sample solution and standard solution as directed under Ultraviolet-visible Spectrophotometry *<2.24>*.

Dissolution rate (%) with respect to the labeled amount of ticlopidine hydrochloride ($C_{14}H_{14}ClNS.HCl$)
$= M_S \times A_T/A_S \times V'/V \times 1/C \times 45$

M_S: Amount (mg) of ticlopidine hydrochloride for assay taken, calculated on the anhydrous basis
C: Labeled amount (mg) of ticlopidine hydrochloride ($C_{14}H_{14}ClNS.HCl$) in 1 tablet

Assay To 20 tablets of Ticlopidine Hydrochloride Tablets, add 400 mL of a mixture of water and methanol (1:1), sonicate until the tablets are completely disintegrated, and add the mixture of water and methanol (1:1) to make exactly 500 mL. Filter this solution through a membrane filter with a pore size not exceeding 0.45 μm, discard the first 10 mL of the filtrate, pipet *V* mL of the subsequent filtrate, equivalent to about 20 mg of ticlopidine hydrochloride ($C_{14}H_{14}ClNS.HCl$), add exactly 4 mL of the internal standard solution, then add the mixture of water and methanol (1:1) to make 100 mL. To 2 mL of this solution add the mixture of water and methanol (1:1) to make 20 mL, and use this solution as the sample solution. Separately, weigh accurately about 25 mg of ticlopidine hydrochloride for assay (separately determine the water *<2.48>* in the same manner as Ticlopidine Hydrochloride), dissolve in a suitable amount of a mixture of water and methanol (1:1), add exactly 5 mL of the internal standard solution, then add the mixture of water and methanol (1:1) to make 50 mL. Pipet 2 mL of this solution, add a mixture of water and methanol (1:1) to make 50 mL, and use this solution as the standard solution. Perform the test with 10 μL each of the sample solution and standard solution as directed under Liquid Chromatography *<2.01>* according to the following conditions, and calculate the ratios, Q_T and Q_S, of the peak area of ticlopidine to that of the internal standard.

Amount (mg) of ticlopidine hydrochloride ($C_{14}H_{14}ClNS.HCl$) in 1 tablet
$= M_S \times Q_T/Q_S \times 1/V \times 20$

M_S: Amount (mg) of ticlopidine hydrochloride for assay taken, calculated on the anhydrous basis

Internal standard solution—A solution of butyl parahydroxybenzoate in a mixture of water and methanol (1:1) (1 in 200).

Operating conditions—

Detector: An ultraviolet absorption photometer (wavelength: 233 nm).

Column: A stainless steel column 4.6 mm in inside diameter and 15 cm in length, packed with octadecylsilanized silica gel for liquid chromatography (5 μm in particle diameter).

Column temperature: A constant temperature of about 40°C.

Mobile phase: A mixture of methanol and 0.05 mol/L phosphate buffer solution (pH 3.5) (7:3).

Flow rate: Adjust so that the retention time of ticlopidine is about 8 minutes.

System suitability—

System performance: When the procedure is run with 10 μL of the standard solution under the above operating conditions, the internal standard and ticlopidine are eluted in this order with the resolution between these peaks being not less than 3.

System repeatability: When the test is repeated 6 times with 10 μL of the standard solution under the above operating conditions, the relative standard deviation of the ratio of the peak area of ticlopidine to that of the internal standard is not more than 1.0%.

Containers and storage Containers—Well-closed containers.

Timepidium Bromide Hydrate

チメピジウム臭化物水和物

$C_{17}H_{22}BrNOS_2.H_2O$: 418.41
(5*RS*)-3-(Dithien-2-ylmethylene)-5-methoxy-1,1-dimethylpiperidinium bromide monohydrate
[*35035-05-3*, anhydride]

Timepidium Bromide Hydrate contains not less than 98.5% of timepidium bromide ($C_{17}H_{22}BrNOS_2$: 400.40), calculated on the anhydrous basis.

Description Timepidium Bromide Hydrate occurs as white, crystals or crystalline powder.

It is very soluble in methanol and in acetic acid (100), freely soluble in ethanol (99.5), sparingly soluble in water and in acetic anhydride, and practically insoluble in diethyl ether.

The pH of a solution of 1.0 g of Timepidium Bromide Hydrate in 100 mL of freshly boiled and cooled water is between 5.3 and 6.3.

A solution of Timepidium Bromide Hydrate in methanol (1 in 20) shows no optical rotation.

Identification **(1)** To 1 mL of a solution of Timepidium Bromide Hydrate (1 in 100) add 1 mL of ninhydrin-sulfuric acid TS: a red purple color develops.

(2) Determine the absorption spectrum of a solution of Timepidium Bromide Hydrate (1 in 50,000) as directed under Ultraviolet-visible Spectrophotometry 〈*2.24*〉, and compare the spectrum with the Reference Spectrum: both spectra exhibit similar intensities of absorption at the same wavelengths.

(3) Determine the infrared absorption spectrum of Timepidium Bromide Hydrate as directed in the potassium bromide disk method under the Infrared Spectrophotometry 〈*2.25*〉, and compare the spectrum with the Reference Spectrum: both spectra exhibit similar intensities of absorption at the same wave numbers.

(4) A solution of Timepidium Bromide Hydrate (1 in 100) responds to Qualitative Tests 〈*1.09*〉 (1) for Bromide.

Purity **(1)** Clarity and color of solution—Dissolve 0.10 g of Timepidium Bromide Hydrate in 10 mL of water: the solution is clear and colorless.

(2) Heavy metals 〈*1.07*〉—Proceed with 1.0 g of Timepidium Bromide Hydrate according to Method 2, and perform the test. Prepare the control solution with 2.0 mL of Standard Lead Solution (not more than 20 ppm).

(3) Related substances—Dissolve 0.10 g of Timepidium Bromide Hydrate in 10 mL of methanol, and use this solution as the sample solution. Pipet 1 mL of the sample solution, and add methanol to make exactly 100 mL. Pipet 1 mL of this solution, add methanol to make exactly 10 mL, and use this solution as the standard solution. Perform the test with these solutions as directed under Thin-layer Chromatography 〈*2.03*〉. Spot 10 μL each of the sample solution and standard solution on a plate of silica gel with fluorescent indicator for thin-layer chromatography. Develop the plate with a mixture of chloroform, methanol, water, acetic acid (100) and ethyl acetate (5:4:1:1:1) to a distance of about 13 cm, and air-dry the plate. Examine under ultraviolet light (main wavelength: 254 nm): the spots other than the principal spot obtained from the sample solution are not more intense than the spot from the standard solution.

Water 〈*2.48*〉 3.5 – 5.0% (0.4 g, volumetric titration, direct titration).

Residue on ignition 〈*2.44*〉 Not more than 0.1% (1 g).

Assay Weigh accurately about 0.6 g of Timepidium Bromide Hydrate, dissolve in 60 mL of a mixture of acetic anhydride and acetic acid (100) (2:1), and titrate 〈*2.50*〉 with 0.1 mol/L perchloric acid VS (potentiometric titration). Perform a blank determination in the same manner, and make any necessary correction.

Each mL of 0.1 mol/L perchloric acid VS
= 40.04 mg of $C_{17}H_{22}BrNOS_2$

Containers and storage Containers—Tight containers.
Storage—Light-resistant.

Timolol Maleate

チモロールマレイン酸塩

$C_{13}H_{24}N_4O_3S \cdot C_4H_4O_4$: 432.49

(2*S*)-1-[(1,1-Dimethylethyl)amino]-3-(4-morpholin-4-yl-1,2,5-thiadiazol-3-yloxy)propan-2-ol monomaleate

[*26921-17-5*]

Timolol Maleate, when dried, contains not less than 98.0% and not more than 101.0% of timolol maleate ($C_{13}H_{24}N_4O_3S.C_4H_4O_4$).

Description Timolol Maleate occurs as a white to pale yellow-white crystalline powder.

It is freely soluble in acetic acid (100), and soluble in water and in ethanol (99.5).

It dissolves in 0.1 mol/L hydrochloric acid TS.

Melting point: about 197°C (with decomposition).

Identification **(1)** Determine the absorption spectrum of a solution of Timolol Maleate in 0.1 mol/L hydrochloric acid TS (3 in 100,000) as directed under Ultraviolet-visible Spectrophotometry 〈*2.24*〉, and compare the spectrum with the Reference Spectrum: both spectra exhibit similar intensities of absorption at the same wavelengths.

(2) Determine the infrared absorption spectrum of Timolol Maleate as directed in the potassium bromide disk method under Infrared Spectrophotometry 〈*2.25*〉, and compare the spectrum with the Reference Spectrum: both spectra exhibit similar intensities of absorption at the same wave numbers.

(3) To 5 mL of a solution of Timolol Maleate (1 in 500) add 1 drop of potassium permanganate TS: the red color of the TS disappears immediately.

Optical rotation 〈*2.49*〉 $[\alpha]_D^{20}$: −5.7 – −6.2° (after drying, 1.25 g, 1 mol/L hydrochloric acid TS, 25 mL, 100 mm).

pH 〈*2.54*〉 The pH of a solution prepared by dissolving 1.0 g of Timolol Maleate in 20 mL of water is between 3.8 and 4.3.

Purity **(1)** Clarity and color of solution—Dissolve 1.0 g of Timolol Maleate in 20 mL of water: the solution is clear, and its absorbance at 440 nm, determined as directed under Ultraviolet-visible Spectrophotometry 〈*2.24*〉, is not more than 0.05.

(2) Heavy metals 〈*1.07*〉—Proceed with 2.0 g of Timolol Maleate according to Method 4, and perform the test. Prepare the control solution with 2.0 mL of Standard Lead Solution (not more than 10 ppm).

(3) Related substances—Dissolve 30 mg of Timolol Maleate in 20 mL of the mobile phase, and use this solution as the sample solution. Pipet 1 mL of the sample solution, add the mobile phase to make exactly 100 mL, and use this solution as the standard solution. Perform the test with exactly 25 μL each of the sample solution and standard solution as directed under Liquid Chromatography 〈*2.01*〉 according to the following conditions, and determine each peak area by the automatic integration method: the area of the peak other than timolol and maleic acid obtained from the sample solution is not larger than 1/5 times the peak area of timolol from the standard solution, and the total area of the peaks other than the peak of timolol and maleic acid is not larger than 1/2 times the peak area of timolol from the standard solution.

Operating conditions—

Detector: An ultraviolet absorption photometer (wavelength: 280 nm).

Column: A stainless steel column 4.6 mm in inside diameter and 25 cm in length, packed with phenylsilanized silica gel for liquid chromatography (5 μm in particle diameter).

Column temperature: A constant temperature of about 40°C.

Mobile phase: Dissolve 1.9 g of sodium 1-hexanesulfonate in 1800 mL of water, add 6.0 mL of triethylamine and 8.0 mL of formic acid, adjust to pH 3.0 with formic acid, and add water to make 2000 mL. To 1400 mL of this solution add 500 mL of methanol and 100 mL of acetonitrile.

Flow rate: Adjust so that the retention time of timolol is about 18 minutes.

Time span of measurement: About 2 times as long as the retention time of timolol, beginning after the solvent peak.

System suitability—

Test for required detectability: To exactly 1 mL of the standard solution add the mobile phase to make exactly 10 mL. Confirm that the peak area of timolol obtained with 25 μL of this solution is equivalent to 7 to 13% of that with 25 μL of the standard solution.

System performance: When the procedure is run with 25 μL of the sample solution under the above operating conditions, the number of theoretical plates and the symmetry factor of the peak of timolol are not less than 1500 and not more than 2.5, respectively.

System repeatability: When the test is repeated 6 times with 25 μL of the standard solution under the above operating conditions, the relative standard deviation of the peak area of timolol is not more than 2.0%.

Loss on drying <*2.41*> Not more than 0.5% (1 g, in vacuum, 100°C, 3 hours).

Residue on ignition <*2.44*> Not more than 0.1% (1 g).

Assay Weigh accurately about 0.8 g of Timolol Maleate, previously dried, dissolve in 90 mL of acetic acid (100), and titrate <*2.50*> with 0.1 mol/L perchloric acid VS (potentiometric titration). Perform a blank determination in the same manner, and make any necessary correction.

Each mL of 0.1 mol/L perchloric acid VS
= 43.25 mg of $C_{13}H_{24}N_4O_3S.C_4H_4O_4$

Containers and storage Containers—Tight containers.

Tinidazole

チニダゾール

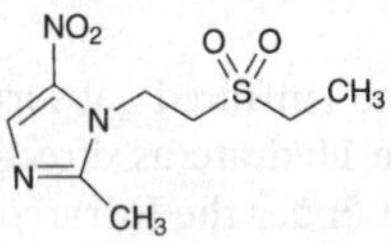

$C_8H_{13}N_3O_4S$: 247.27

1-[2-(Ethylsulfonyl)ethyl]-2-methyl-5-nitro-1*H*-imidazole

[*19387-91-8*]

Tinidazole, when dried, contains not less than 98.5% and not more than 101.0% of tinidazole ($C_8H_{13}N_3O_4S$).

Description Tinidazole occurs as a light yellow crystalline powder.

It is soluble in acetic anhydride and in acetone, sparingly soluble in methanol, slightly soluble in ethanol (99.5), and very slightly soluble in water.

Identification **(1)** Determine the absorption spectrum of a solution of Tinidazole in methanol (1 in 50,000) as directed under Ultraviolet-visible Spectrophotometry <*2.24*>, and compare the spectrum with the Reference Spectrum: both spectra exhibit similar intensities of absorption at the same wavelengths.

(2) Determine the infrared absorption spectrum of Tinidazole as directed in the potassium bromide disk method under Infrared Spectrophotometry <*2.25*>, and compare the spectrum with the Reference Spectrum: both spectra exhibit similar intensities of absorption at the same wave numbers.

Melting point <*2.60*> 125 – 129°C

Purity **(1)** Sulfate <*1.14*>—To 2.0 g of Tinidazole add 100 mL of water, boil for 5 minutes, cool, add water to make 100 mL, and filter. Take 25 mL of the filtrate, and add 1 mL of dilute hydrochloric acid and water to make 50 mL. Use this solution as the test solution, and perform the test. Prepare the control solution with 0.45 mL of 0.005 mol/L sulfuric acid VS (not more than 0.043%).

(2) Heavy metals <*1.07*>—Proceed with 1.0 g of Tinidazole according to Method 4, and perform the test. Prepare the control solution with 2.0 mL of Standard Lead Solution (not more than 20 ppm).

(3) Arsenic <*1.11*>—Prepare the test solution with 2.0 g of Tinidazole according to Method 3, and perform the test (not more than 1 ppm).

(4) Related substances—Dissolve 50 mg of Tinidazole in 2 mL of acetone, and use this solution as the sample solution. Pipet 1 mL of the sample solution, add acetone to make exactly 200 mL, and use this solution as the standard solution. Perform the test with these solutions as directed under Thin-layer Chromatography <*2.03*>. Spot 10 μL each of the sample solution and standard solution on a plate of silica gel with fluorescent indicator for thin-layer chromatography. Develop the plate with a mixture of ethyl acetate and diethylamine (19:1) to a distance of about 10 cm, air-dry the plate, heat the plate at 100°C for 5 minute, and cool. Examine under ultraviolet light (main wavelength: 254 nm): the spots other than the principal spot obtained from the sample solution are not more intense than the spot from the standard solution.

Loss on drying <*2.41*> Not more than 1.0% (1 g, 105°C,

2 hours).

Residue on ignition 〈*2.44*〉 Not more than 0.1% (1 g).

Assay Weigh accurately about 0.35 g of Tinidazole, previously dried, dissolve in 50 mL of acetic anhydride, and titrate 〈*2.50*〉 with 0.1 mol/L perchloric acid VS (potentiometric titration). Perform a blank determination in the same manner, and make any necessary correction.

Each mL of 0.1 mol/L perchloric acid VS
= 24.73 mg of $C_8H_{13}N_3O_4S$

Containers and storage Containers—Tight containers.
Storage—Light-resistant.

Tipepidine Hibenzate

チペピジンヒベンズ酸塩

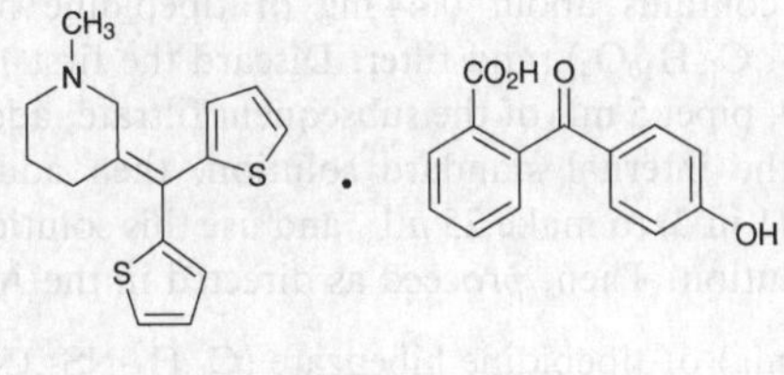

$C_{15}H_{17}NS_2.C_{14}H_{10}O_4$: 517.66
3-(Dithien-2-ylmethylene)-1-methylpiperidine mono[2-(4-hydroxybenzoyl)benzoate]
[*31139-87-4*]

Tipepidine Hibenzate, when dried, contains not less than 98.5% of tipepidine hibenzate ($C_{15}H_{17}NS_2.C_{14}H_{10}O_4$).

Description Tipepidine Hibenzate occurs as a white to light yellow crystalline powder. It is odorless and tasteless.

It is freely soluble in acetic acid (100), slightly soluble in methanol and in ethanol (95), very slightly soluble in water, and practically insoluble in diethyl ether.

Identification **(1)** Dissolve 0.01 g of Tipepidine Hibenzate in 5 mL of sulfuric acid: an orange-red color develops.

(2) Dissolve 0.3 g of Tipepidine Hibenzate in 10 mL of sodium hydroxide TS and 5 mL of water, and extract with two 20-mL portions of chloroform. Wash the chloroform extracts with 10 mL of water, and filter the chloroform layer. Evaporate the filtrate on a water bath to dryness, and dissolve the residue in 0.5 mL of 1 mol/L hydrochloric acid TS and 5 mL of water. To 2 mL of this solution add 5 mL of Reinecke salt TS: a light red precipitate is formed.

(3) Determine the absorption spectrum of a solution of Tipepidine Hibenzate in ethanol (99.5) (1 in 100,000) as directed under Ultraviolet-visible Spectrophotometry 〈*2.24*〉, and compare the spectrum with the Reference Spectrum; both spectra exhibit similar intensities of absorption at the same wavelengths.

(4) Determine the infrared absorption spectrum of Tipepidine Hibenzate, previously dried, as directed in the potassium bromide disk method under Infrared Spectrophotometry 〈*2.25*〉, and compare the spectrum with the Reference Spectrum: both spectra exhibit similar intensities of absorption at the same wave numbers.

Melting point 〈*2.60*〉 189 - 193°C

Purity **(1)** Clarity and color of solution—Dissolve 1.0 g of Tipepidine Hibenzate in 10 mL of acetic acid (100): the solution is clear. Perform the test with this solution as directed under Ultraviolet-visible Spectrophotometry 〈*2.24*〉: its absorbance at 400 nm is not more than 0.16.

(2) Heavy metals 〈*1.07*〉—Proceed with 2.0 g of Tipepidine Hibenzate according to Method 2, and perform the test. Prepare the control solution with 2.0 mL of Standard Lead Solution (not more than 10 ppm).

(3) Arsenic 〈*1.11*〉—Prepare the test solution with 1.0 g of Tipepidine Hibenzate according to Method 3, and perform the test (not more than 2 ppm).

(4) Related substances—(i) Dissolve 10 mg of Tipepidine Hibenzate in 20 mL of the mobile phase, and use this solution as the sample solution. Pipet 1 mL of the sample solution, add the mobile phase to make exactly 100 mL, and use this solution as the standard solution. Perform the test with exactly 20 μL each of the sample solution and standard solution as directed under Liquid Chromatography 〈*2.01*〉 according to the following conditions. Determine each peak area by the automatic integration method: the total area of peaks other than hibenzic acid and tipepidine obtained from the sample solution is not larger than the peak area of the tipepidine from the standard solution.

Operating conditions—

Detector: An ultraviolet absorption photometer (wavelength: 254 nm).

Column: A stainless steel column 4.6 mm in inside diameter and 15 cm in length, packed with octadecylsilanized silica gel for liquid chromatography (5 μm in particle diameter).

Column temperature: A constant temperature of about 50°C.

Mobile phase: A mixture of a solution of ammonium acetate (1 in 100) and tetrahydrofuran (32:13).

Flow rate: Adjust so that the retention time of tipepidine is about 12 minutes.

Time span of measurement: As long as the retention time of tipepidine, beginning after the solvent peak.

System suitability—

Test for required detectability: To exactly 2 mL of the standard solution add the mobile phase to make exactly 20 mL. Confirm that the peak area of tipepidine obtained with 20 μL of this solution is equivalent to 7 to 13% of that with 20 μL of the standard solution.

System performance: Dissolve 10 mg of Tipepidine Hibenzate and 3 mg of propyl parahydroxybenzoate in 100 mL of the mobile phase. When the procedure is run with 20 μL of this solution under the above operating conditions, hibenzic acid, tipepidine and propyl parahydroxybenzoate are eluted in this order with the resolution between the peaks of tipepidine and propyl parahydroxybenzoate being not less than 3.

System repeatability: When the test is repeated 6 times with 20 μL of the standard solution under the above operating conditions, the relative standard deviation of the peak area of tipepidine is not more than 1.5%.

(ii) Dissolve 10 mg of Tipepidine Hibenzate in 20 mL of the mobile phase, and use this solution as the sample solution. Pipet 1 mL of the sample solution, add the mobile phase to make exactly 100 mL, and use this solution as the standard solution. Perform the test with exactly 20 μL each of the sample solution and standard solution as directed under Liquid Chromatography 〈*2.01*〉 according to the following conditions, and determine each peak area by the automatic integration method: the total area of peaks other than hibenzic acid and tipepidine obtained from the sample solution is not larger than 1/2 times the peak area of the tipepidine from the standard solution.

Operating conditions—

Detector: An ultraviolet absorption photometer (wavelength: 254 nm).

Column: A stainless steel column 4.6 mm in inside diameter and 15 cm in length, packed with octadecylsilanized silica gel for liquid chromatography (5 μm in particle diameter).

Column temperature: A constant temperature of about 40°C.

Mobile phase: A mixture of methanol and a solution of ammonium acetate (1 in 500) (13:7).

Flow rate: Adjust so that the retention time of tipepidine is about 10 minutes.

Time span of measurement: Two times as long as the retention time of tipepidine, beginning after the peak of tipepidine.

System suitability—

Test for required detectability: To exactly 2 mL of the standard solution add the mobile phase to make exactly 20 mL. Confirm that the peak area of tipepidine obtained with 20 μL of this solution is equivalent to 7 to 13% of that with 20 μL of the standard solution.

System performance: Dissolve 12 mg of Tipepidine Hibenzate and 4 mg of xanthene in 50 mL of the mobile phase. When the procedure is run with 10 μL of this solution under the above operating conditions, hibenzic acid, tipepidine and xanthene are eluted in this order with the resolution between the peaks of tipepidine and xanthene being not less than 3.

System repeatability: When the test is repeated 6 times with 20 μL of the standard solution under the above operating conditions, the relative standard deviation of the peak area of tipepidine is not more than 3.0%.

Loss on drying <*2.41*> Not more than 0.5% (1 g, 60°C, in vacuum, phosphorus (V) oxide, 3 hours).

Residue on ignition <*2.44*> Not more than 0.1% (1 g).

Assay Weigh accurately about 1 g of Tipepidine Hibenzate, previously dried, dissolve in 40 mL of acetic acid (100), and titrate <*2.50*> with 0.1 mol/L perchloric acid VS until the color of the solution changes from purple through blue to green (indicator: 3 drops of crystal violet TS). Perform a blank determination in the same manner, and make any necessary correction.

Each ml of 0.1 mol/L perchloric acid VS
= 51.77 mg of $C_{15}H_{17}NS_2.C_{14}H_{10}O_4$

Containers and storage Containers—Well-closed containers.

Storage—Light-resistant.

Tipepidine Hibenzate Tablets

チペピジンヒベンズ酸塩錠

Tipepidine Hibenzate Tablets contain not less than 95.0% and not more than 105.0% of the labeled amount of tipepidine hibenzate ($C_{15}H_{17}NS_2.C_{14}H_{10}O_4$: 517.66).

Method of preparation Prepare as directed under Tablets, with Tipepidine Hibenzate.

Identification **(1)** To a quantity of powdered Tipepidine Hibenzate Tablets, equivalent to 44 mg of Tipepidine Hibenzate, add 5 mL of water, shake for 1 minute, add 10 mL of sodium hydroxide TS, and extract with two 20-mL portions of chloroform. Combine the extracts, wash with 10 mL of water, and filter the chloroform layer. Evaporate the filtrate on a water bath to dryness, dissolve the residue in 0.2 mL of 1 mol/L hydrochloric acid TS and 2 mL of water, and add 5 mL of Reinecke salt TS: a light red precipitate is formed.

(2) To a quantity of powdered Tipepidine Hibenzate Tablets, equivalent to 11 mg of Tipepidine Hibenzate, add 30 mL of ethanol (99.5), and warm for 10 minutes with occasional shaking. After cooling, add ethanol (99.5) to make 50 mL, and filter. To 1 mL of the filtrate add ethanol (99.5) to make 20 mL, and determine the absorption spectrum of this solution as directed under Ultraviolet-visible Spectrophotometry <*2.24*>: it exhibits a maximum between 280 nm and 286 nm.

Uniformity of dosage units <*6.02*> Perform the test according to the following method: it meets the requirement of the Content uniformity test.

To 1 tablet of Tipepidine Hibenzate Tablets add 5 mL of diluted acetic acid (100) (1 in 2) and 15 mL of methanol per 11 mg of tipepidine hibenzate ($C_{15}H_{17}NS_2.C_{14}H_{10}O_4$), and warm for 15 minutes with occasional shaking. After cooling, add diluted methanol (1 in 2) to make exactly V mL so that each mL contains about 0.44 mg of tipepidine hibenzate ($C_{15}H_{17}NS_2.C_{14}H_{10}O_4$), and filter. Discard the first 10 mL of the filtrate, pipet 5 mL of the subsequent filtrate, add exactly 5 mL of the internal standard solution, then add diluted methanol (1 in 2) to make 25 mL, and use this solution as the sample solution. Then, proceed as directed in the Assay.

Amount (mg) of tipepidine hibenzate ($C_{15}H_{17}NS_2.C_{14}H_{10}O_4$)
$= M_S \times Q_T/Q_S \times V/50$

M_S: Amount (mg) of tipepidine hibenzate for assay taken

Internal standard solution—A solution of dibucaine hydrochloride in methanol (1 in 2000).

Dissolution <*6.10*> When the test is performed at 50 revolutions per minute according to the Paddle method, using 900 mL of water as the dissolution medium, the dissolution rate in 30 minutes of Tipepidine Hibenzate Tablets is not less than 80%.

Start the test with 1 tablet of Tipepidine Hibenzate Tablets, withdraw not less than 20 mL of the medium at the specified minute after starting the test, filter, discard not less than 10 mL of the first filtrate, and use the subsequent filtrate as the sample solution. Separately, weigh accurately about 0.11 g of tipepidine hibenzate for assay, previously dried in a desiccator (in vacuum, phosphorus (V) oxide, 60° C) for 3 hours, and dissolve in 80 mL of diluted ethanol (3 in 4) by warming occasionally. After cooling, add diluted ethanol (3 in 4) to make exactly 100 mL, then pipet 20 mL of this solution, add water to make exactly 900 mL, and use this solution as the standard solution. Determine the absorbances, A_{T1} and A_{S1}, at 286 nm, and A_{T2} and A_{S2}, at 360 nm of the sample solution and standard solution as directed under Ultraviolet-visible Spectrophotometry <*2.24*>.

Dissolution rate (%) with respect to the labeled amount of tipepidine hibenzate ($C_{15}H_{17}NS_2.C_{14}H_{10}O_4$)
$= M_S \times (A_{T1} - A_{T2}/A_{S1} - A_{S2}) \times 1/C \times 20$

M_S: Amount (mg) of tipepidine hibenzate for assay taken
C: Labeled amount (mg) of tipepidine hibenzate ($C_{15}H_{17}NS_2.C_{14}H_{10}O_4$) in 1 tablet

Assay Weigh accurately and powder not less than 20 Tipepidine Hibenzate Tablets. Weigh accurately a portion of the powder, equivalent to about 22 mg of tipepidine hibenzate ($C_{15}H_{17}NS_2.C_{14}H_{10}O_4$), add 10 mL of diluted acetic acid (100) (1 in 2) and 30 mL of methanol, and warm for 10 minutes with occasional shaking. After cooling, add diluted methanol (1 in 2) to make exactly 50 mL, and filter. Discard the first 10 mL of the filtrate, pipet 5 mL of the subsequent filtrate, add exactly 5 mL of the internal standard solution, then add diluted methanol (1 in 2) to make 25 mL, and use this solution as the sample solution. Separately, weigh accurately about 22 mg of tipepidine hibenzate for assay, previously dried in a desiccator (in vacuum, phosphorus (V) oxide, 60°C) for 3 hours, dissolve in 10 mL of diluted acetic acid (100) (1 in 2) and 30 mL of methanol, and add diluted methanol (1 in 2) to make exactly 50 mL. Pipet 5 mL of this solution, add exactly 5 mL of the internal standard solution, then add diluted methanol (1 in 2) to make exactly 25 mL, and use this solution as the standard solution. Perform the test with 20 µL each of the sample solution and standard solution as directed under Liquid Chromatography *<2.01>* according to the following conditions, and calculate the ratios, Q_T and Q_S, of the peak area of tipepidine to that of the internal standard, respectively.

Amount (mg) of tipepidine hibenzate ($C_{15}H_{17}NS_2.C_{14}H_{10}O_4$)
$= M_S \times Q_T/Q_S$

M_S: Amount (mg) of tipepidine hibenzate for assay taken

Internal standard solution—A solution of dibucaine hydrochloride in methanol (1 in 2000).

Operating conditions—

Detector: An ultraviolet absorption photometer (wavelength: 254 nm).

Column: A stainless steel column 4.6 mm in inside diameter and 15 cm in length, packed with octadecylsilanized silica gel for liquid chromatography (5 µm in particle diameter).

Column temperature: A constant temperature of about 40°C.

Mobile phase: A mixture of a solution of sodium lauryl sulfate in diluted phosphoric acid (1 in 1000) (1 in 500), acetonitrile and 2-propanol (3:2:1).

Flow rate: Adjust the flow rate so that the retention time of tipepidine is about 7 minutes.

System suitability—

System performance: When the procedure is run with 20 µL of the standard solution under the above operating conditions, tipepidine and the internal standard are eluted in this order with the resolution between these peaks being not less than 10.

System repeatability: When the test is repeated 6 times with 20 µL of the standard solution under the above operating conditions, the relative standard deviation of the ratios of the peak area of tipepidine to that of the internal standard is not more than 1.0%.

Containers and storage Containers—Tight containers.
Storage—Light-resistant.

Titanium Oxide

酸化チタン

TiO_2: 79.87

Titanium Oxide, when dried, contains not less than 98.5% of titanium oxide (TiO_2).

Description Titanium Oxide occurs as a white powder. It is odorless and tasteless.

It is practically insoluble in water, in ethanol (99.5) and in diethyl ether.

It dissolves in hot sulfuric acid and in hydrofluoric acid, and does not dissolve in hydrochloric acid, in nitric acid and in dilute sulfuric acid.

When fused by heating with potassium hydrogen sulfate, with potassium hydroxide, or with potassium carbonate, it changes to soluble salts.

Shake 1 g of Titanium Oxide with 10 mL of water: the mixture is neutral.

Identification Heat 0.5 g of Titanium Oxide with 5 mL of sulfuric acid until white fumes are evolved, cool, add cautiously water to make 100 mL, and filter. To 5 mL of the filtrate add 2 to 3 drops of hydrogen peroxide TS: a yellow-red color develops.

Purity **(1)** Lead—Place 1.0 g of Titanium Oxide in a platinum crucible, add 10.0 g of potassium hydrogen sulfate, heat gently with caution at the beginning, then raise the temperature gradually, and heat strongly with occasional shaking until the contents fuse to yield a clear liquid. Cool, add 30 mL of a solution of diammonium hydrogen citrate (9 in 20) and 50 mL of water, dissolve by heating on a water bath, cool, add water to make 100 mL, and use this solution as the sample stock solution. Take 25 mL of the sample stock solution to a separator, add 10 mL of a solution of ammonium sulfate (2 in 5) and 5 drops of thymol blue TS, neutralize with ammonia TS, and add 2.5 mL of ammonia TS. To this solution add exactly 20 mL of a solution of dithizone in *n*-butyl acetate (1 in 500), shake for 10 minutes, and use this *n*-butyl acetate solution as the sample solution. Separately, place 6.0 mL of Standard Lead Solution in a platinum crucible, proceed as directed in the sample solution, and use this solution as the standard solution. Determine the absorbances of the sample solution and standard solution as directed under Atomic Absorption Spectrophotometry *<2.23>* according to the following conditions: the absorbance of the sample solution is smaller than that of the standard solution (not more than 60 ppm).

Gas: Combustible gas—Acetylene gas or hydrogen gas.
Supporting gas—Air.

Lamp: Lead hollow-cathode lamp.

Wavelength: 283.3 nm.

(2) Arsenic *<1.11>*—Perform the test with 20 mL of the sample stock solution obtained in (1) as the test solution: the color is not deeper than the following color standard.

Color standard: Proceed in the same manner without Titanium Oxide, transfer 20 mL of the obtained solution to a generator bottle, add 2.0 mL of Standard Arsenic Solution, and proceed in the same manner as the test with the test solution (not more than 10 ppm).

(3) Water-soluble substances—Shake thoroughly 4.0 g of Titanium Oxide with 50 mL of water, and allow to stand overnight. Shake thoroughly with 2 mL of ammonium chloride TS, add further 2 mL of ammonium chloride TS if necessary, and allow titanium oxide to settle. Add water to make 200 mL, shake thoroughly, and filter through double filter paper. Discard the first 10 mL of the filtrate, evaporate 100 mL of the clear filtrate on a water bath, and heat strongly at 800°C to constant mass: the mass of the residue is not more than 5.0 mg.

Loss on drying *<2.41>* Not more than 0.5% (1 g, 105°C, 3 hours).

Assay Weigh accurately about 0.2 g of Titanium Oxide, previously dried, transfer to a crucible, and add 3 g of potassium disulfate. Cover, and heat gently at first, gradually raise the temperature, and then heat the fused contents for 30 minutes. Continue heating for 30 minutes at a higher temperature to make the fused mixture a deep yellow-red, almost clear liquid. Cool, transfer the contents of the crucible to a 250-mL beaker, wash the crucible with a mixture of

75 mL of water and 2.5 mL of sulfuric acid into the beaker, and heat on a water bath until the solution becomes almost clear. Dissolve 2 g of L-tartaric acid in the solution, add 2 to 3 drops of bromothymol blue TS, neutralize with ammonia TS, and acidify with 1 to 2 mL of diluted sulfuric acid (1 in 2). Pass hydrogen sulfide sufficiently through the solution, add 30 mL of ammonia TS, again saturate the solution with hydrogen sulfide, allow to stand for 10 minutes, and filter. Wash the precipitate on the filter paper with ten 25-mL portions of a mixture of ammonium L-tartrate solution (1 in 100) and ammonium sulfide TS (9:1). When the precipitate is filtered and washed, prevent iron (II) sulfide from oxidation by filling the solution on the filter paper. Combine the filtrate and the washings, add 40 mL of diluted sulfuric acid (1 in 2), and boil to expel hydrogen sulfide. Cool, and dilute with water to make 400 mL. Add gradually 40 mL of cupferron TS to the solution with stirring, and allow to stand. After sedimentation of a yellow precipitate, add again cupferron TS until a white precipitate is produced. Filter by slight suction using quantitative filter paper, wash with twenty portions of diluted hydrochloric acid (1 in 10), and remove water by stronger suction at the last washing. Dry the precipitate together with the filter paper at 70°C, transfer to a tared crucible, and heat very gently at first, and raise the temperature gradually after smoke stops evolving. Heat strongly between 900°C and 950°C to constant mass, cool, and weigh as titanium oxide (TiO_2).

Containers and storage Containers—Well-closed containers.

Tizanidine Hydrochloride

チザニジン塩酸塩

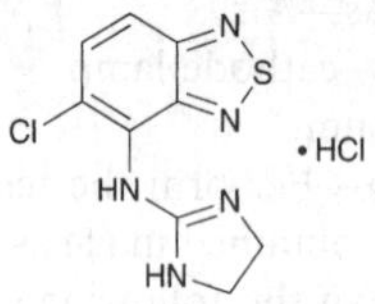

$C_9H_8ClN_5S.HCl$: 290.17
5-Chloro-*N*-(4,5-dihydro-1*H*-imidazol-2-yl)-2,1,3-benzothiadiazole-4-amine monohydrochloride
[*64461-82-1*]

Tizanidine Hydrochloride, when dried, contains not less than 99.0% and not more than 101.0% of tizanidine hydrochloride ($C_9H_8ClN_5S.HCl$).

Description Tizanidine Hydrochloride occurs as a white to light yellow-white crystalline powder.

It is soluble in water, slightly soluble in ethanol (99.5), and practically insoluble in acetic anhydride and in acetic acid (100).

Melting point: about 290°C (with decomposition).

Identification **(1)** Determine the absorption spectrum of a solution of Tizanidine Hydrochloride in diluted 1 mol/L ammonia TS (1 in 10) (1 in 125,000) as directed under Ultraviolet-visible Spectrophotometry *<2.24>*, and compare the spectrum with the Reference Spectrum: both spectra exhibit similar intensities of absorption at the same wavelengths.

(2) Determine the infrared absorption spectrum of Tizanidine Hydrochloride as directed in the potassium chloride disk method under Infrared Spectrophotometry *<2.25>*, and compare the spectrum with the Reference Spectrum: both spectra exhibit similar intensities of absorption at the same wave numbers.

(3) A solution of Tizanidine Hydrochloride (1 in 50) responds to Qualitative Tests *<1.09>* for chloride.

Purity **(1)** Heavy metals *<1.07>*—Proceed with 1.0 g of Tizanidine Hydrochloride according to Method 3, and perform the test. Prepare the control solution with 2.0 mL of Standard Lead Solution (not more than 20 ppm).

(2) Related substances—Dissolve 60 mg of Tizanidine Hydrochloride in 10 mL of a mixture of water and acetonitrile (17:3), and use this solution as the sample solution. Pipet 1 mL of the sample solution, add the mixture of water and acetonitrile (17:3) to make exactly 200 mL, and use this solution as the standard solution. Perform the test with exactly 10 μL of the sample solution and standard solution as directed under Liquid Chromatography *<2.01>* according to the following conditions, and determine each peak area by the automatic integration method: the area of the peak other than tizanidine obtained from the sample solution is not larger than 1/5 times the peak area of tizanidine from the standard solution.

Operating conditions—

Detector: An ultraviolet absorption photometer (wavelength: 230 nm for about 3 minutes after sample injection and 318 nm subsequently).

Column: A stainless steel column 4.6 mm in inside diameter and 12.5 cm in length, packed with octadecylsilanized silica gel for liquid chromatography (5 μm in particle diameter).

Column temperature: A constant temperature of about 25°C.

Mobile phase A: A mixture of water and formic acid (200:1), adjusted to pH 8.5 with ammonia water (28).

Mobile phase B: A mixture of acetonitrile and the mobile phase A (4:1).

Flowing of mobile phase: Control the gradient by mixing the mobile phases A and B as directed in the following table.

Time after injection of sample (min)	Mobile phase A (vol%)	Mobile phase B (vol%)
0 – 10	81 → 68	19 → 32
10 – 13	68	32
13 – 26	68 → 10	32 → 90
26 – 28	10	90

Flow rate: Adjust so that the retention time of tizanidine is about 7 minute.

Time span of measurement: About 4 times as long as the retention time of tizanidine, beginning after the solvent peak.

System suitability—

Test for required detectability: Measure exactly 2 mL of the standard solution, and add the mixture of water and acetonitrile (17:3) to make exactly 10 mL. Confirm that the peak area of tizanidine obtained with 10 μL of this solution is equivalent to 14 to 26% of that with 10 μL of the standard solution.

System performance: Dissolve 2 mg each of Tizanidine Hydrochloride and *p*-toluenesulfonic acid monohydrate in 100 mL of the mixture of water and acetonitrile (17:3). When the procedure is run with 10 μL of this solution under the above operating conditions, *p*-toluenesulfonic acid and tizanidine are eluted in this order with the resolution between these peaks being not less than 10.

System repeatability: When the test is repeated 6 times

with 10 μL of the standard solution under the above operating conditions, the relative standard deviation of the peak area of tizanidine is not more than 2.0%.

Loss on drying 〈*2.41*〉 Not more than 0.2% (1 g, 105°C, 3 hours).

Residue on ignition 〈*2.44*〉 Not more than 0.1% (1 g).

Assay Weigh accurately about 0.2 g of Tizanidine Hydrochloride, previously dried, dissolve in 60 mL of a mixture of acetic anhydride and acetic acid (100) (7:3) with the aid of warming. After cooling, titrate 〈*2.50*〉 with 0.1 mol/L perchloric acid VS (potentiometric titration). Perform a blank determination in the same manner, and make any necessary correction.

Each mL of 0.1 mol/L perchloric acid VS
= 29.02 mg of $C_9H_8ClN_5S.HCl$

Containers and storage Containers—Well-closed containers.

Tobramycin

トブラマイシン

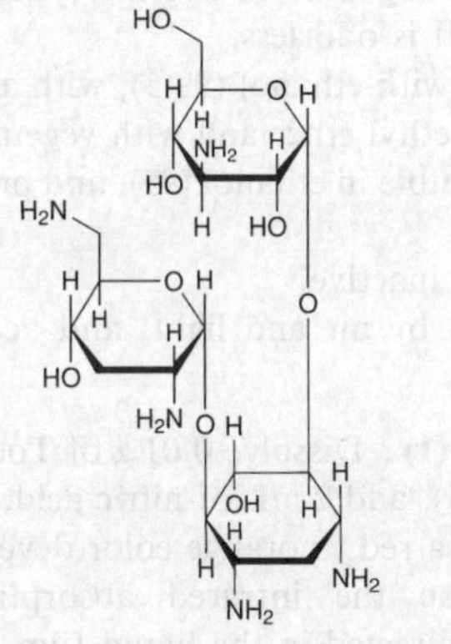

$C_{18}H_{37}N_5O_9$: 467.51
3-Amino-3-deoxy-α-D-glucopyranosyl-(1→6)-[2,6-diamino-2,3,6-trideoxy-α-D-*ribo*-hexopyranosyl-(1→4)]-2-deoxy-D-streptamine
[*32986-56-4*]

Tobramycin is an aminoglycoside substance having antibacterial activity produced by the growth of *Streptomyces tenebrarius*.

It contains not less than 900 μg (potency) and not more than 1060 μg (potency) per mg, calculated on the anhydrous basis. The potency of Tobramycin is expressed as mass (potency) of tobramycin ($C_{18}H_{37}N_5O_9$).

Description Tobramycin occurs as a white to pale yellow-white powder.

It is very soluble in water, freely soluble in formamide, slightly soluble in methanol, and very slightly soluble in ethanol (95).

It is hygroscopic.

Identification (1) Determine the ^1H spectrum of a solution of Tobramycin in heavy water for nuclear magnetic resonance spectroscopy (1 in 125) as directed under Nuclear Magnetic Resonance Spectroscopy 〈*2.21*〉, using sodium 3-trimethylsilylpropanesulfonate for nuclear magnetic resonance spectroscopy as an internal reference compound: it exhibits a doublet signal A at around δ 5.1 ppm, a multiplet signal B between δ 2.6 ppm and δ 4.0 ppm, and a multiplet signal C between δ 1.0 ppm and δ 2.1 ppm. The ratio of the integrated intensity of these signals, A:B:C, is about 1:8:2.

(2) Dissolve 10 mg each of Tobramycin and Tobramycin RS in 1 mL of water, and use these solutions as the sample solution and standard solution. Perform the test with these solutions as directed under Thin-layer Chromatography 〈*2.03*〉. Spot 4 μL of the sample solution and standard solution on a plate of silica gel for thin-layer chromatography. Develop the plate with a mixture of ammonia TS, 1-butanol and methanol (5:5:2) to a distance of about 10 cm, and air-dry the plate. Spray evenly ninhydrin TS on the plate, and heat the plate at 100°C for 5 minutes: the *R*f values of the principal spots obtained from the sample solution and the standard solution are the same.

Optical rotation 〈*2.49*〉 $[\alpha]_D^{20}$: +138 – +148° (1 g calculated on the anhydrous basis, water, 25 mL, 100 mm).

pH 〈*2.54*〉 The pH of a solution obtained by dissolving 0.10 g of Tobramycin in 10 mL of water is between 9.5 and 11.5.

Purity (1) Clarity and color of solution—Dissolve 1.0 g of Tobramycin in 10 mL of water: the solution is clear, and its absorbance at 400 nm, determined as directed under Ultraviolet-visible Spectrophotometry 〈*2.24*〉, is not more than 0.05.

(2) Heavy metals 〈*1.07*〉—Proceed with 1.0 g of Tobramycin according to Method 2, and perform the test. Prepare the control solution with 3.0 mL of Standard Lead Solution (not more than 30 ppm).

(3) Related substances—Dissolve 80 mg of Tobramycin in 10 mL of diluted ammonia solution (28) (1 in 250), and use this solution as the sample solution. Pipet 1 mL of the sample solution, add diluted ammonia solution (28) (1 in 250) to make exactly 100 mL, and use this solution as the standard solution. Perform the test with these solutions as directed under Thin-layer Chromatography 〈*2.03*〉. Spot 5 μL of the sample solution and standard solution on a plate of silica gel for thin-layer chromatography. Develop the plate with a mixture of ammonia solution (28), ethanol (95) and 2-butanone (1:1:1) to a distance of about 10 cm, air-dry the plate, then further dry at 110°C for 10 minutes. Immediately spray evenly a mixture of water and sodium hypochlorite TS (4:1) on the plate, air-dry the plate, then spray potassium iodide-starch TS on the plate: the spot other than the principal spot obtained from the sample solution is not more intense than the spot from the standard solution.

Water 〈*2.48*〉 Not more than 11.0% (0.1 g, volumetric titration, direct titration). Use a mixture of formamide for water determination and methanol for water determination (3:1) instead of methanol for water determination.

Residue on ignition 〈*2.44*〉 Not more than 1.0% (0.5 g).

Assay Perform the test according to the Cylinder-plate method as directed under Microbial Assay for Antibiotics 〈*4.02*〉 according to the following conditions.

(i) Test organism—*Bacillus subtilis* ATCC 6633

(ii) Culture medium—Use the medium i in 1) under (1) Agar media for seed and base layer.

(iii) Standard solutions—Weigh accurately an amount of Tobramycin RS, equivalent to about 25 mg (potency), dissolve in 0.1 mol/L phosphate buffer solution (pH 8.0) to make exactly 25 mL, and use this solution as the standard stock solution. Keep the standard stock solution between 5°C and 15°C, and use within 30 days. Take exactly a suitable amount of the standard stock solution before use, add

0.1 mol/L phosphate buffer solution (pH 8.0) to make solutions so that each mL contains 8 μg (potency) and 2 μg (potency), and use these solutions as the high concentration standard solution and the low concentration standard solution, respectively.

(iv) Sample solutions—Weigh accurately an amount of Tobramycin, equivalent to about 25 mg (potency), and dissolve in 0.1 mol/L phosphate buffer solution (pH 8.0) to make exactly 25 mL. Take exactly a suitable amount of this solution, add 0.1 mol/L phosphate buffer solution (pH 8.0) to make solutions so that each mL contains 8 μg (potency) and 2 μg (potency), and use these solutions as the high concentration sample solution and the low concentration sample solution, respectively.

Containers and storage Containers—Tight containers.

Tobramycin Injection

トブラマイシン注射液

Tobramycin Injection is an aqueous injection.

It contains not less than 90.0% and not more than 110.0% of the labeled potency of tobramycin ($C_{18}H_{37}N_5O_9$: 467.51).

Method of preparation Prepare as directed under Injections, with Tobramycin.

Description Tobramycin Injection occurs as a colorless or very pale yellow, clear liquid.

Identification To a volume of Tobramycin Injection, equivalent to 10 mg (potency) of Tobramycin, add water to make 1 mL, and use this solution as the sample solution. Separately, dissolve 10 mg (potency) of Tobramycin RS in 1 mL of water, and use this solution as the standard solution. Then, proceed as directed in the Identification (2) under Tobramycin.

Osmotic pressure ratio Being specified separately when the drug is granted approval based on the Law.

pH <*2.54*> 5.0 – 7.0

Bacterial endotoxins <*4.01*> Less than 0.50 EU/mg (potency).

Extractable volume <*6.05*> It meets the requirement.

Foreign insoluble matter <*6.06*> Perform the test according to Method 1: it meets the requirement.

Insoluble particulate matter <*6.07*> It meets the requirement.

Sterility <*4.06*> Perform the test according to the Membrane filtration method: it meets the requirement.

Assay Perform the test according to the Cylinder-plate method as directed under Microbial Assay for Antibiotics <*4.02*> according to the following conditions.

(i) Test organism, culture medium, and standard solutions—Proceed as directed in the Assay under Tobramycin.

(ii) Sample solutions—To exactly 5 mL of Tobramycin Injection add 0.1 mol/L phosphate buffer solution (pH 8.0) so that each mL contains 1 mg (potency) of Tobramycin. Take exactly a suitable amount of this solution, add 0.1 mol/L phosphate buffer solution (pH 8.0) to make solutions so that each mL contains 8 μg (potency) and 2 μg (potency), and use these solutions as the concentration sample solution high and the low concentration sample solution, respectively.

Containers and storage Containers—Hermetic containers.

Tocopherol

Vitamin E

トコフェロール

$C_{29}H_{50}O_2$: 430.71

2,5,7,8-Tetramethyl-2-(4,8,12-trimethyltridecyl)chroman-6-ol

[*10191-41-0*]

Tocopherol contains not less than 96.0% and not more than 102.0% of *dl*-α-tocopherol ($C_{29}H_{50}O_2$).

Description Tocopherol is a clear, yellow to red-brown, viscous liquid. It is odorless.

It is miscible with ethanol (99.5), with acetone, with chloroform, with diethyl ether and with vegetable oils.

It is freely soluble in ethanol (95), and practically insoluble in water.

It is optically inactive.

It is oxidized by air and light, and acquires a dark red color.

Identification **(1)** Dissolve 0.01 g of Tocopherol in 10 mL of ethanol (99.5), add 2 mL of nitric acid, and heat at 75°C for 15 minutes: a red to orange color develops.

(2) Determine the infrared absorption spectrum of Tocopherol as directed in the liquid film method under Infrared Spectrophotometry <*2.25*>, and compare the spectrum with the Reference Spectrum or the spectrum of Tocopherol RS: both spectra exhibit similar intensities of absorption at the same wave numbers.

Absorbance <*2.24*> $E^{1\%}_{1\,cm}$ (292 nm): 71.0 – 76.0 (10 mg, ethanol (99.5), 200 mL).

Refractive index <*2.45*> n^{20}_{D}: 1.503 – 1.507

Specific gravity <*2.56*> d^{20}_{20}: 0.947 – 0.955

Purity **(1)** Clarity and color of solution—Dissolve 0.10 g of Tocopherol in 10 mL of ethanol (99.5): the solution is clear and has no more color than Matching Fluid C.

(2) Heavy metals <*1.07*>—Proceed with 1.0 g of Tocopherol according to Method 4, and perform the test. Prepare the control solution with 2.0 mL of Standard Lead Solution (not more than 20 ppm).

Assay Dissolve about 50 mg each of Tocopherol and Tocopherol RS, accurately weighed, in ethanol (99.5) to make exactly 50 mL, and use these solutions as the sample solution and standard solution. Perform the test with exactly 20 μL each of these solutions as directed under Liquid Chromatography <*2.01*> according to the following conditions, and determine the peak heights, H_T and H_S, of tocopherol in each solution.

$$\text{Amount (mg) of tocopherol } (C_{29}H_{50}O_2) = M_S \times H_T/H_S$$

M_S: Amount (mg) of Tocopherol RS taken

Operating conditions—

Detector: An ultraviolet absorption photometer (wavelength: 292 nm).

Column: A stainless steel column 4.6 mm in inside diameter and 15 cm in length, packed with octadecylsilanized silica gel for liquid chromatography (5 μm in particle diameter).

Column temperature: A constant temperature of about 35°C.

Mobile phase: A mixture of methanol and water (49:1).

Flow rate: Adjust so that the retention time of tocopherol is about 10 minutes.

System suitability—

System performance: Dissolve 0.05 g each of Tocopherol and tocopherol acetate in 50 mL of ethanol (99.5). When the procedure is run with 20 μL of this solution under the above operating conditions, tocopherol and tocopherol acetate are eluted in this order with the resolution between these peaks being not less than 2.6.

System repeatability: When the test is repeated 5 times with 20 μL of the standard solution under the above operating conditions, the relative standard deviation of the peak heights of tocopherol is not more than 0.8%.

Containers and storage Containers—Tight containers.

Storage—Light-resistant, and well-filled, or under nitrogen atmosphere.

Tocopherol Acetate

Vitamin E Acetate

トコフェロール酢酸エステル

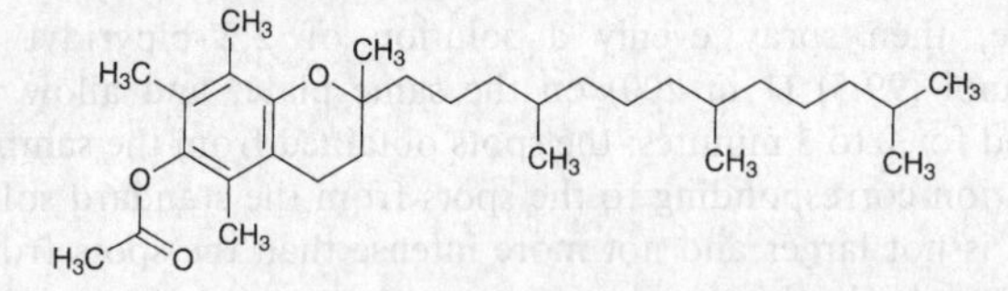

$C_{31}H_{52}O_3$: 472.74

2,5,7,8-Tetramethyl-2-(4,8,12-trimethyltridecyl)chroman-6-yl acetate

[7695-91-2]

Tocopherol Acetate contains not less than 96.0% and not more than 102.0% of *dl*-α-tocopherol acetate ($C_{31}H_{52}O_3$).

Description Tocopherol Acetate is a clear, colorless or yellow, viscous and odorless liquid.

It is miscible with ethanol (99.5), with acetone, with chloroform, with diethyl ether, with hexane and with vegetable oils.

It is freely soluble in ethanol (95), and practically insoluble in water.

It is optically inactive.

It is affected by air and light.

Identification **(1)** Dissolve 0.05 g of Tocopherol Acetate in 10 mL of ethanol (99.5), add 2 mL of nitric acid, and heat at 75°C for 15 minutes: a red to orange color is produced.

(2) Determine the infrared absorption spectrum of Tocopherol Acetate as directed in the liquid film method under Infrared Spectrophotometry <*2.25*>, and compare the spectrum with the Reference Spectrum or the spectrum of Tocopherol Acetate RS: both spectra exhibit similar intensities of absorption at the same wave numbers.

Absorbance <*2.24*> $E^{1\%}_{1\,cm}$ (284 nm): 41.0 – 45.0 (10 mg, ethanol (99.5), 100 mL).

Refractive index <*2.45*> n^{20}_{D}: 1.494 – 1.499

Specific gravity <*2.56*> d^{20}_{20}: 0.952 – 0.966

Purity **(1)** Clarity and color of solution—Dissolve 0.10 g of Tocopherol Acetate in 10 mL of ethanol (99.5): the solution is clear, and has no more color than the following control solution.

Control solution: To 0.5 mL of Iron (III) Chloride CS add 0.5 mol/L hydrochloric acid TS to make 100 mL.

(2) Heavy metals <*1.07*>—Carbonize 1.0 g of Tocopherol Acetate by gentle heating. Cool, add 10 mL of a solution of magnesium nitrate hexahydrate in ethanol (95) (1 in 10), and ignite the ethanol to burn. Cool, add 1 mL of sulfuric acid, proceed according to Method 4, and perform the test. Prepare the control solution with 2.0 mL of Standard Lead Solution (20 ppm).

(3) α-Tocopherol—Dissolve 0.10 g of Tocopherol Acetate in exactly 10 mL of hexane, and use this solution as the sample solution. Separately, dissolve 50 mg of Tocopherol RS in hexane to make exactly 100 mL. Pipet 1 mL of this solution, add hexane to make exactly 10 mL, and use this solution as the standard solution. Perform the test with these solutions as directed under Thin-layer Chromatography <*2.03*>. Spot 10 μL each of the sample solution and standard solution on a plate of silica gel for thin-layer chromatography. Develop the plate with a mixture of toluene and acetic acid (100) (19:1) to a distance of about 10 cm, and air-dry the plate. Spray evenly a solution of iron (III) chloride hexahydrate in ethanol (99.5) (1 in 500) on the plate, then spray evenly a solution of 2,2′-bipyridyl in ethanol (99.5) (1 in 200) on the same plate, and allow to stand for 2 to 3 minutes: the spot obtained from the sample solution corresponding to that from the standard solution is not larger and not more intense than the spot from the standard solution.

Assay Dissolve 50 mg each of Tocopherol Acetate and Tocopherol Acetate RS, accurately weighed, in ethanol (99.5) to make exactly 50 mL, and use these solutions as the sample solution and standard solution. Perform the test with exactly 20 μL each of these solutions as directed under Liquid Chromatography <*2.01*> according to the following conditions, and determine the peak heights, H_T and H_S, of tocopherol acetate in each solution.

$$\text{Amount (mg) of tocopherol acetate } (C_{31}H_{52}O_3) = M_S \times H_T/H_S$$

M_S: Amount (mg) of Tocopherol Acetate RS taken

Operating conditions—

Detector: An ultraviolet absorption photometer (wavelength: 284 nm).

Column: A stainless steel column 4.6 mm in inside diameter and 15 cm in length, packed with octadecylsilanized silica gel (5 μm in particle diameter).

Column temperature: A constant temperature of about 35°C.

Mobile phase: A mixture of methanol and water (49:1).

Flow rate: Adjust so that the retention time of tocopherol acetate is about 12 minutes.

System suitability—

System performance: Dissolve 0.05 g each of Tocopherol Acetate and tocopherol in 50 mL of ethanol (99.5). When the procedure is run with 20 μL of this solution under the above operating conditions, tocopherol and tocopherol acetate are eluted in this order with the resolution between these peaks being not less than 2.6.

System repeatability: When the test is repeated 5 times with 20 μL of the standard solution under the above operating conditions, the relative standard deviation of the peak heights of tocopherol acetate is not more than 0.8%.

Containers and storage Containers—Tight containers.

Storage—Light-resistant.

Tocopherol Calcium Succinate

Vitamin E Calcium Succinate

トコフェロールコハク酸エステルカルシウム

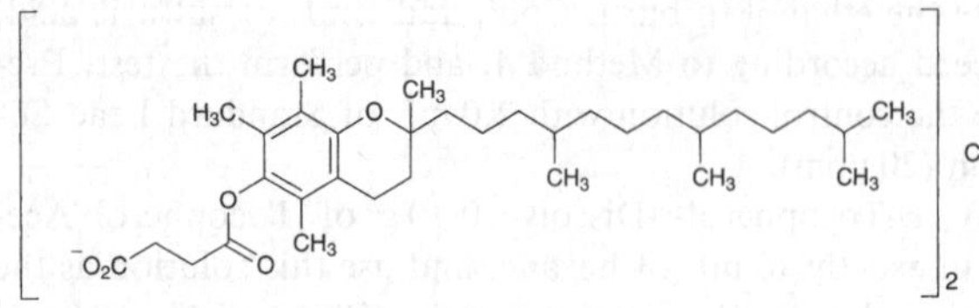

$C_{66}H_{106}CaO_{10}$: 1099.62

Monocalcium bis{3-[2,5,7,8-tetramethyl-2-(4,8,12-trimethyltridecyl)chroman-6-yloxycarbonyl]propanoate}

[*14638-18-7*]

Tocopherol Calcium Succinate, when dried, contains not less than 96.0% and not more than 102.0% of *dl*-α-tocopherol calcium succinate ($C_{66}H_{106}CaO_{10}$).

Description Tocopherol Calcium Succinate occurs as a white to yellowish white powder. It is odorless.

It is freely soluble in chloroform and in carbon tetrachloride, and practically insoluble in water, in ethanol (95) and in acetone.

Shake 1 g of Tocopherol Calcium Succinate with 7 mL of acetic acid (100): it dissolves, and produces a turbidity after being allowed to stand for a while.

It dissolves in acetic acid (100).

It is optically inactive.

Identification **(1)** Dissolve 0.05 g of Tocopherol Calcium Succinate in 1 mL of acetic acid (100), add 9 mL of ethanol (99.5), and mix. To this solution add 2 mL of fuming nitric acid, and heat at 75°C for 15 minutes: a red to orange color develops.

(2) Dissolve 0.08 g of Tocopherol Calcium Succinate, previously dried, in 0.2 mL of carbon tetrachloride. Determine the infrared absorption spectrum of the solution as directed in the liquid film method under Infrared Spectrophotometry *<2.25>*, and compare the spectrum with the Reference Spectrum: both spectra exhibit similar intensities of absorption at the same wave numbers.

(3) Dissolve 5 g of Tocopherol Calcium Succinate in 30 mL of chloroform, add 10 mL of hydrochloric acid, shake for 10 minutes, then draw off the water layer, and neutralize with ammonia TS: the solution responds to Qualitative Tests *<1.09>* for calcium salt.

Absorbance *<2.24>* $E^{1\%}_{1\,cm}$ (286 nm): 36.0 – 40.0 (10 mg, chloroform, 100 mL).

Purity **(1)** Clarity and color of solution—Dissolve 0.10 g of Tocopherol Calcium Succinate in 10 mL of chloroform: the solution is clear, and has no more color than the following control solution.

Control solution: To 0.5 mL of Iron (III) Chloride CS add 0.5 mol/L hydrochloric acid TS to make 100 mL.

(2) Alkalinity—To 0.20 g of Tocopherol Calcium Succinate add 10 mL of diethyl ether, 2 mL of water, 1 drop of phenolphthalein TS and 0.10 mL of 0.1 mol/L hydrochloric acid VS, and shake: no red color develops in the water layer.

(3) Chloride *<1.03>*—Dissolve 0.10 g of Tocopherol Calcium Succinate in 4 mL of acetic acid (100), add 20 mL of water and 50 mL of diethyl ether, shake thoroughly, and collect the water layer. To the diethyl ether layer add 10 mL of water, shake, and collect the water layer. Combine the water layers, add 6 mL of dilute nitric acid and water to make 50 mL, and perform the test using this solution as the test solution. Prepare the control solution in the same manner using 0.60 mL of 0.01 mol/L hydrochloric acid VS in place of Tocopherol Calcium Succinate (not more than 0.212%).

(4) Heavy metals *<1.07>*—Proceed with 1.0 g of Tocopherol Calcium Succinate according to Method 4, and perform the test. Prepare the control solution with 2.0 mL of Standard Lead Solution (not more than 20 ppm).

(5) Arsenic *<1.11>*—Prepare the test solution with 1.0 g of Tocopherol Calcium Succinate according to Method 3, and perform the test (not more than 2 ppm).

(6) α-Tocopherol—Dissolve 0.10 g of Tocopherol Calcium Succinate in exactly 10 mL of chloroform, and use this solution as the sample solution. Separately, dissolve 50 mg of Tocopherol RS in chloroform to make exactly 100 mL. Pipet 1 mL of this solution, add chloroform to make exactly 10 mL, and use this solution as the standard solution. Perform the test with these solutions as directed under Thin-layer Chromatography *<2.03>*. Spot 10 μL each of the sample solution and standard solution on a plate of silica gel for thin-layer chromatography. Develop the plate with a mixture of toluene and acetic acid (100) (19:1) to a distance of about 10 cm, and air-dry the plate. Spray evenly a solution of iron (III) chloride hexahydrate in ethanol (99.5) (1 in 500) on the plate, then spray evenly a solution of 2,2′-bipyridyl in ethanol (99.5) (1 in 200) on the same plate, and allow to stand for 2 to 3 minutes: the spots obtained from the sample solution corresponding to the spots from the standard solution is not larger and not more intense than the spots from the standard solution.

Loss on drying *<2.41>* Not more than 2.0% (1 g, in vacuum, phosphorus (V) oxide, 24 hours).

Assay Weigh accurately about 50 mg each of Tocopherol Calcium Succinate and Tocopherol Succinate RS, previously dried, dissolve in a mixture of ethanol (99.5) and diluted acetic acid (100) (1 in 5) (9:1) to make exactly 50 mL, and use these solutions as the sample solution and standard solution. Pipet exactly 20 μL each of the sample solution and standard solution, and perform the test as directed under Liquid Chromatography *<2.01>* according to the following operating conditions. Determine the peak heights, H_T and H_S, of tocopherol succinate in each solution.

Amount (mg) of tocopherol calcium succinate ($C_{66}H_{106}CaO_{10}$)

$$= M_S \times H_T/H_S \times 1.036$$

M_S: Amount (mg) of Tocopherol Succinate RS taken

Operating conditions—

Detector: An ultraviolet absorption photometer (wavelength: 284 nm).

Column: A stainless steel column about 4 mm in inside diameter and 15 to 30 cm in length, packed with octadecylsilanized silica gel (5 to 10 μm in particle diameter).

Column temperature: Room temperature.

Mobile phase: A mixture of methanol, water and acetic acid (100) (97:2:1).

Flow rate: Adjust so that the retention time of tocopherol succinate is about 8 minutes.

Selection of column: Dissolve 0.05 g each of tocopherol succinate and tocopherol in 50 mL of a mixture of ethanol (99.5) and diluted acetic acid (100) (1 in 5) (9:1). Proceed with 20 μL of this solution under the above operating conditions, and calculate the resolution. Use a column giving elution of tocopherol succinate and tocopherol in this order with the resolution between these peaks being not less than 2.0.

System repeatability: Repeat the test 5 times with 20 μL of the standard solution under the above operating conditions: the relative standard deviation of the peak height of tocopherol succinate is not more than 0.8%.

Containers and storage Containers—Tight containers.

Storage—Light-resistant.

Tocopherol Nicotinate

Vitamin E Nicotinate

トコフェロールニコチン酸エステル

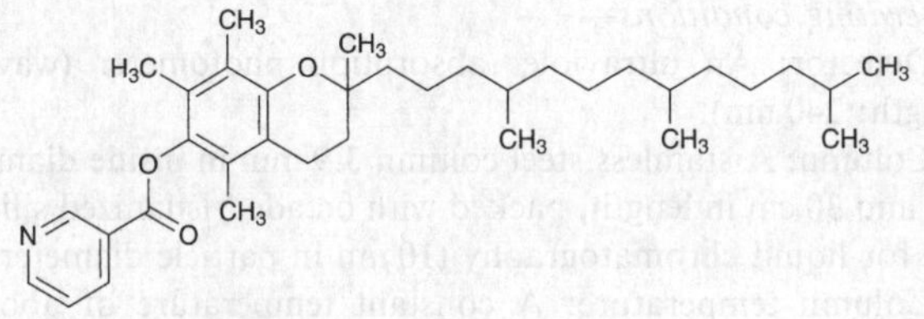

$C_{35}H_{53}NO_3$: 535.80

2,5,7,8-Tetramethyl-2-(4,8,12-trimethyltridecyl)chroman-6-yl nicotinate

[51898-34-1]

Tocopherol Nicotinate contains not less than 96.0% of *dl*-α-tocopherol nicotinate ($C_{35}H_{53}NO_3$).

Description Tocopherol Nicotinate occurs as a yellow to orange-yellow, liquid or solid.

It is freely soluble in ethanol (99.5), and practically insoluble in water.

A solution of Tocopherol Nicotinate in ethanol (99.5) (1 in 10) shows no optical rotation.

It is affected by light.

Identification **(1)** Determine the absorption spectrum of a solution of Tocopherol Nicotinate in ethanol (99.5) (1 in 20,000) as directed under Ultraviolet-visible Spectrophotometry *<2.24>*, and compare the spectrum with the Reference Spectrum or the spectrum of a solution of Tocopherol Nicotinate RS prepared in the same manner as the sample solution: both spectra exhibit similar intensities of absorption at the same wavelengths.

(2) Determine the infrared spectrum of Tocopherol Nicotinate, if necessary melt by warming, as directed in the liquid film method under the Infrared Spectrophotometry *<2.25>*, and compare the spectrum with the Reference Spectrum or the spectrum of Tocopherol Nicotinate RS: both spectra exhibit similar intensities of absorption at the same wave numbers.

Purity **(1)** Heavy metals *<1.07>*—Proceed with 1.0 g of Tocopherol Nicotinate according to Method 4, and perform the test. Prepare the control solution with 2.0 mL of Standard Lead Solution (not more than 20 ppm).

(2) Arsenic *<1.11>*—Prepare the test solution with 1.0 g of Tocopherol Nicotinate according to Method 4, and perform the test (not more than 2 ppm).

(3) Related substances—Dissolve 0.05 g of Tocopherol Nicotinate in 50 mL of ethanol (99.5), and use this solution as the sample solution. Pipet 7 mL of the sample solution, add ethanol (99.5) to make exactly 200 mL, and use this solution as the standard solution. Perform the test with exactly 10 μL each of the sample solution and standard solution as directed under Liquid Chromatography *<2.01>* according to the following conditions. Determine each peak area by the automatic integration method: the total area of the peaks other than tocopherol nicotinate obtained from the sample solution is not larger than the peak area of tocopherol nicotinate from the standard solution, and the area of a peak which has a retention time 0.8 to 0.9 times that of tocopherol nicotinate from the sample solution is not larger than 4/7 times the peak area of tocopherol nicotinate from the standard solution.

Operating conditions—

Detector, column, and column temperature: Proceed as directed in the operating conditions in the Assay.

Mobile phase: A mixture of methanol and water (19:1).

Flow rate: Adjust so that the retention time of tocopherol nicotinate is about 20 minutes.

Time span of measurement: About 1.5 times as long as the retention time of tocopherol nicotinate, beginning after the solvent peak.

System suitability—

Test for required detectability: To exactly 1 mL of the sample solution add ethanol (99.5) to make exactly 100 mL, and use this solution as the solution for system suitability test. Pipet 1 mL of the solution for system suitability test, add ethanol (99.5) to make exactly 10 mL. Confirm that the peak area of tocopherol nicotinate obtained with 10 μL of this solution is equivalent to 7 to 13% of that with 10 μL of the solution for system suitability test.

System performance: Dissolve 0.05 g of Tocopherol Nicotinate and 0.25 g of tocopherol in 100 mL of ethanol (99.5). When the procedure is run with 10 μL of this solution under the above operating conditions, tocopherol and tocopherol nicotinate are eluted in this order with the resolution between these peaks being not less than 8.

System repeatability: When the test is repeated 6 times with 10 μL of the standard solution under the above operating conditions, the relative standard deviation of the peak areas of tocopherol nicotinate is not more than 2.0%.

Assay Weigh accurately about 50 mg each of Tocopherol Nicotinate and Tocopherol Nicotinate RS, dissolve each in ethanol (99.5) to make exactly 50 mL, and use these solutions as the sample solution and the standard solution, respectively. Perform the test with exactly 5 μL each of the sample solution and standard solution as directed under Liquid Chromatography *<2.01>* according to the following conditions, and determine the peak areas, A_T and A_S, of tocopherol nicotinate in each solution.

$$\text{Amount (mg) of tocopherol nicotinate } (C_{35}H_{53}NO_3) = M_S \times A_T/A_S$$

M_S: Amount (mg) of Tocopherol Nicotinate RS taken

Operating conditions—

Detector: An ultraviolet absorption photometer (wavelength: 264 nm).

Column: A stainless steel column 4.6 mm in inside diameter and 15 cm in length, packed with octadecylsilanized silica

gel for liquid chromatography (5 μm in particle diameter).

Column temperature: A constant temperature of about 35°C.

Mobile phase: Methanol.

Flow rate: Adjust so that the retention time of tocopherol nicotinate is about 10 minutes.

System suitability—

System performance: Dissolve 0.05 g of Tocopherol Nicotinate and 0.25 g of tocopherol in 100 mL of ethanol (99.5). When the procedure is run with 5 μL of this solution under the above operating conditions, tocopherol and tocopherol nicotinate are eluted in this order with the resolution between these peaks being not less than 3.

System repeatability: When the test is repeated 6 times with 5 μL of the standard solution under the above operating conditions: the relative standard deviation of the peak areas of tocopherol nicotinate is not more than 0.8%

Containers and storage Containers—Tight containers.

Storage—Light-resistant.

Todralazine Hydrochloride Hydrate

トドララジン塩酸塩水和物

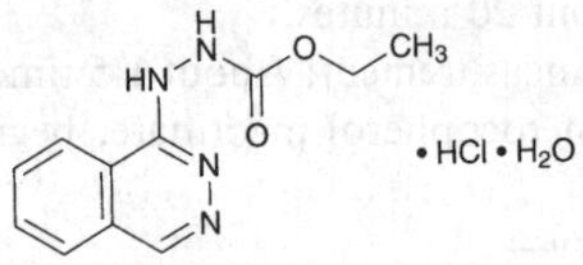

$C_{11}H_{12}N_4O_2.HCl.H_2O$: 286.71

Ethyl 2-(phthalazin-1-yl)hydrazinecarboxylate monohydrochloride monohydrate

[*3778-76-5*, anhydride]

Todralazine Hydrochloride Hydrate contains not less than 98.5% of todralazine hydrochloride ($C_{11}H_{12}N_4O_2.HCl$: 268.70), calculated on the anhydrous basis.

Description Todralazine Hydrochloride Hydrate occurs as white, crystals or crystalline powder. It has a slight, characteristic odor, and has a bitter taste.

It is very soluble in formic acid, freely soluble in methanol, soluble in water, sparingly soluble in ethanol (95), and practically insoluble in diethyl ether.

The pH of a solution of 1.0 g of Todralazine Hydrochloride Hydrate in 200 mL of water is between 3.0 and 4.0.

Identification **(1)** To 2 mL of a solution of Todralazine Hydrochloride Hydrate (1 in 200) add 5 mL of silver nitrate-ammonia TS: the solution becomes turbid, and a black precipitate is formed.

(2) Determine the absorption spectrum of a solution of Todralazine Hydrochloride Hydrate in 0.1 mol/L hydrochloric acid TS (3 in 100,000) as directed under Ultraviolet-visible Spectrophotometry *<2.24>*, and compare the spectrum with the Reference Spectrum: both spectra exhibit similar intensities of absorption at the same wavelengths.

(3) Determine the infrared absorption spectrum of Todralazine Hydrochloride Hydrate as directed in the potassium chloride disk method under the Infrared Spectrophotometry *<2.25>*, and compare the spectrum with the Reference Spectrum: both spectra exhibit similar intensities of absorption at the same wave numbers.

(4) A solution of Todralazine Hydrochloride Hydrate (1 in 50) responds to Qualitative Tests *<1.09>* (1) for chloride.

Purity **(1)** Clarity and color of solution—Dissolve 0.30 g of Todralazine Hydrochloride Hydrate in 10 mL of water: the solution is clear and colorless to pale yellow.

(2) Sulfate *<1.14>*—Proceed the test with 2.0 g of Todralazine Hydrochloride Hydrate. Prepare the control solution with 0.50 mL of 0.005 mol/L sulfuric acid VS (not more than 0.012%).

(3) Heavy metals *<1.07>*—Proceed with 1.0 g of Todralazine Hydrochloride Hydrate according to Method 2, and perform the test. Prepare the control solution with 2.0 mL of Standard Lead Solution (not more than 20 ppm).

(4) Arsenic *<1.11>*—Prepare the test solution with 1.0 g of Todralazine Hydrochloride Hydrate according to Method 1, and perform the test (not more than 2 ppm).

(5) Related substances—Dissolve 50 mg of Todralazine Hydrochloride Hydrate in 100 mL of the mobile phase, and use this solution as the sample solution. Pipet 1 mL of the sample solution, add the mobile phase to make exactly 200 mL, and use this solution as the standard solution. Perform the test with exactly 10 μL each of the sample solution and standard solution as directed under Liquid Chromatography *<2.01>* according to the following conditions. Determine each peak area by the automatic integration method: the total area of the peaks other than todralazine obtained from the sample solution is not larger than the peak area of todralazine from the standard solution.

Operating conditions—

Detector: An ultraviolet absorption photometer (wavelength: 240 nm).

Column: A stainless steel column 3.9 mm in inside diameter and 30 cm in length, packed with octadecylsilanized silica gel for liquid chromatography (10 μm in particle diameter).

Column temperature: A constant temperature of about 25°C.

Mobile phase: Dissolve 1.10 g of sodium 1-heptane sulfonate in 1000 mL of diluted methanol (2 in 5). Adjust the pH of the solution to between 3.0 and 3.5 with acetic acid (100).

Flow rate: Adjust so that the retention time of todralazine is about 8 minutes.

Time span of measurement: About twice as long as the retention time of todralazine, beginning after the solvent peak.

System suitability—

Test for required detectability: To exactly 5 mL of the standard solution add the mobile phase to make exactly 25 mL. Confirm that the peak area of todralazine obtained with 10 μL of this solution is equivalent to 15 to 25% of that with 10 μL of the standard solution.

System performance: Dissolve 5 mg each of Todralazine Hydrochloride Hydrate and potassium hydrogen phthalate in 100 mL of the mobile phase. When the procedure is run with 10 μL of this solution under the above operating conditions, phthalic acid and todralazine are eluted in this order with the resolution between these peaks being not less than 8.

System repeatability: When the test is repeated 6 times with 10 μL of the standard solution under the above operating conditions, the relative standard deviation of the peak areas of todralazine is not more than 2.0%.

Water *<2.48>* 6.0 – 7.5% (0.5 g, volumetric titration, direct titration).

Residue on ignition *<2.44>* Not more than 0.1% (1 g).

Assay Weigh accurately about 0.4 g of Todralazine Hydrochloride Hydrate, dissolve in 5 mL of formic acid, add 70 mL of acetic anhydride, and titrate *<2.50>* with 0.1 mol/L perchloric acid VS (potentiometric titration). Perform a blank determination in the same manner, and make any necessary correction.

Each mL of 0.1 mol/L perchloric acid VS
= 26.87 mg of $C_{11}H_{12}N_4O_2.HCl$

Containers and storage Containers—Tight containers.

Tofisopam

トフィソパム

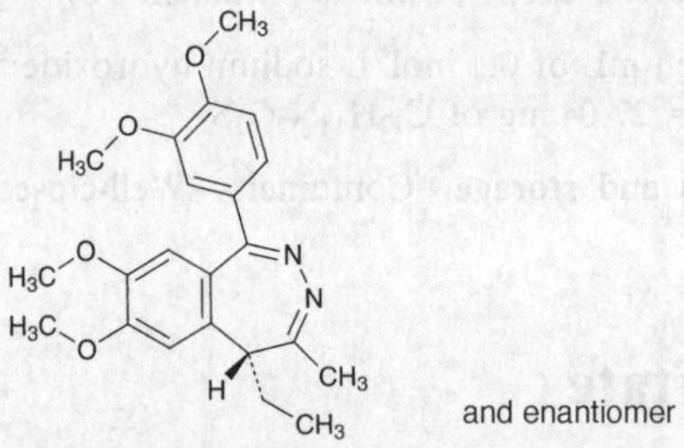

and enantiomer

$C_{22}H_{26}N_2O_4$: 382.45
(5*RS*)-1-(3,4-Dimethoxyphenyl)-5-ethyl-7,8-dimethoxy-4-methyl-5*H*-2,3-benzodiazepine
[*22345-47-7*]

Tofisopam, when dried, contains not less than 98.0% of tofisopam ($C_{22}H_{26}N_2O_4$).

Description Tofisopam occurs as a pale yellow-white crystalline powder.

It is freely soluble in acetic acid (100), soluble in acetone, sparingly soluble in ethanol (95), slightly soluble in diethyl ether, and practically insoluble in water.

A solution of Tofisopam in ethanol (95) (1 in 100) shows no optical rotation.

Identification **(1)** Determine the absorption spectrum of a solution of Tofisopam in ethanol (95) (1 in 100,000) as directed under Ultraviolet-visible Spectrophotometry *<2.24>*, and compare the spectrum with the Reference Spectrum: both spectra exhibit similar intensities of absorption at the same wavelengths.

(2) Determine the infrared absorption spectrum of Tofisopam, previously dried, as directed in the potassium bromide disk method under Infrared Spectrophotometry *<2.25>*, and compare the spectrum with the Reference Spectrum: both spectra exhibit similar intensities of absorption at the same wave numbers.

Melting point *<2.60>* 155 – 159°C

Purity **(1)** Heavy metals *<1.07>*—Proceed with 1.0 g of Tofisopam according to Method 2, and perform the test. Prepare the control solution with 1.0 mL of Standard Lead Solution (not more than 10 ppm).

(2) Arsenic *<1.11>*—Prepare the test solution with 1.0 g of Tofisopam according to Method 3, and perform the test (not more than 2 ppm).

(3) Related substances—Dissolve 0.05 g of Tofisopam in 10 mL of acetone, and use this solution as the sample solution. Pipet 1 mL of the sample solution, add acetone to make exactly 25 mL, pipet 1 mL of this solution, add acetone to make exactly 20 mL, and use this solution as the standard solution. Perform the test with these solutions as directed under Thin-layer Chromatography *<2.03>*. Spot 10 μL each of the sample solution and standard solution on a plate of silica gel with fluorescent indicator for thin-layer chromatography. Develop the plate with a mixture of ethyl acetate, acetone, methanol and formic acid (24:12:2:1) to a distance of about 10 cm, and air-dry the plate. Examine under ultraviolet light (main wavelength: 254 nm): the spots other than the principal spot obtained from the sample solution are not more intense than the spot from the standard solution.

Loss on drying *<2.41>* Not more than 0.5% (1 g, in vacuum, silica gel, 60°C, 3 hours).

Residue on ignition *<2.44>* Not more than 0.1% (1 g).

Assay Weigh accurately about 0.2 g of Tofisopam, previously dried, dissolve in 50 mL of acetic acid (100), and titrate *<2.50>* with 0.1 mol/L perchloric acid VS (potentiometric titration). Perform a blank determination in the same manner, and make any necessary correction.

Each mL of 0.1 mol/L perchloric acid VS
= 38.25 mg of $C_{22}H_{26}N_2O_4$

Containers and storage Containers—Tight containers.
Storage—Light-resistant.

Tolbutamide

トルブタミド

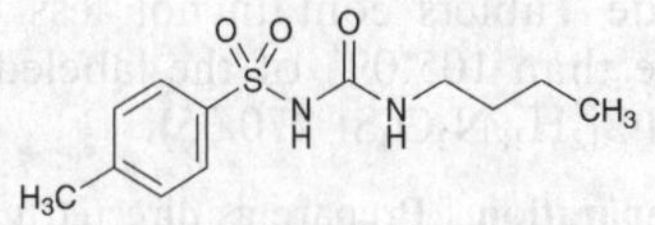

$C_{12}H_{18}N_2O_3S$: 270.35
N-(Butylcarbamoyl)-4-methylbenzenesulfonamide
[*64-77-7*]

Tolbutamide, when dried, contains not less than 99.0% of tolbutamide ($C_{12}H_{18}N_2O_3S$).

Description Tolbutamide occurs as white, crystals or crystalline powder. It is odorless or has a slight, characteristic odor. It is tasteless.

It is soluble in ethanol (95), slightly soluble in diethyl ether, and practically insoluble in water.

Identification **(1)** Boil 0.2 g of Tolbutamide with 8 mL of diluted sulfuric acid (1 in 3) under a reflux condenser for 30 minutes. Cool the solution in ice water, collect the precipitated crystals, recrystallize from water, and dry at 105°C for 3 hours: the crystals melt *<2.60>* between 135°C and 139°C.

(2) Render the filtrate obtained in (1) alkaline with about 20 mL of a solution of sodium hydroxide (1 in 5), and heat: an ammonia-like odor is perceptible.

Melting point *<2.60>* 126 – 132°C

Purity **(1)** Acidity—Warm 3.0 g of Tolbutamide with 150 mL of water at 70°C for 5 minutes, allow to stand for 1 hour in ice water, and filter. To 25 mL of the filtrate add 2 drops of methyl red TS and 0.20 mL of 0.1 mol/L sodium hydroxide VS: a yellow color develops.

(2) Chloride *<1.03>*—To 40 mL of the filtrate obtained in (1) add 6 mL of dilute nitric acid and water to make 50 mL. Perform the test using this solution as the test solution. Prepare the control solution with 0.25 mL of 0.01 mol/L hydrochloric acid VS (not more than 0.011%).

(3) Sulfate *<1.14>*—To 40 mL of the filtrate obtained in (1) add 1 mL of dilute hydrochloric acid and water to make

50 mL. Perform the test using this solution as the test solution. Prepare the control solution with 0.35 mL of 0.005 mol/L sulfuric acid VS (not more than 0.021%).

(4) Heavy metals *<1.07>*—Proceed with 2.0 g of Tolbutamide according to Method 2, and perform the test. Prepare the control solution with 2.0 mL of Standard Lead Solution (not more than 10 ppm).

Loss on drying *<2.41>* Not more than 0.5% (1 g, 105°C, 3 hours).

Residue on ignition *<2.44>* Not more than 0.1% (1 g).

Assay Weigh accurately about 0.5 g of Tolbutamide, previously dried, and dissolve in 30 mL of neutralized ethanol. Add 20 mL of water, and titrate *<2.50>* with 0.1 mol/L sodium hydroxide VS (indicator: 3 drops of phenolphthalein TS).

Each mL of 0.1 mol/L sodium hydroxide VS
= 27.04 mg of $C_{12}H_{18}N_2O_3S$

Containers and storage Containers—Well-closed containers.

Tolbutamide Tablets

トルブタミド錠

Tolbutamide Tablets contain not less than 95.0% and not more than 105.0% of the labeled amount of tolbutamide ($C_{12}H_{18}N_2O_3S$: 270.35).

Method of preparation Prepare as directed under Tablets, with Tolbutamide.

Identification Shake a quantity of powdered Tolbutamide Tablets, equivalent to 0.5 g of Tolbutamide, with 50 mL of chloroform, filter, and evaporate the filtrate to dryness. Proceed with the residue as directed in the Identification under Tolbutamide.

Uniformity of dosage units *<6.02>* It meets the requirement of the Mass variation test.

Dissolution *<6.10>* When the test is performed at 100 revolutions per minute according to the Paddle method, using 900 mL of phosphate buffer solution (pH 7.4) as the dissolution medium, the dissolution rate in 30 minutes of Tolbutamide Tablets is not less than 80%.

Start the test with 1 tablet of Tolbutamide Tablets, withdraw not less than 20 mL of the medium at the specified minute after starting the test, and filter through a membrane filter with a pore size not exceeding 0.8 μm. Discard not less than 10 mL of the first filtrate, pipet V mL of the subsequent filtrate, add water to make exactly V' mL so that each mL contains about 10 μg of tolbutamide ($C_{12}H_{18}N_2O_3S$), and use this solution as the sample solution. Separately, weigh accurately about 50 mg of Tolbutamide RS, previously dried at 105°C for 3 hours, dissolve in 10 mL of methanol, and add the dissolution medium to make exactly 100 mL. Pipet 2 mL of this solution, add water to make exactly 100 mL, and use this solution as the standard solution. Perform the test with the sample solution and standard solution as directed under Ultraviolet-visible Spectrophotometry *<2.24>*, using water as the control, and determine the absorbances, A_T and A_S, at 226 nm.

Dissolution rate (%) with respect to the labeled amount of tolbutamide ($C_{12}H_{18}N_2O_3S$)
$= M_S \times A_T/A_S \times V'/V \times 1/C \times 18$

M_S: Amount (mg) of Tolbutamide RS taken
C: Labeled amount (mg) of tolbutamide ($C_{12}H_{18}N_2O_3S$) in 1 tablet

Assay Weigh accurately and powder not less than 20 Tolbutamide Tablets. Weigh accurately a portion of the powder, equivalent to about 0.5 g of tolbutamide ($C_{12}H_{18}N_2O_3S$), dissolve in 50 mL of neutralized ethanol, add 25 mL of water, and titrate *<2.50>* with 0.1 mol/L sodium hydroxide VS (indicator: 3 drops of phenolphthalein TS).

Each mL of 0.1 mol/L sodium hydroxide VS
= 27.04 mg of $C_{12}H_{18}N_2O_3S$

Containers and storage Containers—Well-closed containers.

Tolnaftate

トルナフタート

$C_{19}H_{17}NOS$: 307.41
O-Naphthalen-2-yl *N*-methyl-*N*-(3-methylphenyl)thiocarbamate
[2398-96-1]

Tolnaftate, when dried, contains not less than 98.0% of tolnaftate ($C_{19}H_{17}NOS$).

Description Tolnaftate occurs as a white powder. It is odorless.

It is freely soluble in chloroform, sparingly soluble in diethyl ether, slightly soluble in methanol and in ethanol (95), and practically insoluble in water.

Identification **(1)** To 0.2 g of Tolnaftate add 20 mL of potassium hydroxide-ethanol TS and 5 mL of water, and heat under a reflux condenser for 3 hours. After cooling, to 10 mL of this solution add 2 mL of acetic acid (100), and shake with 1 mL of lead (II) acetate TS: a black precipitate is formed.

(2) Determine the absorption spectrum of a solution of Tolnaftate in methanol (1 in 100,000) as directed under Ultraviolet-visible Spectrophotometry *<2.24>*, and compare the spectrum with the Reference Spectrum or the spectrum of a solution of Tolnaftate RS prepared in the same manner as the sample solution: both spectra exhibit similar intensities of absorption at the same wavelengths.

(3) Determine the infrared absorption spectrum of Tolnaftate, previously dried, as directed in the potassium bromide disk method under Infrared Spectrophotometry *<2.25>*, and compare the spectrum with the Reference Spectrum or the spectrum of previously dried Tolnaftate RS: both spectra exhibit similar intensities of absorption at the same wave numbers.

Melting point *<2.60>* 111 – 114°C (after drying).

Purity **(1)** Heavy metals *<1.07>*—Carbonize 1.0 g of Tolnaftate by gentle heating. After cooling, add 5 mL of nitric acid and 1 mL of sulfuric acid, and heat until white fumes are evolved. After cooling, add 2 mL of nitric acid, and heat until white fumes are evolved. After cooling, add 2 mL of nitric acid and 0.5 mL of perchloric acid, and heat gradually until white fumes are evolved. Repeat this procedure twice, and heat until white fumes are no longer evolved. Incinerate the residue by igniting between 500°C and 600°C for 1 hour. Proceed according to Method 2, and perform the test with 50 mL of the test solution so obtained. Prepare the control solution as follows: to 11 mL of nitric acid add 1 mL of sulfuric acid, 1 mL of perchloric acid and 2 mL of hydrochloric acid, proceed in the same manner as the test solution, and add 2.0 mL of Standard Lead Solution and water to make 50 mL (not more than 20 ppm).

(2) Related substances—Dissolve 0.50 g of Tolnaftate in 10 mL of chloroform, and use this solution as the sample solution. Pipet 2 mL of the sample solution, and add chloroform to make exactly 100 mL. Pipet 5 mL of this solution, add chloroform to make exactly 100 mL, and use this solution as the standard solution. Perform the test with these solutions as directed under Thin-layer Chromatography <*2.03*>. Spot 10 μL each of the sample solution and standard solution on a plate of silica gel with fluorescent indicator for thin-layer chromatography. Develop the plate with toluene to a distance of about 10 cm, and air-dry the plate. Allow the plate to stand in iodine vapor for 5 minutes, and examine under ultraviolet light (wavelength: 254 nm): the spots other than the principal spot obtained from the sample solution are not more intense than the spot from the standard solution.

Loss on drying <*2.41*> Not more than 0.5% (1 g, in vacuum at a pressure not exceeding 0.67 kPa, 65°C, 3 hours).

Residue on ignition <*2.44*> Weigh accurately about 2 g of Tolnaftate, and carbonize by gradual heating. Moisten the substance with 1 mL of sulfuric acid, heat gradually until white fumes are no longer evolved, and ignite between 450°C and 550°C for about 2 hours to constant mass: the residue is not more than 0.1%.

Assay Weigh accurately about 50 mg of Tolnaftate and Tolnaftate RS, previously dried, dissolve each in 200 mL of methanol by warming in a water bath, cool, and add methanol to make exactly 250 mL. Pipet 5 mL each of the solutions, to each add methanol to make exactly 100 mL, and use these solutions as the sample solution and the standard solution, respectively. Determine the absorbances, A_T and A_S, of the sample solution and standard solution at 257 nm as directed under Ultraviolet-visible Spectrophotometry <*2.24*>.

Amount (mg) of tolnaftate ($C_{19}H_{17}NOS$) = $M_S \times A_T/A_S$

M_S: Amount (mg) of Tolnaftate RS taken

Containers and storage Containers—Tight containers.

Tolnaftate Solution

トルナフタート液

Tolnaftate Solution contains not less than 90.0% and not more than 110.0% of the labeled amount of tolnaftate ($C_{19}H_{17}NOS$: 307.41).

Method of preparation Prepare as directed under Liquids and Solutions for Cutaneous Application, with Tolnaftate.

Identification **(1)** Spot 1 drop of Tolnaftate Solution on filter paper. Spray hydrogen hexachloroplatinate (IV)-potassium iodide TS on the paper: a light yellow color develops in the spot.

(2) To a volume of Tolnaftate Solution, equivalent to 0.02 g of Tolnaftate, add chloroform to make 10 mL, and use this solution as the sample solution. Separately, dissolve 0.02 g of Tolnaftate RS in 10 mL of chloroform, and use this solution as the standard solution. Perform the test with these solutions as directed under Thin-layer Chromatography <*2.03*>. Spot 10 μL each of the sample solution and standard solution on a plate of silica gel with fluorescent indicator for thin-layer chromatography. Develop the plate with toluene to a distance of about 12 cm, and air-dry the plate. Examine under ultraviolet light (main wavelength: 254 nm): the spot obtained from the sample solution and that from the standard solution show the same *Rf* value.

Assay Pipet a volume of Tolnaftate Solution, equivalent to about 20 mg of tolnaftate ($C_{19}H_{17}NOS$), add exactly 4 mL of the internal standard solution, then add chloroform to make 50 mL, and use this solution as the sample solution. Separately, weigh accurately about 0.4 g of Tolnaftate RS, previously dried in vacuum at a pressure not exceeding 0.67 kPa at 65°C for 3 hours, and dissolve in chloroform to make exactly 100 mL. Pipet 5 mL of this solution, add exactly 4 mL of the internal standard solution, then add chloroform to make 50 mL, and use this solution as the standard solution. Perform the test with 10 μL each of the sample solution and standard solution as directed under Liquid Chromatography <*2.01*> according to the following conditions, and calculate the ratios, Q_T and Q_S, of the peak area of tolnaftate to that of the internal standard.

Amount (mg) of tolnaftate ($C_{19}H_{17}NOS$)
$= M_S \times Q_T/Q_S \times 1/20$

M_S: Amount (mg) of Tolnaftate RS taken

Internal standard solution—A solution of diphenyl phthalate in chloroform (3 in 200).

Operating conditions—

Detector: An ultraviolet absorption photometer (wavelength: 254 nm).

Column: A stainless steel column about 4 mm in inside diameter and 15 to 30 cm in length, packed with octadecylsilanized silica gel for liquid chromatography (5 to 10 μm in particle diameter).

Column temperature: A constant temperature of about 25°C.

Mobile phase: A mixture of methanol and water (7:3).

Flow rate: Adjust so that the retention time of tolnaftate is about 14 minutes.

Selection of column: Proceed with 10 μL of the standard solution under the above operating conditions, and calculate the resolution. Use a column giving elution of the internal standard and tolnaftate in this order with the resolution between these peaks being not less than 5.

Containers and storage Containers—Tight containers.

Tolperisone Hydrochloride

トルペリゾン塩酸塩

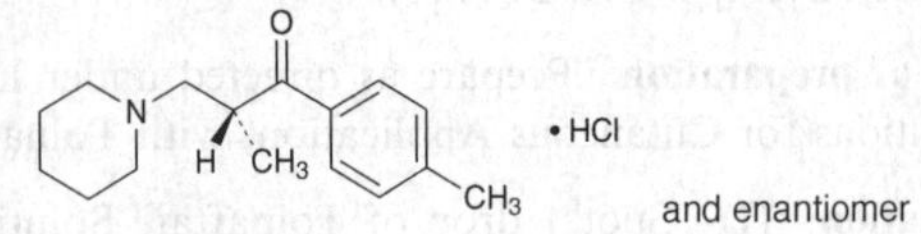

and enantiomer

$C_{16}H_{23}NO.HCl$: 281.82
(2*RS*)-2-Methyl-1-(4-methylphenyl)-3-piperidin-1-ylpropan-1-one monohydrochloride
[*3644-61-9*]

Tolperisone Hydrochloride, when dried, contains not less than 98.5% of tolperisone hydrochloride ($C_{16}H_{23}NO.HCl$).

Description Tolperisone Hydrochloride occurs as a white crystalline powder. It has a slight, characteristic odor.

It is very soluble in acetic acid (100), freely soluble in water and in ethanol (95), soluble in acetic anhydride, slightly soluble in acetone, and practically insoluble in diethyl ether.

The pH of a solution of 1.0 g of Tolperisone Hydrochloride in 20 mL of water is between 4.5 and 5.5.

It is hygroscopic.

Melting point: 167 – 174°C

Identification **(1)** Dissolve 0.2 g of Tolperisone Hydrochloride in 2 mL of ethanol (95), add 2 mL of 1,3-dinitrobenzene TS and 2 mL of sodium hydroxide TS, and heat: a red color develops.

(2) To 5 mL of a solution of Tolperisone Hydrochloride (1 in 20) add 2 to 3 drops of iodine TS: a red-brown precipitate is produced.

(3) Dissolve 0.5 g of Tolperisone Hydrochloride in 5 mL of water, add 2 mL of ammonia TS, and filter. Acidify 5 mL of the filtrate with dilute nitric acid: the solution responds to Qualitative Tests <*1.09*> for chloride.

Absorbance <*2.24*> $E^{1\%}_{1\,cm}$ (257 nm): 555 – 585 (after drying, 5 mg, ethanol (95), 500 mL).

Purity **(1)** Clarity and color of solution—Dissolve 1.0 g of Tolperisone Hydrochloride in 10 mL of water: the solution is clear and colorless.

(2) Sulfate <*1.14*>—Perform the test with 4.0 g of Tolperisone Hydrochloride. Prepare the control solution with 0.40 mL of 0.005 mol/L sulfuric acid VS (not more than 0.005%).

(3) Heavy metals <*1.07*>—Proceed with 1.0 g of Tolperisone Hydrochloride according to Method 2, and perform the test. Prepare the control solution with 2.0 mL of Standard Lead Solution (not more than 20 ppm).

(4) Piperidine hydrochloride—Dissolve 0.20 g of Tolperisone Hydrochloride in water to make exactly 10 mL, and use this solution as the sample solution. Separately, dissolve 20 mg of piperidine hydrochloride in water to make exactly 1000 mL, and use this solution as the standard solution. Transfer 5.0 mL each of the sample solution and standard solution to different separators, add 0.1 mL each of a solution of copper (II) sulfate pentahydrate (1 in 20), then add 0.1 mL each of ammonia solution (28) and exactly 10 mL each of a mixture of isooctane and carbon disulfide (3:1), and shake vigorously for 30 minutes. Immediately after allowing to stand, separate the isooctane-carbon disulfide mixture layer, and dehydrate with anhydrous sodium sulfate. Perform the test with these solutions as directed under Ultraviolet-visible Spectrophotometry <*2.24*>: the absorbance of the sample solution at 438 nm is not more than that of the standard solution.

Loss on drying <*2.41*> Not more than 0.5% (1 g, in vacuum, silica gel, 3 hours).

Residue on ignition <*2.44*> Not more than 0.1% (1 g).

Assay Weigh accurately about 0.5 g of Tolperisone Hydrochloride, previously dried, dissolve in 70 mL of a mixture of acetic anhydride and acetic acid (100) (7:3), and titrate <*2.50*> with 0.1 mol/L perchloric acid VS (potentiometric titration). Perform a blank determination in the same manner, and make any necessary correction.

Each mL of 0.1 mol/L perchloric acid VS
= 28.18 mg $C_{16}H_{23}NO.HCl$

Containers and storage Containers—Well-closed containers.

Tosufloxacin Tosilate Hydrate

トスフロキサシントシル酸塩水和物

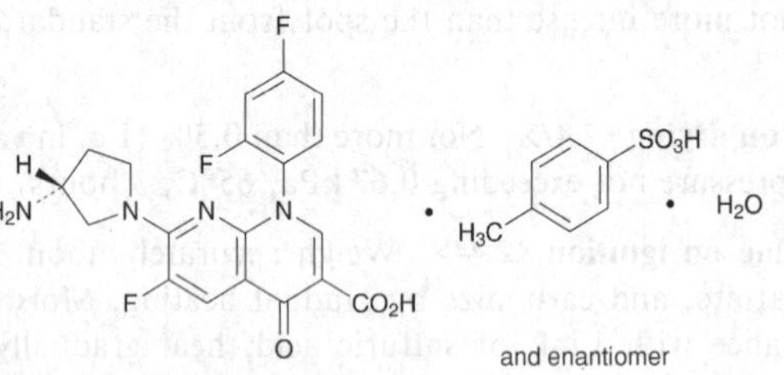

and enantiomer

$C_{19}H_{15}F_{3}N_{4}O_{3}.C_{7}H_{8}O_{3}S.H_{2}O$: 594.56
7-[(3*RS*)-3-Aminopyrrolidin-1-yl]-1-(2,4-difluorophenyl)-6-fluoro-4-oxo-1,4-dihydro-1,8-naphthyridine-3-carboxylic acid mono-4-toluenesulfonate monohydrate
[*115964-29-9*, anhydride]

Tosufloxacin Tosilate Hydrate contains not less than 98.5% and not more than 101.0% of tosufloxacin tosilate ($C_{19}H_{15}F_{3}N_{4}O_{3}.C_{7}H_{8}O_{3}S$: 576.54), calculated on the anhydrous basis.

Description Tosufloxacin Tosilate Hydrate occurs as a white to pale yellowish white crystalline powder.

It is freely soluble in *N*,*N*-dimethylformamide, sparingly soluble in methanol, and practically insoluble in water and in ethanol (99.5).

A solution of Tosufloxacin Tosilate Hydrate in methanol (1 in 100) shows no optical rotation.

Melting point: about 254°C (with decomposition).

Identification **(1)** Tosufloxacin Tosilate Hydrate shows a light bluish-white fluorescence under ultraviolet light (main wavelength 254 nm).

(2) Proceed 10 mg of Tosufloxacin Tosilate Hydrate as directed under Oxygen Flask Combustion Method <*1.06*>, using a mixture of 0.5 mL of 0.01 mol/L sodium hydroxide TS and 20 mL of water as the absorbing liquid: the solution responds to Qualitative Tests <*1.09*> (2) for fluoride.

(3) Determine the absorption spectrum of a solution of Tosufloxacin Tosilate Hydrate in a mixture of methanol and sodium hydroxide TS (49:1) (1 in 100,000) as directed under

Ultraviolet-visible Spectrophotometry <*2.24*>, and compare the spectrum with the Reference Spectrum or the spectrum of a solution of Tosufloxacin Tosilate RS prepared in the same manner as the sample solution: both spectra exhibit similar intensities of absorption at the same wavelengths.

(4) Determine the infrared absorption spectrum of Tosufloxacin Tosilate Hydrate as directed in the paste method under Infrared Spectrophotometry <*2.25*>, and compare the spectrum with the Reference Spectrum or the spectrum of Tosufloxacin Tosilate RS: both spectra exhibit similar intensities of absorption at the same wave numbers.

Purity **(1)** Chloride <*1.03*>—Dissolve 1.0 g of Tosufloxacin Tosilate Hydrate in 40 mL of *N,N*-dimethylformamide, and add 6 mL of dilute nitric acid and *N,N*-dimethylformamide to make 50 mL. Perform the test using this solution as the test solution. Prepare the control solution with 0.20 mL of 0.01 mol/L hydrochloric acid VS, 6 mL of dilute nitric acid and *N,N*-dimethylformamide to make 50 mL (not more than 0.007%).

(2) Heavy metals <*1.07*>—Proceed with 1.0 g of Tosufloxacin Tosilate Hydrate according to Method 4, and perform the test. Prepare the control solution with 2.0 mL of Standard Lead Solution (not more than 20 ppm).

(3) Arsenic <*1.11*>—Prepare the test solution with 1.0 g of Tosufloxacin Tosilate Hydrate according to Method 4, and perform the test under the condition of the ignition temperature being between 750°C and 850°C, and add 10 mL of diluted hydrochloric acid to residue (not more than 2 ppm).

(4) Related substances—Dissolve 10 mg of Tosufloxacin Tosilate Hydrate in 12 mL of mobile phase B, add water to make 25 mL, and use this solution as the sample solution. Pipet 5 mL of the sample solution, and add mobile phase A to make exactly 100 mL. Pipet 2 mL of this solution, add mobile phase A to make exactly 50 mL, and use this solution as the standard solution. Perform the test with exactly 20 μL each of the sample solution and standard solution as directed under Liquid Chromatography <*2.01*> according to the following conditions. Determine each peak area by the automatic integration method: the area of each peak other than tosylic acid and tosufloxacin obtained from the sample solution is not larger than 3/4 times the peak area of tosufloxacin from the standard solution, and the total area of the peaks other than tosylic acid and tosufloxacin from the sample solution is not larger than 2.5 times the peak area of tosufloxacin from the standard solution.

Operating conditions—

Detector: An ultraviolet absorption photometer (wavelength: 272 nm).

Column: A stainless steel column 3.0 mm in inside diameter and 15 cm in length, packed with octadecylsilanized silica gel for liquid chromatography (5 μm in particle diameter).

Column temperature: A constant temperature of about 35°C.

Mobile phase A: To 300 to 500 mL of water add slowly 100 mL of methanesulfonic acid under ice-cooling, add slowly 100 mL of triethylamine under ice-cooling too, and add water to make 1000 mL. To 10 mL of this solution add 143 mL of water, 40 mL of acetonitrile and 7 mL of 1 mol/L dipotassium hydrogen phosphate TS for buffer solution.

Mobile phase B: To 300 to 500 mL of water add slowly 100 mL of methanesulfonic acid under ice-cooling, add slowly 100 mL of triethylamine under ice-cooling too, and add water to make 1000 mL. To 10 mL of this solution add 100 mL of acetonitrile, 83 mL of water and 7 mL of 1 mol/L dipotassium hydrogen phosphate TS for buffer solution.

Flowing of mobile phase: Control the gradient by mixing the mobile phases A and B as directed in the following table.

Time after injection of sample (min)	Mobile phase A (vol%)	Mobile phase B (vol%)
0 – 1	100	0
1 – 16	100 → 0	0 → 100
16 – 35	0	100

Flow rate: 0.5 mL per minute.

Time span of measurement: About 5 times as long as the retention time of tosufloxacin.

System suitability—

Test for required detectability: Pipet 5 mL of the standard solution, and add mobile phase A to make exactly 20 mL. Confirm that the peak area of tosufloxacin obtained with 20 μL of this solution is equivalent to 18 to 32% of the peak area of tosufloxacin with 20 μL of the standard solution.

System performance: When the procedure is run with 20 μL of the standard solution under the above operating conditions, the number of theoretical plates and symmetry factor of the peak of tosufloxacin are not less than 10,000 and not more than 1.5, respectively.

System repeatability: When the test is repeated 6 times with 20 μL of the standard solution under the above operating conditions, the relative standard deviation of the peak area of tosufloxacin is not more than 2.0%.

Water <*2.48*> 2.5 – 3.5% (30 mg, coulometric titration).

Assay Weigh accurately about 30 mg each of Tosufloxacin Tosilate Hydrate and Tosufloxacin Tosilate RS (separately determine the water <*2.48*> in the same manner as Tosufloxacin Tosilate Hydrate), and dissolve each in methanol to make exactly 100 mL. Pipet 20 mL each of these solutions, to each add exactly 4 mL of the internal standard solution and methanol to make 100 mL, and use these solutions as the sample solution and the standard solution, respectively. Perform the test with 10 μL each of the sample solution and standard solution as directed under Liquid Chromatography <*2.01*> according to the following conditions, and calculate the ratios, Q_T and Q_S, of the peak area of tosufloxacin to that of the internal standard.

$$\text{Amount (mg) of tosufloxacin tosilate } (C_{19}H_{15}F_3N_4O_3.C_7H_8O_3S) = M_S \times Q_T/Q_S$$

M_S: Amount (mg) of Tosufloxacin Tosilate RS taken, calculated on the anhydrous basis

Internal standard solution—A solution of methyl parahydroxybenzoate in methanol (1 in 800).

Operating conditions—

Detector: An ultraviolet absorption photometer (wavelength: 270 nm).

Column: A stainless steel column 4.6 mm in inside diameter and 15 cm in length, packed with octadecylsilanized silica gel for liquid chromatography (5 μm in particle diameter).

Column temperature: A constant temperature of about 40°C.

Mobile phase: To a mixture of 0.02 mol/L phosphate buffer solution (pH 3.5) and a solution of dibutylamine in methanol (1 in 2500) (3:1) add diluted phosphoric acid (1 in 10) to adjust the pH to 3.5.

Flow rate: Adjust so that the retention time of tosufloxacin is about 20 minutes.

System suitability—

System performance: When the procedure is run with 10

μL of the standard solution under the above operating conditions, the internal standard and tosufloxacin are eluted in this order with the resolution between these peaks being not less than 2.5.

System repeatability: When the test is repeated 6 times with 10 μL of the standard solution under the above operating conditions, the relative standard deviation of the ratio of the peak area of tosufloxacin to that of the internal standard is not more than 1.0%.

Containers and storage Containers—Tight containers.

Tosufloxacin Tosilate Tablets

トスフロキサシントシル酸塩錠

Tosufloxacin Tosilate Tablets contain not less than 95.0% and not more than 105.0% of the labeled amount of tosufloxacin tosilate hydrate ($C_{19}H_{15}F_3N_4O_3.C_7H_8O_3S.H_2O$: 594.56).

Method of preparation Prepare as directed under Tablets, with Tosufloxacin Tosilate Hydrate.

Identification To a quantity of powdered Tosufloxacin Tosilate Tablets, equivalent to 75 mg of Tosufloxacin Tosilate Hydrate, add 200 mL of a mixture of methanol and sodium hydroxide TS (49:1), shake well, and centrifuge. To 2 mL of the supernatant liquid add 100 mL of a mixture of methanol and sodium hydroxide TS (49:1). Determine the absorption spectrum of this solution as directed under Ultraviolet-visible Spectrophotometry <*2.24*>: it exhibits maxima between 260 nm and 264 nm, between 341 nm and 345 nm, and between 356 nm and 360 nm.

Uniformity of dosage units <*6.02*> Perform the Mass variation test, or the Content uniformity test according to the following method: it meets the requirement.

To 1 tablet of Tosufloxacin Tosilate Tablets add V/10 mL of water and shake until the tablet is disintegrated. Add methanol to make exactly V mL so that each mL contains about 1.5 mg of tosufloxacin tosilate hydrate ($C_{19}H_{15}F_3N_4O_3.C_7H_8O_3S.H_2O$). Shake this solution for 10 minutes, and centrifuge. Pipet 4 mL of the supernatant liquid, add exactly 4 mL of the internal standard solution and methanol to make 100 mL, and use this solution as the sample solution. Proceed as directed in the Assay.

Amount (mg) of tosufloxacin tosilate hydrate ($C_{19}H_{15}F_3N_4O_3.C_7H_8O_3S.H_2O$)
$$= M_S \times Q_T/Q_S \times V/20 \times 1.031$$

M_S: Amount (mg) of Tosufloxacin Tosilate RS taken, calculated on the anhydrous basis

Internal standard solution—A solution of methyl parahydroxybenzoate in methanol (1 in 800).

Dissolution <*6.10*> When the test is performed at 50 revolutions per minute according to the Paddle method, using 900 mL of water as the dissolution medium, the dissolution rate in 90 minutes of Tosufloxacin Tosilate Tablets is not less than 65%.

Start the test with 1 tablet of Tosufloxacin Tosilate Tablets, withdraw not less than 20 mL of the medium at the specified minute after starting the test, and filter through a membrane filter with a pore size not exceeding 0.5 μm. Discard not less than 10 mL of the first filtrate, pipet V mL of the subsequent filtrate, add 0.05 mol/L acetic acid-sodium acetate buffer solution (pH 4.0) to make exactly V' mL so that each mL contains about 17 μg of tosufloxacin tosilate hydrate ($C_{19}H_{15}F_3N_4O_3.C_7H_8O_3S.H_2O$), and use this solution as the sample solution. Separately, weigh accurately about 21 mg of Tosufloxacin Tosilate RS (separately determine the water <*2.48*> in the same manner as Tosufloxacin Tosilate Hydrate), and dissolve in *N,N*-dimethylformamide to make exactly 25 mL. Pipet 2 mL of this solution, add 0.05 mol/L acetic acid-sodium acetate buffer solution (pH 4.0) to make exactly 100 mL, and use this solution as the standard solution. Perform the test with the sample solution and standard solution as directed under Ultraviolet-visible Spectrophotometry <*2.24*>, using 0.05 mol/L acetic acid-sodium acetate buffer solution (pH 4.0) as the blank, and determine the absorbances, A_T and A_S, at 346 nm.

Dissolution rate (%) with respect to the labeled amount of tosufloxacin tosilate hydrate ($C_{19}H_{15}F_3N_4O_3.C_7H_8O_3S.H_2O$)
$$= M_S \times A_T/A_S \times V'/V \times 1/C \times 72 \times 1.031$$

M_S: Amount (mg) of Tosufloxacin Tosilate RS taken, calculated on the anhydrous basis
C: Labeled amount (mg) of tosufloxacin tosilate hydrate ($C_{19}H_{15}F_3N_4O_3.C_7H_8O_3S.H_2O$) in 1 tablet

Assay Weigh accurately the mass of not less than 20 Tosufloxacin Tosilate Tablets, and powder. Weigh accurately a portion of the powder, equivalent to about 0.15 g of tosufloxacin tosilate hydrate ($C_{19}H_{15}F_3N_4O_3.C_7H_8O_3S.H_2O$), add 10 mL of water and methanol to make exactly 100 mL, shake for 10 minutes, and centrifuge. Pipet 4 mL of the supernatant liquid, add exactly 4 mL of the internal standard solution and methanol to make 100 mL, and use this solution as the sample solution. Separately, weigh accurately about 30 mg of Tosufloxacin Tosilate RS (separately determine the water <*2.48*> in the same manner as Tosufloxacin Tosilate Hydrate), add 2 mL of water, and dissolve in methanol to make exactly 100 mL. Pipet 20 mL of this solution, add exactly 4 mL of the internal standard solution and methanol to make 100 mL, and use this solution as the standard solution. Perform the test with 10 μL each of the sample solution and standard solution as directed under Liquid Chromatography <*2.01*> according to the following conditions, and calculate the ratios, Q_T and Q_S, of the peak area of tosufloxacin to that of the internal standard.

Amount (mg) of tosufloxacin tosilate hydrate ($C_{19}H_{15}F_3N_4O_3.C_7H_8O_3S.H_2O$)
$$= M_S \times Q_T/Q_S \times 5 \times 1.031$$

M_S: Amount (mg) of Tosufloxacin Tosilate RS taken, calculated on the anhydrous basis

Internal standard solution—A solution of methyl parahydroxybenzoate in methanol (1 in 800).

Operating conditions—

Proceed as directed in the operating conditions in the Assay under Tosufloxacin Tosilate Hydrate.

System suitability—

Proceed as directed in the system suitability in the Assay under Tosufloxacin Tosilate Hydrate.

Containers and storage Containers—Well-closed containers.

Tramadol Hydrochloride

トラマドール塩酸塩

$C_{16}H_{25}NO_2.HCl$: 299.84
(1*RS*,2*RS*)-2-[(Dimethylamino)methyl]-1-(3-methoxyphenyl)cyclohexanol monohydrochloride
[*36282-47-0*]

Tramadol Hydrochloride contains not less than 99.0% and not more than 101.0% of tramadol hydrochloride ($C_{16}H_{25}NO_2.HCl$), calculated on the anhydrous basis.

Description Tramadol Hydrochloride occurs as a white crystalline powder.

It is very soluble in water, and freely soluble in methanol, in ethanol (95) and in acetic acid (100).

A solution of Tramadol Hydrochloride (1 in 20) shows no optical rotation.

Melting point: 180 – 184°C

Tramadol Hydrochloride shows crystal polymorphism.

Identification **(1)** Determine the absorption spectrum of a solution of Tramadol Hydrochloride in ethanol (95) (1 in 10,000) as directed under Ultraviolet-visible Spectrophotometry <*2.24*>, and compare the spectrum with the Reference Spectrum: both spectra exhibit similar intensities of absorption at the same wavelengths.

(2) Determine the infrared absorption spectrum of Tramadol Hydrochloride as directed in the potassium chloride disk method under Infrared Spectrophotometry <*2.25*>, and compare the spectrum with the Reference Spectrum: both spectra exhibit similar intensities of absorption at the same wave numbers.

(3) A solution of Tramadol Hydrochloride (1 in 100) responds to Qualitative Tests <*1.09*> (2) for chloride.

Purity **(1)** Acidity or alkalinity—Dissolve 1.0 g of Tramadol Hydrochloride in water to make 20 mL. To 10 mL of this solution add 0.2 mL of methyl red TS for acidity or alkalinity test and 0.2 mL of 0.01 mol/L hydrochloric acid VS: a red color develops. To this solution add 0.01 mol/L sodium hydroxide VS until the color of the solution changes from red to yellow: the consumed volume is not more than 0.4 mL.

(2) Heavy metals <*1.07*>—Proceed with 1.0 g of Tramadol Hydrochloride according to Method 1, and perform the test. Prepare the control solution with 2.0 mL of Standard Lead Solution (not more than 20 ppm).

(3) Related substances—(i) Dissolve 0.10 g of Tramadol Hydrochloride in 2 mL of methanol, and use this solution as the sample solution. Pipet 1 mL of the sample solution, add methanol to make exactly 500 mL, and use this solution as the standard solution. Perform the test with these solutions as directed under Thin-layer Chromatography <*2.03*>. Spot 10 μL each of the sample solution and standard solution on a plate of silica gel with fluorescent indicator for thin-layer chromatography. Allow the plate to stand in ammonia vapor for 20 minutes, develop with a mixture of toluene, isopropanol and ammonia solution (28) (80:19:1) to a distance of about 15 cm, and air-dry the plate. Allow the plate to stand in iodine vapor for 1 hour, and examine under ultraviolet light (main wavelength: 254 nm): the spot at the *R*f value of about 0.5 obtained from the sample solution is not more intense than the spot from the standard solution.

(ii) Dissolve 0.15 g of Tramadol Hydrochloride in 100 mL of the mobile phase, and use this solution as the sample solution. Pipet 1 mL of the sample solution, add the mobile phase to make exactly 100 mL, and use this solution as the standard solution. Perform the test with exactly 20 μL each of the sample solution and standard solution as directed under Liquid Chromatography <*2.01*> according to the following conditions. Determine each peak area by the automatic integration method: the area of the peak having the relative retention time of about 0.9 to tramadol obtained from the sample solution is not larger than 1/5 times the peak area of tramadol from the standard solution, the area of the peak other than tramadol and the peak mentioned above from the sample solution is not larger than 1/10 times the peak area of tramadol from the standard solution, and the total area of the peaks other than tramadol from the sample solution is not larger than 2/5 times the peak area of tramadol from the standard solution.

Operating conditions—

Detector: An ultraviolet absorption photometer (wavelength: 270 nm).

Column: A stainless steel column 4.0 mm in inside diameter and 25 cm in length, packed with octylsilanized silica gel for liquid chromatography (5 μm in particle diameter).

Column temperature: A constant temperature of about 25°C.

Mobile phase: A mixture of diluted trifluoroacetic acid (1 in 500) and acetonitrile (141:59).

Flow rate: Adjust so that the retention time of tramadol is about 5 minutes.

Time span of measurement: About 4 times as long as the retention time of tramadol, beginning after the solvent peak.

System suitability—

Test for required detectability: Pipet 1 mL of the standard solution, add the mobile phase to make exactly 20 mL. Confirm that the peak area of tramadol obtained with 20 μL of this solution is equivalent to 3.5 to 6.5% of that with 20 μL of the standard solution.

System performance: When the procedure is run with 20 μL of the standard solution under the above operating conditions, the number of theoretical plates and the symmetry factor of the peak of tramadol are not less than 5000 and not more than 1.5, respectively.

System repeatability: When the test is repeated 6 times with 20 μL of the standard solution under the above operating conditions, the relative standard deviation of the peak area of tramadol is not more than 2.0%.

Water <*2.48*> Not more than 0.5% (1 g, volumetric titration, direct titration).

Residue on ignition <*2.44*> Not more than 0.1% (1 g).

Assay Weigh accurately about 0.18 g of Tramadol Hydrochloride, dissolve in 25 mL of acetic acid(100), add 10 mL of acetic anhydride, and titrate <*2.50*> with 0.1 mol/L perchloric acid VS (potentiometric titration). Perform a blank determination in the same manner, and make any necessary correction.

Each mL of 0.1 mol/L perchloric acid VS
= 29.98 mg of $C_{16}H_{25}NO_2.HCl$

Containers and storage Containers—Tight containers.

Tranexamic Acid

トラネキサム酸

$C_8H_{15}NO_2$: 157.21
trans-4-(Aminomethyl)cyclohexanecarboxylic acid
[1197-18-8]

Tranexamic Acid, when dried, contains not less than 98.0% and not more than 101.0% of tranexamic acid ($C_8H_{15}NO_2$).

Description Tranexamic Acid occurs as white, crystals or crystalline powder.

It is freely soluble in water, and practically insoluble in ethanol (99.5).

Identification Determine the infrared absorption spectrum of Tranexamic Acid as directed in the potassium bromide disk method under Infrared Spectrophotometry *<2.25>*, and compare the spectrum with the Reference Spectrum or the spectrum of Tranexamic Acid RS: both spectra exhibit similar intensities of absorption at the same wave numbers.

pH *<2.54>* The pH of a solution prepared by dissolving 1.0 g of Tranexamic Acid in 20 mL of water is between 7.0 and 8.0.

Purity **(1)** Clarity and color of solution—Dissolve 1.0 g of Tranexamic Acid in 10 mL of water: the solution is clear and colorless.

(2) Chloride *<1.03>*—Perform the test with 1.0 g of Tranexamic Acid. Prepare the control solution with 0.40 mL of 0.01 mol/L hydrochloric acid VS (not more than 0.014%).

(3) Heavy metals—Dissolve 2.0 g of Tranexamic Acid in water to make 20 mL, and use this solution as the sample stock solution. To 12 mL of the sample stock solution add 2 mL of hydrochloric acid-ammonium acetate buffer solution (pH 3.5), mix, add 1.2 mL of thioacetamide TS, mix immediately, and use this solution as the sample solution. Separately, proceed in the same manner as above with a mixture of 1 mL of Standard Lead Solution, 2 mL of the sample stock solution and 9 mL of water, and use the solution so obtained as the standard solution. Separately, proceed in the same manner with a mixture of 10 mL of water and 2 mL of the sample stock solution, and use the solution so obtained as the control solution. Conform that the color of the standard solution is slightly darker than that of the control solution. Compare the sample solution and the standard solution 2 minutes after they are prepared: the color of the sample solution is not more intense than that of the standard solution (not more than 10 ppm).

(4) Arsenic *<1.11>*—Prepare the test solution by dissolving 1.0 g of Tranexamic Acid in 10 mL of water, and perform the test (not more than 2 ppm).

(5) Related substances—Dissolve 0.20 g of Tranexamic Acid in 20 mL of water, and use this solution as the sample solution. Pipet 5 mL of the sample solution, and add water to make exactly 100 mL. Pipet 1 mL of this solution, add water to make exactly 10 mL, and use this solution as the standard solution. Perform the test with exactly 20 μL each of the sample solution and standard solution as directed under Liquid Chromatography *<2.01>* according to the following conditions, and determine each peak area by the automatic integration method: the area multiplied by correction factor 1.2 of the peak, having the relative retention time of about 1.5 to tranexamic acid obtained from sample solution, is not larger than 2/5 times the peak area of tranexamic acid from the standard solution, and the area of the peak, having the relative retention time of about 2.1, is not larger than 1/5 times the peak area of tranexamic acid from the standard solution. The area of each peak other than tranexamic acid and the peaks mentioned above is not larger than 1/5 times the peak area of tranexamic acid from the standard solution. For the area of the peaks, having the relative retention time of about 1.1 and about 1.3, multiply their correction factors 0.005 and 0.006, respectively. The total area of the peaks other than tranexamic acid from the sample solution is not larger than the peak area of tranexamic acid from the standard solution.

Operating conditions—

Detector, column, column temperature, mobile phase, and flow rate: Proceed as directed in the operating conditions in the Assay.

Time span of measurement: About 3 times as long as the retention time of tranexamic acid, beginning after the solvent peak.

System suitability—

System performance: Proceed as directed in the system suitability in the Assay.

Test for required detectability: To exactly 5 mL of the standard solution add water to make exactly 25 mL. Confirm that the peak area of tranexamic acid obtained with 20 μL of this solution is equivalent to 14 to 26% of that with 20 μL of the standard solution.

System repeatability: When the test is repeated 6 times with 20 μL of the standard solution under the above operating conditions, the relative standard deviation of the peak area of tranexamic acid is not more than 7%.

Loss on drying *<2.41>* Not more than 0.5% (1 g, 105°C, 2 hours).

Residue on ignition *<2.44>* Not more than 0.1% (1 g).

Assay Weigh accurately about 50 mg each of Tranexamic Acid and Tranexamic Acid RS, previously dried, dissolve in water to make exactly 25 mL, and use these solutions as the sample solution and standard solution. Perform the test with exactly 20 μL each of the sample solution and standard solution as directed under Liquid Chromatography *<2.01>* according to the following conditions, and determine the peak areas, A_T and A_S, of tranexamic acid in each solution.

Amount (mg) of tranexamic acid ($C_8H_{15}NO_2$)
$= M_S \times A_T/A_S$

M_S: Amount (mg) of Tranexamic Acid RS taken

Operating conditions—

Detector: An ultraviolet absorption photometer (wavelength: 220 nm).

Column: A stainless steel column 6.0 mm in inside diameter and 25 cm in length, packed with octadecylsilanized silica gel for liquid chromatography (5 μm in particle diameter).

Column temperature: A constant temperature of about 25°C.

Mobile phase: Dissolve 11.0 g of anhydrous sodium dihydrogen phosphate in 500 mL of water, and add 5 mL of triethylamine and 1.4 g of sodium lauryl sulfate. Adjust the pH to 2.5 with phosphoric acid or diluted phosphoric acid (1 in 10), add water to make 600 mL, and add 400 mL of methanol.

Flow rate: Adjust so that the retention time of tranexamic acid is about 20 minutes.

System suitability—

System performance: To 5 mL of the standard solution add 1 mL of a solution of 4-(aminomethyl)benzoic acid (1 in 10,000) and water to make 50 mL. When the procedure is run with 20 μL of this solution under the above operating conditions, tranexamic acid and 4-(aminomethyl)benzoic acid are eluted in this order with the resolution between these peaks being not less than 5.

System repeatability: When the test is repeated 6 times with 20 μL of the standard solution under the above operating conditions, the relative standard deviation of the peak area of tranexamic acid is not more than 0.6%.

Containers and storage Containers—Well-closed containers.

Tranexamic Acid Capsules

トラネキサム酸カプセル

Tranexamic Acid Capsules contain not less than 95.0% and not more than 105.0% of the labeled amount of tranexamic acid ($C_8H_{15}NO_2$: 157.21).

Method of preparation Prepare as directed under Capsules, with Tranexamic Acid.

Identification Take an amount of powdered contents of Tranexamic Acid Capsules, equivalent to 0.5 g of Tranexamic Acid, add 50 mL of water, shake well, and filter. To 5 mL of the filtrate add 1 mL of ninhydrin TS, and heat for 3 minutes: a dark purple color develops.

Uniformity of dosage units <*6.02*> It meets the requirement of the Mass variation test.

Dissolution <*6.10*> When the test is performed at 50 revolutions per minute according to the Paddle method using the sinker, using 900 mL of water as the dissolution medium, the dissolution rate in 15 minutes of Tranexamic Acid Capsules is not less than 80%.

Start the test with 1 tablet of Tranexamic Acid Capsules, withdraw not less than 20 mL of the medium at the specified minute after starting the test, and filter through a membrane filter with a pore size not exceeding 0.45 μm. Discard not less than 10 mL of the first filtrate, pipet V mL of the subsequent filtrate, add water to make exactly V' mL so that each mL contains about 0.28 mg of tranexamic acid ($C_8H_{15}NO_2$), and use this solution as the sample solution. Separately, weigh accurately about 28 mg of Tranexamic Acid RS, previously dried at 105°C for 2 hours, dissolve in water to make exactly 100 mL, and use this solution as the standard solution. Perform the test with exactly 10 μL each of the sample solution and standard solution as directed under Liquid Chromatography <*2.01*> according to the following conditions, and determine the peak areas, A_T and A_S, of tranexamic acid in each solution.

Dissolution rate (%) with respect to the labeled amount of tranexamic acid ($C_8H_{15}NO_2$)

$$= M_S \times A_T/A_S \times V'/V \times 1/C \times 900$$

M_S: Amount (mg) of Tranexamic Acid RS taken

C: Labeled amount (mg) of tranexamic acid ($C_8H_{15}NO_2$) in 1 capsule

Operating conditions—

Detector: An ultraviolet absorption photometer (wavelength: 220 nm).

Column: A stainless steel column 4.6 mm in inside diameter and 15 cm in length, packed with octadecylsilanized silica gel for liquid chromatography (5 μm in particle diameter).

Column temperature: A constant temperature of about 25°C.

Mobile phase: Dissolve 11.0 g of anhydrous sodium dihydrogen phosphate in 500 mL of water, and add 10 mL of triethylamine and 1.4 g of sodium lauryl sulfate. Adjust the pH to 2.5 with phosphoric acid, add water to make 600 mL, and add 400 mL of methanol.

Flow rate: Adjust so that the retention time of tranexamic acid is about 8 minutes.

System suitability—

System performance: When the procedure is run with 10 μL of the standard solution under the above operating conditions, the number of theoretical plates and the symmetry factor of the peak of tranexamic acid are not less than 4000 and not more than 2.0, respectively.

System repeatability: When the test is repeated 6 times with 10 μL of the standard solution under the above operating conditions, the relative standard deviation of the peak area of tranexamic acid is not more than 2.0%.

Assay Weigh accurately the mass of the contents of not less than 20 Tranexamic Acid Capsules, and powder. Weigh accurately an amount of the powder, equivalent to about 0.1 g of tranexamic acid ($C_8H_{15}NO_2$), add 30 mL of water, shake well, and add water to make exactly 50 mL. Centrifuge, filter the supernatant liquid through a membrane filter with pore size of not more than 0.45 μm, discard the first 10 mL of the filtrate, and use the subsequent filtrate as the sample solution. Separately, weigh accurately about 50 mg of Tranexamic Acid RS, previously dried at 105°C for 2 hours, dissolve in water to make exactly 25 mL, and use this solution as the standard solution. Perform the test with exactly 30 μL each of the sample solution and standard solution as directed under Liquid Chromatography <*2.01*> according to the following conditions, and determine the peak areas, A_T and A_S, of tranexamic acid in each solution.

Amount (mg) of tranexamic acid ($C_8H_{15}NO_2$)

$$= M_S \times A_T/A_S \times 2$$

M_S: Amount (mg) of Tranexamic Acid RS taken

Operating conditions—

Detector, column, and mobile phase: Proceed as directed in the operating conditions in the Assay under Tranexamic Acid.

Column temperature: A constant temperature of about 35°C.

Flow rate: Adjust so that the retention time of tranexamic acid is about 16 minutes.

System suitability—

System performance: To 5 mL of the standard solution add 1 mL of a solution of 4-(aminomethyl)benzoic acid (1 in 10,000) and water to make 50 mL. When the procedure is run with 30 μL of this solution under the above operating conditions, tranexamic acid and 4-(aminomethyl)benzoic acid are eluted in this order with the resolution between these peaks being not less than 3.

System repeatability: When the test is repeated 6 times

with 30 μL of the standard solution under the above operating conditions, the relative standard deviation of the peak area of tranexamic acid is not more than 1.0%.

Containers and storage Containers—Tight containers.

Tranexamic Acid Injection

トラネキサム酸注射液

Tranexamic Acid Injection is an aqueous injection. It contains not less than 95.0% and not more than 105.0% of the labeled amount of tranexamic acid ($C_8H_{15}NO_2$: 157.21).

Method of preparation Prepare as directed under Injections, with Tranexamic Acid.

Description Tranexamic Acid Injection is a clear and colorless liquid.

Identification To a volume of Tranexamic Acid Injection, equivalent to 50 mg of Tranexamic Acid, add water to make 5 mL, add 1 mL of ninhydrin TS, and heat: a dark purple color develops.

pH <*2.54*> 7.0 – 8.0

Bacterial endotoxins <*4.01*> Not more than 0.12 EU/mg.

Extractable volume <*6.05*> It meets the requirement.

Foreign insoluble matter <*6.06*> Perform the test according to Method 1: it meets the requirement.

Insoluble particulate matter <*6.07*> It meets the requirement.

Sterility <*4.06*> Perform the test according to the Membrane filtration method: it meets the requirement.

Assay Pipet a volume of Tranexamic Acid Injection, equivalent to about 0.1 g of tranexamic acid ($C_8H_{15}NO_2$), add water to make exactly 50 mL, and use this solution as the sample solution. Separately, weigh accurately about 50 mg of Tranexamic Acid RS, previously dried at 105°C for 2 hours, dissolve in water to make exactly 25 mL, and use this solution as the standard solution. Perform the test with exactly 30 μL each of the sample solution and standard solution as directed under Liquid Chromatography <*2.01*> according to the following conditions, and determine the peak areas, A_T and A_S, of tranexamic acid in each solution.

$$\text{Amount (mg) of tranexamic acid } (C_8H_{15}NO_2) = M_S \times A_T/A_S \times 2$$

M_S: Amount (mg) of Tranexamic Acid RS taken

Operating conditions—

Detector, column, and mobile phase: Proceed as directed in the operating conditions in the Assay under Tranexamic Acid.

Column temperature: A constant temperature of about 35°C.

Flow rate: Adjust so that the retention time of tranexamic acid is about 16 minutes.

System suitability—

System performance: To 5 mL of the standard solution add 1 mL of a solution of 4-(aminomethyl)benzoic acid (1 in 10,000) and water to make 50 mL. When the procedure is run with 30 μL of this solution under the above operating conditions, tranexamic acid and 4-(aminomethyl)benzoic acid are eluted in this order with the resolution between these peaks being not less than 3.

System repeatability: When the test is repeated 6 times with 30 μL of the standard solution under the above operating conditions, the relative standard deviation of the peak area of tranexamic acid is not more than 1.0%.

Containers and storage Containers—Hermetic containers.

Tranexamic Acid Tablets

トラネキサム酸錠

Tranexamic Acid Tablets contain not less than 95.0% and not more than 105.0% of the labeled amount of tranexamic acid ($C_8H_{15}NO_2$: 157.21).

Method of preparation Prepare as directed under Tablets, with Tranexamic Acid.

Identification To an amount of powdered Tranexamic Acid Tablets, equivalent to 0.5 g of Tranexamic Acid, add 50 mL of water, shake well, and filter. To 5 mL of the filtrate add 1 mL of ninhydrin TS, and heat for 3 minutes: a dark purple color develops.

Uniformity of dosage units <*6.02*> It meets the requirement of the Mass variation test.

Dissolution Being specified separately when the drug is granted approval based on the Law.

Assay Weigh accurately the mass of not less than 20 Tranexamic Acid Tablets, and powder. Weigh accurately a quantity of the powder, equivalent to about 5 g of tranexamic acid ($C_8H_{15}NO_2$), add 150 mL of water, disintegrate the tablets completely by sonicating, and add water to make exactly 200 mL. Centrifuge, pipet 4 mL of the supernatant liquid, and add water to make exactly 50 mL. Filter through a membrane filter with a pore size of not more than 0.45 μm, discard the first 10 mL of the filtrate, and use the subsequent filtrate as the sample solution. Separately, weigh accurately about 50 mg of Tranexamic Acid RS, previously dried at 105 °C for 2 hours, dissolve in water to make exactly 25 mL, and use this solution as the standard solution. Perform the test with exactly 30 μL each of the sample solution and standard solution as directed under Liquid Chromatography <*2.01*> according to the following conditions, and determine the peak areas, A_T and A_S, of tranexamic acid in each solution.

$$\text{Amount (mg) of tranexamic acid } (C_8H_{15}NO_2) = M_S \times A_T/A_S \times 100$$

M_S: Amount (mg) of Tranexamic Acid RS taken

Operating conditions—

Detector, column, and mobile phase: Proceed as directed in the operating conditions in the Assay under Tranexamic Acid.

Column temperature: A constant temperature of about 35°C.

Flow rate: Adjust so that the retention time of tranexamic acid is about 16 minutes.

System suitability—

System performance: To 5 mL of the standard solution add 1 mL of a solution of 4-(aminomethyl)benzoic acid (1 in 10,000) and water to make 50 mL. When the procedure is run with 30 μL of this solution under the above operating conditions, tranexamic acid and 4-(aminomethyl)benzoic acid are eluted in this order with the resolution between these peaks being not less than 3.

System repeatability: When the test is repeated 6 times with 30 μL of the standard solution under the above operating conditions, the relative standard deviation of the peak area of tranexamic acid is not more than 1.0%.

Containers and storage Containers—Tight containers.

Tranilast

トラニラスト

$C_{18}H_{17}NO_5$: 327.33

2-{[(2*E*)-3-(3,4-Dimethoxyphenyl)prop-2-enoyl]amino}benzoic acid

[*53902-12-8*]

Tranilast, when dried, contains not less than 99.0% and not more than 101.0% of tranilast ($C_{18}H_{17}NO_5$).

Description Tranilast occurs as light yellow, crystals or crystalline powder.

It is freely soluble in *N,N*-dimethylformamide, slightly soluble in acetonitrile, in methanol and in ethanol (99.5), and practically insoluble in water.

It gradually becomes light yellow-brown on exposure to light.

It shows crystal polymorphism.

Identification **(1)** Determine the absorption spectrum of a solution of Tranilast in methanol (1 in 200,000) as directed under Ultraviolet-visible Spectrophotometry 〈*2.24*〉, and compare the spectrum with the Reference Spectrum: both spectra exhibit similar intensities of absorption at the same wavelengths.

(2) Determine the infrared absorption spectrum of Tranilast, previously dried, as directed in the potassium bromide disk method under Infrared Spectrophotometry 〈*2.25*〉, and compare the spectrum with the Reference Spectrum: both spectra exhibit similar intensities of absorption at the same wave numbers.

Melting point 〈*2.60*〉 207 – 210°C

Purity **(1)** Heavy metals 〈*1.07*〉—Proceed with 2.0 g of Tranilast according to Method 2, and perform the test. Prepare the control solution with 2.0 mL of Standard Lead Solution (not more than 10 ppm).

(2) Related substances—Conduct this procedure without exposure to light, using light-resistant vessels. Dissolve 50 mg of Tranilast in 50 mL of acetonitrile, and use this solution as the sample solution. Pipet 1 mL of the sample solution, and add acetonitrile to make exactly 50 mL. Pipet 1 mL of this solution, add acetonitrile to make exactly 20 mL, and use this solution as the standard solution. Perform the test with exactly 5 μL each of the sample solution and standard solution as directed under Liquid Chromatography 〈*2.01*〉 according to the following conditions. Determine each peak area by the automatic integration method: the area of the peak other than tranilast obtained from the sample solution is not larger than the peak area of tranilast from the standard solution.

Operating conditions—

Detector: An ultraviolet absorption photometer (wavelength: 255 nm).

Column: A stainless steel column 4.6 mm in inside diameter and 15 cm in length, packed with octadecylsilanized silica gel for liquid chromatography (5 μm in particle diameter).

Column temperature: A constant temperature of about 25°C.

Mobile phase: A mixture of diluted acetic acid (100) (1 in 100) and acetonitrile (3:2).

Flow rate: Adjust so that the retention time of tranilast is about 7 minutes.

Time span of measurement: About 4 times as long as the retention time of tranilast, beginning after the solvent peak.

System suitability—

System performance: When the procedure is run with 5 μL of the standard solution under the above operating conditions, the number of theoretical plates and the symmetry factor of the peak of tranilast are not less than 5000 and not more than 1.5, respectively.

System repeatability: When the test is repeated 6 times with 5 μL of the standard solution under the above operating conditions, the relative standard deviation of the peak area of tranilast is not more than 3.0%.

(3) Chloroform—Weigh accurately about 1 g of Tranilast, dissolve in exactly 5 mL of a solution, prepared by adding *N,N*-dimethylformamide to exactly 1 mL of the internal standard solution to make exactly 100 mL, and use this solution as the sample solution. Separately, weigh accurately about 3 g of chloroform, and add *N,N*-dimethylformamide to make exactly 100 mL. Pipet 1 mL of this solution, add exactly 1 mL of the internal standard solution, add *N,N*-dimethylformamide to make 100 mL, and use this solution as the standard solution. Perform the test with 1 μL each of the sample solution and standard solution as directed under Gas Chromatography 〈*2.02*〉 according to the following conditions, and calculate the ratios, Q_T and Q_S, of the peak area of chloroform to that of the internal standard: the amount of chloroform is not more than 0.006%.

$$\text{Amount (\%) of chloroform} = M_S/M_T \times Q_T/Q_S \times 1/20$$

M_S: Amount (g) of chloroform taken

M_T: Amount (g) of Tranilast taken

*Internal standard solution—*A solution of trichloroethylene in *N,N*-dimethylformamide (1 in 50).

Operating conditions—

Detector: A hydrogen flame-ionization detector.

Column: A glass column 3 mm in inside diameter and 1 m in length, packed with porous styrene-divinylbenzene copolymer for gas chromatography (0.3 – 0.4 μm in mean pore size, not exceeding 50 m²/g) (150 – 180 μm in particle diameter).

Column temperature: A constant temperature of about 160°C.

Carrier gas: Nitrogen.

Flow rate: Adjust so that the retention time of chloroform is about 2 minutes.

System suitability—

System performance: When the procedure is run with 1 μL of the standard solution under the above operating conditions, chloroform and the internal standard are eluted in this order with the resolution between these peaks being not less than 3.

System repeatability: When the test is repeated 6 times with 1 μL of the standard solution under the above operating conditions, the relative standard deviation of the ratio of the peak area of chloroform to that of the internal standard is not more than 1.0%.

Loss on drying ⟨*2.41*⟩ Not more than 0.3% (1 g, 105°C, 3 hours).

Residue on ignition ⟨*2.44*⟩ Not more than 0.2% (1 g).

Assay Weigh accurately about 0.4 g of Tranilast, previously dried, dissolve in 25 mL of *N,N*-dimethylformamide, add 25 mL of water, and titrate ⟨*2.50*⟩ with 0.1 mol/L sodium hydroxide VS, until a 30-seconds persistent light-red color is obtained (indicator: 3 drops of phenolphthalein TS). Perform a blank determination in the same manner, and make any necessary correction.

Each mL of 0.1 mol/L sodium hydroxide VS
= 32.73 mg of $C_{18}H_{17}NO_5$

Containers and storage Containers—Well-closed containers.

Storage—Light-resistant.

Tranilast Capsules

トラニラストカプセル

Tranilast Capsules contain not less than 95.0% and not more than 105.0% of the labeled amount of tranilast ($C_{18}H_{17}NO_5$: 327.33).

Method of preparation Prepare as directed under Capsules, with Tranilast.

Identification To an amount of the content of Tranilast Capsules, equivalent to 0.1 g of Tranilast, add 180 mL of diethyl ether, shake thoroughly, filter, and evaporate the filtrate to dryness on a water bath. Determine the absorption spectrum of a solution of the residue in methanol (1 in 200,000) as directed under Ultraviolet-visible Spectrophotometry ⟨*2.24*⟩: it exhibits a maximum between 333 nm and 337 nm.

Uniformity of dosage units ⟨*6.02*⟩ Perform the Mass variation test, or the Content uniformity test according to the following method: it meets the requirement.

Conduct this procedure using light-resistant vessels. Shake the contents and the empty capsule shell of 1 Tranilast Capsules with a mixture of 0.05 mol/L phosphate buffer solution (pH 7.0) and acetonitrile (7:3) to make exactly *V* mL so that each mL contains about 0.5 mg of tranilast ($C_{18}H_{17}NO_5$), and filter through a membrane filter with a pore size not exceeding 0.45 μm. Discard the first 10 mL of the filtrate, pipet 10 mL of the subsequent filtrate, add exactly 10 mL of the internal standard solution, then add a mixture of 0.05 mol/L phosphate buffer solution (pH 7.0) and acetonitrile (7:3) to make 50 mL, and use this solution as the sample solution. Then, proceed as directed in the Assay.

Amount (mg) of tranilast ($C_{18}H_{17}NO_5$)
$= M_S \times Q_T/Q_S \times V/50$

M_S: Amount (mg) of tranilast for assay taken

Internal standard solution—Ethyl parahydroxybenzoate in a mixture of 0.05 mol/L phosphate buffer solution (pH 7.0) and acetonitrile (7:3) (1 in 5000).

Dissolution ⟨*6.10*⟩ When the test is performed at 75 revolutions per minute according to the Paddle method using the sinker, using 900 mL of disodium hydrogen phosphate-citric acid buffer solution (pH 5.5) as the dissolution medium, the dissolution rate in 60 minutes of Tranilast Capsules is not less than 75%.

Conduct this procedure without exposure to light, using light-resistant vessels. Start the test with 1 capsule of Tranilast Capsules, withdraw not less than 20 mL of the medium at the specified minute after starting the test, and filter through a membrane filter with a pore size not exceeding 0.45 μm. Discard not less than 10 mL of the first filtrate, pipet *V* mL of the subsequent filtrate, add 2nd fluid for dissolution test to make exactly *V′* mL so that each mL contains about 5.6 μg of tranilast ($C_{18}H_{17}NO_5$), and use this solution as the sample solution. Separately, weigh accurately about 28 mg of tranilast for assay, previously dried at 105°C for 3 hours, and dissolve in 2nd fluid for dissolution test to make exactly 100 mL. Pipet 5 mL of this solution, and add 2nd fluid for dissolution test to make exactly 50 mL. Then, pipet 5 mL of this solution, add 2nd fluid for dissolution test to make exactly 25 mL, and use this solution as the standard solution. Determine the absorbances, A_T and A_S, at 332 nm of the sample solution and standard solution as directed under Ultraviolet-visible Spectrophotometry ⟨*2.24*⟩.

Dissolution rate (%) with respect to the labeled amount of tranilast ($C_{18}H_{17}NO_5$)
$= M_S \times A_T/A_S \times V'/V \times 1/C \times 18$

M_S: Amount (mg) of tranilast for assay taken
C: Labeled amount (mg) of tranilast ($C_{18}H_{17}NO_5$) in 1 capsule

Assay Conduct this procedure using light-resistant vessels. Weigh accurately the mass of the contents of not less than 20 Tranilast Capsules, and powder. Weigh accurately a portion of the powder, equivalent to about 0.1 g of tranilast ($C_{18}H_{17}NO_5$), shake with a suitable amount of a mixture of 0.05 mol/L phosphate buffer solution (pH 7.0) and acetonitrile (7:3), then add the same mixture to make exactly 200 mL, and filter through a membrane filter with a pore size not exceeding 0.45 μm. Discard the first 10 mL of the filtrate, pipet 10 mL of the subsequent filtrate, add exactly 10 mL of the internal standard solution, then add a mixture of 0.05 mol/L phosphate buffer solution (pH 7.0) and acetonitrile (7:3) to make 50 mL, and use this solution as the sample solution. Separately, weigh accurately about 25 mg of tranilast for assay, previously dried at 105°C for 3 hours, and dissolve in a mixture of 0.05 mol/L phosphate buffer solution (pH 7.0) and acetonitrile (7:3) to make exactly 50 mL. Pipet 10 mL of this solution, add exactly 10 mL of the internal standard solution, then add a mixture of 0.05 mol/L phosphate buffer solution (pH 7.0) and acetonitrile (7:3) to make 50 mL, and use this solution as the standard solution. Perform the test with 5 μL each of the sample solution and standard solution as directed under Liquid Chromatography ⟨*2.01*⟩ according to the following conditions, and calculate the ratios, Q_T and Q_S, of the peak area of tranilast to that of the internal standard.

Amount (mg) of tranilast ($C_{18}H_{17}NO_5$)
$= M_S \times Q_T/Q_S \times 4$

M_S: Amount (mg) of tranilast for assay taken

Internal standard solution—Ethyl parahydroxybenzoate in a mixture of 0.05 mol/L phosphate buffer solution (pH 7.0) and acetonitrile (7:3) (1 in 5000).

Operating conditions—

Detector: An ultraviolet absorption photometer (wavelength: 255 nm).

Column: A stainless steel column 4.6 mm in inside diameter and 15 cm in length, packed with octadecylsilanized silica gel for liquid chromatography (5 μm in particle diameter).

Column temperature: A constant temperature of about 25°C.

Mobile phase: A mixture of diluted acetic acid (100) (1 in 100) and acetonitrile (3:2).

Flow rate: Adjust so that the retention time of tranilast is about 7 minutes.

System suitability—

System performance: When the procedure is run with 5 μL of the standard solution under the above operating conditions, the internal standard and tranilast are eluted in this order with the resolution between these peaks being not less than 8.

System repeatability: When the test is repeated 6 times with 5 μL of the standard solution under the above operating conditions, the relative standard deviation of the ratio of the peak area of tranilast to that of the internal standard is not more than 1.0%.

Containers and storage Containers—Tight containers.

Storage—Light-resistant.

Tranilast Fine Granules

トラニラスト細粒

Tranilast Fine Granules contain not less than 95.0% and not more than 105.0% of the labeled amount of tranilast ($C_{18}H_{17}NO_5$: 327.33).

Method of preparation Prepare as directed under Granules, with Tranilast.

Identification To an amount of Tranilast Fine Granules, equivalent to 0.1 g of Tranilast, add 180 mL of diethyl ether, shake thoroughly, filter, and evaporate the filtrate to dryness on a water bath. Determine the absorption spectrum of a solution of the residue in methanol (1 in 200,000) as directed under Ultraviolet-visible Spectrophotometry <*2.24*>: it exhibits a maximum between 333 nm and 337 nm.

Uniformity of dosage units <*6.02*> Perform the test according to the following method: Tranilast Fine Granules in single-dose packages meet the requirement of the Content uniformity test.

Conduct this procedure using light-resistant vessels. Shake the total content of 1 package of Tranilast Fine Granules with a mixture of 0.05 mol/L phosphate buffer solution (pH 7.0) and acetonitrile (7:3) to make exactly V mL so that each mL contains about 0.5 mg of tranilast ($C_{18}H_{17}NO_5$), and filter through a membrane filter with a pore size not exceeding 0.45 μm. Discard the first 10 mL of the filtrate, pipet 10 mL of the subsequent filtrate, add exactly 10 mL of the internal standard solution, then add a mixture of 0.05 mol/L phosphate buffer solution (pH 7.0) and acetonitrile (7:3) to make 50 mL, and use this solution as the sample solution. Then, proceed as directed in the Assay.

$$\text{Amount (mg) of tranilast } (C_{18}H_{17}NO_5) = M_S \times Q_T/Q_S \times V/50$$

M_S: Amount (mg) of tranilast for assay taken

*Internal standard solution—*Ethyl parahydroxybenzoate in a mixture of 0.05 mol/L phosphate buffer solution (pH 7.0) and acetonitrile (7:3) (1 in 5000).

Dissolution <*6.10*> When the test is performed at 50 revolutions per minute according to the Paddle method, using 900 mL of disodium hydrogen phosphate-citric acid buffer solution (pH 5.5) as the dissolution medium, the dissolution rate in 30 minutes of Tranilast Fine Granules is not less than 75%.

Conduct this procedure without exposure to light, using light-resistant vessels. Start the test with an accurately weighed amount of Tranilast Fine Granules, equivalent to about 0.1 g of tranilast ($C_{18}H_{17}NO_5$), withdraw not less than 20 mL of the medium at the specified minute after starting the test, and filter through a membrane filter with a pore size not exceeding 0.45 μm. Discard not less than 10 mL of the first filtrate, pipet 5 mL of the subsequent filtrate, add 2nd fluid for dissolution test to make exactly 100 mL, and use this solution as the sample solution. Separately, weigh accurately about 28 mg of tranilast for assay, previously dried at 105°C for 3 hours, and dissolve in 2nd fluid for dissolution test to make exactly 100 mL. Pipet 5 mL of this solution, and add 2nd fluid for dissolution test to make exactly 50 mL. Then, pipet 5 mL of this solution, add 2nd fluid for dissolution test to make exactly 25 mL, and use this solution as the standard solution. Determine the absorbances, A_T and A_S, at 332 nm of the sample solution and standard solution as directed under Ultraviolet-visible Spectrophotometry <*2.24*>.

$$\text{Dissolution rate (\%) with respect to the labeled amount of tranilast } (C_{18}H_{17}NO_5) = M_S/M_T \times A_T/A_S \times 1/C \times 360$$

M_S: Amount (mg) of tranilast for assay taken

M_T: Amount (g) of Tranilast Fine Granules taken

C: Labeled amount (mg) of tranilast ($C_{18}H_{17}NO_5$) in 1 g

Assay Conduct this procedure using light-resistant vessels. Powder Tranilast Fine Granules. Weigh accurately a portion of the powder, equivalent to about 0.1 g of tranilast ($C_{18}H_{17}NO_5$), shake with a suitable amount of a mixture of 0.05 mol/L phosphate buffer solution (pH 7.0) and acetonitrile (7:3), then add the same mixture to make exactly 200 mL, and filter through a membrane filter with a pore size not exceeding 0.45 μm. Discard the first 10 mL of the filtrate, pipet 10 mL of the subsequent filtrate, add exactly 10 mL of the internal standard solution, then add a mixture of 0.05 mol/L phosphate buffer solution (pH 7.0) and acetonitrile (7:3) to make 50 mL, and use this solution as the sample solution. Separately, weigh accurately about 25 mg of tranilast for assay, previously dried at 105°C for 3 hours, and dissolve in a mixture of 0.05 mol/L phosphate buffer solution (pH 7.0) and acetonitrile (7:3) to make exactly 50 mL. Pipet 10 mL of this solution, add exactly 10 mL of the internal standard solution, then add a mixture of 0.05 mol/L phosphate buffer solution (pH 7.0) and acetonitrile (7:3) to make 50 mL, and use this solution as the standard solution. Perform the test with 5 μL each of the sample solution and standard solution as directed under Liquid Chromatography <*2.01*> according to the following conditions, and calculate the ratios, Q_T and Q_S, of the peak area of tranilast to that of the internal standard.

$$\text{Amount (mg) of tranilast } (C_{18}H_{17}NO_5) = M_S \times Q_T/Q_S \times 4$$

M_S: Amount (mg) of tranilast for assay taken

*Internal standard solution—*Ethyl parahydroxybenzoate in a mixture of 0.05 mol/L phosphate buffer solution (pH 7.0) and acetonitrile (7:3) (1 in 5000).

Operating conditions—

Detector: An ultraviolet absorption photometer (wave-

length: 255 nm).

Column: A stainless steel column 4.6 mm in inside diameter and 15 cm in length, packed with octadecylsilanized silica gel for liquid chromatography (5 μm in particle diameter).

Column temperature: A constant temperature of about 25°C.

Mobile phase: A mixture of diluted acetic acid (100) (1 in 100) and acetonitrile (3:2).

Flow rate: Adjust so that the retention time of tranilast is about 7 minutes.

System suitability—

System performance: When the procedure is run with 5 μL of the standard solution under the above operating conditions, the internal standard and tranilast are eluted in this order with the resolution between these peaks being not less than 8.

System repeatability: When the test is repeated 6 times with 5 μL of the standard solution under the above operating conditions, the relative standard deviation of the ratio of the peak area of tranilast to that of the internal standard is not more than 1.0%.

Containers and storage Containers—Tight containers.

Storage—Light-resistant.

Tranilast Ophthalmic Solution

トラニラスト点眼液

Tranilast Ophthalmic Solution is an aqueous ophthalmic preparation.

It contains not less than 95.0% and not more than 105.0% of the labeled amount of tranilast ($C_{18}H_{17}NO_5$: 327.33).

Method of preparation Prepare as directed under Ophthalmic Liquids and Solutions, with Tranilast.

Description Tranilast Ophthalmic Solution occurs as a clear and pale yellow liquid.

Identification When add 2 mL of dilute hydrochloric acid to a volume of Tranilast Ophthalmic Solution, equivalent to about 50 mg of Tranilast, a white precipitate is produced. Collect the precipitate by filtration, wash the precipitate with two 10-mL portions of water, and dry at 105°C for 3 hours. Dissolve 5 mg of the precipitate in methanol to make 100 mL. To 5 mL of this solution add methanol to make 50 mL, and determine the absorption spectrum of this solution as directed under Ultraviolet-visible Spectrophotometry <*2.24*>: it exhibits a maximum between 333 nm and 337 nm.

Osmotic pressure ratio Being specified separately when the drug is granted approval based on the Law.

pH Being specified separately when the drug is granted approval based on the Law.

Foreign insoluble matter <*6.11*> It meets the requirement.

Insoluble particulate matter <*6.08*> It meets the requirement.

Sterility <*4.06*> Perform the test according to the Membrane filtration method: it meets the requirement.

Assay Conduct this procedure using light-resistant vessels. To exactly a volume of Tranilast Ophthalmic Solution, equivalent to about 5 mg of tranilast ($C_{18}H_{17}NO_5$), add exactly 10 mL of the internal standard solution, then add ethanol (99.5) to make 50 mL, and use this solution as the sample solution. Separately, weigh accurately about 25 mg of tranilast for assay, previously dried at 105°C for 3 hours, and dissolve in ethanol (99.5) to make exactly 50 mL. Pipet 10 mL of this solution, add exactly 10 mL of the internal standard solution, then add ethanol (99.5) to make 50 mL, and use this solution as the standard solution. Perform the test with 5 μL each of the sample solution and standard solution as directed under Liquid Chromatography <*2.01*> according to the following conditions, and calculate the ratios, Q_T and Q_S, of the peak area of tranilast to that of the internal standard.

$$\text{Amount (mg) of tranilast } (C_{18}H_{17}NO_5) = M_S \times Q_T/Q_S \times 1/5$$

M_S: Amount (mg) of tranilast for assay taken

*Internal standard solution—*A solution of ethyl parahydroxybenzoate in ethanol (99.5) (1 in 5000).

Operating conditions—

Detector: An ultraviolet absorption photometer (wavelength: 255 nm).

Column: A stainless steel column 4.6 mm in inside diameter and 15 cm in length, packed with octadecylsilanized silica gel for liquid chromatography (5 μm in particle diameter).

Column temperature: A constant temperature of about 25°C.

Mobile phase: A mixture of diluted acetic acid (100) (1 in 100) and acetonitrile (3:2).

Flow rate: Adjust so that the retention time of tranilast is about 7 minutes.

System suitability—

System performance: When the procedure is run with 5 μL of the standard solution under the above operating conditions, the internal standard and tranilast are eluted in this order with the resolution between these peaks being not less than 8.

System repeatability: When the test is repeated 6 times with 5 μL of the standard solution under the above operating conditions, the relative standard deviation of the ratio of the peak area of tranilast to that of the internal standard is not more than 1.0%.

Containers and storage Containers—Tight containers.

Storage—Light-resistant.

Tranilast for Syrup

シロップ用トラニラスト

Tranilast for Syrup is a preparation for syrup, which is suspended before use.

It contains not less than 95.0% and not more than 105.0% of the labeled amount of tranilast ($C_{18}H_{17}NO_5$: 327.33).

Method of preparation Prepare as directed under Syrups, with Tranilast.

Identification To an amount of Tranilast for Syrup, equivalent to 0.1 g of Tranilast, add 180 mL of diethyl ether, shake thoroughly, filter, and evaporate the filtrate to dryness on a water bath. Determine the absorption spectrum of a solution of the residue in methanol (1 in 200,000) as directed under Ultraviolet-visible Spectrophotometry <*2.24*>: it exhibits a maximum between 333 nm and 337 nm.

Uniformity of dosage units <*6.02*> Perform the test according to the following method: Tranilast for Syrup in single-dose packages meet the requirement of the Content uniformity test.

Conduct this procedure using light-resistant vessels. Shake the total content of 1 package of Tranilast for Syrup with a mixture of 0.05 mol/L phosphate buffer solution (pH 7.0) and acetonitrile (7:3), then add the same mixture to make exactly V mL so that each mL contains about 0.5 mg of tranilast ($C_{18}H_{17}NO_5$), and filter through a membrane filter with a pore size not exceeding 0.45 μm. Discard the first 10 mL of the filtrate, pipet 10 mL of the subsequent filtrate, add exactly 10 mL of the internal standard solution, then add a mixture of 0.05 mol/L phosphate buffer solution (pH 7.0) and acetonitrile (7:3) to make 50 mL, and use this solution as the sample solution. Then, proceed as directed in the Assay.

$$\text{Amount (mg) of tranilast } (C_{18}H_{17}NO_5) = M_S \times Q_T/Q_S \times V/50$$

M_S: Amount (mg) of tranilast for assay taken

Internal standard solution—Ethyl parahydroxybenzoate in a mixture of 0.05 mol/L phosphate buffer solution (pH 7.0) and acetonitrile (7:3) (1 in 5000).

Dissolution *<6.10>* When the test is performed at 50 revolutions per minute according to the Paddle method, using 900 mL of disodium hydrogen phosphate-citric acid buffer solution (pH 5.5) as the dissolution medium, the dissolution rate in 60 minutes of Tranilast for Syrup is not less than 75%.

Conduct this procedure without exposure to light, using light-resistant vessels. Start the test with an accurately weighed amount of Tranilast for Syrup, equivalent to about 0.1 g of tranilast ($C_{18}H_{17}NO_5$), withdraw not less than 20 mL of the medium at the specified minute after starting the test, and filter through a membrane filter with a pore size not exceeding 0.45 μm. Discard not less than 10 mL of the first filtrate, pipet 5 mL of the subsequent filtrate, add 2nd fluid for dissolution test to make exactly 100 mL, and use this solution as the sample solution. Separately, weigh accurately about 28 mg of tranilast for assay, previously dried at 105°C for 3 hours, and dissolve in 2nd fluid for dissolution test to make exactly 100 mL. Pipet 5 mL of this solution, and add 2nd fluid for dissolution test to make exactly 50 mL. Then, pipet 5 mL of this solution, add 2nd fluid for dissolution test to make exactly 25 mL, and use this solution as the standard solution. Determine the absorbances, A_T and A_S, at 332 nm of the sample solution and standard solution as directed under Ultraviolet-visible Spectrophotometry *<2.24>*.

$$\text{Dissolution rate (\%) with respect to the labeled amount of tranilast } (C_{18}H_{17}NO_5) = M_S/M_T \times A_T/A_S \times 1/C \times 360$$

M_S: Amount (mg) of tranilast for assay taken
M_T: Amount (g) of Tranilast for Syrup taken
C: Labeled amount (mg) of tranilast ($C_{18}H_{17}NO_5$) in 1 g

Assay Conduct this procedure using light-resistant vessels. Powder Tranilast for Syrup. Weigh accurately the a portion of the powder, equivalent to about 0.1 g of tranilast ($C_{18}H_{17}NO_5$), shake with a suitable amount of a mixture of 0.05 mol/L phosphate buffer solution (pH 7.0) and acetonitrile (7:3), then add the same mixture to make exactly 200 mL, and filter through a membrane filter with a pore size not exceeding 0.45 μm. Discard the first 10 mL of the filtrate, pipet 10 mL of the subsequent filtrate, add exactly 10 mL of the internal standard solution, then add a mixture of 0.05 mol/L phosphate buffer solution (pH 7.0) and acetonitrile (7:3) to make 50 mL, and use this solution as the sample solution. Separately, weigh accurately about 25 mg of tranilast for assay, previously dried at 105°C for 3 hours, and dissolve in a mixture of 0.05 mol/L phosphate buffer solution (pH 7.0) and acetonitrile (7:3) to make exactly 50 mL. Pipet 10 mL of this solution, add exactly 10 mL of the internal standard solution, then add a mixture of 0.05 mol/L phosphate buffer solution (pH 7.0) and acetonitrile (7:3) to make exactly 50 mL, and use this solution as the standard solution. Perform the test with 5 μL each of the sample solution and standard solution as directed under Liquid Chromatography *<2.01>* according to the following conditions, and calculate the ratios, Q_T and Q_S, of the peak area of tranilast to that of the internal standard.

$$\text{Amount (mg) of tranilast } (C_{18}H_{17}NO_5) = M_S \times Q_T/Q_S \times 4$$

M_S: Amount (mg) of tranilast for assay taken

Internal standard solution—Ethyl parahydroxybenzoate in a mixture of 0.05 mol/L phosphate buffer solution (pH 7.0) and acetonitrile (7:3) (1 in 5000).

Operating conditions—

Detector: An ultraviolet absorption photometer (wavelength: 255 nm).

Column: A stainless steel column 4.6 mm in inside diameter and 15 cm in length, packed with octadecylsilanized silica gel for liquid chromatography (5 μm in particle diameter).

Column temperature: A constant temperature of about 25°C.

Mobile phase: A mixture of diluted acetic acid (100) (1 in 100) and acetonitrile (3:2).

Flow rate: Adjust so that the retention time of tranilast is about 7 minutes.

System suitability—

System performance: When the procedure is run with 5 μL of the standard solution under the above operating conditions, the internal standard and tranilast are eluted in this order with the resolution between these peaks being not less than 8.

System repeatability: When the test is repeated 6 times with 5 μL of the standard solution under the above operating conditions, the relative standard deviation of the ratio of the peak area of tranilast to that of the internal standard is not more than 1.0%.

Containers and storage Containers—Tight containers.

Storage—Light-resistant.

Trapidil

トラピジル

$C_{10}H_{15}N_5$: 205.26

7-Diethylamino-5-methyl[1,2,4]triazolo[1,5-*a*]pyrimidine
[15421-84-8]

Trapidil, when dried, contains not less than 98.5% of trapidil ($C_{10}H_{15}N_5$).

Description Trapidil occurs as a white to pale yellow-white crystalline powder.

It is very soluble in water and in methanol, freely soluble in ethanol (95), in acetic anhydride and in acetic acid (100), and sparingly soluble in diethyl ether.

The pH of a solution of 1.0 g of Trapidil in 100 mL of water is between 6.5 and 7.5.

Identification **(1)** To 5 mL of a solution of Trapidil (1 in 50) add 3 drops of Dragendorff's TS: an orange color develops.

(2) Determine the absorption spectrum of a solution of Trapidil (1 in 125,000) as directed under Ultraviolet-visible Spectrophotometry <*2.24*>, and compare the spectrum with the Reference Spectrum: both spectra exhibit similar intensities of absorption at the same wavelengths.

Absorbance <*2.24*> $E^{1\%}_{1\,\text{cm}}$ (307 nm): 860 – 892 (after drying, 20 mg, water, 2500 mL).

Melting point <*2.60*> 101 – 105°C

Purity **(1)** Clarity and color of solution—Dissolve 2.5 g of Trapidil in 10 mL of water: the solution is clear and colorless to pale yellow.

(2) Chloride <*1.03*>—Perform the test with 0.5 g of Trapidil. Prepare the control solution with 0.25 mL of 0.01 mol/L hydrochloric acid VS (not more than 0.018%).

(3) Ammonium—Place 0.05 g of Trapidil in a glass-stoppered conical flask, thoroughly moisten with 10 drops of sodium hydroxide TS, and stopper the flask. Allow it to stand at 37°C for 15 minutes: the gas evolved does not change moistened red litmus paper to blue.

(4) Heavy metals <*1.07*>—Dissolve 1.0 g of Trapidil in 40 mL of water, and add 1.5 mL of dilute hydrochloric acid, 2 mL of dilute acetic acid and water to make 50 mL. Perform the test using this solution as the test solution. Prepare the control solution as follows: to 1.0 mL of Standard Lead Solution add 2 mL of dilute acetic acid and water to make 50 mL (not more than 10 ppm).

(5) Arsenic <*1.11*>—Prepare the test solution with 1.0 g of Trapidil according to Method 1, and perform the test (not more than 2 ppm).

(6) Related substances—Dissolve 0.10 g of Trapidil in 4 mL of methanol, and use this solution as the sample solution. Pipet 1 mL of the sample solution, and add methanol to make exactly 20 mL. Pipet 1 mL of this solution, add methanol to make exactly 100 mL, and use this solution as the standard solution. Perform the test with these solutions as directed under Thin-layer Chromatography <*2.03*>. Spot 20 μL each of the sample solution and standard solution on a plate of silica gel for thin-layer chromatography. Develop the plate with a mixture of chloroform, ethanol (95) and acetic acid (100) (85:13:2) to a distance of about 10 cm, and air-dry the plate. Allow the plate to stand in iodine vapor for 60 minutes: the spots other than the principal spot obtained from the sample solution are not more intense than the spot from the standard solution.

Loss on drying <*2.41*> Not more than 0.5% (1 g, in vacuum, silica gel, 60°C, 3 hours).

Residue on ignition <*2.44*> Not more than 0.1% (1 g).

Assay Weigh accurately about 0.2 g of Trapidil, previously dried, dissolve in 20 mL of acetic acid (100), and titrate <*2.50*> with 0.1 mol/L perchloric acid VS (potentiometric titration). Perform a blank determination in the same manner, and make any necessary correction.

Each mL of 0.1 mol/L perchloric acid VS
= 20.53 mg of $C_{10}H_{15}N_5$

Containers and storage Containers—Tight containers.

Trehalose Hydrate

トレハロース水和物

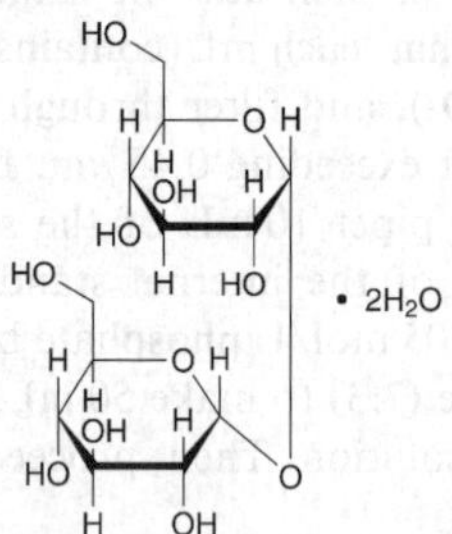

$C_{12}H_{22}O_{11}.2H_2O$: 378.33
α-D-Glucopyranosyl α-D-glucopyranoside dihydrate
[*6138-23-4*]

Trehalose Hydrate contains not less than 98.0% and not more than 101.0% of trehalose ($C_{12}H_{22}O_{11}$: 342.30), calculated on the anhydrous basis.

Description Trehalose Hydrate occurs as white crystals or crystalline powder.

It is freely soluble in water, and slightly soluble in methanol and in ethanol (99.5).

Identification **(1)** To 1 mL of a solution of Trehalose Hydrate (2 in 5) add 5 – 6 drops of a solution of 1-naphthol in ethanol (95) (1 in 20), shake thoroughly, and add gently 2 mL of sulfuric acid: a purple color appears at the zone of contact.

(2) Mix 2 mL of a solution of Trehalose Hydrate (1 in 25) with 1 mL of dilute hydrochloric acid, and allow standing for 20 minutes at room temperature. Then add 4 mL of sodium hydroxide TS and 2 mL of a solution of glycine (1 in 25), and heat in a water bath for 10 minutes: no brown color appears.

(3) Determine the infrared absorption spectrum of Trehalose Hydrate as directed in the potassium bromide disk method under Infrared Spectrophotometry <*2.25*>, and compare the spectrum with the Reference Spectrum or the spectrum of Trehalose RS: both spectra exhibit similar intensities of absorption at the same wave numbers.

Optical rotation <*2.49*> $[\alpha]^{20}_{D}$: +197 – +201° (10 g calculated on the anhydrous basis, water, 100 mL, 100 mm).

pH <*2.54*> The pH of a solution of 1 g of Trehalose Hydrate in 10 mL of water is between 4.5 and 6.5.

Purity **(1)** Chloride <*1.03*>—Perform the test with 2.0 g of Trehalose Hydrate. Prepare the control solution with 1.0 mL of 0.01 mol/L hydrochloric acid VS (not more than 0.018%).

(2) Sulfate <*1.14*>—Perform the test with 2.0 g of Trehalose Hydrate. Prepare the control solution with 1.0 mL of 0.005 mol/L sulfuric acid VS (not more than 0.024%).

(3) Heavy metals <*1.07*>—Proceed with 5.0 g of Trehalose Hydrate according to Method 1, and perform the test. Prepare the control solution with 2.5 mL of Standard Lead Solution (not more than 5 ppm).

(4) Related substances—Dissolve 0.5 g of Trehalose Hydrate in 10 mL of water, and use this solution as the sample solution. Pipet 1 mL of the sample solution, add water to make exactly 100 mL, and use this solution as the standard solution. Perform the test with exactly 20 μL each of the sample solution and standard solution as directed under Liquid Chromatography *<2.01>* according to the following conditions. Determine each peak area by the automatic integration method: the total area of the peaks which are eluted before the peak of trehalose and the total area of the peaks which are eluted after the peak of trehalose obtained from the sample solution are both not larger than 1/2 times the peak area of trehalose from the standard solution.

Operating conditions—

Detector, column, column temperature, mobile phase, and flow rate: Proceed as directed in the operating conditions under the Assay.

Time span of measurement: About 2 times as long as the retention time of trehalose.

System suitability—

System performance: Proceed as directed in the system suitability in the Assay.

Test for required detectability: To exactly 1 mL of the standard solution add water to make exactly 10 mL. Confirm that the peak area of trehalose obtained with 20 μL of this solution is equivalent to 7 to 13% of that with 20 μL of the standard solution.

System repeatability: To exactly 5 mL of the standard solution add water to make exactly 10 mL. When the test is repeated 6 times with 20 μL of this solution under the above operating conditions, the relative standard deviation of the peak area of trehalose is not more than 1.0%.

(5) Dextrin, soluble starch, and sulfite—Dissolve 1.0 g of Trehalose Hydrate in 10 mL of water and add 1 drop of iodine TS: a yellow color appears, which is changed to blue on addition of 1 drop of starch TS.

(6) Nitrogen—Perform the test with accurately weighed Trehalose Hydrate of about 5 g as directed under Nitrogen Determination *<1.08>*, using 30 mL of sulfuric acid for the degradation and adding 45 mL of sodium hydroxide solution (2 in 5): the amount of nitrogen (N: 14.01) is not more than 0.005%.

Water *<2.48>* Not less than 9.0% and not more than 11.0% (0.1 g, volumetric titration, direct titration).

Residue on ignition *<2.44>* Not more than 0.1% (2 g).

Assay Weigh accurately about 0.2 g each of Trehalose Hydrate and Trehalose RS (separately determine the water *<2.48>* in the same manner as Trehalose Hydrate), dissolve each in 6 mL of water, add exactly 2 mL each of the internal standard solution, add water to make them 20 mL, and use these solutions as the sample solution and the standard solution, respectively. Perform the test with 20 μL each of the sample solution and standard solution as directed under Liquid Chromatography *<2.01>* according to the following conditions, and calculate the ratios, Q_T and Q_S, of the peak area of trehalose to that of the internal standard.

Amount (mg) of trehalose ($C_{12}H_{22}O_{11}$) = $M_S \times Q_T/Q_S$

M_S: Amount (mg) of Trehalose RS taken, calculated on the anhydrous basis

Internal standard solution—A solution of glycerin (1 in 10).

Operating conditions—

Detector: A differential refractometer.

Column: A stainless steel column 8 mm in inside diameter and 30 cm in length, packed with strongly acidic ion-exchange resin for liquid chromatography consist of styrene-divinylbenzene copolymer carrying sulfonic acid groups (6 μm in particle diameter).

Column temperature: A constant temperature of about 80°C.

Mobile phase: Water.

Flow rate: Adjust so that the retention time of trehalose is about 15 minutes.

System suitability—

System performance: Dissolve 0.1 g each of maltotriose and glucose in 10 mL of the standard solution, add 1 mL of the internal standard solution, and add water to make 20 mL. When the procedure is run with 20 μL of this solution under the above operating conditions, maltotriose, trehalose, glucose and the internal standard are eluted in this order, and the resolution between the peaks of maltotriose and trehalose is not less than 1.5, the resolution between the peaks of trehalose and glucose is not less than 4, and the resolution between the peaks of glucose and the internal standard is not less than 3.

System repeatability: When the test is repeated 6 times with 20 μL of the standard solution under the above operating conditions, the relative standard deviation of the ratio of the peak area of trehalose to that of the internal standard is not more than 1.0%.

Containers and storage Containers—Tight containers.

Trepibutone

トレピブトン

$C_{16}H_{22}O_6$: 310.34

4-Oxo-4-(2,4,5-triethoxyphenyl)butanoic acid

[*41826-92-0*]

Trepibutone, when dried, contains not less than 98.5% of trepibutone ($C_{16}H_{22}O_6$).

Description Trepibutone occurs as white to yellowish white, crystals or crystalline powder. It is odorless, and is tasteless or has a slight, characteristic aftertaste.

It is soluble in acetone, sparingly soluble in ethanol (95), slightly soluble in diethyl ether, and practically insoluble in water.

It dissolves in sodium hydroxide TS.

Identification **(1)** Determine the absorption spectrum of a solution of Trepibutone in diluted dilute sodium hydroxide TS (1 in 10) (1 in 100,000) as directed under Ultraviolet-visible Spectrophotometry *<2.24>*, and compare the spectrum with the Reference Spectrum: both spectra exhibit similar intensities of absorption at the same wavelengths.

(2) Determine the ^1H spectrum of a solution of Trepibutone in deuterated chloroform for the nuclear magnetic resonance spectroscopy (1 in 10), using tetramethylsilane for the nuclear magnetic resonance spectroscopy as an internal reference compound, as directed under Nuclear Magnetic Resonance Spectroscopy *<2.21>*: it exhibits a sharp multiplet signal A at around δ 1.5 ppm, a triplet signal B at around δ 2.7 ppm, a triplet signal C at around δ 3.3 ppm, a multiplet signal D at around δ 4.2 ppm, a sharp singlet signal E at around δ 6.4 ppm, a sharp singlet signal F at around δ 7.4 ppm, and a singlet signal G at around δ 10.5 ppm. The ratio of integrated intensity of each signal, A:B:C:D:E:F:G, is about 9:2:2:6:1:1:1.

Melting point <*2.60*> 146 – 150°C

Purity (1) Chloride <*1.03*>—Dissolve 0.5 g of Trepibutone in 30 mL of acetone, and add 6 mL of dilute nitric acid and water to make 50 mL. Perform the test using this solution as the test solution. Prepare the control solution as follows: to 0.30 mL of 0.01 mol/L hydrochloric acid VS add 30 mL of acetone, 6 mL of dilute nitric acid and water to make 50 mL (not more than 0.021%).

(2) Heavy metals <*1.07*>—Proceed with 1.0 g of Trepibutone according to Method 2, and perform the test. Prepare the control solution with 2.0 mL of Standard Lead Solution (not more than 20 ppm).

(3) Related substances—Dissolve 0.10 g of Trepibutone in 10 mL of acetone, and use this solution as the sample solution. Pipet 2 mL of the sample solution, add acetone to make exactly 100 mL. To exactly 10 mL of this solution add acetone to make exactly 100 mL, and use this solution as the standard solution. Perform the test with these solutions as directed under Thin-layer Chromatography <*2.03*>. Spot 10 μL each of the sample solution and standard solution on a plate of silica gel with fluorescent indicator for thin-layer chromatography. Develop the plate with a mixture of isopropylether, acetone, water and formic acid (100:30:3:3) to a distance of about 10 cm, and air-dry the plate. Examine under ultraviolet light (main wavelength: 254 nm): the spots other than the principal spot obtained from the sample solution are not more intense than the spot from the standard solution.

Loss on drying <*2.41*> Not more than 0.5% (1 g, 105°C, 4 hours).

Residue on ignition <*2.44*> Not more than 0.1% (1 g).

Assay Weigh accurately about 0.5 g of Trepibutone, previously dried, dissolve in 50 mL of ethanol (95), add 50 mL of water, and titrate <*2.50*> with 0.1 mol/L sodium hydroxide VS (indicator: 5 drops of phenolphthalein TS). Perform a blank determination in the same manner, and make any necessary correction.

Each mL of 0.1 mol/L sodium hydroxide VS
= 31.03 mg of $C_{16}H_{22}O_6$

Containers and storage Containers—Tight containers.
Storage—Light-resistant.

Triamcinolone

トリアムシノロン

$C_{21}H_{27}FO_6$: 394.43
9-Fluoro-11β,16α,17,21-tetrahydroxypregna-1,4-diene-3,20-dione
[*124-94-7*]

Triamcinolone, when dried, contains not less than 97.0% and not more than 103.0% of triamcinolone ($C_{21}H_{27}FO_6$).

Description Triamcinolone occurs as a white crystalline powder.

It is freely soluble in *N*,*N*-dimethylformamide, slightly soluble in methanol and in ethanol (95), and practically insoluble in water.

Melting point: about 264°C (with decomposition).

It shows crystal polymorphism.

Identification (1) Dissolve 1 mg of Triamcinolone in 6 mL of ethanol (95), add 5 mL of 2,6-di-*tert*-butylcresol TS and 5 mL of sodium hydroxide TS, and heat on a water bath for 30 minutes under a reflux condenser: a red-purple color develops.

(2) Add 5 mL of water and 1 mL of Fehling's TS to 0.01 g of Triamcinolone, and heat: a red precipitate is produced.

(3) Proceed with 0.01 g of Triamcinolone as directed under Oxygen Flask Combustion Method <*1.06*>, using a mixture of 0.5 mL of 0.01 mol/L sodium hydroxide TS and 20 mL of water as the absorbing liquid: the solution responds to Qualitative Tests <*1.09*> for fluoride.

(4) Determine the infrared absorption spectrum of Triamcinolone, previously dried, as directed in the potassium bromide disk method under Infrared Spectrophotometry <*2.25*>, and compare the spectrum with the Reference Spectrum or the spectrum of previously dried Triamcinolone RS: both spectra exhibit similar intensities of absorption at the same wave numbers. If any difference appears between the spectra, dissolve 0.1 g each of Triamcinolone and Triamcinolone RS in 7 mL of a mixture of 2-propanol and water (2:1), respectively, by warming. Allow the solutions to cool in ice to effect crystals, filter, then wash the formed crystals with two 10-mL portions of water, and repeat the test on the dried crystals.

Optical rotation <*2.49*> $[\alpha]_D^{20}$: +65 – +71° (after drying, 0.1 g, *N*,*N*-dimethylformamide, 10 mL, 100 mm).

Purity Heavy metals <*1.07*>—Proceed with 0.5 g of Triamcinolone according to Method 2, and perform the test. Prepare the control solution with 1.5 mL of Standard Lead Solution (not more than 30 ppm).

Loss on drying <*2.41*> Not more than 2.0% (0.5 g, in vacuum, phosphorus (V) oxide, 60°C, 3 hours).

Residue on ignition <*2.44*> Not more than 0.3% (0.5 g, platinum crucible).

Assay Dissolve about 20 mg each of Triamcinolone and Triamcinolone RS, previously dried and accurately weighed, in a solution of L-ascorbic acid in methanol (1 in 1000) to make exactly 50 mL. Pipet 5 mL each of these solutions, add exactly 5 mL each of the internal standard solution, add a solution of L-ascorbic acid in methanol (1 in 1000) to make 20 mL, and use these solutions as the sample solution and standard solution. Perform the test with 10 μL each of the sample solution and standard solution as directed under Liquid Chromatography <*2.01*> according to the following conditions, and calculate the ratios, Q_T and Q_S, of the peak height of triamcinolone to that of the internal standard.

Amount (mg) of triamcinolone ($C_{21}H_{27}FO_6$) = $M_S \times Q_T/Q_S$

M_S: Amount (mg) of Triamcinolone RS taken

Internal standard solution—Dissolve 15 mg of methyl parahydroxybenzoate in a solution of L-ascorbic acid in methanol (1 in 1000) to make 100 mL.

Operating conditions—

Detector: An ultraviolet absorption photometer (wavelength: 254 nm).

Column: A stainless steel column 4.0 mm in inside diame-

ter and 15 cm in length, packed with octadecylsilanized silica gel (5 μm in particle diameter).

Column temperature: A constant temperature of about 25°C.

Mobile phase: A mixture of water and acetonitrile (3:1).

Flow rate: Adjust so that the retention time of triamcinolone is about 10 minutes.

System suitability—

System performance: When the procedure is run with 10 μL of the standard solution under the above operating conditions, triamcinolone and the internal standard are eluted in this order with the resolution between these peaks being not less than 2.0.

System repeatability: When the test is repeated 6 times with 10 μL of the standard solution under the above operating conditions, the relative standard deviation of the ratios of the peak height of triamcinolone to that of the internal standard is not more than 1.5%.

Containers and storage Containers—Tight containers.

Storage—Light-resistant.

Triamcinolone Acetonide

トリアムシノロンアセトニド

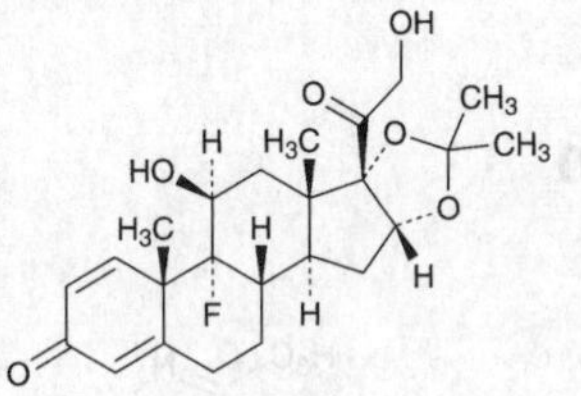

$C_{24}H_{31}FO_6$: 434.50

9-Fluoro-11β,21-dihydroxy-16α,17-(1-methylethylidenedioxy)pregna-1,4-diene-3,20-dione

[76-25-5]

Triamcinolone Acetonide, when dried, contains not less than 97.0% and not more than 103.0% of triamcinolone acetonide ($C_{24}H_{31}FO_6$).

Description Triamcinolone Acetonide occurs as a white crystalline powder.

It is sparingly soluble in ethanol (99.5) and in acetone, slightly soluble in methanol, and practically insoluble in water.

Melting point: about 290°C (with decomposition).

It shows crystal polymorphism.

Identification **(1)** Dissolve 2 mg of Triamcinolone Acetonide in 40 mL of ethanol (95), add 5 mL of 2,6-di-*tert*-butylcresol TS and 5 mL of sodium hydroxide TS, and heat on a water bath under a reflux condenser for 20 minutes: a green color develops.

(2) Add 5 mL of water and 1 mL of Fehling's TS to 0.01 g of Triamcinolone Acetonide, and heat: a red precipitate is produced.

(3) Proceed with 0.01 g of Triamcinolone Acetonide as directed under Oxygen Flask Combustion Method <*1.06*>, using a mixture of 0.5 mL of 0.01 mol/L sodium hydroxide TS and 20 mL of water as the absorbing liquid: the solution responds to Qualitative Tests <*1.09*> for fluoride.

(4) Determine the absorption spectrum of a solution of Triamcinolone Acetonide in ethanol (95) (1 in 100,000) as directed under Ultraviolet-visible Spectrophotometry <*2.24*>, and compare the spectrum with the Reference Spectrum or the spectrum of a solution of Triamcinolone Acetonide RS prepared in the same manner as the sample solution: both spectra exhibit similar intensities of absorption at the same wavelengths.

(5) Determine the infrared absorption spectrum of Triamcinolone Acetonide, previously dried, as directed in the potassium bromide disk method under the Infrared Spectrophotometry <*2.25*>, and compare the spectrum with the Reference Spectrum or the spectrum of previously dried Triamcinolone Acetonide RS: both spectra exhibit similar intensities of absorption at the same wave numbers. If any difference appears between the spectra, dissolve 0.1 g each of Triamcinolone Acetonide and Triamcinolone Acetonide RS in 20 mL of ethanol (95), respectively, then evaporate the ethanol to dryness, and repeat the test on the dried residue.

Optical rotation <*2.49*> $[\alpha]_D^{25}$: +110 – +120° (after drying, 0.1 g, ethanol (99.5), 10 mL, 100 mm).

Purity **(1)** Heavy metals <*1.07*>—Proceed with 0.5 g of Triamcinolone Acetonide according to Method 2, and perform the test. Prepare the control solution with 1.5 mL of Standard Lead Solution (not more than 30 ppm).

(2) Related substances—Dissolve 40 mg of Triamcinolone Acetonide in 4 mL of acetone, and use this solution as the sample solution. Pipet 1 mL of the sample solution, add acetone to make exactly 100 mL, and use this solution as the standard solution. Perform the test with these solutions as directed under Thin-layer Chromatography <*2.03*>. Spot 20 μL each of the sample solution and standard solution on a plate of silica gel with fluorescent indicator for thin-layer chromatography. Develop the plate with a mixture of chloroform and methanol (93:7) to a distance of about 10 cm, and air-dry the plate. Examine under ultraviolet light (main wavelength: 254 nm): the spots other than the principal spot obtained from the sample solution are not more intense than the spot from the standard solution.

Loss on drying <*2.41*> Not more than 2.0% (0.5 g, in vacuum, phosphorus (V) oxide, 60°C, 3 hours).

Residue on ignition <*2.44*> Not more than 0.2% (0.5 g, platinum crucible).

Assay Dissolve about 20 mg each of Triamcinolone Acetonide and Triamcinolone Acetonide RS, previously dried and accurately weighed, in methanol to make exactly 50 mL. Pipet 10 mL each of these solutions, add exactly 10 mL each of the internal standard solution, then add the mobile phase to make 50 mL, and use these solutions as the sample solution and standard solution. Perform the test with 20 μL each of these solutions as directed under Liquid Chromatography <*2.01*> according to the following conditions, and calculate the ratios, Q_T and Q_S, of the peak height of triamcinolone acetonide to that of the internal standard.

Amount (mg) of triamcinolone acetonide ($C_{24}H_{31}FO_6$)
$= M_S \times Q_T/Q_S$

M_S: Amount (mg) of Triamcinolone Acetonide RS taken

Internal standard solution—A solution of prednisolone in methanol (1 in 5000).

Operating conditions—

Detector: An ultraviolet absorption photometer (wavelength: 240 nm).

Column: A stainless steel column 4.6 mm in inside diameter and 30 cm in length, packed with octadecylsilanized silica gel (10 μm in particle diameter).

Column temperature: A constant temperature of about 25°C.

Mobile phase: A mixture of water and acetonitrile (3:1).

Flow rate: Adjust so that the retention time of triamcinolone acetonide is about 13 minutes.

System suitability—

System performance: When the procedure is run with 10 μL of the standard solution under the above operating conditions, the internal standard and triamcinolone acetonide are eluted in this order with the resolution between these peaks being not less than 6.

System repeatability: When the test is repeated 6 times with 10 μL of the standard solution under the above operating conditions, the relative standard deviation of the ratios of the peak height of triamcinolone acetonide to that of the internal standard is not more than 1.0%.

Containers and storage Containers—Tight containers.

Storage—Light-resistant.

Triamterene

トリアムテレン

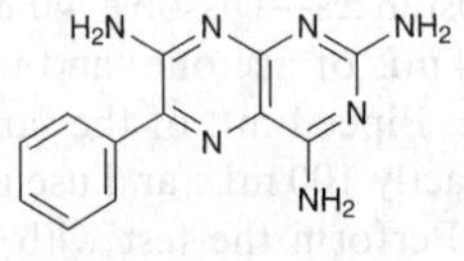

$C_{12}H_{11}N_7$: 253.26

6-Phenylpteridine-2,4,7-triamine

[396-01-0]

Triamterene, when dried, contains not less than 98.5% of triamterene ($C_{12}H_{11}N_7$).

Description Triamterene occurs as a yellow crystalline powder. It is odorless, and tasteless.

It is sparingly soluble in dimethylsulfoxide, very slightly soluble in acetic acid (100), and practically insoluble in water, in ethanol (95), and in diethyl ether.

It dissolves in nitric acid and in sulfuric acid, but does not dissolve in dilute nitric acid, in dilute sulfuric acid and in dilute hydrochloric acid.

Identification **(1)** To 0.01 g of Triamterene add 10 mL of water, heat, and filter after cooling: the filtrate shows a purple fluorescence. To 2 mL of the filtrate add 0.5 mL of hydrochloric acid: the fluorescence disappears.

(2) The filtrate obtained in (1) responds to Qualitative Tests *<1.09>* for primary aromatic amines.

(3) Dissolve 0.01 g of Triamterene in 100 mL of acetic acid (100), and to 10 mL of the solution add water to make 100 mL. Determine the absorption spectrum of the solution as directed under Ultraviolet-visible Spectrophotometry *<2.24>*, and compare the spectrum with the Reference Spectrum: both spectra exhibit similar intensities of absorption at the same wavelengths.

Purity **(1)** Heavy metals *<1.07>*—Proceed with 1.0 g of Triamterene according to Method 2, and perform the test. Prepare the control solution with 2.0 mL of Standard Lead Solution (not more than 20 ppm).

(2) Arsenic *<1.11>*—Prepare the test solution with 1.0 g of Triamterene according to Method 3, and perform the test (not more than 2 ppm).

(3) Related substances—Dissolve 0.10 g of Triamterene in 20 mL of dimethylsulfoxide. To 2 mL of this solution add methanol to make 50 mL, and use this solution as the sample solution. Pipet 1 mL of the sample solution, add methanol to make exactly 200 mL, and use this solution as the standard solution. Perform the test with these solutions as directed under Thin-layer Chromatography *<2.03>*. Spot 5 μL each of the sample solution and standard solution on a plate of silica gel for thin-layer chromatography. Develop the plate with a mixture of ethyl acetate, ammonia solution (28) and methanol (9:1:1) to a distance of about 10 cm, and air-dry the plate. Examine the plate under ultraviolet light (main wavelength: 365 nm): the spots other than the principal spot obtained from the sample solution are not more intense than the spot from the standard solution.

Loss on drying *<2.41>* Not more than 0.5% (1 g, 105°C, 4 hours).

Residue on ignition *<2.44>* Not more than 0.10% (1 g).

Assay Weigh accurately about 0.15 g of Triamterene, previously dried, and dissolve in 100 mL of acetic acid (100) by warming. Titrate *<2.50>* with 0.05 mol/L perchloric acid VS (indicator: 2 drops of crystal violet TS). Perform a blank determination in the same manner, and make any necessary correction.

Each mL of 0.05 mol/L perchloric acid VS
= 12.66 mg of $C_{12}H_{11}N_7$

Containers and storage Containers—Well-closed containers.

Triazolam

トリアゾラム

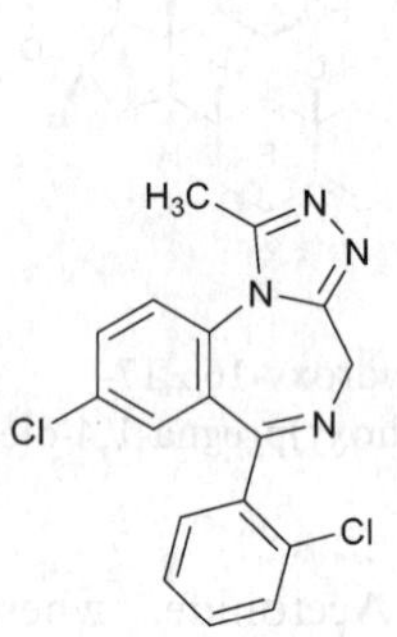

$C_{17}H_{12}Cl_2N_4$:343.21

8-Chloro-6-(2-chlorophenyl)-1-methyl-4*H*-[1,2,4]triazolo[4,3-*a*][1,4]benzodiazepine

[28911-01-5]

Triazolam, when dried, contains not less than 98.0% and not more than 102.0% of triazolam ($C_{17}H_{12}Cl_2N_4$).

Description Triazolam occurs as a white crystalline powder.

It is sparingly soluble in *N*,*N*-dimethylformamide, slightly soluble in ethanol (95), and practically insoluble in water.

It shows crystal polymorphism.

Identification **(1)** Determine the absorption spectrum of a solution of Triazolam in ethanol (95) (1 in 200,000) as directed under Ultraviolet-visible Spectrophotometry *<2.24>*, and compare the spectrum with the Reference Spectrum or the spectrum of a solution of Triazolam RS prepared in the same manner as the sample solution: both spectra exhibit similar intensities of absorption at the same wavelengths.

(2) Determine the infrared absorption spectrum of Triazolam, previously dried, as directed in the paste method under Infrared Spectrophotometry *<2.25>*, and compare the spectrum with the Reference Spectrum or the spectrum of dried Triazolam RS: both spectra exhibit similar intensities of absorption at the same wave numbers.

(3) Perform the test with Triazolam as directed under Flame Coloration Test *<1.04>* (2): a green to blue-green color appears.

Melting point *<2.60>* 239 – 243°C.

Purity **(1)** Chloride *<1.03>*—To 1.0 g of Triazolam add 50 mL of water, and allow to stand for 1 hour while occasional shaking, and filter. Discard the first 10 mL of the filtrate, pipet 25 mL of the subsequent filtrate, and add 6 mL of dilute nitric acid and water to make 50 mL. Perform the test using this solution as the test solution. Prepare the control solution with 0.40 mL of 0.01 mol/L hydrochloric acid VS (not more than 0.028%).

(2) Heavy metals—Being specified separately when the drug is granted approval based on the Law.

(3) Related substances—Dissolve 0.14 g of Triazolam in 10 mL of *N*,*N*-dimethylformamide, and use this solution as the sample solution. Pipet 1 mL of the sample solution, add *N*,*N*-dimethylformamide to make exactly 100 mL, and use this solution as the standard solution. Perform the test with exactly 12 μL each of the sample solution and standard solution as directed under Liquid Chromatography *<2.01>* according to the following conditions. Determine each peak area by the automatic integration method: the area of peak other than triazolam obtained from the sample solution is not larger than 1/5 times the peak area of triazolam from the standard solution, and the total area of the peaks other than triazolam is not larger than the peak area of triazolam from the standard solution. For the areas of the peaks, related substance A having the relative retention time of about 0.7 to triazolam, related substance B having the relative retention time of about 1.5, and related substance C having the relative retention time of about 2.4, multiply their correction factors, 1.8, 0.6 and 4.3, respectively.

Operating conditions—

Detector, column, column temperature, mobile phase A, mobile phase B, flowing of mobile phase, and flow rate: Proceed as directed in the operating conditions in the Assay.

Time span of measurement: For 39 minutes after injection, beginning after the solvent peak.

System suitability—

Test for required detectability: Pipet 1 mL of the standard solution, and add *N*,*N*-dimethylformamide to make exactly 10 mL. Confirm that the peak area of triazolam obtained with 12 μL of this solution is equivalent to 7 to 13% of that with 12 μL of the standard solution.

System performance: When the procedure is run with 12 μL of the standard solution under the above operating conditions, the number of theoretical plates and the symmetry factor of the peak of triazolam are not less than 4500 and not more than 1.6, respectively.

System repeatability: When the test is repeated 6 times with 12 μL of the standard solution under the above operating conditions, the relative standard deviation of the peak area of triazolam is not more than 2.0%.

Loss on drying *<2.41>* Not more than 0.5% (1 g, 105°C, 4 hours).

Residue on ignition *<2.44>* Not more than 0.3% (1 g).

Assay Weigh accurately about 55 mg each of Triazolam and Triazolam RS, previously dried, dissolve each in *N*,*N*-dimethylformamide to make exactly 50 mL, and use these solutions as the sample solution and the standard solution, respectively. Perform the test with 12 μL each of the sample solution and standard solution as directed under Liquid Chromatography *<2.01>* according to the following conditions, and determine the peak areas, A_T and A_S, of triazolam in each solution.

$$\text{Amount (mg) of triazolam } (C_{17}H_{12}Cl_2N_4) = M_S \times A_T/A_S$$

M_S: Amount (mg) of Triazolam RS taken

Operating conditions—

Detector: An ultraviolet absorption photometer (wavelength: 254 nm).

Column: A stainless steel column 4.6 mm in inside diameter and 25 cm in length, packed with phenylsilanized silica gel for liquid chromatography (5 μm in particle diameter).

Column temperature: A constant temperature of about 40°C.

Mobile phase A: A mixture of methanol and diluted acetic acid-ammonium acetate buffer solution (pH 4.5) (1 in 10) (14:11).

Mobile phase B: A mixture of methanol and diluted acetic acid-ammonium acetate buffer solution (pH 4.5) (1 in 10) (19:1).

Flowing of mobile phase: Control the gradient by mixing the mobile phases A and B as directed in the following table.

Time after injection of sample (min)	Mobile phase A (vol%)	Mobile phase B (vol%)
0 – 14	98	2
14 – 34	98 → 1	2 → 99
34 – 39	1	99

Flow rate: 2.0 mL per minute.

System suitability—

System performance: When the procedure is run with 12 μL of the standard solution under the above operating conditions, the number of theoretical plates and the symmetry factor of the peak of triazolam are not less than 4500 and not more than 2.0, respectively.

System repeatability: When the test is repeated 6 times with 12 μL of the standard solution under the above operating conditions, the relative standard deviation of the peak area of triazolam is not more than 1.0%.

Containers and storage Containers—Tight containers.

Others

Related substance A:

3-Amino-6-chloro-4-(2-chlorophenyl)-2-methyl-3,4-dihydroquinazolin-4-ol

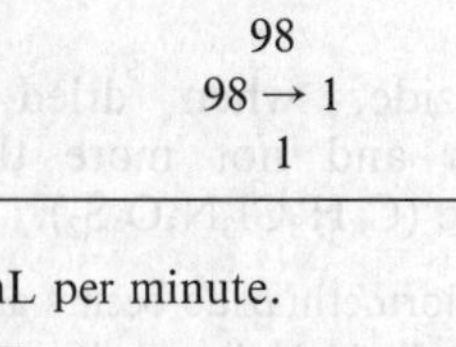

Related substance B:

8-Chloro-6-(2-chlorophenyl)-1-ethenyl-4*H*-[1,2,4]triazolo[4,3-*a*][1,4]benzodiazepine

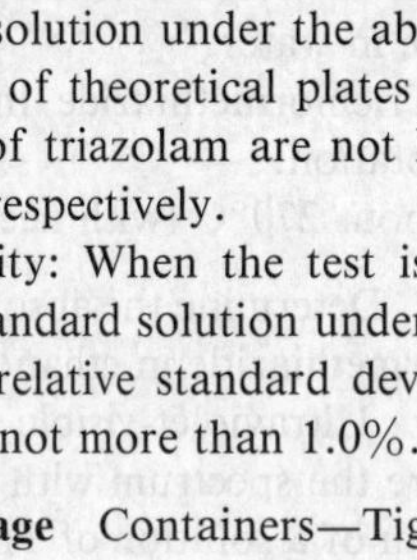

Related substance C:
8-Chloro-6-(2-chlorophenyl)-6-methoxy-1-methyl-4*H*,6*H*-[1,2,4]triazolo[4,3-*a*][4,1]benzoxazepine

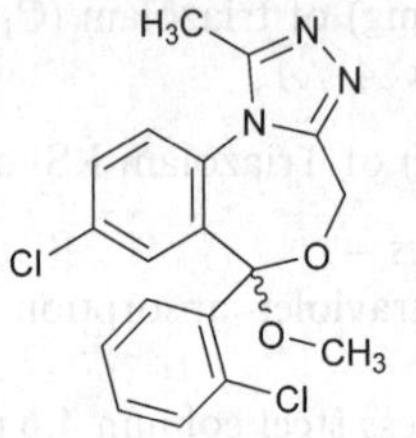

Trichlormethiazide

トリクロルメチアジド

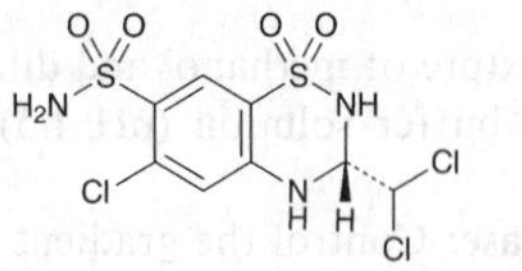

and enantiomer

$C_8H_8Cl_3N_3O_4S_2$: 380.66
(3*RS*)-6-Chloro-3-dichloromethyl-3,4-dihydro-2*H*-1,2,4-benzothiadiazine-7-sulfonamide 1,1-dioxide
[*133-67-5*]

Trichlormethiazide, when dried, contains not less than 97.5% and not more than 102.0% of trichlormethiazide ($C_8H_8Cl_3N_3O_4S_2$).

Description Trichlormethiazide occurs as a white powder.

It is freely soluble in *N*,*N*-dimethylformamide and in acetone, slightly soluble in acetonitrile and in ethanol (95), and practically insoluble in water.

A solution of Trichlormethiazide in acetone (1 in 50) shows no optical rotation.

Melting point: about 270°C (with decomposition).

Identification **(1)** Determine the absorption spectrum of a solution of Trichlormethiazide in ethanol (95) (3 in 250,000) as directed under Ultraviolet-visible Spectrophotometry <*2.24*>, and compare the spectrum with the Reference Spectrum or the spectrum of a solution of Trichlormethiazide RS prepared in the same manner as the sample solution: both spectra exhibit similar intensities of absorption at the same wavelengths.

(2) Determine the infrared absorption spectrum of Trichlormethiazide as directed in the potassium bromide disk method under Infrared Spectrophotometry <*2.25*>, and compare the spectrum with the Reference Spectrum or the spectrum of Trichlormethiazide RS: both spectra exhibit similar intensities of absorption at the same wave numbers.

(3) Perform the test with Trichlormethiazide as directed under Flame Coloration Test <*1.04*> (2): a green color appears.

Purity **(1)** Chloride <*1.03*>—Dissolve 1.0 g of Trichlormethiazide in 30 mL of acetone, add 6 mL of dilute nitric acid and water to make 50 mL, and perform the test using this solution as the test solution. Prepare the control solution as follows: to 1.0 mL of 0.01 mol/L hydrochloric acid VS add 30 mL of acetone, 6 mL of dilute nitric acid and water to make 50 mL (not more than 0.036%).

(2) Sulfate <*1.14*>—Dissolve 1.0 g of Trichlormethiazide in 30 mL of acetone, add 1 mL of dilute hydrochloric acid and water to make 50 mL, and perform the test using this solution as the test solution. Prepare the control solution as follows: to 1.0 mL of 0.005 mol/L sulfuric acid VS add 30 mL of acetone, 1 mL of dilute hydrochloric acid and water to make 50 mL (not more than 0.048%).

(3) Heavy metals <*1.07*>—Proceed with 1.0 g of Trichlormethiazide according to Method 2, and perform the test. Prepare the control solution with 2.0 mL of Standard Lead Solution (not more than 20 ppm).

(4) Arsenic <*1.11*>—Prepare the test solution with 0.6 g of Trichlormethiazide according to Method 5, using 20 mL of *N*,*N*-dimethylformamide, and perform the test (not more than 3.3 ppm).

(5) Related substances—Dissolve 25 mg of Trichlormethiazide in 50 mL of acetonitrile, and use the solution as the sample solution. Perform the test with 10 μL of the sample solution as directed under Liquid Chromatography <*2.01*> according to the following conditions. Determine each peak area by the automatic integration method, and calculate the amount of related substances by the area percentage method: the amount of 4-amino-6-chlorobenzene-1,3-disulfonamide, having the relative retention time of about 0.3 to trichlormethiazide, is not more than 2.0%, and the total amount of the related substances is not more than 2.5%.

Operating conditions—

Detector: An ultraviolet absorption photometer (wavelength: 268 nm).

Column: A stainless steel column 4.6 mm in inside diameter and 15 cm in length, packed with phenylsilanized silica gel for liquid chromatography (5 μm in particle diameter).

Column temperature: A constant temperature of about 25°C.

Mobile phase A: A mixture of diluted phosphoric acid (1 in 1000) and acetonitrile (3:1).

Mobile phase B: A mixture of acetonitrile and diluted phosphoric acid (1 in 1000) (3:1).

Flowing of mobile phase: Control the gradient by mixing the mobile phases A and B as directed in the following table.

Time after injection of sample (min)	Mobile phase A (vol%)	Mobile phase B (vol%)
0 – 10	100	0
10 – 20	100 → 0	0 → 100

Flow rate: 1.5 mL per minute.

Time span of measurement: About 2.5 times as long as the retention time of trichlormethiazide, beginning after the solvent peak.

System suitability—

Test for required detectability: To exactly 1 mL of the sample solution add acetonitrile to make exactly 50 mL, and use this solution as the solution for system suitability test. Pipet 1 mL of the solution for system suitability test, and add acetonitrile to make exactly 20 mL. Confirm that the peak area of trichlormethiazide obtained with 10 μL of this solution is equivalent to 3.5 to 6.5% of that with 10 μL of the solution for system suitability test.

System performance: To 5 mL of the solution for system suitability test add 5 mL of water, and warm in a water bath at 60°C for 30 minutes. When the procedure is run with 10 μL of this solution, after cooling, under the above operating conditions, 4-amino-6-chlorobenzene-1,3-disulfonamide and trichlormethiazide are eluted in this order, the relative retention time of 4-amino-6-chlorobenzene-1,3-disulfonamide to trichlormethiazide is about 0.3, and the number of theoretical plates and the symmetry factor of the peak of trichlormethiazide are not less than 5000 and not more than 1.2, respectively.

System repeatability: When the test is repeated 3 times with 10 μL of the solution for system suitability test under the above operating conditions, the relative standard deviation of the peak area of trichlormethiazide is not more than 2.0%.

Loss on drying <*2.41*> Not more than 0.5% (1 g, 105°C, 3 hours).

Residue on ignition <*2.44*> Not more than 0.1% (1 g).

Assay Weigh accurately about 25 mg of Trichlormethiazide and Trichlormethiazide RS, previously dried, and dissolve separately in exactly 20 mL of the internal standard solution. To 1 mL of these solutions add acetonitrile to make 20 mL, and use these solutions as the sample solution and standard solution. Perform the test with 10 μL each of the sample solution and standard solution as directed under Liquid Chromatography <*2.01*> according to the following conditions, and calculate the ratios, Q_T and Q_S, of the peak area of trichlormethiazide to that of the internal standard.

Amount (mg) of trichlormethiazide ($C_8H_8Cl_3N_3O_4S_2$)
$= M_S \times Q_T/Q_S$

M_S: Amount (mg) of Trichlormethiazide RS taken

Internal standard solution—A solution of 3-nitrophenol in acetonitrile (1 in 800).

Operating conditions—

Detector: An ultraviolet absorption photometer (wavelength: 268 nm).

Column: A stainless steel column 4.6 mm in inside diameter and 15 cm in length, packed with phenylsilanized silica gel for liquid chromatography (5 μm in particle diameter).

Column temperature: A constant temperature of about 25°C.

Mobile phase: A mixture of diluted phosphoric acid (1 in 1000) and acetonitrile (3:1).

Flow rate: Adjust so that the retention time of trichlormethiazide is about 8 minutes.

System suitability—

System performance: When the procedure is run with 10 μL of the standard solution under the above operating conditions, the internal standard and trichlormethiazide are eluted in this order with the resolution between these peaks being not less than 2.0.

System repeatability: When the test is repeated 6 times with 10 μL of the standard solution under the above operating conditions, the relative standard deviation of the ratio of the peak area of trichlormethiazide to that of the internal standard is not more than 1.0%.

Containers and storage Containers—Well-closed containers.

Trichlormethiazide Tablets

トリクロルメチアジド錠

Trichlormethiazide Tablets contain not less than 93.0% and not more than 107.0% of the labeled amount of trichlormethiazide ($C_8H_8Cl_3N_3O_4S_2$: 380.66).

Method of preparation Prepare as directed under Tablets, with Trichlormethiazide.

Identification To an amount of powdered Trichlormethiazide Tablets, equivalent to 4 mg of Trichlormethiazide, add 10 mL of acetone, shake vigorously for 5 minutes, centrifuge, and use the supernatant liquid as the sample solution. Separately, dissolve 4 mg of Trichlormethiazide RS in 10 mL of acetone, and use this solution as the standard solution. Perform the test with these solutions as directed under Thin-layer Chromatography <*2.03*>. Spot 5 μL each of the sample solution and standard solution on a plate of silica gel with fluorescent indicator for thin-layer chromatography. Develop the plate with a mixture of ethyl acetate, hexane and methanol (10:4:1) to a distance of about 10 cm, and air-dry the plate. Examine under ultraviolet light (main wavelength: 254 nm): the principal spots from the sample solution and the standard solution show the same *Rf* value.

Purity Related substances—Powder a suitable amount of Trichlormethiazide Tablets in an agate mortar. Take an amount of the powder, equivalent to 10 mg of Trichlormethiazide, add 20 mL of acetonitrile, shake vigorously for 15 minutes, centrifuge, and use the supernatant liquid as the sample solution. Perform the test with 10 μL of the sample solution as directed under Liquid Chromatography <*2.01*> according to the following conditions, determine each peak area by the automatic integration method, and calculate the amount of each related substance by the area percentage method: the amount of 4-amino-6-chlorobenzene-1,3-disulfoneamide, having the relative retention time of about 0.3 to trichlormethiazide, is not more than 4.0%, and the total amount of the peaks other than trichlormethiazide is not more than 5.0%.

Operating conditions—

Detector: An ultraviolet absorption photometer (wavelength: 268 nm).

Column: A stainless steel column 4.6 mm in inside diameter and 15 cm in length, packed with phenylsilanized silica gel for liquid chromatography (5 μm in particle diameter).

Column temperature: A constant temperature of about 25°C.

Mobile phase A: A mixture of diluted phosphoric acid (1 in 1000) and acetonitrile (3:1).

Mobile phase B: A mixture of acetonitrile and diluted phosphoric acid (1 in 1000) (3:1).

Flowing of mobile phase: Control the gradient by mixing the mobile phases A and B as directed in the following table.

Time after injection of sample (min)	Mobile phase A (vol%)	Mobile phase B (vol%)
0 – 10	100	0
10 – 20	100 → 0	0 → 100

Flow rate: 1.5 mL per minute.

Time span of measurement: About 2.5 times as long as the retention time of trichlormethiazide, beginning after the solvent peak.

System suitability—

Test for required detectability: Dissolve 25 mg of Trichlormethiazide in 50 mL of acetonitrile. To 1 mL of this solution add acetonitrile to make 50 mL, and use this solution as the solution for system suitability test. Pipet 1 mL of the solution for system suitability test, and add acetonitrile to make exactly 20 mL. Confirm that the peak area of trichlormethiazide obtained with 10 μL of this solution is equivalent to 3.5 to 6.5% of that with 10 μL of the solution for system suitability test.

System performance: To 5 mL of the solution for system suitability test add 5 mL of water, and warm in a water bath of 60°C for 30 minutes. When the procedure is run with 10 μL of this solution, after cooling, under the above operating conditions, 4-amino-6-chlorobenzene-1,3-disulfonamide and trichlormethiazide are eluted in this order, the relative retention time of 4-amino-6-chlorobenzene-1,3-disulfonamide to trichlormethiazide is about 0.3, and the number of theoretical plates and the symmetry factor of the peak of trichlormethiazide are not less than 5000 and not more than 1.2, respectively.

System repeatability: When the test is repeated 3 times with 10 μL of the solution for system suitability test under the above operating conditions, the relative standard deviation of the peak area of trichlormethiazide is not more than 2.0%.

Uniformity of dosage units <*6.02*> Perform the test according to the following method: it meets the requirement of the Content uniformity test.

To 1 tablet of Trichlormethiazide Tablets add V/5 mL of diluted phosphoric acid (1 in 50), and disintegrate the tablet. Add 2V/5 mL of acetonitrile, shake vigorously for 15 minutes, add the mobile phase to make exactly V mL so that each mL contains about 40 μg of trichlormethiazide ($C_8H_8Cl_3N_3O_4S_2$). Filter this solution through a membrane filter with a pore size not exceeding 0.45 μm, discard the first 4 mL of the filtrate, and use the subsequent filtrate as the sample solution. Then, proceed as directed in the Assay.

Amount (mg) of trichlormethiazide ($C_8H_8Cl_3N_3O_4S_2$)
$= M_S \times A_T/A_S \times V/500$

M_S: Amount (mg) of Trichlormethiazide RS taken

Dissolution <*6.10*> When the test is performed at 50 revolutions per minute according to the Paddle method, using 900 mL of water as the dissolution medium, the dissolution rate in 15 minutes of Trichlormethiazide Tablets is not less than 75%.

Start the test with 1 tablet of Trichlormethiazide Tablets, withdraw not less than 20 mL of the medium at the specified minute after starting the test, and filter through a membrane filter with a pore size not exceeding 0.45 μm. Discard not less than 10 mL of the first filtrate, pipet V mL of the subsequent filtrate, add diluted phosphoric acid (1 in 50) to make exactly V' mL so that each mL contains about 1.1 μg of trichlormethiazide ($C_8H_8Cl_3N_3O_4S_2$), and use this solution as the sample solution. Separately, weigh accurately about 22 mg of Trichlormethiazide RS, previously dried at 105°C for 3 hours, and dissolve in acetonitrile to make exactly 200 mL. Pipet 2 mL of this solution, add diluted phosphoric acid (1 in 50) to make exactly 200 mL, and use this solution as the standard solution. Perform the test with exactly 40 μL each of the sample solution and standard solution as directed under Liquid Chromatography <*2.01*> according to the following conditions, and determine the peak areas, A_{Ta} and A_{Sa}, of trichlormethiazide obtained with the sample solution and standard solution, and the area, A_{Tb}, of the peak, having the relative retention time of about 0.3 to trichlormethiazide, obtained with the sample solution.

Dissolution rate (%) with respect to the labeled amount of trichlormethiazide ($C_8H_8Cl_3N_3O_4S_2$)
$= M_S \times (A_{Ta} + 0.95A_{Tb})/A_{Sa} \times V'/V \times 1/C \times 9/2$

M_S: Amount (mg) of Trichlormethiazide RS taken
C: Labeled amount (mg) of trichlormethiazide ($C_8H_8Cl_3N_3O_4S_2$) in 1 tablet

Operating conditions—

Proceed as directed in the operating conditions in the Assay.

System suitability—

System performance: Dissolve 25 mg of Trichlormethiazide in 50 mL of acetonitrile. To 1 mL of this solution add acetonitrile to make 50 mL. To 5 mL of this solution add 5 mL of water, and warm at 60°C in a water bath for 30 minutes. After cooling, when the procedure is run with 10 μL of this solution under the above operating conditions, 4-amino-6-chlorobenzene-1,3-disulfonamide and trichlormethiazide are eluted in this order, the relative retention time of 4-amino-6-chlorobenzene-1,3-disulfonamide to trichlormethiazide is about 0.3, and the number of theoretical plates and the symmetry factor of the peak of trichlormethiazide are not less than 5000 and not more than 1.2, respectively.

System repeatability: When the test is repeated 6 times with 40 μL of the standard solution under the above operating conditions, the relative standard deviation of the peak area of trichlormethiazide is not more than 2.0%.

Assay To 10 Trichlormethiazide Tablets add V/10 mL of diluted phosphoric acid (1 in 50), and disintegrate the tablets. Add V/2 mL of acetonitrile, shake vigorously for 15 minutes, add the mobile phase to make exactly V mL so that each mL contains about 0.2 mg of trichlormethiazide ($C_8H_8Cl_3N_3O_4S_2$), and centrifuge. Pipet 5 mL of the supernatant liquid, add the mobile phase to make exactly 25 mL, and filter through a membrane filter with a pore size not exceeding 0.45 μm. Discard the first 4 mL of the filtrate, and use the subsequent filtrate as the sample solution. Separately, weigh accurately about 20 mg of Trichlormethiazide RS, previously dried at 105°C for 3 hours, and dissolve in the mobile phase to make exactly 100 mL. Pipet 5 mL of this solution, add the mobile phase to make exactly 25 mL, and use this solution as the standard solution. Perform the test with exactly 20 μL each of the sample solution and standard solution as directed under Liquid Chromatography <*2.01*> according to the following conditions, and determine the peak areas, A_T and A_S, of trichlormethiazide in each solution.

Amount (mg) of trichlormethiazide ($C_8H_8Cl_3N_3O_4S_2$) in 1 tablet
$= M_S \times A_T/A_S \times V/1000$

M_S: Amount (mg) of Trichlormethiazide RS taken

Operating conditions—

Proceed as directed in the operating conditions in the Assay under Trichlormethiazide.

System suitability—

System performance: When the procedure is run with 20 μL of the standard solution under the above operating conditions, the number of theoretical plates and the symmetry factor of the peak of trichlormethiazide are not less than 5000 and not more than 1.2, respectively.

System repeatability: When the test is repeated 6 times with 20 μL of the standard solution under the above operating conditions, the relative standard deviation of the peak area of trichlormethiazide is not more than 1.0%.

Containers and storage Containers—Tight containers.

Trichomycin

トリコマイシン

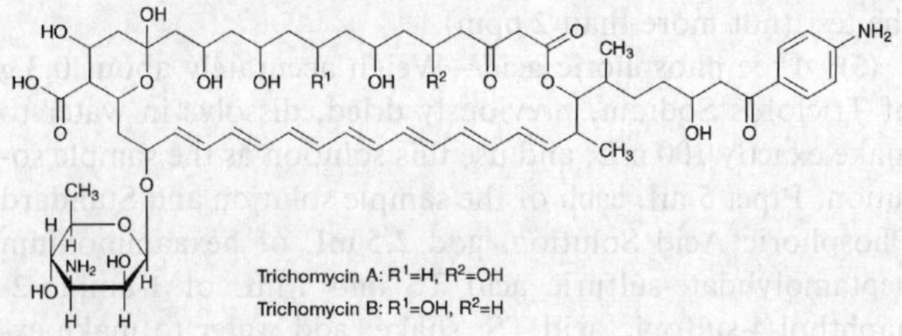

Trichomycin A: R^1=H, R^2=OH
Trichomycin B: R^1=OH, R^2=H

Trichomycin A
33-(3-Amino-3,6-dideoxy-β-D-mannopyranosyloxy)-17-[6-(4-aminophenyl)-4-hydroxy-1-methyl-6-oxohexyl]-1,3,5,9,11,37-hexahydroxy-18-methyl-13,15-dioxo-16,39-dioxabicyclo[33.3.1]nonatriaconta-19,21,23,25,27,29,31-heptaene-36-carboxylic acid
[*12698-99-6*]
Trichomycin B
33-(3-Amino-3,6-dideoxy-β-D-mannopyranosyloxy)-17-[6-(4-aminophenyl)-4-hydroxy-1-methyl-6-oxohexyl]-1,3,5,7,9,37-hexahydroxy-18-methyl-13,15-dioxo-16,39-dioxabicyclo[33.3.1]nonatriaconta-19,21,23,25,27,29,31-heptaene-36-carboxylic acid
[*12699-00-2*]
[*1394-02-1*, Trichomycin]

Trichomycin is a mixture of polyene macrolide substances having antifungal and antiprotozoal activities produced by the growth of *Streptomyces hachijoensis*.

It contains not less than 7000 Units per mg, calculated on the dried basis. The potency of Trichomycin is expressed as unit based on the amount of trichomycin. One unit of Trichomycin is equivalent to 0.05 μg of trichomycin.

Description Trichomycin occurs as a yellow to yellow-brown powder.

It is practically insoluble in water, in ethanol (99.5) and in tetrahydrofuran.

It dissolves in dilute sodium hydroxide TS.

It is hygroscopic.

Identification **(1)** To 2 mg of Trichomycin add 2 mL of sulfuric acid: a blue color appears, and the color is changed to a blue-purple after allowing to stand.

(2) Dissolve 1 mg of Trichomycin in 50 mL of a solution of sodium hydroxide (1 in 200). Determine the absorption spectrum of this solution as directed under Ultraviolet-visible Spectrophotometry <*2.24*>: it exhibits maxima between 359 nm and 365 nm, between 378 nm and 384 nm, and between 400 nm and 406 nm.

Content ratio of the active principle Conduct this procedure without exposure to light, using light-resistant vessels. Dissolve 10 mg of Trichomycin in 50 mL of a mixture of tetrahydrofuran for liquid chromatography and water (3:1), and use this solution as the sample solution. Perform the test with 5 μL of the sample solution as directed under Liquid Chromatography <*2.01*> according to the following conditions, determine the peak areas by the automatic integration method, and calculate the amount of trichomycin A and trichomycin B by the area percentage method: the amount of trichomycin A is between 20% and 40%, and that of trichomycin B is between 15% and 25%. The relative retention time of trichomycin B to trichomycin A is about 1.2.

Operating conditions—

Detector: An ultraviolet absorption photometer (wavelength: 360 nm).

Column: A stainless steel column 4.6 mm in inside diameter and 15 cm in length, packed with octadecylsilanized silica gel for liquid chromatography (5 μm in particle diameter).

Column temperature: A constant temperature of about 25°C.

Mobile phase: Dissolve 3.4 g of potassium dihydrogen phosphate and 1.7 g of sodium lauryl sulfate in a mixture of 600 mL of water and 400 mL of acetonitrile for liquid chromatography.

Flow rate: Adjust so that the retention time of trichomycin A is about 8 minutes.

Time span of measurement: About 4 times as long as the retention time of trichomycin A.

System suitability—

Test for required detectability: Measure 5 mL of the sample solution, add a mixture of tetrahydrofuran for liquid chromatography and water (3:1) to make 50 mL, and use this solution as the solution for system suitability test. Pipet 5 mL of the solution for system suitability test, and add a mixture of tetrahydrofuran for liquid chromatography and water (3:1) to make exactly 30 mL. Confirm that the peak area of trichomycin A obtained with 5 μL of this solution is equivalent to 12 to 22% of that with 5 μL of the solution for system suitability test.

System performance: When the procedure is run with 5 μL of the solution for system suitability test under the above operating conditions, trichomycin A and trichomycin B are eluted in this order with the resolution between these peaks being not less than 2.5.

System repeatability: When the test is repeated 6 times with 5 μL of the solution for system suitability test under the above operating conditions, the relative standard deviation of the peak area of trichomycin A is not more than 2.0%.

Loss on drying <*2.41*> Not more than 5.0% (1 g, in vacuum, 60°C, 3 hours).

Assay Conduct this procedure without exposure to light, using light-resistant vessels. Weigh accurately an amount of Trichomycin and Trichomycin RS, equivalent to about 150,000 units, dissolve them separately in a mixture of tetrahydrofuran for liquid chromatography and water (3:1) to make exactly 100 mL, and use these solutions as the sample solution and standard solution. Perform the test with exactly 20 μL each of the sample solution and standard solution as directed under Liquid Chromatography <*2.01*> according to the following conditions, and determine the peak areas, A_T and A_S, of trichomycin in each solution.

$$\text{Amount (unit) of trichomycin} = M_S \times A_T/A_S$$

M_S: Amount (unit) of Trichomycin RS taken

Operating conditions—

Detector: An ultraviolet absorption photometer (wavelength: 360 nm).

Column: A stainless steel column 4.6 mm in inside diameter and 15 cm in length, packed with silica gel for liquid chromatography (10 μm in particle diameter).

Column temperature: A constant temperature of about 25°C.

Mobile phase: Dissolve 15 g of ammonium acetate in 120 mL of water, and add 1000 mL of acetonitrile for liquid chromatography and 700 mL of methanol.

Flow rate: Adjust so that the retention time of trichomycin is about 6 minutes.

System suitability—

System performance: Dissolve 5 mg of Trichomycin and 1 mg of berberine chloride hydrate in 100 mL of a mixture of tetrahydrofuran for liquid chromatography and water (3:1). When the procedure is run with 20 μL of this solution under the above operating conditions, berberine and trichomycin are eluted in this order with the resolution between these peaks being not less than 4.

System repeatability: When the test is repeated 6 times with 20 μL of the standard solution under the above operating conditions, the relative standard deviation of the peak area of trichomycin is not more than 2.0%.

Containers and storage Containers—Tight containers.

Storage—Light-resistant, and in a cold place.

Triclofos Sodium

トリクロホスナトリウム

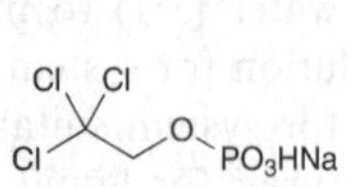

$C_2H_3Cl_3NaO_4P$: 251.37

Monosodium 2,2,2-trichloroethyl monohydrogen phosphate

[*7246-20-0*]

Triclofos Sodium, when dried, contains not less than 97.0% and not more than 102.0% of triclofos sodium ($C_2H_3Cl_3NaO_4P$), and not less than 41.0% and not more than 43.2% of chlorine (Cl: 35.45).

Description Triclofos Sodium is a white crystalline powder.

It is freely soluble in water, slightly soluble in ethanol (95), and practically insoluble in diethyl ether.

It is hygroscopic.

Identification **(1)** Determine the infrared absorption spectrum of Triclofos Sodium as directed in the potassium bromide disk method under Infrared Spectrophotometry <*2.25*>, and compare the spectrum with the Reference Spectrum: both spectra exhibit similar intensities of absorption at the same wave numbers.

(2) To 0.5 g of Triclofos Sodium add 10 mL of nitric acid, evaporate on a water bath to dryness, and ignite further over a flame. Dissolve the residue in 5 mL of water, and filter it necessary: the filtrate responds to Qualitative Tests <*1.09*> for sodium salt.

(3) To 0.1 g of Triclofos Sodium add 1 g of anhydrous sodium carbonate, and heat for 10 minutes. After cooling, dissolve the residue in 40 mL of water, filter if necessary, and render the filtrate acidic with dilute nitric acid: the solution responds to Qualitative Tests <*1.09*> (2) for chloride. The remainder of the filtrate responds to Qualitative Tests <*1.09*> (1) for chloride and to Qualitative Tests <*1.09*> for phosphate.

pH <*2.54*> Dissolve 1.0 g of Triclofos Sodium in 50 mL of water: the pH of this solution is between 3.0 and 4.5.

Purity **(1)** Clarity and color of solution—Dissolve 1.0 g of Triclofos Sodium in 50 mL of water: the solution is clear and colorless.

(2) Chloride <*1.03*>—Perform the test with 0.20 g of Triclofos Sodium. Prepare the control solution with 1.0 mL of 0.01 mol/L hydrochloric acid VS (not more than 0.178%).

(3) Heavy metals <*1.07*>—Proceed with 1.0 g of Triclofos Sodium according to Method 1, and perform the test. Prepare the control solution with 2.0 mL of Standard Lead Solution (not more than 20 ppm).

(4) Arsenic <*1.11*>—Prepare the test solution with 1.0 g of Triclofos Sodium according to Method 1, and perform the test (not more than 2 ppm).

(5) Free phosphoric acid—Weigh accurately about 0.3 g of Triclofos Sodium, previously dried, dissolve in water to make exactly 100 mL, and use this solution as the sample solution. Pipet 5 mL each of the sample solution and Standard Phosphoric Acid Solution, add 2.5 mL of hexaammonium heptamolybdate-sulfuric acid TS and 1 mL of 1-amino-2-naphthol-4-sulfonic acid TS, shake, add water to make exactly 25 mL, and allow to stand at 20°C for 30 minutes. Perform the test with these solutions, using a solution obtained in the same manner with 5 mL of water as the blank, as directed under Ultraviolet-visible Spectrophotometry <*2.24*>. Determine the absorbances, A_T and A_S, of each solution from the sample solution and Standard Phosphoric Acid Solution at 740 nm: the content of the free phosphoric acid is not more than 1.0%.

$$\text{Content (\%) of the free phosphoric acid } (H_3PO_4) = 1/M \times A_T/A_S \times 258.0$$

M: Amount (mg) of Triclofos Sodium taken

Loss on drying <*2.41*> Not more than 5.0% (1 g, in vacuum, 100°C, 3 hours).

Assay **(1)** Triclofos sodium—Weigh accurately about 0.2 g of Triclofos Sodium, previously dried, place in a Kjeldahl flask, add 2 mL of sulfuric acid and 2.5 mL of nitric acid, and heat until brown gas are not evolved. After cooling, add 1 mL of nitric acid, heat until white fumes are produced, and cool. Repeat this procedure until the solution becomes colorless. Transfer this solution to a flask using 150 mL of water, add 50 mL of molybdenum (VI) oxide-citric acid TS, heat gently to boil, add gradually 25 mL of quinoline TS with stirring, and heat on a water bath for 5 minutes. After cooling, filter the precipitate, and wash repeatedly with water until the washing does not indicate acidity. Transfer the precipitate to a flask using 100 mL of water, add exactly 50 mL of 0.5 mol/L sodium hydroxide VS, dissolve, and titrate <*2.50*> with 0.5 mol/L hydrochloric acid VS until the color of the solution changes from purple to yellow (indicator: 3 drops of phenolphthalein-thymol blue TS). Perform a blank determination in the same manner.

$$\text{Each mL of 0.5 mol/L sodium hydroxide VS} = 4.834 \text{ mg of } C_2H_3Cl_3NaO_4P$$

(2) Chlorine—Weigh accurately about 10 mg of Triclofos Sodium, previously dried, perform the test according to the procedure of determination for chlorine as directed under Oxygen Flask Combustion Method <*1.06*>, using 1 mL of sodium hydroxide TS and 20 mL of water as the absorbing liquid.

Containers and storage Containers—Tight containers.

Triclofos Sodium Syrup

トリクロホスナトリウムシロップ

Triclofos Sodium Syrup contains not less than 90.0% and not more than 110.0% of the labeled amount of triclofos sodium ($C_2H_3Cl_3NaO_4P$: 251.37).

Method of preparation Prepare as directed under Syrups, with Triclofos Sodium.

Identification **(1)** Weigh a portion of Triclofos Sodium Syrup, equivalent to 0.25 g of Triclofos Sodium, add 40 mL of water, shake well, add 5 mL of diluted sulfuric acid (3 in 50), and extract with 25 mL of 3-methyl-1-butanol. Take 5 mL of the extract, evaporate on a water bath to dryness, and add 1 mL of diluted sulfuric acid (1 in 2) and 1 mL of a solution of potassium permanganate (1 in 20) to the residue. Heat in a water bath for 5 minutes, add 7 mL of water, and then add a solution of oxalic acid dihydrate (1 in 20) until the color of the solution disappears. To 1 mL of this solution add 1 mL of pyridine and 1 mL of a solution of sodium hydroxide (1 in 5), and heat in a water bath, while shaking, for 1 minute: a light red color develops in the pyridine layer.

(2) Take 10 mL of the extract obtained in (1), evaporate on a water bath to dryness, add 1 g of anhydrous sodium carbonate to the residue, and heat for 10 minutes. After cooling, dissolve the residue in 40 mL of water, filter if necessary, and render the filtrate acidic with dilute nitric acid: the solution responds to Qualitative Tests <*1.09*> (2) for chloride. The remainder of the filtrate responds to Qualitative Tests <*1.09*> (1) for chloride and to Qualitative Tests <*1.09*> for phosphate.

pH <*2.54*> 6.0 – 6.5

Assay Weigh accurately a portion of Triclofos Sodium Syrup, equivalent to 0.13 g of Triclofos Sodium, add 15 mL of water, 1 mL of sodium hydroxide TS and 15 mL of diethyl ether, shake for 1 minute, and separate the water layer. Wash the diethyl ether layer with 1 mL of water, and combine the washing with above water layer. To this solution add 2.5 mL of diluted sulfuric acid (3 in 50), and extract with four 10-mL portions of 3-methyl-1-butanol. Combine the 3-methyl-1-butanol extracts, and add 3-methyl-1-butanol to make exactly 50 mL. Measure exactly 10 mL each of this solution, and dilute potassium hydroxide-ethanol TS, place in a glass ampule, fire-seal, mix, and heat at 120°C for 2 hours in an autoclave. After cooling, transfer the contents to a flask, add 20 mL of diluted nitric acid (63 in 500) and exactly 25 mL of 0.02 mol/L silver nitrate VS, shake well, and titrate <*2.50*> the excess silver nitrate with 0.02 mol/L ammonium thiocyanate VS (indicator: 2 to 3 drops of ammonium iron (III) sulfate TS). Perform a blank determination in the same manner.

Each mL of 0.02 mol/L silver nitrate VS
= 1.676 mg of $C_2H_3Cl_3NaO_4P$

Containers and storage Containers—Tight containers.
Storage—In a cold place.

Trientine Hydrochloride

トリエンチン塩酸塩

$H_2N-CH_2CH_2-NH-CH_2CH_2-NH-CH_2CH_2-NH_2 \cdot 2HCl$

$C_6H_{18}N_4.2HCl$: 219.16
N, *N'*-Bis(2-aminoethyl)ethane-1,2-diamine dihydrochloride
[*38260-01-4*]

Trientine Hydrochloride contains not less than 97.0% and not more than 101.0% of trientine hydrochloride ($C_6H_{18}N_4.2HCl$), calculated on the dried basis.

Description Trientine Hydrochloride occurs as white to pale yellow, crystals or crystalline powder. It is odorless or has slightly an ammonia-like odor.

It is freely soluble in water, soluble in methanol, and slightly soluble in ethanol (99.5).

It is hygroscopic.

Melting point: about 121°C.

Identification **(1)** Determine the infrared absorption spectrum of Trientine Hydrochloride, previously dried, as directed in the paste method under Infrared Spectrophotometry <*2.25*>, and compare the spectrum with the Reference Spectrum: both spectra exhibit similar intensities of absorption at the same wave numbers.

(2) A solution of Trientine Hydrochloride (1 in 100) responds to Qualitative Tests <*1.09*> (2) for chloride.

pH <*2.54*> The pH of a solution obtained by dissolving 1 g of Trientine Hydrochloride in 100 mL of water is between 7.0 and 8.5.

Purity **(1)** Heavy metals <*1.07*>—Proceed with 2.0 g of Trientine Hydrochloride according to Method 4, and perform the test. Prepare the control solution with 2.0 mL of Standard Lead solution (not more than 10 ppm).

(2) Related substances—Dissolve 0.30 g of Trientine Hydrochloride in 100 mL of methanol, and use this solution as the sample solution. Pipet 1 mL of the sample solution, add methanol to make exactly 100 mL, and use this solution as the standard solution. Perform the test with these solutions as directed under Thin-layer Chromatography <*2.03*>. Spot 3 μL each of the sample solution and standard solution on two plates of silica gel for thin-layer chromatography. Develop the one plate with a mixture of 2-propanol and ammonia solution (28) (3:2) to a distance of about 6 cm, and air-dry the plate. Spray evenly ninhydrin-butanol TS on the plate, and heat the plate at 130°C for 5 minutes: the spots other than the principal spot and the spot nearby the starting point obtained from the sample solution is not more intense than the spot from the standard solution. Develop another plate with a mixture of ammonia solution (28), diethylether, acetonitrile, and ethanol (99.5) (10:4:3:3) to a distance of about 6 cm, and air-dry the plate. Spray evenly ninhydrin-butanol TS on the plate, and heat the plate at 130°C for 5 minutes: the spot nearby the starting point from the sample solution is not more intense than the spot from the standard solution.

Loss on drying <*2.41*> Not more than 2.0% (1 g, reduced pressure not exceeding 0.67 kPa, 40°C, 4 hours).

Residue on ignition <*2.44*> Not more than 0.1% (1 g).

Assay Weigh accurately about 0.22 g of Trientine Hydrochloride, and dissolve in 10 mL of 0.1 mol/L hydrochloric acid VS, 2 mL of a solution of sodium nitrate (9 in 20), 10 mL of acetic acid-ammonium acetate buffer solution (pH 4.8) and 50 mL of water. Titrate <*2.50*> with 0.1 mol/L copper (II) nitrate VS (potentiometric titration) using a copper electrode as the indicator electrode, a complex type silver-silver chloride electrode as the reference electrode, and potassium chloride solution (1 in 4) as the inner solution. Perform a blank determination in the same manner, and make any necessary correction.

Each mL of 0.1 mol/L copper (II) nitrate VS
= 21.92 mg of $C_6H_{18}N_4.2HCl$

Containers and storage Containers—Tight containers.

Storage—Light-resistant, substituted by argon gas, at 2 – 8°C.

Trientine Hydrochloride Capsules

トリエンチン塩酸塩カプセル

Trientine Hydrochloride Capsules contain not less than 90.0% and not more than 110.0% of the labeled amount of trientine hydrochloride ($C_6H_{18}N_4.2HCl$: 219.16).

Method of preparation Prepare as directed under Capsules, with Trientine Hydrochloride.

Identification Take out the contents of Trientine Hydrochloride Capsules, dry under reduced pressure not exceeding 0.67 kPa at 40°C for 4 hours, and determine the infrared absorption spectrum as directed in the paste method under Infrared Spectrophotometry <*2.25*>: it exhibits absorption at the wave numbers of about 3220 cm^{-1}, 2120 cm^{-1}, 1641 cm^{-1}, 1620 cm^{-1}, 1556 cm^{-1}, 1502 cm^{-1} and 1116 cm^{-1}.

Uniformity of dosage units <*6.02*> It meets the requirement of the Mass variation test.

Dissolution <*6.10*> When the test is performed at 50 revolutions per minute according to the Paddle method using the sinker, using 900 mL of water as the dissolution medium, the dissolution rate in 15 minutes of Trientine Hydrochloride Capsules is not less than 85%.

Start the test with 1 capsule of Trientine Hydrochloride Capsules, withdraw not less than 25 mL of the medium at the specified minute after starting the test, and filter through a membrane filter with a pore size not exceeding 0.45 μm. Discard not less than 10 mL of the first filtrate, pipet *V* mL of the subsequent filtrate, add water to make exactly *V′* mL so that each mL contains about 0.28 mg of trientine hydrochloride ($C_6H_{18}N_4.2HCl$), and use this solution as the sample solution. Separately, weigh accurately about 28 mg of trientine hydrochloride for assay, previously dried under reduced pressure not exceeding 0.67 kPa at 40°C for 4 hours, dissolve in water to make exactly 100 mL, and use this solution as the standard solution. Pipet 10 mL each of the sample solution and standard solution separately, add exactly 5 mL of a mixture of disodium hydrogen phosphate-citric acid buffer solution (pH 8.2) and cupper (II) sulfate pentahydrate solution (1 in 20) (4:1). Determine the absorbances, A_{T1} and A_{S1} at 580 nm, and A_{T2} and A_{S2} at 410 nm, of these solutions as directed under Ultraviolet-visible Spectrophotometry <*2.24*> using a solution obtained in the same manner with 10 mL of water as the blank.

Dissolution rate (%) with respect to the labeled amount of trientine hydrochloride ($C_6H_{18}N_4.2HCl$)
$= M_s \times (A_{T1} - A_{T2})/(A_{S1} - A_{S2}) \times V'/V \times 1/C \times 900$

M_S: Amount (mg) of trientine hydrochloride for assay taken

C: Labeled amount (mg) of trientine hydrochloride ($C_6H_{18}N_4.2HCl$) in 1 capsule

Assay Take out the contents of not less than 20 Trientine Hydrochloride Capsules, weigh accurately the mass of the contents, and powder. Weigh accurately a portion of the powder, equivalent to about 0.25 g of trientine hydrochloride ($C_6H_{18}N_4.2HCl$), add 70 mL of methanol, dissolve by sonicating if necessary, and add methanol to make exactly 100 mL. Filter through a membrane filter with a pore size not exceeding 0.45 μm, discard the first 10 mL of the filtrate, and use the subsequent filtrate as the sample solution. Separately, weigh accurately about 0.25 g of trientine hydrochloride for assay, previously dried under reduced pressure not exceeding 0.67 kPa at 40°C for 4 hours, dissolve in methanol to make exactly 100 mL, and use this solution as the standard solution. Pipet 5 mL each of the sample solution and standard solution separately, add exactly 10 mL of disodium hydrogen phosphate-citric acid buffer solution (pH 8.2) and exactly 1 mL of cupper (II) sulfate pentahydrate solution (1 in 20), and shake. Determine the absorbances, A_T and A_S, at 580 nm of these solutions, obtained with the sample solution and the standard solution, as directed under Ultraviolet-visible Spectrophotometry <*2.24*>, using a solution obtained in the same manner with 5 mL of methanol as a blank.

Amount (mg) of trientine hydrochloride ($C_6H_{18}N_4.2HCl$)
$= M_S \times A_T/A_S$

M_S: Amount (mg) of trientine hydrochloride for assay taken

Containers and storage Containers—Tight containers.

Storage—At 2 – 8°C.

Trihexyphenidyl Hydrochloride

トリヘキシフェニジル塩酸塩

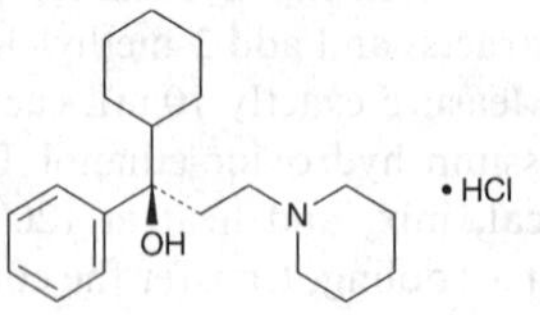

and enantiomer

$C_{20}H_{31}NO.HCl$: 337.93
(1*RS*)-1-Cyclohexyl-1-phenyl-3-(piperidin-1-yl)propan-1-ol monohydrochloride
[*52-49-3*]

Trihexyphenidyl Hydrochloride, when dried, contains not less than 98.5% of trihexyphenidyl hydrochloride ($C_{20}H_{31}NO.HCl$).

Description Trihexyphenidyl Hydrochloride occurs as a white crystalline powder. It is odorless, and has a bitter taste.

It is soluble in ethanol (95), sparingly soluble in acetic acid (100), slightly soluble in water, very slightly soluble in acetic anhydride, and practically insoluble in diethyl ether.

Melting point: about 250°C (with decomposition).

Identification **(1)** Dissolve 1 g of Trihexyphenidyl Hydrochloride in 100 mL of water by warming, and cool. Use this solution as the sample solution. To 5 mL of the sample solution add 1 mL of a solution of 2,4,6-trinitrophenol in chloroform (1 in 50), and shake vigorously: a yellow precipitate is formed.

(2) To 20 mL of the sample solution obtained in (1) add 2 mL of sodium hydroxide TS: a white precipitate is formed. Collect the precipitate, wash with a small amount of water, recrystallize from methanol, and dry in a desiccator (in vacuum, silica gel) for 2 hours: the crystals so obtained melt <*2.60*> between 113°C and 117°C.

(3) The sample solution obtained in (1) responds to Qualitative Tests <*1.09*> (2) for chloride.

pH <*2.54*> Dissolve 1.0 g of Trihexyphenidyl Hydrochloride in 100 mL of water by warming, and cool: the pH of this solution is between 5.0 and 6.0.

Purity **(1)** Clarity and color of solution—Dissolve 1.0 g of Trihexyphenidyl Hydrochloride in 100 mL of water by warming: the solution is clear and colorless.

(2) Heavy metals <*1.07*>—Dissolve 1.5 g of Trihexyphenidyl Hydrochloride in 60 mL of water by warming on a water bath at 80°C, cool, and filter. To 40 mL of the filtrate add 2 mL of dilute acetic acid and water to make 50 mL, and perform the test using this solution as the test solution. Prepare the control solution with 2.0 mL of Standard Lead Solution, 2 mL of dilute acetic acid and water to make 50 mL (not more than 20 ppm).

(3) Piperidylpropiophenone—Dissolve 0.10 g of Trihexyphenidyl Hydrochloride in 40 mL of water and 1 mL of 1 mol/L hydrochloric acid TS by warming, cool, and add water to make exactly 100 mL. Determine the absorbance of this solution at 247 nm as directed under Ultraviolet-visible Spectrophotometry <*2.24*>: the absorbance is not more than 0.50.

Loss on drying <*2.41*> Not more than 0.5% (1 g, 105°C, 3 hours).

Residue on ignition <*2.44*> Not more than 0.1% (1 g).

Assay Weigh accurately about 0.5 g of Trihexyphenidyl Hydrochloride, previously dried, dissolve in 50 mL of a mixture of acetic anhydride and acetic acid (100) (1:1), and titrate <*2.50*> with 0.1 mol/L perchloric acid-1,4-dioxane VS (potentiometric titration). Perform a blank determination in the same manner, and make any necessary correction.

Each mL of 0.1 mol/L perchloric acid-dioxane VS
= 33.79 mg of $C_{20}H_{31}NO.HCl$

Containers and storage Containers—Tight containers.

Trihexyphenidyl Hydrochloride Tablets

トリヘキシフェニジル塩酸塩錠

Trihexyphenidyl Hydrochloride Tablets contain not less than 93.0% and not more than 107.0% of the labeled amount of trihexyphenidyl hydrochloride ($C_{20}H_{31}NO.HCl$: 337.93).

Method of preparation Prepare as directed under Tablets, with Trihexyphenidyl Hydrochloride.

Identification **(1)** Weigh a quantity of powdered Trihexyphenidyl Hydrochloride Tablets, equivalent to 0.1 g of Trihexyphenidyl Hydrochloride, add 30 mL of chloroform, shake, and filter. Evaporate the filtrate on a water bath to dryness. Dissolve the residue in 10 mL of water by warming, cool, and use this solution as the sample solution. With 5 mL of the sample solution, proceed as directed in the Identification (1) under Trihexyphenidyl Hydrochloride.

(2) Shake a quantity of powdered Trihexyphenidyl Hydrochloride Tablets, equivalent to 0.01 g of Trihexyphenidyl Hydrochloride, with 5 mL of chloroform, filter, and use the filtrate as the sample solution. Dissolve 0.02 g of Trihexyphenidyl Hydrochloride RS in 10 mL of chloroform, and use this solution as the standard solution. Perform the test with these solutions as directed under Thin-layer Chromatography <*2.03*>. Spot 10 μL each of the sample solution and standard solution on a plate of silica gel for thin-layer chromatography. Develop the plate with a mixture of chloroform and methanol (9:1) to a distance of about 10 cm, and air-dry the plate. Spray evenly hydrogen hexachloroplatinate (IV)-potassium iodide TS on the plate: the spots from the sample solution and the standard solution show a blue-purple color and the same *R*f value.

(3) The sample solution obtained in (1) responds to Qualitative Tests <*1.09*> (2) for chloride.

Uniformity of dosage units <*6.02*> Perform the test according to the following method: it meets the requirement of the Content uniformity test.

To 1 tablet of Trihexyphenidyl Hydrochloride Tablets add 2 mL of dilute hydrochloric acid and 60 mL of water, disintegrate by vigorous shaking for 10 minutes, and warm on a water bath with occasional shaking for 10 minutes. Cool, add 2 mL of methanol, and add water to make exactly *V* mL so that each mL contains about 20 μg of trihexyphenidyl hydrochloride ($C_{20}H_{31}NO.HCl$). Centrifuge, if necessary, and use the supernatant liquid as the sample solution. Separately, dissolve about 20 mg of Trihexyphenidyl Hydrochloride RS (determine previously its loss on drying <*2.41*> under the same conditions as Trihexyphenidyl Hydrochloride) in methanol to make exactly 20 mL. Pipet 2 mL of this solution, and add 2 mL of dilute hydrochloric acid and water to make exactly 100 mL, and use this solution as the standard solution. Pipet 10 mL each of the sample solution and standard solution, transfer to glass-stoppered centrifuge tubes, add exactly 10 mL of bromocresol purple-dipotassium hydrogenphosphate-citric acid TS and 15 mL of chloroform, stopper tightly, shake well, and centrifuge. Pipet 10 mL each of the chloroform layers, add chloroform to make exactly 50 mL. Determine the absorbances, A_T and A_S, of the subsequent solutions of the sample solution and standard solution at 408 nm as directed under Ultraviolet-visible Spectrophotometry <*2.24*>, respectively.

Amount (mg) of trihexyphenidyl hydrochloride ($C_{20}H_{31}NO.HCl$)
$= M_S \times A_T/A_S \times V/1000$

M_S: Amount (mg) of Trihexyphenidyl Hydrochloride RS taken, calculated on the dried basis

Dissolution <*6.10*> When the test is performed at 50 revolutions per minute according to the Paddle method, using 900 mL of 2nd fluid for dissolution test as the dissolution medium, the dissolution rate in 30 minutes of Trihexyphenidyl Hydrochloride Tablets is not less than 70%.

Start the test with 1 tablet of Trihexyphenidyl Hydrochloride Tablets, withdraw not less than 30 mL of the medium at the specified minute after starting the test, and filter through a membrane filter with a pore size not exceeding 0.8 μm. Discard not less than 10 mL of the first filtrate, pipet *V* mL of the subsequent filtrate, add the dissolution medium to make exactly V' mL so that each mL contains about 2.2 μg of trihexyphenidyl hydrochloride ($C_{20}H_{31}NO.HCl$), and use this solution as the sample solution. Separately, weigh accurately about 10 mg of Trihexyphenidyl Hydrochloride RS, previously dried at 105°C for 3 hours, and dissolve in the dissolution medium to make exactly 100 mL. Pipet 2 mL of this solution, add the dissolution medium to make exactly 100 mL, and use this solution as the standard solution. Pipet 20 mL each of the sample solution, the standard solution and the dissolution medium, add exactly 1 mL of diluted acetic acid (31) (1 in 10), and immediately add 5 mL of bromocresol green-sodium hydroxide-acetic acid-sodium acetate TS, and shake. Then, add exactly 10 mL each of dichloromethane, shake well, centrifuge, and take the dichloromethane layer. Determine the absorbances, A_T, A_S and A_B, of these dichloromethane layers at 415 nm as directed under Ultraviolet-visible Spectrophotometry <*2.24*>, using dichloromethane as the blank.

Dissolution rate (%) with respect to the labeled amount of trihexyphenidyl hydrochloride ($C_{20}H_{31}NO.HCl$)

$$= M_S \times (A_T - A_B)/(A_S - A_B) \times V'/V \times 1/C \times 18$$

M_S: Amount (mg) of Trihexyphenidyl Hydrochloride RS taken

C: Labeled amount (mg) of trihexyphenidyl hydrochloride ($C_{20}H_{31}NO.HCl$) in 1 tablet

Assay Weigh accurately and powder not less than 20 Trihexyphenidyl Hydrochloride Tablets. Weigh accurately a portion of the powder, equivalent to about 5 mg of trihexyphenidyl hydrochloride ($C_{20}H_{31}NO.HCl$), dissolve in 2 mL of dilute hydrochloric acid and 60 mL of water by warming on a water bath for 10 minutes with occasional shaking. After cooling, add 2 mL of methanol and water to make exactly 100 mL, and use this solution as the sample solution. Dissolve about 50 mg of Trihexyphenidyl Hydrochloride RS (determine previously its loss on drying <*2.41*> under the same conditions as Trihexyphenidyl Hydrochloride), weighed accurately, in methanol, add methanol to make exactly 20 mL. Pipet 2 mL of this solution, add 2 mL of dilute hydrochloric acid and water to make exactly 100 mL, and use this solution as the standard solution. Pipet 10 mL each of the sample solution and standard solution into glass-stoppered centrifuge tubes, add exactly 10 mL each of bromocresol purple-dipotassium hydrogenphosphate-citric acid TS and 15 mL each of chloroform, stopper tightly, shake thoroughly, and centrifuge. Pipet 10 mL each of the chloroform layers, and add chloroform to make exactly 50 mL. Determine the absorbances, A_T and A_S, of the subsequent solutions of the sample solution and standard solution at 408 nm as directed under Ultraviolet-visible Spectrophotometry <*2.24*>, respectively.

Amount (mg) of trihexyphenidyl hydrochloride ($C_{20}H_{31}NO.HCl$)

$$= M_S \times A_T/A_S \times 1/10$$

M_S: Amount (mg) of Trihexyphenidyl Hydrochloride RS taken, calculated on the dried basis

Containers and storage Containers—Tight containers.

Trimebutine Maleate

トリメブチンマレイン酸塩

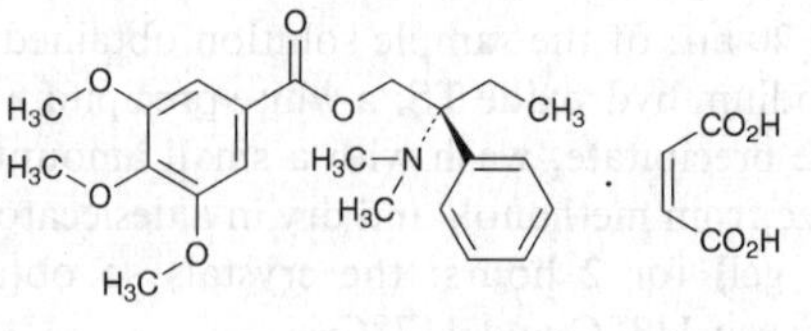

$C_{22}H_{29}NO_5.C_4H_4O_4$: 503.54
(2*RS*)-2-Dimethylamino-2-phenylbutyl 3,4,5-trimethoxybenzoate monomaleate
[*34140-59-5*]

Trimebutine Maleate, when dried, contains not less than 98.5% and not more than 101.0% of trimebutine maleate ($C_{22}H_{29}NO_5.C_4H_4O_4$).

Description Trimebutine Maleate occurs as white, crystals or crystalline powder.

It is freely soluble in *N,N*-dimethylformamide and in acetic acid (100), soluble in acetonitrile, and slightly soluble in water and in ethanol (99.5).

It dissolves in 0.01 mol/L hydrochloric acid TS.

A solution of Trimebutine Maleate in *N,N*-dimethylformamide (1 in 20) shows no optical rotation.

Identification **(1)** Determine the absorption spectrum of a solution of Trimebutine Maleate in 0.01 mol/L hydrochloric acid TS (1 in 50,000) as directed under Ultraviolet-visible Spectrophotometry <*2.24*>, and compare the spectrum with the Reference Spectrum: both spectra exhibit similar intensities of absorption at the same wavelengths.

(2) Determine the infrared absorption spectrum of Trimebutine Maleate as directed in the potassium bromide disk method under Infrared Spectrophotometry <*2.25*>, and compare the spectrum with the Reference Spectrum: both spectra exhibit similar intensities of absorption at the same wave numbers.

Melting point <*2.60*> 131 – 135°C

Purity **(1)** Heavy metals <*1.07*>—Proceed with 2.0 g of Trimebutine Maleate according to Method 2, and perform the test. Prepare the control solution with 2.0 mL of Standard Lead Solution (not more than 10 ppm).

(2) Arsenic <*1.11*>—Prepare the test solution with 2.0 g of Trimebutine Maleate according to Method 3, and perform the test (not more than 1 ppm).

(3) Related substances—Dissolve 0.10 g of Trimebutine Maleate in 100 mL of a mixture of 0.01 mol/L hydrochloric acid TS and acetonitrile (13:7), and use this solution as the sample solution. Pipet 1 mL of the sample solution, add a mixture of 0.01 mol/L hydrochloric acid TS and acetonitrile (13:7) to make exactly 250 mL, and use this solution as the standard solution. Perform the test with exactly 20 μL each of the sample solution and standard solution as directed under Liquid Chromatography <*2.01*> according to the following conditions, and determine each peak area by the automatic integration method: the area of the peak other than maleic acid and trimebutine obtained from the sample solution is not larger than 1/2 times the peak area of trimebutine from the standard solution, and the total area of the peaks other than maleic acid and trimebutine is not larger than the peak area of trimebutine from the standard solution.

Operating conditions—

Detector: An ultraviolet absorption photometer (wavelength: 254 nm).

Column: A stainless steel column 4.6 mm in inside diameter and 15 cm in length, packed with octadecylsilanized silica gel for liquid chromatography (5 μm in particle diameter).

Column temperature: A constant temperature of about 40°C.

Mobile phase: To 650 mL of diluted perchloric acid (17 in 20,000), previously adjusted the pH to 3.0 with a solution of ammonium acetate (1 in 1000), add 1 g of sodium 1-pentanesulfonate to dissolve. To 650 mL of this solution add 350 mL of acetonitrile.

Flow rate: Adjust so that the retention time of trimebutine is about 9 minutes.

Time span of measurement: About 2 times as long as the retention time of trimebutine, beginning after the peak of maleic acid.

System suitability—

Test for required detectability: Measure exactly 5 mL of the standard solution, and add a mixture of 0.01 mol/L hydrochloric acid TS and acetonitrile (13:7) to make exactly 20 mL. Confirm that the peak area of trimebutine obtained with 20 μL of this solution is equivalent to 20 to 30% of that with 20 μL of the standard solution.

System performance: Dissolve 40 mg of Trimebutine Maleate and 20 mg of imipramine hydrochloride in 100 mL of a mixture of 0.01 mol/L hydrochloric acid TS and acetonitrile (13:7). When the procedure is run with 20μL of this solution under the above operating conditions, trimebutine and imipramine are eluted in this order with the resolution between these peaks being not less than 2.5.

System repeatability: When the test is repeated 6 times with 20 μL of the standard solution under the above operating conditions, the relative standard deviation of the peak area of trimebutine is not more than 5%.

Loss on drying <*2.41*> Not more than 0.5% (1 g, 105°C, 3 hours).

Residue on ignition <*2.44*> Not more than 0.1% (1 g).

Assay Weigh accurately about 0.8 g of Trimebutine Maleate, previously dried, dissolve in 70 mL of acetic acid (100), and titrate <*2.50*> with 0.1 mol/L perchloric acid VS until the color of the solution changes from purple through blue to blue-green (indicator: 3 drops of crystal violet TS). Perform a blank determination in the same manner, and make any necessary correction.

Each mL of 0.1 mol/L perchloric acid VS
= 50.35 mg of $C_{22}H_{29}NO_5.C_4H_4O_4$

Containers and storage Containers—Well-closed containers.

Trimetazidine Hydrochloride

トリメタジジン塩酸塩

$C_{14}H_{22}N_2O_3.2HCl$: 339.26

1-(2,3,4-Trimethoxybenzyl)piperazine dihydrochloride

[*13171-25-0*]

Trimetazidine Hydrochloride contains not less than 98.0% and not more than 101.0% of trimetazidine hydrochloride ($C_{14}H_{22}N_2O_3.2HCl$), calculated on the anhydrous basis.

Description Trimetazidine Hydrochloride occurs as a white crystalline powder.

It is very soluble in water and in formic acid, sparingly soluble in methanol, and slightly soluble in ethanol (99.5).

The pH of a solution of 1.0 g of Trimetazidine Hydrochloride in 20 mL of water is between 2.3 and 3.3.

Melting point: about 227°C (with decomposition).

Identification **(1)** Determine the absorption spectrum of a solution of Trimetazidine Hydrochloride in 0.1 mol/L hydrochloric acid TS (1 in 6250) as directed under Ultraviolet-visible Spectrophotometry <*2.24*>, and compare the spectrum with the Reference Spectrum: both spectra exhibit similar intensities of absorption at the same wavelengths.

(2) Determine the infrared absorption spectrum of Trimetazidine Hydrochloride as directed in the potassium chloride disk method under Infrared Spectrophotometry <*2.25*>, and compare the spectrum with the Reference Spectrum: both spectra exhibit similar intensities of absorption at the same wave numbers.

(3) A solution of Trimetazidine Hydrochloride (1 in 50) responds to Qualitative Tests <*1.09*> for chloride.

Purity **(1)** Heavy metals <*1.07*>—Proceed with 2.0 g of Trimetazidine Hydrochloride according to Method 2, and perform the test. Prepare the control solution with 2.0 mL of Standard Lead Solution (not more than 10 ppm).

(2) Related substances—Dissolve 0.2 g of Trimetazidine Hydrochloride in 50 mL of water, and use this solution as the sample solution. Pipet 2 mL of the sample solution, add water to make exactly 20 mL. Pipet 2 mL of this solution, add water to make exactly 100 mL, and use this solution as the standard solution. Perform the test with exactly 10 μL each of the sample solution and standard solution as directed under Liquid Chromatography <*2.01*> according to the following conditions, and determine each peak area by the automatic integration method: the area of the peak other than trimetazidine obtained from the sample solution is not larger than 1.5 times that of trimetazidine from the standard solution, and the total area of the peaks other than trimetazidine from the sample solution is not larger than 2.5 times the peak area of trimetazidine from the standard solution.

Operating conditions—

Detector: An ultraviolet absorption photometer (wavelength: 240 nm).

Column: A stainless steel column 4.6 mm in inside diameter and 15 cm in length, packed with octadecylsilanized silica gel for liquid chromatography (5 μm in particle diameter).

Column temperature: A constant temperature of about

40°C.

Mobile phase A: Dissolve 2.87 g of sodium 1-heptanesulfonate in water to make 1000 mL, and adjust the pH to 3.0 with diluted phosphoric acid (1 in 10). Mix 3 volumes of this solution and 2 volumes of methanol.

Mobile phase B: Methanol.

Flowing of mobile phase: Control the gradient by mixing the mobile phases A and B as directed in the following table.

Time after injection of sample (min)	Mobile phase A (vol%)	Mobile phase B (vol%)
0 – 50	95 → 75	5 → 25

Flow rate: Adjust so that the retention time of trimetazidine is about 25 minutes.

Time span of measurement: About 2 times as long as the retention time of trimetazidine, beginning after the solvent peak.

System suitability—

Test for required detectability: Pipet 5 mL of the standard solution, and add water to make exactly 20 mL. Confirm that the peak area of trimetazidine obtained with 10 μL of this solution is equivalent to 18 to 32% of that with 10 μL of the standard solution.

System performance: When the procedure is run with 10 μL of the standard solution under the above operating conditions, the number of theoretical plates and the symmetry factor of the peak of trimetazidine are not less than 15,000 and not more than 1.5, respectively.

System repeatability: When the test is repeated 6 times with 10 μL of the standard solution under the above operating conditions, the relative standard deviation of the peak area of trimetazidine is not more than 2.0%.

Water <*2.48*> Not more than 1.5% (2 g, volumetric titration, direct titration).

Residue on ignition <*2.44*> Not more than 0.1% (1 g).

Assay Weigh accurately about 0.12 g of Trimetazidine Hydrochloride, dissolve in 5 mL of formic acid, add exactly 15 mL of 0.1 mol/L perchloric acid VS, and heat at 90 – 100°C for 30 minutes. After cooling, add 45 mL of acetic acid (100), and titrate <*2.50*> the excess perchloric acid with 0.1 mol/L sodium acetate VS (potentiometric titration). Perform a blank determination in the same manner.

Each mL of 0.1 mol/L perchloric acid VS
= 16.96 mg of $C_{14}H_{22}N_2O_3.2HCl$

Containers and storage Containers—Tight containers.

Trimetazidine Hydrochloride Tablets

トリメタジジン塩酸塩錠

Trimetazidine Hydrochloride Tablets contain not less than 94.0% and not more than 106.0% of the labeled amount of trimetazidine hydrochloride ($C_{14}H_{22}N_2O_3.2HCl$: 339.26).

Method of preparation Prepare as directed under Tablets, with Trimetazidine Hydrochloride.

Identification Shake a quantity of powdered Trimetazidine Hydrochloride Tablets, equivalent to 10 mg of Trimetazidine Hydrochloride, with 10 mL of a mixture of ethanol (95) and water (3:1), and filter. Evaporate the filtrate on a water bath, add 2 mL of water to the residue, and shake. To 1 mL of this solution add 1 mL of *p*-benzoquinone TS, boil gently for 2 to 3 minutes, and cool: a red color develops.

Uniformity of dosage units <*6.02*> Perform the test according to the following method: it meets the requirement of the Content uniformity test.

To 1 tablet of Trimetazidine Hydrochloride Tablets add 15 mL of a mixture of 0.1 mol/L hydrochloric acid TS and ethanol (99.5) (1:1) to disintegrate the tablet, and sonicate for 10 minutes. Shake the solution for 10 minutes, and add the mixture of 0.1 mol/L hydrochloric acid TS and ethanol (99.5) (1:1) to make exactly 20 mL. Centrifuge, pipet *V* mL of the supernatant liquid, equivalent to about 0.75 mg of trimetazidine hydrochloride ($C_{14}H_{22}N_2O_3.2HCl$), add exactly 5 mL of the internal standard solution, add 0.1 mol/L hydrochloric acid TS to make 50 mL, and use this solution as the sample solution. Separately, weigh accurately about 30 mg of trimetazidine hydrochloride for assay (separately determine the water <*2.48*> in the same manner as Trimetazidine Hydrochloride), and dissolve in the mixture of 0.1 mol/L hydrochloric acid TS and ethanol (99.5) (1:1) to make exactly 200 mL. Pipet 5 mL of this solution, add exactly 5 mL of the internal standard solution and 0.1 mol/L hydrochloric acid TS to make 50 mL, and use this solution as the standard solution. Proceed as directed in the Assay.

$$\text{Amount (mg) of trimetazidine hydrochloride } (C_{14}H_{22}N_2O_3.2HCl) = M_S \times Q_T/Q_S \times 1/2V$$

M_S: Amount (mg) of trimetazidine hydrochloride for assay taken, calculated on the anhydrous basis

Internal standard solution—A solution of parahydroxybenzoic acid in the mixture of 0.1 mol/L hydrochloric acid TS and ethanol (99.5) (1:1) (7 in 40,000).

Dissolution <*6.10*> When the test is performed at 50 revolutions per minute according to the Paddle method, using 900 mL of water as the dissolution medium, the dissolution rate in 45 minutes of Trimetazidine Hydrochloride Tablets is not less than 80%.

Start the test with 1 tablet of Trimetazidine Hydrochloride Tablets, withdraw not less than 20 mL of the medium at the specified minute after starting the test, and filter through a membrane filter with a pore size not exceeding 0.45 μm. Discard not less than 10 mL of the first filtrate, pipet *V* mL of the subsequent filtrate, and add water to make exactly *V′* mL so that each mL contains about 3.3 μg of trimetazidine hydrochloride ($C_{14}H_{22}N_2O_3.2HCl$). Pipet 3 mL of this solution, add exactly 3 mL of 0.1 mol/L hydrochloric acid TS, and use this solution as the sample solution. Separately, weigh accurately about 17 mg of trimetazidine hydrochloride for assay (separately determine the water <*2.48*> in the same manner as Trimetazidine Hydrochloride), and dissolve in water to make exactly 100 mL. Pipet 5 mL of this solution, and add water to make exactly 50 mL. Pipet 5 mL of this solution, and add water to make exactly 25 mL. Pipet 3 mL of this solution, add exactly 3 mL of 0.1 mol/L hydrochloric acid TS, and use this solution as the standard solution. Perform the test with exactly 50 μL each of the sample solution and standard solution as directed under Liquid Chromatography <*2.01*> according to the following conditions, and determine the peak areas, A_T and A_S, of trimetazidine in each solution.

Dissolution rate (%) with respect to the labeled amount of trimetazidine hydrochloride ($C_{14}H_{22}N_2O_3.2HCl$)

$$= M_S \times A_T/A_S \times V'/V \times 1/C \times 18$$

M_S: Amount (mg) of trimetazidine hydrochloride for assay taken, calculated on the anhydrous basis

C: Labeled amount (mg) of trimetazidine hydrochloride ($C_{14}H_{22}N_2O_3.2HCl$) in 1 tablet

Operating conditions—

Proceed as directed in the operating conditions in the Assay.

System suitability—

System performance: When the procedure is run with 50 μL of the standard solution under the above operating conditions, the number of theoretical plates and the symmetry factor of the peak of trimetazidine are not less than 5000 and not more than 1.5, respectively.

System repeatability: When the test is repeated 6 times with 50 μL of the standard solution under the above operating conditions, the relative standard deviation of the peak area of trimetazidine is not more than 1.5%.

Assay Weigh accurately not less than 20 tablets of Trimetazidine Hydrochloride Tablets, and powder. Weigh accurately a portion of the powder, equivalent to about 3 mg of trimetazidine hydrochloride ($C_{14}H_{22}N_2O_3.2HCl$), add about 15 mL of a mixture of 0.1 mol/L hydrochloric acid TS and ethanol (99.5) (1:1), and sonicate for 10 minutes. Then shake for 10 minutes, add the mixture of 0.1 mol/L hydrochloric acid TS and ethanol (99.5) (1:1) to make exactly 20 mL, and centrifuge. To exactly 5 mL of the supernatant liquid add exactly 5 mL of the internal standard solution and 0.1 mol/L hydrochloric acid TS to make 50 mL, and use this solution as the sample solution. Separately, weigh accurately about 30 mg of trimetazidine hydrochloride for assay (separately determine the water *<2.48>* in the same manner as Trimetazidine Hydrochloride), and dissolve in the mixture of 0.1 mol/L hydrochloric acid TS and ethanol (99.5) (1:1) to make exactly 200 mL. To exactly 5 mL of this solution add exactly 5 mL of the internal standard solution and 0.1 mol/L hydrochloric acid TS to make 50 mL, and use this solution as the standard solution. Perform the test with 10 μL each of the sample solution and standard solution as directed under Liquid Chromatography *<2.01>* according to the following conditions, and calculate the ratios, Q_T and Q_S, of the peak area of trimetazidine to that of the internal standard.

Amount (mg) of trimetazidine hydrochloride

$$(C_{14}H_{22}N_2O_3.2HCl) = M_S \times Q_T/Q_S \times 1/10$$

M_S: Amount (mg) of trimetazidine hydrochloride for assay taken, calculated on the anhydrous basis

Internal standard solution—A solution of parahydroxybenzoic acid in the mixture of 0.1 mol/L hydrochloric acid TS and ethanol (99.5) (1:1) (7 in 40,000).

Operating conditions—

Detector: An ultraviolet absorption photometer (wavelength: 230 nm).

Column: A stainless steel column 4.6 mm in inside diameter and 15 cm in length, packed with octadecylsilanized silica gel for liquid chromatography (5 μm in particle diameter).

Column temperature: A constant temperature of about 40°C.

Mobile phase: A mixture of 0.05 mol/L potassium dihydrogen phosphate TS (pH 3.0) and methanol (17:3).

Flow rate: Adjust so that the retention time of trimetazidine is about 7 minutes.

System suitability—

System performance: When the procedure is run with 10 μL of the standard solution under the above operating conditions, trimetazidine and the internal standard are eluted in this order with the resolution between these peaks being not less than 3.

System repeatability: When the test is repeated 6 times with 10 μL of the standard solution under the above operating conditions, the relative standard deviation of the ratio of the peak area of trimetazidine to that of the internal standard is not more than 1.0%.

Containers and storage Containers—Tight containers.

Trimethadione

トリメタジオン

$C_6H_9NO_3$: 143.14

3,5,5-Trimethyl-1,3-oxazolidine-2,4-dione

[127-48-0]

Trimethadione, when dried, contains not less than 98.0% of trimethadione ($C_6H_9NO_3$).

Description Trimethadione occurs as white, crystals or crystalline powder. It has a camphor-like odor.

It is very soluble in ethanol (95) and in chloroform, freely soluble in diethyl ether, and soluble in water.

Identification **(1)** To 5 mL of a solution of Trimethadione (1 in 50) add 2 mL of barium hydroxide TS: a precipitate is formed immediately.

(2) Determine the infrared absorption spectrum of a solution of Trimethadione in chloroform (1 in 50) as directed in the solution method under Infrared Spectrophotometry *<2.25>*, using a 0.1-mm fixed sodium chloride cell, and compare the spectrum with the Reference Spectrum: both spectra exhibit similar intensities of absorption at the same wave numbers.

Melting point *<2.60>* 45 - 47°C

Purity Heavy metals *<1.07>*—Proceed with 2.0 g of Trimethadione according to Method 1, and perform the test. Prepare the control solution with 2.0 mL of Standard Lead Solution (not more than 10 ppm).

Loss on drying *<2.41>* Not more than 0.5% (1 g, silica gel, 6 hours).

Residue on ignition *<2.44>* Not more than 0.1% (1 g).

Assay Weigh accurately about 0.4 g of Trimethadione, previously dried, in a glass-stoppered conical flask, dissolve in 5 mL of ethanol (95), add exactly measured 50 mL of 0.1 mol/L sodium hydroxide VS, stopper, and allow to stand for 15 minutes with occasional shaking. Titrate *<2.50>* the excess sodium hydroxide with 0.1 mol/L hydrochloric acid VS (indicator: 4 drops of cresol red TS). Perform a blank determination in the same manner.

Each mL of 0.1 mol/L sodium hydroxide VS
= 14.31 mg of $C_6H_9NO_3$

Containers and storage Containers—Tight containers.

Storage—Not exceeding 30°C.

Trimetoquinol Hydrochloride Hydrate

トリメトキノール塩酸塩水和物

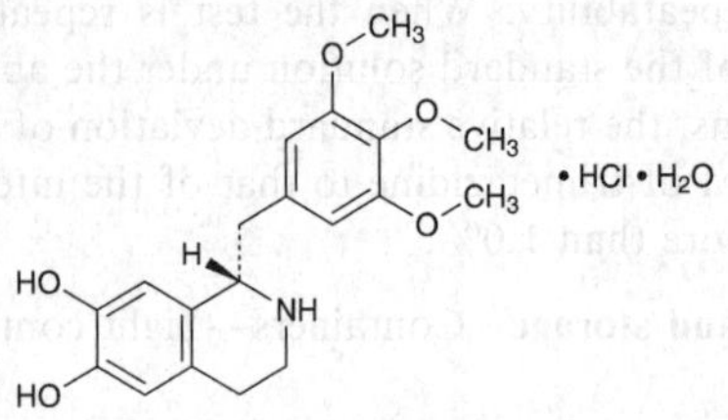

$C_{19}H_{23}NO_5.HCl.H_2O$: 399.87
(1*S*)-1-(3,4,5-Trimethoxybenzyl)-1,2,3,4-tetrahydroisoquinoline-6,7-diol monohydrochloride monohydrate
[*18559-59-6*, anhydride]

Trimetoquinol Hydrochloride Hydrate contains not less than 98.5% and not more than 101.0% of trimetoquinol hydrochloride ($C_{19}H_{23}NO_5.HCl$: 381.85), calculated on the anhydrous basis.

Description Trimetoquinol Hydrochloride Hydrate occurs as white, crystals or crystalline powder.

It is freely soluble in methanol, and sparingly soluble in water and in ethanol (99.5).

Melting point: about 151°C (with decomposition, after drying in vacuum, 105°C, 4 hours).

Identification (1) Determine the absorption spectrum of a solution of Trimetoquinol Hydrochloride Hydrate in 0.01 mol/L hydrochloric acid TS (1 in 20,000) as directed under Ultraviolet-visible Spectrophotometry <*2.24*>, and compare the spectrum with the Reference Spectrum: both spectra exhibit similar intensities of absorption at the same wavelengths.

(2) Determine the infrared absorption spectrum of Trimetoquinol Hydrochloride Hydrate as directed in the potassium chloride disk method under Infrared Spectrophotometry <*2.25*>, and compare the spectrum with the Reference Spectrum: both spectra exhibit similar intensities of absorption at the same wave numbers.

(3) A solution of Trimetoquinol Hydrochloride Hydrate (1 in 50) responds to Qualitative Tests <*1.09*> (1) for chloride.

Optical rotation <*2.49*> $[\alpha]_D^{20}$: −16 − −19° (0.25 g calculated on the anhydrous basis, water, after warming and cooling, 25 mL, 100 mm).

pH <*2.54*> Dissolve 1.0 g of Trimetoquinol Hydrochloride Hydrate in 100 mL of water by warming, and cool: the pH of this solution is between 4.5 and 5.5.

Purity (1) Clarity and color of solution—Dissolve 0.10 g of Trimetoquinol Hydrochloride Hydrate in 10 mL of water by warming: the solution is clear and colorless.

(2) Sulfate <*1.14*>—Perform the test with 0.5 g of Trimetoquinol Hydrochloride Hydrate. Prepare the control solution with 0.40 mL of 0.005 mol/L sulfuric acid VS (not more than 0.038%).

(3) Heavy metals <*1.07*>—Proceed with 1.0 g of Trimetoquinol Hydrochloride Hydrate according to Method 2, and perform the test. Prepare the control solution with 2.0 mL of Standard Lead Solution (not more than 20 ppm).

(4) Related substances—Dissolve 50 mg of Trimetoquinol Hydrochloride Hydrate in 50 mL of the mobile phase, and use this solution as the sample solution. Pipet 1 mL of the sample solution, add the mobile phase to make exactly 100 mL, and use this solution as the standard solution. Perform the test with exactly 20 μL each of the sample solution and standard solution as directed under Liquid Chromatography <*2.01*> according to the following conditions. Determine each peak area by the automatic integration method: the total area of the peaks other than trimetoquinol obtained from the sample solution is not larger than the peak area of trimetoquinol from the standard solution.

Operating conditions—

Detector: An ultraviolet absorption photometer (wavelength: 283 nm).

Column: A stainless steel column 4.6 mm in inside diameter and 15 cm in length, packed with octadecylsilanized silica gel for liquid chromatography (5 μm in particle diameter).

Column temperature: A constant temperature of about 40°C.

Mobile phase: Dissolve 2 g of potassium dihydrogen phosphate and 2 g of sodium 1-pentane sulfonate in 1000 mL of water. Adjust with phosphoric acid to a pH between 2.8 and 3.2, and filter through a membrane filter with a pore size of 0.4 μm. Add 200 mL of acetonitrile to 800 mL of the filtrate.

Flow rate: Adjust so that the retention time of trimetoquinol is about 7 minutes.

Time span of measurement: About twice as long as the retention time of trimetoquinol, beginning after the solvent peak.

System suitability—

Test for required detectability: To exactly 2 mL of the standard solution add the mobile phase to make exactly 20 mL. Confirm that the peak area of trimetoquinol obtained with 20 μL of this solution is equivalent to 7 to 13% of that with 20 μL of the standard solution.

System performance: Dissolve 5 mg of Trimetoquinol Hydrochloride Hydrate and 1 mg of procaine hydrochloride in 50 mL of the mobile phase. When the procedure is run with 20 μL of this solution under the above operating conditions, procaine and trimetoquinol are eluted in this order with the resolution between these peaks being not less than 4.

System repeatability: When the test is repeated 6 times with 20 μL of the standard solution under the above operating conditions, the relative standard deviation of the peak area of trimetoquinol is not more than 2.0%.

Water <*2.48*> 3.5 – 5.5% (0.3 g, volumetric titration, direct titration).

Residue on ignition <*2.44*> Not more than 0.1% (1 g).

Assay Weigh accurately about 0.5 g of Trimetoquinol Hydrochloride Hydrate, dissolve in 2 mL of 0.1 mol/L hydrochloric acid VS and 70 mL of ethanol (99.5) with thorough shaking, and titrate <*2.50*> with 0.1 mol/L potassium hydroxide-ethanol VS (potentiometric titration). Calculate the consumed volume of 0.1 mol/L potassium hydroxide-ethanol VS between the first inflection point and of the second inflection point.

Each mL of 0.1 mol/L potassium hydroxide-ethanol VS
= 38.19 mg of $C_{19}H_{23}NO_5.HCl$

Containers and storage Containers—Well-closed containers.

Storage—Light-resistant.

Dental Triozinc Paste

歯科用トリオジンクパスタ

Dental Triozinc Paste consists of a powder containing Paraformaldehyde, Thymol, anhydrous zinc sulfate and Zinc Oxide, and a solution containing Cresol, Potash Soap and Glycerin. Suitable amounts of the two components are triturated before use.

Method of preparation

(1) The powder

Paraformaldehyde, finely powdered	10 g
Thymol, finely powdered	3 g
Zinc Sulfate Hydrate	9 g
Zinc Oxide	82 g
To make about	100 g

Heat Zinc Sulfate Hydrate at about 250°C to obtain anhydrous zinc sulfate, cool, and pulverize to a fine powder. Mix homogeneously this powder with Thymol, Paraformaldehyde, and Zinc Oxide.

(2) The solution

Cresol	40 g
Potash Soap	40 g
Glycerin	20 g
To make	100 g

Dissolve Potash Soap in a mixture of Cresol and Glycerin.

Description The powder occurs as a fine, white powder, having a characteristic odor. The solution is a clear, yellow-brown to red-brown, viscous liquid, having the odor of cresol.

Containers and storage Containers—Tight containers.

Tropicamide

トロピカミド

and enantiomer

$C_{17}H_{20}N_2O_2$: 284.35
(2*RS*)-*N*-Ethyl-3-hydroxy-2-phenyl-*N*-(pyridin-4-ylmethyl)propanamide
[*1508-75-4*]

Tropicamide, when dried, contains not less than 98.5% of tropicamide ($C_{17}H_{20}N_2O_2$).

Description Tropicamide occurs as a white crystalline powder. It is odorless, and has a bitter taste.

It is freely soluble in ethanol (95) and in chloroform, slightly soluble in water and in diethyl ether, and practically insoluble in petroleum ether.

It dissolves in dilute hydrochloric acid.

The pH of a solution of 1.0 g of Tropicamide in 500 mL of water is between 6.5 and 8.0.

Identification (1) To 5 mg of Tropicamide add 0.5 mL of a solution of ammonium vanadate (V) in sulfuric acid, (1 in 200), and heat: a blue-purple color develops.

(2) Dissolve 5 mg of Tropicamide in 1 mL of ethanol (95) and 1 mL of water, add 0.1 g of 1-chloro-2,4-dinitrobenzene, and heat on a water bath for 5 minutes. Cool, and add 2 to 3 drops of a solution of sodium hydroxide (1 in 10) and 3 mL of ethanol (95): a red-purple color develops.

Absorbance <*2.24*> $E^{1\%}_{1\,cm}$ (255 nm): 166 – 180 (after drying, 5 mg, 2 mol/L hydrochloric acid TS, 200 mL).

Melting point <*2.60*> 96 – 99°C

Purity (1) Chloride <*1.03*>—Dissolve 1.0 g of Tropicamide in 30 mL of ethanol (95), add 6 mL of dilute nitric acid and water to make 50 mL, and perform the test using this solution as the test solution. Prepare the control solution with 0.45 mL of 0.01 mol/L hydrochloric acid VS, 30 mL of ethanol (95), 6 mL of dilute nitric acid, and add water to make 50 mL (not more than 0.016%).

(2) Heavy metals <*1.07*>—Dissolve 1.0 g of Tropicamide in 30 mL of ethanol (95), add 2 mL of dilute acetic acid and water to make 50 mL, and perform the test using this solution as the test solution. Prepare the control solution with 2.0 mL of Standard Lead Solution, 30 mL of ethanol (95), 2 mL of dilute acetic acid and water to make 50 mL (not more than 20 ppm).

(3) *N*-Ethyl-*γ*-picolylamine—Dissolve 0.10 g of Tropicamide in 5 mL of water by heating, add 1 mL of a solution of acetaldehyde (1 in 20), and shake well. Add 1 to 2 drops of sodium pentacyanonitrosylferrate (III) TS and 1 to 2 drops of sodium hydrogen carbonate TS, and shake: no blue color develops.

(4) Tropic acid—To 10 mg of Tropicamide add 5 mg of sodium tetraborate decahydrate and 7 drops of 4-dimethylaminobenzaldehyde TS, and heat in a water bath for 3 minutes. Cool in ice water, and add 5 mL of acetic anhydride: no red-purple color develops.

Loss on drying <*2.41*> Not more than 0.30% (1 g, in vacuum, silica gel, 24 hours).

Residue on ignition <*2.44*> Not more than 0.1% (1 g).

Assay Weigh accurately about 0.5 g of Tropicamide, previously dried, dissolve in 50 mL of acetic acid (100), and titrate <*2.50*> with 0.1 mol/L perchloric acid VS (indicator: 3 drops of crystal violet TS). Perform a blank determination in the same manner, and make any necessary correction.

Each mL of 0.1 mol/L perchloric acid VS
= 28.44 mg of $C_{17}H_{20}N_2O_2$

Containers and storage Containers—Tight containers.
Storage—Light-resistant.

Troxipide

トロキシピド

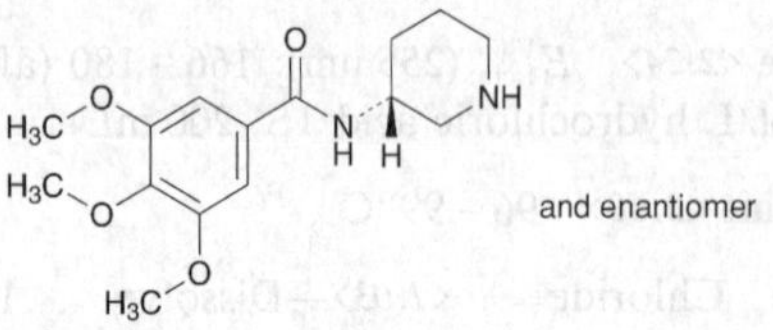

and enantiomer

$C_{15}H_{22}N_2O_4$: 294.35
3,4,5-Trimethoxy-*N*-[(3*RS*)-piperidin-3-yl]benzamide
[*30751-05-4*]

Troxipide, when dried, contains not less than 98.5% and not more than 101.0% of troxipide ($C_{15}H_{22}N_2O_4$).

Description Troxipide occurs as a white crystalline powder.

It is freely soluble in acetic acid (100), soluble in methanol, sparingly soluble in ethanol (99.5) and slightly soluble in water.

It dissolves in 0.1 mol/L hydrochloric acid TS.

A solution of Troxipide in 1 mol/L hydrochloric acid TS (1 in 5) shows no optical rotation.

Identification **(1)** Determine the absorption spectrum of a solution of Troxipide in 0.1 mol/L hydrochloric acid TS (1 in 62,500) as directed under Ultraviolet-visible Spectrophotometry <*2.24*>, and compare the spectrum with the Reference Spectrum or the spectrum of a solution of Troxipide RS prepared in the same manner as the sample solution: both spectra exhibit similar intensities of absorption at the same wavelengths.

(2) Determine the infrared absorption spectrum of Troxipide as directed in the potassium bromide disk method under Infrared Spectrophotometry <*2.25*>, and compare the spectrum with the Reference Spectrum or the spectrum of Troxipide RS: both spectra exhibit similar intensities of absorption at the same wave numbers.

Melting point <*2.60*> 177 - 181°C

Purity **(1)** Chloride <*1.03*>—Dissolve 1.0 g of Troxipide in 30 mL of methanol, and add 6 mL of dilute nitric acid and water to make 50 mL. Perform the test using this solution as the test solution. Prepare the control solution as follows: to 0.25 mL of 0.01 mol/L hydrochloric acid VS add 30 mL of methanol, 6 mL of dilute nitric acid and water to make 50 mL (not more than 0.009%).

(2) Heavy metals <*1.07*>—Moisten 2.0 g of Troxipide with 1 mL of sulfuric acid, and gently heat until charred. After cooling, add 2 mL of nitric acid, carefully heat until white fumes are no longer evolved, and perform the test according to Method 2. Prepare the control solution as follows: evaporate 1 mL of sulfuric acid, 2 mL of nitric acid and 2 mL of hydrochloric acid on a water bath and then on a sand bath to dryness, and moisten the residue with 3 drops of hydrochloric acid. Proceed in the same manner for the preparation of the test solution, and add 2.0 mL of Standard Lead Solution and water to make 50 mL (not more than 10 ppm).

(3) Related substances—Dissolve 0.20 g of Troxipide in 10 mL of methanol, and use this solution as the sample solution. Pipet 2 mL of the sample solution, and add methanol to make exactly 100 mL. Pipet 2 mL of this solution, add methanol to make exactly 20 mL, and use this solution as the standard solution. Perform the test with these solutions as directed under Thin-layer Chromatography <*2.03*>. Spot 5 μL each of the sample solution and standard solution on a plate of silica gel with fluorescent indicator for thin-layer chromatography. Develop the plate with a mixture of methanol, ethyl acetate, water, hexane and ammonia water (28) (20:20:5:5:1) to a distance of about 10 cm, and air-dry the plate. Examine under ultraviolet light (main wavelength: 254 nm): the number of the spots other than the principal spot obtained from the sample solution is not more than three, and they are not more intense than the spot from the standard solution.

Loss on drying <*2.41*> Not more than 1.0% (1 g, 105°C, 2 hours).

Residue on ignition <*2.44*> Not more than 0.1% (1 g).

Assay Weigh accurately about 0.6 g of Troxipide, previously dried, dissolve in 40 mL of acetic acid (100), and titrate <*2.50*> with 0.1 mol/L perchloric acid VS (potentiometric titration). Perform a blank determination in the same manner, and make any necessary correction.

Each mL of 0.1 mol/L perchloric acid VS
= 29.44 mg of $C_{15}H_{22}N_2O_4$

Containers and storage Containers—Tight containers.

Troxipide Fine Granules

トロキシピド細粒

Troxipide Fine Granules contain not less than 93.0% and not more than 107.0% of the labeled amount of troxipide ($C_{15}H_{22}N_2O_4$: 294.35).

Method of preparation Prepare as directed under Granules, with Troxipide.

Identification To a quantity of Troxipide Fine Granules, equivalent to 20 mg of Troxipide, add 100 mL of 0.1 mol/L hydrochloric acid TS, stir, and filter. To 4 mL of the filtrate add 0.1 mol/L hydrochloric acid TS to make 50 mL. Determine the absorption spectrum of this solution as directed under Ultraviolet-visible Spectrophotometry <*2.24*>: it exhibits a maximum between 256 nm and 260 nm.

Uniformity of dosage units <*6.02*> Perform the test according to the following method: Troxipide Fine Granules in single-dose packages meet the requirement of the Content uniformity test.

To the total amount of the content of 1 package of Troxipide Fine Granules, add 80 mL of 0.1 mol/L hydrochloric acid TS, stir for 10 minutes, and add 0.1 mol/L hydrochloric acid TS to make exactly V mL so that each mL contains about 1 mg of troxipide ($C_{15}H_{22}N_2O_4$). Centrifuge this solution, pipet 2 mL of the supernatant liquid, add exactly 3 mL of the internal standard solution, and water to make 100 mL, and use this solution as the sample solution. Proceed as directed in the Assay.

Amount (mg) of troxipide ($C_{15}H_{22}N_2O_4$)
$= M_S \times Q_T/Q_S \times V/25$

M_S: Amount (mg) of Troxipide RS taken

Internal standard solution—A solution of 4-aminoacetophenone in 0.1 mol/L hydrochloric acid TS (3 in 2000).

Dissolution <*6.10*> When the test is performed at 50 revolutions per minute according to the Paddle method, using 900 mL of water as the dissolution medium, the dissolution rate in 60 minutes of Troxipide Fine Granules is not less than 85%.

Weigh accurately an amount of Troxipide Fine Granules, equivalent to about 0.1 g of troxipide ($C_{15}H_{22}N_2O_4$), withdraw not less than 20 mL of the medium at the specified minute after starting the test, and filter through a membrane filter with a pore size not exceeding 0.8 μm. Discard not less than 10 mL of the first filtrate, pipet 4 mL of the subsequent filtrate, add water to make exactly 20 mL, and use this solution as the sample solution. Separately, weigh accurately about 20 mg of Troxipide RS, previously dried at 105°C for 2 hours, and dissolve in water to make exactly 200 mL. Pipet 4 mL of this solution, add water to make exactly 20 mL, and use this solution as the standard solution. Perform the test with the sample solution and standard solution as directed under Ultraviolet-visible Spectrophotometry *<2.24>*, and determine the absorbances, A_T and A_S, at 258 nm.

Dissolution rate (%) with respect to the labeled amount of troxipide ($C_{15}H_{22}N_2O_4$)
$= M_S/M_T \times A_T/A_S \times 1/C \times 450$

M_S: Amount (mg) of Troxipide RS taken
M_T: Amount (mg) of Troxipide Fine Granules taken
C: Labeled amount (mg) of troxipide ($C_{15}H_{22}N_2O_4$) in 1 g

Assay Weigh accurately an amount of Troxipide Fine Granules, equivalent to about 0.5 g of troxipide ($C_{15}H_{22}N_2O_4$), add 200 mL of 0.1 mol/L hydrochloric acid TS, stir for 10 minutes, and add 0.1 mol/L hydrochloric acid TS to make exactly 250 mL. Centrifuge this solution, pipet 5 mL of the supernatant liquid, add 0.1 mol/L hydrochloric acid TS to make exactly 10 mL. Pipet 2 mL of this solution, add exactly 3 mL of the internal standard solution, and water to make 100 mL, and use this solution as the sample solution. Separately, weigh accurately about 25 mg of Troxipide RS, previously dried at 105°C for 2 hours, and dissolve in 0.1 mol/L hydrochloric acid TS to make exactly 25 mL. Pipet 2 mL of this solution, add exactly 3 mL of the internal standard solution, and water to make 100 mL, and use this solution as the standard solution. Perform the test with 20 μL each of the sample solution and standard solution as directed under Liquid Chromatography *<2.01>* according to the following conditions, and calculate the ratios, Q_T and Q_S, of the peak area of troxipide to that of the internal standard.

Amount (mg) of troxipide ($C_{15}H_{22}N_2O_4$)
$= M_S \times Q_T/Q_S \times 20$

M_S: Amount (mg) of Troxipide RS taken

Internal standard solution—A solution of 4-aminoacetophenone in 0.1 mol/L hydrochloric acid TS (3 in 2000).
Operating conditions—

Detector: An ultraviolet absorption photometer (wavelength: 258 nm).

Column: A stainless steel column 4.6 mm in inside diameter and 15 cm in length, packed with octadecylsilanized silica gel for liquid chromatography (5 μm in particle diameter).

Column temperature: A constant temperature of about 30°C.

Mobile phase: To diluted phosphoric acid (1 in 500) add diethylamine to adjust the pH to 3.0. To 1500 mL of this solution add 100 mL of methanol and 50 mL of tetrahydrofuran.

Flow rate: Adjust so that the retention time of troxipide is about 7 minutes.

System suitability—

System performance: When the procedure is run with 20 μL of standard solution under the above operating conditions, troxipide and the internal standard are eluted in this order with the resolution between these peaks being not less than 3.

System repeatability: When the test is repeated 6 times with 20 μL of the standard solution under the above operating conditions, the relative standard deviation of the ratio of the peak area of troxipide to that of the internal standard is not more than 1.0%.

Containers and storage Containers—Tight containers.

Troxipide Tablets

トロキシピド錠

Troxipide Tablets contain not less than 95.0% and not more than 105.0% of the labeled amount of troxipide ($C_{15}H_{22}N_2O_4$: 294.35).

Method of preparation Prepare as directed under Tablets, with Troxipide.

Identification Weigh accurately an amount of powdered Troxipide Tablets, equivalent to 0.1 g of Troxipide, add 250 mL of 0.1 mol/L hydrochloric acid TS, shake, and filter. To 4 mL of the filtrate add 0.1 mol/L hydrochloric acid TS to make 100 mL. Determine the absorption spectrum of this solution as directed under Ultraviolet-visible Spectrophotometry *<2.24>*: it exhibits maximum between 256 nm and 260 nm.

Uniformity of dosage units *<6.02>* Perform the Mass variation test, or the Content uniformity test according to the following method: it meets the requirement.

To 1 tablet of Troxipide Tablets add 90 mL of 0.1 mol/L hydrochloric acid TS, shake well to disintegrate, shake for another 10 minutes, and add 0.1 mol/L hydrochloric acid TS to make exactly V mL so that each mL contains about 1 mg of troxipide ($C_{15}H_{22}N_2O_4$). Centrifuge this solution, pipet 2 mL of the supernatant liquid, add exactly 3 mL of the internal standard solution, add water to make 100 mL, and use this solution as the sample solution. Proceed as directed in the Assay.

Amount (mg) of troxipide ($C_{15}H_{22}N_2O_4$)
$= M_S \times Q_T/Q_S \times V/25$

M_S: Amount (mg) of Troxipide RS taken

Internal standard solution—A solution of 4-aminoacetophenone in 0.1 mol/L hydrochloric acid TS (3 in 2000).

Dissolution *<6.10>* When the test is performed at 50 revolutions per minute according to the Paddle method, using 900 mL of water as the dissolution medium, the dissolution rate in 30 minutes of Troxipide Tablets is not less than 70%.

Start the test with 1 tablet of Troxipide Tablets, withdraw not less than 20 mL of the medium at the specified minute after starting the test, and filter through a membrane filter with a pore size not exceeding 0.8 μm. Discard not less than 10 mL of the first filtrate, pipet V mL of the subsequent filtrate, add water to make exactly V' mL so that each mL contains about 22 μg of troxipide ($C_{15}H_{22}N_2O_4$), and use this solution as the sample solution. Separately weigh accurately about 20 mg of Troxipide RS, previously dried at 105°C for 2 hours, and dissolve in water to make exactly 200 mL. Pipet 4 mL of this solution, add water to make exactly 20 mL, and use this solution as the standard solution. Perform the test with the sample solution and standard solution as directed under Ultraviolet-visible Spectrophotometry *<2.24>*, and determine the absorbances, A_T and A_S, at 258 nm.

Dissolution rate (%) with respect to the labeled amount of troxipide ($C_{15}H_{22}N_2O_4$)
$= M_S \times A_T/A_S \times V'/V \times 1/C \times 90$

M_S: Amount (mg) of Troxipide RS taken
C: Labeled amount (mg) of Troxipide ($C_{15}H_{22}N_2O_4$) in 1 tablet

Assay Weigh accurately the mass of not less than 20 Troxipide Tablets, and powder. Weigh accurately a portion of the powder, equivalent to about 1 g of troxipide ($C_{15}H_{22}N_2O_4$), add 150 mL of 0.1 mol/L hydrochloric acid TS, shake for 30 minutes, add 0.1 mol/L hydrochloric acid TS to make exactly 250 mL. Centrifuge this solution, pipet 5 mL of the supernatant liquid, and add 0.1 mol/L hydrochloric acid TS to make exactly 20 mL. Pipet 2 mL of this solution, add exactly 3 mL of the internal standard solution and water to make 100 mL, and use this solution as the sample solution. Separately, weigh accurately about 25 mg of Troxipide RS, previously dried at 105°C for 2 hours, and dissolve in 0.1 mol/L hydrochloric acid TS to make exactly 25 mL. Pipet 2 mL of this solution, add exactly 3 mL of the internal standard solution and water to make 100 mL, and use this solution as the standard solution. Perform the test with 20 μL each of the sample solution and standard solution as directed under Liquid Chromatography *<2.01>* according to the following conditions, and calculate the ratios, Q_T and Q_S, of the peak area of troxipide to that of the internal standard.

Amount (mg) of troxipide ($C_{15}H_{22}N_2O_4$)
$= M_S \times Q_T/Q_S \times 40$

M_S: Amount (mg) of Troxipide RS taken

Internal standard solution—A solution of 4-aminoacetophenone in 0.1 mol/L hydrochloric acid TS (3 in 2000).
Operating conditions—

Detector: An ultraviolet absorption photometer (wavelength: 258 nm).

Column: A stainless steel column 4.6 mm in inside diameter and 15 cm in length, packed with octadecylsilanized silica gel for liquid chromatography (5 μm in particle diameter).

Column temperature: A constant temperature of about 30°C.

Mobile phase: To 1500 mL of diluted phosphoric acid (1 in 500) add diethylamine to adjust the pH to 3.0. To 1500 mL of this solution add 100 mL of methanol and 50 mL of tetrahydrofuran.

Flow rate: Adjust so that the retention time of troxipide is about 7 minutes.
System suitability—

System performance: When the procedure is run with 20 μL of the standard solution under the above operating conditions, troxipide and the internal standard are eluted in this order with the resolution between these peaks being not less than 3.

System repeatability: When the test is repeated 6 times with 20 μL of the standard solution under the above operating conditions, the relative standard deviation of the ratio of the peak area of troxipide to that of the internal standard is not more than 1.0%.

Containers and storage Containers—Tight containers.

L-Tryptophan

L-トリプトファン

$C_{11}H_{12}N_2O_2$: 204.23
(2*S*)-2-Amino-3-(indol-3-yl)propanoic acid
[73-22-3]

L-Tryptophan, when dried, contains not less than 98.5% of L-tryptophan ($C_{11}H_{12}N_2O_2$).

Description L-Tryptophan occurs as white to yellowish white, crystals or crystalline powder. It is odorless, and has a slightly bitter taste.

It is freely soluble in formic acid, slightly soluble in water, and very slightly soluble in ethanol (95).

It dissolves in dilute hydrochloric acid.

Identification Determine the infrared absorption spectrum of L-Tryptophan, previously dried, as directed in the potassium bromide disk method under Infrared Spectrophotometry *<2.25>*, and compare the spectrum with the Reference Spectrum: both spectra exhibit similar intensities of absorption at the same wave numbers.

Optical rotation *<2.49>* $[\alpha]_D^{20}$: −30.0 – −33.0° Weigh accurately about 0.25 g of L-Tryptophan, previously dried, and dissolve in 20 mL of water by warming. After cooling, add water to make exactly 25 mL, and determine the optical rotation of the solution in a 100-mm cell.

pH *<2.54>* Dissolve 1.0 g of L-Tryptophan in 100 mL of water by warming, and cool: the pH of this solution is between 5.4 and 6.4.

Purity (1) Clarity of solution—Dissolve 0.20 g of L-Tryptophan in 10 mL of 2 mol/L hydrochloric acid TS: the solution is clear.

(2) Chloride *<1.03>*—Dissolve 0.5 g of L-Tryptophan in 6 mL of dilute nitric acid, and add water to make 50 mL. Perform the test using this solution as the test solution. Prepare the control solution with 0.30 mL of 0.01 mol/L hydrochloric acid VS (not more than 0.021%).

(3) Sulfate *<1.14>*—Dissolve 0.6 g of L-Tryptophan in 40 mL of water and 1 mL of dilute hydrochloric acid, and add water to make 50 mL. Perform the test using this solution as the test solution. Prepare the control solution with 0.35 mL of 0.005 mol/L sulfuric acid VS (not more than 0.028%).

(4) Ammonium *<1.02>*—Perform the test with 0.25 g of L-Tryptophan. Prepare the control solution with 5.0 mL of Standard Ammonium Solution (not more than 0.02%).

(5) Heavy metals *<1.07>*—Proceed with 1.0 g of L-Tryptophan according to Method 4, and perform the test. Prepare the control solution with 2.0 mL of Standard Lead Solution (not more than 20 ppm).

(6) Arsenic *<1.11>*—Dissolve 1.0 g of L-Tryptophan in 3 mL of 1 mol/L hydrochloric acid TS and 2 mL of water by heating, and perform the test with this solution as the test solution (not more than 2 ppm).

(7) Related substances—Dissolve 0.30 g of L-Tryptophan in 1 mL of 1 mol/L hydrochloric acid TS, add water to make 50 mL, and use this solution as the sample solution. Pipet 1

mL of the sample solution, and add water to make exactly 50 mL. Pipet 5 mL of this solution, add water to make exactly 20 mL, and use this solution as the standard solution. Perform the test with these solutions as directed under Thin-layer Chromatography <*2.03*>. Spot 5 μL each of the sample solution and standard solution on a plate of silica gel for thin-layer chromatography. Develop the plate with a mixture of 1-butanol, water and acetic acid (100) (3:1:1) to a distance of about 10 cm, and dry the plate at 80°C for 30 minutes. Spray evenly a solution of ninhydrin in acetone (1 in 50) on the plate, and heat the plate at 80°C for 5 minutes: the spots other than the principal spot obtained from the sample solution are not more intense than the spot from the standard solution.

Loss on drying <*2.41*> Not more than 0.30% (1 g, 105°C, 3 hours).

Residue on ignition <*2.44*> Not more than 0.1% (1 g).

Assay Weigh accurately about 0.2 g of L-Tryptophan, previously dried, dissolve in 3 mL of formic acid, add 50 mL of acetic acid (100), and titrate <*2.50*> with 0.1 mol/L perchloric acid VS (potentiometric titration). Perform a blank determination in the same manner, and make any necessary correction.

Each mL of 0.1 mol/L perchloric acid VS
= 20.42 mg of $C_{11}H_{12}N_2O_2$

Containers and storage Containers—Tight containers.
Storage—Light-resistant.

Tulobuterol

ツロブテロール

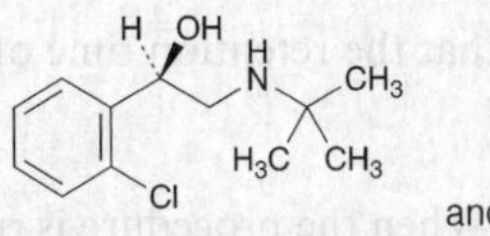

and enantiomer

$C_{12}H_{18}ClNO$: 227.73
(1*RS*)-1-(2-Chlorophenyl)-2-(1,1-dimethylethyl)aminoethanol
[*41570-61-0*]

Tulobuterol contains not less than 98.5% and not more than 101.0% of tulobuterol ($C_{12}H_{18}ClNO$), calculated on the anhydrous basis.

Description Tulobuterol occurs as white, crystals or crystalline powder.

It is very soluble in methanol, freely soluble in ethanol (99.5) and in acetic acid (100), and practically insoluble in water.

It dissolves in 0.1 mol/L hydrochloric acid TS.

It gradually sublimes at 40°C.

A solution of Tulobuterol in methanol (1 in 20) shows no optical rotation.

Identification **(1)** Determine the absorption spectrum of a solution of Tulobuterol in 0.1 mol/L hydrochloric acid TS (3 in 5000) as directed under Ultraviolet-visible Spectrophotometry <*2.24*>, and compare the spectrum with the Reference Spectrum: both spectra exhibit similar intensities of absorption at the same wavelengths.

(2) Determine the infrared absorption spectrum of Tulobuterol as directed in the potassium bromide disk method under Infrared Spectrophotometry <*2.25*>, and compare the spectrum with the Reference Spectrum: both spectra exhibit similar intensities of absorption at the same wave numbers.

Melting point <*2.60*> 90 – 93°C

Purity **(1)** Heavy metals <*1.07*>—Proceed with 2.0 g of Tulobuterol according to Method 2, and perform the test. Prepare the control solution with 1.0 mL of Standard Lead Solution (not more than 5 ppm).

(2) Related substances—Dissolve 25 mg of Tulobuterol in 50 mL of the mobile phase, and use this solution as the sample solution. Pipet 1 mL of the sample solution, add the mobile phase to make exactly 100 mL. Pipet 5 mL of this solution, add the mobile phase to make exactly 50 mL, and use this solution as the standard solution. Perform the test with exactly 25 μL each of the sample solution and standard solution as directed under Liquid Chromatography <*2.01*> according to the following conditions, and determine each peak area by the automatic integration method: each peak area other than tulobuterol obtained from the sample solution is not larger than the peak area of tulobuterol from the standard solution, and the total area of the peaks other than tulobuterol from the sample solution is not larger than 5 times the peak area of tulobuterol from the standard solution.

Operating conditions—

Detector: An ultraviolet absorption photometer (wavelength: 215 nm).

Column: A stainless steel column 4.6 mm in inside diameter and 15 cm in length, packed with octadecylsilanized silica gel for liquid chromatography (5 μm in particle diameter).

Column temperature: A constant temperature of about 30°C.

Mobile phase: Dissolve 3 g of sodium 1-octanesulfonate in 900 mL of water, and add 5 mL of diluted phosphoric acid (1 in 150). To 650 mL of this solution add 350 mL of acetonitrile for liquid chromatography.

Flow rate: Adjust so that the retention time of tulobuterol is about 7 minutes.

Time span of measurement: About 5 times as long as the retention time of tulobuterol, beginning after the solvent peak.

System suitability—

System performance: To 1 mL of the sample solution add the mobile phase to make 100 mL. To 5 mL of this solution add the mobile phase to make 10 mL, and use this solution as the solution for system suitability test. When the procedure is run with 25 μL of the solution for system suitability test under the above operating conditions, the number of theoretical plates and the symmetry factor of the peak of tulobuterol are not less than 5000 and not more than 2.0, respectively.

System repeatability: When the test is repeated 6 times with 25 μL of the solution for system suitability test under the above operating conditions, the relative standard deviation of the peak area of tulobuterol is not more than 2.0%.

(3) Boron—Put 50 mg of Tulobuterol and 3.0 mL of Standard Boron Solution separately in platinum crucibles, and add 5 mL of potassium carbonate-sodium carbonate TS to them. After evaporating to dryness on a water bath, dry them at 120°C for 1 hour, and immediately incinerate by ignition. After cooling, add 0.5 mL of water and 3 mL of curcumin TS to the residue in the crucibles, and warm gently on a water bath for 5 minutes. After cooling, add 3 mL of acetic acid-sulfuric acid TS, and allow to stand for 30 minutes. Then add ethanol (95) to make them exactly 100 mL, filter, discard the first 10 mL of the filtrate, and use these subsequent filtrates as the sample solution and the standard solution, respectively. Perform the test with these solutions as directed under Ultraviolet-visible Spectrophotometry <*2.24*> using methanol (95) as a blank: the absorbance at 555 nm of the sample solution is not more than that of the standard solution.

Water <*2.48*> Not more than 0.2% (2 g, volumetric titration, direct titration).

Residue on ignition <*2.44*> Not more than 0.1% (1 g).

Assay Weigh accurately about 0.5 g of Tulobuterol, dissolve in 20 mL of acetic acid (100), and titrate <*2.50*> with 0.1 mol/L perchloric acid VS until the color of the solution changes from purple to blue-green through blue (indicator: 2 drops of crystal violet TS). Perform a blank determination in the same manner, and make any necessary correction.

Each mL of 0.1 mol/L perchloric acid VS
= 22.77 mg of $C_{12}H_{18}ClNO$

Containers and storage Containers—Tight containers.

Tulobuterol Transdermal Tape

ツロブテロール経皮吸収型テープ

Tulobuterol Transdermal Tape contains not less than 90.0% and not more than 110.0% of the labeled amount of tulobuterol ($C_{12}H_{18}ClNO$: 227.73).

Method of preparation Prepare as directed under Tapes/Plasters, with Tulobuterol.

Identification After removing the liner from an amount of Tulobuterol Transdermal Tape, equivalent to 20 mg of Tulobuterol, shake with 10 mL of hexane. Take the supernatant liquid to an another vessel, shake with 10 mL of 0.1 mol/L hydrochloric acid TS, centrifuge, and take the aqueous layer. To 3 mL of the layer add 0.1 mol/L hydrochloric acid TS to make 10 mL, and determine the absorption spectrum of this solution as directed under Ultraviolet-visible Spectrophotometry <*2.24*>: it exhibits maxima between 261 nm and 263 nm and between 265 nm and 267 nm, and a shoulder between 271 nm and 273 nm.

Uniformity of dosage units <*6.02*> Perform the test according to the following method: it meets the requirement of the Content uniformity test.

After removing the liner from 1 tape of Tulobuterol Transdermal Tape, add exactly V mL of the internal standard solution so that each mL contains about 0.25 mg of tulobuterol ($C_{12}H_{18}ClNO$), shake, and use the supernatant liquid as the sample solution. Separately, weigh accurately about 20 mg of tulobuterol for assay (separately determine the water <*2.48*> in the same manner as Tulobuterol), and dissolve in the internal standard solution to make exactly 20 mL. Pipet 5 mL of this solution, add the internal standard solution to make exactly 20 mL, and use this solution as the standard solution. Then, proceed as directed in the Assay.

Amount (mg) of tulobuterol ($C_{12}H_{18}ClNO$)
$= M_S \times Q_T/Q_S \times V/80$

M_S: Amount (mg) of tulobuterol for assay taken, calculated on the anhydrous basis

Internal standard solution—A solution of benzyl benzoate in hexane (1 in 4000).

Adhesive strength Being specified separately when the drug is granted approval based on the Law.

Drug release Being specified separately when the drug is granted approval based on the Law.

Assay After removing the liner from 10 tapes of Tulobuterol Transdermal Tape, add V mL of hexane so that each mL contains 0.5 mg of tulobuterol ($C_{12}H_{18}ClNO$), then add exactly V/10 mL of the internal standard solution, shake, and use the supernatant liquid as the sample solution. Separately, weigh accurately about 50 mg of tulobuterol for assay (separately determine the water <*2.48*> in the same manner as Tulobuterol), and dissolve in hexane to make exactly 100 mL. Pipet 10 mL of this solution, add exactly 1 mL of the internal standard solution, and use this solution as the standard solution. Perform the test with 1 μL each of the sample solution and standard solution as directed under Gas Chromatography <*2.02*> according to the following conditions, and calculate the ratios, Q_T and Q_S, of the peak area of tulobuterol to that of the internal standard.

Amount (mg) of tulobuterol ($C_{12}H_{18}ClNO$) in 1 tape
$= M_S \times Q_T/Q_S \times V/1000$

M_S: Amount (mg) of tulobuterol for assay taken, calculated on the anhydrous basis

Internal standard solution—A solution of benzyl benzoate in hexane (1 in 200).

Operating conditions—

Detector: A hydrogen flame-ionization detector.

Column: A fused-silica column 0.53 mm in inside diameter and 30 m in length, coated the inside surface with methyl silicon polymer for gas chromatography in 1.5 μm thickness.

Column temperature: A constant temperature of about 180°C.

Carrier gas: Nitrogen.

Flow rate: Adjust so that the retention time of tulobuterol is about 3 minutes.

System suitability—

System performance: When the procedure is run with 1 μL of the standard solution under the above operating conditions, tulobuterol and the internal standard are eluted in this order with the resolution between these peaks being not less than 4.

System repeatability: When the test is repeated 6 times with 1 μL of the standard solution under the above operating conditions, the relative standard deviation of the peak area of tulobuterol is not more than 2.0%.

Containers and storage Containers—Tight containers.

Tulobuterol Hydrochloride

ツロブテロール塩酸塩

and enantiomer

$C_{12}H_{18}ClNO.HCl$: 264.19
(1*RS*)-1-(2-Chlorophenyl)-2-
(1,1-dimethylethyl)aminoethanol monohydrochloride
[*56776-01-3*]

Tulobuterol Hydrochloride, when dried, contains not less than 98.5% and not more than 101.0% of tulobuterol hydrochloride ($C_{12}H_{18}ClNO.HCl$).

Description Tulobuterol Hydrochloride occurs as white, crystals or crystalline powder.

It is very soluble in methanol, freely soluble in water, in ethanol (95) and in acetic acid (100), sparingly soluble in acetic anhydride.

A solution of Tulobuterol Hydrochloride (1 in 20) shows no optical rotation.

Melting point: about 163°C.

Identification **(1)** Determine the absorption spectrum of a solution of Tulobuterol Hydrochloride (1 in 2500) as directed under Ultraviolet-visible Spectrophotometry <*2.24*>, and compare the spectrum with the Reference Spectrum: both spectra exhibit similar intensities of absorption at the same wavelengths.

(2) Determine the infrared absorption spectrum of Tulobuterol Hydrochloride, previously dried, as directed in the potassium bromide disk method under Infrared Spectrophotometry <*2.25*>, and compare the spectrum with the Reference Spectrum: both spectra exhibit similar intensities of absorption at the same wave numbers.

(3) A solution of Tulobuterol Hydrochloride (1 in 20) responds to Qualitative Tests <*1.09*> for chloride.

Purity **(1)** Clarity and color of solution—Dissolve 1.0 g of Tulobuterol Hydrochloride in 10 mL of water: the solution is clear and colorless.

(2) Heavy metals <*1.07*>—Proceed with 2.0 g of Tulobuterol Hydrochloride according to Method 1, and perform the test. Prepare the control solution with 2.0 mL of Standard Lead Solution (not more than 10 ppm).

(3) Related substances—Dissolve 30 mg of Tulobuterol Hydrochloride in 50 mL of the mobile phase, and use this solution as the sample solution. Pipet 1 mL of the sample solution, add the mobile phase to make exactly 100 mL. Pipet 5 mL of this solution, add the mobile phase to make exactly 50 mL, and use this solution as the standard solution. Perform the test with exactly 25 μL each of the sample solution and standard solution as directed under Liquid Chromatography <*2.01*> according to the following conditions, and determine each peak area by the automatic integration method: the area of the peak other than tulobuterol obtained from the sample solution is not larger than the peak area of tulobuterol from the standard solution, and the total area of the peaks other than the peak of tulobuterol from the sample solution is not larger than 5 times the peak area of tulobuterol from the standard solution.

Operating conditions—

Detector: An ultraviolet absorption photometer (wavelength: 215 nm).

Column: A stainless steel column 4.6 mm in inside diameter and 15 cm in length, packed with octadecylsilanized silica gel for liquid chromatography (5 μm in particle diameter).

Column temperature: A constant temperature of about 30°C.

Mobile phase: Dissolve 3 g of sodium 1-octanesulfonate in 900 mL of water, and add 5 mL of diluted phosphoric acid (1 in 150). To 650 mL of this solution add 350 mL of acetonitrile for liquid chromatography.

Flow rate: Adjust so that the retention time of tulobuterol is about 7 minutes.

Time span of measurement: About 5 times as long as the retention time of tulobuterol, beginning after the solvent peak.

System suitability—

System performance: To 1 mL of the sample solution add the mobile phase to make 100 mL. To 5 mL of this solution add the mobile phase to make 10 mL, and use this solution as the solution for system suitability test. When the procedure is run with 25 μL of the solution for system suitability test under the above operating conditions, the number of theoretical plates and the symmetry factor of the peak of tulobuterol are not less than 5000 and not more than 2.0, respectively.

System repeatability: When the test is repeated 6 times with 25 μL of the solution for system suitability test under the above operating conditions, the relative standard deviation of the peak area of tulobuterol is not more than 2.0%.

Loss on drying <*2.41*> Not more than 0.5% (0.5 g, in vacuum, 60°C, 4 hours).

Residue on ignition <*2.44*> Not more than 0.1% (1 g).

Assay Weigh accurately about 0.5 g of Tulobuterol Hydrochloride, previously dried, dissolve in 80 mL of a mixture of acetic anhydride and acetic acid (100) (7:3), and titrate <*2.50*> with 0.1 mol/L perchloric acid VS (potentiometric titration). Perform a blank determination in the same manner, and make any necessary correction.

Each mL of 0.1 mol/L perchloric acid VS
= 26.42 mg of $C_{12}H_{18}ClNO.HCl$

Containers and storage Containers—Tight containers.

L-Tyrosine

L-チロシン

$C_9H_{11}NO_3$: 181.19
(2*S*)-2-Amino-3-(4-hydroxyphenyl)propanoic acid
[*60-18-4*]

L-Tyrosine, when dried, contains not less than 99.0% and not more than 101.0% of L-tyrosine ($C_9H_{11}NO_3$).

Description L-Tyrosine occurs as white, crystals or a crystalline powder.

It is freely soluble in formic acid, and practically insoluble in water and in ethanol (99.5).

It dissolves in dilute hydrochloric acid and in ammonia TS.

Identification (1) Determine the absorption spectrum of a solution of L-Tyrosine in 0.1 mol/L hydrochloric acid (1 in 10,000) as directed under Ultraviolet-visible Spectrophotometry <*2.24*>, and compare the spectrum with the Reference Spectrum: both spectra exhibit similar intensities of absorption at the same wavelengths.

(2) Determine the infrared absorption spectrum of L-Tyrosine as directed in the potassium bromide disk method under Infrared Spectrophotometry <*2.25*>, and compare the spectrum with the Reference Spectrum: both spectra exhibit similar intensities of absorption at the same wave numbers.

Optical rotation <*2.49*> $[\alpha]_D^{20}$: $-10.5 - -12.5°$ (after drying, 2.5 g, 1 mol/L hydrochloric acid TS, 50 mL, 100 mm).

Purity (1) Clarity and color of solution—Dissolve 1.0 g of L-Tyrosine in 20 mL of 1 mol/L hydrochloric acid TS by warming: the solution is clear and colorless.

(2) Chloride <*1.03*>—Dissolve 0.5 g of L-Tyrosine in 12 mL of dilute nitric acid and 20 mL of water, and add water to make 50 mL. Perform the test using this solution as the test solution. Prepare the control solution as follows: To 0.30 mL of 0.01 mol/L hydrochloric acid VS add 12 mL of dilute nitric acid and water to make 50 mL (not more than 0.021%).

(3) Sulfate <*1.14*>—Dissolve 0.6 g of L-Tyrosine in 5 mL of dilute hydrochloric acid, and add water to make 45 mL. Perform the test using this solution as the test solution. Prepare the control solution as follows: To 0.35 mL of 0.005 mol/L sulfuric acid VS add 5 mL of dilute hydrochloric acid and water to make 45 mL. To the test solution and the control solution add 5 mL of barium chloride TS (not more than 0.028%).

(4) Ammonium <*1.02*>—Perform the test with 0.25 g of L-Tyrosine. Prepare the control solution with 5.0 mL of Standard Ammonium Solution (not more than 0.02%).

(5) Heavy metals <*1.07*>—Proceed with 1.0 g of L-Tyrosine according to Method 4, and perform the test. Prepare the control solution with 1.0 mL of Standard Lead Solution (not more than 10 ppm).

(6) Iron <*1.10*>—Prepare the test solution with 1.0 g of L-Tyrosine according to Method 3, and perform the test according to Method A. Prepare the control solution with 1.0 mL of Standard Iron Solution (not more than 10 ppm).

(7) Related substances—Dissolve 0.20 g of L-Tyrosine in 10 mL of diluted ammonia solution (28) (1 in 2), add water to make 20 mL, and use this solution as the sample solution. Pipet 1 mL of the sample solution, add water to make exactly 10 mL, pipet 1 mL of this solution, add water to make exactly 50 mL, and use this solution as the standard solution. Perform the test with these solutions as directed under Thin-layer Chromatography <*2.03*>. Spot 5 μL each of the sample solution and standard solution on a plate of silica gel for thin-layer chromatography. Then develop with a mixture of 1-propanol and ammonia solution (28) (67:33) to a distance of about 10 cm, and dry the plate at 80°C for 30 minutes. Spray evenly a solution of ninhydrin in a mixture of methanol and acetic acid (100) (97:3) (1 in 100) on the plate, and then heat the plate at 80°C for 10 minutes: the spot other than the principal spot obtained from the sample solution is not more intense than the spot from the standard solution.

Loss on drying <*2.41*> Not more than 0.3% (1 g, 105°C, 3 hours).

Residue on ignition <*2.44*> Not more than 0.1% (1 g).

Assay Weigh accurately about 0.18 g of L-Tyrosine previously dried, dissolve in 6 mL of formic acid, add 50 mL of acetic acid (100), and titrate <*2.50*> with 0.1 mol/L perchloric acid VS (potentiometric titration). Perform a blank determination in the same manner, and make any necessary correction.

Each mL of 0.1 mol/L perchloric acid VS
= 18.12 mg of $C_9H_{11}NO_3$

Containers and storage Containers—Tight containers.

Ubenimex

ウベニメクス

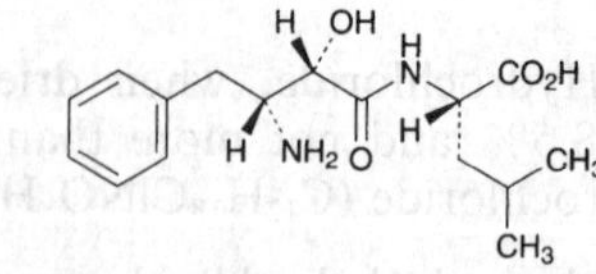

$C_{16}H_{24}N_2O_4$: 308.37
(2*S*)-2-[(2*S*,3*R*)-3-Amino-2-hydroxy-4-phenylbutanoylamino]-4-methylpentanoic acid
[*58970-76-6*]

Ubenimex, when dried, contains not less than 98.5% and not more than 101.0% of ubenimex ($C_{16}H_{24}N_2O_4$).

Description Ubenimex occurs as a white crystalline powder.

It is freely soluble in acetic acid (100), slightly soluble in water, and very slightly soluble in ethanol (99.5).

It dissolves in 1 mol/L hydrochloric acid TS.

Melting point: about 230°C (with decomposition).

Identification (1) Determine the absorption spectrum of a solution of Ubenimex (1 in 2000) as directed under Ultraviolet-visible Spectrophotometry <*2.24*>, and compare the spectrum with the Reference Spectrum: both spectra exhibit similar intensities of absorption at the same wavelengths.

(2) Determine the infrared absorption spectrum as directed in the potassium bromide disk method under Infrared Spectrophotometry <*2.25*>, and compare the spectrum with the Reference Spectrum: both spectra exhibit similar intensities of absorption at the same wave numbers.

Optical rotation <*2.49*> $[\alpha]_D^{20}$: $-15.5 - -17.5°$ (after drying, 0.5 g, 1 mol/L hydrochloric acid TS, 50 mL, 100 mm).

Purity (1) Heavy metals <*1.07*>—Proceed with 2.0 g of Ubenimex according to Method 2, and perform the test. Prepare the control solution with 2.0 mL of Standard Lead Solution (not more than 10 ppm).

(2) Related substances—Dissolve 30 mg of Ubenimex in 10 mL of the mobile phase A, and use this solution as the sample solution. Pipet 2 mL of the sample solution, add the mobile phase A to make exactly 200 mL, and use this solution as the standard solution. Perform the test with exactly 20 μL each of the sample solution and standard solution as directed under Liquid Chromatography <*2.01*> according to the following conditions, and determine each peak area by the automatic integration method: the area of the peak other than ubenimex obtained from the sample solution is not larger than 1/2 times the peak area of ubenimex from the standard solution. Furthermore, the total area of the peaks other than ubenimex from the sample solution is not larger than the peak area of ubenimex from the standard solution.

Operating conditions—

Detector: An ultraviolet absorption photometer (wave-

length: 220 nm).

Column: A stainless steel column 4.6 mm in inside diameter and 25 cm in length, packed with octadecylsilanized silica gel for liquid chromatography (5 μm in particle diameter).

Column temperature: A constant temperature of about 25°C.

Mobile phase A: A mixture of diluted 0.1 mol/L potassium dihydrogen phosphate TS (13 in 20) and acetonitrile for liquid chromatography (17:3).

Mobile phase B: A mixture of acetonitrile for liquid chromatography and diluted 0.1 mol/L potassium dihydrogen phosphate TS (13 in 20) (2:1).

Flowing of mobile phase: Control the gradient by mixing the mobile phases A and B as directed in the following table.

Time after injection of sample (min)	Mobile phase A (vol%)	Mobile phase B (vol%)
0 – 20	100	0
20 – 60	100 → 0	0 → 100
60 – 70	0	100

Flow rate: Adjust so that the retention time of ubenimex is about 14 minutes.

Time span of measurement: About 5 times as long as the retention time of ubenimex, beginning after the solvent peak.

System suitability—

Test for required detectability: Pipet 1 mL of the standard solution, and add the mobile phase A to make exactly 10 mL. Confirm that the peak area of ubenimex obtained with 20 μL of this solution is equivalent to 7 to 13% of that with 20 μL of the standard solution.

System performance: When the procedure is run with 20 μL of the standard solution under the above operating conditions, the number of theoretical plates and the symmetry factor of the peak of ubenimex are not less than 5000 and not more than 2.0, respectively.

System repeatability: When the test is repeated 6 times with 20 μL of the standard solution under the above operating conditions, the relative standard deviation of the peak area of ubenimex is not more than 2.0%.

Loss on drying <2.41> Not more than 0.5% (0.5 g, in vacuum, 80°C, 4 hours).

Residue on ignition <2.44> Not more than 0.1% (1 g).

Assay Weigh accurately about 0.5 g of Ubenimex, previously dried, dissolve in 60 mL of acetic acid (100), and titrate <2.50> with 0.1 mol/L perchloric acid VS (potentiometric titration). Perform a blank determination in the same manner, and make any necessary correction.

Each mL of 0.1 mol/L perchloric acid VS
= 30.84 mg of $C_{16}H_{24}N_2O_4$

Containers and storage Containers—Tight containers.

Ubenimex Capsules

ウベニメクスカプセル

Ubenimex Capsules contain not less than 93.0% and not more than 107.0% of the labeled amount of ubenimex ($C_{16}H_{24}N_2O_4$: 308.37).

Method of preparation Prepare as directed under Capsules, with Ubenimex.

Identification To a quantity of the contents of Ubenimex Capsules, equivalent to 25 mg of Ubenimex, add water to make 50 mL, shake well, and filter. Determine the absorption spectrum of the filtrate as directed under Ultraviolet-visible Spectrophotometry <2.24>: it exhibits maxima between 250 nm and 254 nm, between 255 nm and 259 nm, and between 261 nm and 265 nm.

Uniformity of dosage units <6.02> Perform the test according to the following method: it meets the requirement of the Content uniformity test.

To 1 capsule of Ubenimex Capsules add 30 mL of a mixture of water and acetonitrile (7:3), shake well for 30 minutes, and add a mixture of water and acetonitrile (7:3) to make exactly 50 mL. Centrifuge this solution and filter the supernatant liquid through a membrane filter with a pore size not exceeding 0.45 μm. Discard the first 5 mL of the filtrate, pipet V mL of the subsequent filtrate, equivalent to about 3 mg of ubenimex ($C_{16}H_{24}N_2O_4$), add exactly 4 mL of the internal standard solution, add a mixture of water and acetonitrile (7:3) to make 50 mL, and use this solution as the sample solution. Separately, weigh accurately about 20 mg of ubenimex for assay, previously dried at 80°C for 4 hours under reduced pressure, and dissolve in a mixture of water and acetonitrile (7:3) to make exactly 100 mL. Pipet 15 mL of this solution, add exactly 4 mL of the internal standard solution, add a mixture of water and acetonitrile (7:3) to make 50 mL, and use this solution as the standard solution. Perform the test with 20 μL each of the sample solution and standard solution as directed under Liquid Chromatography <2.01> according to the following conditions, and calculate the ratios, Q_T and Q_S, of the peak area of ubenimex to that of the internal standard.

Amount (mg) of ubenimex ($C_{16}H_{24}N_2O_4$)
$= M_S \times Q_T/Q_S \times 1/V \times 15/2$

M_S: Amount (mg) of ubenimex for assay taken

Internal standard solution—A solution of ethyl parahydroxybenzoate in a mixture of water and acetonitrile (7:3) (1 in 2000).

Operating conditions—

Proceed as directed in the operating conditions in the Assay.

System suitability—

System performance: When the procedure is run with 20 μL of the standard solution under the above operating conditions, ubenimex and the internal standard are eluted in this order with the resolution between these peaks being not less than 10.

System repeatability: When the test is repeated 6 times with 20 μL of the standard solution under the above operating conditions, the relative standard deviation of the ratio of the peak area of ubenimex to that of the internal standard is not more than 2.0%.

Dissolution <6.10> When the test is performed at 50 revolutions per minute according to the Paddle method using the sinker, using 900 mL of water as the dissolution medium, the dissolution rate in 30 minutes of Ubenimex Capsules is not less than 70%.

Start the test with 1 capsule of Ubenimex Capsules, withdraw not less than 20 mL of the medium at the specified minute after starting the test, and filter through a membrane filter with a pore size not exceeding 0.45 μm. Discard not less than 10 mL of the first filtrate, pipet V mL of the subsequent filtrate, add a mixture of water and acetonitrile (7:3) to make exactly V' mL so that each mL contains about 11 μg of ubenimex ($C_{16}H_{24}N_2O_4$), and use this solution as the sample solution. Separately, weigh accurately about 22 mg of ubenimex for assay, previously dried at 80°C for 4 hours under reduced pressure, and dissolve in a mixture of water and acetonitrile (7:3) to make exactly 100 mL. Pipet 5 mL of this solution, add a mixture of water and acetonitrile (7:3) to make exactly 100 mL, and use this solution as the standard solution. Perform the test with exactly 50 μL each of the sample solution and standard solution as directed under Liquid Chromatography <2.01> according to the following conditions, and determine the peak areas, A_T and A_S, of ubenimex in each solution.

Dissolution rate (%) with respect to the labeled amount of ubenimex ($C_{16}H_{24}N_2O_4$)
$= M_S \times A_T/A_S \times V'/V \times 1/C \times 45$

M_S: Amount (mg) of ubenimex for assay taken
C: Labeled amount (mg) of ubenimex ($C_{16}H_{24}N_2O_4$) in 1 capsule

Operating conditions—

Proceed as directed in the operating conditions in the Assay.

System suitability—

System performance: When the procedure is run with 50 μL of the standard solution under the above operating conditions, the number of theoretical plates and symmetry factor of the peak of Ubenimex are not less than 3000 and not more than 2.0, respectively.

System repeatability: When the test is repeated 6 times with 50 μL of the standard solution under the above operating conditions, the relative standard deviation of the peak area of Ubenimex is not more than 2.0%.

Assay To 10 Ubenimex capsules add 140 mL of a mixture of water and acetonitrile (7:3), shake well for 30 minutes, and add a mixture of water and acetonitrile (7:3) to make exactly 200 mL. Centrifuge this solution, and filter. Discard the first 20 mL of the filtrate, pipet a volume of the subsequent filtrate, equivalent to about 7.5 mg of ubenimex ($C_{16}H_{24}N_2O_4$), add exactly 10 mL of the internal standard solution, add a mixture of water and acetonitrile (7:3) to make 50 mL, and use this solution as the sample solution. Separately, weigh accurately about 30 mg of ubenimex for assay, previously dried at 80°C for 4 hours under reduced pressure, dissolve in a mixture of water and acetonitrile (7:3) to make exactly 20 mL. Pipet 5 mL of this solution, add exactly 10 mL of the internal standard solution, and a mixture of water and acetonitrile (7:3) to make 50 mL, and use this solution as the standard solution. Perform the test with 20 μL each of the sample solution and standard solution as directed under Liquid Chromatography <2.01> according to the following conditions, and calculate the ratios, Q_T and Q_S, of the peak area of ubenimex to that of the internal standard.

Amount (mg) of ubenimex ($C_{16}H_{24}N_2O_4$)
$= M_S \times Q_T/Q_S \times 1/4$

M_S: Amount (mg) of ubenimex for assay taken

Internal standard solution—A solution of ethyl parahydroxybenzoate in mixture of water and acetonitrile (7:3) (1 in 2000).

Operating conditions—

Detector: An ultraviolet absorption photometer (wavelength: 200 nm).

Column: A stainless steel column 4.6 mm in inside diameter and 15 cm in length, packed with octadecylsilanized silica gel for liquid chromatography (5 μm in particle diameter).

Column temperature: A constant temperature of about 30°C.

Mobile phase: A mixture of diluted phosphoric acid (1 in 100) and acetonitrile for liquid chromatography (83:17).

Flow rate: Adjust so that the retention time of ubenimex is about 8 minutes.

System suitability—

System performance: When the procedure is run with 20 μL of the standard solution under the above operating conditions, ubenimex and the internal standard are eluted in this order with the resolution between these peaks being not less than 10.

System repeatability: When the test is repeated 6 times with 20 μL of the standard solution under the above operating conditions, the relative standard deviation of the ratio of the peak area of ubenimex to that of the internal standard is not more than 1.0%.

Containers and storage Containers—Tight containers.

Ubidecarenone

ユビデカレノン

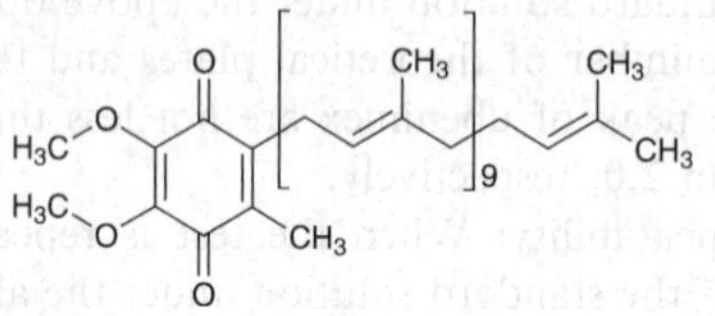

$C_{59}H_{90}O_4$: 863.34
(2*E*,6*E*,10*E*,14*E*,18*E*,22*E*,26*E*,30*E*,34*E*,38*E*)-2-(3,7,11,15,19,23,27,31,35,39-Decamethyltetraconta-2,6,10,14,18,22,26,30,34,38-decaen-1-yl)-5,6-dimethoxy-3-methyl-1,4-benzoquinone
[*303-98-0*]

Ubidecarenone contains not less than 98.0% of ubidecarenone ($C_{59}H_{90}O_4$), calculated on the anhydrous basis.

Description Ubidecarenone occurs as a yellow to orange crystalline powder. It is odorless and has no taste.

It is soluble in diethyl ether, very slightly soluble in ethanol (99.5), and practically insoluble in water.

It is gradually decomposed and colored by light.

Melting point: about 48°C.

Identification **(1)** Dissolve 0.05 g of Ubidecarenone in 1 mL of diethyl ether, and add 10 mL of ethanol (99.5). To 2 mL of this solution add 3 mL of ethanol (99.5) and 2 mL of dimethyl malonate, then add dropwise 1 mL of a solution of potassium hydroxide (1 in 5), and mix: a blue color appears.

(2) Determine the infrared absorption spectrum of Ubidecarenone as directed in the potassium bromide disk method under Infrared Spectrophotometry <2.25>, and compare the spectrum with the Reference Spectrum or the spectrum of Ubidecarenone RS: both spectra exhibit similar intensities of absorption at the same wave numbers.

Purity (1) Heavy metals <*1.07*>—Proceed with 1.0 g of Ubidecarenone according to Method 4, and perform the test. Prepare the control solution with 2.0 mL of Standard Lead Solution (not more than 20 ppm).

(2) Related substances—Dissolve 0.05 g of Ubidecarenone in 50 mL of ethanol (99.5) by warming at about 50°C for 2 minutes, and after cooling use this solution as the sample solution. To exactly 1 mL of the sample solution add ethanol (99.5) to make exactly 100 mL, and use this solution as the standard solution. Perform the test with exactly 5 μL each of the sample solution and standard solution as directed under Liquid Chromatography <*2.01*> according to the following conditions. Determine each peak area of both solutions by the automatic integration method: the total area of the peaks other than ubidecarenone obtained from the sample solution is not larger than the peak area of ubidecarenone from the standard solution.

Operating conditions—

Detector, column, column temperature, mobile phase, flow rate, and selection of column: Proceed as directed in the operating conditions in the Assay.

Detection sensitivity: Adjust so that the peak height of ubidecarenone obtained from 5 μL of the standard solution is between 20 mm and 40 mm.

Time span of measurement: About 2 times of the retention time of ubidecarenone, beginning after the solvent peak.

Water <*2.48*> Not more than 0.20% (1 g, volumetric titration, direct titration).

Residue on ignition <*2.44*> Not more than 0.1% (1 g).

Assay Weigh accurately about 50 mg each of Ubidecarenone and Ubidecarenone RS (separately determined the water <*2.48*> in the same manner as Ubidecarenone) dissolve each in 40 mL of ethanol (99.5) by warming at about 50°C for 2 minutes, and after cooling add ethanol (99.5) to make exactly 50 mL each, and use these solutions as the sample solution and standard solution. Perform the test with exactly 5 μL each of the sample solution and standard solution as directed under Liquid Chromatography <*2.01*> according to the following conditions, and determine peak areas, A_T and A_S, of ubidecarenone in each solution.

$$\text{Amount (mg) of ubidecarenone } (C_{59}H_{90}O_4) = M_S \times A_T/A_S$$

M_S: Amount (mg) of Ubidecarenone RS taken, calculated on the anhydrous basis

Operating conditions—

Detector: An ultraviolet absorption photometer (wavelength: 275 nm).

Column: A stainless steel column about 5 mm in inside diameter and about 15 cm in length, packed with octadecylsilanized silica gel for liquid chromatography (5 μm in particle diameter).

Column temperature: A constant temperature of about 35°C.

Mobile phase: A mixture of methanol and ethanol (99.5) (13:7).

Flow rate: Adjust so that the retention time of ubidecarenone is about 10 minutes.

Selection of column: Dissolve 0.01 g each of Ubidecarenone and ubiquinone-9 in 20 mL of ethanol (99.5) by warming at about 50°C for 2 minutes. After cooling, proceed with 5 μL of this solution under the above operating conditions, and calculate the resolution. Use a column giving elution of ubiquinone-9 and ubidecarenone in this order with the resolution between these peaks being not less than 4.

System repeatability: Repeat the test 5 times with the standard solution under the above operating conditions: the relative standard deviation of the peak areas of ubidecarenone is not more than 0.8%.

Containers and storage Containers—Tight containers.

Storage—Light-resistant.

Ulinastatin

ウリナスタチン

Ulinastatin is a solution of a glycoprotein having trypsin inhibiting activity, which is separated and purified from human urine.

It contains ulinastatin of not less than 45,000 Units per mL and not less than 2500 Units per mg protein.

Description Ulinastatin occurs as a light brown to brown, clear liquid.

Identification (1) Dilute a suitable volume of Ulinastatin with water to make a solution containing 4000 Units of ulinastatin per mL. To 1 mL of this solution add 1 mL of a solution of phenol (1 in 20), then carefully add 5 mL of sulfuric acid, and mix: an orange to red-orange color develops.

(2) Dilute a suitable volume of Ulinastatin with water to make a solution containing 2000 units per mL. Determine the absorption spectrum of the solution as directed under Ultraviolet-visible Spectrophotometry <*2.24*>, and compare the spectrum with the Reference Spectrum: both spectra exhibit similar intensities of absorption at the same wavelengths.

(3) Dilute a suitable volume of Ulinastatin with 2,2′,2″-nitrilotriethanol buffer solution (pH 7.8) to make a solution containing 500 Units of ulinastatin per mL, and use this solution as the sample solution. Use the same buffer solution as the control solution. To 0.1 mL each of the sample solution and control solution add 1.6 mL of the same buffer solution and 0.2 mL of trypsin TS for test of ulinastatin, mix, and allow them to stand in a water bath at 25°C for 1 minute. Then add 1 mL of *N*-α-benzoyl-L-arginine-4-nitroanilide TS, mix, and allow them to stand at 25°C for 2 minutes: the solution obtained with the sample solution develops no color while that obtained with the control solution develops a yellow color.

(4) To 1.5 g of Powdered Agar add 100 mL of boric acid-sodium hydroxide buffer solution (pH 8.4), dissolve by warming in a water bath, then pour immediately into a Petri dish placed horizontally so that the agar layer is about 2 mm in thickness. After the agar becomes hard, bore two wells about 2.5 mm in diameter with a separation of 6 mm from each other. In one of the wells place 10 μL of a solution of Ulinastatin containing 500 Units per mL in boric acid-sodium hydroxide buffer solution (pH 8.4), and in the other well place 10 μL of anti-ulinastatin rabbit serum, cover the dish to avoid drying of the agar, and allow to stand for overnight at a room temperature: a clear precipitin line appears between the wells.

pH <*2.54*> 6.0 – 8.0

Specific activity When calculated from the results obtained by the Assay and the following method, the specific activity is not less than 2500 Units per 1 mg protein.

(i) Sample solution—To an exactly measured volume of Ulinastatin, equivalent to about 10,000 Units, add water to make exactly 20 mL.

(ii) Standard solutions—Weigh accurately about 10 mg of bovine serum albumin for test of ulinastatin, and dissolve in water to make exactly 20 mL. To a suitable volume of this solution add water to make four solutions containing exactly 300, 200, 100 and 50 μg of the bovine serum albumin for test of ulinastatin per mL, respectively.

(iii) Procedure—Pipet 0.5 mL each of the sample solution and standard solutions, put them in glass test tubes about 18 mm in internal diameter and about 130 mm in length, add exactly 5 mL of alkaline copper TS, mix, and allow the tubes to stand in a water bath at 30°C for 10 minutes. Then add exactly 0.5 mL of diluted Folin's TS (1 in 2), mix, and warm in the water bath for 20 minutes. Determine the absorbances of these solutions at 750 nm as directed under Ultraviolet-visible Spectrophotometry <2.24> using a solution obtained in the same manner with 0.5 mL of water as the blank.

Plot the absorbances of the standard solutions on the vertical axis and their protein concentrations on the horizontal axis to prepare a calibration curve, and calculate the protein content of the sample solution from its absorbance by using this curve. Then calculate the amount of protein per mL of Ulinastatin.

Purity (1) Heavy metals <1.07>—Proceed with 10 mL of Ulinastatin according to Method 2, and perform the test. Prepare the control solution with 1.0 mL of Standard Lead Solution (not more than 1 ppm).

(2) Related substances—To a suitable volume of Ulinastatin add water to make a solution containing exactly 12,500 Units per mL, and use this solution as the sample stock solution. To exactly 0.25 mL of the sample stock solution add exactly 0.2 mL of glycerin and exactly 0.05 mL of 0.05% bromophenol blue TS, mix, and use this solution as the sample solution. Separately, to exactly 1 mL of the sample stock solution add water to make exactly 100 mL. To exactly 0.25 mL of this solution add exactly 0.2 mL of glycerin and exactly 0.05 mL of 0.05% bromophenol blue TS, mix, and use this solution as the standard solution. Perform the following test with the sample solution and standard solution: the bands other than the principal band obtained from the sample solution are not more intense than the band obtained from the standard solution in the electrophoretogram.

(i) Tris buffer solution A for polyacrylamide gel electrophoresis Dissolve 18.2 g of 2-amino-2-hydroxymethyl-1,3-propanediol in 80 mL of water, adjust to pH 8.8 with 6 mol/L hydrochloric acid TS, and add water to make 100 mL.

(ii) Tris buffer solution B for polyacrylamide gel electrophoresis Dissolve 6.0 g of 2-amino-2-hydroxymethyl-1,3-propanediol in 80 mL of water, adjust to pH 8.8 with 6 mol/L hydrochloric acid TS, and add water to make 100 mL.

(iii) Tris buffer solution C for polyacrylamide gel electrophoresis Dissolve 3.0 g of 2-amino-2-hydroxymethyl-1,3-propanediol and 14.4 g of glycine in water to make 1000 mL.

(iv) Acrylamide solution for polyacrylamide gel electrophoresis Dissolve 30 g of acrylamide and 0.8 g of *N,N'*-methylenebisacrylamide in water to make 100 mL.

(v) Gel for separation Mix gently 15 mL of tris buffer solution A for polyacrylamide gel electrophoresis, 20 mL of acrylamide solution for polyacrylamide gel electrophoresis, 24.5 mL of water, 0.022 mL of *N,N,N',N'*-tetramethylethylenediamine, 0.32 mL of 10% ammonium peroxodisulfate TS and 0.3 mL of 1 mol/L sodium sulfite TS, pour into a plate for slab gel preparation, then cover the gel mixture with a layer of water, and allow to set for 1 hour.

(vi) Gel for concentration Remove the water layer on the gel for separation, and pour a mixture of 2.5 mL of tris buffer solution B for polyacrylamide gel electrophoresis, 2.66 mL of acrylamide solution for polyacrylamide gel electrophoresis, 14.6 mL of water, 0.01 mL of *N,N,N',N'*-tetramethylethylenediamine, 0.2 mL of 10% ammonium peroxodisulfate TS and 0.04 mL of 1 mol/L sodium sulfite TS on the gel. Then position a plastic sample well former so that the height of the gel for concentration is about 15 mm, and allow to set for 2 hours.

(vii) Procedure

Electrophoresis Set the gel in an apparatus for slab gel electrophoresis, and fill the upper and lower reservoirs with tris buffer solution C for polyacrylamide gel electrophoresis. Introduce carefully 10 μL each of the sample solution and standard solution into the wells using a different well for each solution, and allow electrophoresis to proceed using the electrode of the lower reservoir as the anode. Switch off the power supply when the bromophenol blue band has migrated to about 10 mm from the bottom of the gel.

Staining Dissolve 2.0 g of Coomassie brilliant blue R-250 in a mixture of 400 mL of methanol and 100 mL of acetic acid (100), add water to make 1000 mL, and use this solution as the staining solution. Stain the gel for 2 hours in the staining solution warmed to 40°C.

Decolorization To 100 mL of methanol and 75 mL of acetic acid (100) add water to make 1000 mL, and use this solution as the rinsing solution. Immerse the gel removed from the staining solution in the rinsing solution to decolorise.

(3) Kallidinogenase—Dilute a suitable volume of Ulinastatin with water so that each mL of the solution contains about 50,000 Units, and use this solution as the sample solution. Take exactly 0.4 mL of the sample solution into a test tube, add exactly 0.5 mL of tris buffer solution (pH 8.2), mix, and allow the tube to stand in a water bath at 37 ± 0.2°C for 5 minutes. Add exactly 0.1 mL of substrate TS for kallidinogenase assay (4), mix, allow the tube to stand in the water bath of 37 ± 0.2°C for exactly 30 minutes, then add exactly 0.1 mL of diluted acetic acid (100) (1 in 2), mix, and use this solution as the test solution. Separately, take exactly 0.4 mL of the sample solution in a test tube, add exactly 0.5 mL of tris buffer solution (pH 8.2), mix, and allow the tube to stand in the water bath of 37 ± 0.2°C for 35 minutes. Then add exactly 0.1 mL of diluted acetic acid (100) (1 in 2), mix, add exactly 0.1 mL of substrate TS for kallidinogenase assay (4), mix, and use this solution as the control solution. Determine the absorbances of the test solution and the control solution at 405 nm as directed under Ultraviolet-visible Spectrophotometry <2.24> using water as the blank, and calculate the difference between them: the difference is not more than 0.050.

Molecular mass Dilute a suitable volume of Ulinastatin with the mobile phase so that each mL of the solution contains about 6500 Units, and use this solution as the sample solution. Separately, dissolve 1.0 mg each of γ-globulin (molecular mass: 160,000), bovine serum albumin for test of ulinastatin (molecular mass: 67,000), and myoglobin (molecular mass: 17,000) in about 1 mL of the mobile phase, and use this solution as the molecular mass reference solution. Perform the test with 50 μL each of the sample solution and molecular mass reference solution as directed under Liquid Chromatography <2.01> according to the following conditions. Prepare a calibration curve by plotting the logarithm of molecular masses on the vertical axis and the retention times (minute) of the molecular mass reference substances on the horizontal axis, and determine the molecular mass of the sample using the calibration curve and the retention time obtained with the sample solution: the molecular mass is 67,000 ± 5000.

Operating conditions—

Detector: An ultraviolet absorption photometer (wavelength: 280 nm).

Column: A stainless steel column about 7 mm in inside diameter and about 60 cm in length, packed with porous silica gel for liquid chromatography (10 - 12 μm in particle diameter).

Column temperature: A constant temperature of about 25°C.

Mobile phase: Dissolve 16.33 g of potassium dihydrogenphosphate and 124.15 g of ethylene glycol in water to make 1000 mL. If necessary, adjust to pH 4.0 with phosphoric acid.

Flow rate: Adjust so that the retention time of bovine serum albumin is about 36 minutes.

Selection of column: Proceed with 50 μL of the molecular mass reference solution according to the above operating conditions, and calculate the resolution. Use a column from which γ-globulin, bovine serum albumin and myoglobin are eluted in this order with the resolution between their peaks being not less than 1.5, respectively.

Antigenicity Dilute a suitable volume of Ulinastatin with isotonic sodium chloride solution so that each mL of the solution contains 15,000 Units, and use this solution as the sample solution. Inject 0.10 mL of the sample solution on 3 occasions at intervals of 2 days intraperitoneally to each of 4 well-nourished, healthy guinea pigs weighing 250 to 300 g. Inject 0.10 mL of horse serum intraperitoneally to each of 4 guinea pigs of another group as a control. Inject 0.20 mL of the sample solution intravenously into each of 2 guinea pigs of the first group 14 days after the first intraperitoneal injection and into each of the remaining 2 guinea pigs 21 days after the injection, and inject 0.20 mL of horse serum intravenously in the same manner into each guinea pig of the second group. Observe the signs of respiratory distress, collapse or death of the animals for 30 minutes after each intravenous injection and 24 hours later: the animals of the first group exhibit none of the signs mentioned above, and all the animals of the second group exhibit symptoms of respiratory distress or collapse and not less than 3 animals are killed.

Toxicity Inject intravenously 0.50 mL of Ulinastatin into each of five well-fed, healthy albino mice weighing 18 to 25 g: no mouse dies within 48 hours after injection. If any mouse dies within 48 hours, repeat the test using 5 albino mice weighing 19 to 21 g: all the animals survive for 48 hours.

Assay Measure exactly a suitable volume of Ulinastatin, dilute with 2,2′,2″-nitrilotriethanol buffer solution (pH 7.8) so that each mL of the solution contains about 150 Units, and use this solution as the sample solution. Separately, dilute a suitable volume of Ulinastatin RS with 2,2′,2″-nitrilotriethanol buffer solution (pH 7.8) so that each mL of the solution contains exactly 300, 200, 100, 50 or 0 Units, and use these solutions as the standard solutions. 2,2′,2″-Nitrilotriethanol buffer solution (pH 7.8) and *N*-α-benzoyl-L-arginine-4-nitroanilide TS are warmed in a water bath of 25 ± 1°C for use as described below. Take exactly 0.1 mL each of the sample solution and the standard solutions in test tubes, add exactly 1.6 mL of 2,2′,2″-nitrilotriethanol buffer solution (pH 7.8) mix, and put the tubes in the water bath of 25 ± 1°C. One minute after addition of the buffer solution add exactly 0.2 mL of ice-cooled trypsin TS for test of ulinastatin, mix, and put the tubes again in the water bath. One minute later add exactly 1 mL of *N*-α-benzoyl-L-arginine-4-nitroanilide TS, mix, and then put the tubes in the water bath. Exactly 2 minutes later add exactly 0.1 mL of diluted acetic acid (100) (1 in 2) to stop the enzyme reaction, and determine the absorbances of the solutions so obtained at 405 nm as directed under Ultraviolet-visible Spectrophotometry <*2.24*> using water as the blank. Prepare a calibration curve using the absorbances obtained with the standard solutions, and calculate ulinastatin Units in the sample solution from its absorbance by using this curve.

Containers and storage Containers—Tight containers.

Storage—Not exceeding at −20°C.

Urapidil

ウラピジル

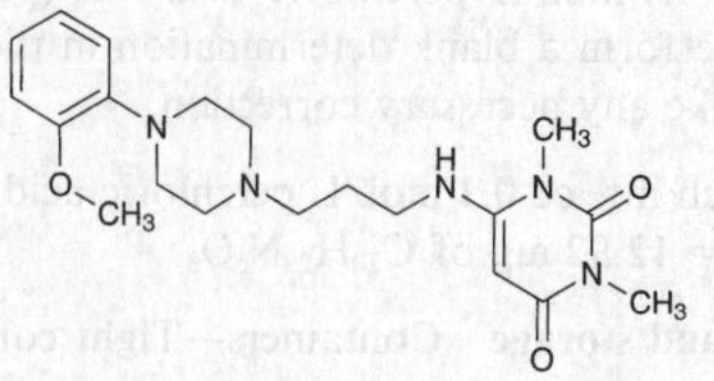

$C_{20}H_{29}N_5O_3$: 387.48

6-{3-[4-(2-Methoxyphenyl)piperazin-1-yl]propylamino}-1,3-dimethyluracil

[34661-75-1]

Urapidil, when dried, contains not less than 98.0% and not more than 101.0% of urapidil ($C_{20}H_{29}N_5O_3$).

Description Urapidil occurs as white to pale yellow-white, crystals or crystalline powder. It has a bitter taste.

It is freely soluble in acetic acid (100), sparingly soluble in ethanol (95) and in acetone, and very slightly soluble in water.

Identification **(1)** Determine the absorption spectrum of a solution of Urapidil in ethanol (95) (1 in 100,000) as directed under Ultraviolet-visible Spectrophotometry <*2.24*>, and compare the spectrum with the Reference Spectrum: both spectra exhibit similar intensities of absorption at the same wavelengths.

(2) Determine the infrared absorption spectrum of Urapidil as directed in the potassium bromide disk method under Infrared Spectrophotometry <*2.25*>, and compare the spectrum with the Reference Spectrum: both spectra exhibit similar intensities of absorption at the same wave numbers.

Melting point <*2.60*> 156 - 161°C

Purity **(1)** Chloride <*1.03*>—Dissolve 3.0 g of Urapidil in 40 mL of acetone and 6 mL of dilute nitric acid, add water to make 50 mL, and perform the test using this solution as the test solution. Prepare the control solution as follows. To 0.25 mL of 0.01 mol/L hydrochloric acid VS add 40 mL of acetone, 6 mL of dilute nitric acid and water to make 50 mL (not more than 0.003%).

(2) Heavy metals <*1.07*>—Proceed with 1.0 g of Urapidil according to Method 4, and perform the test. Prepare the control solution with 2.0 mL of Standard Lead Solution (not more than 20 ppm).

(3) Related substances—Dissolve 40 mg of Urapidil in 5 mL of ethanol (95), and use this solution as the sample solution. Pipet 1 mL of the sample solution, add ethanol (95) to make exactly 200 mL, and use this solution as the standard solution. Perform the test with these solutions as directed under Thin-layer Chromatography *<2.03>*. Spot 5 μL each of the sample solution and standard solution on a plate of silica gel with fluorescent indicator for thin-layer chromatography, develop with a mixture of ethyl acetate, ethanol (95) and ammonia water (28) (22:13:1) to a distance of about 15 cm, and air-dry the plate. Examine under ultraviolet light (main wavelength: 254 nm): the spot other than the principal spot obtained from the sample solution appears not more than one and it is not more intense than the spot from the standard solution.

Loss on drying *<2.41>* Not more than 0.5% (1 g, 105°C, 3 hours).

Residue on ignition *<2.44>* Not more than 0.2% (1 g).

Assay Weigh accurately about 70 mg of Urapidil, previously dried, dissolve in 80 mL of acetic acid (100), and titrate *<2.50>* with 0.1 mol/L perchloric acid VS (potentiometric titration). Perform a blank determination in the same manner, and make any necessary correction.

Each mL of 0.1 mol/L perchloric acid VS
= 12.92 mg of $C_{20}H_{29}N_5O_3$

Containers and storage Containers—Tight containers.

Urea

尿素

CH_4N_2O: 60.06
Urea
[57-13-6]

Urea contains not less than 99.0% of urea (CH_4N_2O).

Description Urea occurs as colorless to white, crystals or crystalline powder. It is odorless, and has a cooling, saline taste.

It is very soluble in water, freely soluble in boiling ethanol (95), soluble in ethanol (95), and very slightly soluble in diethyl ether.

A solution of Urea (1 in 100) is neutral.

Identification **(1)** Heat 0.5 g of Urea: it liquefies and the odor of ammonia is perceptible. Continue heating until the liquid becomes turbid, then cool. Dissolve the resulting lump in a mixture of 10 mL of water and 2 mL of sodium hydroxide TS, and add 1 drop of copper (II) sulfate TS: a reddish purple color develops.

(2) Dissolve 0.1 g of Urea in 1 mL of water, and add 1 mL of nitric acid: a white, crystalline precipitate is formed.

Melting point *<2.60>* 132.5 – 134.5°C

Purity **(1)** Chloride *<1.03>*—Perform the test with 2.0 g of Urea. Prepare the control solution with 0.40 mL of 0.01 mol/L hydrochloric acid VS (not more than 0.007%).

(2) Sulfate *<1.14>*—Perform the test with 2.0 g of Urea. Prepare the control solution with 0.40 mL of 0.005 mol/L sulfuric acid VS (not more than 0.010%).

(3) Heavy metals *<1.07>*—Proceed with 1.0 g of Urea according to Method 1, and perform the test. Prepare the control solution with 2.0 mL of Standard Lead Solution (not more than 20 ppm).

(4) Ethanol-insoluble substances—Dissolve 5.0 g of Urea in 50 mL of warm ethanol (95), filter through a tared glass filter (G4), wash the residue with 20 mL of warm ethanol (95), and dry at 105°C for 1 hour: the mass of the residue is not more than 2.0 mg.

Residue on ignition *<2.44>* Not more than 0.1% (1 g).

Assay Weigh accurately about 0.2 g of Urea, and dissolve in water to make exactly 200 mL. Measure exactly 5 mL of this solution into a Kjeldahl flask, and proceed as directed under Nitrogen Determination *<1.08>*.

Each mL of 0.005 mol/L sulfuric acid VS
= 0.3003 mg of CH_4N_2O

Containers and storage Containers—Well-closed containers.

Urokinase

ウロキナーゼ

[9010-53-1]

Urokinase is an enzyme, obtained from human urine, that activates plasminogen, and has the molecular mass of about 54,000.

It is a solution using a suitable buffer solution as the solvent.

It contains not less than 60,000 Units per mL, and not less than 120,000 Units per mg of protein.

Description Urokinase is a clear and colorless liquid.

The pH is between 5.5 and 7.5.

Identification **(1)** Dissolve 0.07 g of fibrinogen in 10 mL of phosphate buffer solution (pH 7.4). To this solution add 1 mL of a solution of thrombin containing 10 Units per mL in isotonic sodium chloride solution, mix, place in a Petri dish about 90 mm in inside diameter, and keep horizontally until the solution is coagulated. On the surface drop 10 μL of a solution of Urokinase containing 100 Units per mL in gelatin-tris buffer solution, and stand for overnight: lysis circle appears.

(2) Dissolve 1.0 g of Powdered Agar in 100 mL of boric acid-sodium hydroxide buffer solution (pH 8.4) by warming, and pour the solution into a Petri dish until the height come to about 2 mm. After cooling, make two wells of 2.5 mm in diameter with the space of 6 mm. To each well place separately 10 μL of a solution of Urokinase containing 30,000 Units per mL in isotonic sodium chloride solution and 10 μL of anti-urokinase serum, and stand for overnight: a clear precipitin line appears.

Purity **(1)** Heavy metals *<1.07>*—Proceed with 2.0 mL of Urokinase according to Method 2, and perform the test. Prepare the control solution with 2.0 mL of Standard Lead Solution (not more than 10 ppm).

(2) Blood group substances—Dilute Urokinase with isotonic sodium chloride solution so that each mL of the solution contains 12,000 Units, and use this solution as the sample solution. To anti-A type antibody for blood typing add isotonic sodium chloride solution to dilute each 32, 64, 128, 256, 512 and 1024 times, place separately 25 μL each of these solutions in six wells on the first and second lane of a V-shaped 96-wells microplate. Next, add 25 μL of the sample solution into the six wells on the first lane and 25 μL of isotonic sodium chloride solution into the six wells of the second lane, mix, and allow to stand for 30 minutes. To each well add 50 μL of A-type erythrocyte suspension, mix, allow to stand for 2 hours, and compare the agglutination of erythrocyte in both lanes: dilution factor of anti-A type antibody of the wells which show the agglutination is equal in both lanes.

Perform the same test by using anti-B type antibody for blood typing and B-type erythrocyte suspension.

Abnormal toxicity Dilute Urokinase with isotonic sodium chloride solution so that each mL of the solution contains 12,000 Units, and use this solution as the sample solution. Inject 5.0 mL of the sample solution into the peritoneal cavity of each of 2 or more of well-nourished, healthy guinea pigs weighing about 350 g. Observe the conditions of the animals for more than 7 days: all the animals exhibit no abnormalities.

High-molecular mass urokinase Dilute Urokinase with gelatin-phosphate buffer solution so that each mL of the solution contains 10,000 Units, and use this solution as the sample solution. Perform the test with 100 μL of the sample solution as directed under Liquid Chromatography <*2.01*> according to the following conditions. Determine the peak areas of two peaks eluted closely at about 35 minutes having smaller retention time, A_a, and larger retention time, A_b, by the automatic integration method: the value, $A_a/(A_a + A_b)$, is not less than 0.85.

Operating conditions—

Apparatus: Use a pumping system for the mobile phase, a sample injection port, a column, a pumping system for the reaction reagent, a reaction coil, a reaction chamber, a spectrofluorometer and a recorder. Attach a 3-way tube to the outlet for the mobile phase of the column, connect the pumping system for the reaction reagent and the reaction coil, and join outlet of the reaction coil to the spectrofluorometer.

Detector: Spectrofluorometer (excitation wavelength: 365 nm, fluorescence wavelength: 460 nm).

Column: A stainless steel column 7.5 mm in inside diameter and 60 cm in length, packed with porous silica gel for liquid chromatography (10 to 12 μm in particle diameter).

Column temperature: A constant temperature of about 20°C.

Reaction coil: A stainless steel column 0.25 mm in inside diameter and 150 cm in length.

Reaction coil temperature: 37°C.

Mobile phase: Gelatin-phosphate buffer solution.

Flow rate of mobile phase: 0.5 mL per minute.

Reaction reagent: 7-(Glutarylglycyl-L-arginylamino)-4-methylcoumarin TS.

Flow rate of reaction reagent: 0.75 mL per minute.

Selection of column: Adjust the pH of Urokinase to 7.5 with sodium hydroxide TS, allow to stand at 37°C for over 24 hours, and add gelatin-phosphate buffer solution to make the solution containing 20,000 Units per mL. Proceed with 100 μL of this solution under the above operating conditions, and calculate the resolution. Use a column giving elution of high molecular mass urokinase (molecular mass: 54,000) and low molecular mass urokinase (molecular mass: 33,000) in this order with the resolution between these peaks being not less than 1.0.

Assay **(1)** Urokinase—Pipet 1 mL of Urokinase, dilute exactly with gelatin-tris buffer solution so that each mL of the solution contains about 30 Units, and use this solution as the sample solution. Add exactly 2 mL of gelatin-tris buffer solution to contents of one ampoule of High-Molecular Mass Urokinase RS to dissolve, pipet 1 mL of this solution, dilute exactly with gelatin-tris buffer solution so that each mL of the solution contains about 30 Units, and use this solution as the standard solution. Place 1.0 mL of L-pyroglutamylglycyl-L-arginine-*p*-nitroaniline hydrochloride TS in two silicon-coated test tubes about 10 mm in inside diameter, warm them in a water bath at 35 ± 0.2°C for 5 minutes, add separately 0.50 mL each of the sample solution and standard solution, warm in a water bath at 35 ± 0.2°C for exactly 30 minutes, then add 0.50 mL of diluted acetic acid (100) (2 in 5). Determine the absorbances, A_T and A_S, of these solutions at 405 nm as directed under Ultraviolet-visible Spectrophotometry <*2.24*>, using water as the blank. Separately place 1.0 mL of L-pyroglutamylglycyl-L-arginine-*p*-nitroaniline hydrochloride TS in two test tubes, add 0.50 mL of diluted acetic acid (100) (2 in 5), and 0.50 mL each of the sample solution and standard solution. Determine the absorbances, A_{T0} and A_{S0}, of these solutions at 405 nm as the same manner, using water as the blank.

$$\text{Amount (Units) of Urokinase} = (A_T - A_{T0})/(A_S - A_{S0}) \times a \times b$$

a: Amount (Units) of urokinase in 1 mL of the standard solution

b: Total volume (mL) of the sample solution

(2) Protein—Measure exactly a volume of Urokinase, equivalent to about 15 mg of protein, and perform the test as directed under Nitrogen Determination <*1.08*>.

Each mL of 0.005 mol/L sulfuric acid VS
= 0.8754 mg of protein

Containers and storage Containers—Tight containers.

Storage—Not exceeding −20°C.

Ursodeoxycholic Acid

ウルソデオキシコール酸

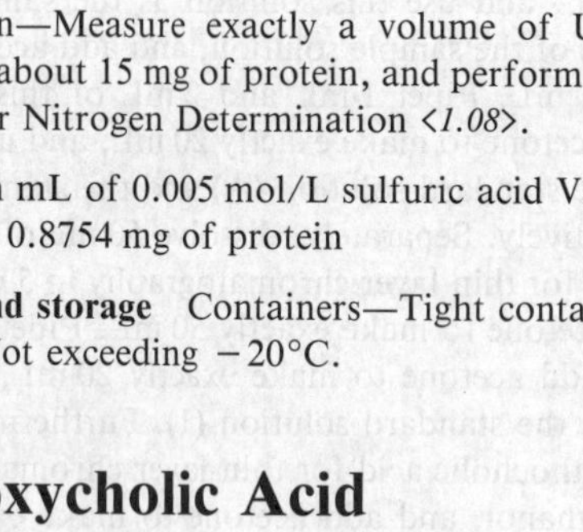

$C_{24}H_{40}O_4$: 392.57

3α,7β-Dihydroxy-5β-cholan-24-oic acid

[128-13-2]

Ursodeoxycholic Acid, when dried, contains not less than 98.5% and not more than 101.0% of ursodeoxycholic acid ($C_{24}H_{40}O_4$).

Description Ursodeoxycholic Acid occurs as a white, crystal or powder, with bitter taste.

It is freely soluble in methanol, in ethanol (99.5) and in acetic acid (100), and practically insoluble in water.

Identification Determine the infrared absorption spectrum of Ursodeoxycholic Acid as directed in the potassium bromide disk method under Infrared Spectrophotometry <2.25>, and compare the spectrum with the Reference Spectrum: both spectra exhibit similar intensities of absorption at the same wave numbers.

Optical rotation <2.49> $[\alpha]_D^{20}$: +59.0 – +62.0° (after drying, 1 g, ethanol (99.5), 25 mL, 100 mm).

Melting point <2.60> 201 – 205°C

Purity **(1)** Sulfate <1.14>—Dissolve 2.0 g of Ursodeoxycholic Acid in 20 mL of acetic acid (100), add water to make 200 mL, and allow to stand for 10 minutes. Filter this solution, discard the first 10 mL of the filtrate, and use the subsequent filtrate as the sample solution. To 40 mL of the sample solution add 1 mL of dilute hydrochloric acid and water to make 50 mL. Perform the test using this solution as the test solution. Prepare the control solution with 0.40 mL of 0.005 mol/L sulfuric acid VS by adding 4 mL of acetic acid (100), 1 mL of dilute hydrochloric acid and water to make 50 mL (not more than 0.048%).

(2) Heavy metals <1.07>—Proceed with 1.0 g of Ursodeoxycholic Acid according to Method 2 and perform the test. Prepare the control solution with 2.0 mL of Standard Lead Solution (not more than 20 ppm).

(3) Barium—To 2.0 g of Ursodeoxycholic Acid add 100 mL of water and 2 mL of hydrochloric acid, boil for 2 minutes, allow it to cool, filter, and wash the filter with water until to get 100 mL of the filtrate. To 10 mL of the filtrate add 1 mL of dilute sulfuric acid: no turbidity appears.

(4) Related substances—Dissolve 0.10 g of Ursodeoxycholic Acid in 1 mL of methanol, add acetone to make exactly 10 mL, and use this solution as the sample solution. Pipet 1 mL of the sample solution, and add acetone to make exactly 100 mL. Pipet 1 mL and 2 mL of this solution, to each add acetone to make exactly 20 mL, and use these solutions as the standard solution (A) and the standard solution (B), respectively. Separately, dissolve 50 mg of chenodeoxycholic acid for thin-layer chromatography in 5 mL of methanol, add acetone to make exactly 50 mL. Pipet 2 mL of this solution, add acetone to make exactly 20 mL, and use this solution as the standard solution (1). Furthermore, dissolve 25 mg of lithocholic acid for thin-layer chromatography in 5 mL of methanol, and add acetone to make exactly 50 mL. Pipet 2 mL of this solution, and add acetone to make exactly 20 mL. Pipet 2 mL of this solution, add acetone to make exactly 10 mL, and use this solution as the standard solution (2). Perform the test with these solutions as directed under Thin-layer Chromatography <2.03>. Spot 10 μL each of the sample solution, standard solutions (1), (2), (A) and (B) on a plate of silica gel for thin-layer chromatography. Develop the plate with a mixture of isooctane, ethanol (99.5), ethyl acetate and acetic acid (100) (10:6:3:1) to a distance of about 15 cm, and air-dry the plate. Dry the plate further at 120°C for 30 minutes, and immediately spray evenly the solution which was prepared by dissolving 5 g of phosphomolybdic acid *n*-hydrate in about 50 mL of ethanol (99.5), to which 5 mL of sulfuric acid is dropped in and add ethanol (99.5) to make 100 mL, and heat the plate at 120°C for 3 to 5 minutes: the spots from the sample solution corresponding to the spots from the standard solution (1) and (2) are not more intense than the spots from the standard solutions (1) and (2), the spots other than the principal spot and those spots mentioned above from the sample solution are not intense than the spots from the standard solution (B), and the total amount of the spots other than the principal spot and those spots mentioned above from the sample solution, which is calculated by the comparison with the spots from the standard solutions (A) and (B), is not more than 0.25%.

Loss on drying <2.41> Not more than 1.0% (1 g, 105°C, 2 hours).

Residue on ignition <2.44> Not more than 0.2% (1 g).

Assay Weigh accurately about 0.5 g of Ursodeoxycholic Acid, previously dried, dissolve in 40 mL of ethanol (95) and 20 mL of water, and titrate <2.50> with 0.1 mol/L sodium hydroxide VS (potentiometric titration). Perform a blank determination in the same manner, and make any necessary correction.

Each mL of 0.1 mol/L sodium hydroxide VS
= 39.26 mg of $C_{24}H_{40}O_4$

Containers and storage Containers—Well-closed containers.

Ursodeoxycholic Acid Granules

ウルソデオキシコール酸顆粒

Ursodeoxycholic Acid Granules contain not less than 95.0% and not more than 105.0% of the labeled amount of ursodeoxycholic acid ($C_{24}H_{40}O_4$: 392.57).

Method of preparation Prepare as directed under Granules, with Ursodeoxycholic Acid.

Identification To a quantity of powdered Ursodeoxycholic Acid Granules, equivalent to 20 mg of Ursodeoxycholic Acid, add 10 mL of methanol, and shake for 20 minutes. Centrifuge this solution, pipet 4 mL of the supernatant liquid, and evaporate the methanol under reduced pressure. To the residue add 4 mL of acetone, disperse by sonication, centrifuge, and use the supernatant liquid as the sample solution. Separately, dissolve 10 mg of ursodeoxycholic acid in 5 mL of acetone, and use this solution as the standard solution. Perform the test with these solutions as directed under Thin-layer Chromatography <2.03>. Spot 10 μL of the sample solution and standard solution on a plate of silica gel for thin-layer chromatography. Develop the plate with a mixture of isooctane, ethanol (99.5), ethyl acetate and acetic acid (100) (10:6:3:1) to a distance of about 15 cm, and air-dry the plate. Dry the plate further at 120°C for 30 minutes, immediately splay evenly a solution of phosphomolybdic acid *n*-hydrate in ethanol (99.5) (1 in 5), and heat the plate at 120°C for 3 to 5 minutes: the principle spot obtained from the sample solution and the spot from the standard solution show a blue color and the same *Rf* value.

Dissolution <6.10> When the test is performed at 50 revolutions per minute according to the Paddle method, using 900 mL of 2nd fluid for dissolution test as the dissolution medium, the dissolution rate in 15 minutes of Ursodeoxycholic Acid Granules is not less than 80%.

Start the test with an accurately weigh amount of Ursodeoxycholic Acid Granules, equivalent to about 50 mg of ursodeoxycholic acid ($C_{24}H_{40}O_4$), withdraw not less than 20 mL of the medium at the specified minute after starting the test, and filter through a membrane filter with a pore size not exceeding 0.45 μm. Discard not less than 10 mL of the first filtrate, use the subsequent filtrate as the sample solution. Separately, weigh accurately about 22 mg of ursodeoxycholic acid for assay, previously dried at 105°C for 2 hours, and dissolve in acetonitrile to make exactly 100 mL. Pipet 5 mL of this solution, add the dissolution medium to make exactly 20 mL, and use this solution as the standard solution. Perform the test with exactly 100 μL each of the sample solution and standard solution as directed under Liquid Chromatography <*2.01*> according to the following conditions, and determine the peak areas, A_T and A_S, of ursodeoxycholic acid in each solution.

Dissolution rate (%) with respect to the labeled amount of ursodeoxycholic acid ($C_{24}H_{40}O_4$)
$= M_S/M_T \times A_T/A_S \times 1/C \times 225$

M_S: Amount (mg) of ursodeoxycholic acid for assay taken
M_T: Amount (g) of Ursodeoxycholic Acid Granules taken
C: Labeled amount (mg) of ursodeoxycholic acid ($C_{24}H_{40}O_4$) in 1 g

Operating conditions—

Proceed as directed in the operating conditions in the Assay.

System suitability—

System performance: When the procedure is run with 100 μL of the standard solution under the above operating conditions, the number of theoretical plates and symmetry factor of the peak of ursodeoxycholic acid are not less than 3000 and not more than 2.0, respectively.

System repeatability: When the test is repeated 6 times with 100 μL of the standard solution under the above operating conditions, the relative standard deviation of the peak area of ursodeoxycholic acid is not more than 2.0%.

Assay Weigh accurately an amount of powdered Ursodeoxycholic Acid Granules, equivalent to about 0.1 g of ursodeoxycholic acid ($C_{24}H_{40}O_4$), add exactly 20 mL of the internal standard solution, shake for 10 minutes, and centrifuge. Filter the supernatant liquid through a membrane filter with a pore size not exceeding 0.45 μm, and use the filtrate as the sample solution. Separately, weigh accurately about 0.1 g of ursodeoxycholic acid for assay, previously dried at 105°C for 2 hours, dissolve in exactly 20 mL of the internal standard solution, and use this solution as the standard solution. Perform the test with 10 μL each of the sample solution and standard solution as directed under Liquid Chromatography <*2.01*> according to the following conditions, and calculate the ratios, Q_T and Q_S, of the peak area of ursodeoxycholic acid to that of the internal standard.

Amount (mg) of ursodeoxycholic acid ($C_{24}H_{40}O_4$)
$= M_S \times Q_T/Q_S$

M_S: Amount (mg) of ursodeoxycholic acid for assay taken

Internal standard solution—A solution of ethyl benzoate in diluted methanol (4 in 5) (7 in 200,000).

Operating conditions—

Detector: An ultraviolet absorption photometer (wavelength: 210 nm).

Column: A stainless steel column 4.6 mm in inside diameter and 15 cm in length, packed with octadecylsilanized silica gel for liquid chromatography (5 μm in particle diameter).

Column temperature: A constant temperature of about 40°C.

Mobile phase: A mixture of diluted phosphoric acid (1 in 500) and acetonitrile for liquid chromatography (11:9).

Flow rate: Adjust so that the retention time of ursodeoxycholic acid is about 6 minutes.

System suitability—

System performance: When the procedure is run with 10 μL of the standard solution under the above operating conditions, ursodeoxycholic acid and the internal standard are eluted in this order with the resolution between these peaks being not less than 8.

System repeatability: When the test is repeated 6 times with 10 μL of the standard solution under the above operating conditions, the relative standard deviation of the ratio of the peak area of ursodeoxycholic acid to that of the internal standard is not more than 1.0%.

Containers and storage Containers—Tight containers.

Ursodeoxycholic Acid Tablets

ウルソデオキシコール酸錠

Ursodeoxycholic Acid Tablets contain not less than 95.0% and not more than 105.0% of the labeled amount of Ursodeoxycholic Acid ($C_{24}H_{40}O_4$: 392.57).

Method of preparation Prepare as directed under Tablets, with Ursodeoxycholic Acid.

Identification To a quantity of powdered Ursodeoxycholic Acid Tablets, equivalent to 20 mg of Ursodeoxycholic Acid, add 10 mL of methanol, and shake for 20 minutes. Centrifuge this solution, pipet 4 mL of the supernatant liquid, and evaporate the methanol under reduced pressure. To the residue add 4 mL of acetone, disperse by sonication, centrifuge, and use the supernatant liquid as the sample solution. Separately, dissolve 10 mg of ursodeoxycholic acid in 5 mL of acetone, and use this solution as the standard solution. Perform the test with these solutions as directed under Thin-layer Chromatography <*2.03*>. Spot 10 μL each of the sample solution and standard solution on a plate of silica gel for thin-layer chromatography. Develop the plate with a mixture of isooctane, ethanol (99.5), ethyl acetate and acetic acid (100) (10:6:3:1) to a distance of about 15 cm, and air-dry the plate. Dry the plate further at 120°C for 30 minutes, and immediately splay evenly a solution of phosphomolybdic acid *n*-hydrate in ethanol (95) (1 in 5) on the plate, and heat at 120°C for 3 to 5 minutes: the principal spot obtained from the sample solution and the spot obtained from the standard solution show a blue color and the same *R*f value.

Uniformity of dosage units <*6.02*> Perform the Mass variation test, or the Content uniformity test according to the following method: it meets the requirement.

Take 1 tablet of Ursodeoxycholic Acid Tablets and add exactly V mL of the internal standard solution so that each mL contains about 5 mg of ursodeoxycholic acid ($C_{24}H_{40}O_4$), disperse by sonicating, then agitate to mix for 10 minutes and then centrifuge. Filter the supernatant liquid through a membrane filter with a pore size not exceeding 0.45 μm, and use the filtrate as the sample solution. Then, proceed as directed in the Assay.

Amount (mg) of ursodeoxycholic acid ($C_{24}H_{40}O_4$)
$= M_S \times Q_T/Q_S \times V/20$

M_S: Amount (mg) of ursodeoxycholic acid for assay taken

Internal standard solution—A solution of ethyl benzoate in diluted methanol (4 in 5) (7 in 200,000).

Dissolution <*6.10*> When the test is performed at 50 revolutions per minute according to the Paddle method, using 900 mL of 2nd fluid for dissolution test as the dissolution medium, the dissolution rates in 30 minutes of a 50-mg tablet and in 45 minutes of a 100-mg tablet are not less than 80% and not less than 70%, respectively.

Start the test with 1 tablet of Ursodeoxycholic Acid Tablets, withdraw not less than 20 mL of the medium at the specified minute after starting the test, and filter through a membrane filter with a pore size not exceeding 0.45 μm. Discard not less than 10 mL of the first filtrate and pipet V mL of the subsequent filtrate. Add the dissolution medium to make exactly V' mL so that each mL contains about 56 μg of ursodeoxycholic acid ($C_{24}H_{40}O_4$), and use the solution as the sample solution. Separately weigh accurately about 22 mg of ursodeoxycholic acid for assay, previously dried at 105°C for 2 hours, and dissolve in acetonitrile to make exactly 100 mL. Pipet 5 mL of this solution, add the dissolution medium to make exactly 20 mL, and use this solution as the standard solution. Perform the test with exactly 100 μL each of sample solution and standard solution as directed under Liquid Chromatography *<2.01>* according to the following conditions, and determine the peak areas, A_T and A_S, of ursodeoxycholic acid in each solution.

Dissolution rate (%) with respect to the labeled amount of ursodeoxycholic acid ($C_{24}H_{40}O_4$)
$$= M_S \times A_T/A_S \times V'/V \times 1/C \times 225$$

M_S: Amount (mg) of ursodeoxycholic acid for assay taken
C: Labeled amount (mg) of ursodeoxycholic acid in 1 tablet ($C_{24}H_{40}O_4$)

Operating conditions—

Proceed as directed in the operating conditions in the Assay.

System suitability—

System performance: When the procedure is run with 100 μL of the standard solution under the above operating condition, the number of theoretical plates and symmetry factor of the peak of ursodeoxycholic acid are not less than 3000 and not more than 2.0, respectively.

System repeatability: When the test is repeated 6 times with 100 μL of the standard solution under the above operating conditions, the relative standard deviation of the peak area of ursodeoxycholic acid is not more than 2.0%.

Assay Weigh accurately the mass of not less than 20 Ursodeoxycholic Acid Tablets, and powder. Weigh accurately a portion of the powder, equivalent to about 0.1 g of ursodeoxycholic acid ($C_{24}H_{40}O_4$), add exactly 20 mL of the internal standard solution, shake for 10 minutes, and centrifuge. Filter the supernatant liquid through a membrane filter with a pore size not exceeding 0.45 μm, and use the filtrate as the sample solution. Separately, weigh accurately about 0.1 g of ursodeoxycholic acid for assay, previously dried at 105°C for 2 hours, dissolve in exactly 20 mL of the internal standard solution, and use this solution as the standard solution. Perform the test with 10 μL each of the sample solution and standard solution as directed under Liquid Chromatography *<2.01>* according to the following conditions, and calculate the ratios, Q_T and Q_S, of the peak area of ursodeoxycholic acid to that of the internal standard.

Amount (mg) of ursodeoxycholic acid ($C_{24}H_{40}O_4$)
$$= M_S \times Q_T/Q_S$$

M_S: Amount (mg) of ursodeoxycholic acid for assay taken

Internal standard solution—A solution of ethyl benzoate in diluted methanol (4 in 5) (7 in 200,000).

Operating conditions—

Detector: An ultraviolet absorption photometer (wavelength: 210 nm).

Column: A stainless steel column 4.6 mm in inside diameter and 15 cm in length, packed with octadecylsilanized silica gel for liquid chromatography (5 μm in particle diameter).

Column temperature: A constant temperature of about 40°C.

Mobile phase: A mixture of diluted phosphoric acid (1 in 500) and acetonitrile for liquid chromatography (11:9).

Flow rate: Adjust so that the retention time of ursodeoxycholic acid is about 6 minutes.

System suitability—

System performance: When the procedure is run with 10 μL of the standard solution according to the above operating conditions, ursodeoxycholic acid and the internal standard are eluted in this order with the resolution between these peaks being not less than 8.

System repeatability: When the test is repeated 6 times with 10 μL of the standard solution under the above operating conditions, the relative standard deviation of the ratio of the peak area of ursodeoxycholic acid to that of the internal standard is not more than 1.0%.

Containers and storage Containers—Tight containers.

Valaciclovir Hydrochloride

バラシクロビル塩酸塩

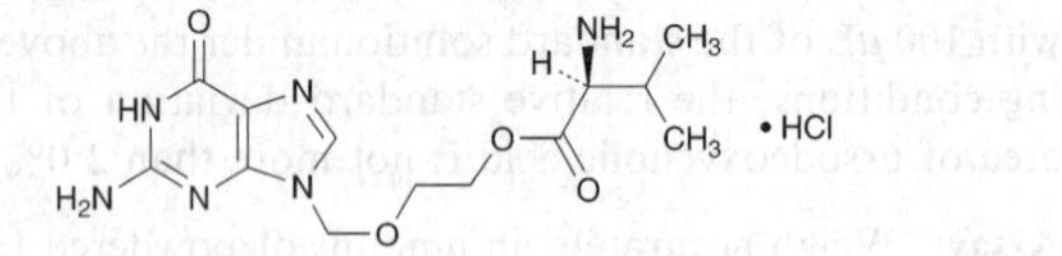

$C_{13}H_{20}N_6O_4.HCl$: 360.80
2-[(2-Amino-1,6-dihydro-6-oxo-9*H*-purin-9-yl)methoxy]ethyl L-valinate monohydrochloride
[124832-27-5]

Valaciclovir Hydrochloride contains not less than 95.0% and not more than 101.0% of valaciclovir hydrochloride ($C_{13}H_{20}N_6O_4.HCl$), calculated on the anhydrous basis.

Description Valaciclovir Hydrochloride occurs as a white to pale yellow-white crystalline powder.

It is freely soluble in water, and very slightly soluble in ethanol (99.5).

It dissolves in 0.05 mol/L hydrochloric acid TS.

Optical rotation $[\alpha]^{20}_{D}$: − 7.1 − − 11.1° (1 g, water, 20 mL, 100 mm).

It shows crystal polymorphism.

Identification **(1)** Determine the absorption spectrum of a solution of Valaciclovir Hydrochloride in 0.05 mol/L hydrochloric acid TS (3 in 200,000) as directed under Ultraviolet-visible Spectrophotometry *<2.24>*, and compare the spectrum with the Reference Spectrum or the spectrum of a solution of Valaciclovir Hydrochloride RS prepared in the same manner as the sample solution: both spectra exhibit similar intensities of absorption at the same wavelengths.

(2) Determine the infrared absorption spectrum of Valaciclovir Hydrochloride as directed in the potassium chloride disk method under Infrared Spectrophotometry *<2.25>*, and compare the spectrum with the Reference Spectrum or the spectrum of Valaciclovir Hydrochloride RS: both spectra exhibit similar intensities of absorption at the same wave numbers. If any difference appears between the spectra, suspend Valaciclovir Hydrochloride in a mixture of ethanol (99.5) and water (45:2), and heat under reflux for 24 hours while stirring. After cooling to room temperature, collect the obtained solid by filtration, dry at 60°C for 1 hour under reduced pressure, and perform the same test with the solid.

(3) A solution of Valaciclovir Hydrochloride (1 in 25) responds to Qualitative Tests *<1.09>* for chloride.

Purity (1) Heavy metals *<1.07>*—Proceed with 2.0 g of Valaciclovir Hydrochloride according to Method 4, and perform the test. Prepare the control solution with 4.0 mL of Standard Lead Solution (not more than 20 ppm).

(2) Palladium—Dissolve exactly 0.100 g of Valaciclovir Hydrochloride in a solution of hydrochloric acid in dimethylsulfoxide (1 in 50) to make exactly 10 mL, and use this solution as the sample solution. Separately, to exactly 6 mL of Standard Palladium Solution for ICP Analysis add a solution of hydrochloric acid in dimethylsulfoxide (1 in 50) to make exactly 100 mL. Pipet 5 mL of this solution, add a solution of hydrochloric acid in dimethylsulfoxide (1 in 50) to make exactly 50 mL. Pipet 5 mL of this solution, add a solution of hydrochloric acid in dimethylsulfoxide (1 in 50) to make exactly 50 mL. Pipet 5 mL of this solution, add a solution of hydrochloric acid in dimethylsulfoxide (1 in 50) to make exactly 50 mL, and use this solution as the standard solution. Perform the test with the sample solution and standard solution as directed under Inductively Coupled Plasma-Atomic Emission Spectrometry *<2.63>* according to the following conditions: the emission intensity obtained from the sample solution is not more than that from the standard solution (not more than 6 ppm).

Operating conditions—

Wavelength: 340.458 nm.

(3) Related substances—(i) To 0.25 g of Valaciclovir Hydrochloride add 2 mL of water, and sonicate for 20 minutes. After cooling, add methanol to make exactly 10 mL, if necessary, filter, through a membrane filter with a pore size not exceeding 0.45 μm. Discard the first 1 mL of the filtrate, and use the subsequent filtrate as the sample solution. Pipet 1 mL of the sample solution, add methanol to make exactly 100 mL, and use this solution as the standard stock solution. Pipet 1 mL and 0.5 mL of the standard stock solution, add methanol to make them exactly 10 mL, and use these solutions as the standard solution (1) and the standard solution (2), respectively. Perform the test with these solutions as directed under Thin-layer Chromatography *<2.03>*. Spot 4 μL each of the sample solution and the standard solutions (1) and (2) on a plate of silica gel with fluorescent indicator for thin-layer chromatography, develop the plate with a mixture of chloroform, methanol, tetrahydrofuran, dichloromethane and ammonia solution (28) (46:34:12:8:3) to a distance of about 8 cm, and air-dry the plate. Examine under ultraviolet light (main wavelength: 254 nm): the spot, having an *Rf* value of about 0.47, obtained from the sample solution is not more intense than the spot from the standard solution (1), and the spot, having an *Rf* value of about 0.67, from the sample solution is not more intense than the spot from the standard solution (2). Furthermore, when spray evenly a solution of fluorescamine in acetone (1 in 10,000) on the plate, and examine under ultraviolet light (main wavelength: 366 nm): the spot, having an *Rf* value of about 0.63, from the sample solution is not more intense than the spot from the standard solution (1).

(ii) Dissolve 40 mg of Valaciclovir Hydrochloride in 100 mL of a mixture of water and ethanol (95) (4:1), and use this solution as the sample solution. Perform the test with 10 μL of the sample solution as directed under Liquid Chromatography *<2.01>* according to the following conditions, determine each peak area by the automatic integration method, and calculate their amount by the area percentage method: the amount of the peaks, having a relative retention time of about 0.54, about 1.06, about 1.17, about 1.61, about 1.66 and about 1.98 to valaciclovir, is not more than 0.1%, 0.2%, 0.5%, 0.8%, 0.2% and 0.3%, respectively, and the amount of the peaks other than valaciclovir, the peaks mentioned above, guanine (relative retention time is about 0.31), aciclovir (relative retention time is about 0.42) and the peak (relative retention time is about 1.09) is not more than 0.05%, and their total amount is not more than 0.2%.

Operating conditions—

Detector: An ultraviolet absorption photometer (wavelength: 254 nm).

Column: A stainless steel column 4.6 mm in inside diameter and 25 cm in length, packed with phenylsilanized silica gel for liquid chromatography (5 μm in particle diameter).

Column temperature: A constant temperature of about 15°C.

Mobile phase A: Dissolve 3 g of trifluoroacetic acid in water to make 1000 mL.

Mobile phase B: Dissolve 3 g of trifluoroacetic acid in methanol to make 1000 mL.

Flowing of mobile phase: Control the gradient by mixing the mobile phases A and B as directed in the following table.

Time after injection of sample (min)	Mobile phase A (vol%)	Mobile phase B (vol%)
0 – 5	90	10
5 – 35	90 → 60	10 → 40

Flow rate: 0.8 mL per minute.

Time span of measurement: 35 minutes, beginning after the solvent peak.

System suitability—

Test for required detectability: To 1 mL of the sample solution add a mixture of water and ethanol (95) (4:1) to make 100 mL, and use this solution as the solution for system suitability test. Pipet 1 mL of the solution for system suitability test, add a mixture of water and ethanol (95) (4:1) to make exactly 20 mL. Confirm that the peak area of valaciclovir obtained with 10 μL of this solution is equivalent to 3.5 to 6.5% of that with 10 μL of the solution for system suitability test.

System performance: When the procedure is run with 10 μL of the solution for system suitability test under the above operating conditions, the number of theoretical plates and the symmetry factor of the peak of valaciclovir are not less than 25,000 and not more than 2.0, respectively.

System repeatability: When the test is repeated 6 times with 10 μL of the solution for system suitability test under the above operating conditions, the relative standard deviation of the peak area of valaciclovir is not more than 2.0%.

(iii) Perform the test with 10 μL of the sample solution obtained in the Assay as directed under Liquid Chromatography *<2.01>* according to the following conditions. Determine each peak area by the automatic integration method, and calculate their amounts by the area percentage method: the amount of the peaks, having a relative retention time of about 0.14 and about 0.42 to valaciclovir, is not more than 2.0% and not more than 0.2%, respectively. For the amounts of the peaks, having a relative retention time of about 0.14 and about 0.42 to valaciclovir, multiply their correction factors, 0.66 and 0.89, respectively.

Operating conditions—

Proceed as directed in the operating conditions in the

Assay.

System suitability—

Test for required detectability: Pipet 1 mL of the sample solution add 0.05 mol/L hydrochloric acid TS to make exactly 100 mL, and use this solution as the solution for system suitability test. To exactly 5 mL of the solution for system suitability test add 0.05 mol/L hydrochloric acid TS to make exactly 50 mL. Confirm that the peak area of valaciclovir obtained with 10 μL of this solution is equivalent to 0.07 to 0.13% of that with 10 μL of the sample solution.

System performance: When the procedure is run with 10 μL of the solution for system suitability test under the above operating conditions, the number of theoretical plates and the symmetry factor of the peak of valaciclovir are not less than 700 and not more than 1.5, respectively.

System repeatability: When the test is repeated 6 times with 10 μL of the solution for system suitability test under the above operating conditions, the relative standard deviation of the peak area of valaciclovir is not more than 2.0%.

(iv) The total amount of the related substances obtained in (i), (ii) and (iii) is not more than 2.0%.

(4) Enantiomer—When perform the test according to (3) (iii), the amount of the peak of the enantiomer, having the relative retention time of about 0.57 to valaciclovir, is not more than 3.0%.

Water <*2.48*> Not more than 1.7% (0.2 g, coulometric titration).

Residue on ignition <*2.44*> Not more than 0.1% (2 g).

Assay Weigh accurately about 25 mg each of Valaciclovir Hydrochloride and Valaciclovir Hydrochloride RS (separately determine the water <*2.48*> and the residual solvent in the same manners as Valaciclovir Hydrochloride), dissolve them separately in 0.05 mol/L hydrochloric acid TS to make exactly 50 mL, and use these solutions as the sample solution and the standard solution, respectively. Perform the test with exactly 10 μL each of the sample solution and standard solution as directed under Liquid Chromatography <*2.01*> according to the following conditions, and determine the peak areas, A_T and A_S, of valaciclovir in each solution.

Amount (mg) of valaciclovir hydrochloride ($C_{13}H_{20}N_6O_4.HCl$)
$$= M_S \times A_T/A_S$$

M_S: Amount (mg) of Valaciclovir Hydrochloride RS taken, calculated on the anhydrous and residual solvent-free basis

Operating conditions—

Detector: An ultraviolet absorption photometer (wavelength: 254 nm).

Column: A stainless steel column 4 mm in inside diameter and 15 cm in length, packed with 18-crown ether-immobilized silica gel for liquid chromatography (5 μm in particle diameter).

Column temperature: A constant temperature of about 10°C.

Mobile phase: To 950 mL of water add 5 mL of perchloric acid and 30 mL of methanol.

Flow rate: Adjust so that the retention time of valaciclovir is about 21 minutes.

System suitability—

System performance: When the procedure is run with 10 μL of the standard solution under the above operating conditions, the number of theoretical plates and the symmetry factor of the peak of valaciclovir are not less than 700 and not more than 1.5, respectively.

System repeatability: When the test is repeated 6 times with 10 μL of the standard solution under the above operating conditions, the relative standard deviation of the peak area of valaciclovir is not more than 1.0%.

Containers and storage Containers—Well-closed containers.

Valaciclovir Hydrochloride Tablets

バラシクロビル塩酸塩錠

Valaciclovir Hydrochloride Tablets contain not less than 95.0% and not more than 105.0% of the labeled amount of valaciclovir ($C_{13}H_{20}N_6O_4$: 324.34).

Method of preparation Prepare as directed under Tablets, with Valaciclovir Hydrochloride.

Identification Powder Valaciclovir Hydrochloride Tablets. To a portion of the powder, equivalent to 50 mg of valaciclovir ($C_{13}H_{20}N_6O_4$), add 90 mL of 0.1 mol/L hydrochloric acid TS, shake, and filter through a membrane filter with a pore size not exceeding 0.45 μm. Discard the first 1 mL of the filtrate, and to 2 mL of the subsequent filtrate add diluted phosphoric acid (1 in 1000) to make 100 mL. Determine the absorption spectrum of this solution as directed under Ultraviolet-visible Spectrophotometry <*2.24*>: it exhibits a maximum between 251 nm and 255 nm and a shoulder between 277 nm and 287 nm.

Uniformity of dosage units <*6.02*> It meets the requirement of the Mass variation test.

Dissolution <*6.10*> When the test is performed at 50 revolutions per minute according to the Paddle method, using 900 mL of 1st fluid for dissolution test as the dissolution medium, the dissolution rate in 30 minutes of Valaciclovir Hydrochloride Tablets is not less than 75%.

Start the test with 1 tablet of Valaciclovir Hydrochloride Tablets, withdraw not less than 10 mL of the medium at the specified minute after starting the test, and filter through a membrane filter with a pore size not exceeding 0.45 μm. Discard not less than 1 mL of the first filtrate, pipet V mL of the subsequent filtrate, add diluted phosphoric acid (1 in 1000) to make exactly V' mL so that each mL contains about 11 μg of valaciclovir ($C_{13}H_{20}N_6O_4$), and use this solution as the sample solution. Separately, weigh accurately about 30 mg of Valaciclovir Hydrochloride RS (separately determine the water <*2.48*> and the residual solvent in the same manners as Valaciclovir Hydrochloride), and dissolve in diluted phosphoric acid (1 in 1000) to make exactly 250 mL. Pipet 5 mL of this solution, add diluted phosphoric acid (1 in 1000) to make exactly 50 mL, and use this solution as the standard solution. Determine the absorbances, A_T and A_S, at 254 nm of the sample solution and standard solution as directed under Ultraviolet-visible Spectrophotometry <*2.24*>, using diluted phosphoric acid (1 in 1000) as the blank.

Dissolution rate (%) with respect to the labeled amount of valaciclovir ($C_{13}H_{20}N_6O_4$)
$$= M_S \times A_T/A_S \times V'/V \times 1/C \times 36 \times 0.899$$

M_S: Amount (mg) of Valaciclovir Hydrochloride RS taken, calculated on the anhydrous and residual solvent-free basis

C: Labeled amount (mg) of valaciclovir ($C_{13}H_{20}N_6O_4$) in 1 tablet

Assay Weigh accurately the mass of not less than 20 Valaciclovir Hydrochloride Tablets, and powder. Weigh accurately a portion of the powder, equivalent to about 1 g of valaciclovir ($C_{13}H_{20}N_6O_4$), add 120 mL of 0.1 mol/L hydrochloric acid TS, and sonicate for 10 minutes. Add 0.1 mol/L hydrochloric acid TS to make exactly 200 mL. Filter this solution through a membrane filter with a pore size not exceeding 0.45 μm. Discard the first 1 mL of the filtrate, pipet 2 mL of the subsequent filtrate, add diluted phosphoric acid (1 in 1000) to make exactly 100 mL, and use this solution as the sample solution. Separately, weigh accurately about 30 mg of Valaciclovir Hydrochloride RS (separately determine the water <*2.48*> and the residual solvent in the same manners as Valaciclovir Hydrochloride), dissolve in diluted phosphoric acid (1 in 1000) to make exactly 250 mL, and use this solution as the standard solution. Perform the test with exactly 10 μL each of the sample solution and standard solution as directed under Liquid Chromatography <*2.01*> according to the following conditions, and determine the peak areas, A_T and A_S, of valaciclovir in each solution.

Amount (mg) of valaciclovir ($C_{13}H_{20}N_6O_4$)
$= M_S \times A_T/A_S \times 40 \times 0.899$

M_S: Amount (mg) of Valaciclovir Hydrochloride RS taken, calculated on the anhydrous and residual solvent-free basis

Operating conditions—

Detector: An ultraviolet absorption photometer (wavelength: 254 nm).

Column: A stainless steel column 4 mm in inside diameter and 15 cm in length, packed with 18-crown ether-immobilized silica gel for liquid chromatography (5 μm in particle diameter).

Column temperature: A constant temperature of about 10°C.

Mobile phase: A mixture of diluted phosphoric acid (1 in 1000) and methanol (19:1).

Flow rate: Adjust so that the retention time of valaciclovir is about 4.5 minutes.

System suitability—

System performance: When the procedure is run with 10 μL of the standard solution under the above operating conditions, the number of theoretical plates and the symmetry factor of the peak of valaciclovir are not less than 600 and not more than 2.0, respectively.

System repeatability: When the test is repeated 6 times with 10 μL of the standard solution under the above operating conditions, the relative standard deviation of the peak area of valaciclovir is not more than 1.0%.

Containers and storage Containers—Well-closed containers.

L-Valine

L-バリン

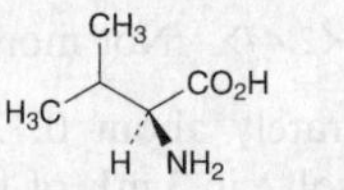

$C_5H_{11}NO_2$: 117.15
(2*S*)-2-Amino-3-methylbutanoic acid
[*72-18-4*]

L-Valine, when dried, contains not less than 98.5% of L-valine ($C_5H_{11}NO_2$).

Description L-Valine occurs as white, crystals or crystalline powder. It is odorless or has a faint characteristic odor, and has a slightly sweet taste, which becomes bitter.

It is freely soluble in formic acid, soluble in water, and practically insoluble in ethanol (95).

It dissolves in dilute hydrochloric acid.

Identification Determine the infrared absorption spectrum of L-Valine, previously dried, as directed in the potassium bromide disk method under Infrared Spectrophotometry <*2.25*>, and compare the spectrum with the Reference Spectrum: both spectra exhibit similar intensities of absorption at the same wave numbers.

Optical rotation <*2.49*> $[\alpha]_D^{20}$: +26.5 – +29.0° (after drying, 2 g, 6 mol/L hydrochloric acid TS, 25 mL, 100 mm).

pH <*2.54*> Dissolve 0.5 g of L-Valine in 20 mL of water: the pH of this solution is between 5.5 and 6.5.

Purity (1) Clarity and color of solution—Dissolve 0.5 g of L-Valine in 20 mL of water: the solution is clear and colorless.

(2) Chloride <*1.03*>—Perform the test with 0.5 g of L-Valine. Prepare the control solution with 0.30 mL of 0.01 mol/L hydrochloric acid VS (not more than 0.021%).

(3) Sulfate <*1.14*>—Perform the test with 0.6 g of L-Valine. Prepare the control solution with 0.35 mL of 0.005 mol/L sulfuric acid VS (not more than 0.028%).

(4) Ammonium <*1.02*>—Perform the test with 0.25 g of L-Valine. Prepare the control solution with 5.0 mL of Standard Ammonium Solution (not more than 0.02%).

(5) Heavy metals <*1.07*>—Proceed with 1.0 g of L-Valine according to Method 1, and perform the test. Prepare the control solution with 2.0 mL of Standard Lead Solution (not more than 20 ppm).

(6) Arsenic <*1.11*>—Proceed with 1.0 g of L-Valine, prepare the test solution according to Method 2, and perform the test (not more than 2 ppm).

(7) Related substances—Dissolve 0.10 g of L-Valine in 25 mL of water, and use this solution as the sample solution. Pipet 1 mL of the sample solution, and add water to make exactly 50 mL. Pipet 5 mL of this solution, add water to make exactly 20 mL, and use this solution as the standard solution. Perform the test with these solutions as directed under Thin-layer Chromatography <*2.03*>. Spot 5 μL each of the sample solution and standard solution on a plate of silica gel for thin-layer chromatography. Develop the plate with a mixture of 1-butanol, water and acetic acid (100) (3:1:1) to a distance of about 10 cm, and dry the plate at 80°C for 30 minutes. Spray evenly a solution of ninhydrin in acetone (1 in 50) on the plate, and heat the plate at 80°C for 5 minutes: the spots other than the principal spot obtained from the

sample solution are not more intense than the spot from the standard solution.

Loss on drying <*2.41*> Not more than 0.30% (1 g, 105°C, 3 hours).

Residue on ignition <*2.44*> Not more than 0.1% (1 g).

Assay Weigh accurately about 0.12 g of L-Valine, previously dried, and dissolve in 3 mL of formic acid, add 50 mL of acetic acid (100), and titrate <*2.50*> with 0.1 mol/L perchloric acid VS (potentiometric titration). Perform a blank determination in the same manner, and make any necessary correction.

Each mL of 0.1 mol/L perchloric acid VS
= 11.72 mg of $C_5H_{11}NO_2$

Containers and storage Containers—Tight containers.

Valsartan

バルサルタン

$C_{24}H_{29}N_5O_3$: 435.52
(2*S*)-3-Methyl-2-(*N*-{[2′-(1*H*-tetrazol-5-yl)biphenyl-4-yl]methyl}pentanamido)butanoic acid
[*137862-53-4*]

Valsartan contains not less than 98.0% and not more than 102.0% of valsartan ($C_{24}H_{29}N_5O_3$), calculated on the anhydrous and residual solvent-free basis.

Description Valsartan occurs as a white powder.

It is very soluble in methanol and in ethanol (99.5), and practically insoluble in water.

Identification (1) Determine the absorption spectrum of a solution of Valsartan in methanol (1 in 62,500) as directed under Ultraviolet-visible Spectrophotometry <*2.24*>, and compare the spectrum with the Reference Spectrum or the spectrum of a solution of Valsartan RS prepared in the same manner as the sample solution: both spectra exhibit similar intensities of absorption at the same wavelengths.

(2) Determine the infrared absorption spectrum of Valsartan as directed in the potassium bromide disk method under Infrared Spectrophotometry <*2.25*>, and compare the spectrum with the Reference Spectrum or the spectrum of Valsartan RS: both spectra exhibit similar intensities of absorption at the same wave numbers.

Optical rotation <*2.49*> $[\alpha]_D^{20}$: −64 – −69° (0.5 g calculated on the anhydrous and residual solvent-free basis, methanol, 50 mL, 100 mm).

Purity (1) Heavy metals <*1.07*>—Proceed with 2.0 g of Valsartan according to Method 4, and perform the test. Prepare the control solution with 2.0 mL of Standard Lead Solution (not more than 10 ppm).

(2) Related substances—Dissolve 50 mg of Valsartan in 100 mL of the mobile phase, and use this solution as the sample solution. Pipet 1 mL of the sample solution, add the mobile phase to make exactly 100 mL, and use this solution as the standard solution. Perform the test with exactly 10 μL each of the sample solution and standard solution as directed under Liquid Chromatography <*2.01*> according to the following conditions, and determine each peak area by the automatic integration method: the area of the peak, having the relative retention time of about 0.8 to valsartan, obtained from the sample solution is not larger than 1/5 times the peak area of valsartan from the standard solution, the area of the peak other than valsartan and the peak mentioned above from the sample solution is not larger than 1/10 times the peak area of valsartan from the standard solution, and the total area of the peaks other than valsartan from the sample solution is not larger than 3/10 times the peak area of valsartan from the standard solution.

Operating conditions—

Detector, column, column temperature, mobile phase and flow rate: Proceed as directed in the operating conditions in the Assay.

Time span of measurement: About 6 times as long as the retention time of valsartan, beginning after the solvent peak.

System suitability—

Test for required detectability: To exactly 1 mL of the standard solution add the mobile phase to make exactly 20 mL. Confirm that the peak area of valsartan obtained with 10 μL of this solution is equivalent to 3.5 to 6.5% of that with 10 μL of the standard solution.

System performance: When the procedure is run with 10 μL of the standard solution under the above operating conditions, the number of theoretical plates and the symmetry factor of the peak of valsartan are not less than 1500 and not more than 1.5, respectively.

System repeatability: When the test is repeated 6 times with 10 μL of the standard solution under the above operating conditions, the relative standard deviation of the peak area of valsartan is not more than 2.0%.

(3) Enantiomer—Dissolve 75 mg of Valsartan in 100 mL of the mobile phase. To 5 mL of this solution add the mobile phase to make 25 mL, and use this solution as the sample solution. Pipet 1 mL of the sample solution, add the mobile phase to make exactly 100 mL, and use this solution as the standard solution. Perform the test with exactly 10 μL each of the sample solution and standard solution as directed under Liquid Chromatography <*2.01*> according to the following conditions, and determine each peak area by the automatic integration method: the peak area of the enantiomer, having the relative retention time of about 0.6 to valsartan, obtained from the sample solution is not larger than the peak area of valsartan from the standard solution.

Operating conditions—

Detector: An ultraviolet absorption photometer (wavelength: 227 nm).

Column: A stainless steel column 4 mm in inside diameter and 10 cm in length, packed with α_1-acid glycoprotein binding silica gel for liquid chromatography (5 μm in particle diameter).

Column temperature: A constant temperature of about 35°C.

Mobile phase: Dissolve 14.68 g of disodium hydrogen phosphate dodecahydrate and 3.81 g of potassium dihydrogen phosphate in 1000 mL of water. To 490 mL of this solution add 10 mL of 2-propanol.

Flow rate: Adjust so that the retention time of valsartan is about 10 minutes.

The JP Drugs are to be tested according to the provisions given in the pertinent monographs, General Notices, General Rules for Crude Drugs, General Rules for Preparations, and General Tests for their conformity to the Japanese Pharmacopoeia. (See the General Notices 5.)

System suitability—

System performance: Dissolve about 75 mg of Valsartan, previously allowed to stand at 105°C for 30 minutes, in the mobile phase to make 100 mL. To 5 mL of this solution add the mobile phase to make 25 mL. When the procedure is run with 10 μL of this solution under the above operating conditions, the enantiomer and valsartan are eluted in this order with the resolution between these peaks being not less than 1.5.

System repeatability: When the test is repeated 6 times with 10 μL of the standard solution under the above operating conditions, the relative standard deviation of the peak area of valsartan is not more than 5%.

Water <*2.48*> Not more than 2.0% (0.1 g, coulometric titration).

Residue on ignition <*2.44*> Not more than 0.1% (1 g).

Assay Weigh accurately about 50 mg each of Valsartan and Valsartan RS (separately determine the water <*2.48*> and the residual solvent in the same manner as Valsartan), and dissolve them separately in the mobile phase to make exactly 100 mL. Pipet 5 mL each of these solutions, add exactly 3 mL of the internal standard solution, and add the mobile phase to make 50 mL, and use these solutions as the sample solution and the standard solution, respectively. Perform the test with 10 μL each of the sample solution and standard solution as directed under Liquid Chromatography <*2.01*> according to the following conditions, and calculate the ratios, Q_T and Q_S, of the peak area of valsartan to that of the internal standard.

$$\text{Amount (mg) of valsartan } (C_{24}H_{29}N_5O_3) = M_S \times Q_T/Q_S$$

M_S: Amount (mg) of Valsartan RS taken, calculated on the anhydrous and residual solvent-free basis

Internal standard solution—A solution of diclofenac sodium in the mobile phase (1 in 1000).

Operating conditions—

Detector: An ultraviolet absorption photometer (wavelength: 225 nm).

Column: A stainless steel column 3 mm in inside diameter and 12.5 cm in length, packed with octadecylsilanized silica gel for liquid chromatography (5 μm in particle diameter).

Column temperature: A constant temperature of about 25°C.

Mobile phase: A mixture of water, acetonitrile, and acetic acid (100) (500:500:1).

Flow rate: Adjust so that the retention time of valsartan is about 5 minutes.

System suitability—

System performance: When the procedure is run with 10 μL of the standard solution under the above operating conditions, valsartan and the internal standard are eluted in this order with the resolution between these peaks being not less than 5.

System repeatability: When the test is repeated 6 times with 10 μL of the standard solution under the above operating conditions, the relative standard deviation of the ratio of the peak area of valsartan to that of the internal standard is not more than 1.0%.

Containers and storage Containers—Tight containers.

Valsartan Tablets

バルサルタン錠

Valsartan Tablets contain not less than 95.0% and not more than 105.0% of the labeled amount of valsartan ($C_{24}H_{29}N_5O_3$: 435.52).

Method of preparation Prepare as directed under Tablets, with Valsartan.

Identification Determine the absorption spectra of the sample solution and the standard solution in the range 220 to 350 nm, which are obtained in the Uniformity of dosage units, as directed under Ultraviolet-visible Spectrophotometry <*2.24*>, and compare the spectrums with each other: both spectra exhibit similar intensities of absorption at the same wavelengths.

Uniformity of dosage units <*6.02*> Perform the Mass variation test, or the Content uniformity test according to the following method: it meets the requirement.

To 1 tablet of Valsartan Tablets add V/10 mL of water, and shake until the tablet is disintegrated. Add V/2 mL of methanol, shake thoroughly, add methanol to make exactly V mL so that each mL contains about 0.4 mg of valsartan ($C_{24}H_{29}N_5O_3$) for 20-mg tablet and 40-mg tablet, or contains about 0.8 mg of valsartan ($C_{24}H_{29}N_5O_3$) for 80-mg tablet and 160-mg tablet, and centrifuge. Pipet V' mL of the supernatant liquid, equivalent to 0.8 mg of valsartan ($C_{24}H_{29}N_5O_3$), add methanol to make exactly 50 mL, and use this solution as the sample solution. Separately, weigh accurately about 40 mg of Valsartan RS (separately determine the water <*2.48*> and the residual solvent in the same manner as Valsartan), dissolve in 10 mL of water, and add methanol to make exactly 100 mL. Pipet 2 mL of this solution, add methanol to make exactly 50 mL, and use this solution as the standard solution. Determine the absorbances, A_T and A_S, at 250 nm of the sample solution and standard solution as directed under Ultraviolet-visible Spectrophotometry <*2.24*>.

$$\text{Amount (mg) of valsartan } (C_{24}H_{29}N_5O_3) = M_S \times A_T/A_S \times V/V' \times 1/50$$

M_S: Amount (mg) of Valsartan RS taken, calculated on the anhydrous and residual solvent-free basis

Dissolution <*6.10*> When the test is performed at 50 revolutions per minute according to the Paddle method, using 900 mL of water as the dissolution medium, the dissolution rate of a 20-mg tablet, 40-mg tablet and 80-mg tablet in 30 minutes are not less than 75%, 75% and 80%, respectively, and of a 160-mg tablet in 45 minutes is not less than 75%.

Start the test with 1 tablet of Valsartan Tablets, withdraw not less than 20 mL of the medium at the specified minute after starting the test, and filter through a membrane filter with a pore size not exceeding 0.5 μm. Discard not less than 10 mL of the first filtrate, pipet V mL of the subsequent filtrate, add water to make exactly V' mL so that each mL contains about 22 μg of valsartan ($C_{24}H_{29}N_5O_3$), and use this solution as the sample solution. Separately, weigh accurately about 22 mg of Valsartan RS (separately determine the water <*2.48*> and the residual solvent in the same manners as Valsartan), and dissolve in methanol to make exactly 50 mL. Pipet 5 mL of this solution, add water to make exactly 100 mL, and use this solution as the standard solution. Determine the absorbances, A_T and A_S, at 250 nm of the sample solution and standard solution as directed under Ultraviolet-visible Spectrophotometry <2.24>, using water as the control.

Dissolution rate (%) with respect to the labeled amount of valsartan ($C_{24}H_{29}N_5O_3$)

$$= M_S \times A_T/A_S \times V'/V \times 1/C \times 90$$

M_S: Amount (mg) of Valsartan RS taken, calculated on the anhydrous and residual solvent-free basis

C: Labeled amount (mg) of valsartan ($C_{24}H_{29}N_5O_3$) in 1 tablet

Assay Weigh accurately the mass of not less than 20 Valsartan Tablets, and powder. Weigh accurately a portion of the powder, equivalent to about 50 mg of valsartan ($C_{24}H_{29}N_5O_3$), add 60 mL of the mobile phase, shake thoroughly, add the mobile phase to make exactly 100 mL, and centrifuge. Pipet 5 mL of the supernatant liquid, add exactly 3 mL of the internal standard solution, add the mobile phase to make 50 mL, and use this solution as the sample solution. Separately, weigh accurately about 50 mg of Valsartan RS (separately, determine the water <2.48> and the residual solvent in the same manner as Valsartan), and dissolve in the mobile phase to make exactly 100 mL. Pipet 5 mL of this solution, add exactly 3 mL of the internal standard solution, add the mobile phase to make 50 mL, and use this solution as the standard solution. Perform the test with 10 μL each of the sample solution and standard solution as directed under Liquid Chromatography <2.01> according to the following conditions, and calculate the ratios, Q_T and Q_S, of the peak area of valsartan to that of the internal standard.

Amount (mg) of valsartan ($C_{24}H_{29}N_5O_3$)

$$= M_S \times Q_T/Q_S$$

M_S: Amount (mg) of Valsartan RS taken, calculated on the anhydrous and residual solvent-free basis

Internal standard solution—A solution of diclofenac sodium in the mobile phase (1 in 1000).

Operating conditions—

Detector: An ultraviolet absorption photometer (wavelength: 225 nm).

Column: A stainless steel column 3 mm in inside diameter and 12.5 cm in length, packed with octadecylsilanized silica gel for liquid chromatography (5 μm in particle diameter).

Column temperature: A constant temperature of about 25°C.

Mobile phase: A mixture of water, acetonitrile, and acetic acid (100) (500:500:1).

Flow rate: Adjust so that the retention time of valsartan is about 5 minutes.

System suitability—

System performance: When the procedure is run with 10 μL of the standard solution under the above operating conditions, valsartan and the internal standard are eluted in this order with the resolution between these peaks being not less than 5.

System repeatability: When the test is repeated 6 times with 10 μL of the standard solution under the above operating conditions, the relative standard deviation of the ratio of the peak area of valsartan to that of the internal standard is not more than 1.0%.

Containers and storage Containers—Tight containers.

Valsartan and Hydrochlorothiazide Tablets

バルサルタン・ヒドロクロロチアジド錠

Valsartan and Hydrochlorothiazide Tablets contain not less than 95.0% and not more than 105.0% of the labeled amount of valsartan ($C_{24}H_{29}N_5O_3$: 435.52) and hydrochlorothiazide ($C_7H_8ClN_3O_4S_2$: 297.74).

Method of preparation Prepare as directed under Tablets, with Valsartan and Hydrochlorothiazide.

Identification (1) To a quantity of powdered Valsartan and Hydrochlorothiazide Tablets, equivalent to 80 mg of Valsartan, add 5 mL of acetone, shake, centrifuge, and use the supernatant liquid as the sample solution. Separately, dissolve 16 mg of valsartan in 1 mL of acetone, and use this solution as the standard solution. Perform the test with these solutions as directed under Thin-layer Chromatography <2.03>. Spot 5 μL each of the sample solution and standard solution on a plate of silica gel with fluorescent indicator for thin-layer chromatography. Develop the plate with a mixture of ethyl acetate, hexane and acetic acid (100) (15:5:2) to a distance of about 10 cm, and air-dry the plate. Examine under ultraviolet light (main wavelength: 254 nm): one of the two spots obtained from the sample solution and the spot from the standard solution show the same *Rf* value.

(2) To a quantity of powdered Valsartan and Hydrochlorothiazide Tablets, equivalent to 6.25 mg of Hydrochlorothiazide, add 5 mL of acetone, shake, centrifuge, and use the supernatant liquid as the sample solution. Separately, dissolve 12.5 mg of hydrochlorothiazide in 10 mL of acetone, and use this solution as the standard solution. Perform the test with these solutions as directed under Thin-layer Chromatography <2.03>. Spot 5 μL each of the sample solution and standard solution on a plate of silica gel with fluorescent indicator for thin-layer chromatography. Develop the plate with a mixture of ethyl acetate, hexane and acetic acid (100) (15:5:2) to a distance of about 10 cm, and air-dry the plate. Examine under ultraviolet light (main wavelength: 254 nm): one of the two spots obtained from the sample solution and the spot from the standard solution show the same *Rf* value.

Uniformity of dosage units <6.02> (1) Valsartan—Perform the Mass variation test, or the Content uniformity test according to the following method: it meets the requirement.

To 1 tablet of Valsartan and Hydrochlorothiazide Tablets add 10 mL of water, and shake until the tablet is disintegrated. Add 10 mL of acetonitrile, shake thoroughly, and add a mixture of water and acetonitrile (1:1) to make exactly 50 mL. Centrifuge this solution, pipet V mL of the supernatant liquid, add a mixture of water and acetonitrile (1:1) to make exactly V' mL so that each mL contains about 0.4 mg of valsartan ($C_{24}H_{29}N_5O_3$), and use this solution as the sample solution. Proceed as directed in the Assay (1).

Amount (mg) of valsartan ($C_{24}H_{29}N_5O_3$)

$$= M_S \times A_T/A_S \times V'/V \times 1/2$$

M_S: Amount (mg) of Valsartan RS taken, calculated on the anhydrous and residual solvent-free basis

(2) Hydrochlorothiazide—Perform the test according to the following method: it meets the requirement of the Content uniformity test.

To 1 tablet of Valsartan and Hydrochlorothiazide Tablets add 10 mL of water, and shake until the tablet is disintegrated. Add 10 mL of acetonitrile, shake thoroughly, and add a mixture of water and acetonitrile (1:1) to make exactly 50 mL. Centrifuge this solution, pipet V mL of the supernatant liquid, add a mixture of water and acetonitrile (1:1) to make exactly V' mL so that each mL contains about 31 μg of hydrochlorothiazide ($C_7H_8ClN_3O_4S_2$), and use this solution as the sample solution. Proceed as directed in the Assay (2).

Amount (mg) of hydrochlorothiazide ($C_7H_8ClN_3O_4S_2$)
$= M_S \times A_T/A_S \times V'/V \times 1/8$

M_S: Amount (mg) of Hydrochlorothiazide RS taken

Dissolution ⟨*6.10*⟩ (1) Valsartan—When the test is performed at 50 revolutions per minute according to the Paddle method, using 900 mL of water as the dissolution medium, the dissolution rate in 30 minutes of Valsartan and Hydrochlorothiazide Tablets is not less than 75%.

Start the test with 1 tablet of Valsartan and Hydrochlorothiazide Tablets, withdraw not less than 20 mL of the medium at the specified minute after starting the test, and filter through a membrane filter with a pore size not exceeding 0.45 μm. Discard not less than 5 mL of the first filtrate, pipet V mL of the subsequent filtrate, and add water to make exactly V' mL so that each mL contains about 89 μg of valsartan ($C_{24}H_{29}N_5O_3$). Pipet 5 mL of this solution, add methanol to make exactly 10 mL, and use this solution as the sample solution. Separately, weigh accurately about 45 mg of Valsartan RS (separately determine the water ⟨*2.48*⟩ and the residual solvent in the same manner as Valsartan), and dissolve in methanol to make exactly 50 mL. Pipet 10 mL of this solution, add exactly 100 mL of water, then add methanol to make exactly 200 mL, and use this solution as the standard solution. Perform the test with exactly 10 μL each of the sample solution and standard solution as directed under Liquid Chromatography ⟨*2.01*⟩ according to the following conditions, and determine the peak areas, A_T and A_S, of valsartan in each solution.

Dissolution rate (%) with respect to the labeled amount of valsartan ($C_{24}H_{29}N_5O_3$)
$= M_S \times A_T/A_S \times V'/V \times 1/C \times 180$

M_S: Amount (mg) of Valsartan RS taken, calculated on the anhydrous and residual solvent-free basis
C: Labeled amount (mg) of valsartan ($C_{24}H_{29}N_5O_3$) in 1 tablet

Operating conditions—

Detector: An ultraviolet absorption photometer (wavelength: 225 nm).

Column: A stainless steel column 3.0 mm in inside diameter and 12.5 cm in length, packed with octadecylsilanized silica gel for liquid chromatography (5 μm in particle diameter).

Column temperature: A constant temperature of about 25°C.

Mobile phase: Dissolve 14.68 g of disodium hydrogen phosphate dodecahydrate and 3.81 g of potassium dihydrogen phosphate in 1000 mL of water. To 4 volumes of this solution add 1 volume of acetonitrile.

Flow rate: Adjust so that the retention time of valsartan is about 6 minutes.

System suitability—

System performance: When the procedure is run with 10 μL of the standard solution under the above operating conditions, the number of theoretical plates and the symmetry factor of the peak of valsartan are not less than 500, and not less than 0.7 and not more than 1.5, respectively.

System repeatability: When the test is repeated 6 times with 10 μL of the standard solution under the above operating conditions, the relative standard deviation of the peak area of valsartan is not more than 1.0%.

(2) Hydrochlorothiazide—When the test is performed at 50 revolutions per minute according to the Paddle method, using 900 mL of water as the dissolution medium, the dissolution rate in 15 minutes of Valsartan and Hydrochlorothiazide Tablets is not less than 85%.

Start the test with 1 tablet of Valsartan and Hydrochlorothiazide Tablets, withdraw not less than 20 mL of the medium at the specified minute after starting the test, and filter through a membrane filter with a pore size not exceeding 0.45 μm. Discard not less than 5 mL of the first filtrate, pipet V mL of the subsequent filtrate, add water to make exactly V' mL so that each mL contains about 6.9 μg of hydrochlorothiazide ($C_7H_8ClN_3O_4S_2$), and use this solution as the sample solution. Separately, weigh accurately about 14 mg of Hydrochlorothiazide RS, previously dried at 105°C for 2 hours, and dissolve in methanol to make exactly 100 mL. Pipet 5 mL of this solution, add water to make exactly 100 mL, and use this solution as the standard solution. Perform the test with exactly 10 μL each of the sample solution and standard solution as directed under Liquid Chromatography ⟨*2.01*⟩ according to the following conditions, and determine the peak areas, A_T and A_S, of hydrochlorothiazide in each solution.

Dissolution rate (%) with respect to the labeled amount of hydrochlorothiazide ($C_7H_8ClN_3O_4S_2$)
$= M_S \times A_T/A_S \times V'/V \times 1/C \times 45$

M_S: Amount (mg) of Hydrochlorothiazide RS taken
C: Labeled amount (mg) of hydrochlorothiazide ($C_7H_8ClN_3O_4S_2$) in 1 tablet

Operating conditions—

Proceed as directed in the operating conditions in (1).

System suitability—

System performance: When the procedure is run with 10 μL of the standard solution under the above operating conditions, the number of theoretical plates and the symmetry factor of the peak of hydrochlorothiazide are not less than 3000 and not more than 2.0, respectively.

System repeatability: When the test is repeated 6 times with 10 μL of the standard solution under the above operating conditions, the relative standard deviation of the peak area of hydrochlorothiazide is not more than 1.0%.

Assay (1) Valsartan—Weigh accurately the mass of not less than 20 tablets of Valsartan and Hydrochlorothiazide Tablets, and powder. Weigh accurately a portion of the powder, equivalent to about 80 mg of valsartan ($C_{24}H_{29}N_5O_3$), add 10 mL of water, and shake. Add 10 mL of acetonitrile, shake thoroughly, add a mixture of water and acetonitrile (1:1) to make exactly 50 mL, and centrifuge. Pipet 5 mL of the supernatant liquid, add a mixture of water and acetonitrile (1:1) to make exactly 20 mL, and use this solution as the sample solution. Separately, weigh accurately about 40 mg of Valsartan RS (separately determine the water ⟨*2.48*⟩ and the residual solvent in the same manner as Valsartan), dissolve in a mixture of water and acetonitrile (1:1) to make exactly 25 mL, and use this solution as the valsartan standard stock solution. Pipet 5 mL of the valsartan standard stock solution, add a mixture of water and acetonitrile (1:1) to make exactly 20 mL, and use this solution as the standard solution. Perform the test with exactly 10 μL each of the sample solution and standard solution as directed under Liquid Chromatography ⟨*2.01*⟩ according to the following conditions, and determine the peak areas, A_T and A_S, of valsartan in each solution.

Amount (mg) of valsartan ($C_{24}H_{29}N_5O_3$)
$= M_S \times A_T/A_S \times 2$

M_S: Amount (mg) of Valsartan RS taken, calculated on the anhydrous and residual solvent-free basis

Operating conditions—

Detector: An ultraviolet absorption photometer (wavelength: 271 nm).

Column: A stainless steel column 3.0 mm in inside diameter and 12.5 cm in length, packed with octadecylsilanized silica gel for liquid chromatography (5 μm in particle diameter).

Column temperature: A constant temperature of about 25°C.

Mobile phase A: A mixture of water, acetonitrile and trifluoroacetic acid (900:100:1).

Mobile phase B: A mixture of acetonitrile, water and trifluoroacetic acid (900:100:1).

Flowing of mobile phase: Control the gradient by mixing the mobile phases A and B as directed in the following table.

Time after injection of sample (min)	Mobile phase A (vol%)	Mobile phase B (vol%)
0 - 25	90 → 10	10 → 90

Flow rate: Adjust so that the retention time of valsartan is about 16 minutes.

System suitability—

System performance: Dissolve 1 mg of 4-amino-6-chlorobenzene-1,3-disulfonamide in a mixture of water and acetonitrile (1:1) to make 200 mL. To 1 mL of this solution, 5 mL of the valsartan standard stock solution and 5 mL of the hydrochlorothiazide standard stock solution in (2) add a mixture of water and acetonitrile (1:1) to make 20 mL. When the procedure is run with 10 μL of this solution under the above operating conditions, 4-amino-6-chlorobenzene-1,3-disulfonamide, hydrochlorothiazide and valsartan are eluted in this order with the resolution between the peaks of 4-amino-6-chlorobenzene-1,3-disulfonamide and hydrochlorothiazide being not less than 1.5.

System repeatability: When the test is repeated 6 times with 10 μL of the standard solution under the above operating conditions, the relative standard deviation of the peak area of valsartan is not more than 1.0%.

(2) Hydrochlorothiazide—Weigh accurately the mass of not less than 20 tablets of Valsartan and Hydrochlorothiazide Tablets, and powder. Weigh accurately a portion of the powder, equivalent to about 6.25 mg of hydrochlorothiazide ($C_7H_8ClN_3O_4S_2$), add 10 mL of water, and shake. Add 10 mL of acetonitrile, shake thoroughly, add a mixture of water and acetonitrile (1:1) to make exactly 50 mL, and centrifuge. Pipet 5 mL of the supernatant liquid, add a mixture of water and acetonitrile (1:1) to make exactly 20 mL, and use this solution as the sample solution. Separately, weigh accurately about 12.5 mg of Hydrochlorothiazide RS, previously dried at 105°C for 2 hours, and dissolve in a mixture of water and acetonitrile (1:1) to make exactly 50 mL, and use this solution as the hydrochlorothiazide standard stock solution. Pipet 2.5 mL of the hydrochlorothiazide standard stock solution, add a mixture of water and acetonitrile (1:1) to make exactly 20 mL, and use this solution as the standard solution. Perform the test with exactly 10 μL each of the sample solution and standard solution as directed under Liquid Chromatography <2.01> according to the following conditions, and determine the peak areas, A_T and A_S, of hydrochlorothiazide in each solution.

Amount (mg) of hydrochlorothiazide ($C_7H_8ClN_3O_4S_2$)
$= M_S \times A_T/A_S \times 1/2$

M_S: Amount (mg) of Hydrochlorothiazide RS taken

Operating conditions—

Proceed as directed in the operating conditions in (1).

System suitability—

System performance: Dissolve 1 mg of 4-amino-6-chlorobenzene-1,3-disulfonamide in a mixture of water and acetonitrile (1:1) to make 200 mL. To 1 mL of this solution, 5 mL of the valsartan standard stock solution in (1) and 5 mL of the hydrochlorothiazide standard stock solution add a mixture of water and acetonitrile (1:1) to make 20 mL. When the procedure is run with 10 μL of this solution under the above operating conditions, 4-amino-6-chlorobenzene-1,3-disulfonamide, hydrochlorothiazide and valsartan are eluted in this order with the resolution between the peaks of 4-amino-6-chlorobenzene-1,3-disulfonamide and hydrochlorothiazide being not less than 1.5.

System repeatability: When the test is repeated 6 times with 10 μL of the standard solution under the above operating conditions, the relative standard deviation of the peak area of hydrochlorothiazide is not more than 1.0%.

Vancomycin Hydrochloride

バンコマイシン塩酸塩

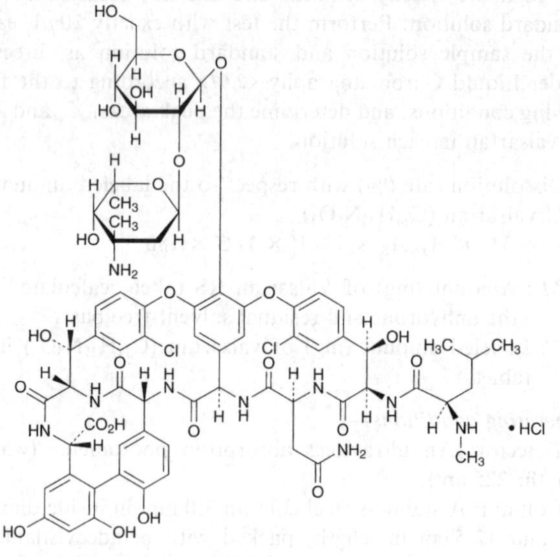

$C_{66}H_{75}Cl_2N_9O_{24}$.HCl: 1485.71

(1*S*,2*R*,18*R*,19*R*,22*S*,25*R*,28*R*,40*S*)-50-[3-Amino-2,3,6-trideoxy-3-*C*-methyl-α-L-*lyxo*-hexopyranosyl-(1→2)-β-D-glucopyranosyloxy]-22-carbamoylmethyl-5,15-dichloro-2,18,32,35,37-pentahydroxy-19-[(2*R*)-4-methyl-2-(methylamino)pentanoylamino]-20,23,26,42,44-pentaoxo-7,13-dioxa-21,24,27,41,43-pentaazaoctacyclo[26.14.2.2^{3,6}.2^{14,17}.1^{8,12}.1^{29,33}.0^{10,25}.0^{34,39}]pentaconta-3,5,8,10,12(50),14,16,29,31,33(49),34,36,38,45,47-pentadecaene-40-carboxylic acid monohydrochloride

[1404-93-9]

Vancomycin Hydrochloride is the hydrochloride of a glycopeptide substance having antibacterial activity produced by the growth of *Streptomyces orientalis.*

It contains not less than 1000 μg (potency) and not more than 1200 μg (potency) per mg, calculated on the anhydrous basis. The potency of Vancomycin Hydrochloride is expressed as mass (potency) of vancomycin ($C_{66}H_{75}Cl_2N_9O_{24}$: 1449.25).

Description Vancomycin Hydrochloride occurs as a white powder.

It is freely soluble in water, soluble in formamide, slightly soluble in methanol, very slightly soluble in ethanol (95), and practically insoluble in acetonitrile.

It is hygroscopic.

Identification **(1)** Determine the absorption spectrum of a solution of Vancomycin Hydrochloride (1 in 10,000) as directed under Ultraviolet-visible Spectrophotometry <*2.24*>, and compare the spectrum with the Reference Spectrum or the spectrum of a solution of Vancomycin Hydrochloride RS prepared in the same manner as the sample solution: both spectra exhibit similar intensities of absorption at the same wavelengths.

(2) Determine the infrared absorption spectrum of Vancomycin Hydrochloride as directed in the potassium bromide disk method under Infrared Spectrophotometry <*2.25*>, and compare the spectrum with the Reference Spectrum or the spectrum of Vancomycin Hydrochloride RS: both spectra exhibit similar intensities of absorption at the same wave numbers.

(3) Dissolve 20 mg of Vancomycin Hydrochloride in 10 mL of water, and add 1 drop of silver nitrate TS: a white turbidity is produced.

Optical rotation <*2.49*> $[\alpha]_D^{20}$: −30 − −40° (0.2 g calculated on the anhydrous basis, water, 20 mL, 100 mm).

pH <*2.54*> The pH of a solution obtained by dissolving 0.25 g of Vancomycin Hydrochloride in 5 mL of water is between 2.5 and 4.5.

Purity **(1)** Heavy metals <*1.07*>—Proceed with 1.0 g of Vancomycin Hydrochloride according to Method 2, and perform the test. Prepare the control solution with 2.0 mL of Standard Lead Solution (not more than 20 ppm).

(2) Related substances—Dissolve 0.10 g of Vancomycin Hydrochloride in 10 mL of the mobile phase A, and use this solution as the sample solution. Pipet 1 mL of the sample solution, add the mobile phase A to make exactly 25 mL, and use this solution as the standard solution. Perform the test with exactly 20 μL each of the sample solution and standard solution as directed under the Liquid Chromatography <*2.01*> according to the following conditions. If necessary, proceed with 20 μL of the mobile phase A in the same manner to compensate for the base line. Determine each peak area by the automatic integration method: the area of each peak other than vancomycin obtained from the sample solution is not larger than the peak area of vancomycin from the standard solution, and the total area of the peaks other than vancomycin from the sample solution is not larger than 3 times of the peak area of vancomycin from the standard solution.

Operating conditions—

Detector: An ultraviolet absorption photometer (wavelength: 280 nm).

Column: A stainless steel column 4.6 mm in inside diameter and 25 cm in length, packed with octadecylsilanized silica gel for liquid chromatography (5 μm in particle diameter).

Column temperature: A constant temperature of about 25°C.

Mobile phase A: A mixture of triethylamine buffer solution (pH 3.2), acetonitrile and tetrahydrofuran (92:7:1). Adjust the amount of acetonitrile so that the retention time of vancomycin is 7.5 to 10.5 minutes.

Mobile phase B: A mixture of triethylamine buffer solution (pH 3.2), acetonitrile and tetrahydrofuran (70:29:1).

Flowing of mobile phase: Control the gradient by mixing the mobile phases A and B as directed in the following table.

Time after injection of sample (min)	Mobile phase A (vol%)	Mobile phase B (vol%)
0 – 12	100	0
12 – 20	100 → 0	0 → 100
20 – 22	0	100

Flow rate: 1.5 mL per minute.

Time span of measurement: As long as about 2.5 times of the retention time of vancomycin, beginning after the solvent peak.

System suitability—

Test for required detectability: Confirm that the peak area of vancomycin obtained with 20 μL of the standard solution is equivalent to 3 to 5% of that with 20 μL of the sample solution.

System performance: Dissolve 5 mg of Vancomycin Hydrochloride in 10 mL of water, heat at 65°C for 48 hours, and cool to the ordinal temperature. When the procedure is run with 20 μL of this solution under the above operating conditions, related substance 1, vancomycin and related substance 2 are eluted in this order, the resolution between the peaks of the related substance 1 and vancomycin is not less than 3, the number of theoretical plates of the peak of vancomycin is not less than 1500, and the related substance 2 is eluted between 15 minutes and 18 minutes.

System repeatability: When the test is repeated 5 times with 20 μL of the standard solution under the above operating conditions, the relative standard deviation of the peak area of vancomycin is not more than 2.0%.

Water <*2.48*> Not more than 5.0% (0.1 g, volumetric titration, direct titration. Use a mixture of formamide for water determination and methanol for water determination (3:1)).

Residue on ignition <*2.44*> Not more than 1.0% (1 g).

Assay Perform the test according to the Cylinder-plate method as directed under Microbial Assay for Antibiotics <*4.02*> according to the following conditions.

(i) Test organism—*Bacillus subtilis* ATCC 6633

(ii) Culture medium—Use the medium i in 1) under (1) Agar media for seed and base layer. Adjust the pH of the medium so that it will be 6.2 to 6.4 after sterilization.

(iii) Standard solutions—Weigh accurately an amount of Vancomycin Hydrochloride RS, equivalent to about 25 mg (potency), dissolve in water to make exactly 25 mL, and use this solution as the standard stock solution. Keep the standard stock solution at 5°C or below, and use within 7 days. Take exactly a suitable amount of the standard stock solution before use, add 0.1 mol/L phosphate buffer solution (pH 4.5) to make solutions so that each mL contains 100 μg (potency) and 25 μg (potency), and use these solutions as the high concentration standard solution and the low concentration standard solution, respectively.

(iv) Sample solutions—Weigh accurately an amount of Vancomycin Hydrochloride, equivalent to about 25 mg (potency), and dissolve in water to make exactly 25 mL. Take exactly a suitable amount of this solution, add 0.1 mol/L phosphate buffer solution (pH 4.5) to make solutions so that each mL contains 100 μg (potency) and 25 μg (potency), and use these solutions as the high concentration sample solution and the low concentration sample solution, respectively.

Containers and storage Containers—Tight containers.

Vancomycin Hydrochloride for Injection

注射用バンコマイシン塩酸塩

Vancomycin Hydrochloride for Injection is a preparation for injection which is dissolved before use.

It contains not less than 90.0% and not more than 115.0% of the labeled potency of vancomycin ($C_{66}H_{75}Cl_2N_9O_{24}$: 1449.25).

Method of preparation Prepare as directed under Injections, with Vancomycin Hydrochloride.

Description Vancomycin Hydrochloride for Injection occurs as white masses or a white powder.

Identification **(1)** Dissolve an amount of Vancomycin Hydrochloride for Injection, equivalent to 5 mg (potency) of Vancomycin Hydrochloride, in 50 mL of water, and determine the absorption spectrum of this solution as directed under Ultraviolet-visible Spectrophotometry <*2.24*>: it exhibits a maximum between 279 nm and 283 nm.

(2) Dissolve an amount of Vancomycin Hydrochloride for Injection, equivalent to 20 mg (potency) of Vancomycin Hydrochloride, in 10 mL of water, and add 1 drop of silver nitrate TS: a white turbidity is produced.

pH <*2.54*> The pH of a solution prepared by dissolving an amount of Vancomycin Hydrochloride for Injection, equivalent to 0.5 g (potency) of Vancomycin Hydrochloride, in 10 mL of water is between 2.5 and 4.5.

Purity **(1)** Clarity and color of solution—Dissolve an amount of Vancomycin Hydrochloride for Injection, equivalent to 0.5 g (potency) of Vancomycin Hydrochloride, in 10 mL of water: the solution is clear and colorless to pale yellow, and the absorbance of the solution, determined at 465 nm as directed under Ultraviolet-visible Spectrophotometry <*2.24*>, is not more than 0.05.

(2) Related substances—Dissolve an amount of Vancomycin Hydrochloride for Injection, equivalent to 0.1 g (potency) of Vancomycin Hydrochloride, in 10 mL of the mobile phase A, and use this solution as the sample solution.

Proceed as directed in the Purity (2) under Vancomycin Hydrochloride.

Water <*2.48*> Not more than 5.0% (0.1 g, volumetric titration, direct titration. Use a mixture of formamide for water determination and methanol for water determination (3:1)).

Bacterial endotoxins <*4.01*> Less than 0.25 EU/mg (potency).

Uniformity of dosage units <*6.02*> It meets the requirement of the Mass variation test.

Foreign insoluble matter <*6.06*> Perform the test according to the Method 2: it meets the requirement.

Insoluble particulate matter <*6.07*> It meets the requirement.

Sterility <*4.06*> Perform the test according to the Membrane filtration method: it meets the requirement.

Assay Perform the test according to the Cylinder-plate method as directed under Microbial Assay for Antibiotics <*4.02*> according to the following conditions.

(i) Test organism, culture medium, and standard solutions—Proceed as directed in the Assay under Vancomycin Hydrochloride.

(ii) Sample solutions—Weigh accurately the contents of not less than 10 Vancomycin Hydrochloride for Injection. Weigh accurately an amount of the content, equivalent to about 25 mg (potency) of Vancomycin Hydrochloride, and dissolve in water to make exactly 25 mL. Take exactly a suitable amount of this solution, add 0.1 mol/L phosphate buffer solution (pH 4.5) to make solutions so that each mL contains 100 μg (potency) and 25 μg (potency), and use these solutions as the high concentration sample solution and the low concentration sample solution, respectively.

Containers and storage Containers—Hermetic containers.

Vasopressin Injection

バソプレシン注射液

Cys-Tyr-Phe-Gln-Asn-Cys-Pro-Arg-Gly-NH_2

$C_{46}H_{65}N_{15}O_{12}S_2$: 1084.23
[*113-79-1*]

Vasopressin Injection is an aqueous injection.

It is a synthetic vasopressin consisting of 9 amino acid residues.

It contains not less than 90.0% and not more than 120.0% of the labeled units of vasopressin ($C_{46}H_{65}N_{15}O_{12}S_2$).

Method of preparation Prepare as directed under Injections, with vasopressin.

Description Vasopressin Injection is a clear and colorless liquid.

pH <*2.54*> 3.0 – 4.0

Purity Related substances—To a suitable amount of Vasopressin Injection add diluted acetic acid (100) (1 in 400) so that each mL contains 20 Units of vasopressin ($C_{46}H_{65}N_{15}O_{12}S_2$), and use this solution as the sample solution. Perform the test with 20 μL of the sample solution as directed under Liquid Chromatography <*2.01*> according to the following conditions. Determine each peak area by the automatic integration method, and calculate the amount of them by the area percentage method: the amount of the peak eluted before vasopressin is not more than 2.0%, and the total amount of the peaks other than vasopressin is not more than 10.0%.

Operating conditions—

Detector: An ultraviolet absorption photometer (wavelength: 220 nm).

Column: A stainless steel column 4.6 mm in inside diameter and 15 cm in length, packed with octadecylsilanized silica gel for liquid chromatography (3 μm in particle diameter).

Column temperature: A constant temperature of about 40°C.

Mobile phase A: Dissolve 6.6 g of diammonium hydrogen phosphate in 950 mL of water, adjust to pH 3.0 with phosphoric acid, and add water to make 1000 mL. To 950 mL of this solution add 50 mL of acetonitrile.

Mobile phase B: Dissolve 6.6 g of diammonium hydrogen

phosphate in 950 mL of water, adjust to pH 3.0 with phosphoric acid, and add water to make 1000 mL. To 450 mL of this solution add 550 mL of acetonitrile.

Flowing of mobile phase: Control the gradient by mixing the mobile phases A and B as directed in the following table.

Time after injection of sample (min)	Mobile phase A (vol%)	Mobile phase B (vol%)
0 – 45	90	10
45 – 90	90 → 30	10 → 70
90 – 100	30	70

Flow rate: About 0.6 mL per minute.

Time span of measurement: About 3 times as long as the retention time of vasopressin.

System suitability—

Test for required detectability: To 1 mL of the sample solution add diluted acetic acid (100) (1 in 400) to make 100 mL, and use this solution as the solution for system suitability test. Pipet 1 mL of the solution for system suitability test, and add diluted acetic acid (100) (1 in 400) to make exactly 10 mL. Confirm that the peak area of vasopressin obtained with 20 μL of this solution is equivalent to 7 to 13% of that with 20 μL of the solution for system suitability test.

System performance: When the procedure is run with 20 μL of the solution for system suitability test under the above operating conditions, the number of theoretical plates and the symmetry factor of the peak of vasopressin are not less than 17,500 and not more than 1.5, respectively.

System repeatability: When the test is repeated 6 times with 20 μL of the solution for system suitability test under the above operating conditions, the relative standard deviation of the peak area of vasopressin is not more than 2.0%.

Bacterial endotoxins *<4.01>* Less than 15 EU/ Unit.

Extractable volume *<6.05>* It meets the requirement.

Foreign insoluble matter *<6.06>* Perform the test according to Method 1: it meets the requirement.

Insoluble particulate matter *<6.07>* It meets the requirement.

Sterility *<4.06>* Perform the test according to the Membrane filtration method: it meets the requirement.

Assay Pipet V mL of Vasopressin Injection, equivalent to about 40 units of vasopressin, add diluted acetic acid (100) (1 in 400) to make exactly 25 mL, and use this solution as the sample solution. Separately, dissolve Vasopressin RS in diluted acetic acid (100) (1 in 400) so that each mL contains about 100 units of vasopressin, then dilute exactly with diluted acetic acid (100) (1 in 400) so that each mL contains about 1.6 units of vasopressin, and use this solution as the standard solution. Perform the test with exactly 20 μL each of the sample solution and standard solution as directed under Liquid Chromatography *<2.01>* according to the following conditions, and determine the peak areas, A_T and A_S, of vasopressin in each solution.

Amount (Unit) of vasopressin in 1 mL of Vasopressin Injection
$$= M_S \times A_T/A_S \times 25/V$$

M_S: Amount (unit) of vasopressin in 1 mL of the standard solution

Operating conditions—

Detector: An ultraviolet absorption photometer (wavelength: 220 nm).

Column: A stainless steel column 4.6 mm in inside diameter and 25 cm in length, packed with octadecylsilanized silica gel for liquid chromatography (5 μm in particle diameter).

Column temperature: A constant temperature of about 40°C.

Mobile phase: Dissolve 6.6 g of diammonium hydrogen phosphate in 950 mL of water, adjust to pH 3.0 with phosphoric acid, and add water to make 1000 mL. To 870 mL of this solution add 130 mL of acetonitrile.

Flow rate: About 1 mL per minute.

System suitability—

System performance: When the procedure is run with 20 μL of the standard solution under the above operating conditions, the number of theoretical plates and the symmetry factor of the peak of vasopressin are not less than 9500 and not more than 1.5, respectively.

System repeatability: When the test is repeated 6 times with 20 μL of the standard solution under the above operating conditions, the relative standard deviation of the peak area of vasopressin is not more than 2.0%.

Containers and storage Containers—Hermetic containers.

Storage—In a cold place, and avoid freezing.

Verapamil Hydrochloride

ベラパミル塩酸塩

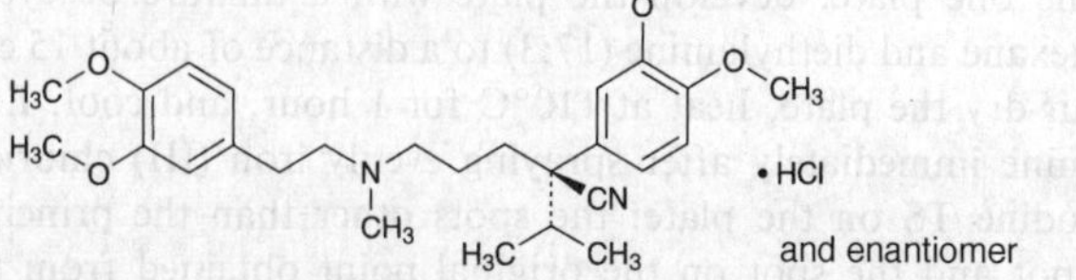

and enantiomer

$C_{27}H_{38}N_2O_4$.HCl: 491.06

(2*RS*)-5-[(3,4-Dimethoxyphenethyl)methylamino]-2-(3,4-dimethoxyphenyl)-2-(1-methylethyl)pentanenitrile monohydrochloride

[*152-11-4*]

Verapamil Hydrochloride, when dried, contains not less than 98.5% and not more than 101.0% of verapamil hydrochloride ($C_{27}H_{38}N_2O_4$.HCl).

Description Verapamil Hydrochloride occurs as a white crystalline powder.

It is freely soluble in methanol and in acetic acid (100), soluble in ethanol (95) and in acetic anhydride, and sparingly soluble in water.

Identification **(1)** To 2 mL of a solution of Verapamil Hydrochloride (1 in 50) add 5 drops of Reinecke salt TS: a light red precipitate is produced.

(2) Determine the absorption spectrum of a solution of Verapamil Hydrochloride in 0.01 mol/L hydrochloric acid TS (1 in 50,000) as directed under Ultraviolet-visible Spectrophotometry *<2.24>*, and compare the spectrum with the Reference Spectrum: both spectra exhibit similar intensities of absorption at the same wavelengths.

(3) Determine the infrared absorption spectrum of Verapamil Hydrochloride, previously dried, as directed in the potassium chloride disk method under Infrared Spectrophotometry *<2.25>*, and compare the spectrum with the Reference Spectrum: both spectra exhibit similar intensities of absorption at the same wave numbers.

(4) A solution of Verapamil Hydrochloride (1 in 50)

responds to Qualitative Tests <*1.09*> for chloride.

Melting point <*2.60*> 141 – 145°C

pH <*2.54*> Dissolve 1.0 g of Verapamil Hydrochloride in 20 mL of freshly boiled and cooled water by warming, and cool: the pH of this solution is between 4.5 and 6.5.

Purity **(1)** Clarity and color of solution—Dissolve 1.0 g of Verapamil Hydrochloride in 20 mL of water by warming: the solution is clear and colorless.

(2) Heavy metals <*1.07*>—Proceed with 1.0 g of Verapamil Hydrochloride according to Method 2, and perform the test. Prepare the control solution with 2.0 mL of Standard Lead Solution (not more than 20 ppm).

(3) Arsenic <*1.11*>—Prepare the test solution with 1.0 g of Verapamil Hydrochloride according to Method 3, and perform the test (not more than 2 ppm).

(4) Related substances—Dissolve 0.50 g of Verapamil Hydrochloride in 10 mL of methanol, and use this solution as the sample solution. Pipet 1 mL of the sample solution, add methanol to make exactly 100 mL, and use this solution as the standard stock solution. Pipet 5 mL of the standard stock solution, add methanol to make exactly 100 mL, and use this solution as the standard solution (1). Separately, pipet 5 mL of the standard stock solution, add methanol to make exactly 50 mL, and use this solution as the standard solution (2). Perform the test with these solutions as directed under Thin-layer Chromatography <*2.03*>. Spot 10 μL each of the sample solution and standard solutions (1) and (2) on two plates of silica gel for thin-layer chromatography. With the one plate, develop the plate with a mixture of cyclohexane and diethylamine (17:3) to a distance of about 15 cm, air-dry the plate, heat at 110°C for 1 hour, and cool. Examine immediately after spraying evenly iron (III) chloride-iodine TS on the plate: the spots other than the principal spot and the spot on the original point obtained from the sample solution, are not more intense than the spot from the standard solution (2), and the number of them which are more intense than the spot from the standard solution (1) is not more than 3. With another plate, develop the plate with a mixture of toluene, methanol, acetone and acetic acid (100) (14:4:1:1), and perform the test in the same manner.

Loss on drying <*2.41*> Not more than 1.0% (1 g, 105°C, 2 hours).

Residue on ignition <*2.44*> Not more than 0.1% (1 g).

Assay Weigh accurately about 0.7 g of Verapamil Hydrochloride, previously dried, dissolve in 50 mL of a mixture of acetic anhydride and acetic acid (100) (7:3), and titrate <*2.50*> with 0.1 mol/L perchloric acid VS (potentiometric titration). Perform a blank determination in the same manner, and make any necessary correction.

Each mL of 0.1 mol/L perchloric acid VS
= 49.11 mg of $C_{27}H_{38}N_2O_4.HCl$

Containers and storage Containers—Well-closed containers.

Storage—Light-resistant.

Verapamil Hydrochloride Injection

ベラパミル塩酸塩注射液

Verapamil Hydrochloride Injection is an aqueous injection.

It contains not less than 93.0% and not more than 107.0% of the labeled amount of verapamil hydrochloride ($C_{27}H_{38}N_2O_4.HCl$: 491.06).

Method of preparation Prepare as directed under Injections, with Verapamil Hydrochloride.

Description Verapamil Hydrochloride Injection is a clear, colorless liquid.

Identification To 1 mL of the sample solution obtained in the Assay, add 0.02 mol/L hydrochloric acid TS to make 50 mL, and determine the absorption spectrum of this solution as directed under Ultraviolet-visible Spectrophotometry <*2.24*>: it exhibits maxima between 227 nm and 231 nm, and between 276 nm and 280 nm.

pH Being specified separately when the drug is granted approval based on the Law.

Bacterial endotoxins <*4.01*> Less than 12 EU/mg.

Extractable volume <*6.05*> It meets the requirement.

Foreign insoluble matter <*6.06*> Perform the test according to Method 1: it meets the requirement.

Insoluble particulate matter <*6.07*> It meets the requirement.

Sterility <*4.06*> Perform the test according to the Membrane filtration method: it meets the requirement.

Assay Pipet a volume of Verapamil Hydrochloride Injection, equivalent to about 10 mg of verapamil hydrochloride ($C_{27}H_{38}N_2O_4.HCl$), add 0.02 mol/L hydrochloric acid TS to make exactly 10 mL, and use this solution as the sample solution. Separately, weigh accurately about 50 mg of verapamil hydrochloride for assay, previously dried at 105°C for 2 hours, dissolve in 0.02 mol/L hydrochloric acid TS to make exactly 50 mL, and use this solution as the standard solution. Perform the test with exactly 10 μL each of the sample solution and standard solution as directed under Liquid Chromatography <*2.01*> according to the following conditions, and determine the peak areas, A_T and A_S, of verapamil in each solution.

Amount (mg) of verapamil hydrochloride
($C_{27}H_{38}N_2O_4.HCl$)
$= M_S \times A_T/A_S \times 1/5$

M_S: Amount (mg) of verapamil hydrochloride for assay taken

Operating conditions—

Detector: An ultraviolet absorption photometer (wavelength: 279 nm).

Column: A stainless steel column 4.6 mm in inside diameter and 15 cm in length, packed with octadecylsilanized silica gel for liquid chromatography (5 μm in particle diameter).

Column temperature: A constant temperature of about 40°C.

Mobile phase: A mixture of methanol, water and perchloric acid (550:450:1).

Flow rate: Adjust so that the retention time of verapamil is about 5 minutes.

System Suitability—

System performance: When the procedure is run with 10 μL of the standard solution under the above operating conditions, the number of theoretical plates and the symmetry factor of the peak of verapamil are not less than 2000 and not more than 2.0, respectively.

System repeatability: When the test is repeated 6 times with 10 μL of the standard solution under the above operating conditions, the relative standard deviation of the peak area of verapamil is not more than 1.0%.

Containers and storage Containers—Hermetic containers, and colored containers may be used.

Storage—Light-resistant.

Verapamil Hydrochloride Tablets

ベラパミル塩酸塩錠

Verapamil Hydrochloride Tablets contain not less than 95.0% and not more than 105.0% of the labeled amount of verapamil hydrochloride ($C_{27}H_{38}N_2O_4.HCl$: 491.06).

Method of preparation Prepare as directed under Tablets, with Verapamil Hydrochloride.

Identification To 2.5 mL of the sample solution obtained in the Assay add the mixture of methanol and 0.1 mol/L hydrochloric acid TS (3:1) to make 100 mL, and determine the absorption spectrum of this solution as directed under Ultraviolet-visible Spectrophotometry *<2.24>*: it exhibits maxima between 228 nm and 232 nm, and between 277 nm and 281 nm.

Uniformity of dosage units *<6.02>* Perform the Mass variation test, or the Content uniformity test according to the following method: it meets the requirement.

To 1 tablet of Verapamil Hydrochloride Tablets add $7V/10$ mL of a mixture of methanol and 0.1 mol/L hydrochloric acid TS (3:1), and sonicate until the tablet is disintegrated. After cooling, add a mixture of methanol and 0.1 mol/L hydrochloric acid TS (3:1) to make exactly V mL so that each mL contains about 0.8 mg of verapamil hydrochloride ($C_{27}H_{38}N_2O_4.HCl$). Centrifuge this solution, and use the supernatant liquid as the sample solution. Then, proceed as directed in the Assay.

Amount (mg) of verapamil hydrochloride ($C_{27}H_{38}N_2O_4.HCl$)

$$= M_S \times A_T/A_S \times V/50$$

M_S: Amount (mg) of verapamil hydrochloride for assay taken

Disintegration *<6.09>* It meets the requirement.

Assay To 25 Verapamil Hydrochloride Tablets, add $7V/10$ mL a mixture of methanol and 0.1 mol/L hydrochloric acid TS (3:1), and sonicate until the tablets are disintegrated. Further, sonicate for about 5 minutes. After cooling, add a mixture of methanol and 0.1 mol/L hydrochloric acid TS (3:1) to make exactly V mL so that each mL contains about 2 mg of verapamil hydrochloride ($C_{27}H_{38}N_2O_4.HCl$). Centrifuge this solution, pipet 10 mL of the supernatant liquid, add a mixture of methanol and 0.1 mol/L hydrochloric acid TS (3:1) to make exactly 25 mL, and use this solution as the sample solution. Separately, weigh accurately about 40 mg of verapamil hydrochloride for assay, previously dried at 105°C for 2 hours, dissolve in a mixture of methanol and 0.1 mol/L hydrochloric acid TS (3:1) to make exactly 50 mL, and use this solution as the standard solution. Perform the test with exactly 10 μL each of the sample solution and standard solution as directed under Liquid Chromatography *<2.01>* according to the following conditions, and determine the peak areas, A_T and A_S, of verapamil in each solution.

Amount (mg) of verapamil hydrochloride ($C_{27}H_{38}N_2O_4.HCl$) in 1 tablet

$$= M_S \times A_T/A_S \times V/500$$

M_S: Amount (mg) of verapamil hydrochloride for assay taken

Operating conditions—

Detector: An ultraviolet absorption photometer (wavelength: 280 nm).

Column: A stainless steel column 4.6 mm in inside diameter and 15 cm in length, packed with octadecylsilanized silica gel for liquid chromatography (5 μm in particle diameter).

Column temperature: A constant temperature of about 40°C.

Mobile phase: A mixture of methanol, water and perchloric acid (550:450:1).

Flow rate: Adjust so that the retention time of verapamil is about 5 minutes.

System suitability—

System performance: When the procedure is run with 10 μL of the standard solution under the above operating conditions, the number of theoretical plates and the symmetry factor of the peak of verapamil are not less than 2000 and not more than 2.0, respectively.

System repeatability: When the test is repeated 6 times with 10 μL of the standard solution under the above operating conditions, the relative standard deviation of the peak area of verapamil is not more than 1.0%.

Containers and storage Containers—Tight containers.

Vinblastine Sulfate

ビンブラスチン硫酸塩

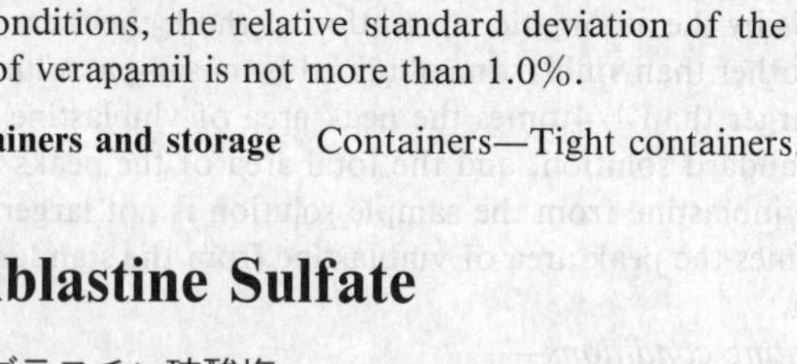

Methyl (3a*R*,4*R*,5*S*,5a*R*,10b*R*,13a*R*)-4-acetoxy-3a-ethyl-9-[(5*S*,7*R*,9*S*)-5-ethyl-5-hydroxy-9-methoxycarbonyl-1,4,5,6,7,8,9,10-octahydro-3,7-methano-3-azacycloundecino[5,4-*b*]indol-9-yl]-5-hydroxy-8-methoxy-6-methyl-3a,4,5,5a,6,11,12,13a-octahydro-1*H*-indolizino[8,1-*cd*]carbazole-5-carboxylate monosulfate
[143-67-9]

Vinblastine Sulfate contains not less than 96.0% and not more than 102.0% of vinblastine sulfate ($C_{46}H_{58}N_4O_9.H_2SO_4$), calculated on the dried basis.

Description Vinblastine Sulfate occurs as a white to pale yellow powder.

It is soluble in water, sparingly soluble in methanol, and

practically insoluble in ethanol (99.5).

It is hygroscopic.

Optical rotation $[\alpha]_D^{20}$: −28 − −35° (20 mg calculated on the dried basis, methanol, 10 mL, 100 mm).

Identification **(1)** Determine the absorption spectrum of a solution of Vinblastine Sulfate (1 in 50,000) as directed under Ultraviolet-visible Spectrophotometry <*2.24*>, and compare the spectrum with the Reference Spectrum or the spectrum of a solution of Vinblastine Sulfate RS prepared in the same manner as the sample solution: both spectra exhibit similar intensities of absorption at the same wavelengths.

(2) Determine the infrared absorption spectrum of Vinblastine Sulfate as directed in the potassium bromide disk method under Infrared Spectrophotometry <*2.25*>, and compare the spectrum with the Reference Spectrum or the spectrum of Vinblastine Sulfate RS: both spectra exhibit similar intensities of absorption at the same wave numbers.

(3) A solution of Vinblastine Sulfate (1 in 100) responds to Qualitative Tests <*1.09*> for sulfate.

pH <*2.54*> Dissolve 15 mg of Vinblastine Sulfate in 10 mL of water: the pH of this solution is between 3.5 and 5.0.

Purity **(1)** Clarity and color of solution—Dissolve 50 mg of Vinblastine Sulfate in 10 mL of water: the solution is clear and colorless.

(2) Related substances—Dissolve about 4 mg of Vinblastine Sulfate in 10 mL of water, and use this solution as the sample solution. Pipet 1 mL of the sample solution, add water to make exactly 25 mL, and use this solution as the standard solution. Perform the test with exactly 200 μL each of the sample solution and standard solution as directed under Liquid Chromatography <*2.01*> according to the following conditions, and determine each peak area of these solutions by the automatic integration method: the area of the peak other than vinblastine obtained from sample solution is not larger than 1/4 times the peak area of vinblastine from the standard solution, and the total area of the peaks other than vinblastine from the sample solution is not larger than 3/4 times the peak area of vinblastine from the standard solution.

Operating conditions—

Detector, column, column temperature, mobile phase, and flow rate: Proceed as directed in the operating conditions in the Assay.

Time span of measurement: About 4 times as long as the retention time of vinblastine, beginning after the solvent peak.

System suitability—

System performance: Proceed as directed in the system suitability in the Assay.

Test for required detectability: To exactly 2.5 mL of the standard solution add water to make exactly 100 mL. Confirm that the peak area of vinblastine obtained with 200 μL of this solution is equivalent to 1.7 to 3.3% of that with 200 μL of the standard solution.

System repeatability: When the test is repeated 6 times with 200 μL of the standard solution under the above operating conditions, the relative standard deviation of the peak area of vinblastine is not more than 1.5%.

Loss on drying Perform the test with about 10 mg of Vinblastine Sulfate as directed in Thermogravimetry under Thermal Analysis <*2.52*> according to the following conditions: not more than 15.0%.

Operating conditions—

Heating rate: 5°C per minute.

Temperature range: room temperature to 200°C.

Atmospheric gas: dried Nitrogen.

Flow rate of atmospheric gas: 40 mL per minute.

Assay Weigh accurately about 10 mg each of Vinblastine Sulfate and Vinblastine Sulfate RS (previously determine the loss on drying under the same conditions as Vinblastine Sulfate), dissolve in water to make exactly 25 mL, and use these solutions as the sample solution and the standard solution, respectively. Perform the test with exactly 20 μL each of the sample solution and standard solution as directed under Liquid Chromatography <*2.01*> according to the following conditions, and determine the peak areas, A_T and A_S, of vinblastine in each solution.

Amount (mg) of vinblastine sulfate ($C_{46}H_{58}N_4O_9.H_2SO_4$)
$= M_S \times A_T/A_S$

M_S: Amount (mg) of Vinblastine Sulfate RS taken, calculated on the dried basis

Operating conditions—

Detector: An ultraviolet absorption photometer (wavelength: 262 nm).

Column: A stainless steel column 4.6 mm in inside diameter and 15 cm in length, packed with octadecylsilanized silica gel for liquid chromatography (5 μm in particle diameter).

Column temperature: A constant temperature of about 25°C.

Mobile phase: To 7 mL of diethylamine add water to make 500 mL, and adjust the pH to 7.5 with phosphoric acid. To 380 mL of this solution add 620 mL of a mixture of methanol and acetonitrile (4:1).

Flow rate: Adjust so that the retention time of vinblastine is about 8 minutes.

System suitability—

System performance: Dissolve 10 mg each of Vinblastine Sulfate and vincristine sulfate in 25 mL of water. When the procedure is run with 20 μL of this solution under the above operating conditions, vincristine and vinblastine are eluted in this order with the resolution between these peaks being not less than 4.

System repeatability: When the test is repeated 6 times with 20 μL of the standard solution under the above operating conditions, the relative standard deviation of the peak area of vinblastine is not more than 1.0%.

Containers and storage Containers—Tight containers.

Storage—Light-resistant, at not exceeding −20°C.

Vinblastine Sulfate for Injection

注射用ビンブラスチン硫酸塩

Vinblastine Sulfate for Injection is a preparation for injection, which is dissolved before use.

It contains not less than 90.0% and not more than 110.0% of the labeled amount of vinblastine sulfate ($C_{46}H_{58}N_4O_9.H_2SO_4$: 909.05).

Method of preparation Prepare as directed under Injections, with Vinblastine Sulfate.

Description Vinblastine Sulfate for Injection occurs as white to pale yellow, light masses or powder.

It is freely soluble in water.

The pH of a solution (1 in 1000) is 3.5 – 5.0.

Identification Proceed as directed in the Identification (1) under Vinblastine Sulfate.

Purity Related substances—Dissolve 4 mg of Vinblastine Sulfate for Injection in 10 mL of water, and use this solution as the sample solution. Pipet 1 mL of the sample solution, add water to make exactly 25 mL, and use this solution as the standard solution. Perform the test with exactly 200 μL each of the sample solution and standard solution as directed under Liquid Chromatography *<2.01>* according to the following conditions, and determine each peak area by the automatic integration method: the area of the peak other than vinblastine obtained from the sample solution is not larger than 1/2 times the peak area of vinblastine from the standard solution, and the total area of the peaks other than vinblastine from the sample solution is not larger than 2 times the peak area of vinblastine from the standard solution.

Operating conditions—

Perform as directed in the operating conditions in Purity (2) under Vinblastine Sulfate.

System suitability—

Perform as directed in the system suitability in Purity (2) under Vinblastine Sulfate.

Bacterial endotoxins *<4.01>* Less than 10 EU/mg.

Uniformity of dosage units *<6.02>* Perform the test according to the following method: it meets the requirement of the Content uniformity test.

Dissolve 1 Vinblastine Sulfate for Injection in water to make exactly *V* mL so that each mL contains about 0.4 mg of vinblastine sulfate ($C_{46}H_{58}N_4O_9.H_2SO_4$), and use this solution as the sample solution. Separately, weigh accurately about 10 mg of Vinblastine Sulfate RS (previously determine the loss on drying under the same conditions as Vinblastine Sulfate), dissolve in water to make exactly 25 mL, and use this solution as the standard solution. Proceed as directed in the Assay under Vinblastine Sulfate.

Amount (mg) of vinblastine sulfate ($C_{46}H_{58}N_4O_9.H_2SO_4$)
$= M_S \times A_T/A_S \times 25/V$

M_S: Amount (mg) of Vinblastine Sulfate RS taken, calculated on the dried basis

Foreign insoluble matter *<6.06>* Perform the test according to Method 2: it meets the requirement.

Insoluble particulate matter *<6.07>* It meets the requirement.

Sterility *<4.06>* Perform the test according to the Membrane filtration method: it meets the requirement.

Assay Take an amount of Vinblastine Sulfate for Injection, equivalent to 0.10 g of vinblastine sulfate ($C_{46}H_{58}N_4O_9.H_2SO_4$), dissolve each content with a suitable amount of water, transfer into a 100-mL volumetric flask, wash each container with water, transfer the washings into the volumetric flask, and add water to make exactly 100 mL. Pipet 10 mL of this solution, add water to make exactly 25 mL, and use this solution as the sample solution. Separately, weigh accurately about 10 mg of Vinblastine Sulfate RS (previously determine the loss on drying under the same conditions as Vinblastine Sulfate), dissolve in water to make exactly 25 mL, and use this solution as the standard solution. Proceed as directed in the Assay under Vinblastine Sulfate.

Amount (mg) of vinblastine sulfate ($C_{46}H_{58}N_4O_9.H_2SO_4$)
$= M_S \times A_T/A_S \times 10$

M_S: Amount (mg) of Vinblastine Sulfate RS taken, calculated on the dried basis

Containers and storage Containers—Hermetic containers, and colored containers may be used.

Storage—Light-resistant, at 2 to 8°C.

Vincristine Sulfate

ビンクリスチン硫酸塩

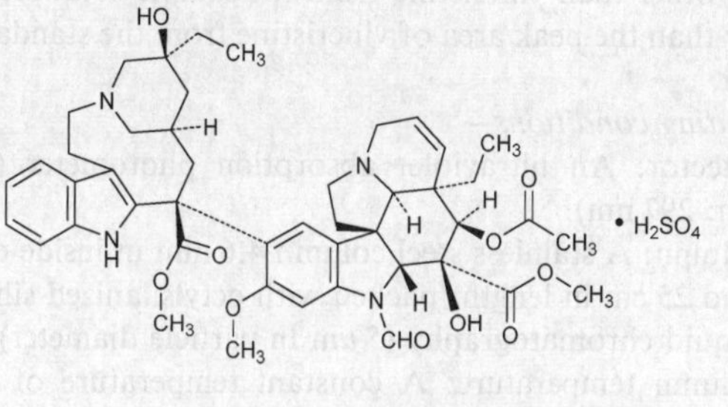

Methyl (3a*R*,4*R*,5*S*,5a*R*,10b*R*,13a*R*)-4-acetoxy-3a-ethyl-9-[(5*S*,7*R*,9*S*)-5-ethyl-5-hydroxy-9-methoxycarbonyl-1,4,5,6,7,8,9,10-octahydro-3,7-methano-3-azacycloundecino[5,4-*b*]indol-9-yl]-6-formyl-5-hydroxy-8-methoxy-3a,4,5,5a,6,11,12,13a-octahydro-1*H*-indolizino[8,1-*cd*]carbazole-5-carboxylate monosulfate
[*2068-78-2*]

Vincristine Sulfate contains not less than 95.0% and not more than 105.0% of vincristine sulfate ($C_{46}H_{56}N_4O_{10}.H_2SO_4$), calculated on the dried basis.

Description Vincristine Sulfate occurs as a white to light yellow-white powder.

It is very soluble in water, and practically insoluble in ethanol (99.5).

It is hygroscopic.

Optical rotation $[\alpha]_D^{20}$: +28.5 – +35.5° (0.2 g calculated on the dried basis, water, 10 mL, 100 mm).

Identification **(1)** Determine the absorption spectrum of a solution of Vincristine Sulfate (1 in 50,000) as directed under Ultraviolet-visible Spectrophotometry *<2.24>*, and compare the spectrum with the Reference Spectrum or the spectrum of a solution of Vincristine Sulfate RS prepared in the same manner as the sample solution: both spectra exhibit similar intensities of absorption at the same wavelengths.

(2) Determine the infrared absorption spectrum of Vincristine Sulfate as directed in the potassium bromide disk method under Infrared Spectrophotometry *<2.25>*, and compare the spectrum with the Reference Spectrum or the spectrum of Vincristine Sulfate RS: both spectra exhibit similar intensities of absorption at the same wave numbers.

(3) A solution of Vincristine Sulfate (1 in 100) responds to Qualitative Tests *<1.09>* for sulfate.

pH *<2.54>* Dissolve 10 mg of Vincristine Sulfate in 10 mL of water: the pH of this solution is between 3.5 and 4.5.

Purity **(1)** Clarity and color of solution—Dissolve 50 mg of Vincristine Sulfate in 10 mL of water: the solution is clear and colorless.

(2) Related substances—Dissolve 10 mg of Vincristine Sulfate in 10 mL of water, and use this solution as the sample solution. Pipet 2 mL of the sample solution, add water to make exactly 50 mL, and use this solution as the standard solution. Perform the test with exactly 200 μL each of the sample solution and standard solution as directed under Liquid Chromatography *<2.01>* according to the following conditions. Determine each peak area by the automatic integration method: the peak area of desacetyl vincristine and vinblastine, having the relative retention times of about 0.9

and about 1.6 to vincristine, respectively, obtained from the sample solution are not larger than 1/8 times and 3/20 times, respectively, the peak area of vincristine from the standard solution, and the area of the peak other than vincristine, desacetyl vincristine and vinblastine from the sample solution is not larger than 1/4 times the peak area of vincristine from standard solution. Furthermore, the total area of the peaks other than vincristine from the sample solution is not larger than the peak area of vincristine from the standard solution.

Operating conditions—

Detector: An ultraviolet absorption photometer (wavelength: 297 nm).

Column: A stainless steel column 4.6 mm in inside diameter and 25 cm in length, packed with octylsilanized silica gel for liquid chromatography (5 μm in particle diameter).

Column temperature: A constant temperature of about 40°C.

Mobile phase A: methanol.

Mobile phase B: A mixture of water and diethylamine (197:3), adjusted the pH to 7.5 with phosphoric acid.

Flowing of mobile phase: Control the gradient by mixing the mobile phases A and B as directed in the following table.

Time after injection of sample (min)	Mobile phase A (vol%)	Mobile phase B (vol%)
0 - 12	62	38
12 - 27	62 → 92	38 → 8

Flow rate: Adjust so that the retention time of vincristine is about 15 minutes.

Time span of measurement: About 1.7 times as long as the retention time of vincristine, beginning after the solvent peak.

System suitability—

Test for required detectability: Pipet 5 mL of the standard solution, and add water to make exactly 200 mL. Confirm that the peak area of vincristine obtained with 200 μL of this solution is equivalent to 1.75 to 3.25% of that with 200 μL of the standard solution.

System performance: Dissolve 15 mg each of Vincristine Sulfate and vinblastine sulfate in 100 mL of water. When the procedure is run with 200 μL of this solution under the above operating conditions, vincristine and vinblastine are eluted in this order with the resolution between these peaks being not less than 4.

System repeatability: When the test is repeated 6 times with 200 μL of the standard solution under the above operating conditions, the relative standard deviation of the peak area of vincristine is not more than 1.5%.

Loss on drying Perform the test with about 10 mg of Vincristine Sulfate as directed in Thermogravimetry under Thermal Analysis *<2.52>* according to the following conditions: not more than 12.0%.

Operating conditions—

Heating rate: 5°C per minute.

Temperature range: room temperature to 200°C.

Atmospheric gas: dried nitrogen.

Flow rate of atmospheric gas: 40 mL per minute.

Assay Weigh accurately about 10 mg each of Vincristine Sulfate and Vincristine Sulfate RS (separately determine the loss on drying under the same conditions as Vincristine Sulfate), dissolve each in water to make exactly 10 mL, and use these solutions as the sample solution and the standard solution, respectively. Perform the test with exactly 10 μL each of the sample solution and standard solution as directed under Liquid Chromatography *<2.01>* according to the following conditions, and determine the peak areas, A_T and A_S, of vincristine in each solution.

Amount (mg) of vincristine sulfate ($C_{46}H_{56}N_4O_{10}.H_2SO_4$)
$= M_S \times A_T/A_S$

M_S: Amount (mg) of Vincristine Sulfate RS taken, calculated on the dried basis

Operating conditions—

Detector: An ultraviolet absorption photometer (wavelength: 297 nm).

Column: A stainless steel column 4.6 mm in inside diameter and 25 cm in length, packed with octylsilanized silica gel for liquid chromatography (5 μm in particle diameter).

Column temperature: A constant temperature of about 25°C.

Mobile phase: Adjust the pH to 7.5 of a mixture of water and diethylamine (59:1) with phosphoric acid. To 300 mL of this solution add 700 mL of methanol.

Flow rate: Adjust so that the retention time of vincristine is about 7 minutes.

System suitability—

System performance: Dissolve 5 mg each of Vincristine Sulfate and vinblastine sulfate in 5 mL of water. When the procedure is run with 10 μL of this solution under the above operating conditions, vincristine and vinblastine are eluted in this order with the resolution between these peaks being not less than 4.

System repeatability: When the test is repeated 6 times with 10 μL of the standard solution under the above operating conditions, the relative standard deviation of the peak area of vincristine is not more than 1.0%.

Containers and storage Containers—Tight containers.

Storage—Light-resistant, and at not exceeding −20°C.

Vitamin A Oil

ビタミンA油

Vitamin A Oil is synthetic vitamin A esters diluted with fixed oils.

It contains not less than 30,000 vitamin A Units per g.

It may contain suitable antioxidants.

It contains not less than 90.0% and not more than 120.0% of the labeled units of vitamin A.

Description Vitamin A Oil is a yellow to yellow-brown, clear or slightly turbid oil. It is odorless or has a faint, characteristic odor.

It is decomposed upon exposure to air or light.

Identification Dissolve Vitamin A Oil, Retinol Acetate RS and Retinol Palmitate RS, equivalent to 15,000 Units, in 5 mL of petroleum ether, and use these solutions as the sample solution, the standard solution (1) and the standard solution (2), respectively. Perform the test with these solutions as directed under Thin-layer Chromatography *<2.03>*. Spot 5 μL each of the sample solution and standard solutions (1) and (2) on a plate of silica gel for thin-layer chromatography. Develop with a mixture of cyclohexane and diethyl ether (12:1) to a distance of about 10 cm, and air-dry the plate. Spray evenly antimony (III) chloride TS: the principal spot obtained from the sample solution has the same color tone and the same *Rf* value with the blue spot from the standard solution (1) or the standard solution (2).

Purity **(1)** Acidity—Dissolve 1.2 g of Vitamin A Oil in 30 mL of a mixture of neutralized ethanol and diethyl ether (1:1), boil gently for 10 minutes under a reflux condenser, cool, and add 5 drops of phenolphthalein TS and 0.60 mL of 0.1 mol/L sodium hydroxide VS: a red color develops.

(2) Rancidity—No unpleasant odor of rancid oil is perceptible by warming Vitamin A Oil.

Assay Proceed as directed in Method 1-1 under Vitamin A Assay *<2.55>*.

Containers and storage Containers—Tight containers.

Storage—Light-resistant, and almost well-filled, or under Nitrogen atmosphere.

Voglibose

ボグリボース

$C_{10}H_{21}NO_7$: 267.28
3,4-Dideoxy-4-[2-hydroxy-1-(hydroxymethyl)ethylamino]-2-*C*-(hydroxymethyl)-D-*epi*-inositol
[83480-29-9]

Voglibose contains not less than 99.5% and not more than 101.0% of voglibose ($C_{10}H_{21}NO_7$), calculated on the anhydrous basis.

Description Voglibose occurs as white, crystals or crystalline powder.

It is very slightly soluble in water, freely soluble in acetic acid (100), slightly soluble in methanol, and very slightly soluble in ethanol (99.5).

It dissolves in 0.1 mol/L hydrochloric acid TS.

Identification **(1)** Determine the infrared absorption spectrum of Voglibose as directed in the potassium bromide disk method under Infrared Spectrophotometry *<2.25>*, and compare the spectrum with the Reference Spectrum: both spectra exhibit similar intensities of absorption at the same wave numbers.

(2) Determine the ^1H spectrum of a solution of Voglibose in heavy water for nuclear magnetic resonance spectroscopy (3 in 70) as directed under Nuclear Magnetic Resonance Spectroscopy *<2.21>*, using sodium 3-trimethylsilylpropionate-d_4 for nuclear magnetic resonance spectroscopy as an internal reference compound: it exhibits 2 doublet signals A at about δ 1.5 ppm, 2 doublet signals B at about δ 2.1 ppm, a multiplet signal C at about δ 2.9 ppm, and a multiplet signal D between δ 3.4 ppm and δ 3.9 ppm. The area intensity ratio of each signal, A:B:C:D, is about 1:1:1:10.

Optical rotation *<2.49>* $[\alpha]_D^{20}$: +45 – +48° (0.2 g calculated on the anhydrous basis, 0.1 mol/L hydrochloric acid TS, 20 mL, 100 mm).

pH *<2.54>* Dissolve 1.0 g of Voglibose in 10 mL of water: the pH of the solution is between 9.8 and 10.4.

Melting point *<2.60>* 163 – 168°C

Purity **(1)** Heavy metals *<1.07>*—Proceed with 1.0 g of Voglibose according to Method 1, and perform the test. Adjust the pH of the test solution between 3.0 and 3.5 with dilute hydrochloric acid instead of dilute acetic acid. Prepare the control solution with 1.0 mL of Standard Lead Solution (not more than 10 ppm).

(2) Related substances—Dissolve 50 mg of Voglibose in 50 mL of the mobile phase, and use this solution as the sample solution. Pipet 1 mL of the sample solution, add the mobile phase to make exactly 100 mL, and use this solution as the standard solution. Perform the test with exactly 50 μL each of the sample solution and standard solution as directed under Liquid Chromatography *<2.01>* according to the following conditions, and determine each peak area by the automatic integration method: the total area of the peaks other than voglibose obtained from sample solution is not larger than 1/5 times the peak area of voglibose from the standard solution. For the area of the peaks, having the relative retention time of about 1.7, about 2.0 and about 2.3 to voglibose, multiply their correction factors, 2, 2 and 2.5, respectively.

Operating conditions—

Apparatus: Use an apparatus consisting of 2 pumps for the mobile phase and reaction reagent transportation, sample injection port, column, reaction coil, cooling coil, detector and recording device, and the reaction coil and cooling coil maintained at a constant temperature.

Detector: Fluorophotometer (excitation wavelength: 350 nm, fluorescence wavelength: 430 nm).

Column: A stainless steel column 4.6 mm in inside diameter and 25 cm in length, packed with pentaethylenehexaaminated polyvinyl alcohol polymer bead for liquid chromatography (5 μm in particle diameter).

Column temperature: A constant temperature of about 25°C.

Reaction coil: A polytetrafluoroethylene tube 0.5 mm in inside diameter and 20 m in length.

Cooling coil: A polytetrafluoroethylene tube 0.3 mm in inside diameter and 2 m in length.

Mobile phase: To 1.56 g of sodium dihydrogen phosphate dihydrate add water to make 500 mL. To this solution add a solution, prepared by dissolving 3.58 g of disodium hydrogen phosphate dodecahydrate in water to make 500 mL, to adjust to pH 6.5. To 370 mL of this solution add 630 mL of acetonitrile.

Reaction reagent: Dissolve 6.25 g of taurine and 2.56 g of sodium periodate in water to make 1000 mL.

Reaction temperature: A constant temperature of about 100°C.

Cooling temperature: A constant temperature of about 15°C.

Flow rate of mobile phase: Adjust so that the retention time of voglibose is about 20 minutes.

Flow rate of reaction reagent: Same as the flow rate of the mobile phase.

Time span of measurement: About 2.5 times as long as the retention time of voglibose, beginning after the solvent peak.

System suitability—

Test for required detectability: Pipet 10 mL of the standard solution, and add the mobile phase to make exactly 100 mL. Confirm that the peak area of voglibose obtained with 50 μL of this solution is equivalent to 7 to 13% of that with 50 μL of the standard solution.

System performance: When the procedure is run with 50 μL of the standard solution under the above operating conditions, the number of theoretical plates and the symmetry

factor of the peak of voglibose are not less than 7000 and between 0.8 and 1.2, respectively.

System repeatability: When the test is repeated 6 times with 50 μL of the standard solution under the above operating conditions, the relative standard deviation of the peak area of voglibose is not more than 3.0%.

Water *<2.48>* Not more than 0.2% (0.5 g, coulometric titration).

Residue on ignition *<2.44>* Not more than 0.1% (1 g).

Assay Weigh accurately about 0.4 g of Voglibose, dissolve in 80 mL of acetic acid (100), and titrate *<2.50>* with 0.1 mol/L perchloric acid VS (potentiometric titration). Perform a blank determination in the same manner, and make any necessary correction.

$$\text{Each mL of 0.1 mol/L perchloric acid VS} = 26.73 \text{ mg of } C_{10}H_{21}NO_7$$

Containers and storage Containers—Tight containers.

Voglibose Tablets

ボグリボース錠

Voglibose Tablets contain not less than 95.0% and not more than 105.0% of the labeled amount of voglibose ($C_{10}H_{21}NO_7$: 267.28).

Method of preparation Prepare as directed under Tablets, with Voglibose.

Identification Shake vigorously an amount of powdered Voglibose Tablets, equivalent to 5 mg of Voglibose, with 40 mL of water, and centrifuge. Transfer the supernatant liquid to a chromatographic column [prepared by pouring 1.0 mL of strongly acidic ion-exchange resin (H type) for column chromatography (100 to 200 μm in particle diameter) into a chromatographic column 8 mm in inside diameter and 130 mm in height], and allow to flow at a rate of about 5 mL per minute. Then wash the column with 200 mL of water, and allow to flow with 10 mL of diluted ammonia TS (1 in 4) at a rate of about 5 mL per minute. Filter the effluent solution 2 times through a membrane filter with a pore size not exceeding 0.22 μm. Evaporate the filtrate to dryness at 50°C under reduced pressure, dissolve the residue with 0.5 mL of a mixture of water and methanol (1:1), and use this solution as the sample solution. Separately, dissolve 20 mg of voglibose for assay in 2 mL of the mixture of water and methanol (1:1), and use this solution as the standard solution. Perform the test with these solutions as directed under Thin-layer Chromatography *<2.03>*. Spot 20 μL each of the sample solution and standard solution on a plate of silica gel for thin-layer chromatography. Develop the plate with a mixture of acetone, ammonia water (28) and water (5:3:1) to a distance of about 12 cm, air-dry the plate, and allow to stand in iodine vapors: the principal spot obtained from the sample solution and the spot from the standard solution show a yellow-brown color, and the same *Rf* value.

Uniformity of dosage units *<6.02>* Perform the test according to the following method: it meets the requirement of the Content uniformity test.

To 1 tablet of Voglibose Tablets add exactly *V* mL of the mobile phase so that the solution contains about 40 μg of voglibose ($C_{10}H_{21}NO_7$) per mL, disintegrate the tablet completely by shaking, and centrifuge. Filter the supernatant liquid through a membrane filter with a pore size not exceeding 0.45 μm. Discard the first 1 mL of the filtrate, and use the subsequent filtrate as the sample solution. Proceed as directed in the Assay.

$$\text{Amount (g) of voglibose } (C_{10}H_{21}NO_7) = M_S \times A_T/A_S \times V/500$$

M_S: Amount (mg) of voglibose for assay taken, calculated on the anhydrous basis

Dissolution *<6.10>* When the test is performed at 50 revolutions per minute according to the Paddle method, using 900 mL of water as the dissolution medium, the dissolution rate in 30 minutes of Voglibose Tablets is not less than 85%.

Start the test with 1 tablet of Voglibose Tablets, withdraw not less than 20 mL of the medium at the specified minute after starting the test, and filter through a membrane filter with a pore size not exceeding 0.45 μm. Discard not less than 10 mL of the first filtrate, pipet *V* mL of the subsequent filtrate, add the mobile phase to make exactly *V′* mL so that each mL contains about 0.11 μg of voglibose ($C_{10}H_{21}NO_7$), and use this solution as the sample solution. Separately, weigh accurately about 22 mg of voglibose for assay (separately determine the water *<2.48>* in the same manner as Voglibose), and dissolve in water to make exactly 100 mL. Pipet 5 mL of this solution, and add water to make exactly 100 mL. Pipet 2 mL of this solution, and add water to make exactly 100 mL. Pipet 10 mL of this solution, add the mobile phase to make exactly 20 mL, and use this solution as the standard solution. Perform the test with exactly 100 μL each of the sample solution and standard solution as directed under Liquid Chromatography *<2.01>* according to the following conditions, and determine the peak areas, A_T and A_S, of voglibose in each solution.

$$\text{Dissolution rate (\%) with respect to the labeled amount of voglibose } (C_{10}H_{21}NO_7) = M_S \times A_T/A_S \times V'/V \times 1/C \times 9/20$$

M_S: Amount (mg) of voglibose for assay taken

C: Labeled amount (mg) of voglibose ($C_{10}H_{21}NO_7$) in 1 tablet

Operating conditions—

Apparatus, detector, column, column temperature, reaction coil, cooling coil, reaction reagent, reaction temperature, and flow rate of reaction reagent: Proceed as directed in the operating conditions in the Assay.

Mobile phase: Dissolve 1.56 g of sodium dihydrogen phosphate dihydrate in 500 mL of water. To this solution add a suitable amount of a solution, prepared by dissolving 3.58 g of disodium hydrogen phosphate decahydrate in 500 mL of water, to adjust to pH 6.5. To 500 mL of this solution add 500 mL of acetonitrile.

Cooling temperature: A constant temperature of about 25°C.

Flow rate of mobile phase: Adjust so that the retention time of voglibose is about 6 minutes.

System suitability—

System performance: When the procedure is run with 100 μL of the standard solution under the above operating conditions, the number of theoretical plates and the symmetry factor of the peak of voglibose are not less than 2000 and not more than1.5, respectively.

System repeatability: When the test is repeated 6 times with 100 μL of the standard solution under the above operating conditions, the relative standard deviation of the peak area of voglibose is not more than 3.0%.

Assay To 20 tables of Voglibose Tablets add 80 mL of the mobile phase, and completely disintegrate by shaking. To an exact volume of the solution, equivalent to about 4 mg of voglibose ($C_{10}H_{21}NO_7$), add the mobile phase to make exactly 100 mL, and centrifuge. Filter the supernatant liquid through a membrane filter with a pore size not exceeding 0.45 μm. Discard the first 1 mL of the filtrate, and use the subsequent filtrate as the sample solution. Separately, weigh accurately about 20 mg of voglibose for assay (previously determine the water *<2.48>* in the same manner as Voglibose), and dissolve in the mobile phase to make exactly 25 mL. Pipet 5 mL of this solution, add the mobile phase to make exactly 100 mL, and use this solution as the standard solution. Perform the test with exactly 50 μL each of the sample solution and standard solution as directed under Liquid Chromatography *<2.01>* according to the following conditions, and determine the peak areas, A_T and A_S, of voglibose in each solution.

$$\text{Amount (mg) of voglibose } (C_{10}H_{21}NO_7) = M_S \times A_T/A_S \times 1/500$$

M_S: Amount of voglibose for assay taken, calculated on the dried basis

Operating conditions—

Apparatus: Use an apparatus consisting of 2 pumps for the mobile phase and reaction reagent transportation, sample injection port, column, reaction coil, cooling coil, detector and recording device, and the reaction coil and cooling coil maintained at a constant temperature.

Detector: Fluorophotometer (excitation wavelength: 350 nm, fluorescence wavelength: 430 nm).

Column: A stainless steel column 4 mm in inside diameter and 15 cm in length, packed with aminopropylsilanized silica gel for liquid chromatography (5 μm in particle diameter).

Column temperature: A constant temperature of about 25°C.

Reaction coil: A polytetrafluoroethylene tube 0.5 mm in inside diameter and 20 m in length.

Cooling coil: A polytetrafluoroethylene tube 0.3 mm in inside diameter and 2 m in length.

Mobile phase: To 1.56 g of sodium dihydrogen phosphate dihydrate add water to make 500 mL. To this solution add a solution, prepared by dissolving 3.58 g of disodium hydrogen phosphate dodecahydrate in water to make 500 mL, to adjust to pH 6.5. To 300 mL of this solution add 600 mL of acetonitrile.

Reaction reagent: Dissolve 6.25 g of taurine and 2.56 g of sodium periodate in water to make 1000 mL.

Reaction temperature: A constant temperature of about 100°C.

Cooling temperature: A constant temperature of about 15°C.

Flow rate of mobile phase: Adjust so that the retention time of voglibose is about 20 minutes.

Flow rate of reaction reagent: Same as the flow rate of the mobile phase.

System suitability—

System performance: Dissolve 2 mg of voglibose for assay and 0.2 g of lactose monohydrate in 5 mL of water, and add the mobile phase to make 50 mL. When the procedure is run with 50 μL of this solution under the above operating conditions, lactose and voglibose are eluted in this order with the resolution between these peaks being not less than 4.

System repeatability: When the test is repeated 6 times with 50 μL of the standard solution under the above operating conditions, the relative standard deviation of the peak area of voglibose is not more than 2.0%.

Containers and storage Containers—Tight containers.

Voriconazole

ボリコナゾール

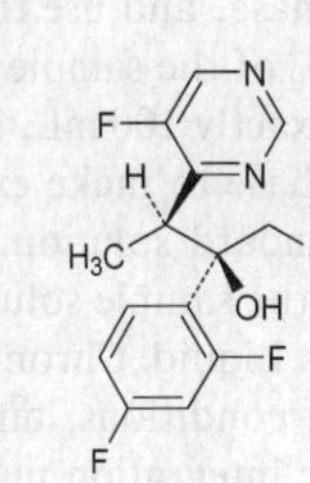

$C_{16}H_{14}F_3N_5O$: 349.31

(2*R*,3*S*)-2-(2,4-Difluorophenyl)-3-(5-fluoropyrimidin-4-yl)-1-(1*H*-1,2,4-triazol-1-yl)butan-2-ol

[*137234-62-9*]

Voriconazole contains not less than 98.0% and not more than 102.0% of $C_{16}H_{14}F_3N_5O$, calculated on the anhydrous basis.

Description Voriconazole is a white crystalline powder.

It is freely soluble in methanol and in acetonitrile, soluble in ethanol (99.5), and very slightly soluble in water.

It dissolves in 1 mol/L hydrochloric acid TS.

Optical rotation $[\alpha]^{25}_{365}$: −374 – −404°(50 mg calculated on the anhydrous basis, methanol, 25 mL, 100 mm).

Identification **(1)** Determine the absorption spectrum of a solution of Voriconazole in methanol (1 in 40,000) as directed under Ultraviolet-visible Spectrophotometry *<2.24>*, and compare the spectrum with the Reference Spectrum or the spectrum of a solution of Voriconazole RS prepared in the same manner as the sample solution: both spectra exhibit similar intensities of absorption at the same wavelengths.

(2) Determine the infrared absorption spectrum of Voriconazole as directed in the potassium bromide disk method under Infrared Spectrophotometry *<2.25>*, and compare the spectrum with the Reference Spectrum or the spectrum of Voriconazole RS: both spectra exhibit similar intensities of absorption at the same wave numbers.

Purity **(1)** Heavy metals—Take 2.0 g of Voriconazole in a porcelain crucible, moisten with an appropriate amount of sulfuric acid, cover the crucible loosely, and ignite at a low temperature until charred. After cooling, add 2 mL of nitric acid and 5 drops of sulfuric acid to the content of the crucible, heat gently the crucible until white fumes are no longer evolved, then ignite at 500 – 600°C. After cooling, add 4 mL of 6 mol/L hydrochloric acid TS, evaporate to dryness on a water bath, moisten the residue with 1 drop of hydrochloric acid, add 10 mL of boiling water, and heat for 2 minutes. After cooling, add appropriate drops of ammonia TS until litmus paper changes to blue, add water to make 15 mL, and adjust the pH between 3.0 and 4.0 with dilute acetic acid. Filter if necessary, wash the crucible and the filter paper with 10 mL of water, put the filtrate and washings to a Nessler tube, add water to make 40 mL, and use this solution as the sample solution. Separately, put 2.0 mL of Standard Lead Solution in another Nessler tube, add water to make 25 mL, adjust the pH between 3.0 and 4.0 with dilute acetic acid or ammonia TS, then add water to make 40 mL, and use this solution as the control solution. To each of the sample solution and control solution add 2 mL of acetate buffer solution (pH 3.5), then add 1.2 mL of thioacetamide-alkaline glycerin TS, and add water to make 50 mL. After allowing to stand for 2 minutes, observe vertically both tubes against a white background: the color obtained with the test solution is not more intense than that with the control solution (not more than 10 ppm).

(2) Related substances—Dissolve 50 mg of Voriconazole in 100 mL of the mobile phase, and use this solution as the sample solution. Pipet 1 mL of the sample solution, and add the mobile phase to make exactly 100 mL. Pipet 1 mL of this solution, add the mobile phase to make exactly 10 mL, and use this solution as the standard solution. Perform the test with exactly 20 μL each of the sample solution and standard solution as directed under Liquid Chromatography <*2.01*> according to the following conditions, and determine each peak area by the automatic integration method: the area of the peaks other than voriconazole obtained from the sample solution is not larger than the peak area of voriconazole from the standard solution. The total area of the peaks other than voriconazole from the sample solution is not larger than 4 times the peak area of voriconazole from the standard solution. For the area of the peak, having a relative retention time of about 0.26, about 0.32, and about 0.61 to voriconazole, multiply the correction factor, 0.7, 0.7 and 2.1, respectively.

Operating conditions—

Detector, column, column temperature, mobile phase, and flow rate: Proceed as directed in the operating conditions in the Assay.

Time span of measurement: About 2.7 times as long as the retention time of voriconazole.

System suitability—

System performance: Suspend 0.1 g of Voriconazole in 10 mL of sodium hydroxide solution (1 in 25), add the mobile phase to make 20 mL, and allow to stand for 30 minutes. To 1 mL of this solution add the mobile phase to make 100 mL. When the procedure is run with 20 μL of this solution under the above operating conditions, the resolution between the peaks, having the relative retention times of about 0.26 and about 0.32 to voriconazole, is not less than 1.7.

System repeatability: When the test is repeated 6 times with 20 μL of the solution prepared by adding the mobile phase to 5 mL of the standard solution to make 10 mL under the above operating conditions, the relative standard deviation of the peak area of voriconazole is not more than 10.0%.

(3) Enantiomer—Dissolve 25 mg of Voriconazole in 2 mL of acetonitrile, add the mobile phase to make 50 mL, and use this solution as the sample solution. Pipet 1 mL of the sample solution, and add the mobile phase to make exactly 100 mL. Pipet 1 mL of this solution, add the mobile phase to make exactly 10 mL, and use this solution as the standard solution. Perform the test with exactly 20 μL each of the sample solution and standard solution as directed under Liquid Chromatography <*2.01*> according to the following conditions, and determine each peak area by the automatic integration method: the area of the peak of the enantiomer, having the relative retention time of about 1.3 to voriconazole, obtained from the sample solution is not larger than 1.2 times the peak area of voriconazole from the standard solution.

Operating conditions—

Detector: An ultraviolet absorption photometer (wavelength: 256 nm).

Column: A stainless steel column 4.6 mm in inside diameter and 25 cm in length, packed with 2-hydroxypropyl-β-cyclodextrinized silica gel for liquid chromatography (5 μm in particle diameter).

Column temperature: A constant temperature of about 30°C.

Mobile phase: Dissolve 0.77 g of ammonium acetate in 1000 mL of water, and adjust to pH 5.0 with acetic acid (100). To 820 mL of this solution add 180 mL of acetonitrile.

Flow rate: Adjust so that the retention time of voriconazole is about 6 minutes.

System suitability—

System performance: When the procedure is run with 20 μL of the standard solution under the above operating conditions, the number of theoretical plates and the symmetry factor of the peak of voriconazole are not less than 2500 and not more than 2.0, respectively.

System repeatability: When the test is repeated 6 times with 20 μL of a solution, prepared by adding the mobile phase to 5 mL of the standard solution to make 10 mL, under the above operating conditions, the relative standard deviation of the peak area of voriconazole is not more than 5.0%.

Water <*2.48*> Not more than 0.2% (1.0 g, volumetric titration, direct titration).

Residue on ignition <*2.44*> Not more than 0.1% (1 g, a platinum crucible).

Assay Weigh accurately about 50 mg each of Voriconazole and Voriconazole RS (separately determine the water <*2.48*> in the same manner as Voriconazole), dissolve each in the mobile phase to make exactly 100 mL. Pipet 5 mL each of these solutions, add each the mobile phase to make exactly 100 mL, and use these solutions as the sample solution and the standard solution, respectively. Perform the test with exactly 20 μL each of the sample solution and standard solution as directed under Liquid Chromatography <*2.01*> according to the following conditions, and determine the peak areas, A_T and A_S, of voriconazole in each solution.

$$\text{Amount (mg) of voriconazole } (C_{16}H_{14}F_3N_5O) = M_S \times A_T/A_S$$

M_S: Amount (mg) of Voriconazole RS taken, calculated on the anhydrous basis

Operating conditions—

Detector: An ultraviolet absorption photometer (wavelength: 256 nm).

Column: A stainless steel column 3.9 mm in inside diameter and 15 cm in length, packed with octadecylsilanized silica gel for liquid chromatography (4 μm in particle diameter).

Column temperature: A constant temperature of about 35°C.

Mobile phase: Dissolve 1.9 g of ammonium formate in 1000 mL of water, and adjust to pH 4.0 with formic acid. To 550 mL of this solution add 300 mL of methanol and 150 mL of acetonitrile.

Flow rate: Adjust so that the retention time of voriconazole is about 8 minutes.

System suitability—

System performance: When the procedure is run with 20 μL of the standard solution under the above operating conditions, the number of theoretical plates and the symmetry factor of the peak of voriconazole are not less than 3500 and not more than 1.7, respectively.

System repeatability: When the test is repeated 6 times with 20 μL of the standard solution under the above operating conditions, the relative standard deviation of the peak area of voriconazole is not more than 1.0%.

Containers and storage Containers—Well-closed containers.

Voriconazole for Injection

注射用ボリコナゾール

Voriconazole for Injection is a preparation for injection which is dissolved before use.

It contains not less than 93.0% and not more than 105.0% of the labeled amount of voriconazole ($C_{16}H_{14}F_3N_5O$: 349.31). Correct the amount obtained in the Assay with T value.

Method of preparation Prepare as directed under Injections, with Voriconazole.

Description Voriconazole for Injection is white, masses or powder.

Identification To 5 mL of the sample solution obtained in the Assay add the mobile phase in the Assay to make 25 mL. Determine the absorption spectrum of this solution as directed under Ultraviolet-visible Spectrophotometry <*2.24*>: it exhibits a maximum between 254 nm and 258 nm.

pH Being specified separately when the drug is granted approval based on the Law.

Purity **(1)** Related substances—Dissolve the content of 1 container of Voriconazole for Injection in water so that each mL contains about 10 mg of voriconazole ($C_{16}H_{14}F_3N_5O$). To 5 mL of this solution add the mobile phase to make 100 mL, and use this solution as the sample solution. Pipet 5 mL of the sample solution, and add the mobile phase to make exactly 50 mL. Pipet 2 mL of this solution, add the mobile phase to make exactly 100 mL, and use this solution as the standard solution. Perform the test with exactly 20 μL each of the sample solution and standard solution as directed under Liquid Chromatography <*2.01*> according to the following conditions. Determine each peak area by the automatic integration method: the area of the peak, having the relative retention time of about 0.26 to voriconazole, obtained from the sample solution is not larger than 2.5 times the peak area of voriconazole from the standard solution, the area of the peak, having the relative retention time of about 0.32, from the sample solution is not larger than the peak area of voriconazole from the standard solution, the area of the peak, having the relative retention time of about 0.5, from the sample solution is not larger than 2 times the peak area of voriconazole from the standard solution, and the area of the peak other than voriconazole, the peak having the relative retention time of about 0.61 and the peaks mentioned above from the sample solution is not larger than the peak area of voriconazole from the standard solution. Furthermore, the total area of the peaks other than voriconazole and the peak having the relative retention time of about 0.61 from the sample solution is not larger than 7 times the peak area of voriconazole from the standard solution. For the areas of the peaks, having the relative retention times of about 0.26, about 0.32 and about 0.5, multiply their correction factors, 0.7, 0.7 and 1.2, respectively.

Operating conditions—

Detector, column, column temperature, mobile phase and flow rate: Proceed as directed in the operating conditions in the Assay.

Time span of measurement: About 1.3 times as long as the retention time of voriconazole.

System suitability—

System performance: Suspend 0.1 g of voriconazole in 10 mL of a solution of sodium hydroxide (1 in 25), add the mobile phase to make 20 mL, and allow to stand for 30 minutes. To 1 mL of this solution add the mobile phase to make 100 mL. When the procedure is run with 20 μL of this solution under the above operating conditions, the resolution between the peaks, having the relative retention times about 0.26 and about 0.32 to voriconazole, is not less than 1.5.

System repeatability: To 5 mL of the standard solution add the mobile phase to make 10 mL. When the test is repeated 6 times with 20 μL of this solution under the above operating conditions, the relative standard deviation of the peak area of voriconazole is not more than 5.0%.

(2) Enantiomer—Dissolve the content of 1 container of Voriconazole for Injection in the mobile phase so that each mL contains about 1 mg of voriconazole ($C_{16}H_{14}F_3N_5O$). To 5 mL of this solution add the mobile phase to make 10 mL, and use this solution as the sample solution. Pipet 1 mL of the sample solution, and add the mobile phase to make exactly 100 mL. Pipet 1 mL of this solution, add the mobile phase to make exactly 10 mL, and use this solution as the standard solution. Perform the test with exactly 20 μL each of the sample solution and standard solution as directed under Liquid Chromatography <*2.01*> according to the following conditions. Determine each peak area by the automatic integration method: the area of the peak of the enantiomer, having the relative retention time of about 1.3 to voriconazole, obtained from the sample solution is not larger than 4 times the peak area of voriconazole from the standard solution.

Operating conditions—

Proceed as directed in the operating conditions in the Purity (3) under Voriconazole.

System suitability—

Proceed as directed in the system suitability in the Purity (3) under Voriconazole.

Bacterial endotoxins <*4.01*> Less than 1.5 EU/mg.

Uniformity of dosage units <*6.02*> It meets the requirement of the Mass variation test (T: 106.0%).

Foreign insoluble matter <*6.06*> Perform the test according to Method 2: it meets the requirement.

Insoluble particulate matter <*6.07*> It meets the requirement.

Sterility <*4.06*> Perform the test according to the Membrane filtration method: it meets the requirement.

Assay Take 10 containers of Voriconazole for Injection, dissolve the contents of each in the mobile phase, combine the solutions, and add the mobile phase to make exactly 1000 mL. Pipet 5 mL of this solution, add the mobile phase to make exactly 100 mL, and use this solution as the sample solution. Separately, weigh accurately about 50 mg of Voriconazole RS (separately determine the water <*2.48*> in the same manner as Voriconazole), and dissolve in the mobile phase to make exactly 50 mL. Pipet 5 mL of this solution, add the mobile phase to make exactly 50 mL, and use this solution as the standard solution. Perform the test with exactly 20 μL each of the sample solution and standard solution as directed under Liquid Chromatography <*2.01*> according to the following conditions, and determine the peak areas, A_T and A_S, of voriconazole in each solution.

Amount (mg) of voriconazole ($C_{16}H_{14}F_3N_5O$) in 1 container of Voriconazole for Injection

$= M_S \times A_T/A_S \times 4$

M_S: Amount (mg) of Voriconazole RS taken, calculated on the anhydrous basis

Operating conditions—

Detector: An ultraviolet absorption photometer (wavelength: 256 nm).

Column: A stainless steel column 3.9 mm in inside diameter and 15 cm in length, packed with octadecylsilanized silica gel for liquid chromatography (4 μm in particle diameter).

Column temperature: A constant temperature of about 35°C.

Mobile phase: Dissolve 1.9 g of ammonium formate in 1000 mL of water, and adjust to pH 4.0 with formic acid. To 550 mL of this solution add 300 mL of methanol and 150 mL of acetonitrile.

Flow rate: Adjust so that the retention time of voriconazole is about 9 minutes.

System suitability—

System performance: When the procedure is run with 20 μL of the standard solution under the above operating conditions, the number of theoretical plates and the symmetry factor of the peak of voriconazole are not less than 5000 and not more than 1.7, respectively.

System repeatability: When the test is repeated 6 times with 20 μL of the standard solution under the above operating conditions, the relative standard deviation of the peak area of voriconazole is not more than 1.0%.

Containers and storage Containers—Hermetic containers.

Voriconazole Tablets

ボリコナゾール錠

Voriconazole Tablets contain not less than 95.0% and not more than 105.0% of the labeled amount of voriconazole ($C_{16}H_{14}F_3N_5O$: 349.31).

Method of preparation Prepare as directed under Tablets, with Voriconazole.

Identification To 5 mL of the sample solution obtained in the Assay add the mobile phase in the Assay to make 25 mL. Determine the absorption spectrum of this solution as directed under Ultraviolet-visible Spectrophotometry *<2.24>*: it exhibits a maximum between 254 nm and 258 nm.

Uniformity of dosage units *<6.02>* Perform the Mass variation test, or the Content uniformity test according to the following method: it meets the requirement.

To 1 tablet of Voriconazole Tablets add small amount of water to disintegrate the tablet, add $V/2$ mL of the mobile phase, stir for 20 minutes, and add the mobile phase to make exactly V mL so that each mL contains about 1 mg of voriconazole ($C_{16}H_{14}F_3N_5O$). Centrifuge, pipet 5 mL of the supernatant liquid, add the mobile phase to make exactly 50 mL, and use this solution as the sample solution. Then, proceed as directed in the Assay.

Amount (mg) of voriconazole ($C_{16}H_{14}F_3N_5O$)

$= M_S \times A_T/A_S \times V/20$

M_S: Amount (mg) of Voriconazole RS taken, calculated on the anhydrous basis

Dissolution *<6.10>* When the test is performed at 50 revolutions per minute according to the Paddle method, using 900 mL of 1st fluid for dissolution test as the dissolution medium, the value Q in 30 minutes of Voriconazole Tablets is 80%.

Start the test with 1 tablet of Voriconazole Tablets, withdraw not less than 20 mL of the medium at the specified minute after starting the test, and filter through a membrane filter with a pore size not exceeding 0.45 μm. Discard not less than 10 mL of the first filtrate, pipet V mL of the subsequent filtrate, add the dissolution medium to make exactly V' mL so that each mL contains about 22 μg of voriconazole ($C_{16}H_{14}F_3N_5O$), and use this solution as the sample solution. Separately, weigh accurately about 18 mg of Voriconazole RS (separately determine the water *<2.48>* in the same manner as Voriconazole), dissolve in 2 mL of methanol, and add the dissolution medium to make exactly 200 mL. Pipet 10 mL of this solution, add the dissolution medium to make exactly 50 mL, and use this solution as the standard solution. Determine the absorbances, A_T and A_S, at 256 nm of the sample solution and standard solution as directed under Ultraviolet-visible Spectrophotometry *<2.24>*, using the dissolution medium as the blank.

Dissolution rate (%) with respect to the labeled amount of voriconazole ($C_{16}H_{14}F_3N_5O$)

$= M_S \times A_T/A_S \times V'/V \times 1/C \times 90$

M_S: Amount (mg) of Voriconazole RS taken, calculated on the anhydrous basis

C: Labeled amount (mg) of voriconazole ($C_{16}H_{14}F_3N_5O$) in 1 tablet

Assay Weigh accurately the mass of not less than 20 Voriconazole Tablets, and powder. Weigh accurately a portion of the powder, equivalent to about 50 mg of voriconazole ($C_{16}H_{14}F_3N_5O$), add the mobile phase, stir, and add the mobile phase to make exactly 50 mL. Centrifuge, pipet 5 mL of the supernatant liquid, add the mobile phase to make exactly 50 mL, and use this solution as the sample solution. Separately, weigh accurately about 20 mg of Voriconazole RS (separately determine the water *<2.48>* in the same manner as Voriconazole), and dissolve in the mobile phase to make exactly 200 mL, and use this solution as the standard solution. Perform the test with exactly 20 μL each of the sample solution and standard solution as directed under Liquid Chromatography *<2.01>* according to the following conditions, and determine the peak areas, A_T and A_S, of voriconazole in each solution.

Amount (mg) of voriconazole ($C_{16}H_{14}F_3N_5O$)

$= M_S \times A_T/A_S \times 5/2$

M_S: Amount (mg) of Voriconazole RS taken, calculated on the anhydrous basis

Operating conditions—

Detector: An ultraviolet absorption photometer (wavelength: 256 nm).

Column: A stainless steel column 3.9 mm in inside diameter and 15 cm in length, packed with octadecylsilanized silica gel for liquid chromatography (4 μm in particle diameter).

Column temperature: A constant temperature of about 35°C.

Mobile phase: Dissolve 1.9 g of ammonium formate in 1000 mL of water, and adjust to pH 4.0 with formic acid. To 550 mL of this solution add 300 mL of methanol and 150 mL of acetonitrile.

Flow rate: Adjust so that the retention time of voriconazole is about 9 minutes.

System suitability—

System performance: When the procedure is run with 20 μL of the standard solution under the above operating conditions, the number of theoretical plates and the symmetry factor of the peak of voriconazole are not less than 5000 and not more than 1.7, respectively.

System repeatability: When the test is repeated 6 times with 20 μL of the standard solution under the above operating conditions, the relative standard deviation of the peak area of voriconazole is not more than 1.0%.

Containers and storage Containers—Tight containers.

Warfarin Potassium

ワルファリンカリウム

and enantiomer

$C_{19}H_{15}KO_4$: 346.42
Monopotassium (1*RS*)-2-oxo-3-(3-oxo-1-phenylbutyl)chromen-4-olate
[*2610-86-8*]

Warfarin Potassium, when dried, contains not less than 98.0% and not more than 102.0% of warfarin potassium ($C_{19}H_{15}KO_4$).

Description Warfarin Potassium occurs as a white crystalline powder.

It is very soluble in water, and freely soluble in ethanol (95).

It dissolves in sodium hydroxide TS.

The pH of a solution prepared by dissolving 1.0 g of Warfarin Potassium in 100 mL of water is between 7.2 and 8.3.

It is colored to light yellow by light.

A solution of Warfarin Potassium (1 in 10) shows no optical rotation.

Identification **(1)** Determine the absorption spectrum of a solution of Warfarin Potassium in 0.02 mol/L potassium hydroxide TS (1 in 100,000) as directed under Ultraviolet-visible Spectrophotometry <*2.24*>, and compare the spectrum with the Reference Spectrum or the spectrum of a solution of Warfarin Potassium RS prepared in the same manner as the sample solution: both spectra exhibit similar intensities of absorption at the same wavelengths.

(2) Determine the infrared absorption spectrum of Warfarin Potassium, previously dried, as directed in the potassium bromide disk method under Infrared Spectrophotometry <*2.25*>, and compare the spectrum with the Reference Spectrum or the spectrum of Warfarin Potassium RS: both spectra exhibit similar intensities of absorption at the same wave numbers.

(3) A solution of Warfarin Potassium (1 in 250) responds to Qualitative Tests <*1.09*> (1) for potassium salt.

Purity **(1)** Alkaline colored substances—Dissolve 1.0 g of Warfarin Potassium in a solution of sodium hydroxide (1 in 20) to make exactly 10 mL, and determine the absorbance at 385 nm within 15 minutes as directed under Ultraviolet-visible Spectrophotometry <*2.24*>, using a solution of sodium hydroxide (1 in 20) as a blank: it does not exceed 0.20.

(2) Heavy metals <*1.07*>—Dissolve 2.0 g of Warfarin Potassium in 30 mL of ethanol (95), add 2 mL of dilute acetic acid and ethanol (95) to make 50 mL. Perform the test using this solution as the test solution. Prepare the control solution with 2.0 mL of Standard Lead Solution, 2 mL of dilute acetic acid and ethanol (95) to make 50 mL (not more than 10 ppm).

(3) Related substances—Dissolve 0.10 g of Warfarin Potassium in 100 mL of a mixture of water and methanol (3:1), and use this solution as the sample solution. Pipet 1 mL of the sample solution, add the mixture of water and methanol (3:1) to make exactly 100 mL, and use this solution as the standard solution. Perform the test with exactly 20 μL each of the sample solution and standard solution as directed under Liquid Chromatography <*2.01*> according to the following conditions, and determine each peak area by the automatic integration method: each peak area other than warfarin obtained from the sample solution is not larger than 1/10 times the peak area of warfarin from the standard solution, and the total area of the peaks other than warfarin from the sample solution is not larger than 1/2 times the peak area of warfarin from the standard solution.

Operating conditions—

Detector, column, column temperature, mobile phase, and flow rate: Proceed as directed in the operating conditions in the Assay.

Time span of measurement: About 2 times as long as the retention time of warfarin, beginning after the solvent peak.

System suitability—

Test for required detectability: To exactly 1 mL of the standard solution add the mixture of water and methanol (3:1) to make exactly 20 mL. Confirm that the peak area of warfarin obtained with 20 μL of this solution is equivalent to 3.5 to 6.5% of that with 20 μL of the standard solution.

System performance: Dissolve 20 mg of propyl parahydroxybenzoate in 50 mL of methanol, and add water to make 200 mL. To 5 mL of this solution add 4 mL of a solution of Warfarin Potassium in the mixture of water and methanol (3:1) (1 in 2000), and add the mixture of water and methanol (3:1) to make 100 mL. When the procedure is run with 20 μL of this solution under the above operating conditions, propyl parahydroxybenzoate and warfarin are eluted in this order with the resolution between these peaks being not less than 7 and the symmetry factor is not more than 1.5.

System repeatability: When the test is repeated 6 times with 20 μL of the standard solution under the above operating conditions, the relative standard deviation of the peak area of warfarin is not more than 2.0%.

Loss on drying <*2.41*> Not more than 4.5% (1 g, 105°C, 3 hours).

Assay Weigh accurately about 25 mg each of Warfarin Potassium and Warfarin Potassium RS, previously dried, and separately dissolve in the mixture of water and methanol (3:1) to make exactly 50 mL. Pipet 10 mL each of these solutions, add the mixture of water and methanol (3:1) to make exactly 50 mL, and use these solutions as the sample solution and standard solution. Perform the test with exactly 20 μL each of the sample solution and standard solution as directed under Liquid Chromatography <*2.01*> according to the following conditions, and determine the peak areas, A_T and A_S, of warfarin in each solution.

$$\text{Amount (mg) of warfarin potassium } (C_{19}H_{15}KO_4) = M_S \times A_T/A_S$$

M_S: Amount (mg) of Warfarin Potassium RS taken

Operating conditions—

Detector: An ultraviolet absorption photometer (wavelength: 260 nm).

Column: A stainless steel column 4.6 mm in inside diameter and 25 cm in length, packed with cyanopropylsilanized silica gel for liquid chromatography (5 μm in particle diameter).

Column temperature: A constant temperature of about 40°C.

Mobile phase: A mixture of water, acetonitrile and acetic acid (100) (68:32:1).

Flow rate: Adjust so that the retention time of warfarin is about 10 minutes.

System suitability—

System performance: When the procedure is run with 20 μL of the standard solution under the above operating conditions, the number of theoretical plates and the symmetry factor of the peak of warfarin are not less than 8000 and not more than 1.5, respectively.

System repeatability: When the test is repeated 6 times with 20 μL of the standard solution under the above operating conditions, the relative standard deviation of the peak area of warfarin is not more than 1.0%.

Containers and storage Containers—Tight containers.
Storage—Light-resistant.

Warfarin Potassium Tablets

ワルファリンカリウム錠

Warfarin Potassium Tablets contain not less than 95.0% and not more than 105.0% of the labeled amount of warfarin potassium ($C_{19}H_{15}KO_4$: 346.42).

Method of preparation Prepare as directed under Tablets, with Warfarin Potassium.

Identification **(1)** Determine the absorption spectrum of the solution T_2 obtained in the Assay, using 0.02 mol/L potassium hydroxide TS as the blank, as directed under Ultraviolet-visible Spectrophotometry <2.24>: it exhibits a maximum between 306 nm and 310 nm, and a minimum between 258 nm and 262 nm. Separately, determine the absorption spectrum of the solution T_1 obtained in the Assay, using 0.02 mol/L hydrochloric acid TS as the blank, as directed under Ultraviolet-visible Spectrophotometry <2.24>: it exhibits maxima between 281 nm and 285 nm and between 303 nm and 307 nm, and a minimum between 243 nm and 247 nm.

(2) Weigh a quantity of Warfarin Potassium Tablets, equivalent to 0.01 g of Warfarin Potassium, add 10 mL of acetone, shake, and filter. Heat the filtrate on a water bath to evaporate the acetone. To the residue add 10 mL of diethyl ether and 2 mL of dilute hydrochloric acid, and shake: the aqueous layer responds to Qualitative Tests <1.09> (1) for potassium salt.

Uniformity of dosage units <6.02> Perform the test according to the following method: it meets the requirement of the Content uniformity test.

Powder 1 tablet of Warfarin Potassium Tablets, add 40 mL of water, and shake vigorously for 30 minutes. Add water to make exactly V mL of this solution containing about 20 μg of warfarin potassium ($C_{19}H_{15}KO_4$) per ml. Filter this solution, discard the first 5 mL of the filtrate, and use the subsequent filtrate as the sample solution. Separately, weigh accurately about 40 mg of Warfarin Potassium RS, previously dried at 105°C for 3 hours, and dissolve in water to make exactly 100 mL. Pipet 5 mL of this solution, add water to make exactly 100 mL, and use this solution as the standard solution. Pipet 20 mL each of the sample solution and standard solution, add 0.05 mol/L hydrochloric acid TS to make exactly 25 mL, and use these solutions as the solution T_1 and the solution S_1, respectively. Separately, pipet 20 mL each of the sample solution and standard solution, add 0.05 mol/L potassium hydroxide TS to make exactly 25 mL, and use these solutions as the solution T_2 and the solution S_2, respectively. Determine the absorbances, A_T and A_S, of the solution T_1 and the solution S_1 at 272 nm as directed under Ultraviolet-visible Spectrophotometry <2.24>, using the solution T_2 and the solution S_2 as the blank, respectively.

$$\text{Amount (mg) of warfarin potassium } (C_{19}H_{15}KO_4) = M_S \times A_T/A_S \times V/2000$$

M_S: Amount (mg) of Warfarin Potassium RS taken

Dissolution <6.10> When the test is performed at 50 revolutions per minute according to the Paddle method, using 900 mL of water as the dissolution medium, the dissolution rates in 15 minutes of 0.5-mg, 1-mg and 2-mg tablet and in 30 minutes of 5-mg tablet of Warfarin Potassium Tablets are not less than 80%.

Start the test with 1 tablet of Warfarin Potassium Tablets, withdraw not less than 20 mL of the medium at the specified minute after starting the test, and filter through a membrane filter with a pore size not exceeding 0.45 μm. Discard not less than 10 mL of the first filtrate, pipet V mL of the subsequent filtrate, add water to make exactly V' mL so that each mL contains about 0.56 μg of warfarin potassium ($C_{19}H_{15}KO_4$), and use this solution as the sample solution. Separately, weigh accurately about 22 mg of Warfarin Potassium RS, previously dried at 105°C for 3 hours, and dissolve in water to make exactly 100 mL. Pipet 5 mL of this solution, and add water to make exactly 100 mL. Pipet 5 mL of this solution, add water to make exactly 100 mL, and use this solution as the standard solution. Perform the test with exactly 100 μL each of the sample solution and standard solution as directed under Liquid Chromatography <2.01> according to the following conditions, and determine the peak areas, A_T and A_S, of warfarin in each solution.

$$\text{Dissolution rate (\%) with respect to the labeled amount of warfarin potassium } (C_{19}H_{15}KO_4) = M_S \times A_T/A_S \times V'/V \times 1/C \times 9/4$$

M_S: Amount (mg) of Warfarin Potassium RS taken
C: Labeled amount (mg) of warfarin potassium ($C_{19}H_{15}KO_4$) in 1 tablet

Operating conditions—

Detector: An ultraviolet absorption photometer (wavelength: 283 nm).

Column: A stainless steel column 4.6 mm in inside diameter and 15 cm in length, packed with octadecylsilanized silica gel for liquid chromatography (5 μm in particle diameter).

Column temperature: A constant temperature of about 35°C.

Mobile phase: A mixture of methanol, water and phosphoric acid (700:300:1).

Flow rate: Adjust so that the retention time of warfarin is about 6 minutes.

System suitability—

System performance: When the procedure is run with 100 μL of the standard solution under the above conditions, the number of theoretical plates and the symmetry factor of the peak of warfarin are not less than 2000 and not more than 2.0, respectively.

System repeatability: When the test is repeated 6 times with 100 μL of the standard solution under the above operating conditions, the relative standard deviation of the peak area of warfarin is not more than 2.0%.

Assay Weigh accurately and powder not less than 20 Warfarin Potassium Tablets. Weigh accurately a portion of the powder, equivalent to about 4 mg of warfarin potassium ($C_{19}H_{15}KO_4$), add 80 mL of water, shake vigorously for 15 minutes, and add water to make exactly 100 mL. Filter this solution, discard the first 10 mL of the filtrate, and use the subsequent filtrate as the sample solution. Separately, weigh accurately about 80 mg of Warfarin Potassium RS, previously dried at 105°C for 3 hours, and dissolve in water to make exactly 100 mL. Pipet 5 mL of this solution, add water to make exactly 100 mL, and use this solution as the standard solution. Pipet 10 mL each of the sample solution and standard solution, add 0.02 mol/L hydrochloric acid TS to make exactly 20 mL, and use these solutions as the solution T_1 and the solution S_1, respectively. Separately, pipet 10 mL each of the sample solution and standard solution, add 0.02 mol/L potassium hydroxide TS to make exactly 20 mL, and use these solutions as the solution T_2 and the solution S_2, respectively. Determine the absorbances, A_T and A_S, of the solution T_1 and the solution S_1 at 272 nm as directed under Ultraviolet-visible Spectrophotometry <*2.24*>, using the solution T_2 and the solution S_2 as the blank, respectively.

Amount (mg) of warfarin potassium ($C_{19}H_{15}KO_4$)
$= M_S \times A_T/A_S \times 1/20$

M_S: Amount (mg) of Warfarin Potassium RS taken

Containers and storage Containers—Tight containers.

Storage—Light-resistant.

Water

常水

H_2O: 18.02

Water must meet the Quality Standards of Drinking water provided under the Article 4 of the Water Supply Law (the Ministry of Health, Labour and Welfare Ministerial Ordinance No.101, 2003). In the case that Water is prepared at individual facilities using well water or industrial water as source water, it must meet the following additional requirement as well as the Quality Standards of Drinking water.

Purity Ammonium <*1.02*>—Perform the test with 30 mL of Water as directed under Ammonium Limit Test. Prepare the control solution as follows: to 0.15 mL of Standard Ammonium Solution add water for ammonium limit test to make 30 mL (not more than 0.05 mg/L).

Purified Water

精製水

Purified Water is prepared from Water by ion-exchange, distillation, reverse osmosis or ultrafiltration, or by a combination of these processes.

It must be used immediately after preparation. However, it may be stored temporarily, if adequate countermeasures for preventing microbial proliferation are taken.

Description Purified Water is a clear and colorless liquid, having no odor.

Purity Total organic carbon <*2.59*>—Not more than 0.50 mg/L.

Conductivity <*2.51*> When the test is performed according to the following method, the conductivity (25°C) is not more than 2.1 $\mu S \cdot cm^{-1}$.

Transfer a suitable amount of Purified Water to a beaker, and stir the water specimen. Adjust the temperature to 25 ± 1°C, and begin agitating the water specimen vigorously, while observing its conductivity periodically. When the change in conductivity becomes not greater than 0.1 $\mu S \cdot cm^{-1}$ per 5 minutes, adopt the observed value as the conductivity of the water specimen.

Purified Water in Containers

精製水(容器入り)

Purified Water in Containers is prepared from Purified Water by introducing it in a tight container.

It is allowable to describe it as "Purified Water" on the label.

Description Purified Water in Containers is a clear and colorless liquid, having no odor.

Purity Potassium permanganate-reducing substances—To 100 mL of Purified Water in Containers add 10 mL of dilute sulfuric acid, boil, then add 0.10 mL of 0.02 mol/L potassium permanganate VS, and boil again for 10 minutes: the red color of the solution does not disappear.

Conductivity <*2.51*> When the test is performed according to the following method, the conductivity (25°C) is not more than 25 $\mu S \cdot cm^{-1}$ for containers with a nominal volume of 10 mL or less, and not more than 5 $\mu S \cdot cm^{-1}$ for containers with a nominal volume greater than 10 mL.

Transfer a suitable amount of Purified Water in Containers to a beaker, and stir the water specimen. Adjust the temperature to 25 ± 1°C, and begin agitating the water specimen vigorously, while observing its conductivity periodically. When the change in conductivity becomes not greater than 0.1 $\mu S \cdot cm^{-1}$ per 5 minutes, adopt the observed value as the conductivity of the water specimen.

Microbial limit <*4.05*> The acceptance criteria of TAMC is 10^2 CFU/mL. Perform the test using soybean-casein digest agar medium.

Containers and storage Containers—Tight containers.

Sterile Purified Water in Containers

滅菌精製水(容器入り)

Sterile Purified Water in Containers is prepared from Purified Water by introducing it into a hermetic container, sealing up the container, then sterilizing the product, or by making it sterile using a suitable method, introducing the sterilized water into a sterile hermetic container by applying aseptic manipulation, then sealing up the container.

Description Sterile Purified Water in Containers is a clear and colorless liquid, having no odor.

Purity Potassium permanganate-reducing substances—To 100 mL of Sterile Purified Water in Containers add 10 mL of dilute sulfuric acid, boil, then add 0.10 mL of 0.02 mol/L potassium permanganate VS, and boil again for 10 minutes: the red color of the solution does not disappear.

Conductivity <*2.51*> When the test is performed according to the following method, the conductivity (25°C) is not more than 25 $\mu S \cdot cm^{-1}$ for containers with a nominal volume of 10 mL or less, and not more than 5 $\mu S \cdot cm^{-1}$ for containers with a nominal volume greater than 10 mL.

Transfer a suitable amount of Sterile Purified Water in Containers to a beaker, and stir the water specimen. Adjust the temperature to 25 ± 1°C, and begin agitating the water specimen vigorously, while observing its conductivity periodically. When the change in conductivity becomes not greater than 0.1 $\mu S \cdot cm^{-1}$ per 5 minutes, adopt the observed value as the conductivity of the water specimen.

Sterility <*4.06*> It meets the requirements.

Containers and storage Containers—Hermetic containers. Plastic containers for aqueous injections can be used in place of hermetic containers.

Water for Injection

注射用水

Water for Injection is prepared by distillation or by reverse osmosis and/or ultrafiltration, either: from the water which is obtained by appropriate pretreatments such as ion-exchange or reverse osmosis on Water: or from Purified Water.

When Water for Injection is prepared by the reverse osmosis and/or ultrafiltration (methods for refining water by using a reverse osmosis membrane module, an ultrafiltration membrane module capable of removing substances having molecular masses of 6,000 and above, or a module using both types of membranes), care must be taken to avoid microbial contamination of the water processing system, and to provide water with equivalent quality to that prepared by distillation consistently.

Water for Injection must be used immediately after preparation. However, it may be stored temporarily, if adequate countermeasures able to prevent microbial proliferation stringently, such as circulating it in a loop at a high temperature, are established.

Description Water for Injection is a clear and colorless liquid, having no odor.

Purity Total organic carbon <*2.59*>—Not more than 0.50 mg/L.

Conductivity <*2.51*> When the test is performed according to the following method, the conductivity (25°C) is not more than 2.1 $\mu S \cdot cm^{-1}$.

Transfer a suitable amount of Water for Injection to a beaker, and stir the water specimen. Adjust the temperature to 25 ± 1°C, and begin agitating the water specimen vigorously, while observing its conductivity periodically. When the change in conductivity becomes not greater than 0.1 $\mu S \cdot cm^{-1}$ per 5 minutes, adopt the observed value as the conductivity of the water specimen.

Bacterial endotoxins <*4.01*> Less than 0.25 EU/mL.

Sterile Water for Injection in Containers

注射用水(容器入り)

Sterile Water for Injection in Containers is prepared from Water for Injection by introducing it into a hermetic container, sealing up the container, then sterilizing the product, or by making it sterile using a suitable method, introducing the sterilized water into a sterile hermetic container by applying aseptic manipulation, then sealing up the container.

It is allowable to describe it as ''Water for Injection'' on the label.

For Sterile Water for Injection in Containers prepared from Water for Injection obtained by distillation, an alternative name of ''Distilled Water for Injection'' may be used.

Description Sterile Water for Injection in Containers is a clear and colorless liquid, having no odor.

Purity Potassium permanganate-reducing substances—To 100 mL of Sterile Water for Injection in Containers add 10 mL of dilute sulfuric acid, boil, then add 0.10 mL of 0.02 mol/L potassium permanganate VS, and boil again for 10 minutes: the red color of the solution does not disappear.

Conductivity <*2.51*> When the test is performed according to the following method, the conductivity (25°C) is not more than 25 $\mu S \cdot cm^{-1}$ for containers with a nominal volume of 10 mL or less, and not more than 5 $\mu S \cdot cm^{-1}$ for containers with a nominal volume greater than 10 mL.

Transfer a suitable amount of Sterile Water for Injection in Containers to a beaker, and stir the water specimen. Adjust the temperature to 25 ± 1°C, and begin agitating the water specimen vigorously, while observing its conductivity periodically. When the change in conductivity becomes not greater than 0.1 $\mu S \cdot cm^{-1}$ per 5 minutes, adopt the observed value as the conductivity of the water specimen.

Bacterial endotoxins <*4.01*> Less than 0.25 EU/mL.

Foreign insoluble matter <*6.06*> Perform the test according to Method 1: it meets the requirement.

Insoluble particulate matter <*6.07*> It meets the requirement.

Sterility <*4.06*> It meets the requirement.

Containers and storage Containers—Hermetic containers. Plastic containers for aqueous injections can be used in place of hermetic containers.

White Ointment

白色軟膏

Method of preparation

White Beeswax	50 g
Sorbitan Sesquioleate	20 g
White Petrolatum	a sufficient quantity
To make	1000 g

Prepare as directed under Ointments, with the above materials.

Description White Ointment is white in color. It has a slight, characteristic odor.

Containers and storage Containers—Tight containers.

Whole Human Blood

人全血液

Whole Human Blood is a liquid for injection which is prepared by mixing human blood cells and an anticoagulant solution for storage.

It conforms to the requirements of Whole Human Blood in the Minimum Requirements for Biological Products.

Description Whole Human Blood is a deep red liquid from which the erythrocytes settle upon standing, leaving a yellow supernatant layer. A gray layer which mainly consists of leucocytes may appear on the surface of the settled erythrocyte layer. The supernatant layer may become turbid in the presence of fat, or may show the faint color of hemoglobin.

Wine

ブドウ酒

Wine is an alcoholic liquid obtained by fermenting the juice of the fruits of *Vitis vinifera* Linné (*Vitaceae*) or allied plants.

It contains not less than 11.0 vol% and not more than 14.0 vol% of ethanol (C_2H_6O: 46.07) (by specific gravity), and not less than 0.10 w/v% and not more than 0.40 w/v% of L-tartaric acid ($C_4H_6O_6$: 150.09).

It contains no artificial sweetener and no artificial coloring agent.

Description Wine is a light yellow or reddish purple to red-purple liquid. It has a characteristic and aromatic odor. It has a slightly astringent and faintly irritating taste.

Optical rotation <*2.49*> Boil 160 mL of Wine, neutralize with potassium hydroxide TS, and concentrate to 80 mL on a water bath. Cool, dilute with water to 160 mL, add 16 mL of lead subacetate TS, shake well, and filter. To 100 mL of the filtrate add 10 mL of a saturated solution of sodium sulfate decahydrate, shake well, filter, and use the filtrate as the sample solution. Allow 20 mL of the sample solution to stand for 24 hours, add 0.5 g of activated charcoal, shake, stopper, and allow to stand for 10 minutes. Filter, and observe the optical rotation of the filtrate in a 200-mm cell. Multiply the optical rotation observed by 1.21, and designate as the optical rotation of Wine: it is between −0.3° and +0.3°.

Specific gravity <*2.56*> d^{20}_{20}: 0.990 – 1.010

Purity (1) Total acid [as L-tartaric acid ($C_4H_6O_6$)]—To exactly 10 mL of Wine add 250 mL of freshly boiled and cooled water, and titrate <*2.50*> with 0.1 mol/L sodium hydroxide VS (indicator: 1 mL of phenolphthalein TS).

Each mL of 0.1 mol/L sodium hydroxide VS
= 7.504 mg of $C_4H_6O_6$

Total acid is not less than 0.40 w/v% and not more than 0.80 w/v%.

(2) Volatile acid [as acetic acid ($C_2H_4O_2$: 60.05)]—Transfer 100 mL of Wine to a beaker, add 1 mL of 1 mol/L sodium hydroxide VS and the same volume of 1 mol/L sodium hydroxide VS as that of 0.1 mol/L sodium hydroxide VS titrated in (1) to make the solution alkaline, and concentrate to 50 mL on a water bath. Cool, add water to make 100 mL, transfer to a 1000-mL distillation flask, containing previously added 100 g of sodium chloride. Wash the beaker with 100 mL of water, and combine the washings in the distillation flask. Add 5 mL of a solution of L-tartaric acid (3 in 20), and distil with steam cautiously to maintain the volume of the solution in the flask until 450 mL of the distillate is obtained for 45 minutes. Dilute the distillate to exactly 500 mL with water, and use this solution as the sample solution. Titrate <*2.50*> a 250-mL portion of the sample solution with 0.1 mol/L sodium hydroxide VS (indicator: 5 drops of phenolphthalein TS). Perform a blank determination in the same manner, and make any necessary correction.

Each mL of 0.1 mol/L sodium hydroxide VS
= 6.005 mg of $C_2H_4O_2$

The volatile acid is not more than 0.15 w/v%.

(3) Sulfur dioxide—Stopper a 750-mL round-bottomed flask with a stopper having two holes. Through one hole, insert a glass tube A extending nearly to the bottom of the flask. Through the other hole, insert a glass tube B ending to the neck of the flask. Connect the tube B to a Liebig's condenser, and the end of the condenser to a joint of which inner diameter is 5 mm at the lower end. Connect the other end of the joint with a holed rubber stopper to a U tube having three bulbs as shown in the Figure. Pass carbon dioxide washed with a solution of potassium permanganate (3 in 100) through the tube A. Displace the air in the apparatus by carbon dioxide, and place 50 mL of a freshly prepared and diluted starch TS (1 in 5) and 1 g of potassium iodide in the U tube. From the other end of the U tube, add 1 to 2 drops of 0.01 mol/L iodine VS from a burette. While passing carbon dioxide, remove the stopper of the flask a little, add exactly 25 mL of Wine, 180 mL of freshly boiled and cooled water, 0.2 g of tannic acid, and 30 mL of phosphoric acid, and stopper again. Pass carbon dioxide for further 15 minutes, heat the distillation flask with caution so that 40 to 50 drops of the distillate may be obtained in 1 minute. When the color of starch TS in the U tube is discharged, add 0.01 mol/L iodine VS dropwise from a burette so that the color of the starch TS remains light blue to blue during the distillation. Read the volume of 0.01 mol/L iodine VS consumed when exactly 60 minutes have passed after the beginning of distillation. In this case, however, the coloration of starch TS produced by 1 drop of 0.01 mol/L iodine VS should persist at least for 1 minute.

Each mL of 0.01 mol/L iodine VS = 0.6406 mg of SO_2

The amount of sulfur dioxide (SO_2: 64.06) does not exceed 7.5 mg.

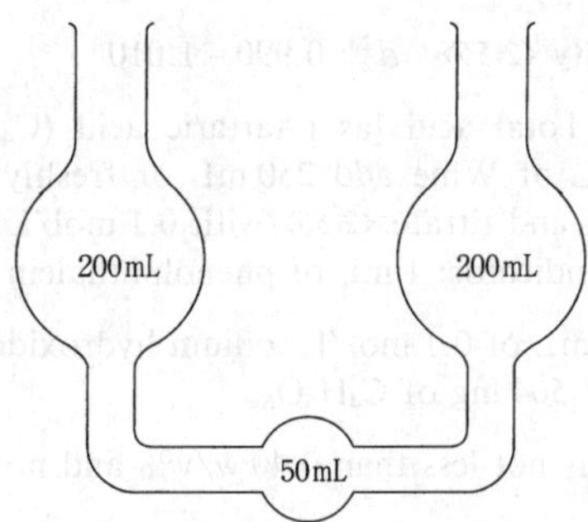

(4) Total sulfuric acid—Transfer 10 mL of Wine to a beaker, boil, and add 50 mL of a solution prepared by dissolving 5.608 g of barium chloride dihydrate in 50 mL of hydrochloric acid and water to make 1000 mL. Cover the beaker, and heat on a water bath for 2 hours, supplying the water lost by distillation. Cool, centrifuge, and decant the supernatant liquid in another beaker. To this solution add 1 to 2 drops of dilute sulfuric acid, and allow to stand for 1 hour: a white precipitate is formed.

(5) Arsenic *<1.11>*—Evaporate 10 mL of Wine on a water bath to dryness. Prepare the test solution with the residue according to Method 3, and perform the test (not more than 0.2 ppm).

(6) Glycerin—Pipet 100 mL of Wine into a 150-mL porcelain dish, and concentrate on a water bath to 10 mL. Add 1 g of sea sand (No. 1), and make the solution strongly alkaline by adding a solution prepared by dissolving 4 g of calcium hydroxide in 6 mL of water. Heat on a water bath with constant stirring and pushing down any material adhering to the wall of the dish until the contents of the dish become soft masses. Cool, add 5 mL of ethanol (99.5), and grind to a gruel-like substance. Heat on a water bath, add 10 to 20 mL of ethanol (99.5) while agitating, boil, and transfer to a 100-mL volumetric flask. Wash the dish with seven 10-mL portions of hot ethanol (99.5), combine the washings with the contents of the flask, cool, and add ethanol (99.5) to make exactly 100 mL. Filter through a dry filter paper, evaporate 90 mL of the filtrate on a water bath, taking care not to boil the solution during the evaporation. Dissolve the residue in a small amount of ethanol (99.5), transfer to a 50-mL glass-stoppered volumetric cylinder, wash with several portions of ethanol (99.5), and add the washings to the solution in the cylinder to make 15 mL. Add three 7.5-mL portions of dehydrated diethyl ether, shake vigorously each time, and allow to stand. When the solution becomes quite clear, transfer to a tared, flat weighing bottle. Wash the volumetric cylinder with 5 mL of a mixture of dehydrated diethyl ether and ethanol (99.5) (3:2). Transfer the washings to the weighing bottle, and evaporate carefully on a water bath. When the liquid becomes sticky, dry at 105°C for 1 hour, and cool in a desiccator (silica gel), and weigh: the mass of the residue is not less than 0.45 g and not more than 0.90 g.

(7) Reducing sugars—To a 25-mL portion of the sample solution obtained in the Optical rotation add 50 mL of boiling Fehling's TS, and heat for exactly 2 minutes. Filter the separated precipitates by a tared glass filter by suction, wash successively with hot water, with ethanol (95) and with diethyl ether, and continue to dry the precipitates by suction. Heat the filter gently at first, and then strongly until the precipitates become completely black. Cool the precipitates in a desiccator (silica gel), and weigh as copper (II) oxide: the mass of cupric oxide does not exceed 0.325 g.

(8) Sucrose—Transfer a 50-mL portion of the sample solution obtained in the Optical rotation to a 100-mL flask, neutralize with diluted hydrochloric acid (1 in 30), followed by further addition of 5 mL of diluted hydrochloric acid (1 in 30). Heat in a water bath for 30 minutes, cool, neutralize with a solution of potassium hydroxide (1 in 100), add 4 drops of sodium carbonate TS, filter into a 100-mL volumetric flask, wash with water, combine the washings with the filtrate, and add water to make 100 mL. To 25 mL of this solution add 50 mL of boiling Fehling's TS, and proceed as directed in (7), and weigh as copper (II) oxide. From the number obtained by multiplying the mass (g) of copper (II) oxide by 2, deduct the amount (g) of copper (II) oxide determined in (7), and multiply again the number so obtained by 1.2: the number obtained does not exceed 0.104 (g).

(9) Benzoic acid, cinnamic acid and salicylic acid—Transfer exactly 50 mL of the sample solution obtained in (2) to a separator, add 10 g of sodium chloride and 2 mL of dilute hydrochloric acid, and extract with three 10-mL portions of diethyl ether. Combine the diethyl ether extracts, wash with two 5-mL portions of water, and extract with three 10-mL portions of 0.1 mol/L sodium hydroxide VS. Combine the alkaline extracts, evaporate the diethyl ether by warming on a water bath, cool, neutralize with 1 mol/L hydrochloric acid VS, and add 5 mL of potassium chloride-hydrochloric acid buffer solution and water to make exactly 50 mL. Perform the test as directed under Ultraviolet-visible Spectrophotometry *<2.24>* with this solution, using a solution prepared in the same manner instead of the sample solution as the blank: the absorbance does not exceed 0.15 at a wavelength between 220 nm and 340 nm.

(10) Boric acid—Transfer 50 mL of Wine to a porcelain dish, add 5 mL of sodium carbonate TS, evaporate on a water bath to dryness, and ignite: a half portion of the residue does not respond to Qualitative Tests *<1.09>* (1) for borate. Dissolve another half portion of the residue in 5 mL of hydrochloric acid: it does not respond to Qualitative Tests *<1.09>* (2) for borate.

(11) Methanol—Wine meets the requirements of Methanol Test *<1.12>*, when proceeding with exactly 1 mL of ethanol layer obtained by Method 1 of Alcohol Number Determination *<1.01>* and distilling without adding water after shaking with 0.5 g of calcium carbonate.

(12) Formaldehyde—To 25 mL of Wine add 5 g of sodium chloride and 0.2 g of L-tartaric acid, distil, and obtain 15 mL of the distillate. To 5 mL of the distillate add 5 mL of acetyl acetone TS, mix, and heat on a water bath for 10 minutes: the solution has no more color than that of the following control solution.

Control solution: Using 5 mL of water instead of the distillate, perform the test in the same manner.

Extract content 1.9 - 3.5 w/v% Pipet 25 mL of Wine to a 200-mL tared beaker containing 10 g of sea sand (No. 1), previously dried at 105°C for 2.5 hours, and evaporate to dryness on a water bath. Dry the residue at 105°C for 2 hours, cool in a desiccator (silica gel), and weigh.

Total ash 0.13 - 0.40 w/v% Pipet 50 mL of Wine to a tared porcelain dish, and evaporate to dryness on a water bath. Ignite the residue to the constant mass, cool, and weigh.

Assay **(1)** Ethanol—Pipet Wine into a 100-mL volumetric flask at 15°C, transfer to a 300- to 500-mL flask, and wash this volumetric flask with two 15-mL portions of water. Add the washings to the sample in the flask, connect the flask to a distillation tube having a trap, and distil using the volumetric flask as a receiver. When about 80 mL of the distillate is obtained (it takes about 20 minutes), stop the distillation, allow to stand in water at 15°C for 30 minutes, and add water to make exactly 100 mL. Shake well, and determine the specific gravity at 15°C under Specific Gravity <*2.56*> (Method 3 may be used): the specific gravity d^{15}_{15} is between 0.98217 and 0.98547.

(2) L-Tartaric acid—Pipet 100 mL of Wine, add 2 mL of acetic acid (100), 0.5 mL of a solution of potassium acetate (1 in 5) and 15 g of powdered potassium chloride, and shake vigorously to dissolve as much as possible. Add 10 mL of ethanol (95), rub the inner wall of the beaker strongly for 1 minute to induce the crystallization, and allow to stand between 0°C and 5°C for more than 15 hours. Filter the crystals by suction, wash successively the beaker and the crystals with 3-mL portions of a solution prepared by dissolving 15 g of powdered potassium chloride in 120 mL of diluted ethanol (1 in 6), and repeat the washings five times. Transfer the crystals together with the filter paper to a beaker, wash the filter with 50 mL of hot water, combine the washings in the beaker, and dissolve the crystals by heating. Titrate <*2.50*> the solution with 0.2 mol/L sodium hydroxide VS immediately (indicator: 1 mL of phenolphthalein TS). The number obtained by adding 0.75 to the amount (mL) of 0.2 mol/L sodium hydroxide VS consumed represents the amount (mL) of 0.2 mol/L sodium hydroxide VS consumed.

Each mL of 0.2 mol/L sodium hydroxide VS
= 30.02 mg of $C_4H_6O_6$

Containers and storage Containers—Tight containers.

Xylitol

キシリトール

$C_5H_{12}O_5$: 152.15
meso-Xylitol
[87-99-0]

Xylitol, when dried, contains not less than 98.0% of xylitol ($C_5H_{12}O_5$).

Description Xylitol occurs as white, crystals or powder. It is odorless and has a sweet taste.

It is very soluble in water, slightly soluble in ethanol (95).

It is hygroscopic.

Identification **(1)** To 1 mL of a solution of Xylitol (1 in 2) add 2 mL of iron (II) sulfate TS and 1 mL of a solution of sodium hydroxide (1 in 5): blue-green color is produced without turbidity.

(2) Determine the infrared absorption spectrum of Xylitol, previously dried, as directed in the potassium bromide disk method under Infrared Spectrophotometry <*2.25*>, and compare the spectrum with the Reference Spectrum: both spectra exhibit similar intensities of absorption at the same wave numbers.

pH <*2.54*> Dissolve 5.0 g of Xylitol in 10 mL of freshly boiled and cooled water: the pH of this solution is between 5.0 and 7.0.

Melting point <*2.60*> 93.0 – 95.0°C

Purity **(1)** Clarity and color of solution—Dissolve 5 g of Xylitol in 10 mL of water: the solution is clear and colorless.

(2) Chloride <*1.03*>—Perform the test with 2.0 g of Xylitol. Prepare the control solution with 0.30 mL of 0.01 mol/L hydrochloric acid VS (not more than 0.005%).

(3) Sulfate <*1.14*>—Perform the test with 4.0 g of Xylitol. Prepare the control solution with 0.50 mL of 0.005 mol/L sulfuric acid VS (not more than 0.006%).

(4) Heavy metals <*1.07*>—Proceed with 4.0 g of Xylitol according to Method 1, and perform the test. Prepare the control solution with 2.0 mL of Standard Lead Solution (not more than 5 ppm).

(5) Nickel—Dissolve 0.5 g of Xylitol in 5 mL of water, add 3 drops of dimethylglyoxime TS and 3 drops of ammonia TS, and allow to stand for 5 minutes: no red color is produced.

(6) Arsenic <*1.11*>—Prepare the test solution with 1.5 g of Xylitol according to Method 1, and perform the test (not more than 1.3 ppm).

(7) Sugars—Dissolve 5.0 g of Xylitol in 15 mL of water, add 4.0 mL of dilute hydrochloric acid, and heat in a water bath for 3 hours under a reflux condenser. After cooling, neutralize with sodium hydroxide TS (indicator: 2 drops of methyl orange TS). Then add water to make 50 mL, transfer 10 mL of this solution to a flask, add 10 mL of water and 40 mL of Fehling's TS, boil gently for 3 minutes, and allow to stand to precipitate copper (I) oxide. Remove the supernatant liquid through a glass filter (G4), and wash the precipitate with warm water until the last washing does not show alkalinity. Filter these washings through the glass filter mentioned above. Dissolve the precipitate in the flask in 20 mL of iron (III) sulfate TS, filter the solution through the glass filter mentioned above, wash with water, combine the washings with the filtrate, heat at 80°C, and titrate <*2.50*> with 0.02 mol/L potassium permanganate VS: not more than 1.0 mL of 0.02 mol/L potassium permanganate VS is consumed.

Loss on drying <*2.41*> Not more than 1.0% (1 g, in vacuum, phosphorus (V) oxide, 24 hours).

Residue on ignition <*2.44*> Not more than 0.1% (1 g).

Assay Weigh accurately about 0.2 g of Xylitol, previously dried, dissolve in water to make exactly 100 mL. Pipet 10 mL of this solution into an iodine flask, add 50 mL of potassium periodate TS exactly, and heat in a water bath for 15 minutes. After cooling, add 2.5 g of potassium iodide, stopper, shake well, allow to stand for 5 minutes in a dark place, and titrate <*2.50*> with 0.1 mol/L sodium thiosulfate VS (indicator: 3 mL of starch TS). Perform a blank determination in the same manner.

Each mL of 0.1 mol/L sodium thiosulfate VS
= 1.902 mg of $C_5H_{12}O_5$

Containers and storage Containers—Tight containers.

Xylitol Injection

キシリトール注射液

Xylitol Injection is an aqueous injection.

It contains not less than 95.0% and not more than 105.0% of the labeled amount of xylitol ($C_5H_{12}O_5$: 152.15).

Method of preparation Prepare as directed under Injections, with Xylitol.

No preservative may be added.

Description Xylitol Injection is a clear, colorless liquid. It has a sweet taste.

Identification Measure a volume of Xylitol Injection, equivalent to 0.1 g of Xylitol, add water to make 10 mL, and use this solution as the sample solution. Separately, dissolve 0.1 g of xylitol in 10 mL of water, and use this solution as the standard solution. Perform the test with these solutions as directed under Thin-layer Chromatography <*2.03*>. Spot 2 μL each of the sample solution and standard solution on a plate of silica gel for thin-layer chromatography. Develop the plate with a mixture of ethanol (95), ammonia solution (28) and water (25:4:3) to a distance of about 10 cm, and air-dry the plate. Spray evenly silver nitrate-ammonia TS, and dry the plate at 105°C for 15 minutes: the spots from the sample solution and standard solution show a black-brown color and the same *R*f value.

pH <*2.54*> 4.5 - 7.5

Bacterial endotoxins <*4.01*> Less than 0.50 EU/mL.

Extractable volume <*6.05*> It meets the requirement.

Foreign insoluble matter <*6.06*> Perform the test according to Method 1: it meets the requirement.

Insoluble particulate matter <*6.07*> It meets the requirement.

Sterility <*4.06*> Perform the test according to the Membrane filtration method: it meets the requirement.

Assay Measure exactly a volume of Xylitol Injection, equivalent to about 5 g of xylitol ($C_5H_{12}O_5$), and add water to make exactly 250 mL. Measure exactly 10 mL of this solution, and add water to make exactly 100 mL. Then, pipet 10 mL of this solution into an iodine flask, and proceed as directed in the Assay under Xylitol.

Each mL of 0.1 mol/L sodium thiosulfate VS
= 1.902 mg of $C_5H_{12}O_5$

Containers and storage Containers—Hermetic containers. Plastic containers for aqueous injections may be used.

Dried Yeast

乾燥酵母

Dried Yeast is dried and powdered cells of yeast belonging to *Saccharomyces*.

It contains not less than 400 mg of protein and not less than 100 μg of thiamine compounds [as thiamine chloride hydrochloride ($C_{12}H_{17}ClN_4OS.HCl$: 337.27)] in each 1 g.

Description Dried Yeast occurs as a light yellow-white to brown powder. It has a characteristic odor and taste.

Identification Dried Yeast, when examined under a microscope <*5.01*>, shows isolated cells, spheroidal or oval in shape, and 6 to 12 μm in length.

Purity **(1)** Rancidity—Dried Yeast is free from any unpleasant or rancid odor or taste.

(2) Starch—Add iodine TS to Dried Yeast, and examine microscopically <*5.01*>: no or only a few granules are tinted black-purple.

Loss on drying <*2.41*> Not more than 8.0% (1 g, 100°C, 8 hours).

Total ash <*5.01*> Not more than 9.0% (1 g).

Assay **(1)** Protein—Weigh accurately about 50 mg of Dried Yeast and perform the test as directed under Nitrogen Determination <*1.08*>.

Amount (mg) of protein in 1 g of Dried Yeast
$= N \times 6.25 \times 1/M$

N: Amount (mg) of nitrogen (N)
M: Amount (g) of Dried Yeast taken

(2) Thiamine—Weigh accurately about 1 g of Dried Yeast, add 1 mL of dilute hydrochloric acid and 80 mL of water, and heat in a water bath at 80 to 85°C for 30 minutes with occasional shaking. After cooling, add water to make exactly 100 mL, and centrifuge for 10 minutes. Pipet 4 mL of the supernatant liquid, add exactly 5 mL of acetic acid-sodium acetate TS and exactly 1 mL of enzyme TS, and allow to stand at 45 to 50°C for 3 hours. Place exactly 2 mL of this solution onto a chromatographic column prepared by pouring 2.5 mL of a weakly acidic CM-bridged cellulose cation exchanger (H type) (40 to 110 μm in particle diameter) into a chromatographic tube about 1 cm in inside diameter and about 17 cm in length, and elute at the flow rate of about 0.5 mL per minute. Wash the upper part of the column with a small amount of water, and wash the column with two 10-mL portions of water at the flow rate of about 1 mL per minute. Elute the column with two 2.5-mL portions of diluted phosphoric acid (1 in 50) at the flow rate of about 0.5 mL per minute, and combine the eluate. To the eluate add exactly 1 mL of the internal standard solution and 0.01 g of sodium 1-octanesulfonate, and after dissolving, use this solution as the sample solution. Separately, weigh accurately about 15 mg of Thiamine Chloride Hydrochloride RS (previously determine the water <*2.48*> in the same manner as Thiamine Chloride Hydrochloride), dissolve in 0.001 mol/L hydrochloric acid TS to make exactly 100 mL. Pipet 1 mL of this solution, and add the mobile phase to make exactly 100 mL. Pipet 1 mL of this solution, add exactly 1 mL of the internal standard solution and 3 mL of the mobile phase, and use this solution as the standard solution. Perform the test with 200 μL each of the sample solution and standard solution as directed under Liquid Chromatography <*2.01*> according to the following conditions, and calculate the ratios, Q_T and Q_S, of the peak area of thiamine to that of the internal standard.

$$\text{Amount } (\mu g) \text{ of thiamine in 1 g of Dried Yeast} = M_S/M_T \times Q_T/Q_S \times 12.5$$

M_S: Amount (mg) of Thiamine Chloride Hydrochloride RS taken, calculated on the anhydrous basis
M_T: Amount (g) of the Dried Yeast taken

Internal standard solution—Dissolve 0.01 g of phenacetin in acetonitrile to make 100 mL, and to 1 mL of this solution add diluted acetonitrile (1 in 5) to make 100 mL.
Operating conditions—

Detector: An ultraviolet absorption photometer (wavelength: 254 nm).

Column: A stainless steel column about 4 mm in inside diameter and 15 to 30 cm in length, packed with octadecylsilanized silica gel for liquid chromatography (5 to 10 μm in particle diameter).

Column temperature: A constant temperature of about 40°C.

Mobile phase: Dissolve 2.7 g of potassium dihydrogenphosphate in 1000 mL of water, and adjust the pH to 3.5 with diluted phosphoric acid (1 in 10). Dissolve 1.6 g of sodium 1-octanesulfonate in 800 mL of this solution, and add 200 mL of acetonitrile.

Flow rate: Adjust so that the retention time of thiamine is about 8 minutes.

Selection of column: Proceed with 200 μL of the standard solution under the above operating conditions, and calculate the resolution. Use a column giving elution of thiamine and the internal standard in this order with the resolution between these peaks being not less than 8.

Containers and storage Containers—Tight containers.

Zaltoprofen

ザルトプロフェン

$C_{17}H_{14}O_3S$: 298.36
(2*RS*)-2-(10-Oxo-10,11-dihydrodibenzo[*b*, *f*]thiepin-2-yl)propanoic acid
[*74711-43-6*]

Zaltoprofen, when dried, contains not less than 99.0% and not more than 101.0% of zaltoprofen ($C_{17}H_{14}O_3S$).

Description Zaltoprofen occurs as white to light yellow, crystals or crystalline powder.

It is freely soluble in acetone, soluble in methanol and in ethanol (99.5), and practically insoluble in water.

It is gradually decomposed by light.

A solution of Zaltoprofen in acetone (1 in 10) shows no optical rotation.

Identification **(1)** To 0.2 g of Zaltoprofen add 0.5 g of sodium hydroxide, heat gradually to melt, and then carbonize. After cooling, add 5 mL of diluted hydrochloric acid (1 in 2): the gas evolved darkens moisten lead (II) acetate paper.

(2) Determine the absorption spectrum of a solution of Zaltoprofen in ethanol (99.5) (1 in 100,000) as directed under Ultraviolet-visible Spectrophotometry <*2.24*>, and compare the spectrum with the Reference Spectrum: both spectra exhibit similar intensities of absorption at the same wavelengths.

(3) Determine the infrared absorption spectrum of Zaltoprofen as directed in the potassium bromide disk method under Infrared Spectrophotometry <*2.25*>, and compare the spectrum with the Reference Spectrum: both spectra exhibit similar intensities of absorption at the same wave numbers.

Melting point <*2.60*> 135 – 139°C

Purity **(1)** Heavy metals <*1.07*>—Proceed with 2.0 g of Zaltoprofen according to Method 4, and perform the test. Prepare the control solution with 2.0 mL of Standard Lead Solution (not more than 10 ppm).

(2) Arsenic <*1.11*>—Prepare the test solution with 1.0 g of Zaltoprofen according to Method 3, using 10 mL of a solution of magnesium nitrate hexahydrate in ethanol (95) (2 in 25), and perform the test (not more than 2 ppm).

(3) Related substances—Dissolve 50 mg of Zaltoprofen in 50 mL of the mobile phase, and use this solution as the sample solution. Pipet 1 mL of the sample solution, and add the mobile phase to make exactly 50 mL. Pipet 1 mL of this solution, add the mobile phase to make exactly 20 mL, and use this solution as the standard solution. Perform the test with exactly 20 μL each of the sample solution and standard solution as directed under Liquid Chromatography <*2.01*> according to the following conditions, and determine each peak area by the automatic integration method: the area of the peak other than zaltoprofen and the peak having the relative retention time of about 0.7 to zaltoprofen obtained from the sample solution is not larger than the peak area of zaltoprofen from the standard solution.
Operating conditions—

Detector: An ultraviolet absorption photometer (wavelength: 240 nm).

Column: A stainless steel column 4.6 mm in inside diameter and 15 cm in length, packed with octadecylsilanized silica gel for liquid chromatography (5 μm in particle diameter).

Column temperature: A constant temperature of about 25°C.

Mobile phase: A mixture of acetonitrile, water and acetic acid (100) (300:200:1).

Flow rate: Adjust so that the retention time of zaltoprofen is about 4 minutes.

Time span of measurement: About 15 times as long as the retention time of zaltoprofen, beginning after the solvent peak.
System suitability—

Test for required detectability: To exactly 2 mL of the standard solution add the mobile phase to make exactly 20 mL. Confirm that the peak area of zaltoprofen obtained with 20 μL of this solution is equivalent to 8 to 12% of that with 20 μL of the standard solution.

System performance: Dissolve 25 mg of zaltoprofen and 50 mg of isopropyl benzoate in 100 mL of ethanol (99.5). Pipet 1 mL of this solution, and add the mobile phase to make exactly 50 mL. When the procedure is run with 20 μL of this solution under the above operating conditions, zaltoprofen and isopropyl benzoate are eluted in this order with the resolution between these peaks being not less than 6.

System repeatability: When the test is repeated 6 times with 20 μL of the standard solution under the above operating conditions, the relative standard deviation of the peak

area of zaltoprofen is not more than 2.0%.

Loss on drying <*2.41*> Not more than 0.5% (1 g, 105°C, 4 hours).

Residue on ignition <*2.44*> Not more than 0.1% (1 g).

Assay Weigh accurately about 0.5 g of Zaltoprofen, previously dried, dissolve in 50 mL of methanol, and titrate <*2.50*> with 0.1 mol/L sodium hydroxide VS (potentiometric titration). Perform a blank determination in the same manner, and make any necessary correction.

Each mL of 0.1 mol/L sodium hydroxide VS
= 29.84 mg of $C_{17}H_{14}O_3S$

Containers and storage Containers—Tight containers.
Storage—Light-resistant.

Zaltoprofen Tablets

ザルトプロフェン錠

Zaltoprofen Tablets contain not less than 95.0% and not more than 105.0% of the labeled amount of zaltoprofen ($C_{17}H_{14}O_3S$: 298.36).

Method of preparation Prepare as directed under Tablets, with Zaltoprofen.

Identification Powder a suitable amount of Zaltoprofen Tablets. To a portion of the powder, equivalent to 80 mg of Zaltoprofen, add 30 mL of ethanol (99.5), shake well, and centrifuge. To 1 mL of the supernatant liquid add ethanol (99.5) to make 20 mL. To 2 mL of this solution add ethanol (99.5) to make 25 mL, and determine the absorption spectrum of this solution as directed under Ultraviolet-visible Spectrophotometry <*2.24*>: it exhibits maxima between 227 nm and 231 nm and between 329 nm and 333 nm, and a shoulder between 238 nm and 248 nm.

Uniformity of dosage units <*6.02*> Perform the Mass variation test, or the Content uniformity test according to the following method: it meets the requirement.

To 1 tablet of Zaltoprofen Tablets add 4 mL of water, and shake to disintegrate. Add a suitable amount of ethanol (95), shake, then add ethanol (95) to make exactly V mL so that each mL contains about 4 mg of zaltoprofen ($C_{17}H_{14}O_3S$), and centrifuge. Pipet 2 mL of the supernatant liquid, add exactly 10 mL of the internal standard solution and ethanol (95) to make 50 mL, and use this solution as the sample solution. Proceed as directed in the Assay.

Amount (mg) of zaltoprofen ($C_{17}H_{14}O_3S$)
$= M_S \times Q_T/Q_S \times V/20$

M_S: Amount (mg) of zaltoprofen for assay taken

Internal standard solution—A solution of benzyl benzoate in acetonitrile (1 in 1000).

Dissolution <*6.10*> When the test is performed at 50 revolutions per minute according to the Paddle method, using 900 mL of 2nd fluid for dissolution test as the dissolution medium, the dissolution rate in 30 minutes of Zaltoprofen Tablets is not less than 75%.

Start the test with 1 tablet of Zaltoprofen Tablets, withdraw not less than 20 mL of the medium at the specified minute after starting the test, and filter through a membrane filter with a pore size not exceeding 0.45 μm. Discard not less than 10 mL of the first filtrate, pipet V mL of the subsequent filtrate, add the dissolution medium to make exactly V' mL so that each mL contains about 44 μg of zaltoprofen ($C_{17}H_{14}O_3S$), and use this solution as the sample solution. Separately, weigh accurately about 22 mg of zaltoprofen for assay, previously dried at 105°C for 4 hours, dissolve in 20 mL of ethanol (99.5), and add the dissolution medium to make exactly 100 mL. Pipet 4 mL of this solution, add the dissolution medium to make exactly 20 mL, and use this solution as the standard solution. Determine the absorbances, A_T and A_S, of the sample solution and standard solution at 340 nm as directed under Ultraviolet-visible Spectrophotometry <*2.24*>, using the dissolution medium as the control.

Dissolution rate (%) with respect to the labeled amount of zaltoprofen ($C_{17}H_{14}O_3S$)
$= M_S \times A_T/A_S \times V'/V \times 1/C \times 180$

M_S: Amount (mg) of zaltoprofen for assay taken
C: Labeled amount (mg) of zaltoprofen for assay in 1 tablet

Assay To 10 tablets of Zaltoprofen Tablets add 40 mL of water, shake to disintegrate, then add a suitable amount of ethanol (95), shake, add ethanol (95) to make exactly 200 mL, and centrifuge. Pipet an amount of the supernatant liquid, equivalent to about 8 mg of zaltoprofen ($C_{17}H_{14}O_3S$), add exactly 10 mL of the internal standard solution and ethanol (95) to make 50 mL, and use this solution as the sample solution. Separately, weigh accurately about 80 mg of zaltoprofen for assay, previously dried at 105°C for 4 hours, add 4 mL of water and ethanol (95) to make exactly 20 mL. Pipet 2 mL of this solution, add exactly 10 mL of the internal standard solution and ethanol (95) to make 50 mL, and use this solution as the standard solution. Perform the test with 5 μL each of the sample solution and standard solution as directed under Liquid Chromatography <*2.01*> according to the following conditions, and calculate the ratios, Q_T and Q_S, of the peak area of zaltoprofen to that of the internal standard.

Amount (mg) of zaltoprofen ($C_{17}H_{14}O_3S$)
$= M_S \times Q_T/Q_S \times 1/10$

M_S: Amount (mg) of zaltoprofen for assay taken

Internal standard solution—A solution of benzyl benzoate in acetonitrile (1 in 1000).

Operating conditions—

Detector: An ultraviolet absorption photometer (wavelength: 240 nm).

Column: A stainless steel column 4.6 mm in inside diameter and 15 cm in length, packed with octadecylsilanized silica gel for liquid chromatography (5 μm in particle diameter).

Column temperature: A constant temperature of about 25°C.

Mobile phase: A mixture of acetonitrile, water and acetic acid (100) (300:200:1).

Flow rate: Adjust so that the retention time of zaltoprofen is about 4 minutes.

System suitability—

System performance: When the procedure is run with 5 μL of the standard solution under the above operating conditions, zaltoprofen and the internal standard are eluted in this order with the resolution between these peaks being not less than 10.

System repeatability: When the test is repeated 6 times with 5 μL of the standard solution under the above operating conditions, the relative standard deviation of the ratio of the peak area of zaltoprofen to that of the internal standard is not more than 1.0%.

Containers and storage Containers—Tight containers.

Zidovudine

ジドブジン

$C_{10}H_{13}N_5O_4$: 267.24
3′-Azido-3′-deoxythymidine
[*30516-87-1*]

Zidovudine contains not less than 97.0% and not more than 102.0% of zidovudine ($C_{10}H_{13}N_5O_4$), calculated on the anhydrous basis.

Description Zidovudine occurs as a white to pale yellow-white powder.

It is freely soluble in methanol, soluble in ethanol (99.5), and sparingly soluble in water.

It gradually turns yellow-brown on exposure to light.

Melting point: about 124°C.

It shows crystal polymorphism.

Identification Determine the infrared absorption spectrum of Zidovudine as directed in the potassium bromide disc method under Infrared Spectrophotometry <*2.25*>, and compare the spectrum with the Reference Spectrum or the spectrum of Zidovudine RS: both spectra exhibit similar intensities of absorption at the same wave numbers. If any difference appears between the spectra, dissolve Zidovudine and Zidovudine RS separately in a small amount of water and dry them in a desiccator (in vacuum, phosphorus (V) oxide), and perform the test with the residues.

Optical rotation <*2.49*> $[\alpha]_D^{25}$: +60.5 – +63.0° (0.5 g calculated on the anhydrous basis, ethanol (99.5), 50 mL, 100 mm).

Purity (1) Heavy metals <*1.07*>— Proceed with 1.0 g of Zidovudine according to Method 4, and perform the test. Prepare the control solution with 2.0 mL of Standard Lead Solution (not more than 20 ppm).

(2) 1-[(2*R*,5*S*)-2,5-Dihydro-5-(hydroxymethyl)-2-furyl] thymine, triphenylmethanol, and other related substances—Dissolve 0.20 g of Zidovudine in methanol to make exactly 10 mL, and use this solution as the sample solution. Separately, add 1 mL of the sample solution to 20 mg each of thymine for liquid chromatography, 1-[(2*R*,5*S*)-2,5-dihydro-5-(hydroxymethyl)-2-furyl]thymine for thin-layer chromatography, and triphenylmethanol for thin-layer chromatography, and add methanol to dissolve to make exactly 100 mL. Pipet 5 mL of this solution, add methanol to make exactly 10 mL, and use this solution as the standard solution. Perform the test with these solutions as directed under Thin-layer Chromatography <*2.03*>. Spot 10 μL each of the sample solution and standard solution on a plate of silica gel with fluorescent indicator for thin-layer chromatography. Develop the plate with a mixture of chloroform and methanol (9:1) to a distance of about 12 cm, and air-dry the plate. Examine under ultraviolet light (main wavelength: 254 nm): the spot obtained from the sample solution that corresponds to the position of the 1-[(2*R*,5*S*)-2,5-dihydro-5-(hydroxymethyl)-2-furyl]thymine from the standard solution is not more intense than the spot from the standard solution, and the spot other than the principal spot and spots other than thymine and 1-[(2*R*,5*S*)-2,5-dihydro-5-(hydroxymethyl)-2-furyl]thymine from the sample solution is not more intense than zidovudine spot from the standard solution. However, the 3 spots from the standard solution appear in ascending order of *R*f value thymine, 1-[(2*R*,5*S*)-2,5-dihydro-5-(hydroxymethyl)-2-furyl]thymine, and zidovudine. Furthermore, spray evenly on the plate a solution of vanillin in sulfuric acid (1 in 100): the spot from the sample solution corresponding to the spot of triphenylmethanol from the standard solution is not more intense than the spot from the standard solution.

(3) Thymine, 3′-chloro-3′-deoxythymidine, and other related substances—Use the sample solution obtained in the Assay as the sample solution. Separately, weigh accurately about 20 mg of thymine for liquid chromatography, dissolve in 100 mL of methanol, and add the mobile phase to make exactly 250 mL. Pipet 5 mL of this solution, add the mobile phase to make exactly 50 mL, and use this solution as the standard solution. Perform the test with exactly 10 μL each of the sample solution and standard solution as directed under Liquid Chromatography <*2.01*> according to the following conditions. Determine the peak areas, A_T and A_S, of thymine in each solution, and calculate the amount of thymine using the following formula: the amount is not more than 2.0%. Also, determine the peak area of each peak obtained from the sample solution by the automatic integration method, and calculate the amounts of related substances other than thymine by the area percentage method: the amount of 3′-chloro-3′-deoxythymidine, whose relative retention time to zidovudine is 1.2, is not more than 1.0%, and is not more than 0.5% for all other related substances. Finally, the total amount of thymine, 3′-chloro-3′-deoxythymidine, and all related substances obtained above is not more than 3.0%.

$$\text{Amount (\%) of thymine} = M_S/M_T \times A_T/A_S \times 10$$

M_S: Amount (mg) of thymine for liquid chromatography taken

M_T: Amount (mg) of Zidovudine taken

Operating conditions—

Detector, column, column temperature, mobile phase, and flow rate: Proceed as directed in the operating conditions in the Assay.

Time span of measurement: About 2 times as long as the retention time of zidovudine, beginning after the solvent peak.

System suitability—

System performance and system repeatability: Proceed as directed in the system suitability in the Assay.

Test for required detectability: Pipet 2 mL of the sample solution, add the mobile phase to make exactly 100 mL, and use this solution as the solution for system suitability test. Pipet 1 mL of the solution for system suitability test, and add the mobile phase to make exactly 20 mL. Confirm that the peak area of zidovudine obtained with 10 μL of this solution is equivalent to 3.5 to 6.5% of that with 10 μL of the solution for system suitability test.

Water <*2.48*> Not more than 1.0% (0.25 g, coulometric titration).

Residue on ignition <*2.44*> Not more than 0.2% (0.5 g).

Assay Weigh accurately about 50 mg of Zidovudine and Zidovudine RS (separately determine the water <*2.48*> in the same manner as Zidovudine), and dissolve in the mobile phase to make exactly 50 mL. Pipet 10 mL of each solution, add the mobile phase to make them exactly 50 mL, and use these solutions as the sample solution and the standard solution, respectively. Perform the test with exactly 10 μL each of the sample solution and standard solution as directed under Liquid Chromatography <*2.01*> according to the following conditions. Determine the peak areas, A_T and A_S, of zidovudine in each solution.

Amount (mg) of zidovudine ($C_{10}H_{13}N_5O_4$) = $M_S \times A_T/A_S$

M_S: Amount (mg) of Zidovudine RS taken, calculated on the anhydrous basis

Operating conditions—

Detector: An ultraviolet absorption photometer (wavelength: 265 nm).

Column: A stainless steel column 4.6 mm in inside diameter and 25 cm in length, packed with octadecylsilanized silica gel for liquid chromatography (particle diameter: 5 μm).

Column temperature: A constant temperature of about 25°C.

Mobile phase: A mixture of water and methanol (4:1).

Flow rate: Adjust so that the retention time of zidovudine is about 15 minutes.

System suitability—

System performance: Dissolve 50 mg of Zidovudine in 50 mL of the mobile phase. Separately, dissolve 5 mg of 3′-chloro-3′-deoxythymidine for liquid chromatography in 50 mL of the mobile phase. Mix 10 mL and 1 mL of these solutions, respectively, and add the mobile phase to make 50 mL. When the procedure is run with 10 μL of this solution under the above conditions, zidovudine and 3′-chloro-3′-deoxythymidine are eluted in this order with the resolution between these peaks being not less than 1.4, and the symmetry factor of the peak of zidovudine is not more than 1.5.

System repeatability: When the test is repeated 6 times with 10 μL of the standard solution under the above conditions, the relative standard deviation of the peak area of zidovudine is not more than 2.0%.

Containers and storage Containers—Tight containers.

Storage—Light-resistant.

Zinc Chloride

塩化亜鉛

$ZnCl_2$: 136.29

Zinc Chloride contains not less than 97.0% of zinc chloride ($ZnCl_2$).

Description Zinc Chloride occurs as white, crystalline powder, rods, or masses. It is odorless.

It is very soluble in water, and freely soluble in ethanol (95), and its solution may sometimes be slightly turbid. The solution becomes clear on addition of a small amount of hydrochloric acid.

The pH of a solution of 1.0 g of Zinc Chloride in 2 mL of water is between 3.3 and 5.3.

It is deliquescent.

Identification A solution of Zinc Chloride (1 in 30) responds to Qualitative Tests <*1.09*> for zinc salt and chloride.

Purity (1) Clarity and color of solution—Dissolve 1.0 g of Zinc Chloride in 10 mL of water and 2 drops of hydrochloric acid: the solution has no color, and is clear.

(2) Sulfate <*1.14*>—Perform the test with 2.0 g of Zinc Chloride. Prepare the control solution with 0.40 mL of 0.005 mol/L sulfuric acid VS (not more than 0.010%).

(3) Ammonium—Dissolve 0.5 g of Zinc Chloride in 5 mL of water, and warm with 10 mL of a solution of sodium hydroxide (1 in 6): the evolving gas does not change moistened red litmus paper to blue.

(4) Heavy metals—Dissolve 0.5 g of Zinc Chloride in 5 mL of water in a Nessler tube, shake thoroughly with 15 mL of potassium cyanide TS, add 1 drop of sodium sulfide TS, allow to stand for 5 minutes, and immediately observe from the top downward against a white background: the solution has no more color than the following control solution.

Control solution: To 2.5 mL of Standard Lead Solution add 3 mL of water and 15 mL of potassium cyanide TS, shake thoroughly, and add 1 drop of sodium sulfide TS (not more than 50 ppm).

(5) Alkali earth metals and alkali metals—Dissolve 2.0 g of Zinc Chloride in 120 mL of water, add ammonium sulfide TS to complete precipitation, add water to make 200 mL, shake thoroughly, and filter through dry filter paper. Discard the first 20 mL of the filtrate, take the following 100 mL of the filtrate, evaporate with 3 drops of sulfuric acid to dryness, and heat the residue strongly at 600°C to constant mass: the mass is not more than 10.0 mg.

(6) Arsenic <*1.11*>—Prepare the test solution with 0.40 g of Zinc Chloride according to Method 1, and perform the test (not more than 5 ppm).

(7) Oxychloride—Shake gently 0.25 g of Zinc Chloride with 5 mL of water and 5 mL of ethanol (95), and add 0.3 mL of 1 mol/L hydrochloric acid VS: the solution is clear.

Assay Weigh accurately about 0.3 g of Zinc Chloride, add 0.4 mL of dilute hydrochloric acid and water to make exactly 200 mL. Measure exactly 20 mL of the solution, add 80 mL of water, 2 mL of ammonia-ammonium chloride buffer solution (pH 10.7) and titrate <*2.50*> with 0.01 mol/L disodium dihydrogen ethylenediamine tetraacetate VS (indicator: 0.04 g of eriochrome black T-sodium chloride indicator).

Each mL of 0.01 mol/L disodium dihydrogen ethylenediamine tetraacetate VS
= 1.363 mg of $ZnCl_2$

Containers and storage Containers—Tight containers.

Zinc Oxide

酸化亜鉛

ZnO: 81.38

Zinc Oxide, when ignited, contains not less than 99.0% of zinc oxide (ZnO).

Description Zinc Oxide occurs as a white, amorphous powder. It is odorless and tasteless.

It is practically insoluble in water, in ethanol (95), in acetic acid (100) and in diethyl ether.

It dissolves in dilute hydrochloric acid and in sodium hydroxide TS.

It gradually absorbs carbon dioxide from air.

Identification (1) Heat Zinc Oxide strongly: a yellow color develops on strong heating, and disappears on cooling.

(2) A solution of Zinc Oxide in dilute hydrochloric acid (1 in 10) responds to Qualitative Tests <*1.09*> for zinc salt.

Purity **(1)** Carbonate, and clarity and color of solution—Mix 2.0 g of Zinc Oxide with 10 mL of water, add 30 mL of dilute sulfuric acid, and heat on a water bath with stirring: no effervescence occurs, and the solution obtained is clear and colorless.

(2) Alkalinity—To 1.0 g of Zinc Oxide add 10 mL of water, and boil for 2 minutes. Cool, filter through a glass filter (G3), and to the filtrate add 2 drops of phenolphthalein TS and 0.20 mL of 0.1 mol/L hydrochloric acid VS: no color develops.

(3) Sulfate <*1.14*>—Shake 0.5 g of Zinc Oxide with 40 mL of water, and filter. Take 20 mL of the filtrate, add 1 mL of dilute hydrochloric acid and water to make 50 mL, and perform the test using this solution as the test solution. Prepare the control solution with 0.50 mL of 0.005 mol/L sulfuric acid VS (not more than 0.096%).

(4) Iron—Dissolve 1.0 g of Zinc Oxide in 50 mL of diluted hydrochloric acid (1 in 2), dissolve 0.1 g of ammonium peroxodisulfate in this solution, and extract with 20 mL of 4-methyl-2-pentanone. Add 30 mL of acetic acid-sodium acetate buffer solution for Iron Limit Test (pH 4.5) to the 4-methyl-2-pentanone layer, extract again, and use the layer of the buffer solution as the test solution. Separately, perform the test in the same manner with 1.0 mL of Standard Iron Solution, and use the layer so obtained as the control solution. Add 2 mL each of L-ascorbic acid solution for Iron Limit Test (1 in 100) to the test solution and the control solution, respectively, mix, allow to stand for 30 minutes, add 5 mL of a solution of 2,2′-bipyridyl in ethanol (95) (1 in 200) and water to make 50 mL. After allowing to stand for 30 minutes, compare the color of the both liquids against a white back: the color of the liquid from the test solution is not stronger than that from the control solution (not more than 10 ppm).

(5) Lead—To 2.0 g of Zinc Oxide add 20 mL of water, then add 5 mL of acetic acid (100) with stirring, and heat on a water bath until solution is complete. Cool, and add 5 drops of potassium chromate TS: no turbidity is produced.

(6) Arsenic <*1.11*>—Dissolve 0.5 g of Zinc Oxide in 5 mL of dilute hydrochloric acid, use this solution as the test solution, and perform the test (not more than 4 ppm).

Loss on ignition <*2.43*> Not more than 1.0% (1 g, 850°C, 1 hour).

Assay Weigh accurately about 0.8 g of Zinc Oxide, previously ignited at 850°C for 1 hour, dissolve in 2 mL of water and 3 mL of hydrochloric acid, and add water to make exactly 100 mL. Pipet 10 mL of this solution, add 80 mL of water, then add a solution of sodium hydroxide (1 in 50) until a slight precipitate is produced. Add 5 mL of ammonia-ammonium chloride buffer solution (pH 10.7), and titrate <*2.50*> with 0.05 mol/L disodium dihydrogen ethylenediamine tetraacetate VS (indicator: 0.04 g of eriochrome black T-sodium chloride indicator).

Each mL of 0.05 mol/L disodium dihydrogen ethylenediamine tetraacetate VS
= 4.069 mg of ZnO

Containers and storage Containers—Tight containers.

Zinc Oxide Oil

チンク油

Zinc Oxide Oil contains not less than 45.0% and not more than 55.0% of zinc oxide (ZnO: 81.38).

Method of preparation

Zinc Oxide	500 g
Fixed oil	a sufficient quantity
To make	1000 g

Mix the above ingredients. An appropriate quantity of Castor Oil or polysorbate 20 may be used partially in place of fixed oil.

Description Zinc Oxide Oil is a white to whitish, slimy substance, separating a part of its ingredients when stored for a prolonged period.

Identification Mix thoroughly, and place 0.5 g of Zinc Oxide Oil in a crucible, heat gradually raising the temperature until the mass is thoroughly charred, and then ignite it strongly: a yellow color is produced, and disappears on cooling. To the residue add 10 mL of water and 5 mL of dilute hydrochloric acid, shake well, and filter. To the filtrate add 2 to 3 drops of potassium hexacyanoferrate (II) TS: a white precipitate is formed (zinc oxide).

Assay Weigh accurately about 0.8 g of Zinc Oxide Oil, mixed well, place in a crucible, heat gradually raising the temperature until the mass is thoroughly charred, and then ignite until the residue becomes yellow, and cool. Dissolve the residue in 1 mL of water and 1.5 mL of hydrochloric acid, and add water to make exactly 100 mL. Pipet 20 mL of this solution, add 80 mL of water, and add a solution of sodium hydroxide (1 in 50) until a small amount of precipitates begins to form in the solution. Add 5 mL of ammonia-ammonium chloride buffer solution (pH 10.7), and titrate <*2.50*> with 0.05 mol/L disodium dihydrogen ethylenediamine tetraacetate VS (indicator: 0.04 g of eriochrome black T-sodium chloride indicator).

Each mL of 0.05 mol/L disodium dihydrogen ethylenediamine tetraacetate VS
= 4.069 mg of ZnO

Containers and storage Containers—Tight containers.

Zinc Oxide Ointment

亜鉛華軟膏

Zinc Oxide Ointment contains not less than 18.5% and not more than 21.5% of zinc oxide (ZnO: 81.38).

Method of preparation

Zinc Oxide	200 g
Liquid Paraffin	30 g
White Ointment	a sufficient quantity
To make	1000 g

Prepare as directed under Ointments, with the above ingredients. White Beeswax, Sorbitan Sesquioleate or White Petrolatum may be used instead of White Ointment.

Description Zinc Oxide Ointment is white in color.

Identification Place 1 g of Zinc Oxide Ointment in a crucible, melt by warming, heat gradually raising the temperature until the mass is thoroughly charred, and then ignite it strongly: a yellow color is produced, and disappears on cooling. To the residue add 10 mL of water and 5 mL of dilute hydrochloric acid, shake well, and filter. To the filtrate add 2 to 3 drops of potassium hexacyanoferrate (II) TS: a white precipitate is formed (zinc oxide).

Purity Calcium, magnesium and other foreign inorganic matters—Place 2.0 g of Zinc Oxide Ointment in a crucible, melt by warming, and heat gradually raising the temperature, until the mass is thoroughly charred. Ignite the mass strongly until the residue becomes uniformly yellow, and cool. Add 6 mL of dilute hydrochloric acid, and heat on a water bath for 5 to 10 minutes: the solution is colorless and clear. Filter the solution, add 10 mL of water to the filtrate, and add ammonia TS until the precipitate first formed redissolves. Add 2 mL each of ammonium oxalate TS and disodium hydrogenphosphate TS to this solution: the solution remains unchanged or becomes very slightly turbid within 5 minutes.

Assay Weigh accurately about 2 g of Zinc Oxide Ointment, place in a crucible, melt by warming, heat gradually raising the temperature until the mass is thoroughly charred, and then ignite until the residue becomes uniformly yellow, and cool. Dissolve the residue in 1 mL of water and 1.5 mL of hydrochloric acid, and add water to make exactly 100 mL. Add 80 mL of water to exactly 20 mL of this solution, and add a solution of sodium hydroxide (1 in 50) until a small amount of precipitates begins to form in the solution. Add 5 mL of ammonia-ammonium chloride buffer solution (pH 10.7), and titrate <2.50> with 0.05 mol/L disodium dihydrogen ethylenediamine tetraacetate VS (indicator: 0.04 g of eriochrome black T-sodium chloride indicator).

Each mL of 0.05 mol/L disodium dihydrogen ethylenediamine tetraacetate VS
= 4.069 mg of ZnO

Containers and storage Containers—Tight containers.

Zinc Oxide Starch Powder

亜鉛華デンプン

Method of preparation

Zinc Oxide	500 g
Starch	a sufficient quantity
	To make 1000 g

Prepare as directed under Powders, with the above ingredients.

Description Zinc Oxide Starch Powder occurs as a white powder.

Identification **(1)** Place 1 g of Zinc Oxide Starch Powder in a crucible, heat gradually, raising the temperature until it is charred, and then ignite strongly: a yellow color develops, and disappears on cooling. To the residue add 10 mL of water and 5 mL of dilute hydrochloric acid, shake well, and filter. To the filtrate add 2 to 3 drops of potassium hexacyanoferrate (II) TS: a white precipitate is formed (zinc oxide).

(2) Shake throughly 1 g of Oxide Starch Powder with 10 mL of water and 5 mL of dilute hydrochloric acid, and filter. Boil the residue on a filter paper with 10 mL of water, cool, and add 1 drop of iodine TS: a dark blue-purple color is produced (starch).

Containers and storage Containers—Tight containers.

Zinc Sulfate Hydrate

硫酸亜鉛水和物

$ZnSO_4.7H_2O$: 287.55

Zinc Sulfate Hydrate contains not less than 99.0% and not more than 102.0% of zinc sulfate hydrate ($ZnSO_4.7H_2O$).

Description Zinc Sulfate Hydrate occurs as colorless crystals or white crystalline powder.

It is very soluble in water, and very slightly soluble in ethanol (99.5).

It effloresces in dry air.

Identification **(1)** A solution of Zinc Sulfate Hydrate (1 in 20) responds to Qualitative Tests <*1.09*> for zinc salt.

(2) A solution of Zinc Sulfate Hydrate (1 in 20) responds to Qualitative Tests <*1.09*> for sulfate.

pH <*2.54*> Dissolve 1.0 g of Zinc Sulfate Hydrate in 20 mL of water: the pH of the solution is between 4.4 and 6.0.

Purity **(1)** Clarity and color of solution—Dissolve 0.25 g of Zinc Sulfate Hydrate in 5 mL of water: the solution is clear and colorless.

(2) Heavy metals <*1.07*>—Dissolve 1.0 g of Zinc Sulfate Hydrate in 10 mL of water contained in a Nessler tube. Add 20 mL of potassium cyanide TS, and mix well. Add 2 drops of sodium sulfide TS, and allow the mixture to stand for 5 minutes. Observe vertically against a white background, the color of the solution is not more intense than the following control solution.

Control solution: To 1.0 mL of Standard Lead Solution add 10 mL of water and 20 mL of potassium cyanide TS, and mix well. Add 2 drops of sodium sulfide TS (not more than 10 ppm).

(3) Alkali earth metals and alkali metals—Dissolve 2.0 g of Zinc Sulfate Hydrate in 150 mL of water, add a suitable amount of ammonium sulfide TS to complete the precipitation, and add water to make exactly 200 mL. Shake well, and filter through a dry filter paper. Discard the first 20 mL of the filtrate, take exactly 100 mL of the subsequent filtrate, evaporate to dryness, and ignite as directed under Residue on Ignition <*2.44*>: the mass of the residue is not more than 5.0 mg.

(4) Arsenic <*1.11*>—Prepare the test solution with 1.0 g of Zinc Sulfate Hydrate according to Method 1, and perform the test (not more than 2 ppm).

Loss on drying <*2.41*> Not less than 35.5% and not more than 38.5% (1 g, 105°C, 3 hours).

Assay Weigh accurately about 0.3 g of Zinc Sulfate Hydrate, and dissolve in water to make exactly 100 mL. Measure exactly 25 mL of this solution, add 100 mL of water and 2 mL of ammonia-ammonium chloride buffer solution (pH 10.7), and titrate <*2.50*> with 0.01 mol/L disodium dihydorogen ethylenediamine tetraacetate VS (indicator: 0.04 g of eriochrome black T-sodium chloride indicator).

Each mL of 0.01 mol/L disodium dihydrogen ethylenediamine tetraacetate VS
= 2.876 mg of $ZnSO_4.7H_2O$

Containers and storage Containers—Tight containers.

Zinc Sulfate Ophthalmic Solution

硫酸亜鉛点眼液

Zinc Sulfate Ophthalmic Solution contains not less than 0.27 w/v% and not more than 0.33 w/v% of zinc sulfate hydrate ($ZnSO_4.7H_2O$: 287.55).

Method of preparation

Zinc Sulfate Hydrate	3 g
Boric Acid	20 g
Sodium Chloride	5 g
Fennel Oil	2 mL
Purified Water or Purified Water in Containers	a sufficient quantity
	To make 1000 mL

Prepare as directed under Ophthalmic Liquids and Solutions, with the above ingredients.

Description Zinc Sulfate Ophthalmic Solution is a clear, colorless liquid.

Identification **(1)** Zinc Sulfate Ophthalmic Solution responds to Qualitative Tests 〈*1.09*〉 for zinc salt.

(2) Zinc Sulfate Ophthalmic Solution responds to Qualitative Tests 〈*1.09*〉 for borate.

(3) Zinc Sulfate Ophthalmic Solution responds to Qualitative Tests 〈*1.09*〉 for chloride.

Assay Pipet 25 mL of Zinc Sulfate Ophthalmic Solution, add 100 mL of water and 2 mL of ammonia-ammonium chloride buffer solution (pH 10.7), and titrate 〈*2.50*〉 with 0.01 mol/L disodium dihydrogen ethylenediamine tetraacetate VS (indicator: 0.04 g of eriochrome black T-sodium chloride indicator).

Each mL of 0.01 mol/L disodium dihydrogen ethylenediamine tetraacetate VS
= 2.876 mg of $ZnSO_4.7H_2O$

Containers and storage Containers—Tight containers.

Zolpidem Tartrate

ゾルピデム酒石酸塩

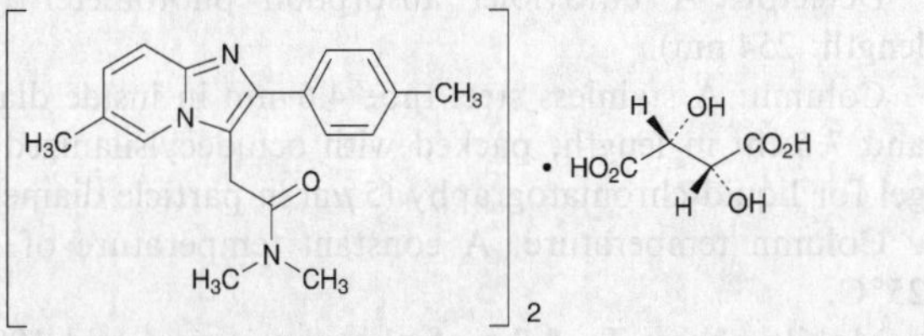

$(C_{19}H_{21}N_3O)_2.C_4H_6O_6$: 764.87
N,*N*,6-Trimethyl-2-(4-methylphenyl)imidazo[1,2-*a*]pyridine-3-acetamide hemi-(2*R*,3*R*)-tartrate
[*99294-93-6*]

Zolpidem Tartrate contains not less than 98.5% and not more than 101.0% of zolpidem tartrate [$(C_{19}H_{21}N_3O)_2.C_4H_6O_6$], calculated on the anhydrous basis.

Description Zolpidem Tartrate occurs as a white crystalline powder.

It is freely soluble in acetic acid (100), soluble in *N*,*N*-dimethylformamide and in methanol, sparingly soluble in water, and slightly soluble in ethanol (99.5) and in acetic anhydride.

It dissolves in 0.1 mol/L hydrochloric acid TS.

It gradually changes to yellow in color on exposure to light.

Optical rotation $[\alpha]_D^{20}$: about +1.8° (1 g, *N*,*N*-dimethylformamide, 20 mL, 100 mm).

Identification **(1)** Dissolve 50 mg of Zolpidem Tartrate in 5 mL of acetic acid (100) and add 3 drops of Dragendorff's TS: an orange precipitate is formed.

(2) Determine the absorption spectrum of a solution of Zolpidem Tartrate in 0.1 mol/L hydrochloric acid TS (1 in 100,000) as directed under Ultraviolet-visible Spectrophotometry 〈*2.24*〉, and compare the spectrum with the Reference Spectrum: both spectra exhibit similar intensities of absorption at the same wavelengths.

(3) Determine the infrared absorption spectrum of Zolpidem Tartrate as directed in the potassium bromide disk method under Infrared Spectrophotometry 〈*2.25*〉, and compare the spectrum with the Reference Spectrum: both spectra exhibit similar intensities of absorption at the same wave numbers.

(4) A solution of 1.0 g of Zolpidem Tartrate in 10 mL of methanol by warming, responds to Qualitative Tests 〈*1.09*〉 (3) for tartrate.

Purity **(1)** Heavy metals 〈*1.07*〉—Proceed with 2.0 g of Zolpidem Tartrate according to Method 4, and perform the test. Prepare the control solution with 2.0 mL of Standard Lead Solution (not more than 10 ppm).

(2) Related substances—Dissolve 10 mg of Zolpidem Tartrate in 20 mL of methanol and use this solution as the sample solution. Pipet 1 mL of the sample solution, and add methanol to make exactly 100 mL. Pipet 2 mL of this solution, add methanol to make exactly 20 mL, and use this solution as the standard solution. Perform the test with exactly 5 μL each of the sample solution and standard solution as directed under Liquid Chromatography 〈*2.01*〉 according to the following conditions. Determine each peak area of both solutions by the automatic integration method: each area of the peak other than zolpidem obtained from the sample solution is not larger than the peak area of zolpidem from the standard solution.

Operating conditions—

Detector: A ultraviolet absorption photometer (wavelength: 254 nm).

Column: A stainless steel tube 4.6 mm in inside diameter and 7.5 cm in length, packed with octadecylsilanized silica gel for liquid chromatography (5 μm in particle diameter).

Column temperature: A constant temperature of about 25°C.

Mobile phase: To 4.9 g of phosphoric acid add 1000 mL of water, and adjust the pH to 5.5 with triethylamine. To 11 volumes of this solution add 5 volumes of methanol and 4 volumes of acetonitrile.

Flow rate: Adjust so that the retention time of zolpidem is about 5 minutes.

Time span of measurement: About 5 times as long as the retention time of zolpidem.

System suitability—

System performance: Dissolve 10 mg each of Zolpidem Tartrate and benzyl parahydroxybenzoate in 100 mL of methanol. When the procedure is run with 5 μL of this solution under the above operating conditions, zolpidem and benzyl parahydroxybenzoate are eluted in this order with the resolution between these peaks being not less than 9.

System repeatability: When the test is repeated 6 times with 5 μL of the standard solution under the above operating conditions, the relative standard deviation of the peak area of zolpidem is not more than 5.0%.

Water *<2.48>* Not more than 3.0% (0.5 g, volumetric titration, direct titration).

Residue on ignition *<2.44>* Not more than 0.1% (1 g).

Assay Weigh accurately about 0.4 g of Zolpidem Tartrate, dissolve in 100 mL of a mixture of acetic anhydride and acetic acid (100) (7:3) and titrate *<2.50>* with 0.1 mol/L perchloric acid VS (potentiometric titration). Perform a blank determination in the same manner, and make any necessary correction.

Each mL of 0.1 mol/L perchloric acid VS
$= 38.24$ mg of $(C_{19}H_{21}N_3O)_2.C_4H_6O_6$

Containers and storage Containers—Tight containers.

Storage conditions—Light-resistant.

Zolpidem Tartrate Tablets

ゾルピデム酒石酸塩錠

Zolpidem Tartrate Tablets contain not less than 95.0% and not more than 105.0% of the labeled amount of zolpidem tartrate [$(C_{19}H_{21}N_3O)_2.C_4H_6O_6$: 764.87].

Method of preparation Prepare as directed under Tablets, with Zolpidem Tartrate.

Identification To 1 tablet of Zolpidem Tartrate Tablets add 100 mL of 0.1 mol/L hydrochloric acid TS, shake for 30 minutes, and filter. Discard the first 20 mL of the filtrate, to a volume of the subsequent filtrate, equivalent to 1 mg of Zolpidem Tartrate, add 0.1 mol/L hydrochloric acid TS to make 100 mL, and determine the absorption spectrum of this solution as directed under Ultraviolet-visible Spectrophotometry *<2.24>*: it exhibits maxima between 235 nm and 239 nm and between 292 nm and 296 nm.

Uniformity of dosage units *<6.02>* Perform the test according to the following method: it meets the requirements of the Content uniformity test.

To 1 tablet of Zolpidem Tartrate Tablets add $V/10$ mL of 0.1 mol/L hydrochloric acid TS, and disintegrate the tablet by shaking for 15 minutes. Add $2V/5$ mL of methanol, then add exactly $V/10$ mL of the internal standard solution, shake for 15 minutes, and add methanol to make V mL so that each mL contains about 0.1 mg of zolpidem tartrate [$(C_{19}H_{21}N_3O)_2.C_4H_6O_6$]. Centrifuge this solution, and use the supernatant liquid as the sample solution. Separately, weigh accurately about 25 mg of zolpidem tartrate for assay (separately determine the water *<2.48>* in the same manner as Zolpidem Tartrate), and dissolve in 25 mL of 0.1 mol/L hydrochloric acid TS, add exactly 25 mL of the internal standard solution, then add methanol to make 250 mL, and use this solution as the standard solution. Then, proceed as directed in the Assay.

Amount (mg) of zolpidem tartrate [$(C_{19}H_{21}N_3O)_2.C_4H_6O_6$]
$= M_S \times Q_T/Q_S \times V/250$

M_S: Amount (mg) of zolpidem tartrate for assay taken, calculated on the anhydrous basis

*Internal standard solution—*A solution of benzyl parahydroxybenzoate in methanol (1 in 1000).

Dissolution *<6.10>* When the test is performed at 50 revolutions per minute according to the Paddle method, using 900 mL of water as the dissolution medium, the dissolution rate in 15 minutes of Zolpidem Tartrate Tablets is not less than 80%.

Start the test with 1 tablet of Zolpidem Tartrate Tablets, withdraw not less than 20 mL of the medium at the specified minute after starting the test, and filter through a membrane filter with a pore size not exceeding 0.45 μm. Discard not less than 10 mL of the first filtrate, pipet V mL of the subsequent filtrate, add 2nd fluid for dissolution test to make exactly V' mL so that each mL contains about 2.8 μg of zolpidem tartrate [$(C_{19}H_{21}N_3O)_2.C_4H_6O_6$], and use this solution as the sample solution. Separately, weigh accurately about 22 mg of zolpidem tartrate for assay (separately determine the water *<2.48>* in the same manner as Zolpidem Tartrate), and dissolve in water to make exactly 100 mL. Pipet 5 mL of this solution, and add water to make exactly 200 mL. Pipet 25 mL of this solution, add 2nd fluid for dissolution test to make exactly 50 mL, and use this solution as the standard solution. Determine the absorbances, A_T and A_S, of the sample solution and standard solution at 242 nm as directed under Ultraviolet-visible Spectrophotometry *<2.24>* using diluted 2nd fluid for dissolution test (1 in 2) as the blank.

Dissolution rate (%) with respect to the labeled amount of zolpidem tartrate [$(C_{19}H_{21}N_3O)_2.C_4H_6O_6$]
$= M_S \times A_T/A_S \times V'/V \times 1/C \times 45/4$

M_S: Amount (mg) of zolpidem tartrate for assay taken, calculated on the anhydrous basis

C: Labeled amount (mg) of zolpidem tartrate [$(C_{19}H_{21}N_3O)_2.C_4H_6O_6$] in 1 tablet

Assay To 20 Zolpidem Tartrate Tablets add $V/10$ mL of 0.1 mol/L hydrochloric acid TS, and disintegrate the tablet by shaking for 15 minutes. Add $2V/5$ mL of methanol, then add exactly $V/10$ mL of the internal standard solution, shake for 15 minutes, and add methanol to make V mL so that each mL contains about 1 mg of zolpidem tartrate [$(C_{19}H_{21}N_3O)_2.C_4H_6O_6$]. Centrifuge this solution, add to 1 mL of the supernatant liquid add a mixture of methanol and 0.1 mol/L hydrochloric acid TS (9:1) to make 10 mL, and use this solution as the sample solution. Separately, weigh accurately about 25 mg of zolpidem tartrate for assay (separately determine the water <*2.48*> in the same manner as Zolpidem Tartrate), and dissolve in 25 mL of 0.1 mol/L hydrochloric acid TS, add exactly 2.5 mL of the internal standard solution, then add methanol to make 250 mL, and use this solution as the standard solution. Perform the test with 5 μL each of the sample solution and standard solution as directed under Liquid Chromatography <*2.01*>, and calculate the ratios, Q_T and Q_S, of the peak area of zolpidem to that of the internal standard.

Amount (mg) of zolpidem tartrate [$(C_{19}H_{21}N_3O)_2.C_4H_6O_6$] in 1 tablet of Zolpidem Tartrate Tablets
$= M_S \times Q_T/Q_S \times V/500$

M_S: Amount (mg) of zolpidem tartrate for assay taken, calculated on the anhydrous basis

Internal standard solution—A solution of benzyl parahydroxybenzoate in methanol (1 in 100).

Operating conditions—

Detector: An ultraviolet absorption photometer (wavelength: 254 nm).

Column: A stainless steel column 4.6 mm in inside diameter and 75 mm in length, packed with octadecylsilanized silica gel for liquid chromatography (5 μm in particle diameter).

Column temperature: A constant temperature of about 25°C.

Mobile phase: To 4.9 g of phosphoric acid add 1000 mL of water, and adjust to pH 5.5 with triethylamine. To 550 mL of this solution add 250 mL of methanol and 200 mL of acetonitrile.

Flow rate: Adjust so that the retention time of zolpidem is about 5 minutes.

System suitability—

System performance: When the procedure is run with 5 μL of the standard solution under the above operating conditions, zolpidem and the internal standard are eluted in this order with the resolution between these peaks being not less than 9.

System repeatability: When the test is repeated 6 times with 5 μL of the standard solution under the above operating conditions, the relative standard deviation of the ratio of the peak area of zolpidem to that of the internal standard is not more than 1.0%.

Containers and storage Containers—Well-closed containers.

Zonisamide

ゾニサミド

$C_8H_8N_2O_3S$: 212.23
1,2-Benzisoxazol-3-ylmethanesulfonamide
[*68291-97-4*]

Zonisamide, when dried, contains not less than 98.0% and not more than 101.0% of zonisamide ($C_8H_8N_2O_3S$).

Description Zonisamide occurs as white to pale yellow, crystals or crystalline powder.

It is freely soluble in acetone and in tetrahydrofuran, sparingly soluble in methanol, slightly soluble in ethanol (99.5), and very slightly soluble in water.

Identification (1) Determine the absorption spectrum of a solution of Zonisamide in methanol (3 in 200,000) as directed under Ultraviolet-visible Spectrophotometry <*2.24*>, and compare the spectrum with the Reference Spectrum or the spectrum of a solution of Zonisamide RS prepared in the same manner as the sample solution: both spectra exhibit similar intensities of absorption at the same wavelengths.

(2) Determine the infrared absorption spectrum of Zonisamide, previously dried, as directed in the potassium bromide disk method under Infrared Spectrophotometry <*2.25*>, and compare the spectrum with the Reference Spectrum or the spectrum of dried Zonisamide RS: both spectra exhibit similar intensities of absorption at the same wave numbers.

Melting point <*2.60*> 164 – 168°C

Purity (1) Chloride <*1.03*>—Dissolve 1.0 g of Zonisamide in 30 mL of acetone, and add 6 mL of dilute nitric acid and water to make 50 mL. Perform the test using this solution as the test solution. Prepare the control solution as follows: to 1.0 mL of 0.01 mol/L hydrochloric acid VS add 30 mL of acetone, 6 mL of dilute nitric acid and water to make 50 mL (not more than 0.036%).

(2) Sulfate <*1.14*>—Dissolve 1.0 g of Zonisamide in 30 mL of acetone, and add 1 mL of dilute hydrochloric acid and water to make 50 mL. Perform the test using this solution as the test solution. Prepare the control solution as follows: to 1.0 mL of 0.005 mol/L sulfuric acid VS add 30 mL of acetone, 1 mL of dilute hydrochloric acid and water to make 50 mL (not more than 0.048%).

(3) Heavy metals <*1.07*>—Proceed with 2.0 g of Zonisamide according to Method 4, and perform the test. Prepare the control solution with 2.0 mL of Standard Lead Solution (not more than 10 ppm).

(4) Related substances—Dissolve 25 mg of Zonisamide in 8 mL of tetrahydrofuran, add water to make 50 mL, and use this solution as the sample solution. Pipet 1 mL of the sample solution, add the mobile phase to make exactly 200 mL, and use this solution as the standard solution. Perform the test with exactly 10 μL each of the sample solution and standard solution as directed under Liquid Chromatography <*2.01*> according to the following conditions. Determine each peak area by the automatic integration method: the area of the peak other than zonisamide obtained from the sample

solution is not larger than 1/5 times the peak area of zonisamide from the standard solution.

Operating conditions—

Detector, column, column temperature, mobile phase, and flow rate: Proceed as directed in the operating conditions in the Assay.

Time span of measurement: About 2 times as long as the retention time of zonisamide, beginning after the solvent peak.

System suitability—

Test for required detectability: Pipet 3 mL of the standard solution, add the mobile phase to make exactly 50 mL. Confirm that the peak area of zonisamide obtained with 10 μL of this solution is equivalent to 4.2 to 7.8% of that with 10 μL of the standard solution.

System performance: When the procedure is run with 10 μL of the standard solution under the above operating conditions, the number of theoretical plates and the symmetry factor of the peak of zonisamide are not less than 8000 and not more than 1.5, respectively.

System repeatability: When the test is repeated 6 times with 10 μL of the standard solution under the above operating conditions, the relative standard deviation of the peak area of zonisamide is not more than 2.0%.

Loss on drying <*2.41*> Not more than 0.5% (1 g, 105°C, 3 hours).

Residue on ignition <*2.44*> Not more than 0.1% (1 g).

Assay Weigh accurately about 0.1 g of Zonisamide, previously dried, and dissolve in methanol to make exactly 100 mL. Pipet 5 mL of this solution, add exactly 5 mL of the internal standard solution, add the mobile phase to make 100 mL, and use this solution as the sample solution. Separately, weigh accurately about 50 mg of Zonisamide RS, previously dried, and dissolve in methanol to make exactly 50 mL. Pipet 5 mL of this solution, add exactly 5 mL of the internal standard solution, add the mobile phase to make 100 mL, and use this solution as the standard solution. Perform the test with 10 μL each of the sample solution and standard solution as directed under Liquid Chromatography <*2.01*> according to the following conditions, and calculate the ratios, Q_T and Q_S, of the peak area of zonisamide to that of the internal standard.

$$\text{Amount (mg) of zonisamide } (C_8H_8N_2O_3S) = M_S \times Q_T/Q_S \times 2$$

M_S: Amount (mg) of Zonisamide RS taken

Internal standard solution—A solution of 4-aminoacetophenone in methanol (1 in 1000).

Operating conditions—

Detector: An ultraviolet absorption photometer (wavelength: 239 nm).

Column: A stainless steel column 5 mm in inside diameter and 15 cm in length, packed with octadecylsilanized silica gel for liquid chromatography (5 μm in particle diameter).

Column temperature: A constant temperature of about 40°C.

Mobile phase: A mixture of water and tetrahydrofuran (5:1).

Flow rate: Adjust so that the retention time of zonisamide is about 11 minutes.

System suitability—

System performance: When the procedure is run with 10 μL of the standard solution under the above operating conditions, the internal standard and zonisamide are eluted in this order with the resolution between these peaks being not less than 5.

System repeatability: When the test is repeated 6 times with 10 μL of the standard solution under the above operating conditions, the relative standard deviation of the ratio of the peak area of zonisamide to that of the internal standard is not more than 1.0%.

Containers and storage Containers—Tight containers.

Zonisamide Tablets

ゾニサミド錠

Zonisamide Tablets contain not less than 95.0% and not more than 105.0% of the labeled amount of zonisamide ($C_8H_8N_2O_3S$: 212.23).

Method of preparation Prepare as directed under Tablets, with Zonisamide.

Identification To 5 mL of the sample solution obtained in the Assay add 5 mL of methanol. Determine the absorption spectrum of this solution as directed under Ultraviolet-visible Spectrophotometry <*2.24*>: it exhibits maxima between 237 nm and 241 nm, between 243 nm and 247 nm, and between 282 nm and 286 nm.

Uniformity of dosage unit <*6.02*> Perform the Mass variation test, or the Content uniformity test according to the following method: it meets the requirement.

To 1 tablet of Zonisamide Tablets add V/25 mL of water, disintegrate completely by sonicating, add 7V/10 mL of methanol, and shake for 15 minutes. Add methanol to make exactly V mL so that each mL contains about 0.5 mg of zonisamide ($C_8H_8N_2O_3S$). Centrifuge this solution, pipet 3 mL of the supernatant liquid, add methanol to make exactly 50 mL, and use this solution as the sample solution. Then, proceed as directed in the Assay.

$$\text{Amount (mg) of zonisamide } (C_8H_8N_2O_3S) = M_S \times A_T/A_S \times V/75$$

M_S: Amount (mg) of Zonisamide RS taken

Dissolution <*6.10*> When the test is performed at 50 revolutions per minute according to the Paddle method, using 900 mL of water as the dissolution medium, the dissolution rate in 45 minutes of 25-mg tablet is not less than 75%, and those in 10 minutes and 45 minutes of 100-mg tablet are not more than 65% and not less than 70%, respectively.

Start the test with 1 tablet of Zonisamide Tablets. In the case of 25-mg tablets, withdraw not less than 20 mL of the medium at the specified minutes after starting the test. In the case of 100-mg tablets, withdraw exactly 20 mL of the medium at the specified minutes after starting the test, and supply exactly 20 mL of water warmed to 37 ± 0.5°C immediately after withdrawing of the medium every time. Filter these media through a membrane filter with a pore size not exceeding 0.45 μm. Discard not less than 10 mL of the first filtrate, pipet V mL of the subsequent filtrate, add water to make exactly V' mL so that each mL contains about 22 μg of zonisamide ($C_8H_8N_2O_3S$), and use this solution as the sample solution. Separately, weigh accurately about 22 mg of Zonisamide RS, previously dried at 105°C for 3 hours, and dissolve in water to make exactly 100 mL. Pipet 5 mL of this solution, add water to make exactly 50 mL, and use this solution as the standard solution. Determine the absorbances, $A_{T(n)}$ and A_S, of the sample solution and standard solution at 285 nm as directed under Ultraviolet-visible Spectrophotometry <2.24>.

Dissolution rate (%) with respect to the labeled amount of zonisamide ($C_8H_8N_2O_3S$) on the nth medium withdrawing (n = 1, 2)

$$= M_S \times \left\{\frac{A_{T(n)}}{A_S} + \sum_{i=1}^{n-1}\left(\frac{A_{T(i)}}{A_S} \times \frac{1}{45}\right)\right\} \times \frac{V'}{V} \times \frac{1}{C} \times 90$$

M_S: Amount (mg) of Zonisamide RS taken

C: Labeled amount (mg) of zonisamide ($C_8H_8N_2O_3S$) in 1 tablet

Assay Weigh accurately the mass of not less than 20 Zonisamide Tablets, and powder. Weigh accurately a portion of the powder, equivalent to about 75 mg of zonisamide ($C_8H_8N_2O_3S$), and moisten with 2 mL of water. Add 70 mL of methanol, shake for 15 minutes, and add methanol to make exactly 100 mL. Centrifuge this solution, pipet 2 mL of the supernatant liquid, add methanol to make exactly 50 mL, and use this solution as the sample solution. Separately, weigh accurately about 38 mg of Zonisamide RS, previously dried at 105°C for 3 hours, dissolve in 1 mL of water and methanol to make exactly 50 mL. Pipet 2 mL of this solution, add methanol to make exactly 50 mL, and use this solution as the standard solution. Determine the absorbances, A_T and A_S, of the sample solution and standard solution at 284 nm as directed under Ultraviolet-visible Spectrophotometry <2.24>.

$$\text{Amount (mg) of zonisamide } (C_8H_8N_2O_3S) = M_S \times A_T/A_S \times 2$$

M_S: Amount (mg) of Zonisamide RS taken

Containers and storage Containers—Tight containers.

Zopiclone

ゾピクロン

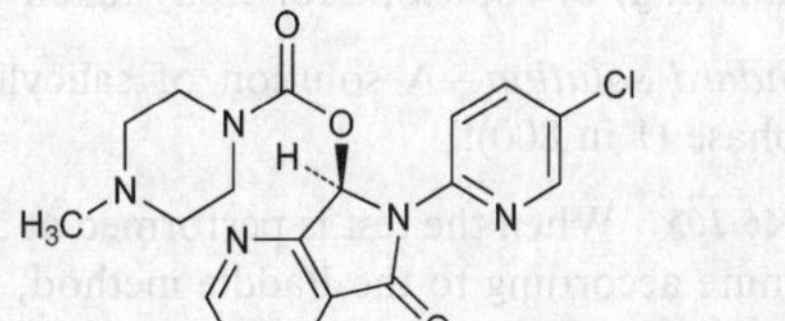

and enantiomer

$C_{17}H_{17}ClN_6O_3$: 388.81

(5*RS*)-6-(5-Chloropyridin-2-yl)-7-oxo-6,7-dihydro-5*H*-pyrrolo[3,4-*b*]pyrazin-5-yl 4-methylpiperazine-1-carboxylate

[*43200-80-2*]

Zopiclone contains not less than 99.0% and not more than 101.0% of zopiclone ($C_{17}H_{17}ClN_6O_3$), calculated on the dried basis.

Description Zopiclone occurs as a white to pale yellow crystalline powder.

It is slightly soluble in ethanol (99.5), and practically insoluble in water.

It dissolves in 0.1 mol/L hydrochloric acid TS.

It is gradually colored to pale brown by light.

A solution of Zopiclone in 0.1 mol/L hydrochloric acid TS (1 in 40) shows no optical rotation.

Melting point: 175 - 178°C

Zopiclone shows crystal polymorphism.

Identification (1) Determine the absorption spectrum of a solution of Zopiclone in 0.1 mol/L hydrochloric acid TS (1 in 100,000) as directed under Ultraviolet-visible Spectrophotometry <2.24>, and compare the spectrum with the Reference Spectrum: both spectra exhibit similar intensities of absorption at the same wavelengths.

(2) Determine the infrared absorption spectrum of Zopiclone as directed in the potassium bromide disk method under Infrared Spectrophotometry <2.25>, and compare the spectrum with the Reference Spectrum: both spectra exhibit similar intensities of absorption at the same wave numbers. If any difference appears between the spectra, dissolve Zopiclone in 21 times its mass of 2-propanol, heat under a reflux condenser for 15 minutes, and gradually cool to 5°C or below. Maintain the temperature for more than 2 hours, filter this solution, wash the residue with 2-propanol, dry, and perform the test using the residue.

Purity (1) Heavy metals <1.07>—Proceed with 2.0 g of Zopiclone according to Method 2, and perform the test. Prepare the control solution with 4.0 mL of Standard Lead Solution (not more than 20 ppm).

(2) Related substances—Conduct this procedure using light-resistant vessels. Dissolve 40 mg of Zopiclone in 100 mL of the mobile phase, and use this solution as the sample solution. Pipet 1 mL of the sample solution, add the mobile phase to make exactly 100 mL, and use this solution as the standard solution. Perform the test with exactly 20 μL each of the sample solution and standard solution as directed under Liquid Chromatography <2.01> according to the following conditions, and determine each peak area by the automatic integration method: the peak areas of related substance A, having the relative retention time of about 0.1 to zopiclone, related substance B, having the relative retention time of about 0.2, related substance C, having the relative retention time of about 0.5, related substance D, having the relative retention time of about 0.9 and the peaks other than mentioned above, obtained from the sample solution, are not larger than 1/10 times the peak area of zopiclone from the standard solution. For the peak areas of related substances A and B, multiply their correction factors, 0.7, and 0.6, respectively.

Operating conditions—

Detector: An ultraviolet absorption photometer (wavelength: 303 nm).

Column: A stainless steel column 4.6 mm in inside diameter and 25 cm in length, packed with octadecylsilanized silica gel for liquid chromatography (5 μm in particle diameter).

Column temperature: A constant temperature of about 30°C.

Mobile phase: Dissolve 1.20 g of sodium dihydrogen phosphate and 8.2 g of sodium lauryl sulfate in 1000 mL of water, and adjust to pH 3.5 with diluted phosphoric acid (1 in 10). To 620 mL of this solution add 380 mL of acetonitrile, and adjust to pH 4.0 with 8 mol/L sodium hydroxide TS or diluted phosphoric acid (1 in 10).

Flow rate: 1.5 mL per minute.

Time span of measurement: About 1.5 times as long as the retention time of zopiclone, beginning after the solvent peak.

System suitability—

Test for required detectability: Pipet 1 mL of the standard solution, and add the mobile phase to make exactly 20 mL. Confirm that the peak area of zopiclone obtained with 20 μL of this solution is equivalent to 3.5 to 6.5% of that with 20 μL of the standard solution.

System performance: When the procedure is run with 20 μL of the standard solution under the above operating conditions, the number of theoretical plates and the symmetry factor of the peak of zopiclone are not less than 7500 and not more than 1.5, respectively.

System repeatability: When the test is repeated 6 times with 20 μL of the standard solution under the above operating conditions, the relative standard deviation of the peak area of zopiclone is not more than 3.0%.

Loss on drying *<2.41>* Not more than 0.5% (2 g, in vacuum, 100°C, 24 hours).

Residue on ignition *<2.44>* Not more than 0.1% (1 g).

Assay Weigh accurately about 0.3 g of Zopiclone, dissolve in 50 mL of a mixture of acetic anhydride and acetic acid (100) (4:1), and titrate *<2.50>* with 0.1 mol/L perchloric acid VS (potentiometric titration). Perform a blank determination in the same manner, and make any necessary correction.

Each mL of 0.1 mol/L perchloric acid VS
= 38.88 mg of $C_{17}H_{17}ClN_6O_3$

Containers and storage Containers—Well-closed containers.

Storage—Light-resistant.

Others

Related substance A:
(7*RS*)-6-(5-Chloropyridin-2-yl)-7-hydroxy-6,7-dihydro-5*H*-pyrrolo[3,4-*b*]pyrazin-5-one

and enantiomer

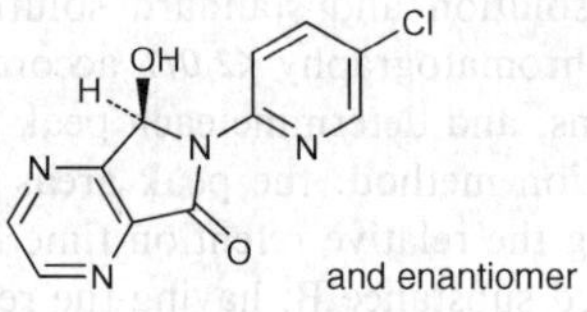

Related substance B:
6-(5-Chloropyridin-2-yl)-6,7-dihydro-5*H*-pyrrolo[3,4-*b*]pyrazin-5-one

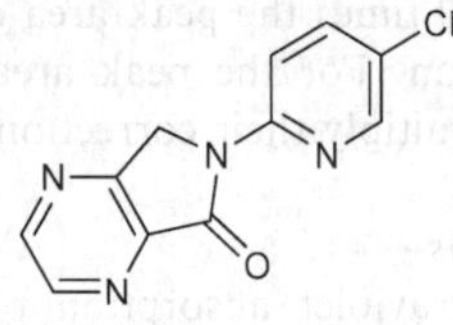

Related substance C:
(5*RS*)-7-Oxo-6-(pyridin-2-yl)-6,7-dihydro-5*H*-pyrrolo[3,4-*b*]pyrazin-5-yl 4-methylpiperazine-1-carboxylate

and enantiomer

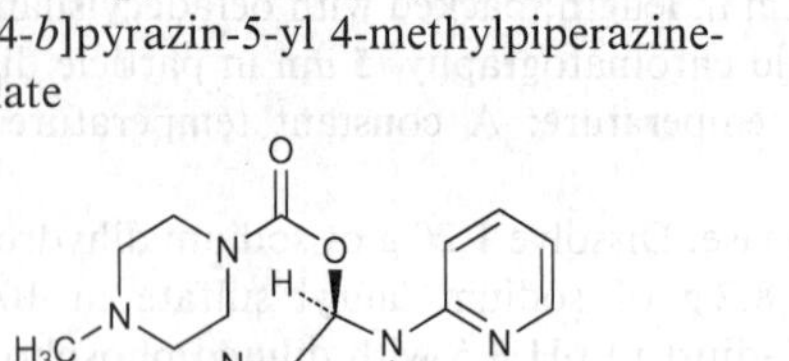

Related substance D:
(5*RS*)-6-(5-Chloropyridin-2-yl)-7-oxo-6,7-dihydro-5*H*-pyrrolo[3,4-*b*]pyrazin-5-yl 4-methylpiperazine-1-carboxylate 4-oxide

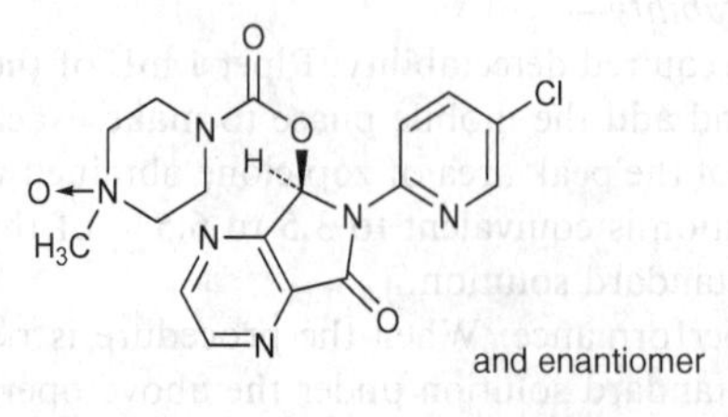

and enantiomer

Zopiclone Tablets

ゾピクロン錠

Zopiclone Tablets contain not less than 95.0% and not more than 105.0% of the labeled amount of zopiclone ($C_{17}H_{17}ClN_6O_3$: 388.81).

Method of preparation Prepare as directed under Tablets, with Zopiclone.

Identification To a quantity of powdered Zopiclone Tablets, equivalent to 30 mg of Zopiclone, add 60 mL of 0.1 mol/L hydrochloric acid TS, shake thoroughly, add 0.1 mol/L hydrochloric acid TS to make 100 mL, and filter. To 2 mL of the filtrate add 0.1 mol/L hydrochloric acid TS to make 50 mL. Determine the absorption spectrum of this solution as directed under Ultraviolet-visible Spectrophotometry *<2.24>*: it exhibits maxima between 214 nm and 218 nm, and between 302 nm and 306 nm.

Uniformity of dosage units *<6.02>* Perform the test according to the following method: it meets the requirement of the Content uniformity test.

To 1 tablet of Zopiclone Tablets add the mobile phase, sonicate while occasional shaking to disintegrate the tablet, add the mobile phase to make exactly 50 mL, and filter through a membrane filter with a pore size not exceeding 0.45 μm. Discard the first 10 mL of the filtrate, pipet V mL of the subsequent filtrate, add exactly $V'/10$ mL of the internal standard solution, add the mobile phase to make V' mL so that each mL contains about 0.1 mg of zopiclone ($C_{17}H_{17}ClN_6O_3$), and use this solution as the sample solution. Then, proceed as directed in the Assay.

Amount (mg) of zopiclone ($C_{17}H_{17}ClN_6O_3$)
$= M_S \times Q_T/Q_S \times V'/V \times 1/10$

M_S: Amount (mg) of zopiclone for assay taken

Internal standard solution—A solution of salicylic acid in the mobile phase (1 in 800).

Dissolution *<6.10>* When the test is performed at 50 revolutions per minute according to the Paddle method, using 900 mL of 0.05 mol/L acetic acid-sodium acetate buffer solution (pH 4.0) as the dissolution medium, the dissolution rate in 30 minutes of Zopiclone Tablets is not less than 80%.

Start the test with 1 tablet of Zopiclone Tablets, withdraw not less than 20 mL of the medium at the specified minute after starting the test, and filter through a membrane filter with a pore size not exceeding 0.45 μm. Discard not less than 10 mL of the first filtrate, pipet V mL of the subsequent filtrate, add the dissolution medium to make exactly V' mL so that each mL contains about 8.3 μg of zopiclone ($C_{17}H_{17}ClN_6O_3$), and use this solution as the sample solution. Separately, weigh accurately about 21 mg of zopiclone for assay (separately determine the loss on drying *<2.41>* in the same conditions as Zopiclone), and dissolve in the dissolution medium to make exactly 100 mL. Pipet 4 mL of this solution, add the dissolution medium to make exactly 100 mL, and use this solution as the standard solution. Determine the absorbances, A_T and A_S, of the sample solution and standard solution at 304 nm as directed under Ultraviolet-visible Spectrophotometry *<2.24>*.

Dissolution rate (%) with respect to the labeled amount of zopiclone ($C_{17}H_{17}ClN_6O_3$)
$= M_S \times A_T/A_S \times V'/V \times 1/C \times 36$

M_S: Amount (mg) of zopiclone for assay taken, calculated on the dried basis
C: Labeled amount (mg) of zopiclone ($C_{17}H_{17}ClN_6O_3$) in 1 tablet

Assay To 20 tablets of Zopiclone Tablets add the mobile phase, sonicate while occasional shaking to disintegrate the tablets, add the mobile phase to make exactly 500 mL, and filter through a membrane filter with a pore size not exceeding 0.45 μm. Discard the first 10 mL of the filtrate, pipet V mL of the subsequent filtrate, add exactly $V'/10$ mL of the internal standard solution, add the mobile phase to make V' mL so that each mL contains about 0.1 mg of zopiclone ($C_{17}H_{17}ClN_6O_3$), and use this solution as the sample solution. Separately, weigh accurately about 50 mg of zopiclone for assay (separately determine the loss on drying <*2.41*> in the same conditions as Zopiclone), and dissolve in the mobile phase to make exactly 20 mL. Pipet 4 mL of this solution, add exactly 10 mL of the internal standard solution, add the mobile phase to make 100 mL, and use this solution as the standard solution. Perform the test with 10 μL each of the sample solution and standard solution as directed under Liquid Chromatography <*2.01*> according to the following conditions, and calculate the ratios, Q_T and Q_S, of the peak area of zopiclone to that of the internal standard.

Amount (mg) of zopiclone ($C_{17}H_{17}ClN_6O_3$) in 1 tablet of Zopiclone Tablet
$$= M_S \times Q_T/Q_S \times V'/V \times 1/20$$

M_S: Amount (mg) of zopiclone for assay taken, calculated on the dried basis

Internal standard solution—A solution of salicylic acid in the mobile phase (1 in 800).
Operating conditions—
Detector: An ultraviolet absorption photometer (wavelength: 304 nm).
Column: A stainless steel column 4.6 mm in inside diameter and 15 cm in length, packed with octadecylsilanized silica gel for liquid chromatography (5 μm in particle diameter).
Column temperature: A constant temperature of about 30°C.
Mobile phase: To 378 mL of diluted acetic acid (100) (57 in 5000), add 222 mL of a solution of sodium acetate trihydrate (17 in 625), and add 400 mL of acetonitrile.
Flow rate: Adjust so that the retention time of zopiclone is about 9.5 minutes.
System suitability—
System performance: When the procedure is run with 10 μL of the standard solution under the above operating conditions, the internal standard and zopiclone are eluted in this order with the resolution between these peaks being not less than 5.
System repeatability: When the test is repeated 6 times with 10 μL of the standard solution under the above operating conditions, the relative standard deviation of the ratio of the peak area of zopiclone to that of the internal standard is not more than 1.0%.

Containers and storage Containers—Tight containers.
Storage—Light-resistant.

JP XVIII

THE JAPANESE PHARMACOPOEIA

EIGHTEENTH EDITION

〈II〉

Official from June 7, 2021

English Version

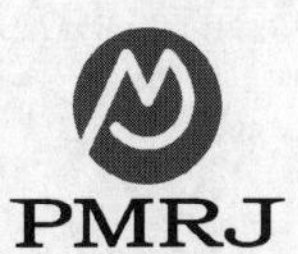

PHARMACEUTICAL AND MEDICAL DEVICE
REGULATORY SCIENCE SOCIETY OF JAPAN

Published 2022 by

PHARMACEUTICAL AND MEDICAL DEVICE
REGULATORY SCIENCE SOCIETY OF JAPAN

2–12–15, Shibuya, Shibuya-ku, Tokyo, 150–0002 JAPAN

Distributed by

YAKUJI NIPPO, LTD.

1, Kanda Izumicho, Chiyoda-ku, Tokyo, 101–8648 JAPAN

Notice: This *English Version* of the Japanese Pharmacopoeia is published for the convenience of users unfamiliar with the Japanese language. When and if any discrepancy arises between the Japanese original and its English translation, the former is authentic.

ISBN978-4-8408-1589-5 C3047

Printed in Japan

JP XVIII
TOTAL CONTENTS

I

II

Crude Drugs and Related Drugs

Acacia

Gummi Arabicum

アラビアゴム

Acacia is the secretions obtained from the stems and branches of *Acacia senegal* Willdenow or other species of the same genus (*Leguminosae*).

Description Colorless or light yellow-brown, translucent or somewhat opaque spheroidal tears, or angular fragments with numerous fissures on the surface; very brittle; the fractured surface glassy and occasionally iridescent.

Odorless; tasteless, but produces a mucilaginous sensation on the tongue.

Pulverized Acacia (1.0 g) dissolves almost completely in 2.0 mL of water, and the solution is acid.

It is practically insoluble in ethanol (95).

Identification To 1 g of pulverized Acacia add 25 mL of water and 1 mL of sulfuric acid, and heat under a reflux condenser for 60 minutes. After cooling, add gently 2.0 g of anhydrous sodium carbonate. To 1 mL of this solution add 9 mL of methanol, mix well, centrifuge, and use the supernatant liquid as the sample solution. Separately, dissolve 10 mg each of D-galactose, L-arabinose and L-rhamnose monohydrate in 1 mL water separately, add methanol to make 10 mL, and use these solutions as the standard solutions (1), (2) and (3), respectively. Perform the test with these solutions as directed under Thin-layer chromatography *<2.03>*. Spot 2 μL each of the sample solution and standard solutions (1), (2) and (3) on a plate of silica gel for thin-layer chromatography. Develop the plate with a mixture of ethyl acetate, methanol, acetic acid (100) and water (12:3:3:2) to a distance of about 7 cm, and air-dry the plate. Spray evenly 1-naphthol-sulfuric acid TS on the plate, and heat the plate at 105°C for 2 minutes: the three spots obtained from the sample solution are the same with each spot from the standard solutions (1), (2) and (3) in the color tone and the *R*f value, respectively.

Purity **(1)** Insoluble residue—To 5.0 g of pulverized Acacia add 100 mL of water and 10 mL of dilute hydrochloric acid, and dissolve by gentle boiling for 15 minutes with swirling. Filter the warm mixture through a tared glass filter (G3), wash the residue thoroughly with hot water, and dry at 105°C for 5 hours: the mass of the residue does not exceed 10.0 mg.

(2) Tannin-bearing gums—To 10 mL of a solution of Acacia (1 in 50) add 3 drops of iron (III) chloride TS: no dark green color is produced.

(3) Glucose—Use the sample solution obtained in the Identification as the sample solution. Separately, dissolve 10 mg of glucose in 1 mL of water, add methanol to make 10 mL, and use this solution as the standard solution. Perform the test with these solutions as directed under Thin-layer Chromatography *<2.03>*. Spot 10 μL each of the sample solution and standard solution on a plate of silica gel for thin-layer chromatography, develop the plate with a mixture of acetone and water (9:1) to a distance of about 10 cm, and air-dry the plate. Spray evenly 1-naphthol-sulfuric acid TS on the plate, and heat the plate at 105°C for 5 minutes: no spot obtained from the sample solution is observed at the position corresponding to the spot from the standard solution.

Loss on drying *<5.01>* Not more than 17.0% (6 hours).

Total ash *<5.01>* Not more than 4.0%.

Acid-insoluble ash *<5.01>* Not more than 0.5%.

Containers and storage Containers—Well-closed containers.

Powdered Acacia

Gummi Arabicum Pulveratum

アラビアゴム末

Powdered Acacia is the powder of Acacia.

Description Powdered Acacia occurs as a white to light yellowish white powder. It is odorless, tasteless, but produces a mucilaginous sensation on the tongue.

Under a microscope *<5.01>*, Powdered Acacia, immersed in olive oil or liquid paraffin, reveals colorless, angular fragments or nearly globular grains. Usually starch grains or vegetable tissues are not observed or very trace, if any.

Powdered Acacia (1.0 g) dissolves almost completely in 2.0 mL of water, and the solution is acid.

It is practically insoluble in ethanol (95).

Identification To 1 g of Powdered Acacia add 25 mL of water and 1 mL of sulfuric acid, and heat under a reflux condenser for 60 minutes. After cooling, add gently 2.0 g of anhydrous sodium carbonate. To 1 mL of this solution add 9 mL of methanol, mix well, centrifuge, and use the supernatant liquid as the sample solution. Separately, dissolve 10 mg each of D-galactose, L-arabinose and L-rhamnose monohydrate in 1 mL water, add methanol to make 10 mL, and use these solutions as the standard solutions, (1), (2) and (3), respectively. Perform the test with these solutions as directed under Thin-layer Chromatography *<2.03>*. Spot 2 μL each of the sample solution and standard solutions (1), (2) and (3) on a plate of silica gel for thin-layer chromatography. Develop the plate with a mixture of ethyl acetate, methanol, acetic acid (100) and water (12:3:3:2) to a distance of about 7 cm, and air-dry the plate. Spray evenly 1-naphthol-sulfuric acid TS on the plate, and heat the plate at 105°C for 2 minutes: the three spots obtained from the sample solution are the same with each spot from the standard solutions (1), (2) and (3) in the color tone and the *R*f value, respectively.

Purity **(1)** Insoluble residue—To 5.0 g of Powdered Acacia add 100 mL of water and 10 mL of dilute hydrochloric acid, and dissolve by gentle boiling for 15 minutes with swirling. Filter the warm mixture through a tared glass filter (G3), wash the residue thoroughly with hot water, and dry at 105°C for 5 hours: the mass of the residue does not exceed 10.0 mg.

(2) Tannin-bearing gums—To 10 mL of a solution of Powdered Acacia (1 in 50) add 3 drops of iron (III) chloride TS: no dark green color is produced.

(3) Glucose—Use the sample solution obtained in the Identification as the sample solution. Separately, dissolve 10 mg of glucose in 1 mL of water, add methanol to make 10 mL, and use this solution as the standard solution. Perform the test with these solutions as directed under Thin-layer Chromatography <*2.03*>. Spot 10 μL each of the sample solution and standard solution on a plate of silica gel for thin-layer chromatography, develop the plate with a mixture of acetone and water (9:1) to a distance of about 10 cm, and air-dry the plate. Spray evenly 1-naphthol-sulfuric acid TS on the plate, and heat the plate at 105°C for 5 minutes: no spot obtained from the sample solution is observed at the position corresponding to the spot from the standard solution.

Loss on drying <*5.01*> Not more than 15.0% (6 hours).

Total ash <*5.01*> Not more than 4.0%.

Acid-insoluble ash <*5.01*> Not more than 0.5%.

Containers and storage Containers—Tight containers.

Achyranthes Root

Achyranthis Radix

ゴシツ

Achyranthes Root is the root of *Achyranthes bidentata* Blume or *Achyranthes fauriei* H. Léveillé et Vaniot (*Amaranthaceae*).

Description Main root or main root with some lateral roots, with or without short remains of rhizome at the crown; main root, long cylindrical and sometimes somewhat tortuous, 15 - 90 cm in length, 0.3 - 0.7 cm in diameter; externally grayish yellow to yellow-brown, with numerous longitudinal wrinkles, and with scattering scars of lateral roots. Fractured surface is flat; grayish white to light brown on the circumference, and with yellow-white xylem in the center. Hard and brittle, or flexible.

Odor, slight; taste, slightly sweet, and mucilaginous.

Under a microscope <*5.01*>, a transverse section reveals a rather distinct cambium separating the cortex from the xylem; small protoxylem located at the center of the xylem, and surrounded by numerous vascular bundles arranged on several concentric circles; parenchyma cells containing sand crystals of calcium oxalate; starch grains absent.

Identification Shake vigorously 0.5 g of pulverized Achyranthes Root with 10 mL of water: a lasting fine foam is produced.

Purity **(1)** Heavy metals <*1.07*>—Proceed with 3.0 g of pulverized Achyranthes Root according to Method 3, and perform the test. Prepare the control solution with 3.0 mL of Standard Lead Solution (not more than 10 ppm).

(2) Arsenic <*1.11*>—Prepare the test solution with 0.40 g of pulverized Achyranthes Root according to Method 4, and perform the test (not more than 5 ppm).

(3) Stem—When perform the test of foreign matter <*5.01*>, the amount of stems contained in Achyranthes Root does not exceed 5.0%.

(4) Foreign matter <*5.01*>—The amount of foreign matter other than stems contained in Achyranthes Root does not exceed 1.0%.

Loss on drying <*5.01*> Not more than 17.0% (6 hours).

Total ash <*5.01*> Not more than 10.0%.

Acid-insoluble ash <*5.01*> Not more than 1.5%.

Containers and storage Containers—Well-closed containers.

Agar

Agar

カンテン

Agar is the solid residue obtained by freezing dehydration of a mucilage derived from *Gelidium elegans* Kuetzing, other species of the same genus (*Gelidiaceae*), or other red algae (*Rhodophyta*).

Description White, translucent rectangular column, string or flakes. Rectangular column about 26 cm in length, 4 cm square in cross section; a string of about 35 cm in length and about 3 mm in width; flakes about 3 mm in length; externally, with wrinkles and somewhat lustrous, light and pliable.

Odorless; tasteless and mucilaginous.

It is practically insoluble in organic solvents.

A boiling solution of Agar (1 in 100) is neutral.

Identification **(1)** To a fragment of Agar add dropwise iodine TS: a dark blue to reddish purple color develops.

(2) Dissolve 1 g of Agar in 65 mL of water by boiling for 10 minutes with constant stirring, and add a sufficient amount of hot water to make up the water lost by evaporation: the solution is clear. Cool the solution between 30°C and 39°C: the solution forms a firm, resilient gel, which does not melt below 85°C.

Purity **(1)** Sulfuric acid—Dissolve 1.0 g of Agar in 100 mL of water by boiling: the solution is not acidic.

(2) Sulfurous acid and starch—To 5 mL of the solution obtained in (1) add 2 drops of iodine TS: the solution is not decolorized immediately, and does not show a blue color.

(3) Insoluble matter—To 7.5 g of Agar add 500 mL of water, boil for 15 minutes, and add water to make exactly 500 mL. Measure exactly 100 mL of the solution, add 100 mL of hot water, heat to boiling, filter while hot through a tared glass filter (G3), wash the residue with a small amount of hot water, and dry the residue at 105°C for 3 hours: the mass of the residue is not more than 15.0 mg.

(4) Water absorption—To 5.0 g of Agar add water to make 100 mL, shake well, allow to stand at 25°C for 24 hours, and filter through moistened glass wool in a 100-mL graduated cylinder: the volume of the filtrate is not more than 75 mL.

Loss on drying <*5.01*> Not more than 22.0% (6 hours).

Total ash <*5.01*> Not more than 4.5%.

Acid-insoluble ash <*5.01*> Not more than 0.5%.

Containers and storage Containers—Well-closed containers.

Powdered Agar

Agar Pulveratum

カンテン末

Powdered Agar is the powder of Agar.

Description Powdered Agar appears as a white powder, is odorless, and is tasteless and mucilaginous.

Under a microscope *<5.01>*, Powdered Agar, immersed in olive oil or liquid paraffin, reveals angular granules with striations or nearly spheroidal granules 5 to 60 μm in diameter.

It becomes transparent in chloral hydrate TS.

It is practically insoluble in organic solvents.

A boiling solution of Powdered Agar (1 in 100) is neutral.

Identification **(1)** To a part of Powdered Agar add dropwise iodine TS: a dark blue to reddish purple color develops.

(2) Dissolve 1 g of Powdered Agar in 65 mL of water by boiling for 10 minutes with constant stirring, and add a sufficient amount of hot water to maintain the original volume lost by evaporation: the solution is clear. Cool the solution between 30°C and 39°C: the solution forms a firm, resilient gel, which does not melt below 85°C.

Purity **(1)** Sulfuric acid—Dissolve 1.0 g of Powdered Agar in 100 mL of water by boiling: the solution is not acid.

(2) Sulfurous acid and starch—To 5 mL of the solution obtained in (1) add 2 drops of iodine TS: the solution is not decolorized immediately, and does not show a blue color.

(3) Insoluble matter—To 7.5 g of Powdered Agar add 500 mL of water, boil for 15 minutes, and add water to make exactly 500 mL. Take exactly 100 mL of the solution, add 100 mL of hot water, heat to boiling, filter while hot through a tared glass filter (G3), wash the residue with a small amount of hot water, and dry the residue at 105°C for 3 hours: the mass of the residue is not more than 15.0 mg.

(4) Water absorption—To 5.0 g of Powdered Agar add water to make 100 mL, shake well, allow to stand at 25°C for 24 hours, and filter through moistened glass wool in a 100-mL graduated cylinder: the volume of the filtrate is not more than 75 mL.

Loss on drying *<5.01>* Not more than 22.0% (6 hours).

Total ash *<5.01>* Not more than 4.5%.

Acid-insoluble ash *<5.01>* Not more than 0.5%.

Containers and storage Containers—Tight containers.

Akebia Stem

Akebiae Caulis

モクツウ

Akebia Stem is the climbing stem of *Akebia quinata* Decaisne or *Akebia trifoliata* Koidzumi (*Lardizabalaceae*), usually cut transversely.

Description Circular or ellipsoidal sections 0.2 – 0.3 cm in thickness, and 1 – 3 cm in diameter; phloem on both fractured surfaces is dark grayish brown; xylem reveals light brown vessel portions and grayish white medullary rays lined alternately and radially; pith light grayish yellow, and distinct; flank grayish brown, and with circular or transversely elongated elliptical lenticels.

Almost odorless; slightly acrid taste.

Under a microscope *<5.01>*, a transverse section reveals ring layers mainly consisting of fiber bundles with crystal cells and stone cell groups and surrounding the outside of the phloem in arc shape. Medullary rays of the cortex consisting of sclerenchyma cells containing solitary crystals; portion near cambium is distinct; cells around the pith remarkably thick-walled; xylem medullary rays and parenchyma cells around the pith contain solitary crystals of calcium oxalate and starch grains less than 8 μm in diameter.

Identification To 0.5 g of pulverized Akebia Stem add 10 mL of water, boil, allow to cool, and shake vigorously: lasting fine foams are produced.

Total ash *<5.01>* Not more than 10.0%.

Containers and storage Containers—Well-closed containers.

Alisma Tuber

Alismatis Tuber

タクシャ

Alisma Tuber is the tuber of *Alisma orientale* Juzepczuk (*Alismataceae*), from which periderm has been usually removed.

Description Spherical or conical tubers, 3 – 8 cm in length, 3 – 5 cm in diameter, sometimes a 2- to 4-branched irregular tuber; externally light grayish brown to light yellow-brown, and slightly annulate; many remains of root appearing as small warty protrusions; fractured surface nearly dense, the outer portion grayish brown, and the inner part white to light yellow-brown in color; rather light in texture and difficult to break.

Slight odor and slightly bitter taste.

Identification To 1.0 g of pulverized Alisma Tuber add 10 mL of diethyl ether, shake for 10 minutes, centrifuge, and use the supernatant liquid as the sample solution. Use alisma tuber triterpenes TS for identification as the standard solution. Perform the test with these solutions as directed under Thin-layer Chromatography *<2.03>*. Spot 5 μL of the sample solution and 1 μL of the standard solution on a plate of silica gel for thin-layer chromatography. Develop the plate with a mixture of ethyl acetate, hexane and acetic acid (100) (10:10:3) to a distance of about 7 cm, and air-dry the plate. Spray evenly vanillin-sulfuric acid-ethanol TS for spraying on the plate, and heat the plate at 105°C for 5 minutes: one of the several spots obtained from the sample solution has the same color tone and *R*f value with a spot among the three spots from the standard solution.

Purity **(1)** Heavy metals *<1.07>*—Proceed with 1.0 g of pulverized Alisma Tuber according to Method 3, and perform the test. Prepare the control solution with 2.0 mL of Standard Lead Solution (not more than 20 ppm).

(2) Arsenic *<1.11>*—Prepare the test solution with 0.40 g of pulverized Alisma Tuber according to Method 4, and perform the test (not more than 5 ppm).

Total ash *<5.01>* Not more than 5.0%.

Acid-insoluble ash *<5.01>* Not more than 0.5%.

Containers and storage Containers—Well-closed contain-

ers.

Powdered Alisma Tuber

Alismatis Tuber Pulveratum

タクシャ末

Powdered Alisma Tuber is the powder of Alisma Rhizome.

Description Powdered Alisma Tuber occurs as a light grayish brown powder, and has a slight odor and a slightly bitter taste.

Under a microscope <*5.01*>, Powdered Alisma Tuber reveals mainly starch grains, fragments of parenchyma containing them, parenchyma cells containing yellow contents, and fragments of vascular bundles. Starch grains, spheroidal to ellipsoidal simple grains, 3 - 15 μm in diameter.

Identification To 1.0 g of Powdered Alisma Tuber add 10 mL of diethyl ether, shake for 10 minutes, centrifuge, and use the supernatant liquid as the sample solution. Use alisma tuber triterpenes TS for identification as the standard solution. Perform the test with these solutions as directed under Thin-layer Chromatography <*2.03*>. Spot 5 μL of the sample solution and 1 μL of the standard solution on a plate of silica gel for thin-layer chromatography. Develop the plate with a mixture of ethyl acetate, hexane and acetic acid (100) (10:10:3) to a distance of about 7 cm, and air-dry the plate. Spray evenly vanillin-sulfuric acid-ethanol TS for spraying on the plate, and heat the plate at 105°C for 5 minutes: one of the several spots obtained from the sample solution has the same color tone and *R*f value with a spot among the three spots from the standard solution.

Purity **(1)** Heavy metals <*1.07*>—Proceed with 1.0 g of Powdered Alisma Tuber according to Method 3, and perform the test. Prepare the control solution with 2.0 mL of Standard Lead Solution (not more than 20 ppm).

(2) Arsenic <*1.11*>—Prepare the test solution with 0.40 g of Powdered Alisma Tuber according to Method 4, and perform the test (not more than 5 ppm).

Total ash <*5.01*> Not more than 5.0%.

Acid-insoluble ash <*5.01*> Not more than 0.5%.

Containers and storage Containers—Well-closed containers.

Aloe

Aloe

アロエ

Aloe is the dried juice of the leaves mainly of *Aloe ferox* Miller, or of interspecific hybrids of the species with *Aloe africana* Miller or *Aloe spicata* Baker (*Liliaceae*).

It contains not less than 4.0% of barbaloin, calculated on the basis of dried material.

Description Aloe occurs as blackish brown to dark brown, irregular masses; sometimes the external surface covered with a yellow powder; the fractured surface smooth and glassy.

Odor, characteristic; taste, extremely bitter.

Identification **(1)** Dissolve 0.5 g of pulverized Aloe in 50 mL of water by warming. After cooling, add 0.5 g of siliceous earth, and filter. Perform the following tests using the filtrate as the sample solution.

(i) Dissolve 0.2 g of sodium tetraborate decahydrate in 5 mL of the sample solution by warming in a water bath. Add a few drops of this solution into 30 mL of water, and shake: a green fluorescence is produced.

(ii) Shake 2 mL of the sample solution with 2 mL of nitric acid: a yellow-brown color which changes gradually to green is produced. Then warm this colored solution in a water bath: the color of the solution changes to red-brown.

(2) To 0.2 g of pulverized Aloe add 10 mL of methanol, shake for 5 minutes, filter, and use the filtrate as the sample solution. Separately, dissolve 1 mg of barbaloin for thin-layer chromatography in 1 mL of methanol, and use this solution as the standard solution. Perform the test with these solutions as directed under Thin-layer Chromatography <*2.03*>. Spot 10 μL each of the sample solution and standard solution on a plate of silica gel for thin-layer chromatography. Develop the plate with a mixture of ethyl acetate, acetone, water and acetic acid (100) (20:5:2:2) to a distance of about 10 cm, and air-dry the plate. Examine under ultraviolet light (main wavelength: 365 nm): one of the several spots obtained from the sample solution and a red fluorescent spot from the standard solution show the same color tone and the same *R*f value.

Purity **(1)** Resin—Warm 0.5 g of pulverized Aloe with 10 mL of diethyl ether on a water bath, and filter. Wash the residue and the filter paper with 3 mL of diethyl ether. Combine the filtrate and the washing, and evaporate the solvent: the mass of the residue is not more than 5.0 mg.

(2) Ethanol-insoluble substances—Heat 1.0 g of pulverized Aloe with 50 mL of ethanol (95) for 30 minutes under a reflux condenser. Filter the warm mixture through a tared glass filter (G4), and wash the residue on the filter with ethanol (95) until the last washing becomes colorless. Dry the residue at 105°C for 5 hours, and weigh: the mass of the residue is not more than 0.10 g.

Loss on drying <*5.01*> Not more than 12.0%.

Total ash <*5.01*> Not more than 2.0%.

Extract content <*5.01*> Water-soluble extract: not less than 40.0%.

Assay Weigh accurately about 0.1 g of pulverized Aloe, add 40 mL of methanol, and heat under a reflex condenser for 30 minutes. After cooling, filter, and add methanol to the filtrate to make exactly 50 mL. Pipet 5 mL of the solution, add methanol to make exactly 10 mL, and use this solution as the sample solution. Separately, weigh accurately about 10 mg of barbaloin for assay, previously dried in a desiccator (in vacuum, phosphorus (V) oxide) for 24 hours, add 40 mg of oxalic acid dihydrate, and dissolve in methanol to make exactly 100 mL. Pipet 5 mL of the solution, add methanol to make exactly 10 mL, and use this solution as the standard solution. Perform the test with exactly 5 μL each of the sample solution and standard solution as directed under Liquid Chromatography <*2.01*> according to the following conditions, and determine the peak areas, A_T and A_S, of barbaloin in each solution.

$$\text{Amount (mg) of barbaloin} = M_S \times A_T/A_S \times 1/2$$

M_S: Amount (mg) of barbaloin for assay taken

Operating conditions—

Detector: An ultraviolet absorption photometer (wavelength: 360 nm).

Column: A stainless steel column 6 mm in inside diameter and 15 cm in length, packed with octadecylsilanized silica gel for liquid chromatography (5 μm in particle diameter).

Column temperature: A constant temperature of about 30°C.

Mobile phase: A mixture of water, acetonitrile and acetic acid (100) (74:26:1).

Flow rate: Adjust so that the retention time of barbaloin is about 12 minutes.

System suitability—

System performance: Dissolve 10 mg of barbaloin for assay add 40 mg of oxalic acid dihydrate, in methanol to make 100 mL. To 5 mL of the solution add 1 mL of a solution of ethenzamide in methanol (1 in 2000) and methanol to make 10 mL. When the procedure is run with 5 μL of this solution under the above operating conditions except the wavelength of 300 nm, barbaloin and ethenzamide are eluted in this order with the resolution between these peaks being not less than 2.0.

System repeatability: When the test is repeated 6 times with 5 μL of the standard solution under the above operating conditions, the relative standard deviation of the peak area of barbaloin is not more than 1.5%.

Containers and storage Containers—Well-closed containers.

Powdered Aloe

Aloe Pulverata

アロエ末

Powdered Aloe is the powder of Aloe.

It contains not less than 4.0% of barbaloin, calculated on the basis of dried material.

Description Powdered Aloe occurs as a dark brown to yellowish dark brown powder. It has a characteristic odor and an extremely bitter taste.

Under a microscope *<5.01>*, Powdered Aloe, immersed in olive oil or liquid paraffin, reveals greenish yellow to reddish brown, angular or rather irregular fragments.

Identification (1) Dissolve 0.5 g of Powdered Aloe in 50 mL of water by warming. After cooling, add 0.5 g of siliceous earth, and filter. Perform the following tests with the filtrate as the sample solution.

(i) Dissolve 0.2 g of sodium tetraborate decahydrate in 5 mL of the sample solution by warming in a water bath. Add a few drops of this solution into 30 mL of water, and shake: a green fluorescence is produced.

(ii) Shake 2 mL of the sample solution with 2 mL of nitric acid: a yellow-brown color which changes gradually to green is produced. Then warm this colored solution in a water bath: the color of the solution changes to red-brown.

(2) To 0.2 g of Powdered Aloe add 10 mL of methanol, shake for 5 minutes, filter, and use the filtrate as the sample solution. Separately, dissolve 1 mg of barbaloin for thin-layer chromatography in 1 mL of methanol, and use this solution as the standard solution. Perform the test with these solutions as directed under Thin-layer Chromatography *<2.03>*. Spot 10 μL each of the sample solution and standard solution on a plate of silica gel for thin-layer chromatography. Develop the plate with a mixture of ethyl acetate, acetone, water and acetic acid (100) (20:5:2:2) to a distance of about 10 cm, and air-dry the plate. Examine under ultraviolet light (main wavelength: 365 nm): one of the several spots obtained from the sample solution has the same color tone and the same *Rf* value with the red fluorescent spot from the standard solution.

Purity (1) Resin—Warm 0.5 of Powdered Aloe with 10 mL of diethyl ether on a water bath, and filter. Wash the residue and the filter paper with 3 mL of diethyl ether. Combine the filtrate and the washing, and evaporate the solvent: the mass of the residue does not exceed 5.0 mg.

(2) Ethanol-insoluble substances—Heat 1.0 g of Powdered Aloe with 50 mL of ethanol (95) for 30 minutes under a reflux condenser. Filter the warm mixture through a tared glass filter (G4), and wash the residue on the filter with ethanol (95) until the last washing becomes colorless. Dry the residue at 105°C for 5 hours, and weigh: the mass of the residue is not more than 0.10 g.

Loss on drying *<5.01>* Not more than 12.0%.

Total ash *<5.01>* Not more than 2.0%.

Extract content *<5.01>* Water-soluble extract: not less than 40.0%.

Assay Weigh accurately about 0.1 g of Powdered Aloe, add 40 mL of methanol, and heat under a reflex condenser for 30 minutes. After cooling, filter, and add methanol to the filtrate to make exactly 50 mL. Pipet 5 mL of the solution, add methanol to make exactly 10 mL, and use this solution as the sample solution. Separately, weigh accurately about 10 mg of barbaloin for assay, previously dried in a desiccator (in vacuum, phosphorus (V) oxide) for 24 hours, add 40 mg of oxalic acid dihydrate, and dissolve in methanol to make exactly 100 mL. Pipet 5 mL of the solution, add methanol to make exactly 10 mL, and use this solution as the standard solution. Perform the test with exactly 5 μL each of the sample solution and standard solution as directed under Liquid Chromatography *<2.01>* according to the following conditions, and determine the peak areas, A_T and A_S, of barbaloin in each solution.

$$\text{Amount (mg) of barbaloin} = M_S \times A_T/A_S \times 1/2$$

M_S: Amount (mg) of barbaloin for assay taken

Operating conditions—

Detector: An ultraviolet absorption photometer (wavelength: 360 nm).

Column: A stainless steel column about 6 mm in inside diameter and about 15 cm in length, packed with octadecylsilanized silica gel for liquid chromatography (5 μm in particle diameter).

Column temperature: A constant temperature of about 30°C.

Mobile phase: A mixture of water, acetonitrile and acetic acid (100) (74:26:1).

Flow rate: Adjust so that the retention time of barbaloin is about 12 minutes.

System suitability—

System performance: To about 10 mg of barbaloin for assay add 40 mg of oxalic acid dihydrate, and dissolve in methanol to make 100 mL. To 5 mL of the solution add 1 mL of a solution of ethenzamide in methanol (1 in 2000) and methanol to make 10 mL. When the procedure is run with 5 μL of this solution under the above operating conditions except the wavelength of 300 nm, barbaloin and ethenzamide are eluted in this order with the resolution between these peaks being not less than 2.0.

System repeatability: When the test is repeated 6 times with 5 μL of the standard solution under the above operating conditions, the relative standard deviation of the peak area of barbaloin is not more than 1.5%.

Containers and storage Containers—Tight containers.

Alpinia Officinarum Rhizome

Alpiniae Officinarum Rhizoma

リョウキョウ

Alpinia Officinarum Rhizome is the rhizome of *Alpinia officinarum* Hance (*Zingiberaceae*).

Description Alpinia Officinarum Rhizome is a slightly curved and cylindrical rhizome, sometimes branched; 2 - 8 cm in length, 0.6 - 1.5 cm in diameter; externally red-brown to dark brown with fine striped lines, grayish white nodes and several traces of rootlet; hard to break; fracture surface, light brown in color and thickness of cortex is approximately the same as that of stele.

Odor, characteristic; taste, extremely pungent.

Under a microscope <*5.01*>, a transverse section reveals epidermal cells often containing oil-like substances; cortex, endodermis and stele present beneath the epidermis; cortex and stele divided by endodermis; vascular bundles surrounded by fibers, scattered throughout the cortex and stele, cortex and stele composed of parenchyma interspersed with oil cells; parenchyma cells containing solitary crystals of calcium oxalate and starch grains, starch grains generally simple (sometimes 2- to 8-compound), narrowly ovate, ellipsoidal or ovate, 10 - 40 μm in diameter and with an eccentric navel.

Identification To 0.5 g of pulverized Alpinia Officinarum Rhizome add 5 mL of acetone, shake for 5 minutes, filter, and use the filtrate as the sample solution. Perform the test with the sample solution as directed under Thin-layer Chromatography <*2.03*>. Spot 5 μL of the sample solution on a plate of silica gel with fluorescent indicator for thin-layer chromatography, develop the plate with a mixture of cyclohexane, ethyl acetate and acetic acid (100) (12:8:1) to a distance of about 7 cm, and air-dry the plate. Examine under ultraviolet light (main wavelength: 254 nm): two spots appear at an *R*f value of about 0.4.

Purity **(1)** Heavy metals <*1.07*>—Proceed with 3.0 g of pulverized Alpinia Officinarum Rhizome according to Method 3, and perform the test. Prepare the control solution with 3.0 mL of Standard Lead Solution (not more than 10 ppm).

(2) Arsenic <*1.11*>—Prepare the test solution with 0.40 g of pulverized Alpinia Officinarum Rhizome according to Method 4, and perform the test (not more than 5 ppm).

Loss on drying <*5.01*> Not more than 15.0% (6 hours).

Total ash <*5.01*> Not more than 7.5%.

Acid-insoluble ash <*5.01*> Not more than 1.5%.

Extract content <*5.01*> Dilute ethanol-extract: not less than 14.0%.

Containers and storage Containers—Well-closed containers.

Aluminum Silicate Hydrate with Silicon Dioxide

Kasseki

カッセキ

Aluminum Silicate Hydrate with Silicon Dioxide is a mineral substance, mainly composed of aluminum silicate hydrate and silicon dioxide.

It is not the same substance with the mineralogical talc.

Description Aluminum Silicate Hydrate with Silicon Dioxide occurs as white to light red powdered crystalline masses, which becomes easily fine powder on crushing. The powder is roughish and easily adheres to skin, and becomes slightly darken and obtains plasticity when moisten with water.

It has a characteristic odor and almost tasteless. It feels like as sand of fine grains by chewing.

Under a microscope <*5.01*>, the powder of Aluminum Silicate Hydrate with Silicon Dioxide, thoroughly grained between a slide glass and a cover glass together with mounting medium, shows numbers of round to polygonal crystals not smaller than 10 μm in diameter.

Identification To 0.5 g of powdered Aluminum Silicate Hydrate with Silicon Dioxide add 3 mL of diluted sulfuric acid (1 in 3), heat until white vapors evolve, then after cooling add 20 mL of water, and filter. The filtrate neutralized to be a weak acidity with ammonia TS responds to Qualitative Tests <*1.09*> (1), (2) and (4) for aluminum salt.

Purity **(1)** Heavy metals <*1.07*>—To 1.5 g of Aluminum Silicate Hydrate with Silicon Dioxide add 50 mL of water and 5 mL of hydrochloric acid, and boil gently for 20 minutes while thorough shaking. After cooling, centrifuge, and separate the supernatant liquid. Wash the precipitate twice with 10 mL portions of water, centrifuging each time, and combine the supernatant liquids. Add ammonia solution (28) dropwise to the combined liquid until a slight precipitate form, then add, while shaking vigorously, dilute hydrochloric acid dropwise to dissolve the precipitate. Add 0.45 g of hydroxylammonium chloride to this solution, heat, then after cooling add 0.45 g of sodium acetate trihydrate and 6 mL of dilute acetic acid, and add water to make 150 mL. Perform the test with 50 mL of this solution as the test solution. Prepare the control solution by adding to 2.0 mL of Standard Lead Solution, 0.15 g of hydroxylammonium chloride, 0.15 g of sodium acetate trihydrate and 2 mL of dilute acetic acid, and add water to make 50 mL (not more than 40 ppm).

(2) Arsenic <*1.11*>—To 1.0 g of Aluminum Silicate Hydrate with Silicon Dioxide add 5 mL of dilute hydrochloric acid, heat gently until boiling begins while shaking thoroughly, then cool quickly, and centrifuge. To the precipitate add 5 mL of dilute hydrochloric acid, shake thoroughly, centrifuge, and take the supernatant liquid. Repeat this operation with 10 mL of water, combine all the extracts, and concentrate the extract to make 5 mL by heating on a water bath. Perform the test using this solution as the test solution (not more than 2 ppm).

Containers and storage Containers—Well-closed containers.

Amomum Seed

Amomi Semen

シュクシャ

Amomum Seed is the seed mass of *Amomum villosum* Loureiro var. *xanthioides* T. L. Wu et S. J. Chen, *Amomum villosum* Loureiro var. *villosum* or *Amomum longiligulare* T. L. Wu (*Zingiberaceae*).

Description Approximately spherical or ellipsoidal mass, 1 - 1.5 cm in length, 0.8 - 1 cm in diameter; externally grayish brown to dark brown, and with white powder in those dried by spreading lime over the seeds; the seed mass is divided into three loculi by thin membranes, and each loculus contains 10 to 20 seeds joining by aril; each seed is polygonal and spherical, 0.3 - 0.5 cm in length, about 0.3 cm in diameter, externally dark brown, with numerous, fine protrusions; hard tissue; under a magnifying glass, a longitudinal section along the raphe reveals oblong section, with deeply indented hilum and with slightly indented chalaza; white perisperm covering light yellow endosperm and long embryo.

Characteristic aroma when cracked, and taste acrid.

Identification To 1.0 g of coarse powdered Amomum Seed add 20 mL of hexane, shake for 10 minutes, centrifuge, and use the supernatant liquid as the sample solution. Separately, use a mixture of hexane and borneol acetate (1000:1) as the standard solution. Perform the test with these solutions as directed under Thin-layer Chromatography <*2.03*>. Spot 10 μL of the sample solution and 2 μL of the standard solution on a plate of silica gel for thin-layer chromatography. Develop the plate with a mixture of hexane, diethyl ether and methanol (15:5:1) to a distance of about 7 cm, and air-dry the plate. Spray evenly 4-methoxybenzaldehyde-sulfuric acid TS on the plate, and heat the plate at 105°C for 5 minutes: one of the several spots obtained from the sample solution has the same color tone and *R*f value with the spot from the standard solution.

Total ash <*5.01*> Not more than 9.0%.

Acid-insoluble ash <*5.01*> Not more than 3.0%.

Essential oil content <*5.01*> Perform the test with 30.0 g of pulverized Amomum Seed: the volume of essential oil is not less than 0.6 mL.

Containers and storage Containers—Well-closed containers.

Powdered Amomum Seed

Amomi Semen Pulveratum

シュクシャ末

Powdered Amomum Seed is the powder of Amomum Seed.

Description Powdered Amomum Seed occurs as a grayish brown powder, and has a characteristic aroma and an acrid taste.

Under a microscope <*5.01*>, Powdered Amomum Seed reveals fragments of wavy perisperm cells filled with starch grains and containing in each cell a calcium oxalate crystal; yellow and long epidermal cells of seed coat and fragments of thin-walled tissue perpendicular to them; fragments of groups of brown, thick-walled polygonal stone cells.

Identification To 2.0 g of Powdered Amomum Seed add 20 mL of hexane, shake for 10 minutes, centrifuge, and use the supernatant liquid as the sample solution. Separately, use a mixture of hexane and borneol acetate (1000:1) as the standard solution. Perform the test with these solutions as directed under Thin-layer Chromatography <*2.03*>. Spot 10 μL of the sample solution and 2 μL of the standard solution on a plate of silica gel for thin-layer chromatography. Develop the plate with a mixture of hexane, diethyl ether and methanol (15:5:1) to a distance of about 7 cm, and air-dry the plate. Spray evenly 4-methoxybenzaldehyde-sulfuric acid TS on the plate, and heat the plate at 105°C for 5 minutes: one of the several spots obtained from the sample solution has the same color tone and *R*f value with the spot from the standard solution.

Total ash <*5.01*> Not more than 9.0%.

Acid-insoluble ash <*5.01*> Not more than 3.0%.

Essential oil content <*5.01*> Perform the test with 30.0 g of Powdered Amomum Seed: the volume of essential oil is not less than 0.4 mL.

Containers and storage Containers—Tight containers.

Anemarrhena Rhizome

Anemarrhenae Rhizoma

チモ

Anemarrhena Rhizome is the rhizome of *Anemarrhena asphodeloides* Bunge (*Liliaceae*).

Description Rather flat and cord-like rhizome, 3 - 15 cm in length, 0.5 - 1.5 cm in diameter, slightly bent and branched; externally yellow-brown to brown; on the upper surface, a longitudinal furrow and hair-like remains or scars of leaf sheath forming fine ring-nodes; on the lower surface, scars of root appearing as numerous round spot-like hollows; light and easily broken. Under a magnifying glass, a light yellow-brown transverse section reveals an extremely narrow cortex; stele porous, with many irregularly scattered vascular bundles.

Odor, slight; taste, slightly sweet and mucous, followed by bitterness.

Identification **(1)** Shake vigorously 0.5 g of pulverized Anemarrhena Rhizome with 10 mL of water in a test tube: a lasting fine foam is produced. Filter the mixture, and to 2 mL of the filtrate add 1 drop of iron (III) chloride TS: a dark green precipitate is produced.

(2) To 1 g of pulverized Anemarrhena Rhizome add 10 mL of 1 mol/L hydrochloric acid TS, and heat under a reflux condenser for 30 minutes. After cooling, centrifuge, and remove the supernatant liquid. To the residue add 10 mL of diethyl ether, shake for 10 minutes, centrifuge, and use the supernatant liquid as the sample solution. Separately, dissolve 1 mg of sarsasapogenin for thin-layer chromatography in 1 mL of methanol, and use this solution as the standard solution. Perform the test with these solutions as directed under Thin-layer Chromatography <*2.03*>. Spot 5 μL each of the sample solution and standard solution on a plate of silica gel for thin-layer chromatography. Develop the plate with a mixture of hexane and acetone (7:3) to a distance of about 7 cm, and air-dry the plate. Spray evenly vanillin-sulfuric acid-ethanol TS for spraying on the plate, and heat the plate at 105°C for 2 minutes: one of the several spots obtained from the sample solution has the same color tone and *Rf* value with the spot from the standard solution.

Purity (1) Heavy metals *<1.07>*—Proceed with 3.0 g of pulverized Anemarrhena Rhizome according to Method 3, and perform the test. Prepare the control solution with 3.0 mL of Standard Lead Solution (not more than 10 ppm).

(2) Arsenic *<1.11>*—Prepare the test solution with 0.40 g of pulverized Anemarrhena Rhizome according to Method 4, and perform the test (not more than 5 ppm).

(3) Foreign matter *<5.01>*—The amount of fiber, originating from the dead leaves, and other foreign matters contained in Anemarrhena Rhizome is not more than 3.0%.

Total ash *<5.01>* Not more than 7.0%.

Acid-insoluble ash *<5.01>* Not more than 2.5%.

Containers and storage Containers—Well-closed containers.

Angelica Dahurica Root

Angelicae Dahuricae Radix

ビャクシ

Angelica Dahurica Root is the root of *Angelica dahurica* Bentham et Hooker filius ex Franchet et Savatier (*Umbelliferae*).

Description Main root from which many long roots are branched out and nearly fusiform and conical in whole shape, 10 - 25 cm in length; externally grayish brown to dark brown, with longitudinal wrinkles, and with numerous scars of rootlets laterally elongated and protruded. A few remains of leaf sheath at the crown and ring-nodes closely protruded near the crown. In a transverse section, the outer region is grayish white in color, and the central region is sometimes dark brown in color.

Odor, characteristic; taste, slightly bitter.

Identification To 0.2 g of pulverized Angelica Dahurica Root add 5 mL of ethanol (95), shake for 5 minutes, and filter. Examine the filtrate under ultraviolet light (main wavelength: 365 nm): a blue to blue-purple fluorescence develops.

Purity (1) Heavy metals *<1.07>*—Proceed with 3.0 g of pulverized Angelica Dahurica Root according to Method 3, and perform the test. Prepare the control solution with 3.0 mL of Standard Lead Solution (not more than 10 ppm).

(2) Arsenic *<1.11>*—Prepare the test solution with 0.40 g of pulverized Angelica Dahurica Root according to Method 4, and perform the test (not more than 5 ppm).

(3) Leaf sheath—When perform the test of foreign matter *<5.01>*, the amount of leaf sheath contained in Angelica Dahurica Root does not exceed 3.0%.

(4) Foreign matter *<5.01>*—The amount of foreign matter other than leaf sheath contained in Angelica Dahurica Root is not more than 1.0%.

Total ash *<5.01>* Not more than 7.0%.

Acid-insoluble ash *<5.01>* Not more than 2.0%.

Extract content *<5.01>* Dilute ethanol-soluble extract: not less than 25.0%.

Containers and storage Containers—Well-closed containers.

Apricot Kernel

Armeniacae Semen

キョウニン

Apricot Kernel is the seed of *Prunus armeniaca* Linné, *Prunus armeniaca* Linné var. *ansu* Maximowicz or *Prunus sibirica* Linné (*Rosaceae*).

It contains not less than 2.0% of amygdalin, calculated on the basis of dried material.

Description Flattened, somewhat asymmetric ovoid seed, 1.1 - 1.8 cm in length, 0.8 - 1.3 cm in width, 0.4 - 0.7 cm in thickness; sharp at one end and rounded at the other end where chalaza situated; seed coat brown and its surface being powdery with rubbing easily detachable stone cells of epidermis; numerous vascular bundles running from chalaza throughout the seed coat, appearing as thin vertical furrows; seed coat and thin semitransparent white albumen easily separate from cotyledon when soaked in boiling water; cotyledon, white in color.

Almost odorless; taste, bitter and oily.

Under a microscope *<5.01>*, surface of epidermis reveals stone cells on veins protruded by vascular bundles, forming round polygon to ellipse and approximately uniform in shape, with uniformly thickened cell walls, and 60 - 90 μm in diameter; in lateral view, stone cell appearing obtusely triangular and its cell wall extremely thickened at the apex.

Identification (1) When Apricot Kernel is knocked and ground together with water, the odor of benzaldehyde is produced.

(2) To 1.0 g of ground Apricot Kernel add 10 mL of methanol, immediately heat under a reflux condenser for 10 minutes, cool, filter, and use the filtrate as the sample solution. Separately, dissolve 2 mg of amygdalin for thin-layer chromatography in 1 mL of methanol, and use this solution as the standard solution. Perform the test with these solutions as directed under Thin-layer Chromatography *<2.03>*. Spot 20 μL each of the sample solution and standard solution on a plate of silica gel for thin-layer chromatography. Develop the plate with a mixture of ethyl acetate, methanol and water (20:5:4) to a distance of about 7 cm, and air-dry the plate. Examine under ultraviolet light (main wavelength: 365 nm): a spot with a bluish white fluorescence appears at an *Rf* value of about 0.7. Spray evenly thymol-sulfuric acid-methanol TS for spraying upon the plate, and heat the plate at 105°C for 5 minutes: one of the several spots from the sample solution has the same color tone and *Rf* value with the spot from the standard solution.

Purity (1) Rancidity—Grind Apricot Kernel with hot water: no unpleasant odor of rancid oil is perceptible.

(2) Foreign matter *<5.01>*—When perform the test with not less than 250 g of Apricot Kernel, it contains not more than 0.10% of fragments of endocarp.

Loss on drying *<5.01>* Not more than 7.0% (6 hours).

Assay Weigh accurately 0.5 g of ground Apricot Kernel, add 40 mL of diluted methanol (9 in 10), heat immediately under a reflux condenser for 30 minutes, and cool. Filter the mixture, add diluted methanol (9 in 10) to make exactly 50 mL. Pipet 5 mL of this solution, add water to make exactly 10 mL, filter, and use the filtrate as the sample solution. Separately, weigh accurately about 10 mg of amygdalin for assay, previously dried in a desiccator (silica gel) for not less than 24 hours, dissolve in diluted methanol (1 in 2) to make exactly 50 mL, and use this solution as the standard solution. Perform the test with exactly 10 μL each of the sample solution and standard solution as directed under Liquid Chromatography ⟨*2.01*⟩ according to the following conditions, and determine the peak areas, A_T and A_S, of amygdalin in each solution.

$$\text{Amount (mg) of amygdalin} = M_S \times A_T/A_S \times 2$$

M_S: Amount (mg) of amygdalin for assay taken

Operating conditions—

Detector: An ultraviolet absorption photometer (wavelength: 210 nm).

Column: A stainless steel column 4.6 mm in inside diameter and 15 cm in length, packed with octadecylsilanized silica gel for liquid chromatography (5 μm in particle diameter).

Column temperature: A constant temperature of about 45°C.

Mobile phase: A mixture of 0.05 mol/L sodium dihydrogen phosphate TS and methanol (5:1).

Flow rate: 0.8 mL per minute (the retention time of amygdalin is about 12 minutes).

System suitability—

System performance: When the procedure is run with 10 μL of the standard solution under the above operating conditions, the number of theoretical plates and the symmetry factor of the peak of amygdalin are not less than 5000 and not more than 1.5, respectively.

System repeatability: When the test is repeated 6 times with 10 μL of the standard solution under the above operating conditions, the relative standard deviation of the peak area of amygdalin is not more than 1.5%.

Containers and storage Containers—Well-closed containers.

Apricot Kernel Water

キョウニン水

Apricot Kernel Water contains not less than 0.09 w/v% and not more than 0.11 w/v% of hydrogen cyanide (HCN: 27.03).

Method of preparation Prepare by one of the following methods.

(1) To Apricot Kernels, previously crushed and pressed to remove fixed oils as much as possible, add a suitable amount of Water, Purified Water or Purified Water in Containers, and carry out steam distillation. Determine the amount of hydrogen cyanide in the distillate by the method as directed in the Assay, and carry on the distillation until the content of hydrogen cyanide in the distillate is about 0.14 w/v%. To the distillate add Ethanol in about 1/3 of the volume of the distillate, and dilute with a mixture of Purified Water or Purified Water in Containers and Ethanol (3:1) until the content of hydrogen cyanide meets the specification.

(2) Dissolve 7.5 mL of freshly prepared mandelonitrile in 1000 mL of a mixture of Purified Water or Purified Water in Containers and Ethanol (3:1), mix well, and filter. Determine the amount of hydrogen cyanide in the solution as directed in the Assay, and, if the amount is more than that specified above, dilute the solution to the specified concentration by the addition of the mixture of Purified Water or Purified Water in Containers and Ethanol (3:1).

Description Apricot Kernel Water is a clear, colorless or pale yellow liquid. It has an odor of benzaldehyde and a characteristic taste.

pH: 3.5 – 5.0

Identification To 2 mL of Apricot Kernel Water add 1 mL of ammonia TS, and allow to stand for 10 minutes: a slight turbidity is produced. Allow to stand for 20 minutes: the turbidity is intensified.

Specific gravity ⟨*2.56*⟩ d_{20}^{20}: 0.968 – 0.978

Purity **(1)** Sulfate ⟨*1.14*⟩—Add a few drops of 0.1 mol/L sodium hydroxide VS to 5.0 mL of Apricot Kernel Water to make slightly alkaline, evaporate on a water bath to dryness, and ignite between 450°C and 550°C. Dissolve the residue in 1.0 mL of dilute hydrochloric acid, and add water to make 50 mL. Perform the test using this solution as the test solution. Prepare the control solution with 0.50 mL of 0.005 mol/L sulfuric acid VS (not more than 0.005%).

(2) Heavy metals ⟨*1.07*⟩—Evaporate 50 mL of Apricot Kernel Water on a water bath to dryness, ignite between 450°C and 550°C, dissolve the residue in 5 mL of dilute acetic acid with warming, add water to make exactly 50 mL, and filter. Remove the first 10 mL of the filtrate, dilute the subsequent 20 mL to 50 mL with water, and perform the test using this solution as the test solution. Prepare the control solution as follows: to 2.0 mL of Standard Lead Solution add 2 mL of dilute acetic acid and water to make 50 mL (not more than 1 ppm).

(3) Free hydrogen cyanide—To 10 mL of Apricot Kernel Water add 0.8 mL of 0.1 mol/L silver nitrate VS and 2 to 3 drops of nitric acid at 15°C, filter, and add 0.1 mol/L silver nitrate VS to the filtrate: no change occurs.

(4) Residue on evaporation—Evaporate 5.0 mL of Apricot Kernel Water to dryness, and dry the residue at 105°C for 1 hour: the mass of the residue is not more than 1.0 mg.

Assay Measure exactly 25 mL of Apricot Kernel Water, add 100 mL of water, 2 mL of potassium iodide TS and 1 mL of ammonia TS, and titrate ⟨*2.50*⟩ with 0.1 mol/L silver nitrate VS until a yellow turbidity persists.

Each mL of 0.1 mol/L silver nitrate VS
= 5.405 mg of HCN

Containers and storage Containers—Tight containers.
Storage—Light-resistant.

Aralia Rhizome

Araliae Cordatae Rhizoma

ドクカツ

Aralia Rhizome is usually the rhizome of *Aralia cordata* Thunberg (*Araliaceae*).

Description Aralia Rhizome is curved, irregular cylindrical to masses occasionally with remains of short roots. 4 – 12 cm in length, 2.5 – 7 cm in diameter, often cut crosswise or lengthwise. 1 to several, enlarged dents by remains of stems on the upper part or rarely 1.5 - 2.5 cm in diameter, remains of short stem. The outer surface is dark brown to yellow-brown, with longitudinally wrinkles, bases or dents of root. The transverse section of rhizome reveals dark brown to yellow-brown, scattered brownish small spots with oil canals, and with numerous splits.

Odor, characteristic; taste, slightly bitter.

Under a microscope *<5.01>*, a transverse section of rhizome reveals the outermost layer to be cork layer, rarely composed of cork stone cells, followed these appeared several cellular layers of collenchyma. Vascular bundle and medullary rays is distinct, pith broad. Phloem fibre bundles are sometimes observed at the outer portion of phloem. Oil canals composed of schizogenous intercellular space in cortex and pith. Cortex composed of vessels, xylem fibres, and occasionally thick-wall xylem parenchyma. Vascular bundles scattered on the pith. And, parenchymatous cells observed rosette aggregates of calcium oxalate. Starch grains composed of simple grains, 2- to 6- compound grains.

Identification To 1 g of pulverized Aralia Rhizome add 10 mL of methanol, shake for 5 minutes, filter, and use the filtrate as the sample solution. Perform the test with the sample solution as directed under Thin-layer Chromatography *<2.03>*. Spot 5 μL of the sample solution on a plate of silica gel for thin-layer chromatography, develop the plate with a mixture of hexane, ethyl acetate and acetic acid (100) (30:10:1) to a distance of about 7 cm, and air-dry the plate. Spray evenly vanillin-sulfuric acid-ethanol TS for spraying on the plate, and heat the plate at 105°C for 5 minutes: a purple spot appears at an *R*f value of about 0.5.

Purity Heavy metals *<1.07>*—Proceed with 1.0 g of pulverized Aralia Rhizome according to Method 3, and perform the test. Prepare the control solution with 2.0 mL of Standard Lead Solution (not more than 20 ppm).

Loss on drying *<5.01>* Not more than 12.0%.

Total ash *<5.01>* Not more than 9.0%.

Acid-insoluble ash *<5.01>* Not more than 1.5%.

Extract content *<5.01>* Dilute ethanol-soluble extract: not less than 15.0%.

Containers and storage Containers—Well-closed containers.

Areca

Arecae Semen

ビンロウジ

Areca is the seed of *Areca catechu* Linné (*Palmae*).

Description Rounded-conical or flattened nearly spherical seed 1.5 - 3.5 cm high and 1.5 - 3 cm in diameter; hilum at the center of its base and usually forming a dent; externally grayish red-brown to grayish yellow-brown, with a network of pale lines; hard in texture; cross section dense in texture, exhibiting a marbly appearance of grayish brown seed coat alternating with white albumen; center of the seed often hollow.

Odor, slight; taste, astringent and slightly bitter.

Identification To 1.0 g of pulverized Areca add 5 mL of 0.01 mol/L hydrochloric acid TS and 5 mL of ethyl acetate, shake for 15 minutes, centrifuge, and remove the ethyl acetate layer. To the aqueous layer add 1 mL of sodium hydroxide TS and 5 mL of ethyl acetate, shake for 15 minutes, centrifuge, and use the ethyl acetate layer as the sample solution. Separately, dissolve 1 mg of arecoline hydrobromide for thin-layer chromatography in 5 mL of methanol, and use this solution as the standard solution. Perform the test with these solutions as directed under Thin-layer Chromatography *<2.03>*. Spot 5 μL each of the sample solution and standard solution on a plate of silica gel for thin-layer chromatography. Develop the plate with a mixture of acetone, water and acetic acid (100) (10:6:1) to a distance of about 7 cm, and air-dry the plate. Spray evenly Dragendorff's TS, air-dry, then spray evenly sodium nitrite TS: one of the spot among the several spots obtained from the sample solution has the same color tone and *R*f value with the spot from the standard solution. The color of this spot fades immediately and then disappears after air-drying.

Purity **(1)** Pericarp—When perform the test of foreign matter *<5.01>*, the amount of pericarp contained in Areca is not more than 2.0%.

(2) Foreign matter *<5.01>*—The amount of foreign matter other than the pericarp contained in Areca does not exceed 1.0%.

Total ash *<5.01>* Not more than 2.5%.

Containers and storage Containers—Well-closed containers.

Artemisia Capillaris Flower

Artemisiae Capillaris Flos

インチンコウ

Artemisia Capillaris Flower is the capitulum of *Artemisia capillaris* Thunberg (*Compositae*).

Description Capitulum, of ovoid to spherical, about 1.5 - 2 mm in length, about 2 mm in diameter, with linear leaves and pedicels. Outer surface of capitulum, light green to light yellow-brown in color; outer surface of leaf, green to green-brown; outer surface of pedicel, green-brown to dark brown. Under a magnifying glass, at the capitulum, involucral scale in 3 - 4 succubous rows; outer scale, of ovate with obtuse; inner scale, of elliptical, 1.5 mm in length, longer than outer one, with keel midrib and thin membranous margin. Floret, tubular; marginal flower, of female; disk flower, of hermaphrodite. Achene, of obovoid, 0.8 mm in length. Light in texture.

Odor, characteristic, slight; taste, slightly acrid, which gives slightly numbing sensation to the tongue.

Identification To 0.5 g of pulverized Artemisia Capillaris Flower add 10 mL of methanol, shake for 3 minutes, filter, and use the filtrate as the sample solution. Perform the test with the sample solution as directed under Thin-layer Chromatography *<2.03>*. Spot 5 μL of the sample solution on a plate of silica gel for thin-layer chromatography. Develop the plate with a mixture of acetone and hexane (1:1) to a distance of about 7 cm, and air-dry the plate. Examine under ultraviolet light (main wavelength: 365 nm): a principal spot with a blue fluorescence appears at an *R*f value of about 0.5.

Purity Stem—When perform the test of foreign matter *<5.01>*, Artemisia Capillaris Flower does not contain any stem more than 2 mm in diameter.

Loss on drying <5.01> Not more than 12.0% (6 hours).

Total ash <5.01> Not more than 9.0%.

Acid-insoluble ash <5.01> Not more than 2.0%.

Extract content <5.01> Dilute ethanol-soluble extract: not less than 15.0%.

Containers and storage Containers—Well-closed containers.

Artemisia Leaf

Artemisiae Folium

ガイヨウ

Artemisia leaf is the leaf and twig of *Artemisia princeps* Pampanini or *Artemisia montana* Pampanini (*Compositae*).

Description Wrinkled leaves and their fragments, frequently with thin stems. The upper surface of leaf dark green, the lower surface covered densely with grayish white cotton-like hairs. When smoothed by immersion in water, unfolded laminas 4 – 15 cm long, 4 – 12 cm wide, 1- to 2-pinnately cleft or pinnately parted. Segments in 2 to 4 pairs, oblong-lanceolate to oblong, apex acuminate sometimes obtuse, margins irregularly lobed or entire. Small sized leaves tri-cleft or entire, lanceolate.

Order, characteristic; taste, slightly bitter.

Under a microscope <5.01>, a transverse section of leaf reveals several-cells-layered collenchyma beneath epidermis of midvein; vascular bundles at the central portion of midvein, occasionally fiber bundles adjacent to phloem and xylem; laminas composed of upper epidermis, palisade tissue, spongy tissue and lower epidermis, long soft hairs, T-shaped hairs and glandular hairs on epidermis of laminas; epidermal cells contain tannin-like substances, parenchyma cells contain oil-like substances and tannin-like substances.

Identification To 0.5 g of pulverized Artemisia Leaf (the parts like a floccose substance which are not easily pulverized may be removed) add 5 mL of a mixture of methanol and water (3:2), shake for 10 minutes, centrifuge, and use the supernatant liquid as the sample solution. Separately, dissolve 1 mg each of umbelliferone for thin-layer chromatography and scopoletin for thin-layer chromatography in 10 mL each of methanol, and use these solutions as the standard solution (1) and the standard solution (2), respectively. Perform the test with these solutions as directed under Thin-layer Chromatography <2.03>. Spot 10 μL of the sample solution and 5 μL each of the standard solutions (1) and (2) on a plate of silica gel for thin-layer chromatography. Develop the plate with a mixture of ethyl acetate, hexane and acetic acid (100) (20:10:1) to a distance of about 7 cm, and air-dry the plate. Examine under ultraviolet light (main wavelength: 365 nm): two of the several spots obtained from the sample solution have the same color tone and *R*f value with the corresponding blue-white fluorescent spots from the standard solutions (1) and (2).

System suitability—(Ultraviolet light (main wavelength: 365 nm)).

To 1 mL of the standard solution (1) add methanol to make 10 mL. Confirm that when perform the test with 1 μL of this solution under the above conditions, a bluish white fluorescent spot is detectable.

Purity *Artemisia argyi*—To 0.5 g of powdered Artemisia Leaf (the parts like a floccose substance which are not easily pulverized may be removed) add 5 mL of a mixture of methanol and water (3:2), shake for 10 minutes, centrifuge, and use the supernatant liquid as the sample solution. Separately, to 0.5 g of artemisia·argyi for purity test add 5 mL of a mixture of methanol and water (3:2), shake for 10 minutes, centrifuge, and use the supernatant liquid as the standard solution. Perform the test with these solutions as directed under Thin-layer Chromatography <2.03>. Spot 10 μL each of the sample solution and standard solution on a plate of silica gel for thin-layer chromatography. Develop the plate with a mixture of ethyl acetate, hexane and acetic acid (100) (20:10:1) to a distance of about 7 cm, and air-dry the plate. Spray evenly dilute sulfuric acid on the plate, heat the plate at 105°C for 5 minutes, and examine under ultraviolet light (main wavelength: 365 nm): no spot appears from the sample solution at the position of the green fluorescent spot (*R*f value of about 0.5) obtained from the standard solution.

Loss on drying <5.01> Not more than 14.0%.

Total ash <5.01> Not more than 13.0%.

Acid-insoluble ash <5.01> Not more than 3.0%.

Extract content <5.01> Dilute ethanol-soluble extract: not less than 16.0%.

Containers and storage Containers—Well-closed containers.

Asiasarum Root

Asiasari Radix

サイシン

Asiasarum Root is the root and rhizome of *Asiasarum heterotropoides* F. Maekawa var. *mandshuricum* F. Maekawa or *Asiasarum sieboldii* F. Maekawa (*Aristolochiaceae*).

Description Asiasarum Root is a nearly cylindrical rhizome with numerous thin and long roots, externally light brown to dark brown. The root, about 15 cm in length, about 0.1 cm in diameter, with shallow longitudinal wrinkles on the surface, and brittle. The rhizome, 2 – 4 cm in length, 0.2 – 0.3 cm in diameter, often branched, with longitudinal wrinkles on the surface; internode short; each node has several scars of petiole and peduncle, and several thin and long roots.

Odor, characteristic; taste, acrid, which gives slightly numbing sensation to the tongue.

Identification To 1 g of pulverized Asiasarum Root add 10 mL of diethyl ether, shake for 10 minutes, centrifuge, and use the supernatant liquid as the sample solution. Separately, dissolve 1 mg of asarinin for thin-layer chromatography in 1 mL of methanol, and use this solution as the standard solution. Perform the test with these solutions as directed under Thin-layer Chromatography <2.03>. Spot 10 μL of the sample solution and 5 μL of the standard solution on a plate of silica gel for thin-layer chromatography. Develop the plate with a mixture of hexane and ethyl acetate (2:1) to a distance of about 7 cm, and air-dry the plate. Spray evenly dilute sulfuric acid on the plate, and heat the plate at 105°C for 5 minutes: one of the several spots obtained from the sample solution has the same color tone and *Rf* value with the spot from the standard solution.

Purity (1) Heavy metals *<1.07>*—Proceed with 1.0 g of pulverized Asiasarum Root according to Method 3, and perform the test. Prepare the control solution with 2.0 mL of Standard Lead Solution (not more than 20 ppm).

(2) Arsenic *<1.11>*—Prepare the test solution with 0.40 g of pulverized Asiasarum Root according to Method 4, and perform the test (not more than 5 ppm).

(3) Terrestrial part—When perform the test of foreign matter *<5.01>*, any terrestrial parts are not found.

(4) Foreign matter *<5.01>*—The amount of foreign matter other than terrestrial part contained in Asiasarum Root is not more than 1.0%.

(5) Aristolochic acid I—To exactly 2.0 g of pulverized Asiasarum Root add exactly 50 mL of diluted methanol (3 in 4), shake for 15 minutes, filter, and use the filtrate as the sample solution. Separately, dissolve exactly 1.0 mg of aristolochic acid I for crude drugs purity test in diluted methanol (3 in 4) to make exactly 100 mL. Pipet 1 mL of this solution, add diluted methanol (3 in 4) to make exactly 25 mL, and use this solution as the standard solution. Perform the test with exactly 20 μL each of the sample solution and standard solution as directed under Liquid Chromatography *<2.01>*, according to the following conditions: the sample solution shows no peak at the retention time corresponding to aristolochic acid I from the standard solution. If the sample solution shows such a peak, repeat the test under different conditions to confirm that the peak in question is not aristolochic acid I.

Operating conditions—

Detector: An ultraviolet or visible absorption photometer (wavelength: 400 nm).

Column: A stainless steel column 4.6 mm in inside diameter and 25 cm in length, packed with octadecylsilanized silica gel for liquid chromatography (5 μm in particle diameter).

Column temperature: A constant temperature of about 40°C.

Mobile phase: A mixture of a solution prepared by dissolving 7.8 g of sodium dihydrogen phosphate dihydrate and 2 mL of phosphoric acid in water to make 1000 mL and acetonitrile (11:9).

Flow rate: Adjust so that the retention time of aristolochic acid I is about 15 minutes.

System suitability—

Test for required detectability: Measure exactly 1 mL of the standard solution, and add diluted methanol (3 in 4) to make exactly 10 mL. Confirm that the ratio, S/N, of the signal (S) and noise (N) of aristolochic acid I obtained with 20 μL of this solution is not less than 3.

System repeatability: When the test is repeated 6 times with 20 μL of the standard solution under the above operating conditions, the relative standard deviation of the peak area of aristolochic acid I is not more than 5.0%.

(6) Total BHC's and total DDT's *<5.01>*—Not more than 0.2 ppm, respectively.

Total ash *<5.01>* Not more than 10.0%.

Acid-insoluble ash *<5.01>* Not more than 3.0%.

Essential oil content *<5.01>* Perform the test with 30.0 g of pulverized Asiasarum Root: the volume of essential oil is not less than 0.6 mL.

Containers and storage Containers—Well-closed containers.

Asparagus Root

Asparagi Radix

テンモンドウ

Asparagus Root is the root of *Asparagus cochinchinensis* Merrill (*Liliaceae*), from which most of the velamen is removed, after being passed through hot water or steamed.

Description Fusiform to cylindrical tubers, 5 - 15 cm in length, 5 - 20 mm in diameter; externally light yellow-brown to light brown, translucent and often with longitudinal wrinkles; flexible, or hard and easily broken in texture; fractured surface, grayish yellow, glossy and horny.

Odor, characteristic; taste, sweet at first, followed by a slightly bitter aftertaste.

Under a microscope *<5.01>*, a transverse section reveals stone cells and their groups scattered on outer layer of cortex; mucilaginous cells containing raphides of calcium oxalate in the parenchyma cells of cortex and stele; no starch grains.

Identification To 1 g of the coarse cutting of Asparagus Root add 5 mL of a mixture of 1-butanol and water (40:7), shake for 30 minutes, filter, and use the filtrate as the sample solution. Perform the test with the sample solution as directed under Thin-layer Chromatography *<2.03>*. Spot 10 μL of the sample solution on a plate of silica gel for thin-layer chromatography, develop the plate with a mixture of 1-butanol, water and acetic acid (100) (10:6:3) to a distance of about 7 cm, and air-dry the plate. Spray evenly dilute sulfuric acid on the plate, and heat the plate at 105°C for 2 minutes: the spot of a red-brown at first then changes to brown color appears at an *Rf* value of about 0.4.

Purity (1) Heavy metals *<1.07>*—Proceed with 3.0 g of pulverized Asparagus Root according to Method 3, and perform the test. Prepare the control solution with 3.0 mL of Standard Lead Solution (not more than 10 ppm).

(2) Arsenic *<1.11>*—Prepare the test solution with 0.40 g of pulverized Asparagus Root according to Method 4, and perform the test (not more than 5 ppm).

Loss on drying *<5.01>* Not more than 18.0% (6 hours).

Total ash *<5.01>* Not more than 3.0%.

Containers and storage Containers—Well-closed containers.

Astragalus Root

Astragali Radix

オウギ

Astragalus Root is the root of *Astragalus membranaceus* Bunge or *Astragalus mongholicus* Bunge (*Leguminosae*).

Description Nearly cylindrical root, 30 - 100 cm in length, 0.7 - 2 cm in diameter, with small bases of lateral root dispersed on the surface, twisted near the crown; externally light grayish yellow to light yellow-brown, and covered with irregular, dispersed longitudinal wrinkles and horizontal lenticel-like patterns; difficult to break; fractured surface fibrous. Under a magnifying glass, a transverse section reveals an outer layer composed of periderm; cortex light yellowish white, xylem light yellow, and zone near the cambium somewhat brown in color; thickness of cortex from about one-third to one-half of the diameter of xylem; white medullary ray from xylem to cortex in thin root, but often appearing as radiating cracks in thick root; usually pith unobservable.

Odor, slight; taste, sweet.

Identification To 1 g of pulverized Astragalus Root add 5 mL of potassium hydroxide TS and 5 mL of acetonitrile in a glass-stoppered centrifuge tube. After shaking this for 10 minutes, centrifuge, and use the acetonitrile layer as the sample solution. Separately, dissolve 1 mg of astragaloside IV for thin-layer chromatography in 10 mL of methanol, and use this solution as the standard solution. Perform the test with these solutions as directed under Thin-layer Chromatography *<2.03>*. Spot 10 μL each of the sample solution and standard solution on a plate of silica gel for thin-layer chromatography. Develop the plate with a mixture of ethyl acetate, methanol and water (20:5:4) to a distance of about 7 cm, and air-dry the plate. Spray evenly dilute sulfuric acid on the plate, heat the plate at 105°C for 5 minutes, and examine under ultraviolet light (main wavelength: 365 nm): one of the several spots obtained from the sample solution has the same color tone and *R*f value with the yellow-brown fluorescent spot from the standard solution.

Purity **(1)** Heavy metals *<1.07>*—Proceed with 3.0 g of pulverized Astragalus Root according to Method 3, and perform the test. Prepare the control solution with 3.0 mL of Standard Lead Solution (not more than 10 ppm).

(2) Arsenic *<1.11>*—Prepare the test solution with 0.40 g of pulverized Astragalus Root according to Method 4, and perform the test (not more than 5 ppm).

(3) Root of *Hedysarum* species and others—Under a microscope *<5.01>*, a vertical section of Astragalus Root reveals no crystal fiber containing solitary crystals of calcium oxalate outside the fiber bundle.

(4) Total BHC's and total DDT's *<5.01>*—Not more than 0.2 ppm, respectively.

Loss on drying *<5.01>* Not more than 13.0% (6 hours).

Total ash *<5.01>* Not more than 5.0%.

Acid-insoluble ash *<5.01>* Not more than 1.0%.

Containers and storage Containers—Well-closed containers.

Atractylodes Lancea Rhizome

Atractylodis Lanceae Rhizoma

ソウジュツ

Atractylodes Lancea Rhizome is the rhizome of *Atractylodes lancea* De Candolle, *Atractylodes chinensis* Koidzumi or their interspecific hybrids (*Compositae*).

Description Irregularly curved, cylindrical rhizome, 3 - 10 cm in length, 1 - 2.5 cm in diameter; externally dark grayish brown to dark yellow-brown; a transverse section nearly orbicular, with light brown to red-brown secretes as fine points. Often white cotton-like crystals produced on its surface.

Odor, characteristic; taste, slightly bitter.

Under a microscope *<5.01>*, a transverse section usually reveals periderm with stone cells; parenchyma of cortex, usually without any fiber bundle; oil sacs, containing light brown to yellow-brown substances, located at the end region of medullary rays; xylem exhibits vessels surrounded by fiber bundles and arranged radially on the region adjoining the cambium; pith and medullary rays exhibit the same oil sacs as in the cortex; parenchyma cells contain spherocrystals of inulin and small needle crystals of calcium oxalate.

Identification To 2.0 g of pulverized Atractylodes Lancea Rhizome add 5 mL of hexane, shake for 5 minutes, filter, and use the filtrate as the sample solution. Perform the test with the sample solution as directed under Thin-layer Chromatography *<2.03>*. Spot 10 μL of the sample solution on a plate of silica gel for thin-layer chromatography, develop the plate with a mixture of hexane and acetic acid (100) (10:1) to a distance of about 7 cm, and air-dry the plate. Spray evenly 4-dimethylaminobenzaldehyde TS for spraying on the plate, and heat the plate at 105°C for 5 minutes: a grayish green spot appears at an *R*f value of about 0.5.

Purity **(1)** Heavy metals *<1.07>*—Proceed with 3.0 g of pulverized Atractylodes Lancea Rhizome according to Method 3, and perform the test. Prepare the control solution with 3.0 mL of Standard Lead Solution (not more than 10 ppm).

(2) Arsenic *<1.11>*—Prepare the test solution with 0.40 g of pulverized Atractylodes Lancea Rhizome according to Method 4, and perform the test (not more than 5 ppm).

Total ash *<5.01>* Not more than 7.0%.

Acid-insoluble ash *<5.01>* Not more than 1.5%.

Essential oil content *<5.01>* Perform the test with 50.0 g of pulverized Atractylodes Lancea Rhizome: the volume of essential oil is not less than 0.7 mL.

Containers and storage Containers—Well-closed containers.

Powdered Atractylodes Lancea Rhizome

Atractylodis Lanceae Rhizoma Pulveratum

ソウジュツ末

Powdered Atractylodes Lancea Rhizome is the powder of Atractylodes Lancea Rhizome.

Description Powdered Atractylodes Lancea Rhizome occurs as a yellow-brown powder. It has a characteristic odor, and a slightly bitter taste.

Under a microscope *<5.01>*, Powdered Atractylodes Lancea Rhizome reveals mainly parenchyma cells, spherocrystals of inulin, fragments of parenchyma cells containing small needle crystals of calcium oxalate as their contents; and further fragments of light yellow thick-walled fibers, stone cells and cork cells; a few fragments of reticulate and scalariform vessels, and small yellow-brown secreted masses or oil drops; starch grains absent.

Identification To 2.0 g of Powdered Atractylodes Lancea Rhizome add 5 mL of hexane, shake for 5 minutes, filter, and use the filtrate as the sample solution. Perform the test with the sample solution as directed under Thin-layer Chromatography <2.03>. Spot 10 μL of the sample solution on a plate of silica gel for thin-layer chromatography, develop the plate with a mixture of hexane and acetic acid (100) (10:1) to a distance of about 7 cm, and air-dry the plate. Spray evenly 4-dimethylaminobenzaldehyde TS for spraying on the plate, and heat the plate at 105°C for 5 minutes: a grayish green spot appears at an *R*f value of about 0.5.

Purity **(1)** Heavy metals <1.07>—Proceed with 3.0 g of Powdered Atractylodes Lancea Rhizome according to Method 3, and perform the test. Prepare the control solution with 3.0 mL of Standard Lead Solution (not more than 10 ppm).

(2) Arsenic <1.11>—Prepare the test solution with 0.40 g of Powdered Atractylodes Lancea Rhizome according to Method 4, and perform the test (not more than 5 ppm).

Total ash <5.01> Not more than 7.0%.

Acid-insoluble ash <5.01> Not more than 1.5%.

Essential oil content <5.01> Perform the test with 50.0 g of Powdered Atractylodes Lancea Rhizome: the volume of essential oil is not less than 0.5 mL.

Containers and storage Containers—Tight containers.

Atractylodes Rhizome

Atractylodis Rhizoma

ビャクジュツ

Atractylodes Rhizome is the rhizome of 1) *Atractylodes japonica* Koidzumi ex Kitamura (*Compositae*) (Wa-byakujutsu) or 2) *Atractylodes macrocephala* Koidzumi (*Atractylodes ovata* De Candolle) (*Compositae*) (Kara-byakujutsu).

Description **1)** Wa-byakujutsu—Periderm-removed rhizome is irregular masses or irregularly curved cylinder, 3 – 8 cm in length, 2 – 3 cm in diameter; externally light grayish yellow to light yellowish white, with scattered grayish brown parts. The rhizome covered with periderm is externally grayish brown, often with node-like protuberances and coarse wrinkles. Difficult to break, and the fractured surface is fibrous. A transverse section, with fine dots of light yellow-brown to brown secrete.

Odor, characteristic; taste, somewhat bitter.

Under a microscope <5.01>, a transverse section reveals periderm with stone cell layers; fiber bundles in the parenchyma of the cortex, often adjoined to the outside of the phloem; oil sacs containing light brown to brown substances, situated at the outer end of medullary rays; in the xylem, radially lined vessels, surrounding large pith, and distinct fiber bundle surrounding the vessels; in pith and in medullary rays, oil sacs similar to those in cortex, and in parenchyma, crystals of inulin and small needle crystals of calcium oxalate.

2) Kara-byakujutsu—Irregularly enlarged mass, 4 – 8 cm in length, 2 – 5 cm in diameter; externally grayish yellow to dark brown, having sporadic, knob-like small protrusions. Difficult to break; fractured surface has a light brown to dark brown xylem remarkably fibrous.

Odor, characteristic; taste, somewhat sweet, but followed by slight bitterness.

Under a microscope <5.01>, a transverse section usually reveals periderm with stone cells, absence of fibers in the cortex; oil sacs containing yellow-brown contents in phloem ray and also at the outer end of it; xylem with radially lined vessels surrounding large pith, and distinct fiber bundle surrounding the vessels; pith and medullary ray exhibit oil sacs as in cortex; parenchyma contains crystals of inulin and small needle crystals of calcium oxalate.

Identification To 2.0 g of pulverized Atractylodes Rhizome add 5 mL of hexane, shake for 5 minutes, filter, and use the filtrate as the sample solution. Perform the test with the sample solution as directed under Thin-layer Chromatography <2.03>. Spot 10 μL of the sample solution on a plate of silica gel for thin-layer chromatography. Develop the plate with a mixture of hexane and acetic acid (100) (10:1) to a distance of about 7 cm, and air-dry the plate. Spray evenly 4-dimethylaminobenzaldehyde TS for spraying on the plate, and heat the plate at 105°C for 5 minutes: a red-purple spot appears at an *R*f value of about 0.6.

Purity **(1)** Heavy metals <1.07>—Proceed with 1.0 g of pulverized Atractylodes Rhizome according to Method 3, and perform the test. Prepare the control solution with 2.0 mL of Standard Lead Solution (not more than 20 ppm).

(2) Arsenic <1.11>—Prepare the test solution with 0.40 g of pulverized Atractylodes Rhizome according to Method 4, and perform the test (not more than 5 ppm).

(3) Atractylodes lancea rhizome—When proceed as directed in the Identification, using exactly 5 mL of hexane, any grayish green spot does not appear at an *R*f value of about 0.5, immediately below the red-purple spot appeared at an *R*f value of about 0.6.

Total ash <5.01> Not more than 7.0%.

Acid-insoluble ash <5.01> Not more than 1.0%.

Essential oil content <5.01> Perform the test with 50.0 g of pulverized Atractylodes Rhizome: the volume of essential oil is not less than 0.5 mL.

Containers and storage Containers—Well-closed containers.

Powdered Atractylodes Rhizome

Atractylodis Rhizoma Pulveratum

ビャクジュツ末

Powdered Atractylodes Rhizome is the powder of Atractylodes Rhizome.

Description Powdered Atractylodes Rhizome occurs as a light brown to yellow-brown powder, and has a characteristic odor and a slightly bitter or slightly sweet taste, followed by a slightly bitter aftertaste.

Under a microscope <5.01>, Powdered Atractylodes Rhizome reveals mainly parenchyma cells, crystals of inulin and fragments of parenchyma cells containing small needle crystals of calcium oxalate; fragments of light yellow thick-walled fibers, stone cells and cork cells; a few fragments of reticulate and scalariform vessels; small yellow-brown secrete masses or oil droplets; starch grains absent.

Identification To 2.0 g of Powdered Atractylodes Rhizome add 5 mL of hexane, shake for 5 minutes, filter, and use the filtrate as the sample solution. Perform the test with the sample solution as directed under Thin-layer Chromatography <2.03>. Spot 10 μL of the sample solution on a plate of silica gel for thin-layer chromatography. Develop the plate with a mixture of hexane and acetic acid (100) (10:1) to a distance of about 7 cm, and air-dry the plate. Spray evenly 4-dimethylaminobenzaldehyde TS for spraying on the plate, and heat the plate at 105°C for 5 minutes: a red-purple spot appears at an *R*f value of about 0.6.

Purity **(1)** Heavy metals <1.07>—Proceed with 1.0 g of Powdered Atractylodes Rhizome according to Method 3, and perform the test. Prepare the control solution with 2.0 mL of Standard Lead Solution (not more than 20 ppm).

(2) Arsenic <1.11>—Prepare the test solution with 0.40 g of Powdered Atractylodes Rhizome according to Method 4, and perform the test (not more than 5 ppm).

(3) Atractylodes lancea rhizome—When proceed as directed in the Identification, using exactly 5 mL of hexane, any grayish green spot does not appear at an *R*f value of about 0.5, immediately below the red-purple spot appeared at an *R*f value of about 0.6.

Total ash <5.01> Not more than 7.0%.

Acid-insoluble ash <5.01> Not more than 1.0%.

Essential oil content <5.01> Perform the test with 50.0 g of Powdered Atractylodes Rhizome: the volume of essential oil is not less than 0.4 mL.

Containers and storage Containers—Tight containers.

Bakumondoto Extract

麦門冬湯エキス

Bakumondoto Extract contains not less than 1.2 mg of ginesenoside Rb_1 ($C_{54}H_{92}O_{23}$: 1109.29), and not less than 14 mg and not more than 42 mg of glycyrrhizic acid ($C_{42}H_{62}O_{16}$: 822.93), per extract prepared with the amount specified in the Method of preparation.

Method of preparation

	1)
Ophiopogon Root	10 g
Pinellia Tuber	5 g
Brown Rice	5 g
Jujube	3 g
Ginseng	2 g
Glycyrrhiza	2 g

Prepare a dry extract or viscous extract as directed under Extracts, according to the prescription 1), using the crude drugs shown above.

Description Bakumondoto Extract occurs as a light yellow to light brown powder or black-brown viscous extract. It has a slight odor, and a sweet taste.

Identification **(1)** Shake 2.0 g of the dry extract (or 6.0 g of the viscous extract) with 10 mL of water, add 5 mL of 1-butanol, shake, centrifuge, remove the 1-butanol layer, and use the aqueous layer as the sample solution. Separately, heat 3.0 g of pulverized ophiopogon root in 50 mL of water under a reflux condenser for 1 hour. After cooling, shake 20 mL of the extract with 5 mL of 1-butanol, centrifuge, remove the 1-butanol layer, and use the aqueous layer as the standard solution. Perform the test with these solutions as directed under Thin-layer Chromatography <2.03>. Spot 2 μL of the sample solution and 5 μL of the standard solution as bands on the original line on a plate of silica gel for thin-layer chromatography. Develop the plate with a mixture of ethanol (99.5), water and acetic acid (100) (120:80:1) to a distance of about 7 cm, and air-dry the plate. Spray evenly 4-methoxybenzaldehyde-sulfuric acid TS on the plate, and heat the plate at 105°C for 5 minutes: one of the several spots obtained from the sample solution has the same color tone and *R*f value with the dark blue-green spot (*R*f value: about 0.3) from the standard solution (Ophiopogon Root).

(2) Shake 5.0 g of the dry extract (or 15 g of the viscous extract) with 15 mL of water, add 5 mL of diethyl ether, shake, centrifuge, and use the diethyl ether layer as the sample solution. Separately, dissolve 1 mg of cycloartenyl ferulate for thin-layer chromatography in 1 mL of ethyl acetate, and use this solution as the standard solution. Perform the test with these solutions as directed under Thin-layer Chromatography <2.03>. Spot 30 μL of the sample solution and 5 μL of the standard solution on a plate of silica gel for thin-layer chromatography. Develop the plate with a mixture of hexane, acetone and acetic acid (100) (50:20:1) to a distance of about 7 cm, and air-dry the plate. Examine under ultraviolet light (main wavelength: 365 nm): one of the several spots obtained from the sample solution has the same color tone and *R*f value with the blue-white fluorescent spot from the standard solution. Or examine under ultraviolet light (main wavelength: 365 nm) after spraying evenly a mixture of sulfuric acid and ethanol (99.5) (1:1) on the plate, and heating the plate at 105°C for 5 minutes: one of the several spots obtained from the sample solution has the same color tone and *R*f value with the yellow fluorescent spot from the standard solution (Brown Rice).

(3) Shake 2.0 g of the dry extract (or 6.0 g of the viscous extract) with 10 mL of sodium hydroxide TS, add 5 mL of 1-butanol, shake, centrifuge, and use the 1-butanol layer as the sample solution. Separately, dissolve 1 mg of Ginsenoside Rb_1 RS or ginsenoside Rb_1 for thin-layer chromatography in 1 mL of methanol, and use this solution as the standard solution. Perform the test with these solutions as directed under Thin-layer Chromatography <2.03>. Spot 10 μL of the sample solution and 2 μL of the standard solution on a plate of silica gel for thin-layer chromatography. Develop the plate with a mixture of ethyl acetate, 1-propanol, water and acetic acid (100) (7:5:4:1) to a distance of about 7 cm, and air-dry the plate. Spray evenly vanillin-sulfuric acid-ethanol TS for spraying on the plate, heat the plate at 105°C for 5 minutes, and allow to cool: one of the several spots obtained from the sample solution has the same color tone and *R*f value with the blue-purple spot from the standard solution (Ginseng).

(4) Shake 1.0 g of the dry extract (or 3.0 g of the viscous extract) with 10 mL of water, add 10 mL of 1-butanol, shake, centrifuge, and use the 1-butanol layer as the sample solution. Separately, dissolve 1 mg of liquiritin for thin-layer chromatography in 1 mL of methanol, and use this solution as the standard solution. Perform the test with these solutions as directed under Thin-layer Chromatography <2.03>. Spot 1 μL each of the sample solution and standard solution on a plate of silica gel for thin-layer chromatography. Develop the plate with a mixture of ethyl acetate, methanol and water (20:3:2) to a distance of about 7 cm, and air-dry the plate. Spray evenly dilute sulfuric acid on the plate, heat the plate at 105°C for 5 minutes, and examine under ultraviolet light (main wavelength: 365 nm): one of the several spots obtained from the sample solution has the same color tone and *R*f value with the yellow-green fluorescent spot from the standard solution (Glycyrrhiza).

Purity (1) Heavy metals *<1.07>*—Prepare the test solution with 1.0 g of the dry extract (or an amount of the viscous extract, equivalent to 1.0 g of dried substance) as directed under Extracts (4), and perform the test (not more than 30 ppm).

(2) Arsenic *<1.11>*—Prepare the test solution with 0.67 g of the dry extract (or an amount of the viscous extract, equivalent to 0.67 g of dried substance) according to Method 3, and perform the test (not more than 3 ppm).

Loss on drying *<2.41>* The dry extract: Not more than 7.0% (1 g, 105°C, 5 hours).

The viscous extract: Not more than 66.7% (1 g, 105°C, 5 hours).

Total ash *<5.01>* Not more than 10.0%, calculated on the dried basis.

Assay (1) Ginsenoside Rb_1—Weigh accurately about 2 g of the dry extract (or an amount of the viscous extract, equivalent to about 2 g of dried substance), add 30 mL of diluted methanol (3 in 5), shake for 15 minutes, centrifuge, and separate the supernatant liquid. To the residue add 15 mL of diluted methanol (3 in 5), and repeat the same procedure. Combine all of the supernatant liquid, and add diluted methanol (3 in 5) to make exactly 50 mL. Pipet 10 mL of this solution, add 3 mL of sodium hydroxide TS, allow to stand for 30 minutes, then add 3 mL of 1 mol/L hydrochloric acid TS, and add water to make exactly 20 mL. Apply exactly 5 mL of this solution to a column [about 10 mm in inside diameter, packed with 0.36 g of octadecylsilanized silica gel for pre-treatment (55 – 105 μm in particle size), and washed just before using with methanol and then diluted methanol (3 in 10)], and wash the column in sequence with 2 mL of diluted methanol (3 in 10), 1 mL of sodium carbonate TS and 10 mL of diluted methanol (3 in 10). Finally, elute with methanol to collect exactly 5 mL, and use this as the sample solution. Separately, weigh accurately about 10 mg of Ginsenoside Rb_1 RS (separately determine the water *<2.48>* by coulometric titration, using 10 mg), and dissolve in methanol to make exactly 100 mL. Pipet 10 mL of this solution, add methanol to make exactly 50 mL, and use this solution as the standard solution. Perform the test with exactly 20 μL each of the sample solution and standard solution as directed under Liquid Chromatography *<2.01>* according to the following conditions, and determine the peak areas, A_T and A_S, of ginsenoside Rb_1 in each solution.

$$\text{Amount (mg) of ginsenoside } Rb_1 \ (C_{54}H_{92}O_{23}) = M_S \times A_T/A_S \times 1/5$$

M_S: Amount (mg) of Ginsenoside Rb_1 RS taken, calculated on the anhydrous basis

Operating conditions—

Detector: An ultraviolet absorption photometer (wavelength: 203 nm).

Column: A stainless steel column 4.6 mm in inside diameter and 25 cm in length, packed with carbamoyl group bound silica gel for liquid chromatography (5 μm in particle diameter).

Column temperature: A constant temperature of about 60°C.

Mobile phase: A mixture of acetonitrile, water and phosphoric acid (400:100:1).

Flow rate: 1.0 mL per minute (the retention time of ginsenoside Rb_1 is about 16 minutes).

System suitability—

System performance: When the procedure is run with 20 μL of the standard solution under the above operating conditions, the number of theoretical plates and the symmetry factor of the peak of ginsenoside Rb_1 are not less than 5000 and not more than 1.5, respectively.

System repeatability: When the test is repeated 6 times with 20 μL of the standard solution under the above operating conditions, the relative standard deviation of the peak area of ginsenoside Rb_1 is not more than 1.5%.

(2) Glycyrrhizic acid—Weigh accurately about 0.5 g of the dry extract (or an amount of the viscous extract, equivalent to about 0.5 g of the dried substance), add exactly 50 mL of diluted methanol (1 in 2), shake for 15 minutes, filter, and use the filtrate as the sample solution. Separately, weigh accurately about 10 mg of Glycyrrhizic Acid RS (separately determine the water *<2.48>* by coulometric titration, using 10 mg), dissolve in diluted methanol (1 in 2) to make exactly 100 mL, and use this solution as the standard solution. Perform the test with exactly 10 μL each of the sample solution and standard solution as directed under Liquid Chromatography *<2.01>* according to the following conditions, and determine the peak areas, A_T and A_S, of glycyrrhizic acid in each solution.

$$\text{Amount (mg) of glycyrrhizic acid } (C_{42}H_{62}O_{16}) = M_S \times A_T/A_S \times 1/2$$

M_S: Amount (mg) of Glycyrrhizic Acid RS taken, calculated on the anhydrous basis

Operating conditions—

Detector: An ultraviolet absorption photometer (wavelength: 254 nm).

Column: A stainless steel column 4.6 mm in inside diameter and 15 cm in length, packed with octadecylsilanized silica gel for liquid chromatography (5 μm in particle diameter).

Column temperature: A constant temperature of about 40°C.

Mobile phase: Dissolve 3.85 g of ammonium acetate in 720 mL of water, and add 5 mL of acetic acid (100) and 280 mL of acetonitrile.

Flow rate: 1.0 mL per minute (the retention time of glycyrrhizic acid is about 15 minutes).

System suitability—

System performance: Dissolve 5 mg of monoammonium glycyrrhizinate for resolution check in 20 mL of dilute ethanol. When the procedure is run with 10 μL of this solution under the above operating conditions, the resolution between the peak having the relative retention time of about 0.9 to glycyrrhizic acid and the peak of glycyrrhizic acid is not less than 1.5.

System repeatability: When the test is repeated 6 times with 10 μL of the standard solution under the above operating conditions, the relative standard deviation of the peak area of glycyrrhizic acid is not more than 1.5%.

Containers and storage Containers—Tight containers.

Bear Bile

Fel Ursi

ユウタン

Bear Bile is the dried bile of *Ursus arctos* Linné or allied animals (*Ursidae*).

Description Indefinite small masses; externally yellow-brown to dark yellow-brown; easily broken; fractured surface has a glassy luster, and is not wet.

Usually in a gall sac, occasionally taken out, the gall sac consists of a fibrous and strong membrane, 9 - 15 cm in length and 7 - 9 cm in width; externally dark brown and translucent.

Odor, slight and characteristic; taste, extremely bitter.

Identification To 0.1 g of pulverized Bear Bile, add 5 mL of methanol, warm in a water bath for 10 minutes. After cooling, filter, and use the filtrate as the sample solution. Separately, dissolve 10 mg of sodium tauroursodeoxycholate for thin-layer chromatography in 5 mL of methanol, and use this solution as the standard solution. Perform the test with these solutions as directed under Thin-layer Chromatography *<2.03>*. Spot 5 μL each of the sample solution and standard solution on a plate of silica gel for thin-layer chromatography. Develop the plate with a mixture of acetic acid (100), toluene and water (10:10:1) to a distance of about 10 cm, and air-dry the plate. Spray evenly diluted sulfuric acid on the plate, and heat the plate at 105°C for 10 minutes: one of the several spots obtained from the sample solution has the same color tone and *R*f value with the spot from the standard solution.

Purity Other animal biles—Use the sample solution obtained in the Identification as the sample solution. Separately, dissolve 10 mg of sodium glycocholate for thin-layer chromatography and 20 mg of powdered porcine bile for thin-layer chromatography in 5 mL each of methanol, and use these solutions as the standard solution (1) and (2), respectively. Perform the test with these solutions as directed in the Identification: no spot obtained from the sample solution appears at the position of the spot from the standard solution (1) and no grayish brown to black spot appears at the position of the spot at an *R*f value of about 0.3 from the standard solution (2).

Containers and storage Containers—Well-closed containers.

Bearberry Leaf

Uvae Ursi Folium

ウワウルシ

Bearberry Leaf is the leaf of *Arctostaphylos uva-ursi* Sprengel (*Ericaceae*).

It contains not less than 7.0% of arbutin.

Description Obovate to spatulate leaves, 1 - 3 cm in length, 0.5 - 1.5 cm in width; upper surface yellow-green to dark green; lower surface light yellow-green; margin entire; apex obtuse or round, sometimes retuse; base cuneate; petiole very short; lamina thick with characteristic reticulate venation, and easily broken.

Odor, slight; taste, slightly bitter and astringent.

Under a microscope *<5.01>*, the transverse section reveals thick cuticule; parenchyma cells of palisade tissue and sponge tissue being similar in form; in the vascular bundle, medullary ray consisting of 2 to 7 rows of one-cell line, appearing as bones of Japanese fan; polygonal solitary crystals and clustered crystals of calcium oxalate present sparsely in cells on both outer and inner sides of the vascular bundle, but no crystals in mesophyll.

Identification **(1)** Macerate 0.5 g of pulverized Bearberry Leaf with 10 mL of boiling water, shake the mixture for a few minutes, allow to cool, and filter. Place 1 drop of the filtrate on filter paper, and add 1 drop of iron (III) chloride TS: a dark purple color appears.

(2) To 0.2 g of pulverized Bearberry Leaf add 10 mL of a mixture of ethanol (95) and water (7:3), shake for 5 minutes, filter, and use the filtrate as the sample solution. Separately, dissolve 1 mg of arbutin for thin-layer chromatography in 1 mL of a mixture of ethanol (95) and water (7:3), and use this solution as the standard solution. Perform the test with these solutions as directed under Thin-layer Chromatography *<2.03>*. Spot 10 μL each of the sample solution and standard solution on a plate of silica gel for thin-layer chromatography. Develop the plate with a mixture of ethyl formate, water and formic acid (8:1:1) to a distance of about 7 cm, and air-dry the plate. Spray evenly dilute sulfuric acid upon the plate, and heat the plate at 105°C for 10 minutes: one of the several spots obtained from the sample solution and the spot from the standard solution show the same color tone and the *R*f value.

Purity **(1)** Twig—When perform the test of foreign matter *<5.01>*, the amount of twigs contained in Bearberry Leaf does not exceed 4.5%.

(2) Foreign matter *<5.01>*—The amount of foreign matter other than twigs contained in Bearberry Leaf does not exceed 2.0%.

Total ash *<5.01>* Not more than 4.0%.

Acid-insoluble ash *<5.01>* Not more than 1.5%.

Assay Weigh accurately about 0.5 g of pulverized Bearberry Leaf in a glass-stoppered centrifuge tube, add 40 mL of water, shake for 30 minutes, centrifuge, and separate the supernatant liquid. To the residue add 40 mL of water, and proceed in the same manner. To the combined extracts add water to make exactly 100 mL, and use this solution as the sample solution. Separately, weigh accurately about 40 mg of arbutin for assay, previously dried for 12 hours (in vacuum, silica gel), dissolve in water to make exactly 100 mL, and use this solution as the standard solution. Perform the test with exactly 10 μL each of the sample solution and standard solution as directed under Liquid Chromatography *<2.01>* according to the following conditions. Determine the peak areas, A_T and A_S, of arbutin in each solution.

$$\text{Amount (mg) of arbutin} = M_S \times A_T/A_S$$

M_S: Amount (mg) of arbutin for assay taken

Operating conditions—

Detector: An ultraviolet spectrophotometer (wavelength: 280 nm).

Column: A stainless steel column 4 - 6 mm in inside diameter and 15 - 25 cm in length, packed with octadecylsilanized silica gel (5 - 10 μm in particle diameter).

Column temperature: A constant temperature of about 20°C.

Mobile phase: A mixture of water, methanol and 0.1 mol/L hydrochloric acid TS (94:5:1).

Flow rate: Adjust so that the retention time of arbutin is about 6 minutes.

System suitability—

System performance: Dissolve 50 mg each of arbutin for assay, hydroquinone and gallic acid in water to make 100 mL. When the procedure is run with 10 μL of this solution under the above operating conditions, arbutin, hydroquinone and gallic acid are eluted in this order with the resolutions among these peaks being not less than 1.5.

System repeatability: When the test is repeated 5 times with 10 μL of the standard solution under the above operating conditions, the relative standard deviation of the peak area of arbutin is not more than 1.5%.

Containers and storage Containers—Well-closed containers.

Beef Tallow

Sevum Bovinum

牛脂

Beef Tallow is a purified fat obtained by wet steam rendering from the fresh fatty tissues of *Bos taurus* Linné var. *domesticus* Gmelin (*Bovidae*).

Description Beef Tallow occurs as a white, uniform mass. It has a characteristic odor and a mild taste.

It is freely soluble in diethyl ether and in petroleum ether, very slightly soluble in ethanol (95), and practically insoluble in water.

It is breakable at a low temperature, but softens above 30°C.

Melting point: 42 – 50°C

Acid value 〈*1.13*〉 Not more than 2.0.

Saponification value 〈*1.13*〉 193 – 200

Iodine value 〈*1.13*〉 33 – 50 (When the sample is insoluble in 20 mL of cyclohexane, dissolve it by shaking a glass-stoppered flask in warm water. Then, if insoluble, increase the volume of solvent.)

Purity **(1)** Moisture and coloration—Beef Tallow (5.0 g), melted by heating on a water bath, forms a clear liquid, from which no water separates. In a 10-mm thick layer of the liquid, it is colorless or slightly yellow.

(2) Alkalinity—To 2.0 g of Beef Tallow add 10 mL of water, melt by heating on a water bath, and shake vigorously. After cooling, add 1 drop of phenolphthalein TS to the separated aqueous layer: no color develops.

(3) Chloride—To 1.5 g of Beef Tallow add 30 mL of ethanol (95), heat for 10 minutes under a reflux condenser, and filter after cooling. To 20 mL of the filtrate add 5 drops of a solution of silver nitrate in ethanol (95) (1 in 50): the turbidity of the mixture does not exceed that of the following control solution.

Control solution: To 1.0 mL of 0.01 mol/L hydrochloric acid VS add ethanol (95) to make 20 mL, then add 5 drops of an ethanolic solution of silver nitrate (1 in 50).

Containers and storage Containers—Well-closed containers.

White Beeswax

Cera Alba

サラシミツロウ

White Beeswax is bleached Yellow Beeswax.

Description White Beeswax occurs as white to yellowish white masses. It has a characteristic odor. It is comparatively brittle when cooled, and the fractured surface is granular, and non-crystalline.

It is slightly soluble in diethyl ether, and practically insoluble in water and in ethanol (99.5).

Acid value 〈*1.13*〉 5 – 9 or 17 – 22 Weigh accurately about 6 g of White Beeswax, place in a glass-stoppered 250-mL flask, and add 50 mL of ethanol (99.5). Warm the mixture to dissolve the wax, add mL of phenolphthalein TS, and proceed as directed in the Acid value. Perform a blank determination using solvent which is not previously neutralized, and make any necessary correction.

Saponification value 〈*1.13*〉 80 – 100 Weigh accurately about 3 g of White Beeswax, place in a glass-stoppered 250-mL flask, and add exactly 25 mL of 0.5 mol/L potassium hydroxide-ethanol VS and 50 mL of ethanol (95), heat under a reflux condenser for 4 hours, and proceed as directed in the Saponification value.

Melting point 〈*1.13*〉 60 – 67°C

Purity Paraffin, fat, Japan wax or resin—Melt White Beeswax at the lowest possible temperature, drip the liquid into a vessel containing ethanol (95) to form granules, and allow them to stand in air for 24 hours. Drop the granules into two mixtures of ethanol (95) and water, one adjusted so as to have a specific gravity of 0.95 and the other 0.97: the granules sink or are suspended in the mixture with the specific gravity of 0.95, and float or are suspended in the other mixture.

Containers and storage Containers—Well-closed containers.

Yellow Beeswax

Cera Flava

ミツロウ

Yellow Beeswax is the purified wax obtained from honeycombs such as those of *Apis mellifera* Linné or *Apis cerana* Fabricius (*Apidae*).

Description Yellow Beeswax occurs as light yellow to brownish yellow masses. It has a characteristic odor, which is not rancid.

It is comparatively brittle when cooled, and the fractured surface is granular, and non-crystalline.

Acid value 〈*1.13*〉 5 – 9 or 17 – 22 Weigh accurately about 6 g of Yellow Beeswax, place in a glass-stoppered 250-mL flask, and add 50 mL of ethanol (99.5). Warm the mixture to dissolve the wax, add 1 mL of phenolphthalein TS, and proceed as directed in the Acid value. Perform a blank determination using solvent which is not previously neutralized, and make any necessary correction.

Saponification value <1.13> 80 – 100 Weigh accurately about 3 g of Yellow Beeswax, place in a 250-mL glass-stoppered flask, and add 25 mL of 0.5 mol/L potassium hydroxide-ethanol and 50 mL of ethanol (95), heat under a reflux condenser for 4 hours, and proceed as directed in the Saponification value.

Melting point <1.13> 60 – 67°C

Purity Paraffin, fat, Japan wax or resin—Melt Yellow Beeswax at the lowest possible temperature, drip the liquid into a glass vessel containing ethanol (95) to form granules, and allow them to stand in air for 24 hours. Drop the granules into two mixtures of ethanol (95) and water, one adjusted so as to have a specific gravity of 0.95 and the other 0.97: the granules sink or are suspended in the mixture with the specific gravity of 0.95, and float or are suspended in the other mixture.

Containers and storage Containers—Well-closed containers.

Belladonna Root

Belladonnae Radix

ベラドンナコン

Belladonna Root is the root of *Atropa belladonna* Linné (*Solanaceae*).

When dried, it contains not less than 0.4% of hyoscyamine ($C_{17}H_{23}NO_3$: 289.37).

Description Cylindrical root, usually 10 – 30 cm in length, 0.5 – 4 cm in diameter; often cut crosswise or lengthwise; externally grayish brown to grayish yellow-brown, with longitudinal wrinkles; periderm often removed; fractured surface is light yellow to light yellow-brown in color and is powdery.

Almost odorless.

Identification Place 2.0 g of pulverized Belladonna Root in a glass-stoppered centrifuge tube, add 30 mL of ammonia TS, and centrifuge after irradiation of ultrasonic waves for 5 minutes. Transfer the supernatant liquid to a separator, add 40 mL of ethyl acetate, and shake. Drain off the ethyl acetate layer, add 3 g of anhydrous sodium sulfate to the ethyl acetate, shake, and filter after the ethyl acetate becomes clear. Evaporate the solvent of the filtrate to dryness under low pressure (in vacuo), dissolve the residue in 1 mL of ethanol (95), and use this solution as the sample solution. Separately, dissolve 2 mg of Atropine Sulfate RS or atropine sulfate hydrate for thin-layer chromatography in 1 mL of ethanol (95), and use this solution as the standard solution. Perform the test with these solutions as directed under Thin-layer Chromatography <2.03>. Spot 5 μL each of the sample solution and standard solutions on a plate of silica gel for thin-layer chromatography. Develop the plate with a mixture of acetone, water and ammonia water (28) (90:7:3) to a distance of about 7 cm, and air-dry the plate. Spray evenly Dragendorff's TS on the plate: the principal spot obtained from the sample solution is the same in color tone and *R*f value with the spot from the standard solution.

Purity **(1)** Stem and crown—When perform the test of foreign matter <5.01>, the amount of stem and crowns contained in Belladonna Root does not exceed 10.0%.

(2) Foreign matter <5.01>—The amount of foreign matter other than stems and crowns contained in Belladonna Root does not exceed 2.0%.

Total ash <5.01> Not more than 6.0%.

Acid-insoluble ash <5.01> Not more than 4.0%.

Assay Weigh accurately about 0.7 g of pulverized Belladonna Root, previously dried at 60°C for 8 hours, place in a glass-stoppered centrifuge tube, and moisten with 15 mL of ammonia TS. To this add 25 mL of diethyl ether, stopper the centrifuge tube tightly, shake for 15 minutes, centrifuge, and separate the diethyl ether layer. To the residue add 25 mL of diethyl ether, proceed in the same manner, and repeat this procedure twice. Combine all the extracts, and evaporate the solvent on a water bath. Dissolve the residue in 5 mL of the mobile phase, add exactly 3 mL of the internal standard solution, and add the mobile phase to make 25 mL. Filter this solution through a filter of a porosity of not more than 0.8 μm, discard the first 2 mL of the filtrate, and use the subsequent filtrate as the sample solution. Separately, weigh accurately about 25 mg of Atropine Sulfate RS (previously determine the loss on drying <2.41> under the same conditions as Atropine Sulfate Hydrate), dissolve in the mobile phase to make exactly 25 mL, and use this solution as the standard stock solution. Pipet 5 mL of the standard stock solution, add exactly 3 mL of the internal standard solution, then add the mobile phase to make 25 mL, and use this solution as the standard solution. Perform the test with exactly 10 μL each of the sample solution and standard solution as directed under Liquid Chromatography <2.01> according to the following conditions. Calculate the ratios, Q_T and Q_S, of the peak area of hyoscyamine (atropine), to that of the internal standard.

$$\text{Amount (mg) of hyoscyamine } (C_{17}H_{23}NO_3) = M_S \times Q_T/Q_S \times 1/5 \times 0.855$$

M_S: Amount (mg) of Atropine Sulfate RS taken, calculated on the dried basis

Internal standard solution—A solution of brucine dihydrate in the mobile phase (1 in 2500).

Operating conditions—

Detector: An ultraviolet absorption spectrometer (wavelength: 210 nm).

Column: A stainless steel column about 4 mm in inside diameter and about 15 cm in length, packed with octadecylsilanized silica gel for liquid chromatography (5 μm in particle diameter).

Column temperature: A constant temperature of about 20°C.

Mobile phase: Dissolve 6.8 g of potassium dihydrogen phosphate in 900 mL of water, add 10 mL of triethylamine, adjust with phosphoric acid to pH 3.5, and add water to make 1000 mL, and mix this solution with acetonitrile (9:1).

Flow rate: Adjust so that the retention time of atropine is about 14 minutes.

System suitability—

System performance: When the procedure is run with 10 μL of the standard solution under the above operating conditions, atropine and the internal standard are eluted in this order with the resolution between these peaks being not less than 4.

Containers and storage Containers—Well-closed containers.

Belladonna Extract

ベラドンナエキス

Belladonna Extract contains not less than 0.85% and not more than 1.05% of hyoscyamine ($C_{17}H_{23}NO_3$: 289.37).

Method of preparation To 1000 g of a coarse powder of Belladonna Root add 4000 mL of 35 vol% Ethanol, and digest for 3 days. Press the mixture, add 2000 mL of 35 vol% Ethanol to the residue, and digest again for 2 days. Combine all the extracts, and allow to stand for 2 days. Filter, and prepare the viscous extract as directed under Extracts. An appropriate quantity of Ethanol and Purified Water or Purified Water in Containers may be used in place of 35 vol% Ethanol.

Description Belladonna Extract has a dark brown color, a characteristic odor and a bitter taste.

Identification Mix 0.5 g of Belladonna Extract with 30 mL of ammonia TS in a flask, transfer the mixture to a separator, then add 40 mL of ethyl acetate, and shake the mixture. Drain off the ethyl acetate layer, add 3 g of anhydrous sodium sulfate to the ethyl acetate, shake, and filter after the ethyl acetate becomes clear. Evaporate the solvent to dryness under low pressure (in vacuo), dissolve the residue in 1 mL of ethanol (95), and use this solution as the sample solution. Proceed as directed in the Identification under Belladonna Root.

Purity Heavy metals *<1.07>*—Prepare the test solution with 1.0 g of Belladonna Extract as directed under the Extracts (4), and perform the test (not more than 30 ppm).

Assay Weigh accurately about 0.4 g of Belladonna Extract, place in a glass-stoppered centrifuge tube, add 15 mL of ammonia TS, and shake. Add 25 mL of diethyl ether, stopper tightly, shake for 15 minutes, centrifuge, and separate the diethyl ether layer. Repeat this procedure twice with the aqueous layer, using 25 mL each of diethyl ether. Combine the extracts, and evaporate the solvent on a water bath. Dissolve the residue in 5 mL of the mobile phase, add exactly 3 mL of the internal standard solution, and add the mobile phase to make exactly 25 mL. Proceed as directed under Belladonna Root.

$$\text{Amount (mg) of hyoscyamine } (C_{17}H_{23}NO_3) = M_S \times Q_T/Q_S \times 1/5 \times 0.855$$

M_S: Amount (mg) of Atropine Sulfate RS taken, calculated on the dried basis

Internal standard solution—A solution of brucine dihydrate in the mobile phase (1 in 2500).

Containers and storage Containers—Tight containers.

Storage—Light-resistant, and in a cold place.

Belladonna Total Alkaloids

ベラドンナ総アルカロイド

Belladonna Total Alkaloids contains not less than 95.0% and not more than 99.0% of hyoscyamine ($C_{17}H_{23}NO_3$: 289.37), not less than 1.3% and not more than 3.9% of scopolamine ($C_{17}H_{21}NO_4$: 303.35), and not less than 99.0% and not more than 102.0% of the total alkaloids (hyoscyamine and scopolamine), calculated on the dried basis.

Method of preparation Belladonna Total Alkaloids is prepared by purification of the extract from Belladonna Root with water or aqueous ethanol.

Description Belladonna Total Alkaloids occurs as white, crystals or crystalline powder.

It is very soluble in methanol, freely soluble in ethanol (99.5), and slightly soluble in water.

Identification Dissolve 2 mg of Belladonna Total Alkaloids in 1 mL of ethanol (95), and use this solution as the sample solution. Then proceed as directed in the Identification under Belladonna Root.

Optical rotation *<2.49>* $[\alpha]_D^{20}$: −18.5 – −22.0° (after drying, 1 g, ethanol (99.5), 25 mL, 100 mm).

Purity **(1)** Heavy metals *<1.07>*—Place 1.0 g of Belladonna Total Alkaloids in a porcelain crucible, and mix with 1.2 mL of dilute hydrochloric acid. Mix with 10 mL of a solution of magnesium nitrate hexahydrate in ethanol (95) (1 in 10), and after evaporating the solvent on a boiling water bath, carbonize by gradual heating. Then proceed according to Method 4, and perform the test. The control solution is prepared as follows: Mix 1.2 mL of dilute hydrochloric acid with 10 mL of a solution of magnesium nitrate hexahydrate in ethanol (95) (1 in 10), and evaporate the solvent on a boiling water bath. After cooling, add 1 mL of sulfuric acid, then proceed according to Method 4, and add 2.0 mL of Standard Lead Solution and water to make 50 mL (not more than 20 ppm).

(2) Arsenic *<1.11>*—Prepare the test solution with 2.0 g of Belladonna Total Alkaloids according to Method 4, and perform the test (not more than 1 ppm).

Loss on drying *<2.41>* Not more than 1.0% (1 g, in vacuum, 60°C, 6 hours).

Residue on ignition *<2.44>* Not more than 0.2% (0.5 g).

Assay Weigh accurately about 25 mg of Belladonna Total Alkaloids, and dissolve in methanol to make exactly 25 mL. Pipet 5 mL of this solution, add exactly 3 mL of the internal standard solution and the mobile phase to make 25 mL, and use this solution as the sample solution. Separately, weigh accurately about 25 mg of Atropine Sulfate RS (separately determine the loss on drying *<2.41>* under the same conditions as Atropine Sulfate Hydrate), dissolve in the mobile phase to make exactly 25 mL, and use this solution as the standard stock solution (1). Also, weigh accurately about 25 mg of Scopolamine Hydrobromide RS (separately determine the loss on drying *<2.41>* under the same conditions as Scopolamine Hydrobromide Hydrate), and dissolve in the mobile phase to make exactly 25 mL. Pipet 3 mL of this solution, add the mobile phase to make exactly 25 mL, and use this solution as the standard stock solution (2). Take exactly 5 mL of standard stock solution (1), add exactly 2 mL of the standard stock solution (2), and add exactly 3 mL of the internal standard solution. To this solution add the mobile phase to make 25 mL, and use this solution as the standard solution. Perform the test with 10 μL each of the sample solution and standard solution as directed under Liquid Chromatography <2.01> according to the following conditions, and calculate the ratios, Q_{TA} and Q_{SA}, of the peak area of hyoscyamine (atropine) to that of the internal standard and the ratios, Q_{TS} and Q_{SS}, of the peak area of scopolamine to that of the internal standard. Then calculate the amounts of hyoscyamine and scopolamine using the following equations. The amount of the total alkaloids is obtained as the sum of them.

The amount (mg) of hyoscyamine ($C_{17}H_{23}NO_3$)
$= M_{SA} \times Q_{TA}/Q_{SA} \times 0.855$

The amount (mg) of scopolamine ($C_{17}H_{21}NO_4$)
$= M_{SS} \times Q_{TS}/Q_{SS} \times 6/125 \times 0.789$

M_{SA}: The amount (mg) of Atropine Sulfate RS taken, calculated on the dried basis

M_{SS}: The amount (mg) of Scopolamine Hydrobromide RS taken, calculated on the dried basis

Internal standard solution: A solution of brucine *n*-hydrate in the mobile phase (1 in 2500).

Operating conditions—

Detector: An ultraviolet absorption photometer (wavelength: 210 nm).

Column: A stainless steel column 4.6 mm in inside diameter and 15 cm in length, packed with octadecylsilanized silica gel for liquid chromatography (5 μm in particle diameter).

Column temperature: A constant temperature of around 20°C.

Mobile phase: Dissolve 6.8 g of potassium dihydrogen phosphate in 900 mL of water, add 10 mL of triethylamine, adjust to pH 3.5 with phosphoric acid, and add water to make 1000 mL. To 900 mL of this solution add 100 mL of acetonitrile.

Flow rate: Adjust so that the retention time of atropine is about 14 minutes.

System suitability—

System performance: When the procedure is run with 10 μL of the standard solution under the above operating conditions, scopolamine, atropine and the internal standard are eluted in this order, and the resolutions between scopolamine and atropine, and atropine and the internal standard are not less than 11 and not less than 4, respectively.

System repeatability: When the test is repeated 6 times with 10 μL of the standard solution under the above operating conditions, the relative standard deviation of the ratio of the peak area of scopolamine to that of the internal standard is not more than 1.5%.

Containers and storage Containers—Tight containers.

Storage—Light-resistant.

Benincasa Seed

Benincasae Semen

トウガシ

Benincasa seed is the seed of 1) *Benincasa cerifera* Savi or 2) *Benincasa cerifera* Savi forma *emarginata* K. Kimura et Sugiyama (*Cucurbitaceae*).

Description 1) *Benincasa cerifera* origin—Flattened, ovate to orbicular ovate seed, 10 - 13 mm in length, 6 - 7 mm in width, about 2 mm in thickness; slightly acute at base; hilum and germ pore form two protrusions; externally light grayish yellow to light yellowish brown; prominent band along with marginal edge of seed; under a magnifying glass, surface of the seed is with fine wrinkles and minute hollows.

Odorless; bland taste and slightly oily.

Under a microscope <5.01>, a transverse section reveals the outermost layer of seed coat composed of a single-layered and palisade like epidermis, the epidermis obvious at prominent band along with marginal edge of seed; hypodermis composed of slightly sclerified parenchyma beneath epidermis; inside of the parenchyma several layers of stone cells lie; the innermost layer of seed coat composed of parenchyma several cells thick; perisperm coated with cuticle, composed of parenchyma several cells thick; endosperm composed of a row of compressed cells; cotyledon contains oil drops and aleurone grains, occasionally starch grains.

2) *Benincasa cerifera* forma *emarginata* origin—Flattened, ovate to ellipsoidal seed, 9 - 12 mm in length, 5 - 6 mm in width, about 2 mm in thickness; hilum and germ pore form two protrusions as in 1); externally light grayish yellow, smooth, no prominent band along with marginal edge of seed.

Odorless; bland taste and slightly oily.

Under a microscope <5.01>, a transverse section reveals the outermost layer composed of a single-layered epidermis coated with cuticle, often detached; hypodermis composed of slightly sclerified parenchyma beneath epidermis; inside of the parenchyma several layers of stone cells lie; the innermost layer of seed coat composed of parenchyma several cells thick; perisperm coated with cuticle, composed of parenchyma several cells thick; endosperm composed of a row of compressed cells; cotyledon contains oil drops and aleurone grains, occasionally starch grains.

Identification To 0.5 g of pulverized Benincasa Seed add 10 mL of a mixture of methanol and water (4:1), shake for 10 minutes, filter, and use the filtrate as the sample solution. Perform the test with the sample solution as directed under Thin-layer Chromatography <2.03>. Spot 20 μL of the sample solution on a plate of silica gel for thin-layer chromatography, develop the plate with a mixture of 1-butanol, water and acetic acid (100) (8:6:3) to a distance of about 7 cm, and air-dry the plate. Examine under ultraviolet light (main wavelength: 365 nm): two blue-white fluorescent spots appear at an *Rf* value of about 0.4, and the spot having the smaller *Rf* value shows more intense fluorescence.

Purity Foreign matter <5.01>—It contains not more than 2.0%.

Loss on drying <5.01> Not more than 11.0% (6 hours).

Total ash <5.01> Not more than 5.0%.

Acid-insoluble ash <*5.01*> Not more than 1.5%.

Extract content <*5.01*> Dilute ethanol-soluble extract: not less than 3.0%.

Containers and storage Containers—Well-closed containers.

Benzoin

Benzoinum

アンソッコウ

Benzoin is the resin obtained from *Styrax benzoin* Dryander or other species of the same genus (*Styracaceae*).

Description Benzoin occurs as grayish brown to dark red-brown blocks varying in size; the fractured surface exhibiting whitish to light yellow-red grains in the matrix; hard and brittle at ordinary temperature but softened by heat.

Odor, characteristic and aromatic; taste, slightly pungent and acrid.

Identification **(1)** Heat a fragment of Benzoin in a test tube: it evolves an irritating vapor, and a crystalline sublimate is produced.

(2) Digest 0.5 g of Benzoin with 10 mL of diethyl ether, decant 1 mL of the diethyl ether into a porcelain dish, and add 2 to 3 drops of sulfuric acid: a deep red-brown to deep red-purple color develops.

Purity Ethanol-insoluble substances—Boil gently 1.0 g of Benzoin with 30 mL of ethanol (95) for 15 minutes under a reflux condenser. After cooling, collect the insoluble substances through a tared glass filter (G3), and wash with three 5-mL portions of ethanol (95). Dry the residue at 105°C for 4 hours: the mass of the residue does not exceed 0.30 g.

Total ash <*5.01*> Not more than 2.0%.

Acid-insoluble ash <*5.01*> Not more than 1.0%.

Containers and storage Containers—Well-closed containers.

Bitter Cardamon

Alpiniae Fructus

ヤクチ

Bitter Cardamon is the fruit of *Alpinia oxyphylla* Miquel (*Zingiberaceae*).

Description Spherical to fusiform fruit, with both ends somewhat pointed; 1 - 2 cm in length, 0.7 - 1 cm in width; externally brown to dark brown, with numerous longitudinal, knob-like protruding lines; pericarp 0.3 - 0.5 mm in thickness, closely adhering to the seed mass, and difficult to separate; inside divided vertically into three loculi by thin membranes, each loculus containing 5 to 8 seeds adhering by aril; seeds irregularly polygonal, about 3.5 mm in diameter, brown to dark brown in color, and hard in texture.

Odor, characteristic; taste, slightly bitter.

Total ash <*5.01*> Not more than 10.0%.

Acid-insoluble ash <*5.01*> Not more than 2.5%.

Essential oil content <*5.01*> Perform the test with 50.0 g of pulverized Bitter Cardamon: the volume of essential oil is not less than 0.4 mL.

Containers and storage Containers—Well-closed containers.

Bitter Orange Peel

Aurantii Pericarpium

トウヒ

Bitter Orange Peel is the pericarp of the ripe fruit of *Citrus aurantium* Linné or *Citrus aurantium* Linné var. *daidai* Makino (*Rutaceae*).

Description Usually quartered sections of a sphere, sometimes warped or flattened, 4 - 8 cm in length, 2.5 - 4.5 cm in width and 0.5 - 0.8 cm in thickness; the outer surface is dark red-brown to grayish yellow-brown, with numerous small dents associated with oil sacs; the inner surface is white to light grayish yellow-red, with irregular indented reticulation left by vascular bundles; light and brittle in texture.

Odor, characteristic aroma; taste, bitter, somewhat mucilaginous and slightly pungent.

Identification To 1.0 g of Bitter Orange Peel add 10 mL of ethanol (95), allow to stand for 30 minutes with occasional shaking, filter, and use the filtrate as the sample solution. Separately, dissolve 10 mg of naringin for thin-layer chromatography in 10 mL of ethanol (95), and use this solution as the standard solution. Perform the test with these solutions as directed under Thin-layer Chromatography <*2.03*>. Spot 10 μL each of the sample solution and standard solution on a plate of silica gel for thin-layer chromatography. Develop the plate with a mixture of ethyl acetate, ethanol (99.5) and water (8:2:1) to a distance of about 10 cm, and air-dry the plate. Spray evenly dilute 2,6-dibromo-*N*-chloro-1,4-benzoquinone monoimine TS on the plate, and allow to stand in ammonia gas: one of the several spots obtained from the sample solution and a grayish green spot from the standard solution show the same color tone and the same *R*f value.

Loss on drying <*5.01*> Not more than 14.0% (6 hours).

Total ash <*5.01*> Not more than 5.5%.

Acid-insoluble ash <*5.01*> Not more than 0.5%.

Essential oil content <*5.01*> Perform the test with 50.0 g of pulverized Bitter Orange Peel provided that 1 mL of silicon resin is previously added to the test sample in the flask: the volume of essential oil is not less than 0.2 mL.

Containers and storage Containers—Well-closed containers.

Bitter Tincture

Tinctura Amara

苦味チンキ

Method of preparation

Bitter Orange Peel, in coarse powder	50 g
Swertia Herb, in coarse powder	5 g
Japanese Zanthoxylum Peel, in coarse powder	5 g
70 vol% Ethanol	a sufficient quantity
To make	1000 mL

Prepare as directed under Tinctures, with the above ingredients. An appropriate quantity of Ethanol and Purified Water or Purified Water in Containers may be used in place of 70 vol% Ethanol.

Description Bitter Tincture is a yellow-brown liquid. It has a characteristic aroma and a bitter taste.

Specific gravity d^{20}_{20}: about 0.90

Identification (1) To 1 mL of Bitter Tincture add 5 mL of methanol, then add 0.1 g of magnesium in ribbon form and 1 mL of hydrochloric acid, and allow to stand: the solution is red-purple in color.

(2) Use Bitter Tincture as the sample solution. Separately, to 0.5 g of pulverized Bitter Orange Peel add 10 mL of methanol, shake for 5 minutes, filter, and use the filtrate as the standard solution (1). Proceed with 0.5 g each of pulverized Swertia Herb and Japanese Zanthoxylum Peel in the same manner, and use the solutions so obtained as the standard solution (2) and the standard solution (3). Perform the test with these solutions as directed under Thin-layer Chromatography <2.03>. Spot 10 μL of the sample solution and 5 μL each of standard solutions (1), (2) and (3) on a plate of silica gel with fluorescent indicator for thin-layer chromatography. Develop the plate with a mixture of ethyl acetate, ethanol (99.5) and water (8:2:1) to a distance of about 7 cm, and air-dry the plate. Examine the plate under ultraviolet light (main wavelength: 254 nm): one of the several spots obtained from the sample solution has the same *R*f value with the clear spot at an *R*f value of about 0.7 from the standard solution (3). Spray evenly vanillin-sulfuric acid-ethanol TS for spraying on the plate, and heat the plate at 105°C for 5 minutes: two of the several spots from the sample solution show the same color tone and *R*f value with the clear spot at an *R*f value of about 0.4 from the standard solution (1), and the clear spot at an *R*f value of about 0.35 from the standard solution (2).

Alcohol number <*1.01*> Not less than 6.9 (Method 2).

Containers and storage Containers—Tight containers.

Bofutsushosan Extract

防風通聖散エキス

Bofutsushosan Extract contains not less than 9 mg and not more than 36 mg of paeoniflorin ($C_{23}H_{28}O_{11}$: 480.46), not less than 4 mg and not more than 12 mg of total alkaloids (ephedrine and pseudoephedrine), not less than 54 mg and not more than 162 mg of baicalin ($C_{21}H_{18}O_{11}$: 446.36), and not less than 13 mg and not more than 39 mg of glycyrrhizic acid ($C_{42}H_{62}O_{16}$: 822.93), per extract prepared with the amount specified in the Method of preparation.

Method of preparation

	1)	2)	3)	4)	5)	6)
Japanese Angelica Root	1.2 g	1.2 g	1.2 g	1.2 g	1.2 g	1.2 g
Peony Root	1.2 g	1.2 g	1.2 g	1.2 g	1.2 g	1.2 g
Cnidium Rhizome	1.2 g	1.2 g	1.2 g	1.2 g	1.2 g	1.2 g
Gardenia Fruit	1.2 g	1.2 g	1.2 g	1.2 g	1.2 g	1.2 g
Forsythia Fruit	1.2 g	1.2 g	1.2 g	1.2 g	1.2 g	1.2 g
Mentha Herb	1.2 g	1.2 g	1.2 g	1.2 g	1.2 g	1.2 g
Ginger	0.3 g	0.3 g	0.4 g	0.4 g	1.2 g	0.3 g
Schizonepeta Spike	1.2 g	1.2 g	1.2 g	1.2 g	1.2 g	1.2 g
Saposhnikovia Root and Rhizome	1.2 g	1.2 g	1.2 g	1.2 g	1.2 g	—
Glehnia Root and Rhizome	—	—	—	—	—	1.2 g
Ephedra Herb	1.2 g	1.2 g	1.2 g	1.2 g	1.2 g	1.2 g
Rhubarb	1.5 g	1.5 g	1.5 g	1.5 g	1.5 g	1.5 g
Sodium Sulfate	—	1.5 g	—	1.5 g	—	—
Anhydrous Sodium Sufate	0.7 g	—	0.75 g	—	1.5 g	0.75 g
Atractylodes Rhizome	2 g	2 g	2 g	2 g	2 g	2 g
Platycodon Root	2 g	2 g	2 g	2 g	2 g	2 g
Scutellaria Root	2 g	2 g	2 g	2 g	2 g	2 g
Glycyrrhiza	2 g	2 g	2 g	2 g	2 g	2 g
Gypsum	2 g	2 g	2 g	2 g	2 g	2 g
Aluminum Silicate Hydrate with Silicon Dioxide	3 g	3 g	3 g	3 g	3 g	3 g

Prepare a dry extract or viscous extract as directed under Extracts, according to the prescription 1) to 6), using the crude drugs shown above.

Description Bofutsushosan Extract is a yellow-brown to brown powder or black-brown viscous extract. It has a slightly odor and a sweet and slightly bitter taste.

Identification (1) To 2.0 g of the dry extract (or 6.0 g of the viscous extract) add 10 mL of water, shake, then add 10 mL of diethyl ether, shake, and centrifuge. Separate the diethyl ether layer, add 10 mL of sodium hydroxide TS, shake, centrifuge, and use the diethy ether layer as the sample solution. Separately, use (*Z*)-ligustilide TS for thin-layer chromatography as the standard solution. Perform the test with these solutions as directed under Thin-layer Chromatography <*2.03*>. Spot 20 μL of the sample solution and 10 μL of the standard solution on a plate of silica gel for thin-layer chromatography. Develop the plate with a mixture of butyl acetate and hexane (2:1) to a distance of about 7 cm, and air-dry the plate. Examine under ultraviolet light (main wavelength: 365 nm): one of the several spots obtained from the sample solution has the same color tone and *Rf* value with the blue-white fluorescent spot from the standard solution (Japanese Angelica Root; Cnidium Rhizome).

(2) To 1.0 g of the dry extract (or 3.0 g of the viscous extract) add 10 mL of water, shake, then add 10 mL of 1-butanol, shake, centrifuge, and use the 1-butanol layer as the sample solution. Separately, dissolve 1 mg of paeoniflorin for thin-layer chromatography in 1 mL of methanol, and use this solution as the standard solution. Perform the test with these solutions as directed under Thin-layer Chromatography <*2.03*>. Spot 10 μL of the sample solution and 5 μL of the standard solution on a plate of silica gel for thin-layer chromatography. Develop the plate with a mixture of ethyl acetate, methanol and ammonia solution (28) (6:3:2) to a distance of about 7 cm, and air-dry the plate. Spray evenly 4-methoxybenzaldehyde-sulfuric acid TS on the plate, heat the plate at 105°C for 1 minute: one of the spot among the several spots obtained from the sample solution has the same color tone and *Rf* value with the red-purple to purple spot from the standard solution (Peony Root).

(3) To 1.0 g of the dry extract (or 3.0 g of the viscous extract) add 10 mL of water, shake, then add 10 mL of 1-butanol, shake, centrifuge, and use the 1-butanol layer as the sample solution. Separately, dissolve 1 mg of geniposide for thin-layer chromatography in 1 mL of methanol, and use this solution as the standard solution. Perform the test with these solutions as directed under Thin-layer Chromatography <*2.03*>. Spot 10 μL of the sample solution and 5 μL of the standard solution on a plate of silica gel for thin-layer chromatography. Develop the plate with a mixture of ethyl acetate, methanol and ammonia solution (28) (6:3:2) to a distance of about 7 cm, and air-dry the plate. Spray evenly 4-methoxybenzaldehyde-sulfric acid TS on the plate, and heat the plate at 105°C for 1 minute: one of the spot among the several spots obtained from the sample solution has the same color tone and *Rf* value with the red-purple to purple spot from the standard solution (Gardenia Fruit).

(4) To 1.0 g of the dry extract (or 3.0 g of the viscous extract) add 10 mL of water, shake, then add 5 mL of 1-butanol, shake, centrifuge, and use the 1-butanol layer as the sample solution. Separately, to 1.0 g of pulverized forsythia fruit add 10 mL of methanol, shake, centrifuge, and use the supernatant liquid as the standard solution. Perform the test with these solutions as directed under Thin-layer Chromatography <*2.03*>. Spot 20 μL of the sample solution and 10 μL of the standard solution as bands on the original line on a plate of silica gel for thin-layer chromatography. Develop the plate with a mixture of ethyl acetate, methanol and ammonia solution (28) (10:2:1) to a distance of about 7 cm, and air-dry the plate. Spray evenly 4-methoxybenzaldehyde-sulfric acid TS on the plate, heat the plate at 105°C for 5 minutes, and allow to cool: one of the spot among the several spots obtained from the sample solution has the same color tone and *Rf* value with the red-purple spot (*Rf* value: about 0.4) from the standard solution (Forsythia Fruit).

(5) To 2.0 g of the dry extract (or 6.0 g of the viscous extract) add 10 mL of diluted phosphoric acid (1 in 30), shake, then add 15 mL of ethyl acetate, shake, centrifuge, and use the ethyl acetate layer as the sample solution. Separately, shake 0.2 g of pulverized mentha herb with 10 mL of diluted phosphoric acid (1 in 30), add 15 mL of ethyl acetate, shake, centrifuge, and use the ethyl acetate layer as the standard solution. Perform the test with these solutions as directed under Thin-layer Chromatography <*2.03*>. Spot 20 μL each of the sample solution and standard solution on a plate of silica gel for thin-layer chromatography. Develop the plate with a mixture of acetone, ethyl acetate, water, and acetic acid (100) (10:10:3:1) to a distance of about 7 cm, and air-dry the plate. Spray evenly 2,6-dibromo-*N*-chloro-1,4-benzoquinone monoimine TS on the plate, heat the plate at 105°C for 5 minutes: one of the spot among the several spots obtained from the sample solution has the same color tone and *Rf* value with the red-brown spot (*Rf* value: around 0.4) from the standard solution (Mentha Herb).

(6) Perform the test according to the following (i) or (ii) (Ginger).

(i) To 1.0 g of the dry extract (or 3.0 g of the viscous extract) add 10 mL of water, shake, then add 25 mL of diethyl ether, shake, and centrifuge. Separate the diethyl ether layer, evaporate the solvent under low pressure (in vacuo), dissolve the residue in 2 mL of diethyl ether, and use the solution as the sample solution. Separately, dissolve 1 mg of [6]-gingerol for thin-layer chromatography in 1 mL of methanol, and use this solution as the standard solution. Perform the test with these solutions as directed under Thin-layer Chromatography <*2.03*>. Spot 20 μL of the sample solution and 5 μL of the standard solution on a plate of silica gel for thin-layer chromatography. Develop the plate with a mixture of ethyl acetate and hexane (1:1) to a distance of about 7 cm, and air-dry the plate. Spray evenly 4-dimethylaminobenzaldehyde TS for spraying on the plate, heat the plate at 105°C for 5 minutes, allow to cool, and spray water: one of the spot among the several spots obtained from the sample solution has the same color tone and *Rf* value with the blue-green to grayish green spot from the standard solution.

(ii) To 1.0 g of the dry extract (or 3.0 g of the viscous extract) add 10 mL of water, shake, then add 25 mL of diethyl ether, shake, and centrifuge. Separate the diethyl ether layer, evaporate the solvent under low pressure (in vacuo), dissolve the residue in 2 mL of diethyl ether, and use the solution as the sample solution. Separately, dissolve 1 mg of [6]-shogaol for thin-layer chromatography in 1 mL of methanol, and use this solution as the standard solution. Perform the test with these solutions as directed under Thin-layer Chromatography <*2.03*>. Spot 20 μL of the sample solution and 5 μL of the standard solution on a plate of silica gel for thin-layer chromatography. Develop the plate with a mixture of ethyl acetate and hexane (1:1) to a distance of about 7 cm, and air-dry the plate. Spray evenly 4-dimethylaminobenzaldehyde TS for spraying on the plate, heat the plate at 105°C for 5 minutes, allow to cool, and spray water: one of the spot among the several spots obtained from the sample solution has the same color tone and *Rf* value with the blue-green to grayish green spot from the standard solution.

(7) To 1.0 g of the dry extract (or 3.0 g of the viscous extract) add 10 mL of 0.1 mol/L hydrochloric acid TS, shake, then add 25 mL of diethyl ether, shake, and centrifuge. Separate the diethyl ether layer, evaporate the solvent under low pressure (in vacuo), add 1 mL of methanol to the residue, and use the solution as the sample solution. Separately, dissolve 1 mg of rosmarinic acid for thin-layer chromatography in 1 mL of methanol, and use this solution as the standard solution. Perform the test with these solutions as directed under Thin-layer Chromatography <*2.03*>. Spot 5 μL each of the sample solution and standard solution on a plate of silica gel for thin-layer chromatography. Develop the plate with a mixture of ethyl acetate, water and acetic acid (100) (60:1:1) to a distance of about 10 cm, and air-dry the plate. Spray evenly iron (III) chloride-methanol TS on the plate: one of the several spots obtained from the sample solution has the same color tone and *Rf* value with the greenish brown spot from the standard solution (Schizonepeta Spike; Mentha Herb).

(8) For preparation prescribed Saposhnikovia Root and Rhizome—To 2.0 g of the dry extract (or 6.0 g of the viscous extract) add 10 mL of sodium hydroxide TS, shake, then add 5 mL of 1-butanol, shake, centrifuge, and use the 1-butanol layer as the sample solution. Separately, dissolve 1 mg of 4′-*O*-glycosyl-5-*O*-methylvisamminol for thin-layer chromatography in 1 mL of methanol, and use this solution as the standard solution. Perform the test with these solutions as directed under Thin-layer Chromatography <*2.03*>. Spot 10 μL of the sample solution and 5 μL of the standard solution on a plate of silica gel for thin-layer chromatography. Develop the plate with a mixture of ethyl acetate, 1-propanol, water and acetic acid (100) (7:5:4:1) to a distance of about 7 cm, and air-dry the plate. Spray evenly dilute sulfuric acid on the plate, heat the plate at 105°C for 2 minutes, then examine under ultraviolet light (main wavelength: 365 nm): one of the several spots obtained from the sample solution has the same color tone and *R*f value with the blue-white fluorescent spot from the standard solution (Saposhnikovia Root and Rhizome).

(9) For preparation prescribed Glehnia Root and Rhizome—To 0.5 g of the dry extract (or 1.5 g of the viscous extract) add 5 mL of ethyl acetate, and heat under a reflux condenser for 30 minutes. After cooling, filter, and use the filtrate as the sample solution. Separately, dissolve 1 mg of scopoletin for thin-layer chromatography in 10 mL of methanol, and use this solution as the standard solution. Perform the test with these solutions as directed under Thin-layer Chromatography <*2.03*>. Spot 20 μL of the sample solution and 2 μL of the standard solution on a plate of silica gel for thin-layer chromatography. Develop the plate with a mixture of ethyl acetate and hexane (3:1) to a distance of about 7 cm, and air-dry the plate. Spray evenly dilute sulfuric acid on the plate, heat the plate at 105°C for 5 minutes, and examine under ultraviolet light (main wavelength: 365 nm): one of the several spots obtained from the sample solution has the same color tone and *R*f value with the blue-white fluorescent spot from the standard solution (Glehnia Root and Rhizome).

(10) To 1.0 g of the dry extract (or 3.0 g of the viscous extract) add 10 mL of sodium hydroxide TS, shake, then add 10 mL of diethyl ether, shake, centrifuge, and use the diethyl ether layer as the sample solution. Perform the test with the sample solution as directed under Thin-layer Chromatography <*2.03*>. Spot 15 μL of the sample solution on a plate of silica gel for thin-layer chromatography. Develop the plate with a mixture of 1-propanol, ethyl acetate, water and acetic acid (100) (4:4:2:1) to a distance of about 7 cm, and air-dry the plate. Spray evenly ninhydrin-ethanol TS for spraying on the plate, and heat the plate at 105°C for 5 minutes: a red-purple spot is observed at about 0.5 of *R*f value (Ephedra Herb).

(11) To 1.0 g of the dry extract (or 3.0 g of the viscous extract) add 10 mL of water, shake, then add 25 mL of diethyl ether, shake, and centrifuge. Separate the diethyl ether layer, evaporate the solvent under low pressure (in vacuo), dissolve the residue in 2 mL of diethyl ether, and use this solution as the sample solution. Separately, dissolve 1 mg of rhein for thin-layer chromatography in 10 mL of acetone, and use this solution as the standard solution. Perform the test with these solutions as directed under Thin-layer Chromatography <*2.03*>. Spot 10 μL of the sample solution and 5 μL of the standard solution on a plate of silica gel for thin-layer chromatography. Develop the plate with a mixture of ethyl acetate, methanol and water (20:3:2) to a distance of about 7 cm, and air-dry the plate. Examine under ultraviolet light (main wavelength: 365 nm): one of the spot among the several spots obtained from the sample solution has the same color tone and *R*f value with the orange fluorescent spot from the standard solution (Rhubarb).

(12) To 1.0 g of the dry extract (or 3.0 g of the viscous extract) add 10 mL of water, shake, then add 25 mL of diethyl ether, shake, and centrifuge. Separate the diethyl ether layer, evaporate the solvent under low pressure (in vacuo), then dissolve the residue in 2 mL of diethyl ether, and use this solution as the sample solution. Separately, dissolve 1 mg of atractylenolide III for thin-layer chromatography in 2 mL of methanol, and use this solution as the standard solution. Perform the test with these solutions as directed under Thin-layer Chromatography <*2.03*>. Spot 20 μL of the sample solution and 5 μL of the standard solution on a plate of silica gel for thin-layer chromatography. Develop the plate with a mixture of hexane and ethyl acetate (2:1) to a distance of about 7 cm, and air- dry the plate. Spray evenly 1-naphthol-sulfuric acid TS on the plate, heat the plate at 105°C for 5 minutes, and allow to cool: one of the spot among the several spots obtained from the sample solution has the same color tone and *R*f value with the red to red-purple spot from the standard solution (Atractylodes Rhizome).

(13) To 2.0 g of the dry extract (or 6.0 g of the viscous extract) add 10 mL of sodium carbonate TS, shake, then add 5 mL of 1-butanol, shake, centrifuge, and use the 1-butanol layer as the sample solution. Separately, to 2.0 g of pulverized platycodon root add 10 mL of sodium carbonate TS, shake, then add 5 mL of 1-butanol, shake, centrifuge, and use the 1-butanol layer as the standard solution. Perform the test with these solutions as directed under Thin-layer Chromatography <*2.03*>. Spot 10 μL each of the sample solution and standard solution on a plate of silica gel for thin-layer chromatography. Develop the plate with a mixture of 1-propanol, ethyl acetate and water (4:4:3) to a distance of about 10 cm, and air-dry the plate. Spray evenly 1,3-naphthalenediol TS on the plate, heat the plate at 105°C for 5 minutes: one of the spot among the several spots obtained from the sample solution has the same color tone and *R*f value with the blue-purple spot (*R*f value: about 0.4) from the standard solution (Platycodon Root).

(14) To 1.0 g of the dry extract (or 3.0 g of the viscous extract) add 10 mL of water, centrifuge, then add 25 mL of diethyl ether, shake, and centrifuge. Separate the diethyl ether layer, evaporate the solvent under low pressure (in vacuo), dissolve the residue in 2 mL of diethyl ether, and use the solution as the sample solution. Separately, dissolve 1 mg of wogonin for thin-layer chromatography in 1 mL of methanol, and use this solution as the standard solution. Perform the test with these solutions as directed under Thin-layer Chromatography <*2.03*>. Spot 20 μL of the sample solution and 2 μL of the standard solution on a plate of silica gel for thin-layer chromatography. Develop the plate with a mixture of ethyl acetate, hexane and acetic acid (100) (10:10:1) to a distance of about 7 cm, and air-dry the plate. Spray evenly iron (III) chloride-methanol TS on the plate: one of the spot among the several spots obtained from the sample solution has the same color tone and *R*f value with the yellow-brown to grayish brown spot from the standard solution (Scutellaria Root).

(15) To 1.0 g of the dry extract (or 3.0 g of the viscous extract) add 10 mL of water, shake, then add 10 mL of 1-butanol, shake, centrifuge, and use the 1-butanol layer as the sample solution. Separately, dissolve 1 mg of liquiritin for thin-layer chromatography in 1 mL of methanol, and use this solution as the standard solution. Perform the test with these solutions as directed under Thin-layer Chromatography <*2.03*>. Spot 1 μL each of the sample solution and standard solution on a plate of silica gel for thin-layer chromatography. Develop the plate with a mixture of ethyl acetate, methanol and water (20:3:2) to a distance of about 7 cm, and air-dry the plate. Spray evenly dilute sulfuric acid on the plate, heat the plate at 105°C for 5 minutes, and examine under ultraviolet light (main wavelength: 365 nm): one of the several spots obtained from the sample solution has the same color tone and *R*f value with the yellow-green fluorescent spot from the standard solution (Glycyrrhiza).

(16) Place 2.0 g of the dry extract (or 6.0 g of the viscous extract) in a porcelain crucible, ignite to incinerate at 550°C, then to the residue add 60 mL of water, shake, centrifuge, and use the supernatant as the sample solution. Add ammonium oxalate TS to the sample solution: a white precipitate is formed. The precipitate does not dissolve in diluted acetic acid, but dissolve on the addition of diluted hydrochloric acid (Gypsum).

(17) Place 2.0 g of the dry extract (or 6.0 g of the viscous extract) in a porcelain crucible, ignite to incinerate at 550°C. To the residue add 60 mL of water, shake well, centrifuge, and use the supernatant as the sample solution. The sample solution responds to the Qualitative Tests <*1.09*> (1) for sulfate (Gypsum; Sodium Sulfate or Anhydrous Sodium Sulfate).

(18) Place 2.0 g of the dry extract (or 6.0 g of the viscous extract) in a crucible, and ignite at 550°C for 5 hours to incinerate. To the residue add 3 mL of diluted sulfuric acid (1 in 3), and heat until white fumes are evolved. After cooling, add 20 mL of water, shake, and filter. To 5 mL of the filtrate add ammonia TS until a white gelatinous precipitate is formed, centrifuge, and remove the supernatant liquid. To the residue add 5 mL of water, shake, centrifuge, and remove the supernatant liquid. Then, to the residue add 5 mL of water, shake, centrifuge, and remove the supernatant liquid. To the obtained residue add 5 drops of alizarin red S TS, and shake occasionally in lukewarm water: the residue shows red to red-brown in color (Kasseki).

Purity **(1)** Heavy metals <*1.07*>—Prepare the test solution with 1.0 g of the dry extract (or an amount of the viscous extract, equivalent to 1.0 g of the dried substance) as directed under Extracts (4), and perform the test (not more than 30 ppm).

(2) Arsenic <*1.11*>—Prepare the test solution with 0.67 g of the dry extract (or an amount of the viscous extract, equivalent to 0.67 g of the dried substance) according to Method 3, and perform the test (not more than 3 ppm).

Loss on drying <*2.41*> The dry extract: Not more than 9.0% (1 g, 105°C, 5 hours).

The viscous extract: Not more than 66.7% (1 g, 105°C, 5 hours).

Total ash <*5.01*> Not less than 10.0% and more than 22.0%, calculated on the dried basis.

Assay **(1)** Paeoniflorin—Weigh accurately about 0.5 g of the dry extract (or an amount of the viscous extract, equivalent to about 0.5 g of the dried substance), add exactly 50 mL of diluted methanol (1 in 2), shake for 15 minutes, and filter. Pipet 5 mL of the filtrate, elute through a column packed with 2 g of polyamide for column chromatography using 20 mL of water, then add 1 mL of acetic acid (100), add water to make exactly 25 mL, and use this solution as the sample solution. Separately, weigh accurately about 10 mg of Paeoniflorin RS (separately determine the water <*2.48*> by coulometric titration, using 10 mg), and dissolve in diluted methanol (1 in 2) to make exactly 100 mL. Pipet 5 mL of this solution, add diluted methanol (1 in 2) to make exactly 20 mL, and use this solution as the standard solution. Perform the test with exactly 10 μL each of the sample solution and standard solution as directed under Liquid Chromatography <*2.01*> according to the following conditions, and determine the peak areas, A_T and A_S, of paeoniflorin in each solution.

$$\text{Amount (mg) of paeoniflorin } (C_{23}H_{28}O_{11}) = M_S \times A_T/A_S \times 5/8$$

M_S: Amount (mg) of Paeoniflorin RS taken, calculated on the anhydrous basis

Operating conditions—

Detector: An ultraviolet absorption photometer (wavelength: 232 nm).

Column: A stainless steel column 4.6 mm in inside diameter and 15 cm in length, packed with octadecylsilanized silica gel for liquid chromatography (5 μm in particle diameter).

Column temperature: A constant temperature of about 20°C.

Mobile phase: A mixture of water, acetonitrile and phosphoric acid (850:150:1).

Flow rate: 1.0 mL per minute (the retention time of paeoniflorin is about 9 minutes).

System suitability—

System performance: Dissolve 1 mg each of Paeoniflorin RS and albiflorin in diluted methanol (1 in 2) to make 10 mL. When the procedure is run with 10 μL of this solution under the above operating conditions, albiflorin and paeoniflorin are eluted in this order with the resolution between these peaks being not less than 2.5.

System repeatability: When the test is repeated 6 times with 10 μL of the standard solution under the above operating conditions, the relative standard deviation of the peak area of paeoniflorin is not more than 1.5%.

(2) Total alkaloids (ephedrine and pseudoephedrine)—Weigh accurately about 0.5 g of the dry extract (or an amount of the viscous extract, equivalent to about 0.5 g of the dried substance), add 20 mL of diethyl ether, shake, then add 3.0 mL of 0.1 mol/L hydrochloric acid TS, and shake for 10 minutes. After centrifugation, remove the diethyl ether layer, add 20 mL of diethyl ether, proceed in the same manner as above, and remove the diethyl ether layer. To the aqueous layer add 1.0 mL of ammonia TS and 20 mL of diethyl ether, shake for 30 minutes, centrifuge, and separate the diethyl ether layer. In addition, repeat twice in the same manner for the aqueous layer using 1.0 mL of ammonia TS and 20 mL of diethyl ether. Combine all the extracts, evaporate the solvent under low pressure (in vacuo), dissolve the residue in diluted methanol (1 in 2) to make exactly 50 mL, centrifuge, and use the supernatant liquid as the sample solution. Separately, weigh accurately about 10 mg of ephedrine hydrochloride for assay of crude drug, previously dried at 105°C for 3 hours, dissolve in diluted methanol (1 in 2) to make exactly 100 mL. Pipet 10 mL of this solution, add diluted methanol (1 in 2) to make exactly 50 mL, and use this solution as the standard solution. Perform the test with exactly 10 μL each of the sample solution and standard solution as directed under Liquid Chromatography <*2.01*> according to the following conditions. Determine the peak areas, A_{TE} and A_{TP}, of ephedrine and pseudoephedrine obtained with the sample solution, and the peak area, A_S, of ephedrine obtained with the standard solution.

Amount (mg) of total alkaloids (ephedrine and pseudoephedrine)

$$= M_S \times (A_{TE} + A_{TP})/A_S \times 1/10 \times 0.819$$

M_S: Amount (mg) of ephedrine hydrochloride for assay of crude drug taken

Operating conditions—

Detector: An ultraviolet absorption photometer (wavelength: 210 nm).

Column: A stainless steel column 4.6 mm in inside diameter and 15 cm in length, packed with octadecylsilanized silica gel for liquid chromatography (5 μm in particle diameter).

Column temperature: A constant temperature of about 40°C.

Mobile phase: To 5 g of sodium lauryl sulfate add 350 mL of acetonitrile, shake, then add 650 mL of water and 1 mL of phosphoric acid.

Flow rate: 1.0 mL per minute (the retention time of ephedrine is about 27 minutes).

System suitability—

System performance: Dissolve 1 mg each of ephedrine hydrochloride for assay of crude drug and pseudoephedrine hydrochloride in diluted methanol (1 in 2) to make 10 mL. When the procedure is run with 10 μL of this solution under the above operating conditions, pseudoephedrine and ephedrine are eluted in this order with the resolution between these peaks being not less than 1.5.

System repeatability: When the test is repeated 6 times with 10 μL of the standard solution under the above operating conditions, the relative standard deviation of the peak area of ephedrine is not more than 1.5%.

(3) Baicalin—Weigh accurately about 0.1 g of the dry extract (or an amount of the viscous extract, equivalent to about 0.1 g of the dried substance), add exactly 50 mL of diluted methanol (7 in 10), shake for 15 minutes, filter, and use the filtrate as the sample solution. Separately, weigh accurately about 10 mg of Baicalin RS (separately determine the water <*2.48*> by coulometric titration, using 10 mg), dissolve in methanol to make exactly 100 mL. Pipet 5 mL of this solution, add diluted methanol (7 in 10) to make exactly 10 mL, and use this solution as the standard solution. Perform the test with exactly 10 μL each of the sample solution and standard solution as directed under Liquid Chromatography <*2.01*> according to the following conditions, and determine the peak areas, A_T and A_S, of baicalin in each solution.

$$\text{Amount (mg) of baicalin } (C_{21}H_{18}O_{11}) = M_S \times A_T/A_S \times 1/4$$

M_S: Amount (mg) of Baicalin RS taken, calculated on the anhydrous basis

Operating conditions—

Detector: An ultraviolet absorption photometer (wavelength: 277 nm).

Column: A stainless steel column 4.6 mm in inside diameter and 15 cm in length, packed with octadecylsilanized silica gel for liquid chromatography (5 μm in particle diameter).

Column temperature: A constant temperature of about 40°C.

Mobile phase: A mixture of diluted phosphoric acid (1 in 200) and acetonitrile (19:6).

Flow rate: 1.0 mL per minute (the retention time of baicalin is about 10 minutes).

System suitability—

System performance: When the procedure is run with 10 μL of the standard solution under the above operating conditions, the number of theoretical plates and the symmetry factor of the peak of baicalin are not less than 5000 and not more than 1.5, respectively.

System repeatability: When the test is repeated 6 times with 10 μL of the standard solution under the above operating conditions, the relative standard deviation of the peak area of baicalin is not more than 1.5%.

(4) Glycyrrhizic acid—Weigh accurately about 0.5 g of the dry extract (or an amount of the viscous extract, equivalent to about 0.5 g of the dried substance), add 20 mL of ethyl acetate and 10 mL of water, and shake for 10 minutes. After centrifugation, remove the ethyl acetate layer, add 20 mL of ethyl acetate, proceed in the same manner as described above, and remove the ethyl acetate layer. To the aqueous layer add 10 mL of methanol, shake for 30 minutes, centrifuge, and take the supernatant liquid. To the residue add 20 mL of diluted methanol (1 in 2), shake for 5 minutes, centrifuge, and take the supernatant liquid. Combine these supernatant liquids, add diluted methanol (1 in 2) to make exactly 50 mL, and use this solution as the sample solution. Separately, weigh accurately about 10 mg of Glycyrrhizic Acid RS (separately determine the water <*2.48*> by coulometric titration, using 10 mg), dissolve in diluted methanol (1 in 2) to make exactly 100 mL, and use this solution as the standard solution. Perform the test with exactly 10 μL each of the sample solution and standard solution as directed under Liquid Chromatography <*2.01*> according to the following conditions, and determine the peak areas, A_T and A_S, of glycyrrhizic acid in each solution.

$$\text{Amount (mg) of glycyrrhizic acid } (C_{42}H_{62}O_{16}) = M_S \times A_T/A_S \times 1/2$$

M_S: Amount (mg) of Glycyrrhizic Acid RS taken, calculated on the anhydrous basis

Operating conditions—

Detector: An ultraviolet absorption photometer (wavelength: 254 nm).

Column: A stainless steel column 4.6 mm in inside diameter and 15 cm in length, packed with octadecylsilanized silica gel for liquid chromatography (5 μm in particle diameter).

Column temperature: A constant temperature of about 40°C.

Mobile phase: Dissolve 3.85 g of ammonium acetate in 720 mL of water, and add 5 mL of acetic acid (100) and 280 mL of acetonitrile.

Flow rate: 1.0 mL per minute (the retention time of glycyrrhizic acid is about 15 minutes).

System suitability—

System performance: Dissolve 5 mg of monoammonium glycyrrhizinate for resolution check in 20 mL of dilute ethanol. When the procedure is run with 10 μL of this solution under the above operating conditions, the resolution between the peak having the relative retention time of about 0.9 to glycyrrhizic acid and the peak of glycyrrhizic acid is not less than 1.5.

System repeatability: When the test is repeated 6 times with 10 μL of the standard solution under the above operating conditions, the relative standard deviation of the peak area of glycyrrhizic acid is not more than 1.5%.

Containers and storage Containers—Tight containers.

Boiogito Extract

防已黄耆湯エキス

Boiogito Extract contains not less than 4 mg and not more than 16 mg of sinomenine, and not less than 10 mg and not more than 30 mg of glycyrrhizic acid ($C_{42}H_{62}O_{16}$: 822.93), per extract prepared with the amount specified in the Method of preparation.

Method of preparation

	1)	2)	3)
Sinomenium Stem and Rhizome	5 g	5 g	5 g
Astragalus Root	5 g	5 g	5 g
Atractylodes Rhizome	3 g	3 g	—
Atractylodes Lancea Rhizome	—	—	3 g
Ginger	0.8 g	1 g	1 g
Jujube	3 g	3 g	3 g
Glycyrrhiza	1.5 g	1.5 g	1.5 g

Prepare a dry extract or viscous extract as directed under Extracts, according to the prescription 1) to 3), using the crude drugs shown above. Or, prepare a dry extract by adding Light Anhydrous Silicic Acid to an extractive, prepared as directed under Extracts, according to the prescription 3), using the crude drugs shown above.

Description Boiogito Extract is a light yellow-brown to reddish brown powder or black-brown viscous extract. It has a slightly odor, and a sweet taste at first and then a slight hot and bitter taste later.

Identification (1) To 2.0 g of the dry extract (or 6.0 g of the viscous extract) add 15 mL of sodium hydroxide TS, shake, centrifuge, and separate the supernatant liquid. To this liquid add 10 mL of 1-butanol, shake, centrifuge, and separate 1-butanol layer. To this liquid add 10 mL of water, shake, centrifuge, separate the 1-butanol layer, then evaporate the solvent under low pressure (in vacuo), dissolve the residue in 1 mL of methanol, and use the solution as the sample solution. Separately, dissolve 1 mg of sinomenine for thin-layer chromatography in 1 mL of methanol, and use this solution as the standard solution. Perform the test with these solutions as directed under Thin-layer Chromatography <*2.03*>. Spot 10 μL of the sample solution and 2 μL of the standard solution on a plate of silica gel for thin-layer chromatography. Develop the plate with a mixture of ethyl acetate, 1-propanol, water and acetic acid (100) (7:5:4:1) to a distance of about 7 cm, and air-dry the plate. Spray evenly 4-dimethylaminobenzaldehyde TS for spraying on the plate, heat the plate at 105°C for 5 minutes, and allow to cool: one of the several spots obtained from the sample solution has the same color tone and *Rf* value with the red to red-brown spot from the standard solution (Sinomenium Stem and Rhizome).

(2) To 2.0 g of the dry extract (or 6.0 g of the viscous extract) add 15 mL of sodium hydroxide TS, shake, centrifuge, and separate the supernatant liquid. To this liquid add 10 mL of 1-butanol, shake, centrifuge, and separate 1-butanol layer. To the aqueous layer add 10 mL of 1-butanol, and proceed in the same manner as above. Combine the 1-butanol layers, add 10 mL of water, shake, centrifuge, separate the 1-butanol layer, and evaporate the solvent under low pressure (in vacuo). Dissolve the residue in exactly 1 mL of methanol, and use this solution as the sample solution. Separately, dissolve 1.0 mg of astragaloside IV for thin-layer chromatography in exactly 10 mL of methanol, and use this solution as the standard solution. Perform the test with these solutions as directed under Thin-layer Chromatography <*2.03*>. Spot 5 μL of the sample solution and standard solution on a plate of silica gel for thin-layer chromatography. Develop the plate with a mixture of ethyl acetate, 1-propanol, water and acetic acid (100) (7:5:4:1) to a distance of about 10 cm, and air-dry the plate. Spray evenly 4-dimethylaminobenzaldehyde TS for spraying on the plate, heat the plate at 105°C for 5 minutes, and allow to cool: one of the several spots obtained from the sample solution has the same color tone and *Rf* value with the red-brown spot obtained from the standard solution, and the spot is larger and more intense than the spot from the standard solution (Astragalus Root).

(3) For preparation prescribed Atractylodes Rhizome—To 1.0 g of the dry extract (or 3.0 g of the viscous extract) add 10 mL of water, shake, then add 25 mL of diethyl ether, and shake. Separate the diethyl ether layer, evaporate the solvent under low pressure (in vacuo), then dissolve the residue in 2 mL of diethyl ether, and use the solution as the sample solution. Separately, dissolve 1 mg of Atractylenolide III for thin-layer chromatography in 2 mL of methanol, and use this solution as the standard solution. Perform the test with these solutions as directed under Thin-layer Chromatography <*2.03*>. Spot 10 μL of the sample solution and 5 μL of the standard solution on a plate of silica gel for thin-layer chromatography. Develop the plate with a mixture of ethyl acetate and hexane (1:1) to a distance of about 7 cm, and air-dry the plate. Spray evenly 1-naphthol-sulfuric acid TS on the plate, heat the plate at 105°C for 5 minutes, and allow to cool: one of the several spots obtained from the sample solution has the same color tone and *Rf* value with the red to red-purple spot from the standard solution (Atractylodes Rhizome).

(4) For preparation prescribed Atractylodes Lancea Rhizome—To 2.0 g of the dry extract (or 6.0 g of the viscous extract) add 10 mL of water, shake, then add 25 mL of hexane, and shake. Separate the hexane layer, evaporate the solvent under low pressure (in vacuo), then add 0.5 mL of hexane to the residue, and use this solution as the sample solution. Perform the test with the sample solution as directed under Thin-layer Chromatography <*2.03*>. Spot 10 μL of the sample solution on a plate of silica gel with fluorescent indicator for thin-layer chromatography. Develop the plate with a mixture of hexane and acetone (7:1) to a distance of about 7 cm, and air-dry the plate. Examine under ultraviolet light (main wavelength: 254 nm): a dark purple spot is observed at an *Rf* value of about 0.5. The spot shows a greenish brown color after being sprayed evenly 4-dimethylamino-benzaldehyde TS for spraying on the plate, heated at 105°C for 5 minutes, and allowed to cool (Atractylodes Lancea Rhizome).

(5) To 1.0 g of the dry extract (or 3.0 g of the viscous extract) add 10 mL of water, shake, then add 25 mL of diethyl ether, and shake. Separate the diethyl ether layer, evaporate the solvent under low pressure (in vacuo), then dissolve the residue in 2 mL of diethyl ether, and use the solution as the sample solution. Separately, dissolve 1 mg of [6]-gingerol for thin-layer chromatography in 1 mL of methanol, and use this solution as the standard solution. Perform the test with these solutions as directed under Thin-layer Chromatography <*2.03*>. Spot 20 μL of the sample solution and 5 μL of the standard solution on a plate of silica gel for thin-layer chromatography. Develop the plate with a mixture of ethyl acetate and hexane (1:1) to a distance of about 7 cm, and air-dry the plate. Spray evenly 4-dimethylaminobenzaldehyde TS on the plate, heat the plate at 105°C for 5 minutes, allow to cool, and spray water: one of the several spots obtained from the sample solution has the same color tone and *R*f value with the blue-green to grayish green spot from the standard solution (Ginger).

(6) To 1.0 g of the dry extract (or 3.0 g of the viscous extract) add 10 mL of water, shake, then add 10 mL of 1-butanol, shake, centrifuge, and use the 1-butanol layer as the sample solution. Separately, dissolve 1 mg of liquiritin for thin-layer chromatography in 1 mL of methanol, and use this solution as the standard solution. Perform the test with these solutions as directed under Thin-layer Chromatography <*2.03*>. Spot 1 μL each of the sample solution and standard solution on a plate of silica gel for thin-layer chromatography. Develop the plate with a mixture of ethyl acetate, methanol and water (20:3:2) to a distance of about 7 cm, and air-dry the plate. Spray evenly dilute sulfuric acid on the plate, heat the plate at 105°C for 5 minutes, and examine under ultraviolet light (main wavelength: 365 nm): one of the several spots obtained from the sample solution has the same color tone and *R*f value with the yellow-green fluorescent spot from the standard solution (Glycyrrhiza).

Purity (1) Heavy metals <*1.07*>—Prepare the test solution with 1.0 g of the dry extract (or an amount of the viscous extract, equivalent to 1.0 g of the dried substance) as directed under Extracts (4), and perform the test (not more than 30 ppm).

(2) Arsenic <*1.11*>—Prepare the test solution with 0.67 g of the dry extract (or an amount of the viscous extract, equivalent to 0.67 g of the dried substance) according to Method 3, and perform the test (not more than 3 ppm).

Loss on drying <*2.41*> The dry extract: Not more than 11.0% (1 g, 105°C, 5 hours).

The viscous extract: Not more than 66.7% (1 g, 105°C, 5 hours).

Total ash <*5.01*> Not less than 8.0%, calculated on the dried basis. However, for the dry extract prepared by adding Light Anhydrous Silicic Acid, between 9.0% and 18.0%.

Assay (1) Sinomenine—Weigh accurately about 0.5 g of the dry extract (or an amount of the viscous extract, equivalent to about 0.5 g of the dried substance), add 20 mL of diethyl ether, shake, then add 5.0 mL of 0.1 mol/L hydrochloric acid TS, and shake for 10 minutes, centrifuge, and remove the diethyl ether layer. To the aqueous layer add 20 mL of diethyl ether, and proceed in the same manner as described above. To the aqueous layer add 5.0 mL of diluted sodium hydroxide TS (1 in 10) and 10 mL of methanol, shake for 15 minutes, centrifuge, and take the supernatant liquid. To the residue add 20 mL of diluted methanol (1 in 2), shake for 15 minutes, centrifuge, and take the supernatant liquid. Combine all the supernatant liquids, add diluted methanol (1 in 2) to make exactly 50 mL, and use this solution as the sample solution. Separately, weigh accurately about 5 mg of sinomenine for assay, dissolve in diluted methanol (1 in 2) to make exactly 100 mL, and use this solution as the standard solution. Perform the test with exactly 10 μL each of the sample solution and standard solution as directed under Liquid Chromatography <*2.01*> according to the following conditions, and determine the peak areas, A_T and A_S, of sinomenine in each solution.

$$\text{Amount (mg) of sinomenine} = M_S \times A_T/A_S \times 1/2$$

M_S: Amount (mg) of sinomenine for assay taken

Operating conditions—

Detector: An ultraviolet absorption photometer (wavelength: 254 nm).

Column: A stainless steel column 4.6 mm in inside diameter and 15 cm in length, packed with octadecylsilanized silica gel for liquid chromatography (5 μm in particle diameter).

Column temperature: A constant temperature of about 30°C.

Mobile phase: To 3 g of sodium lauryl sulfate add 350 mL of acetonitrile, shake, then add 650 mL of water and 1 mL of phosphoric acid to dissolve lauryl sulfate.

Flow rate: 1.0 mL per minute (the retention time of sinomenine is about 18 minutes).

System suitability—

System performance: When the procedure is run with 10 μL each of the sample solution, the sinomenine standard solution and the glycyrrhizic acid standard solution obtained in Assay (2) under the above operating conditions, peaks of sinomenine and glycyrrhizic acid are observed in the sample solution, glycyrrhizic acid and sinomenine are eluted in this order with the resolution between these peaks being not less than 4.5. Furthermore, except for the peak of glycyrrhizic acid, distinct peaks are observed before and after the peak of sinomenine, and the resolutions between sinomenine and these peaks are respectively not less than 1.5.

System repeatability: When the test is repeated 6 times with 10 μL of the standard solution under the above operating conditions, the relative standard deviation of the peak area of sinomenine is not more than 1.5%.

(2) Glycyrrhizic acid—Weigh accurately about 0.5 g of the dry extract (or an amount of the viscous extract, equivalent to about 0.5 g of the dried substance), add exactly 50 mL of diluted methanol (1 in 2), shake for 15 minutes, filter, and use the filtrate as the sample solution. Separately, weigh accurately about 10 mg of Glycyrrhizic Acid RS (separately determine the water <*2.48*> by coulometric titration, using 10 mg), dissolve in diluted methanol (1 in 2) to make exactly 100 mL, and use this solution as the standard solution. Perform the test with exactly 10 μL each of the sample solution and standard solution as directed under Liquid Chromatography <*2.01*> according to the following conditions, and determine the peak areas, A_T and A_S, of glycyrrhizic acid in each solution.

$$\text{Amount (mg) of glycyrrhizic acid } (C_{42}H_{62}O_{16}) = M_S \times A_T/A_S \times 1/2$$

M_S: Amount (mg) of Glycyrrhizic Acid RS taken, calculated on the anhydrous basis

Operating conditions—

Detector: An ultraviolet absorption photometer (wavelength: 254 nm).

Column: A stainless steel column 4.6 mm in inside diameter and 15 cm in length, packed with octadecylsilanized silica gel for liquid chromatography (5 μm in particle diameter).

Column temperature: A constant temperature of about 40°C.

Mobile phase: Dissolve 3.85 g of ammonium acetate in 720 mL of water, and add 5 mL of acetic acid (100) and 280 mL of acetonitrile.

Flow rate: 1.0 mL per minute (the retention time of glycyrrhizic acid is about 15 minutes).

System suitability—

System performance: Dissolve 5 mg of monoammonium glycyrrhizinate for resolution check in 20 mL of dilute ethanol. When the procedure is run with 10 μL of this solu tion under the above operating conditions, the resolution between the peak having the relative retention time of about 0.9 to glycyrrhizic acid and the peak of glycyrrhizic acid is not less than 1.5.

System repeatability: When the test is repeated 6 times with 10 μL of the standard solution under the above operating conditions, the relative standard deviation of the peak area of glycyrrhizic acid is not more than 1.5%.

Containers and storage Containers—Tight containers.

Brown Rice

Oryzae Fructus

コウベイ

Brown Rice is the fruit of *Oryza sativa* Linné (*Gramineae*).

Description Brown Rice occurs as ellipsoidal, slightly flattened, 4 - 6 mm in length; externally translucent, light yellowish white to light brown. Slightly cave in and a white embryo at one end; a brown small dent of scar of style at the other end; few longitudinally striates on the surface.

Odor, slight; taste, slightly sweet.

Under a microscope <*5.01*>, a transverse section of the caryopsis reveals the outermost layer composed of pericarp; vascular bundles in the pericarp; seed coat adhering closely to the pericarp; in the interior, 1 or 2 cellular layered aleuron layers; parenchymatous cells of endosperm contain simple or compound starch grains.

Identification **(1)** To 0.1 g of pulverized Brown Rice add 50 mL of water, and heat in a water bath for 5 minutes. After cooling, add 1 drops of iodine TS, and shake: a blue-purple color develops.

(2) To 1 g of pulverized Brown Rice add 5 mL of ethyl acetate, shake for 10 minutes, centrifuge, and use the supernatant liquid as the sample solution. Separately, dissolve 1 mg of cycloartenyl ferulate for thin-layer chromatography in 1 mL of ethyl acetate, and use this solution as the standard solution. Perform the test with these solutions as directed under Thin-layer chromatography <*2.03*>. Spot 10 μL of the sample solution and 5 μL of the standard solution on a plate of silica gel for thin-layer chromatography. Develop the plate with a mixture of hexane and acetone (5:2) to a distance of about 7 cm, and air-dry the plate. Examine under ultraviolet light (main wavelength: 365 nm): one of the several spots obtained from the sample solution has the same color tone and *R*f value with the blue-purple fluorescent spot obtained from the standard solution.

Total ash <*5.01*> Not more than 1.5%.

Containers and storage Containers—Well-closed containers.

Bupleurum Root

Bupleuri Radix

サイコ

Bupleurum Root is the root of *Bupleurum falcatum* Linné (*Umbelliferae*).

It contains not less than 0.35% of the total saponin (saikosaponin a and saikosaponin d), calculated on the basis of dried material.

Description Long cone or column shape, single or branched root, 10 - 20 cm in length, 0.5 - 1.5 cm in diameter; occasionally with remains of stem on the crown; externally light brown to brown and sometimes with deep wrinkles; easily broken, and fractured surface somewhat fibrous. Under a magnifying glass, a transverse section reveals the thickness of cortex reaching 1/3 - 1/2 of the radius and tangentially extended clefts in cortex.

Odor, characteristic, and taste, slightly bitter.

Under a microscope <*5.01*>, a transverse section reveals the cortex scattered with a good many oil canals 15 - 35 μm in diameter; in xylem, vessels lined radially or in a staircase pattern, and fiber bundles scattered; in the pith at the crown, the same oil canals as in the cortex; parenchyma cells containing starch grains and oil droplets. Starch grains composed of simple grains, 2 - 10 μm in diameter, or compound grains.

Identification **(1)** Shake vigorously 0.5 g of pulverized Bupleurum Root with 10 mL of water: lasting fine foams are produced.

(2) To 1.0 g of the pulverized Bupleurum Root, add 10 mL of methanol, and boil gently under a reflux condenser for 15 minutes. After cooling, filter, and use the filtrate as the sample solution. Separately, dissolve 1 mg of saikosaponin a for thin-layer chromatography in 1 mL of methanol, and use this solution as the standard solution. Perform the test with these solutions as directed under Thin-layer Chromatography <*2.03*>. Spot 10 μL each of the sample solution and standard solution on a plate of silica gel for thin-layer chromatography. Develop the plate with a mixture of ethyl acetate, ethanol (99.5) and water (8:2:1) to a distance of about 10 cm, and air-dry the plate. Spray evenly 4-dimethylaminobenzaldehyde TS on the plate, and heat the plate at 105°C for 5 minutes: one of the several spots obtained from the sample solution has the same color tone and *R*f value with the spot from the standard solution, accompanied by the adjacent yellow-red spot above.

Purity **(1)** Heavy metals <*1.07*>—Proceed with 3.0 g of pulverized Bupleurum Root according to Method 3, and perform the test. Prepare the control solution with 3.0 mL of Standard Lead Solution (not more than 10 ppm).

(2) Arsenic <*1.11*>—Prepare the test solution with 0.40 g of pulverized Bupleurum Root according to Method 4, and perform the test (not more than 5 ppm).

(3) Stem and leaf—When perform the test of foreign matter <*5.01*>, the amount of the stems and leaves contained in Bupleurum Root does not exceed 10.0%.

(4) Foreign matter <*5.01*>—The amount of foreign matter other than stems and leaves contained in Bupleurum Root does not exceed 1.0%.

Loss on drying <*5.01*> Not more than 12.5% (6 hours).

Total ash <*5.01*> Not more than 6.5%.

Acid-insoluble ash ⟨5.01⟩ Not more than 2.0%.

Extract content ⟨5.01⟩ Dilute ethanol-soluble extract: not less than 11.0%.

Assay Weigh accurately about 1 g of pulverized Bupleurum Root, transfer in a glass-stoppered centrifuge tube, add 20 mL of diluted methanol (9 in 10), shake for 15 minutes, centrifuge, and separate the supernatant liquid. Perform the same procedure with the residue using two 15-mL potions of diluted methanol (9 in 10), combine all the extracts, and add diluted methanol (9 in 10) to make exactly 50 mL. Pipet 5 mL of this solution, add 2.5 mL of dilute sodium hydroxide TS, heat in a water bath at 50°C for 1 hour, and add 7.5 mL of phosphate buffer solution for assay of bupleurum root. Allow this solution to flow through a chromatographic column [about 10 mm inside diameter containing 0.36 g of octadecylsilanized silica gel for pretreatment (55 to 105 μm in particle diameter), conditioned with 10 mL of methanol then 10 mL of water just before use]. Wash the column with 10 mL of diluted methanol (7 in 20), then flow with methanol to get exactly 10 mL of effluent solution, and use this as the sample solution. Use saikosamponins a and d standard TS for assay as the standard solution. Perform the test with exactly 20 μL each of the sample solution and standard solution as directed under Liquid Chromatography ⟨2.01⟩ according to the following conditions, and determine the peak areas, A_{TA} and A_{SA}, of saikosaponin a and A_{TD} and A_{SD}, of saikosaponin d in each solusion. Calculate the amount of saikosaponin a and saikosaponin d by the following equation, and designate the total as the amount of total saponin.

Amount (mg) of saikosaponin a $= M_{SA} \times A_{TA}/A_{SA} \times 1/2$

M_{SA}: Amount (mg) of saikosaponin a for assay taken

Amount (mg) of saikosaponin d $= M_{SD} \times A_{TD}/A_{SD} \times 1/2$

M_{SD}: Amount (mg) of saikosaponin d for assay taken

Operating conditions—

Detector: An ultraviolet absorption photometer (wavelength: 206 nm).

Column: A stainless steel column 4.6 mm in inside diameter and 15 cm in length, packed with octadecylsilanized silica gel (5 μm in particle diameter).

Column temperature: A constant temperature of about 50°C.

Mobile phase: A mixture of water and acetonitrile (3:2).

Flow rate: Adjust so that the retention time of saikosaponin a is about 8 minutes.

System suitability—

System performance: When the procedure is run with 20 μL of the standard solution under the above operating conditions, saikosaponin a and saikosaponin d are eluted in this order, and the numbers of theoretical plates and the symmetry factors of their peaks are not less than 4000 and not more than 1.4, respectively.

System repeatability: When the test is repeated 6 times with 20 μL of the standard solution under the above operating conditions, the relative standard deviations of the peak area of saikosaponin a and saikosaponin d are not more than 1.5%, respectively.

Containers and storage Containers—Well-closed containers.

Burdock Fruit

Arctii Fructus

ゴボウシ

Burdock Fruit is the fruit of *Arctium lappa* Linné (*Compositae*).

Description Burdock Fruit is slightly curved, long obovate achene, 5 – 7 mm in length, 2.0 – 3.2 mm in width, 0.8 to 1.5 mm in thickness; externally grayish brown to brown, with black spots; hollow about 1 mm in diameter at one broad end; flat, indistinct, longitudinal ridge at the other narrow end. 100 fruits weigh 1.0 – 1.5 g.

Practically odorless; taste, bitter and oily.

Under a microscope ⟨5.01⟩, transverse section reveals an exocarp composed of an epidermis, mesocarp of slightly sclerified parenchyma, and endocarp of a single cellular layer of stone cells; seed coat composed of radially elongated, sclerified epidermis, and parenchyma of several cellular layers; parenchymatous cells of the mesocarp contain a brown substance; stone cells of endocarp contain solitary, discrete crystals of calcium oxalate; cotyledons with starch grains, oil drops, aleurone grains, and minute crystals of calcium oxalate.

Identification To 0.5 g of pulverized Burdock Fruit add 20 mL of methanol, shake for 10 minutes, filter, and use filtrate as the sample solution. Perform the test with the sample solution as directed under Thin-layer Chromatography ⟨2.03⟩. Spot 5 μL of the sample solution on a plate of silica gel for thin-layer chromatography, develop the plate with a mixture of acetone, ethyl acetate and water (15:10:1) to a distance of about 7 cm, and air-dry the plate. Spray evenly dilute sulfuric acid on the plate, and heat the plate at 105°C for 5 minutes: a red-purple spot appears at an *R*f value of about 0.4.

Loss on drying ⟨5.01⟩ Not more than 12.0% (6 hours).

Total ash ⟨5.01⟩ Not more than 7.0%.

Acid-insoluble ash ⟨5.01⟩ Not more than 1.0%.

Extract content ⟨5.01⟩ Dilute ethanol-extract: not less than 15.0%.

Containers and storage Containers—Well-closed containers.

Byakkokaninjinto Extract

白虎加人参湯エキス

Byakkokaninjinto Extract contains not less than 9 mg and not more than 36 mg of mangiferin, not less than 13 mg and not more than 39 mg of glycyrrhizic acid ($C_{42}H_{62}O_{16}$: 822.93), and not less than 0.9 mg (for preparation prescribed 1.5 g of Ginseng) or not less than 1.8 mg (for preparation prescribed 3 g of Ginseng) of ginsenoside Rb_1 ($C_{54}H_{92}O_{23}$: 1109.29), per extract prepared with the amount specified in the Method of preparation.

Method of preparation

	1)	2)
Anemarrhena Rhizome	5 g	5 g
Gypsum	15 g	15 g
Glycyrrhiza	2 g	2 g
Brown Rice	8 g	8 g
Ginseng	1.5 g	3 g

Prepare a dry extract or viscous extract as directed under Extracts, according to the prescription 1) or 2), using the crude drugs shown above.

Description Byakkokaninjinto Extract occurs as a very pale yellow-brown to light brown powder or blackish brown viscous extract. It has a slight odor, and has a slightly sweet and slightly bitter taste.

Identification **(1)** To 2.0 g of the dry extract (or 6.0 g of the viscous extract) add 10 mL of sodium hydroxide TS, shake, then add 5 mL of 1-butanol, shake, centrifuge, and use the 1-butanol layer as the sample solution. Separately, to 1 g of pulverized Anemarrhena Rhizome add 10 mL of water, shake, then add 10 mL of 1-butanol, shake, centrifuge, and use the 1-butanol layer as the standard solution. Perform the test with these solutions as directed under Thin-layer Chromatography <*2.03*>. Spot 5 μL of the sample solution and 1 μL of the standard solution on a plate of silica gel for thin-layer chromatography. Develop the plate with a mixture of ethyl acetate, 1-propanol, water and acetic acid (100) (7:5:4:1) to a distance of about 7 cm, and air-dry the plate. Spray evenly 4-dimethylaminobenzaldehyde TS for spraying on the plate, and heat the plate at 105°C for 2 minutes, and allow to cool: one of the several spots obtained from the sample solution has the same color tone and *R*f value with the yellowish red to dark red spot (at an *R*f value of about 0.3) from the standard solution (Anemarrhena Rhizome).

(2) Place 2.0 g of the dry extract (or 6.0 g of the viscous extract) in a porcelain crucible, and ignite to incinerate at 500 - 550°C. To the residue add 60 mL of water, shake, centrifuge, and use the supernatant as the sample solution. Add ammonium oxalate TS to the sample solution: a white precipitate is formed. The precipitate does not dissolve in diluted acetic acid, but dissolves on the addition of diluted hydrochloric acid (Gypsum).

(3) To 1.0 g of the dry extract (or 3.0 g of the viscous extract) add 10 mL of water, shake, then add 10 mL of 1-butanol, shake, centrifuge, and use the 1-butanol layer as the sample solution. Separately, dissolve 1 mg of liquiritin for thin-layer chromatography in 1 mL of methanol, and use this solution as the standard solution. Perform the test with these solutions as directed under Thin-layer Chromatography <*2.03*>. Spot 1 μL each of the sample solution and standard solution on a plate of silica gel for thin-layer chromatography. Develop the plate with a mixture of ethyl acetate, methanol and water (20:3:2) to a distance of about 7 cm, and air-dry the plate. Spray evenly dilute sulfuric acid on the plate, heat the plate at 105°C for 5 minutes, and examine under ultraviolet light (main wavelength: 365 nm): one of the several spots obtained from the sample solution has the same color tone and *R*f value with the yellow-green fluorescent spot from the standard solution (Glycyrrhiza).

(4) To 5.0 g of the dry extract (or 15 g of the viscous extract) add 15 mL of water, shake, then add 5 mL of diethyl ether, shake, centrifuge, and use the diethyl ether layer as the sample solution. Separately, dissolve 1 mg of cycloartenyl ferulate for thin-layer chromatography in 1 mL of ethyl acetate, and use this solution as the standard solution. Perform the test with these solutions as directed under Thin-layer Chromatography <*2.03*>. Spot 30 μL of the sample solution and 5 μL of the standard solution on a plate of silica gel for thin-layer chromatography. Develop the plate with a mixture of hexane, acetone and acetic acid (100) (50:20:1) to a distance of about 7 cm, and air-dry the plate. Spray evenly a mixture of sulfuric acid and ethanol (99.5) (1:1), heat the plate at 105°C for 5 minutes, and examine under ultraviolet light (main wavelength: 365 nm): one of the several spots obtained from the sample solution has the same color tone and *R*f value with the light yellow-white to yellow fluorescent spot from the standard solution. (Brown Rice).

(5) To 2.0 g of the dry extract (or 6.0 g of the viscous extract) add 10 mL of sodium hydroxide TS, shake, then add 5 mL of 1-butanol, shake, centrifuge, and use the 1-butanol layer as the sample solution. Separately, dissolve 1 mg of Ginsenoside Rg_1 RS or ginsenoside Rg_1 for thin-layer chromatography in 1 mL of methanol, and use this solution as the standard solution. Perform the test with these solutions as directed under Thin-layer Chromatography <*2.03*>. Spot 10 μL of the sample solution and 5 μL of the standard solution on a plate of silica gel for thin-layer chromatography. Develop the plate with a mixture of ethyl acetate, 1-propanol, water and acetic acid (100) (7:5:4:1) to a distance of about 7 cm, and air-dry the plate. Spray evenly vanillin-sulfuric acid-ethanol TS for spraying on the plate, heat the plate at 105°C for 5 minutes, and allow to cool: one of the several spots obtained from the sample solution has the same color tone and *R*f value with the blue-purple to dark purple spot from the standard solution (Ginseng).

Purity **(1)** Heavy metals <*1.07*>—Prepare the test solution with 1.0 g of the dry extract (or an amount of the viscous extract, equivalent to 1.0 g of the dried substance) as directed under Extracts (4), and perform the test (not more than 30 ppm).

(2) Arsenic <*1.11*>—Prepare the test solution with 0.67 g of the dry extract (or an amount of the viscous extract, equivalent to 0.67 g of the dried substance) according to Method 3, and perform the test (not more than 3 ppm).

Loss on drying <*2.41*> The dry extract: Not more than 10.0% (1 g, 105°C, 5 hours).

The viscous extract: Not more than 66.7% (1 g, 105°C, 5 hours).

Total ash <*5.01*> Not more than 20.0%, calculated on the dried basis.

Assay **(1)** Mangiferin—Weigh accurately about 0.5 g of the dry extract (or an amount of the viscous extract, equivalent to about 0.5 g of the dried substance), add exactly 50 mL of diluted methanol (1 in 2), shake for 15 minutes, centrifuge, and use the supernatant as the sample solution. Separately, weigh accurately about 10 mg of mangiferin for assay, dissolve in diluted methanol (1 in 2) to make exactly 200 mL, and use this solution as the standard solution. Perform the test with exactly 10 μL each of the sample solution and standard solution as directed under Liquid Chromatography <*2.01*> according to the following conditions, and determine the peak areas, A_T and A_S, of mangiferin in each solution.

$$\text{Amount (mg) of mangiferin} = M_S \times A_T/A_S \times 1/4$$

M_S: Amount (mg) of mangiferin for assay taken, calculated on the basis of the content obtained by qNMR

Operating conditions—

Detector: An ultraviolet absorption photometer (wavelength: 367 nm).

Column: A stainless steel column 4.6 mm in inside diameter and 15 cm in length, packed with octadecylsilanized silica gel for liquid chromatography (5 μm in particle diameter).

Column temperature: A constant temperature of about 40°C.

Mobile phase: A mixture of water, acetonitrile and phosphoric acid (1780:220:1).

Flow rate: 1.0 mL per minute.

System suitability—

System performance: When the procedure is run with 10 μL of the standard solution under the above operating conditions, the number of theoretical plates and the symmetry factor of the peak of mangiferin are not less than 5000 and not more than 1.5, respectively.

System repeatability: When the test is repeated 6 times with 10 μL of the standard solution under the above operating conditions, the relative standard deviation of the peak area of mangiferin is not more than 1.5%.

(2) Glycyrrhizic acid—Weigh accurately about 0.5 g of the dry extract (or an amount of the viscous extract, equivalent to about 0.5 g of the dried substance), add exactly 50 mL of diluted methanol (1 in 2), shake for 15 minutes, filter, and use the filtrate as the sample solution. Separately, weigh accurately about 10 mg of Glycyrrhizic Acid RS (separately determine the water <*2.48*> by coulometric titration, using 10 mg), dissolve in diluted methanol (1 in 2) to make exactly 100 mL, and use this solution as the standard solution. Perform the test with exactly 10 μL each of the sample solution and standard solution as directed under Liquid Chromatography <*2.01*> according to the following conditions, and determine the peak areas, A_T and A_S, of glycyrrhizic acid in each solution.

$$\text{Amount (mg) of glycyrrhizic acid } (C_{42}H_{62}O_{16}) = M_S \times A_T/A_S \times 1/2$$

M_S: Amount (mg) of Glycyrrhizic Acid RS taken, calculated on the anhydrous basis

Operating conditions—

Detector: An ultraviolet absorption photometer (wavelength: 254 nm).

Column: A stainless steel column 4.6 mm in inside diameter and 15 cm in length, packed with octadecylsilanized silica gel for liquid chromatography (5 μm in particle diameter).

Column temperature: A constant temperature of about 40°C.

Mobile phase: Dissolve 3.85 g of ammonium acetate in 720 mL of water, and add 5 mL of acetic acid (100) and 280 mL of acetonitrile.

Flow rate: 1.0 mL per minute.

System suitability—

System performance: Dissolve 5 mg of monoammonium glycyrrhizinate for resolution check in 20 mL of dilute ethanol. When the procedure is run with 10 μL of this solution under the above operating conditions, the resolution between the peak having the relative retention time of about 0.9 to glycyrrhizic acid and the peak of glycyrrhizic acid is not less than 1.5.

System repeatability: When the test is repeated 6 times with 10 μL of the standard solution under the above operating conditions, the relative standard deviation of the peak area of glycyrrhizic acid is not more than 1.5%.

(3) Ginsenoside Rb_1—Weigh accurately about 1 g of the dry extract (or an amount of the viscous extract, equivalent to about 1 g of the dried substance), add 25 mL of diluted methanol (3 in 5), shake for 30 minutes, then allow to stand, and separate the supernatant liquid. To the residue add 8 mL of water, shake for 15 minutes, then add 12 mL of methanol, shake for 15 minutes, centrifuge, and separate the supernatant liquid. Combine all the supernatant liquids, and add diluted methanol (3 in 5) to make exactly 50 mL. Pipet 10 mL of this solution, add 3 mL of sodium hydroxide TS, allow to stand for 30 minutes, then add 3 mL of 1 mol/L hydrochloric acid TS, and add water to make exactly 20 mL. Apply exactly 10 mL of this solution to a column [about 10 mm in inside diameter, packed with 0.36 g of octadecylsilanized silica gel for pre-treatment (55 – 105 μm in particle size), and washed just before using with methanol and then diluted methanol (3 in 10)], and wash the column in sequence with 2 mL of diluted methanol (3 in 10), 1 mL of sodium carbonate TS and 10 mL of diluted methanol (3 in 10). Finally, elute with methanol to collect exactly 5 mL, and use this solution as the sample solution. Separately, weigh accurately about 10 mg of Ginsenoside Rb_1 RS (separately determine the water <*2.48*> by coulometric titration, using 10 mg), and dissolve in methanol to make exactly 100 mL. Pipet 10 mL of this solution, add methanol to make exactly 50 mL, and use this solution as the standard solution. Perform the test with exactly 20 μL each of the sample solution and standard solution as directed under Liquid Chromatography <*2.01*> according to the following conditions, and determine the peak areas, A_T and A_S, of ginsenoside Rb_1 in each solution.

$$\text{Amount (mg) of ginsenoside Rb}_1 (C_{54}H_{92}O_{23}) = M_S \times A_T/A_S \times 1/10$$

M_S: Amount (mg) of Ginsenoside Rb_1 RS taken, calculated on the anhydrous basis

For the prescription 1)

Operating conditions—

Detector: An ultraviolet absorption photometer (wavelength: 203 nm).

Column: A stainless steel column 4.6 mm in inside diameter and 15 cm in length, packed with carbamoyl group bound silica gel for liquid chromatography (3.5 μm in particle diameter).

Column temperature: A constant temperature of about 60°C.

Mobile phase: A mixture of acetonitrile, water and phosphoric acid (1700:300:1).

Flow rate: 1.0 mL per minute.

System suitability—

System performance: When the procedure is run with 20 μL of the standard solution under the above operating conditions, the number of theoretical plates and the symmetry factor of the peak of ginsenoside Rb_1 are not less than 5000 and not more than 1.5, respectively.

System repeatability: When the test is repeated 6 times with 20 μL of the standard solution under the above operating conditions, the relative standard deviation of the peak area of ginsenoside Rb_1 is not more than 1.5%.

For the prescription 2)

Operating conditions—

Detector, column temperature, and flow rate: Proceed as directed in the operating conditions in the prescription 1).

Column: A stainless steel column 4.6 mm in inside diameter and 25 cm in length, packed with carbamoyl group bound silica gel for liquid chromatography (5 μm in particle diameter).

Mobile phase: A mixture of acetonitrile, water and phosphoric acid (400:100:1).

System suitability—

System performance and system repeatability: Proceed as directed in the system suitability in the prescription 1).

Containers and storage Containers—Tight containers.

Cacao Butter

Oleum Cacao

カカオ脂

Cacao Butter is the fat obtained from the seed of *Theobroma cacao* Linné (*Sterculiaceae*).

Description Cacao Butter occurs as a yellow-white, hard, brittle mass. It has a slight, chocolate-like odor, and has no odor of rancidity.

It is freely soluble in diethyl ether and in petroleum ether, soluble in boiling ethanol (99.5), and very slightly soluble in ethanol (95).

Congealing point of the fatty acids: 45 – 50°C

Melting point 31 – 35°C (Cram the sample into a capillary tube without melting the sample).

Specific gravity <*1.13*> d^{40}_{20}: 0.895 – 0.904

Acid value <*1.13*> Not more than 3.0.

Saponification value <*1.13*> 188 – 195

Iodine value <*1.13*> 35 – 43

Containers and storage Containers—Well-closed containers.

Calumba

Calumbae Radix

コロンボ

Calumba is the cross-sectioned root of *Jateorhiza columba* Miers (*Menispermaceae*).

Description Disk-like slices, 0.5 – 2 cm in thickness, 3 – 8 cm in diameter; mostly with concave center and slightly waved; side surface grayish brown in color, with irregular wrinkles; cut surface light yellow and powdery, with pale and dark radiating stripes; cortex rather yellowish; cambium and its neighborhood light grayish brown, warty protrusions in the center; hard in texture, but brittle.

Odor characteristic; taste, bitter.

Identification To 3 g of pulverized Calumba add 30 mL of water, allow to stand for 5 minutes with occasional shaking, and filter. To 2 mL of the filtrate add gently 1 mL of sulfuric acid, and after cooling, add carefully chlorine TS to make two layers: a light red to red color develops at the zone of contact.

Purity **(1)** Heavy metals <*1.07*>—Proceed with 2.0 g of pulverized Calumba according to Method 3, and perform the test. Prepare the control solution with 3.0 mL of Standard Lead Solution (not more than 15 ppm).

(2) Arsenic <*1.11*>—Prepare the test solution with 0.40 g of pulverized Calumba according to Method 4, and perform the test (not more than 5 ppm).

Total ash <*5.01*> Not more than 7.5%.

Containers and storage Containers—Well-closed containers.

Powdered Calumba

Calumbae Radix Pulverata

コロンボ末

Powdered Calumba is the powder of Calumba.

Description Powdered Calumba occurs as a grayish yellow powder, and has a characteristic odor and a bitter taste.

Under a microscope <*5.01*>, Powdered Calumba reveals numerous starch grains, fragments of parenchyma cells containing them; fragments of cork cells, stone cells, fibers, substitute fibers, vessels, tracheids, and also solitary crystals of calcium oxalate; starch grains consisting of solitary grains or 2- to 3-compound grains; hilum, unevenly scattered, usually 25 – 50 μm, but up to 90 μm in diameter.

Identification To 3 g of Powdered Calumba add 30 mL of water, allow to stand for 5 minutes with occasional shaking, and filter. To 2 mL of the filtrate add gently 1 mL of sulfuric acid, and after cooling, add carefully chlorine TS to make two layers: a light red to red color develops at the zone of contact.

Purity **(1)** Heavy metals <*1.07*>—Proceed with 2.0 g of Powdered Calumba according to Method 3, and perform the test. Prepare the control solution with 3.0 mL of Standard Lead Solution (not more than 15 ppm).

(2) Arsenic <*1.11*>—Prepare the test solution with 0.40 g of Powdered Calumba according to Method 4, and perform the test (not more than 5 ppm).

Total ash <*5.01*> Not more than 7.5%.

Containers and storage Containers—Well-closed containers.

Camellia Oil

Oleum Camelliae

ツバキ油

Camellia Oil is the fixed oil obtained from the peeled seeds of *Camellia japonica* Linné (*Theaceae*).

Description Camellia Oil is a colorless or pale yellow, clear oil. It is nearly odorless and tasteless.

It is miscible with diethyl ether and with petroleum ether.

It is slightly soluble in ethanol (95).

It congeals partly at −10°C, and completely at −15°C.

Specific gravity d^{25}_{25}: 0.910 – 0.914

Identification To 2 mL of Camellia Oil add dropwise 10 mL of a mixture of fuming nitric acid, sulfuric acid, and water (1:1:1), previously cooled to room temperature: a bluish green color develops at the zone of contact.

Acid value <*1.13*> Not more than 2.8.

Saponification value <*1.13*> 188 – 194

Unsaponifiable matters *<1.13>* Not more than 1.0%.

Iodine value *<1.13>* 78 – 83

Containers and storage Containers—Tight containers.

Capsicum

Capsici Fructus

トウガラシ

Capsicum is the fruit of *Capsicum annuum* Linné (*Solanaceae*).

It contains not less than 0.10% of total capsaicins ((*E*)-capsaicin and dihydrocapsaicin), calculated on the basis of dried material.

Description Elongated conical to fusiform fruit, often bent, 3 – 10 cm in length, about 0.8 cm in width; outer surface lustrous and dark red to dark yellow-red; interior of pericarp hollow and usually divided into two loculi, containing numerous seeds nearly circular and compressed, light yellow-red, about 0.5 cm in diameter.

Usually it remains of calyx and peduncle.

Odor, slight and characteristic; taste, hot and acrid.

Identification To 1.0 g of pulverized Capsicum add 5 mL of ethanol (95), shake for 10 minutes, centrifuge, and use the supernatant liquid as the sample solution. Separately, dissolve 1 mg of (*E*)-capsaicin for thin-layer chromatography in 1 mL of ethanol (95), and use this solution as the standard solution. Perform the test with these solutions as directed under Thin-layer Chromatography *<2.03>*. Spot 10 μL each of the sample solution and standard solution on a plate of silica gel for thin-layer chromatography. Develop the plate with a mixture of hexane, ethyl acetate and formic acid (10:9:1) to a distance of about 7 cm, and air-dry the plate. Spray evenly 2,6-dibromo-*N*-chloro-1,4-benzoquinone monoimine TS on the plate, and expose to an ammonia vapor: a spot obtained from the sample solution and a blue spot from the standard solution show the same color tone and the same *R*f value.

Purity Foreign matter *<5.01>*—The amount of foreign matter contained in Capsicum does not exceed 1.0%.

Loss on drying *<5.01>* Not more than 14.0% (6 hours).

Total ash *<5.01>* Not more than 8.0%.

Acid-insoluble ash *<5.01>* Not more than 1.2%.

Assay Weigh accurately about 0.5 g of moderately fine powder of Capsicum in a glass-stoppered centrifuge tube, add 30 mL of methanol, shake for 15 minutes, centrifuge, and separate the supernatant liquid. To the residue add 10 mL of methanol, shake for 5 minutes, centrifuge, and separate the supernatant liquid. Repeat this procedure again, combine all the extracts, add methanol to make exactly 50 mL, and use this solution as the sample solution. Separately, weigh accurately about 10 mg of (*E*)-capsaicin for assay, previously dried in a desiccator (in vacuum, phosphorus (V) oxide, 40°C) for 5 hours, and dissolve in methanol to make exactly 50 mL. Pipet 2 mL of this solution, add methanol to make exactly 25 mL, and use this solution as the standard solution. Perform the test with exactly 20 μL each of the sample solution and standard solution as directed under Liquid Chromatography *<2.01>* according to the following conditions, and determine the peak areas, A_{TC} and A_{TD}, of (*E*)-capsaicin and dihydrocapsaicin (the relative retention time to (*E*)-capsaicin is about 1.3) obtained with the sample solution, and the peak area, A_S, of (*E*)-capsaicin obtained with the standard solution.

$$\text{Amount (mg) of total capsaicins} = M_S \times (A_{TC} + A_{TD})/A_S \times 0.08$$

M_S: Amount (mg) of (*E*)-capsaicin for assay taken

Operating conditions—

Detector: An ultraviolet absorption photometer (wavelength: 281 nm).

Column: A stainless steel column 4.6 mm in inside diameter and 25 cm in length, packed with phenylated silica gel for liquid chromatography (5 μm in particle diameter).

Column temperature: A constant temperature of about 30°C.

Mobile phase: A mixture of diluted phosphoric acid (1 in 1000) and acetonitrile (3:2).

Flow rate: Adjust so that the retention time of (*E*)-capsaicin is about 20 minutes.

System suitability—

System performance: Dissolve 1 mg each of (*E*)-capsaicin for assay and 4-hydroxy-3-methoxybenzyl nonylic acid amide in methanol to make 50 mL. When the procedure is run with 20 μL of this solution under the above operating conditions, 4-hydroxy-3-methoxybenzyl nonylic acid amide and (*E*)-capsaicin are eluted in this order with the resolution between these peaks being not less than 1.5.

System repeatability: When the test is repeated 6 times with 20 μL of the standard solution under the above operating conditions, the relative standard deviation of the peak areas of (*E*)-capsaicin is not more than 1.5%.

Containers and storage Containers—Well-closed containers.

Powdered Capsicum

Capsici Fructus Pulveratus

トウガラシ末

Powdered Capsicum is the powder of Capsicum.

It contains not less than 0.10% of total capsaicins ((*E*)-capsaicin and dihydrocapsaicin), calculated on the basis of dried material.

Description Powdered Capsicum occurs as a yellow-red powder. It has a slight, characteristic odor and a hot, acrid taste.

Under a microscope *<5.01>*, Powdered Capsicum reveals fragments of parenchyma containing oil droplets and yellow-red chromoplasts; fragments of epidermis from outer surface of pericarp with thick cuticle; fragments of stone cells from inner surface of pericarp, with wavy curved side walls; fragments of thin vessels; fragments of seed coat with thick wall, and fragments of parenchyma consisting of small cells of endosperm containing fixed oil and aleuron grains.

Identification To 1.0 g of Powdered Capsicum add 5 mL of ethanol (95), shake for 10 minutes, centrifuge, and use the supernatant liquid as the sample solution. Separately, dissolve 1 mg of (*E*)-capsaicin for thin-layer chromatography in 1 mL of ethanol (95), and use this solution as the standard solution. Perform the test with these solutions as directed under Thin-layer Chromatography *<2.03>*. Spot 10 μL each of the sample solution and standard solution on a plate of silica gel for thin-layer chromatography. Develop the plate with a mixture of hexane, ethyl acetate and formic acid (10:9:1) to a distance of about 7 cm, and air-dry the plate. Spray evenly 2,6-dibromo-*N*-chloro-1,4-benzoquinone monoimine TS on the plate, and expose to an ammonia vapor: a spot obtained from the sample solution and blue spot obtained from the standard solution show the same in color tone and *R*f value.

Loss on drying <*5.01*> Not more than 14.0% (6 hours).

Total ash <*5.01*> Not more than 8.0%.

Acid-insoluble ash <*5.01*> Not more than 1.2%.

Assay Weigh accurately about 0.5 g of Powdered Capsicum in a glass-stoppered centrifuge tube, add 30 mL of methanol, shake for 15 minutes, centrifuge, and separate the supernatant liquid. To the residue add 10 mL of methanol, shake for 5 minutes, centrifuge, and separate the supernatant liquid. Repeat this procedure again, combine all the extracts, add methanol to make exactly 50 mL, and use this solution as the sample solution. Separately, weigh accurately about 10 mg of (*E*)-capsaicin for assay, previously dried in a desiccator (in vacuum, phosphorus (V) oxide, 40°C) for 5 hours, and dissolve in methanol to make exactly 50 mL. Pipet 2 mL of this solution, add methanol to make exactly 25 mL, and use this solution as the standard solution. Perform the test with exactly 20 μL each of the sample solution and standard solution as directed under Liquid Chromatography <*2.01*> according to the following conditions, and determine the peak areas, A_{TC} and A_{TD}, of (*E*)-capsaicin and dihydrocapsaicin (the relative retention time to (*E*)-capsaicin is about 1.3) obtained with the sample solution, and the peak area, A_S, of (*E*)-capsaicin obtained with the standard solution.

$$\text{Amount (mg) of total capsaicins} = M_S \times (A_{TC} + A_{TD})/A_S \times 0.08$$

M_S: Amount (mg) of (*E*)-capsaicin for assay taken

Operating conditions—

Detector: An ultraviolet absorption photometer (wavelength: 281 nm).

Column: A stainless steel column 4.6 mm in inside diameter and 25 cm in length, packed with phenylated silica gel for liquid chromatography (5 μm in particle diameter).

Column temperature: A constant temperature of about 30°C.

Mobile phase: A mixture of diluted phosphoric acid (1 in 1000) and acetonitrile (3:2).

Flow rate: Adjust so that the retention time of (*E*)-capsaicin is about 20 minutes.

System suitability—

System performance: Dissolve 1 mg each of (*E*)-capsaicin for assay and 4-hydroxy-3-methoxybenzyl nonylic acid amide in methanol to make 50 mL. When the procedure is run with 20 μL of this solution under the above operating conditions, 4-hydroxy-3-methoxybenzyl nonylic acid amide and (*E*)-capsaicin are eluted in this order with the resolution between these peaks being not less than 1.5.

System repeatability: When the test is repeated 6 times with 20 μL of the standard solution under the above operating conditions, the relative standard deviation of the peak areas of (*E*)-capsaicin is not more than 1.5%.

Containers and storage Containers—Well-closed containers.

Capsicum Tincture

トウガラシチンキ

Capsicum Tincture contains not less than 0.010 w/v% of total capsaicins ((*E*)-capsaicin and dihydrocapsaicin).

Method of preparation

Capsicum, in moderately fine cutting	100 g
Ethanol	a sufficient quantity
To make	1000 mL

Prepare as directed under Tinctures, with the above ingredients.

Description Capsicum Tincture is a yellow-red liquid. It has a burning, pungent taste.

Specific gravity d^{20}_{20}: about 0.82

Identification Proceed as directed in the Identification under Capsicum, using Capsicum Tincture as the sample solution. Spot 20 μL each of the sample solution and standard solution.

Alcohol number <*1.01*> Not less than 9.7 (Method 2).

Assay Pipet 2 mL of Capsicum Tincture, add methanol to make exactly 20 mL, and use this solution as the sample solution. Separately, weigh accurately about 10 mg of (*E*)-capsaicin for assay, previously dried in a desiccator (in vacuum, phosphorus (V) oxide, 40°C) for 5 hours, dissolve in methanol to make exactly 50 mL. Pipet 2 mL of this solution, add methanol to make exactly 25 mL, and use this solution as the standard solution. Perform the test with exactly 20 μL each of the sample solution and standard solution as directed under Liquid Chromatography <*2.01*> according to the following conditions, and determine the peak areas, A_{TC} and A_{TD}, of (*E*)-capsaicin and dihydrocapsaicin (the relative retention time to (*E*)-capsaicin is about 1.3) obtained with the sample solution, and the peak area, A_S, of (*E*)-capsaicin obtained with the standard solution.

$$\text{Amount (mg) of total capsaicins} = M_S \times (A_{TC} + A_{TD})/A_S \times 0.032$$

M_S: Amount (mg) of (*E*)-capsaicin for assay taken

Operating conditions—

Detector: An ultraviolet absorption photometer (wavelength: 281 nm).

Column: A stainless steel column 4.6 mm in inside diameter and 25 cm in length, packed with phenylated silica gel for liquid chromatography (5 μm in particle diameter).

Column temperature: A constant temperature of about 30°C.

Mobile phase: A mixture of diluted phosphoric acid (1 in 1000) and acetonitrile (3:2).

Flow rate: Adjust so that the retention time of (*E*)-capsaicin is about 20 minutes.

System suitability—

System performance: Dissolve 1 mg each of (*E*)-capsaicin for assay and 4-hydroxy-3-methoxybenzyl nonylic acid amide in methanol to make 50 mL. When the procedure is run with 20 μL of this solution under the above operating conditions, 4-hydroxy-3-methoxybenzyl nonylic acid amide and (*E*)-capsaicin are eluted in this order with the resolution between these peaks being not less than 1.5.

System repeatability: When the test is repeated 6 times

with 20 μL of the standard solution under the above operating conditions, the relative standard deviation of the peak areas of (*E*)-capsaicin is not more than 1.5%.

Containers and storage Containers—Tight containers.
Storage—Light-resistant.

Capsicum and Salicylic Acid Spirit

トウガラシ·サリチル酸精

Method of preparation

Capsicum Tincture	40 mL
Salicylic Acid	50 g
Liquefied Phenol	20 mL
Castor Oil	100 mL
aromatic substance	a suitable quantity
Ethanol	a sufficient quantity
	To make 1000 mL

Prepare as directed under Spirits, with the above ingredients.

Description Capsicum and Salicylic Acid Spirit is a light brown-yellow liquid.

Specific gravity d_{20}^{20}: about 0.84

Identification **(1)** Shake 10 mL of Capsicum and Salicylic Acid Spirit with 15 mL of sodium hydrogen carbonate TS and 10 mL of diethyl ether, and separate the aqueous layer. To 1 mL of the solution add hydrochloric acid-potassium chloride buffer solution (pH 2.0) to make 200 mL, and to 5 mL of this solution add 5 mL of a solution of iron (III) nitrate enneahydrate (1 in 200): a red-purple color is produced (salicylic acid).

(2) To 0.5 mL of Capsicum and Salicylic Acid Spirit add 20 mL of water and 5 mL of dilute hydrochloric acid, extract with 20 mL of diethyl ether, wash the diethyl ether extract with two 5-mL portions of sodium hydrogen carbonate TS, and then extract with 20 mL of dilute sodium hydroxide TS. To 1 mL of the extract add 1 mL of sodium nitrite TS and 1 mL of dilute hydrochloric acid, shake, and allow to stand for 10 minutes. Add 3 mL of sodium hydroxide TS: a yellow color is produced (phenol).

(3) To 0.2 mL of Capsicum and Salicylic Acid Spirit add 5 mL of dilute hydrochloric acid, extract with 5 mL of chloroform, and use the extract as the sample solution. Dissolve 0.01 g of salicylic acid and 0.02 g of phenol in 5 mL and 25 mL of chloroform, respectively, and use both solutions as the standard solution (1) and the standard solution (2). Perform the test with these solutions as directed under Thin-layer Chromatography <*2.03*>. Spot 5 μL of the sample solution and standard solutions (1) and (2) on a plate of silica gel with fluorescent indicator for thin-layer chromatography. Develop the plate with a mixture of chloroform, acetone and acetic acid (100) (45:5:1) to a distance of about 10 cm, and air-dry the plate. Examine under ultraviolet light (main wavelength: 254 nm): two spots of the several spots obtained from the sample solution exhibit the same *Rf* values as those from standard solution (1) and standard solution (2). Spray evenly iron (III) chloride TS upon the plate: one of the several spots from the sample solution has the same color tone and *R*f value with the spot from the standard solution (1).

Alcohol number <*1.01*> Not less than 8.1 (Method 2). Prepare the sample solution as follows: Pipet 5 mL of Capsicum and Salicylic Acid Spirit at 15 ± 2°C into a glass-stoppered, conical flask containing exactly 45 mL of water while shaking vigorously, allow to stand, and filter the lower layer. Discard the first 15 mL of the filtrate. Pipet 25 mL of the subsequent filtrate, add exactly 10 mL of the internal standard solution, and add water to make exactly 100 mL.

Containers and storage Containers—Tight containers.

Cardamon

Cardamomi Fructus

ショウズク

Cardamon is the fruit of *Elettaria cardamomum* Maton (*Zingiberaceae*). The capsules are removed from the seeds before use.

Description Nearly ellipsoidal, 1 – 2 cm in length, 0.5 – 1 cm in diameter; externally, light yellow with three blunt ridges and many longitudinal lines; 0.1 – 0.2-cm beak at one end; pericarp thin, light and fibrous; interior longitudinally divided into three loculi by thin membranes, each loculus containing 3 to 7 seeds joining by aril; seed irregularly angular ovoid, 0.3 – 0.4 cm in length, dark brown to blackish brown; the dorsal side convex, the ventral side longitudinally grooved; external surface coarsely tuberculated.

Seed has a characteristic aroma, and pungent, slightly bitter taste; pericarp, slight characteristic odor and practically tasteless.

Total ash <*5.01*> Not more than 6.0% (seed).

Acid-insoluble ash <*5.01*> Not more than 4.0% (seed).

Essential oil content <*5.01*> Perform the test with 30.0 g of the pulverized seeds of Cardamon: the volume of essential oil is not less than 1.0 mL.

Containers and storage Containers—Well-closed containers.

Carnauba Wax

Cera Carnauba

カルナウバロウ

Carnauba Wax is the wax obtained from the leaves of *Copernicia cerifera* Martius (*Palmae*).

Description Carnauba Wax occurs as light yellow to light brown, hard and brittle masses or white to light yellow powder. It has a slight, characteristic odor. It is tasteless.

It is practically insoluble in water, in ethanol (95), in diethyl ether and in xylene.

Specific gravity d_{20}^{20}: 0.990 – 1.002

Melting point: 80 – 86°C

Acid value <*1.13*> Not more than 10.0. Use a mixture of xylene and ethanol (95) (2:1) as solvent.

Saponification value <*1.13*> 78 – 95 Weigh accurately about 3 g of Carnauba Wax in a 300-mL flask, add 25 mL of xylene, and dissolve by warming. To this solution add 50 mL of ethanol (95) and exactly 25 mL of 0.5 mol/L potassium hydroxide-ethanol VS, and proceed as directed in the Saponification value. The time of heating should be 2 hours and the titration should be done by warming.

Iodine value 〈*1.13*〉 5 – 14 (Dissolve the sample by shaking a glass-stoppered flask in warm water.)

Containers and storage Containers—Well-closed containers.

Cassia Seed

Cassiae Semen

ケツメイシ

Cassia Seed is the seed of *Cassia obtusifolia* Linné or *Cassia tora* Linné (*Leguminosae*).

Description Short cylindrical seed, 3 – 6 mm in length, 2 – 3.5 mm in diameter; acuminate at one end and flat at the other; externally green-brown to brown and lustrous, with light yellow-brown longitudinal lines or bands on both sides; hard in texture; cross section round or obtuse polygonal; under a magnifying glass, albumen enclosing a bent, dark-colored cotyledon.

When ground, characteristic odor and taste.

Identification To 1.0 g of pulverized Cassia Seed add 10 mL of diluted methanol (4 in 5), heat on a water bath for 5 minutes, and filter. Evaporate the solvent of the filtrate, dissolve the residue in 5 mL of water, add 2 mL of ethyl acetate, and shake for 10 minutes. Centrifuge this solution, and use the ethyl acetate layer as the sample solution. Perform the test with the sample solution as directed under Thin-layer Chromatography 〈*2.03*〉. Spot 10 μL of the sample solution on a plate of silica gel for thin-layer chromatography. Develop the plate with a mixture of diethyl ether, cyclohexane and formic acid (5:5:1) to a distance of about 7 cm, and air-dry the plate. Spray evenly potassium hydroxide-ethanol TS on the plate: an orange to yellow-brown spot appears at an *R*f value of about 0.35.

Purity Foreign matter 〈*5.01*〉—The amount of foreign matter contained in Cassia Seed does not exceed 1.0%.

Total ash 〈*5.01*〉 Not more than 5.0%.

Containers and storage Containers—Well-closed containers.

Castor Oil

Oleum Ricini

ヒマシ油

Castor Oil is the fixed oil obtained by compression from the seeds of *Ricinus communis* Linné (*Euphorbiaceae*).

Description Castor Oil is a colorless or pale yellow, clear, viscous oil. It has a slight, characteristic odor, and has a bland at first, and afterwards slightly acrid taste.

It is miscible with ethanol (99.5) and with diethyl ether.

It is freely soluble in ethanol (95), and practically insoluble in water.

When cooled to 0°C, it becomes more viscous, and turbidity is gradually formed.

Identification To 3 g of Castor Oil add 1 g of potassium hydroxide, and heat the mixture carefully to fuse: a characteristic odor is perceptible. Dissolve the fused matter in 30 mL of water, add an excess of magnesium oxide, and filter. Acidify the filtrate with hydrochloric acid: white crystals is produced.

Specific gravity 〈*1.13*〉 d^{25}_{25}: 0.953 – 0.965

Acid value 〈*1.13*〉 Not more than 1.5.

Saponification value 〈*1.13*〉 176 – 187

Hydroxyl value 〈*1.13*〉 155 – 177

Iodine value 〈*1.13*〉 80 – 90

Purity Adulteration—Shake to mix 1.0 g of Castor Oil with 4.0 mL of ethanol (95): it dissolves clearly. Add 15 mL of ethanol (95): no turbidity is produced.

Containers and storage Containers—Tight containers.

Aromatic Castor Oil

加香ヒマシ油

Method of preparation

Castor Oil	990 mL
Orange Oil	5 mL
Mentha Oil	5 mL
To make	1000 mL

Mix the above ingredients.

Description Aromatic Castor Oil is a colorless or yellowish, clear, viscous liquid. It has an aromatic odor.

Identification To 3 g of Aromatic Castor Oil add 1 g of potassium hydroxide, and heat the mixture carefully to fuse: a characteristic odor is perceptible. Dissolve the fused matter in 30 mL of water, add an excess of magnesium oxide, and filter. Acidify the filtrate with hydrochloric acid: white crystals are produced.

Containers and storage Containers—Tight containers.

Catalpa Fruit

Catalpae Fructus

キササゲ

Catalpa Fruit is the fruit of *Catalpa ovata* G. Don or *Catalpa bungei* C. A. Meyer (*Bignoniaceae*).

Description Slender stick-like fruit, 30 – 40 cm in length and about 0.5 cm in diameter; externally, dark brown; inner part contains numerous seeds; seed compressed or semitubular, about 3 cm in length and about 0.3 cm in width, externally grayish brown; hairs, about 1 cm in length, attached to both ends of seed; pericarp, thin and brittle.

Odor, slight; taste, slightly astringent.

Identification To 1.0 g of pulverized Catalpa Fruit add 20 mL of water, warm on a water bath for 5 minutes, and filter immediately. Transfer the filtrate to a separator, and extract with two 20-mL portions of 1-butanol. Combine the extracts, evaporate the solvent under low pressure (in vacuo) on a water bath, dissolve the residue in 1 mL of methanol, and use this solution as the sample solution. Separately, dissolve 1 mg of parahydroxybenzoic acid in 1 mL of methanol, and use this solution as the standard solution. Perform the test with these solutions as directed under Thin-layer Chromatography <*2.03*>. Spot 5 μL each of the sample solution and standard solution on a plate of silica gel with fluorescent indicator for thin-layer chromatography. Develop the plate with a mixture of ethyl acetate, ethanol (99.5) and water (20:2:1) to a distance of about 10 cm, and air-dry the plate. Examine under ultra-violet light (main wavelength: 254 nm): one of the several spots obtained from the sample solution and a dark purple spot from the standard solution show the same color tone and the same *R*f value. Prescribe that the moving distance of the spot corresponding to parahydroxybenzoic acid from the sample solution is 1: a dark purple spot develops at the relative moving distance of about 0.3.

Purity Peduncle—When perform the test of foreign matter <*5.01*>, the amount of peduncles contained in Catalpa Fruit does not exceed 5.0%.

Total ash <*5.01*> Not more than 6.0%.

Acid-insoluble ash <*5.01*> Not more than 0.5%.

Extract content <*5.01*> Dilute ethanol-soluble extract: not less than 8.0%.

Containers and storage Containers—Well-closed containers.

Cherry Bark

Pruni Cortex

オウヒ

Cherry Bark is the bark of *Prunus jamasakura* Siebold ex Koidzumi or *Prunus verecunda* Koehne (*Rosaceae*).

Description Flat or semi-tubular pieces of bark; 3 – 6 mm thick, externally light brown to brown, internal surface smooth, grayish brown to brown, occasionally periderm peeled off; the bark with periderm externally rough and lenticels observed; internal surface with many fine longitudinal lines; transversely cut surface grayish brown to brown, fibrous.

Odor, slightly characteristics; taste, slightly bitter and astringent.

Under a microscope <*5.01*>, a transverse section reveals cork layer containing solitary crystals and rosette aggregates of calcium oxalate in the bark with periderm; in secondary cortex many stone cells and idioblasts arranged irregularly and parenchyma cells containing solitary crystals and rosette aggregates of calcium oxalate dotted; groups of phloem fibers lined alternately with the other tissue of phloem between rays.

Identification Shake 1 g of pulverized Cherry Bark with 10 mL of dilute hydrochloric acid, and heat in a boiling water bath for 10 minutes. After cooling, add 5 mL of diethyl ether, shake for 10 minutes, centrifuge, and use the diethyl ether layer as the sample solution. Perform the test with the sample solution as directed under Thin-layer Chromatography <*2.03*>. Spot 10 μL of the sample solution on a plate of silica gel for thin-layer chromatography. Develop the plate with a mixture of ethyl acetate, hexane and acetic acid (100) (20:20:1) to a distance of about 7 cm, and air-dry the plate. Spray evenly vanillin-sulfuric acid-ethanol TS for spraying on the plate, and heat the plate at 105°C for 5 minutes: a crimson spot appears at an *R*f value of about 0.5.

Loss on drying <*5.01*> Not more than 13.0% (6 hours).

Total ash <*5.01*> Not more than 6.5%.

Acid-insoluble ash <*5.01*> Not more than 0.5%.

Containers and storage Containers—Well-closed containers.

Chotosan Extract

釣藤散エキス

Chotosan Extract contains not less than 24 mg and not more than 72 mg of hesperidin, not less than 6 mg and not more than 18 mg of glycyrrhizic acid ($C_{42}H_{62}O_{16}$: 822.93), and not less than 0.3 mg of the total alkaloid (rhyncophylline and hirsutine), per extract prepared with the amount specified in the Method of preparation.

Method of preparation

	1)	2)
Uncaria Hook	3 g	3 g
Citrus Unshiu Peel	3 g	3 g
Pinellia Tuber	3 g	3 g
Ophiopogon Root	3 g	3 g
Poria Sclerotium	3 g	3 g
Ginseng	2 g	3 g
Saposhnikovia Root and Rhizome	2 g	3 g
Chrysanthemum Flower	2 g	3 g
Glycyrrhiza	1 g	1 g
Ginger	1 g	1 g
Gypsum	5 g	3 g

Prepare a dry extract or viscous extract as directed under Extracts, according to the prescription 1) or 2), using the crude drugs shown above.

Description Chotosan Extract is a light brown to yellow-brown powder or black-brown viscous extract. It has a slight odor, and has a pungent and slightly sweet first, then bitter taste.

Identification **(1)** Shake 2.0 g of the dry extract (or 6.0 g of the viscous extract) with 20 mL of water and 2 mL of ammonia TS, add 20 mL of diethyl ether, and shake. Separate the diethyl ether layer, evaporate the solvent under low pressure (in vacuo), add 1 mL of methanol to the residue, and use this solution as the sample solution. Separately, dissolve 1 mg each of rhyncophylline for thin-layer chromatography and hirsutine for thin-layer chromatography in 1 mL of methanol, and use this solution as the standard solution. Perform the test with these solutions as directed under Thin-layer Chromatography <*2.03*>. Spot 10 μL of the sample solution and 2 μL of the standard solution on a plate of silica gel with fluorescent indicator for thin-layer chromatography. Develop the plate with a mixture of ethyl acetate, 1-propanol, water and acetic acid (100) (7:5:4:1) to a distance of about 7 cm, and air-dry the plate. Examine under ultraviolet light (main wavelength: 254 nm): one of the several spots obtained from the sample solution has the same color tone and *R*f value with one of the two dark purple spots from the standard solution (Uncaria Hook).

(2) Shake 2.0 g of the dry extract (or 6.0 g of the viscous extract) with 10 mL of water, add 10 mL of 1-butanol, shake, centrifuge, and use the 1-butanol layer as the sample solution. Separately, dissolve 1 mg of hesperidin for thin-layer chromatography in 1 mL of methanol, and use this solution as the standard solution. Perform the test with these solutions as directed under Thin-layer Chromatography <*2.03*>. Spot 20 μL of the sample solution and 10 μL of the standard solution on a plate of silica gel for thin-layer chromatography. Develop the plate with a mixture of ethyl acetate, acetone, water and acetic acid (100) (10:6:3:1) to a distance of about 7 cm, and air-dry the plate. Spray evenly 2,6-dibromo-*N*-chloro-1,4-benzoquinone monoimine TS on the plate, and allow to stand in an ammonia gas: one of the several spots obtained from the sample solution has the same color tone and *Rf* value with the blue spot from the standard solution (Citrus Unshiu Peel).

(3) Shake 2.0 g of the dry extract (or 6.0 g of the viscous extract) with 10 mL of water, add 5 mL of 1-butanol, shake, centrifuge, remove the 1-butanol layer, and use the aqueous layer as the sample solution. Separately, heat 3.0 g of pulverized ophiopogon root in 50 mL of water under a reflux condenser for 1 hour. After cooling, shake 20 mL of the extract with 5 mL of 1-butanol, centrifuge, remove the 1-butanol layer, and use the aqueous layer as the standard solution. Perform the test with these solutions as directed under Thin-layer Chromatography <*2.03*>. Spot 2 μL of the sample solution and 5 μL of the standard solution as bands on the original line on a plate of silica gel for thin-layer chromatography. Develop the plate with a mixture of ethanol (99.5), water and acetic acid (100) (120:80:1) to a distance of about 7 cm, and air-dry the plate. Spray evenly 4-methoxybenzaldehyde-sulfuric acid TS on the plate, and heat the plate at 105°C for 5 minutes: one of the several spots obtained from the sample solution has the same color tone and *Rf* value with the dark blue-green spot (around *Rf* value 0.3) from the standard solution (Ophiopogon Root).

(4) Shake 2.0 g of the dry extract (or 6.0 g of the viscous extract) with 10 mL of sodium hydroxide TS, add 5 mL of 1-butanol, shake, centrifuge, and use the 1-butanol layer as the sample solution. Separately, dissolve 1 mg of Ginsenoside Rb_1 RS or ginsenoside Rb_1 for thin-layer chromatography in 1 mL of methanol, and use this solution as the standard solution. Perform the test with these solutions as directed under Thin-layer Chromatography <*2.03*>. Spot 10 μL of the sample solution and 2 μL of the standard solution on a plate of silica gel for thin-layer chromatography. Develop the plate with a mixture of ethyl acetate, 1-propanol, water and acetic acid (100) (7:5:4:1) to a distance of about 7 cm, and air-dry the plate. Spray evenly vanillin-sulfuric acid-ethanol TS for spraying on the plate, heat the plate at 105°C for 5 minutes, and allow to cool: one of the several spots obtained from the sample solution has the same color tone and *Rf* value with the blue-purple spot from the standard solution (Ginseng).

(5) Shake 2.0 g of the dry extract (or 6.0 g of the viscous extract) with 10 mL of sodium hydroxide TS, add 5 mL of 1-butanol, shake, centrifuge, and use the 1-butanol layer as the sample solution. Separately, dissolve 1 mg of 4′-*O*-glycosyl-5-*O*-methylvisamminol for thin-layer chromatography in 1 mL of methanol, and use this solution as the standard solution. Perform the test with these solutions as directed under Thin-layer Chromatography <*2.03*>. Spot 5 μL each of the sample solution and standard solution on a plate of silica gel with fluorescent indicator for thin-layer chromatography. Develop the plate with a mixture of 1-butanol, water and acetic acid (100) (7:2:1) to a distance of about 7 cm, and air-dry the plate. Examine under ultraviolet light (main wavelength: 254 nm): one of the several spots obtained from the sample solution has the same color tone and *Rf* value with the blue spot from the standard solution (Saposhnikovia Root and Rhizome).

(6) Shake 2.0 g of the dry extract (or 6.0 g of the viscous extract) with 10 mL of water, add 20 mL of diethyl ether, and shake. Separate the diethyl ether layer, evaporate the solvent under low pressure (in vacuo), add 1 mL of methanol to the residue, and use this solution as the sample solution. Separately, dissolve 1 mg of luteolin for thin-layer chromatography in 1 mL of methanol, and use this solution as the standard solution. Perform the test with these solutions as directed under Thin-layer Chromatography <*2.03*>. Spot 10 μL of the sample solution and 3 μL of the standard solution on a plate of silica gel for thin-layer chromatography. Develop the plate with a mixture of ethyl acetate, hexane and formic acid (5:5:1) to a distance of about 7 cm, and air-dry the plate. Spray evenly iron (III) chloride-methanol TS on the plate: one of the several spots obtained from the sample solution has the same color tone and *Rf* value with the yellow-brown spot from the standard solution (Chrysanthemum Flower).

(7) Shake 2.0 g of the dry extract (or 6.0 g of the viscous extract) with 10 mL of water, add 10 mL of 1-butanol, shake, centrifuge, and use the 1-butanol layer as the sample solution. Separately, dissolve 1 mg of liquiritin for thin-layer chromatography in 1 mL of methanol, and use this solution as the standard solution. Perform the test with these solutions as directed under Thin-layer Chromatography <*2.03*>. Spot 1 μL each of the sample solution and standard solution on a plate of silica gel for thin-layer chromatography. Develop the plate with a mixture of ethyl acetate, methanol and water (20:3:2) to a distance of about 7 cm, and air-dry the plate. Spray evenly dilute sulfuric acid on the plate, heat the plate at 105°C for 5 minutes, and examine under ultraviolet light (main wavelength: 365 nm): one of the several spots obtained from the sample solution has the same color tone and *Rf* value with the yellow-green fluorescent spot from the standard solution (Glycyrrhiza).

(8) Shake 1.0 g of the dry extract (or 3.0 g of the viscous extract) with 10 mL of water, add 25 mL of diethyl ether, and shake. Separate the diethyl ether layer, evaporate the solvent under low pressure (in vacuo), add 2 mL of diethyl ether to the residue, and use this solution as the sample solution. Separately, dissolve 1 mg of [6]-gingerol for thin-layer chromatography in 1 mL of methanol, and use this solution as the standard solution. Perform the test with these solutions as directed under Thin-layer Chromatography <*2.03*>. Spot 10 μL of the sample solution and 5 μL of the standard solution on a plate of silica gel for thin-layer chromatography. Develop the plate with a mixture of ethyl acetate and hexane (1:1) to a distance of about 7 cm, and air-dry the plate. Spray evenly vanillin-sulfuric acid TS on the plate, heat the plate at 105°C for 5 minutes: one of the several spots obtained from the sample solution has the same color tone and *Rf* value with the red-purple spot from the standard solution (Ginger).

(9) Shake 1.0 g of a dry extract (or 3.0 g of the viscous extract) with 30 mL of methanol, centrifuge, and separate the supernatant liquid. Shake the residue with 30 mL of water, centrifuge, and separate the supernatant liquid. Add ammonium oxalate TS to this solution: a white precipitate is formed, and it does not dissolve by addition of dilute acetic acid, but it dissolve by addition of dilute hydrochloric acid. (Gypsum)

Purity (1) Heavy metals <*1.07*>—Prepare the test solution with 1.0 g of the dry extract (or an amount of the viscous extract, equivalent to 1.0 g of the dried substance) as directed under Extracts (4), and perform the test (not more than 30 ppm).

(2) Arsenic <*1.11*>—Prepare the test solution with 0.67 g of the dry extract (or an amount of the viscous extract, equivalent to 0.67 g of the dried substance) according to Method 3, and perform the test (not more than 3 ppm).

Loss on drying <*2.41*> The dry extract: Not more than 7.5% (1 g, 105°C, 5 hours).

The viscous extract: Not more than 66.7% (1 g, 105°C, 5 hours).

Total ash <*5.01*> Not more than 15.0%, calculated on the dried basis.

Assay (1) Hesperidin—Weigh accurately about 0.1 g of the dry extract (or an amount of the viscous extract, equivalent to about 0.1 g of dried substance), add exactly 50 mL of diluted tetrahydrofuran (1 in 4), shake for 30 minutes, centrifuge, and use the supernatant liquid as the sample solution. Separately, weigh accurately about 10 mg of hesperidin for assay, previously dried in a desiccator (silica gel) for 24 hours, dissolve in methanol to make exactly 100 mL. Pipet 10 mL of this solution, add diluted tetrahydrofuran (1 in 4) to make exactly 100 mL, and use this solution as the standard solution. Perform the test with exactly 10 μL each of the sample solution and standard solution as directed under Liquid Chromatography <*2.01*> according to the following conditions, and determine the peak areas, A_T and A_S, of hesperidin in each solution.

$$\text{Amount (mg) of hesperidin} = M_S \times A_T/A_S \times 1/20$$

M_S: Amount (mg) of hesperidin for assay taken

Operating conditions—

Detector: An ultraviolet absorption photometer (wavelength: 285 nm).

Column: A stainless steel column 4.6 mm in inside diameter and 15 cm in length, packed with octadecylsilanized silica gel for liquid chromatography (5 μm in particle diameter).

Column temperature: A constant temperature of about 40°C.

Mobile phase: A mixture of water, acetonitrile and acetic acid (100) (82:18:1).

Flow rate: 1.0 mL per minute (the retention time of hesperidin is about 15 minutes).

System suitability—

System performance: Dissolve 1 mg each of hesperidin for assay and naringin for thin-layer chromatography in diluted methanol (1 in 2) to make 100 mL. When the procedure is run with 10 μL of this solution under the above operating conditions, naringin and hesperidin are eluted in this order with the resolution between these peaks being not less than 1.5.

System repeatability: When the test is repeated 6 times with 10 μL of the standard solution under the above operating conditions, the relative standard deviation of the peak area of hesperidin is not more than 1.5%.

(2) Glycyrrhizic acid—Weigh accurately about 0.5 g of the dry extract (or an amount of the viscous extract, equivalent to about 0.5 g of the dried substance), add 20 mL of ethyl acetate and 10 mL of water, and shake for 10 minutes. After centrifugation, remove the ethyl acetate layer, add 20 mL of ethyl acetate, proceed in the same manner as described above, and remove the ethyl acetate layer. To the resultant aqueous layer add 10 mL of methanol, shake for 30 minutes, centrifuge, and take the supernatant liquid. To the residue add 20 mL of diluted methanol (1 in 2), shake for 5 minutes, centrifuge, and take the supernatant liquid. Combine these supernatant liquids, add diluted methanol (1 in 2) to make exactly 50 mL, and use this solution as the sample solution. Separately, weigh accurately about 10 mg of Glycyrrhizic Acid RS (separately determine the water <*2.48*> by coulometric titration, using 10 mg), dissolve in diluted methanol (1 in 2) to make exactly 100 mL, and use this solution as the standard solution. Perform the test with exactly 10 μL each of the sample solution and standard solution as directed under Liquid Chromatography <*2.01*> according to the following conditions, and determine the peak areas, A_T and A_S, of glycyrrhizic acid in each solution.

$$\text{Amount (mg) of glycyrrhizic acid } (C_{42}H_{62}O_{16}) = M_S \times A_T/A_S \times 1/2$$

M_S: Amount (mg) of Glycyrrhizic Acid RS taken, calculated on the anhydrous basis

Operating conditions—

Detector: An ultraviolet absorption photometer (wavelength: 254 nm).

Column: A stainless steel column 4.6 mm in inside diameter and 15 cm in length, packed with octadecylsilanized silica gel for liquid chromatography (5 μm in particle diameter).

Column temperature: A constant temperature of about 40°C.

Mobile phase: Dissolve 3.85 g of ammonium acetate in 720 mL of water, and add 5 mL of acetic acid (100) and 280 mL of acetonitrile.

Flow rate: 1.0 mL per minute (the retention time of glycyrrhizic acid is about 15 minutes).

System suitability—

System performance: Dissolve 5 mg of monoammonium glycyrrhizinate for resolution check in 20 mL of dilute ethanol. When the procedure is run with 10 μL of this solution under the above operating conditions, the resolution between the peak having the relative retention time of about 0.9 to glycyrrhizic acid and the peak of glycyrrhizic acid is not less than 1.5.

System repeatability: When the test is repeated 6 times with 10 μL of the standard solution under the above operating conditions, the relative standard deviation of the peak area of glycyrrhizic acid is not more than 1.5%.

(3) Total alkaloid (rhyncophylline and hirsutine)—Weigh accurately about 1 g of the dry extract (or an amount of the viscous extract, equivalent to about 1 g of dried substance), add 20 mL of diethyl ether, shake, add 3 mL of 1 mol/L hydrochloric acid TS and 7 mL of water, shake for 10 minutes, centrifuge, and remove the diethyl ether layer. To the aqueous layer add 20 mL of diethyl ether, and repeat the above process. To the aqueous layer add 10 mL of sodium hydroxide TS and 20 mL of diethyl ether, shake for 10 minutes, centrifuge, and separate the diethyl ether layer. To the residue add 20 mL of diethyl ether, proceed in the same manner, and repeat the procedure twice. Combine all the extracts, evaporate the solvent under low pressure (in vacuo) at not more than 40°C, and dissolve the residue in the mobile phase to make exactly 10 mL, and use this solution as the sample solution. Separately, weigh accurately about 5 mg of rhyncophylline for assay and about 5 mg of hirsutine for assay, and dissolve in a mixture of methanol and dilute acetic acid (7:3) to make exactly 100 mL. Pipet 10 mL of this solution, add a mixture of methanol and dilute acetic acid (7:3) to make exactly 50 mL, and use this solution as the standard solution. Perform the test with exactly 10 μL each

of the sample solution and standard solution as directed under Liquid Chromatography <*2.01*> according to the following conditions, and determine the peak areas of rhyncophylline and hirsutine, A_{TR} and A_{TH}, and A_{SR} and A_{SH}, in each solution.

Amount (mg) of the total alkaloid (rhyncophylline and hirsutine)

$$= M_{SR} \times A_{TR}/A_{SR} \times 1/50 + M_{SH} \times A_{TH}/A_{SH} \times 1/50$$

M_{SR}: Amount (mg) of rhyncophylline for assay taken
M_{SH}: Amount (mg) of hirsutine for assay taken

Operating conditions—

Detector: An ultraviolet absorption photometer (wavelength: 245 nm).

Column: A stainless steel column 4.6 mm in inside diameter and 15 cm in length, packed with octadecylsilanized silica gel for liquid chromatography (5 μm in particle diameter).

Column temperature: A constant temperature of about 40°C.

Mobile phase: Dissolve 5 g of sodium lauryl sulfate in 1150 mL of acetonitrile and 1350 mL of water, mix with 1 mL of phosphoric acid.

Flow rate: 1.0 mL per minute (the retention time of rhyncophylline is about 12 minutes and that of hirsutine is about 27 minutes).

System suitability—

System performance: When the procedure is run with 10 μL of the standard solution under the above operating conditions, the number of theoretical plates and the symmetry factor of the peak of rhyncophylline and hirsutine are not less than 5000 and not more than 1.5, respectively.

System repeatability: When the test is repeated 6 times with 10 μL of the standard solution under the above operating conditions, the relative standard deviations of the peak area of rhyncophylline and hirsutine are not more than 1.5%, respectively.

Containers and storage Containers—Tight containers.

Chrysanthemum Flower

Chrysanthemi Flos

キクカ

Chrysanthemum Flower is the capitulum of 1) *Chrysanthemum indicum* Linné or 2) *Chrysanthemum morifolium* Ramatuelle (*Compositae*).

Description **1)** *Chrysanthemum indicum* origin—Capitulum, 3 - 10 mm in diameter; involucre, consisting of 3 to 5 rows of involucral scales, often with peduncle; the outer involucral scale, linear to lanceolate; inner involucral scale, narrow ovate to ovate; ligulate flower, in a single circle, yellow to light yellow-brown in color; tubular flowers, numerous, light yellow-brown; outer surface of involucre, yellow-brown to brown; light in texture and easy to break.

Odor, characteristic; taste, slightly bitter.

2) *Chrysanthemum morifolium* origin—Capitulum, 15 - 40 mm in diameter; involucre, consisting of 3 to 4 rows of involucral scales, often with peduncle; the outer involucral scale, linear to lanceolate; inner involucral scale, narrow ovate to ovate; ligulate flowers, numerous, white to yellow in color; tubular flowers, small in number, light yellow-brown, occasionally degenerate; outer surface of involucre, green-brown to brown; light in texture and easy to break.

Odor, characteristic; taste, slightly bitter.

Identification To 1 g of pulverized Chrysanthemum Flower add 20 mL of methanol, shake for 10 minutes, and filter. Evaporate the filtrate to dryness, dissolve the residue in 1 mL of methanol, and use this solution as the sample solution. Separately, dissolve 1 mg of luteolin for thin-layer chromatography in 1 mL of methanol, and use this solution as the standard solution. Perform the test with these solutions as directed under Thin-layer Chromatography <*2.03*>. Spot 10 μL each of the sample solution and standard solution on a plate of silica gel for thin-layer chromatography, develop the plate with a mixture of ethyl acetate, 2-butanone, water and formic acid (25:3:1:1) to a distance of about 7 cm, and air-dry the plate. Spray evenly iron (III) chloride-methanol TS on the plate: one of the several spots obtained from the sample solution has the same color tone and *R*f value with the spot from the standard solution.

Loss on drying <*5.01*> Not more than 15.0% (6 hours).

Total ash <*5.01*> Not more than 8.5%.

Acid-insoluble ash <*5.01*> Not more than 1.0%.

Extract content <*5.01*> Dilute ethanol-soluble extract: not less than 30.0%.

Containers and storage Containers—Well-closed containers.

Cimicifuga Rhizome

Cimicifugae Rhizoma

ショウマ

Cimicifuga Rhizome is the rhizome of *Cimicifuga dahurica* Maximowicz, *Cimicifuga heracleifolia* Komarov, *Cimicifuga foetida* Linné or *Cimicifuga simplex* Turczaninow (*Ranunculaceae*).

Description Knotted, irregularly shaped rhizome, 6 - 18 cm in length, 1 - 2.5 cm in diameter; externally dark brown to blackish brown, with many remains of roots, often with scars of terrestrial stems; the center of the scar dented, and the circumference being pale in color and showing a radial pattern; fractured surface fibrous; pith dark brown in color and often hollow; light and hard in texture.

Almost odorless; taste, bitter and slightly astringent.

Identification Dissolve 1 g of pulverized Cimicifuga Rhizome add 5 mL of dilute hydrochloric acid and 5 mL of diethyl ether, shake for 10 minutes, centrifuge, and use the diethy ether layer as the sample solution. Use (*E*)-isoferulic acid-(*E*)-ferulic acid TS for thin-layer chromatography as the standard solution. Perform the test with these solutions as directed under Thin-layer Chromatography <*2.03*>. Spot 10 μL of the sample solution and 2 μL of the standard solution on a plate of silica gel for thin-layer chromatography. Develop the plate with a mixture of ethyl acetate, hexane and acetic acid (100) (30:10:1) to a distance of about 7 cm, and air-dry the plate. Examine under ultraviolet light (main wavelength: 365 nm): one of the spot among the several spots obtained from the sample solution has the same color tone and *R*f value with the blue fluorescent spot from the standard solution.

Purity **(1)** Heavy metals <*1.07*>—Proceed with 3.0 g of pulverized Cimicifuga Rhizome according to Method 3, and

perform the test. Prepare the control solution with 3.0 mL of Standard Lead Solution (not more than 10 ppm).

(2) Arsenic *<1.11>*—Prepare the test solution with 0.40 g of pulverized Cimicifuga Rhizome according to Method 4, and perform the test (not more than 5 ppm).

(3) Rhizome of *Astilbe thunbergii* Miquel—Under a microscope *<5.01>*, pulverized Cimicifuga Rhizome does not contain crystal druses in the parenchyma.

Total ash *<5.01>* Not more than 9.0%.

Acid-insoluble ash *<5.01>* Not more than 1.5%.

Extract content *<5.01>* Dilute ethanol-soluble extract: not less than 18.0%.

Containers and storage Containers—Well-closed containers.

Cinnamon Bark

Cinnamomi Cortex

ケイヒ

Cinnamon Bark is the bark of the trunk of *Cinnamomum cassia* J. Presl (*Lauraceae*), or such bark from which a part of the periderm has been removed.

Description Usually semi-tubular or tubularly rolled pieces of bark, 0.1 - 0.5 cm in thickness, 5 - 50 cm in length, 1.5 - 5 cm in diameter; the outer surface dark red-brown, and the inner surface red-brown and smooth; brittle; the fractured surface is slightly fibrous, red-brown, exhibiting a light brown, thin layer.

Characteristic aroma; taste, sweet and pungent at first, later rather mucilaginous and slightly astringent.

Under a microscope *<5.01>*, a transverse section of Cinnamon Bark reveals a primary cortex and a secondary cortex divided by an almost continuous ring consisting of stone cells; nearly round bundles of fibers in the outer region of the ring; cell wall of each stone cell often thickened in a U-shape; secondary cortex lacking stone cells, and with a small number of sclerenchymatous fibers coarsely scattered; parenchyma scattered with oil cells, mucilage cells and cells containing starch grains; medullary rays with cells containing fine needles of calcium oxalate.

Identification To 2.0 g of pulverized Cinnamon Bark add 10 mL of diethyl ether, shake for 3 minutes, filter, and use the filtrate as the sample solution. Perform the test with this solution as directed under Thin-layer Chromatography *<2.03>*. Spot 10 μL of the sample solution on a plate of silica gel with fluorescent indicator for thin-layer chromatography. Develop the plate with a mixture of hexane and ethyl acetate (2:1) to a distance of about 7 cm, and air-dry the plate. Examine under ultraviolet light (main wavelength: 254 nm): a purple spot develops at an *R*f value of about 0.4. Spray evenly 2,4-dinitrophenylhydrazine TS upon the spot: a yellow-orange color develops.

Purity Total BHC's and total DDT's *<5.01>*—Not more than 0.2 ppm, respectively.

Loss on drying *<5.01>* Not more than 15.5% (6 hours).

Total ash *<5.01>* Not more than 6.0%.

Essential oil content *<5.01>* Perform the test with 50.0 g of pulverized Cinnamon Bark provided that 1 mL of silicon resin is previously added to the sample in the flask: the volume of essential oil is not less than 0.5 mL.

Containers and storage Containers—Well-closed containers.

Powdered Cinnamon Bark

Cinnamomi Cortex Pulveratus

ケイヒ末

Powdered Cinnamon Bark is the powder of Cinnamon Bark.

Description Powdered Cinnamon Bark is red-brown to brown in color. It has a characteristic aroma and a sweet, pungent taste with a slightly mucilaginous and astringent aftertaste.

Under a microscope *<5.01>*, Powdered Cinnamon Bark reveals starch grains, fragments of parenchyma cells containing them; fragments of fibers, oil cells containing yellow-brown oil droplets, stone cells, cork stone cells, cork tissue, and fine crystals of calcium oxalate. Starch grains are simple and compound grains 6 to 20 μm in diameter.

Identification To 2.0 g of Powdered Cinnamon Bark add 10 mL of diethyl ether, shake for 3 minutes, filter, and use the filtrate as the sample solution. Perform the test with this solution as directed under Thin-layer Chromatography *<2.03>*. Spot 10 μL of the sample solution on a plate of silica gel with fluorescent indicator for thin-layer chromatography. Develop the plate with a mixture of hexane and ethyl acetate (2:1) to a distance of about 7 cm, and air-dry the plate. Examine under ultraviolet light (main wavelength: 254 nm): a purple spot develops at an *R*f value of about 0.4. Spray 2,4-dinitrophenylhydrazine TS upon the spot: a yellow orange color develops.

Purity **(1)** Petiole—Under a microscope *<5.01>*, Powdered Cinnamon Bark does not reveal epidermal cells, hairs, cells containing chlorophyll granules, and fragments of vascular bundle.

(2) Total BHC's and total DDT's *<5.01>*—Not more than 0.2 ppm, respectively.

Loss on drying *<5.01>* Not more than 15.0% (6 hours).

Total ash *<5.01>* Not more than 6.0%.

Essential oil content *<5.01>* Perform the test with 50.0 g of Powdered Cinnamon Bark provided that 1 mL of silicon resin is previously added to the sample in the flask: the volume of essential oil is not less than 0.35 mL.

Containers and storage Containers—Tight containers.

Cinnamon Oil

Oleum Cinnamomi

ケイヒ油

Cinnamon Oil is the essential oil distilled with steam from the leaves and twigs or bark of *Cinnamomum cassia* J. Presl or from the bark of *Cinnamomum zeylanicum* Nees (*Lauraceae*).

It contains not less than 60 vol% of the total aldehydes.

Description Cinnamon Oil is a yellow to brown liquid. It has a characteristic, aromatic odor and a sweet, pungent taste.

It is clearly miscible with ethanol (95) and with diethyl ether.

It is practically insoluble in water.

It is weakly acidic. Upon aging or long exposure to air, it darkens and becomes viscous.

Specific gravity d_{20}^{20}: 1.010 - 1.065

Identification Shake 4 drops of Cinnamon Oil with 4 drops of nitric acid: the mixture forms white to light yellow crystals at a temperature below 5°C.

Purity **(1)** Rosin—Mix 1.0 mL of Cinnamon Oil with 5 mL of ethanol (95), then add 3 mL of freshly prepared, saturated ethanol solution of lead (II) acetate trihydrate: no precipitate is produced.

(2) Heavy metals *<1.07>*—Proceed with 1.0 mL of Cinnamon Oil according to Method 2, and perform the test. Prepare the control solution with 4.0 mL of Standard Lead Solution (not more than 40 ppm).

Assay Pipet 5.0 mL of Cinnamon Oil into a cassia flask, add 70 mL of sodium hydrogensulfite TS, and heat the mixture in a water bath with frequent shaking to dissolve completely. To this solution add sodium hydrogensulfite TS to raise the lower level of the oily layer within the graduate portion of the neck. Allow to stand for 2 hours, and measure the volume (mL) of the separated oily layer.

$$\text{Total aldehydes (vol\%)} = \{5.0 - (\text{volume of separated oily layer})\} \times 20$$

Containers and storage Containers—Tight containers.

Storage—Light-resistant.

Cistanche Herb

Cistanchis Herba

ニクジュヨウ

Cistanche Herb is stout stem of 1) *Cistanche salsa* G. Beck, 2) *Cistanche deserticola* Y. C. Ma or 3) *Cistanche tubulosa* Wight (*Orobanchaceae*), spadix removed in case flowers open.

Description **1)** *Cistanche salsa* origin—Flatly cylindrical, 5 - 25 cm in length, 1 - 2.5 cm in diameter; the one end mostly slightly narrow and curved; external surface brown to blackish brown, covered with thick scales; fleshy and solid, slightly soft and oily, hardly broken; fractured surface yellow-brown to brown, vascular bundles light brown and arranged in a wavy ring.

Odor, characteristic; taste, slightly sweet, followed by slight bitterness.

Under a microscope *<5.01>* a transverse section of middle part reveals the outermost part is an epidermis coated with cuticle; cortex composed of parenchyma; collateral vascular bundles fusiform or rhombic and arranged in a wavy ring in the inner portion of cortex; groups of cells with slightly thickened cell walls sometimes attached outside of phloem of collateral vascular bundles, and exhibit tail like form; pith composed of parenchyma; parenchyma contains starch grains or gelatinized starch.

2) *Cistanche deserticola* origin—Flatly cylindrical, and approximate to 1), but large in size, 5 - 50 cm in length, 1 - 8 cm in diameter.

Odor, characteristic; taste, slightly sweet, followed by slight bitterness.

Under a microscope *<5.01>* a transverse section of middle part reveals, approximate to 1).

3) *Cistanche tubulosa* origin—Flatly fusiform to cylindrical, slightly curved, 5 - 25 cm in length, 2 - 9 cm in diameter; external surface brown to blackish brown, covered with thick scales; solid in texture and firm, hardly broken; fractured surface light grayish brown to yellow-brown, vascular bundles yellow-white and scattered throughout the surface.

Odor, characteristic; taste, slightly sweet, followed by slight bitterness.

Under a microscope *<5.01>* a transverse section of middle part reveals, approximate to 1) and 2), but collateral vascular bundles distributed throughout the parenchyma from marginal region to the center of transverse section; cells with slightly thickened cell walls observed sometimes around collateral vascular bundles, but exhibit no tail like form;

Identification To 1 g of pulverized Cistanche Herb add 5 mL of water and 5 mL of 1-butanol, shake for 15 minutes, centrifuge, and use the 1-butanol layer as the sample solution. Separately, dissolve 1 mg of verbascoside for thin-layer chromatography in 1 mL of methanol, and use this solution as the standard solution. Perform the test with these solutions as directed under Thin-layer Chromatography *<2.03>*. Spot 20 μL of the sample solution and 10 μL of the standard solution on a plate of silica gel for thin-layer chromatography. Develop the plate with a mixture of ethyl acetate, methanol and water (20:3:2) to a distance of about 7 cm, and air-dry the plate. Spray evenly 2,6-dibromo-*N*-chlolo-1,4-benzoquinone monoimine TS on the plate, and allow to stand in an ammonia gas: one of the several spots obtained from the sample solution has the same color tone and *R*f value with the spot from the standard solution.

Purity **(1)** Heavy metals *<1.07>*—Proceed with 3.0 g of pulverized Cistanche Herb according to Method 3, and perform the test. Prepare the control solution with 3.0 mL of Standard Lead Solution (not more than 10 ppm).

(2) Arsenic *<1.11>*—Prepare the test solution with 0.40 g of pulverized Cistanche Herb according to Method 4, and perform the test (not more than 5 ppm).

Loss on drying *<5.01>* Not more than 20.0%.

Total ash *<5.01>* Not more than 11.0%.

Acid-insoluble ash *<5.01>* Not more than 2.0%.

Extract content *<5.01>* Dilute ethanol-soluble extract: not less than 35.0%.

Containers and storage Containers—Well-closed containers.

Citrus Unshiu Peel

Citri Unshiu Pericarpium

チンピ

Citrus Unshiu Peel is the pericarp of the ripe fruit of *Citrus unshiu* Marcowicz or *Citrus reticulata* Blanco (*Rutaceae*).

It contains not less than 4.0% of hesperidin, calculated on the basis of dried material.

Description Irregular pieces of pericarp, about 2 mm in thickness; externally yellow-red to dark yellow-brown, with numerous small dents associated with oil sacs; internally white to light grayish yellow-brown; light and brittle in texture.

Odor, characteristic aroma; taste, bitter and slightly pungent.

Identification To 0.5 g of pulverized Citrus Unshiu Peel add 10 mL of methanol, warm on a water bath for 2 minutes, and filter. To 5 mL of the filtrate add 0.1 g of magnesium in ribbon-form and 1 mL of hydrochloric acid, and allow to stand: a red-purple color develops.

Purity Total BHC's and total DDT's *<5.01>*—Not more than 0.2 ppm, respectively.

Loss on drying *<5.01>* Not more than 13.0% (6 hours).

Total ash *<5.01>* Not more than 4.0%.

Extract content *<5.01>* Dilute ethanol-soluble extract: not less than 30.0%.

Essential oil content *<5.01>* Perform the test with 50.0 g of pulverized Citrus Unshiu Peel provided that 1 mL of silicon resin is previously added to the sample in the flask: the volume of essential oil is not less than 0.2 mL.

Assay Weigh accurately about 0.1 g of pulverized Citrus Unshiu Peel, add 30 mL of methanol, heat under a reflux condenser for 15 minutes, centrifuge after cooling, and separate the supernatant liquid. To the residue add 20 mL of methanol, and proceed in the same manner. Combine the extracts, and add methanol to make exactly 50 mL. Pipet 5 mL of this solution, add water to make exactly 10 mL, and use this solution as the sample solution. Separately, weigh accurately about 10 mg of hesperidin for assay, previously dried in a desiccator (silica gel) for not less than 24 hours, and dissolve in methanol to make exactly 100 mL. Pipet 5 mL of this solution, add water to make exactly 10 mL, and use this solution as the standard solution. Perform the test with exactly 10 μL each of the sample solution and standard solution as directed under Liquid Chromatography *<2.01>* according to the following conditions, and determine the peak areas, A_T and A_S, of hesperidin in each solution.

$$\text{Amount (mg) of hesperidin} = M_S \times A_T/A_S \times 1/2$$

M_S: Amount (mg) of hesperidin for assay taken

Operating conditions—

Detector: An ultraviolet absorption photometer (wavelength: 285 nm).

Column: A stainless steel column 4.6 mm in inside diameter and 15 cm in length, packed with octadecylsilanized silica gel for liquid chromatography (5 μm in particle diameter).

Column temperature: A constant temperature of about 40°C.

Mobile phase: A mixture of water, acetonitrile and acetic acid (100) (82:18:1).

Flow rate: 1.0 mL per minute (the retention time of hesperidin is about 15 minutes).

System suitability—

System performance: Dissolve 1 mg each of hesperidin for assay and naringin for thin-layer chromatography in 10 mL of methanol, and add water to make 20 mL. When the procedure is run with 10 μL of this solution under the above operating conditions, naringin and hesperidin are eluted in this order with the resolution between these peaks being not less than 1.5.

System repeatability: When the test is repeated 6 times with 10 μL of the standard solution under the above operating conditions, the relative standard deviation of the peak area of hesperidin is not more than 1.5%.

Containers and storage Containers—Well-closed containers.

Clematis Root

Clematidis Radix

イレイセン

Clematis Root is the root with rhizome of *Clematis mandshurica* Ruprecht, *Clematis chinensis* Osbeck or *Clematis hexapetala* Pallas (*Ranunculaceae*).

Description Clematis Root consists of short rhizome and numerous slender roots. The root, 10 – 20 cm in length, 1 – 2 mm in diameter, externally brown to blackish brown, with fine longitudinal wrinkles, brittle. The cortex easily separable from central cylinder; root, grayish white to light yellow-brown in the transverse section, light grayish yellow to yellow in the central cylinder; under a magnifying glass, central cylinder almost round, slight 2 – 4 sinuses on xylem. The rhizome, 2 – 4 cm in length, 5 – 20 mm in diameter, externally light grayish brown to grayish brown; cortex peeled off and fibrous, often with rising node; apex having the residue of lignified stem.

Odor, slight; practically tasteless.

Under a microscope, *<5.01>* transverse section of root reveals an epidermis in the outermost layer; with exodermis lying just inside of the epidermis; cortex and stele divided by endodermis; cortex composed of parenchymatous tissue; xylem with 2 – 4 small concavities where phloem is present; parenchymatous cells contain both simple and 2- to 8-compound starch grains.

Identification **(1)** To 0.5 g of pulverized Clematis Root add 10 mL of water, and boil for 2 to 3 minutes. After cooling, shake vigorously: lasting fine foams appear.

(2) To 0.5 g of pulverized Clematis Root add 3 mL of acetic anhydride, warm on a water bath for 2 minutes, and filter. To the filtrate add 1 mL of sulfuric acid gently: a brown color appears at the zone of contact.

Purity **(1)** Heavy metals *<1.07>*—Proceed with 1.0 g of pulverized Clematis Root according to Method 3, and perform the test. Prepare the control solution with 2.0 mL of Standard Lead Solution (not more than 20 ppm).

(2) Arsenic *<1.11>*—Prepare the test solution with 0.40 g of pulverized Clematis Root according to Method 4, and perform the test (not more than 5 ppm).

Loss on drying *<5.01>* Not more than 13.0% (6 hours).

Total ash <*5.01*> Not more than 8.5%.

Acid-insoluble ash <*5.01*> Not more than 3.0%.

Extract content <*5.01*> Dilute ethanol-soluble extract: not less than 15.0%.

Containers and storage Containers—Well-closed containers.

Clove

Caryophylli Flos

チョウジ

Clove is the flowering bud of *Syzygium aromaticum* Merrill et Perry (*Eugenia caryophyllata* Thunberg) (*Myrtaceae*).

Description Dark brown to dark red buds, 1 - 1.8 cm in length, consisting of slightly compressed and four-sided receptacle, crowned by 4 thick sepals and 4 nearly spherical, membranous, imbricated petals, enclosing numerous stamens and a single style.

Odor, strong and characteristic; taste, pungent, which gives numbing sensation to the tongue.

Identification To 1.5 g of pulverized Clove add 20 mL of ethyl acetate, shake for 5 minutes, filter, and use the filtrate as the sample solution. Separately, dissolve 5 mg of eugenol for thin-layer chromatography in 1 mL of methanol, and use this solution as the standard solution. Perform the test with these solutions as directed under Thin-layer Chromatography <*2.03*>. Spot 1 μL each of the sample solution and standard solution on a plate of silica gel for thin-layer chromatography. Develop the plate with a mixture of hexane and acetone (2:1) to a distance of about 7 cm, and air-dry the plate. Spray evenly vanillin-sulfuric acid-ethanol TS for spraying on the plate, and heat the plate at 105°C for 5 minutes: one of the several spots obtained from the sample solution has the same color tone and *R*f value with the spot from the standard solution.

Purity **(1)** Stem—When perform the test of foreign matter <*5.01*>, the amount of the stem contained in Clove does not exceed 5.0%.

(2) Foreign matter <*5.01*>—The amount of foreign matter other than the stem contained in Clove does not exceed 1.0%.

Total ash <*5.01*> Not more than 7.0%.

Acid-insoluble ash <*5.01*> Not more than 0.5%.

Essential oil content <*5.01*> Perform the test with 10.0 g of pulverized Clove: the volume of essential oil is not less than 1.6 mL.

Containers and storage Containers—Well-closed containers.

Powdered Clove

Caryophylli Flos Pulveratus

チョウジ末

Powdered Clove is the powder of Clove.

Description Powdered Clove occurs as a dark brown powder. It has a strong, characteristic odor and a pungent taste, leaving a sensation of numbness on the tongue.

Under a microscope <*5.01*>, Powdered Clove reveals epidermal tissue with stomata, collenchyma, parenchyma with oil sacs, and spongy parenchyma or its fragments; furthermore, a few fusiform thick-walled fibers, spiral vessels 6 - 10 μm in diameter, anther and pollen grains, and rosette aggregates of calcium oxalate 10 - 15 μm in diameter. Epidermis of anther shows characteristically reticulated walls; pollen grains tetrahedral 10 - 20 μm in diameter; rosette aggregates of calcium oxalate arranged in crystal cell rows, or contained in collenchyma cells and parenchyma cells.

Identification To 1.5 g of Powdered Clove add 20 mL of ethyl acetate, shake for 5 minutes, filter, and use the filtrate as the sample solution. Separately, dissolve 5 mg of eugenol for thin-layer chromatography in 1 mL of methanol, and use this solution as the standard solution. Perform the test with these solutions as directed under Thin-layer Chromatography <*2.03*>. Spot 1 μL each of the sample solution and standard solution on a plate of silica gel for thin-layer chromatography. Develop the plate with a mixture of hexane and acetone (2:1) to a distance of about 7 cm, and air-dry the plate. Spray evenly vanillin-sulfuric acid-ethanol TS for spraying on the plate, and heat the plate at 105°C for 5 minutes: one of the several spots obtained from the sample solution has the same color tone and *R*f value with the spot from the standard solution.

Purity Foreign matter <*5.01*>—Under a microscope, Powdered Clove does not contain stone cells or starch grains.

Total ash <*5.01*> Not more than 7.0%.

Acid-insoluble ash <*5.01*> Not more than 0.5%.

Essential oil content <*5.01*> Perform the test with 10.0 g of Powdered Clove: the volume of essential oil is not less than 1.3 mL.

Containers and storage Containers—Tight containers.

Clove Oil

Oleum Caryophylli

チョウジ油

Clove Oil is the volatile oil distilled with steam from the flower buds or leaves of *Syzygium aromaticum* Merrill et Perry (*Eugenia caryophyllata* Thunberg) (*Myrtaceae*).

It contains not less than 80.0 vol% of total eugenol.

Description Clove Oil is a colorless or light yellow-brown, clear liquid. It has a characteristic aroma and a burning taste.

It is miscible with ethanol (95) and with diethyl ether.

It is slightly soluble in water.

It acquires a brown color upon aging or by air.

Identification (1) To 5 drops of Clove Oil add 10 mL of calcium hydroxide TS, and shake vigorously: the oil forms a flocculent mass, and a white to light yellow color develops.

(2) Dissolve 2 drops of Clove Oil in 4 mL of ethanol (95), and add 1 to 2 drops of iron (III) chloride TS: a green color is produced.

Refractive index <*2.45*> n_D^{20}: 1.527 – 1.537

Specific gravity <*1.13*> d_{20}^{20}: 1.040 – 1.068

Purity (1) Clarity of solution—Dissolve 1.0 mL of Clove Oil in 2.0 mL of diluted ethanol (7 in 10): the solution is clear.

(2) Water-soluble phenols—To 1.0 mL of Clove Oil add 20 mL of boiling water, shake vigorously, filter the aqueous layer after cooling, and add 1 to 2 drops of iron (III) chloride TS: a yellow-green, but no blue or violet, color develops.

(3) Heavy metals <*1.07*>—Proceed with 1.0 mL of Clove Oil according to Method 2, and perform the test. Prepare the control solution with 4.0 mL of Standard Lead Solution (not more than 40 ppm).

(4) Optical rotation <*2.49*> α_D^{20}: 0 – −1.5° (100 mm).

Assay Take 10.0 mL of Clove Oil in a Cassia flask, add 70 mL of sodium hydroxide TS, shake for 5 minutes and warm for 10 minutes in a water bath with occasional shaking, add sodium hydroxide TS to the volume after cooling, and allow to stand for 18 hours. Measure the volume (mL) of the separated oily layer.

Total eugenol (vol%)
= {10 − (volume of separated oily layer)} × 10

Containers and storage Containers—Tight containers.

Storage—Light-resistant.

Cnidium Monnieri Fruit

Cnidii Monnieris Fructus

ジャショウシ

Cnidium Monnieri Fruit is the fruit of *Cnidium monnieri* Cusson (*Umbelliferae*).

Description Elliptical cremocarp, often each mericarp separated; 2 – 3 mm in length, 1 – 2 mm in width; externally light brown to brown, each mericarp usually with five winged longitudinal ridges; inner surface of mericarp almost flat.

Odor, characteristic; it gives characteristic aroma, later a slight sensation of numbness on chewing.

Under a microscope <*5.01*>, a transverse section reveals one oil canal between longitudinal ridges, usually two oil canals in the inner part of mericarp facing to gynophore; longitudinal ridges composed of slightly lignified parenchymatous cells, with vascular bundles in the base; epidermal cells and parenchymatous cells of longitudinal ridges contain solitary crystals of calcium oxalate; parenchymatous cells of albumen contain oil drops and aleurone grains, and occasionally starch grains.

Identification To 1 g of pulverized Cnidium Monnieri Fruit add 10 mL of ethyl acetate, shake for 10 minutes, filter, and use the filtrate as the sample solution. Separately, dissolve 1 mg of osthole for thin-layer chromatography in 2 mL of methanol, and use this solution as the standard solution. Perform the test with these solutions as directed under Thin-layer Chromatography <*2.03*>. Spot 5 μL each of the sample solution and standard solution on a plate of silica gel for thin-layer chromatography, develop the plate with a mixture of hexane and ethyl acetate (2:1) to a distance of about 7 cm, and air-dry the plate. Examine under ultraviolet light (main wavelength: 365 nm): one of the several spots obtained from the sample solution has the same color tone and the *Rf* value with the blue-white fluorescent spot from the standard solution.

Loss on drying <*5.01*> Not more than 12.0% (6 hours).

Total ash <*5.01*> Not more than 17.0%.

Acid-insoluble ash <*5.01*> Not more than 6.0%.

Extract content <*5.01*> Dilute ethanol-soluble extract: not less than 8.0%.

Containers and storage Containers—Well-closed containers.

Cnidium Rhizome

Cnidii Rhizoma

センキュウ

Cnidium Rhizome is the rhizome of *Cnidium officinale* Makino (*Umbelliferae*), usually passed through hot water.

Description Irregular massive rhizome, occasionally cut lengthwise; 5 – 10 cm in length, and 3 – 5 cm in diameter; externally grayish brown to dark brown, with gathered nodes, and with knobbed protrusions on the node; margin of the vertical section irregularly branched; internally grayish white to grayish brown, translucent and occasionally with hollows; dense and hard in texture.

Odor, characteristic; taste, slightly bitter.

Under a microscope <*5.01*>, a transverse section reveals cortex and pith with scattered oil canals; in the xylem, thick-walled and lignified xylem fibers appear in groups of various sizes; starch grains usually gelatinized, but rarely remaining as grains of 5 – 25 μm in diameter; crystals of calcium oxalate not observable.

Identification To 1 g of pulverized Cnidium Rhizome add 5 mL of methanol and 0.1 mL of sodium hydroxide TS, shake for 10 minutes, centrifuge, and use the supernatant liquid as the sample solution. Separately, use (*Z*)-ligustilide TS for thin-layer chromatography as the standard solution (1). Dissolve 1 mg of (*E*)-ferulic acid in 2 mL of methanol and use this solution as the standard solution (2). Perform the test with these solutions as directed under Thin-layer Chromatography <*2.03*>. Spot 20 μL of the sample solution and 5 μL each of the standard solution (1) and the standard solution (2) on a plate of silica gel for thin-layer chromatography. Develop the plate with a mixture of hexane, acetone and acetic acid (100) (30:25:1) to a distance of about 7 cm, and air-dry the plate. Examine under ultraviolet light (main wavelength: 365 nm): one of the several spots obtained from the sample solution has the same color tone and *Rf* value with the blue-white fluorescent spot from the standard solution (1). Spray evenly 4-dimethylaminobenzaldehyde TS for spraying on the plate, heat the plate at 105°C for 5 minutes and allow to cool: one of the several spots from the sample solution has the same color tone and *R*f value with the spot from the standard solution (2).

Purity (1) Heavy metals <*1.07*>—Proceed with 3.0 g of pulverized Cnidium Rhizome according to Method 3, and perform the test. Prepare the control solution with 3.0 mL of Standard Lead Solution (not more than 10 ppm).

(2) Arsenic <*1.11*>—Prepare the test solution with 0.40 g of pulverized Cnidium Rhizome according to Method 4, and perform the test (not more than 5 ppm).

Total ash <*5.01*> Not more than 6.0%.

Acid-insoluble ash <*5.01*> Not more than 1.0%.

Containers and storage Containers—Well-closed containers.

Powdered Cnidium Rhizome

Cnidii Rhizoma Pulveratum

センキュウ末

Powdered Cnidium Rhizome is the powder of Cnidium Rhizome.

Description Powdered Cnidium Rhizome occurs as a gray to light grayish brown powder. It has a characteristic odor and a slightly bitter taste.

Under a microscope <*5.01*>, Powdered Cnidium Rhizome reveals colorless and gelatinized starch masses, and fragments of parenchyma containing them; fragments of scalariform and reticulate vessels 15 - 30 μm in diameter; fragments of thick-walled and lignified xylem fibers 20 - 60 μm in diameter; fragments of yellow brown cork tissue; fragments of secretory tissue.

Identification To 1 g of Powdered Cnidium Rhizome add 5 mL of methanol and 0.1 mL of sodium hydroxide TS, shake for 10 minutes, centrifuge, and use the supernatant liquid as the sample solution. Separately, use (*Z*)-ligustilide TS for thin-layer chromatography as the standard solution (1). Dissolve 1 mg of (*E*)-ferulic acid in 2 mL of methanol and use this solution as the standard solution (2). Perform the test with these solutions as directed under Thin-layer Chromatography <*2.03*>. Spot 20 μL of the sample solution and 5 μL each of the standard solution (1) and the standard solution (2) on a plate of silica gel for thin-layer chromatography. Develop the plate with a mixture of hexane, acetone and acetic acid (100) (30:25:1) to a distance of about 7 cm, and air-dry the plate. Examine under ultraviolet light (main wavelength: 365 nm): one of the several spots obtained from the sample solution has the same color tone and *R*f value with the blue-white fluorescent spot from the standard solution (1). Spray evenly 4-dimethylaminobenzaldehyde TS for spraying on the plate, heat the plate at 105°C for 5 minutes and allow to cool: one of the several spots from the sample solution has the same color tone and *R*f value with the spot from the standard solution (2).

Purity (1) Heavy metals <*1.07*>—Proceed with 3.0 g of Powdered Cnidium Rhizome according to Method 3, and perform the test. Prepare the control solution with 3.0 mL of Standard Lead Solution (not more than 10 ppm).

(2) Arsenic <*1.11*>—Prepare the test solution with 0.40 g of Powdered Cnidium Rhizome according to Method 4, and perform the test (not more than 5 ppm).

(3) Foreign matter—Under a microscope <*5.01*>, Powdered Cnidium Rhizome does not contain a large quantity of starch grains, stone cells, crystals of calcium oxalate or other foreign matter.

Total ash <*5.01*> Not more than 6.0%.

Acid-insoluble ash <*5.01*> Not more than 1.0%.

Containers and storage Containers—Tight containers.

Storage—Light-resistant.

Coconut Oil

Oleum Cocois

ヤシ油

Coconut oil is the fixed oil obtained from the seeds of *Cocos nucifera* Linné (*Palmae*).

Description Coconut Oil is a white to light yellow mass or a colorless or light yellow, clear oil. It has a slight, characteristic odor and a mild taste.

It is freely soluble in diethyl ether and in petroleum ether. It is practically insoluble in water.

At a temperature below 15°C, it congeals to a hard and brittle solid.

Melting point: 20 - 28°C

Acid value <*1.13*> Not more than 0.2.

Saponification value <*1.13*> 246 - 264

Unsaponifiable matter <*1.13*> Not more than 1.0%.

Iodine value <*1.13*> 7 - 11

Containers and storage Containers—Tight containers.

Codonopsis Root

Codonopsis Radix

トウジン

Codonopsis Root is the root of *Codonopsis pilosula* Nannfeldt or *Codonopsis tangshen* Oliver (*Campanulaceae*).

Description Codonopsis Root nearly cylindrical, 8 - 30 cm in length, 0.5 - 2.5 cm in diameter; gradually slender to the apex, often branched; outer surface light yellow to grayish brown; from the base to central part with ring-like wrinkles, and longitudinal wrinkles entirely obvious; numerous projections composed of scars of stems at the crown, with a round dent at the distal end; blackish brown and tremellose secretion often at the scars of lateral roots; flexible and easily bendable or hard and easily breakable in texture; in cut surface yellow-white to light brown in cortex, light yellow in xylem, sometimes with slit in cortex.

Odor, slight and characteristic; taste, slightly sweet.

Under a microscope <*5.01*>, a transverse section reveals cork layer at the outermost portion, outer 1- to 10-layer consisting of cork stone cells; groups of laticifers containing light yellow substances arranged radially in phloem, intercellular spaces usually observed; vessels of xylem arranged radially; starch grains and crystals of inulin usually contained in phloem parenchyma cells.

Identification To 2.0 g of pulverized Codonopsis Root add 50 mL of water, and heat in a water bath for 1 hour. After cooling, filter, and wash the filtrate with two 20-mL portions of ethyl acetate. Separate the aqueous layer, extract with two 30-mL portions of water saturated 1-butanol. Combine the 1-butanol layers, and evaporate the solvent in a water bath under low pressure (in vacuo). Dissolve the residue in 1 mL of methanol, and use this solution as the sample solution. Perform the test with the sample solution as directed under Thin-layer Chromatography *<2.03>*. Spot 5 μL of the sample solution on a plate of silica gel for thin-layer chromatography. Develop the plate with a mixture of 1-propanol, water and ethyl acetate (6:5:2) to a distance of about 10 cm, and air-dry the plate. Spray evenly naphthoresorcin-phosphoric acid TS on the plate, and heat the plate at 105°C for 10 minutes: an orange to red-purple spot at an *R*f value of about 0.5 is observed.

Purity **(1)** Heavy metals *<1.07>*—Proceed with 3.0 g of pulverized Codonopsis Root according to Method 3, and perform the test. Prepare the control solution with 3.0 mL of Standard Lead Solution (not more than 10 ppm).

(2) Arsenic *<1.11>*—Prepare the test solution with 0.40 g of pulverized Codonopsis Root according to Method 4, and perform the test (not more than 5 ppm).

Loss on drying *<5.01>* Not more than 23.0% (6 hours).

Total ash *<5.01>* Not more than 5.0%.

Acid-insoluble ash *<5.01>* Not more than 1.5%.

Extract content *<5.01>* Dilute ethanol-soluble extract: not less than 25.0%.

Containers and storage Containers—Well-closed containers.

Coix Seed

Coicis Semen

ヨクイニン

Coix Seed is the seed of *Coix lachryma-jobi* Linné var. *mayuen* Stapf (*Gramineae*), from which the seed coat has been removed.

Description Ovoid or broad ovoid seed, about 6 mm in length, and about 5 mm in width; with a slightly hollowed apex and base; dorsal side distended; ventral side longitudinally and deeply furrowed in the center; dorsal side mostly white in color and powdery; in the furrow on the ventral surface, attached brown, membranous pericarp and seed coat. Under a magnifying glass, the cross section reveals light yellow scutellum in the hollow of the ventral side. Hard in texture.

Odor, slight; taste, slightly sweet; adheres to the teeth on chewing.

Identification To a transverse section of Coix Seed add iodine TS dropwise: a dark red-brown color develops in the endosperm, and a dark gray color develops in the scutellum.

Loss on drying *<5.01>* Not more than 14.0% (6 hours).

Total ash *<5.01>* Not more than 3.0%.

Containers and storage Containers—Well-closed containers.

Powdered Coix Seed

Coicis Semen Pulveratum

ヨクイニン末

Powdered Coix Seed is the powder of Coix Seed.

Description Powdered Coix Seed occurs as a brownish, grayish white to grayish yellow-white powder, and has a slight odor and a slightly sweet taste.

Under a microscope *<5.01>*, Powdered Coix Seed reveals starch grains, and fragments of endosperm containing them; fragments of tissue accompanied with epidermal cells of pericarp composed of yellowish and oblong cells, and fragments of parenchyma cells containing fixed oil, aleuron grains and starch grains; a very few fragments of spiral vessels. Starch grains are simple and 2-compound grains, simple grain nearly equidiameter to obtuse polygon, 10 – 20 μm in diameter, and have a stellate cleft-like hilum in the center. Spherical starch grains, coexisting with aleuron grains, are spherical simple grains, 3 – 7 μm in diameter.

Identification Place a small amount of Powdered Coix Seed on a slide glass, add dropwise iodine TS, and examine under a microscope *<5.01>*: nearly equidiameter and obtuse polygonal simple starch grains, usually 10 – 15 μm in diameter, and compound starch grains have a reddish brown color. Small spheroidal starch grains, coexisting with fixed oil and with aleuron grains in parenchymatous cells, have a blue-purple color.

Purity Foreign matter—Under a microscope *<5.01>*, Powdered Coix Seed reveals no fragments of tissue having silicified cell wall, no stone cells, no fragments of other thick-walled and lignified cells, no fragments of reticulate, scalariform and pitted vessels, no fragments of fibers and hairs, and no large starch grains, more than 10 μm in diameter, appearing blue-purple upon addition of iodine TS.

Loss on drying *<5.01>* Not more than 14.0% (6 hours).

Total ash *<5.01>* Not more than 3.0%.

Containers and storage Containers—Tight containers.

Condurango

Condurango Cortex

コンズランゴ

Condurango is the bark of the trunk of *Marsdenia cundurango* Reichenbach filius (*Asclepiadaceae*).

Description Tubular or semi-tubular pieces of bark, 0.1 – 0.6 cm in thickness, 4 – 15 cm in length; outer surface grayish brown to dark brown, nearly smooth and with numerous lenticels, or more or less scaly and rough; inner surface light grayish brown and longitudinally striate; fractured surface fibrous on the outer region and generally granular in the inner region.

Odor, slight; taste, bitter.

Under a microscope *<5.01>*, a transverse section reveals a cork layer composed of several cellular layers of thin-walled cells; primary cortex with numerous stone cell groups; secondary cortex with phloem fiber bundles scattered inside the starch sheath consisting of one-cellular layer; articulate latex tubes scattered in both cortices; parenchyma cells containing starch grains or rosette aggregates of calcium oxalate; starch grain 3 - 20 μm in diameter.

Identification Digest 1 g of pulverized Condurango in 5 mL of water, and filter: the clear filtrate becomes turbid on heating, but becomes clear again upon cooling.

Purity Foreign matter <*5.01*>—The xylem and other foreign matter contained in Condurango do not exceed 2.0%.

Total ash <*5.01*> Not more than 12.0%.

Containers and storage Containers—Well-closed containers.

Condurango Fluidextract

コンズランゴ流エキス

Method of preparation Take moderately fine powder of Condurango, and prepare the fluidextract as directed under Fluidextracts using a suitable quantity of a mixture of Purified Water or Purified Water in Containers, Ethanol and Glycerin (5:3:2) as the first solvent, and a suitable quantity of a mixture of Purified Water or Purified Water in Containers and Ethanol (3:1) as the second solvent.

Description Condurango Fluidextract is a brown liquid. It has a characteristic odor and a bitter taste.

Identification Mix 1 mL of Condurango Fluidextract with 5 mL of water, filter, if necessary, and heat the clear solution: turbidity is produced. However, it becomes almost clear upon cooling.

Purity Heavy metals <*1.07*>—Prepare the test solution with 1.0 g of Condurango Fluidextract as direct under the Fluidextracts (4), and perform the test (not more than 30 ppm).

Containers and storage Containers—Tight containers.

Coptis Rhizome

Coptidis Rhizoma

オウレン

Coptis Rhizome is the rhizome of *Coptis japonica* Makino, *Coptis chinensis* Franchet, *Coptis deltoidea* C. Y. Cheng et Hsiao or *Coptis teeta* Wallich (*Ranunculaceae*), from which the roots have been removed practically.

It contains not less than 4.2% of berberine [as berberine chloride ($C_{20}H_{18}ClNO_4$: 371.81)], calculated on the basis of dried material.

For Coptis Rhizome used only for extracts or infusions and decoctions, the label states the restricted utilization forms.

Description Irregular, cylindrical rhizome, 2 - 4 cm, rarely up to 10 cm in length, 0.2 - 0.7 cm in diameter, slightly curved and often branched; externally grayish yellow-brown, with ring nodes, and with numerous remains of rootlets; generally remains of petiole at one end; fractured surface rather fibrous; cork layer light grayish brown, cortex and pith are yellow-brown to reddish yellow-brown, xylem is yellow to reddish yellow in color.

Odor, slight; taste, extremely bitter and lasting; it colors the saliva yellow on chewing.

Under a microscope <*5.01*>, a transverse section of Coptis Rhizome reveals a cork layer composed of thin-walled cork cells; cortex parenchyma usually exhibiting groups of stone cells near the cork layer and yellow phloem fibers near the cambium; xylem consisting chiefly of vessels, tracheids and xylem fibers; medullary ray distinct; pith large; in pith, stone cells or stone cells with thick-walled and lignified cells are sometimes recognized; parenchyma cells contain minute starch grains.

Identification **(1)** To 0.5 g of pulverized Coptis Rhizome add 10 mL of water, allow to stand for 10 minutes with occasional shaking, and filter. To 2 to 3 drops of the filtrate add 1 mL of hydrochloric acid and 1 to 2 drops of hydrogen peroxide TS, and shake: a red-purple color develops.

(2) To 0.5 g of pulverized Coptis Rhizome add 20 mL of methanol, shake for 2 minutes, filter, and use the filtrate as the sample solution. Separately, dissolve 1 mg of Berberine Chloride RS or berberin chloride hydrate for thin-layer chromatography in 1 mL of methanol, and use this solution as the standard solution. Perform the test with these solutions as directed under Thin-layer Chromatography <*2.03*>. Spot 5 μL each of the sample solution and standard solution on a plate of silica gel for thin-layer chromatography. Develop the plate with a mixture of 1-butanol, water and acetic acid (100) (7:2:1) to a distance of about 7 cm, and air-dry the plate. Examine under ultraviolet light (main wavelength: 365 nm): one of the several spots obtained from the sample solution and a yellow to yellow-green fluorescence spot from the standard solution show the same color tone and the same Rf value.

Purity **(1)** Heavy metals <*1.07*>—Proceed with 1.0 g of pulverized Coptis Rhizome according to Method 3, and perform the test. Prepare the control solution with 2.0 mL of Standard Lead Solution (not more than 20 ppm). When the decision is difficult by this method, perform the test as directed under Atomic Absorption Spectrophotometry <*2.23*>. Put 5.0 g of pulverized Coptis Rhizome in a platinum, quartz or porcelain crucible, heat gently, and then incinerate by ignition between 450°C and 550°C. After cooling, add a small amount of 2 mol/L nitric acid TS, filter if necessary, and wash the crucible and filter several times with small portions of 2 mol/L nitric acid TS. Combine the filtrate and the washings, add 2 mol/L nitric acid TS to make exactly 20 mL, and use this solution as the sample solution. Separately, to 2.5 mL of Standard Lead Solution add 2 mol/L nitric acid TS to make exactly 20 mL, and use this solution as the standard solution. Perform the test with the sample solution and the standard solution according to the following conditions: the absorbance of the sample solution is not more than that of the standard solution (not more than 5 ppm).

Gas: Combustible gas—Acetylene or hydrogen.
Supporting gas—Air.

Lamp: A lead hollow-cathode lamp.

Wavelength: 283.3 nm.

The procedure and permissible limit for Coptis Rhizome labeled to be used for extracts or infusions and decoctions are as follows.

To 4.0 g of moderately fine cuttings of Coptis Rhizome add 80 mL of water, and heat until the amount becomes about 40 mL with occasional stirring. After cooling, filter, and proceed with the filtrate according to Method 3, and perform the test. Prepare the control solution with 2.0 mL of

Standard Lead Solution (not more than 5 ppm).

(2) Arsenic <*1.11*>—Prepare the test solution with 0.40 g of pulverized Coptis Rhizome according to Method 4, and perform the test (not more than 5 ppm).

Loss on drying <*5.01*> Not more than 11.0% (6 hours).

Total ash <*5.01*> Not more than 4.0%.

Acid-insoluble ash <*5.01*> Not more than 1.0%.

Assay Weigh accurately about 0.5 g of pulverized Coptis Rhizome, add 30 mL of a mixture of methanol and dilute hydrochloric acid (100:1), heat under a reflux condenser for 30 minutes, cool, and filter. Repeat the above procedure twice with the residue, using 30-mL and 20-mL portions of a mixture of methanol and dilute hydrochloric acid (100:1). To the last residue add 10 mL of methanol, shake well, and filter. Combine the whole filtrates, add methanol to make exactly 100 mL, and use this solution as the sample solution. Separately, weigh accurately about 10 mg of Berberine Chloride RS (previously determine the water <*2.48*> in the same manner as Berberine Chloride Hydrate), dissolve in methanol to make exactly 100 mL, and use this solution as the standard solution. Perform the test with exactly 20 μL each of the sample solution and standard solution as directed under Liquid Chromatography <*2.01*> according to the following conditions, and determine the peak areas, A_T and A_S, of berberine in each solution.

Amount (mg) of berberine [as berberine chloride ($C_{20}H_{18}ClNO_4$)]
$= M_S \times A_T/A_S$

M_S: Amount (mg) of Berberine Chloride RS taken, calculated on the anhydrous basis

Operating conditions—

Detector: An ultraviolet absorption photometer (wavelength: 345 nm).

Column: A stainless steel column 4 to 6 mm in inside diameter and 15 to 25 cm in length, packed with octadecylsilanized silica gel (5 to 10 μm in particle diameter).

Column temperature: A constant temperature of about 40°C.

Mobile phase: Dissolve 3.4 g of potassium dihydrogenphosphate and 1.7 g of sodium lauryl sulfate in 1000 mL of a mixture of water and acetonitrile (1:1).

Flow rate: Adjust so that the retention time of berberine is about 10 minutes.

System suitability—

System performance: Dissolve 1 mg each of Berberine Chloride RS and palmatine chloride in methanol to make 10 mL. When the procedure is run with 20 μL of this solution under the above operating conditions, palmatine and berberine are eluted in this order with the resolution between these peaks being not less than 1.5.

System repeatability: When the test is repeated 5 times with 20 μL of the standard solution under the above operating conditions, the relative standard deviation of the peak area of berberine is not more than 1.5%.

Containers and storage Containers—Well-closed containers.

Powdered Coptis Rhizome

Coptidis Rhizoma Pulveratum

オウレン末

Powdered Coptis Rhizome is the powder of Coptis Rhizome.

It contains not less than 4.2% of berberine [as berberine chloride ($C_{20}H_{18}ClNO_4$: 371.81)], calculated on the basis of dried material.

Description Powdered Coptis Rhizome occurs as a yellow-brown to grayish yellow-brown powder. It has a slight odor and an extremely bitter, lasting taste, and colors the saliva yellow on chewing.

Under a microscope <*5.01*>, almost all elements are yellow in color; it reveals mainly fragments of vessels, tracheids and xylem fibers; parenchyma cells containing starch grains; polygonal cork cells. Usually, round to obtuse polygonal stone cells and their groups, and phloem fibers, 10 - 20 μm in diameter, and fragments of their bundles. Sometimes, polygonal and elongated epidermal cells, originated from the petiole, having characteristically thickened cell walls. Starch grains are single grains 1 - 7 μm in diameter.

Identification **(1)** To 0.5 g of Powdered Coptis Rhizome add 10 mL of water, allow to stand for 10 minutes with occasional shaking, and filter. To 2 to 3 drops of the filtrate add 1 mL of hydrochloric acid and 1 to 2 drops of hydrogen peroxide TS, and shake: a red-purple color develops.

(2) To 0.5 g of Powdered Coptis Rhizome add 20 mL of methanol, shake for 2 minutes, filter, and use the filtrate as the sample solution. Separately, dissolve 1 mg of Berberine Chloride RS or berberine chloride hydrate for thin-layer chromatography in 1 mL of methanol, and use this solution as the standard solution. Perform the test with these solutions as directed under Thin-layer Chromatography <*2.03*>. Spot 5 μL each of the sample solution and standard solution on a plate of silica gel for thin-layer chromatography. Develop the plate with a mixture of 1-butanol, water and acetic acid (100) (7:2:1) to a distance of about 7 cm, and air-dry the plate. Examine under ultraviolet light (main wavelength: 365 nm): one of the spot among the several spots from the sample solution and a yellow to yellow-green fluorescence spot from the standard solution show the same color tone and the same *Rf* value.

Purity **(1)** Heavy metals <*1.07*>—Proceed with 1.0 g of Powdered Coptis Rhizome according to Method 3, and perform the test. Prepare the control solution with 2.0 mL of Standard Lead Solution (not more than 20 ppm). When the decision is difficult by this method, perform the test as directed under Atomic Absorption Spectrophotometry <*2.23*>. Put 5.0 g of Powdered Coptis Rhizome in a platinum, quartz or porcelain crucible, heat gently, and then incinerate by ignition between 450°C and 550°C. After cooling, add a small amount of 2 mol/L nitric acid TS, filter if necessary, and wash the crucible and filter several times with small portions of 2 mol/L nitric acid TS. Combine the filtrate and the washings, add 2 mol/L nitric acid TS to make exactly 20 mL, and use this solution as the sample solution. Separately, to 2.5 mL of Standard Lead Solution add 2 mol/L nitric acid TS to make exactly 20 mL, and use this solution as the standard solution. Perform the test with the sample solution and the standard solution according to the following conditions: the absorbance of the sample solution is not more than that of the standard solution (not more than 5 ppm).

Gas: Combustible gas—Acetylene or hydrogen.

Supporting gas—Air.

Lamp: A lead hollow-cathode lamp.

Wavelength: 283.3 nm.

(2) Arsenic <*1.11*>—Prepare the test solution with 0.40 g of Powdered Coptis Rhizome according to Method 4, and perform the test (not more than 5 ppm).

(3) Phellodendron bark—Under a microscope <*5.01*>, crystal cell rows or mucilage masses are not observable. Stir 0.5 g of Powdered Coptis Rhizome with 2 mL of water: the solution does not become gelatinous.

(4) Curcuma—Place Powdered Coptis Rhizome on a filter paper, drop diethyl ether on it, and allow to stand. Remove the powder from the filter paper, and drop 1 drop of potassium hydroxide TS: no red-purple color develops. Under a microscope <*5.01*>, Powdered Coptis Rhizome does not contain gelatinized starch or secretory cells containing yellow-red resin.

Loss on drying <*5.01*> Not more than 11.0% (6 hours).

Total ash <*5.01*> Not more than 4.0%.

Acid-insoluble ash <*5.01*> Not more than 1.0%.

Assay Weigh accurately about 0.5 g of Powdered Coptis Rhizome, add 30 mL of a mixture of methanol and dilute hydrochloric acid (100:1), heat under a reflux condenser for 30 minutes, cool, and filter. Repeat the above procedure twice with the residue, using 30-mL and 20-mL portions of a mixture of methanol and dilute hydrochloric acid (100:1). To the last residue add 10 mL of methanol, shake well, and filter. Combine the whole filtrates, add methanol to make exactly 100 mL, and use this solution as the sample solution. Separately, weigh accurately about 10 mg of Berberine Chloride RS (previously determine the water <*2.48*> in the same manner as Berberine Chloride Hydrate), dissolve in methanol to make exactly 100 mL, and use this solution as the standard solution. Perform the test with exactly 20 μL each of the sample solution and standard solution as directed under Liquid Chromatography <*2.01*> according to the following conditions, and determine the peak areas, A_T and A_S, of berberine in each solution.

Amount (mg) of berberine [as berberine chloride ($C_{20}H_{18}ClNO_4$)]
$= M_S \times A_T/A_S$

M_S: Amount (mg) of Berberine Chloride RS taken, calculated on the anhydrous basis

Operating conditions—

Detector: An ultraviolet absorption photometer (wavelength: 345 nm).

Column: A stainless steel column 4 to 6 mm in inside diameter and 15 to 25 cm in length, packed with octadecylsilanized silica gel (5 to 10 μm in particle diameter).

Column temperature: A constant temperature of about 40°C.

Mobile phase: Dissolve 3.4 g of potassium dihydrogenphosphate and 1.7 g of sodium lauryl sulfate in 1000 mL of a mixture of water and acetonitrile (1:1).

Flow rate: Adjust so that the retention time of berberine is about 10 minutes.

System suitability—

System performance: Dissolve 1 mg each of Berberine Chloride RS and palmatine chloride in methanol to make 10 mL. When the procedure is run with 20 μL of this solution under the above operating conditions, palmatine and berberine are eluted in this order with the resolution between these peaks being not less than 1.5.

System repeatability: When the test is repeated 5 times with 20 μL of the standard solution under the above operating conditions, the relative standard deviation of the peak area of berberine is not more than 1.5%.

Containers and storage Containers—Well-closed containers.

Corn Oil

Oleum Maydis

トウモロコシ油

Corn Oil is the fixed oil obtained from the embryo of *Zea mays* Linné (*Gramineae*).

Description Corn Oil is a clear, light yellow oil. It is odorless or has a slight odor, and a mild taste.

It is miscible with diethyl ether and with petroleum ether.

It is slightly soluble in ethanol (95), and practically insoluble in water.

At −7°C, it congeals to an unguentary mass.

Specific gravity d_{25}^{25}: 0.915 – 0.921

Acid value <*1.13*> Not more than 0.2.

Saponification value <*1.13*> 187 – 195

Unsaponifiable matter <*1.13*> Not more than 1.5%.

Iodine value <*1.13*> 103 – 130

Containers and storage Containers—Tight containers.

Cornus Fruit

Corni Fructus

サンシュユ

Cornus Fruit is the pulp of the pseudocarp of *Cornus officinalis* Siebold et Zuccarini (*Cornaceae*).

It contains not less than 0.4% of loganin, calculated on the basis of dried material.

Description Flattened oblong, 1.5 – 2 cm in length, about 1 cm in width; externally dark red-purple to dark purple, lustrous, and with coarse wrinkles; a crack-like scar formed by removal of true fruits; a scar of calyx at one end, and a scar of peduncle at the other; soft in texture.

Odor, slight; taste, acid and occasionally slightly sweet.

Identification To 1 g of coarse cuttings of Cornus Fruit add 10 mL of methanol, shake for 5 minutes, filter, and use the filtrate as the sample solution. Separately, dissolve 1 mg of loganin for thin-layer chromatography in 2 mL of methanol, and use this solution as the standard solution. Perform the test with these solutions as directed under Thin-layer Chromatography <*2.03*>. Spot 10 μL each of the sample solution and standard solution on a plate of silica gel for thin-layer chromatography. Develop the plate with a mixture of ethyl acetate, water and formic acid (6:1:1) to a distance of about 10 cm, and air-dry the plate. Spray evenly 4-methoxybenzaldehyde-sulfuric acid TS on the plate, and heat the plate at 105°C for 5 minutes: one of the several spots obtained from the sample solution has the same color tone and Rf value with the spot from the standard solution. Further, a spot, slightly different in color tone from the above-mentioned spot, is found immediately below of the spot.

Purity (1) Foreign matter <*5.01*>—The amount of its peduncles and other foreign matter contained in Cornus Fruit does no exceed 2.0%.

(2) Total BHC's and total DDT's <*5.01*>—Not more than 0.2 ppm, respectively.

Total ash <*5.01*> Not more than 5.0%.

Extract content <*5.01*> Dilute ethanol-soluble extract: not less than 35.0%.

Assay Weigh accurately about 1 g of fine cuttings of Cornus Fruit (separately determine the loss on drying <*5.01*>), put in a glass-stoppered centrifuge tube, add 30 mL of diluted methanol (1 in 2), shake for 20 minutes, centrifuge, and take the supernatant liquid. To the residue add 30 mL of diluted methanol (1 in 2), and repeat the above process twice more. Combine all the extacts, add diluted methanol (1 in 2) to make exactly 100 mL, and use this solution as the sample solution. Separately, weigh accurately about 10 mg of loganin for assay, dissolve in diluted methanol (1 in 2) to make exactly 100 mL, and use this solution as the standard solution. Perform the test with exactly 10 μL each of the sample solution and standard solution as directed under Liquid Chromatography <*2.01*> according to the following conditions, and determine the peak areas, A_T and A_S, of loganin in each solution.

$$\text{Amount (mg) of loganin} = M_S \times A_T/A_S$$

M_S: Amount (mg) of loganin for assay taken

Operating conditions—

Detector: An ultraviolet absorption photometer (wavelength: 238 nm).

Column: A stainless steel column 4.6 mm in inside diameter and 15 cm in length, packed with octadecylsilanized silica gel for liquid chromatography (5 μm in particle diameter).

Column temperature: A constant temperature of about 50°C.

Mobile phase: A mixture of water, acetonitrile and methanol (55:4:1).

Flow rate: Adjust so that the retention time of loganin is about 25 minutes.

System suitability—

System performance: When the procedure is run with 10 μL of the standard solution under the above operating conditions, the number of theoretical plates and the symmetry factor of the peak of loganin are not less than 5000 and not more than 1.5, respectively.

System repeatability: When the test is repeated 6 times with 10 μL of the standard solution under the above operating conditions, the relative standard deviation of the peak area of loganin is not more than 1.5%.

Containers and storage Containers—Well-closed containers.

Corydalis Tuber

Corydalis Tuber

エンゴサク

Corydalis Tuber is the tuber of *Corydalis turtschaninovii* Basser forma *yanhusuo* Y. H. Chou et C. C. Hsu (*Papaveraceae*), usually after being passed through hot water.

It contains not less than 0.08% of dehydrocorydaline [as dehydrocorydaline nitrate ($C_{22}H_{24}N_2O_7$)], calculated on the basis of dried material.

Description Nearly flattened spherical, 1 - 2 cm in diameter, and with stem scar at one end; externally grayish yellow to grayish brown; hard in texture; fractured surface is yellow and smooth or grayish yellow-green in color and granular.

Almost odorless; taste, bitter.

Identification To 2 g of pulverized Corydalis Tuber add 10 mL of methanol, shake for 15 minutes, filter, and use the filtrate as the sample solution. Separately, dissolve 1 mg of dehydrocorydaline nitrate for thin-layer chromatography in 20 mL of methanol, and use this solution as the standard solution. Perform the test with these solutions as directed under Thin-layer Chromatography <*2.03*>. Spot 10 μL each of the sample solution and standard solution on a plate of silica gel for thin-layer chromatography, develop the plate with a mixture of methanol, ammonium acetate solution (3 in 10) and acetic acid (100) (20:1:1) to a distance of about 10 cm, and air-dry the plate. Examine under ultraviolet light (main wavelength: 365 nm): one of the several spots obtained from the sample solution has the same color tone and Rf value with the yellow-green fluorescent spot from the standard solution, and a yellow fluorescent spot appears at the lower side of the spot. Separately, spray evenly Dragendorff's TS for spraying on the plate, air-dry, and then spray sodium nitrite TS: a brown spot appears at an Rf value of about 0.6.

Purity (1) Heavy metals <*1.07*>—Proceed with 3.0 g of pulverized Corydalis Tuber according to Method 3, and perform the test. Prepare the control solution with 3.0 mL of Standard Lead Solution (not more than 10 ppm).

(2) Arsenic <*1.11*>—Prepare the test solution with 0.40 g of pulverized Corydalis Tuber according to Method 4, and perform the test (not more than 5 ppm).

Loss on drying <*5.01*> Not more than 15.0%.

Total ash <*5.01*> Not more than 3.0%.

Assay Weigh accurately about 1 g of pulverized Corydalis Tuber, add 30 mL of a mixture of methanol and dilute hydrochloric acid (3:1), heat under a reflux condenser for 30 minutes, and filter after cooling. To the residue add 15 mL of a mixture of methanol and dilute hydrochloric acid (3:1), and repeat the above procedure. Combine all the filtrates, add a mixture of methanol and dilute hydrochloric acid (3:1) to make exactly 50 mL, and use this solution as the sample solution. Separately, weigh accurately about 10 mg of dehydrocorydaline nitrate for assay, previously dried in a desiccator (silica gel) for not less than 1 hour, dissolve in a mixture of methanol and dilute hydrochloric acid (3:1) to make exactly 200 mL, and use this solution as the standard solution. Perform the test with exactly 5 μL each of the sample solution and standard solution as directed under Liquid Chromatography <*2.01*> according to the following conditions, and determine the peak areas, A_T and A_S, of dehydrocorydaline in each solution.

Amount (mg) of dehydrocorydaline [as dehydrocorydaline nitrate ($C_{22}H_{24}N_2O_7$)]
$= M_S \times A_T/A_S \times 1/4$

M_S: Amount (mg) of dehydrocorydaline nitrate for assay taken

Operating conditions—

Detector: An ultraviolet absorption photometer (wavelength: 340 nm).

Column: A stainless steel column 4.6 mm in inside diameter and 15 cm in length, packed with octadecylsilanized silica gel for liquid chromatography (5 μm in particle diameter).

Column temperature: A constant temperature of about 40°C.

Mobile phase: Dissolve 17.91 g of disodium hydrogen phosphate dodecahydrate in 970 mL of water, and adjust to pH 2.2 with phosphoric acid. To this solution add 14.05 g of sodium perchlorate, dissolve, and add water to make exactly 1000 mL. To this solution add 450 mL of acetonitrile, then dissolve 0.20 g of sodium lauryl sulfate.

Flow rate: Adjust so that the retention time of dehydrocorydaline is about 24 minutes.

System suitability—

System performance: Dissolve 1 mg each of dehydrocorydaline nitrate for assay and berberine chloride hydrate in 20 mL of a mixture of water and acetonitrile (20:9). When the procedure is run with 5 μL of this solution under the above operating conditions, berberine and dehydrocorydaline are eluted in this order with the resolution between these peaks being not less than 1.5.

System repeatability: When the test is repeated 6 times with 5 μL of the standard solution under the above operating conditions, the relative standard deviation of the peak areas of dehydrocorydaline is not more than 1.5%.

Containers and storage Containers—Well-closed containers.

Powdered Corydalis Tuber

Corydalis Tuber Pulveratum

エンゴサク末

Powdered Corydalis Tuber is the powder of Corydalis Tuber.

It contains not less than 0.08% of dehydrocorydaline [as dehydrocorydaline nitrate ($C_{22}H_{24}N_2O_7$)], calculated on the basis of dried material.

Description Powdered Corydalis Tuber occurs as a greenish yellow to grayish yellow powder. Almost odorless; taste, bitter.

Under a microscope <*5.01*>, Powdered Corydalis Tuber reveals mainly, masses of gelatinized starch or light yellow to colorless parenchymatous cells containing starch grains, fragments of cork layers, light yellow stone cells, sclerenchymatous cells, reticulate vessels, spiral vessels and ring vessels; starch grains observed simple grains and 2- to 3-compound grains.

Identification To 2 g of Powdered Corydalis Tuber add 10 mL of methanol, shake for 15 minutes, filter, and use the filtrate as the sample solution. Separately, dissolve 1 mg of dehydrocorydaline nitrate for thin-layer chromatography in 20 mL of methanol, and use this solution as the standard solution. Perform the test with these solutions as directed under Thin-layer Chromatography <*2.03*>. Spot 10 μL each of the sample solution and standard solution on a plate of silica gel for thin-layer chromatography, develop the plate with a mixture of methanol, ammonium acetate solution (3 in 10) and acetic acid (100) (20:1:1) to a distance of about 10 cm, and air-dry the plate. Examine under ultraviolet light (main wavelength: 365 nm): one of the several spots obtained from the sample solution has the same color tone and *Rf* value with the yellow-green fluorescent spot from the standard solution, and a yellow fluorescent spot appears at the lower side of the spot. Separately, spray evenly Dragendorff's TS for spraying on the plate, air-dry, and then spray sodium nitrite TS: a brown spot appears at an *Rf* value of about 0.6.

Purity (1) Heavy metals <*1.07*>—Proceed with 3.0 g of Powdered Corydalis Tuber according to Method 3, and perform the test. Prepare the control solution with 3.0 mL of Standard Lead Solution (not more than 10 ppm).

(2) Arsenic <*1.11*>—Prepare the test solution with 0.40 g of Powdered Corydalis Tuber according to Method 4, and perform the test (not more than 5 ppm).

Loss on drying <*5.01*> Not more than 15.0%.

Total ash <*5.01*> Not more than 3.0%.

Assay Weigh accurately about 1 g of Powdered Corydalis Tuber, add 30 mL of a mixture of methanol and dilute hydrochloric acid (3:1), heat under a reflux condenser for 30 minutes, and filter after cooling. To the residue add 15 mL of the mixture of methanol and dilute hydrochloric acid (3:1), and proceed in the same way as above. Combine all the filtrates, add the mixture of methanol and dilute hydrochloric acid (3:1) to make exactly 50 mL, and use this solution as the sample solution. Separately, weigh accurately about 10 mg of dehydrocorydaline nitrate for assay, previously dried in a desiccator (silica gel) for not less than 1 hour, dissolve in the mixture of methanol and dilute hydrochloric acid (3:1) to make exactly 200 mL, and use this solution as the standard solution. Perform the test with exactly 5 μL each of the sample solution and standard solution as directed under Liquid Chromatography <*2.01*> according to the following conditions, and determine the peak areas, A_T and A_S, of dehydrocorydaline in each solution.

Amount (mg) of dehydrocorydaline [as dehydrocorydaline nitrate ($C_{22}H_{24}N_2O_7$)]
$= M_S \times A_T/A_S \times 1/4$

M_S: Amount (mg) of dehydrocorydaline nitrate for assay taken

Operating conditions—

Detector: An ultraviolet absorption photometer (wavelength: 340 nm).

Column: A stainless steel column 4.6 mm in inside diameter and 15 cm in length, packed with octadecylsilanized silica gel for liquid chromatography (5 μm in particle diameter).

Column temperature: A constant temperature of about 40°C.

Mobile phase: Dissolve 17.91 g of disodium hydrogen phosphate dodecahydrate in 970 mL of water, and adjust to pH 2.2 with phosphoric acid. To this solution add 14.05 g of sodium perchlorate, dissolve, and add water to make exactly 1000 mL. Add 450 mL of acetonitrile, and dissolve 0.20 g of sodium lauryl sulfate in this solution.

Flow rate: Adjust so that the retention time of dehydrocorydaline is about 24 minutes.

System suitability—

System performance: Dissolve 1 mg of dehydrocorydaline nitrate for assay and 1 mg of berberine chloride hydrate in 20 mL of a mixture of water and acetonitrile (20:9). When the procedure is run with 5 μL of this solution under the above operating conditions, berberine and dehydrocorydaline are eluted in this order with the resolution between these peaks being not less than 1.5.

System repeatability: When the test is repeated 6 times with 5 μL of the standard solution under the above operating conditions, the relative standard deviation of the peak area of dehydrocorydaline is not more than 1.5%.

Containers and storage Containers—Well-closed containers.

Crataegus Fruit

Crataegi Fructus

サンザシ

Crataegus Fruit is the pseudocarp of **1)** *Crataegus cuneata* Siebold et Zuccarini or **2)** *Crataegus pinnatifida* Bunge var. *major* N. E. Brown (*Rosaceae*) without any treatment or cut crosswise or lengthwise.

Description

1) *Crataegus cuneata* origin—Nearly spherical fruits, 8 – 14 mm in diameter; externally yellow-brown to grayish brown, with fine reticulated wrinkles, remained dent of 4 – 6 mm in diameter at one end, often the base of calyx around the dent, short peduncle or scar at the other end. True fruits, usually five loculus, often split five, mericarp, 5 – 8 mm in length, light brown, usually, containing one seed into each mericarp.

Almost odorless; taste, slightly acid.

Under a microscope *<5.01>*, a transverse section of central parts reveals in the outermost layer composed of epidermis to be covered with comparatively thick cuticle layer, cuticle intrude into lateral cell walls of epidermis, and reveal wedge-like. Cell of the epidermis or 2- to 3-cellular layer of parenchyma cells beneath these observed contents of yellow-brown to red-brown in color followed these appeared parenchyma. Vascular bundles and numerous stone cells appear single or gathered 2 to several cells scattered on the parenchyma, and observed solitary crystals and clustera crystals of calcium oxalate. Pericarp of true fruits composed of mainly sclerenchyma cells, seed covered with seed coats, perisperm, endosperm, cotyledon observed inside seed coats; sclerenchyma cells of true fruits and cells of seed coats containing solitary crystals of calcium oxalate.

2) *Crataegus pinnatifida* var. *major* origin—Approximate to 1), but it is large in size, 17 – 23 mm in diameter, the outer surface red-brown and lustrous, spot-like scars of hairs are distinct. At one end remained dent, 7 – 9 mm in diameter, mericarp, 10 – 12 mm in length, yellow-brown in color, usually ripe seeds are absent.

Odor, characteristic; taste, acid.

Under a microscope *<5.01>*, a transverse section of the central parts approximate to 1), but it contains a few stone cells in parenchyma.

Identification

1) *Crataegus cuneata* origin—To 1.0 g of pulverized Crataegus Fruit add 5 mL of methanol, shake for 30 minutes, centrifuge, and use the supernatant liquid as the sample solution. Separately, dissolve 1 mg of rutin for thin-layer chromatography in 20 mL of methanol, and use this solution as the standard solution. Perform the test with these solutions as directed under Thin-layer Chromatography *<2.03>*. Spot 10 μL each of the sample solution and standard solution on a plate of silica gel for thin-layer chromatography, develop the plate with a mixture of ethyl acetate, 2-butanone, water and formic acid (5:3:1:1) to a distance of about 10 cm, and air-dry the plate. Spray evenly dilute sulfuric acid on the plate, heat the plate at 105°C for 5 minutes, and examine under ultraviolet light (main wavelength: 365 nm): one of the several spots obtained from the sample solution has the same color tone and *R*f value with the green fluorescent spot from the standard solution, and one or two similar green fluorescent spots are found at an *R*f value of about 0.5. These spots disappear gradually by allowing to cool, and appear again by heating.

2) *Crataegus pinnatifida* var. *major* origin—To 1 g of pulverized Crataegus Fruit add 5 mL of methanol, shake for 30 minutes, centrifuge, and use the supernatant liquid as the sample solution. Separately, dissolve 1 mg of hyperoside for thin-layer chromatography in 20 mL of methanol, and use this solution as the standard solution. Perform the test with these solutions as directed under Thin-layer Chromatography *<2.03>*. Spot 10 μL each of the sample solution and standard solution on a plate of silica gel for thin-layer chromatography, develop the plate with a mixture of ethyl acetate, 2-butanone, water and formic acid (5:3:1:1) to a distance of about 10 cm, and air-dry the plate. Spray evenly dilute sulfuric acid on the plate, heat the plate at 105°C for 5 minutes, and examine under ultraviolet light (main wavelength: 365 nm): one of the several spots obtained from the sample solution has the same color tone and *R*f value with the green fluorescent spot from the standard solution, and a similar fluorescent spot is found just above the spot. These spots disappear gradually by allowing to cool, and appear again by heating.

Loss on drying *<5.01>* Not more than 17.0%.

Total ash *<5.01>* Not more than 4.0%.

Extract content *<5.01>* Dilute ethanol-soluble extract: not less than 8.0%.

Containers and storage Containers—Well-closed containers.

Curcuma Rhizome

Curcumae Rhizoma

ガジュツ

Curcuma Rhizome is the rhizome of 1) *Curcuma zedoaria* Roscoe, 2) *Curcuma phaeocaulis* Valeton or 3) *Curcuma kwangsiensis* S. G. Lee et C. F. Liang (*Zingiberaceae*), usually after being passed through hot water.

Description Nearly ovoid to oblong-ovoid or conical rhizome, 2 – 8 cm in length, 1.5 – 4 cm in diameter; externally grayish yellow-brown to grayish brown; nodes protruded as rings; internode of 0.3 – 0.8 cm, with scars of roots, and small protrusions consisting of scars of branched rhizomes; hard in texture; a transverse section reveals cortex and stele distinctly; cortex 2 – 5 mm in thickness; a transverse section, grayish brown in rhizome of 1) *Curcuma zedoria* origin, light yellow to grayish yellow or light yellow-green to grayish yellow-green in 2) *Curcuma phaeocaulis* origin and purplish brown to dark purple-brown in 3) *Curcuma kwangsiensis* origin, and sometimes lustrous.

Odor, characteristic; taste, pungent, bitter and cool feeling on chewing.

Under a microscope <*5.01*>, a transverse section of central part reveals the outermost layer usually consisting of a cork layer 4 - 10 cells thick; cortex and stele divided by endodermis, composed of parenchyma cells, vascular bundles scattered; small sized vascular bundles line up beneath the endodermis; oil cells contain yellow-brown to dark brown oily substances, scattered in parenchyma; parenchyma contains gelatinized starch and rarely crystals of calcium oxalate.

Identification To 2.0 g of pulverized Curcuma Rhizome add 5 mL of water, shake, then add 5 mL of hexane, shake for 10 minutes, centrifuge, and use the hexane layer as the sample solution. Perform the test with this solution as directed under Thin-layer Chromatography <*2.03*>. Spot 5 μL of the sample solution on a plate of silica gel for thin-layer chromatography. Develop the plate with a mixture of hexane and ethyl acetate (4:1) to a distance of about 7 cm, and air-dry the plate. Spray evenly 4-methoxybezaldehyde-sulfuric acid TS on the plate, and heat the plate at 105°C for 5 minutes: a deep blue to dark brown spot and a red-brown to brown spot appear at *R*f values of about 0.3 and about 0.2, respectively.

Purity **(1)** Heavy metals <*1.07*>—Proceed with 1.0 g of pulverized Curcuma Rhizome according to Method 3, and perform the test. Prepare the control solution with 1.0 mL of Standard Lead Solution (not more than 10 ppm).

(2) Arsenic <*1.11*>—Prepare the test solution with 0.40 g of pulverized Curcuma Rhizome according to Method 4, and perform the test (not more than 5 ppm).

Total ash <*5.01*> Not more than 7.0%.

Essential oil content <*5.01*> Perform the test with 50.0 g of pulverized Curcuma Rhizome, provided that 1 mL of silicon resin is previously added to the sample in the flask: the volume of essential oil is not less than 0.5 mL.

Containers and storage Containers—Well-closed containers.

Cyperus Rhizome

Cyperi Rhizoma

コウブシ

Cyperus Rhizome is the rhizome of *Cyperus rotundus* Linné (*Cyperaceae*).

Description Fusiform rhizome, 1.5 - 2.5 cm in length, 0.5 - 1 cm in diameter; externally grayish brown to grayish blackish brown, with 5 to 8 irregular ring nodes, and with hair-like fiber bundles on each node; hard in texture. The transverse section red-brown to light yellow in color, with waxy luster; thickness of cortex approximately equal to or slightly smaller than the diameter of stele. Under a magnifying glass, a cut surface reveals fiber bundles as brown spots lined in rings along circumference; here and there in the cortex, vascular bundles appear as red-brown spots, and numerous secretory cells scattered as minute yellow-brown spots; in the stele, numerous vascular bundles scattered as spots or lines.

Characteristic odor and taste.

Identification To 2.0 g of pulverized Cyperus Rhizome add 10 mL of diethyl ether, shake for 5 minutes, filter, and use the filtrate as the sample solution. Perform the test with the sample solution as directed under Thin-layer Chromatography <*2.03*>. Spot 5 μL of the sample solution on a plate of silica gel for thin-layer chromatography. Develop the plate with a mixture of diethyl ether, cyclohexane and formic acid (10:10:1) to a distance of about 7 cm, and air-dry the plate. Spray evenly 4-dimethylaminobenzaldehyde TS for spraying on the plate, and heat the plate at 105°C for 5 minutes: a red-purple spot appears at an *R*f value of about 0.35.

Purity **(1)** Heavy metals <*1.07*>—Proceed with 3.0 g of pulverized Cyperus Rhizome according to Method 3, and perform the test. Prepare the control solution with 3.0 mL of Standard Lead Solution (not more than 10 ppm).

(2) Arsenic <*1.11*>—Prepare the test solution with 0.40 g of pulverized Cyperus Rhizome according to Method 4, and perform the test (not more than 5 ppm).

Total ash <*5.01*> Not more than 3.0%.

Essential oil content <*5.01*> Perform the test with 50.0 g of pulverized Cyperus Rhizome, provided that 1 mL of silicon resin is previously added on the sample in the flask: the volume of essential oil is not less than 0.3 mL.

Containers and storage Containers—Well-closed containers.

Powdered Cyperus Rhizome

Cyperi Rhizoma Pulveratum

コウブシ末

Powdered Cyperus Rhizome is the powder of Cyperus Rhizome.

Description Powdered Cyperus Rhizome occurs as a light red-brown powder, and has a characteristic odor and taste.

Under a microscope <*5.01*>, Powdered Cyperus Rhizome reveals fragments of polygonal parenchyma cells, scalariform vessels, and seta-like fibers; a large quantity of starch, mostly gelatinized; an extremely small number of stone cells.

Identification To 2.0 g of Powdered Cyperus Rhizome add 10 mL of diethyl ether, shake for 5 minutes, filter, and use the filtrate as the sample solution. Perform the test with the sample solution as directed under Thin-layer Chromatography <*2.03*>. Spot 5 μL of the sample solution on a plate of silica gel for thin-layer chromatography. Develop the plate with a mixture of diethyl ether, cyclohexane and formic acid (10:10:1) to a distance of about 7 cm, and air-dry the plate. Spray evenly 4-dimethylaminobenzaldehyde TS for spraying on the plate, and heat the plate at 105°C for 5 minutes: a red-purple spot appears at an *R*f value of about 0.35.

Purity **(1)** Heavy metals <*1.07*>—Proceed with 3.0 g of Powdered Cyperus Rhizome according to Method 3, and perform the test. Prepare the control solution with 3.0 mL of Standard Lead Solution (not more than 10 ppm).

(2) Arsenic <*1.11*>—Prepare the test solution with 0.40 g of Powdered Cyperus Rhizome according to Method 4, and perform the test (not more than 5 ppm).

(3) Foreign matter—Under a microscope <*5.01*>, Powdered Cyperus Rhizome does not show extremely lignified cells, except stone cells, and crystals.

Total ash <*5.01*> Not more than 3.0%.

Acid-insoluble ash <*5.01*> Not more than 1.5%.

Essential oil content <*5.01*> Perform the test with 50.0 g of Powdered Cyperus Rhizome provided that 1 mL of silicon resin is previously added on the sample in the flask: the volume of essential oil is not less than 0.2 mL.

Containers and storage Containers—Tight containers.

Daiokanzoto Extract

大黄甘草湯エキス

Daiokanzoto Extract contains not less than 3.5 mg of sennoside A ($C_{42}H_{38}O_{20}$: 862.74), and not less than 7 mg and not more than 21 mg (for preparation prescribed 1 g of Glycyrrhiza) or not less than 14 mg and not more than 42 mg (for preparation prescribed 2 g of Glycyrrhiza) of glycyrrhizic acid ($C_{42}H_{62}O_{16}$: 822.93), per extract prepared with the amount specified in the Method of preparation.

Method of preparation

	1)	2)
Rhubarb	4 g	4 g
Glycyrrhiza	1 g	2 g

Prepare a dry extract as directed under Extracts, according to the prescription 1) or 2), using the crude drugs shown above.

Description Daiokanzoto Extract occurs as a brown powder. It has a characteristic odor and an astringent first then slightly sweet taste.

Identification **(1)** To 1.0 g of Daiokanzoto Extract add 10 mL of water, shake, then add 10 mL of diethyl ether, shake, centrifuge, and use the diethyl ether layer as the sample solution. Separately, dissolve 1 mg of rhein for thin-layer chromatography in 10 mL of acetone, and use this solution as the standard solution. Perform the test with these solutions as directed under Thin-layer Chromatography <*2.03*>. Spot 5 μL each of the sample solution and standard solution on a plate of silica gel for thin-layer chromatography. Develop the plate with a mixture of ethyl acetate, methanol and water (20:3:2) to a distance of about 7 cm, and air-dry the plate. Examine under ultraviolet light (main wavelength: 365 nm): one of the several spots obtained from the sample solution has the same color tone and *R*f value with the orange fluorescent spot from the standard solution (Rhubarb).

(2) To 0.5 g of Daiokanzoto Extract add 10 mL of water, shake, then add 10 mL of 1-butanol, shake, centrifuge, and use the 1-butanol layer as the sample solution. Separately, dissolve 1 mg of liquiritin for thin-layer chromatography in 1 mL of methanol, and use this solution as the standard solution. Perform the test with these solutions as directed under Thin-layer Chromatography <*2.03*>. Spot 1 μL each of the sample solution and standard solution on a plate of silica gel for thin-layer chromatography. Develop the plate with a mixture of ethyl acetate, methanol and water (20:3:2) to a distance of about 7 cm, and air-dry the plate. Spray evenly dilute sulfuric acid on the plate, heat the plate at 105°C for 5 minutes, and examine under ultraviolet light (main wavelength: 365 nm): one of the several spots obtained from the sample solution has the same color tone and *R*f value with the yellow-green fluorescent spot from the standard solution (Glycyrrhiza).

Purity **(1)** Heavy metals <*1.07*>—Prepare the test solution with 1.0 g of Daiokanzoto Extract as directed under Extract (4), and perform the test (not more than 30 ppm).

(2) Arsenic <*1.11*>—Prepare the test solution with 0.67 g of Daiokanzoto Extract according to Method 3, and perform the test (not more than 3 ppm).

Loss on drying <*2.41*> Not more than 7.0% (1 g, 105°C, 5 hours).

Total ash <*5.01*> Not more than 10.0%.

Assay **(1)** Sennoside A—Weigh accurately about 0.2 g of Daiokanzoto Extract, add 20 mL of ethyl acetate and 10 mL of water, shake for 10 minutes, centrifuge, and remove the ethyl acetate layer. To the aqueous layer add 20 mL of ethyl acetate, shake for 10 minutes, centrifuge, and remove the ethyl acetate layer. To the aqueous layer add 10 mL of methanol, shake for 30 minutes, centrifuge, and take the supernatant liquid. To the residue add 20 mL of diluted methanol (1 in 2), shake for 5 minutes, centrifuge, and take the supernatant liquid. Combine these supernatant liquids, add diluted methanol (1 in 2) to make exactly 50 mL, and use this solution as the sample solution. Separately, weigh accurately about 5 mg of Sennoside A RS (separately determine the water <*2.48*> by coulometric titration, using 10 mg), dissolve in diluted methanol (1 in 2) to make exactly 200 mL, and use this solution as the standard solution. Perform the test with exactly 10 μL each of the sample solution and standard solution as directed under Liquid Chromatography <*2.01*> according to the following conditions, and determine the peak areas, A_T and A_S, of sennoside A in each solution.

$$\text{Amount (mg) of sennoside A } (C_{42}H_{38}O_{20}) = M_S \times A_T/A_S \times 1/4$$

M_S: Amount (mg) of Sennoside A RS taken, calculated on the anhydrous basis

Operating conditions—

Detector: An ultraviolet absorption photometer (wavelength: 340 nm).

Column: A stainless steel column 4.6 mm in inside diameter and 15 cm in length, packed with octadecylsilanized silica gel for liquid chromatography (5 μm in particle diameter).

Column temperature: A constant temperature of about 30°C.

Mobile phase: A mixture of water, acetonitrile and phosphoric acid (2460:540:1).

Flow rate: 1.0 mL per minute (the retention time of sennoside A is about 14 minutes.)

System suitability—

System performance: When the procedure is run with 10 μL of the standard solution under the above operating conditions, the number of theoretical plates and the symmetry factor of the peak of sennoside A are not less than 5000 and not more than 1.5, respectively.

System repeatability: When the test is repeated 6 times with 10 μL of the standard solution under the above operating conditions, the relative standard deviation of the peak area of sennoside A is not more than 1.5%.

(2) Glycyrrhizic acid—Weigh accurately about 0.2 g of

Daiokanzoto Extract, add 20 mL of ethyl acetate and 10 mL of water, and shake for 10 minutes. After centrifugation, remove the ethyl acetate layer, add 20 mL of ethyl acetate, proceed in the same manner as described above, and remove the ethyl acetate layer. To the aqueous layer add 10 mL of methanol, shake for 30 minutes, centrifuge, and take the supernatant liquid. To the residue add 20 mL of diluted methanol (1 in 2), shake for 5 minutes, centrifuge, and take the supernatant liquid. Combine these supernatant liquids, add diluted methanol (1 in 2) to make exactly 50 mL, and use this solution as the sample solution. Separately, weigh accurately about 10 mg of Glycyrrhizic Acid RS (separately determine the water <*2.48*> by coulometric titration, using 10 mg), dissolve in diluted methanol (1 in 2) to make exactly 100 mL, and use this solution as the standard solution. Perform the test with exactly 10 μL each of the sample solution and standard solution as directed under Liquid Chromatography <*2.01*> according to the following conditions, and determine the peak areas, A_T and A_S, of glycyrrhizic acid in each solution.

$$\text{Amount (mg) of glycyrrhizic acid } (C_{42}H_{62}O_{16}) = M_S \times A_T/A_S \times 1/2$$

M_S: Amount (mg) of Glycyrrhizic Acid RS taken, calculated on the anhydrous basis

Operating conditions—

Detector: An ultraviolet absorption photometer (wavelength: 254 nm).

Column: A stainless steel column 4.6 mm in inside diameter and 15 cm in length, packed with octadecylsilanized silica gel for liquid chromatography (5 μm in particle diameter).

Column temperature: A constant temperature of about 40°C.

Mobile phase: Dissolve 3.85 g of ammonium acetate in 720 mL of water, and add 5 mL of acetic acid (100) and 280 mL of acetonitrile.

Flow rate: 1.0 mL per minute (the retention time of glycyrrhizic acid is about 15 minutes).

System suitability—

System performance: Dissolve 5 mg of monoammonium glycyrrhizinate for resolution check in 20 mL of dilute ethanol. When the procedure is run with 10 μL of this solution under the above operating conditions, the resolution between the peak having the relative retention time of about 0.9 to glycyrrhizic acid and the peak of glycyrrhizic acid is not less than 1.5.

System repeatability: When the test is repeated 6 times with 10 μL of the standard solution under the above operating conditions, the relative standard deviation of the peak area of glycyrrhizic acid is not more than 1.5%.

Containers and storage Containers—Tight containers.

Daisaikoto Extract

大柴胡湯エキス

Daisaikoto Extract contains not less than 1.8 mg and not more than 7.2 mg of saikosaponin b_2, not less than 80 mg and not more than 240 mg of baicalin ($C_{21}H_{18}O_{11}$: 446.36), and not less than 26 mg and not more than 78 mg of paeoniflorin ($C_{23}H_{28}O_{11}$: 480.46), per extract prepared with the amount specified in the Method of preparation.

Method of preparation

	1)	2)	3)	4)	5)
Bupleurum Root	6 g	6 g	6 g	6 g	6 g
Pinellia Tuber	4 g	4 g	4 g	3 g	4 g
Scutellaria Root	3 g	3 g	3 g	3 g	3 g
Peony Root	3 g	3 g	3 g	3 g	3 g
Jujube	3 g	3 g	3 g	3 g	3 g
Immature Orange	2 g	2 g	2 g	2 g	2 g
Ginger	1 g	1 g	2 g	1 g	1.5 g
Rhubarb	1 g	2 g	1 g	1 g	2 g

Prepare a dry extract or viscous extract as directed under Extracts, according to the prescription 1) to 5), using the crude drugs shown above.

Description Daisaikoto Extract occurs as light yellow-brown to brown powder or black-brown viscous extract, having a slightly order, and a hot first, then a bitter taste.

Identification **(1)** Shake 1.0 g of the dry extract (or 3.0 g of the viscous extract) with 10 mL of water, add 10 mL of 1-butanol, shake, centrifuge, and use the 1-butanol layer as the sample solution. Separately, dissolve 1 mg of saikosaponin b_2 for thin-layer chromatography in 1 mL of methanol, and use this solution as the standard solution. Perform the test with these solutions as directed under Thin-layer Chromatography <*2.03*>. Spot 10 μL of the sample solution and 2 μL of the standard solution on a plate of silica gel for thin-layer chromatography. Develop the plate with a mixture of ethyl acetate, ethanol (99.5) and water (8:2:1) to a distance of about 7 cm, and air-dry the plate. Spray evenly 4-dimethylaminobenzaldehyde TS for spraying on the plate, and heat the plate at 105°C for 5 minutes. Examine under ultraviolet light (main wavelength: 365 nm): one of the several spots obtained from the sample solution has the same color tone and *Rf* value with the yellow fluorescent spot from the standard solution (Bupleurum Root).

(2) Shake 1.0 g of the dry extract (or 3.0 g of the viscous extract) with 10 mL of water, add 25 mL of diethyl ether, shake, and centrifuge. Separate the diethyl ether layer, evaporate the solvent under low pressure (in vacuo), add 2 mL of diethyl ether to the residue, and use this solution as the sample solution. Separately, dissolve 1 mg of wogonin for thin-layer chromatography in 1 mL of methanol, and use this solution as the standard solution. Perform the test with these solutions as directed under Thin-layer Chromatography <*2.03*>. Spot 20 μL of the sample solution and 5 μL of the standard solution on a plate of silica gel for thin-layer chromatography. Develop the plate with a mixture of ethyl acetate, hexane and acetic acid (100) (10:10:1) to a distance of about 7 cm, and air-dry the plate. Spray evenly iron (III) chloride-methanol TS on the plate: one of the several spots obtained from the sample solution has the same color tone and *Rf* value with the yellow-brown to grayish brown spot from the standard solution (Scutellaria Root).

(3) Shake 1.0 g of the dry extract (or 3.0 g of the viscous extract) with 10 mL of water, add 10 mL of 1-butanol, shake, centrifuge, and use the 1-butanol layer as the sample solution. Separately, dissolve 1 mg of Paeoniflorin RS or paeoniflorin for thin-layer chromatography in 1 mL of methanol, and use this solution as the standard solution. Perform the test with these solutions as directed under Thin-layer Chromatography <*2.03*>. Spot 5 μL each of the sample solution and standard solution on a plate of silica gel for thin-layer chromatography. Develop the plate with a mixture of ethyl acetate, methanol and ammonia solution (28) (6:3:2) to a distance of about 7 cm, and air-dry the plate. Spray evenly 4-methoxybenzoaldehyde-sulfuric acid TS on the plate, heat the plate at 105°C for 2 minutes: one of the several spots obtained from the sample solution has the same color tone and *R*f value with the red-purple to purple spot from the standard solution (Peony Root).

(4) Shake 1.0 g of the dry extract (or 3.0 g of the viscous extract) with 10 mL of water, add 10 mL of 1-butanol, shake, centrifuge, and use the 1-butanol layer as the sample solution. Separately, to 1.0 g of pulverized immature orange add 10 mL of methanol, shake, centrifuge, and use the supernatant liquid as the standard solution. Perform the test with these solutions as directed under Thin-layer Chromatography <*2.03*>. Spot 10 μL of the sample solution and 5 μL of the standard solution on a plate of silica gel for thin-layer chromatography. Develop the plate with a mixture of ethyl acetate, 1-propanol, water and acetic acid (100) (7:5:4:1) to a distance of about 10 cm, and air-dry the plate. Spray evenly 2,6-dibromo-*N*-chloro-1,4-benzoquinone monoimine TS on the plate, and allow to stand in an ammonia gas: two consecutive spots at *R*f values of about 0.7 obtained from the sample solution have respectively the same color tone and *R*f value with the blue-green spot and blue spot underneath from the standard solution (Immature Orange).

(5) Shake 1.0 g of the dry extract (or 3.0 g of the viscous extract) with 10 mL of water, add 25 mL of diethyl ether, shake, and centrifuge. Separate the diethyl ether layer, evaporate the solvent under low pressure (in vacuo), add 2 mL of diethyl ether to the residue, and use this solution as the sample solution. Separately, dissolve 1 mg of [6]-gingerol for thin-layer chromatography in 1 mL of methanol, and use this solution as the standard solution. Perform the test with these solutions as directed under Thin-layer Chromatography <*2.03*>. Spot 10 μL of the sample solution and 5 μL of the standard solution on a plate of silica gel for thin-layer chromatography. Develop the plate with a mixture of ethyl acetate and hexane (1:1) to a distance of about 7 cm, and air-dry the plate. Spray evenly 4-dimethylaminobenzaldehyde TS for spraying on the plate, heat the plate at 105°C for 5 minutes, allow to cool, and spray water: one of the several spots obtained from the sample solution has the same color tone and *R*f value with the blue-green to grayish green spot from the standard solution (Ginger).

(6) Shake 1.0 g of the dry extract (or 3.0 g of the viscous extract) with 10 mL of water, add 25 mL of diethyl ether, shake, and centrifuge. Separate the diethyl ether layer, evaporate the solvent under low pressure (in vacuo), add 2 mL of diethyl ether to the residue, and use this solution as the sample solution. Separately, dissolve 1 mg of rhein for thin-layer chromatography in 10 mL of acetone, and use this solution as the standard solution. Perform the test with these solutions as directed under Thin-layer Chromatography <*2.03*>. Spot 10 μL of the sample solution and 5 μL of the standard solution on a plate of silica gel for thin-layer chromatography. Develop the plate with a mixture of ethyl acetate, methanol and water (20:3:2) to a distance of about 7 cm, and air-dry the plate. Examine under ultraviolet light (main wavelength: 365 nm): one of the several spots obtained from the sample solution has the same color tone and *R*f value with the orange fluorescent spot from the standard solution (Rhubarb).

Purity **(1)** Heavy metals <*1.07*>—Prepare the test solution with 1.0 g of the dry extract (or an amount of the viscous extract, equivalent to 1.0 g of dried substance) as directed under Extracts (4), and perform the test (not more than 30 ppm).

(2) Arsenic <*1.11*>—Prepare the test solution with 0.67 g of the dry extract (or an amount of the viscous extract, equivalent to 0.67 g of dried substance) according to Method 3, and perform the test (not more than 3 ppm).

Loss on drying <*2.41*> The dry extract: Not more than 11.0% (1 g, 105°C, 5 hours).

The viscous extract: Not more than 66.7% (1 g, 105°C, 5 hours).

Total ash <*5.01*> Not more than 9.0%, calculated on the dried basis.

Assay **(1)** Saikosaponin b_2—Weigh accurately about 0.5 g of the dry extract (or an amount of the viscous extract, equivalent to about 0.5 g of the dried substance), add 20 mL of diethyl ether and 10 mL of water, and shake for 10 minutes. After centrifugation, remove the diethyl ether layer, add 20 mL of diethyl ether, proceed in the same manner as described above, and remove the diethyl ether layer. To the aqueous layer add 10 mL of methanol, shake for 30 minutes, centrifuge, and separate the supernatant liquid. To the residue add 20 mL of diluted methanol (1 in 2), shake for 5 minutes, centrifuge, separate the supernatant liquid, combine these supernatant liquids, add diluted methanol (1 in 2) to make exactly 50 mL, and use this solution as the sample solution. Separately, use saikosaponin b_2 standard TS for assay as the standard solution. Perform the test with exactly 10 μL each of the sample solution and standard solution as directed under Liquid Chromatography <*2.01*> according to the following conditions, and determine the peak areas, A_T and A_S, of saikosaponin b_2 in each solution.

$$\text{Amount (mg) of saikosaponin } b_2 = C_S \times A_T/A_S \times 50$$

C_S: Concentration (mg/mL) of saikosaponin b_2 in saikosaponin b_2 standard TS for assay

Operating conditions—

Detector: An ultraviolet absorption photometer (wavelength: 254 nm).

Column: A stainless steel column 4.6 mm in inside diameter and 15 cm in length, packed with octadecylsilanized silica gel for liquid chromatography (5 μm in particle diameter).

Column temperature: A constant temperature of about 40°C.

Mobile phase: A mixture of 0.05 mol/L sodium dihydrogen phosphate TS and acetonitrile (5:3).

Flow rate: 1.0 mL per minute (the retention time of saikosaponin b_2 is about 12 minutes).

System suitability—

System performance: When the procedure is run with 10 μL of the standard solution under the above operating conditions, the number of theoretical plates and the symmetry factor of the peak of saikosaponin b_2 are not less than 5000 and not more than 1.5, respectively.

System repeatability: When the test is repeated 6 times with 10 μL of the standard solution under the above operating conditions, the relative standard deviation of the peak area of saikosaponin b_2 is not more than 1.5%.

(2) Baicalin—Weigh accurately about 0.1 g of the dry extract (or an amount of the viscous extract, equivalent to about 0.1 g of the dried substance), add exactly 50 mL of diluted methanol (7 in 10), shake for 15 minutes, filter, and use the filtrate as the sample solution. Separately, weigh accurately about 10 mg of Baicalin RS (separately determine the water <*2.48*> by coulometric titration, using 10 mg), dissolve in methanol to make exactly 100 mL. Pipet 5 mL of this solution, add diluted methanol (7 in 10) to make exactly

10 mL, and use this solution as the standard solution. Perform the test with exactly 10 μL each of the sample solution and standard solution as directed under Liquid Chromatography <*2.01*> according to the following conditions, and determine the peak areas, A_T and A_S, of baicalin in each solution.

$$\text{Amount (mg) of baicalin } (C_{21}H_{18}O_{11}) = M_S \times A_T/A_S \times 1/4$$

M_S: Amount (mg) of Baicalin RS taken, calculated on the anhydrous basis

Operating conditions—

Detector: An ultraviolet absorption photometer (wavelength: 277 nm).

Column: A stainless steel column 4.6 mm in inside diameter and 15 cm in length, packed with octadecylsilanized silica gel for liquid chromatography (5 μm in particle diameter).

Column temperature: A constant temperature of about 40°C.

Mobile phase: A mixture of diluted phosphoric acid (1 in 200) and acetonitrile (19:6).

Flow rate: 1.0 mL per minute (the retention time of baicalin is about 10 minutes).

System suitability—

System performance: When the procedure is run with 10 μL of the standard solution under the above operating conditions, the number of theoretical plates and the symmetry factor of the peak of baicalin are not less than 5000 and not more than 1.5, respectively.

System repeatability: When the test is repeated 6 times with 10 μL of the standard solution under the above operating conditions, the relative standard deviation of the peak area of baicalin is not more than 1.5%.

(3) Paeoniflorin—Weigh accurately about 0.5 g of the dry extract (or an amount of the viscous extract, equivalent to about 0.5 g of the dried substance), add exactly 50 mL of diluted methanol (1 in 2), shake for 15 minutes, and filter. Pipet 5 mL of the filtrate, flow through in a column packed with 2 g of polyamide for column chromatography, elute with 20 mL of water, add 1 mL of acetic acid (100), to the effluent, then add water to make exactly 25 mL, and use this as the sample solution. Separately, weigh accurately about 10 mg of Paeoniflorin RS (separately determine the water <*2.48*> by coulometric titration, using 10 mg), and dissolve in diluted methanol (1 in 2) to make exactly 100 mL. Pipet 5 mL of this solution, add diluted methanol (1 in 2) to make exactly 20 mL, and use this solution as the standard solution. Perform the test with exactly 10 μL each of the sample solution and standard solution as directed under Liquid Chromatography <*2.01*> according to the following conditions, and determine the peak areas, A_T and A_S, of paeoniflorin in each solution.

$$\text{Amount (mg) of paeoniflorin } (C_{23}H_{28}O_{11}) = M_S \times A_T/A_S \times 5/8$$

M_S: Amount (mg) of Paeoniflorin RS taken, calculated on the anhydrous basis

Operating conditions—

Detector: An ultraviolet absorption photometer (wavelength: 232 nm).

Column: A stainless steel column 4.6 mm in inside diameter and 15 cm in length, packed with octadecylsilanized silica gel for liquid chromatography (5 μm in particle diameter).

Column temperature: A constant temperature of about 20°C.

Mobile phase: A mixture of water, acetonitrile and phosphoric acid (850:150:1).

Flow rate: 1.0 mL per minute (the retention time of paeoniflorin is about 9 minutes).

System suitability—

System performance: Dissolve 1 mg each of Paeoniflorin RS and albiflorin in diluted methanol (1 in 2) to make 10 mL. When the procedure is run with 10 μL of this solution under the above operating conditions, albiflorin and paeoniflorin are eluted in this order with the resolution between these peaks being not less than 2.5.

System repeatability: When the test is repeated 6 times with 10 μL of the standard solution under the above operating conditions, the relative standard deviation of the peak area of paeoniflorin is not more than 1.5%.

Containers and storage Containers—Tight containers.

Digenea

Digenea

マクリ

Digenea is the whole algae of *Digenea simplex* C. Agardh (*Rhodomelaceae*).

Description Rounded, string-like algae, 2 - 3 mm in diameter; externally, dark red-purple to dark grayish red or grayish brown; a few branched rods irregularly forked, covered with short hairy twigs; calcified weeds and other small algae often attached.

Odor, seaweed-like; taste, disagreeable and slightly salty.

Identification To 2 g of pulverized Digenea add 10 mL of dilute ethanol, shake for 15 minutes, filter, and use the filtrate as the sample solution. Separately, dissolve 5 mg of kainic acid in 10 mL of dilute ethanol, and use this solution as the standard solution. Perform the test with these solutions as directed under Thin-layer Chromatography <*2.03*>. Spot 5 μL each of the sample solution and standard solution on a plate of silica gel for thin-layer chromatography. Develop the plate with a mixture of ethyl formate, water and formic acid (5:1:1) to a distance of about 7 cm, and air-dry the plate. Spray evenly ninhydrin-ethanol TS for spraying on the plate, and heat the plate at 105°C for 5 minutes: one of the several spots obtained from the sample solution has the same color tone and *R*f value with the spot from the standard solution.

Purity Foreign matter <*5.01*>—The amount of other algae in Digenea does not exceed 20.0%.

Loss on drying <*5.01*> Not more than 22.0%.

Acid-insoluble ash <*5.01*> Not more than 8.0%.

Containers and storage Containers—Well-closed containers.

Dioscorea Rhizome

Dioscoreae Rhizoma

サンヤク

Dioscorea Rhizome is the rhizome (rhizophore) of *Dioscorea japonica* Thunberg or *Dioscorea batatas* Decaisne (*Dioscoreaceae*), from which the periderm has been removed.

Description Cylindrical or irregular cylindrical rhizome, 5 – 15 cm in length, 1 – 4 cm in diameter, occasionally longitudinally split or transversely cut; externally whitish to yellowish white; fractured surface, whitish, smooth and powdery; hard in texture but breakable.

Practically odorless and tasteless.

Identification **(1)** To the cut surface of Dioscorea Rhizome add diluted iodine TS (1 in 50) dropwise: a dark purple to dark blue color develops.

(2) To 0.2 g of pulverized Dioscorea Rhizome add 2 mL of acetic anhydride, warm on a water bath for 2 minutes, and filter. To 1 mL of the filtrate add 0.5 mL of sulfuric acid carefully to make two layers: a red-brown to purple-brown color appears at the zone of contact.

(3) To 1 g of pulverized Dioscorea Rhizome add 4 mL of a mixture of methanol and water (4:1), shake for 10 minutes, centrifuge, and use the supernatant liquid as the sample solution. Separately, dissolve 1 mg of allantoin for thin-layer chromatography in 2 mL of a mixture of methanol and water (4:1), and use this solution as the standard solution. Perform the test with these solutions as directed under Thin-layer Chromatography <*2.03*>. Spot 5 μL of the sample solution and 2 μL of the standard solution on a plate of silica gel for thin-layer chromatography. Develop the plate with a mixture of ethyl acetate, methanol and water (7:3:1) to a distance of about 7 cm, and air-dry the plate. Spray evenly a solution of 0.2 g of 4-dimethylaminocinnamaldehyde in 10 mL of 6 mol/L hydrochloric acid TS and 10 mL of ethanol (99.5) on the plate, and heat the plate at 105°C for 2 minutes: one of the several spots obtained from the sample solution has the same color tone and *R*f value with the spot from the standard solution.

Purity **(1)** Heavy metals <*1.07*>—Proceed with 3.0 g of pulverized Dioscorea Rhizome according to Method 3, and perform the test. Prepare the control solution with 3.0 mL of Standard Lead Solution (not more than 10 ppm).

(2) Arsenic <*1.11*>—Prepare the test solution with 0.40 g of pulverized Dioscorea Rhizome according to Method 4, and perform the test (not more than 5 ppm).

Loss on drying <*5.01*> Not more than 14.0% (6 hours).

Total ash <*5.01*> Not more than 6.0%.

Acid-insoluble ash <*5.01*> Not more than 0.5%.

Containers and storage Containers—Well-closed containers.

Powdered Dioscorea Rhizome

Dioscoreae Rhizoma Pulveratum

サンヤク末

Powdered Dioscorea Rhizome is the powder of Dioscorea Rhizome.

Description Powdered Dioscorea Rhizome occurs as nearly yellowish white to white; odorless and tasteless.

Under a microscope <*5.01*>, Dioscorea rhizome powder reveals starch grains; fragments of parenchyma cells containing starch grains; raphides of calcium oxalate, 100 to 200 μm in length and its containing mucilage cells; ring and scalariform vessels, 15 to 35 μm in diameter; starch grain isosceles deltoid or oblong, solitary, 18 to 35 μm, hilum and striation being distinct.

Identification **(1)** To 0.2 g of Powdered Dioscorea Rhizome add 2 mL of acetic anhydride, warm on a water bath for 2 minutes, and filter. To 1 mL of the filtrate add carefully 0.5 mL of sulfuric acid to make two layers: a red-brown to purple-brown color develops at the zone of contact.

(2) To 1 g of Powdered Dioscorea Rhizome add 4 mL of a mixture of methanol and water (4:1), shake for 10 minutes, centrifuge, and use the supernatant liquid as the sample solution. Separately, dissolve 1 mg of allantoin for thin-layer chromatography in 2 mL of a mixture of methanol and water (4:1), and use this solution as the standard solution. Perform the test with these solutions as directed under Thin-layer Chromatography <*2.03*>. Spot 5 μL of the sample solution and 2 μL of the standard solution on a plate of silica gel for thin-layer chromatography. Develop the plate with a mixture of ethyl acetate, methanol and water (7:3:1) to a distance of about 7 cm, and air-dry the plate. Spray evenly a solution of 0.2 g of 4-dimethylaminocinnamaldehyde in 10 mL of 6 mol/L hydrochloric acid TS and 10 mL of ethanol (99.5) on the plate, and heat the plate at 105°C for 2 minutes: one of the several spots obtained from the sample solution has the same color tone and *R*f value with the spot from the standard solution.

Purity **(1)** Heavy metals <*1.07*>—Proceed with 3.0 g of Powdered Dioscorea Rhizome according to Method 3, and perform the test. Prepare the control solution with 3.0 mL of Standard Lead Solution (not more than 10 ppm).

(2) Arsenic <*1.11*>—Prepare the test solution with 0.40 g of Powdered Dioscorea Rhizome according to Method 4, and perform the test (not more than 5 ppm).

Loss on drying <*5.01*> Not more than 14.0% (6 hours).

Total ash <*5.01*> Not more than 6.0%.

Acid-insoluble ash <*5.01*> Not more than 0.5%.

Containers and storage Containers—Tight containers.

Dolichos Seed

Dolichi Semen

ヘンズ

Dolichos Seed is the seed of *Dolichos lablab* Linné (*Leguminosae*).

Description Flattened ellipsoidal to flattened orbicular-ovate seed, 9 - 14 mm in length, 6 - 10 mm in width, 4 - 7 mm in thickness; externally light yellowish white to light yellow, smooth and somewhat lustrous; caruncle white, like a half-moon, protrudent at one side; hard in texture.

Almost odorless; taste, slightly sweet and acid.

Under a microscope <*5.01*>, a transverse section reveals the outermost layer of seed coat composed of a single layer of palisade like epidermal cells coated with cuticle; beneath epidermis a single layer of sclerenchymatous and sandglass like cells; inside of the layer mentioned above parenchyma lie, the innermost portion of the parenchyma decayed; cotyledons occur inside of the seed coat; the outermost layer of cotyledon composed of a single layer of epidermal cells, inner part of cotyledon mainly parenchyma, containing aleurone grains and oil drops, and occasionally starch grains.

Identification To 3 g of pulverized Dolichos Seed add 30 mL of methanol, shake for 10 minutes, centrifuge, and take the supernatant liquid. Evaporate the solvent of the supernatant liquid, add 30 mL of water and 50 mL of ethyl acetate to the residue, shake, and take the ethyl acetate layer. To the ethyl acetate add 10 g of anhydrous sodium sulfate, shake, and filter. Evaporate the solvent of the filtrate, add 1 mL of ethyl acetate to the residue, and use this solution as the sample solution. Perform the test with the sample solution as directed under Thin-layer Chromatography <*2.03*>. Spot 20 μL of the sample solution on a plate of silica gel for thin-layer chromatography, develop the plate with a mixture of ethyl acetate and acetic acid (100) (100:1) to a distance of about 10 cm, and air-dry the plate. Examine under ultraviolet light (main wavelength: 365 nm): a blue-white fluorescent spot appears at an *R*f value of about 0.4.

Loss on drying <*5.01*> Not more than 14.0% (6 hours).

Total ash <*5.01*> Not more than 4.5%.

Extract content <*5.01*> Dilute ethanol-soluble extract: not less than 9.0%.

Containers and storage Containers—Well-closed containers.

Eleutherococcus Senticosus Rhizome

Eleutherococci senticosi Rhizoma

シゴカ

Eleutherococcus Senticosus Rhizome is the rhizome of *Eleutherococcus senticosus* Maximowicz (*Acanthopanax senticosus* Harms) (*Araliaceae*), often with root.

Description Slightly curved subcolumnar rhizome, 15 - 30 cm in length, 1 - 2.5 cm in diameter; externally grayish brown and slightly rough; transversely cut surface light brown, cortex thin, xylem thick with a pith in center; extremely hard in texture.

Odor, slightly characteristics; tasteless or slightly sweet, astringency.

Under a microscope <*5.01*>, a transverse section reveals the outermost layer consisting of a cork layer 3 - 7 cells thick; oil canals scattered in parenchyma; fiber bundles lined stepwise in phloem; phloem and xylem separated clearly by cambium; xylem composed of vessels, xylem fibers and xylem parenchyma; ray composed of 2 - 6 rows of cells; pith composed of parenchyma; parenchyma of cortex and ray contain aggregate crystals of calcium oxalate; occasionally starch grains in ray, parenchyma of cortex and xylem.

Identification To 0.5 g of pulverized Eleutherococcus Senticosus Rhizome add 20 mL of diluted methanol (1 in 2), shake for 15 minutes, centrifuge, and use the supernatant liquid as the sample solution. Separately, dissolve 1 mg of eleutheroside B for liquid chromatography in diluted methanol (1 in 2) to make 20 mL. To 2 mL of this solution add diluted methanol (1 in 2) to make 20 mL, and use this solution as the standard solution. Perform the test with 10 μL each of the sample solution and standard solution as directed under Liquid Chromatography <*2.01*> according to the following conditions: the peak corresponding to eleutheroside B in the chromatogram obtained from the sample solution shows the same retention time with the peak of eleutheroside B in the chromatogram from the standard solution.

Operating conditions—

Detector: An ultraviolet absorption photometer (wavelength: 265 nm).

Column: A stainless steel column 4.6 mm in inside diameter and 15 cm in length, packed with octadecylsilanized silica gel for liquid chromatography (5 μm in particle diameter).

Column temperature: A constant temperature of about 50°C.

Mobile phase: A mixture of water and acetonitrile (9:1).

Flow rate: Adjust so that the retention time of eleutheroside B is about 10 minutes.

System suitability—

System performance: When the procedure is run with 10 μL of the standard solution under the above operating conditions, the number of theoretical plates and the symmetry factor of the peak of eleutheroside B are not less than 5000 and not more than 1.5, respectively.

Purity (1) Heavy metals <*1.07*>—Proceed with 3.0 g of pulverized Eleutherococcus Senticosus Rhizome according to Method 3, and perform the test. Prepare the control solution with 3.0 mL of Standard Lead Solution (not more than 10 ppm).

(2) Arsenic <*1.11*>—Prepare the test solution with 0.40 g of pulverized Eleutherococcus Senticosus Rhizome according to Method 4, and perform the test (not more than 5 ppm).

Loss on drying <*5.01*> Not more than 13.0% (6 hours).

Total ash <*5.01*> Not more than 6.0%.

Acid-insoluble ash <*5.01*> Not more than 1.0%.

Extract content <*5.01*> Dilute ethanol-soluble extract: not less than 2.5%.

Containers and storage Containers—Well-closed containers.

Ephedra Herb

Ephedrae Herba

マオウ

Ephedra Herb is the terrestrial stem of *Ephedra sinica* Stapf, *Ephedra intermedia* Schrenk et C.A. Meyer or *Ephedra equisetina* Bunge (*Ephedraceae*).

Ephedra Herb contains not less than 0.7% of total alkaloids (as ephedrine and pseudoephedrine), calculated on the basis of dried material.

Description Thin cylindrical or ellipsoidal cylinder, 0.1 – 0.2 cm in diameter; 3 – 5 cm in length of internode; light green to yellow-green; numerous parallel vertical furrows on the surface; scaly leaves at the node portion; leaves, 0.2 – 0.4 cm in length, light brown to brown in color, usually being opposite at every node, adhering at the base to form a tubular sheath around the stem. Under a magnifying glass, the transverse section of the stem appears as circle and ellipse, the outer portion grayish green to yellow-green in color, and the center filled with a red-purple substance or hollow. When fractured at internode, the outer part is fibrous and easily split vertically.

Odor, slight; taste, astringent and slightly bitter, giving a slight sensation of numbness on the tongue.

Identification To 0.5 g of pulverized Ephedra Herb add 10 mL of methanol, shake for 2 minutes, filter, and use the filtrate as the sample solution. Perform the test with the sample solution as directed under Thin-layer Chromatography <2.03>. Spot 10 μL of the sample solution on a plate of silica gel for thin-layer chromatography. Develop the plate with a mixture of 1-butanol, water and acetic acid (100) (7:2:1) to a distance of about 7 cm, and air-dry the plate. Spray evenly ninhydrin-ethanol TS for spraying, and heat the plate at 105°C for 5 minutes: a red-purple spot appears at an *R*f value of about 0.35.

Purity (1) Woody stem—When perform the test of foreign matter <5.01>, the amount of the woody stems contained in Ephedra Herb does not exceed 5.0%.

(2) Foreign matter <5.01>—The amount of foreign matter other than woody stems contained in Ephedra Herb does not exceed 1.0%.

Loss on drying <5.01> Not more than 12.5% (6 hours).

Total ash <5.01> Not more than 11.0%.

Acid-insoluble ash <5.01> Not more than 2.0%.

Assay Weigh accurately about 0.5 g of moderately fine powder of Ephedra Herb, place in a glass-stoppered centrifuge tube, add 20 mL of diluted methanol (1 in 2), shake for 30 minutes, centrifuge, and separate the supernatant liquid. To the residue add 20 mL of diluted methanol (1 in 2), proceed in the same manner, and repeat this procedure twice. Combine all the extracts, add diluted methanol (1 in 2) to make exactly 100 mL, and use this solution as the sample solution. Separately, weigh accurately about 50 mg of ephedrine hydrochloride for assay of crude drugs, previously dried at 105°C for 3 hours, and dissolve in diluted methanol (1 in 2) to make exactly 20 mL. Pipet 2 mL of the solution, add diluted methanol (1 in 2) to make exactly 100 mL, and use this solution as the standard solution. Perform the test with exactly 10 μL each of the sample solution and standard solution as directed under Liquid Chromatography <2.01> according to the following conditions. Determine the peak areas, A_{TE} and A_{TP}, of ephedrine and pseudoephedrine (the relative retention time to ephedrine is about 0.9) obtained from the sample solution, and the peak area, A_S, of ephedrine obtained from the standard solution.

Amount (mg) of total alkaloids (ephedrine and pseudoephedrine)

$$= M_S \times (A_{TE} + A_{TP})/A_S \times 1/10 \times 0.819$$

M_S: Amount (mg) of ephedrine hydrochloride for assay of crude drugs taken

Operating conditions—

Detector: An ultraviolet absorption photometer (wavelength: 210 nm).

Column: A stainless steel column 4.6 mm in inside diameter and 15 cm in length, packed with octadecylsilanized silica gel for liquid chromatography (5 μm in particle diameter).

Column temperature: A constant temperature of about 40°C.

Mobile phase: To 5 g of sodium lauryl sulfate add 350 mL of acetonitrile, shake, and add 650 mL of water and 1 mL of phosphoric acid to dissolve lauryl sulfate.

Flow rate: Adjust so that the retention time of ephedrine is about 27 minutes.

System suitability—

System performance: Dissolve 1 mg of ephedrine hydrochloride for assay of crude drugs and 1 mg of pseudoephedrine hydrochloride in diluted methanol (1 in 2) to make 10 mL. When the procedure is run with 10 μL of this solution under the above operating conditions, pseudoephedrine and ephedrine are eluted in this order with the resolution between these peaks being not less than 1.5.

System repeatability: When the test is repeated 6 times with 10 μL of the standard solution under the above operating conditions, the relative standard deviation of the peak area of ephedrine is not more than 1.5%.

Containers and storage Containers—Well-closed containers.

Epimedium Herb

Epimedii Herba

インヨウカク

Epimedium Herb is the terrestrial part of *Epimedium koreanum* Nakai, *Epimedium grandiflorum* Morren var. *thunbergianum* Nakai, *Epimedium pubescens* Maximowicz, *Epimedium brevicornu* Maximowicz, *Epimedium wushanense* T. S. Ying, *Epimedium sagittatum* Maximowicz or *Epimedium sempervirens* Nakai (*Berberidaceae*).

Description Epimedium Herb is composed of a stem and a ternate to triternate compound leaf; leaflet ovate to broadly ovate or ovate-lanceolate, 3 – 20 cm in length, 2 – 8 cm in width, petiolule 1.5 – 7 cm in length, apex of leaflet acuminate, needle hair on margin 0.1 – 0.2 cm in length, base of leaflet cordate to deeply cordate, lateral leaflet asymmetry; upper surface green to green-brown, sometimes lustrous, lower surface light green to grayish green-brown, often pilose, especially on vein densely pilose, papery or coriaceous; petiole and stem cylindrical, light yellowish brown to slightly purplish and light green-brown, easily broken.

Odor, slight; taste, slightly bitter.

Under a microscope <5.01>, a transverse section of the leaf reveals 3 - 6 vascular bundles in midvein; mesophyll composed of upper epidermis, single-layered palisade, spongy tissue and lower epidermis; leaf margins orbicular or oblong, sclerenchymatous; multi-cellular hairs on epidermis; 8 - 20 vascular bundles in petiole and 6 - 15 vascular bundles in petiolule. Under a microscope <5.01>, a transverse section of the stem reveals a single to several-layered hypodermis, cortex of 4 - 10 cellular layers of sclerenchyma, vascular bundle 13 - 30 in number, oblong to obovate.

Identification To 2 g of pulverized Epimedium Herb add 20 mL of methanol, shake for 15 minutes, filter, and use the filtrate as the sample solution. Separately, dissolve 1 mg of icariin for thin-layer chromatography in 1 mL of methanol, and use this solution as the standard solution. Perform the test with these solutions as directed under Thin-layer Chromatography <2.03>. Spot 10 μL each of the sample solution and standard solution on a plate of silica gel with fluorescent indicator for thin-layer chromatography. Develop the plate with a mixture of ethyl acetate, ethanol (99.5) and water (8:2:1) to a distance of about 7 cm, and air-dry the plate. Examine under ultraviolet light (main wavelength: 254 nm): one of the several spots obtained from the sample solution has the same color tone and Rf value with the spot from the standard solution.

Loss on drying <5.01> Not more than 12.5% (6 hours).

Total ash <5.01> Not more than 8.5%.

Acid-insoluble ash <5.01> Not more than 2.0%.

Extract content <5.01> Dilute ethanol-soluble extract: not less than 17.0%.

Containers and storage Containers—Well-closed containers.

Eucalyptus Oil

Oleum Eucalypti

ユーカリ油

Eucalyptus Oil is the essential oil distilled with steam from the leaves of *Eucalyptus globulus* Labillardière or allied plants (*Myrtaceae*).

It contains not less than 70.0% of cineol.

Description Eucalyptus Oil is a clear, colorless or pale yellow liquid. It has a characteristic, aromatic odor and a pungent taste.

It is neutral.

Identification Shake 1 mL of Eucalyptus Oil vigorously with 1 mL of phosphoric acid, and allow to stand: the solution congeals within 30 minutes.

Refractive index <2.45> n_D^{20}: 1.458 - 1.470

Specific gravity <1.13> d_{20}^{20}: 0.907 - 0.927

Purity (1) Clarity of solution—Mix 1.0 mL of Eucalyptus Oil with 5 mL of diluted ethanol (7 in 10): the solution is clear.

(2) Heavy metals <1.07>—Proceed with 1.0 mL of Eucalyptus Oil according to Method 2, and perform the test. Prepare the control solution with 4.0 mL of Standard Lead Solution (not more than 40 ppm).

Assay Weigh accurately about 0.1 g each of Eucalyptus Oil and cineol for assay, and dissolve each in hexane to make exactly 25 mL. Pipet 5 mL each of these solutions, add exactly 5 mL of the internal standard solution to each, then add hexane to make 100 mL, and use these solutions as the sample solution and the standard solution, respectively. Perform the test with 2 μL each of the sample solution and standard solution as directed under Gas Chromatography <2.02> according to the following conditions. Calculate the ratios, Q_T and Q_S, of the peak area of cineol to that of the internal standard.

$$\text{Amount (mg) of cineol} = M_S \times Q_T/Q_S$$

M_S: Amount (mg) of cineol for assay taken

Internal standard solution—A solution of anisole in hexane (1 in 250).

Operating conditions—

Detector: A hydrogen flame-ionization detector.

Column: A glass column 3 mm in inside diameter and 5 m in length, packed with silanized porous silica gel for gas chromatography coated in 5% with alkylene glycol phthalate ester for gas chromatography (150 to 180 μm in particle diameter).

Column temperature: A constant temperature of about 120°C.

Carrier gas: Nitrogen.

Flow rate: Adjust so that the retention time of cineol is about 11 minutes.

System suitability—

System performance: Dissolve 0.1 g each of cineol for assay and limonene in 25 mL of hexane. To 1 mL of this solution add hexane to make 20 mL. When the procedure is run with 2 μL of this solution under the above operating conditions, limonene and cineol are eluted in this order with the resolution between these peaks being not less than 1.5.

System repeatability: When the test is repeated 6 times with 2 μL of the standard solution under the above operating conditions, the relative standard deviation of the ratio of the peak area of cineol to that of the internal standard is not more than 1.0%.

Containers and storage Containers—Tight containers.

Storage—Light-resistant.

Eucommia Bark

Eucommiae Cortex

トチュウ

Eucommia Bark is the bark of *Eucommia ulmoides* Oliver (*Eucommiaceae*).

Description Eucommia Bark is a semi-tubular or plate-like bark, 2 - 6 mm in thickness; externally pale grayish brown to grayish brown, and rough in texture, sometimes red-brown due to the cork layer falling off; internally dark violet, smooth and covered with a linear pattern that runs longitudinally, silk-like threads of gutta-percha (a thermoplastic rubber-like substance) appearing when broken.

It has a faint but characteristic odor and taste.

Under a microscope <5.01>, transverse section reveals parenchymatous cells containing gutta-percha; phloem with stone-cell and fiber layers; rays in rows of 2 - 3 cells; calcium oxalate crystals absent.

Identification Put 1 g of pulverized Eucommia Bark in a glass-stoppered centrifuge tube, add 10 mL of water and 20 mL of diethyl ether, shake for 15 minutes, and centrifuge. Take the diethyl ether layer so obtained, evaporate the solvent on a water bath, and add 1 mL of ethanol (99.5) to the residue: colloidal substances appear.

Loss on drying 〈*5.01*〉 Not more than 12.0% (6 hours).

Total ash 〈*5.01*〉 Not more than 8.0%.

Acid-insoluble ash 〈*5.01*〉 Not more than 5.0%.

Extract content 〈*5.01*〉 Dilute ethanol-soluble extract: not less than 7.0%.

Containers and storage Containers—Well-closed containers.

Euodia Fruit

Euodiae Fructus

ゴシュユ

Euodia Fruit is the fruit of *Euodia officinalis* Dode (*Evodia officinalis* Dode), *Euodia bodinieri* Dode (*Evodia bodinieri* Dode) or *Euodia ruticarpa* Hooker filius et Thomson (*Evodia rutaecarpa* Bentham) (Rutaceae).

Description Flattened spheroidal or globular fruit, 2 – 5 mm in diameter; externally dark brown to grayish brown, with many oil sacs appearing as hollow pits, and often with peduncle, 2 – 5 mm in length, covered densely with hairs; pericarp in matured split to five loculi, and each loculus containing obovoid or globular seeds of a lustrous brown to black-brown or bluish black color.

Odor, characteristic; taste, acrid, followed by a lasting bitterness.

Identification To 1.0 g of pulverized Euodia Fruit add 10 mL of methanol, shake for 10 minutes, centrifuge, and use the supernatant liquid as the sample solution. Perform the test with the sample solution as directed under Thin-layer Chromatography 〈*2.03*〉. Spot 10 μL of the sample solution on a plate of silica gel for thin-layer chromatography. Develop the plate with a mixture of acetone, 2-propanol, water and formic acid (7:7:1:1) to a distance of about 7 cm, and air-dry the plate. Examine under ultraviolet light (main wavelength: 365 nm): a blue-white fluorescent spot is observed at an *R*f value of about 0.6. The spot shows a yellow-red color after being sprayed evenly Dragendorff's TS for spraying.

Purity **(1)** Peduncle—The amount of peduncles contained in Euodia Fruit does not exceed 5.0%.

(2) Foreign matter 〈*5.01*〉—The amount of foreign matter other than peduncles contained in Euodia Fruit does not exceed 1.0%.

Total ash 〈*5.01*〉 Not more than 8.0%.

Containers and storage Containers—Well-closed containers.

Fennel

Foeniculi Fructus

ウイキョウ

Fennel is the fruit of *Foeniculum vulgare* Miller (*Umbelliferae*).

Description Cylindrical cremocarp, 3.5 – 8 mm in length, 1 – 2.5 mm in width; externally grayish yellow-green to grayish yellow; two mericarps closely attached with each other, and with five longitudinal ridges; cremocarp often with pedicel 2 – 10 mm in length.

Characteristic odor and taste.

Under a microscope 〈*5.01*〉, ridges near the ventral side are far protruded than those on the dorsal side; one large oil canal between each ridge, and two oil canals on the ventral side.

Identification To 0.5 g of pulverized Fennel add 10 mL of hexane, allow to stand for 5 minutes with occasional shaking, filter, and use the filtrate as the sample solution. Perform the test with the sample solution as directed under Thin-layer Chromatography 〈*2.03*〉. Spot 5 μL of the sample solution on a plate of silica gel with fluorescent indicator for thin-layer chromatography. Develop the plate with a mixture of hexane and ethyl acetate (20:1) to a distance of about 7 cm, and air-dry the plate. Examine under ultraviolet light (main wavelength: 254 nm): a spot with a dark purple color appears at an *R*f value of about 0.4.

Purity **(1)** Peduncle—When perform the test of foreign matter 〈*5.01*〉, the amount of peduncles contained in Fennel does not exceed 3.0%.

(2) Foreign matter 〈*5.01*〉—The amount of foreign matter other than the peduncle contained in Fennel does not exceed 1.0%.

Total ash 〈*5.01*〉 Not more than 10.0%.

Acid-insoluble ash 〈*5.01*〉 Not more than 1.5%.

Essential oil content 〈*5.01*〉 Perform the test with 50.0 g of pulverized Fennel: the volume of essential oil is not less than 0.7 mL.

Containers and storage Containers—Well-closed containers.

Powdered Fennel

Foeniculi Fructus Pulveratus

ウイキョウ末

Powdered Fennel is the powder of Fennel.

Description Powdered Fennel occurs as a greenish light brown to greenish brown, and is a characteristic odor and taste.

Under a microscope 〈*5.01*〉, Powdered Fennel reveals fragments of parenchyma cells of perisperm containing aleurone grain, fragments of parenchyma cells of endosperm containing fatty oil, fragments of sclerenchyma with characteristic simple pits, fragments of oil canal within yellow-brown material, fragments of endocarp shown scalariform, spiral vessels, fragments of epidermis or epidermis with stomata.

Identification To 0.5 g of Powdered Fennel add 10 mL of hexane, allow to stand for 5 minutes with occasional shaking, filter, and use the filtrate as the sample solution. Perform the test with the sample solution as directed under Thin-layer Chromatography <2.03>. Spot 5 μL of the sample solution on a plate prepared with silica gel with fluorescent indicator for thin-layer chromatography. Then develop the plate with a mixture of hexane and ethyl acetate (20:1) to a distance of about 7 cm, and air-dry the plate. Examine under ultraviolet light (main wavelength: 254 nm): a spot with dark purple color appears at an *R*f value of about 0.4.

Total ash <5.01> Not more than 10.0%.

Acid-insoluble ash <5.01> Not more than 1.5%.

Essential oil content <5.01> Perform the test with 50.0 g of Powdered Fennel: the volume of essential oil is not less than 0.45 mL.

Containers and storage Containers—Tight containers.

Fennel Oil

Oleum Foeniculi

ウイキョウ油

Fennel Oil is the essential oil distilled with steam from the fruit of *Foeniculum vulgare* Miller (*Umbelliferae*) or of *Illicium verum* Hooker filius (*Illiciaceae*).

Description Fennel Oil is a colorless to pale yellow liquid. It has a characteristic, aromatic odor and a sweet taste with a slight, bitter aftertaste.

It is miscible with ethanol (95) and with diethyl ether.

It is practically insoluble in water.

When cold, white crystals or crystalline masses may often separate from the oil.

Identification Dissolve 0.30 g of Fennel Oil in 20 mL of hexane, pipet 1 mL of this solution, add hexane to make exactly 10 mL, and use this solution as the sample solution. Perform the test with the sample solution as directed under Thin-layer Chromatography <2.03>. Spot 5 μL of the sample solution on a plate of silica gel with fluorescent indicator for thin-layer chromatography. Develop the plate with a mixture of hexane and ethyl acetate (20:1) to a distance of about 7 cm, and air-dry the plate. Examine under ultraviolet light (main wavelength: 254 nm): a spot with a dark purple color appears at the *R*f value of about 0.4.

Refractive index <2.45> n_D^{20}: 1.528 – 1.560

Specific gravity <1.13> d_{20}^{20}: 0.955 – 0.995

Purity **(1)** Clarity of solution—To 1.0 mL of Fennel Oil add 3 mL of ethanol (95): the solution is clear. To this solution add 7 mL of ethanol (95): the solution remains clear.

(2) Heavy metals <1.07>—Proceed with 1.0 mL of Fennel Oil according to Method 2, and perform the test. Prepare the control solution with 4.0 mL of Standard Lead Solution (not more than 40 ppm).

Containers and storage Containers—Tight containers.

Storage—Light-resistant.

Foeniculated Ammonia Spirit

アンモニア・ウイキョウ精

Method of preparation

Ammonia Water	170 mL
Fennel Oil	30 mL
Ethanol	a sufficient quantity
To make	1000 mL

Prepare as directed under Spirits, with the above ingredients. A sufficient quantity of ammonia solution (28) and Purified Water or Purified Water in Containers may be used in place of Ammonia Water.

Description Foeniculated Ammonia Spirit is a colorless to yellow liquid, having a characteristic odor. It has a slightly sweet, pungent taste.

Specific gravity d_{20}^{20}: about 0.85

Alcohol number <1.01> Not less than 7.8 (Method 2).

Containers and storage Containers—Tight containers.

Forsythia Fruit

Forsythiae Fructus

レンギョウ

Forsythia Fruit is the fruit of *Forsythia suspensa* Vahl (*Oleaceae*).

Description Ovoid to long ovoid capsule, 1.5 – 2.5 cm in length, 0.5 – 1 cm in width, with acute apex, and sometimes with a peduncle at the base; externally light gray to dark brown, scattered with light gray and small ridged dots, and with two longitudinal furrows; a capsule dehiscing along the longitudinal furrows has the apexes bent backward; the inner surface of dehisced pericarp is yellow-brown in color, with a longitudinal partition-wall in the middle; seeds, slender and oblong, 0.5 – 0.7 cm in length, and usually with a wing.

Odor, slight; taste, slightly bitter.

Identification To 1.0 g of pulverized Forsythia Fruit add 10 mL of methanol, shake for 10 minutes, centrifuge, and use the supernatant liquid as the sample solution. Perform the test with the sample solution as directed under Thin-layer Chromatography <2.03>. Spot 10 μL of the sample solution on a plate of silica gel for thin-layer chromatography. Develop the plate with a mixture of ethyl acetate, methanol and water (20:3:1) to a distance of about 7 cm, and air-dry the plate. Spray evenly 4-methoxybenzaldehyde-sulfuric acid TS on the plate, and heat the plate at 105°C for 5 minutes: a red-purple to red-brown spot is observed at an *R*f value of about 0.3.

Purity **(1)** Branchlet—When perform the test of foreign matter <5.01>, the amount of branchlets contained in Forsythia Fruit does not exceed 5.0%.

(2) Foreign matter <5.01>—The amount of foreign matter other than branchlets contained in Forsythia Fruit does not exceed 1.0%.

Total ash <5.01> Not more than 5.0%.

Extract content <5.01> Dilute ethanol-soluble extract: not less than 10.0%.

Containers and storage Containers—Well-closed containers.

Fritillaria Bulb

Fritillariae Bulbus

バイモ

Fritillaria Bulb is the bulb of *Fritillaria verticillata* Willdenow var. *thunbergii* Baker (*Liliaceae*).

Description Fritillaria Bulb is a depressed spherical bulb, 2 – 3 cm in diameter, 1 – 2 cm in height, consisting of 2 thickened scaly leaves often separated; externally and internally white to light yellow-brown in color; inside base is in a slightly dark color; the bulb sprinkled with lime before drying is dusted with white powder; fractured surface, white in color and powdery.

Odor, slight and characteristic; taste, bitter.

Under a microscope <*5.01*>, a transverse section reveals the outermost layer to be composed of an epidermis; numerous vascular bundles scattered throughout the parenchyma inside of the epidermis; parenchyma filled with starch grains; starch grains are mainly simple (rarely 2- to 3-compound), 5 – 60 μm in diameter, narrowly ovate to ovate or triangular to obovate, stratiform figure obvious; epidermal cells and parenchyma cells near the vessels contain solitary crystals of calcium oxalate.

Identification Put 2 g of pulverized Fritillaria Bulb in a glass-stoppered centrifuge tube, add 10 mL of ammonia TS and 20 mL of a mixture of ethyl acetate and diethyl ether (1:1), shake for 20 minutes, and centrifuge. Take the upper layer, add 20 g of anhydrous sodium sulfate to the layer, shake, and filter. Evaporate the solvent of the filtrate, dissolve the residue in 1 mL of ethanol (99.5), and use this solution as the sample solution. Perform the test with the sample solution as directed under Thin-layer Chromatography <*2.03*>. Spot 10 μL of the sample solution on a plate of silica gel for thin-layer chromatography, develop the plate with a mixture of ethyl acetate, methanol and ammonia solution (28) (17:2:1) to a distance of about 7 cm, and air-dry the plate. Spray evenly Dragendorff's TS for spraying on the plate: spots of a yellow-red color appear at *R*f values of about 0.4 and about 0.6.

Purity (1) Heavy metals <*1.07*>—Proceed with 3.0 g of pulverized Fritillaria Bulb according to Method 3, and perform the test. Prepare the control solution with 3.0 mL of Standard Lead Solution (not more than 10 ppm).

(2) Arsenic <*1.11*>—Prepare the test solution with 0.40 g of pulverized Fritillaria Bulb according to Method 4, and perform the test (not more than 5 ppm).

Loss on drying <*5.01*> Not more than 16.0% (6 hours).

Total ash <*5.01*> Not more than 6.5%.

Acid-insoluble ash <*5.01*> Not more than 1.0%.

Extract content <*5.01*> Dilute ethanol-soluble extract: not less than 8.0%.

Containers and storage Containers—Well-closed containers.

Gambir

Gambir

アセンヤク

Gambir is the dried aqueous extract prepared from the leaves and young twigs of *Uncaria gambir* Roxburgh (*Rubiaceae*).

Description Brown to dark brown, brittle mass; inside light brown.

Odor, slight; taste, extremely astringent and bitter.

Identification (1) To 0.2 g of pulverized Gambir add 10 mL of water, warm in a water bath for 5 minutes with occasional shaking, and filter. Cool the filtrate, and add 2 to 3 drops of gelatin TS: a white turbidity or precipitate is produced.

(2) Shake 0.1 g of pulverized Gambir with 20 mL of dilute ethanol for 2 minutes, and filter. Mix 1 mL of the filtrate with 9 mL of dilute ethanol, and to the solution add 1 mL of vanillin-hydrochloric acid TS: a light red to red-brown color develops.

Total ash <*5.01*> Not more than 6.0%.

Acid-insoluble ash <*5.01*> Not more than 1.5%.

Extract content <*5.01*> Dilute ethanol-soluble extract: not less than 70.0%.

Containers and storage Containers—Well-closed containers.

Powdered Gambir

Gambir Pulveratum

アセンヤク末

Powdered Gambir is the powder of Gambir.

Description Powdered Gambir occurs as a red-brown to dark brown powder. It has a slight odor, and an extremely astringent and bitter taste.

Under a microscope <*5.01*>, Powdered Gambir, immersed in olive oil or liquid paraffin, consists of masses of needle crystals or yellow-brown to red-brown angular fragments, and reveals epidermal tissue and thick-walled hairs.

Identification (1) To 0.2 g of Powdered Gambir add 10 mL of water, warm in a water bath for 5 minutes with occasional shaking, and filter. Cool the filtrate, and add 2 to 3 drops of gelatin TS: a white turbidity or precipitate is produced.

(2) Shake 0.1 g of Powdered Gambir with 20 mL of dilute ethanol for 2 minutes, and filter. Mix 1 mL of the filtrate with 9 mL of dilute ethanol, and to the solution add 1 mL of vanillin-hydrochloric acid TS: a light red to red-brown color develops.

Total ash <*5.01*> Not more than 6.0%.

Acid-insoluble ash <*5.01*> Not more than 1.5%.

Extract content <*5.01*> Dilute ethanol-soluble extract: not less than 70.0%.

Containers and storage Containers—Well-closed contain-

ers.

Gardenia Fruit

Gardeniae Fructus

サンシシ

Gardenia Fruit is the fruit of *Gardenia jasminoides* Ellis (*Rubiaceae*), sometimes after being passed through hot water or steamed.

It contains not less than 2.7% of geniposide, calculated on the basis of dried material.

Description Nearly long ovoid to ovoid fruit, 1 - 5 cm in length, 1 - 1.5 cm in width; externally yellow-brown to yellow-red, usually having 6, rarely 5 or 7, markedly raised ridges; calyx or its scar at one end, and sometimes peduncle at the other end; inner surface of pericarp yellow-brown, smooth and lustrous; internally divided into two loculi, containing a mass of seeds in yellow-red to dark red placenta; seed nearly circular, flat, about 0.5 cm in major axis, black-brown or yellow-red.

Odor, slight; taste, bitter.

Identification **(1)** To 1.0 g of pulverized Gardenia Fruit, previously dried in a desiccator (silica gel) for 24 hours, add 100 mL of hot water, warm the mixture between 60°C and 70°C for 30 minutes with frequent shaking, and filter after cooling. To 1.0 mL of the filtrate add water to make 10 mL: the color of the resulting solution is yellow and is not lighter than that of the following control solution.

Control solution: Dissolve 9.8 mg of carbazochrome sodium sulfonate trihydrate in water to make exactly 10 mL. Pipet 1 mL of this solution, and add water to make exactly 50 mL.

(2) To 1.0 g of pulverized Gardenia Fruit add 20 mL of methanol, warm for 3 minutes on a water bath, cool, filter, and use the filtrate as the sample solution. Separately, dissolve 1 mg of geniposide for thin-layer chromatography in 1 mL of methanol, and use this solution as the standard solution. Perform the test with these solutions as directed under Thin-layer Chromatography <*2.03*>. Spot 5 μL each of the sample solution and standard solution on a plate of silica gel for thin-layer chromatography. Develop the plate with a mixture of ethyl acetate and methanol (3:1) to a distance of about 7 cm, and air-dry the plate. Spray evenly 4-methoxybenzaldehyde-sulfuric acid TS on the plate, and heat the plate at 105°C for 10 minutes: one of the several spots obtained from the sample solution has the same color tone and *Rf* value with the spot from the standard solution.

Loss on drying <*5.01*> Not more than 13.0%.

Total ash <*5.01*> Not more than 6.0%.

Assay Weigh accurately about 0.5 g of pulverized Gardenia Fruit, transfer into a glass-stoppered centrifuge tube, add 40 mL of diluted methanol (1 in 2), shake for 15 minutes, centrifuge, and take the supernatant liquid. To the residue add 40 mL of diluted methanol (1 in 2), and repeat the same procedure as above. Combine the extracts so obtained, and add diluted methanol (1 in 2) to make exactly 100 mL. Pipet 5 mL of the solution, add methanol to make exactly 20 mL, use this solution as the sample solution. Separately, weigh accurately about 10 mg of geniposide for assay, and dissolve in methanol to make exactly 100 mL. Pipet 5 mL of the solution, add methanol to make exactly 10 mL, and use this solution as the standard solution. Perform the test with exactly 10 μL each of the sample solution and standard solution as directed under Liquid Chromatography <*2.01*> according to the following conditions, and determine the peak areas, A_T and A_S, of geniposide in each solution.

$$\text{Amount (mg) of geniposide} = M_S \times A_T/A_S \times 2$$

M_S: Amount (mg) of geniposide for assay taken, calculated on the basis of the content obtained by qNMR

Operating conditions—

Detector: An ultraviolet absorption photometer (wavelength: 240 nm).

Column: A stainless steel column 6 mm in inside diameter and 15 cm in length, packed with octadecylsilanized silica gel for liquid chromatography (5 μm in particle diameter).

Column temperature: A constant temperature of about 30°C.

Mobile phase: A mixture of water and acetonitrile (22:3).

Flow rate: Adjust so that the retention time of geniposide is about 15 minutes.

System suitability—

System performance: Dissolve 1 mg each of geniposide for assay and caffeine in methanol to make 15 mL. When the procedure is run with 10 μL of this solution under the above operating conditions, caffeine and geniposide are eluted in this order with the resolution between these peaks being not less than 3.5.

System repeatability: When the test is repeated 6 times with 10 μL of the standard solution under the above operating conditions, the relative standard deviation of the peak area of geniposide is not more than 1.5%.

Containers and storage Containers—Well-closed containers.

Powdered Gardenia Fruit

Gardeniae Fructus Pulveratus

サンシシ末

Powdered Gardenia Fruit is the powder of Gardenia Fruit.

It contains not less than 2.7% of geniposide, calculated on the basis of dried material.

Description Powdered Gardenia Fruit occurs as a yellow-brown powder, and has a slight odor and a bitter taste.

Under a microscope <*5.01*>, Powdered Gardenia Fruit reveals fragments of yellow-brown epidermis consisting of polygonal epidermal cells in surface view; unicellular hairs, spiral and ring vessels, stone cells often containing crystals of calcium oxalate; fragments of thin-walled parenchyma containing yellow pigments, oil drops and rosette aggregates of calcium oxalate (the above elements from fruit receptacle and pericarp); fragments of large and thick-walled epidermis of seed coat, containing a red-brown substance; fragments of endosperm filled with aleuron grains (the above elements from seed).

Identification **(1)** To 1.0 g of Powdered Gardenia Fruit, previously dried in a desiccator (silica gel) for 24 hours, add 100 mL of hot water, warm the mixture between 60°C and 70°C for 30 minutes with frequent shaking, and filter after cooling. To 1.0 mL of the filtrate add water to make 10 mL: the color of the resulting solution is yellow and is not lighter than that of the following control solution.

Control solution: Dissolve 9.8 mg of carbazochrome sodium sulfonate trihydrate in water to make exactly 10 mL. Pipet 1 mL of this solution, and add water to make exactly 50 mL.

(2) To 1.0 g of Powdered Gardenia Fruit add 20 mL of methanol, warm for 3 minutes on a water bath, cool, filter, and use the filtrate as the sample solution. Separately, dissolve 1 mg of geniposide for thin-layer chromatography in 1 mL of methanol, and use this solution as the standard solution. Perform the test with these solutions as directed under Thin-layer Chromatography <2.03>. Spot 5 μL each of the sample solution and standard solution on a plate of silica gel for thin-layer chromatography. Develop the plate with a mixture of ethyl acetate and methanol (3:1) to a distance of about 7 cm, and air-dry the plate. Spray evenly 4-methoxybenzaldehyde-sulfuric acid TS on the plate, and heat the plate at 105°C for 10 minutes: one of the several spots obtained from the sample solution has the same color tone and *Rf* value with the spot from the standard solution.

Loss on drying <5.01> Not more than 13.0%.

Total ash <5.01> Not more than 6.0%.

Assay Weigh accurately about 0.5 g of Powdered Gardenia Fruit, transfer into a glass-stoppered centrifuge tube, add 40 mL of diluted methanol (1 in 2), shake for 15 minutes, centrifuge, and take the supernatant liquid. To the residue add 40 mL of diluted methanol (1 in 2), and repeat the same procedure as above. Combine the extracts so obtained, and add diluted methanol (1 in 2) to make exactly 100 mL. Pipet 5 mL of the solution, add methanol to make exactly 20 mL, use this solution as the sample solution. Separately, weigh accurately about 10 mg of geniposide for assay, and dissolve in methanol to make exactly 100 mL. Pipet 5 mL of the solution, add methanol to make exactly 10 mL, and use this solution as the standard solution. Perform the test with exactly 10 μL each of the sample solution and standard solution as directed under Liquid Chromatography <2.01> according to the following conditions, and determine the peak areas, A_T and A_S, of geniposide in each solution.

$$\text{Amount (mg) of geniposide} = M_S \times A_T/A_S \times 2$$

M_S: Amount (mg) of geniposide for assay taken, calculated on the basis of the content obtained by qNMR

Operating conditions—

Detector: An ultraviolet absorption photometer (wavelength: 240 nm).

Column: A stainless steel column 6 mm in inside diameter and 15 cm in length, packed with octadecylsilanized silica gel for liquid chromatography (5 μm in particle diameter).

Column temperature: A constant temperature of about 30°C.

Mobile phase: A mixture of water and acetonitrile (22:3).

Flow rate: Adjust so that the retention time of geniposide is about 15 minutes.

System suitability—

System performance: Dissolve 1 mg each of geniposide for assay and caffeine in methanol to make 15 mL. When the procedure is run with 10 μL of this solution under the above operating conditions, caffeine and geniposide are eluted in this order with the resolution between these peaks being not less than 3.5.

System repeatability: When the test is repeated 6 times with 10 μL of the standard solution under the above operating conditions, the relative standard deviation of the peak area of geniposide is not more than 1.5%.

Containers and storage Containers—Well-closed containers.

Gastrodia Tuber

Gastrodiae Tuber

テンマ

Gastrodia Tuber is the tuber of *Gastrodia elata* Blume (*Orchidaceae*), after being passed through hot water or steamed.

Description Gastrodia Tuber is an irregularly curved and flattened cylindrical to flattened fusiform tuber, 5 – 15 cm in length, 2 – 5 cm in diameter, 1 – 2 cm in thickness; externally light yellow-brown to light yellow-white; with ring nodes, and irregular longitudinal wrinkles; hard in texture; fractured surface, dark brown to yellow-brown in color, with luster, horny and gluey.

Odor, characteristic; practically tasteless.

Under a microscope <5.01>, a transverse section reveals parenchyma cells containing raphides of calcium oxalate; starch grain absent.

Identification To 1 g of pulverized Gastrodia Tuber add 5 mL of methanol, shake for 15 minutes, and filter. Evaporate the filtrate to dryness, dissolve the residue in 1 mL of methanol, and use this solution as the sample solution. Perform the test with the sample solution as directed under Thin-layer Chromatography <2.03>. Spot 10 μL of the sample solution on a plate of silica gel for thin-layer chromatography, develop the plate with a mixture of ethyl acetate, methanol and water (8:2:1) to a distance of about 7 cm, and air-dry the plate. Spray evenly dilute sulfuric acid on the plate, and heat the plate at 105°C for 5 minutes: a red-purple to light brown spot appears at an *Rf* value of about 0.4.

Purity **(1)** Heavy metals <1.07>—Proceed with 3.0 g of pulverized Gastrodia Tuber according to Method 3, and perform the test. Prepare the control solution with 3.0 mL of Standard Lead Solution (not more than 10 ppm).

(2) Arsenic <1.11>—Prepare the test solution with 0.40 g of pulverized Gastrodia Tuber according to Method 4, and perform the test (not more than 5 ppm).

Loss on drying <5.01> Not more than 16.0% (6 hours).

Total ash <5.01> Not more than 4.0%.

Extract content <5.01> Dilute ethanol-soluble extract: not less than 16.0%.

Containers and storage Containers—Well-closed containers.

Gentian

Gentianae Radix

ゲンチアナ

Gentian is the root and rhizome of *Gentiana lutea* Linné (*Gentianaceae*).

Description Nearly cylindrical pieces, 10 – 50 cm in length, 2 – 4 cm in diameter; externally dark brown; the rhizome short, with fine, transverse wrinkles, and sometimes with buds and remains of leaves at the upper edge. The root longitudinally and deeply wrinkled, and more or less twisted; fractured surface yellow-brown and not fibrous, and a cambium and its neighborhood tinged dark brown.

Odor, characteristic; taste, sweet at first, later persistently bitter.

Under a microscope <*5.01*>, a transverse section of the root reveals several cellular layers of collenchyma adjoined internally to 4 to 6 cellular layers of thin-walled cork; secondary cortex with irregularly distributed phloem; xylem consisting chiefly of parenchyma, with individual or clustered vessels and tracheids, and exhibiting some sieve tubes of xylem; parenchyma of the xylem and the cortex containing oil droplets, minute needle crystals of calcium oxalate and very rarely starch grains 10 - 20 μm in diameter.

Identification (1) Place 0.1 g of pulverized Gentian, previously dried in a desiccator (silica gel) for 48 hours, on a slide glass, put a glass ring 10 mm in both inside diameter and in height on it, then cover with another slide, and heat gently and gradually: pale yellow crystals are sublimed on the upper slide. The crystals are insoluble in water and in ethanol (95), and soluble in potassium hydroxide TS.

(2) To 0.5 g of pulverized Gentian add 10 mL of methanol, shake for 5 minutes, filter, and use the filtrate as the sample solution. Separately, dissolve 1 mg of gentiopicroside for thin-layer chromatography in 1 mL of methanol, and use this solution as the standard solution. Perform the test with these solutions as directed under Thin-layer Chromatography <*2.03*>. Spot 10 μL each of the sample solution and standard solution on a plate of silica gel with fluorescent indicator for thin-layer chromatography. Develop the plate with a mixture of ethyl acetate, ethanol (99.5) and water (8:2:1) to a distance of about 10 cm, and air-dry the plate. Examine under ultraviolet light (main wavelength: 254 nm): one of the several spots obtained from the sample solution and a spot from the standard solution show the same color tone and the same *R*f value.

Purity (1) Heavy metals <*1.07*>—Proceed with 1.0 g of pulverized Gentian according to Method 3, and perform the test. Prepare the control solution with 2.0 mL of Standard Lead Solution (not more than 20 ppm).

(2) Arsenic <*1.11*>—Prepare the test solution with 0.40 g of pulverized Gentian according to Method 4, and perform the test (not more than 5 ppm).

Total ash <*5.01*> Not more than 6.0%.

Acid-insoluble ash <*5.01*> Not more than 3.0%.

Containers and storage Containers—Well-closed containers.

Powdered Gentian

Gentianae Radix Pulverata

ゲンチアナ末

Powdered Gentian is the powder of Gentian.

Description Powdered Gentian occurs as a yellow-brown powder, and has a characteristic odor. It has a sweet taste at first, which later becomes persistently bitter.

Under a microscope <*5.01*>, Powdered Gentian reveals parenchyma cells containing oil droplets and minute needle crystals, vessels, tracheids, cork tissues, and crystals of calcium oxalate. Vessels are chiefly reticulate vessels and scalariform vessels, 20 - 80 μm in diameter. Starch grains are observed very rarely, in simple grains about 10 - 20 μm in diameter.

Identification (1) Place 0.1 g of Powdered Gentian, previously dried in a desiccator (silica gel) for 48 hours, on a slide glass, put a glass ring 10 mm in both inside diameter and in height on it, then cover with another slide glass, and heat gently and gradually: light yellow crystals are sublimed on the upper glass. The crystals are insoluble in water and in ethanol (95), and soluble in potassium hydroxide TS.

(2) To 0.5 g of Powdered Gentian add 10 mL of methanol, shake for 5 minutes, filter, and use the filtrate as the sample solution. Separately, dissolve 1 mg of gentiopicroside for thin-layer chromatography in 1 mL of methanol, and use this solution as the standard solution. Perform the test with these solutions as directed under Thin-layer Chromatography <*2.03*>. Spot 10 μL each of the sample solution and standard solution on a plate of silica gel with fluorescent indicator for thin-layer chromatography. Develop the plate with a mixture of ethyl acetate, ethanol (99.5) and water (8:2:1) to a distance of about 10 cm, and air-dry the plate. Examine under ultraviolet light (main wavelength: 254 nm): one of the several spots obtained from the sample solution and a spot from the standard solution show the same color tone and the same *R*f value.

Purity (1) Heavy metals <*1.07*>—Proceed with 1.0 g of Powdered Gentian according to Method 3, and perform the test. Prepare the control solution with 2.0 mL of Standard Lead Solution (not more than 20 ppm).

(2) Arsenic <*1.11*>—Prepare the test solution with 0.40 g of Powdered Gentian according to Method 4, and perform the test (not more than 5 ppm).

(3) Foreign matter—Under a microscope <*5.01*>, stone cell and fiber are not observed.

Total ash <*5.01*> Not more than 6.0%.

Acid-insoluble ash <*5.01*> Not more than 3.0%.

Containers and storage Containers—Tight containers.

Gentian and Sodium Bicarbonate Powder

ゲンチアナ・重曹散

Method of preparation

Powdered Gentian	300 g
Sodium Bicarbonate	700 g
To make	1000 g

Prepare as directed under Powders, with the above ingredients.

Description Gentian and Sodium Bicarbonate Powder occurs as a light yellow-brown powder, and has a bitter taste.

Identification (1) To 2 g of Gentian and Sodium Bicarbonate Powder add 10 mL of water, stir, and filter: the filtrate responds to the Qualitative Tests <*1.09*> (1) for bicarbonate.

(2) To 1.5 g of Gentian and Sodium Bicarbonate Powder add 10 mL of methanol, shake for 5 minutes, filter, and use the filtrate as the sample solution. Separately, dissolve 1 mg of gentiopicroside for thin-layer chromatography in 1 mL of

methanol, and use this solution as the standard solution. Perform the test with these solutions as directed under Thin-layer Chromatography <*2.03*>. Spot 5 μL each of the sample solution and standard solution on a plate of silica gel with fluorescent indicator for thin-layer chromatography. Develop the plate with a mixture of ethyl acetate, ethanol (99.5) and water (8:2:1) to a distance of about 10 cm, and air-dry the plate. Examine under ultraviolet light (main wavelength: 254 nm): one of the several spots obtained from the sample solution and a spot from the standard solution show the same color tone and the same *R*f value.

Containers and storage Containers—Well-closed containers.

Geranium Herb

Geranii Herba

ゲンノショウコ

Geranium Herb is the terrestrial part of *Geranium thunbergii* Siebold et Zuccarini (*Geraniaceae*).

Description Stem with leaves opposite; stem, slender and long, green-brown; stem and leaf covered with soft hairs; leaf divided palmately into 3 to 5 lobes, and 2 - 4 cm in length, grayish yellow-green to grayish brown; each lobe oblong to obovate, and its upper margin crenate.

Odor, slight; taste, astringent.

Identification Boil 0.1 g of Geranium Herb with 10 mL of water, filter, and to the filtrate add 1 drop of iron (III) chloride TS: a blackish blue color develops.

Purity Foreign matter <*5.01*>—The amount of the root and other foreign matter contained in Geranium Herb does not exceed 2.0%.

Total ash <*5.01*> Not more than 10.0%.

Acid-insoluble ash <*5.01*> Not more than 1.5%.

Extract content <*5.01*> Dilute ethanol-soluble extract: not less than 15.0%.

Containers and storage Containers—Well-closed containers.

Powdered Geranium Herb

Geranii Herba Pulverata

ゲンノショウコ末

Powdered Geranium Herb is the powder of Geranium Herb.

Description Powdered Geranium Herb occurs as a grayish green to light yellow-brown powder. It has a slight odor and an astringent taste.

Under a microscope <*5.01*>, Powdered Geranium Herb reveals mainly fibers, spiral vessels, pitted vessels, and unicellular hairs; furthermore, multicellular glandular hairs, epidermis with stomata, fragments of palisade tissue, rosette aggregates of calcium oxalate, and starch grains. Fiber is thick-walled, with somewhat distinct pits; unicellular hair shows small point-like protrusions on the surface; palisade tissue consisting of circular parenchyma cells in surface view, each cell containing one rosette aggregate of calcium oxalate which is about 20 μm in diameter. Starch grains consisting of simple grains but rarely of 2-compound grains, ovoid to spherical, 5 - 30 μm in diameter, with distinct hilum.

Identification Boil 0.1 g of Powdered Geranium Herb with 10 mL of water, filter, and to the filtrate add 1 drop of iron (III) chloride TS: a dark blue color develops.

Purity Foreign matter—Under a microscope <*5.01*>, Powdered Geranium Herb reveals no stone cells.

Total ash <*5.01*> Not more than 10.0%.

Acid-insoluble ash <*5.01*> Not more than 1.5%.

Extract content <*5.01*> Dilute ethanol-soluble extract: not less than 15.0%.

Containers and storage Containers—Well-closed containers.

Ginger

Zingiberis Rhizoma

ショウキョウ

Ginger is the rhizome, with (unpeeled) or without (peeled) the periderm, of *Zingiber officinale* Roscoe (*Zingiberaceae*).

It contains not less than 0.3% of [6]-gingerol, calculated on the basis of dried material.

Description Irregularly compressed and often branched massive rhizome or a part of it; the branched parts are slightly curved ovoid or oblong-ovoid, 2 - 4 cm in length, and 1 - 2 cm in diameter; external surface grayish white to light grayish brown, and often with white powder; fractured surface is somewhat fibrous, powdery, light yellowish brown; under a magnifying glass, a transverse section reveals cortex and stele distinctly divided; vascular bundles and secretes scattered all over the surface as small dark brown dots.

Odor, characteristic; taste, extremely pungent.

Under a microscope <*5.01*>, a transverse section reveals cork layer, cortex, endodermis and stele in this order from the outside, cork layer often peeled off; cortex and stele, divided by an endodermis, composed of parenchyma; vascular bundles surrounded by fibers scattered in cortex and stele; oil cells contain yellow oily substances, scattered in parenchyma; parenchyma cells contain solitary crystals of calcium oxalate; starch grains in parenchyma cells mainly simple, ovoid, triangular ovoid, ellipsoidal or spherical, with abaxial hilum, usually 10 - 30 μm in long axis.

Identification To 2 g of pulverized Ginger add 5 mL of diethyl ether, shake for 10 minutes, filter, and use the filtrate as the sample solution. Separately, dissolve 1 mg of [6]-gingerol for thin-layer chromatography in 2 mL of methanol, and use this solution as the standard solution. Perform the test with these solutions as directed under Thin-layer Chromatography <*2.03*>. Spot 10 μL each of the sample solution and standard solution on a plate of silica gel for thin-layer chromatography. Develop the plate with a mixture of ethyl acetate and hexane (1:1) to a distance of about 7 cm, and air-dry the plate. Spray evenly 4-dimethylaminobenzaldehyde TS for spraying on the plate, heat the plate at 105°C for 5 minutes, and allow to cool: one of the several spots obtained from the sample solution and the spot from the standard solution show the same color tone and *R*f value.

Purity (1) Heavy metals <*1.07*>—Proceed with 3.0 g of pulverized Ginger according to Method 3, and perform the test. Prepare the control solution with 3.0 mL of Standard Lead Solution (not more than 10 ppm).

(2) Arsenic <*1.11*>—Prepare the test solution with 0.40 g of pulverized Ginger according to Method 4, and perform the test (not more than 5 ppm).

Total ash <*5.01*> Not more than 8.0%.

Assay Weigh accurately about 1 g of pulverized Ginger (separately determine the loss on drying <*5.01*>, at 105°C for 5 hours), place in a centrifuge tube, add 30 mL of a mixture of methanol and water (3:1), shake for 20 minutes, centrifuge, and separate the supernatant liquid. To the residue add 30 mL of a mixture of methanol and water (3:1), and repeat the extraction twice more. To the combined all extracts add a mixture of methanol and water (3:1) to make exactly 100 mL, use this solution as the sample solution. Separately, weigh accurately about 5 mg of [6]-gingerol for assay, dissolve in a mixture of methanol and water (3:1) to make exactly 100 mL, and use this solution as the standard solution. Perform the test with exactly 10 μL each of the sample solution and standard solution as directed under Liquid Chromatography <*2.01*> according to the following conditions, and determine the peak areas, A_T and A_S, of [6]-gingerol in each solution.

$$\text{Amount (mg) of [6]-gingerol} = M_S \times A_T/A_S$$

M_S: Amount (mg) of [6]-gingerol for assay taken

Operating conditions—

Detector: An ultraviolet absorption photometer (wavelength: 205 nm).

Column: A stainless steel column 4.6 mm in inside diameter and 15 cm in length, packed with octadecylsilanized silica gel for liquid chromatography (5 μm in particle diameter).

Column temperature: A constant temperature of about 40°C.

Mobile phase: A mixture of water and acetonitrile and phosphoric acid (3800:2200:1).

Flow rate: Adjust so that the retention time of [6]-gingerol is about 19 minutes.

System suitability—

System performance: When the procedure is run with 10 μL of the standard solution under the above operating conditions, the number of theoretical plates and the symmetry factor of the peak of [6]-gingerol are not less than 5000 and not more than 1.5, respectively.

System repeatability: When the test is repeated 6 times with 10 μL of the standard solution under the above operating conditions, the relative standard deviation of the peak area of [6]-gingerol is not more than 1.5%.

Containers and storage Containers—Well-closed containers.

Powdered Ginger

Zingiberis Rhizoma Pulveratum

ショウキョウ末

Powdered Ginger is the powder of Ginger.

It contains not less than 0.20% of [6]-gingerol, calculated on the basis of dried material.

Description Powdered Ginger occurs as a light grayish brown to light grayish yellow powder. It has a characteristic odor and an extremely pungent taste.

Under a microscope <*5.01*>, Powdered Ginger reveals mainly starch grains and parenchyma cells containing them; also, parenchyma cells containing yellow-brown to dark brown oily substances or single crystals of calcium oxalate; fragments of fibers with distinct pits; fragments of spiral, ring and reticulate vessels, and rarely fragments of cork tissue; starch grains composed of simple, compound or half-compound grains, ovoid, triangular ovoid, ellipsoidal or spherical, with abaxial hilum, usually 10 - 30 μm in long axis.

Identification To 2 g of Powdered Ginger add 5 mL of diethyl ether, shake for 10 minutes, filter, and use the filtrate as the sample solution. Separately, dissolve 1 mg of [6]-gingerol for thin-layer chromatography in 2 mL of methanol, and use this solution as the standard solution. Perform the test with these solutions as directed under Thin-layer Chromatography <*2.03*>. Spot 10 μL each of the sample solution and standard solution on a plate of silica gel for thin-layer chromatography. Develop the plate with a mixture of ethyl acetate and hexane (1:1) to a distance of about 7 cm, and air-dry the plate. Spray evenly 4-dimethylaminobenzaldehyde TS for spraying on the plate, heat the plate at 105°C for 5 minutes, and allow to cool: one of the several spots obtained from the sample solution and the spot from the standard solution show the same color tone and *R*f value.

Purity (1) Heavy metals <*1.07*>—Proceed with 3.0 g of Powdered Ginger according to Method 3, and perform the test. Prepare the control solution with 3.0 mL of Standard Lead Solution (not more than 10 ppm).

(2) Arsenic <*1.11*>—Prepare the test solution with 0.40 g of Powdered Ginger according to Method 4, and perform the test (not more than 5 ppm).

(3) Foreign matter—Under a microscope <*5.01*>, Powdered Ginger does not show stone cells, lignified parenchyma cells and other foreign matter.

Total ash <*5.01*> Not more than 8.0%.

Assay Weigh accurately about 1 g of Powdered Ginger (separately determine the loss on drying <*5.01*>, at 105°C for 5 hours), place in a centrifuge tube, add 30 mL of a mixture of methanol and water (3:1), shake for 20 minutes, centrifuge, and separate the supernatant liquid. To the residue add 30 mL of a mixture of methanol and water (3:1), and repeat the extraction twice more. To the combined all extracts add a mixture of methanol and water (3:1) to make exactly 100 mL, use this solution as the sample solution. Separately, weigh accurately about 5 mg of [6]-gingerol for assay, dissolve in a mixture of methanol and water (3:1) to make exactly 100 mL, and use this solution as the standard solution. Perform the test with exactly 10 μL each of the sample solution and standard solution as directed under Liquid Chromatography <*2.01*> according to the following conditions, and determine the peak areas, A_T and A_S, of [6]-gingerol in each solution.

$$\text{Amount (mg) of [6]-gingerol} = M_S \times A_T/A_S$$

M_S: Amount (mg) of [6]-gingerol for assay taken

Operating conditions—

Detector: An ultraviolet absorption photometer (wavelength: 205 nm).

Column: A stainless steel column 4.6 mm in inside diameter and 15 cm in length, packed with octadecylsilanized silica gel for liquid chromatography (5 μm in particle diameter).

Column temperature: A constant temperature of about 40°C.

Mobile phase: A mixture of water and acetonitrile and phosphoric acid (3800:2200:1).

Flow rate: Adjust so that the retention time of [6]-gingerol is about 19 minutes.

System suitability—

System performance: When the procedure is run with 10 μL of the standard solution under the above operating conditions, the number of theoretical plates and the symmetry factor of the peak of [6]-gingerol are not less than 5000 and not more than 1.5, respectively.

System repeatability: When the test is repeated 6 times with 10 μL of the standard solution under the above operating conditions, the relative standard deviation of the peak area of [6]-gingerol is not more than 1.5%.

Containers and storage Containers—Tight containers.

Ginseng

Ginseng Radix

ニンジン

Ginseng is the root of *Panax ginseng* C. A. Meyer (*Panax schinseng* Nees) (*Araliaceae*), from which rootlets have been removed, or the root that has been quickly passed through hot water.

It contains not less than 0.10% of ginsenoside Rg_1 ($C_{42}H_{72}O_{14}$: 801.01) and not less than 0.20% of ginsenoside Rb_1 ($C_{54}H_{92}O_{23}$: 1109.29), calculated on the basis of dried material.

Description Thin and long cylindrical to fusiform root, often branching 2 to 5 lateral roots from the middle; 5 - 20 cm in length, main root 0.5 - 3 cm in diameter; externally light yellow-brown to light grayish brown, with longitudinal wrinkles and scars of rootlets; sometimes crown somewhat constricted and with short remains of rhizome; fractured surface practically flat, light yellow-brown in color, and brown in the neighborhood of the cambium.

Odor, characteristic; taste, at first slightly sweet, followed by a slight bitterness.

Identification **(1)** On a section of Ginseng add dilute iodine TS dropwise: a dark blue color is produced on the surface.

(2) To 2.0 g of pulverized Ginseng add 10 mL of water and 10 mL of 1-butanol, shake for 15 minutes, centrifuge, and use the 1-butanol layer as the sample solution. Separately, dissolve 1 mg of ginsenoside Rg_1 for thin-layer chromatography in 1 mL of methanol, and use this solution as the standard solution. Perform the test with these solutions as directed under Thin-layer Chromatography <2.03>. Spot 5 μL of the sample solution and 2 μL of the standard solution on a plate of silica gel for thin-layer chromatography. Develop the plate with a mixture of ethyl acetate, methanol and water (14:5:4) to a distance of about 7 cm, and air-dry the plate. Spray evenly vanillin-sulfuric acid-ethanol TS for spraying on the plate, and heat the plate at 105°C for 10 minutes: one of the several spots obtained from the sample solution has the same color tone and *R*f value with the spot from the standard solution.

Purity **(1)** Heavy metals <1.07>—Proceed with 1.0 g of pulverized Ginseng according to Method 4, and perform the test. Prepare the control solution with 1.5 mL of Standard Lead Solution (not more than 15 ppm).

(2) Arsenic <1.11>—Prepare the test solution with 1.0 g of pulverized Ginseng according to Method 4, and perform the test (not more than 2 ppm).

(3) Foreign matter <5.01>—The amount of stems and other foreign matter contained in Ginseng does not exceed 2.0%.

(4) Total BHC's and total DDT's <5.01>—Not more than 0.2 ppm, respectively.

Loss on drying <5.01> Not more than 14.0% (6 hours).

Total ash <5.01> Not more than 4.2%.

Extract content <5.01> Dilute ethanol-soluble extract: not less than 14.0%.

Assay **(1)** Ginsenoside Rg_1—Weigh accurately about 1.0 g of pulverized Ginseng, put in a glass-stoppered centrifuge tube, add 30 mL of diluted methanol (3 in 5), shake for 15 minutes, centrifuge, and separate the supernatant liquid. Repeat the procedure with the residue using 15 mL of diluted methanol (3 in 5), combine the supernatant liquids, and add diluted methanol (3 in 5) to make exactly 50 mL. Pipet 10 mL of this solution, add 3 mL of dilute sodium hydroxide TS, allow to stand for 30 minutes, add 3 mL of 0.1 mol/L hydrochloric acid TS and diluted methanol (3 in 5) to make exactly 20 mL, and use this solution as the sample solution. Separately, weigh accurately about 10 mg of Ginsenoside Rg_1 RS (separately determine the water <2.48> by coulometric titration, using 10 mg), dissolve in diluted methanol (3 in 5) to make exactly 100 mL, and use this solution as the standard solution. Perform the test with exactly 10 μL each of the sample solution and standard solution as directed under Liquid Chromatography <2.01> according to the following conditions, and determine the peak areas, A_T and A_S, of ginsenoside Rg_1 in each solution.

$$\text{Amount (mg) of ginsenoside } Rg_1\ (C_{42}H_{72}O_{14}) = M_S \times A_T/A_S$$

M_S: Amount (mg) of Ginsenoside Rg_1 RS taken, calculated on the anhydrous basis

Operating conditions—

Detector: An ultraviolet absorption photometer (wavelength: 203 nm).

Column: A stainless steel column 4.6 mm in inside diameter and 15 cm in length, packed with octadecylsilanized silica gel for liquid chromatography (5 μm in particle diameter).

Column temperature: A constant temperature of about 30°C.

Mobile phase: A mixture of water and acetonitrile (4:1).

Flow rate: Adjust so that the retention time of ginsenoside Rg_1 is about 25 minutes.

System suitability—

System performance: Dissolve 1 mg each of Ginsenoside Rg_1 RS and ginsenoside Re in diluted methanol (3 in 5) to make 10 mL. When the procedure is run with 10 μL of this solution under the above operating conditions, ginsenoside Rg_1 and ginsenoside Re are eluted in this order with the resolution between these peaks being not less than 1.5.

System repeatability: When the test is repeated 6 times with 10 μL of the standard solution under the above operating conditions, the relative standard deviation of the peak area of ginsenoside Rg_1 is not more than 1.5%.

(2) Ginsenoside Rb_1—Use the sample solution obtained in (1) as the sample solution. Separately, weigh accurately about 10 mg of Ginsenoside Rb_1 RS (separately determine the water <*2.48*> by coulometric titration, using 10 mg), dissolve in diluted methanol (3 in 5) to make exactly 100 mL, and use this solution as the standard solution. Perform the test with exactly 10 μL each of the sample solution and standard solution as directed under Liquid Chromatography <*2.01*> according to the following conditions, and determine the peak areas, A_T and A_S, of ginsenoside Rb_1 in each solution.

$$\text{Amount (mg) of ginsenoside Rb}_1\ (C_{54}H_{92}O_{23}) = M_S \times A_T/A_S$$

M_S: Amount (mg) of Ginsenoside Rb_1 RS taken, calculated on the anhydrous basis

Operating conditions—

Detector: An ultraviolet absorption photometer (wavelength: 203 nm).

Column: A stainless steel column 4.6 mm in inside diameter and 15 cm in length, packed with octadecylsilanized silica gel for liquid chromatography (5 μm in particle diameter).

Column temperature: A constant temperature of about 40°C.

Mobile phase: A mixture of water and acetonitrile (7:3).

Flow rate: Adjust so that the retention time of ginsenoside Rb_1 is about 20 minutes.

System suitability—

System performance: Dissolve 1 mg each of Ginsenoside Rb_1 RS and ginsenoside Rc in diluted methanol (3 in 5) to make 10 mL. When the procedure is run with 10 μL of this solution under the above operating conditions, ginsenoside Rb_1 and ginsenoside Rc are eluted in this order with the resolution between these peaks being not less than 3.

System repeatability: When the test is repeated 6 times with 10 μL of the standard solution under the above operating conditions, the relative standard deviation of the peak area of ginsenoside Rb_1 is not more than 1.5%.

Containers and storage Containers—Well-closed containers.

Powdered Ginseng

Ginseng Radix Pulverata

ニンジン末

Powdered Ginseng is the powder of Ginseng.

It contains not less than 0.10% of ginsenoside Rg_1 ($C_{42}H_{72}O_{14}$: 801.01) and not less than 0.20% of ginsenoside Rb_1 ($C_{54}H_{92}O_{23}$: 1109.29), calculated on the basis of dried material.

Description Powdered Ginseng occurs as a light yellow-white to light yellow-brown powder. It has characteristic odor and is a slight sweet taste followed by a slight bitterness.

Under a microscope <*5.01*>, Powdered Ginseng reveals round to rectangular parenchyma cells containing starch grains, occasionally gelatinized starch, vessels, secretory cell, sclerenchyma cell, big and thin-walled cork cell; crystals of calcium oxalate and starch. Vessels are reticulate vessel fragments, scalariform vessel and spiral vessel, 15 - 40 μm in diameter. Secretory cell containing a mass of yellow glistened contents; rosette aggregate of calcium oxalate, 20 - 60 μm in diameter, and 1 - 5 μm in diameter, rarely up to 30 μm in diameter of its single crystal; sclerenchymatous cells and thin-walled cork cells. Starch grains are observed in simple grain and 2 to 6-compound grain, simple grain, 3 - 20 μm in diameter.

Identification To 2.0 g of Powdered Ginseng add 10 mL of water and 10 mL of 1-butanol, shake for 15 minutes, centrifuge, and use the 1-butanol layer as the sample solution. Separately, dissolve 1 mg of ginsenoside Rg_1 for thin-layer chromatography in 1 mL of methanol, and use this solution as the standard solution. Perform the test with these solutions as directed under Thin-layer Chromatography <*2.03*>. Spot 5 μL of the sample solution and 2 μL of the standard solution on a plate of silica gel for thin-layer chromatography. Develop the plate with a mixture of ethyl acetate, methanol and water (14:5:4) to a distance of about 7 cm, and air-dry the plate. Spray evenly vanillin-sulfuric acid-ethanol TS for spraying on the plate, and heat the plate at 105°C for 10 minutes: one of the several spots obtained from the sample solution has the same color tone and *Rf* value with the spot from the standard solution.

Purity **(1)** Heavy metals <*1.07*>—Proceed with 1.0 g of Powdered Ginseng according to Method 4, and perform the test. Prepare the control solution with 1.5 mL of Standard Lead Solution (not more than 15 ppm).

(2) Arsenic <*1.11*>—Prepare the test solution with 1.0 g of Powdered Ginseng according to Method 4, and perform the test (not more than 2 ppm).

(3) Total BHC's and total DDT's <*5.01*>—Not more than 0.2 ppm, respectively.

Loss on drying <*5.01*> Not more than 13.0% (6 hours).

Total ash <*5.01*> Not more than 4.2%.

Acid-insoluble ash <*5.01*> Not more than 0.5%.

Extract content <*5.01*> Dilute ethanol-soluble extract; not less than 14.0%.

Assay **(1)** Ginsenoside Rg_1—Weigh accurately about 1.0 g of Powdered Ginseng, put in a glass-stoppered centrifuge tube, add 30 mL of diluted methanol (3 in 5), shake for 15 minutes, centrifuge, and separate the supernatant liquid. Repeat the procedure with the residue using 15 mL of diluted methanol (3 in 5), combine the supernatant liquids, and add diluted methanol (3 in 5) to make exactly 50 mL. Pipet 10 mL of this solution, add 3 mL of dilute sodium hydroxide TS, allow to stand for 30 minutes, add 3 mL of 0.1 mol/L hydrochloric acid TS and diluted methanol (3 in 5) to make exactly 20 mL, and use this solution as the sample solution. Separately, weigh accurately about 10 mg of Ginsenoside Rg_1 RS (separately determine the water <*2.48*> by coulometric titration, using 10 mg), dissolve in diluted methanol (3 in 5) to make exactly 100 mL, and use this solution as the standard solution. Perform the test with exactly 10 μL each of the sample solution and standard solution as directed under Liquid Chromatography <*2.01*> according to the following conditions, and determine the peak areas, A_T and A_S, of ginsenoside Rg_1 in each solution.

Amount (mg) of ginsenoside Rg_1 ($C_{42}H_{72}O_{14}$)
$= M_S \times A_T/A_S$

M_S: Amount (mg) of Ginsenoside Rg_1 RS taken, calculated on the anhydrous basis

Operating conditions—

Detector: An ultraviolet absorption photometer (wavelength: 203 nm).

Column: A stainless steel column 4.6 mm in inside diameter and 15 cm in length, packed with octadecylsilanized silica gel for liquid chromatography (5 μm in particle diameter).

Column temperature: A constant temperature of about 30°C.

Mobile phase: A mixture of water and acetonitrile (4:1).

Flow rate: Adjust so that the retention time of ginsenoside Rg_1 is about 25 minutes.

System suitability—

System performance: Dissolve 1 mg each of Ginsenoside Rg_1 RS and ginsenoside Re in diluted methanol (3 in 5) to make 10 mL. When the procedure is run with 10 μL of this solution under the above operating conditions, ginsenoside Rg_1 and ginsenoside Re are eluted in this order with the resolution between these peaks being not less than 1.5.

System repeatability: When the test is repeated 6 times with 10 μL of the standard solution under the above operating conditions, the relative standard deviation of the peak area of ginsenoside Rg_1 is not more than 1.5%.

(2) Ginsenoside Rb_1—Use the sample solution obtained in (1) as the sample solution. Separately, weigh accurately about 10 mg of Ginsenoside Rb_1 RS (separately determined the water *<2.48>* by coulometric titration, using 10 mg), dissolve in diluted methanol (3 in 5) to make exactly 100 mL, and use this solution as the standard solution. Perform the test with exactly 10 μL each of the sample solution and standard solution as directed under Liquid Chromatography *<2.01>* according to the following conditions, and determine the peak areas, A_T and A_S, of ginsenoside Rb_1 in each solution.

Amount (mg) of ginsenoside Rb_1 ($C_{54}H_{92}O_{23}$)
$= M_S \times A_T/A_S$

M_S: Amount (mg) of Ginsenoside Rb_1 RS taken, calculated on the anhydrous basis

Operating conditions—

Detector: An ultraviolet absorption photometer (wavelength: 203 nm).

Column: A stainless steel column 4.6 mm in inside diameter and 15 cm in length, packed with octadecylsilanized silica gel for liquid chromatography (5 μm in particle diameter).

Column temperature: A constant temperature of about 40°C.

Mobile phase: A mixture of water and acetonitrile (7:3).

Flow rate: Adjust so that the retention time of ginsenoside Rb_1 is about 20 minutes.

System suitability—

System performance: Dissolve 1 mg each of Ginsenoside Rb_1 RS and ginsenoside Rc in diluted methanol (3 in 5) to make 10 mL. When the procedure is run with 10 μL of this solution under the above operating conditions, ginsenoside Rb_1 and ginsenoside Rc are eluted in this order with the resolution between these peaks being not less than 3.

System repeatability: When the test is repeated 6 times with 10 μL of the standard solution under the above operating conditions, the relative standard deviation of the peak area of ginsenoside Rb_1 is not more than 1.5%.

Containers and storage Containers—Tight containers.

Glehnia Root and Rhizome

Glehniae Radix cum Rhizoma

ハマボウフウ

Glehnia Root and Rhizome is the root and rhizome of *Glehnia littoralis* Fr. Schmidt ex Miquel (*Umbelliferae*).

Description Cylindrical to long conical root or rhizome, 10 – 20 cm in length, 0.5 – 1.5 cm in diameter; externally light yellow-brown to red-brown. Rhizome short, with fine ring nodes; roots having longitudinal wrinkles and numerous, dark red-brown, warty protrusions or transversely elongated protuberances. Brittle and easily breakable. A transverse section white and powdery, and under a magnifying glass, oil canals scattered as brown dots.

Odor, slight; taste, slightly sweet.

Purity **(1)** Heavy metals *<1.07>*—Proceed with 3.0 g of pulverized Glehnia Root and Rhizome according to Method 3, and perform the test. Prepare the control solution with 3.0 mL of Standard Lead Solution (not more than 10 ppm).

(2) Arsenic *<1.11>*—Prepare the test solution with 0.40 g of pulverized Glehnia Root and Rhizome according to Method 4, and perform the test (not more than 5 ppm).

Total ash *<5.01>* Not more than 6.0%.

Acid-insoluble ash *<5.01>* Not more than 1.5%.

Containers and storage Containers—Well-closed containers.

Glycyrrhiza

Glycyrrhizae Radix

カンゾウ

Glycyrrhiza is the root and stolon, with (unpeeled) or without (peeled) the periderm, of *Glycyrrhiza uralensis* Fisher or *Glycyrrhiza glabra* Linné (*Leguminosae*).

It contains not less than 2.0% of glycyrrhizic acid ($C_{42}H_{62}O_{16}$: 822.93), calculated on the basis of dried material.

Description Nearly cylindrical pieces, 0.5 – 3 cm in diameter, over 1 m in length; externally dark brown to red-brown, longitudinally wrinkled, and often having lenticels, small buds and scaly leaves; peeled Glycyrrhiza is externally light yellow and fibrous. The transverse section reveals a rather clear border between cortex and xylem, and a radial structure which often has radiating splits. Glycyrrhiza originated from stolon has a pith, but those from root has no pith.

Odor, slight; taste, sweet.

Under a microscope *<5.01>*, a transverse section reveals multicellular layers of yellow-brown cork layers, and 1- to 3-cellular layer of cork cortex inside the cork layer; the secondary cortex exhibiting medullary rays and phloems radiated alternately; the phloem exhibiting fiber bundles with thick but incompletely lignified cell walls, surrounded by crystal cells; peeled Glycyrrhiza sometimes lacks a part of secondary cortex; the xylem exhibiting large yellow vessels and medullary rays in 3 to 10 rows radiated alternately; the vessels accompanied with xylem fibers surrounded by crystal cells, and with xylem parenchyma cells; the parenchymatous pith only in Glycyrrhiza originated from stolon. The parenchyma cells contain starch grains and often solitary crystals of calcium oxalate. Under a microscope <*5.01*>, a vertical section reveals crystal cells row observed along with phloem fibers or xylem fibers.

Identification To 2 g of pulverized Glycyrrhiza add 10 mL of a mixture of ethanol (95) and water (7:3), heat by shaking on a water bath for 5 minutes, cool, filter, and use the filtrate as the sample solution. Separately, dissolve 5 mg of Glycyrrhizic Acid RS or glycyrrhizic acid for thin-layer chromatography in 1 mL of a mixture of ethanol (95) and water (7:3), and use this solution as the standard solution. Perform the test with these solutions as directed under Thin-layer Chromatography <*2.03*>. Spot 2 μL each of the sample solution and standard solution on a plate of silica gel with fluorescent indicator for thin-layer chromatography. Develop the plate with a mixture of 1-butanol, water and acetic acid (100) (7:2:1) to a distance of about 7 cm, and air-dry the plate. Examine under ultraviolet light (main wavelength: 254 nm): one of the several spots obtained from the sample solution and a spot from the standard solution show the same color tone and the same *R*f value.

Purity **(1)** Heavy metals <*1.07*>—Proceed with 3.0 g of pulverized Glycyrrhiza according to Method 3, and perform the test. Prepare the control solution with 3.0 mL of Standard Lead Solution (not more than 10 ppm).

(2) Arsenic <*1.11*>—Prepare the test solution with 0.40 g of pulverized Glycyrrhiza according to Method 4, and perform the test (not more than 5 ppm).

(3) Total BHC's and total DDT's <*5.01*>—Not more than 0.2 ppm, respectively.

Loss on drying <*5.01*> Not more than 12.0% (6 hours).

Total ash <*5.01*> Not more than 7.0%.

Acid-insoluble ash <*5.01*> Not more than 2.0%.

Extract content <*5.01*> Dilute ethanol-soluble extract: not less than 25.0%.

Assay Weigh accurately about 0.5 g of pulverized Glycyrrhiza in a glass-stoppered centrifuge tube, add 70 mL of dilute ethanol, shake for 15 minutes, centrifuge, and separate the supernatant liquid. To the residue add 25 mL of dilute ethanol, and proceed in the same manner. Combine all the extracts, add dilute ethanol to make exactly 100 mL, and use this solution as the sample solution. Separately, weigh accurately about 25 mg of Glycyrrhizic Acid RS (separately determine the water <*2.48*> by coulometric titration, using 10 mg), dissolve in dilute ethanol to make exactly 100 mL, and use this solution as the standard solution. Perform the test with exactly 10 μL each of the sample solution and standard solution as directed under Liquid Chromatography <*2.01*> according to the following conditions, and determine the peak areas, A_T and A_S, of glycyrrhizic acid in each solution.

$$\text{Amount (mg) of glycyrrhizic acid } (C_{42}H_{62}O_{16}) = M_S \times A_T/A_S$$

M_S: Amount (mg) of Glycyrrhizic Acid RS taken, calculated on the anhydrous basis

Operating conditions—

Detector: An ultraviolet absorption photometer (wavelength: 254 nm).

Column: A stainless steel column 4.6 mm in inside diameter and 15 cm in length, packed with octadecylsilanized silica gel for liquid chromatography (5 μm in particle diameter).

Column temperature: A constant temperature of about 40°C.

Mobile phase: Dissolve 3.85 g of ammonium acetate in 720 mL of water, and add 5 mL of acetic acid (100) and 280 mL of acetonitrile.

Flow rate: Adjust so that the retention time of glycyrrhizic acid is about 15 minutes.

System suitability—

System performance: Dissolve 5 mg of monoammonium glycyrrhizinate for resolution check in 20 mL of dilute ethanol. When the procedure is run with 10 μL of this solution under the above operating conditions, the resolution between the peak with the relative retention time of about 0.9 to glycyrrhizic acid and the peak of glycyrrhizic acid is not less than 1.5.

System repeatability: When the test is repeated 6 times with 10 μL of the standard solution under the above operating conditions, the relative standard deviation of the peak area of glycyrrhizic acid is not more than 1.5%.

Containers and storage Containers—Well-closed containers.

Powdered Glycyrrhiza

Glycyrrhizae Radix Pulverata

カンゾウ末

Powdered Glycyrrhiza is the powder of Glycyrrhiza.

It contains not less than 2.0% of glycyrrhizic acid ($C_{42}H_{62}O_{16}$: 822.93), calculated on the basis of dried material.

Description Powdered Glycyrrhiza is light yellow-brown or light yellow to grayish yellow (powder of peeled Glycyrrhiza) in color. It has a slight odor and a sweet taste.

Under a microscope <*5.01*>, Powdered Glycyrrhiza reveals mainly yellow sclerenchymatous fiber bundles accompanied with crystal cell rows; vessels, 80 - 200 μm in diameter, with pitted, reticulate and scalariform pits, and with round perforations; parenchyma cells, containing starch grains and solitary crystals of calcium oxalate, their fragments, and cork tissues; but powder of peeled Glycyrrhiza shows no cork tissue; if any, a very few. Starch grains are simple grains, 2 - 20 μm in diameter; solitary crystals of calcium oxalate, 10 - 30 μm in a diameter.

Identification To 2 g of Powdered Glycyrrhiza add 10 mL of a mixture of ethanol (95) and water (7:3), heat by shaking on a water bath for 5 minutes, cool, filter, and use the filtrate as the sample solution. Separately, dissolve 5 mg of Glycyrrhizic Acid RS or glycyrrhizic acid for thin-layer chromatography in 1 mL of a mixture of ethanol (95) and water (7:3), and use this solution as the standard solution. Perform the test with these solutions as directed under Thin-layer Chromatography <*2.03*>. Spot 2 μL each of the sample solution and standard solution on a plate of silica gel with fluorescent indicator for thin-layer chromatography. Develop the plate with a mixture of 1-butanol, water and acetic acid (100) (7:2:1) to a distance of about 7 cm, and air-dry the plate. Examine under ultraviolet light (main wavelength: 254 nm): one of the several spots obtained from the sample solution and a spot from the standard solution show the same color tone and the same *R*f value.

Purity (1) Heavy metals <*1.07*>—Proceed with 3.0 g of Powdered Glycyrrhiza according to Method 3, and perform the test. Prepare the control solution with 3.0 mL of Standard Lead Solution (not more than 10 ppm).

(2) Arsenic <*1.11*>—Prepare the test solution with 0.40 g of Powdered Glycyrrhiza according to Method 4, and perform the test (not more than 5 ppm).

(3) Foreign matter—Under a microscope <*5.01*>, Powdered Glycyrrhiza shows no stone cells.

(4) Total BHC's and total DDT's <*5.01*>—Not more than 0.2 ppm, respectively.

Loss on drying <*5.01*> Not more than 12.0% (6 hours).

Total ash <*5.01*> Not more than 7.0%.

Acid-insoluble ash <*5.01*> Not more than 2.0%.

Extract content <*5.01*> Dilute ethanol-soluble extract: not less than 25.0%.

Assay Weigh accurately about 0.5 g of Powdered Glycyrrhiza in a glass-stoppered centrifuge tube, add 70 mL of dilute ethanol, shake for 15 minutes, centrifuge, and separate the supernatant liquid. To the residue add 25 mL of dilute ethanol, and proceed in the same manner. Combine all the extracts, add dilute ethanol to make exactly 100 mL, and use this solution as the sample solution. Separately, weigh accurately about 25 mg of Glycyrrhizic Acid RS (separately determine the water <*2.48*> by coulometric titration, using 10 mg), dissolve in dilute ethanol to make exactly 100 mL, and use this solution as the standard solution. Perform the test with exactly 10 μL each of the sample solution and standard solution as directed under Liquid Chromatography <*2.01*> according to the following conditions, and determine the peak areas, A_T and A_S, of glycyrrhizic acid in each solution.

Amount (mg) of glycyrrhizic acid ($C_{42}H_{62}O_{16}$)
$= M_S \times A_T/A_S$

M_S: Amount (mg) of Glycyrrhizic Acid RS taken, calculated on the anhydrous basis

Operating conditions—

Detector: An ultraviolet absorption photometer (wavelength: 254 nm).

Column: A stainless steel column 4.6 mm in inside diameter and 15 cm in length, packed with octadecylsilanized silica gel for liquid chromatography (5 μm in particle diameter).

Column temperature: A constant temperature of about 40°C.

Mobile phase: Dissolve 3.85 g of ammonium acetate in 720 mL of water, and add 5 mL of acetic acid (100) and 280 mL of acetonitrile.

Flow rate: Adjust so that the retention time of glycyrrhizic acid is about 15 minutes.

System suitability—

System performance: Dissolve 5 mg of monoammonium glycyrrhizinate for resolution check in 20 mL of dilute ethanol. When the procedure is run with 10 μL of this solution under the above operating conditions, the resolution between the peak with the relative retention time of about 0.9 to glycyrrhizic acid and the peak of glycyrrhizic acid is not less than 1.5.

System repeatability: When the test is repeated 6 times with 10 μL of the standard solution under the above operating conditions, the relative standard deviation of the peak area of glycyrrhizic acid is not more than 1.5%.

Containers and storage Containers—Well-closed containers.

Glycyrrhiza Extract

カンゾウエキス

Glycyrrhiza Extract contains not less than 3.6% of glycyrrhizic acid ($C_{42}H_{62}O_{16}$: 822.93).

Method of preparation 1) To 1 kg of fine cuttings of Glycyrrhiza or the root and stolon of *Glycyrrhiza glabra* Linné (*Leguminosae*) which meets the requirement of Glycyrrhiza add 5 L of Water, Purified Water or Purified Water in Containers, and macerate for 2 days. Filter the macerated solution through a cloth filter. Add 3 L of Water, Purified Water or Purified Water in Containers to the residue, macerate again for 12 hours, and filter through a cloth filter. Evaporate the combined filtrates until the whole volume becomes 3 L. After cooling, add 1 L of Ethanol, and allow to stand in a cold place for 2 days. Filter, and evaporate the filtrate to a viscous extract.

2) Take Glycyrrhiza or the root and stolon of *Glycyrrhiza glabra* Linné (*Leguminosae*) which meets the requirement of Glycyrrhiza, pulverized to suitable sizes, and prepare the viscous extract as directed under Extracts using Water, Purified Water or Purified Water in Containers as the solvent. Immediately before making a millet jelly-like consistency for the viscous extract, add Ethanol, Anhydrous Ethanol or ethanol (99.5) to the extract, allow it to stand in a cold place, filter, and concentrate the filtrate to prepare.

Description Glycyrrhiza Extract is a brown to blackish brown, viscous extract, and has a characteristic odor and a sweet taste.

It dissolves in water, forming a clear solution, or with a slight turbidity.

Identification To 0.8 g of Glycyrrhiza Extract add 10 mL of a mixture of ethanol (95) and water (7:3), shake for 2 minutes, centrifuge, and use the supernatant liquid as the sample solution. Proceed as directed in the Identification under Glycyrrhiza.

Purity (1) Heavy metals <*1.07*>—Prepare the test solution with 1.0 g of Glycyrrhiza Extract as directed under the Extracts (4), and perform the test (not more than 30 ppm).

(2) Insoluble matter—Dissolve 2.0 g of Glycyrrhiza Extract in 18 mL of water, and filter. To 10 mL of the filtrate add 5 mL of ethanol (95): a clear solution results.

Assay Weigh accurately about 0.15 g of Glycyrrhiza Extract, place in a glass-stoppered centrifuge tube, add 25 mL of dilute ethanol, and heat at 50°C for 30 minutes with occasional shaking. Cool, centrifuge, and take the supernatant liquid. To the residue add 20 mL of dilute ethanol, and proceed in the same manner. Combine all the extracts, add dilute ethanol to make exactly 100 mL, and use this solution as the sample solution. Separately, weigh accurately about 20 mg of Glycyrrhizic Acid RS (separately determine the water <*2.48*> by coulometric titration, using 10 mg), dissolve in dilute ethanol to make exactly 100 mL, and use this solution as the standard solution. Perform the test with exactly 10 μL each of the sample solution and standard solution as directed under Liquid Chromatography <*2.01*> according to the following conditions, and determine the peak areas, A_T and A_S, of glycyrrhizic acid in each solution.

Amount (mg) of glycyrrhizic acid ($C_{42}H_{62}O_{16}$)
$= M_S \times A_T/A_S$

M_S: Amount (mg) of Glycyrrhizic Acid RS taken, calculated on the anhydrous basis

Operating conditions—

Detector: An ultraviolet absorption photometer (wavelength: 254 nm).

Column: A stainless steel column 4.6 mm in inside diameter and 15 cm in length, packed with octadecylsilanized silica gel for liquid chromatography (5 μm in particle diameter).

Column temperature: A constant temperature of about 40°C.

Mobile phase: Dissolve 3.85 g of ammonium acetate in 720 mL of water, and add 5 mL of acetic acid (100) and 280 mL of acetonitrile.

Flow rate: Adjust so that the retention time of glycyrrhizic acid is about 15 minutes.

System suitability—

System performance: Dissolve 5 mg of monoammonium glycyrrhizinate for resolution check in 20 mL of dilute ethanol. When the procedure is run with 10 μL of this solution under the above operating conditions, the resolution between the peak with the relative retention time of about 0.9 to glycyrrhizic acid and the peak of glycyrrhizic acid is not less than 1.5.

System repeatability: When the test is repeated 6 times with 10 μL of the standard solution under the above operating conditions, the relative standard deviation of the peak area of glycyrrhizic acid is not more than 1.5%.

Containers and storage Containers—Tight containers.

Crude Glycyrrhiza Extract

カンゾウ粗エキス

Crude Glycyrrhiza Extract contains not less than 4.8% of glycyrrhizic acid ($C_{42}H_{62}O_{16}$: 822.93).

Method of preparation Take Glycyrrhiza or the root and stolon of *Glycyrrhiza glabra* Linné (*Leguminosae*) which meets the requirement of Glycyrrhiza, pulverized to suitable sizes, and prepare the dry extracts as directed under Extracts using Water, Purified Water or Purified Water in Containers as the solvent.

Description Crude Glycyrrhiza Extract occurs as lustrous, dark yellow-red to black-brown plates, rods or masses. It is comparatively brittle when cold, and the fractured surface is dark yellow-red, shell-like, and lustrous. It softens when warmed.

It has a characteristic odor and a sweet taste.

It dissolves in water with turbidity.

Identification To 0.6 g of Crude Glycyrrhiza Extract add 10 mL of a mixture of ethanol (95) and water (7:3), dissolve by warming if necessary, cool, centrifuge, and use the supernatant liquid as the sample solution. Proceed as directed in the Identification under Glycyrrhiza.

Purity (1) Heavy metals <*1.07*>—Prepare the test solution with 1.0 g of Crude Glycyrrhiza Extract as directed in the Extracts (4) under General Rules for Preparations, and perform the test (not more than 30 ppm).

(2) Water-insoluble substances—Boil 5.0 g of pulverized Crude Glycyrrhiza Extract with 100 mL of water. After cooling, filter the mixture through tared filter paper, wash with water, and dry the residue at 105°C for 5 hours: the mass of the residue is not more than 1.25 g.

(3) Foreign matter—The filtrate obtained in (2) does not have a strong bitter taste.

(4) Starch—To about 1 g of pulverized Crude Glycyrrhiza Extract add water to make 20 mL, shake the mixture thoroughly, and filter. Examine the insoluble substance on the filter paper under a microscope: the residue contains no starch grains.

Total ash <*5.01*> Not more than 12.0% (1 g).

Assay Weigh accurately about 0.15 g of Crude Glycyrrhiza Extract, place in a glass-stoppered centrifuge tube, add 25 mL of dilute ethanol, and heat at 50°C for 30 minutes with occasional shaking. Cool, centrifuge, and take the supernatant liquid. To the residue add 20 mL of dilute ethanol, and proceed in the same manner. Combine all the extracts, add dilute ethanol to make exactly 100 mL, and use this solution as the sample solution. Separately, weigh accurately about 20 mg of Glycyrrhizic Acid RS (separately determine the water <*2.48*> by coulometric titration, using 10 mg), dissolve in dilute ethanol to make exactly 100 mL, and use this solution as the standard solution. Perform the test with exactly 10 μL each of the sample solution and standard solution as directed under Liquid Chromatography <*2.01*> according to the following conditions, and determine the peak areas, A_T and A_S, of glycyrrhizic acid in each solution.

$$\text{Amount (mg) of glycyrrhizic acid } (C_{42}H_{62}O_{16}) = M_S \times A_T/A_S$$

M_S: Amount (mg) of Glycyrrhizic Acid RS taken, calculated on the anhydrous basis

Operating conditions—

Detector: An ultraviolet absorption photometer (wavelength: 254 nm).

Column: A stainless steel column 4.6 mm in inside diameter and 15 cm in length, packed with octadecylsilanized silica gel for liquid chromatography (5 μm in particle diameter).

Column temperature: A constant temperature of about 40°C.

Mobile phase: Dissolve 3.85 g of ammonium acetate in 720 mL of water, and add 5 mL of acetic acid (100) and 280 mL of acetonitrile.

Flow rate: Adjust so that the retention time of glycyrrhizic acid is about 15 minutes.

System suitability—

System performance: Dissolve 5 mg of monoammonium glycyrrhizinate for resolution check in 20 mL of dilute ethanol. When the procedure is run with 10 μL of this solution under the above operating conditions, the resolution between the peak with the relative retention time of about 0.9 to glycyrrhizic acid and the peak of glycyrrhizic acid is not less than 1.5.

System repeatability: When the test is repeated 6 times with 10 μL of the standard solution under the above operating conditions, the relative standard deviation of the peak area of glycyrrhizic acid is not more than 1.5%.

Containers and storage Containers—Tight containers.

Goreisan Extract

五苓散エキス

Goreisan Extract contains not less than 0.3 mg and not more than 1.2 mg (for preparation prescribed 1.5 g of Cinnamon Bark) or not less than 0.4 mg and not more than 1.6 mg (for preparation prescribed 2 g of Cinnamon Bark) or not less than 0.5 mg and not more than 2.0 mg (for preparation prescribed 2.5 g of Cinnamon Bark) or not less than 0.6 mg and not more than 2.4 mg (for preparation prescribed 3 g of Cinnamon Bark) of (*E*)-cinnamic acid, per extract prepared with the amount specified in the Method of preparation.

Method of preparation

	1)	2)	3)	4)	5)
Alisma Tuber	5 g	6 g	6 g	4 g	6 g
Polyporus Sclerotium	3 g	4.5 g	4.5 g	3 g	4.5 g
Poria Sclerotium	3 g	4.5 g	4.5 g	3 g	4.5 g
Atractylodes Rhizome	3 g	4.5 g	4.5 g	—	—
Atractylodes Lancea Rhizome	—	—	—	3 g	4.5 g
Cinnamon Bark	2 g	2.5 g	3 g	1.5 g	3 g

Prepare a dry extract or viscous extract as directed under Extracts, according to the prescription 1) to 5), using the crude drugs shown above.

Description Goreisan Extract occurs as a light red-brown to light brown powder, or a black-brown viscous extract. It has a characteristic odor, and a slightly sweet first, bitter, then acrid taste.

Identification **(1)** Weigh exactly 2.0 g of the dry extract (or 6.0 g of the viscous extract), add 20 mL of water and 2 mL of ammonia solution (28), and shake. Add 20 mL of a mixture of hexane and ethyl acetate (20:1), shake, centrifuge, and separate the upper layer. Add 20 mL of a mixture of hexane and ethyl acetate (20:1) to the aqueous layer, shake, centrifuge, and separate the upper layer. Combine these extracts, evaporate the solvent under low pressure (in vacuo), add exactly 2 mL of methanol to the residue, and use this solution as the sample solution. Separately, weigh exactly 10 mg of alisol A for thin-layer chromatography, and dissolve in exactly 10 mL of methanol. Pipet 1 mL of this solution, add methanol to make exactly 50 mL, and use this solution as the standard solution. Perform the test with these solutions as directed under Thin-layer Chromatography <*2.03*>. Spot 2 μL each of the sample solution and standard solution on a plate of silica gel for thin-layer chromatography. Develop the plate with a mixture of ethyl formate, water and formic acid (30:1:1) to a distance of about 7 cm, and air-dry the plate. Spray evenly 4-methoxybenzaldehyde-sulfuric acid-acetic acid TS on the plate, heat the plate at 105°C for 5 minutes, allow to cool, and examine under ultraviolet light (main wavelength: 365 nm): one of the several spots obtained from the sample solution has the same color tone and *R*f value with the yellow fluorescent spot from the standard solution, and it is larger and more intense than the spot from the standard solution (Alisma Tuber).

(2) For preparation prescribed Atractylodes Rhizome—Shake 1.0 g of the dry extract (or 3.0 g of the viscous extract) with 10 mL of water, add 25 mL of diethyl ether, and shake. Separate the diethyl ether layer, evaporate the solvent under low pressure (in vacuo), add 2 mL of diethyl ether to the residue, and use this solution as the sample solution. Separately, dissolve 1 mg of atractylenolide III for thin-layer chromatography in 2 mL of methanol, and use this solution as the standard solution. Perform the test with these solutions as directed under Thin-layer Chromatography <*2.03*>. Spot 5 μL each of the sample solution and standard solution on a plate of silica gel for thin-layer chromatography. Develop the plate with a mixture of hexane and ethyl acetate (2:1) to a distance of about 7 cm, and air-dry the plate. Spray evenly 1-naphthol-sulfuric acid TS on the plate, heat the plate at 105°C for 5 minutes, and allow to cool: one of the several spots obtained from the sample solution has the same color tone and *R*f value with the red to red-purple spot from the standard solution (Atractylodes Rhizome).

(3) For preparation prescribed Atractylodes Lancea Rhizome—Shake 2.0 g of the dry extract (or 6.0 g of the viscous extract) with 10 mL of water, add 25 mL of hexane, and shake. Separate the hexane layer, and evaporate the solvent under low pressure (in vacuo), add 0.5 mL of hexane to the residue, and use this solution as the sample solution. Perform the test with the sample solution as directed under Thin-layer Chromatography <*2.03*>. Spot 20 μL of the sample solution on a plate of silica gel with fluorescent indicator for thin-layer chromatography. Develop the plate with a mixture of hexane and acetone (7:1) to a distance of about 7 cm, and air-dry the plate. Examine under ultraviolet light (main wavelength: 254 nm): a dark purple spot is observed at an *R*f value of about 0.5. The spot shows a green-brown color after being sprayed evenly 4-dimethylaminobenzaldehyde TS for spraying, heated at 105°C for 5 minutes, and allowed to cool (Atractylodes Lancea Rhizome).

(4) Perform the test according to the following i) or ii) (Cinnamon Bark).

i) Put 10 g of the dry extract (or 30 g of the viscous extract) in a 300-mL hard-glass flask, add 100 mL of water and 1 mL of silicone resin, connect an apparatus for essential oil determination, and heat to boil under a reflux condenser. The graduated tube of the apparatus is to be previously filled with water to the standard line, and 2 mL of hexane is added to the graduated tube. After heating under reflux for 1 hour, separate the hexane layer, and use the layer as the sample solution. Separately, dissolve 1 mg of (*E*)-cinnamaldehyde for thin-layer chromatography in 1 mL of methanol, and use this solution as the standard solution. Perform the test with these solutions as directed under Thin-layer Chromatography <*2.03*>. Spot 50 μL of the sample solution and 2 μL of the standard solution on a plate of silica gel for thin-layer chromatography. Develop the plate with a mixture of hexane, diethyl ether and methanol (15:5:1) to a distance of about 7 cm, and air-dry the plate. Spray evenly 2,4-dinitrophenylhydradine TS on the plate: one of the several spots obtained from the sample solution has the same color tone and *R*f value with the yellow-orange spot from the standard solution.

ii) Shake 2.0 g of the dry extract (or 6.0 g of the viscous extract) with 10 mL of water, add 5 mL of hexane, and shake. Centrifuge this solution, and use the hexane layer as the sample solution. Separately, dissolve 1 mg of (*E*)-2-methoxycinnamaldehyde for thin-layer chromatography in 1 mL of methanol, and use this solution as the standard solution. Perform the test with these solutions as directed under Thin-layer Chromatography <*2.03*>. Spot 20 μL of the sample solution and 2 μL of the standard solution on a plate of silica gel for thin-layer chromatography. Develop the plate with a mixture of hexane and ethyl acetate (2:1) to a distance of about 7 cm, and air-dry the plate. Examine under ultraviolet light (main wavelength: 365 nm): one of the several spots obtained from the sample solution has the same color tone and *R*f value with the blue-white fluorescent spot from the standard solution.

Purity (1) Heavy metals <*1.07*>—Prepare the test solution with 1.0 g of the dry extract (or an amount of the viscous extract, equivalent to 1.0 g of the dried substance) as directed under Extracts (4), and perform the test (not more than 30 ppm).

(2) Arsenic <*1.11*>—Prepare the test solution with 0.67 g of the dry extract (or an amount of the viscous extract, equivalent to 0.67 g of the dried substance) according to Method 3, and perform the test (not more than 3 ppm).

Loss on drying <*2.41*> The dry extract: Not more than 10.0% (1 g, 105°C, 5 hours).

The viscous extract: Not more than 66.7% (1 g, 105°C, 5 hours).

Total ash <*5.01*> Not more than 10.0%, calculated on the dried basis.

Assay Conduct this procedure using light-resistant vessels. Weigh accurately about 0.5 g of the dry extract (or an amount of the viscous extract, equivalent to about 0.5 g of the dried substance), add exactly 50 mL of diluted methanol (1 in 2), shake for 15 minutes, filter, and use the filtrate as the sample solution. Separately, weigh accurately about 10 mg of (*E*)-cinnamic acid for assay, and dissolve in diluted methanol (1 in 2) to make exactly 100 mL. Pipet 10 mL of this solution, add diluted methanol (1 in 2) to make exactly 100 mL, and use this solution as the standard solution. Perform the test with exactly 10 μL each of the sample solution and standard solution as directed under Liquid Chromatography <*2.01*> according to the following conditions, and determine the peak areas, A_T and A_S, of (*E*)-cinnamic acid in each solution.

$$\text{Amount (mg) of } (E)\text{-cinnamic acid} = M_S \times A_T/A_S \times 1/20$$

M_S: Amount (mg) of (*E*)-cinnamic acid for assay taken, calculated on the basis of the content obtained by qNMR

Operating conditions—

Detector: An ultraviolet absorption photometer (wavelength: 273 nm).

Column: A stainless steel column 4.6 mm in inside diameter and 15 cm in length, packed with octadecylsilanized silica gel for liquid chromatography (5 μm in particle diameter).

Column temperature: A constant temperature of about 40°C.

Mobile phase: A mixture of water, acetonitrile and phosphoric acid (750:250:1).

Flow rate: 1.0 mL per minute (the retention time of (*E*)-cinnamic acid is about 12 minutes).

System suitability—

System performance: When the procedure is run with 10 μL of the standard solution under the above operating conditions, the number of theoretical plates and the symmetry factor of the peak of (*E*)-cinnamic acid are not less than 5000 and not more than1.5, respectively.

System repeatability: When the test is repeated 6 times with 10 μL of the standard solution under the above operating conditions, the relative standard deviation of the peak area of (*E*)-cinnamic acid is not more than 1.5%.

Containers and storage Containers—Tight containers.

Goshajinkigan Extract

牛車腎気丸エキス

Goshajinkigan Extract contains not less than 4 mg and not more than 16 mg of loganin, not less than 6 mg and not more than 18 mg of paeoniflorin ($C_{23}H_{28}O_{11}$: 480.46), and not less than 0.2 mg (for preparation prescribed Powdered Processed Aconite Root 1) of total alkaloids (as benzoylmesaconine hydrochloride and 14-anisoylaconine hydrochloride, or as benzoylmesaconine hydrochloride and benzoylhypaconine hydrochloride) or not less than 0.1 mg (for preparation prescribed Powdered Processed Aconite Root 2) of total alkaloids (as benzoylmesaconine hydrochloride and benzoylhypaconine hydrochloride), per extract prepared with the amount specified in the Method of preparation.

Method of preparation

	1)	2)
Rehmannia Root	5 g	5 g
Cornus Fruit	3 g	3 g
Dioscorea Rhizome	3 g	3 g
Alisma Tuber	3 g	3 g
Poria Sclerotium	3 g	3 g
Moutan Bark	3 g	3 g
Cinnamon Bark	1 g	1 g
Powdered Processed Aconite Root (Powdered Processed Aconite Root 1)	1 g	—
Powdered Processed Aconite Root (Powdered Processed Aconite Root 2)	—	1 g
Achyranthes Root	3 g	3 g
Plantago Seed	3 g	3 g

Prepare a dry extract or viscous extract as directed under Extracts, according to the prescription 1) or 2), using the crude drugs shown above.

Description Goshajinkigan Extract occurs as a brown to dark brown powder or black-brown viscous extract. It has slightly a characteristic odor and an acid taste.

Identification (1) To 1.0 g of the dry extract (or 3.0 g of the viscous extract), add 10 mL of water, shake, then add 30 mL of methanol, shake, centrifuge, and use the supernatant liquid as the sample solution. Perform the test with the sample solution as directed under Thin-layer Chromatography <*2.03*>. Spot 5 μL of the sample solution on a plate of silica gel for thin-layer chromatography. Develop the plate with a mixture of water, methanol and 1-butanol (1:1:1) to a distance of about 7 cm, and air-dry the plate. Spray evenly 4-methoxybenzaldehyde-sulfuric acid TS on the plate, heat the plate at 105°C for 5 minutes, and allow to cool; a dark-green spot is observed at an *R*f value of about 0.6 (Rehmannia Root).

(2) To 2.0 g of the dry extract (or 6.0 g of the viscous extract), add 10 mL of water, shake, then add 5 mL of 1-butanol, shake, centrifuge, and use the 1-butanol layer as the sample solution. Separately, dissolve 1 mg of loganin for thin-layer chromatography in 1 mL of methanol, and use this solution as the standard solution. Perform the test with these solutions as directed under Thin-layer Chromatography <*2.03*>. Spot 10 μL of the sample solution and 2 μL of the standard solution on a plate of silica gel for thin-layer

chromatography. Develop the plate with a mixture of ethyl acetate, water and formic acid (6:1:1) to a distance of about 10 cm, and air-dry the plate. Spray evenly 4-methoxybezaldehyde-sulfuric acid TS on the plate, and heat the plate at 105°C for 2 minutes: one of the several spots obtained from the sample solution has the same color tone and *R*f value with the purple spot from the standard solution (Cornus Fruit).

(3) To 2.0 g of the dry extract (or 6.0 g of the viscous extract), add 10 mL of sodium carbonate TS, shake, then add 10 mL of diethyl ether, shake, centrifuge, and use the diethyl ether layer as the sample solution. Separately, dissolve 1 mg of alisol A for thin-layer chromatography in 1 mL of methanol, and use this solution as the standard solution. Perform the test with these solutions as directed under Thin-layer Chromatography <*2.03*>. Spot 20 μL of the sample solution and 2 μL of the standard solution on a plate of silica gel for thin-layer chromatography. Develop the plate with a mixture of ethyl acetate, hexane and acetic acid (100) (10:10:3) to a distance of about 7 cm, and air-dry the plate. Spray evenly 4-methoxybenzaldehyde-sulfuric acid-acetic acid TS on the plate, heat the plate at 105°C for 5 minutes, and allow to cool, and examine under ultraviolet light (main wavelength: 365 nm): one of the several spots obtained from the sample solution has the same color tone and *R*f value with the yellow fluorescent spot from the standard solution (Alisma Tuber).

(4) To 2.0 g of the dry extract (or 6.0 g of the viscous extract), add 10 mL of water, shake, then add 5 mL of diethyl ether, shake, centrifuge, and use the diethyl ether layer as the sample solution. Separately, dissolve 1 mg of paeonol for thin-layer chromatography in 1 mL of methanol, and use this solution as the standard solution. Perform the test with these solutions as directed under Thin-layer Chromatography <*2.03*>. Spot 20 μL of the sample solution and 2 μL of the standard solution on a plate of silica gel for thin-layer chromatography. Develop the plate with a mixture of hexane and diethyl ether (5:3) to a distance of about 7 cm, and air-dry the plate. Spray evenly 4-methoxybenzaldehyde-sulfuric acid TS on the plate, and heat the plate at 105°C for 5 minutes: one of the several spots obtained from the sample solution has the same color tone and *R*f value with the orange spot from the standard solution (Moutan Bark).

(5) Perform the test according to the following i) or ii) (Cinnamon Bark).

i) Put 10 g of the dry extract (or 30 g of the viscous extract) in a 300-mL hard-glass flask, add 100 mL of water and 1 mL of silicone resin, connect an apparatus for essential oil determination, and heat to boil under a reflux condenser. The graduated tube of the apparatus is to be previously filled with water to the standard line, and 2 mL of hexane is added to the graduated tube. After heating under reflux for 1 hour, separate 1 mL of the hexane layer, add 0.5 mL of sodium hydroxide TS, shake, centrifuge, and use the hexane layer as the sample solution. Separately, dissolve 1 mg of (*E*)-cinnamaldehyde for thin-layer chromatography in 1 mL of methanol, and use this solution as the standard solution. Perform the test with these solutions as directed under Thin-layer Chromatography <*2.03*>. Spot 50 μL of the sample solution and 2 μL of the standard solution on a plate of silica gel for thin-layer chromatography. Develop the plate with a mixture of hexane, diethyl ether and methanol (15:5:1) to a distance of about 7 cm, and air-dry the plate. Spray evenly 2,4-dinitrophenylhydrazine TS on the plate: one of the several spots obtained from the sample solution has the same color tone and *R*f value with the yellow-orange spot from the standard solution.

ii) To 2.0 g of the dry extract (or 6.0 g of the viscous extract), add 10 mL of water, shake, then add 5 mL of hexane, shake, centrifuge, and use the hexane layer as the sample solution. Separately, dissolve 1 mg of (*E*)-2-methoxycinnamaldehyde for thin-layer chromatography in 1 mL of methanol, and use this solution as the standard solution. Perform the test with these solutions as directed under Thin-layer Chromatography <*2.03*>. Spot 20 μL of the sample solution and 2 μL of the standard solution on a plate of silica gel for thin-layer chromatography. Develop the plate with a mixture of hexane and ethyl acetate (2:1) to a distance of about 7 cm, and air-dry the plate. Examine under ultraviolet light (main wavelength: 365 nm): one of the several spots obtained from the sample solution has the same color tone and *R*f value with the blue-white fluorescent spot from the standard solution.

(6) To 3.0 g of the dry extract (or 9.0 g of the viscous extract), add 20 mL of diethyl ether and 2 mL of ammonia TS, shake for 10 minutes, and centrifuge. Separate the diethyl ether layer, evaporate the solvent under low pressure (in vacuo), add 1 mL of acetonitrile to the residue, and use this solution as the sample solution. Separately, dissolve 1 mg of benzoylmesaconine hydrochloride for thin-layer chromatography in 10 mL of ethanol (99.5), and use this solution as the standard solution. Perform the test with these solutions as directed under Thin-layer Chromatography <*2.03*>. Spot 20 μL of the sample solution and 10 μL of the standard solution on a plate of silica gel for thin-layer chromatography. Develop the plate with a mixture of 1-butanol, water and acetic acid (100) (4:2:1) to a distance of about 7 cm, and air-dry the plate. Spray evenly Dragendorff's TS for spraying on the plate, and air-dry the plate. Then spray evenly sodium nitrite TS on the plate: one of the several spots obtained from the sample solution has the same color tone and *R*f value with the yellow-brown spot from the standard solution (Powdered Processed Aconite Root).

(7) To 2.0 g of the dry extract (or 6.0 g of the viscous extract), add 10 mL of water, shake, then add 5 mL of 1-butanol, shake, centrifuge, and use the 1-butanol layer as the sample solution. Separately, to 0.3 g of pulverized plantago seed for thin-layer chromatography, add 1 mL of methanol, warm on a water bath for 3 minutes, centrifuge after cooling, and use the supernatant liquid as the standard solution. Perform the test with these solutions as directed under Thin-layer Chromatography <*2.03*>. Spot 10 μL each of the sample solution and standard solution on a plate of silica gel for thin-layer chromatography. Develop the plate with a mixture of acetone, ethyl acetate, water and acetic acid (100) (10:10:3:1) to a distance of about 7 cm, and air-dry the plate. Spray evenly 4-methoxybenzaldehyde-sulfuric acid TS on the plate, and heat the plate at 105°C for 5 minutes: one of the several spots obtained from the sample solution has the same color tone and *R*f value with the deep blue spot (*R*f value: about 0.3) from the standard solution (Plantago Seed).

(8) To 2.0 g of the dry extract (or 6.0 g of the viscous extract), add 10 mL of water, shake, then add 5 mL of 1-butanol, shake, centrifuge, and use the 1-butanol layer as the sample solution. Separately, to 2 g of achyranthes root for thin-layer chromatography, add 10 mL of water, shake, then add 10 mL of 1-butanol, shake, centrifuge, and use the 1-butanol layer as the standard solution. Perform the test with these solutions as directed under Thin-layer Chromatography <*2.03*>. Spot 20 μL each of the sample solution and standard solution on a plate of silica gel for thin-layer chromatography. Develop the plate with a mixture of 1-propanol, ethyl acetate and water (4:4:3) to a distance of about 10 cm, and air-dry the plate. Spray evenly diluted sulfuric acid on the plate and heat the plate at 105°C for 5 minutes: one of the several spots obtained from the sample solution has the same color tone and *Rf* value (around 0.4) with the dark red spot from the standard solution (Achyranthes Root).

Purity **(1)** Heavy metals <*1.07*>—Prepare the test solution with 1.0 g of the dry extract (or an amount of the viscous extract, equivalent to 1.0 g of the dried substance) as directed under the Extracts (4), and perform the test (not more than 30 ppm).

(2) Arsenic <*1.11*>—Prepare the test solution with 0.67 g of the dry extract (or an amount of the viscous extract, equivalent to 0.67 g of the dried substance) according to Method 3, and perform the test (not more than 3 ppm).

(3) Aconitum diester alkaloids (aconitine, jesaconitine, hypaconitine and mesaconitine)—Weigh accurately 1.0 g of the dry extract (or an amount of the viscous extract, equivalent to 1.0 g of the dried substance), add 20 mL of diethyl ether, shake, then add 3.0 mL of 0.1 mol/L hydrochloric acid TS and shake for 10 minutes. Centrifuge this solution, remove the diethyl ether layer, then add 20 mL of diethyl ether, proceed in the same manner as described above, and remove the diethyl ether layer. To the aqueous layer, add 1.0 mL of ammonia TS and 20 mL of diethyl ether, shake for 30 minutes, centrifuge, and take the diethyl ether layer. To the aqueous layer, add 1.0 mL of ammonia TS and 20 mL of diethyl ether, and repeat the above process twice more. Combine all the extracts, and evaporate to dryness under low pressure (in vacuo). Dissolve the residue with exactly 10 mL of a mixture of phosphate buffer solution for processed aconite root and acetonitrile (1:1). Centrifuge this solution, and use the supernatant liquid as the sample solution. Separately, pipet 1 mL of aconitum diester alkaloids standard solution for purity, add a mixture of phosphate buffer solution for processed aconite root and acetonitrile (1:1) to make exactly 10 mL, and use this solution as the standard solution. Perform the test with exactly 40 μL each of the sample solution and standard solution as directed under Liquid Chromatography <*2.01*> according to the following conditions: the heights of the peaks corresponding to aconitine, jesaconitine, hypaconitine and mesaconitine from the sample solution are not higher than the respective heights corresponding to aconitine, jesaconitine, hypaconitine and mesaconitine from the standard solution.

Operating conditions—

Detector: An ultraviolet absorption photometer (wavelength: 231 nm for aconitine, hypaconitine and mesaconitine; 254 nm for jesaconitine).

Column: A stainless steel column 4.6 mm in inside diameter and 15 cm in length, packed with octadecylsilanized silica gel for liquid chromatography (5 μm in particle diameter).

Column temperature: A constant temperature of about 40°C.

Mobile phase: A mixture of phosphate buffer for processed aconite root and tetrahydrofuran (183:17).

Flow rate: 1.0 mL per minute (the retention time of mesaconitine is about 31 minutes).

System suitability—

System performance: When the procedure is run with 20 μL of aconitum diester alkaloids standard solution for purity under the above operating conditions, using 254 nm, mesaconitine, hypaconitine, aconitine and jesaconitine are eluted in this order, and each resolution between their peaks is not less than 1.5 respectively.

System repeatability: When the test is repeated 6 times with 20 μL of the standard solution under the above operating conditions, using 231 nm, the relative standard deviation of the peak height of mesaconitine is not more than 1.5%.

Loss on drying <*2.41*> The dry extract: Not more than 9.0% (1 g, 105°C, 5 hours).

The viscous extract: Not more than 66.7% (1 g, 105°C, 5 hours).

Total ash <*5.01*> Not more than 9.0%, calculated on the dried basis.

Assay **(1)** Loganin—Weigh accurately about 0.5 g of the dry extract (or an amount of the viscous extract, equivalent to about 0.5 g of the dried substance), add exactly 50 mL of diluted methanol (1 in 2), shake for 15 minutes, filter, and use the filtrate as the sample solution. Separately, weigh accurately about 10 mg of loganin for assay, dissolve in diluted methanol (1 in 2) to make exactly 100 mL, and use this solution as the standard solution. Perform the test with exactly 10 μL each of the sample solution and standard solution as directed under Liquid Chromatography <*2.01*> according to the following conditions, and determine the peak areas, A_T and A_S, of loganin in each solution.

$$\text{Amount (mg) of loganin} = M_S \times A_T/A_S \times 1/2$$

M_S: Amount (mg) of loganin for assay taken

Operating conditions—

Detector: An ultraviolet absorption photometer (wavelength: 238 nm).

Column: A stainless steel column 4.6 mm in inside diameter and 15 cm in length, packed with octadecylsilanized silica gel for liquid chromatography (5 μm in particle diameter).

Column temperature: A constant temperature of about 50°C.

Mobile phase: A mixture of water, acetonitrile and methanol (55:4:1).

Flow rate: 1.2 mL per minute (the retention time of loganin is about 25 minutes).

System suitability—

System performance: When the procedure is run with 10 μL of the standard solution under the above operating conditions, the number of theoretical plates and symmetry factor of the peak of loganin are not less than 5000 and not more than 1.5, respectively.

System repeatability: When the test is repeated 6 times with 10 μL of the standard solution under the above operating conditions, the relative standard deviation of the peak area of loganin is not more than 1.5%.

(2) Paeoniflorin—Weigh accurately about 0.5 g of the dry extract (or an amount of the viscous extract, equivalent to about 0.5 g of the dried substance), add exactly 50 mL of diluted methanol (1 in 2), shake for 15 minutes, filter, and use the filtrate as the sample solution. Separately, weigh accurately about 10 mg of Paeoniflorin RS (separately determine the water <*2.48*> by coulometric titration, using 10 mg), and dissolve in diluted methanol (1 in 2) to make exactly 100 mL, and use this solution as the standard solution. Perform the test with exactly 10 μL each of the sample solution and standard solution as directed under Liquid Chromatography <*2.01*> according to the following conditions, and determine the peak areas, A_T and A_S, of paeoniflorin in each solution.

$$\text{Amount (mg) of paeoniflorin } (C_{23}H_{28}O_{11}) = M_S \times A_T/A_S \times 1/2$$

M_S: Amount (mg) of Paeoniflorin RS taken, calculated on the anhydrous basis

Operating conditions—

Detector: An ultraviolet absorption photometer (wavelength: 232 nm).

Column: A stainless steel column 4.6 mm in inside diameter and 15 cm in length, packed with octadecylsilanized silica gel for liquid chromatography (5 μm in particle diameter).

Column temperature: A constant temperature of about 20°C.

Mobile phase: A mixture of water, acetonitrile and phosphoric acid (850:150:1).

Flow rate: 1.0 mL per minute (the retention time of paeoniflorin is about 9 minutes).

System suitability—

System performance: Dissolve 1 mg each of Paeoniflorin RS and albiflorin in diluted methanol (1 in 2) to make 10 mL. When the procedure is run with 10 μL of this solution under the above operating conditions, albiflorin and paeoniflorin are eluted in this order with the resolution between these peaks being not less than 2.5.

System repeatability: When the test is repeated 6 times with 10 μL of the standard solution under the above operating conditions, the relative standard deviation of the peak area of paeoniflorin is not more than 1.5%.

(3) Total alkaloids—Weigh accurately about 1 g of the dry extract (or an amount of the viscous extract, equivalent to about 1 g of the dried substance), add 20 mL of diethyl ether, shake, then add 3.0 mL of 0.1 mol/L hydrochloric acid TS, and shake for 10 minutes. Centrifuge this solution, remove the diethyl ether layer, then add 20 mL of diethyl ether, proceed in the same manner as described above, and remove the diethyl ether layer. To the aqueous layer, add 1.0 mL of ammonia TS and 20 mL of diethyl ether, shake for 30 minutes, centrifuge, and take the diethyl ether layer. To the aqueous layer, add 1.0 mL of ammonia TS and 20 mL of diethyl ether, and repeat the above process twice more. Combine all the extracts, and evaporate to dryness under low pressure (in vacuo). Dissolve the residue with a mixture of phosphate buffer solution for processed aconite root and acetonitrile (1:1) to make exactly 10 mL. Centrifuge this solution, and use the supernatant liquid as the sample solution. Perform the test with exactly 20 μL each of the sample solution and the aconitum monoester alkaloids standard solution TS for assay as directed under Liquid Chromatography *<2.01>* according to the following conditions. Determine the peak areas of benzoylmesaconine, benzoylhypaconine and 14-anisoylaconine, A_{TM} and A_{SM}, A_{TH} and A_{SH}, as well as A_{TA} and A_{SA}, in each solution, respectively.

Amount (mg) of benzoylmesaconine hydrochloride
$= C_{SM} \times A_{TM}/A_{SM} \times 10$

Amount (mg) of benzoylhypaconine hydrochloride
$= C_{SH} \times A_{TH}/A_{SH} \times 10$

Amount (mg) of 14-anisoylaconine hydrochloride
$= C_{SA} \times A_{TA}/A_{SA} \times 10$

C_{SM}: Concentration (mg/mL) of benzoylmesaconine hydrochloride for assay in aconitum monoester alkaloids standard solution TS for assay
C_{SH}: Concentration (mg/mL) of benzoylhypaconine hydrochloride for assay in aconitum monoester alkaloids standard solution TS for assay
C_{SA}: Concentration (mg/mL) of 14-anisoylaconine hydrochloride for assay in aconitum monoester alkaloids standard solution TS for assay

Operating conditions—

Detector: An ultraviolet absorption photometer (wavelength: 231 nm for benzoylmesaconine and benzoylhypaconine; 254 nm for 14-anisoylaconine).

Column: A stainless steel column 4.6 mm in inside diameter and 15 cm in length, packed with octadecylsilanized silica gel for liquid chromatography (5 μm in particle diameter).

Column temperature: A constant temperature of about 40°C.

Mobile phase: A mixture of phosphate buffer solution for processed aconite root and tetrahydrofuran (183:17).

Flow rate: 1.0 mL per minute (the retention time of benzoylmesaconine is about 15 minutes).

System suitability—

System performance: When the procedure is run with 20 μL of the aconitum monoester alkaloids standard solution TS for assay under the above operating conditions, the number of theoretical plates and the symmetry factor of the peak of benzoylmesaconine are not less than 5000 and not more than 1.5, respectively.

System repeatability: When the test is repeated 6 times with 20 μL of the aconitum monoester alkaloids standard solution TS for assay under the above operating conditions, the relative standard deviation of the peak areas of benzoylmesaconine, benzoylhypaconine and 14-anisoylaconine is not more than 1.5%.

Containers and storage Containers—Tight containers.

Goshuyuto Extract

呉茱萸湯エキス

Goshuyuto Extract contains not less than 0.3 mg (for preparation prescribed 3 g of Euodia Fruit) or not less than 0.4 mg (for preparation prescribed 4 g of Euodia Fruit) of evodiamine, not less than 0.5 mg and not more than 2.0 mg (for preparation prescribed 1 g of Ginger) or not less than 0.7 mg and not more than 2.8 mg (for preparation prescribed 1.5 g of Ginger) of [6]-gingerol, and not less than 1.2 mg (for preparation prescribed 2 g of Ginseng) or not less than 1.8 mg (for preparation prescribed 3 g of Ginseng) of ginsenoside Rb_1 ($C_{54}H_{92}O_{23}$: 1109.29), per extract prepared with the amount specified in the Method of preparation.

Method of preparation

	1)	2)	3)
Euodia Fruit	3 g	4 g	3 g
Ginger	1 g	1.5 g	1.5 g
Ginseng	2 g	3 g	2 g
Jujube	4 g	3 g	4 g

Prepare a dry extract or viscous extract as directed under Extracts, according to the prescription 1) to 3), using the crude drugs shown above.

Description Goshuyuto Extract occurs as a light brown to light red-yellow powder, or a black-brown viscous extract. It has a slight odor and a hot and bitter taste.

Identification **(1)** To 1.0 g of the dry extract (or 3.0 g of the viscous extract) add 10 mL of sodium hydroxide TS, shake, add 5 mL of 1-butanol, shake, centrifuge, and use the 1-butanol layer as the sample solution. Separately, to 1 g of pulverized euodia fruit add 10 mL of methanol, shake, centrifuge, and use the supernatant liquid as the standard solution. Perform the test with these solutions as directed under

Thin-layer Chromatography <*2.03*>. Spot 1 μL each of the sample solution and standard solution on a plate of silica gel for thin-layer chromatography. Develop the plate with a mixture of acetone, 2-propanol, water and formic acid (7:7:1:1) to a distance of about 7 cm, and air-dry the plate. Examine under ultraviolet light (main wavelength: 365 nm): one of the several spots obtained from the sample solution has the same color tone and *R*f value with the blue-white fluorescent spot (*R*f value: about 0.5) from the standard solution (Euodia Fruit).

(2) To 1.0 g of the dry extract (or 3.0 g of the viscous extract) add 10 mL of water, shake, add 25 mL of diethyl ether, and shake. Separate the diethyl ether layer, evaporate the solvent under low pressure (in vacuo), add 2 mL of diethyl ether to the residue, and use this solution as the sample solution. Separately, dissolve 1 mg of [6]-gingerol for thin-layer chromatography in 1 mL of methanol, and use this solution as the standard solution. Perform the test with these solutions as directed under Thin-layer Chromatography <*2.03*>. Spot 10 μL of the sample solution and 5 μL of the standard solution on a plate of silica gel for thin-layer chromatography. Develop the plate with a mixture of ethyl acetate and hexane (1:1) to a distance of about 7 cm, and air-dry the plate. Spray evenly 4-dimethylaminobenzaldehyde TS for spraying on the plate, heat the plate at 105°C for 5 minutes, allow to cool, and spray water: one of the several spots obtained from the sample solution has the same color tone and *R*f value with the blue-green to grayish green spot from the standard solution (Ginger).

(3) To 1.0 g of the dry extract (or 3.0 g of the viscous extract) add 10 mL of sodium hydroxide TS, shake, add 5 mL of 1-butanol, shake, centrifuge, and use the 1-butanol layer as the sample solution. Separately, dissolve 1 mg of Ginsenoside Rb_1 RS or ginsenoside Rb_1 for thin-layer chromatography in 1 mL of methanol, and use this solution as the standard solution. Perform the test with these solutions as directed under Thin-layer Chromatography <*2.03*>. Spot 5 μL each of the sample solution and standard solution on a plate of silica gel for thin-layer chromatography. Develop the plate with a mixture of ethyl acetate, 1-propanol, water and acetic acid (100) (7:5:4:1) to a distance of about 7 cm, and air-dry the plate. Spray evenly vanillin-sulfuric acid-ethanol TS for spraying on the plate, heat the plate at 105°C for 5 minutes, and allow to cool: one of the several spots obtained from the sample solution has the same color tone and *R*f value with the blue-purple spot from the standard solution (Ginseng).

Purity (1) Heavy metals <*1.07*>—Prepare the test solution with 1.0 g of the dry extract (or an amount of the viscous extract, equivalent to 1.0 g of the dried substance) as directed under Extracts (4), and perform the test (not more than 30 ppm).

(2) Arsenic <*1.11*>—Prepare the test solution with 0.67 g of the dry extract (or an amount of the viscous extract, equivalent to 0.67 g of the dried substance) according to Method 3, and perform the test (not more than 3 ppm).

Loss on drying <*2.41*> The dry extract: Not more than 11.0% (1 g, 105°C, 5 hours).

The viscous extract: Not more than 66.7% (1 g, 105°C, 5 hours).

Total ash <*5.01*> Not more than 10.0%, calculated on the dried basis.

Assay (1) Evodiamine—Weigh accurately about 0.5 g of the dry extract (or an amount of the viscous extract, equivalent to about 0.5 g of the dried substance), add exactly 50 mL of diluted methanol (7 in 10), shake for 30 minutes, filter, and use the filtrate as the sample solution. Separately, weigh accurately about 10 mg of evodiamine for assay, and dissolve in methanol to make exactly 200 mL, and use this solution as the standard solution. Perform the test with exactly 10 μL each of the sample solution and standard solution as directed under Liquid Chromatography <*2.01*> according to the following conditions, and determine the peak areas, A_T and A_S, of evodiamine in each solution.

$$\text{Amount (mg) of evodiamine} = M_S \times A_T/A_S \times 1/4$$

M_S: Amount (mg) of evodiamine for assay taken, calculated on the basis of the content obtained by qNMR

Operating conditions—

Detector: An ultraviolet absorption photometer (wavelength: 282 nm).

Column: A stainless steel column 4.6 mm in inside diameter and 15 cm in length, packed with octadecylsilanized silica gel for liquid chromatography (5 μm in particle diameter).

Column temperature: A constant temperature of about 40°C.

Mobile phase: A mixture of water, acetonitrile and phosphoric acid (620:380:1).

Flow rate: 1.0 mL per minute (the retention time of evodiamine is about 18 minutes).

System suitability—

System performance: When the procedure is run with 10 μL of the standard solution under the above operating conditions, the number of theoretical plates and the symmetry factor of the peak of evodiamine are not less than 5000 and not more than 1.5, respectively.

System repeatability: When the test is repeated 6 times with 10 μL of the standard solution under the above operating conditions, the relative standard deviation of the peak area of evodiamine is not more than 1.5%.

(2) [6]-Gingerol—Weigh accurately about 0.5 g of the dry extract (or an amount of the viscous extract, equivalent to about 0.5 g of the dried substance), add exactly 50 mL of diluted methanol (7 in 10), shake for 30 minutes, filter, and use the filtrate as the sample solution. Separately, weigh accurately about 10 mg of [6]-gingerol for assay, dissolve in methanol to make exactly 100 mL. Pipet 5 mL of this solution, add methanol to make exactly 50 mL, and use this solution as the standard solution. Perform the test with exactly 10 μL each of the sample solution and standard solution as directed under Liquid Chromatography <*2.01*> according to the following conditions, and determine the peak areas, A_T and A_S, of [6]-gingerol in each solution.

$$\text{Amount (mg) of [6]-gingerol} = M_S \times A_T/A_S \times 1/20$$

M_S: Amount (mg) of [6]-gingerol for assay taken

Operating conditions—

Detector, column, column temperature and mobile phase: Proceed as directed in the operating conditions in (1).

Flow rate: 1.0 mL per minute (the retention time of [6]-gingerol is about 14 minutes).

System suitability—

System performance: When the procedure is run with 10 μL of the standard solution under the above operating conditions, the number of theoretical plates and the symmetry factor of the peak of [6]-gingerol are not less than 5000 and not more than 1.5, respectively.

System repeatability: When the test is repeated 6 times with 10 μL of the standard solution under the above operat-

ing conditions, the relative standard deviation of the peak area of [6]-gingerol is not more than 1.5%.

(3) Ginsenoside Rb_1—Weigh accurately about 2 g of the dry extract (or an amount of the viscous extract, equivalent to about 2 g of the dried substance), add 30 mL of diluted methanol (3 in 5), shake for 15 minutes, centrifuge, and separate the supernatant liquid. To the residue add 15 mL of diluted methanol (3 in 5), and repeat the same procedure. Combine all the supernatant liquids, and add diluted methanol (3 in 5) to make exactly 50 mL. Pipet 10 mL of this solution, add 3 mL of sodium hydroxide TS, allow to stand for 30 minutes, then add 3 mL of 1 mol/L hydrochloric acid TS, and add water to make exactly 20 mL. Apply exactly 5 mL of this solution to a column [about 10 mm in inside diameter, packed with 0.36 g of octadecylsilanized silica gel for pre-treatment (55 – 105 μm in particle size), and washed just before using with methanol and then diluted methanol (3 in 10)], and wash the column in sequence with 2 mL of diluted methanol (3 in 10), 1 mL of sodium carbonate TS and 10 mL of diluted methanol (3 in 10). Finally, elute with methanol to collect exactly 5 mL, and use this as the sample solution. Separately, weigh accurately about 10 mg of Ginsenoside Rb_1 RS (separately determine the water <*2.48*> by coulometric titration, using 10 mg), and dissolve in methanol to make exactly 100 mL. Pipet 10 mL of this solution, add methanol to make exactly 50 mL, and use this solution as the standard solution. Perform the test with exactly 20 μL each of the sample solution and standard solution as directed under Liquid Chromatography <*2.01*> according to the following conditions, and determine the peak areas, A_T and A_S, of ginsenoside Rb_1 in each solution.

$$\text{Amount (mg) of ginsenoside Rb}_1\ (C_{54}H_{92}O_{23}) = M_S \times A_T/A_S \times 1/5$$

M_S: Amount (mg) of Ginsenoside Rb_1 RS taken, calculated on the anhydrous basis

Operating conditions—

Detector: An ultraviolet absorption photometer (wavelength: 203 nm).

Column: A stainless steel column 4.6 mm in inside diameter and 25 cm in length, packed with carbamoyl group bound silica gel for liquid chromatography (5 μm in particle diameter).

Column temperature: A constant temperature of about 60°C.

Mobile phase: A mixture of acetonitrile, water and phosphoric acid (400:100:1).

Flow rate: 1.0 mL per minute.

System suitability—

System performance: When the procedure is run with 20 μL of the standard solution under the above operating conditions, the number of theoretical plates and the symmetry factor of the peak of ginsenoside Rb_1 are not less than 5000 and not more than 1.5, respectively.

System repeatability: When the test is repeated 6 times with 20 μL of the standard solution under the above operating conditions, the relative standard deviation of the peak area of ginsenoside Rb_1 is not more than 1.5%.

Containers and storage Containers—Tight containers.

Gypsum

Gypsum Fibrosum

セッコウ

Gypsum is natural hydrous calcium sulfate. It possibly corresponds to the formula $CaSO_4.2H_2O$.

Description Gypsum occurs as lustrous, white, heavy, fibrous, crystalline masses, which easily split into needles or very fine crystalline powder.

It is odorless and tasteless.

It is slightly soluble in water.

Identification To 1 g of pulverized Gypsum add 20 mL of water, allow to stand with occasional shaking for 30 minutes, and filter: the filtrate responds to the Qualitative Tests <*1.09*> (2) and (3) for calcium salt and to the Qualitative Tests <*1.09*> for sulfate.

Purity **(1)** Heavy metals <*1.07*>—Boil 4.0 g of pulverized Gypsum with 4 mL of acetic acid (100) and 96 mL of water for 10 minutes, cool, add water to make exactly 100 mL, and filter. Perform the test using 50 mL of the filtrate as the test solution. Prepare the control solution as follows: to 4.0 mL of Standard Lead Solution add 2 mL of dilute acetic acid and water to make 50 mL (not more than 20 ppm).

(2) Arsenic <*1.11*>—Prepare the test solution with 0.40 g of pulverized Gypsum according to Method 2, and perform the test (not more than 5 ppm).

Containers and storage Containers—Well-closed containers.

Exsiccated Gypsum

Gypsum Exsiccatum

焼セッコウ

Exsiccated Gypsum possibly corresponds to the formula $CaSO_4.\frac{1}{2}H_2O$.

Description Exsiccated Gypsum occurs as a white to grayish white powder. It is odorless and tasteless.

It is slightly soluble in water, and practically insoluble in ethanol (95).

It absorbs moisture slowly on standing in air to lose its solidifying property.

When it is heated to yield an anhydrous compound at a temperature above 200°C, it loses its solidifying property.

Identification Shake 1 g of Exsiccated Gypsum with 20 mL of water for 5 minutes, and filter: the filtrate responds to the Qualitative Tests <*1.09*> (2) and (3) for calcium salt and to the Qualitative Tests <*1.09*> for sulfate.

Purity Alkalinity—Take 3.0 g of Exsiccated Gypsum in a glass-stoppered test tube, add 10 mL of water and 1 drop of phenolphthalein TS, and shake vigorously: no red color develops.

Solidification To 10.0 g of Exsiccated Gypsum add 10 mL of water, stir immediately for 3 minutes, and allow to stand: the period until water no longer separates, when the material is pressed with a finger, is not more than 10 minutes from the time when the water was added.

Containers and storage Containers—Tight containers.

Hachimijiogan Extract

八味地黄丸エキス

Hachimijiogan Extract contains not less than 4 mg and not more than 16 mg of loganin, not less than 6 mg and not more than 18 mg (for preparation prescribed 3 g of Moutan Bark) or not less than 5 mg and not more than 15 mg (for preparation prescribed 2.5 g of Moutan Bark) of paeoniflorin ($C_{23}H_{28}O_{11}$: 480.46), and not less than 0.7 mg (for preparation prescribed 1 g of Processed Aconite Root 1) of total alkaloids (as benzoylmesaconine hydrochloride and 14-anisoylaconine hydrochloride), or not less than 0.2 mg (for preparation prescribed 1 g of Powdered Processed Aconite Root 1) of total alkaloids (as benzoylmesaconine hydrochloride and 14-anisoylaconine hydrochloride, or as benzoylmesaconine hydrochloride and benzoylhypaconine hydrochloride), or not less than 0.1 mg (for preparation prescribed 1 g of Powdered Processed Aconite Root 2) of total alkaloids (as benzoylmesaconine hydrochloride and benzoylhypaconine hydrochloride), or not less than 0.1 mg (for preparation prescribed 0.5 g of Powdered Processed Aconite Root 1) of total alkaloids (as benzoylmesaconine hydrochloride and 14-anisoylaconine hydrochloride, or as benzoylmesaconine hydrochloride and benzoylhypaconine hydrochloride), per extract prepared with the amount specified in the Method of preparation.

Method of preparation

	1)	2)	3)	4)
Rehmannia Root	5 g	5 g	5 g	6 g
Cornus Fruit	3 g	3 g	3 g	3 g
Dioscorea Rhizome	3 g	3 g	3 g	3 g
Alisma Tuber	3 g	3 g	3 g	3 g
Poria Sclerotium	3 g	3 g	3 g	3 g
Moutan Bark	3 g	3 g	3 g	2.5 g
Cinnamon Bark	1 g	1 g	1 g	1 g
Processed Aconite Root (Processed Aconite Root 1)	1 g	—	—	—
Powdered Processed Aconite Root (Powdered Processed Aconite Root 1)	—	1 g	—	0.5 g
Powdered Processed Aconite Root (Powdered Processed Aconite Root 2)	—	—	1 g	—

Prepare a dry extract or viscous extract as directed under Extracts, according to the prescription 1) to 4), using the crude drugs shown above.

Description Hachimijiogan Extract occurs as a grayish brown to brown powder or black-brown viscous extract. It has a characteristic odor and a slightly bitter and acid taste.

Identification **(1)** To 1.0 g of the dry extract (or 3.0 g of the viscous extract), add 10 mL of water, shake, then add 30 mL of methanol, shake, centrifuge, and use the supernatant liquid as the sample solution. Perform the test with the sample solution as directed under Thin-layer Chromatography <*2.03*>. Spot 5 μL of the sample solution on a plate of silica gel for thin-layer chromatography. Develop the plate with a mixture of water, methanol and 1-butanol (1:1:1) to a distance of about 7 cm, and air-dry the plate. Spray evenly 4-methoxybenzaldehyde-sulfuric acid TS on the plate, heat the plate at 105°C for 5 minutes, and allow to cool; a dark green spot is observed at an *Rf* value of about 0.6 (Rehmannia Root).

(2) To 2.0 g of the dry extract (or 6.0 g of the viscous extract), add 10 mL of water, shake, then add 5 mL of 1-butanol, shake, centrifuge, and use the 1-butanol layer as the sample solution. Separately, dissolve 1 mg of loganin for thin-layer chromatography in 1 mL of methanol, and use this solution as the standard solution. Perform the test with these solutions as directed under Thin-layer Chromatography <*2.03*>. Spot 10 μL of the sample solution and 2 μL of the standard solution on a plate of silica gel for thin-layer chromatography. Develop the plate with a mixture of ethyl acetate, water and formic acid (6:1:1) to a distance of about 10 cm, and air-dry the plate. Spray evenly 4-methoxybezaldehyde-sulfuric acid TS on the plate, and heat the plate at 105°C for 2 minutes: one of the several spots obtained from the sample solution has the same color tone and *Rf* value with the purple spot from the standard solution (Cornus Fruit).

(3) To 2.0 g of the dry extract (or 6.0 g of the viscous extract), add 10 mL of sodium carbonate TS, shake, then add 10 mL of diethyl ether, shake, centrifuge, and use the diethyl ether layer as the sample solution. Separately, dissolve 1 mg of alisol A for thin-layer chromatography in 1 mL of methanol, and use this solution as the standard solution. Perform the test with these solutions as directed under Thin-layer Chromatography <*2.03*>. Spot 20 μL of the sample solution and 2 μL of the standard solution on a plate of silica gel for thin-layer chromatography. Develop the plate with a mixture of ethyl acetate, hexane and acetic acid (100) (10:10:3) to a distance of about 7 cm, and air-dry the plate. Spray evenly 4-methoxybenzaldehyde-sulfuric acid-acetic acid TS on the plate, heat the plate at 105°C for 5 minutes, allow to cool, and examine under ultraviolet light (main wavelength: 365 nm): one of the several spots obtained from the sample solution has the same color tone and *Rf* value with the yellow fluorescent spot from the standard solution (Alisma Tuber).

(4) To 2.0 g of the dry extract (or 6.0 g of the viscous extract), add 10 mL of water, shake, then add 5 mL of diethyl ether, shake, centrifuge, and use the diethyl ether layer as the sample solution. Separately, dissolve 1 mg of paeonol for thin-layer chromatography in 1 mL of methanol, and use this solution as the standard solution. Perform the test with these solutions as directed under Thin-layer Chromatography <*2.03*>. Spot 20 μL of the sample solution and 2 μL of the standard solution on a plate of silica gel for thin-layer chromatography. Develop the plate with a mixture of hexane and diethyl ether (5:3) to a distance of about 7 cm, and air-dry the plate. Spray evenly 4-methoxybenzaldehyde-sulfuric acid TS on the plate, and heat the plate at 105°C for 5 minutes: one of the several spots obtained from the sample solution has the same color tone and *Rf* value with the orange spot from the standard solution (Moutan Bark).

(5) Perform the test according to the following i) or ii) (Cinnamon Bark).

i) Put 10 g of the dry extract (or 30 g of the viscous extract) in a 300-mL hard-glass flask, add 100 mL of water and 1 mL of silicone resin, connect an apparatus for essential oil determination, and heat to boil under a reflux condenser. The graduated tube of the apparatus is to be previously filled with water to the standard line, and 2 mL of hexane is added to the graduated tube. After heating under reflux for 1 hour, separate 1 mL of the hexane layer, add 0.5 mL of sodium hydroxide TS, shake, centrifuge, and use the hexane layer as the sample solution. Separately, dissolve 1 mg of (*E*)-cinnamaldehyde for thin-layer chromatography in 1 mL of methanol, and use this solution as the standard solution. Perform the test with these solutions as directed under Thin-layer Chromatography <*2.03*>. Spot 50 μL of the sample solution and 2 μL of the standard solution on a plate of silica gel for thin-layer chromatography. Develop the plate with a mixture of hexane, diethyl ether and methanol (15:5:1) to a distance of about 7 cm, and air-dry the plate. Spray evenly 2,4-dinitrophenylhydrazine TS on the plate: one of the several spots obtained from the sample solution has the same color tone and *R*f value with the yellow-orange spot from the standard solution.

ii) To 2.0 g of the dry extract (or 6.0 g of the viscous extract), add 10 mL of water, shake, then add 5 mL of hexane, shake, centrifuge, and use the hexane layer as the sample solution. Separately, dissolve 1 mg of (*E*)-2-methoxycinnamaldehyde for thin-layer chromatography in 1 mL of methanol, and use this solution as the standard solution. Perform the test with these solutions as directed under Thin-layer Chromatography <*2.03*>. Spot 20 μL of the sample solution and 2 μL of the standard solution on a plate of silica gel for thin-layer chromatography. Develop the plate with a mixture of hexane and ethyl acetate (2:1) to a distance of about 7 cm, and air-dry the plate. Examine under ultraviolet light (main wavelength: 365 nm): one of the several spots obtained from the sample solution has the same color tone and *R*f value with the blue-white fluorescent spot from the standard solution.

(6) To 3.0 g of the dry extract (or 9.0 g of the viscous extract), add 20 mL of diethyl ether and 2 mL of ammonia TS, shake for 10 minutes and centrifuge. Separate the diethyl ether layer, evaporate the diethyl ether layer under low pressure (in vacuo), add 1 mL of acetonitrile to the residue, and use this solution as the sample solution. Separately, dissolve 1 mg of benzoylmesaconine hydrochloride for thin-layer chromatography in 10 mL of ethanol (99.5), and use this solution as the standard solution. Perform the test with these solutions as directed under Thin-layer Chromatography <*2.03*>. Spot 20 μL of the sample solution and 10 μL of the standard solution on a plate of silica gel for thin-layer chromatography. Develop the plate with a mixture of 1-butanol, water and acetic acid (100) (4:2:1) to a distance of about 7 cm, and air-dry the plate. Spray evenly Dragendorff's TS for spraying on the plate, and air-dry the plate. Then spray evenly sodium nitrite TS on the plate: one of the several spots obtained from the sample solution has the same color tone and *R*f value with the yellow-brown spot from the standard solution (Processed Aconite Root or Powdered Processed Aconite Root).

Purity **(1)** Heavy metals <*1.07*>—Prepare the test solution with 1.0 g of the dry extract (or an amount of the viscous extract, equivalent to 1.0 g of the dried substance) as directed under the Extracts (4), and perform the test (not more than 30 ppm).

(2) Arsenic <*1.11*>—Prepare the test solution with 0.67 g of the dry extract (or an amount of the viscous extract, equivalent to 0.67 g of the dried substance) according to Method 3, and perform the test (not more than 3 ppm).

(3) Aconitum diester alkaloids (aconitine, jesaconitine, hypaconitine and mesaconitine)—Weigh accurately 1.0 g of the dry extract (or an amount of the viscous extract, equivalent to 1.0 g of the dried substance), add 20 mL of diethyl ether, shake, then add 3.0 mL of 0.1 mol/L hydrochloric acid TS and shake for 10 minutes. Centrifuge this solution, remove the diethyl ether layer, then add 20 mL of diethyl ether, proceed in the same manner as described above, and remove the diethyl ether layer. To the aqueous layer, add 1.0 mL of ammonia TS and 20 mL of diethyl ether, shake for 30 minutes, centrifuge, and take the diethyl ether layer. To the aqueous layer, add 1.0 mL of ammonia TS and 20 mL of diethyl ether, and repeat the above process twice more. Combine all the extracts, and evaporate the solvent under low pressure (in vacuo). Dissolve the residue with exactly 10 mL of a mixture of phosphate buffer solution for processed aconite root and acetonitrile (1:1), centrifuge this solution, and use the supernatant liquid as the sample solution. Separately, pipet exactly 1 mL of aconitum diester alkaloids standard solution for purity, add a mixture of phosphate buffer solution for processed aconite root and acetonitrile (1:1) to make exactly 10 mL, and use this solution as the standard solution. Perform the test with exactly 40 μL each of the sample solution and standard solution as directed under Liquid Chromatography <*2.01*> according to the following conditions: the heights of the peaks corresponding to aconitine, jesaconitine, hypaconitine and mesaconitine from the sample solution are not higher than the respective heights corresponding to aconitine, jesaconitine, hypaconitine and mesaconitine from the standard solution.

Operating conditions—

Detector: An ultraviolet absorption photometer (wavelength: 231 nm for aconitine, hypaconitine and mesaconitine; 254 nm for jesaconitine).

Column: A stainless steel column 4.6 mm in inside diameter and 15 cm in length, packed with octadecylsilanized silica gel for liquid chromatography (5 μm in particle diameter).

Column temperature: A constant temperature of about 40°C.

Mobile phase: A mixture of phosphate buffer for processed aconite root and tetrahydrofuran (183:17).

Flow rate: 1.0 mL per minute (the retention time of mesaconitine is about 31 minutes).

System suitability—

System performance: When the procedure is run with 20 μL of aconitum diester alkaloids standard solution for purity under the above operating conditions, using 254 nm, mesaconitine, hypaconitine, aconitine and jesaconitine are eluted in this order, and each resolution between their peaks is not less than 1.5, respectively.

System repeatability: When the test is repeated 6 times with 20 μL of the standard solution under the above operating conditions, using 231 nm, the relative standard deviation of the peak height of mesaconitine is not more than 1.5 %.

Loss on drying <*2.41*> The dry extract: Not more than 8.5% (1 g, 105°C, 5 hours).

The viscous extract: Not more than 66.7% (1 g, 105°C, 5 hours).

Total ash <*5.01*> Not more than 10.0%, calculated on the dried basis.

Assay **(1)** Loganin—Weigh accurately about 0.5 g of the dry extract (or an amount of the viscous extract, equivalent to about 0.5 g of the dried substance), add exactly 50 mL of diluted methanol (1 in 2), shake for 15 minutes, filter, and use the filtrate as the sample solution. Separately, weigh accurately about 10 mg of loganin for assay, dissolve in diluted methanol (1 in 2) to make exactly 100 mL, and use this solution as the standard solution. Perform the test with exactly 10 μL each of the sample solution and standard solution as directed under Liquid Chromatography <*2.01*> according to the following conditions, and determine the peak areas, A_T and A_S, of loganin in each solution.

Amount (mg) of loganin $= M_S \times A_T/A_S \times 1/2$

M_S: Amount (mg) of loganin for assay taken

Operating conditions—

Detector: An ultraviolet absorption photometer (wavelength: 238 nm).

Column: A stainless steel column 4.6 mm in inside diameter and 15 cm in length, packed with octadecylsilanized silica gel for liquid chromatography (5 μm in particle diameter).

Column temperature: A constant temperature of about 50°C.

Mobile phase: A mixture of water, acetonitrile and methanol (55:4:1).

Flow rate: 1.2 mL per minute (the retention time of loganin is about 25 minutes).

System suitability—

System performance: When the procedure is run with 10 μL of the standard solution under the above operating conditions, the number of theoretical plates and symmetry factor of the peak of loganin are not less than 5000 and not more than 1.5, respectively.

System repeatability: When the test is repeated 6 times with 10 μL of the standard solution under the above operating conditions, the relative standard deviation of the peak area of loganin is not more than 1.5%.

(2) Paeoniflorin—Weigh accurately about 0.5 g of the dry extract (or an amount of the viscous extract, equivalent to about 0.5 g of the dried substance), add exactly 50 mL of diluted methanol (1 in 2), shake for 15 minutes, filter, and use the filtrate as the sample solution. Separately, weigh accurately about 10 mg of Paeoniflorin RS (separately determine the water *<2.48>* by coulometric titration, using 10 mg), and dissolve in diluted methanol (1 in 2) to make exactly 100 mL, and use this solution as the standard solution. Perform the test with exactly 10 μL each of the sample solution and standard solution as directed under Liquid Chromatography *<2.01>* according to the following conditions, and determine the peak areas, A_T and A_S, of paeoniflorin in each solution.

Amount (mg) of paeoniflorin ($C_{23}H_{28}O_{11}$)
$= M_S \times A_T/A_S \times 1/2$

M_S: Amount (mg) of Paeoniflorin RS taken, calculated on the anhydrous basis

Operating conditions—

Detector: An ultraviolet absorption photometer (wavelength: 232 nm).

Column: A stainless steel column 4.6 mm in inside diameter and 15 cm in length, packed with octadecylsilanized silica gel for liquid chromatography (5 μm in particle diameter).

Column temperature: A constant temperature of about 20°C.

Mobile phase: A mixture of water, acetonitrile and phosphoric acid (850:150:1).

Flow rate: 1.0 mL per minute (the retention time of paeoniflorin is about 9 minutes).

System suitability—

System performance: Dissolve 1 mg each of Paeoniflorin RS and albiflorin in diluted methanol (1 in 2) to make 10 mL. When the procedure is run with 10 μL of this solution under the above operating conditions, albiflorin and paeoniflorin are eluted in this order with the resolution between these peaks being not less than 2.5.

System repeatability: When the test is repeated 6 times with 10 μL of the standard solution under the above operating conditions, the relative standard deviation of the peak area of paeoniflorin is not more than 1.5%.

(3) Total alkaloids—Weigh accurately about 1 g of the dry extract (or an amount of the viscous extract, equivalent to about 1 g of the dried substance), add 20 mL of diethyl ether, shake, then add 3.0 mL of 0.1 mol/L hydrochloric acid TS, and shake for 10 minutes. Centrifuge this solution, remove the diethyl ether layer, then add 20 mL of diethyl ether, proceed in the same manner as described above, and remove the diethyl ether layer. To the aqueous layer, add 1.0 mL of ammonia TS and 20 mL of diethyl ether, shake for 30 minutes, centrifuge, and take the diethyl ether layer. To the aqueous layer, add 1.0 mL of ammonia TS and 20 mL of diethyl ether, and repeat the above process twice more. Combine all the extracts, and evaporate the solvent under low pressure (in vacuo). Dissolve the residue with a mixture of phosphate buffer solution for processed aconite root and acetonitrile (1:1) to make exactly 10 mL. Centrifuge this solution, and use the supernatant liquid as the sample solution. Perform the test with exactly 20 μL each of the sample solution and the aconitum monoester alkaloids standard solution TS for assay as directed under Liquid Chromatography *<2.01>* according to the following conditions. Determine the peak areas of benzoylmesaconine, benzoylhypaconine and 14-anisoylaconine, A_{TM} and A_{SM}, A_{TH} and A_{SH}, as well as A_{TA} and A_{SA}, in each solution, respectively.

Amount (mg) of benzoylmesaconine hydrochloride
$= C_{SM} \times A_{TM}/A_{SM} \times 10$

Amount (mg) of benzoylhypaconine hydrochloride
$= C_{SH} \times A_{TH}/A_{SH} \times 10$

Amount (mg) of 14-anisoylaconine hydrochloride
$= C_{SA} \times A_{TA}/A_{SA} \times 10$

C_{SM}: Concentration (mg/mL) of benzoylmesaconine hydrochloride for assay in aconitum monoester alkaloids standard solution TS for assay

C_{SH}: Concentration (mg/mL) of benzoylhypaconine hydrochloride for assay in aconitum monoester alkaloids standard solution TS for assay

C_{SA}: Concentration (mg/mL) of 14-anisoylaconine hydrochloride for assay in aconitum monoester alkaloids standard solution TS for assay

Operating conditions—

Detector: An ultraviolet absorption photometer (wavelength: 231 nm for benzoylmesaconine and benzoylhypaconine; 254 nm for 14-anisoylaconine).

Column: A stainless steel column 4.6 mm in inside diameter and 15 cm in length, packed with octadecylsilanized silica gel for liquid chromatography (5 μm in particle diameter).

Column temperature: A constant temperature of about 40°C.

Mobile phase: A mixture of phosphate buffer solution for processed aconite root and tetrahydrofuran (183:17).

Flow rate: 1.0 mL per minute (the retention time of benzoylmesaconine is about 15 minutes).

System suitability—

System performance: When the procedure is run with 20 μL of the aconitum monoester alkaloids standard solution TS for assay under the above operating conditions, the number of theoretical plates and the symmetry factor of the peak of benzoylmesaconine are not less than 5000 and not more than 1.5, respectively.

System repeatability: When the test is repeated 6 times with 20 μL of the aconitum monoester alkaloids standard solution TS for assay under the above operating conditions, the relative standard deviation of the peak areas of benzoylmesaconine, benzoylhypaconine and 14-anisoylaconine is not more than 1.5%.

Containers and storage Containers—Tight containers.

Hangekobokuto Extract

半夏厚朴湯エキス

Hangekobokuto Extract contains not less than 2 mg and not more than 6 mg of magnolol, not less than 4 mg (for preparation prescribed 2 g of Perilla Herb) or not less than 6 mg (for preparation prescribed 3 g of Perilla Herb) of rosmarinic acid, and not less than 0.6 mg and not more than 2.4 mg (for preparation prescribed 1 g of Ginger) or not less than 0.8 mg and not more than 3.2 mg (for preparation prescribed 1.3 g of Ginger) or not less than 0.9 mg and not more than 3.6 mg (for preparation prescribed 1.5 g of Ginger) of [6]-gingerol, per extract prepared with the amount specified in the Method of preparation.

Method of preparation

	1)	2)	3)	4)
Pinellia Tuber	6 g	6 g	6 g	6 g
Poria Sclerotium	5 g	5 g	5 g	5 g
Magnolia bark	3 g	3 g	3 g	3 g
Perilla Herb	2 g	3 g	2 g	2 g
Ginger	1 g	1 g	1.3 g	1.5 g

Prepare a dry extract or viscous extract as directed under Extracts, according to the prescription 1) to 4), using the crude drugs shown above.

Description Hangekobokuto Extract is a light brown to dark brown powder or black-brown viscous extract. It has a characteristic odor and has a bitter and astringent taste first then pungent later.

Identification **(1)** Shake 1.0 g of the dry extract (or 3.0 g of the viscous extract) with 10 mL of water, add 25 mL of diethyl ether, and shake. Separate the diethyl ether layer, evaporate the solvent under low pressure (in vacuo), add 2 mL of diethyl ether to the residue, and use this solution as the sample solution. Separately, dissolve 1 mg of magnolol for thin-layer chromatography in 1 mL of methanol, and use this solution as the standard solution. Perform the test with these solutions as directed under Thin-layer Chromatography <*2.03*>. Spot 5 μL each of the sample solution and standard solution on a plate of silica gel with fluorescent indicator for thin-layer chromatography. Develop the plate with a mixture of ethyl acetate and hexane (1:1) to a distance of about 7 cm, and air-dry the plate. Examine under ultraviolet light (main wavelength: 254 nm): one of the several spots obtained from the sample solution has the same color tone and *Rf* value with the dark purple spot from the standard solution (Magnolia Bark).

(2) Shake 1.0 g of the dry extract (or 3.0 g of the viscous extract) with 10 mL of 0.1 mol/L hydrochloric acid TS, add 25 mL of diethyl ether, and shake. Separate the diethyl ether layer, evaporate the solvent under low pressure (in vacuo), add 1 mL of methanol to the residue, and use this solution as the sample solution. Separately, dissolve 1 mg of rosmarinic acid for thin-layer chromatography in 1 mL of methanol, and use this solution as the standard solution. Perform the test with these solutions as directed under Thin-layer Chromatography <*2.03*>. Spot 5 μL each of the sample solution and standard solution on a plate of silica gel for thin-layer chromatography. Develop the plate with a mixture of ethyl acetate, water and formic acid (60:1:1) to a distance of about 7 cm, and air-dry the plate. Spray evenly iron (III) chloride-methanol TS on the plate: one of the several spots obtained from the sample solution has the same color tone and *Rf* value with the dark purple spot from the standard solution (Perilla Herb).

(3) Shake 1.0 g of the dry extract (or 3.0 g of the viscous extract) with 10 mL of water, add 25 mL of diethyl ether, and shake. Separate the diethyl ether layer, evaporate the solvent under low pressure (in vacuo), add 2 mL of diethyl ether to the residue, and use this solution as the sample solution. Separately, dissolve 1 mg of [6]-gingerol for thin-layer chromatography in 1 mL of methanol, and use this solution as the standard solution. Perform the test with these solutions as directed under Thin-layer Chromatography <*2.03*>. Spot 5 μL each of the sample solution and standard solution on a plate of silica gel for thin-layer chromatography. Develop the plate with a mixture of hexane and acetone (2:1) to a distance of about 7 cm, and air-dry the plate. Spray evenly 4-dimethylaminobenzaldehyde TS for spraying on the plate, heat the plate at 105°C for 5 minutes, allow to cool, and spray water: one of the several spots obtained from the sample solution has the same color tone and *Rf* value with the blue-green to grayish green spot from the standard solution (Ginger).

Purity **(1)** Heavy metals <*1.07*>—Prepare the test solution with 1.0 g of the dry extract (or an amount of the viscous extract, equivalent to 1.0 g of the dried substance) as directed under the Extracts (4), and perform the test (not more than 30 ppm).

(2) Arsenic <*1.11*>—Prepare the test solution with 0.67 g of the dry extract (or an amount of the viscous extract, equivalent to 0.67 g of the dried substance) according to Method 3, and perform the test (not more than 3 ppm).

Loss on drying <*2.41*> The dry extract: Not more than 11.0% (1 g, 105°C, 5 hours).

The viscous extract: Not more than 66.7% (1 g, 105°C, 5 hours).

Total ash <*5.01*> Not more than 14.0%, calculated on the dried basis.

Assay **(1)** Magnolol—Weigh accurately about 0.5 g of the dry extract (or an amount of the viscous extract, equivalent to about 0.5 g of the dried substance), add exactly 50 mL of diluted methanol (7 in 10), shake for 15 minutes, filter, and use the filtrate as the sample solution. Separately, weigh accurately about 10 mg of magnolol for assay, and dissolve in diluted methanol (7 in 10) to make exactly 100 mL. Pipet 5 mL of this solution, add diluted methanol (7 in 10) to make exactly 20 mL, and use this solution as the standard solution. Perform the test with exactly 10 μL each of the sample solution and standard solution as directed under Liquid Chromatography <*2.01*> according to the following conditions, and determine the peak areas, A_T and A_S, of magnolol in each solution.

$$\text{Amount (mg) of magnolol} = M_S \times A_T/A_S \times 1/8$$

M_S: Amount (mg) of magnolol for assay taken, calculated on the basis of the content obtained by qNMR

Operating conditions—

Detector: An ultraviolet absorption photometer (wave-

length: 289 nm).

Column: A stainless steel column 4.6 mm in inside diameter and 15 cm in length, packed with octadecylsilanized silica gel for liquid chromatography (5 μm in particle diameter).

Column temperature: A constant temperature of about 40°C.

Mobile phase: A mixture of water, acetonitrile and acetic acid (100) (50:50:1).

Flow rate: 1.0 mL per minute (the retention time of magnolol is about 15 minutes).

System suitability—

System performance: Dissolve 1 mg each of magnolol for assay and honokiol in diluted methanol (7 in 10) to make 10 mL. When the procedure is run with 10 μL of this solution under the above operating conditions, honokiol and magnolol are eluted in this order with the resolution between these peaks being not less than 2.5.

System repeatability: When the test is repeated 6 times with 10 μL of the standard solution under the above operating conditions, the relative standard deviation of the peak area of magnolol is not more than 1.5%.

(2) Rosmarinic acid—Conduct this procedure using light-resistant vessels. Weigh accurately about 0.5 g of the dry extract (or an amount of the viscous extract, equivalent to about 0.5 g of the dried substance), add exactly 50 mL of diluted methanol (7 in 10), shake for 15 minutes, filter, and use the filtrate as the sample solution. Separately, weigh accurately about 10 mg of rosmarinic acid for assay, dissolve in diluted methanol (7 in 10) to make exactly 200 mL, and use this solution as the standard solution. Perform the test with exactly 10 μL each of the sample solution and standard solution as directed under Liquid Chromatography <*2.01*> according to the following conditions, and determine the peak areas, A_T and A_S, of rosmarinic acid in each solution.

Amount (mg) of rosmarinic acid = $M_S \times A_T/A_S \times 1/4$

M_S: Amount (mg) of rosmarinic acid for assay taken, calculated on the basis of the content obtained by qNMR

Operating conditions—

Detector: An ultraviolet absorption photometer (wavelength: 330 nm).

Column: A stainless steel column 4.6 mm in inside diameter and 15 cm in length, packed with octadecylsilanized silica gel for liquid chromatography (5 μm in particle diameter).

Column temperature: A constant temperature of about 30°C.

Mobile phase: A mixture of water, acetonitrile and phosphoric acid (800:200:1).

Flow rate: 1.0 mL per minute (the retention time of rosmarinic acid is about 11 minutes).

System suitability—

System performance: When the procedure is run with 10 μL of the standard solution under the above operating conditions, the number of theoretical plates and the symmetry factor of the peak of rosmarinic acid are not less than 5000 and not more than 1.5, respectively.

System repeatability: When the test is repeated 6 times with 10 μL of the standard solution under the above operating conditions, the relative standard deviation of the peak area of rosmarinic acid is not more than 1.5%.

(3) [6]-Gingerol—Weigh accurately about 0.5 g of the dry extract (or an amount of the viscous extract, equivalent to about 0.5 g of the dried substance), add exactly 50 mL of diluted methanol (7 in 10), shake for 15 minutes, filter, and use the filtrate as the sample solution. Separately, weigh accurately about 10 mg of [6]-gingerol for assay, dissolve in methanol to make exactly 100 mL. Pipet 5 mL of this solution, add methanol to make exactly 50 mL, and use this solution as the standard solution. Perform the test with exactly 10 μL each of the sample solution and standard solution as directed under Liquid Chromatography <*2.01*> according to the following conditions, and determine the peak areas, A_T and A_S, of [6]-gingerol in each solution.

Amount (mg) of [6]-gingerol = $M_S \times A_T/A_S \times 1/20$

M_S: Amount (mg) of [6]-gingerol for assay taken

Operating conditions—

Detector: An ultraviolet absorption photometer (wavelength: 282 nm).

Column: A stainless steel column 4.6 mm in inside diameter and 15 cm in length, packed with octadecylsilanized silica gel for liquid chromatography (5 μm in particle diameter).

Column temperature: A constant temperature of about 30°C.

Mobile phase: A mixture of water, acetonitrile and phosphoric acid (620:380:1).

Flow rate: 1.0 mL per minute (the retention time of [6]-gingerol is about 15 minutes).

System suitability—

System performance: When the procedure is run with 10 μL of the standard solution under the above operating conditions, the number of theoretical plates and the symmetry factor of the peak of [6]-gingerol are not less than 5000 and not more than 1.5, respectively.

System repeatability: When the test is repeated 6 times with 10 μL of the standard solution under the above operating conditions, the relative standard deviation of the peak area of [6]-gingerol is not more than 1.5%.

Containers and storage Containers—Tight containers.

Hangeshashinto Extract

半夏瀉心湯エキス

Hangeshashinto Extract contains not less than 70 mg and not more than 210 mg (for preparation prescribed 2.5 g of Scutellaria Root) or not less than 80 mg and not more than 240 mg (for preparation prescribed 3 g of Scutellaria Root) of baicalin ($C_{21}H_{18}O_{11}$: 446.36), not less than 18 mg and not more than 54 mg (for preparation prescribed 2.5 g of Glycyrrhiza) or not less than 20 mg and not more than 60 mg (for preparation prescribed 3 g of Glycyrrhiza) of glycyrrhizic acid ($C_{42}H_{62}O_{16}$: 822.93), and not less than 7 mg and not more than 21 mg of berberine [as berberine chloride ($C_{20}H_{18}ClNO_4$: 371.81)], per extract prepared with the amount specified in the Method of preparation.

Method of preparation

	1)	2)	3)
Pinellia Tuber	5 g	6 g	5 g
Scutellaria Root	2.5 g	3 g	2.5 g
Processed Ginger	2.5 g	3 g	—
Ginger	—	—	2.5 g
Ginseng	2.5 g	3 g	2.5 g
Glycyrrhiza	2.5 g	3 g	2.5 g
Jujube	2.5 g	3 g	2.5 g
Coptis Rhizome	1 g	1 g	1 g

Prepare a dry extract or viscous extract as directed under Extracts, according to the prescription 1), 2) or 3), using the crude drugs shown above.

Description Hangeshashinto Extract is a light yellow to yellow-brown powder or black-brown viscous extract. It has a slightly odor and a hotter, bitter and slightly sweet taste.

Identification **(1)** Shake 1.0 g of the dry extract (or 3.0 g of the viscous extract) with 10 mL of water, add 25 mL of diethyl ether, and shake. Take the diethyl ether layer, evaporate the solvent under low pressure (in vacuo), add 2 mL of diethyl ether to the residue, and use this solution as the sample solution. Separately, dissolve 1 mg of wogonin for thin-layer chromatography in 1 mL of methanol, and use this solution as the standard solution. Perform the test with these solutions as directed under Thin-layer Chromatography <*2.03*>. Spot 10 μL of the sample solution and 5 μL of the standard solution on a plate of silica gel for thin-layer chromatography. Develop the plate with a mixture of ethyl acetate, hexane and acetic acid (100) (10:10:1) to a distance of about 7 cm, and air-dry the plate. Spray evenly iron (III) chloride-methanol TS on the plate: one of the several spots obtained from the sample solution has the same color tone and *R*f value with the yellow-brown spot from the standard solution (Scutellaria Root).

(2) For preparation prescribed Processed Ginger—Shake 1.0 g of the dry extract (or 3.0 g of the viscous extract) with 10 mL of water, add 25 mL of diethyl ether, and shake. Separate the diethyl ether layer, evaporate the solvent under low pressure (in vacuo), add 2 mL of diethyl ether to the residue, and use this solution as the sample solution. Separately, dissolve 1 mg of [6]-shogaol for thin-layer chromatography in 1 mL of methanol, and use this solution as the standard solution. Perform the test with these solutions as directed under Thin-layer Chromatography <*2.03*>. Spot 20 μL of the sample solution and 1 μL of the standard solution on a plate of silica gel for thin-layer chromatography. Develop the plate with a mixture of cyclohexane and ethyl acetate (2:1) to a distance of about 7 cm, and air-dry the plate. Spray evenly 4-dimethylaminobenzaldehyde TS for spraying on the plate, heat the plate at 105°C for 5 minutes, allow to cool, and spray water: one of the several spots obtained from the sample solution has the same color tone and *R*f value with the blue-green to grayish green spot from the standard solution (Processed Ginger).

(3) For preparation prescribed Ginger—Shake 1.0 g of the dry extract (or 3.0 g of the viscous extract) with 10 mL of water, add 25 mL of diethyl ether, and shake. Separate the diethyl ether layer, evaporate the solvent under low pressure (in vacuo), add 2 mL of diethyl ether to the residue, and use this solution as the sample solution. Separately, dissolve 1 mg of [6]-gingerol for thin-layer chromatography in 1 mL of methanol, and use this solution as the standard solution. Perform the test with these solutions as directed under Thin-layer Chromatography <*2.03*>. Spot 10 μL of the sample solution and 5 μL of the standard solution on a plate of silica gel for thin-layer chromatography. Develop the plate with a mixture of ethyl acetate and hexane (1:1) to a distance of about 7 cm, and air-dry the plate. Spray evenly 4-dimethylaminobenzaldehyde TS for spraying on the plate, heat the plate at 105°C for 5 minutes, allow to cool, and spray water: one of the several spots obtained from the sample solution has the same color tone and *R*f value with the blue-green to grayish green spot from the standard solution (Ginger).

(4) Shake 2.0 g of the dry extract (or 6.0 g of the viscous extract) with 10 mL of sodium hydroxide TS, add 5 mL of 1-butanol, shake, centrifuge, and use the 1-butanol layer as the sample solution. Separately, dissolve 1 mg of Ginsenoside Rg_1 RS or ginsenoside Rg_1 for thin-layer chromatography in 1 mL of methanol, and use this solution as the standard solution. Perform the test with these solutions as directed under Thin-layer Chromatography <*2.03*>. Spot 10 μL of the sample solution and 2 μL of the standard solution on a plate of silica gel for thin-layer chromatography. Develop the plate with a mixture of ethyl acetate, 1-propanol, water and acetic acid (100) (7:5:4:1) to a distance of about 7 cm, and air-dry the plate. Spray evenly vanillin-sulfuric acid-ethanol TS for spraying on the plate, heat the plate at 105°C for 5 minutes, and allow to cool: one of the several spots obtained from the sample solution has the same color tone and *R*f value with the purple spot from the standard solution (Ginseng).

(5) Shake 1.0 g of the dry extract (or 3.0 g of the viscous extract) with 10 mL of water, add 5 mL of 1-butanol, shake, centrifuge, and use the 1-butanol layer as the sample solution. Separately, dissolve 1 mg of liquiritin for thin-layer chromatography in 1 mL of methanol, and use this solution as the standard solution. Perform the test with these solutions as directed under Thin-layer Chromatography <*2.03*>. Spot 1 μL each of the sample solution and standard solution on a plate of silica gel for thin-layer chromatography. Develop the plate with a mixture of ethyl acetate, methanol and water (20:3:2) to a distance of about 7 cm, and air-dry the plate. Spray evenly dilute sulfuric acid on the plate, heat the plate at 105°C for 5 minutes, and examine under ultraviolet light (main wavelength: 365 nm): one of the several spots obtained from the sample solution has the same color tone and *R*f value with the yellow-green fluorescent spot from the standard solution (Glycyrrhiza).

(6) Shake 0.5 g of the dry extract (or 1.5 g of the viscous extract) with 10 mL of methanol, centrifuge, and use the supernatant liquid as the sample solution. Separately, dissolve 1 mg of coptisine chloride for thin-layer chromatography in 5 mL of methanol, and use this solution as the standard solution. Perform the test with these solutions as directed under Thin-layer Chromatography <*2.03*>. Spot 5 μL each of the sample solution and standard solution on a plate of silica gel for thin-layer chromatography. Develop the plate with a mixture of ethyl acetate, ammonia solution (28) and methanol (15:1:1) to a distance of about 7 cm, and air-dry the plate. Examine under ultraviolet light (main wavelength: 365 nm): one of the several spots obtained from the sample solution has the same color tone and *R*f value with the yellow fluorescent spot from the standard solution (Coptis Rhizome).

Purity **(1)** Heavy metals <*1.07*>—Prepare the test solution with 1.0 g of the dry extract (or an amount of the viscous extract, equivalent to 1.0 g of the dried substance) as directed under Extracts (4), and perform the test (not more than 30 ppm).

(2) Arsenic <*1.11*>—Prepare the test solution with 0.67 g of the dry extract (or an amount of the viscous extract, equivalent to 0.67 g of the dried substance) according to Method 3, and perform the test (not more than 3 ppm).

Loss on drying <*2.41*> The dry extract—Not more than 9.5% (1 g, 105°C, 5 hours).

The viscous extract—Not more than 66.7% (1 g, 105°C, 5 hours).

Total ash <*5.01*> Not more than 10.0%, calculated on the dried basis.

Assay **(1)** Baicalin—Weigh accurately about 0.1 g of the dry extract (or an amount of the viscous extract, equivalent to about 0.1 g of the dried substance), add exactly 50 mL of diluted methanol (7 in 10), shake for 15 minutes, filter, and use the filtrate as the sample solution. Separately, weigh accurately about 10 mg of Baicalin RS (separately determine the water <*2.48*> by coulometric titration, using 10 mg), and dissolve in methanol to make exactly 100 mL. Pipet 5 mL of this solution, add diluted methanol (7 in 10) to make exactly 10 mL, and use this solution as the standard solution. Perform the test with exactly 10 μL each of the sample solution and standard solution as directed under Liquid Chromatography <*2.01*> according to the following conditions, and determine the peak areas, A_T and A_S, of baicalin in each solution.

$$\text{Amount (mg) of baicalin } (C_{21}H_{18}O_{11}) = M_S \times A_T/A_S \times 1/4$$

M_S: Amount (mg) of Baicalin RS taken, calculated on the anhydrous basis

Operating conditions—

Detector: An ultraviolet absorption photometer (wavelength: 277 nm).

Column: A stainless steel column 4.6 mm in inside diameter and 15 cm in length, packed with octadecylsilanized silica gel for liquid chromatography (5 μm in particle diameter).

Column temperature: A constant temperature of about 40°C.

Mobile phase: A mixture of diluted phosphoric acid (1 in 200) and acetonitrile (19:6).

Flow rate: 1.0 mL per minute (the retention time of baicalin is about 10 minutes).

System suitability—

System performance: When the procedure is run with 10 μL of the standard solution under the above operating conditions, the number of theoretical plates and the symmetry factor of the peak of baicalin are not less than 5000 and not more than 1.5, respectively.

System repeatability: When the test is repeated 6 times with 10 μL of the standard solution under the above operating conditions, the relative standard deviation of the peak area of baicalin is not more than 1.5%.

(2) Glycyrrhizic acid—Perform the test according to the following i) or ii).

i) Weigh accurately about 0.5 g of the dry extract (or an amount of the viscous extract, equivalent to about 0.5 g of the dried substance), add exactly 50 mL of diluted methanol (1 in 2), shake for 15 minutes, filter, and use the filtrate as the sample solution. Separately, weigh accurately about 10 mg of Glycyrrhizic Acid RS (separately determine the water <*2.48*> by coulometric titration, using 10 mg), dissolve in diluted methanol (1 in 2) to make exactly 100 mL, and use this solution as the standard solution. Perform the test with exactly 10 μL each of the sample solution and standard solution as directed under Liquid Chromatography <*2.01*> according to the following conditions, and determine the peak areas, A_T and A_S, of glycyrrhizic acid in each solution.

$$\text{Amount (mg) of glycyrrhizic acid } (C_{42}H_{62}O_{16}) = M_S \times A_T/A_S \times 1/2$$

M_S: Amount (mg) of Glycyrrhizic Acid RS taken, calculated on the anhydrous basis

Operating conditions—

Detector: An ultraviolet absorption photometer (wavelength: 254 nm).

Column: A stainless steel column 4.6 mm in inside diameter and 15 cm in length, packed with octadecylsilanized silica gel for liquid chromatography (5 μm in particle diameter).

Column temperature: A constant temperature of about 40°C.

Mobile phase: Dissolve 3.85 g of ammonium acetate in 720 mL of water, and add 5 mL of acetic acid (100) and 280 mL of acetonitrile.

Flow rate: 1.0 mL per minute (the retention time of glycyrrhizic acid is about 15 minutes).

System suitability—

System performance: Dissolve 5 mg of monoammonium glycyrrhizinate for resolution check in 20 mL of dilute ethanol. When the procedure is run with 10 μL of this solution under the above operating conditions, the resolution between the peak having the relative retention time of about 0.9 to glycyrrhizic acid and the peak of glycyrrhizic acid is not less than 1.5. Dissolve 1 mg of baicalein for resolution check in 50 mL of methanol. To 2 mL of this solution add 2 mL of the standard solution. When the procedure is run with 10 μL of this solution under the above operating conditions, the resolution between the peaks of glycyrrhizic acid and baicalein is not less than 1.5.

System repeatability: When the test is repeated 6 times with 10 μL of the standard solution under the above operating conditions, the relative standard deviation of the peak area of glycyrrhizic acid is not more than 1.5%.

ii) Weigh accurately about 0.5 g of the dry extract (or an amount of the viscous extract, equivalent to about 0.5 g of the dried substance), add 20 mL of ethyl acetate and 10 mL of water, and shake for 10 minutes. After centrifugation, remove the ethyl acetate layer, add 20 mL of ethyl acetate, proceed in the same manner as described above, and remove the ethyl acetate layer. To the aqueous layer add 10 mL of methanol, shake for 30 minutes, centrifuge, and take the supernatant liquid. To the residue add 20 mL of diluted methanol (1 in 2), shake for 5 minutes, centrifuge, and take the supernatant liquid. Combine these supernatant liquids, add diluted methanol (1 in 2) to make exactly 50 mL, and use this solution as the sample solution. Separately, weigh accurately about 10 mg of Glycyrrhizic Acid RS (separately determine the water <*2.48*> by coulometric titration, using 10 mg), dissolve in diluted methanol (1 in 2) to make exactly 100 mL, and use this solution as the standard solution. Perform the test with exactly 10 μL each of the sample solution and standard solution as directed under Liquid Chromatography <*2.01*> according to the following conditions, and determine the peak areas, A_T and A_S, of glycyrrhizic acid in each solution.

$$\text{Amount (mg) of glycyrrhizic acid } (C_{42}H_{62}O_{16}) = M_S \times A_T/A_S \times 1/2$$

M_S: Amount (mg) of Glycyrrhizic Acid RS taken, calculated on the anhydrous basis

Operating conditions—

Proceed as directed in the operating conditions in i).

System suitability—

System repeatability: Proceed as directed in the system suitability in i).

System performance: Dissolve 5 mg of monoammonium glycyrrhizinate for resolution check in 20 mL of dilute ethanol. When the procedure is run with 10 μL of this solution under the above operating conditions, the resolution between the peak having the relative retention time of about 0.9 to glycyrrhizic acid and the peak of glycyrrhizic acid is not less than 1.5.

(3) Berberine—Weigh accurately about 0.2 g of the dry

extract (or an amount of the viscous extract, equivalent to about 0.2 g of the dried substance), add exactly 50 mL of the mobile phase, shake for 15 minutes, filter, and use the filtrate as the sample solution. Separately, weigh accurately about 10 mg of Berberine Chloride RS (separately determine the water <*2.48*> in the same manner as Berberine Chloride Hydrate), dissolve in the mobile phase to make exactly 100 mL, and use this solution as the standard solution. Perform the test with exactly 10 μL each of the sample solution and standard solution as directed under Liquid Chromatography <*2.01*> according to the following conditions, and determine the peak areas, A_T and A_S, of berberine in each solution.

Amount (mg) of berberine chloride ($C_{20}H_{18}ClNO_4$)
$= M_S \times A_T/A_S \times 1/2$

M_S: Amount (mg) of Berberine Chloride RS taken, calculated on the anhydrous basis

Operating conditions—

Detector: An ultraviolet absorption photometer (wavelength: 345 nm).

Column: A stainless steel column 4.6 mm in inside diameter and 15 cm in length, packed with octadecylsilanized silica gel for liquid chromatography (5 μm in particle diameter).

Column temperature: A constant temperature of about 30°C.

Mobile phase: Dissolve 3.4 g of potassium dihydrogen phosphate and 1.7 g of sodium lauryl sulfate in 1000 mL of a mixture of water and acetonitrile (1:1).

Flow rate: 1.0 mL per minute (the retention time of berberine is about 8 minutes).

System suitability—

System performance: Dissolve 1 mg each of Berberine Chloride RS and palmatine chloride in the mobile phase to make 10 mL. When the procedure is run with 10 μL of this solution under the above operating conditions, palmatine and berberine are eluted in this order with the resolution between these peaks being not less than 1.5.

System repeatability: When the test is repeated 6 times with 10 μL of the standard solution under the above operating conditions, the relative standard deviation of the peak area of berberine is not more than 1.5%.

Containers and storage Containers—Tight containers.

Hedysarum Root

Hedysari Radix

シンギ

Hedysarum Root is the root of *Hedysarum polybotrys* Handel-Mazzetti (*Leguminosae*).

Description Hedysarum Root is nearly cylindrical, 20 - 100 cm in length, 0.5 - 2.5 cm in diameter; outer surface yellow-brown to red-brown, with irregular longitudinal wrinkles; often horizontal lenticels and scars of lateral roots; periderm peeled easily, internally light yellow-brown to light red-brown; soft in texture, flexible and difficult to break; fractured surface fibrous, powdery; in transverse section nearly white in cortex, brownish around cambium, light yellow-brown in xylem; ray obvious.

Odor, slightly characteristic; taste, slightly sweet.

Under a microscope <*5.01*>, a transverse section reveals cork layer 6 - 8 cells layered, 2 - 4 cells layered parenchyma cells with sparingly thick wall inside the cork layer; ray obvious in secondary cortex and often appearing cracked tissue in outer portion of secondary cortex; phloem fiber bungles arranged stepwise in phloem; ray obvious in xylem, reticulate, scalariform, pitted, and spiral vessels; xylem tissues around vessels; thin walled cells containing solitary crystals of calcium oxalate in peripheral region of phloem fibers and xylem fibers and appearing as crystal cell rows in a longitudinal section; solitary crystals of calcium oxalate 7 - 20 μm in diameter, starch grains simple or 2- to 8-compound grains in parenchyma.

Identification To 1.0 g of pulverized Hedysarum Root add 10 mL of methanol, shake for 10 minutes, and filter. Evaporate the solvent of the filtrate under low pressure (in vacuo), add 1 mL of methanol to the residue, and use this solution as the sample solution. Perform the test with the sample solution as directed under Thin-layer Chromatography <*2.03*>. Spot 10 μL of the sample solution on a plate of silica gel for thin-layer chromatography. Develop the plate with a mixture of hexane, 2-butanone and formic acid (60:40:1) to a distance of about 7 cm, and air-dry the plate. Examine under ultraviolet light (main wavelength: 365 nm): a blue-white fluorescent spot at an *R*f value of about 0.4 is observed.

Purity **(1)** Heavy metals <*1.07*>—Proceed with 3.0 g of pulverized Hedysarum Root according to Method 3, and perform the test. Prepare the control solution with 3.0 mL of Standard Lead Solution (not more than 10 ppm).

(2) Arsenic <*1.11*>—Prepare the test solution with 0.40 g of pulverized Hedysarum Root according to Method 4, and perform the test (not more than 5 ppm).

Loss on drying <*5.01*> Not more than 16.0% (6 hours).

Total ash <*5.01*> Not more than 5.5%.

Acid-insoluble ash <*5.01*> Not more than 1.0%.

Extract content <*5.01*> Dilute ethanol-soluble extract: not less than 25.0%.

Containers and storage Containers—Well-closed containers.

Hemp Fruit

Cannabis Fructus

マシニン

Hemp Fruit is the fruit of *Cannabis sativa* Linné (*Moraceae*).

Description Hemp Fruit is a slightly compressed void fruit, 4 - 5 mm in length, 3 - 4 mm in diameter; externally grayish green to grayish brown; pointed at one end, a scar of gynophore at the other end, and ridge on both sides; outer surface lustrous with white mesh-like pattern; slightly hard pericarp; seed, slightly green in color and internally has grayish white albumen; 100 fruits weigh 1.6 - 2.7 g.

Practically odorless, aromatic on chewing; taste, mild and oily.

Under a microscope <*5.01*>, a transverse section reveals the exocarp composed of an epidermis; mesocarp composed of parenchyma, a pigment cell layer and rows of short, small cells; endocarp made up of a single cellular layer of radially elongated stone cells; seed coat comprises a tubular cellular layer and spongy tissue. Inside of the seed; exosperm consists of one cellular layer of parenchymatous cells, endosperm of one to several cellular layers of parenchymatous cells; most of the embryo composed of parenchyma, vascular bundles occurring in the center of hypocotyls and cotyledons; embryo parenchyma contains aleurone grains and oil drops.

Identification To 0.3 g of pulverized Hemp Fruit add 3 mL of methanol, shake for 10 minutes, centrifuge, and use the supernatant liquid as the sample solution. Perform the test with the sample solution as directed under Thin-layer Chromatography <*2.03*>. Spot 5 μL of the sample solution on a plate of silica gel for thin-layer chromatography, develop the plate with a mixture of hexane and ethyl acetate (9:2) to a distance of about 7 cm, and air-dry the plate. Spray evenly vanillin-sulfuric acid-ethanol TS for spraying on the plate, and heat the plate at 105°C for 5 minutes: a dark blue-purple spot appears at an *Rf* value of about 0.6.

Purity Bract—When perform the test of foreign matter <*5.01*>, Hemp Fruit does not contain bract.

Loss on drying <*5.01*> Not more than 9.0% (6 hours).

Total ash <*5.01*> Not more than 7.0%.

Acid-insoluble ash <*5.01*> Not more than 2.0%.

Containers and storage Containers—Well-closed containers.

Hochuekkito Extract

補中益気湯エキス

Hochuekkito Extract contains not less than 16 mg and not more than 64 mg of hesperidin, not less than 0.3 mg and not more than 1.2 mg (for preparation prescribed 1 g of Bupleurum Root) or not less than 0.6 mg and not more than 2.4 mg (for preparation prescribed 2 g of Bupleurum Root) of saikosaponin b_2, and not less than 10 mg and not more than 30 mg of glycyrrhizic acid ($C_{42}H_{62}O_{16}$: 822.93), per extract prepared with the amount specified in the Method of preparation.

Method of preparation

	1)	2)	3)	4)	5)	6)
Ginseng	4 g	4 g	4 g	4 g	4 g	4 g
Atractylodes Rhizome	4 g	—	4 g	—	4 g	4 g
Atractylodes Lancea Rhizom	—	4 g	—	4 g	—	—
Astragalus Root	4 g	4 g	4 g	4 g	3 g	4 g
Japanese Angelica Root	3 g	3 g	3 g	3 g	3 g	3 g
Citrus Unshiu Peel	2 g	2 g	2 g	2 g	2 g	2 g
Jujube	2 g	2 g	2 g	2 g	2 g	2 g
Bupleurum Root	2 g	2 g	1 g	1 g	2 g	1 g
Glycyrrhiza	1.5 g	1.5 g	1.5 g	1.5 g	1.5 g	1.5 g
Ginger	0.5 g	0.5 g	0.5 g	0.5 g	0.5 g	—
Processed Ginger	—	—	—	—	—	0.5 g
Cimicifuga Rhizome	1 g	1 g	0.5 g	0.5 g	1 g	0.5 g

Prepare a dry extract or viscous extract as directed under Extracts, according to the prescription 1) to 6), using the crude drugs shown above.

Description Hochuekkito Extract occurs as a light brown to brown powder or black-brown viscous extract. It has a slight odor, and a sweet and bitter taste.

Identification **(1)** To 2.0 g of the dry extract (or 6.0 g of the viscous extract) add 10 mL of sodium hydroxide TS, shake, then add 5 mL of 1-butanol, and shake. Centrifuge this solution, and use the 1-butanol layer as the sample solution. Separately, dissolve 1 mg of Ginsenoside Rb_1 RS or ginsenoside Rb_1 for thin-layer chromatography in 1 mL of methanol, and use this solution as the standard solution. Perform the test with these solutions as directed under Thin-layer Chromatography <*2.03*>. Spot 5 μL each of the sample solution and standard solution on a plate of silica gel for thin-layer chromatography. Develop the plate with a mixture of ethyl acetate, 1-propanol, water and acetic acid (100) (7:5:4:1) to a distance of about 7 cm, and air-dry the plate. Spray evenly vanillin-sulfuric acid-ethanol TS for spraying on the plate, heat the plate at 105°C for 5 minutes, and allow to cool: one of the several spots obtained from the sample solution has the same color tone and *Rf* value with the blue-purple spot from the standard solution (Ginseng).

(2) For preparation prescribed Atractylodes Rhizome—To 3.0 g of the dry extract (or 9.0 g of the viscous extract) add 30 mL of water, shake, then add 50 mL of diethyl ether, shake, and separate the diethyl ether layer. Evaporate the solvent under low pressure (in vacuo), add 1 mL of diethyl ether to the residue, and use this solution as the sample solution. Separately, dissolve 1 mg of atractylenolide III for thin-layer chromatography in 1 mL of methanol, and use this solution as the standard solution. Perform the test with these solutions as directed under Thin-layer Chromatography <*2.03*>. Spot 5 μL of the sample solution and 10 μL of the standard solution on a plate of silica gel for thin-layer chromatography. Develop the plate with a mixture of ethyl acetate and hexane (1:1) to a distance of about 7 cm, and air-dry the plate. Spray evenly 1-naphthol-sulfuric acid TS on the plate, heat the plate at 105°C for 5 minutes, and allow to cool: one of the several spots obtained from the sample solution has the same color tone and *Rf* value with the red spot from the standard solution (Atractylodes Rhizome).

(3) For preparation prescribed Atractylodes Lancea Rhizome—To 2.0 g of the dry extract (or 6.0 g of the viscous extract) add 10 mL of water, shake, then add 25 mL of hexane, shake, and separate the hexane layer. Evaporate the solvent under low pressure (in vacuo), add 2 mL of hexane to the residue, and use this solution as the sample solution. Perform the test with the sample solution as directed under Thin-layer Chromatography <*2.03*>. Spot 20 μL of the sample solution on a plate of silica gel with fluorescent indicator for thin-layer chromatography. Develop the plate with a mixture of hexane and acetone (7:1) to a distance of about 7 cm, and air-dry the plate. Examine under ultraviolet light (main wavelength: 254 nm): a dark purple spot is observed at an *Rf* value of about 0.5. The spot shows a greenish brown color after being sprayed evenly 4-dimethylaminobenzaldehyde TS for spraying, heated the plate at 105°C for 5 minutes, and allowed to cool (Atractylodes Lancea Rhizome).

(4) To 3.0 g of the dry extract (or 9.0 g of the viscous extract) add 40 mL of a solution of potassium hydroxide in methanol (1 in 50), shake for 15 minutes, centrifuge, and evaporate the solvent under low pressure (in vacuo). Add 30 mL of water and 20 mL of diethyl ether to the residue, shake, remove the diethyl ether layer, and separate the aqueous layer. To the aqueous layer add 20 mL of 1-butanol, shake, and separate the 1-butanol layer. To the 1-butanol layer add 20 mL of water, shake, separate the 1-butanol layer, evaporate the solvent under low pressure (in vacuo), add 1 mL of methanol to the residue, and use this solution as the sample solution. Separately, dissolve 1 mg of astragaloside IV for thin-layer chromatography in 1 mL of methanol, and use this solution as the standard solution. Perform the test with these solutions as directed under Thin-layer Chromatography <*2.03*>. Spot 5 μL each of the sample solution and standard solution on a plate of octadecylsilanized silica gel for thin-layer chromatography. Develop the plate with a mixture of methanol, water, 1-butanol and acetic acid (100) (60:30:10:1) to a distance of about 7 cm, and air-dry the plate. Spray evenly 4-dimethylaminobenzaldehyde TS for spraying on the plate, and heat the plate at 105°C for 5 minutes: one of the several spots obtained from the sample solution has the same color tone and *R*f value with the red-brown spot from the standard solution (Astragalus Root).

(5) To 3.0 g of the dry extract (or 9.0 g of the viscous extract) add 30 mL of water, shake, then add 50 mL of diethyl ether, shake, and separate the diethyl ether layer. Evaporate the solvent under low pressure (in vacuo), add 1 mL of diethyl ether to the residue, and use this solution as the sample solution. Separately, use (*Z*)-ligustilide TS for thin-layer chromatography as the standard solution. Perform the test with these solutions as directed under Thin-layer Chromatography <*2.03*>. Spot 10 μL each of the sample solution and standard solution on a plate of silica gel for thin-layer chromatography. Develop the plate with a mixture of ethyl acetate and hexane (1:1) to a distance of about 7 cm, and air-dry the plate. Examine under ultraviolet light (main wavelength: 365 nm): one of the several spots obtained from the sample solution has the same color tone and *R*f value with the blue-white fluorescent spot from the standard solution (Japanese Angelica Root).

(6) To 2.0 g of the dry extract (or 6.0 g of the viscous extract) add 30 mL of water, shake, then add 50 mL of 1-butanol, shake, and separate the 1-butanol layer. Evaporate the solvent under low pressure (in vacuo), add 3 mL of methanol to the residue, and use this solution as the sample solution. Separately, dissolve 1 mg of hesperidin for thin-layer chromatography in 2 mL of methanol, and use this solution as the standard solution. Perform the test with these solutions as directed under Thin-layer Chromatography <*2.03*>. Spot 2 μL of the sample solution and 20 μL of the standard solution on a plate of silica gel for thin-layer chromatography. Develop the plate with a mixture of ethyl acetate, acetone, water and acetic acid (100) (10:6:3:1) to a distance of about 7 cm, and air-dry the plate. Spray evenly 2,6-dibromo-*N*-chloro-1,4-benzoquinone monoimine TS on the plate, and expose to ammonia vapor: one of the several spots obtained from the sample solution has the same color tone and *R*f value with the blue spot from the standard solution (Citrus Unshiu Peel).

(7) To 2.0 g of the dry extract (or 6.0 g of the viscous extract) add 10 mL of sodium hydroxide TS, shake, then add 5 mL of 1-butanol, and shake. Centrifuge this solution, and use the 1-butanol layer as the sample solution. Separately, dissolve 1 mg of saikosaponin b_2 for thin-layer chromatography in 1 mL of methanol, and use this solution as the standard solution. Perform the test with these solutions as directed under Thin-layer Chromatography <*2.03*>. Spot 5 μL of the sample solution and 2 μL of the standard solution on a plate of silica gel for thin-layer chromatography. Develop the plate with a mixture of ethyl acetate, ethanol (99.5) and water (8:2:1) to a distance of about 7 cm, and air-dry the plate. Spray evenly 4-dimethylaminobenzaldehyde TS for spraying on the plate, heat the plate at 105°C for 5 minutes, and examine under ultraviolet light (main wavelength: 365 nm): one of the several spots obtained from the sample solution has the same color tone and *R*f value with the yellow fluorescent spot from the standard solution (Bupleurum Root).

(8) To 2.0 g of the dry extract (or 6.0 g of the viscous extract) add 30 mL of water, shake, then add 50 mL of 1-butanol, shake, and separate the 1-butanol layer. Evaporate the solvent under low pressure (in vacuo), add 3 mL of methanol to the residue, and use this solution as the sample solution. Separately, dissolve 1 mg of liquiritin for thin-layer chromatography in 1 mL of methanol, and use this solution as the standard solution. Perform the test with these solutions as directed under Thin-layer Chromatography <*2.03*>. Spot 1 μL each of the sample solution and standard solution on a plate of silica gel for thin-layer chromatography. Develop the plate with a mixture of ethyl acetate, methanol and water (20:3:2) to a distance of about 7 cm, and air-dry the plate. Spray evenly dilute sulfuric acid on the plate, heat the plate at 105°C for 5 minutes, and examine under ultraviolet light (main wavelength: 365 nm): one of the several spots obtained from the sample solution has the same color tone and *R*f value with the yellow-green fluorescent spot from the standard solution (Glycyrrhiza).

(9) For preparation prescribed Ginger—To 3.0 g of the dry extract (or 9.0 g of the viscous extract) add 30 mL of water, shake, then add 50 mL of diethyl ether, shake, and separate the diethyl ether layer. Evaporate the solvent under low pressure (in vacuo), add 1 mL of diethyl ether to the residue, and use this solution as the sample solution. Separately, dissolve 1 mg of [6]-gingerol for thin-layer chromatography in 1 mL of methanol, and use this solution as the standard solution. Perform the test with these solutions as directed under Thin-layer Chromatography <*2.03*>. Spot 5 μL each of the sample solution and standard solution on a plate of silica gel for thin-layer chromatography. Develop the plate with a mixture of ethyl acetate and hexane (1:1) to a distance of about 7 cm, and air-dry the plate. Spray evenly 4-dimethylaminobenzaldehyde TS for spraying on the plate, heat the plate at 105°C for 5 minutes, allow to cool, and spray water: one of the several spots obtained from the sample solution has the same color tone and *R*f value with the blue-green to grayish green spot from the standard solution (Ginger).

(10) For preparation prescribed Processed Ginger—Put 10 g of the dry extract (or 30 g of the viscous extract) in a 300-mL hard-glass flask, add 100 mL of water and 1 mL of silicone resin, connect an apparatus for essential oil determination, and heat to boil under a reflux condenser. The graduated tube of the apparatus is previously filled with water to the standard line, and 2 mL of hexane is added to the graduated tube. After heating under reflux for 1 hour, separate the hexane layer, and use the layer as the sample solution. Separately, dissolve 1 mg of [6]-shogaol for thin-layer chromatography in 1 mL of methanol, and use this solution as the standard solution. Perform the test with these solutions as directed under Thin-layer Chromatography <*2.03*>. Spot 60 μL of the sample solution and 10 μL of the standard solution on a plate of silica gel for thin-layer chromatography. Develop the plate with a mixture of cyclohexane and ethyl acetate (2:1) to a distance of about 7 cm, and air-dry the plate. Spray evenly 4-dimethylaminobenzaldehyde TS for spraying on the plate, heat the plate at 105°C for 5 minutes, allow to cool, and spray water: one of the several spots obtained from the sample solution has the same color tone and *R*f value with the blue-green to grayish green spot from the standard solution (Processed Ginger).

(11) To 2.0 g of the dry extract (or 6.0 g of the viscous extract) add 30 mL of water, shake, then add 50 mL of 1-butanol, shake, and separate the 1-butanol layer. Evaporate the solvent under low pressure (in vacuo), add 3 mL of methanol to the residue, and use this solution as the sample solution. Use (*E*)-isoferulic acid-(*E*)-ferulic acid TS for thin-layer chromatography as the standard solution. Perform the test with these solutions as directed under Thin-layer Chromatography <*2.03*>. Spot 5 μL of the sample solution and 2 μL of the standard solution on a plate of silica gel for thin-layer chromatography. Develop the plate with a mixture of ethyl acetate, acetone and water (20:12:3) to a distance of about 7 cm, and air-dry the plate. Spray evenly sulfuric acid on the plate, heat the plate at 105°C for 5 minutes, and examine under ultraviolet light (main wavelength: 365 nm): one of the several spots obtained from the sample solution has the same color tone and *R*f value with the light yellow-white fluorescent spot from the standard solution (Cimicifuga Rhizome).

Purity **(1)** Heavy metals <*1.07*>—Prepare the test solution with 1.0 g of the dry extract (or an amount of the viscous extract, equivalent to 1.0 g of the dried substance) as directed in the Extracts (4), and perform the test (not more than 30 ppm).

(2) Arsenic <*1.11*>—Prepare the test solution with 0.67 g of the dry extract (or an amount of the viscous extract, equivalent to 0.67 g of the dried substance) according to Method 3, and perform the test (not more than 3 ppm).

Loss on drying <*2.41*> The dry extract: Not more than 11.5% (1 g, 105°C, 5 hours).

The viscous extract: Not more than 66.7% (1g, 105°C, 5 hours).

Total ash <*5.01*> Not more than 9.0%, calculated on the dried basis.

Assay **(1)** Hesperidin—Weigh accurately about 0.1 g of the dry extract (or an amount of the viscous extract, equivalent to about 0.1 g of the dried substance), add exactly 50 mL of diluted tetrahydrofuran (1 in 4), shake for 30 minutes, centrifuge, and use the supernatant liquid as the sample solution. Separately, weigh accurately about 10 mg of hesperidin for assay, previously dried in a desiccator (silica gel) for not less than 24 hours, and dissolve in methanol to make exactly 100 mL. Pipet 10 mL of this solution, add diluted tetrahydrofuran (1 in 4) to make exactly 100 mL, and use this solution as the standard solution. Perform the test with exactly 10 μL each of the sample solution and standard solution as directed under Liquid Chromatography <*2.01*> according to the following conditions, and determine the peak areas, A_T and A_S, of hesperidin in each solution.

$$\text{Amount (mg) of hesperidin} = M_S \times A_T/A_S \times 1/20$$

M_S: Amount (mg) of hesperidin for assay taken

Operating conditions—

Detector: An ultraviolet absorption photometer (wavelength: 285 nm).

Column: A stainless steel column 4.6 mm in inside diameter and 15 cm in length, packed with octadecylsilanized silica gel for liquid chromatography (5 μm in particle diameter).

Column temperature: A constant temperature of about 40°C.

Mobile phase: A mixture of water, acetonitrile and acetic acid (100) (82:18:1).

Flow rate: 1.0 mL per minute (the retention time of hesperidin is about 15 minutes).

System suitability—

System performance: Dissolve 1 mg each of hesperidin for assay and naringin for thin-layer chromatography in diluted methanol (1 in 2) to make 100 mL. When the procedure is run with 10 μL of this solution under the above operating conditions, naringin and hesperidin are eluted in this order with the resolution between these peaks being not less than 1.5.

System repeatability: When the test is repeated 6 times with 10 μL of the standard solution under the above operating conditions, the relative standard deviation of the peak area of hesperidin is not more than 1.5%.

(2) Saikosaponin b_2—Weigh accurately about 0.5 g of the dry extract (or an amount of the viscous extract, equivalent to about 0.5 g of the dried substance), add exactly 50 mL of diluted methanol (1 in 2), shake for 15 minutes, filter, and use the filtrate as the sample solution. Separately, use saikosaponin b_2 standard TS for assay as the standard solution. Perform the test with exactly 10 μL each of the sample solution and standard solution as directed under Liquid Chromatography <*2.01*> according to the following conditions, and determine the peak areas, A_T and A_S, of saikosaponin b_2 in each solution.

$$\text{Amount (mg) of saikosaponin } b_2 = C_S \times A_T/A_S \times 50$$

C_S: Concentration (mg/mL) of saikosaponin b_2 in saikosaponin b_2 standard TS for assay

Operating conditions—

Detector: An ultraviolet absorption photometer (wavelength: 254 nm).

Column: A stainless steel column 4.6 mm in inside diameter and 15 cm in length, packed with octadecylsilanized silica gel for liquid chromatography (5 μm in particle diameter).

Column temperature: A constant temperature of about 40°C.

Mobile phase: A mixture of 0.05 mol/L sodium dihydrogen phosphate TS and acetonitrile (5:3).

Flow rate: 1.0 mL per minute (the retention time of saikosaponin b_2 is about 12 minutes).

System suitability—

System performance: When the procedure is run with 10 μL of the standard solution under the above operating conditions, the number of theoretical plates and the symmetry factor of the peak of saikosaponin b_2 are not less than 5000 and not more than 1.5, respectively.

System repeatability: When the test is repeated 6 times with 10 μL of the standard solution under the above operating conditions, the relative standard deviation of the peak area of saikosaponin b_2 is not more than 1.5%.

(3) Glycyrrhizic acid—Weigh accurately about 0.5 g of the dry extract (or an amount of the viscous extract, equivalent to about 0.5 g of the dried substance), add 20 mL of ethyl acetate and 10 mL of water, and shake for 10 minutes. After centrifugation, remove the ethyl acetate layer, add 20 mL of ethyl acetate, proceed in the same manner as described above, and remove the ethyl acetate layer. To the aqueous layer add 10 mL of methanol, shake for 30 minutes, centrifuge, and take the supernatant liquid. To the residue add 20 mL of diluted methanol (1 in 2), shake for 5 minutes, centrifuge, and take the supernatant liquid. Combine these supernatant liquids, add diluted methanol (1 in 2) to make exactly 50 mL, and use this solution as the sample solution. Separately, weigh accurately about 10 mg of Glycyrrhizic Acid RS (separately determine the water <*2.48*> by coulometric titration, using 10 mg), dissolve in diluted methanol (1 in 2) to make exactly 100 mL, and use this solution as the standard solution. Perform the test with exactly 10 μL each of the sample solution and standard solution as directed under Liquid Chromatography <*2.01*> according to the following conditions, and determine the peak areas, A_T and A_S, of glycyrrhizic acid in each solution.

Amount (mg) of glycyrrhizic acid ($C_{42}H_{62}O_{16}$)
$= M_S \times A_T/A_S \times 1/2$

M_S: Amount (mg) of Glycyrrhizic Acid RS taken, calculated on the anhydrous basis

Operating conditions—

Detector: An ultraviolet absorption photometer (wavelength: 254 nm).

Column: A stainless steel column 4.6 mm in inside diameter and 15 cm in length, packed with octadecylsilanized silica gel for liquid chromatography (5 μm in particle diameter).

Column temperature: A constant temperature of about 40°C.

Mobile phase: Dissolve 3.85 g of ammonium acetate in 720 mL of water, and add 5 mL of acetic acid (100) and 280 mL of acetonitrile.

Flow rate: 1.0 mL per minute (the retention time of glycyrrhizic acid is about 15 minutes).

System suitability—

System performance: Dissolve 5 mg of monoammonium glycyrrhizinate for resolution check in 20 mL of dilute ethanol. When the procedure is run with 10 μL of this solution under the above operating conditions, the resolution between the peak having the relative retention time of about 0.9 to glycyrrhizic acid and the peak of glycyrrhizic acid is not less than 1.5.

System repeatability: When the test is repeated 6 times with 10 μL of the standard solution under the above operating conditions, the relative standard deviation of the peak area of glycyrrhizic acid is not more than 1.5%.

Containers and storage Containers—Tight containers.

Honey

Mel

ハチミツ

Honey is the saccharine substances obtained from the honeycomb of *Apis mellifera* Linné or *Apis cerana* Fabricius (*Apidae*).

Description Honey is a light yellow to light yellow-brown, syrupy liquid. Usually it is transparent, but often opaque with separated crystals.

It has a characteristic odor and a sweet taste.

Specific gravity <*2.56*> Mix 50.0 g of Honey with 100 mL of water: the specific gravity of the solution is not less than d^{20}_{20}: 1.111.

Purity **(1)** Acidity—Mix 10 g of Honey with 50 mL of water, and titrate <*2.50*> with 1 mol/L potassium hydroxide VS (indicator: 2 drops of phenolphthalein TS): not more than 0.5 mL is required.

(2) Sulfate—Mix 1.0 g of Honey with 2.0 mL of water, and filter. To the filtrate add 2 drops of barium chloride TS: the solution does not show any change immediately.

(3) Ammonia-coloring substances—Mix 1.0 g of Honey with 2.0 mL of water, and filter. To the filtrate add 2 mL of ammonia TS: the solution does not show any change immediately.

(4) Resorcinol-coloring substances—Mix well 5 g of Honey with 15 mL of diethyl ether, filter, and evaporate the diethyl ether solution at ordinary temperature. To the residue add 1 to 2 drops of resorcinol TS: a yellow-red color may develop in the solution of resorcinol and in the residue, and a red to red-purple color which does not persist more than 1 hour.

(5) Starch or dextrin—(i) Shake 7.5 g of Honey with 15 mL of water, warm the mixture on a water bath, and add 0.5 mL of tannic acid TS. After cooling, filter, and to 1.0 mL of the filtrate add 1.0 mL of ethanol (99.5) containing 2 drops of hydrochloric acid: no turbidity is produced.

(ii) To 2.0 g of Honey add 10 mL of water, warm in a water bath, mix, and allow to cool. Shake 1.0 mL of the mixture with 1 drop of iodine TS: no blue, green or red-brown color develops.

(6) Foreign matter—Mix 1.0 g of Honey with 2.0 mL of water, centrifuge the mixture, and examine the precipitate microscopically <*5.01*>: no foreign substance except pollen grains is observable.

Total ash <*5.01*> Not more than 0.4%.

Containers and storage Containers—Tight containers.

Houttuynia Herb

Houttuyniae Herba

ジュウヤク

Houttuynia Herb is the terrestrial part of *Houttuynia cordata* Thunberg (*Saururaceae*), collected during the flowering season.

Description Stem with alternate leaves and spikes; stem light brown, with longitudinal furrows and protruded nodes; when soaked in water and smoothed out, leaves wide ovate and cordate, 3 – 8 cm in length, 3 – 6 cm in width; light green-brown; margin entire, apex acuminate; petiole long, and membranous stipule at the base; spike, 1 – 3 cm in length, with numerous light yellow-brown achlamydeous florets, and the base enclosed by 4 long ovate, light yellow to light yellow-brown involucres.

Odor, slight; taste, slight.

Identification Heat 2 g of pulverized Houttuynia Herb with 20 mL of ethyl acetate under a reflux condenser for 15 minutes, and filter. Evaporate the filtrate to dryness, add 10 mL of water to the residue, warm the mixture on a water bath for 2 minutes, and, after cooling, filter. Shake well the filtrate with 20 mL of ethyl acetate in a separator, take 15 mL of ethyl acetate solution, and evaporate the solution on a water bath to dryness. Dissolve the residue in 5 mL of methanol, add 0.1 g of magnesium ribbon and 1 mL of hydrochloric acid, and allow the mixture to stand: a light red to red color develops.

Purity Foreign matter <*5.01*>—The amount of the rhizome, roots and other foreign matter contained in Houttuynia Herb is not more than 2.0%.

Total ash <*5.01*> Not more than 14.0%.

Acid-insoluble ash <*5.01*> Not more than 3.0%.

Extract content <*5.01*> Dilute ethanol-soluble extract: not less than 10.0%.

Containers and storage Containers—Well-closed containers.

Immature Orange

Aurantii Fructus Immaturus

キジツ

Immature Orange is the immature fruit or the fruit cut crosswise of *Citrus aurantium* Linné var. *daidai* Makino, *Citrus aurantium* Linné or *Citrus natsudaidai* Hayata (*Rutaceae*).

Description Nearly spherical fruit, 1 - 2 cm in diameter, or semispherical, 1.5 - 4.5 cm in diameter; external surface, deep green-brown to brown, and without luster, with numerous small dents associated with oil sacs; the outer portion of transverse section exhibits pericarp and mesocarp about 0.4 cm in thickness, yellow-brown in color in the region contacting epidermis, and light grayish brown color in the other parts; the central portion is radially divided into 8 to 16 small loculi; each loculus is brown and indented, often containing immature seeds.

Odor, characteristic; taste, bitter.

Identification To 0.5 g of pulverized Immature Orange add 10 mL of methanol, boil gently for 2 minutes, and filter. To 5 mL of the filtrate add 0.1 g of magnesium ribbon and 1 mL of hydrochloric acid, and allow to stand: a red-purple color develops.

Total ash <*5.01*> Not more than 7.0%.

Containers and storage Containers—Well-closed containers.

Imperata Rhizome

Imperatae Rhizoma

ボウコン

Imperata Rhizome is the rhizome of *Imperata cylindrica* Beauvois (*Gramineae*), from which rootlets and scale leaves have been removed.

Description Long and thin cylindrical rhizome, 0.3 - 0.5 cm in diameter; sometimes branched; externally yellow-white, with slight longitudinal wrinkles, and with nodes at 2 - 3 cm intervals; difficult to break; fractured surface fibrous. Cross section irregularly round; thickness of cortex is slightly smaller than the diameter of the stele; pith often forms a hollow. Under a magnifying glass, a transverse section reveals cortex, yellow-white, and with scattered brown spots; stele, yellow-brown in color.

Almost odorless, and tasteless at first, but later slightly sweet.

Identification To 1 g of pulverized Imperata Rhizome add 20 mL of hexane, allow the mixture to stand for 30 minutes with occasional shaking, and filter. Evaporate the solvent of the filtrate under low pressure (in vacuo), dissolve the residue in 5 mL of acetic anhydride, place 0.5 mL of this solution in a test tube, and add carefully 0.5 mL of sulfuric acid to make two layers: a red-brown color develops at the zone of contact, and the upper layer acquires a blue-green to blue-purple color.

Purity (1) Heavy metals <*1.07*>—Proceed with 3.0 g of pulverized Imperata Rhizome according to Method 3, and perform the test. Prepare the control solution with 3.0 mL of Standard Lead Solution (not more than 10 ppm).

(2) Arsenic <*1.11*>—Prepare the test solution with 0.40 g of pulverized Imperata Rhizome according to Method 4, and perform the test (not more than 5 ppm).

(3) Rootlet and scaly leaf—When perform the test of foreign matter <*5.01*>, the amount of the rootlets and scaly leaves contained in Imperata Rhizome is not more than 3.0 %.

(4) Foreign matter <*5.01*>—The amount of foreign matter other than rootlets and scaly leaves is not more than 1.0%.

Total ash <*5.01*> Not more than 5.0%.

Acid-insoluble ash <*5.01*> Not more than 1.5%.

Containers and storage Containers—Well-closed containers.

Ipecac

Ipecacuanhae Radix

トコン

Ipecac is the root and rhizome of *Cephaelis ipecacuanha* A. Richard or *Cephaelis acuminata* Karsten (*Rubiaceae*).

It contains not less than 2.0% of the total alkaloids (emetine and cephaeline), calculated on the basis of dried material.

Description Slender, curved, cylindrical root, 3 - 15 cm in length, 0.3 - 0.9 cm in diameter; mostly twisted, and sometimes branched; outer surface gray, dark grayish brown, red-brown in color and irregularly annulated; when root fractured, cortex easily separable from the xylem; the cortex on the fractured surface is grayish brown, and the xylem is light brown in color: thickness of cortex up to about two-thirds of radius in thickened portion. Scales in rhizome opposite.

Odor, slight; powder irritates the mucous membrane of the nose; taste, slightly bitter and unpleasant.

Under a microscope <*5.01*>, the transverse section of Ipecac reveals a cork layer, consisting of brown thin-walled cork cells; in the cortex, sclerenchyma cells are absent; in the xylem, vessels and tracheids arranged alternately; parenchyma cells filled with starch grains and sometimes with raphides of calcium oxalate.

Identification To 0.5 g of pulverized Ipecac add 2.5 mL of hydrochloric acid, allow to stand for 1 hour with occasional shaking, and filter. Collect the filtrate into an evaporating dish, and add a small pieces of chlorinated lime: circumference of it turns red.

Purity (1) Heavy metals <*1.07*>—Proceed with 3.0 g of pulverized Ipecac according to Method 3, and perform the test. Prepare the control solution with 3.0 mL of Standard Lead Solution (not more than 10 ppm).

(2) Arsenic <*1.11*>—Prepare the test solution with 0.40 g of pulverized Ipecac according to Method 4, and perform the test (not more than 5 ppm).

Loss on drying <*5.01*> Not more than 12.0% (6 hours).

Total ash <5.01> Not more than 5.0%.

Acid-insoluble ash <5.01> Not more than 2.0%.

Assay Weigh accurately about 0.5 g of pulverized Ipecac, in a glass-stoppered centrifuge tube, add 30 mL of 0.01 mol/L hydrochloric acid TS, shake for 15 minutes, centrifuge, and separate the supernatant liquid. Repeat this procedure twice with the residue using 30-mL portions of 0.01 mol/L hydrochloric acid TS. Combine all the extracts, add 0.01 mol/L hydrochloric acid TS to make exactly 100 mL, and use this solution as the sample solution. Separately, weigh accurately about 10 mg of emetine hydrochloride for assay, previously dried in a desiccator (in vacuum, phosphorus (V) oxide, 50°C) for 5 hours, dissolve in 0.01 mol/L hydrochloric acid TS to make exactly 100 mL, and use this solution as the standard solution. Perform the test with exactly 10 μL each of the sample solution and standard solution as directed under Liquid Chromatography <2.01> according to the following conditions. Determine the peak areas, A_{TE} and A_{TC}, of emetine and cephaeline obtained with the sample solution, and the peak area, A_{SE}, of emetine obtained with the standard solution.

Amount (mg) of total alkaloids (emetine and cephaeline)
$$= M_S \times \{A_{TE} + (A_{TC} \times 0.971)\}/A_{SE} \times 0.868$$

M_S: Amount (mg) of emetine hydrochloride for assay taken

Operating conditions—

Detector: An ultraviolet absorption photometer (wavelength: 283 nm).

Column: A stainless steel column 4.6 mm in inside diameter and 15 cm in length, packed with octadecylsilanized silica gel for liquid chromatography (5 μm in particle diameter).

Column temperature: A constant temperature of about 50°C.

Mobile phase: Dissolve 2.0 g of sodium 1-heptane sulfonate in 500 mL of water, adjust the pH 4.0 with acetic acid (100), and add 500 mL of methanol.

Flow rate: Adjust so that the retention time of emetine is about 14 minutes.

System suitability—

System performance: Dissolve 1 mg each of emetine hydrochloride for assay and cephaeline hydrobromide in 0.01 mol/L hydrochloric acid TS to make 10 mL. When the procedure is run with 10 μL of this solution under the above operating conditions, cephaeline and emetine are eluted in this order with the resolution between these peaks being not less than 5.

System repeatability: When the test is repeated 6 times with 10 μL of the standard solution under the above operating conditions, the relative standard deviation of the peak area of emetine is not more than 1.5%.

Containers and storage Containers—Well-closed containers.

Powdered Ipecac

Ipecacuanhae Radix Pulverata

トコン末

Powdered Ipecac is the powder of Ipecac or its powder diluted with Potato Starch.

It contains not less than 2.0% and not more than 2.6% of the total alkaloids (emetine and cephaeline), calculated on the basis of dried material.

Description Powdered Ipecac occurs as a light grayish yellow to light brown powder. It has a slight odor, which is irritating to the nasal mucosa, and has a somewhat bitter and unpleasant taste.

Under a microscope <5.01>, Powdered Ipecac reveals starch grains and needle crystals of calcium oxalate; fragments of parenchyma cells containing starch grains or the needle crystals; substitute fibers,thin-walled cork tissue; vessels and tracheids with simple or bordered pits; a few wood fibers and wood parenchyma. Starch grains inherent in Ipecac, mainly 2 – 8-compound grains, rarely simple grains 4 – 22 μm in diameter; and needle crystals of calcium oxalate 25 – 60 μm in length.

Identification To 0.5 g of Powdered Ipecac add 2.5 mL of hydrochloric acid, allow to stand for 1 hour with occasional shaking, and filter. Collect the filtrate into an evaporating dish, and add a small pieces of chlorinated lime: circumference of it turns red.

Purity **(1)** Heavy metals <1.07>—Proceed with 3.0 g of Powdered Ipecac according to Method 3, and perform the test. Prepare the control solution with 3.0 mL of Standard Lead Solution (not more than 10 ppm).

(2) Arsenic <1.11>—Prepare the test solution with 0.40 g of Powdered Ipecac according to Method 4, and perform the test (not more than 5 ppm).

(3) Foreign matter—Under a microscope <5.01>, groups of stone cells and sclerenchymatous fibers are not observed.

Loss on drying <5.01> Not more than 12.0% (6 hours).

Total ash <5.01> Not more than 5.0%.

Acid-insoluble ash <5.01> Not more than 2.0%.

Assay Weigh accurately about 0.5 g of Powdered Ipecac, transfer into a glass-stoppered centrifuge tube, add 30 mL of 0.01 mol/L hydrochloric acid TS, shake for 15 minutes, centrifuge, and separate the supernatant liquid. Repeat this procedure twice with the residue using 30-mL portions of 0.01 mol/L hydrochloric acid TS. Combine all the extracts, add 0.01 mol/L hydrochloric acid TS to make exactly 100 mL, and use this solution as the sample solution. Separately, weigh accurately about 10 mg of emetine hydrochloride for assay, previously dried in a desiccator (in vacuum, phosphorus (V) oxide, 50°C) for 5 hours, dissolve in 0.01 mol/L hydrochloric acid TS to make exactly 100 mL, and use this solution as the standard solution. Perform the test with exactly 10 μL each of the sample solution and standard solution as directed under Liquid Chromatography <2.01> according to the following conditions. Determine the peak areas, A_{TE} and A_{TC}, of emetine and cephaeline obtained with the sample solution, and the peak area, A_{SE}, of emetine obtained with the standard solution.

Amount (mg) of total alkaloids (emetine and cephaeline)
$= M_S \times \{A_{TE} + (A_{TC} \times 0.971)\}/A_{SE} \times 0.868$

M_S: Amount (mg) of emetine hydrochloride for assay taken

Operating conditions—

Detector: An ultraviolet absorption photometer (wavelength: 283 nm).

Column: A stainless steel column 4.6 mm in inside diameter and 15 cm in length, packed with octadecylsilanized silica gel for liquid chromatography (5 μm in particle diameter).

Column temperature: A constant temperature of about 50°C.

Mobile phase: Dissolve 2.0 g of sodium 1-heptane sulfonate in 500 mL of water, adjust the pH 4.0 with acetic acid (100), and add 500 mL of methanol.

Flow rate: Adjust so that the retention time of emetine is about 14 minutes.

System suitability—

System performance: Dissolve 1 mg each of emetine hydrochloride for assay and cephaeline hydrobromide in 10 mL of 0.01 mol/L hydrochloric acid TS. When the procedure is run with 10 μL of this solution under the above operating conditions, cephaeline and emetine are eluted in this order with the resolution between these peaks being not less than 5.

System repeatability: When the test is repeated 6 times with 10 μL of the standard solution under the above operating conditions, the relative standard deviation of the peak area of emetine is not more than 1.5%.

Containers and storage Containers—Well-closed containers.

Ipecac Syrup

トコンシロップ

Ipecac Syrup is a syrup containing not less than 0.12 g and not more than 0.15 g of the total alkaloids (emetine and cephaeline) per 100 mL.

Method of preparation Take coarse powder of Ipecac, prepare the fluidextract as directed under Fluidextracts using a mixture of Ethanol and Purified Water or Purified Water in Containers (3:1), and evaporate the mixture under low pressure (in vacuo) or add a suitable amount of Ethanol or Purified Water or Purified Water in Containers if necessary to get a solution containing 1.7 to 2.1 g of the total alkaloids (emetine and cephaeline) per 100 mL. To 70 mL of this solution add 100 mL of Glycerin and Simple Syrup to make 1000 mL, as directed under Syrups.

Description Ipecac Syrup is a yellow-brown, viscous liquid. It has a sweet taste and a bitter aftertaste.

Identification Take 2 mL of Ipecac Syrup into an evaporating dish, mix with 1 mL of hydrochloric acid, and add small pieces of chlorinated lime: circumference of it turns orange.

Purity Ethanol—Take exactly 5 mL of Ipecac Syrup, add exactly 5 mL of the internal standard solution and water to make 50 mL, and use this solution as the sample solution. Separately, pipet 5 mL of ethanol (99.5), and add water to make exactly 100 mL. To exactly 5 mL of this solution add exactly 5 mL of the internal standard solution and water to make 50 mL, and use this solution as the standard solution. Perform the test with 2 μL each of the sample solution and standard solution as directed under Gas Chromatography <2.02> according to the following conditions, and calculate the rate of peak height of ethanol to that of the internal standard, Q_T and Q_S: Q_T is not larger than Q_S.

Internal standard solution—A solution of acetonitrile (1 in 20).

Operating conditions–

Detector: A hydrogen flame-ionization detector.

Column: A glass-column about 3 mm in inside diameter and about 1.5 m in length, packed with ethylvinylbenzene-divinylbenzene porous co-polymer for gas chromatography (150 to 180 μm in particle diameter).

Column temperature: A constant temperature of between 105°C and 115°C.

Carrier gas: Nitrogen.

Flow rate: Adjust so that the retention time of ethanol is 5 to 10 minutes.

System suitability—

System performance: When the procedure is run with 2 μL of the standard solution under the above operating conditions, ethanol and the internal standard are eluted in this order with the resolution between these peaks being not less than 1.5.

Microbial limit *<4.05>* The acceptance criteria of TAMC and TYMC are 10^3 CFU/mL and 10^2 CFU/mL, respectively. *Escherichia coli*, *Salmonella*, *Pseudomonas aeruginosa* and *Staphylococcus aureus* are not observed.

Assay Take exactly 5 mL of Ipecac Syrup, add 0.01 mol/L hydrochloric acid TS to make exactly 50 mL, and use the solution as the sample solution. Separately, weigh accurately about 10 mg of emetine hydrochloride for assay, previously dried in a desiccator (in vacuum, phosphorus (V) oxide, 50°C) for 5 hours, dissolve in 0.01 mol/L hydrochloric acid TS to make exactly 100 mL, and use this solution as the standard solution. Perform the test with exactly 10 μL each of the sample solution and standard solution as directed under Liquid Chromatography *<2.01>* according to the following conditions. Determine the peak areas, A_{TE} and A_{TC}, of emetine and cephaeline with the sample solution, and the peak area, A_{SE}, of emetine with the standard solution.

Amount (mg) of total alkaloids (emetine and cephaeline)
$= M_S \times \{A_{TE} + (A_{TC} \times 0.971)\}/A_{SE} \times 1/2 \times 0.868$

M_S: Amount (mg) of emetine hydrochloride for assay taken

Operating conditions—

Detector: An ultraviolet absorption photometer (wavelength: 283 nm).

Column: A stainless steel column 4.6 mm in inside diameter and 15 cm in length, packed with octadecylsilanized silica gel for liquid chromatography (5 μm in particle diameter).

Column temperature: A constant temperature of about 50°C.

Mobile phase: Dissolve 2.0 g of sodium l-heptane sulfonate in 500 mL of water, adjust the pH to 4.0 with acetic acid (100), and add 500 mL of methanol.

Flow rate: Adjust so that the retention time of emetine is about 14 minutes.

System suitability—

System performance: Dissolve 1 mg each of emetine hydrochloride for assay and cephaeline hydrobromide in 10 mL of 0.01 mol/L hydrochloric acid TS. When the procedure is run with 10 μL of this solution under the above operating conditions, cephaeline and emetine are eluted in this order with the resolution between these peaks being not less than 5.

System repeatability: When the test is repeated 6 times with 10 μL of the standard solution under the above operat-

ing conditions, the relative standard deviation of the peak area of emetine is not more than 1.5%.

Containers and storage Containers—Tight containers.
Storage—Light-resistant.

Japanese Angelica Root

Angelicae Acutilobae Radix

トウキ

Japanese Angelica Root is the root of *Angelica acutiloba* Kitagawa or *Angelica acutiloba* Kitagawa var. *sugiyamae* Hikino (*Umbelliferae*), usually after being passed through hot water.

Description Thick and short main root, with numerous branched roots, nearly fusiform; 10 – 25 cm in length; externally dark brown to red-brown, with longitudinal wrinkles and horizontal protrusions composed of numerous scars of fine rootlets; fractured surface is dark brown to yellow-brown in color, and smooth; and with a little remains of leaf sheath at the crown.

Odor, characteristic; taste, slightly sweet, followed by slight pungency.

Under a microscope <*5.01*>, a transverse section reveals 4 to 10 cellular layers of cork, with several cellular layers of collenchyma inside of the layer; the cortex exhibits many oil canals surrounded by secretory cells and often large hollows appear; boundary of cortex and xylem is distinct; in the xylem, numerous vessels radiate alternately with medullary rays; vessels in the outer part of the xylem are singly or in several groups, and disposed rather densely in a cuneiform pattern, but vessels in the region of the center are scattered very sparsely; starch grains are simple grains, not more than 20 μm in diameter, and rarely 2- to 5-compound grains, some times up to 25 μm in diameter; starch grains often gelatinized.

Identification To 1.0 g of pulverized Japanese Angelica Root add 5 mL of methanol, shake for 10 minutes, centrifuge, and use the supernatant liquid as the sample solution. Separately, use (*Z*)-ligustilide TS for thin-layer chromatography as the standard solution (1). Dissolve 1 mg of scopoletin for thin-layer chromatography in 10 mL of methanol, and use this solution as the standard solution (2). Perform the test with these solutions as directed under Thin-layer Chromatography <*2.03*>. Spot 10 μL of the sample solution and 5 μL each of the standard solutions (1) and (2) on a plate of silica gel for thin-layer chromatography. Develop the plate with a mixture of hexane, acetone and acetic acid (100) (30:25:1) to a distance of about 7 cm, and air-dry the plate. Examine under ultraviolet light (main wavelength: 365 nm): two of the several spots obtained from the sample solution have the same color tones and *R*f values with the corresponding blue-white fluorescent spots from the standard solutions (1) and (2).

Purity **(1)** Heavy metals <*1.07*>—Proceed with 3.0 g of pulverized Japanese Angelica Root according to Method 3, and perform the test. Prepare the control solution with 3.0 mL of Standard Lead Solution (not more than 10 ppm).

(2) Arsenic <*1.11*>—Prepare the test solution with 0.40 g of pulverized Japanese Angelica Root according to Method 4, and perform the test (not more than 5 ppm).

(3) Leaf sheath—When perform the test of foreign matter <*5.01*>, the amount of leaf sheath contained in Japanese Angelica Root does not exceed 3.0%.

(4) Foreign matter <*5.01*>—The amount of foreign matter other than leaf sheath contained in Japanese Angelica Root does not exceed 1.0%.

Total ash <*5.01*> Not more than 7.0%.

Acid-insoluble ash <*5.01*> Not more than 1.0%.

Extract content <*5.01*> Dilute ethanol-soluble extract: not less than 35.0%.

Containers and storage Containers—Well-closed containers.

Powdered Japanese Angelica Root

Angelicae Acutilobae Radix Pulverata

トウキ末

Powdered Japanese Angelica Root is the powder of Japanese Angelica Root.

Description Powdered Japanese Angelica Root occurs as a light grayish brown powder. It has a characteristic odor and a slight, sweet taste with a slightly pungent aftertaste.

Under a microscope <*5.01*>, Powdered Japanese Angelica Root reveals starch grains or masses of gelatinized starch, and fragments of parenchyma containing them; fragments of light yellow-brown cork tissue; fragments of rather thick-walled collenchyma and phloem tissue; fragments of oil canal surrounded by secretory cells; fragments, 20 – 60 μm in diameter, of scalariform and reticulate vessels with simple perforation; starch grains composed of simple grains not more than 20 μm in diameter, and rarely 2- to 5-compound grains, sometimes comes up to 25 μm.

Identification To 1.0 g of Powdered Japanese Angelica Root add 5 mL of methanol, shake for 10 minutes, centrifuge, and use the supernatant liquid as the sample solution. Separately, use (*Z*)-ligustilide TS for thin-layer chromatography as the standard solution (1). Dissolve 1 mg of scopoletin for thin-layer chromatography in 10 mL of methanol, and use this solution as the standard solution (2). Perform the test with these solutions as directed under Thin-layer Chromatography <*2.03*>. Spot 10 μL of the sample solution and 5 μL each of the standard solutions (1) and (2) on a plate of silica gel for thin-layer chromatography. Develop the plate with a mixture of hexane, acetone and acetic acid (100) (30:25:1) to a distance of about 7 cm, and air-dry the plate. Examine under ultraviolet light (main wavelength: 365 nm): two of the several spots obtained from the sample solution have the same color tones and *R*f values with the corresponding blue-white fluorescent spots from the standard solutions (1) and (2).

Purity **(1)** Heavy metals <*1.07*>—Proceed with 3.0 g of Powdered Japanese Angelica Root according to Method 3, and perform the test. Prepare the control solution with 3.0 mL of Standard Lead Solution (not more than 10 ppm).

(2) Arsenic <*1.11*>—Prepare the test solution with 0.40 g of Powdered Japanese Angelica Root according to Method 4, and perform the test (not more than 5 ppm).

(3) Foreign matter—Under a microscope <*5.01*>, Powdered Japanese Angelica Root does not show remarkably lignified sclerenchymatous cells.

Total ash <*5.01*> Not more than 7.0%.

Acid-insoluble ash <*5.01*> Not more than 1.0%.

Extract content <*5.01*> Dilute ethanol-soluble extract: not less than 35.0%.

Containers and storage Containers—Tight containers.
Storage—Light-resistant.

Japanese Gentian

Gentianae Scabrae Radix

リュウタン

Japanese Gentian is the root and rhizome of *Gentiana scabra* Bunge, *Gentiana manshurica* Kitagawa or *Gentiana triflora* Pallas (*Gentianaceae*).

Description Irregular, cylindrical, short rhizome with numerous, slender roots around, and externally yellow-brown to grayish yellow-brown. The root is 10 - 15 cm in length, about 0.3 cm in diameter, and has longitudinal, coarse wrinkles on the outer surface; flexible; fractured surface, smooth and yellow-brown in color. The rhizome is about 2 cm in length, about 0.7 cm in diameter, and has buds or short remains of stems at the top.

Odor, slight; taste, extremely bitter and lasting.

Under a microscope <*5.01*>, a transverse section of the young root reveals epidermis, exodermis and a few cellular layers of primary cortex; usually, the outermost layer is endodermis consisting of characteristic cells divided into a few daughter cells, often with collenchyma of 1 to 2 cellular layers contacting the inner side; secondary cortex having rents here and there, and irregularly scattered sieve tubes; vessels arranged rather radially in xylem, sieve tubes existing in xylem; the rhizome has a large pith, rarely with sieve tubes; parenchyma cells contain small needle, plate or sand crystals of calcium oxalate and oil drops; starch grains usually absent.

Identification To 0.5 g of pulverized Japanese Gentian add 10 mL of methanol, shake for 20 minutes, filter, and use the filtrate as the sample solution. Separately, dissolve 1 mg of gentiopicroside for thin-layer chromatography in 1 mL of methanol, and use this solution as the standard solution. Perform the test with these solutions as directed under Thin-layer Chromatography <*2.03*>. Spot 10 μL each of the sample solution and standard solution on a plate of silica gel with fluorescent indicator for thin-layer chromatography. Develop the plate with a mixture of ethyl acetate, ethanol (99.5) and water (8:2:1) to a distance of about 7 cm, and air-dry the plate. Examine under ultraviolet light (main wavelength: 254 nm): one of the several spots obtained from the sample solution has the same color tone and the same *Rf* value with the spot from the standard solution.

Purity (1) Heavy metals <*1.07*>—Proceed with 3.0 g of pulverized Japanese Gentian according to Method 3, and perform the test. Prepare the control solution with 3.0 mL of Standard Lead Solution (not more than 10 ppm).

(2) Arsenic <*1.11*>—Prepare the test solution with 0.40 g of pulverized Japanese Gentian according to Method 4, and perform the test (not more than 5 ppm).

Total ash <*5.01*> Not more than 7.0%.

Acid-insoluble ash <*5.01*> Not more than 3.0%.

Containers and storage Containers—Well-closed containers.

Powdered Japanese Gentian

Gentianae Scabrae Radix Pulverata

リュウタン末

Powdered Japanese Gentian is the powder of Japanese Gentian.

Description Powdered Japanese Gentian occurs as a grayish yellow-brown powder. It has a slight odor and a lasting, extremely bitter taste.

Under a microscope <*5.01*>, Powdered Japanese Gentian reveals fragments of parenchyma cells containing oil droplets and fine crystals, fragments of endodermis divided into daughter cells with suberized cell wall, exodermis, and vessels; vessels mainly reticulate vessels and scalariform vessels, 20 - 30 μm in diameter.

Identification To 0.5 g of Powdered Japanese Gentian add 10 mL of methanol, shake for 20 minutes, filter, and use the filtrate as the sample solution. Separately, dissolve 1 mg of gentiopicroside for thin-layer chromatography in 1 mL of methanol, and use this solution as the standard solution. Perform the test with these solutions as directed under Thin-layer Chromatography <*2.03*>. Spot 10 μL each of the sample solution and standard solution on a plate of silica gel with fluorescent indicator for thin-layer chromatography. Develop the plate with a mixture of ethyl acetate, ethanol (99.5) and water (8:2:1) to a distance of about 7 cm, and air-dry the plate. Examine under ultraviolet light (main wavelength: 254 nm): one of the several spots obtained from the sample solution and a spot from the standard solution show the same color tone and the same *Rf* value.

Purity (1) Heavy metals <*1.07*>—Proceed with 3.0 g of Powdered Japanese Gentian according to Method 3, and perform the test. Prepare the control solution with 3.0 mL of Standard Lead Solution (not more than 10 ppm).

(2) Arsenic <*1.11*>—Prepare the test solution with 0.40 g of Powdered Japanese Gentian according to Method 4, and perform the test (not more than 5 ppm).

(3) Foreign matter—Under a microscope <*5.01*>, Powdered Japanese Gentian usually reveals no stone cells and fibers. No starch grains; if any, very few.

Total ash <*5.01*> Not more than 7.0%.

Acid-insoluble ash <*5.01*> Not more than 3.0%.

Containers and storage Containers—Well-closed containers.

Japanese Valerian

Valerianae Fauriei Radix

カノコソウ

Japanese Valerian is the root and rhizome of *Valeriana fauriei* Briquet (*Valerianaceae*).

Description Obovoid, short rhizome with numerous, fine and long roots; externally dark brown to grayish brown. The root, 10 - 15 cm in length, 0.1 - 0.3 cm in diameter; externally, with fine longitudinal wrinkles; brittle. The rhizome, 1 - 2 cm in length, 1 - 2 cm in diameter, with buds and remains of stem at the crown; hard in texture and difficult to break; flank of rhizome sometimes accompanied with stolons having thick and short or thin, long and extremely small, scaly leaves. Under a magnifying glass, the transverse section reveals a thick, light grayish brown cortex, and a grayish brown stele.

Odor, strong and characteristic; taste, slightly bitter.

Purity **(1)** Heavy metals *<1.07>*—Proceed with 3.0 g of pulverized Japanese Valerian according to Method 3, and perform the test. Prepare the control solution with 3.0 mL of Standard Lead Solution (not more than 10 ppm).

(2) Arsenic *<1.11>*—Prepare the test solution with 0.40 g of pulverized Japanese Valerian according to Method 4, and perform the test (not more than 5 ppm).

Total ash *<5.01>* Not more than 10.0%.

Acid-insoluble ash *<5.01>* Not more than 5.0%.

Essential oil content *<5.01>* Perform the test with 50.0 g of pulverized Japanese Valerian provided that 1 mL of silicon resin is previously added to the sample in the flask: the volume of essential oil is not less than 0.3 mL.

Containers and storage Containers—Tight containers.

Powdered Japanese Valerian

Valerianae Fauriei Radix Pulverata

カノコソウ末

Powdered Japanese Valerian is the powder of Japanese Valerian.

Description Powdered Japanese Valerian occurs as a dark grayish brown powder. It is somewhat moist to the touch. It has a strong, characteristic odor and a slightly bitter taste.

Under a microscope *<5.01>*, Powdered Japanese Valerian reveals starch grains and fragments of parenchyma cells containing them; fragments of pitted vessels, reticulate vessels, ring vessels, and spiral vessels; fragments of exodermis containing oil droplets and composed of cells suberized and divided into daughter cells; fragments of yellow stone cells from the rhizome and the stolon; and very rarely, some fragments of epidermis and phloem fibers. Starch grains, simple grains 10 - 20 μm in diameter and 2- to 4-compound grains; oil droplets stained red with sudan III TS.

Purity **(1)** Heavy metals *<1.07>*—Proceed with 3.0 g of Powdered Japanese Valerian according to Method 3, and perform the test. Prepare the control solution with 3.0 mL of Standard Lead Solution (not more than 10 ppm).

(2) Arsenic *<1.11>*—Prepare the test solution with 0.40 g of Powdered Japanese Valerian according to Method 4, and perform the test (not more than 5 ppm).

Total ash *<5.01>* Not more than 10.0%.

Acid-insoluble ash *<5.01>* Not more than 5.0%.

Essential oil content *<5.01>* Perform the test with 50.0 g of Powdered Japanese Valerian provided that 1 mL of silicon resin is previously added to the sample in the flask: the volume of essential oil is not less than 0.2 mL.

Containers and storage Containers—Tight containers.

Japanese Zanthoxylum Peel

Zanthoxyli Piperiti Pericarpium

サンショウ

Japanese Zanthoxylum Peel is the pericarps of the ripe fruit of *Zanthoxylum piperitum* De Candolle (*Rutaceae*), from which the seeds separated from the pericarps have been mostly removed.

Description Pericarps of capsules of 2 or 3 flattened spheroidal mericarps, which are dehiscent in 2 pieces about 5 mm in diameter; the outer surface of pericarp, dark yellow-red to dark red-brown, with numerous dented spots originated from oil sacs; the inner surface, light yellow-white.

Odor, characteristically aromatic; taste, acrid, which gives numbing sensation to the tongue.

Under a microscope *<5.01>*, a transverse section of Japanese Zanthoxylum Peel reveals the external epidermis and the adjoined unicellular layer containing red-brown tannin; the mesocarp holds oil sacs being up to approximately 500 μm in diameter and sporadically vascular bundles consisting mainly of spiral vessels; the endocarp consists of stone cell layers; inner epidermal cells very small.

Identification To 2 g of pulverized Japanese Zanthoxylum Peel add 10 mL of water, shake for 5 minutes, add 5 mL of diethyl ether, shake, centrifuge, and use the diethyl ether layer as the sample solution. Perform the test with the sample solution as directed under Thin-layer Chromatography *<2.03>*. Spot 10 μL of the sample solution on a plate of silica gel with fluorescent indicator for thin-layer chromatography. Develop the plate with a mixture of ethyl acetate, hexane, methanol and acetic acid (100) (20:20:1:1) to a distance of about 7 cm, and air-dry the plate. Examine under ultraviolet light (main wavelength: 254 nm): a spot with an *R*f value of about 0.3 is observed.

Purity **(1)** Seed—When perform the test of foreign matter *<5.01>*, the amount of the seeds contained in Japanese Zanthoxylum Peel does not exceed 20.0%.

(2) Peduncle and twig—The amount of the peduncles and twigs contained in Japanese Zanthoxylum Peel does not exceed 5.0%.

(3) Foreign matter *<5.01>*—The amount of foreign matter other than peduncles and twigs contained in Japanese Zanthoxylum Peel does not exceed 1.0%.

Total ash *<5.01>* Not more than 8.0%.

Acid-insoluble ash *<5.01>* Not more than 1.5%.

Essential oil content *<5.01>* Perform the test with 30.0 g of pulverized Japanese Zanthoxylum Peel: the volume of essential oil is not less than 1.0 mL.

Containers and storage Containers—Well-closed containers.

Powdered Japanese Zanthoxylum Peel

Zanthoxyli Piperiti Pericarpium Pulveratum

サンショウ末

Powdered Japanese Zanthoxylum Peel is the powder of Japanese Zanthoxylum Peel.

Description Powdered Japanese Zanthoxylum Peel occurs as a dark yellow-brown powder. It has a strong, characteristic aroma and an acrid taste, leaving a sensation of numbness on the tongue.

Under a microscope <*5.01*>, Powdered Japanese Zanthoxylum Peel reveals fragments of inner tissue of endocarp consisting of stone cells with cell walls about 2.5 μm in thickness; fragments of spiral and ring vessels 10 - 15 μm in diameter; fragments of oil sacs containing essential oil or resin; fragments of epidermal cells, polygonal in surface view, containing tannin; numerous oil drops; masses of tannin, colored red by adding vanillin-hydrochloric acid TS.

Identification To 2 g of Powdered Japanese Zanthoxylum Peel add 10 mL of water, shake for 5 minutes, add 5 mL of diethyl ether, shake, centrifuge, and use the diethyl ether layer as the sample solution. Perform the test with the sample solution as directed under Thin-layer Chromatography <*2.03*>. Spot 10 μL of the sample solution on a plate of silica gel with fluorescent indicator for thin-layer chromatography. Develop the plate with a mixture of ethyl acetate, hexane, methanol and acetic acid (100) (20:20:1:1) to a distance of about 7 cm, and air-dry the plate. Examine under ultraviolet light (main wavelength: 254 nm): a spot with an *R*f value of about 0.3 is observed.

Total ash <*5.01*> Not more than 8.0%.

Acid-insoluble ash <*5.01*> Not more than 1.5%.

Essential oil content <*5.01*> Perform the test with 30.0 g of Powdered Japanese Zanthoxylum Peel: the volume of essential oil is not less than 0.8 mL.

Containers and storage Containers—Tight containers.

Jujube

Ziziphi Fructus

タイソウ

Jujube is the fruit of *Ziziphus jujuba* Miller var. *inermis* Rehder (*Rhamnaceae*).

Description Ellipsoidal or broad ovoid fruit, 2 - 3 cm in length, 1 - 2 cm in diameter; externally red-brown with coarse wrinkles, or dark grayish red with fine wrinkles, and both lustrous; both ends slightly dented, with a scar of style on one end and a scar of peduncle on the other; epicarp thin and leather; mesocarp thick, dark grayish brown in color, spongy, soft and adhesive; endocarp extremely hard, fusiform, and divided into two loculi; seeds flat and ovoid.

Odor, slight and characteristic; taste, sweet.

Purity **(1)** Rancidity—Jujube has no unpleasant, rancid odor and taste.

(2) Total BHC's and total DDT's <*5.01*> Not more than 0.2 ppm, respectively.

Total ash <*5.01*> Not more than 3.0%.

Containers and storage Containers—Well-closed containers.

Jujube Seed

Ziziphi Semen

サンソウニン

Jujube Seed is the seed of *Ziziphus jujuba* Miller var. *spinosa* Hu ex H. F. Chow (*Rhamnaceae*).

Description Jujube Seed is a compressed ovate to orbicular, lenticular seed, 5 - 9 mm in length, 4 - 6 mm in width, 2 - 3 mm in thickness, externally brown to dark red-brown, glossy; hilum at one end, chalaza at the other end; seed coat sightly flexible, covering, milky white endosperm and light yellow embryo. 100 seeds weigh 3.0 - 4.5 g.

Odor, slightly oily; taste, mild and slightly oily.

Under a microscope <*5.01*>, transverse section reveals seed coat composed of an upper epidermis, parenchyma and lower epidermis; upper epidermal cells sclerified and elongated in radial direction; lower epidermis covered with cuticle; endosperm composed of parenchyma, containing aggregated crystals of calcium oxalate, aleurone grains and starch grains; cotyledons composed of parenchyma that contains aleurone grains, starch grains and oil drops.

Identification To 2 g of pulverized Jujube Seed add 10 mL of methanol, and heat under a reflux condenser for 10 minutes. After cooling, filter, and use the filtrate as the sample solution. Perform the test with the sample solution as directed under Thin-layer Chromatography <*2.03*>. Spot 10 μL of the sample solution on a plate of silica gel with fluorescent indicator for thin-layer chromatography, develop the plate with a mixture of acetone, ethyl acetate, water and acetic acid (100) (10:10:3:1) to a distance of about 7 cm, and air-dry the plate. Examine under ultraviolet light (main wavelength: 254 nm): two spots appear at the *R*f value of about 0.3 and about 0.4, and these spots exhibit a blue-white fluorescence when examined under ultraviolet light (main wavelength: 365 nm) after spraying evenly dilute sulfuric acid on the plate and heating at 105°C for 5 minutes.

Purity Foreign matter <*5.01*>—Jujube Seed contains not more than 1.0% of the endocarp and other foreign matters.

Loss on drying <*5.01*> Not more than 11.0% (6 hours).

Total ash <*5.01*> Not more than 5.0%.

Extract content <*5.01*> Dilute ethanol-soluble extract: not less than 8.5%.

Containers and storage Containers—Well-closed containers.

Juzentaihoto Extract

十全大補湯エキス

Juzentaihoto Extract contains not less than 1.5 mg (for preparation prescribed 2.5 g of Ginseng) or not less than 1.8 mg (for preparation prescribed 3 g of Ginseng) of ginsenoside Rb_1 ($C_{54}H_{92}O_{23}$: 1109.29), not less than 26 mg and not more than 78 mg of paeoniflorin ($C_{23}H_{28}O_{11}$: 480.46), and not less than 6 mg and not more than 18 mg (for preparation prescribed 1 g of Glycyrrhiza) or not less than 10 mg and not more than 30 mg (for preparation prescribed 1.5 g of Glycyrrhiza) of glycyrrhizic acid ($C_{42}H_{62}O_{16}$: 822.93), per extract prepared with the amount specified in the Method of preparation.

Method of preparation

	1)	2)	3)	4)
Ginseng	3 g	3 g	2.5 g	3 g
Astragalus Root	3 g	3 g	2.5 g	3 g
Atractylodes Rhizome	3 g	—	3.5 g	3 g
Atractylodes Lancea Rhizome	—	3 g	—	—
Poria Sclerotium	3 g	3 g	3.5 g	3 g
Japanese Angelica Root	3 g	3 g	3.5 g	3 g
Peony Root	3 g	3 g	3 g	3 g
Rehmannia Root	3 g	3 g	3.5 g	3 g
Cnidium Rhizome	3 g	3 g	3 g	3 g
Cinnamon Bark	3 g	3 g	3 g	3 g
Glycyrrhiza	1.5 g	1.5 g	1 g	1g

Prepare a dry extract or viscous extract as directed under Extracts, according to the prescription 1) to 4), using the crude drugs shown above.

Description Juzentaihoto Extract is a light brown to brown powder or black-brown viscous extract. It has a slight odor and a sweet and bitter taste.

Identification **(1)** Shake 2.0 g of the dry extract (or 6.0 g of the viscous extract) with 15 mL of sodium hydroxide TS, centrifuge, and separate the supernatant liquid. To the liquid add 10 mL of 1-butanol, shake, centrifuge, and separate the 1-butanol layer. To the 1-butanol layer add 10 mL of water, shake, centrifuge, and separate the 1-butanol layer. Evaporate the solvent under low pressure (in vacuo), add 1 mL of methanol to the residue, and use this solution as the sample solution. Separately, dissolve 1 mg of Ginsenoside Rb_1 RS or ginsenoside Rb_1 for thin-layer chromatography in 1 mL of methanol, and use this solution as the standard solution. Perform the test with these solutions as directed under Thin-layer Chromatography <*2.03*>. Spot 10 μL of the sample solution and 2 μL of the standard solution on a plate of silica gel for thin-layer chromatography. Develop the plate with a mixture of ethyl acetate, 1-propanol, water and acetic acid (100) (7:5:4:1) to a distance of about 7 cm, and air-dry the plate. Spray evenly 4-dimethylaminobenzaldehyde TS for spraying on the plate, heat the plate at 105°C for 5 minutes, and allow to cool: one of the several spots obtained from the sample solution has the same color tone and *R*f value with the dark brown spot from the standard solution (Ginseng).

(2) Shake 2.0 g of the dry extract (or 6.0 g of the viscous extract) with 15 mL of sodium hydroxide TS, centrifuge, and separate the supernatant liquid. To the liquid add 10 mL of 1-butanol, shake, centrifuge, and separate the 1-butanol layer. To the 1-butanol layer add 10 mL of water, shake, centrifuge, and separate the 1-butanol layer. Evaporate the solvent under low pressure (in vacuo), add 1 mL of methanol to the residue, and use this solution as the sample solution. Separately, dissolve 1 mg of astragaloside IV for thin-layer chromatography in 1 mL of methanol, and use this solution as the standard solution. Perform the test with these solutions as directed under Thin-layer Chromatography <*2.03*>. Spot 10 μL of the sample solution and 2 μL of the standard solution on a plate of silica gel for thin-layer chromatography. Develop the plate with a mixture of ethyl acetate, 1-propanol, water and acetic acid (100) (7:5:4:1) to a distance of about 7 cm, and air-dry the plate. Spray evenly 4-dimethylaminobenzaldehyde TS for spraying on the plate, heat the plate at 105°C for 5 minutes, and allow to cool: one of the several spots obtained from the sample solution has the same color tone and *R*f value with the red-brown spot from the standard solution (Astragalus Root).

(3) For preparation prescribed Atractylodes Rhizome—Shake 1.0 g of the dry extract (or 3.0 g of the viscous extract) with 10 mL of water, add 5 mL of diethyl ether, shake, and centrifuge. Use the diethyl ether layer as the sample solution. Separately, dissolve 1 mg of atractylenolide III for thin-layer chromatography in 1 mL of methanol, and use this solution as the standard solution. Perform the test with these solutions as directed under Thin-layer Chromatography <*2.03*>. Spot 10 μL each of the sample solution and standard solution on a plate of silica gel for thin-layer chromatography. Develop the plate with a mixture of ethyl acetate and hexane (1:1) to a distance of about 7 cm, and air-dry the plate. Spray evenly 1-naphthol-sulfuric acid TS on the plate, heat the plate at 105°C for 5 minutes, and allow to cool: one of the several spots obtained from the sample solution has the same color tone and *R*f value with the red spot from the standard solution (Atractylodes Rhizome).

(4) For preparation prescribed Atractylodes Lancea Rhizome—Shake 5.0 g of the dry extract (or 15.0 g of the viscous extract) with 10 mL of water, add 25 mL of hexane, and shake. Separate the hexane layer, evaporate the solvent under low pressure (in vacuo), add 2 mL of hexane to the residue, and use this solution as the sample solution. Perform the test with the sample solution as directed under Thin-layer Chromatography <*2.03*>. Spot 40 μL of the sample solution on a plate of silica gel with fluorescent indicator for thin-layer chromatography. Develop the plate with a mixture of hexane and acetone (7:1) to a distance of about 7 cm, and air-dry the plate. Examine under ultraviolet light (main wavelength: 254 nm): a dark purple spot is observed at an *R*f value of about 0.5. The spot shows a greenish brown color after being sprayed evenly 4-dimethylaminobenzaldehyde TS for spraying, heated at 105°C for 5 minutes, and allowed to cool (Atractylodes Lancea Rhizome).

(5) Shake 1.0 g of the dry extract (or 3.0 g of the viscous extract) with 15 mL of water and 5 mL of 0.1 mol/L hydrochloric acid TS, add 25 mL of diethyl ether, and shake. Separate the diethyl ether layer, evaporate the solvent under low pressure (in vacuo), then add 2 mL of diethyl ether to the residue, and use this solution as the sample solution. Separately, use (*Z*)-ligustilide TS for thin-layer chromatography as the standard solution. Perform the test with these solutions as directed under Thin-layer Chromatography <*2.03*>. Spot 10 μL each of the sample solution and standard solution on a plate of silica gel for thin-layer chromatography. Develop the plate with a mixture of ethyl acetate and hexane (1:1) to a distance of about 7 cm, and air-dry the plate. Examine under ultraviolet light (main wavelength: 365

nm): one of the several spots obtained from the sample solution has the same color tone and *R*f value with the blue-white fluorescent spot from the standard solution (Cnidium Rhizome; Japanese Angelica Root).

(6) Shake 1.0 g of the dry extract (or 3.0 g of the viscous extract) with 10 mL of water, add 10 mL of 1-butanol, shake, centrifuge, and use the 1-butanol layer as the sample solution. Separately, dissolve 1 mg of Paeoniflorin RS or paeoniflorin for thin-layer chromatography in 1 mL of methanol, and use this solution as the standard solution. Perform the test with these solutions as directed under Thin-layer Chromatography *<2.03>*. Spot 5 μL each of the sample solution and standard solution on a plate of silica gel for thin-layer chromatography. Develop the plate with a mixture of ethyl acetate, methanol and water (20:3:2) to a distance of about 7 cm, and air-dry the plate. Spray evenly 4-methoxybenzaldehyde-sulfuric acid TS on the plate, and heat the plate at 105°C for 5 minutes: one of the several spots obtained from the sample solution has the same color tone and *R*f value with the purple spot from the standard solution (Peony Root).

(7) Shake 1.0 g of the dry extract (or 3.0 g of the viscous extract) with 10 mL of water, add 30 mL of methanol, shake, centrifuge, and use the supernatant liquid as the sample solution. Perform the test with the sample solution as directed under Thin-layer Chromatography *<2.03>*. Spot 5 μL of the sample solution on a plate of silica gel for thin-layer chromatography. Develop the plate with a mixture of water, methanol and 1-butanol (1:1:1) to a distance of about 7 cm, and air-dry the plate. Spray evenly 4-methoxybenzaldehyde-sulfuric acid TS on the plate, heat the plate at 105°C for 5 minutes, and allow to cool: a dark green spot is observed at an *R*f value of about 0.6 (Rehmannia Root).

(8) Perform the test according to the following i) or ii) (Cinnamon Bark).

i) Put 10 g of the dry extract (or 30 g of the viscous extract) in a 300-mL hard-glass flask, add 100 mL of water and 1 mL of silicone resin, connect an apparatus for essential oil determination, and heat to boil under a reflux condenser. The graduated tube of the apparatus is to be previously filled with water to the standard line, and 2 mL of hexane is added to the graduated tube. After heating under reflux for 1 hour, separate the hexane layer, and use the layer as the sample solution. Separately, dissolve 1 mg of (*E*)-cinnamaldehyde for thin-layer chromatography in 1 mL of methanol, and use this solution as the standard solution. Perform the test with these solutions as directed under Thin-layer Chromatography *<2.03>*. Spot 50 μL of the sample solution and 2 μL of the standard solution on a plate of silica gel for thin-layer chromatography. Develop the plate with a mixture of hexane, diethyl ether and methanol (15:5:1) to a distance of about 7 cm, and air-dry the plate. Spray evenly 2,4-dinitrophenylhydrazine TS on the plate: one of the several spots obtained from the sample solution has the same color tone and *R*f value with the yellow-orange spot from the standard solution.

ii) Shake 2.0 g of the dry extract (or 6.0 g of the viscous extract) with 10 mL of water, add 5 mL of hexane, shake, centrifuge, and use the hexane layer as the sample solution. Separately, dissolve 1 mg of (*E*)-2-methoxycinnamaldehyde for thin-layer chromatography in 1 mL of methanol, and use this solution as the standard solution. Perform the test with these solutions as directed under Thin-layer Chromatography *<2.03>*. Spot 20 μL of the sample solution and 2 μL of the standard solution on a plate of silica gel for thin-layer chromatography. Develop the plate with a mixture of hexane and ethyl acetate (2:1) to a distance of about 7 cm, and air-dry the plate. Examine under ultraviolet light (main wavelength: 365 nm): one of the several spots obtained from the sample solution has the same color tone and *R*f value with the blue-white fluorescent spot from the standard solution.

(9) Shake 1.0 g of the dry extract (or 3.0 g of the viscous extract) with 10 mL of water, add 10 mL of 1-butanol, shake, centrifuge, and use the 1-butanol layer as the sample solution. Separately, dissolve 1 mg of liquiritin for thin-layer chromatography in 1 mL of methanol, and use this solution as the standard solution. Perform the test with these solutions as directed under Thin-layer Chromatography *<2.03>*. Spot 1 μL each of the sample solution and standard solution on a plate of silica gel for thin-layer chromatography. Develop the plate with a mixture of ethyl acetate, methanol and water (20:3:2) to a distance of about 7 cm, and air-dry the plate. Spray evenly dilute sulfuric acid on the plate, heat the plate at 105°C for 5 minutes, and examine under ultraviolet light (main wavelength: 365 nm): one of the several spots obtained from the sample solution has the same color tone and *R*f value with the yellow-green fluorescent spot from the standard solution (Glycyrrhiza).

Purity **(1)** Heavy metals *<1.07>*—Prepare the test solution with 1.0 g of the dry extract (or an amount of the viscous extract, equivalent to 1.0 g of the dried substance) as directed under Extracts (4), and perform the test (not more than 30 ppm).

(2) Arsenic *<1.11>*—Prepare the test solution with 0.67 g of the dry extract (or an amount of the viscous extract, equivalent to 0.67 g of the dried substance) according to Method 3, and perform the test (not more than 3 ppm).

Loss on drying *<2.41>* The dry extract: Not more than 9.5% (1 g, 105°C, 5 hours).

The viscous extract: Not more than 66.7% (1 g, 105°C, 5 hours).

Total ash *<5.01>* Not more than 10.0%, calculated on the dried basis.

Assay **(1)** Ginsenoside Rb_1—Weigh accurately about 2 g of the dry extract (or an amount of the viscous extract, equivalent to about 2 g of the dried substance), add 30 mL of diluted methanol (3 in 5), shake for 15 minutes, centrifuge, and separate the supernatant liquid. To the residue add 15 mL of diluted methanol (3 in 5), and repeat the same procedure. Combine the supernatant liquids, add diluted methanol (3 in 5) to make exactly 50 mL. Pipet 10 mL of this solution, add 3 mL of sodium hydroxide TS, allow to stand for 30 minutes, then add 3 mL of 1 mol/L hydrochloric acid TS, and add water to make exactly 20 mL. Apply exactly 5 mL of this solution to a column (about 10 mm in inside diameter and packed with 0.36 g of octadecylsilanized silica gel for pre-treatment (55 - 105 μm in particle size), washed just before use with methanol and then with diluted methanol (3 in 10)), and wash the column in sequence with 2 mL of diluted methanol (3 in 10), 1 mL of sodium carbonate TS and 10 mL of diluted methanol (3 in 10). Finally, elute with methanol to collect exactly 5 mL, and use this as the sample solution. Separately, weigh accurately about 10 mg of Ginsenoside Rb_1 RS (separately determine the water *<2.48>* by coulometric titration, using 10 mg), and dissolve in methanol to make exactly 100 mL. Pipet 10 mL of this solution, add methanol to make exactly 50 mL, and use this solution as the standard solution. Perform the test with exactly 20 μL each of the sample solution and standard solution as directed under Liquid Chromatography *<2.01>* according to the following conditions, and determine the peak areas, A_T and A_S, of ginsenoside Rb_1 in each solution.

$$\text{Amount (mg) of ginsenoside Rb}_1\ (C_{54}H_{92}O_{23}) = M_S \times A_T/A_S \times 1/5$$

M_S: Amount (mg) of Ginsenoside Rb_1 RS taken, calculated on the anhydrous basis

Operating conditions—

Detector: An ultraviolet absorption photometer (wavelength: 203 nm).

Column: A stainless steel column 4.6 mm in inside diameter and 25 cm in length, packed with carbamoyl groups bound silica gel for liquid chromatography (5 μm in particle diameter).

Column temperature: A constant temperature of about 60°C.

Mobile phase: A mixture of acetonitrile, water and phosphoric acid (400:100:1).

Flow rate: 1.0 mL per minute (the retention time of ginsenoside Rb_1 is about 16 minutes).

System suitability—

System performance: When the procedure is run with 20 μL of the standard solution under the above operating conditions, the number of theoretical plates and the symmetry factor of the peak of ginsenoside Rb_1 are not less than 5000 and not more than 1.5, respectively.

System repeatability: When the test is repeated 6 times with 20 μL of the standard solution under the above operating conditions, the relative standard deviation of the peak area of ginsenoside Rb_1 is not more than 1.5%.

(2) Paeoniflorin—Weigh accurately about 0.5 g of the dry extract (or an amount of the viscous extract, equivalent to about 0.5 g of the dried substance), add exactly 50 mL of diluted methanol (1 in 2), shake for 15 minutes, filter, and use the filtrate as the sample solution. Separately, weigh accurately about 10 mg of Paeoniflorin RS (separately determine the water <*2.48*> by coulometric titration, using 10 mg), dissolve in diluted methanol (1 in 2) to make exactly 100 mL, and use this solution as the standard solution. Perform the test with exactly 10 μL each of the sample solution and standard solution as directed under Liquid Chromatography <*2.01*> according to the following conditions, and determine the peak areas, A_T and A_S, of paeoniflorin in each solution.

$$\text{Amount (mg) of paeoniflorin}\ (C_{23}H_{28}O_{11}) = M_S \times A_T/A_S \times 1/2$$

M_S: Amount (mg) of Paeoniflorin RS taken, calculated on the anhydrous basis

Operating conditions—

Detector: An ultraviolet absorption photometer (wavelength: 232 nm).

Column: A stainless steel column 4.6 mm in inside diameter and 15 cm in length, packed with octadecylsilanized silica gel for liquid chromatography (5 μm in particle diameter).

Column temperature: A constant temperature of about 20°C.

Mobile phase: A mixture of water, acetonitrile and phosphoric acid (850:150:1).

Flow rate: 1.0 mL per minute (the retention time of paeoniflorin is about 9 minutes).

System suitability—

System performance: Dissolve 1 mg each of Paeoniflorin RS and albiflorin in diluted methanol (1 in 2) to make 10 mL. When the procedure is run with 10 μL of this solution under the above operating conditions, albiflorin and paeoniflorin are eluted in this order with the resolution between these peaks being not less than 2.5.

System repeatability: When the test is repeated 6 times with 10 μL of the standard solution under the above operating conditions, the relative standard deviation of the peak area of paeoniflorin is not more than 1.5%.

(3) Glycyrrhizic acid—Perform the test according to the following i) or ii).

i) Weigh accurately about 0.5 g of the dry extract (or an amount of the viscous extract, equivalent to about 0.5 g of the dried substance), add exactly 50 mL of diluted methanol (1 in 2), shake for 15 minutes, filter, and use the filtrate as the sample solution. Separately, weigh accurately about 10 mg of Glycyrrhizic Acid RS (separately determine the water <*2.48*> by coulometric titration, using 10 mg), dissolve in diluted methanol (1 in 2) to make exactly 100 mL, and use this solution as the standard solution. Perform the test with exactly 10 μL each of the sample solution and standard solution as directed under Liquid Chromatography <*2.01*> according to the following conditions, and determine the peak areas, A_T and A_S, of glycyrrhizic acid in each solution.

$$\text{Amount (mg) of glycyrrhizic acid}\ (C_{42}H_{62}O_{16}) = M_S \times A_T/A_S \times 1/2$$

M_S: Amount (mg) of Glycyrrhizic Acid RS taken, calculated on the anhydrous basis

Operating conditions—

Detector: An ultraviolet absorption photometer (wavelength: 254 nm).

Column: A stainless steel column 4.6 mm in inside diameter and 15 cm in length, packed with octadecylsilanized silica gel for liquid chromatography (5 μm in particle diameter).

Column temperature: A constant temperature of about 40°C.

Mobile phase: Dissolve 3.85 g of ammonium acetate in 720 mL of water, and add 5 mL of acetic acid (100) and 280 mL of acetonitrile.

Flow rate: 1.0 mL per minute (the retention time of glycyrrhizic acid is about 15 minutes).

System suitability—

System performance: Dissolve 5 mg of monoammonium glycyrrhizinate for resolution check in 20 mL of dilute ethanol. When the procedure is run with 10 μL of this solution under the above operating conditions, the resolution between the peak having the relative retention time of about 0.9 to glycyrrhizic acid and the peak of glycyrrhizic acid is not less than 1.5. Dissolve 1 mg of (*E*)-cinnamaldehyde for thin-layer chromatography in 50 mL of methanol. To 2 mL of this solution add 2 mL of the standard solution. When the procedure is run with 10 μL of this solution under the above operating conditions, the resolution between the peaks of glycyrrhizic acid and (*E*)-cinnamaldehyde is not less than 1.5.

System repeatability: When the test is repeated 6 times with 10 μL of the standard solution under the above operating conditions, the relative standard deviation of the peak area of glycyrrhizic acid is not more than 1.5%.

ii) Weigh accurately about 0.5 g of the dry extract (or an amount of the viscous extract, equivalent to about 0.5 g of the dried substance), add 20 mL of ethyl acetate and 10 mL of water, and shake for 10 minutes. After centrifugation, remove the ethyl acetate layer, add 20 mL of ethyl acetate, proceed in the same manner as described above, and remove the ethyl acetate layer. To the aqueous layer add 10 mL of methanol, shake for 30 minutes, centrifuge, and take the supernatant liquid. To the residue add 20 mL of diluted methanol (1 in 2), shake for 5 minutes, centrifuge, and take the supernatant liquid. Combine these supernatant liquids, add diluted methanol (1 in 2) to make exactly 50 mL, and use this solution as the sample solution. Separately, weigh accurately about 10 mg of Glycyrrhizic Acid RS (separately determine the water <*2.48*> by coulometric titration, using 10 mg), dissolve in diluted methanol (1 in 2) to make exactly 100 mL, and use this solution as the standard solution. Perform the test with exactly 10 μL each of the sample solution and standard solution as directed under Liquid Chromatography <*2.01*> according to the following conditions, and determine the peak areas, A_T and A_S, of glycyrrhizic acid in each solution.

$$\text{Amount (mg) of glycyrrhizic acid } (C_{42}H_{62}O_{16}) = M_S \times A_T/A_S \times 1/2$$

M_S: Amount (mg) of Glycyrrhizic Acid RS taken, calculated on the anhydrous basis

Operating conditions—

Proceed as directed in the operating conditions in i).

System suitability—

System repeatability: Proceed as directed in the system suitability in i).

System performance: Dissolve 5 mg of monoammonium glycyrrhizinate for resolution check in 20 mL of dilute ethanol. When the procedure is run with 10 μL of this solution under the above operating conditions, the resolution between the peak having the relative retention time of about 0.9 to glycyrrhizic acid and the peak of glycyrrhizic acid is not less than 1.5.

Containers and storage Containers—Tight containers.

Kakkonto Extract

葛根湯エキス

Kakkonto Extract contains not less than 7 mg and not more than 21 mg (for preparation prescribed 3 g of Ephedra Herb) or not less than 10 mg and not more than 30 mg (for preparation prescribed 4 g of Ephedra Herb) of total alkaloids (ephedrine and pseudoephedrine), not less than 14 mg and not more than 56 mg (for preparation prescribed 2 g of Peony Root) or not less than 21 mg and not more than 84 mg (for preparation prescribed 3 g of Peony Root) of paeoniflorin ($C_{23}H_{28}O_{11}$: 480.46), and not less than 15 mg and not more than 45 mg of glycyrrhizic acid ($C_{42}H_{62}O_{16}$: 822.93), per extract prepared with the amount specified in the Method of preparation.

Method of preparation

	1)	2)	3)	4)
Pueraria Root	8 g	4 g	4 g	4 g
Ephedra Herb	4 g	4 g	3 g	3 g
Jujube	4 g	3 g	3 g	3 g
Cinnamon Bark	3 g	2 g	2 g	2 g
Peony Root	3 g	2 g	2 g	2 g
Glycyrrhiza	2 g	2 g	2 g	2 g
Ginger	1 g	1 g	1 g	2 g

Prepare a dry extract or viscous extract as directed under Extracts, according to the prescription 1) to 4), using the crude drugs shown above.

Description Kakkonto Extract occurs as a light brown to brown powder or black-brown viscous extract. It has a characteristic odor, and a sweet first, then hot, and slightly bitter taste.

Identification **(1)** To 1.0 g of the dry extract (or 3.0 g of the viscous extract) add 10 mL of water, shake, then add 10 mL of 1-butanol, shake, centrifuge, and use the 1-butanol layer as the sample solution. Separately, dissolve 1 mg of Puerarin RS or puerarin for thin-layer chromatography in 1 mL of methanol, and use this solution as the standard solution. Perform the test with these solutions as directed under Thin-layer Chromatography <*2.03*>. Spot 5 μL each of the sample solution and standard solution on a plate of silica gel for thin-layer chromatography. Develop the plate with a mixture of ethyl acetate, methanol and water (20:3:2) to a distance of about 7 cm, and air-dry the plate. Examine under ultraviolet light (main wavelength: 365 nm): one of the several spots obtained from the sample solution has the same color tone and *Rf* value with the blue-white fluorescent spot from the standard solution (Pueraria Root).

(2) To 1.0 g of the dry extract (or 3.0 g of the viscous extract) add 10 mL of water, shake, then add 10 mL of 1-butanol, shake, centrifuge, and use the 1-butanol layer as the sample solution. Perform the test with the sample solution as directed under Thin-layer Chromatography <*2.03*>. Spot 5 μL of the sample solution on a plate of silica gel for thin-layer chromatography. Develop the plate with a mixture of 1-propanol, ethyl acetate, water and acetic acid (100) (4:4:2:1) to a distance of about 7 cm, and air-dry the plate. Spray evenly ninhydrin-ethanol TS for spraying on the plate, and heat the plate at 105°C for 5 minutes: a red-purple spot is observed at an *Rf* value of about 0.5 (Ephedra Herb).

(3) Perform the test according to the following i) or ii) (Cinnamon Bark).

i) Put 10 g of the dry extract (or 30 g of the viscous extract) in a 300-mL hard-glass flask, add 100 mL of water and 1 mL of silicone resin, connect an apparatus for essential oil determination, and heat to boil under a reflux condenser. The graduated tube of the apparatus is to be previously filled with water to the standard line, and 2 mL of hexane is added to the graduated tube. After heating under reflux for 1 hour, separate the hexane layer, and use the layer as the sample solution. Separately, dissolve 1 mg of (*E*)-cinnamaldehyde for thin-layer chromatography in 1 mL of methanol, and use this solution as the standard solution. Perform the test with these solutions as directed under Thin-layer Chromatography <*2.03*>. Spot 20 μL of the sample solution and 2 μL of the standard solution on a plate of silica gel for thin-layer chromatography. Develop the plate with a mixture of hexane and ethyl acetate (2:1) to a distance of about 7 cm, and air-dry the plate. Spray evenly 2,4-dinitrophenylhydrazine TS on the plate: one of the several spots obtained from the sample solution has the same color tone and *Rf* value with the yellow-orange spot from the standard solution.

ii) To 2.0 g of the dry extract (or 6.0 g of the viscous extract), add 10 mL of water, shake, then add 5 mL of hexane, shake, centrifuge, and use the hexane layer as the sample solution. Separately, dissolve 1 mg of (*E*)-2-methoxycinnamaldehyde for thin-layer chromatography in 1 mL of methanol, and use this solution as the standard solution. Perform the test with these solutions as directed under Thin-layer Chromatography <*2.03*>. Spot 40 μL of the sample solution and 2 μL of the standard solution on a plate of silica gel for thin-layer chromatography. Develop the plate with a mixture of hexane and ethyl acetate (2:1) to a distance of about 7 cm, and air-dry the plate. Examine under ultraviolet light (main wavelength: 365 nm): one of the several spots obtained from the sample solution has the same color tone and *Rf* value with the blue-white fluorescent spot from the standard solution.

(4) To 1.0 g of the dry extract (or 3.0 g of the viscous extract) add 10 mL of water, shake, then add 10 mL of 1-butanol, shake, centrifuge, and use the 1-butanol layer as the sample solution. Separately, dissolve 1 mg of Paeoniflorin RS or paeoniflorin for thin-layer chromatog-raphy in 1 mL of methanol, and use this solution as the standard solution. Perform the test with these solutions as directed under Thin-layer Chromatography <*2.03*>. Spot 5 μL each of the sample solution and standard solution on a plate of silica gel for thin-layer chromatography. Develop the plate with a mixture of ethyl acetate, methanol and water (20:3:2) to a distance of about 7 cm, and air-dry the plate. Spray evenly 4-methoxybenzaldehyde-sulfuric acid TS on the plate, and heat the plate at 105°C for 5 minutes: one of the several spots obtained from the sample solution has the same color tone and *R*f value with the purple spot from the standard solution (Peony Root).

(5) To 1.0 g of the dry extract (or 3.0 g of the viscous extract) add 10 mL of water, shake, then add 10 mL of 1-butanol, shake, centrifuge, and use the 1-butanol layer as the sample solution. Separately, dissolve 1 mg of liquiritin for thin-layer chromatography in 1 mL of methanol, and use this solution as the standard solution. Perform the test with these solutions as directed under Thin-layer Chromatography <*2.03*>. Spot1 μL each of the sample solution and standard solution on a plate of silica gel for thin-layer chromatography. Develop the plate with a mixture of ethyl acetate, methanol and water (20:3:2) to a distance of about 7 cm, and air-dry the plate. Spray evenly dilute sulfuric acid on the plate, heat the plate at 105°C for 5 minutes, and examine under ultraviolet light (main wavelength: 365 nm): one of the several spots obtained from the sample solution has the same color tone and *R*f value with the yellow-green fluorescent spot from the standard solution (Glycyrrhiza).

(6) To 1.0 g of the dry extract (or 3.0 g of the viscous extract) add 10 mL of water, shake, then add 25 mL of diethyl ether, shake, and separate the diethyl ether layer. Evaporate the solvent under low pressure (in vacuo), add 2 mL of diethyl ether to the residue, and use this solution as the sample solution. Separately, dissolve 1 mg of [6]-gingerol for thin-layer chromatography in 1 mL of methanol, and use this solution as the standard solution. Perform the test with these solutions as directed under Thin-layer Chromatography <*2.03*>. Spot 10 μL of the sample solution and 5 μL of the standard solution on a plate of silica gel for thin-layer chromatography. Develop the plate with a mixture of ethyl acetate and hexane (1:1) to a distance of about 7 cm, and air-dry the plate. Spray evenly 4-dimethylaminobenzaldehyde TS for spraying on the plate, heat the plate at 105°C for 5 minutes, allow to cool, and spray water: one of the several spots obtained from the sample solution has the same color tone and *R*f value with the blue-green to grayish green spot from the standard solution (Ginger).

Purity **(1)** Heavy metals <*1.07*>—Prepare the test solution with 1.0 g of the dry extract (or an amount of the viscous extract, equivalent to 1.0 g of the dried substance) as directed in the Extracts (4), and perform the test (not more than 30 ppm).

(2) Arsenic <*1.11*>—Prepare the test solution with 0.67 g of the dry extract (or an amount of the viscous extract, equivalent to 0.67 g of the dried substance) according to Method 3, and perform the test (not more than 3 ppm).

Loss on drying <*2.41*> The dry extract: Not more than 10.0% (1 g, 105°C, 5 hours).

The viscous extract: Not more than 66.7% (1 g, 105°C, 5 hours).

Total ash <*5.01*> Not more than 10.0%, calculated on the dried basis.

Assay **(1)** Total alkaloids (ephedrine and pseudoephedrine)—Weigh accurately about 0.5 g of the dry extract (or an amount of the viscous extract, equivalent to about 0.5 g of the dried substance), add 20 mL of diethyl ether, shake, then add 3.0 mL of 0.1 mol/L hydrochloric acid TS, and shake for 10 minutes. After centrifugation, remove the diethyl ether layer, add 20 mL of diethyl ether, proceed in the same manner as described above, and remove the diethyl ether layer. To the aqueous layer add 1.0 mL of ammonia TS and 20 mL of diethyl ether, shake for 30 minutes, centrifuge, and separate the diethyl ether layer. In addition, repeat twice in the same manner for the aqueous layer using 1.0 mL of ammonia TS and 20 mL of diethyl ether. Combine all the extracts, evaporate the solvent under low pressure (in vacuo), dissolve the residue in diluted methanol (1 in 2) to make exactly 50 mL. Centrifuge this solution, and use the supernatant liquid as the sample solution. Separately, weigh accurately about 10 mg of ephedrine hydrochloride for assay of crude drugs, previously dried at 105°C for 3 hours, and dissolve in diluted methanol (1 in 2) to make exactly 100 mL. Pipet 10 mL of this solution, add diluted methanol (1 in 2) to make exactly 50 mL, and use this solution as the standard solution. Perform the test with exactly 10 μL each of the sample solution and standard solution as directed under Liquid Chromatography <*2.01*> according to the following conditions. Determine the peak areas, A_{TE} and A_{TP}, of ephedrine and pseudoephedrine obtained with the sample solution, and the peak area, A_S, of ephedrine with the standard solution.

Amount (mg) of total alkaloids (ephedrine and pseudoephedrine)
$= M_S \times (A_{TE} + A_{TP})/A_S \times 1/10 \times 0.819$

M_S: Amount (mg) of ephedrine hydrochloride for assay of crude drugs taken

Operating conditions—

Detector: An ultraviolet absorption photometer (wavelength: 210 nm).

Column: A stainless steel column 4.6 mm in inside diameter and 15 cm in length, packed with octadecylsilanized silica gel for liquid chromatography (5 μm in particle diameter).

Column temperature: A constant temperature of about 40°C.

Mobile phase: To 5 g of sodium lauryl sulfate add 350 mL of acetonitrile, shake, and add 650 mL of water and 1 mL of phosphoric acid to dissolve sodium lauryl sulfate.

Flow rate: 1.0 mL per minute (the retention time of ephedrine is about 27 minutes).

System suitability—

System performance: Dissolve 1 mg each of ephedrine hydrochloride for assay of crude drugs and pseudoephedrine hydrochloride in diluted methanol (1 in 2) to make 10 mL. When the procedure is run with 10 μL of this solution under the above operating conditions, pseudoephedrine and ephedrine are eluted in this order with the resolution between these peaks being not less than 1.5.

System repeatability: When the test is repeated 6 times with 10 μL of the standard solution under the above operating conditions, the relative standard deviation of the peak area of ephedrine is not more than 1.5%.

(2) Paeoniflorin—Weigh accurately about 0.5 g of the dry extract (or an amount of the viscous extract, equivalent to about 0.5 g of the dried substance), add exactly 50 mL of diluted methanol (1 in 2), shake for 15 minutes, and filter. Pipet 5 mL of the filtrate, flow through in a column packed with 2 g of polyamide for column chromatography, elute with 20 mL of water, add 1 mL of acetic acid (100) and water to make exactly 25 mL, and use this solution as the sample solution. Separately, weigh accurately about 10 mg of Paeoniflorin RS (separately determine the water *<2.48>* by coulometric titration, using 10 mg), and dissolve in diluted methanol (1 in 2) to make exactly 100 mL. Pipet 5 mL of this solution, add diluted methanol (1 in 2) to make exactly 20 mL, and use this solution as the standard solution. Perform the test with exactly 10 μL each of the sample solution and standard solution as directed under Liquid Chromatography *<2.01>* according to the following conditions, and determine the peak areas, A_T and A_S, of paeoniflorin in each solution.

Amount (mg) of paeoniflorin ($C_{23}H_{28}O_{11}$)
$= M_S \times A_T/A_S \times 5/8$

M_S: Amount (mg) of Paeoniflorin RS taken, calculated on the anhydrous basis

Operating conditions—

Detector: An ultraviolet absorption photometer (wavelength: 232 nm).

Column: A stainless steel column 4.6 mm in inside diameter and 15 cm in length, packed with octadecylsilanized silica gel for liquid chromatography (5 μm in particle diameter).

Column temperature: A constant temperature of about 20°C.

Mobile phase: A mixture of water, acetonitrile and phosphoric acid (850:150:1).

Flow rate: 1.0 mL per minute (the retention time of paeoniflorin is about 9 minutes).

System suitability—

System performance: Dissolve 1 mg each of Paeoniflorin RS and albiflorin in diluted methanol (1 in 2) to make 10 mL. When the procedure is run with 10 μL of this solution under the above operating conditions, albiflorin and paeoniflorin are eluted in this order with the resolution between these peaks being not less than 2.5.

System repeatability: When the test is repeated 6 times with 10 μL of the standard solution under the above operating conditions, the relative standard deviation of the peak area of paeoniflorin is not more than 1.5%.

(3) Glycyrrhizic acid—Perform the test according to the following i) or ii).

i) Weigh accurately about 0.5 g of the dry extract (or an amount of the viscous extract, equivalent to about 0.5 g of the dried substance), add exactly 50 mL of diluted methanol (1 in 2), shake for 15 minutes, filter, and use the filtrate as the sample solution. Separately, weigh accurately about 10 mg of Glycyrrhizic Acid RS (separately determine the water *<2.48>* by coulometric titration, using 10 mg), dissolve in diluted methanol (1 in 2) to make exactly 100 mL, and use this solution as the standard solution. Perform the test with exactly 10 μL each of the sample solution and standard solution as directed under Liquid Chromatography *<2.01>* according to the following conditions, and determine the peak areas, A_T and A_S, of glycyrrhizic acid in each solution.

Amount (mg) of glycyrrhizic acid ($C_{42}H_{62}O_{16}$)
$= M_S \times A_T/A_S \times 1/2$

M_S: Amount (mg) of Glycyrrhizic Acid RS taken, calculated on the anhydrous basis

Operating conditions—

Detector: An ultraviolet absorption photometer (wavelength: 254 nm).

Column: A stainless steel column 4.6 mm in inside diameter and 15 cm in length, packed with octadecylsilanized silica gel for liquid chromatography (5 μm in particle diameter).

Column temperature: A constant temperature of about 40°C.

Mobile phase: Dissolve 3.85 g of ammonium acetate in 720 mL of water, and add 5 mL of acetic acid (100) and 280 mL of acetonitrile.

Flow rate: 1.0 mL per minute (the retention time of glycyrrhizic acid is about 15 minutes).

System suitability—

System performance: Dissolve 5 mg of monoammonium glycyrrhizinate for resolution check in 20 mL of dilute ethanol. When the procedure is run with 10 μL of this solution under the above operating conditions, the resolution between the peak having the relative retention time of about 0.9 to glycyrrhizic acid and the peak of glycyrrhizic acid is not less than 1.5. Dissolve 1 mg of (*E*)-cinnamaldehyde for thin-layer chromatography in 50 mL of methanol. To 2 mL of this solution add 2 mL of the standard solution. When the procedure is run with 10 μL of this solution under the above operating conditions, the resolution between the peaks of glycyrrhizic acid and (*E*)-cinnamaldehyde is not less than 1.5.

System repeatability: When the test is repeated 6 times with 10 μL of the standard solution under the above operating conditions, the relative standard deviation of the peak area of glycyrrhizic acid is not more than 1.5%.

ii) Weigh accurately about 0.5 g of the dry extract (or an amount of the viscous extract, equivalent to about 0.5 g of the dried substance), add 20 mL of ethyl acetate and 10 mL of water, and shake for 10 minutes. After centrifugation, remove the ethyl acetate layer, add 20 mL of ethyl acetate, proceed in the same manner as described above, and remove the ethyl acetate layer. To the aqueous layer add 10 mL of methanol, shake for 30 minutes, centrifuge, and take the supernatant liquid. To the residue add 20 mL of diluted methanol (1 in 2), shake for 5 minutes, centrifuge, and take the supernatant liquid. Combine these supernatant liquids, add diluted methanol (1 in 2) to make exactly 50 mL, and use this solution as the sample solution. Separately, weigh accurately about 10 mg of Glycyrrhizic Acid RS (separately determine the water *<2.48>* by coulometric titration, using 10 mg), dissolve in diluted methanol (1 in 2) to make exactly 100 mL, and use this solution as the standard solution. Perform the test with exactly 10 μL each of the sample solution and standard solution as directed under Liquid Chromatography *<2.01>* according to the following conditions, and determine the peak areas, A_T and A_S, of glycyrrhizic acid in each solution.

Amount (mg) of glycyrrhizic acid ($C_{42}H_{62}O_{16}$)
$= M_S \times A_T/A_S \times 1/2$

M_S: Amount (mg) of Glycyrrhizic Acid RS taken, calculated on the anhydrous basis

Operating conditions—

Proceed as directed in the operating conditions in i).

System suitability—

System repeatability: Proceed as directed in the system suitability in i).

System performance: Dissolve 5 mg of monoammonium glycyrrhizinate for resolution check in 20 mL of dilute ethanol. When the procedure is run with 10 μL of this solution under the above operating conditions, the resolution between the peak having the relative retention time of about

0.9 to glycyrrhizic acid and the peak of glycyrrhizic acid is not less than 1.5.

Containers and storage Containers—Tight containers.

Kakkontokasenkyushin'i Extract

葛根湯加川芎辛夷エキス

Kakkontokasenkyushin'i Extract contains not less than 9.5 mg and not more than 28.5 mg (for preparation prescribed 3 g of Ephedra Herb) or not less than 13 mg and not more than 39 mg (for preparation prescribed 4 g of Ephedra Herb) of total alkaloids (ephedrine and pseudoephedrine), not less than 17 mg and not more than 51 mg of paeoniflorin ($C_{23}H_{28}O_{11}$: 480.46), not less than 14 mg and not more than 42 mg of glycyrrhizic acid ($C_{42}H_{62}O_{16}$: 822.93), and not less than 1.5 mg and not more than 6 mg (for preparation prescribed 2 g of Magnolia Flower) or not less than 2 mg and not more than 8 mg (for preparation prescribed 3 g of Magnolia Flower) of magnoflorine [as magnoflorine iodide ($C_{20}H_{24}INO_4$: 469.31)], per extract prepared with the amount specified in the Method of preparation.

Method of preparation

	1)	2)
Pueraria Root	4 g	4 g
Ephedra Herb	4 g	3 g
Jujube	3 g	3 g
Cinnamon Bark	2 g	2 g
Peony Root	2 g	2 g
Glycyrrhiza	2 g	2 g
Ginger	1 g	1 g
Cnidium Rhizome	3 g	2 g
Magnolia Flower	3 g	2 g

Prepare a dry extract or viscous extract as directed under Extracts, according to the prescription 1) or 2), using the crude drugs shown above.

Description Kakkontokasenkyushin'i Extract occurs as a light brown to brown powder or black-brown viscous extract, having a characteristic order, and a sweet first, then a bitter and hot taste.

Identification **(1)** Shake 1.0 g of the dry extract (or 3.0 g of the viscous extract) with 10 mL of water, add 10 mL of 1-butanol, shake, centrifuge, and use the 1-butanol layer as the sample solution. Separately, dissolve 1 mg of Puerarin RS or puerarin for thin-layer chromatography in 1 mL of methanol, and use this solution as the standard solution. Perform the test with these solutions as directed under Thin-layer Chromatography <*2.03*>. Spot 5 μL each of the sample solution and standard solution on a plate of silica gel for thin-layer chromatography. Develop the plate with a mixture of ethyl acetate, methanol and water (20:3:2) to a distance of about 7 cm, and air-dry the plate. Examine under ultraviolet light (main wavelength: 365 nm): one of the several spots obtained from the sample solution has the same color tone and *R*f value with the blue-white fluorescent spot from the standard solution (Pueraria Root).

(2) Shake 1.0 g of the dry extract (or 3.0 g of the viscous extract) with 10 mL of water, add 10 mL of 1-butanol, shake, centrifuge, and use the 1-butanol layer as the sample solution. Perform the test with the sample solution as directed under Thin-layer Chromatography <*2.03*>. Spot 5 μL of the sample solution on a plate of silica gel for thin-layer chromatography. Develop the plate with a mixture of 1-propanol, ethyl acetate, water and acetic acid (100) (4:4:2:1) to a distance of about 7 cm, and air-dry the plate. Spray evenly ninhydrin-ethanol TS for spraying on the plate, and heat the plate at 105°C for 5 minutes: a red-purple spot is observed at an *R*f value of about 0.5 (Ephedra Herb).

(3) Perform the test according to the following (i) or (ii) (Cinnamon Bark).

(i) Put 10 g of the dry extract (or 30 g of the viscous extract) in a 300-mL hard-glass flask, add 100 mL of water and 1 mL of silicone resin, connect the apparatus for essential oil determination, and heat to boil under a reflux condenser. The graduated tube of the apparatus is to be previously filled with water to the standard line, and 2 mL of hexane is added to the graduated tube. After heating under reflux for 1 hour, separate the hexane layer, and use the layer as the sample solution. Separately, dissolve 1 mg of (*E*)-cinnamaldehyde for thin-layer chromatography in 1 mL of methanol, and use this solution as the standard solution. Perform the test with these solutions as directed under Thin-layer Chromatography <*2.03*>. Spot 40 μL of the sample solution and 2 μL of the standard solution on a plate of silica gel for thin-layer chromatography. Develop the plate with a mixture of hexane and ethyl acetate (2:1) to a distance of about 7 cm, and air-dry the plate. Spray evenly 2,4-dinitrophenylhydrazine TS on the plate: one of the several spots obtained from the sample solution has the same color tone and *R*f value with the yellow-orange spot from the standard solution.

(ii) Shake 2.0 g of the dry extract (or 6.0 g of the viscous extract) with 10 mL of water, then add 5 mL of hexane, shake, centrifuge, and use the hexane layer as the sample solution. Separately, dissolve 1 mg of (*E*)-2-methoxycinnamaldehyde for thin-layer chromatography in 1 mL of methanol, and use this solution as the standard solution. Perform the test with these solutions as directed under Thin-layer Chromatography <*2.03*>. Spot 40 μL of the sample solution and 2 μL of the standard solution on a plate of silica gel for thin-layer chromatography. Develop the plate with a mixture of hexane and ethyl acetate (2:1) to a distance of about 7 cm, and air-dry the plate. Examine under ultraviolet light (main wavelength: 365 nm): one of the several spots obtained from the sample solution has the same color tone and *R*f value with the blue-white fluorescent spot from the standard solution.

(4) Shake 1.0 g of the dry extract (or 3.0 g of the viscous extract) with 10 mL of water, add 10 mL of 1-butanol, shake, centrifuge, and use the 1-butanol layer as the sample solution. Separately, dissolve 1 mg of Paeoniflorin RS or paeoniflorin for thin-layer chromatography in 1 mL of methanol, and use this solution as the standard solution. Perform the test with these solutions as directed under Thin-layer Chromatography <*2.03*>. Spot 5 μL each of the sample solution and standard solution on a plate of silica gel for thin-layer chromatography. Develop the plate with a mixture of ethyl acetate, methanol and ammonia solution (28) (6:3:2) to a distance of about 7 cm, and air-dry the plate. Spray evenly 4-methoxybenzoaldehyde-sulfuric acid TS on the plate, and heat the plate at 105°C for 2 minutes: one of the several spots obtained from the sample solution has the same color tone and *R*f value with the red-purple to purple spot from the standard solution (Peony Root).

(5) Shake 1.0 g of the dry extract (or 3.0 g of the viscous extract) with 10 mL of water, add 10 mL of 1-butanol, shake, centrifuge, and use the 1-butanol layer as the sample solution. Separately, dissolve 1 mg of liquiritin for thin-layer chromatography in 1 mL of methanol, and use this solution as the standard solution. Perform the test with these solutions as directed under Thin-layer Chromatography <*2.03*>. Spot 1 μL each of the sample solution and standard solution on a plate of silica gel for thin-layer chromatography. Develop the plate with a mixture of ethyl acetate, methanol and water (20:3:2) to a distance of about 7 cm, and air-dry the plate. Spray evenly dilute sulfuric acid on the plate, heat the plate at 105°C for 5 minutes, and examine under ultraviolet light (main wavelength: 365 nm): one of the several spots obtained from the sample solution has the same color tone and *R*f value with the yellow-green fluorescent spot from the standard solution (Glycyrrhiza).

(6) Shake 1.0 g of the dry extract (or 3.0 g of the viscous extract) with 10 mL of water, add 25 mL of diethyl ether, and shake. Separate the diethyl ether layer, evaporate the solvent under low pressure (in vacuo), add 2 mL of diethyl ether to the residue, and use this solution as the sample solution. Separately, dissolve 1 mg of [6]-gingerol for thin-layer chromatography in 1 mL of methanol, and use this solution as the standard solution. Perform the test with these solutions as directed under Thin-layer Chromatography <*2.03*>. Spot 10 μL of the sample solution and 5 μL of the standard solution on a plate of silica gel for thin-layer chromatography. Develop the plate with a mixture of ethyl acetate and hexane (1:1) to a distance of about 7 cm, and air-dry the plate. Spray evenly 4-dimethylaminobenzaldehyde TS for spraying on the plate, heat the plate at 105°C for 5 minutes, allow to cool, and spray water: one of the several spots obtained from the sample solution has the same color tone and *R*f value with the blue-green to grayish green spot from the standard solution (Ginger).

(7) Shake 1.0 g of the dry extract (or 3.0 g of the viscous extract) with 15 mL of water and 5 mL of 0.1 mol/L hydrochloric acid TS, and then shake with 25 mL of diethyl ether. Separate the diethyl ether layer, evaporate the solvent under low pressure (in vacuo), then dissolve the residue in 2 mL of diethyl ether, and use this solution as the sample solution. Separately, use (*Z*)-ligustilide TS for thin-layer chromatography as the standard solution. Perform the test with these solutions as directed under Thin-layer Chromatography <*2.03*>. Spot 10 μL each of the sample solution and standard solution on a plate of silica gel for thin-layer chromatography. Develop the plate with a mixture of ethyl acetate and hexane (1:1) to a distance of about 7 cm, and air-dry the plate. Examine under ultraviolet light (main wavelength: 365 nm): one of the several spots obtained from the sample solution has the same color tone and *R*f value with the blue-white fluorescent spot from the standard solution (Cnidium Rhizome).

(8) Shake 1.0 g of the dry extract (or 3.0 g of the viscous extract) with 10 mL of water, add 25 mL of diethyl ether, and shake. Separate the diethyl ether layer, evaporate the solvent under low pressure (in vacuo), add 2 mL of diethyl ether to the residue, and use this solution as the sample solution. Separately, to 1 g of powdered magnolia flower add 10 mL of methanol, shake, centrifuge, and use the supernatant liquid as the standard solution. Perform the test with these solutions as directed under Thin-layer Chromatography <*2.03*>. Spot 5 μL of the sample solution and 10 μL of the standard solution on a plate of silica gel for thin-layer chromatography. Develop the plate with a mixture of ethyl acetate and hexane (3:1) to a distance of about 7 cm, and air-dry the plate. Spray evenly dilute sulfuric acid on the plate, and heat the plate at 105°C for 5 minutes: one of the several spots obtained from the sample solution has the same color tone and *R*f value with the brown spot (*R*f value: about 0.4) from the standard solution (Magnolia Flower).

Purity **(1)** Heavy metals <*1.07*>—Prepare the test solution with 1.0 g of the dry extract (or an amount of the viscous extract, equivalent to 1.0 g of dried substance) as directed in Extracts (4), and perform the test (not more than 30 ppm).

(2) Arsenic <*1.11*>—Prepare the test solution with 0.67 g of the dry extract (or an amount of the viscous extract, equivalent to 0.67 g of dried substance) according to Method 3, and perform the test (not more than 3 ppm).

Loss on drying <*2.41*> The dry extract: Not more than 10.0% (1 g, 105°C, 5 hours).

The viscous extract: Not more than 66.7% (1 g, 105°C, 5 hours).

Total ash <*5.01*> Not more than 10.0%, calculated on the dried basis.

Assay **(1)** Total alkaloids (ephedrine and pseudoephedrine)—Weigh accurately about 0.5 g of the dry extract (or an amount of the viscous extract, equivalent to about 0.5 g of the dried substance), add 20 mL of diethyl ether, shake, then add 3.0 mL of 0.1 mol/L hydrochloric acid TS, and shake for 10 minutes. After centrifugation, remove the diethyl ether layer, add 20 mL of diethyl ether, proceed in the same manner as described above, and remove the diethyl ether layer. To the aqueous layer add 1.0 mL of ammonia TS and 20 mL of diethyl ether, shake for 30 minutes, centrifuge, and separate the diethyl ether layer. In addition, repeat twice in the same manner for the aqueous layer using 1.0 mL of ammonia TS and 20 mL of diethyl ether. Combine the extracts, evaporate the solvent under low pressure (in vacuo), dissolve the residue in diluted methanol (1 in 2) to make exactly 50 mL, centrifuge, and use the supernatant liquid as the sample solution. Separately, weigh accurately about 10 mg of ephedrine hydrochloride for assay of crude drugs, previously dried at 105°C for 3 hours, dissolve in diluted methanol (1 in 2) to make exactly 100 mL. Pipet 10 mL of this solution, add diluted methanol (1 in 2) to make exactly 50 mL, and use this solution as the standard solution. Perform the test with exactly 10 μL each of the sample solution and standard solution as directed under Liquid Chromatography <*2.01*> according to the following conditions, and determine the peak areas, A_{TE} and A_{TP}, of ephedrine and pseudoephedrine with the sample solution, and peak area, A_S, of ephedrine with standard solution.

Amount (mg) of total alkaloids (ephedrine and pseudoephedrine)

$$= M_S \times (A_{TE} + A_{TP})/A_S \times 1/10 \times 0.819$$

M_S: Amount (mg) of ephedrine hydrochloride for assay of crude drugs taken

Operating conditions—

Detector: An ultraviolet absorption photometer (wavelength: 210 nm).

Column: A stainless steel column 4.6 mm in inside diameter and 15 cm in length, packed with octadecylsilanized silica gel for liquid chromatography (5 μm in particle diameter).

Column temperature: A constant temperature of about 40°C.

Mobile phase: To 5 g of sodium lauryl sulfate add 350 mL of acetonitrile, shake, then add 650 mL of water and 1 mL of phosphoric acid to dissolve lauryl sulfate.

Flow rate: 1.0 mL per minute (the retention time of ephedrine is about 27 minutes).

System suitability—

System performance: Dissolve 1 mg each of ephedrine hydrochloride for assay of crude drugs and pseudoephedrine hydrochloride in diluted methanol (1 in 2) to make 10 mL. When the procedure is run with 10 μL of this solution under the above operating conditions, pseudoephedrine and ephedrine are eluted in this order with the resolution between these peaks being not less than 1.5.

System repeatability: When the test is repeated 6 times with 10 μL of the standard solution under the above operating conditions, the relative standard deviation of the peak area of ephedrine is not more than 1.5%.

(2) Paeoniflorin—Weigh accurately about 0.5 g of the dry extract (or an amount of the viscous extract, equivalent to about 0.5 g of the dried substance), add exactly 50 mL of diluted methanol (1 in 2), shake for 15 minutes, and filter. Pipet 5 mL of the filtrate, flow through in a column packed with 2 g of polyamide for column chromatography, elute with 20 mL of water, add 1 mL of acetic acid (100) to the effluent, then add water to make exactly 25 mL, and use this solution as the sample solution. Separately, weigh accurately about 10 mg of Paeoniflorin RS (separately determine the water <*2.48*> by coulometric titration, using 10 mg), and dissolve in diluted methanol (1 in 2) to make exactly 100 mL. Pipet 5 mL of this solution, add diluted methanol (1 in 2) to make exactly 20 mL, and use this solution as the standard solution. Perform the test with exactly 10 μL each of the sample solution and standard solution as directed under Liquid Chromatography <*2.01*> according to the following conditions, and determine the peak areas, A_T and A_S, of paeoniflorin in each solution.

$$\text{Amount (mg) of paeoniflorin } (C_{23}H_{28}O_{11}) = M_S \times A_T/A_S \times 5/8$$

M_S: Amount (mg) of Paeoniflorin RS taken, calculated on the anhydrous basis

Operating conditions—

Detector: An ultraviolet absorption photometer (wavelength: 232 nm).

Column: A stainless steel column 4.6 mm in inside diameter and 15 cm in length, packed with octadecylsilanized silica gel for liquid chromatography (5 μm in particle diameter).

Column temperature: A constant temperature of about 20°C.

Mobile phase: A mixture of water, acetonitrile and phosphoric acid (850:150:1).

Flow rate: 1.0 mL per minute (the retention time of paeoniflorin is about 9 minutes).

System suitability—

System performance: Dissolve 1 mg each of Paeoniflorin RS and albiflorin in diluted methanol (1 in 2) to make 10 mL. When the procedure is run with 10 μL of this solution under the above operating conditions, albiflorin and paeoniflorin are eluted in this order with the resolution between these peaks being not less than 2.5.

System repeatability: When the test is repeated 6 times with 10 μL of the standard solution under the above operating conditions, the relative standard deviation of the peak area of paeoniflorin is not more than 1.5%.

(3) Glycyrrhizic acid—Perform the test according to the following i) or ii).

i) Weigh accurately about 0.5 g of the dry extract (or an amount of the viscous extract, equivalent to about 0.5 g of the dried substance), add exactly 50 mL of diluted methanol (1 in 2), shake for 15 minutes, filter, and use the filtrate as the sample solution. Separately, weigh accurately about 10 mg of Glycyrrhizic Acid RS (separately determine the water <*2.48*> by coulometric titration, using 10 mg), dissolve in diluted methanol (1 in 2) to make exactly 100 mL, and use this solution as the standard solution. Perform the test with exactly 10 μL each of the sample solution and standard solution as directed under Liquid Chromatography <*2.01*> according to the following conditions, and determine the peak areas, A_T and A_S, of glycyrrhizic acid in each solution.

$$\text{Amount (mg) of glycyrrhizic acid } (C_{42}H_{62}O_{16}) = M_S \times A_T/A_S \times 1/2$$

M_S: Amount (mg) of Glycyrrhizic Acid RS taken, calculated on the anhydrous basis

Operating conditions—

Detector: An ultraviolet absorption photometer (wavelength: 254 nm).

Column: A stainless steel column 4.6 mm in inside diameter and 15 cm in length, packed with octadecylsilanized silica gel for liquid chromatography (5 μm in particle diameter).

Column temperature: A constant temperature of about 40°C.

Mobile phase: Dissolve 3.85 g of ammonium acetate in 720 mL of water, and add 5 mL of acetic acid (100) and 280 mL of acetonitrile.

Flow rate: 1.0 mL per minute (the retention time of glycyrrhizic acid is about 15 minutes).

System suitability—

System performance: Dissolve 5 mg of monoammonium glycyrrhizinate for resolution check in 20 mL of dilute ethanol. When the procedure is run with 10 μL of this solution under the above operating conditions, the resolution between the peak having the relative retention time of about 0.9 to glycyrrhizic acid and the peak of glycyrrhizic acid is not less than 1.5. Dissolve 1 mg of (*E*)-cinnamaldehyde for thin-layer chromatography in 50 mL of methanol. To 2 mL of this solution add 2 mL of the standard solution. When the procedure is run with 10 μL of this solution under the above operating conditions, the resolution between the peaks of glycyrrhizic acid and (*E*)-cinnamaldehyde is not less than 1.5.

System repeatability: When the test is repeated 6 times with 10 μL of the standard solution under the above operating conditions, the relative standard deviation of the peak area of glycyrrhizic acid is not more than 1.5%.

ii) Weigh accurately about 0.5 g of the dry extract (or an amount of the viscous extract, equivalent to about 0.5 g of the dried substance), add 20 mL of ethyl acetate and 10 mL of water, and shake for 10 minutes. After centrifugation, remove the ethyl acetate layer, add 20 mL of ethyl acetate, proceed in the same manner as described above, and remove the ethyl acetate layer. To the aqueous layer add 10 mL of methanol, shake for 30 minutes, centrifuge, and take the supernatant liquid. To the residue add 20 mL of diluted methanol (1 in 2), shake for 5 minutes, centrifuge, and take the supernatant liquid. Combine these supernatant liquids, add diluted methanol (1 in 2) to make exactly 50 mL, and use this solution as the sample solution. Separately, weigh accurately about 10 mg of Glycyrrhizic Acid RS (separately determine the water <*2.48*> by coulometric titration, using 10 mg), dissolve in diluted methanol (1 in 2) to make exactly 100 mL, and use this solution as the standard solution. Perform the test with exactly 10 μL each of the sample solution and standard solution as directed under Liquid Chromatography <*2.01*> according to the following conditions, and determine the peak areas, A_T and A_S, of glycyrrhizic acid in each solution.

Amount (mg) of glycyrrhizic acid ($C_{42}H_{62}O_{16}$)
$= M_S \times A_T/A_S \times 1/2$

M_S: Amount (mg) of Glycyrrhizic Acid RS taken, calculated on the anhydrous basis

Operating conditions—

Proceed as directed in the operating conditions in i).

System suitability—

System repeatability: Proceed as directed in the system suitability in i).

System performance: Dissolve 5 mg of monoammonium glycyrrhizinate for resolution check in 20 mL of dilute ethanol. When the procedure is run with 10 μL of this solution under the above operating conditions, the resolution between the peak having the relative retention time of about 0.9 to glycyrrhizic acid and the peak of glycyrrhizic acid is not less than 1.5.

(4) Magnoflorine—Weigh accurately about 0.5 g of the dry extract (or an amount of the viscous extract, equivalent to about 0.5 g of the dried substance), add 20 mL of diethyl ether, shake, add 3.0 mL of diluted sodium hydroxide TS (1 in 10), shake for 10 minutes, centrifuge, and remove the diethyl ether layer. Add 20 mL of diethyl ether, proceed in the same manner as described above, and remove the diethyl ether layer. To the aqueous layer add 3.0 mL of 0.1 mol/L hydrochloric acid TS and 20 mL of diluted methanol (1 in 2), shake for 15 minutes, centrifuge, and separate the supernatant liquid. To the residue add 20 mL of diluted methanol (1 in 2) shake for 15 minutes, centrifuge, and separate the supernatant liquid. Combine the previous supernatant liquids, add diluted methanol (1 in 2) to make exactly 50 mL, and use this solution as the sample solution. Separately, weigh accurately about 10 mg of magnoflorine iodide for assay, and dissolve in diluted methanol (1 in 2) to make exactly 100 mL. Pipet 5 mL of this solution, add diluted methanol (1 in 2) to make exactly 50 mL, and use this solution as the standard solution. Perform the test with exactly 20 μL each of the sample solution and standard solution as directed under Liquid Chromatography *<2.01>* according to the following conditions, and determine the peak areas, A_T and A_S, of magnoflorine in each solution.

Amount (mg) of magnoflorine [as magnoflorine iodide ($C_{20}H_{24}INO_4$)]
$= M_S \times A_T/A_S \times 1/20$

M_S: Amount (mg) of magnoflorine iodide for assay taken, calculated on the basis of the content obtained by qNMR

Operating conditions—

Detector: An ultraviolet absorption photometer (wavelength: 303 nm).

Column: A stainless steel column 4.6 mm in inside diameter and 15 cm in length, packed with octadecylsilanized silica gel for liquid chromatography (5 μm in particle diameter).

Column temperature: A constant temperature of about 40°C.

Mobile phase: To 5 g of sodium lauryl sulfate add 350 mL of acetonitrile, shake, then add 650 mL of water and 1 mL of phosphoric acid to dissolve lauryl sulfate.

Flow rate: 1.0 mL per minute (the retention time of magnoflorine is about 20 minutes).

System suitability—

System performance: When the procedure is run with 20 μL of the standard solution under the above operating conditions, the number of theoretical plates and the symmetry factor of the peak of magnoflorine are not less than 5000 and not more than 1.5, respectively.

System repeatability: When the test is repeated 6 times with 20 μL of the standard solution under the above operating conditions, the relative standard deviation of the peak area of magnoflorine is not more than 1.5%.

Containers and storage Containers—Tight containers.

Kamikihito Extract

加味帰脾湯エキス

Kamikihito Extract contains not less than 0.8 mg and not more than 3.2 mg of saikosaponin b_2, not less than 27 mg and not more than 81 mg of geniposide, and not less than 6 mg and not more than 18 mg of glycyrrhizic acid ($C_{42}H_{62}O_{16}$: 822.93), per extract prepared with the amount specified in the Method of preparation.

Method of preparation

	1)	2)	3)	4)
Ginseng	3 g	3 g	3 g	3 g
Atractylodes Rhizome	3 g			3 g
Atractylodes Lancea Rhizome		3 g	3 g	
Poria Sclerotium	3 g	3 g	3 g	3 g
Jujube Seed	3 g	3 g	3 g	3 g
Longan Aril	3 g	3 g	3 g	3 g
Astragalus Root	2 g	3 g	2 g	3 g
Japanese Angelica Root	2 g	2 g	2 g	2 g
Polygala Root	1.5 g	2 g	1 g	2 g
Bupleurum Root	3 g	3 g	3 g	3 g
Gardenia Fruit	2 g	2 g	2 g	2 g
Glycyrrhiza	1 g	1 g	1 g	1 g
Saussurea Root	1 g	1 g	1 g	1 g
Jujube	1.5 g	2 g	1 g	2 g
Ginger	0.5 g	1 g	1 g	0.5g
Moutan Bark				2 g

Prepare a dry extract or viscous extract as directed under Extracts, according to the preparation 1) to 4), using the crude drugs shown above. Or, prepare a dry extract by adding Light Anhydrous Silicic Acid to an extractive prepared as directed under Extracts, according to the preparation 2, using the crude drugs shown above.

Description Kamikihito Extract is a light yellow-brown to brown powder or black-brown viscous extract. It has a slightly odor, and a slightly sweet, hot and bitter taste.

Identification **(1)** To 3.0 g of the dry extract (or 9.0 g of the viscous extract) add 15 mL of sodium hydroxide TS, shake, centrifuge, and separate the supernatant liquid. To the liquid add 10 mL of 1-butanol, shake, centrifuge, and separate the 1-butanol layer. To this layer add 10 mL of water, shake, centrifuge, and separate the 1-butanol layer. Evaporate the solvent under low pressure (in vacuo), dissolve the residue in 2 mL of methanol, and use the solution as the sample solution. Separately, dissolve 1 mg of ginsenoside Rb_1 for thin-layer chromatography in 1 mL of methanol, and use this solution as the standard solution. Perform the test with these solutions as directed under Thin-layer Chromatography *<2.03>*. Spot 10 μL of the sample solution and 5 μL of the standard solution on a plate of silica gel for thin-layer chromatography. Develop the plate with a mixture of ethyl acetate, 1-propanol, water and acetic acid (100)

(7:5:4:1) to a distance of about 7 cm, and air-dry the plate. Spray evenly vanillin-sulfuric acid-ethanol TS for spraying on the plate, heat the plate at 105°C for 5 minutes, and allow to cool: one of the several spots obtained from the sample solution has the same color tone and *R*f value with the blue-purple spot from the standard solution (Ginseng).

(2) For preparation prescribed Atractylodes Rhizome—To 3.0 g of the dry extract (or 9.0 g of the viscous extract) add 15 mL of water, shake, then add 25 mL of diethyl ether, and shake. Separate the diethyl ether layer, evaporate the solvent under low pressure (in vacuo), then dissolve the residue in 2 mL of diethyl ether, and use the solution as the sample solution. Separately, dissolve 1 mg of atractylenolide III for thin-layer chromatography in 1 mL of methanol, and use this solution as the standard solution. Perform the test with these solutions as directed under Thin-layer Chromatography *<2.03>*. Spot 10 μL each of the sample solution and standard solution on a plate of silica gel for thin-layer chromatography. Develop the plate with a mixture of ethyl acetate and hexane (1:1) to a distance of about 7 cm, and air-dry the plate. Spray evenly 1-naphthol-sulfuric acid TS on the plate, heat the plate at 105°C for 5 minutes, and allow to cool: one of the several spots obtained from the sample solution has the same color tone and *R*f value with the red to red-purple spot from the standard solution (Atractylodes Rhizome).

(3) For preparation prescribed Atractylodes Lancea Rhizome—To 3.0 g of the dry extract (or 9.0 g of the viscous extract) add 10 mL of water, shake, then add 25 mL of hexane, and shake. Separate the hexane layer, evaporate the solvent under low pressure (in vacuo), then dissolve the residue in 2 mL of hexane, and use the solution as the sample solution. Perform the test with the sample solution as directed under Thin-layer Chromatography *<2.03>*. Spot 10 μL of the sample solution on a plate of silica gel with fluorescent indicator for thin-layer chromatography. Develop the plate with a mixture of hexane and acetone (7:1) to a distance of about 7 cm, and air-dry the plate. Examine under ultraviolet light (main wavelength: 254 nm): a dark violet spot is observed at an *R*f value of about 0.5, and this spot exhibits greenish brown when the plate is sprayed evenly 4-dimethylaminobenzaldehyde TS for spraying, heated the plate at 105°C for 5 minutes, and allowed to cool (Atractylodes Lancea Rhizome).

(4) To 3.0 g of the dry extract (or 9.0 g of the viscous extract) add 15 mL of sodium hydroxide TS, shake, centrifuge, and separate the supernatant liquid. To the liquid add 10 mL of 1-butanol, shake, centrifuge, and separate 1-butanol layer. To the 1-butanol layer add 10 mL of water, shake, centrifuge, separate the 1-butanol layer, and evaporate the solvent under low pressure (in vacuo). Dissolve the residue in 2 mL of methanol, and use this solution as the sample solution. Separately, dissolve 1 mg of astragaloside IV for thin-layer chromatography in 1 mL of methanol, and use this solution as the standard solution. Perform the test with these solutions as directed under Thin-layer Chromatography *<2.03>*. Spot 10 μL of the sample solution and 2 μL of the standard solution on a plate of silica gel for thin-layer chromatography. Develop the plate with a mixture of 2-propanol, water and ammonia solution (28) (9:2:1) to a distance of about 10 cm, and air-dry the plate. Spray evenly vanillin-sulfuric acid-ethanol TS for spraying on the plate, heat the plate at 105°C for 5 minutes, and allow to cool: one of the several spots obtained from the sample solution has the same color tone and *R*f value with the blue-green to blue-purple spot from the standard solution (Astragalus Root).

(5) To 3.0 g of the dry extract (or 9.0 g of the viscous extract) add 15 mL of water, shake, then add 25 mL of diethyl ether, and shake. Separate the diethyl ether layer, evaporate the solvent under low pressure (in vacuo), then add 2 mL of diethyl ether to the residue, and use the solution as the sample solution. Separately, use (*Z*)-ligustilide TS for thin-layer chromatography as the standard solution. Perform the test with these solutions as directed under Thin-layer Chromatography *<2.03>*. Spot 10 μL of the sample solution and 2 μL of the standard solution on a plate of silica gel for thin-layer chromatography. Develop the plate with a mixture of butyl acetate and hexane (2:1) to a distance of about 7 cm, and air-dry the plate. Examine the plate under ultraviolet light (main wavelength: 365 nm): one of the several spots obtained from the sample solution has the same color tone and *R*f value with the blue-white fluorescent spot from the standard solution (Japanese Angelica Root).

(6) To 2.0 g of the dry extract (or 6.0 g of the viscous extract) add 30 mL of 1 mol/L hydrochloric acid TS, and heat for 10 minutes. After cooling, to 10 mL of this solution add 10 mL of ethyl acetate, shake, centrifuge, and use the ethyl acetate layer as the sample solution. Separately, to 2.0 g of a powder of polygala root add 30 mL of 1 mol/L hydrochloric acid TS, and heat for 10 minutes. After cooling, to 10 mL of this solution add 10 mL of ethyl acetate, shake, centrifuge, and use the ethyl acetate layer as the standard solution. Perform the test with these solutions as directed under Thin-layer Chromatography *<2.03>*. Spot 20 μL of the sample solution and 5 μL of the standard solution on a plate of silica gel for thin-layer chromatography. Develop the plate with a mixture of ethyl acetate, 1-propanol and acetic acid (100) (7:5:1) to a distance of about 7 cm, and air-dry the plate. Spray evenly 4-methoxybenzaldehyde-sulfric acid TS on the plate, heat the plate at 105°C for 1 minute, and observe while hot: one of the several spots obtained from the sample solution has the same color tone and *R*f value with the purplish red spot (at an *R*f value of about 0.5) from the standard solution (Polygala Root).

(7) To 3.0 g of the dry extract (or 9.0 g of the viscous extract) add 15 mL of sodium hydroxide TS, shake, centrifuge, and separate the supernatant liquid. To the liquid add 10 mL of 1-butanol, shake, centrifuge, and separate the 1-butanol layer. To this layer add 10 mL of water, shake, centrifuge, and separate the 1-butanol layer. Evaporate the solvent under low pressure (in vacuo), dissolve the residue in 2 mL of methanol, and use this solution as the sample solution. Separately, dissolve 1 mg of saikosaponin b_2 for thin-layer chromatography in 1 mL of methanol, and use this solution as the standard solution. Perform the test with these solutions as directed under Thin-layer Chromatography *<2.03>*. Spot 10 μL of the sample solution and 2 μL of the standard solution on a plate of silica gel for thin-layer chromatography. Develop the plate with a mixture of ethyl acetate, ethanol (99.5) and water (8:2:1) to a distance of about 7 cm, and air-dry the plate. Spray evenly 4-dimethylaminobenzaldehyde TS for spraying on the plate, heat the plate at 105°C for 5 minutes, and examine under ultraviolet light (main wavelength: 365 nm): one of the several spots obtained from the sample solution has the same color tone and *R*f value with the yellow fluorescent spot from the standard solution (Bupleurum Root).

(8) To 1.0 g of the dry extract (or 3.0 g of the viscous extract) add 10 mL of water, shake, add 10 mL of 1-butanol, shake, centrifuge, and use the 1-butanol layer as the sample solution. Separately, dissolve 1 mg of geniposide for thin-layer chromatography in 1 mL of methanol, and use this solution as the standard solution. Perform the test with these solutions as directed under Thin-layer Chromatography

<2.03>. Spot 5 μL each of the sample solution and standard solution on a plate of silica gel for thin-layer chromatography. Develop the plate with a mixture of ethyl acetate, methanol, ammonia solution (28) (6:3:2) to a distance of about 7 cm, and air-dry the plate. Spray evenly 4-methoxybenzaldehyde-sulfuric acid TS on the plate, and heat the plate at 105°C for 5 minute: one of the several spots obtained from the sample solution has the same color tone and *Rf* value with the dark purple spot from the standard solution (Gardenia Fruit).

(9) To 1.0 g of the dry extract (or 3.0 g of the viscous extract) add 10 mL of water, shake, add 10 mL of 1-butanol, shake, centrifuge, and use the 1-butanol layer as the sample solution. Separately, dissolve 1 mg of liquiritin for thin-layer chromatography in 1 mL of methanol, and use this solution as the standard solution. Perform the test with these solutions as directed under Thin-layer Chromatography <2.03>. Spot 1 μL each of the sample solution and standard solution on a plate of silica gel for thin-layer chromatography. Develop the plate with a mixture of ethyl acetate, methanol and water (20:3:2) to a distance of about 7 cm, and air-dry the plate. Spray evenly dilute sulfuric acid on the plate, heat the plate at 105°C for 5 minutes, and examine under ultraviolet light (main wavelength: 365 nm): one of the several spots obtained from the sample solution has the same color tone and *Rf* value with the yellow-green fluorescent spot from the standard solution (Glycyrrhiza).

(10) To 3.0 g of the dry extract (or 9.0 g of the viscous extract) add 15 mL of water, shake, add 25 mL of diethyl ether, and shake. Separate the diethyl ether layer, evaporate the solvent under low pressure (in vacuo), dissolve the residue in 2 mL of diethyl ether, and use this solution as the sample solution. Separately, to 1.0 g of a powder of saussurea root add 10 mL of methanol, shake, centrifuge, and use the supernatant liquid as the standard solution. Perform the test with these solutions as directed under Thin-layer Chromatography <2.03>. Spot 10 μL of the sample solution and 5 μL of the standard solution on a plate of silica gel for thin-layer chromatography. Develop the plate with a mixture of hexane and acetone (7:3) to a distance of about 7 cm, and air-dry the plate. Spray evenly vanillin-sulfuric acid-ethanol TS for spraying on the plate, heat the plate at 105°C for 2 minutes, and allow to cool: one of the several spots obtained from the sample solution has the same color tone and *Rf* value with the blue spot from the standard solution (Saussurea Root).

(11) To 3.0 g of the dry extract (or 9.0 g of the viscous extract) add 15 mL of water, shake, add 25 mL of diethyl ether, and shake. Separate the diethyl ether layer, evaporate the solvent under low pressure (in vacuo), dissolve the residue in 2 mL of diethyl ether, and use this solution as the sample solution. Separately, dissolve 1 mg of [6]-gingerol for thin-layer chromatography in 1 mL of methanol, and use this solution as the standard solution. Perform the test with these solutions as directed under Thin-layer Chromatography <2.03>. Spot 10 μL of the sample solution and 5 μL of the standard solution on a plate of silica gel for thin-layer chromatography. Develop the plate with a mixture of ethyl acetate and hexane (1:1) to a distance of about 7 cm, and air-dry the plate. Spray evenly 4-dimethylaminobenzaldehyde TS for spraying on the plate, heat the plate at 105°C for 5 minutes, allow to cool, and spray water: one of the several spots obtained from the sample solution has the same color tone and *Rf* value with the blue-green to grayish green spot from the standard solution (Ginger).

(12) For preparation prescribed Moutan Bark—To 3.0 g of the dry extract (or 9.0 g of the viscous extract) add 15 mL of water, shake, add 25 mL of diethyl ether, and shake. Separate the diethyl ether layer, evaporate the solvent under low pressure (in vacuo), dissolve the residue in 2 mL of diethyl ether, and use this solution as the sample solution. Separately, dissolve 1 mg of paeonol for thin-layer chromatography in 1 mL of methanol, and use this solution as the standard solution. Perform the test with these solutions as directed under Thin-layer Chromatography <2.03>. Spot 20 μL of the sample solution and 10 μL of the standard solution on a plate of silica gel for thin-layer chromatography. Develop the plate with a mixture of hexane and diethyl ether (5:3) to a distance of about 7 cm, and air-dry the plate. Spray evenly 4-methoxybenzaldehyde-sulfuric acid TS on the plate, heat the plate at 105°C for 5 minutes, and allow to cool: one of the several spots obtained from the sample solution has the same color tone and *Rf* value with the orange spot from the standard solution (Moutan Bark).

Purity **(1)** Heavy metals <1.07>—Prepare the test solution with 1.0 g of the dry extract (or an amount of the viscous extract, equivalent to 1.0 g of the dried substance) as directed under Extracts (4), and perform the test (not more than 30 ppm).

(2) Arsenic <1.11>—Prepare the test solution with 0.67 g of the dry extract (or an amount of the viscous extract, equivalent to 0.67 g of the dried substance) according to Method 3, and perform the test (not more than 3 ppm).

Loss on drying <2.41> The dry extract: Not more than 10.0% (1 g, 105°C, 5 hours).

The viscous extract: Not more than 66.7% (1 g, 105°C, 5 hours).

Total ash <5.01> Not less than 8.0%, calculated on the dried basis. However, for the dry extract prepared by adding Light Anhydrous Silicic Acid, between 9.0% and 18.0%.

Assay **(1)** Saikosaponin b_2—Weigh accurately about 0.5 g of the dry extract (or an amount of the viscous extract, equivalent to about 0.5 g of the dried substance), add 20 mL of diethyl ether and 10 mL of water, and shake for 10 minutes. Centrifuge, remove the diethyl ether layer, then add 20 mL of diethyl ether, proceed in the same manner as above, and remove the diethyl ether layer. To the aqueous layer add 10 mL of methanol, shake for 30 minutes, centrifuge, and separate the supernatant liquid. To the residue add 20 mL of diluted methanol (1 in 2), shake for 5 minutes, centrifuge, and separate the supernatant liquid. Combine all the supernatant liquids, add diluted methanol (1 in 2) to make exactly 50 mL, and use this solution as the sample solution. Separately, use saikosaponin b_2 standard TS for assay as the standard solution. Perform the test with exactly 10 μL each of the sample solution and standard solution as directed under Liquid Chromatography <2.01> according to the following conditions, and determine the peak areas, A_T and A_S, of saikosaponin b_2 in each solution.

$$\text{Amount (mg) of saikosaponin } b_2 = C_S \times A_T/A_S \times 50$$

C_S: Concentration (mg/mL) of saikosaponin b_2 in saikosaponin b_2 standard TS for assay

Operating conditions—

Detector: An ultraviolet absorption photometer (wavelength: 254 nm).

Column: A stainless steel column 4.6 mm in inside diameter and 15 cm in length, packed with octadecylsilanized silica gel for liquid chromatography (5 μm in particle diameter).

Column temperature: A constant temperature of about 40°C.

Mobile phase: A mixture of 0.05 mol/L sodium dihydrogen phosphate TS and acetonitrile (5:3).

Flow rate: 1.0 mL per minute (retention time of saikosaponin b_2 is about 12 minutes).

System suitability—

System performance: When the procedure is run with 10 μL of the standard solution under the above operating conditions, the number of theoretical plates and the symmetry factor of the peak of saikosaponin b_2 are not less than 5000 and not more than 1.5, respectively.

System repeatability: When the test is repeated 6 times with 10 μL of the standard solution under the above operating conditions, the relative standard deviation of the peak area of saikosaponin b_2 is not more than 1.5%.

(2) Geniposide—Weigh accurately about 0.5 g of the dry extract (or an amount of the viscous extract, equivalent to about 0.5 g of the dried substance), add exactly 50 mL of diluted methanol (1 in 2), shake for 15 minutes, filter, and use the filtrate as the sample solution. Separately, weigh accurately about 10 mg of geniposide for assay, dissolve in diluted methanol (1 in 2) to make exactly 100 mL, and use this solution as the standard solution. Perform the test with exactly 10 μL each of the sample solution and standard solution as directed under Liquid Chromatography <*2.01*> according to the following conditions, and determine the peak areas, A_T and A_S, of geniposide in each solution.

$$\text{Amount (mg) of geniposide} = M_S \times A_T/A_S \times 1/2$$

M_S: Amount (mg) of geniposide for assay taken, calculated on the basis of the content obtained by qNMR

Operating conditions—

Detector: An ultraviolet absorption photometer (wavelength: 240 nm).

Column: A stainless steel column 4.6 mm in inside diameter and 15 cm in length, packed with octadecylsilanized silica gel for liquid chromatography (5 μm in particle diameter).

Column temperature: A constant temperature of about 40°C.

Mobile phase: A mixture of water, acetonitrile and phosphoric acid (900:100:1).

Flow rate: 1.0 mL per minute (retention time of geniposide is about 10 minutes).

System suitability—

System performance: When the procedure is run with 10 μL of the standard solution under the above operating conditions, the number of theoretical plates and the symmetry factor of the peak of geniposide are not less than 5000 and not more than 1.5, respectively.

System repeatability: When the test is repeated 6 times with 10 μL of the standard solution under the above operating conditions, the relative standard deviation of the peak area of geniposide is not more than 1.5%.

(3) Glycyrrhizic acid—Weigh accurately about 0.5 g of the dry extract (or an amount of the viscous extract, equivalent to about 0.5 g of the dried substance), add 20 mL of diethyl ether and 10 mL of water, and shake for 10 minutes. After centrifugation, remove the diethyl ether layer, add 20 mL of diethyl ether, proceed in the same manner as described above, and remove the diethyl ether layer. To the aqueous layer add 10 mL of methanol, shake for 30 minutes, centrifuge, and take the supernatant liquid. To the residue add 20 mL of diluted methanol (1 in 2), shake for 5 minutes, centrifuge, and take the supernatant liquid. Combine these supernatant liquids, add diluted methanol (1 in 2) to make exactly 50 mL, and use this solution as the sample solution. Separately, weigh accurately about 10 mg of Glycyrrhizic Acid RS (separately determine the water <*2.48*> by coulometric titration, using 10 mg), dissolve in diluted methanol (1 in 2) to make exactly 100 mL, and use this solution as the standard solution. Perform the test with exactly 10 μL each of the sample solution and standard solution as directed under Liquid Chromatography <*2.01*> according to the following conditions, and determine the peak areas, A_T and A_S, of glycyrrhizic acid in each solution.

$$\text{Amount (mg) of glycyrrhizic acid } (C_{42}H_{62}O_{16}) = M_S \times A_T/A_S \times 1/2$$

M_S: Amount (mg) of Glycyrrhizic Acid RS taken, calculated on the anhydrous basis

Operating conditions—

Detector: An ultraviolet absorption photometer (wavelength: 254 nm).

Column: A stainless steel column 4.6 mm in inside diameter and 15 cm in length, packed with octadecylsilanized silica gel for liquid chromatography (5 μm in particle diameter).

Column temperature: A constant temperature of about 40°C.

Mobile phase: Dissolve 3.85 g of ammonium acetate in 720 mL of water, and add 5 mL of acetic acid (100) and 280 mL of acetonitrile.

Flow rate: 1.0 mL per minute (the retention time of glycyrrhizic acid is about 15 minutes).

System suitability—

System performance: Dissolve 5 mg of monoammonium glycyrrhizinate for resolution check in 20 mL of dilute ethanol. When the procedure is run with 10 μL of this solution under the above operating conditions, the resolution between the peak having the relative retention time of about 0.9 to glycyrrhizic acid and the peak of glycyrrhizic acid is not less than 1.5.

System repeatability: When the test is repeated 6 times with 10 μL of the standard solution under the above operating conditions, the relative standard deviation of the peak area of glycyrrhizic acid is not more than 1.5%.

Containers and storage Containers—Tight containers.

Kamishoyosan Extract

加味逍遙散エキス

Kamishoyosan Extract contains not less than 28 mg and not more than 84 mg of paeoniflorin ($C_{23}H_{28}O_{11}$: 480.46), not less than 25 mg and not more than 75 mg of geniposide, and not less than 10 mg and not more than 30 mg (for preparation prescribed 1.5 g of Glycyrrhiza) or not less than 13 mg and not more than 39 mg (for preparation prescribed 2 g of Glycyrrhiza) of glycyrrhizic acid ($C_{42}H_{62}O_{16}$: 822.93), per extract prepared with the amount specified in the Method of preparation.

Method of preparation

	1)	2)	3)	4)	5)	6)
Japanese Angelica Root	3 g	3 g	3 g	3 g	3 g	3 g
Peony Root	3 g	3 g	3 g	3 g	3 g	3 g
Atractylodes Rhizome	3 g	—	3 g	—	3 g	3 g
Atractylodes Lancea Rhizome	—	3 g	—	3 g	—	—
Poria Sclerotium	3 g	3 g	3 g	3 g	3 g	3 g
Bupleurum Root	3 g	3 g	3 g	3 g	3 g	3 g
Moutan Bark	2 g	2 g	2 g	2 g	2 g	2 g
Gardenia Fruit	2 g	2 g	2 g	2 g	2 g	2 g
Glycyrrhiza	2 g	2 g	1.5 g	1.5 g	1.5 g	1.5 g
Ginger	1 g	1 g	1 g	1 g	1.5 g	0.5 g
Mentha Herb	1 g	1 g	1 g	1 g	1 g	1 g

Prepare a dry extract or viscous extract as directed under Extracts, according to the prescription 1) to 6), using the crude drugs shown above.

Description Kamishoyosan Extract occurs as a yellow-brown to brown powder or black-brown viscous extract. It has slightly a characteristic odor, and a sweet, slightly hot, then bitter taste.

Identification **(1)** To 2.0 g of the dry extract (or 6.0 g of the viscous extract) add 10 mL of water, shake, then add 5 mL of diethyl ether, shake, centrifuge, and use the diethyl ether layer as the sample solution. Separately, use (*Z*)-ligustilide TS for thin-layer chromatography as the standard solution. Perform the test with these solutions as directed under Thin-layer Chromatography <*2.03*>. Spot 10 μL each of the sample solution and standard solution on a plate of silica gel for thin-layer chromatography. Develop the plate with a mixture of ethyl acetate and hexane (1:1) to a distance of about 7 cm, and air-dry the plate. Examine under ultraviolet light (main wavelength: 365 nm): one of the several spots obtained from the sample solution has the same color tone and *Rf* value with the blue-white fluorescent spot from the standard solution (Japanese Angelica Root).

(2) To 1.0 g of the dry extract (or 3.0 g of the viscous extract) add 10 mL of water, shake, then add 10 mL of methanol, shake, centrifuge, and use the supernatant liquid as the sample solution. Separately, dissolve 1 mg of albiflorin in 1 mL of methanol, and use this solution as the standard solution. Perform the test with these solutions as directed under Thin-layer Chromatography <*2.03*>. Spot 10 μL each of the sample solution and standard solution on a plate of silica gel for thin-layer chromatography. Develop the plate with a mixture of ethyl acetate, methanol and ammonia solution (28) (6:3:2) to a distance of about 10 cm, and air-dry the plate. Spray evenly 4-methoxybenzaldehyde-sulfuric acid TS on the plate, heat the plate at 105°C for 5 minutes, allow to cool for more than 30 minutes, and examine under ultraviolet light (main wavelength: 365 nm): one of the several spots obtained from the sample solution has the same color tone and *Rf* value with the orange fluorescent spot from the standard solution (Peony Root).

(3) For preparation prescribed Atractylodes Rhizome—To 2.0 g of the dry extract (or 6.0 g of the viscous extract) add 10 mL of water, shake, then add 5 mL of diethyl ether, shake, centrifuge, and use the diethyl ether layer as the sample solution. Separately, dissolve 1 mg of atractylenolide III for thin-layer chromatography in 1 mL of methanol, and use this solution as the standard solution. Perform the test with these solutions as directed under Thin-layer Chromatography <*2.03*>. Spot 10 μL each of the sample solution and standard solution on a plate of silica gel for thin-layer chromatography. Develop the plate with a mixture of ethyl acetate and hexane (1:1) to a distance of about 7 cm, and air-dry the plate. Spray evenly 1-naphthol-sulfuric acid TS on the plate, heat the plate at 105°C for 5 minutes, and allow to cool: one of the several spots obtained from the sample solution has the same color tone and *Rf* value with the red spot from the standard solution (Atractylodes Rhizome).

(4) For preparation prescribed Atractylodes Lancea Rhizome—To 2.0 g of the dry extract (or 6.0 g of the viscous extract) add 10 mL of water, shake, then add 25 mL of hexane, and shake. Separate the hexane layer, evaporate the solvent under low pressure (in vacuo), add 2 mL of hexane to the residue, and use this solution as the sample solution. Perform the test with the sample solution as directed under Thin-layer Chromatography <*2.03*>. Spot 20 μL of the sample solution on a plate of silica gel with fluorescent indicator for thin-layer chromatography. Develop the plate with a mixture of hexane and acetone (7:1) to a distance of about 7 cm, and air-dry the plate. Examine under ultraviolet light (main wavelength: 254 nm): a dark purple spot is observed at an *Rf* value of about 0.5. The spot shows a greenish brown color after being sprayed evenly 4-dimethylaminobenzaldehyde TS for spraying, heat the plate at 105°C for 5 minutes, and allowed to cool (Atractylodes Lancea Rhizome).

(5) To 2.0 g of the dry extract (or 6.0 g of the viscous extract) add 10 mL of sodium hydroxide TS, shake, then add 5 mL of 1-butanol, shake, centrifuge, and use the 1-butanol layer as the sample solution. Separately, dissolve 1 mg of saikosaponin b_2 for thin-layer chromatography in 1 mL of methanol, and use this solution as the standard solution. Perform the test with these solutions as directed under Thin-layer Chromatography <*2.03*>. Spot 10 μL of the sample solution and 2 μL of the standard solution on a plate of silica gel for thin-layer chromatography. Develop the plate with a mixture of ethyl acetate, ethanol (99.5) and water (8:2:1) to a distance of about 7 cm, and air-dry the plate. Spray evenly 4-dimethylaminobenzaldehyde TS for spraying on the plate, heat the plate at 105°C for 5 minutes, and examine under ultraviolet light (main wavelength: 365 nm): one of the several spots obtained from the sample solution has the same color tone and *Rf* value with the yellow fluorescent spot from the standard solution (Bupleurum Root).

(6) To 2.0 g of the dry extract (or 6.0 g of the viscous extract) add 10 mL of water, shake, then add 15 mL of diethyl ether, and shake. Separate the diethyl ether layer, evaporate the solvent under low pressure (in vacuo), add 1 mL of diethyl ether to the residue, and use this solution as the sample solution. Separately, dissolve 1 mg of paeonol for thin-layer chromatography in 1 mL of methanol, and use this solution as the standard solution. Perform the test with these solutions as directed under Thin-layer Chromatography <*2.03*>. Spot 10 μL each of the sample solution and standard solution on a plate of silica gel for thin-layer chromatography. Develop the plate with a mixture of hexane and diethyl ether (5:3) to a distance of about 7 cm, and air-dry the plate. Spray evenly 4-methoxybenzaldehyde-sulfuric acid TS on the plate, and heat the plate at 105°C for 5 minutes: one of the several spots obtained from the sample solution has the same color tone and *Rf* value with the orange spot from the standard solution (Moutan Bark).

(7) To 2.0 g of the dry extract (or 6.0 g of the viscous extract) add 10 mL of water, shake, then add 5 mL of 1-butanol, shake, centrifuge, and use the 1-butanol layer as the sample solution. Separately, dissolve 1 mg of geniposide for thin-layer chromatography in 1 mL of methanol, and use this solution as the standard solution. Perform the test with these solutions as directed under Thin-layer Chromatography <*2.03*>. Spot 10 μL each of the sample solution and standard solution on a plate of silica gel for thin-layer chromatography. Develop the plate with a mixture of ethyl acetate, methanol and ammonia solution (28) (6:3:2) to a distance of about 7 cm, and air-dry the plate. Spray evenly 4-methoxybenzaldehyde-sulfric acid TS on the plate, and heat the plate at 105°C for 5 minutes: one of the several spots obtained from the sample solution has the same color tone and *R*f value with the purple spot from the standard solution (Gardenia Fruit).

(8) To 2.0 g of the dry extract (or 6.0 g of the viscous extract) add 10 mL of water, shake, then add 5 mL of 1-butanol, shake, centrifuge, and use the 1-butanol layer as the sample solution. Separately, dissolve 1 mg of liquiritin for thin-layer chromatography in 1 mL of methanol, and use this solution as the standard solution. Perform the test with these solutions as directed under Thin-layer Chromatography <*2.03*>. Spot 1 μL each of the sample solution and standard solution on a plate of silica gel for thin-layer chromatography. Develop the plate with a mixture of ethyl acetate, methanol and water (20:3:2) to a distance of about 7 cm, and air-dry the plate. Spray evenly dilute sulfuric acid on the plate, heat the plate at 105°C for 5 minutes, and examine under ultraviolet light (main wavelength: 365 nm): one of the several spots obtained from the sample solution has the same color tone and *R*f value with the yellow-green fluorescent spot from the standard solution (Glycyrrhiza).

(9) To 2.0 g of the dry extract (or 6.0 g of the viscous extract) add 10 mL of water, shake, then add 5 mL of diethyl ether, shake, centrifuge, and use the diethyl ether layer as the sample solution. Separately, dissolve 1 mg of [6]-gingerol for thin-layer chromatography in 1 mL of methanol, and use this solution as the standard solution. Perform the test with these solutions as directed under Thin-layer Chromatography <*2.03*>. Spot 10 μL each of the sample solution and standard solution on a plate of silica gel for thin-layer chromatography. Develop the plate with a mixture of ethyl acetate and hexane (1:1) to a distance of about 7 cm, and air-dry the plate. Spray evenly 4-dimethylaminobenzaldehyde TS for spraying on the plate, heat the plate at 105°C for 5 minutes, allow to cool, and spray water: one of the several spots obtained from the sample solution has the same color tone and *R*f value with the blue-green to grayish green spot from the standard solution (Ginger).

(10) To 2.0 g of the dry extract (or 6.0 g of the viscous extract) add 10 mL of diluted phosphoric acid (1 in 30), shake, then add 15 mL of ethyl acetate, shake, centrifuge, and use the ethyl acetate layer as the sample solution. Separately, shake 0.2 g of pulverized mentha herb with 10 mL of diluted phosphoric acid (1 in 30), add 15 mL of ethyl acetate, shake, centrifuge, and use the ethyl acetate layer as the standard solution. Perform the test with these solutions as directed under Thin-layer Chromatography <*2.03*>. Spot 20 μL each of the sample solution and standard solution on a plate of silica gel for thin-layer chromatography. Develop the plate with a mixture of acetone, ethyl acetate, water and acetic acid (100) (10:10:3:1) to a distance of about 7 cm, and air-dry the plate. Spray evenly 2,6-dibromo-*N*-chloro-1,4-benzoquinone monoimine TS on the plate, heat the plate at 105°C for 5 minutes: one of the several spots obtained from the sample solution has the same color tone and *R*f value with the red-brown spot (around *R*f value 0.4) from the standard solution (Mentha Herb).

Purity **(1)** Heavy metals <*1.07*>—Prepare the test solution with 1.0 g of the dry extract (or an amount of the viscous extract, equivalent to 1.0 g of the dried substance) as directed under the Extracts (4), and perform the test (not more than 30 ppm).

(2) Arsenic <*1.11*>—Prepare the test solution with 0.67 g of the dry extract (or an amount of the viscous extract, equivalent to 0.67 g of the dried substance) according to Method 3, and perform the test (not more than 3 ppm).

Loss on drying <*2.41*> The dry extract: Not more than 9.0% (1 g, 105°C, 5 hours).

The viscous extract: Not more than 66.7% (1 g, 105°C, 5 hours).

Total ash <*5.01*> Not more than 10.0%, calculated on the dried basis.

Assay **(1)** Paeoniflorin—Weigh accurately about 0.5 g of the dry extract (or an amount of the viscous extract, equivalent to about 0.5 g of the dried substance), add exactly 50 mL of diluted methanol (1 in 2), shake for 15 minutes, filter, and use the filtrate as the sample solution. Separately, weigh accurately about 10 mg of Paeoniflorin RS (separately determine the water <*2.48*> by coulometric titration, using 10 mg), and dissolve in diluted methanol (1 in 2) to make exactly 100 mL, and use this solution as the standard solution. Perform the test with exactly 10 μL each of the sample solution and standard solution as directed under Liquid Chromatography <*2.01*> according to the following conditions, and determine the peak areas, A_T and A_S, of paeoniflorin in each solution.

$$\text{Amount (mg) of paeoniflorin } (C_{23}H_{28}O_{11}) = M_S \times A_T/A_S \times 1/2$$

M_S: Amount (mg) of Paeoniflorin RS taken, calculated on the anhydrous basis

Operating conditions—

Detector: An ultraviolet absorption photometer (wavelength: 232 nm).

Column: A stainless steel column 4.6 mm in inside diameter and 15 cm in length, packed with octadecylsilanized silica gel for liquid chromatography (5 μm in particle diameter).

Column temperature: A constant temperature of about 20°C.

Mobile phase: A mixture of water, acetonitrile and phosphoric acid (850:150:1).

Flow rate: 1.0 mL per minute (the retention time of paeoniflorin is about 9 minutes).

System suitability—

System performance: Dissolve 1 mg each of Paeoniflorin RS and albiflorin in diluted methanol (1 in 2) to make 10 mL. When the procedure is run with 10 μL of this solution under the above operating conditions, albiflorin and paeoniflorin are eluted in this order with the resolution between these peaks being not less than 2.5.

System repeatability: When the test is repeated 6 times with 10 μL of the standard solution under the above operating conditions, the relative standard deviation of the peak area of paeoniflorin is not more than 1.5%.

(2) Geniposide—Weigh accurately about 0.5 g of the dry extract (or an amount of the viscous extract, equivalent to about 0.5 g of the dried substance), add exactly 50 mL of diluted methanol (1 in 2), shake for 15 minutes, filter, and use the filtrate as the sample solution. Separately, weigh accurately about 10 mg of geniposide for assay, dissolve in diluted methanol (1 in 2) to make exactly 100 mL, and use this solution as the standard solution. Perform the test with exactly 10 μL each of the sample solution and standard solution as directed under Liquid Chromatography <2.01> according to the following conditions, and determine the peak areas, A_T and A_S, of geniposide in each solution.

$$\text{Amount (mg) of geniposide} = M_S \times A_T/A_S \times 1/2$$

M_S: Amount (mg) of geniposide for assay taken, calculated on the basis of the content obtained by qNMR

Operating conditions—

Detector: An ultraviolet absorption photometer (wavelength: 240 nm).

Column: A stainless steel column 4.6 mm in inside diameter and 15 cm in length, packed with octadecylsilanized silica gel for liquid chromatography (5 μm in particle diameter).

Column temperature: A constant temperature of about 40°C.

Mobile phase: A mixture of water, acetonitrile and phosphoric acid (900:100:1).

Flow rate: 1.0 mL per minute (the retention time of geniposide is about 10 minutes).

System suitability—

System performance: When the procedure is run with 10 μL of the standard solution under the above operating conditions, the number of theoretical plates and the symmetry factor of the peak of geniposide are not less than 5000 and not more than 1.5, respectively.

System repeatability: When the test is repeated 6 times with 10 μL of the standard solution under the above operating conditions, the relative standard deviation of the peak area of geniposide is not more than 1.5%.

(3) Glycyrrhizic acid—Weigh accurately about 0.5 g of the dry extract (or an amount of the viscous extract, equivalent to about 0.5 g of the dried substance), add 20 mL of ethyl acetate and 10 mL of water, and shake for 10 minutes. After centrifugation, remove the ethyl acetate layer, add 20 mL of ethyl acetate, proceed in the same manner as described above, and remove the ethyl acetate layer. To the aqueous layer add 10 mL of methanol, shake for 30 minutes, centrifuge, and take the supernatant liquid. To the residue add 20 mL of diluted methanol (1 in 2), shake for 5 minutes, centrifuge, and take the supernatant liquid. Combine these supernatant liquids, add diluted methanol (1 in 2) to make exactly 50 mL, and use this solution as the sample solution. Separately, weigh accurately about 10 mg of Glycyrrhizic Acid RS (separately determine the water <2.48> by coulometric titration, using 10 mg), dissolve in diluted methanol (1 in 2) to make exactly 100 mL, and use this solution as the standard solution. Perform the test with exactly 10 μL each of the sample solution and standard solution as directed under Liquid Chromatography <2.01> according to the following conditions, and determine the peak areas, A_T and A_S, of glycyrrhizic acid in each solution.

$$\text{Amount (mg) of glycyrrhizic acid } (C_{42}H_{62}O_{16}) = M_S \times A_T/A_S \times 1/2$$

M_S: Amount (mg) of Glycyrrhizic Acid RS taken, calculated on the anhydrous basis

Operating conditions—

Detector: An ultraviolet absorption photometer (wavelength: 254 nm).

Column: A stainless steel column 4.6 mm in inside diameter and 15 cm in length, packed with octadecylsilanized silica gel for liquid chromatography (5 μm in particle diameter).

Column temperature: A constant temperature of about 40°C.

Mobile phase: Dissolve 3.85 g of ammonium acetate in 720 mL of water, and add 5 mL of acetic acid (100) and 280 mL of acetonitrile.

Flow rate: 1.0 mL per minute (the retention time of glycyrrhizic acid is about 15 minutes).

System suitability—

System performance: Dissolve 5 mg of monoammonium glycyrrhizinate for resolution check in 20 mL of dilute ethanol. When the procedure is run with 10 μL of this solution under the above operating conditions, the resolution between the peak having the relative retention time of about 0.9 to glycyrrhizic acid and the peak of glycyrrhizic acid is not less than 1.5.

System repeatability: When the test is repeated 6 times with 10 μL of the standard solution under the above operating conditions, the relative standard deviation of the peak area of glycyrrhizic acid is not more than 1.5%.

Containers and storage Containers—Tight containers.

Keishibukuryogan Extract

桂枝茯苓丸エキス

Keishibukuryogan Extract contains not less than 0.6 mg and not more than 2.4 mg (for preparation prescribed 3 g of Cinnamon Bark) or not less than 0.8 mg and not more than 3.2 mg (for preparation prescribed 4 g of Cinnamon Bark) of (*E*)-cinnamic acid, not less than 30 mg and not more than 90 mg (for preparation prescribed 3 g each of Moutan Bark and Peony Root) or not less than 40 mg and not more than 120 mg (for preparation prescribed 4 g each of Moutan Bark and Peony Root) of paeoniflorin ($C_{23}H_{28}O_{11}$: 480.46), and not less than 21 mg and not more than 63 mg (for preparation prescribed 3 g of Peach Kernel) or not less than 28 mg and not more than 84 mg (for preparation prescribed 4 g of Peach Kernel) of amygdalin, per extract prepared with the amount specified in the Method of preparation.

Method of preparation

	1)	2)
Cinnamon Bark	4 g	3 g
Poria Sclerotium	4 g	3 g
Moutan Bark	4 g	3 g
Peach Kernel	4 g	3 g
Peony Root	4 g	3 g

Prepare a dry extract or viscous extract as directed under Extracts, according to the prescription 1) using the crude drugs shown above, or prepare a dry extract by adding Light Anhydrous Silicic Acid to an extractive, prepared as directed under Extracts, according to the prescription 2), using the crude drugs shown above.

Description Keishibukuryogan Extract is a light brown to brown powder or black-brown viscous extract. It has a characteristic odor and has a taste slightly sweet first then bitter later.

Identification **(1)** Shake 1.0 g of the dry extract (or 3.0 g of the viscous extract) with 10 mL of water, add 25 mL of diethyl ether, and shake. Separate the diethyl ether layer, evaporate the solvent under low pressure (in vacuo), dissolve the residue in 2 mL of diethyl ether, and use this solution as the sample solution. Separately, dissolve 1 mg of (*E*)-

cinnamic acid for thin-layer chromatography in 1 mL of methanol, and use this solution as the standard solution. Perform the test with these solutions as directed under Thin-layer Chromatography <*2.03*>. Spot 5 μL each of the sample solution and standard solution on a plate of silica gel with fluorescent indicator for thin-layer chromatography. Develop the plate with a mixture of hexane, ethyl acetate, formic acid and water (60:40:4:1) to a distance of about 7 cm, and air-dry the plate. Examine under ultraviolet light (main wavelength: 254 nm): one of the several spots obtained from the sample solution has the same color tone and *R*f value with the blue-purple spot from the standard solution (Cinnamon Bark).

(2) Shake 1.0 g of the dry extract (or 3.0 g of the viscous extract) with 10 mL of water, add 25 mL of diethyl ether, and shake. Separate the diethyl ether layer, evaporate the solvent under low pressure (in vacuo), dissolve the residue in 2 mL of diethyl ether, and use this solution as the sample solution. Separately, dissolve 1 mg of paeonol for thin-layer chromatography in 1 mL of methanol, and use this solution as the standard solution. Perform the test with these solutions as directed under Thin-layer Chromatography <*2.03*>. Spot 10 μL each of the sample solution and standard solution on a plate of silica gel for thin-layer chromatography. Develop the plate with a mixture of hexane and diethyl ether (5:3) to a distance of about 7 cm, and air-dry the plate. Spray evenly 4-methoxybenzaldehyde-sulfuric acid TS on the plate, and heat the plate at 105°C for 5 minutes: one of the several spots obtained from the sample solution has the same color tone and *R*f value with the orange spot from the standard solution (Moutan Bark).

(3) Shake 1.0 g of the dry extract (or 3.0 g of the viscous extract) with 10 mL of methanol, filter, and use the filtrate as the sample solution. Separately, dissolve 2 mg of amygdalin for thin-layer chromatography in 1 mL of methanol, and use this solution as the standard solution. Perform the test with these solutions as directed under Thin-layer Chromatography <*2.03*>. Spot 5 μL each of the sample solution and standard solution on a plate of silica gel for thin-layer chromatography. Develop the plate with a mixture of 1-propanol, ethyl acetate and water (4:4:3) to a distance of about 7 cm, and air-dry the plate. Spray evenly 4-methoxybenzaldehyde-sulfuric acid TS on the plate, and heat the plate at 105°C for 10 minutes: one of the several spots obtained from the sample solution has the same color tone and *R*f value with the green-brown spot from the standard solution (Peach Kernel).

(4) Shake 1.0 g of the dry extract (or 3.0 g of the viscous extract) with 10 mL of water, add 10 mL of methanol, shake, centrifuge, and use the supernatant liquid as the sample solution. Separately, dissolve 1 mg of albiflorin in 1 mL of methanol, and use this solution as the standard solution. Perform the test with these solutions as directed under Thin-layer Chromatography <*2.03*>. Spot 5 μL each of the sample solution and standard solution on a plate of silica gel for thin-layer chromatography. Develop the plate with a mixture of ethyl acetate, methanol and ammonia solution (28) (6:3:2) to a distance of about 10 cm, and air-dry the plate. Spray evenly 4-methoxybenzaldehyde-sulfuric acid TS on the plate, heat the plate at 105°C for 5 minutes, allow to cool for more than 30 minutes, and examine under ultraviolet light (main wavelength: 365 nm): one of the several spots obtained from the sample solution has the same color tone and *R*f value with the orange fluorescent spot from the standard solution (Peony Root).

Purity **(1)** Heavy metals <*1.07*>—Prepare the test solution with 1.0 g of the dry extract (or an amount of the viscous extract, equivalent to 1.0 g of the dried substance) as directed under the Extracts (4), and perform the test (not more than 30 ppm).

(2) Arsenic <*1.11*>—Prepare the test solution with 0.67 g of the dry extract (or an amount of the viscous extract, equivalent to 0.67 g of the dried substance) according to Method 3, and perform the test (not more than 3 ppm).

Loss on drying <*2.41*> The dry extract: Not more than 10.0% (1 g, 105°C, 5 hours).

The viscous extract: Not more than 66.7% (1 g, 105°C, 5 hours).

Total ash <*5.01*> Not more than 10.0%, calculated on the dried basis. However, for the dry extract prepared by adding Light Anhydrous Silicic Acid, between 9.0% and 18.0%.

Assay **(1)** (*E*)-Cinnamic acid—Conduct this procedure using light-resistant vessels. Weigh accurately about 0.5 g of the dry extract (or an amount of the viscous extract, equivalent to about 0.5 g of the dried substance), add exactly 50 mL of diluted methanol (1 in 2), shake for 15 minutes, filter, and use the filtrate as the sample solution. Separately, weigh accurately about 10 mg of (*E*)-cinnamic acid for assay, and dissolve in diluted methanol (1 in 2) to make exactly 100 mL. Pipet 10 mL of this solution, add diluted methanol (1 in 2) to make exactly 100 mL, and use this solution as the standard solution. Perform the test with exactly 10 μL each of the sample solution and standard solution as directed under Liquid Chromatography <*2.01*> according to the following conditions, and determine the peak areas, A_T and A_S, of (*E*)-cinnamic acid in each solution.

$$\text{Amount (mg) of } (E)\text{-cinnamic acid} = M_S \times A_T/A_S \times 1/20$$

M_S: Amount (mg) of (*E*)-cinnamic acid for assay taken, calculated on the basis of the content obtained by qNMR

Operating conditions—

Detector: An ultraviolet absorption photometer (wavelength: 273 nm).

Column: A stainless steel column 4.6 mm in inside diameter and 15 cm in length, packed with octadecylsilanized silica gel for liquid chromatography (5 μm in particle diameter).

Column temperature: A constant temperature of about 40°C.

Mobile phase: A mixture of water, acetonitrile and phosphoric acid (750:250:1).

Flow rate: 1.0 mL per minute (the retention time of (*E*)-cinnamic acid is about 12 minutes).

System suitability—

System performance: When the procedure is run with 10 μL of the standard solution under the above operating conditions, the number of theoretical plates and the symmetry factor of the peak of (*E*)-cinnamic acid are not less than 5000 and not more than 1.5, respectively.

System repeatability: When the test is repeated 6 times with 10 μL of the standard solution under the above operating conditions, the relative standard deviation of the peak area of (*E*)-cinnamic acid is not more than 1.5%.

(2) Paeoniflorin—Weigh accurately about 0.5 g of the dry extract (or an amount of the viscous extract, equivalent to about 0.5 g of the dried substance), add exactly 50 mL of diluted methanol (1 in 2), shake for 15 minutes, filter, and use the filtrate as the sample solution. Separately, weigh accurately about 10 mg of Paeoniflorin RS (separately determine the water <*2.48*> by coulometric titration, using 10 mg), dissolve in diluted methanol (1 in 2) to make exactly 50 mL, and use this solution as the standard solution. Perform the test with exactly 10 μL each of the sample solution and standard solution as directed under Liquid Chromatography <*2.01*> according to the following conditions, and determine the peak areas, A_T and A_S, of paeoniflorin in each solution.

$$\text{Amount (mg) of paeoniflorin } (C_{23}H_{28}O_{11}) = M_S \times A_T/A_S$$

M_S: Amount (mg) of Paeoniflorin RS taken, calculated on the anhydrous basis

Operating conditions—

Detector: An ultraviolet absorption photometer (wavelength: 232 nm).

Column: A stainless steel column 4.6 mm in inside diameter and 15 cm in length, packed with octadecylsilanized silica gel for liquid chromatography (5 μm in particle diameter).

Column temperature: A constant temperature of about 20°C.

Mobile phase: A mixture of water, acetonitrile and phosphoric acid (850:150:1).

Flow rate: 1.0 mL per minute (the retention time of paeoniflorin is about 9 minutes).

System suitability—

System performance: Dissolve 1 mg each of Paeoniflorin RS and albiflorin in diluted methanol (1 in 2) to make 10 mL. When the procedure is run with 10 μL of this solution under the above operating conditions, albiflorin and paeoniflorin are eluted in this order with the resolution between these peaks being not less than 2.5.

System repeatability: When the test is repeated 6 times with 10 μL of the standard solution under the above operating conditions, the relative standard deviation of the peak area of paeoniflorin is not more than 1.5%.

(3) Amygdalin—Weigh accurately about 0.5 g of the dry extract (or an amount of the viscous extract, equivalent to about 0.5 g of the dried substance), add exactly 50 mL of diluted methanol (1 in 2), shake for 15 minutes, filter, and use the filtrate as the sample solution. Separately, weigh accurately about 10 mg of amygdalin for assay, previously dried in a desiccator (silica gel) for not less than 24 hours, dissolve in diluted methanol (1 in 2) to make exactly 50 mL, and use this solution as the standard solution. Perform the test with exactly 10 μL each of the sample solution and standard solution as directed under Liquid Chromatography <*2.01*> according to the following conditions, and determine the peak areas, A_T and A_S, of amygdalin in each solution.

$$\text{Amount (mg) of amygdalin} = M_S \times A_T/A_S$$

M_S: Amount (mg) of amygdalin for assay taken

Operating conditions—

Detector: An ultraviolet absorption photometer (wavelength: 210 nm).

Column: A stainless steel column 4.6 mm in inside diameter and 15 cm in length, packed with octadecylsilanized silica gel for liquid chromatography (5 μm in particle diameter).

Column temperature: A constant temperature of about 45°C.

Mobile phase: A mixture of 0.05 mol/L sodium dihydrogen phosphate TS and methanol (5:1).

Flow rate: 0.8 mL per minute (the retention time of amygdalin is about 12 minutes).

System suitability—

System performance: When the procedure is run with 10 μL of the standard solution under the above operating conditions, the number of theoretical plates and the symmetry factor of the peak of amygdalin are not less than 5000 and not more than 1.5, respectively.

System repeatability: When the test is repeated 6 times with 10 μL of the standard solution under the above operating conditions, the relative standard deviation of the peak area of amygdalin is not more than 1.5%.

Containers and storage Containers—Tight containers.

Koi

Koi

コウイ

Koi is a saccharized substance obtained by hydrolysis of the starch of *Zea mays* Linné (*Gramineae*), *Manihot esculenta* Crantz (*Euphorbiaceae*), *Solanum tuberosum* Linné (*Solanaceae*), *Ipomoea batatas* Poiret (*Convolvulaceae*) or *Oryza sativa* Linné (*Gramineae*), or the seed of *Oryza sativa* Linné from which the seed coat is removed.

Koi is prepared by the following processes 1 or 2, and contains mainly maltose, sometimes glucose and maltotriose also.

Process 1. Saccharize starch with hydrochloric acid, oxalic acid, amylase or wort, then concentrate to dryness, and powder.

Process 2. To starch or a paste of starch prepared by adding water and heating, add hydrochloric acid, oxalic acid, amylase or wort to saccharize, and dry or concentrate.

Koi prepared by Process 1 is termed ''Koi 1'' and by Process 2 is termed ''Koi 2''. The label states the process.

Description

Koi 1: A white crystalline powder. It is odorless and has a sweet taste.

Koi 2: Colorless or brown, clear or semi-translucent, masses or viscous liquid. It is odorless and has a sweet taste.

Identification Dissolve exactly 0.50 g of Koi in a mixture of water and methanol (1:1) to make exactly 50 mL, and use this solution as the sample solution. Separately, dissolve exactly 20.0 mg of maltose hydrate in a mixture of water and methanol (1:1) to make exactly 5 mL, and use this solution as the standard solution. Perform the test with these solutions as directed under Thin-layer Chromatography <*2.03*>. Spot 1 μL each of the sample solution and standard solution on a plate of silica gel for thin-layer chromatography in equal size of circular spot each other. Develop the plate with a mixture of 2-butanone, water and acetic acid (100) (3:1:1) to a distance of about 7 cm, and dry at 105°C for 10 minutes the plate. Spray evenly 2,3,5-triphenyl-2*H*-tetrazolium chloride-methanol TS for spraying on the plate, and heat the plate at 105°C for 5 minutes: one of the several spots obtained from the sample solution has the same color tone and *Rf* value with the orange spot obtained from the standard solution, and it is larger and more intense than the spot from the standard solution.

Purity **(1)** Clarity of solution—A solution obtained by dissolving 2.0 g of Koi in 20 mL of hot water is practically clear.

(2) Heavy metals <*1.07*>

Koi 1: Proceed with 1.0 g of Koi 1 according to Method

1, and perform the test. Prepare the control solution with 1.0 mL of Standard Lead Solution (not more than 10 ppm).

Koi 2: Proceed with 1.0 g of Koi 2 according to Method 2, and perform the test. Prepare the control solution with 1.0 mL of Standard Lead Solution (not more than 10 ppm).

(3) Arsenic *<1.11>*—Prepare the test solution with 1.0 g of Koi according to Method 3, and perform the test (not more than 2 ppm).

Loss on drying *<5.01>*

Koi 1: Not more than 3.0% (1 g, 80°C, 4 hours).

Koi 2: Not more than 15.0% (1 g, 80°C, 4 hours). In the case where the sample is in masses, crush the masses, weigh accurately the mass, and put in a desiccator. In the case in viscous liquid, put in a weighing bottle to spread about 1 mm thick, weigh accurately the mass, and put the bottle in a desiccator.

Total ash *<5.01>* Not more than 0.5%.

Containers and storage Containers—Well-closed containers.

Hydrous Lanolin

加水ラノリン

Hydrous Lanolin is Purified Lanolin to which water is added. It contains not less than 70% and not more than 75% of Purified Lanolin (as determined by the test for Residue on evaporation).

Description Hydrous Lanolin is a yellow-white, ointment-like substance, and has a slight, characteristic odor, which is not rancid.

It is soluble in diethyl ether and in cyclohexane, with the separation of water.

When melted by heating on a water bath, it separates into a clear oily layer and a clear aqueous layer.

Melting point: about 39°C.

Identification Dissolve 1 g of Hydrous Lanolin in 50 mL of cyclohexane, and remove the separated water. Superimpose carefully 1 mL of the cyclohexane solution on 2 mL of sulfuric acid: a red-brown color develops at the zone of contact, and sulfuric acid layer shows a green fluorescence.

Acid value *<1.13>* Not more than 1.0.

Iodine value 18 – 36 Heat a suitable amount of Hydrous Lanolin on a water bath to remove its almost moisture, then weigh accurately about 0.8 g of the treated Hydrous Lanolin in a glass-stoppered 500-mL flask, and add 10 mL of cyclohexane to dissolve, and add exactly 25 mL of Hanus's TS, and mix well. If a clear solution is not obtained, add more cyclohexane to make clear, and allow the mixture to stand for 1 hour between 20°C and 30°C in a light-resistant, well-closed container while occasional shaking. Add 20 mL of a solution of potassium iodide (1 in 10) and 100 mL of water, shake, and titrate *<2.50>* the liberated iodine with 0.1 mol/L sodium thiosulfate VS (indicator: 1 mL of starch TS). Perform a blank determination in the same manner.

$$\text{Iodine value} = (a - b) \times 1.269/M$$

M: amount (g) of Hydrous Lanolin taken

a: Volume (mL) of 0.1 mol/L sodium thiosulfate VS consumed in the blank determination

b: Volume (mL) of 0.1 mol/L sodium thiosulfate VS consumed in the titration

Purity **(1)** Acidity or alkalinity—To 5 g of Hydrous Lanolin add 25 mL of water, boil for 10 minutes, and cool. Add water to restore the previous mass, and separate the aqueous layer: the aqueous layer is neutral.

(2) Chloride *<1.03>*—To 2.0 g of Hydrous Lanolin add 40 mL of water, boil for 10 minutes, and cool. Add water to restore the previous mass, and filter. To 20 mL of the filtrate add 6 mL of dilute nitric acid and water to make 50 mL. Use this solution as the test solution, and perform the test. Prepare the control solution with 1.0 mL of 0.01 mol/L hydrochloric acid VS (not more than 0.036%).

(3) Ammonia—To 10 mL of the aqueous layer obtained in (1) add 1 mL of sodium hydroxide TS, and boil: the gas evolved does not turn moistened red litmus paper to blue.

(4) Water-soluble organic substances—To 5 mL of the aqueous layer obtained in (1) add 0.25 mL of 0.002 mol/L potassium permanganate VS, and allow to stand for 5 minutes: the red color of the solution does not disappear.

(5) Petrolatum—Dissolve 1.0 g of the dried residue obtained in the Residue on evaporation in 10 mL of a mixture of tetrahydrofuran and isooctane (1:1), and use this solution as the sample solution. Add dissolve 20 mg of vaseline in 10 mL of a mixture of tetrahydrofuran and isooctane (1:1), and use this solution as the standard solution. Perform the test with these solutions as directed under Thin-layer Chromatography *<2.03>*. Spot 25 μL each of the sample solution and standard solution on a plate of silica gel for thin-layer chromatography. Develop the plate with isooctane to a distance of about 10 cm, and air-dry the plate. Spray evenly diluted sulfuric acid (1 in 2) on the plate, heat the plate at 80°C for 5 minutes, cool, and examine under ultraviolet light (main wavelength: 365 nm): no fluorescent spot is observed in the same level with the spot of standard solution. For this test use a thin-layer plate previously developed with isooctane to the upper end, dried in air, and heated at 110°C for 60 minutes.

Residue on evaporation Weigh accurately about 12.5 g of Hydrous Lanolin, dissolve in 50 mL of diethyl ether, put it in a separator, transfer the separated aqueous layer to another separator, add 10 mL of diethyl ether, shake, and combine the diethyl ether layer and diethyl ether in the first separator. Shake the diethyl ether layer with 3 g of anhydrous sodium sulfate, and filter through dry filter paper. Wash the separator and the filter paper with two 20-mL portions of diethyl ether, combine the washings with the filtrate, evaporate on a water bath until the odor of diethyl ether is no longer perceptible, and dry in a desiccator (in vacuum, silica gel) for 24 hours: the content is not less than 70% and not more than 75%.

Containers and storage Containers—Well-closed containers.

Storage—Not exceeding 30°C.

Purified Lanolin

Adeps Lanae Purificatus

精製ラノリン

Purified Lanolin is the purified product of the fat-like substance obtained from the wool of *Ovis aries* Linné (*Bovidae*).

Description Purified Lanolin is a light yellow to yellowish brown, viscous, ointment-like substance, and has a faint, characteristic but not rancid odor.

It is very soluble in diethyl ether and in cyclohexane, freely soluble in tetrahydrofuran and in toluene, and very slightly soluble in ethanol (95). It is practically insoluble in water, but miscible without separation with about twice its mass of water, retaining ointment-like viscosity.

Melting point: 37 - 43°C

Identification Superimpose carefully 1 mL of a solution of Purified Lanolin in cyclohexane (1 in 50) on 2 mL of sulfuric acid: a red-brown color develops at the zone of contact, and the sulfuric acid layer shows a green fluorescence.

Acid value <*1.13*> Not more than 1.0.

Iodine value 18 - 36 Weigh accurately about 0.8 g of Purified Lanolin in a glass-stoppered 500-mL flask, add 20 mL of cyclohexane to dissolve, and add exactly 25 mL of Hanus' TS, and mix well. If a clear solution is not obtained, add more cyclohexane to make clear, and allow the mixture to stand for 1 hour between 20°C and 30°C in light-resistant, well-closed containers, with occasional shaking. Add 20 mL of a solution of potassium iodide (1 in 10) and 100 mL of water, shake, and titrate the liberated iodine with 0.1 mol/L sodium thiosulfate VS (indicator: 1 mL of starch TS). Perform a blank determination in the same manner.

$$\text{Iodine value} = (a - b) \times 1.269/M$$

M: amount (g) of Purified Lanolin taken
a: Volume (mL) of 0.1 mol/L sodium thiosulfate VS used in the blank determination
b: Volume (mL) of 0.1 mol/L sodium thiosulfate VS used in the titration of the sample

Purity **(1)** Acid or alkali—To 5 g of Purified Lanolin add 25 mL of water, boil for 10 minutes, and cool. Add water to restore the previous mass, and separate the aqueous layer: the aqueous layer is neutral.

(2) Chloride <*1.03*>—To 2.0 g of Purified Lanolin add 40 mL of water, boil for 10 minutes, and cool. Add water to restore the previous mass, and filter. To 20 mL of the filtrate add 6 mL of dilute nitric acid and water to make 50 mL. Use this solution as the test solution, and perform the test. Prepare the control solution with 1.0 mL of 0.01 mol/L hydrochloric acid VS (not more than 0.036%).

(3) Ammonia—To 10 mL of the aqueous layer obtained in (1) add 1 mL of sodium hydroxide TS, and boil: the gas evolved does not turn moistened red litmus paper to blue.

(4) Water-soluble organic substances—To 5 mL of the aqueous layer obtained in (1) add 0.25 mL of 0.002 mol/L potassium permanganate VS, and allow to stand for 5 minutes: the red color of the solution does not disappear.

(5) Petrolatum—Dissolve 1.0 g of Purified Lanolin in 10 mL of a mixture of tetrahydrofuran and isooctane (1:1), and use this solution as the sample solution. And dissolve 20 mg of vaseline in 10 mL of a mixture of tetrahydrofuran and isooctane (1:1), and use this solution as the standard solution. Perform the test with the sample solution as directed under Thin-layer Chromatography <*2.03*>. Spot 25 μL each of the sample solution and standard solution on a plate of silica gel for thin-layer chromatography. Develop the plate with isooctane to a distance of about 10 cm, and air-dry the plate. Spray evenly diluted sulfuric acid (1 in 2) on the plate, heat the plate at 80°C for 5 minutes, cool, and examine under ultraviolet light (main wavelength: 365 nm): no fluorescent spot is observable same level of the spot of standard solution. Use a thin-layer plate previously developed with isooctane to the upper end, dried in air, and heated at 110°C for 60 minutes.

Loss on drying <*2.41*> Not more than 0.5% (1 g, 105°C, 2 hours).

Total ash <*5.01*> Not more than 0.1%.

Containers and storage Containers—Well-closed containers.

Storage—Not exceeding 30°C.

Lard

Adeps Suillus

豚脂

Lard is the fat obtained from *Sus scrofa* Linné var. *domesticus* Gray (*Suidae*).

Description Lard occurs as a white, soft, unctuous mass, and has a faint, characteristic odor and a bland taste.

It is freely soluble in diethyl ether and in petroleum ether, very slightly soluble in ethanol (95), and practically insoluble in water.

Melting point: 36 - 42°C

Congealing point of the fatty acids: 36 - 42°C

Acid value <*1.13*> Not more than 2.0.

Saponification value <*1.13*> 195 - 203

Iodine value <*1.13*> 46 - 70

Purity **(1)** Moisture and coloration—Melt 5 g of Lard by heating on a water bath: it forms a clear liquid, from which no water separates. Observe the liquid in a layer 10 mm thick: the liquid is colorless to slightly yellow.

(2) Alkalinity—To 2.0 g of Lard add 10 mL of water, melt by warming on a water bath, and shake vigorously. After cooling, add 1 drop of phenolphthalein TS to the separated aqueous layer: the layer is colorless.

(3) Chloride <*1.03*>—To 1.5 g of Lard add 30 mL of ethanol (95), heat under a reflux condenser for 10 minutes, and filter after cooling. To 20 mL of the filtrate add 5 drops of a solution of silver nitrate in ethanol (95) (1 in 50): the opalescence of the mixture does not exceed that of the following control solution.

Control solution: To 1.0 mL of 0.01 mol/L hydrochloric acid VS add ethanol (95) to make 20 mL, and add 5 drops of a solution of silver nitrate in ethanol (95) (1 in 50).

(4) Beef tallow—Dissolve 5 g of Lard in 20 mL of diethyl ether, stopper lightly with absorbent cotton, and allow to stand at 20°C for 18 hours. Collect the separated crystals, moisten them with ethanol (95), and examine under a microscope of 200 magnifications: the crystals are in the form of rhomboidal plates grouped irregularly, and do not contain prisms or needles grouped in fan-shaped clusters.

Containers and storage Containers—Well-closed containers.

Storage—Not exceeding 30°C.

Leonurus Herb

Leonuri Herba

ヤクモソウ

Leonurus Herb is the aerial part of *Leonurus japonicus* Houttuyn or *Leonurus sibiricus* Linné (*Labiatae*), collected during the flowering season.

Description Stem, leaves, and flowers usually cross sectioned, stems square, 0.2 – 3 cm in diameter, yellow-green to green-brown in color, covered densely with white short hairs; the pith white, a great parts of central of cut surface. Light in texture. Leaves opposite, petiolated, 3-dissected to 3-incised, each lobe splits pinnately, and end lobes reveals linear-lanceolate, acute or acuminate, the upper surface light green, the lower surface bristle with white short hairs, grayish green. Flower, verticillate; sepal, tubular, and the upper end acerate with five lobes; light green to light green-brown in color, corolla labiate, light red-purple to light brown.

Odor, slightly; taste, slightly bitter, astringent.

Under a microscope ⟨*5.01*⟩, a transverse section of stem reveals four ridges, a part of the ridge of *Leonurus sibiricus* Linné protruding knobby. Epidermis, observed non-glandular hairs from 1 to 3 cells, glandular hairs with head of 1 to 4 celled or glandular scale with 8 cells. Each ridge parts, beneath epidermis, collenchyma developed, development of xylem fibers remarkably. Cortex composed of several cellular layers parenchymatous cells. Collateral vascular bundle arranged in a circle. Phloem fibers observed at the outer portion of phloem. Parenchymatous cells of cortex and pith observe needle crystals or plate-like crystals of calcium oxalate.

Identification To 1 g of pulverized Leonurus Herb add 10 mL of methanol, shake for 10 minutes, centrifuge, and use the supernatant liquid as the sample solution. Perform the test with the sample solution as directed under Thin-layer Chromatography ⟨*2.03*⟩. Spot 10 μL of the sample solution on a plate of silica gel for thin-layer chromatography, develop the plate with a mixture of water and methanol (1:1) to a distance of about 7 cm, and air-dry the plate. Spray evenly Dragendorff's TS followed by immediate spraying of sodium nitrite TS on the plate: a grayish brown spot appears at an *R*f value of about 0.5, which color fades soon and then disappears after air-drying the plate.

Loss on drying ⟨*5.01*⟩ Not more than 12.0%.

Total ash ⟨*5.01*⟩ Not more than 10.0%.

Acid-insoluble ash ⟨*5.01*⟩ Not more than 2.0%.

Extract content ⟨*5.01*⟩ Dilute ethanol-soluble extract: not less than 12.0%.

Containers and storage Containers—Well-closed containers.

Lilium Bulb

Lilii Bulbus

ビャクゴウ

Lilium Bulb is the scaly leaves of *Lilium lancifolium* Thunberg, *Lilium brownii* F.E.Brown var. *colchesteri* Wilson, *Lilium brownii* F.E.Brown or *Lilium pumilum* De Candolle (*Liliaceae*), usually with the application of steaming.

Description Lilium Bulb reveals oblong with narrowed apex, lanceolate, or narrowly triangular boat-shaped, translucent, 1.3 – 6 cm in length, 0.5 – 2.0 cm in diameter, externally milky white to light yellow-brown occasionally purplish in color, nearly smooth; central portion somewhat thickened, circumferential portion thin, slightly waved, occasionally rolled inside; usually several lines of vascular bundles longitudinally in parallel are seen through parenchyma; hard in texture, easy to break; fractured surface horny and flat.

Almost odorless; taste, slightly acid and bitter.

Under a microscope ⟨*5.01*⟩, the surface reveals epidermal cells rectangular to almost square, stomata nearly circular, the cells adjacent to stomata mostly 4 in number. Under a microscope ⟨*5.01*⟩, a transverse section reveals the outermost layer composed of epidermal cells covered with smooth cuticle; epidermis circular to quadrangular parenchymatous cells distributed evenly, palisade tissue not observed; in parenchyma of mesophyll collateral vascular bundles extended from adaxial side to abaxial side of scaly leaves are arranged almost in a transverse line; starch grains contained in parenchymatous cells, usually gelatinized.

Identification To 3 g of pulverized Lilium Bulb add 10 mL of 1-butanol, shake, add 10 mL of water, shake for 30 minutes, and centrifuge. Evaporate the solvent under low pressure (in vacuo), add 1 mL of methanol to the residue, shake gently, and use the supernatant liquid so obtained as the sample solution. Perform the test with the sample solution as directed under Thin-layer Chromatography ⟨*2.03*⟩. Spot 10 μL of the sample solution on a plate of silica gel with fluorescent indicator for thin-layer chromatography. Develop the plate with a mixture of ethyl acetate, methanol and water (12:2:1) to a distance of about 7 cm, and air-dry the plate. Examine under ultraviolet light (main wavelength: 254 nm): two spots appear at an *R*f value of about 0.3. When examine these spots under ultraviolet light (main wavelength: 365 nm) after spraying with sodium carbonate TS, they appear as blue-purple fluorescent spots.

Loss on drying ⟨*5.01*⟩ Not more than 16.0%.

Total ash ⟨*5.01*⟩ Not more than 4.5%.

Extract content ⟨*5.01*⟩ Dilute ethanol-soluble extract: not less than 8.0%.

Containers and storage Containers—Well-closed containers.

Lindera Root

Linderae Radix

ウヤク

Lindera Root is the root of *Lindera strychnifolia* Fernandez-Villar (*Lauraceae*).

Description Fusiform or rosary-like root, 10 - 15 cm in length, 10 - 25 mm in diameter; externally yellow-brown to brown, with a few scars of rootlets; a transversely cut surface reveals cortex brown, xylem light yellow-brown, concentric circles and radially arranged lines brown; dense and hard in texture.

Odor, camphor-like; taste, bitter.

Under a microscope <*5.01*>, a transverse section of the root with periderm reveals a cork layer several cells thick, partially consisting of cork stone cells; cortex parenchyma sometimes contains oil cells and fibers; in xylem, vessels-xylem fibers and rays are arranged alternately; parenchyatous cells of cortex and xylem contain sandy and columnar crystals of calcium oxalate, simple starch grains 1 - 15 μm in diameter, and 2- to 4- compound starch grains.

Identification To 3 g of pulverized Lindera Root add 40 mL of hexane, and heat under a reflux condenser for 30 minutes. After cooling, filter, to the residue add 10 mL of ammonia TS and 30 mL of a mixture of ethyl acetate and diethyl ether (1:1), shake vigorously for 20 minutes, and centrifuge. Separate the upper layer, add 10 g of anhydrous sodium sulfate, shake, and filter. Evaporate the solvent of the filtrate, dissolve the residue with 0.5 mL of ethanol (99.5), and use this solution as the sample solution. Perform the test with the sample solution as directed under Thin-layer Chromatography <*2.03*>. Spot 20 μL of the sample solution on a plate of silica gel for thin-layer chromatography, develop the plate with a mixture of ethyl acetate, methanol and ammonia water (28) (10:2:1) to a distance of about 10 cm, and air-dry the plate. Spray evenly Dragendorff's TS for spraying on the plate: a yellow-brown spot appears at an *R*f value of about 0.4.

Purity **(1)** Heavy metals <*1.07*>—Proceed with 3.0 g of pulverized Lindera Root according to Method 3, and perform the test. Prepare the control solution with 3.0 mL of Standard Lead Solution (not more than 10 ppm).

(2) Arsenic <*1.11*>—Prepare the test solution with 0.40 g of pulverized Lindera Root according to Method 4, and perform the test (not more than 5 ppm).

Loss on drying <*5.01*> Not more than 14.0% (6 hours).

Total ash <*5.01*> Not more than 2.5%.

Extract content <*5.01*> Dilute ethanol-soluble extract: not less than 6.0%.

Containers and storage Containers—Well-closed containers.

Lithospermum Root

Lithospermi Radix

シコン

Lithospermum Root is the root of *Lithospermum erythrorhizon* Siebold et Zuccarini (*Boraginaceae*).

Description Rather slender conical root, often branched, 6 - 10 cm in length, 0.5 - 1.5 cm in diameter; externally dark purple, coarse in texture, thin and easily peeled; mostly with twisted and deep longitudinal furrows, which sometimes reach to xylem; sometimes remains of stem at the crown; easily broken; fractured surface granular and with many clefts. Under a magnifying glass, a transverse section reveals a dark purple color at the outer portion of cortex, and light brown inner portion making irregular wave; xylem yellowish in color; the center of the crown is often cracked, and the surrounding part red-purple.

Odor, slight; taste, slightly sweet.

Identification **(1)** Heat 0.5 g of pulverized Lithospermum Root in a test tube: red vapor evolves, which condenses on the wall of the upper part of the tube into red-brown oil drops.

(2) Shake 0.5 g of pieces or powder of Lithospermum Root with 1 mL of ethanol (95), and to the red solution thereby obtained add 1 drop of sodium hydroxide TS: the red color changes to blue-purple. To this solution add 1 to 2 drops of dilute hydrochloric acid: the color turns red again.

(3) To 0.5 g of pulverized Lithospermum Root add 5 mL of ethanol (95), shake for 30 minutes, filter, and evaporate the solvent of the filtrate at a temperature not higher than 40°C under low pressure (in vacuo). Add 1 mL of ethanol (95) to the residue, and use this solution as the sample solution. Perform the test with the sample solution as directed under Thin-layer Chromatography <*2.03*>. Spot 5 μL of the sample solution on a plate of silica gel for thin-layer chromatography. Develop the plate with a mixture of ethyl acetate and ethanol (95) (3:1) to a distance of about 7 cm, and air-dry the plate: a red-purple spot appears at an *R*f value of about 0.75.

Purity **(1)** Heavy metals <*1.07*>—Proceed with 2.0 g of pulverized Lithospermum Root according to Method 3, and perform the test. Prepare the control solution with 3.0 mL of Standard Lead Solution (not more than 15 ppm).

(2) Arsenic <*1.11*>—Prepare the test solution with 0.40 g of pulverized Lithospermum Root according to Method 4, and perform the test (not more than 5 ppm).

Total ash <*5.01*> Not more than 11.0%.

Acid-insoluble ash <*5.01*> Not more than 3.5%.

Containers and storage Containers—Well-closed containers.

Longan Aril

Longan Arillus

リュウガンニク

Longan Aril is the aril of *Euphoria longana* Lamarck (*Sapindaceae*).

Description Depressed ellipsoidal aril, 1 – 2 cm in length, about 1 cm in width; yellow-red-brown to black-brown; soft in texture and mucous; when immersed in water, bell-shaped, with the tip split in several parts.

Odor, characteristic; taste, sweet.

Under a microscope <*5.01*>, a transverse section reveals the outmost layer composed of an epidermis, beneath this observed parenchyma consisting of depressed parenchyma cells; the innermost layer composed of slightly thick-walled epidermis; parenchyma contains red-brown to brown contents as well as solitary crystals, amorphous crystals and sand crystals of calcium oxalate.

Identification To 1 g of coarse cuttings of Longan Aril, add 10 mL of water, shake thoroughly, and filter. To 3 mL of the filtrate, add 3 mL of Fehling solution, and heat on a water bath: a red precipitate is produced.

Total ash <*5.01*> Not more than 5.0%.

Extract content <*5.01*> Dilute ethanol-soluble extract: Not less than 75.0%.

Containers and storage Containers—Well-closed containers.

Longgu

Fossilia Ossis Mastodi

リュウコツ

Longgu is the ossified bone of large mammal, and is mainly composed of calcium carbonate.

For Longgu used only for extracts, infusions and decoctions, the label states the restricted utilization forms.

Description Irregular masses or fragments, occasionally cylindrical masses; externally light grayish white, sometimes with grayish black or yellow-brown spots here and there; the outer part consists of a layer 2 – 10 mm in thickness, and is minute in texture, surrounding the light brown, porous portion; heavy and hard, but somewhat fragile in texture; when crushed, it changes into pieces and powder.

Odorless, tasteless, and strongly adhesive to the tongue on licking.

Identification **(1)** Dissolve 0.5 g of pulverized Longgu in 10 mL of dilute hydrochloric acid: it evolves a gas, and forms a slightly brownish and turbid solution. Pass the gas evolved through calcium hydroxide TS: a white precipitate is produced.

(2) The turbid solution obtained in (1) has a characteristic odor. Filter this solution and neutralize filtrate with ammonia TS: this solution responds to Qualitative Tests <*1.09*> (1), (2) and (3) for calcium salt.

(3) Dissolve 0.1 g of pulverized Longgu in 5 mL of nitric acid by warming, and add hexaammonium heptamolybdate TS: a yellow precipitate is produced.

Purity **(1)** Heavy metals <*1.07*>—To 2.0 g of pulverized Longgu, add 5 mL of water, shake, add gradually 6 mL of hydrochloric acid, evaporate on a water bath to dryness, dissolve the residue in 50 mL of water, and filter. To 25 mL of the filtrate, add 2 mL of dilute acetic acid, 1 drop of ammonia TS and water to make 50 mL. Perform the test with this solution as the test solution. Prepare the control solution as follows: evaporate 3 mL of hydrochloric acid on a water bath to dryness, add 2 mL of dilute acetic acid, 2.0 mL of Standard Lead Solution and water to make 50 mL, and use this solution as the control solution (not more than 20 ppm).

When being shown as extracts, infusions and decoctions on the label, the procedure and the limit are as follows.

To 20.0 g of pulverized Longgu, add 80 mL of water, shake occasionally in a water bath, heat to make about 40 mL, allow to cool, and filter. Proceed with this solution according to Method 3, and perform the test. To the control solution, add 1.0 mL of Standard Lead Solution (not more than 0.5 ppm).

(2) Arsenic <*1.11*>—Prepare the test solution with 0.20 g of pulverized Longgu according to Method 2, and perform the test (not more than 10 ppm).

When being shown the restricted utilization forms as ''extracts, infusions and decoctions only'', the procedure and the limit are as follows.

Put 4.0 g of pulverized Longgu in a centrifuge tube, add 30 mL of water, and heat in a water bath with occasional shaking to make about 15 mL. After cooling, centrifuge, and perform the test using the supernatant liquid as the test solution (not more than 0.5 ppm).

Containers and storage Containers—Well-closed containers.

Powdered Longgu

Fossilia Ossis Mastodi Pulveratum

リュウコツ末

Powdered Longgu is the powder of Longgu.

Description Powdered Longgu occurs as a light grayish white to light grayish brown. It is odorless and tasteless.

Identification **(1)** Dissolve 0.5 g of Powdered Longgu in 10 mL of dilute hydrochloric acid: it evolves a gas, and forms a slightly brownish and turbid solution. Pass the gas evolved through calcium hydroxide TS: a white precipitate is produced.

(2) The turbid solution obtained in (1) has a characteristic odor. Filter this solution, and neutralize filtrate with ammonia TS: the solution responds to Qualitative test <*1.09*> (1), (2) and (3) for calcium salt.

(3) Dissolve 0.1 g of Powdered Longgu in 5 mL of nitric acid by warming, and add hexaammonium heptamolybdate TS: a yellow precipitate is produced.

Purity **(1)** Heavy metals <*1.07*>—To 2.0 g of Powdered Longgu add 5 mL of water, shake to mix, add gradually 6 mL of hydrochloric acid, and evaporate on a water bath to dryness. Dissolve the residue in 50 mL of water, and filter. To 25 mL of the filtrate add 2 mL of dilute acetic acid, 1 drop of ammonia TS and water to make 50 mL. Perform the test using this solution as the test solution. Prepare the control solution as follows: evaporate 3 mL of hydrochloric acid on a water bath to dryness, add 2 mL of dilute acetic acid and 2.0 mL of Standard Lead Solution, and add water to make 50 mL (not more than 20 ppm).

(2) Arsenic <*1.11*>—Prepare the test solution with 0.20 g of Powdered Longgu according to Method 2, and perform the test (not more than 10 ppm).

Containers and storage Containers—Well-closed containers.

Lonicera Leaf and Stem

Lonicerae Folium Cum Caulis

ニンドウ

Lonicera Leaf and Stem is the leaves and stems of *Lonicera japonica* Thunberg (*Caprifoliaceae*).

Description Leaves and opposite leaves on short stem; leaf, ovate and entire, with short petiole, 3 - 7 cm in length, 1 - 3 cm in width; upper surface green-brown, lower surface light grayish green; under a magnifying glass, both surfaces pubescent. Stem, 1 - 4 mm in diameter; externally grayish yellow-brown to purplish brown, a transversely cut surface of stem, round and hollow.

Almost odorless; taste, slightly astringent, followed by a litter bitterness.

Under a microscope <*5.01*>, a transverse section of leaf reveals the outermost layer of upper and lower surfaces to be composed of a single-layered epidermis, uni-cellular non-glandular hairs and multi-cellular glandular hairs on epidermis; in midvein, several-cellular-layered collenchyma present beneath the epidermis and vascular bundles in the center; in mesophyll, palisade layer adjacent to upper epidermis, spongy tissue adjacent to lower epidermis; glandular hairs contain brown secretion, parenchymatous cells contain aggregate crystals of calcium oxalate, and occasionally starch grains.

Identification To 1 g of pulverized Lonicera Leaf and Stem add 5 mL of methanol, shake for 5 minutes, centrifuge, and use the supernatant liquid as the sample solution. Separately, dissolve 1 mg of chlorogenic acid for thin-layer chromatography in 2 mL of methanol, and use this solution as the standard solution (1). Separately, dissolve 1 mg of loganin for thin-layer chromatography in 2 mL of methanol, and use this solution as the standard solution (2). Perform the test with these solutions as directed under Thin-layer Chromatography <*2.03*>. Spot 10 μL each of the sample solution and standard solutions (1) and (2) on a plate of silica gel for thin-layer chromatography. Develop the plate with a mixture of ethyl acetate, water and formic acid (6:1:1) to a distance of about 7 cm, and air-dry the plate. Examine under ultraviolet light (main wavelength: 365 nm): one of the several spots obtained from the sample solution has the same color tone and *R*f value with the blue-white fluorescent spot from the standard solution (1). Spray evenly 4-methoxybenzaldehyde-sulfuric acid TS on the plate, and heat the plate at 105°C for 5 minutes: one of the several spots obtained from the sample solution has the same color tone and *R*f value with the spot from the standard solution (2).

Purity Stem—Lonicera Leaf and Stem does not contains the stems larger than 5 mm in diameter.

Loss on drying <*5.01*> Not more than 12.0% (6 hours).

Total ash <*5.01*> Not more than 9.0%.

Acid-insoluble ash <*5.01*> Not more than 1.0%.

Extract content <*5.01*> Dilute ethanol-soluble extract: not less than 12.0%.

Containers and storage Containers—Well-closed containers.

Loquat Leaf

Eriobotryae Folium

ビワヨウ

Loquat Leaf is the leaf of *Eriobotrya japonica* Lindley (*Rosaceae*).

Description Loquat Leaf is an oblong to wide lanceolate leaf, 12 - 30 cm in length, 4 - 9 cm in width; pointed at the apex and wedge-shaped at the base; roughly serrate leaf with short petiole; occasionally being cut into strips 5 - 10 mm in shorter diameter and several cm in longer diameter; upper surface green to green-brown in color, lower surface light green-brown with light brown woolly hairs; vein, light yellow-brown in color, raised out on the lower surface of the leaf.

Odor, slight; practically tasteless.

Under a microscope <*5.01*>, a transverse section of Loquat Leaf reveals thick cuticle on both surfaces; palisade tissue, mostly 4 to 5 cellular layers with several large cells without chloroplast; at main vein, ring of collateral bundle partly cut by intruding fundamental tissue at xylem side, and group of fiber attaching to phloem; solitary and clustered crystals of calcium oxalate in mesophyll; woolly hair, unicellular and curved, about 25 μm in thickness, and up to 1.5 mm in length.

Identification To 0.3 g of pulverized Loquat Leaf add 10 mL of methanol, warm on a water bath for 5 minutes with occasional shaking, cool, filter, and use the filtrate as the sample solution. Perform the test with the sample solution as directed under Thin-layer Chromatography <*2.03*>. Spot 5 μL of the sample solution on a plate of silica gel for thin-layer chromatography. Develop the plate with a mixture of water and acetonitrile (3:2) to a distance of about 7 cm, and air-dry the plate. Spray evenly dilute sulfuric acid on the plate, and heat the plate at 105°C for 10 minutes: a red-purple principal spot appears at an *R*f value of about 0.5.

Purity Total BHC's and total DDT's <*5.01*>—Not more than 0.2 ppm, respectively.

Loss on drying <*5.01*> Not more than 15.0% (6 hours).

Total ash <*5.01*> Not more than 10.0%.

Extract content <*5.01*> Dilute ethanol-soluble extract: not less than 16.0%.

Containers and storage Containers—Well-closed containers.

Lycium Bark

Lycii Cortex

ジコッピ

Lycium Bark is the root bark of *Lycium chinense* Miller or *Lycium barbarum* Linné (*Solanaceae*).

Description Tubular to semitubular bark, 1 – 6 mm in thickness; externally light brown to light yellow-brown, periderm peeled easily as scale; internally grayish brown, longitudinally striate; brittle in texture; fractured surface, grayish white, not fibrous.

Odor, weak and characteristic; taste, slightly sweet at first.

Under a microscope <*5.01*>, a transverse section reveals periderm composed of a cork layer of several cellular layers of thin-walled cork cells; in cortex parenchyma cells containing sandy crystals of calcium oxalate sparsely distributed, occasionally a few fibers observed; parenchyma cells contain starch grains, 1 – 10 μm in diameter; stone cells very rare.

Identification To 1.0 g of pulverized Lycium Bark add 10 mL of methanol, shake for 15 minutes, filter, and use the filtrate as the sample solution. Perform the test with the sample solution as directed under Thin-layer Chromatography <*2.03*>. Spot 10 μL of the sample solution on a plate of silica gel for thin-layer chromatography. Develop the plate with a mixture of 1-butanol, ammonium acetate solution (1 in 20) and acetic acid (100) (2:1:1) to a distance of about 7 cm, and air-dry the plate. Spray evenly Dragendorff's TS for spraying on the plate, heat the plate at 105°C for 2 minutes, then spray evenly sodium nitrite TS, and allow to stand for 5 minutes: a dark brown principal spot appears at an *R*f value of about 0.4.

Purity **(1)** Heavy metals <*1.07*>—Proceed with 2.0 g of pulverized Lycium Bark according to Method 3, and perform the test. Prepare the control solution with 3.0 mL of Standard Lead Solution (not more than 15 ppm).

(2) Arsenic <*1.11*>—Prepare the test solution with 0.40 g of pulverized Lycium Bark according to Method 4, and perform the test (not more than 5 ppm).

Loss on drying <*5.01*> Not more than 11.5% (6 hours).

Total ash <*5.01*> Not more than 20.0%.

Acid-insoluble ash <*5.01*> Not more than 3.0%.

Extract content <*5.01*> Dilute ethanol-soluble extract: not less than 10.0%.

Containers and storage Containers—Well-closed containers.

Lycium Fruit

Lycii Fructus

クコシ

Lycium Fruit is the fruit of *Lycium chinense* Miller or *Lycium barbarum* Linné (*Solanaceae*).

Description Fusiform fruit with acute apex, 6 – 20 mm in length, 3 – 8 mm in diameter, pericarp red to dark red, externally roughly wrinkled; under a magnifying glass, a transverse section of fruit reveals two locules containing numerous seeds; seed light brown to light yellow-brown, about 2 mm in a diameter, compressed reniform.

Odor, characteristic; taste, sweet, occasionally slightly bitter.

Identification To 1.0 g of pulverized Lycium Fruit add 5 mL of ethyl acetate, shake for 15 minutes, filter, and use the filtrate as the sample solution. Perform the test with the sample solution as directed under Thin-layer Chromatography <*2.03*>. Spot 20 μL of the sample solution on a plate of silica gel for thin-layer chromatography, develop the plate with a mixture of hexane and ethyl acetate (10:1) to a distance of about 7 cm, and air-dry the plate: a yellow principal spot appears at an *R*f value of about 0.6.

Purity Foreign matter <*5.01*>—It contains not more than 2.0% of foreign matter such as peduncle or others.

Total ash <*5.01*> Not more than 8.0%.

Acid-insoluble ash <*5.01*> Not more than 1.0%.

Extract content <*5.01*> Dilute ethanol-soluble extract: not less than 35.0%.

Containers and storage Containers—Well-closed containers.

Magnolia Bark

Magnoliae Cortex

コウボク

Magnolia Bark is the bark of the trunk of *Magnolia obovata* Thunberg (*Magnolia hypoleuca* Siebold et Zuccarini), *Magnolia officinalis* Rehder et Wilson or *Magnolia officinalis* Rehder et Wilson var. *biloba* Rehder et Wilson (*Magnoliaceae*).

It contains not less than 0.8% of magnolol.

Description Plate-like or semi-tubular bark, 2 – 7 mm in thickness; externally grayish white to grayish brown, and rough, sometimes cork layer removed, and externally red-brown; internally light brown to dark purple-brown; cut surface extremely fibrous, and light red-brown to purple-brown.

Odor, slight; taste, bitter.

Under a microscope <*5.01*>, a transverse section reveals a thick cork layer or several thin cork layers, and internally adjoining the circular tissue of stone cells of approximately equal in diameter; primary cortex thin; fiber groups scattered in the pericycle; groups of phloem fibers lined alternately with the other tissue of phloem between medullary rays in the secondary cortex, and then these tissues show a latticework; oil cells scattered in the primary and secondary cortex, but sometimes observed in the narrow medullary rays.

Identification To 1.0 g of pulverized Magnolia Bark add 10 mL of methanol, stir for 10 minutes, centrifuge, and use the supernatant liquid as the sample solution. Perform the test with the sample solution as directed under Thin-layer Chromatography <*2.03*>. Spot 20 μL of the sample solution on a plate of silica gel for thin-layer chromatography. Develop the plate with a mixture of 1-butanol, water and acetic acid (100) (4:2:1) to a distance of about 7 cm, and air-dry the plate. Spray evenly Dragendorff's TS on the plate: a yellow spot appears at an *Rf* value of about 0.3.

Total ash <*5.01*> Not more than 6.0%.

Extract content <*5.01*> Dilute ethanol-soluble extract: not less than 11.0%.

Assay Weigh accurately about 0.5 g of pulverized Magnolia Bark, add 40 mL of diluted methanol (7 in 10), heat under a reflux condenser for 20 minutes, cool, and filter. Repeat the above procedure with the residue, using 40 mL of diluted methanol (7 in 10). Combine the whole filtrates, add diluted methanol (7 in 10) to make exactly 100 mL, and use this solution as the sample solution. Separately, weigh accurately about 10 mg of magnolol for assay, dissolve in diluted methanol (7 in 10) to make exactly 100 mL, and use this solution as the standard solution. Perform the test with exactly 10 μL each of the sample solution and standard solution as directed under Liquid Chromatography <*2.01*> according to the following conditions, and determine the peak areas, A_T and A_S, of magnolol in each solution.

$$\text{Amount (mg) of magnolol} = M_S \times A_T/A_S$$

M_S: Amount (mg) of magnolol for assay taken, calculated on the basis of the content obtained by qNMR

Operating conditions—

Detector: An ultraviolet absorption photometer (wavelength: 289 nm).

Column: A stainless steel column 4 to 6 mm in inside diameter and 15 to 25 cm in length, packed with octadecylsilanized silica gel (5 to 10 μm in particle diameter).

Column temperature: A constant temperature of about 20°C.

Mobile phase: A mixture of water, acetonitrile and acetic acid (100) (50:50:1).

Flow rate: Adjust so that the retention time of magnolol is about 14 minutes.

System suitability—

System performance: Dissolve 1 mg each of magnolol for assay and honokiol in diluted methanol (7 in 10) to make 10 mL. When the procedure is run with 10 μL of this solution under the above operating conditions, honokiol and magnolol are eluted in this order with the resolution between these peaks being not less than 5.

System repeatability: When the test is repeated 6 times with 10 μL of the standard solution under the above operating conditions, the relative standard deviation of the peak area of magnolol is not more than 1.5%.

Containers and storage Containers—Well-closed containers.

Powdered Magnolia Bark

Magnoliae Cortex Pulveratus

コウボク末

Powdered Magnolia Bark is the powder of Magnolia Bark.

It contains not less than 0.8% of magnolol.

Description Powdered Magnolia Bark occurs as a yellow-brown powder, and has a slight odor and a bitter taste.

Under a microscope <*5.01*>, Powdered Magnolia Bark reveals starch grains and parenchyma cells containing them; stone cells of various sizes or its groups; fibers 12 to 25 μm in diameter; yellow-red-brown cork tissue; oil cells containing a yellow-brown to red-brown substance. Simple starch grains about 10 μm in diameter and 2- to 4-compound starch grains.

Identification To 1.0 g of Powdered Magnolia Bark add 10 mL of methanol, shake for 10 minutes, centrifuge, and use the supernatant liquid as the sample solution. Perform the test with the sample solution as directed under Thin-layer Chromatography <*2.03*>. Spot 20 μL of the sample solution on a plate of silica gel for thin-layer chromatography. Develop the plate with a mixture of 1-butanol, water and acetic acid (100) (4:2:1) to a distance of about 7 cm, and air-dry the plate. Spray evenly Dragendorff's TS on the plate: a yellow spot appears at an *Rf* value of about 0.3.

Total ash <*5.01*> Not more than 6.0%.

Extract content <*5.01*> Dilute ethanol-soluble extract: not less than 11.0%.

Assay Weigh accurately about 0.5 g of Powdered Magnolia Bark, add 40 mL of diluted methanol (7 in 10), heat under a reflux condenser for 20 minutes, cool, and filter. Repeat the above procedure with the residue, using 40 mL of diluted methanol (7 in 10). Combine the whole filtrates, add diluted methanol (7 in 10) to make exactly 100 mL, and use this solution as the sample solution. Separately, weigh accurately about 10 mg of magnolol for assay, dissolve in diluted methanol (7 in 10) to make exactly 100 mL, and use this solution as the standard solution. Perform the test with exactly 10 μL each of the sample solution and standard solution as directed under Liquid Chromatography <*2.01*> according to the following conditions, and determine the peak areas, A_T and A_S, of magnolol in each solution.

$$\text{Amount (mg) of magnolol} = M_S \times A_T/A_S$$

M_S: Amount (mg) of magnolol for assay taken, calculated on the basis of the content obtained by qNMR

Operating conditions—

Detector: An ultraviolet absorption photometer (wavelength: 289 nm).

Column: A stainless steel column 4 to 6 mm in inside diameter and 15 to 25 cm in length, packed with octadecylsilanized silica gel (5 to 10 μm in particle diameter).

Column temperature: A constant temperature of about 20°C.

Mobile phase: A mixture of water, acetonitrile and acetic acid (100) (50:50:1).

Flow rate: Adjust so that the retention time of magnolol is about 14 minutes.

System suitability—

System performance: Dissolve 1 mg each of magnolol for assay and honokiol in diluted methanol (7 in 10) to make 10 mL. When the procedure is run with 10 μL of this solution under the above operating conditions, honokiol and magnolol are eluted in this order with the resolution between these peaks being not less than 5.

System repeatability: When the test is repeated 6 times with 10 μL of the standard solution under the above operating conditions, the relative standard deviation of the peak area of magnolol is not more than 1.5%.

Containers and storage Containers—Tight containers.

Magnolia Flower

Magnoliae Flos

シンイ

Magnolia Flower is the flower bud of *Magnolia biondii* Pampanini, *Magnolia heptapeta* Dandy (*Magnolia denudata* Desrousseaux), *Magnolia sprengeri* Pampanini, *Magnolia salicifolia* Maximowicz, or *Magnolia kobus* De Candolle (*Magnoliaceae*).

Description Magnolia Flower is a fusiform flower bud, 15 – 45 mm in length, 6 – 20 mm in diameter at central part; often having ligneous peduncles on base; usually 3 bracts, externally with sparse hairs, brown to dark brown, or with dense hairs, grayish white to light yellow-brown, and the inner surface of 3 bracts smooth and dark brown in color; interior perianth of 9 pieces or 12 pieces, same size or outer three pieces are smaller; 50 – 100 stamens and numerous pistils. Brittle in texture.

Odor, characteristic; taste, acrid and slightly bitter.

Identification To 1 g of pulverized Magnolia Flower add 10 mL of methanol, shake for 15 minutes, filter, and use the filtrate as the sample solution. Perform the test with the sample solution as directed under Thin-layer Chromatography <*2.03*>. Spot 20 μL of the sample solution on a plate of silica gel for thin-layer chromatography, develop the plate with a mixture of ethyl acetate, acetone, water and formic acid (5:3:1:1) to a distance of about 7 cm, and air-dry the plate. Spray evenly Dragendorff's TS for spraying on the plate: a yellow-red spot appears at an *R*f value of about 0.3.

Loss on drying <*5.01*> Not more than 14.0% (6 hours).

Total ash <*5.01*> Not more than 5.5%.

Acid-insoluble ash <*5.01*> Not more than 1.5%.

Extract content <*5.01*> Dilute ethanol-extract: not less than 13.0%.

Essential oil content <*5.01*> Perform the test with 50.0 g of pulverized Magnolia Flower: the volume of essential oil is not less than 0.5 mL.

Containers and storage Containers—Well-closed containers.

Mallotus Bark

Malloti Cortex

アカメガシワ

Mallotus Bark is the bark of *Mallotus japonica* Müeller Argoviensis (*Euphorbiaceae*).

Description Mallotus Bark is flat or semitubular pieces of bark, 1 – 3 mm in thickness; externally greenish gray to brownish gray brow in color, with a vertically striped shape gathering numerous lenticels; internal surface light yellow-brown to grayish brown in color, and smooth with numerous fine striped lines; easy to break; slightly fibrous at fractured surface.

Mallotus Bark has a slight odor, a bitter taste and slightly astringent.

Identification To 0.5 g pulverized Mallotus Bark add 10 mL of methanol, warm on a water bath for 5 minutes, filter, and use the filtrate as the sample solution. Separately, dissolve 1 mg of bergenin for thin-layer chromatography in 1 mL of methanol, and use this solution as the standard solution. Perform the test with these solutions as directed under Thin-layer Chromatography <*2.03*>. Spot 10 μL each of the sample solution and standard solution on a plate of silica gel with fluorescent indicator for thin-layer chromatography. Develop the plate with a mixture of ethyl acetate, ethanol (99.5) and water (100:17:13) to a distance of about 7 cm, and air-dry the plate. Examine under ultraviolet light (main wavelength: 254 nm): one of the several spots obtained from the sample solution has the same color tone and *R*f value with the spot from the standard solution.

Loss on drying <*5.01*> Not more than 13.0% (6 hours).

Total ash <*5.01*> Not more than 12.0%.

Acid-insoluble ash <*5.01*> Not more than 2.5%.

Extract content <*5.01*> Dilute ethanol-soluble extract: not less than 11.0%.

Containers and storage Containers—Well-closed containers.

Malt

Fructus Hordei Germinatus

バクガ

Malt is the dried ripe caryopsis of *Hordeum vulgare* Linné (*Gramineae*), after being germinated.

Description Oval caryopsis, 10 mm in length, 3 – 4 mm in width, furrowed on one surface; externally light yellow, sometimes with plumule at one end, with hairs and sometimes with roots at the other end; cut surface of caryopsis white and powdery; easily broken and light in texture.

Odor, slight; taste, slightly sweet.

Under a microscope <*5.01*>, a transverse section of the caryopsis reveals glume, pericarp, seed coat and endosperm in this order from the outside; 2 – 4 cellular layered aleurone layers on the circumference of endosperm; endosperm filled with starch grains; starch grains as spheroidal or ellipsoidal, large grains about 20 μm and small grains about 2 μm in diameter mixed together.

Identification To 3.0 g of pulverized Malt add 5 mL of methanol, shake for 15 minutes, centrifuge, and use the supernatant liquid as the sample solution. Perform the test with the sample solution as directed under Liquid Chromatography <*2.03*>. Spot 5 μL of the sample solution on a plate of silica gel for thin-layer chromatography. Develop the plate with a mixture of methanol, water and acetic acid (100) (8:1:1) to a distance of about 7 cm, and air-dry the plate. Spray evenly a solution of 0.1 g of 2,3-indolinedione in 50 mL of acetone on the plate, and heat the plate at 105°C for 5 minutes: a blue-purple spot appears at an *R*f value of about 0.4.

Loss on drying <*5.01*> Not more than 11.0%.

Total ash <*5.01*> Not more than 2.6%.

Acid-insoluble ash <*5.01*> Not more than 0.8%.

Extract content <*5.01*> Dilute ethanol-soluble extract: Not less than 15.0%.

Containers and storage Containers—Well-closed containers.

Maoto Extract

麻黄湯エキス

Maoto Extract contains not less than 15 mg and not more than 45 mg of total alkaloids (ephedrine and pseudoephedrine), not less than 48 mg and not more than 192 mg of amygdalin, and not less than 11 mg and not more than 33 mg of glycyrrhizic acid ($C_{42}H_{62}O_{16}$: 822.93), per extract prepared with the amount specified in the Method of preparation.

Method of preparation

	1)
Ephedra Herb	5 g
Apricot Kernel	5 g
Cinnamon Bark	4 g
Glycyrrhiza	1.5 g

Prepare a dry extract or viscous extract as directed under Extracts, according to the prescription 1), using the crude drugs shown above, or prepare a dry extract by adding Light Anhydrous Silicic Acid to an extractive prepared as directed under Extracts, according to the prescription 1), using the crude drugs shown above.

Description Maoto Extract occurs as a light brown powder or black-brown viscous extract, having a slightly order, and a sweet and bitter, then a slightly astringent taste.

Identification **(1)** Shake 1.0 g of the dry extract (or 3.0 g of the viscous extract) with 10 mL of water, add 10 mL of 1-butanol, shake, centrifuge, and use the 1-butanol layer as the sample solution. Perform the test with the sample solution as directed under Thin-layer Chromatography *<2.03>*. Spot 5 μL of the sample solution on a plate of silica gel for thin-layer chromatography. Develop the plate with a mixture of 1-propanol, ethyl acetate, water and acetic acid (100) (4:4:2:1) to a distance of about 7 cm, and air-dry the plate. Spray evenly ninhydrin-ethanol TS for spraying on the plate, and heat the plate at 105°C for 5 minutes: a red-purple spot is observed at an *R*f value of about 0.5 (Ephedra Herb).

(2) Shake 1.0 g of the dry extract (or 3.0 g of the viscous extract) with 10 mL of water, add 10 mL of 1-butanol, shake, centrifuge, and use the 1-butanol layer as the sample solution. Separately, dissolve 2 mg of amygdalin for thin-layer chromatography in 1 mL of methanol, and use this solution as the standard solution. Perform the test with these solutions as directed under Thin-layer Chromatography *<2.03>*. Spot 5 μL each of the sample solution and standard solution on a plate of silica gel for thin-layer chromatography. Develop the plate with a mixture of 1-propanol, ethyl acetate and water (4:4:3) to a distance of about 7 cm, and air-dry the plate. Spray evenly 4-methoxybenzaldehyde-sulfuric acid TS on the plate, and heat the plate at 105°C for 10 minutes: one of the several spots obtained from the sample solution has the same color tone and *R*f value with the green-brown spot from the standard solution (Apricot Kernel).

(3) Perform the test according to the following (i) or (ii) (Cinnamon Bark).

(i) Put 10 g of the dry extract (or 30 g of the viscous extract) in a 300-mL hard-glass flask, add 100 mL of water and 1 mL of silicone resin, connect the apparatus for essential oil determination, and heat to boil under a reflux condenser. The graduated tube of the apparatus is to be previously filled with water to the standard line, and 2 mL of hexane is added to the graduated tube. After heating under reflux for 1 hour, separate the hexane layer, and use the layer as the sample solution. Separately, dissolve 1 mg of (*E*)-cinnamaldehyde for thin-layer chromatography in 1 mL of methanol, and use this solution as the standard solution. Perform the test with these solutions as directed under Thin-layer Chromatography *<2.03>*. Spot 40 μL of the sample solution and 2 μL of the standard solution on a plate of silica gel for thin-layer chromatography. Develop the plate with a mixture of hexane and ethyl acetate (2:1) to a distance of about 7 cm, and air-dry the plate. Spray evenly 2,4-dinitrophenylhydrazine TS on the plate: one of the several spots obtained from the sample solution has the same color tone and *R*f value with the yellow-orange spot from the standard solution.

(ii) Shake 2.0 g of the dry extract (or 6.0 g of the viscous extract) with 10 mL of water, then add 5 mL of hexane, shake, centrifuge, and use the hexane layer as the sample solution. Separately, dissolve 1 mg of (*E*)-2-methoxycinnamaldehyde for thin-layer chromatography in 1 mL of methanol, and use this solution as the standard solution. Perform the test with these solutions as directed under Thin-layer Chromatography *<2.03>*. Spot 40 μL of the sample solution and 2 μL of the standard solution on a plate of silica gel for thin-layer chromatography. Develop the plate with a mixture of hexane and ethyl acetate (2:1) to a distance of about 7 cm, and air-dry the plate. Examine under ultraviolet light (main wavelength: 365 nm): one of the several spots obtained from the sample solution has the same color tone and *R*f value with the blue-white fluorescent spot from the standard solution.

(4) Shake 1.0 g of the dry extract (or 3.0 g of the viscous extract) with 10 mL of water, add 10 mL of 1-butanol, shake, centrifuge, and use the 1-butanol layer as the sample solution. Separately, dissolve 1 mg of liquiritin for thin-layer chromatography in 1 mL of methanol, and use this solution as the standard solution. Perform the test with these solutions as directed under Thin-layer Chromatography *<2.03>*. Spot 1 μL each of the sample solution and standard solution on a plate of silica gel for thin-layer chromatography. Develop the plate with a mixture of ethyl acetate, methanol and water (20:3:2) to a distance of about 7 cm, and air-dry the plate. Spray evenly dilute sulfuric acid on the plate, heat the plate at 105°C for 5 minutes, and examine under ultraviolet light (main wavelength: 365 nm): one of the several spots obtained from the sample solution has the same color tone and *R*f value with the yellow-green fluorescent spot from the standard solution (Glycyrrhiza).

Purity **(1)** Heavy metals *<1.07>*—Prepare the test solution with 1.0 g of the dry extract (or an amount of the viscous extract, equivalent to 1.0 g of dried substance) as directed under Extracts (4), and perform the test (not more than 30 ppm).

(2) Arsenic *<1.11>*—Prepare the test solution with 0.67 g of the dry extract (or an amount of the viscous extract, equivalent to 0.67 g of dried substance) according to Method 3, and perform the test (not more than 3 ppm).

Loss on drying *<2.41>* The dry extract: Not more than 9.5% (1 g, 105°C, 5 hours).

The viscous extract: Not more than 66.7% (1 g, 105°C, 5 hours).

Total ash <*5.01*> Not more than 13.0%, calculated on the dried basis. However, for the dry extract prepared by adding Light Anhydrous Silicic Acid, between 10.0% and 22.0%.

Assay **(1)** Total alkaloids (ephedrine and pseudoephedrine)—Weigh accurately about 0.5 g of the dry extract (or an amount of the viscous extract, equivalent to about 0.5 g of the dried substance), add 20 mL of diethyl ether, shake, then add 3.0 mL of 0.1 mol/L hydrochloric acid TS, and shake for 10 minutes. After centrifugation, remove the diethyl ether layer, add 20 mL of diethyl ether, proceed in the same manner as described above, and remove the diethyl ether layer. To the aqueous layer add 1.0 mL of ammonia TS and 20 mL of diethyl ether, shake for 30 minutes, centrifuge, and separate the diethyl ether layer. In addition, repeat twice in the same manner for the aqueous layer using 1.0 mL of ammonia TS and 20 mL of diethyl ether. Combine all the extracts, evaporate the solvent under low pressure (in vacuo), dissolve the residue in diluted methanol (1 in 2) to make exactly 50 mL, centrifuge, and use the supernatant liquid as the sample solution. Separately, weigh accurately about 10 mg of ephedrine hydrochloride for assay of crude drugs, previously dried at 105°C for 3 hours, dissolve in diluted methanol (1 in 2) to make exactly 100 mL. Pipet 10 mL of this solution, add diluted methanol (1 in 2) to make exactly 50 mL, and use this solution as the standard solution. Perform the test with exactly 10 μL each of the sample solution and standard solution as directed under Liquid Chromatography <*2.01*> according to the following conditions, and determine the peak areas, A_{TE} and A_{TP}, of ephedrine and pseudoephedrine obtained from the sample solution, and peak area, A_S, of ephedrine from the standard solution.

Amount (mg) of total alkaloids (ephedrine and pseudoephedrine)
$= M_S \times (A_{TE} + A_{TP})/A_S \times 1/10 \times 0.819$

M_S: Amount (mg) of ephedrine hydrochloride for assay of crude drugs taken

Operating conditions—

Detector: An ultraviolet absorption photometer (wavelength: 210 nm).

Column: A stainless steel column 4.6 mm in inside diameter and 15 cm in length, packed with octadecylsilanized silica gel for liquid chromatography (5 μm in particle diameter).

Column temperature: A constant temperature of about 40°C.

Mobile phase: To 5 g of sodium lauryl sulfate add 350 mL of acetonitrile, shake, then add 650 mL of water and 1 mL of phosphoric acid to dissolve lauryl sulfate.

Flow rate: 1.0 mL per minute (the retention time of ephedrine is about 27 minutes).

System suitability—

System performance: Dissolve 1 mg each of ephedrine hydrochloride for assay of crude drugs and pseudoephedrine hydrochloride in diluted methanol (1 in 2) to make 10 mL. When the procedure is run with 10 μL of this solution under the above operating conditions, pseudoephedrine and ephedrine are eluted in this order with the resolution between these peaks being not less than 1.5.

System repeatability: When the test is repeated 6 times with 10 μL of the standard solution under the above operating conditions, the relative standard deviation of the peak area of ephedrine is not more than 1.5%.

(2) Amygdalin—Weigh accurately about 0.5 g of the dry extract (or an amount of the viscous extract, equivalent to about 0.5 g of the dried substance), add exactly 50 mL of diluted methanol (1 in 2), shake for 15 minutes, and filter. Pipet 5 mL of the filtrate, flow through in a column packed with 2 g of polyamide for column chromatography, then elute with water to make exactly 20 mL, and use this effluent as the sample solution. Separately, weigh accurately about 10 mg of amygdalin for assay, previously dried in a desiccator (silica gel) for 24 hours or more, and dissolve in diluted methanol (1 in 2) to make exactly 50 mL, and use this solution as the standard solution. Perform the test with exactly 10 μL each of the sample solution and standard solution as directed under Liquid Chromatography <*2.01*> according to the following conditions, and determine the peak areas, A_T and A_S, of amygdalin in each solution.

Amount (mg) of amygdalin $= M_S \times A_T/A_S \times 4$

M_S: Amount (mg) of amygdalin for assay taken

Operating conditions—

Detector: An ultraviolet absorption photometer (wavelength: 210 nm).

Column: A stainless steel column 4.6 mm in inside diameter and 15 cm in length, packed with octadecylsilanized silica gel for liquid chromatography (5 μm in particle diameter).

Column temperature: A constant temperature of about 45°C.

Mobile phase: A mixture of 0.05 mol/L sodium dihydrogen phosphate TS and methanol (5:1).

Flow rate: 0.8 mL per minute (the retention time of amygdalin is about 12 minutes).

System suitability—

System performance: When the procedure is run with 10 μL of the standard solution under the above operating conditions, the number of theoretical plates and the symmetry factor of the peak of amygdalin are not less than 5000 and not more than 1.5, respectively.

System repeatability: When the test is repeated 6 times with 10 μL of the standard solution under the above operating conditions, the relative standard deviation of the peak area of amygdalin is not more than 1.5%.

(3) Glycyrrhizic acid—Perform the test according to the following i) or ii).

i) Weigh accurately about 0.5 g of the dry extract (or an amount of the viscous extract, equivalent to about 0.5 g of the dried substance), add exactly 50 mL of diluted methanol (1 in 2), shake for 15 minutes, filter, and use the filtrate as the sample solution. Separately, weigh accurately about 10 mg of Glycyrrhizic Acid RS (separately determine the water <*2.48*> by coulometric titration, using 10 mg), dissolve in diluted methanol (1 in 2) to make exactly 100 mL, and use this solution as the standard solution. Perform the test with exactly 10 μL each of the sample solution and standard solution as directed under Liquid Chromatography <*2.01*> according to the following conditions, and determine the peak areas, A_T and A_S, of glycyrrhizic acid in each solution.

Amount (mg) of glycyrrhizic acid ($C_{42}H_{62}O_{16}$)
$= M_S \times A_T/A_S \times 1/2$

M_S: Amount (mg) of Glycyrrhizic Acid RS taken, calculated on the anhydrous basis

Operating conditions—

Detector: An ultraviolet absorption photometer (wavelength: 254 nm).

Column: A stainless steel column 4.6 mm in inside diameter and 15 cm in length, packed with octadecylsilanized silica gel for liquid chromatography (5 μm in particle diameter).

Column temperature: A constant temperature of about

40°C.

Mobile phase: Dissolve 3.85 g of ammonium acetate in 720 mL of water, and add 5 mL of acetic acid (100) and 280 mL of acetonitrile.

Flow rate: 1.0 mL per minute (the retention time of glycyrrhizic acid is about 15 minutes).

System suitability—

System performance: Dissolve 5 mg of monoammonium glycyrrhizinate for resolution check in 20 mL of dilute ethanol. When the procedure is run with 10 μL of this solution under the above operating conditions, the resolution between the peak having the relative retention time of about 0.9 to glycyrrhizic acid and the peak of glycyrrhizic acid is not less than 1.5. Dissolve 1 mg of (*E*)-cinnamaldehyde for thin-layer chromatography in 50 mL of methanol. To 2 mL of this solution add 2 mL of the standard solution. When the procedure is run with 10 μL of this solution under the above operating conditions, the resolution between the peaks of glycyrrhizic acid and (*E*)-cinnamaldehyde is not less than 1.5.

System repeatability: When the test is repeated 6 times with 10 μL of the standard solution under the above operating conditions, the relative standard deviation of the peak area of glycyrrhizic acid is not more than 1.5%.

ii) Weigh accurately about 0.5 g of the dry extract (or an amount of the viscous extract, equivalent to about 0.5 g of the dried substance), add 20 mL of ethyl acetate and 10 mL of water, and shake for 10 minutes. After centrifugation, remove the ethyl acetate layer, add 20 mL of ethyl acetate, proceed in the same manner as described above, and remove the ethyl acetate layer. To the aqueous layer add 10 mL of methanol, shake for 30 minutes, centrifuge, and take the supernatant liquid. To the residue add 20 mL of diluted methanol (1 in 2), shake for 5 minutes, centrifuge, and take the supernatant liquid. Combine these supernatant liquids, add diluted methanol (1 in 2) to make exactly 50 mL, and use this solution as the sample solution. Separately, weigh accurately about 10 mg of Glycyrrhizic Acid RS (separately determine the water <*2.48*> by coulometric titration, using 10 mg), dissolve in diluted methanol (1 in 2) to make exactly 100 mL, and use this solution as the standard solution. Perform the test with exactly 10 μL each of the sample solution and standard solution as directed under Liquid Chromatography <*2.01*> according to the following conditions, and determine the peak areas, A_T and A_S, of glycyrrhizic acid in each solution.

Amount (mg) of glycyrrhizic acid ($C_{42}H_{62}O_{16}$)
$= M_S \times A_T/A_S \times 1/2$

M_S: Amount (mg) of Glycyrrhizic Acid RS taken, calculated on the anhydrous basis

Operating conditions—

Proceed as directed in the operating conditions in i).

System suitability—

System repeatability: Proceed as directed in the system suitability in i).

System performance: Dissolve 5 mg of monoammonium glycyrrhizinate for resolution check in 20 mL of dilute ethanol. When the procedure is run with 10 μL of this solution under the above operating conditions, the resolution between the peak having the relative retention time of about 0.9 to glycyrrhizic acid and the peak of glycyrrhizic acid is not less than 1.5.

Containers and storage Containers—Tight containers.

Mentha Herb

Menthae Herba

ハッカ

Mentha Herb is the terrestrial part of *Mentha arvensis* Linné var. *piperascens* Malinvaud (*Labiatae*).

Description Stem with opposite leaves; stem, square, light brown to red-purple in color, and with fine hairs; when smoothed by immersing in water, leaf, ovate to oblong, with acute apex and base, 2 - 8 cm in length, 1 - 2.5 cm in width, margin irregularly serrated; the upper surface, light brown-yellow to light green-yellow, and the lower surface, light green to light green-yellow in color; petiole 0.3 - 1 cm in length. Under a magnifying glass, leaf reveals hairs, glandular hairs and scales.

It has a characteristic aroma and gives a cool feeling on keeping in the mouth.

Identification To 1.0 g of pulverized Mentha Herb add 10 mL of diethyl ether, shake for 10 minutes, centrifuge, and use the supernatant liquid as the sample solution. Separately, dissolve 1 mg of menthol in 1 mL of diethyl ether, and use this solution as the standard solution. Perform the test with these solutions as directed under Thin-layer Chromatography <*2.03*>. Spot 2 μL each of the sample solution and standard solution on a plate of silica gel for thin-layer chromatography. Develop the plate with a mixture of hexane and acetone (7:3) to a distance of about 7 cm, and air-dry the plate. Spray evenly 4-methoxybenzaldehyde-sulfuric acid-acetic acid-ethanol TS for spraying on the plate, and heat the plate at 105°C for 5 minutes: one of the several spots obtained from the sample solution has the same color tone and *R*f value with the spot from the standard solution.

Purity Foreign matter <*5.01*>—The amount of roots and other foreign matter contained in Mentha Herb does not exceed 2.0%.

Loss on drying <*5.01*> Not more than 15.0% (6 hours).

Total ash <*5.01*> Not more than 12.0%.

Acid-insoluble ash <*5.01*> Not more than 2.5%.

Essential oil content <*5.01*> Perform the test with 50.0 g of pulverized Mentha Herb after adding 1 mL of silicone resin to the sample in the flask: the volume of essential oil is not less than 0.4 mL.

Containers and storage Containers—Well-closed containers.

Mentha Oil

Oleum Menthae Japonicae

ハッカ油

Mentha Oil is the essential oil which is distilled with steam from the terrestrial parts of *Mentha arvensis* Linné var. *piperascens* Malinvaud (*Labiatae*), and from which solids are removed after cooling.

It contains not less than 30.0% of menthol.

Description Mentha Oil is a colorless or pale yellow, clear liquid. It has a characteristic, pleasant aroma and has a pungent taste, followed by a cool aftertaste.

It is miscible with ethanol (95), with ethanol (99.5), with warm ethanol (95), and with diethyl ether.

It is practically insoluble in water.

Refractive index <*2.45*> n_D^{20}: 1.455 – 1.467

Optical rotation <*2.49*> α_D^{20}: −17.0 – −36.0° (100 mm).

Specific gravity <*1.13*> d_{25}^{25}: 0.885 – 0.910

Acid value <*1.13*> Not more than 1.0.

Purity **(1)** Clarity and color of solution—To 1.0 mL of Mentha Oil add 3.5 mL of diluted ethanol (7 in 10), and shake: Mentha Oil dissolves clearly. To the solution add 10 mL of ethanol (95): the solution is clear or has no more turbidity, if any, than the following control solution.

Control solution: To 0.70 mL of 0.01 mol/L hydrochloric acid VS add 6 mL of dilute nitric acid and water to make 50 mL, add 1 mL of silver nitrate TS, and allow to stand for 5 minutes.

(2) Heavy metals <*1.07*>—Proceed with 1.0 mL of Mentha Oil according to Method 2, and perform the test. Prepare the control solution with 4.0 mL of Standard Lead Solution (not more than 40 ppm).

Assay Weigh accurately about 5 g of Mentha Oil, and dissolve in ethanol (95) to make exactly 20 mL. Pipet 10 mL of this solution, add exactly 10 mL of the internal standard solution, and use this solution as the sample solution. Separately, weigh accurately about 10 g of *l*-menthol for assay, and dissolve in ethanol (95) to make exactly 100 mL. Pipet 10 mL of this solution, add exactly 10 mL of the internal standard solution, and use this solution as the standard solution. Perform the test with 1 μL each of the sample solution and standard solution as directed under Gas Chromatography <*2.02*> according to the following conditions. Calculate the ratios, Q_T and Q_S, of the peak area of menthol to that of the internal standard.

$$\text{Amount (mg) of menthol} = M_S \times Q_T/Q_S \times 1/5$$

M_S: Amount (mg) of *l*-menthol for assay taken

Internal standard solution—A solution of *n*-ethyl caprylate in ethanol (95) (1 in 25).

Operating conditions—

Detector: A hydrogen flame-ionization detector.

Column: A glass column about 3 mm in inside diameter and about 2 m in length, packed with 25% of polyethylene glycol 6000 for gas chromatography supported on acid-washed 180 – 250 μm siliceous earth for gas chromatography.

Column temperature: A constant temperature of about 150°C.

Carrier gas: Nitrogen.

Flow rate: Adjust so that the retention time of the internal standard is about 10 minutes.

System suitability—

System performance: When the procedure is run with 1 μL of the standard solution under the above operating conditions, the internal standard and *l*-menthol are eluted in this order with the resolution between these peaks being not less than 5.

Containers and storage Containers—Tight containers.

Storage—Light-resistant.

Mentha Water

ハッカ水

Method of preparation

Mentha Oil	2 mL
Purified Water or Purified Water in Containers	a sufficient quantity
To make	1000 mL

Prepare as directed under Aromatic Waters, with the above ingredients.

Description Mentha Water is a clear, colorless liquid, having the odor of mentha oil.

Containers and storage Containers—Tight containers.

Moutan Bark

Moutan Cortex

ボタンピ

Moutan Bark is the root bark of *Paeonia suffruticosa* Andrews (*Paeonia moutan* Sims) (*Paeoniaceae*).

It contains not less than 0.9% of paeonol.

Description Tubular to semi-tubular bark, about 0.5 cm in thickness, 5 – 8 cm in length, 0.8 – 1.5 cm in diameter; externally dark brown to purple-brown, with small and transversely elongated ellipsoidal scars of lateral roots, and with longitudinal wrinkles; internally, light grayish brown to purplish brown and smooth; fractured surface coarse; white crystals often attached on the internal and fractured surfaces.

Odor, characteristic; taste, slightly pungent and bitter.

Identification To 2.0 g of pulverized Moutan Bark add 10 mL of hexane, shake for 3 minutes, filter, and use the filtrate as the sample solution. Separately, dissolve 1 mg of paeonol for thin-layer chromatography in 1 mL of hexane, and use this solution as the standard solution. Perform the test with these solutions as directed under Thin-layer Chromatography <*2.03*>. Spot 10 μL each of the sample solution and standard solution on a plate of silica gel with fluorescent indicator for thin-layer chromatography. Develop the plate with a mixture of ethyl acetate and hexane (1:1) to a distance of about 7 cm, and air-dry the plate. Examine under ultraviolet light (main wavelength: 254 nm): one of the several spots obtained from the sample solution has the same color tone and *R*f value with the spot from the standard solution.

Purity **(1)** Heavy metals <*1.07*>—Proceed with 3.0 g of pulverized Moutan Bark according to Method 3, and perform the test. Prepare the control solution with 3.0 mL of Standard Lead Solution (not more than 10 ppm).

(2) Arsenic <*1.11*>—Prepare the test solution with 0.40 g of pulverized Moutan Bark according to Method 4, and perform the test (not more than 5 ppm).

(3) Xylem—When perform the test of foreign matter <*5.01*>, the amount of the xylem contained in Moutan Bark is not more than 5.0%.

(4) Foreign matter <*5.01*>—The amount of foreign matter other than xylem contained in Moutan Bark is not exceed 1.0%.

(5) Total BHC's and total DDT's <*5.01*>—Not more than 0.2 ppm, respectively.

Total ash <*5.01*> Not more than 6.0%.

Acid-insoluble ash <*5.01*> Not more than 1.0%.

Assay Weigh accurately about 0.3 g of pulverized Moutan Bark, add 40 mL of methanol, heat under a reflux condenser for 30 minutes, cool, and filter. Repeat the above procedure with the residue, using 40 mL of methanol. Combine all the filtrates, add methanol to make exactly 100 mL, then pipet 10 mL of this solution, add methanol to make exactly 25 mL, and use this solution as the sample solution. Separately, weigh accurately about 10 mg of paeonol for assay, dissolve in methanol to make exactly 100 mL, then pipet 10 mL of this solution, add methanol to make exactly 50 mL, and use this solution as the standard solution. Perform the test with exactly 10 μL each of the sample solution and standard solution as directed under Liquid Chromatography <*2.01*> according to the following conditions, and determine the peak areas, A_T and A_S, of paeonol in each solution.

$$\text{Amount (mg) of paeonol} = M_S \times A_T/A_S \times 1/2$$

M_S: Amount (mg) of paeonol for assay taken, calculated on the basis of the content obtained by qNMR

Operating conditions—

Detector: An ultraviolet absorption photometer (wavelength: 274 nm).

Column: A stainless steel column 4 to 6 mm in inside diameter and 15 to 25 cm in length, packed with octadecylsilanized silica gel (5 to 10 μm in particle diameter).

Column temperature: A constant temperature of about 20°C.

Mobile phase: A mixture of water, acetonitrile, and acetic acid (100) (65:35:2).

Flow rate: Adjust so that the retention time of paeonol is about 14 minutes.

System suitability—

System performance: Dissolve 1 mg of paeonol for assay and 5 mg of butyl parahydroxybenzoate for resolution check in methanol to make 25 mL. When the procedure is run with 10 μL of this solution under the above operating conditions, paeonol and butyl parahydroxybenzoate are eluted in this order with the resolution between these peaks being not less than 2.0.

System repeatability: When the test is repeated 6 times with the standard solution under the above operating conditions, the relative standard deviation of the peak area of paeonol is not more than 1.5%.

Containers and storage Containers—Well-closed containers.

Powdered Moutan Bark

Moutan Cortex Pulveratus

ボタンピ末

Powdered Moutan Bark is the powder of Moutan Bark.

It contains not less than 0.6% of paeonol.

Description Powdered Moutan Bark occurs as a light grayish yellow-brown powder. It has a characteristic odor and a slight, pungent and bitter taste.

Under a microscope <*5.01*>, Powdered Moutan Bark reveals starch grains and fragments of parenchyma containing them; fragments of cork tissue containing tannin; fragments of somewhat thick-walled collenchyma, medullary rays, and phloem parenchyma; rosette aggregates of calcium oxalate and also fragments of parenchyma cells containing them. Starch grains are simple or 2- to 10-compound grains, 10 - 25 μm in diameter; rosette aggregates are 20 - 30 μm in diameter.

Identification **(1)** To 2.0 g of Powdered Moutan Bark add 10 mL of hexane, shake for 3 minutes, filter, and use the filtrate as the sample solution. Separately, dissolve 1 mg of paeonol for thin-layer chromatography in 1 mL of hexane, and use this solution as the standard solution. Perform the test with these solutions as directed under Thin-layer Chromatography <*2.03*>. Spot 10 μL each of the sample solution and standard solution on a plate of silica gel with fluorescent indicator for thin-layer chromatography. Develop the plate with a mixture of ethyl acetate and hexane (1:1) to a distance of about 7 cm, and air-dry the plate. Examine under ultraviolet light (main wavelength: 254 nm): one of the several spots obtained from the sample solution has the same color tone and *R*f value with the spot from the standard solution.

(2) Evaporate the solvent to dryness 1 mL of the sample solution obtained in (1), dissolve the residue in 50 mL of ethanol (95), and determine the absorption spectrum of this solution as directed under Ultraviolet-visible Spectrophotometry <*2.24*>: it exhibits maxima at around 228 nm, 274 nm and 313 nm.

Purity **(1)** Heavy metals <*1.07*>—Proceed with 3.0 g of Powdered Moutan Bark according to Method 3, and perform the test. Prepare the control solution with 3.0 mL of Standard Lead Solution (not more than 10 ppm).

(2) Arsenic <*1.11*>—Prepare the test solution with 0.40 g of Powdered Moutan Bark according to Method 4, and perform the test (not more than 5 ppm).

(3) Foreign matter—Under a microscope <*5.01*>, usually vessels and other sclerenchymatous cells are not observable.

(4) Total BHC's and total DDT's <*5.01*>—Not more than 0.2 ppm, respectively.

Total ash <*5.01*> Not more than 6.0%.

Acid-insoluble ash <*5.01*> Not more than 1.0%.

Assay Weigh accurately about 0.5 g of Powdered Moutan Bark, add 40 mL of methanol, heat under a reflux condenser for 30 minutes, cool, and filter. Repeat the above procedure with the residue, using 40 mL of methanol. Combine all the filtrates, add methanol to make exactly 100 mL, then pipet 10 mL of this solution, add methanol to make exactly 25 mL, and use this solution as the sample solution. Separately, weigh accurately about 10 mg of paeonol for assay, dissolve in methanol to make exactly 100 mL, then pipet 10 mL of this solution, add methanol to make exactly 50 mL, and use this solution as the standard solution. Perform the test with exactly 10 μL each of the sample solution and standard solution as directed under Liquid Chromatography <*2.01*> according to the following conditions, and determine the peak areas, A_T and A_S, of paeonol in each solution.

$$\text{Amount (mg) of paeonol} = M_S \times A_T/A_S \times 1/2$$

M_S: Amount (mg) of paeonol for assay taken, calculated on the basis of the content obtained by qNMR

Operating conditions—

Detector: An ultraviolet absorption photometer (wavelength: 274 nm).

Column: A stainless steel column 4 to 6 mm in inside diameter and 15 to 25 cm in length, packed with octadecylsilanized silica gel (5 to 10 μm in particle diameter).

Column temperature: A constant temperature of about 20°C.

Mobile phase: A mixture of water, acetonitrile, and acetic acid (100) (65:35:2).

Flow rate: Adjust so that the retention time of paeonol is about 14 minutes.

System suitability—

System performance: Dissolve 1 mg of paeonol for assay and 5 mg of butyl parahydroxybenzoate for resolution check in methanol to make 25 mL. When the procedure is run with 10 μL of this solution under the above operating conditions, paeonol and butyl parahydroxybenzoate are eluted in this order with the resolution between these peaks being not less than 2.0.

System repeatability: When the test is repeated 6 times with 10 μL of the standard solution under the above operating conditions, the relative standard deviation of the peak area of paeonol is not more than 1.5%.

Containers and storage Containers—Tight containers.

Mukoi-Daikenchuto Extract

無コウイ大建中湯エキス

Mukoi-Daikenchuto Extract contains not less than 1.8 mg of ginsenoside Rb_1 ($C_{54}H_{92}O_{23}$: 1109.29), and not less than 1.4 mg and not more than 4.2 mg of [6]-shogaol, per extract prepared with the amount specified in the Method of preparation.

Method of preparation

	1)
Japanese Zanthoxylum Peel	2 g
Ginseng	3 g
Processed Ginger	5 g

Prepare a dry extract as directed under Extracts, according to the prescription 1), using crude drugs shown above.

Description Mukoi-Daikenchuto Extract is a light brown powder. It has a slight odor, and has a pungent taste.

Identification **(1)** Shake 2.0 g of Mukoi-Daikenchuto Extract with 10 mL of water, add 10 mL of diethyl ether, shake, centrifuge, and use the diethyl ether layer as the sample solution. Separately, shake 2.0 g of pulverized japanese zanthoxylum peel with 10 mL of water, add 5 mL of diethyl ether, shake, centrifuge, and use the diethyl ether layer as the standard solution. Perform the test with these solutions as directed under Thin-layer Chromatography *<2.03>*. Spot 10 μL each of the sample solution and standard solution on a plate of silica gel with fluorescent indicator for thin-layer chromatography. Develop the plate with a mixture of ethyl acetate, hexane, methanol and acetic acid (100) (20:20:1:1) to a distance of about 7 cm, and air-dry the plate. Examine under ultraviolet light (main wavelength: 254 nm): one of the several spots obtained from the sample solution has the same color tone and *R*f value with the dark purple spot (*R*f value: about 0.3) from the standard solution (Japanese Zanthoxylum Peel).

(2) Shake 2.0 g of Mukoi-Daikenchuto Extract with 10 mL of water, add 10 mL of 1-butanol, shake, centrifuge, and use the 1-butanol layer as the sample solution. Separately, dissolve 1 mg of Ginsenoside Rb_1 RS or ginsenoside Rb_1 for thin-layer chromatography in 1 mL of methanol, and use this solution as the standard solution. Perform the test with these solutions as directed under Thin-layer Chromatography *<2.03>*. Spot 10 μL of the sample solution and 2 μL of the standard solution on a plate of silica gel for thin-layer chromatography. Develop the plate with a mixture of ethyl acetate, 1-propanol, water and acetic acid (100) (7:5:4:1) to a distance of about 7 cm, and air-dry the plate. Spray evenly vanillin-sulfuric acid-ethanol TS for spraying on the plate, heat the plate at 105°C for 5 minutes, and allow to cool: one of the several spots obtained from the sample solution has the same color tone and *R*f value with the blue-purple spot from the standard solution (Ginseng).

(3) Shake 2.0 g of Mukoi-Daikenchuto Extract with 10 mL of water, add 10 mL of diethyl ether, shake, centrifuge, and use the diethyl ether layer as the sample solution. Separately, dissolve 1 mg of [6]-shogaol for thin-layer chromatography in 1 mL of methanol, and use this solution as the standard solution. Perform the test with these solutions as directed under Thin-layer Chromatography *<2.03>*. Spot 10 μL of the sample solution and 2 μL of the standard solution on a plate of silica gel for thin-layer chromatography. Develop the plate with a mixture of ethyl acetate and hexane (1:1) to a distance of about 7 cm, and air-dry the plate. Spray evenly 4-dimethylaminobenzaldehyde TS for spraying on the plate, heat the plate at 105°C for 5 minutes, allow to cool, and spray water: one of the several spots obtained from the sample solution has the same color tone and *R*f value with the blue-green to grayish green spot from the standard solution (Processed ginger).

Purity **(1)** Heavy metals *<1.07>*—Prepare the test solution with 2.0 g of Mukoi-Daikenchuto Extract as directed under Extracts (4), and perform the test (not more than 15 ppm).

(2) Arsenic *<1.11>*—Prepare the test solution with 2.0 g of Mukoi-Daikenchuto Extract according to Method 3, and perform the test (not more than 1 ppm).

Loss on drying *<2.41>* Not more than 5.9% (1 g, 105°C, 5 hours).

Total ash *<5.01>* Not more than 10.0%.

Assay **(1)** Ginsenoside Rb_1—Weigh accurately about 2 g of Mukoi-Daikenchuto Extract, add 30 mL of diluted methanol (3 in 5), shake for 15 minutes, centrifuge, and separate the supernatant liquid. To the residue add 15 mL of diluted methanol (3 in 5), and repeat the same procedure. Combine the supernatant liquids, and add diluted methanol (3 in 5) to make exactly 50 mL. Pipet 10 mL of this solution, add 3 mL of sodium hydroxide TS, allow to stand for 30 minutes, add 3 mL of 1 mol/L hydrochloric acid TS, and add water to make exactly 20 mL. Apply exactly 5 mL of this solution to a column [10 mm in inside diameter, packed with 0.36 g of octadecylsilanized silica gel for pre-treatment (55 – 105 μm in particle size), and washed just before using with methanol and then diluted methanol (3 in 10)], and wash the column in sequence with 2 mL of diluted methanol (3 in 10), 1 mL of sodium carbonate TS and 10 mL of diluted methanol (3 in 10). Finally, elute with methanol to collect exactly 5 mL, and use this solution as the sample solution. Separately, weigh accurately about 10 mg of Ginsenoside Rb_1 RS (separately determine the water *<2.48>* by coulometric titration, using 10 mg), and dissolve in methanol to make exactly 100 mL. Pipet 10 mL of this solution, add methanol to make exactly 50 mL, and use this solution as the standard solution. Perform the test with exactly 20 μL each of the sample solution and standard solution as directed under Liquid Chromatography <*2.01*> according to the following conditions, and determine the peak areas, A_T and A_S, of ginsenoside Rb_1 in each solution.

$$\text{Amount (mg) of ginsenoside } Rb_1\ (C_{54}H_{92}O_{23}) = M_S \times A_T/A_S \times 1/5$$

M_S: Amount (mg) of Ginsenoside Rb_1 RS taken, calculated on the anhydrous basis

Operating conditions—

Detector: An ultraviolet absorption photometer (wavelength: 203 nm).

Column: A stainless steel column 4.6 mm in inside diameter and 25 cm in length, packed with carbamoyl group bound silica gel for liquid chromatography (5 µm in particle diameter).

Column temperature: A constant temperature of about 60°C.

Mobile phase: A mixture of acetonitrile, water and phosphoric acid (400:100:1).

Flow rate: 1.0 mL per minute (the retention time of ginsenoside Rb_1 is about 16 minutes).

System suitability—

System performance: When the procedure is run with 20 µL of the standard solution under the above operating conditions, the number of theoretical plates and the symmetry factor of the peak of ginsenoside Rb_1 are not less than 5000 and not more than 1.5, respectively.

System repeatability: When the test is repeated 6 times with 20 µL of the standard solution under the above operating conditions, the relative standard deviation of the peak area of ginsenoside Rb_1 is not more than 1.5%.

(2) [6]-Shogaol—Weigh accurately about 0.5 g of Mukoi-Daikenchuto Extract, add exactly 50 mL of diluted methanol (3 in 4), shake for 15 minutes, centrifuge, and use the supernatant liquid as the sample solution. Separately, weigh accurately about 10 mg of [6]-shogaol for assay, dissolve in diluted methanol (3 in 4) to make exactly 100 mL. Pipet 10 mL of this solution, add diluted methanol (3 in 4) to make exactly 50 mL, and use this solution as the standard solution. Perform the test with exactly 20 µL each of the sample solution and standard solution as directed under Liquid Chromatography <*2.01*> according to the following conditions, and determine the peak areas, A_T and A_S, of [6]-shogaol in each solution.

$$\text{Amount (mg) of [6]-shogaol} = M_S \times A_T/A_S \times 1/10$$

M_S: Amount (mg) of [6]-shogaol for assay taken

Operating conditions—

Detector: An ultraviolet absorption photometer (wavelength: 225 nm).

Column: A stainless steel column 4.6 mm in inside diameter and 15 cm in length, packed with octylsilanized silica gel for liquid chromatography (5 µm in particle diameter).

Column temperature: A constant temperature of about 50°C.

Mobile phase: Dissolve 0.1 g of oxalic acid dihydrate in 600 mL of water, and add 400 mL of acetonitrile.

Flow rate: 1.0 mL per minute (the retention time of [6]-shogaol is about 30 minutes).

System suitability—

System performance: When the procedure is run with 20 µL of the standard solution under the above operating conditions, the number of theoretical plates and the symmetry factor of the peak of [6]-shogaol are not less than 5000 and not more than 1.5, respectively.

System repeatability: When the test is repeated 6 times with 20 µL of the standard solution under the above operating conditions, the relative standard deviation of the peak area of [6]-shogaol is not more than 1.5%.

Containers and storage Containers—Tight containers.

Mulberry Bark

Mori Cortex

ソウハクヒ

Mulberry Bark is the root bark of *Morus alba* Linné (*Moraceae*).

Description Tubular, semi-tubular or cord-like bark, 1 - 6 mm thick, often in fine lateral cuttings; externally, white to yellow-brown; in the case of the bark with periderm, its periderm is yellow-brown in color, easy to peel, with numerous longitudinal, fine wrinkles and numerous red-purple lenticels laterally elongated; inner surface, dark yellow-brown in color and flat; cross section, white to light brown in color, and fibrous.

Odor, slight; taste, slight.

Under a microscope <*5.01*>, a transverse section of bark with periderm reveals 5 to 12 cellular layers of cork cells in the outer portion; phloem fibers or their bundles scattered in the cortex, arranged alternately and stepwise with phloem parenchyma; lactiferous tubes; solitary crystals of calcium oxalate; starch grains as spheroidal or ellipsoidal, simple or compound grains, simple grain 1 - 7 µm in diameter.

Identification Heat 1 g of pulverized Mulberry Bark with 20 mL of hexane under a reflux condenser for 15 minutes, and filter. Evaporate the solvent of the filtrate under low pressure (in vacuo), dissolve the residue in 10 mL of acetic anhydride, place 0.5 mL of the solution in a test tube, and add carefully 0.5 mL of sulfuric acid to make two layers: a red-brown color develops at the zone of contact.

Purity **(1)** Heavy metals <*1.07*>—Proceed with 3.0 g of pulverized Mulberry Bark according to Method 3, and perform the test. Prepare the control solution with 3.0 mL of Standard Lead Solution (not more than 10 ppm).

(2) Arsenic <*1.11*>—Prepare the test solution with 0.40 g of pulverized Mulberry Bark according to Method 4, and perform the test (not more than 5 ppm).

(3) Foreign matter <*5.01*>—The amount of the root xylem and other foreign matter is not more than 1.0%.

Total ash <*5.01*> Not more than 11.0%.

Acid-insoluble ash <*5.01*> Not more than 1.0%.

Containers and storage Containers—Well-closed containers.

Nelumbo Seed

Nelumbinis Semen

レンニク

Nelumbo Seed is the seed of *Nelumbo nucifera* Gaertner (*Nymphaeaceae*), usually with the endocarp, sometime being removed the embryo.

Description Ovoid to ellipsoidal seed, at the base a papillate protuberance surrounded with shallow depression, 1.0 – 1.7 cm in length, 0.5 – 1.2 cm in width; externally light red-brown to light yellow-brown; projection part dark reddish brown; endocarp not lustrous and hardly peeled off; endosperm yellow-white, a green embryo in the center.

Almost odorless; taste, slightly sweet and oily, embryo is extremely bitter.

Under a microscope *<5.01>*, a transverse section of the seed at central portion reveals endocarp composed of parenchyma or endocarp occasionally left out; seed coat composed of epidermis and parenchyma of compressed cells; vascular bundles scattered in parenchyma; endosperm composed of epidermis and parenchyma; aggregate crystals of calcium oxalate and tannin-like substances contained in endocarp remained; parenchymatous cells of seed coat contain tannin-like substances; parenchyma of endosperm contain starch grains.

Identification To 0.5 g of pulverized Nelumbo Seed add 5 mL of water, shake for 5 minutes, and centrifuge. To 0.5 mL of the supernatant liquid add 1 drop of a solution of 1-naphthol in ethanol (99.5) (1 in 5), mix, then add gently 1 mL of sulfuric acid: the solution shows a purple color.

Loss on drying *<5.01>* Not more than 14.0% (6 hours).

Total ash *<5.01>* Not more than 5.0%.

Extract content *<5.01>* Dilute ethanol-soluble extract: not less than 14.5%.

Containers and storage Containers—Well-closed containers.

Notopterygium

Notopterygii Rhizoma

キョウカツ

Notopterygium is the rhizome and root of *Notopterygium incisum* Ting ex H. T. Chang or *Notopterygium forbesii* Boissieu (*Umbelliferae*).

Description Notopterygium is slightly curved, cylindrical to conical, 3 – 10 cm in length, 5 – 20 mm in diameter; rhizome occasionally branched; externally yellow-brown to dark brown. The rhizome with nearly orbicular, hollowed stem scars at the apex, sometimes having short residue of stem; externally node rising, internode short; root scars in warty processes on the node; externally root has coarse longitudinal wrinkles and lateral root scars in warty processes; light and slightly brittle in texture, easy to break. The transverse section of the rhizome reveals numerous radial cracks; cortex yellow-brown to brown; xylem light yellow to light grayish yellow; pith grayish white to light brown. Under a magnifying glass, the rhizome reveals brown, fine points of resin canals in the cortex and pith.

Odor, characteristic; taste, a slight characteristic taste at first, followed by a slightly pungent and slightly numbing aftertaste.

Under a microscope *<5.01>*, transverse section shows the outermost layer to be composed of a cork layer several to a dozen or so cells thick; several-layered collenchyma just inside of the cork layer; oil canals scattered in cortex, large ones more than 300 μm in diameter; intercellular space occurring in radial direction in cortex; oil canals scattered in pith, large ones more than 500 μm in diameter; parenchymatous cells contain simple and 2- to 3-compound starch grains.

Identification To 0.3 g of pulverized Notopterygium add 3 mL of hexane in a glass-stoppered centrifuge tube, shake for 10 minutes, centrifuge, and use the supernatant liquid as the sample solution. Perform the test with the sample solution as directed under Thin-layer Chromatography *<2.03>*. Spot 10 μL of the sample solution on a plate of octadecylsilanized silica gel with fluorescent indicator for thin-layer chromatography, develop the plate with a mixture of methanol and water (9:1) to a distance of about 7 cm, and air-dry the plate. Examine under ultraviolet light (main wavelength: 365 nm): a blue-white fluorescent spot appears at an *R*f value of about 0.5, which shows a dark purple color under ultraviolet light (main wavelength: 254 nm).

Purity **(1)** Heavy metals *<1.07>*—Proceed with 3.0 g of pulverized Notopterygium according to Method 3, and perform the test. Prepare the control solution with 3.0 mL of Standard Lead Solution (not more than 10 ppm).

(2) Arsenic *<1.11>*—Prepare the test solution with 0.40 g of pulverized Notopterygium according to Method 4, and perform the test (not more than 5 ppm).

Loss on drying *<5.01>* Not more than 13.0% (6 hours).

Total ash *<5.01>* Not more than 6.5%.

Acid-insoluble ash *<5.01>* Not more than 1.5%.

Extract content *<5.01>* Dilute ethanol-soluble extract: not less than 20.0%.

Containers and storage Containers—Well-closed containers.

Nuphar Rhizome

Nupharis Rhizoma

センコツ

Nuphar Rhizome is the longitudinally split rhizome of *Nuphar japonica* De Candolle, *Nuphar pumila* De Candolle, or their interspecific hybrids (*Nymphaeaceae*).

Description Usually, longitudinally split irregular column, twisted, bent or somewhat pressed, 20 – 30 cm in length, about 2 cm in width; the outer surface, dark brown, and the cut surface, white to grayish white in color; one side shows nearly round to blunt triangular scars of petiole about 1 cm in diameter, and the other side numerous scars of roots less than 0.3 cm in diameter; light, spongy in texture, and easily broken; fractured surface flat and powdery. Under a magnifying glass, a transverse section reveals a black outer portion, and porous tissue with scattered vascular bundles in the inner portion.

Odor, slight; taste, slightly bitter and unpleasant.

Identification To 1.0 g of pulverized Nuphar Rhizome add 5 mL of methanol, shake for 10 minutes, centrifuge, and use the supernatant liquid as the sample solution. Perform the test with the sample solution as directed under Thin-layer Chromatography <*2.03*>. Spot 5 μL of the sample solution on a plate of silica gel for thin-layer chromatography, develop the plate with a mixture of ethyl acetate, methanol and ammonia solution (28) (20:3:2) to a distance of about 7 cm, and air-dry the plate. Spray evenly Dragendorff's TS for spraying on the plate: a yellow-brown spot appears at an *Rf* value of about 0.4.

Purity **(1)** Heavy metals <*1.07*>—Proceed with 3.0 g of pulverized Nuphar Rhizome according to Method 3, and perform the test. Prepare the control solution with 3.0 mL of Standard Lead Solution (not more than 10 ppm).

(2) Arsenic <*1.11*>—Prepare the test solution with 0.40 g of pulverized Nuphar Rhizome according to Method 4, and perform the test (not more than 5 ppm).

(3) Petiole—When perform the test of foreign matter <*5.01*>, the amount of the petioles contained in Nuphar Rhizome does not exceed 3.0%.

(4) Foreign matter <*5.01*>—The amount of foreign matter other than petioles is not more than 1.0%.

Loss on drying <*5.01*> Not more than 15.0% (6 hours).

Total ash <*5.01*> Not more than 10.0%.

Acid-insoluble ash <*5.01*> Not more than 1.0%.

Containers and storage Containers—Well-closed containers.

Nutmeg

Myristicae Semen

ニクズク

Nutmeg is the seed of *Myristica fragrans* Houttuyn (*Myristicaceae*), usually from which the seed coat is removed.

Description Ovoid-globose to ellipsoidal seeds, 1.5 - 3.0 cm in length, 1.3 - 2.0 cm in diameter; externally grayish brown, with wide and shallow longitudinal furrows and fine wrinkles; usually, reveals a hilum at one end, the hilum grayish white to grayish yellow and slightly protruding, and a chalaza at the other end, the chalaza grayish brown to dark brown and slightly concave; dark brown thin perisperm extending irregularly into the light yellow-white to light brown endosperm, by which cut surface exhibiting a marble-like appearance.

Odor, characteristic and strong; taste, acrid and slightly bitter.

Under a microscope <*5.01*>, a transverse section reveals perisperm composed of outer and inner layers; the outer layer composed of parenchyma containing red-brown to dark red-brown contents; the inner layer, composed of parenchyma filled with red-brown to dark red-brown contents, often extends into endosperm, where numerous oil cells are scattered: several vascular bundles present in the inner layer, the vessels spiral; in parenchyma cells of endosperm, simple or compound starch grains and aleurone grains observed; and in the parenchyma cells in the outer layer of perisperm and the marginal part of endosperm, numerous crystals of calcium oxalate observed.

Identification To 1 g of pulverized Nutmeg add 5 mL of methanol, allow to stand for 10 minutes with occasional shaking, filter, and use the filtrate as the sample solution. Separately, dissolve 2 mg of myristicin for thin-layer chromatography in 1 mL of ethanol (95), and use this solution as the standard solution. Perform the test with these solutions as directed under Thin-layer Chromatography <*2.03*>. Spot 5 μL each of the sample solution and standard solution on a plate of silica gel for thin-layer chromatography. Develop the plate with a mixture of hexane and acetone (9:1) to a distance of about 7 cm, and air-dry the plate. Spray evenly diluted sulfuric acid on the plate, and heat the plate at 105°C for 5 minutes: one of the several spots obtained from the sample solution has the same color tone and *Rf* value with the spot from the standard solution.

Loss on drying <*5.01*> Not more than 16.0% (6 hours).

Total ash <*5.01*> Not more than 2.5%.

Essential oil content <*5.01*> When the test is performed with 10.0 g of pulverized Nutmeg, the essential oil content is not less than 0.5 mL.

Containers and storage Containers—Well-closed containers.

Nux Vomica

Strychni Semen

ホミカ

Nux Vomica is the seed of *Strychnos nux-vomica* Linné (*Loganiaceae*).

When dried, it contains not less than 1.07% of strychnine.

Description Disk, often slightly bent, 1 - 3 cm in diameter, 0.3 - 0.5 cm in thickness; externally light grayish yellow-green to light grayish brown, covered densely with lustrous appressed hairs radiating from the center to the circumference; on both sides, the margin and the central part bulged a little; the dot-like micropyle situated at one point on the margin, and from which usually a raised line runs to the center on one side; extremely hard in texture; when cracked upon soaking in water, the seed coat thin, the interior consisting of two horny, light grayish yellow endosperms, and leaving a central narrow cavity at the center; a white embryo, about 0.7 cm in length, situated at one end between the inner surfaces of the endosperms.

Odorless.

Identification **(1)** To 3 g of pulverized Nux Vomica add 3 mL of ammonia TS and 20 mL of chloroform, macerate for 30 minutes with occasional shaking, and filter. Remove most of the chloroform from the filtrate by warming on a water bath, add 5 mL of diluted sulfuric acid (1 in 10), and warm on a water bath while shaking well until the odor of chloroform is no longer perceptible. After cooling, filter through a pledget of absorbent cotton, and add 2 mL of nitric acid to 1 mL of the filtrate: a red color develops.

(2) To the remaining filtrate obtained in (1) add 1 mL of potassium dichromate TS, and allow to stand for 1 hour: a yellow-red precipitate is produced. Collect the precipitate by filtration, and wash with 1 mL of water. Transfer a part of the precipitate to a small test tube, add 1 mL of water, dissolve by warming, cool, and add 5 drops of sulfuric acid dropwise carefully along the wall of the test tube: the layer of sulfuric acid shows a purple color which turns immediately red to red-brown.

Total ash <*5.01*> Not more than 3.0%.

Assay Weigh accurately about 1 g of pulverized Nux Vomica, previously dried at 60°C for 8 hours, place in a glass-stoppered centrifuge tube, and moisten with 1 mL of ammonia solution (28). To this solution add 20 mL of diethyl ether, stopper the centrifuge tube tightly, shake for 15 minutes, centrifuge, and separate the supernatant liquid. To the residue add 20 mL of diethyl ether, proceed in the same manner, and repeat this procedure three times. Combine all the extracts, and evaporate the solvent on a water bath. Dissolve the residue in 10 mL of the mobile phase, add exactly 10 mL of the internal standard solution, and add the mobile phase to make 100 mL. Filter this solution through a membrane filter with a porosity not more than 0.8 μm, discard the first 2 mL of the filtrate, and use the subsequent filtrate as the sample solution. Separately, weigh accurately about 75 mg of strychnine nitrate for assay (separately determine the loss on drying), and dissolve in the mobile phase to make exactly 50 mL. Pipet 10 mL of this solution, add exactly 10 mL of the internal standard solution, then add the mobile phase to make 100 mL, and use this solution as the standard solution. Perform the test with exactly 5 μL each of the sample solution and standard solution as directed under Liquid Chromatography <*2.01*> according to the following conditions. Calculate the ratio, Q_T and Q_S, of the peak area of strychnine to that of the internal standard.

Amount (mg) of strychnine = $M_S \times Q_T/Q_S \times 1/5 \times 0.841$

M_S: Amount (mg) of strychnine nitrate for assay taken, calculated on the dried basis

Internal standard solution—A solution of barbital sodium in the mobile phase (1 in 500).

Operating conditions—

Detector: An ultraviolet absorption photometer (wavelength: 210 nm).

Column: A stainless steel column about 4 mm in inside diameter and about 15 cm in length, packed with octadecylsilanized silica gel for liquid chromatography (5 μm in particle diameter).

Column temperature: Room temperature.

Mobile phase: Dissolve 6.8 g of potassium dihydrogenphosphate in water to make 1000 mL, and mix with acetonitrile and triethylamine (45:5:1), and adjust the mixture with phosphoric acid to pH 3.0.

Flow rate: Adjust so that the retention time of Strychnine is about 17 minutes.

System suitability—

System performance: When the procedure is run with 5 μL of the standard solution under the above operating conditions, the internal standard and strychnine are eluted in this order with the resolution between these peaks being not less than 1.5.

Containers and storage Containers—Well-closed containers.

Nux Vomica Extract

ホミカエキス

Nux Vomica Extract contains not less than 6.15% and not more than 6.81% of strychnine ($C_{21}H_{22}N_2O_2$: 334.41).

Method of preparation After defatting 1000 g of coarse powder of Nux Vomica with hexane, extract with the percolation method, using a mixture of 750 mL of Ethanol, 10 mL of Acetic Acid and 240 mL of Purified Water or Purified Water in Containers as the first solvent, and 70 vol% ethanol as the second solvent. Combine the extracts, and prepare the dry extract as directed under Extracts. Where, an appropriate quantity of Ethanol and Purified Water or Purified Water in Containers may be used instead of 70 vol% ethanol.

Description Nux Vomica Extract occurs as yellow-brown to brown powder. It has a slight characteristic odor, and an extremely bitter taste.

Identification Extract 0.5 g of Nux Vomica Extract with 0.5 mL of ammonia TS and 10 mL of chloroform with occasional shaking. Filter the chloroform extract, evaporate the filtrate on a water bath until most of the chloroform is removed, and proceed as directed in the Identification under Nux Vomica.

Purity Heavy metals <*1.07*>—Prepare the test solution with 1.0 g of Nux Vomica Extract as directed in the Extracts (4), and perform the test (not more than 30 ppm).

Assay Weigh accurately about 0.2 g of Nux Vomica Extract, place in a glass-stoppered centrifuge tube, add 15 mL of ammonia TS, and shake. Add 20 mL of diethyl ether, stopper tightly, shake for 15 minutes, centrifuge to disperse the diethyl ether layer. To the aqueous layer add 20 mL of diethyl ether, proceed in the same manner, and repeat this procedure three times. Combine the extracts, and evaporate the solvent on a water bath. Dissolve the residue in 10 mL of the mobile phase, add exactly 10 mL of the internal standard solution, and add the mobile phase to make 100 mL. Then, proceed as directed in the Assay under Nux Vomica.

Amount (mg) of strychnine = $M_S \times Q_T/Q_S \times 1/5 \times 0.841$

M_S: Amount (mg) of strychnine nitrate for assay taken, calculated on the dried basis

Internal standard solution—A solution of barbital sodium in the mobile phase (1 in 500).

Containers and storage Containers—Tight containers.

Storage—Light-resistant.

Nux Vomica Extract Powder

ホミカエキス散

Nux Vomica Extract Powder contains not less than 0.61% and not more than 0.68% of strychnine.

Method of preparation

Nux Vomica Extract	100 g
Starch, Lactose Hydrate or their mixture	a sufficient quantity
To make	1000 g

To Nux Vomica Extract add 100 mL of Purified Water or Purified Water in Containers, then warm, and soften with stirring. Cool, add 800 g of Starch, Lactose Hydrate or their mixture little by little, and mix well. Dry, preferably at a low temperature, and dilute with a sufficient additional quantity of Starch, Lactose or their mixture to make 1000 g of the homogeneous powder.

Description Nux Vomica Extract Powder occurs as a yellow-brown to grayish brown powder. It has a slight, characteristic odor and a bitter taste.

Identification **(1)** To 3 g of Nux Vomica Extract Powder add 3 mL of ammonia TS and 20 mL of chloroform, macerate for 30 minutes with occasional shaking, and filter. Remove most of the chloroform from the filtrate by warming on a water bath, add 5 mL of diluted sulfuric acid (1 in 10), and warm on a water bath while shaking well until the odor of chloroform is no longer perceptible. After cooling, filter through a pledget of absorbent cotton, and add 2 mL of nitric acid to 1 mL of the filtrate: a red color develops.

(2) To the remaining filtrate obtained in (1) add 1 mL of potassium dichromate TS, and allow to stand for 1 hour: a yellow-red precipitate is produced. Collect the precipitate by filtration, and wash with 1 mL of water. Transfer a part of the precipitate to a small test tube, add 1 mL of water, dissolve by warming, cool, and add 5 drops of sulfuric acid dropwise carefully along the wall of the test tube: the layer of sulfuric acid shows a purple color which turns immediately red to red-brown.

Assay Weigh accurately about 2.0 g of Nux Vomica Extract Powder, place in a glass-stoppered centrifuge tube, add 15 mL of ammonia TS, and shake. Add 20 mL of diethyl ether, stopper tightly, shake for 15 minutes, centrifuge to separate the diethyl ether layer. To the aqueous layer add 20 mL of diethyl ether, proceed in the same manner, and repeat this procedure three times. Combine the extracts, and evaporate the solvent on a water bath. Dissolve the residue in 10 mL of the mobile phase, add exactly 10 mL of the internal standard solution, and add the mobile phase to make 100 mL. Filter this solution through a membrane filter with a porosity not more than 0.8 μm, discard the first 2 mL of the filtrate, and use the subsequent filtrate as the sample solution. Separately, weigh accurately about 75 mg of strychnine nitrate for assay (separately determine the loss on drying), and dissolve in the mobile phase to make exactly 50 mL. Pipet 10 mL of this solution, add exactly 10 mL of the internal standard solution, then add the mobile phase to make 100 mL, and use this solution as the standard solution. Perform the test with exactly 5 μL each of the sample solution and standard solution as directed under Liquid Chromatography <*2.01*> according to the following conditions. Calculate the ratio, Q_T and Q_S, of the peak area of strychnine to that of the internal standard.

Amount (mg) of strychnine = $M_S \times Q_T/Q_S \times 1/5 \times 0.841$

M_S: Amount (mg) of strychnine nitrate for assay taken, calculated on the dried basis

Internal standard solution—A solution of barbital sodium in the mobile phase (1 in 500).

Operating conditions—

Detector: An ultraviolet absorption photometer (wavelength: 210 nm).

Column: A stainless steel column about 4 mm in inside diameter and about 15 cm in length, packed with octadecylsilanized silica gel for liquid chromatography (5 μm in particle diameter).

Column temperature: Room temperature.

Mobile phase: A mixture of a solution of potassium dihydrogenphosphate (6.8 in 1000), acetonitrile and triethylamine (45:5:1), adjusted the pH to 3.0 with phosphoric acid.

Flow rate: Adjust so that the retention time of strychnine is about 17 minutes.

System suitability—

System performance: When the procedure is run with 5 μL of the standard solution under the above operating conditions, the internal standard and strychnine are eluted in this order with the resolution between these peaks being not less than 1.5.

Containers and storage Containers—Tight containers.

Storage—Light-resistant.

Nux Vomica Tincture

ホミカチンキ

Nux Vomica Tincture contains not less than 0.097 w/v% and not more than 0.116 w/v% of strychnine.

Method of preparation

Nux Vomica, in coarse powder	100 g
70 vol% Ethanol	a sufficient quantity
To make	1000 mL

Prepare as directed under Tinctures, with the above ingredients. May be prepared with an appropriate quantity of Ethanol and Purified Water or Purified Water in Containers.

Description Nux Vomica Tincture is a yellow-brown liquid. It has an extremely bitter taste.

Specific gravity d^{20}_{20}: about 0.90

Identification Heat 20 mL of Nux Vomica Tincture on a water bath to remove ethanol, cool, transfer to a separator, add 2 mL of ammonia TS and 20 mL of chloroform, and shake well for 2 to 3 minutes. Filter the chloroform layer through a pledget of absorbent cotton, warm the filtrate on a water bath to remove most of chloroform, and proceed as directed in the Identification under Nux Vomica.

Alcohol number <*1.01*> Not less than 6.7 (Method 2).

Assay Pipet 3 mL of Nux Vomica Tincture into a glass-stoppered centrifuge tube, add 10 mL of ammonia TS and 20 mL of diethyl ether, stopper tightly, shake for 15 minutes, centrifuge to separate the diethyl ether layer. To the aqueous layer add 20 mL of diethyl ether, proceed in the same manner, and repeat this procedure twice. Combine the extracts, and evaporate the solvent on a water bath. Dissolve the residue with 10 mL of the mobile phase, add exactly 5 mL of the internal standard solution, and add the mobile phase to make 50 mL. Filter the solution through a membrane filter with a pore size not exceeding 0.8-μm, discard the first 2 mL of the filtrate, and use the subsequent filtrate as the sample solution. Separately, weigh accurately about 75 mg of strychnine nitrate for assay (separately determine the loss on drying), and dissolve in the mobile phase to make exactly 100 mL. Pipet 5 mL of this solution, add exactly 5 mL of the internal standard solution, add the mobile phase to make 50 mL, and use this solution as the standard solution. Proceed with the sample solution and the standard solution as directed in the Assay under Nux Vomica.

Amount (mg) of strychnine = $M_S \times Q_T/Q_S \times 1/20 \times 0.841$

M_S: Amount (mg) of strychnine nitrate for assay taken, calculated on the dried basis

Internal standard solution—A solution of barbital sodium in the mobile phase (1 in 500).

Containers and storage Containers—Tight containers.
Storage—Light-resistant.

Olive Oil

Oleum Olivae

オリブ油

Olive Oil is the fixed oil obtained by expression from the ripe fruit of *Olea europaea* Linné (*Oleaceae*).

Description Olive Oil is a light yellow oil. It has a faint odor, which is not rancid, and has a bland taste.

It is miscible with diethyl ether, with petroleum ether.

It is slightly soluble in ethanol (95).

The whole or a part of it congeals between 0°C and 6°C.

Congealing point of the fatty acids: 17 – 26°C

Specific gravity <*1.13*> d^{25}_{25}: 0.908 – 0.914

Acid value <*1.13*> Not more than 1.0.

Saponification value <*1.13*> 186 – 194

Unsaponifiable matters <*1.13*> Not more than 1.5%.

Iodine value <*1.13*> 79 – 88

Purity **(1)** Drying oil—Mix 2 mL of Olive Oil with 10 mL of diluted nitric acid (1 in 4), add 1 g of powdered sodium nitrite little by little with thorough shaking, and allow to stand in a cold place for 4 to 10 hours: the mixture congeals to a white solid.

(2) Peanut oil—Weigh exactly 1.0 g of Olive Oil, dissolve in 60 mL of sulfuric acid-hexane-methanol TS, heat for 2.5 hours under a reflux condenser, cool, transfer to a separator, and add 100 mL of water. Wash the vessel for the reflux extraction with 50 mL of petroleum ether, add the washing to the separator, shake, allow to stand, and separate the petroleum ether layer. Extract the aqueous layer with another 50 mL of petroleum ether, and combine the petroleum ether layer with the former petroleum ether solution. Wash the petroleum ether solution repeatedly with 20-mL portions of water until the washings show no more acidity to methyl orange TS. Then add 5 g of anhydrous sodium sulfate, shake, filter, wash anhydrous sodium sulfate with two 10-mL portions of petroleum ether, and filter the washings using the former separator. Combine all the filtrates, distil the solvent on a water bath, passing nitrogen. Dissolve the residue in acetone to make exactly 20 mL, and use this solution as the sample solution. Separately, dissolve 0.067 g of methyl behenate in acetone to make exactly 50 mL. Pipet 2 mL of this solution, add acetone to make exactly 20 mL, and use this solution as the standard solution. Perform the test with exactly 2 μL each of the sample solution and standard solution as directed under Gas Chromatography <*2.02*> according to the following conditions. Measure the peak heights, H_T and H_S, of methyl behenate of respective solutions: H_T is not higher than H_S.

Operating conditions—

Detector: A hydrogen flame-ionization detector.

Column: A glass column about 3 mm in inside diameter and about 2 m in length, packed with silanized siliceous earth for gas chromatography (150 to 180 μm in particle diameter), coated with polyethylene glycol 20 mol/L in a ratio of 5%.

Column temperature: A constant temperature of about 220°C.

Carrier gas: Nitrogen.

Flow rate: Adjust so that the retention time of methyl behenate is about 18 minutes.

System suitability—

Test for required detectability: Adjust so that the peak height of methyl behenate obtained with 2 μL of the standard solution is 5 to 10 mm.

Containers and storage Containers—Tight containers.

Ophiopogon Root

Ophiopogonis Radix

バクモンドウ

Ophiopogon Root is the enlarged part of the root of *Ophiopogon japonicus* Ker-Gawler (*Liliaceae*).

Description Fusiform root, 1 – 2.5 cm in length, 0.3 – 0.5 cm in diameter, somewhat sharp at one end, and somewhat rounded at the other; externally light yellow to light yellow-brown, with longitudinal wrinkles of various sizes; when fractured, cortex flexible and friable, stele strong; fractured surface of cortex light yellow-brown in color, slightly translucent and viscous.

Odor, slight; taste, slightly sweet and mucous.

Under a microscope <*5.01*>, a transverse section reveals brown, 4- to 5-cellular layer velamen internally adjoining the epidermis; a single-layer exodermis inside the velamen, and cortex of parenchyma cells inside the exodermis; endodermis is distinct; about 20 protoxylems in actionstele; cortex parenchyma contains columnar crystals and raphides of calcium oxalate; oil drops in the exodermis.

Purity **(1)** Heavy metals <*1.07*>—Proceed with 3.0 g of pulverized Ophiopogon Root according to Method 3, and perform the test. Prepare the control solution with 3.0 mL of Standard Lead Solution (not more than 10 ppm).

(2) Arsenic <*1.11*>—Prepare the test solution with 0.40 g of pulverized Ophiopogon Root according to Method 4, and perform the test (not more than 5 ppm).

(3) Rootlets—When perform the test of foreign matter <*5.01*>, the amount of the rootlets contained in Ophiopogon Root is not exceed 1.0%.

Total ash *<5.01>* Not more than 3.0%.

Containers and storage Containers—Well-closed containers.

Powdered Opium

Opium Pulveratum

アヘン末

Powdered Opium is a homogeneous powder of opium obtained from *Papaver somniferum* Linné (*Papaveraceae*). Starch or Lactose Hydrate may be added.

Powdered Opium contains not less than 9.5% and not more than 10.5% of morphine ($C_{17}H_{19}NO_3$: 285.34).

Description Powdered Opium occurs as a yellow-brown to dark brown powder.

Identification **(1)** To 0.1 g of Powdered Opium add 5 mL of diluted ethanol (7 in 10), dissolve by sonicating for 10 minutes, and add diluted ethanol (7 in 10) to make 10 mL. Filter this solution, and use the filtrate as the sample solution. Separately, dissolve 25 mg of Morphine Hydrochloride Hydrate, 12 mg of Codeine Phosphate Hydrate, 2 mg of Papaverine Hydrochloride, and 12 mg of Noscapine Hydrochloride Hydrate separately in 25 mL of diluted ethanol (7 in 10), and use these solutions as the standard solution (1), the standard solution (2), the standard solution (3) and the standard solution (4), respectively. Perform the test with these solutions as directed under Thin-layer Chromatography *<2.03>*. Spot 10 μL each of the sample solution and standard solutions on a plate of silica gel for thin-layer chromatography. Develop the plate with a mixture of acetone, toluene, ethanol (99.5) and ammonia water (28) (20:20:3:1) to a distance of about 10 cm, and air-dry the plate. Spray evenly Dragendorff's TS for spraying on the plate: each spot obtained from the sample solution shows the same color tone and *R*f value of each spot from the standard solution (1), the standard solution (2), the standard solution (3), and the standard solution (4) (morphine, codeine, papaverine and noscapine), respectively.

(2) To 0.1 g of Powdered Opium add 5 mL of water, and shake the mixture for 5 minutes. Filter, to the filtrate add 1 mL of a solution of hydroxylammonium chloride (3 in 10) and 1 drop of iron (III) chloride TS, and shake: a red-brown color is produced. To this solution add immediately 5 mL of diethyl ether, and shake: the diethyl ether layer has no red-purple color (meconic acid).

Loss on drying *<2.41>* Not more than 8.0% (1 g, 105°C, 5 hours).

Assay Place about 5 g of Powdered Opium, accurately weighed, in a mortar, and triturate it with exactly 10 mL of water. Add 2 g of calcium hydroxide and exactly 40 mL of water, and stir the mixture for 20 minutes. Filter, and shake 30 mL of the filtrate with 0.1 g of magnesium sulfate heptahydrate for 1 minute. To the mixture add 0.3 g of calcium hydroxide, shake for 1 minute, and allow to stand for 1 hour. Filter, place 20 mL of the filtrate, exactly measured, in a glass-stoppered flask, and add 10 mL of diethyl ether and 0.3 g of ammonium chloride. Shake vigorously with caution. When crystals begin to separate out, shake for 30 minutes with a mechanical shaker, and set aside overnight at a temperature of 5°C to 10°C. Decant the diethyl ether layer and filter first, and then the aqueous layer through filter paper 7 cm in diameter. Wash the adhering crystals in the flask with three 5-mL portions of water saturated with diethyl ether, and wash the crystals on the filter paper with each of these washings. Wash the top of the glass-stoppered flask and the upper part of the filter paper with final 5 mL of water saturated with diethyl ether. Transfer the crystals and the filter paper to a beaker. Dissolve the crystals remaining in the glass-stoppered flask with the aid of 15 mL of 0.05 mol/L sulfuric acid VS, accurately measured, and pour the solution into the beaker. Wash the glass-stoppered flask with four 5-mL portions of water, and add the washings to the solution in the beaker. Titrate *<2.50>* the excess sulfuric acid with 0.1 mol/L sodium hydroxide VS (indicator: 4 drops of methyl red-methylene blue TS).

Each mL of 0.05 mol/L sulfuric acid VS
= 28.53 mg of $C_{17}H_{19}NO_3$

Containers and storage Containers—Tight containers.

Diluted Opium Powder

アヘン散

Diluted Opium Powder contains not less than 0.90% and not more than 1.10% of morphine ($C_{17}H_{19}NO_3$: 285.34).

Method of preparation

Powdered Opium	100 g
Starch or a suitable diluent	a sufficient quantity
To make	1000 g

Prepare as directed under Powders, with the above ingredients. Lactose Hydrate should not be used.

Description Diluted Opium Powder occurs as a light brown powder.

Identification **(1)** Proceed with 1 g of Diluted Opium Powder as directed in the Identification (1) under Powdered Opium.

(2) Proceed with 1 g of Diluted Opium Powder as directed in the Identification (2) under Powdered Opium.

Assay Place about 50 g of Diluted Opium Powder, accurately weighed, in a glass-stoppered flask, and stir with 250 mL of dilute ethanol in a water bath at 40°C for 1 hour. Filter the mixture through a glass filter (G3). Transfer the residue on the filter to the first glass-stoppered flask, and add 50 mL of dilute ethanol. Stir the mixture in a water bath at 40°C for 10 minutes, and filter through the same glass filter. Repeat the extraction with three 50-mL portions of dilute ethanol. Evaporate the combined filtrate in a mortar to dryness on a water bath. Add 10 mL of ethanol (99.5) to the residue, evaporate to dryness again, and, after cooling, triturate it with exactly 10 mL of water. Proceed with this solution as directed in Assay under Powdered Opium.

Each mL of 0.05 mol/L sulfuric acid VS
= 28.53 mg of $C_{17}H_{19}NO_3$

Containers and storage Containers—Tight containers.

Opium Tincture

アヘンチンキ

Opium Tincture contains not less than 0.93 w/v% and not more than 1.07 w/v% of morphine ($C_{17}H_{19}NO_3$: 285.34).

Method of preparation

Powdered Opium	100 g
35 vol% Ethanol	a sufficient quantity
To make	1000 mL

Prepare as directed under Tinctures, with the above ingredients. May be prepared with an appropriate quantity of Ethanol and Purified Water or Purified Water in Containers in place of 35 vol% Ethanol.

Description Opium Tincture is a dark red-brown liquid. It is affected by light.

Identification (1) To 1 mL of Opium Tincture add diluted ethanol (7 in 10) to make 10 mL, filter, and use the filtrate as the sample solution. Proceed as directed in the Identification (1) under Powdered Opium.

(2) Evaporate 1 mL of Opium Tincture to dryness on a water bath, and proceed with the residue as directed in the Identification (2) under Powdered Opium.

Alcohol number <*1.01*> Not less than 3.5 (Method 1).

Assay Evaporate 50 mL of Opium Tincture, accurately measured, on a water bath to dryness. Add 10 mL of ethanol (99.5) to the residue, evaporate to dryness again, cool, and triturate with exactly 10 mL of water. Proceed with this solution as directed in the Assay under Powdered Opium.

Each mL of 0.05 mol/L sulfuric acid VS
= 28.53 mg of $C_{17}H_{19}NO_3$

Containers and storage Containers—Tight containers.
Storage—Light-resistant.

Opium Ipecac Powder

アヘン・トコン散

Opium Ipecac Powder contains not less than 0.90% and not more than 1.10% of morphine ($C_{17}H_{19}NO_3$: 285.34).

Method of preparation

Powdered Opium	100 g
Powdered Ipecac	100 g
Starch or a suitable ingredient	a sufficient quantity
To make	1000 g

Prepare as directed under Powders, with the above ingredients. Lactose Hydrate should not be used.

Description Opium Ipecac Powder occurs as a light brown powder.

Identification (1) Proceed with 1 g of Opium Ipecac Powder as directed in the Identification (1) under Powdered Opium.

(2) Proceed with 1 g of Opium Ipecac Powder as directed in the Identification (2) under Powdered Opium.

(3) Shake frequently a mixture of 3 g of Opium Ipecac Powder and 5 mL of hydrochloric acid, and allow to stand for 1 hour. Filter the solution into an evaporating dish. Add 5 mg of chlorinated lime to the filtrate: an orange color is produced at the circumference of the chlorinated lime (emetine).

Assay Weigh accurately about 50 g of Opium Ipecac Powder in a glass stoppered flask, add 250 mL of dilute ethanol, warm in a water bath at 40°C for 1 hour with stirring, and filter through a glass filter (G3). Transfer the residue on the filter to the first glass-stoppered flask, add 50 mL of dilute ethanol, warm in a water bath at 40°C for 10 minutes with stirring, and filter through the glass filter. Repeat the extraction with three 50-mL portions of dilute ethanol. Combine all the filtrates in a mortar, evaporate on a water bath to dryness, add 10 mL of ethanol (99.5) to the residue, and evaporate again. After cooling, triturate the residue with an exactly measured 10 mL of water, add 2 g of calcium hydroxide and an exactly measured 40 mL of water, stir the mixture for 20 minutes, and filter. To 30 mL of the filtrate add 0.1 g of magnesium sulfate heptahydrate, shake for 1 minute, then add 0.3 g of calcium hydroxide, shake for 1 minute, allow to stand for 1 hour, and filter. To an exactly measured 20 mL of the filtrate add 5 mL of sodium hydroxide TS, and adjust the pH to between 9.0 and 9.2 with ammonium chloride. Extract the solution successively with 60 mL, 40 mL and 30 mL of a mixture of chloroform and ethanol (95) (3:1). Combine all the extracts, distil, then evaporate the solvent on a water bath. Dissolve the residue in 20 mL of dilute sodium hydroxide TS and 10 mL of diethyl ether with shaking, add 0.5 g of ammonium chloride, shake vigorously with caution, and proceed as directed in the Assay under Powdered Opium.

Each mL of 0.05 mol/L sulfuric acid VS
= 28.53 mg of $C_{17}H_{19}NO_3$

Containers and storage Containers—Tight containers.

Orange Oil

Oleum Aurantii

オレンジ油

Orange Oil is the essential oil obtained by expression from the peel of the edible fruit of *Citrus* species (*Rutaceae*).

Description Orange Oil is a yellow to yellow-brown liquid. It has a characteristic, aromatic odor, and a slightly bitter taste.

It is miscible with an equal volume of ethanol (95) with turbidity.

Refractive index <*2.45*> n_D^{20}: 1.472 – 1.474

Optical rotation <*2.49*> α_D^{20}: +43 – +50° (50 mm).

Specific gravity <*1.13*> d_{20}^{20}: 0.842 – 0.848

Purity Heavy metals <*1.07*>—Proceed with 1.0 mL of Orange Oil according to Method 2, and perform the test. Prepare the control solution with 4.0 mL of Standard Lead Solution (not more than 40 ppm).

Containers and storage Containers—Tight containers.
Storage—Light-resistant.

Orange Peel Syrup

トウヒシロップ

Method of preparation

Orange Peel Tincture	200 mL
Simple Syrup	a sufficient quantity
To make	1000 mL

Prepare as directed under Syrups, with the above ingredients. An appropriate quantity of Sucrose and Purified Water or Purified Water in Containers may be used in place of Simple Syrup.

Description Orange Peel Syrup is a brownish yellow to reddish brown liquid. It has a characteristic odor, a sweet taste and a bitter aftertaste.

Specific gravity d^{20}_{20}: about 1.25

Identification To 25 mL of Orange Peel Syrup add 50 mL of ethyl acetate, shake for 5 minutes, allow to stand until clear ethyl acetate layer separate, and take the ethyl acetate layer, and evaporate on a water bath to dryness. Dissolve the residue in 10 mL of ethanol (95), filter if necessary, and use this solution as the sample solution. Separately, dissolve 10 mg of naringin for thin-layer chromatography in 10 mL of ethanol (95), and use this solution as the standard solution. Perform the test with these solutions as directed under Thin-layer Chromatography <*2.03*>. Spot 10 μL each of the sample solution and standard solution on a plate of silica gel for thin-layer chromatography. Develop the plate with a mixture of ethyl acetate, ethanol (99.5) and water (8:2:1) to a distance of about 10 cm, and air-dry the plate. Spray evenly dilute 2,6-dibromo-*N*-chloro-1,4-benzoquinone monoimine TS on the plate, and allow to stand in ammonia gas: one of the several spots obtained from the sample solution has the same color tone and the same *R*f value with the spot from the standard solution.

Containers and storage Containers—Tight containers.

Orange Peel Tincture

トウヒチンキ

Method of preparation

Bitter Orange Peel, in coarse powder	200 g
70 vol% Ethanol	a sufficient quantity
To make	1000 mL

Prepare as directed under Tinctures, with the above ingredients. An appropriate quantity of Ethanol and Purified Water or Purified Water in Containers may be used in place of 70 vol% Ethanol.

Description Orange Peel Tincture is a yellowish brown liquid. It has a characteristic odor, and a bitter taste.

Specific gravity d^{20}_{20}: about 0.90

Identification To 5.0 mL of Orange Peel Tincture add 5 mL of ethanol (95), filter if necessary, and use the filtrate as the sample solution. Proceed as directed in the Identification under Bitter Orange Peel.

Alcohol number <*1.01*> Not less than 6.6 (Method 2).

Containers and storage Containers—Tight containers.

Orengedokuto Extract

黄連解毒湯エキス

Orengedokuto Extract contains not less than 20 mg and not more than 80 mg of berberine [as berberine chloride ($C_{20}H_{18}ClNO_4$: 371.81)], not less than 80 mg and not more than 240 mg of baicalin ($C_{21}H_{18}O_{11}$: 446.36), and not less than 30 mg and not more than 90 mg (for preparation prescribed 2 g of Gardenia Fruit) or not less than 45 mg and not more than 135 mg (for preparation prescribed 3 g of Gardenia Fruit) of geniposide, per extract prepared with the amount specified in the Method of preparation.

Method of preparation

	1)	2)	3)	4)
Coptis Rhizome	1.5 g	1.5 g	2 g	2 g
Phellodendron Bark	1.5 g	3 g	2 g	1.5 g
Scutellaria Root	3 g	3 g	3 g	3 g
Gardenia Fruit	2 g	3 g	2 g	2 g

Prepare a dry extract or viscous extract as directed under Extracts, according to the prescription 1) to 4), using the crude drugs shown above.

Description Orengedokuto Extract occurs as a yellow-brown to red-brown powder or blackish brown viscous extract. It has a characteristic odor and a very bitter taste.

Identification **(1)** Shake 0.5 g of the dry extract (or 1.5 g of the viscous extract) with 10 mL of methanol, centrifuge, and use the supernatant liquid as the sample solution. Separately, dissolve 1 mg of coptisine chloride for thin-layer chromatography in 5 mL of methanol, and use this solution as the standard solution. Perform the test with these solutions as directed under Thin-layer Chromatography <*2.03*>. Spot 5 μL each of the sample solution and standard solution on a plate of silica gel for thin-layer chromatography. Develop the plate with a mixture of ethyl acetate, ammonia solution (28) and methanol (15:1:1) to a distance of about 7 cm, and air-dry the plate. Examine under ultraviolet light (main wavelength: 365 nm): one of the several spots obtained from the sample solution has the same color tone and *R*f value with the yellow fluorescent spot from the standard solution (Coptis Rhizome).

(2) Shake 0.5 g of the dry extract (or 1.5 g of the viscous extract) with 5 mL of water, then add 25 mL of ethyl acetate, and shake. Separate the ethyl acetate layer, evaporate the solvent under low pressure (in vacuo), add 1 mL of methanol to the residue, and use this solution as the sample solution. Separately, dissolve 1 mg of limonin for thin-layer chromatography in 1 mL of methanol, and use this solution as the standard solution. Perform the test with these solutions as directed under Thin-layer Chromatography <*2.03*>. Spot 10 μL of the sample solution and 5 μL of the standard solution on a plate of silica gel for thin-layer chromatography. Develop the plate with a mixture of ethyl acetate and hexane (5:1) to a distance of about 7 cm, and air-dry the plate. Spray evenly vanillin-sulfuric acid-ethanol TS for spraying on the plate, heat the plate at 105°C for 5 minutes, and allow to cool: one of the several spots obtained from the sample solution has the same color tone and *R*f value with the purple spot from the standard solution (Phellodendron Bark).

(3) Shake 1.0 g of the dry extract (or 3.0 g of the viscous extract) with 10 mL of water, then add 10 mL of diethyl ether, shake, centrifuge, and use the diethyl ether layer as the sample solution. Separately, dissolve 1 mg of wogonin for thin-layer chromatography in 1 mL of methanol, and use this solution as the standard solution. Perform the test with these solutions as directed under Thin-layer Chromatography *<2.03>*. Spot 20 μL of the sample solution and 5 μL of the standard solution on a plate of silica gel for thin-layer chromatography. Develop the plate with a mixture of ethyl acetate, hexane and acetic acid (100) (10:10:1) to a distance of about 7 cm, and air-dry the plate. Spray evenly iron (III) chloride-methanol TS on the plate: one of the several spots obtained from the sample solution has the same color tone and *R*f value with the yellow-brown spot from the standard solution (Scutellaria Root).

(4) Shake 0.5 g of the dry extract (or 1.5 g of the viscous extract) with 10 mL of methanol, centrifuge, and use the supernatant liquid as the sample solution. Separately, dissolve 1 mg of geniposide for thin-layer chromatography in 1 mL of methanol, and use this solution as the standard solution. Perform the test with these solutions as directed under Thin-layer Chromatography *<2.03>*. Spot 5 μL each of the sample solution and standard solution on a plate of silica gel for thin-layer chromatography. Develop the plate with a mixture of ethyl acetate, methanol and water (20:3:2) to a distance of about 7 cm, and air-dry the plate. Spray evenly 4-methoxybenzaldehyde-sulfuric acid TS on the plate, and heat the plate at 105°C for 5 minutes: one of the several spots obtained from the sample solution has the same color tone and *R*f value with the dark purple spot from the standard solution (Gardenia Fruit).

Purity **(1)** Heavy metals *<1.07>*—Prepare the test solution with 1.0 g of the dry extract (or an amount of the viscous extract, equivalent to 1.0 g of dried substance) as directed under Extracts (4), and perform the test (not more than 30 ppm).

(2) Lead—Take 5.0 g of the dry extract (or an amount of the viscous extract, equivalent to 5.0 g of the dried substance) in a platinum, quartz or porcelain crucible, heat gently, and then incinerate by ignition at 450 to 550°C. After cooling, add a small amount of 2 mol/L nitric acid TS, filter if necessary, and wash the crucible and filter several times with small portions of 2 mol/L nitric acid TS. Combine the washings and the filtrate, add 2 mol/L nitric acid TS to make exactly 20 mL, and use this solution as the sample solution. Separately, to 2.5 mL of Standard Lead Solution add 2 mol/L nitric acid TS to make exactly 20 mL, and use this solution as the standard solution. Perform the test with the sample solution and the standard solution as directed under Atomic Absorption Spectrophotometry *<2.23>* according to the following conditions: the absorbance of the sample solution is not more than that of the standard solution (not more than 5 ppm).

Gas: Combustible gas—Acetylene or hydrogen.
Supporting gas—Air.
Lamp: A lead hollow-cathode lamp.
Wavelength: 283.3 nm.

(3) Arsenic *<1.11>*—Prepare the test solution with 0.67 g of the dry extract (or an amount of the viscous extract, equivalent to 0.67 g of dried substance) according to Method 3, and perform the test (not more than 3 ppm).

Loss on drying *<2.41>* The dry extract: Not more than 7.0% (1 g, 105°C, 5 hours).

The viscous extract: Not more than 66.7% (1 g, 105°C, 5 hours).

Total ash *<5.01>* Not more than 12.0%, calculated on the dried basis.

Assay **(1)** Berberine—Weigh accurately about 0.2 g of the dry extract (or an amount of the viscous extract, equivalent to about 0.2 g of dried substance), add exactly 50 mL of the mobile phase, shake for 15 minutes, filter, and use the filtrate as the sample solution. Separately, weigh accurately about 10 mg of Berberine Chloride RS (separately determine the water *<2.48>* in the same manner as Berberine Chloride Hydrate), dissolve in the mobile phase to make exactly 100 mL, and use this solution as the standard solution. Perform the test with exactly 10 μL each of the sample solution and standard solution as directed under Liquid Chromatography *<2.01>* according to the following conditions, and determine the peak areas, A_T and A_S, of berberine in each solution.

Amount (mg) of berberine chloride ($C_{20}H_{18}ClNO_4$)
$= M_S \times A_T/A_S \times 1/2$

M_S: Amount (mg) of Berberine Chloride RS taken, calculated on the anhydrous basis

Operating conditions—

Detector: An ultraviolet absorption photometer (wavelength: 345 nm).

Column: A stainless steel column 4.6 mm in inside diameter and 15 cm in length, packed with octadecylsilanized silica gel for liquid chromatography (5 μm in particle diameter).

Column temperature: A constant temperature of about 30°C.

Mobile phase: Dissolve 3.4 g of potassium dihydrogen phosphate and 1.7 g of sodium lauryl sulfate in 1000 mL of a mixture of water and acetonitrile (1:1).

Flow rate: 1.0 mL per minute (the retention time of berberine is about 8 minutes).

System suitability—

System performance: Dissolve 1 mg each of Berberine Chloride RS and palmatine chloride in the mobile phase to make 10 mL. When the procedure is run with 10 μL of this solution under the above operating conditions, palmatine and berberine are eluted in this order with the resolution between these peaks being not less than 1.5.

System repeatability: When the test is repeated 6 times with 10 μL of the standard solution under the above operating conditions, the relative standard deviation of the peak area of berberine is not more than 1.5%.

(2) Baicalin—Weigh accurately about 0.1 g of the dry extract (or an amount of the viscous extract, equivalent to about 0.1 g of dried substance), add exactly 50 mL of diluted methanol (7 in 10), shake for 15 minutes, and filter. Pipet 5 mL of the filtrate, add diluted methanol (7 in 10) to make exactly 20 mL, and use this solution as the sample solution. Separately, weigh accurately about 10 mg of Baicalin RS (separately determine the water *<2.48>* by coulometric titration, using 10 mg), and dissolve in methanol to make exactly 100 mL. Pipet 5 mL of this solution, add diluted methanol (7 in 10) to make exactly 10 mL, and use this solution as the standard solution. Perform the test with exactly10 μL each of the sample solution and standard solution as directed under Liquid Chromatography *<2.01>* according to the following conditions, and determine the peak areas, A_T and A_S, of baicalin in each solution.

Amount (mg) of baicalin ($C_{21}H_{18}O_{11}$) $= M_S \times A_T/A_S$

M_S: Amount (mg) of Baicalin RS taken, calculated on the anhydrous basis

Operating conditions—

Detector: An ultraviolet absorption photometer (wavelength: 277 nm).

Column: A stainless steel column 4.6 mm in inside diameter and 15 cm in length, packed with octadecylsilanized silica gel for liquid chromatography (5 μm in particle diameter).

Column temperature: A constant temperature of about 40°C.

Mobile phase: A mixture of diluted phosphoric acid (1 in 200) and acetonitrile (19:6).

Flow rate: 1.0 mL per minute (the retention time of baicalin is about 10 minutes).

System suitability—

System performance: When the procedure is run with 10 μL of the standard solution under the above operating conditions, the number of theoretical plates and the symmetry factor of the peak of baicalin are not less than 5000 and not more than 1.5, respectively.

System repeatability: When the test is repeated 6 times with 10 μL of the standard solution under the above operating conditions, the relative standard deviation of the peak area of baicalin is not more than 1.5%.

(3) Geniposide—Weigh accurately about 0.2 g of the dry extract (or an amount of the viscous extract, equivalent to about 0.2 g of dried substance), add exactly 50 mL of diluted methanol (1 in 2), shake for 15 minutes, filter, and use the filtrate as the sample solution. Separately, weigh accurately about 10 mg of geniposide for assay, dissolve in diluted methanol (1 in 2) to make exactly 100 mL, and use this solution as the standard solution. Perform the test with exactly 10 μL each of the sample solution and standard solution as directed under Liquid Chromatography <*2.01*> according to the following conditions, and determine the peak areas, A_T and A_S, of geniposide in each solution.

Amount (mg) of geniposide = $M_S \times A_T/A_S \times 1/2$

M_S: Amount (mg) of geniposide for assay taken, calculated on the basis of the content obtained by qNMR

Operating conditions—

Detector: An ultraviolet absorption photometer (wavelength: 240 nm).

Column: A stainless steel column 4.6 mm in inside diameter and 15 cm in length, packed with octadecylsilanized silica gel for liquid chromatography (5 μm in particle diameter).

Column temperature: A constant temperature of about 40°C.

Mobile phase: A mixture of water, acetonitrile and phosphoric acid (900:100:1).

Flow rate: 1.0 mL per minute (the retention time of geniposide is about 10 minutes).

System suitability—

System performance: When the procedure is run with 10 μL of the standard solution under the above operating conditions, the number of theoretical plates and the symmetry factor of the peak of geniposide are not less than 5000 and not more than 1.5, respectively.

System repeatability: When the test is repeated 6 times with 10 μL of the standard solution under the above operating conditions, the relative standard deviation of the peak area of geniposide is not more than 1.5%.

Containers and storage Containers—Tight containers.

Oriental Bezoar

Bezoar Bovis

ゴオウ

Oriental Bezoar is a stone formed in the gall sac of *Bos taurus* Linné var. *domesticus* Gmelin (*Bovidae*).

It contains not less than 10.0% of bilirubin.

Description Spherical or massive stone, 1 – 4 cm in diameter; externally yellow-brown to red-brown; light, fragile and easily broken. Fractured surface shows yellow-brown to red-brown annular rings, often containing white granular substances or thin layers in these annular rings.

Odor, slight; taste, slightly bitter, followed by slight sweetness.

Identification To 25 mg of pulverized Oriental Bezoar add 10 mL of methanol, shake for 5 minutes, and centrifuge. Take the supernatant liquid, evaporate the solvent under low pressure (in vacuo), dissolve the residue in 0.5 mL of methanol, and use this solution as the sample solution. Separately, dissolve 5 mg each of cholic acid for thin-layer chromatography and deoxycholic acid for thin-layer chromatography in 5 mL of methanol, respectively, and use these solutions as the standard solution (1) and the standard solution (2). Perform the test with these solutions as directed under Thin-layer Chromatography <*2.03*>. Spot 5 μL each of the sample solution, standard solutions (1) and (2) on a plate of silica gel for thin-layer chromatography. Develop the plate with a mixture of ethyl acetate, formic acid and methanol (30:1:1) to a distance of about 7 cm, and air-dry the plate. Spray evenly vanillin-sulfuric acid-ethanol TS for spraying on the plate, and heat the plate at 105°C for 10 minutes: two of the several spots obtained from the sample solution have the same color tone and *Rf* value with each spot from the standard solutions (1) and (2).

Purity **(1)** Synthetic dye—To 2 mg of pulverized Oriental Bezoar add 1 mL dilute hydrochloric acid: no violet color develops.

(2) Starch—To 5 mg of pulverized Oriental Bezoar add 2 mL of water, and heat on a water bath for 5 minutes. Cool and add 2 to 3 drops of iodine TS: no blue-purple color develops.

(3) Sucrose—To 0.02 g of pulverized Oriental Bezoar add 10 mL of water, shake for 15 minutes, and filter. To 1 mL of the filtrate add 2 mL of anthrone TS, and shake: no deep blue-green to dark green color develops.

Total ash <*5.01*> Not more than 10.0%.

Assay Conduct this procedure without exposure to light using light-resistant vessels. The following sample solution and standard solution should be prepared before use. Weigh accurately about 10 mg of pulverized Oriental Bezoar, add 10 mL of a mixture of dimethyl sulfoxide and acetic acid (100) (9:1), warm at 60°C for 20 minutes, and add a mixture of dimethyl sulfoxide and acetic acid (100) (9:1) to make exactly 50 mL. Pipet 5 mL of this solution, add the mobile phase to make exactly 50 mL, filter through a membrane filter, and use the filtrate as the sample solution. Separately, weigh accurately about 10 mg of bilirubin for assay, add about 350 mg of L-ascorbic acid, and dissolve in a mixture of dimethyl sulfoxide and acetic acid (100) (9:1) to make exactly 100 mL. Pipet 5 mL of this solution, add the mobile phase to make exactly 50 mL, and use this solution as the standard solution.

Perform the test with exactly 10 μL each of the sample solution and standard solution as directed under Liquid Chromatography <*2.01*> according to the following conditions, and determine the peak areas, A_T and A_S, of bilirubin in each solution.

$$\text{Amount (mg) of bilirubin} = M_S \times A_T/A_S \times 1/2$$

M_S: Amount (mg) of bilirubin for assay taken

Operating conditions—

Detector: A visible absorption photometer (wavelength: 450 nm).

Column: A stainless steel column 4.6 mm in inside diameter and 15 cm in length, packed with octadecylsilanized silica gel for liquid chromatography (5 μm in particle diameter).

Column temperature: A constant temperature of about 30°C.

Mobile phase: A mixture of acetonitrile and diluted acetic acid (100) (1 in 100) (19:1).

Flow rate: Adjust so that the retention time of bilirubin is about 10 minutes.

System suitability—

System performance: When the procedure is run with 10 μL of the standard solution under the above operating conditions, the number of theoretical plates and the symmetry factor of the peak of bilirubin are not less than 5000 and not more than 1.5, respectively.

System repeatability: When the test is repeated 6 times with 10 μL of the standard solution under the above operating conditions, the relative standard deviation of the peak area of bilirubin is not more than 1.5%.

Containers and storage Containers—Well-closed containers.

Otsujito Extract

乙字湯エキス

Otsujito Extract contains not less than 1.2 mg and not more than 4.8 mg of saikosaponin b_2, not less than 80 mg and not more than 240 mg of baicalin ($C_{21}H_{18}O_{11}$: 446.36), not less than 14 mg and not more than 42 mg (for preparation prescribed 2 g of Glycyrrhiza) or not less than 20 mg and not more than 60 mg (for preparation prescribed 3 g of Glycyrrhiza) of glycyrrhizic acid ($C_{42}H_{62}O_{16}$: 822.93), and not less than 0.5 mg of sennoside A ($C_{42}H_{38}O_{20}$: 862.74) or not less than 1.5 mg of rhein (for preparation prescribed 0.5 g of Rhubarb) or not less than 1 mg of sennoside A ($C_{42}H_{38}O_{20}$: 862.74) or not less than 3 mg of rhein (for preparation prescribed 1 g of Rhubarb), per extract prepared with the amount specified in the Method of preparation.

Method of preparation

	1)	2)	3)
Japanese Angelica Root	6 g	6 g	6 g
Bupleurum Root	5 g	5 g	5 g
Scutellaria Root	3 g	3 g	3 g
Glycyrrhiza	2 g	2 g	3 g
Cimicifuga Rhizome	1.5 g	1 g	1 g
Rhubarb	1 g	0.5 g	1 g

Prepare a dry extract or viscous extract as directed under Extracts, according to the prescription 1) to 3), using the crude drugs shown above.

Description Otsujito Extract occurs as light brown to brown powder or black-brown viscous extract, having a slightly order, and a hot and slight sweet taste.

Identification **(1)** Shake 2.0 g of the dry extract (or 6.0 g of the viscous extract) with 10 mL of water, add 10 mL of diethyl ether, shake, and centrifuge. Separate the diethyl ether layer, add 10 mL of sodium hydroxide TS, shake, centrifuge, and use the diethyl ether layer as the sample solution. Separately, use (*Z*)-ligustilide TS for thin-layer chromatography as the standard solution. Perform the test with these solutions as directed under Thin-layer Chromatography <*2.03*>. Spot 10 μL each of the sample solution and standard solution on a plate of silica gel for thin-layer chromatography. Develop the plate with a mixture of butyl acetate and hexane (2:1) to a distance of about 7 cm, and air-dry the plate. Examine under ultraviolet light (main wavelength: 365 nm): one of the several spots obtained from the sample solution has the same color tone and *R*f value with the blue-white fluorescent spot from the standard solution (Japanese Angelica Root).

(2) Shake 1.0 g of the dry extract (or 3.0 g of the viscous extract) with 10 mL of water, add 10 mL of 1-butanol, shake, centrifuge, and use the 1-butanol layer as the sample solution. Separately, dissolve 1 mg of saikosaponin b_2 for thin-layer chromatography in 1 mL of methanol, and use this solution as the standard solution. Perform the test with these solutions as directed under Thin-layer Chromatography <*2.03*>. Spot 10 μL of the sample solution and 2 μL of the standard solution on a plate of silica gel for thin-layer chromatography. Develop the plate with a mixture of ethyl acetate, ethanol (99.5) and water (8:2:1) to a distance of about 7 cm, and air-dry the plate. Spray evenly 4-dimethylaminobenzaldehyde TS for spraying on the plate, and heat the plate at 105°C for 5 minutes. Examine under ultraviolet light (main wavelength: 365 nm): one of the several spots obtained from the sample solution has the same color tone and *R*f value with the yellow fluorescent spot from the standard solution (Bupleurum Root).

(3) Shake 1.0 g of the dry extract (or 3.0 g of the viscous extract) with 10 mL of water, add 25 mL of diethyl ether, and shake. Separate the diethyl ether layer, evaporate the solvent under low pressure (in vacuo), add 2 mL of diethyl ether to the residue, and use this solution as the sample solution. Separately, dissolve 1 mg of wogonin for thin-layer chromatography in 1 mL of methanol, and use this solution as the standard solution. Perform the test with these solutions as directed under Thin-layer Chromatography <*2.03*>. Spot 20 μL of the sample solution and 5 μL of the standard solution on a plate of silica gel for thin-layer chromatography. Develop the plate with a mixture of ethyl acetate, hexane and acetic acid (100) (10:10:1) to a distance of about 7 cm, and air-dry the plate. Spray evenly iron (III) chloride-methanol TS on the plate: one of the several spots obtained from the sample solution has the same color tone and *R*f value with the yellow-brown to grayish brown spot from the standard solution (Scutellaria Root).

(4) Shake 1.0 g of the dry extract (or 3.0 g of the viscous extract) with 10 mL of water, add 10 mL of 1-butanol, shake, centrifuge, and use the 1-butanol layer as the sample solution. Separately, dissolve 1 mg of liquiritin for thin-layer chromatography in 1 mL of methanol, and use this solution as the standard solution. Perform the test with these solutions as directed under Thin-layer Chromatography <*2.03*>.

Spot 1 μL each of the sample solution and standard solution on a plate of silica gel for thin-layer chromatography. Develop the plate with a mixture of ethyl acetate, methanol and water (20:3:2) to a distance of about 7 cm, and air-dry the plate. Spray evenly dilute sulfuric acid on the plate, heat the plate at 105°C for 5 minutes, and examine under ultraviolet light (main wavelength: 365 nm): one of the several spots obtained from the sample solution has the same color tone and *Rf* value with the yellow-green fluorescent spot from the standard solution (Glycyrrhiza).

(5) Shake 1.0 g of the dry extract (or 3.0 g of the viscous extract) with 10 mL of water, add 10 mL of 1-butanol, shake, centrifuge, and use the 1-butanol layer as the sample solution. Use (*E*)-isoferulic acid-(*E*)-ferulic acid TS for thin-layer chromatography as the standard solution. Perform the test with these solutions as directed under Thin-layer Chromatography <*2.03*>. Spot 10 μL of the sample solution and 2 μL of the standard solution on a plate of silica gel for thin-layer chromatography. Develop the plate with a mixture of ethyl acetate, acetone and water (20:12:3) to a distance of about 7 cm, and air-dry the plate. Spray evenly sulfuric acid on the plate, and heat the plate at 105°C for 5 minutes, and examine under ultraviolet light (main wavelength: 365 nm): one of the several spots obtained from the sample solution has the same color tone and *Rf* value with the light yellow-white fluorescent spot from the standard solution (Cimicifuga Rhizome).

(6) Shake 1.0 g of the dry extract (or 3.0 g of the viscous extract) with 10 mL of water, add 25 mL of diethyl ether, and shake. Separate the diethyl ether layer, evaporate the solvent under low pressure (in vacuo), add 2 mL of diethyl ether to the residue, and use this solution as the sample solution. Separately, dissolve 1 mg of rhein for thin-layer chromatography in 10 mL of acetone, and use this solution as the standard solution. Perform the test with these solutions as directed under Thin-layer Chromatography <*2.03*>. Spot 10 μL of the sample solution and 5 μL of the standard solution on a plate of silica gel for thin-layer chromatography. Develop the plate with a mixture of ethyl acetate, methanol and water (20:3:2) to a distance of about 7 cm, and air-dry the plate. Examine under ultraviolet light (main wavelength: 365 nm): one of the several spots obtained from the sample solution has the same color tone and *Rf* value with the orange fluorescent spot from the standard solution (Rhubarb).

Purity **(1)** Heavy metals <*1.07*>—Prepare the test solution with 1.0 g of the dry extract (or an amount of the viscous extract, equivalent to 1.0 g of dried substance) as directed under Extracts (4), and perform the test (not more than 30 ppm).

(2) Arsenic <*1.11*>—Prepare the test solution with 0.67 g of the dry extract (or an amount of the viscous extract, equivalent to 0.67 g of dried substance) according to Method 3, and perform the test (not more than 3 ppm).

Loss on drying <*2.41*> The dry extract: Not more than 9.5% (1 g, 105°C, 5 hours).

The viscous extract: Not more than 66.7% (1 g, 105°C, 5 hours).

Total ash <*5.01*> Not more than 10.5%, calculated on the dried basis.

Assay **(1)** Saikosaponin b_2—Weigh accurately about 0.5 g of the dry extract (or an amount of the viscous extract, equivalent to about 0.5 g of the dried substance), add 20 mL of diethyl ether and 10 mL of water, shake for 10 minutes, and centrifuge. After removing the diethyl ether layer, add 20 mL of diethyl ether, proceed in the same manner as described above, and remove the diethyl ether layer. To the aqueous layer add 10 mL of methanol, shake for 30 minutes, centrifuge, and separate the supernatant liquid. To the residue add 20 mL of diluted methanol (1 in 2), shake for 5 minutes, centrifuge, separate the supernatant liquid, combine these supernatant liquids, add diluted methanol (1 in 2) to make exactly 50 mL, and use this solution as the sample solution. Separately use saikosaponin b_2 standard TS for assay as the standard solution. Perform the test with exactly 10 μL each of the sample solution and standard solution as directed under Liquid Chromatography <*2.01*> according to the following conditions, and determine the peak areas, A_T and A_S, of saikosaponin b_2 in each solution.

$$\text{Amount (mg) of saikosaponin } b_2 = C_S \times A_T/A_S \times 50$$

C_S: Concentration (mg/mL) of saikosaponin b_2 in saikosaponin b_2 standard TS for assay

Operating conditions—

Detector: An ultraviolet absorption photometer (wavelength: 254 nm).

Column: A stainless steel column 4.6 mm in inside diameter and 15 cm in length, packed with octadecylsilanized silica gel for liquid chromatography (5 μm in particle diameter).

Column temperature: A constant temperature of about 40°C.

Mobile phase: A mixture of 0.05 mol/L sodium dihydrogen phosphate TS and acetonitrile (5:3).

Flow rate: 1.0 mL per minute (the retention time of saikosaponin b_2 is about 12 minutes).

System suitability—

System performance: When the procedure is run with 10 μL of the standard solution under the above operating conditions, the number of theoretical plates and the symmetry factor of the peak of saikosaponin b_2 are not less than 5000 and not more than 1.5, respectively.

System repeatability: When the test is repeated 6 times with 10 μL of the standard solution under the above operating conditions, the relative standard deviation of the peak area of saikosaponin b_2 is not more than 1.5%.

(2) Baicalin—Weigh accurately about 0.1 g of the dry extract (or an amount of the viscous extract, equivalent to about 0.1 g of the dried substance), add exactly 50 mL of diluted methanol (7 in 10), shake for 15 minutes, filter, and use the filtrate as the sample solution. Separately, weigh accurately about 10 mg of Baicalin RS (separately determine the water <*2.48*> by coulometric titration, using 10 mg), dissolve in methanol to make exactly 100 mL. Pipet 5 mL of this solution, add diluted methanol (7 in 10) to make exactly 10 mL, and use this solution as the standard solution. Perform the test with exactly 10 μL each of the sample solution and standard solution as directed under Liquid Chromatography <*2.01*> according to the following conditions, and determine the peak areas, A_T and A_S, of baicalin in each solution.

$$\text{Amount (mg) of baicalin } (C_{21}H_{18}O_{11}) = M_S \times A_T/A_S \times 1/4$$

M_S: Amount (mg) of Baicalin RS taken, calculated on the anhydrous basis

Operating conditions—

Detector: An ultraviolet absorption photometer (wavelength: 277 nm).

Column: A stainless steel column 4.6 mm in inside diameter and 15 cm in length, packed with octadecylsilanized silica gel for liquid chromatography (5 μm in particle diameter).

Column temperature: A constant temperature of about 40°C.

Mobile phase: A mixture of diluted phosphoric acid (1 in 200) and acetonitrile (19:6).

Flow rate: 1.0 mL per minute (the retention time of baicalin is about 10 minutes).

System suitability—

System performance: When the procedure is run with 10 μL of the standard solution under the above operating conditions, the number of theoretical plates and the symmetry factor of the peak of baicalin are not less than 5000 and not more than 1.5, respectively.

System repeatability: When the test is repeated 6 times with 10 μL of the standard solution under the above operating conditions, the relative standard deviation of the peak area of baicalin is not more than 1.5%.

(3) Glycyrrhizic acid—Weigh accurately about 0.5 g of the dry extract (or an amount of the viscous extract, equivalent to about 0.5 g of the dried substance), add 20 mL of diethyl ether and 10 mL of water, shake for 10 minutes, and centrifuge. After removing the diethyl ether layer, add 20 mL of diethyl ether, proceed in the same manner as described above, and remove the diethyl ether layer. To the aqueous layer add 10 mL of methanol, shake for 30 minutes, centrifuge, and take the supernatant liquid. To the residue add 20 mL of diluted methanol (1 in 2), shake for 5 minutes, centrifuge, and take the supernatant liquid. Combine these supernatant liquids, add diluted methanol (1 in 2) to make exactly 50 mL, and use this solution as the sample solution. Separately, weigh accurately about 10 mg of Glycyrrhizic Acid RS (separately determine the water *<2.48>* by coulometric titration, using 10 mg), dissolve in diluted methanol (1 in 2) to make exactly 100 mL, and use this solution as the standard solution. Perform the test with exactly 10 μL each of the sample solution and standard solution as directed under Liquid Chromatography *<2.01>* according to the following conditions, and determine the peak areas, A_T and A_S, of glycyrrhizic acid in each solution.

Amount (mg) of glycyrrhizic acid ($C_{42}H_{62}O_{16}$)
$= M_S \times A_T/A_S \times 1/2$

M_S: Amount (mg) of Glycyrrhizic Acid RS taken, calculated on the anhydrous basis

Operating conditions—

Detector: An ultraviolet absorption photometer (wavelength: 254 nm).

Column: A stainless steel column 4.6 mm in inside diameter and 15 cm in length, packed with octadecylsilanized silica gel for liquid chromatography (5 μm in particle diameter).

Column temperature: A constant temperature of about 40°C.

Mobile phase: Dissolve 3.85 g of ammonium acetate in 720 mL of water, and add 5 mL of acetic acid (100) and 280 mL of acetonitrile.

Flow rate: 1.0 mL per minute (the retention time of glycyrrhizic acid is about 15 minutes).

System suitability—

System performance: Dissolve 5 mg of monoammonium glycyrrhizinate for resolution check in 20 mL of dilute ethanol. When the procedure is run with 10 μL of this solution under the above operating conditions, the resolution between the peak having the relative retention time of about 0.9 to glycyrrhizic acid and the peak of glycyrrhizic acid is not less than 1.5.

System repeatability: When the test is repeated 6 times with 10 μL of the standard solution under the above operating conditions, the relative standard deviation of the peak area of glycyrrhizic acid is not more than 1.5%.

(4) Sennoside A—Weigh accurately about 0.5 g of the dry extract (or an amount of the viscous extract, equivalent to about 0.5 g of the dried substance), add exactly 50 mL of diluted methanol (1 in 2), shake for 15 minutes, and centrifuge. Pipet 10 mL of the supernatant liquid, pour it into a column about 10 mm in inside diameter (previously prepared by packing 0.36 g of strongly basic ion-exchange resin for column chromatography, and washing with 10 mL of methanol and 10 mL of diluted methanol (1 in 2)) to flow out, wash out the column with 10 mL of diluted methanol (1 in 2), then flow out with a mixture of water, methanol and formic acid (25:25:1) to obtain exactly 5 mL of the outflow liquid, and use this liquid as the sample solution. Separately, weigh accurately about 5 mg of Sennoside A RS (separately determine the water *<2.48>* by coulometric titration, using 10 mg), dissolve in diluted methanol (1 in 2) to make exactly 200 mL, and use this solution as the standard solution. Perform the test with exactly 10 μL each of the sample solution and standard solution as directed under Liquid Chromatography *<2.01>* according to the following conditions, and determine the peak areas, A_T and A_S, of sennoside A in each solution.

Amount (mg) of sennoside A ($C_{42}H_{38}O_{20}$)
$= M_S \times A_T/A_S \times 1/8$

M_S: Amount (mg) of Sennoside A RS taken, calculated on the anhydrous basis

Operating conditions—

Detector: An ultraviolet absorption photometer (wavelength: 340 nm).

Column: A stainless steel column 4.6 mm in inside diameter and 15 cm in length, packed with octadecylsilanized silica gel for liquid chromatography (5 μm in particle diameter).

Column temperature: A constant temperature of about 30°C.

Mobile phase: A mixture of water, acetonitrile and phosphoric acid (2460:540:1).

Flow rate: 1.0 mL per minute (the retention time of sennoside A is about 14 minutes).

System suitability—

System performance: When the procedure is run with 10 μL of the standard solution under the above operating conditions, the number of theoretical plates and the symmetry factor of the peak of sennoside A are not less than 5000 and not more than 1.5, respectively.

System repeatability: When the test is repeated 6 times with 10 μL of the standard solution under the above operating conditions, the relative standard deviation of the peak area of sennoside A is not more than 1.5%.

(5) Rhein—Weigh accurately about 0.5 g of the dry extract (or an amount of the viscous extract, equivalent to about 0.5 g of the dried substance), add 80 mL of water, shake, and add water to make exactly 100 mL. Pipet 5 mL of this solution, add 20 mL of iron (III) chloride TS, heat under a reflux condenser for 30 minutes, add 3 mL of hydrochloric acid, and heat in addition under a reflux condenser for 30 minutes. After cooling, extract three times with 25 mL each of diethyl ether, combine all the diethyl ether layers, evaporate the solvent under low pressure (in vacuo), dissolve the residue in methanol to make exactly 10 mL, and use this solution as the sample solution. Separately, weigh accurately about 5 mg of rhein for assay, and dissolve in acetone to make exactly 100 mL. Pipet 10 mL of this solution, add methanol to make exactly 50 mL, and use this solution as the standard solution. Perform the test with exactly 10 μL each of the sample solution and standard solution as directed under Liquid Chromatography *<2.01>* according to the following conditions, and determine the peak areas, A_T and A_S, of rhein in each solution.

$$\text{Amount (mg) of rhein} = M_S \times A_T/A_S \times 2/5$$

M_S: Amount (mg) of rhein for assay taken

Operating conditions—

Detector: An ultraviolet absorption photometer (wavelength: 278 nm).

Column: A stainless steel column 4.6 mm in inside diameter and 25 cm in length, packed with octadecylsilanized silica gel for liquid chromatography (5 μm in particle diameter).

Column temperature: A constant temperature of about 50°C.

Mobile phase: A mixture of water, acetonitrile and phosphoric acid (650:350:1).

Flow rate: 1.0 mL per minute (the retention time of rhein is about 17 minutes).

System suitability—

System performance: When the procedure is run with 10 μL of the standard solution under the above operating conditions, the number of theoretical plates and the symmetry factor of the peak of rhein are not less than 5000 and not more than 1.5, respectively.

System repeatability: When the test is repeated 6 times with 10 μL of the standard solution under the above operating conditions, the relative standard deviation of the peak area of rhein is not more than 1.5%.

Containers and storage Containers—Tight containers.

Oyster Shell

Ostreae Testa

ボレイ

Oyster Shell is the shell of *Ostrea gigas* Thunberg (*Ostreidae*).

Description Irregularly curved, foliaceous or lamellated broken pieces. The unbroken oyster shell forms a bivalve 6 - 10 cm in length and 2 - 5 cm in width. The upper valve is flat and the lower one is somewhat hollow. Both the upper and lower edges of the valve are irregularly curved and bite with each other. The surface of the valve is externally light green-gray-brown and internally milky in color.

Almost odorless and tasteless.

Identification **(1)** Dissolve 1 g of sample pieces of Oyster Shell in 10 mL of dilute hydrochloric acid by heating: it evolves a gas, and forms a very slightly red, turbid solution in which a transparent, thin suspended matter remains. Pass the evolved gas through calcium hydroxide TS: a white precipitate is produced.

(2) The solution obtained in (1) has a slight, characteristic odor. Filter this solution and neutralize with ammonia TS: the solution responds to Qualitative Tests *<1.09>* for calcium salt.

(3) Ignite 1 g of pulverized Oyster Shell: it turns black-brown in color at first, and evolves a characteristic odor. Ignite it further: it becomes almost white.

Purity Barium—Dissolve 1 g of pulverized Oyster Shell in 10 mL of dilute hydrochloric acid: the solution does not respond to Qualitative Tests (1) *<1.09>* for barium salt.

Containers and storage Containers—Well-closed containers.

Powdered Oyster Shell

Ostreae Testa Pulverata

ボレイ末

Powdered Oyster Shell is the powder of Oyster Shell.

Description Powdered Oyster Shell occurs as a grayish white powder. It is almost odorless and tasteless.

Identification **(1)** Dissolve 1 g of Powdered Oyster Shell in 10 mL of dilute hydrochloric acid by heating: it evolves a gas, and forms a very slightly red, turbid solution. Pass the gas evolved through calcium hydroxide TS: a white precipitate is produced.

(2) The solution obtained in (1) has a slight, characteristic odor. Filter this solution, and neutralize with ammonia TS: the solution responds to Qualitative Tests *<1.09>* for calcium salt.

(3) Ignite 1 g of Powdered Oyster Shell: it turns black-brown in color at first evolving a characteristic odor. Ignite it further: it becomes almost white.

Purity **(1)** Water-soluble substances—Shake 3.0 g of Powdered Oyster Shell with 50 mL of freshly boiled and cooled water for 5 minutes, filter, and evaporate 25 mL of the filtrate to dryness. Dry the residue at 105°C for 1 hour, cool, and weigh: the mass of the residue does not exceed 15 mg.

(2) Acid-insoluble substances—To 5.0 g of Powdered Oyster Shell add 100 mL of water, and add hydrochloric acid in small portions with stirring until the solution becomes acid. Boil the acidic mixture with additional 1 mL of hydrochloric acid. After cooling, collect the insoluble substance by filtration, and wash it with hot water until the last washing no longer gives any reaction in Qualitative Tests *<1.09>* (2) for chloride. Ignite the residue and weigh: the mass of the residue does not exceed 25 mg.

(3) Barium—Dissolve 1 g of Powdered Oyster Shell in 10 mL of dilute hydrochloric acid: the solution does not respond to Qualitative Tests *<1.09>* (1) for barium salt.

Loss on drying *<2.41>* Not more than 4.0% (1 g, 180°C, 4 hours).

Containers and storage Containers—Tight containers.

Panax Japonicus Rhizome

Panacis Japonici Rhizoma

チクセツニンジン

Panax Japonicus Rhizome is the rhizome of *Panax japonicus* C. A. Meyer (*Araliaceae*), usually after being treated with hot water.

Description Irregularly cylidrical rhizome with distinct nodes, 3 - 20 cm in length, 1 - 1.5 cm in diameter, internode 1 - 2 cm; externally light yellow-brown, with fine longitudinal wrinkles; stem scars, hollowed at the center, protruding on the upper surface, and root scars protruding as knobs on internodes; easily broken; fractured surface approximately flat, and light yellow-brown in color; horny in texture.

Odor, slight; taste, slightly bitter.

Identification Shake 0.5 g of pulverized Panax Japonicus Rhizome with 10 mL of methanol for 10 minutes, filter, and use the filtrate as the sample solution. Separately, dissolve 2 mg of chikusetsusaponin IV for thin-layer chromatography in 1 mL of methanol, and use this solution as the standard solution. Perform the test with these solutions as directed under Thin-layer Chromatography *<2.03>*. Spot 5 μL each of the sample solution and standard solution on a plate of silica gel for thin-layer chromatography. Develop the plate with a mixture of ethyl acetate, water and formic acid (5:1:1) to a distance of about 7 cm, and air-dry the plate. Spray evenly dilute sulfuric acid on the plate, and heat the plate at 110°C for 5 minutes: one of the several spots obtained from the sample solution shows the same color tone and *R*f value with the spot from the standard solution.

Purity (1) Heavy metals *<1.07>*—Proceed with 3.0 g of pulverized Panax Japonicus Rhizome according to Method 3, and perform the test. Prepare the control solution with 3.0 mL of Standard Lead Solution (not more than 10 ppm).

(2) Arsenic *<1.11>*—Prepare the test solution with 0.40 g of pulverized Panax Japonicus Rhizome according to Method 4, and perform the test (not more than 5 ppm).

Total ash *<5.01>* Not more than 5.0%.

Extract content *<5.01>* Dilute ethanol-soluble extract: not less than 30.0%.

Containers and storage Containers—Well-closed containers.

Powdered Panax Japonicus Rhizome

Panacis Japonici Rhizoma Pulveratum

チクセツニンジン末

Powdered Panax Japonicus Rhizome is the powder of Panax Japonicus Rhizome.

Description Powdered Panax Japonicus Rhizome occurs as a light grayish yellow-brown powder, and has a slight odor and a slightly bitter taste.

Under a microscope *<5.01>*, Powdered Panax Japonicus Rhizome reveals mainly starch grains or gelatinized starch masses, and fragments of parenchyma cells containing them; also fragments of cork tissue, somewhat thick-walled collenchyma, phloem tissue, and reticulate vessels; rarely fragments of scalariform vessels with a simple perforation, fibers and fiber bundles, rosette aggregates of calcium oxalate, and parenchyma cells containing them; yellow to orange-yellow resin; starch grains consisting of simple grains or 2- to 4-compound grains, simple grains, 3 – 18 μm in diameter; rosette aggregates of calcium oxalate are 20 – 60 μm in diameter.

Identification Shake 0.5 g of Powdered Panax Japonicus Rhizome with 10 mL of methanol for 10 minutes, filter, and use the filtrate as the sample solution. Separately, dissolve 2 mg of chikusetsusaponin IV for thin-layer chromatography in 1 mL of methanol, and use this solution as the standard solution. Perform the test with these solutions as directed under Thin-layer Chromatography *<2.03>*. Spot 5 μL each of the sample solution and standard solution on a plate of silica gel for thin-layer chromatography. Develop the plate with a mixture of ethyl acetate, water and formic acid (5:1:1) to a distance of about 7 cm, and air-dry the plate. Spray evenly dilute sulfuric acid on the plate, and heat the plate at 110°C for 5 minutes: one of the several spots obtained from the sample solution shows the same color tone and *R*f value with the spot from the standard solution.

Purity (1) Heavy metals *<1.07>*—Proceed with 3.0 g of Powdered Panax Japonicus Rhizome according to Method 3, and perform the test. Prepare the control solution with 3.0 mL of Standard Lead Solution (not more than 10 ppm).

(2) Arsenic *<1.11>*—Prepare the test solution with 0.40 g of Powdered Panax Japonicus Rhizome according to Method 4, and perform the test (not more than 5 ppm).

Total ash *<5.01>* Not more than 5.0%.

Extract content *<5.01>* Dilute ethanol-soluble extract: not less than 30.0%.

Containers and storage Containers—Well-closed containers.

Peach Kernel

Persicae Semen

トウニン

Peach Kernel is the seed of *Prunus persica* Batsch or *Prunus persica* Batsch var. *davidiana* Maximowicz (*Rosaceae*).

It contains not less than 1.2% of amygdalin, calculated on the basis of dried material.

Description Flattened, asymmetric ovoid seed, 1.2 – 2.0 cm in length, 0.6 – 1.2 cm in width, and 0.3 – 0.7 cm in thickness; somewhat sharp at one end, and round at the other end with chalaza; seed coat red-brown to light brown; externally, its surface being powdery by easily detachable stone cells of epidermis; numerous vascular bundles running and rarely branching from chalaza through the seed coat, and, appearing as dented longitudinal wrinkles; when soaked in boiling water and softened, the seed coat and thin, translucent, white albumen easily separated from the cotyledone; cotyledone white in color.

Almost odorless; taste, slightly bitter and oily.

Under a microscope *<5.01>*, the outer surface of seed coat reveals polygonal, long polygonal, or obtuse triangular stone cells on the protrusion from vascular bundles, shape of which considerably different according to the position, and their cell walls almost equally thickened; in lateral view, appearing as a square, rectangle or obtuse triangle.

Identification To 1.0 g of ground Peach Kernel add 10 mL of methanol, immediately heat under a reflux condenser for 10 minutes, cool, filter, and use the filtrate as the sample solution. Separately, dissolve 2 mg of amygdalin for thin-layer chromatography in 1 mL of methanol, and use this solution as the standard solution. Perform the test with these solutions as directed under Thin-layer Chromatography *<2.03>*. Spot 10 μL each of the sample solution and standard solution on a plate of silica gel for thin-layer chromatography.

Develop the plate with a mixture of ethyl acetate, methanol and water (20:5:4) to a distance of about 7 cm, and air-dry the plate. Spray evenly thymol-sulfuric acid-methanol TS for spraying upon the plate, and heat the plate at 105°C for 5 minutes: one of the several spots obtained from the sample solution has the same color tone and *R*f value with the spot from the standard solution.

Purity (1) Rancidity—Grind Peach Kernel with boiling water: no odor of rancid oil is perceptible.

(2) Foreign matter <*5.01*>—When perform the test with not less than 250 g of Peach Kernel, it contains not more than 0.10% of broken pieces of endocarp.

Loss on drying <*5.01*> Not more than 8.0% (6 hours).

Assay Weigh accurately 0.5 g of ground Peach Kernel, add 40 mL of diluted methanol (9 in 10), heat immediately under a reflux condenser for 30 minutes, and cool. Filter the mixture, add diluted methanol (9 in 10) to make exactly 50 mL. Pipet 5 mL of this solution, add water to make exactly 10 mL, filter, and use the filtrate as the sample solution. Separately, weigh accurately about 10 mg of amygdalin for assay, previously dried in a desiccator (silica gel) for not less than 24 hours, dissolve in diluted methanol (1 in 2) to make exactly 50 mL, and use this solution as the standard solution. Perform the test with exactly 10 μL each of the sample solution and standard solution as directed under Liquid Chromatography <*2.01*> according to the following conditions, and determine the peak areas, A_T and A_S, of amygdalin in each solution.

$$\text{Amount (mg) of amygdalin} = M_S \times A_T/A_S \times 2$$

M_S: Amount (mg) of amygdalin for assay taken

Operating conditions—

Detector: An ultraviolet absorption photometer (wavelength: 210 nm).

Column: A stainless steel column 4.6 mm in inside diameter and 15 cm in length, packed with octadecylsilianized silica gel for liquid chromatography (5 μm in particle diameter).

Column temperature: A constant temperature of about 45°C.

Mobile phase: A mixture of 0.05 mol/L sodium dihydrogen phosphate TS and methanol (5:1).

Flow rate: 0.8 mL per minute (the retention time of amygdalin is about 12 minutes).

System suitability—

System performance: When the procedure is run with 10 μL of the standard solution under the above operating conditions, the number of theoretical plates and the symmetry factor of the peak of amygdalin are not less than 5000 and not more than 1.5, respectively.

System repeatability: When the test is repeated 6 times with 10 μL of the standard solution under the above operating conditions, the relative standard deviation of the peak area of amygdalin is not more than 1.5%.

Containers and storage Containers—Well-closed containers.

Powdered Peach Kernel

Persicae Semen Pulveratum

トウニン末

Powdered Peach Kernel is the powder of the Peach Kernel.

It contains not less than 1.2% of amygdalin, calculated on the basis of dried material.

Description Powdered Peach Kernel occurs as a reddish-light brown to light brown powder. It is almost odorless and is oily and has slightly a bitter taste.

Under a microscope <*5.01*>, Powdered Peach Kernel fragments of outer seed coat epidermis; elliptical to ovoid, containing yellow-brown compound 50 to 80 μm in diameter and stone cell; cap-like shape to ovoid, yellow-brown in color. The stone cell is element of epidermis, 50 to 80 μm in diameter and 70 to 80 μm in height, cell wall of the top, 12 to 25 μm thickness, the base 4 μm in thickness, with obvious and numerous pits. Inner seed coat, yellow-brown, irregular and somewhat long polygon, 15 to 30 μm in diameter; and fragments of cotyledon and albumen containing aleurone grains and fatted oil, Aleurone grains are almost spherical grains, 5 to 10 μm in diameter.

Identification To 1.0 g of Powdered Peach Kernel add 10 mL of methanol, and immediately heat under a reflux condenser for 10 minutes. After cooling, filter, and use the filtrate as the sample solution. Separately, dissolve 2 mg of amygdalin for thin-layer chromatography in 1 mL of methanol, and use this solution as the standard solution. Perform the test with these solutions as directed under Thin-layer Chromatography <*2.03*>. Spot 10 μL each of the sample solution and standard solution on a plate of silica gel for thin-layer chromatography. Develop the plate with a mixture of ethyl acetate, methanol and water (20:5:4) to a distance of about 7 cm, and air-dry the plate. Spray evenly thymol-sulfuric acid-methanol TS for spraying on the plate, and heat the plate at 105°C for 5 minutes: one of the several spots obtained from the sample solution has the same color tone and *R*f value with the spot from the standard solution.

Loss on drying <*5.01*> Not more than 8.5% (6 hours).

Total ash <*5.01*> Not more than 3.5%.

Acid-insoluble ash <*5.01*> Not more than 0.5%.

Assay Weigh accurately 0.5 g of Powdered Peach Kernel, add 40 mL of diluted methanol (9 in 10), heat immediately under a reflux condenser for 30 minutes, and cool. Filter the mixture, add diluted methanol (9 in 10) to make exactly 50 mL. Pipet 5 mL of this solution, add water to make exactly 10 mL, filter, and use the filtrate as the sample solution. Separately, weigh accurately about 10 mg of amygdalin for assay, previously dried in a desiccator (silica gel) for not less than 24 hours, dissolve in diluted methanol (1 in 2) to make exactly 50 mL, and use this solution as the standard solution. Perform the test exactly with 10 μL each of the sample solution and standard solution as directed under Liquid Chromatography <*2.01*> according to the following conditions, and determine the peak areas, A_T and A_S, of amygdalin in each solution.

$$\text{Amount (mg) of amygdalin} = M_S \times A_T/A_S \times 2$$

M_S: Amount (mg) of amygdalin for assay taken

Operating conditions—

Detector: An ultraviolet absorption photometer (wavelength: 210 nm).

Column: A stainless steel column 4.6 mm in inside diameter and 15 cm in length, packed with octadecylsilianized silica gel for liquid chromatography (5 μm in particle diameter).

Column temperature: A constant temperature of about 45°C.

Mobile phase: A mixture of 0.05 mol/L sodium dihydrogen phosphate TS and methanol (5:1).

Flow rate: 0.8 mL per minute (the retention time of amygdalin is about 12 minutes).

System suitability—

System performance: When the procedure is run with 10 μL of the standard solution under the above operating conditions, the number of theoretical plates and the symmetry factor of the peak of amygdalin are not less than 5000 and not more than 1.5, respectively.

System repeatability: When the test is repeated 6 times with 10 μL of the standard solution under the above operating conditions, the relative standard deviation of the peak area of amygdalin is not more than 1.5%.

Containers and storage Containers—Tight containers.

Peanut Oil

Oleum Arachidis

ラッカセイ油

Peanut Oil is the fixed oil obtained from the seeds of *Arachis hypogaea* Linné (*Leguminosae*).

Description Peanut Oil is a pale yellow, clear oil. It is odorless or has a slight odor. It has a mild taste.

It is miscible with diethyl ether and with petroleum ether.

It is slightly soluble in ethanol (95).

Specific gravity d_{25}^{25}: 0.909 – 0.916

Congealing point of the fatty acids: 22 – 33°C

Identification Saponify 5 g of Peanut Oil by boiling with 2.5 mL of sodium hydroxide solution (3 in 10) and 12.5 mL of ethanol (95). Evaporate the ethanol, dissolve the residue in 50 mL of hot water, and add dilute hydrochloric acid in excess until the free fatty acids separate as an oily layer. Cool the mixture, remove the separated fatty acids, and dissolve them in 75 mL of diethyl ether. To the diethyl ether solution add a solution of 4 g of lead (II) acetate trihydrate in 40 mL of ethanol (95), and allow the mixture to stand for 18 hours. Filter the supernatant liquid, transfer the precipitate to the filter with the aid of diethyl ether, and filter by suction. Place the precipitate in a beaker, heat it with 40 mL of dilute hydrochloric acid and 20 mL of water until the oily layer is entirely clear, cool, and decant the aqueous layer. Boil the fatty acids with 50 mL of diluted hydrochloric acid (1 in 100). When the solution prepared by dissolving 0.1 g of the fatty acids in 10 mL of ethanol (95) is not darkened by the addition of 2 drops of sodium sulfide TS, allow the fatty acids to solidify, and press them between dry filter papers to exclude moisture. Dissolve the solid fatty acid in 25 mL of diluted ethanol (9 in 10) with the aid of gentle heat, and then cool to 15°C to crystallize the fatty acids. Recrystallize them from diluted ethanol (9 in 10) and dry in a desiccator (phosphorus (V) oxide, in vacuum) for 4 hours: the melting point <*1.13*> of the dried crystals is between 73°C and 76°C.

Acid value <*1.13*> Not more than 0.2.

Saponification value <*1.13*> 188 – 196

Unsaponifiable matters <*1.13*> Not more than 1.5%.

Iodine value <*1.13*> 84 – 103

Containers and storage Containers—Tight containers.

Peony Root

Paeoniae Radix

シャクヤク

Peony Root is the root of *Paeonia lactiflora* Pallas (*Paeoniaceae*).

It contains not less than 2.0% of paeoniflorin ($C_{23}H_{28}O_{11}$: 480.46), calculated on the basis of dried material.

Description Cylindrical root, 7 – 20 cm in length, 1 – 2.5 cm in diameter; externally brown to light grayish brown, with distinct longitudinal wrinkles, with warty scars of lateral roots, and with laterally elongated lenticels; fractured surface dense in texture, light grayish brown, and with light brown radial lines in xylem.

Odor, characteristic; taste, slightly sweet at first, followed by an astringency and a slight bitterness.

Identification **(1)** Shake 0.5 g of pulverized Peony Root with 30 mL of ethanol (95) for 15 minutes, and filter. Shake 3 mL of the filtrate with 1 drop of iron (III) chloride TS: a blue-purple to blue-green color is produced, and it changes to dark blue-purple to dark green.

(2) To 2 g of pulverized Peony Root add 10 mL of methanol, warm on a water bath for 5 minutes, cool, filter, and use the filtrate as the sample solution. Separately, dissolve 1 mg of Paeoniflorin RS or paeoniflorin for thin-layer chromatography in 1 mL of methanol, and use this solution as the standard solution. Perform the test with these solutions as directed under Thin-layer Chromatography <*2.03*>. Spot 10 μL each of the sample solution and standard solution on a plate of silica gel for thin-layer chromatography. Develop the plate with a mixture of acetone, ethyl acetate and acetic acid (100) (10:10:1) to a distance of about 7 cm, and air-dry the plate. Spray evenly 4-methoxybenzaldehyde-sulfuric acid TS on the plate, and heat the plate at 105°C for 5 minutes: one of the several spots obtained from the sample solution has the same color tone and *R*f value with the spot from the standard solution.

Purity **(1)** Heavy metals <*1.07*>—Proceed with 3.0 g of pulverized Peony Root according to Method 3, and perform the test. Prepare the control solution with 3.0 mL of Standard Lead Solution (not more than 10 ppm).

(2) Arsenic <*1.11*>—Prepare the test solution with 0.40 g of pulverized Peony Root according to Method 4, and perform the test (not more than 5 ppm).

Loss on drying <*5.01*> Not more than 14.0% (6 hours).

Total ash <*5.01*> Not more than 6.5%.

Acid-insoluble ash <*5.01*> Not more than 0.5%.

Assay Weigh accurately about 0.5 g of pulverized Peony Root, add 50 mL of diluted methanol (1 in 2), heat under a reflux condenser for 30 minutes, cool, and filter. To the residue add 50 mL of diluted methanol (1 in 2), and proceed in the same manner. Combine the filtrates, add diluted methanol (1 in 2) to make exactly 100 mL, and use this solution as the sample solution. Separately, weigh accurately about 10 mg of Paeoniflorin RS (separately determine the water <*2.48*> by coulometric titration, using 10 mg), dissolve in diluted methanol (1 in 2) to make exactly 100 mL, and use this solution as the standard solution. Perform the test with exactly 10 μL each of the sample solution and standard solution as directed under Liquid Chromatography <*2.01*> according to the following conditions. Determine the peak areas, A_T and A_S, of paeoniflorin in each solution.

$$\text{Amount (mg) of paeoniflorin } (C_{23}H_{28}O_{11}) = M_S \times A_T/A_S$$

M_S: Amount (mg) of Paeoniflorin RS taken, calculated on the anhydrous basis

Operating conditions—

Detector: An ultraviolet absorption photometer (wavelength: 232 nm).

Column: A stainless steel column 4.6 mm in inside diameter and 15 cm in length, packed with octadecylsilanized silica gel for liquid chromatography (5 μm in particle diameter).

Column temperature: A constant temperature of about 20°C.

Mobile phase: A mixture of water, acetonitrile and phosphoric acid (850:150:1).

Flow rate: Adjust so that the retention time of paeoniflorin is about 10 minutes.

System suitability—

System performance: Dissolve 1 mg each of Paeoniflorin RS and albiflorin in diluted methanol (1 in 2) to make 10 mL. When the procedure is run with 10 μL of this solution under the above operating conditions, albiflorin and paeoniflorin are eluted in this order with the resolution between these peaks being not less than 2.5.

System repeatability: When the test is repeated 6 times with 10 μL of the standard solution under the above operating conditions, the relative standard deviation of the peak area of paeoniflorin is not more than 1.5%.

Containers and storage Containers—Well-closed containers.

Powdered Peony Root

Paeoniae Radix Pulverata

シャクヤク末

Powdered Peony Root is the powder of Peony Root.

It contains not less than 2.0% of paeoniflorin ($C_{23}H_{28}O_{11}$: 480.46), calculated on the basis of dried material.

Description Powdered Peony Root occurs as a light grayish brown powder, and has a characteristic odor and a slightly sweet taste at first, followed by an astringency and a slight bitterness.

Under a microscope <*5.01*>, Powdered Peony Root reveals starch grains and fragments of parenchyma cells containing them; fragments of cork cells, vessels, tracheids and xylem fibers; rosette aggregates of calcium oxalate, and fragments of rows of crystal cells containing them. Starch grains consist of simple grains, 5 – 25 μm in diameter, occasionally 2- to 3-compound grains.

Identification **(1)** Shake 0.5 g of Powdered Peony Root with 30 mL of ethanol (95) for 15 minutes, and filter. To 3 mL of the filtrate add 1 drop of iron (III) chloride TS, and mix: a blue-purple to blue-green color is produced, and thereafter it changes to dark blue-purple to dark green.

(2) To 2 g of Powdered Peony Root add 10 mL of methanol, warm on a water bath for 5 minutes, cool, filter, and use the filtrate as the sample solution. Separately, dissolve 1 mg of Paeoniflorin RS or paeoniflorin for thin-layer chromatography in 1 mL of methanol, and use this solution as the standard solution. Perform the test with these solutions as directed under Thin-layer Chromatography <*2.03*>. Spot 10 μL each of the sample solution and standard solution on a plate of silica gel for thin-layer chromatography. Develop the plate with a mixture of acetone, ethyl acetate and acetic acid (100) (10:10:1) to a distance of about 7 cm, and air-dry the plate. Spray evenly 4-methoxybenzaldehyde-sulfuric acid TS on the plate, and heat the plate at 105°C for 5 minutes: one of the several spots obtained from the sample solution has the same color tone and *Rf* value with the spot from the standard solution.

Purity **(1)** Heavy metals <*1.07*>—Proceed with 3.0 g of Powdered Peony Root according to Method 3, and perform the test. Prepare the control solution with 3.0 mL of Standard Lead Solution (not more than 10 ppm).

(2) Arsenic <*1.11*>—Prepare the test solution with 0.40 g of Powdered Peony Root according to Method 4, and perform the test (not more than 5 ppm).

(3) Foreign matter—Under a microscope <*5.01*>, Powdered Peony Root does not show groups of light yellow stone cells and fibers.

Loss on drying <*5.01*> Not less than 14.0% (6 hours).

Total ash <*5.01*> Not more than 6.5%.

Acid-insoluble ash <*5.01*> Not more than 0.5%.

Assay Weigh accurately about 0.5 g of Powdered Peony Root, add 50 mL of diluted methanol (1 in 2), heat under a reflux condenser for 30 minutes, cool, and filter. To the residue add 50 mL of diluted methanol (1 in 2), and proceed in the same manner. Combine the filtrates, add diluted methanol (1 in 2) to make exactly 100 mL, and use this solution as the sample solution. Separately, weigh accurately about 10 mg of Paeoniflorin RS (separately determine the water <*2.48*> by coulometric titration, using 10 mg), dissolve in diluted methanol (1 in 2) to make exactly 100 mL, and use this solution as the standard solution. Perform the test with exactly 10 μL each of the sample solution and standard solution as directed under Liquid Chromatography <*2.01*> according to the following conditions. Determine the peak areas, A_T and A_S, of paeoniflorin in each solution.

$$\text{Amount (mg) of paeoniflorin } (C_{23}H_{28}O_{11}) = M_S \times A_T/A_S$$

M_S: Amount (mg) of Paeoniflorin RS taken, calculated on the anhydrous basis

Operating conditions—

Detector: An ultraviolet absorption photometer (wavelength: 232 nm).

Column: A stainless steel column 4.6 mm in inside diameter and 15 cm in length, packed with octadecylsilanized silica gel for liquid chromatography (5 μm in particle diameter).

Column temperature: A constant temperature of about 20°C.

Mobile phase: A mixture of water, acetonitrile and phosphoric acid (850:150:1).

Flow rate: Adjust so that the retention time of paeoniflorin is about 10 minutes.

System suitability—

System performance: Dissolve 1 mg each of Paeoniflorin RS and albiflorin in diluted methanol (1 in 2) to make 10 mL. When the procedure is run with 10 μL of this solution under the above operating conditions, albiflorin and paeoniflorin are eluted in this order with the resolution between these peaks being not less than 2.5.

System repeatability: When the test is repeated 6 times with 10 μL of the standard solution under the above operating conditions, the relative standard deviation of the peak area of paeoniflorin is not more than 1.5%.

Containers and storage Containers—Well-closed containers.

Perilla Herb

Perillae Herba

ソヨウ

Perilla Herb is the leaves and the tips of branches of *Perilla frutescens* Britton var. *crispa* W. Deane (*Labiatae*).

It contains not less than 0.07% of perillaldehyde, calculated on the basis of dried material.

Description Usually, contracted and wrinkled leaves, often with thin stems. Both surfaces of the leaf are brownish purple, or the upper surface is grayish green to brownish green, and the lower surface is brownish purple in color. When smoothed by immersion in water, the lamina is ovate to obcordate, 5 - 12 cm in length, 5 - 8 cm in width; the apex, acuminate; the margin, serrate; the base, broadly cuneate; petiole, 3 - 5 cm in length; cross sections of stem and petiole, square. Under a magnifying glass, hairs are observed on both surfaces of the leaf, but abundantly on the vein and sparsely on other parts; small glandular hairs are observed on the lower surface.

Odor, characteristic; taste slightly bitter.

Identification To 0.6 g of pulverized Perilla Herb, add 10 mL of diethyl ether, shake for 15 minutes, filter, and use the filtrate as the sample solution. Separately, dissolve 1 mg of perillaldehyde for thin-layer chromatography in 10 mL of methanol, and use this solution as the standard solution. Perform the test with these solutions as directed under Thin-layer Chromatography <2.03>. Spot 10 μL each of the sample solution and standard solution on a plate of silica gel for thin-layer chromatography. Develop the plate with a mixture of hexane and ethyl acetate (3:1) to a distance of about 7 cm, and air-dry the plate. Spray evenly 4-methoxybenzaldehyde-sulfuric acid-acetic acid-ethanol TS for spray on the plate, and heat the plate at 105°C for 2 minutes: one of the several spots obtained from the sample solution has the same color tone and *R*f value with the spot from the standard solution.

Purity **(1)** Stem—When perform the test of foreign matter <5.01>, Perilla Herb does not contain its stems equal to or greater than 3 mm in diameter.

(2) Foreign matter <5.01>—The amount of foreign matter other than the stems contained in Perilla Herb does not exceed 1.0%.

(3) Total BHC's and total DDT's <5.01>—Not more than 0.2 ppm, respectively.

Loss on drying <5.01> Not more than 13.0% (6 hours).

Total ash <5.01> Not more than 16.0%.

Acid-insoluble ash <5.01> Not more than 2.5%.

Assay Weigh accurately about 0.2 g of freshly prepared pulverized Perilla Herb, put in a glass-stoppered centrifuge tube, add 20 mL of methanol, shake for 10 minutes, centrifuge, and separate the supernatant liquid. To the residue, add 20 mL of methanol, and proceed in the same manner. Combine all the extracts, add methanol to make exactly 50 mL, and use this solution as the sample solution. Separately, weigh accurately about 10 mg of diphenyl sulfone for assay, and dissolve in methanol to make exactly 100 mL. Pipet 10 mL of this solution, add methanol to make exactly 100 mL, and use this solution as the standard solution. Perform the test with exactly 10 μL each of the sample solution and standard solution as directed under Liquid Chromatography <2.01> according to the following conditions, and determine the peak areas, A_T of perillaldehyde and A_s of diphenyl sulfone, in each solution.

$$\text{Amount (mg) of perillaldehyde} = M_S \times A_T/A_S \times 1/20 \times 0.700$$

M_S: Amount (mg) of diphenyl sulfone for assay taken

Operating conditions—

Detector: An ultraviolet absorption photometer (wavelength: 234 nm).

Column: A stainless steel column 4.6 mm in inside diameter and 15 cm in length, packed with octadecylsilanized silica gel for liquid chromatography (5 μm in particle diameter).

Column temperature: A constant temperature of about 40°C.

Mobile phase: A mixture of water and acetonitrile (13:7).

Flow rate: 1.0 mL per minute.

System suitability—

System performance: Dissolve 1 mg of (*E*)-asarone and 1 mg of perillaldehyde for thin-layer chromatography in the standard solution to make 50 mL. When the procedure is run with 10 μL of this solution under the above operating conditions, diphenyl sulfone, perillaldehyde, and (*E*)-asarone are eluted in this order with the resolution between these peaks being not less than 1.5.

System repeatability: When the test is repeated 6 times with 10 μL of the standard solution under the above operating conditions, the relative standard deviation of the peak area of diphenyl sulfone is not more than 1.5%.

Containers and storage Containers—Well-closed containers.

Peucedanum Root

Peucedani Radix

ゼンコ

Peucedanum Root is the root of **1)** *Peucedanum praeruptorum* Dunn (Peucedanum Praeruptorum Root) or **2)** *Angelica decursiva* Franchet et Savatier (*Peucedanum decursivum* Maximowicz) (*Umbelliferae*) (Angelica Decursiva Root).

Description **1)** Peucedanum Praeruptorum Root—Slender obconical to cylindrical root, occasionally dichotomized at the lower part, 3 - 15 cm in length, 0.8 - 1.8 cm in diameter at the crown; externally light brown to dark brown; ring-node-like wrinkles numerous at the crown, sometimes with hair-like remains of leaf sheath; the root having somewhat deep longitudinal wrinkles and scars of cutting off of lateral roots; transverse section surface light brown to whitish in color; brittle in texture.

Odor, characteristic; taste, slightly bitter.

Under a microscope <*5.01*>, a transverse section reveals the outermost layer composed of a cork layer, inner tangential walls of some cork cells thickened; collenchyma just inside of the cork layer; in cortex numerous oil canals scattered and intercellular air spaces observed; occasionally phloem fibers observed at the terminal portion of phloem; vessels and scattered oil canals in xylem; starch grains in parenchyma, 2 to 10 several-compound grains.

2) Angelica Decursiva Root—Similar to 1), but without hair-like remains of leaf sheath at the crown.

Odor, characteristic; taste, slightly bitter.

Under a microscope <*5.01*>, a transverse section reveals, similar to 1), but cell wall of cork cells not thickened, phloem fibers not observed at the terminal portion of phloem, nor oil canals observed in xylem.

Identification **1)** Peucedanum Praeruptorum Root—To 1 g of pulverized Peucedanum Root add 10 mL of methanol, shake for 10 minutes, centrifuge, and use the supernatant liquid as the sample solution. Separately, dissolve 1 mg of (±)-praeruptorin A for thin-layer chromatography in 1 mL of methanol, and use this solution as the standard solution. Perform the test with these solutions as directed under Thin-layer Chromatography <*2.03*>. Spot 10 μL each of the sample solution and standard solution on a plate of silica gel for thin-layer chromatography. Develop the plate with a mixture of diethyl ether and hexane (3:1) to a distance of about 7 cm, and air-dry the plate. Examine under ultraviolet light (main wavelength: 365 nm): one of the several spots obtained from the sample solution has the same color tone and *R*f value with the blue-white to blue-purple fluorescent spot from the standard solution.

2) Angelica Decursiva Root—To 1 g of pulverized Peucedanum Root add 10 mL of methanol, shake for 10 minutes, centrifuge, and use the supernatant liquid as the sample solution. Separately, dissolve 1 mg of nodakenin for thin-layer chromatography in 1 mL of methanol, and use this solution as the standard solution. Perform the test with these solutions as directed under Thin-layer Chromatography <*2.03*>. Spot 10 μL each of the sample solution and standard solution on a plate of silica gel for thin-layer chromatography. Develop the plate with a mixture of ethyl acetate, methanol and water (12:2:1) to a distance of about 7 cm, and air-dry the plate. Examine under ultraviolet light (main wavelength: 365 nm): one of the several spots obtained from the sample solution has the same color tone and *R*f value with the blue-white to blue-purple fluorescent spot from the standard solution.

Purity Heavy metals <*1.07*>—Proceed with 1.0 g of pulverized Peucedanum Root according to Method 3, and perform the test. Prepare the control solution with 2.0 mL of Standard Lead Solution (not more than 20 ppm).

Loss on drying <*5.01*> Not more than 13.0%.

Total ash <*5.01*> Not more than 7.0%.

Acid-insoluble ash <*5.01*> Not more than 2.0%.

Extract content <*5.01*> Dilute ethanol-soluble extract: not less than 20.0%.

Containers and storage Containers—Well-closed containers.

Pharbitis Seed

Pharbitidis Semen

ケンゴシ

Pharbitis Seed is the seed of *Pharbitis nil* Choisy (*Convolvulaceae*).

Description Longitudinally quartered or sexpartite globe, 4 - 6 mm in length, 3 - 5 mm in width; externally black to grayish red-brown or grayish white, smooth, but slightly shrunken and coarsely wrinkled. The transverse section almost fan-shaped, light yellow-brown to light grayish brown, and dense in texture. Under a magnifying glass, the surface of the seed coat reveals dense, short hairs; dented hilum at the bottom of the raphe. Seed coat thin, the outer layer dark gray, and the inner layer light gray; two irregularly folded cotyledons in the transverse section at one end; two septa from the center of the dorsal side to the ridge separating cotyledons but unrecognizable in the transverse section of the other end having hilum; dark gray secretory pits in the section of the cotyledon. 100 seeds weighing about 3.5 g.

When cracked, odor, slight; taste, oily and slightly pungent.

Total ash <*5.01*> Not more than 6.0%.

Containers and storage Containers—Well-closed containers.

Phellodendron Bark

Phellodendri Cortex

オウバク

Phellodendron Bark is the bark of *Phellodendron amurense* Ruprecht or *Phellodendron chinense* Schneider (*Rutaceae*), from which the periderm has been removed.

It contains not less than 1.2% of berberine [as berberine chloride ($C_{20}H_{18}ClNO_4$: 371.81)], calculated on the basis of dried material.

Description Flat or rolled semi-tubular pieces of bark, 2 - 4 mm in thickness; externally grayish yellow-brown to grayish brown, with numerous traces of lenticels; the internal surface yellow to dark yellow-brown in color, with fine vertical lines, and smooth; fractured surface fibrous and bright yellow.

Odor, slight; taste, extremely bitter; mucilaginous; it colors the saliva yellow on chewing.

Under a microscope <*5.01*>, a transverse section reveals primary ray expands outward and looks fan shaped in secondary cortex, and sometimes ray differentiated later converges outward; groups of stone cells yellow and scattered in primary ray; groups of phloem fibers light yellow to yellow, lined alternately with the other tissue of phloem between rays, and then these tissues show obviously latticework; solitary crystals of calcium oxalate, single and compound starch grains observed in parenchyma.

Identification **(1)** To 1 g of pulverized Phellodendron Bark add 10 mL of diethyl ether, allow to stand for 10 minutes with occasional shaking, and filter to remove the diethyl ether. Collect the powder on the filter paper, add 10 mL of ethanol (95), allow to stand for 10 minutes with occasional shaking, and filter. To 2 to 3 drops of the filtrate add 1 mL of hydrochloric acid, add 1 to 2 drops of hydrogen peroxide TS, and shake: a red-purple color develops.

(2) Use the filtrate obtained in (1) as the sample solution. Separately, dissolve 1 mg of Berberine Chloride RS or berberine chloride hydrate for thin-layer chromatography in 1 mL of methanol, and use this solution as the standard solution. Perform the test with these solutions as directed under Thin-layer Chromatography <*2.03*>. Spot 5 μL each of the sample solution and standard solution on a plate of silica gel for thin-layer chromatography. Develop the plate with a mixture of 1-butanol, water and acetic acid (100) (7:2:1) to a distance of about 7 cm, and air-dry the plate. Examine under ultraviolet light (main wavelength: 365 nm): one of the several spots obtained from the sample solution and a spot with yellow to yellow-green fluorescence from the standard solution show the same color tone and the same *R*f value.

(3) Stir up pulverized Phellodendron Bark with water: the solution becomes gelatinous owing to mucilage.

Loss on drying <*5.01*> Not more than 11.0% (6 hours).

Total ash <*5.01*> Not more than 7.5%.

Acid-insoluble ash <*5.01*> Not more than 0.5%.

Assay Weigh accurately about 0.5 g of pulverized Phellodendron Bark, add 30 mL of a mixture of methanol and dilute hydrochloric acid (100:1), heat under a reflux condenser for 30 minutes, cool, and filter. Repeat the above procedure twice with the residue, using 30-mL and 20-mL portions of a mixture of methanol and dilute hydrochloric acid (100:1). To the last residue add 10 mL of methanol, shake well, and filter. Combine the whole filtrates, add methanol to make exactly 100 mL, and use this solution as the sample solution. Separately, weigh accurately about 10 mg of Berberine Chloride RS (separately determine the water <*2.48*> in the same manner as Berberine Chloride Hydrate), dissolve in methanol to make exactly 100 mL, and use this solution as the standard solution. Perform the test with exactly 20 μL each of the sample solution and standard solution as directed under Liquid Chromatography <*2.01*> according to the following conditions, and determine the peak areas, A_T and A_S, of berberine in each solution.

Amount (mg) of berberine [as berberine chloride ($C_{20}H_{18}ClNO_4$)]
$= M_S \times A_T/A_S$

M_S: Amount (mg) of Berberine Chloride RS taken, calculated on the anhydrous basis

Operating conditions—

Detector: An ultraviolet absorption photometer (wavelength: 345 nm).

Column: A stainless steel column 4 to 6 mm in inside diameter and 15 to 25 cm in length, packed with octadecylsilanized silica gel (5 to 10 mm in particle diameter).

Column temperature: A constant temperature of about 40°C

Mobile phase: Dissolve 3.4 g of potassium dihydrogenphosphate and 1.7 g of sodium lauryl sulfate in 1000 mL of a mixture of water and acetonitrile (1:1).

Flow rate: Adjust so that the retention time of berberine is about 10 minutes.

System suitability—

System performance: Dissolve 1 mg each of Berberine Chloride RS and palmatine chloride in methanol to make 10 mL. When the procedure is run with 20 μL of this solution under the above operating conditions, palmatine and berberine are eluted in this order with the resolution between these peaks being not less than 1.5.

System repeatability: When the test is repeated 5 times with 20 μL of the standard solution under the above operating conditions, the relative standard deviation of the peak area of berberine is not more than 1.5%.

Containers and storage Containers—Well-closed containers.

Powdered Phellodendron Bark

Phellodendri Cortex Pulveratus

オウバク末

Powdered Phellodendron Bark is the powder of Phellodendron Bark.

It contains not less than 1.2% of berberine [as berberine chloride ($C_{20}H_{18}ClNO_4$: 371.81)], calculated on the basis of dried material.

Description Powdered Phellodendron Bark occurs as a bright yellow to yellow powder. It has a slight odor and an extremely bitter taste, is mucilaginous, and colors the saliva yellow on chewing.

Under a microscope <*5.01*>, Powdered Phellodendron Bark reveals fragments of yellow, thick-walled fiber bundles or fibers, and fibers often accompanied by crystal cell rows; fewer groups of stone cells together with idioblasts; fragments of parenchyma cells containing starch grains and oil droplets; fragments of medullary ray and phloem; mucilage cells and mucilage masses. Numerous solitary crystals of calcium oxalate, 7 – 20 μm in diameter; starch grains, simple grains and 2- to 4-compound grains, simple grain, 2 - 6 μm in diameter; oil droplets, stained red with sudan III TS.

Identification **(1)** To 1 g of Powdered Phellodendron Bark add 10 mL of diethyl ether, allow to stand for 10 minutes with occasional shaking, and filter to remove the diethyl ether. Collect the powder on the filter paper, add 10 mL of ethanol (95), allow to stand for 10 minutes with occasional shaking, and filter. To 2 to 3 drops of the filtrate add 1 mL of hydrochloric acid, add 1 to 2 drops of hydrogen peroxide TS, and shake: a red-purple color develops.

(2) Use the filtrate obtained in (1) as the sample solution. Separately, dissolve 1 mg of Berberine Chloride RS or berberine chloride hydrate for thin-layer chromatography in 1 mL of methanol, and use this solution as the standard solution. Perform the test with these solutions as directed under Thin-layer Chromatography <*2.03*>. Spot 5 μL each of the sample solution and standard solution on a plate of silica gel for thin-layer chromatography. Develop the plate with a mixture of 1-butanol, water and acetic acid (100) (7:2:1) to a distance of about 7 cm, and air-dry the plate. Examine under ultraviolet light (main wavelength: 365 nm): one of the several spots obtained from the sample solution and a spot with yellow to yellow-green fluorescence from the standard solution show the same color tone and the same *R*f value.

(3) Stir up Powdered Phellodendron Bark with water: the solution becomes gelatinous owing to mucilage.

Purity Curcuma—Place Powdered Phellodendron Bark on filter paper, drop diethyl ether on it, and allow to stand. Take the powder off the filter paper, and drip 1 drop of potassium hydroxide TS: no red-purple color develops. Under a microscope *<5.01>*, Powdered Phellodendron Bark does not contain gelatinized starch or secretory cells containing yellow-red resin.

Loss on drying *<5.01>* Not more than 11.0% (6 hours).

Total ash *<5.01>* Not more than 7.5%.

Acid-insoluble ash *<5.01>* Not more than 0.5%.

Assay Weigh accurately about 0.5 g of Powdered Phellodendron Bark, add 30 mL of a mixture of methanol and dilute hydrochloric acid (100:1), heat under a reflux condenser for 30 minutes, cool, and filter. Repeat the above procedure twice with the residue, using 30-mL and 20-mL portions of a mixture of methanol and dilute hydrochloric acid (100:1). To obtained residue add 10 mL of methanol, shake well, and filter. Combine the whole filtrates, add methanol to make exactly 100 mL, and use this solution as the sample solution. Separately, weigh accurately about 10 mg of Berberine Chloride RS (separately determine the water *<2.48>* in the same manner as Berberine Chloride Hydrate), dissolve in methanol to make exactly 100 mL, and use this solution as the standard solution. Perform the test with exactly 20 μL each of the sample solution and standard solution as directed under Liquid Chromatography *<2.01>* according to the following conditions, and determine the peak areas, A_T and A_S, of berberine in each solution.

Amount (mg) of berberine [as berberine chloride ($C_{20}H_{18}ClNO_4$)]
$= M_S \times A_T/A_S$

M_S: Amount (mg) of Berberine Chloride RS taken, calculated on the anhydrous basis

Operating conditions—

Detector: An ultraviolet absorption photometer (wavelength: 345 nm).

Column: A stainless steel column 4 to 6 mm in inside diameter and 15 to 25 cm in length, packed with octadecylsilanized silica gel for liquid chromatography (5 to 10 μm in particle diameter).

Column temperature: A constant temperature of about 40°C.

Mobile phase: Dissolve 3.4 g of potassium dihydrogenphosphate and 1.7 g of sodium lauryl sulfate in 1000 mL of a mixture of water and acetonitrile (1:1).

Flow rate: Adjust so that the retention time of berberine is about 10 minutes.

System suitability—

System performance: Dissolve 1 mg each of Berberine Chloride RS and palmatine chloride in methanol to make 10 mL. When the procedure is run with 20 μL of this solution under the above operating conditions, palmatine and berberine are eluted in this order with the resolution between these peaks being not less than 1.5.

System repeatability: When the test is repeated 5 times with 20 μL of the standard solution under the above operating conditions, the relative standard deviation of the peak area of berberine is not more than 1.5%.

Containers and storage Containers—Well-closed containers.

Compound Phellodendron Powder for Cataplasm

パップ用複方オウバク散

Method of preparation

Powdered Phellodendron Bark	660 g
Powdered Gardenia Fruit	325 g
d- or *dl*-Camphor	10 g
dl- or *l*-Menthol	5 g
To make	1000 g

Prepare as directed under Powders, with the above ingredients.

Description Compound Phellodendron Powder for Cataplasm occurs as a yellow-brown powder, having a characteristic odor.

Identification Shake thoroughly 0.2 g of Compound Phellodendron Powder for Cataplasm with 5 mL of methanol, filter, and use the filtrate as the sample solution. Separately, dissolve 1 mg of Berberine Chloride RS or berberine chloride hydrate for thin-layer chromatography in 1 mL of methanol, and use the solution as the standard solution. Perform the test with these solutions as directed under Thin-layer Chromatography *<2.03>*. Spot 5 μL each of the sample solution and standard solution on a plate of silica gel for thin-layer chromatography. Develop the plate with a mixture of 1-butanol, water and acetic acid (100) (7:2:1) to a distance of about 10 cm, air-dry the plate. Examine under ultraviolet light (main wavelength: 365 nm): one of the several spots obtained from the sample solution has the same color tone and *R*f value with the yellow to yellow-green fluorescent spot from the standard solution (phellodendron bark).

Containers and storage Containers—Tight containers.

Phellodendron, Albumin Tannate and Bismuth Subnitrate Powder

オウバク・タンナルビン・ビスマス散

Phellodendron, Albumin Tannate and Bismuth Subnitrate Powder contains not less than 12.9% and not more than 16.3% of bismuth (Bi: 208.98).

Method of preparation

Powdered Phellodendron Bark	300 g
Albumin Tannate	300 g
Bismuth Subnitrate	200 g
Scopolia Extract	10 g
Starch, Lactose Hydrate or their mixture	a sufficient quantity
To make	1000 g

Prepare as directed under Powders, with the above ingredients. Scopolia Extract Powder may be used in place of Scopolia Extract.

Description Phellodendron, Albumin Tannate and Bismuth Subnitrate Powder is brownish yellow in color, and has a bitter taste.

Identification **(1)** Shake thoroughly 0.1 g of Phellodendron, Albumin Tannate and Bismuth Subnitrate Powder with 5 mL of methanol, filter, and use the filtrate as the sample solution. Separately, dissolve 1 mg of Berberine Chloride RS or berberine chloride hydrate for thin-layer chromatography in 1 mL of methanol, and use this solution as the standard solution. Perform the test with these solutions as directed under Thin-layer Chromatography *<2.03>*. Spot 5 μL each of the sample solution and standard solution on a plate of silica gel for thin-layer chromatography. Develop the plate with a mixture of 1-butanol, water and acetic acid (100) (7:2:1) to a distance of about 10 cm, air-dry the plate. Examine under ultraviolet light (main wavelength: 365 nm): one spot of the several spots obtained from the sample solution and a spot with yellow to yellow-green fluorescence from the standard solution show the same color tone and the same *R*f value (phellodendron bark).

(2) To 0.3 g of Phellodendron, Albumin Tannate and Bismuth Subnitrate Powder add 20 mL of ethanol (95), heat in a water bath for 3 minutes with shaking, cool, and filter. To 10 mL of the filtrate add 1 drop of iron (III) chloride TS: a blue-green color is produced. Allow to stand: a bluish black precipitate is produced (albumin tannate).

(3) To 0.3 g of Phellodendron, Albumin Tannate and Bismuth Subnitrate Powder add 10 mL of diluted pyridine (1 in 5), warm in a water bath for 3 minutes with shaking, cool, and filter. Add 1 mL of ninhydrin-ascorbic acid TS to the filtrate, and heat in a water bath: a blue color is produced (albumin tannate).

(4) To 0.5 g of Phellodendron, Albumin Tannate and Bismuth Subnitrate Powder add 5 mL of dilute hydrochloric acid and 10 mL of water, warm, shake thoroughly, and filter. The filtrate responds to the Qualitative Tests *<1.09>* for bismuth salt.

Assay Weigh accurately about 0.7 g of Phellodendron, Albumin Tannate and Bismuth Subnitrate Powder, shake well with 10 mL of water and 20 mL of diluted nitric acid (1 in 3), add water to make exactly 100 mL, and filter. Discard the first 20 mL of the filtrate, pipet the subsequent 10 mL of the filtrate, and add water to make exactly 100 mL. Pipet 25 mL of this solution, add diluted nitric acid (1 in 100) to make exactly 100 mL, and use this solution as the sample solution. Separately, weigh accurately about 0.23 g of bismuth nitrate pentahydrate, add 20 mL of diluted nitric acid (1 in 3) and water to make exactly 100 mL. Pipet 10 mL of this solution, and add water to make exactly 100 mL. Pipet 25 mL of this solution, add diluted nitric acid (1 in 100) to make exactly 100 mL, and use this solution as the standard solution. Determine the absorbances, A_T and A_S, of the sample solution and standard solution as directed under Atomic Absorption Spectrophotometry *<2.23>* according to the following conditions. On the other hand, determine the absorbance A_0 of the solution prepared in the same manner using 20 mL of diluted nitric acid (1 in 3) instead of the standard solution.

Gas: Combustible gas—Acetylene.
　Supporting gas—Air.
Lamp: A bismuth hollow-cathode lamp.
Wavelength: 223.1 nm.

$$\text{Amount (mg) of bismuth (Bi)} = M \times (A_T - A_0)/(A_S - A_0) \times 0.431$$

M: Amount (mg) of bismuth nitrate pentahydrate taken

Containers and storage Containers—Well-closed containers.

Picrasma Wood

Picrasmae Lignum

ニガキ

Picrasma Wood is the wood of *Picrasma quassioides* Bennet (*Simaroubaceae*).

Description Light yellow chips, slices or short pieces of wood; a transverse section reveals distinct annual rings and thin medullary rays; tissue dense in texture.

Odorless; taste, extremely bitter and lasting.

Under a microscope *<5.01>*, it reveals medullary rays consisting of 1 - 5 cells wide for transverse section, and 5 - 50 cells high for longitudinal cut surface; vessels of spring wood up to about 150 μm in diameter, but those of autumn wood only one-fifth as wide; vessels, single or in groups, scattered in the xylem parenchyma; wall of wood fibers extremely thickened; medullary rays and xylem parenchyma cells contain rosette aggregates of calcium oxalate and starch grains. Vivid yellow or red-brown, resinous substance often present in the vessels.

Purity Foreign matter *<5.01>*—The amount of foreign matter contained in Picrasma Wood does not exceed 1.0%.

Total ash *<5.01>* Not more than 4.0%.

Containers and storage Containers—Well-closed containers.

Powdered Picrasma Wood

Picrasmae Lignum Pulveratum

ニガキ末

Powdered Picrasma Wood is the powder of Picrasma Wood.

Description Powdered Picrasma occurs as a grayish white to light yellow powder. It is odorless, and has an extremely bitter and lasting taste.

Under a microscope *<5.01>*, Powdered Picrasma Wood reveals fragments of vessels of various sizes, xylem fibers and xylem parenchyma cells; fragments of medullary rays containing starch grains; all tissues lignified; a few crystals of calcium oxalate observed. Starch grains are 5 to 15 μm in diameter.

Total ash *<5.01>* Not more than 4.0%.

Acid-insoluble ash *<5.01>* Not more than 1.0%.

Containers and storage Containers—Well-closed containers.

Pinellia Tuber

Pinelliae Tuber

ハンゲ

Pinellia Tuber is the tuber of *Pinellia ternata* Breitenbach (*Araceae*), from which the cork layer has been removed.

Description Slightly flattened spherical to irregular-shaped tuber; 0.7 - 2.5 cm in diameter and 0.7 - 1.5 cm in height; externally white to grayish white-yellow; the upper end dented, where the stem has been removed, with root scars dented as numerous small spots on the circumference; dense in texture; cross section white and powdery.

Almost odorless; tasteless at first, slightly mucous, but leaving a strong acrid taste.

Under a microscope <*5.01*>, a transverse section reveals mainly tissue of parenchyma filled with starch grains, and scattered with a few mucilage cells containing raphides of calcium oxalate. Starch grains mostly 2- to 3-compound grains, usually 10 - 15 μm in diameter, and simple grains, usually 3 - 7 μm in diameter; raphides of calcium oxalate 25 - 150 μm in length.

Purity (1) Heavy metals <*1.07*>—Proceed with 3.0 g of pulverized Pinellia Tuber according to Method 3, and perform the test. Prepare the control solution with 3.0 mL of Standard Lead Solution (not more than 10 ppm).

(2) Arsenic <*1.11*>—Prepare the test solution with 0.40 g of pulverized Pinellia Tuber according to Method 4, and perform the test (not more than 5 ppm).

(3) Rhizome of Arisaema species and others—Under a microscope <*5.01*>, no mucilage canal is revealed on the outer layer of cortex.

Loss on drying <*5.01*> Not more than 14.0% (6 hours).

Total ash <*5.01*> Not more than 3.5%.

Containers and storage Containers—Well-closed containers.

Plantago Herb

Plantaginis Herba

シャゼンソウ

Plantago Herb is the entire plant of *Plantago asiatica* Linné (*Plantaginaceae*), collected during the flowering season.

Description Usually wrinkled and contracted leaf and spike, grayish green to dark yellow-green in color; when soaked in water and smoothed out, the lamina is ovate to orbicular-ovate, 4 - 15 cm in length, 3 - 8 cm in width; apex acute, and base sharply narrowed; margin slightly wavy, with distinct parallel veins; glabrous or nearly glabrous; petiole is rather longer than the lamina, and its base is slightly expanded with thin-walled leaf-sheath; scape is 10 - 50 cm in length, one-third to one-half of the upper part forming the spike, with dense florets; the lower part of inflorescence often shows pyxidia; roots usually removed, but, if any, fine roots are closely packed.

Odor, slight; practically tasteless.

Identification To 2.0 g of pulverized Plantago Herb add 10 mL of methanol, warm on a water bath for 3 minutes, cool, filter, and use the filtrate as the sample solution. Perform the test with the sample solution as directed under Thin-layer Chromatography <*2.03*>. Spot 10 μL of the sample solution on a plate of silica gel for thin-layer chromatography. Develop the plate with a mixture of 1-butanol, water and acetic acid (100) (7:2:1) to a distance of about 7 cm, and air-dry the plate. Spray evenly iron (III) chloride TS on the plate: a dark blue spot appears at an *Rf* value of about 0.55.

Total ash <*5.01*> Not more than 15.0%.

Acid-insoluble ash <*5.01*> Not more than 4.0%.

Extract content <*5.01*> Dilute ethanol-soluble extract: not less than 14.0%.

Containers and storage Containers—Well-closed containers.

Plantago Seed

Plantaginis Semen

シャゼンシ

Plantago Seed is the seed of *Plantago asiatica* Linné (*Plantaginaceae*).

Description Flattened ellipsoidal seed, 2 - 2.5 mm in length, 0.7 - 1 mm in width, 0.3 - 0.5 mm in thickness; externally brown to yellow-brown and lustrous. Under a magnifying glass, the surface of the seed is practically smooth, with the dorsal side protruding like a bow, and with the ventral side somewhat dented; micropyle and raphe not observable. 100 seeds weigh about 0.05 g.

Almost odorless; taste, slightly bitter and mucous.

Under a microscope <*5.01*>, a transverse section reveals a seed coat consisting of three layers of epidermis composed of cells containing mucilage, a vegetative layer, and a pigment layer of approximately equidiameter cells; in the interior, endosperm thicker than seed coat, enclosing two cotyledons.

Identification (1) To 1 g of Plantago Seed add 2 mL of warm water, and allow the mixture to stand for 10 minutes: the seed coat swells to discharge mucilage.

(2) To 1.0 g of pulverized Plantago Seed add 5 mL of methanol, shake for 10 minutes, centrifuge, and use the supernatant liquid as the sample solution. Separately, to 0.2 g of powdered plantago seed for thin-layer chromatography add 1 mL of methanol, and warm on a water bath for 3 minutes. After cooling, centrifuge, and use the supernatant liquid as the standard solution. Perform the test with these solutions as directed under Thin-layer Chromatography <*2.03*>. Spot 5 μL each of the sample solution and standard solution on a plate of silica gel for thin-layer chromatography. Develop the plate with a mixture of acetone, ethyl acetate, water and acetic acid (100) (10:10:3:1) to a distance of about 7 cm, and air-dry the plate. Spray evenly 4-methoxybenzaldehyde-sulfuric acid TS on the plate, and heat the plate at 105°C for 10 minutes: the spot appeared at an *Rf* value of about 0.25 obtained from the sample solution has the same color tone with the dark blue spot appeared at an *Rf* value of about 0.25 from the standard solution.

Purity Foreign matter <*5.01*>—The amount of foreign matter contained in Plantago Seed does not exceed 2.0%.

Total ash <5.01> Not more than 5.5%.

Acid-insoluble ash <5.01> Not more than 2.0%.

Containers and storage Containers—Well-closed containers.

Platycodon Root

Platycodi Radix

キキョウ

Platycodon Root is the root of *Platycodon grandiflorus* A. De Candolle (*Campanulaceae*).

Description Irregular, somewhat thin and long fusiform to conical root, often branched; externally grayish brown, light brown or white; main root 10 – 15 cm in length, 1 – 3 cm in diameter; the upper end, with dented scars of removed stems; the neighborhood, with fine lateral wrinkles and longitudinal furrows and also slightly constricted; the greater part of the root, except the crown, covered with coarse longitudinal wrinkles, lateral furrows and lenticel-like lateral lines; hard in texture, but brittle; fractured surface not fibrous, often with cracks. Under a magnifying glass, a transverse section reveals cambium and its neighborhood often brown in color; cortex slightly thinner than xylem, almost white and with scattered cracks; xylem white to light brown in color, and the tissue slightly denser than cortex.

Odor, slight; tasteless at first, later acrid and bitter.

Identification (1) Warm 0.2 g of pulverized Platycodon Root with 2 mL of acetic anhydride on a water bath for 2 minutes, and filter. To 1 mL of the filtrate add carefully 0.5 mL of sulfuric acid to make two layers: a red to red-brown color develops at the zone of contact, and the upper layer acquires a blue-green to green color.

(2) To 2.0 g of pulverized Platycodon Root add 20 mL of sodium carbonate TS, and shake. Add 5 mL of 1-butanol, shake for 10 minutes, centrifuge, and use the 1-butanol layer as the sample solution. Separately, dissolve 1 mg of platycodin D for thin-layer chromatography in 1 mL of methanol, and use this solution as the standard solution. Perform the test with these solutions as directed under Thin-layer Chromatography <2.03>. Spot 5 μL each of the sample solution and standard solution on a plate of silica gel for thin-layer chromatography. Develop the plate with a mixture of 1-propanol, ethyl acetate, water and acetic acid (100) (5:3:2:1) to a distance of about 7 cm, and air-dry the plate. Spray evenly dilute sulfuric acid on the plate, and heat the plate at 105°C for 5 minutes: one of the several spots obtained from the sample solution and a spot from the standard solution show the same color tone and the same *R*f value.

Purity (1) Heavy metals <1.07>—Proceed with 3.0 g of pulverized Platycodon Root according to Method 3, and perform the test. Prepare the control solution with 3.0 mL of Standard Lead Solution (not more than 10 ppm).

(2) Arsenic <1.11>—Prepare the test solution with 0.40 g of pulverized Platycodon Root according to Method 4, and perform the test (not more than 5 ppm).

Total ash <5.01> Not more than 4.0%.

Extract content <5.01> Dilute ethanol-soluble extract: not less than 25.0%.

Containers and storage Containers—Well-closed containers.

Powdered Platycodon Root

Platycodi Radix Pulverata

キキョウ末

Powdered Platycodon Root is the powder of Platycodon Root.

Description Powdered Platycodon Root occurs as a light grayish yellow to light grayish brown powder. It has a slight odor, and is tasteless at first, later acrid and bitter.

Under a microscope <5.01>, Powdered Platycodon Root reveals numerous fragments of colorless parenchyma cells; fragments of reticulate vessels and scalariform vessels; fragments of sieve tubes and lactiferous tubes; fragments of cork layer are sometimes observed. Usually, starch grains are not observed, but very rarely simple grain.

Identification (1) Warm 0.2 g of Powdered Platycodon Root with 2 mL of acetic anhydride on a water bath for 2 minutes, and filter. To 1 mL of the filtrate add carefully 0.5 mL of sulfuric acid to make two layers: a red to red-brown color develops at the zone of contact, and the upper layer acquires a blue-green to green color.

(2) To 2.0 g of Powdered Platycodon Root add 20 mL of sodium carbonate TS, and shake. Add 5 mL of 1-butanol, shake for 10 minutes, centrifuge, and use the 1-butanol layer as the sample solution. Separately, dissolve 1 mg of platycodin D for thin-layer chromatography in 1 mL of methanol, and use this solution as the standard solution. Perform the test with these solutions as directed under Thin-layer Chromatography <2.03>. Spot 5 μL each of the sample solution and standard solution on a plate of silica gel for thin-layer chromatography. Develop the plate with a mixture of 1-propanol, ethyl acetate, water and acetic acid (100) (5:3:2:1) to a distance of about 7 cm, and air-dry the plate. Spray evenly dilute sulfuric acid on the plate, and heat the plate at 105°C for 5 minutes: one of the several spots obtained from the sample solution and a spot from the standard solution show the same color tone and the same *R*f value.

Purity (1) Heavy metals <1.07>—Proceed with 3.0 g of Powdered Platycodon Root according to Method 3, and perform the test. Prepare the control solution with 3.0 mL of Standard Lead Solution (not more than 10 ppm).

(2) Arsenic <1.11>—Prepare the test solution with 0.40 g of Powdered Platycodon Root according to Method 4, and perform the test (not more than 5 ppm).

(3) Foreign matter—Under a microscope <5.01>, Powdered Platycodon Root does not show fibers, stone cells or other foreign matter.

Total ash <5.01> Not more than 4.0%.

Acid-insoluble ash <5.01> Not more than 1.0%.

Extract content <5.01> Dilute ethanol-soluble extract: not less than 25.0%.

Containers and storage Containers—Well-closed containers.

Platycodon Fluidextract

キキョウ流エキス

Method of preparation **1)** Take coarse powder of Platycodon Root, and prepare the fluidextract as directed under Fluidextracts using 25 vol% ethanol. An appropriate quantity of Ethanol and Purified Water or Purified Water in Containers may be used in place of 25 vol% ethanol.

2) Take Platycodon Root pulverized to suitable sizes, and prepare the fluidextract as directed under Fluidextracts using 25 vol% ethanol or diluted ethanol (1 in 4) as the solvent.

Description Platycodon Fluidextract is a red-brown liquid. It is miscible with water, producing slight turbidity. It has a mild taste at first, followed by an acrid and bitter taste.

Identification To 2 mL of Platycodon Fluidextract add 20 mL of water and 5 mL of 1-butanol, mix, shake for 10 minutes, centrifuge, and use the 1-butanol layer as the sample solution. Separately, dissolve 1 mg of platycodin D for thin-layer chromatography in 1 mL of methanol, and use this solution as the standard solution. Perform the test with these solutions as directed under Thin-layer Chromatography <*2.03*>. Spot 5 μL each of the sample solution and standard solution on a plate of silica gel for thin-layer chromatography. Develop the plate with a mixture of 1-propanol, ethyl acetate, water and acetic acid (100) (5:3:2:1) to a distance of about 7 cm, and air-dry the plate. Spray evenly dilute sulfuric acid on the plate, and heat the plate at 105°C for 5 minutes: one of the several spots obtained from the sample solution has the same color tone and *R*f value with the spot from the standard solution.

Alcohol number <*1.01*> Apply to Platycodon Fluidextract prepared by the Method of preparation 2). 2.0 - 3.0 (Method 1).

Purity **(1)** Heavy metals <*1.07*>—Prepare the test solution with 1.0 g of Platycodon Fluidextract as directed in the Fluidextracts (4), and perform the test (not more than 30 ppm).

(2) Starch—Mix 1 mL of Platycodon Fluidextract with 4 mL of water, and add 1 drop of dilute iodine TS: no purple or blue color develops.

Content of the active principle Transfer exactly 5 mL of Platycodon Fluidextract to a tared beaker or porcelain dish, evaporate to dryness on a water bath, and dry at 105°C for 5 hours: the mass of the residue is not less than 0.50 g.

Containers and storage Containers—Tight containers.
Storage—Light-resistant.

Pogostemi Herb

Pogostemi Herba

カッコウ

Pogostemon Herb is the terrestrial part of *Pogostemon cablin* Bentham (*Labiatae*).

Description Stems with opposite leaves, leaves wrinkled and shriveled. When smoothed by immersion in water, leaves are obovate to ovate-oblong, 2.5 - 10 cm in length, 2.5 - 7 cm in width, with obtusely serrate margins and petioles at the cuneate bases; the upper surface of leaves dark brown, the lower surface grayish brown, both sides covered densely with hairs. Stems are square, solid, grayish green, covered with grayish white to yellow-white hairs; the pith broad, whitish, spongy. Under a magnifying glass, leaf reveals hairs, glandular hairs and glandular scales.

Odor, distinct; taste, slightly bitter.

Under a microscope <*5.01*>, a transverse section of petiole reveals central portion of the adaxial side protruding remarkably, with collenchyma cells beneath epidermis; vascular bundles at the center divided into two groups. Under a microscope <*5.01*>, a transverse section of the midvein of lamina reveals the adaxial side protruding remarkably, with collenchyma cells beneath epidermis; vascular bundles at the center arranged in fan-shape. Under a microscope <*5.01*>, a transverse section of stem reveals several-cells-layered collenchyma beneath epidermis, occasionally with cork layer developed; beneath cortex, collateral vascular bundles arranged in a circle, phloem fibers in groups observed at the outer portion of phloem; oil droplets observed in parenchymat cells of cortex, needle, solitary or columnar crystals of calcium oxalate in parenchyma cells of pith.

Identification To 0.5 g of pulverized Pogostemon Herb, add 5 mL of methanol, shake for 3 minutes, filter, and use the filtrate as the sample solution. Perform the test with the sample solution as directed under Thin-layer Chromatography <*2.03*>. Spot 5 μL of the sample solution on a plate of silica gel for thin-layer chromatography, develop the plate with a mixture of hexane and acetone (9:1) to a distance of about 7 cm, and air-dry the plate. Spray evenly 4-methoxybenzaldehyde-sulfuric acid TS on the plate, and heat the plate at 105°C for 5 minutes; a blue-purple spot appears at an *R*f value of about 0.4.

Loss on drying <*5.01*> Not more than 15.0% (6 hours).

Total ash <*5.01*> Not more than 13.0%.

Acid-insoluble ash <*5.01*> Not more than 3.0%.

Essential oil content <*5.01*> When the test is performed with 50.0 g of pulverized Pogostemon Herb in a flask with 1 mL of silicon resin added, the essential oil content is not less than 0.3 mL.

Containers and storage Containers—Well-closed containers.

Polygala Root

Polygalae Radix

オンジ

Polygala Root is the root or the root bark of *Polygala tenuifolia* Willdenow (*Polygalaceae*).

Description Thin, long and bent, cylindrical or tubular root; main root, 10 - 20 cm in length, 0.2 - 1 cm in diameter, sometimes with one to several lateral roots; externally light grayish brown, with coarse longitudinal wrinkles, and with deep lateral furrows cracked to some degree here and there; brittle, and fractured surface not fibrous; under a magnifying glass, margin of the transverse section irregularly undulate; cortex, comparatively thick, with large cracks here and there; xylem usually round to elliptical, light brown in color, and often tears in a wedge-like shape.

Odor, slight; taste, slightly acrid.

Identification **(1)** Shake vigorously 0.5 g of pulverized Polygala Root with 10 mL of water: a lasting fine foam is produced.

(2) To 1.0 g of pulverized Polygala Root add 10 mL of a solution of sodium hydroxide (1 in 10), and heat under a reflux condenser for 20 minutes. After cooling, add 10 mL of dilute hydrochloric acid, and shake. After cooling, add 10 mL of 1-butanol, shake for 10 minutes, centrifuge, and use the 1-butanol layer as the sample solution. Perform the test with the sample solution as directed under Thin-layer Chromatography *<2.03>*. Spot 5 μL of the sample solution on a plate of silica gel for thin-layer chromatography. Develop the plate with a mixture of ethyl acetate, methanol, water and acetic acid (100) (20:4:2:1) to a distance of about 7 cm, and air-dry the plate. Spray evenly dilute sulfuric acid on the plate, and heat the plate at 105°C for 10 minutes: a red-brown to light brown spot appears at an *R*f value of about 0.35.

Purity **(1)** Heavy metals *<1.07>*—Proceed with 3.0 g of pulverized Polygala Root according to Method 3, and perform the test. Prepare the control solution with 3.0 mL of Standard Lead Solution (not more than 10 ppm).

(2) Arsenic *<1.11>*—Prepare the test solution with 0.40 g of pulverized Polygala Root according to Method 4, and perform the test (not more than 5 ppm).

(3) Stem—When perform the test of foreign matter *<5.01>*, the amount of the stems contained in Polygala Root does not exceed 10.0%.

(4) Foreign matter *<5.01>*—The amount of foreign matter other than the stems is not more than 1.0%.

(5) Total BHC's and total DDT's *<5.01>*—Not more than 0.2 ppm, respectively.

Total ash *<5.01>* Not more than 6.0%.

Containers and storage Containers—Well-closed containers.

Powdered Polygala Root

Polygalae Radix Pulverata

オンジ末

Powdered Polygala Root is the powder of Polygala Root.

Description Powdered Polygala Root occurs as a light yellow-grayish brown powder. It has a slight odor and a slightly acrid taste.

Under a microscope *<5.01>*, Powdered Polygala Root reveals fragments of cork layers, pitted vessels, reticulate vessels and tracheids; fragments of xylem fibers and xylem parenchyma cells with a small number of simple pits; fragments of parenchyma cells containing substances such as oil droplets, rosette aggregates and solitary crystals of calcium oxalate. Oil drop-like contents stained red with sudan III TS.

Identification **(1)** Shake vigorously 0.5 g of Powdered Polygala Root with 10 mL of water: a lasting fine foam is produced.

(2) To 1.0 g of Powdered Polygala Root add 10 mL of a solution of sodium hydroxide (1 in 10), and heat under a reflux condenser for 20 minutes. After cooling, add 10 mL of dilute hydrochloric acid, and shake. After cooling, add 10 mL of 1-butanol, shake for 10 minutes, centrifuge, and use the 1-butanol layer as the sample solution. Perform the test with the sample solution as directed under Thin-layer Chromatography *<2.03>*. Spot 5 μL of the sample solution on a plate of silica gel for thin-layer chromatography. Develop the plate with a mixture of ethyl acetate, methanol, water and acetic acid (100) (20:4:2:1) to a distance of about 7 cm, and air-dry the plate. Spray evenly dilute sulfuric acid on the plate, and heat the plate at 105°C for 10 minutes: a red-brown to light brown spot appears at an *R*f value of about 0.35.

Purity **(1)** Heavy metals *<1.07>*—Proceed with 3.0 g of Powdered Polygala Root according to Method 3, and perform the test. Prepare the control solution with 3.0 mL of Standard Lead Solution (not more than 10 ppm).

(2) Arsenic *<1.11>*—Prepare the test solution with 0.40 g of Powdered Polygala Root according to Method 4, and perform the test (not more than 5 ppm).

(3) Foreign matter—Under a microscope *<5.01>*, Powdered Polygala Root does not show stone cells or starch grains.

(4) Total BHC's and total DDT's *<5.01>*—Not more than 0.2 ppm, respectively.

Total ash *<5.01>* Not more than 6.0%.

Containers and storage Containers—Well-closed containers.

Polygonatum Rhizome

Polygonati Rhizoma

オウセイ

Polygonatum Rhizome is the rhizome of *Polygonatum kingianum* Collett et Hemsley, *Polygonatum sibiricum* Redouté, *Polygonatum cyrtonema* Hua or *Polygonatum falcatum* A. Gray (*Liliaceae*), usually after being steamed.

Description Irregularly cylindrical rhizome, 3 – 10 cm in length, 0.5 – 3 cm in diameter; or irregular massive rhizome, 5 – 10 cm in length, 2 – 6 cm in diameter, occasionally branched; both rhizomes with many cyclic nodes and longitudinally striate; externally yellow-brown to black-brown; stem scars, round, concave at their center, and protuberant on the upper surface; root scars on the lower surface; cut surface flat and horny.

Odor, slight; taste, slightly sweet.

Under a microscope *<5.01>*, a transverse section of the rhizome reveals an epidermis coated with cuticle; inside of epidermis parenchyma lie; numerous vascular bundles and mucilage cells scattered in parenchyma; vascular bundles collateral or amphivasal concentric; mucilage cells contain raphides of calcium oxalate.

Identification **(1)** To 0.5 g of fine cutted Polygonatum Rhizome add 2 mL of acetic anhydride, warm on a water bath for 2 minutes, and filter. To 1 mL of the filtrate add gently 0.5 mL of sulfuric acid: a red-brown color appears at the zone of contact.

(2) To 1.0 g of fine cutted Polygonatum Rhizome add 10 mL of dilute hydrochloric acid, boil gently for 2 minutes, and filter. Neutralize the filtrate with sodium hydroxide TS. To 3 mL of this solution add 1 mL of Fehling's TS, and warm: red precipitates appear.

Purity (1) Heavy metals <*1.07*>—Proceed with 3.0 g of pulverized Polygonutum Rhizome according to Method 3, and perform the test. Prepare the control solution with 3.0 mL of Standard Lead Solution (not more than 10 ppm).

(2) Arsenic <*1.11*>—Prepare the test solution with 0.40 g of pulverized Polygonutum Rhizome according to Method 4, and perform the test (not more than 5 ppm).

Total ash <*5.01*> Not more than 5.0%.

Acid-insoluble ash <*5.01*> Not more than 1.0%.

Containers and storage Containers—Well-closed containers.

Polygonum Root

Polygoni Multiflori Radix

カシュウ

Polygonum Root is the root of *Polygonum multiflorum* Thunberg (*Polygonaceae*), often being cut into round slices.

Description Polygonum Root is nearly fusiform, 10 - 15 cm in length, 2 - 5 cm in diameter; externally red-brown to dark brown; roughly wrinkled; a cross section light red-brown or light grayish brown, with numerous abnormal vascular bundles scattering irregularly around the large vascular bundles near center; heavy and hard in texture.

Odor, slight and characteristic; taste, astringent and slightly bitter.

Under a microscope <*5.01*>, transverse section reveals the outermost layer to be several cells thick and composed of cork; cork cells contain brown substances; cortex composed of parenchyma; abnormal vascular bundles, exhibiting a ring of cambium; xylem lies inside of the cambium, and phloem outside; fibers lie outside the phloem; central portion of root lignified; parenchymatous cells contain aggregated crystals of calcium oxalate, and both simple and 2- to 8-compound starch grains; navel of starch grain obvious.

Identification To 1 g of pulverized Polygonum Root add 10 mL of methanol, shake for 15 minutes, and filter. Evaporate the filtrate to dryness, dissolve the residue in 2 mL of methanol, and use this as the sample solution. Perform the test with the sample solution as directed under Thin-layer Chromatography <*2.03*>. Spot 5 μL of the sample solution on a plate of silica gel for thin-layer chromatography, develop the plate with a mixture of ethyl acetate, water, methanol and acetic acid (100) (200:10:10:3) to a distance of about 7 cm, and air-dry the plate. Examine under ultraviolet light (main wavelength: 365 nm): a fluorescent blue-white spot appears at an *Rf* value of about 0.3.

Purity (1) Heavy metals <*1.07*>—Proceed with 3.0 g of pulverized Polygonum Root according to Method 3, and perform the test. Prepare the control solution with 3.0 mL of Standard Lead Solution (not more than 10 ppm).

(2) Arsenic <*1.11*>—Prepare the test solution with 0.40 g of pulverized Polygonum Root according to Method 4, and perform the test (not more than 5 ppm).

Loss on drying <*5.01*> Not more than 14.0% (6 hours).

Total ash <*5.01*> Not more than 5.5%.

Extract content <*5.01*> Dilute ethanol-soluble extract: not less than 17.0%.

Containers and storage Containers—Well-closed containers.

Polyporus Sclerotium

Polyporus

チョレイ

Polyporus Sclerotium is the sclerotium of *Polyporus umbellatus* Fries (*Polyporaceae*).

Description Irregularly shaped mass, usually 5 - 15 cm in length; externally black-brown to grayish brown, with numerous dents and coarse wrinkles; breakable; fractured surface rather soft and cork-like, and almost white to light brown in color, and a white speckled pattern on the inner region; light in texture.

Practically odorless and tasteless.

Identification Warm, while shaking, 0.5 g of pulverized Polyporus Sclerotium with 5 mL of acetone on a water bath for 2 minutes, filter, and evaporate the filtrate to dryness. Dissolve the residue in 5 drops of acetic anhydride, and add 1 drop of sulfuric acid: a red-purple color develops, and immediately changes to dark green.

Purity (1) Heavy metals <*1.07*>—Proceed with 3.0 g of pulverized Polyporus Sclerotium according to Method 3, and perform the test. Prepare the control solution with 3.0 mL of Standard Lead Solution (not more than 10 ppm).

(2) Arsenic <*1.11*>—Prepare the test solution with 0.40 g of pulverized Polyporus Sclerotium according to Method 4, and perform the test (not more than 5 ppm).

Total ash <*5.01*> Not more than 16.0%.

Acid-insoluble ash <*5.01*> Not more than 4.0%.

Containers and storage Containers—Well-closed containers.

Powdered Polyporus Sclerotium

Polyporus Pulveratus

チョレイ末

Powdered Polyporus Sclerotium is the powder of the Polyporus Sclerotium.

Description Powdered Polyporus Sclerotium occurs as a light grayish brown to light brown powder. Almost odorless and tasteless.

Under a microscope <*5.01*>, Powdered Polyporus Sclerotium reveals hypha, 1 to 2 μm, rarely up to 13 μm in diameter, and colorless transparent; granule strongly refracting light; and a few mucilage plates; sometimes fragments of false tissue consisting of them; somewhat brown false tissues; and solitary crystal of calcium oxalate. Solitary crystal is 10 to 40 μm in diameter, sometimes 100 μm in diameter.

Identification Warm, while shaking, 0.5 g of Powdered Polyporus Sclerotium with 5 mL of acetone on a water bath for 2 minutes, filter and evaporate the filtrate to dryness. Dissolve the residue in 5 drops of acetic anhydride, and add 1 drop of sulfuric acid: a red-purple color develops, and immediately changes to dark green.

Purity (1) Heavy metals <1.07>—Proceed with 3.0 g of Powdered Polyporus Sclerotium according to Method 3, and perform the test. Prepare the control solution with 3.0 mL of Standard Lead Solution (not more than 10 ppm).

(2) Arsenic <1.11>—Prepare the test solution with 0.40 g of Powdered Polyporus Sclerotium according to Method 4, and perform the test (not more than 5 ppm).

Total ash <5.01> Not more than 16.0%.

Acid-insoluble ash <5.01> Not more than 4.0%.

Containers and storage Containers—Tight containers.

Poria Sclerotium

Poria

ブクリョウ

Poria Sclerotium is the sclerotium of *Wolfiporia cocos* Ryvarden et Gilbertson (*Poria cocos* Wolf) (*Polyporaceae*), from which usually the external layer has been mostly removed.

Description Mass, about 10 - 30 cm in diameter, up to 0.1 - 2 kg in mass; usually it appears as broken or chipped pieces; white or slightly reddish white; sclerotium with remaining outer layer is dark brown to dark red-brown in color, coarse, which fissures; hard in texture, but brittle.

Almost odorless, almost tasteless, and slightly mucous.

Identification (1) Warm 1 g of pulverized Poria Sclerotium with 5 mL of acetone on a water bath for 2 minutes with shaking, and filter. Evaporate the filtrate to dryness, dissolve the residue in 0.5 mL of acetic anhydride, and add 1 drop of sulfuric acid: a light red color develops, which changes immediately to dark green.

(2) To a cut surface or powder of Poria Sclerotium add 1 drop of iodine TS: a deep red-brown color is produced.

Purity (1) Heavy metals <1.07>—Proceed with 3.0 g of pulverized Poria Sclerotium according to Method 3, and perform the test. Prepare the control solution with 3.0 mL of Standard Lead Solution (not more than 10 ppm).

(2) Arsenic <1.11>—Prepare the test solution with 0.40 g of pulverized Poria Sclerotium according to Method 4, and perform the test (not more than 5 ppm).

Total ash <5.01> Not more than 1.0%.

Containers and storage Containers—Well-closed containers.

Powdered Poria Sclerotium

Poria Pulveratum

ブクリョウ末

Powdered Poria Sclerotium is the powder of Poria Sclerotium.

Description Powdered Poria Sclerotium occurs as a white to grayish white powder. It is almost odorless and almost tasteless, but is slightly mucous.

Under a microscope <5.01>, Powdered Poria Sclerotium reveals colorless and transparent hyphae strongly refracting light, and fragments of false tissue consisting of granules and mucilage plates. Thin hyphae, 2 - 4 μm in diameter; thick ones, usually 10 - 20 μm, up to 30 μm.

Identification (1) Warm 1 g of Powdered Poria Sclerotium with 5 mL of acetone on a water bath for 2 minutes with shaking, and filter. Evaporate the filtrate to dryness, dissolve the residue in 0.5 mL of acetic anhydride, and add 1 drop of sulfuric acid: a light red color develops, which changes immediately to dark green.

(2) To Powdered Poria Sclerotium add 1 drop of iodine TS: a deep red-brown color is produced.

Purity (1) Heavy metals <1.07>—Proceed with 3.0 g of Powdered Poria Sclerotium according to Method 3, and perform the test. Prepare the control solution with 3.0 mL of Standard Lead Solution (not more than 10 ppm).

(2) Arsenic <1.11>—Prepare the test solution with 0.40 g of Powdered Poria Sclerotium according to Method 4, and perform the test (not more than 5 ppm).

(3) Foreign matter—Under a microscope <5.01>, Powdered Poria Sclerotium does not show starch grains.

Total ash <5.01> Not more than 1.0%.

Containers and storage Containers—Well-closed containers.

Prepared Glycyrrhiza

Glycyrrhizae Radix Praeparata

シャカンゾウ

Prepared Glycyrrhiza is prepared by roasting Glycyrrhiza.

It contains not less than 2.0% of glycyrrhizic acid ($C_{42}H_{62}O_{16}$: 822.93), calculated on the basis of dried material.

Description Usually cut; external surface dark brown to dark red-brown and with longitudinal wrinkles; cut surface brown to light yellow-brown; in case periderm fallen off, external surface brown to light yellow-brown and fibrous; on transversely cut surface cortex and xylem almost distinctly defined, and exhibits radial structure; sometimes radial cleft observed.

Odor, fragrant; taste sweet, followed by slight bitterness.

Identification To 2.0 g of pulverized Prepared Glycyrrhiza add 10 mL of ethyl acetate, shake for 15 minutes, centrifuge, and separate the ethyl acetate layer. Shake the residue with 5 mL of ethyl acetate and 5 mL of 0.1 mol/L hydrochloric acid TS for 15 minutes, centrifuge, and use the ethyl acetate layer as the sample solution. Perform the test with the sample solution as directed under Thin-layer Chromatography <2.03>. Spot 20 μL of the sample solution on a plate of silica gel for thin-layer chromatography. Develop the plate with a mixture of ethyl acetate, methanol and water (7:2:1) to a distance of about 7 cm, and air-dry the plate. Spray evenly 4-methoxybenzaldehyde-sulfuric acid TS on the plate, heat the plate at 105°C for 3 minutes, and allow to cool: a red-purple spot is observed at an *Rf* value of about 0.6.

Purity (1) Heavy metals <1.07>—Proceed with 3.0 g of pulverized Prepared Glycyrrhiza according to Method 3, and perform the test. Prepare the control solution with 3.0 mL of Standard Lead Solution (not more than 10 ppm).

(2) Arsenic <1.11>—Prepare the test solution with 0.40 g

of pulverized Prepared Glycyrrhiza according to Method 4, and perform the test (not more than 5 ppm).

(3) Total BHC's and total DDT's <*5.01*>—Not more than 0.2 ppm, respectively.

Loss on drying <*5.01*> Not more than 8.0% (6 hours).

Total ash <*5.01*> Not more than 7.0%.

Acid-insoluble ash <*5.01*> Not more than 2.0%.

Extract content <*5.01*> Dilute ethanol-soluble extract: not less than 25.0%.

Assay Weigh accurately about 0.5 g of pulverized Prepared Glycyrrhiza in a glass-stoppered centrifuge tube, add 70 mL of dilute ethanol, shake for 15 minutes, centrifuge, and separate the supernatant liquid. To the residue add 25 mL of dilute ethanol, and proceed in the same manner. Combine all the extracts, add dilute ethanol to make exactly 100 mL, and use this solution as the sample solution. Separately, weigh accurately about 25 mg of Glycyrrhizic Acid RS (separately determine the water <*2.48*> by coulometric titration, using 10 mg), dissolve in dilute ethanol to make exactly 100 mL, and use this solution as the standard solution. Perform the test with exactly 10 μL each of the sample solution and standard solution as directed under Liquid Chromatography <*2.01*> according to the following conditions, and determine the peak areas, A_T and A_S, of glycyrrhizic acid in each solution.

Amount (mg) of glycyrrhizic acid ($C_{42}H_{62}O_{16}$)
$= M_S \times A_T/A_S$

M_S: Amount (mg) of Glycyrrhizic Acid RS taken, calculated on the anhydrous basis

Operating conditions—

Detector: An ultraviolet absorption photometer (wavelength: 254 nm).

Column: A stainless steel column 4.6 mm in inside diameter and 15 cm in length, packed with octadecylsilanized silica gel for liquid chromatography (5 μm in particle diameter).

Column temperature: A constant temperature of about 40°C.

Mobile phase: Dissolve 3.85 g of ammonium acetate in 720 mL of water, and add 5 mL of acetic acid (100) and 280 mL of acetonitrile.

Flow rate: Adjust so that the retention time of glycyrrhizic acid is about 15 minutes.

System suitability—

System performance: Dissolve 5 mg of monoammonium glycyrrhizinate for resolution check in 20 mL of dilute ethanol. When the procedure is run with 10 μL of this solution under the above operating conditions, the resolution between the peak with the relative retention time of about 0.9 to glycyrrhizic acid, and the peak of glycyrrhizic acid is not less than 1.5.

System repeatability: When the test is repeated 6 times with 10 μL of the standard solution under the above operating conditions, the relative standard deviation of the peak area of glycyrrhizic acid is not more than 1.5%.

Containers and storage Containers—Well-closed containers.

Processed Aconite Root

Aconiti Radix Processa

ブシ

Processed Aconite Root is the tuberous root of *Aconitum carmichaeli* Debeaux or *Aconitum japonicum* Thunberg (*Ranunculaceae*) prepared by the following processes.

Process 1: Autoclaving. [Processed Aconite Root 1]

Process 2: Heating or autoclaving after rinsing in salt or rock salt solution. [Processed Aconite Root 2]

Process 3: Treating with calcium hydroxide after rinsing in salt solution. [Processed Aconite Root 3]

Processed Aconite Root 1, Processed Aconite Root 2 and Processed Aconite Root 3 contain the total alkaloid [as benzoyl aconin ($C_{32}H_{45}NO_{10}$: 603.70)] of not less than 0.7% and not more than 1.5%, not less than 0.1% and not more than 0.6%, and not less than 0.5% and not more than 0.9%, calculated on the dried bases, respectively.

The label indicates the treating process.

Description **1)** Processed Aconite Root 1: Cut pieces irregularly polygonal, less than 10 mm in diameter; externally dark grayish brown to black-brown; hard in texture; cut surface flat, light brown to dark brown, usually horny and lustrous.

Odor, weak and characteristic.

Under a microscope <*5.01*>, transverse and longitudinal sections reveal pitted, scaraliform, reticulate and spiral vessels; starch grains in parenchymatous cells usually gelatinized but sometimes not gelatinized; starch grains, simple, spherical or ellipsoid, 2 - 25 μm in diameter, or 2- to a dozen or so- compound, hilum of starch grain distinct.

2) Processed Aconite Root 2: Nearly obconical root, 15 - 30 mm in length, 12 - 16 mm in diameter, slices cut longitudinally or transversely, 20 - 60 mm in length, 15 - 40 mm in width, and 200 - 700 μm in thickness, or cut pieces irregularly polygonal, less than 12 mm in diameter; externally light brown to dark brown or yellow-brown; hard in texture, usually without wrinkles; cut surface flat, light brown to dark brown or yellow-white to light yellow-brown, usually horny, semi-transparent and lustrous.

Odor, weak and characteristic.

Under a microscope <*5.01*>, transverse and longitudinal sections reveal metaderm, primary cortex, endodermis, secondary cortex, cambium, and xylem; primary cortex contains oblong to oblong-square sclerenchymatous cells, 30 - 75 μm in short axis, 60 - 150 μm in long axis; endodermis single layered cell, endodermal cells elongated in tangential direction; cambium, star shaped or irregular polygons to orbicular; a group of vessel in xylem v-shaped; sometimes isolated ring of cambium appears in secondary cortex or in pith; vessels, pitted, scaraliform, reticulate and spiral; starch grains in parenchymatous cells gelatinized.

3) Processed Aconite Root 3: Cut pieces irregularly polygonal, less than 5 mm in diameter; externally grayish brown; hard in texture; cut surface flat, light grayish brown to grayish white, not lustrous.

Odor, weak and characteristic.

Under a microscope <*5.01*>, transverse and longitudinal sections reveal pitted, scaraliform, reticulate and spiral vessels; starch grains, simple, spherical or ellipsoid, 2 - 25 μm in diameter, or 2- to a dozen or so- compound, hilum of starch grain distinct.

Identification To 3 g of pulverized Processed Aconite Root in a glass-stoppered centrifuge tube add 20 mL of diethyl ether and 2 mL of ammonia TS, shake for 10 minutes, centrifuge, and take the diethyl ether layer. Evaporate the solvent under low pressure (in vacuo), dissolve the residue in 1 mL of diethyl ether, and use this solution as the sample solution. Separately, dissolve 1 mg of benzoylmesaconine hydrochloride for thin-layer chromatography in 5 mL of ethanol (99.5), and use this solution as the standard solution. Perform the test with these solutions as directed under Thin-layer Chromatography <*2.03*>. Spot 10 μL each of the sample solution and standard solution on a plate of silica gel for thin-layer chromatography, develop the plate with a mixture of ethyl acetate, ethanol (99.5) and ammonia water (28) (40:3:2) to a distance of about 7 cm, and air-dry the plate. Spray evenly Dragendorff's TS for spraying on the plate, air-dry the plate, and spray evenly sodium nitrite TS: one of the several spots obtained from the sample solution has the same color tone and *R*f value with the spot from the standard solution.

Purity **(1)** Heavy metals <*1.07*>—Proceed with 3.0 g of pulverized Processed Aconite Root according to Method 3, and perform the test. Prepare the control solution with 3.0 mL of Standard Lead Solution (not more than 10 ppm).

(2) Arsenic <*1.11*>—Prepare the test solution with 0.40 g of pulverized Processed Aconite Root according to Method 4, and perform the test (not more than 5 ppm).

(3) Aconitum diester alkaloids (aconitine, jesaconitine, hypaconitine and mesaconitine)—Weigh accurately about 0.5 g of pulverized Processed Aconite Root, put in a glass-stoppered centrifuge tube, suspend in 3.0 mL of water by shaking, and add 1.0 mL of ammonia TS and 20 mL of diethyl ether, shake for 30 minutes, centrifuge, and separate the diethyl ether layer. To the residue add 1.0 mL of ammonia TS and 20 mL of diethyl ether, and repeat the above process twice more. Combine all the extracts, evaporate under low pressure (in vacuo), and dissolve the residue with exactly 10 mL of a mixture of phosphate buffer solution for processed aconite root and acetonitrile (1:1). Centrifuge and use the supernatant liquid as the sample solution. Perform the test with exactly 20 μL each of the sample solution and aconitum diester alkaloids standard solution for purity as directed under Liquid Chromatography <*2.01*> according to the following conditions. Determine the heights of the peaks corresponding to aconitine, H_{TA} and H_{SA}, jesaconitine, H_{TJ} and H_{SJ}, hypaconitine, H_{TH} and H_{SH}, and mesaconitine, H_{TM} and H_{SM}, respectively, and calculate the amounts of them by the following formulae: the amounts of aconitine, jesaconitine, hypaconitine and mesaconitine per g calculated on the dried basis are not more than 60 μg, 60 μg, 280 μg and 140 μg, respectively, and the total amount of them is not more than 450 μg.

$$\text{Amount } (\mu g) \text{ of aconitine} = C_{SA}/M \times H_{TA}/H_{SA} \times 10$$

$$\text{Amount } (\mu g) \text{ of jesaconitine} = C_{SJ}/M \times H_{TJ}/H_{SJ} \times 10$$

$$\text{Amount } (\mu g) \text{ of hypaconitine} = C_{SH}/M \times H_{TH}/H_{SH} \times 10$$

$$\text{Amount } (\mu g) \text{ of mesaconitine} = C_{SM}/M \times H_{TM}/H_{SM} \times 10$$

C_{SA}: Concentration (μg/mL) of aconitine for purity in aconitum diester alkaloids standard solution for purity

C_{SJ}: Concentration (μg/mL) of jesaconitine for purity in aconitum diester alkaloids standard solution for purity

C_{SH}: Concentration (μg/mL) of hypaconitine for purity in aconitum diester alkaloids standard solution for purity

C_{SM}: Concentration (μg/mL) of mesaconitine for purity in aconitum diester alkaloids standard solution for purity

M: Amount (g) of Processed Aconite Root taken, calculated on the dried basis

Operating conditions—

Detector: An ultraviolet absorption photometer (wavelength: 231 nm for aconitine, hypaconitine and mesaconitine; 254 nm for jesaconitine).

Column: A stainless steel column 4.6 mm in inside diameter and 15 cm in length, packed with octadecylsilanized silica gel for liquid chromatography (5 μm in particle diameter).

Column temperature: A constant temperature of about 40°C.

Mobile phase: A mixture of phosphate buffer solution for processed aconite root and tetrahydrofuran (183:17).

Flow rate: Adjust so that the retention time of mesaconitine is about 31 minutes.

System suitability—

System performance: When the procedure is run with 20 μL of aconitum diester alkaloids standard solution for purity under the above operating conditions, using 254 nm, mesaconitine, hypaconitine, aconitine and jesaconitine are eluted in this order, and each resolution between their peaks is not less than 1.5, respectively.

System repeatability: To 1 mL of aconitum diester alkaloids standard solution for purity add a mixture of phosphate buffer solution for processed aconite root and acetonitrile (1:1) to make 10 mL. When the test is repeated 6 times with 20 μL of this solution under the above operating conditions, using 231 nm, the relative standard deviation of the peak height of mesaconitine is not more than 1.5%.

Loss on drying <*5.01*> Not more than 15.0% (6 hours).

Total ash <*5.01*>

Processed Aconite Root 1: Not more than 4.0%.

Processed Aconite Root 2: Not more than 12.0%.

Processed Aconite Root 3: Not more than 19.0%.

Acid-insoluble ash <*5.01*> Not more than 0.9%.

Assay Weigh accurately about 2 g of pulverized Processed Aconite Root, put in a glass-stoppered centrifuge tube, and add 1.6 mL of ammonia TS and 20 mL of diethyl ether, shake for 30 minutes, centrifuge, and separate the diethyl ether layer. To the residue add 0.8 mL of ammonia TS and 20 mL of diethyl ether, and proceed as above. Repeat this process more three times. Combine all the extracts, evaporate the solvent under low pressure (in vacuo), dissolve the residue in 5 mL of ethanol (99.5), add 30 mL of freshly boiled and cooled water, and titrate <*2.50*> with 0.01 mol/L hydrochloric acid VS until the color of the solution changes from green to gray-blue through blue-green (indicator: 3 drops of methyl red-methylene blue TS). Perform a blank determination in the same manner, and make any necessary correction.

Each mL of 0.01 mol/L hydrochloric acid VS
= 6.037 mg of total alkaloid [as benzoylaconine ($C_{32}H_{45}NO_{10}$)]

Containers and storage Containers—Well-closed containers.

Powdered Processed Aconite Root

Aconiti Radix Processa et Pulverata

ブシ末

Powdered Processed Aconite Root is the powder of Processed Aconite Root prepared by the process 1 or process 2, the powder of Processed Aconite Root prepared by process 1, or the powder of Processed Aconite Root prepared by the process 1 to which Corn Starch or Lactose Hydrate is added.

Process 1: Autoclaving. [Powdered Processed Aconite Root 1]

Process 2: Heating or autoclaving after rinsing in salt or rock salt solution. [Powdered Processed Aconite Root 2]

Powdered Processed Aconite Root 1 and Powdered Processed Aconite Root 2 contain the total alkaloid [as benzoyl aconin ($C_{32}H_{45}NO_{10}$: 603.70)] of not less than 0.4% and not more than 1.2%, and not less than 0.1% and not more than 0.3%, calculated on the dried bases, respectively.

The label indicates the treating process.

Description **1)** Powdered Processed Aconite Root 1: Powdered Processed Aconite Root 1 occurs as a light grayish brown powder. It has a characteristic odor.

Under a microscope <*5.01*>, Powered Processed Aconite Root 1 reveals gelatinized starch masses or starch grains and parenchymatous cells containing them, fragments of red-brown metaderm, fragments of pitted, scaraliform, reticulate and spiral vessels; also square to oblong-square sclerenchymatous cells, 30 - 150 μm in diameter, 100 - 250 μm in length, cell wall of sclerenchymatous cells, 6 - 12 μm in thickness; starch grains of *Aconitum carmichaeli Debeaux* or *Aconitum japonicum* Thunberg (*Ranunculaceae*) origin, simple, spherical or ellipsoid, 2 - 25 μm in diameter, or 2- to a dozen or so- compound, hilum of starch grain distinct.

2) Powdered Processed Aconite Root 2: Powdered Processed Aconite Root 2 occurs as a light yellow-white powder. It has a characteristic odor.

Under a microscope <*5.01*>, Powered Processed Aconite Root 2 reveals gelatinized starch masses and parenchymatous cells containing them, fragments of red-brown metaderm, fragments of pitted, scaraliform, reticulate and spiral vessels; also square to oblong-square sclerenchymatous cells, 30 - 150 μm in diameter, 100 - 250 μm in length, cell wall of sclerenchymatous cells, 6 - 12 μm in thickness.

Identification To 3 g of Powdered Processed Aconite Root in a glass-stoppered centrifuge tube add 20 mL of diethyl ether and 2 mL of ammonia TS, shake for 10 minutes, centrifuge, and take the diethyl ether layer. Evaporate the solvent under low pressure (in vacuo), dissolve the residue in 1 mL of diethyl ether, and use this solution as the sample solution. Separately, dissolve 1 mg of benzoylmesaconine hydrochloride for thin-layer chromatography in 5 mL of ethanol (99.5), and use this solution as the standard solution. Perform the test with these solutions as directed under Thin-layer Chromatography <*2.03*>. Spot 10 μL each of the sample solution and standard solution on a plate of silica gel for thin-layer chromatography, develop the plate with a mixture of ethyl acetate, ethanol (99.5) and ammonia water (28) (40:3:2) to a distance of about 7 cm, and air-dry the plate. Spray evenly Dragendorff's TS for spraying on the plate, air-dry the plate, and spray evenly sodium nitrite TS: one of the several spots obtained from the sample solution has the same color tone and *Rf* value with the spot from the standard solution.

Purity **(1)** Heavy metals <*1.07*>—Proceed with 3.0 g of Powdered Processed Aconite Root according to Method 3, and perform the test. Prepare the control solution with 3.0 mL of Standard Lead Solution (not more than 10 ppm).

(2) Arsenic <*1.11*>—Prepare the test solution with 0.40 g of Powdered Processed Aconite Root according to Method 4, and perform the test (not more than 5 ppm).

(3) Aconitum diester alkaloids (aconitine, jesaconitine, hypaconitine and mesaconitine)—Weigh accurately about 0.5 g of Powdered Processed Aconite Root, put in a glass-stoppered centrifuge tube, suspend in 3.0 mL of water by shaking, and add 1.0 mL of ammonia TS and 20 mL of diethyl ether, shake for 30 minutes, centrifuge, and separate the diethyl ether layer. To the residue add 1.0 mL of ammonia TS and 20 mL of diethyl ether, and repeat the above process twice more. Combine all the extracts, evaporate the solvent under low pressure (in vacuo), and dissolve the residue with exactly 10 mL of a mixture of phosphate buffer solution for processed aconite root and acetonitrile (1:1). Centrifuge this solution, and use the supernatant liquid as the sample solution. Perform the test with exactly 20 μL each of the sample solution and aconitum diester alkaloids standard solution for purity as directed under Liquid Chromatography <*2.01*> according to the following conditions. Determine the heights of the peaks corresponding to aconitine, H_{TA} and H_{SA}, jesaconitine, H_{TJ} and H_{SJ}, hypaconitine, H_{TH} and H_{SH}, and mesaconitine, H_{TM} and H_{SM}, respectively, and calculate the amounts of them by the following formulae: the amounts of aconitine, jesaconitine, hypaconitine and mesaconitine per g calculated on the dried basis are not more than 55 μg, 40 μg, 55 μg and 120 μg, respectively, and the total amount of them is not more than 230 μg.

Amount (μg) of aconitine
$= C_{SA}/M \times H_{TA}/H_{SA} \times 10$

Amount (μg) of jesaconitine
$= C_{SJ}/M \times H_{TJ}/H_{SJ} \times 10$

Amount (μg) of hypaconitine
$= C_{SH}/M \times H_{TH}/H_{SH} \times 10$

Amount (μg) of mesaconitine
$= C_{SM}/M \times H_{TM}/H_{SM} \times 10$

C_{SA}: Concentration (μg/mL) of aconitine for purity in aconitum diester alkaloids standard solution for purity

C_{SJ}: Concentration (μg/mL) of jesaconitine for purity in aconitum diester alkaloids standard solution for purity

C_{SH}: Concentration (μg/mL) of hypaconitine for purity in aconitum diester alkaloids standard solution for purity

C_{SM}: Concentration (μg/mL) of mesaconitine for purity in aconitum diester alkaloids standard solution for purity

M: Amount (g) of Powdered Processed Aconitine Root taken, calculated on the dried basis

Operating conditions—

Detector: An ultraviolet absorption photometer (wavelength: 231 nm for aconitine, hypaconitine and mesaconitine; 254 nm for jesaconitine).

Column: A stainless steel column 4.6 mm in inside diameter and 15 cm in length, packed with octadecylsilanized silica gel for liquid chromatography (5 μm in particle diameter).

Column temperature: A constant temperature of about 40°C.

Mobile phase: A mixture of phosphate buffer solution for processed aconite root and tetrahydrofuran (183:17).

Flow rate: Adjust so that the retention time of mesaconitine is about 31 minutes.

System suitability—

System performance: When the procedure is run with 20 μL of aconitum diester alkaloids standard solution for purity under the above operating conditions, using 254 nm, mesaconitine, hypaconitine, aconitine and jesaconitine are eluted in this order, and each resolution between their peaks is not less than 1.5, respectively.

System repeatability: To 1 mL of aconitum diester alkaloids standard solution for purity add a mixture of phosphate buffer solution for processed aconite root and acetonitrile (1:1) to make 10 mL. When the test is repeated 6 times with 20 μL of this solution under the above operating conditions, using 231 nm, the relative standard deviation of the peak height of mesaconitine is not more than 1.5%.

Loss on drying ⟨*5.01*⟩ Not more than 11.0% (6 hours).

Total ash ⟨*5.01*⟩

Powdered Processed Aconite Root 1: Not more than 4.0%.

Powdered Processed Aconite Root 2: Not more than 7.0%.

Acid-insoluble ash ⟨*5.01*⟩ Not more than 0.7%.

Assay Weigh accurately about 2 g of Powdered Processed Aconite Root, put in a glass-stoppered centrifuge tube, and add 1.6 mL of ammonia TS and 20 mL of diethyl ether, shake for 30 minutes, centrifuge, and separate the diethyl ether layer. To the residue add 0.8 mL of ammonia TS and 20 mL of diethyl ether, and proceed as above. Repeat this process more three times. Combine all the extracts, evaporate the solvent under low pressure (in vacuo), dissolve the residue in 5 mL of ethanol (99.5), add 30 mL of freshly boiled and cooled water, and titrate ⟨*2.50*⟩ with 0.01 mol/L hydrochloric acid VS until the color of the solution changes from green to gray-blue through blue-green (indicator: 3 drops of methyl red-methylene blue TS). Perform a blank determination in the same manner, and make any necessary correction.

Each mL of 0.01 mol/L hydrochloric acid VS
= 6.037 mg of total alkaloid [as benzoylaconine ($C_{32}H_{45}NO_{10}$)]

Containers and storage Containers—Well-closed containers.

Processed Ginger

Zingiberis Rhizoma Processum

カンキョウ

Processed Ginger is the rhizome of *Zingiber officinale* Roscoe (*Zingiberaceae*), after being passed through hot water or being steamed.

It contains not less than 0.10% of [6]-shogaol, calculated on the basis of dried material.

Description Irregularly compressed and often branched massive rhizome; branched parts slightly curved ovoid or oblong- ovoid, 2 - 4 cm in length, and 1 - 2 cm in diameter; external surface grayish yellow to grayish yellow-brown, with wrinkles and ring node; fractured surface brown to dark brown, transparent and horny; under a magnifying glass, a transverse cut surface reveals cortex and stele distinctly divided; vascular bundles scattered throughout the surface.

Odor, characteristic; taste, extremely pungent.

Under a microscope ⟨*5.01*⟩, a transverse section reveals cork layer, cortex and stele in this order from the outside; cortex and stele, divided by an endodermis, composed of parenchyma; vascular bundles surrounded by fibers scattered in cortex and stele; oil cells contain yellow oily substances, scattered in parenchyma; parenchyma cells contain solitary crystals of calcium oxalate, and gelatinized starch.

Identification To 2 g of pulverized Processed Ginger add 5 mL of diethyl ether, shake for 10 minutes, filter, and use the filtrate as the sample solution (1). To the residue add 5 mL of methanol, proceed in the same manner as above, and use so obtained solution as the sample solution (2). Separately, dissolve 1 mg of [6]-shogaol for thin-layer chromatography in 2 mL of methanol, and use this solution as the standard solution (1). Separately, dissolve 1 mg of sucrose in 2 mL of methanol, and use this solution as the standard solution (2). Perform the test with these solutions as directed under Thin-layer Chromatography ⟨*2.03*⟩. Spot 10 μL each of the sample solution (1) and standard solution (1) on a plate of silica gel for thin-layer chromatography. Develop the plate with a mixture of ethyl acetate and hexane (1:1) to a distance of about 7 cm, and air-dry the plate. Spray evenly 4-dimethylaminobenzaldehyde TS for spraying on the plate, heat the plate at 105°C for 5 minutes, and allow to cool: one of the several spots obtained from the sample solution (1) has the same color tone and *R*f value with the spot from the standard solution (1). Spot 10 μL each of the sample solution (2) and standard solution (2) on a plate of silica gel for thin-layer chromatography, develop the plate with a mixture of 1-butanol, water and acetic acid (100) (8:5:3) to a distance of about 7 cm, and air-dry the plate. Spray evenly 1,3-naphthalenediol TS on the plate, and heat the plate at 105°C for 5 minutes: one of the several spots obtained from the sample solution (2) has the same color tone and *R*f value with the spot from the standard solution (2).

Purity (1) Heavy metals ⟨*1.07*⟩—Proceed with 1.0 g of pulverized Processed Ginger according to Method 3, and perform the test. Prepare the control solution with 2.0 mL of Standard Lead Solution (not more than 20 ppm).

(2) Arsenic ⟨*1.11*⟩—Prepare the test solution with 0.40 g of pulverized Processed Ginger according to Method 4, and perform the test (not more than 5 ppm).

Loss on drying ⟨*5.01*⟩ Not more than 15.0% (6 hours).

Total ash <*5.01*> Not more than 6.5%.

Acid-insoluble ash <*5.01*> Not more than 1.5%.

Extract content <*5.01*> Dilute ethanol-soluble extract: not less than 8.0%.

Assay Weigh accurately about 1 g of pulverized Processed Ginger, place in a centrifuge tube, add 30 mL of the mobile phase, shake for 20 minutes, centrifuge, and separate the supernatant liquid. To the residue add 30 mL of the mobile phase, and repeat the extraction twice more. To the combined all extracts add the mobile phase to make exactly 100 mL, use this solution as the sample solution. Separately, weigh accurately about 5 mg of [6]-shogaol for assay, dissolve in the mobile phase to make exactly 100 mL, and use this solution as the standard solution. Perform the test with exactly 10 μL each of the sample solution and standard solution as directed under Liquid Chromatography <*2.01*> according to the following conditions, and determine the peak areas, A_T and A_S, of [6]-shogaol in each solution.

$$\text{Amount (mg) of [6]-shogaol} = M_S \times A_T/A_S$$

M_S: Amount (mg) of [6]-shogaol for assay taken

Operating conditions—

Detector: An ultraviolet absorption photometer (wavelength: 225 nm).

Column: A stainless steel column 6 mm in inside diameter and 15 cm in length, packed with octadecylsilanized silica gel for liquid chromatography (5 μm in particle diameter).

Column temperature: A constant temperature of about 40°C.

Mobile phase: A mixture of acetonitrile and water (3:2).

Flow rate: Adjust so that the retention time of [6]-shogaol is about 14 minutes.

System suitability—

System performance: When the procedure is run with 10 μL of the standard solution under the above operating conditions, the number of theoretical plates and the symmetry factor of the peak of [6]-shogaol are not less than 5000 and not more than 1.5, respectively.

System repeatability: When the test is repeated 6 times with 10 μL of the standard solution under the above operating conditions, the relative standard deviation of the peak area of [6]-shogaol is not more than 1.5%.

Containers and storage Containers—Well-closed containers.

Prunella Spike

Prunellae Spica

カゴソウ

Prunella Spike is the spike of *Prunella vulgaris* Linné var. *lilacina* Nakai (*Labiatae*).

Description Spikes in nearly cylindrical and wheat ear-like shape, 3 - 6 cm in length, 1 - 1.5 cm in diameter, externally grayish brown; spikes composed of a floral axis having numerous bracts and calyxes; corollas often remaining on the upper part; a calyx usually enclosing four mericarps; bract, cordate to eccentric, and exhibiting white hairs on the vein, as on the calyx; light in texture.

Almost odorless and tasteless.

Purity (1) Stem—When perform the test of foreign matter <*5.01*>, the amount of the stems contained in Prunella Spike does not exceed 5.0%.

(2) Foreign matter <*5.01*>—The amount of foreign matter other than the stems contained in Prunella Spike does not exceed 1.0%.

Total ash <*5.01*> Not more than 13.0%.

Acid-insoluble ash <*5.01*> Not more than 5.0%.

Containers and storage Containers—Well-closed containers.

Pueraria Root

Puerariae Radix

カッコン

Pueraria Root is the root of *Pueraria lobata* Ohwi (*Leguminosae*), from which periderm has been removed.

It contains not less than 2.0% of puerarin ($C_{21}H_{20}O_9$: 416.38), calculated on the basis of dried material.

Description Usually cut into small pieces of irregular hexagons of about 0.5 cm cube, or cut into longitudinally plate-like pieces 20 - 30 cm in length, 5 - 10 cm in width, and about 1 cm in thickness; externally light grayish yellow to grayish white; transverse section showing concentric annulate ring or part of it formed by abnormal growth of cambium. Under a magnifying glass, phloem light grayish yellow in color; in xylem, numerous vessels appearing as small dots; medullary rays slightly dented; vertical section showing longitudinal patterns formed alternately by fibrous xylem and parenchyma; easily breakable lengthwise, and its section extremely fibrous.

Almost odorless; taste, at first slightly sweet, followed by a slight bitterness.

Under a microscope <*5.01*>, a transverse section reveals fiber bundles accompanied by crystal cells in phloem; distinct vessels and xylem fibers in xylem; starch grains numerous in parenchyma, mainly composed of polygonal simple grains, rarely 2- to 3-compound grains, 2 - 18 μm, mostly 8 - 12 μm, in size, with hilum or cleft in the center, and also with striae.

Identification To 2 g of pulverized Pueraria Root add 10 mL of methanol, shake for 3 minutes, filter, and use the filtrate as the sample solution. Separately, dissolve 1 mg of Puerarin RS or puerarin for thin-layer chromatography in 1 mL of methanol, and use this solution as the standard solution. Perform the test with these solutions as directed under Thin-layer Chromatography <*2.03*>. Spot 2 μL each of the sample solution and standard solution on a plate of silica gel for thin-layer chromatography. Develop the plate with a mixture of ethyl acetate, methanol and water (12:2:1) to a distance of about 7 cm, and air-dry the plate. Examine under ultraviolet light (main wavelength: 365 nm): one of the several spots obtained from the sample solution has the same color tone and *R*f value with the blue-white fluorescent spot from the standard solution.

Purity (1) Heavy metals <*1.07*>—Proceed with 3.0 g of pulverized Pueraria Root according to Method 3, and perform the test. Prepare the control solution with 3.0 mL of Standard Lead Solution (not more than 10 ppm).

(2) Arsenic <*1.11*>—Prepare the test solution with 0.40 g

of pulverized Pueraria Root according to Method 4, and perform the test (not more than 5 ppm).

Loss on drying *<5.01>* Not less than 13.0% (6 hours).

Total ash *<5.01>* Not more than 6.0%.

Assay Weigh accurately about 0.3 g of pulverized Pueraria Root, add 50 mL of diluted methanol (1 in 2), and heat under a reflex condenser for 30 minutes, cool, and filter. To the residue add 50 mL of diluted methanol (1 in 2), and perform as the same as above. Combine the filtrates, add diluted methanol (1 in 2) to make exactly 100 mL, and use this solution as the sample solution. Separately, weigh accurately about 10 mg of Puerarin RS (separately determine the water *<2.48>* by coulometric titration, using 10 mg), add diluted methanol (1 in 2) to make exactly 100 mL, and use this solution as the standard solution. Perform the test with exactly 10 μL each of the sample solution and standard solution as directed under Liquid Chromatography *<2.01>* according to the following conditions, and determine the peak areas, A_T and A_S, of puerarin in each solution.

Amount (mg) of puerarin ($C_{21}H_{20}O_9$) = $M_S \times A_T/A_S$

M_S: Amount (mg) of Puerarin RS taken, calculated on the anhydrous basis

Operating conditions—

Detector: An ultraviolet absorption photometer (wavelength: 250 nm).

Column: A stainless steel column 4.6 mm in inside diameter and 15 cm in length, packed with octadecylsilanized silica gel for liquid chromatography (5 μm in particle diameter).

Column temperature: A constant temperature of about 40°C.

Mobile phase: A mixture of 0.05 mol/L sodium dihydrogen phosphate TS and acetonitrile (9:1).

Flow rate: Adjust so that the retention time of puerarin is about 15 minutes.

System suitability—

System performance: When the procedure is run with 10 μL of the standard solution under the above operating conditions, the number of theoretical plates and the symmetry coefficient of the peak of puerarin are not less than 3000 and not more than 2.0, respectively.

System repeatability: When the test is repeated 6 times with 10 μL of the standard solution under the above operating conditions, the relative standard deviation of the peak area of puerarin is not more than 1.5%.

Containers and storage Containers—Well-closed containers.

Quercus Bark

Quercus Cortex

ボクソク

Quercus Bark is the bark of *Quercus acutissima* Carruthers, *Quercus serrata* Murray, *Quercus mongolica* Fischer ex Ledebour var. *crispula* Ohashi or *Quercus variabilis* Blume (*Fagaceae*).

Description Plate-like or semi-tubular pieces of bark, 5 - 15 mm in thickness; externally grayish brown to dark brown, with thick periderm and longitudinal coarse splits; internally brown to light brown, with longitudinal ridges, the transverse section brown to light brown, white small spots composed of stone cells in groups observed sporadically.

Almost odorless, tasteless.

Under a microscope *<5.01>*, a transverse section reveals a cork layer with scattered cork stone cells; in secondary cortex fiber bundles lined almost stepwise, large groups of stone cells arranged irregularly; in parenchyma aggregated crystals of calcium oxalate scattered; adjacent to stone cells and fiber cells, cells containing solitary crystals of calcium oxalate observed, and these cells form crystal cell rows in a longitudinal section.

Identification To 2 g of pulverized Quercus Bark, add 10 mL of ethyl acetate, shake for 10 minutes, and centrifuge to remove the supernatant liquid. Add 10 mL of acetone to the residue, shake for 10 minutes, centrifuge, and use the supernatant liquid as the sample solution. Perform the test with the sample solution as directed under Thin-layer Chromatography *<2.03>*. Spot 10 μL of the sample solution on a plate of silica gel for thin-layer chromatography, develop the plate with a mixture of ethyl acetate, methanol and water (7:2:1) to a distance of about 10 cm, and air-dry the plate. Examine under ultraviolet light (main wavelength: 365 nm): Two consecutive blue to blue-white fluorescent spots in different color tone are observed at an *R*f value of about 0.4. Then, spray evenly diluted sulfuric acid on the plate, heat the plate at 105°C. Examine under ultraviolet light (main wavelength: 365 nm): one of these spots produces blue to blue-white fluorescence.

Loss on drying *<5.01>* Not more than 11.0% (6 hours).

Total ash *<5.01>* Not more than 8.5%.

Acid-insoluble ash *<5.01>* Not more than 0.5%.

Containers and storage Containers—Well-closed containers.

Rape Seed Oil

Oleum Rapae

ナタネ油

Rape Seed Oil is the fixed oil obtained from the seed of *Brassica napus* Linné or *Brassica rapa* Linné var. *oleifera* De Candolle (*Cruciferae*).

Description Rape Seed Oil is a clear, pale yellow, slightly viscous oil. It is odorless or has a slight odor and a mild taste.

It is miscible with diethyl ether and with petroleum diethyl ether. It is slightly soluble in ethanol (95).

Specific gravity d_{25}^{25}: 0.906 - 0.920

Acid value *<1.13>* Not more than 0.2.

Saponification value *<1.13>* 169 - 195

Unsaponifiable matters *<1.13>* Not more than 1.5%.

Iodine value *<1.13>* 95 - 127

Containers and storage Containers—Tight containers.

Red Ginseng

Ginseng Radix Rubra

コウジン

Red Ginseng is the root of *Panax ginseng* C. A. Meyer (*Panax schinseng* Nees) (*Araliaceae*), after being steamed.

It contains not less than 0.10% of ginsenoside Rg_1 ($C_{42}H_{72}O_{14}$: 801.01) and not less than 0.20% of ginsenoside Rb_1 ($C_{54}H_{92}O_{23}$: 1109.29), calculated on the basis of dried material.

Description Thin and long cylindrical to fusiform root, often branching out into 2 to 5 lateral roots from the middle; 5 - 25 cm in length, main root 0.5 - 3 cm in diameter; externally light yellow-brown to red-brown, and translucent and with longitudinal wrinkles; crown somewhat constricted, and sometimes with short remains of stem; fractured surface flat; horny and hard in texture.

Odor, characteristic; taste, at first slightly sweet, followed by a slight bitterness.

Identification **(1)** To 0.2 g of pulverized Red Ginseng add 2 mL of acetic anhydride, warm on a water bath for 2 minutes, and filter. To 1 mL of the filtrate add gently 0.5 mL of sulfuric acid to make two layers: a red-brown color develops at the zone of contact.

(2) To 2.0 g of pulverized Red Ginseng add 10 mL of water and 10 mL of 1-butanol, shake for 15 minutes, centrifuge, and use the 1-butanol layer as the sample solution. Separately, dissolve 1 mg of ginsenoside Rg_1 for thin-layer chromatography in 1 mL of methanol, and use this solution as the standard solution. Perform the test with these solutions as directed under Thin-layer Chromatography <*2.03*>. Spot 5 μL of the sample solution and 2 μL of the standard solution on a plate of silica gel for thin-layer chromatography. Develop the plate with a mixture of ethyl acetate, methanol and water (14:5:4) to a distance of about 7 cm, and air-dry the plate. Spray evenly vanillin-sulfuric acid-ethanol TS for spraying on the plate, and heat the plate at 105°C for 10 minutes: one of the several spots obtained from the sample solution has the same color tone and *R*f value with the spot from the standard solution.

Purity **(1)** Heavy metals <*1.07*>—Proceed with 1.0 g of pulverized Red Ginseng according to Method 4, and perform the test. Prepare the control solution with 1.5 mL of Standard Lead Solution (not more than 15 ppm).

(2) Arsenic <*1.11*>—Prepare the test solution with 1.0 g of pulverized Red Ginseng according to Method 4, and perform the test (not more than 2 ppm).

(3) Foreign matter <*5.01*>—The amount of stems and other foreign matter contained in Red Ginseng does not exceed 2.0%.

(4) Total BHC's and total DDT's <*5.01*>—Not more than 0.2 ppm, respectively.

Loss on drying <*5.01*> Not more than 15.5% (6 hours).

Total ash <*5.01*> Not more than 4.5%.

Extract content <*5.01*> Dilute ethanol-soluble extract: not less than 18.0%.

Assay **(1)** Ginsenoside Rg_1—Weigh accurately about 1 g of pulverized Red Ginseng, put in a glass-stoppered centrifuge tube, add 30 mL of diluted methanol (3 in 5), shake for 15 minutes, centrifuge, and separate the supernatant liquid. Repeat the procedure with the residue using 15 mL of diluted methanol (3 in 5), combine the supernatant liquids, and add diluted methanol (3 in 5) to make exactly 50 mL. Pipet 10 mL of this solution, add 3 mL of dilute sodium hydroxide TS, allow to stand for 30 minutes, add 3 mL of 0.1 mol/L hydrochloric acid TS and diluted methanol (3 in 5) to make exactly 20 mL, and use this solution as the sample solution. Separately, weigh accurately about 10 mg of Ginsenoside Rg_1 RS (separately determine the water <*2.48*> by coulometric titration, using 10 mg) dissolve in diluted methanol (3 in 5) to make exactly 100 mL, and use this solution as the standard solution. Perform the test with exactly 10 μL each of the sample solution and standard solution as directed under Liquid Chromatography <*2.01*> according to the following conditions, and determine the peak areas, A_T and A_S, of ginsenoside Rg_1 in each solution.

$$\text{Amount (mg) of ginsenoside } Rg_1\ (C_{42}H_{72}O_{14}) = M_S \times A_T/A_S$$

M_S: Amount (mg) of Ginsenoside Rg_1 RS taken, calculated on the anhydrous basis

Operating conditions—

Detector: An ultraviolet absorption photometer (wavelength: 203 nm).

Column: A stainless steel column 4.6 mm in inside diameter and 15 cm in length, packed with octadecylsilanized silica gel for liquid chromatography (5 μm in particle diameter).

Column temperature: A constant temperature of about 30°C.

Mobile phase: A mixture of water and acetonitrile (4:1).

Flow rate: Adjust so that the retention time of ginsenoside Rg_1 is about 25 minutes.

System suitability—

System performance: Dissolve 1 mg each of Ginsenoside Rg_1 RS and ginsenoside Re in diluted methanol (3 in 5) to make 10 mL. When the procedure is run with 10 μL of this solution under the above operating conditions, ginsenoside Rg_1 and ginsenoside Re are eluted in this order with the resolution between these peaks being not less than 1.5.

System repeatability: When the test is repeated 6 times with 10 μL of the standard solution under the above operating conditions, the relative standard deviation of the peak area of ginsenoside Rg_1 is not more than 1.5%.

(2) Ginsenoside Rb_1—Use the sample solution obtained in (1) as the sample solution. Separately, weigh accurately about 10 mg of Ginsenoside Rb_1 RS (separately determine the water <*2.48*> by coulometric titration, using 10 mg), dissolve in diluted methanol (3 in 5) to make exactly 100 mL, and use this solution as the standard solution. Perform the test with exactly 10 μL each of the sample solution and standard solution as directed under Liquid Chromatography <*2.01*> according to the following conditions, and determine the peak areas, A_T and A_S, of ginsenoside Rb_1 in each solution.

$$\text{Amount (mg) of ginsenoside } Rb_1\ (C_{54}H_{92}O_{23}) = M_S \times A_T/A_S$$

M_S: Amount (mg) of Ginsenoside Rb_1 RS taken, calculated on the anhydrous basis

Operating conditions—

Detector: An ultraviolet absorption photometer (wavelength: 203 nm).

Column: A stainless steel column 4.6 mm in inside diameter and 15 cm in length, packed with octadecylsilanized silica gel for liquid chromatography (5 μm in particle diameter).

Column temperature: A constant temperature of about 40°C.

Mobile phase: A mixture of water and acetonitrile (7:3).

Flow rate: Adjust so that the retention time of ginsenoside Rb_1 is about 20 minutes.

System suitability—

System performance: Dissolve 1 mg each of Ginsenoside Rb_1 RS and ginsenoside Rc in diluted methanol (3 in 5) to make 10 mL. When the procedure is run with 10 μL of this solution under the above operating conditions, ginsenoside Rb_1 and ginsenoside Rc are eluted in this order with the resolution between these peaks being not less than 3.

System repeatability: When the test is repeated 6 times with 10 μL of the standard solution under the above operating conditions, the relative standard deviation of the peak area of ginsenoside Rb_1 is not more than 1.5%.

Containers and storage Containers—Well-closed containers.

Rehmannia Root

Rehmanniae Radix

ジオウ

Rehmannia Root is the root of *Rehmannia glutinosa* Liboschitz var. *purpurea* Makino or *Rehmannia glutinosa* Liboschitz (*Scrophulariaceae*), with the application of steaming (prepared one: Juku-jio) or without it (non-prepared one: Kan-jio).

Description **1)** Kan-jio—Massive or fusiform root, narrow at one or both ends, 5 - 10 cm in length, 0.5 - 3.0 cm in diameter, sometimes broken or markedly deformed in shape; externally yellow-brown, black-brown or black, with deep, longitudinal wrinkles and constrictions; soft in texture; transversely cut surface yellow-brown, black-brown, or black and peripheral portion darker.

Odor, characteristic; taste, slightly sweet at first, followed by a slight bitterness.

Under a microscope <*5.01*>, a transverse section reveals 7 - 15 cellular layers of cork layer; cortex composed entirely of parenchyma; cells containing brown secretes scattered in cortex; xylem practically filled with parenchyma; vessels radially lined, mainly reticulate vessels.

2) Juku-jio—Irregularly massive root, or massive or fusiform root, narrow at one or both ends, 5 - 10 cm in length, 0.5 - 3.0 cm in diameter; externally black, usually lustrous, with deep, longitudinal wrinkles and constrictions; soft in texture and mucous; transversely cut surface black.

Odor, characteristic; taste, sweet at first, followed by a slight bitterness.

Under a microscope <*5.01*>, a transverse section reveals 7 - 15 cellular layers of cork layer; cortex composed entirely of parenchyma; cells containing brown secretes scattered in cortex; xylem practically filled with parenchyma, often parenchyma partially broken and gaps observed; vessels radially lined, mainly reticulate vessels.

Identification **1)** Kan-jio—Sake 0.5 g of the fine cutting of Rehmannia Root with 5 mL of water, add 20 mL of methanol, shake for 10 minutes, centrifuge, and use the supernatant liquid as the sample solution. Separately, dissolve 2 mg of stachyose for thin-layer chromatography in 1 mL of a mixture of water and methanol (1:1), and use this solution as the standard solution. Perform the test with these solutions as directed under Thin-layer Chromatography <*2.03*>. Spot 2 μL each of the sample solution and standard solution on a plate of silica gel for thin-layer chromatography. Develop the plate with a mixture of 2-propanol, water and methanol (3:2:2) to a distance of about 7 cm, and air-dry the plate. Spray evenly 1,3-naphthalenediol TS on the plate, heat the plate at 105°C for 5 minutes: one of the several spots obtained from the sample solution has the same color tone and *R*f value with the spot from the standard solution. When further heat for more than 5 minutes, a blue spot is not observed at just lower than the spot mentioned above, or even appears it is only few.

2) Juku-jio—Sake 0.5 g of the fine cutting of Rehmannia Root with 5 mL of water, add 20 mL of methanol, shake for 10 minutes, centrifuge, and use the supernatant liquid as the sample solution. Separately, dissolve 2 mg of fructose for thin-layer chromatography in 1 mL of a mixture of water and methanol (1:1), and use this solution as the standard solution (1). Separately, dissolve 3 mg of manninotriose for thin-layer chromatography in 1 mL of a mixture of water and methanol (1:1), and use this solution as the standard solution (2). Perform the test with these solutions as directed under Thin-layer Chromatography <*2.03*>. Spot 2 μL each of the sample solution and the standard solutions (1) and (2) on a plate of silica gel for thin-layer chromatography. Develop the plate with a mixture of 2-propanol, water and methanol (3:2:2) to a distance of about 7 cm, and air-dry the plate. Spray evenly 1,3-naphthalenediol TS on the plate, heat the plate at 105°C for 10 minutes: the principal spot obtained from the sample solution has the same color tone and *R*f value with the spot from the standard solution (1). Furthermore, one of the several spots from the sample solution has the same color tone and *R*f value with the blue spot from the standard solution (2).

Purity **(1)** Heavy metals <*1.07*>—Proceed with 3.0 g of pulverized Rehmannia Root according to Method 3, and perform the test. Prepare the control solution with 3.0 mL of Standard Lead Solution (not more than 10 ppm).

(2) Arsenic <*1.11*>—Prepare the test solution with 0.40 g of pulverized Rehmannia Root according to Method 4, and perform the test (not more than 5 ppm).

Total ash <*5.01*> Not more than 6.0%.

Acid-insoluble ash <*5.01*> Not more than 2.5%.

Containers and storage Containers—Well-closed containers.

Rhubarb

Rhei Rhizoma

ダイオウ

Rhubarb is usually the rhizome of *Rheum palmatum* Linné, *Rheum tanguticum* Maximowicz, *Rheum officinale* Baillon, *Rheum coreanum* Nakai or their interspecific hybrids (*Polygonaceae*).

It contains not less than 0.25% of sennosides A ($C_{42}H_{38}O_{20}$: 862.74), calculated on the basis of dried material.

Description Ovoid, oblong-ovoid or cylindrical rhizome, often cut crosswise or longitudinally, 4 - 10 cm in diameter, 5 - 15 cm in length. In the case of Rhubarb without most part of cortex, the outer surface is flat and smooth, yellow-brown to light brown in color, and sometimes exhibiting white, fine reticulations; thick and hard in texture. In the case of Rhubarb with cork layer, externally dark brown or red-black, and with coarse wrinkles; rough and brittle in texture. The fractured surface of Rhubarb is not fibrous; transverse section grayish brown, light grayish brown or brown in color, having patterns of black-brown tissue complicated with white and light brown tissues; near the cambium, the patterns often radiate, and in pith, consist of whirls of tissues radiated from the center of a small brown circle 1 - 3 mm in diameter and arranged in a ring or scattered irregularly.

Odor, characteristic; taste, slightly astringent and bitter; when chewed, gritty between the teeth, and coloring the saliva yellow.

Under a microscope <*5.01*>, the transverse section reveals mostly parenchyma cells; small abnormal cambium-rings scattered here and there in the pith; the cambium-rings produce phloem inside and xylem outside, accompanied with 2 to 4 cell rows of medullary rays containing brown-colored substances, and the rays run radiately from the center of the ring towards the outside forming whirls of tissues; parenchyma cells contain starch grains, brown-colored substances or crystal druses of calcium oxalate.

Identification To 1.0 g of pulverized Rhubarb add 10 mL of water, shake, then add 10 mL of diethyl ether, shake, centrifuge, and use the diethyl ether layer as the sample solution. Separately, dissolve 1 mg of rhein for thin-layer chromatography in 10 mL of acetone, and use this solution as the standard solution. Perform the test with these solutions as directed under Thin-layer Chromatography<*2.03*>. Spot 5 μL each of the sample solution and standard solution on a plate of silica gel for thin-layer chromatography. Develop the plate with a mixture of ethyl acetate, methanol and water (20:3:2) to a distance of about 7 cm, and air-dry the plate: one of the several spots obtained from the sample solution has the same color tone and *R*f value with the spot from the standard solution, and the spot develops a red color on spraying sodium carbonate TS.

Purity **(1)** Heavy metals <*1.07*>—Proceed with 3.0 g of pulverized Rhubarb according to Method 3, and perform the test. Prepare the control solution with 3.0 mL of Standard Lead Solution (not more than 10 ppm).

(2) Arsenic <*1.11*>—Prepare the test solution with 0.40 g of pulverized Rhubarb according to Method 4, and perform the test (not more than 5 ppm).

(3) Rhaponticin—To 0.1 g of pulverized Rhubarb add exactly 10 mL of methanol, shake for 15 minutes, filter, and use the filtrate as the sample solution. Separately, dissolve 1 mg of rhaponticin for purity in 1 mL of methanol, and use this solution as the standard solution. Perform the test with these solutions as directed under Thin-layer Chromatography <*2.03*>. Spot 10 μL each of the sample solution and standard solution on a plate of silica gel for thin-layer chromatography. Develop the plate with a mixture of ethyl formate, 2-butanon, water and formic acid (10:7:1:1) to a distance of about 7 cm, and air-dry the plate. Examine under ultraviolet light (main wavelength: 365 nm): the chromatogram obtained from the sample solution shows no spot having the same color tone and *R*f value with the blue fluorescent spot from the standard solution.

Loss on drying <*5.01*> Not more than 13.0% (6 hours).

Total ash <*5.01*> Not more than 13.0%.

Extract content <*5.01*> Dilute ethanol-soluble extract: not less than 30.0%.

Assay Weigh accurately about 0.5 g of pulverized Rhubarb, add exactly 50 mL of a solution of sodium hydrogen carbonate (1 in 1000), shake for 30 minutes, filter, and use the filtrate as the sample solution. Separately, weigh accurately about 10 mg of Sennoside A RS, (separately determine the water <*2.48*> by coulometric titration, using 10 mg) dissolve in a solution of sodium hydrogen carbonate (1 in 1000) to make exactly 50 mL. Pipet 5 mL of this solution, add a solution of sodium hydrogen carbonate (1 in 1000) to make exactly 20 mL and use this solution as the standard solution. Perform the test with exactly 10 μL of the sample solution and standard solution as directed under Liquid Chromatography <*2.01*> according to the following conditions, and determine the peak areas, A_T and A_S, of sennoside A in each solution.

$$\text{Amount (mg) of sennoside A } (C_{42}H_{38}O_{20}) = M_S \times A_T/A_S \times 1/4$$

M_S: Amount (mg) of Sennoside A RS taken, calculated on the anhydrous basis

Operating conditions—

Detector: An ultraviolet absorption photometer (wavelength: 340 nm).

Column: A stainless steel column 4 - 6 mm in inside diameter and 15 cm in length, packed with octadecylsilanized silica gel for liquid chromatography (5 μm in particle diameter).

Column temperature: A constant temperature of about 40°C.

Mobile phase: A mixture of diluted acetic acid (100) (1 in 80) and acetonitrile (4:1).

Flow rate: Adjust so that the retention time of sennoside A is about 15 minutes.

System suitability—

System performance: Dissolve 1 mg each of Sennoside A RS and naringin for thin-layer chromatography in a solution of sodium hydrogen carbonate (1 in 1000) to make 10 mL. When the procedure is run with 20 μL of this solution under the above operating conditions, sennoside A and naringin are eluted in this order with the resolution between these peaks being not less than 3.

System repeatability: When the test is repeated 6 times with 10 μL of the standard solution under the above operating conditions, the relative standard deviation of the peak area of sennoside A is not more than 1.5%.

Containers and storage Containers—Well-closed containers.

Powdered Rhubarb

Rhei Rhizoma Pulveratum

ダイオウ末

Powdered Rhubarb is the powder of Rhubarb.

It contains not less than 0.25% of sennoside A ($C_{42}H_{38}O_{20}$: 862.74), calculated on the basis of dried materials.

Description Powdered Rhubarb occurs as a brown powder. It has a characteristic odor and a slightly astringent and bitter taste; is gritty between the teeth and colors the saliva yellow on chewing.

Under a microscope <5.01>, Powdered Rhubarb reveals starch grains, dark brown substances or druses of calcium oxalate, fragments of parenchyma cells containing them, and reticulate vessels. The starch grains are spherical, simple, or 2- to 4-compound grains. Simple grain, 3 - 18 μm in diameter, rarely 30 μm; crystal druses of calcium oxalate, 30 - 60 μm in diameter, sometimes exceeding 100 μm.

Identification To 1.0 g of Powdered Rhubarb add 10 mL of water, shake, then add 10 mL of diethyl ether, shake, centrifuge, and use the diethyl ether layer as the sample solution. Separately, dissolve 1 mg of rhein for thin-layer chromatography in 10 mL of acetone, and use this solution as the standard solution. Perform the test with these solutions as directed under Thin-layer Chromatography <2.03>. Spot 5 μL each of the sample solution and standard solution on a plate of silica gel for thin-layer chromatography. Develop the plate with a mixture of ethyl acetate, methanol and water (20:3:2) to a distance of about 7 cm, and air-dry the plate: one of the several spots obtained from the sample solution has the same color tone and *R*f value with the spot from the standard solution, and the spot develops a red color on spraying sodium carbonate TS.

Purity (1) Heavy metals <1.07>—Proceed with 3.0 g of Powdered Rhubarb according to Method 3, and perform the test. Prepare the control solution with 3.0 mL of Standard Lead Solution (not more than 10 ppm).

(2) Arsenic <1.11>—Prepare the test solution with 0.40 g of Powdered Rhubarb according to Method 4, and perform the test (not more than 5 ppm).

(3) Rhaponticin—To 0.1 g of Powdered Rhubarb add exactly 10 mL of methanol, shake for 15 minutes, filter, and use the filtrate as the sample solution. Separately, dissolve 1 mg of rhaponticin for purity in 1 mL of methanol, and use this solution as the standard solution. Perform the test with these solutions as directed under Thin-layer Chromatography <2.03>. Spot 10 μL each of the sample solution and standard solution on a plate of silica gel for thin-layer chromatography. Develop the plate with a mixture of ethyl formate, 2-butanon, water and formic acid (10:7:1:1) to a distance of about 7 cm, and air-dry the plate. Examine under ultraviolet light (main wavelength: 365 nm): the chromatogram obtained from the sample solution shows no spot having the same color tone and *R*f value with the blue fluorescent spot from the standard solution.

Loss on drying <5.01> Not more than 13.0% (6 hours).

Total ash <5.01> Not more than 13.0%.

Acid-insoluble ash <5.01> Not more than 2.0%.

Extract content <5.01> Dilute ethanol-soluble extract: not less than 30.0%.

Assay Weigh accurately about 0.5 g of Powdered Rhubarb, add exactly 50 mL of a solution of sodium hydrogen carbonate (1 in 1000), shake for 30 minutes, filter, and use the filtrate as the sample solution. Separately, weigh accurately about 10 mg of Sennoside A RS, (separately determine the water <2.48> by coulometric titration, using 10 mg), dissolve in a solution of sodium hydrogen carbonate (1 in 1000) to make exactly 50 mL. Pipet 5 mL of this solution, add a solution of sodium hydrogen carbonate (1 in 1000) to make exactly 20 mL, and use this solution as the standard solution. Perform the test with exactly 10 μL each of the sample solution and standard solution as directed under Liquid Chromatography <2.01> according to the following conditions, and determine the peak areas, A_T and A_S, of sennoside A in each solution.

$$\text{Amount (mg) of sennoside A } (C_{42}H_{38}O_{20}) = M_S \times A_T/A_S \times 1/4$$

M_S: Amount (mg) of Sennoside A RS taken, calculated on the anhydrous basis

Operating conditions—

Detector: An ultraviolet absorption photometer (wavelength: 340 nm).

Column: A stainless steel column about 4 - 6 mm in inside diameter and 15 cm in length, packed with octadecylsilanized silica gel for liquid chromatography (5 μm in particle diameter).

Column temperature: A constant temperature of about 40°C.

Mobile phase: A mixture of diluted acetic acid (100) (1 in 80) and acetonitrile (4:1).

Flow rate: Adjust so that the retention time of sennoside A is about 15 minutes.

System suitability—

System performance: Dissolve 1 mg each of Sennoside A RS and naringin for thin-layer chromatography in a solution of sodium hydrogen carbonate (1 in 1000) to make 10 mL. When the procedure is run with 20 μL of this solution under the above operating conditions, sennoside A and naringin are eluted in this order with the resolution between these peaks being not less than 3.

System repeatability: When the test is repeated 6 times with 10 μL of the standard solution under the above operating conditions, the relative standard deviation of the peak area of sennoside A is not more than 1.5%.

Containers and storage Containers—Well-closed containers.

Compound Rhubarb and Senna Powder

複方ダイオウ·センナ散

Method of preparation

Powdered Senna Leaves	110 g
Powdered Rhubarb	110 g
Sulfur	555 g
Magnesium Oxide	225 g
To make	1000 g

Prepare as directed under Powders, with the above ingredients.

Description Compound Rhubarb and Senna Powder occurs as a yellow-brown powder, having a characteristic odor and a bitter taste.

Identification To 2 g of Compound Rhubarb and Senna Powder add 50 mL of water, warm on a water bath for 30 minutes, and filter. Add 2 drops of dilute hydrochloric acid to the filtrate, shake with two 20-mL portions of diethyl ether, and remove the diethyl ether layer. Add 5 mL of hydrochloric acid to the aqueous layer, and heat it on a water bath for 30 minutes. Cool, shake with 20 mL of diethyl ether, take the diethyl ether layer, add 10 mL of sodium hydrogen carbonate TS, and shake: the aqueous layer is red in color.

Containers and storage Containers—Well-closed contain-

ers.

Rikkunshito Extract

六君子湯エキス

Rikkunshito Extract contains not less than 2.4 mg of ginsenoside Rb_1 ($C_{54}H_{92}O_{23}$: 1109.29), not less than 16 mg and not more than 48 mg of hesperidin, and not less than 6 mg and not more than 18 mg of glycyrrhizic acid ($C_{42}H_{62}O_{16}$: 822.93), per extract prepared with the amount specified in the Method of preparation.

Method of preparation

	1)	2)
Ginseng	4 g	4 g
Atractylodes Rhizome	4 g	—
Atractylodes Lancea Rhizome	—	4 g
Poria Sclerotium	4 g	4 g
Pinellia Tuber	4 g	4 g
Citrus Unshiu Peel	2 g	2 g
Jujube	2 g	2 g
Glycyrrhiza	1 g	1 g
Ginger	0.5 g	0.5 g

Prepare a dry extract or viscous extract as directed under Extracts, according to the prescription 1) or 2), using the crude drugs shown above.

Description Rikkunshito Extract is a light brown to brown powder or black-brown viscous extract. It has an odor and a sweet and bitter taste.

Identification (1) Shake 2.0 g of the dry extract (or 6.0 g of the viscous extract) with 10 mL of sodium hydroxide TS, add 5 mL of 1-butanol, shake, centrifuge, and use the 1-butanol layer as the sample solution. Separately, dissolve 1 mg of Ginsenoside Rb_1 RS or ginsenoside Rb_1 for thin-layer chromatography in 1 mL of methanol, and use this solution as the standard solution. Perform the test with these solutions as directed under Thin-layer Chromatography *<2.03>*. Spot 10 μL of the sample solution and 2 μL of the standard solution on a plate of silica gel for thin-layer chromatography. Develop the plate with a mixture of ethyl acetate, 1-propanol, water and acetic acid (100) (7:5:4:1) to a distance of about 7 cm, and air-dry the plate. Spray evenly vanillin-sulfuric acid-ethanol TS for spraying on the plate, heat the plate at 105°C for 5 minutes, and allow to cool: one of the several spots obtained from the sample solution has the same color tone and *R*f value with the blue-purple spot from the standard solution (Ginseng).

(2) For preparation prescribed Atractylodes Rhizome—Shake 1.0 g of the dry extract (or 3.0 g of the viscous extract) with 10 mL of water, add 25 mL of diethyl ether, shake, and centrifuge. Separate the diethyl ether layer, evaporate the solvent under low pressure (in vacuo), add 2 mL of diethyl ether to the residue, and use this solution as the sample solution. Separately, dissolve 1 mg of atractylenolide III for thin-layer chromatography in 2 mL of methanol, and use this solution as the standard solution. Perform the test with these solutions as directed under Thin-layer Chromatography *<2.03>*. Spot 5 μL each of the sample solution and standard solution on a plate of silica gel for thin-layer chromatography. Develop the plate with a mixture of ethyl acetate and hexane (1:1) to a distance of about 7 cm, and air-dry the plate. Spray evenly dilute sulfuric acid on the plate, heat the plate at 105°C for 5 minutes, and examine under ultraviolet light (main wavelength: 365 nm): one of the several spots obtained from the sample solution has the same color tone and *R*f value with the blue-white fluorescent spot from the standard solution (Atractylodes Rhizome).

(3) For preparation prescribed Atractylodes Lancea Rhizome—Shake 2.0 g of the dry extract (or 6.0 g of the viscous extract) with 10 mL of water, add 25 mL of hexane, shake, and centrifuge. Separate the hexane layer, evaporate the solvent under low pressure (in vacuo), add 2 mL of hexane to the residue, and use this solution as the sample solution. Perform the test with the sample solution as directed under Thin-layer Chromatography *<2.03>*. Spot 20 μL of the sample solution on a plate of silica gel with fluorescent indicator for thin-layer chromatography. Develop the plate with a mixture of hexane and acetone (7:1) to a distance of about 7 cm, and air-dry the plate. Examine under ultraviolet light (main wavelength: 254 nm): a dark purple spot is observed at an *R*f value of about 0.5. The spot shows a greenish brown color after being sprayed evenly 4-dimethylaminobenzaldehyde TS for spraying, heated at 105°C for 5 minutes, and allowed to cool (Atractylodes Lancea Rhizome).

(4) Shake 1.0 g of the dry extract (or 3.0 g of the viscous extract) with 10 mL of water, add 10 mL of 1-butanol, shake, centrifuge, and use the 1-butanol layer as the sample solution. Separately, dissolve 1 mg of hesperidin for thin-layer chromatography in 1 mL of methanol, and use this solution as the standard solution. Perform the test with these solutions as directed under Thin-layer Chromatography *<2.03>*. Spot 20 μL of the sample solution and 10 μL of the standard solution on a plate of silica gel for thin-layer chromatography. Develop the plate with a mixture of ethyl acetate, acetone, water and acetic acid (100) (10:6:3:1) to a distance of about 7 cm, and air-dry the plate. Spray evenly 2,6-dibromo-*N*-chloro-1,4-benzoquinone monoimine TS on the plate, and allow to stand in an ammonia gas: one of the several spots obtained from the sample solution has the same color tone and *R*f value with the blue spot from the standard solution (Citrus Unshiu Peel).

(5) Shake 1.0 g of the dry extract (or 3.0 g of the viscous extract) with 10 mL of water, add 10 mL of 1-butanol, shake, centrifuge, and use the 1-butanol layer as the sample solution. Separately, dissolve 1 mg of liquiritin for thin-layer chromatography in 1 mL of methanol, and use this solution as the standard solution. Perform the test with these solutions as directed under Thin-layer Chromatography *<2.03>*. Spot 1 μL each of the sample solution and standard solution on a plate of silica gel for thin-layer chromatography. Develop the plate with a mixture of ethyl acetate, methanol and water (20:3:2) to a distance of about 7 cm, and air-dry the plate. Spray evenly dilute sulfuric acid on the plate, heat the plate at 105°C for 5 minutes, and examine under ultraviolet light (main wavelength: 365 nm): one of the several spots obtained from the sample solution has the same color tone and *R*f value with the yellow-green fluorescent spot from the standard solution (Glycyrrhiza).

(6) Shake 1.0 g of the dry extract (or 3.0 g of the viscous extract) with 10 mL of water, add 25 mL of diethyl ether, shake, and centrifuge. Separate the diethyl ether layer, evaporate the solvent under low pressure (in vacuo), add 2 mL of diethyl ether to the residue, and use this solution as the sample solution. Separately, dissolve 1 mg of [6]-gingerol for thin-layer chromatography in 1 mL of methanol, and use this solution as the standard solution. Perform the test with these solutions as directed under Thin-layer Chromatography *<2.03>*. Spot 30 μL of the sample solution and 5 μL of the standard solution on a plate of silica gel for thin-layer chromatography. Develop the plate with a mixture of ethyl acetate and hexane (1:1) to a distance of about 7 cm, and air-dry the plate. Spray evenly 4-dimethylaminobenzaldehyde TS for spraying on the plate, heat the plate at 105°C for 5 minutes, allow to cool, and spray water: one of the several spots obtained from the sample solution has the same color tone and *R*f value with the blue-green to grayish green spot from the standard solution (Ginger).

Purity **(1)** Heavy metals *<1.07>*—Prepare the test solution with 1.0 g of the dry extract (or an amount of the viscous extract, equivalent to 1.0 g of the dried substance) as directed under Extracts (4), and perform the test (not more than 30 ppm).

(2) Arsenic *<1.11>*—Prepare the test solution with 0.67 g of the dry extract (or an amount of the viscous extract, equivalent to 0.67 g of the dried substance) according to Method 3, and perform the test (not more than 3 ppm).

Loss on drying *<2.41>* The dry extract: Not more than 10.0% (1 g, 105°C, 5 hours).

The viscous extract: Not more than 66.7% (1 g, 105°C, 5 hours).

Total ash *<5.01>* Not more than 9.0%, calculated on the dried basis.

Assay **(1)** Ginsenoside Rb_1—Weigh accurately about 2 g of the dry extract (or an amount of the viscous extract, equivalent to about 2 g of the dried substance), add 30 mL of diluted methanol (3 in 5), shake for 15 minutes, centrifuge, and separate the supernatant liquid. To the residue add 15 mL of diluted methanol (3 in 5), repeat the same procedure. Combine the supernatant liquids, add diluted methanol (3 in 5) to make exactly 50 mL. Pipet 10 mL of this solution, add 3 mL of sodium hydroxide TS, allow to stand for 30 minutes, then add 3 mL of 1 mol/L hydrochloric acid TS, and add water to make exactly 20 mL. Apply exactly 5 mL of this solution to a column (about 10 mm in inside diameter and packed with 0.36 g of octadecylsilanized silica gel for pre-treatment (55 – 105 μm in particle size), washed just before use with methanol and then with diluted methanol (3 in 10)), and wash the column in sequence with 2 mL of diluted methanol (3 in 10), 1 mL of sodium carbonate TS and 10 mL of diluted methanol (3 in 10). Finally, elute with methanol to collect exactly 5 mL, and use this as the sample solution. Separately, weigh accurately about 10 mg of Ginsenoside Rb_1 RS (separately determine the water *<2.48>* by coulometric titration, using 10 mg), and dissolve in methanol to make exactly 100 mL. Pipet 10 mL of this solution, add methanol to make exactly 50 mL, and use this solution as the standard solution. Perform the test with exactly 20 μL each of the sample solution and standard solution as directed under Liquid Chromatography *<2.01>* according to the following conditions, and determine the peak areas, A_T and A_S, of ginsenoside Rb_1 in each solution.

Amount (mg) of ginsenoside Rb_1 ($C_{54}H_{92}O_{23}$)
$= M_S \times A_T/A_S \times 1/5$

M_S: Amount (mg) of Ginsenoside Rb_1 RS taken, calculated on the anhydrous basis

Operating conditions—

Detector: An ultraviolet absorption photometer (wavelength: 203 nm).

Column: A stainless steel column 4.6 mm in inside diameter and 25 cm in length, packed with carbamoyl groups bound silica gel for liquid chromatography (5 μm in particle diameter).

Column temperature: A constant temperature of about 60°C.

Mobile phase: A mixture of acetonitrile, water and phosphoric acid (400:100:1).

Flow rate: 1.0 mL per minute (the retention time of ginsenoside Rb_1 is about 16 minutes).

System suitability—

System performance: When the procedure is run with 20 μL of the standard solution under the above operating conditions, the number of theoretical plates and the symmetry factor of the peak of ginsenoside Rb_1 are not less than 5000 and not more than 1.5, respectively.

System repeatability: When the test is repeated 6 times with 20 μL of the standard solution under the above operating conditions, the relative standard deviation of the peak area of ginsenoside Rb_1 is not more than 1.5%.

(2) Hesperidin—Weigh accurately about 0.1 g of the dry extract (or an amount of the viscous extract, equivalent to about 0.1 g of the dried substance), add exactly 50 mL of diluted tetrahydrofuran (1 in 4), shake for 30 minutes, centrifuge, and use the supernatant liquid as the sample solution. Separately, weigh accurately about 10 mg of hesperidin for assay, previously dried in a desiccator (silica gel) for more than 24 hours, dissolve in methanol to make exactly 100 mL. Pipet 10 mL of this solution, add diluted tetrahydrofuran (1 in 4) to make exactly 100 mL, and use this solution as the standard solution. Perform the test with exactly 10 μL each of the sample solution and standard solution as directed under Liquid Chromatography *<2.01>* according to the following conditions, and determine the peak areas, A_T and A_S, of hesperidin in each solution.

Amount (mg) of hesperidin $= M_S \times A_T/A_S \times 1/20$

M_S: Amount (mg) of hesperidin for assay taken

Operating conditions—

Detector: An ultraviolet absorption photometer (wavelength: 285 nm).

Column: A stainless steel column 4.6 mm in inside diameter and 15 cm in length, packed with octadecylsilanized silica gel for liquid chromatography (5 μm in particle diameter).

Column temperature: A constant temperature of about 40°C.

Mobile phase: A mixture of water, acetonitrile and acetic acid (100) (82:18:1).

Flow rate: 1.0 mL per minute (the retention time of hesperidin is about 15 minutes).

System suitability—

System performance: Dissolve 1 mg each of hesperidin for assay and naringin for thin-layer chromatography in diluted methanol (1 in 2) to make 100 mL. When the procedure is run with 10 μL of this solution under the above operating conditions, naringin and hesperidin are eluted in this order with the resolution between these peaks being not less than 1.5.

System repeatability: When the test is repeated 6 times with 10 μL of the standard solution under the above operating conditions, the relative standard deviation of the peak area of hesperidin is not more than 1.5%.

(3) Glycyrrhizic acid—Weigh accurately about 0.5 g of the dry extract (or an amount of the viscous extract, equivalent to about 0.5 g of the dried substance), add exactly 50 mL of diluted methanol (1 in 2), shake for 15 minutes, filter, and use the filtrate as the sample solution. Separately, weigh accurately about 10 mg of Glycyrrhizic Acid RS (separately determine the water *<2.48>* by coulometric titration, using 10 mg), dissolve in diluted methanol (1 in 2) to make exactly 100 mL, and use this solution as the standard solution. Perform the test with exactly 10 μL each of the sample solution and standard solution as directed under Liquid Chromatography <2.01> according to the following conditions, and determine the peak areas, A_T and A_S, of glycyrrhizic acid in each solution.

$$\text{Amount (mg) of glycyrrhizic acid } (C_{42}H_{62}O_{16}) = M_S \times A_T/A_S \times 1/2$$

M_S: Amount (mg) of Glycyrrhizic Acid RS taken, calculated on the anhydrous basis

Operating conditions—

Detector: An ultraviolet absorption photometer (wavelength: 254 nm).

Column: A stainless steel column 4.6 mm in inside diameter and 15 cm in length, packed with octadecylsilanized silica gel for liquid chromatography (5 μm in particle diameter).

Column temperature: A constant temperature of about 40°C.

Mobile phase: Dissolve 3.85 g of ammonium acetate in 720 mL of water, and add 5 mL of acetic acid (100) and 280 mL of acetonitrile.

Flow rate: 1.0 mL per minute (the retention time of glycyrrhizic acid is about 15 minutes).

System suitability—

System performance: Dissolve 5 mg of monoammonium glycyrrhizinate for resolution check in 20 mL of dilute ethanol. When the procedure is run with 10 μL of this solution under the above operating conditions, the resolution between the peak having the relative retention time of about 0.9 to glycyrrhizic acid and the peak of glycyrrhizic acid is not less than 1.5.

System repeatability: When the test is repeated 6 times with 10 μL of the standard solution under the above operating conditions, the relative standard deviation of the peak area of glycyrrhizic acid is not more than 1.5%.

Containers and storage Containers—Tight containers.

Rose Fruit

Rosae Fructus

エイジツ

Rose Fruit is false or true fruit of *Rosa multiflora* Thunberg (*Rosaceae*).

Description The pseudocarp, spherical, ellipsoidal or spheroidal, 5 - 9.5 mm in length, 3.5 - 8 mm in diameter; the external surface red to dark brown in color, smooth and lustrous; often with peduncle about 10 mm in length at one end, and with pentagonal remains of calyx without sepal at the other end; internal wall of receptacle covered densely with silvery hairs; the interior containing 5 - 10 mature nuts; the nut, irregularly angular ovoid, about 4 mm in length, about 2 mm in diameter; external surface, light yellow-brown; obtuse at one end, and slightly acute at the other.

Odor, slight; taste of fruit receptacle, sweet and acid, and of nut, mucilaginous at first, later astringent, bitter and irritative.

Identification Boil gently 1 g of pulverized Rose Fruit with 20 mL of methanol for 2 minutes, and filter. To 5 mL of the filtrate add 0.1 g of magnesium in ribbon form and 0.5 mL of hydrochloric acid, and allow the mixture to stand: a light red to red color develops.

Purity Foreign matter <5.01>—The amount of the peduncle and other foreign matter contained in Rose Fruit is not more than 1.0%.

Total ash <5.01> Not more than 6.0%.

Containers and storage Containers—Well-closed containers.

Powdered Rose Fruit

Rosae Fructus Pulveratus

エイジツ末

Powdered Rose Fruit is the powder of Rose Fruit.

Description Powdered Rose Fruit occurs as a grayish yellow-brown powder. It has a slight odor, and has a slightly mucilaginous, astringent, bitter, and slightly acid taste.

Under a microscope <5.01>, Powdered Rose Fruit reveals fragments of extremely thick-walled hairs 35 - 70 μm in diameter, fragments of epidermis and hypodermis containing brown tannin masses, fragments of thin-walled fundamental tissue containing grayish brown substances, fragments of fine vessels, and solitary or twin crystals or rosette agregates of calcium oxalate (components of fruit receptacle); fragments of sclerenchyma, fiber groups, fine vessels, and fragments of epidermis containing brown tannin and mucilage (components of pericarp); fragments of endosperm composed of polygonal cells containing aleuron grains and fatty oil, fragments of outer epidermis composed of polygonal cells containing tannin, and fragments of inner epidermis composed of elongated cells having wavy lateral walls (components of seed).

Identification Boil gently 1 g of Powdered Rose Fruit with 20 mL of methanol for 2 minutes, and filter. To 5 mL of the filtrate add 0.1 g of magnesium in ribbon form and 0.5 mL of hydrochloric acid, and allow the mixture of stand: a light red to red color develops.

Total ash <5.01> Not more than 6.0%.

Containers and storage Containers—Well-closed containers.

Rosin

Resina Pini

ロジン

Rosin is the resin obtained from the exudation of plants of *Pinus* species (*Pinaceae*) from which essential oil has been removed.

Description Rosin occurs as a light yellow to light brown, glassily transparent, brittle mass, the surfaces of which are often covered with a yellow powder. The fractured surface is shell-like and lustrous.

It has a slight odor.

It melts easily, and burns with a yellow-brown flame.

It is freely soluble in ethanol (95), in acetic acid (100) and in diethyl ether.

A solution of Rosin in ethanol (95) is acidic.

Acid value <*1.13*> 150 – 177

Total ash <*5.01*> Not more than 0.1%.

Containers and storage Containers—Well-closed containers.

Royal Jelly

Apilac

ローヤルゼリー

Royal Jelly is the viscous liquid or its dried substance secreted by the secreting gland on the head of *Apis mellifera* Linné or *Apis cerana* Fabricius (*Apidae*).

It contains not less than 4.0% and not more than 8.0% of 10-hydroxy-2-(*E*)-decenoic acid, calculated on the basis of dried material.

Description Slightly viscous liquid or powder, milky white to light yellow in color. Odor, characteristic; taste, astringent and acid.

Identification To a portion of Royal Jelly, equivalent to 0.2 g of dried substance, add 5 mL of water, 1 mL of dilute hydrochloric acid and 10 mL of diethyl ether, shake for 15 minutes, and centrifuge. Take the diethyl ether layer, evaporate the solvent under low pressure (in vacuo), dissolve the residue in 5 mL of methanol, and use this solution as the sample solution. Separately, dissolve 2 mg of 10-hydroxy-2-(*E*)-decenoic acid for thin-layer chromatography in 1 mL of methanol, and use this solution as the standard solution. Perform the test with these solutions as directed under Thin-layer Chromatography <*2.03*>. Spot 20 μL each of the sample solution and standard solution on a plate of silica gel with fluorescent indicator for thin-layer chromatography, develop the plate with a mixture of 1-propanol and ammonia solution (28) (7:3) to a distance of about 7 cm, and air-dry the plate. Examine under ultraviolet light (main wavelength: 254 nm): the spot obtained from the sample solution has the same color tone and *R*f value with the spot from the standard solution.

Purity **(1)** Heavy metals <*1.07*>—Proceed with a portion of Royal Jelly, equivalent to 1.0 g of the dried substance, according to Method 3, and perform the test. Prepare the control solution with 3.0 mL of Standard Lead Solution (not more than 30 ppm).

(2) Arsenic <*1.11*>—Prepare the test solution with an amount of Royal Jelly, equivalent to 0.40 g of the dried substance according to Method 3, and perform the test (not more than 5 ppm).

Loss on drying <*5.01*> The slightly viscous liquid: Not less than 57.0% and not more than 77.0% (6 hours).

The powder: Not less than 7.0% and not more than 13.0% (6 hours).

Total ash <*5.01*> Not more than 4.0%, calculated on the dried basis.

Acid-insoluble ash <*5.01*> Not more than 0.5%, calculated on the dried basis.

Assay Weigh accurately a portion of Royal Jelly, equivalent to 0.2 g of the dried substance, add 20 mL of methanol, sonicate for 30 minutes, and add methanol to make exactly 50 mL. Centrifuge this solution, pipet 2 mL of the supernatant liquid, add exactly 2 mL of the internal standard solution, then add 25 mL of water and methanol to make 50 mL, and use this solution as the sample solution. Separately, weigh accurately about 10 mg of 10-hydroxy-2-(*E*)-decenoic acid for assay, dissolve in methanol to make exactly 100 mL. Pipet 3 mL of this solution, add exactly 2 mL of the internal standard solution, then add 25 mL of water and methanol to make 50 mL, and use this solution as the standard solution. Perform the test with 10 μL each of the sample solution and standard solution as directed under Liquid Chromatography <*2.01*> according to the following conditions, and calculate the ratios, Q_T and Q_S, of the peak area of 10-hydroxy-2-(*E*)-decenoic acid to that of the internal standard.

$$\text{Amount (mg) of 10-hydroxy-2-}(E)\text{-decenoic acid} = M_S \times Q_T/Q_S \times 3/4$$

M_S: Amount (mg) of 10-hydroxy-2-(*E*)-decenoic acid for assay taken

Internal standard solution—A solution of propyl parahydroxybenzoate in methanol (1 in 5000).

Operating conditions—

Detector: An ultraviolet absorption photometer (wavelength: 215 nm).

Column: A stainless steel column 4.6 mm in inside diameter and 15 cm in length, packed with octadecylsilanized silica gel for liquid chromatography (5 μm in particle diameter).

Column temperature: A constant temperature of about 50°C.

Mobile phase: A mixture of water, methanol for liquid chromatography and phosphoric acid (550:450:1).

Flow rate: Adjust so that the retention time of 10-hydroxy-2-(*E*)-decenoic acid is about 10 minutes.

System suitability—

System performance: When the procedure is run with 10 μL of the standard solution under the above operating conditions, 10-hydroxy-2-(*E*)-decenoic acid and the internal standard are eluted in this order with the resolution between these peaks being not less than 6.

System repeatability: When the test is repeated 6 times with 10 μL of the standard solution under the above operating conditions, the relative standard deviation of the ratio of the peak area of 10-hydroxy-2-(*E*)-decenoic acid to that of the internal standard is not more than 1.0%.

Containers and storage Containers—Tight containers.

Storage—At not exceeding 10°C.

Ryokeijutsukanto Extract

苓桂朮甘湯エキス

Ryokeijutsukanto Extract contains not less than 1 mg and not more than 4 mg of (*E*)-cinnamic acid, and not less than 17 mg and not more than 51 mg of glycyrrhizic acid ($C_{42}H_{62}O_{16}$: 822.93), per extract prepared with the amount specified in the Method of preparation.

Method of preparation

	1)	2)
Poria Sclerotium	6 g	6 g
Cinnamon Bark	4 g	4 g
Atractylodes Rhizome	3 g	—
Atractylodes Lancea Rhizome	—	3 g
Glycyrrhiza	2 g	2 g

Prepare a dry extract or viscous extract as directed under Extracts, according to the prescription 1) or 2), using the crude drugs shown above.

Description Ryokeijutsukanto Extract occurs as a brown powder or black-brown viscous extract. It has an odor, and a sweet first then bitter taste.

Identification **(1)** To 1.0 g of the dry extract (or 3.0 g of the viscous extract) add 10 mL of water, shake, then add 25 mL of diethyl ether, and shake. Separate the diethyl ether layer, evaporate the solvent under low pressure (in vacuo), add 2 mL of diethyl ether to the residue, and use this solution as the sample solution. Separately, dissolve 1 mg of (*E*)-cinnamic acid for thin-layer chromatography in 1 mL of methanol, and use this solution as the standard solution. Perform the test with these solutions as directed under Thin-layer Chromatography *<2.03>*. Spot 5 μL each of the sample solution and standard solution on a plate of silica gel with fluorescent indicator for thin-layer chromatography. Develop the plate with a mixture of hexane, ethyl acetate, formic acid and water (60:40:4:1) to a distance of about 7 cm, and air-dry the plate. Examine under ultraviolet light (main wavelength: 254 nm): one of the several spots obtained from the sample solution has the same color tone and *Rf* value with the blue-purple spot from the standard solution (Cinnamon Bark).

(2) For preparation prescribed Atractylodes Rhizome—To 1.0 g of the dry extract (or 3.0 g of the viscous extract) add 10 mL of water, shake, then add 25 mL of diethyl ether, and shake. Separate the diethyl ether layer, evaporate the solvent under low pressure (in vacuo), add 2 mL of diethyl ether to the residue, and use this solution as the sample solution. Separately, dissolve 1 mg of atractylenolide III for thin-layer chromatography in 2 mL of methanol, and use this solution as the standard solution. Perform the test with these solutions as directed under Thin-layer Chromatography *<2.03>*. Spot 5 μL each of the sample solution and standard solution on a plate of silica gel for thin-layer chromatography. Develop the plate with a mixture of ethyl acetate and hexane (1:1) to a distance of about 7 cm, and air-dry the plate. Spray evenly dilute sulfuric acid on the plate, heat the plate at 105°C for 5 minutes, and examine under ultraviolet light (main wavelength: 365 nm): one of the several spots obtained from the sample solution has the same color tone and *Rf* value with the blue-white fluorescent spot from the standard solution (Atractylodes Rhizome).

(3) For preparation prescribed Atractylodes Lancea Rhizome—To 2.0 g of the dry extract (or 6.0 g of the viscous extract) add 10 mL of water, shake, then add 25 mL of hexane, and shake. Separate the hexane layer, evaporate the solvent under low pressure (in vacuo), add 2 mL of hexane to the residue, and use this solution as the sample solution. Perform the test with the sample solution as directed under Thin-layer Chromatography *<2.03>*. Spot 20 μL of the sample solution on a plate of silica gel with fluorescent indicator for thin-layer chromatography. Develop the plate with a mixture of hexane and acetone (7:1) to a distance of about 7 cm, and air-dry the plate. Examine under ultraviolet light (main wavelength: 254 nm): a dark purple spot is observed at an *Rf* value of about 0.5. The spot shows a greenish brown color after being sprayed evenly 4-dimethylaminobenzaldehyde TS for spraying, heated at 105°C for 5 minutes, and allowed to cool (Atractylodes Lancea Rhizome).

(4) To 1.0 g of the dry extract (or 3.0 g of the viscous extract) add 10 mL of water, shake, then add 10 mL of 1-butanol, and shake. Centrifuge, and use the 1-butanol layer as the sample solution. Separately, dissolve 1 mg of liquiritin for thin-layer chromatography in 1 mL of methanol, and use this solution as the standard solution. Perform the test with these solutions as directed under Thin-layer Chromatography *<2.03>*. Spot 1 μL each of the sample solution and standard solution on a plate of silica gel for thin-layer chromatography. Develop the plate with a mixture of ethyl acetate, methanol and water (20:3:2) to a distance of about 7 cm, and air-dry the plate. Spray evenly dilute sulfuric acid on the plate, heat the plate at 105°C for 5 minutes, and examine under ultraviolet light (main wavelength: 365 nm): one of the several spots obtained from the sample solution has the same color tone and *Rf* value with the yellow-green fluorescent spot from the standard solution (Glycyrrhiza).

Purity **(1)** Heavy metals *<1.07>*—Prepare the test solution with 1.0 g of dry extract (or an amount of the viscous extract, equivalent to 1.0 g of the dried substance) of Ryokeijutsukanto Extract as directed in the Extracts (4), and perform the test (not more than 30 ppm).

(2) Arsenic *<1.11>*—Prepare the test solution with 0.67 g of dry extract (or an amount of the viscous extract, equivalent to 0.67 g of the dried substance) of Ryokeijutsukanto Extract according to Method 3, and perform the test (not more than 3 ppm).

Loss on drying *<2.41>* The dry extract: Not more than 8.5% (1 g, 105°C, 5 hours).

The viscous extract: Not more than 66.7% (1 g 105°C, 5 hours).

Total ash *<5.01>* Not more than 8.0%, calculated on the dried basis.

Assay **(1)** (*E*)-Cinnamic acid—Conduct this procedure using light-resistant vessels. Weigh accurately about 0.5 g of dry extract (or an amount of the viscous extract, equivalent to about 0.5 g of the dried substance) of Ryokeijutsukanto Extract, add exactly 50 mL of diluted methanol (1 in 2), shake for 15 minutes, filter, and use the filtrate as the sample solution. Separately, weigh accurately about 10 mg of (*E*)-cinnamic acid for assay, and dissolve in diluted methanol (1 in 2) to make exactly 100 mL. Pipet 10 mL of this solution, add diluted methanol (1 in 2) to make exactly 100 mL, and use this solution as the standard solution. Perform the test with exactly 10 μL each of the sample solution and standard solution as directed under Liquid Chromatography *<2.01>* according to the following conditions, and determine the peak areas, A_T and A_S, of (*E*)-cinnamic acid in each solution.

$$\text{Amount (mg) of } (E)\text{-cinnamic acid} = M_S \times A_T/A_S \times 1/20$$

M_S: Amount (mg) of (*E*)-cinnamic acid for assay taken, calculated on the basis of the content obtained by qNMR

Operating conditions—

Detector: An ultraviolet absorption photometer (wave-

length: 273 nm).

Column: A stainless steel column 4.6 mm in inside diameter and 15 cm in length, packed with octadecylsilanized silica gel for liquid chromatography (5 μm in particle diameter).

Column temperature: A constant temperature of about 40°C.

Mobile phase: A mixture of water, acetonitrile and phosphoric acid (750:250:1).

Flow rate: 1.0 mL per minute (the retention time of (E)-cinnamic acid is about 12 minutes).

System suitability—

System performance: When the procedure is run with 10 μL of the standard solution under the above operating conditions, the number of theoretical plates and the symmetry factor of the peak of (E)-cinnamic acid are not less than 5000 and not more than 1.5, respectively.

System repeatability: When the test is repeated 6 times with 10 μL of the standard solution under the above operating conditions, the relative standard deviation of the peak area of (E)-cinnamic acid is not more than 1.5%.

(2) Glycyrrhizic acid—Perform the test according to the following i) or ii).

i) Weigh accurately about 0.5 g of the dry extract (or an amount of the viscous extract, equivalent to about 0.5 g of the dried substance), add exactly 50 mL of diluted methanol (1 in 2), shake for 15 minutes, filter, and use the filtrate as the sample solution. Separately, weigh accurately about 10 mg of Glycyrrhizic Acid RS (separately determine the water <*2.48*> by coulometric titration, using 10 mg), dissolve in diluted methanol (1 in 2) to make exactly 100 mL, and use this solution as the standard solution. Perform the test with exactly 10 μL each of the sample solution and standard solution as directed under Liquid Chromatography <*2.01*> according to the following conditions, and determine the peak areas, A_T and A_S, of glycyrrhizic acid in each solution.

$$\text{Amount (mg) of glycyrrhizic acid } (C_{42}H_{62}O_{16}) = M_S \times A_T/A_S \times 1/2$$

M_S: Amount (mg) of Glycyrrhizic Acid RS taken, calculated on the anhydrous basis

Operating conditions—

Detector: An ultraviolet absorption photometer (wavelength: 254 nm).

Column: A stainless steel column 4.6 mm in inside diameter and 15 cm in length, packed with octadecylsilanized silica gel for liquid chromatography (5 μm in particle diameter).

Column temperature: A constant temperature of about 40°C.

Mobile phase: Dissolve 3.85 g of ammonium acetate in 720 mL of water, and add 5 mL of acetic acid (100) and 280 mL of acetonitrile.

Flow rate: 1.0 mL per minute (the retention time of glycyrrhizic acid is about 15 minutes).

System suitability—

System performance: Dissolve 5 mg of monoammonium glycyrrhizinate for resolution check in 20 mL of dilute ethanol. When the procedure is run with 10 μL of this solution under the above operating conditions, the resolution between the peak having the relative retention time of about 0.9 to glycyrrhizic acid and the peak of glycyrrhizic acid is not less than 1.5. Dissolve 1 mg of (E)-cinnamaldehyde for thin-layer chromatography in 50 mL of methanol. To 2 mL of this solution add 2 mL of the standard solution. When the procedure is run with 10 μL of this solution under the above operating conditions, the resolution between the peaks of glycyrrhizic acid and (E)-cinnamaldehyde is not less than 1.5.

System repeatability: When the test is repeated 6 times with 10 μL of the standard solution under the above operating conditions, the relative standard deviation of the peak area of glycyrrhizic acid is not more than 1.5%.

ii) Weigh accurately about 0.5 g of the dry extract (or an amount of the viscous extract, equivalent to about 0.5 g of the dried substance), add 20 mL of ethyl acetate and 10 mL of water, and shake for 10 minutes. After centrifugation, remove the ethyl acetate layer, add 20 mL of ethyl acetate, proceed in the same manner as described above, and remove the ethyl acetate layer. To the aqueous layer add 10 mL of methanol, shake for 30 minutes, centrifuge, and take the supernatant liquid. To the residue add 20 mL of diluted methanol (1 in 2), shake for 5 minutes, centrifuge, and take the supernatant liquid. Combine these supernatant liquids, add diluted methanol (1 in 2) to make exactly 50 mL, and use this solution as the sample solution. Separately, weigh accurately about 10 mg of Glycyrrhizic Acid RS (separately determine the water <*2.48*> by coulometric titration, using 10 mg), dissolve in diluted methanol (1 in 2) to make exactly 100 mL, and use this solution as the standard solution. Perform the test with exactly 10 μL each of the sample solution and standard solution as directed under Liquid Chromatography <*2.01*> according to the following conditions, and determine the peak areas, A_T and A_S, of glycyrrhizic acid in each solution.

$$\text{Amount (mg) of glycyrrhizic acid } (C_{42}H_{62}O_{16}) = M_S \times A_T/A_S \times 1/2$$

M_S: Amount (mg) of Glycyrrhizic Acid RS taken, calculated on the anhydrous basis

Operating conditions—

Proceed as directed in the operating conditions in i).

System suitability—

System repeatability: Proceed as directed in the system suitability in i).

System performance: Dissolve 5 mg of monoammonium glycyrrhizinate for resolution check in 20 mL of dilute ethanol. When the procedure is run with 10 μL of this solution under the above operating conditions, the resolution between the peak having the relative retention time of about 0.9 to glycyrrhizic acid and the peak of glycyrrhizic acid is not less than 1.5.

Containers and storage Containers—Tight containers.

Safflower

Carthami Flos

コウカ

Safflower is the tubulous flower of *Carthamus tinctorius* Linné (*Compositae*) without any treatment or with most of the yellow pigment removed, and sometimes with pressed into a flat slab.

Description Red to red-brown corolla, yellow style and stamen, rarely mixed with immature ovary; total length about 1 cm; corolla, tubular and with 5 lobes; 5 stamens surrounding long pistil; pollen grains yellow and approximately spherical, about 50 μm in diameter, with fine protrusions on the surface. The pressed slab, about 0.5 cm in thickness, consists of a collection of numerous corollas.

Odor, characteristic; taste, slightly bitter.

Identification To 1.0 g of pulverized Safflower add 10 mL of a mixture of acetone and water (4:1), shake for 10 minutes, filter, and use the filtrate as the sample solution. Perform the test with the sample solution as directed under Thin-layer Chromatography <*2.03*>. Spot 5 μL of the sample solution on a plate of silica gel for thin-layer chromatography. Develop the plate with a mixture of ethyl acetate, water, formic acid and methanol (35:15:10:2) to a distance of about 7 cm, and air-dry the plate: a red spot appears at an *R*f value of about 0.5.

Purity Foreign matter <*5.01*>—The amount of ovaries, stems, leaves and other foreign matter contained in Safflower does not exceed 2.0%.

Total ash <*5.01*> Not more than 18.0%.

Containers and storage Containers—Well-closed containers.

Storage—Light-resistant.

Saffron

Crocus

サフラン

Saffron is the stigma of *Crocus sativus* Linné (*Iridaceae*).

Description Thin cord-like stigma, externally dark yellow-red to red-brown, 1.5 - 3.5 cm in length, tripartite or separate; the end of partite part widened and the other end narrowed gradually.

Odor, strong and characteristic; taste, bitter; colors the saliva yellow on chewing.

Under a microscope <*5.01*>, when softened by immersion in water, the upper end has numerous tubular protrusions about 150 μm in length, with a small number of pollen grains.

Identification Use the sample solution obtained in the Purity (1) as the sample solution. Perform the test with this solution as directed under Thin-layer Chromatography <*2.03*>. Spot 5 μL of the sample solution on a plate of silica gel for thin-layer chromatography. Develop the plate with a mixture of ethyl acetate, methanol, water and acetic acid (100) (20:5:4:1) to a distance of about 10 cm, and air-dry the plate: three yellow spots appear at the *R*f values of about 0.1, about 0.25 and about 0.4.

Purity **(1)** Synthetic dye—To 0.10 g of pulverized Saffron add 5 mL of methanol, shake for 10 minutes, centrifuge, and use the supernatant liquid as the sample solution. Perform the test with the sample solution as directed under Thin-layer Chromatography <*2.03*>. Spot 5 μL of the sample solution on a plate of silica gel for thin-layer chromatography. Develop the plate with a mixture of ethyl acetate, methanol, water and acetic acid (100) (20:5:4:1) to a distance of about 10 cm, and air-dry the plate: any spot other than yellow spots does not appear upper in position than a yellow spot at an *R*f value of about 0.4 and any yellow spot does not appear between yellow spots at *R*f values of about 0.25 and about 0.4. Spray evenly diluted sulfuric acid on the plate, and heat the plate at 105°C for 10 minutes: any clear yellow spot does not appear at an *R*f value of less than 0.1, and any orange spot does not appear between blue-purple spots at *R*f values of about 0.1 and about 0.25.

(2) Glycerol, sugar or honey—Saffron has no sweet taste. Press it between two pieces of paper: no spot is left on the paper.

(3) Yellow style—When perform the test of foreign matter <*5.01*>, the yellow style in Saffron does not exceed 10.0%.

Loss on drying <*5.01*> Not more than 12.0% (6 hours).

Total ash <*5.01*> Not more than 7.5%.

Content of the active principle Crocin—Dry Saffron in a desiccator (silica gel) for 24 hours, and powder. To exactly 0.100 g of the powder add 150 mL of warm water, warm the mixture between 60°C and 70°C for 30 minutes with frequent shaking, cool, and filter. Pipet 1 mL of the filtrate, add water to make exactly 10 mL, and use this solution as the sample solution. Separately, dissolve exactly 98 mg of carbazochrome sodium sulfonate trihydrate in water to make exactly 100 mL. Pipet 5 mL of this solution, add water to make exactly 100 mL, and use this solution as the standard solution. Determine the absorbances of the sample solution and standard solution at 438 nm as directed under Ultraviolet-visible Spectrophotometry <*2.24*>: the absorbance of the sample solution is larger than that of the standard solution.

Containers and storage Containers—Well-closed containers.

Storage—Light-resistant.

Saibokuto Extract

柴朴湯エキス

Saibokuto Extract contains not less than 2 mg and not more than 8 mg of saikosaponin b_2, not less than 90 mg and not more than 270 mg of baicalin ($C_{21}H_{18}O_{11}$: 446.36), and not less than 14 mg and not more than 42 mg of glycyrrhizic acid ($C_{42}H_{62}O_{16}$: 822.93), per extract prepared with the amount specified in the Method of preparation.

Method of preparation

	1)	2)
Bupleurum Root	7 g	7 g
Pinellia Tuber	6 g	5 g
Poria Sclerotium	5 g	5 g
Scutellaria Root	3 g	3 g
Magnolia Bark	3 g	3 g
Jujube	3 g	3 g
Ginseng	3 g	3 g
Glycyrrhiza	2 g	2 g
Perilla Herb	2 g	2 g
Ginger	1 g	1 g

Prepare a dry extract or viscous extract as directed under Extracts, according to the prescription 1) or 2), using the crude drugs shown above.

Description Saibokuto Extract is a light brown powder or black-brown viscous extract, having a slightly odor and a slight sweet first, then a bitter taste.

Identification **(1)** Shake 2.0 g of the dry extract (or 6.0 g of the viscous extract) with 10 mL of sodium hydroxide TS, add 5 mL of 1-butanol, shake, centrifuge, and use the 1-

butanol layer as the sample solution. Separately, dissolve 1 mg of saikosaponin b_2 for thin-layer chromatography in 1 mL of methanol, and use this solution as the standard solution. Perform the test with these solutions as directed under Thin-layer Chromatography <*2.03*>. Spot 10 μL of the sample solution and 2 μL of the standard solution on a plate of silica gel for thin-layer chromatography. Develop the plate with a mixture of ethyl acetate, ethanol (99.5) and water (8:2:1) to a distance of about 7 cm, and air-dry the plate. Spray evenly 4-dimethylaminobenzaldehyde TS for spraying on the plate, heat the plate at 105°C for 5 minutes, and examine under ultraviolet light (main wavelength: 365 nm): one of the several spots obtained from the sample solution has the same color tone and *R*f value with the yellow fluorescent spot from the standard solution (Bupleurum Root).

(2) Shake 1.0 g of the dry extract (or 3.0 g of the viscous extract) with 10 mL of water, add 25 mL of diethyl ether, shake, and separate the diethyl ether layer. Evaporate the solvent under low pressure (in vacuo), add 2 mL of diethyl ether to the residue, and use this solution as the sample solution. Separately, dissolve 1 mg of wogonin for thin-layer chromatography in 1 mL of methanol, and use this solution as the standard solution. Perform the test with these solutions as directed under Thin-layer Chromatography <*2.03*>. Spot 20 μL of the sample solution and 2 μL of the standard solution on a plate of silica gel for thin-layer chromatography. Develop the plate with a mixture of ethyl acetate, hexane and acetic acid (100) (10:10:1) to a distance of about 7 cm, and air-dry the plate. Spray evenly iron (III) chloride-methanol TS on the plate: one of the several spots obtained from the sample solution has the same color tone and *R*f value with the yellow-brown spot from the standard solution (Scutellaria Root).

(3) Shake 1.0 g of the dry extract (or 3.0 g of the viscous extract) with 10 mL of water, add 25 mL of diethyl ether, shake, and separate the diethyl ether layer. Evaporate the solvent under low pressure (in vacuo), add 2 mL of diethyl ether to the residue, and use this solution as the sample solution. Separately, dissolve 1 mg of magnolol for thin-layer chromatography in 1 mL of methanol, and use this solution as the standard solution. Perform the test with these solutions as directed under Thin-layer Chromatography <*2.03*>. Spot 5 μL each of the sample solution and standard solution on a plate of silica gel with fluorescent indicator for thin layer chromatography. Develop the plate with a mixture of ethyl acetate and hexane (1:1) to a distance of about 7 cm, and air-dry the plate. Examine under ultraviolet light (main wavelength: 254 nm): one of the several spots obtained from the sample solution has the same color tone and *R*f value with the dark purple spot from the standard solution (Magnolia Bark).

(4) Shake 2.0 g of the dry extract (or 6.0 g of the viscous extract) with 10 mL of sodium hydroxide TS, add 5 mL of 1-butanol, shake, centrifuge, and use the 1-butanol layer as the sample solution. Separately, dissolve 1 mg of Ginsenoside Rb_1 RS or ginsenoside Rb_1 for thin-layer chromatography in 1 mL of methanol, and use this solution as the standard solution. Perform the test with these solutions as directed under Thin-layer Chromatography <*2.03*>. Spot 10 μL of the sample solution and 2 μL of the standard solution on a plate of silica gel for thin-layer chromatography. Develop the plate with a mixture of ethyl acetate, 1-propanol, water and acetic acid (100) (7:5:4:1) to a distance of about 7 cm, and air-dry the plate. Spray evenly vanillin-sulfuric acid-ethanol TS for spraying on the plate, heat the plate at 105°C for 5 minutes, and allow to cool: one of the several spots obtained from the sample solution has the same color tone and *R*f value with the blue-purple spot from the standard solution (Ginseng).

(5) Shake 1.0 g of the dry extract (or 3.0 g of the viscous extract) with 10 mL of water, add 10 mL of 1-butanol, shake, centrifuge, and use the 1-butanol layer as the sample solution. Separately, dissolve 1 mg of liquiritin for thin-layer chromatography in 1 mL of methanol, and use this solution as the standard solution. Perform the test with these solutions as directed under Thin-layer Chromatography <*2.03*>. Spot 1 μL each of the sample solution and standard solution on a plate of silica gel for thin-layer chromatography. Develop the plate with a mixture of ethyl acetate, methanol and water (20:3:2) to a distance of about 7 cm, and air-dry the plate. Spray evenly dilute sulfuric acid on the plate, heat the plate at 105°C for 5 minutes, and examine under ultraviolet light (main wavelength: 365 nm): one of the several spots obtained from the sample solution has the same color tone and *R*f value with the yellow-green fluorescent spot from the standard solution (Glycyrrhiza).

(6) Shake 1.0 g of the dry extract (or 3.0 g of the viscous extract) with 10 mL of 0.1 mol/L hydrochloric acid TS, add 25 mL of diethyl ether, shake, and separate the diethyl ether layer. Evaporate the solvent under low pressure (in vacuo), add 1 mL of methanol to the residue, and use this solution as the sample solution. Separately, dissolve 1 mg of rosmarinic acid for thin-layer chromatography in 1 mL of methanol, and use this solution as the standard solution. Perform the test with these solutions as directed under Thin-layer Chromatography <*2.03*>. Spot 5 μL each of the sample solution and standard solution on a plate of silica gel for thin-layer chromatography. Develop the plate with a mixture of ethyl acetate, water and formic acid (60:1:1) to a distance of about 7 cm, and air-dry the plate. Spray evenly iron (III) chloride-methanol TS on the plate: one of the several spots obtained from the sample solution has the same color tone and *R*f value with the dark purple spot from the standard solution (Perilla Herb).

(7) Shake 1.0 g of the dry extract (or 3.0 g of the viscous extract) with 10 mL of water, add 25 mL of diethyl ether, and shake. Separate the diethyl ether layer, evaporate the solvent under low pressure (in vacuo), add 2 mL of diethyl ether to the residue, and use this solution as the sample solution. Separately, dissolve 1 mg of [6]-gingerol for thin-layer chromatography in 1 mL of methanol, and use this solution as the standard solution. Perform the test with these solutions as directed under Thin-layer Chromatography <*2.03*>. Spot 10 μL of the sample solution and 5 μL of the standard solution on a plate of silica gel for thin-layer chromatography. Develop the plate with a mixture of ethyl acetate and hexane (1:1) to a distance of about 7 cm, and air-dry the plate. Spray evenly 4-dimethylaminobenzaldehyde TS for spraying on the plate, heat the plate at 105°C for 5 minutes, allow to cool, and spray water: one of the several spots obtained from the sample solution has the same color tone and *R*f value with the blue-green to grayish green spot from the standard solution (Ginger).

Purity **(1)** Heavy metals <*1.07*>—Prepare the test solution with 1.0 g of the dry extract (or an amount of the viscous extract, equivalent to 1.0 g of the dried substance) as directed under Extracts (4), and perform the test (not more than 30 ppm).

(2) Arsenic <*1.11*>—Prepare the test solution with 0.67 g of the dry extract (or an amount of the viscous extract, equivalent to 0.67 g of the dried substance) according to Method 3, and perform the test (not more than 3 ppm).

Loss on drying <*2.41*> The dry extract: Not more than

9.0% (1 g, 105°C, 5 hours).

The viscous extract: Not more than 66.7% (1 g, 105°C, 5 hours).

Total ash *<5.01>* Not more than 9.0%, calculated on the dried basis.

Assay **(1)** Saikosaponin b_2—Weigh accurately about 0.5 g of the dry extract (or an amount of the viscous extract, equivalent to about 0.5 g of the dried substance), add exactly 50 mL of diluted methanol (1 in 2), shake for 15 minutes, filter, and use the filtrate as the sample solution. Separately, use saikosaponin b_2 standard TS for assay as the standard solution. Perform the test with exactly 10 μL each of the sample solution and standard solution as directed under Liquid Chromatography *<2.01>* according to the following conditions, and determine the peak areas, A_T and A_S, of saikosaponin b_2 in each solution.

$$\text{Amount (mg) of saikosaponin } b_2 = C_S \times A_T/A_S \times 50$$

C_S: Concentration (mg/mL) of saikosaponin b_2 in saikosaponin b_2 standard TS for assay

Operating conditions—

Detector: An ultraviolet absorption photometer (wavelength: 254 nm).

Column: A stainless steel column 4.6 mm in inside diameter and 15 cm in length, packed with octadecylsilanized silica gel for liquid chromatography (5 μm in particle diameter).

Column temperature: A constant temperature of about 40°C.

Mobile phase: A mixture of 0.05 mol/L sodium dihydrogen phosphate TS and acetonitrile (5:3).

Flow rate: 1.0 mL per minute (the retention time of saikosaponin b_2 is about 12 minutes).

System suitability—

System performance: When the procedure is run with 10 μL of the standard solution under the above operating conditions, the number of theoretical plates and the symmetry factor of the peak of saikosaponin b_2 are not less than 5000 and not more than 1.5, respectively.

System repeatability: When the test is repeated 6 times with 10 μL of the standard solution under the above operating conditions, the relative standard deviation of the peak area of saikosaponin b_2 is not more than 1.5%.

(2) Baicalin—Weigh accurately about 0.1 g of the dry extract (or an amount of the viscous extract, equivalent to about 0.1 g of the dried substance), add exactly 50 mL of diluted methanol (7 in 10), shake for 15 minutes, filter, and use the filtrate as the sample solution. Separately, weigh accurately about 10 mg of Baicalin RS (separately determine the water *<2.48>* by coulometric titration, using 10 mg), and dissolve in methanol to make exactly 100 mL. Pipet 5 mL of this solution, add diluted methanol (7 in 10) to make exactly 10 mL, and use this solution as the standard solution. Perform the test with exactly 10 μL each of the sample solution and standard solution as directed under Liquid Chromatography *<2.01>* according to the following conditions, and determine the peak areas, A_T and A_S, of baicalin in each solution.

$$\text{Amount (mg) of baicalin } (C_{21}H_{18}O_{11}) = M_S \times A_T/A_S \times 1/4$$

M_S: Amount (mg) of Baicalin RS taken, calculated on the anhydrous basis

Operating conditions—

Detector: An ultraviolet absorption photometer (wavelength: 277 nm).

Column: A stainless steel column 4.6 mm in inside diameter and 15 cm in length, packed with octadecylsilanized silica gel for liquid chromatography (5 μm in particle diameter).

Column temperature: A constant temperature of about 40°C.

Mobile phase: A mixture of diluted phosphoric acid (1 in 200) and acetonitrile (19:6).

Flow rate: 1.0 mL per minute (the retention time of baicalin is about 10 minutes).

System suitability—

System performance: When the procedure is run with 10 μL of the standard solution under the above operating conditions, the number of theoretical plates and the symmetry factor of the peak of baicalin are not less than 5000 and not more than 1.5, respectively.

System repeatability: When the test is repeated 6 times with 10 μL of the standard solution under the above operating conditions, the relative standard deviation of the peak area of baicalin is not more than 1.5%.

(3) Glycyrrhizic acid—Perform the test according to the following i) or ii).

i) Weigh accurately about 0.5 g of the dry extract (or an amount of the viscous extract, equivalent to about 0.5 g of the dried substance), add exactly 50 mL of diluted methanol (1 in 2), shake for 15 minutes, filter, and use the filtrate as the sample solution. Separately, weigh accurately about 10 mg of Glycyrrhizic Acid RS (separately determine the water *<2.48>* by coulometric titration, using 10 mg), dissolve in diluted methanol (1 in 2) to make exactly 100 mL, and use this solution as the standard solution. Perform the test with exactly 10 μL each of the sample solution and standard solution as directed under Liquid Chromatography *<2.01>* according to the following conditions, and determine the peak areas, A_T and A_S, of glycyrrhizic acid in each solution.

$$\text{Amount (mg) of glycyrrhizic acid } (C_{42}H_{62}O_{16}) = M_S \times A_T/A_S \times 1/2$$

M_S: Amount (mg) of Glycyrrhizic Acid RS taken, calculated on the anhydrous basis

Operating conditions—

Detector: An ultraviolet absorption photometer (wavelength: 254 nm).

Column: A stainless steel column 4.6 mm in inside diameter and 15 cm in length, packed with octadecylsilanized silica gel for liquid chromatography (5 μm in particle diameter).

Column temperature: A constant temperature of about 40°C.

Mobile phase: Dissolve 3.85 g of ammonium acetate in 720 mL of water, and add 5 mL of acetic acid (100) and 280 mL of acetonitrile.

Flow rate: 1.0 mL per minute (the retention time of glycyrrhizic acid is about 15 minutes).

System suitability—

System performance: Dissolve 5 mg of monoammonium glycyrrhizinate for resolution check in 20 mL of dilute ethanol. When the procedure is run with 10 μL of this solution under the above operating conditions, the resolution between the peak having the relative retention time of about 0.9 to glycyrrhizic acid and the peak of glycyrrhizic acid is not less than 1.5. Dissolve 1 mg of baicalein for resolution check in 50 mL of methanol. To 2 mL of this solution add 2 mL of the standard solution. When the procedure is run with 10 μL of this solution under the above operating conditions, the resolution between the peaks of glycyrrhizic acid and baicalein is not less than 1.5.

System repeatability: When the test is repeated 6 times

with 10 μL of the standard solution under the above operating conditions, the relative standard deviation of the peak area of glycyrrhizic acid is not more than 1.5%.

ii) Weigh accurately about 0.5 g of the dry extract (or an amount of the viscous extract, equivalent to about 0.5 g of the dried substance), add 20 mL of ethyl acetate and 10 mL of water, and shake for 10 minutes. After centrifugation, remove the ethyl acetate layer, add 20 mL of ethyl acetate, proceed in the same manner as described above, and remove the ethyl acetate layer. To the aqueous layer add 10 mL of methanol, shake for 30 minutes, centrifuge, and take the supernatant liquid. To the residue add 20 mL of diluted methanol (1 in 2), shake for 5 minutes, centrifuge, and take the supernatant liquid. Combine these supernatant liquids, add diluted methanol (1 in 2) to make exactly 50 mL, and use this solution as the sample solution. Separately, weigh accurately about 10 mg of Glycyrrhizic Acid RS (separately determine the water *<2.48>* by coulometric titration, using 10 mg), dissolve in diluted methanol (1 in 2) to make exactly 100 mL, and use this solution as the standard solution. Perform the test with exactly 10 μL each of the sample solution and standard solution as directed under Liquid Chromatography *<2.01>* according to the following conditions, and determine the peak areas, A_T and A_S, of glycyrrhizic acid in each solution.

$$\text{Amount (mg) of glycyrrhizic acid } (C_{42}H_{62}O_{16}) = M_S \times A_T/A_S \times 1/2$$

M_S: Amount (mg) of Glycyrrhizic Acid RS taken, calculated on the anhydrous basis

Operating conditions—

Proceed as directed in the operating conditions in i).

System suitability—

System repeatability: Proceed as directed in the system suitability in i).

System performance: Dissolve 5 mg of monoammonium glycyrrhizinate for resolution check in 20 mL of dilute ethanol. When the procedure is run with 10 μL of this solution under the above operating conditions, the resolution between the peak having the relative retention time of about 0.9 to glycyrrhizic acid and the peak of glycyrrhizic acid is not less than 1.5.

Containers and storage Containers—Tight containers.

Saikokeishito Extract

柴胡桂枝湯エキス

Saikokeishito Extract contains not less than 1.5 mg and not more than 6 mg of saikosaponin b_2, not less than 60 mg and not more than 180 mg of baicalin ($C_{21}H_{18}O_{11}$: 446.36), not less than 17 mg and not more than 51 mg (for preparation prescribed 2 g of Peony Root) or not less than 21 mg and not more than 63 mg (for preparation prescribed 2.5 g of Peony Root) of paeoniflorin ($C_{23}H_{28}O_{11}$: 480.46), and not less than 10 mg and not more than 30 mg (for preparation prescribed 1.5 g of Glycyrrhiza) or not less than 14 mg and not more than 42 mg (for preparation prescribed 2 g of Glycyrrhiza) of glycyrrhizic acid ($C_{42}H_{62}O_{16}$: 822.93), per extract prepared with the amount specified in the Method of preparation.

Method of preparation

	1)	2)	3)	4)
Bupleurum Root	5 g	5 g	5 g	5 g
Pinellia Tuber	4 g	4 g	4 g	4 g
Scutellaria Root	2 g	2 g	2 g	2 g
Peony Root	2 g	2.5 g	2 g	2 g
Jujube	2 g	2 g	2 g	2 g
Ginseng	2 g	2 g	2 g	2 g
Cinnamon Bark	2.5 g	2.5 g	2.5 g	2 g
Glycyrrhiza	1.5 g	1.5 g	1.5 g	2 g
Ginger	0.5 g	1 g	1 g	1 g

Prepare a dry extract or viscous extract as directed under Extracts, according to the prescription 1) to 4), using the crude drugs shown above.

Description Saikokeishito Extract is a yellow-brown powder or black-brown viscous extract, having a slightly odor and a slight sweet first, then a bitter and slightly pungent taste.

Identification **(1)** Shake 2.0 g of the dry extract (or 6.0 g of the viscous extract) with 10 mL of sodium hydroxide TS, add 5 mL of 1-butanol, shake, centrifuge, and use the 1-butanol layer as the sample solution. Separately, dissolve 1 mg of saikosaponin b_2 for thin-layer chromatography in 1 mL of methanol, and use this solution as the standard solution. Perform the test with these solutions as directed under Thin-layer Chromatography *<2.03>*. Spot 10 μL of the sample solution and 2 μL of the standard solution on a plate of silica gel for thin-layer chromatography. Develop the plate with a mixture of ethyl acetate, ethanol (99.5) and water (8:2:1) to a distance of about 7 cm, and air-dry the plate. Spray evenly 4-dimethylaminobenzaldehyde TS for spraying on the plate, heat the plate at 105°C for 5 minutes, and examine under ultraviolet light (main wavelength: 365 nm): one of the several spots obtained from the sample solution has the same color tone and *R*f value with the yellow fluorescent spot from the standard solution (Bupleurum Root).

(2) Shake 1.0 g of the dry extract (or 3.0 g of the viscous extract) with 10 mL of water, add 25 mL of diethyl ether, shake, and separate the diethyl ether layer. Evaporate the solvent under low pressure (in vacuo), add 2 mL of diethyl ether to the residue, and use this solution as the sample solution. Separately, dissolve 1 mg of wogonin for thin-layer chromatography in 1 mL of methanol, and use this solution as the standard solution. Perform the test with these solutions as directed under Thin-layer Chromatography *<2.03>*. Spot 20 μL of the sample solution and 2 μL of the standard solution on a plate of silica gel for thin-layer chromatography. Develop the plate with a mixture of ethyl acetate, hexane and acetic acid (100) (10:10:1) to a distance of about 7 cm, and air-dry the plate. Spray evenly iron (III) chloride-methanol TS on the plate: one of the several spots obtained from the sample solution has the same color tone and *R*f value with the yellow-brown spot from the standard solution (Scutellaria Root).

(3) Shake 1.0 g of the dry extract (or 3.0 g of the viscous extract) with 10 mL of water, add 10 mL of 1-butanol, shake, centrifuge, and use the 1-butanol layer as the sample solution. Separately, dissolve 1 mg of Paeoniflorin RS or paeoniflorin for thin-layer chromatography in 1 mL of methanol, and use this solution as the standard solution. Perform the test with these solutions as directed under Thin-layer Chromatography *<2.03>*. Spot 5 μL each of the sample solution and standard solution on a plate of silica gel for thin-layer chromatography. Develop the plate with a mixture of ethyl acetate, methanol and water (20:3:2) to a distance of about 7 cm, and air-dry the plate. Spray evenly 4-methoxybenzaldehyde-sulfuric acid TS on the plate, and heat the plate at 105°C for 5 minutes: one of the several spots obtained from the sample solution has the same color tone and *R*f value with the purple spot from the standard solution (Peony Root).

(4) Shake 2.0 g of the dry extract (or 6.0 g of the viscous extract) with 10 mL of sodium hydroxide TS, add 5 mL of 1-butanol, shake, centrifuge, and use the 1-butanol layer as the sample solution. Separately, dissolve 1 mg of Ginsenoside Rb_1 RS or ginsenoside Rb_1 for thin-layer chromatography in 1 mL of methanol, and use this solution as the standard solution. Perform the test with these solutions as directed under Thin-layer Chromatography <*2.03*>. Spot 10 μL of the sample solution and 2 μL of the standard solution on a plate of silica gel for thin-layer chromatography. Develop the plate with a mixture of ethyl acetate, 1-propanol, water and acetic acid (100) (7:5:4:1) to a distance of about 7 cm, and air-dry the plate. Spray evenly vanillin-sulfuric acid-ethanol TS for spraying on the plate, heat the plate at 105°C for 5 minutes, and allow to cool: one of the several spots obtained from the sample solution has the same color tone and *R*f value with the blue-purple spot from the standard solution (Ginseng).

(5) Perform the test according to the following i) or ii) (Cinnamon Bark).

i) Put 10 g of the dry extract (or 30 g of the viscous extract) in a 300-mL hard-glass flask, add 100 mL of water and 1 mL of silicone resin, connect an apparatus for essential oil determination, and heat to boil under a reflux condenser. The graduated tube of the apparatus is to be previously filled with water to the standard line, and 2 mL of hexane is added to the graduated tube. After heating under reflux for 1 hour, separate the hexane layer, and use this solution as the sample solution. Separately, dissolve 1 mg of (*E*)-cinnamaldehyde for thin-layer chromatography in 1 mL of methanol, and use this solution as the standard solution. Perform the test with these solutions as directed under Thin-layer Chromatography <*2.03*>. Spot 50 μL of the sample solution and 2 μL of the standard solution on a plate of silica gel for thin-layer chromatography. Develop the plate with a mixture of hexane, diethyl ether and methanol (15:5:1) to a distance of about 7 cm, and air-dry the plate. Spray evenly 2,4-dinitrophenylhydradine TS on the plate: one of the several spots obtained from the sample solution has the same color tone and *R*f value with the yellow-orange spot from the standard solution.

ii) Shake 2.0 g of the dry extract (or 6.0 g of the viscous extract) with 10 mL of water, add 5 mL of hexane, shake, centrifuge, and use the supernatant liquid as the sample solution. Separately, dissolve 1 mg of (*E*)-2-methoxycinnamaldehyde for thin-layer chromatography in 1 mL of methanol, and use this solution as the standard solution. Perform the test with these solutions as directed under Thin-layer Chromatography <*2.03*>. Spot 20 μL of the sample solution and 2 μL of the standard solution on a plate of silica gel for thin-layer chromatography. Develop the plate with a mixture of hexane and ethyl acetate (2:1) to a distance of about 7 cm, and air-dry the plate. Examine under ultraviolet light (main wavelength: 365 nm): one of the several spots obtained from the sample solution has the same color tone and *R*f value with the blue-white fluorescent spot from the standard solution.

(6) Shake 1.0 g of the dry extract (or 3.0 g of the viscous extract) with 10 mL of water, add 10 mL of 1-butanol, shake, centrifuge, and use the 1-butanol layer as the sample solution. Separately, dissolve 1 mg of liquiritin for thin-layer chromatography in 1 mL of methanol, and use this solution as the standard solution. Perform the test with these solutions as directed under Thin-layer Chromatography <*2.03*>. Spot 1 μL each of the sample solution and standard solution on a plate of silica gel for thin-layer chromatography. Develop the plate with a mixture of ethyl acetate, methanol and water (20:3:2) to a distance of about 7 cm, and air-dry the plate. Spray evenly dilute sulfuric acid on the plate, heat the plate at 105°C for 5 minutes, and examine under ultraviolet light (main wavelength: 365 nm): one of the several spots obtained from the sample solution has the same color tone and *R*f value with the yellow-green fluorescent spot from the standard solution (Glycyrrhiza).

(7) Shake 1.0 g of the dry extract (or 3.0 g of the viscous extract) with 10 mL of water, add 25 mL of diethyl ether, and shake. Separate the diethyl ether layer, evaporate the solvent under low pressure (in vacuo), add 2 mL of diethyl ether to the residue, and use this solution as the sample solution. Separately, dissolve 1 mg of [6]-gingerol for thin-layer chromatography in 1 mL of methanol, and use this solution as the standard solution. Perform the test with these solutions as directed under Thin-layer Chromatography <*2.03*>. Spot 10 μL of the sample solution and 5 μL of the standard solution on a plate of silica gel for thin-layer chromatography. Develop the plate with a mixture of ethyl acetate and hexane (1:1) to a distance of about 7 cm, and air-dry the plate. Spray evenly 4-dimethylaminobenzaldehyde TS for spraying on the plate, heat the plate at 105°C for 5 minutes, allow to cool, and spray water: one of the several spots obtained from the sample solution has the same color tone and *R*f value with the blue-green to grayish green spot from the standard solution (Ginger).

Purity **(1)** Heavy metals <*1.07*>—Prepare the test solution with 1.0 g of the dry extract (or an amount of the viscous extract, equivalent to 1.0 g of the dried substance) as directed under Extracts (4), and perform the test (not more than 30 ppm).

(2) Lead—Take 5.0 g of the dry extract (or an amount of the viscous extract, equivalent to 5.0 g of the dried substance) in a platinum, quartz or porcelain crucible, heat gently, and then incinerate by ignition at 450 to 550°C. After cooling, add a small amount of 2 mol/L nitric acid TS to the residue, filter if necessary, and wash the crucible several times with small portions of 2 mol/L nitric acid TS. Combine the washings and the filtrate, add 2 mol/L nitric acid TS to make exactly 20 mL, and use this solution as the sample solution. Separately, to 2.5 mL of Standard Lead Solution add 2 mol/L nitric acid TS to make exactly 20 mL, and use this solution as the standard solution. Perform the test with the sample solution and standard solution as directed under Atomic Absorption Spectrophotometry <*2.23*> according to the following conditions: the absorbance of the sample solution is not more than that of the standard solution (not more than 5 ppm).

Gas: Combustible gas—Acetylene or hydrogen.
Supporting gas—Air.
Lamp: A lead hollow-cathode lamp.
Wavelength: 283.3 nm.

(3) Arsenic <*1.11*>—Prepare the test solution with 0.67 g of the dry extract (or an amount of the viscous extract, equivalent to 0.67 g of the dried substance) according to Method 3, and perform the test (not more than 3 ppm).

Loss on drying <*2.41*> The dry extract: Not more than 9.5% (1 g, 105°C, 5 hours).

The viscous extract: Not more than 66.7% (1 g, 105°C, 5 hours).

Total ash <*5.01*> Not more than 10.0%, calculated on the dried basis.

Assay **(1)** Saikosaponin b_2—Weigh accurately about 0.5 g of the dry extract (or an amount of the viscous extract, equivalent to about 0.5 g of the dried substance), add exactly 50 mL of diluted methanol (1 in 2), shake for 15 minutes, filter, and use the filtrate as the sample solution. Separately, use saikosaponin b_2 standard TS for assay as the standard solution. Perform the test with exactly 10 μL each of the sample solution and standard solution as directed under Liquid Chromatography <*2.01*> according to the following conditions, and determine the peak areas, A_T and A_S, of saikosaponin b_2 in each solution.

Amount (mg) of saikosaponin b_2
$= C_S \times A_T/A_S \times 50$

C_S: Concentration (mg/mL) of saikosaponin b_2 in saikosaponin b_2 standard TS for assay

Operating conditions—

Detector: An ultraviolet absorption photometer (wavelength: 254 nm).

Column: A stainless steel column 4.6 mm in inside diameter and 15 cm in length, packed with octadecylsilanized silica gel for liquid chromatography (5 μm in particle diameter).

Column temperature: A constant temperature of about 40°C.

Mobile phase: A mixture of 0.05 mol/L sodium dihydrogen phosphate TS and acetonitrile (5:3).

Flow rate: 1.0 mL per minute (the retention time of saikosaponin b_2 is about 12 minutes).

System suitability—

System performance: When the procedure is run with 10 μL of the standard solution under the above operating conditions, the number of theoretical plates and the symmetry factor of the peak of saikosaponin b_2 are not less than 5000 and not more than 1.5, respectively.

System repeatability: When the test is repeated 6 times with 10 μL of the standard solution under the above operating conditions, the relative standard deviation of the peak area of saikosaponin b_2 is not more than 1.5%.

(2) Baicalin—Weigh accurately about 0.1 g of the dry extract (or an amount of the viscous extract, equivalent to about 0.1 g of the dried substance), add exactly 50 mL of diluted methanol (7 in 10), shake for 15 minutes, filter, and use the filtrate as the sample solution. Separately, weigh accurately about 10 mg of Baicalin RS (separately determine the water <*2.48*> by coulometric titration, using 10 mg), and dissolve in methanol to make exactly 100 mL. Pipet 5 mL of this solution, add diluted methanol (7 in 10) to make exactly 10 mL, and use this solution as the standard solution. Perform the test with exactly 10 μL each of the sample solution and standard solution as directed under Liquid Chromatography <*2.01*> according to the following conditions, and determine the peak areas, A_T and A_S, of baicalin in each solution.

Amount (mg) of baicalin ($C_{21}H_{18}O_{11}$)
$= M_S \times A_T/A_S \times 1/4$

M_S: Amount (mg) of Baicalin RS taken, calculated on the anhydrous basis

Operating conditions—

Detector: An ultraviolet absorption photometer (wavelength: 277 nm).

Column: A stainless steel column 4.6 mm in inside diameter and 15 cm in length, packed with octadecylsilanized silica gel for liquid chromatography (5 μm in particle diameter).

Column temperature: A constant temperature of about 40°C.

Mobile phase: A mixture of diluted phosphoric acid (1 in 200) and acetonitrile (19:6).

Flow rate: 1.0 mL per minute (the retention time of baicalin is about 10 minutes).

System suitability—

System performance: When the procedure is run with 10 μL of the standard solution under the above operating conditions, the number of theoretical plates and the symmetry factor of the peak of baicalin are not less than 5000 and not more than 1.5, respectively.

System repeatability: When the test is repeated 6 times with 10 μL of the standard solution under the above operating conditions, the relative standard deviation of the peak area of baicalin is not more than 1.5%.

(3) Paeoniflorin—Weigh accurately about 0.5 g of the dry extract (or an amount of the viscous extract, equivalent to about 0.5 g of the dried substance), add exactly 50 mL of diluted methanol (1 in 2), shake for 15 minutes, filter, and use the filtrate as the sample solution. Separately, weigh accurately about 10 mg of Paeoniflorin RS (separately determine the water <*2.48*> by coulometric titration, using 10 mg), dissolve in diluted methanol (1 in 2) to make exactly 100 mL, and use this solution as the standard solution. Perform the test with exactly 10 μL each of the sample solution and standard solution as directed under Liquid Chromatography <*2.01*> according to the following conditions, and determine the peak areas, A_T and A_S, of paeoniflorin in each solution.

Amount (mg) of paeoniflorin ($C_{23}H_{28}O_{11}$)
$= M_S \times A_T/A_S \times 1/2$

M_S: Amount (mg) of Paeoniflorin RS taken, calculated on the anhydrous basis

Operating conditions—

Detector: An ultraviolet absorption photometer (wavelength: 232 nm).

Column: A stainless steel column 4.6 mm in inside diameter and 15 cm in length, packed with octadecylsilanized silica gel for liquid chromatography (5 μm in particle diameter).

Column temperature: A constant temperature of about 20°C.

Mobile phase: A mixture of water, acetonitrile and phosphoric acid (850:150:1).

Flow rate: 1.0 mL per minute (the retention time of paeoniflorin is about 9 minutes).

System suitability—

System performance: Dissolve 1 mg each of Paeoniflorin RS and albiflorin in diluted methanol (1 in 2) to make 10 mL. When the procedure is run with 10 μL of this solution under the above operating conditions, albiflorin and paeoniflorin are eluted in this order with the resolution between these peaks being not less than 2.5.

System repeatability: When the test is repeated 6 times with 10 μL of the standard solution under the above operating conditions, the relative standard deviation of the peak area of paeoniflorin is not more than 1.5%.

(4) Glycyrrhizic acid—Perform the test according to the following i) or ii).

i) Weigh accurately about 0.5 g of the dry extract (or an amount of the viscous extract, equivalent to about 0.5 g of the dried substance), add exactly 50 mL of diluted methanol (1 in 2), shake for 15 minutes, filter, and use the filtrate as the sample solution. Separately, weigh accurately about 10 mg of Glycyrrhizic Acid RS (separately determine the water <*2.48*> by coulometric titration, using 10 mg), dissolve in diluted methanol (1 in 2) to make exactly 100 mL, and use this solution as the standard solution. Perform the test with exactly 10 μL each of the sample solution and standard solution as directed under Liquid Chromatography <*2.01*> according to the following conditions, and determine the peak areas, A_T and A_S, of glycyrrhizic acid in each solution.

Amount (mg) of glycyrrhizic acid ($C_{42}H_{62}O_{16}$)
$= M_S \times A_T/A_S \times 1/2$

M_S: Amount (mg) of Glycyrrhizic Acid RS taken, calculated on the anhydrous basis

Operating conditions—

Detector: An ultraviolet absorption photometer (wavelength: 254 nm).

Column: A stainless steel column 4.6 mm in inside diameter and 15 cm in length, packed with octadecylsilanized silica gel for liquid chromatography (5 μm in particle diameter).

Column temperature: A constant temperature of about 40°C.

Mobile phase: Dissolve 3.85 g of ammonium acetate in 720 mL of water, and add 5 mL of acetic acid (100) and 280 mL of acetonitrile.

Flow rate: 1.0 mL per minute (the retention time of glycyrrhizic acid is about 15 minutes).

System suitability—

System performance: Dissolve 5 mg of monoammonium glycyrrhizinate for resolution check in 20 mL of dilute ethanol. When the procedure is run with 10 μL of this solution under the above operating conditions, the resolution between the peak having the relative retention time of about 0.9 to glycyrrhizic acid and the peak of glycyrrhizic acid is not less than 1.5. Dissolve 1 mg of (*E*)-cinnamaldehyde for thin-layer chromatography and 1 mg of baicalein for resolution check in 50 mL of methanol. To 2 mL of this solution add 2 mL of the standard solution. When the procedure is run with 10 μL of this solution under the above operating conditions, two peaks other than glycyrrhizic acid are observed with the resolutions between the peak of glycyrrhizic acid and each of the two peaks being not less than 1.5.

System repeatability: When the test is repeated 6 times with 10 μL of the standard solution under the above operating conditions, the relative standard deviation of the peak area of glycyrrhizic acid is not more than 1.5%.

ii) Weigh accurately about 0.5 g of the dry extract (or an amount of the viscous extract, equivalent to about 0.5 g of the dried substance), add 20 mL of ethyl acetate and 10 mL of water, and shake for 10 minutes. After centrifugation, remove the ethyl acetate layer, add 20 mL of ethyl acetate, proceed in the same manner as described above, and remove the ethyl acetate layer. To the aqueous layer add 10 mL of methanol, shake for 30 minutes, centrifuge, and take the supernatant liquid. To the residue add 20 mL of diluted methanol (1 in 2), shake for 5 minutes, centrifuge, and take the supernatant liquid. Combine these supernatant liquids, add diluted methanol (1 in 2) to make exactly 50 mL, and use this solution as the sample solution. Separately, weigh accurately about 10 mg of Glycyrrhizic Acid RS (separately determine the water <*2.48*> by coulometric titration, using 10 mg), dissolve in diluted methanol (1 in 2) to make exactly 100 mL, and use this solution as the standard solution. Perform the test with exactly 10 μL each of the sample solution and standard solution as directed under Liquid Chromatography <*2.01*> according to the following conditions, and determine the peak areas, A_T and A_S, of glycyrrhizic acid in each solution.

Amount (mg) of glycyrrhizic acid ($C_{42}H_{62}O_{16}$)
$= M_S \times A_T/A_S \times 1/2$

M_S: Amount (mg) of Glycyrrhizic Acid RS taken, calculated on the anhydrous basis

Operating conditions—

Proceed as directed in the operating conditions in i).

System suitability—

System repeatability: Proceed as directed in the system suitability in i).

System performance: Dissolve 5 mg of monoammonium glycyrrhizinate for resolution check in 20 mL of dilute ethanol. When the procedure is run with 10 μL of this solution under the above operating conditions, the resolution between the peak having the relative retention time of about 0.9 to glycyrrhizic acid and the peak of glycyrrhizic acid is not less than 1.5.

Containers and storage Containers—Tight containers.

Saireito Extract

柴苓湯エキス

Saireito Extract contains not less than 2 mg and not more than 8 mg of saikosaponin b_2, not less than 80 mg and not more than 240 mg of baicalin ($C_{21}H_{18}O_{11}$: 446.36), and not less than 14 mg and not more than 42 mg of glycyrrhizic acid ($C_{42}H_{62}O_{16}$: 822.93), per extract prepared with the amount specified in the Method of preparation.

Method of preparation

	1)	2)
Bupleurum Root	7 g	7 g
Pinellia Tuber	5 g	5 g
Ginger	1 g	1 g
Scutellaria Root	3 g	3 g
Jujube	3 g	3 g
Ginseng	3 g	3 g
Glycyrrhiza	2 g	2 g
Alisma Tuber	6 g	5 g
Polyporus Sclerotium	4.5 g	3 g
Poria Sclerotium	4.5 g	3 g
Atractylodes Rhizome	4.5 g	—
Atractylodes Lancea Rhizome	—	3 g
Cinnamon Bark	3 g	2 g

Prepare a dry extract as directed under Extracts, according to the prescription 1) or 2), using the crude drugs shown above.

Description Saireito Extract occurs as a light yellow-brown powder. It has slightly a characteristic odor, and a sweet, then bitter taste.

Identification **(1)** To 2.0 g of Saireito Extract add 10 mL of sodium hydroxide TS, shake, then add 5 mL of 1-butanol, shake, centrifuge, and use the 1-butanol layer as the sample solution. Separately, dissolve 1 mg of saikosaponin b_2 for thin-layer chromatography in 1 mL of methanol, and use this solution as the standard solution. Perform the test with these solutions as directed under Thin-layer Chromatography <2.03>. Spot 10 μL of the sample solution and 2 μL of the standard solution on a plate of silica gel for thin-layer chromatography. Develop the plate with a mixture of ethyl acetate, ethanol (99.5) and water (8:2:1) to a distance of about 7 cm, and air-dry the plate. Spray evenly 4-dimethylaminobenzaldehyde TS for spraying on the plate, heat the plate at 105°C for 5 minutes, and examine under ultraviolet light (main wavelength: 365 nm): one of the several spots obtained from the sample solution has the same color tone and *R*f value with the yellow fluorescent spot from the standard solution (Bupleurum Root).

(2) To 1.0 g of Saireito Extract add 10 mL of water, shake, then add 25 mL of diethyl ether, and shake. Separate the diethyl ether layer, evaporate the solvent under low pressure (in vacuo), add 2 mL of diethyl ether to the residue, and use this solution as the sample solution. Separately, dissolve 1 mg of [6]-gingerol for thin-layer chromatography in 1 mL of methanol, and use this solution as the standard solution. Perform the test with these solutions as directed under Thin-layer Chromatography <2.03>. Spot 15 μL of the sample solution and 5 μL of the standard solution on a plate of silica gel for thin-layer chromatography. Develop the plate with a mixture of ethyl acetate and hexane (1:1) to a distance of about 7 cm, and air-dry the plate. Spray evenly 4-dimethylaminobenzaldehyde TS for spraying on the plate, heat the plate at 105°C for 5 minutes, allow to cool, and spray water: one of the several spots obtained from the sample solution has the same color tone and *R*f value with the blue-green to grayish green spot from the standard solution (Ginger).

(3) To 1.0 g of Saireito Extract add 10 mL of water, shake, then add 25 mL of diethyl ether, and shake. Separate the diethyl ether layer, evaporate the solvent under low pressure (in vacuo), add 2 mL of diethyl ether to the residue, and use this solution as the sample solution. Separately, dissolve 1 mg of wogonin for thin-layer chromatography in 1 mL of methanol, and use this solution as the standard solution. Perform the test with these solutions as directed under Thin-layer Chromatography <2.03>. Spot 20 μL of the sample solution and 2 μL of the standard solution on a plate of silica gel for thin-layer chromatography. Develop the plate with a mixture of ethyl acetate, hexane and acetic acid (100) (10:10:1) to a distance of about 7 cm, air-dry the plate. Spray evenly iron (III) chloride-methanol TS on the plate: one of the several spots obtained from the sample solution has the same color tone and *R*f value with the yellow-brown spot from the standard solution (Scutellaria Root).

(4) To 2.0 g of Saireito Extract add 10 mL of sodium hydroxide TS, shake, then add 5 mL of 1-butanol, shake, centrifuge, and use the 1-butanol layer as the sample solution. Separately, dissolve 1 mg of Ginsenoside Rb_1 RS or ginsenoside Rb_1 for thin-layer chromatography in 1 mL of methanol, and use this solution as the standard solution. Perform the test with these solutions as directed under Thin-layer Chromatography <2.03>. Spot 10 μL of the sample solution and 2 μL of the standard solution on a plate of silica gel for thin-layer chromatography. Develop the plate with a mixture of ethyl acetate, 1-propanol, water and acetic acid (100) (7:5:4:1) to a distance of about 7 cm, and air-dry the plate. Spray evenly vanillin-sulfuric acid-ethanol TS for spraying on the plate, heat the plate at 105°C for 5 minutes, and allow to cool: one of the several spots obtained from the sample solution has the same color tone and *R*f value with the blue-purple spot from the standard solution (Ginseng).

(5) To 2.0 g of Saireito Extract add 10 mL of water, shake, then add 5 mL of 1-butanol, shake, centrifuge, and use the 1-butanol layer as the sample solution. Separately, dissolve 1 mg of liquiritin for thin-layer chromatography in 1 mL of methanol, and use this solution as the standard solution. Perform the test with these solutions as directed under Thin-layer Chromatography <2.03>. Spot 1 μL each of the sample solution and standard solution on a plate of silica gel for thin-layer chromatography. Develop the plate with a mixture of ethyl acetate, methanol and water (20:3:2) to a distance of about 7 cm, and air-dry the plate. Spray evenly dilute sulfuric acid on the plate, heat the plate at 105°C for 5 minutes, and examine under ultraviolet light (main wavelength: 365 nm): one of the several spots obtained from the sample solution has the same color tone and *R*f value with the yellow-green fluorescent spot from the standard solution (Glycyrrhiza).

(6) To 2.0 g of Saireito Extract add 10 mL of sodium carbonate TS, shake, then add 10 mL of diethyl ether, shake, centrifuge, and use the diethyl ether layer as the sample solution. Separately, dissolve 1 mg of alisol A for thin-layer chromatography in 1 mL of methanol, and use this solution as the standard solution. Perform the test with these solutions as directed under Thin-layer Chromatography <2.03>. Spot 20 μL of the sample solution and 2 μL of the standard solution on a plate of silica gel for thin-layer chromatography. Develop the plate with a mixture of ethyl acetate, hexane and acetic acid (100) (10:10:3) to a distance of about 7 cm, and air-dry the plate. Spray evenly 4-methoxybenzaldehyde-sulfuric acid-acetic acid TS on the plate, heat the plate at 105°C for 5 minutes, allow to cool, and examine under ultraviolet light (main wavelength: 365 nm): one of the several spots obtained from the sample solution has the same color tone and *R*f value with the yellow fluorescent spot from the standard solution (Alisma Tuber).

(7) For preparation prescribed Atractylodes Rhizome—To 1.0 g of Saireito Extract add 10 mL of water, shake, then add 25 mL of diethyl ether, and shake. Separate the diethyl ether layer, evaporate the solvent under low pressure (in vacuo), add 2 mL of diethyl ether to the residue, and use this solution as the sample solution. Separately, dissolve 1 mg of atractylenolide III for thin-layer chromatography in 2 mL of methanol, and use this solution as the standard solution. Perform the test with these solutions as directed under Thin-layer Chromatography <2.03>. Spot 5 μL each of the sample solution and standard solution on a plate of silica gel for thin-layer chromatography. Develop the plate with a mixture of ethyl acetate and hexane (1:1) to a distance of about 7 cm, and air-dry the plate. Spray evenly dilute sulfuric acid on the plate, heat the plate at 105°C for 5 minutes, and examine under ultraviolet light (main wavelength: 365 nm): one of the several spots obtained from the sample solution has the same color tone and *R*f value with the blue-white fluorescent spot from the standard solution (Atractylodes Rhizome).

(8) For preparation prescribed Atractylodes Lancea Rhizome—To 2.0 g of Saireito Extract add 10 mL of water, shake, then add 25 mL of hexane, and shake. Separate the hexane layer, evaporate the solvent under low pressure (in vacuo), add 2 mL of hexane to the residue, and use this solution as the sample solution. Perform the test with the sample solution as directed under Thin-layer Chromatography <2.03>. Spot 20 μL of the sample solution on a plate of silica gel with fluorescent indicator for thin-layer chromatography. Develop the plate with a mixture of hexane and acetone (7:1) to a distance of about 7 cm, and air-dry the plate. Examine under ultraviolet light (main wavelength: 254 nm): a dark purple spot is observed at an *R*f value of about 0.5. The spot shows a greenish brown color after being sprayed evenly 4-dimethylaminobenzaldehyde TS for spraying, heated at 105°C for 5 minutes, and allowed to cool (Atractylodes

Lancea Rhizome).

(9) To 1.0 g of Saireito Extract add 10 mL of water, shake, then add 25 mL of diethyl ether, and shake. Separate the diethyl ether layer, evaporate the solvent under low pressure (in vacuo), add 2 mL of diethyl ether to the residue, and use this solution as the sample solution. Separately, dissolve 1 mg of (*E*)-cinnamic acid for thin-layer chromatography in 1 mL of methanol, and use this solution as the standard solution. Perform the test with these solutions as directed under Thin-layer Chromatography <*2.03*>. Spot 40 μL of the sample solution and 2 μL of the standard solution on a plate of silica gel with fluorescent indicator for thin-layer chromatography. Develop the plate with a mixture of hexane, ethyl acetate, formic acid and water (60:40:4:1) to a distance of about 7 cm, and air-dry the plate. Examine under ultraviolet light (main wavelength: 254 nm): one of the several spots obtained from the sample solution has the same color tone and *Rf* value with the dark purple spot from the standard solution (Cinnamon Bark).

Purity **(1)** Heavy metals <*1.07*>—Prepare the test solution with 1.0 g of Saireito Extract as directed under Extract (4), and perform the test (not more than 30 ppm).

(2) Arsenic <*1.11*>—Prepare the test solution with 0.67 g of Saireito Extract according to Method 3, and perform the test (not more than 3 ppm).

Loss on drying <*2.41*> Not more than 10.0% (1 g, 105°C, 5 hours).

Total ash <*5.01*> Not more than 9.0%.

Assay **(1)** Saikosaponin b_2—Weigh accurately about 0.5 g of Saireito Extract, add exactly 50 mL of diluted methanol (1 in 2), shake for 15 minutes, filter, and use the filtrate as the sample solution. Separately, use saikosaponin b_2 standard TS for assay as the standard solution. Perform the test with exactly 10 μL each of the sample solution and standard solution as directed under Liquid Chromatography <*2.01*> according to the following conditions, and determine the peak areas, A_T and A_S, of saikosaponin b_2 in each solution.

Amount (mg) of saikosaponin b_2 = $C_S \times A_T/A_S \times 50$

C_S: Concentration (mg/mL) of saikosaponin b_2 in saikosaponin b_2 standard TS for assay

Operating conditions—

Detector: An ultraviolet absorption photometer (wavelength: 254 nm).

Column: A stainless steel column 4.6 mm in inside diameter and 15 cm in length, packed with octadecylsilanized silica gel for liquid chromatography (5 μm in particle diameter).

Column temperature: A constant temperature of about 40°C.

Mobile phase: A mixture of 0.05 mol/L sodium dihydrogen phosphate TS and acetonitrile (5:3).

Flow rate: 1.0 mL per minute (the retention time of saikosaponin b_2 is about 12 minutes).

System suitability—

System performance: When the procedure is run with 10 μL of the standard solution under the above operating conditions, the number of theoretical plates and the symmetry factor of the peak of saikosaponin b_2 are not less than 5000 and not more than 1.5, respectively.

System repeatability: When the test is repeated 6 times with 10 μL of the standard solution under the above operating conditions, the relative standard deviation of the peak area of saikosaponin b_2 is not more than 1.5%.

(2) Baicalin—Weigh accurately about 0.1 g of Saireito Extract, add exactly 50 mL of diluted methanol (7 in 10), shake for 15 minutes, filter, and use the filtrate as the sample solution. Separately, weigh accurately about 10 mg of Baicalin RS (separately determine the water <*2.48*> by coulometric titration, using 10 mg), and dissolve in methanol to make exactly 100 mL. Pipet 5 mL of this solution, add diluted methanol (7 in 10) to make exactly 10 mL, and use this solution as the standard solution. Perform test with exactly 10 μL each of the sample solution and standard solution as directed under Liquid Chromatography <*2.01*> according to the following conditions, and determine the peak areas, A_T and A_S, of baicalin in each solution.

Amount (mg) of baicalin ($C_{21}H_{18}O_{11}$)
$= M_S \times A_T/A_S \times 1/4$

M_S: Amount (mg) of Baicalin RS taken, calculated on the anhydrous basis

Operating conditions—

Detector: An ultraviolet absorption photometer (wavelength: 277 nm).

Column: A stainless steel column 4.6 mm in inside diameter and 15 cm in length, packed with octadecylsilanized silica gel for liquid chromatography (5 μm in particle diameter).

Column temperature: A constant temperature of about 40°C.

Mobile phase: A mixture of diluted phosphoric acid (1 in 200) and acetonitrile (19:6).

Flow rate: 1.0 mL per minute (the retention time of baicalin is about 10 minutes).

System suitability—

System performance: When the procedure is run with 10 μL of the standard solution under the above operating conditions, the number of theoretical plates and the symmetry factor of the peak of baicalin are not less than 5000 and not more than 1.5, respectively.

System repeatability: When the test is repeated 6 times with 10 μL of the standard solution under the above operating conditions, the relative standard deviation of the peak area of baicalin is not more than 1.5%.

(3) Glycyrrhizic acid—Perform the test according to the following i) or ii).

i) Weigh accurately about 0.5 g of Saireito Extract, add exactly 50 mL of diluted methanol (1 in 2), shake for 15 minutes, filter, and use the filtrate as the sample solution. Separately, weigh accurately about 10 mg of Glycyrrhizic Acid RS (separately determine the water <*2.48*> by coulometric titration, using 10 mg), dissolve in diluted methanol (1 in 2) to make exactly 100 mL, and use this solution as the standard solution. Perform the test with exactly 10 μL each of the sample solution and standard solution as directed under Liquid Chromatography <*2.01*> according to the following conditions, and determine the peak areas, A_T and A_S, of glycyrrhizic acid in each solution.

Amount (mg) of glycyrrhizic acid ($C_{42}H_{62}O_{16}$)
$= M_S \times A_T/A_S \times 1/2$

M_S: Amount (mg) of Glycyrrhizic Acid RS taken, calculated on the anhydrous basis

Operating conditions—

Detector: An ultraviolet absorption photometer (wavelength: 254 nm).

Column: A stainless steel column 4.6 mm in inside diameter and 15 cm in length, packed with octadecylsilanized silica gel for liquid chromatography (5 μm in particle diameter).

Column temperature: A constant temperature of about 40°C.

Mobile phase: Dissolve 3.85 g of ammonium acetate in 720 mL of water, and add 5 mL of acetic acid (100) and 280 mL of acetonitrile.

Flow rate: 1.0 mL per minute (the retention time of glycyrrhizic acid is about 15 minutes).

System suitability—

System performance: Dissolve 5 mg of monoammonium glycyrrhizinate for resolution check in 20 mL of dilute ethanol. When the procedure is run with 10 μL of this solution under the above operating conditions, the resolution between the peak having the relative retention time of about 0.9 to glycyrrhizic acid and the peak of glycyrrhizic acid is not less than 1.5. Dissolve 1 mg of (E)-cinnamaldehyde for thin-layer chromatography and 1 mg of baicalein for resolution check in 50 mL of methanol. To 2 mL of this solution add 2 mL of the standard solution. When the procedure is run with 10 μL of this solution under the above operating conditions, two peaks other than glycyrrhizic acid are observed with the resolutions between the peak of glycyrrhizic acid and each of the two peaks being not less than 1.5.

System repeatability: When the test is repeated 6 times with 10 μL of the standard solution under the above operating conditions, the relative standard deviation of the peak area of glycyrrhizic acid is not more than 1.5%.

ii) Weigh accurately about 0.5 g of Saireito Extract, add 20 mL of ethyl acetate and 10 mL of water, and shake for 10 minutes. After centrifugation, remove the ethyl acetate layer, add 20 mL of ethyl acetate, proceed in the same manner as described above, and remove the ethyl acetate layer. To the aqueous layer add 10 mL of methanol, shake for 30 minutes, centrifuge, and take the supernatant liquid. To the residue add 20 mL of diluted methanol (1 in 2), shake for 5 minutes, centrifuge, and take the supernatant liquid. Combine these supernatant liquids, add diluted methanol (1 in 2) to make exactly 50 mL, and use this solution as the sample solution. Separately, weigh accurately about 10 mg of Glycyrrhizic Acid RS (separately determine the water <2.48> by coulometric titration, using 10 mg), dissolve in diluted methanol (1 in 2) to make exactly 100 mL, and use this solution as the standard solution. Perform the test with exactly 10 μL each of the sample solution and standard solution as directed under Liquid Chromatography <2.01> according to the following conditions, and determine the peak areas, A_T and A_S, of glycyrrhizic acid in each solution.

$$\text{Amount (mg) of glycyrrhizic acid } (C_{42}H_{62}O_{16}) = M_S \times A_T/A_S \times 1/2$$

M_S: Amount (mg) of Glycyrrhizic Acid RS taken, calculated on the anhydrous basis

Operating conditions—

Proceed as directed in the operating conditions in i).

System suitability—

System repeatability: Proceed as directed in the system suitability in i).

System performance: Dissolve 5 mg of monoammonium glycyrrhizinate for resolution check in 20 mL of dilute ethanol. When the procedure is run with 10 μL of this solution under the above operating conditions, the resolution between the peak having the relative retention time of about 0.9 to glycyrrhizic acid and the peak of glycyrrhizic acid is not less than 1.5.

Containers and storage Containers—Tight containers.

Salvia Miltiorrhiza Root

Salviae Miltiorrhizae Radix

タンジン

Salvia Miltiorrhiza Root is the root of *Salvia miltiorrhiza* Bunge (*Labiatae*).

Description Nearly cylindrical root, 5 - 25 cm in length, 0.3 - 1.5 cm in diameter; slightly curved, often with lateral roots; outer surface red-brown, dark red-brown or black-brown; with irregular rough wrinkles; hard in texture, and easily broken; fracture surface fine or rough with clefts; cortex grayish yellow-white or red-brown, xylem light yellow-white or black-brown.

Odor, slight; taste, sweet at first and followed by slight bitterness and astringency.

Under a microscope <5.01>, a transverse section reveals usually cork layer in the outermost part, or rarely parenchyma or endodermis at the outside of the cork layer; several sclerenchyma cells observed or not in secondary cortex; cambium obvious; vessels radially arranged in secondary xylem, sometimes radial lines of vessels unite in the center of root; xylem fibers surrounding vessels; primary xylem divided into 2 - 3; vessels of secondary xylem mainly pitted vessels and reticulate vessels in a longitudinal section.

Identification To 1.0 g of pulverized Salvia Miltiorrhiza Root add 10 mL of diethyl ether, allow to stand for 10 minutes with occasional shaking, and filter. Evaporate the filtrate on a water bath to dryness, dissolve the residue in 1 mL of ethyl acetate, and use this solution as the sample solution. Perform the test with the sample solution as directed under Thin-layer Chromatography <2.03>. Spot 10 μL of the sample solution on a plate of silica gel for thin-layer chromatography. Develop the plate with a mixture of hexane and ethyl acetate (3:1) to a distance of about 10 cm, and air-dry the plate: a red-brown spot at an Rf value of about 0.4 is observed.

Purity (1) Heavy metals <1.07>—Proceed with 3.0 g of pulverized Salvia Miltiorrhiza Root according to Method 3, and perform the test. Prepare the control solution with 3.0 mL of Standard Lead Solution (not more than 10 ppm).

(2) Arsenic <1.11>—Prepare the test solution with 0.40 g of pulverized Salvia Miltiorrhiza Root according to Method 4, and perform the test (not more than 5 ppm).

Loss on drying <5.01> Not more than 16.0% (6 hours).

Total ash <5.01> Not more than 7.5%.

Acid-insoluble ash <5.01> Not more than 2.0%.

Extract content <5.01> Dilute ethanol-soluble extract: not less than 42.0%.

Containers and storage Containers—Well-closed containers.

Saposhnikovia Root and Rhizome

Saposhnikoviae Radix

ボウフウ

Saposhnikovia Root and Rhizome is the root and rhizome of *Saposhnikovia divaricata* Schischkin (*Umbelliferae*).

Description Long and narrow, conical rhizome and root, 15 - 20 cm in length, 0.7 - 1.5 cm in diameter; externally light brown; rhizome reveals dense crosswise wrinkles like ring nodes, and sometimes reveals brown and hair-like remains of leaf sheath; the root reveals many longitudinal wrinkles and scars of rootlets; in a transverse section, cortex is grayish brown in color and reveals many lacunae, and xylem is yellow in color.

Odor, slight; taste, slightly sweet.

Identification To 1.0 g of pulverized Saposhnikovia Root and Rhizome, add 5 mL of methanol, shake for 10 minutes, filter, and use the filtrate as the sample solution. Separately, dissolve 1 mg of 4′-*O*-glucosyl-5-*O*-methylvisamminol for thin-layer chromatography in 1 mL of methanol, and use this solution as the standard solution. Perform the test with these solutions as directed under Thin-layer Chromatography <*2.03*>. Spot 4 μL of the sample solution and 1 μL of the standard solution on a plate of silica gel with fluorescent indicator for thin-layer chromatography. Develop the plate with a mixture of ethyl formate, formic acid, 2-butanone, and water (20:5:5:1) to a distance of about 7 cm, and air-dry the plate. Examine under ultraviolet light (main wavelength: 254 nm): one of the several spots obtained from the sample solution has the same color tone and *R*f value with the spot from the standard solution.

Purity **(1)** Heavy metals <*1.07*>—Proceed with 2.0 g of pulverized Saposhnikovia Root and Rhizome according to Method 3, and perform the test. Prepare the control solution with 3.0 mL of Standard Lead Solution (not more than 15 ppm).

(2) Arsenic <*1.11*>—Prepare the test solution with 0.40 g of pulverized Saposhnikovia Root and Rhizome according to Method 4, and perform the test (not more than 5 ppm).

(3) Foreign matter <*5.01*>—The amount of stems and other foreign matter is not more than 2.0%.

(4) Peucedanum ledebourielloides—Place 1.0 g of pulverized Saposhnikovia Root and Rhizome in a glass-stoppered centrifuge tube, add 5 mL of hexane, shake for 10 minutes, centrifuge, and use the supernatant liquid as the sample solution. Separately, place 1.0 g of peucedanum· ledebourielloides for purity in a glass-stoppered centrifuge tube, add 5 mL of hexane, shake for 10 minutes, centrifuge, and use the supernatant liquid as the standard solution. Perform the test with these solutions as directed under Thin-layer Chromatography <*2.03*>. Spot 5 μL each of the sample solution and standard solution on a plate of silica gel for thin-layer chromatography. Develop the plate with a mixture of hexane, ethyl acetate and acetic acid (100) (20:10:1) to a distance of about 7 cm, and air-dry the plate. Examine under ultraviolet light (main wavelength: 365 nm): the sample solution shows no spot corresponding to the blue fluorescent spot at an *R*f value of about 0.4 obtained from the standard solution.

Total ash <*5.01*> Not more than 7.0%.

Acid-insoluble ash <*5.01*> Not more than 1.5%.

Extract content <*5.01*> Dilute ethanol-soluble extract: not less than 20.0%.

Containers and storage Containers—Well-closed containers.

Sappan Wood

Sappan Lignum

ソボク

Sappan Wood is the duramen of *Caesalpinia sappan* Linné (*Leguminosae*).

Description Chips, slices or short pieces of wood; yellow-red to grayish yellow-brown, sometimes with light brown to grayish white splint woods; hard in texture; a transverse section shows a pattern like annual ring.

Almost odorless; almost tasteless.

Under a microscope <*5.01*>, a transverse section reveals ray composed of 1 - 2 cell rows of slender and long cells; the area between rays filled with fiber cells, and large and oblong vessels scattered there; solitary crystals of calcium oxalate in parenchymatous cells of the innermost of xylem.

Identification To 1 g of pulverized Sappan Wood add 10 mL of methanol, shake for 5 minutes, filter, and use the filtrate as the sample solution. Perform the test with the sample solution as directed under Thin-layer Chromatography <*2.03*>. Spot 5 μL of the sample solution on a plate of silica gel for thin-layer chromatography. Develop the plate with a mixture of ethyl acetate, water, formic acid and 2-propanol (20:1:1:1) to a distance of about 7 cm, and air-dry the plate. Spray evenly sodium carbonate TS on the plate, and air-dry the plate: a red-purple spot appears at an *R*f value of about 0.7.

Purity Put a small piece of Sappan Wood in calcium hydroxide TS: no purple-blue color develops.

Loss on drying <*5.01*> Not more than 11.5% (6 hours).

Total ash <*5.01*> Not more than 2.0%.

Extract content <*5.01*> Dilute ethanol-soluble extract: not less than 7.0%.

Containers and storage Containers—Well-closed containers.

Saussurea Root

Saussureae Radix

モッコウ

Saussurea Root is the root of *Saussurea lappa* Clarke (*Compositae*).

Description Nearly cylindrical roots, 5 - 20 cm in length, 1 - 6 cm in diameter; some of them slightly bent, and sometimes longitudinally cut; scar of stem dented on the top of the root with crown; externally yellow-brown to grayish brown, with coarse longitudinal wrinkles and fine reticulate furrows, and also with remains of lateral roots; sometimes root from which periderm has been removed; hard and dense in texture, and difficult to break. A transverse section is yellow-brown to dark brown, and cambium part has a dark color. Under a magnifying glass, a transverse section reveal obvious medullary rays, large clefts here and there, and brown oil sacs scattered; in old root, pith existing in the center, and often forming a hollow.

Odor, characteristic; taste, bitter.

Identification To 1.0 g of pulverized Saussurea Root add 10 mL of methanol, shake for 10 minutes, centrifuge, and use the supernatant liquid as the sample solution. Perform the test with the sample solution as directed under Thin-layer Chromatography <*2.03*>. Spot 5 μL of the sample solution on a plate of silica gel for thin-layer chromatography. Develop the plate with a mixture of hexane and acetone (7:3) to a distance of about 7 cm, and air-dry the plate. Spray evenly dilute sulfuric acid on the plate, heat the plate at 105°C for 5 minutes, and cool: a red-purple spot at an *R*f value of about 0.5 and a grayish blue to grayish brown spot just below it are observed.

Purity **(1)** Heavy metals <*1.07*>—Proceed with 1.0 g of pulverized Saussurea Root according to Method 3, and perform the test. Prepare the control solution with 2.0 mL of Standard Lead Solution (not more than 20 ppm).

(2) Arsenic <*1.11*>—Prepare the test solution with 0.40 g of pulverized Saussurea Root according to Method 4, and perform the test (not more than 5 ppm).

(3) Foreign matter—Add iodine TS dropwise to a transverse section: no blue-purple color develops.

Total ash <*5.01*> Not more than 4.0%.

Extract content <*5.01*> Dilute ethanol-soluble extract: not less than 17.0%.

Containers and storage Containers—Well-closed containers.

Schisandra Fruit

Schisandrae Fructus

ゴミシ

Schisandra Fruit is the fruit of *Schisandra chinensis* Baillon (*Schisandraceae*).

Description Sap fruit of irregular sphere or spheroid, about 6 mm in diameter; externally dark red to black-brown in color, with wrinkles, and occasionally with white powder; seeds, kidney-shaped, externally yellow-brown to dark red-brown, lustrous, with distinct raphe on the dorsal side; external seed coat easily peeled but internal seed coat adhering closely to the albumen.

Odor, slight; taste, acid, later astringent and bitter.

Identification To 1.0 g of pulverized Schisandra Fruit add 10 mL of methanol, warm on a water bath for 3 minutes with shaking, cool, filter, and use the filtrate as the sample solution. Separately, dissolve 1 mg of schisandrin for thin-layer chromatography in 1 mL of methanol, and use this solution as the standard solution. Perform the test with these solutions as directed under Thin-layer Chromatography <*2.03*>. Spot 5 μL each of the sample solution and standard solution on a plate of silica gel with fluorescent indicator for thin-layer chromatography. Develop the plate with a mixture of ethyl acetate, hexane and acetic acid (100) (10:10:1) to a distance of about 7 cm, and air-dry the plate. Examine under ultraviolet light (main wavelength: 254 nm): one of the several spots obtained from the sample solution has the same color tone and *R*f value with the spot from the standard solution.

Purity Foreign matter <*5.01*>—The amount of fruit receptacle, peduncle and other foreign matter contained in Schisandra Fruit is not more than 1.0%.

Total ash <*5.01*> Not more than 5.0%.

Containers and storage Containers—Well-closed containers.

Schizonepeta Spike

Schizonepetae Spica

ケイガイ

Schizonepeta Spike is the spike of *Schizonepeta tenuifolia* Briquet (*Labiatae*).

Description Oblong spike, 5 – 10 cm in length, 0.5 – 0.8 cm in diameter, purplish green-brown to green-brown in color. Spike, with calyx-tubes containing small labiate flower or often fruits; sometimes leaves under spike; leaf, linear or small lanceolate; stem, prismatic, purple-brown in color. Under a magnifying glass, it reveals short hairs.

It has a characteristic aroma and slightly cool feeling on keeping in the mouth.

Identification To 1 g of pulverized Schizonepeta Spike add 10 mL of ethyl acetate, shake for 15 minutes, filter, and use the filtrate as the sample solution. Perform the test with the sample solution as directed under Thin-layer Chromatography <*2.03*>. Spot 5 μL of the sample solution on a plate of silica gel for thin-layer chromatography. Develop the plate with a mixture of hexane and ethyl acetate (3:1) to a distance of about 7 cm, and air-dry the plate. Spray evenly 4-methoxybenzaldehyde-sulfuric acid TS on the plate, and heat the plate at 105°C for 5 minutes. After cooling for more than 10 minutes under an adequate humidity, examine under ultraviolet light (main wavelength: 365 nm): two spots, one is a blue fluorescent spot with an *R*f value of about 0.5 and the another is a yellow fluorescent spot with an *R*f value of about 0.1, are observed.

Total ash <*5.05*> Not more than 11.0%.

Acid-insoluble ash <*5.05*> Not more than 3.0%.

Extract content <*5.05*> Dilute ethanol-soluble extract: not less than 8.0%.

Containers and storage Containers—Well-closed containers.

Scopolia Rhizome

Scopoliae Rhizoma

ロートコン

Scopolia Rhizome is the rhizome with root of *Scopolia japonica* Maximowicz, *Scopolia carniolica* Jacquin or *Scopolia parviflora* Nakai (*Solanaceae*).

When dried, it contains not less than 0.29% of total

alkaloids [hyoscyamine ($C_{17}H_{23}NO_3$: 289.37) and scopolamine ($C_{17}H_{21}NO_4$: 303.35)].

Description Chiefly irregularly branched, slightly curved rhizome, about 15 cm in length, about 3 cm in diameter, occasionally longitudinally cut; externally grayish brown, with wrinkles; rhizome has constrictions and nodes; rarely, remains of stem at the apex; stem scars at upper side of each node; roots or root scars on both sides and lower surface of rhizome; fractured surface granular, grayish white to light brown in color; cortex a little lighter in color.

Odor characteristic.

Under a microscope <*5.01*>, xylem reveals groups of vessels arranged stepwise between medullary rays; xylem sieve tubes accompanied to the groups of vessels; parenchyma cells contain starch grains, and sometimes sand crystals of calcium oxalate.

Identification **(1)** To 1 g of pulverized Scopolia Rhizome add 10 mL of diethyl ether and 0.5 mL of ammonia TS, shake for 30 minutes, and filter. Wash the residue with 10 mL of diethyl ether, transfer the filtrate and the washing to a separator, add 20 mL of diluted sulfuric acid (1 in 50), shake well, and drain off the acid extract into another separator. Render the solution slightly alkaline with ammonia TS, add 10 mL of diethyl ether, shake well, transfer the diethyl ether layer to a porcelain dish, and evaporate the solvent on a water bath. To the residue add 5 drops of fuming nitric acid, and evaporate the mixture on a water bath to dryness. Cool, dissolve the residue in 1 mL of *N,N*-dimethylformamide, and add 5 to 6 drops of tetraethylammonium hydroxide TS: a red-purple to purple color develops.

(2) Place 2.0 g of pulverized Scopolia Rhizome in a glass-stoppered centrifuge tube, add 30 mL of ammonia TS, sonicate for 5 minutes, and centrifuge. Transfer the supernatant liquid to a separator, add 40 mL of ethyl acetate, and shake. Drain off the ethyl acetate layer, add 3 g of anhydrous sodium sulfate to the ethyl acetate, shake, and filter after the ethyl acetate becomes clear. Evaporate the solvent of the filtrate under low pressure (in vacuo), dissolve the residue in 1 mL of ethanol (95), and use this solution as the sample solution. Separately, dissolve 2 mg of Atropine Sulfate RS or atropine sulfate hydrate for thin-layer chromatography and 1 mg of Scopolamine Hydrobromide RS or scopolamine hydrobromide hydrate for thin-layer chromatography in 1 mL each of ethanol (95), and use these solutions as standard solution (1) and standard solution (2), respectively. Perform the test with these solutions as directed under Thin-layer Chromatography <*2.03*>. Spot 5 μL each of the sample solution, standard solutions (1) and (2) on a plate of silica gel for thin-layer chromatography. Develop the plate with a mixture of acetone, water and ammonia water (28) (90:7:3) to a distance of about 10 cm, and dry the plate at 80°C for 10 minutes. After cooling, spray evenly Dragendorff's TS for spraying on the plate: two principal spots obtained from the sample solution and each spot from the standard solutions show the same color tone and the same *R*f value.

Purity **(1)** Heavy metals <*1.07*>—Proceed with 3.0 g of pulverized Scopolia Rhizome according to Method 3, and perform the test. Prepare the control solution with 4.5 mL of Standard Lead Solution (not more than 15 ppm).

(2) Arsenic <*1.11*>—Prepare the test solution with 0.40 g of pulverized Scopolia Rhizome according to Method 4, and perform the test (not more than 5 ppm).

Total ash <*5.01*> Not more than 7.0%.

Assay Weigh accurately about 0.7 g of pulverized Scopolia Rhizome, previously dried at 60°C for 8 hours, in a glass-stoppered centrifuge tube, and moisten with 15 mL of ammonia TS. To this add 25 mL of diethyl ether, stopper the centrifuge tube tightly, shake for 15 minutes, centrifuge, and separate the diethyl ether layer. To the residue add 25 mL of diethyl ether, proceed in the same manner, and repeat this procedure twice. Combine all the extracts, and evaporate the solvent on a water bath. Dissolve the residue in 5 mL of the mobile phase, add exactly 3 mL of the internal standard solution, and add the mobile phase to make 25 mL. Filter this solution through a filter of a porosity of not more than 0.8 μm, discard the first 2 mL of the filtrate, and use the subsequent filtrate as the sample solution. Separately, weigh accurately about 25 mg of Atropine Sulfate RS (separately determine the loss on drying <*2.41*> under the same conditions as Atropine Sulfate Hydrate), dissolve in the mobile phase to make exactly 25 mL, and use this solution as standard stock solution A. Weigh accurately about 25 mg of Scopolamine Hydrobromide RS (separately determine the loss on drying <*2.41*> under the same conditions as Scopolamine Hydrobromide Hydrate), dissolve in the mobile phase to make exactly 25 mL, and use this solution as standard stock solution B. Pipet 5 mL of standard stock solution A and 1 mL of standard stock solution B, add exactly 3 mL of the internal standard solution, then add 25 mL of the mobile phase, and use this solution as the standard solution. Perform the test with 10 μL each of the sample solution and standard solution as directed under Liquid Chromatography <*2.01*> according to the following conditions. Calculate the ratios, Q_{TA} and Q_{SA}, of the peak area of hyoscyamine (atropine), and the ratios, Q_{TS} and Q_{SS}, of the peak area of scopolamine to that of the internal standard in each solution, calculate the amounts of hyoscyamine and scopolamine by the following equation, and designate the total as the amount of total alkaloids.

Amount (mg) of hyoscyamine ($C_{17}H_{23}NO_3$)
$= M_{SA} \times Q_{TA}/Q_{SA} \times 1/5 \times 0.855$

Amount (mg) of scopolamine ($C_{17}H_{21}NO_4$)
$= M_{SS} \times Q_{TS}/Q_{SS} \times 1/25 \times 0.789$

M_{SA}: Amount (mg) of Atropine Sulfate RS taken, calculated on the dried basis

M_{SS}: amount (mg) of Scopolamine Hydrobromide RS taken, calculated on the dried basis

Internal standard solution—A solution of brucine dihydrate in the mobile phase (1 in 2500).

Operating conditions—

Detector: An ultraviolet absorption spectrometer (wavelength: 210 nm).

Column: A stainless steel column 4 mm in inside diameter and 15 cm in length, packed with octadesilcylanized silica gel for liquid chromatography (5 μm in particle diameter).

Column temperature: A constant temperature of about 20°C.

Mobile phase: Dissolve 6.8 g of potassium dihydrogenphosphate in 900 mL of water, add 10 mL of triethylamine, adjust with phosphoric acid to pH 3.5, and add water to make 1000 mL. To 9 parts of this solution add 1 part of acetonitrile.

Flow rate: Adjust so that the retention time of scopolamine is about 8 minutes.

System suitability—

System performance: When the procedure is run with 10 μL of the standard solution under the above operating conditions, scopolamine, atropine and the internal standard are eluted in this order with the resolution between the peaks of scopolamine and atropine being not less than 11, and with the resolution between the peaks of atropine and the internal standard being not less than 4.

Containers and storage Containers—Well-closed containers.

Scopolia Extract

ロートエキス

Scopolia Extract contains not less than 0.90% and not more than 1.09% of total alkaloids [hyoscyamine ($C_{17}H_{23}NO_3$: 289.37) and scopolamine ($C_{17}H_{21}NO_4$: 303.35)].

Method of preparation Extract the coarse powder of Scopolia Rhizome with 35 vol% ethanol, Water, Purified Water or Purified Water in Containers, and prepare the viscous extract as directed under Extracts.

Description Scopolia Extract is brown to dark brown in color. It has a characteristic odor, and a bitter taste.

It dissolves in water with a slight turbidity.

Identification **(1)** Dissolve 4 g of Scopolia Extract in 10 mL of water, add 8 mL of ammonia TS and 80 mL of diethyl ether, stopper tightly, shake for 1 hour, add 2.5 g of powdered tragacanth, shake vigorously, allow to stand for 5 minutes, and separate the diethyl ether layer into a porcelain dish. Evaporate the diethyl ether on a water bath, add 5 drops of fuming nitric acid, and evaporate on a water bath to dryness. After cooling, dissolve the residue in 1 mL of *N*,*N*-dimethylformamide, and add 5 to 6 drops of tetraethylammonium hydroxide TS: a red-purple to purple color develops.

(2) Mix 0.5 g of Scopolia Extract with 30 mL of ammonia TS in a flask, and transfer the mixture to a separator. Add 40 mL of ethyl acetate to the separator, and shake the mixture. After drain off the ethyl acetate layer, add 3 g of anhydrous sodium sulfate to the ethyl acetate, shake, and filter after the ethyl acetate becomes clear. Evaporate the solvent of the filtrate under low pressure (in vacuo), dissolve the residue in 1 mL of ethanol (95), and use this solution as the sample solution. Proceed as directed in Identification (2) under Scopolia Rhizome.

Purity Heavy metals <*1.07*>—Prepare the test solution with 1.0 g of Scopolia Extract as directed in the Extracts (4), and perform the test (not more than 30 ppm).

Assay Weigh accurately about 0.4 g of Scopolia Extract, place in a glass-stoppered centrifuge tube, add 15 mL of ammonia TS, and shake. Add 25 mL of diethyl ether, stopper tightly, shake for 15 minutes, centrifuge, and separate the diethyl ether layer. Repeat this procedure twice with the aqueous layer, using 25 mL each of diethyl ether. Combine all the extracts, and evaporate the solvent on a water bath. Dissolve the residue in 5 mL of the mobile phase, add exactly 3 mL of the internal standard solution, and add the mobile phase to make 25 mL. Proceed as directed under Scopolia Rhizome.

Amount (mg) of hyoscyamine ($C_{17}H_{23}NO_3$)
$= M_{SA} \times Q_{TA}/Q_{SA} \times 1/5 \times 0.855$

Amount (mg) of scopolamine ($C_{17}H_{21}NO_4$)
$= M_{SS} \times Q_{TS}/Q_{SS} \times 1/25 \times 0.789$

M_{SA}: Amount (mg) of Atropine Sulfate RS taken, calculated on the dried basis

M_{SS}: Amount (mg) of Scopolamine Hydrobromide RS taken, calculated on the dried basis

Internal standard solution—A solution of brucine dihydrate in the mobile phase (1 in 2500).

Containers and storage Containers—Tight containers.

Storage—Light-resistant, and in a cold place.

Scopolia Extract Powder

ロートエキス散

Scopolia Extract Powder contains not less than 0.085% and not more than 0.110% of total alkaloids [hyoscyamine ($C_{17}H_{23}NO_3$: 289.37) and scopolamine ($C_{17}H_{21}NO_4$: 303.35)].

Method of preparation

Scopolia Extract	100 g
Starch, Lactose Hydrate or their mixture	a sufficient quantity
To make	1000 g

To Scopolia Extract add 100 mL of Purified Water or Purified Water in Containers, then warm and soften the mixture with stirring. Cool, add 800 g of starch, Lactose Hydrate or their mixture little by little, and mix well. Dry preferably at a low temperature, and dilute with a sufficient additional quantity of starch, Lactose Hydrate or their mixture to make 1000 g of homogeneous powder.

Description Scopolia Extract Powder is a brownish yellow to grayish yellow-brown powder. It has a faint, characteristic odor and a slightly bitter taste.

Identification **(1)** To 20 g of Scopolia Extract Powder add 15 mL of water and 8 mL of ammonia TS, mix homogeneously, add 100 mL of diethyl ether and 7 g of sodium chloride, stopper tightly, shake for 1 hour, add 5 g of powdered tragacanth, and shake vigorously. Allow to stand for 5 minutes, take the clearly separated diethyl ether layer, and filter. Proceed with the filtrate as directed in the Identification (1) under Scopolia Extract.

(2) Place 5.0 g of Scopolia Extract Powder in a glass-stoppered centrifuge tube, add 30 mL of ammonia TS, sonicate for 5 minutes, and centrifuge. Transfer the supernatant liquid to a separator, add 40 mL of ethyl acetate, and shake. Drain off the ethyl acetate layer, add 3 g of anhydrous sodium sulfate to the ethyl acetate, shake, and filter after the ethyl acetate becomes clear. Evaporate the solvent of the filtrate under low pressure (in vacuo), dissolve the residue in 1 mL of ethanol (95), and use this solution as the sample solution. Proceed as directed in the Identification (2) under Scopolia Rhizome.

Assay Weigh accurately about 4 g of Scopolia Extract Powder, place in a glass-stoppered centrifuge tube, add 15 mL of ammonia TS, and shake. Add 25 mL of diethyl ether, stopper tightly, shake for 15 minutes, centrifuge to take the diethyl ether layer. To the aqueous layer add 25 mL of diethyl ether, proceed in the same manner, and repeat this procedure three times. Combine all the extracts, and evaporate the solvent on a water bath. Dissolve the residue in 5 mL of the mobile phase, add exactly 3 mL of the internal standard solution, and add the mobile phase to make 25 mL. Filter this solution through a membrane filter with a pore size not exceeding 0.8 μm, discard the first 2 mL of the filtrate, and use the subsequent filtrate as the sample solution. Separately, weigh accurately about 25 mg of Atropine Sulfate RS (separately determine the loss on drying <*2.41*> under the same manner as Atropine Sulfate Hydrate), dissolve in the mobile phase to make exactly 25 mL, and use this solution as standard stock solution A. Weigh accurately about 25 mg of Scopolamine Hydrobromide RS (separately determine the loss on drying <*2.41*> under the same manner as Scopolamine Hydrobromide Hydrate), dissolve in the mobile phase to make exactly 25 mL, and use this solution as standard stock solution B. Pipet 5 mL of the standard stock solution A and 1 mL of the standard stock solution B, add exactly 3 mL of the internal standard solution, then add the mobile phase to make 25 mL, and use this solution as the standard solution. Perform the test with 10 μL each of the sample solution and standard solution as directed under Liquid Chromatography <*2.01*> according to the following conditions. Calculate the ratios, Q_{TA} and Q_{SA}, of the peak area of hyoscyamine (atropine), and ratios, Q_{TS} and Q_{SS}, of the peak area of scopolamine to that of the internal standard in each solution, calculate the amounts of hyoscyamine and scopolamine by the following equation, and designate the total as the amount of total alkaloids.

$$\text{Amount (mg) of hyoscyamine } (C_{17}H_{23}NO_3) = M_{SA} \times Q_{TA}/Q_{SA} \times 1/5 \times 0.855$$

$$\text{Amount (mg) of scopolamine } (C_{17}H_{21}NO_4) = M_{SS} \times Q_{TS}/Q_{SS} \times 1/25 \times 0.789$$

M_{SA}: Amount (mg) of Atropine Sulfate RS taken, calculated on the dried basis

M_{SS}: Amount (mg) of Scopolamine Hydrobromide RS taken, calculated on the dried basis

Internal standard solution—A solution of brucine dihydrate in the mobile phase (1 in 2500).

Operating conditions—

Detector: An ultraviolet absorption spectrometer (wavelength: 210 nm).

Column: A stainless steel column about 4 mm in inside diameter and about 15 cm in length, packed with octadecylsilanized silica gel for liquid chromatography (5 μm in particle diameter).

Column temperature: A constant temperature of about 20°C.

Mobile phase: A mixture of a solution obtained by dissolving 6.8 g of potassium dihydrogenphosphate in 900 mL of water, adding 10 mL of triethylamine, adjusting the pH to 3.5 with phosphoric acid, and adding water to make 1000 mL, and acetonitrile (9:1).

Flow rate: Adjust so that the retention time of scopolamine is about 8 minutes.

System suitability—

System performance: When the procedure is run with 10 μL of the standard solution under the above operating conditions, scopolamine, atropine and the internal standard are eluted in this order with the resolution between the peaks of scopolamine and atropine being not less than 11, and the resolution between the peaks of atropine and the internal standard being not less than 4.

Containers and storage Containers—Tight containers.

Scopolia Extract and Carbon Powder

ロートエキス·カーボン散

Method of preparation

Scopolia Extract	5 g
Medicinal Carbon	550 g
Natural Aluminum Silicate	345 g
Starch, Lactose Hydrate or their mixture	a sufficient quantity
To make	1000 g

Prepare before use as directed under Powders, with the above ingredients. May be prepared with an equivalent amount of Scopolia Extract Powder in place of Scopolia Extract.

Description Scopolia Extract and Carbon Powder is easily dustable and black in color. It is tasteless.

Containers and storage Containers—Well-closed containers.

Compound Scopolia Extract and Diastase Powder

複方ロートエキス·ジアスターゼ散

Method of preparation

Scopolia Extract	8 g
Diastase	200 g
Precipitate Calcium Carbonate	300 g
Sodium Bicarbonate	250 g
Magnesium Oxide	100 g
Powdered Gentian	50 g
Starch, Lactose Hydrate or their mixture	a sufficient quantity
To make	1000 g

Prepare before use as directed under Powders, with the above ingredients. May be prepared with an equivalent amount of Scopolia Extract Powder in place of Scopolia Extract.

Description Compound Scopolia Extract and Diastase Powder is light yellow in color. It has a bitter taste.

Containers and storage Containers—Well-closed containers.

Scopolia Extract and Ethyl Aminobenzoate Powder

ロートエキス·アネスタミン散

Scopolia Extract and Ethyl Aminobenzoate Powder contains not less than 22.5% and not more than 27.5% of ethyl aminobenzoate ($C_9H_{11}NO_2$: 165.19).

Method of preparation

Scopolia Extract	10 g
Ethyl Aminobenzoate	250 g
Magnesium Oxide	150 g
Sodium Bicarbonate	500 g
Starch, Lactose Hydrate or their mixture	a sufficient quantity
To make	1000 g

Prepare as directed under Powders, with the above ingredients. May be prepared with an equivalent amount of Scopolia Extract Powder in place of Scopolia Extract.

Description Scopolia Extract and Ethyl Aminobenzoate Powder is slightly brownish white in color. It has a slightly bitter taste, leaving a sensation of numbness on the tongue.

Identification **(1)** To 2 g of Scopolia Extract and Ethyl Aminobenzoate Powder add 20 mL of diethyl ether, shake, and filter through a glass filter (G4). Wash the residue with three 10-mL portions of diethyl ether, combine the filtrate and the washings, evaporate to dryness, and perform the following test with the residue (ethyl aminobenzoate).

(i) Dissolve 0.01 g of the residue in 1 mL of dilute hydrochloric acid and 4 mL of water: the solution responds to Qualitative Tests <*1.09*> for primary aromatic amines.

(ii) Dissolve 0.1 g of the residue in 5 mL of water with the aid of dilute hydrochloric acid added dropwise, and add iodine TS dropwise: a brown precipitate is produced.

(iii) Warm 0.05 g of the residue with 2 drops of acetic acid (31) and 5 drops of sulfuric acid: the odor of ethyl acetate is perceptible.

(2) To the diethyl ether-insoluble residue obtained in (1) add 30 mL of water, shake gently, and filter: the filtrate responds to Qualitative Tests <*1.09*> for sodium salt and for bicarbonate.

(3) To the water-insoluble residue obtained in (2) add 10 mL of dilute hydrochloric acid, shake, and filter: the filtrate responds to Qualitative Tests <*1.09*> for magnesium salt.

(4) Place 30 g of Scopolia Extract and Ethyl Aminobenzoate Powder in a glass-stoppered conical flask, add 100 mL of water, shake for 30 minutes, and filter immediately by suction through a glass filter (G3). Transfer the residue in the flask to the same glass filter with the filtrate, and filter the residue by suction while pressing vigorously the residue on the same glass filter. Place 75 mL of the filtrate in a 300-mL beaker, and add cautiously 10 mL of diluted sulfuric acid (1 in 3). Add 0.2 mL of bromocresol green TS to this solution, and add dilute sulfuric acid dropwise while shaking thoroughly, until the color of the solution changes from green to yellow-green. After cooling, place this solution in a separator, wash with two 25-mL portions of a mixture of hexane and diethyl ether (1:1) by shaking well, and place the aqueous layer in another separator. Make slightly alkaline with ammonia TS, add immediately 30 mL of diethyl ether, and shake well. Wash the diethyl ether layer with two 10-mL portions of a saturated solution of sodium chloride, separate the diethyl ether layer, add 3 g of anhydrous sodium sulfate, shake, and filter through a pledget of cotton. Evaporate the filtrate to dryness, dissolve the residue in 0.2 mL of ethanol (95), and use this solution as the sample solution. Separately, dissolve 2 mg of Atropine Sulfate RS or atropine sulfate hydrate for thin-layer chromatography and 1 mg of Scopolamine Hydrobromide RS or scopolamine hydrobromide hydrate for thin-layer chromatography in 1 mL each of ethanol (95), and use these solutions as standard solution (1) and standard solution (2), respectively. Perform the test with these solutions as directed under Thin-layer Chromatography <*2.03*>. Spot 10 μL each of the sample solution, standard solution (1) and (2) on a plate of silica gel for thin-layer chromatography. Develop the plate with a mixture of acetone, water and ammonia solution (28) (90:7:3) to a distance of about 10 cm, and dry the plate at 80°C for 10 minutes. After cooling, spray evenly Dragendorff's TS for spraying on the plate: two principal spots obtained from the sample solution show the same color tone and the same *R*f value with each spot from the standard solutions, respectively.

Assay Weigh accurately about 0.3 g of Scopolia Extract and Ethyl Aminobenzoate Powder, transfer to a Soxhlet extractor, extract with 100 mL of diethyl ether for 1 hour, and evaporate the solvent on a water bath. Dissolve the residue in 25 mL of 1 mol/L hydrochloric acid TS, and add water to make exactly 100 mL. Pipet 5 mL of this solution, add water to make exactly 250 mL, and use this solution as the sample solution. Weigh accurately about 75 mg of Ethyl Aminobenzoate RS, previously dried in a desiccator (silica gel) for 3 hours, dissolve in 25 mL of 1 mol/L hydrochloric acid TS, and add water to make exactly 100 mL. Pipet 5 mL of this solution, add water to make exactly 250 mL, and use this solution as the standard solution. Pipet 5 mL each of the sample solution and standard solution, to each add 10 mL of 1 mol/L hydrochloric acid TS, then add 1 mL of a solution of sodium nitrite (1 in 200), prepared before use, and allow to stand for 5 minutes with occasional shaking. Add 5 mL of ammonium amidosulfate TS, shake well, and allow to stand for 10 minutes. Add 2 mL of *N*-*N*-diethyl-*N*′-1-naphthylethylenediamine oxalate-acetone TS, mix immediately, and add water to make exactly 50 mL. Allow to stand for 2 hours, determine the absorbances, A_T and A_S, of these solutions at 550 nm, as directed under Ultraviolet-visible Spectrophotometry <*2.24*> using a blank prepared in the same manner with 5 mL of water in place of the sample solution.

Amount (mg) of ethyl aminobenzoate ($C_9H_{11}NO_2$)
$= M_S \times A_T/A_S$

M_S: Amount (mg) of Ethyl Aminobenzoate RS taken

Containers and storage Containers—Well-closed containers.

Scopolia Extract and Tannic Acid Suppositories

ロートエキス·タンニン坐剤

Method of preparation

Scopolia Extract	0.5 g
Tannic Acid	1 g
Cacao Butter or a suitable base	a sufficient quantity

Prepare 10 suppositories as directed under Suppositories, with the above ingredients.

Description Scopolia Extract and Tannic Acid Suppositories are light brown in color.

Identification **(1)** To 2 Scopolia Extract and Tannic Acid Suppositories add 20 mL of diethyl ether, and dissolve the base of suppositories with shaking for 10 minutes. Shake thoroughly the mixture with 15 mL of water, separate the aqueous layer, and filter. To the filtrate add 10 mL of chloroform, shake well, and separate the chloroform layer. Take 5 mL of the chloroform solution, add 5 mL of ammonia TS, shake, and allow to stand: the ammonia layer shows a blue-green fluorescence.

(2) To 1 mL of the aqueous layer obtained in (1) after extraction with diethyl ether, add 2 drops of iron (III) chloride TS: a blue-black color develops. Allow to stand: a blue-black precipitate is formed (tannic acid).

Containers and storage Containers—Well-closed containers.

Scutellaria Root

Scutellariae Radix

オウゴン

Scutellaria Root is the root of *Scutellaria baicalensis* Georgi (*Labiatae*), from which the periderm has been removed.

It contains not less than 10.0% of baicalin ($C_{21}H_{18}O_{11}$: 446.36), calculated on the basis of dried material.

Description Cone-shaped, cylindrical, semitubular or flattened root, 5 - 20 cm in length, 0.5 - 3 cm in diameter; externally yellow-brown, with coarse and marked longitudinal wrinkles, and with scattered scars of lateral root and remains of brown periderm; scars of stem or remains of stem at the crown; sometimes central portion of xylem rotted, often forming a hollow; hard in texture and easily broken; fractured surface fibrous and yellow in color.

Almost odorless; taste, slightly bitter.

Under a microscope *<5.01>*, a transverse section reveals a remaining cork layer 6 - 20 cells thick, coritical layer composed of parenchyma, sclerenchyma cells scattered in cortex; xylem composed of parenchyma, vessels and small amount of xylem fibers observed in xylem; vessels usually in groups and arranged in tangential direction, radial direction or in irregular form; in case where central portion of xylem rotted, cork layer observed around hollow; parenchyma cells of coritical layer and xylem contain simple and compound starch grains.

Identification **(1)** Heat gently 0.5 g of pulverized Scutellaria Root with 20 mL of diethyl ether under a reflux condenser for 5 minutes, cool, and filter. Evaporate the solvent of the filtrate, dissolve the residue in 10 mL of ethanol (95), and to 3 mL of the solution add 1 to 2 drops of dilute iron (III) chloride TS: a grayish green color develops, and it changes to purple-brown.

(2) To 1 g of pulverized Scutellaria Root add 25 mL of methanol, shake for 15 minutes, filter, and use the filtrate as the sample solution. Separately, dissolve 1 mg of Baicalin RS or baicalin for thin-layer chromatography in 1 mL of methanol, and use this solution as the standard solution. Perform the test with these solutions as directed under Thin-layer Chromatography *<2.03>*. Spot 5 μL each of the sample solution and standard solution on a plate of silica gel for thin-layer chromatography. Develop the plate with a mixture of 1-butanol, water and acetic acid (100) (4:2:1) to a distance of about 7 cm, and air-dry the plate. Spray evenly iron (III) chloride-methanol TS on the plate: one of the several spots obtained from the sample solution has the same color tone and *R*f value with the spot from the standard solution.

Purity **(1)** Heavy metals *<1.07>*—Proceed with 3.0 g of pulverized Scutellaria Root according to Method 3, and perform the test. Prepare the control solution with 3.0 mL of Standard Lead Solution (not more than 10 ppm).

(2) Arsenic *<1.11>*—Prepare the test solution with 0.40 g of pulverized Scutellaria Root according to Method 4, and perform the test (not more than 5 ppm).

Loss on drying *<5.01>* Not more than 12.0% (6 hours).

Total ash *<5.01>* Not more than 6.0%.

Assay Weigh accurately about 0.5 g of pulverized Scutellaria Root, add 30 mL of diluted methanol (7 in 10), heat under a reflux condenser for 30 minutes, and cool. Transfer the mixture to a glass-stoppered centrifuge tube, centrifuge, and separate the supernatant liquid. Wash the vessel for the reflux extraction with 30 mL of diluted methanol (7 in 10), transfer the washings to the glass-stoppered centrifuge tube, centrifuge after shaking for 5 minutes, and separate the supernatant liquid. To the residue add 30 mL of diluted methanol (7 in 10), shake for 5 minutes, centrifuge, and separate the supernatant liquid. Combine all the extracts, add diluted methanol (7 in 10) to make exactly 100 mL, then pipet 2 mL of this solution, add diluted methanol (7 in 10) to make exactly 20 mL, and use this solution as the sample solution. Separately, weigh accurately about 10 mg of Baicalin RS (separately determine the water *<2.48>* by coulometric titration, using 10 mg), and dissolve in methanol to make exactly 100 mL. Pipet 5 mL of the solution, add diluted methanol (7 in 10) to make exactly 10 mL, and use this solution as the standard solution. Perform the test with exactly 10 μL each of the sample solution and standard solution as directed under Liquid Chromatography *<2.01>* according to the following conditions. Determine the peak areas, A_T and A_S, of baicalin in each solution.

$$\text{Amount (mg) of baicalin } (C_{21}H_{18}O_{11}) = M_S \times A_T/A_S \times 5$$

M_S: Amount (mg) of Baicalin RS taken, calculated on the anhydrous basis

Operating conditions—

Detector: An ultraviolet absorption photometer (wavelength: 277 nm).

Column: A stainless steel column 4.6 mm in inside diameter and 15 cm in length, packed with octadecylsilanized silica

gel for liquid chromatography (5 μm in particle diameter).

Column temperature: A constant temperature of about 50°C.

Mobile phase: A mixture of diluted phosphoric acid (1 in 146) and acetonitrile (18:7).

Flow rate: Adjust so that the retention time of baicalin is about 6 minutes.

System suitability—

System performance: Dissolve 1 mg of Baicalin RS and 2 mg of methyl parahydroxybenzoate for resolution check in methanol to make 100 mL. When the procedure is run with 10 μL of this solution under the above operating conditions, baicalin and methyl parahydroxybenzoate are eluted in this order with the resolution between these peaks being not less than 3.

System repeatability: When the test is repeated 6 times with 10 μL of the standard solution under the above operating conditions, the relative standard deviation of the peak area of baicalin is not more than 1.5%.

Containers and storage Containers—Well-closed containers.

Powdered Scutellaria Root

Scutellariae Radix Pulverata

オウゴン末

Powdered Scutellaria Root is the powder of Scutellaria Root.

It contains not less than 10.0% of baicalin ($C_{21}H_{18}O_{11}$: 446.36), calculated on the basis of dried material.

Description Powdered Scutellaria Root occurs as a yellow-brown powder. It is almost odorless, and has a slight, bitter taste.

Under a microscope *<5.01>*, Powdered Scutellaria Root reveals fragments of parenchyma cells containing small amount of simple and compound starch grains, fragments of short reticulate vessel elements and fusiform, stick-like and ellipsoidal to spherical sclerenchyma cells; also a few fragments of spiral vessels and xylem fibers are observed.

Identification **(1)** Heat gently 0.5 g of Powdered Scutellaria Root with 20 mL of diethyl ether under a reflux condenser for 5 minutes, cool, and filter. Evaporate the filtrate, dissolve the residue in 10 mL of ethanol (95), and to 3 mL of the solution add 1 to 2 drops of dilute iron (III) chloride TS: a grayish green color develops, and it changes to purple-brown later.

(2) To 1 g of Powdered Scutellaria Root add 25 mL of methanol, shake for 15 minutes, filter, and use the filtrate as the sample solution. Separately, dissolve 1 mg of Baicalin RS or baicalin for thin-layer chromatography in 1 mL of methanol, and use this solution as the standard solution. Perform the test with these solutions as directed under Thin-layer Chromatography *<2.03>*. Spot 5 μL each of the sample solution and standard solution on a plate of silica gel for thin-layer chromatography. Develop the plate with a mixture of 1-butanol, water and acetic acid (100) (4:2:1) to a distance of about 7 cm, and air-dry the plate. Spray evenly iron (III) chloride-methanol TS on the plate: one of the several spots obtained from the sample solution has the same color tone and *Rf* value with the spot from the standard solution.

Purity **(1)** Heavy metals *<1.07>*—Proceed with 3.0 g of Powdered Scutellaria Root according to Method 3, and perform the test. Prepare the control solution with 3.0 mL of Standard Lead Solution (not more than 10 ppm).

(2) Arsenic *<1.11>*—Prepare the test solution with 0.40 g of Powdered Scutellaria Root according to Method 4, and perform the test (not more than 5 ppm).

(3) Foreign matter—Under a microscope *<5.01>*, Powdered Scutellaria Root does not show crystals of calcium oxalate.

Loss on drying *<5.01>* Not more than 12.0% (6 hours).

Total ash *<5.01>* Not more than 6.0%.

Acid-insoluble ash *<5.01>* Not more than 1.0%.

Assay Weigh accurately about 0.5 g of Powdered Scutellaria Root, add 30 mL of diluted methanol (7 in 10), heat under a reflux condenser for 30 minutes, and cool. Transfer the mixture to a glass-stoppered centrifuge tube, centrifuge, and separate the supernatant liquid. Wash the vessel for the reflux extraction with 30 mL of diluted methanol (7 in 10), transfer the washings to the glass-stoppered centrifuge tube, centrifuge after shaking for 5 minutes, and separate the supernatant liquid. To the residue add 30 mL of diluted methanol (7 in 10), shake for 5 minutes, centrifuge, and separate the supernatant liquid. Combine all the extracts, add diluted methanol (7 in 10) to make exactly 100 mL, then pipet 2 mL of this solution, add diluted methanol (7 in 10) to make exactly 20 mL, and use this solution as the sample solution. Separately, weigh accurately about 10 mg of Baicalin RS (separately determine the water *<2.48>* by coulometric titration, using 10 mg), and dissolve in methanol to make exactly 100 mL. Pipet 5 mL of the solution, add diluted methanol (7 in 10) to make exactly 10 mL, and use this solution as the standard solution. Perform the test with exactly 10 μL each of the sample solution and standard solution as directed under Liquid Chromatography *<2.01>* according to the following conditions. Determine the peak areas, A_T and A_S, of baicalin in each solution.

$$\text{Amount (mg) of baicalin } (C_{21}H_{18}O_{11}) = M_S \times A_T/A_S \times 5$$

M_S: Amount (mg) of Baicalin RS taken, calculated on the anhydrous basis

Operating conditions—

Detector: An ultraviolet absorption photometer (wavelength: 277 nm).

Column: A stainless steel column 4.6 mm in inside diameter and 15 cm in length, packed with octadecylsilanized silica gel for liquid chromatography (5 μm in particle diameter).

Column temperature: A constant temperature of about 50°C.

Mobile phase: A mixture of diluted phosphoric acid (1 in 146) and acetonitrile (18:7).

Flow rate: Adjust so that the retention time of baicalin is about 6 minutes.

System suitability—

System performance: Dissolve 1 mg of Baicalin RS and 2 mg of methyl parahydroxybenzoate for resolution check in methanol to make 100 mL. When the procedure is run with 10 μL of this solution under the above operating conditions, baicalin and methyl parahydroxybenzoate are eluted in this order with the resolution between these peaks being not less than 3.

System repeatability: When the test is repeated 6 times with 10 μL of the standard solution under the above operat-

ing conditions, the relative standard deviation of the peak area of baicalin is not more than 1.5%.

Containers and storage Containers—Well-closed containers.

Senega

Senegae Radix

セネガ

Senega is the root of *Polygala senega* Linné or *Polygala senega* Linné var. *latifolia* Torrey et Gray (*Polygalaceae*).

Description Slender, conical root often branched, 3 - 10 cm in length; main root 0.5 - 1.5 cm in diameter; externally light grayish brown to grayish brown; with many longitudinal wrinkles and sometimes with twisted protruding lines; tuberously enlarged crown, with remains of stems and red buds; branched rootlets twisted; a transverse section reveals grayish brown cortex and yellowish white xylem; usually round, and sometimes cuneate to semicircular; cortex on the opposite side is thickened.

Odor, characteristic, resembling the aroma of methyl salicylate; taste, sweet at first but leaving an acrid taste.

Under a microscope <*5.01*>, a transverse section of the main root reveals a cork layer consisting of several cell rows of light brown cork cells; secondary cortex composed of parenchyma cells and phloen, traversed by medullary rays, 1 to 3 cells wide; medullary rays on xylem not distinct. Its parenchyma cells contain oil droplets, but starch grains and calcium oxalate crystals are absent.

Identification (1) Shake vigorously 0.5 g of pulverized Senega with 10 mL of water: a lasting fine foam is produced.

(2) Shake 0.5 g of pulverized Senega with 30 mL of water for 15 minutes, and filter. Take 1 mL of the filtrate, mix with 50 mL of water, and determine the absorption spectrum of the solution as directed under Ultraviolet-visible Spectrophotometry <*2.24*>: it exhibits a maximum at about 317 nm.

Purity (1) Heavy metals <*1.07*>—Proceed with 3.0 g of pulverized Senega according to Method 3, and perform the test. Prepare the control solution with 3.0 mL of Standard Lead Solution (not more than 10 ppm).

(2) Arsenic <*1.11*>—Prepare the test solution with 0.40 g of pulverized Senega according to Method 4, and perform the test (not more than 5 ppm).

(3) Stem—When perform the test of foreign matter <*5.01*>, the amount of the stems contained in Senega does not exceed 2.0%.

(4) Foreign matter <*5.01*>—The amount of foreign matter other than the stems is not more than 1.0%.

Loss on drying <*5.01*> Not more than 13.0% (6 hours).

Total ash <*5.01*> Not more than 5.0%.

Acid-insoluble ash <*5.01*> Not more than 2.0%.

Extract content <*5.01*> Dilute ethanol-soluble extract: not less than 30.0%.

Containers and storage Containers—Well-closed containers.

Powdered Senega

Senegae Radix Pulverata

セネガ末

Powdered Senega is the powder of Senega.

Description Powdered Senega occurs as a light brown powder, and has a characteristic odor resembling the aroma of methyl salicylate; taste, sweet at first, but later acrid.

Under a microscope <*5.01*>, Powdered Senega reveals fragments of pitted vessels, reticulate vessels and tracheids; fragments of xylem fibers with oblique pits; fragments of xylem parenchyma cells with simple pits; fragments of phloem parenchyma containing oily droplets; fragments of exodermis often composed of cells suberized and divided into daughter cells; oily droplets stained red by sudan III TS. The parenchyma cells of Powdered Senega do not contain starch grains and crystals of calcium oxalate.

Identification (1) Shake vigorously 0.5 g of Powdered Senega with 10 mL of water: a lasting fine foam is produced.

(2) Shake 0.5 g of Powdered Senega with 30 mL of water for 15 minutes, and filter. Take 1 mL of the filtrate, mix with 50 mL of water, and determine the absorption spectrum of the solution as directed under Ultraviolet-visible Spectrophotometry <*2.24*>: it exhibits a maximum at about 317 nm.

Purity (1) Heavy metals <*1.07*>—Proceed with 3.0 g of Powdered Senega according to Method 3, and perform the test. Prepare the control solution with 3.0 mL of Standard Lead Solution (not more than 10 ppm).

(2) Arsenic <*1.11*>—Prepare the test solution with 0.40 g of Powdered Senega according to Method 4, and perform the test (not more than 5 ppm).

(3) Foreign matter—Under a microscope <*5.01*>, stone cells, starch grains or crystals of calcium oxalate are not observed.

Loss on drying <*5.01*> Not more than 13.0% (6 hours).

Total ash <*5.01*> Not more than 5.0%.

Acid-insoluble ash <*5.01*> Not more than 2.0%.

Extract content <*5.01*> Dilute ethanol-soluble extract: not less than 30.0%.

Containers and storage Containers—Well-closed containers.

Senega Syrup

セネガシロップ

Method of preparation

Senega, in moderately fine cutting	40 g
Sucrose	780 g
10 vol% Ethanol	a sufficient quantity
Purified Water or Purified Water in Containers	a sufficient quantity
To make	1000 mL

Add 400 mL of 10 vol% ethanol to Senega, and macerate for one or two days. Filter the extract, wash the residue with a small amount of 10 vol% Ethanol, filter, and combine the filtrate of the extracts and washings until total volume measures about 500 mL. Dissolve Sucrose in the mixture, by warming if necessary, and dilute to 1000 mL with Purified Water or Purified Water in Containers. May be prepared with an appropriate quantity of Ethanol and Purified Water or Purified Water in Containers in place of 10 vol% Ethanol.

Description Senega Syrup is a yellow-brown, viscous liquid. It has a characteristic odor resembling methyl salicylate and a sweet taste.

Identification Add 5 mL of water to 1 mL of Senega Syrup, and shake: lasting small bubbles are produced.

Containers and storage Containers—Tight containers.

Senna Leaf

Sennae Folium

センナ

Senna Leaf is the leaflets of *Cassia angustifolia* Vahl or *Cassia acutifolia* Delile (*Leguminosae*).

It contains not less than 1.0% of total sennosides [sennoside A ($C_{42}H_{38}O_{20}$: 862.74) and sennoside B ($C_{42}H_{38}O_{20}$: 862.74)], calculated on the basis of dried material.

Description Lanceolate to narrow lanceolate leaflets, 1.5 - 5 cm in length, 0.5 - 1.5 cm in width, light grayish yellow to light grayish yellow-green in color; margin entire, apex acute, base asymmetric, petiole short; under a magnifying glass, vein marked, primary lateral veins running toward the apex along the margin and joining the lateral vein above; lower surface having slight hairs.

Odor slight; taste, bitter.

Under a microscope <*5.01*>, a transverse section of Senna Leaf reveals epidermis with thick cuticle, with numerous stomata, and with thick-walled, warty unicellular hairs; epidermal cells are often separated into two loculi by a septum which is in parallel with the surface of the leaf, and contain mucilage in the inner loculus; palisade of a single cellular layer under each epidermis; spongy tissue, consisting of 3 to 4 cellular layers, and containing clustered or solitary crystals of calcium oxalate; cells adjacent to vascular bundle, forming crystal cell rows.

Identification (1) Macerate 0.5 g of pulverized Senna Leaf in 10 mL of diethyl ether for 2 minutes, and filter. Add 5 mL of ammonia TS to the filtrate: a yellow-red color is produced in the aqueous layer. To the residue of maceration add 10 mL of water, and macerate for 2 minutes. Filter, and add 5 mL of ammonia TS: a yellow-red color is produced in the aqueous layer.

(2) To 2 g of pulverized Senna Leaf add 40 mL of a mixture of tetrahydrofuran and water (7:3), shake for 30 minutes, and centrifuge. Transfer the supernatant liquid to a separator, add 13 g of sodium chloride, and shake for 30 minutes. Separate the aqueous layer with undissolved sodium chloride, and adjust to pH 1.5 with 1 mol/L hydrochloric acid TS. Transfer this solution to another separator, shake with 30 mL of tetrahydrofuran for 10 minutes, separate the tetrahydrofuran layer, and use the tetrahydrofuran layer as the sample solution. Separately, dissolve 1 mg of Sennoside A RS or sennoside A for thin-layer chromatography in 1 mL of a mixture of tetrahydrofuran and water (7:3), and use this solution as the standard solution. Perform the test with these solutions as directed under Thin-layer Chromatography <*2.03*>. Spot 10 μL each of the sample solution and standard solution on a plate of silica gel for thin-layer chromatography. Develop the plate with a mixture of 1-propanol, ethyl acetate, water and acetic acid (100) (40:40:30:1) to a distance of about 7 cm, and air-dry the plate. Examine under ultraviolet light (main wavelength: 365 nm): one of the several spots obtained from the sample solution has the same color tone and *R*f value with the red fluorescent spot from the standard solution.

Purity (1) Rachis and fruit—When perform the test of foreign matter <*5.01*>, the amount of rachis and fruits contained in Senna Leaf does not exceed 5.0%.

(2) Foreign matter <*5.01*>—The amount of foreign matter other than rachis and fruits contained in Senna Leaf does not exceed 1.0%.

(3) Total BHC's and total DDT's <*5.01*>—Not more than 0.2 ppm, respectively.

Loss on drying <*5.01*> Not more than 12.0% (6 hours).

Total ash <*5.01*> Not more than 12.0%.

Acid-insoluble ash <*5.01*> Not more than 2.0%.

Assay Weigh accurately about 0.5 g of pulverized Senna Leaf in a glass-stoppered centrifuge tube, add 25 mL of diluted methanol (7 in 10), shake for 30 minutes, centrifuge, and separate the supernatant liquid. To the residue add 10 mL of diluted methanol (7 in 10), shake for 10 minutes, centrifuge, and separate the supernatant liquid. Repeat this procedure once more, combine all the extracts, add diluted methanol (7 in 10) to make exactly 50 mL, and use this solution as the sample solution. Separately, weigh accurately about 10 mg of Sennoside A RS (separately determine the water <*2.48*> by coulometric titration, using 10 mg), dissolve in a solution of sodium hydrogen carbonate (1 in 100) to make exactly 20 mL, and use this solution as standard stock solution (1). Weigh accurately about 10 mg of Sennoside B RS (separately determine the water <*2.48*> by coulometric titration, using 10 mg), dissolve in a solution of sodium hydrogen carbonate (1 in 100) to make exactly 20 mL, and use this solution as standard stock solution (2). Pipet 5 mL of the standard stock solution (1) and 10 mL of the standard stock solution (2), add methanol to make exactly 50 mL, and use this solution as the standard solution. Perform the test with exactly 10 μL each of the sample solution and standard solution as directed under Liquid Chromatography <*2.01*> according to the following conditions. Determine the peak areas, A_{Ta} and A_{Sa}, of sennoside A, and the peak areas, A_{Tb} and A_{Sb}, of sennoside B in each solution, calculate the amounts of sennoside A and sennoside B by the following equations, and designate the total as the amount of total sennosides.

$$\text{Amount (mg) of sennoside A } (C_{42}H_{38}O_{20}) = M_{Sa} \times A_{Ta}/A_{Sa} \times 1/4$$

$$\text{Amount (mg) of sennoside B } (C_{42}H_{38}O_{20}) = M_{Sb} \times A_{Tb}/A_{Sb} \times 1/2$$

M_{Sa}: Amount (mg) of Sennoside A RS taken, calculated on the anhydrous basis

M_{Sb}: Amount (mg) of Sennoside B RS taken, calculated on the anhydrous basis

Operating conditions—

Detector: An ultraviolet absorption photometer (wavelength: 340 nm).

Column: A stainless steel column 4.6 mm in inside diameter and 15 cm in length, packed with octadecylsilanized silica gel for liquid chromatography (5 μm in particle diameter).

Column temperature: A constant temperature of about 50°C.

Mobile phase: Dissolve 2.45 g of tetra-*n*-heptylammonium bromide in 1000 mL of a mixture of diluted 1 mol/L acetic acid-sodium acetate buffer solution (pH 5.0) (1 in 10) and acetonitrile (17:8).

Flow rate: Adjust so that the retention time of sennoside A is about 26 minutes.

System suitability—

System performance: When the procedure is run with 10 μL of the standard solution under the above operating conditions, sennoside B and sennoside A are eluted in this order with the resolution between these peaks being not less than 15, and the number of theoretical plates of the peak of sennoside A being not less than 8000.

System repeatability: When the test is repeated 6 times with 10 μL of the standard solution under the above operating conditions, the relative standard deviation of the peak area of sennoside A is not more than 1.5%.

Containers and storage Containers—Well-closed containers.

Powdered Senna Leaf

Sennae Folium Pulveratum

センナ末

Powdered Senna Leaf is the powder of Senna Leaf.

It contains not less than 1.0% of total sennosides [sennoside A ($C_{42}H_{38}O_{20}$: 862.74) and sennoside B ($C_{42}H_{38}O_{20}$: 862.74)], calculated on the basis of dried material.

Description Powdered Senna Leaf occurs as a light yellow to light grayish yellow-green powder. It has a slight odor and a bitter taste.

Under a microscope <*5.01*>, Powdered Senna Leaf reveals fragments of vessels and vein tissue accompanied with crystal cell rows; fragments of thick-walled, bent, unicellular hairs; fragments of palisade and spongy tissue; clustered and solitary crystals of calcium oxalate, 10 to 20 μm in diameter.

Identification **(1)** Macerate 0.5 g of Powdered Senna Leaf in 10 mL of diethyl ether for 2 minutes, and filter. Add 5 mL of ammonia TS to the filtrate: a yellow-red color is produced in the aqueous layer. To the residue of maceration add 10 mL of water, and macerate for 2 minutes. Filter, and add 5 mL of ammonia TS: a yellow-red color is produced in the aqueous layer.

(2) To 2 g of Powdered Senna Leaf add 40 mL of a mixture of tetrahydrofuran and water (7:3), shake for 30 minutes, and centrifuge. Transfer the supernatant liquid to a separator, add 13 g of sodium chloride, and shake for 30 minutes. Separate the aqueous layer with undissolved sodium chloride, and adjust to pH 1.5 with 1 mol/L hydrochloric acid TS. Transfer this solution to another separator, shake with 30 mL of tetrahydrofuran for 10 minutes, separate the tetrahydrofuran layer, and use the tetrahydrofuran layer as the sample solution. Separately, dissolve 1 mg of Sennoside A RS or sennoside A for thin-layer chromatography in 1 mL of a mixture of tetrahydrofuran and water (7:3), and use this solution as the standard solution. Perform the test with these solutions as directed under Thin-layer Chromatography <*2.03*>. Spot 10 μL each of the sample solution and standard solutions on a plate of silica gel for thin-layer chromatography. Develop the plate with a mixture of 1-propanol, ethyl acetate, water and acetic acid (100) (40:40:30:1) to a distance of about 7 cm, and air-dry the plate. Examine under ultraviolet light (main wavelength: 365 nm): one of the several spots obtained from the sample solution has the same color tone and *Rf* value with the red fluorescent spot from the standard solution.

Purity **(1)** Foreign matter <*5.01*>—Under a microscope, stone cells and thick fibers are not observable.

(2) Total BHC's and total DDT's <*5.01*>—Not more than 0.2 ppm, respectively.

Loss on drying <*5.01*> Not more than 12.0% (6 hours).

Total ash <*5.01*> Not more than 12.0%.

Acid-insoluble ash <*5.01*> Not more than 2.0%.

Assay Weigh accurately about 0.5 g of Powdered Senna Leaf in a glass-stoppered centrifuge tube, add 25 mL of diluted methanol (7 in 10), shake for 30 minutes, centrifuge, and separate the supernatant liquid. To the residue add 10 mL of diluted methanol (7 in 10), shake for 10 minutes, centrifuge, and separate the supernatant liquid. Repeat this procedure once more, combine all the extracts, add diluted methanol (7 in 10) to make exactly 50 mL, and use this solution as the sample solution. Separately, weigh accurately about 10 mg of Sennoside A RS (separately determine the water <*2.48*> by coulometric titration, using 10 mg), dissolve in a solution of sodium hydrogen carbonate (1 in 100) to make exactly 20 mL, and use this solution as standard stock solution (1). Weigh accurately about 10 mg of Sennoside B RS (separately determine the water <*2.48*> by coulometric titration, using 10 mg), dissolve in a solution of sodium hydrogen carbonate (1 in 100) to make exactly 20 mL, and use this solution as standard stock solution (2). Pipet 5 mL of the standard stock solution (1) and 10 mL of the standard stock solution (2), add methanol to make exactly 50 mL, and use this solution as the standard solution. Perform the test with exactly 10 μL each of the sample solution and standard solution as directed under Liquid Chromatography <*2.01*> according to the following conditions. Determine the peak areas, A_{Ta} and A_{Sa}, of sennoside A, and the peak areas, A_{Tb} and A_{Sb}, of sennoside B in each solution, calculate the amounts of sennoside A and sennoside B by the following equations, and designate the total as the amount of total sennoside.

$$\text{Amount (mg) of sennoside A } (C_{42}H_{38}O_{20}) = M_{Sa} \times A_{Ta}/A_{Sa} \times 1/4$$

$$\text{Amount (mg) of sennoside B } (C_{42}H_{38}O_{20}) = M_{Sb} \times A_{Tb}/A_{Sb} \times 1/2$$

M_{Sa}: Amount (mg) of Sennoside A RS taken, calculated on the anhydrous basis

M_{Sb}: Amount (mg) of Sennoside B RS taken, calculated on the anhydrous basis

Operating conditions—

Detector: An ultraviolet absorption photometer (wavelength: 340 nm).

Column: A stainless steel column 4.6 mm in inside diameter and 15 cm in length, packed with octadecylsilanized silica gel for liquid chromatography (5 μm in particle diameter).

Column temperature: A constant temperature of about 50°C.

Mobile phase: Dissolve 2.45 g of tetra-*n*-heptylammonium bromide in 1000 mL of a mixture of diluted 1 mol/L acetic acid-sodium acetate buffer solution (pH 5.0) (1 in 10) and acetonitrile (17:8).

Flow rate: Adjust so that the retention time of sennoside A is about 26 minutes.

System suitability—

System performance: When the procedure is run with 10 μL of the standard solution under the above operating conditions, sennoside B and sennoside A are eluted in this order with the resolution between these peaks being not less than 15, and the number of theoretical plates of the peak of sennoside A being not less than 8000.

System repeatability: When the test is repeated 6 times with 10 μL of the standard solution under the above operating conditions, the relative standard deviation of the peak area of sennoside A is not more than 1.5%.

Containers and storage Containers—Well-closed containers.

Sesame

Sesami Semen

ゴマ

Sesame is the seed of *Sesamum indicum* Linné (*Pedaliaceae*).

Description Ovate to spatulate seed, 3 – 4 mm in length, about 2 mm in width, about 1 mm in thickness; externally dark brown to black, rarely light brown to brown. Under a magnifying glass, thin ridges are observed on edges. 100 seeds weigh about 0.2 – 0.3 g.

Odorless; taste, slightly sweet and oily.

Under a microscope 〈*5.01*〉, transverse section reveals a seed coat consisting of palisade epidermis and flattened parenchyma; in the interior, endosperm and cotyledon; epidermal cells contain orbicular crystals of calcium oxalate and black pigment; parenchymatous cells of endosperm and cotyledon contain oil drops and aleurone grains.

Identification Grind a suitable amount of Sesame. To 1.0 g of the ground add 10 mL of methanol, shake for 10 minutes, centrifuge, and use the supernatant liquid as the sample solution. Separately, dissolve 1 mg of sesamin for thin-layer chromatography in 5 mL of methanol, and use this solution as the standard solution. Perform the test with these solutions as directed under Thin-layer Chromatography 〈*2.03*〉. Spot 5 μL each of the sample solution and standard solution on a plate of silica gel for thin-layer chromatography. Develop the plate with a mixture of hexane, ethyl acetate and acetic acid (100) (10:5:1) to a distance of about 7 cm, and air-dry the plate. Spray evenly dilute sulfuric acid on the plate, and heat the plate at 105°C for 5 minutes: one of the several spots obtained from the sample solution has the same color tone and *Rf* value with the spot from the standard solution.

Total ash 〈*5.01*〉 Not more than 6.0%.

Acid-insoluble ash 〈*5.01*〉 Not more than 0.5%.

Containers and storage Containers—Well-closed containers.

Sesame Oil

Oleum Sesami

ゴマ油

Sesame Oil is the fixed oil obtained from the seeds of *Sesamum indicum* Linné (*Pedaliaceae*).

Description Sesame Oil is a clear, pale yellow oil. It is odorless or has a faint, characteristic odor, and has a bland taste.

It is miscible with diethyl ether and with petroleum ether.

It is slightly soluble in ethanol (95).

It congeals between 0°C and −5°C.

Congealing point of the fatty acids: 20 – 25°C

Identification To 1 mL of Sesame Oil add 0.1 g of sucrose and 10 mL of hydrochloric acid, and shake for 30 seconds: the acid layer becomes light red and changes to red on standing.

Specific gravity 〈*1.13*〉 d_{25}^{25}: 0.914 – 0.921

Acid value 〈*1.13*〉 Not more than 0.2.

Saponification value 〈*1.13*〉 187 – 194

Unsaponifiable matters 〈*1.13*〉 Not more than 2.0%.

Iodine value 〈*1.13*〉 103 – 118

Containers and storage Containers—Tight containers.

Shakuyakukanzoto Extract

芍薬甘草湯エキス

Shakuyakukanzoto Extract contains not less than 50 mg and not more than 150 mg of paeoniflorin ($C_{23}H_{28}O_{11}$: 480.46), and not less than 40 mg and not more than 120 mg of glycyrrhizic acid ($C_{42}H_{62}O_{16}$: 822.93), per extract prepared with the amount specified in the Method of preparation.

Method of preparation

	1)	2)
Peony Root	6 g	5 g
Glycyrrhiza	6 g	5 g

Prepare a dry extract or viscous extract as directed under Extracts, according to the prescription 1) or 2), using the crude drugs shown above.

Description Shakuyakukanzoto Extract occurs as a light brown powder or brown viscous extract. It has slightly an odor, and a sweet taste.

Identification (1) Shake 0.5 g of the dry extract (or 1.5 g of the viscous extract) with 10 mL of water, then add 10 mL of 1-butanol, shake, centrifuge, and use the 1-butanol layer as the sample solution. Separately, dissolve 1 mg of Paeoniflorin RS or paeoniflorin for thin-layer chromatography in 1 mL of methanol, and use this solution as the standard solution. Perform the test with these solutions as directed under Thin-layer Chromatography 〈*2.03*〉. Spot 5 μL each of the sample solution and standard solution on a plate of silica gel for thin-layer chromatography. Develop the plate with a mixture of ethyl acetate, methanol and water (20:3:2) to a distance of about 7 cm, and air-dry the plate. Spray evenly 4-methoxybenzaldehyde-sulfuric acid TS on the plate, and heat the plate at 105°C for 5 minutes: one of the several spots obtained from the sample solution has the same color tone and *R*f value with the purple spot from the standard solution (Peony Root).

(2) Shake 0.5 g of the dry extract (or 1.5 g of the viscous extract) with 10 mL of water, then add 10 mL of 1-butanol, shake, centrifuge, and use the 1-butanol layer as the sample solution. Separately, dissolve 1 mg of liquiritin for thin-layer chromatography in 1 mL of methanol, and use this solution as the standard solution. Perform the test with these solutions as directed under Thin-layer Chromatography *<2.03>*. Spot 1 μL each of the sample solution and standard solution on a plate of silica gel for thin-layer chromatography. Develop the plate with a mixture of ethyl acetate, methanol and water (20:3:2) to a distance of about 7 cm, and air-dry the plate. Spray evenly dilute sulfuric acid on the plate, heat the plate at 105°C for 5 minutes, and examine under ultraviolet light (main wavelength: 365 nm): one of the several spots obtained from the sample solution has the same color tone and *R*f value with the yellow-green fluorescent spot from the standard solution (Glycyrrhiza).

Purity **(1)** Heavy metals *<1.07>*—Prepare the test solution with 1.0 g of the dry extract (or an amount of the viscous extract, equivalent to 1.0 g of dried substance) as directed under Extracts (4), and perform the test (not more than 30 ppm).

(2) Arsenic *<1.11>*—Prepare the test solution with 1.0 g of the dry extract (or an amount of the viscous extract, equivalent to 1.0 g of dried substance) according to Method 3, and perform the test (not more than 2 ppm).

Loss on drying *<2.41>* The dry extract: Not more than 8.0% (1 g, 105°C, 5 hours).

The viscous extract: Not more than 66.7% (1 g, 105°C, 5 hours).

Total ash *<5.01>* Not more than 9.0%, calculated on the dried basis.

Assay **(1)** Paeoniflorin—Weigh accurately about 0.2 g of the dry extract (or an amount of the viscous extract, equivalent to 0.2 g of dried substance), add exactly 50 mL of diluted methanol (1 in 2), shake for 15 minutes, filter, and use the filtrate as the sample solution. Separately, weigh accurately about 10 mg of Paeoniflorin RS (separately determine the water *<2.48>* by coulometric titration, using 10 mg), dissolve in diluted methanol (1 in 2) to make exactly 100 mL, and use this solution as the standard solution. Perform the test with exactly 10 μL each of the sample solution and standard solution as directed under Liquid Chromatography *<2.01>* according to the following conditions, and determine the peak areas, A_T and A_S, of paeoniflorin in each solution.

$$\text{Amount (mg) of paeoniflorin } (C_{23}H_{28}O_{11}) = M_S \times A_T/A_S \times 1/2$$

M_S: Amount (mg) of Paeoniflorin RS taken, calculated on the anhydrous basis

Operating conditions—

Detector: An ultraviolet absorption photometer (wavelength: 232 nm).

Column: A stainless steel column 4.6 mm in inside diameter and 15 cm in length, packed with octadecylsilanized silica gel for liquid chromatography (5 μm in particle diameter).

Column temperature: A constant temperature of about 20°C.

Mobile phase: A mixture of water, acetonitrile and phosphoric acid (850:150:1).

Flow rate: 1.0 mL per minute (the retention time of paeoniflorin is about 9 minutes).

System suitability—

System performance: Dissolve 1 mg each of Paeoniflorin RS and albiflorin in diluted methanol (1 in 2) to make 10 mL. When the procedure is run with 10 μL of this solution under the above operating conditions, albiflorin and paeoniflorin are eluted in this order with the resolution between these peaks being not less than 2.5.

System repeatability: When the test is repeated 6 times with 10 μL of the standard solution under the above operating conditions, the relative standard deviation of the peak area of paeoniflorin is not more than 1.5%.

(2) Glycyrrhizic acid—Weigh accurately about 0.2 g of the dry extract (or an amount of the viscous extract, equivalent to about 0.2 g of the dried substance), add exactly 50 mL of diluted methanol (1 in 2), shake for 15 minutes, filter, and use the filtrate as the sample solution. Separately, weigh accurately about 10 mg of Glycyrrhizic Acid RS (separately determine the water *<2.48>* by coulometric titration, using 10 mg), dissolve in diluted methanol (1 in 2) to make exactly 100 mL, and use this solution as the standard solution. Perform the test with exactly 10 μL each of the sample solution and standard solution as directed under Liquid Chromatography *<2.01>* according to the following conditions, and determine the peak areas, A_T and A_S, of glycyrrhizic acid in each solution.

$$\text{Amount (mg) of glycyrrhizic acid } (C_{42}H_{62}O_{16}) = M_S \times A_T/A_S \times 1/2$$

M_S: Amount (mg) of Glycyrrhizic Acid RS taken, calculated on the anhydrous basis

Operating conditions—

Detector: An ultraviolet absorption photometer (wavelength: 254 nm).

Column: A stainless steel column 4.6 mm in inside diameter and 15 cm in length, packed with octadecylsilanized silica gel for liquid chromatography (5 μm in particle diameter).

Column temperature: A constant temperature of about 40°C.

Mobile phase: Dissolve 3.85 g of ammonium acetate in 720 mL of water, and add 5 mL of acetic acid (100) and 280 mL of acetonitrile.

Flow rate: 1.0 mL per minute (the retention time of glycyrrhizic acid is about 15 minutes).

System suitability—

System performance: Dissolve 5 mg of monoammonium glycyrrhizinate for resolution check in 20 mL of dilute ethanol. When the procedure is run with 10 μL of this solution under the above operating conditions, the resolution between the peak having the relative retention time of about 0.9 to glycyrrhizic acid and the peak of glycyrrhizic acid is not less than 1.5.

System repeatability: When the test is repeated 6 times with 10 μL of the standard solution under the above operating conditions, the relative standard deviation of the peak area of glycyrrhizic acid is not more than 1.5%.

Containers and storage Containers—Tight containers.

Shimbuto Extract

真武湯エキス

Shimbuto Extract contains not less than 26 mg and not more than 78 mg of paeoniflorin ($C_{23}H_{28}O_{11}$: 480.46), not less than 0.5 mg and not more than 2.0 mg (for preparation prescribed 0.8 g of Ginger) or not less than 0.6 mg and not more than 2.4 mg (for preparation prescribed 1 g of Ginger) or not less than 0.9 mg and not more than 3.6 mg (for preparation prescribed 1.5 g of Ginger) of [6]-gingerol, and not less than 0.7 mg (for preparation prescribed 1 g of Processed Aconite Root 1) of total alkaloids (as benzoylmesaconine hydrochloride and 14-anisoylaconine hydrochloride) or not less than 0.2 mg (for preparation prescribed 1 g of Powdered Processed Aconite Root 1) of total alkaloids (as benzoylmesaconine hydrochloride and 14-anisoylaconine hydrochloride, or as benzoylmesaconine hydrochloride and benzoylhypaconine hydrochloride) or not less than 0.1 mg (for preparation prescribed 1 g of Powdered Processed Aconite Root 2) of total alkaloids (as benzoylmesaconine hydrochloride and 14-benzoylhypacomine hydrochloride) or not less than 0.1 mg (for preparation prescribed 0.5 g of Powdered Processed Aconite Root 1) of total alkaloids (as benzoylmesaconine hydrochloride and 14-anisoylaconine hydrochloride, or as benzoylmesaconine hydrochloride and benzoylhypaconine hydrochloride), per extract prepared with the amount specified in the Method of preparation.

Method of preparation

	1)	2)	3)	4)
Poria Sclerotium	5 g	5 g	5 g	4 g
Peony Root	3 g	3 g	3 g	3 g
Atractylodes Rhizome	3 g	—	3 g	—
Atractylodes Lancea Rhizome	—	3 g	—	3 g
Ginger	1 g	1 g	0.8 g	1.5 g
Processed Aconite Root (Processed Aconite Root 1)	1 g	—	—	—
Powdered Processed Aconite Root (Powdered Processed Aconite Root 1)	—	1 g	—	0.5 g
Powdered Processed Aconite Root (Powdered Processed Aconite Root 2)	—	—	1 g	—

Prepare a dry extract as directed under Extracts, according to the prescription 1) to 4), using the crude drugs shown above.

Description Shimbuto Extract occurs as light yellow-brown to brown powder. It has a characteristic odor and a hot and bitter taste.

Identification (1) To 2.0 g of Shimbuto Extract, add 10 mL of water, shake, then add 5 mL of 1-butanol, shake, centrifuge, and use the 1-butanol layer as the sample solution. Separately, dissolve 1 mg of Paeoniflorin RS or paeoniflorin for thin-layer chromatography in 1 mL of methanol, and use this solution as the standard solution. Perform the test with these solutions as directed under Thin-layer Chromatography <*2.03*>. Spot 5 μL each of the sample solution and standard solution on a plate of silica gel for thin-layer chromatography. Develop the plate with a mixture of ethyl acetate, methanol and water (20:3:2) to a distance of about 7 cm, and air-dry the plate. Spray evenly 4-methoxybenzaldehyde-sulfuric acid TS on the plate, and heat the plate at 105°C for 5 minutes: one of the several spots obtained from the sample solution has the same color tone and *R*f value with the purple spot from the standard solution (Peony Root).

(2) For preparation prescribed Atractylodes Rhizome—To 1.0 g of Shimbuto Extract, add 10 mL of water, shake, then add 25 mL of diethyl ether, and shake. Separate the diethyl ether layer, evaporate the solvent under low pressure (in vacuo), add 2 mL of diethyl ether to the residue, and use this solution as the sample solution. Separately, dissolve 1 mg of atractylenolide III for thin-layer chromatography in 2 mL of methanol, and use this solution as the standard solution. Perform the test with these solutions as directed under Thin-layer Chromatography <*2.03*>. Spot 5 μL each of the sample solution and standard solution on a plate of silica gel for thin-layer chromatography. Develop the plate with a mixture of ethyl acetate and hexane (1:1) to a distance of about 7 cm, and air-dry the plate. Spray evenly diluted sulfuric acid on the plate, heat the plate at 105°C for 5 minutes, and examine under ultraviolet light (main wavelength: 365 nm): one of the several spots obtained from the sample solution has the same color tone and *R*f value with the blue-white fluorescent spot from the standard solution (Atractylodes Rhizome).

(3) For preparation prescribed Atractylodes Lancea Rhizome—To 2.0 g of Shimbuto Extract, add 10 mL of water, shake, then add 25 mL of hexane, and shake. Separate the hexane layer, evaporate the solvent under low pressure (in vacuo), add 2 mL of hexane to the residue, and use this solution as the sample solution. Perform the test with the sample solution as directed under Thin-layer Chromatography <*2.03*>. Spot 20 μL of the sample solution on a plate of silica gel with fluorescent indicator for thin-layer chromatography. Develop the plate with a mixture of hexane and acetone (7:1) to a distance of about 7 cm, and air-dry the plate. Examine under ultraviolet light (main wavelength: 254 nm): a dark purple spot is observed at an *R*f value of about 0.5. The spot shows a greenish brown color after being sprayed evenly 4-dimethylaminobenzaldehyde TS for spraying, heated at 105°C for 5 minutes, and allowed to cool (Atractylodes Lancea Rhizome).

(4) To 1.0 g of Shimbuto Extract, add 10 mL of water, shake, then add 25 mL of diethyl ether, and shake. Separate the diethyl ether layer, evaporate the solvent under low pressure (in vacuo), add 2 mL of diethyl ether to the residue, and use this solution as the sample solution. Separately, dissolve 1 mg of [6]-gingerol for thin-layer chromatography in 1 mL of methanol, and use this solution as the standard solution. Perform the test with these solutions as directed under Thin-layer Chromatography <*2.03*>. Spot 10 μL of the sample solution and 5 μL of the standard solution on a plate of silica gel for thin-layer chromatography. Develop the plate with a mixture of ethyl acetate and hexane (1:1) to a distance of about 7 cm, and air-dry the plate. Spray evenly 4-dimethylaminobenzaldehyde TS for spraying on the plate, heat the plate at 105°C for 5 minutes, allow to cool, and spray water: one of the several spots obtained from the sample solution has the same color tone and *R*f value with the blue-green to grayish green spot from the standard solution (Ginger).

(5) To 3.0 g of Shimbuto Extract, add 20 mL of diethyl ether and 2 mL of ammonia TS, shake for 10 minutes, centrifuge, and take the diethyl ether layer. Evaporate the solvent under low pressure (in vacuo), add 1 mL of acetonitrile to the residue, and use this solution as the sample solution. Separately, dissolve 1 mg of benzoylmesaconine hydrochloride for thin-layer chromatography in 10 mL of ethanol (99.5), and use this solution as the standard solution. Perform the test with these solutions as directed under Thin-layer Chromatography <*2.03*>. Spot 20 μL of the sample solution and 10 μL of the standard solution on a plate of silica gel for thin-layer chromatography. Develop the plate with a mixture of 1-butanol, water and acetic acid (100) (4:2:1) to a distance of about 7 cm, and air-dry the plate. Spray evenly Dragendorff's TS for spraying on the plate, and air-dry the plate. Then spray evenly sodium nitrite TS on the plate: one of the several spots obtained from the sample solution has the same color tone and *Rf* value with the yellow-brown spot from the standard solution (Processed Aconite Root or Powdered Processed Aconite Root).

Purity **(1)** Heavy metals <*1.07*>—Prepare the test solution with 1.0 g of Shimbuto Extract as directed in the Extracts (4), and perform the test (not more than 30 ppm).

(2) Arsenic <*1.11*>—Prepare the test solution with 0.67 g of Shimbuto Extract according to Method 3, and perform the test (not more than 3 ppm).

(3) Aconitum diester alkaloids (aconitine, jesaconitine, hypaconitine and mesaconitine)—Weigh accurately 1.0 g of Shimbuto Extract, add 20 mL of diethyl ether, shake, then add 3.0 mL of 0.1 mol/L hydrochloric acid TS and shake for 10 minutes. Centrifuge this solution, remove the diethyl ether layer, then add 20 mL of diethyl ether, proceed in the same manner as described above, and remove the diethyl ether layer. To the aqueous layer, add 1.0 mL of ammonia TS and 20 mL of diethyl ether, shake for 30 minutes, centrifuge, and take the diethyl ether layer. To the aqueous layer, add 1.0 mL of ammonia TS and 20 mL of diethyl ether, proceed in the same manner, and repeat the procedure twice. Combine all the extracts, and evaporate the solvent under low pressure (in vacuo). Dissolve the residue with exactly 10 mL of a mixture of phosphate buffer solution for processed aconite root and acetonitrile (1:1). Centrifuge this solution, and use the supernatant liquid as the sample solution. Separately, pipet 1 mL of aconitum diester alkaloids standard solution for purity, add a mixture of phosphate buffer solution for processed aconite root and acetonitrile (1:1) to make exactly 10 mL, and use this solution as the standard solution. Perform the test with exactly 40 μL each of the sample solution and standard solution as directed under Liquid Chromatography <*2.01*> according to the following conditions: the heights of the peaks corresponding to aconitine, jesaconitine, hypaconitine and mesaconitine from the sample solution are not higher than the respective heights corresponding to aconitine, jesaconitine, hypaconitine and mesaconitine from the standard solution.

Operating conditions—

Detector: An ultraviolet absorption photometer (wavelength: 231 nm for aconitine, hypaconitine and mesaconitine; 254 nm for jesaconitine).

Column: A stainless steel column 4.6 mm in inside diameter and 15 cm in length, packed with octadecylsilanized silica gel for liquid chromatography (5 μm in particle diameter).

Column temperature: A constant temperature of about 40°C.

Mobile phase: A mixture of phosphate buffer for processed aconite root and tetrahydrofuran (183:17).

Flow rate: 1.0 mL per minute (the retention time of mesaconitine is about 31 minutes).

System suitability—

System performance: When the procedure is run with 20 μL of aconitum diester alkaloids standard solution for purity under the above operating conditions, using 254 nm, mesaconitine, hypaconitine, aconitine and jesaconitine are eluted in this order, and each resolution between these peaks is not less than 1.5, respectively.

System repeatability: When the test is repeated 6 times with 20 μL of the standard solution under the above operating conditions, using 231 nm, the relative standard deviation of the peak height of mesaconitine is not more than 1.5%.

Loss on drying <*2.41*> Not more than 7.0% (1 g, 105°C, 5 hours).

Total ash <*5.01*> Not more than 10.0%.

Assay **(1)** Paeoniflorin—Weigh accurately about 0.5 g of Shimbuto Extract, add exactly 50 mL of diluted methanol (1 in 2), shake for 15 minutes, filter, and use the filtrate as the sample solution. Separately, weigh accurately about 10 mg of Paeoniflorin RS (separately determine the water <*2.48*> by coulometric titration, using 10 mg), and dissolve in diluted methanol (1 in 2) to make exactly 100 mL, and use this solution as the standard solution. Perform the test with exactly 10 μL each of the sample solution and standard solution as directed under Liquid Chromatography <*2.01*> according to the following conditions, and determine the peak areas, A_T and A_S, of paeoniflorin in each solution.

$$\text{Amount (mg) of paeoniflorin } (C_{23}H_{28}O_{11}) = M_S \times A_T/A_S \times 1/2$$

M_S: Amount (mg) of Paeoniflorin RS taken, calculated on the anhydrous basis

Operating conditions—

Detector: An ultraviolet absorption photometer (wavelength: 232 nm).

Column: A stainless steel column 4.6 mm in inside diameter and 15 cm in length, packed with octadecylsilanized silica gel for liquid chromatography (5 μm in particle diameter).

Column temperature: A constant temperature of about 20°C.

Mobile phase: A mixture of water, acetonitrile and phosphoric acid (850:150:1).

Flow rate: 1.0 mL per minute (the retention time of paeoniflorin is about 9 minutes).

System suitability—

System performance: Dissolve 1 mg each of Paeoniflorin RS and albiflorin in diluted methanol (1 in 2) to make 10 mL. When the procedure is run with 10 μL of this solution under the above operating conditions, albiflorin and paeoniflorin are eluted in this order with the resolution between these peaks being not less than 2.5.

System repeatability: When the test is repeated 6 times with 10 μL of the standard solution under the above operating conditions, the relative standard deviation of the peak area of paeoniflorin is not more than 1.5%.

(2) [6]-gingerol—Weigh accurately about 0.5 g of Shimbuto Extract, add exactly 50 mL of diluted methanol (7 in 10), shake for 15 minutes, filter, and use the filtrate as the sample solution. Separately, weigh accurately about 10 mg of [6]-gingerol for assay, dissolve in diluted methanol to make exactly 100 mL. Pipet 5 mL of this solution, add methanol to make exactly 50 mL, and use this solution as the standard solution. Perform the test with exactly 10 μL each of the sample solution and standard solution as directed under Liquid Chromatography <*2.01*> according to the following conditions, and determine the peak areas, A_T and A_S, of [6]-gingerol in each solution.

Amount (mg) of [6]-gingerol = $M_S \times A_T/A_S \times 1/20$

M_S: Amount (mg) of [6]-gingerol for assay taken

Operating conditions—

Detector: An ultraviolet absorption photometer (wavelength: 282 nm).

Column: A stainless steel column 4.6 mm in inside diameter and 15 cm in length, packed with octadecylsilanized silica gel for liquid chromatography (5 μm in particle diameter).

Column temperature: A constant temperature of about 30°C.

Mobile phase: A mixture of water, acetonitrile and phosphoric acid (620:380:1).

Flow rate: 1.0 mL per minute (the retention time of [6]-gingerol is about 15 minutes).

System suitability—

System performance: When the procedure is run with 10 μL of the standard solution under the above operating conditions, the number of theoretical plates and the symmetry factor of the peak of [6]-gingerol are not less than 5000 and not more than 1.5, respectively.

System repeatability: When the test is repeated 6 times with 10 μL of the standard solution under the above operating conditions, the relative standard deviation of the peak area of [6]-gingerol is not more than 1.5%.

(3) Total alkaloids—Weigh accurately about 1 g of Shimbuto Extract, add 20 mL of diethyl ether, shake, then add 3.0 mL of 0.1 mol/L hydrochloric acid TS, and shake for 10 minutes. Centrifuge this solution, remove the diethyl ether layer, then add 20 mL of diethyl ether, proceed in the same manner as described above, and remove the diethyl ether layer. To the aqueous layer, add 1.0 mL of ammonia TS and 20 mL of diethyl ether, shake for 30 minutes, centrifuge, and take the diethyl ether layer. To the aqueous layer, add 1.0 mL of ammonia TS and 20 mL of diethyl ether, and repeat the above process twice more. Combine all the extracts, and evaporate the solvent under low pressure (in vacuo). Dissolve the residue with a mixture of phosphate buffer solution for processed aconite root and acetonitrile (1:1) to make exactly 10 mL. Centrifuge this solution, and use the supernatant liquid as the sample solution. Perform the test with exactly 20 μL each of the sample solution and the aconitum monoester alkaloids standard solution TS for assay as directed under Liquid Chromatography <2.01> according to the following conditions. Determine the peak areas of benzoylmesaconine, benzoylhypaconine and 14-anisoylaconine, A_{TM} and A_{SM}, A_{TH} and A_{SH}, as well as A_{TA} and A_{SA}, in each solution, respectively.

Amount (mg) of benzoylmesaconine hydrochloride
$= C_{SM} \times A_{TM}/A_{SM} \times 10$

Amount (mg) of benzoylhypaconine hydrochloride
$= C_{SH} \times A_{TH}/A_{SH} \times 10$

Amount (mg) of 14-anisoylaconine hydrochloride
$= C_{SA} \times A_{TA}/A_{SA} \times 10$

C_{SM}: Concentration (mg/mL) of benzoylmesaconine hydrochloride for assay in aconitum monoester alkaloids standard solution TS for assay

C_{SH}: Concentration (mg/mL) of benzoylhypaconine hydrochloride for assay in aconitum monoester alkaloids standard solution TS for assay

C_{SA}: Concentration (mg/mL) of 14-anisoylaconine hydrochloride for assay in aconitum monoester alkaloids standard solution TS for assay

Operating conditions—

Detector: An ultraviolet absorption photometer (wavelength: 231 nm for benzoylmesaconine and benzoylhypaconine; 254 nm for 14-anisoylaconine).

Column: A stainless steel column 4.6 mm in inside diameter and 15 cm in length, packed with octadecylsilanized silica gel for liquid chromatography (5 μm in particle diameter).

Column temperature: A constant temperature of about 40°C.

Mobile phase: A mixture of phosphate buffer solution for processed aconite root and tetrahydrofuran (183:17).

Flow rate: 1.0 mL per minute (the retention time of benzoylmesaconine is about 15 minutes).

System suitability—

System performance: When the procedure is run with 20 μL of the aconitum monoester alkaloids standard solution TS for assay under the above operating conditions, the number of theoretical plates and the symmetry factor of the peak of benzoylmesaconine are not less than 5000 and not more than 1.5, respectively.

System repeatability: When the test is repeated 6 times with 20 μL of the aconitum monoester alkaloids standard solution TS for assay under the above operating conditions, the relative standard deviation of the peak areas of benzoylmesaconine, benzoylhypaconine and 14-anisoylaconine is not more than 1.5%.

Containers and storage Containers—Tight containers.

Shosaikoto Extract

小柴胡湯エキス

Shosaikoto Extract contains not less than 2 mg and not more than 8 mg of saikosaponin b_2, not less than 80 mg and not more than 240 mg of baicalin ($C_{21}H_{18}O_{11}$: 446.36), and not less than 14 mg and not more than 42 mg of glycyrrhizic acid ($C_{42}H_{62}O_{16}$: 822.93), per extract prepared with the amount specified in the Method of preparation.

Method of preparation

	1)	2)
Bupleurum Root	7 g	6 g
Pinellia Tuber	5 g	5 g
Ginger	1 g	1 g
Scutellaria Root	3 g	3 g
Jujube	3 g	3 g
Ginseng	3 g	3 g
Glycyrrhiza	2 g	2 g

Prepare a dry extract or viscous extract as directed under Extracts, according to the prescription 1) or 2), using the crude drugs shown above.

Description Shosaikoto Extract occurs as a light brown to grayish brown powder or black-grayish brown viscous extract. It has a slight odor, and a sweet first then slightly pungent and bitter taste.

Identification **(1)** Shake 2.0 g of the dry extract (or 6.0 g of the viscous extract) with 10 mL of sodium hydroxide TS, then add 5 mL of 1-butanol, shake, centrifuge, and use the 1-butanol layer as the sample solution. Separately, dissolve 1 mg of saikosaponin b_2 for thin-layer chromatography in 1 mL of methanol, and use this solution as the standard solution. Perform the test with these solutions as directed under Thin-layer Chromatography <*2.03*>. Spot 10 μL of the sample solution and 2 μL of the standard solution on a plate of silica gel for thin-layer chromatography. Develop the plate with a mixture of ethyl acetate, ethanol (99.5) and water (8:2:1) to a distance of about 7 cm, and air-dry the plate. Spray evenly 4-dimethylaminobenzaldehyde TS for spraying on the plate, heat the plate at 105°C for 5 minutes, and examine under ultraviolet light (main wavelength: 365 nm): one of the several spots obtained from the sample solution has the same color tone and *R*f value with the yellow fluorescent spot from the standard solution (Bupleurum Root).

(2) Shake 1.0 g of the dry extract (or 3.0 g of the viscous extract) with 10 mL of water, then add 25 mL of diethyl ether, and shake. Separate the diethyl ether layer, evaporate the solvent under low pressure (in vacuo), add 2 mL of diethyl ether to the residue, and use this solution as the sample solution. Separately, dissolve 1 mg of [6]-gingerol for thin-layer chromatography in 1 mL of methanol, and use this solution as the standard solution. Perform the test with these solutions as directed under Thin-layer Chromatography <*2.03*>. Spot 15 μL of the sample solution and 5 μL of the standard solution on a plate of silica gel for thin-layer chromatography. Develop the plate with a mixture of ethyl acetate and hexane (1:1) to a distance of about 7 cm, and air-dry the plate. Spray evenly 4-dimethylaminobenzaldehyde TS for spraying on the plate, heat the plate at 105°C for 5 minutes, allow to cool, and spray water: one of the several spots obtained from the sample solution has the same color tone and *R*f value with the blue-green to grayish green spot from the standard solution (Ginger).

(3) Shake 1.0 g of the dry extract (or 3.0 g of the viscous extract) with 10 mL of water, then add 25 mL of diethyl ether, and shake. Separate the diethyl ether layer, evaporate the solvent under low pressure (in vacuo), add 2 mL of diethyl ether to the residue, and use this solution as the sample solution. Separately, dissolve 1 mg of wogonin for thin-layer chromatography in 1 mL of methanol, and use this solution as the standard solution. Perform the test with these solutions as directed under Thin-layer Chromatography <*2.03*>. Spot 20 μL of the sample solution and 2 μL of the standard solution on a plate of silica gel for thin-layer chromatography. Develop the plate with a mixture of ethyl acetate, hexane and acetic acid (100) (10:10:1) to a distance of about 7 cm, air-dry the plate. Spray evenly iron (III) chloride-methanol TS on the plate: one of the several spots obtained from the sample solution has the same color tone and *R*f value with the yellow-brown spot from the standard solution (Scutellaria Root).

(4) Shake 2.0 g of the dry extract (or 6.0 g of the viscous extract) with 10 mL of sodium hydroxide TS, then add 5 mL of 1-butanol, shake, centrifuge, and use the 1-butanol layer as the sample solution. Separately, dissolve 1 mg of Ginsenoside Rb_1 RS or ginsenoside Rb_1 for thin-layer chromatography in 1 mL of methanol, and use this solution as the standard solution. Perform the test with these solutions as directed under Thin-layer Chromatography <*2.03*>. Spot 10 μL of the sample solution and 2 μL of the standard solution on a plate of silica gel for thin-layer chromatography. Develop the plate with a mixture of ethyl acetate, 1-propanol, water and acetic acid (100) (7:5:4:1) to a distance of about 7 cm, and air-dry the plate. Spray evenly vanillin-sulfuric acid-ethanol TS for spraying on the plate, heat the plate at 105°C for 5 minutes, and allow to cool: one of the several spots obtained from the sample solution has the same color tone and *R*f value with the blue-purple spot from the standard solution (Ginseng).

(5) Shake 2.0 g of the dry extract (or 6.0 g of the viscous extract) with 10 mL of water, then add 5 mL of 1-butanol, shake, centrifuge, and use the 1-butanol layer as the sample solution. Separately, dissolve 1 mg of liquiritin for thin-layer chromatography in 1 mL of methanol, and use this solution as the standard solution. Perform the test with these solutions as directed under Thin-layer Chromatography <*2.03*>. Spot 1 μL each of the sample solution and standard solution on a plate of silica gel for thin-layer chromatography. Develop the plate with a mixture of ethyl acetate, methanol and water (20:3:2) to a distance of about 7 cm, and air-dry the plate. Spray evenly dilute sulfuric acid on the plate, heat the plate at 105°C for 5 minutes, and examine under ultraviolet light (main wavelength: 365 nm): one of the several spots obtained from the sample solution has the same color tone and *R*f value with the yellow-green fluorescent spot from the standard solution (Glycyrrhiza).

Purity **(1)** Heavy metals <*1.07*>—Prepare the test solution with 1.0 g of the dry extract (or an amount of the viscous extract, equivalent to about 1.0 g of dried substance) as directed under Extracts (4), and perform the test (not more than 30 ppm).

(2) Arsenic <*1.11*>—Prepare the test solution with 0.67 g of the dry extract (or an amount of the viscous extract, equivalent to about 0.67 g of dried substance) according to Method 3, and perform the test (not more than 3 ppm).

Loss on drying <*2.41*> The dry extract: Not more than 10.0% (1 g, 105°C, 5 hours).

The viscous extract: Not more than 66.7% (1 g, 105°C, 5 hours).

Total ash <*5.01*> Not more than 10.0%, calculated on the dried basis.

Assay **(1)** Saikosaponin b_2—Weigh accurately about 0.5 g of the dry extract (or an amount of the viscous extract, equivalent to about 0.5 g of dried substance), add exactly 50 mL of diluted methanol (1 in 2), shake for 15 minutes, filter, and use the filtrate as the sample solution. Separaterly, use saikosaponin b_2 standard TS for assay as the standard solution. Perform the test with exactly 10 μL each of the sample solution and standard solution as directed under Liquid Chromatography <*2.01*> according to the following conditions, and determine the peak areas, A_T and A_S, of saikosaponin b_2 in each solution.

Amount (mg) of saikosaponin $b_2 = C_S \times A_T/A_S \times 50$

C_S: Concentration (mg/mL) of saikosaponin b_2 in saikosaponin b_2 standard TS for assay

Operating conditions—

Detector: An ultraviolet absorption photometer (wavelength: 254 nm).

Column: A stainless steel column 4.6 mm in inside diameter and 15 cm in length, packed with octadecylsilanized silica gel for liquid chromatography (5 μm in particle diameter).

Column temperature: A constant temperature of about 40°C.

Mobile phase: A mixture of 0.05 mol/L sodium dihydrogen phosphate TS and acetonitrile (5:3).

Flow rate: 1.0 mL per minute (the retention time of saikosaponin b_2 is about 12 minutes).

System suitability—

System performance: When the procedure is run with 10 μL of the standard solution under the above operating conditions, the number of theoretical plates and the symmetry factor of the peak of saikosaponin b_2 are not less than 5000

and not more than 1.5, respectively.

System repeatability: When the test is repeated 6 times with 10 μL of the standard solution under the above operating conditions, the relative standard deviation of the peak area of saikosaponin b_2 is not more than 1.5%.

(2) Baicalin—Weigh accurately about 0.1 g of the dry extract (or an amount of the viscous extract, equivalent to about 0.1 g of dried substance), add exactly 50 mL of diluted methanol (7 in 10), shake for 15 minutes, filter, and use the filtrate as the sample solution. Separately, weigh accurately about 10 mg of Baicalin RS (separately determine the water <*2.48*> by coulometric titration, using 10 mg), and dissolve in methanol to make exactly 100 mL. Pipet 5 mL of this solution, add diluted methanol (7 in 10) to make exactly 10 mL, and use this solution as the standard solution. Perform the test with exactly 10 μL each of the sample solution and standard solution as directed under Liquid Chromatography <*2.01*> according to the following conditions, and determine the peak areas, A_T and A_S, of baicalin in each solution.

$$\text{Amount (mg) of baicalin } (C_{21}H_{18}O_{11}) = M_S \times A_T/A_S \times 1/4$$

M_S: Amount (mg) of Baicalin RS taken, calculated on the anhydrous basis

Operating conditions—

Detector: An ultraviolet absorption photometer (wavelength: 277 nm).

Column: A stainless steel column 4.6 mm in inside diameter and 15 cm in length, packed with octadecylsilanized silica gel for liquid chromatography (5 μm in particle diameter).

Column temperature: A constant temperature of about 40°C.

Mobile phase: A mixture of diluted phosphoric acid (1 in 200) and acetonitrile (19:6).

Flow rate: 1.0 mL per minute (the retention time of baicalin is about 10 minutes).

System suitability—

System performance: When the procedure is run with 10 μL of the standard solution under the above operating conditions, the number of theoretical plates and the symmetry factor of the peak of baicalin are not less than 5000 and not more than 1.5, respectively.

System repeatability: When the test is repeated 6 times with 10 μL of the standard solution under the above operating conditions, the relative standard deviation of the peak area of baicalin is not more than 1.5%.

(3) Glycyrrhizic acid—Perform the test according to the following i) or ii).

i) Weigh accurately about 0.5 g of the dry extract (or an amount of the viscous extract, equivalent to about 0.5 g of dried substance), add exactly 50 mL of diluted methanol (1 in 2), shake for 15 minutes, filter, and use the filtrate as the sample solution. Separately, weigh accurately about 10 mg of Glycyrrhizic Acid RS (separately determine the water <*2.48*> by coulometric titration, using 10 mg), dissolve in diluted methanol (1 in 2) to make exactly 100 mL, and use this solution as the standard solution. Perform the test with exactly 10 μL each of the sample solution and standard solution as directed under Liquid Chromatography <*2.01*> according to the following conditions, and determine the peak areas, A_T and A_S, of glycyrrhizic acid in each solution.

$$\text{Amount (mg) of glycyrrhizic acid } (C_{42}H_{62}O_{16}) = M_S \times A_T/A_S \times 1/2$$

M_S: Amount (mg) of Glycyrrhizic Acid RS taken, calculated on the anhydrous basis

Operating conditions—

Detector: An ultraviolet absorption photometer (wavelength: 254 nm).

Column: A stainless steel column 4.6 mm in inside diameter and 15 cm in length, packed with octadecylsilanized silica gel for liquid chromatography (5 μm in particle diameter).

Column temperature: A constant temperature of about 40°C.

Mobile phase: Dissolve 3.85 g of ammonium acetate in 720 mL of water, and add 5 mL of acetic acid (100) and 280 mL of acetonitrile.

Flow rate: 1.0 mL per minute (the retention time of glycyrrhizic acid is about 15 minutes).

System suitability—

System performance: Dissolve 5 mg of monoammonium glycyrrhizinate for resolution check in 20 mL of dilute ethanol. When the procedure is run with 10 μL of this solution under the above operating conditions, the resolution between the peak having the relative retention time of about 0.9 to glycyrrhizic acid and the peak of glycyrrhizic acid is not less than 1.5. Dissolve 1 mg of baicalein for resolution check in 50 mL of methanol. To 2 mL of this solution add 2 mL of the standard solution. When the procedure is run with 10 μL of this solution under the above operating conditions, the resolution between the peaks of glycyrrhizic acid and baicalein is not less than 1.5.

System repeatability: When the test is repeated 6 times with 10 μL of the standard solution under the above operating conditions, the relative standard deviation of the peak area of glycyrrhizic acid is not more than 1.5%.

ii) Weigh accurately about 0.5 g of the dry extract (or an amount of the viscous extract, equivalent to about 0.5 g of the dried substance), add 20 mL of ethyl acetate and 10 mL of water, and shake for 10 minutes. After centrifugation, remove the ethyl acetate layer, add 20 mL of ethyl acetate, proceed in the same manner as described above, and remove the ethyl acetate layer. To the aqueous layer add 10 mL of methanol, shake for 30 minutes, centrifuge, and take the supernatant liquid. To the residue add 20 mL of diluted methanol (1 in 2), shake for 5 minutes, centrifuge, and take the supernatant liquid. Combine these supernatant liquids, add diluted methanol (1 in 2) to make exactly 50 mL, and use this solution as the sample solution. Separately, weigh accurately about 10 mg of Glycyrrhizic Acid RS (separately determine the water <*2.48*> by coulometric titration, using 10 mg), dissolve in diluted methanol (1 in 2) to make exactly 100 mL, and use this solution as the standard solution. Perform the test with exactly 10 μL each of the sample solution and standard solution as directed under Liquid Chromatography <*2.01*> according to the following conditions, and determine the peak areas, A_T and A_S, of glycyrrhizic acid in each solution.

$$\text{Amount (mg) of glycyrrhizic acid } (C_{42}H_{62}O_{16}) = M_S \times A_T/A_S \times 1/2$$

M_S: Amount (mg) of Glycyrrhizic Acid RS taken, calculated on the anhydrous basis

Operating conditions—

Proceed as directed in the operating conditions in i).

System suitability—

System repeatability: Proceed as directed in the system suitability in i).

System performance: Dissolve 5 mg of monoammonium glycyrrhizinate for resolution check in 20 mL of dilute ethanol. When the procedure is run with 10 μL of this solution under the above operating conditions, the resolution between the peak having the relative retention time of about 0.9 to glycyrrhizic acid and the peak of glycyrrhizic acid is not less than 1.5.

Containers and storage Containers—Tight containers.

Shoseiryuto Extract

小青竜湯エキス

Shoseiryuto Extract contains not less than 8 mg and not more than 24 mg of the total alkaloids (ephedrine and pseudoephedrine), not less than 26 mg and not more than 78 mg of paeoniflorin ($C_{23}H_{28}O_{11}$: 480.46), and not less than 14 mg and not more than 42 mg of glycyrrhizic acid ($C_{42}H_{62}O_{16}$: 822.93), per extract prepared with the amount specified in the Method of preparation.

Method of preparation

	1)	2)
Ephedra Herb	3 g	3 g
Peony Root	3 g	3 g
Processed Ginger	3 g	—
Ginger	—	3 g
Glycyrrhiza	3 g	3 g
Cinnamon Bark	3 g	3 g
Asiasarum Root	3 g	3 g
Schisandra Fruit	3 g	3 g
Pinellia Tuber	6 g	6 g

Prepare a dry extract or viscous extract as directed under Extracts, according to the prescription 1) or 2), using the crude drugs shown above.

Description Shoseiryuto Extract occurs as a light brown to brown powder or black-brown viscous extract. It has a characteristic odor and a acid first then pungent taste.

Identification **(1)** Shake 1.0 g of dry extract (or 3.0 g of the viscous extract) with 10 mL of water, add 10 mL of 1-butanol and shake, centrifuge, and use the 1-butanol layer as the sample solution. Perform the test with the sample solution as directed under Thin-layer Chromatography <*2.03*>. Spot 5 μL of the sample solution on a plate of silica gel for thin-layer chromatography. Develop the plate with a mixture of 1-propanol, ethyl acetate, water and acetic acid(100) (4:4:2:1) to a distance of about 7 cm, and air-dry the plate. Spray evenly ninhydrin-ethanol TS for spraying on the plate, and heat the plate at 105°C for 5 minutes: a red-purple spot is observed at an *Rf* value of about 0.5 (Ephedra Herb).

(2) Shake 1.0 g of the dry extract (or 3.0 g of the viscous extract) with 10 mL of water, add 10 mL of 1-butanol, shake, centrifuge, and use the 1-butanol layer as the sample solution. Separately, dissolve 1 mg of Paeoniflorin RS or paeoniflorin for thin-layer chromatography in 1 mL of methanol, and use this solution as the standard solution. Perform the test with these solutions as directed under Thin-layer Chromatography <*2.03*>. Spot 5 μL each of the sample solution and standard solution on a plate of silica gel for thin-layer chromatography. Develop the plate with a mixture of ethyl acetate, methanol and water (20:3:2) to a distance of about 7 cm, and air-dry the plate. Spray evenly 4-methoxybenzaldehyde-sulfuric acid TS on the plate, and heat the plate at 105°C for 5 minutes: one of the several spots obtained from the sample solution has the same color tone and *Rf* value with the purple spot from the standard solution (Peony Root).

(3) For preparation prescribed Processed Ginger—Shake 1.0 g of the dry extract (or 3.0 g of the viscous extract) with 10 mL of water, add 25 mL of diethyl ether, and shake. Separate the diethyl ether layer, evaporate the solvent under low pressure (in vacuo), add 2 mL of diethyl ether to the residue, and use this solution as the sample solution. Separately, dissolve 1 mg of [6]-shogaol for thin-layer chromatography in 1 mL of methanol, and use this solution as the standard solution. Perform the test with these solutions as directed under Thin-layer Chromatography <*2.03*>. Spot 20 μL of the sample solution and 1 μL of the standard solution on a plate of silica gel for thin-layer chromatography. Develop the plate with a mixture of cyclohexane and ethyl acetate (2:1) to a distance of about 7 cm, and air-dry the plate. Spray evenly 4-dimethylaminobenzaldehyde TS for spraying on the plate, heat the plate at 105°C for 5 minutes, allow to cool, and spray water: one of the several spots obtained from the sample solution has the same color tone and *Rf* value with the blue-green to grayish green spot from the standard solution (Processed Ginger).

(4) For preparation prescribed Ginger—Shake 1.0 g of the dry extract (or 3.0 g of the viscous extract) with 10 mL of water, add 25 mL of diethyl ether, and shake. Separate the diethyl ether layer, evaporate the solvent under low pressure (in vacuo), add 2 mL of diethyl ether to the residue, and use this solution as the sample solution. Separately, dissolve 1 mg of [6]-gingerol for thin-layer chromatography in 1 mL of methanol, and use this solution as the standard solution. Perform the test with these solutions as directed under Thin-layer Chromatography <*2.03*>. Spot 10 μL of the sample solution and 5 μL of the standard solution on a plate of silica gel for thin-layer chromatography. Develop the plate with a mixture of ethyl acetate and hexane (1:1) to a distance of about 7 cm, and air-dry the plate. Spray evenly 4-dimethylaminobenzaldehyde TS for spraying on the plate, heat the plate at 105°C for 5 minutes, allow to cool, and spray water: one of the several spots obtained from the sample solution has the same color tone and *Rf* value with the blue-green to grayish green spot from the standard solution (Ginger).

(5) Shake 1.0 g of the dry extract (or 3.0 g of the viscous extract) with 10 mL of water, add 10 mL of 1-butanol, shake, centrifuge, and use the 1-butanol layer as the sample solution. Separately, dissolve 1 mg of liquiritin for thin-layer chromatography in 1 mL of methanol, and use this solution as the standard solution. Perform the test with these solutions as directed under Thin-layer Chromatography <*2.03*>. Spot 1 μL each of the sample solution and standard solution on a plate of silica gel for thin-layer chromatography. Develop the plate with a mixture of ethyl acetate, methanol and water (20:3:2) to a distance of about 7 cm, and air-dry the plate. Spray evenly dilute sulfuric acid on the plate, heat the plate at 105°C for 5 minutes, and examine under ultraviolet light (main wavelength: 365 nm): one of the several spots obtained from the sample solution has the same color tone and *Rf* value with the yellow-green fluorescent spot from the standard solution (Glycyrrhiza).

(6) Perform the test according to the following i) or ii) (Cinnamon Bark).

i) Put 10 g of the dry extract (or 30 g of the viscous extract) in a 300-mL hard-glass flask, add 100 mL of water and 1 mL of silicone resin, connect the apparatus for essential oil determination, and heat under a reflux condenser. The graduated tube of the apparatus is to be previously filled with water to the standard line, and 2 mL of hexane is added to the graduated tube. After heating under reflux for 1 hour, separate the hexane layer, and use the layer as the sample solution. Separately, dissolve 1 mg of (*E*)-cinnamaldehyde for thin-layer chromatography in 1 mL of methanol, and use this solution as the standard solution. Perform the test with these solutions as directed under Thin-layer Chromatography <*2.03*>. Spot 20 μL of the sample solution and 2 μL the standard solution on a plate of silica gel for thin-layer chromatography. Develop the plate with a mixture of hexane and ethyl acetate (2:1) to a distance of about 7 cm, and air-dry the plate. Spray evenly 2,4-dinitrophenylhydrazine TS on the plate: one of the several spots obtained from the sample solution has the same color tone and *R*f value with the yellow-orange spot from the standard solution.

ii) Shake 2.0 g of the dry extract (or 6.0 g of the viscous extract) with 10 mL of water, then add 5 mL of hexane, shake, centrifuge, and use the hexane layer as the sample solution. Separately, dissolve 1 mg of (*E*)-2-methoxycinnamaldehyde for thin-layer chromatography in 1 mL of methanol, and use this solution as the standard solution. Perform the test with these solutions as directed under Thin-layer Chromatography <*2.03*>. Spot 20 μL of the sample solution and 2 μL the standard solution on a plate of silica gel for thin-layer chromatography. Develop the plate with a mixture of hexane and ethyl acetate (2:1) to a distance of about 7 cm, and air-dry the plate. Examine under ultraviolet light (main wavelength: 365 nm): one of the several spots obtained from the sample solution has the same color tone and *R*f value with the blue-white fluorescent spot from the standard solution.

(7) Shake 1.0 g of the dry extract (or 3.0 g of the viscous extract) with 10 mL of water, then add 25 mL of diethyl ether, and shake. Separate the diethyl ether layer, evaporate the solvent under low pressure (in vacuo), add 2 mL of diethyl ether to the residue, and use this solution as the sample solution. Separately, dissolve 1 mg of asarinin for thin-layer chromatography in 1 mL of methanol, and use this solution as the standard solution. Perform the test with these solutions as directed under Thin-layer Chromatography <*2.03*>. Spot 20 μL of the sample solution and 5 μL of the standard solution on a plate of silica gel for thin-layer chromatography. Develop the plate with a mixture of hexane and ethyl acetate (2:1) to a distance of about 7 cm, and air-dry the plate. Spray evenly dilute sulfuric acid on the plate, and heat the plate at 105°C for 5 minutes: one of the several spots obtained from the sample solution has the same color tone and *R*f value with the yellow-brown spot from the standard solution (Asiasarum Root).

(8) Shake 1.0 g of the dry extract (or 3.0 g of the viscous extract) with 10 mL of sodium hydroxide TS, then add 25 mL of diethyl ether, and shake. Separate the diethyl ether layer, evaporate the solvent under low pressure (in vacuo), add 2 mL of diethyl ether to the residue, and use this solution as the sample solution. Separately, dissolve 1 mg of schisandrin for thin-layer chromatography in 1 mL of methanol, and use this solution as the standard solution. Perform the test with these solutions as directed under Thin-layer Chromatography <*2.03*>. Spot 10 μL of the sample solution and 5 μL of the standard solution on a plate of silica gel with fluorescent indicator for thin-layer chromatography. Develop the plate with a mixture of ethyl acetate, hexane and acetic acid (100) (10:10:1) to a distance of about 7 cm, and air-dry the plate. Examine under ultraviolet light (main wavelength: 254 nm): one of the several spots obtained from the sample solution has the same color tone and *R*f value with the blue-purple spot from the standard solution (Schisandra Fruit).

Purity **(1)** Heavy metals <*1.07*>—Prepare the test solution with 1.0 g of the dry extract (or an amount of the viscous extract, equivalent to 1.0 g of dried substance) as directed under Extracts (4), and perform the test (not more than 30 ppm).

(2) Cadmium—Take 5.0 g of the dry extract (or an amount of the viscous extract, equivalent to 5.0 g of the dried substance) in a platinum, quartz or porcelain crucible, heat weakly, then incinerate by ignition at 450°C. After cooling, add a small amount of 2 mol/L nitric acid TS to the residue, filter if necessary, wash the crucible several times with small portions of 2 mol/L nitric acid TS, combine the filtrate and washings, add 2 mol/L nitric acid TS to make exactly 20 mL, and use this solution as the sample solution. Separately, to 5.0 mL of Standard Cadmium Solution add 2 mol/L nitric acid TS to make exactly 20 mL, and use this solution as the standard solution. Perform the test with the sample solution and standard solution as directed under Atomic Absorption Spectrophotometry <*2.23*>: the absorbance of the sample solution is not more than that of the standard solution (not more than 1 ppm).

Gas: Combustible gas—Acetylene or hydrogen.

Supporting gas—Air.

Lamp: Cadmium hollow-cathode lamp.

Wavelength: 228.8 nm.

(3) Arsenic <*1.11*>—Prepare the test solution with 0.67 g of the dry extract (or an amount of the viscous extract, equivalent to 0.67 g of dried substance) according to Method 3, and perform the test (not more than 3 ppm).

Loss on drying <*2.41*> The dry extract: Not more than 10.0% (1 g, 105°C, 5 hours).

The viscous extract: Not more than 66.7% (1 g, 105°C, 5 hours).

Total ash <*5.01*> Not more than 12.0%, calculated on the dried basis.

Assay **(1)** Total alkaloids (ephedrine and pseudoephedrine)—Weigh accurately about 0.5 g of the dry extract (or an amount of the viscous extract, equivalent to about 0.5 g of dried substance), add 20 mL of diethyl ether, shake, then add 3.0 mL of 0.1 mol/L hydrochloric acid TS, and shake for 10 minutes. After centrifugation, remove the diethyl ether layer, add 20 mL of diethyl ether, proceed in the same manner as described above, and remove the diethyl ethler layer. To the aqueous layer add 1.0 mL of ammonia TS and 20 mL of diethyl ether, shake for 30 minutes, centrifuge, and separate the diethyl ether layer. In addition, repeat twice in the same manner for the aqueous layer using 1.0 mL of ammonia TS and 20 mL of diethyl ether. Combine all the extracts, evaporate the solvent under low pressure (in vacuo), dissolve the residue in diluted methanol (1 in 2) to make exactly 50 mL. Centrifuge this solution, and use the supernatant liquid as the sample solution. Separately, weigh accurately about 10 mg of ephedrine hydrochloride for assay of crude drugs, previously dried at 105°C for 3 hours, and dissolve in diluted methanol (1 in 2) to make exactly 100 mL. Pipet 10 mL of this solution, add diluted methanol (1 in 2) to make exactly 50 mL, and use this solution as the standard solution. Perform the test with exactly 10 μL each of the sample solution and standard solution as directed under Liquid Chromatography <*2.01*> according to the following conditions. Determine the peak areas, A_{TE} and A_{TP}, of ephedrine and pseudoephedrine obtained from the sample solution, and the peak area, A_S, of ephedrine from the standard solution.

Amount (mg) of total alkaloids (ephedrine and pseudoephedrine)
$= M_S \times (A_{TE} + A_{TP})/A_S \times 1/10 \times 0.819$

M_S: Amount (mg) of ephedrine hydrochloride for assay of crude drugs taken

Operating conditions—

Detector: An ultraviolet absorption photometer (wavelength: 210 nm).

Column: A stainless steel column 4.6 mm in inside diameter and 15 cm in length, packed with octadecylsilanized silica gel for liquid chromatography (5 μm in particle diameter).

Column temperature: A constant temperature of about 40°C.

Mobile phase: To 5 g of sodium lauryl sulfate add 350 mL of acetonitrile, shake, and add 650 mL of water and 1 mL of phosphoric acid to dissolve lauryl sulfate.

Flow rate: 1.0 mL per minute (the retention time of ephedrine is about 27 minutes).

System suitability—

System performance: Dissolve 1 mg each of ephedrine hydrochloride for assay of crude drugs and pseudoephedrine hydrochloride in diluted methanol (1 in 2) to make 10 mL. When the procedure is run with 10 μL of this solution under the above operating conditions, pseudoephedrine and ephedrine are eluted in this order with the resolution between these peaks being not less than 1.5.

System repeatability: When the test is repeated 6 times with 10 μL of the standard solution under the above operating conditions, the relative standard deviation of the peak area of ephedrine is not more than 1.5%.

(2) Paeoniflorin—Weigh accurately about 0.5 g of the dry extract (or an amount of the viscous extract, equivalent to about 0.5 g of dried substance), add exactly 50 mL of diluted methanol (1 in 2), shake for 15 minutes, filter, and use the filtrate as the sample solution. Separately, weigh accurately about 10 mg of Paeoniflorin RS, (separately determined the water *<2.48>* by coulometric titration, using 10 mg), dissolve in diluted methanol (1 in 2) to make exactly 100 mL, and use this solution as the standard solution. Perform the test with exactly 10 μL each of the sample solution and standard solution as directed under Liquid Chromatography *<2.01>* according to the following conditions, and determine the peak areas, A_T and A_S, of paeoniflorin in each solution.

Amount (mg) of paeoniflorin ($C_{23}H_{28}O_{11}$)
$= M_S \times A_T/A_S \times 1/2$

M_S: Amount (mg) of Paeoniflorin RS taken, calculated on the anhydrous basis

Operating conditions—

Detector: An ultraviolet absorption photometer (wavelength: 232 nm).

Column: A stainless steel column 4.6 mm in inside diameter and 15 cm in length, packed with octadecylsilanized silica gel for liquid chromatography (5 μm in particle diameter).

Column temperature: A constant temperature of about 20°C.

Mobile phase: A mixture of water, acetonitrile and phosphoric acid (850:150:1).

Flow rate: 1.0 mL per minute (the retention time of paeoniflorin is about 9 minutes).

System suitability—

System performance: Dissolve 1 mg each of Paeoniflorin RS and albiflorin in diluted methanol (1 in 2) to make 10 mL. When the procedure is run with 10 μL of this solution under the above operating conditions, albiflorin and paeoniflorin are eluted in this order with the resolution between these peaks being not less than 2.5.

System repeatability: When the test is repeated 6 times with 10 μL of the standard solution under the above operating conditions, the relative standard deviation of the peak area of paeoniflorin is not more than 1.5%.

(3) Glycyrrhizic acid—Perform the test according to the following i) or ii).

i) Weigh accurately about 0.5 g of the dry extract (or an amount of the viscous extract, equivalent to about 0.5 g of the dried substance), add exactly 50 mL of diluted methanol (1 in 2), shake for 15 minutes, filter, and use the filtrate as the sample solution. Separately, weigh accurately about 10 mg of Glycyrrhizic Acid RS, (separately determine the water *<2.48>* by coulometric titration, using 10 mg), dissolve in diluted methanol (1 in 2) to make exactly 100 mL, and use this solution as the standard solution. Perform the test with exactly 10 μL each of the sample solution and standard solution as directed under Liquid Chromatography *<2.01>* according to the following conditions, and determine the peak areas, A_T and A_S, of glycyrrhizic acid in each solution.

Amount (mg) of glycyrrhizic acid ($C_{42}H_{62}O_{16}$)
$= M_S \times A_T/A_S \times 1/2$

M_S: Amount (mg) of Glycyrrhizic Acid RS taken, calculated on the anhydrous basis

Operating conditions—

Detector: An ultraviolet absorption photometer (wavelength: 254 nm).

Column: A stainless steel column 4.6 mm in inside diameter and 15 cm in length, packed with octadecylsilanized silica gel for liquid chromatography (5 μm in particle diameter).

Column temperature: A constant temperature of about 40°C.

Mobile phase: Dissolve 3.85 g of ammonium acetate in 720 mL of water, and add 5 mL of acetic acid (100) and 280 mL of acetonitrile.

Flow rate: 1.0 mL per minute (the retention time of glycyrrhizic acid is about 15 minutes).

System suitability—

System performance: Dissolve 5 mg of monoammonium glycyrrhizinate for resolution check in 20 mL of dilute ethanol. When the procedure is run with 10 μL of this solution under the above operating conditions, the resolution between the peak having the relative retention time of about 0.9 to glycyrrhizic acid and the peak of glycyrrhizic acid is not less than 1.5. Dissolve 1 mg of (*E*)-cinnamaldehyde for thin-layer chromatography in 50 mL of methanol. To 2 mL of this solution add 2 mL of the standard solution. When the procedure is run with 10 μL of this solution under the above operating conditions, the resolution between the peaks of glycyrrhizic acid and (*E*)-cinnamaldehyde is not less than 1.5.

System repeatability: When the test is repeated 6 times with 10 μL of the standard solution under the above operating conditions, the relative standard deviation of the peak area of glycyrrhizic acid is not more than 1.5%.

ii) Weigh accurately about 0.5 g of the dry extract (or an amount of the viscous extract, equivalent to about 0.5 g of the dried substance), add 20 mL of diethyl ether and 10 mL of water, and shake for 10 minutes. After centrifugation, remove the diethyl ether layer, add 20 mL of diethyl ether, proceed in the same manner as described above, and remove the diethyl ether layer. To the aqueous layer add 10 mL of methanol, shake for 30 minutes, centrifuge, and take the supernatant liquid. To the residue add 20 mL of diluted methanol (1 in 2), shake for 5 minutes, centrifuge, and take the supernatant liquid. Combine these supernatant liquids, add diluted methanol (1 in 2) to make exactly 50 mL, and use this solution as the sample solution. Separately, weigh accurately about 10 mg of Glycyrrhizic Acid RS (separately determine the water <2.48> by coulometric titration, using 10 mg), dissolve in diluted methanol (1 in 2) to make exactly 100 mL, and use this solution as the standard solution. Perform the test with exactly 10 μL each of the sample solution and standard solution as directed under Liquid Chromatography <2.01> according to the following conditions, and determine the peak areas, A_T and A_S, of glycyrrhizic acid in each solution.

$$\text{Amount (mg) of glycyrrhizic acid } (C_{42}H_{62}O_{16}) = M_S \times A_T/A_S \times 1/2$$

M_S: Amount (mg) of Glycyrrhizic Acid RS taken, calculated on the anhydrous basis

Operating conditions—

Proceed as directed in the operating conditions in i).

System suitability—

System repeatability: Proceed as directed in the system suitability in i).

System performance: Dissolve 5 mg of monoammonium glycyrrhizinate for resolution check in 20 mL of dilute ethanol. When the procedure is run with 10 μL of this solution under the above operating conditions, the resolution between the peak having the relative retention time of about 0.9 to glycyrrhizic acid and the peak of glycyrrhizic acid is not less than 1.5.

Containers and storage Containers—Tight containers.

Simple Ointment

単軟膏

Method of preparation

Yellow Beeswax	330 g
Fixed oil	a sufficient quantity
To make	1000 g

Prepare as directed under Ointments, with the above ingredients.

Description Simple Ointment is yellow in color. It has a slight, characteristic odor.

Containers and storage Containers—Tight containers.

Sinomenium Stem and Rhizome

Sinomeni Caulis et Rhizoma

ボウイ

Sinomenium Stem and Rhizome is the climbing stem and rhizome of *Sinomenium acutum* Rehder et Wilson (*Menispermaceae*), usually cut transversely.

Description Round or elliptic sections, 0.2 - 0.4 cm in thickness, 1 - 4.5 cm in diameter; cortex on both fractured surfaces, light brown to dark brown; in xylem, grayish brown vessel portions and dark brown medullary rays lined alternately and radially; flank, dark gray, with longitudinal wrinkles and warty protrusions.

Almost odorless; taste, bitter.

Under a microscope <5.01>, a transverse section reveals extremely thick-walled stone cells in primary cortex and pericycle; irregular-sized vessels lined nearly stepwise in the vessel portion; cells of medullary ray mostly not lignified, and extremely thick-walled and large stone cells scattered here and there; primary cortex containing needle crystals of calcium oxalate; medullary rays containing starch gains, mainly simple grain, 3 - 20 μm in diameter, and small needle crystals of calcium oxalate.

Identification To 1.0 g of pulverized Sinomenium Stem and Rhizome add 5 mL of methanol, shake for 10 minutes, filter, and use the filtrate as the sample solution. Separately, dissolve 1 mg of sinomenine for thin-layer chromatography in 1 mL of methanol, and use this solution as the standard solution. Perform the test with these solutions as directed under Thin-layer Chromatography <2.03>. Spot 10 μL of the sample solution and 5 μL of the standard solution on a plate of silica gel for thin-layer chromatography. Develop the plate with a mixture of ethyl formate, 1-propanol, water and acetic acid (100) (3:3:2:2) to a distance of about 7 cm, and air-dry the plate. Spray evenly Dragendorff's TS for spraying on the plate, air-dry the plate, and spray evenly sodium nitrite TS on the plate: one of the several spots obtained from the sample solution and the spot from the standard solution show the same color tone and the same *R*f value. Further, a spot with the same color tone appears immediately below the spot.

Total ash <5.01> Not more than 7.0%.

Acid-insoluble ash <5.01> Not more than 0.5%.

Containers and storage Containers—Well-closed containers.

Smilax Rhizome

Smilacis Rhizoma

サンキライ

Smilax Rhizome is the rhizome of *Smilax glabra* Roxburgh (*Liliaceae*).

Description Flattened and irregular cylindrical tuber, often with node-like branches; usually 5 - 15 cm in length, 2 - 5 cm in diameter; the outer surface grayish yellow-brown to yellow-brown, and the upper surface scattered with knotty remains of stem; transverse section irregular elliptical to obtuse triangular, whitish to reddish white, consisting of extremely thin cortex and mostly of stele.

Odor, slight; almost tasteless.

Under a microscope <5.01>, a transverse section reveals a 2- to 3-cell-wide cork layer, with extremely narrow cortical layer, usually consisting of a 2- to 4-cell-wide, thick-walled parenchyma cells, showing large mucilage cells here and there; mucilage cell containing raphides of calcium oxalate; stele consisting chiefly of parenchyma cells, and scattered with vascular bundles; parenchyma cells containing starch grains composed mostly of simple grains, 12 - 36 μm in diameter, and sometimes mixed with 2- to 4-compound grains.

Purity (1) Heavy metals <1.07>—Proceed with 3.0 g of pulverized Smilax Rhizome according to Method 3, and perform the test. Prepare the control solution with 3.0 mL of Standard Lead Solution (not more than 10 ppm).

(2) Arsenic ⟨*1.11*⟩—Prepare the test solution with 0.40 g of pulverized Smilax Rhizome according to Method 4, and perform the test (not more than 5 ppm).

Total ash ⟨*5.01*⟩ Not more than 5.0%.

Containers and storage Containers—Well-closed containers.

Powdered Smilax Rhizome

Smilacis Rhizoma Pulveratum

サンキライ末

Powdered Smilax Rhizome is the powder of Smilax Rhizome.

Description Powdered Smilax Rhizome occurs as a light yellow-brown powder, and has a slight odor, and is practically tasteless.

Under a microscope ⟨*5.01*⟩, Powdered Smilax Rhizome reveals starch grains and fragments of parenchyma cells containing them; fragments of raphides of calcium oxalate contained in mucilage masses; fragments of lignified parenchyma cells of cortical layer; fragments of cork cells and scalariform vessels; starch grains composed mostly of simple grains, and mixed with a few 2- to 4-compound grains 12 – 36 μm in diameter.

Purity **(1)** Heavy metals ⟨*1.07*⟩—Proceed with 3.0 g of Powdered Smilax Rhizome according to Method 3, and perform the test. Prepare the control solution with 3.0 mL of Standard Lead Solution (not more than 10 ppm).

(2) Arsenic ⟨*1.11*⟩—Prepare the test solution with 0.40 g of Powdered Smilax Rhizome according to Method 4, and perform the test (not more than 5 ppm).

(3) Foreign matter—Under a microscope ⟨*5.01*⟩, Powdered Smilax Rhizome does not show a large quantity of stone cells or thick-walled fibers.

Total ash ⟨*5.01*⟩ Not more than 5.0%.

Containers and storage Containers—Well-closed containers.

Sodium Bicarbonate and Bitter Tincture Mixture

苦味重曹水

Method of preparation

Sodium Bicarbonate	30 g
Bitter Tincture	20 mL
Water, Purified Water or Purified Water in Containers	a sufficient quantity
To make	1000 mL

Prepare before use, with the above ingredients.

Description Sodium Bicarbonate and Bitter Tincture Mixture is a clear, yellowish liquid, having a bitter taste.

Containers and storage Containers—Tight containers.

Anhydrous Sodium Sulfate

Sal Mirabilis Anhydricus

無水ボウショウ

Na_2SO_4: 142.04

[7757-82-6]

Anhydrous Sodium Sulfate is mainly sodium sulfate (Na_2SO_4) containing no water of crystallization.

It, when dried, contains not less than 99.0% of sodium sulfate (Na_2SO_4).

Description Anhydrous Sodium Sulfate occurs as white, crystals or powder. It is odorless and has a salty and slightly bitter taste.

It is freely soluble in water, and practically insoluble in ethanol (99.5).

Identification **(1)** A solution of Anhydrous Sodium Sulfate (1 in 20) responds to Qualitative Tests ⟨*1.09*⟩ (1) for sodium salt.

(2) A solution of Anhydrous Sodium Sulfate (1 in 20) responds to Qualitative Tests ⟨*1.09*⟩ (1) for sulfate.

Purity **(1)** Acidity or alkalinity—Dissolve 0.5 g of Anhydrous Sodium Sulfate in 5 mL of freshly boiled and cooled water: the solution is clear and colorless, and neutral.

(2) Chloride ⟨*1.03*⟩—Perform the test with 0.5 g of previously dried Anhydrous Sodium Sulfate. Prepare the control solution with 0.5 mL of 0.01 mol/L hydrochloric acid VS (not more than 0.036%).

(3) Heavy metals ⟨*1.07*⟩—Proceed with 2.0 g of previously dried Anhydrous Sodium Sulfate according to Method 1, and perform the test. Prepare the control solution with 2.0 mL of Standard Lead Solution (not more than 10 ppm).

(4) Arsenic ⟨*1.11*⟩—Prepare the test solution with 1.0 g of previously dried Anhydrous Sodium Sulfate according to Method 1, and perform the test (not more than 2 ppm).

Loss on drying ⟨*2.41*⟩ Not more than 0.5% (4 g, 105°C, 4 hours).

Assay Weigh accurately about 0.4 g of previously dried Anhydrous Sodium Sulfate, dissolve in 200 mL of water, add 1 mL of hydrochloric acid, boil, and gradually add 8 mL of barium chloride TS. Heat the solution in a water bath for 1 hour. After cooling, filter through a filter paper for quantitative analysis (No.5C), wash the residue on the filter paper with water until the washings do not give the turbidity with silver nitrate TS. After drying the residue together with the paper, ignite at 500 – 800°C to constant mass, and weigh the mass of the residue as the amount of barium sulfate ($BaSO_4$: 233.39).

$$\text{Amount (mg) of sodium sulfate } (Na_2SO_4) = \text{amount (mg) of barium sulfate } (BaSO_4) \times 0.609$$

Containers and storage Containers—Well-closed containers.

Sodium Sulfate Hydrate

Sal Mirabilis

ボウショウ

$Na_2SO_4.10H_2O$: 322.19
[7727-73-3]

Sodium Sulfate Hydrate is mainly decahydrate of sodium sulfate (Na_2SO_4).

It, when dried, contains not less than 99.0% of sodium sulfate (Na_2SO_4: 142.04).

Description Sodium Sulfate Hydrate occurs as colorless or white, crystals or crystalline powder. It is odorless and has a cooling and salty taste.

It is freely soluble in water, and practically insoluble in ethanol (99.5).

It is quickly efflorescent in air, soluble in its own water of crystallization at about 33°C and lost the water at 100°C.

Identification **(1)** A solution of Sodium Sulfate Hydrate (1 in 20) responds to Qualitative Tests <*1.09*> (1) for sodium salt.

(2) A solution of Sodium Sulfate Hydrate (1 in 20) responds to Qualitative Tests <*1.09*> (1) for sulfate.

Purity **(1)** Acidity or alkalinity—Dissolve 0.5 g of Sodium Sulfate Hydrate in 5 mL of freshly boiled and cooled water: the solution is clear and colorless, and neutral.

(2) Chloride <*1.03*>—Perform the test with 0.5 g of previously dried Sodium Sulfate Hydrate. Prepare the control solution with 0.5 mL of 0.01 mol/L hydrochloric acid VS (not more than 0.036%).

(3) Heavy metals <*1.07*>—Proceed with 2.0 g of previously dried Sodium Sulfate Hydrate according to Method 1, and perform the test. Prepare the control solution with 2.0 mL of Standard Lead Solution (not more than 10 ppm).

(4) Arsenic <*1.11*>—Prepare the test solution with 1.0 g of previously dried Sodium Sulfate Hydrate according to Method 1, and perform the test (not more than 2 ppm).

Loss on drying <*2.41*> 51.0 – 57.0% (4 g, 105°C, 4 hours).

Assay Weigh accurately about 0.4 g of previously dried Sodium Sulfate Hydrate, dissolve in 200 mL of water, add 1 mL of hydrochloric acid, boil, and gradually add 8 mL of barium chloride TS. Heat the solution in a water bath for 1 hour. After cooling, filter through a filter paper for quantitative analysis (No.5C), wash the residue on the filter paper with water until the washings do not give the turbidity with silver nitrate TS. After drying the residue together with the paper, ignite at 500 – 800°C to constant mass, and weigh the mass of the residue as the amount of barium sulfate ($BaSO_4$: 233.39).

Amount (mg) of sodium sulfate (Na_2SO_4)
= amount (mg) of barium sulfate ($BaSO_4$) × 0.609

Containers and storage Containers—Well-closed containers.

Sophora Root

Sophorae Radix

クジン

Sophora Root is the root of *Sophora flavescens* Aiton (*Leguminosae*) or often such root from which the periderm has been removed.

Description Cylindrical root, 5 – 20 cm in length, 2 – 3 cm in diameter; externally dark brown to yellow-brown, with distinct longitudinal wrinkles, and with laterally extended lenticels; root without periderm, externally yellow-white, with somewhat fibrous surface; under a magnifying glass, the transverse section, light yellow-brown; cortex, 0.1 – 0.2 cm in thickness, slightly tinged with dark color near cambium, forming a crack between xylem.

Odor, slight; taste, extremely bitter and lasting.

Identification To 1.0 g of pulverized Sophora Root add 10 mL of methanol, shake for 10 minutes, filter, and use the filtrate as the sample solution. Perform the test with the sample solution as directed under Thin-layer Chromatography <*2.03*>. Spot 1 μL of the sample solution on a plate of silica gel for thin-layer chromatography, develop the plate with a mixture of ethanol (99.5), ethyl acetate and ammonia solution (28) (3:2:1) to a distance of about 7 cm, and air-dry the plate. Spray evenly Dragendorff's TS for spraying on the plate, and air-dry the plate. Then spray evenly sodium nitrite TS on the plate: two brown spots appear at an *R*f value of about 0.5.

Purity **(1)** Heavy metals <*1.07*>—Proceed with 3.0 g of pulverized Sophora Root according to Method 3, and perform the test. Prepare the control solution with 3.0 mL of Standard Lead Solution (not more than 10 ppm).

(2) Arsenic <*1.11*>—Prepare the test solution with 0.40 g of pulverized Sophora Root according to Method 4, and perform the test (not more than 5 ppm).

(3) Stem—When perform the test of foreign matter <*5.01*>, the amount of its stems contained in Sophora Root does not exceed 10.0%.

(4) Foreign matter <*5.01*>—The amount of foreign matter other than stems is not more than 1.0%.

Total ash <*5.01*> Not more than 6.0%.

Acid-insoluble ash <*5.01*> Not more than 1.5%.

Containers and storage Containers—Well-closed containers.

Powdered Sophora Root

Sophorae Radix Pulverata

クジン末

Powdered Sophora Root is the powder of Sophora Root.

Description Powdered Sophora Root occurs as a light brown powder. It has a slight odor, and an extremely bitter and lasting taste.

Under a microscope <*5.01*>, Powdered Sophora Root reveals mainly starch grains and fragments of parenchyma cells containing them, fibers, bordered pitted vessels, reticulate vessels; a few fragments of corky tissue and solitary crystals of calcium oxalate. Starch grains usually composed of 2- to 4-compound grains 15 - 20 μm in diameter, and simple grains 2 - 5 μm in diameter.

Identification To 1.0 g of Powdered Sophora Root add 10 mL of methanol, shake for 10 minutes, filter, and use the filtrate as the sample solution. Perform the test with the sample solution as directed under Thin-layer Chromatography *<2.03>*. Spot 1 μL of the sample solution on a plate of silica gel for thin-layer chromatography, develop the plate with a mixture of ethanol (99.5), ethyl acetate, and ammonia solution (28) (3:2:1) to a distance of about 7 cm, and air-dry the plate. Spray evenly Dragendorff's TS for spraying on the plate, and air-dry the plate. Then spray evenly sodium nitrite TS on the plate: two brown spots appear at an *Rf* value of about 0.5.

Purity **(1)** Heavy metals *<1.07>*—Proceed with 3.0 g of Powdered Sophora Root according to Method 3, and perform the test. Prepare the control solution with 3.0 mL of Standard Lead Solution (not more than 10 ppm).

(2) Arsenic *<1.11>*—Prepare the test solution with 0.40 g of Powdered Sophora Root according to Method 4, and perform the test (not more than 5 ppm).

Total ash *<5.01>* Not more than 6.0%.

Acid-insoluble ash *<5.01>* Not more than 1.5%.

Containers and storage Containers—Well-closed containers.

Soybean Oil

Oleum Sojae

ダイズ油

Soybean Oil is the fixed oil obtained from the seeds of *Glycine max* Merrill (*Leguminosae*).

Description Soybean Oil is a clear, pale yellow oil. It is odorless or has a slight odor, and has a bland taste.

It is miscible with diethyl ether and with petroleum ether.

It is slightly soluble in ethanol (95), and practically insoluble in water.

It congeals between −10°C and −17°C.

Congealing point of the fatty acids: 22 - 27°C

Specific gravity *<1.13>* d^{25}_{25}: 0.916 - 0.922

Acid value *<1.13>* Not more than 0.2.

Saponification value *<1.13>* 188 - 195

Unsaponifiable matter *<1.13>* Not more than 1.0%.

Iodine value *<1.13>* 126 - 140

Containers and storage Containers—Tight containers.

Sweet Hydrangea Leaf

Hydrangeae Dulcis Folium

アマチャ

Sweet Hydrangea Leaf is the leaf and twig of *Hydrangea macrophylla* Seringe var. *thunbergii* Makino (*Saxifragaceae*), usually crumpled.

Description Usually wrinkled and contracted leaf, dark green to dark yellow-green in color. When soaked in water and smoothed out, it is lanceolate to acuminately ovate, 5 - 15 cm in length, 2 - 10 cm in width; margin serrated, base slightly wedged; coarse hair on both surfaces, especially on the veins; lateral veins not reaching the margin but curving upwards and connecting with each other; petiole short and less than one-fifth of the length of lamina.

Odor, slight; taste, characteristically sweet.

Identification To 1.0 g of pulverized Sweet Hydrangea Leaf add 10 mL of methanol, shake for 10 minutes, centrifuge, and use the supernatant liquid as the sample solution. Separately, dissolve 2 mg of sweet hydrangea leaf dihydroisocoumarin for thin-layer chromatography in 1 mL of methanol, and use this solution as the standard solution. Perform the test with these solutions as directed under Thin-layer Chromatography *<2.03>*. Spot 5 μL each of the sample solution and standard solution on a plate of silica gel with fluorescent indicator for thin-layer chromatography. Develop the plate with a mixture of diethyl ether, hexane and formic acid (5:5:1) to a distance of about 7 cm, and air-dry the plate. Examine under ultraviolet light (main wavelength: 254 nm): two of the several spots obtained from the sample solution have the same color tone and *Rf* value with the spots from the standard solution.

Purity **(1)** Stem—When perform the test of foreign matter *<5.01>*, the amount of stems contained in Sweet Hydrangea Leaf does not exceed 3.0%.

(2) Foreign matter *<5.01>*—The amount of foreign matter other than stems contained in Sweet Hydrangea Leaf does not exceed 1.0%.

Loss on drying *<5.01>* Not more than 13.0% (6 hours).

Total ash *<5.01>* Not more than 12.0%.

Acid-insoluble ash *<5.01>* Not more than 2.5%.

Containers and storage Containers—Well-closed containers.

Powdered Sweet Hydrangea Leaf

Hydrangeae Dulcis Folium Pulveratum

アマチャ末

Powdered Sweet Hydrangea Leaf is the powder of Sweet Hydrangea Leaf.

Description Powdered Sweet Hydrangea Leaf occurs as a dark yellow-green powder, and has a faint odor and a characteristic, sweet taste.

Under a microscope *<5.01>*, Powdered Sweet Hydrangea Leaf reveals fragments of epidermis with wavy lateral cell wall; stomata with two subsidiary cells; unicellular and thin-walled hair with numerous protrusions of the surface, 150 – 300 μm in length; fragments of palisade tissue and spongy tissue; fragments of vascular bundle and mucilage cells containing raphides of calcium oxalate 50 – 70 μm in length.

Identification To 1.0 g of Powdered Sweet Hydrangea Leaf add 10 mL of methanol, shake for 10 minutes, centrifuge, and use the supernatant liquid as the sample solution. Separately, dissolve 2 mg of sweet hydrangea leaf dihydroisocoumarin for thin-layer chromatography in 1 mL of methanol, and use this solution as the standard solution. Perform the test with these solutions as directed under Thin-layer Chromatography ⟨*2.03*⟩. Spot 5 μL each of the sample solution and standard solution on a plate of silica gel with fluorescent indicator for thin-layer chromatography. Develop the plate with a mixture of diethyl ether, hexane and formic acid (5:5:1) to a distance of about 7 cm, and air-dry the plate. Examine under ultraviolet light (main wavelength: 254 nm): two of the several spots obtained from the sample solution have the same color tone and *R*f value with the spots from the standard solution.

Purity Foreign matter ⟨*5.01*⟩—Under a microscope, Powdered Sweet Hydrangea Leaf does not show stone cells, a large quantity of fibers or starch grains.

Loss on drying ⟨*5.01*⟩ Not more than 12.0% (6 hours).

Total ash ⟨*5.01*⟩ Not more than 12.0%.

Acid-insoluble ash ⟨*5.01*⟩ Not more than 2.5%.

Containers and storage Containers—Well-closed containers.

Swertia Herb

Swertiae Herba

センブリ

Swertia Herb is the whole herb of *Swertia japonica* Makino (*Gentianaceae*) collected during the blooming season.

It contains not less than 2.0% of swertiamarin ($C_{16}H_{22}O_{10}$: 374.34), calculated on the basis of dried material.

Description Herb, 10 – 50 cm in length, having flowers, opposite leaves, stems, and, usually, with short, lignified roots; stems square, about 2 mm in diameter, often with branches; the leaves and stems dark green to dark purple or yellow-brown in color; the flowers white to whitish, and the roots yellow-brown. When smoothed by immersing in water, leaves, linear or narrow lanceolate, 1 – 4 cm in length, 0.1 – 0.5 cm in width, entire, and sessile; corolla split deeply as five lobes; the lobes narrow, elongated ellipse shape, and under a magnifying glass, with two elliptical nectaries juxtaposed at the base of the inner surface; the margin of lobe resembles eyelashes; the five stamens grow on the tube of the corolla and stand alternately in a row with corolla-lobes; peduncle distinct.

Odor, slight; taste, extremely bitter and persisting.

Identification To 0.5 g of pulverized Swertia Herb add 10 mL of methanol, shake for 5 minutes, filter, and use the filtrate as the sample solution. Separately, dissolve 1 mg of Swertiamarin RS or swertiamarin for thin-layer chromatography in 1 mL of methanol, and use this solution as the standard solution. Perform the test with these solutions as directed under Thin-layer Chromatography ⟨*2.03*⟩. Spot 5 μL each of the sample solution and standard solution on a plate of silica gel for thin-layer chromatography. Develop the plate with a mixture of ethyl acetate, ethanol (99.5) and water (8:2:1) to a distance of about 7 cm, and air-dry the plate. Spray evenly vanillin-sulfuric acid-ethanol TS for spraying on the plate, and heat the plate at 105°C for 5 minutes: one of the several spots obtained from the sample solution and the spot from the standard solution show the same color tone and *R*f value.

Purity Foreign matter ⟨*5.01*⟩—The amount of straw and other foreign matters contained in Swertia Herb is not more than 1.0%.

Loss on drying ⟨*5.01*⟩ Not more than 12.0% (6 hours).

Total ash ⟨*5.01*⟩ Not more than 6.5%.

Extract content ⟨*5.01*⟩ Dilute ethanol-soluble extract: not less than 20.0%.

Assay Weigh accurately about 1 g of moderately fine powder of Swertia Herb in a glass-stoppered centrifuge tube, add 40 mL of methanol, shake for 15 minutes, centrifuge, and separate the supernatant liquid. To the residue add 40 mL of methanol, and proceed in the same manner. Combine the extracts, and add methanol to make exactly 100 mL. Pipet 5 mL of the solution, add the mobile phase to make exactly 20 mL, and use this solution as the sample solution. Separately, weigh accurately about 10 mg of Swertiamarin RS (separately determine the water ⟨*2.48*⟩ by coulometric titration, using 10 mg), dissolve in methanol to make exactly 20 mL. Pipet 5 mL of the solution, add the mobile phase to make exactly 20 mL, and use this solution as the standard solution. Perform the test with exactly 10 μL each of the sample solution and standard solution as directed under Liquid Chromatography ⟨*2.01*⟩ according to the following conditions, and determine the peak areas, A_T and A_S, of swertiamarin in each solution.

$$\text{Amount (mg) of swertiamarin } (C_{16}H_{22}O_{10}) = M_S \times A_T/A_S \times 5$$

M_S: Amount (mg) of Swertiamarin RS taken, calculated on the anhydrous basis

Operating conditions—

Detector: An ultraviolet absorption photometer (wavelength: 238 nm).

Column: A stainless steel column 4.6 mm in inside diameter and 15 cm in length, packed with octadecylsilanized silica gel for liquid chromatography (5 μm in particle diameter).

Column temperature: A constant temperature of about 50°C.

Mobile phase: A mixture of water and acetonitrile (91:9).

Flow rate : Adjust so that the retention time of swertiamarin is about 12 minutes.

System suitability—

System performance: Dissolve 1 mg each of Swertiamarin RS and theophylline in the mobile phase to make 10 mL. When the procedure is run with 10 μL of this solution under the above operating conditions, theophylline and swertiamarin are eluted in this order with the resolution of these peaks being not less than 10.

System repeatability: When the test is repeated 6 times with 10 μL of the standard solution under the above operating conditions, the relative standard deviation of the peak areas of swertiamarin is not more than 1.5%.

Containers and storage Containers—Well-closed containers.

Powdered Swertia Herb

Swertiae Herba Pulverata

センブリ末

Powdered Swertia Herb is the powder of Swertia Herb.

It contains not less than 2.0% of swertiamarin ($C_{16}H_{22}O_{10}$: 374.34), calculated on the basis of dried material.

Description Powdered Swertia Herb occurs as a grayish yellow-green to yellow-brown powder. It has a slight odor, and extremely bitter, persistent taste.

Under a microscope <*5.01*>, Powdered Swertia Herb reveals xylem tissues with fibers (components of stems and roots); assimilation tissues (components of leaves and calyces); striated epidermis (components of stems and peduncles); tissues of corollas and filaments with spiral vessels; cells of anthers and their inner walls; spherical pollen grains with granular patterns (components of flowers), about 30 μm in diameter; starch grains are simple grain, about 6 μm in diameter, and very few.

Identification To 0.5 g of Powdered Swertia Herb add 10 mL of methanol, shake for 5 minutes, filter, and use the filtrate as the sample solution. Separately, dissolve 1 mg of Swertiamarin RS or swertiamarin for thin-layer chromatography in 1 mL of methanol, and use this solution as the standard solution. Perform the test with these solutions as directed under Thin-layer Chromatography <*2.03*>. Spot 5 μL each of the sample solution and standard solution on a plate of silica gel for thin-layer chromatography. Develop the plate with a mixture of ethyl acetate, ethanol (99.5) and water (8:2:1) to a distance of about 7 cm, and air-dry the plate. Spray evenly vanillin-sulfuric acid-ethanol TS for spraying on the plate, and heat the plate at 105°C for 5 minutes: one of the several spots obtained from the sample solution and the spot from the standard solution show the same color tone and *R*f value.

Purity Foreign matter—Under a microscope <*5.01*>, crystals of calcium oxalate, a large quantity of starch grains and groups of stone cells are not observable.

Loss on drying <*5.01*> Not more than 12.0% (6 hours).

Total ash <*5.01*> Not more than 6.5%.

Acid-insoluble ash <*5.01*> Not more than 2.0%.

Extract content <*5.01*> Dilute ethanol-soluble extract: not less than 20.0%.

Assay Weigh accurately about 1 g of Powdered Swertia Herb in a glass-stoppered centrifuge tube, add 40 mL of methanol, shake for 15 minutes, centrifuge, and separate the supernatant liquid. To the residue add 40 mL of methanol, and proceed in the same manner. Combine the extracts, and add methanol to make exactly 100 mL. Pipet 5 mL of the solution, add the mobile phase to make exactly 20 mL, and use this solution as the sample solution. Separately, weigh accurately about 10 mg of Swertiamarin RS (separately determine the water <*2.48*> by coulometric titration, using 10 mg), dissolve in methanol to make exactly 20 mL. Pipet 5 mL of the solution, add the mobile phase to make exactly 20 mL, and use this solution as the standard solution. Perform the test with exactly 10 μL each of the sample solution and standard solution as directed under Liquid Chromatography <*2.01*> according to the following conditions, and determine the peak areas, A_T and A_S, of swertiamarin in each solution.

$$\text{Amount (mg) of swertiamarin } (C_{16}H_{22}O_{10}) = M_S \times A_T/A_S \times 5$$

M_S: Amount (mg) of Swertiamarin RS taken, calculated on the anhydrous basis

Operating conditions—

Detector: An ultraviolet absorption photometer (wavelength: 238 nm).

Column: A stainless steel column 4.6 mm in inside diameter and 15 cm in length, packed with octadecylsilanized silica gel for liquid chromatography (5 μm in particle diameter).

Column temperature: A constant temperature of about 50°C.

Mobile phase: A mixture of water and acetonitrile (91:9).

Flow rate: Adjust so that the retention time of swertiamarin is about 12 minutes.

System suitability—

System performance: Dissolve 1 mg each of Sweriamarin RS and theophylline in the mobile phase to make 10 mL. When the procedure is run with 10 μL of this solution under the above operating conditions, theophylline and swertiamarin are eluted in this order with the resolution of these peaks being not less than 10.

System repeatability: When the test is repeated 6 times with 10 μL of the standard solution under the above operating conditions, the relative standard deviation of the peak areas of swertiamarin is not more than 1.5%.

Containers and storage Containers—Well-closed containers.

Swertia and Sodium Bicarbonate Powder

センブリ・重曹散

Method of preparation

Powdered Swertia Herb	30 g
Sodium Bicarbonate	700 g
Starch, Lactose Hydrate or their mixture	a sufficient quantity
	To make 1000 g

Prepare as directed under Powders, with the above ingredients.

Description Swertia and Sodium Bicarbonate Powder occurs as a light grayish yellow powder, having a bitter taste.

Identification **(1)** To 10 g of Swertia and Sodium Bicarbonate Powder add 10 mL of ethanol (95), shake for 15 minutes, filter, and use the filtrate as the sample solution. Separately, dissolve 2 mg of Swertiamarin RS or swertiamarin for thin-layer chromatography in 1 mL of ethanol (95), and use this solution as the standard solution. Perform the test with these solutions as directed under Thin-layer Chromatography <*2.03*>. Spot 10 μL of the sample solution and 5 μL of the standard solution on a plate of silica gel for thin-layer chromatography. Proceed as directed in the Identification under Powdered Swertia Herb.

(2) To 0.5 g of Swertia and Sodium Bicarbonate Powder add 10 mL of water. After stirring, centrifuge the mixture with 500 revolutions per minute. Smear, using a small glass rod, the slide glass with a small amount of the precipitate, add 1 drop of a mixture of water and glycerin (1:1), and put a cover glass on it so that the tissue section spreads evenly without overlapping each other, taking precaution against inclusion of bubbles, and use this as the preparation for microscopic examination. If the precipitate separates into two layers, proceed with the upper layer in the same manner, and use as the preparation for microscopic examination. Heat the preparation for microscopic examination in a short time: the preparation reveals the yellow-green to yellow-brown, approximately spherical pollen grains with granular patterns under a microscope <*5.01*>. The pollen grains are 25 – 34 μm in diameter.

(3) The supernatant liquid obtained in (2) by centrifuging responds to Qualitative Tests <*1.09*> (1) for bicarbonate.

Containers and storage Containers—Well-closed containers.

Toad Cake

Bufonis Crustum

センソ

Toad Cake is the parotoid secretion of *Bufo gargarizans* Cantor or *Bufo melanostictus* Schneider (*Bufonidae*).

When dried, it contains not less than 5.8% of bufo steroid (bufalin, cinobufagin and resibufogenin).

Description A round disk with slightly dented bottom and protuberant surface, about 8 cm in diameter, about 1.5 cm in thickness, the mass of one disk being about 80 to 90 g; or a round disk with almost flattened surfaces on both sides, about 3 cm in diameter, and about 0.5 cm in thickness, the mass of one disk being about 8 g; externally red-brown to black-brown, somewhat lustrous, approximately uniform and horny, hard in texture, and difficult to break; fractured surface nearly flat, and edges of broken pieces red-brown and translucent.

Odorless.

Identification To 0.3 g of pulverized Toad Cake add 3 mL of acetone, shake for 10 minutes, filter, and use the filtrate as the sample solution. Separately, dissolve 1 mg of resibufogenin for thin-layer chromatography in 2 mL of acetone, and use this solution as the standard solution. Perform the test with these solutions as directed under Thin-layer Chromatography <*2.03*>. Spot 10 μL each of the sample solution and standard solution on a plate of silica gel for thin-layer chromatography, develop the plate with a mixture of cyclohexane and acetone (3:2) to a distance of about 10 cm, and air-dry the plate. Spray evenly dilute sulfuric acid on the plate, and heat the plate at 105°C for 5 minutes: one of the several spots obtained from the sample solution has the same color tone and *Rf* value with the spot from the standard solution.

Total ash <*5.01*> Not more than 5.0%.

Acid-insoluble ash <*5.01*> Not more than 2.0%.

Assay Weigh accurately about 0.5 g of pulverized Toad Cake, previously dried in a desiccator (silica gel) for 24 hours, add 50 mL of methanol, heat under a reflux condenser for 1 hour, cool, and filter. Wash the residue with 30 mL of methanol, and combine the washing and filtrate. To this solution add methanol to make exactly 100 mL. Pipet 10 mL of this solution, add exactly 5 mL of the internal standard solution, add methanol to make 25 mL, and use this solution as the sample solution. Separately, weigh accurately about 10 mg, about 20 mg and about 20 mg of bufalin for assay, cinobufagin for assay and resibufogenin for assay, respectively, previously dried in a desiccator (silica gel) for 24 hours, and dissolve in methanol to make exactly 100 mL. Pipet 10 mL of this solution, proceed in the same manner as the sample solution, and use this solution as the standard solution. Perform the test with 10 μL each of the sample solution and standard solution as directed under Liquid Chromatography <*2.01*> according to the following conditions. Calculate the ratios, Q_{TB} and Q_{SB}, of the peak area of bufalin, Q_{TC} and Q_{SC}, of the peak area of cinobufagin, and Q_{TR} and Q_{SR}, of the peak area of resibufogenin, respectively, to that of the internal standard, and designate the total amount as an amount of bufosteroid.

$$\text{Amount (mg) of bufalin} = M_{SB} \times Q_{TB}/Q_{SB}$$

$$\text{Amount (mg) of cinobufagin} = M_{SC} \times Q_{TC}/Q_{SC}$$

$$\text{Amount (mg) of resibufogenin} = M_{SR} \times Q_{TR}/Q_{SR}$$

M_{SB}: Amount (mg) of bufalin for assay taken
M_{SC}: Amount (mg) of cinobufagin for assay taken
M_{SR}: Amount (mg) of resibufogenin for assay taken

Internal standard solution—A solution of indometacin in methanol (1 in 4000).

Operating conditions—

Detector: An ultraviolet spectrophotometer (wavelength: 300 nm).

Column: A stainless steel column 4 to 6 mm in inside diameter and 15 to 30 cm in length, packed with octadecylsilanized silica gel for liquid chromatography (5 to 10 μm in particle diameter).

Column temperature: A constant temperature of about 40°C.

Mobile phase: A mixture of diluted phosphoric acid (1 in 1000) and acetonitrile (11:9).

Flow rate: Adjust so that the retention time of the internal standard is 16 to 19 minutes.

System suitability—

System performance: When the procedure is run with 10 μL of the standard solution under the above operating conditions, bufalin, cinobufagin, resibufogenin and the internal standard are eluted in this order with the resolution among these peaks being not less than 1.5.

Containers and storage Containers—Well-closed containers.

Tokakujokito Extract

桃核承気湯エキス

Tokakujokito Extract contains not less than 38 mg and not more than 152 mg of amygdalin, not less than 1 mg and not more than 4 mg of (*E*)-cinnamic acid, not less than 3 mg of sennosides A ($C_{42}H_{38}O_{20}$: 862.74) or not less than 9 mg of rhein, and not less than 10 mg and not more than 30 mg of glycyrrhizic acid ($C_{42}H_{62}O_{16}$: 822.93), per extract prepared with the amount specified in the Method of preparation.

Method of preparation

	1)	2)	3)
Peach Kernel	5 g	5 g	5 g
Cinnamon Bark	4 g	4 g	4 g
Rhubarb	3 g	3 g	3 g
Glycyrrhiza	1.5 g	1.5 g	1.5 g
Anhydrous Sodium Sulfate	1 g	0.9 g	
Sodium Sulfate			2 g

Prepare a dry extract as directed under Extracts, according to the prescription 1) to 3), using the crude drugs shown above. Or, prepare a dry extract by adding Light Anhydrous Silicic Acid to an extractive, prepared as directed under Extracts, according to the prescription 2), using the crude drugs shown above.

Description Tokakujokito Extract occurs as a green-yellow-brown to dark brown powder. It has characteristic odor and, salty, slightly astringent, and then slightly sweet taste.

Identification **(1)** To 1.0 g of Tokakujokito Extract add 10 mL of water, shake, then add 10 mL of 1-butanol, shake, centrifuge, and use the 1-butanol layer as the sample solution. Separately, dissolve 2 mg of amygdalin for thin-layer chromatography in 1 mL of methanol, and use this solution as the standard solution. Perform the test with these solutions as directed under Thin-layer Chromatography <*2.03*>. Spot 5 μL each of the sample solution and standard solution on a plate of silica gel for thin-layer chromatography. Develop the plate with a mixture of 1-propanol, ethyl acetate and water (4:4:3) to a distance of about 7 cm, and air-dry the plate. Spray evenly 4-methoxybenzaldehyde-sulfuric acid TS on the plate, and heat the plate at 105°C for 10 minutes: one of the several spots obtained from the sample solution has the same color tone and *R*f value with the green-brown spot from the standard solution (Peach Kernel).

(2) Perform the test according to the following (i) or (ii) (Cinnamon Bark).

(i) Put 10 g of Tokakujokito Extract in a 300-mL of hard-glass flask, add 100 mL of water and 1 mL of silicone resin, connect the apparatus for essential oil determination, and heat to boil under a reflux condenser. The graduated tube of the apparatus is to be previously filled with water to the standard line, and 2 mL of hexane is added to the graduated tube. After heating under reflux for 1 hour, separate the hexane layer, and use this solution as the sample solution. Separately, dissolve 1 mg of (*E*)-cinnamaldehyde for thin-layer chromatography in 1 mL of methanol, and use this solution as the standard solution. Perform the test with these solutions as directed under Thin-layer Chromatography <*2.03*>. Spot 40 μL of the sample solution and 2 μL of the standard solution on a plate of silica gel for thin-layer chromatography. Develop the plate with a mixture of hexane and ethyl acetate (2:1) to a distance of about 7 cm, and air-dry the plate. Spray evenly 2,4-dinitrophenylhydrazine TS on the plate: one of the several spots obtained from the sample solution has the same color tone and *R*f value with the yellow-orange spot from the standard solution.

(ii) To 2.0 g of Tokakujokito Extract add 10 mL of water, shake, then add 5 mL of hexane, shake, centrifuge, and use the hexane layer as the sample solution. Separately, dissolve 1 mg of (*E*)-2-methoxycinnamaldehyde for thin-layer chromatography in 1 mL of methanol, and use this solution as the standard solution. Perform the test with these solutions as directed under Thin-layer Chromatography <*2.03*>. Spot 40 μL of the sample solution and 2 μL of the standard solution on a plate of silica gel for thin-layer chromatography. Develop the plate with a mixture of hexane and ethyl acetate (2:1) to a distance of about 7 cm, and air-dry the plate. Examine under ultraviolet light (main wavelength: 365 nm): one of the several spots obtained from the sample solution has the same color tone and *R*f value with the bluish white fluorescent spot from the standard solution.

(3) To 1.0 g of Tokakujokito Extract add 10 mL of water, shake, then add 10 mL of diethyl ether, shake, centrifuge, and use the diethyl ether layer as the sample solution. Separately, dissolve 1 mg of rhein for thin-layer chromatography in 10 mL of acetone, and use this solution as the standard solution. Perform the test with these solutions as directed under Thin-layer Chromatography <*2.03*>. Spot 10 μL of the sample solution and 5 μL of the standard solution on a plate of silica gel for thin-layer chromatography. Develop the plate with a mixture of ethyl acetate, methanol and water (20:3:2) to a distance of about 7 cm, and air-dry the plate. Examine under ultraviolet light (main wavelength: 365 nm): one of the several spots obtained from the sample solution has the same color tone and *R*f value with the orange fluorescent spot from the standard solution (Rhubarb).

(4) To 1.0 g of Tokakujokito Extract add 10 mL of water, shake, then add 10 mL of 1-butanol, shake, centrifuge, and use the 1-butanol layer as the sample solution. Separately, dissolve 1 mg of liquiritin for thin-layer chromatography in 1 mL of methanol, and use this solution as the standard solution. Perform the test with these solutions as directed under Thin-layer Chromatography <*2.03*>. Spot 1 μL each of the sample solution and standard solution on a plate of silica gel for thin-layer chromatography. Develop the plate with a mixture of ethyl acetate, methanol and water (20:3:2) to a distance of about 7 cm, and air-dry the plate. Spray evenly dilute sulfuric acid on the plate, heat the plate at 105°C for 5 minutes, and examine under ultraviolet light (main wavelength: 365 nm): one of the several spots obtained from the sample solution has the same color tone and *R*f value with the yellow-green fluorescent spot from the standard solution (Glycyrrhiza).

Purity **(1)** Heavy metals <*1.07*>—Prepare the test solution with 1.0 g of Tokakujokito Extract as directed in Extracts (4), and perform the test (not more than 30 ppm).

(2) Arsenic <*1.11*>—Prepare the test solution with 0.67 g of Tokakujokito Extract according to Method 3, and perform the test (not more than 3 ppm).

Loss on drying <*2.41*> The dry extract: Not more than 8.0% (1 g, 105°C, 5 hours).

Total ash <*5.01*> Not less than 20.0% and more than 40.0%.

Assay **(1)** Amygdalin—Weigh accurately about 0.5 g of

Tokakujokito Extract, add exactly 50 mL of diluted methanol (1 in 2), shake for 15 minutes, and filter. Pipet 5 mL of the filtrate, elute through a column prepared previously with 2 g of polyamide for column chromatography using water to make exactly 20 mL of effluent , and use this solution as the sample solution. Separately, weigh accurately about 10 mg of amygdalin for assay, previously dried in a desiccator (silica gel) for 24 hours or more, and dissolve in diluted methanol (1 in 2) to make exactly 50 mL, and use this solution as the standard solution. Perform the test with exactly 10 μL each of the sample solution and standard solution as directed under Liquid Chromatography <*2.01*> according to the following conditions, and determine the peak areas, A_T and A_S, of amygdalin in each solution.

$$\text{Amount (mg) of amygdalin} = M_S \times A_T/A_S \times 4$$

M_S: Amount (mg) of amygdalin for assay taken

Operation conditions—

Detector: An ultraviolet absorption photometer (wavelength: 210 nm).

Column: A stainless steel column 4.6 mm in inside diameter and 15 cm in length, packed with octadecylsilanized silica gel for liquid chromatography (5 μm in particle diameter).

Column temperature: A constant temperature of about 45°C.

Mobile phase: A mixture of 0.05 mol/L sodium dihydrogen phosphate TS and methanol (5:1).

Flow rate: 0.8 mL per minute (the retention time of amygdalin is about 12 minutes).

Systemic suitability—

System performance: When the procedure is run with 10 μL of the standard solution under the above operating conditions, the number of theoretical plates and the symmetry factor of the peak of amygdalin are not less than 5000 and not more than 1.5, respectively.

System repeatability: When the test is repeated 6 times with 10 μL of the standard solution under the above operating conditions, the relative standard deviation of the peak area of amygdalin is not more than 1.5%.

(2) (*E*)-Cinnamic acid—Conduct this procedure using light-resistant vessels. Weigh accurately about 0.5 g of Tokakujokito Extract, add 20 mL of diethyl ether and 10 mL of water, shake for 10 minutes, centrifuge, and separate the diethyl ether layer. To the aqueous layer add 20 mL of diethyl ether, proceed in the same manner as above, and repeat this procedure two more times. Combine all the extracts, evaporate the solvent under low pressure (in vacuo), dissolve the residue in diluted methanol (1 in 2) to make exactly 50 mL, and use this solution as the sample solution. Separately, weigh accurately about 10 mg of (*E*)-cinnamic acid for assay, and dissolve in diluted methanol (1 in 2) to make exactly 100 mL. Pipet 10 mL of this solution, add diluted methanol (1 in 2) to make exactly 100 mL, and use this solution as the standard solution. Perform the test with exactly 10 μL each of the sample solution and standard solution as directed under Liquid Chromatography <*2.01*> according to the following conditions, and determine the peak areas, A_T and A_S, of (*E*)-cinnamic acid in each solution.

$$\text{Amount (mg) of } (E)\text{-cinnamic acid} = M_S \times A_T/A_S \times 1/20$$

M_S: Amount (mg) of (*E*)-cinnamic acid for assay taken, calculated on the basis of the content obtained by qNMR

Operating conditions—

Detector: An ultraviolet absorption photometer (wavelength: 273 nm).

Column: A stainless steel column 4.6 mm in inside diameter and 15 cm in length, packed with octadecylsilanized silica gel for liquid chromatography (5 μm in particle diameter).

Column temperature: A constant temperature of about 40°C.

Mobile phase: A mixture of water, acetonitrile and phosphoric acid (800:200:1).

Flow rate: 1.0 mL per minute (the retention time of (*E*)-cinnamic acid is about 22 minutes).

System suitability—

System performance: When the procedure is run with 10 μL of the standard solution under the above operating conditions, the number of theoretical plates and the symmetry factor of the peak of (*E*)-cinnamic acid are not less than 5000 and not more than 1.5, respectively.

System repeatability: When the test is repeated 6 times with 10 μL of the standard solution under the above operating conditions, the relative standard deviation of the peak area of (*E*)-cinnamic acid is not more than 1.5%.

(3) Sennoside A—Weigh accurately about 0.5 g of Tokakujokito Extract, add 20 mL of ethyl acetate and 10 mL of water, shake for 10 minutes, centrifuge, remove the ethyl acetate layer, then add 20 mL of ethyl acetate, proceed in the same manner as above, and remove the ethyl acetate layer. To the aqueous layer obtained add 10 mL of methanol, shake for 30 minutes, centrifuge, and separate the supernatant liquid. To the residue add 20 mL of diluted methanol (1 in 2), shake for 5 minutes, centrifuge, and separate the supernatant liquid. Combine all the supernatant liquids, add diluted methanol (1 in 2) to make exactly 50 mL, and use this solution as the sample solution. Separately, weigh accurately about 5 mg of Sennoside A RS (separately determine the water <*2.48*> by coulometric titration, using 10 mg), dissolve in diluted methanol (1 in 2) to make exactly 200 mL, and use this solution as the standard solution. Perform the test with exactly 10 μL each of the sample solution and standard solution as directed under Liquid Chromatography <*2.01*> according to the following conditions, and determine the peak areas, A_T and A_S, of sennoside A in each solution.

$$\text{Amount (mg) of sennoside A } (C_{42}H_{38}O_{20}) = M_S \times A_T/A_S \times 1/4$$

M_S: Amount (mg) of Sennoside A RS taken, calculated on the anhydrous basis

Operating conditions—

Detector: An ultraviolet absorption photometer (wavelength: 340 nm).

Column: A stainless steel column 4.6 mm in inside diameter and 15 cm in length, packed with octadecylsilanized silica gel for liquid chromatography (5 μm in particle diameter).

Column temperature: A constant temperature of about 50°C.

Mobile phase: A mixture of water, acetonitrile and phosphoric acid (840:160:1).

Flow rate: 1.0 mL per minute (the retention time of sennoside A is about 20 minutes).

System suitability—

System performance: When the procedure is run with 10 μL of the standard solution under the above operating conditions, the number of theoretical plates and the symmetry factor of the peak of sennoside A are not less than 5000 and not more than 1.5, respectively.

System repeatability: When the test is repeated 6 times with 10 μL of the standard solution under the above operating conditions, the relative standard deviation of the peak

area of sennoside A is not more than 1.5%.

(4) Rhein—Weigh accurately about 0.5 g of Tokakujokito Extract, add 80 mL of water, shake, and add water to make exactly 100 mL. Pipet 5 mL of this solution, add 20 mL of iron (III) chloride TS, heat under a reflux condenser for 30 minutes, add 3 mL of hydrochloric acid, and heat in addition under a reflux condenser for 30 minutes. After cooling, extract three times with 25 mL each of diethyl ether, combine all the extracts, evaporate the solvent under low pressure (in vacuo), dissolve the residue to make exactly 20 mL, and use this solution as the sample solution. Separately, weigh accurately about 5 mg of rhein for assay, and dissolve in acetone to make exactly 100 mL. Pipet 10 mL of this solution, add methanol to make exactly 50 mL, and use this solution as the standard solution. Perform the test with exactly 10 μL each of the sample solution and standard solution as directed under Liquid Chromatography <*2.01*> according to the following conditions, and determine the peak areas, A_T and A_S, of rhein in each solution.

$$\text{Amount (mg) of rhein} = M_S \times A_T/A_S \times 4/5$$

M_S: Amount (mg) of rhein for assay taken, calculated on the basis of the content obtained by qNMR

Operating conditions—

Detector: An ultraviolet absorption photometer (wavelength: 278 nm).

Column: A stainless steel column 4.6 mm in inside diameter and 25 cm in length, packed with octadecylsilanized silica gel for liquid chromatography (5 μm in particle diameter).

Column temperature: A constant temperature of about 50°C.

Mobile phase: A mixture of water, acetonitrile and phosphoric acid (650:350:1).

Flow rate: 1.0 mL per minute (the retention time of rhein is about 17 minutes).

System suitability—

System performance: When the procedure is run with 10 μL of the standard solution under the above operating conditions, the number of theoretical plates and the symmetry factor of the peak of rhein are not less than 5000 and not more than 1.5, respectively.

System repeatability: When the test is repeated 6 times with 10 μL of the standard solution under the above operating conditions, the relative standard deviation of the peak area of rhein is not more than 1.5%.

(5) Glycyrrhizic acid—Weigh accurately about 0.5 g of Tokakujokito Extract, add 20 mL of ethyl acetate and 10 mL of water, and shake for 10 minutes. After centrifugation remove the ethyl acetate layer, add 20 mL of ethyl acetate, proceed in the same manner as described above, and remove the ethyl acetate layer. To the aqueous layer add 10 mL of methanol, shake for 30 minutes, centrifuge, and take the supernatant liquid. To the residue add 20 mL of diluted methanol (1 in 2), shake for 5 minutes, centrifuge, and take the supernatant liquid. Combine these supernatant liquids, add diluted methanol (1 in 2) to make exactly 50 mL, and use this solution as the sample solution. Separately, weigh accurately about 10 mg of Glycyrrhizic Acid RS (separately determine the water <*2.48*> by coulometric titration, using 10 mg), dissolve in diluted methanol (1 in 2) to make exactly 100 mL, and use this solution as the standard solution. Perform the test with exactly 10 μL each of the sample solution and standard solution as directed under Liquid Chromatography <*2.01*> according to the following conditions, and determine the peak areas, A_T and A_S, of glycyrrhizic acid in each solution.

$$\text{Amount (mg) of glycyrrhizic acid } (C_{42}H_{62}O_{16}) = M_S \times A_T/A_S \times 1/2$$

M_S: Amount (mg) of Glycyrrhizic Acid RS taken, calculated on the anhydrous basis

Operating conditions—

Detector: An ultraviolet absorption photometer (wavelength: 254 nm).

Column: A stainless steel column 4.6 mm in inside diameter and 15 cm in length, packed with octadecylsilanized silica gel for liquid chromatography (5 μm in particle diameter).

Column temperature: A constant temperature of about 40°C.

Mobile phase: Dissolve 3.85 g of ammonium acetate in 720 mL of water, and add 5 mL of acetic acid (100) and 280 mL of acetonitrile.

Flow rate: 1.0 mL per minute (the retention time of glycyrrhizic acid is about 15 minutes).

System suitability—

System performance: Dissolve 5 mg of monoammonium glycyrrhizinate for resolution check in 20 mL of dilute ethanol. When the procedure is run with 10 μL of this solution under the above operating conditions, the resolution between the peak having the relative retention time of about 0.9 to glycyrrhizic acid and the peak of glycyrrhizic acid is not less than 1.5.

System repeatability: When the test is repeated 6 times with 10 μL of the standard solution under the above operating conditions, the relative standard deviation of the peak area of glycyrrhizic acid is not more than 1.5%.

Containers and storage Containers—Tight containers.

Tokishakuyakusan Extract

当帰芍薬散エキス

Tokishakuyakusan Extract contains not less than 0.6 mg and not more than 2.4 mg of (*E*)-ferulic acid, not less than 34 mg and not more than 102 mg (for preparation prescribed 4 g of Peony Root) or not less than 51 mg and not more than153 mg (for preparation prescribed 6 g of Peony Root) of paeoniflorin ($C_{23}H_{28}O_{11}$: 480.46), and not less than 0.4 mg of atractylenolide III (for preparation prescribed Atractylodes Rhizome) or not less than 0.1 mg of atractylodin (for preparation prescribed Atractylodes Lancea Rhizome), per extract prepared with the amount specified in the Method of preparation.

Method of preparation

	1)	2)	3)	4)
Japanese Angelica Root	3 g	3 g	3 g	3 g
Cnidium Rhizome	3 g	3 g	3 g	3 g
Peony Root	6 g	6 g	4 g	4 g
Poria Sclerotium	4 g	4 g	4 g	4 g
Atractylodes Rhizome	4 g	4 g	4 g	—
Atractylodes Lancea Rhizome	—	—	—	4 g
Alisma Tuber	4 g	5 g	4 g	4 g

Prepare a dry extract or viscous extract as directed under Extracts, according to the preparation 1) to 4), using the crude drugs shown above.

Description Tokishakuyakusan Extract is a light brown to brown powder or black-brown viscous extract. It has a characteristic odor, and a slight sweet taste at first and a bitter taste later.

Identification (1) Shake 1.0 g of the dry extract (or 3.0 g of the viscous extract) with 15 mL of water and 5 mL of 0.1 mol/L hydrochloric acid TS, then add 25 mL of diethyl ether, and shake. Separate the diethyl ether layer, evaporate the solvent under low pressure (in vacuo), add 2 mL of diethyl ether to the residue, and use this solution as the sample solution. Separately, use (*Z*)-ligustilide TS for thin-layer chromatography as the standard solution. Perform the test with these solutions as directed under Thin-layer Chromatography <*2.03*>. Spot 10 μL each of the sample solution and standard solution on a plate of silica gel for thin-layer chromatography, develop the plate with a mixture of ethyl acetate and hexane (1:1) to a distance of about 7 cm, and air-dry the plate. Examine under ultraviolet light (main wavelength: 365 nm): one of the several spots obtained from the sample solution has the same color tone and *R*f value with the blue-white fluorescent spot from the standard solution (Japanese Angelica Root; Cnidium Rhizome).

(2) Shake 1.0 g of the dry extract (or 3.0 g of the viscous extract) with 10 mL of water, add 10 mL of 1-butanol, shake, centrifuge, and use the 1-butanol layer as the sample solution. Separately, dissolve 1 mg of Paeoniflorin RS or paeoniflorin for thin-layer chromatography in 1 mL of methanol, and use this solution as the standard solution. Perform the test with these solutions as directed under Thin-layer Chromatography <*2.03*>. Spot 5 μL each of the sample solution and standard solution on a plate of silica gel for thin-layer chromatography. Develop the plate with a mixture of ethyl acetate, methanol and water (20:3:2) to a distance of about 7 cm, and air-dry the plate. Spray evenly 4-methoxybenzaldehyde-sulfuric acid TS on the plate, and heat the plate at 105°C for 5 minutes: one of the several spots obtained from the sample solution has the same color tone and *R*f value with the purple spot from the standard solution (Peony Root).

(3) For preparation prescribed Atractylodes Rhizome—Shake 1.0 g of the dry extract (or 3.0 g of the viscous extract) with 10 mL of water, add 25 mL of diethyl ether, and shake. Separate the diethyl ether layer, evaporate the solvent under low pressure (in vacuo), add 2 mL of diethyl ether to the residue, and use this solution as the sample solution. Separately, dissolve 1 mg of atractylenolide III for thin-layer chromatography in 2 mL of methanol, and use this solution as the standard solution. Perform the test with these solutions as directed under Thin-layer Chromatography <*2.03*>. Spot 5 μL each of the sample solution and standard solution on a plate of silica gel for thin-layer chromatography. Develop the plate with a mixture of ethyl acetate and hexane (1:1) to a distance of about 7 cm, and air-dry the plate. Spray evenly dilute sulfuric acid on the plate, heat the plate at 105°C for 5 minutes, and examine under ultraviolet light (main wavelength: 365 nm): one of the several spots obtained from the sample solution has the same color tone and *R*f value with the blue-white fluorescent spot from the standard solution (Atractylodes Rhizome).

(4) For preparation prescribed Atractylodes Lancea Rhizome—Shake 2.0 g of the dry extract (or 6.0 g of the viscous extract) with 10 mL of water, add 25 mL of hexane, and shake. Separate the hexane layer, evaporate the solvent under low pressure (in vacuo), add 0.5 mL of hexane to the residue, and use this solution as the sample solution. Perform the test with the sample solution as directed under Thin-layer Chromatography <*2.03*>. Spot 20 μL of the sample solution on a plate of silica gel with fluorescent indicator for thin-layer chromatography. Develop the plate with a mixture of hexane and acetone (7:1) to a distance of about 7 cm, and air-dry the plate. Examine under ultraviolet light (main wavelength: 254 nm): a dark purple spot is observed at an *R*f value of about 0.5. The spot shows a greenish brown color after being sprayed evenly 4-dimethylaminobenzaldehyde TS for spraying, heated at 105°C for 5 minutes, and allowed to cool (Atractylodes Lancea Rhizome).

(5) Shake 2.0 g of the dry extract (or 6.0 g of the viscous extract) with 20 mL of water and 2 mL of ammonia solution (28), add 20 mL of a mixture of hexane and ethyl acetate (20:1), shake, and centrifuge. Separate the upper layer, evaporate the solvent under low pressure (in vacuo), add 2 mL of methanol to the residue, and use this solution as the sample solution. Separately, dissolve 1 mg of alisol A for thin-layer chromatography in 1 mL of methanol, and use this solution as the standard solution. Perform the test with these solutions as directed under Thin-layer Chromatography <*2.03*>. Spot 10 μL each of the sample solution and standard solution on a plate of silica gel for thin-layer chromatography. Develop the plate with a mixture of ethyl formate, water and formic acid (30:1:1) to a distance of about 7 cm, and air-dry the plate. Spray evenly 4-methoxybenzaldehyde-sulfuric acid-acetic acid TS on the plate, heat the plate at 105°C for 5 minutes, allow to cool, and examine under ultraviolet light (main wavelength: 365 nm): one of the several spots obtained from the sample solution has the same color tone and *R*f value with the yellow fluorescent spot from the standard solution (Alisma Tuber).

Purity (1) Heavy metals <*1.07*>—Prepare the test solution with 1.0 g of the dry extract (or an amount of the viscous extract, equivalent to 1.0 g of the dried substance) as directed under Extracts (4), and perform the test (not more than 30 ppm).

(2) Arsenic <*1.11*>—Prepare the test solution with 0.67 g of the dry extract (or an amount of the viscous extract, equivalent to 0.67 g of the dried substance) according to Method 3, and perform the test (not more than 3 ppm).

Loss on drying <*2.41*> The dry extract: Not more than 9.5% (1 g, 105°C, 5 hours).

The viscous extract: Not more than 66.7% (1 g, 105°C, 5 hours).

Total ash <*5.01*> Not more than 10.0%, calculated on the dried basis.

Assay (1) (*E*)-Ferulic acid—Conduct this procedure without exposure to light, using light-resistant vessels. Weigh accurately about 0.5 g of the dry extract (or an amount of the viscous extract, equivalent to about 0.5 g of the dried substance), add exactly 50 mL of diluted methanol (1 in 2), shake for 15 minutes, filter, and use the filtrate as the sample solution. Separately, weigh accurately about 10 mg of (*E*)-ferulic acid for assay, and dissolve in diluted methanol (1 in 2) to make exactly 100 mL. Pipet 2 mL of this solution, add diluted methanol (1 in 2) to make exactly 50 mL, and use this solution as the standard solution. Perform the test with exactly 10 μL each of the sample solution and standard solution as directed under Liquid Chromatography <*2.01*> according to the following conditions, and determine the peak areas, A_T and A_S, of (*E*)-ferulic acid in each solution.

Amount (mg) of (*E*)-ferulic acid $= M_S \times A_T/A_S \times 1/50$

M_S: Amount (mg) of (*E*)-ferulic acid for assay taken

Operating conditions—

Detector: An ultraviolet absorption photometer (wavelength: 320 nm).

Column: A stainless steel column 4.6 mm in inside diameter and 15 cm in length, packed with octadecylsilanized silica gel for liquid chromatography (5 μm in particle diameter).

Column temperature: A constant temperature of about 40°C.

Mobile phase: Dissolve 7.8 g of sodium dihydrogen phosphate in 1000 mL of water, and add 2 mL of phosphoric acid. To 850 mL of this solution add 150 mL of acetonitrile.

Flow rate: 1.0 mL per minute [the retention time of (*E*)-ferulic acid is about 10 minutes].

System suitability—

System performance: When the procedure is run with 10 μL of the standard solution under the above operating conditions, the number of theoretical plates and the symmetry factor of the peak of (*E*)-ferulic acid are not less than 5000 and not more than 1.5, respectively.

System repeatability: When the test is repeated 6 times with 10 μL of the standard solution under the above operating conditions, the relative standard deviation of the peak area of (*E*)-ferulic acid is not more than 1.5%.

(2) Paeoniflorin—Weigh accurately about 0.5 g of the dry extract (or an amount of the viscous extract, equivalent to about 0.5 g of the dried substance), add exactly 50 mL of diluted methanol (1 in 2), shake for 15 minutes, filter, and use the filtrate as the sample solution. Separately, weigh accurately about 10 mg of Paeoniflorin RS (separately determine the water <*2.48*> by coulometric titration, using 10 mg), dissolve in diluted methanol (1 in 2) to make exactly 100 mL, and use this solution as the standard solution. Perform the test with exactly 10 μL each of the sample solution and standard solution as directed under Liquid Chromatography <*2.01*> according to the following conditions, and determine the peak areas, A_T and A_S, of paeoniflorin in each solution.

$$\text{Amount (mg) of paeoniflorin } (C_{23}H_{28}O_{11}) = M_S \times A_T/A_S \times 1/2$$

M_S: Amount (mg) of Paeoniflorin RS taken, calculated on the anhydrous basis

Operating conditions—

Detector: An ultraviolet absorption photometer (wavelength: 232 nm).

Column: A stainless steel column 4.6 mm in inside diameter and 15 cm in length, packed with octadecylsilanized silica gel for liquid chromatography (5 μm in particle diameter).

Column temperature: A constant temperature of about 20°C.

Mobile phase: A mixture of water, acetonitrile and phosphoric acid (850:150:1).

Flow rate: 1.0 mL per minute (the retention time of paeoniflorin is about 9 minutes).

System suitability—

System performance: Dissolve 1 mg of albiflorin in 10 mL of the standard solution. When the procedure is run with 10 μL of this solution under the above operating conditions, albiflorin and paeoniflorin are eluted in this order with the resolution between these peaks being not less than 2.5.

System repeatability: When the test is repeated 6 times with 10 μL of the standard solution under the above operating conditions, the relative standard deviation of the peak area of paeoniflorin is not more than 1.5%.

(3) Atractylenolide III—Weigh accurately about 0.5 g of the dry extract (or an amount of the viscous extract, equivalent to about 0.5 g of the dried substance), add exactly 50 mL of diluted methanol (1 in 2), shake for 15 minutes, filter, and use the filtrate as the sample solution. Separately, weigh accurately about 10 mg of atractylenolide III for assay, previously dried in a desiccator (silica gel) for more than 24 hours, and dissolve in methanol to make exactly 100 mL. Pipet 5 mL of this solution, add diluted methanol (1 in 2) to make exactly 100 mL, and use this solution as the standard solution. Perform the test with exactly 10 μL each of the sample solution and standard solution as directed under Liquid Chromatography <*2.01*> according to the following conditions, and determine the peak areas, A_T and A_S, of atractylenolide III in each solution.

$$\text{Amount (mg) of atractylenolide III} = M_S \times A_T/A_S \times 1/40$$

M_S: Amount (mg) of atractylenolide III for assay taken

Operating conditions—

Detector: An ultraviolet absorption photometer (wavelength: 210 nm).

Column: A stainless steel column 4.6 mm in inside diameter and 15 cm in length, packed with octadecylsilanized silica gel for liquid chromatography (5 μm in particle diameter).

Column temperature: A constant temperature of about 40°C.

Mobile phase: A mixture of water, acetonitrile and phosphoric acid (550:450:1).

Flow rate: 1.0 mL per minute (the retention time of atractylenolide III is about 10 minutes).

System suitability—

System performance: When the procedure is run with 10 μL of the standard solution under the above operating conditions, the number of theoretical plates and the symmetry factor of the peak of atractylenolide III are not less than 5000 and not more than 1.5, respectively.

System repeatability: When the test is repeated 6 times with 10 μL of the standard solution under the above operating conditions, the relative standard deviation of the peak area of atractylenolide III is not more than 1.5%.

(4) Atractylodin—Conduct this procedure without exposure to light, using light-resistant vessels. Weigh accurately about 0.5 g of the dry extract (or an amount of the viscous extract, equivalent to about 0.5 g of the dried substance), add exactly 50 mL of methanol, shake for 15 minutes, filter, and use the filtrate as the sample solution. Perform the test with exactly 10 μL each of the sample solution and atractylodin TS for assay as directed under Liquid Chromatography <*2.01*> according to the following conditions, and determine the peak areas, A_T and A_S, of atractylodin in each solution.

$$\text{Amount (mg) of atractylodin} = C_S \times A_T/A_S \times 50$$

C_S: Concentration (mg/mL) of atractylodin in atractylodin TS for assay

Operating conditions—

Detector: An ultraviolet absorption photometer (wavelength: 340 nm).

Column: A stainless steel column 4.6 mm in inside diameter and 15 cm in length, packed with octadecylsilanized silica gel for liquid chromatography (5 μm in particle diameter).

Column temperature: A constant temperature of about 40°C.

Mobile phase: To 330 mL of a mixture of water and phosphoric acid (55:1) add 670 mL of acetonitrile.

Flow rate: 1.0 mL per minute (the retention time of atractylodin is about 13 minutes).

System suitability—

System performance: When the procedure is run with 10 μL of atractylodin TS for assay under the above operating conditions, the number of theoretical plates and the symmetry factor of the peak of atractylodin are not less than 5000 and not more than 1.5, respectively.

System repeatability: When the test is repeated 6 times with 10 μL of atractylodin TS for assay under the above operating conditions, the relative standard deviation of the peak area of atractylodin is not more than 1.5%.

Containers and storage Containers—Tight containers.

Tragacanth

Tragacantha

トラガント

Tragacanth is the exudation obtained from the trunks of *Astragalus gummifer* Labillardiére or other species of the same genus (*Leguminosae*).

Description Tragacanth occurs as curved, flattened or lamellate fragments, 0.5 – 3 mm in thickness. It is white to light yellow in color, translucent, and horny in texture. It is easily broken, and swells in water.

Odorless; tasteless and mucilaginous.

Identification **(1)** To 1 g of pulverized Tragacanth add 50 mL of water: a nearly uniform, slightly turbid mucilage is formed.

(2) To pulverized Tragacanth add dilute iodine TS, and examine the mixture microscopically ⟨*5.01*⟩: a few blue-colored starch grains are observable.

Purity Karaya gum—Boil 1 g of Tragacanth with 20 mL of water until a mucilage is formed, add 5 mL of hydrochloric acid, and again boil the mixture for 5 minutes: no light red to red color develops.

Total ash ⟨*5.01*⟩ Not more than 4.0%.

Containers and storage Containers—Well-closed containers.

Powdered Tragacanth

Tragacantha Pulverata

トラガント末

Powdered Tragacanth is the powder of Tragacanth.

Description Powdered Tragacanth occurs as a white to yellowish white powder. It is odorless, tasteless and mucilaginous.

Under a microscope ⟨*5.01*⟩, it, immersed in olive oil or liquid paraffin, reveals numerous angular fragments with a small amount of the circular or irregular lamellae or of starch grains. Starch grains are spherical to elliptical, mostly simple and occasionally 2- to 4-compound grains, simple grain, 3 – 25 μm in diameter. The fragments are swollen and altered with water.

Identification **(1)** To 1 g of Powdered Tragacanth add 50 mL of water: a nearly uniform, slightly turbid mucilage is formed.

(2) To Powdered Tragacanth add dilute iodine TS, and examine the mixture microscopically ⟨*5.01*⟩: a few blue-colored starch grains are observable.

Purity Karaya gum—Boil 1 g of Powdered Tragacanth with 20 mL of water until a mucilage is formed, add 5 mL of hydrochloric acid, and again boil the mixture for 5 minutes: no light red to red color develops.

Total ash ⟨*5.01*⟩ Not more than 4.0%.

Containers and storage Containers—Tight containers.

Tribulus Fruit

Tribuli Fructus

シツリシ

Tribulus Fruit is the fruit of *Tribulus terrestris* Linné (*Zygophyllaceae*).

Description Pentagonal star shaped fruit, composed of five mericarps, 7 – 12 mm in diameter, often each mericarp separated; externally grayish green to grayish brown; a pair of longer and shorter spines on surface of each mericarp, the longer spine 3 – 7 mm in length, the shorter one 2 – 5 mm in length, numerous small processes on ridge; pericarp hard in texture, cut surface light yellow; each mericarp contains 1 – 3 seeds.

Almost odorless; taste, mild at first, followed by bitterness.

Under a microscope ⟨*5.01*⟩, a transverse section reveals epicarp composed of an epidermis; mesocarp composed of parenchyma and sclerenchyma layer; endocarp composed of several-cellular-layered fiber cells; a single-layer of cell between mesocarp and endocarp contain solitary crystals of calcium oxalate; cotyledons of seed contain oil drops and aleurone grains, and occasionally starch grains.

Identification To 2 g of pulverized Tribulus Fruit add 5 mL of methanol, shake for 10 minutes, filter, and use the filtrate as the sample solution. Perform the test with the sample solution as directed under Thin-layer Chromatography ⟨*2.03*⟩. Spot 10 μL of the sample solution on a plate of silica gel for thin-layer chromatography, develop the plate with a mixture of ethyl acetate and water (40:1) to a distance of about 7 cm, and air-dry the plate. Spray evenly dilute sulfuric acid on the plate, heat the plate at 105°C for 5 minutes, and examine under ultraviolet light (main wavelength: 365 nm): a bluish white fluorescent spot appears at an *R*f value of about 0.4.

Purity **(1)** Peduncle—When perform the test of foreign matter ⟨*5.01*⟩, the amount of peduncle contained in Tribulus Fruit does not exceed 4.0%.

(2) Foreign matters ⟨*5.01*⟩—Not more than 1.0% of foreign matters other than peduncle.

Loss on drying ⟨*5.01*⟩ Not more than 11.0% (6 hours).

Total ash ⟨*5.01*⟩ Not more than 13.0%.

Acid-insoluble ash ⟨*5.01*⟩ Not more than 1.5%.

Extract content ⟨*5.01*⟩ Dilute ethanol-soluble extract: not less than 8.5%.

Containers and storage Containers—Well-closed containers.

Trichosanthes Root

Trichosanthis Radix

カロコン

Trichosanthes Root is the root of *Trichosanthes kirilowii* Maximowicz, *Trichosanthes kirilowii* Maximowicz var. *japonica* Kitamura or *Trichosanthes bracteata* Voigt (*Cucurbitaceae*), from which the cork layer is mostly removed.

Description Irregular cylindrical root, 5 - 10 cm in length, 3 - 5 cm in diameter, often cut lengthwise; externally light yellow-white, and with irregular pattern of vascular bundles appearing as brownish yellow lines; fractured surface somewhat fibrous and light yellow in color; under a magnifying glass, the transverse section reveals wide medullary rays and brownish yellow spots or small holes formed by vessels.

Almost odorless; taste, slightly bitter.

Identification To 2.0 g of pulverized Trichosanthes Root add 5 mL of methanol, shake for 10 minutes, centrifuge, and use the supernatant liquid as the sample solution. Perform the test with the sample solution as directed under Thin-layer Chromatography <*2.03*>. Spot 10 μL of the sample solution on a plate of silica gel for thin-layer chromatography. Develop the plate with a mixture of hexane, ethyl acetate and acetic acid (100) (20:10:1) to a distance of about 7 cm, and air-dry the plate. Spray evenly dilute sulfuric acid on the plate, heat the plate at 105°C for 10 minutes, and examine under ultraviolet light (main wavelength: 365 nm): a light yellow to light yellow-green fluorescent spot appears at an *R*f value of about 0.4.

Purity **(1)** Heavy metals <*1.07*>—Proceed with 3.0 g of pulverized Trichosanthes Root according to Method 3, and perform the test. Prepare the control solution with 3.0 mL of Standard Lead Solution (not more than 10 ppm).

(2) Arsenic <*1.11*>—Prepare the test solution with 0.40 g of pulverized Trichosanthes Root according to Method 4, and perform the test (not more than 5 ppm).

Total ash <*5.01*> Not more than 4.0%.

Containers and storage Containers—Well-closed containers.

Turmeric

Curcumae Longae Rhizoma

ウコン

Turmeric is the rhizome of *Curcuma longa* Linné (*Zingiberaceae*) with or without cork layers, usually with the application of blanching.

It contains not less than 1.0% and not more than 5.0% of total curcuminoids (curcumin, demethoxycurcumin and bisdemethoxycurcumin), calculated on the basis of dried material.

Description Turmeric is a main rhizome or a lateral rhizome; main rhizome, nearly ovoid, about 3 cm in diameter, about 4 cm in length; lateral rhizome, cylindrical, with round tips, curved, about 1 cm in diameter, 2 - 6 cm in length; both main and lateral rhizomes with cyclic nodes; rhizome with cork layer, yellow-brown, lustrous; rhizome without cork layer, dark yellow-red, with yellow-red powders on surface; hard in texture, not easily broken; transversely cut surface yellow-brown to red-brown, lustrous like wax.

Odor, characteristic; taste, slightly bitter and stimulant, it colors a saliva yellow on chewing.

Under a microscope <*5.01*>, a transverse section reveals the outermost layer to be composed of a cork layer 4 - 10 cells thick; sometimes a cork layer partly remains; cortex and stele, divided by an endodermis, composed of parenchyma, vascular bundles scattered; oil cells scattered in parenchyma; parenchymatous cells contain yellow substances, sandy and solitary crystals of calcium oxalate, and gelatinized starch.

Identification **(1)** To 0.5 g of pulverized Turmeric, add 20 mL of methanol, shake for 15 minutes, filter, and use the filtrate as the sample solution. Perform the test with the sample solution as directed under Thin-layer Chromatography <*2.03*>. Spot 5 μL of the sample solution on a plate of silica gel for thin-layer chromatography. Develop the plate with a mixture of ethyl acetate, hexane and acetic acid (100) (11:9:1) to a distance about 7 cm, and air-dry the plate: a yellow spot appears at an *R*f value of about 0.4.

(2) To 0.2 g of pulverized Turmeric, add 25 mL of a mixture of methanol and acetic acid (100) (99:1), centrifuge after shaking for 20 minutes. Perform the test with the supernatant liquid as directed in the Assay, and determine the peak areas of curcumin, demethoxycurcumin and bisdemethoxycurcumin: the peak area of curcumin is larger than the peak area of demethoxycurcumin and is larger than 0.69 times the peak area of bisdemethoxycurcumin.

Purity **(1)** Heavy metals <*1.07*>—Proceed with 3.0 g of pulverized Turmeric according to Method 3, and perform the test. Prepare the control solution with 3.0 mL of Standard Lead Solution (not more than 10 ppm).

(2) Arsenic <*1.11*>—Prepare the test solution with 0.40 g of pulverized Turmeric according to Method 4, and perform the test (not more than 5 ppm).

Loss on drying <*5.01*> Not more than 17.0% (6 hours).

Total ash <*5.01*> Not more than 7.5%.

Acid-insoluble ash <*5.01*> Not more than 1.0%.

Extract content <*5.01*> Dilute ethanol-soluble extract: not less than 9.0%.

Assay Weigh accurately about 0.2 g of pulverized Turmeric, add 25 mL of a mixture of methanol and acetic acid (100) (99:1), shake for 20 minutes, centrifuge, and separate the supernatant liquid. To the residue, add 25 mL of a mixture of methanol and acetic acid (100) (99:1), and proceed in the same manner as described above. Combine all the extracts, add methanol to make exactly 50 mL, and use this solution as the sample solution. Separately, weigh accurately about 10 mg of curcumin for assay, and dissolve in methanol to make exactly 50 mL. Pipet 10 mL of this solution, add methanol to make exactly 50 mL, and use this solution as the standard solution. Perform the test with exactly 10 μL each of the sample solution and standard solution as described under Liquid Chromatography <*2.01*> according to the following conditions, and determine the peak areas, A_{TC}, A_{TD} and A_{TD} of curcumin, demethoxycurcumin and bisdemethoxycurcumin in the sample solution as well as the peak area A_S of curcumin in the standard solution.

Amount (mg) of total curcuminoids (curcumin, demethoxycurcumin and bisdemethoxycurcumin)
$= M_S \times (A_{TC} + A_{TD} + A_{TB} \times 0.69)/A_S \times 1/5$

M_S: Amount (mg) of curcumin for assay taken

Operating conditions—

Detector: An ultraviolet absorption photometer (wavelength: 245 nm).

Column: A stainless steel column 4.6 mm in inside diameter and 15 cm in length, packed with octadecylsilianized silica gel for liquid chromatography (5 μm in particle diameter).

Column temperature: A constant temperature of about 40°C.

Mobile phase: A mixture of water, acetonitrile and acetic acid (100) (56:43:1).

Flow rate: 1.0 mL per minute (the retention time of curcumin is about 11 minutes).

System suitability—

System performance: Dissolve 1 mg each of curcumin for assay, demethoxycurcumin and bisdemethoxycurcumin in methanol to make 5 mL. When the procedure is run with 10 μL of this solution under the above operating conditions, bisdemethoxycurcumin, demethoxycurcumin and curcumin are eluted in this order with the resolution among these peaks being not less than 1.5.

System repeatability: When the test is repeated 6 times with 10 μL of the standard solution under the above operating conditions, the relative standard deviation of curcumin is not more than 1.5%.

Containers and storage Containers—Well-closed containers.

Powdered Turmeric

Curcumae Longae Rhizoma Pulveratum

ウコン末

Powdered Turmeric is the powder of Turmeric.

It contains not less than 1.0% and not more than 5.0% of total curcuminoids (curcumin, demethoxycurcumin and bisdemethoxycurcumin), calculated on the basis of dried material.

Description Powdered Turmeric occurs as a yellow-brown to dark yellow-brown powder. It has a characteristic odor and a bitter, stimulant taste, and colors the saliva yellow on chewing.

Under a microscope <5.01>, all elements are yellow in color; it reveals parenchymatous cells containing mainly masses of gelatinized starch or yellow substances, also fragments of scalariform vessels; fragments of cork layers, epidermis, thick-walled xylem parenchymatous cells, and non-glandular hairs are occasionally observed.

Identification **(1)** To 0.5 g of Powdered Turmeric, add 20 mL of methanol, shake for 15 minutes, filter, and use the filtrate as the sample solution. Perform the test with the sample solution as directed under Thin-layer Chromatography <2.03>. Spot 5 μL of the sample solution on a plate of silica gel for thin-layer chromatography. Develop the plate with a mixture of ethyl acetate, hexane and acetic acid (100) (11:9:1) to a distance about 7 cm, and air-dry the plate: a yellow spot appears at an *R*f value of about 0.4.

(2) To 0.2 g of Powdered Turmeric, add 25 mL of a mixture of methanol and acetic acid (100) (99:1), centrifuge after shaking for 20 minutes. Perform the test with the supernatant liquid as directed in the Assay, and determine the peak areas of curcumin, demethoxycurcumin and bisdemethoxycurcumin: the peak area of curcumin is larger than the peak area of demethoxycurcumin and is larger than 0.69 times the peak area of bisdemethoxycurcumin.

Purity **(1)** Heavy metals <1.07>—Proceed with 3.0 g of Powdered Turmeric according to Method 3, and perform the test. Prepare the control solution with 3.0 mL of Standard Lead Solution (not more than 10 ppm).

(2) Arsenic <1.11>—Prepare the test solution with 0.40 g of Powdered Turmeric according to Method 4, and perform the test (not more than 5 ppm).

Loss on drying <5.01> Not more than 17.0% (6 hours).

Total ash <5.01> Not more than 7.5%.

Acid-insoluble ash <5.01> Not more than 1.0%.

Extract content <5.01> Dilute ethanol-soluble extract: not less than 9.0%.

Assay Weigh accurately about 0.2 g of Powdered Turmeric, add 25 mL of a mixture of methanol and acetic acid (100) (99:1), shake for 20 minutes, centrifuge, and separate the supernatant liquid. To the residue, add 25 mL of a mixture of methanol and acetic acid (100) (99:1), and proceed in the same manner as described above. Combine all the extracts, add methanol to make exactly 50 mL, and use this solution as the sample solution. Separately, weigh accurately about 10 mg of curcumin for assay, and dissolve in methanol to make exactly 50 mL. Pipet 10 mL of this solution, add methanol to make exactly 50 mL, and use this solution as the standard solution. Perform the test with exactly 10 μL each of the sample solution and standard solution as described under Liquid Chromatography <2.01> according to the following conditions, and determine the peak areas, A_{TC}, A_{TD} and A_{TB} of curcumin, demethoxycurcumin and bisdemethoxycurcumin in the sample solution as well as the peak area A_S of curcumin in the standard solution.

Amount (mg) of total curcuminoids (curcumin, demethoxycurcumin and bisdemethoxycurcumin)
$= M_S \times (A_{TC} + A_{TD} + A_{TB} \times 0.69)/A_S \times 1/5$

M_S: Amount (mg) of curcumin for assay taken

Operating conditions—

Detector: An ultraviolet absorption photometer (wavelength: 245 nm).

Column: A stainless steel column 4.6 mm in inside diameter and 15 cm in length, packed with octadecylsilianized silica gel for liquid chromatography (5 μm in particle diameter).

Column temperature: A constant temperature of about 40°C.

Mobile phase: A mixture of water, acetonitrile and acetic acid (100) (56:43:1).

Flow rate: 1.0 mL/per minute (the retention time of curcumin is about 11 minutes).

System suitability—

System performance: Dissolve 1 mg each of curcumin for assay, demethoxycurcumin and bisdemethoxycurcumin in methanol to make 5 mL. When the procedure is run with 10 μL of this solution under the above operating conditions, bisdemethoxycurcumin, demethoxycurcumin and curcumin are eluted in this order with the resolution among these peaks being not less than 1.5.

System repeatability: When the test is repeated 6 times with 10 μL of the standard solution under the above operating conditions, the relative standard deviation of curcumin is not more than 1.5%.

Containers and storage Containers—Well-closed containers.

Turpentine Oil

Oleum Terebinthinae

テレビン油

Turpentine Oil is the essential oil distilled with steam from the wood or balsam of *Pinus* species (*Pinaceae*).

Description Turpentine Oil is a clear, colorless to pale yellow liquid. It has a characteristic odor and a pungent, bitter taste.

Turpentine Oil (1 mL) is miscible with 5 mL of ethanol (95) and this solution is neutral.

Refractive index *<2.45>* n_D^{20}: 1.465 - 1.478

Specific gravity *<1.13>* d_{20}^{20}: 0.860 - 0.875

Purity **(1)** Foreign matter—Turpentine Oil has no offensive odor. Shake 5 mL of Turpentine Oil with 5 mL of a solution of potassium hydroxide (1 in 6): the aqueous layer does not show a yellow-brown to dark brown color.

(2) Hydrochloric acid-coloring substances—Shake 5 mL of Turpentine Oil with 5 mL of hydrochloric acid, and allow to stand for 5 minutes: the hydrochloric acid layer is light yellow and not brown in color.

(3) Mineral oil—Place 5 mL of Turpentine Oil in a Cassia flask, cool to a temperature not exceeding 15°C, add dropwise 25 mL of fuming sulfuric acid while shaking, warm between 60°C and 65°C for 10 minutes, and add sulfuric acid to raise the lower level of the oily layer to the graduated portion of the neck: not more than 0.1 mL of oil separates.

Distilling range *<2.57>* 150 - 170°C, not less than 90 vol%.

Containers and storage Containers—Tight containers.

Storage—Light-resistant.

Uncaria Hook

Uncariae Uncis Cum Ramulus

チョウトウコウ

Uncaria Hook is, hook or the hook-bearing stem of *Uncaria rhynchophylla* Miquel, *Uncaria sinensis* Haviland or *Uncaria macrophylla* Wallich (*Rubiaceae*), sometimes after being passed through hot water or steamed.

Uncaria Hook contains not less than 0.03% of total alkaloids (rhynchophylline and hirsutine), calculated on the basis of dried material.

Description Uncaria Hook is uncinate hook or short stem with opposite or single hook; the hook, 1 - 4 cm in length, curved and acuminate; externally red-brown to dark brown or grayish brown, some one with hairs, the transverse section oblong to elliptical, light brown; stem thin and prismatic square to cylindrical, 2 - 5 mm in diameter, externally, red-brown to dark brown or grayish brown; the transverse section, square to elliptical; the pith light brown, square to elliptical; hard in texture.

Odorless and practically tasteless.

Under a microscope *<5.01>*, a transverse section of the hook reveals vascular bundles in the cortex, unevenly distributed and arranged in a ring. Parenchyma cells in the secondary cortex containing sand crystals of calcium oxalate.

Identification To 1.0 g of pulverized Uncaria Hook add 10 mL of water and 1 mL of ammonia TS, shake, then add 10 mL of diethyl ether, shake for 10 minutes, centrifuge, and use the diethyl ether layer as the sample solution. Separately, dissolve 1 mg each of rhyncophylline for thin-layer chromatography and hirsutine for thin-layer chromatography in 1 mL of methanol, and use this solution as the standard solution. Perform the test with these solutions as directed under Thin-layer Chromatography *<2.03>*. Spot 10 μL of the sample solution and 2 μL of the standard solution on a plate of silica gel for thin-layer chromatography. Develop the plate with a mixture of ethyl acetate, methanol and water (7:2:1) to a distance of about 7 cm, and air-dry the plate. Spray evenly Dragendorff's TS for spraying on the plate, and air-dry the plate. Then spray evenly sodium nitrite TS on the plate: one of the several spots obtained from the sample solution has the same color tone and *Rf* value with one of the spots from the standard solution.

Loss on drying *<5.01>* Not more than 12.0% (6 hours).

Total ash *<5.01>* Not more than 4.0%.

Extract content *<5.01>* Dilute ethanol-soluble extract: not less than 8.5%.

Assay Weigh accurately about 0.2 g of moderately fine powder of Uncaria Hook, transfer into a glass-stoppered centrifuge tube, add 30 mL of a mixture of methanol and dilute acetic acid (7:3), shake for 30 minutes, centrifuge, and separate the supernatant liquid. To the residue add two 10-mL portions of a mixture of methanol and dilute acetic acid (7:3), proceed in the same manner, and combine all of the supernatant liquid. To the combined liquid add a mixture of methanol and dilute acetic acid (7:3) to make exactly 50 mL, and use this as the sample solution. Separately, weigh accurately about 5 mg of rhynchophylline for assay, previously dried in a desiccator (silica gel) for 24 hours, and dissolve in a mixture of methanol and dilute acetic acid (7:3) to make exactly 100 mL. Pipet 1 mL of this solution, add a mixture of methanol and dilute acetic acid (7:3) to make exactly 10 mL, and use this solution as the standard solution (1). Separately, dissolve 1 mg of hirsutine in 100 mL of a mixture of methanol and dilute acetic acid (7:3), and use this solution as the standard solution (2). Perform the test with exactly 20 μL each of the sample solution and standard solutions (1) and (2) as directed under Liquid Chromatography *<2.01>* according to the following conditions. Determine the peak areas, A_{Ta} and A_{Tb}, of rhynchophylline and hirsutine obtained from the sample solution, and the peak area, A_S, of rhynchophylline from the standard solution (1).

Amount (mg) of total alkaloids (rhynchophylline and hirsutine)

$$= M_S \times (A_{Ta} + 1.405 A_{Tb})/A_S \times 1/20$$

M_S: Amount (mg) of rhynchophylline for assay taken

Operating conditions—

Detector: An ultraviolet absorption photometer (wavelength: 245 nm).

Column: A stainless steel column 4.6 mm in inside diameter and 25 cm in length, packed with octadecylsilanized silica gel for liquid chromatography (5 μm in particle diameter).

Column temperature: A constant temperature of about 40°C.

Mobile phase: Dissolve 3.85 g of ammonium acetate in 200 mL of water, add 10 mL of acetic acid (100) and water to make 1000 mL, and add 350 mL of acetonitrile.

Flow rate: Adjust so that the retention time of rhynchophylline is about 17 minutes.

System suitability—

System performance: Dissolve 5 mg of rhynchophylline for assay in 100 mL of a mixture of methanol and dilute acetic acid (7:3). To 5 mL of this solution add 1 mL of ammonia solution (28), and reflux for 10 minutes or warm at about 50°C for 2 hours. After cooling, to 1 mL of the solution so obtained add a mixture of methanol and dilute acetic acid (7:3) to make 5 mL. When the procedure is run with 20 μL of this solution under the above operating conditions, the peak of isorhynchophylline is appears in addition to the peak of rhynchophylline, and the resolution between these peaks is not less than 1.5.

System repeatability: When the test is repeated 6 times with 20 μL of the standard solution (1) under the above operating conditions, the relative standard deviation of the peak areas of rhynchophylline is not more than 1.5%.

Containers and storage Containers—Well-closed containers.

Unseiin Extract

温清飲エキス

Unseiin Extract contains not less than 24 mg and not more than 72 mg (for preparation prescribed 3 g of Peony Root) or not less than 32 mg and not more than 96 mg (for preparation prescribed 4 g of Peony Root) of paeoniflorin ($C_{23}H_{28}O_{11}$: 480.46), not less than 39 mg and not more than 117 mg (for preparation prescribed 1.5 g of Scutellaria Root), or not less than 78 mg and not more than 234 mg (for preparation prescribed 3 g of Scutellaria Root) of baicalin ($C_{21}H_{18}O_{11}$: 446.36), and not less than 20 mg and not more than 60 mg of berberine [as berberine chloride ($C_{20}H_{18}ClNO_4$: 371.81)], per extract prepared with the amount specified in the Method of preparation.

Method of preparation

	1)	2)	3)
Japanese Angelica Root	4 g	4 g	3 g
Rehmannia Root	4 g	4 g	3 g
Peony Root	3 g	4 g	3 g
Cnidium Rhizome	3 g	4 g	3 g
Scutellaria Root	3 g	3 g	1.5 g
Gardenia Fruit	2 g	2 g	1.5 g
Coptis Rhizome	1.5 g	1.5 g	1.5 g
Phellodendron Bark	1.5 g	1.5 g	1.5 g

Prepare a dry extract or viscous extract as directed under Extracts, according to the prescription 1) to 3), using the crude drugs shown above.

Description Unseiin Extract occurs as a yellow-brown to very dark brown powder or black-brown viscous extract. It has a slight odor, and has a slightly sweet taste at first, followed by a pungent taste.

Identification **(1)** To 1.0 g of the dry extract (or 3.0 g of the viscous extract) add 15 mL of water and 5 mL of 0.1 mol/L hydrochloric acid TS, shake, then add 25 mL of diethyl ether, and shake. Separate the diethyl ether layer, evaporate the solvent under low pressure (in vacuo), add 2 mL of diethyl ether to the residue, and use this solution as the sample solution. Separately, use (*Z*)-ligustilide TS for thin-layer chromatography as the standard solution. Perform the test with these solutions as directed under Thin layer Chromatography <*2.03*>. Spot 10 μL each of the sample solution and standard solution on a plate of silica gel for thin-layer chromatography. Develop the plate with a mixture of butyl acetate and hexane (2:1) to a distance of about 7 cm, and air-dry the plate. Examine under ultraviolet light (main wavelength: 365 nm): one of the several spots obtained from the sample solution has the same color tone and *R*f value with the blue-white fluorescent spot from the standard solution (Japanese Angelica Root and Cnidium Rhizome).

(2) To 0.5 g of the dry extract (or 1.5 g of the viscous extract) add 10 mL of methanol, shake, centrifuge, and use the supernatant liquid as the sample solution. Separately, dissolve 1 mg of Paeoniflorin RS or paeoniflorin for thin-layer chromatography in 1 mL of methanol, and use this solution as the standard solution. Perform the test with these solutions as directed under Thin-layer Chromatography <*2.03*>. Spot 5 μL each of the sample solution and standard solution on a plate of silica gel for thin-layer chromatography. Develop the plate with a mixture of ethyl acetate, methanol and water (20:3:2) to a distance of about 7 cm, and air-dry the plate. Spray evenly 4-methoxybenzaldehyde-sulfuric acid TS on the plate, and heat the plate at 105°C for 1 minute: one of the several spots obtained from the sample solution has the same color tone and *R*f value with the red-purple to purple spot from the standard solution (Peony Root).

(3) To 1.0 g of the dry extract (or 3.0 g of the viscous extract) add 10 mL of water, shake, then add 25 mL of diethyl ether, and shake. Separate the diethyl ether layer, evaporate the solvent under low pressure (in vacuo), then add 2 mL of diethyl ether to the residue, and use this solution as the sample solution. Separately, dissolve 1 mg of wogonin for thin-layer chromatography in 1 mL of methanol, and use this solution as the standard solution. Perform the test with these solutions as directed under Thin-layer Chromatography <*2.03*>. Spot 20 μL of the sample solution and 5 μL of the standard solution on a plate of silica gel for thin-layer chromatography. Develop the plate with a mixture of ethyl acetate, hexane and acetic acid (100) (10:10:1) to a distance of about 7 cm, and air-dry the plate. Spray evenly iron (III) chloride-methanol TS on the plate: one of the several spots obtained from the sample solution has the same color tone and *R*f value with the yellow-brown to grayish brown spot from the standard solution (Scutellaria Root).

(4) To 0.5 g of the dry extract (or 1.5 g of the viscous extract) add 10 mL of methanol, shake, centrifuge, and use the supernatant liquid as the sample solution. Separately, dissolve 1 mg of geniposide for thin-layer chromatography in 1 mL of methanol, and use this solution as the standard solution. Perform the test with these solutions as directed under Thin-layer Chromatography <*2.03*>. Spot 5 μL each of the sample solution and standard solution on a plate of silica gel for thin-layer chromatography. Develop the plate with a mixture of ethyl acetate, methanol and water (20:3:2) to a distance of about 7 cm, and air-dry the plate. Spray evenly 4-methoxybenzaldehyde-sulfric acid TS on the plate, and heat the plate at 105°C for 1 minute: one of the several spots obtained from the sample solution has the same color tone and *Rf* value with the purple to dark purple spot from the standard solution (Gardenia Fruit).

(5) To 0.5 g of the dry extract (or 1.5 g of the viscous extract) add 10 mL of methanol, shake, centrifuge, and use the supernatant liquid as the sample solution. Separately, dissolve 1 mg of coptisine chloride for thin-layer chromatography in 5 mL of methanol, and use this solution as the standard solution. Perform the test with these solutions as directed under Thin-layer Chromatography <*2.03*>. Spot 2 μL each of the sample solution and standard solution on a plate of silica gel for thin-layer chromatography. Develop the plate with a mixture of ethyl acetate, ammonia solution (28) and methanol (15:1:1) to a distance of about 7 cm, and air-dry the plate. Examine under ultraviolet light (main wavelength: 365 nm): one of the several spots obtained from the sample solution has the same color tone and *Rf* value with the yellow fluorescent spot from the standard solution (Coptis Rhizome).

(6) To 1.0 g of dry extract (or 3.0 g of the viscous extract) add 10 mL of water, shake, then add 25 mL of diethyl ether, and shake. Separate the diethyl ether layer, evaporate the solvent under low pressure (in vacuo), then add 2 mL of diethyl ether to the residue, and use this solution as the sample solution. Separately, dissolve 1 mg of limonin for thin-layer chromatography in 1 mL of methanol, and use this solution as the standard solution. Perform the test with these solutions as directed under Thin-layer Chromatography <*2.03*>. Spot 10 μL of the sample solution and 5 μL of the standard solution on a plate of silica gel for thin-layer chromatography. Develop the plate with a mixture of ethyl acetate, hexane and acetic acid (100) (10:5:1) to a distance of about 7 cm, and air-dry the plate. Spray evenly vanillin-sulfuric acid-ethanol TS for spraying on the plate, heat the plate at 105°C for 5 minutes, and allow to cool: one of the several spots obtained from the sample solution has the same color tone and *Rf* value with the purple to dark purple spot from the standard solution (Phellodendron Bark).

Purity **(1)** Heavy metals <*1.07*>—Prepare the test solution with 1.0 g of the dry extract (or an amount of the viscous extract, equivalent to 1.0 g of the dried substance) as directed under Extracts (4), and perform the test (not more than 30 ppm).

(2) Arsenic <*1.11*>—Prepare the test solution with 0.67 g of the dry extract (or an amount of the viscous extract, equivalent to 0.67 g of the dried substance) according to Method 3, and perform the test (not more than 3 ppm).

Loss on drying <*2.41*> The dry extract: Not more than 10.0% (1 g, 105°C, 5 hours).

The viscous extract: Not more than 66.7% (1 g, 105°C, 5 hours).

Total ash <*5.01*> Not more than 9.0%, calculated on the dried basis.

Assay **(1)** Paeoniflorin—Weigh accurately about 0.5 g of the dry extract (or an amount of the viscous extract, equivalent to about 0.5 g of the dried substance), add exactly 50 mL of diluted methanol (1 in 2), shake for 15 minutes, and filter. Pipet 5 mL of the filtrate, flow through in a column packed with 2 g of polyamide for column chromatography, elute with 20 mL of water, then add 1 mL of acetic acid (100) to the eluate, add water to make exactly 25 mL, and use this solution as the sample solution. Separately, weigh accurately about 10 mg of Paeoniflorin RS (separately determine the water <*2.48*> by coulometric titration, using 10 mg), and dissolve in diluted methanol (1 in 2) to make exactly 100 mL. Pipet 5 mL of this solution, add diluted methanol (1 in 2) to make exactly 20 mL, and use this solution as the standard solution. Perform the test with exactly 10 μL each of the sample solution and standard solution as directed under Liquid Chromatography <*2.01*> according to the following conditions, and determine the peak areas, A_T and A_S, of paeoniflorin in each solution.

$$\text{Amount (mg) of paeoniflorin } (C_{23}H_{28}O_{11}) = M_S \times A_T/A_S \times 5/8$$

M_S: Amount (mg) of Paeoniflorin RS taken, calculated on the anhydrous basis

Operating conditions—

Detector: An ultraviolet absorption photometer (wavelength: 232 nm).

Column: A stainless steel column 4.6 mm in inside diameter and 15 cm in length, packed with octadecylsilanized silica gel for liquid chromatography (5 μm in particle diameter).

Column temperature: A constant temperature of about 20°C.

Mobile phase: A mixture of water, acetonitrile and phosphoric acid (850:150:1).

Flow rate: 1.0 mL per minute.

System suitability—

System performance: Dissolve 1 mg each of Paeoniflorin RS and albiflorin in diluted methanol (1 in 2) to make 10 mL. When the procedure is run with 10 μL of this solution under the above operating conditions, albiflorin and paeoniflorin are eluted in this order with the resolution between these peaks being not less than 2.5.

System repeatability: When the test is repeated 6 times with 10 μL of the standard solution under the above operating conditions, the relative standard deviation of the peak area of paeoniflorin is not more than 1.5%.

(2) Baicalin—Weigh accurately about 0.1 g of the dry extract (or an amount of the viscous extract, equivalent to about 0.1 g of the dried substance), add exactly 50 mL of diluted methanol (7 in 10), shake for 15 minutes, filter, and use the filtrate as the sample solution. Separately, weigh accurately about 10 mg of Baicalin RS (separately determine the water <*2.48*> by coulometric titration, using 10 mg), and dissolve in methanol to make exactly 100 mL. Pipet 5 mL of this solution, add diluted methanol (7 in 10) to make exactly 10 mL, and use this solution as the standard solution. Perform the test with exactly 10 μL each of the sample solution and standard solution as directed under Liquid Chromatography <*2.01*> according to the following conditions, and determine the peak areas, A_T and A_S, of baicalin in each solution.

$$\text{Amount (mg) of baicalin } (C_{21}H_{18}O_{11}) = M_S \times A_T/A_S \times 1/4$$

M_S: Amount (mg) of Baicalin RS taken, calculated on the anhydrous basis

Operating conditions—

Detector: An ultraviolet absorption photometer (wavelength: 277 nm).

Column: A stainless steel column 4.6 mm in inside diameter and 15 cm in length, packed with octadecylsilanized silica gel for liquid chromatography (5 μm in particle diameter).

Column temperature: A constant temperature of about 40°C.

Mobile phase: A mixture of diluted phosphoric acid (1 in 200) and acetonitrile (19:6).

Flow rate: 1.0 mL per minute.

System suitability—

System performance: When the procedure is run with 10 μL of the standard solution under the above operating conditions, the number of theoretical plates and the symmetry factor of the peak of baicalin are not less than 5000 and not more than 1.5, respectively.

System repeatability: When the test is repeated 6 times with 10 μL of the standard solution under the above operating conditions, the relative standard deviation of the peak area of baicalin is not more than 1.5%.

(3) Berberine—Weigh accurately about 0.2 g of the dry extract (or an amount of the viscous extract, equivalent to about 0.2 g of the dried substance), add exactly 50 mL of the mobile phase, shake for 15 minutes, filter, and use the filtrate as the sample solution. Separately, weigh accurately about 10 mg of Berberine Chloride RS (separately determine the water *<2.48>* in the same manner as Berberine Chloride Hydrate), dissolve in the mobile phase to make exactly 100 mL, and use this solution as the standard solution. Perform the test with exactly 10 μL each of the sample solution and standard solution as directed under Liquid Chromatography *<2.01>* according to the following conditions, and determine the peak areas, A_T and A_S, of berberine in each solution.

Amount (mg) of berberine chloride ($C_{20}H_{18}ClNO_4$)
$= M_S \times A_T/A_S \times 1/2$

M_S: Amount (mg) of Berberine Chloride RS taken, calculated on the anhydrous basis

Operating conditions—

Detector: An ultraviolet absorption photometer (wavelength: 345 nm).

Column: A stainless steel column 4.6 mm in inside diameter and 15 cm in length, packed with octadecylsilanized silica gel for liquid chromatography (5 μm in particle diameter).

Column temperature: A constant temperature of about 30°C.

Mobile phase: Dissolve 3.4 g of potassium dihydrogen phosphate and 1.7 g of sodium lauryl sulfate in 1000 mL of a mixture of water and acetonitrile (1:1).

Flow rate: 1.0 mL per minute.

System suitability—

System performance: Dissolve 1 mg each of Berberine Chloride RS and palmatine chloride in the mobile phase to make 10 mL. When the procedure is run with 10 μL of this solution under the above operating conditions, palmatine and berberine are eluted in this order with the resolution between these peaks being not less than 1.5.

System repeatability: When the test is repeated 6 times with 10 μL of the standard solution under the above operating conditions, the relative standard deviation of the peak area of berberine is not more than 1.5%.

Containers and storage Containers—Tight containers.

Uva Ursi Fluidextract

ウワウルシ流エキス

Uva Ursi Fluidextract contains not less than 3.0 w/v% of arbutin.

Method of preparation Prepare an infusion from Bearberry Leaf, in coarse powder, as directed under Fluidextracts, using hot Purified Water or hot Purified Water in Containers. Remove a part of the accompanying tannin, evaporate the mixture under low pressure (in vacuo), if necessary, and add Purified Water or Purified Water in Containers to adjust the percentage. It may contain an appropriate quantity of Ethanol.

Description Uva Ursi Fluidextract is a yellow-brown to dark red-brown liquid, and has a bitter and astringent taste.

It is miscible with water and with ethanol (95).

Identification To 1 mL of Uva Ursi Fluidextract add 30 mL of a mixture of ethanol (95) and water (7:3), shake, filter, and use the filtrate as the sample solution. Proceed as directed in the Identification (2) under Bearberry Leaf.

Purity Heavy metals *<1.07>*—Prepare the test solution with 1.0 g of Uva Ursi Fluidextract as direct under the Fluidextracts (4), and perform the test (not more than 30 ppm).

Assay Pipet 1 mL of Uva Ursi Fluidextract, add water to make exactly 100 mL, and use this solution as the sample solution. Proceed as directed in the Assay under Bearberry Leaf.

Amount (mg) of arbutin $= M_S \times A_T/A_S$

M_S: Amount (mg) of arbutin for assay taken

Containers and storage Containers—Tight containers.

Wood Creosote

Creosotum Ligni

木クレオソート

Wood Creosote is a mixture of phenols obtained from by using wood tar derived from dry distillation of stems and branches of various plants of genus *Pinus* (*Pinaceae*), genus *Cryptomeria* (*Taxodiaceae*), genus *Fagus* (*Fagaceae*), genus *Afzelia* (genus *Intsia*); (*Leguminosae*), genus *Shorea* (*Dipterocarpaceae*) or genus *Tectona* (*Verbenaceae*), followed by distillation and collection at 180 to 230°C, then further purification and then re-distillation.

Wood Creosote contains not less than 23% and not more than 35% of guaiacol ($C_7H_8O_2$: 124.14).

Description Wood Creosote is a colorless or pale yellow, clear liquid. It has a characteristic odor.

It is slightly soluble in water.

It is miscible with methanol and with ethanol (99.5).

Its saturated solution is acidic.

It is highly refractive.

It gradually changes in color by light or by air.

Identification Use the sample solution obtained in the Assay as the sample solution. Separately, dissolve 0.1 g of phenol, *p*-cresol, guaiacol, and 2-methoxy-4-methylphenol in methanol respectively, to make 100 mL. To 10 mL of each solution add methanol to make 50 mL, and use these solutions as standard solution (1), standard solution (2), standard solution (3) and standard solution (4). Perform the test with 10 μL each of the sample solution, standard solution (1), (2), (3) and (4) as directed under Liquid Chromatography *<2.01>* according to the following conditions: the main peaks obtained with the sample solution show the same retention times with those obtained with the standard solutions (1), (2), (3) and (4).

Operating conditions—

Proceed as directed in the operating conditions in the Assay.

Specific gravity <*2.56*> d^{20}_{20}: not less than 1.076.

Purity **(1)** Coal Creosote—Accurately measure 10 mL of Wood Creosote, add methanol to make exactly 20 mL, and use this solution as the sample solution. Separately, to 1 mg each of benzo[*a*]pyrene, benz[*a*]anthracene and dibenz[*a*,*h*]anthracene add a small quantity of ethyl acetate, if necessary, and add methanol to make 100 mL. To 1 mL of this solution add methanol to make 100 mL, and use this solution as the standard solution. Perform the test with exactly 1 μL each of the sample solution and standard solution as directed under Gas Chromatography <*2.02*> according to the following conditions: No peaks are detected with the sample solution for the retention times corresponding to benzo[*a*]pyrene, benz[*a*]anthracene and dibenz[*a*,*h*]anthracene of the standard solution. Change these conditions if any peak is detected for retention times that correspond to benzo[*a*]pyrene, benz[*a*]anthracene or dibenz[*a*,*h*]anthracene, to verify that such a peak does not belong to benzo[*a*]pyrene, benz[*a*]anthracene or dibenz[*a*,*h*]anthracene.

Operating conditions—

Detector: A mass spectrometer (EI).

Monitored ions:

Benz[*a*]anthracene: Molecular ion *m/z* 228, Fragment ion *m/z* 114	About 14 to 20 minutes
Benzo[*a*]pyrene: Molecular ion *m/z* 252, Fragment ion *m/z* 125	About 20 to 25 minutes
Dibenz[*a*,*h*]anthracene: Molecular ion *m/z* 278, Fragment ion *m/z* 139	About 25 to 30 minutes

Column: A quartz tube 0.25 mm in inside diameter and 30 m in length, with internal coating 0.25 - 0.5 μm in thickness made of 5% diphenyl-95% dimethyl polysiloxane for gas chromatography.

Column temperature: Inject sample at a constant temperature in vicinity of 45°C, then raise temperature to 240°C at the rate of 40°C per minute, maintain the temperature at 240°C for 5 minutes, then raise temperature to 300°C at the rate of 4°C per minute, then raise the temperature to 320°C at the rate of 10°C per minute, then maintain temperature at 320°C for 3 minutes.

Injection port temperature: A constant temperature in vicinity of 250°C.

Interface temperature: A constant temperature in vicinity of 300°C.

Carrier gas: Helium.

Flow rate: Adjust so that the retention time of benzo[*a*]pyrene is about 22 minutes.

Splitless.

System suitability—

Test for required detectability: Accurately measure 1 mL of standard solution and add methanol to make exactly 10 mL, and use this solution as the solution for system suitability test. When the test is performed with conditions described above with 1 μL of the solution for system suitability test, the SN ratio of each substance is not less than 3.

System performance: When the procedure is run with conditions described above with 1 μL of the solution for system suitability test, the elution takes place in order of benz[*a*]anthracene, benzo[*a*]pyrene and then dibenz[*a*,*h*]anthracene.

System repeatability: When the test is repeated 6 times with 1 μL of the solution for system suitability test under the above conditions, the relative standard deviation of the peak area of benzo[*a*]pyrene, benz[*a*]anthracene and dibenz[*a*,*h*]anthracene is respectively not more than 10%.

(2) Acenaphthene—To 0.12 g of Wood Creosote add methanol to make exactly 50 mL, and use this solution as the sample solution. Separately, dissolve 25 mg of acenaphthene in methanol to make 50 mL. To 5 mL of this solution add methanol to make 20 mL. To 2 mL of this solution add methanol to make 100 mL, and use this solution as the standard solution. Perform the test with exactly 1 μL each of the sample solution and standard solution as directed under Gas Chromatography <*2.02*> according to the following conditions: No peaks are detected with sample solution for the retention time corresponding to acenaphthene of the standard solution. Change these conditions if any peak is detected for the retention time corresponding to acenaphthene, to verify that such a peak does not belong to athenaphthene.

Operating conditions—

Detector: A hydrogen flame-ionization detector.

Column: A fused silica tube 0.25 mm inside diameter and 60 m in length, with internal coating 0.25 - 0.5 μm in thickness made of polymethylsiloxane for gas chromatography.

Column temperature: Perform injection at a constant temperature in vicinity of 45°C, then raise the temperature by 11.5°C per minute until reaching 160°C, then raise the temperature by 4°C per minute until reaching 180°C, then raise the temperature by 8°C until reaching 270°C, then maintain temperature at 270°C for 3 minutes.

Injection port temperature: 250°C.

Detector temperature: 250°C.

Carrier gas: Helium.

Flow rate: Adjust so that the retention time of acenaphthene is about 18 minutes.

Splitless.

System suitability—

Test for required detectability: Accurately measure 1 mL of the standard solution, add methanol to make exactly 10 mL, and use this solution as the solution for system suitability test. When the procedure is run with conditions described above with 1 μL of solution for system suitability test, the SN ratio of acenaphthene is not less than 3.

System repeatability: When the test is repeated 6 times with 1 μL of the solution for system suitability test under the above operating conditions, the relative standard deviation of the peak area of acenaphthene is not more than 6.0%.

(3) Other impurities

Add 2 mL of petroleum benzin to 1.0 mL of Wood Creosote, then add 2 mL of barium hydroxide test solution, agitate to mix and allow to stand. No blue or muddy brown color develops in the upper layer of the mixture. Furthermore, no red color develops in the lower layer.

Distilling range <*2.57*> 200 - 220°C, not less than 85 vol%.

Assay To about 0.1 g of Wood Creosote, accurately weighed, add methanol to make exactly 50 mL. Pipet 10 mL of this solution add methanol to make exactly 50 mL, and use this solution as the sample solution. Separately, add methanol to about 30 mg of accurately measured guaiacol for assay to make exactly 50 mL. Pipet 10 mL of this solution, add methanol to make exactly 50 mL, and use this solution as the standard solution. Perform the test with 10 μL each of the sample solution and standard solution under Liquid Chromatography <*2.01*> according to the following conditions, and determine the peak areas, A_T and A_S, of guaiacol in each solution.

$$\text{Amount (mg) of guaiacol} = M_S \times A_T/A_S$$

M_S: Amount (mg) of guaiacol for assay taken

Operating conditions—

Detector: An ultraviolet absorption photometer (wavelength: 275 nm).

Column: A stainless steel column 4.6 mm in inside diameter and 15 cm in length, packed with octadecylsilanized silica gel for liquid chromatography (5 μm in particle diameter).

Column temperature: A constant temperature of about 40°C.

Mobile phase: Mixture of water and acetonitrile (4:1).

Flow rate: Adjust so that the retention time of guaiacol is about 9 minutes.

System suitability—

System performance: Dissolve 2 mg each of guaiacol and phenol in methanol to make 10 mL. The procedure is run with conditions described above with 10 μL of this solution, the elution takes place in order of phenol then guaiacol, with the degree in separation of not less than 2.5.

System repeatability: When the test is repeated 6 times with 10 μL of the standard solution under the above operating conditions, the relative standard deviation of the peak area of guaiacol is not more than 1.5%.

Containers and storage Containers—Tight containers.
Storage—Light-resistant.

Yokukansan Extract

抑肝散エキス

Yokukansan Extract contains not less than 0.15 mg of total alkaloids (rhyncophylline and hirsutine), not less than 0.6 mg and not more than 2.4 mg of saikosaponin b_2, and not less than 10 mg and not more than 30 mg of glycyrrhizic acid ($C_{42}H_{62}O_{16}$: 822.93), per extract prepared with the amount specified in the Method of preparation.

Method of preparation

	1)	2)
Japanese Angelica Root	3 g	3 g
Uncaria Hook	3 g	3 g
Cnidium Rhizome	3 g	3 g
Atractylodes Rhizome	4 g	—
Atractylodes Lancea Rhizome	—	4 g
Poria Sclerotium	4 g	4 g
Bupleurum Root	2 g	2 g
Glycyrrhiza	1.5 g	1.5 g

Prepare a dry extract or viscous extract as directed under Extracts, according to the prescription 1) or 2), using the crude drugs shown above.

Description Yokukansan Extract is a light brown to grayish brown powder or a black-brown viscous extract. It has a slightly odor, and a slightly bitter and acid taste.

Identification **(1)** To 2.0 g of the dry extract (or 6.0 g of the viscous extract) add 10 mL of water, shake, then add 10 mL of diethyl ether, shake, and centrifuge. Separate the diethyl ether layer, add 10 mL of sodium hydroxide TS, shake, centrifuge, separate the diethyl ether layer, and use this layer as the sample solution. Separately, use (*Z*)-ligustilide TS for thin-layer chromatography as the standard solution. Perform the test with these solutions as directed under Thin-layer Chromatography <*2.03*>. Spot 10 μL each of the sample solution and standard solution on a plate of silica gel for thin-layer chromatography. Develop the plate with a mixture of butyl acetate and hexane (2:1) to a distance of about 7 cm, and air-dry the plate. Examine under ultraviolet light (main wavelength: 365 nm): one of the several spots obtained from the sample solution has the same color tone and *R*f value with the blue-white fluorescent spot from the standard solution (Japanese Angelica Root; Cnidium Rhizome).

(2) To 2.0 g of the dry extract (or 6.0 g of the viscous extract) add 20 mL of water and 2 mL of ammonia TS, shake, then add 20 mL of diethyl ether, shake, and separate the diethyl ether layer. Evaporate the solvent under low pressure (in vacuo), add 1 mL of methanol to the residue, and use the solution as the sample solution. Separately, dissolve 1 mg each of rhyncophyllin for thin-layer chromatography and hirsutine for thin-layer chromatography in 1 mL of methanol, and use this solution as the standard solution. Perform the test with these solutions as directed under Thin-layer Chromatography <*2.03*>. Spot 20 μL of the sample solution and 2 μL of the standard solution on a plate of silica gel with fluorescent indicator for thin-layer chromatography. Develop the plate with a mixture of ethyl acetate, 1-propanol, water and acetic acid (100) (7:5:4:1) to a distance of about 7 cm, and air-dry the plate. Examine under ultraviolet light (main wavelength: 254 nm): at least one of the several spots obtained from the sample solution has the same color tone and *R*f value with one of the two dark violet spots from the standard solution (Uncaria Hook).

(3) For preparation prescribed Atractylodes Rhizome—To 1.0 g of the dry extract (or 3.0 g of the viscous extract) add 10 mL of water, shake, then add 25 mL of diethyl ether, and shake. Separate the diethyl ether layer, evaporate the solvent under low pressure (in vacuo), dissolve the residue in 2 mL of diethyl ether, and use this solution as the sample solution. Separately, dissolve 1 mg of atractylenoide III for thin-layer chromatography in 2 mL of methanol, and use this solution as the standard solution. Perform the test with these solutions as directed under Thin-layer Chromatography <*2.03*>. Spot 5 μL each of the sample solution and standard solution on a plate of silica gel for thin-layer chromatography. Develop the plate with a mixture of ethyl acetate and hexane (1:1) to a distance of about 7 cm, and air-dry the plate. Spray evenly 1-naphthol-sulfuric acid TS on the plate, heat the plate at 105°C for 5 minutes, and allow to cool: one of the several spots obtained from the sample solution has the same color tone and *R*f value with the red to purple-red spot from the standard solution (Atractylodes Rhizome).

(4) For preparation prescribed Atractylodes Lancea Rhizome—To 2.0 g of the dry extract (or 6.0 g of the viscous extract) add 10 mL of water, shake, then add 25 mL of hexane, and shake. Separate the hexane layer, evaporate the solvent under low pressure (in vacuo), add 2 mL of hexane to the residue, and use this solution as the sample solution. Perform the test with the sample solution as directed under Thin-layer Chromatography <*2.03*>. Spot 20 μL of the sample solution on a plate of silica gel with fluorescent indicator for thin-layer chromatography. Develop the plate with a mixture of hexane and acetone (7:1) to a distance of about 7 cm, and air-dry the plate. Examine under ultraviolet light (main wavelength: 254 nm): a dark purple spot is observed at an *R*f value of about 0.5. The spot shows a greenish brown color after being sprayed evenly 4-dimethylaminobenzaldehyde TS for spraying on the plate, heated at 105°C for 5 minutes, and allowed to cool (Atractylodes Lancea Rhizome).

(5) To 1.0 g of the dry extract (or 3.0 g of the viscous extract) add 10 mL of water, shake, then add 10 mL of 1-butanol, shake, centrifuge, and use the 1-butanol layer as the sample solution. Separately, dissolve 1 mg of saikosaponin b_2 for thin-layer chromatography in 1 mL of methanol, and use this solution as the standard solution. Perform the test with these solutions as directed under Thin-layer Chromatography <*2.03*>. Spot 10 μL of the sample solution and 2 μL of the standard solution on a plate of silica gel for thin-layer chromatography. Develop the plate with a mixture of ethyl acetate, ethanol (99.5) and water (8:2:1) to a distance of about 7 cm, and air-dry the plate. Spray evenly 4-dimethylaminobenzaldehyde TS for spraying on the plate, heat the plate at 105°C for 5 minutes, and examine under ultraviolet light (main wavelength: 365 nm): one of the several spots obtained from the sample solution has the same color tone and *Rf* value with the yellow fluorescent spot from the standard solution (Bupleurum Root).

(6) To 1.0 g of the dry extract (or 3.0 g of the viscous extract) add 10 mL of water, shake, then add 10 mL of 1-butanol, shake, centrifuge, and use the 1-butanol layer as the sample solution. Separately, dissolve 1 mg of liquiritin for thin-layer chromatography in 1 mL of methanol, and use this solution as the standard solution. Perform the test with these solutions as directed under Thin-layer Chromatography <*2.03*>. Spot 1 μL each of the sample solution and standard solution on a plate of silica gel for thin-layer chromatography. Develop the plate with a mixture of ethyl acetate, methanol and water (20:3:2) to a distance of about 7 cm, and air-dry the plate. Spray evenly dilute sulfuric acid on the plate, heat the plate at 105°C for 5 minutes, and examine under ultraviolet light (main wavelength: 365 nm): one of the several spots obtained from the sample solution has the same color tone and *Rf* value with the yellow-green fluorescent spot from the standard solution (Glycyrrhiza).

Purity **(1)** Heavy metals <*1.07*>—Prepare the test solution with 1.0 g of the dry extract (or an amount of the viscous extract, equivalent to 1.0 g of the dried substance) as directed under Extracts (4), and perform the test (not more than 30 ppm).

(2) Arsenic <*1.11*>—Prepare the test solution with 0.67 g of the dry extract (or an amount of the viscous extract, equivalent to 0.67 g of the dried substance) according to Method 3, and perform the test (not more than 3 ppm).

Loss on drying <*2.41*> The dry extract: Not more than 10.0% (1 g, 105°C, 5 hours).

The viscous extract: Not more than 66.7% (1 g, 105°C, 5 hours).

Total ash <*5.01*> Not less than 10.0%, calculated on the dried basis.

Assay **(1)** Total alkaloids (rhyncophylline and hirsutine)—Weigh accurately about 1 g of the dry extract (or an amount of the viscous extract, equivalent to about 1 g of the dried substance), add 20 mL of diethyl ether, shake, then add 3 mL of 1 mol/L hydrochloric acid TS and 7 mL of water, and shake for 10 minutes, centrifuge, and remove the diethyl ether layer. To the aqueous layer add 20 mL of diethyl ether, and proceed in the same manner as above. To the aqueous layer add 10 mL of sodium hydroxide TS and 20 mL of diethyl ether, shake for 10 minutes, centrifuge, and separate the diethyl ether layer. To the aqueous layer add 20 mL of diethyl ether, proceed in the same manner, and repeat this procedure twice. Combine all the extracts, evaporate the solvent under low pressure (in vacuo) at not more than 40°C, dissolve the residue in the mobile phase to make exactly 10 mL, and use this solution as the sample solution. Separately, weigh accurately about 5 mg each of rhyncophylline for assay and hirsutine for assay, dissolve in a mixture of methanol and diluted acetic acid (7:3) to make exactly 100 mL. Pipet 10 mL of this solution, add the mixture of methanol and diluted acetic acid (7:3) to make exactly 50 mL, and use this solution as the standard solution. Perform the test with exactly 10 μL each of the sample solution and standard solution as directed under Liquid Chromatography <*2.01*> according to the following conditions, and determine the peak areas, A_{TR} and A_{TH}, and A_{SR} and A_{SH}, of rhyncophylline and hirsutine in each solution.

Amount (mg) of total alkaloids (rhyncophylline and hirsutine)
$$= (M_{SR} \times A_{TR}/A_{SR} + M_{SH} \times A_{TH}/A_{SH}) \times 1/50$$

M_{SR}: Amount (mg) of rhyncophylline for assay taken
M_{SH}: Amount (mg) of hirsutine for assay taken

Operation conditions—

Detector: An ultraviolet absorption photometer (wavelength: 245 nm).

Column: A stainless steel column 4.6 mm in inside diameter and 15 cm in length, packed with octadecylsilanized silica gel for liquid chromatography (5 μm in particle diameter).

Column temperature: A constant temperature of about 40°C.

Mobile phase: To 1 g of sodium lauryl sulfate add 600 mL of methanol, shake, then add 400 mL of water and 1 mL of phosphoric acid.

Flow rate: 1.0 mL per minute (the retention times of rhyncophylline and hirsutine are about 17 minutes and about 47 minutes, respectively).

Systemic suitability—

System performance: When the procedure is run with 10 μL of the standard solution under the above operating conditions, the number of theoretical plates and the symmetry factor of the peaks of rhyncophylline and hirsutine are not less than 5000 and not more than 1.5, respectively.

System repeatability: When the test is repeated 6 times with 10 μL of the standard solution under the above operating conditions, the relative standard deviation of the peak area of rhyncophylline and hirsutine is not more than 1.5%, respectively.

(2) Saikosaponin b_2—Weigh accurately about 0.5 g of the dry extract (or an amount of the viscous extract, equivalent to about 0.5 g of the dried substance), add 20 mL of diethyl ether and 10 mL of water, and shake for 10 minutes. After centrifugation, remove the diethyl ether layer, add 20 mL of diethyl ether, proceed in the same manner as above, and remove the diethyl ether layer. To the aqueous layer add 10 mL of methanol, shake for 30 minutes, centrifuge, and separate the supernatant liquid. To the residue add 20 mL of diluted methanol (1 in 2), shake for 5 minutes, centrifuge, separate the supernatant liquid, combine all the supernatant liquids, add diluted methanol (1 in 2) to make exactly 50 mL, and use this solution as the sample solution. Separately, use saikosaponin b_2 standard TS for assay as the standard solution. Perform the test with exactly 10 μL each of the sample solution and standard solution as directed under Liquid Chromatography <*2.01*> according to the following conditions, and determine the peak areas, A_T and A_S, of saikosaponin b_2 in each solution.

$$\text{Amount (mg) of saikosaponin } b_2 = C_S \times A_T/A_S \times 50$$

C_S: Concentration (mg/mL) of saikosaponin b_2 in saikosaponin b_2 standard TS for assay

Operation conditions—

Detector: An ultraviolet absorption photometer (wavelength: 254 nm).

Column: A stainless steel column 4.6 mm in inside diameter and 15 cm in length, packed with octadecylsilanized silica gel for liquid chromatography (5 μm in particle diameter).

Column temperature: A constant temperature of about 40°C.

Mobile phase: A mixture of 0.05 mol/L sodium dihydrogen phosphate TS and acetonitrile (5:3).

Flow rate: 1.0 mL per minute (the retention time of saikosaponin b_2 is about 12 minutes).

Systemic suitability—

System performance: When the procedure is run with 10 μL of the standard solution under the above operating conditions, the number of theoretical plates and the symmetry factor of the peak of saikosaponin b_2 are not less than 5000 and not more than 1.5, respectively.

System repeatability: When the test is repeated 6 times with 10 μL of the standard solution under the above operating conditions, the relative standard deviation of the peak area of saikosaponin b_2 is not more than 1.5%.

(3) Glycyrrhizic acid—Weigh accurately about 0.5 g of the dry extract (or an amount of the viscous extract, equivalent to about 0.5 g of the dried substance), add 20 mL of diethyl ether and 10 mL of water, and shake for 10 minutes. After centrifugation, remove the diethyl ether layer, add 20 mL of diethyl ether, proceed in the same manner as described above, and remove the diethyl ether layer. To the aqueous layer add 10 mL of methanol, shake for 30 minutes, centrifuge, and take the supernatant liquid. To the residue add 20 mL of diluted methanol (1 in 2), shake for 5 minutes, centrifuge, and take the supernatant liquid. Combine these supernatant liquids, add diluted methanol (1 in 2) to make exactly 50 mL, and use this solution as the sample solution. Separately, weigh accurately about 10 mg of Glycyrrhizic Acid RS (separately determine the water <*2.48*> by coulometric titration, using 10 mg), dissolve in diluted methanol (1 in 2) to make exactly 100 mL, and use this solution as the standard solution. Perform the test with exactly 10 μL each of the sample solution and standard solution as directed under Liquid Chromatography <*2.01*> according to the following conditions, and determine the peak areas, A_T and A_S, of glycyrrhizic acid in each solution.

Amount (mg) of glycyrrhizic acid ($C_{42}H_{62}O_{16}$)
$= M_S \times A_T/A_S \times 1/2$

M_S: Amount (mg) of Glycyrrhizic Acid RS taken, calculated on the anhydrous basis

Operating conditions—

Detector: An ultraviolet absorption photometer (wavelength: 254 nm).

Column: A stainless steel column 4.6 mm in inside diameter and 15 cm in length, packed with octadecylsilanized silica gel for liquid chromatography (5 μm in particle diameter).

Column temperature: A constant temperature of about 40°C.

Mobile phase: Dissolve 3.85 g of ammonium acetate in 720 mL of water, and add 5 mL of acetic acid (100) and 280 mL of acetonitrile.

Flow rate: 1.0 mL per minute (the retention time of glycyrrhizic acid is about 15 minutes).

System suitability—

System performance: Dissolve 5 mg of monoammonium glycyrrhizinate for resolution check in 20 mL of dilute ethanol. When the procedure is run with 10 μL of this solution under the above operating conditions, the resolution between the peak having the relative retention time of about 0.9 to glycyrrhizic acid and the peak of glycyrrhizic acid is not less than 1.5.

System repeatability: When the test is repeated 6 times with 10 μL of the standard solution under the above operating conditions, the relative standard deviation of the peak area of glycyrrhizic acid is not more than 1.5%.

Containers and storage Containers—Tight containers.

INFRARED REFERENCE SPECTRA

The infrared reference spectra presented here were obtained by the use of Fourier-transform infrared spectrophotometers under the conditions specified in the individual monographs. The horizontal axis indicates the wave numbers (cm^{-1}) and the vertical axis indicates the transmittance (%). A spectrum of polystyrene obtained in the same manner is also presented for reference.

Polystyrene

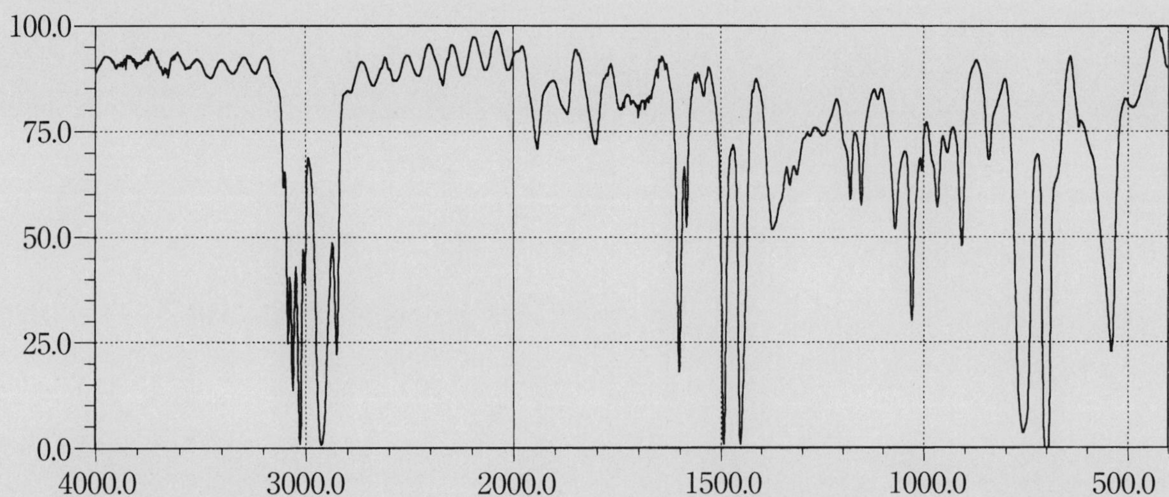

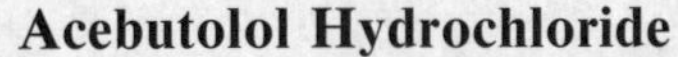

Acebutolol Hydrochloride

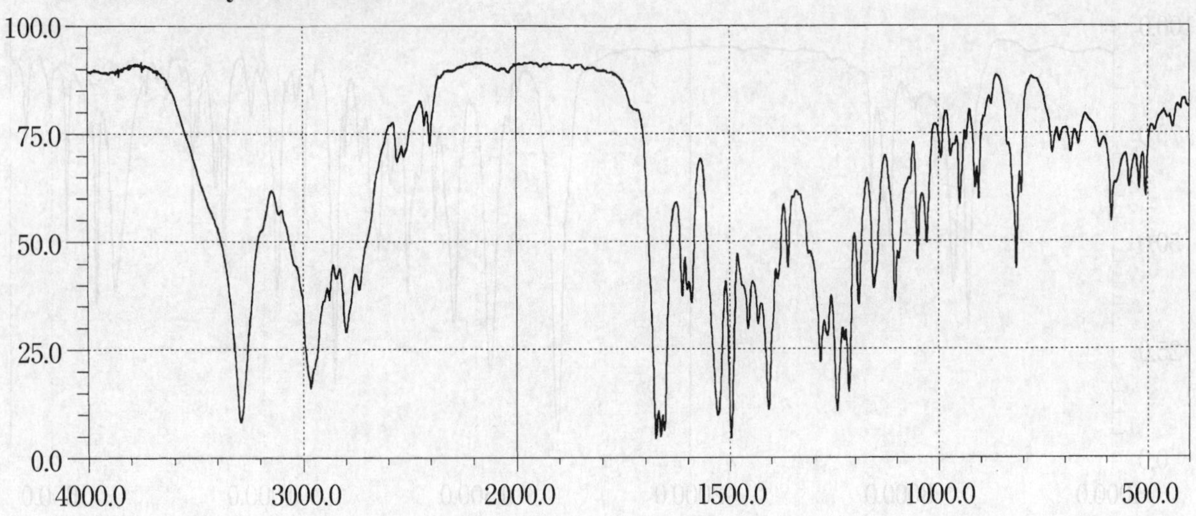

Acemetacin

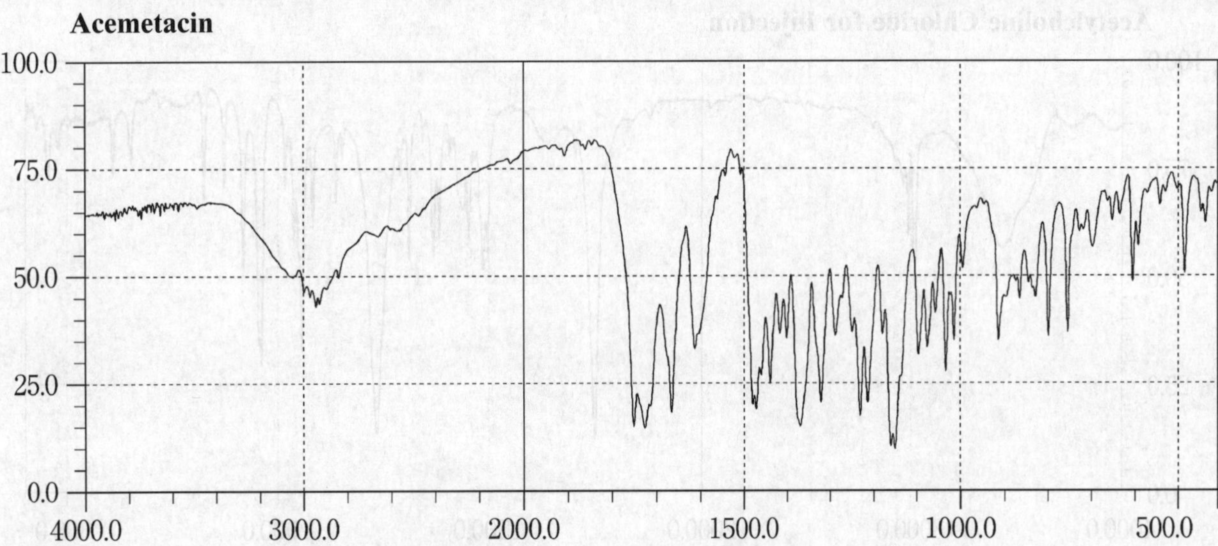

Acetaminophen

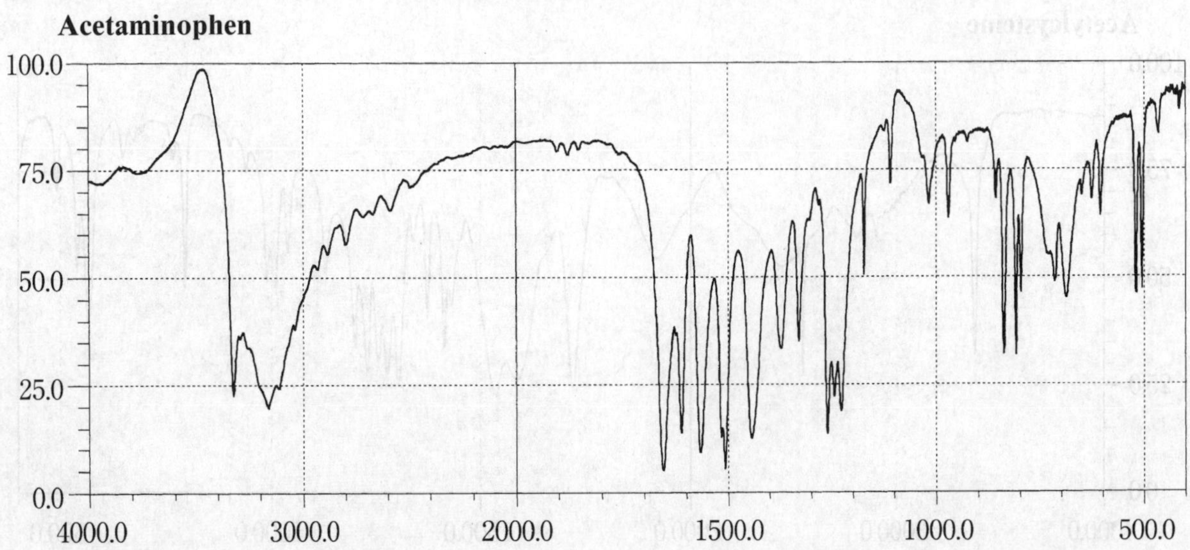

The JP Drugs are to be tested according to the provisions given in the pertinent monographs, General Notices, General Rules for Crude Drugs, General Rules for Preparations, and General Tests for their conformity to the Japanese Pharmacopoeia. (See the General Notices 5.)

Acetohexamide

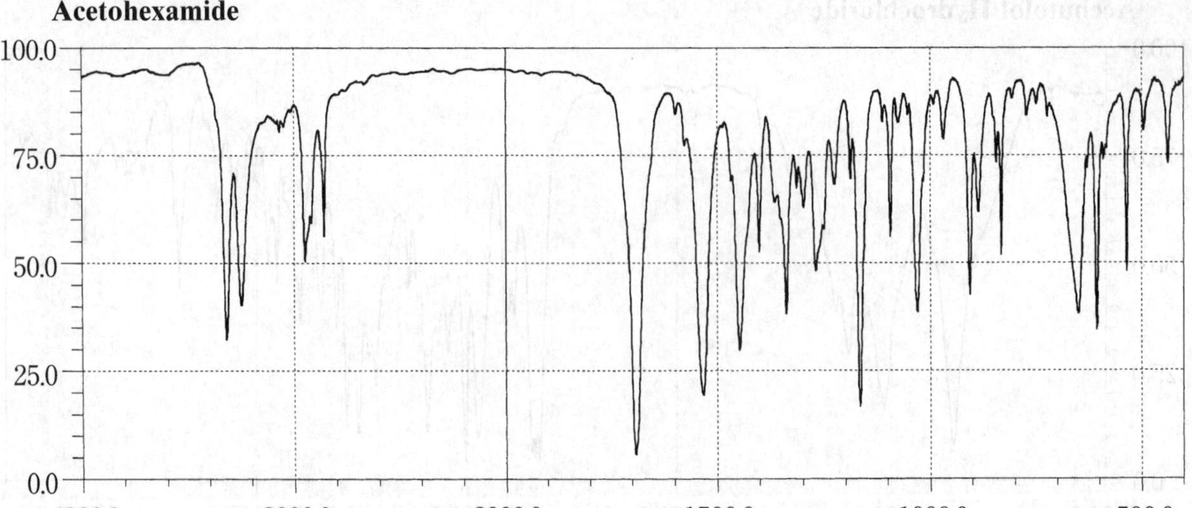

Acetylcholine Chloride for Injection

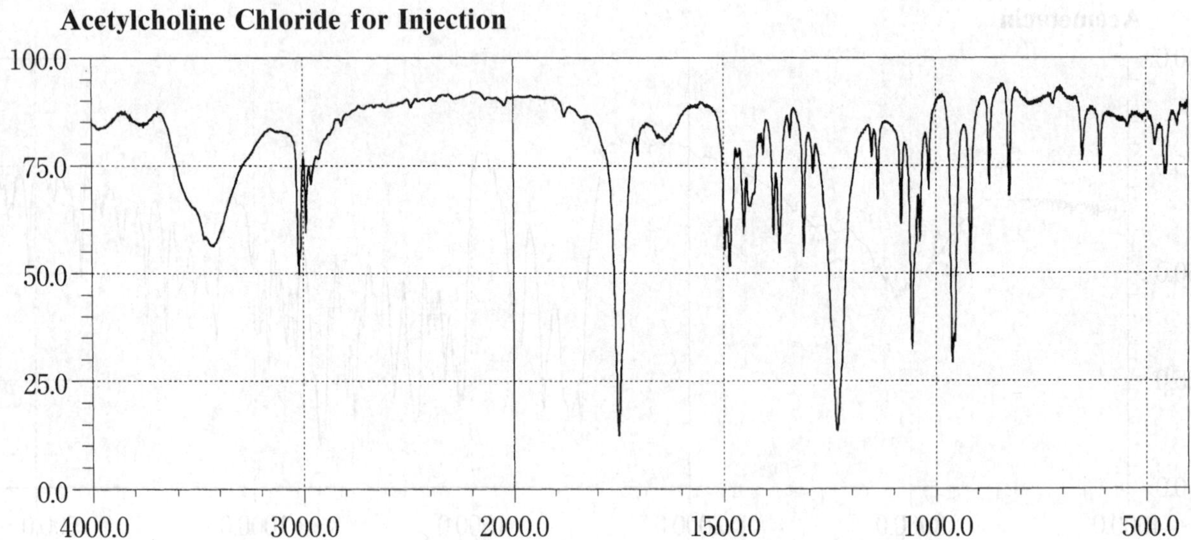

Acetylcysteine

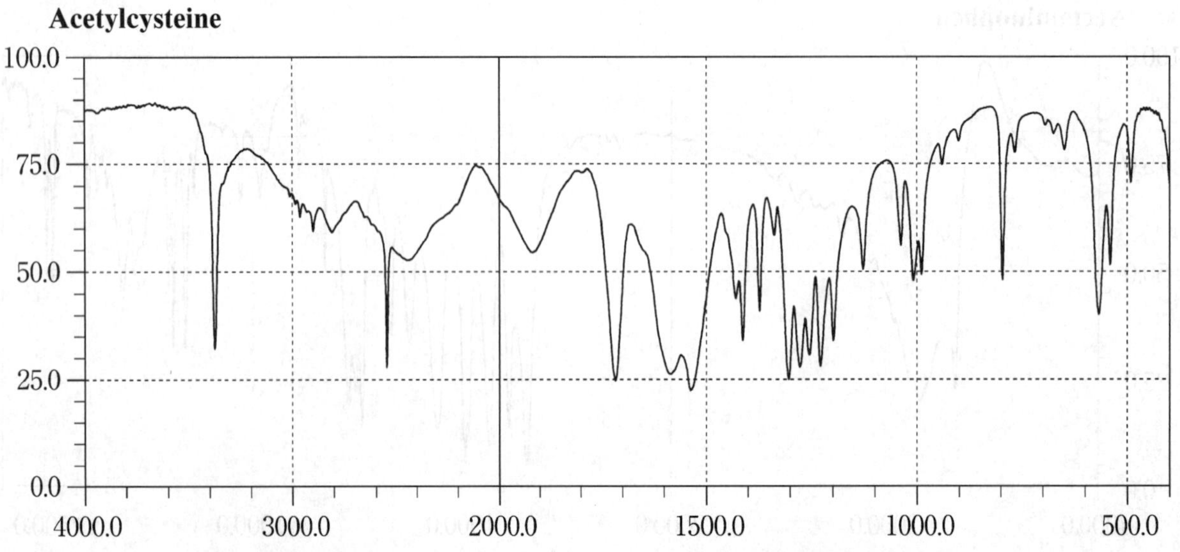

The JP Drugs are to be tested according to the provisions given in the pertinent monographs, General Notices, General Rules for Crude Drugs, General Rules for Preparations, and General Tests for their conformity to the Japanese Pharmacopoeia. (See the General Notices 5.)

Aciclovir

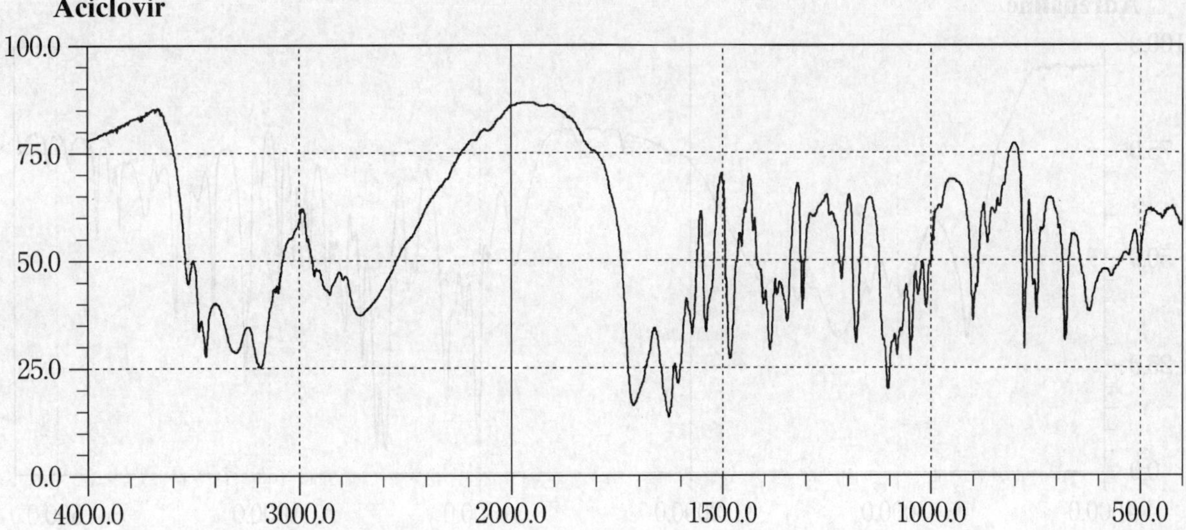

Aclarubicin Hydrochloride

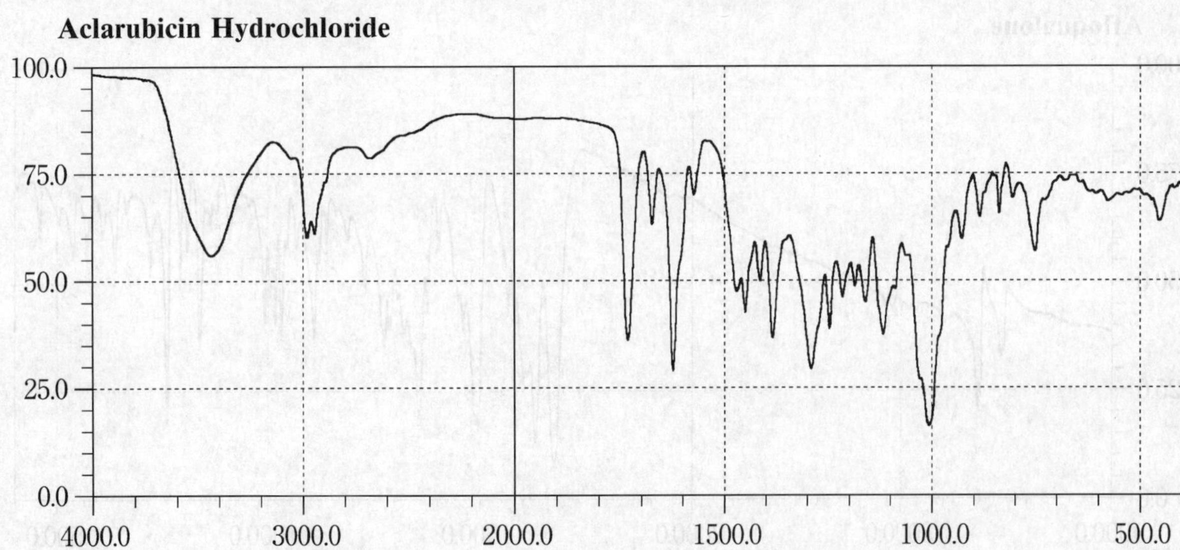

Acrinol Hydrate

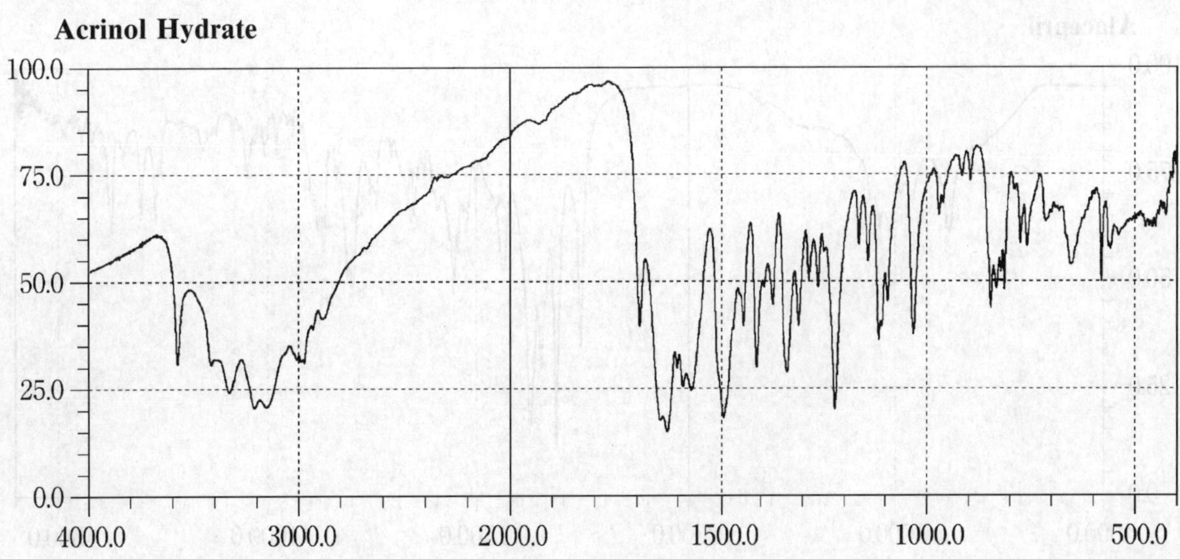

Adrenaline

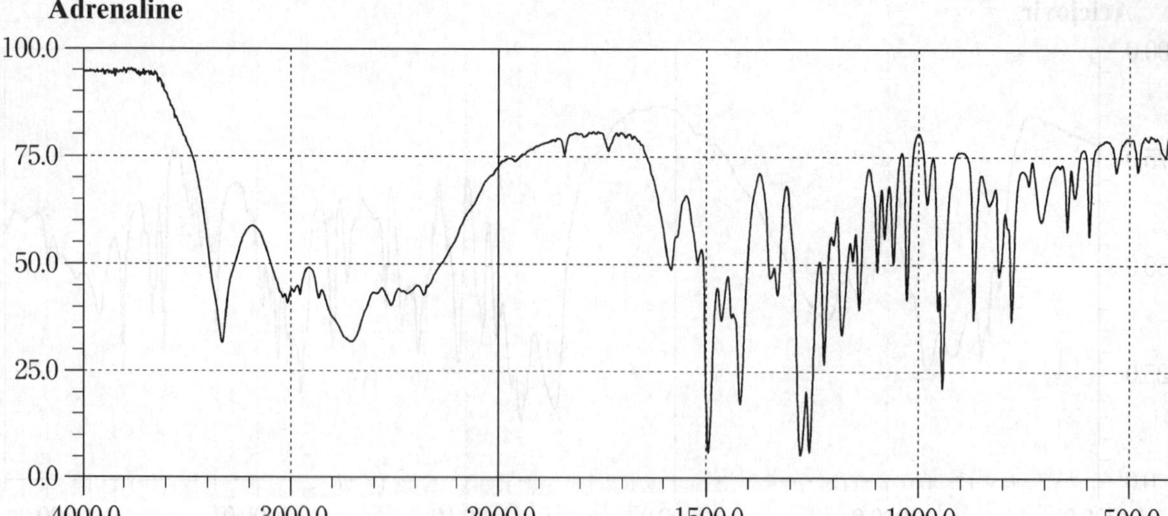

Afloqualone

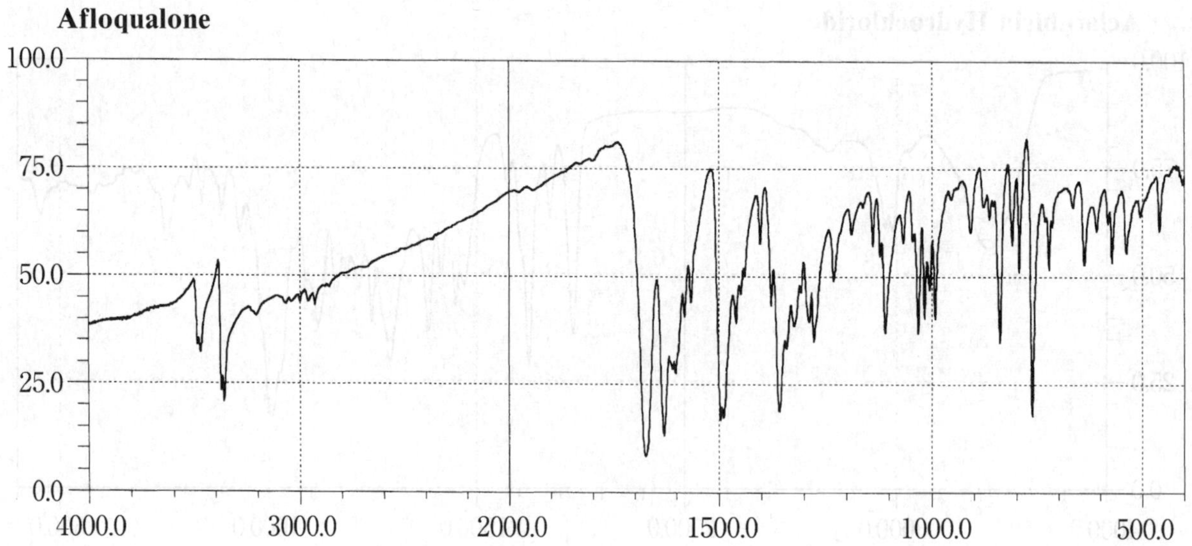

Alacepril

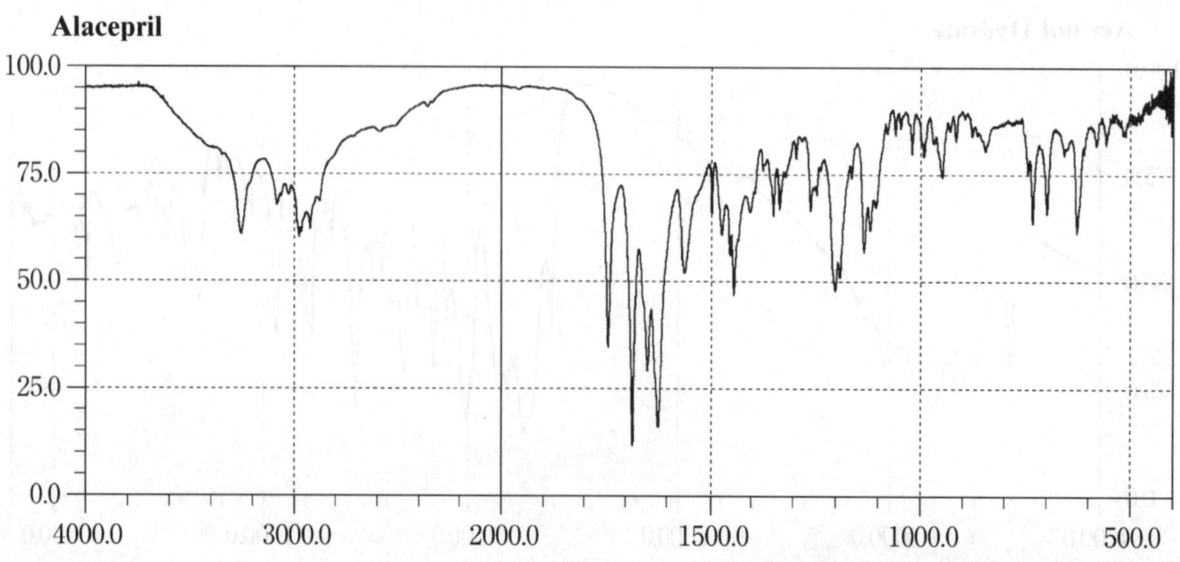

L-Alanine

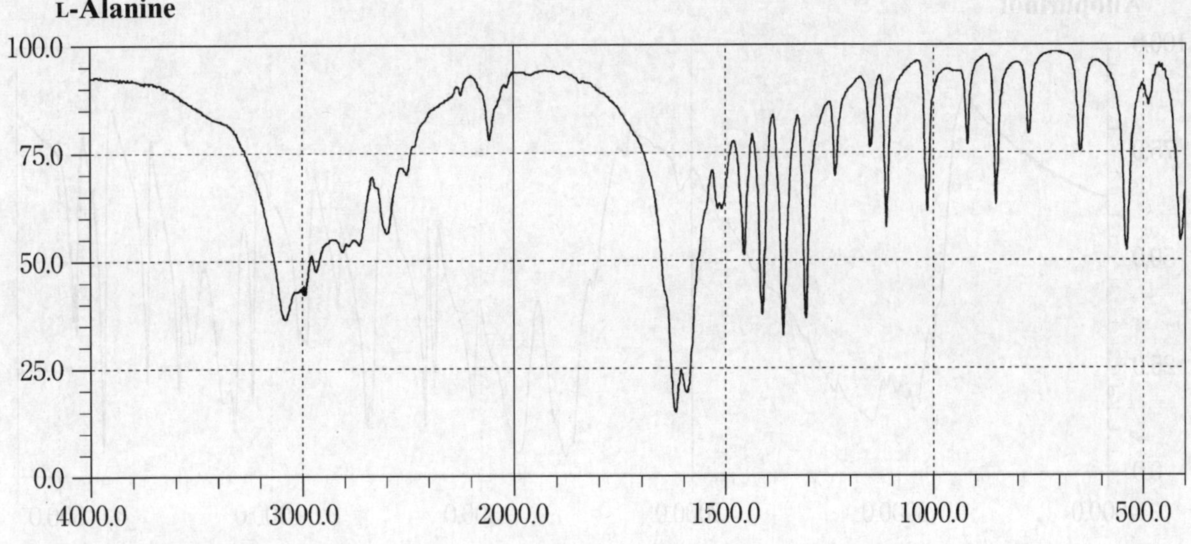

Aldioxa

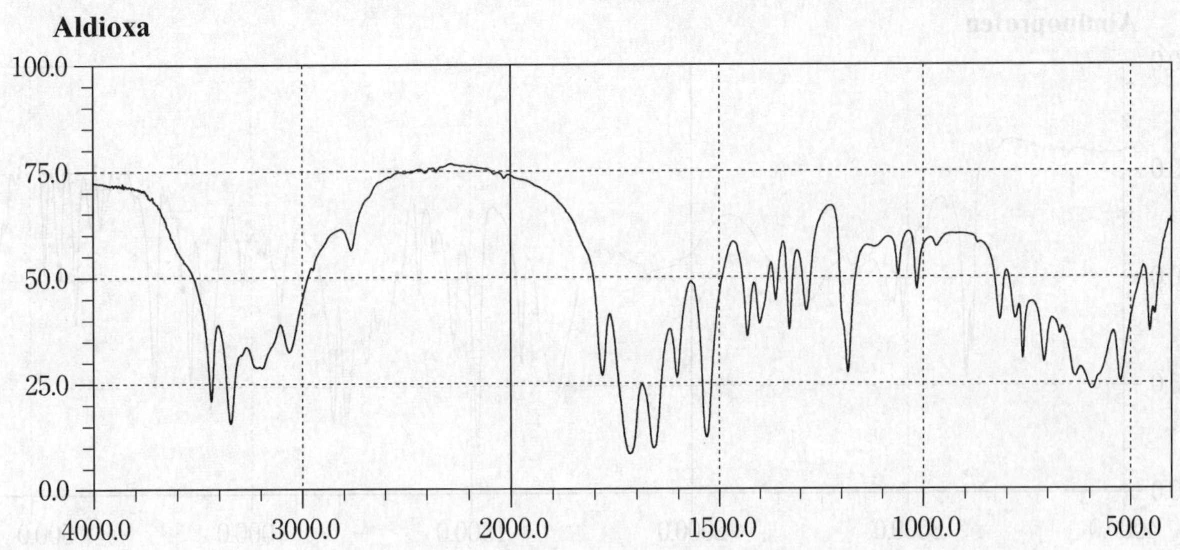

Alendronate Sodium Hydrate

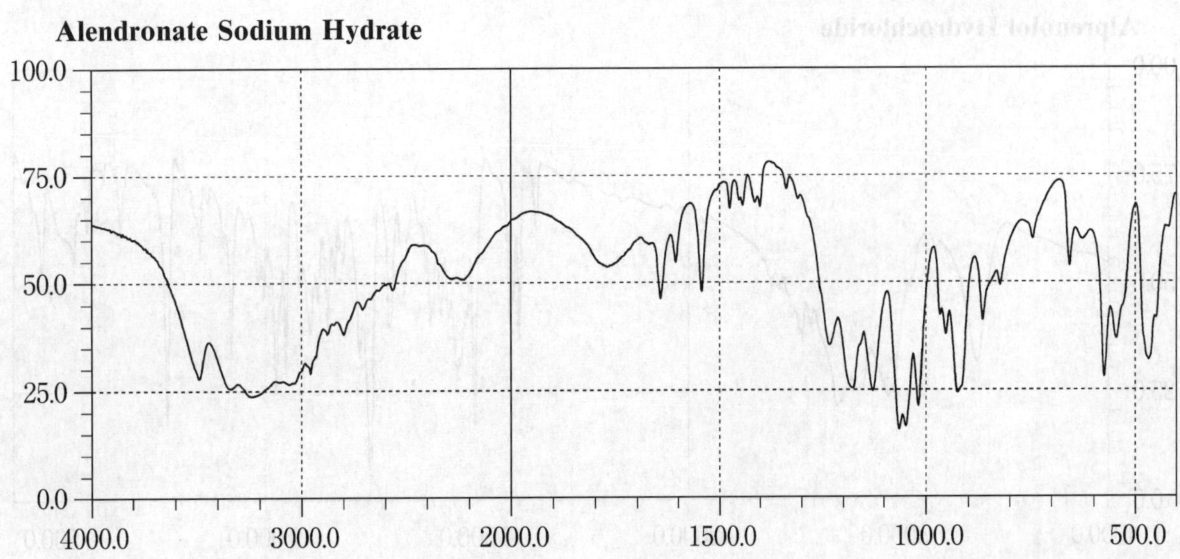

Allopurinol

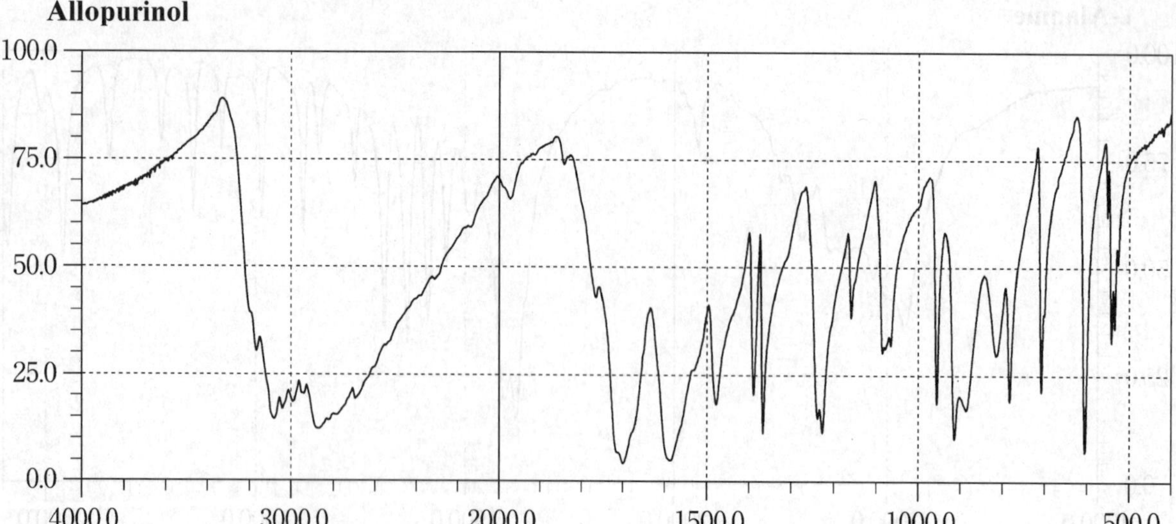

Alminoprofen

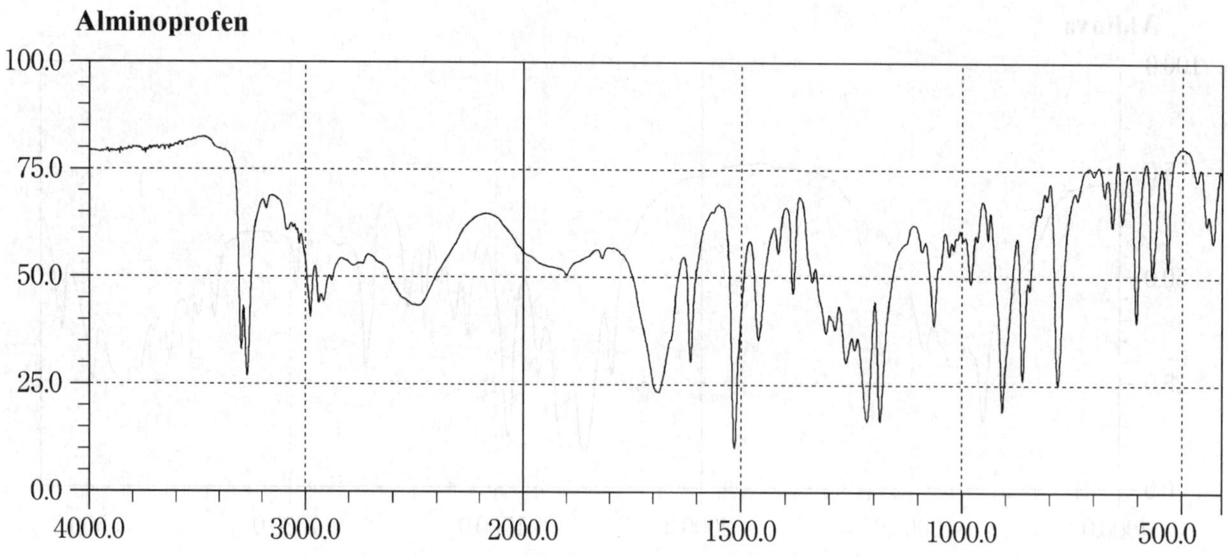

Alprenolol Hydrochloride

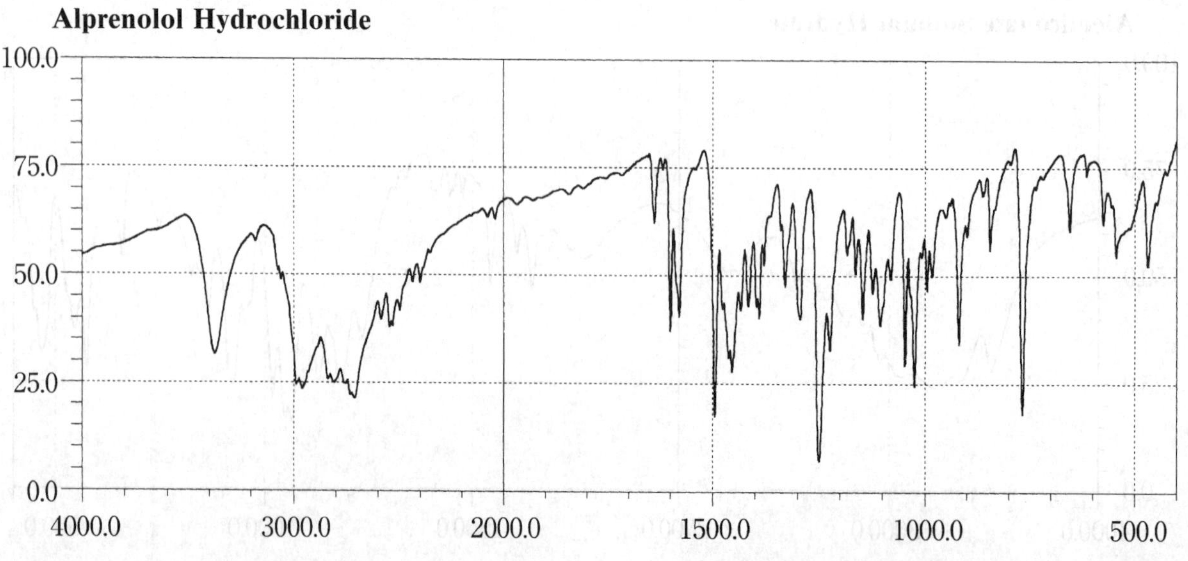

Alprostadil

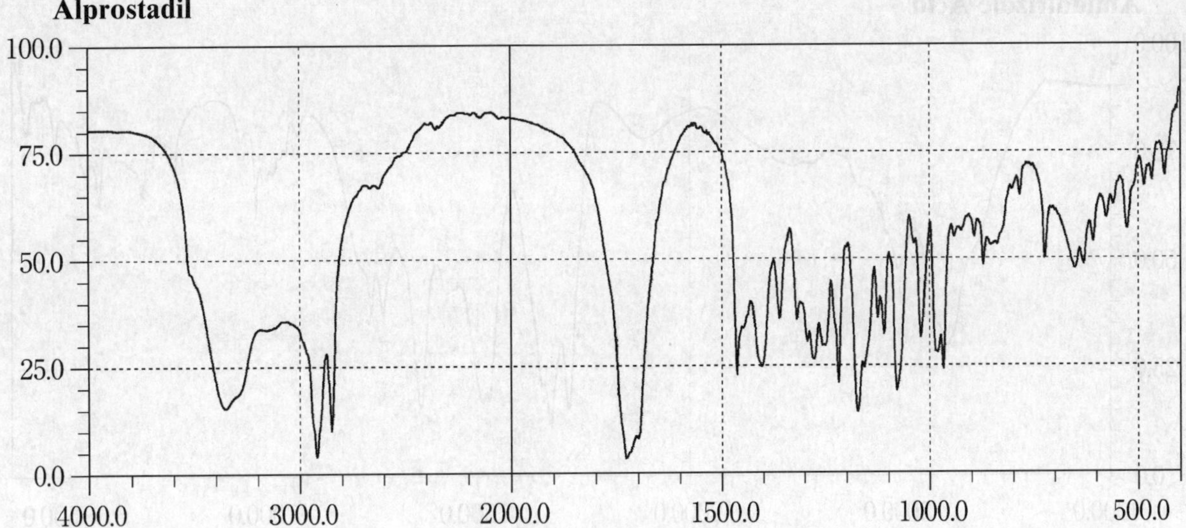

Amantadine Hydrochloride

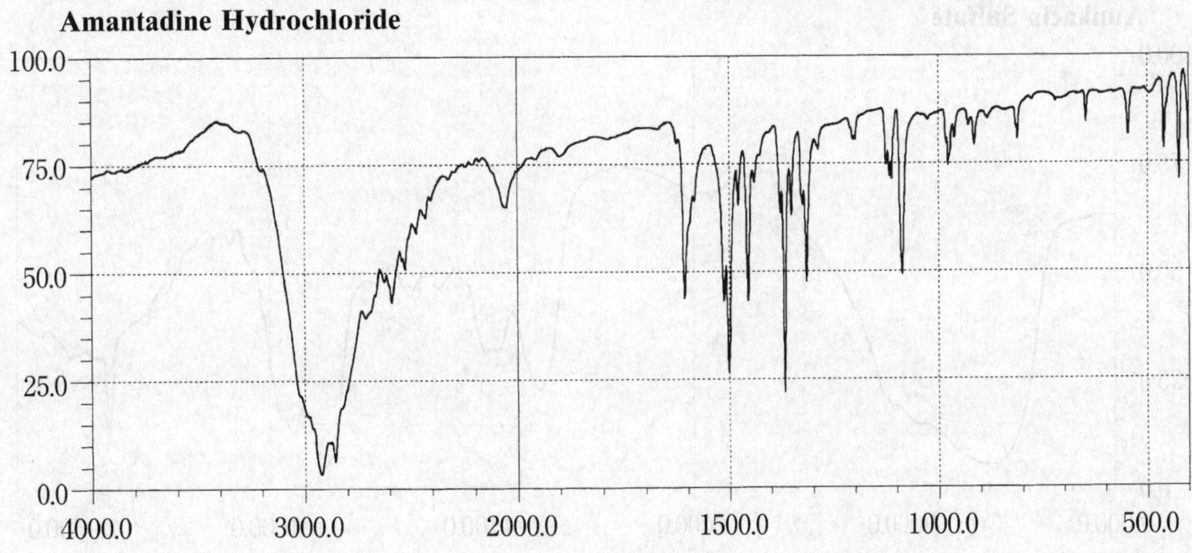

Ambenonium Chloride

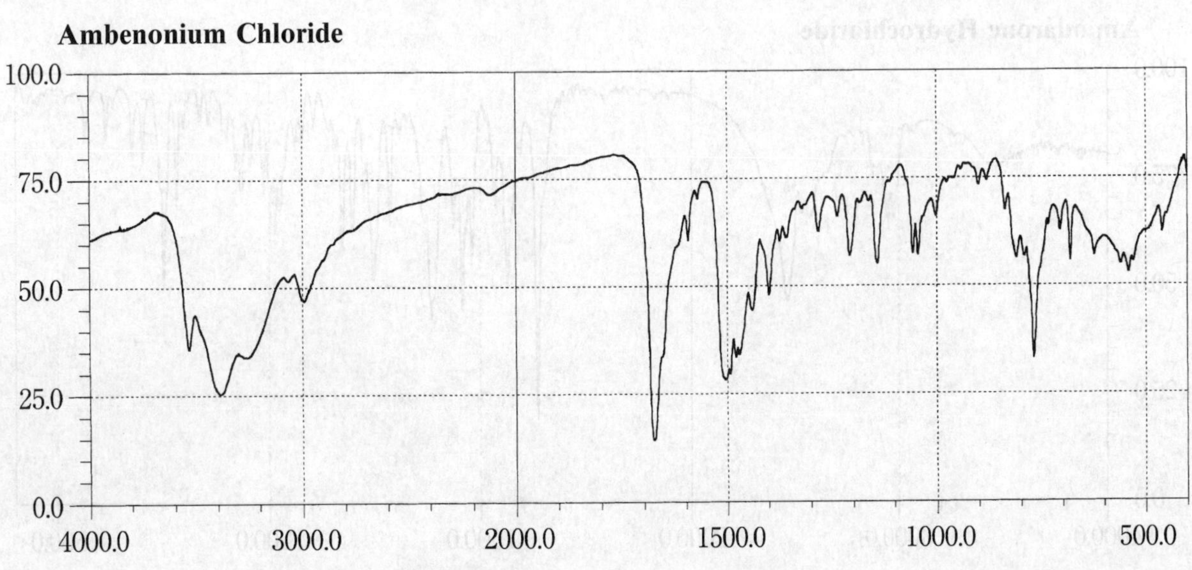

Amidotrizoic Acid

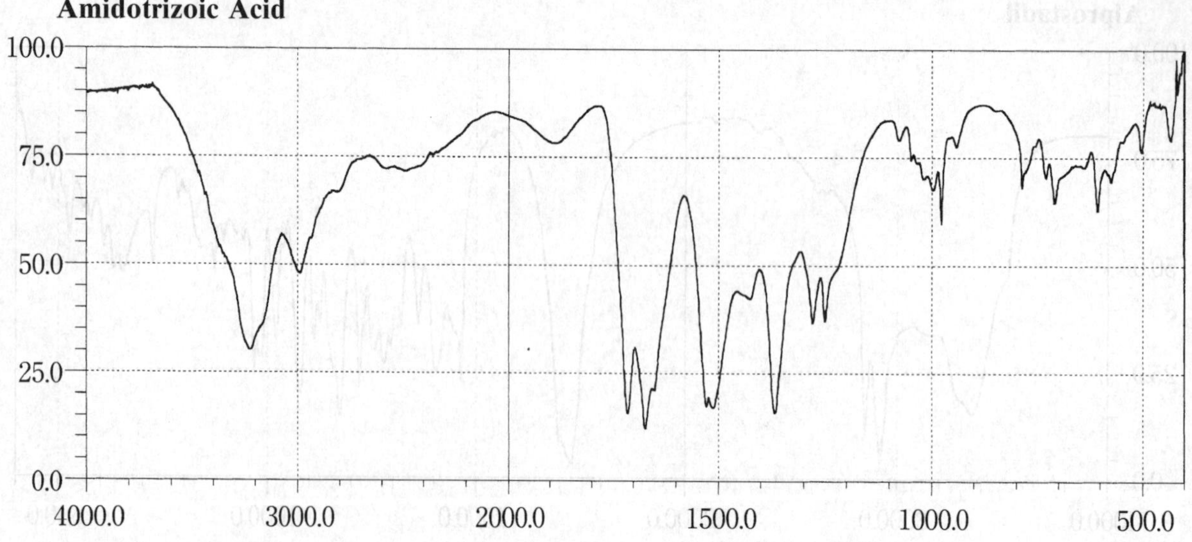

Amikacin Sulfate

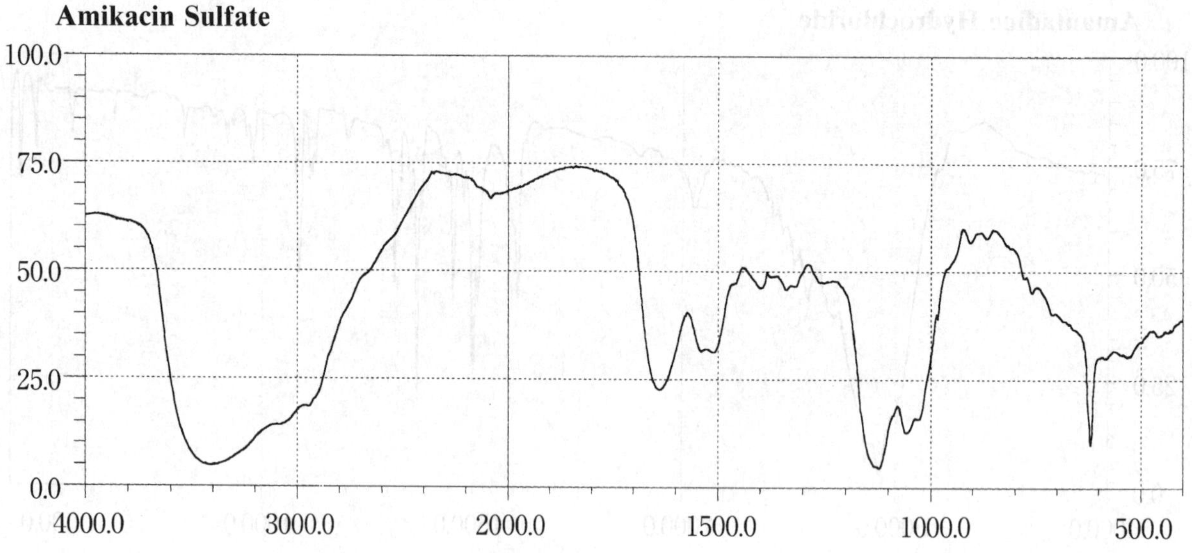

Amiodarone Hydrochloride

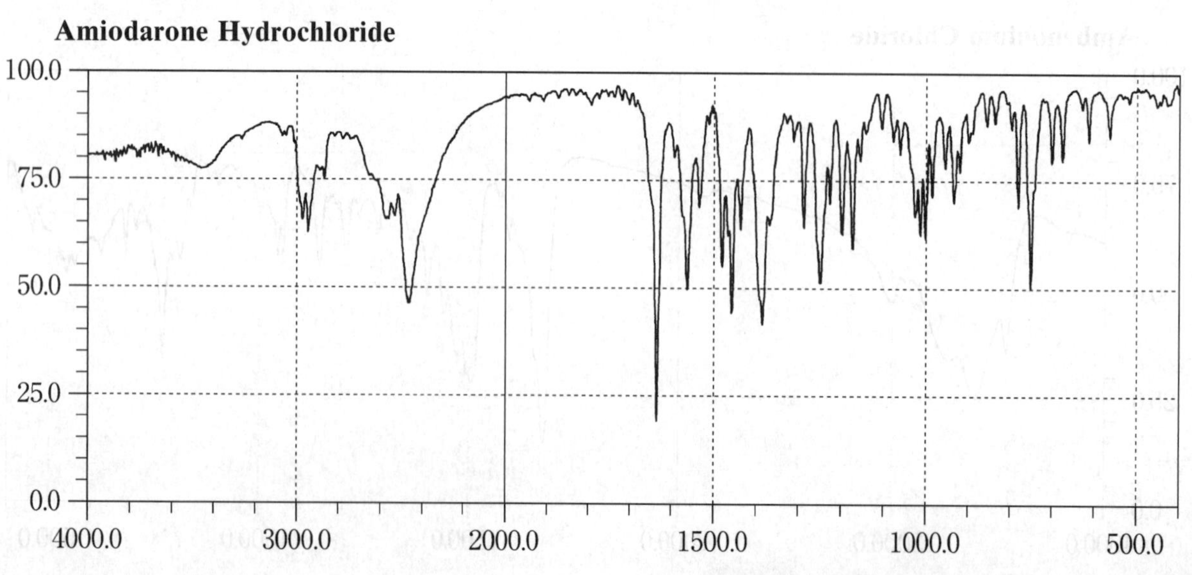

The JP Drugs are to be tested according to the provisions given in the pertinent monographs, General Notices, General Rules for Crude Drugs, General Rules for Preparations, and General Tests for their conformity to the Japanese Pharmacopoeia. (See the General Notices 5.)

Amlexanox

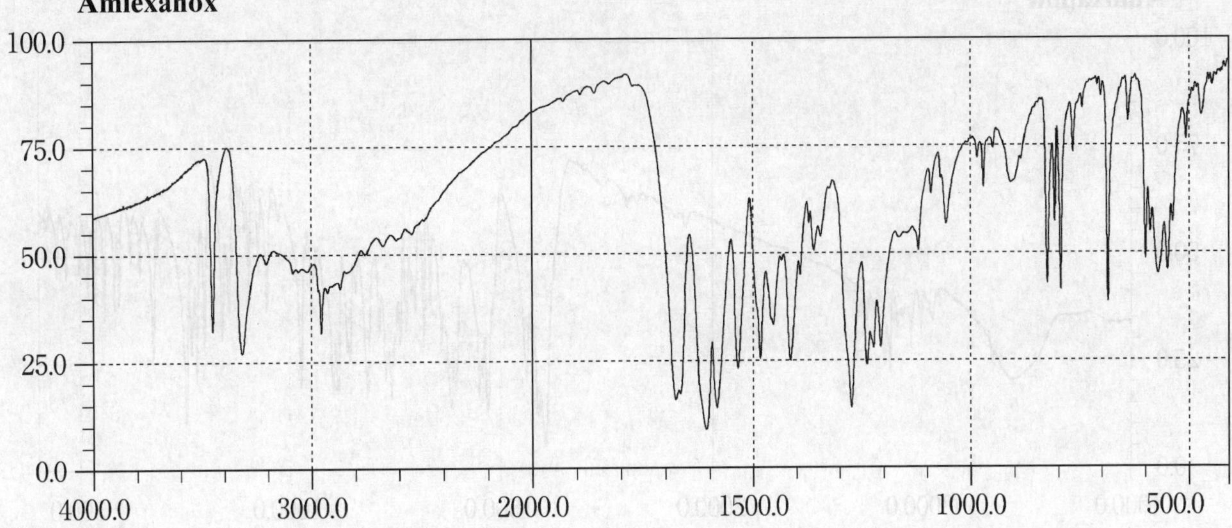

Amlodipine Besilate

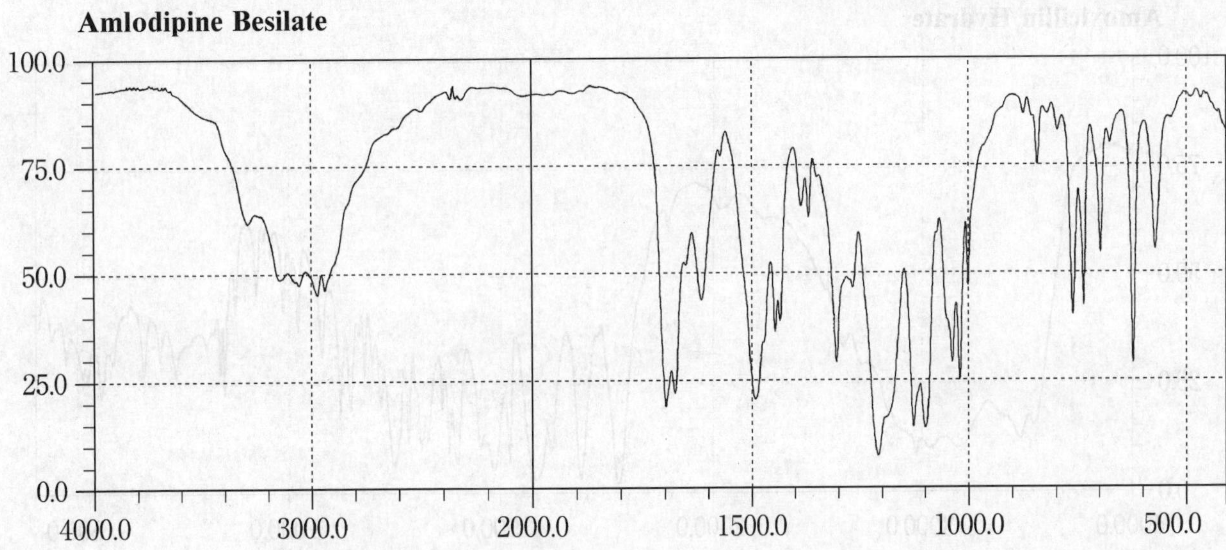

Amosulalol Hydrochloride

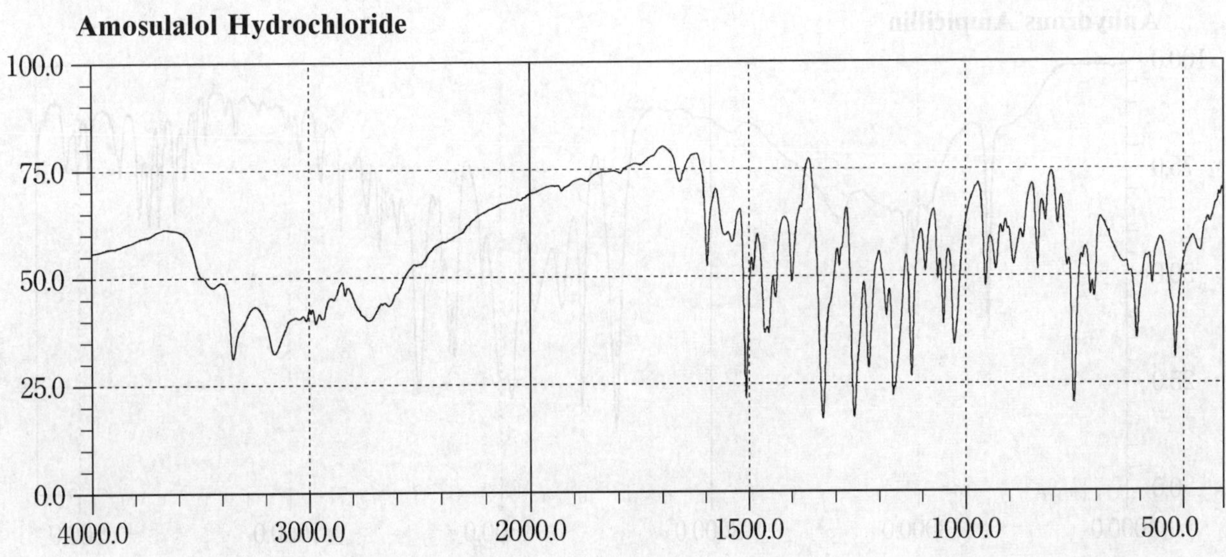

Amoxapine

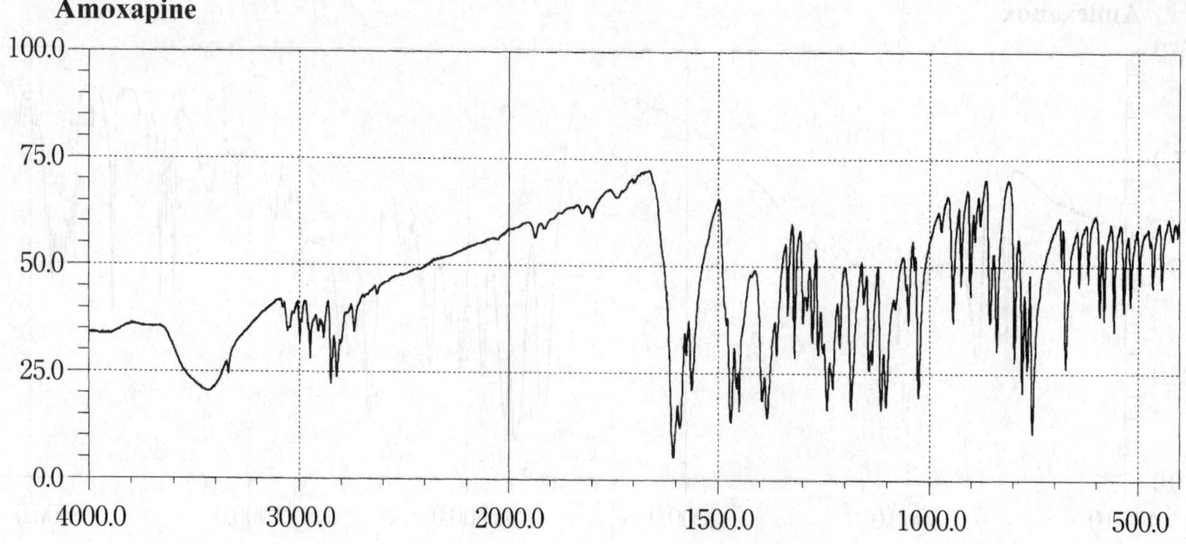

Amoxicillin Hydrate

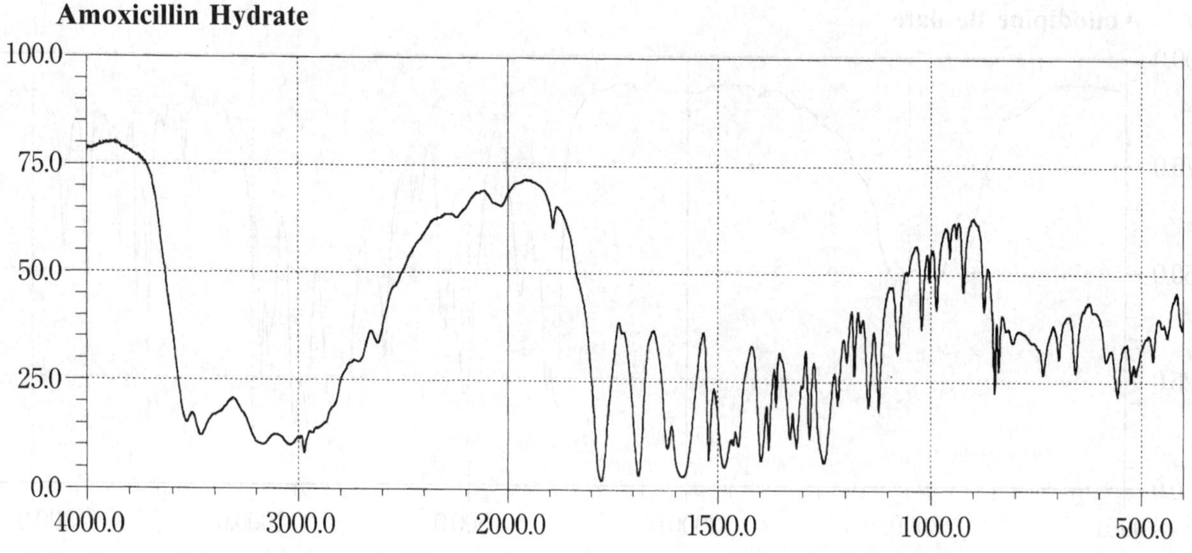

Anhydrous Ampicillin

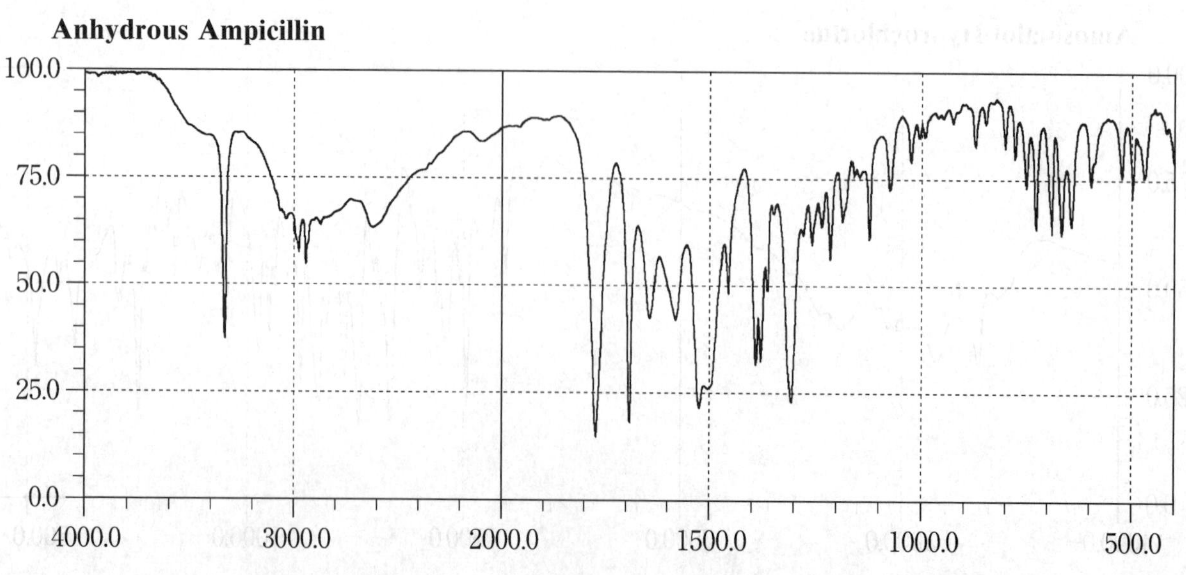

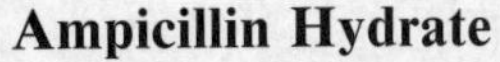

Ampicillin Hydrate

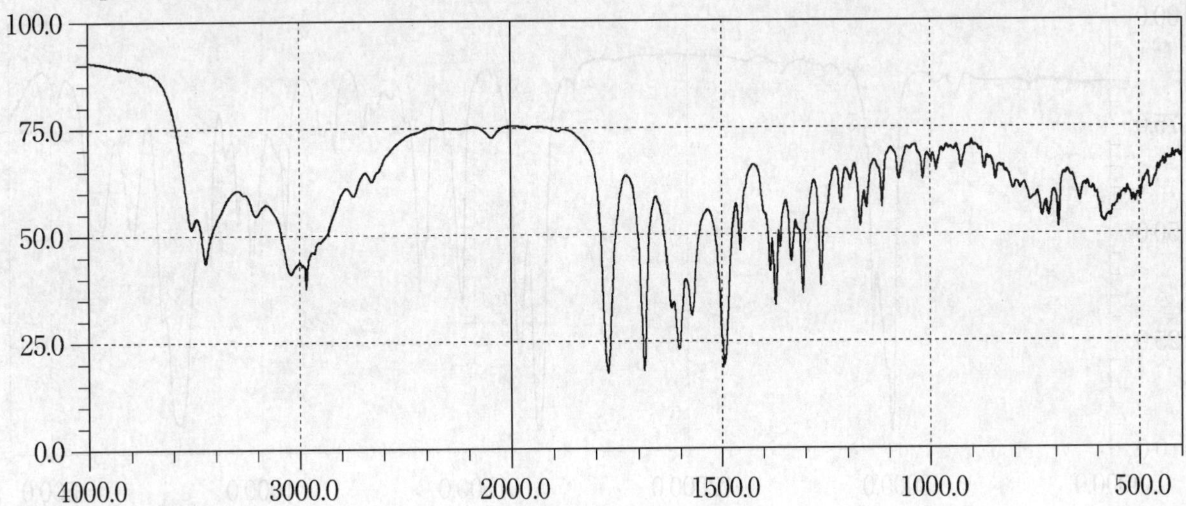

Ampicillin Sodium

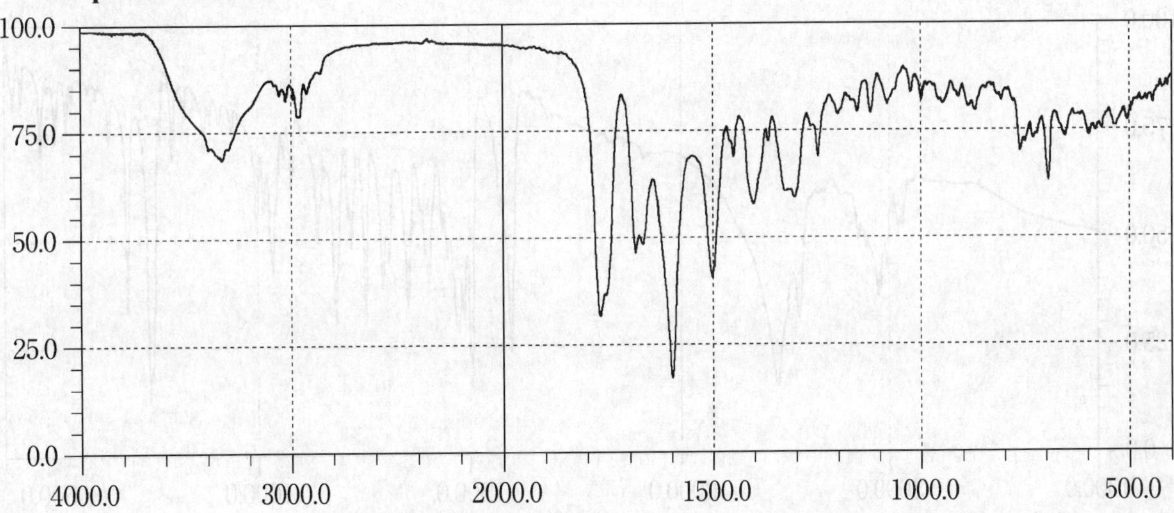

Ampiroxicam

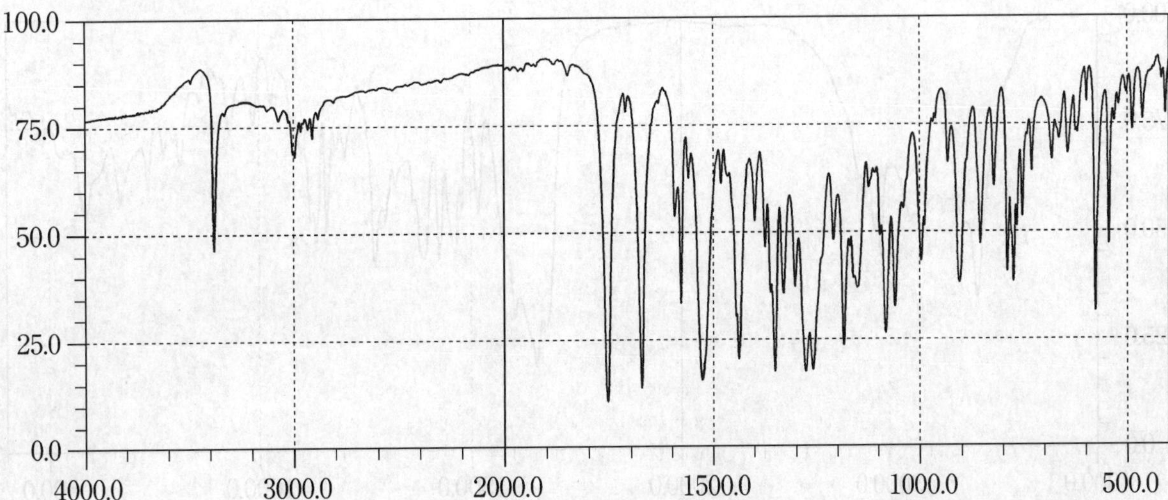

Amyl Nitrite

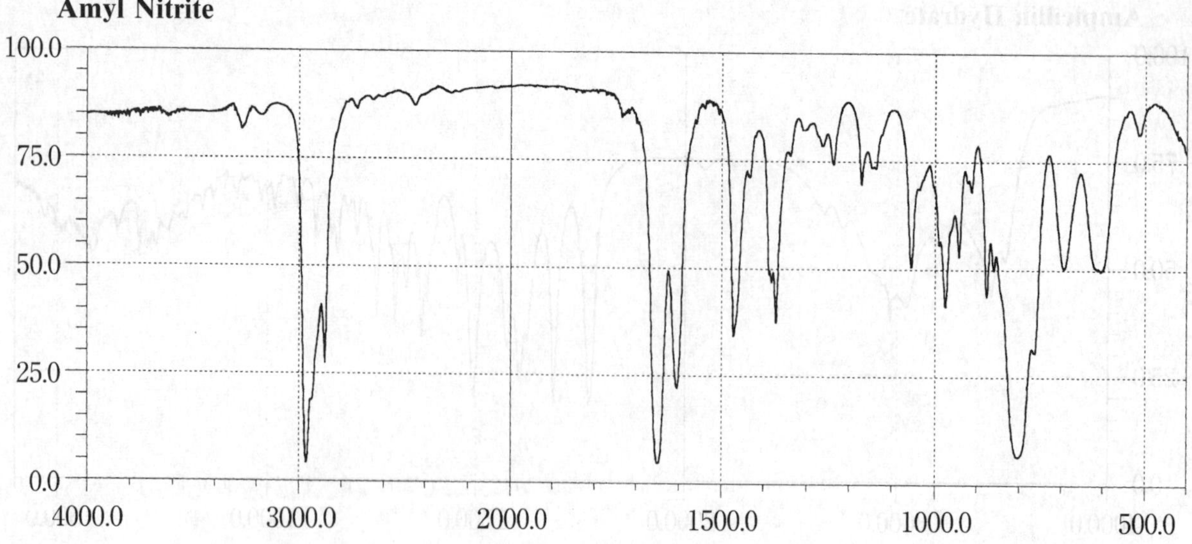

Aprindine Hydrochloride

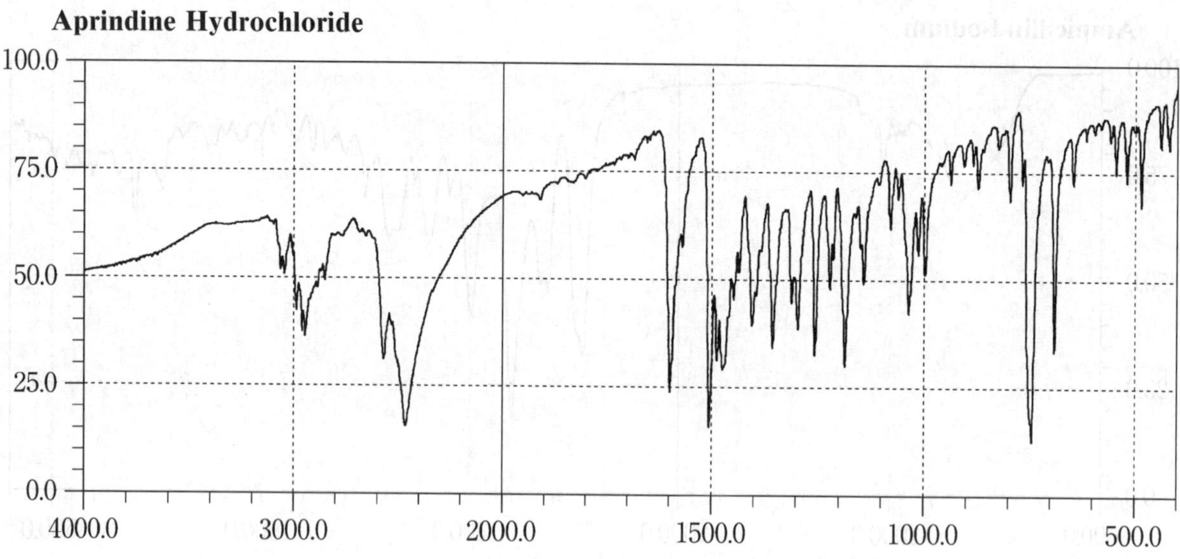

Argatroban Hydrate

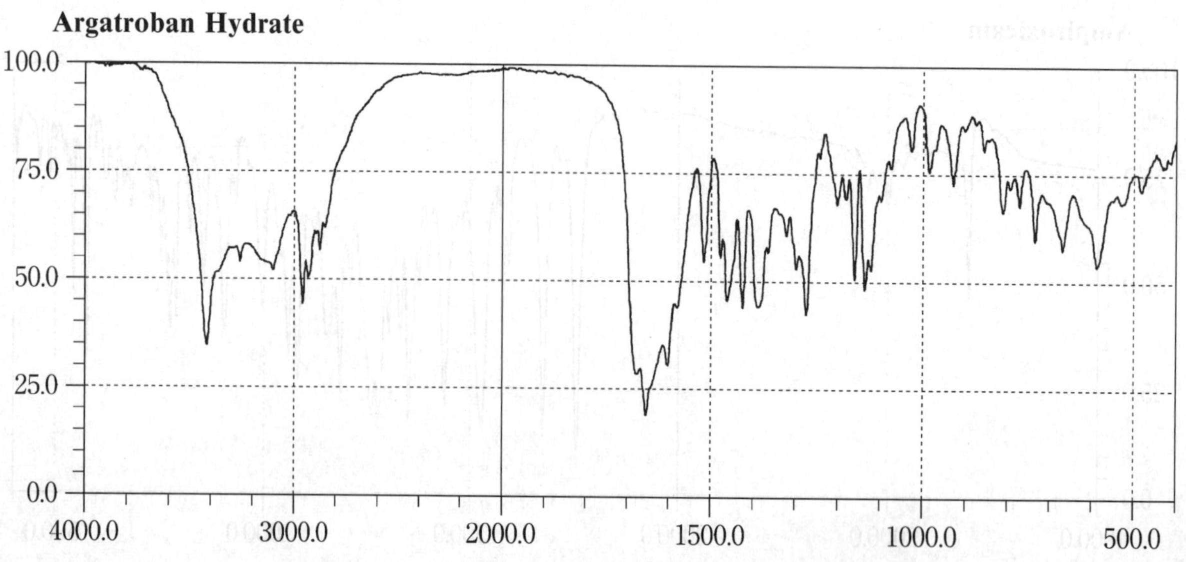

L-Arginine

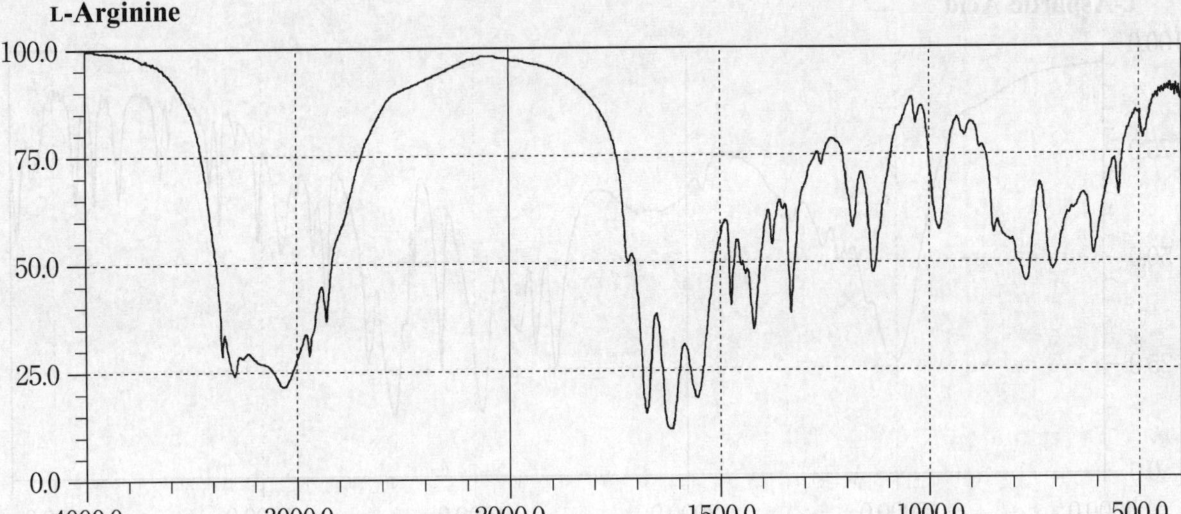

L-Arginine Hydrochloride

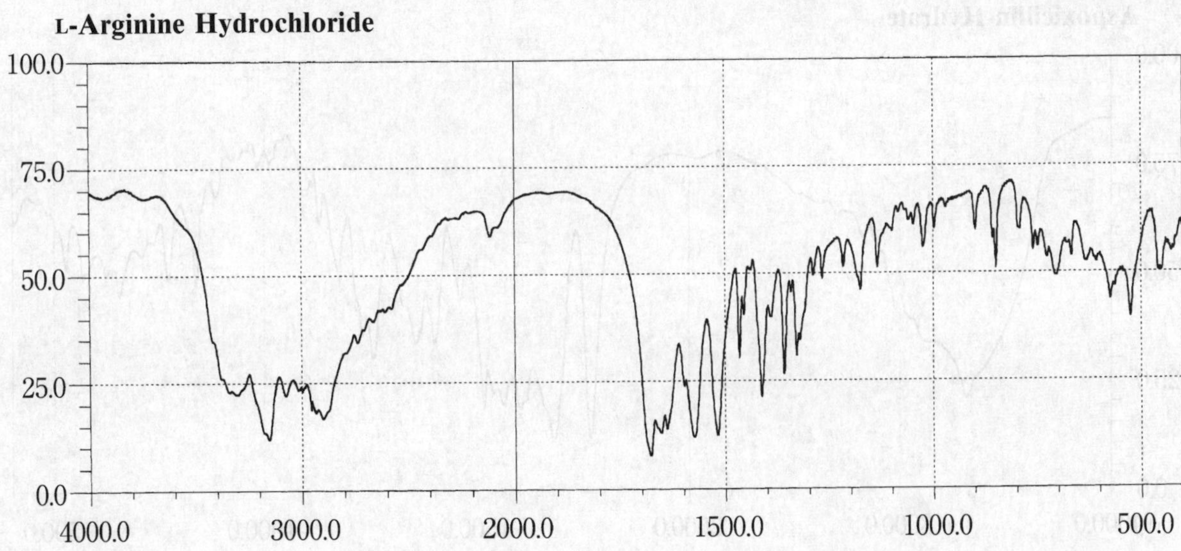

Arotinolol Hydrochloride

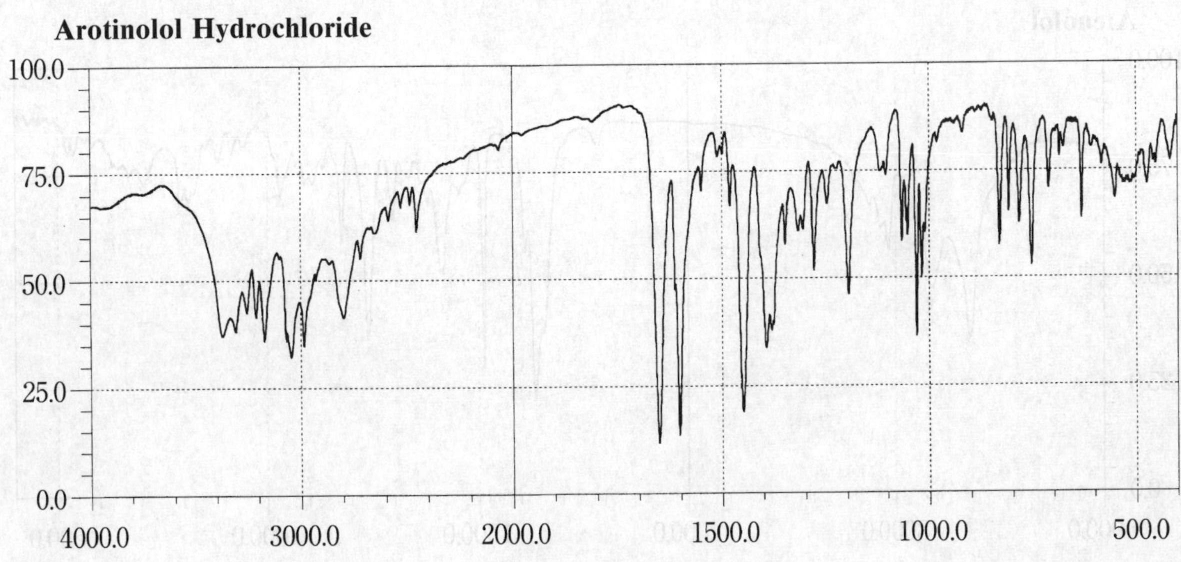

L-Aspartic Acid

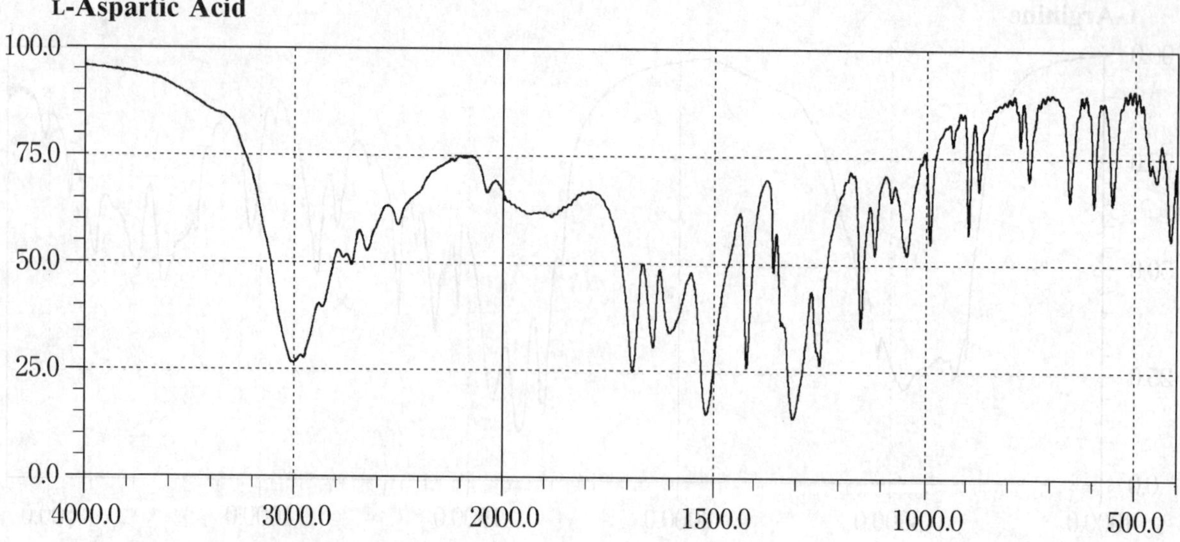

Aspoxicillin Hydrate

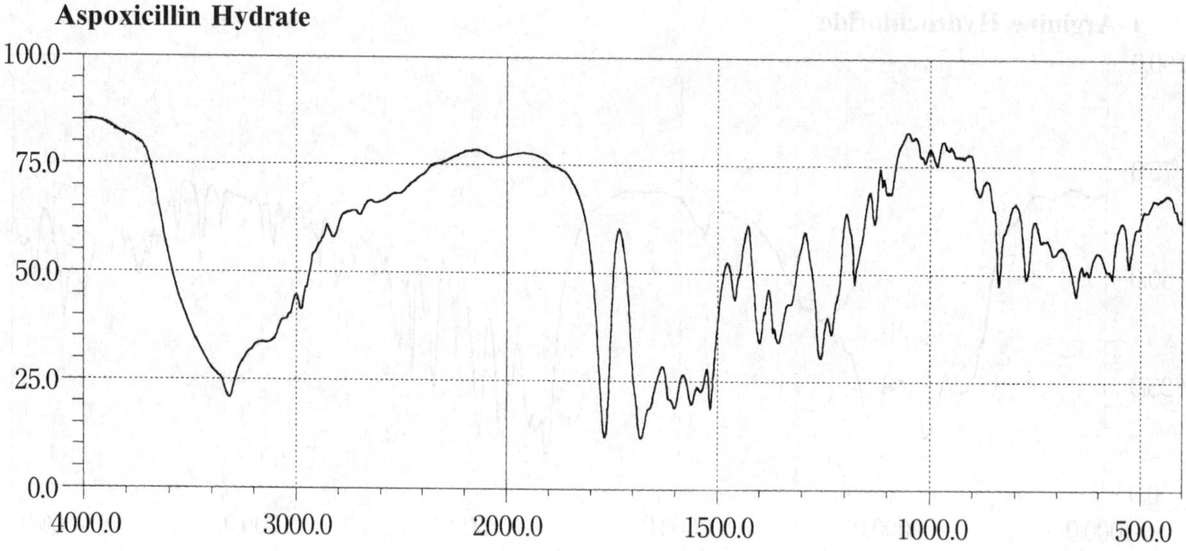

Atenolol

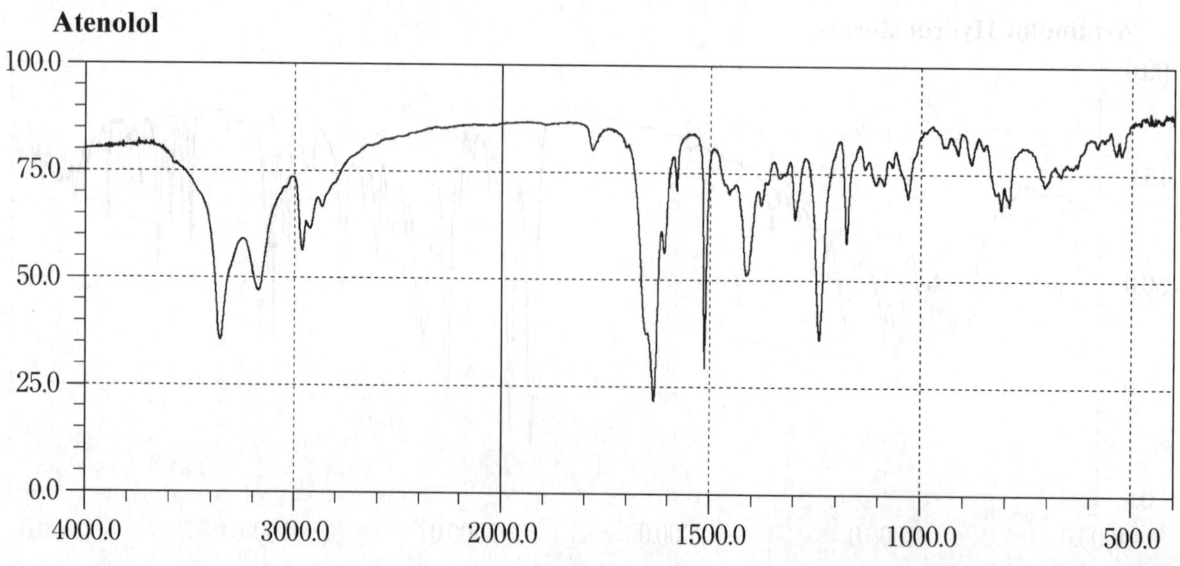

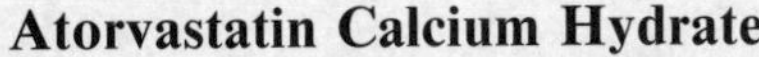

Atorvastatin Calcium Hydrate

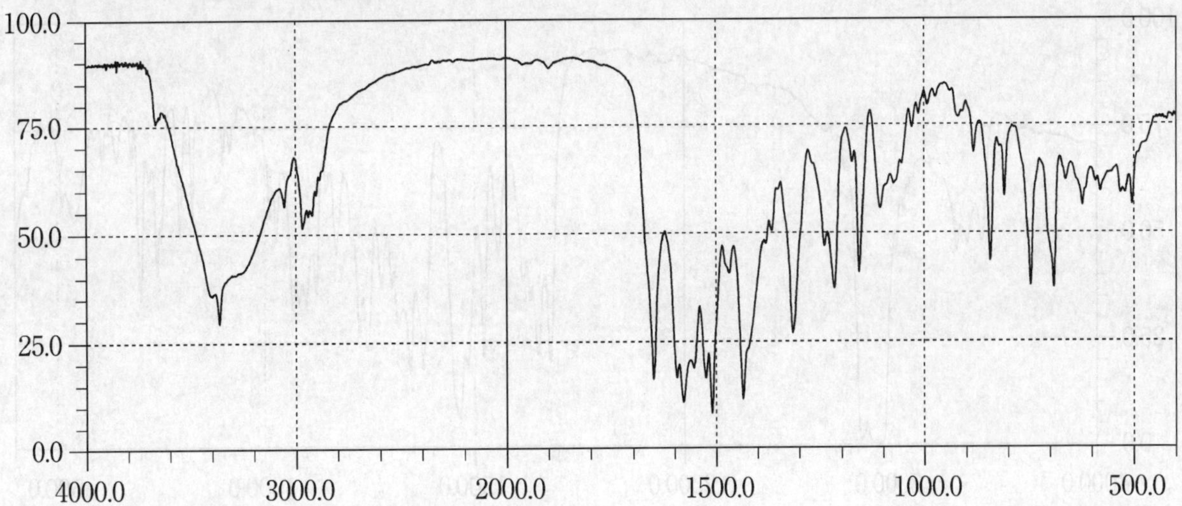

Auranofin

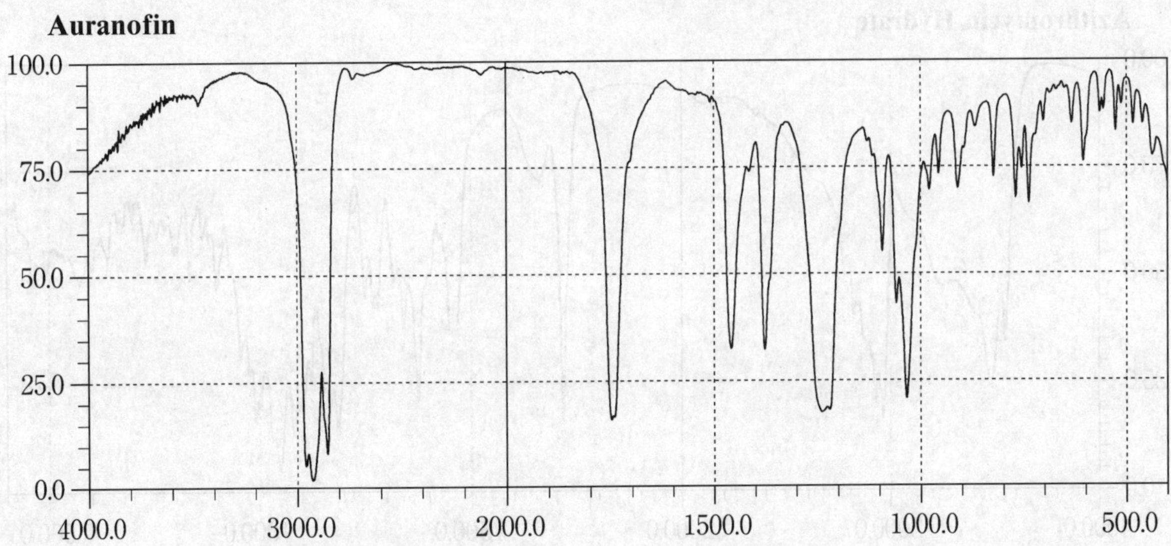

Azelastine Hydrochloride

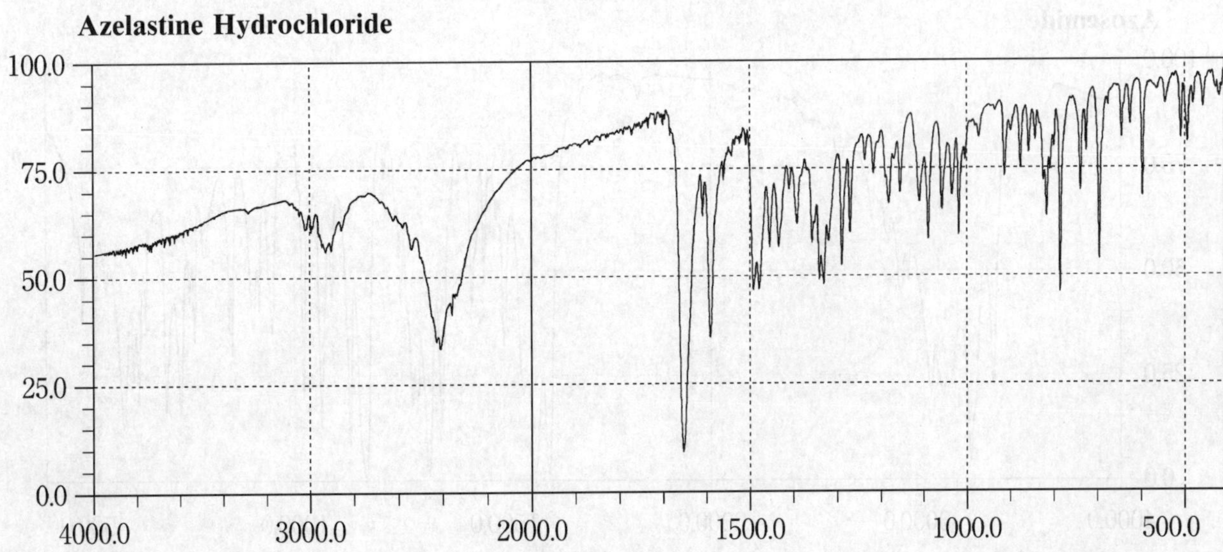

Azelnidipine

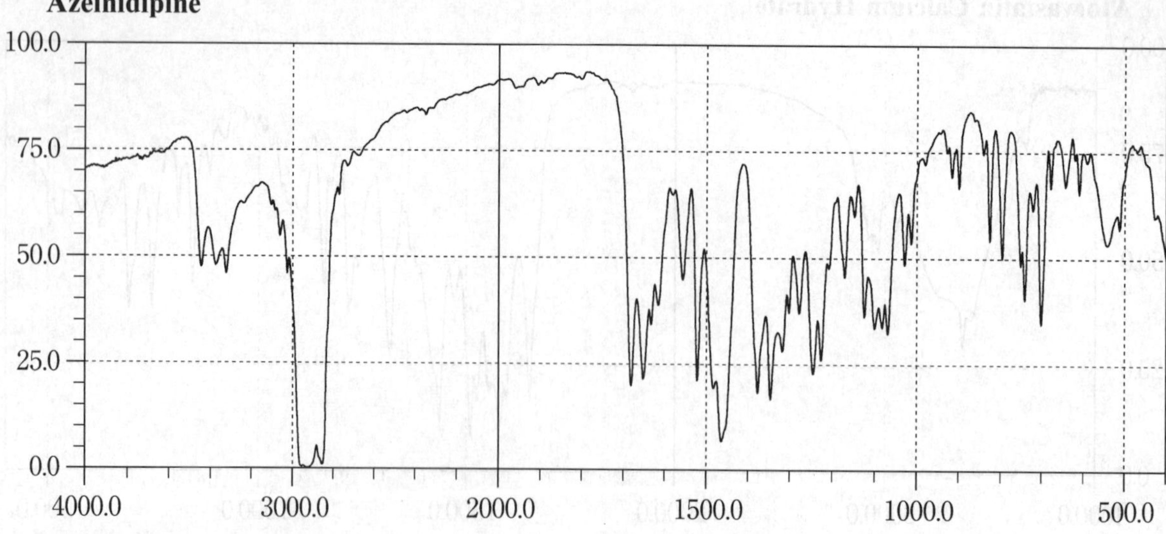

Azithromycin Hydrate

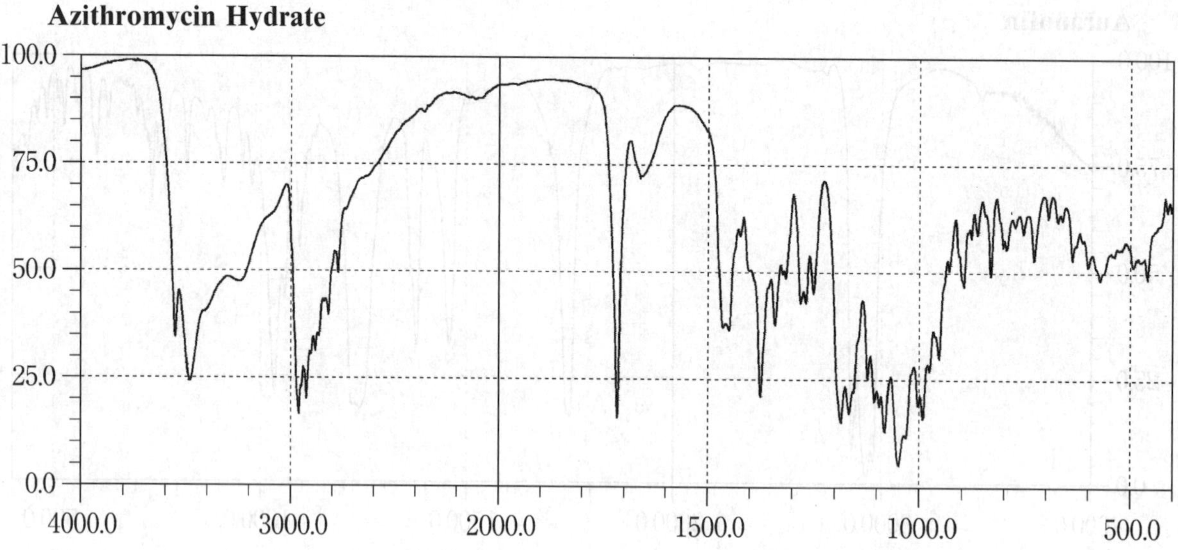

Azosemide

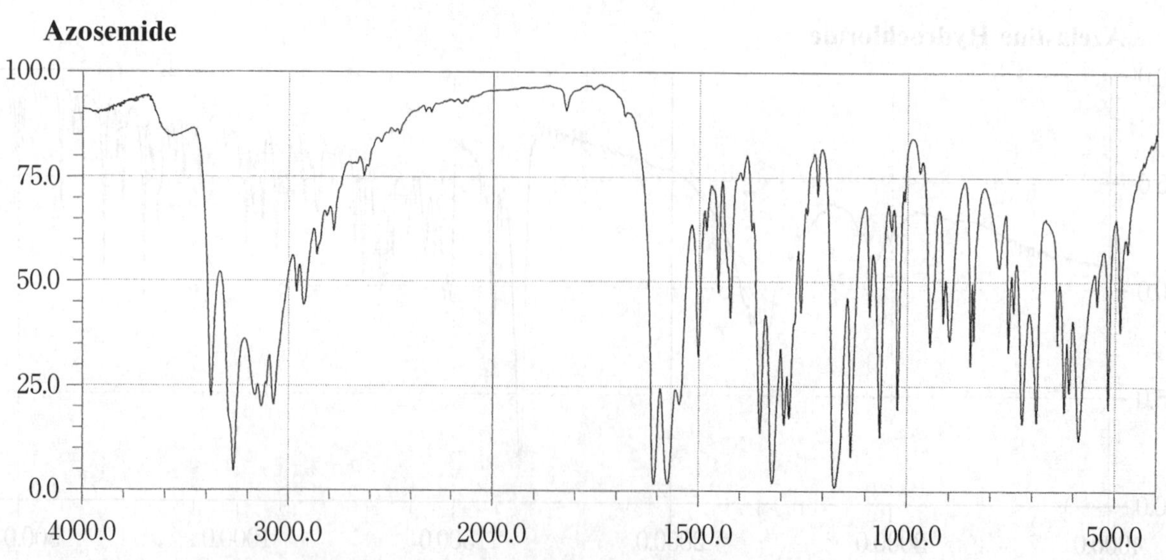

Bacampicillin Hydrochloride

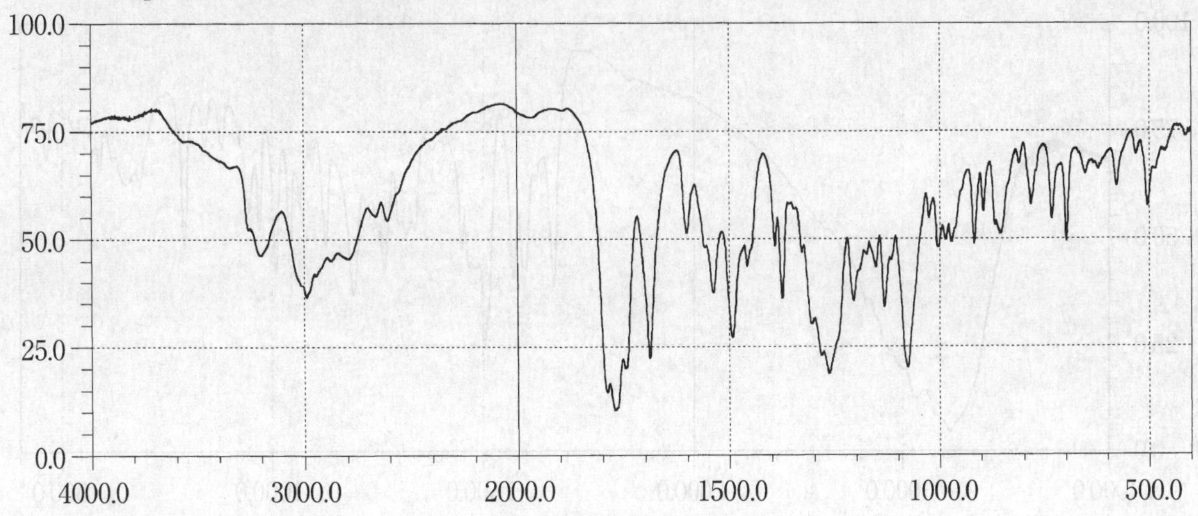

Beclometasone Dipropionate

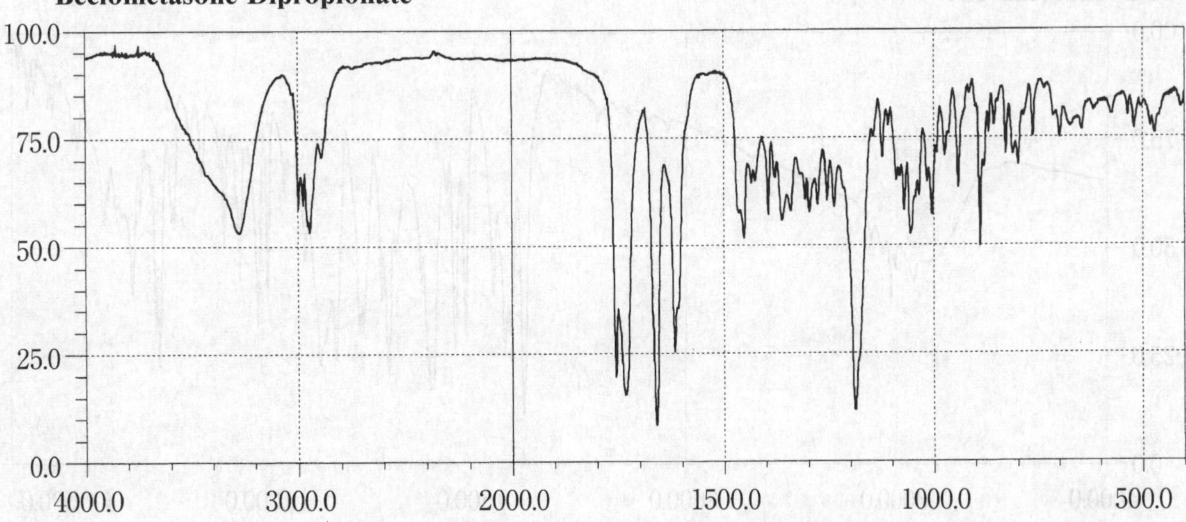

Benidipine Hydrochloride

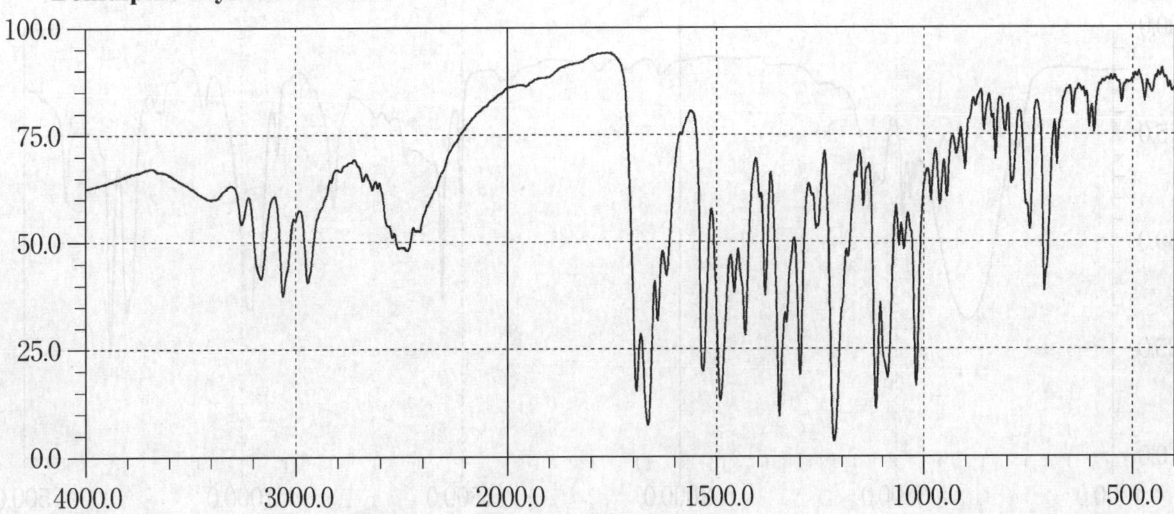

Benserazide Hydrochloride

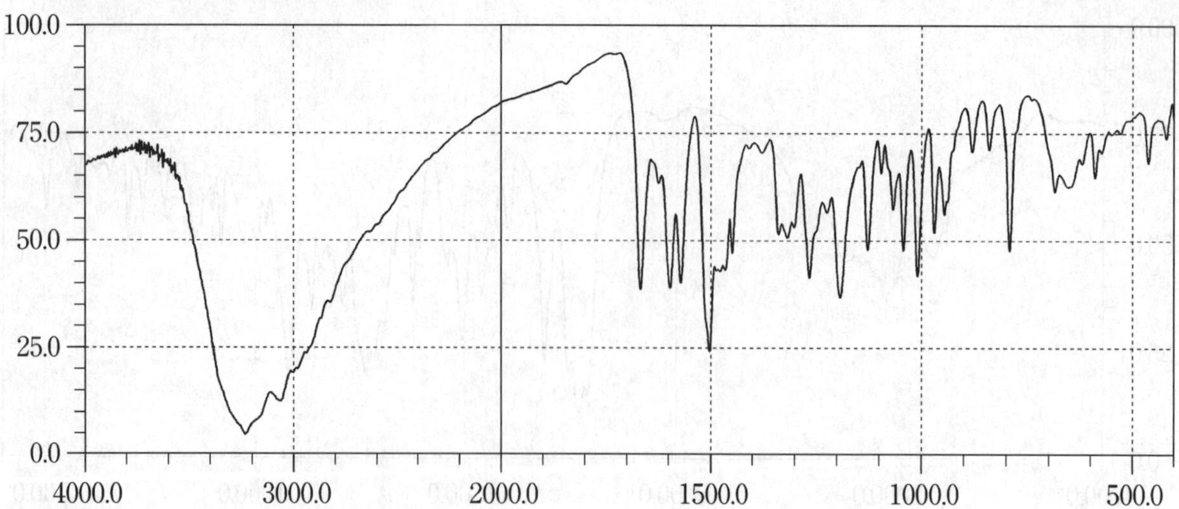

Benzbromarone

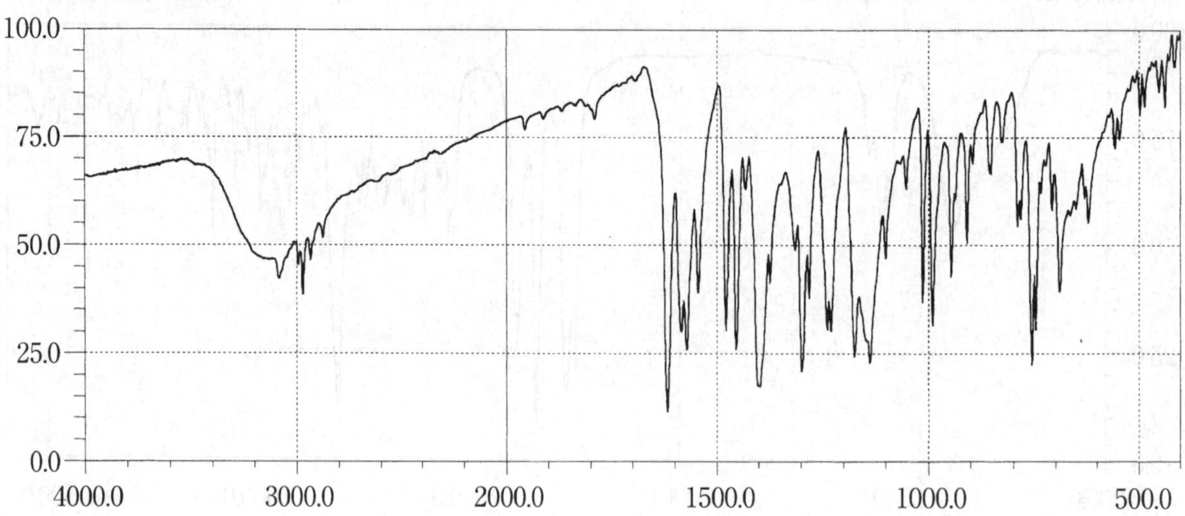

Benzyl Alcohol

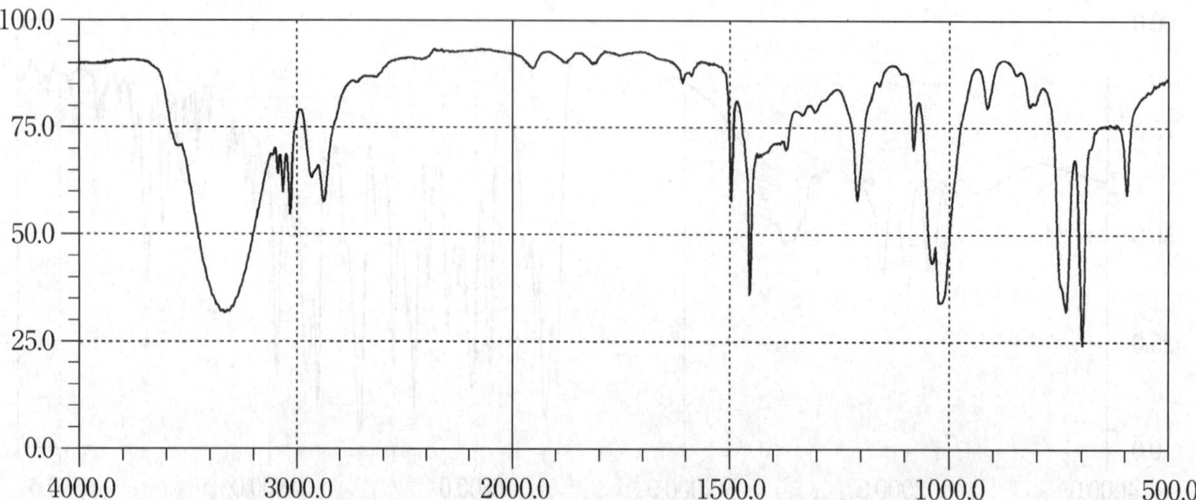

Benzylpenicillin Benzathine Hydrate

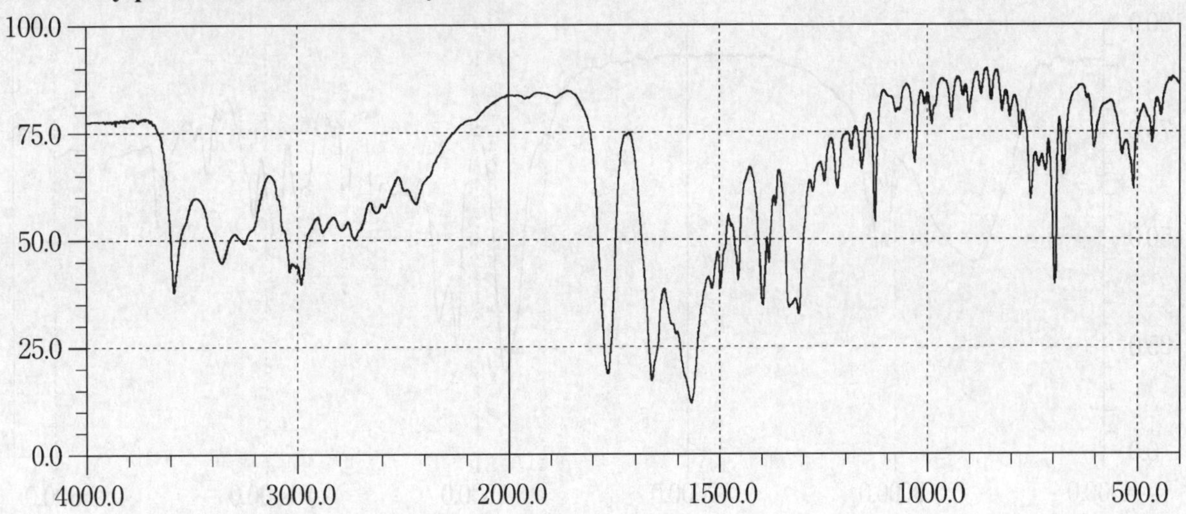

Benzylpenicillin Potassium

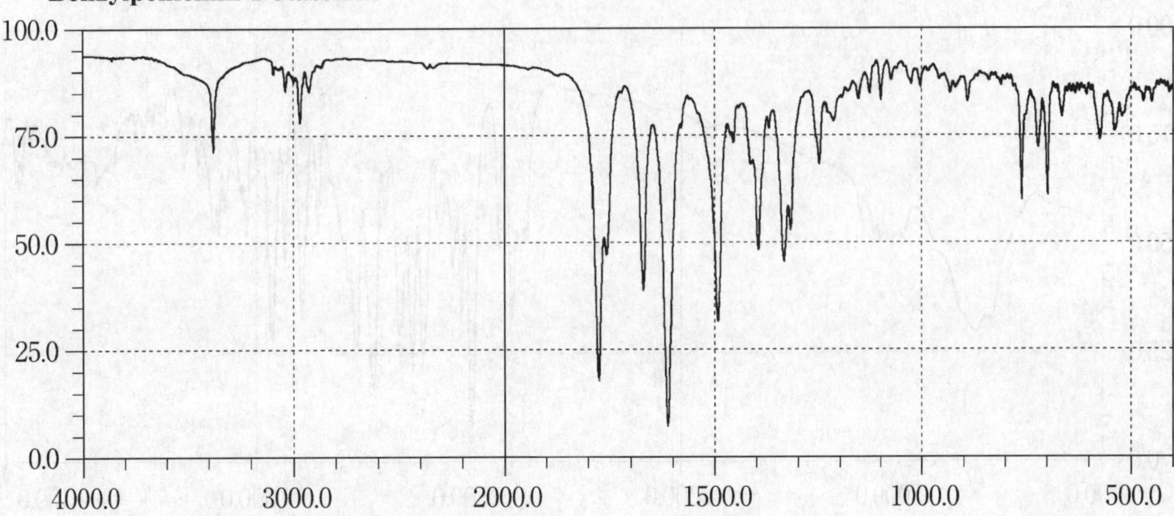

Bepotastine Besilate

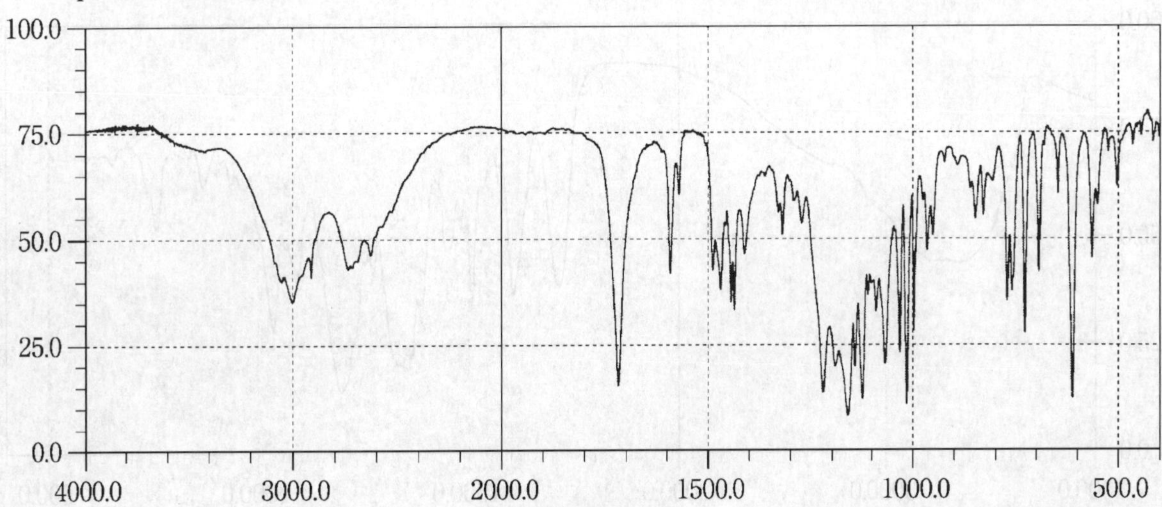

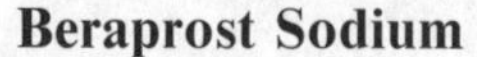

Beraprost Sodium

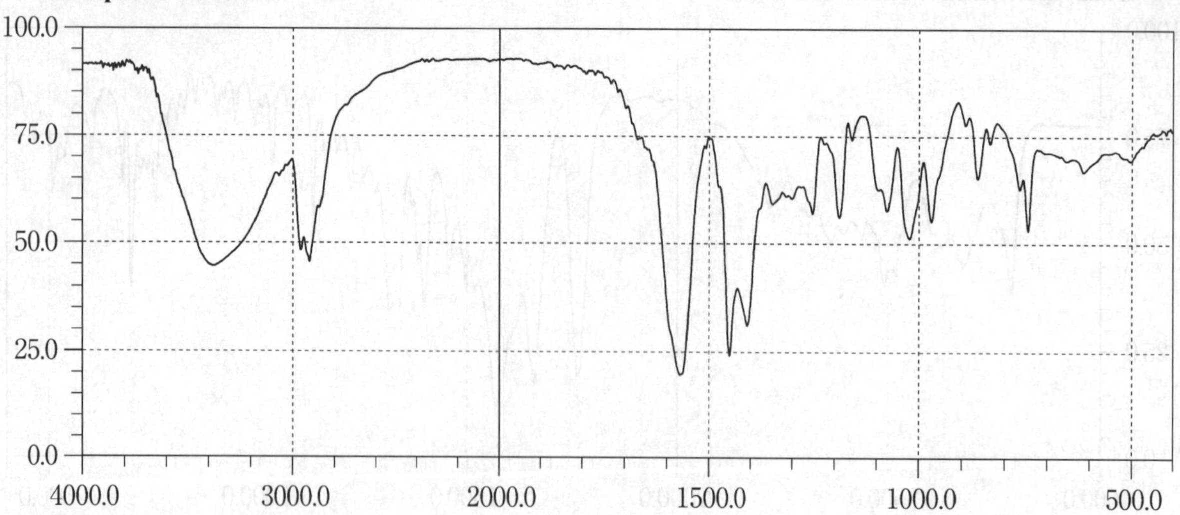

Berberine Chloride Hydrate

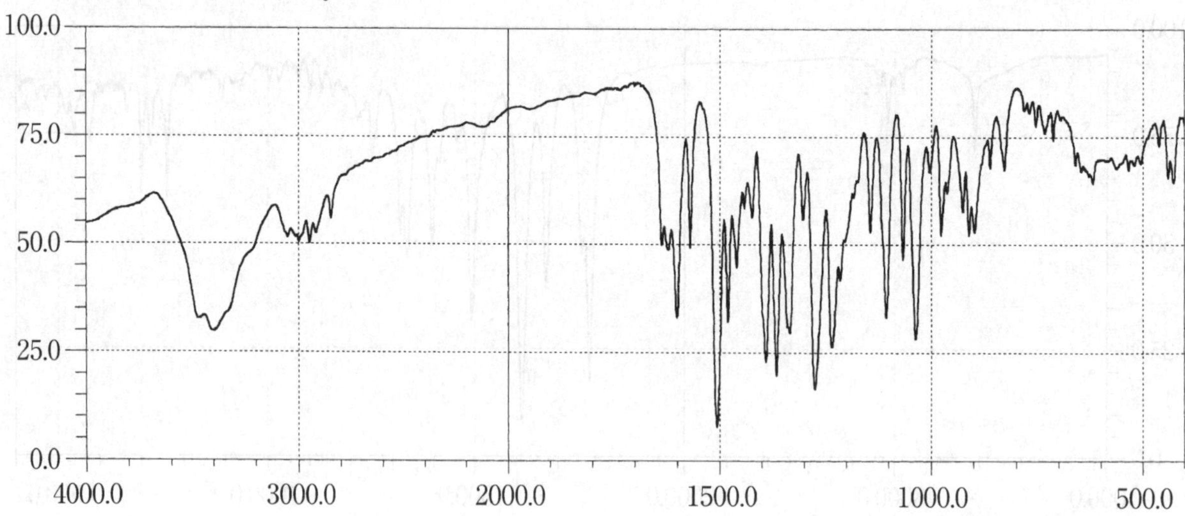

Berberine Tannate

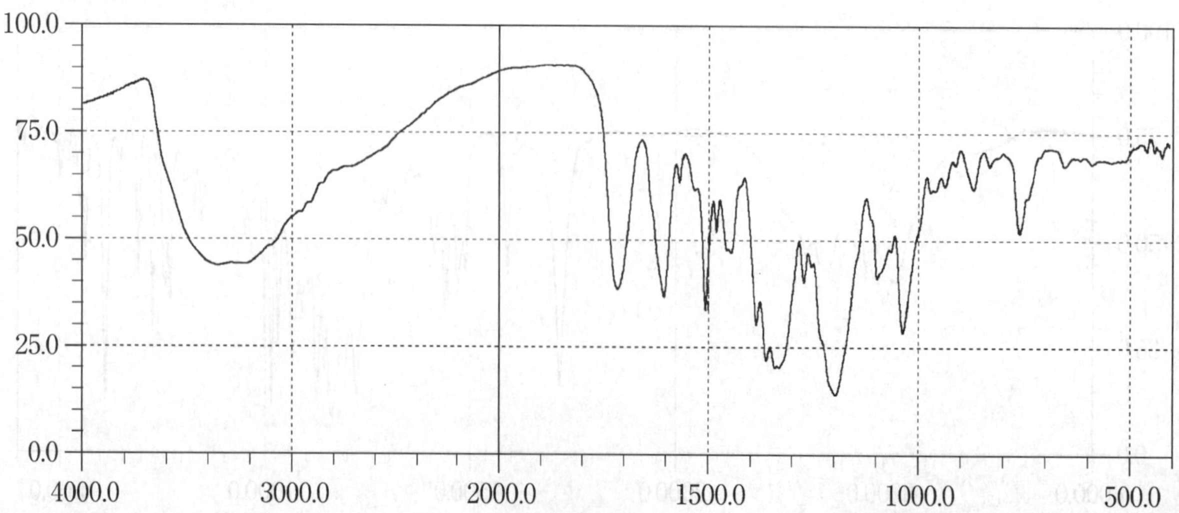

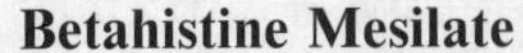

Betahistine Mesilate

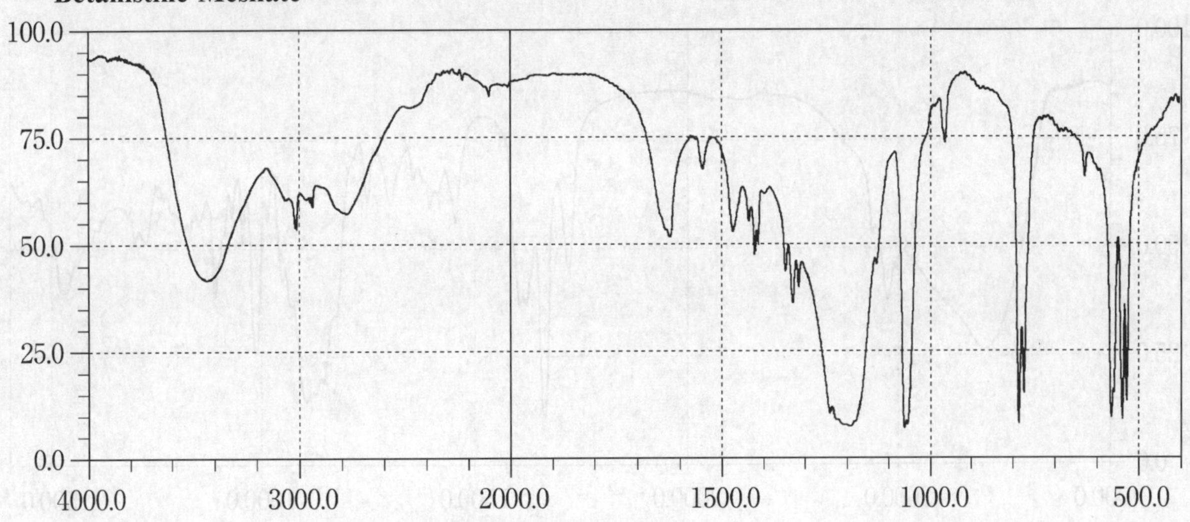

Betamethasone

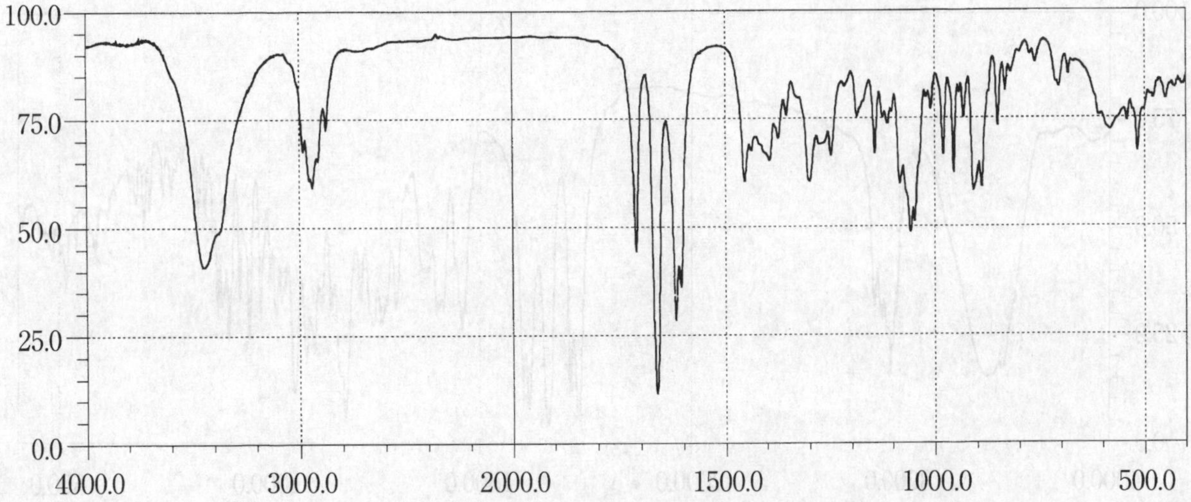

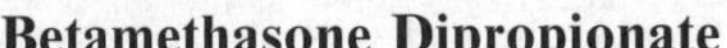

Betamethasone Dipropionate

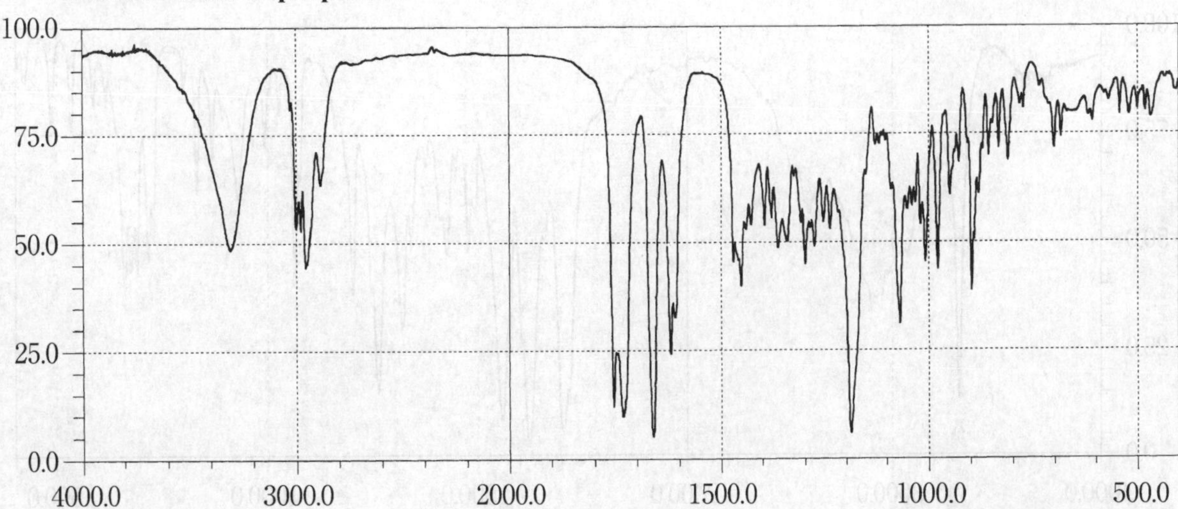

Betamethasone Sodium Phosphate

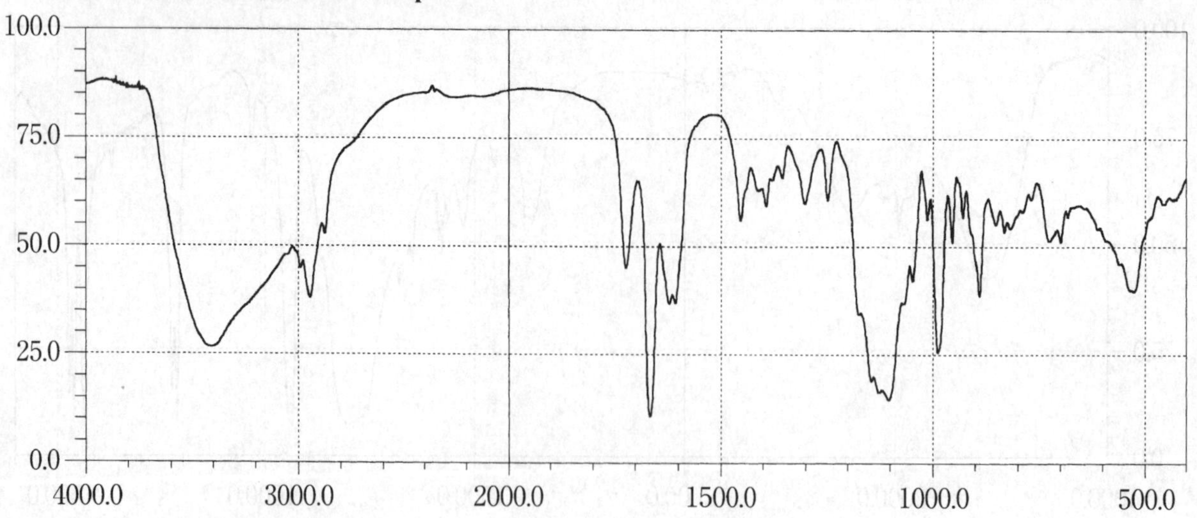

Betamethasone Valerate

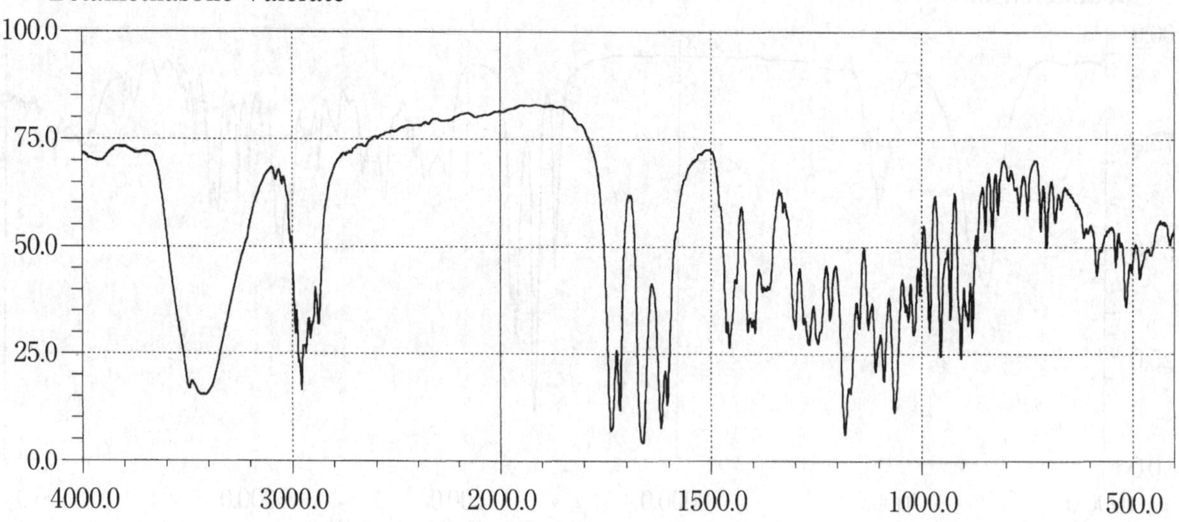

Betamipron

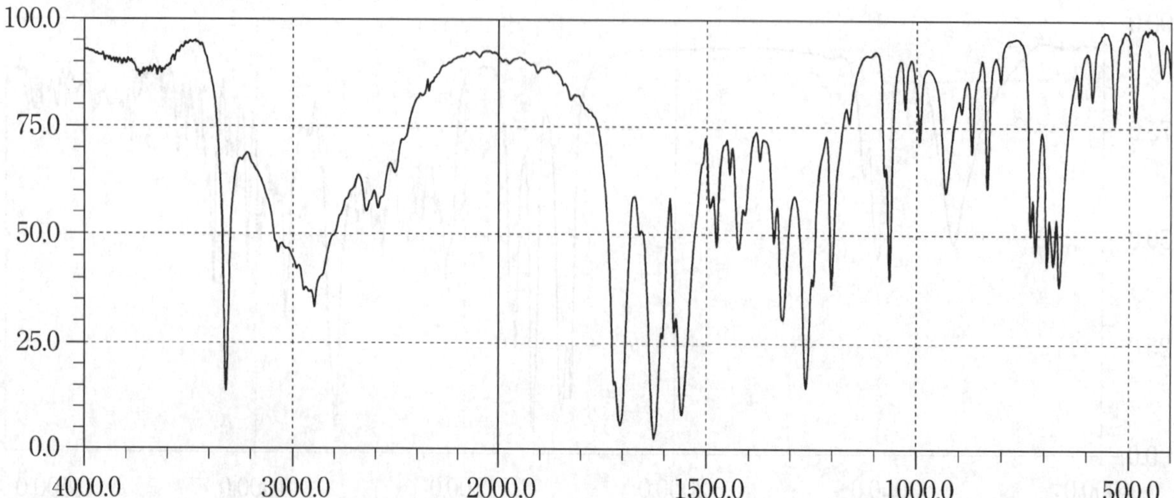

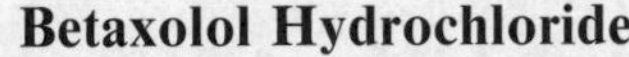

Betaxolol Hydrochloride

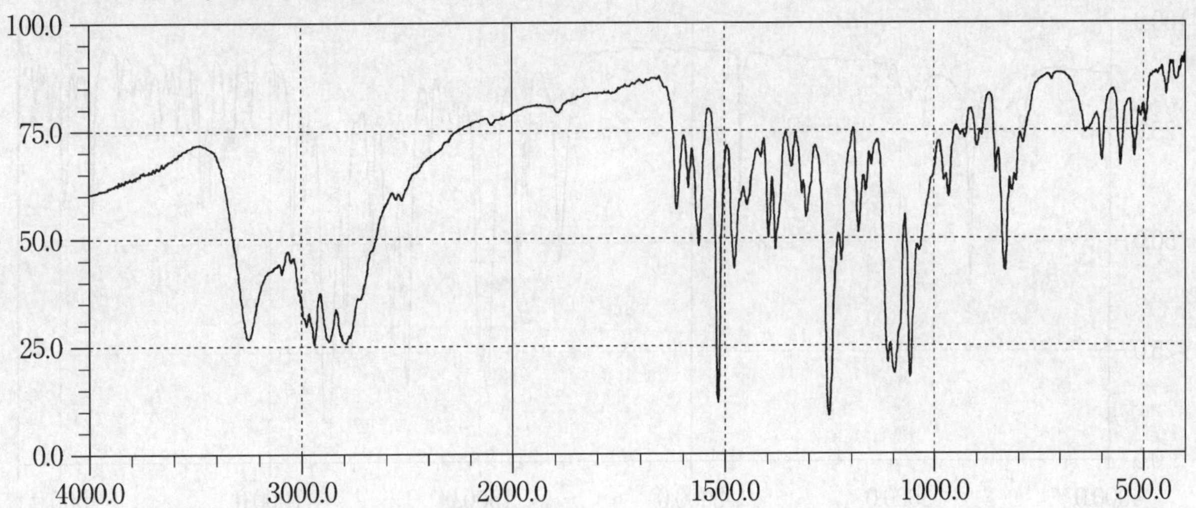

Bethanechol Chloride

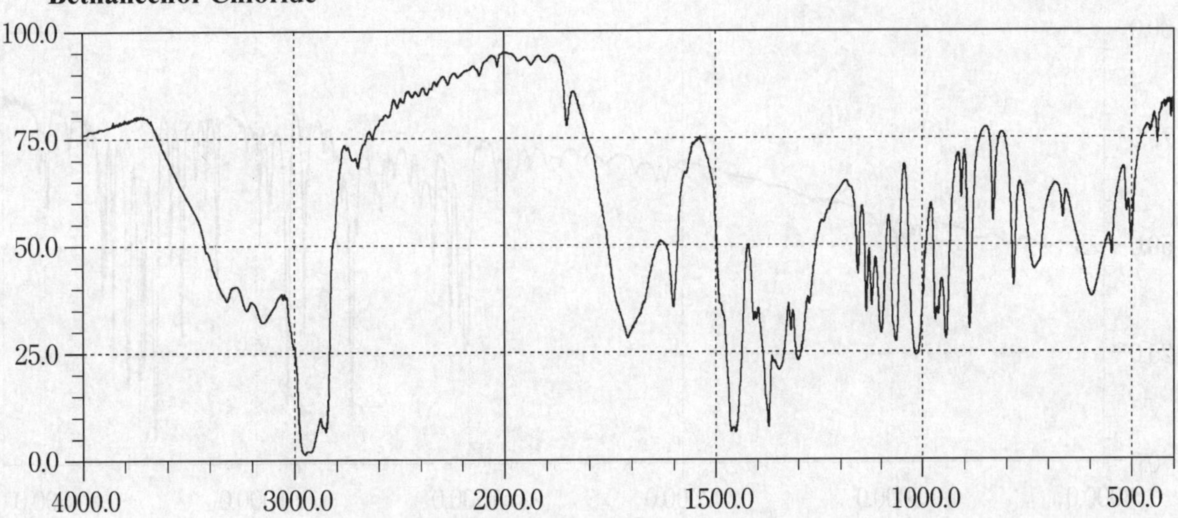

Bezafibrate

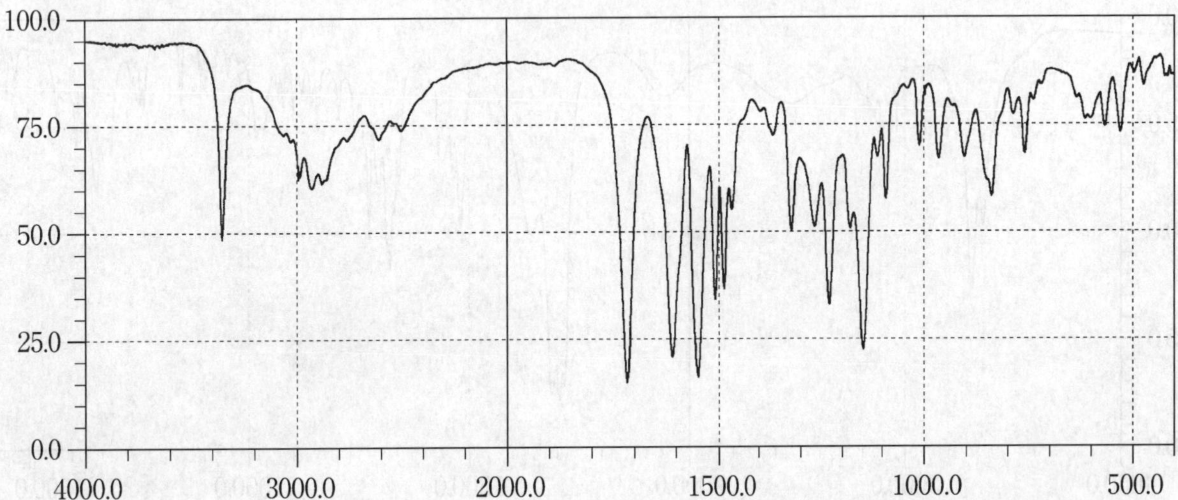

Bicalutamide

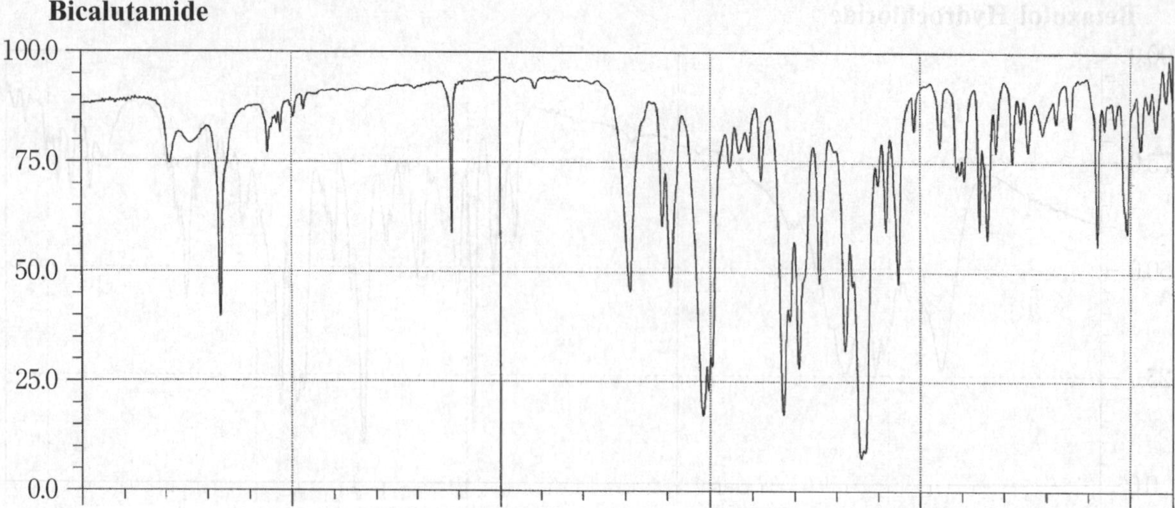

Bifonazole

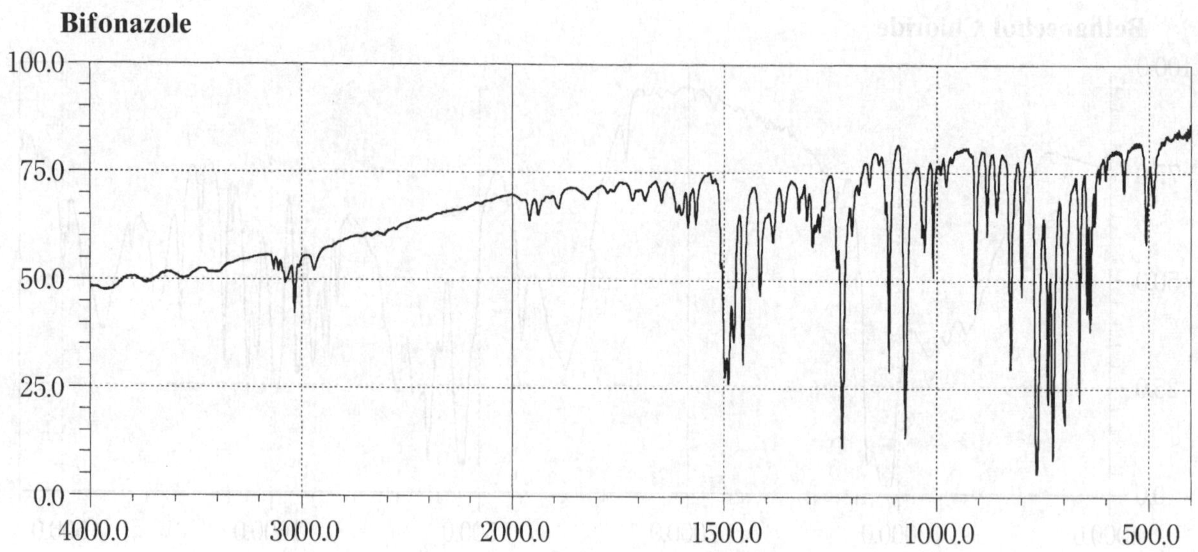

Biotin

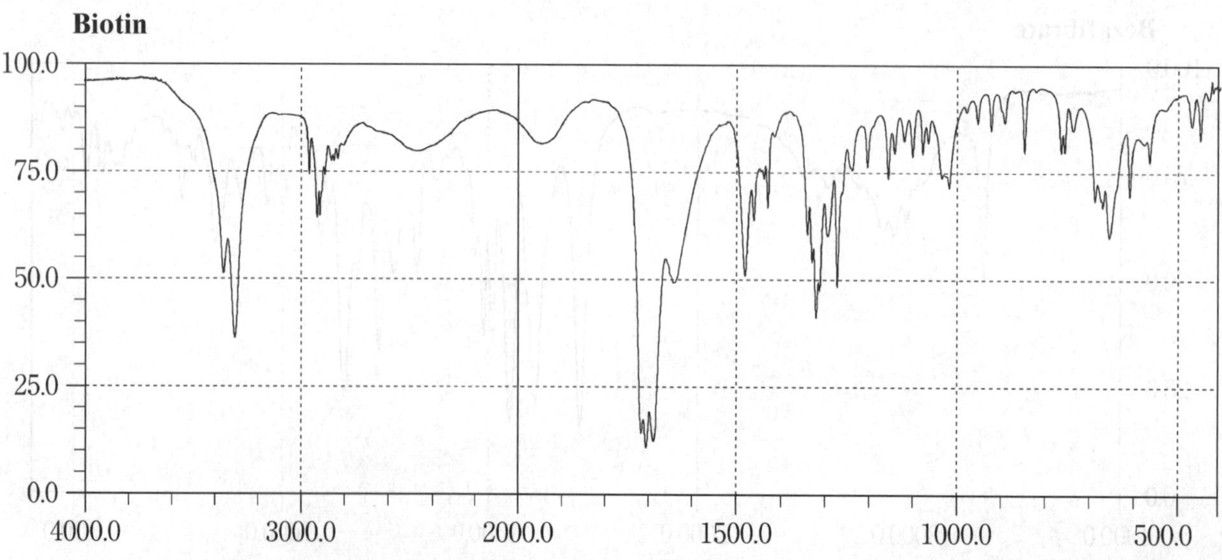

The JP Drugs are to be tested according to the provisions given in the pertinent monographs, General Notices, General Rules for Crude Drugs, General Rules for Preparations, and General Tests for their conformity to the Japanese Pharmacopoeia. (See the General Notices 5.)

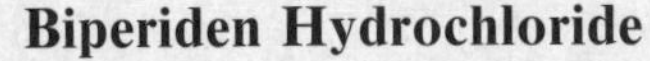

Biperiden Hydrochloride

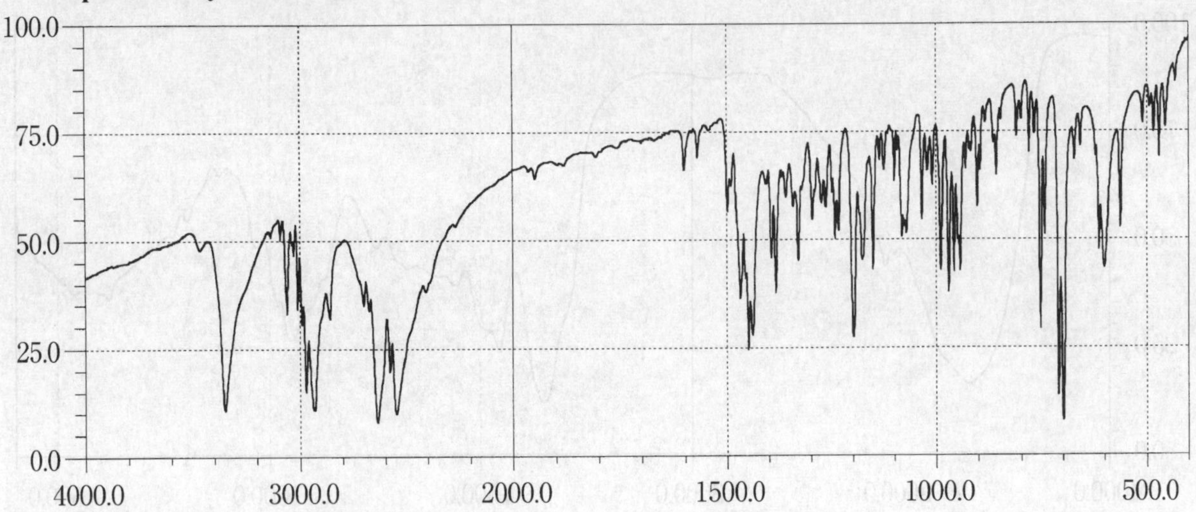

Bisacodyl

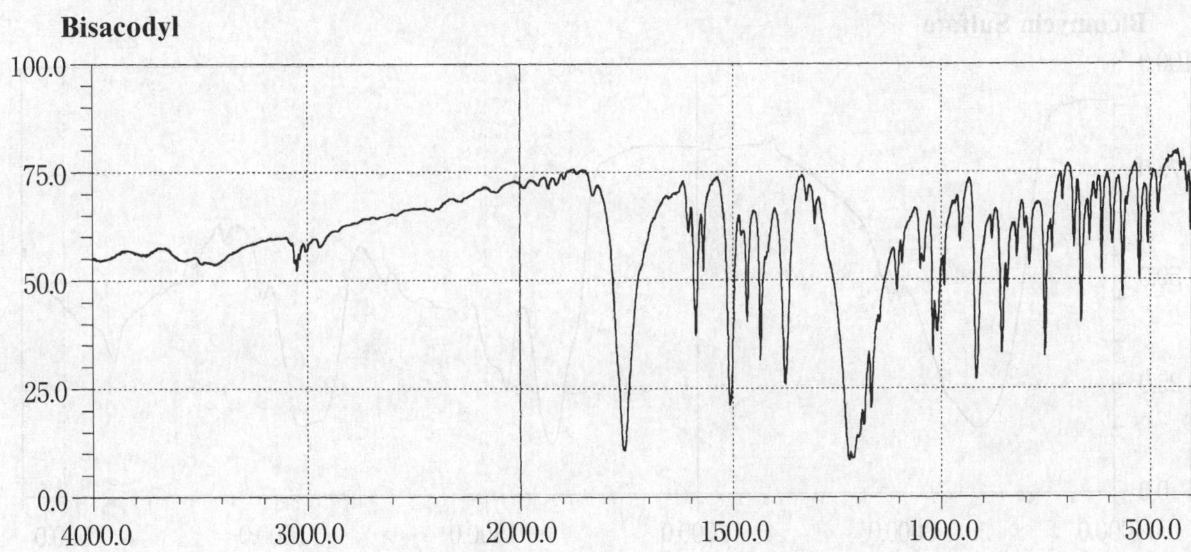

Bisoprolol Fumarate

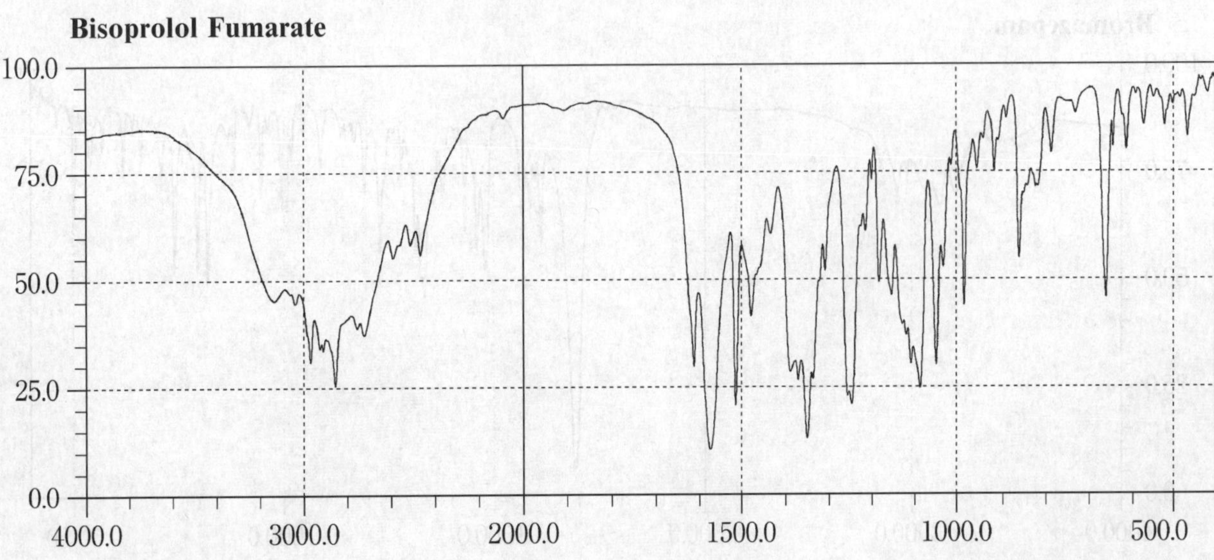

Bleomycin Hydrochloride

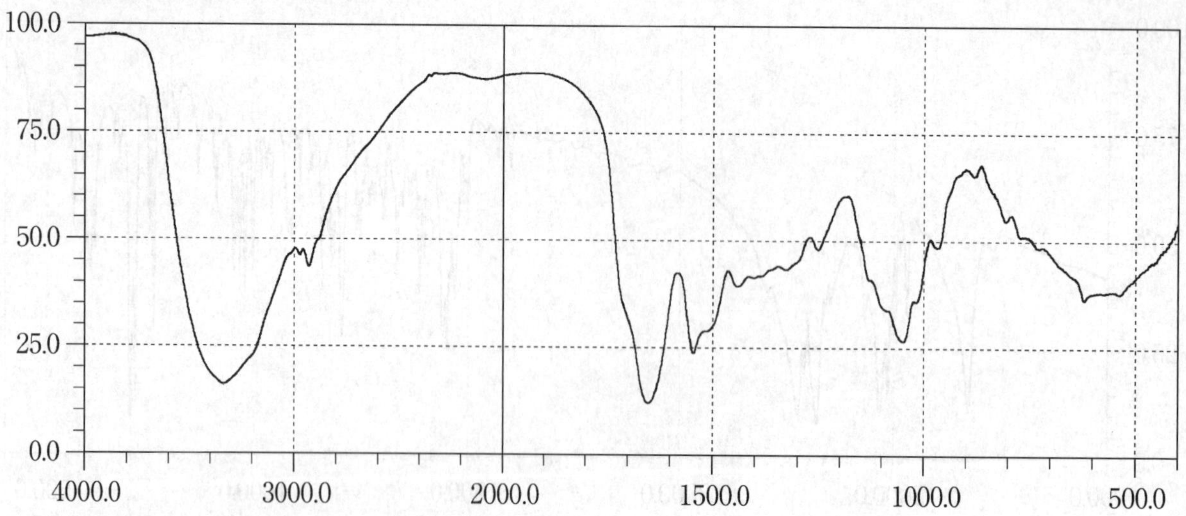

Bleomycin Sulfate

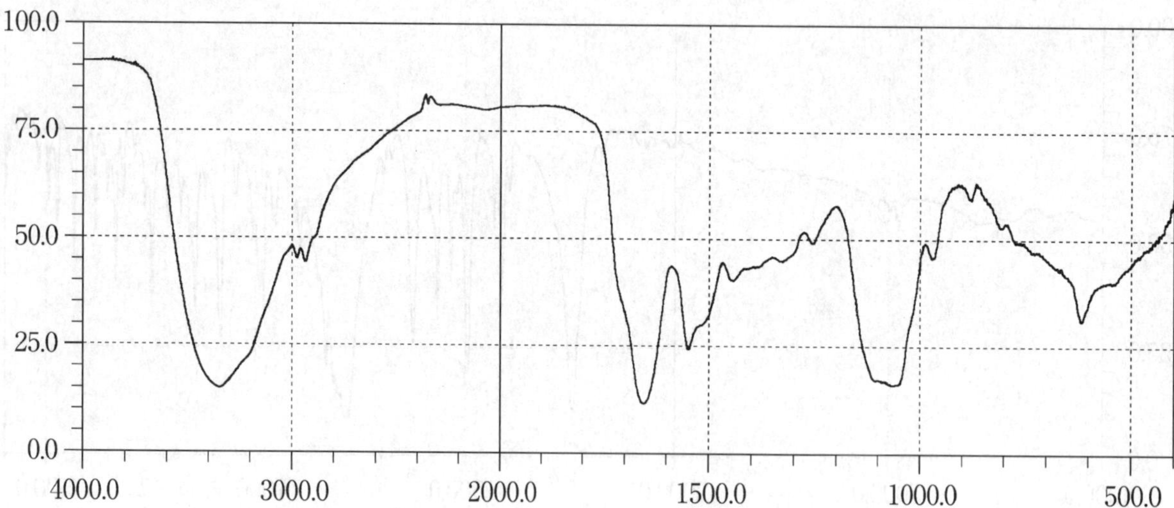

Bromazepam

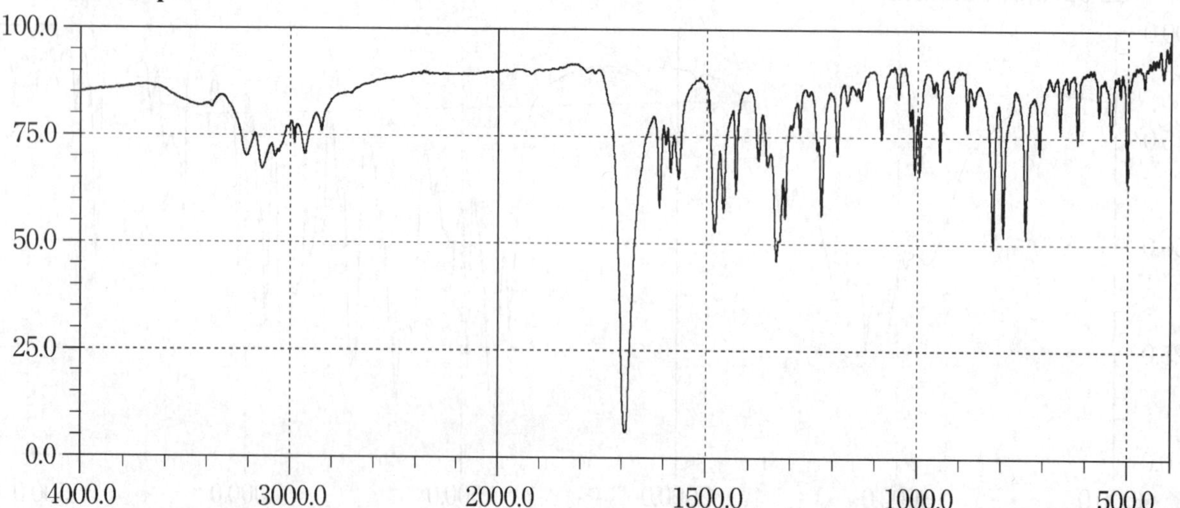

Bromfenac Sodium Hydrate

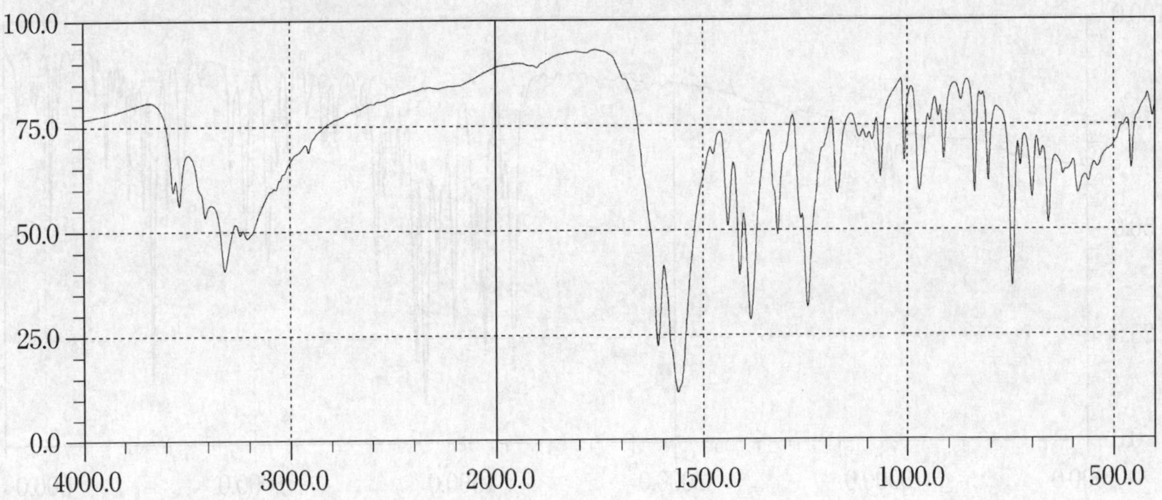

Bromhexine Hydrochloride

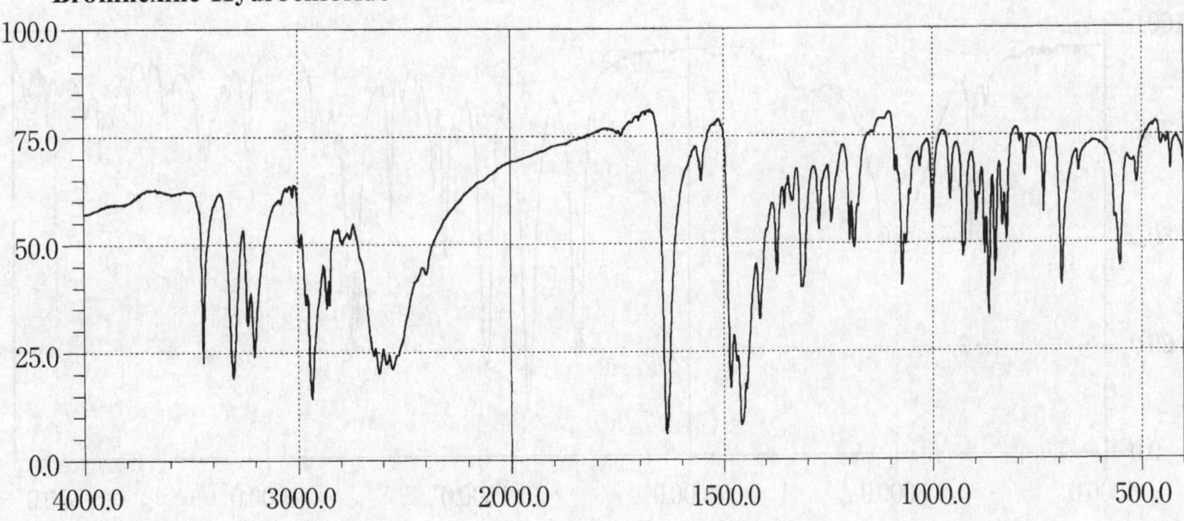

Bromocriptine Mesilate

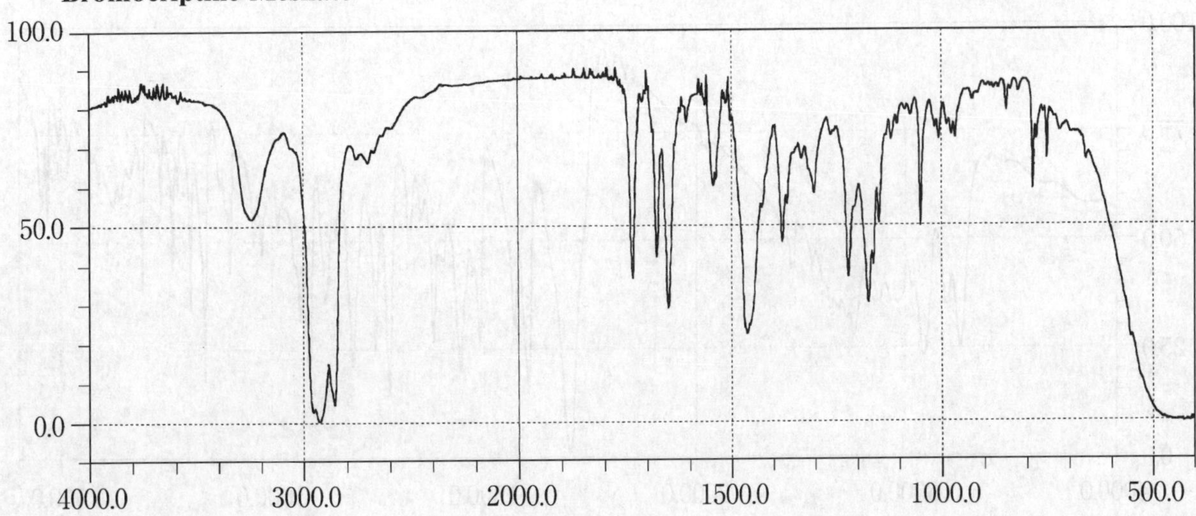

Brotizolam

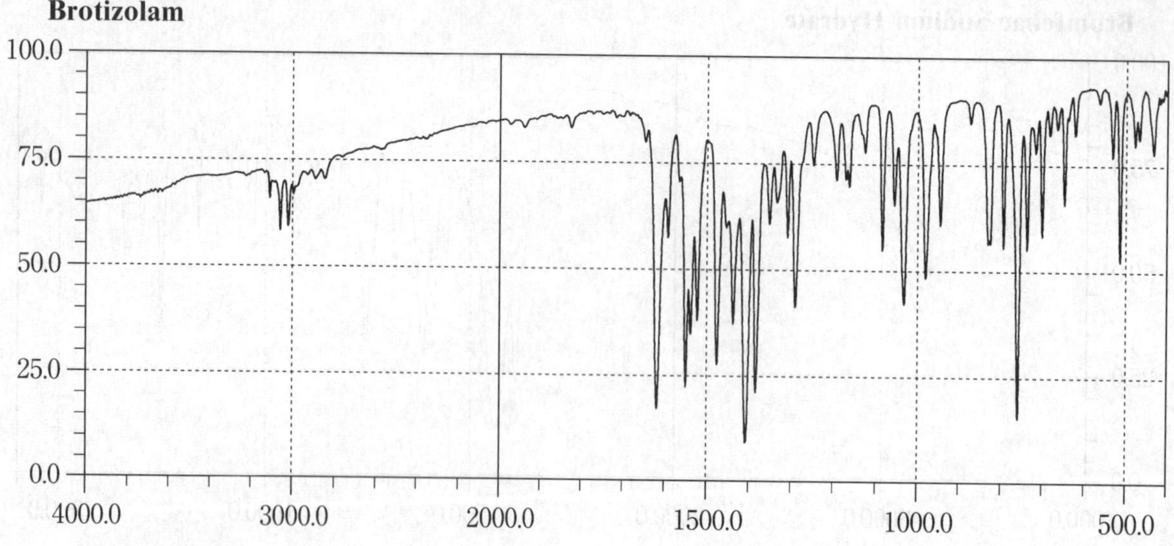

Bucillamine

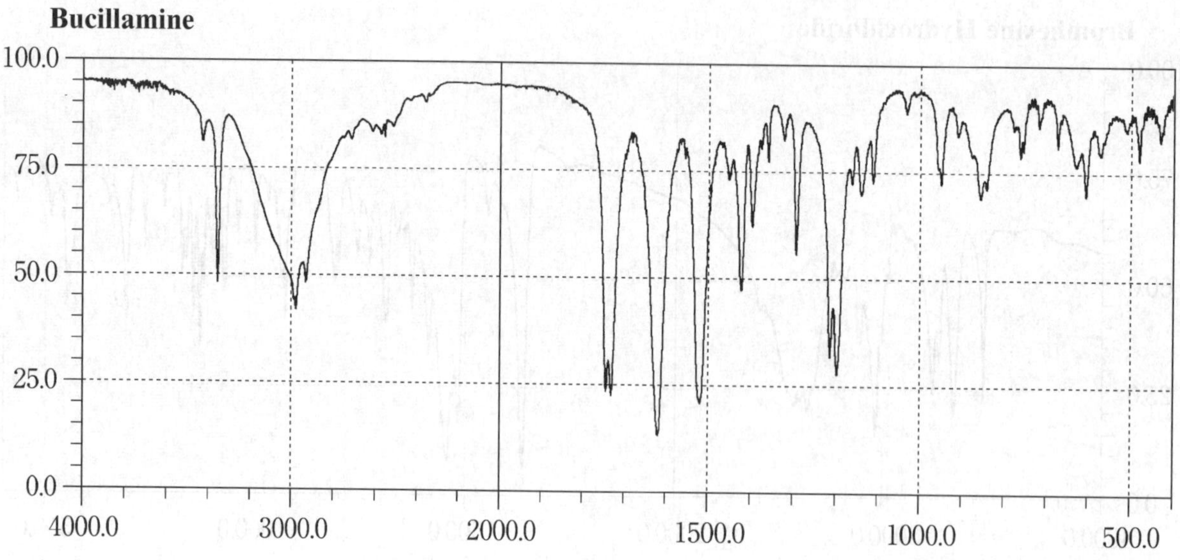

Bucumolol Hydrochloride

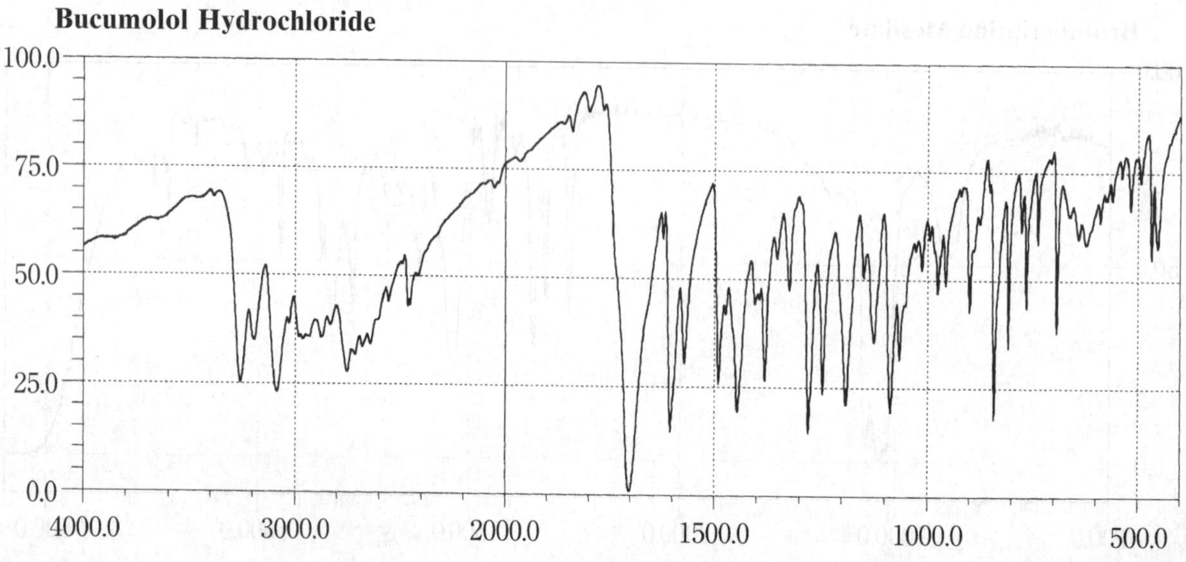

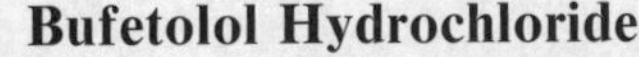

Bufetolol Hydrochloride

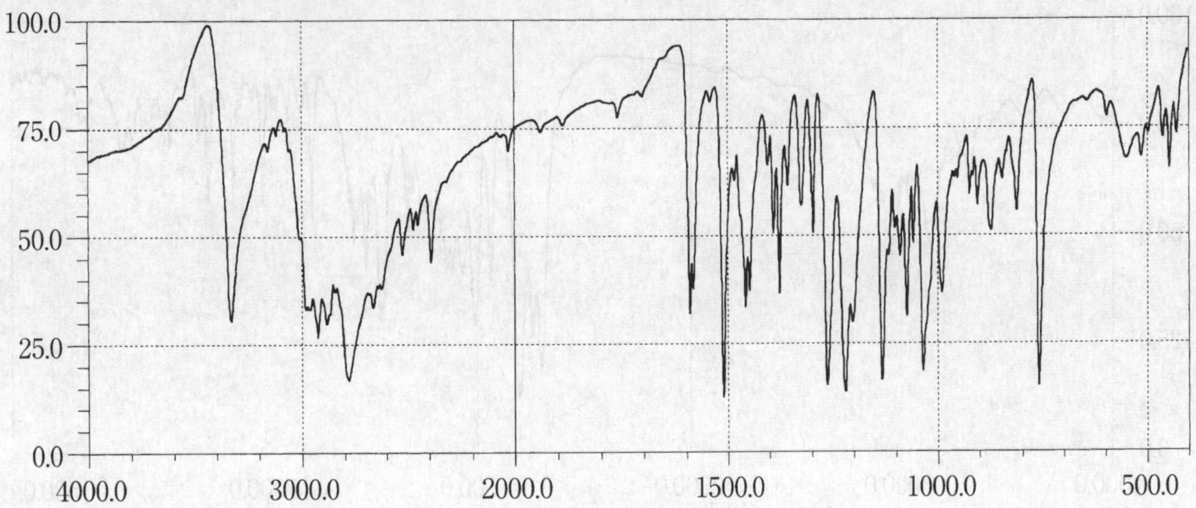

Buformin Hydrochloride

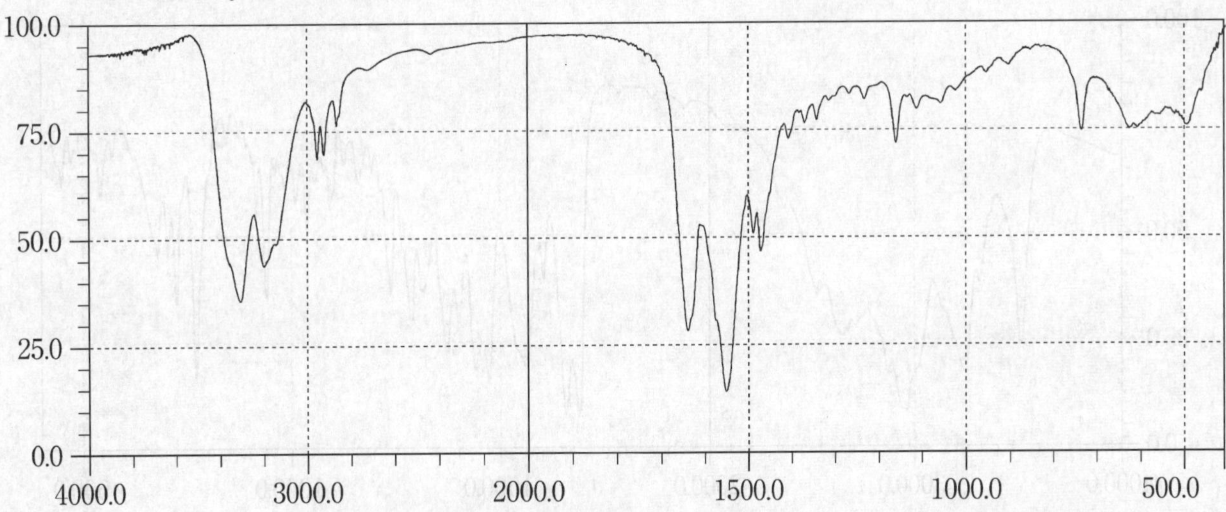

Bumetanide

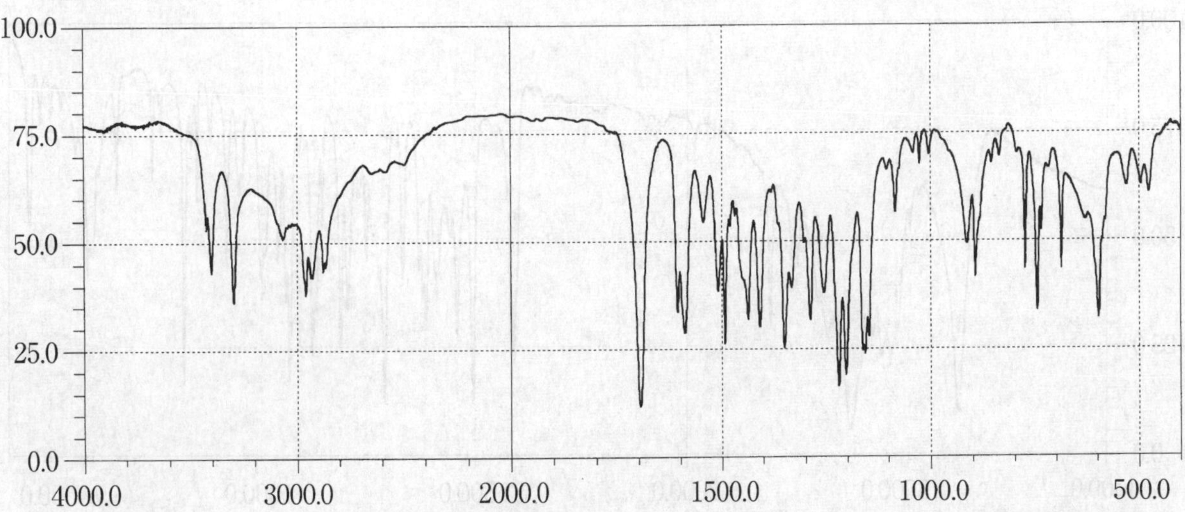

Bunazosin Hydrochloride

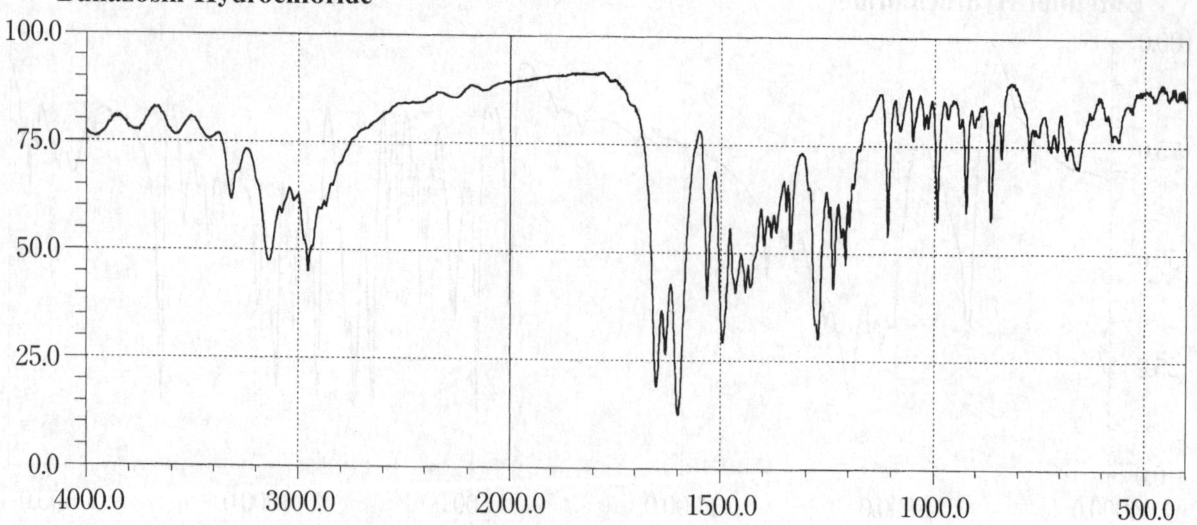

Bupivacaine Hydrochloride Hydrate

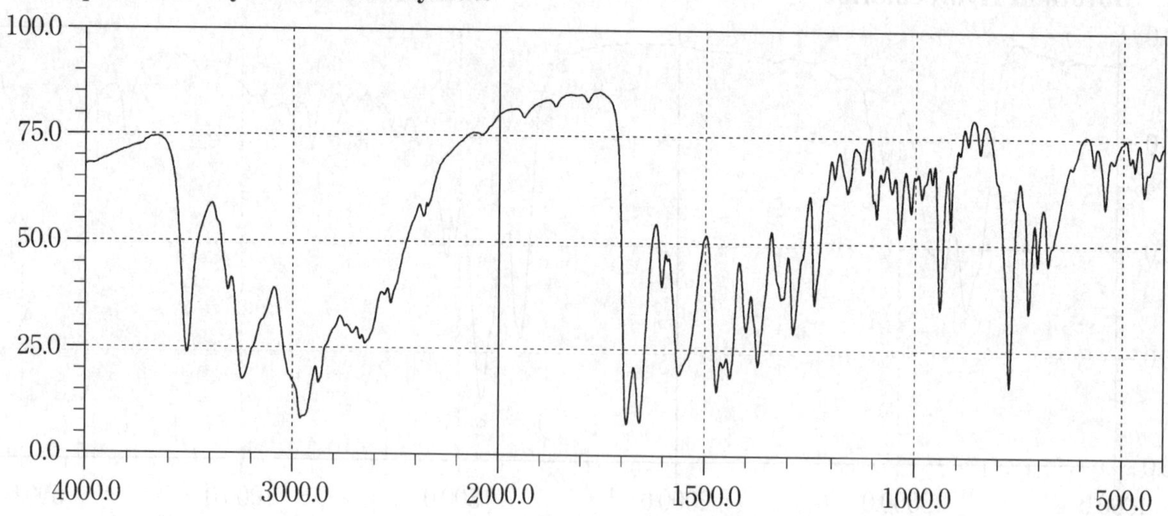

Bupranolol Hydrochloride

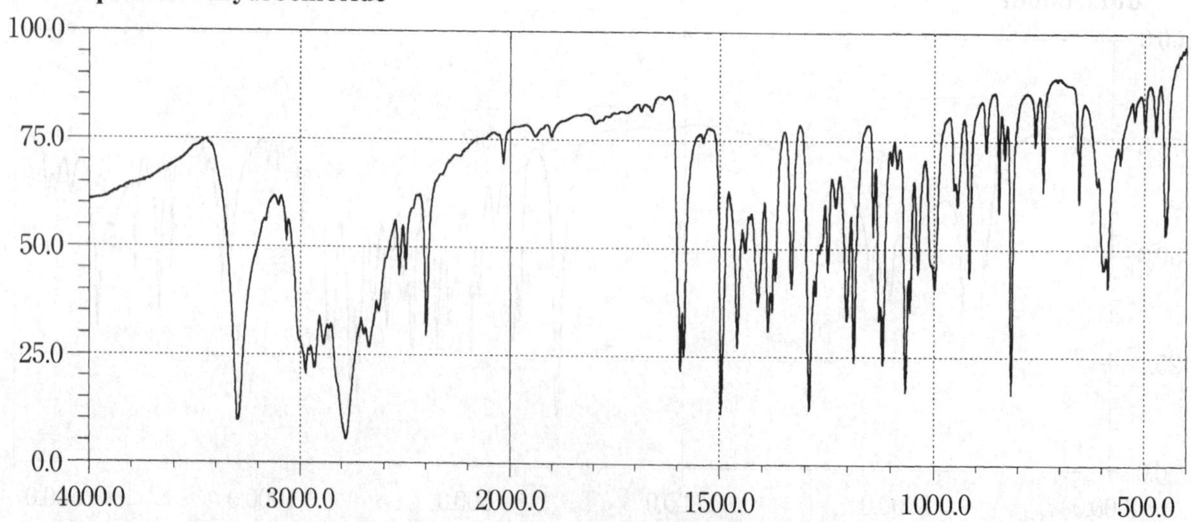

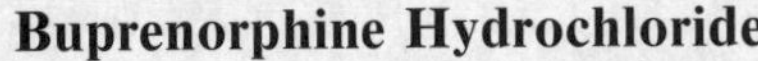

Buprenorphine Hydrochloride

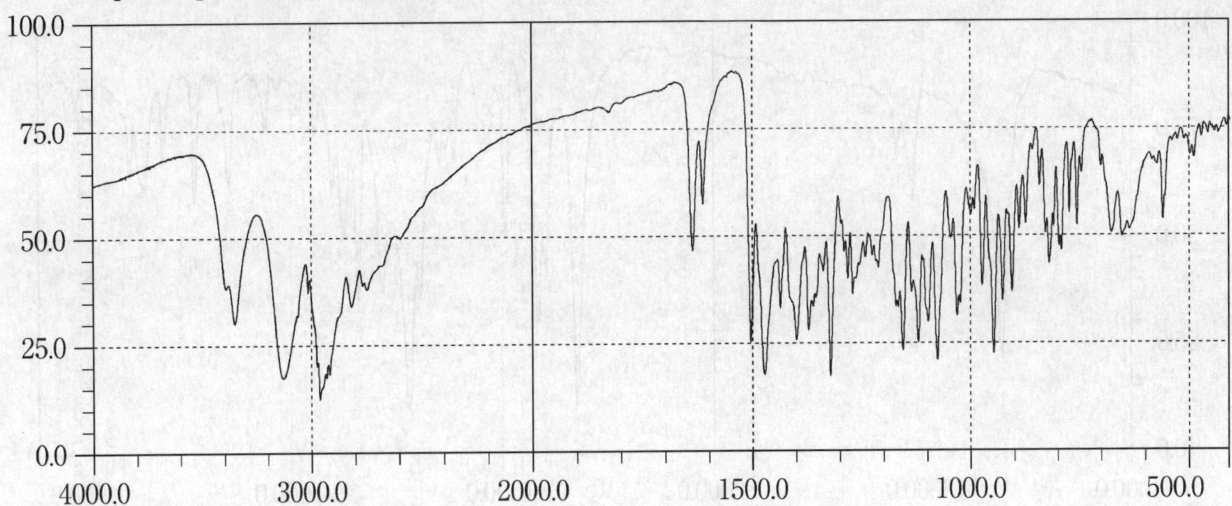

Busulfan

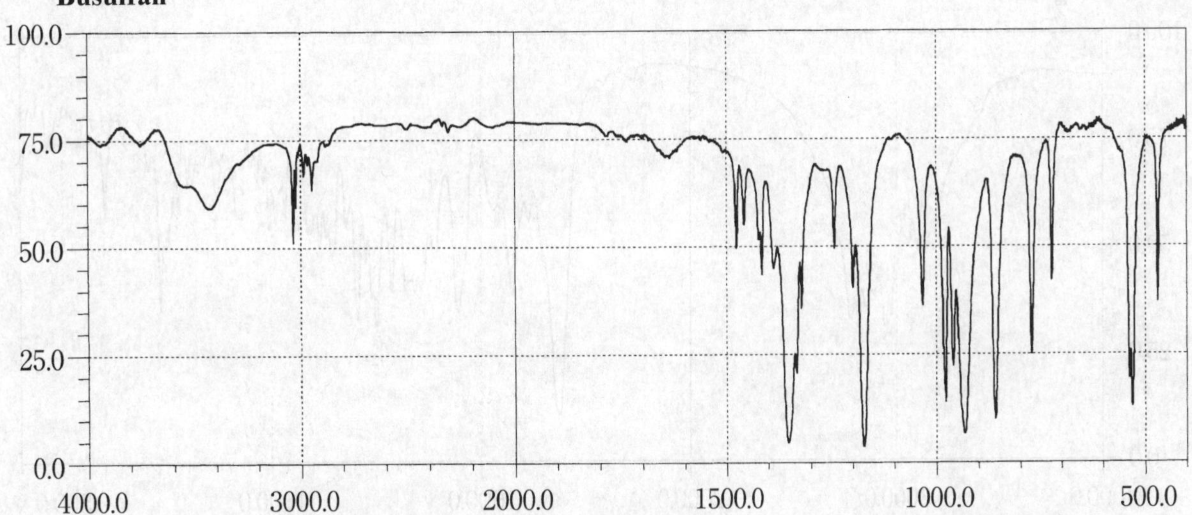

Butenafine Hydrochloride

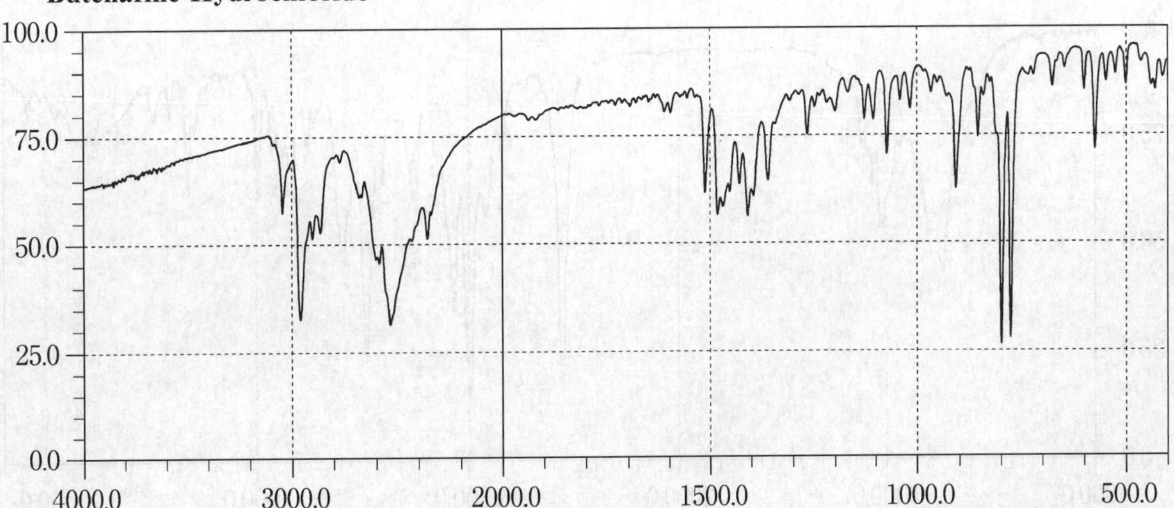

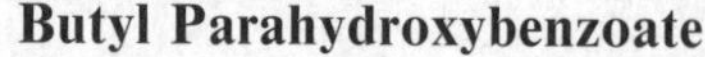

Butyl Parahydroxybenzoate

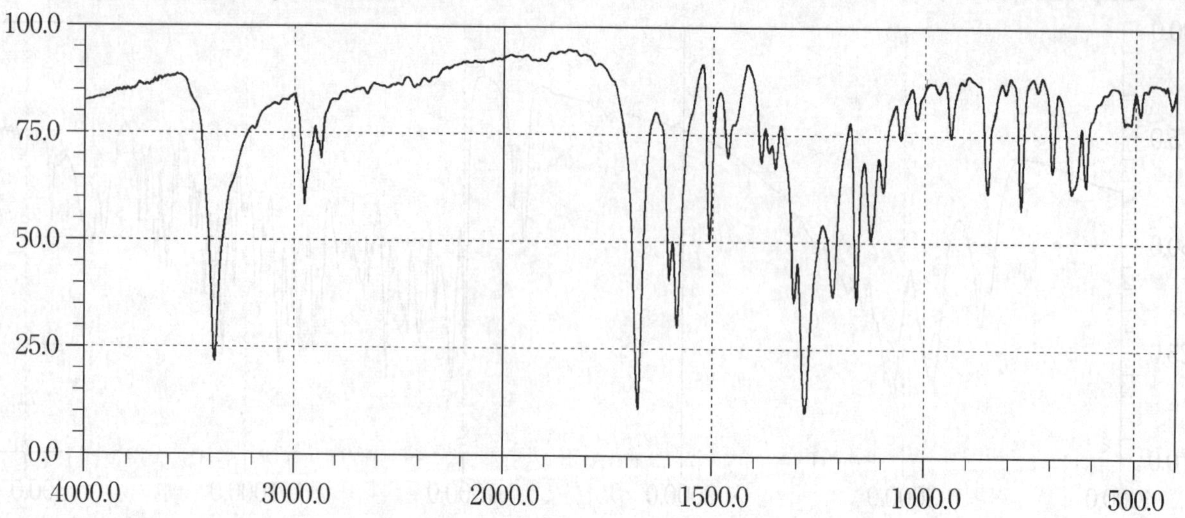

Cabergoline

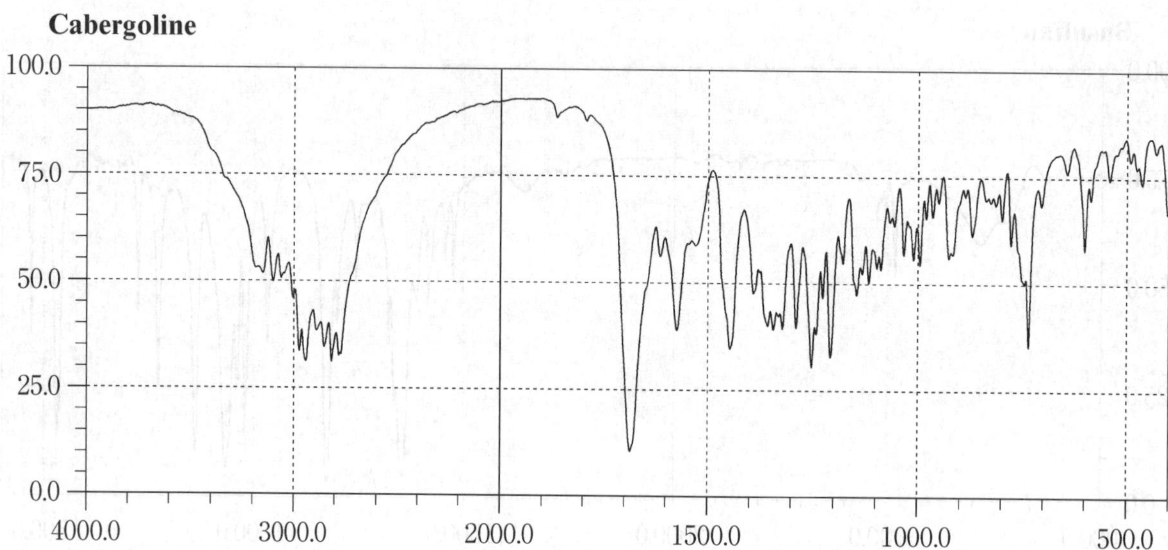

Cadralazine

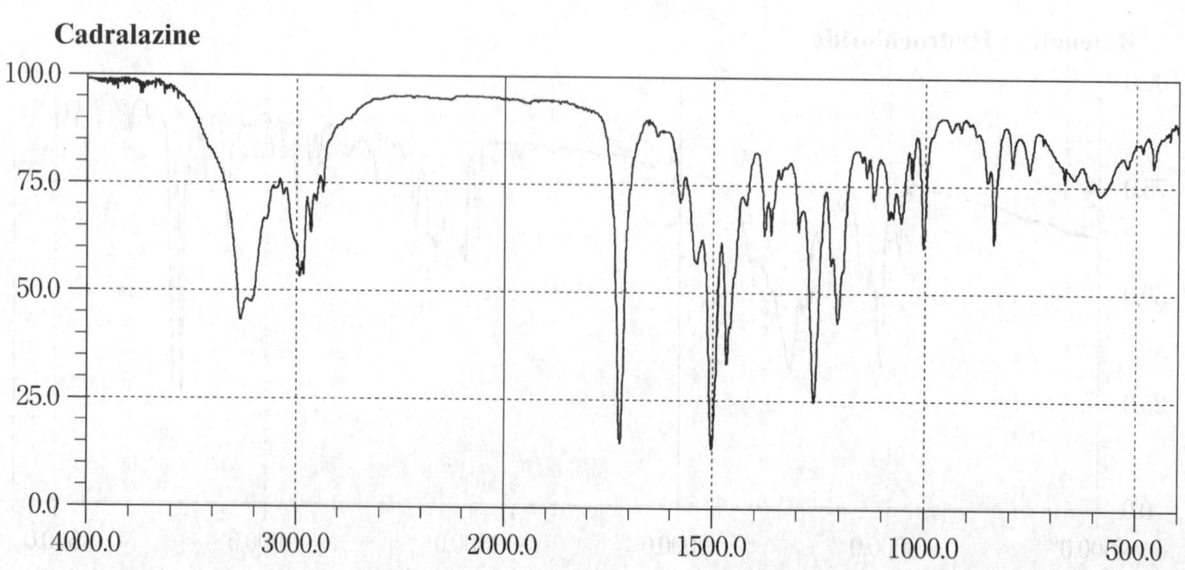

The JP Drugs are to be tested according to the provisions given in the pertinent monographs, General Notices, General Rules for Crude Drugs, General Rules for Preparations, and General Tests for their conformity to the Japanese Pharmacopoeia. (See the General Notices 5.)

Calcium Folinate Hydrate

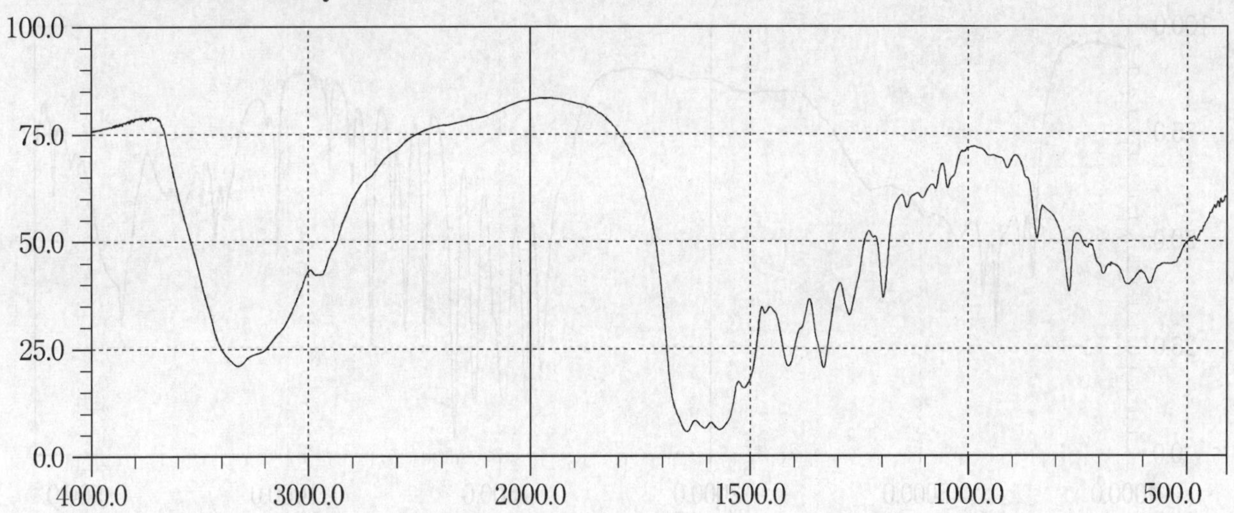

Calcium Levofolinate Hydrate

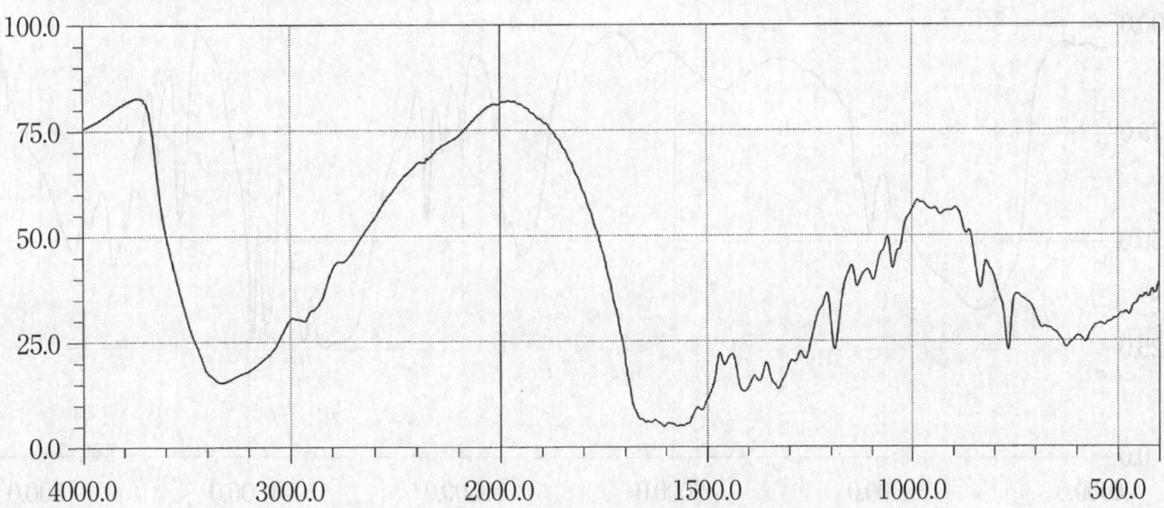

Calcium Pantothenate

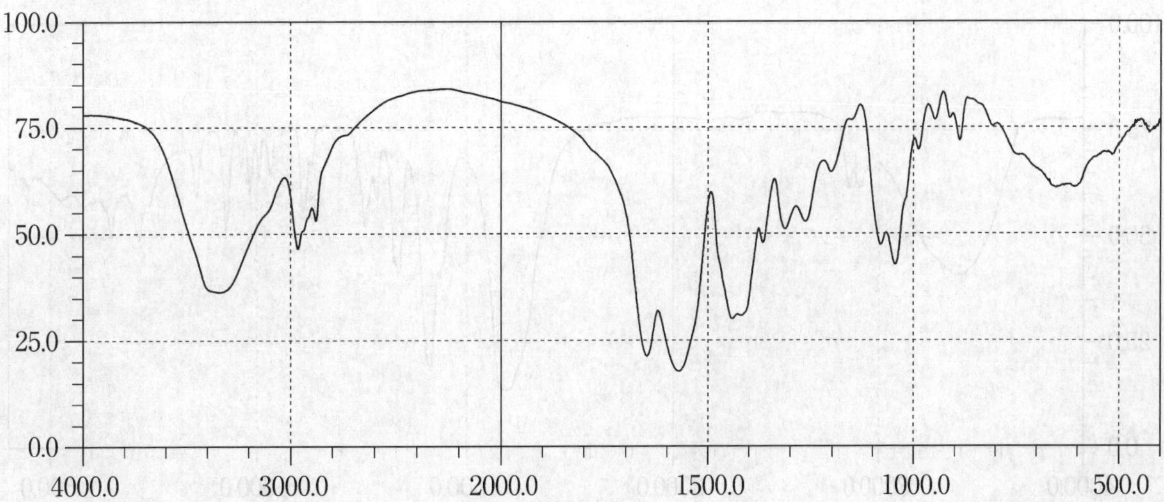

Calcium Paraaminosalicylate Hydrate

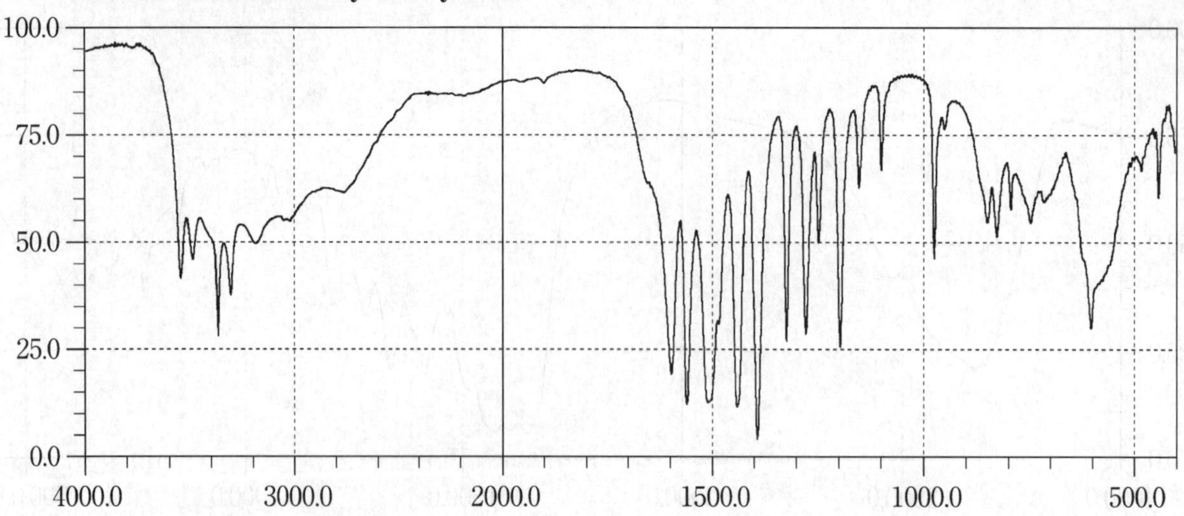

Calcium Polystyrene Sulfonate

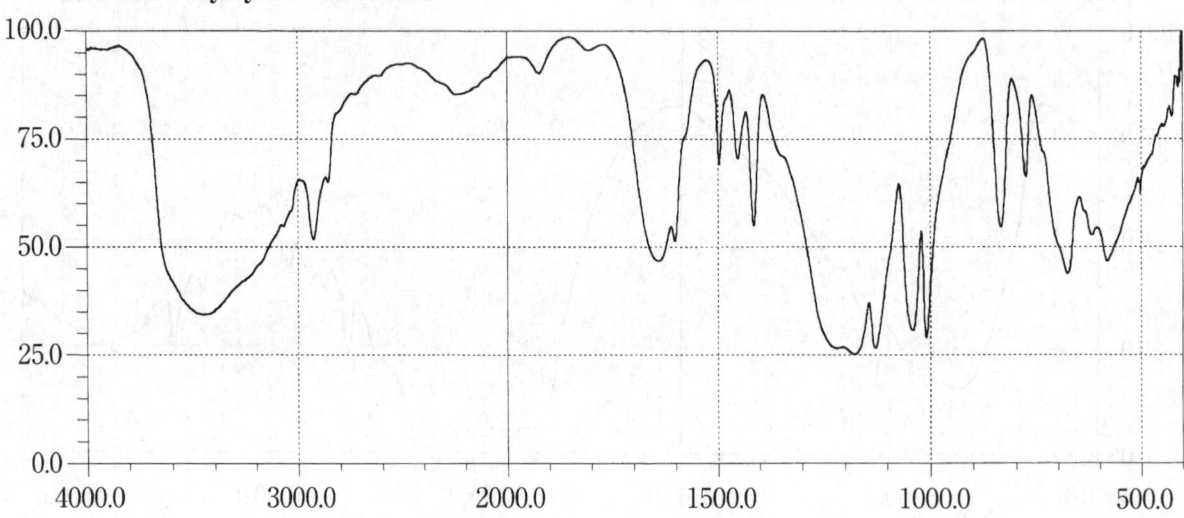

Calcium Sodium Edetate Hydrate

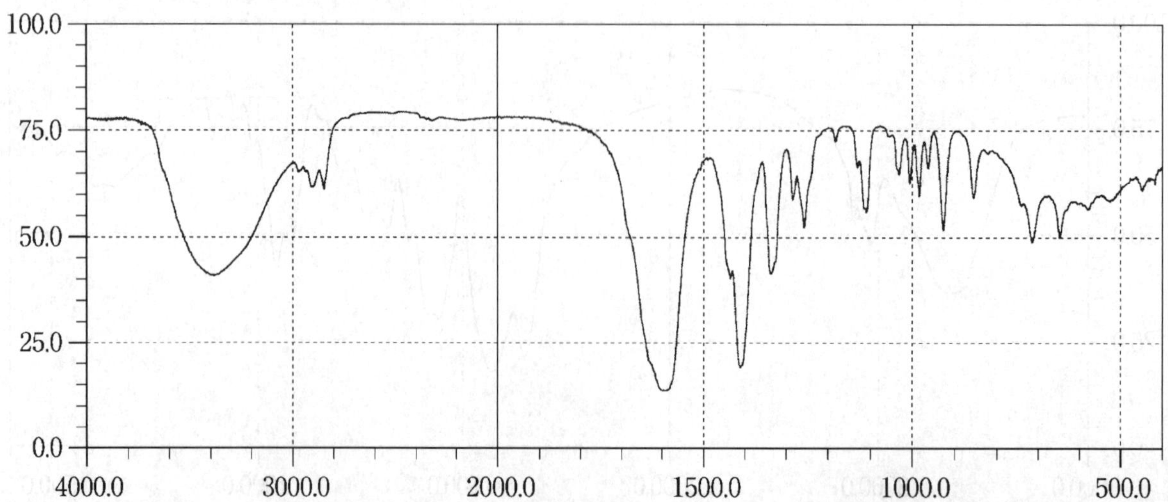

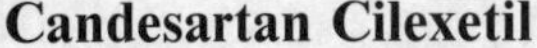

Candesartan Cilexetil

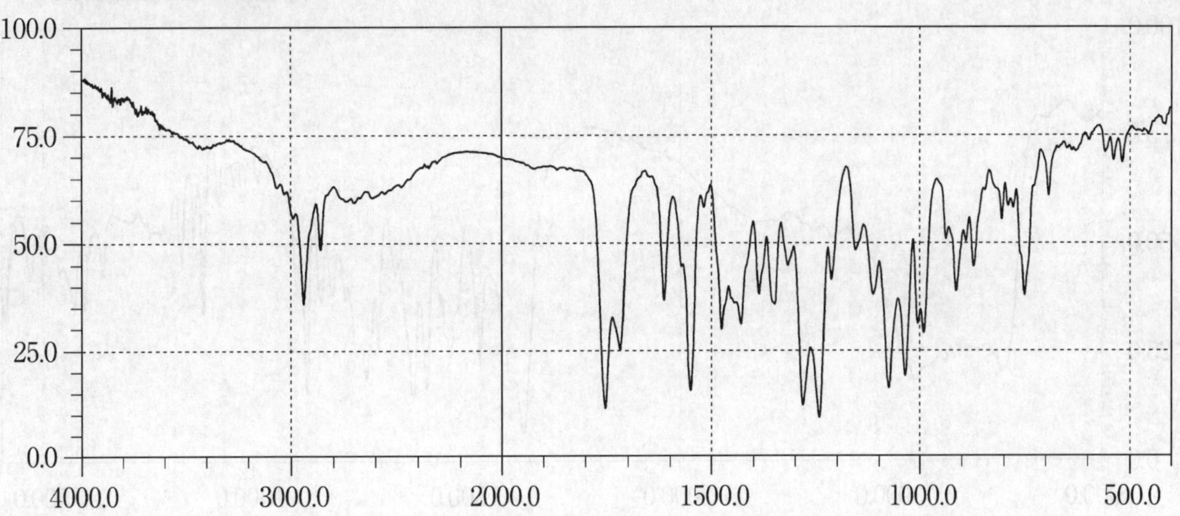

Captopril

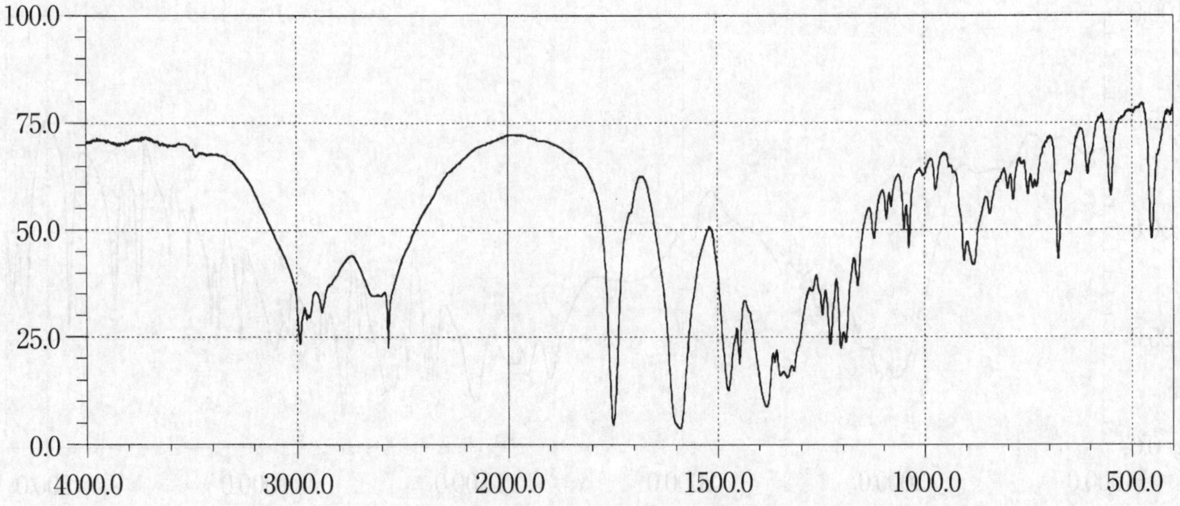

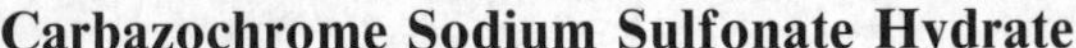

Carbazochrome Sodium Sulfonate Hydrate

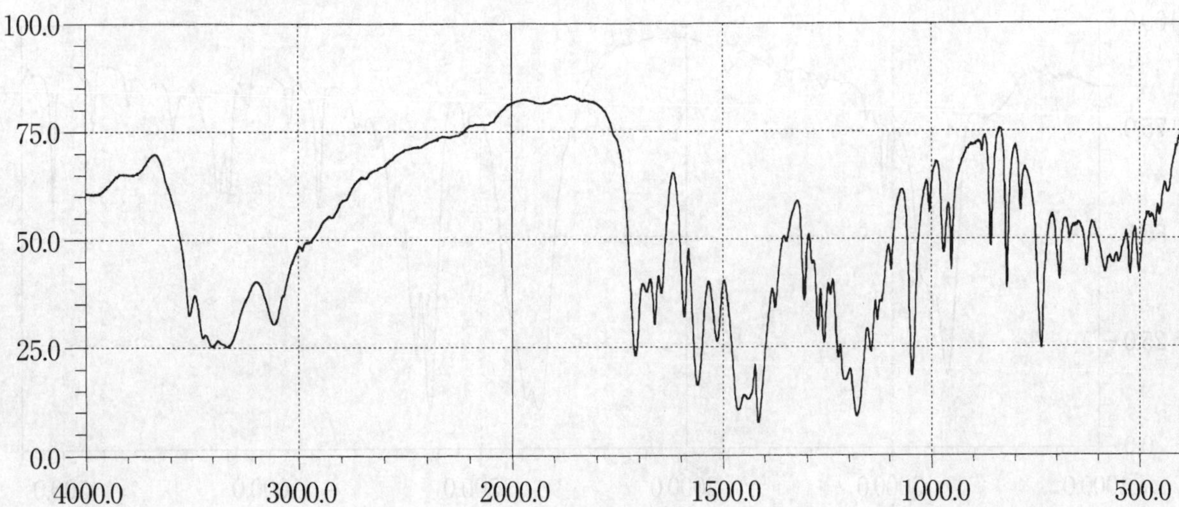

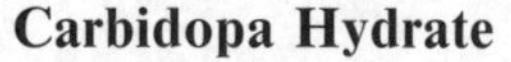

Carbidopa Hydrate

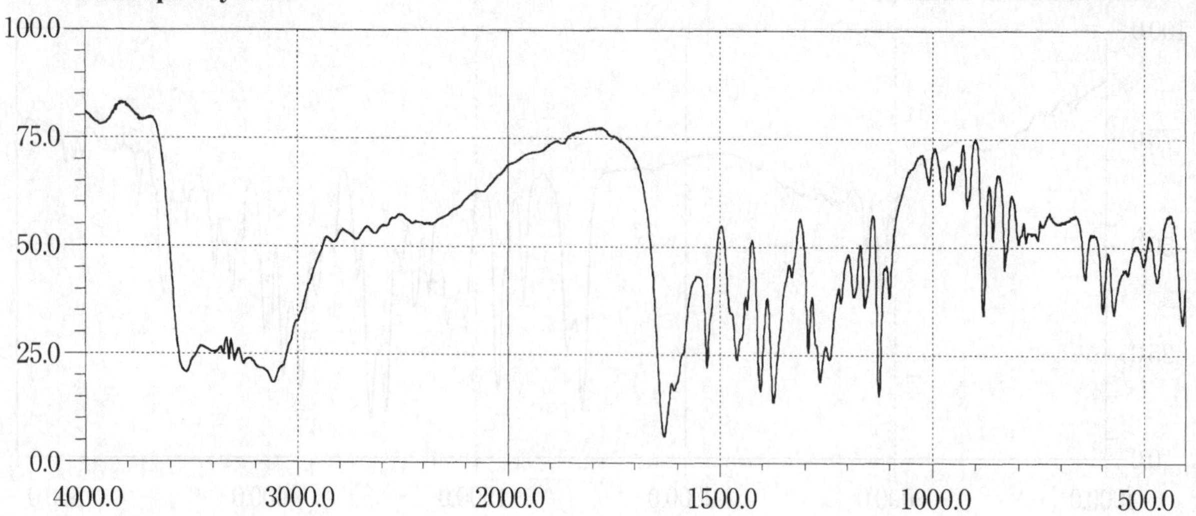

L-Carbocisteine

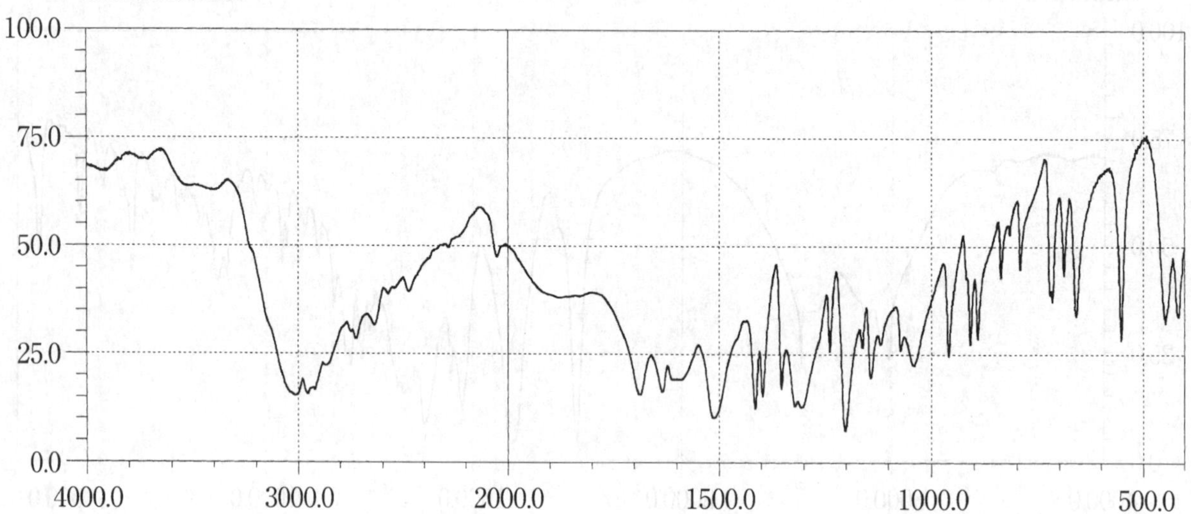

Carboplatin

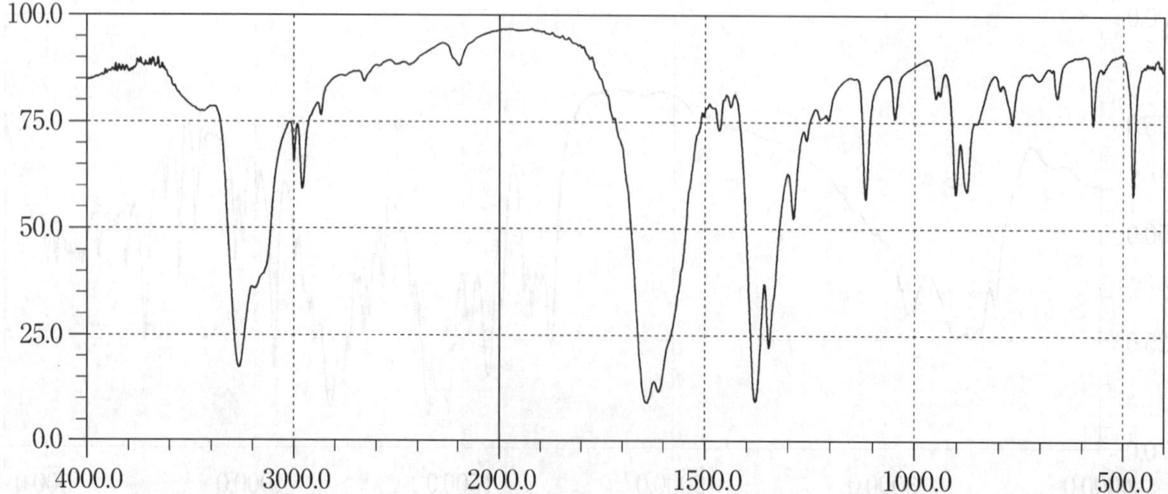

The JP Drugs are to be tested according to the provisions given in the pertinent monographs, General Notices, General Rules for Crude Drugs, General Rules for Preparations, and General Tests for their conformity to the Japanese Pharmacopoeia. (See the General Notices 5.)

Carmellose

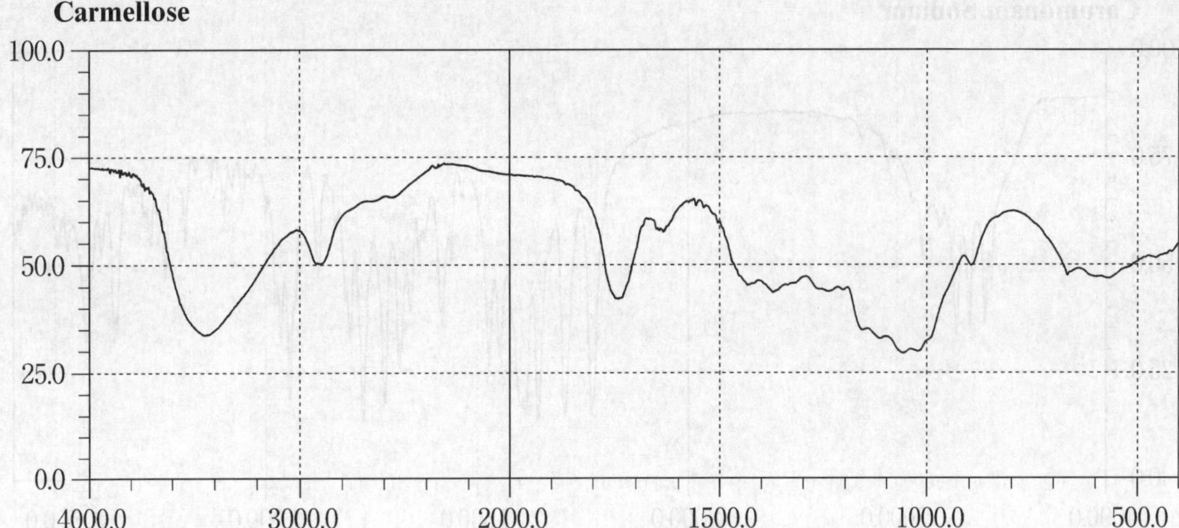

Carmofur

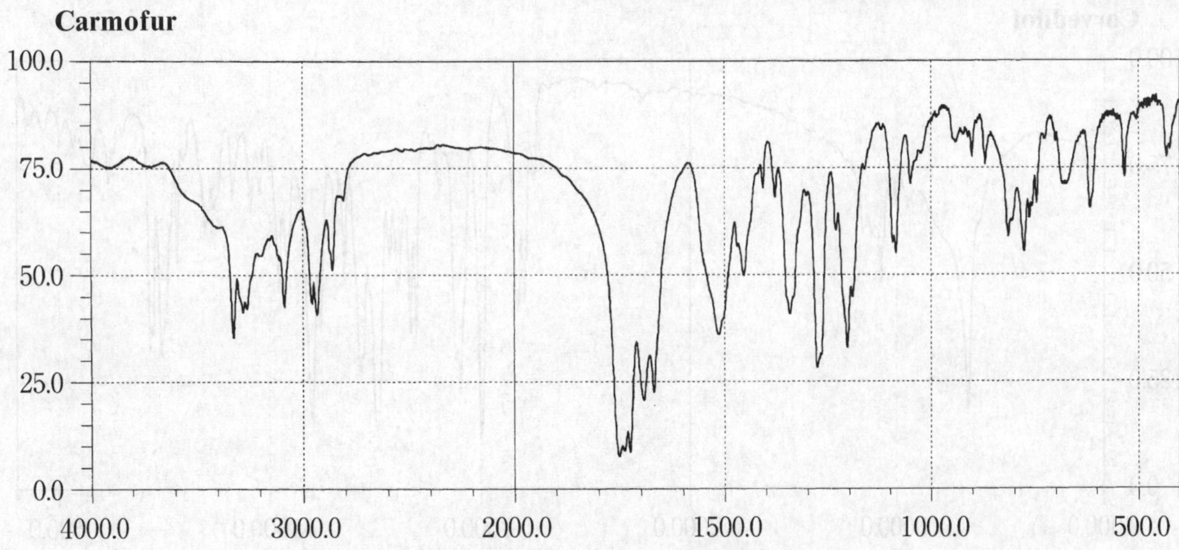

Carteolol Hydrochloride

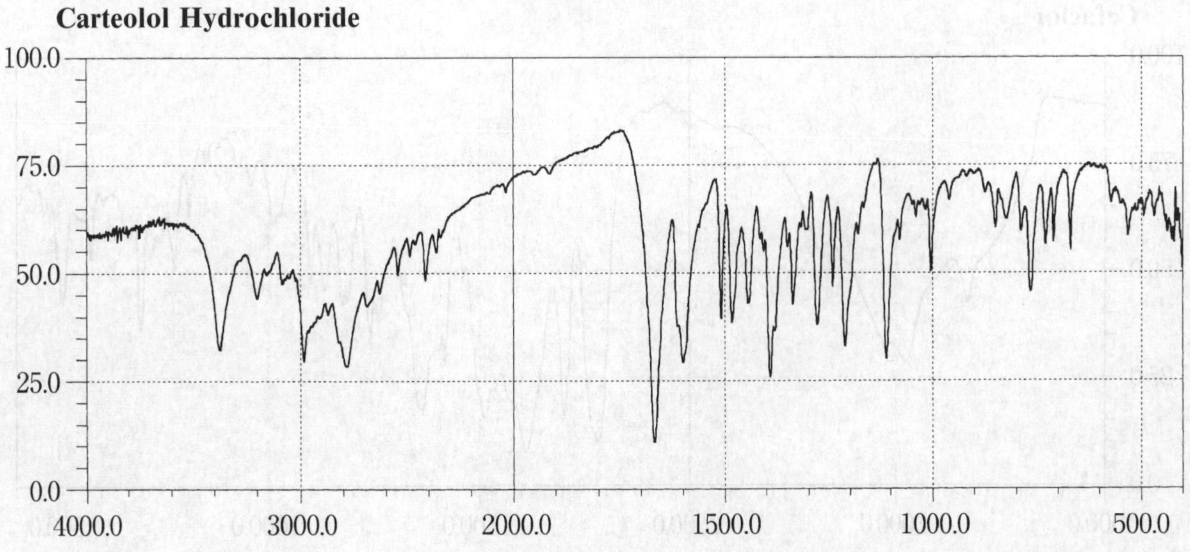

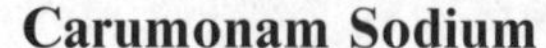

Carumonam Sodium

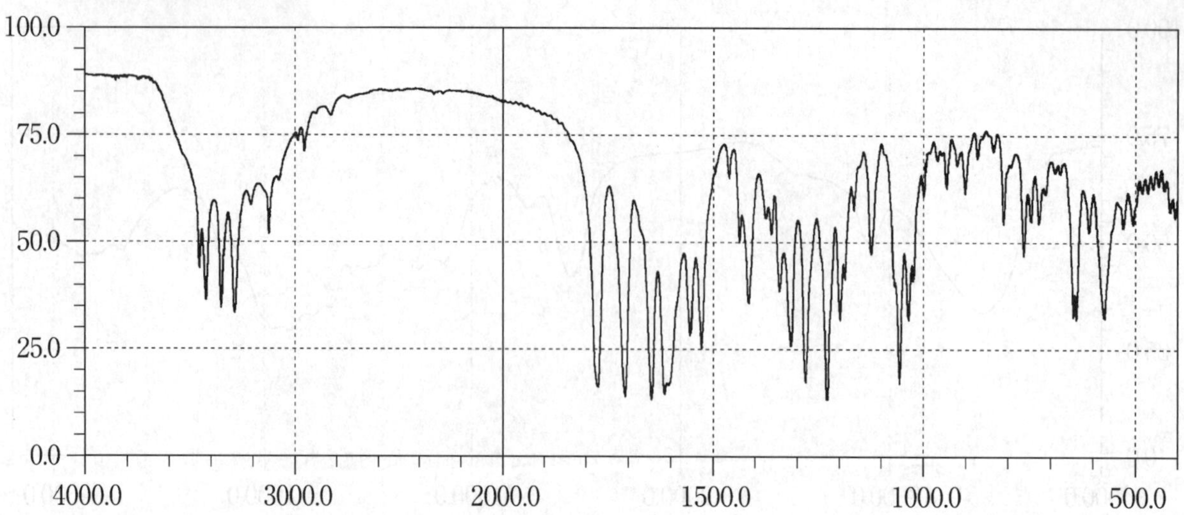

Carvedilol

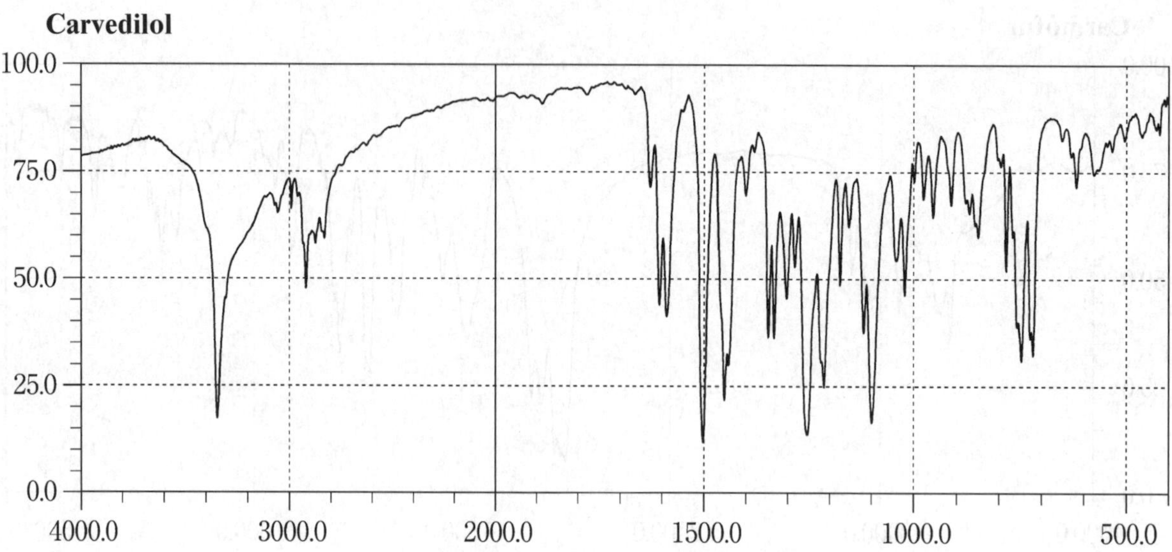

Cefaclor

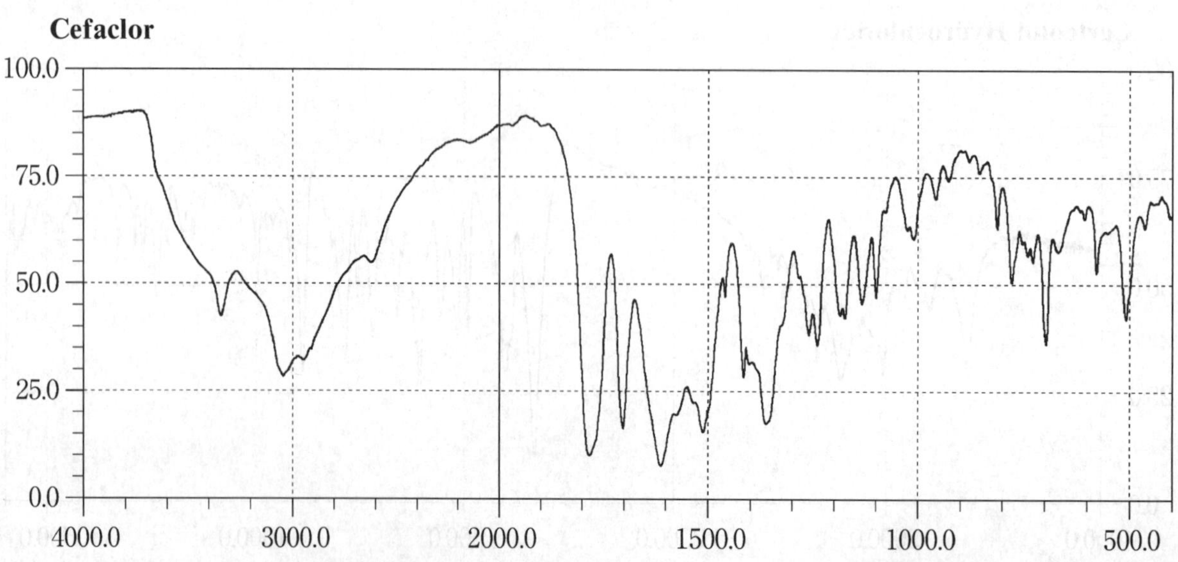

Cefadroxil

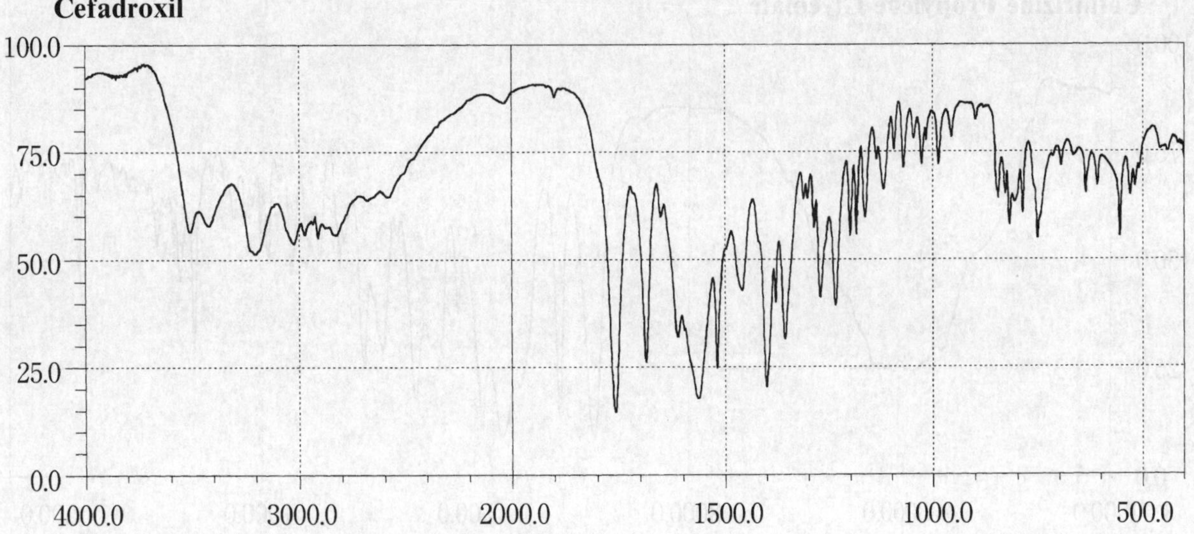

Cefalexin

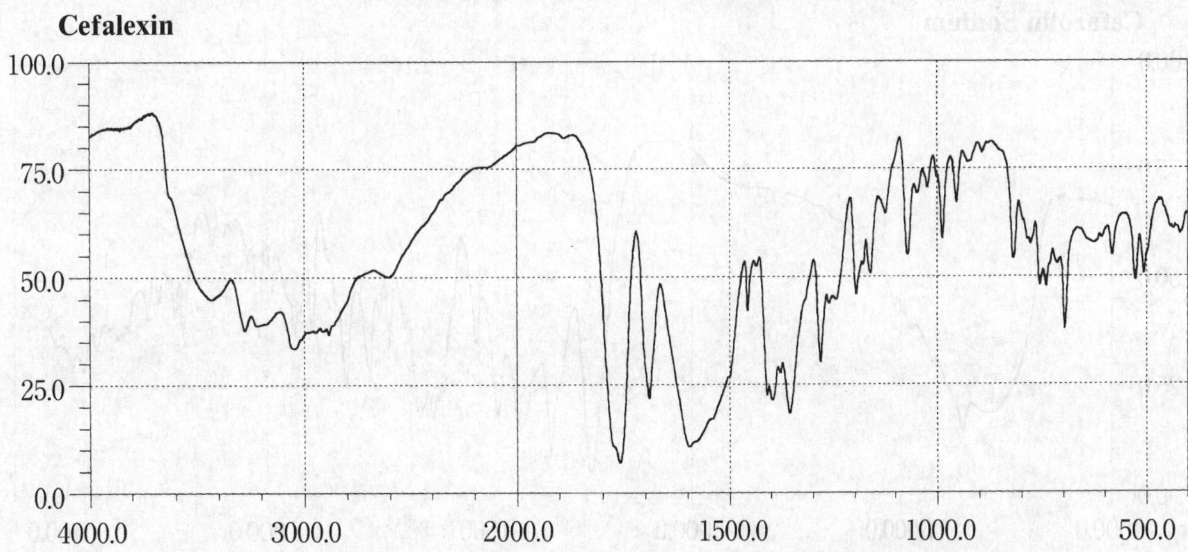

Cefalotin Sodium

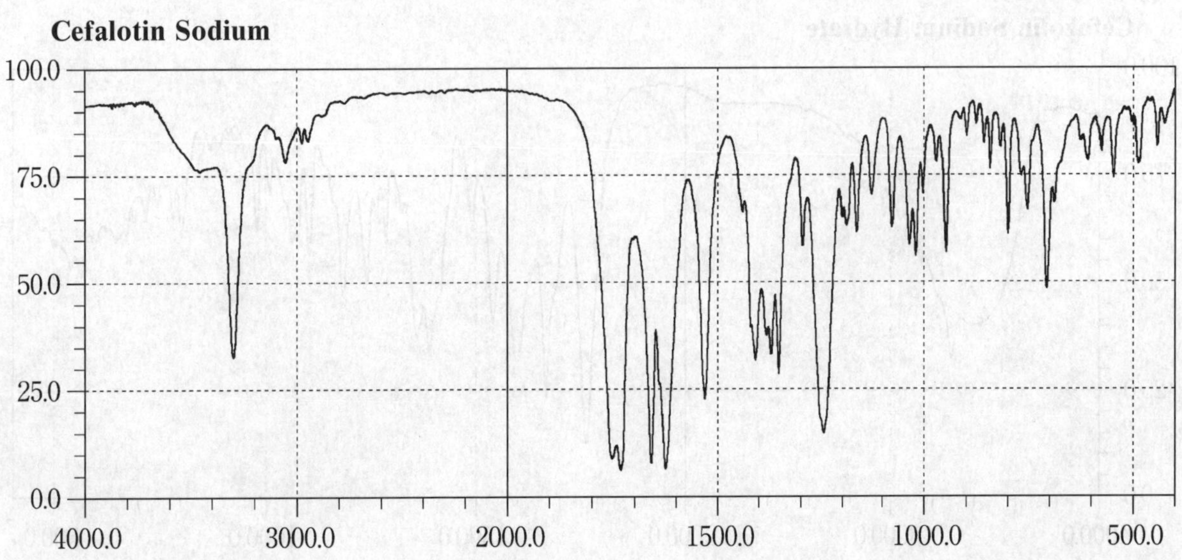

Cefatrizine Propylene Glycolate

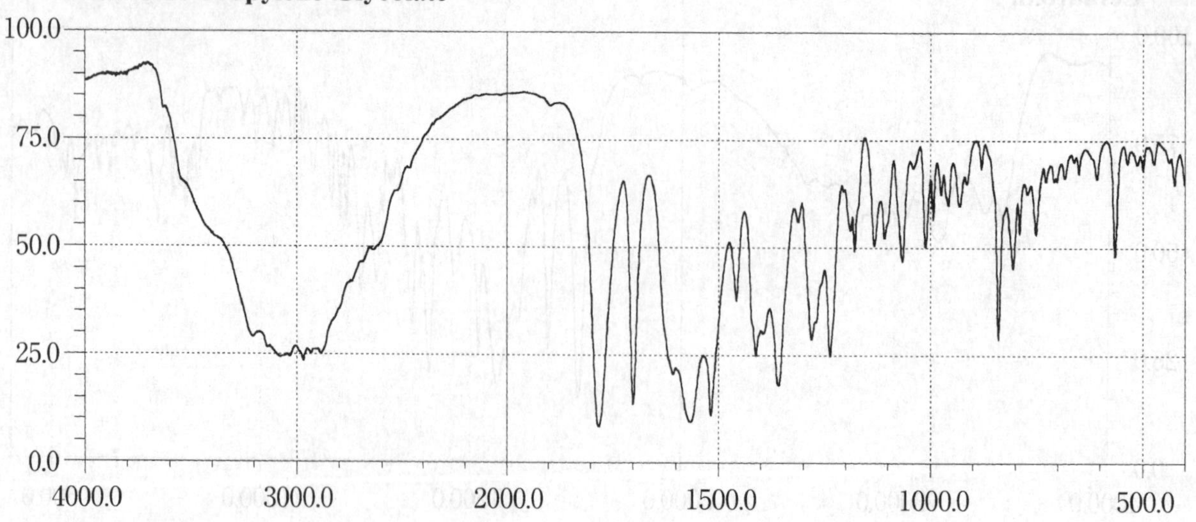

Cefazolin Sodium

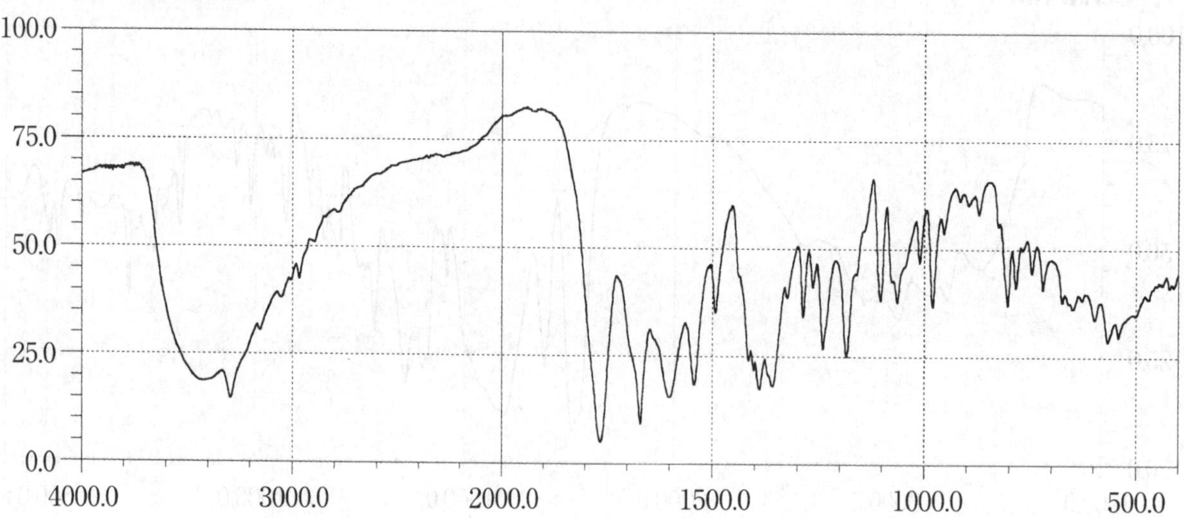

Cefazolin Sodium Hydrate

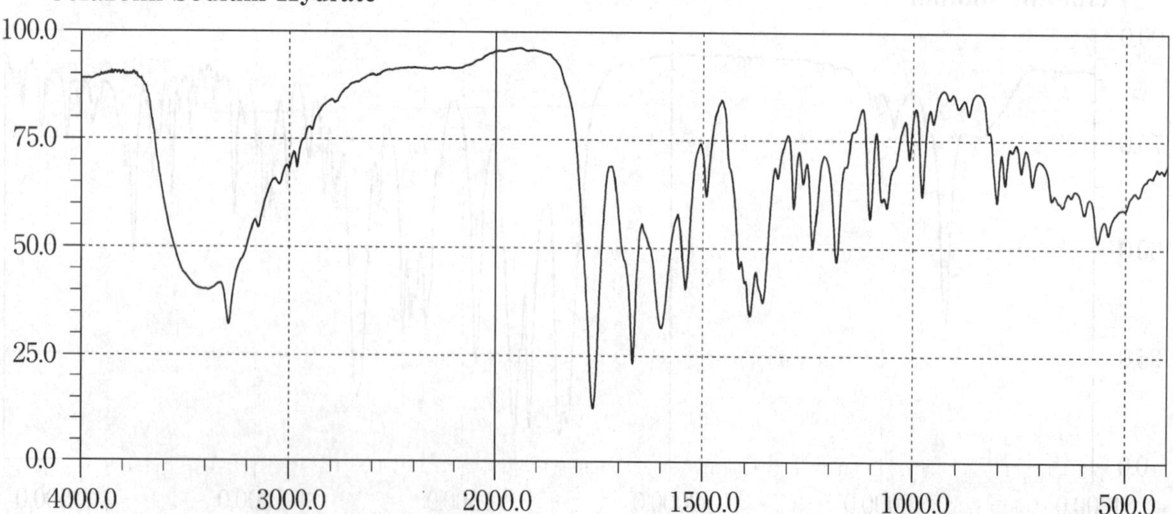

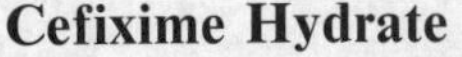

Cefixime Hydrate

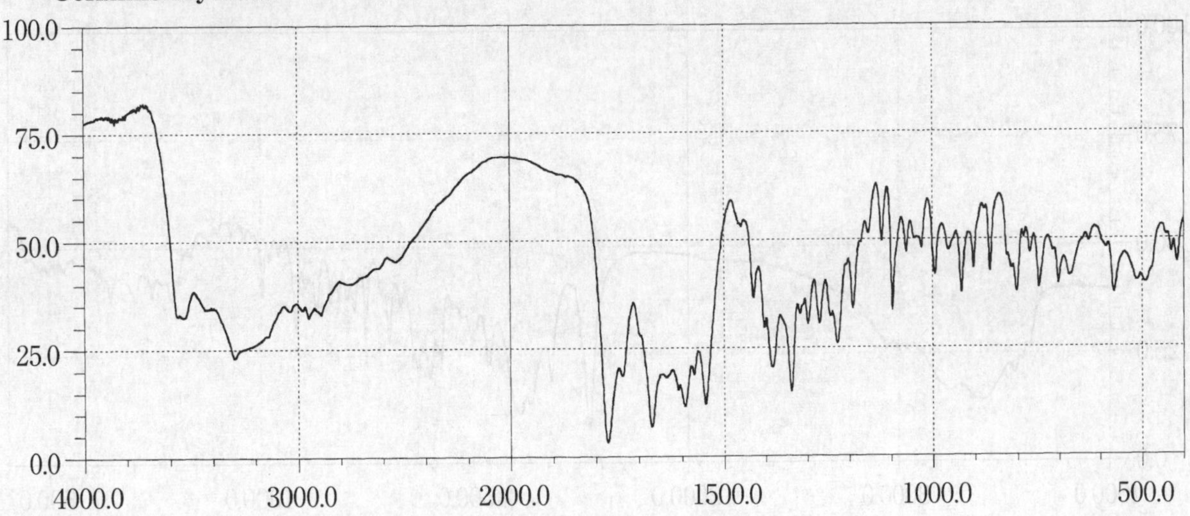

Cefmenoxime Hydrochloride

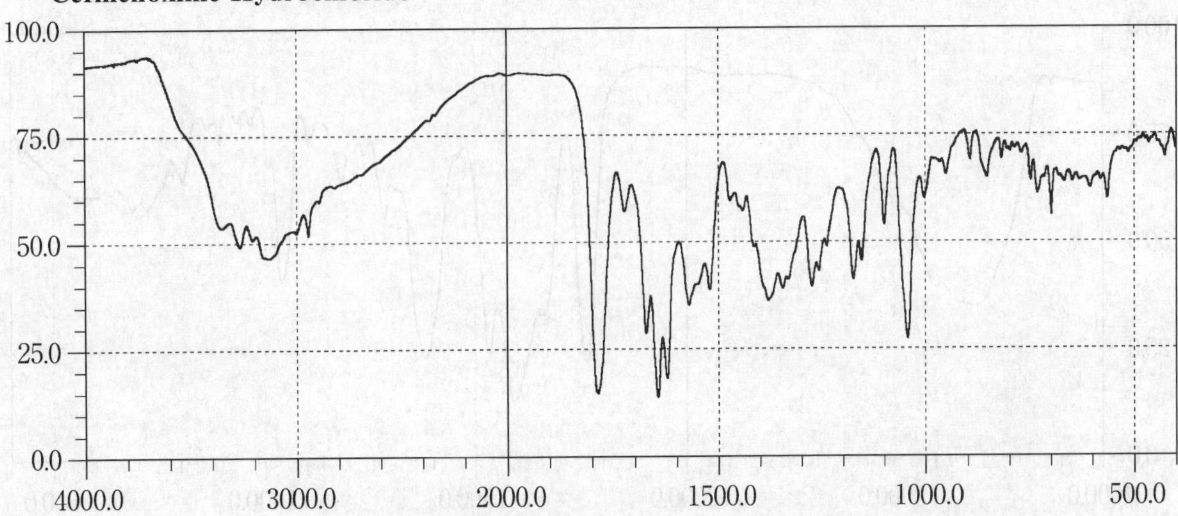

Cefmetazole Sodium

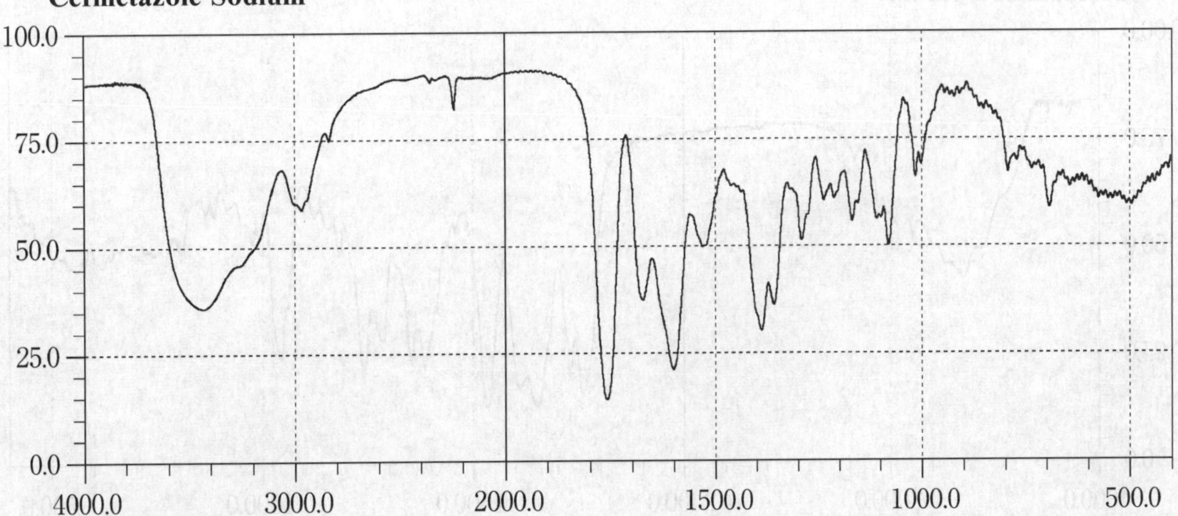

Cefminox Sodium Hydrate

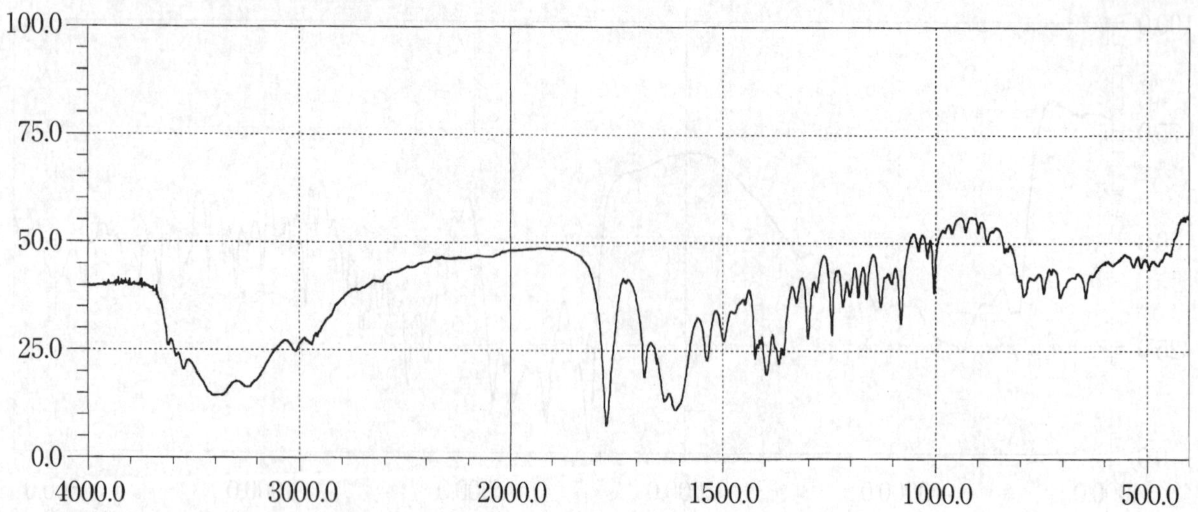

Cefodizime Sodium

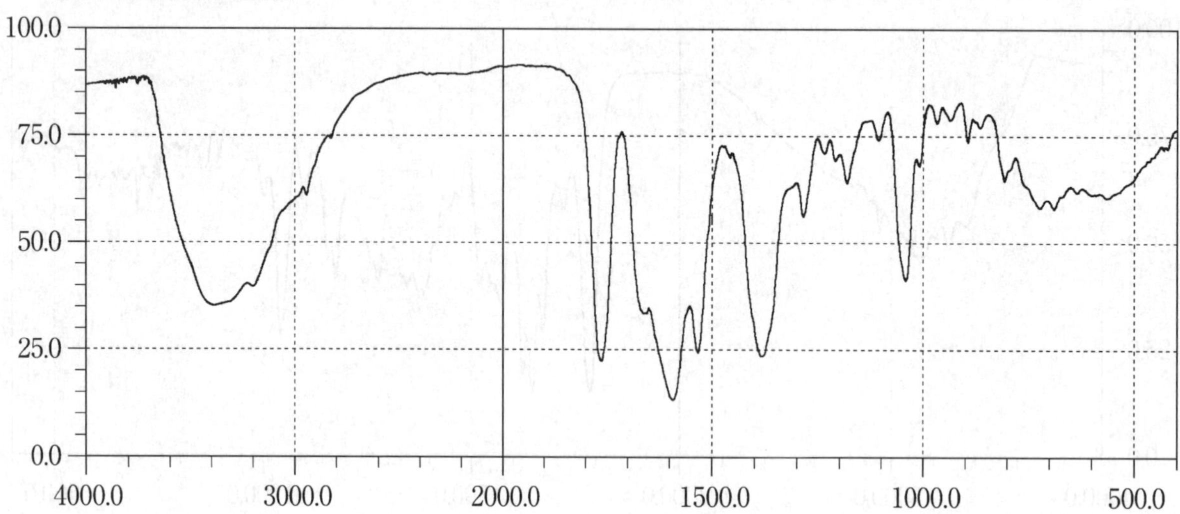

Cefotaxime Sodium

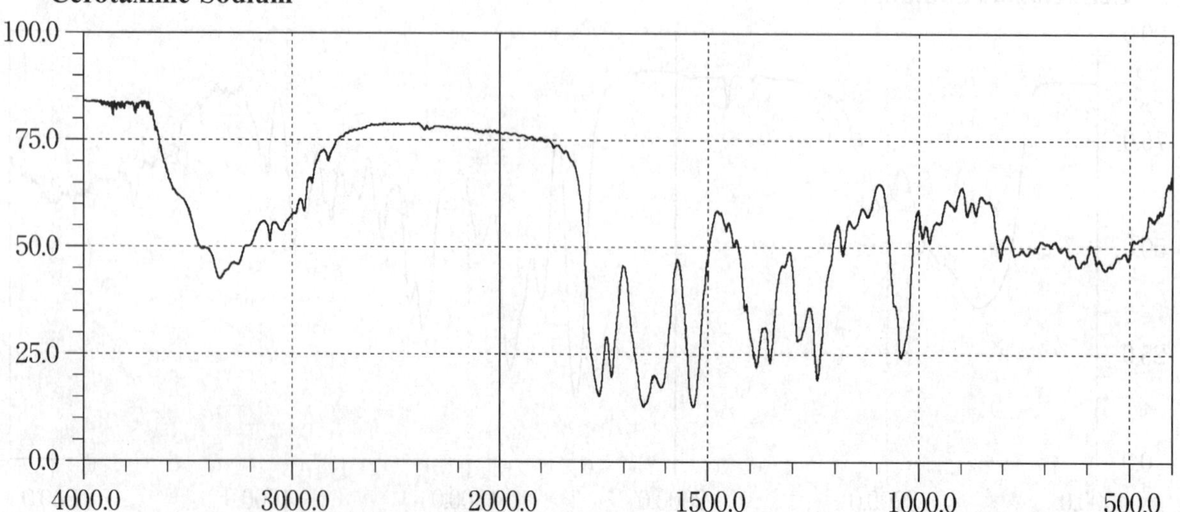

Cefotetan

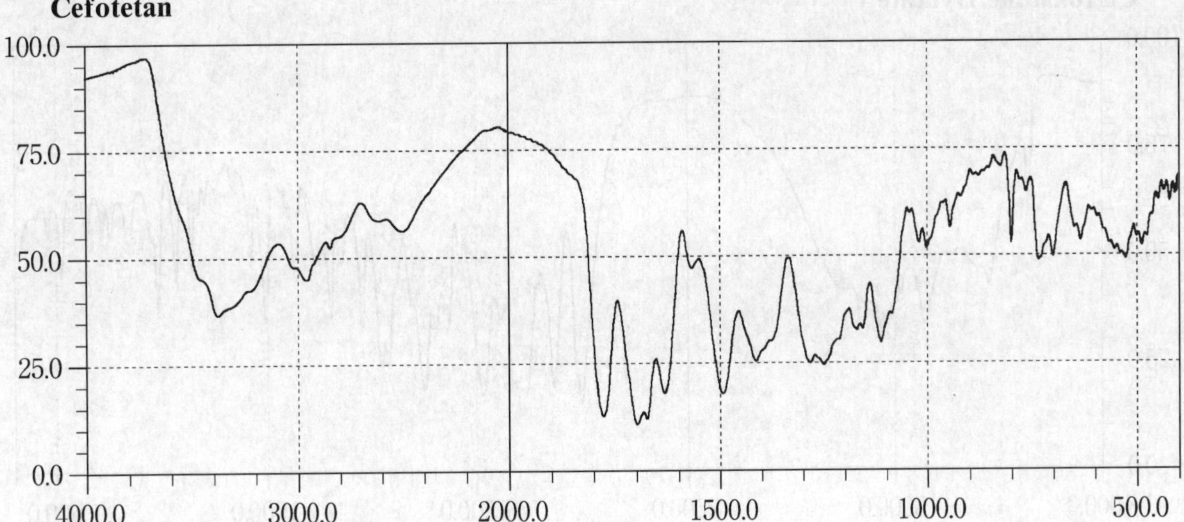

Cefotiam Hydrochloride

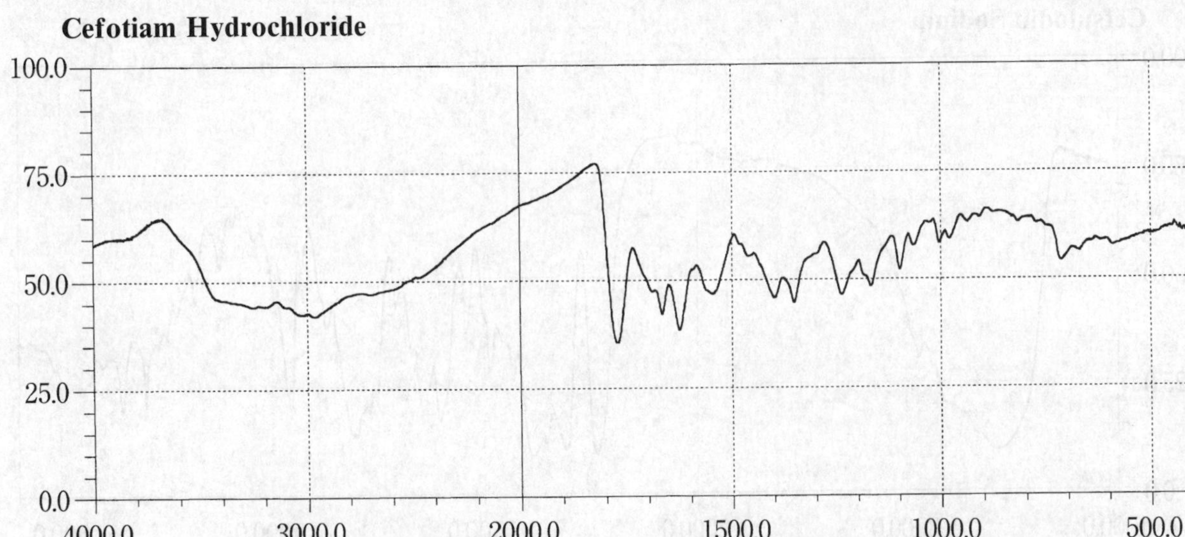

Cefpodoxime Proxetil

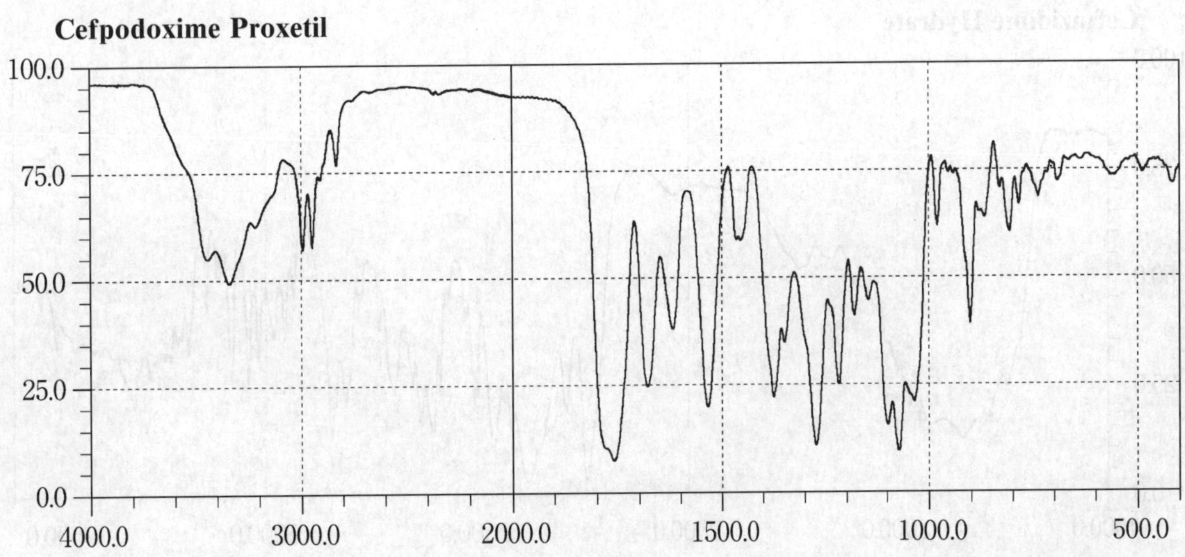

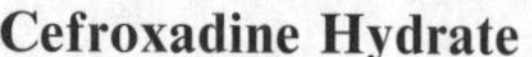

Cefroxadine Hydrate

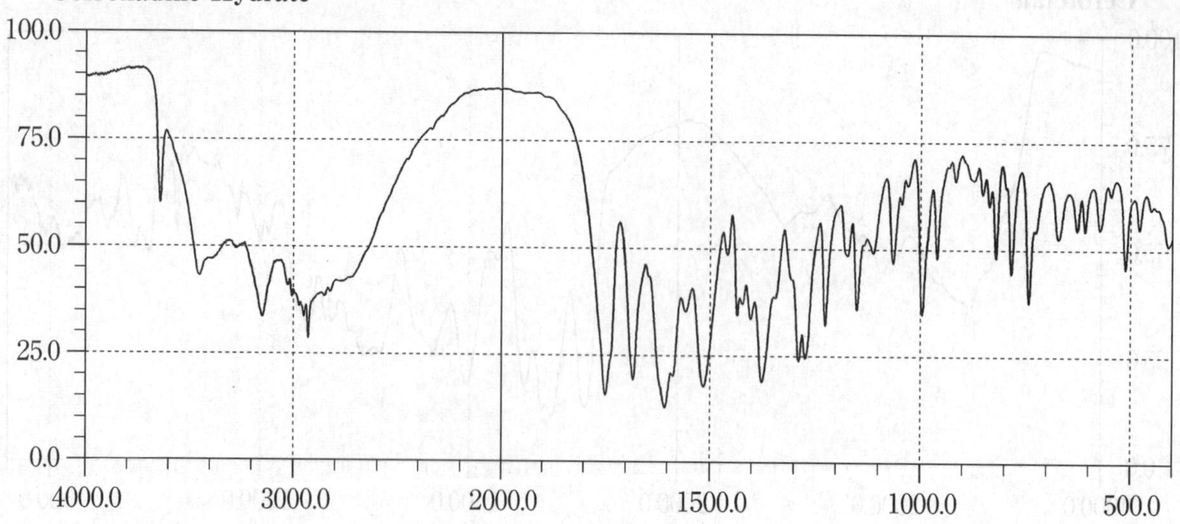

Cefsulodin Sodium

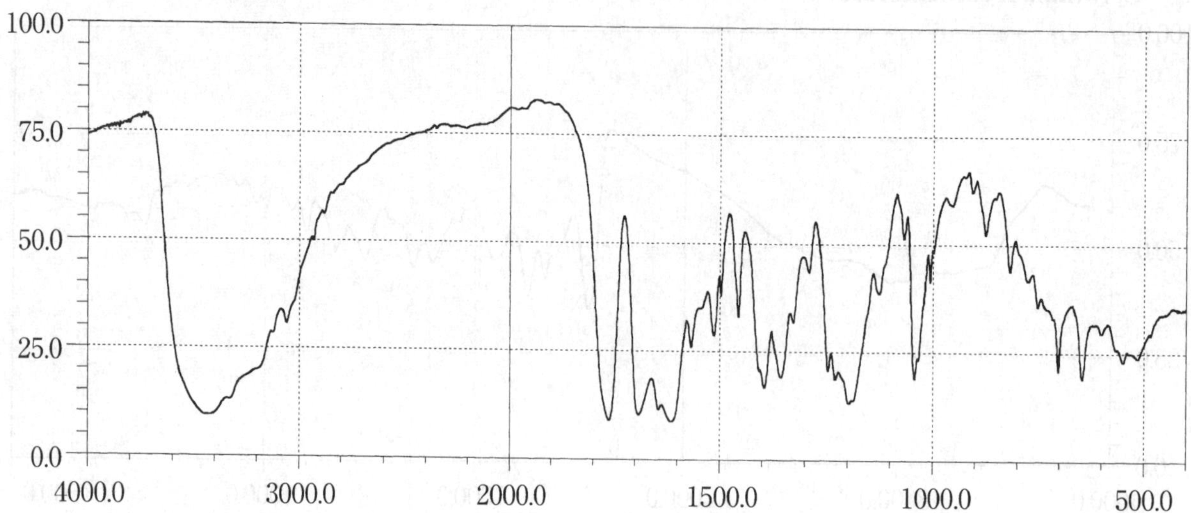

Ceftazidime Hydrate

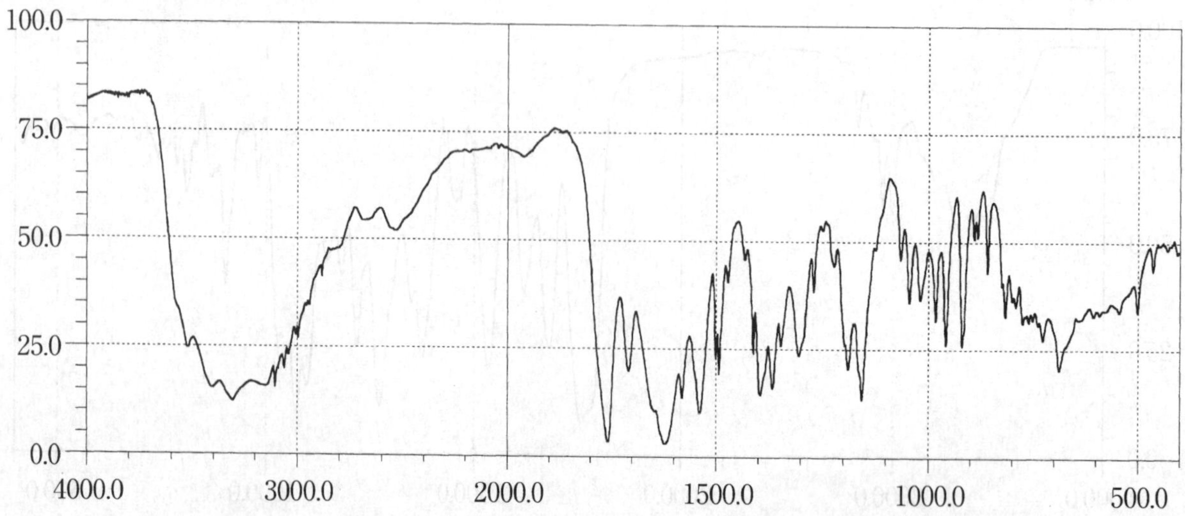

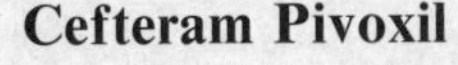

Cefteram Pivoxil

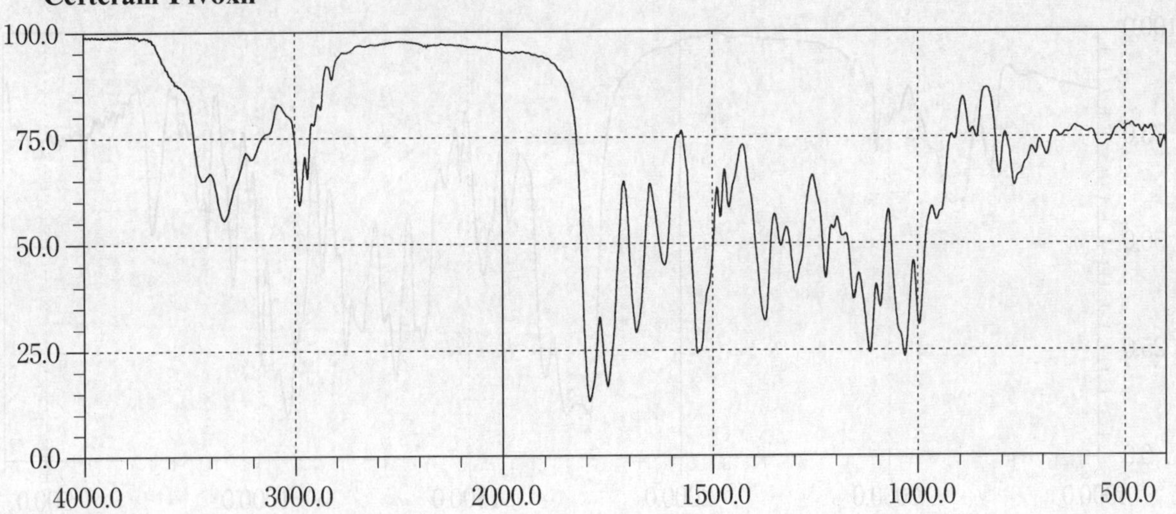

Ceftibuten Hydrate

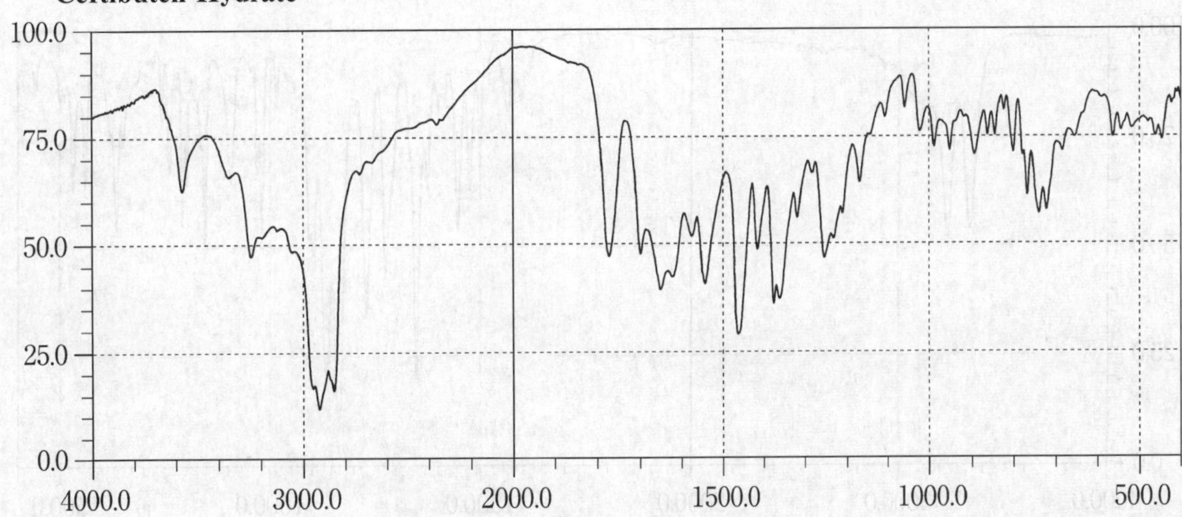

Ceftizoxime Sodium

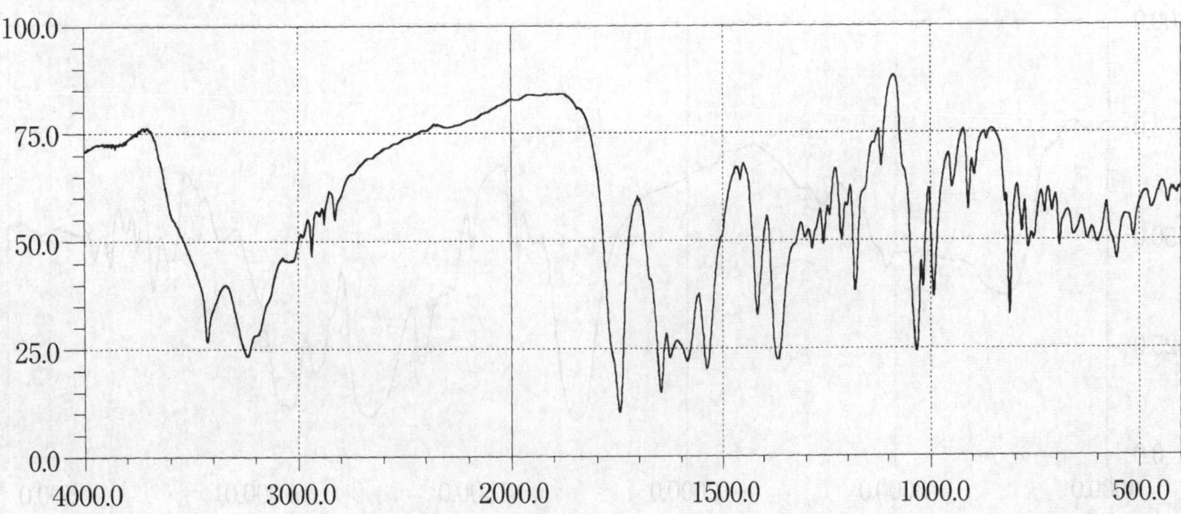

Cefuroxime Axetil

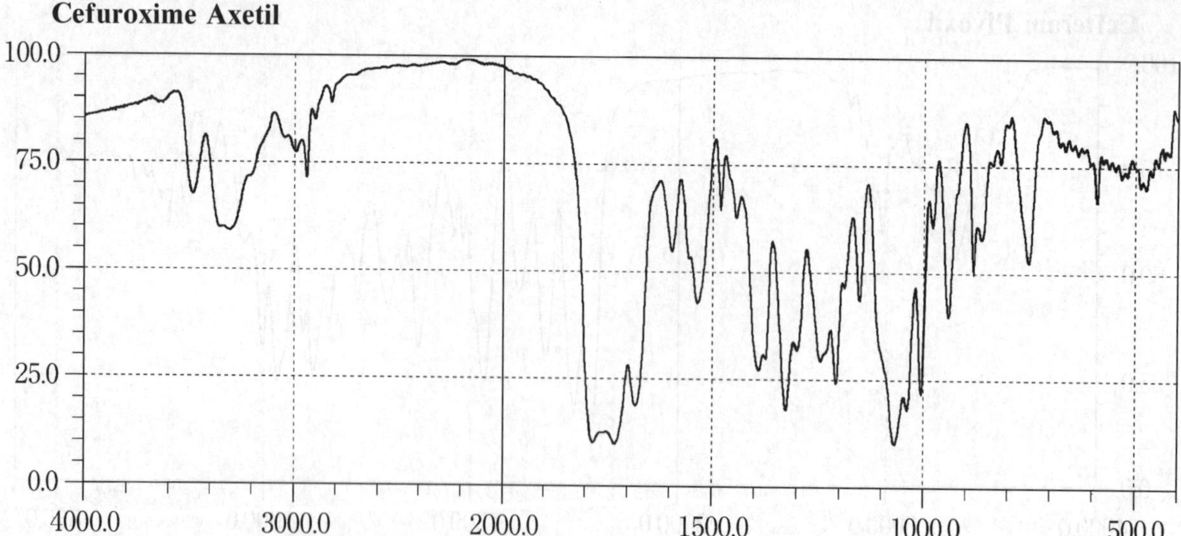

Celecoxib

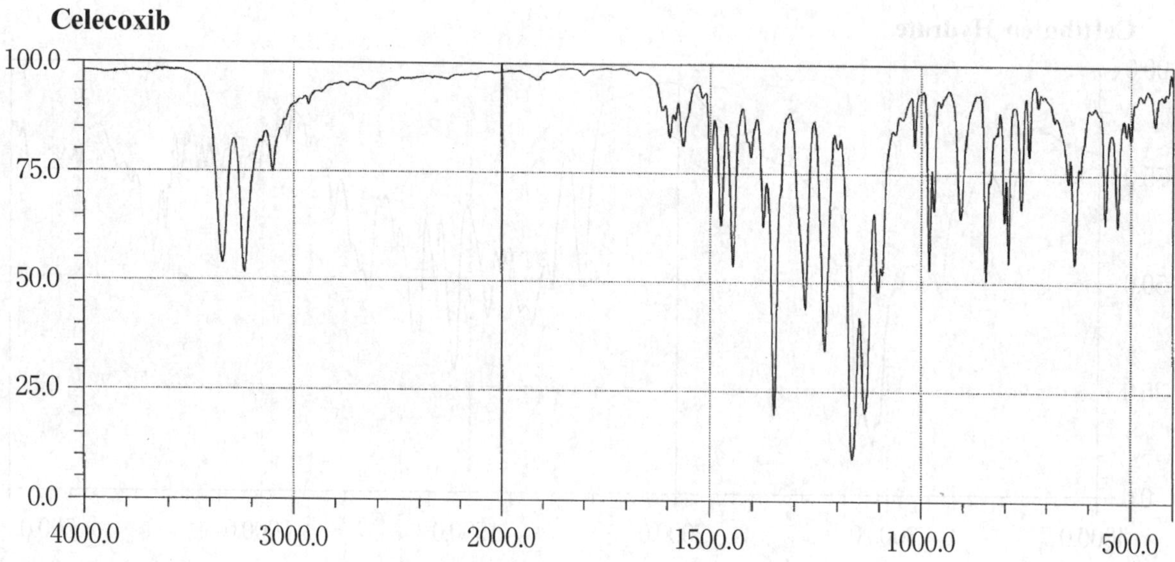

Cellacefate

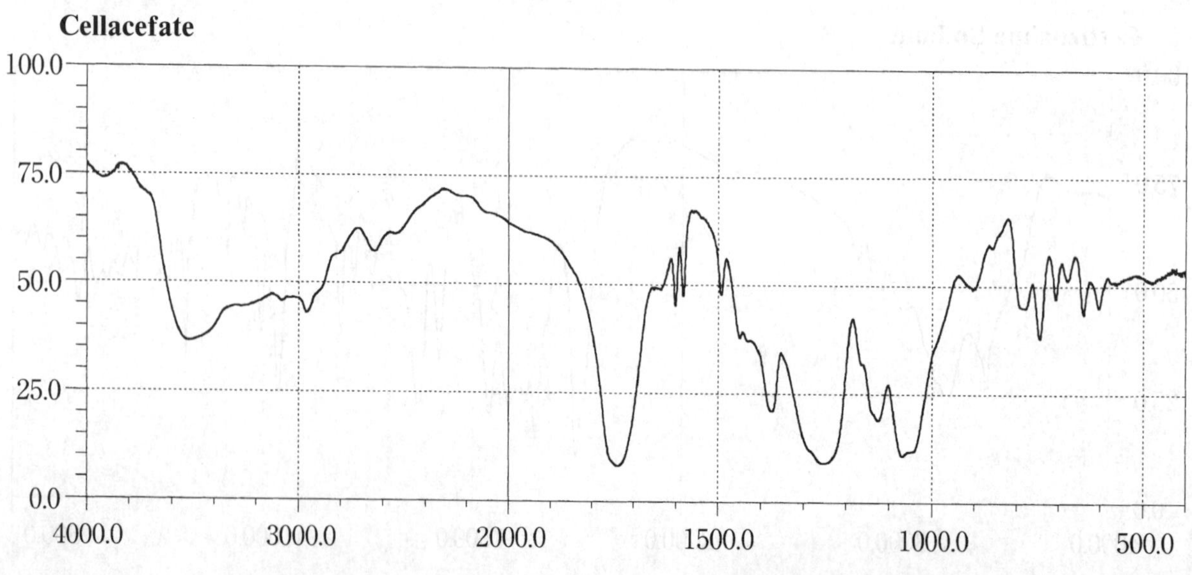

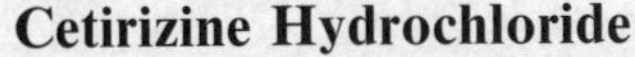

Cetirizine Hydrochloride

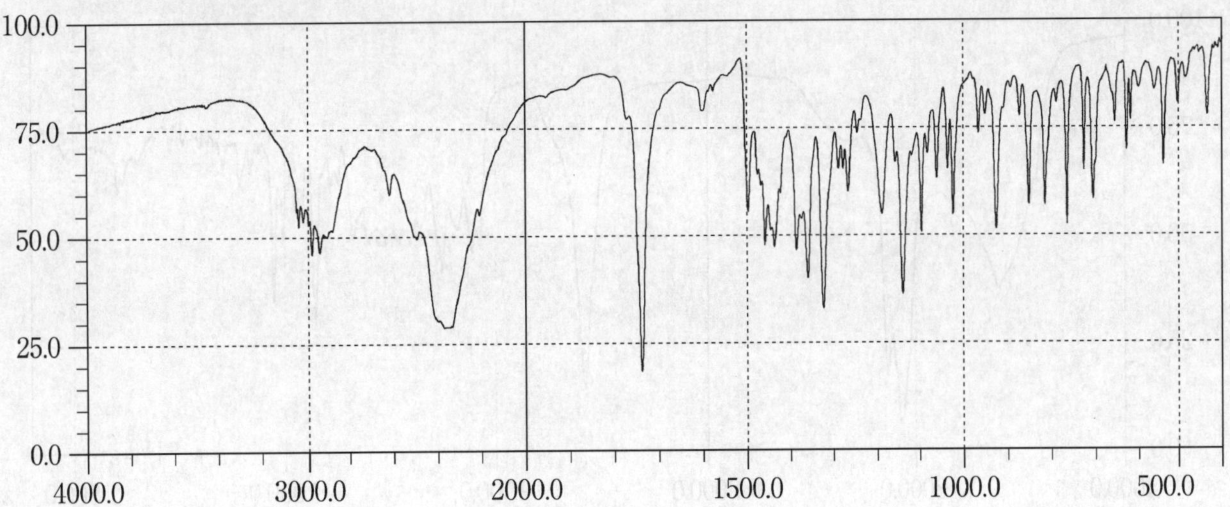

Cetotiamine Hydrochloride Hydrate

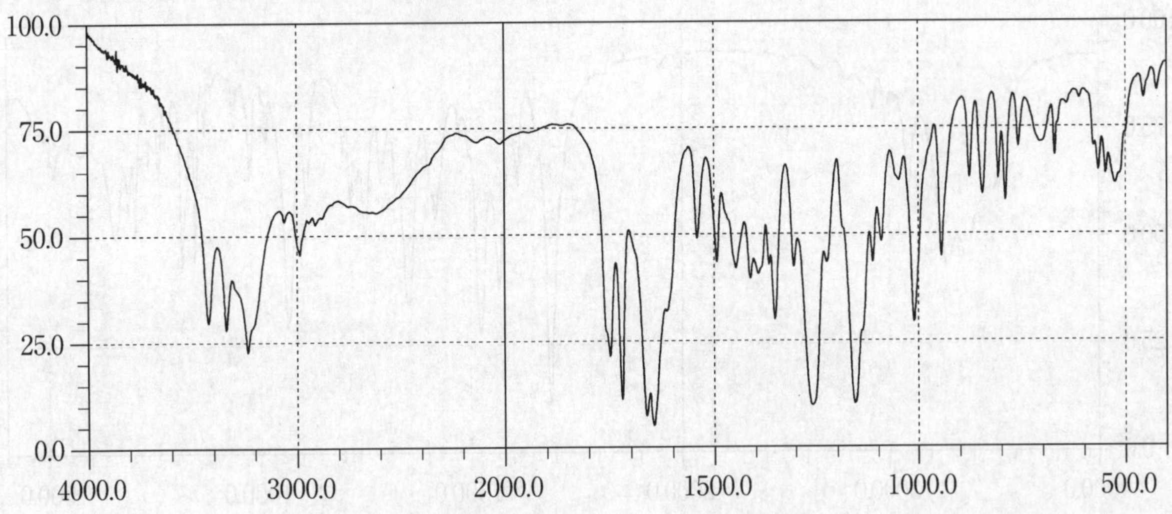

Cetraxate Hydrochloride

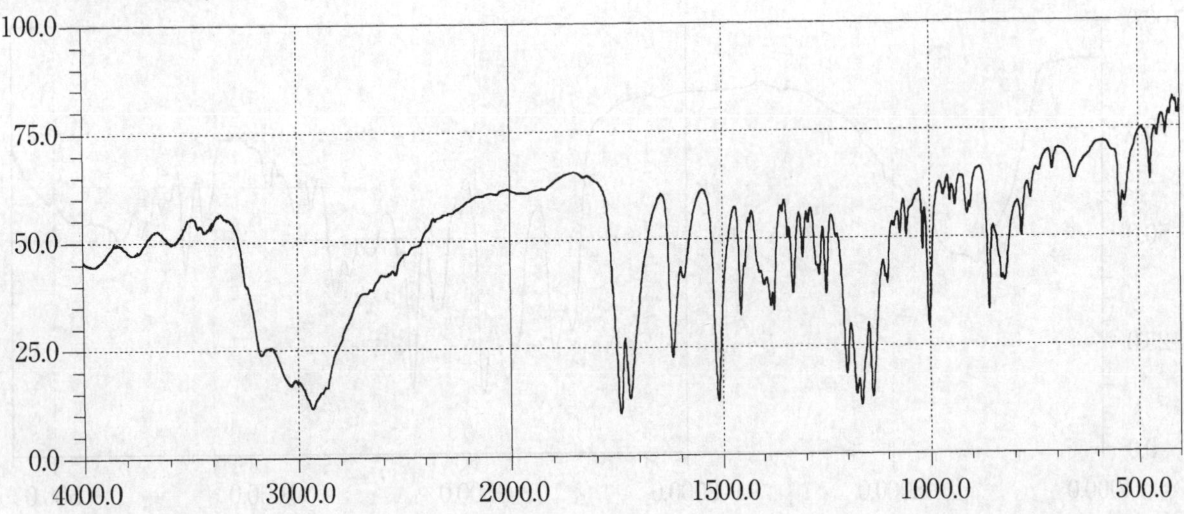

The JP Drugs are to be tested according to the provisions given in the pertinent monographs, General Notices, General Rules for Crude Drugs, General Rules for Preparations, and General Tests for their conformity to the Japanese Pharmacopoeia. (See the General Notices 5.)

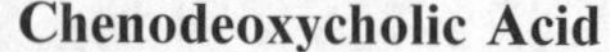

Chenodeoxycholic Acid

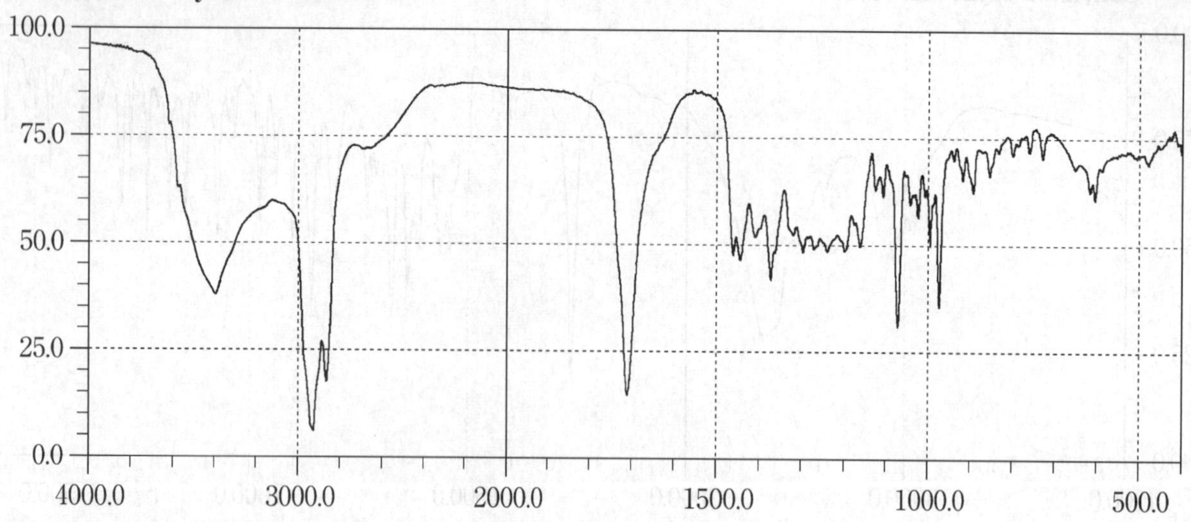

Chloramphenicol

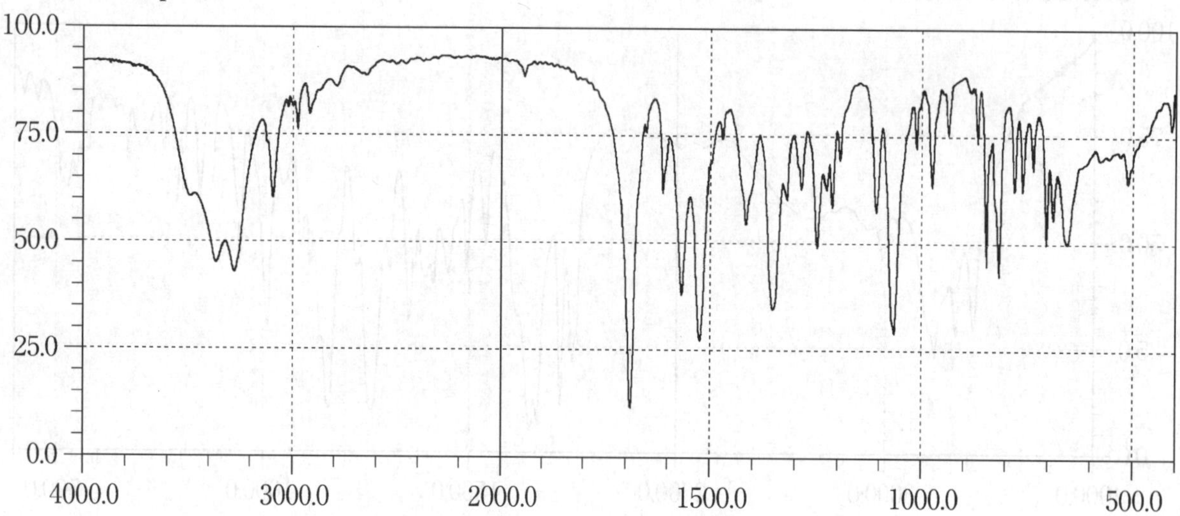

Chloramphenicol Sodium Succinate

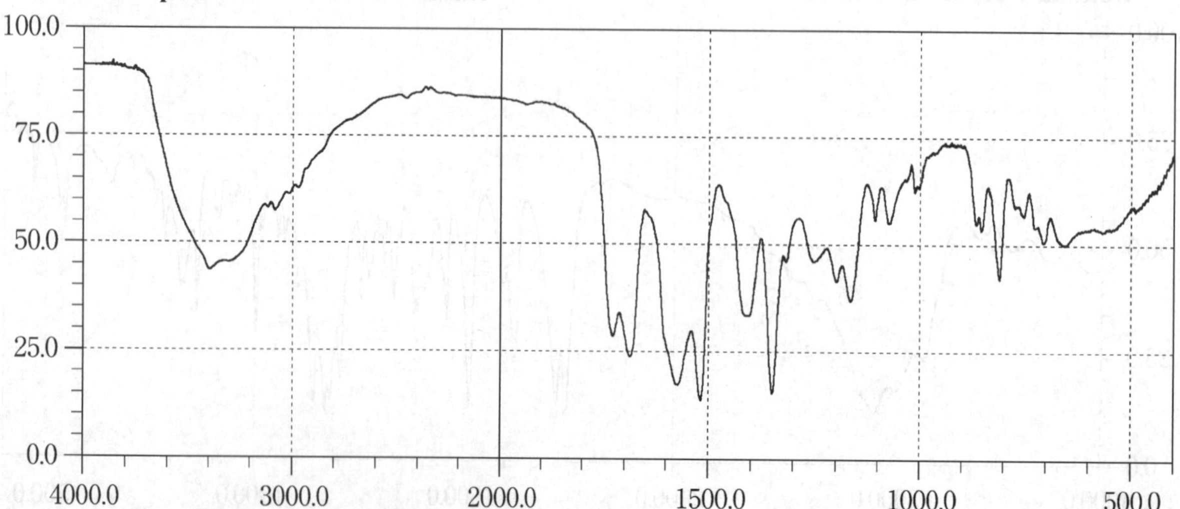

Chlordiazepoxide

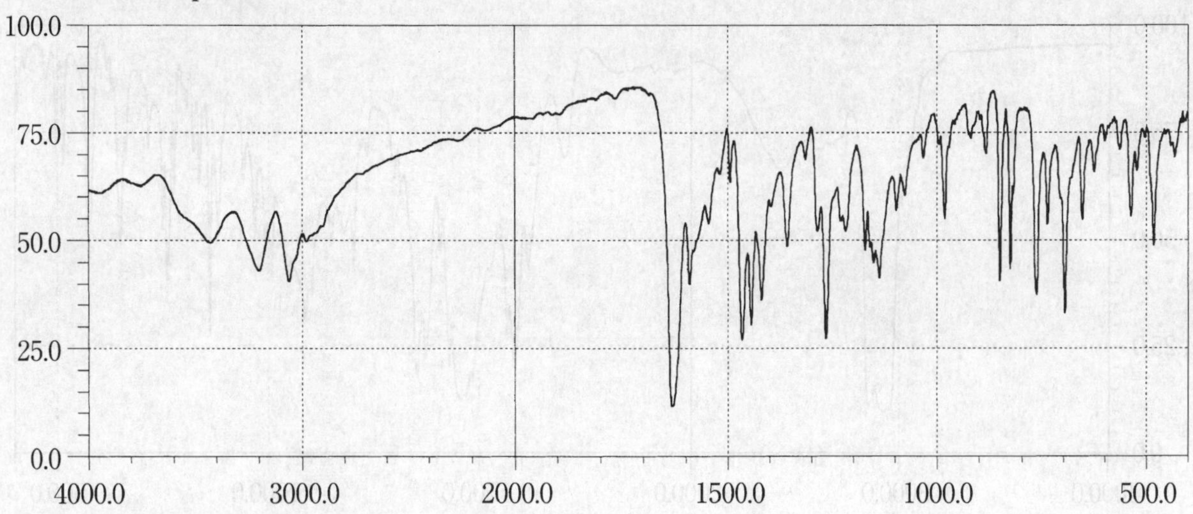

Chlormadinone Acetate

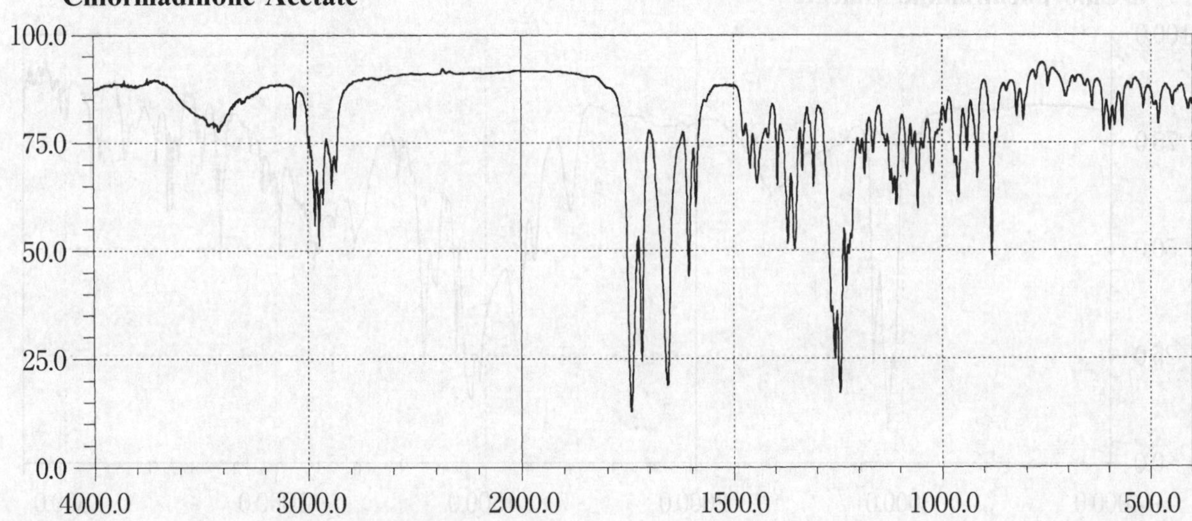

Chlorphenesin Carbamate

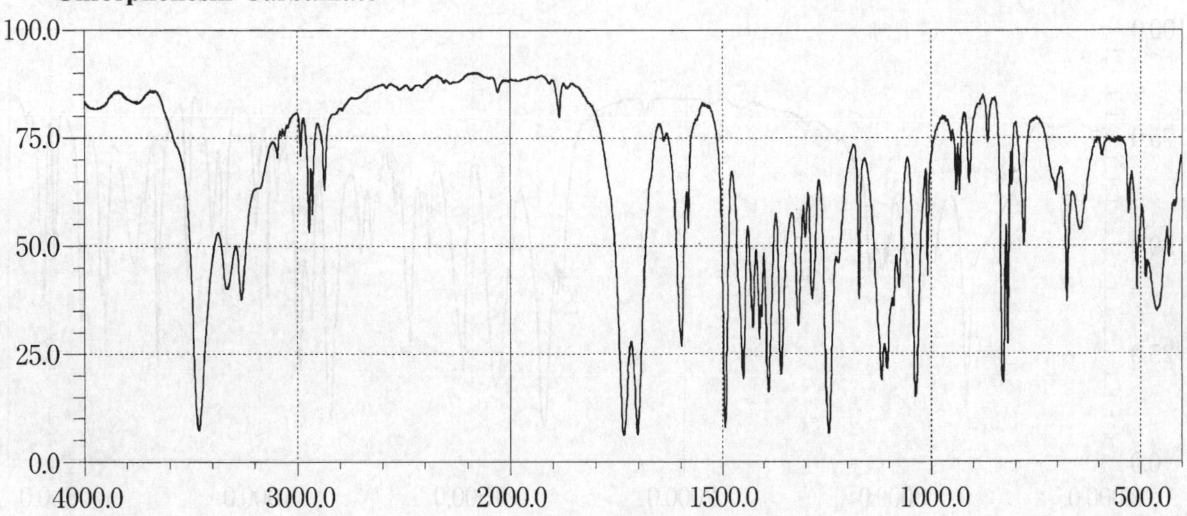

Chlorpheniramine Maleate

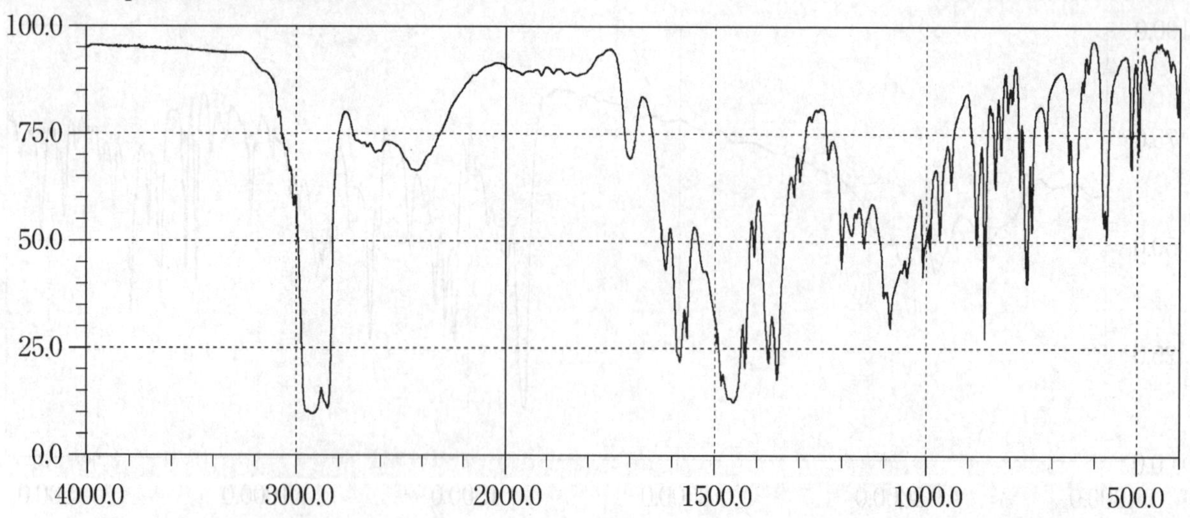

***d*-Chlorpheniramine Maleate**

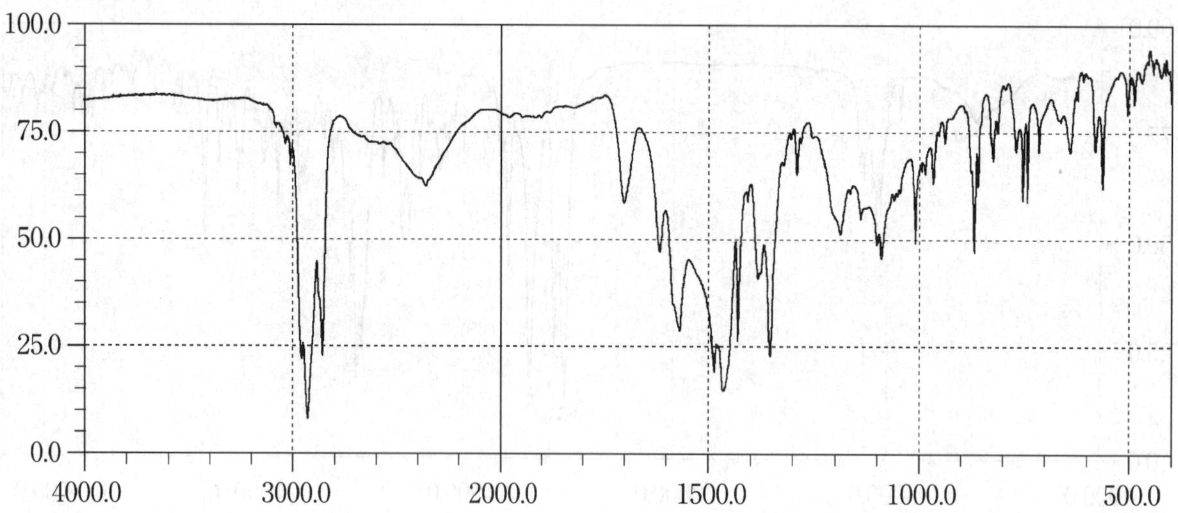

Chlorpropamide

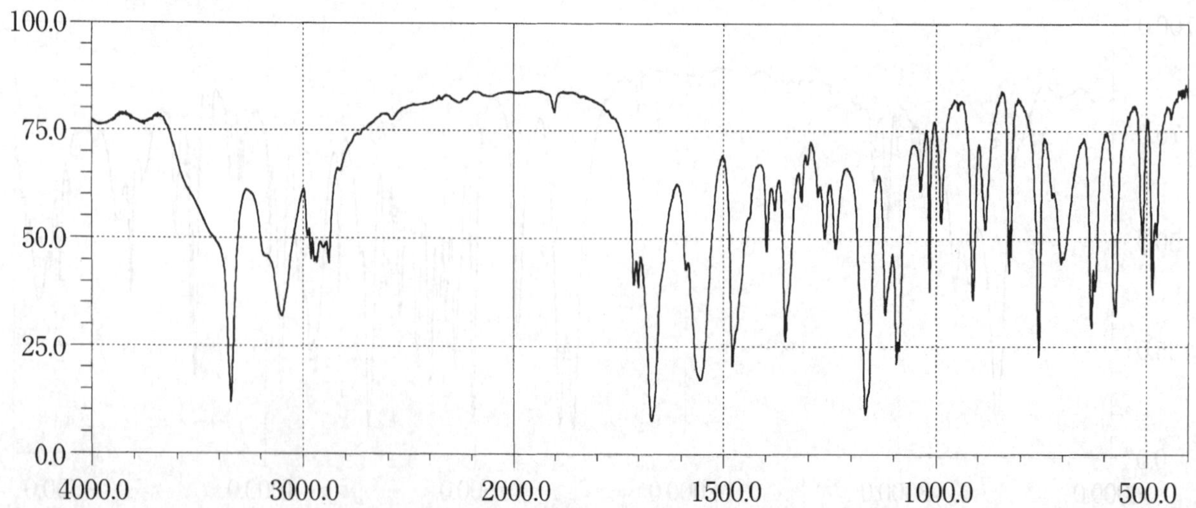

Cholecalciferol

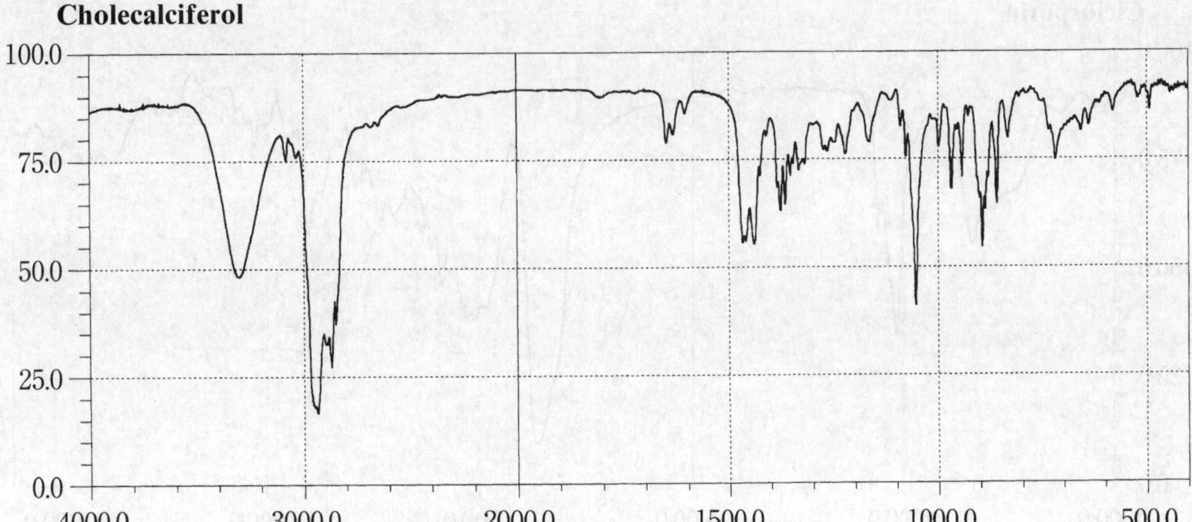

Cibenzoline Succinate

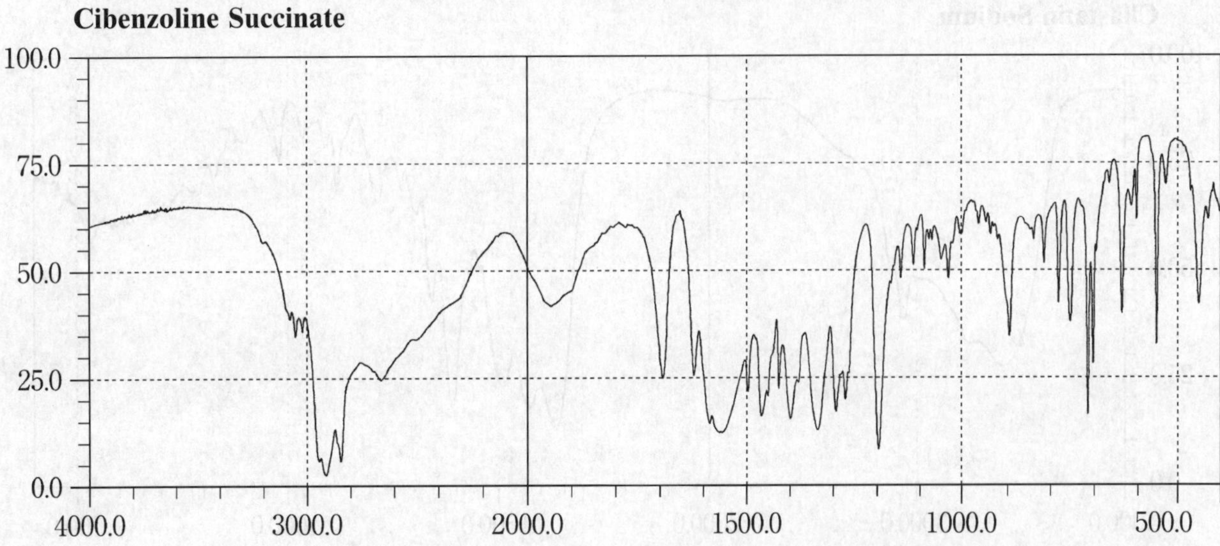

Ciclacillin

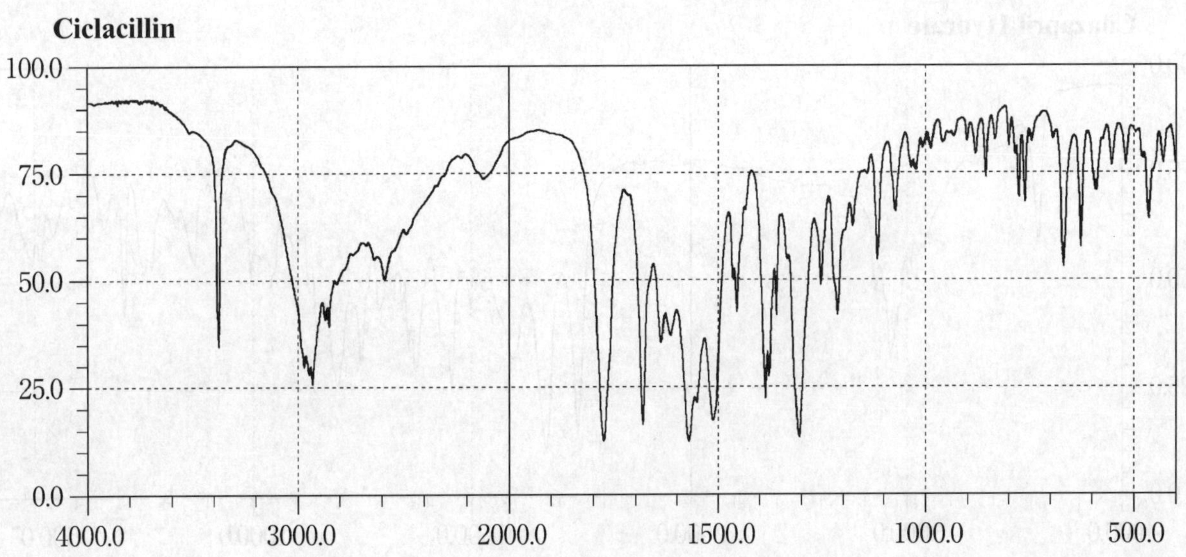

Ciclosporin

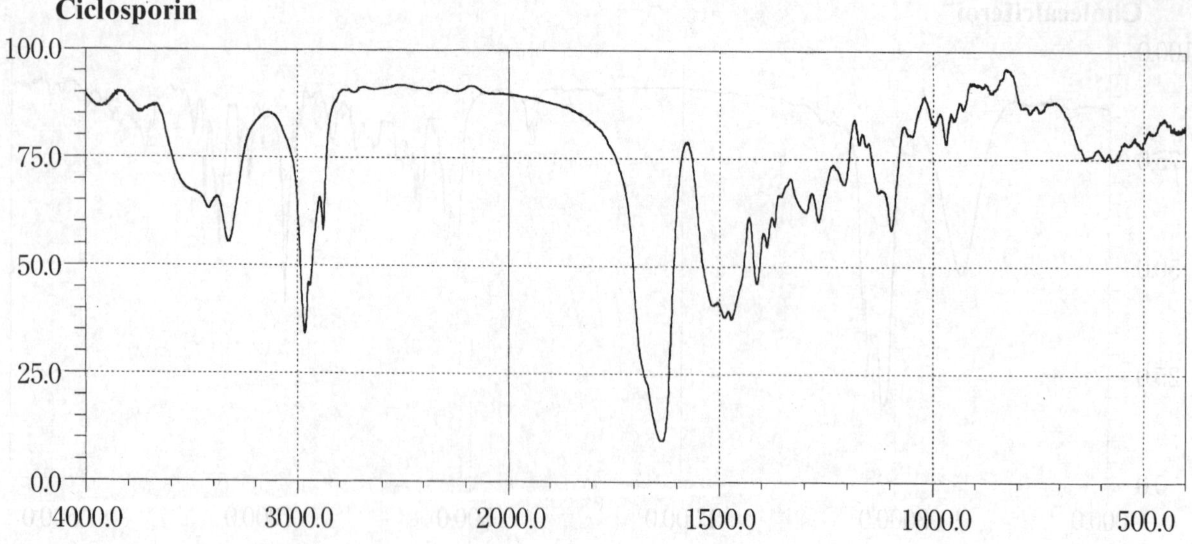

Cilastatin Sodium

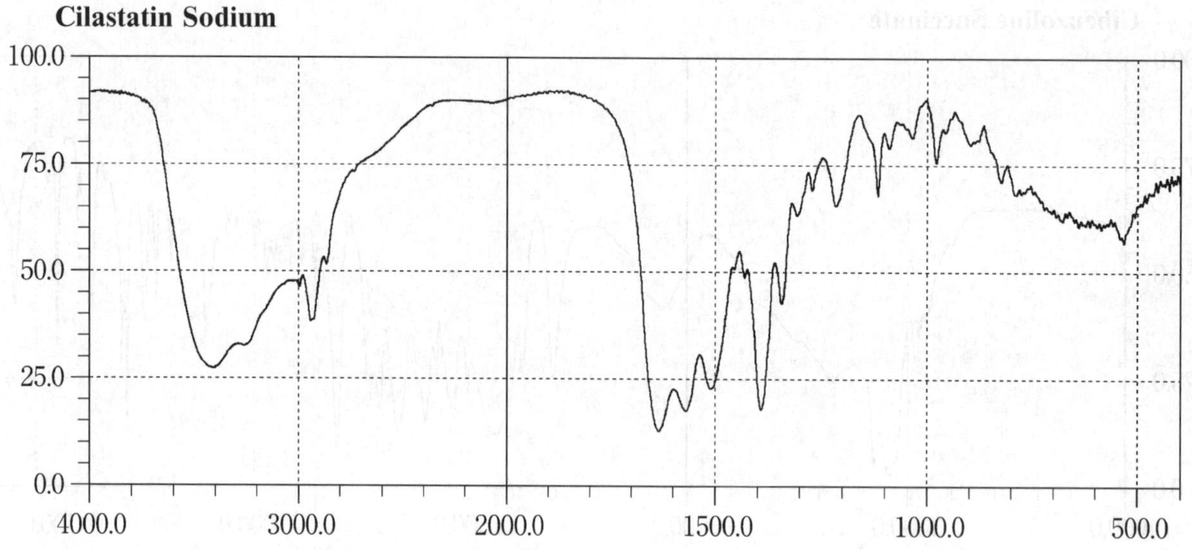

Cilazapril Hydrate

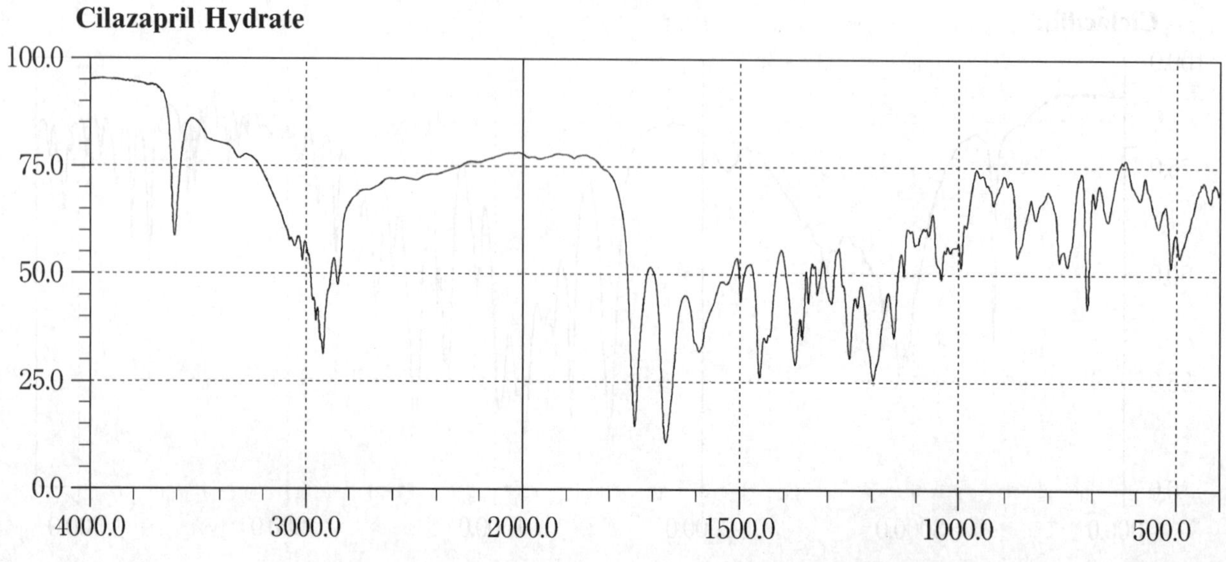

Cilnidipine

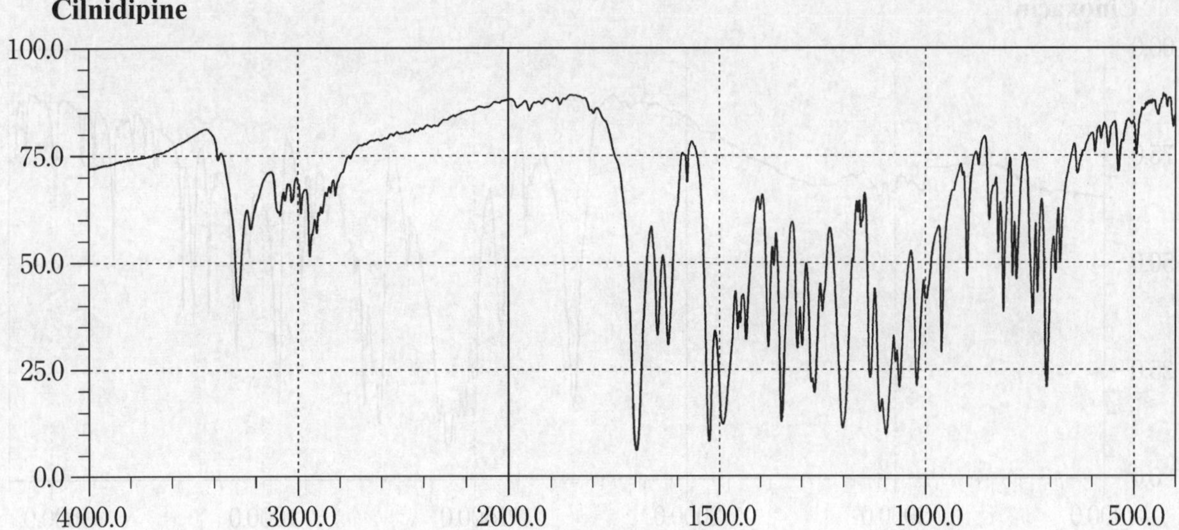

Cilostazol

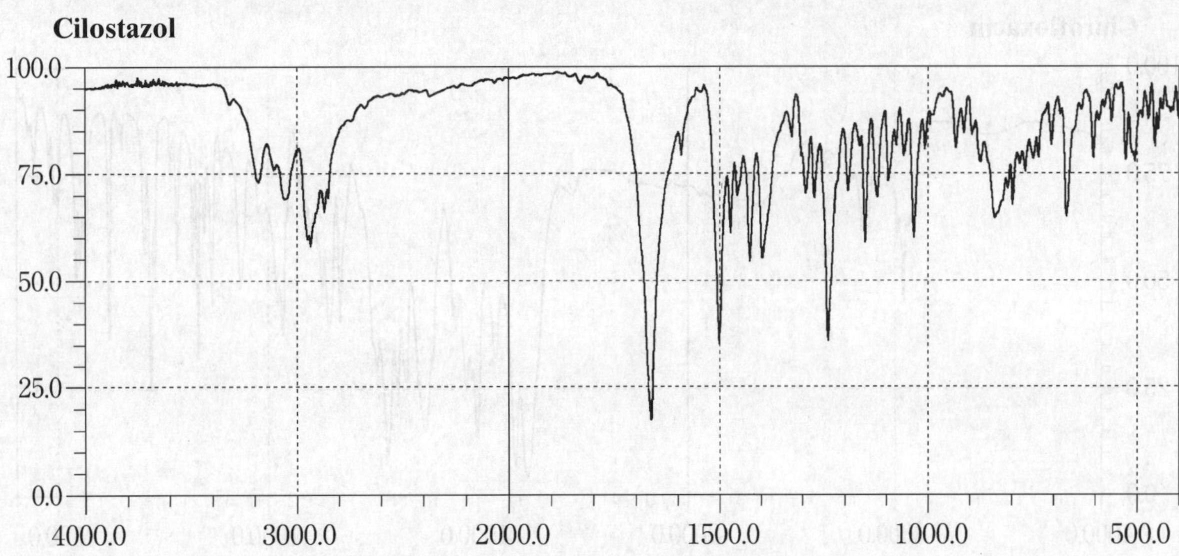

Cimetidine

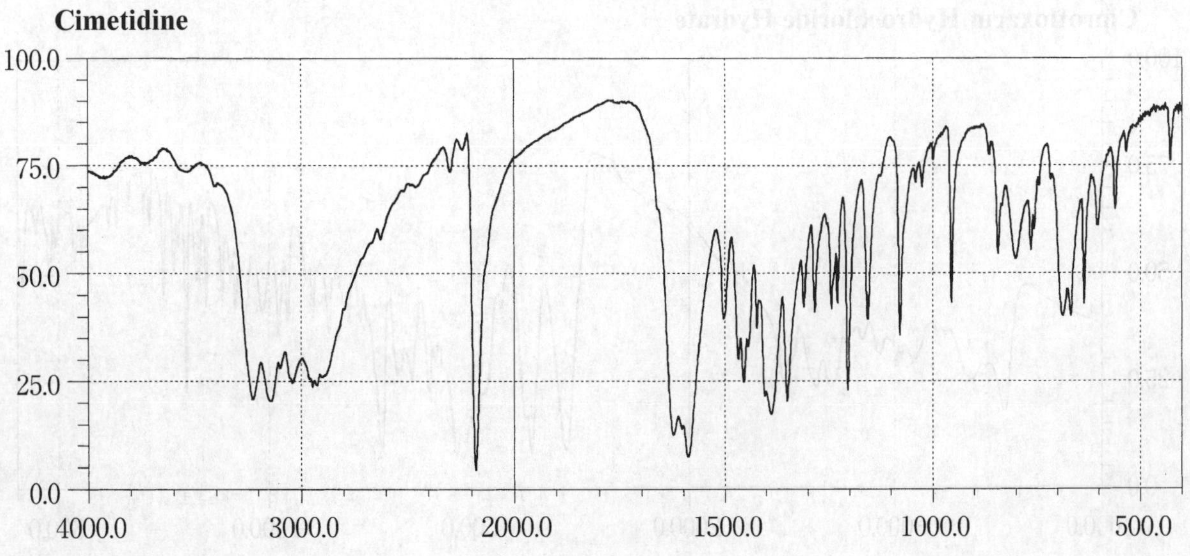

Cinoxacin

100.0
75.0
50.0
25.0
0.0
4000.0 3000.0 2000.0 1500.0 1000.0 500.0

Ciprofloxacin

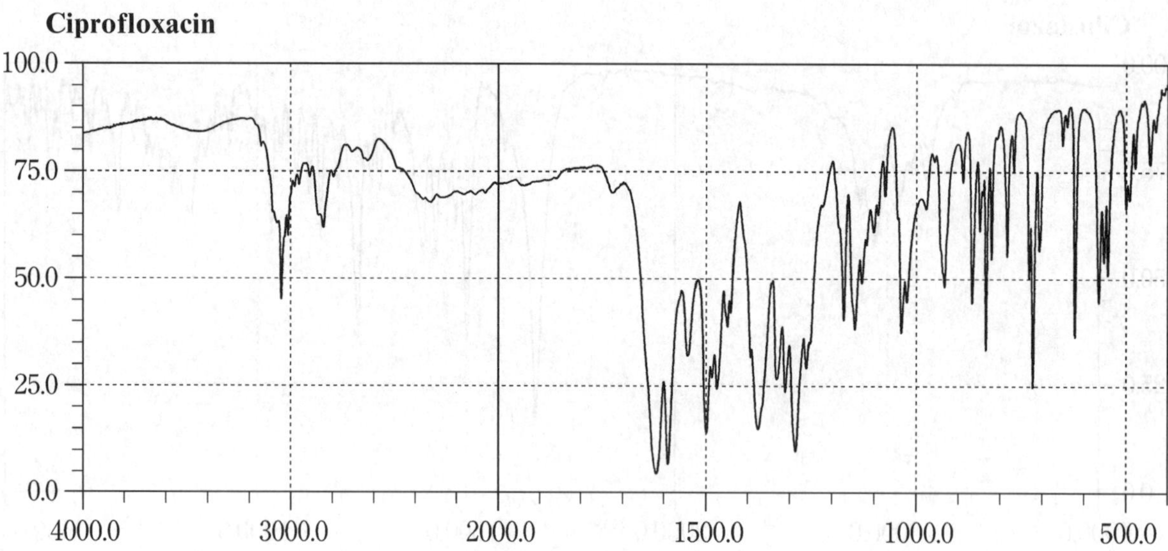

Ciprofloxacin Hydrochloride Hydrate

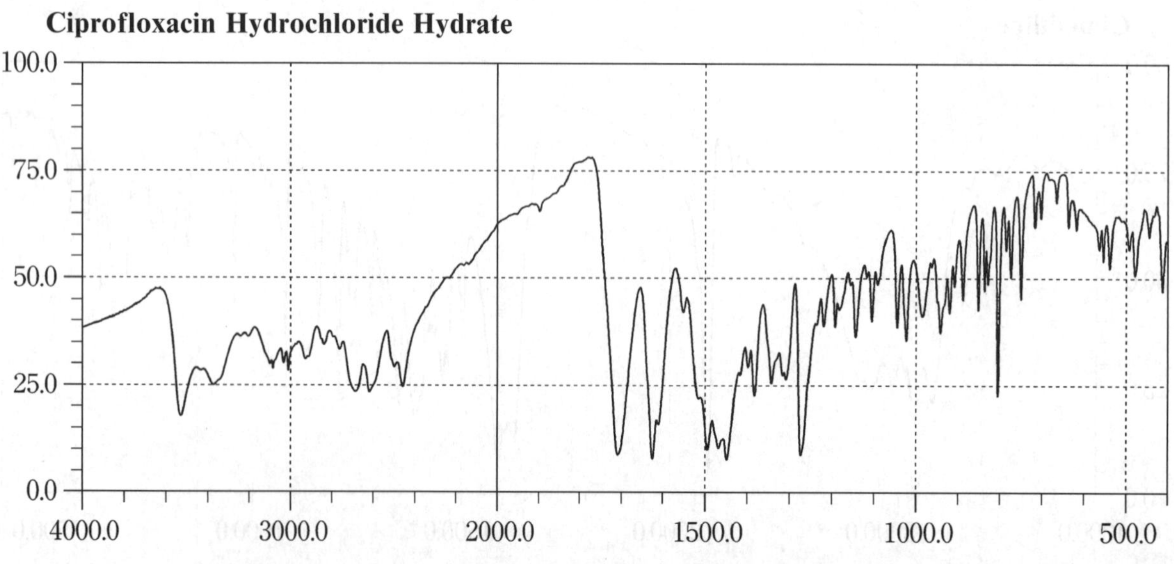

The JP Drugs are to be tested according to the provisions given in the pertinent monographs, General Notices, General Rules for Crude Drugs, General Rules for Preparations, and General Tests for their conformity to the Japanese Pharmacopoeia. (See the General Notices 5.)

Cisplatin

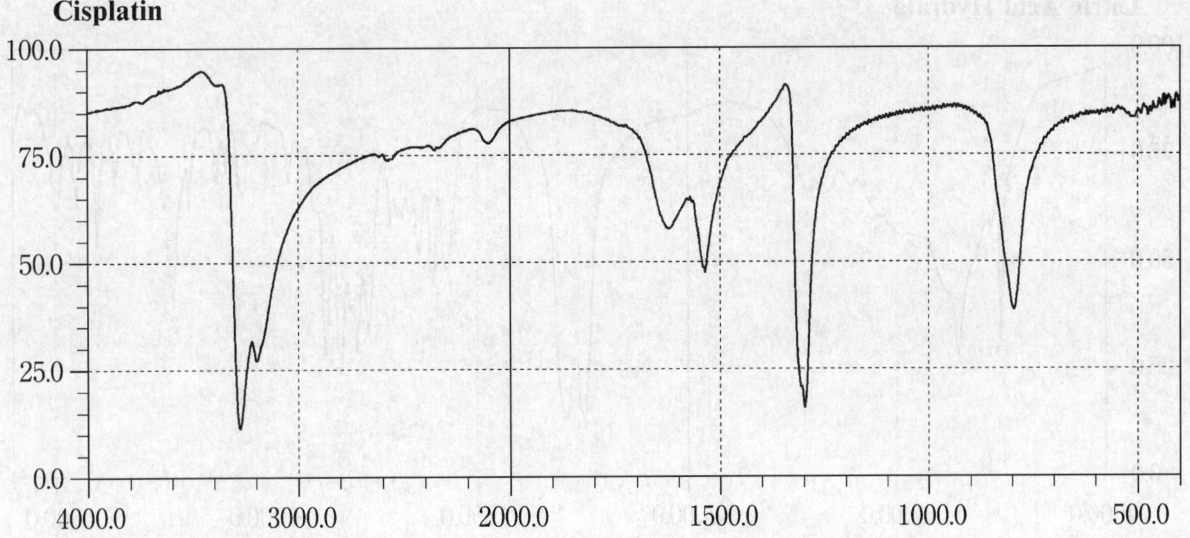

Citicoline

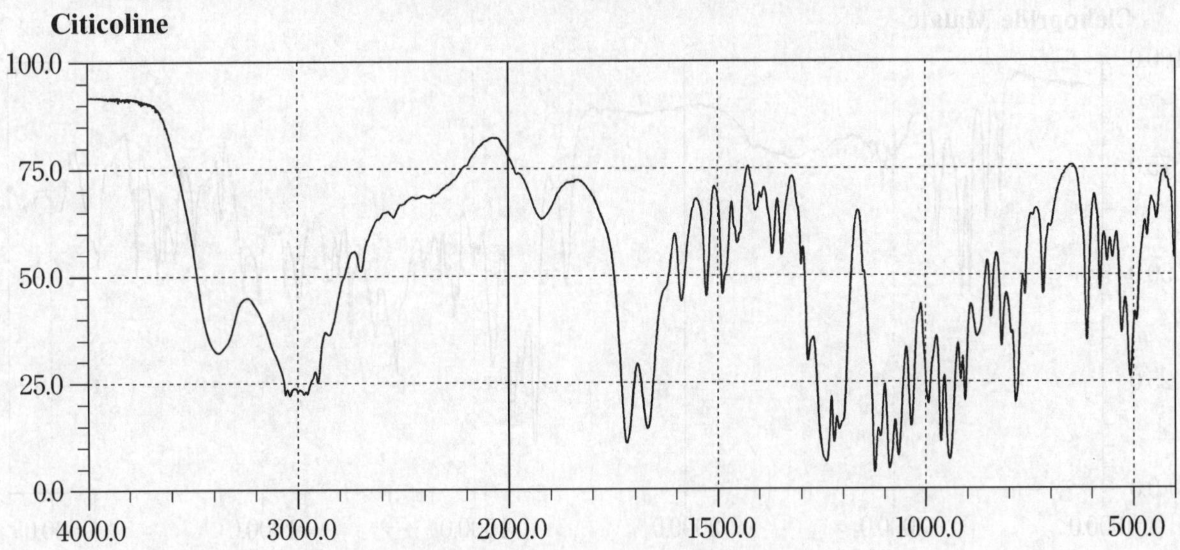

Anhydrous Citric Acid

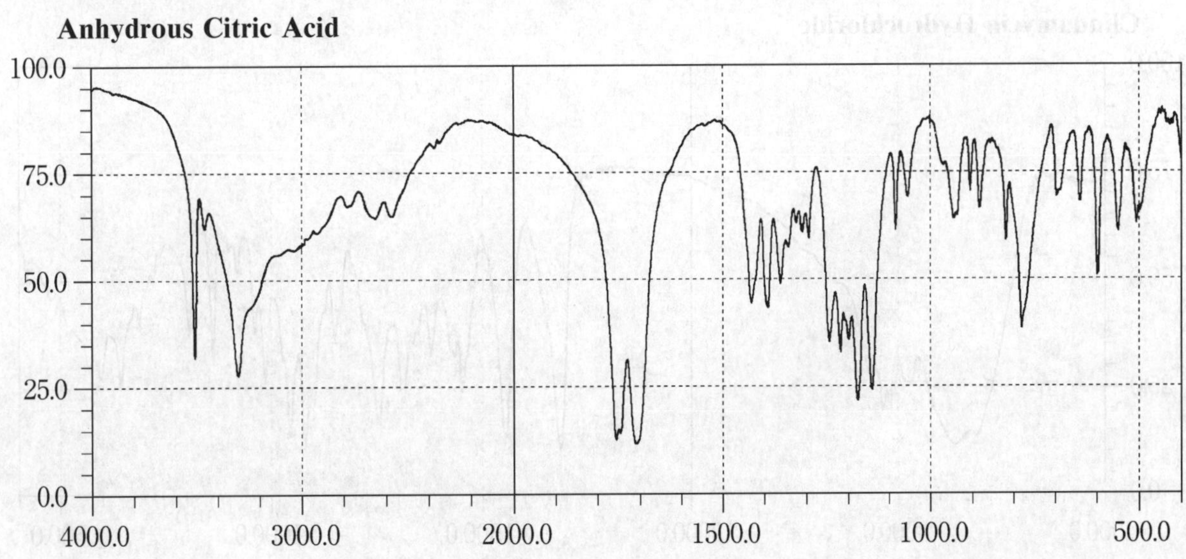

Citric Acid Hydrate

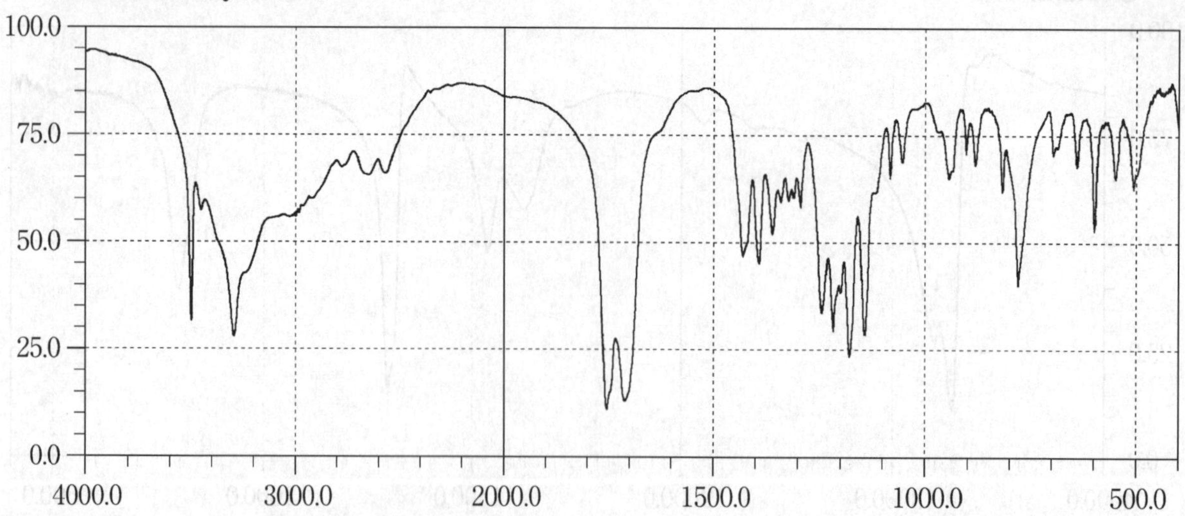

Clebopride Malate

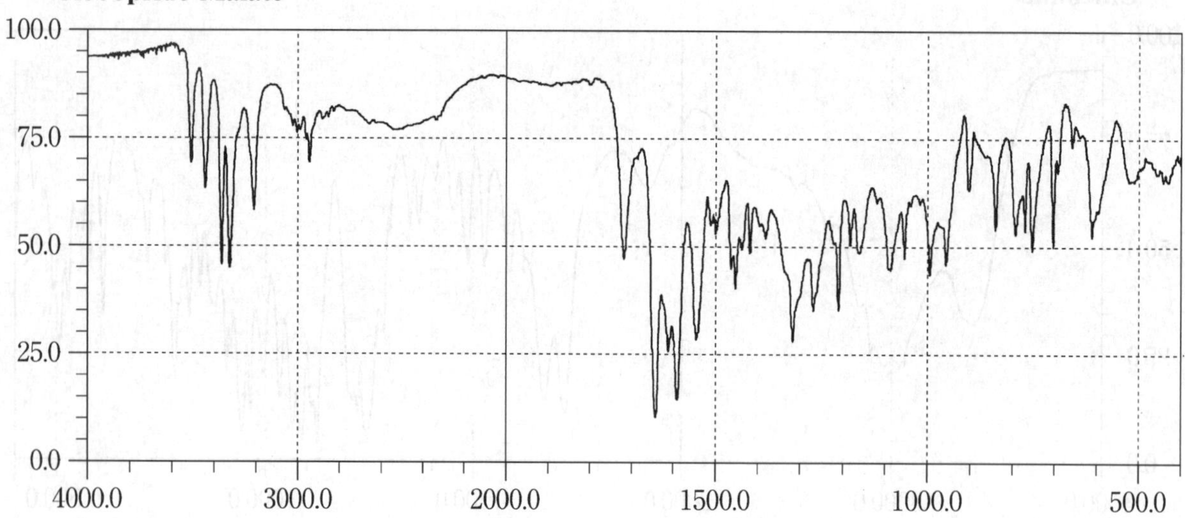

Clindamycin Hydrochloride

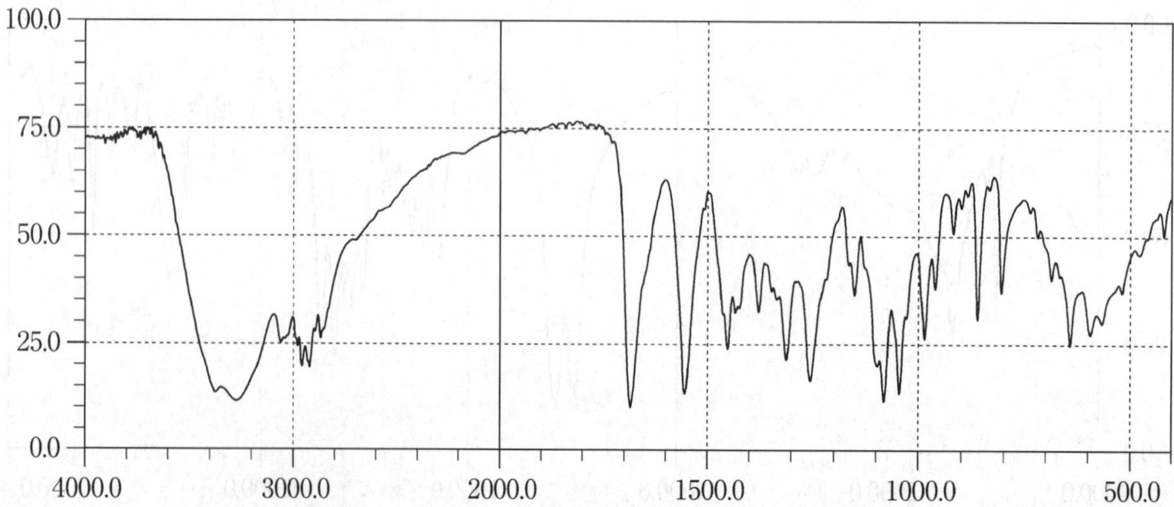

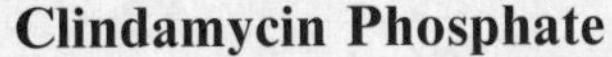
Clindamycin Phosphate

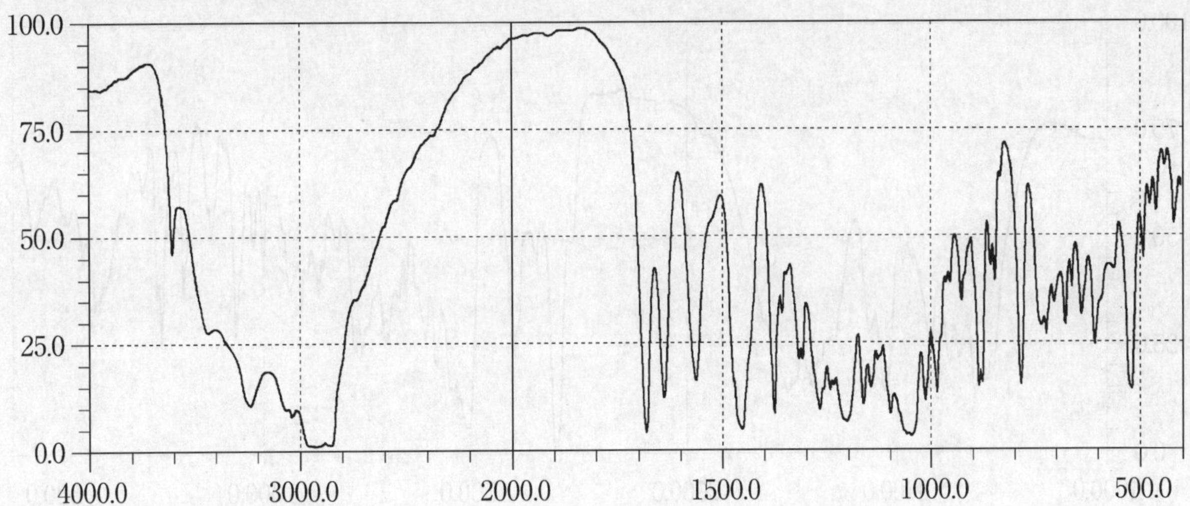

Clinofibrate

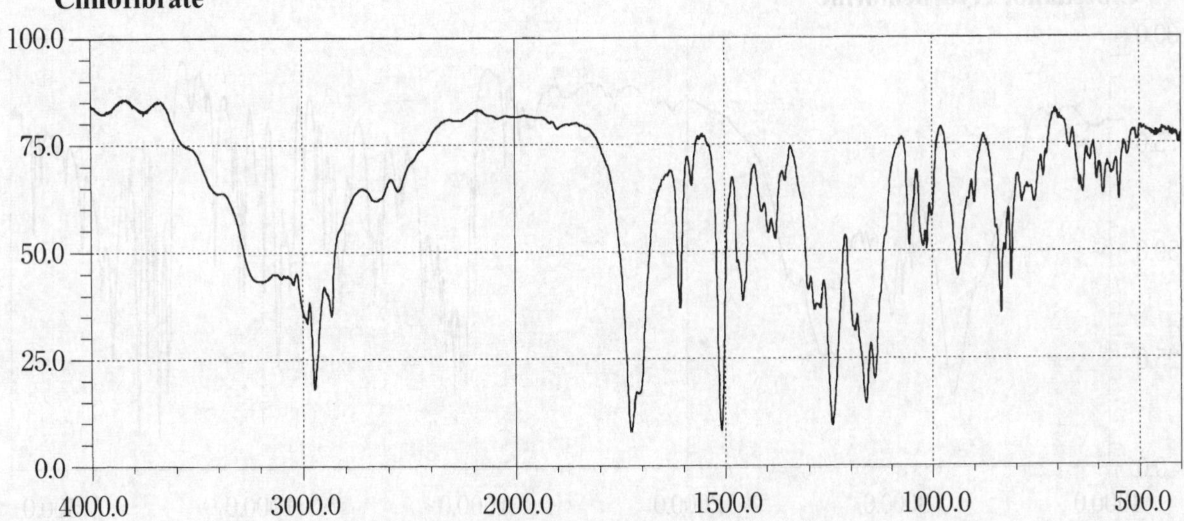

Clobetasol Propionate

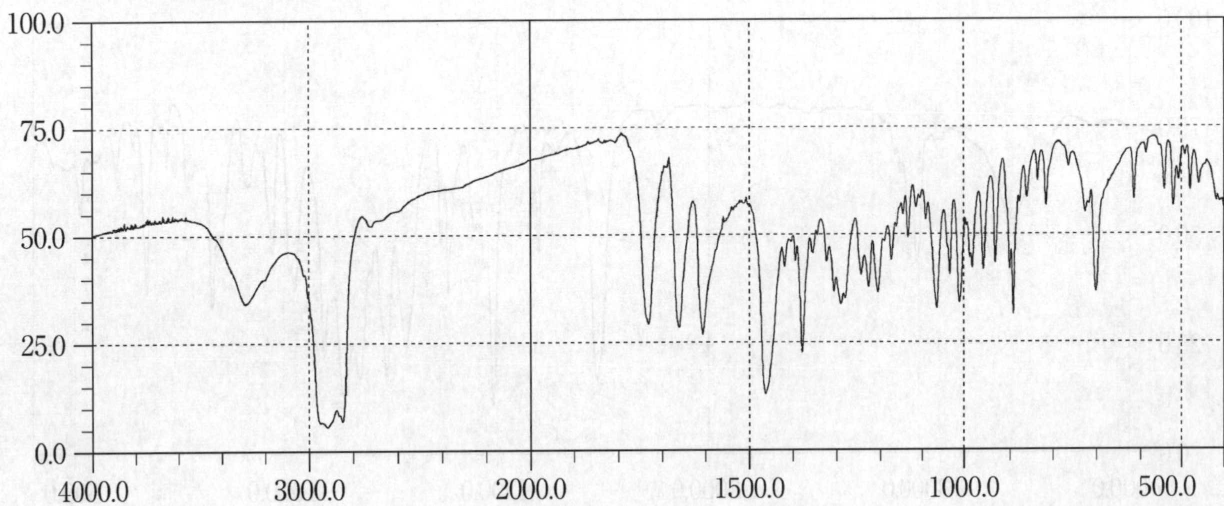

Clocapramine Hydrochloride Hydrate

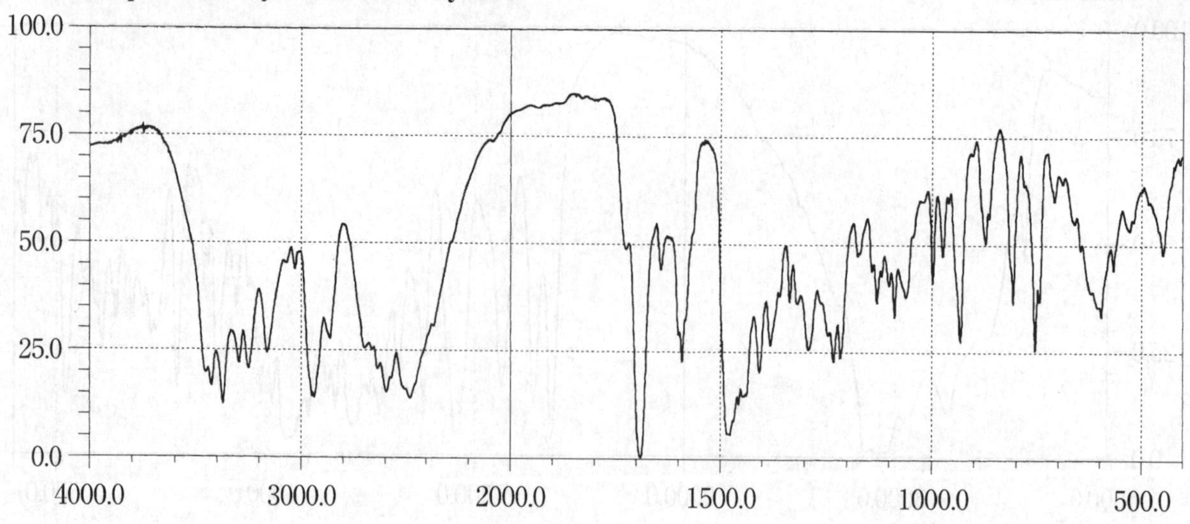

Clofedanol Hydrochloride

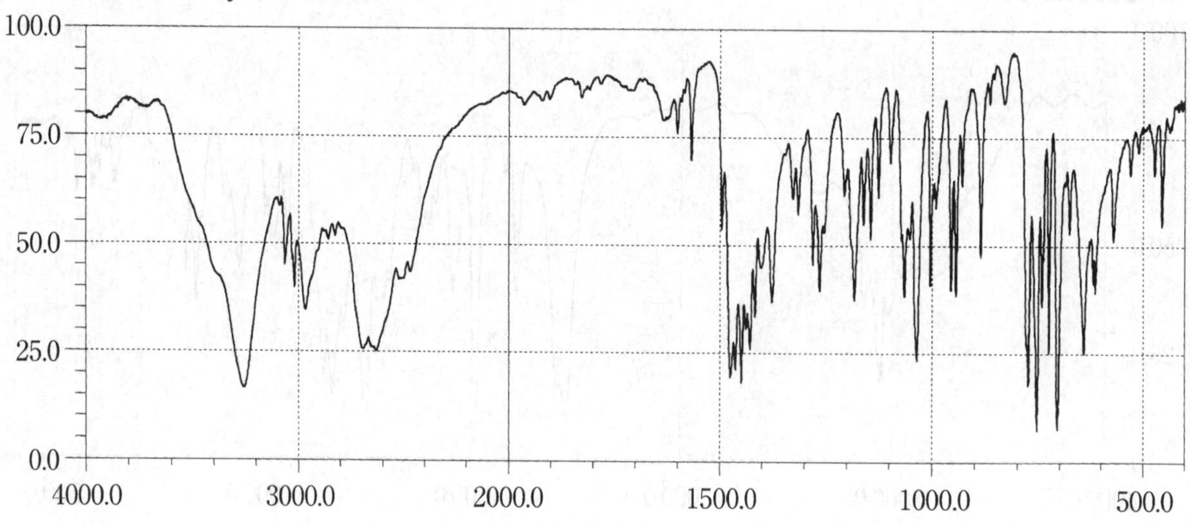

Clofibrate

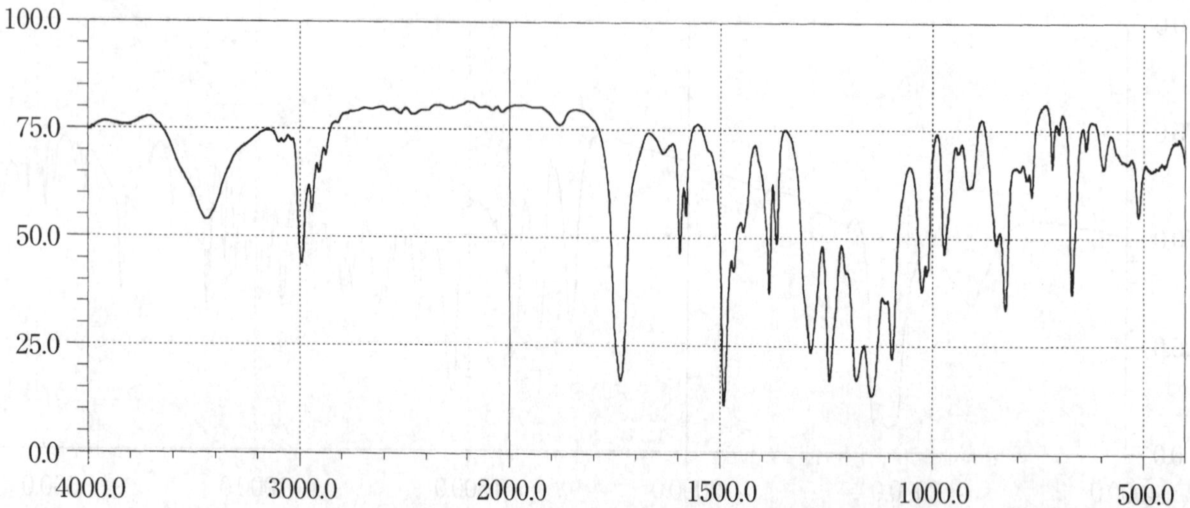

The JP Drugs are to be tested according to the provisions given in the pertinent monographs, General Notices, General Rules for Crude Drugs, General Rules for Preparations, and General Tests for their conformity to the Japanese Pharmacopoeia. (See the General Notices 5.)

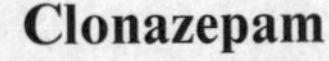

Clonazepam

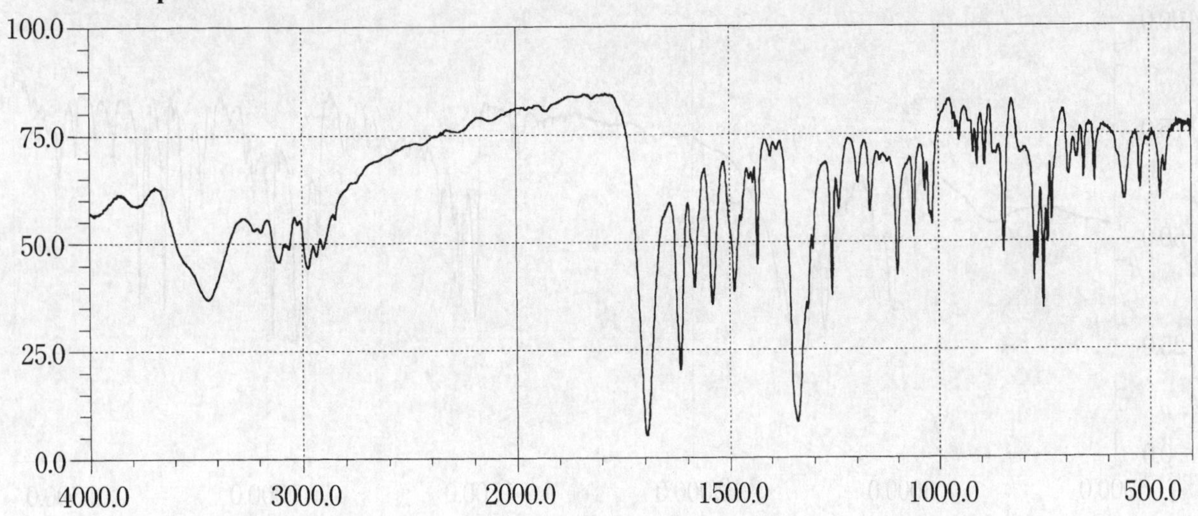

Clonidine Hydrochloride

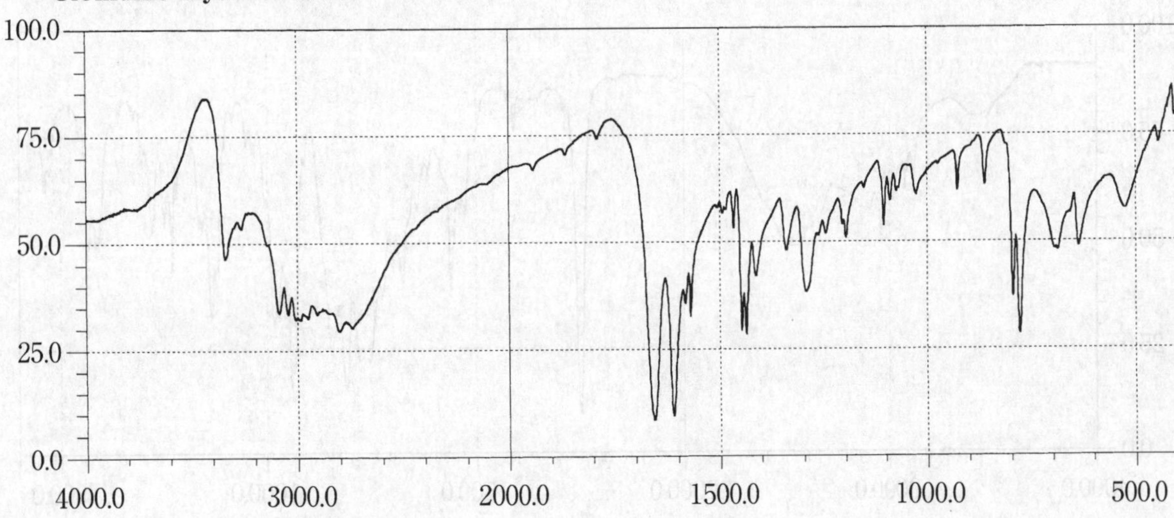

Cloperastine Fendizoate

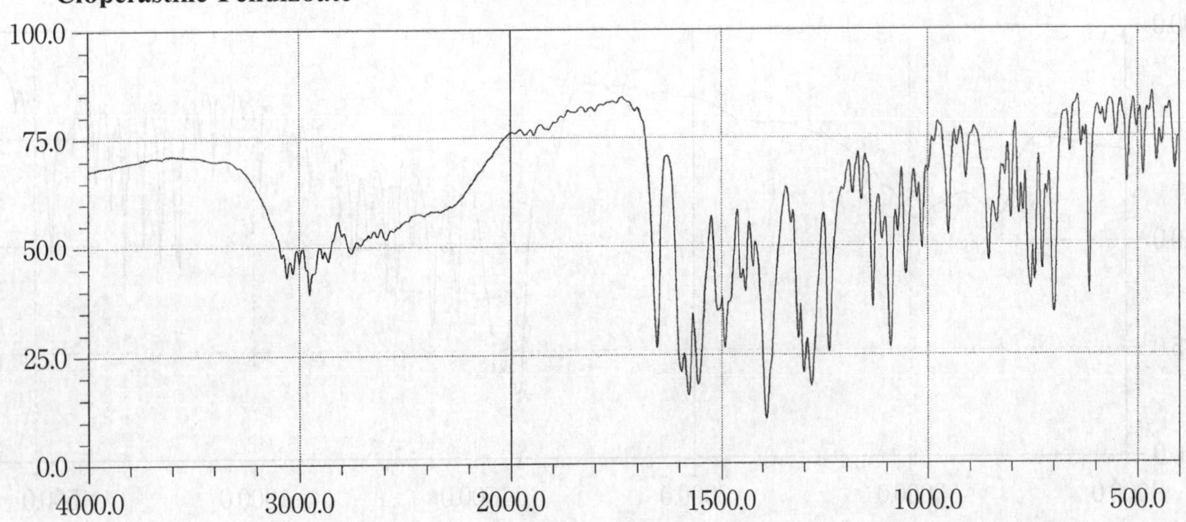

Cloperastine Hydrochloride

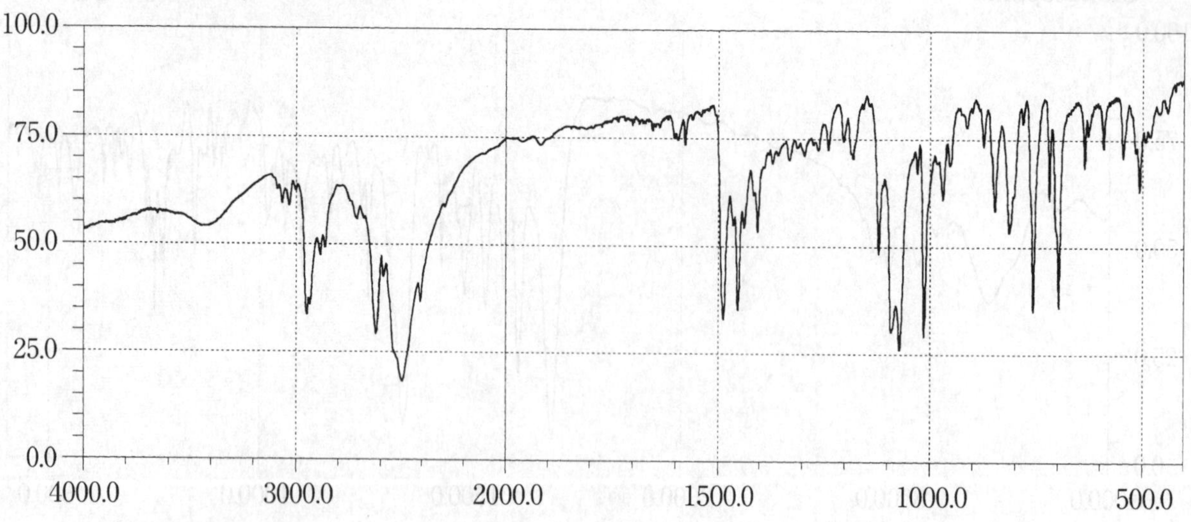

Clopidogrel Sulfate

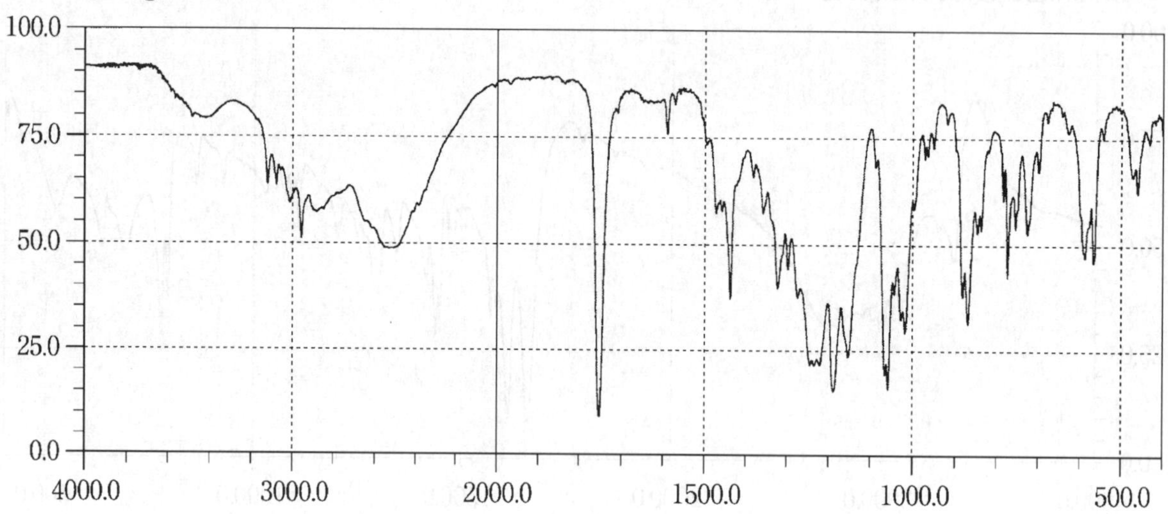

Clorazepate Dipotassium

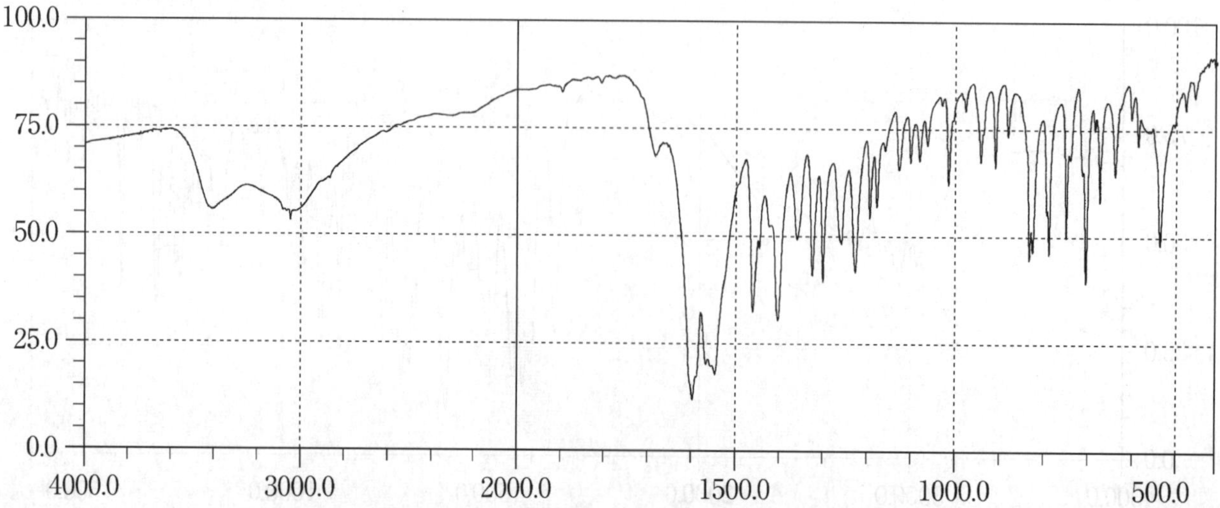

Clotrimazole

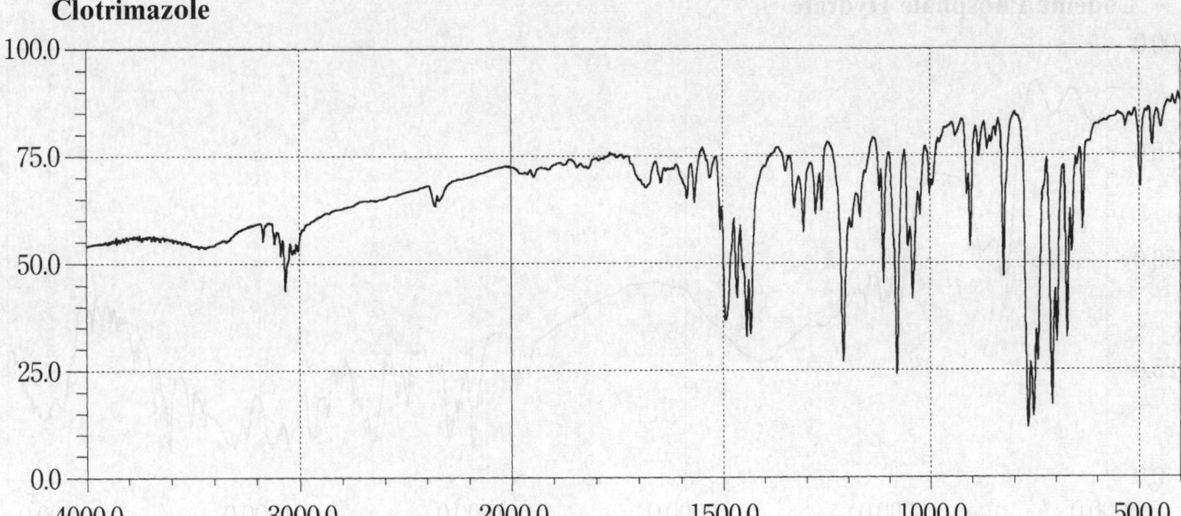

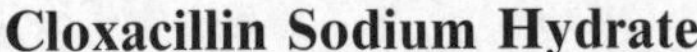

Cloxacillin Sodium Hydrate

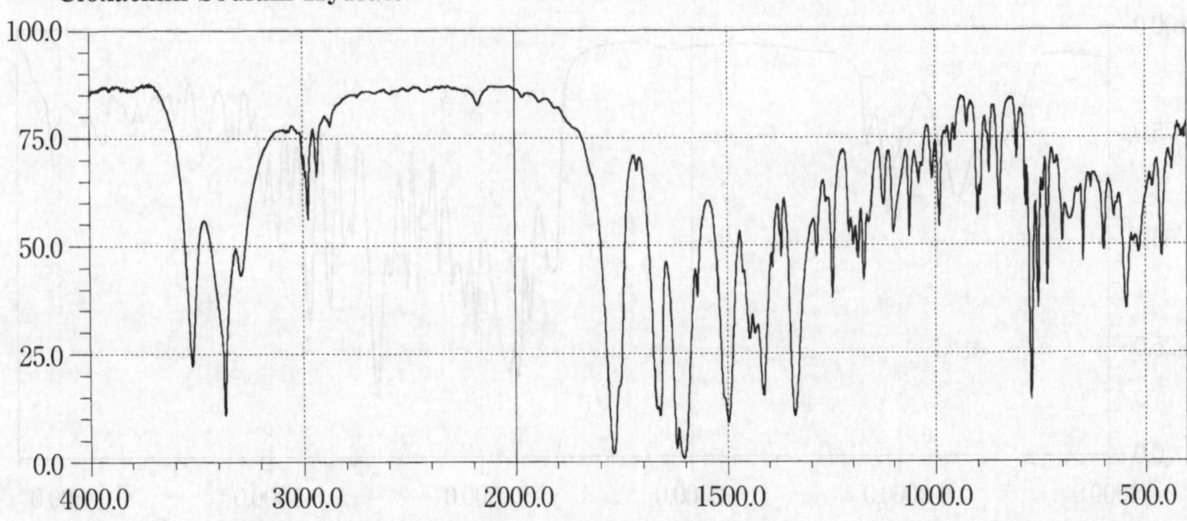

Cocaine Hydrochloride

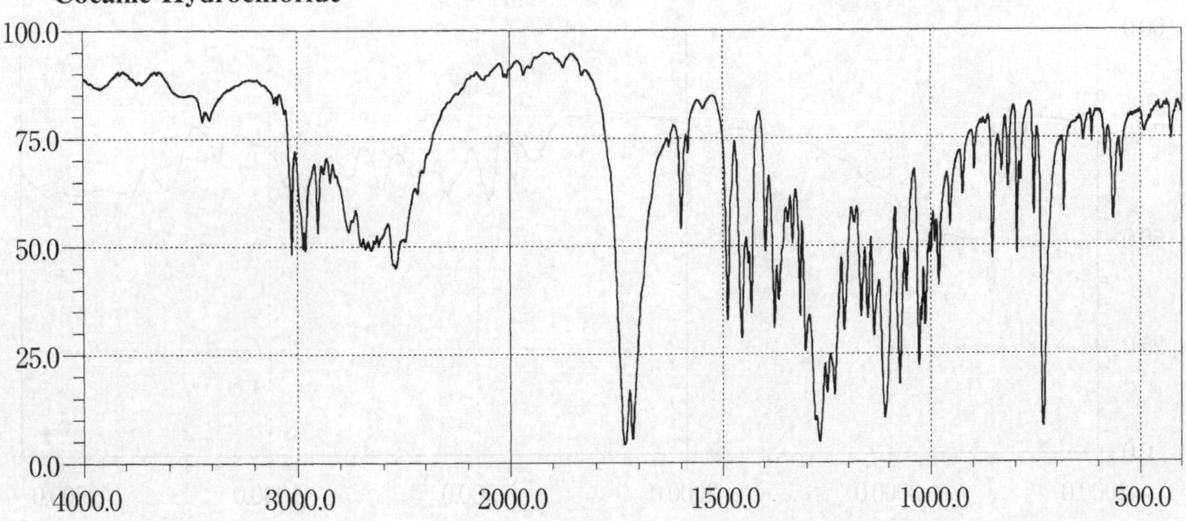

Codeine Phosphate Hydrate

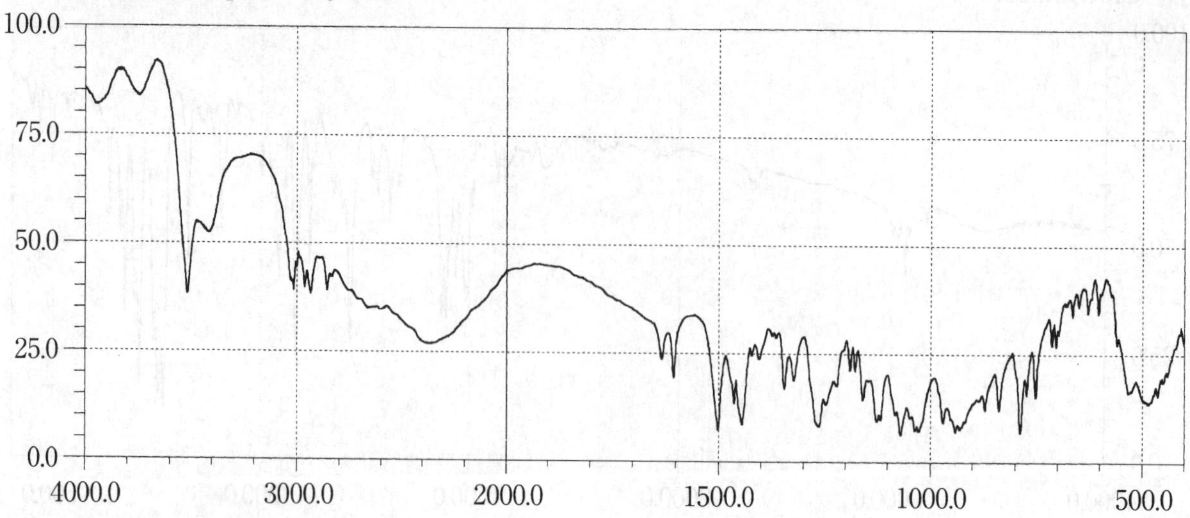

Colchicine

100.0
75.0
50.0
25.0
0.0
4000.0
3000.0
2000.0
1500.0
1000.0
500.0

Colestimide

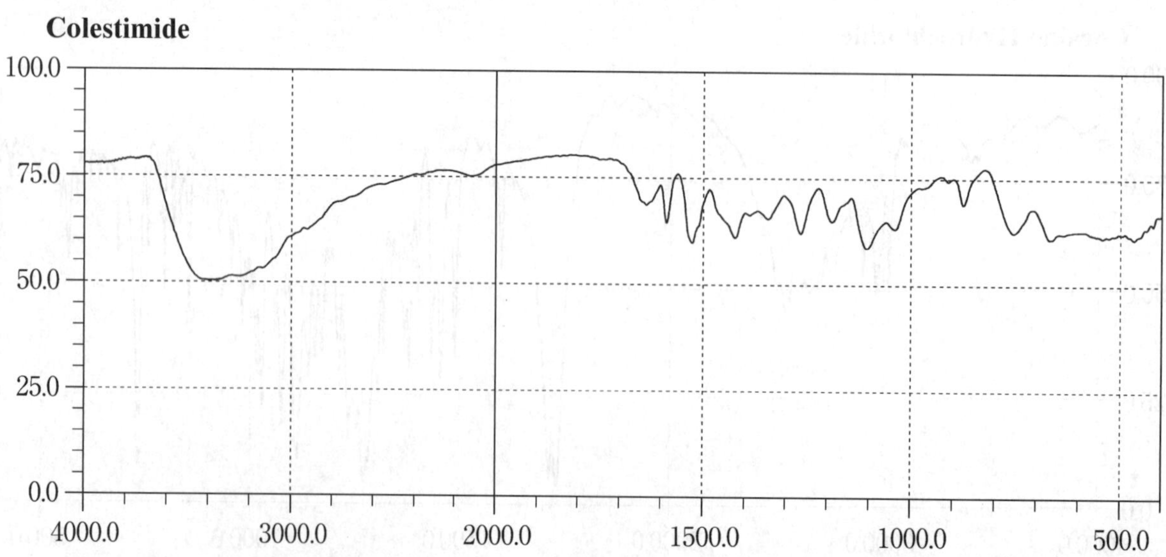

Colistin Sodium Methanesulfonate

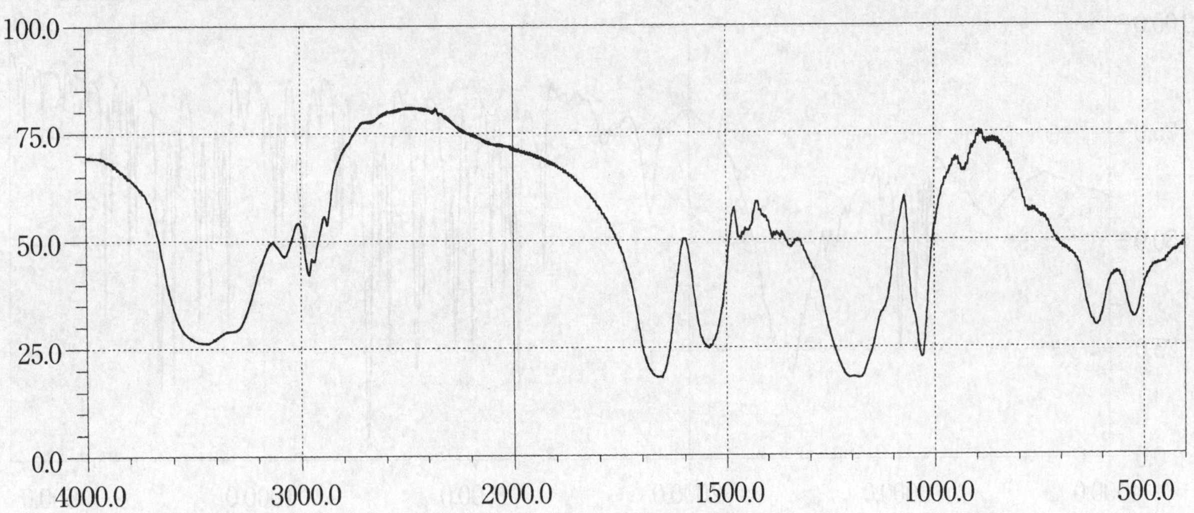

Copovidone

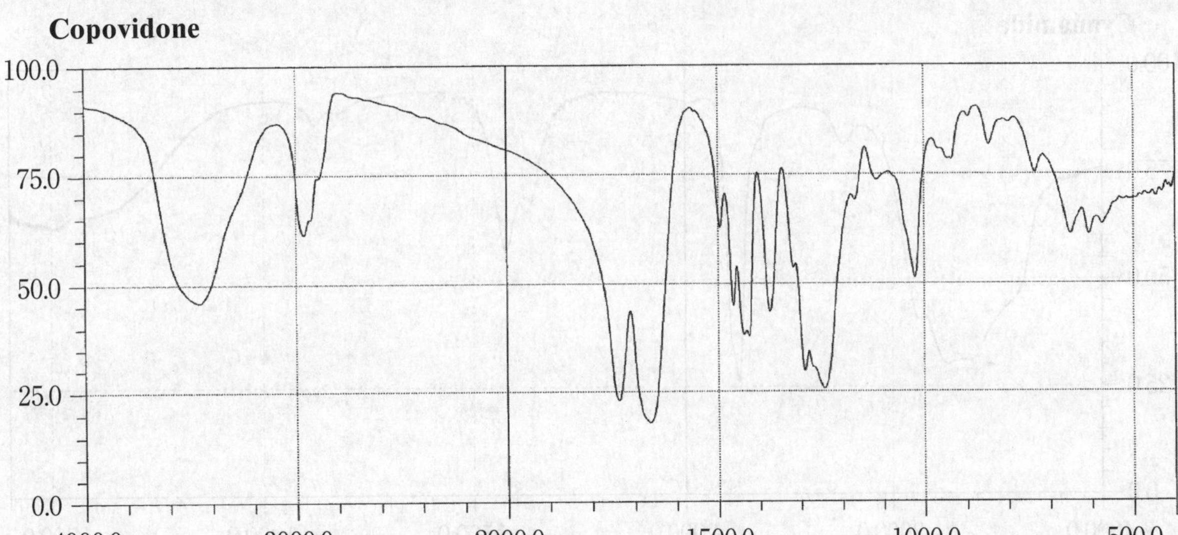

Cortisone Acetate

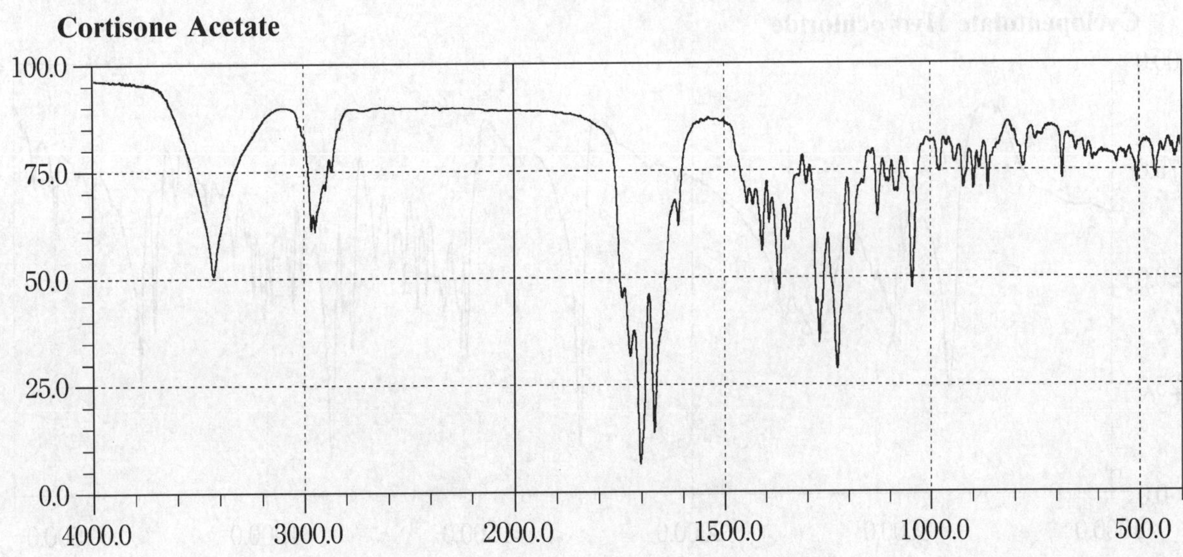

Croconazole Hydrochloride

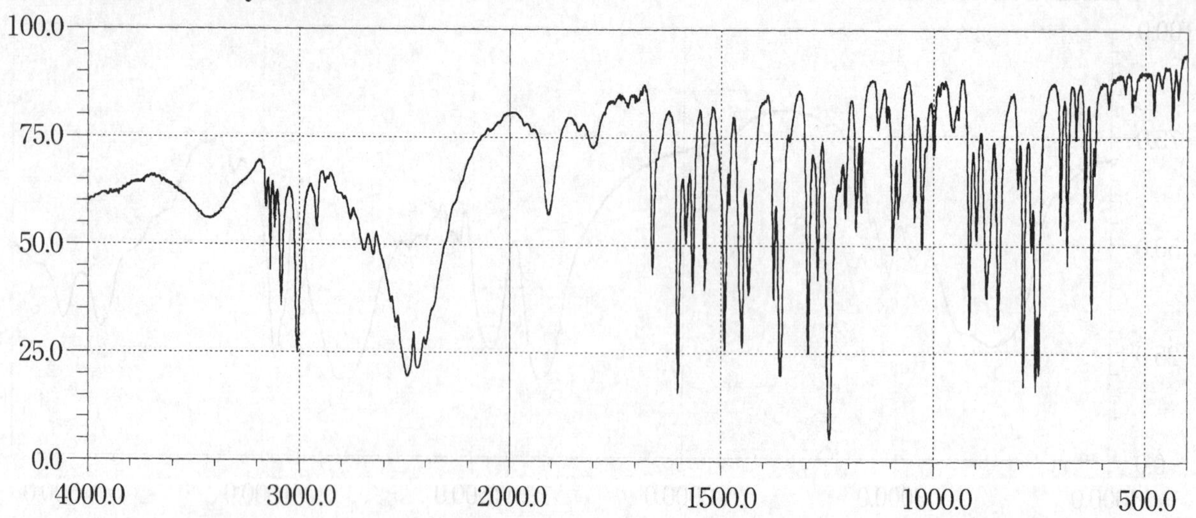

Cyanamide

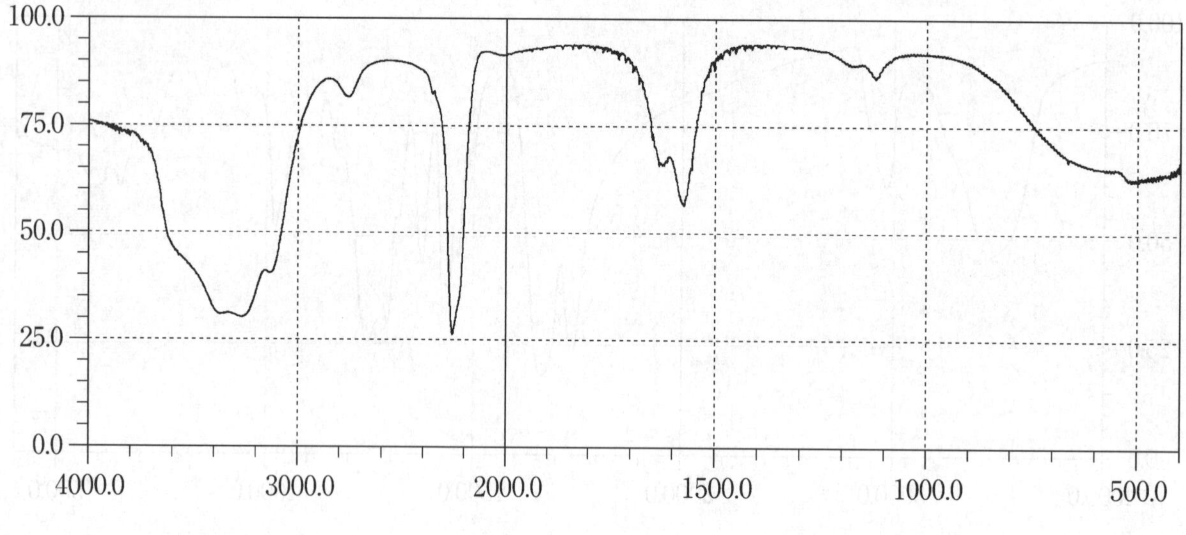

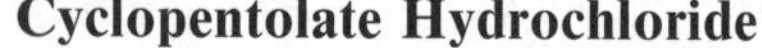

Cyclopentolate Hydrochloride

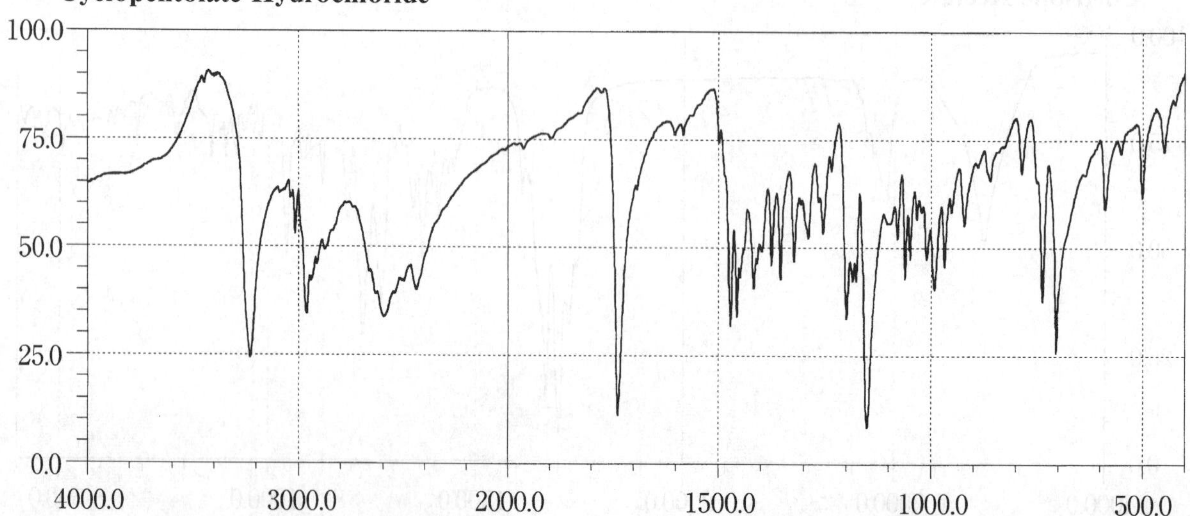

Cycloserine

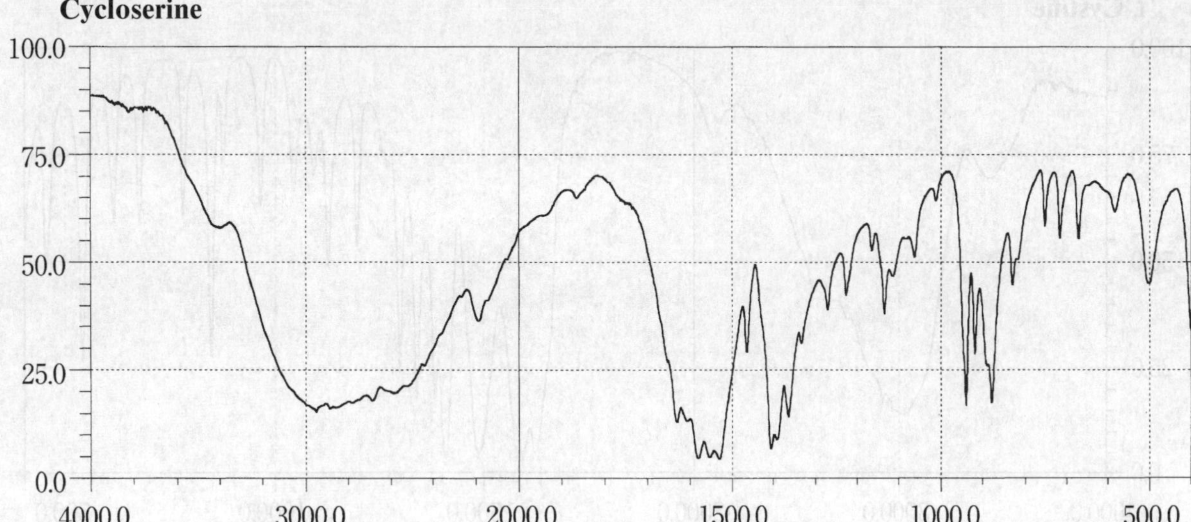

L-Cysteine

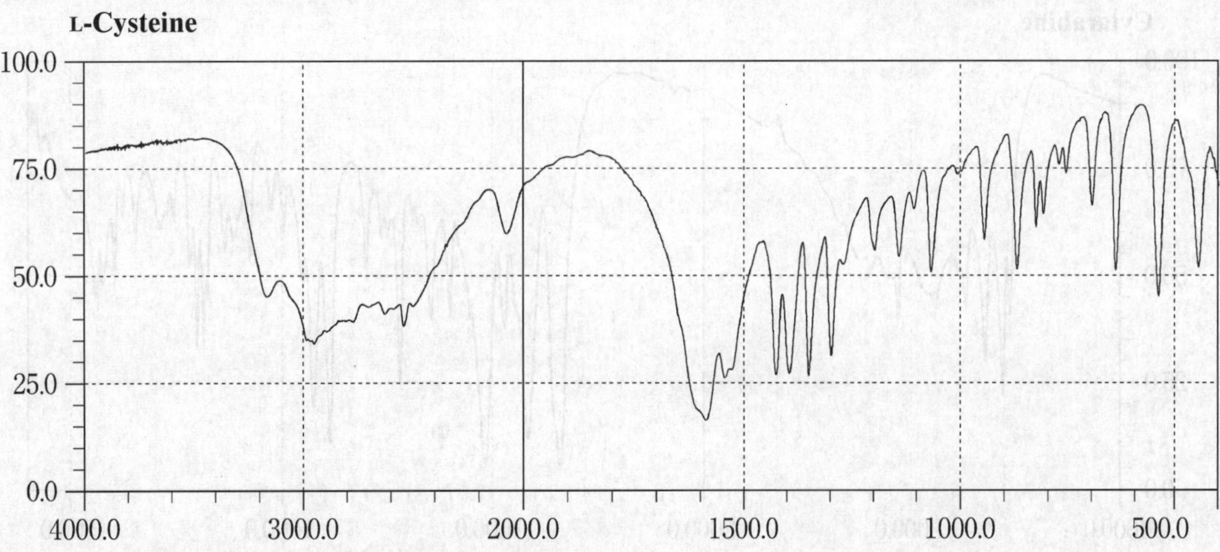

L-Cysteine Hydrochloride Hydrate

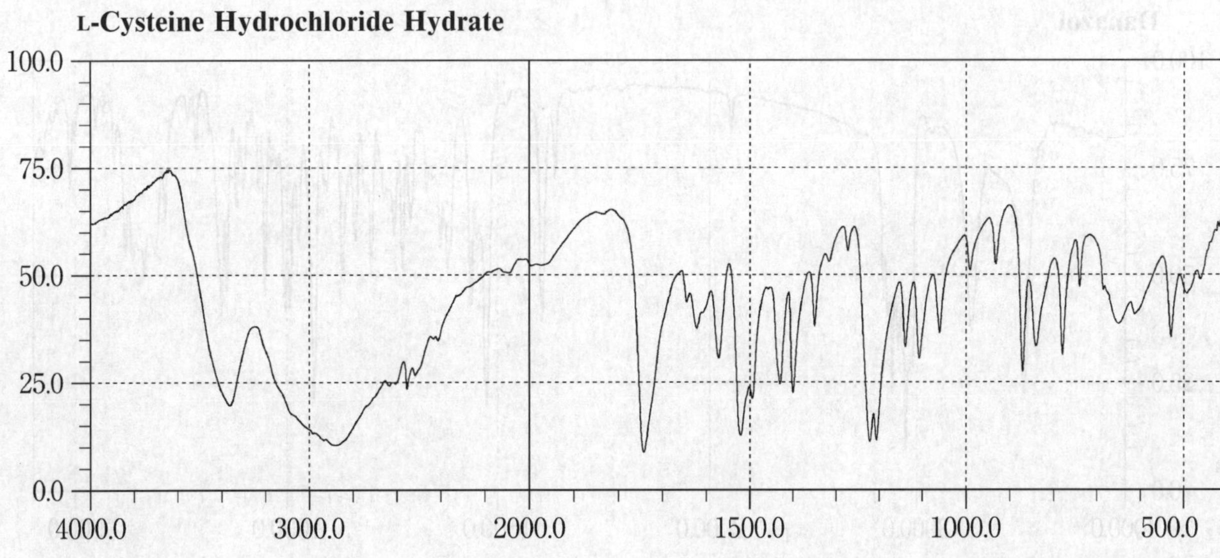

L-Cystine

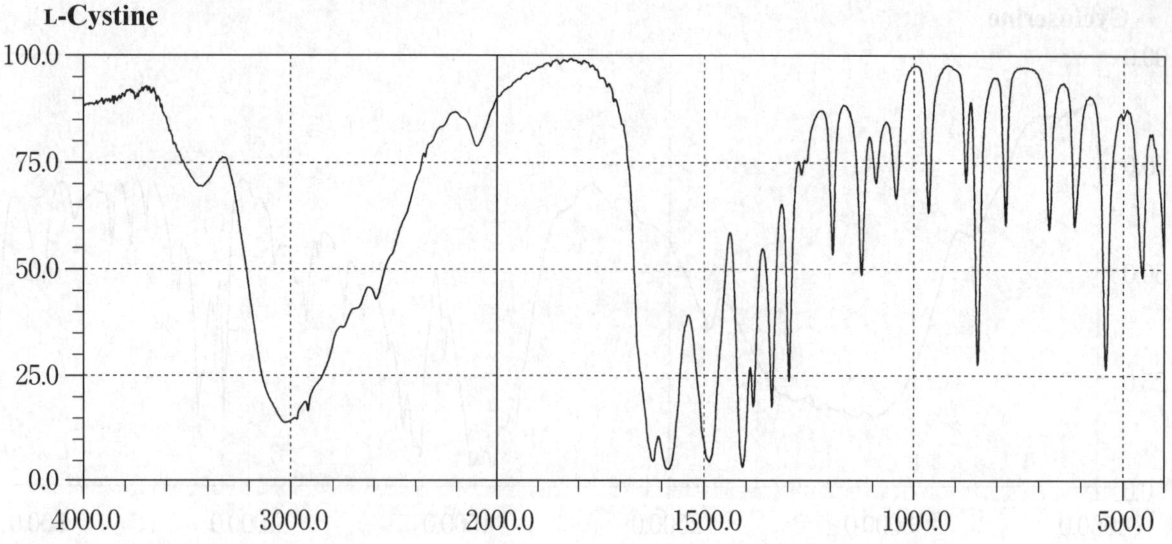

Cytarabine

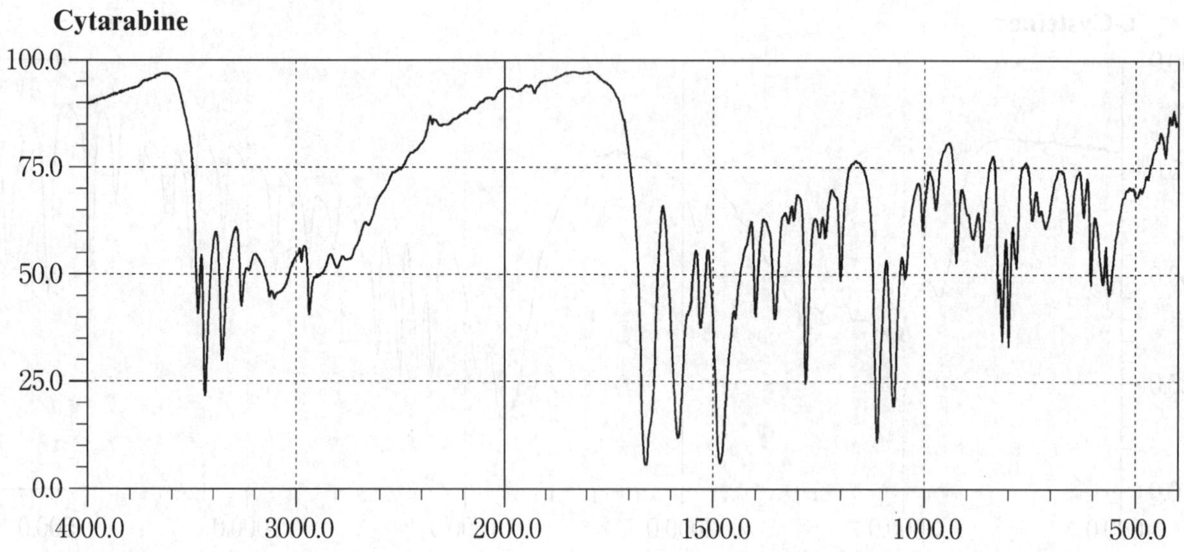

Danazol

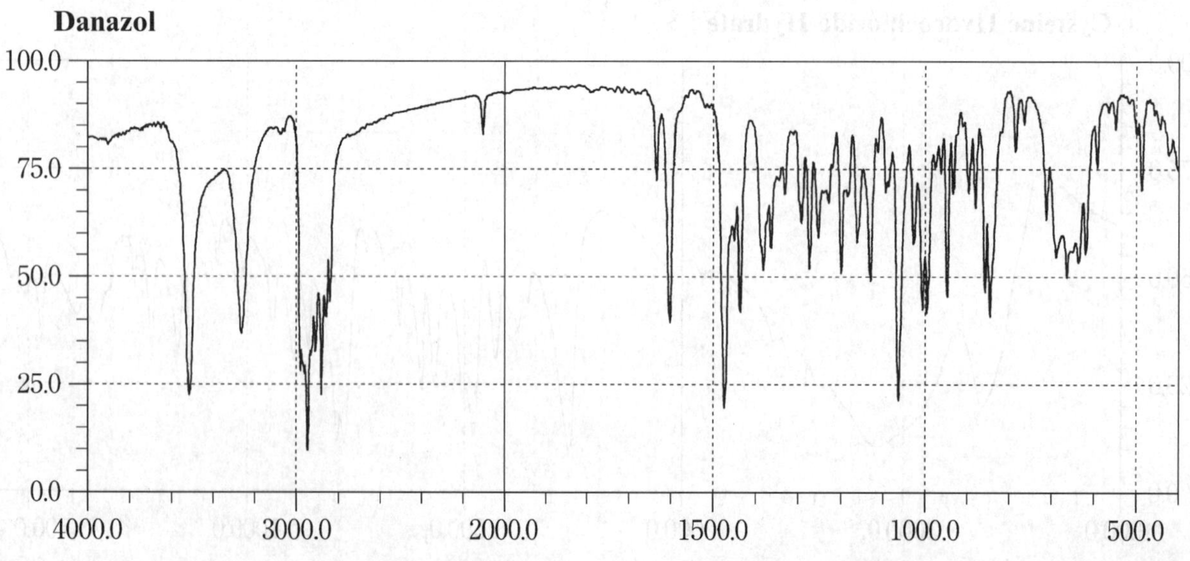

Dantrolene Sodium Hydrate

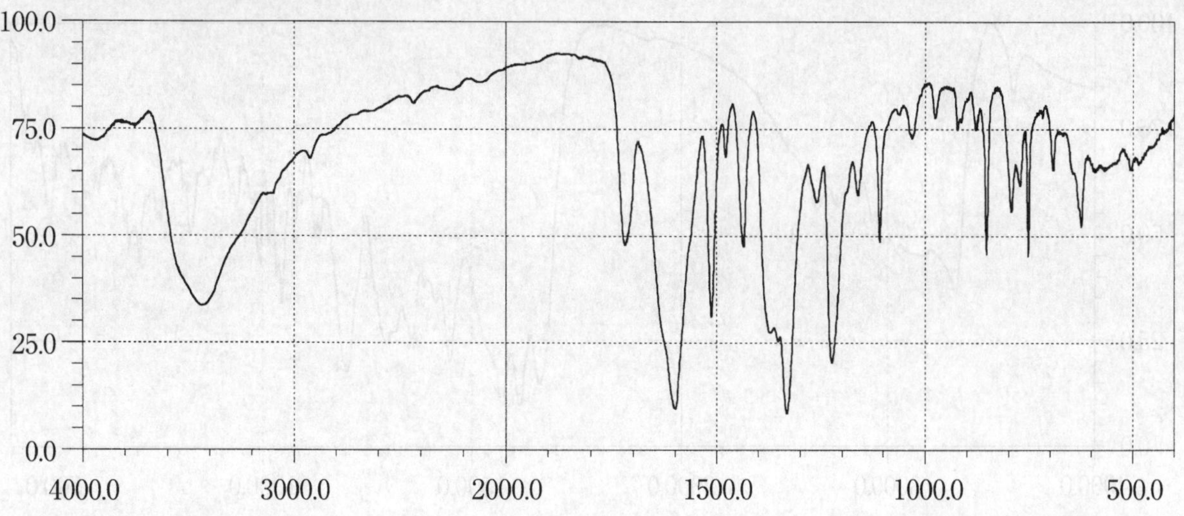

Daunorubicin Hydrochloride

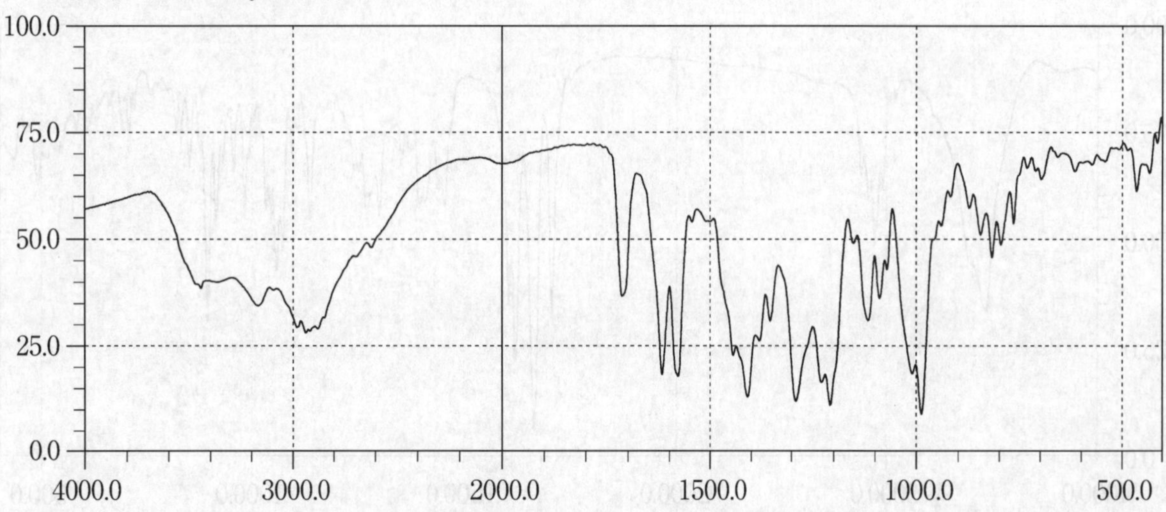

Deferoxamine Mesilate

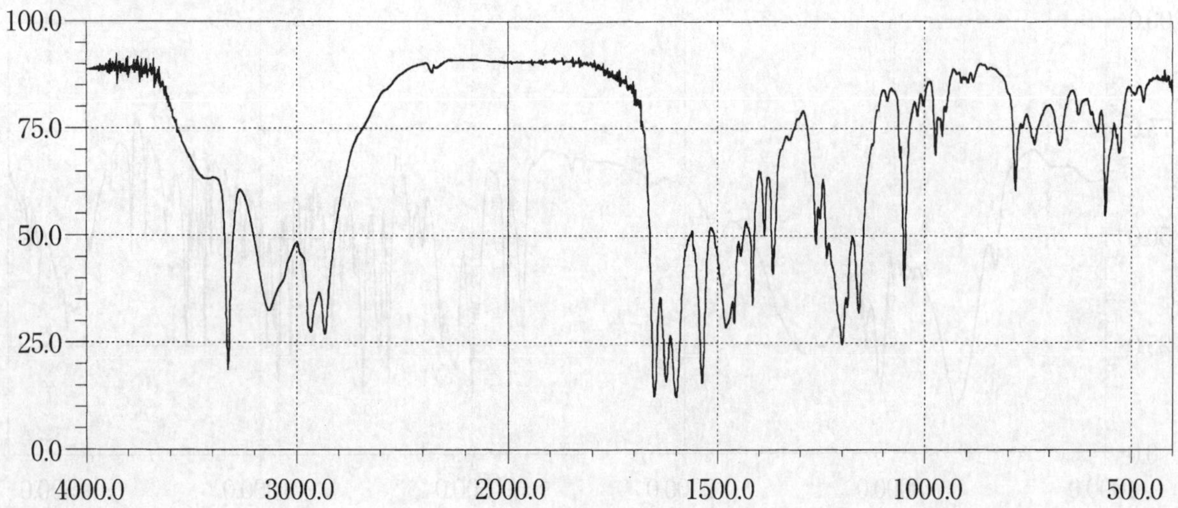

Demethylchlortetracycline Hydrochloride

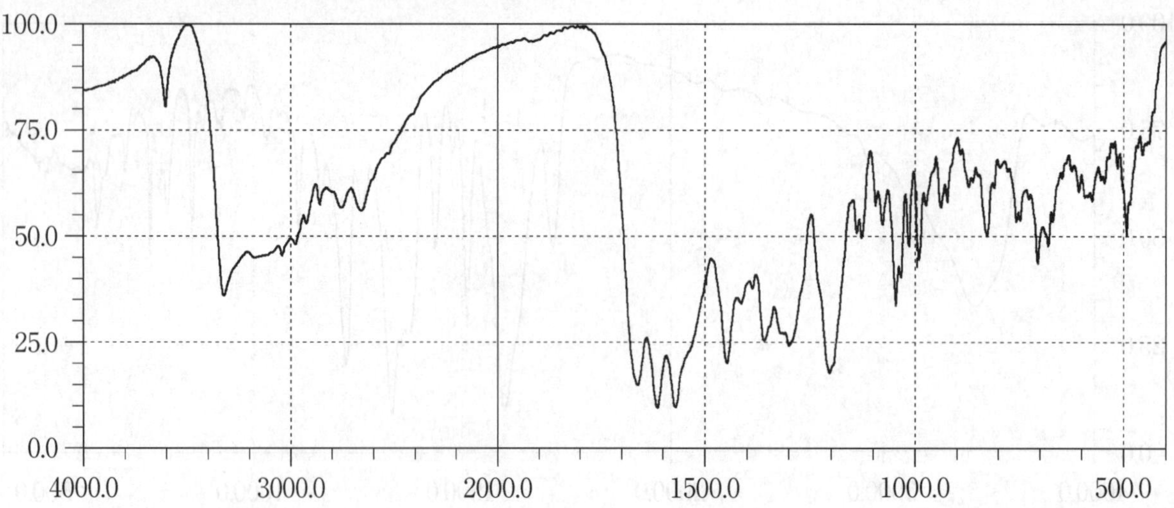

Dexamethasone

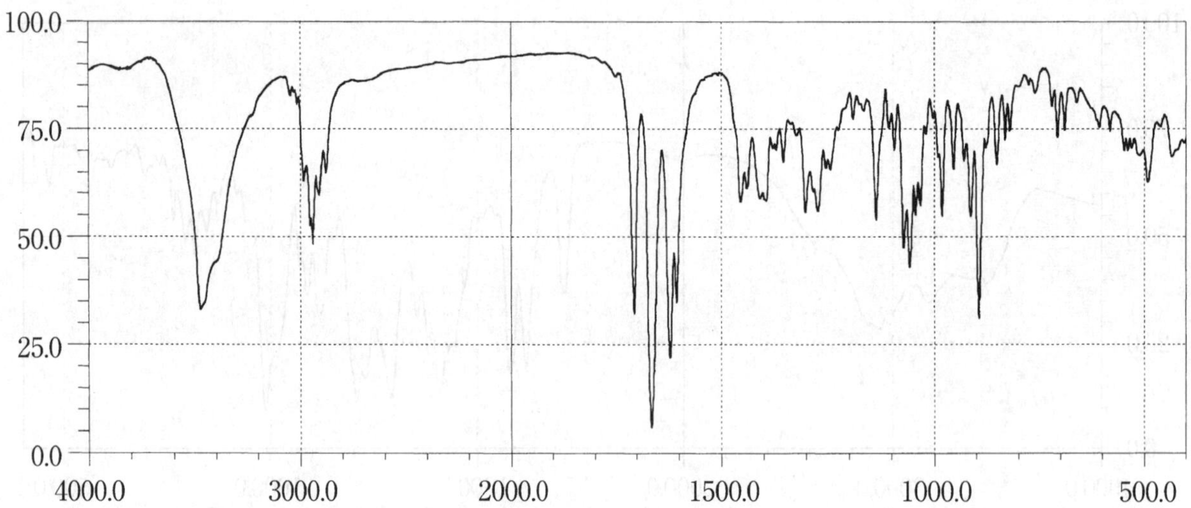

Dextromethorphan Hydrobromide Hydrate

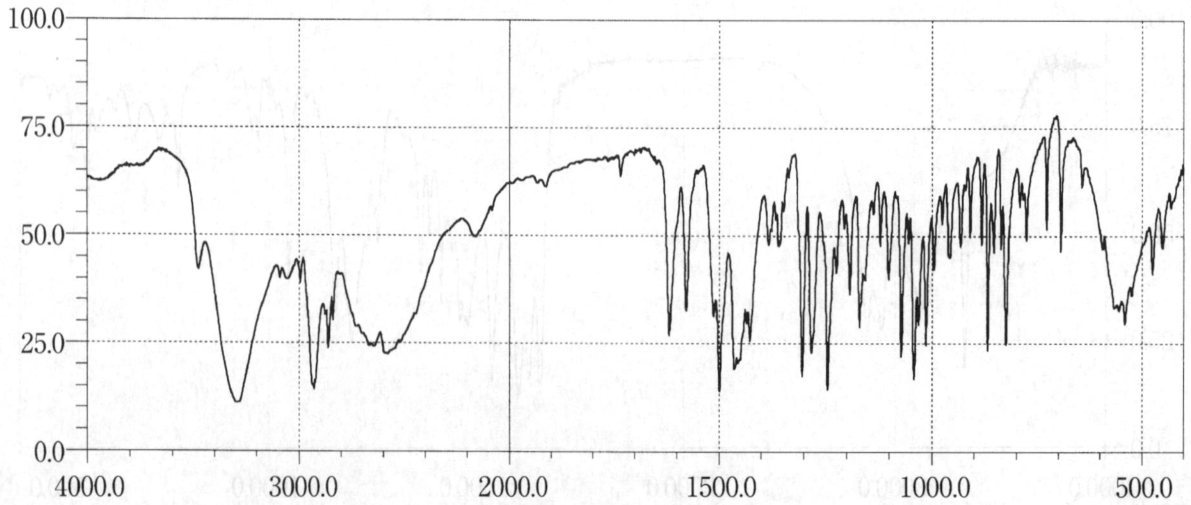

Diazepam

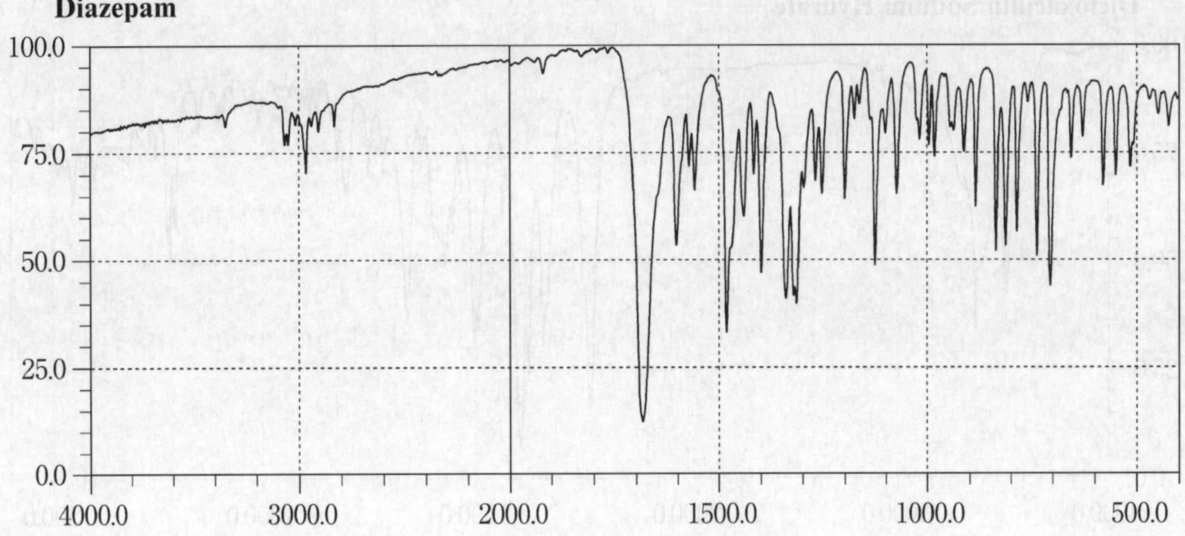

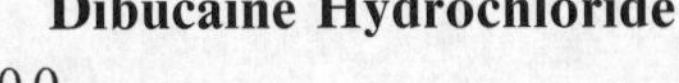
Dibucaine Hydrochloride

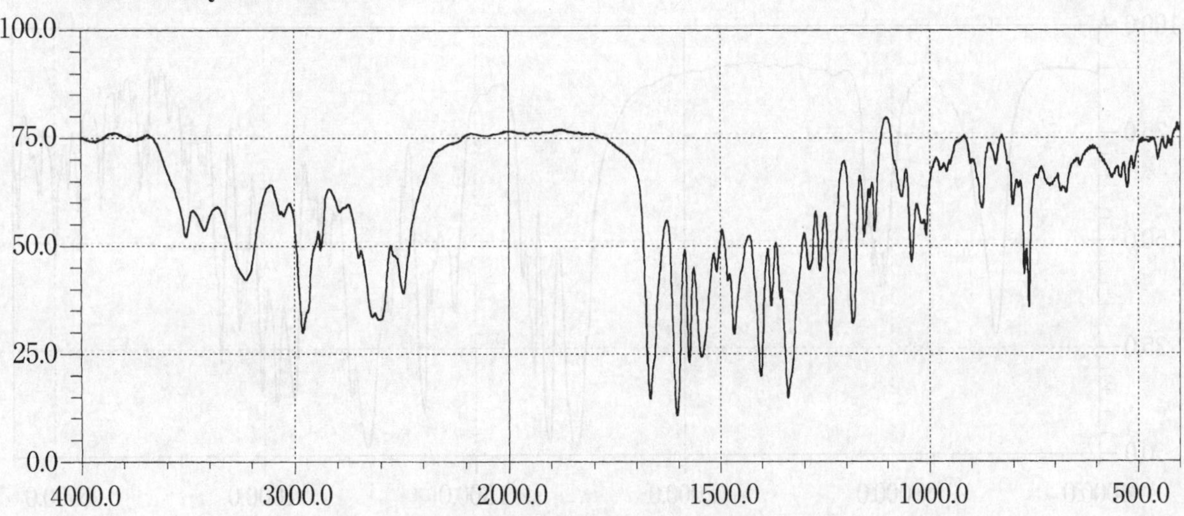

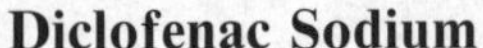
Diclofenac Sodium

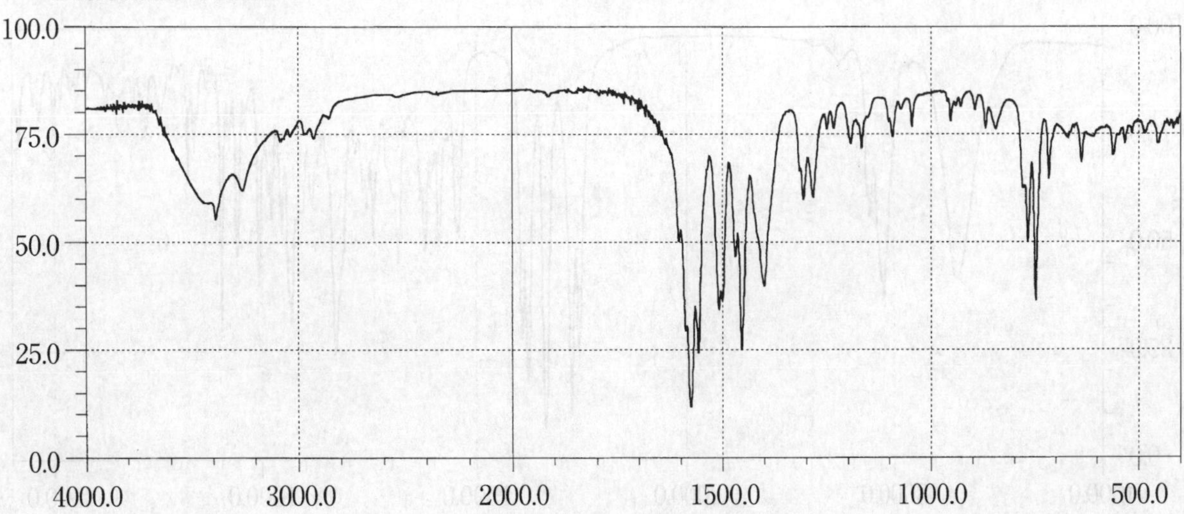

Dicloxacillin Sodium Hydrate

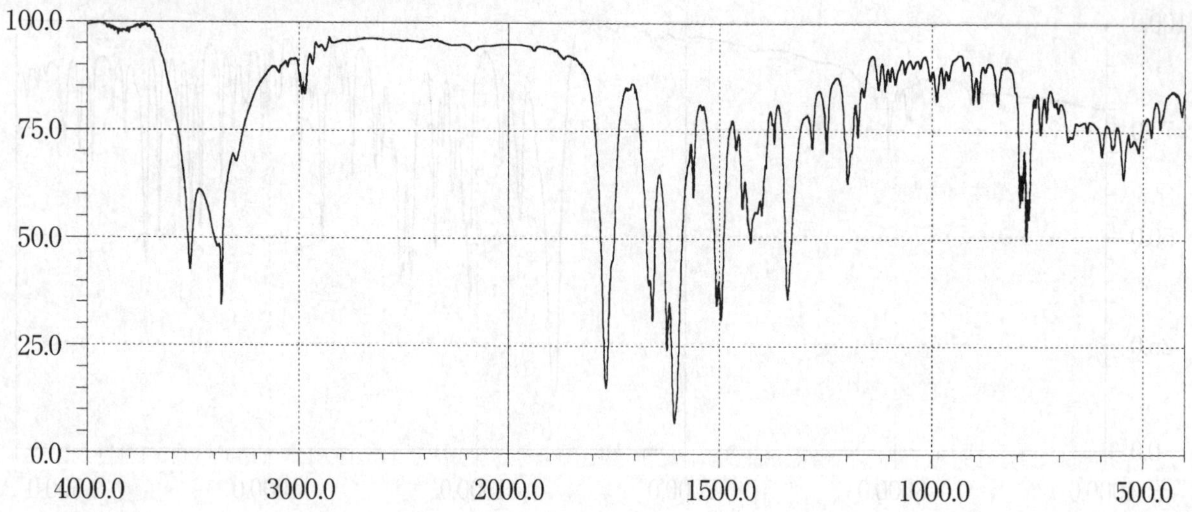

Diflorasone Diacetate

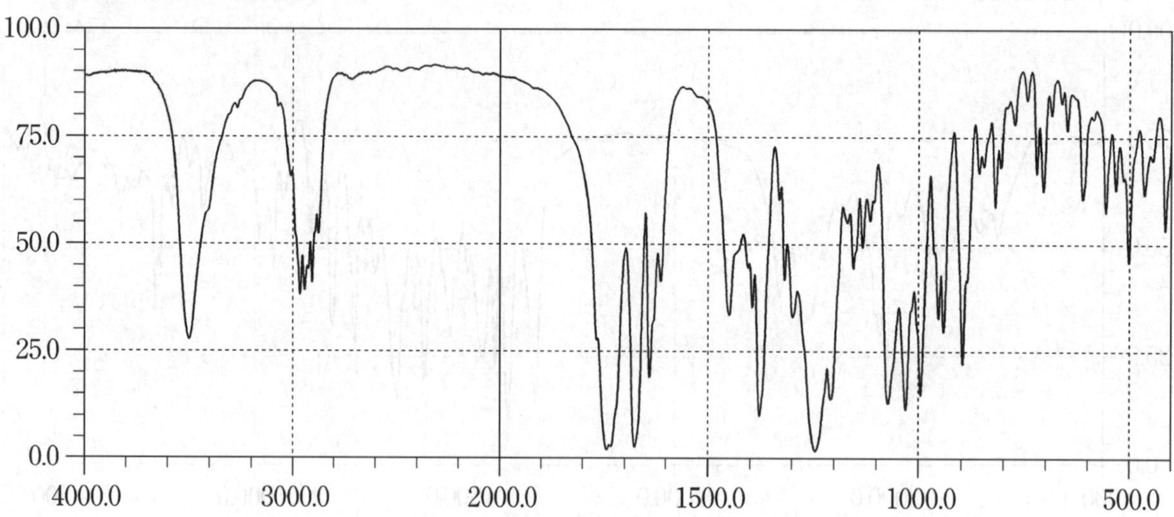

Diflucortolone Valerate

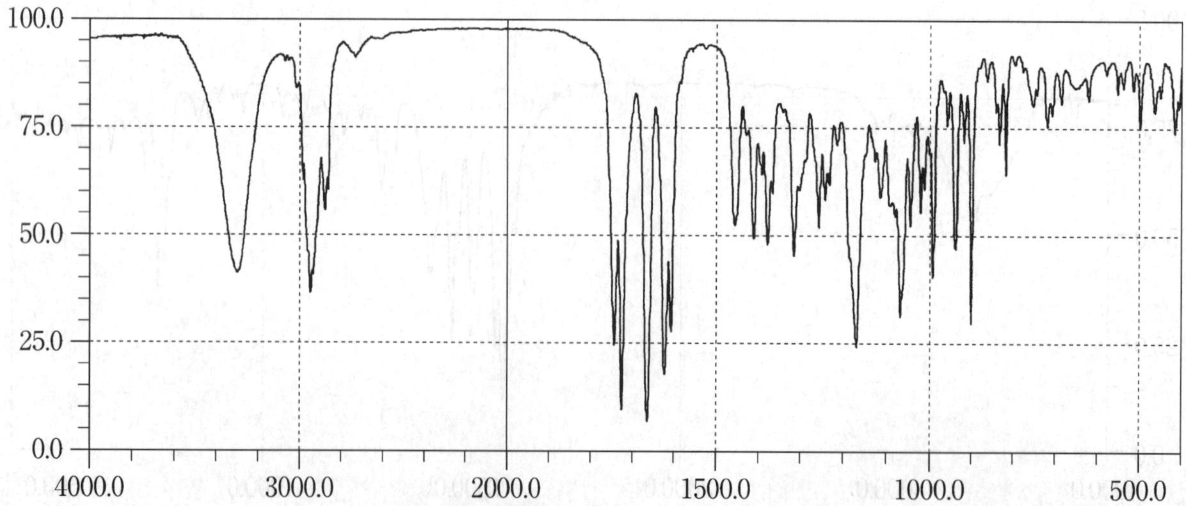

Digoxin

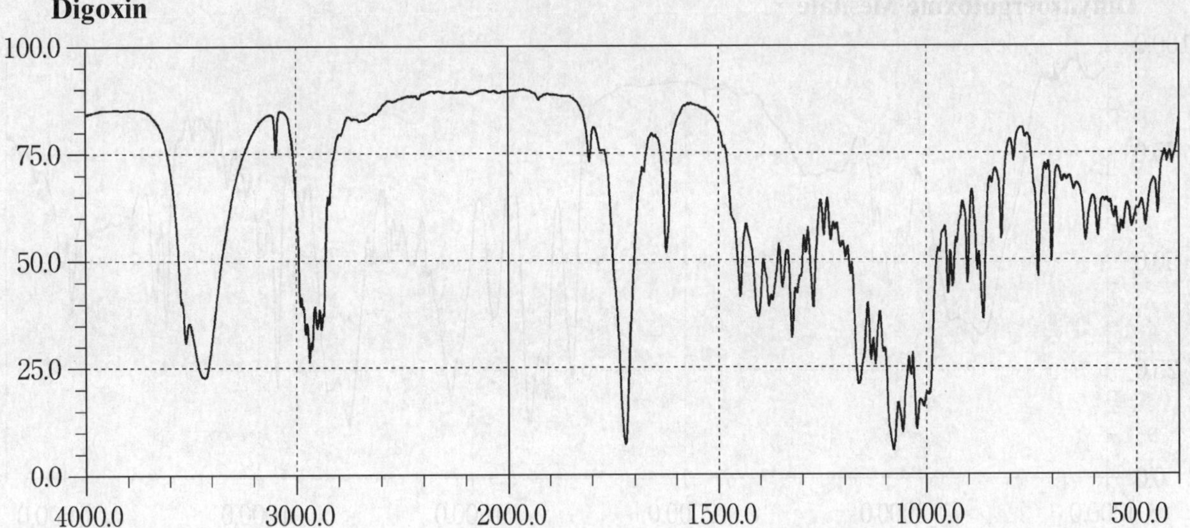

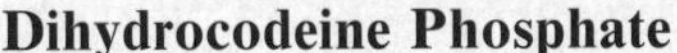

Dihydrocodeine Phosphate

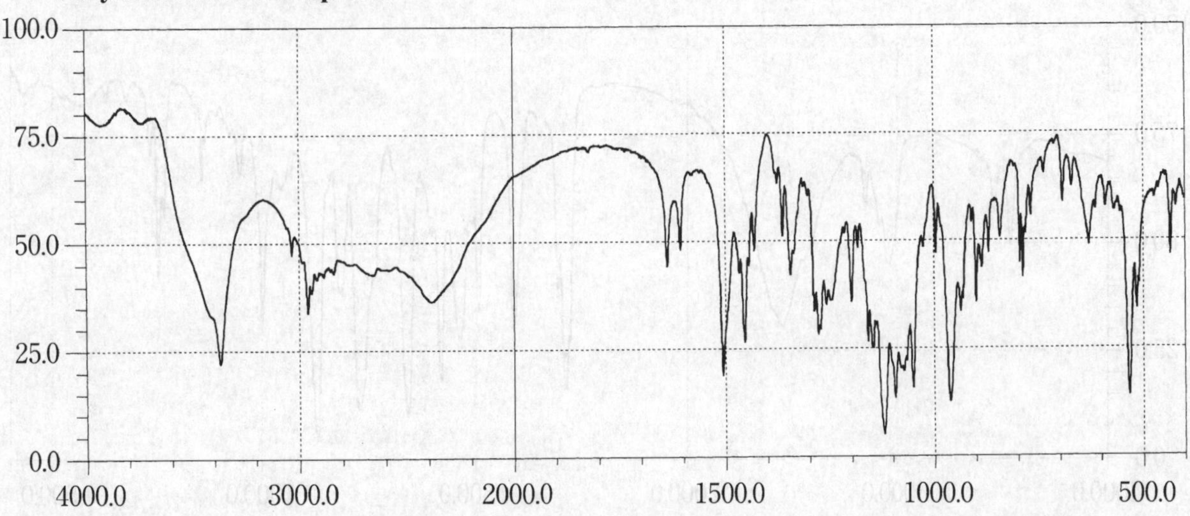

Dihydroergotamine Mesilate

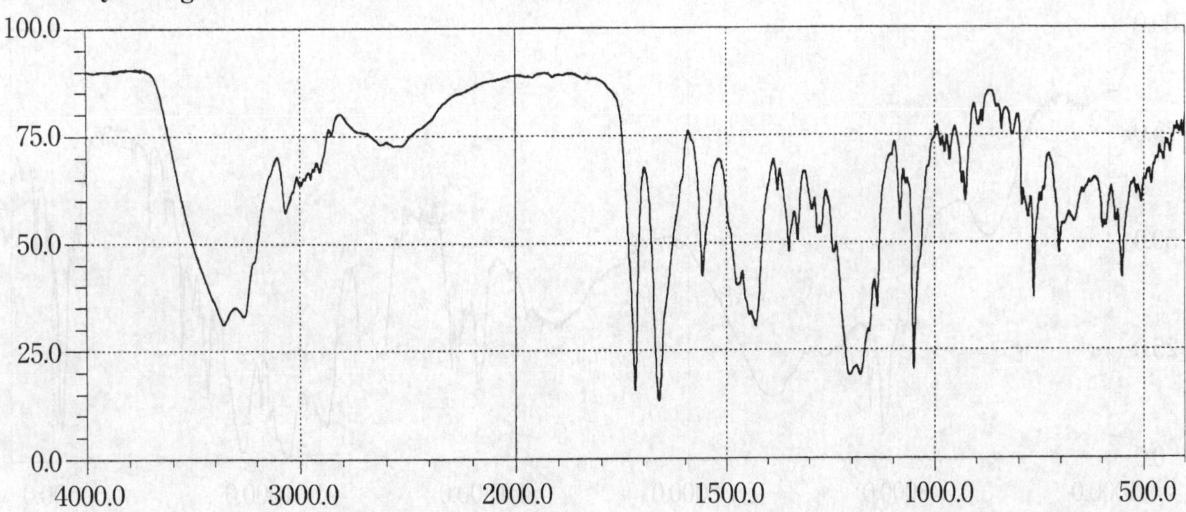

Dihydroergotoxine Mesilate

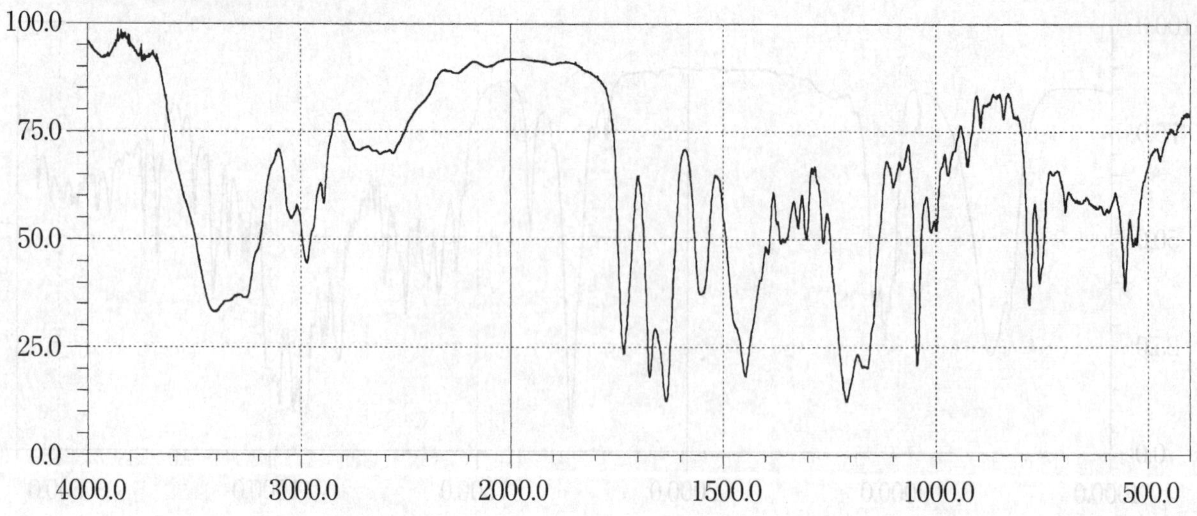

Dilazep Hydrochloride Hydrate

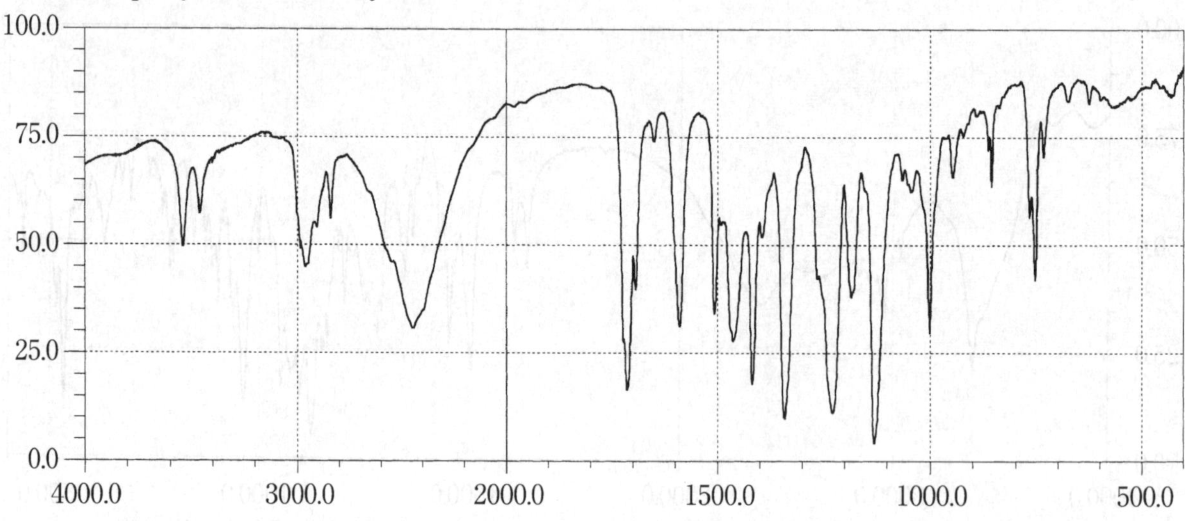

Dimemorfan Phosphate

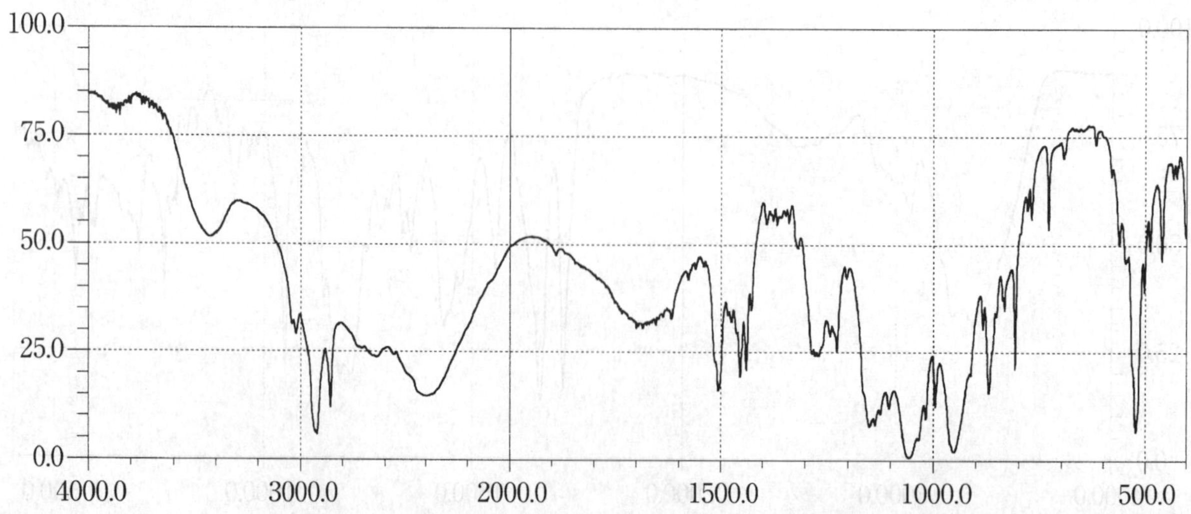

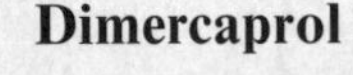

Dimercaprol

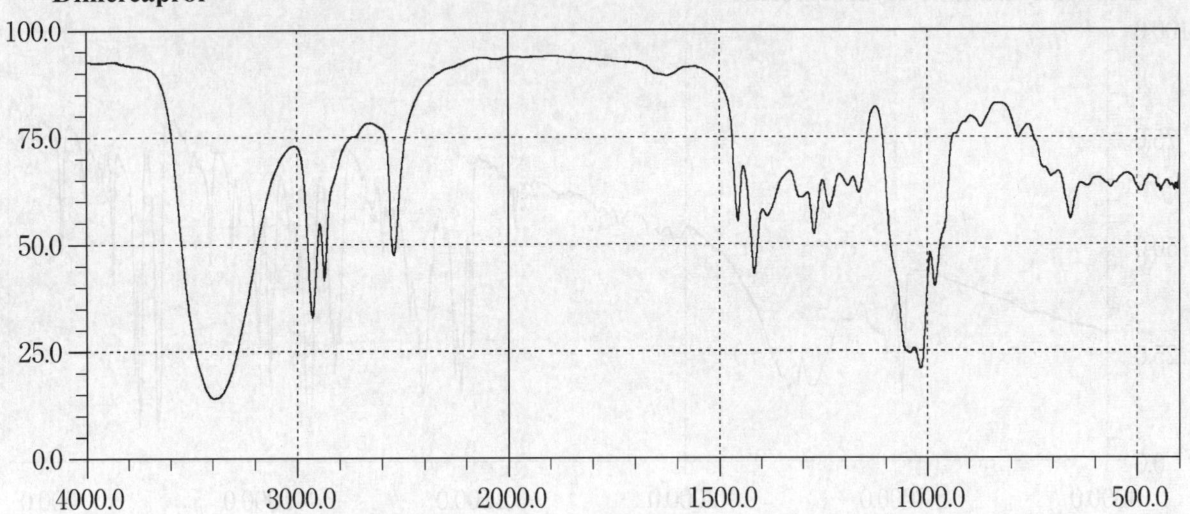

Dimorpholamine

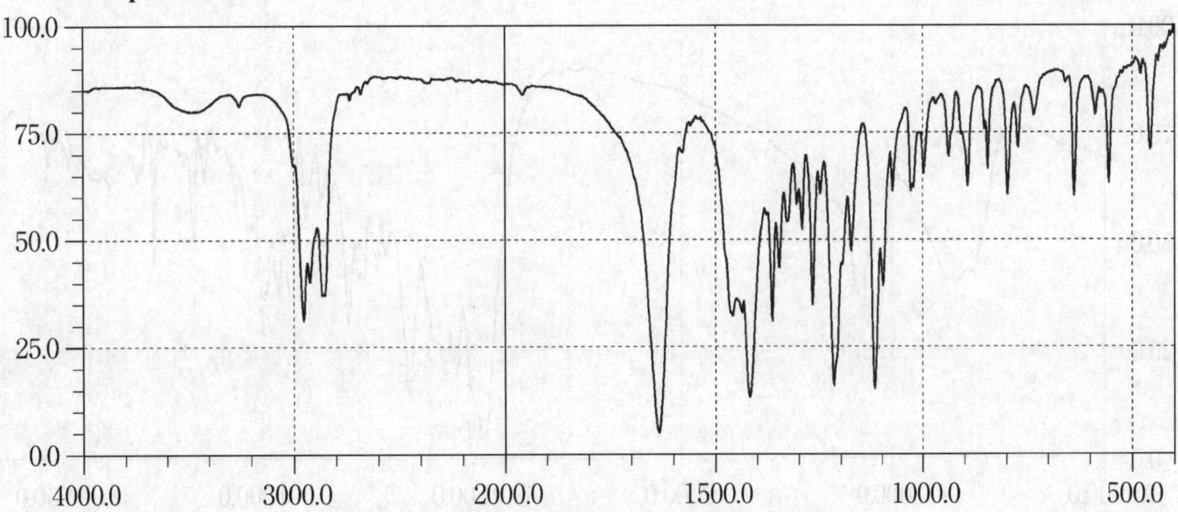

Dinoprost

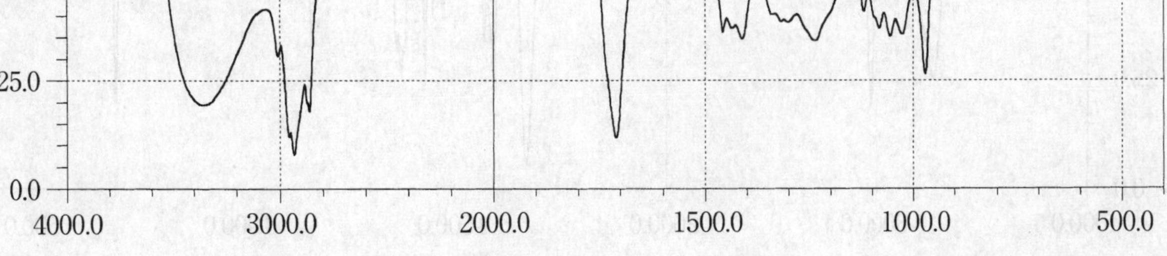

Diphenhydramine Hydrochloride

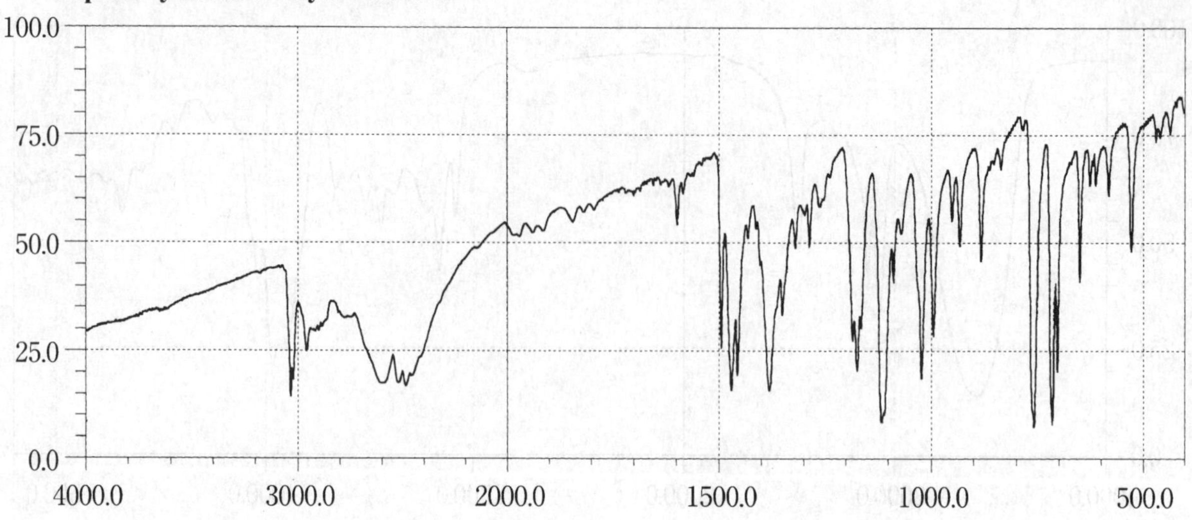

Dipyridamole

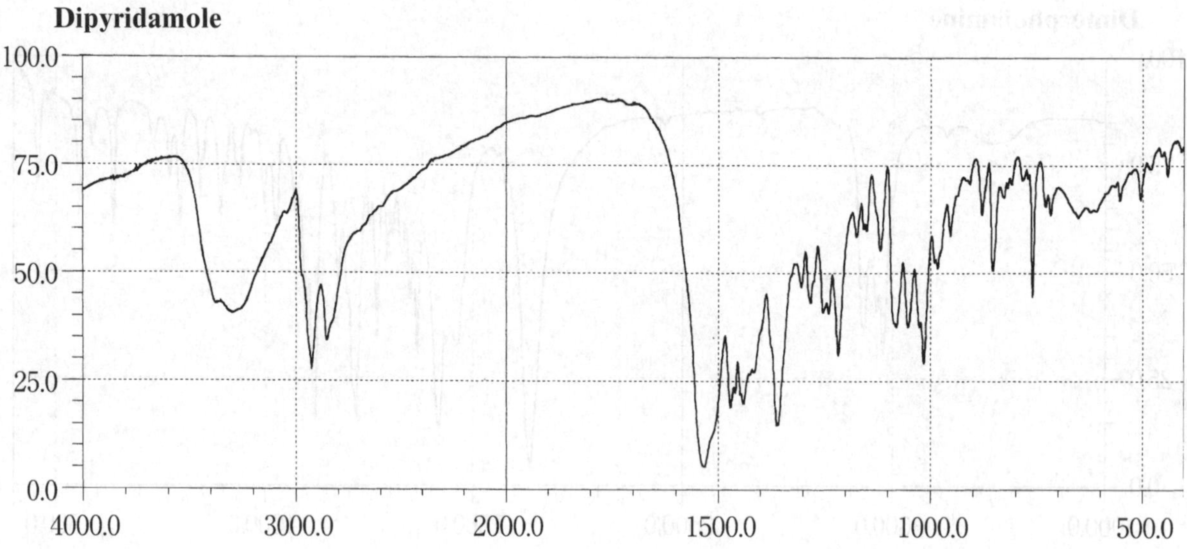

Disopyramide

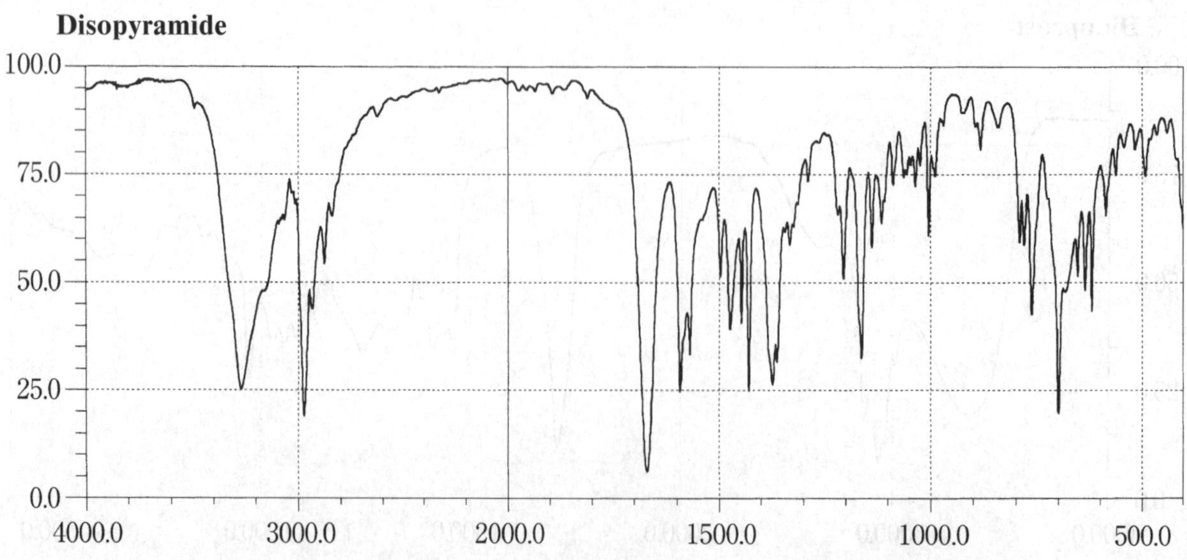

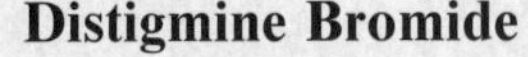

Distigmine Bromide

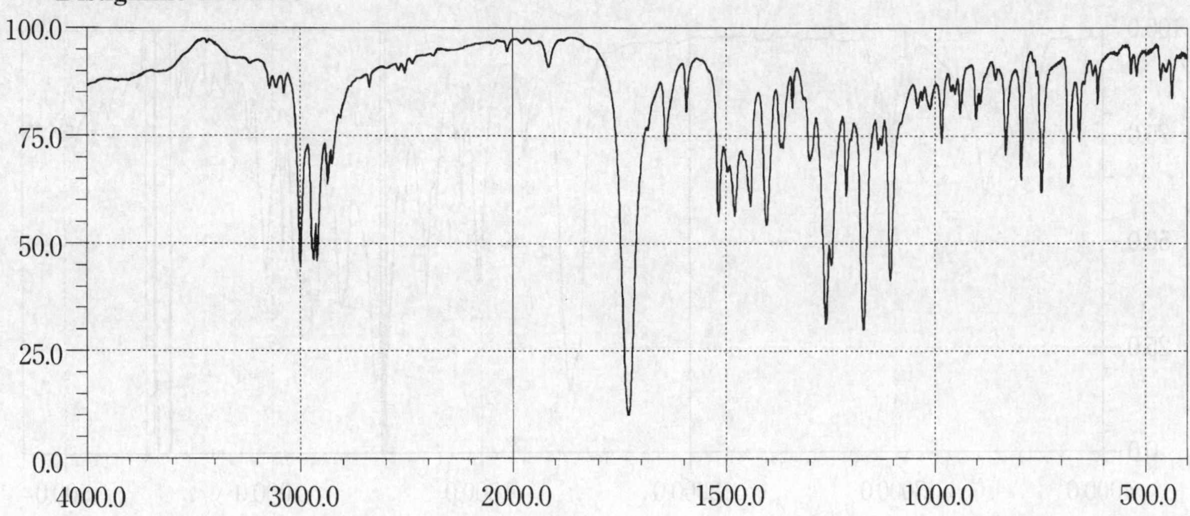

Disulfiram

Dobutamine Hydrochloride

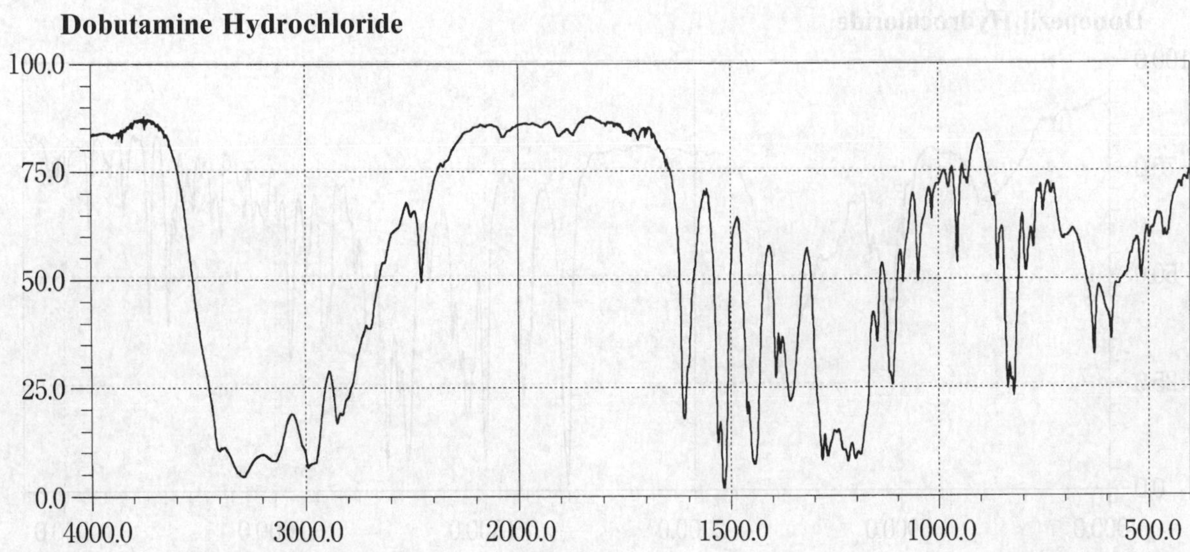

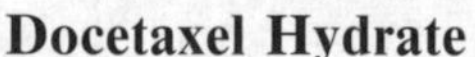

Docetaxel Hydrate

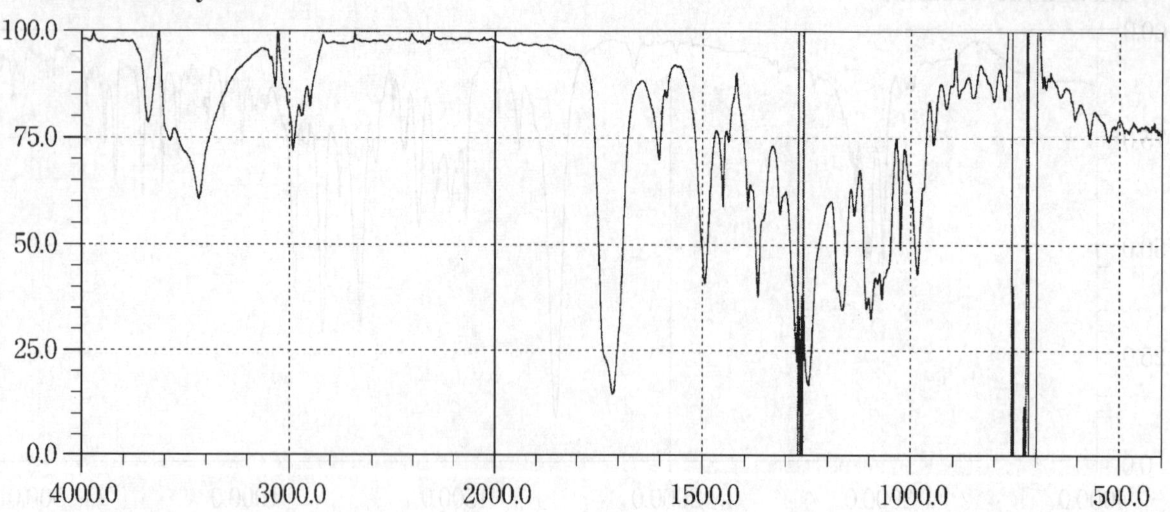

Domperidone

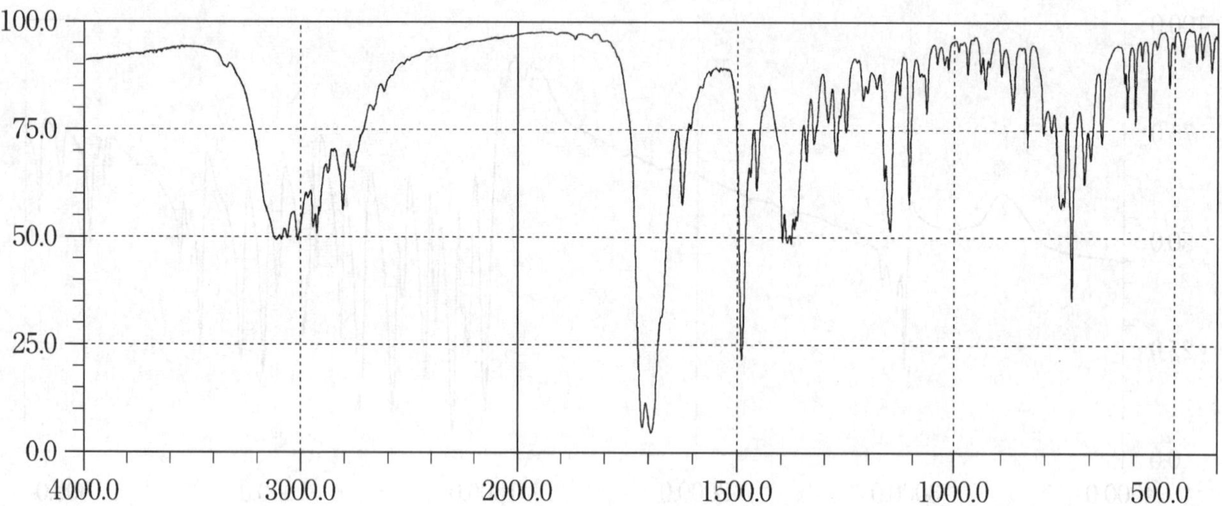

Donepezil Hydrochloride

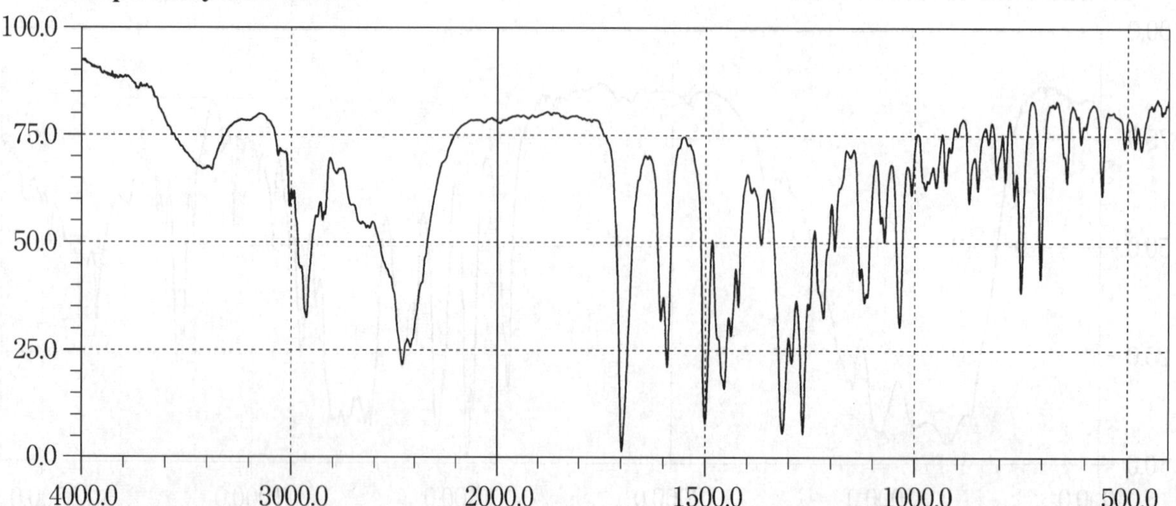

Dopamine Hydrochloride

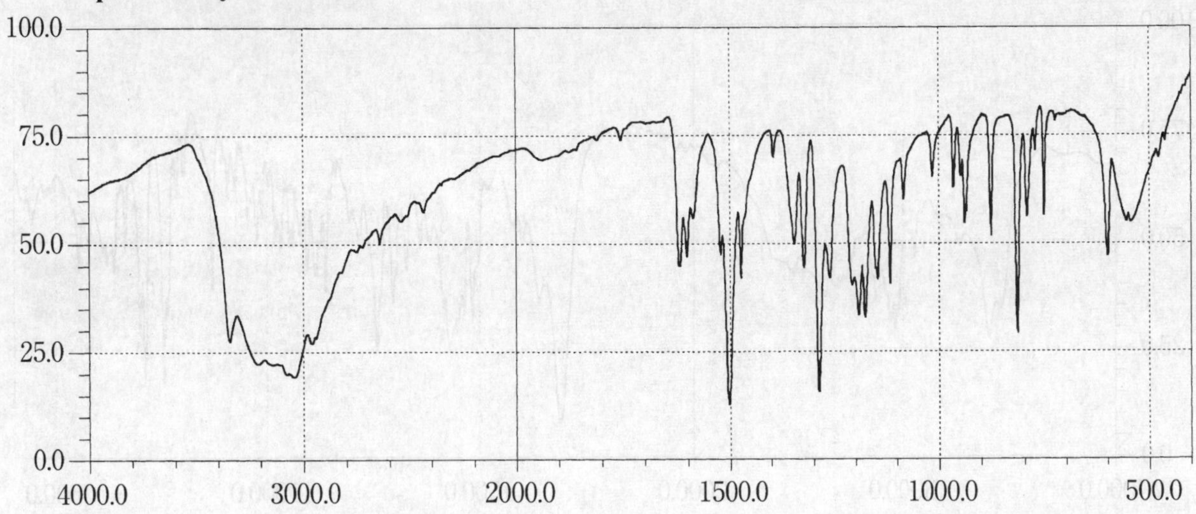

Doripenem Hydrate

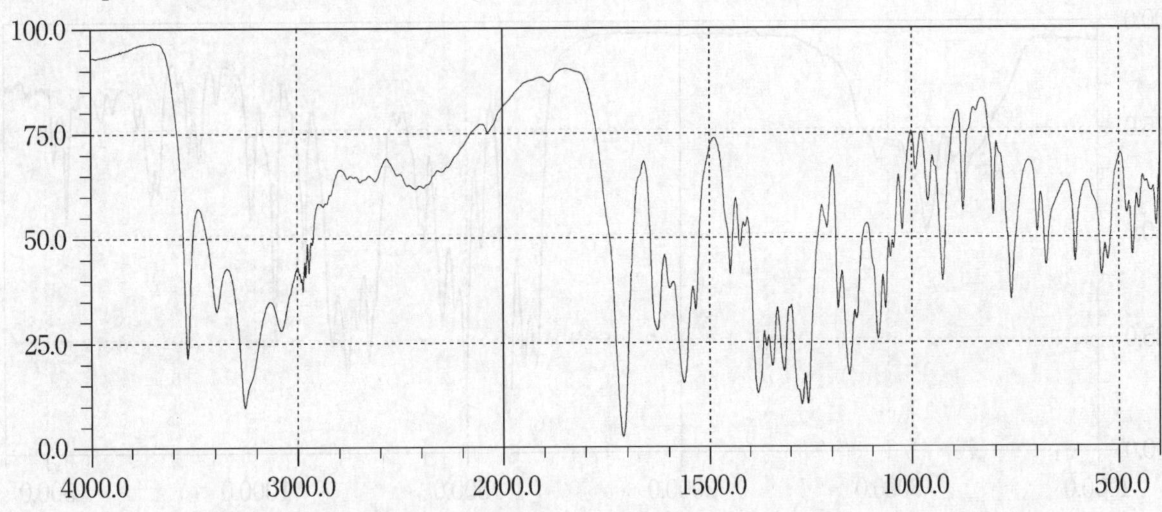

Dorzolamide Hydrochloride

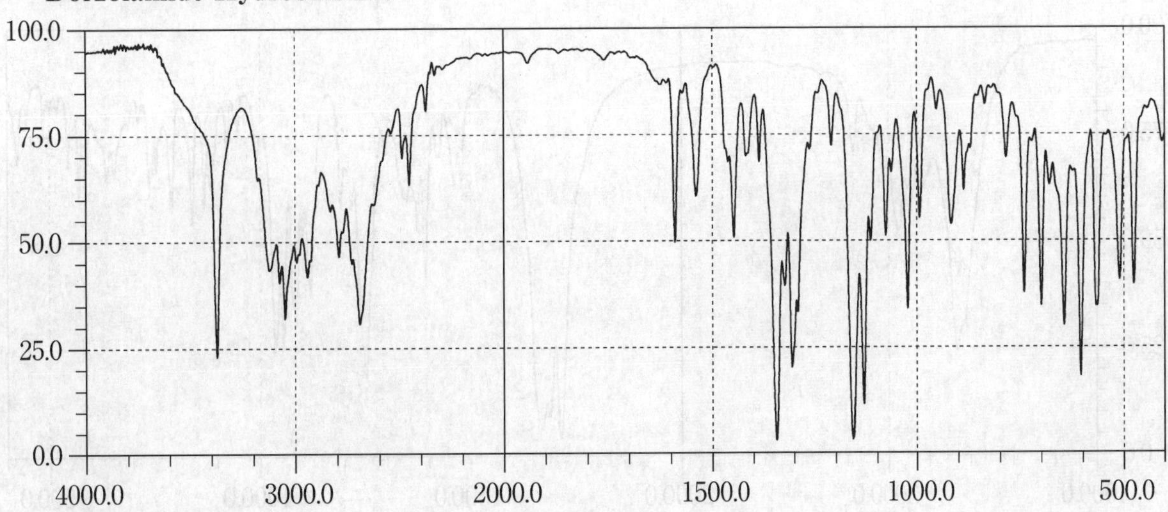

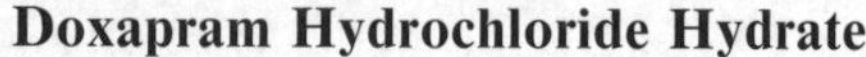

Doxapram Hydrochloride Hydrate

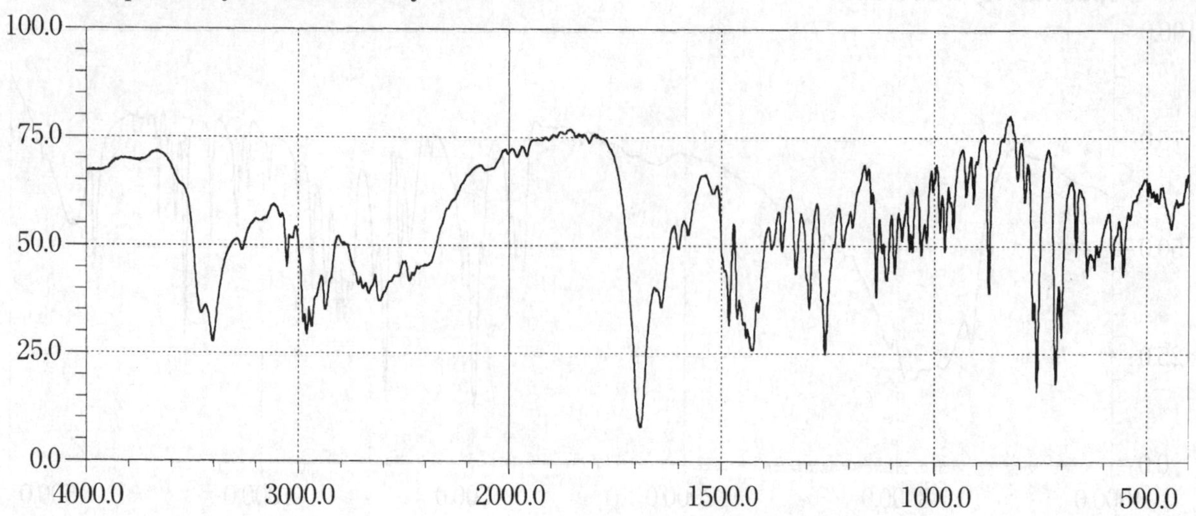

Doxazosin Mesilate

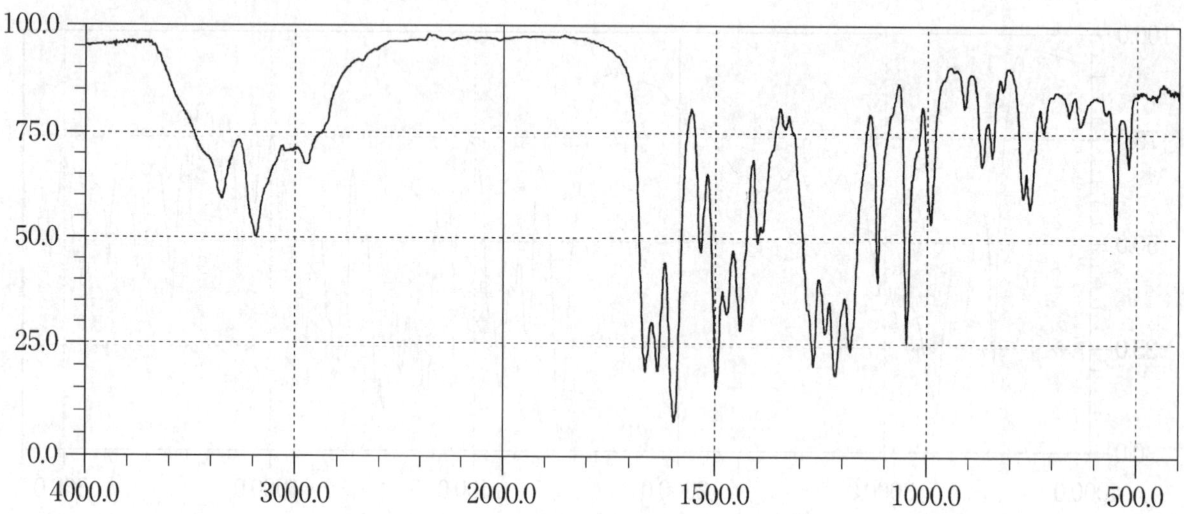

Doxifluridine

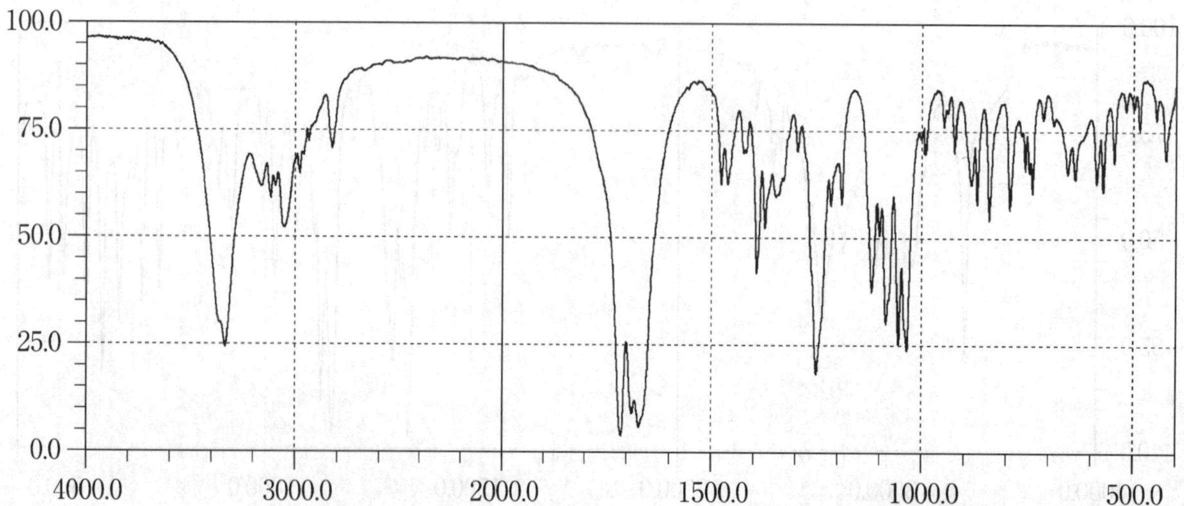

Doxorubicin Hydrochloride

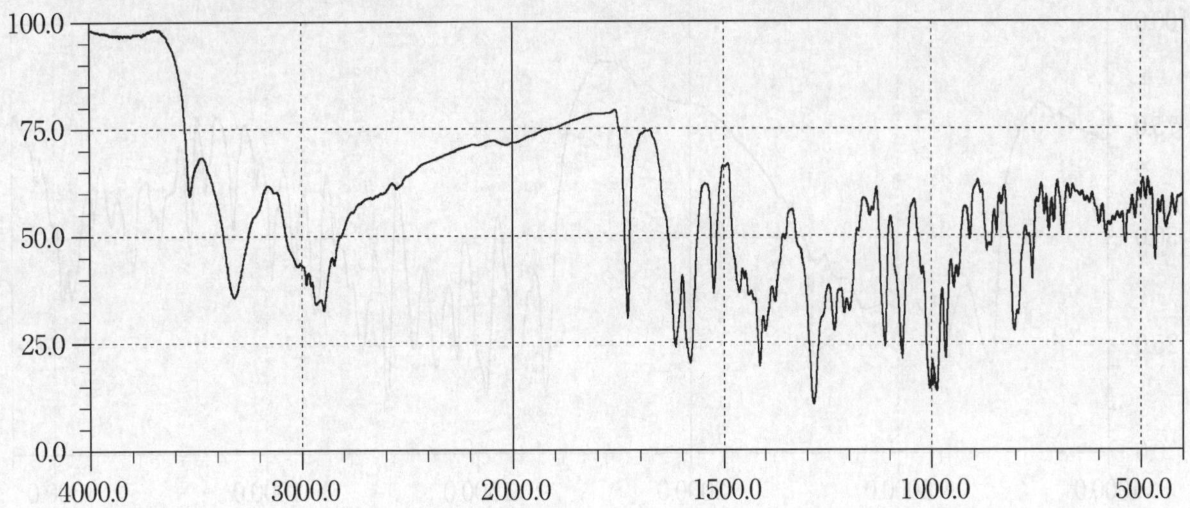

Doxycycline Hydrochloride Hydrate

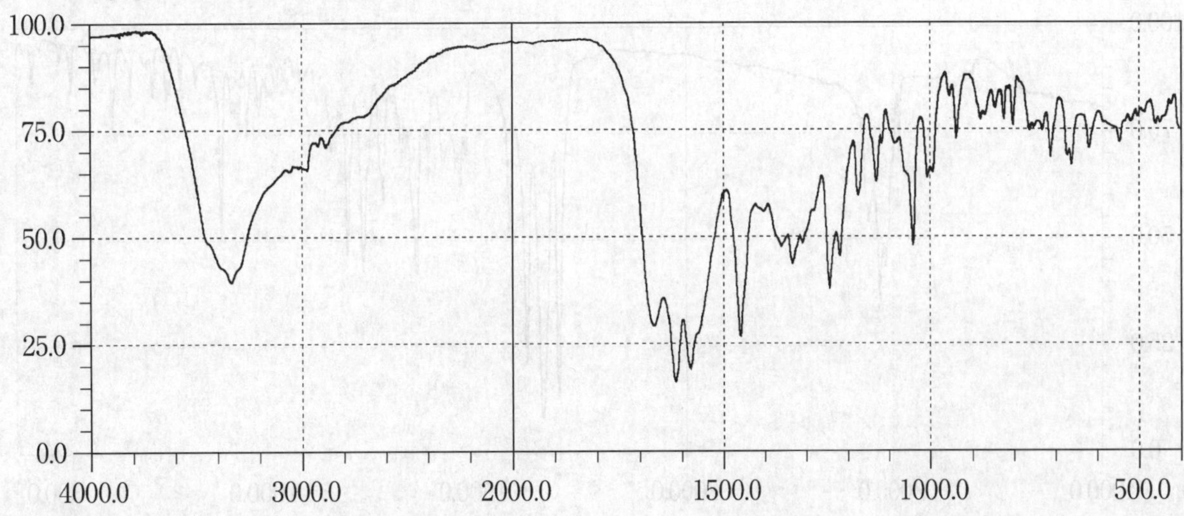

Droperidol

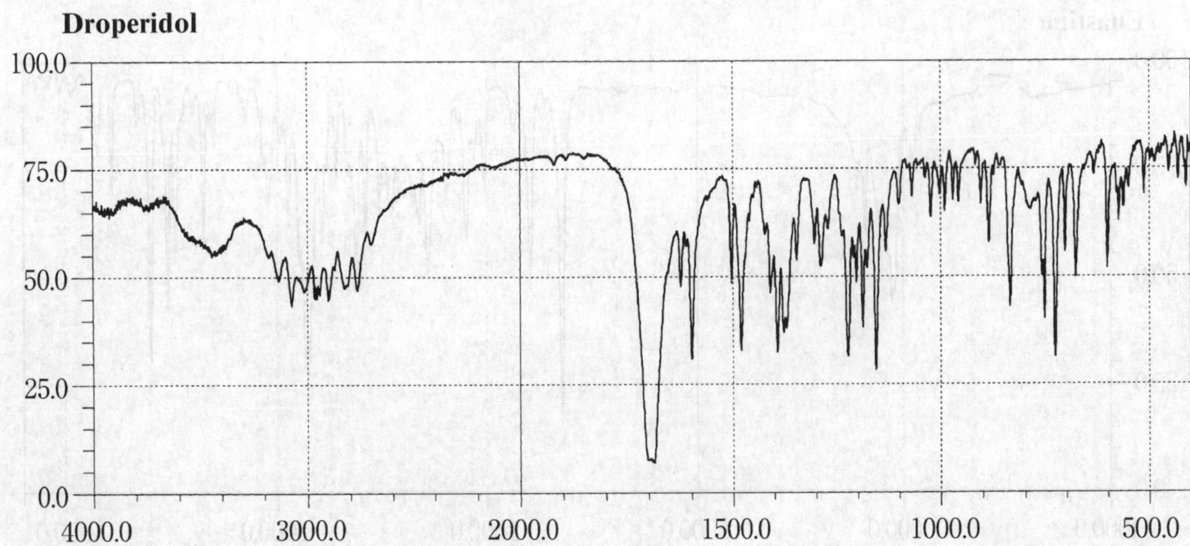

Droxidopa

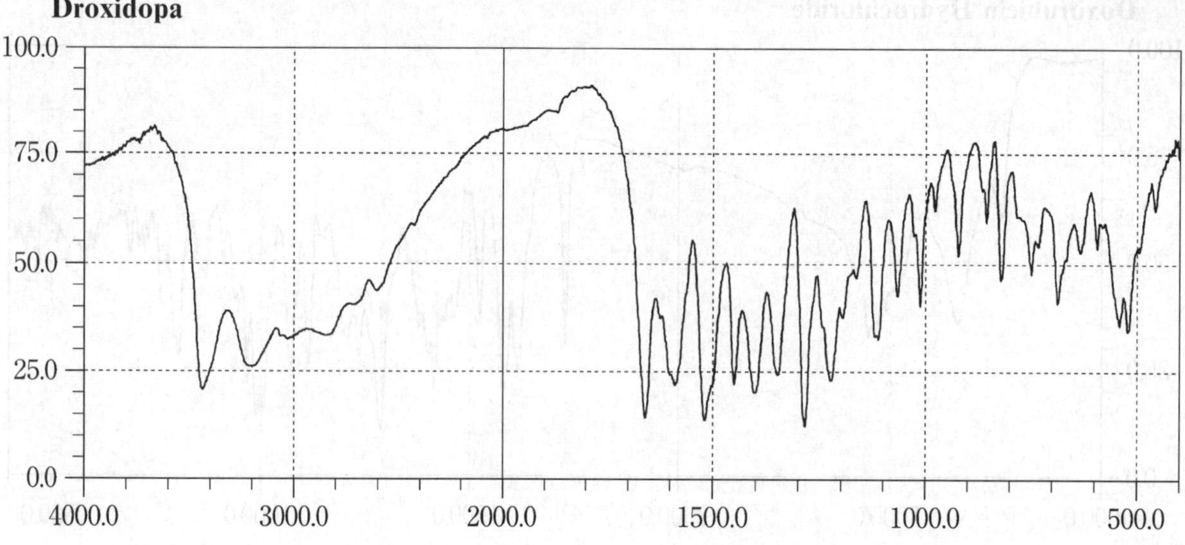

Dydrogesterone

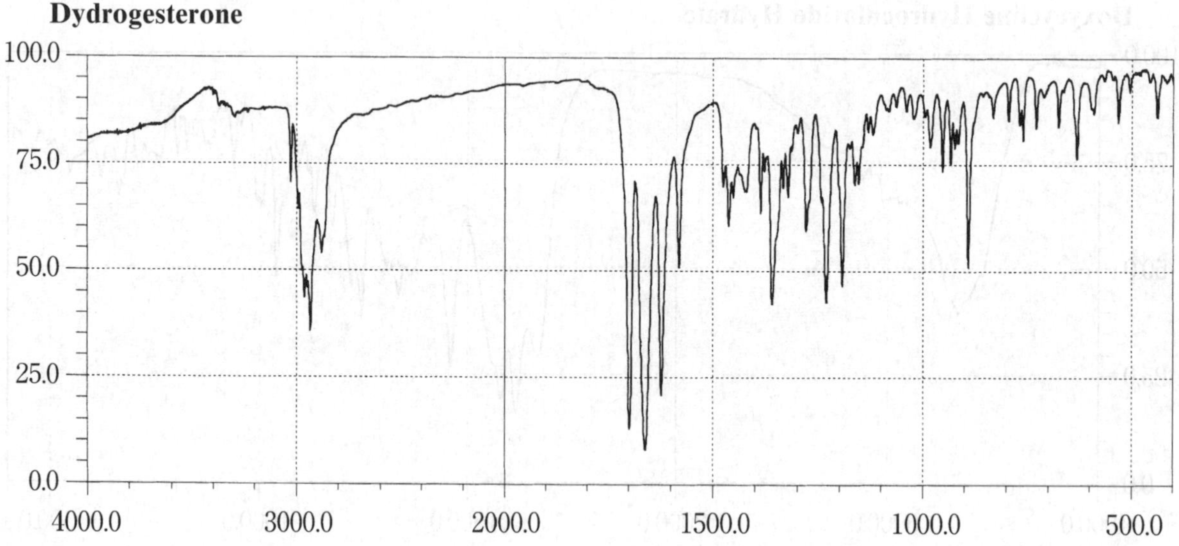

Ebastine

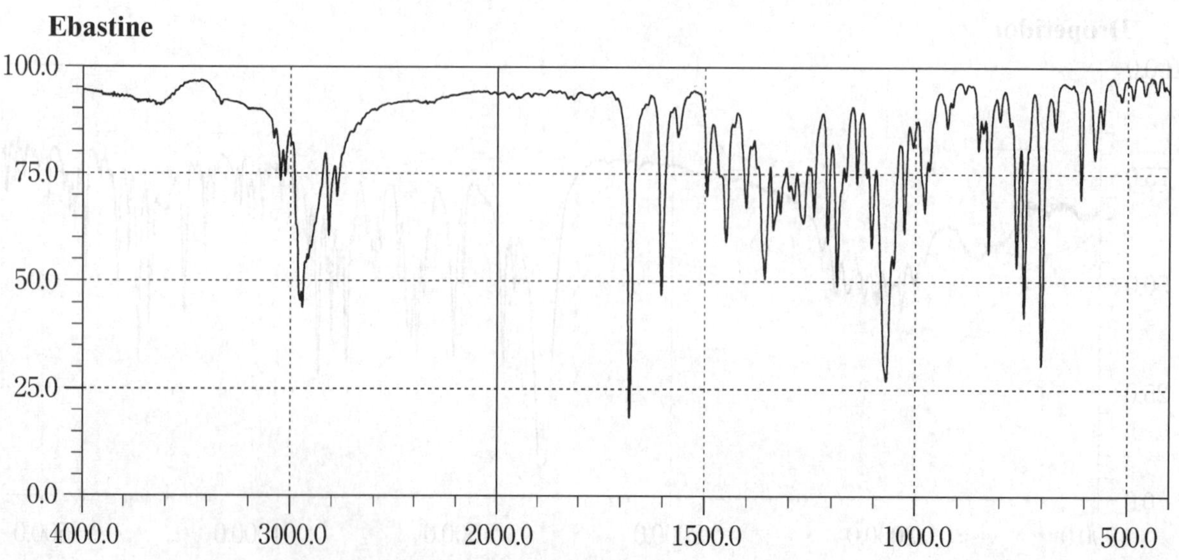

Ecabet Sodium Hydrate

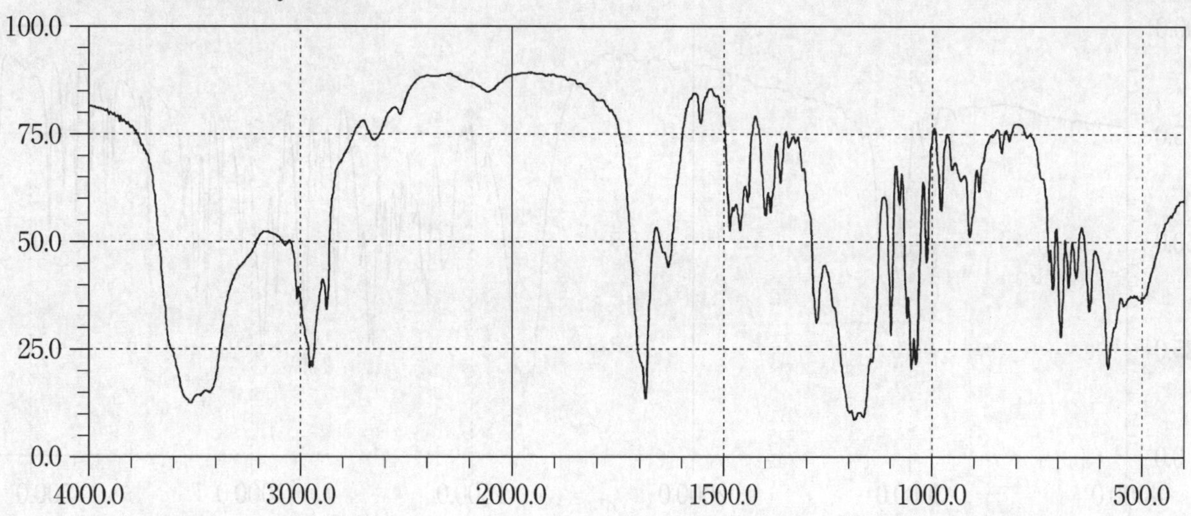

Edaravone

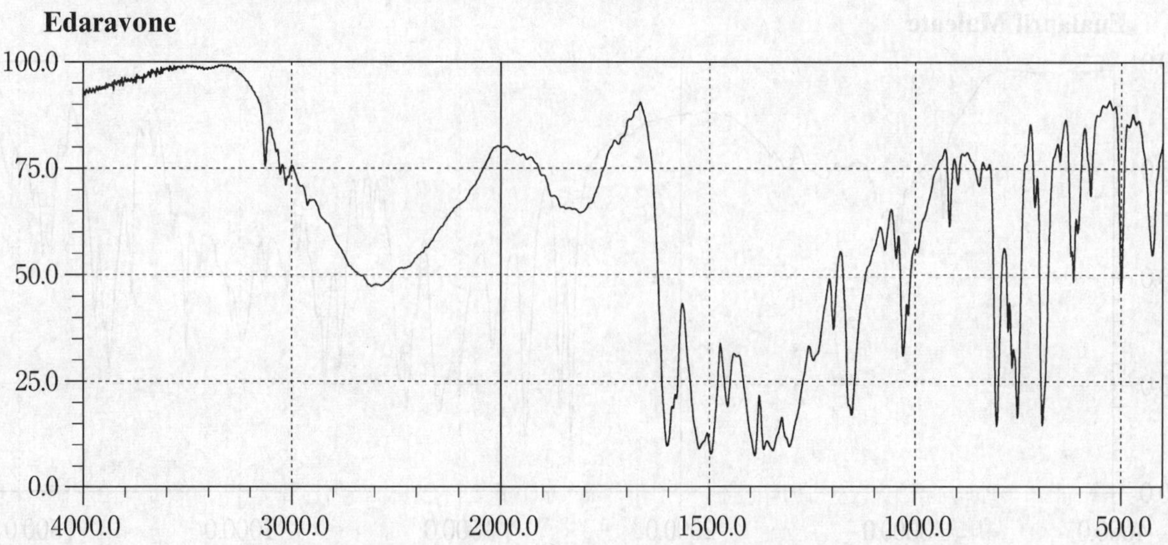

Emedastine Fumarate

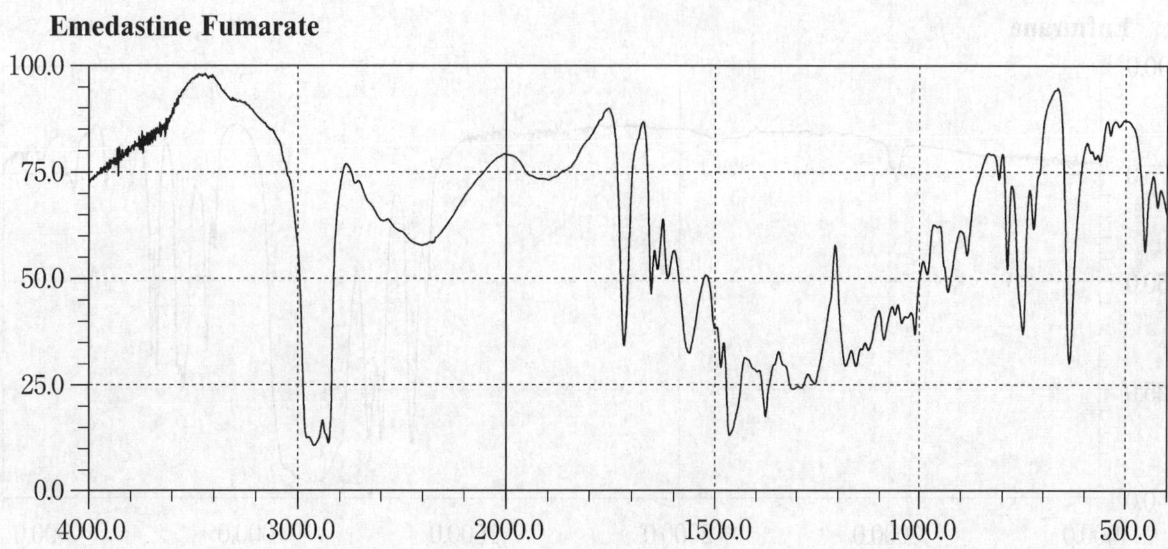

Emorfazone

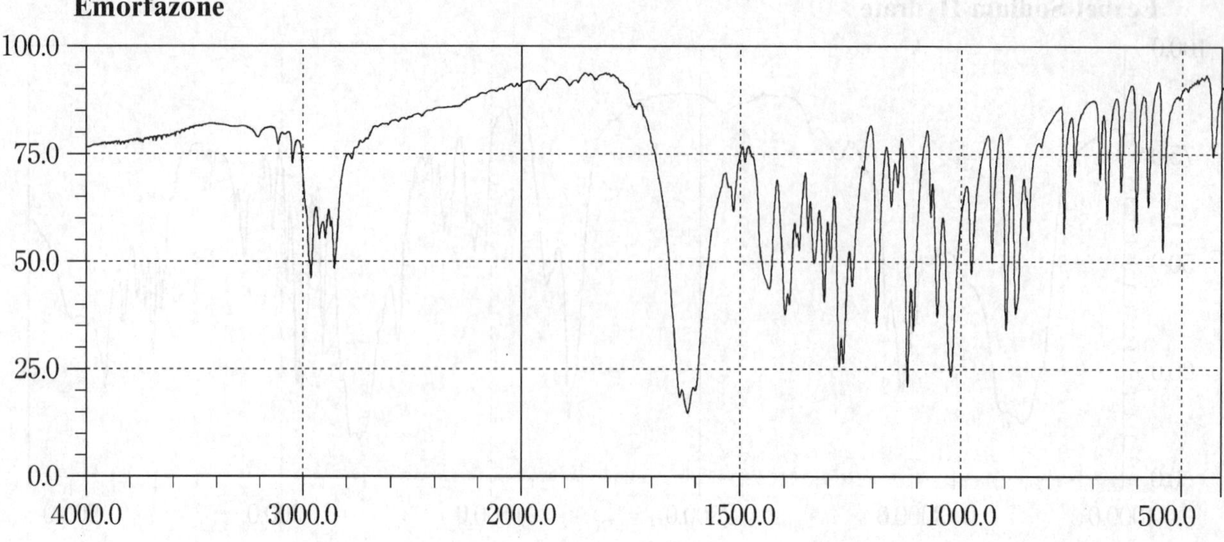

Enalapril Maleate

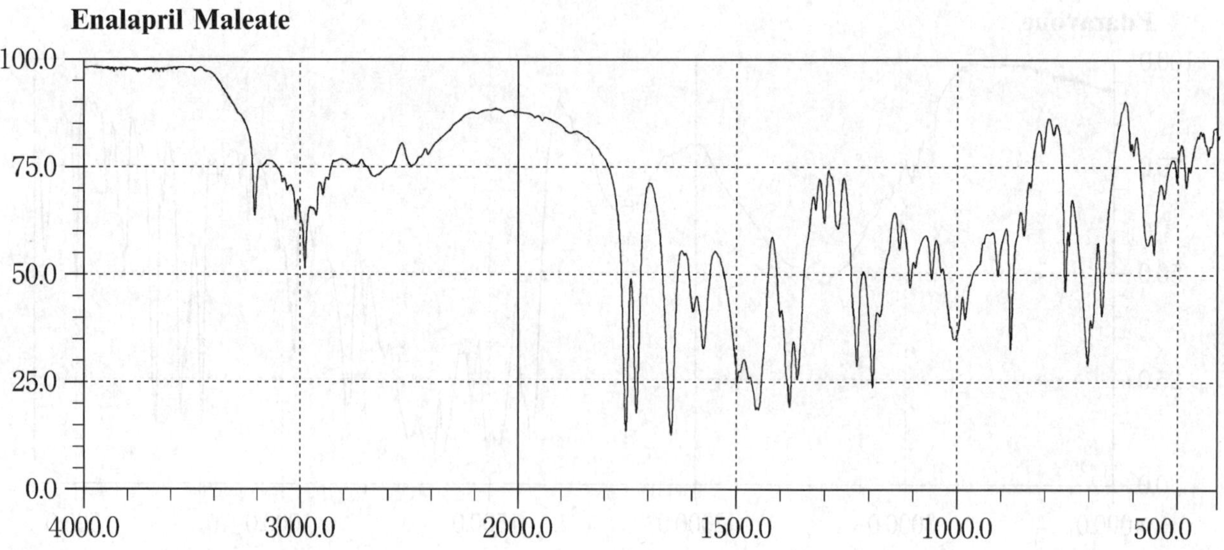

Enflurane

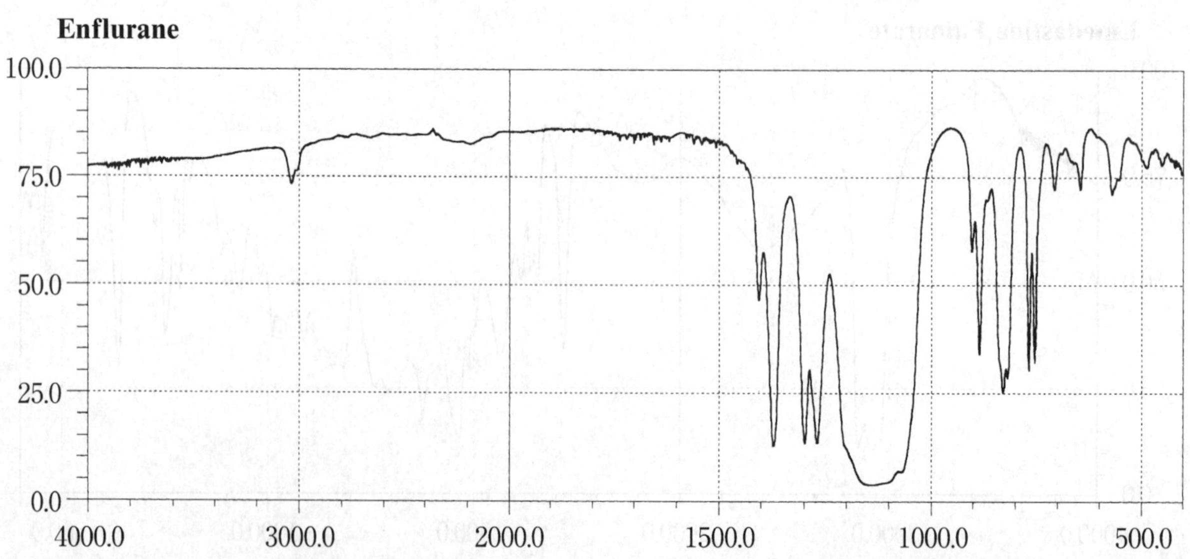

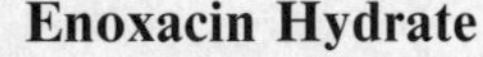

Enoxacin Hydrate

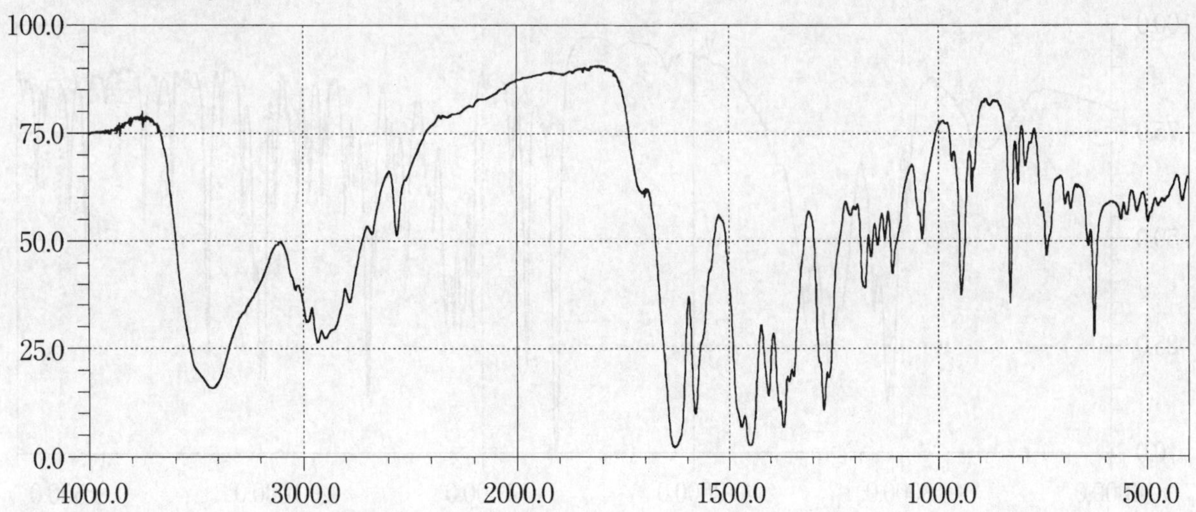

Entacapone

Epalrestat

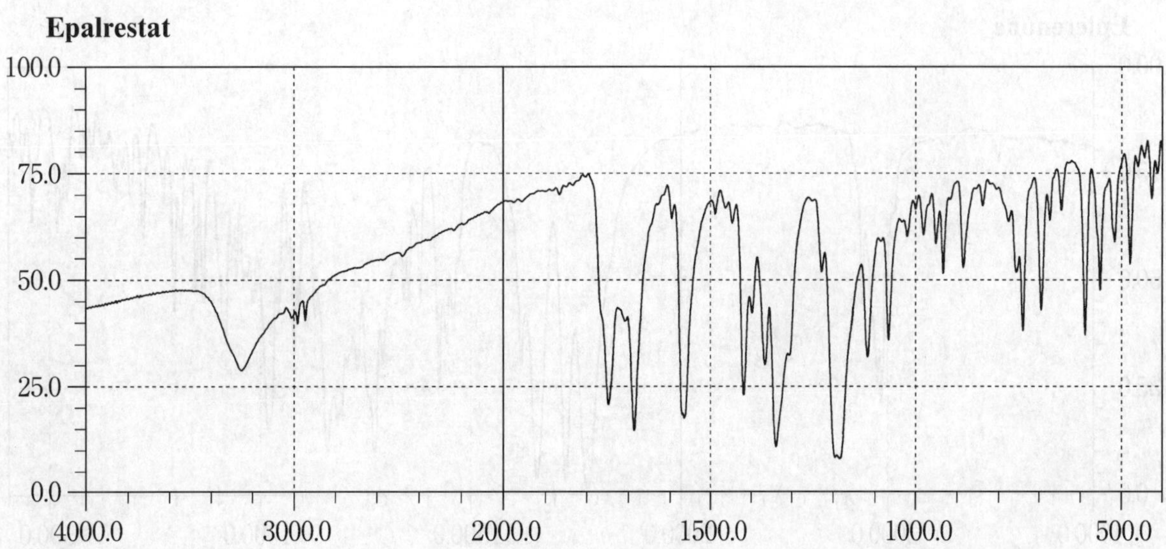

Eperisone Hydrochloride

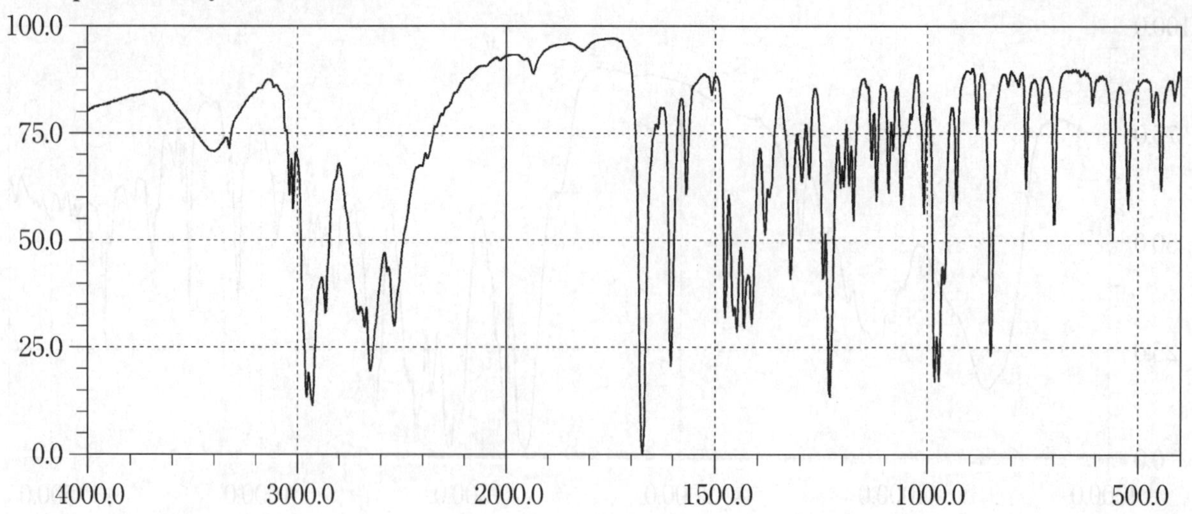

Ephedrine Hydrochloride

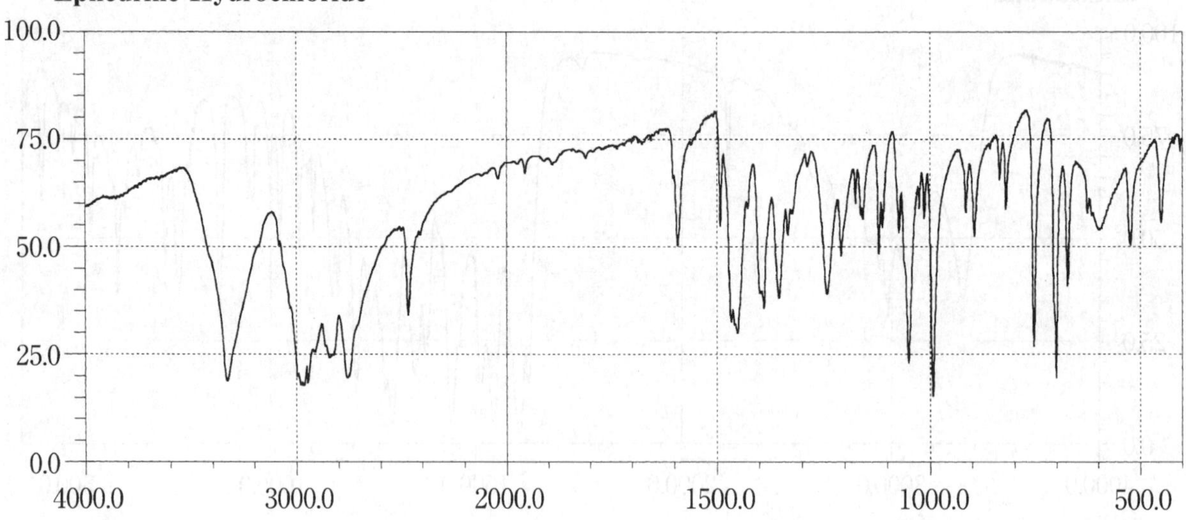

Eplerenone

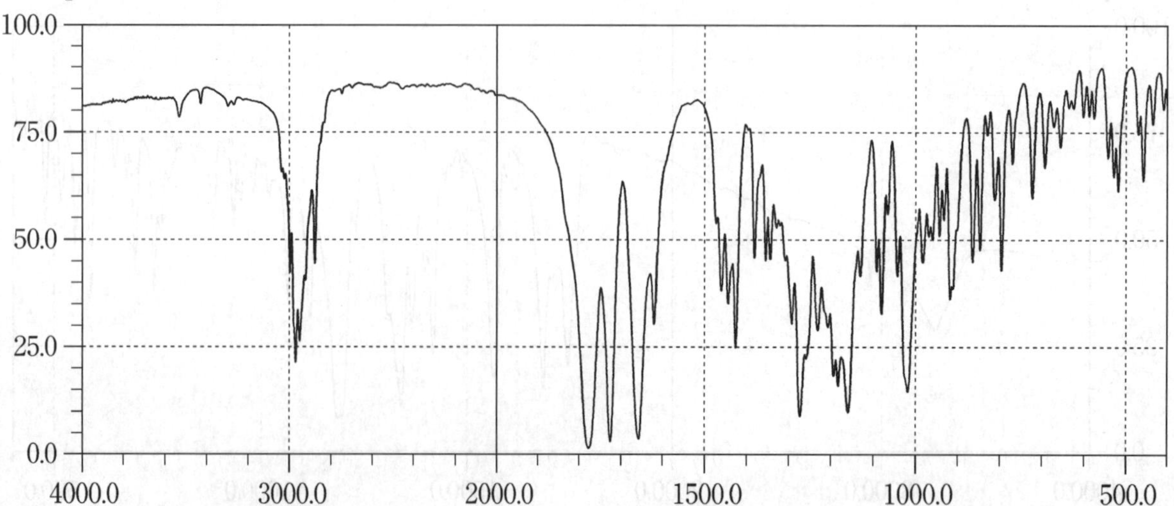

Ergocalciferol

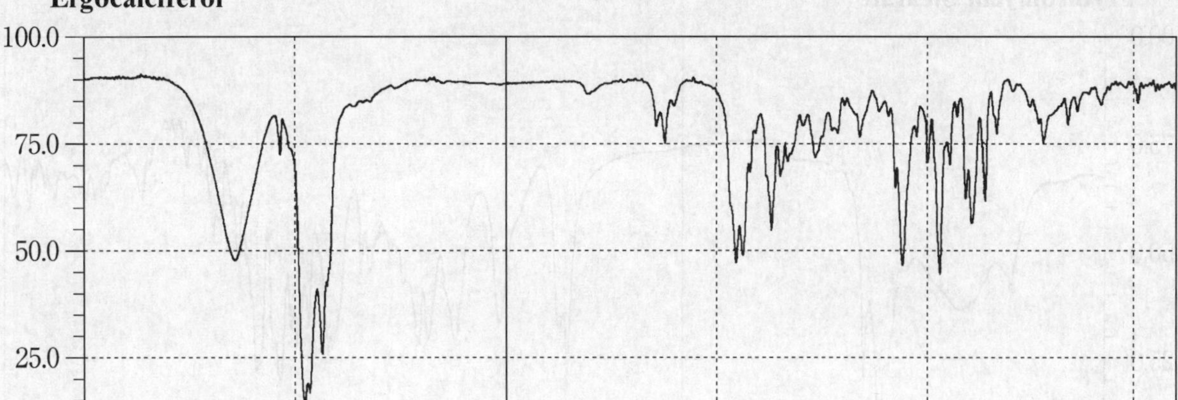

Erythromycin

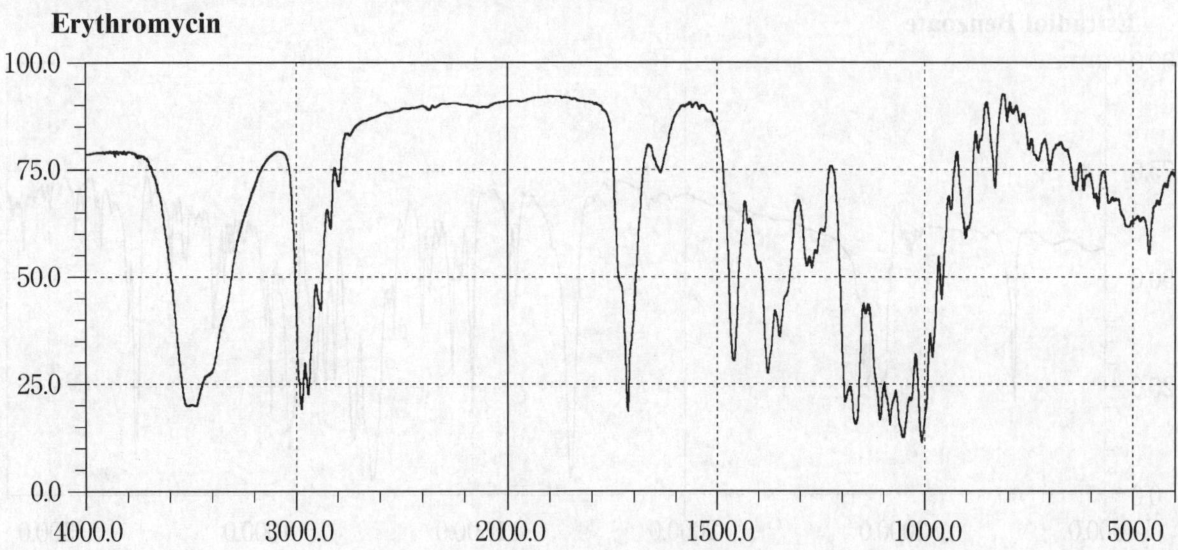

Erythromycin Ethylsuccinate

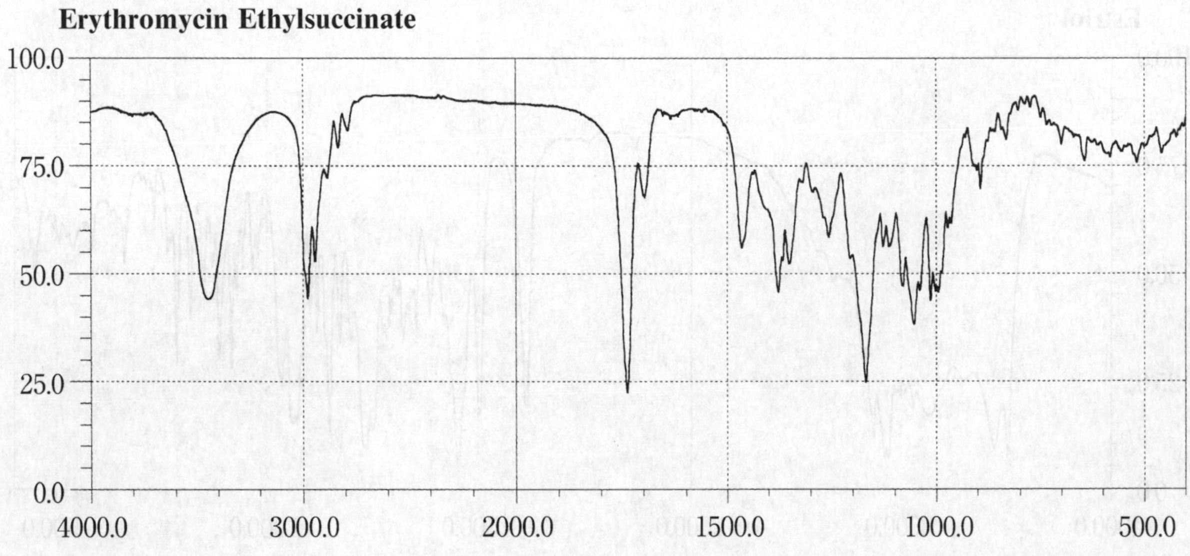

Erythromycin Stearate

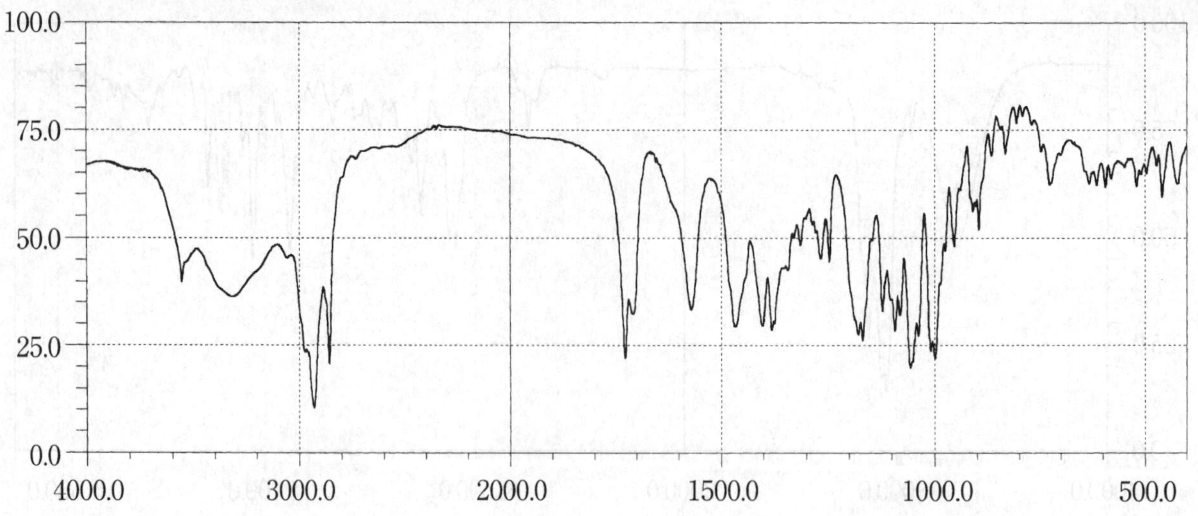

Estradiol Benzoate

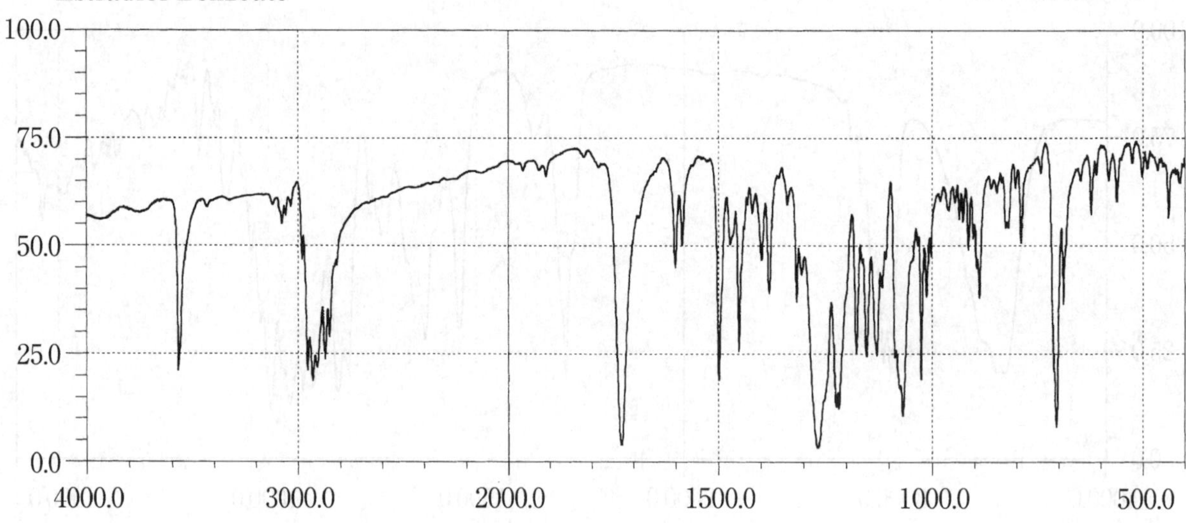

Estriol

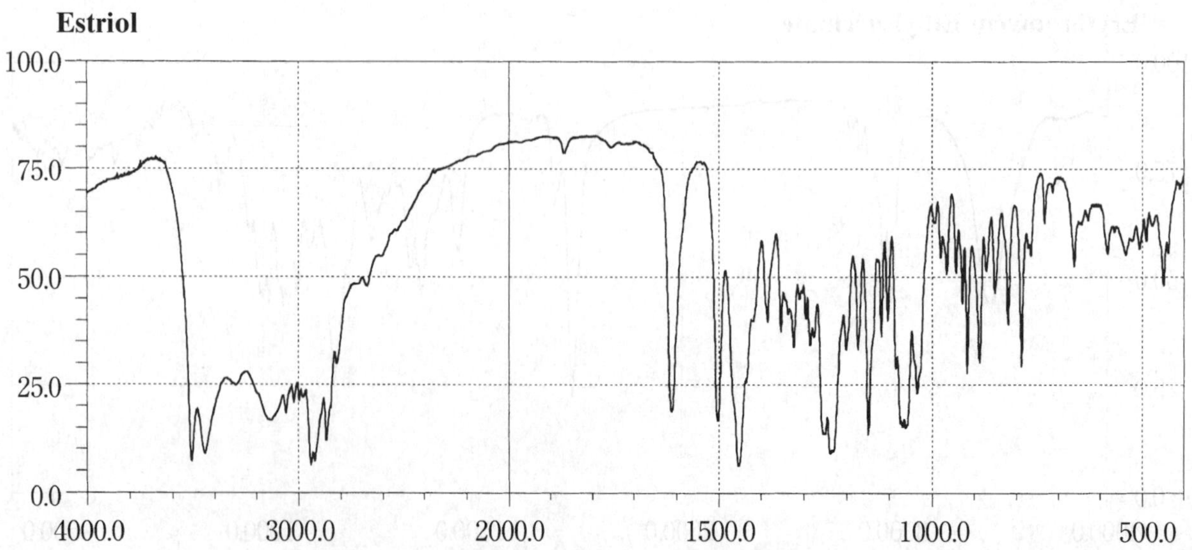

Ethanol

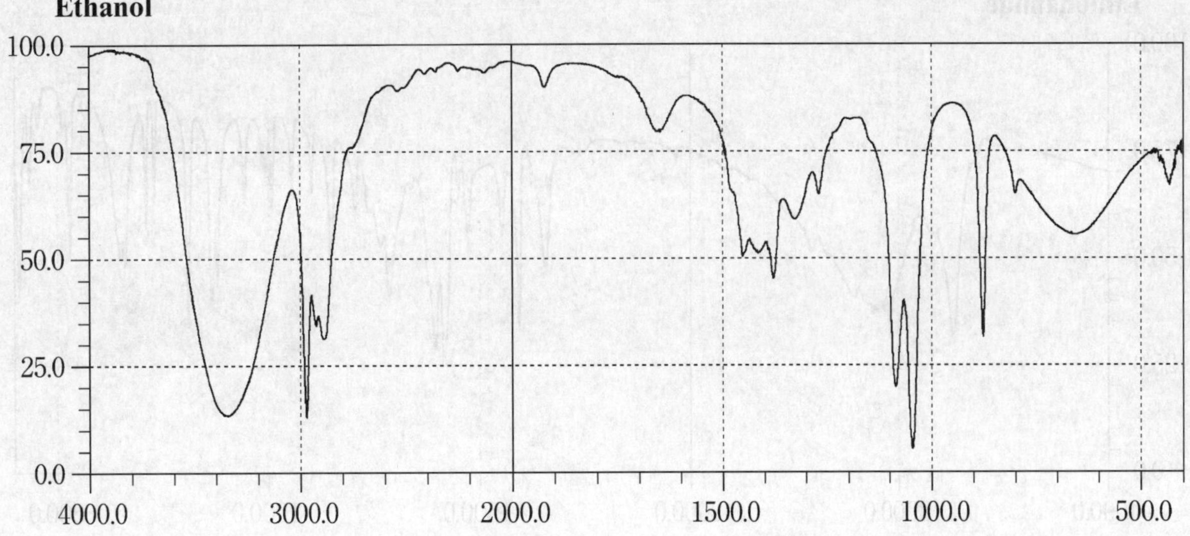

Anhydrous Ethanol

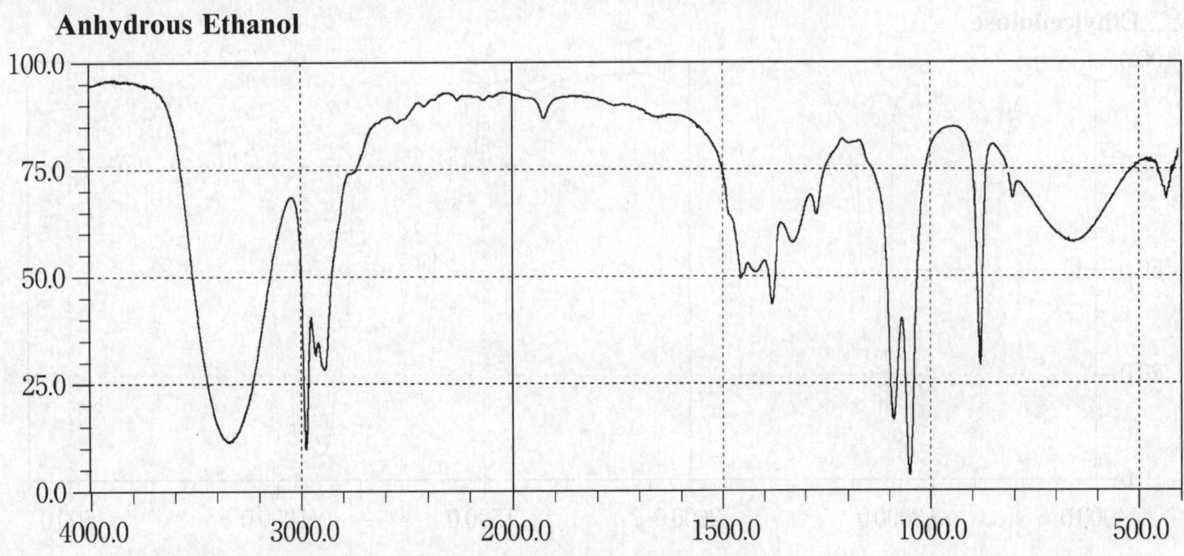

Ethenzamide

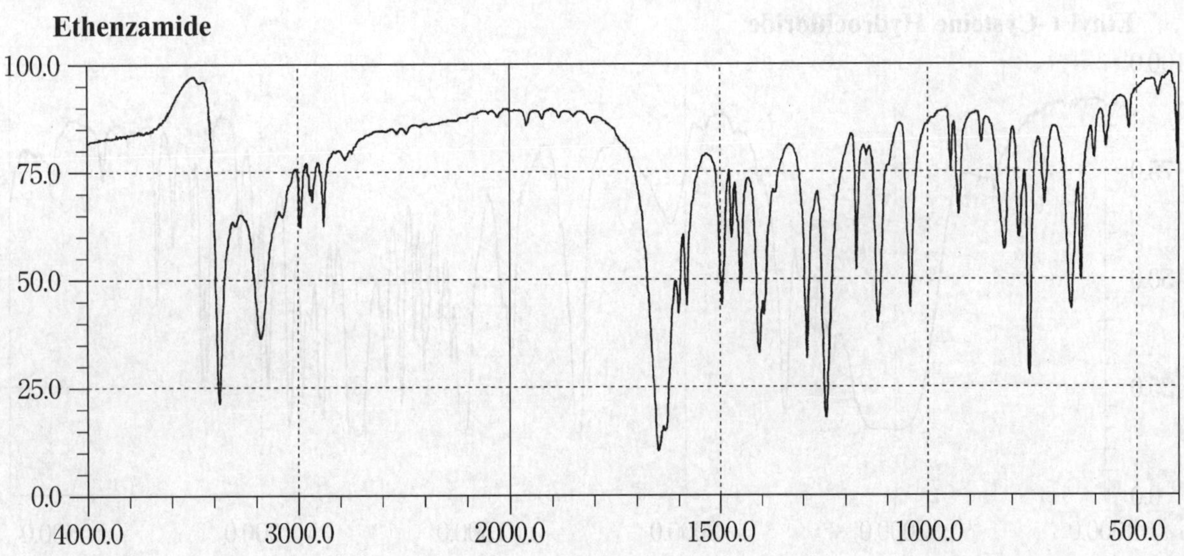

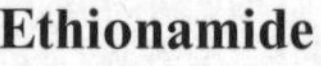

Ethionamide

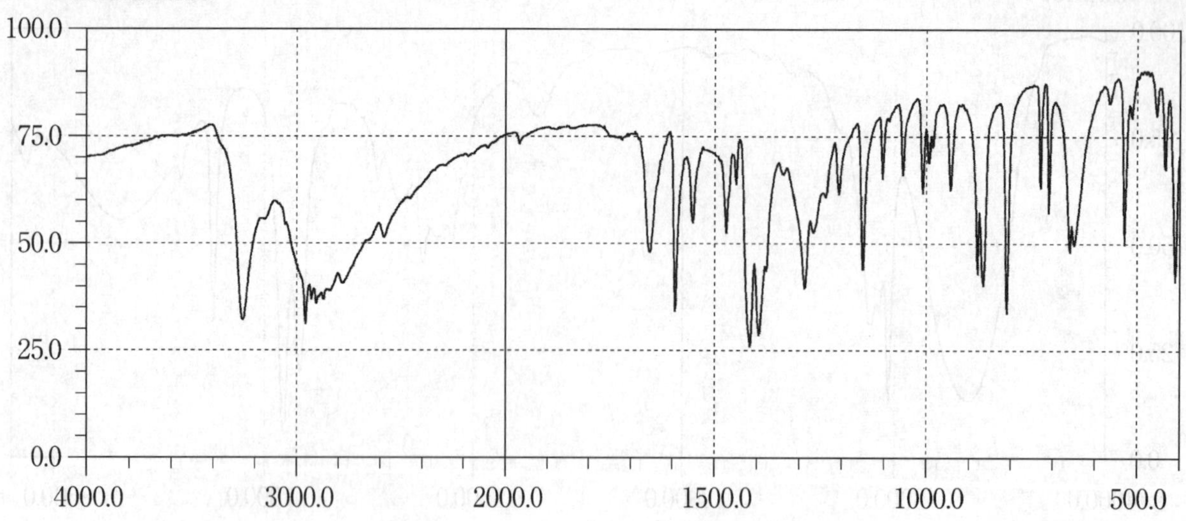

Ethylcellulose

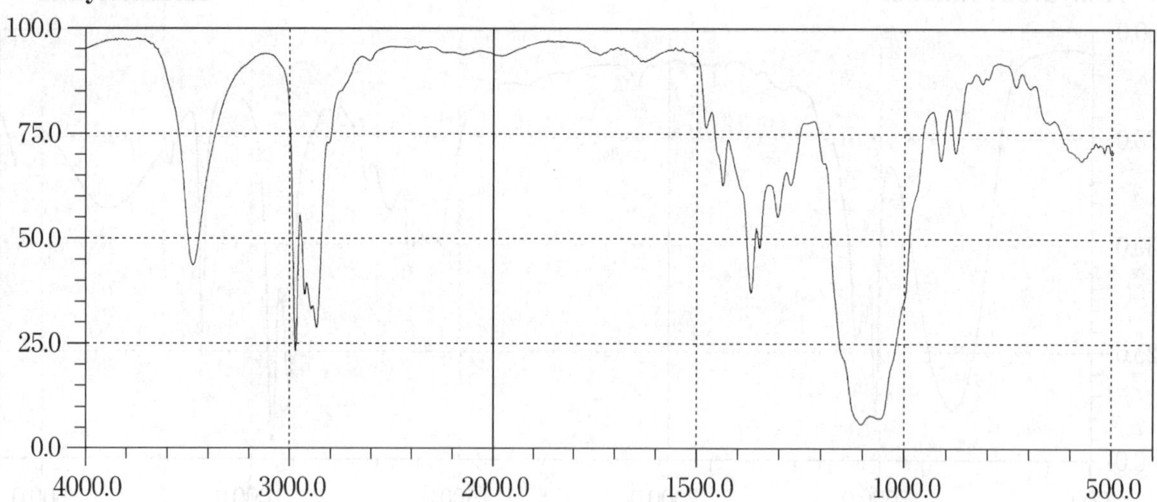

Ethyl L-Cysteine Hydrochloride

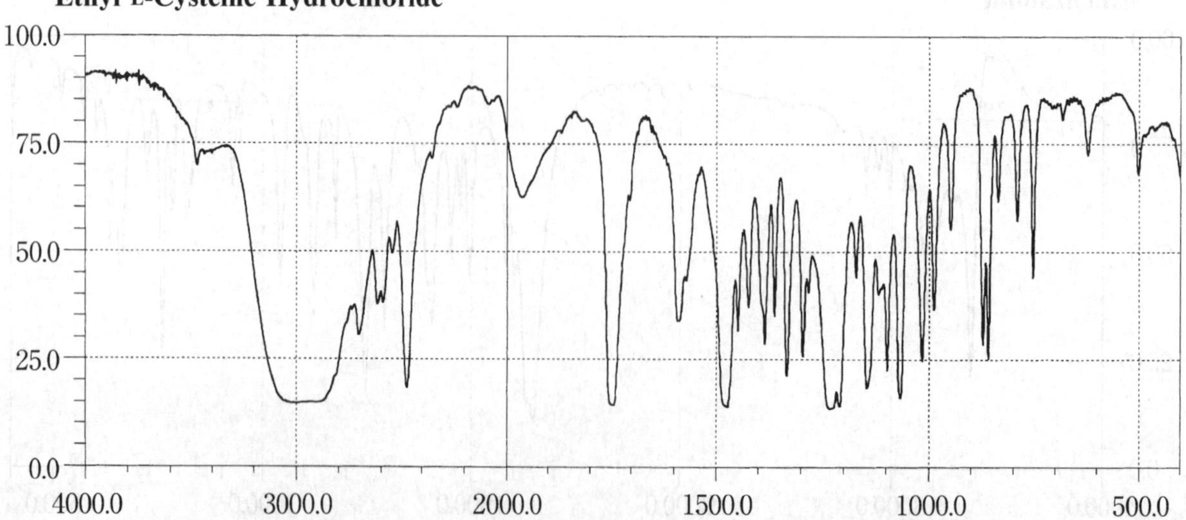

The JP Drugs are to be tested according to the provisions given in the pertinent monographs, General Notices, General Rules for Crude Drugs, General Rules for Preparations, and General Tests for their conformity to the Japanese Pharmacopoeia. (See the General Notices 5.)

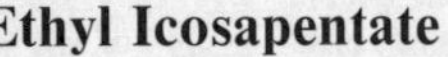

Ethyl Icosapentate

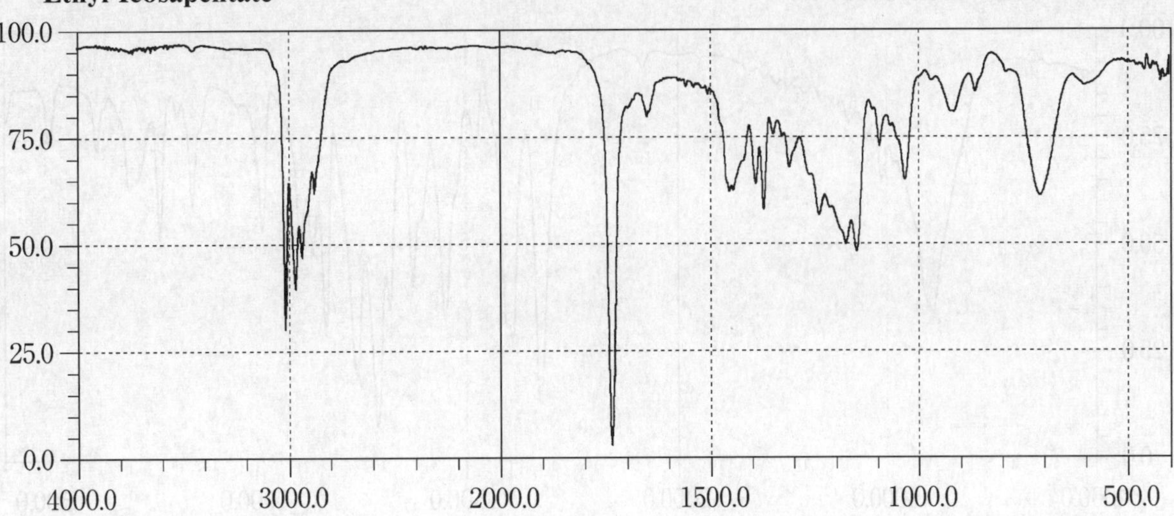

Ethyl Loflazepate

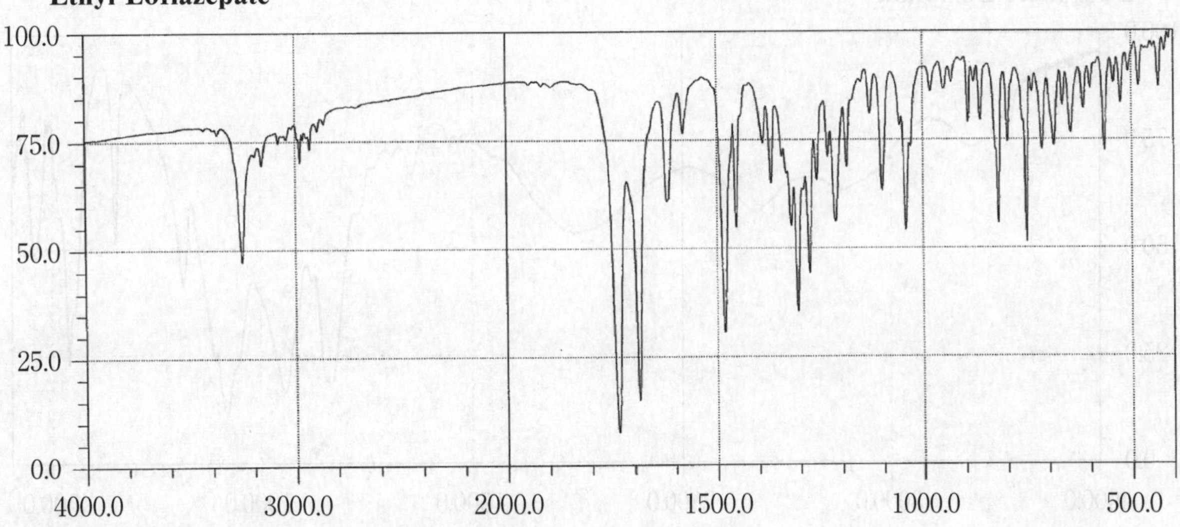

Ethylmorphine Hydrochloride Hydrate

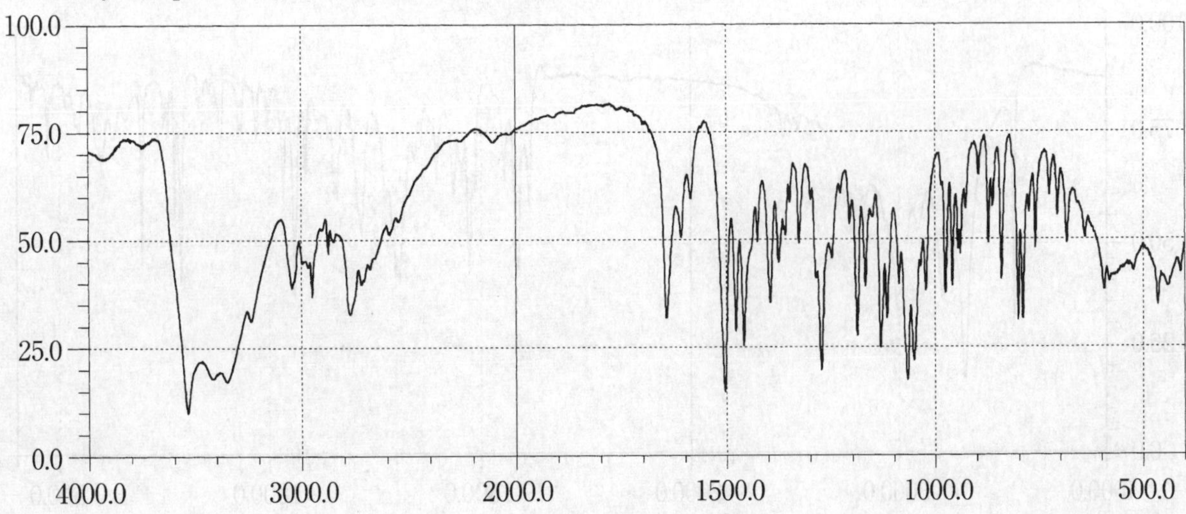

Ethyl Parahydroxybenzoate

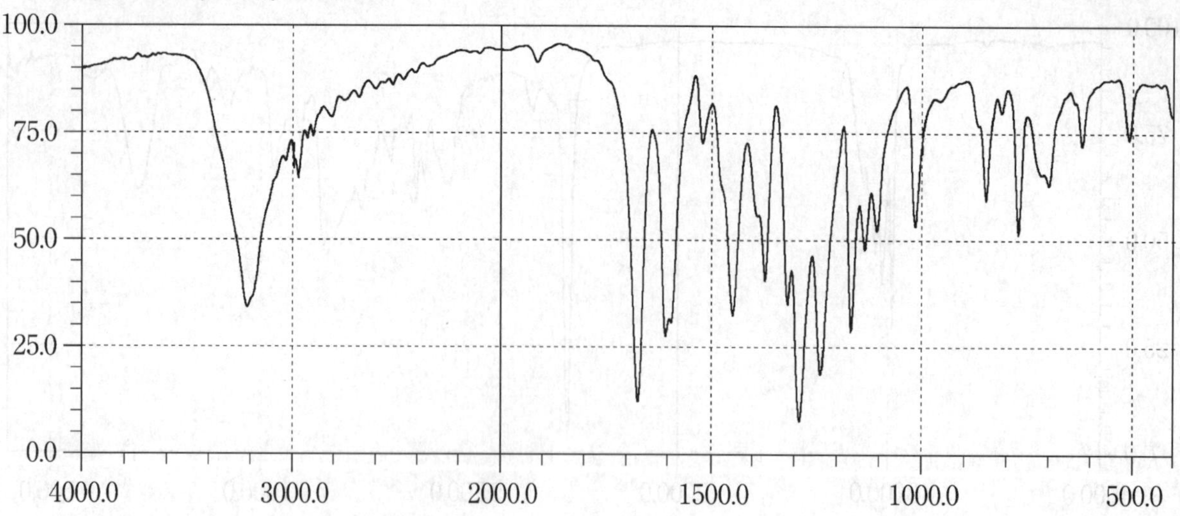

Etidronate Disodium

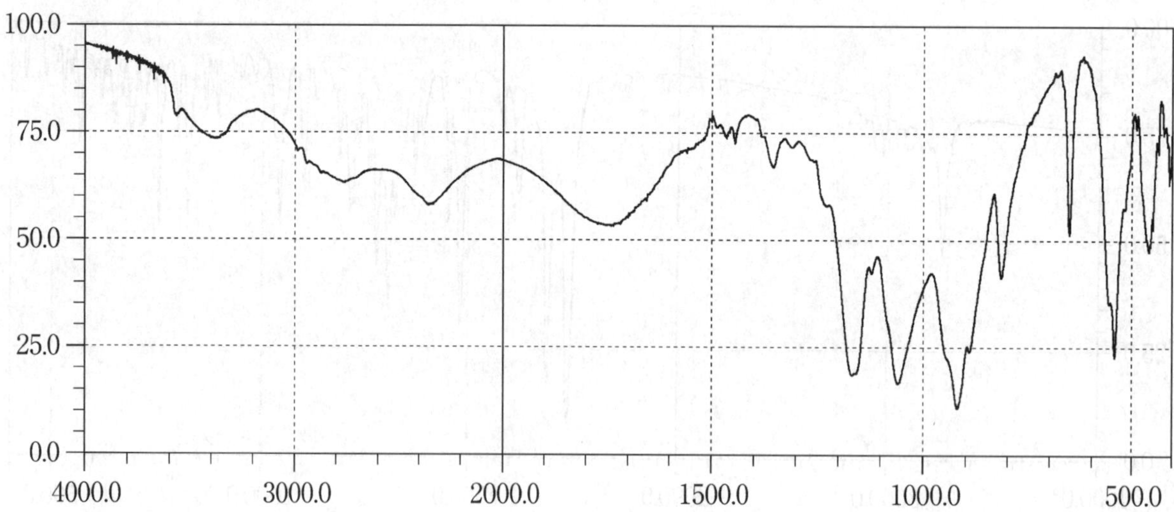

Etilefrine Hydrochloride

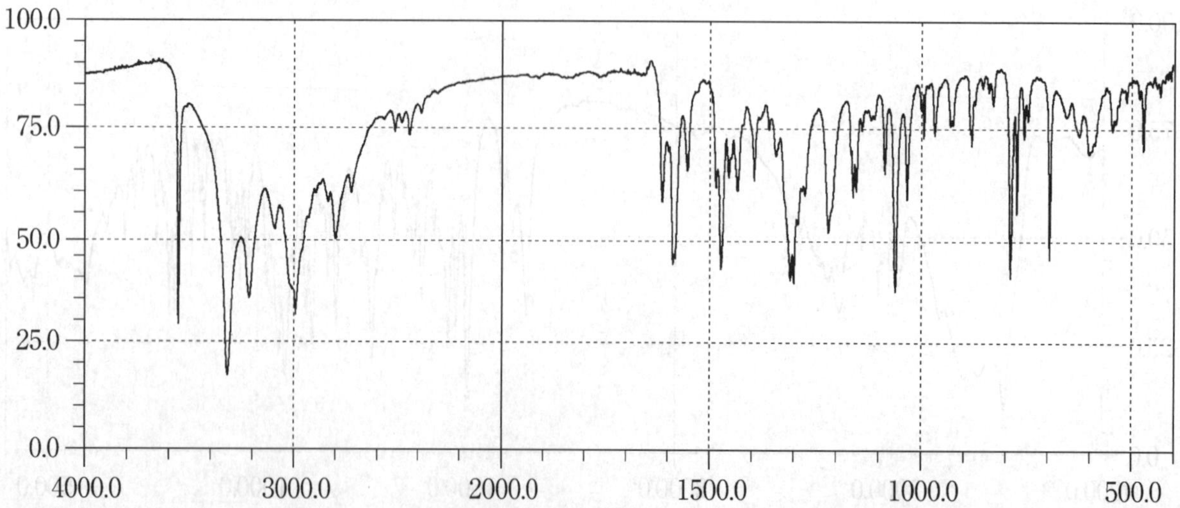

Etizolam

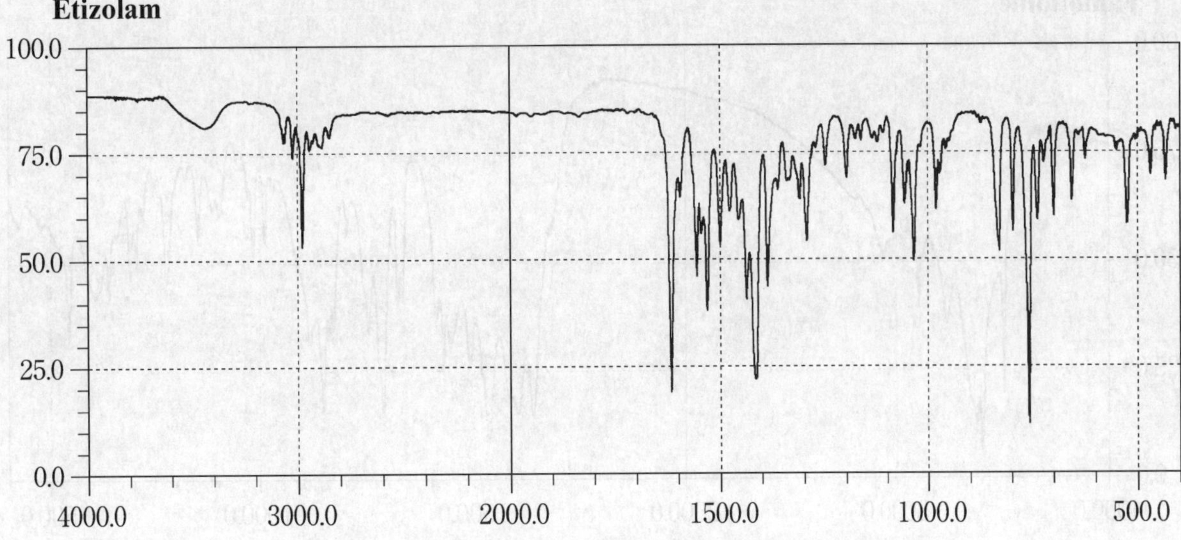

Etodolac

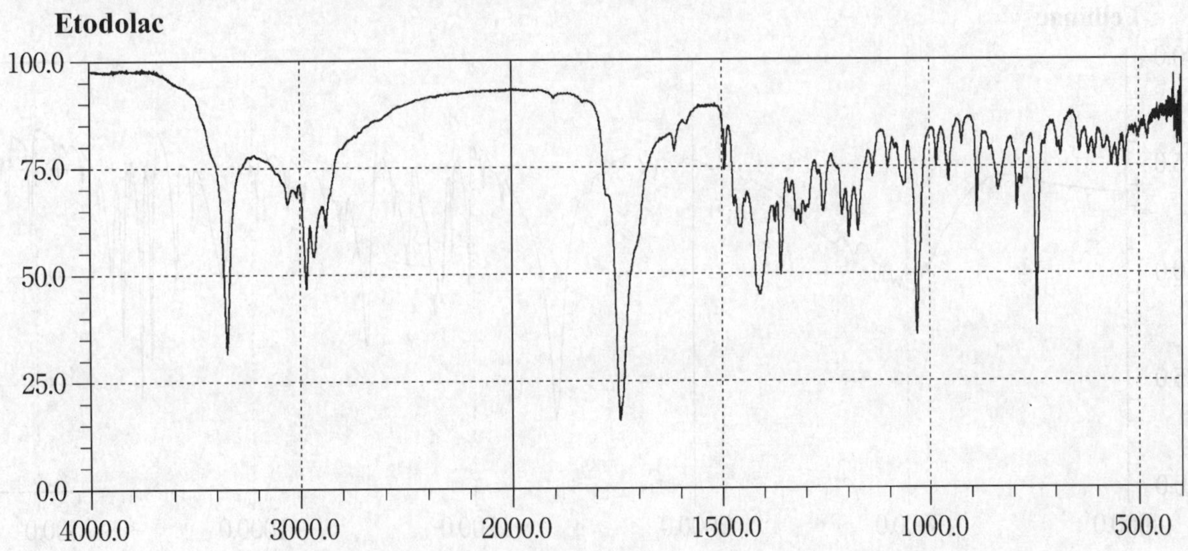

Etoposide

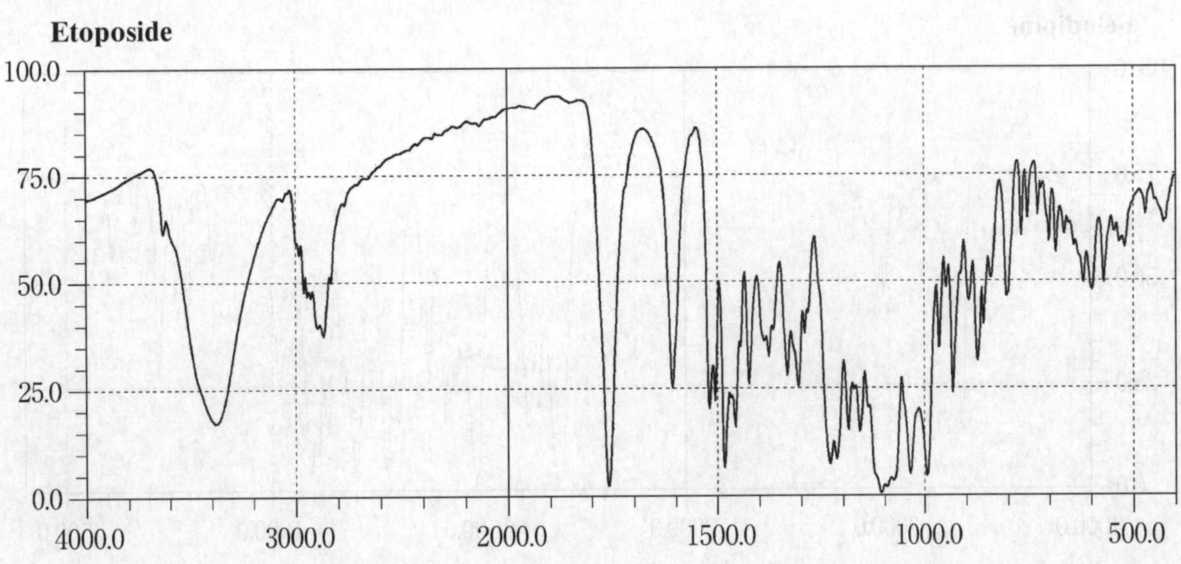

The JP Drugs are to be tested according to the provisions given in the pertinent monographs, General Notices, General Rules for Crude Drugs, General Rules for Preparations, and General Tests for their conformity to the Japanese Pharmacopoeia. (See the General Notices 5.)

Famotidine

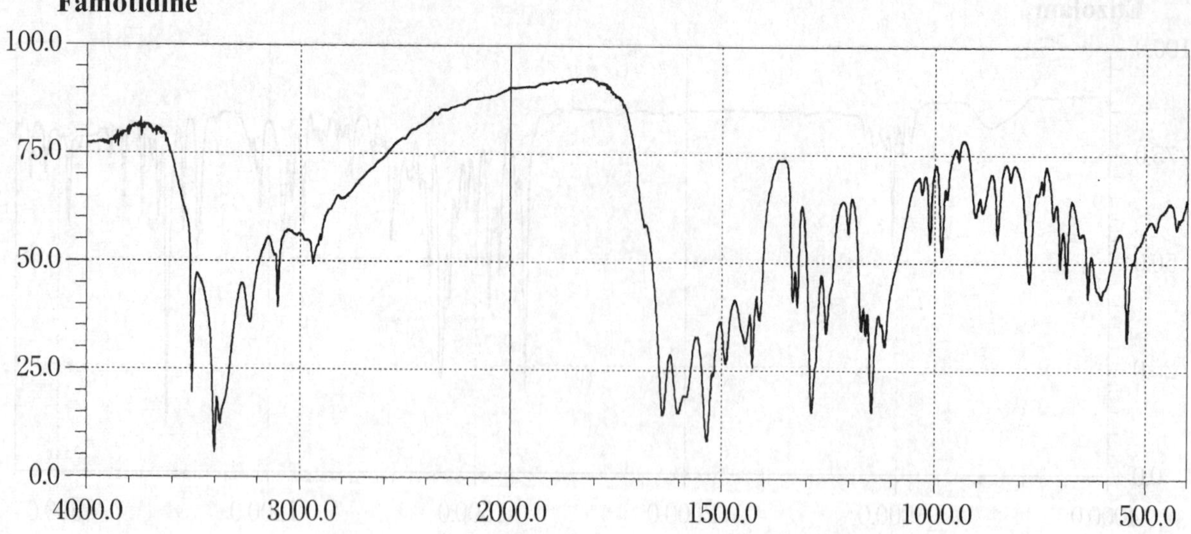

Felbinac

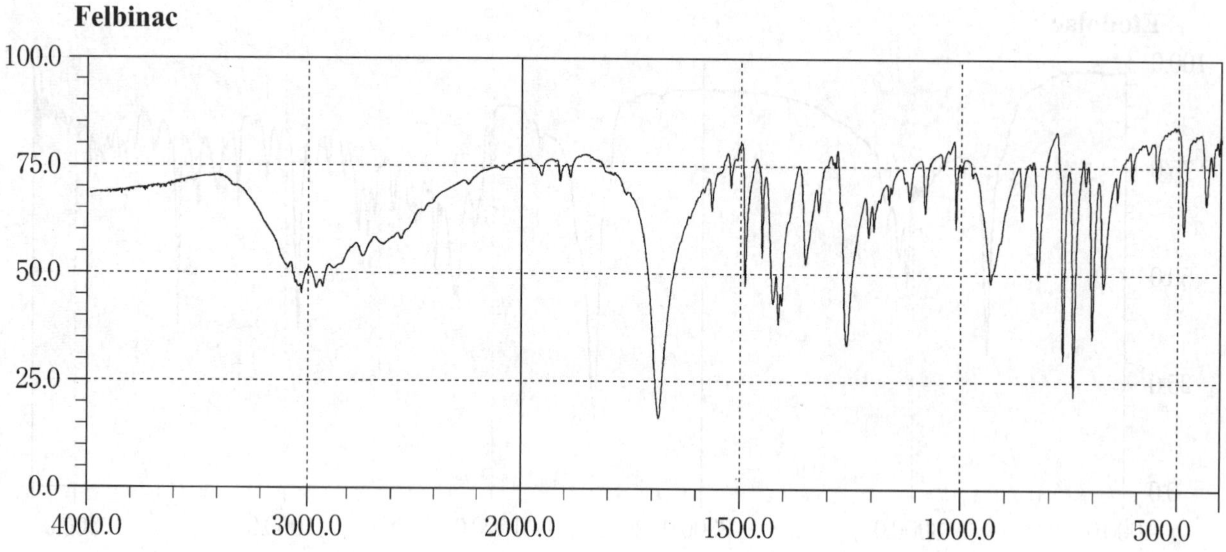

Felodipine

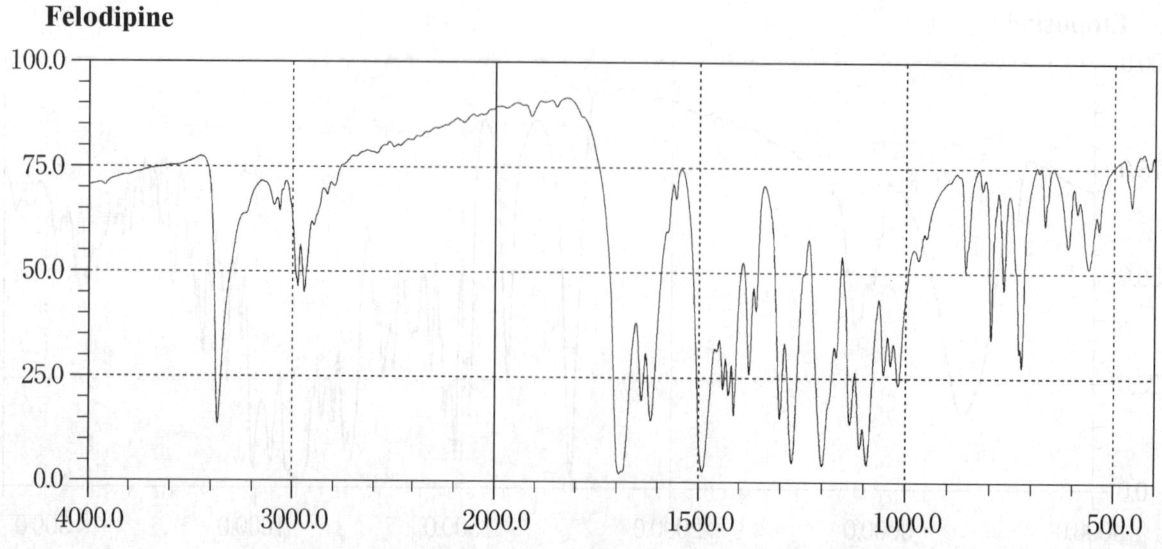

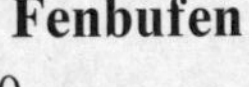

Fenbufen

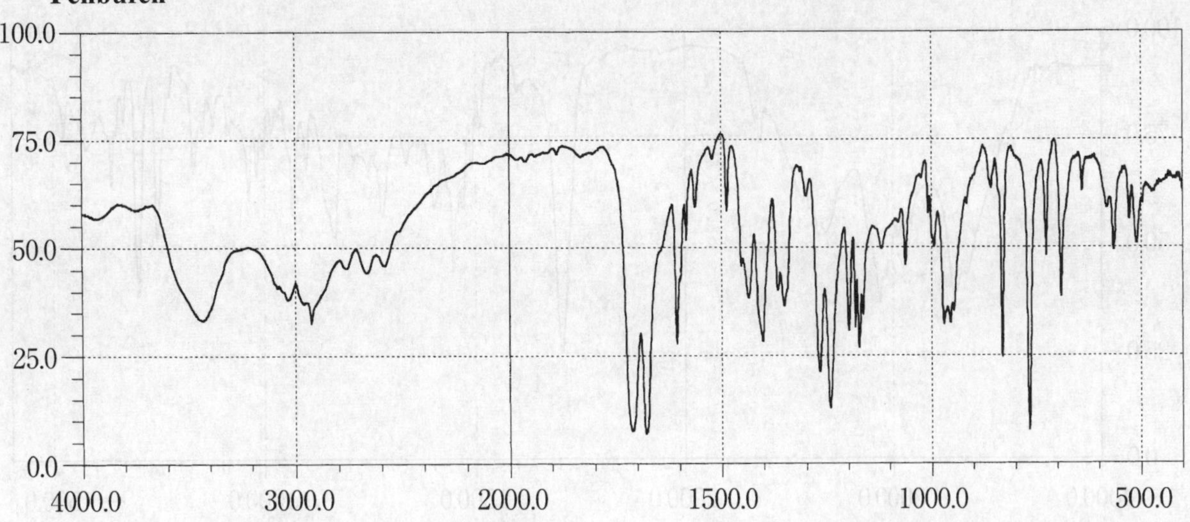

Fenofibrate

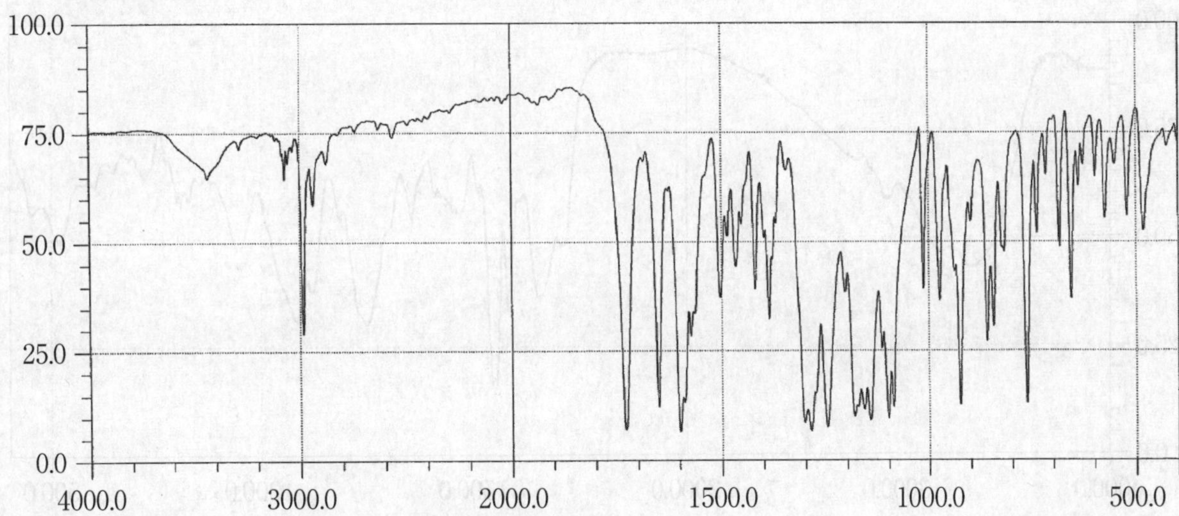

Fentanyl Citrate

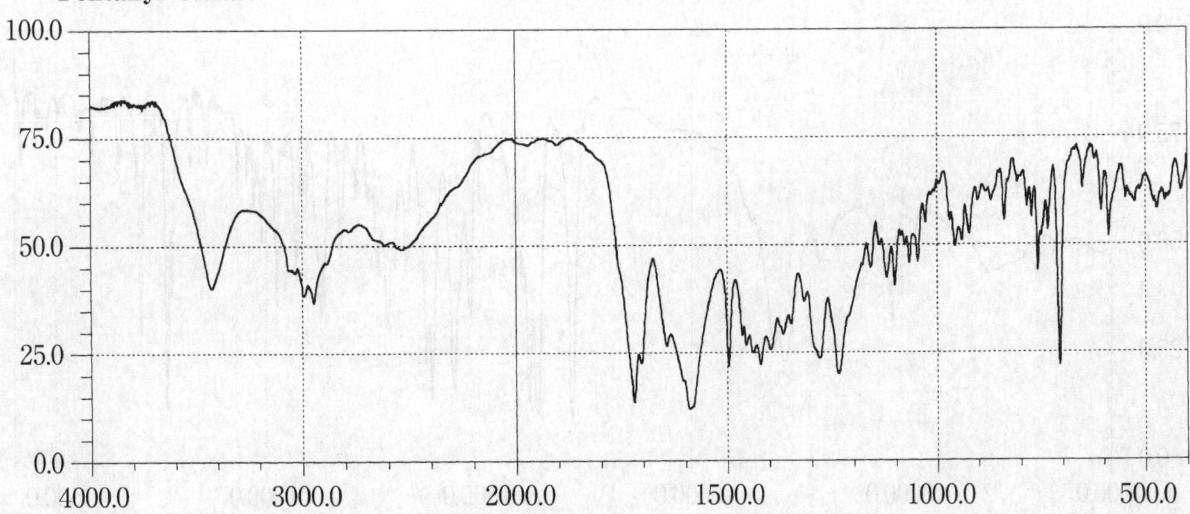

Fexofenadine Hydrochloride

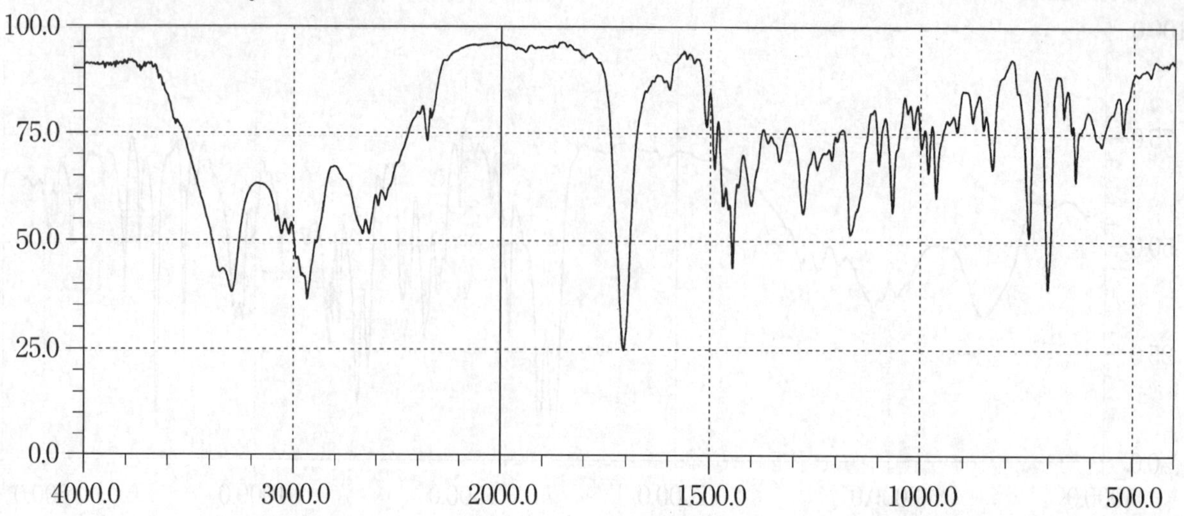

Flavin Adenine Dinucleotide Sodium

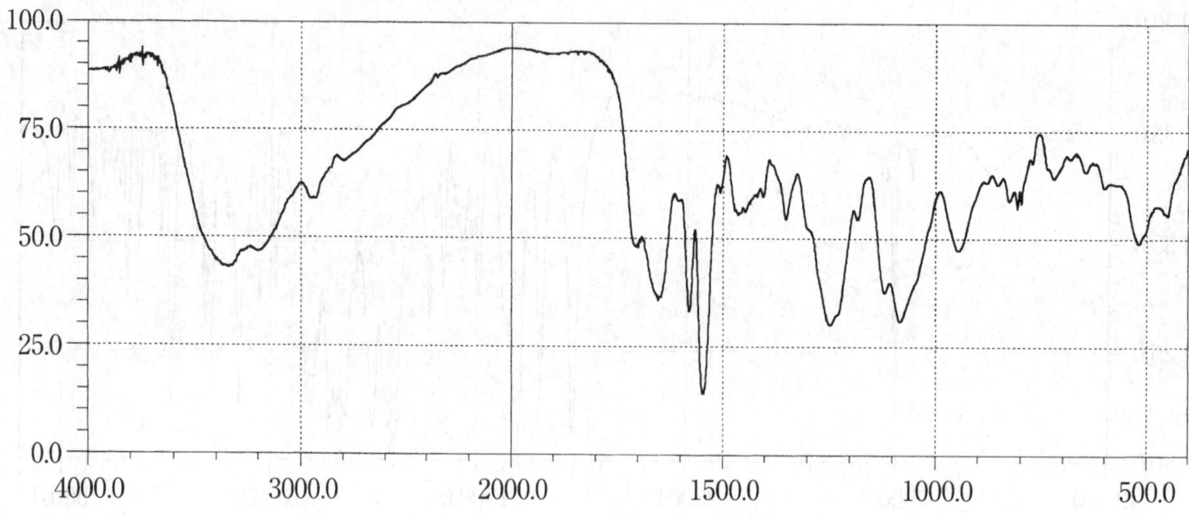

Flavoxate Hydrochloride

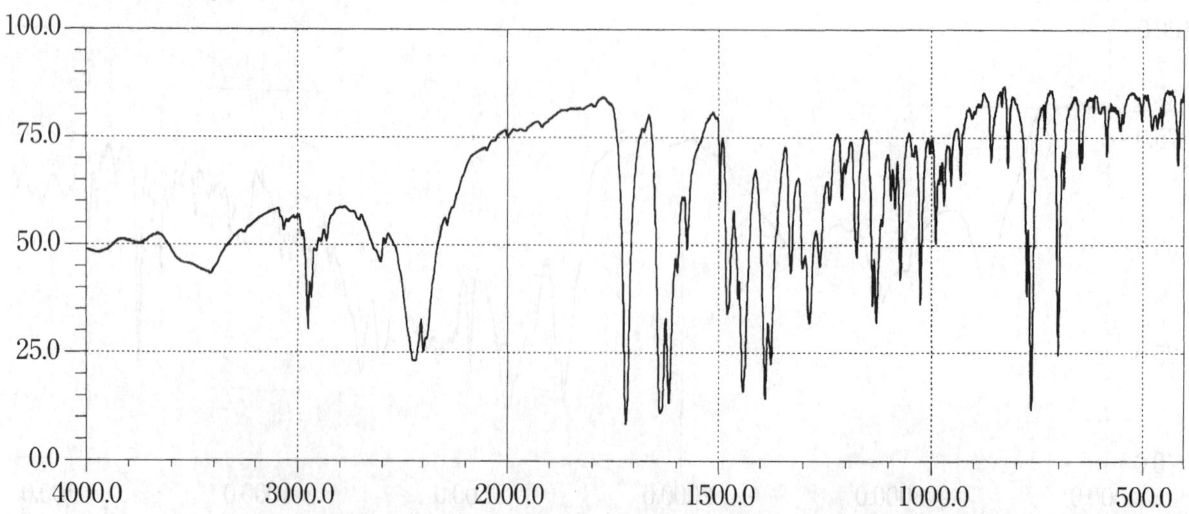

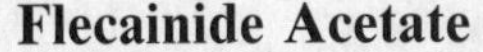

Flecainide Acetate

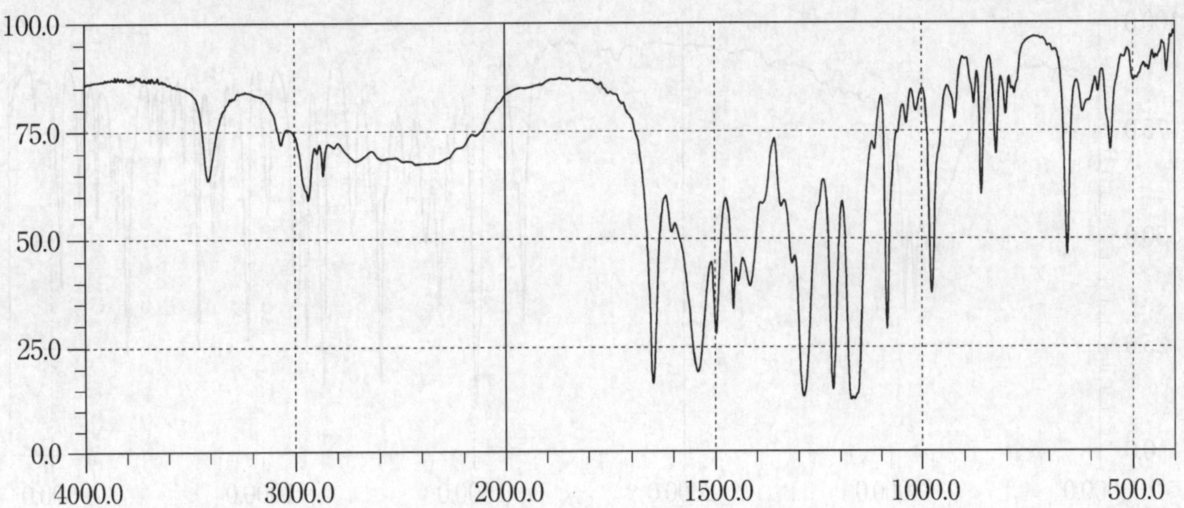

Flomoxef Sodium

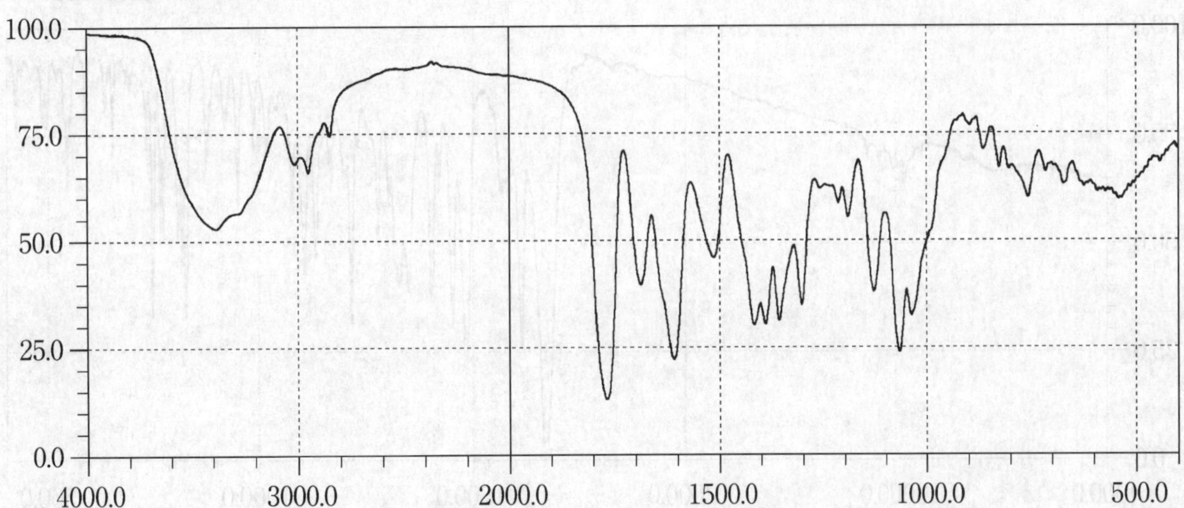

Flopropione

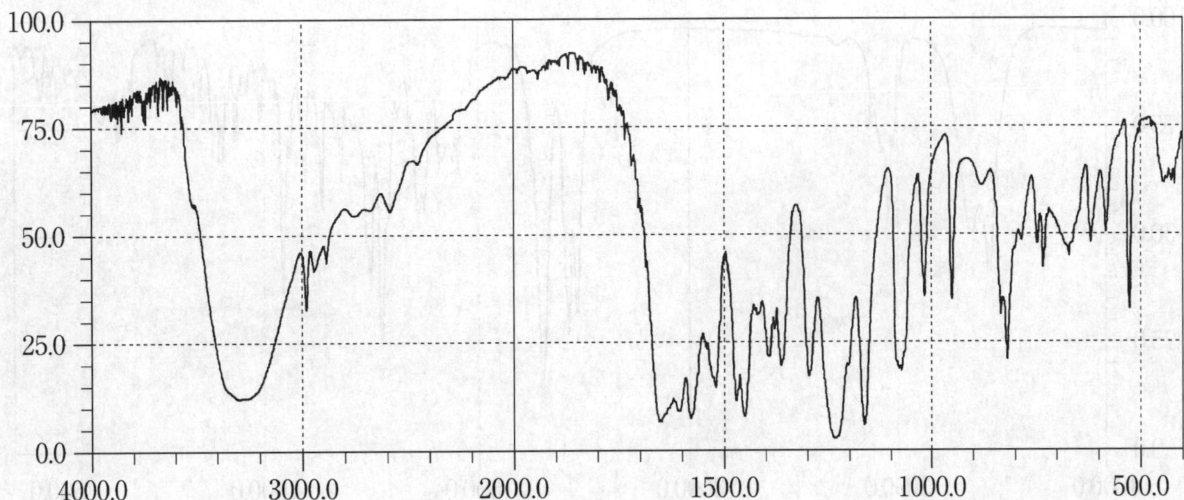

The JP Drugs are to be tested according to the provisions given in the pertinent monographs, General Notices, General Rules for Crude Drugs, General Rules for Preparations, and General Tests for their conformity to the Japanese Pharmacopoeia. (See the General Notices 5.)

Fluconazole

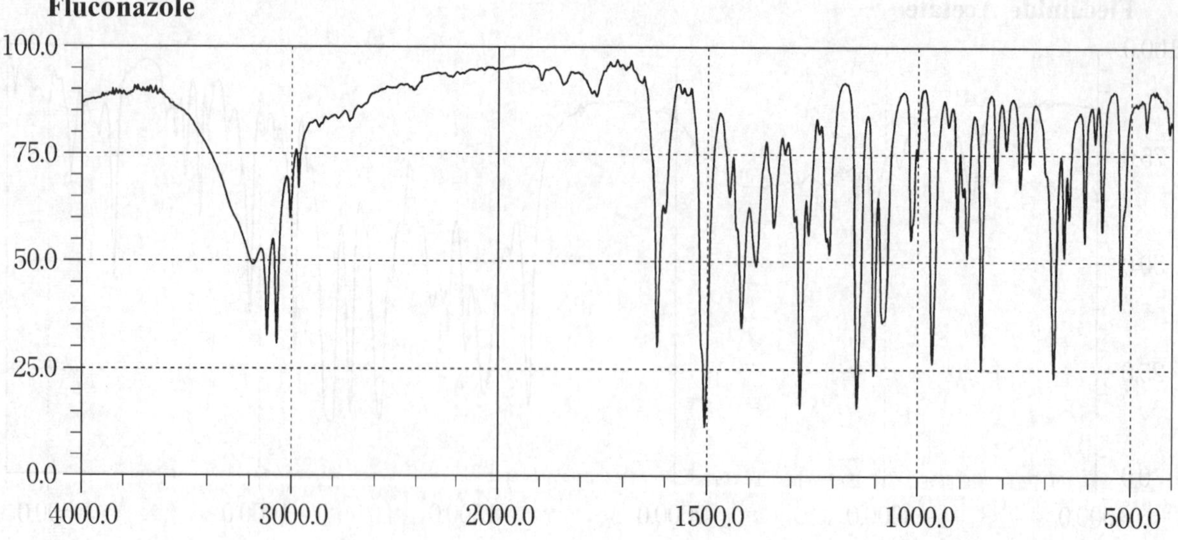

Fludiazepam

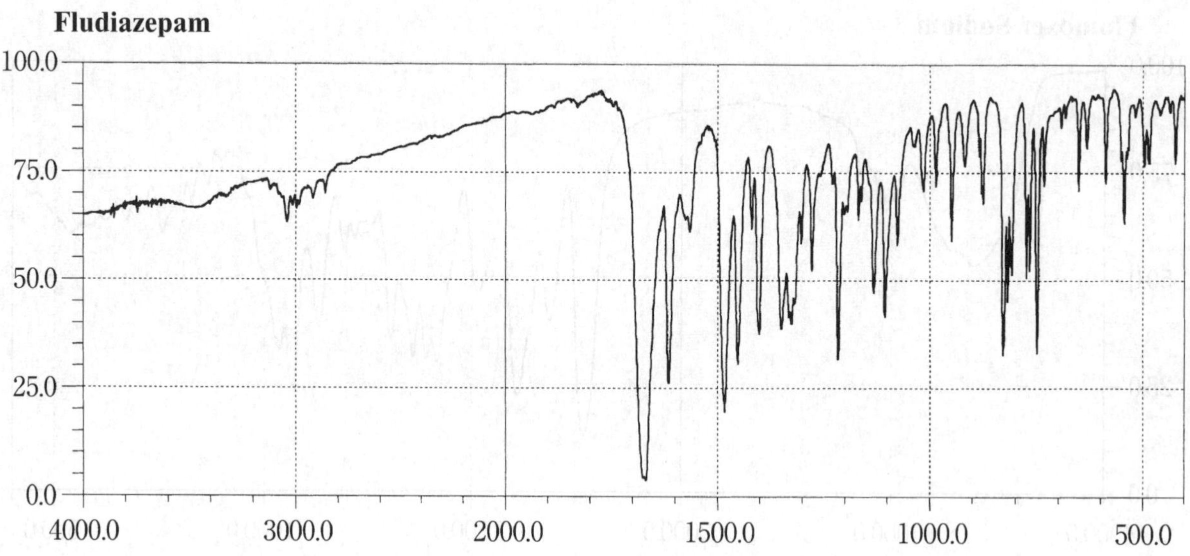

Fludrocortisone Acetate

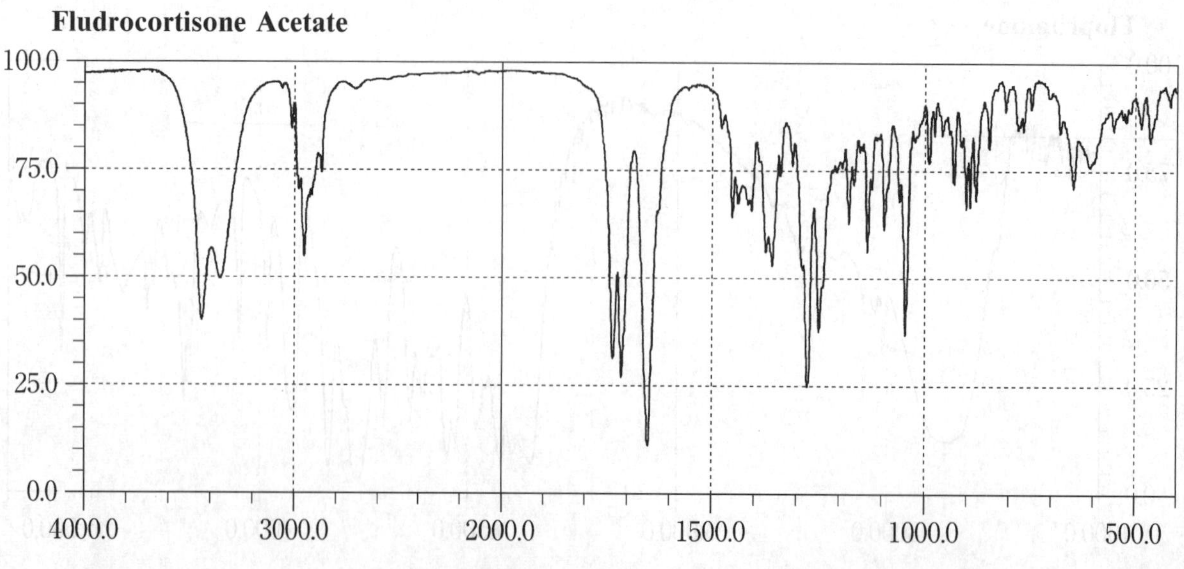

Flunitrazepam

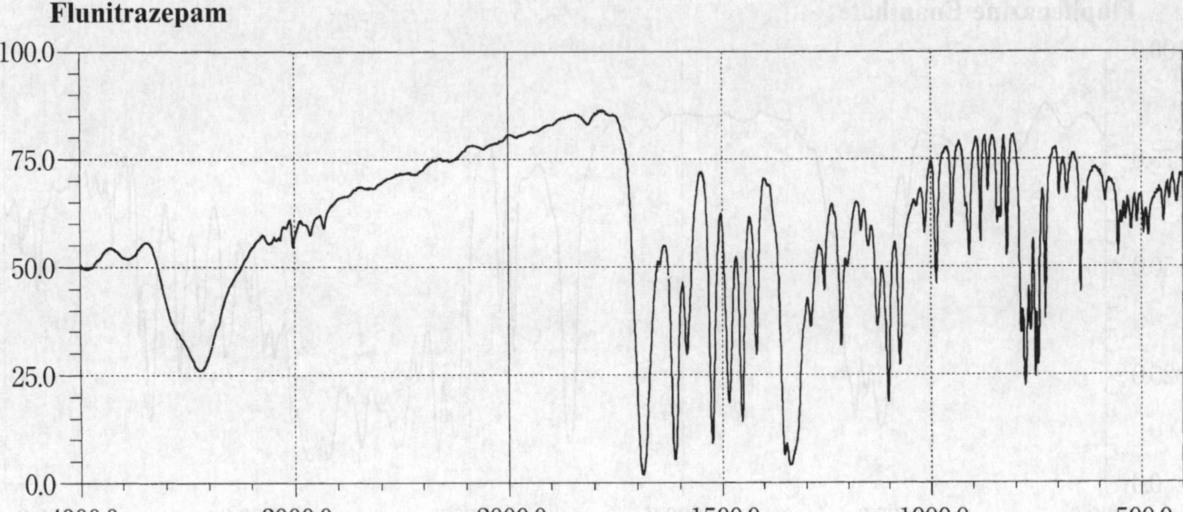

Fluocinolone Acetonide

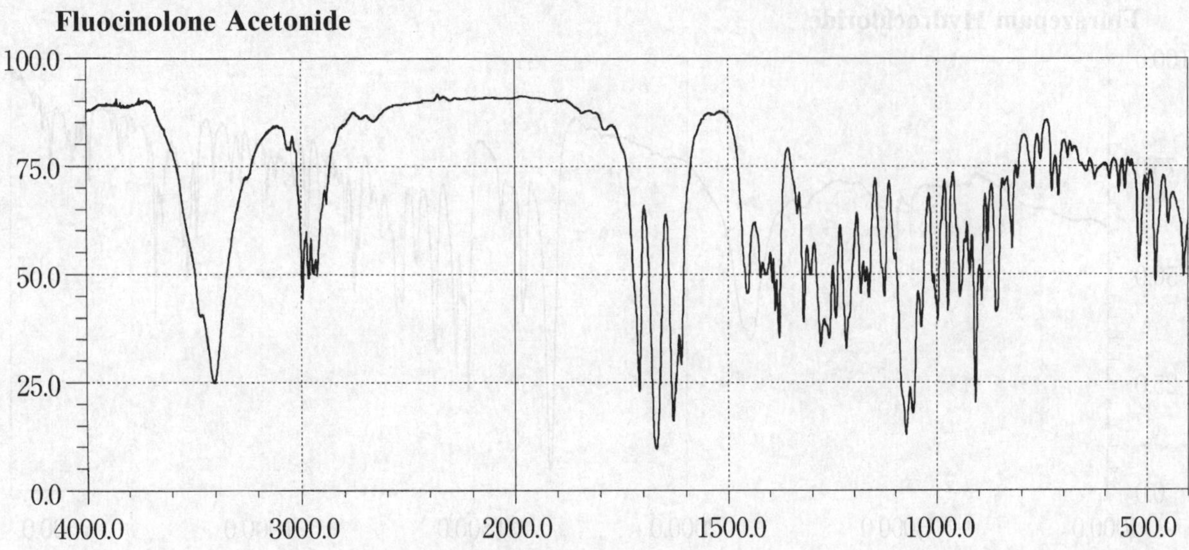

Fluorometholone

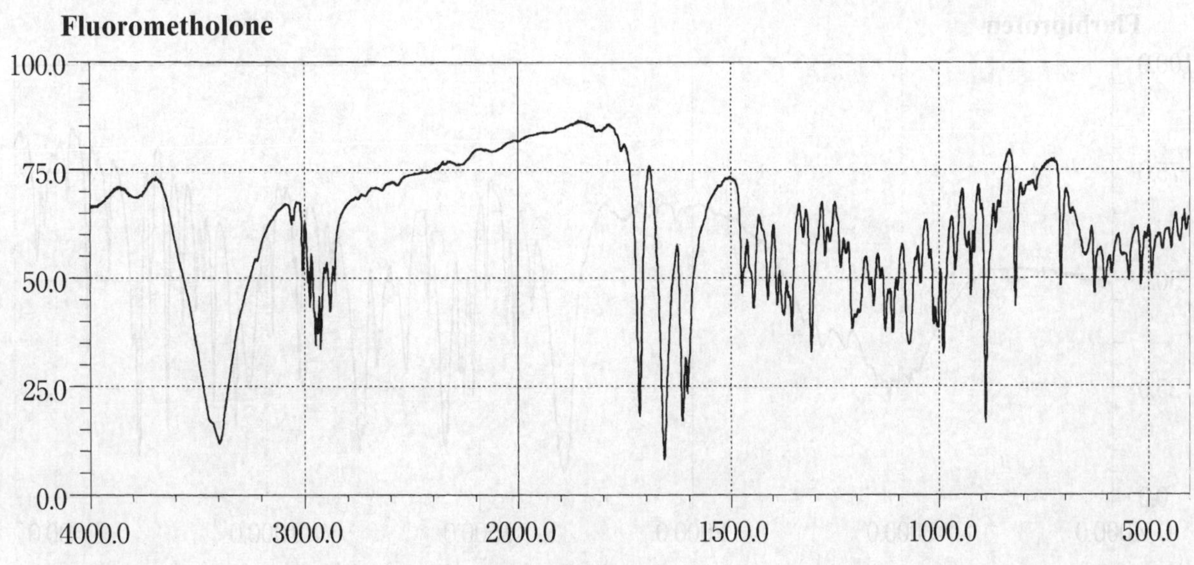

Fluphenazine Enanthate

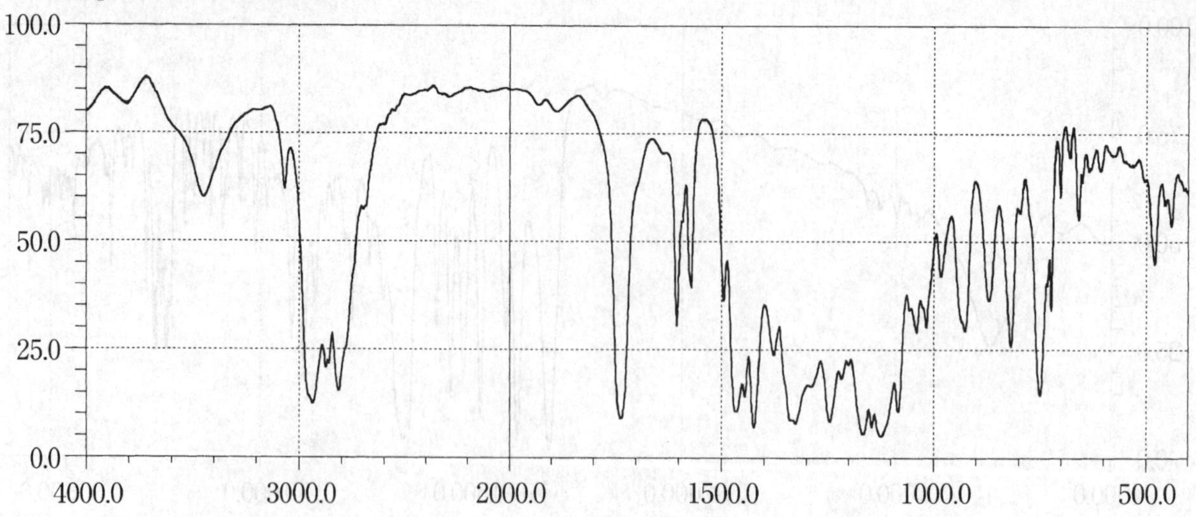

Flurazepam Hydrochloride

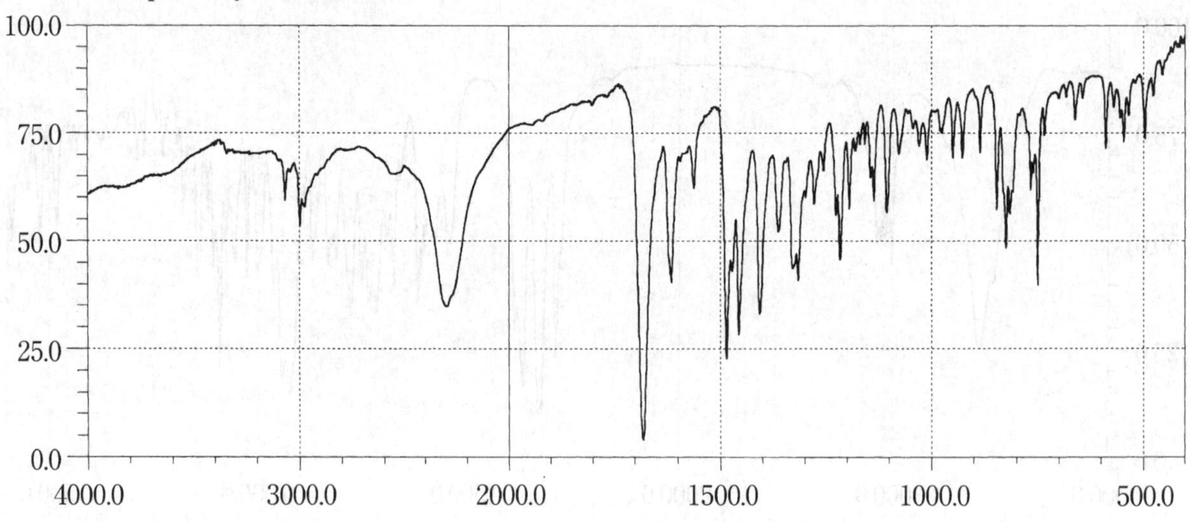

Flurbiprofen

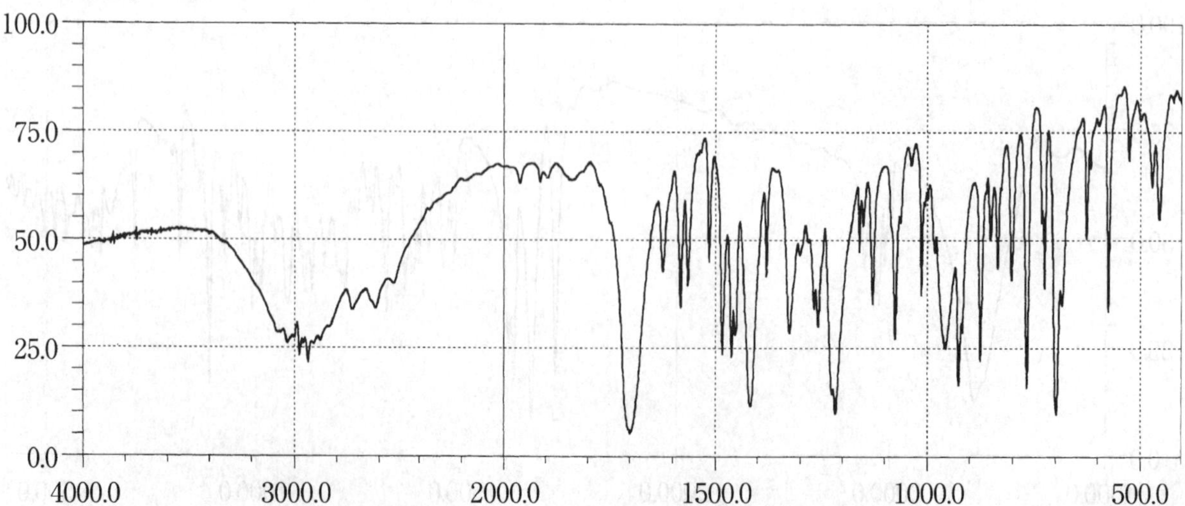

Flutamide

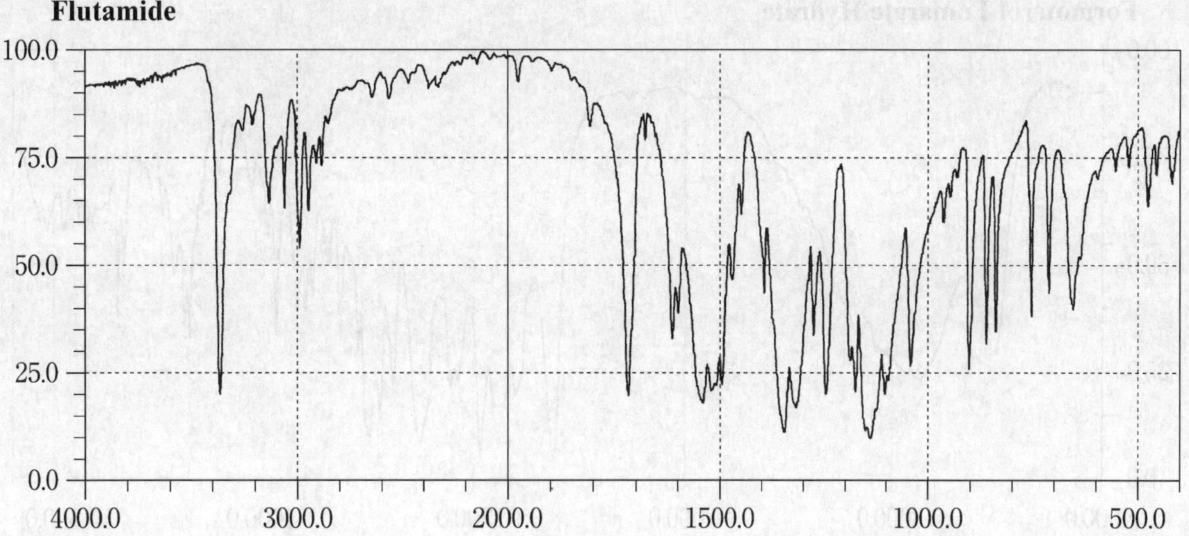

Flutoprazepam

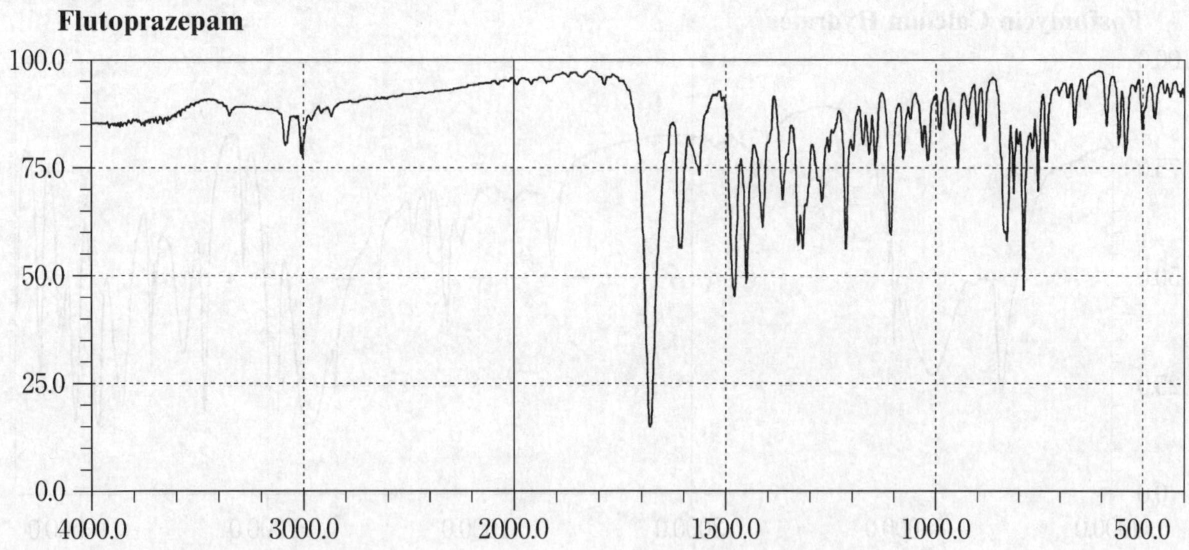

Fluvoxamine Maleate

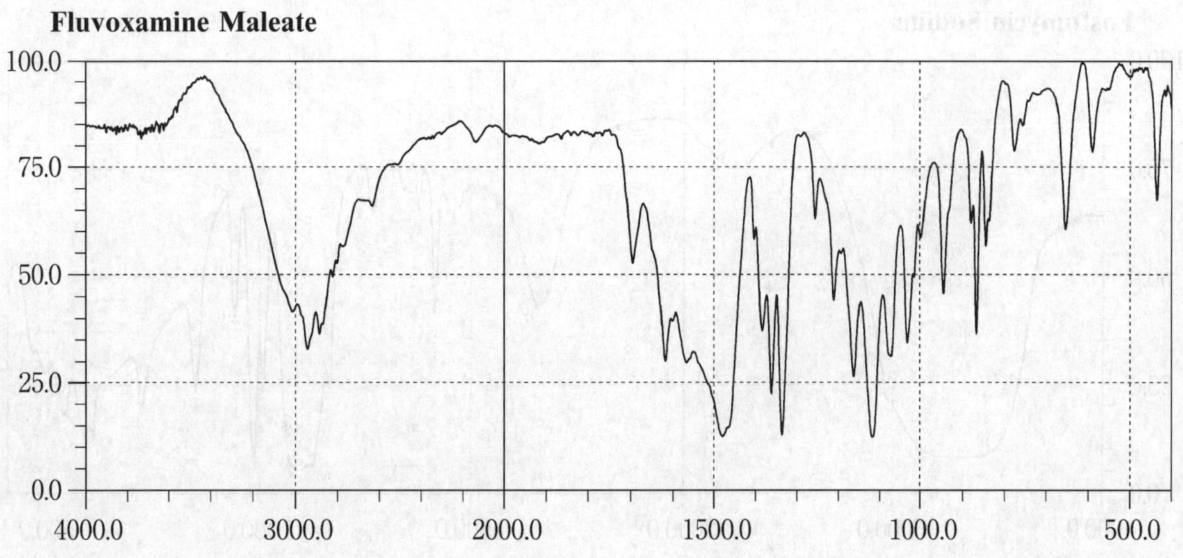

Formoterol Fumarate Hydrate

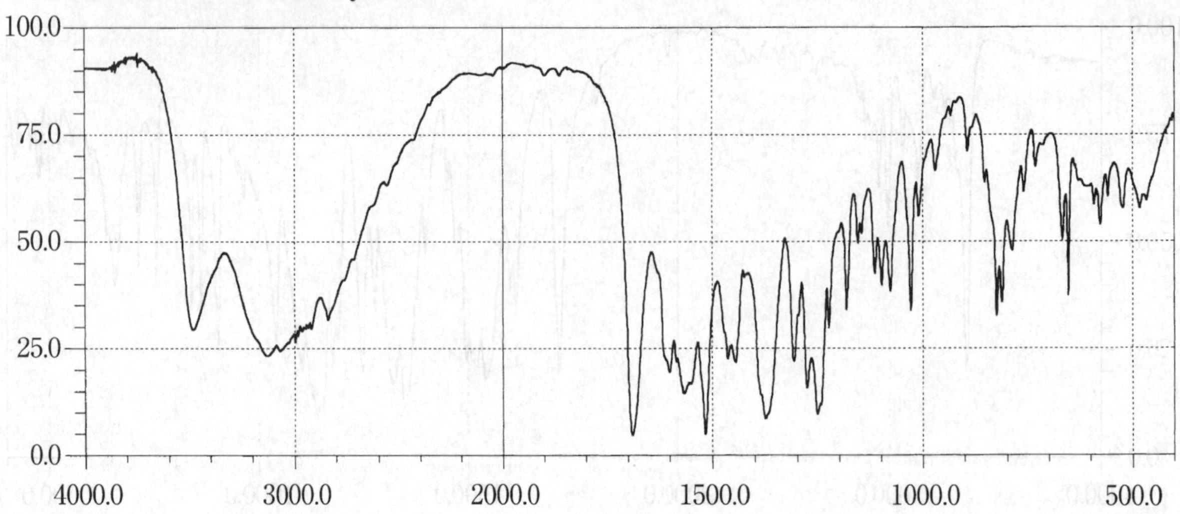

Fosfomycin Calcium Hydrate

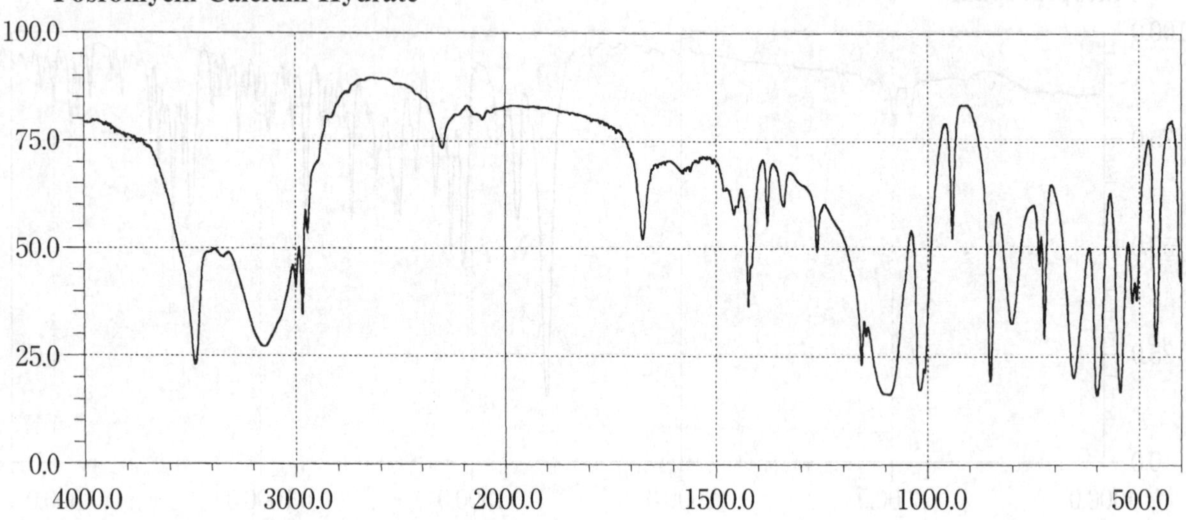

Fosfomycin Sodium

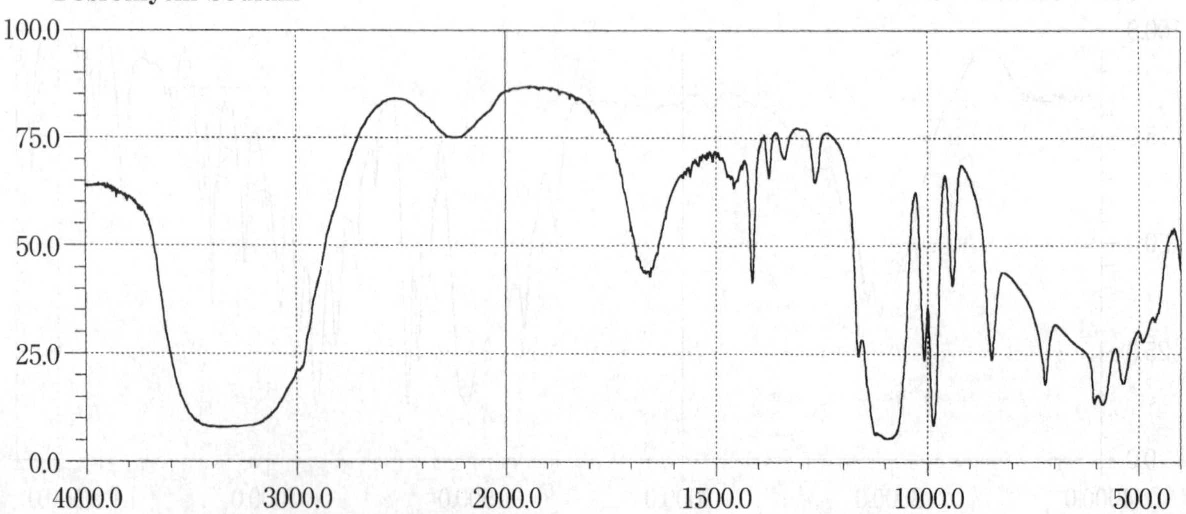

Fructose

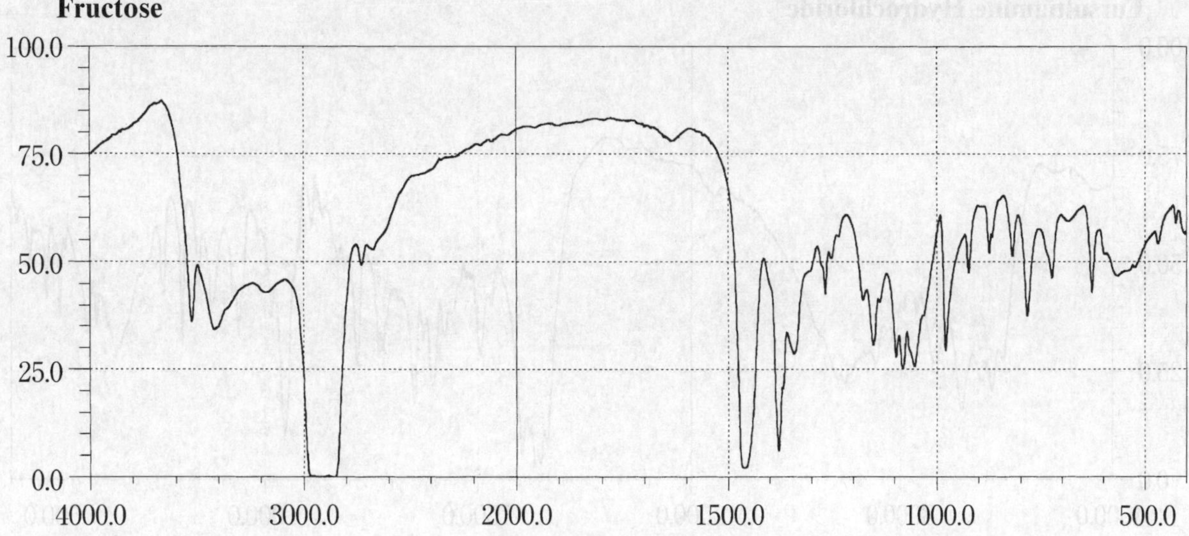

Fudosteine

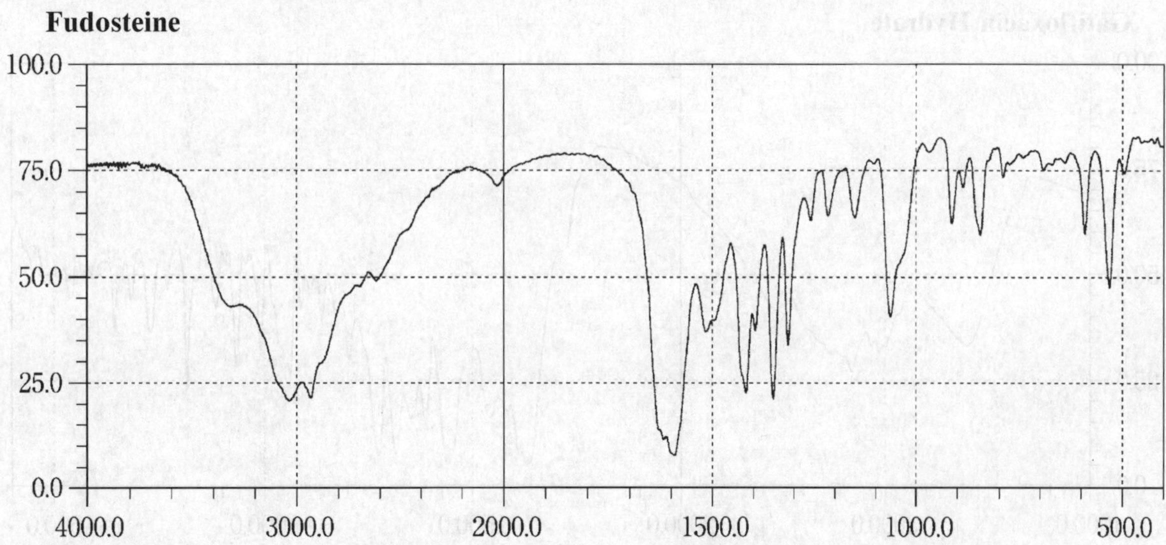

Furosemide

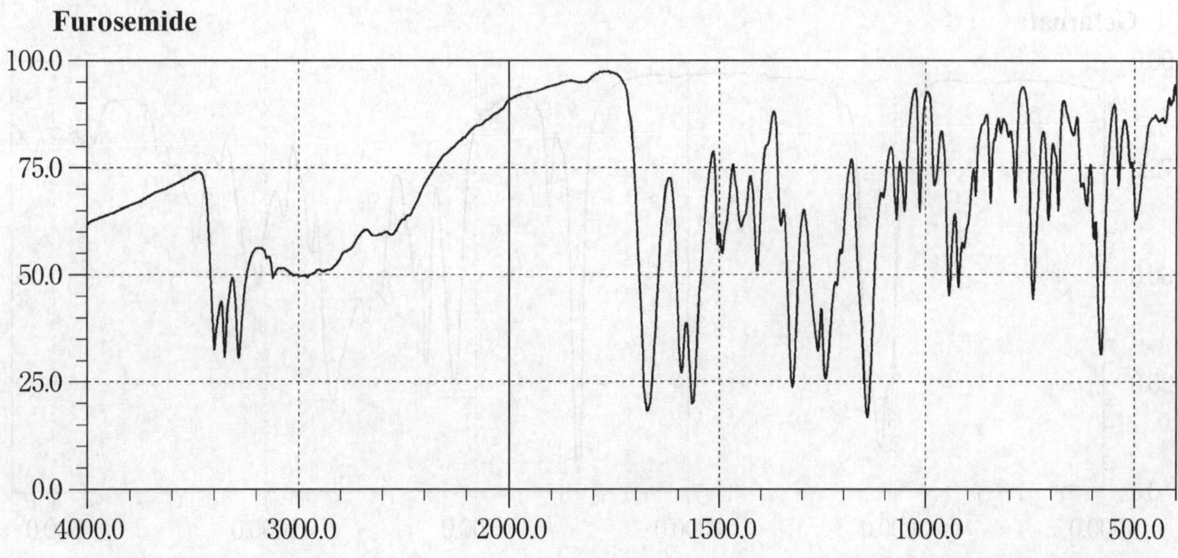

Fursultiamine Hydrochloride

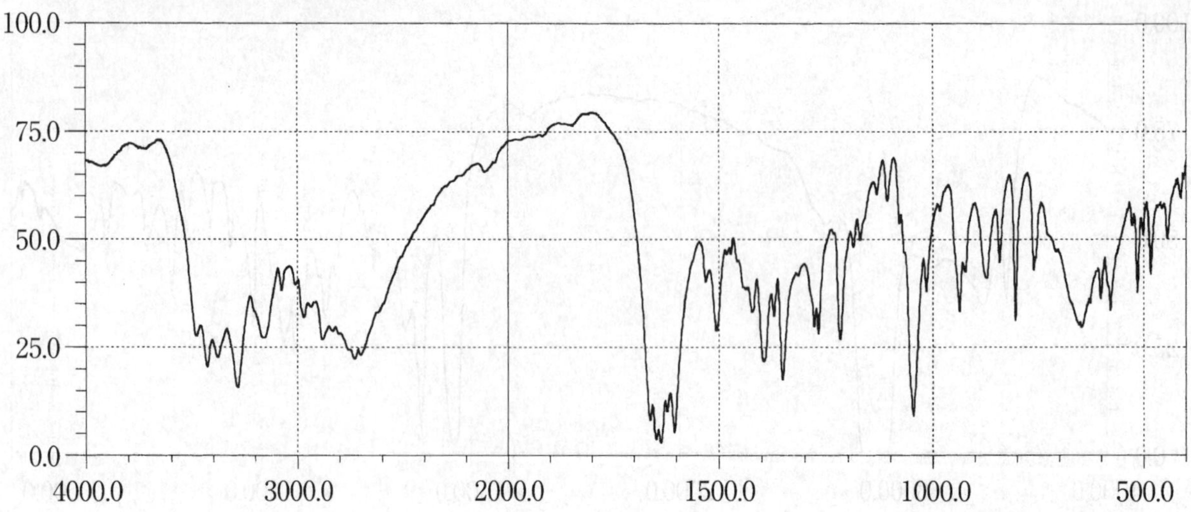

Gatifloxacin Hydrate

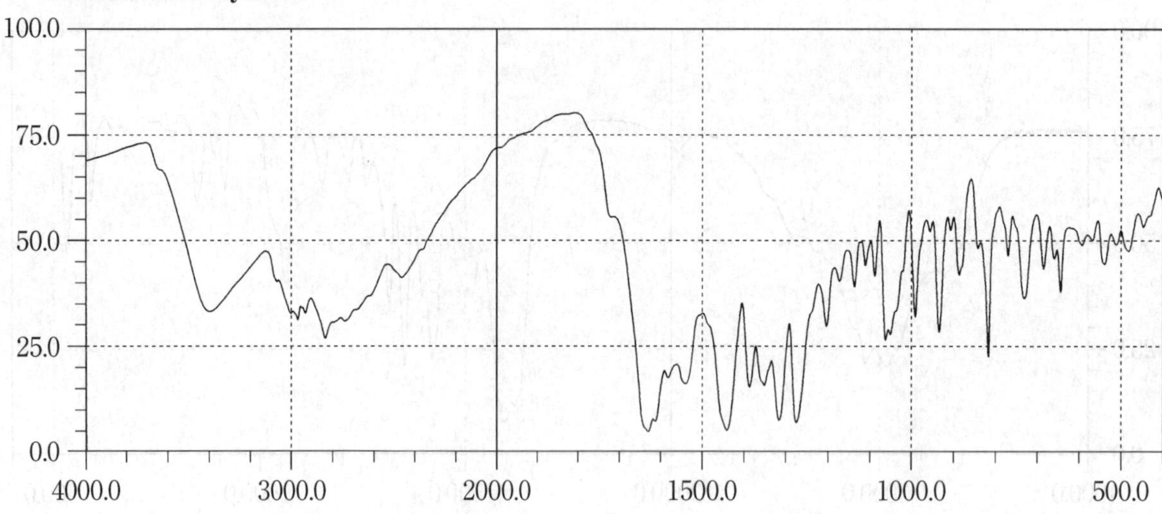

Gefarnate

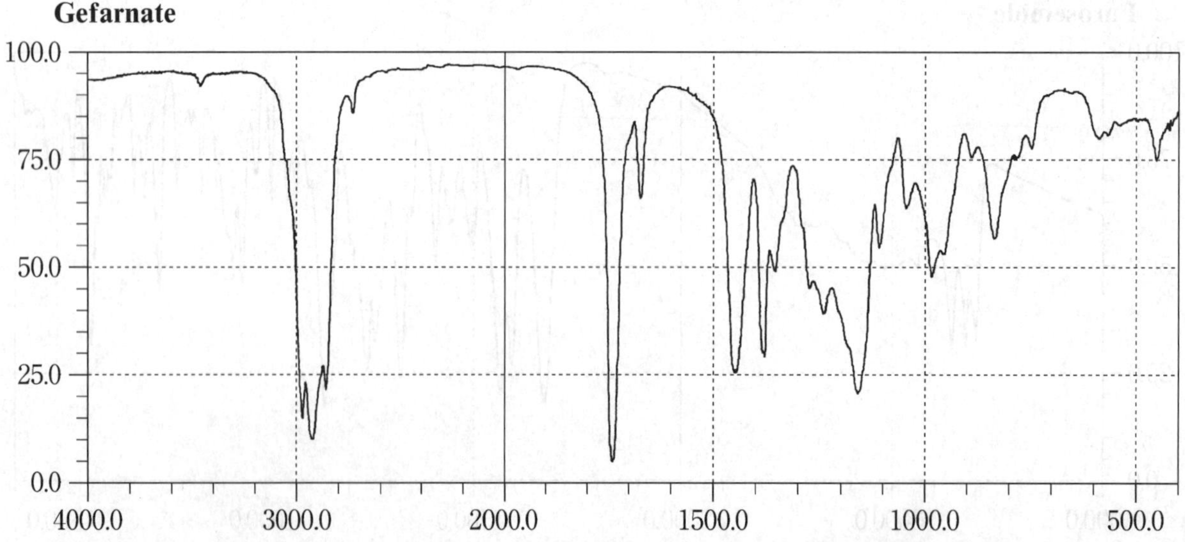

Gefitinib

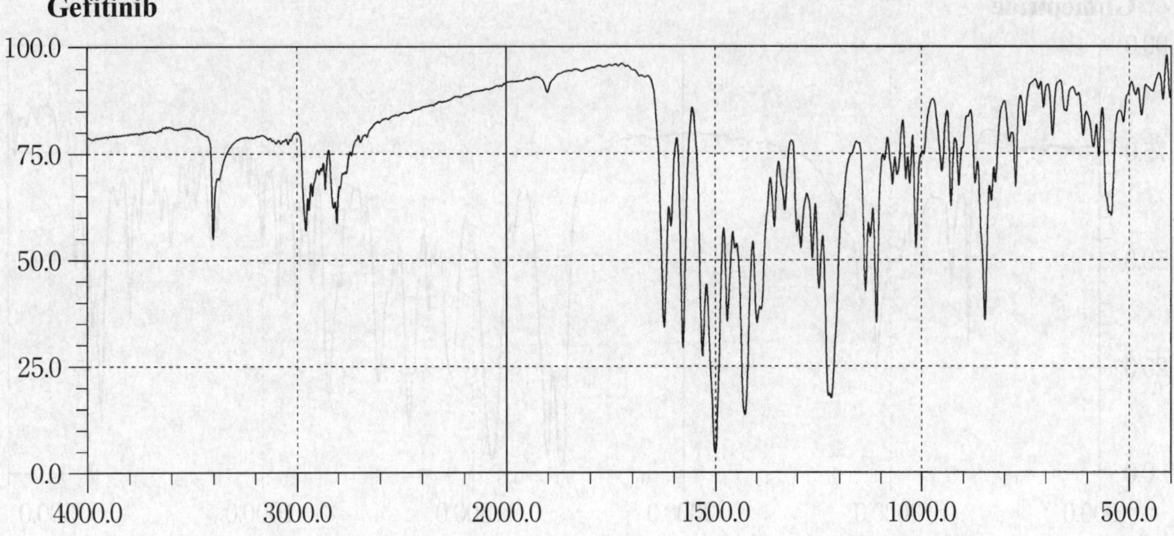

Glibenclamide

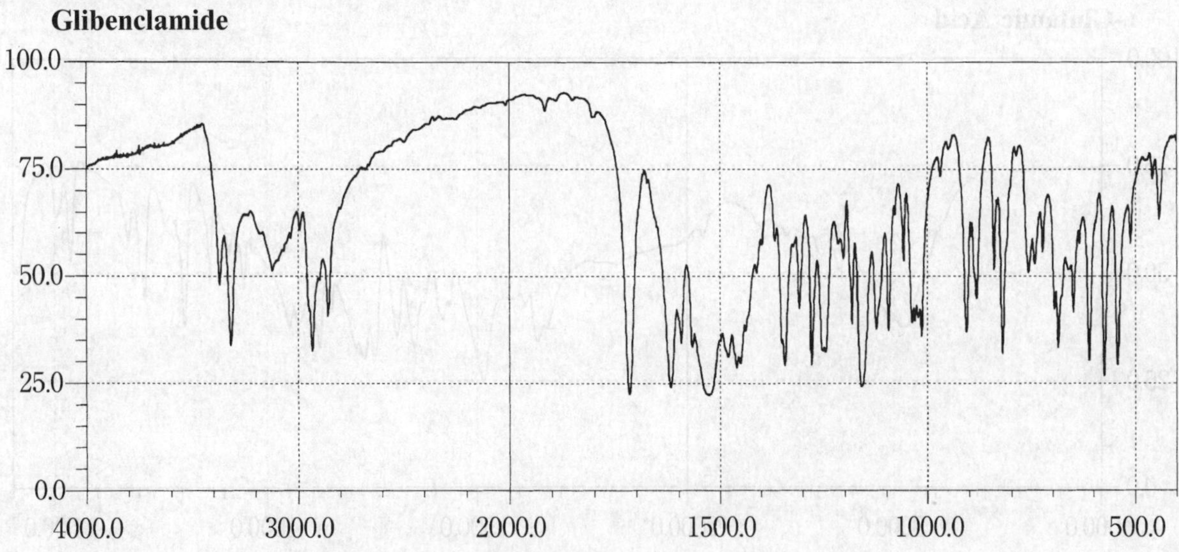

Gliclazide

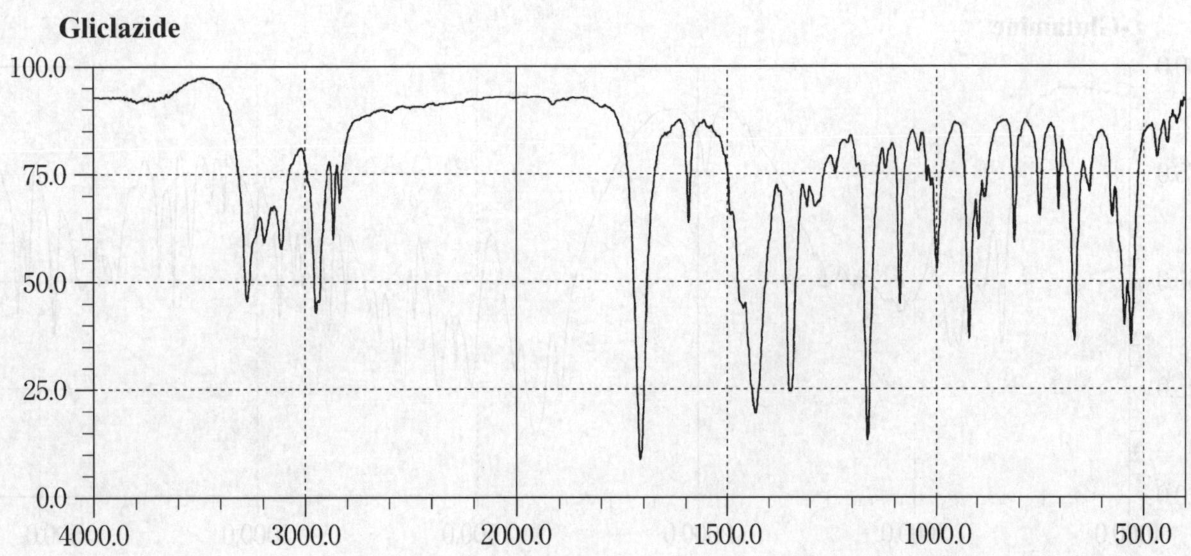

Glimepiride

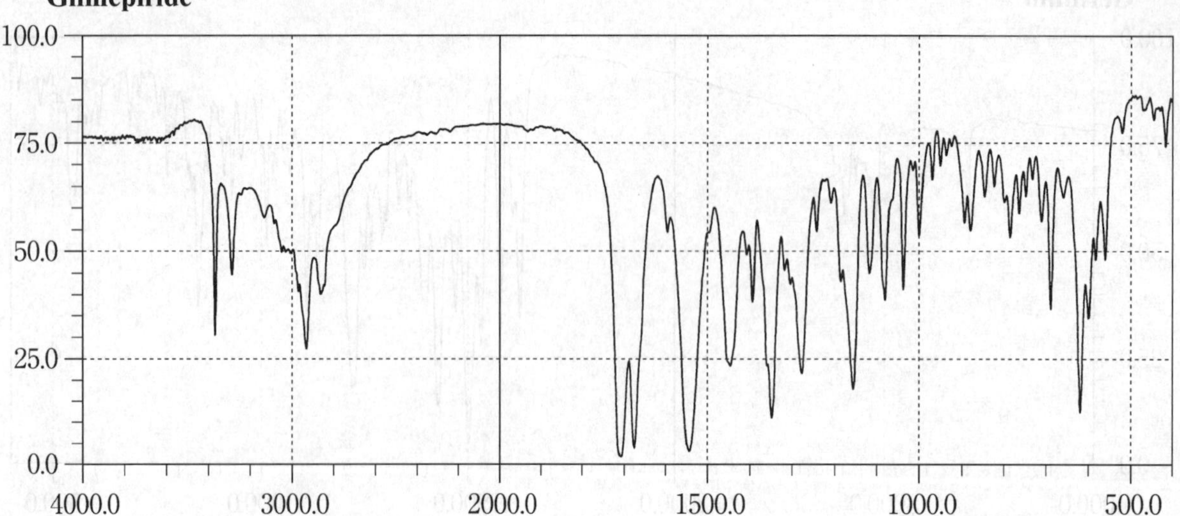

L-Glutamic Acid

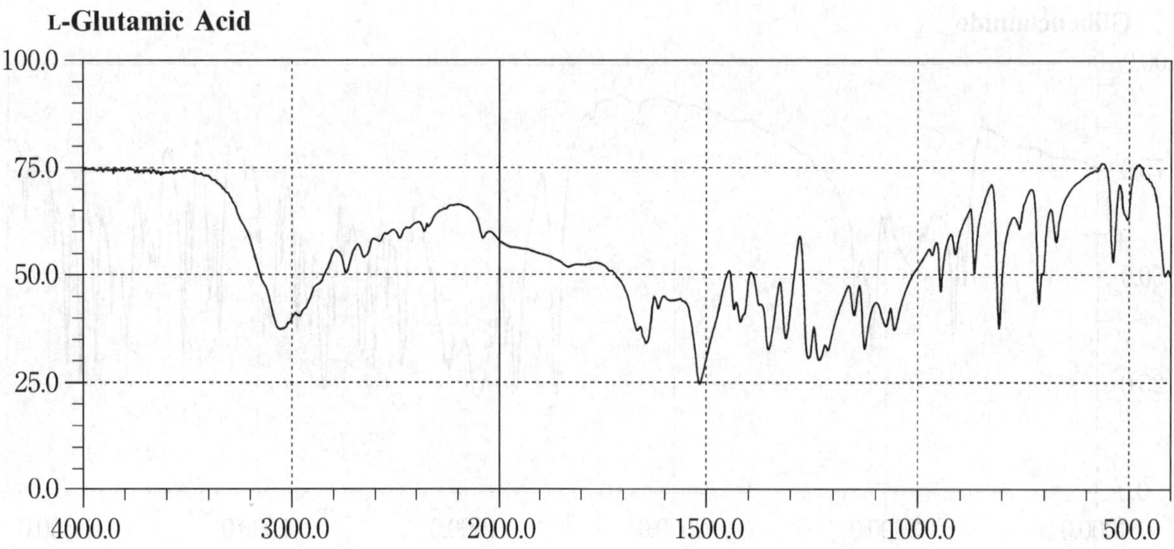

L-Glutamine

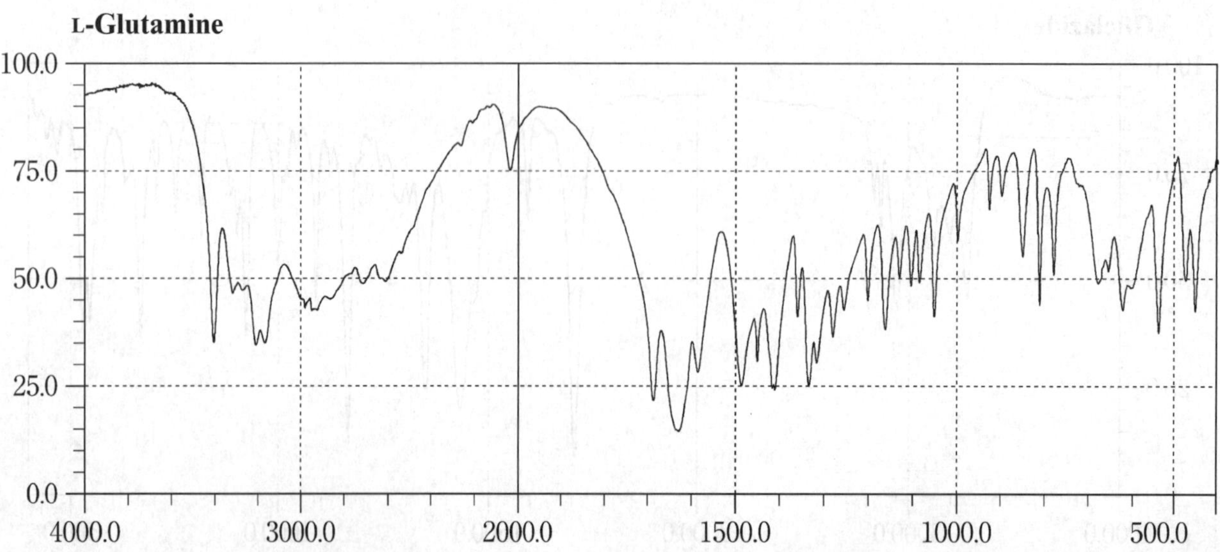

Glutathione

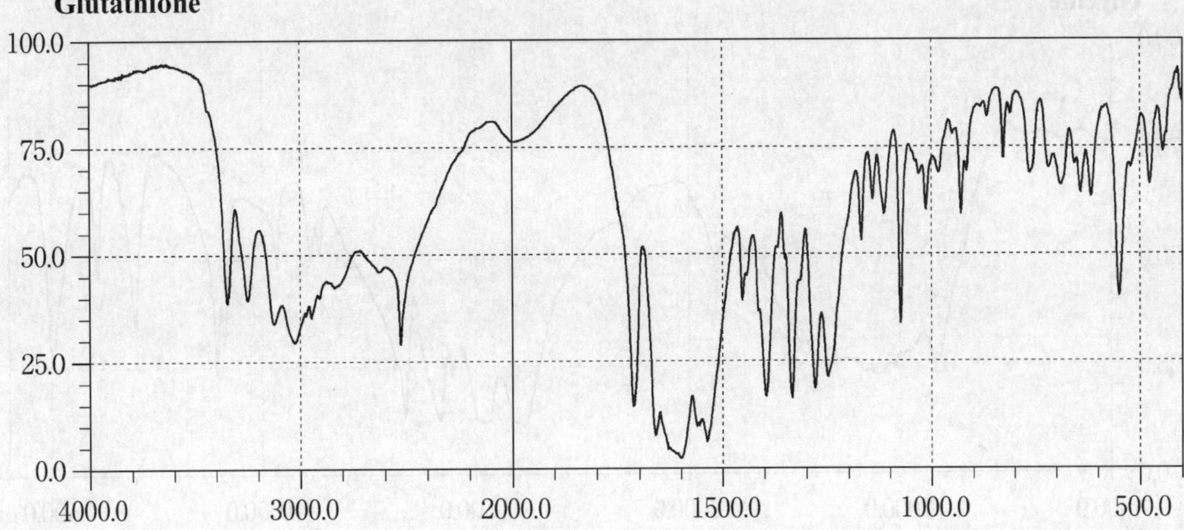

Glycerin

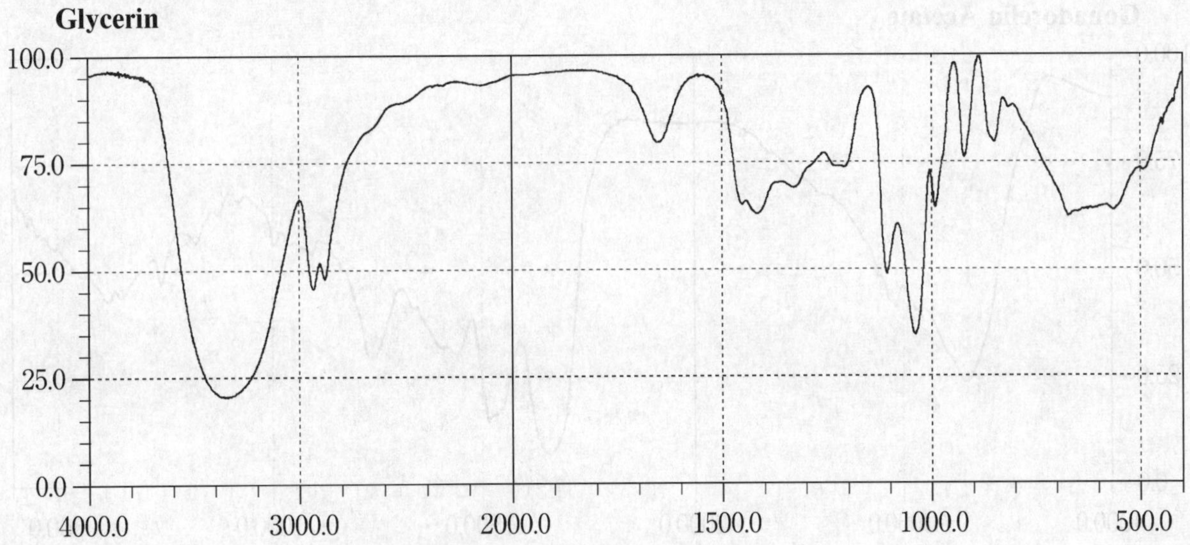

Concentrated Glycerin

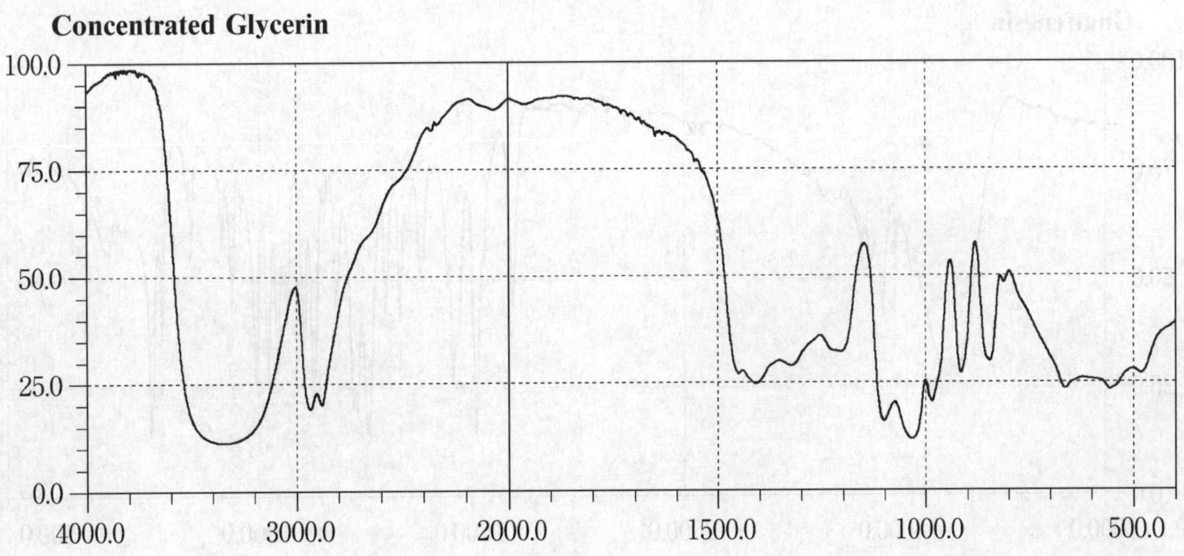

Glycine

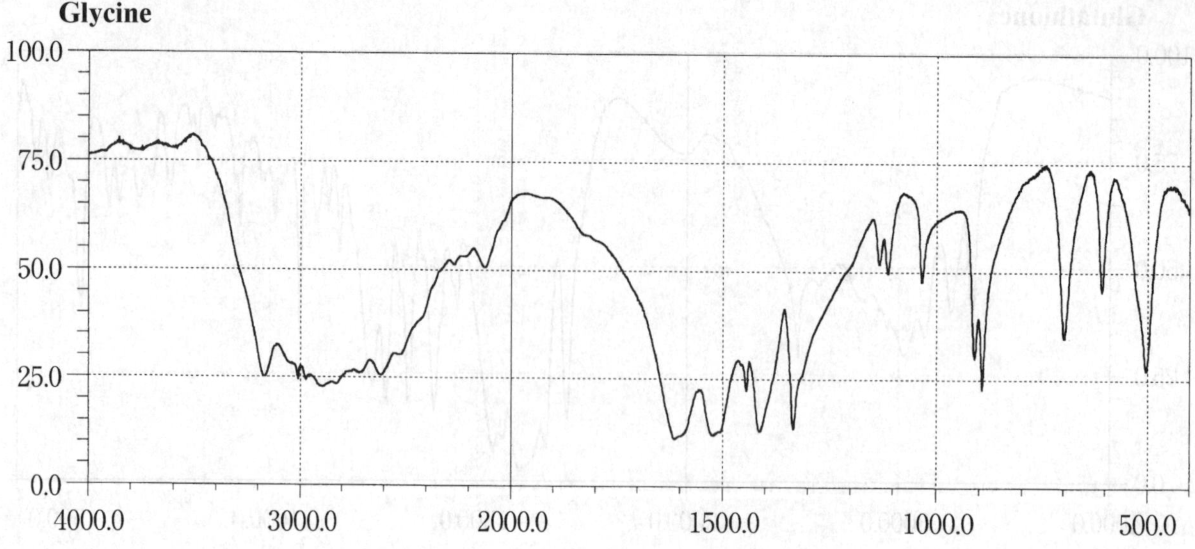

Gonadorelin Acetate

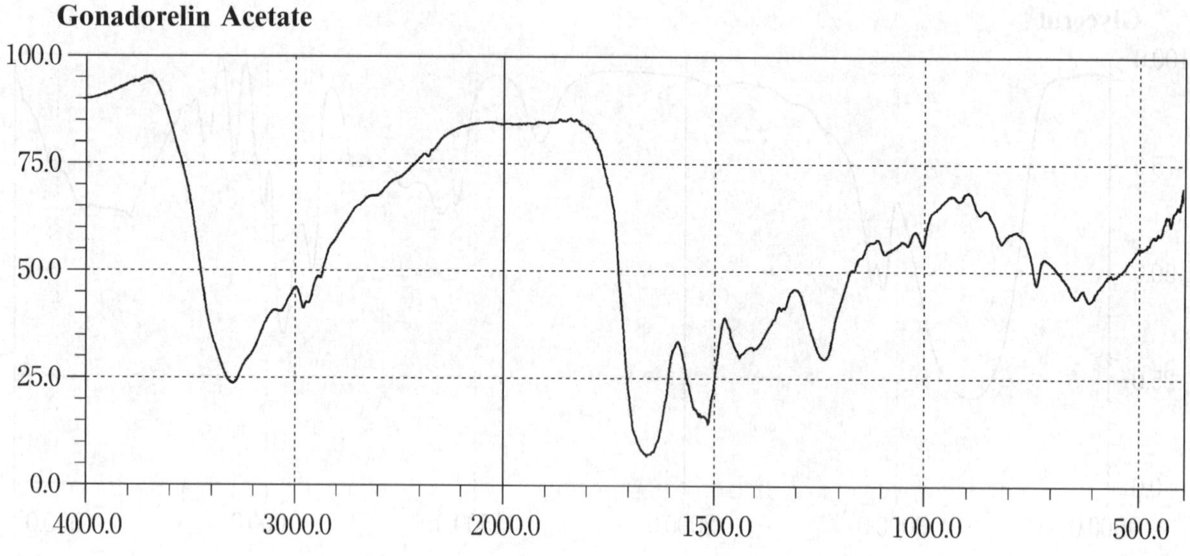

Guaifenesin

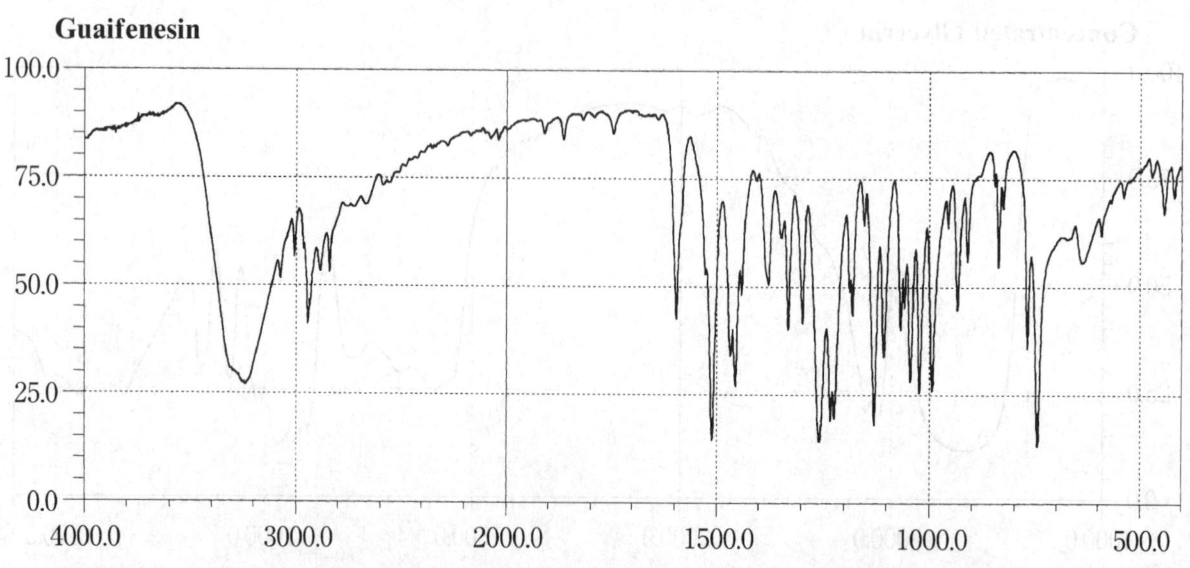

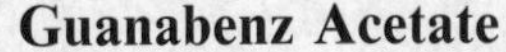

Guanabenz Acetate

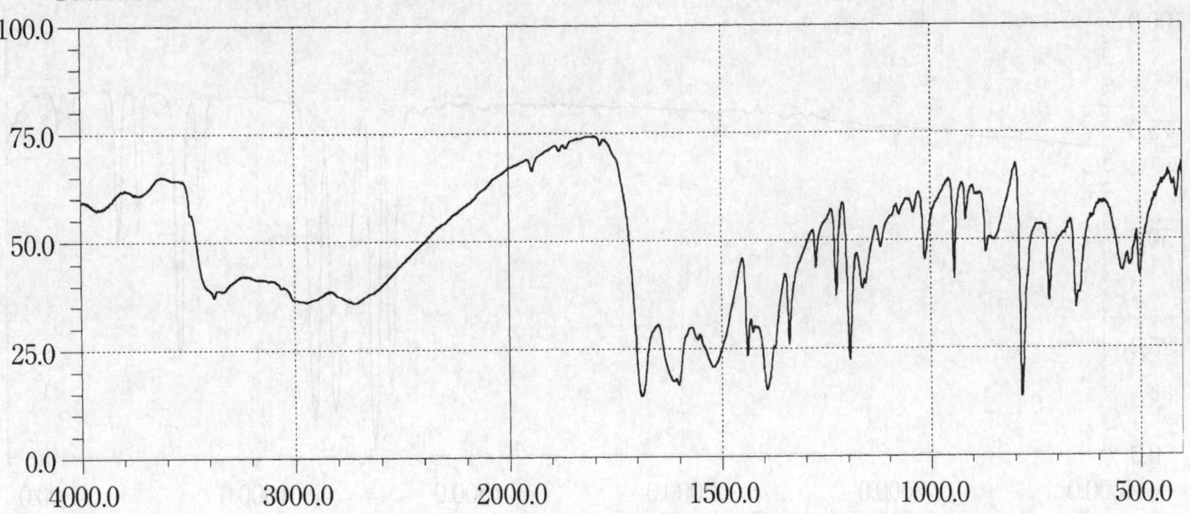

Guanethidine Sulfate

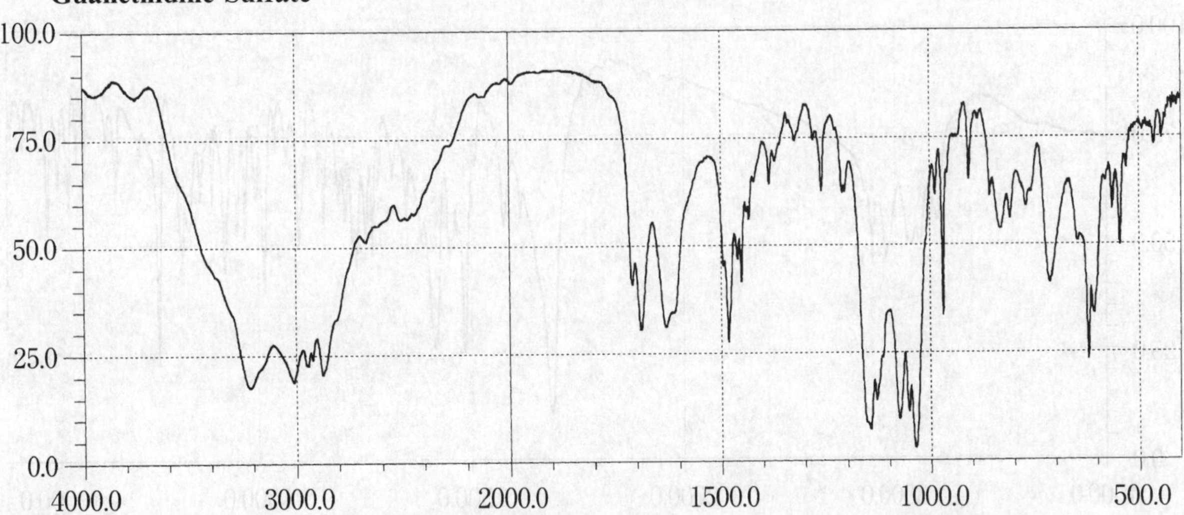

Haloperidol

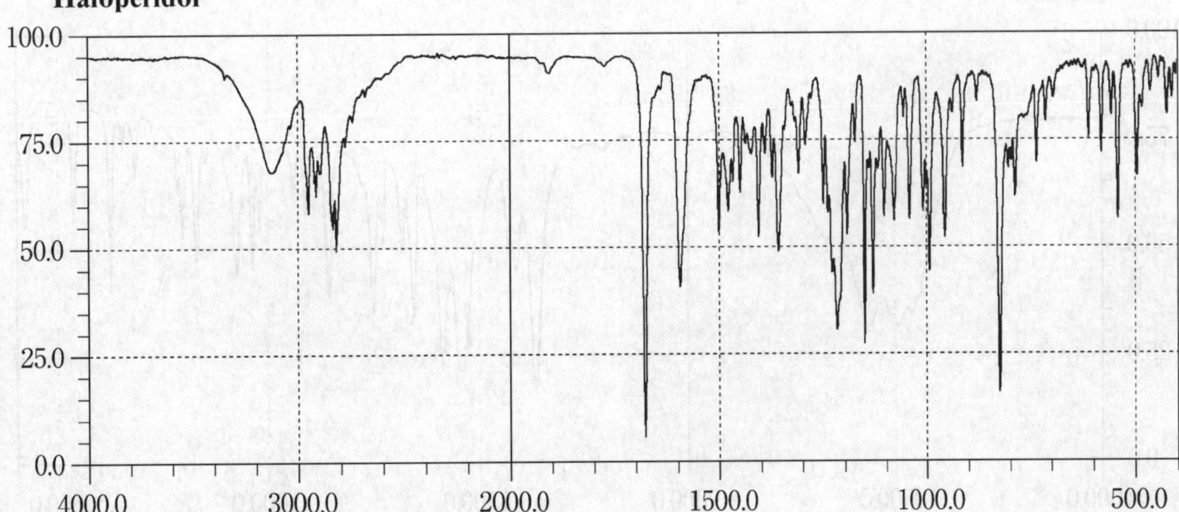

Halothane

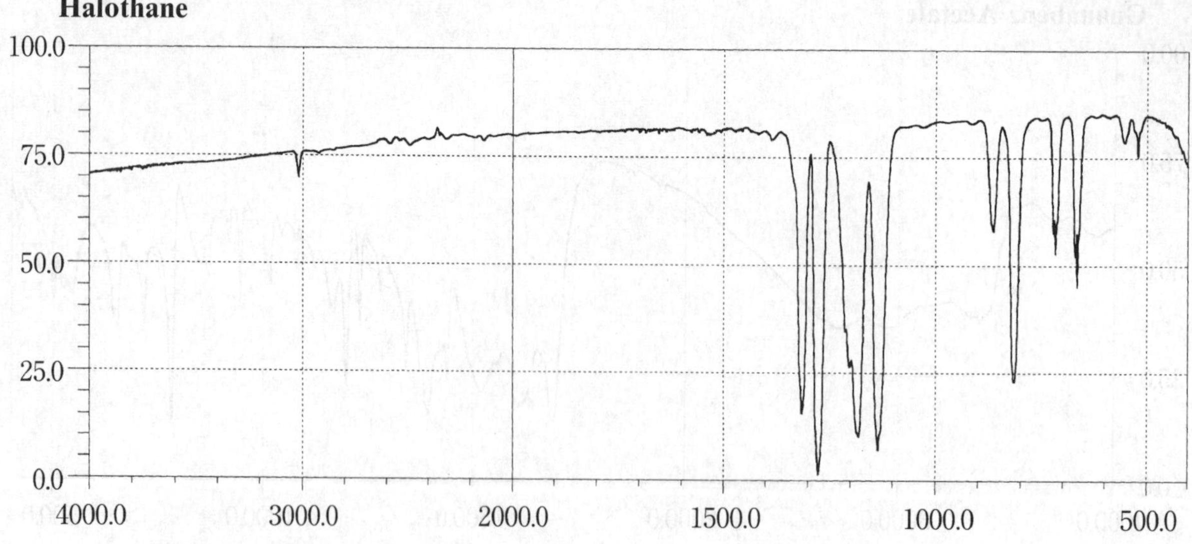

Haloxazolam

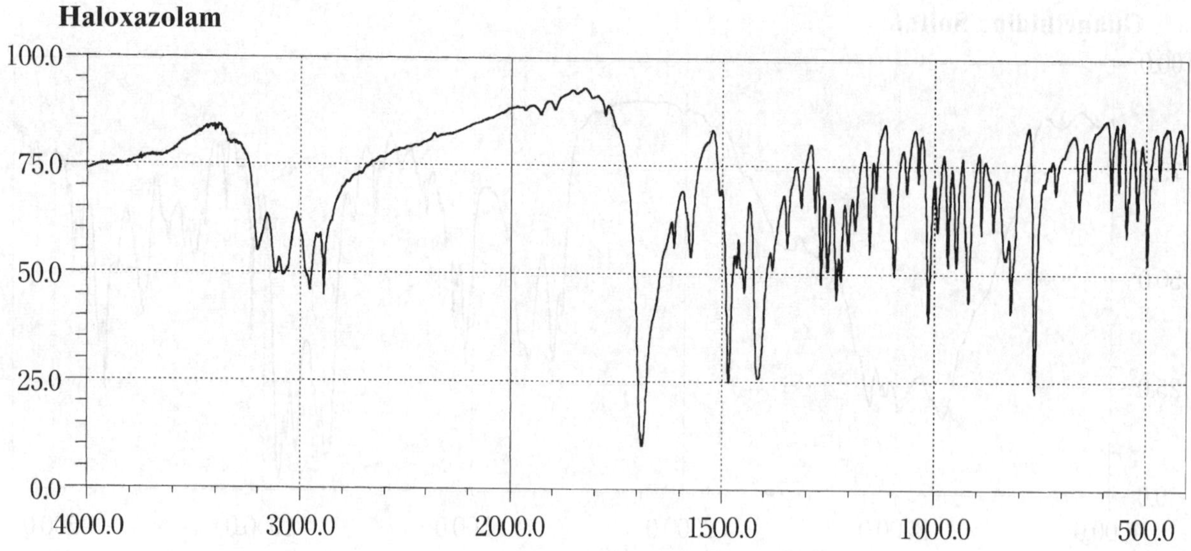

L-Histidine

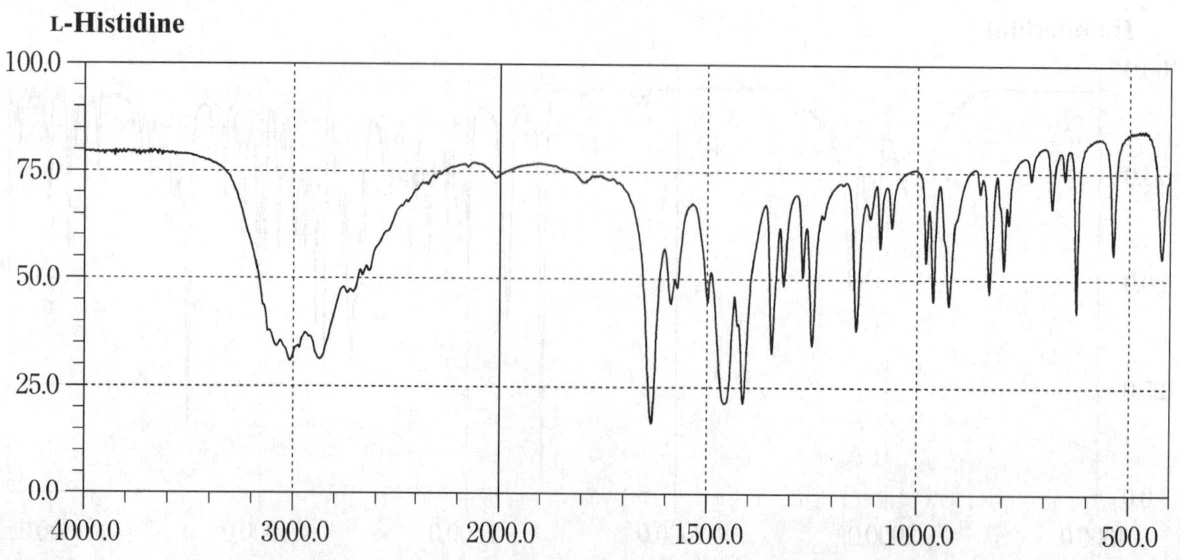

L-Histidine Hydrochloride Hydrate

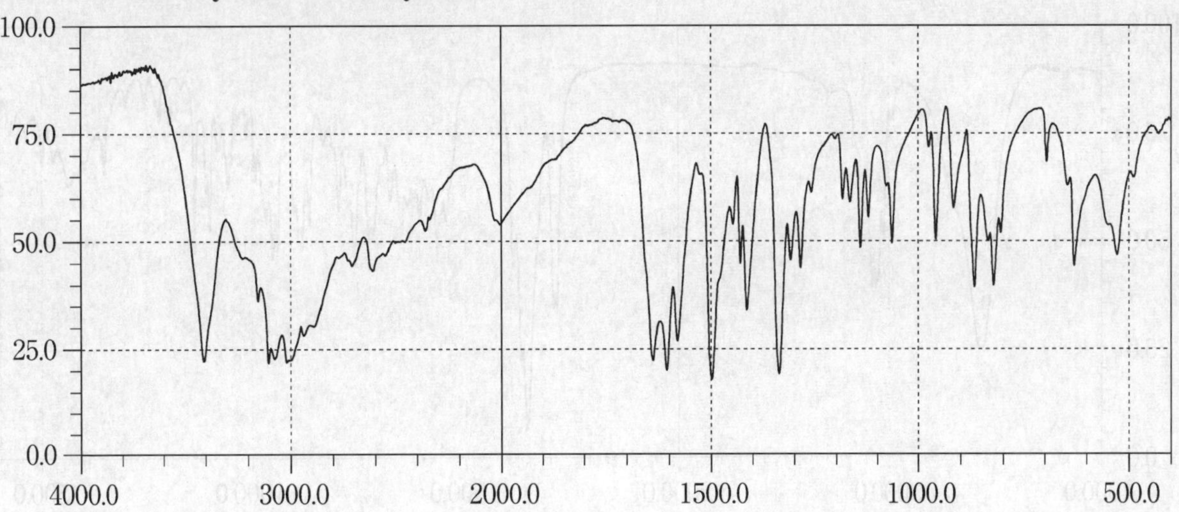

Homochlorcyclizine Hydrochloride

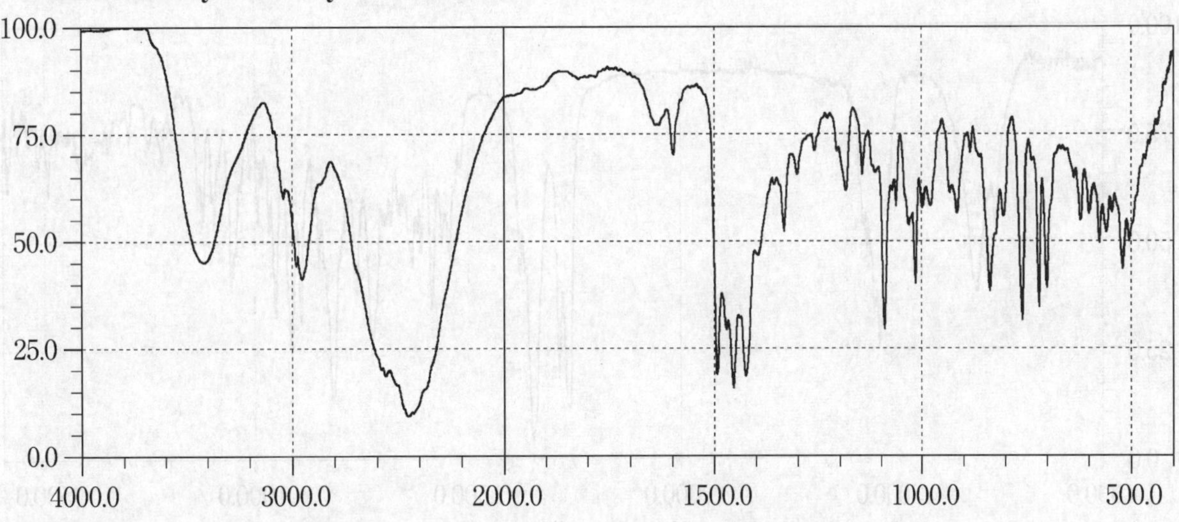

Hydralazine Hydrochloride

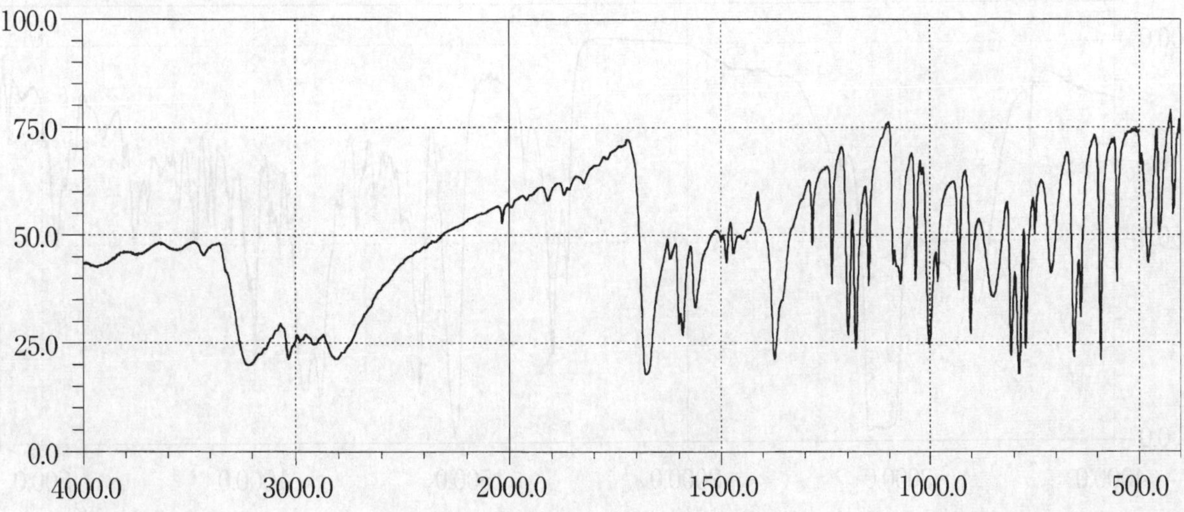

Hydrocortisone

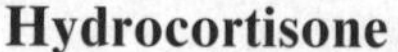

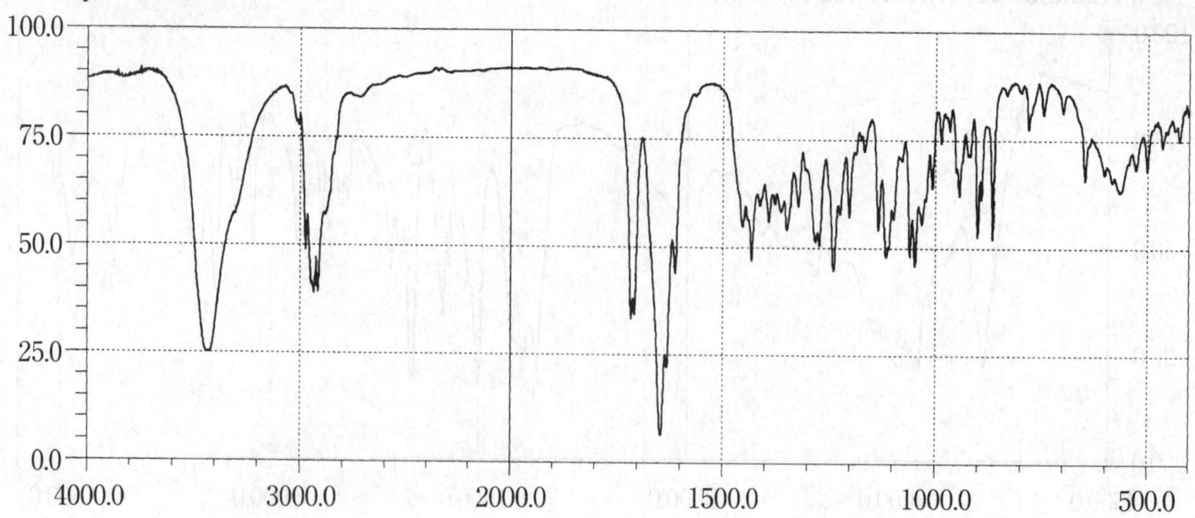

Hydrocortisone Butyrate

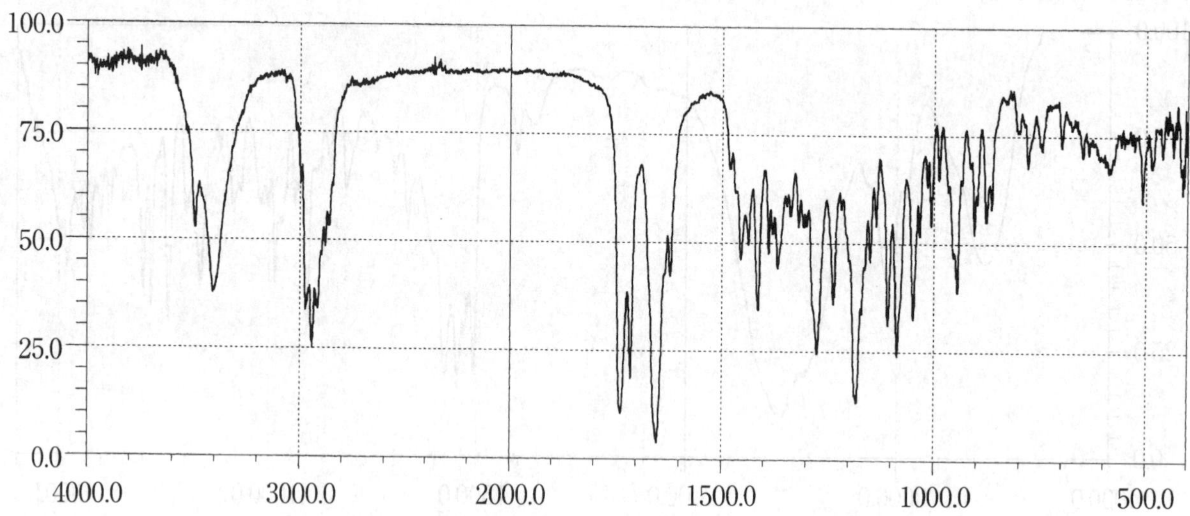

Hydrocortisone Sodium Phosphate

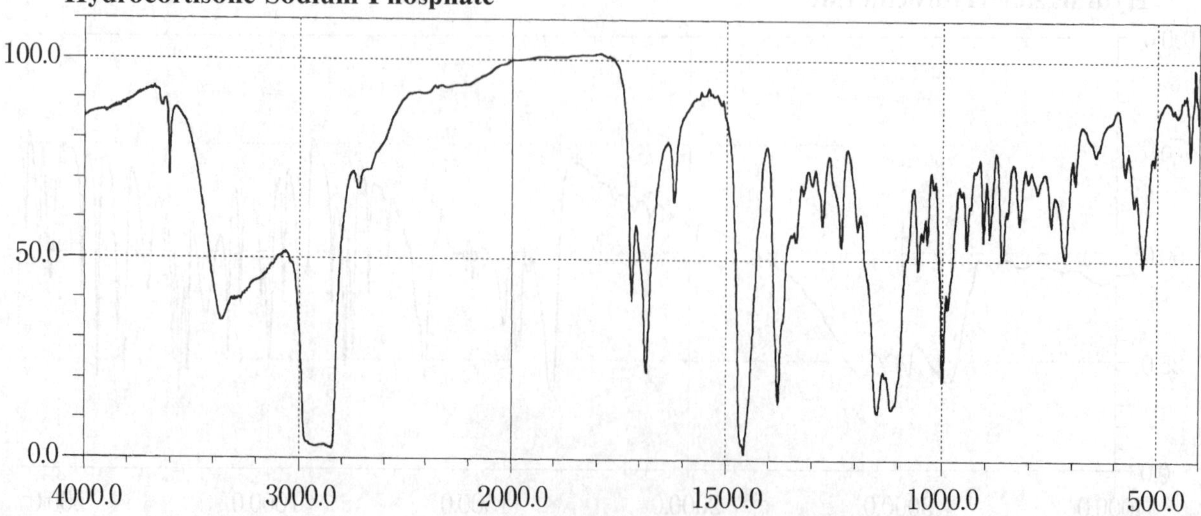

The JP Drugs are to be tested according to the provisions given in the pertinent monographs, General Notices, General Rules for Crude Drugs, General Rules for Preparations, and General Tests for their conformity to the Japanese Pharmacopoeia. (See the General Notices 5.)

Hydrocortisone Sodium Succinate

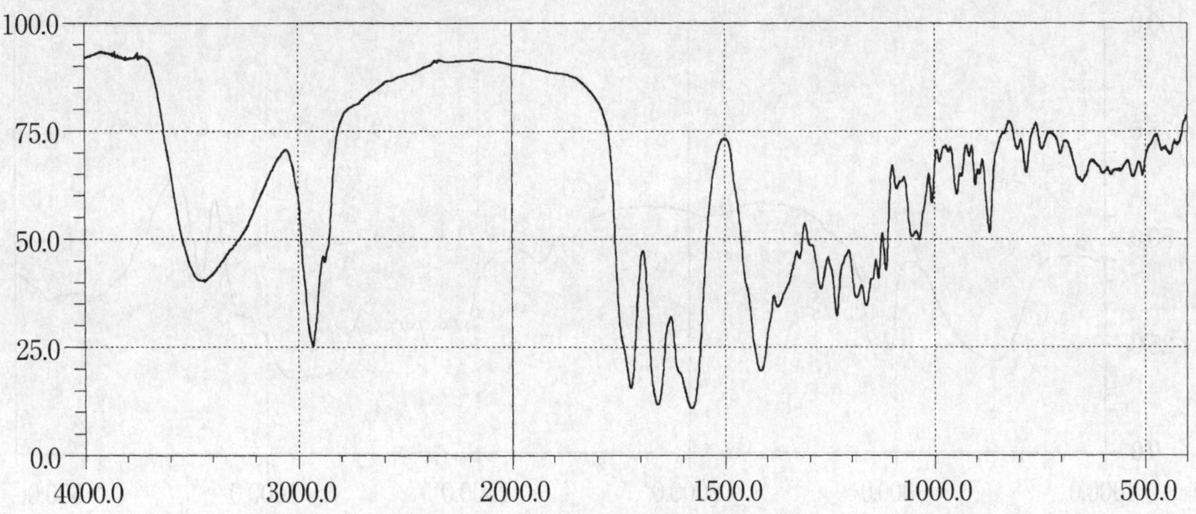

Hydrocortisone Succinate

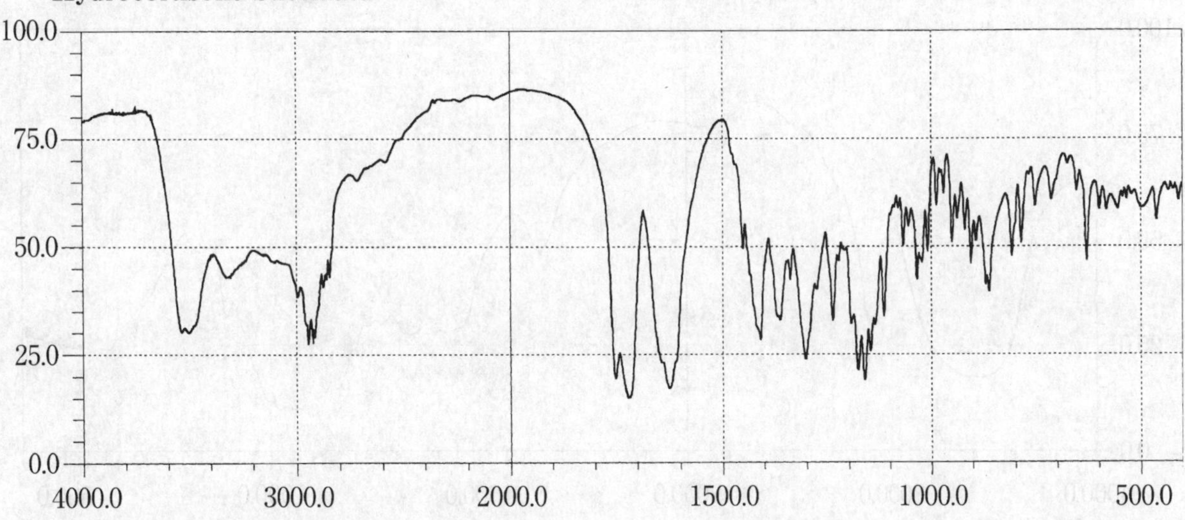

Hydrocotarnine Hydrochloride Hydrate

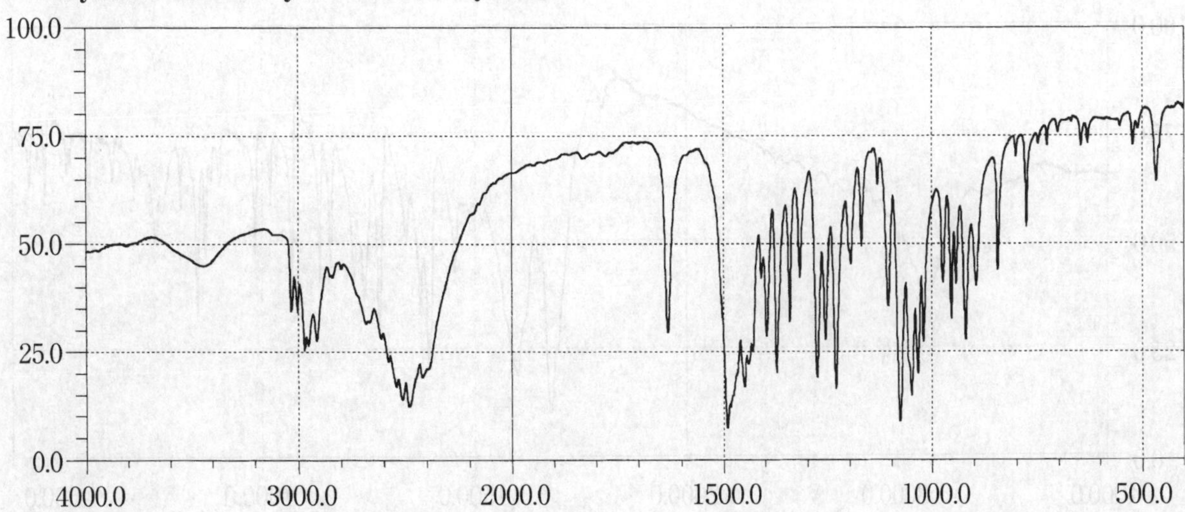

Hydroxypropylcellulose

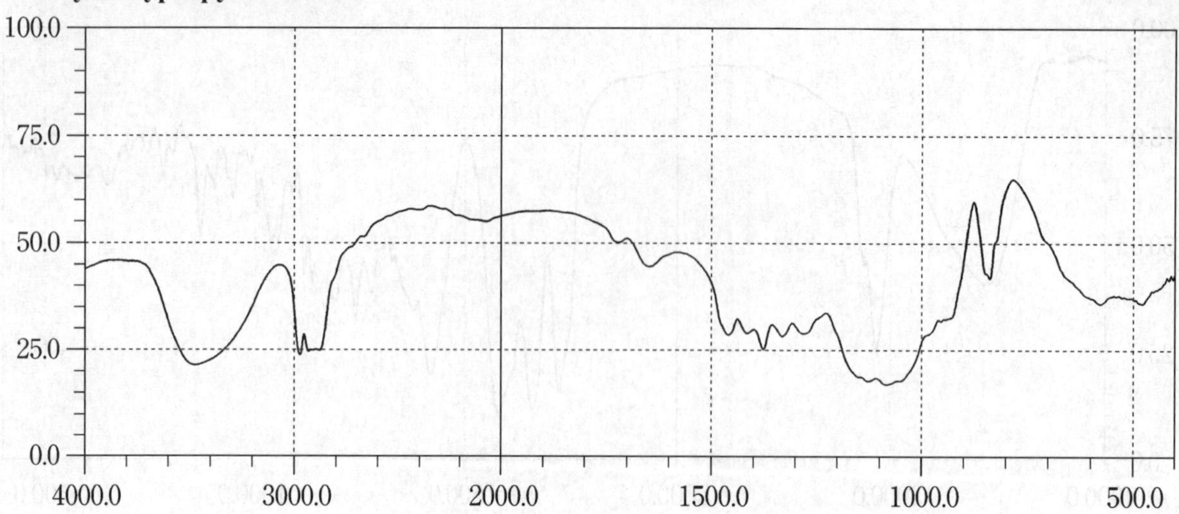

Low Substituted Hydroxypropylcellulose

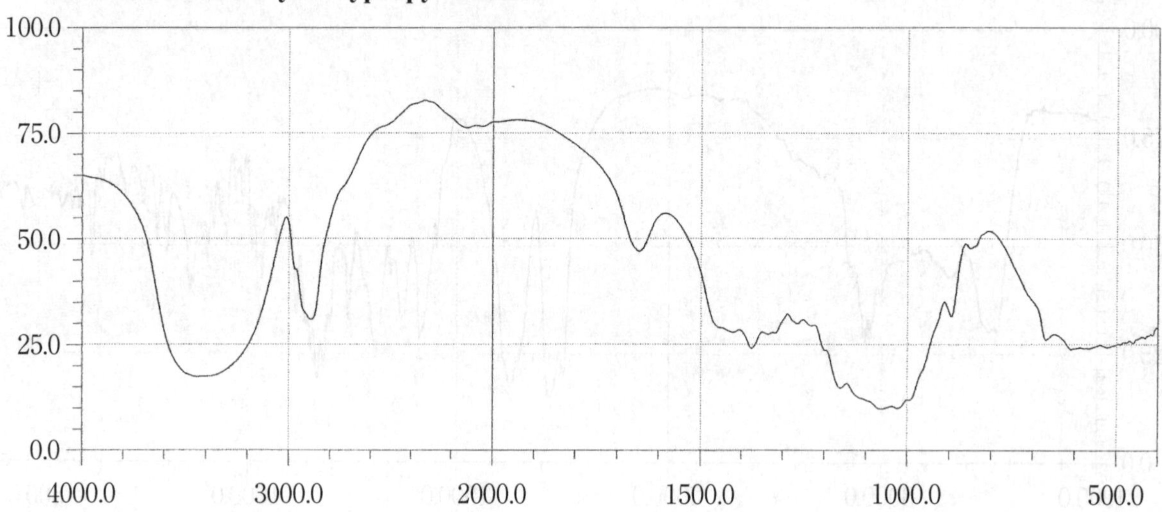

Hymecromone

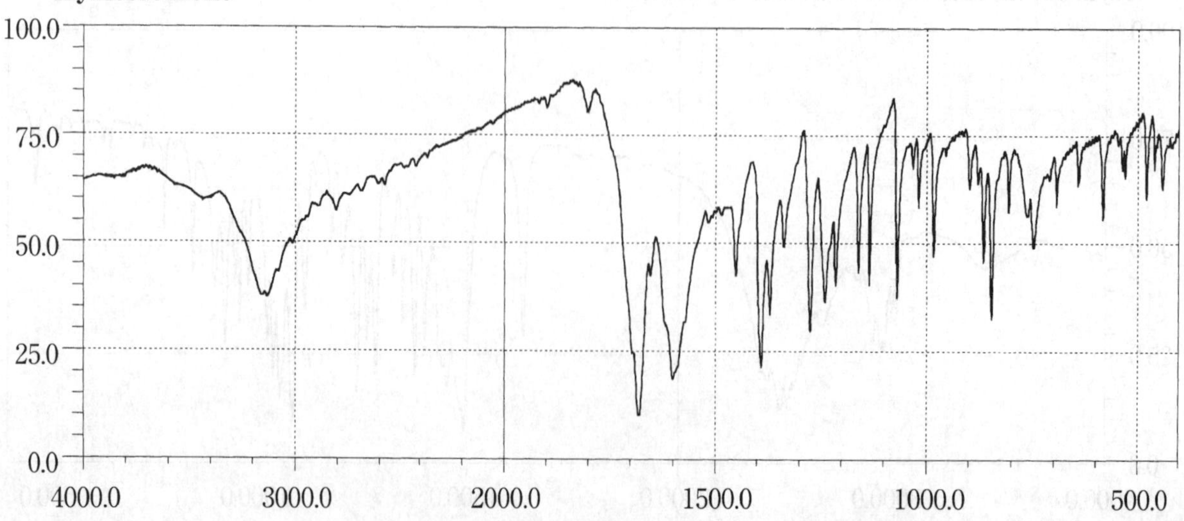

Hypromellose Phthalate (200731)

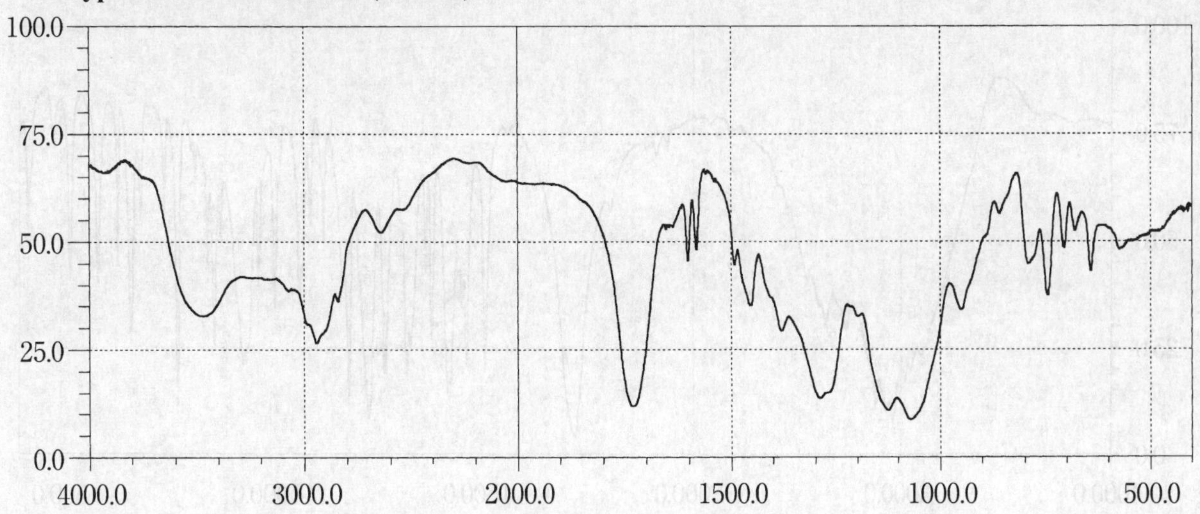

Hypromellose Phthalate (220824)

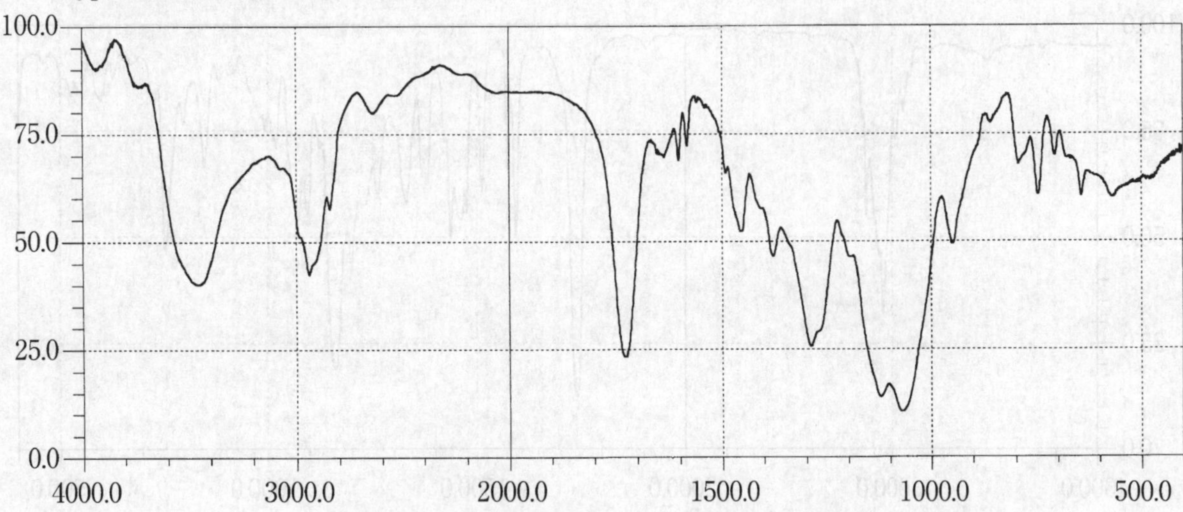

Ibudilast

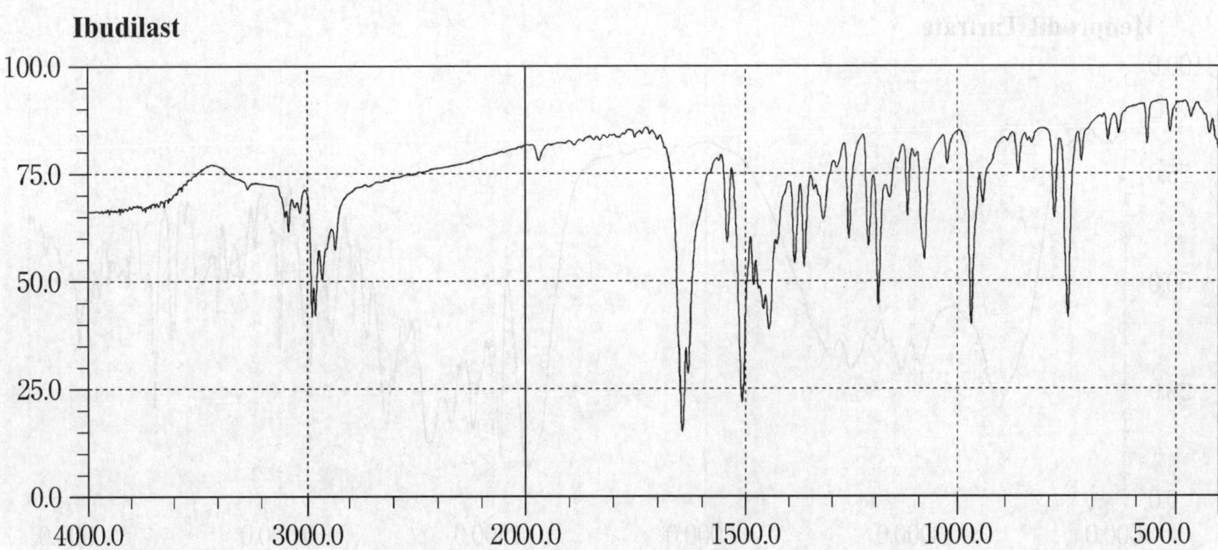

Ibuprofen

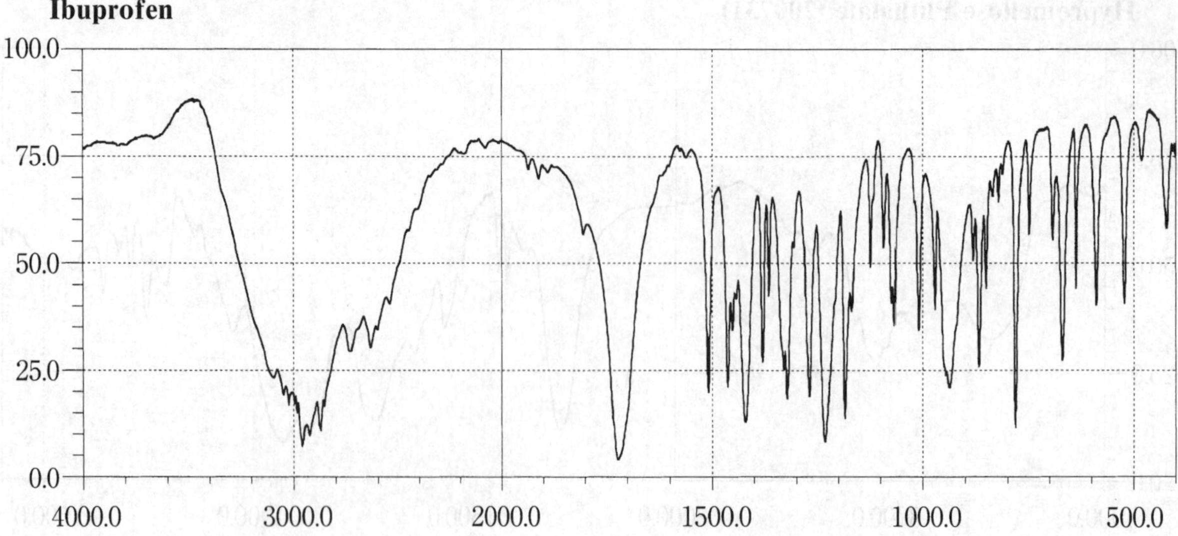

Ibuprofen Piconol

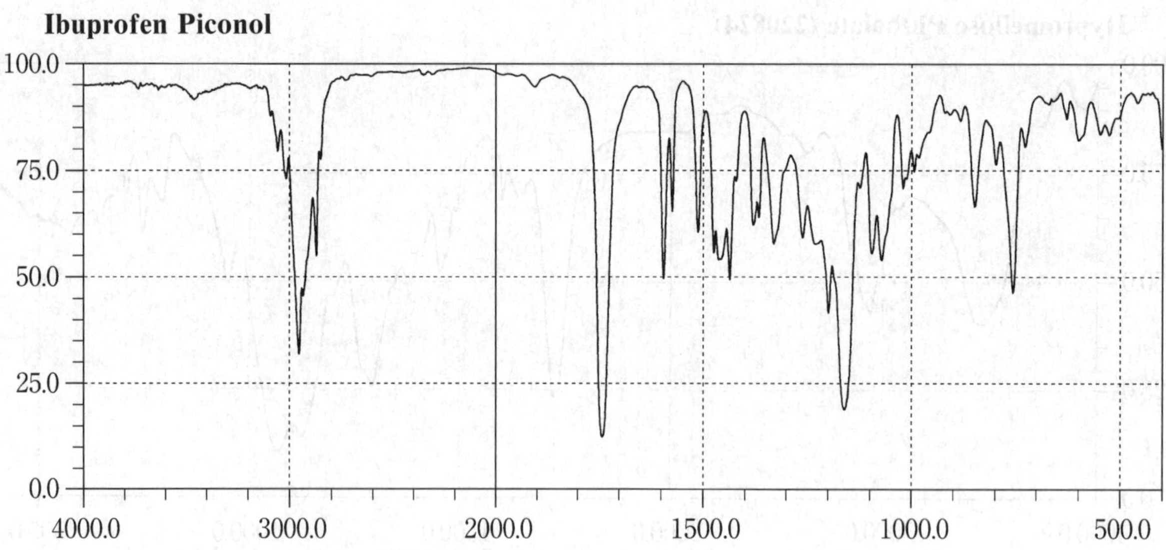

Ifenprodil Tartrate

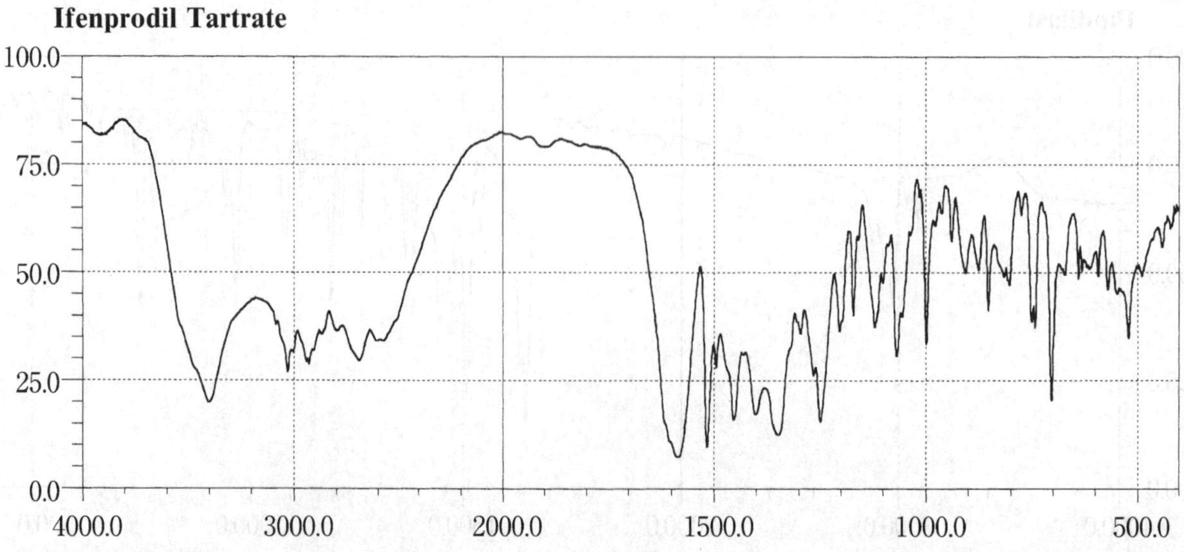

Imidapril Hydrochloride

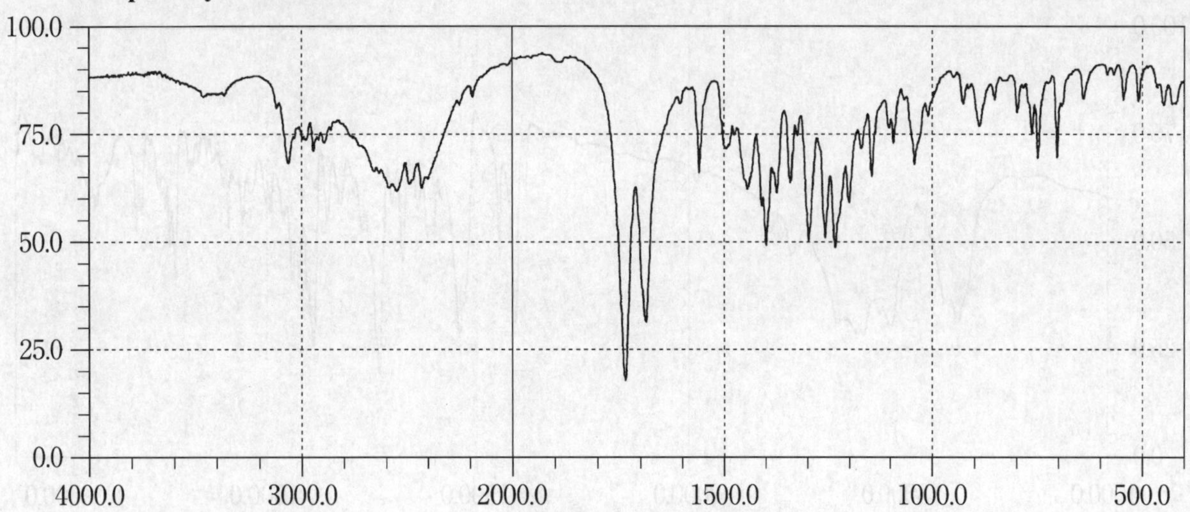

Imipenem Hydrate

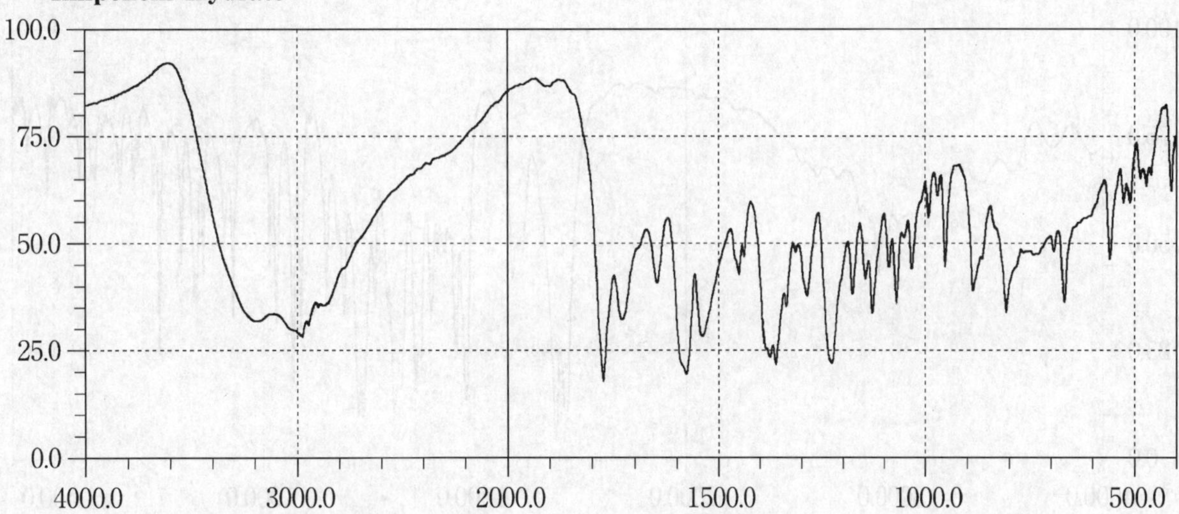

Indapamide

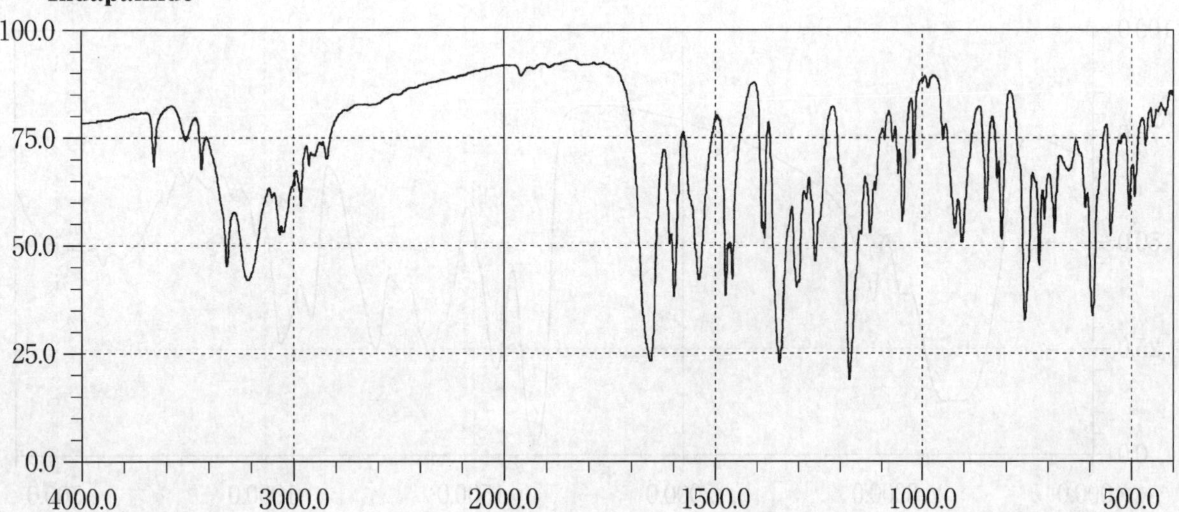

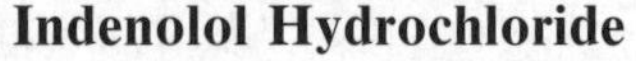

Indenolol Hydrochloride

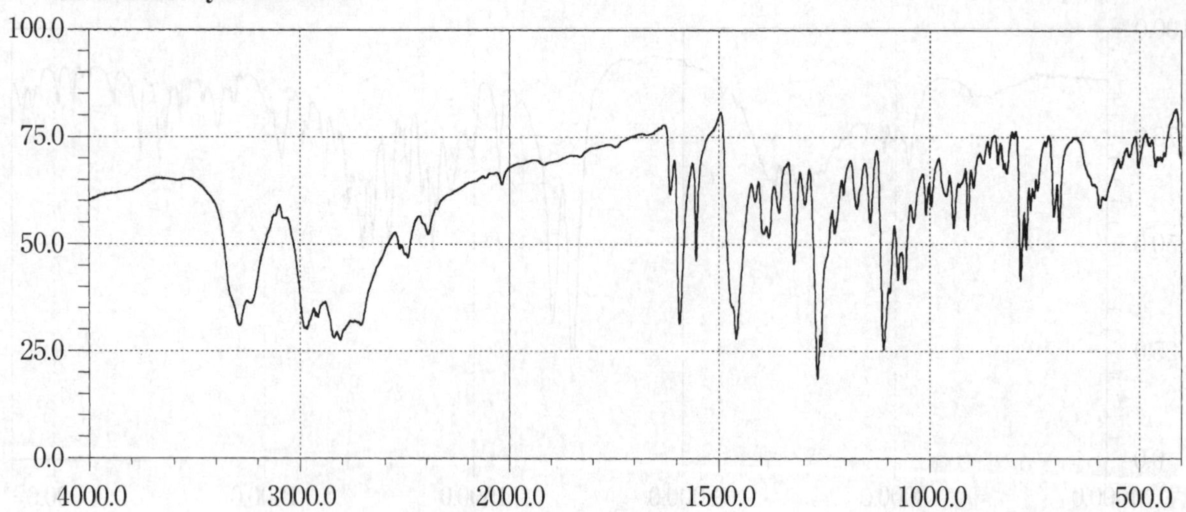

Indometacin

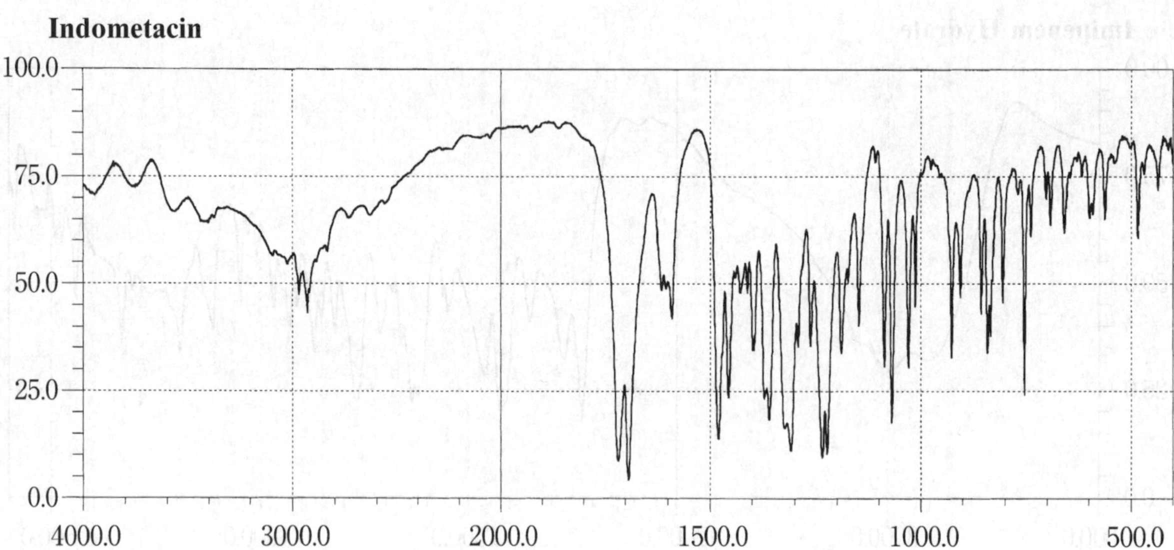

Iohexol

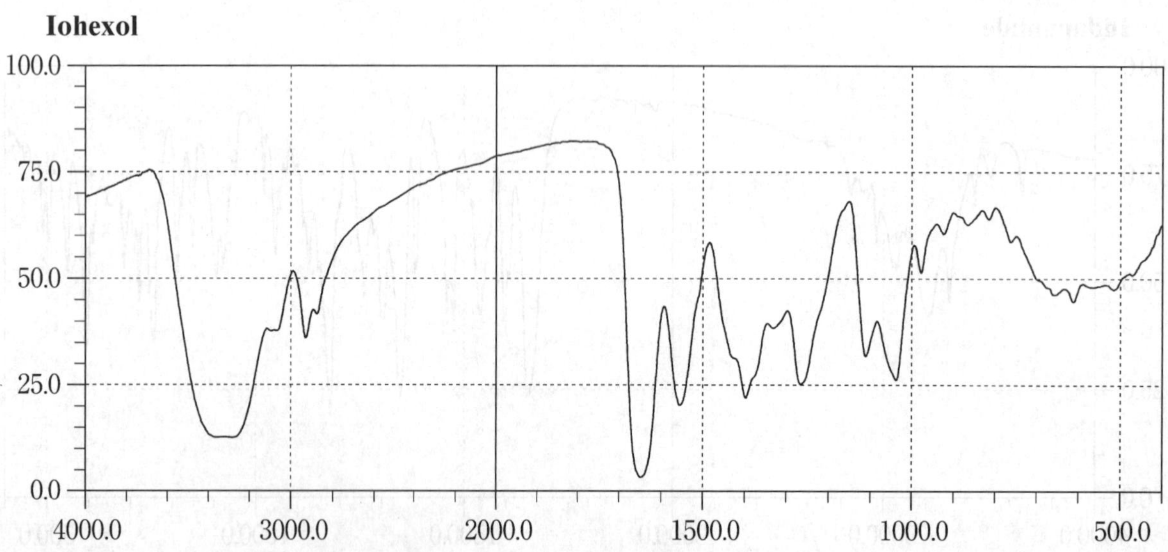

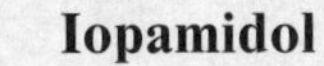

Iopamidol

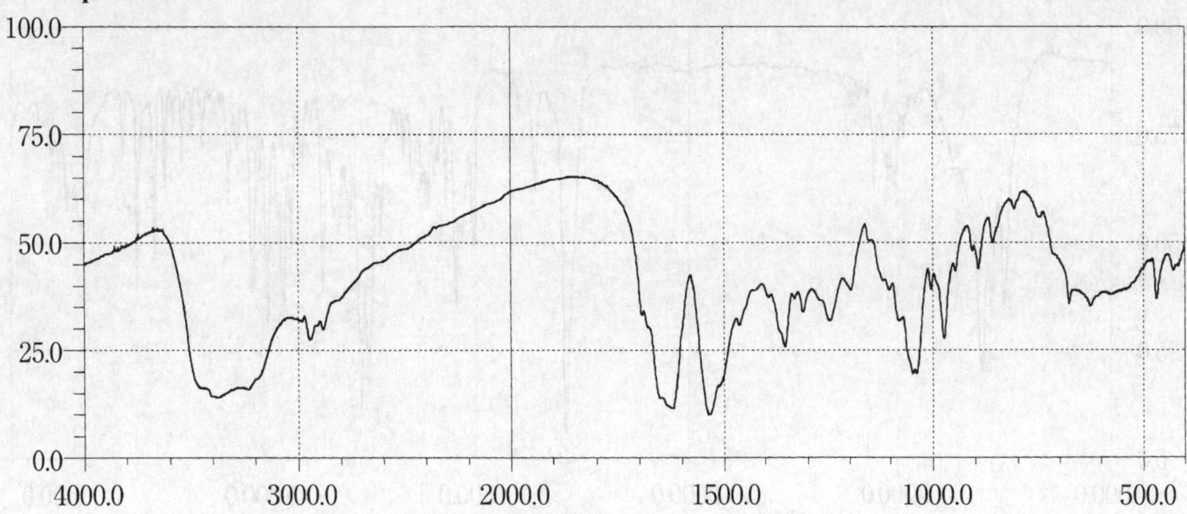

Iotalamic Acid

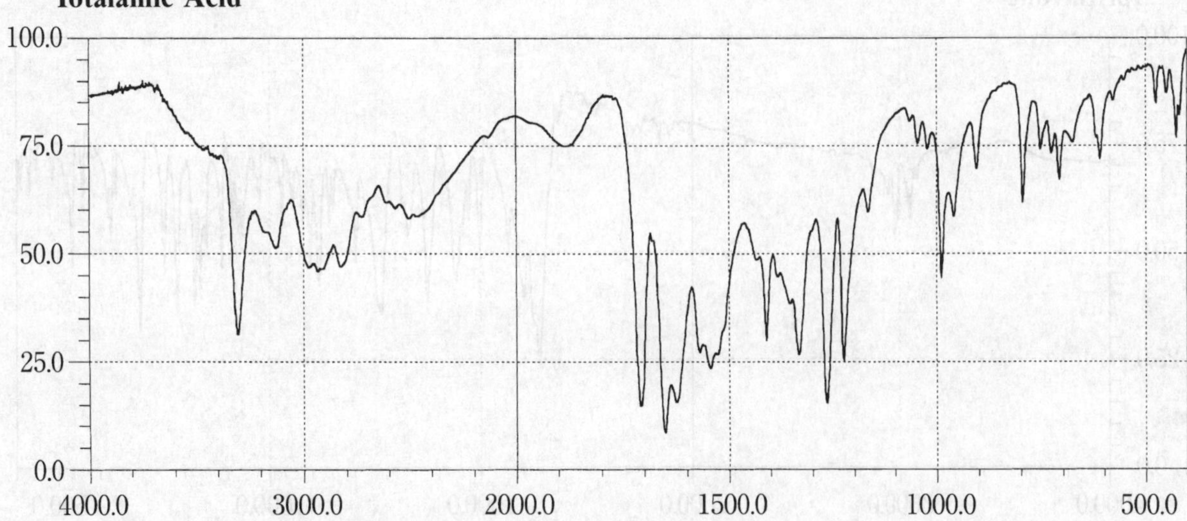

Iotroxic Acid

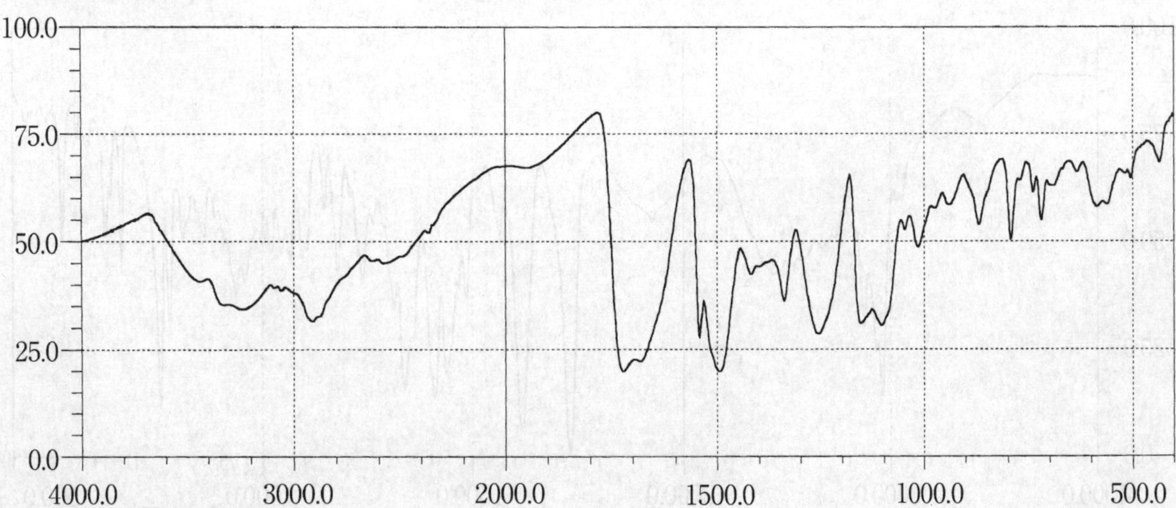

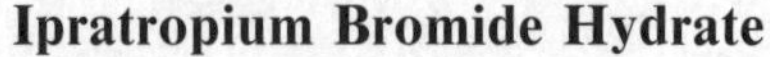

Ipratropium Bromide Hydrate

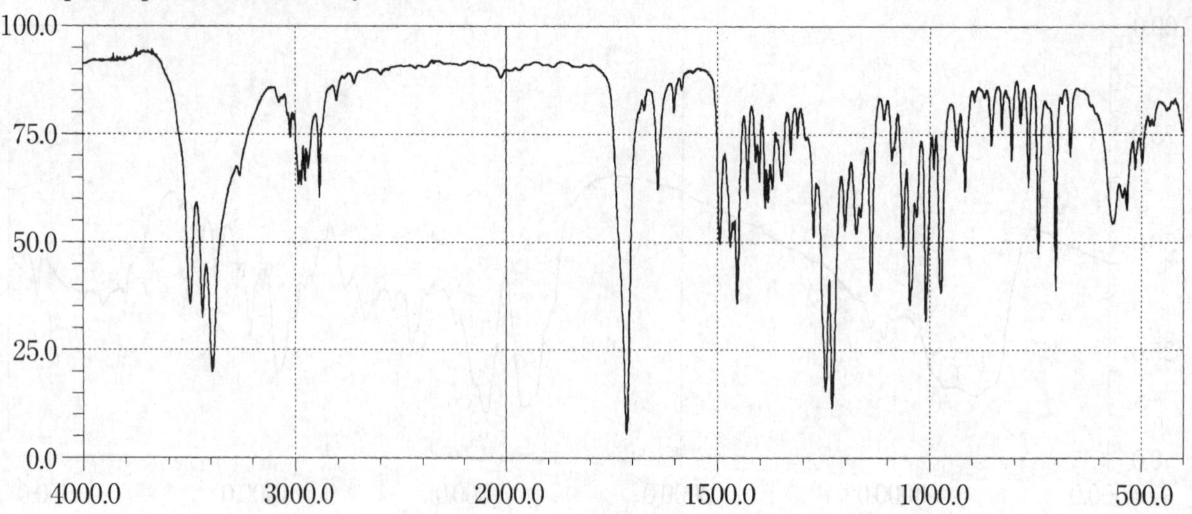

Ipriflavone

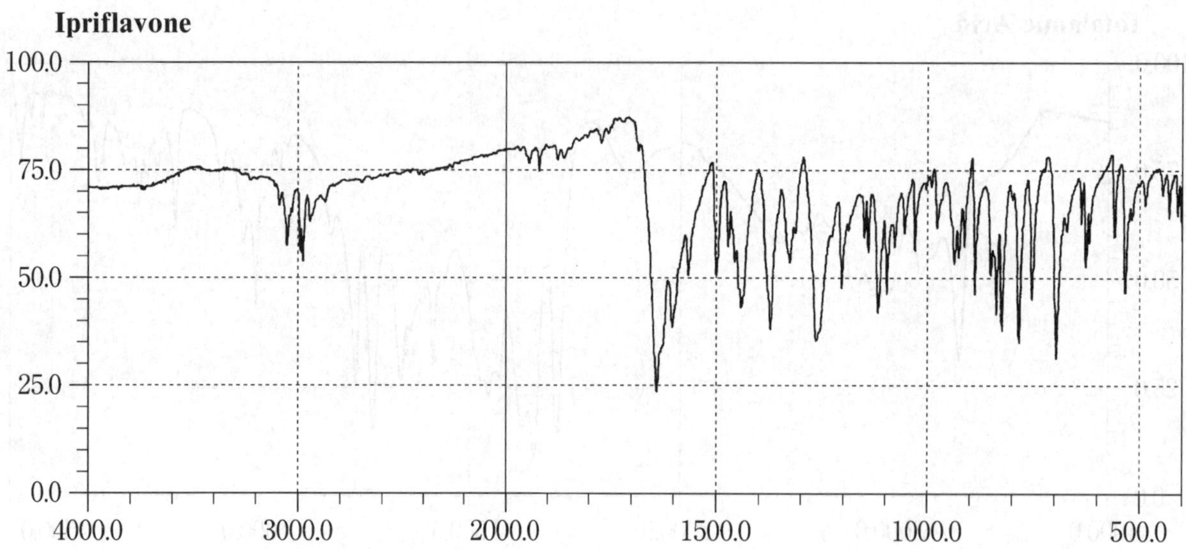

Irbesartan

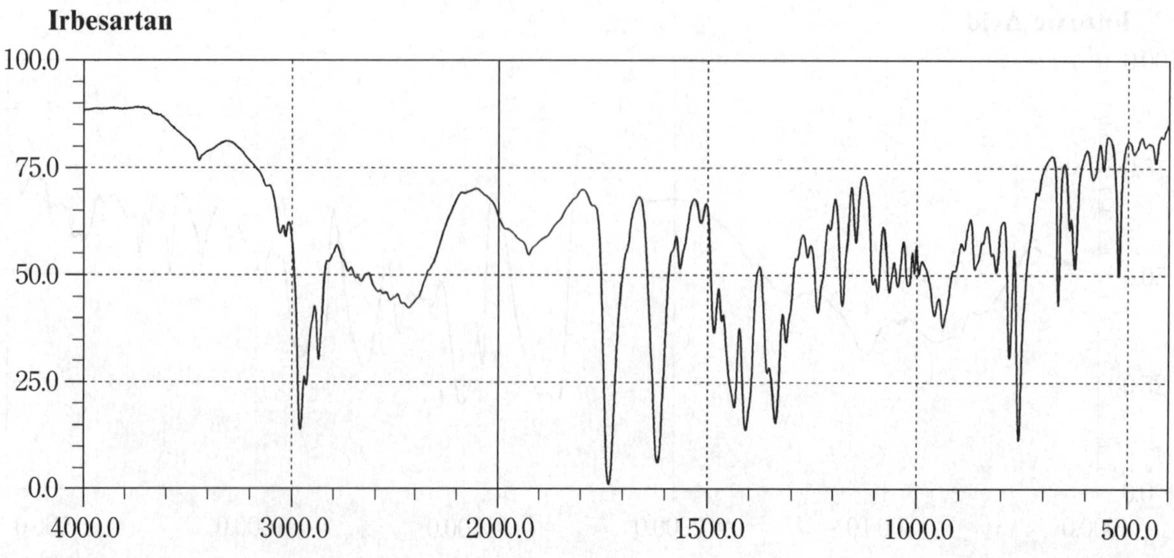

Irinotecan Hydrochloride Hydrate

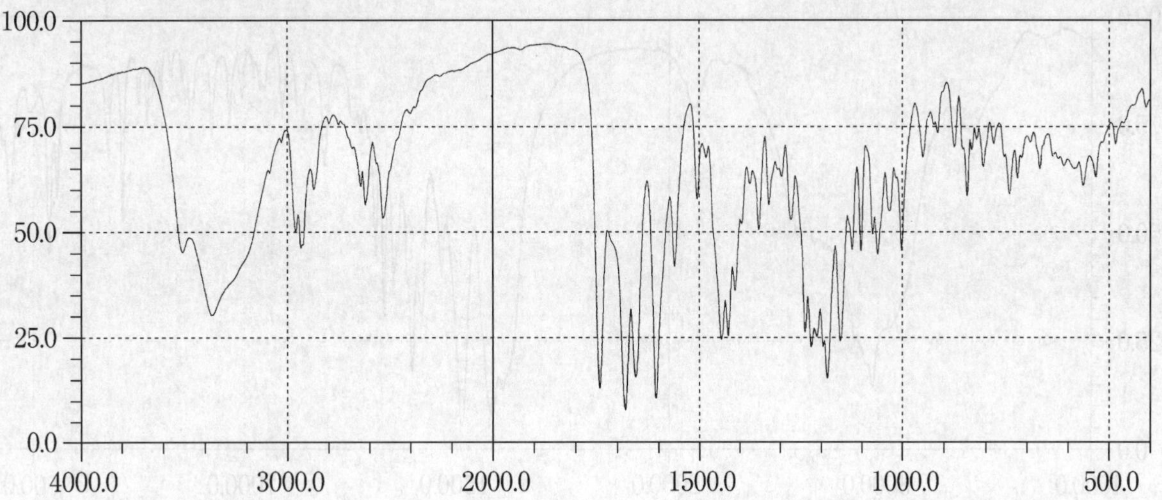

Irsogladine Maleate

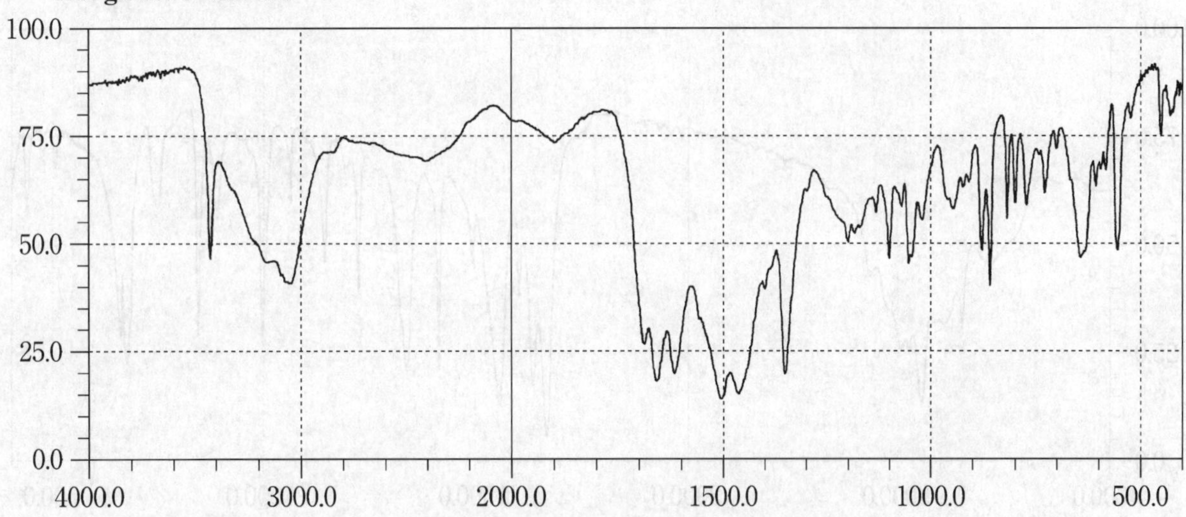

Isoflurane

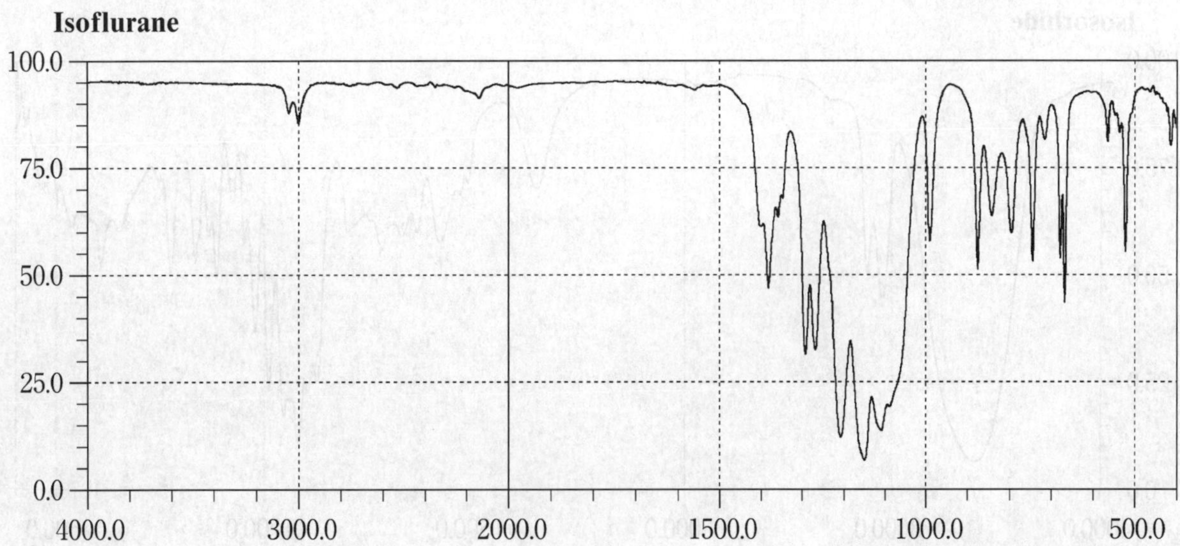

L-Isoleucine

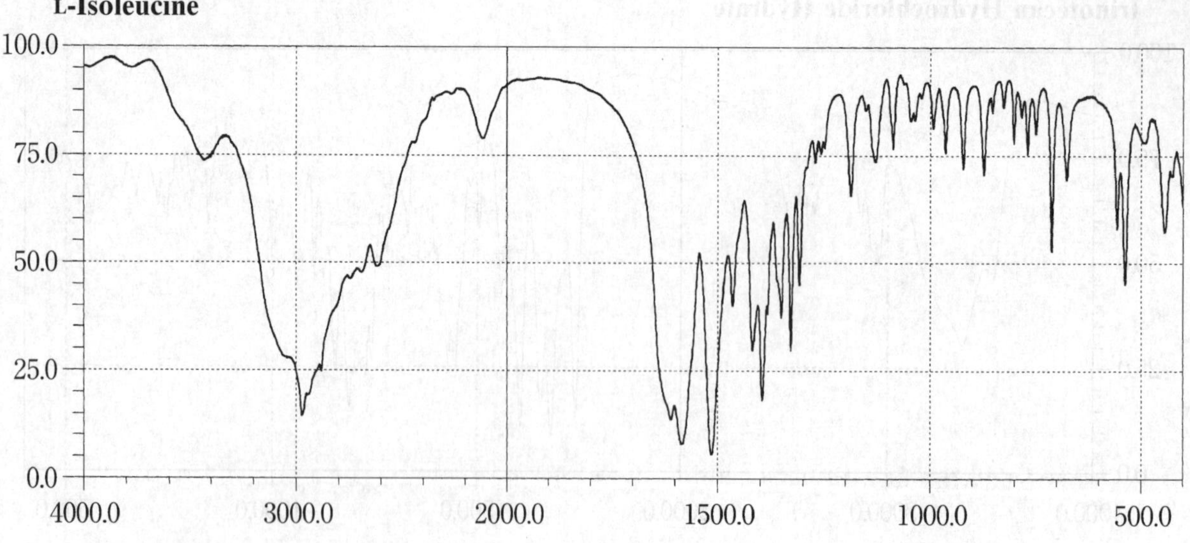

Isoniazid

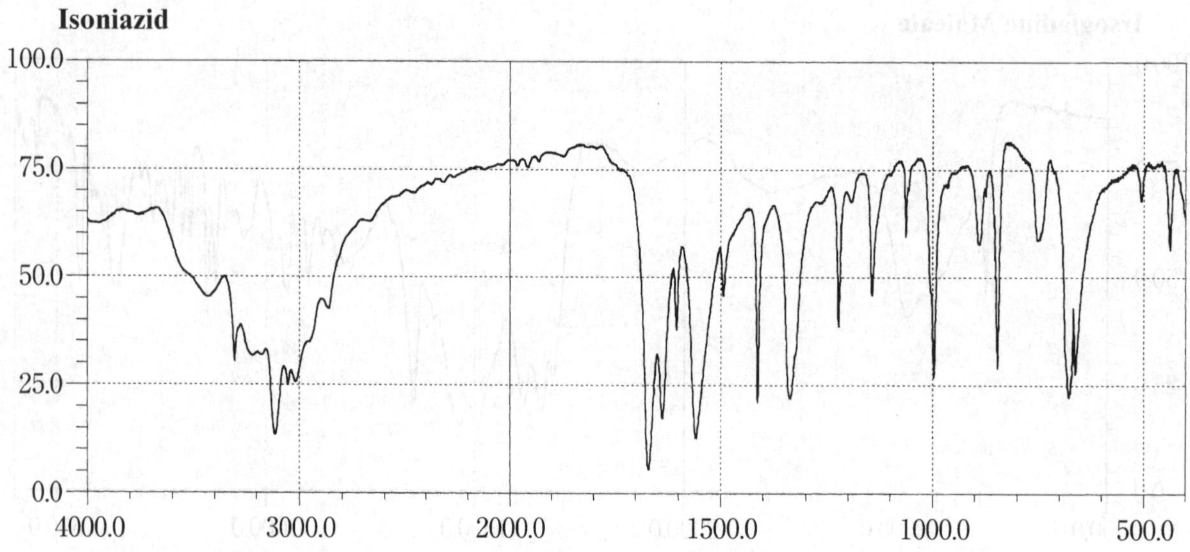

Isosorbide

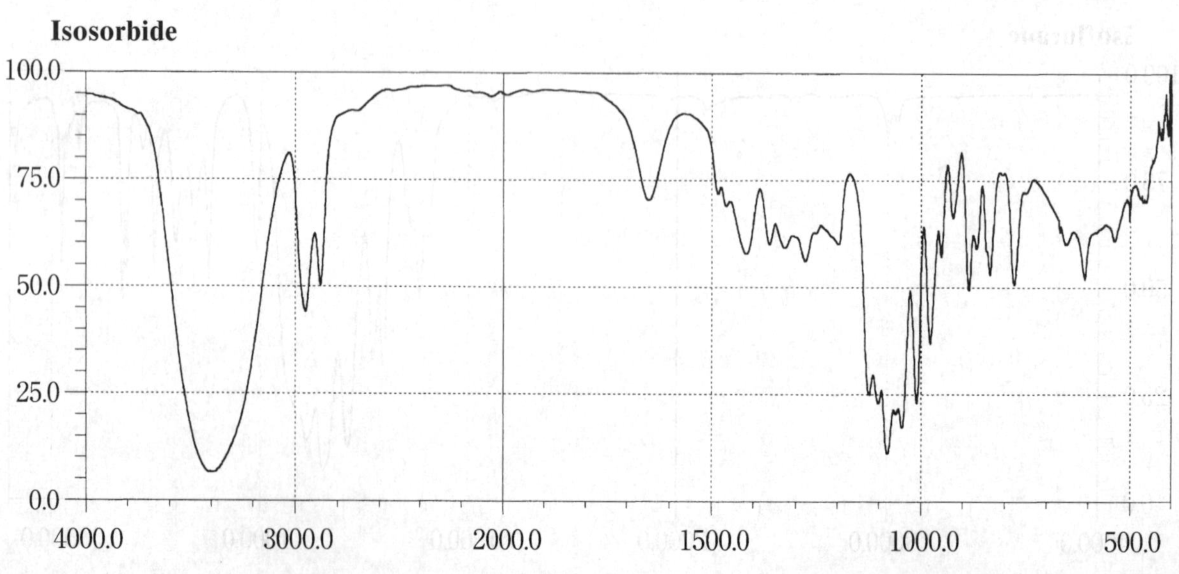

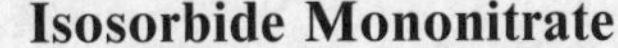

Isosorbide Mononitrate

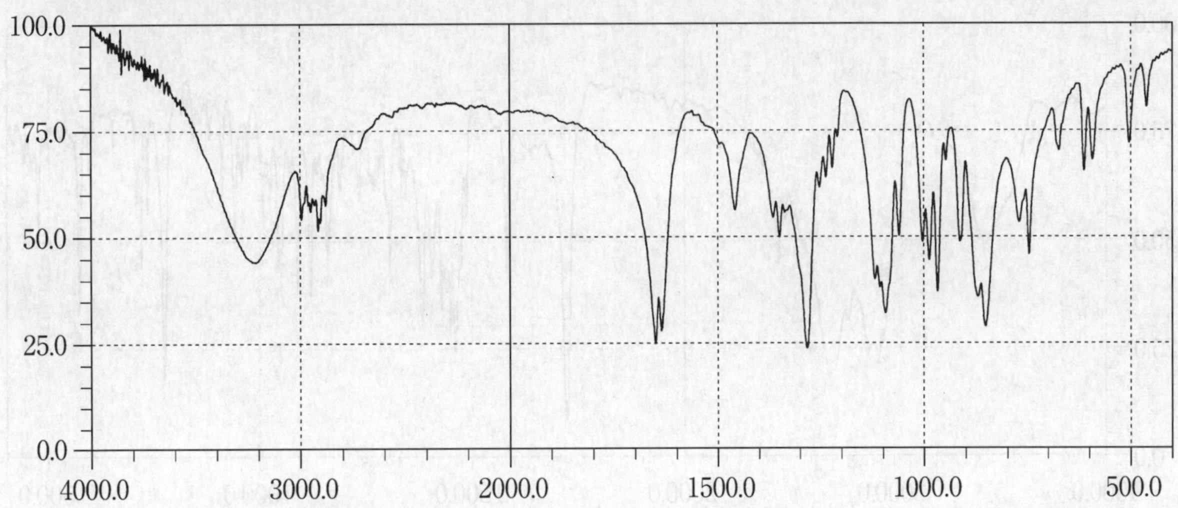

Isoxsuprine Hydrochloride

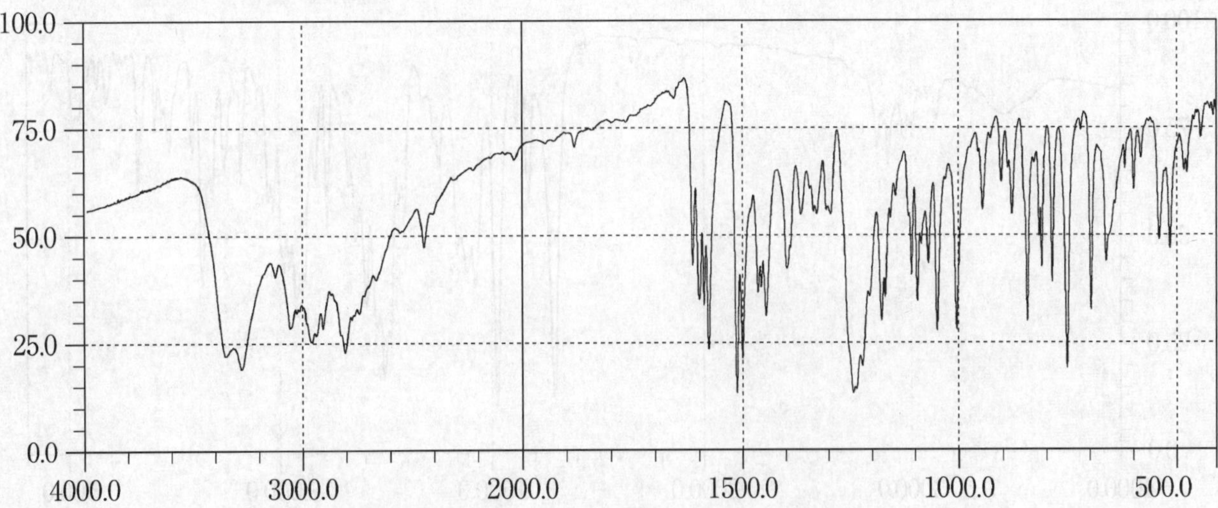

Itraconazole

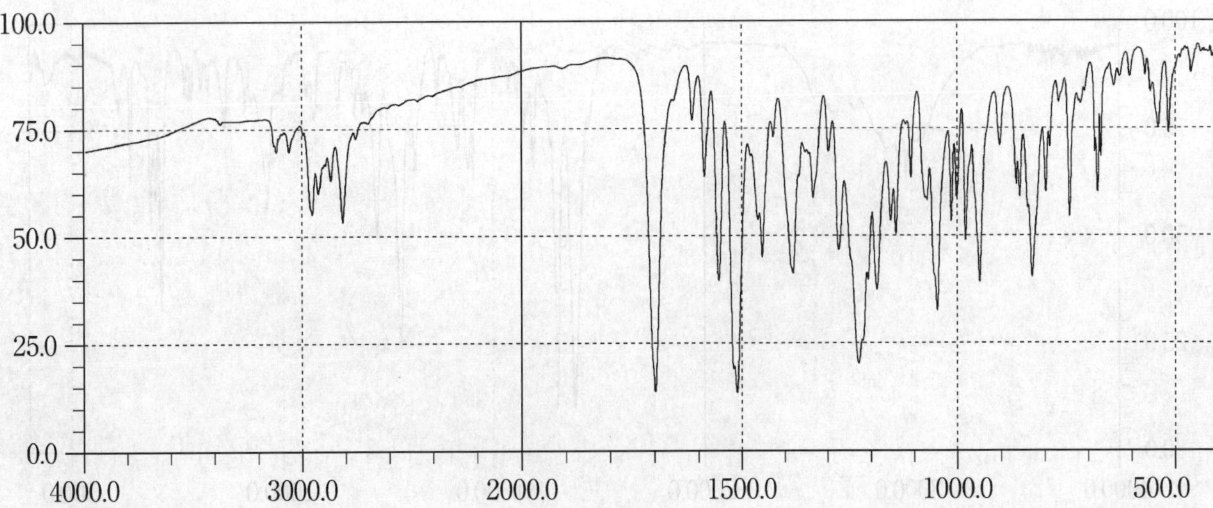

Ketamine Hydrochloride

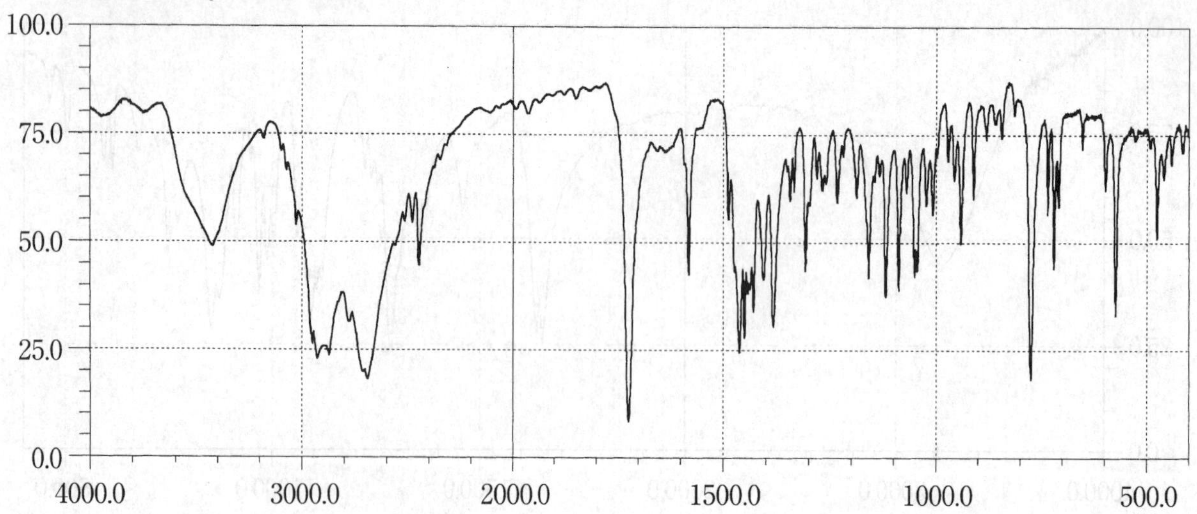

Ketoconazole

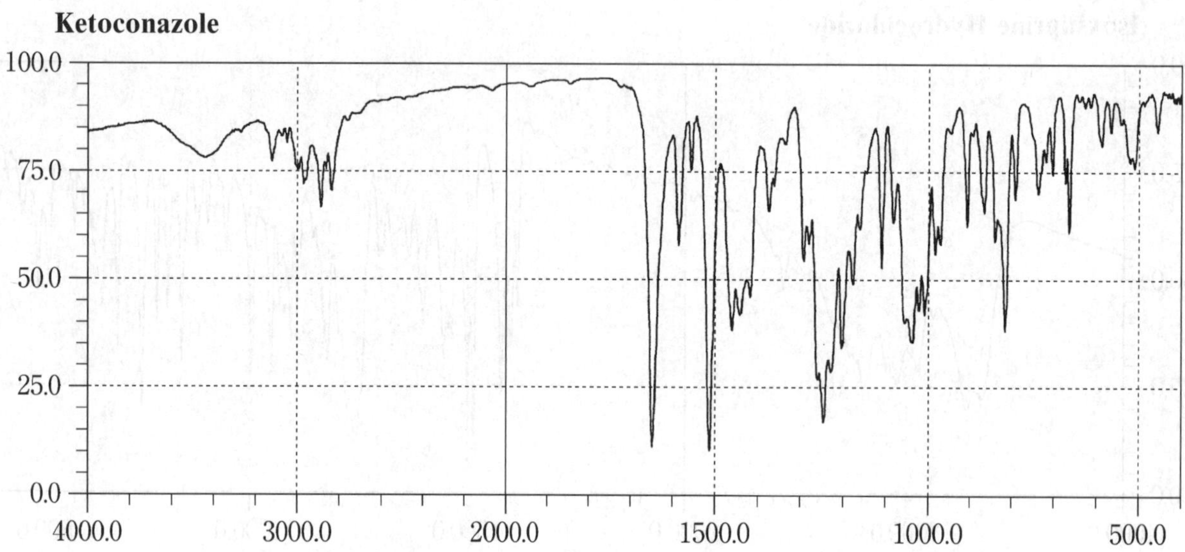

Ketoprofen

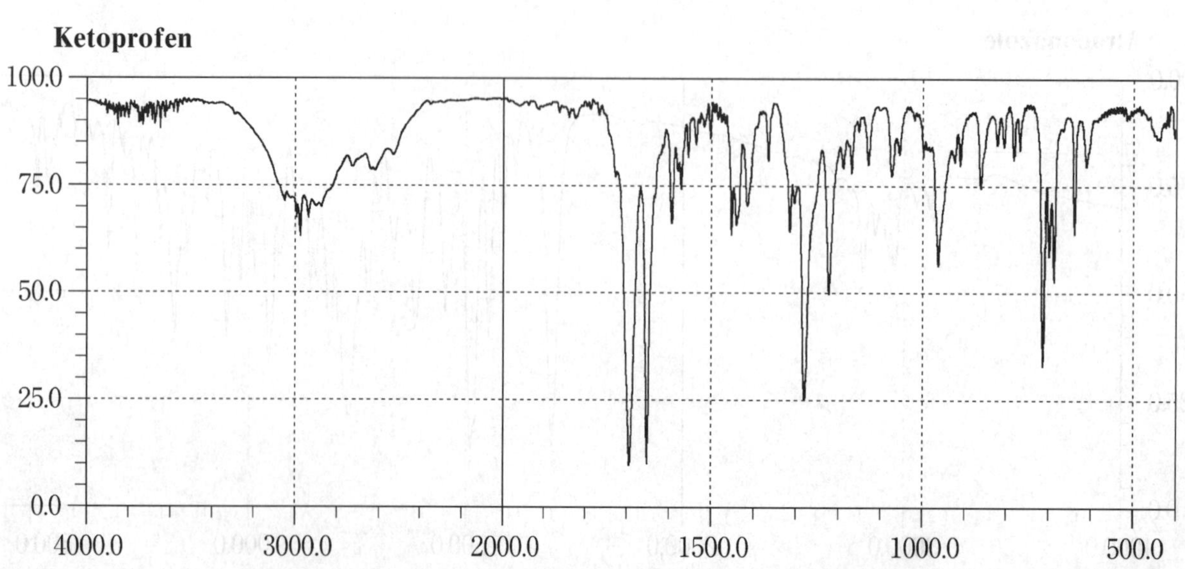

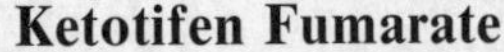

Ketotifen Fumarate

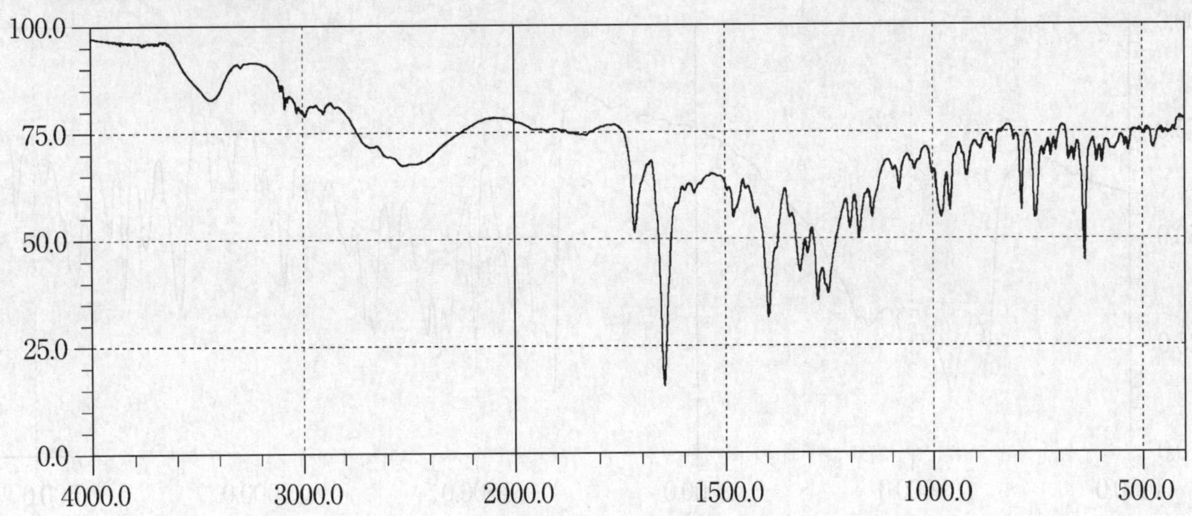

Kitasamycin Acetate

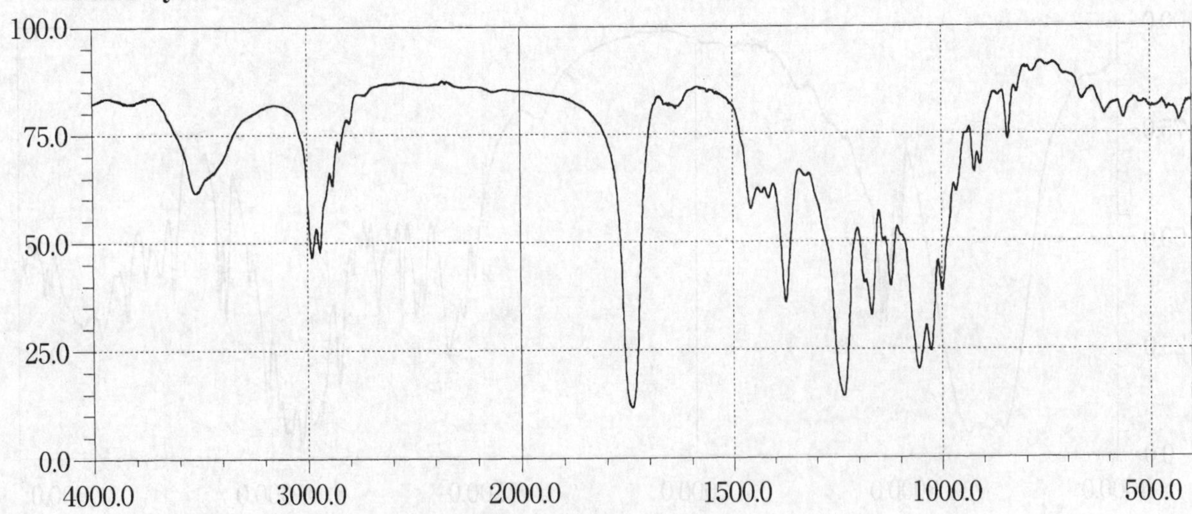

Kitasamycin Tartrate

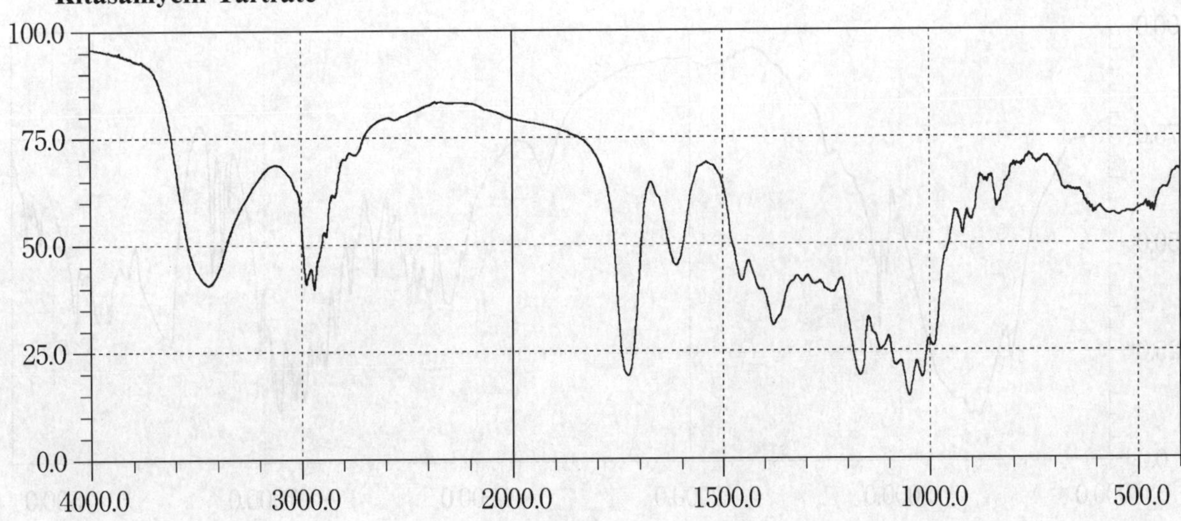

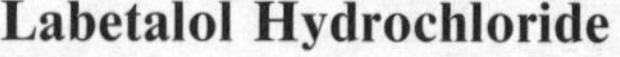

Labetalol Hydrochloride

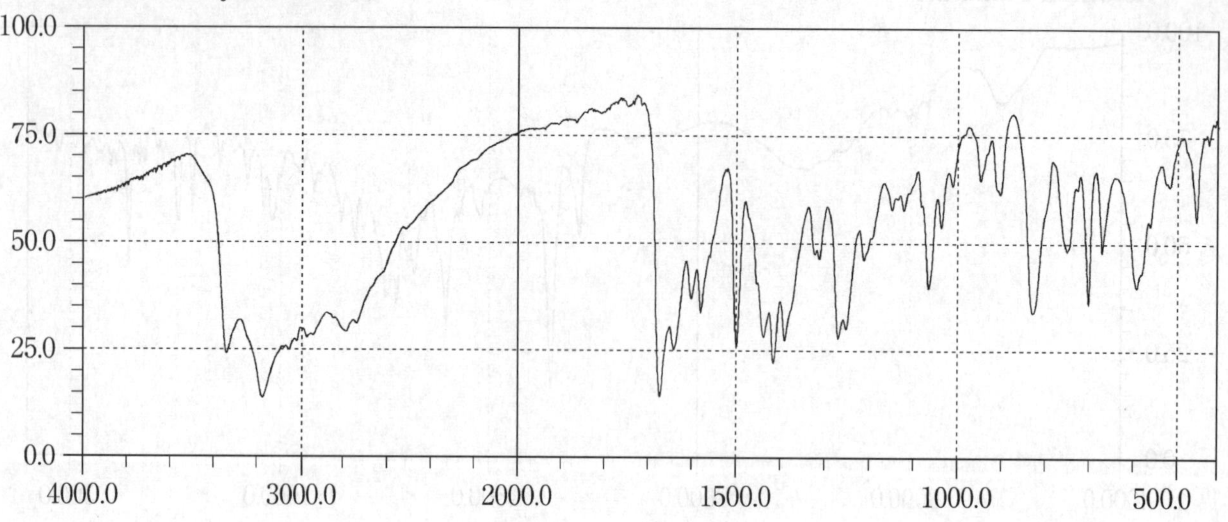

Anhydrous Lactose

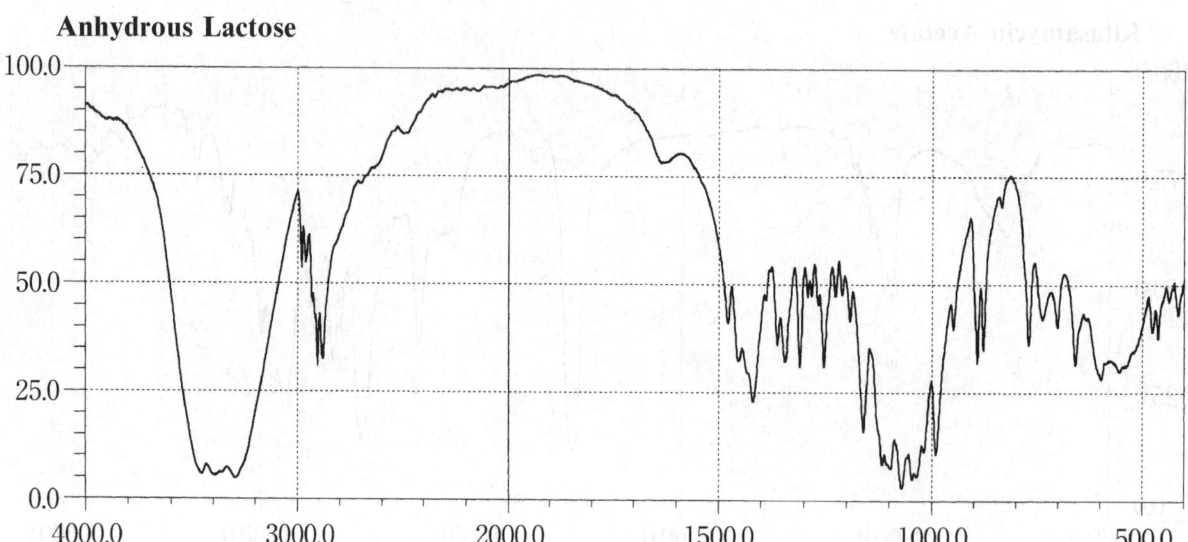

Lactose Hydrate

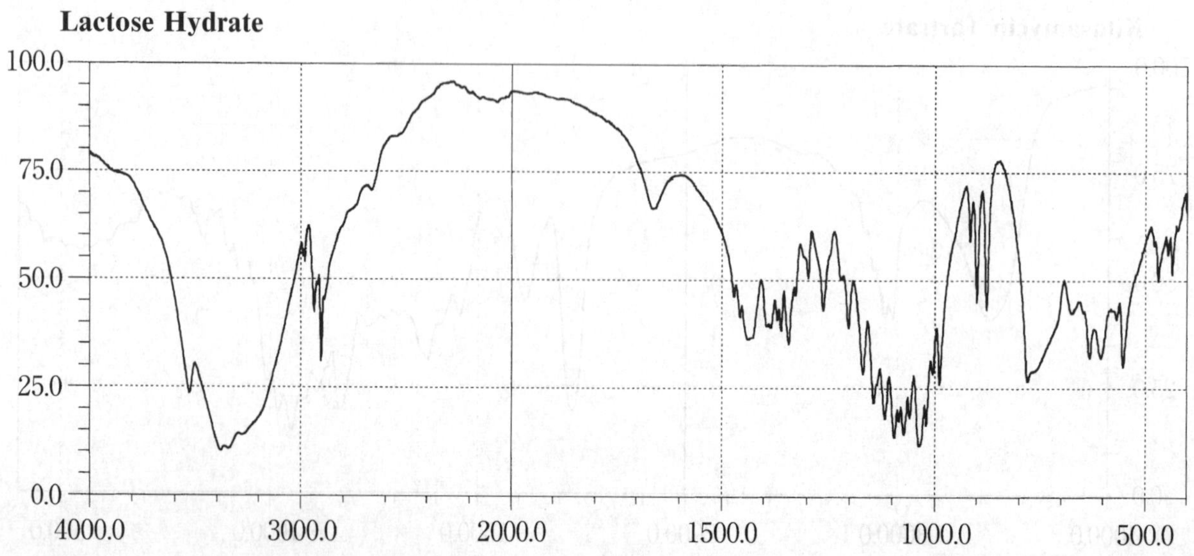

Lafutidine

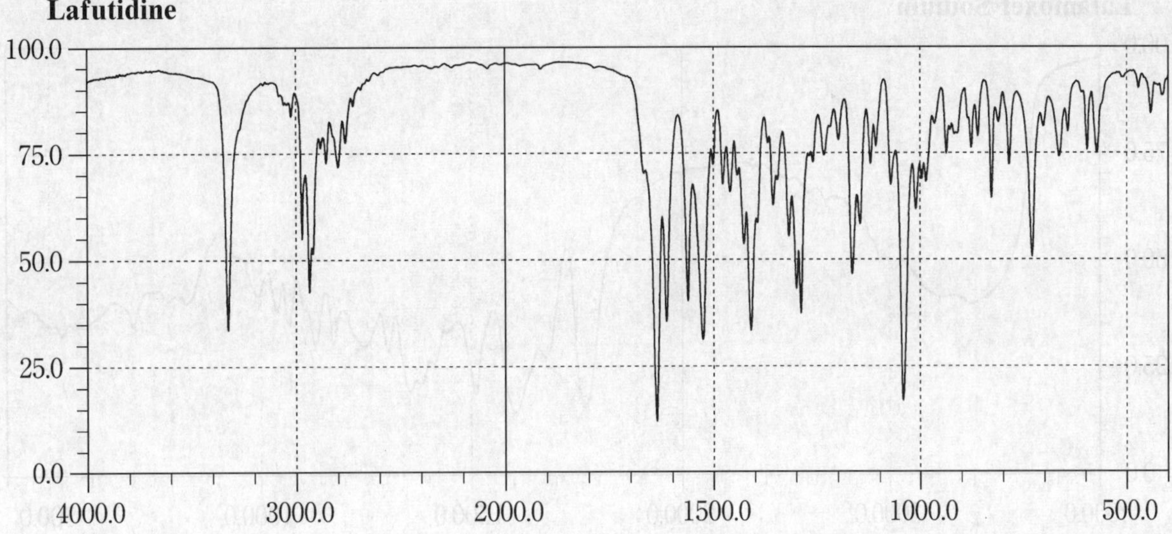

Lanoconazole

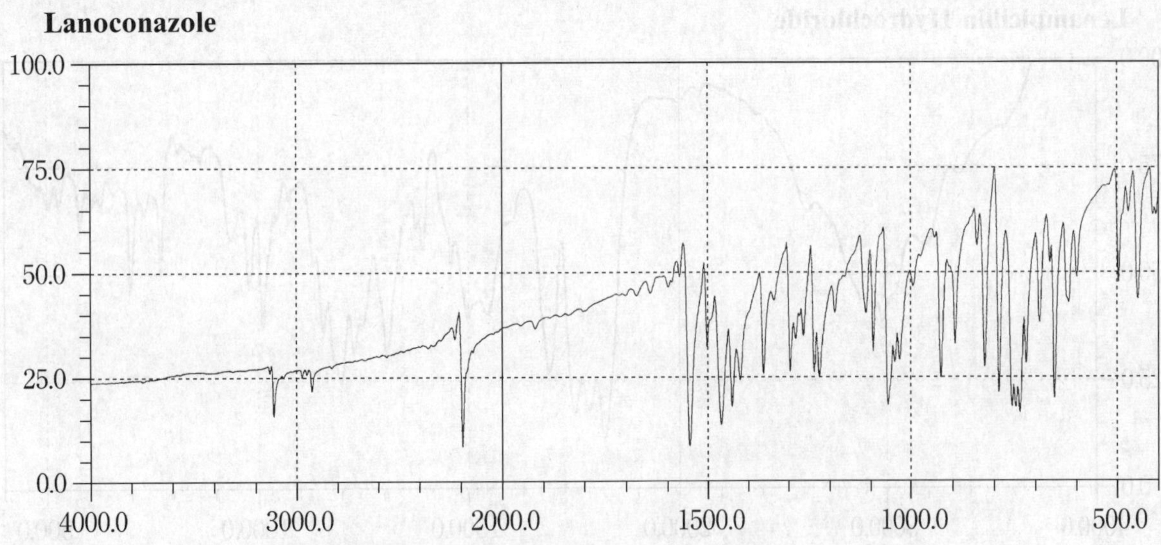

Lansoprazole

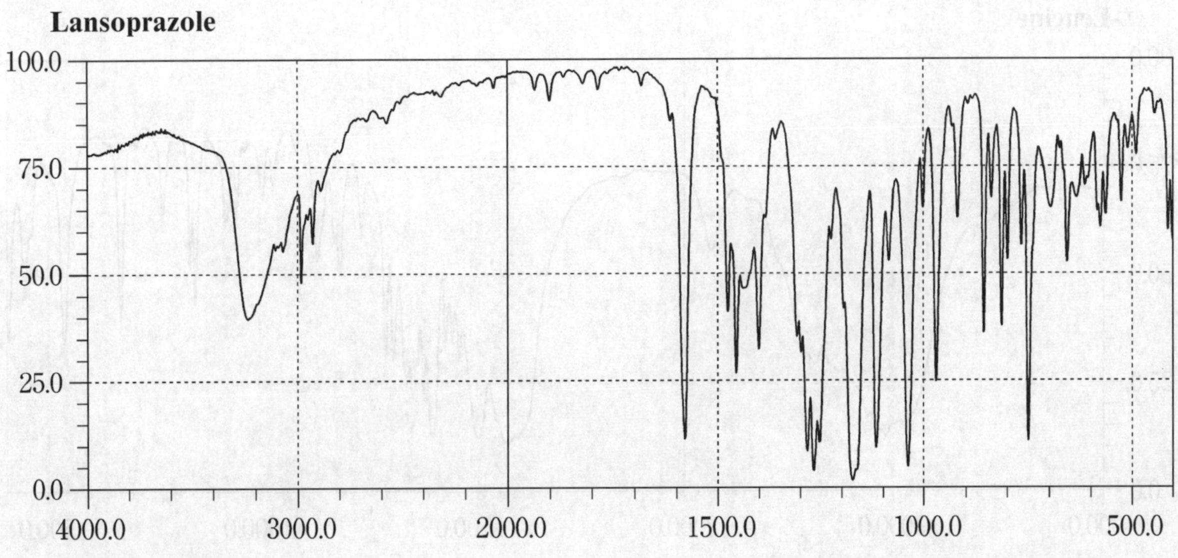

Latamoxef Sodium

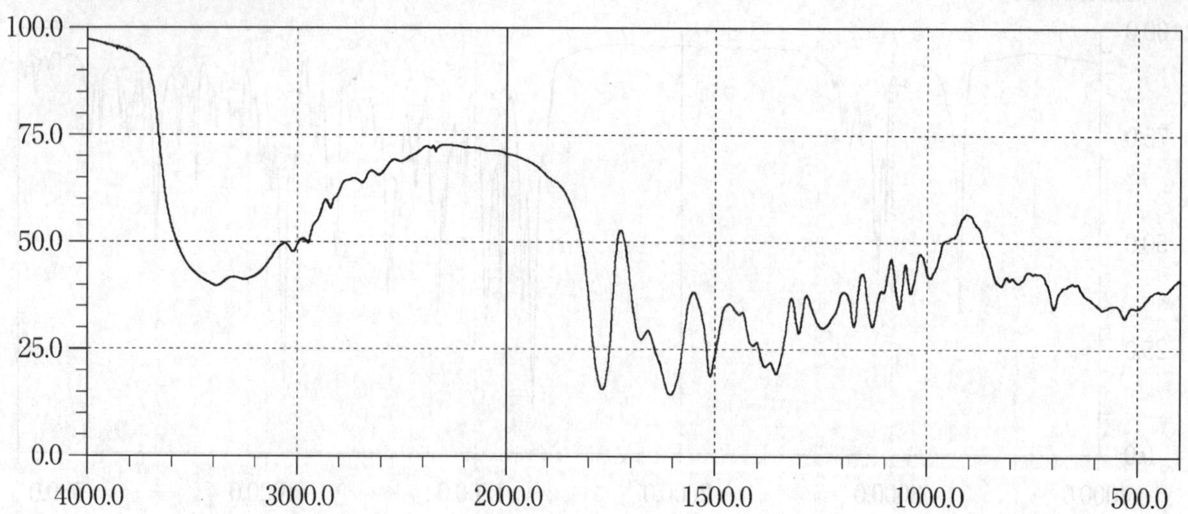

Lenampicillin Hydrochloride

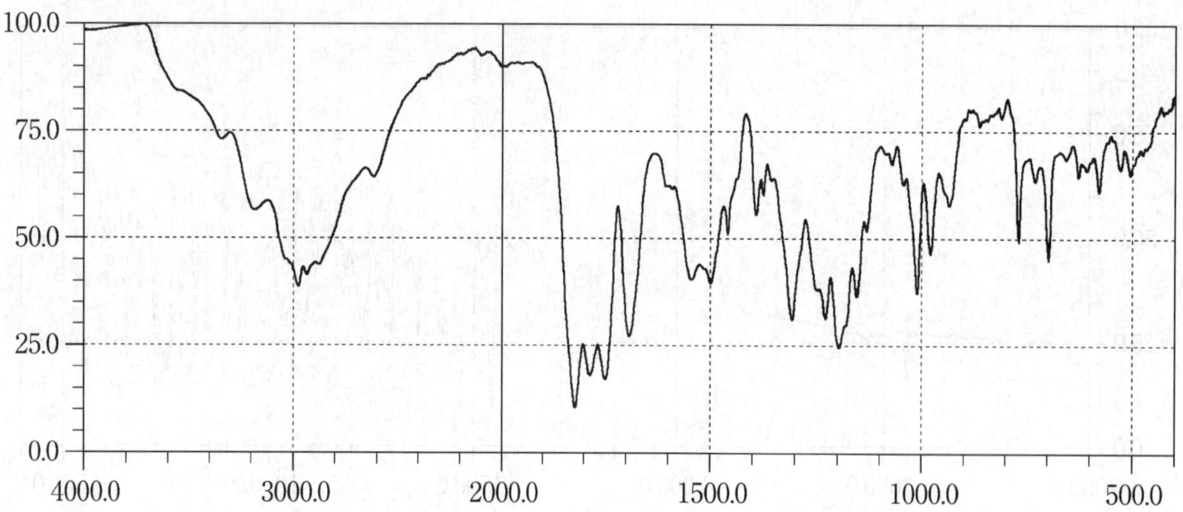

L-Leucine

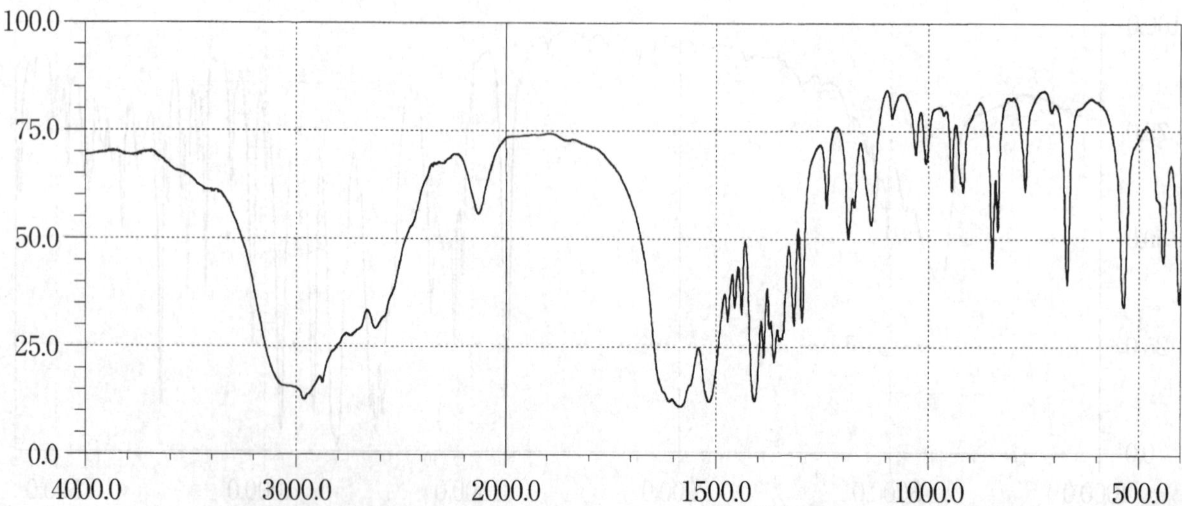

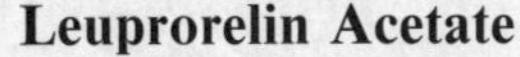

Leuprorelin Acetate

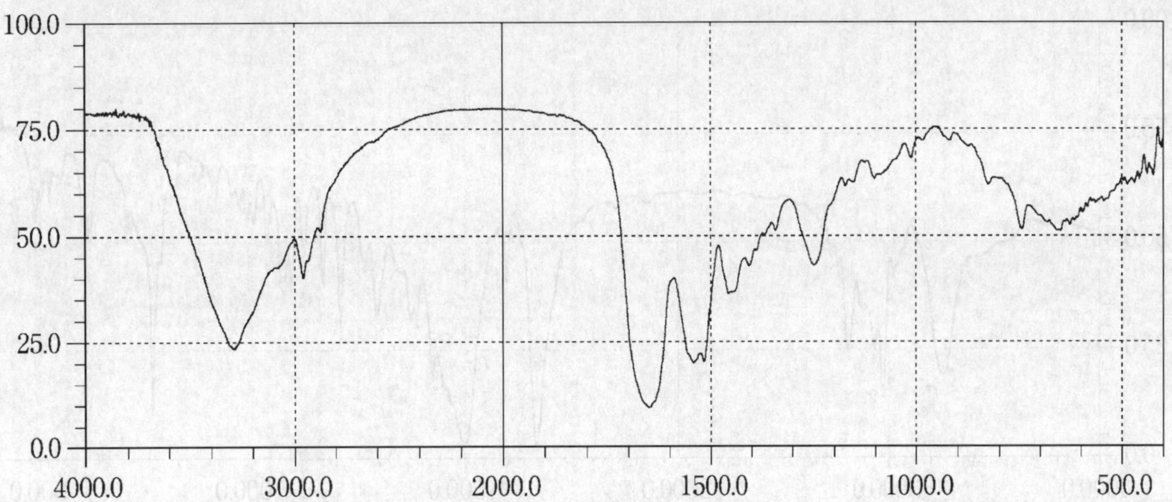

Levallorphan Tartrate

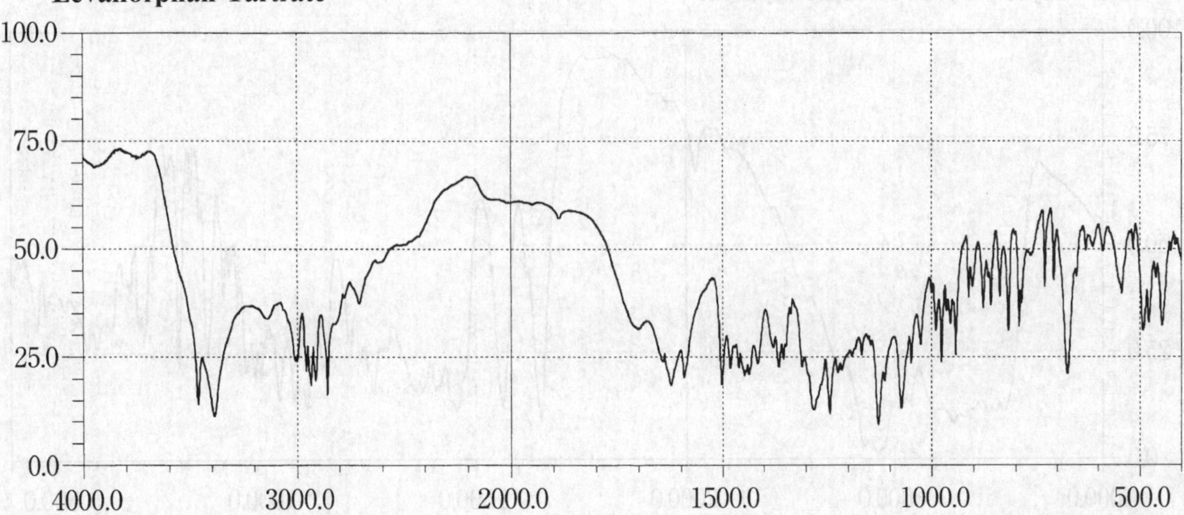

Levofloxacin Hydrate

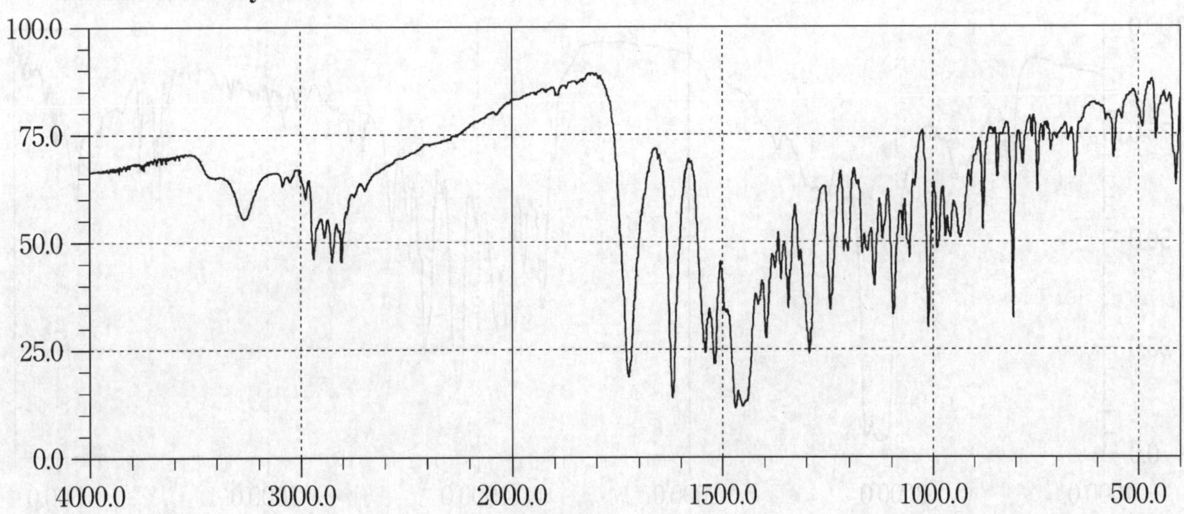

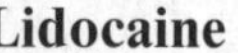

Lidocaine

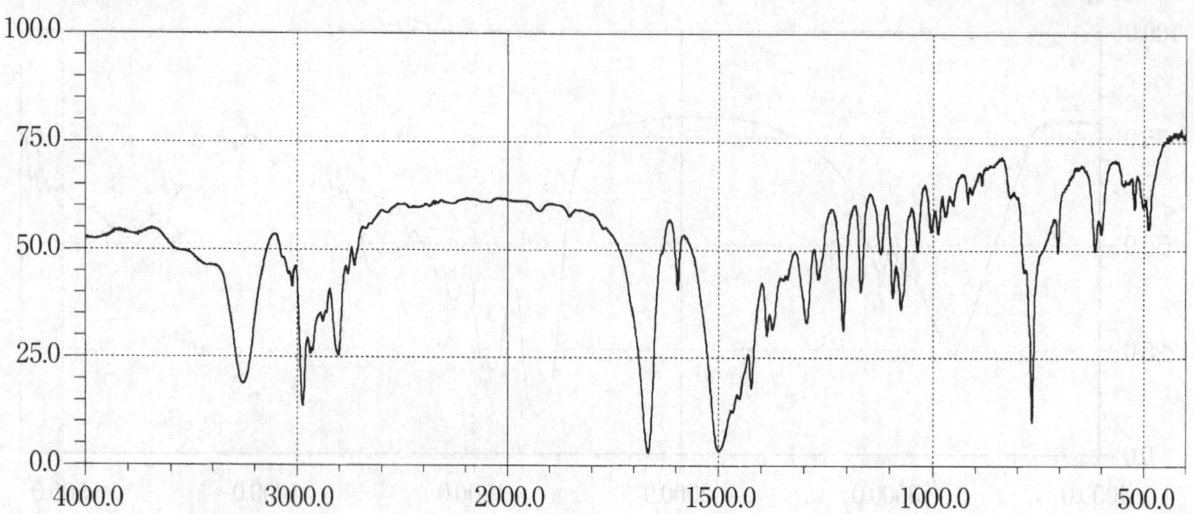

Lincomycin Hydrochloride Hydrate

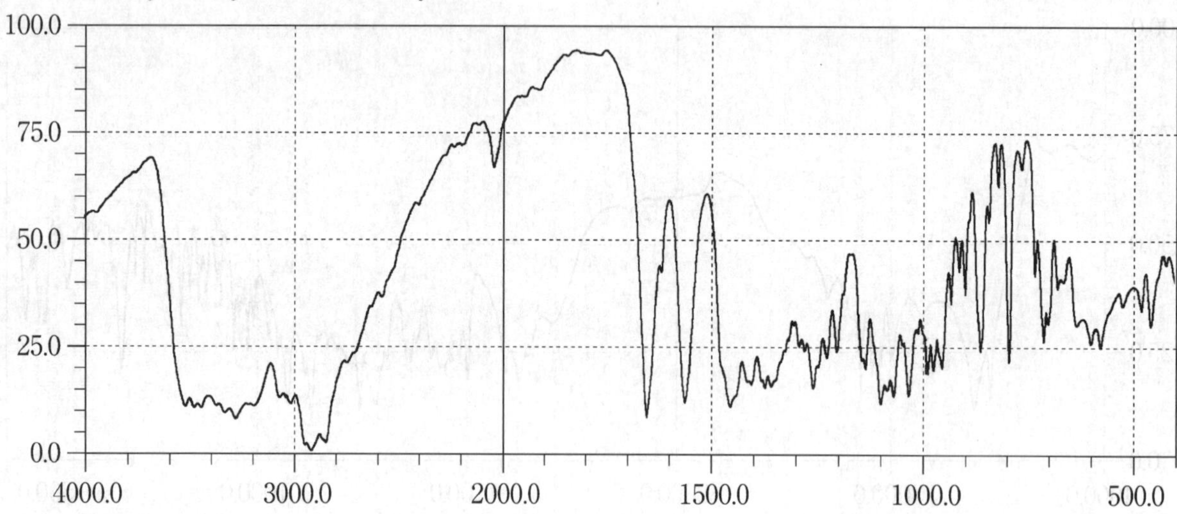

Lisinopril Hydrate

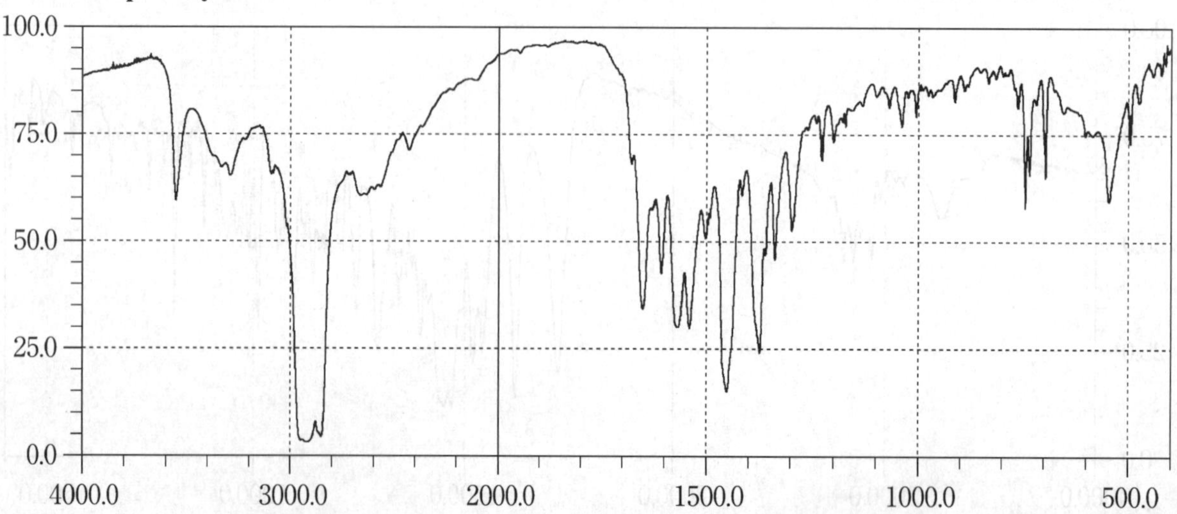

Lobenzarit Sodium

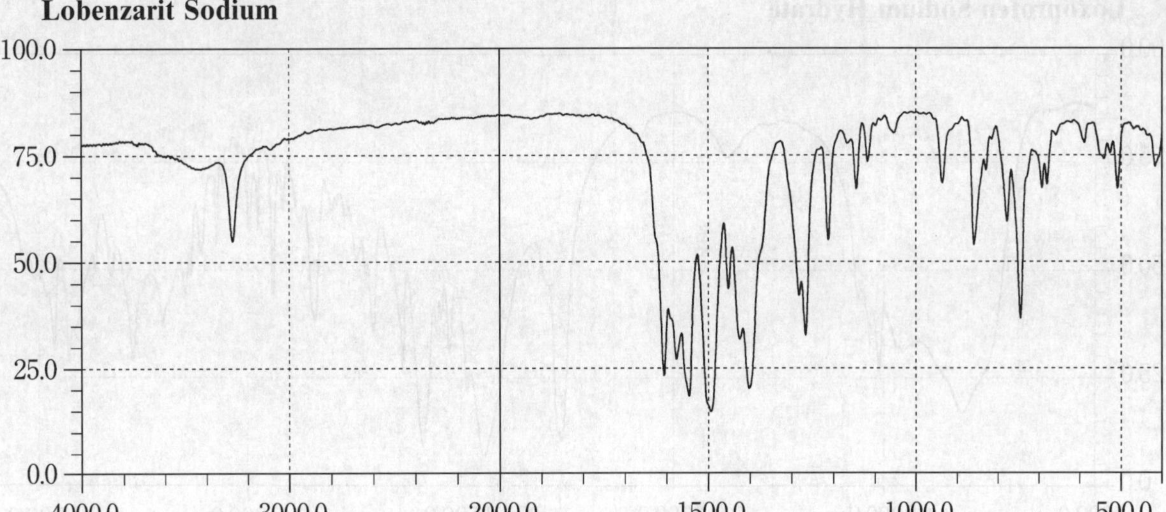

Lorazepam

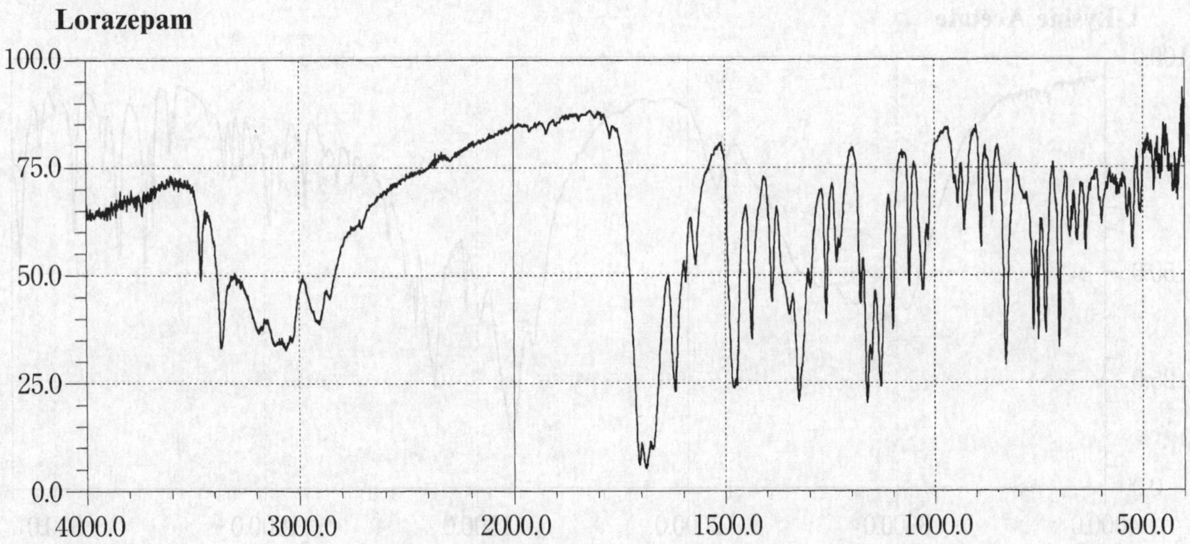

Losartan Potassium

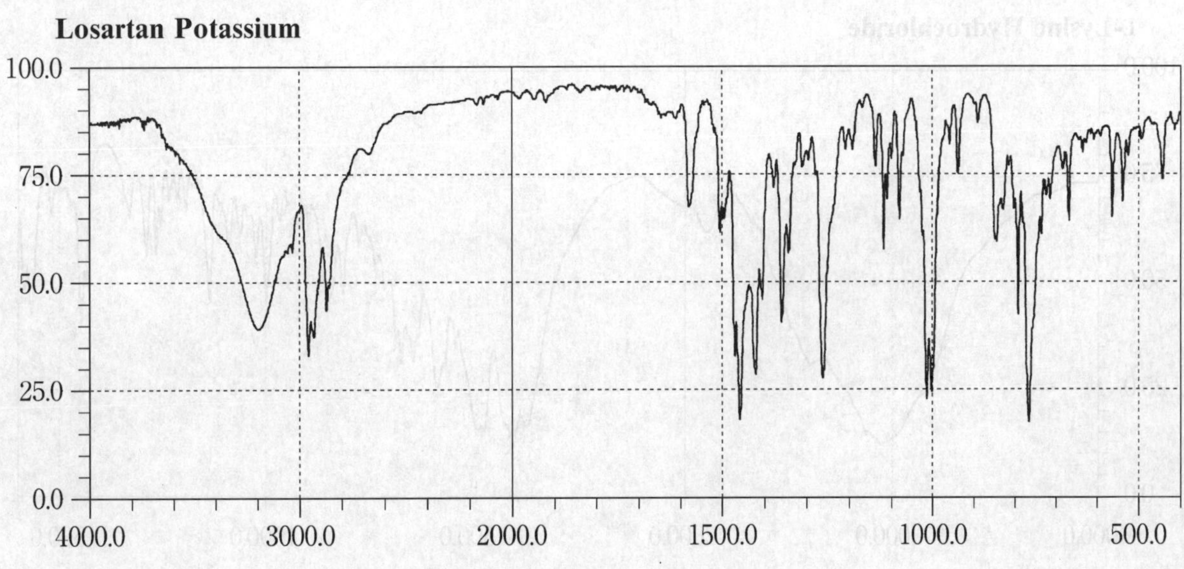

Loxoprofen Sodium Hydrate

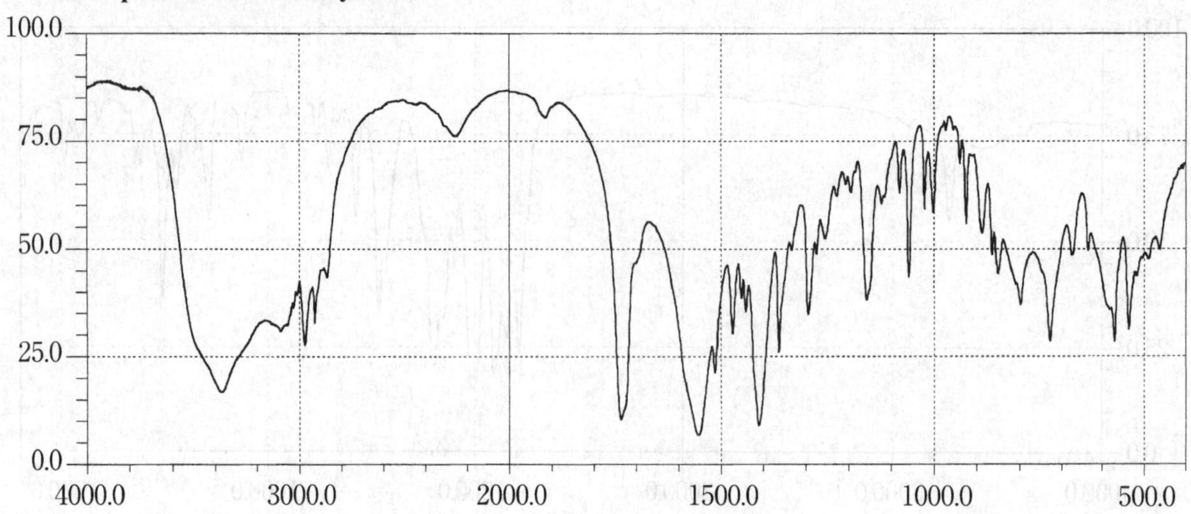

L-Lysine Acetate

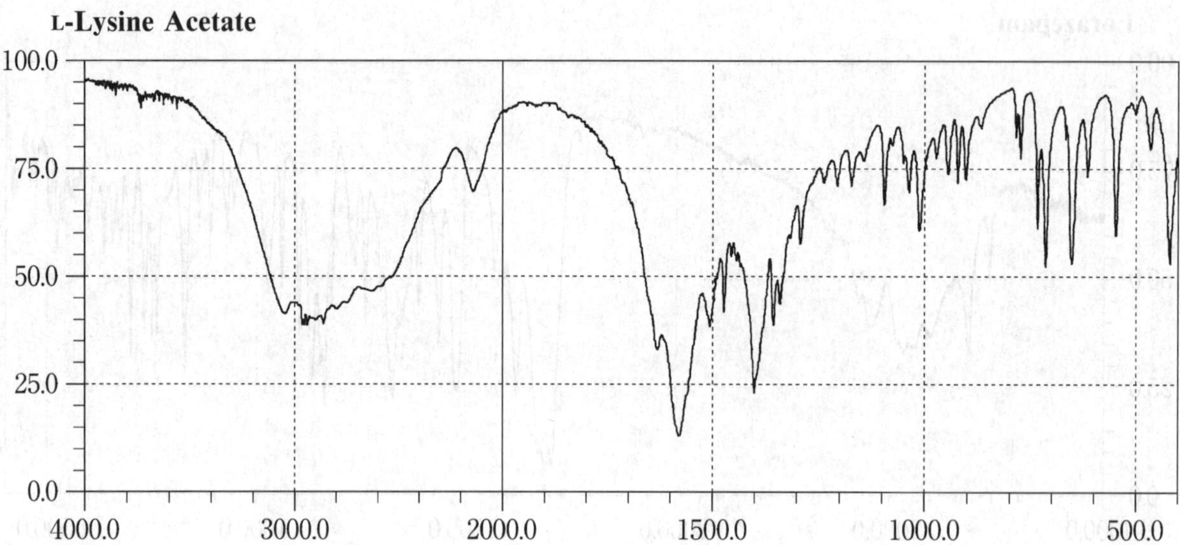

L-Lysine Hydrochloride

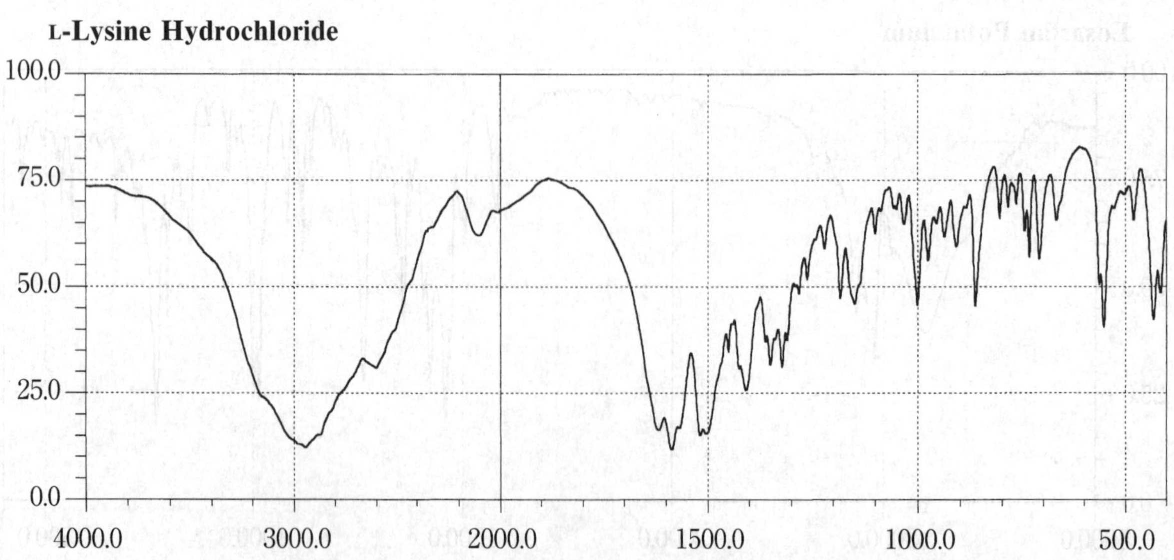

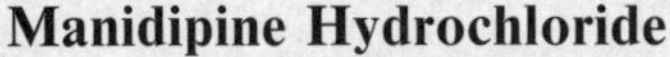

Manidipine Hydrochloride

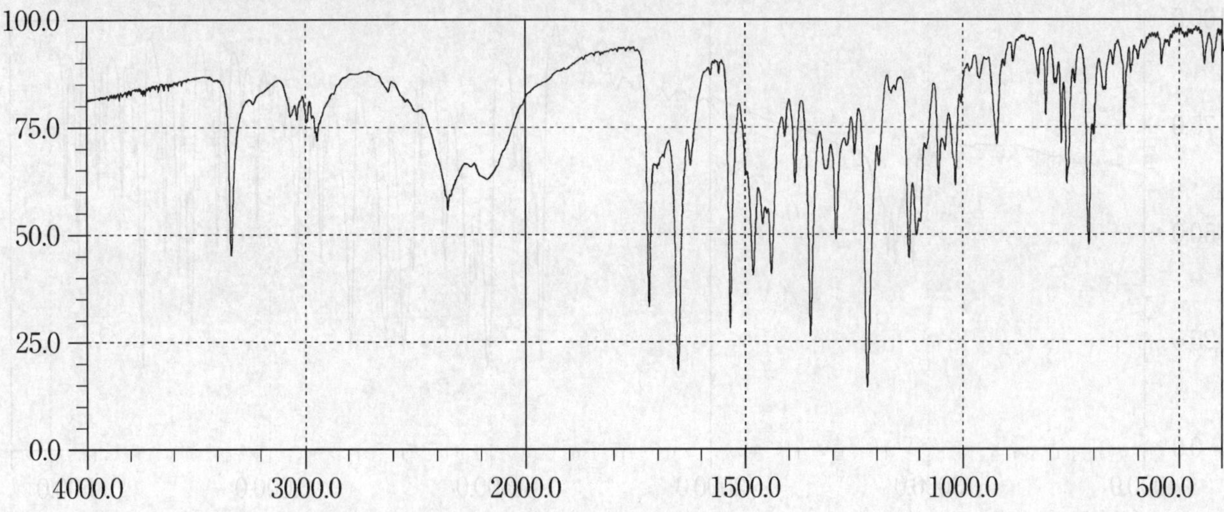

D-Mannitol

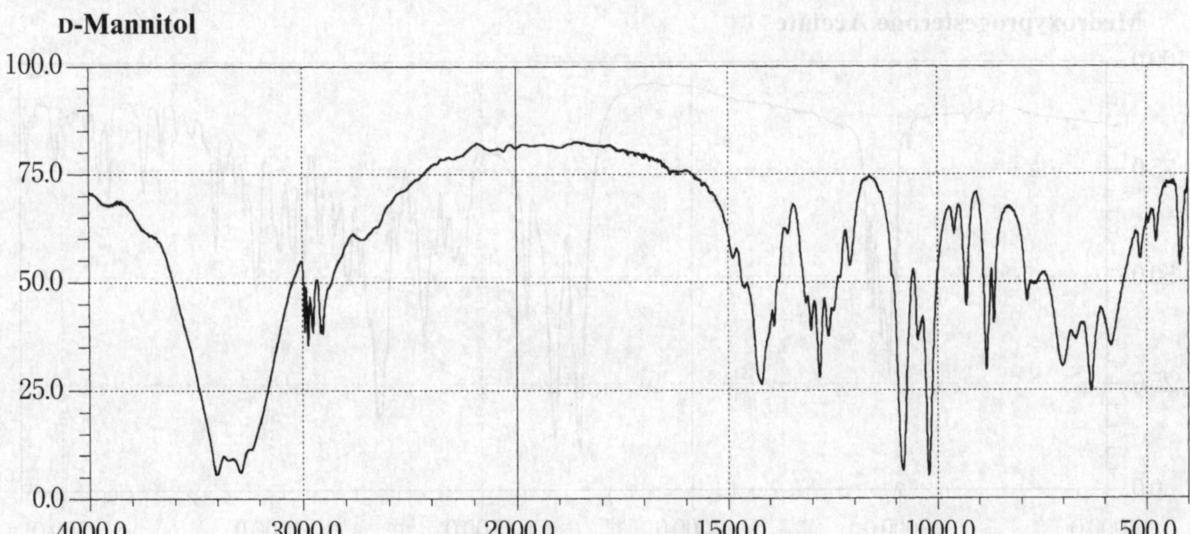

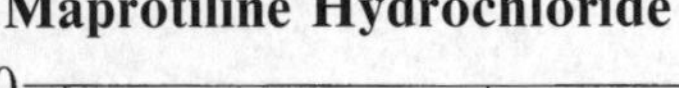

Maprotiline Hydrochloride

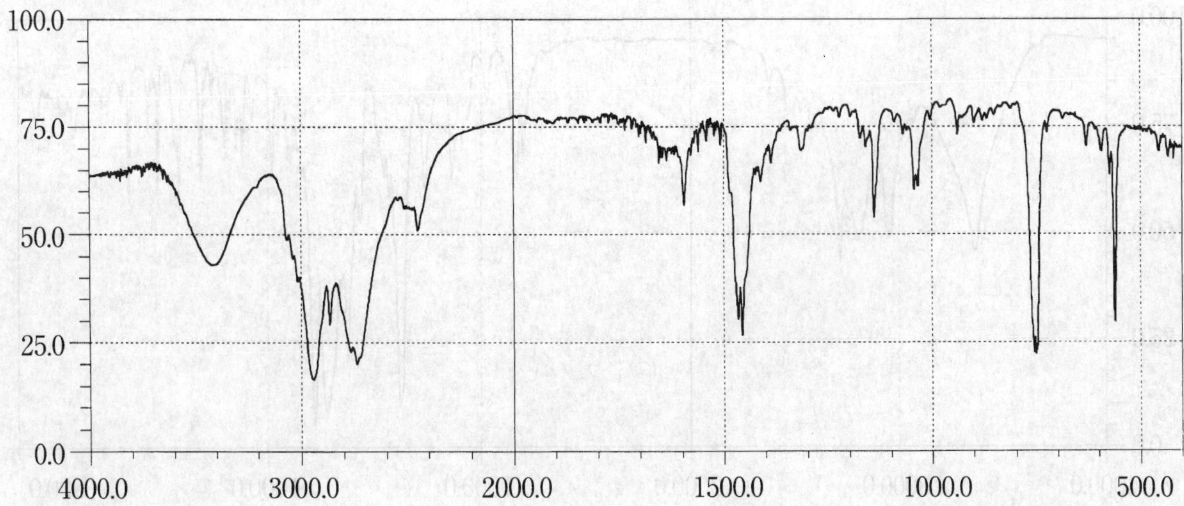

Medazepam

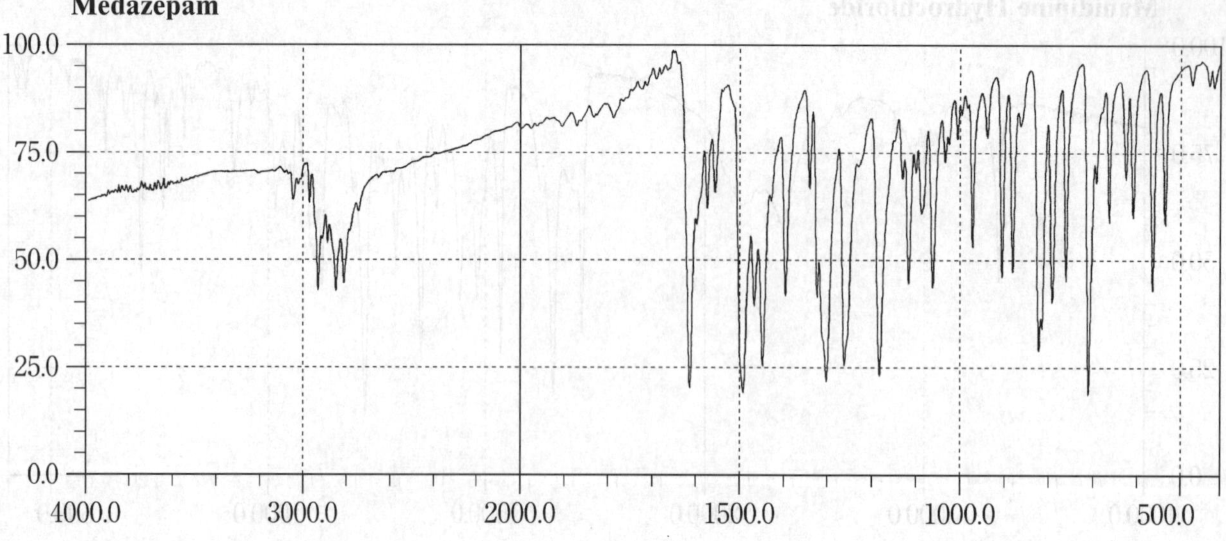

Medroxyprogesterone Acetate

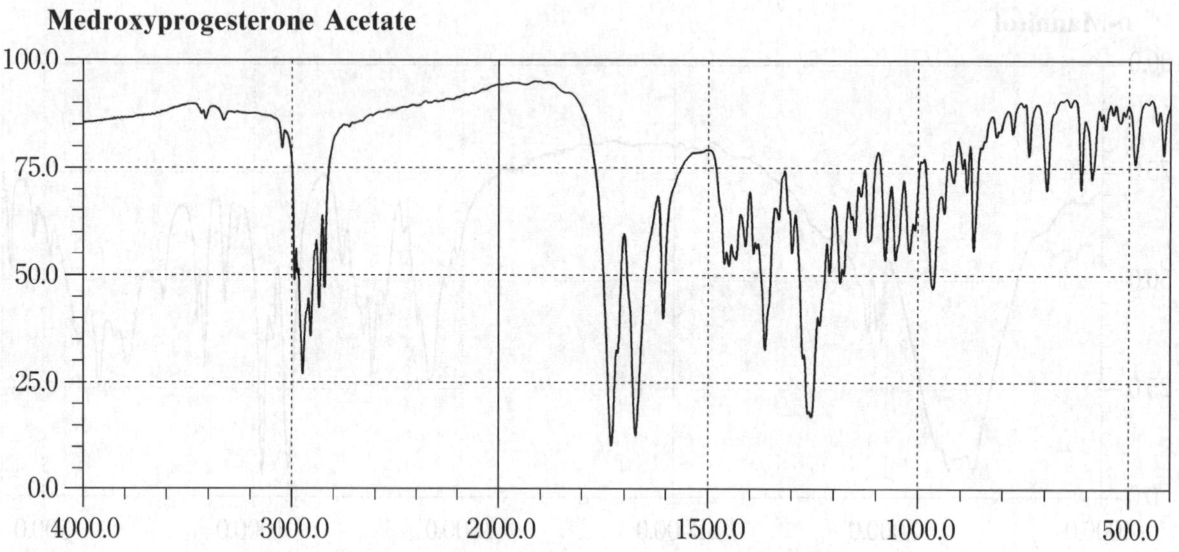

Mefloquine Hydrochloride

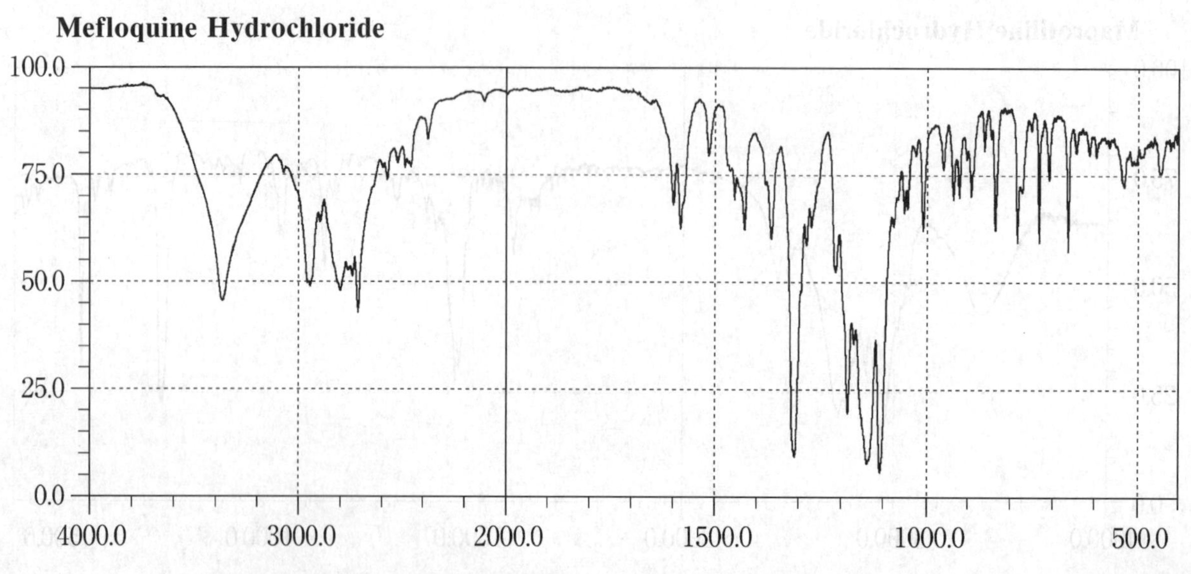

Mefruside

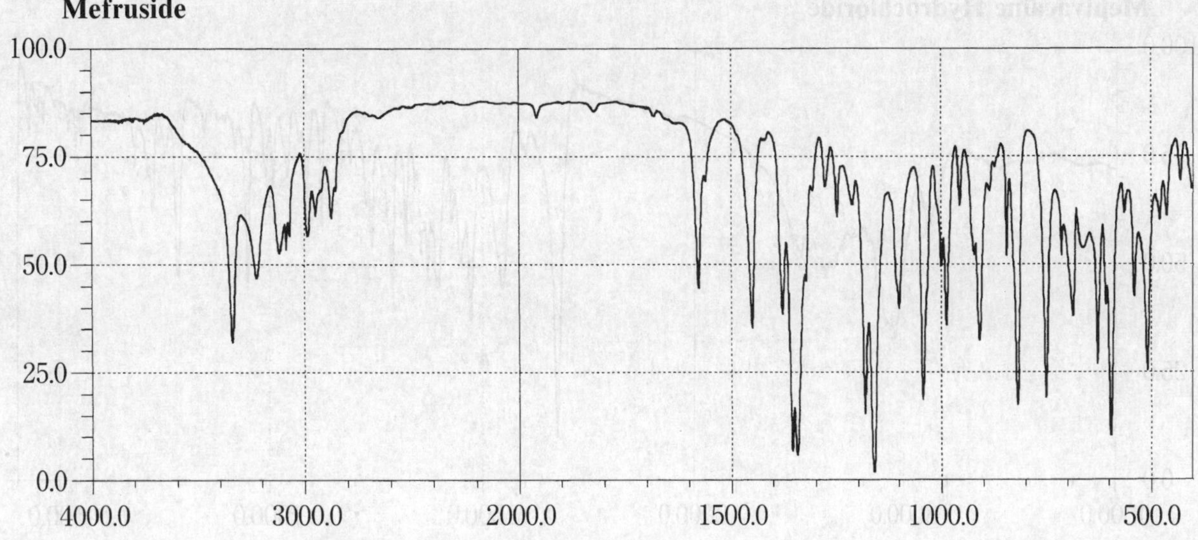

Menatetrenone

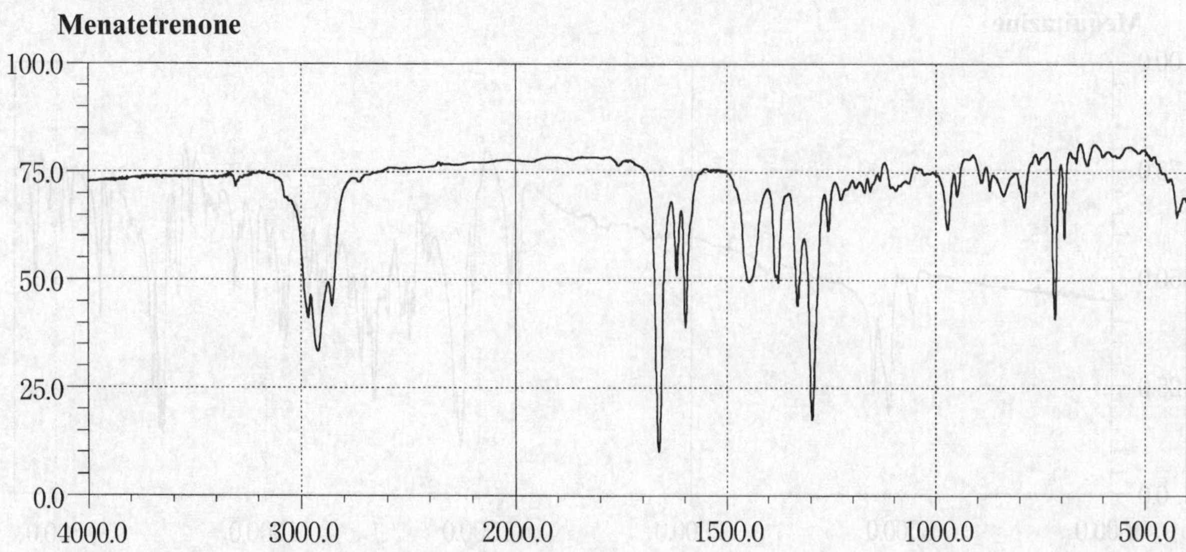

Mepitiostane

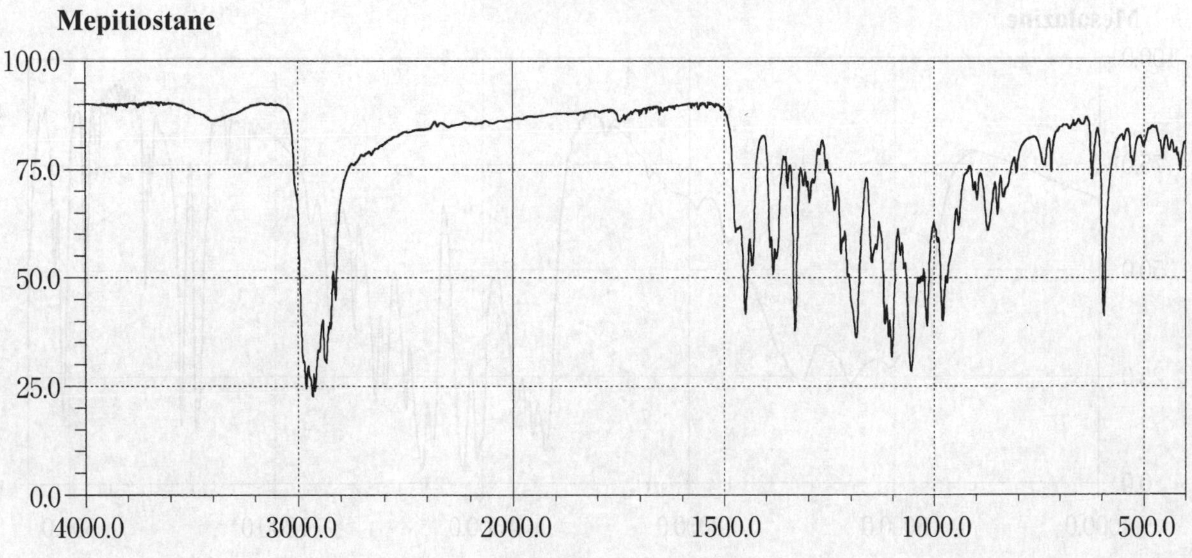

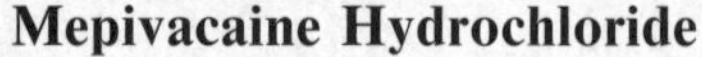

Mepivacaine Hydrochloride

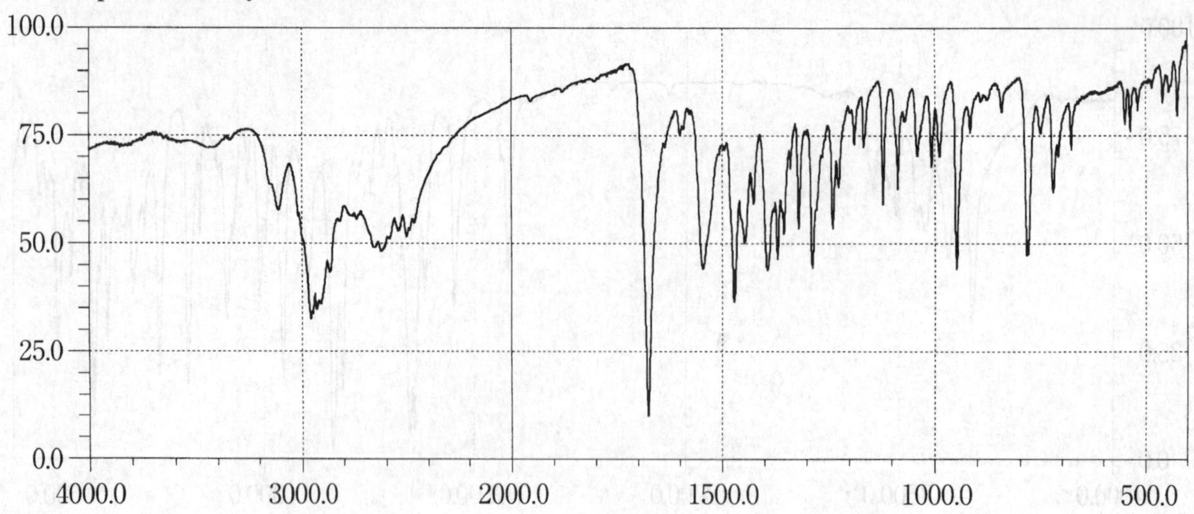

Mequitazine

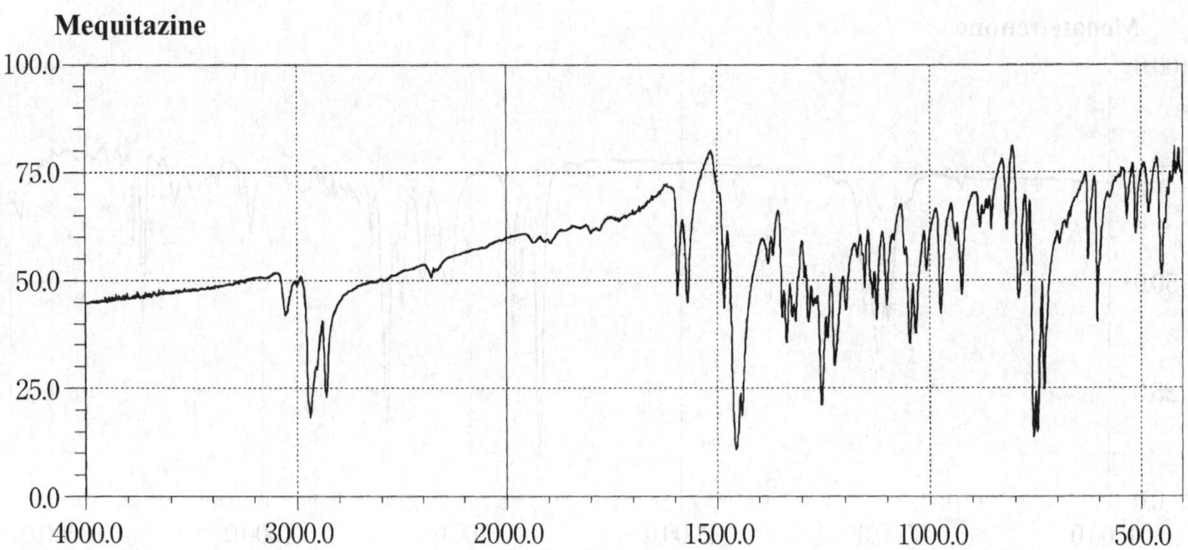

Mesalazine

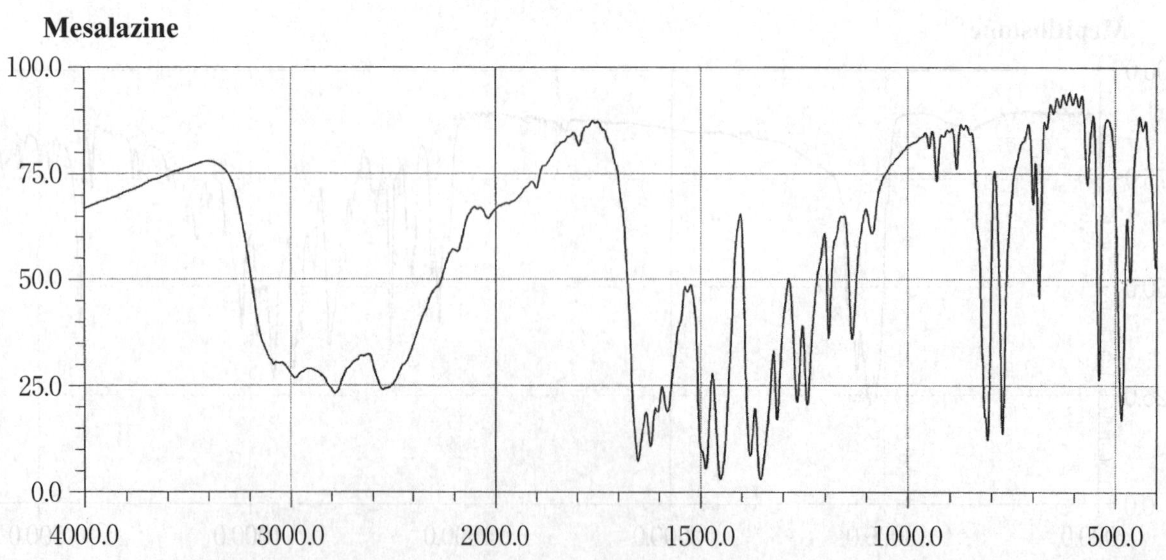

Mestranol

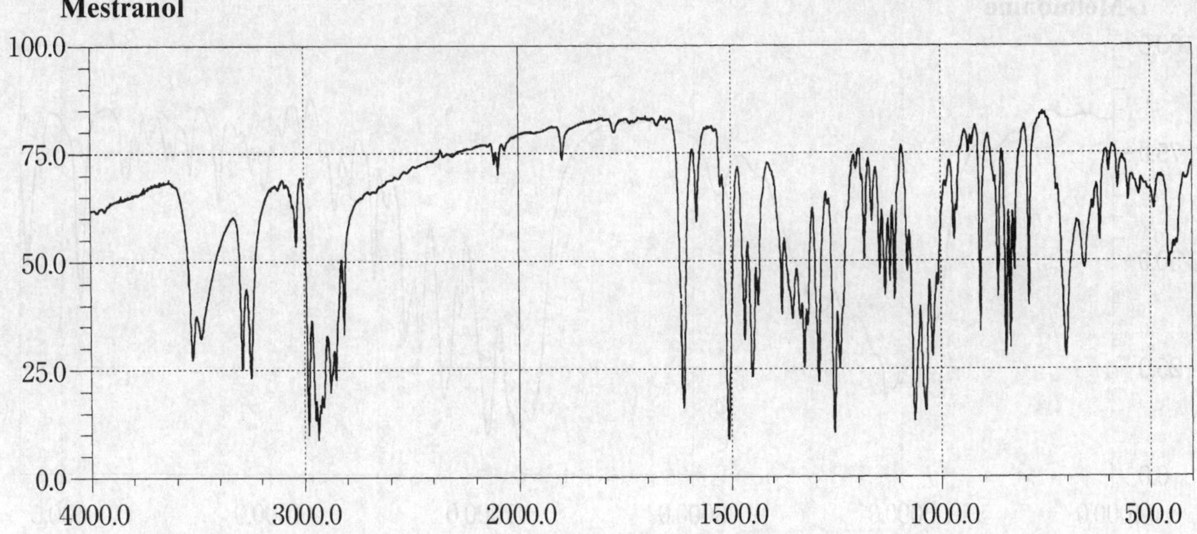

Metenolone Acetate

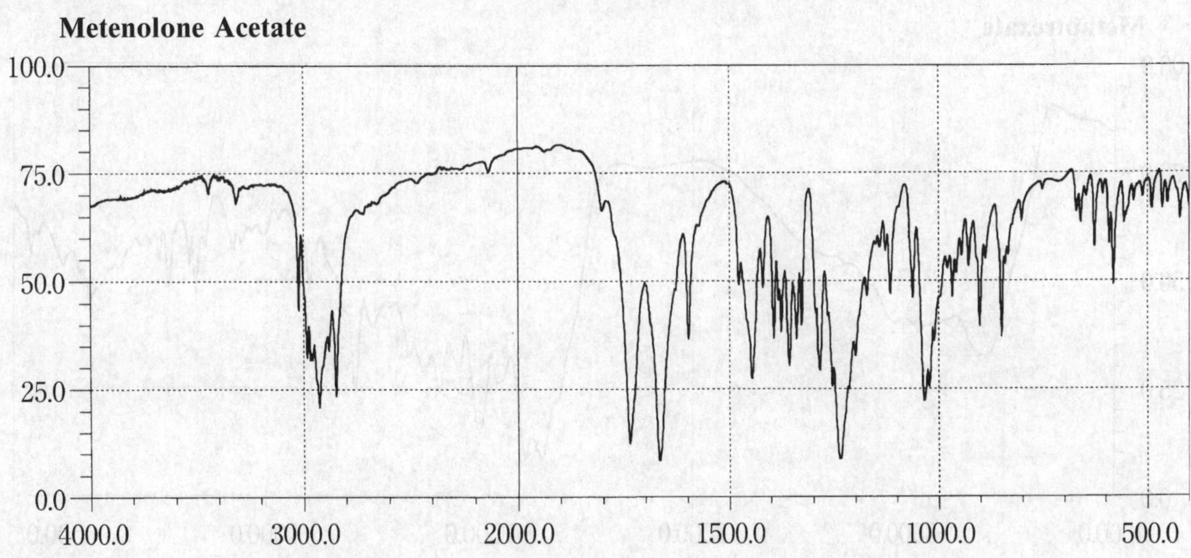

Metformin Hydrochloride

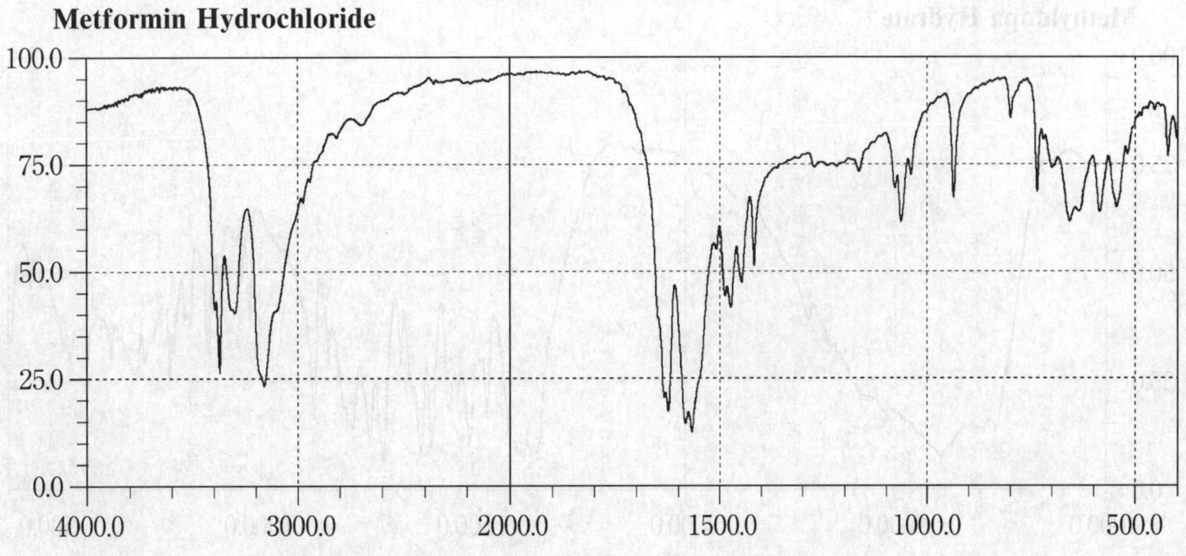

L-Methionine

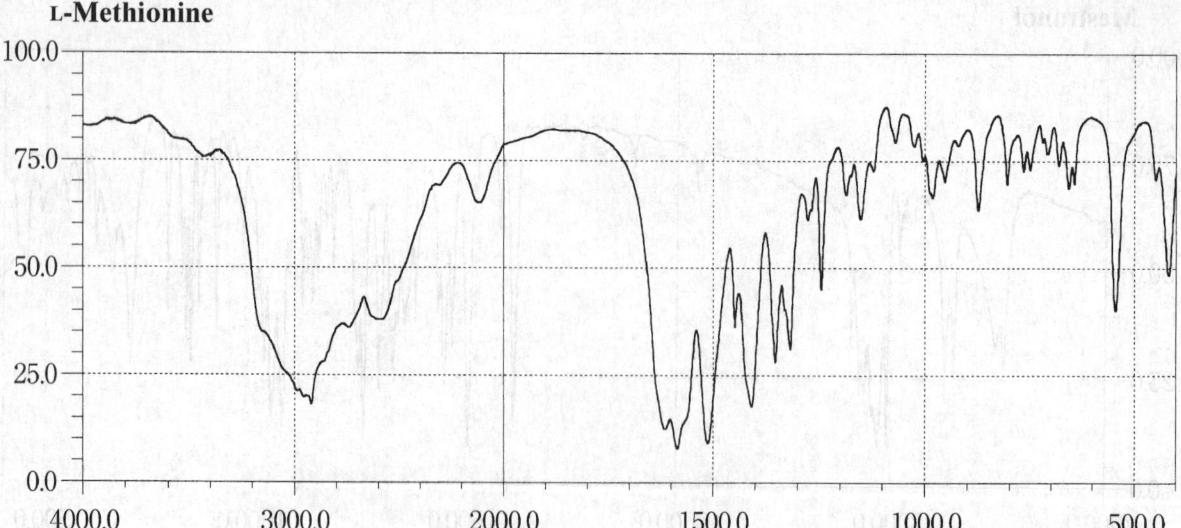

Methotrexate

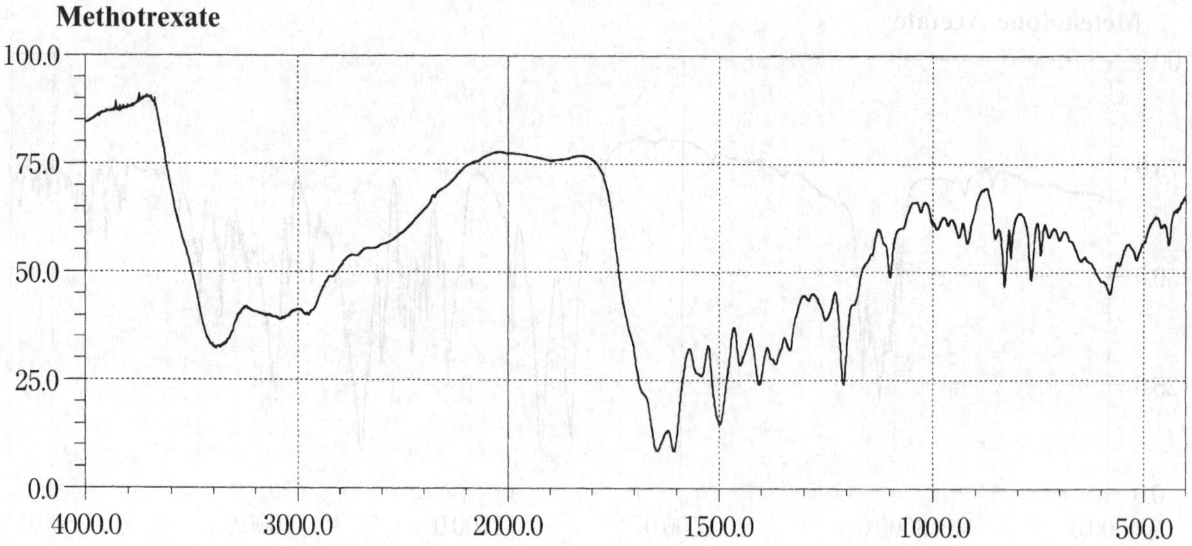

Methyldopa Hydrate

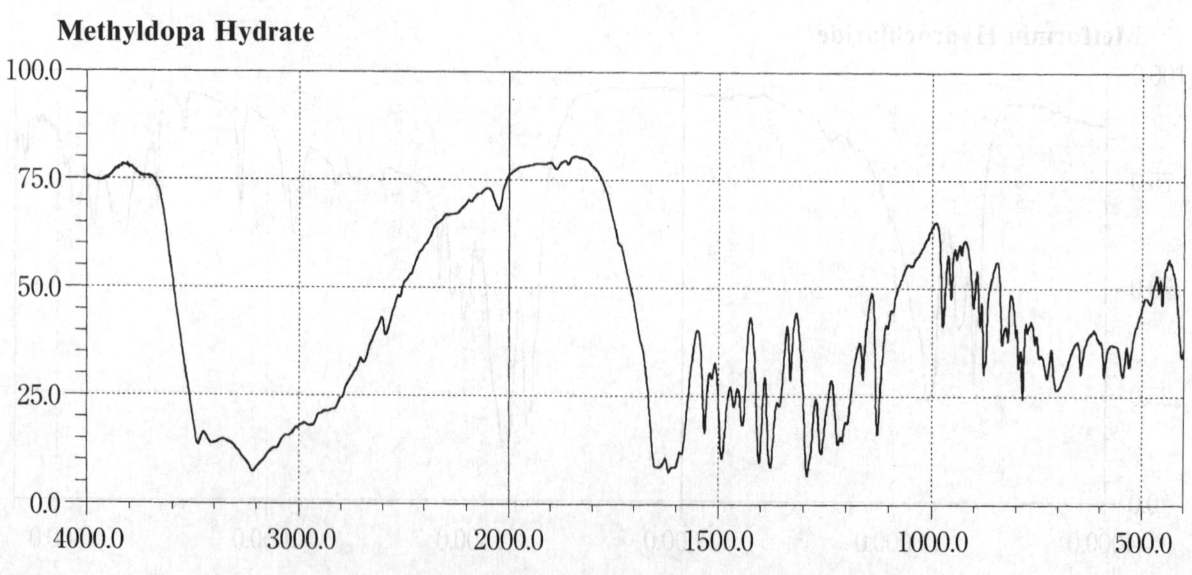

The JP Drugs are to be tested according to the provisions given in the pertinent monographs, General Notices, General Rules for Crude Drugs, General Rules for Preparations, and General Tests for their conformity to the Japanese Pharmacopoeia. (See the General Notices 5.)

dl-Methylephedrine Hydrochloride

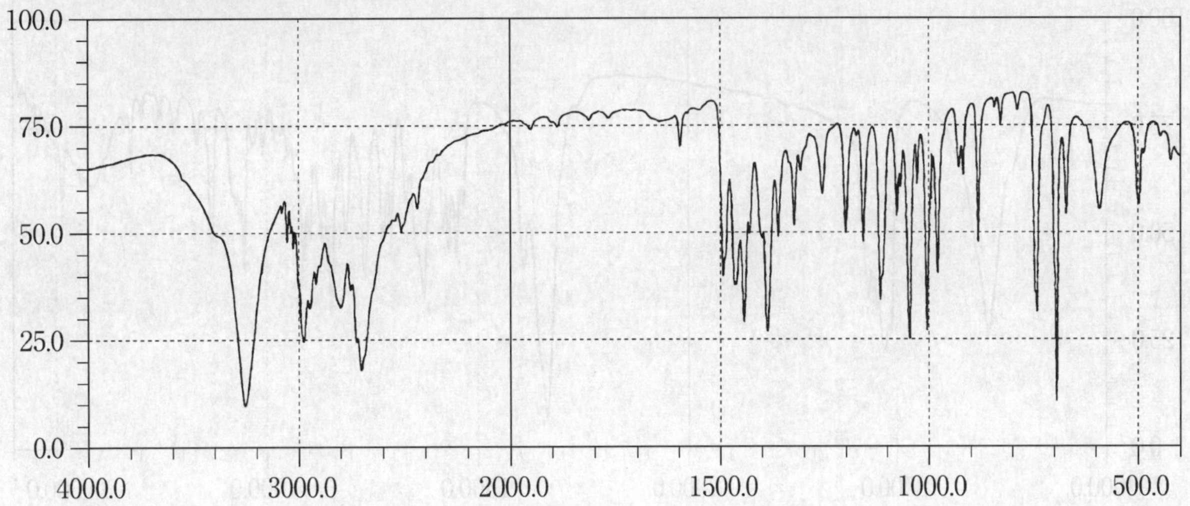

Methyl Parahydroxybenzoate

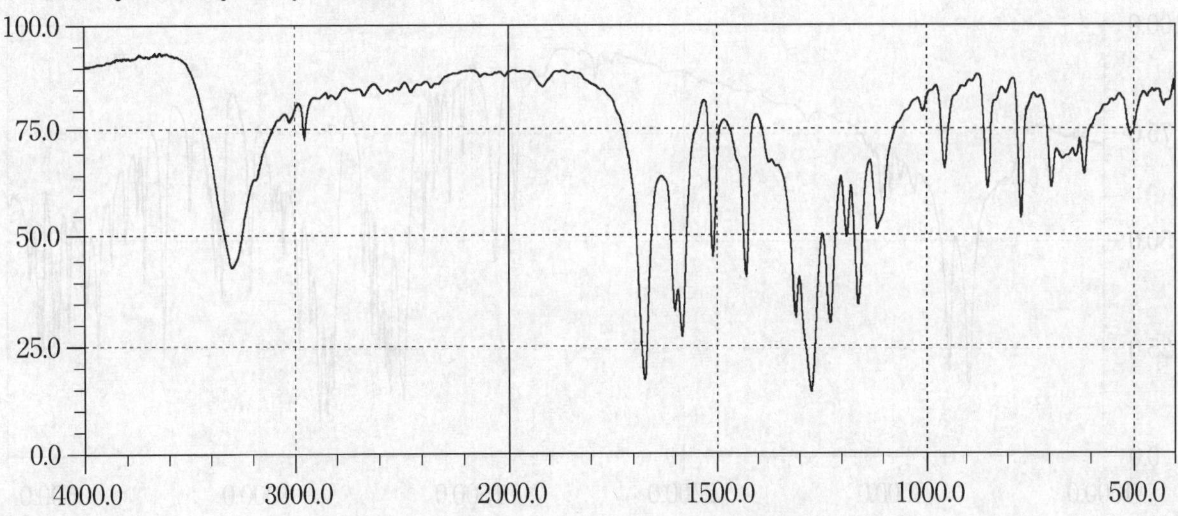

Methylprednisolone Succinate

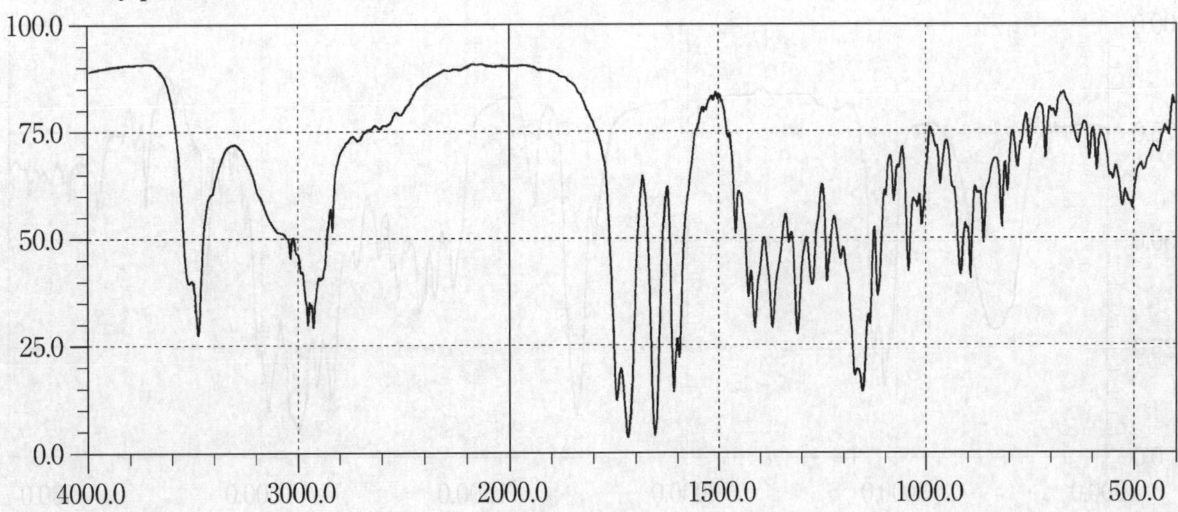

The JP Drugs are to be tested according to the provisions given in the pertinent monographs, General Notices, General Rules for Crude Drugs, General Rules for Preparations, and General Tests for their conformity to the Japanese Pharmacopoeia. (See the General Notices 5.)

Methyltestosterone

100.0
75.0
50.0
25.0
0.0
4000.0 3000.0 2000.0 1500.0 1000.0 500.0

Meticrane

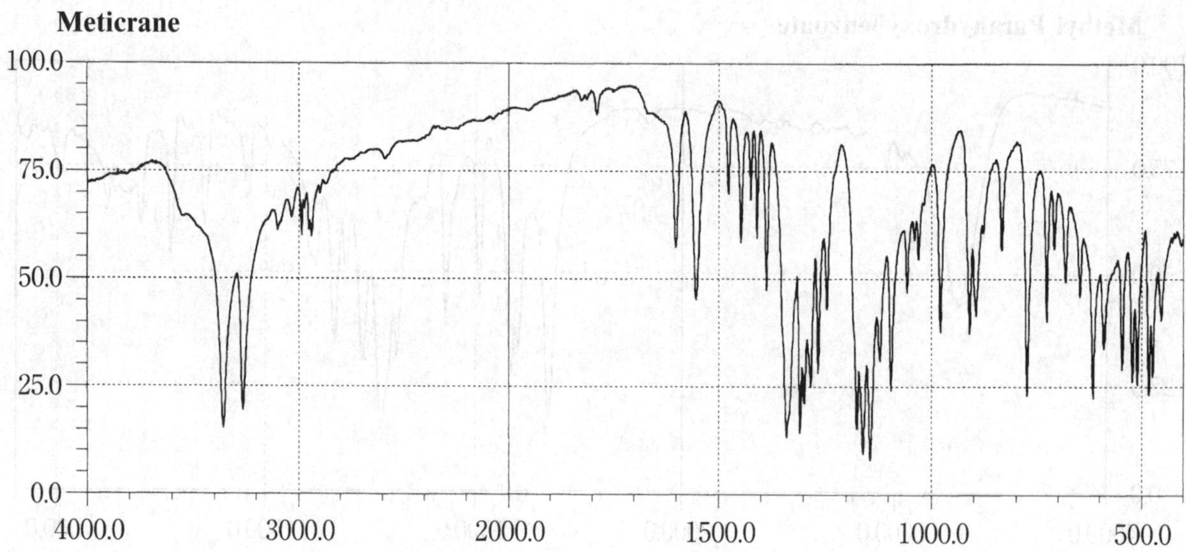

Metildigoxin

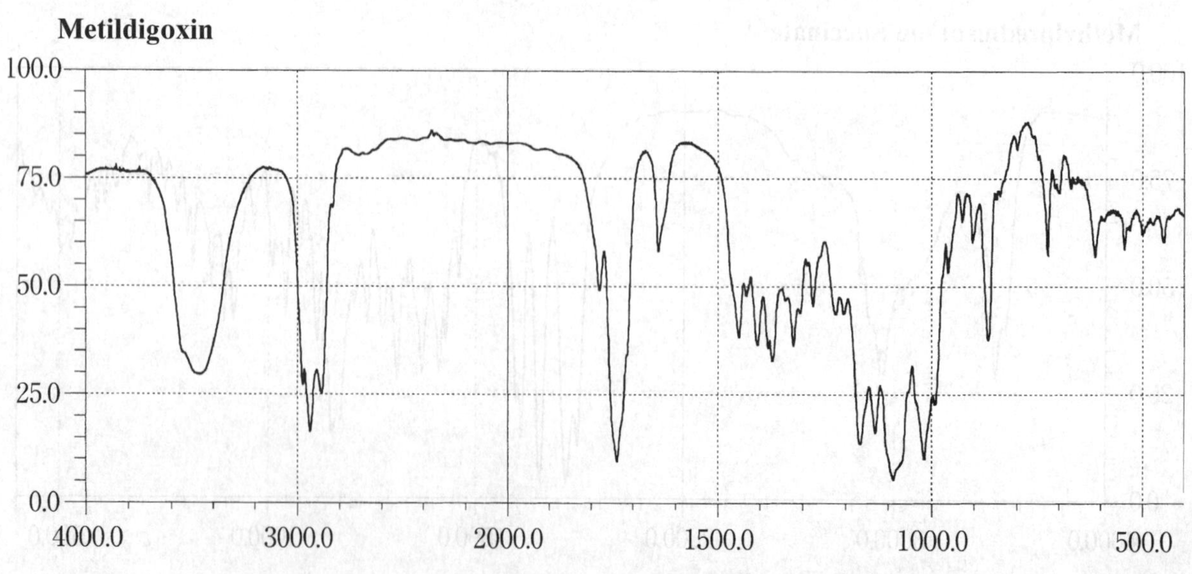

The JP Drugs are to be tested according to the provisions given in the pertinent monographs, General Notices, General Rules for Crude Drugs, General Rules for Preparations, and General Tests for their conformity to the Japanese Pharmacopoeia. (See the General Notices 5.)

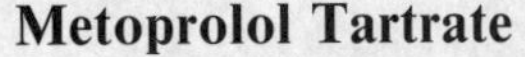

Metoprolol Tartrate

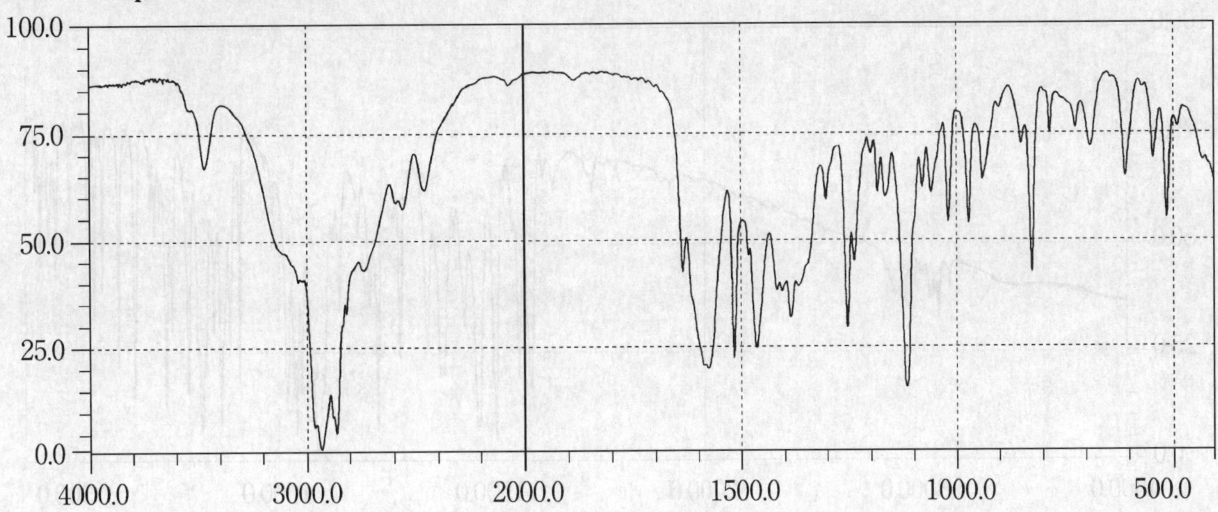

Metronidazole

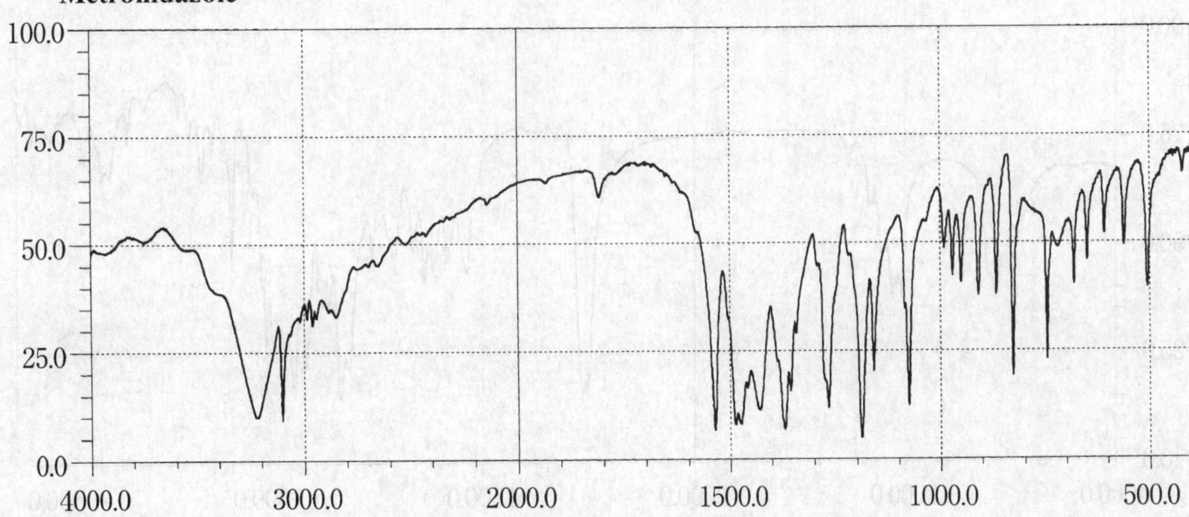

Mexiletine Hydrochloride

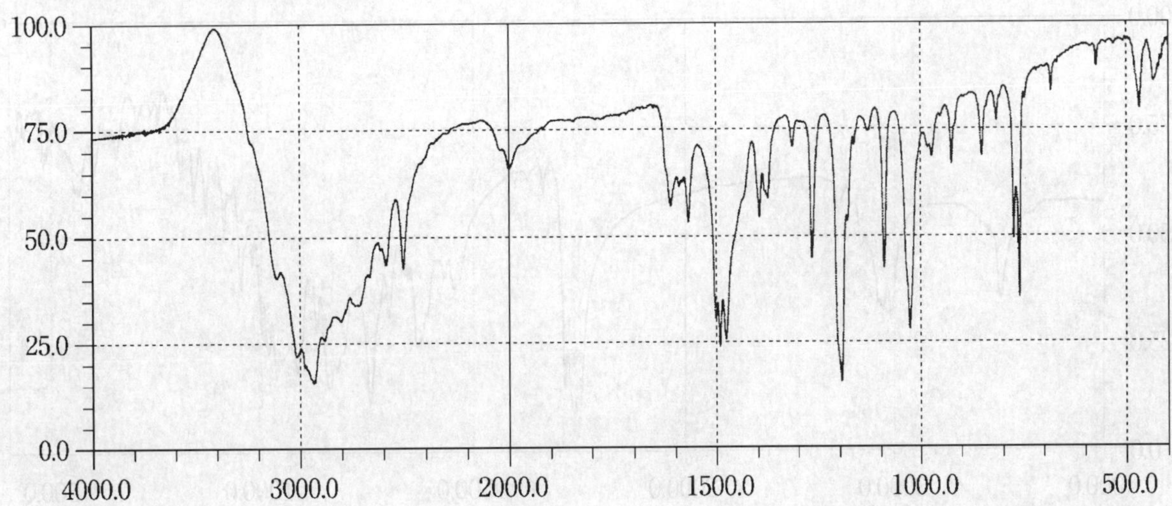

The JP Drugs are to be tested according to the provisions given in the pertinent monographs, General Notices, General Rules for Crude Drugs, General Rules for Preparations, and General Tests for their conformity to the Japanese Pharmacopoeia. (See the General Notices 5.)

Miconazole

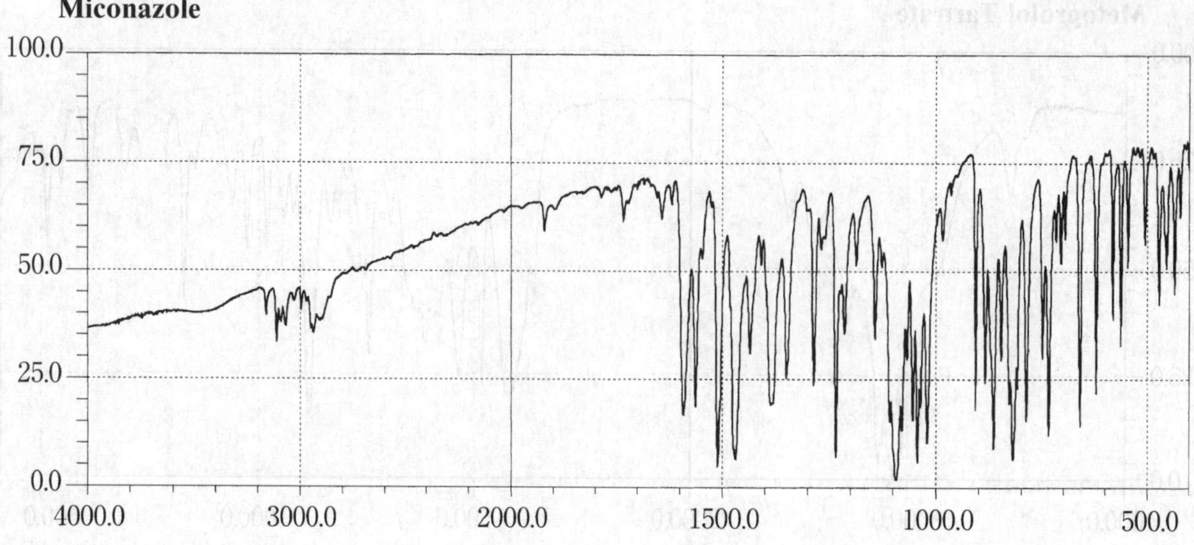

Midecamycin

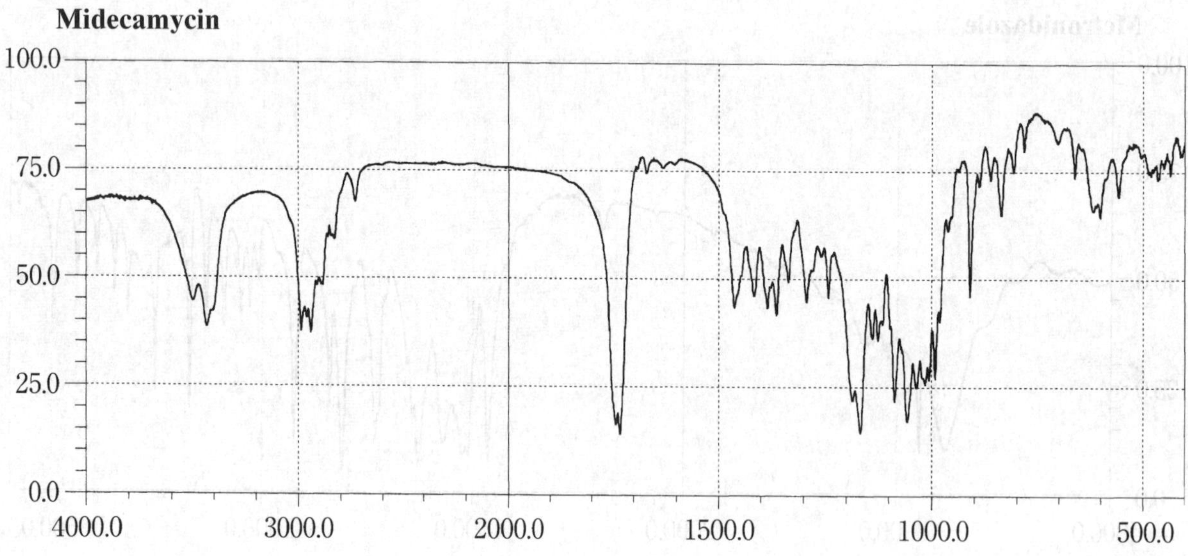

Midecamycin Acetate

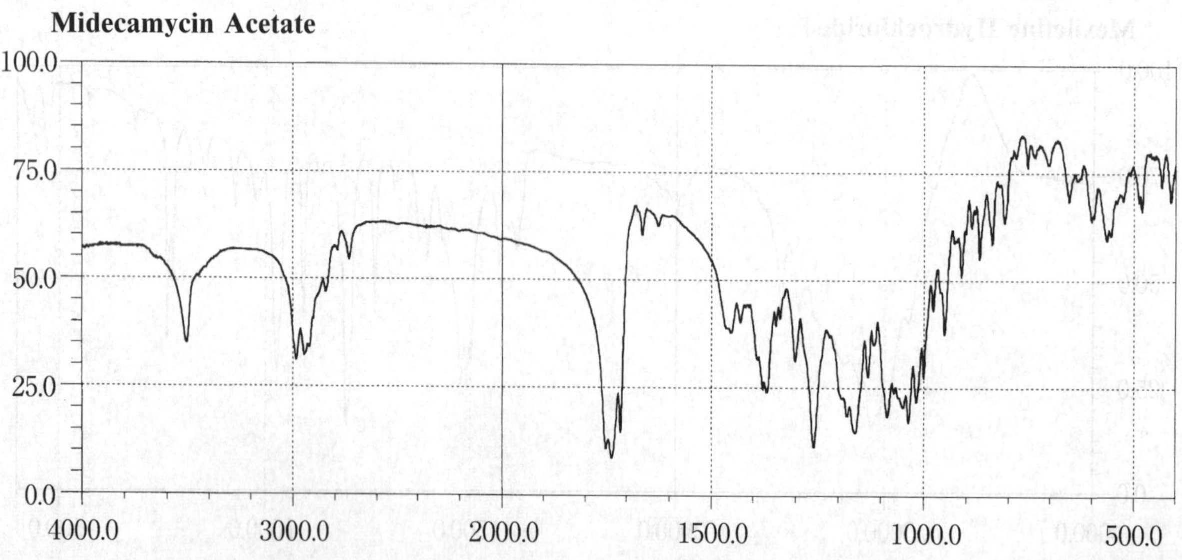

Miglitol

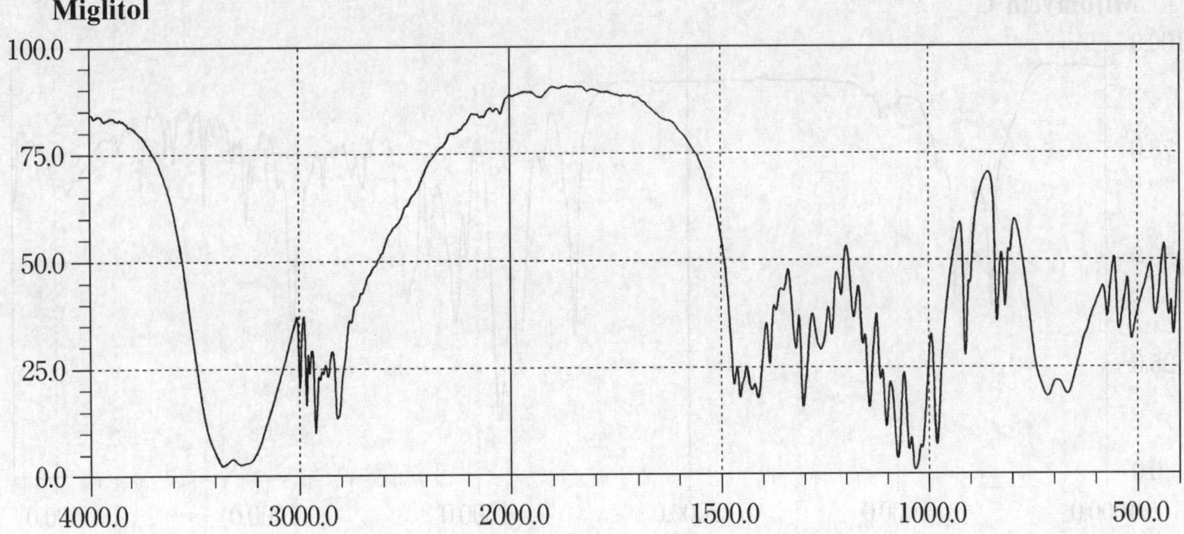

Minocycline Hydrochloride

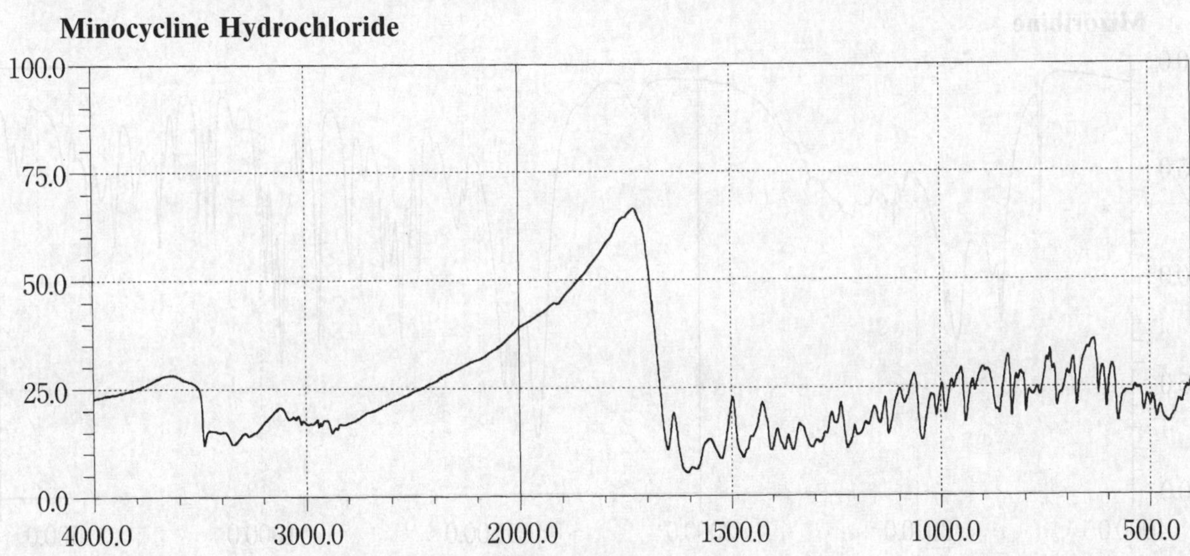

Mitiglinide Calcium Hydrate

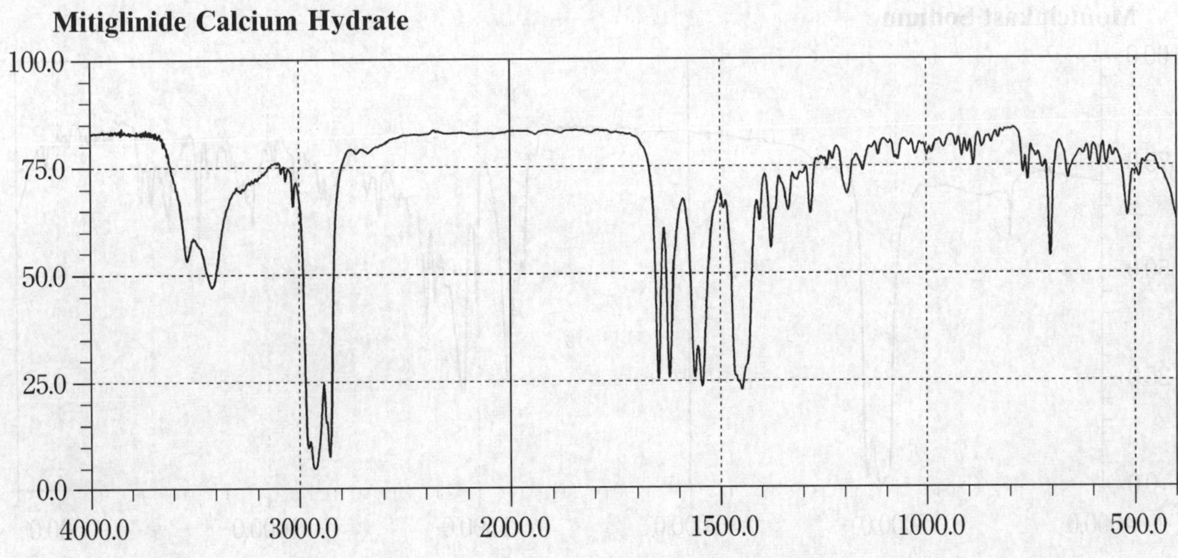

Mitomycin C

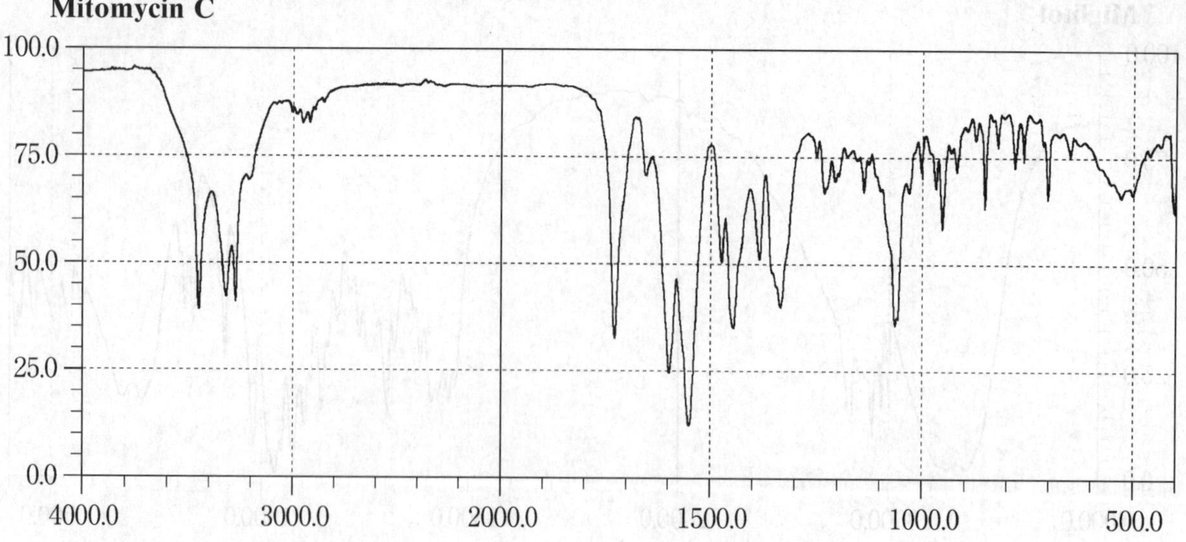

Mizoribine

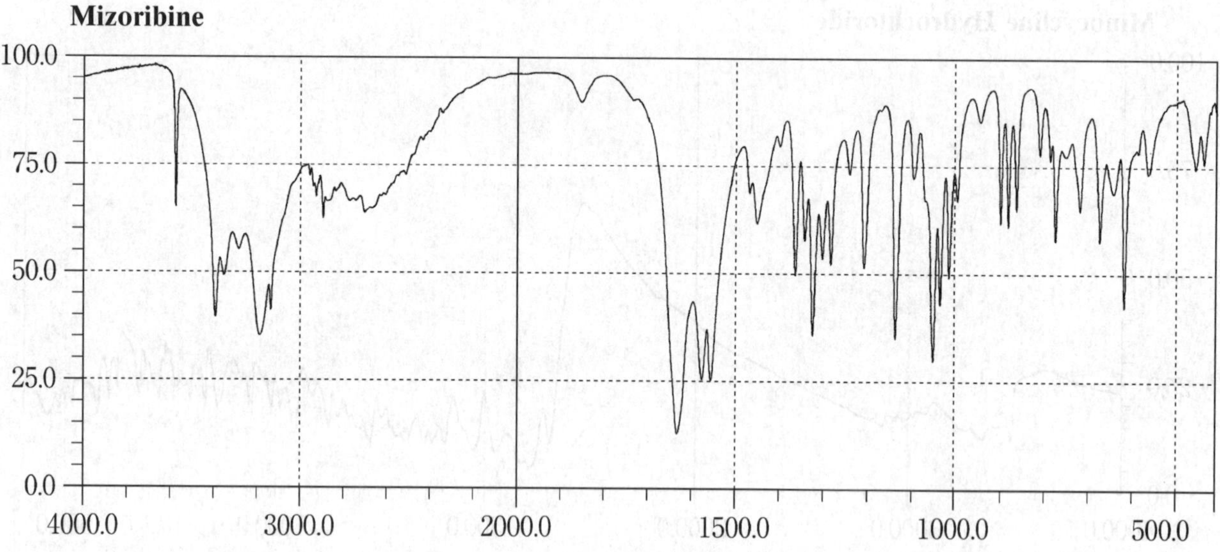

Montelukast Sodium

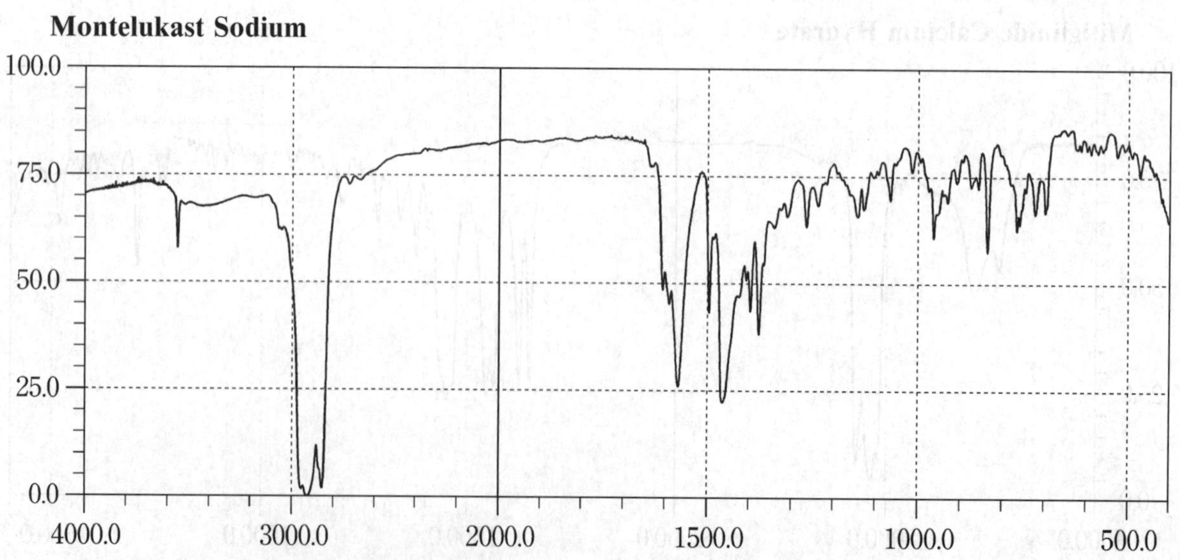

The JP Drugs are to be tested according to the provisions given in the pertinent monographs, General Notices, General Rules for Crude Drugs, General Rules for Preparations, and General Tests for their conformity to the Japanese Pharmacopoeia. (See the General Notices 5.)

Morphine Hydrochloride Hydrate

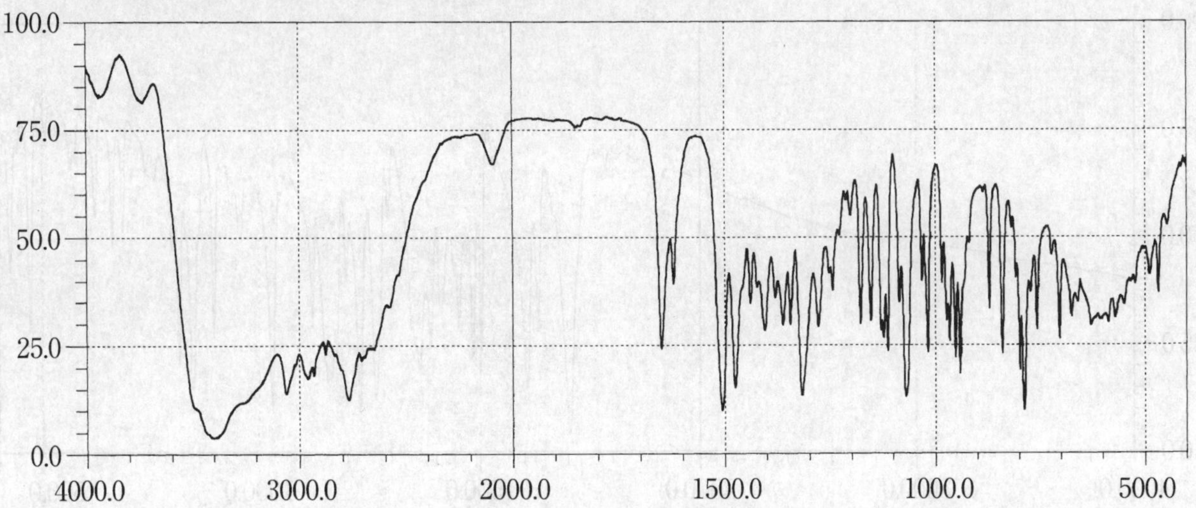

Morphine Sulfate Hydrate

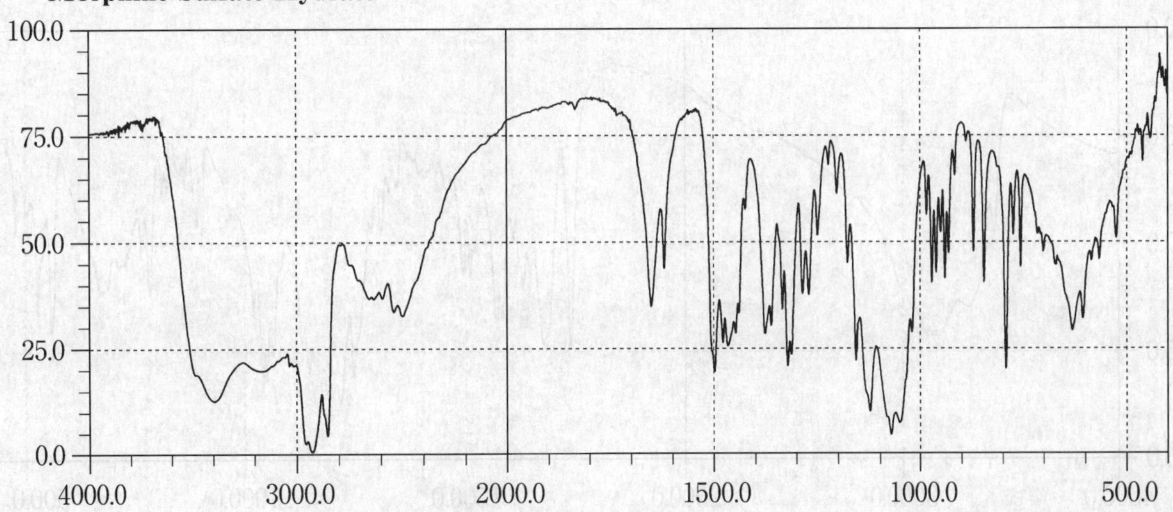

Mosapride Citrate Hydrate

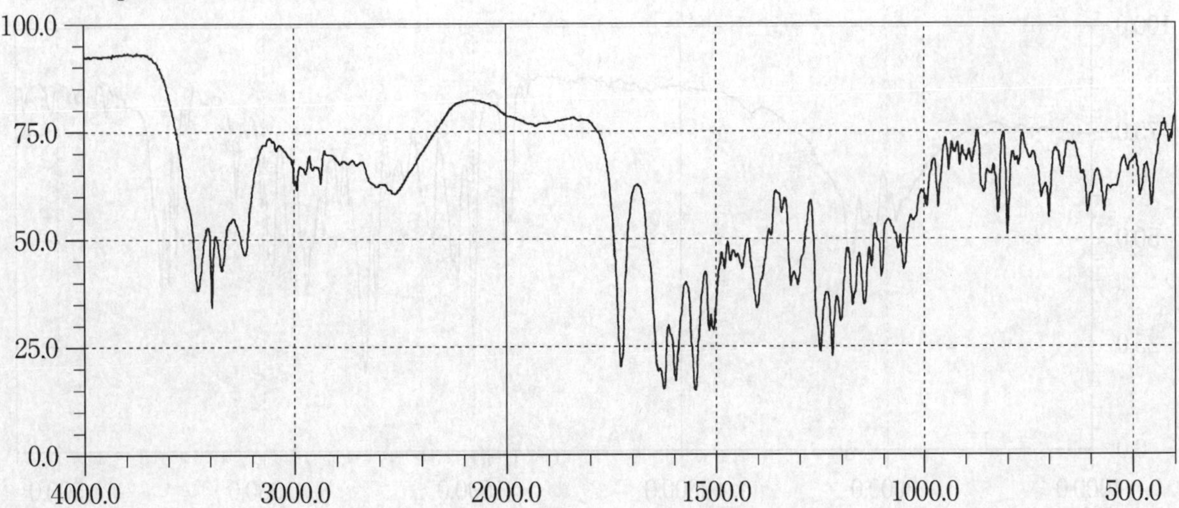

Nabumetone

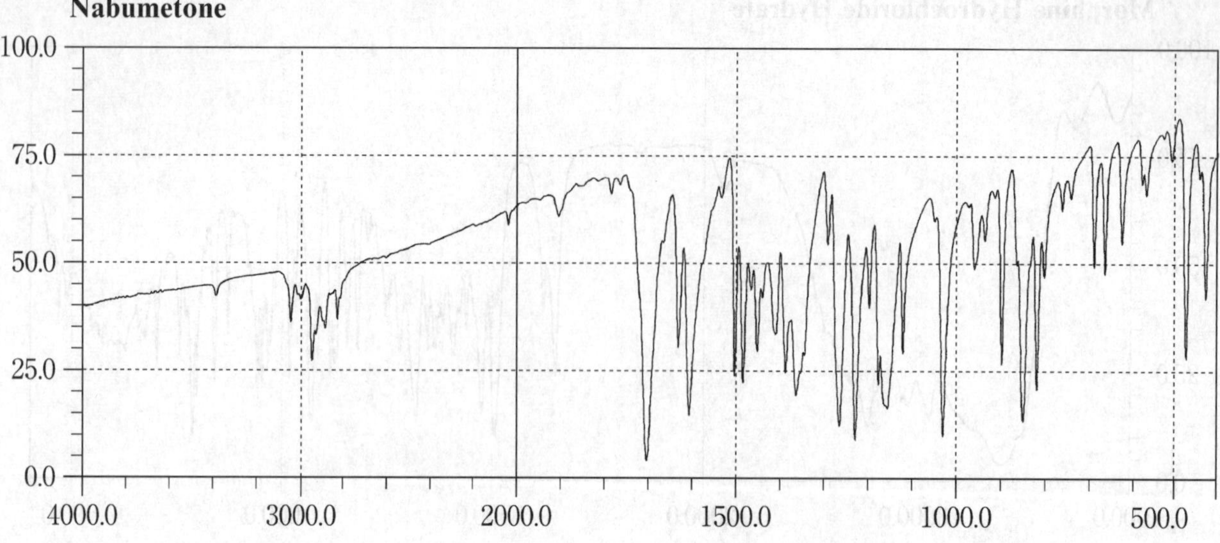

Nafamostat Mesilate

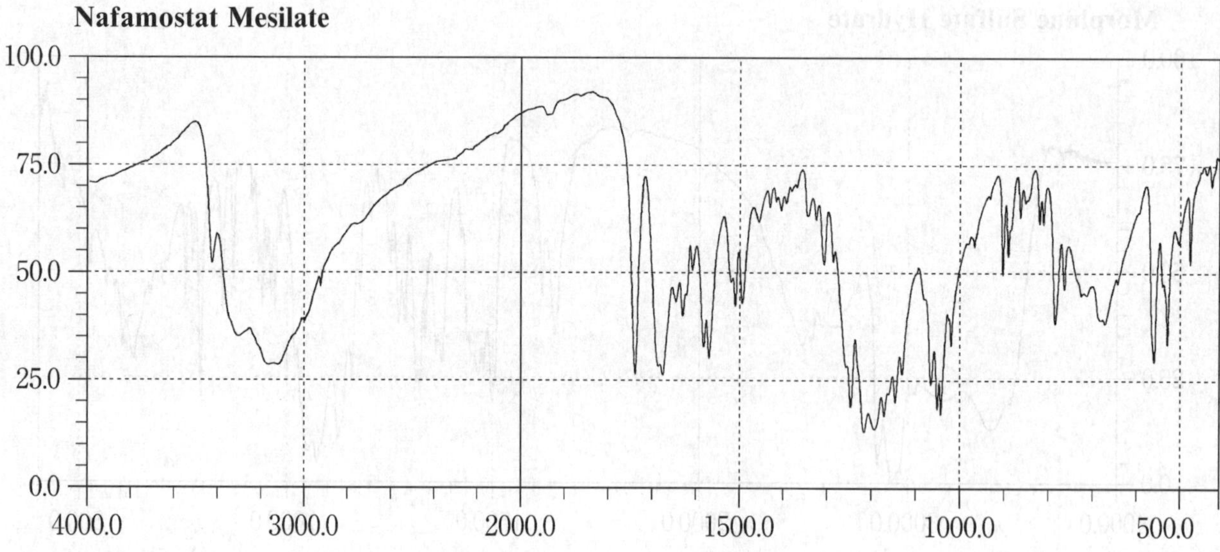

Naftopidil

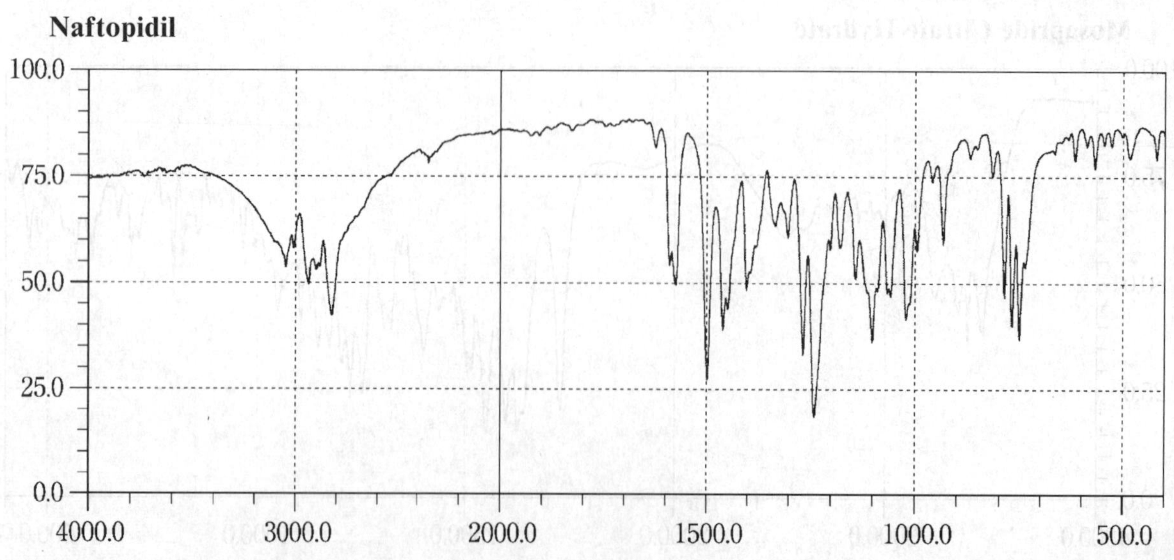

Nalidixic Acid

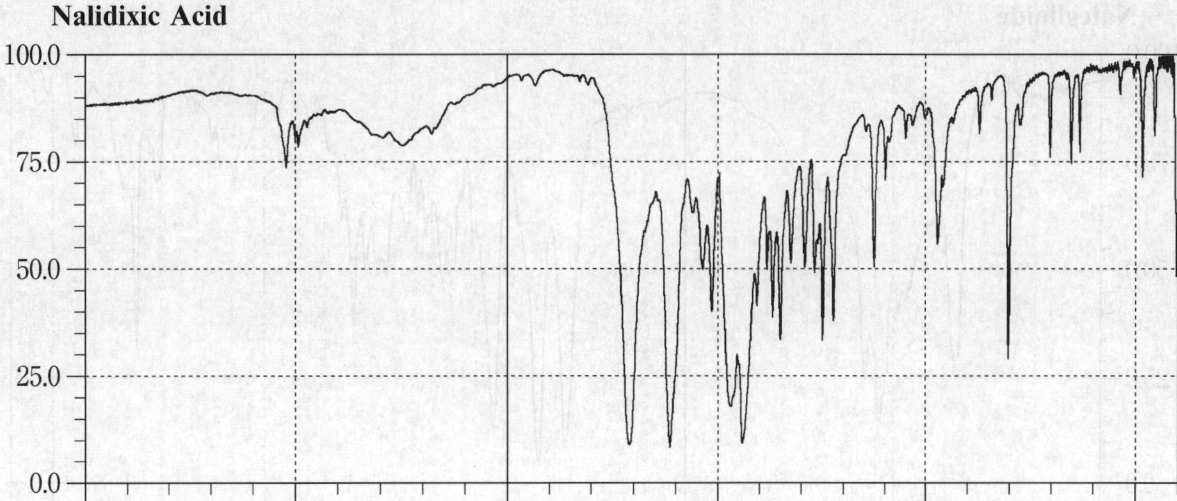

Naloxone Hydrochloride

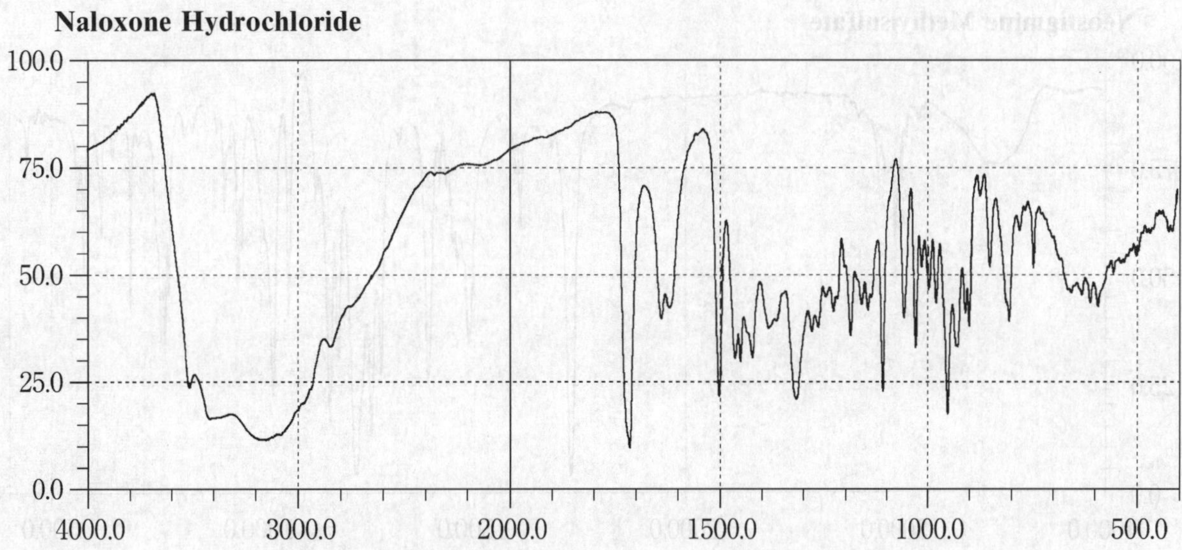

Naproxen

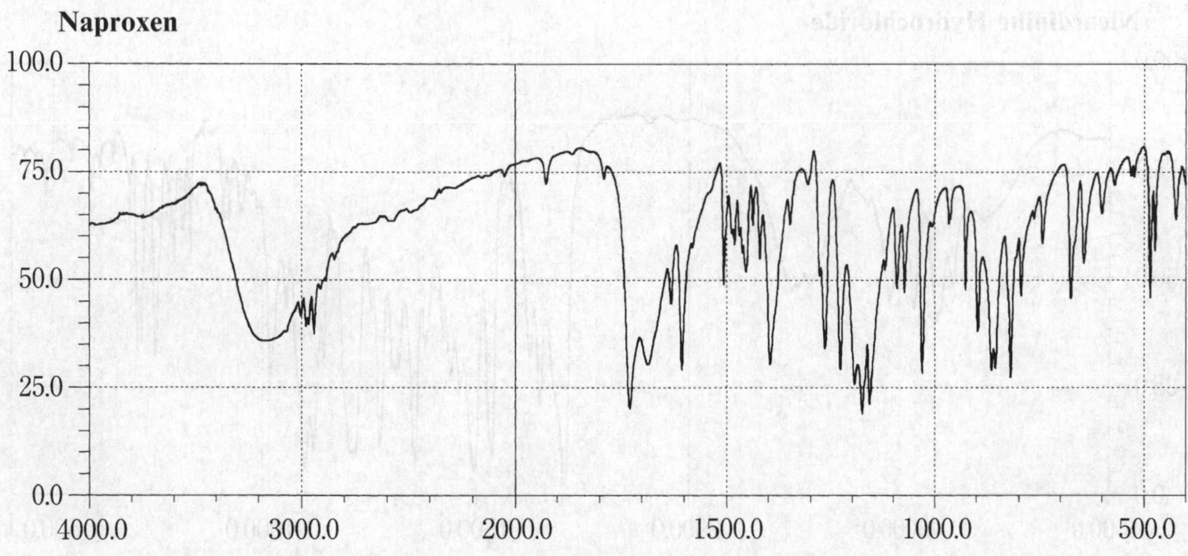

Nateglinide

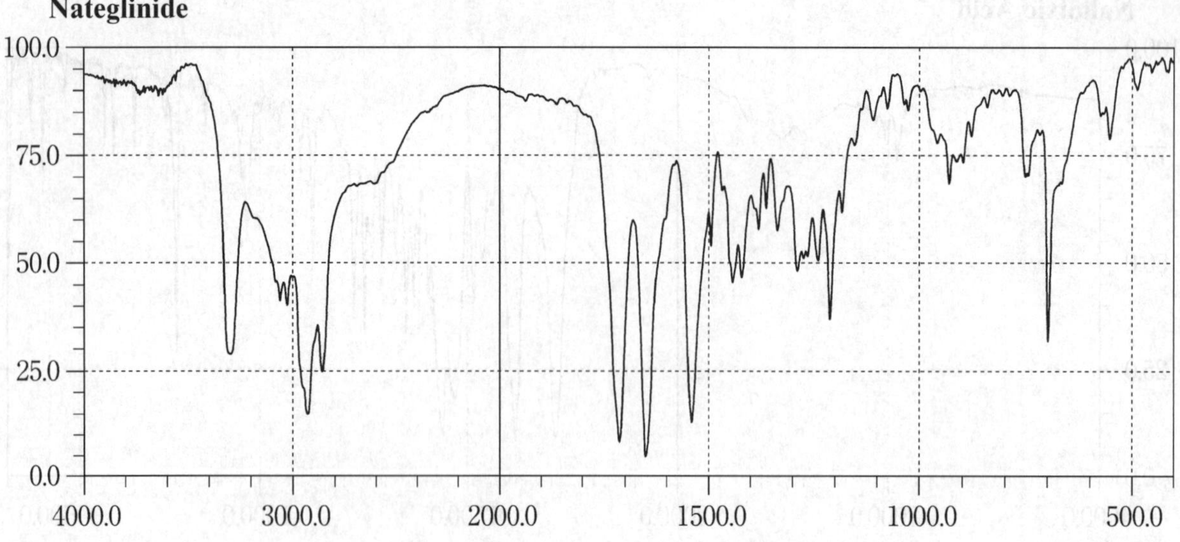

Neostigmine Methylsulfate

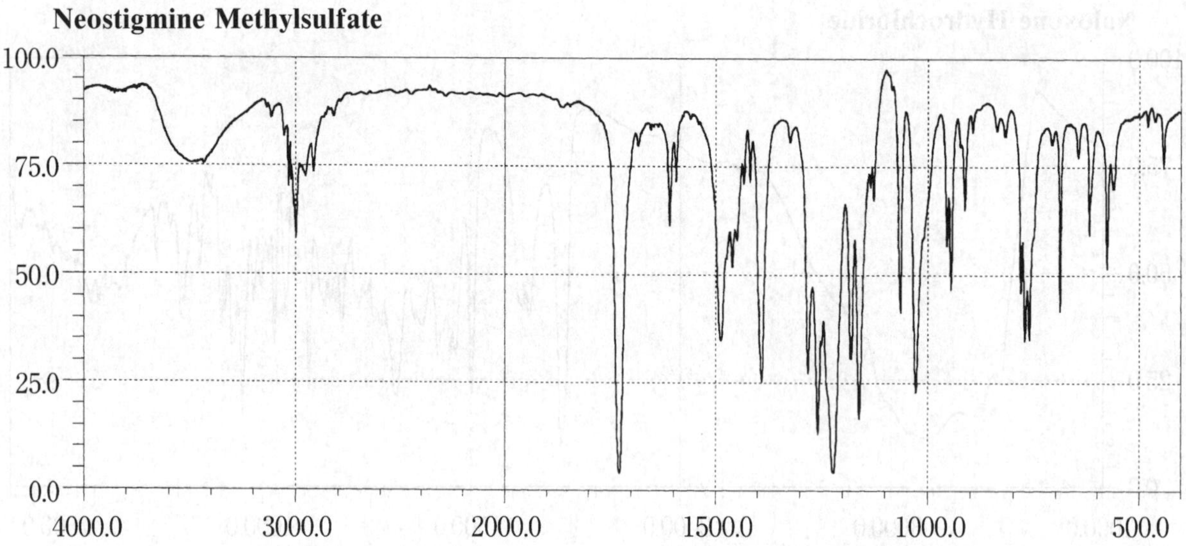

Nicardipine Hydrochloride

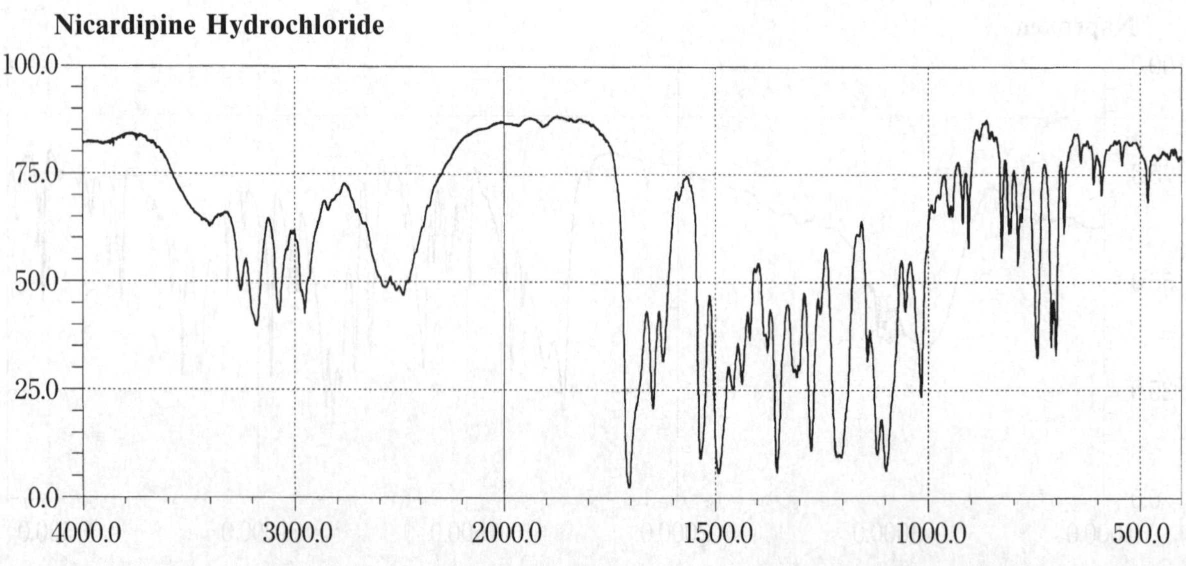

Nicergoline

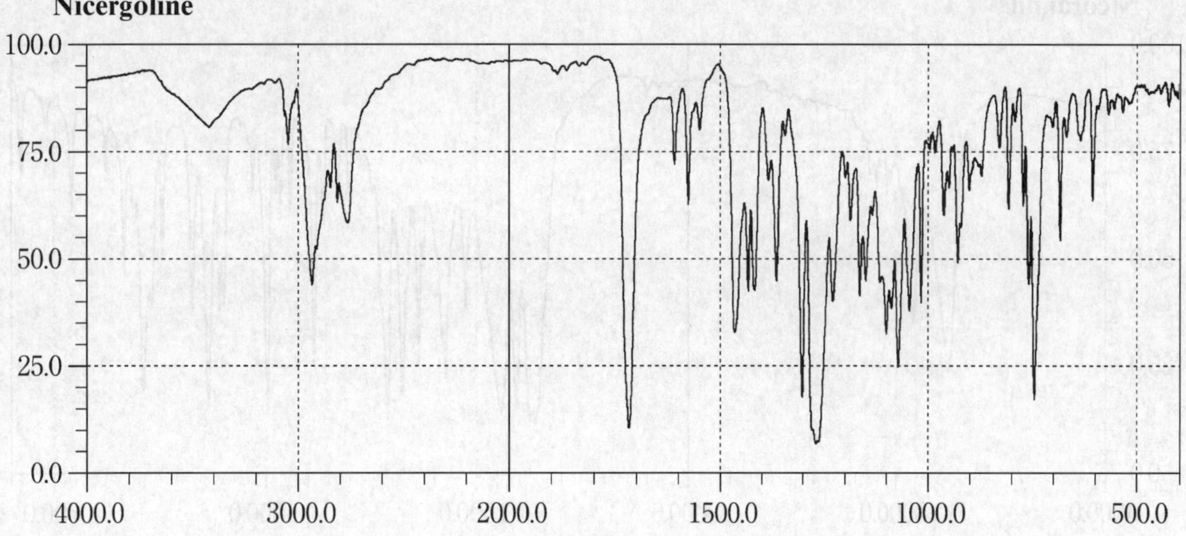

Niceritrol

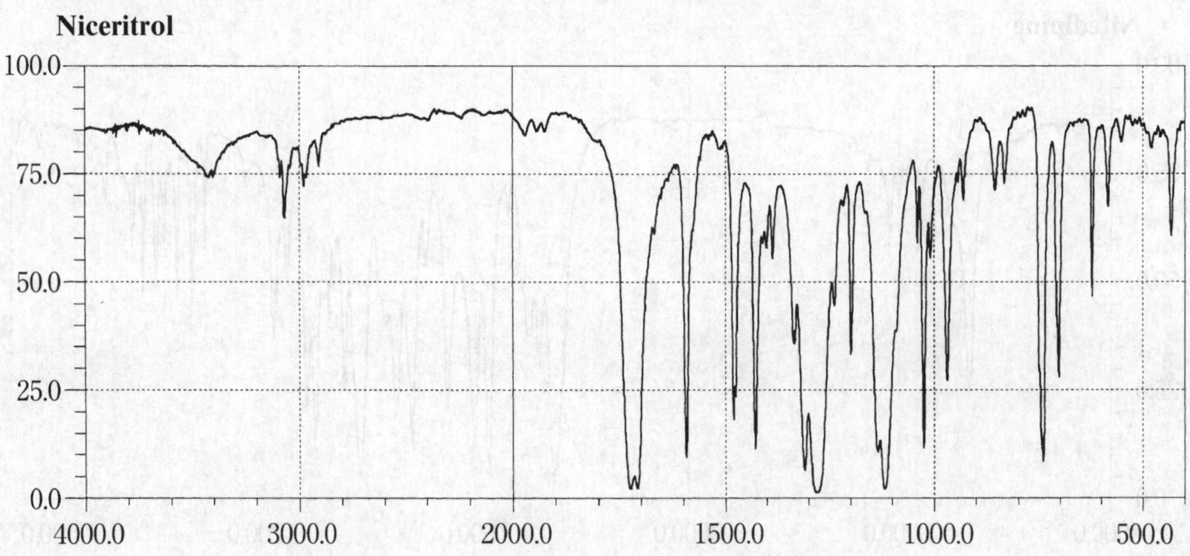

Nicomol

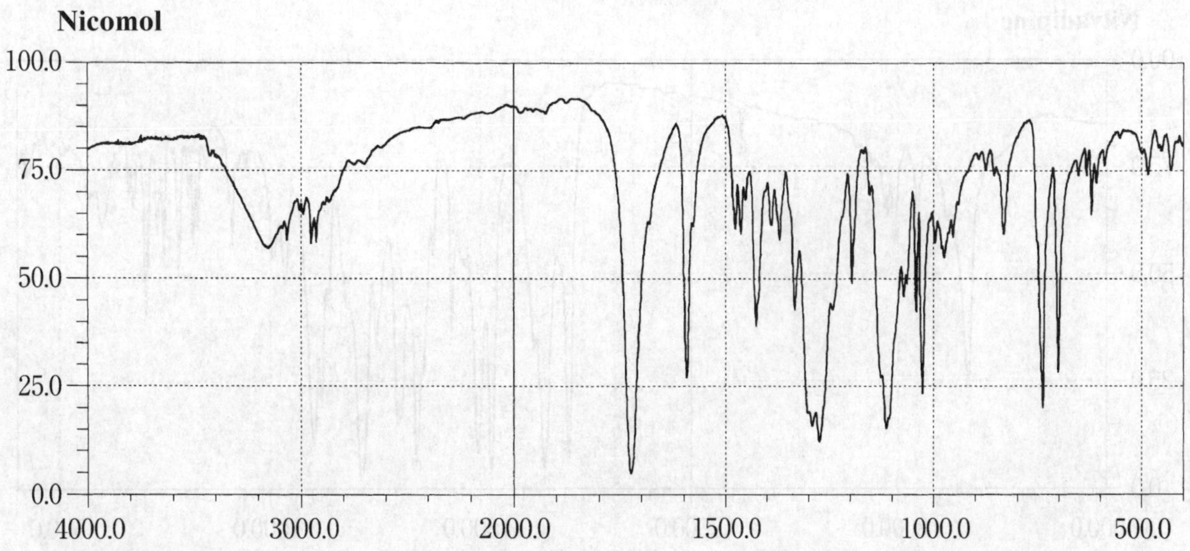

Nicorandil

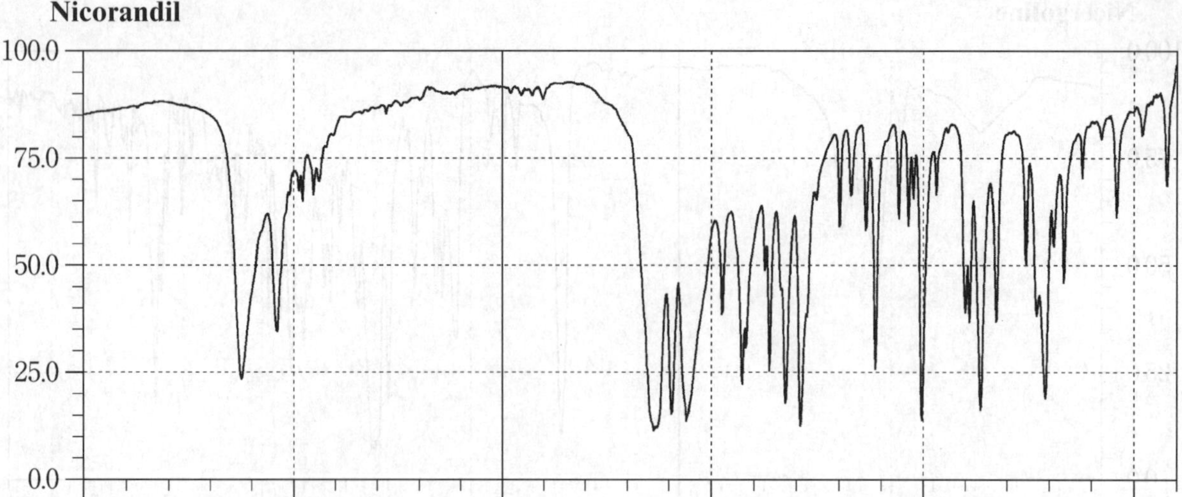

Nifedipine

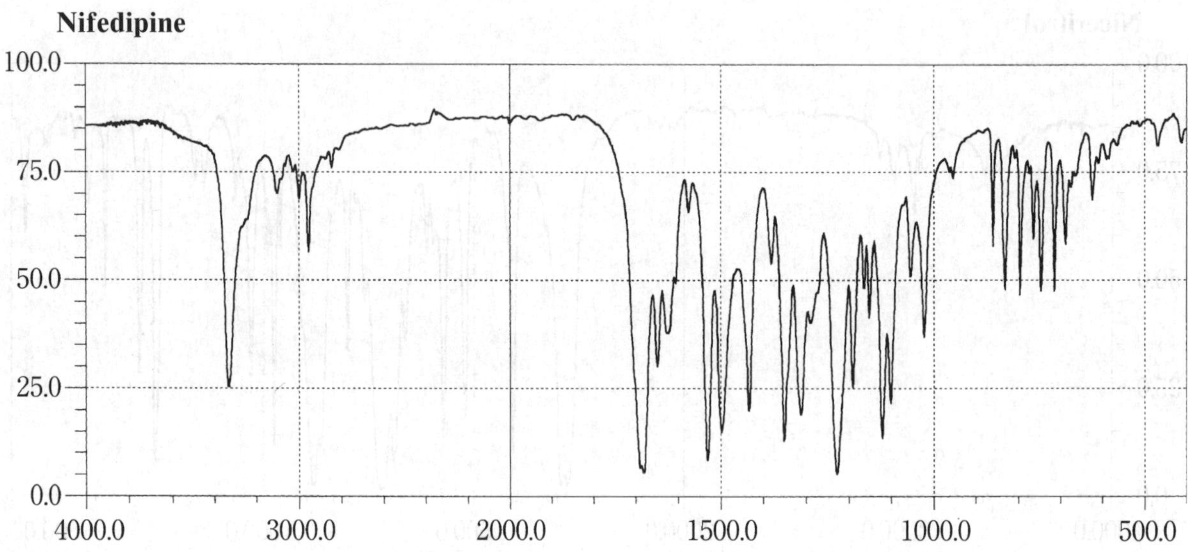

Nilvadipine

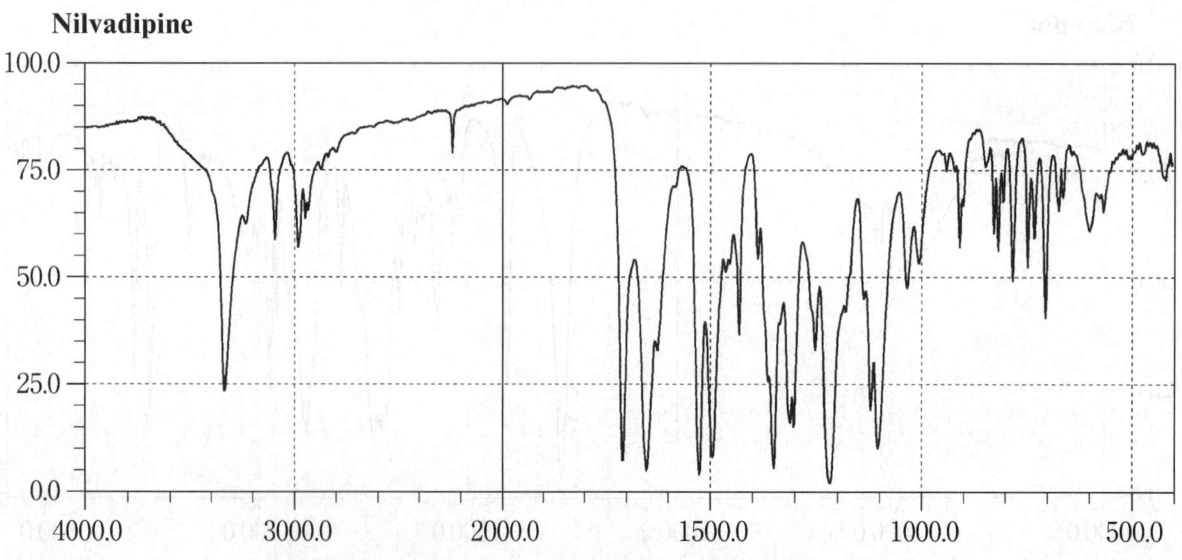

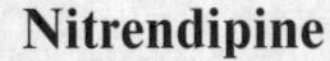

Nitrendipine

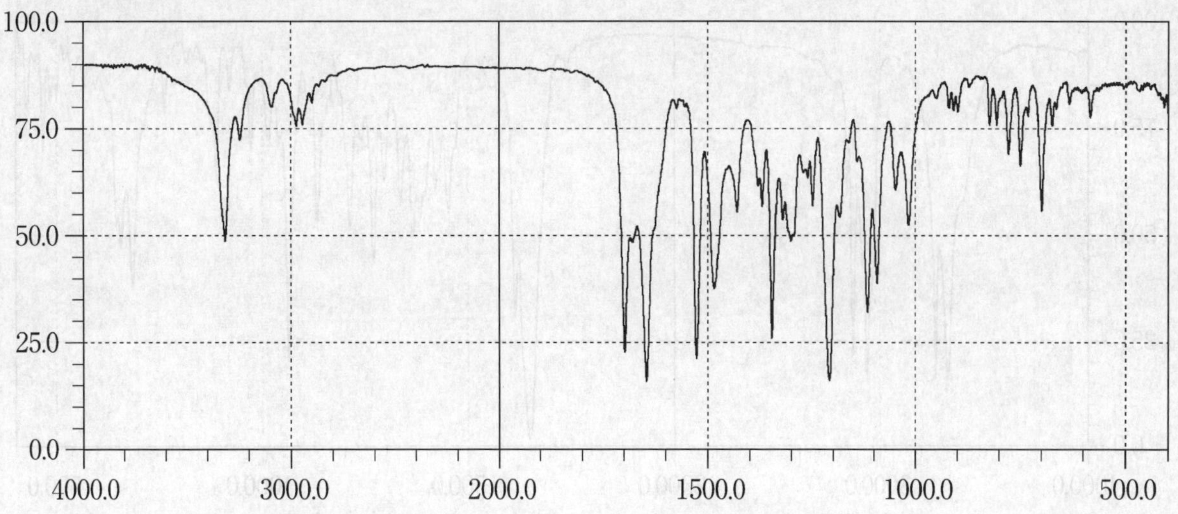

Nizatidine

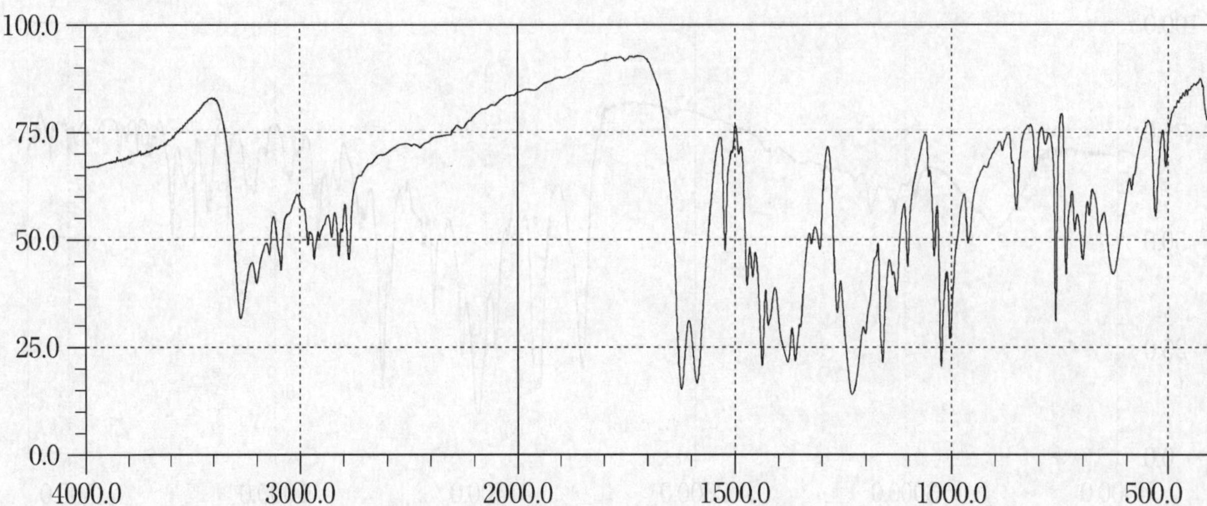

Noradrenaline

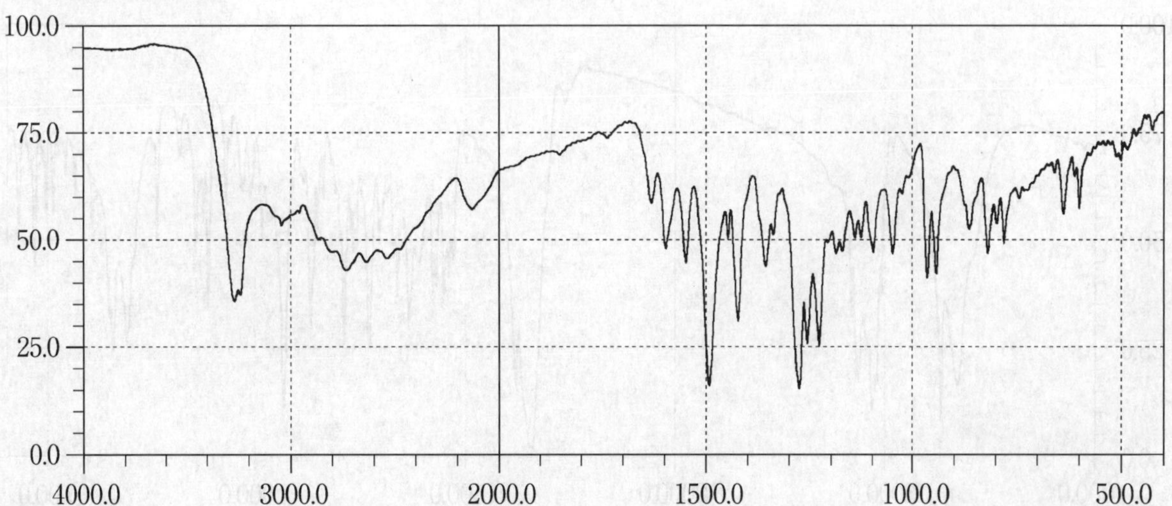

Norethisterone

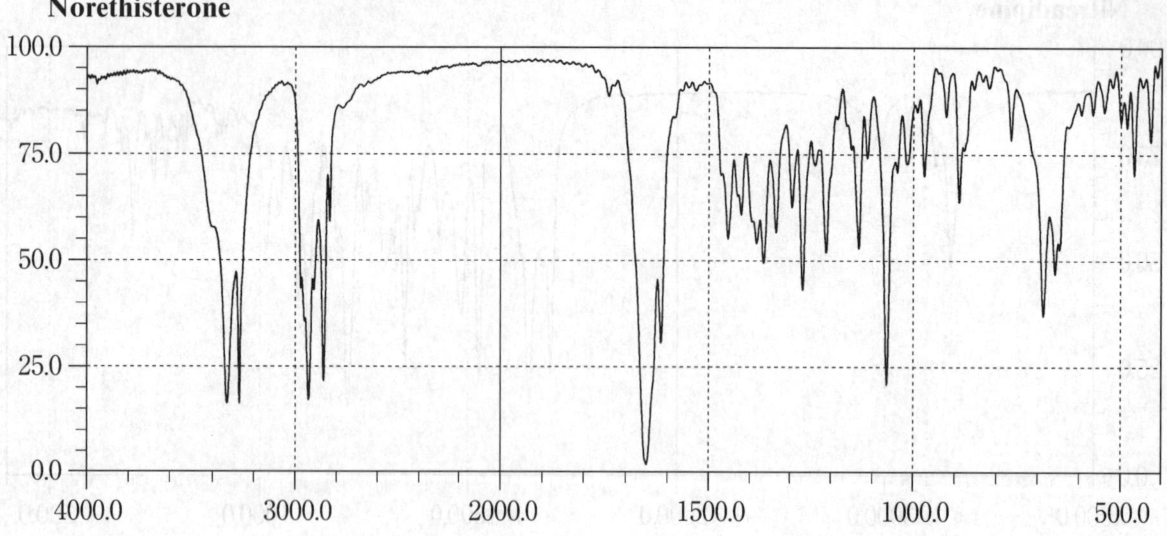

Norfloxacin

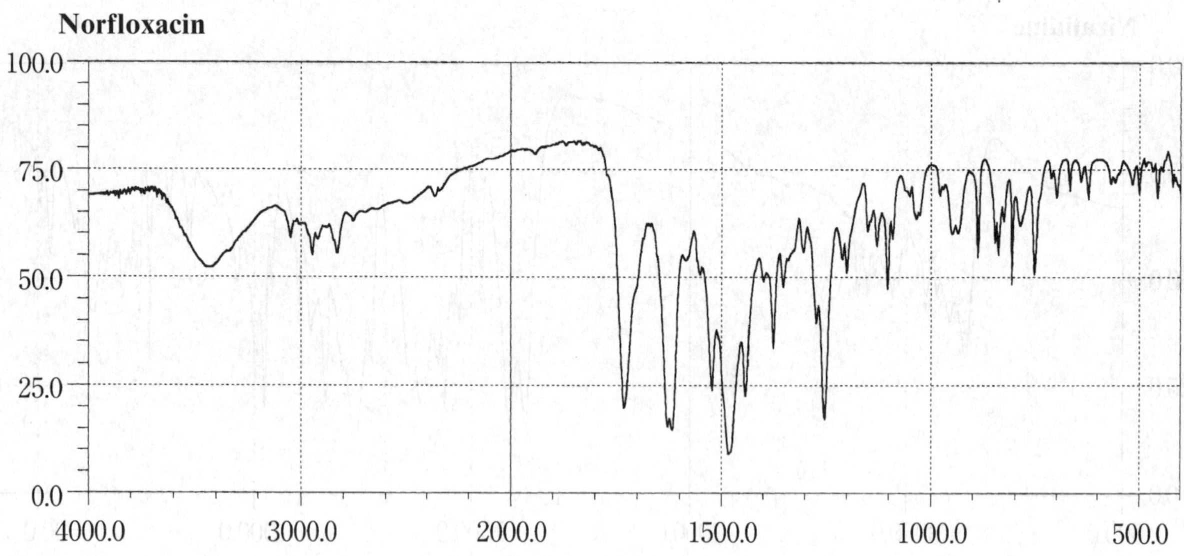

Norgestrel

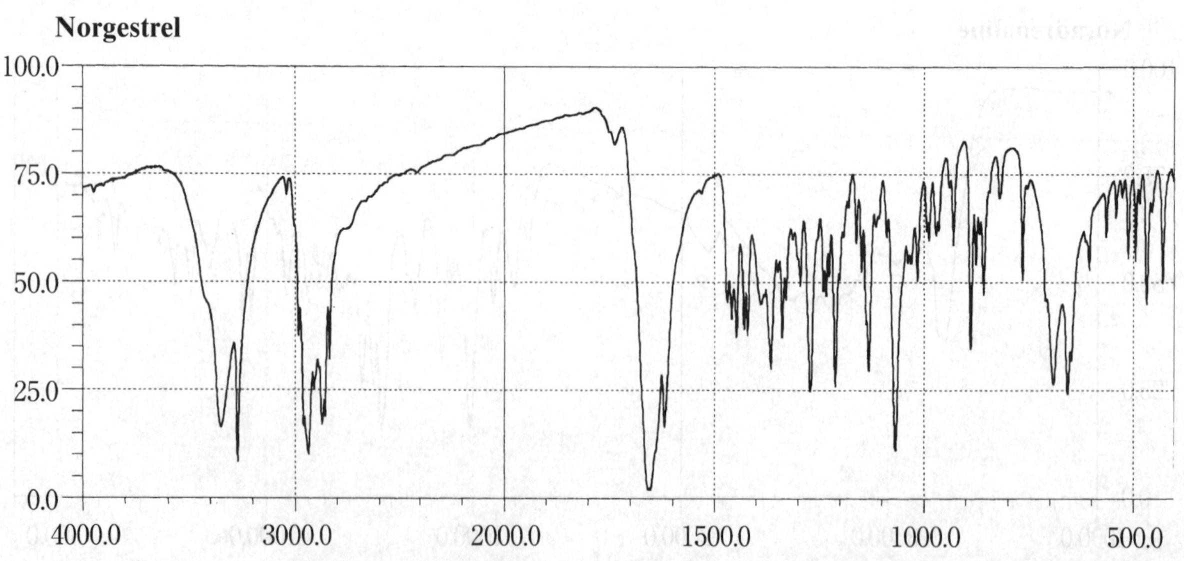

Nortriptyline Hydrochloride

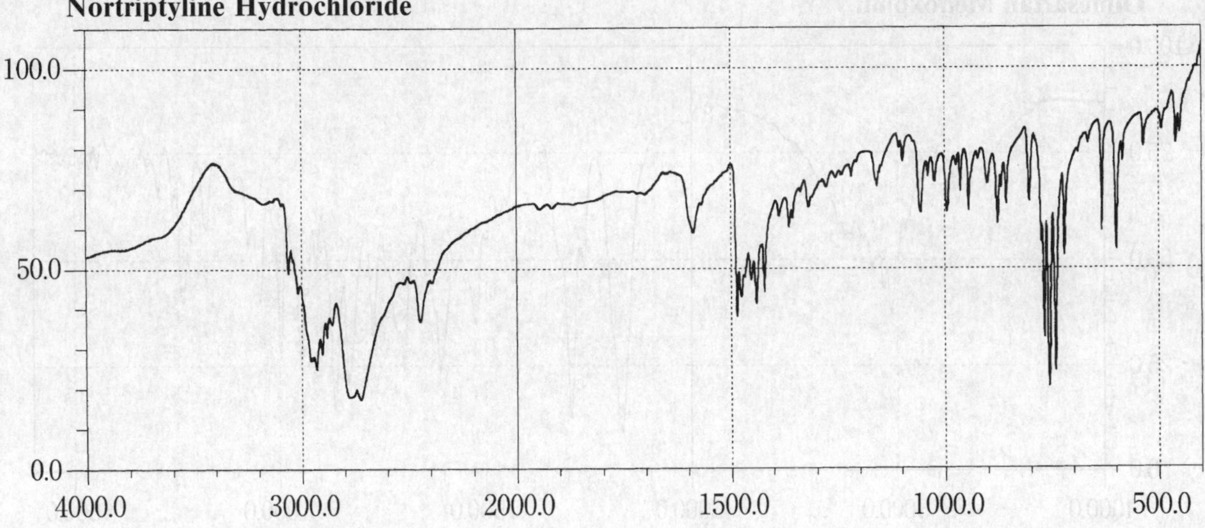

Noscapine

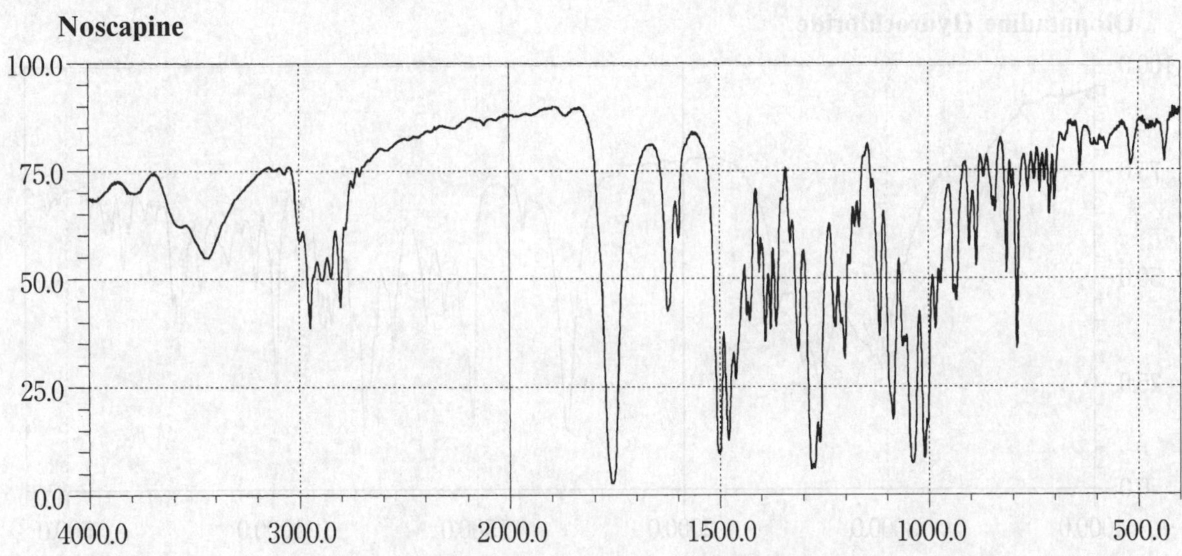

Ofloxacin

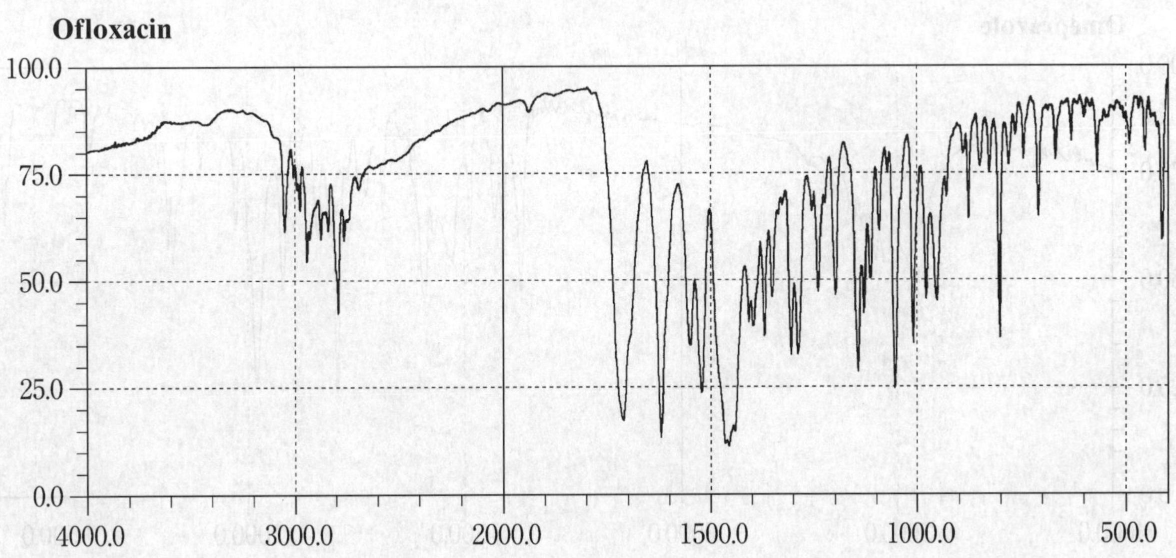

Olmesartan Medoxomil

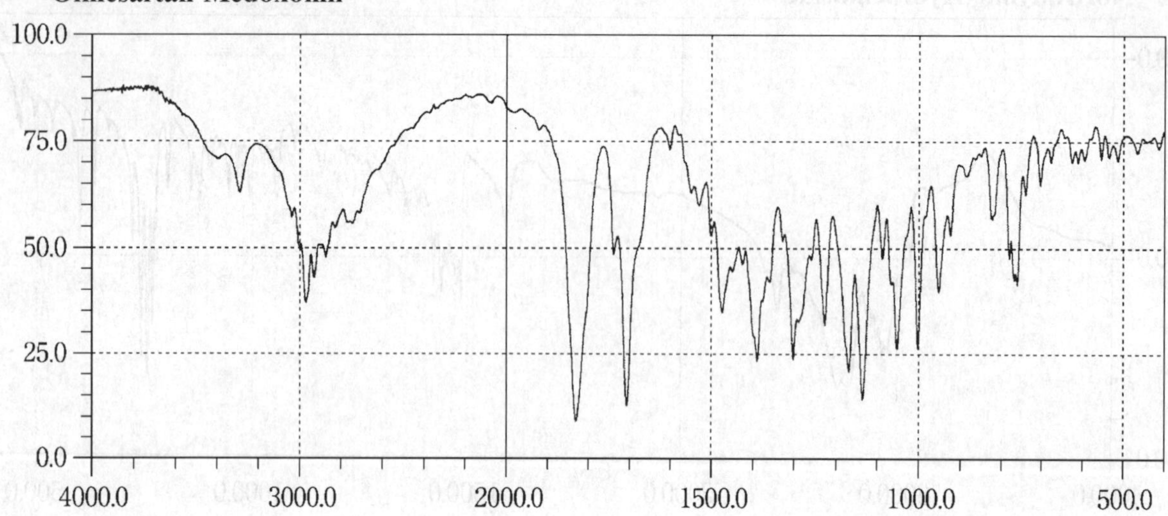

Olopatadine Hydrochloride

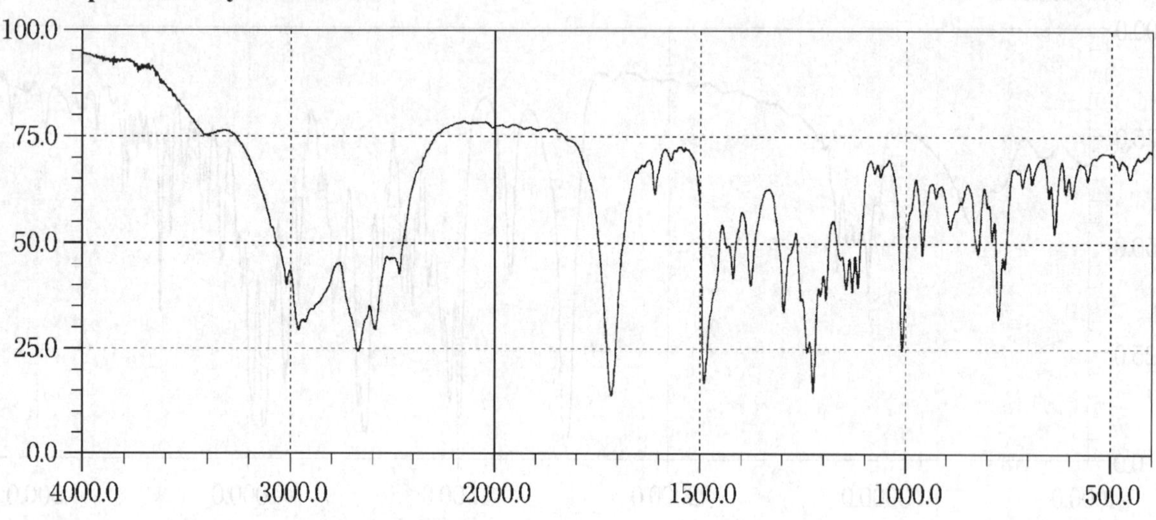

Omeprazole

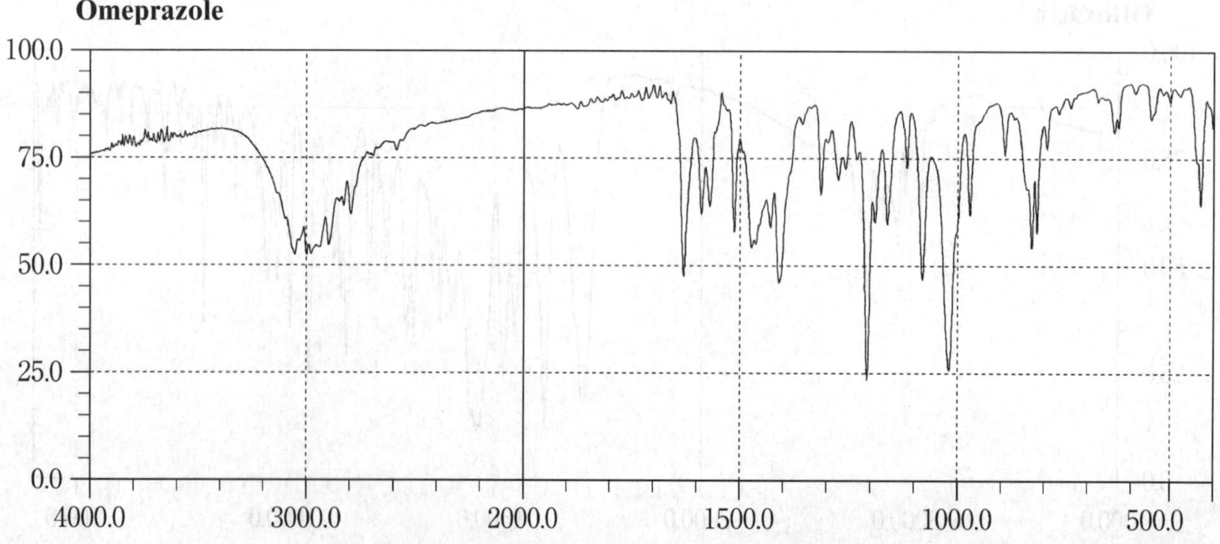

Oxapium Iodide

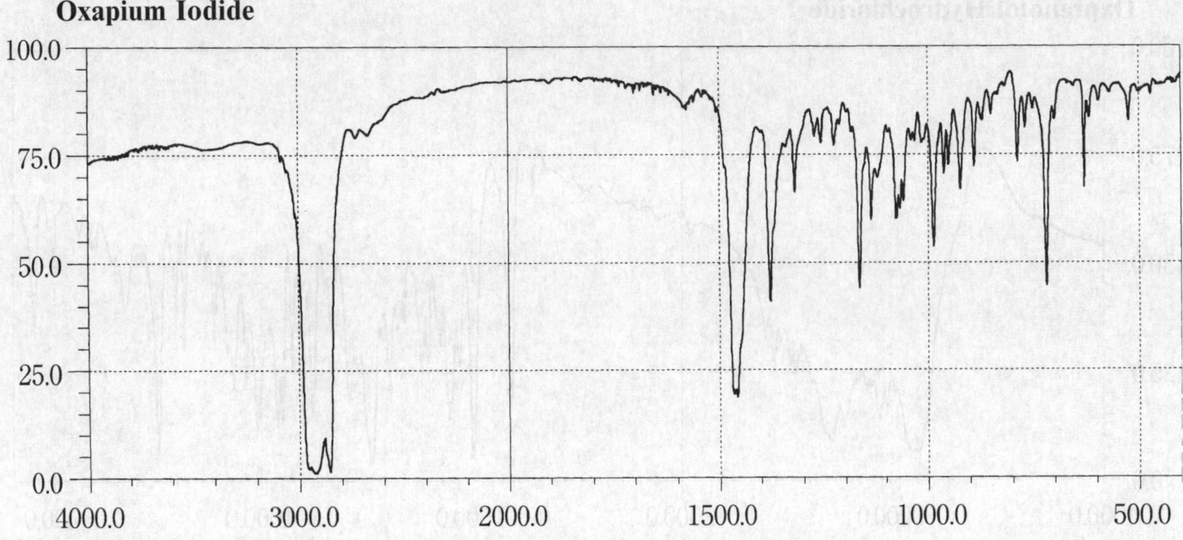

Oxaprozin

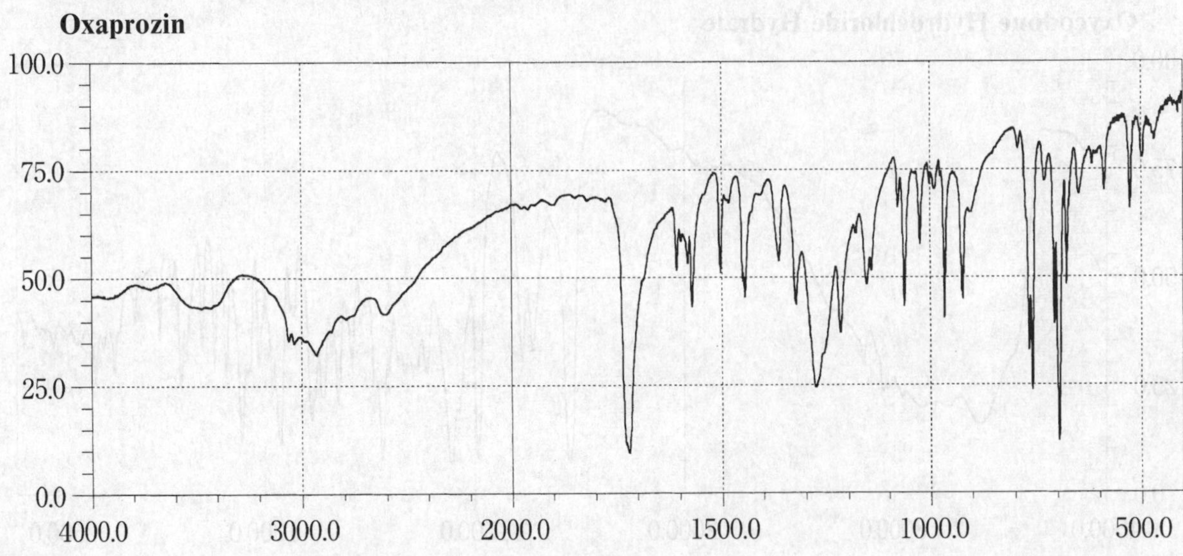

Oxethazaine

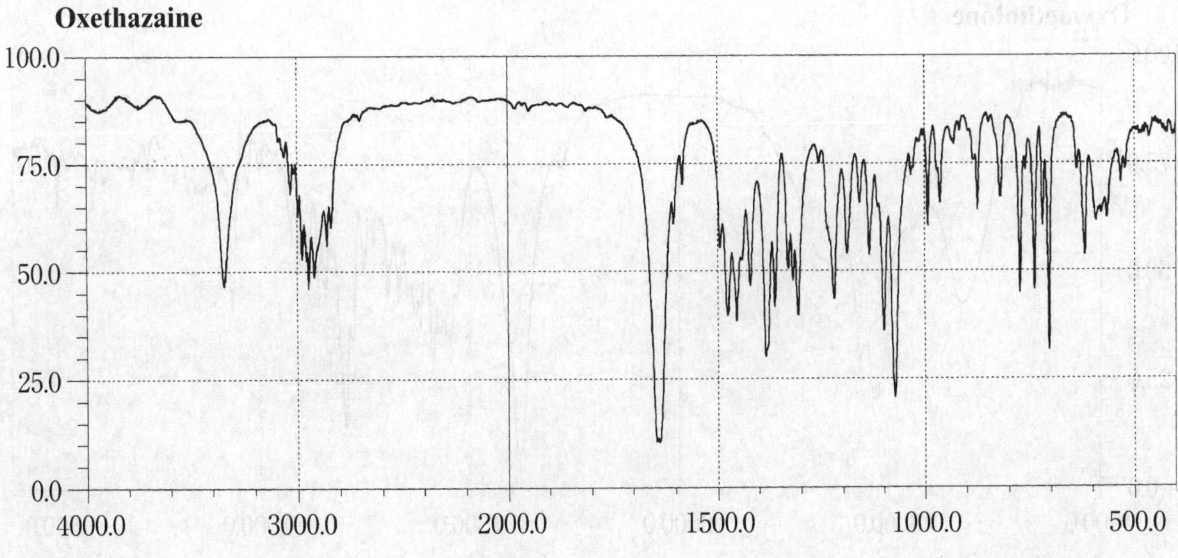

Oxprenolol Hydrochloride

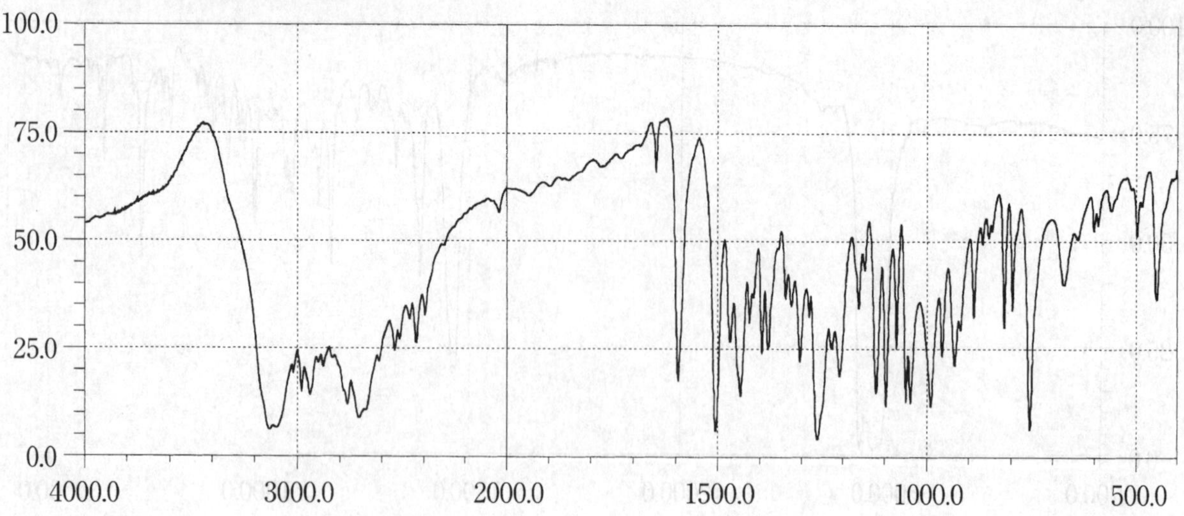

Oxycodone Hydrochloride Hydrate

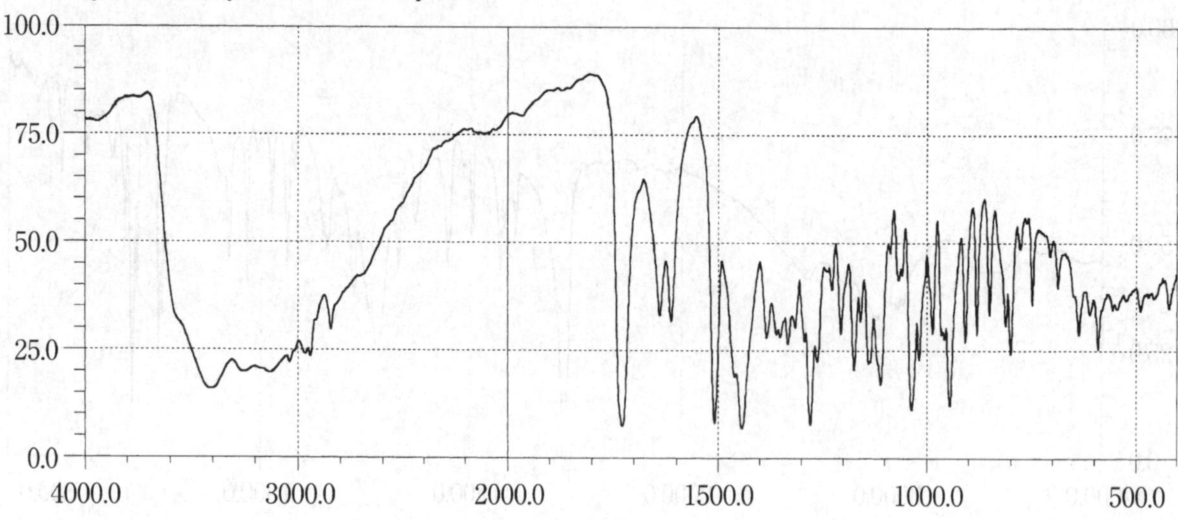

Oxymetholone

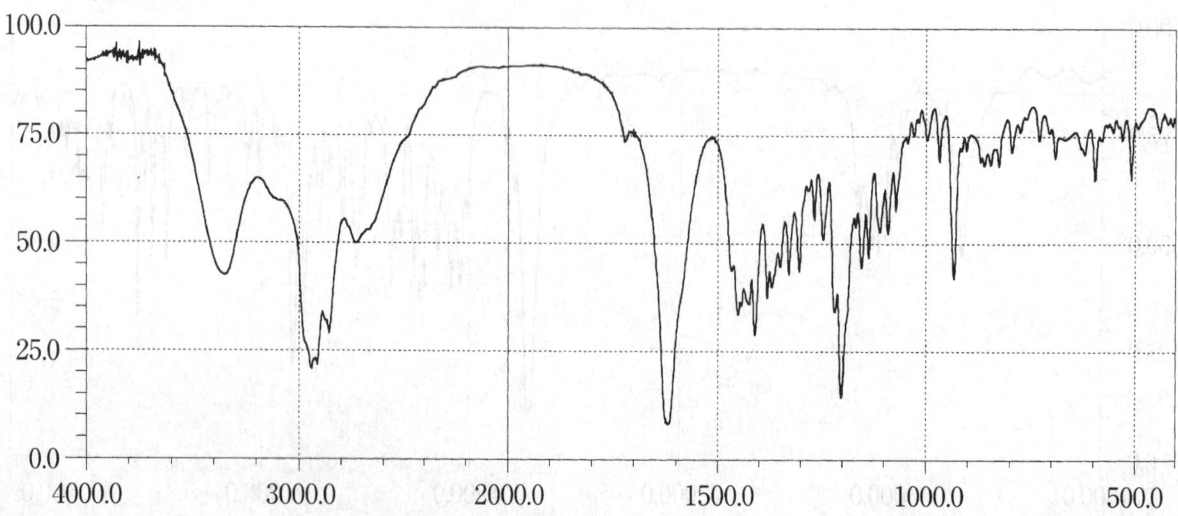

Oxytetracycline Hydrochloride

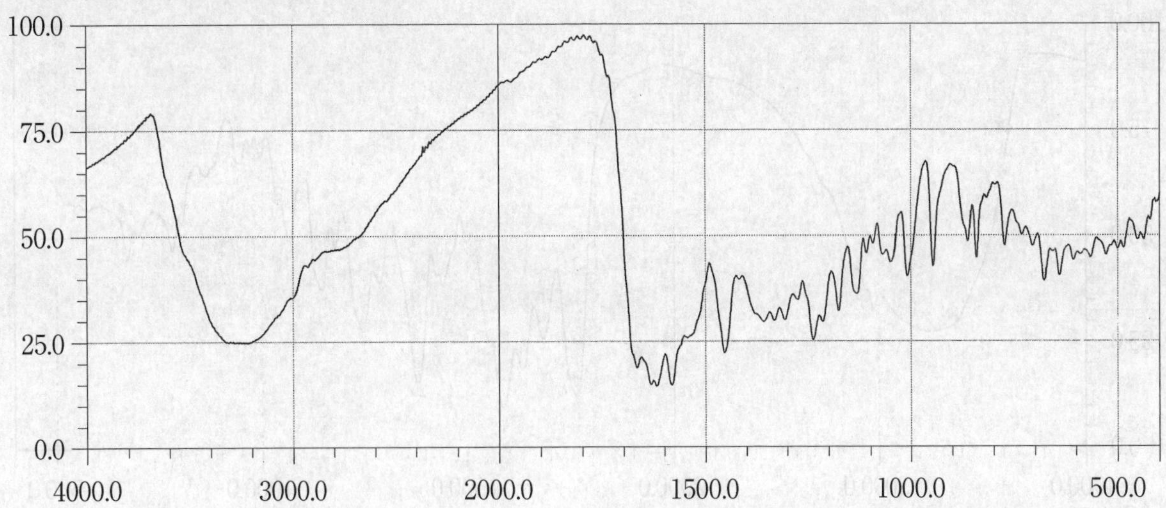

Ozagrel Sodium

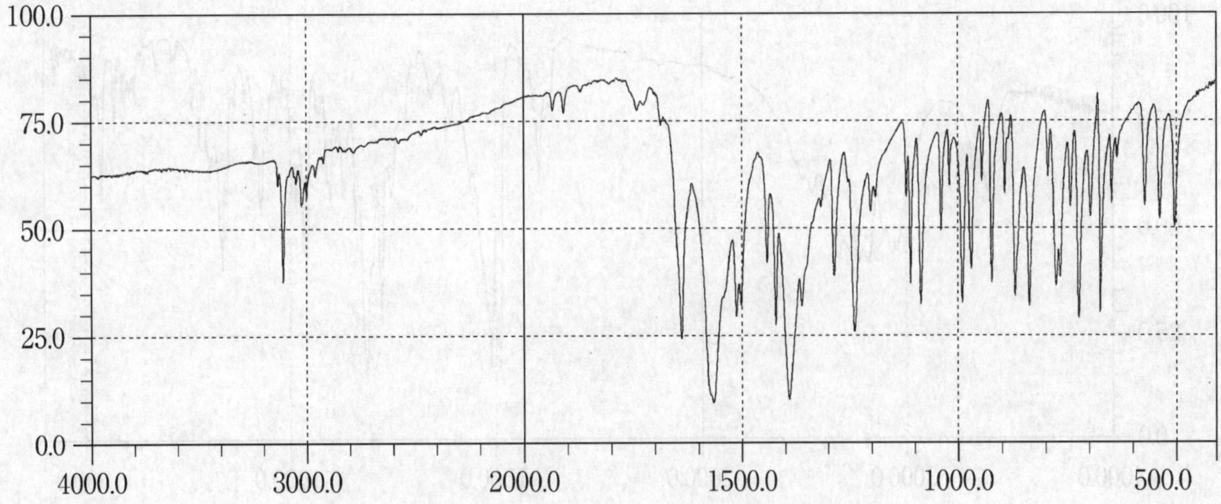

Pancuronium Bromide

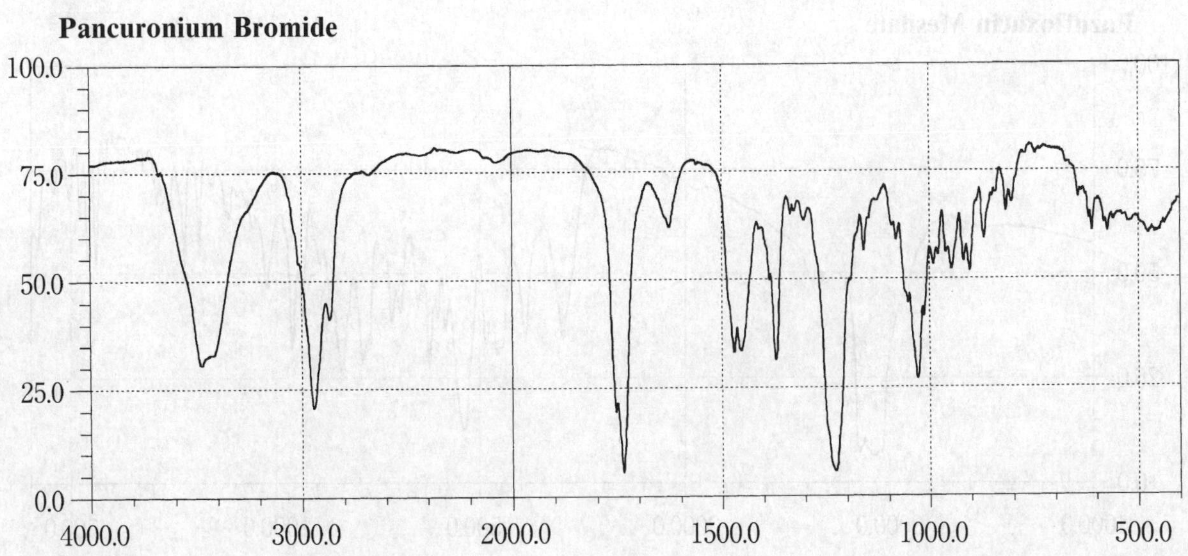

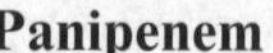

Panipenem

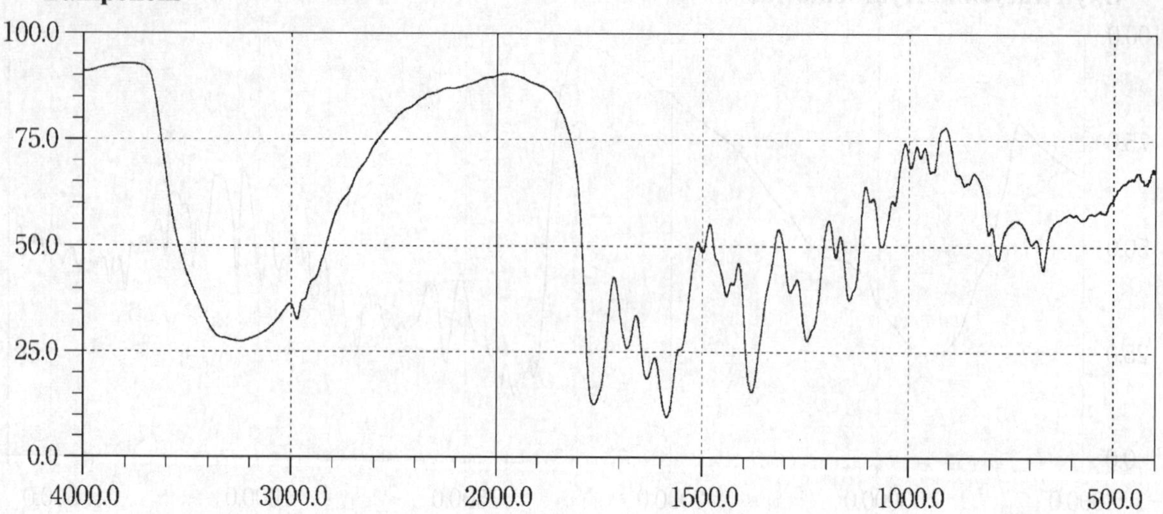

Paroxetine Hydrochloride Hydrate

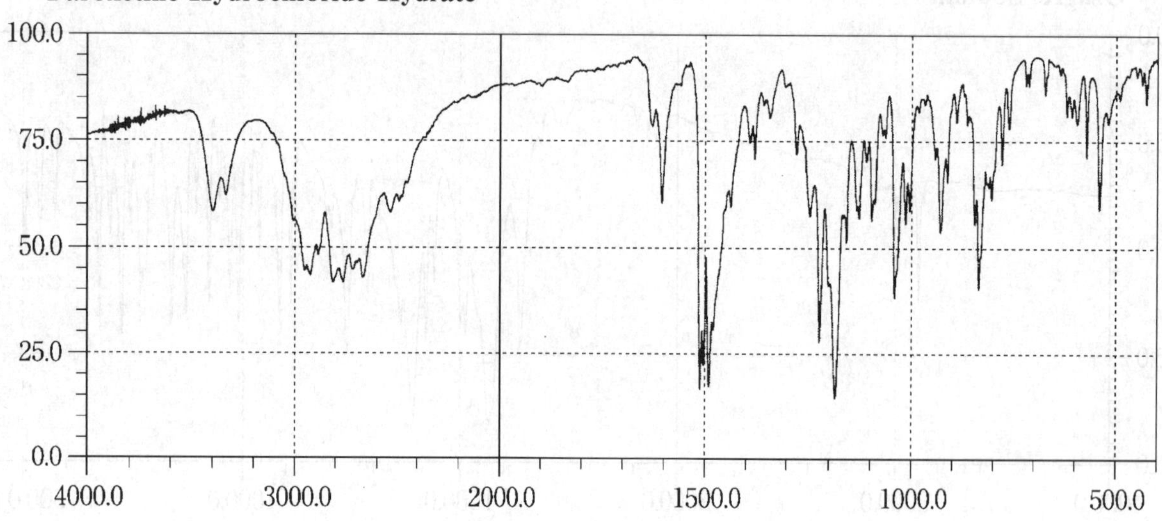

Pazufloxacin Mesilate

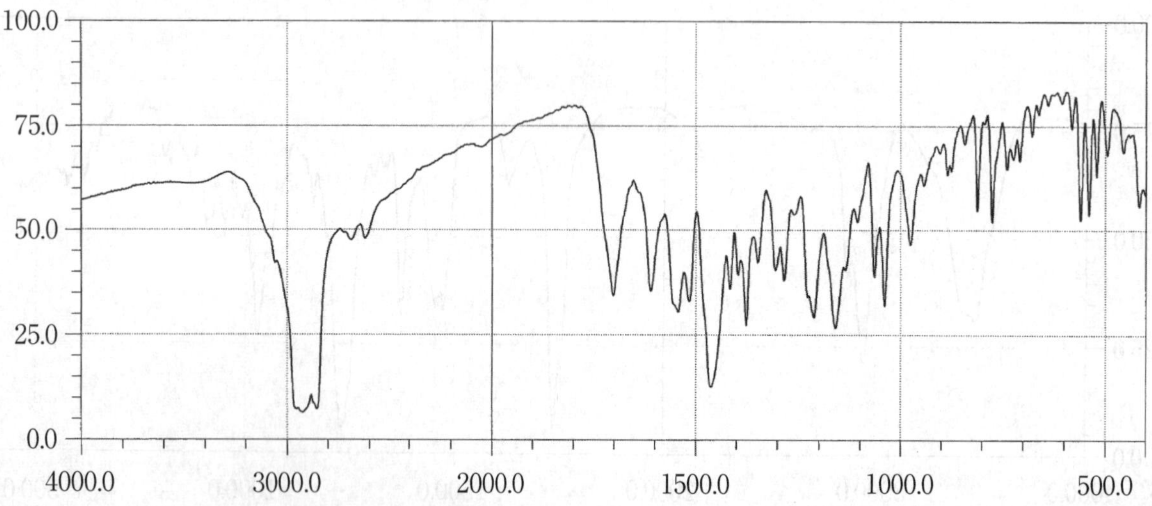

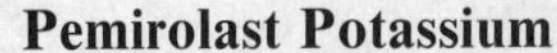

Pemirolast Potassium

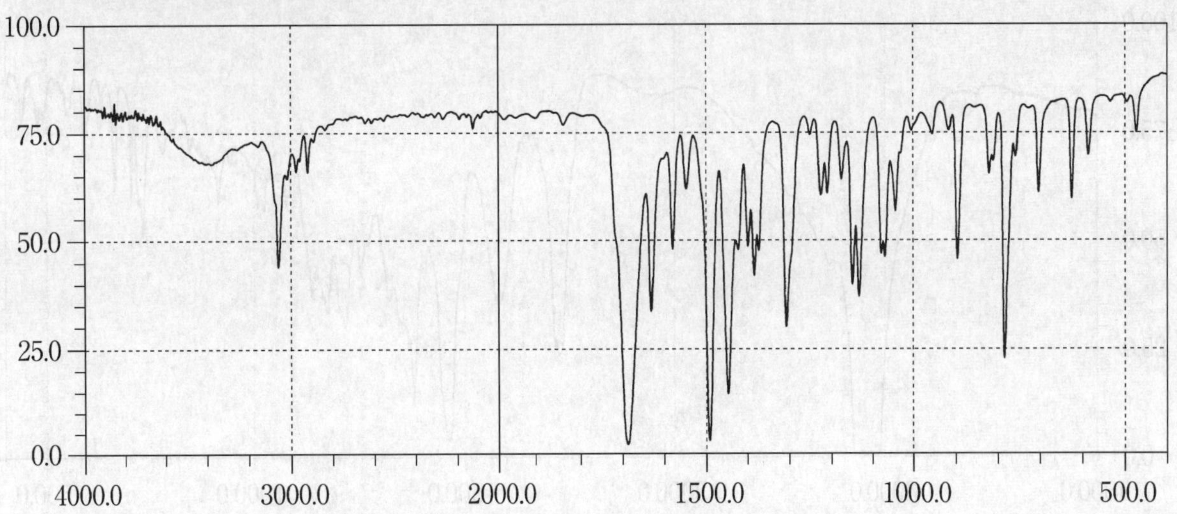

Penbutolol Sulfate

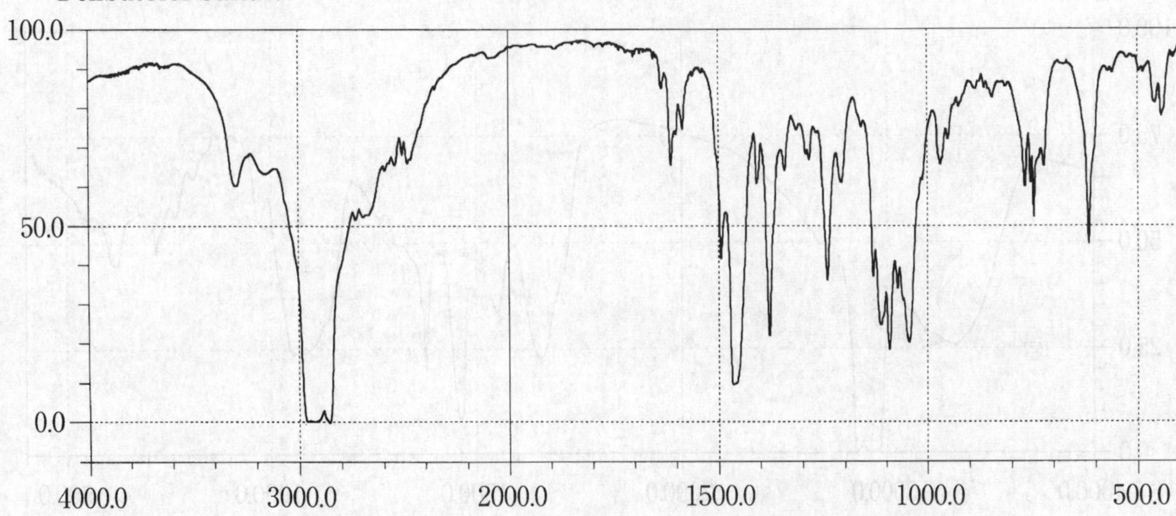

Pentobarbital Calcium

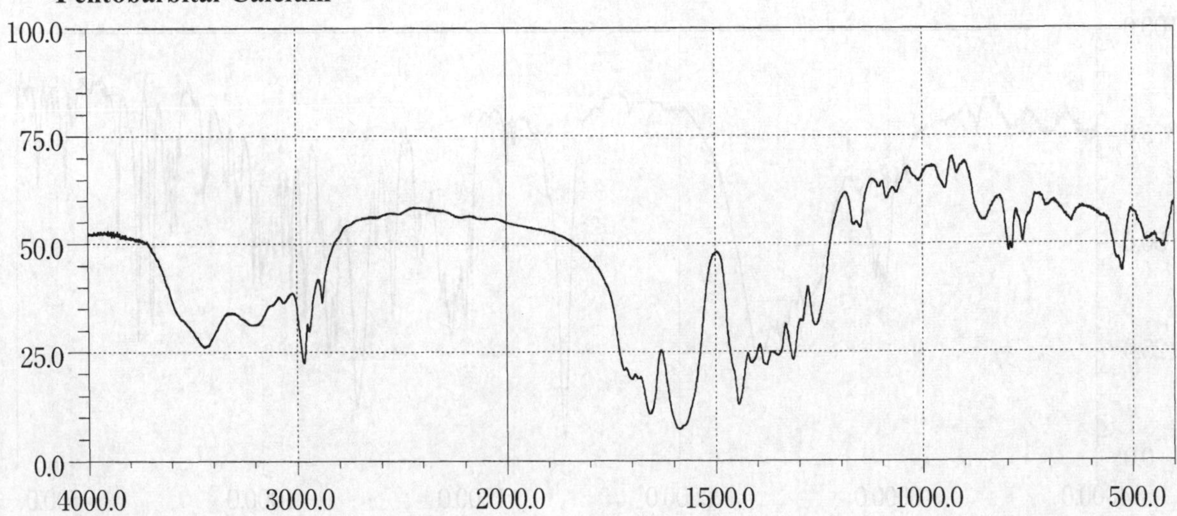

The JP Drugs are to be tested according to the provisions given in the pertinent monographs, General Notices, General Rules for Crude Drugs, General Rules for Preparations, and General Tests for their conformity to the Japanese Pharmacopoeia. (See the General Notices 5.)

Pentoxyverine Citrate

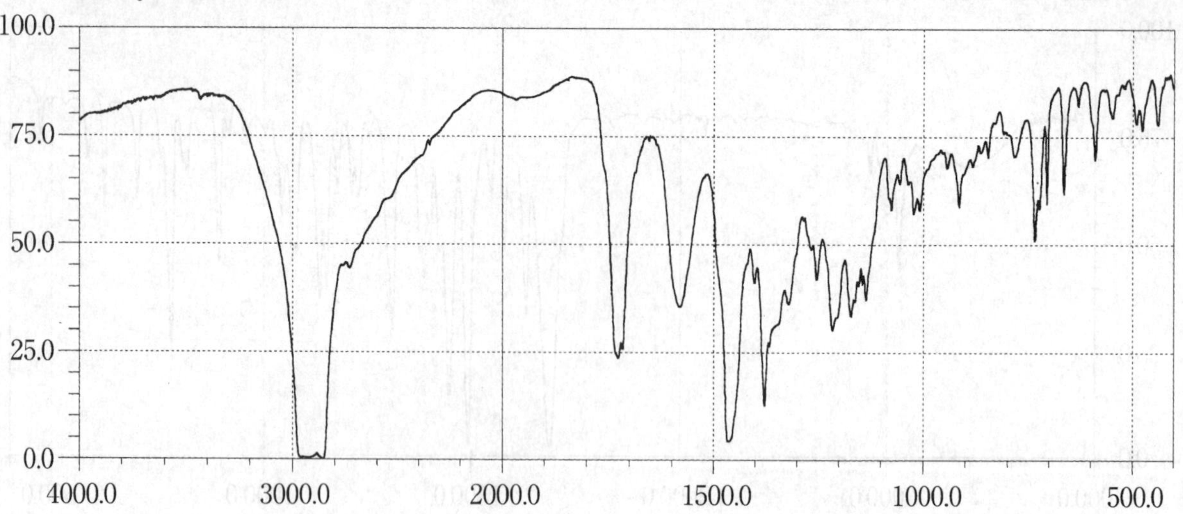

Peplomycin Sulfate

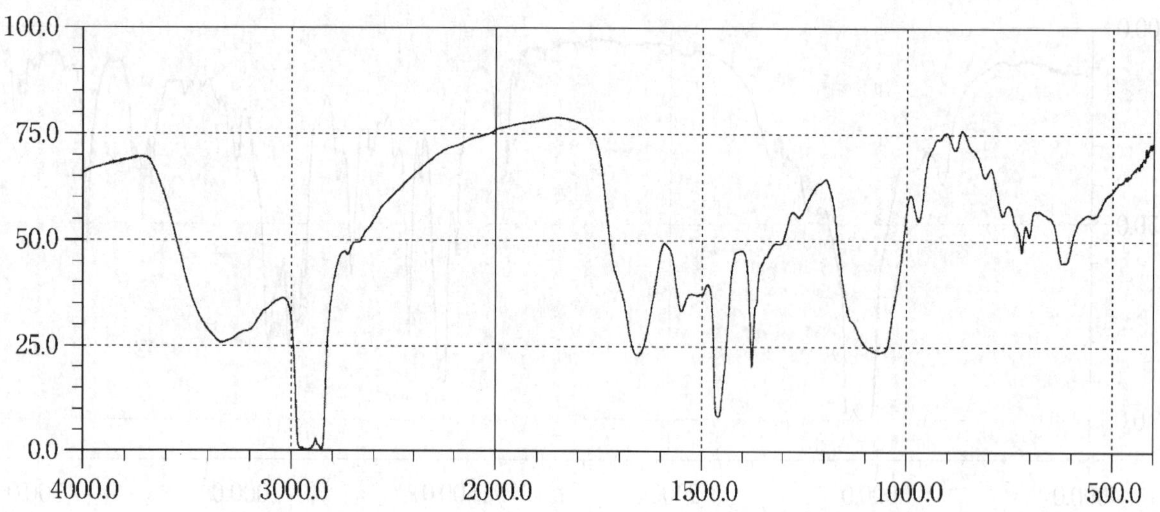

Pethidine Hydrochloride

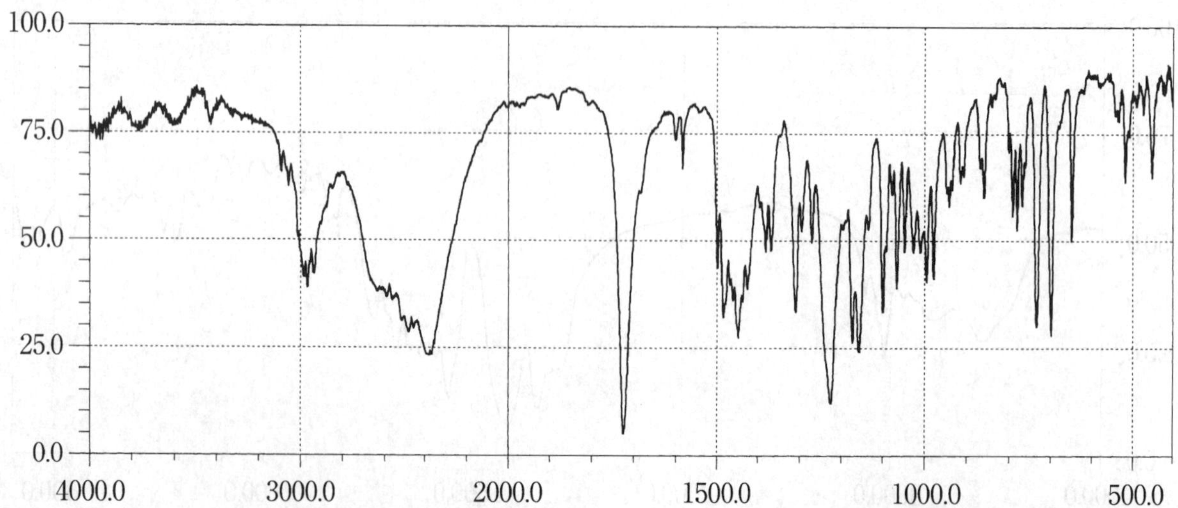

The JP Drugs are to be tested according to the provisions given in the pertinent monographs, General Notices, General Rules for Crude Drugs, General Rules for Preparations, and General Tests for their conformity to the Japanese Pharmacopoeia. (See the General Notices 5.)

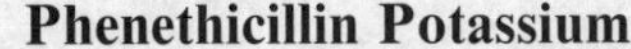

Phenethicillin Potassium

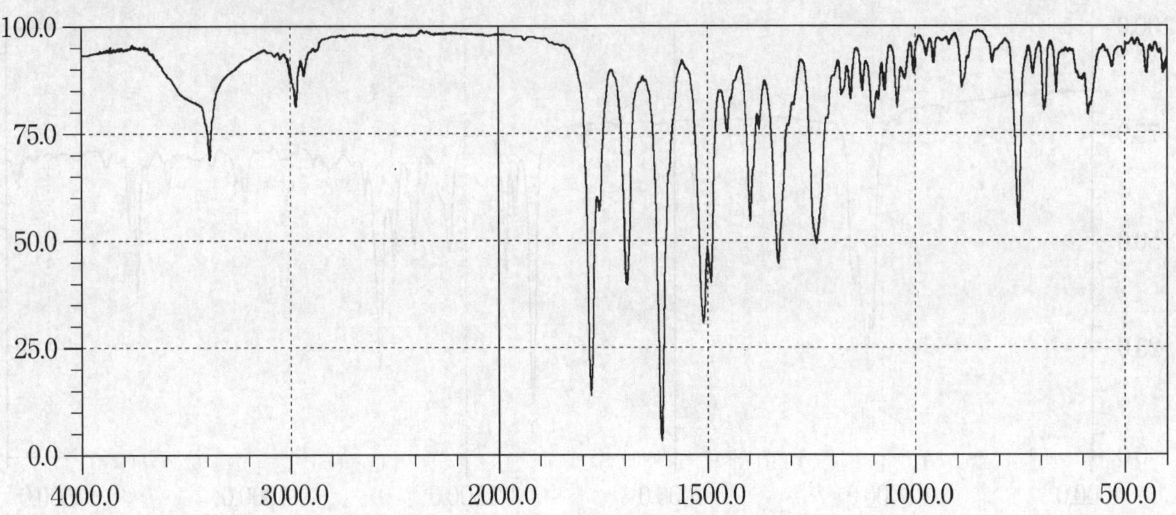

Phenobarbital

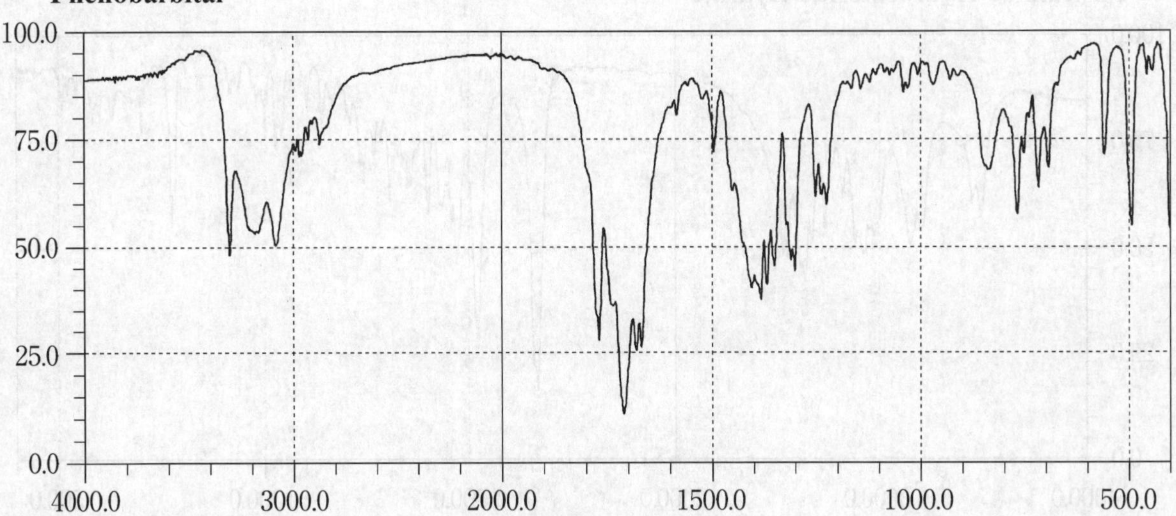

L-Phenylalanine

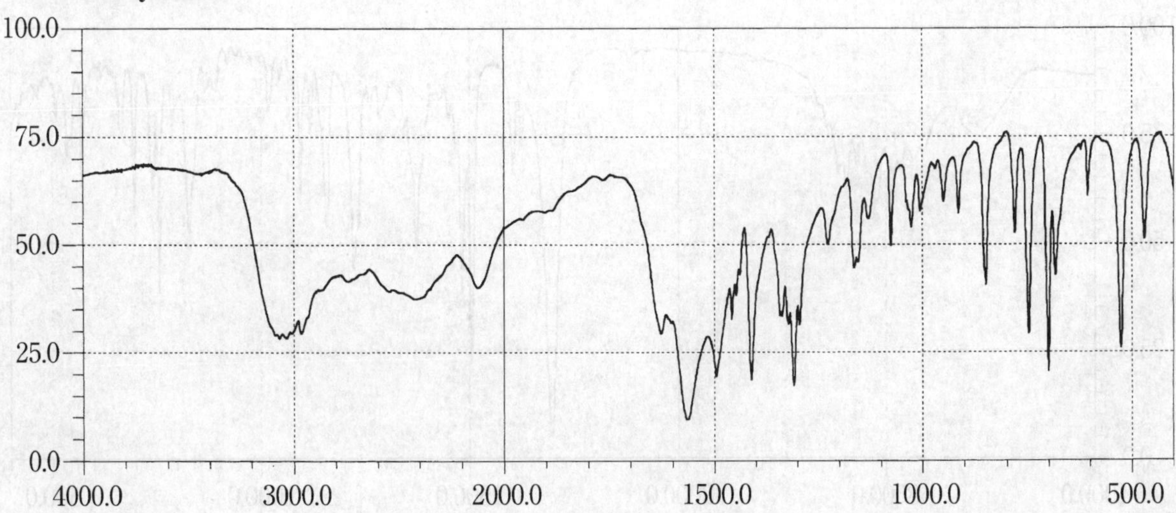

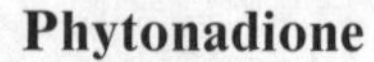

Phytonadione

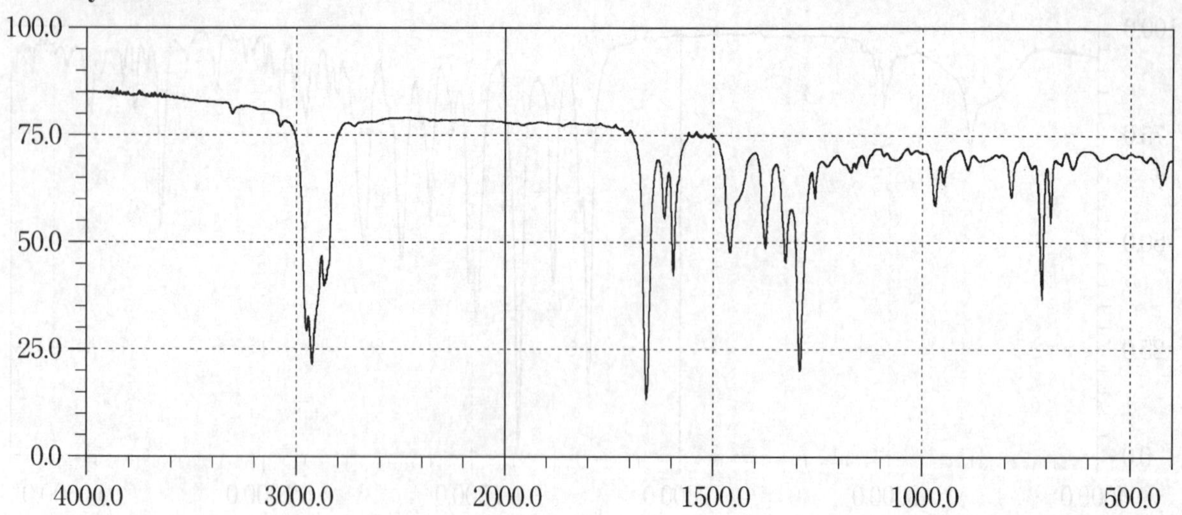

Pilsicainide Hydrochloride Hydrate

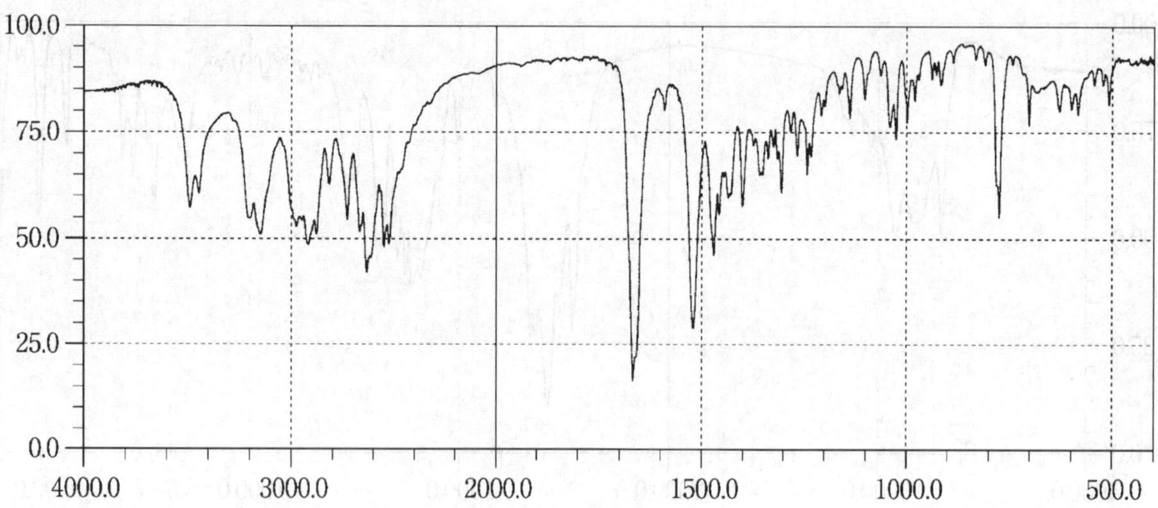

Pimozide

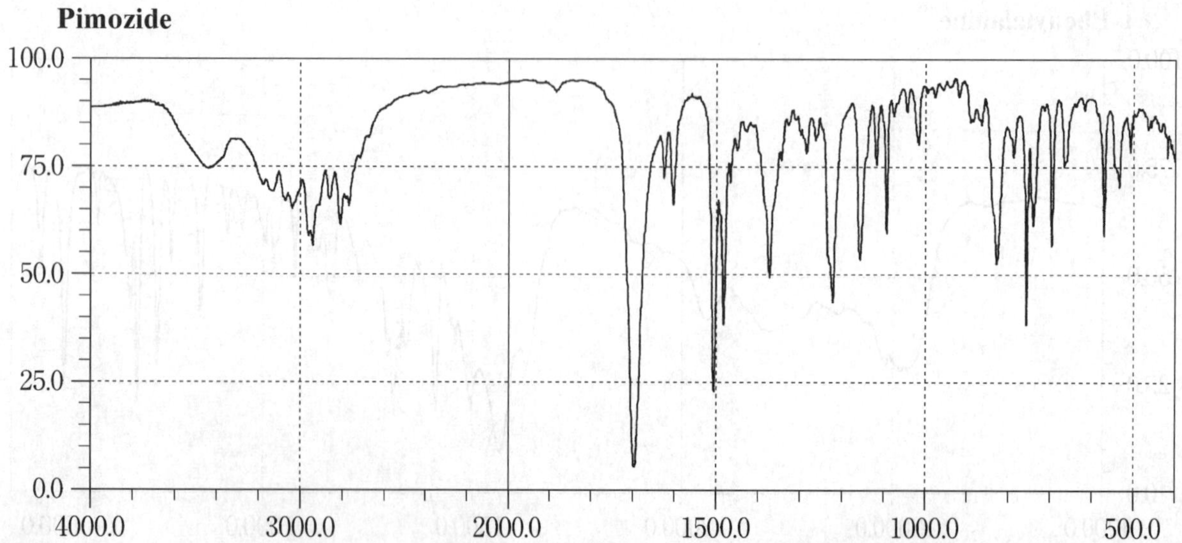

Pindolol

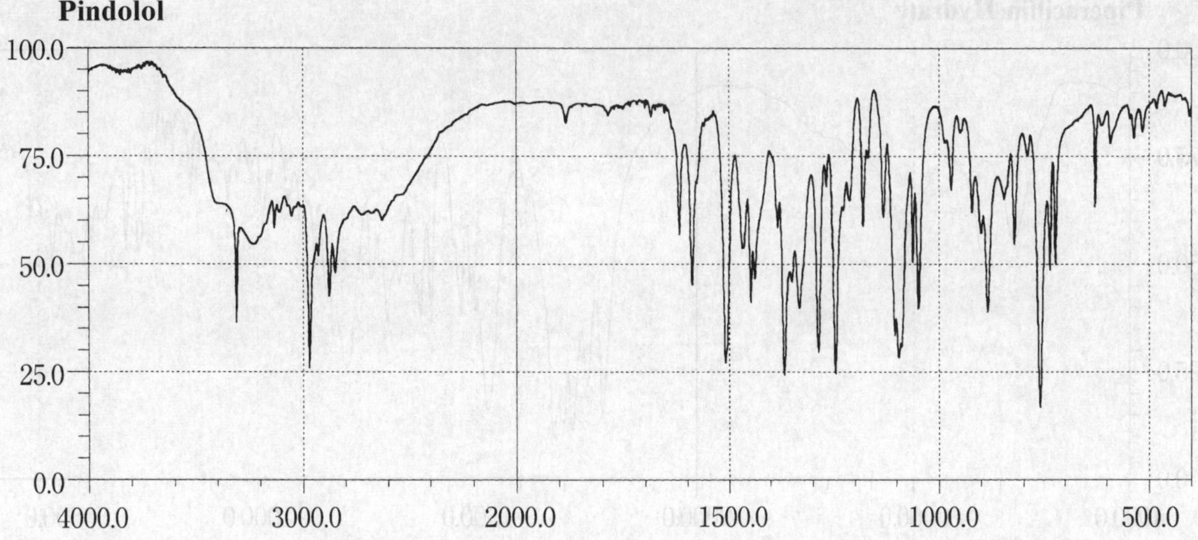

Pioglitazone Hydrochloride

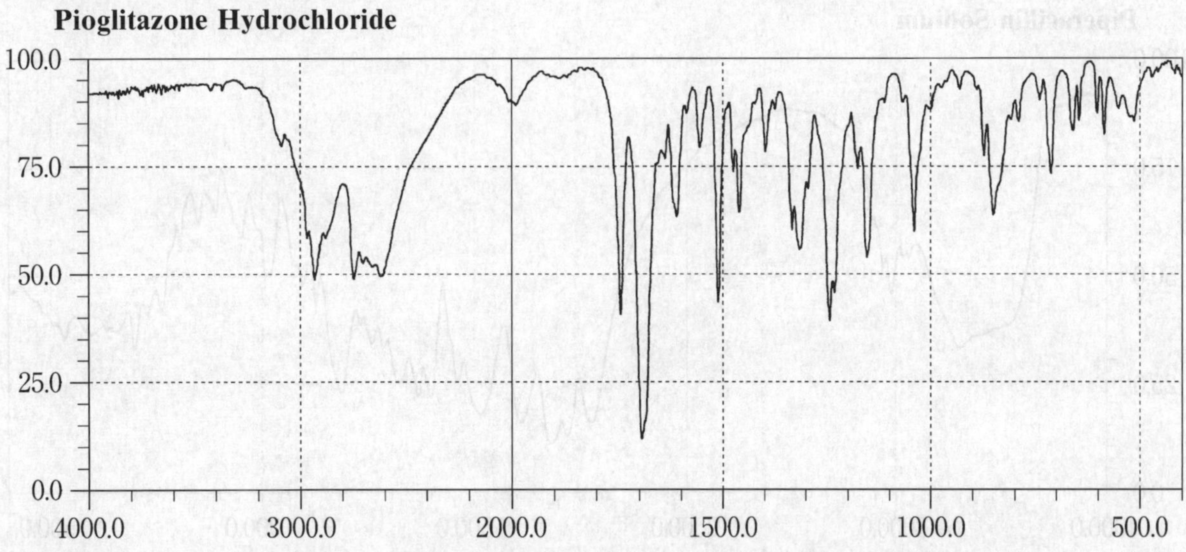

Pipemidic Acid Hydrate

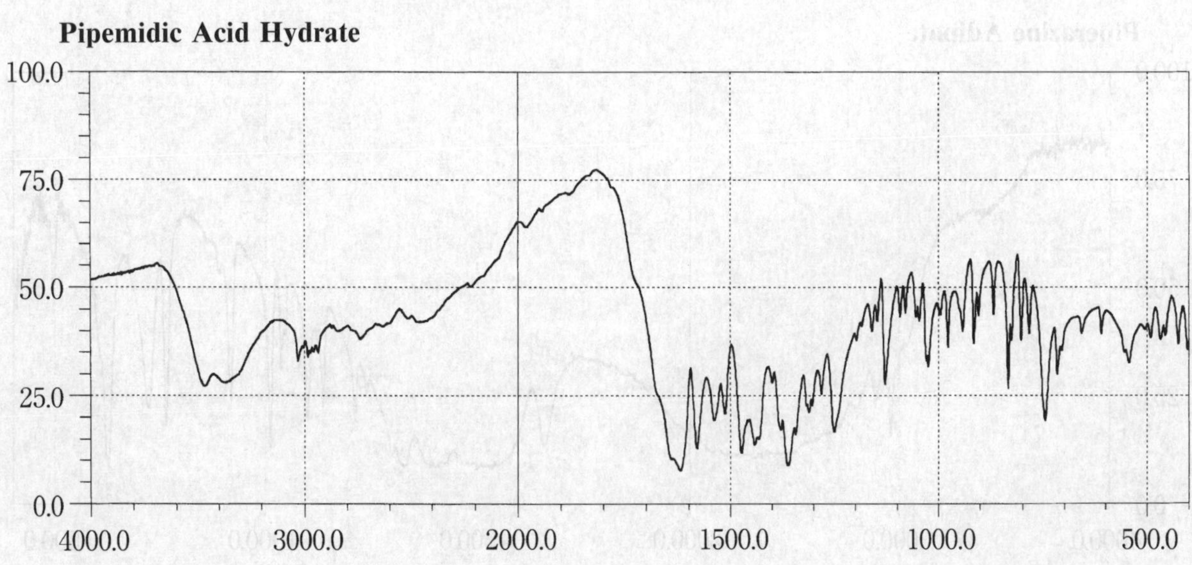

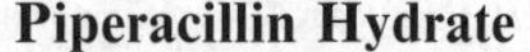

Piperacillin Hydrate

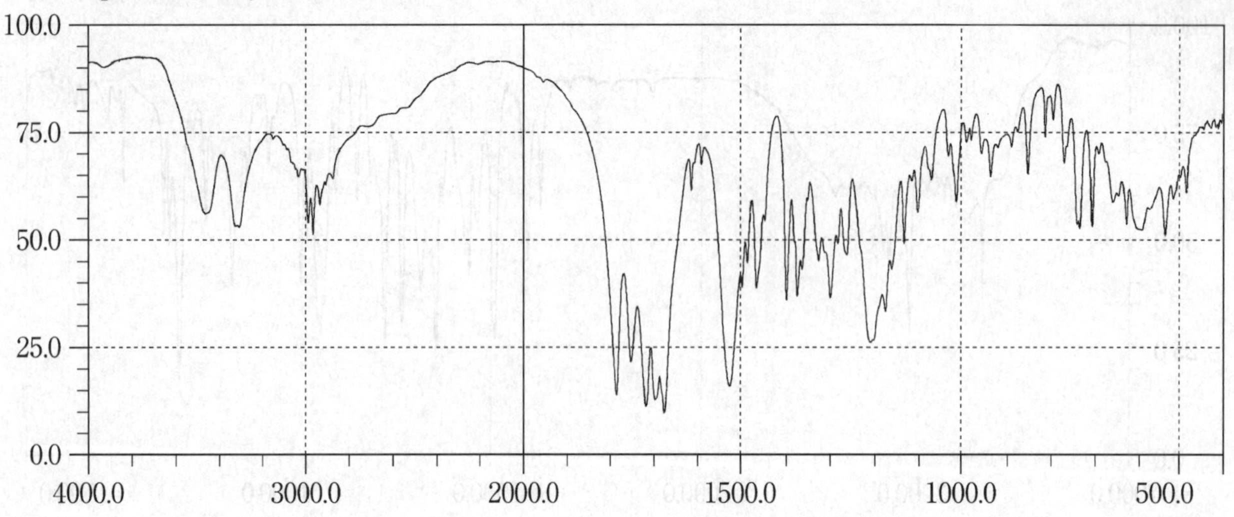

Piperacillin Sodium

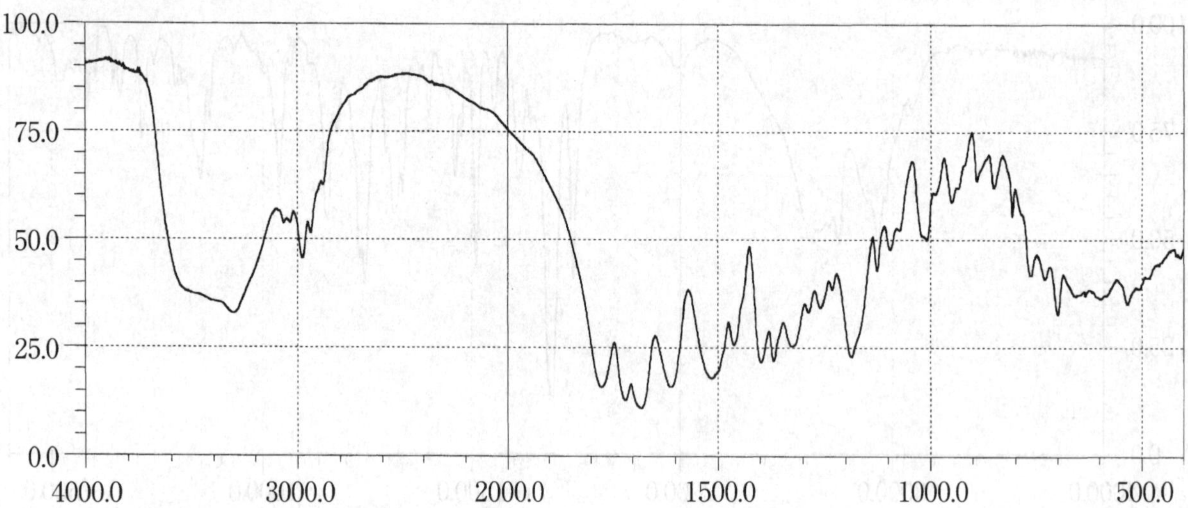

Piperazine Adipate

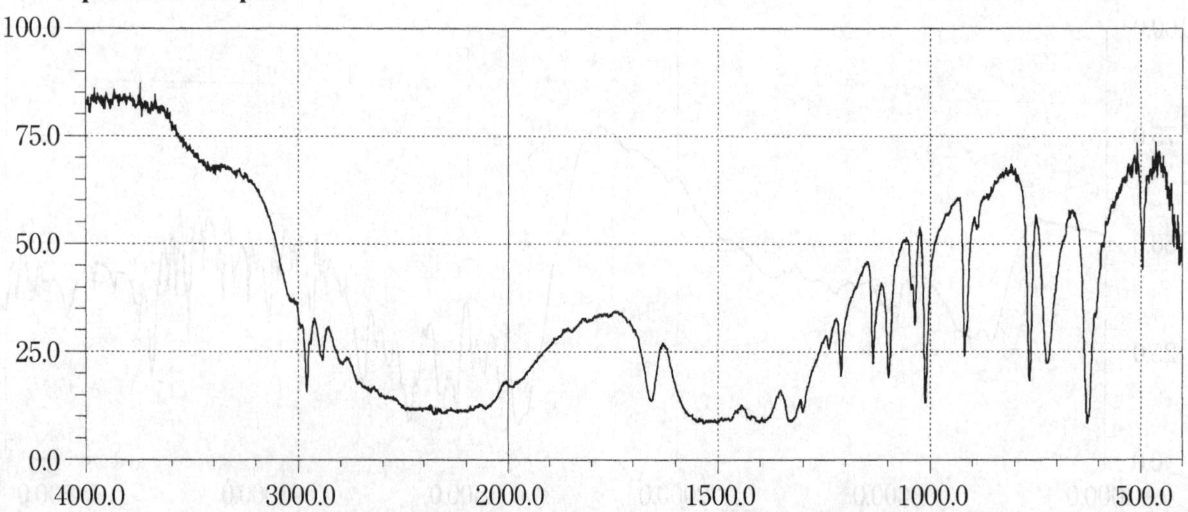

Piperazine Phosphate Hydrate

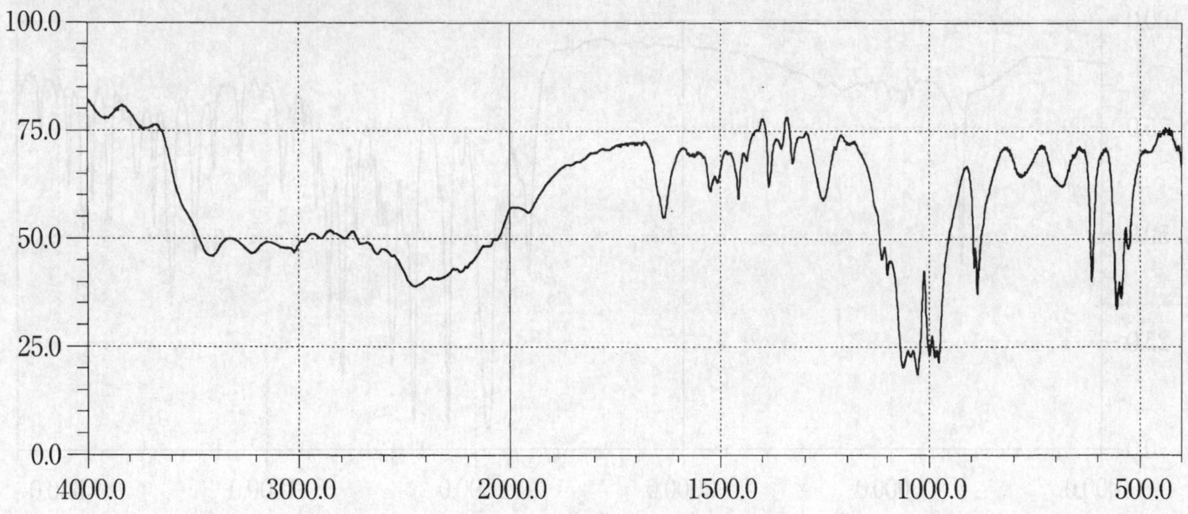

Pirenoxine

Pirenzepine Hydrochloride Hydrate

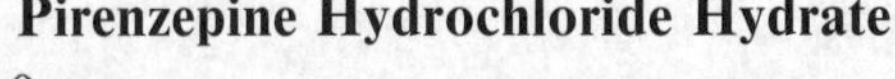

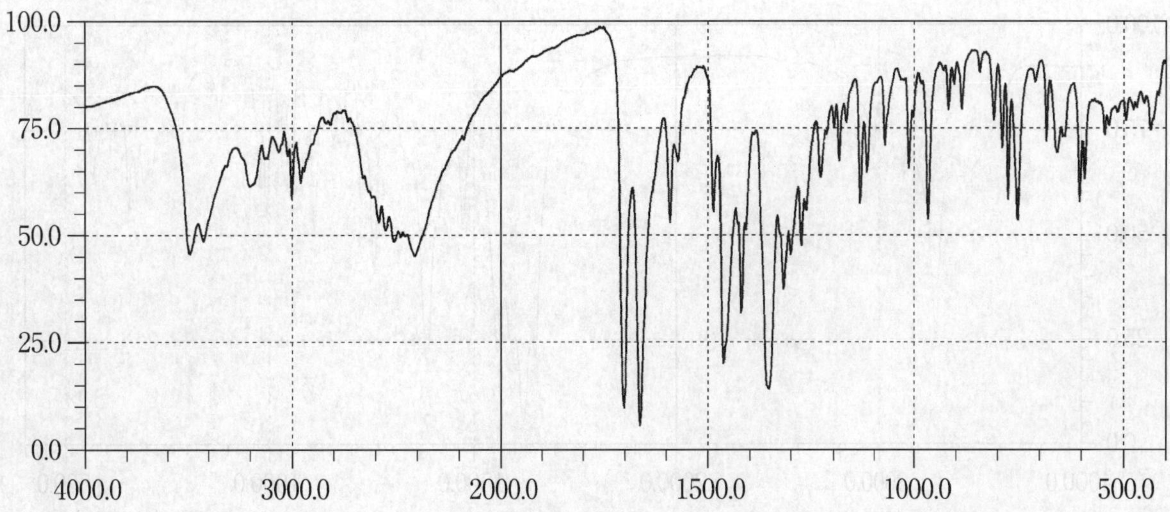

Piroxicam

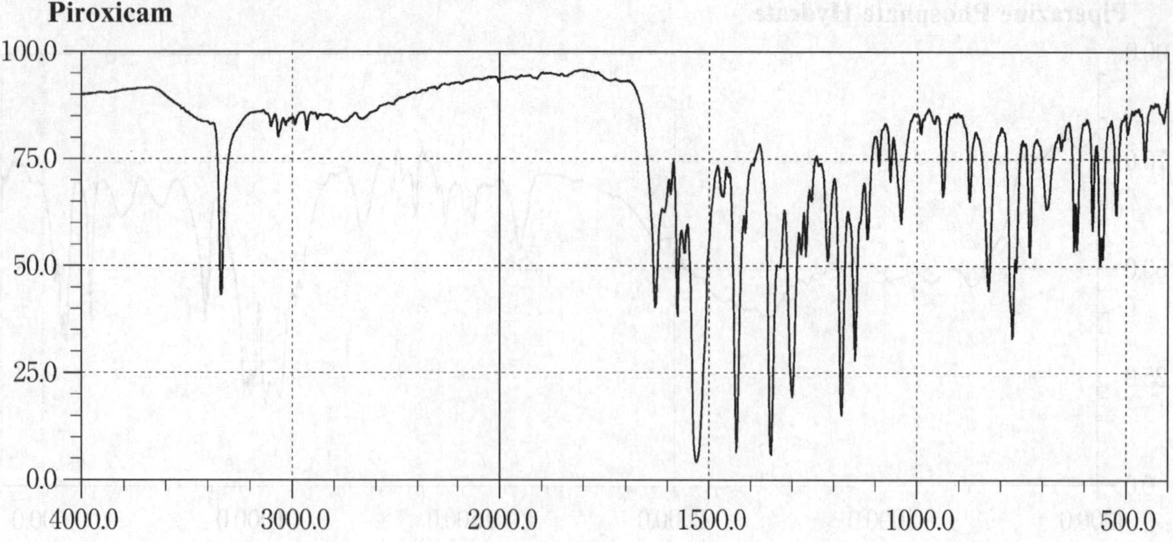

Pivmecillinam Hydrochloride

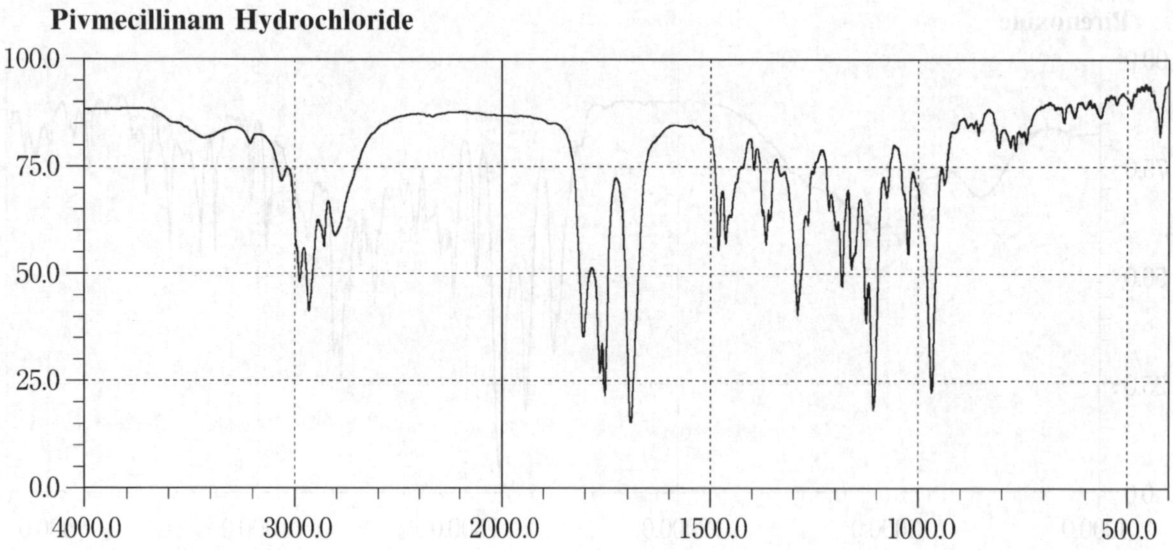

Polaprezinc

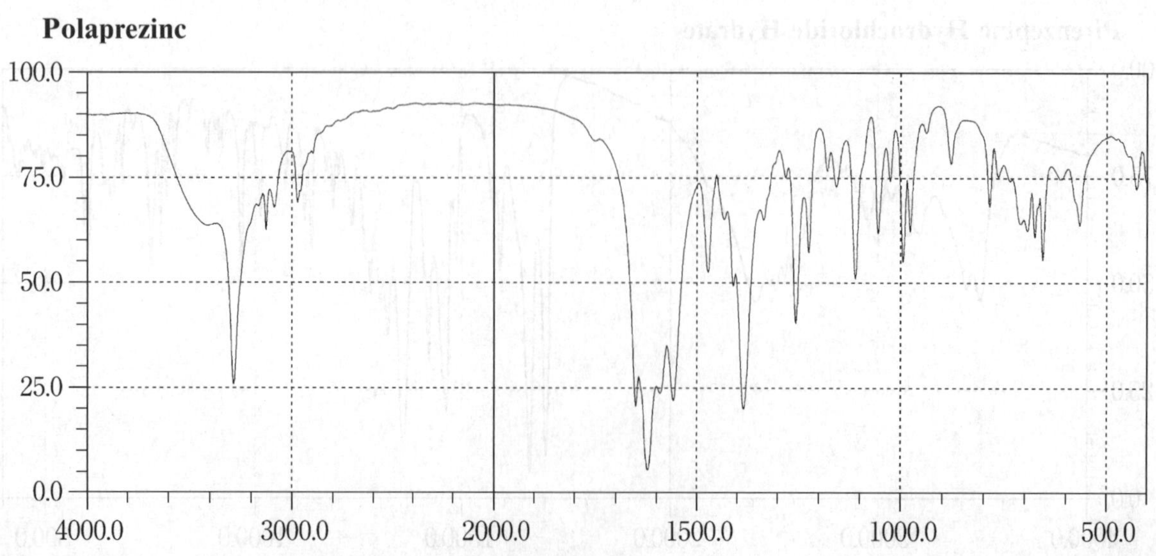

Potassium Canrenoate

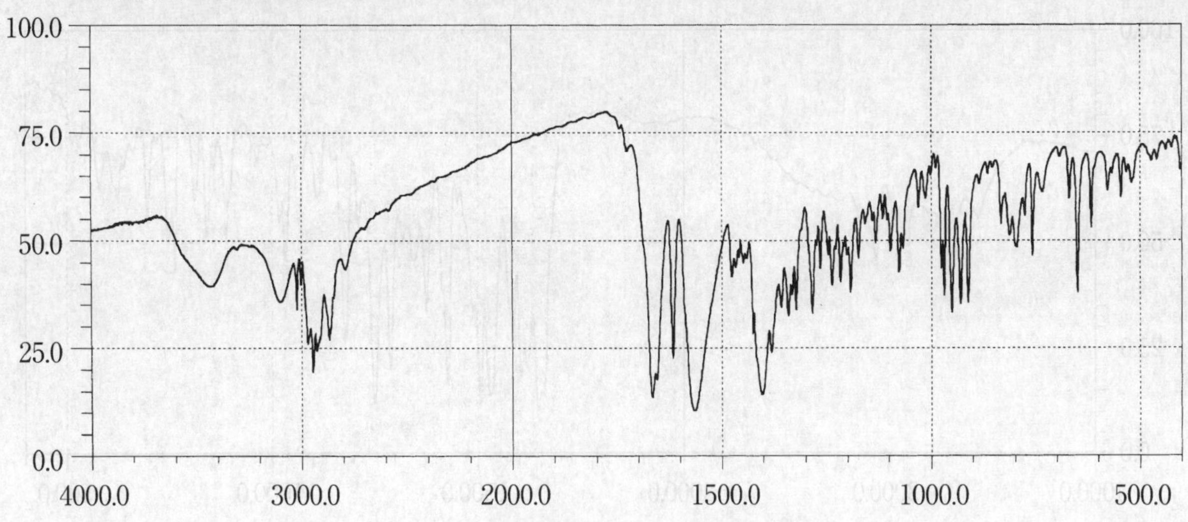

Potassium Clavulanate

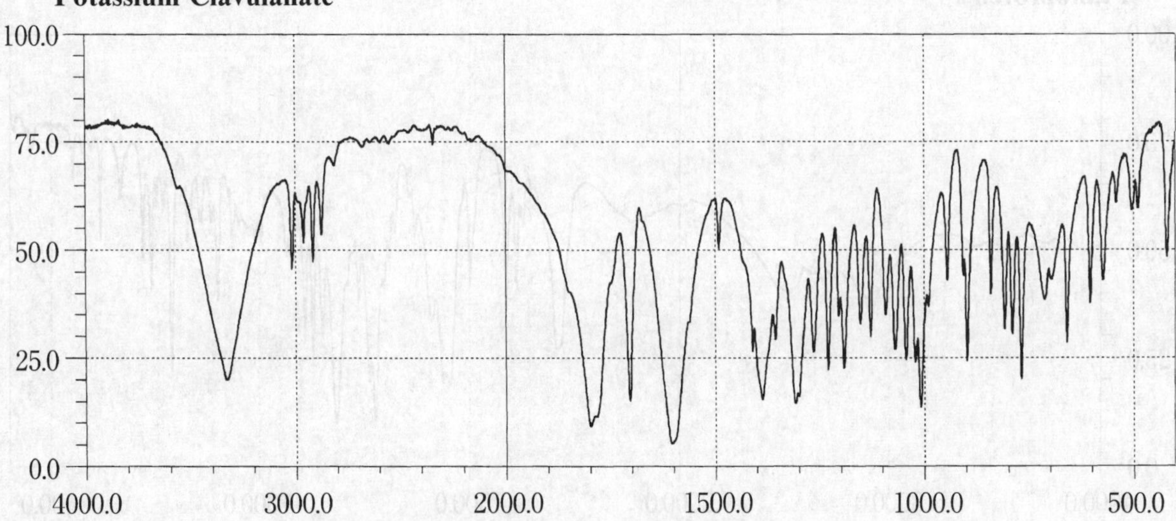

Povidone

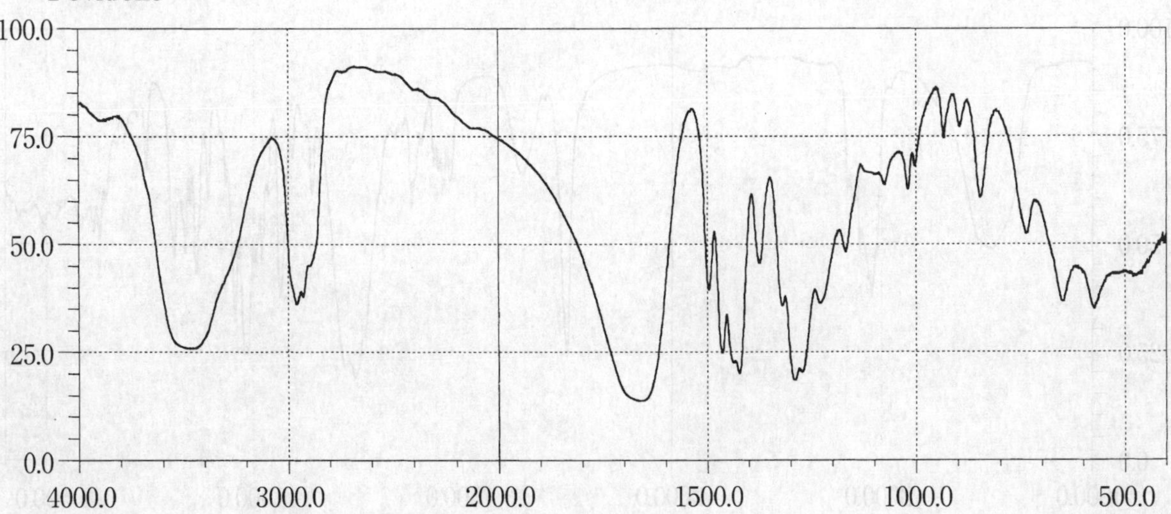

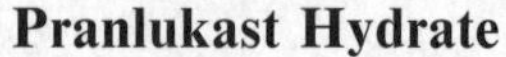

Pranlukast Hydrate

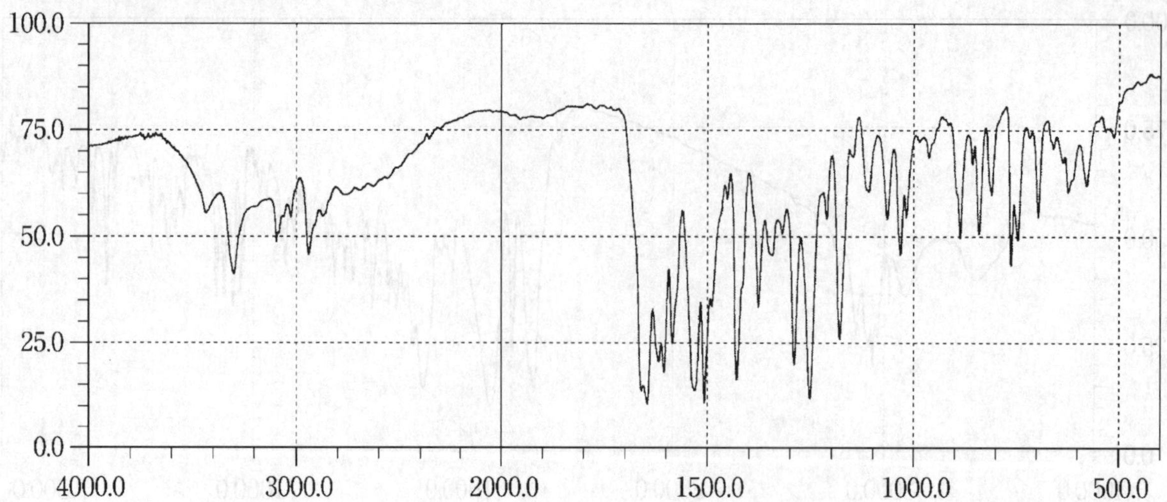

Pranoprofen

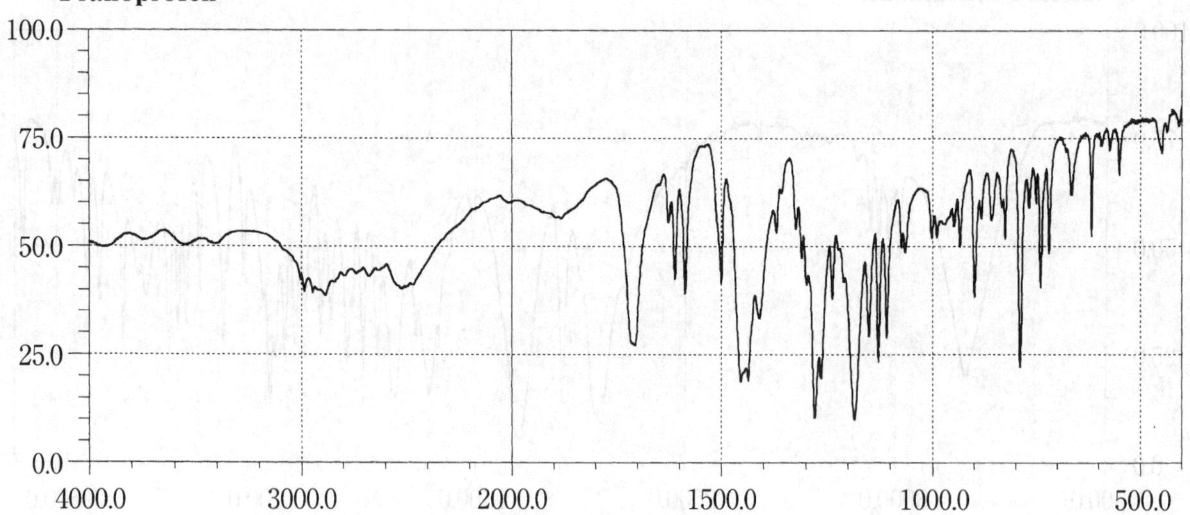

Prasterone Sodium Sulfate Hydrate

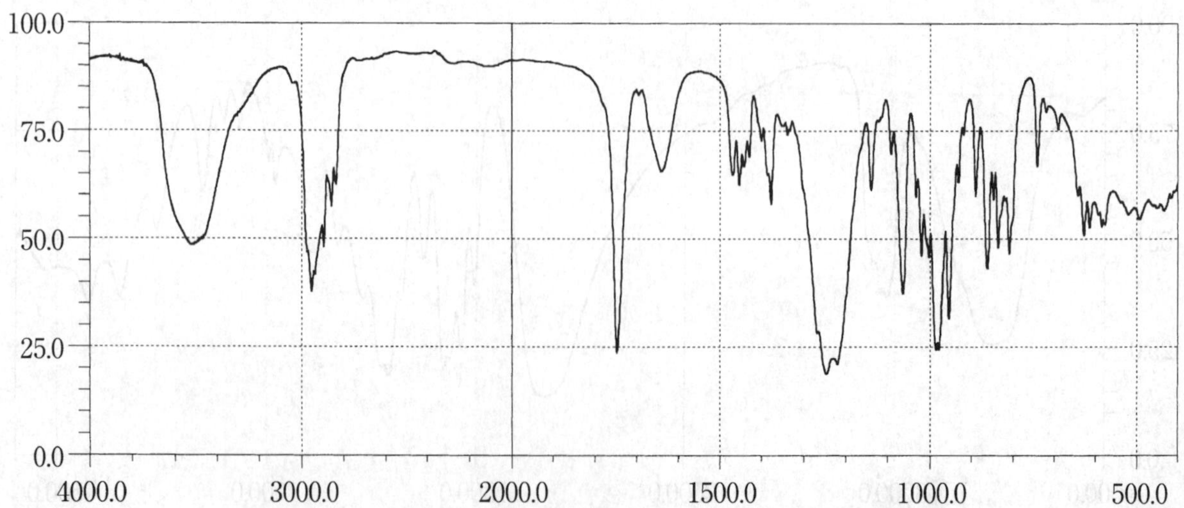

Prazepam

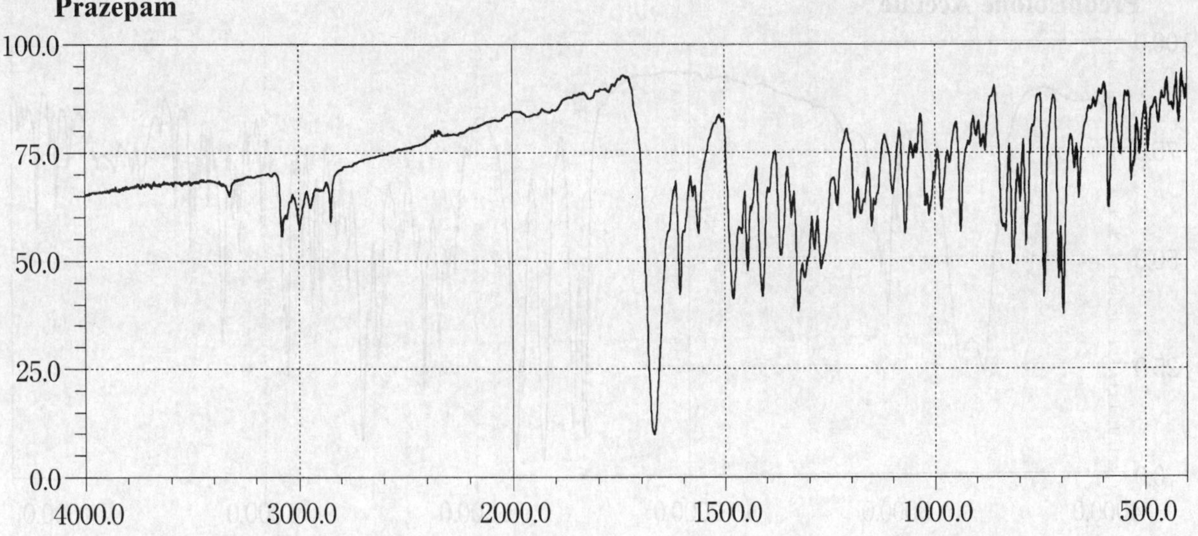

Prazosin Hydrochloride

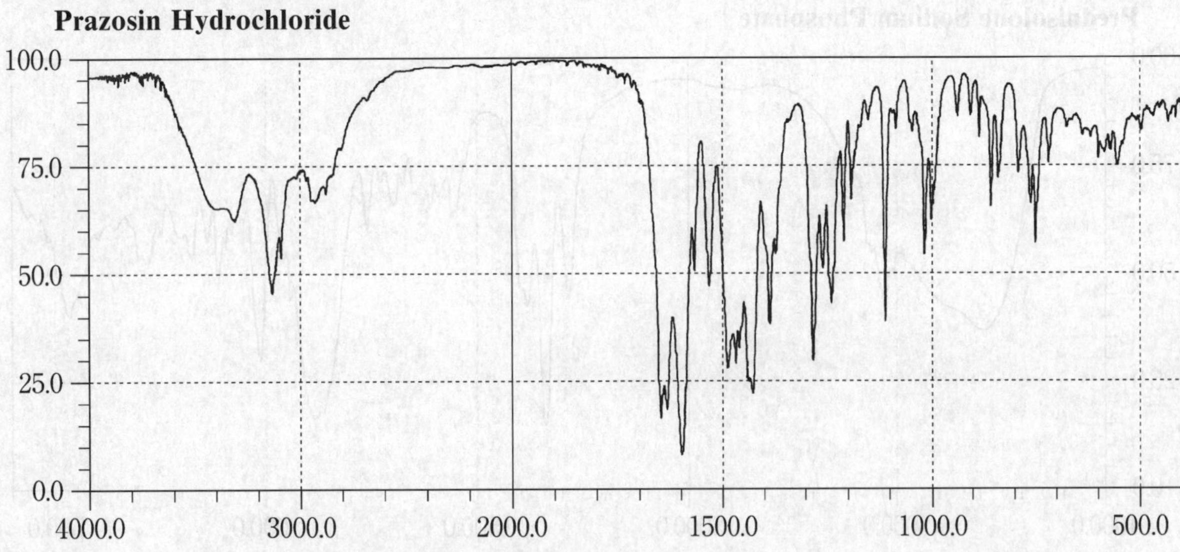

Prednisolone

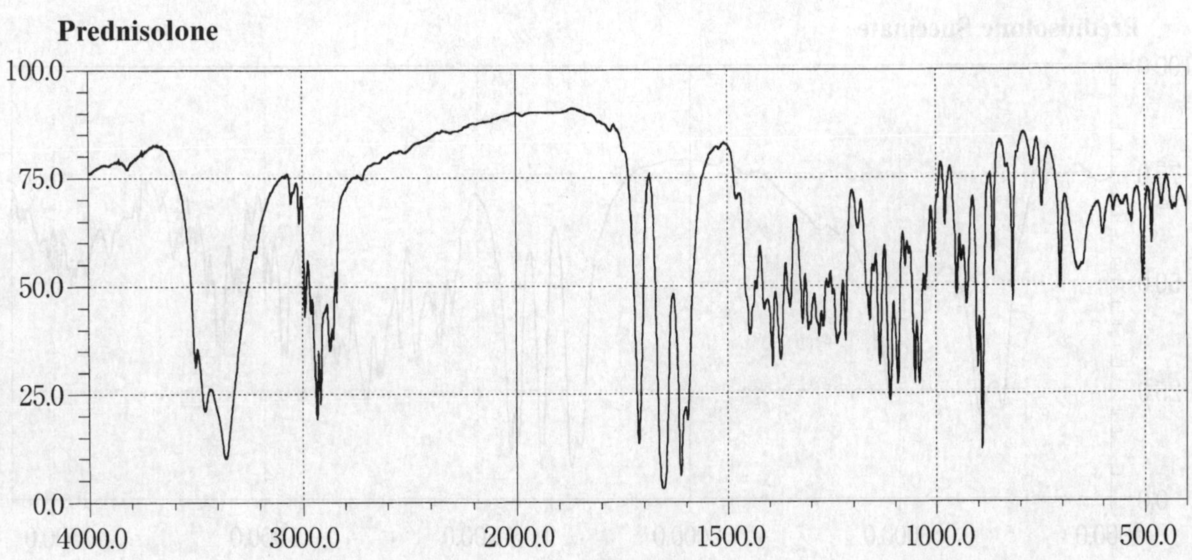

Prednisolone Acetate

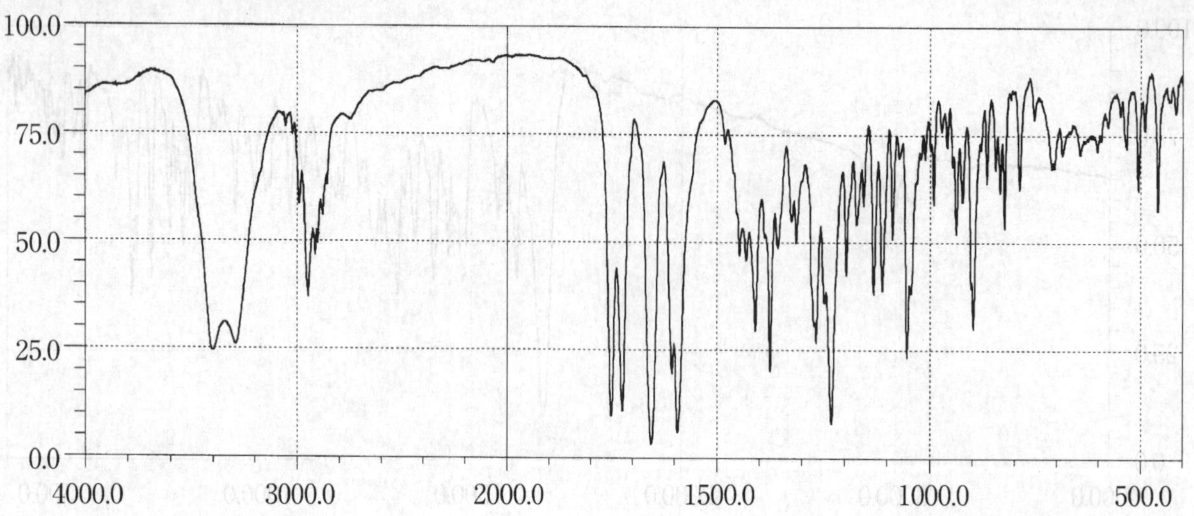

Prednisolone Sodium Phosphate

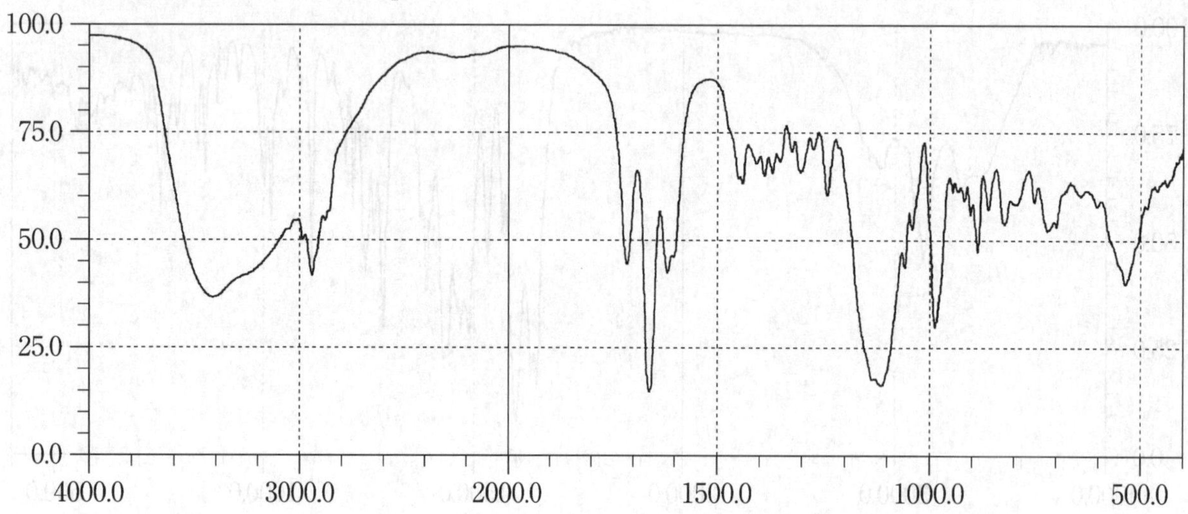

Prednisolone Succinate

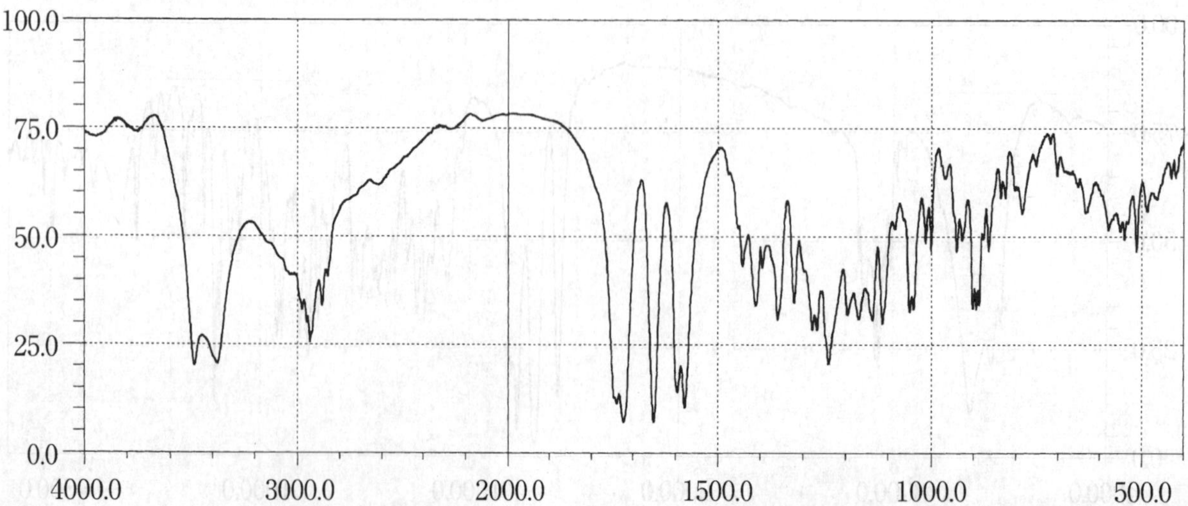

Probucol

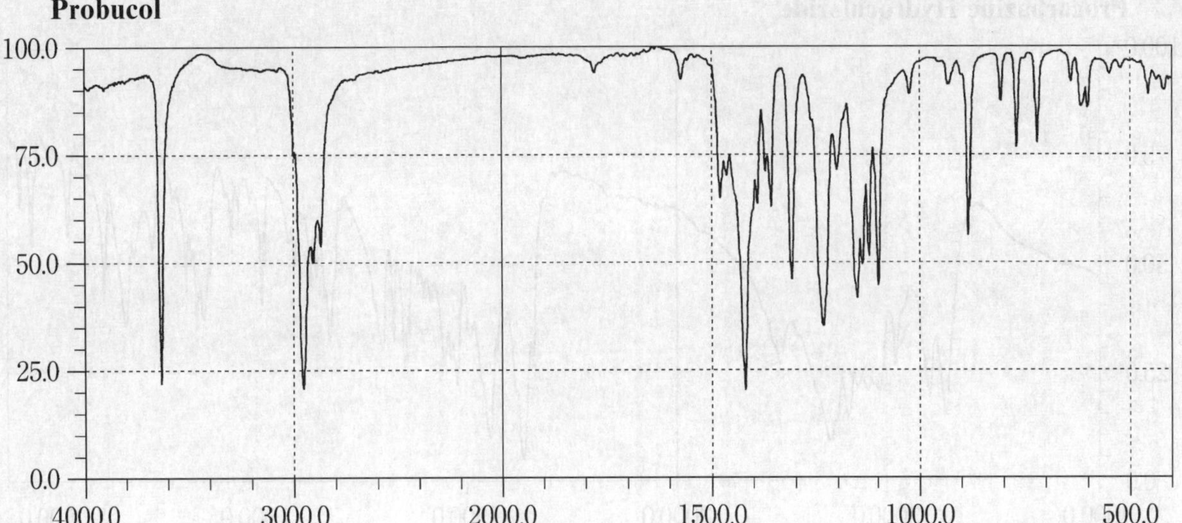

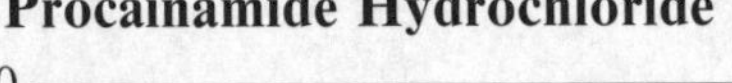

Procainamide Hydrochloride

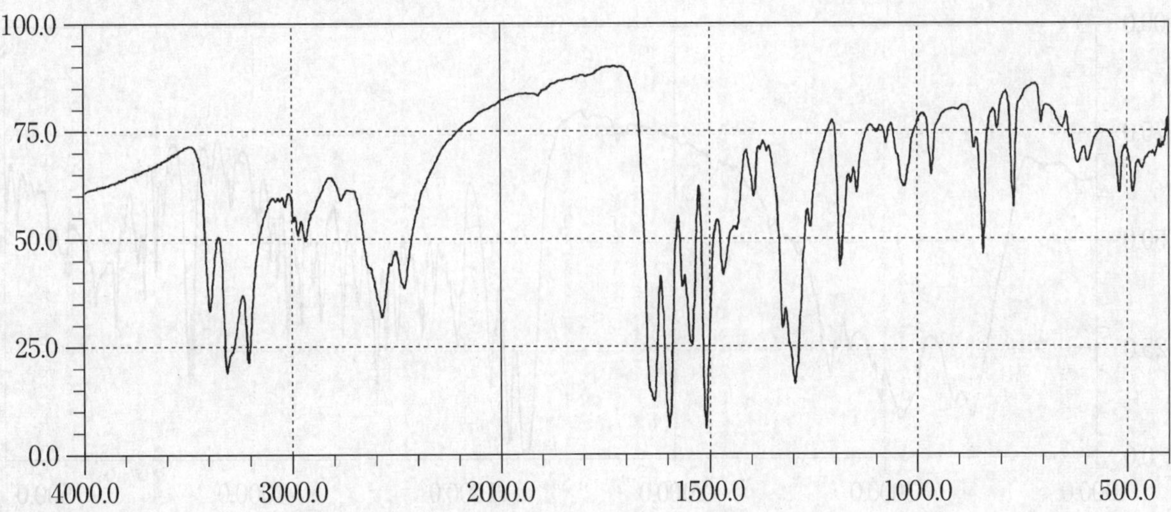

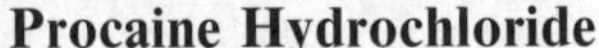

Procaine Hydrochloride

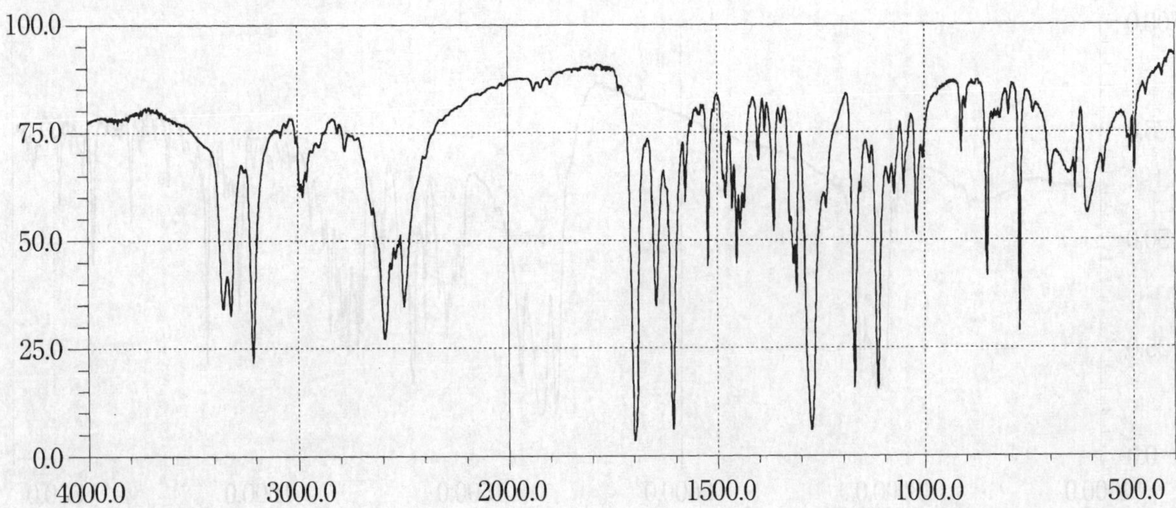

Procarbazine Hydrochloride

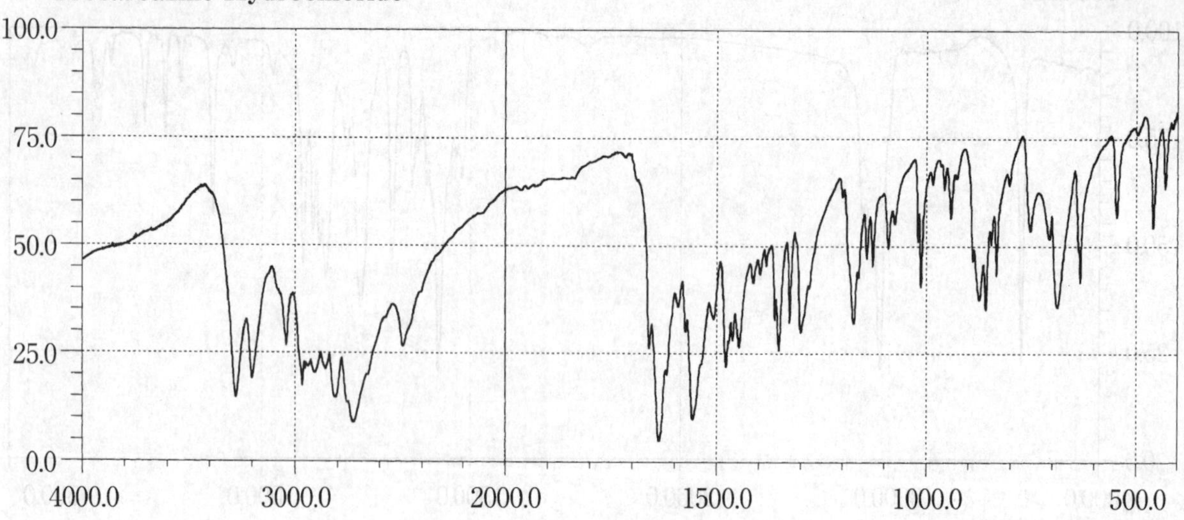

Procaterol Hydrochloride Hydrate

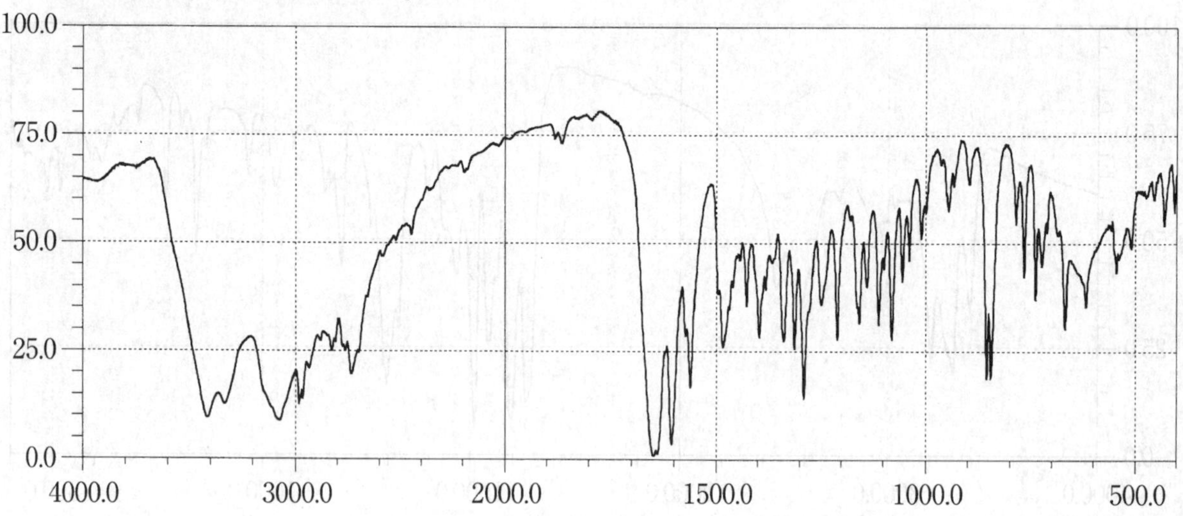

Progesterone

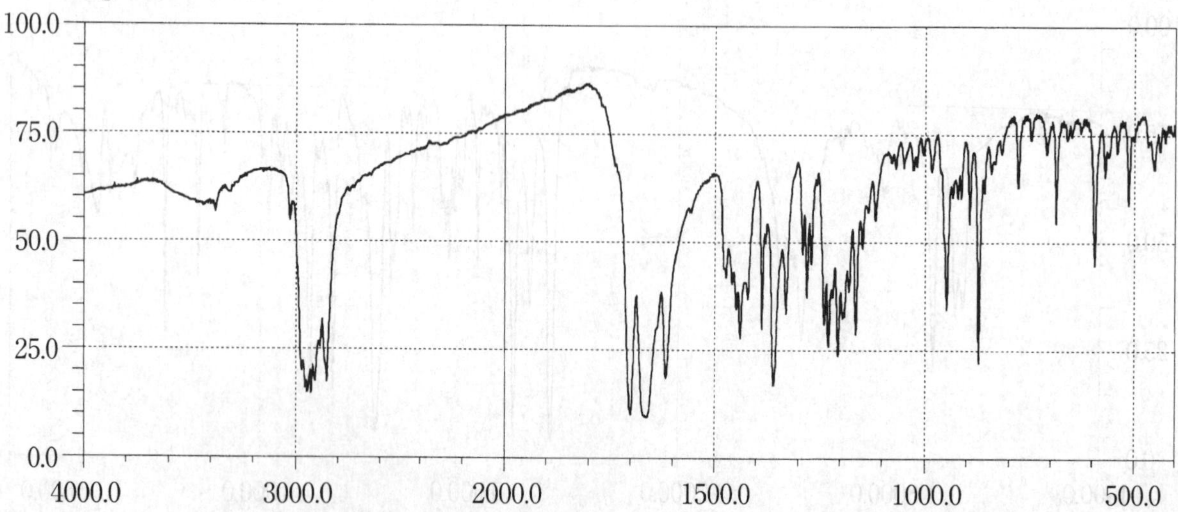

Proglumide

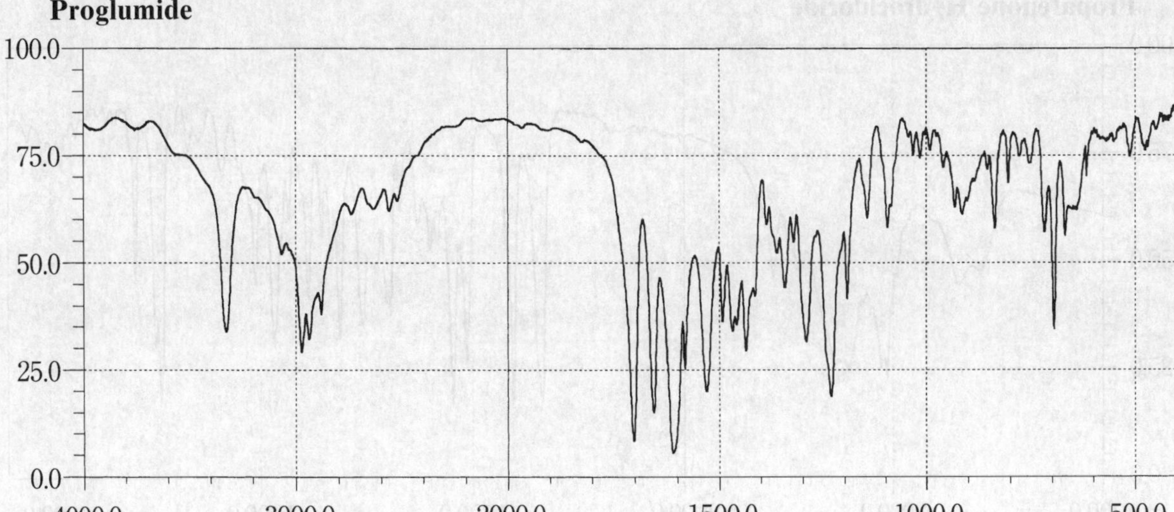

L-Proline

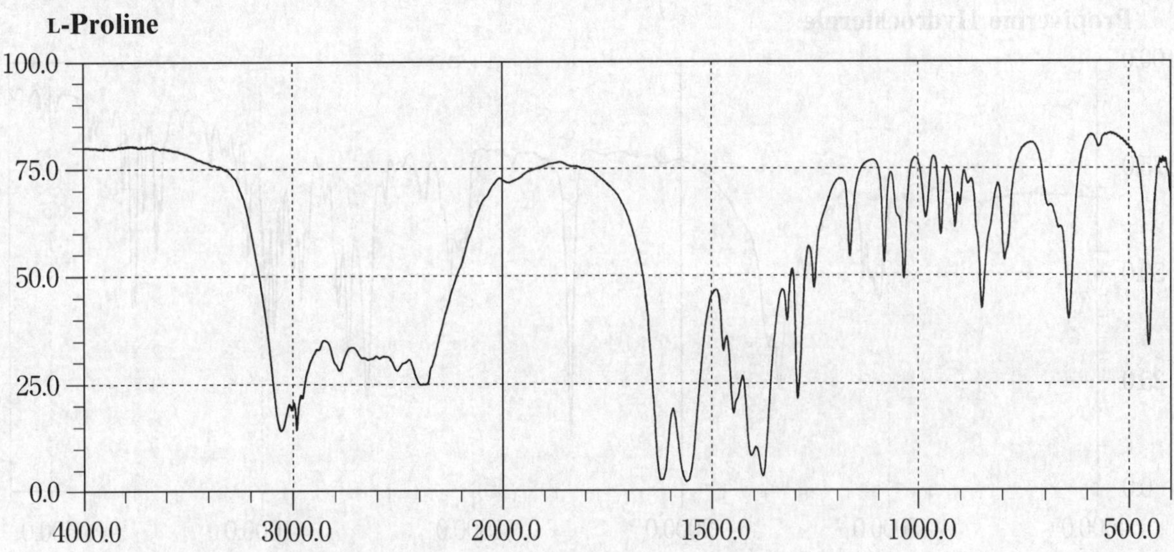

Promethazine Hydrochloride

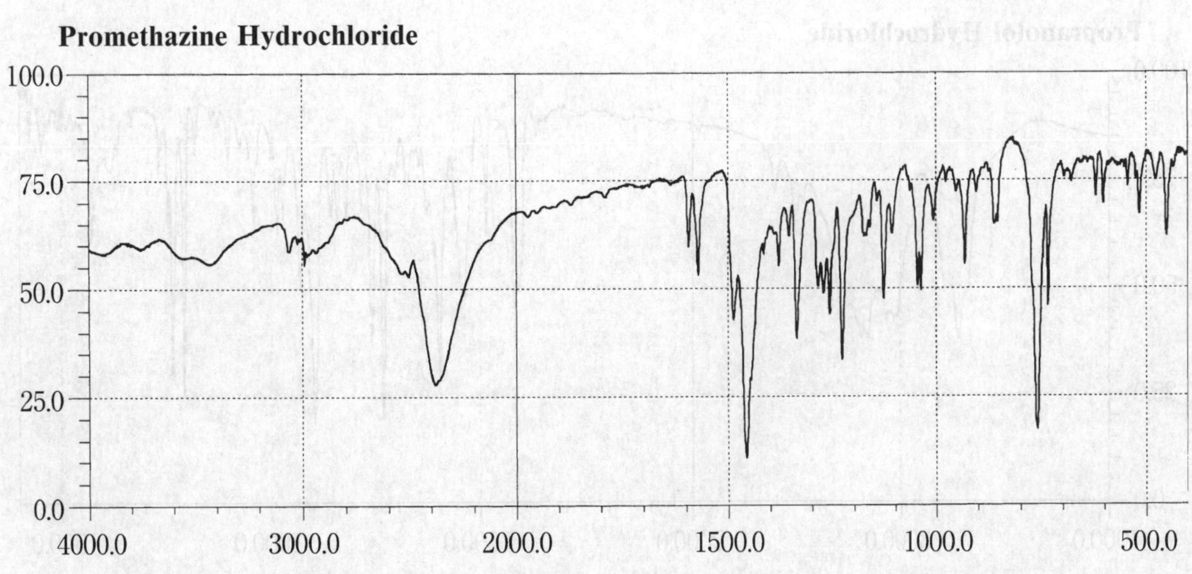

Propafenone Hydrochloride

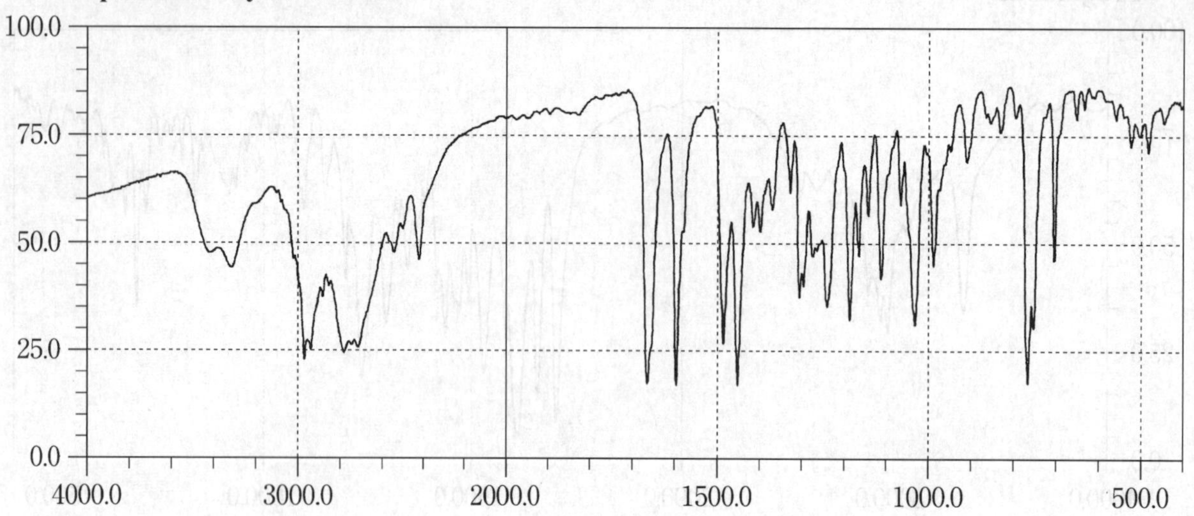

Propiverine Hydrochloride

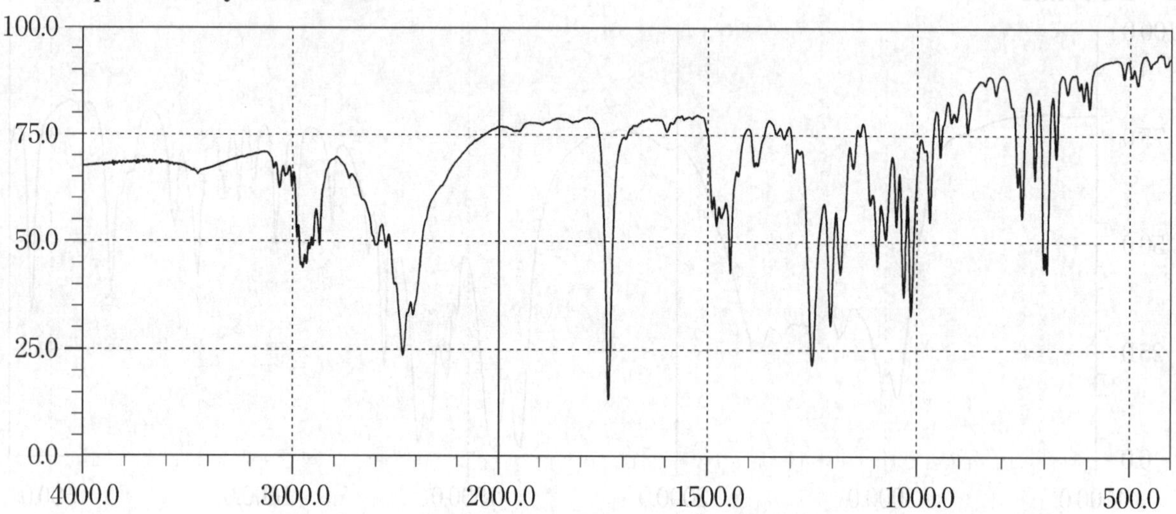

Propranolol Hydrochloride

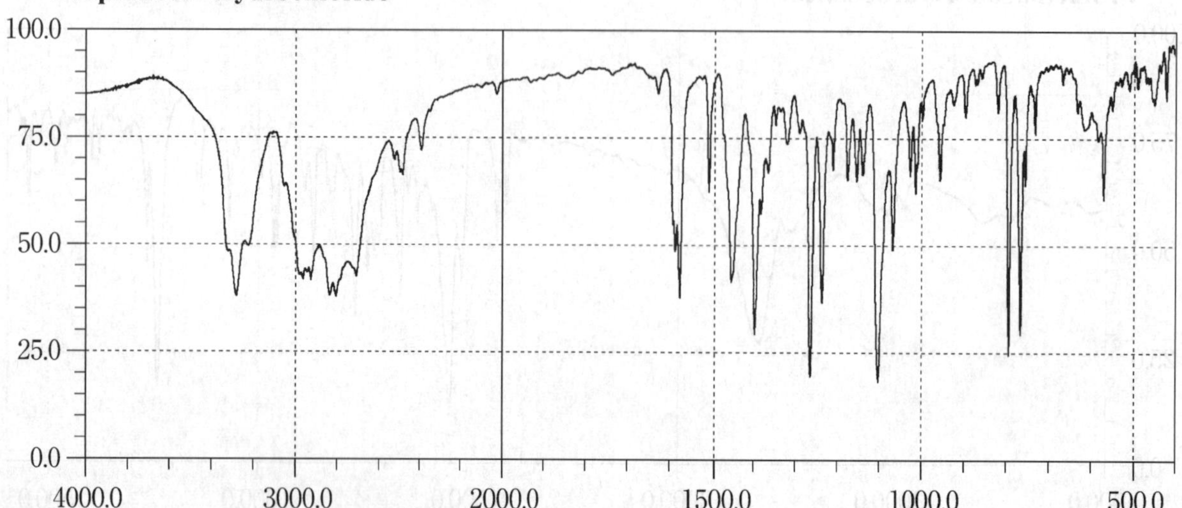

Propyl Parahydroxybenzoate

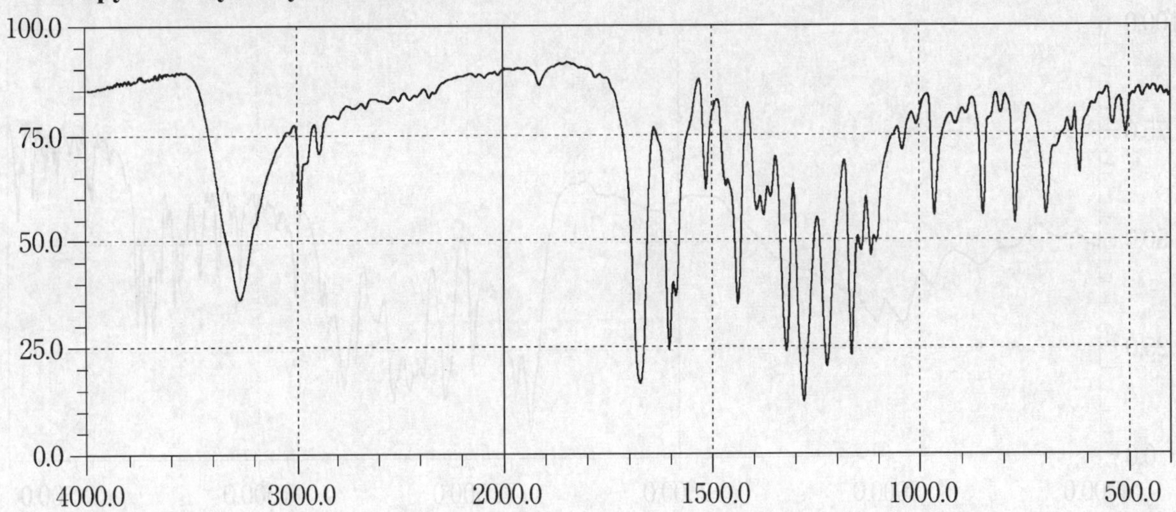

Protirelin

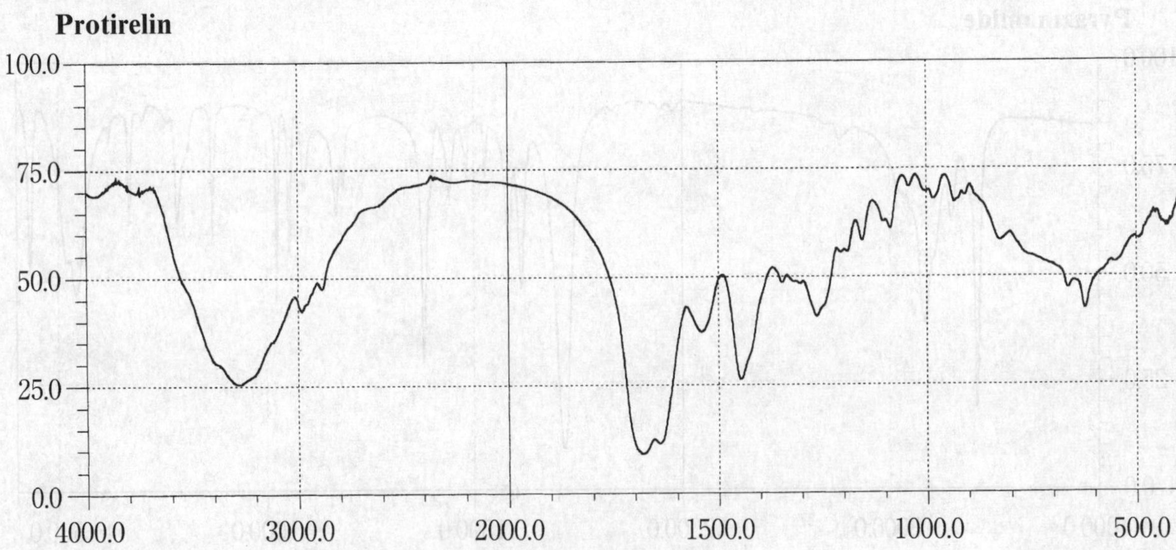

Purified Sodium Hyaluronate

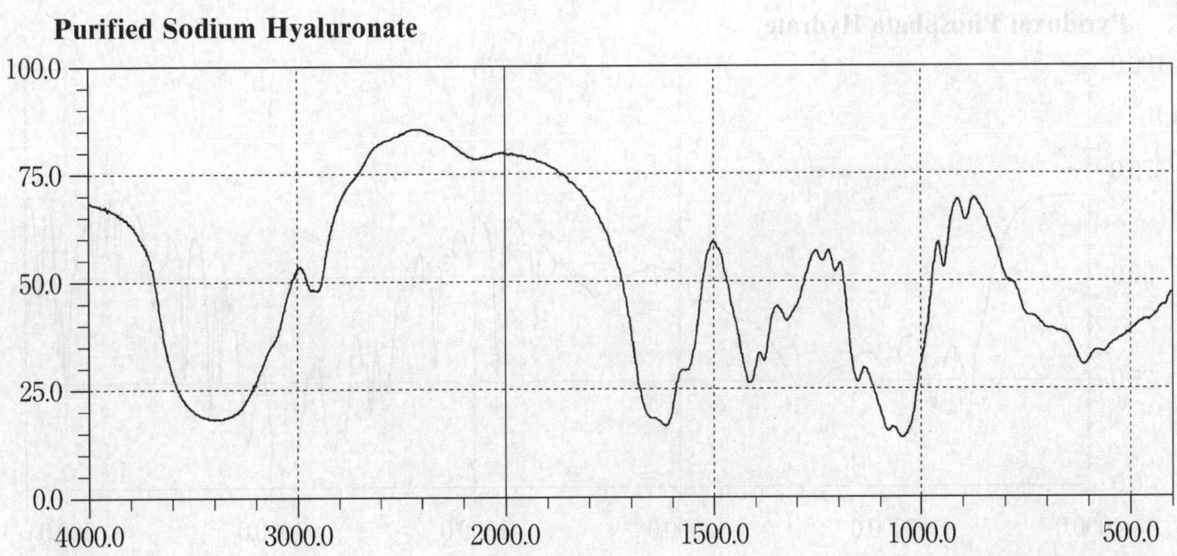

The JP Drugs are to be tested according to the provisions given in the pertinent monographs, General Notices, General Rules for Crude Drugs, General Rules for Preparations, and General Tests for their conformity to the Japanese Pharmacopoeia. (See the General Notices 5.)

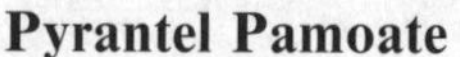

Pyrantel Pamoate

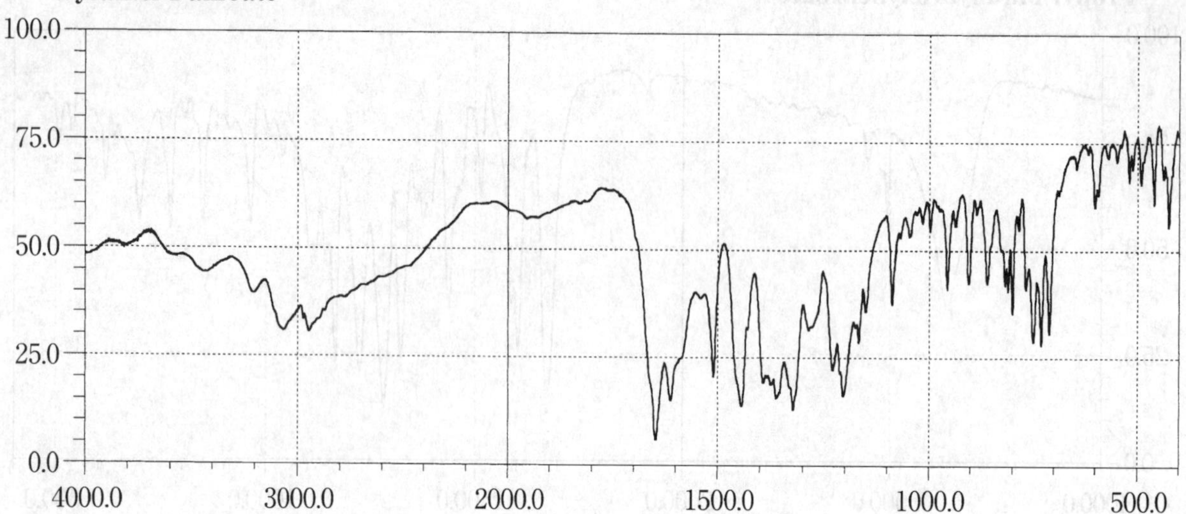

Pyrazinamide

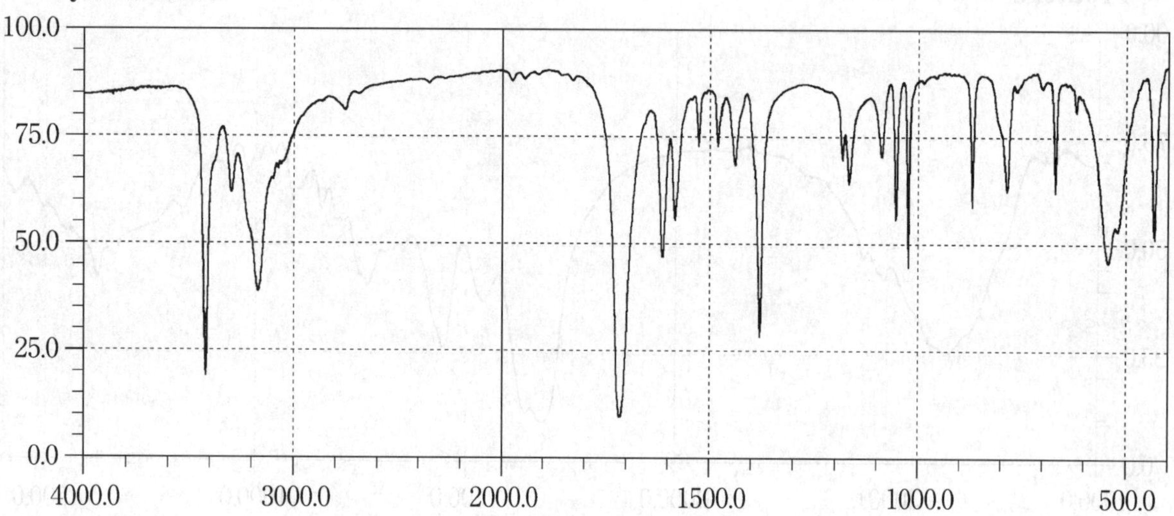

Pyridoxal Phosphate Hydrate

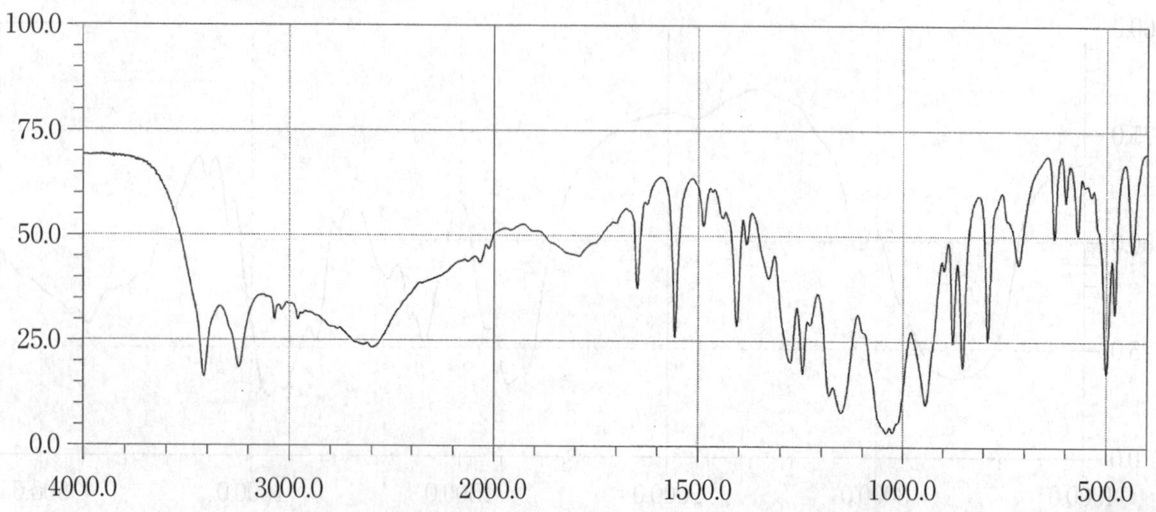

Pyridoxine Hydrochloride

100.0
75.0
50.0
25.0
0.0
4000.0
3000.0
2000.0
1500.0
1000.0
500.0

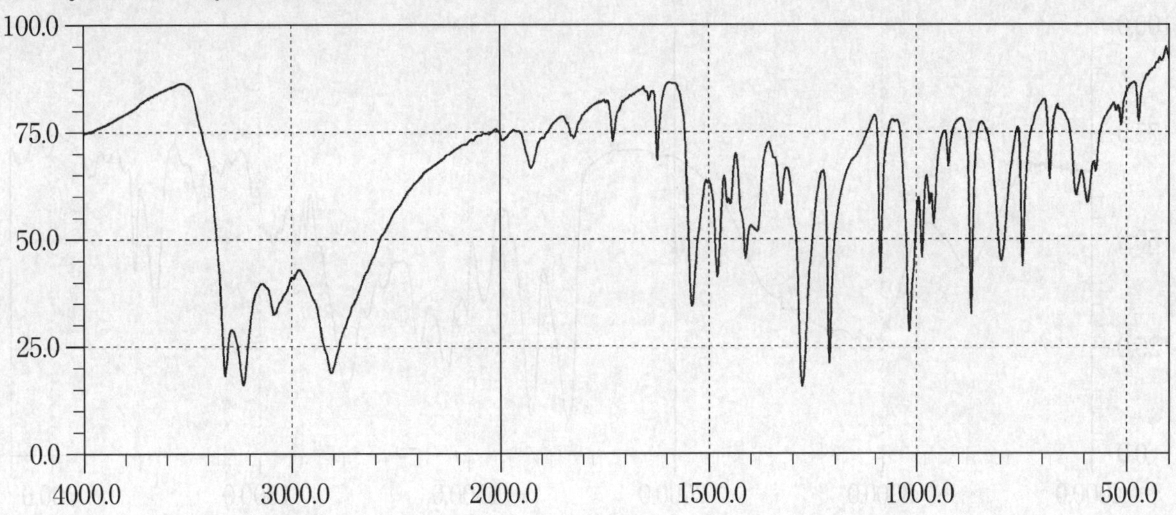

Pyrrolnitrin

100.0
75.0
50.0
25.0
0.0
4000.0
3000.0
2000.0
1500.0
1000.0
500.0

Quetiapine Fumarate

100.0
75.0
50.0
25.0
0.0
4000.0
3000.0
2000.0
1500.0
1000.0
500.0

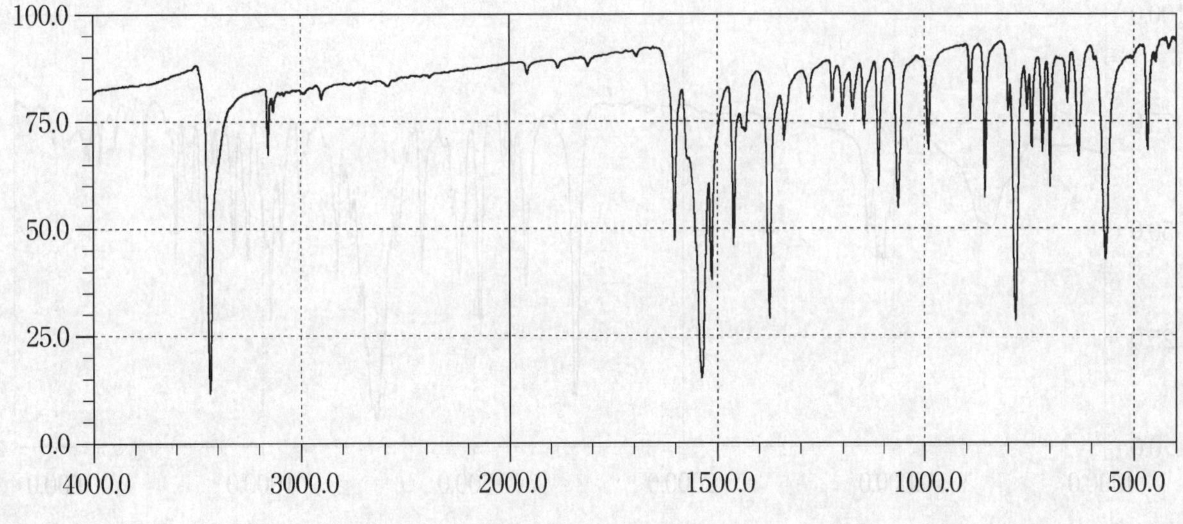

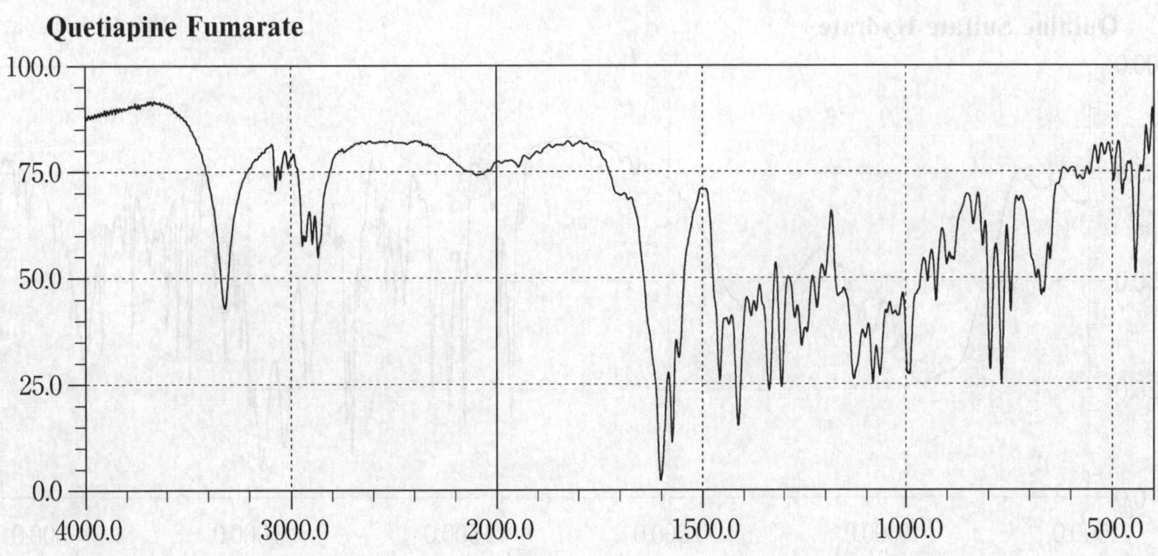

Quinapril Hydrochloride

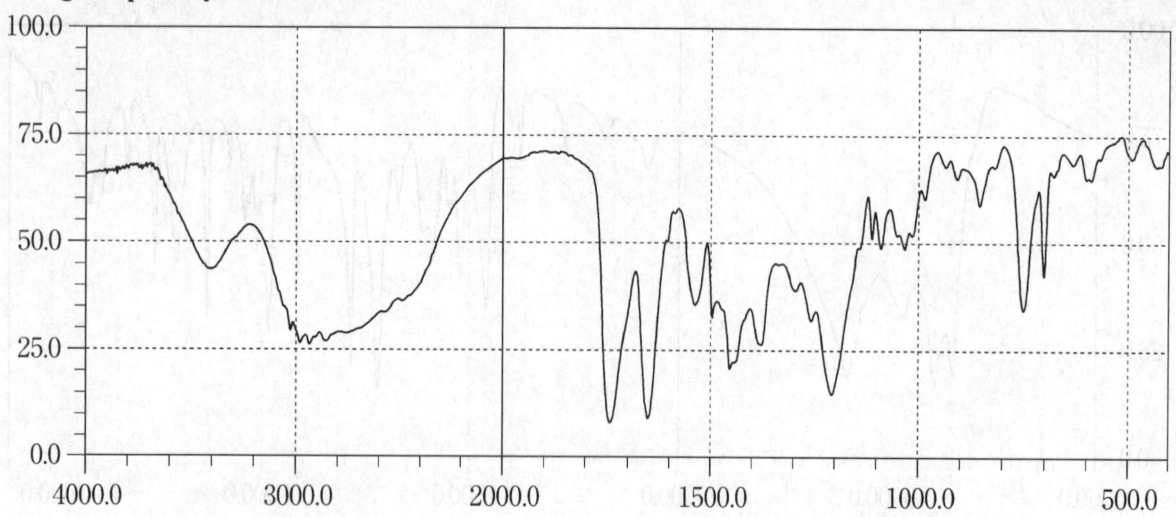

Quinine Ethyl Carbonate

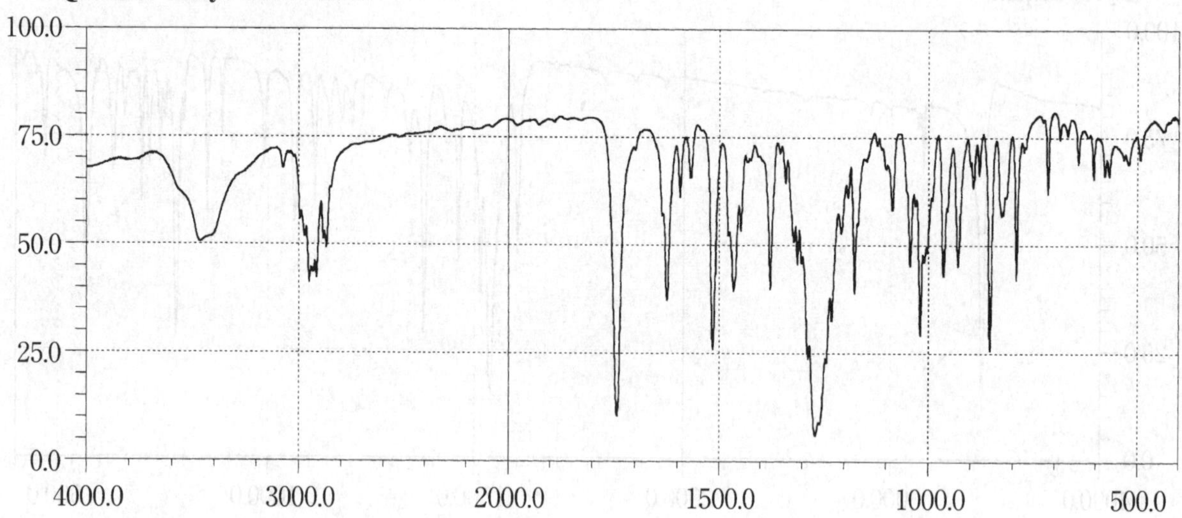

Quinine Sulfate Hydrate

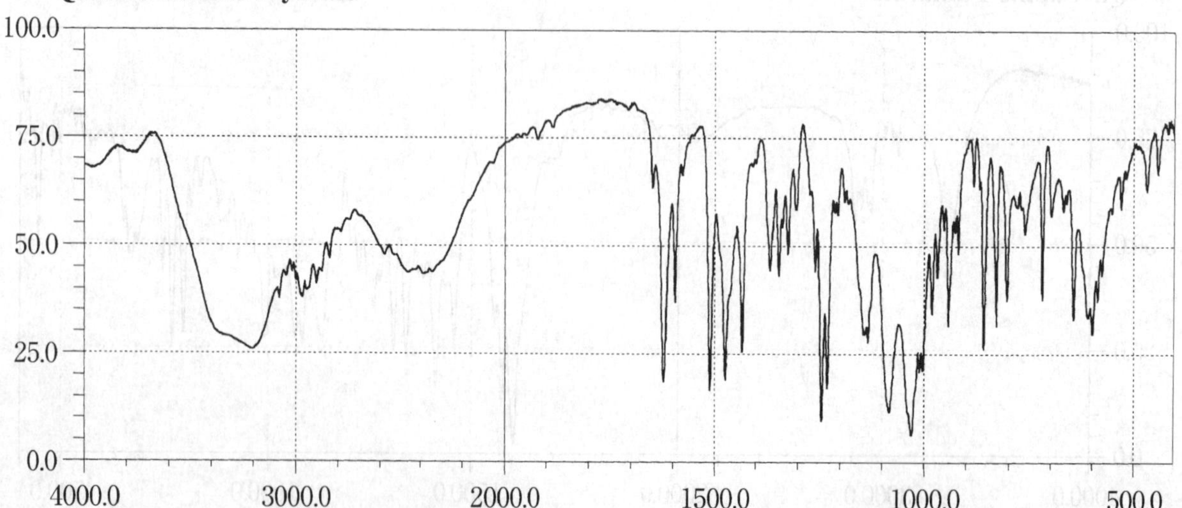

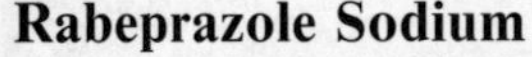

Rabeprazole Sodium

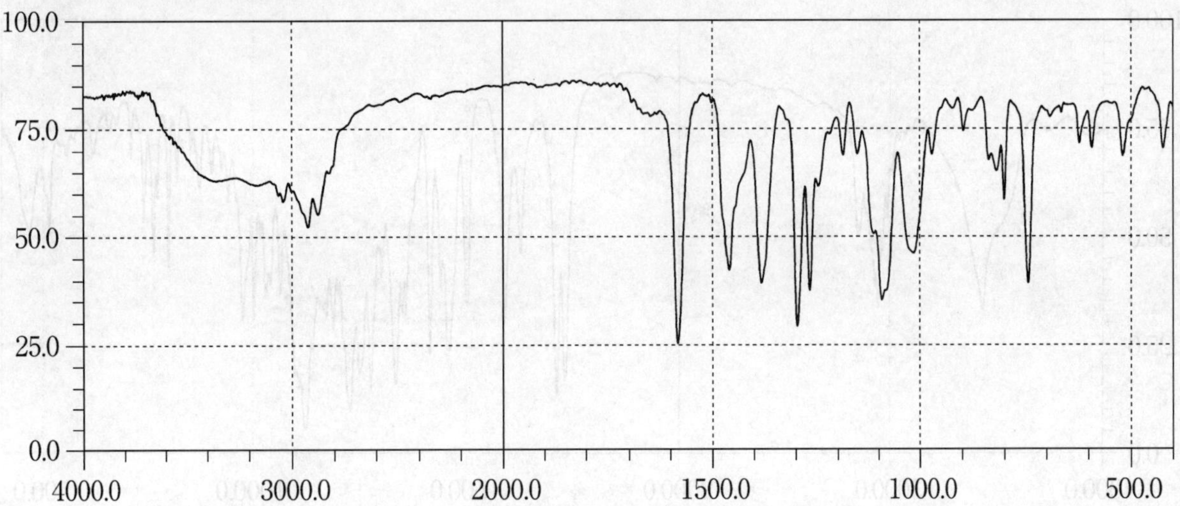

Ranitidine Hydrochloride

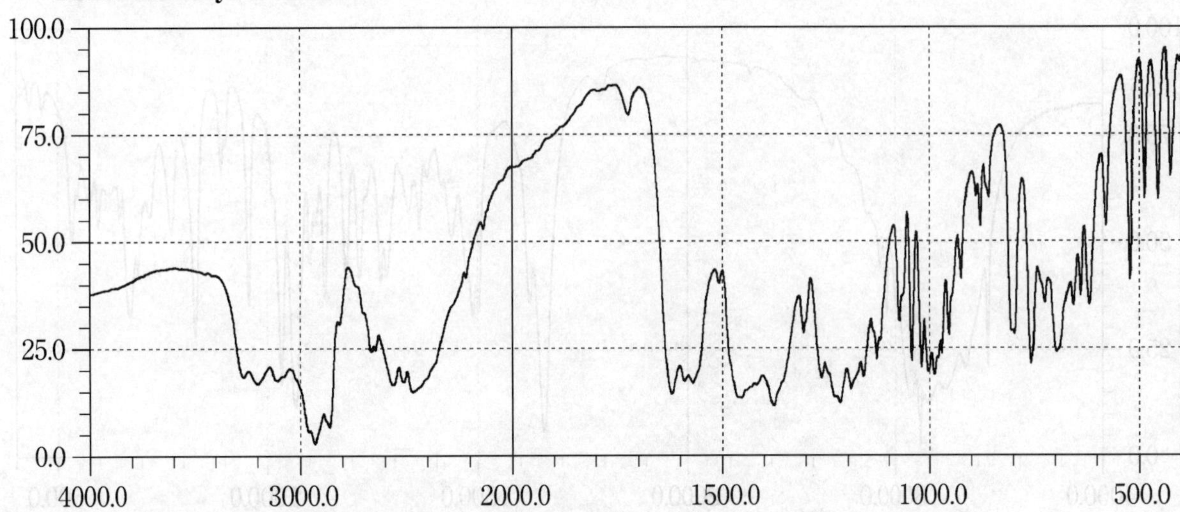

Rebamipide

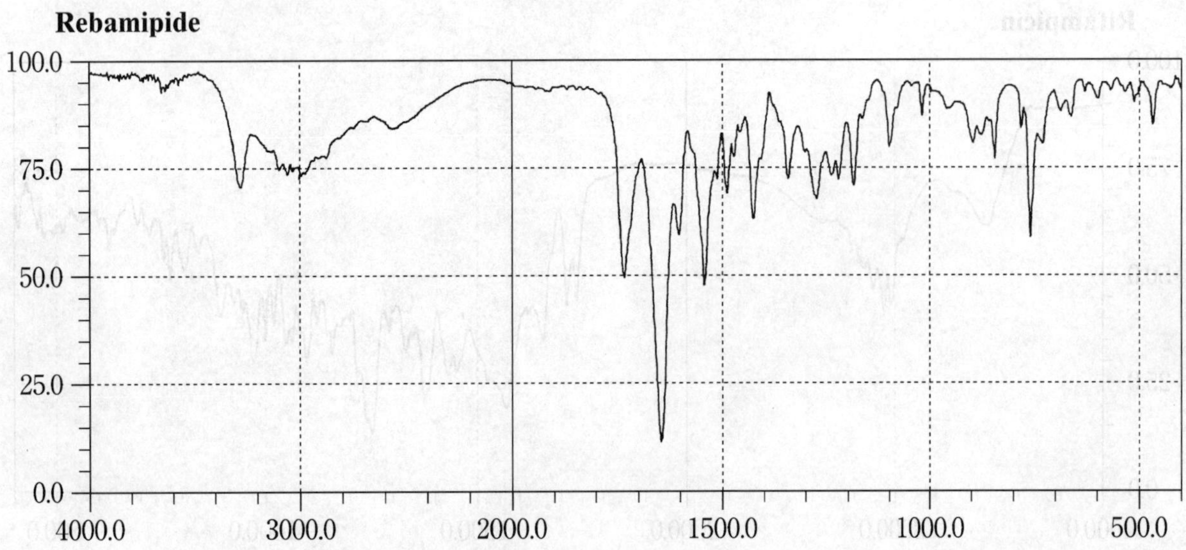

Reserpine

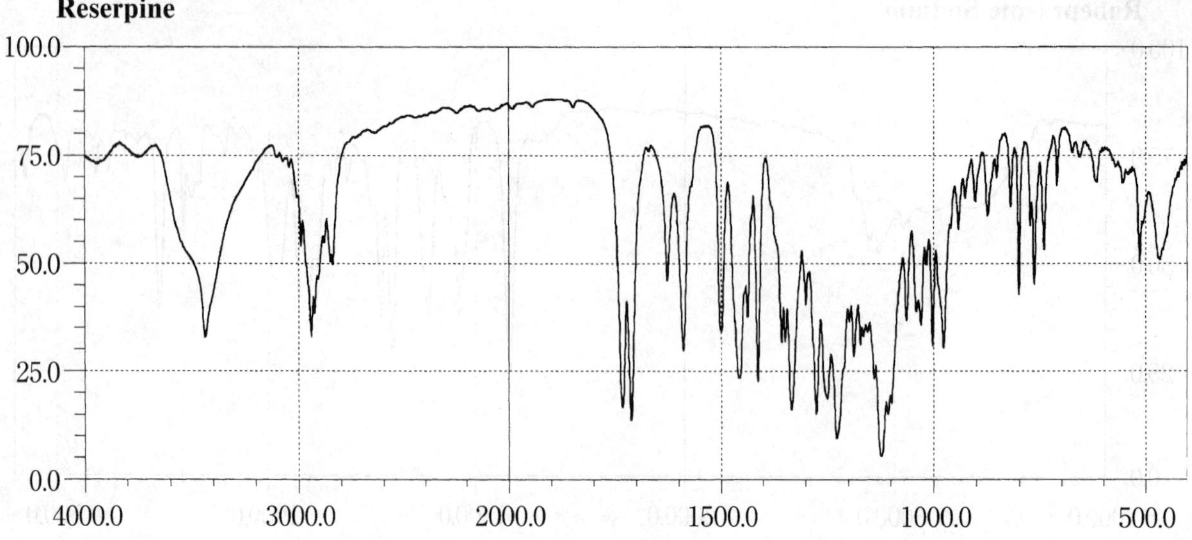

Ribavirin

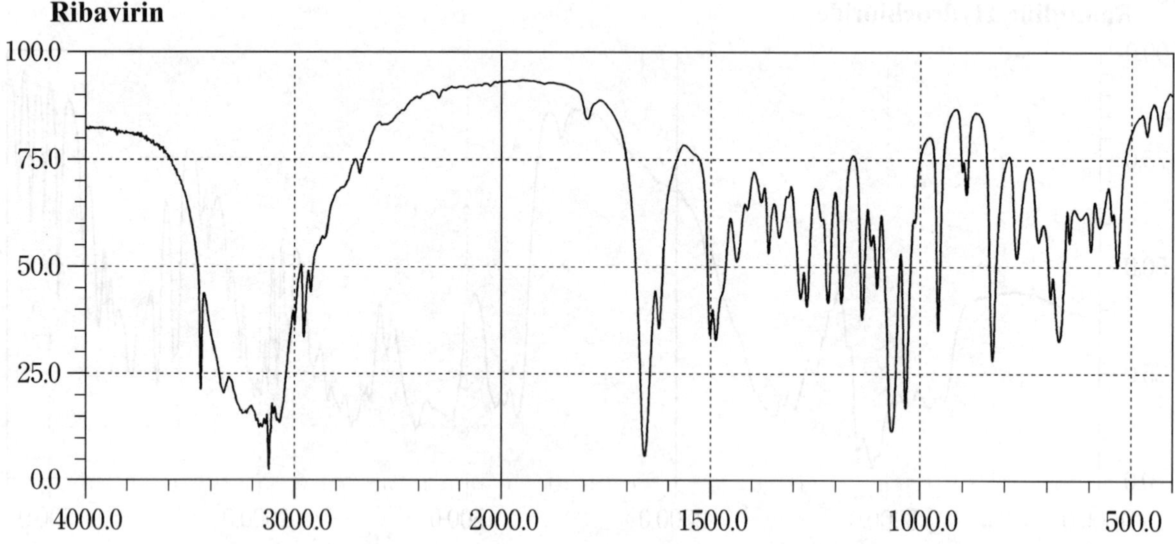

Rifampicin

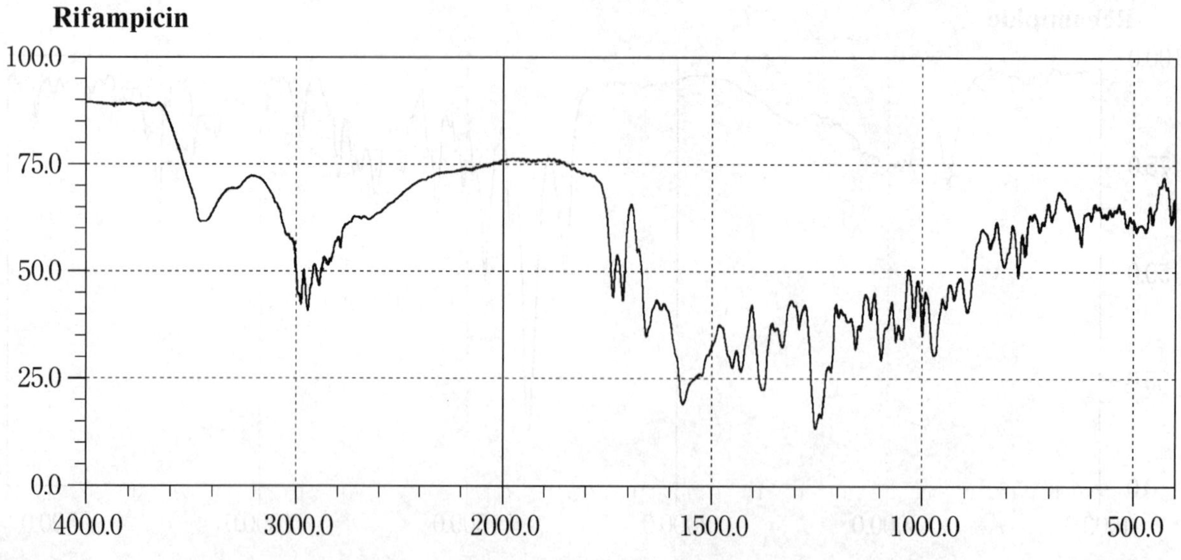

Rilmazafone Hydrochloride Hydrate

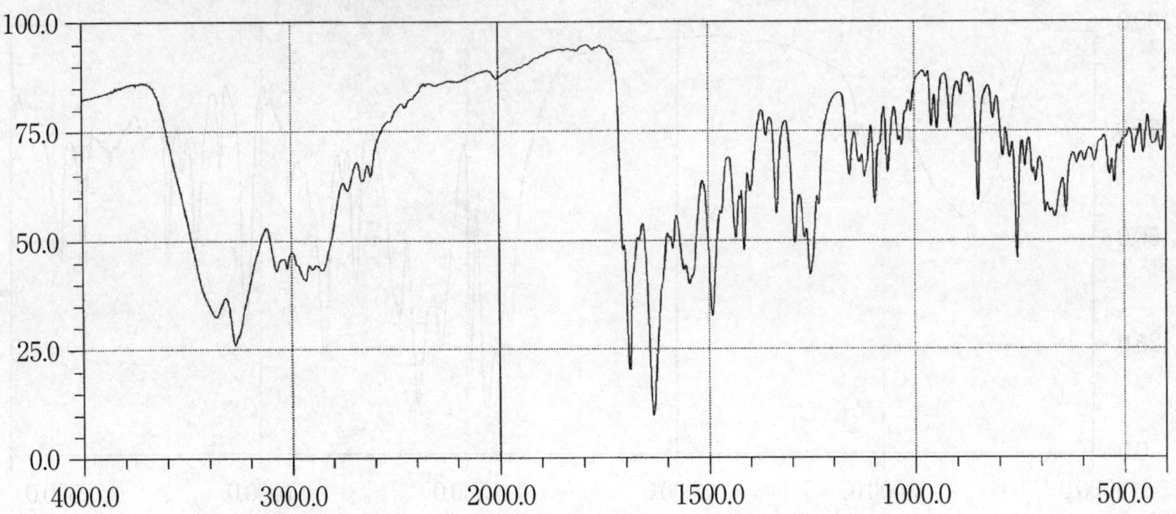

Risperidone

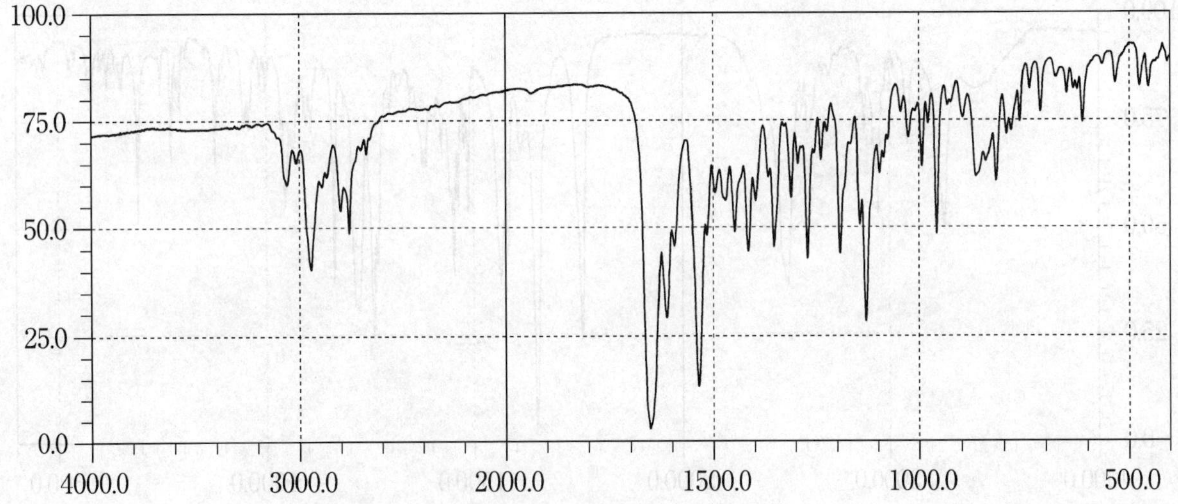

Ritodrine Hydrochloride

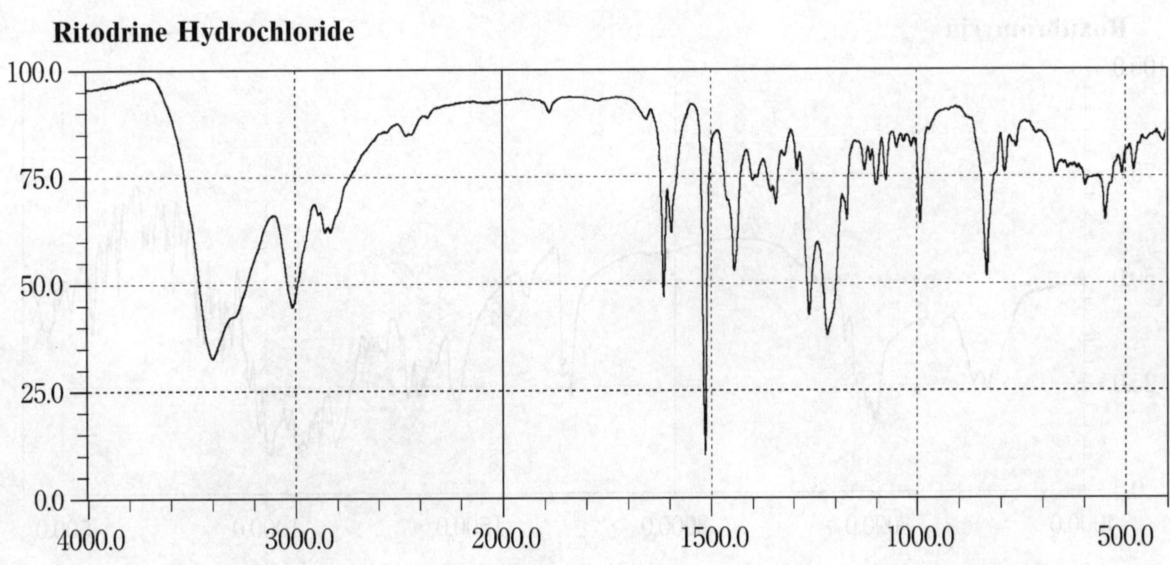

The JP Drugs are to be tested according to the provisions given in the pertinent monographs, General Notices, General Rules for Crude Drugs, General Rules for Preparations, and General Tests for their conformity to the Japanese Pharmacopoeia. (See the General Notices 5.)

Rosuvastatin Calcium

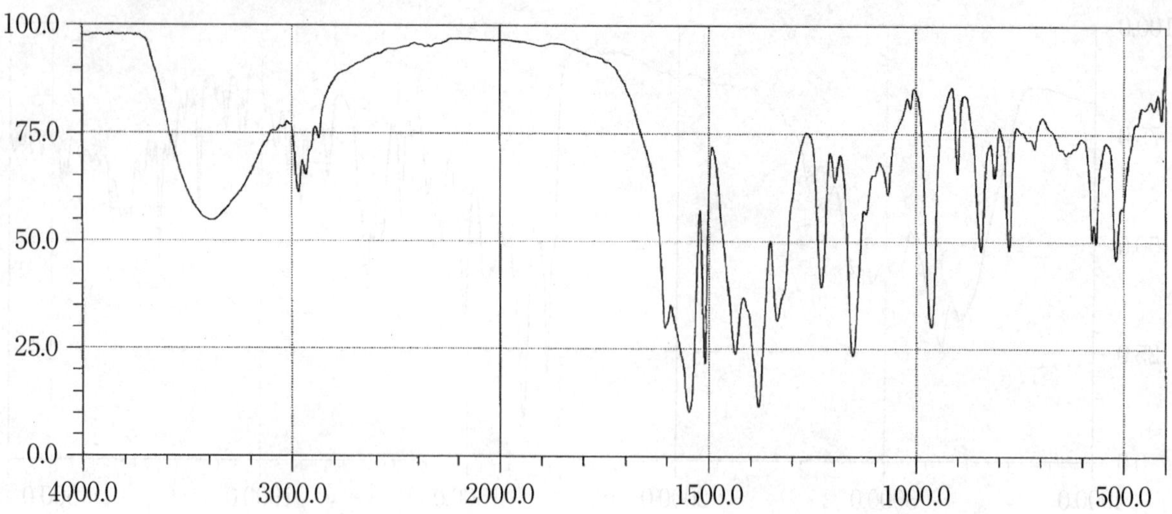

Roxatidine Acetate Hydrochloride

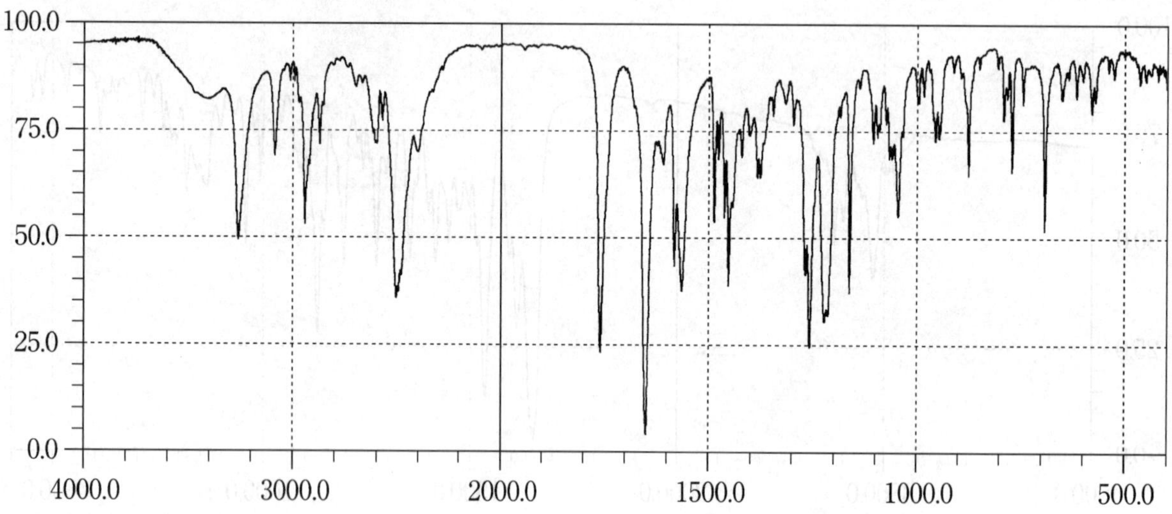

Roxithromycin

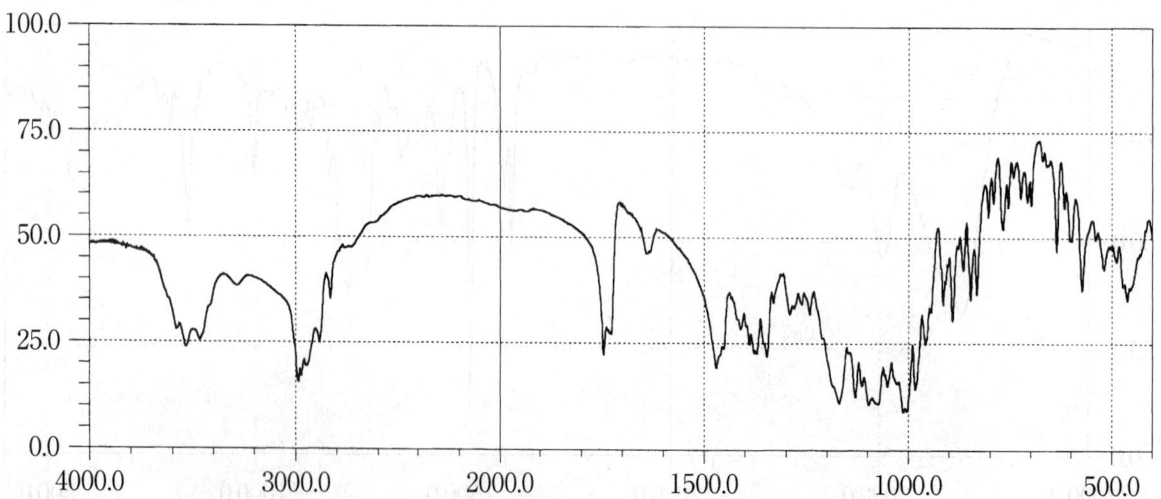

Saccharin

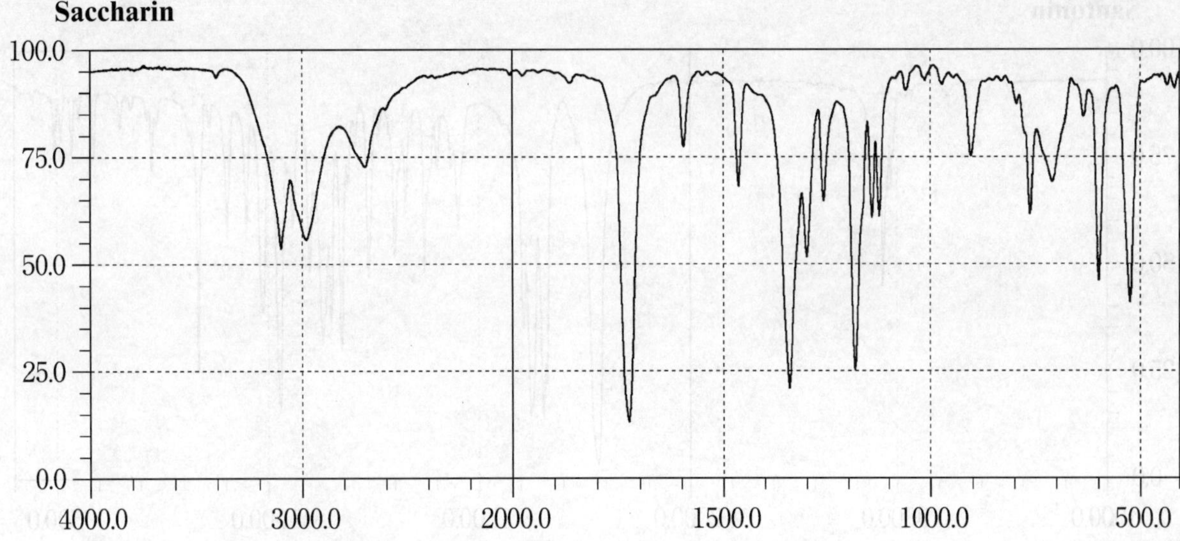

Salbutamol Sulfate

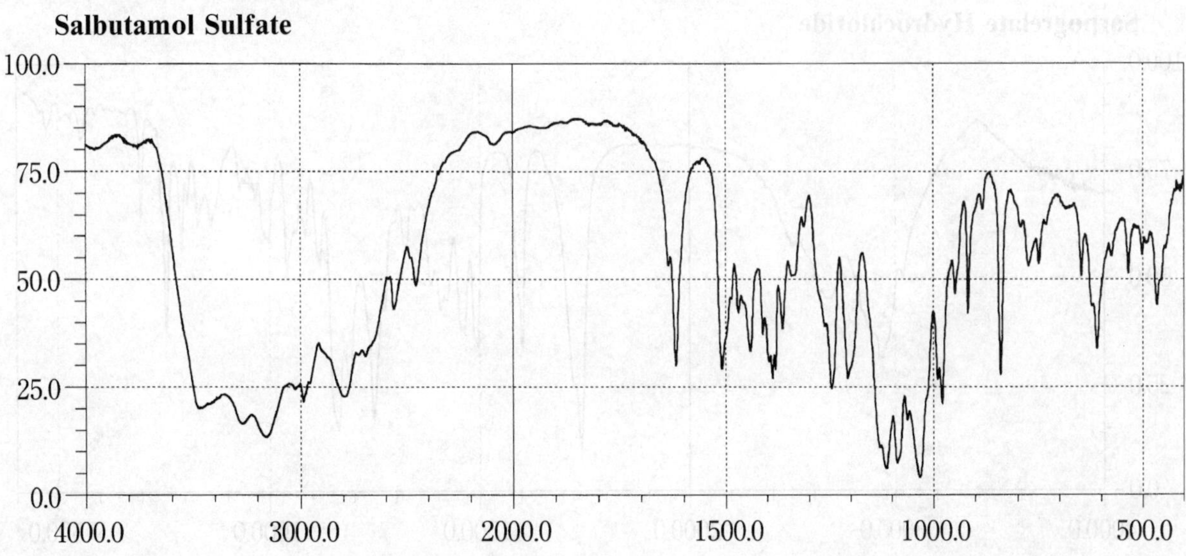

Salicylic Acid

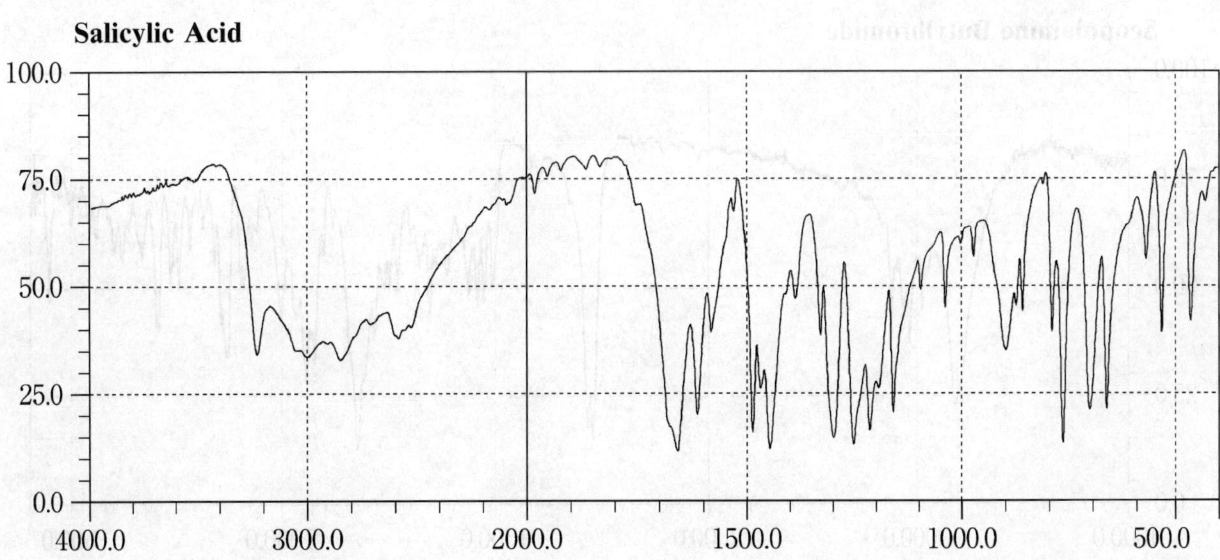

Santonin

100.0
75.0
50.0
25.0
0.0
4000.0 3000.0 2000.0 1500.0 1000.0 500.0

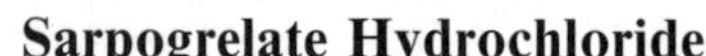

Sarpogrelate Hydrochloride

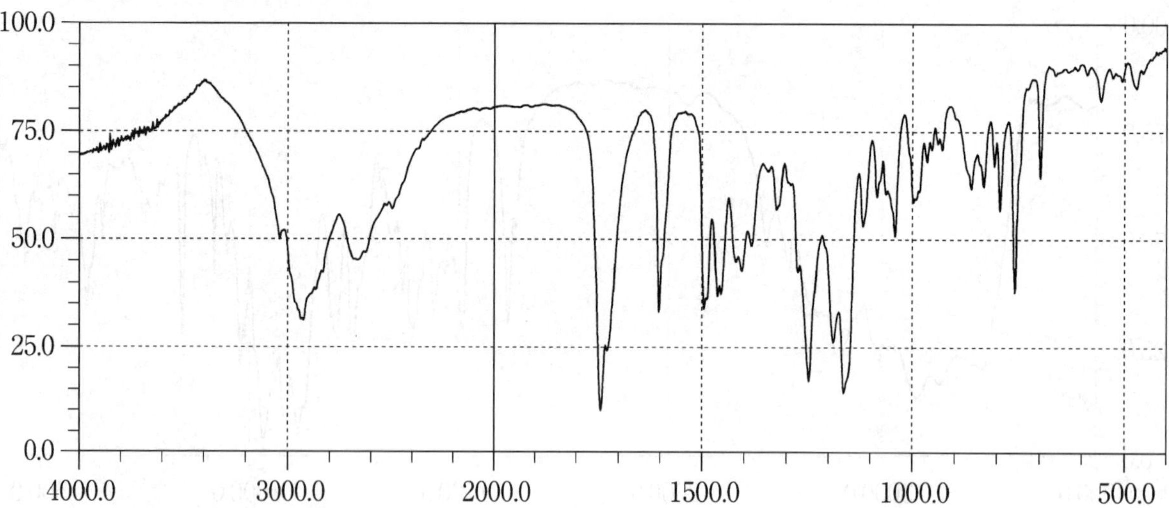

Scopolamine Butylbromide

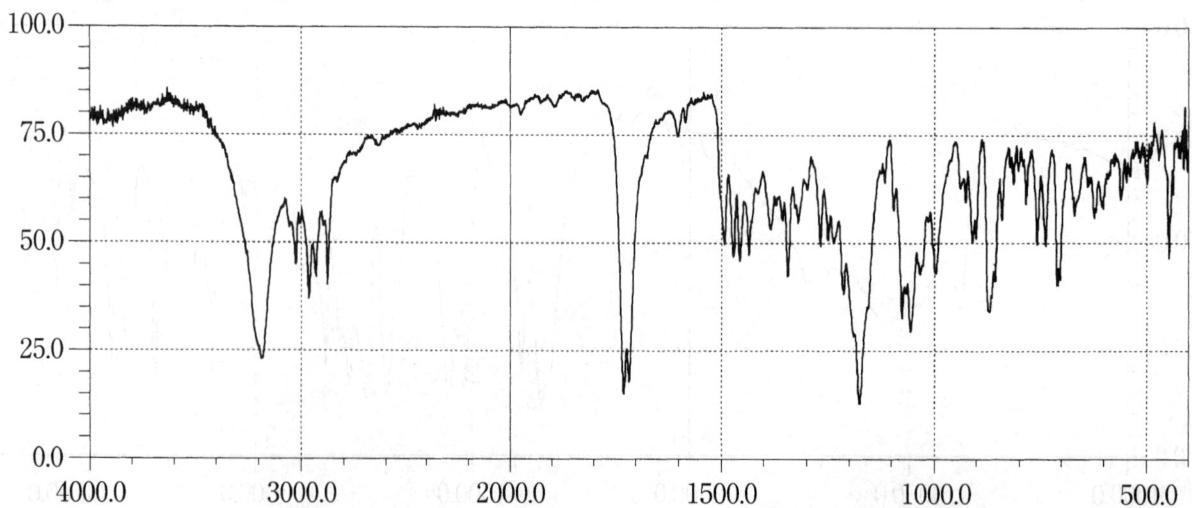

The JP Drugs are to be tested according to the provisions given in the pertinent monographs, General Notices, General Rules for Crude Drugs, General Rules for Preparations, and General Tests for their conformity to the Japanese Pharmacopoeia. (See the General Notices 5.)

L-Serine

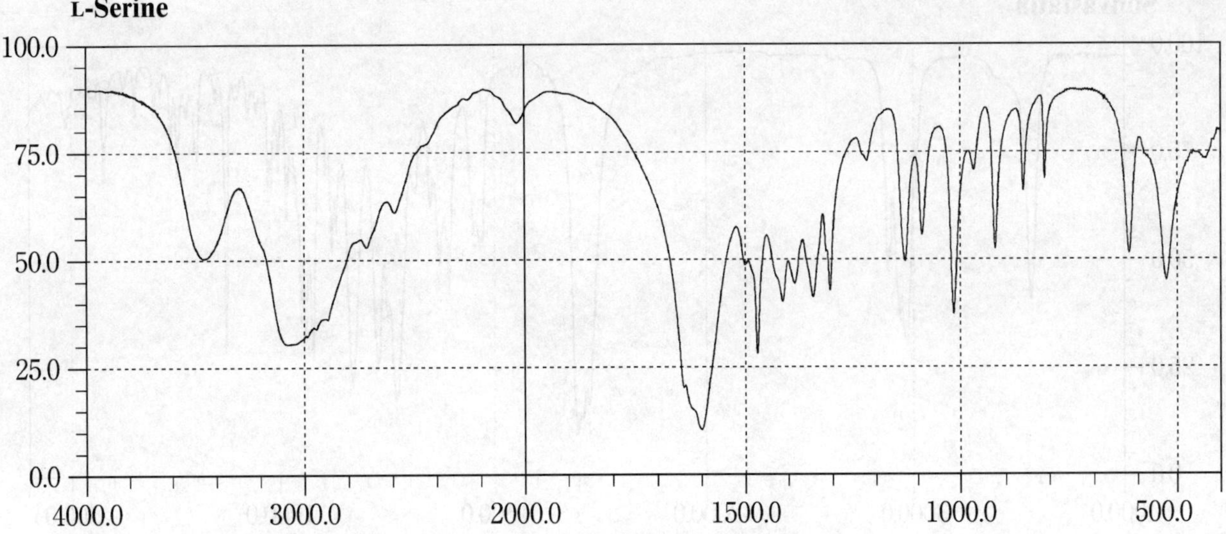

Sevoflurane

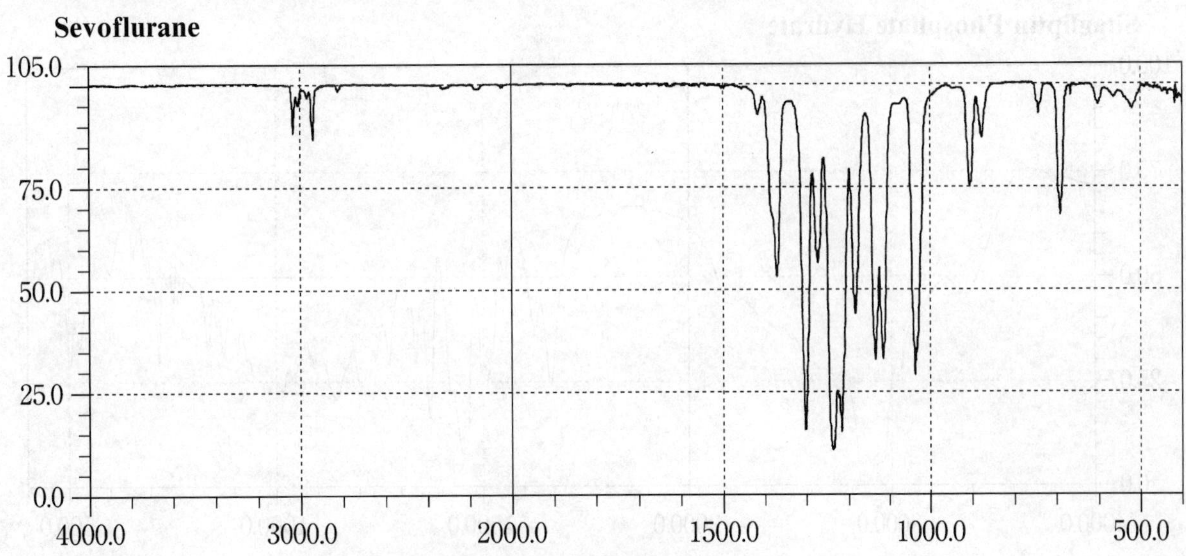

Silodosin

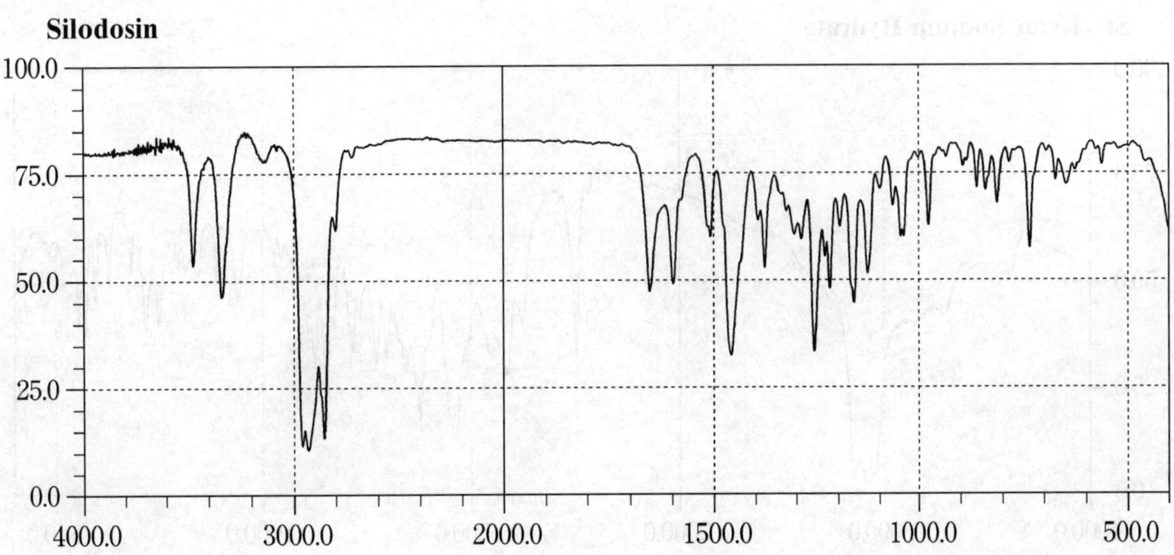

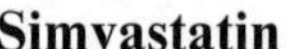

Simvastatin

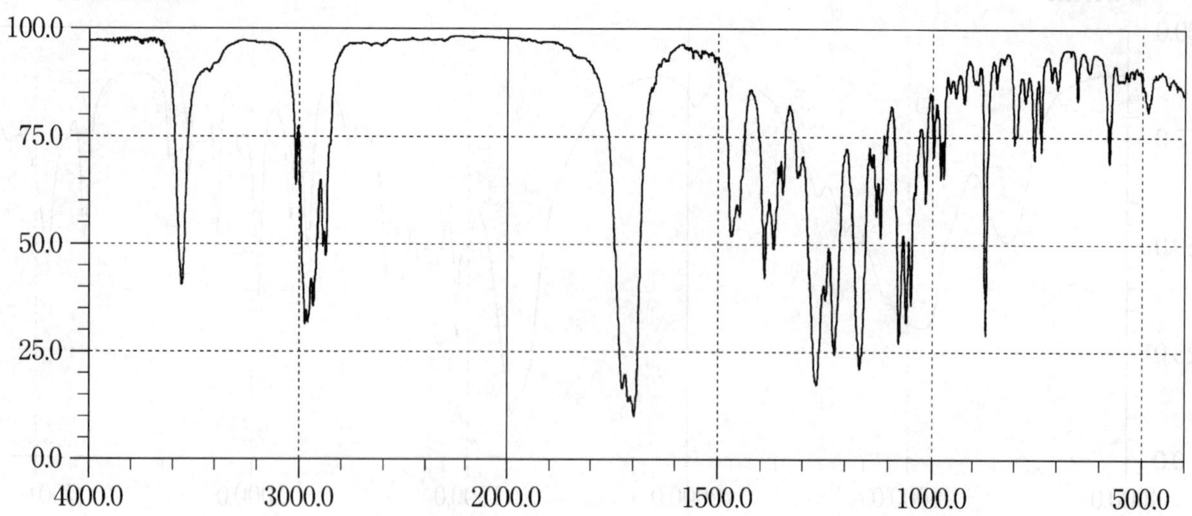

Sitagliptin Phosphate Hydrate

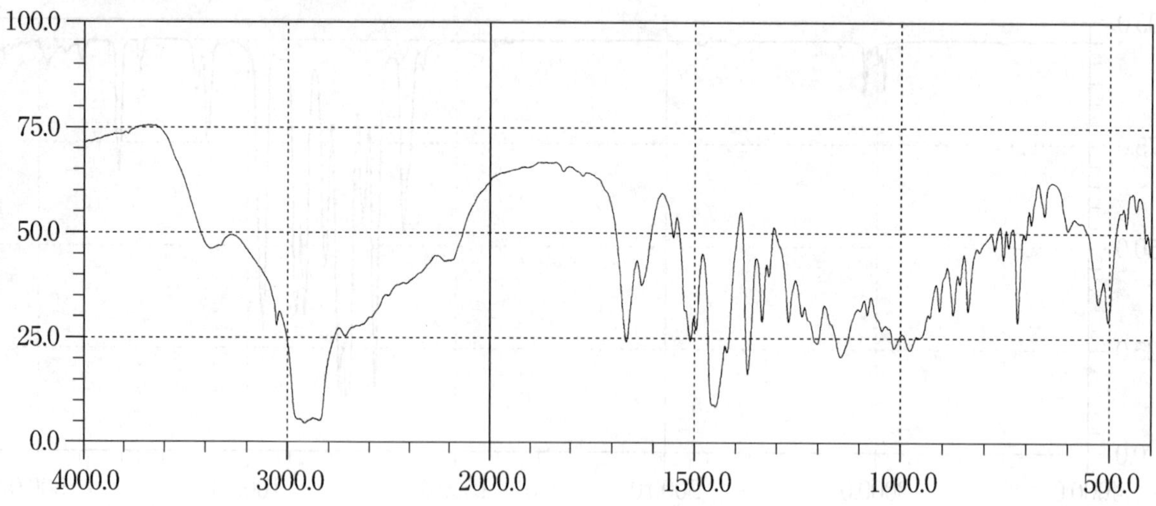

Sivelestat Sodium Hydrate

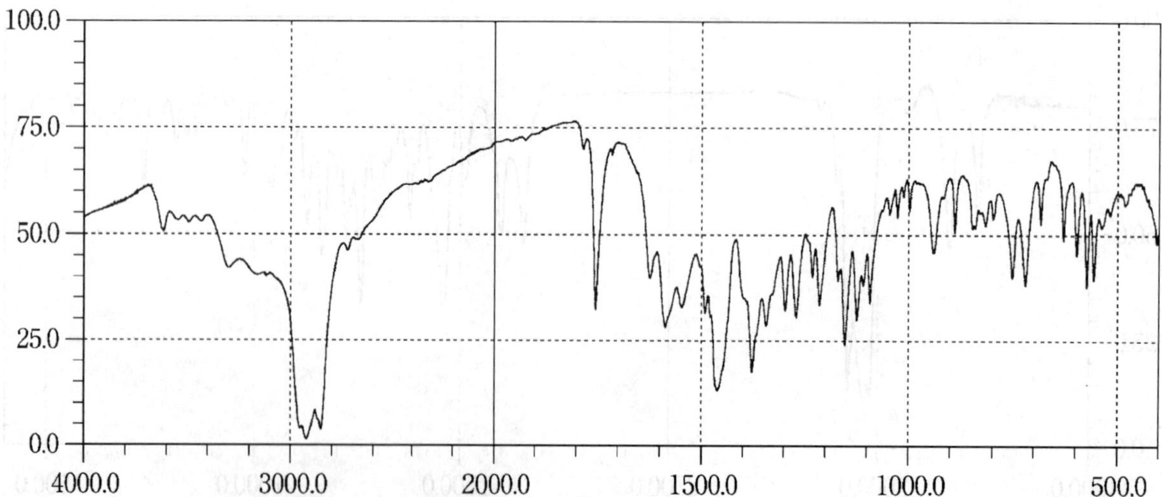

Sodium Fusidate

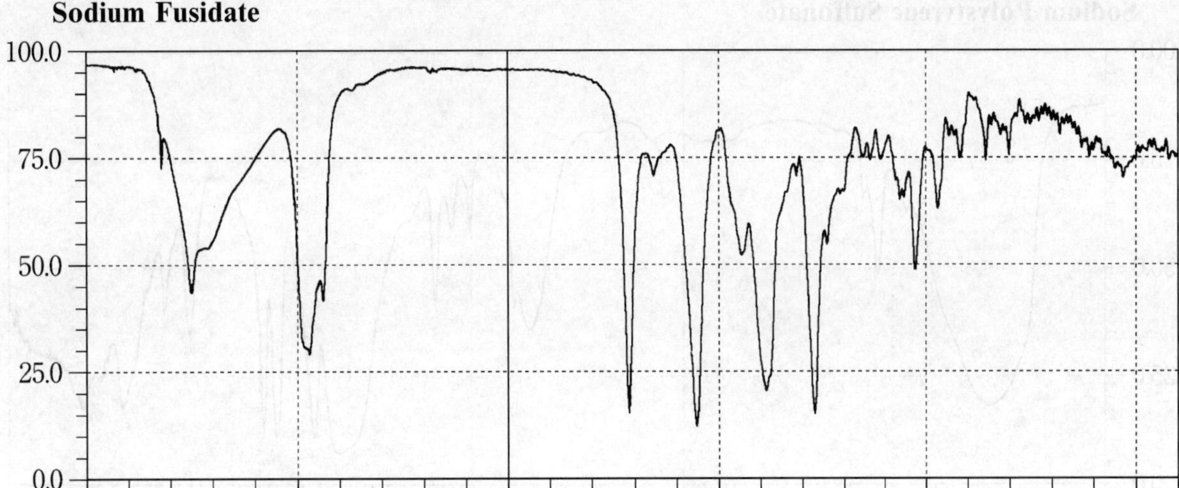

Sodium Lauryl Sulfate

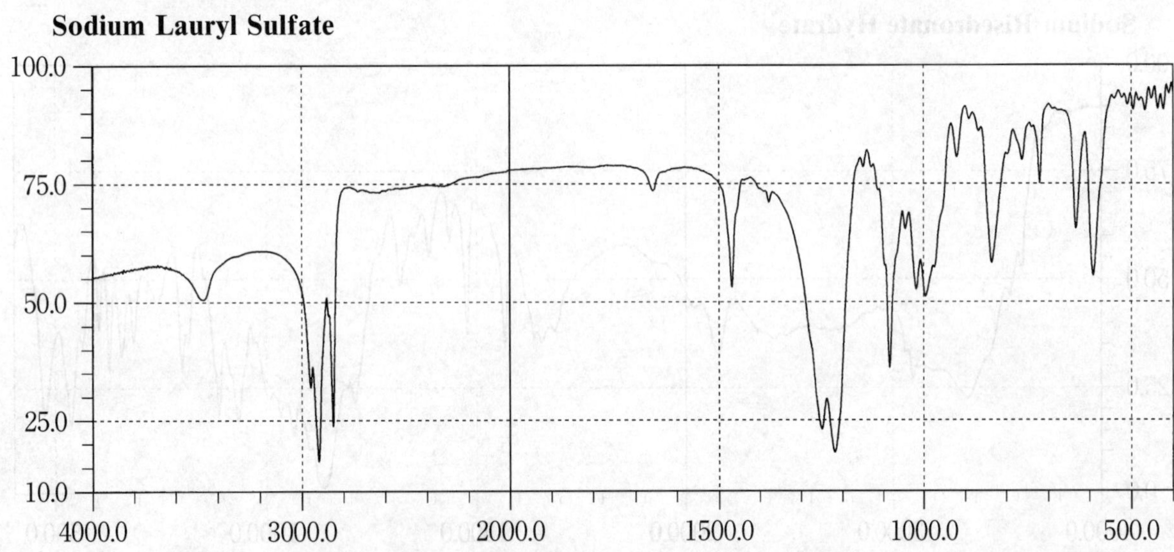

Sodium Picosulfate Hydrate

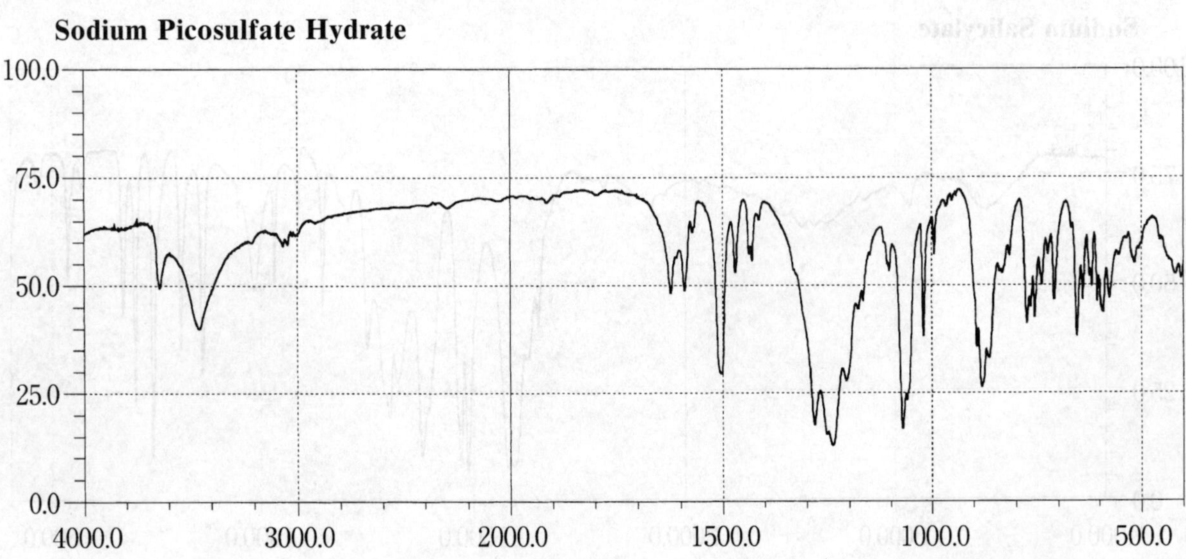

Sodium Polystyrene Sulfonate

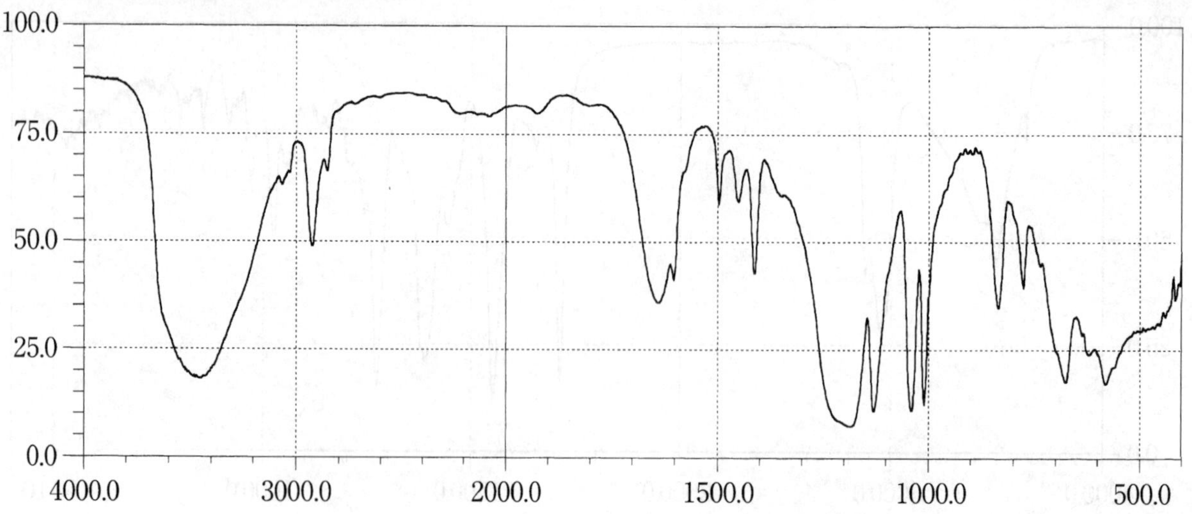

Sodium Risedronate Hydrate

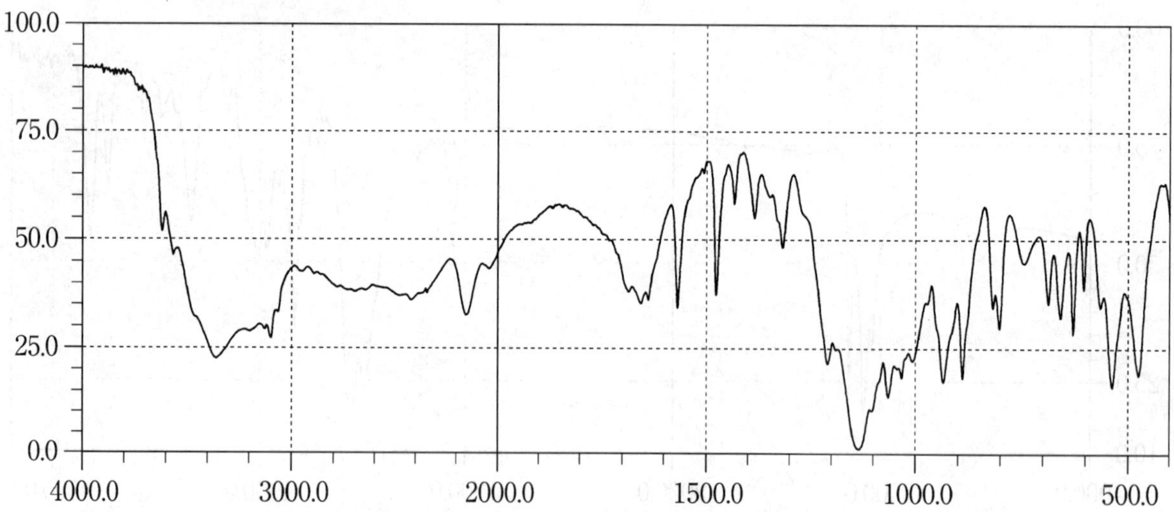

Sodium Salicylate

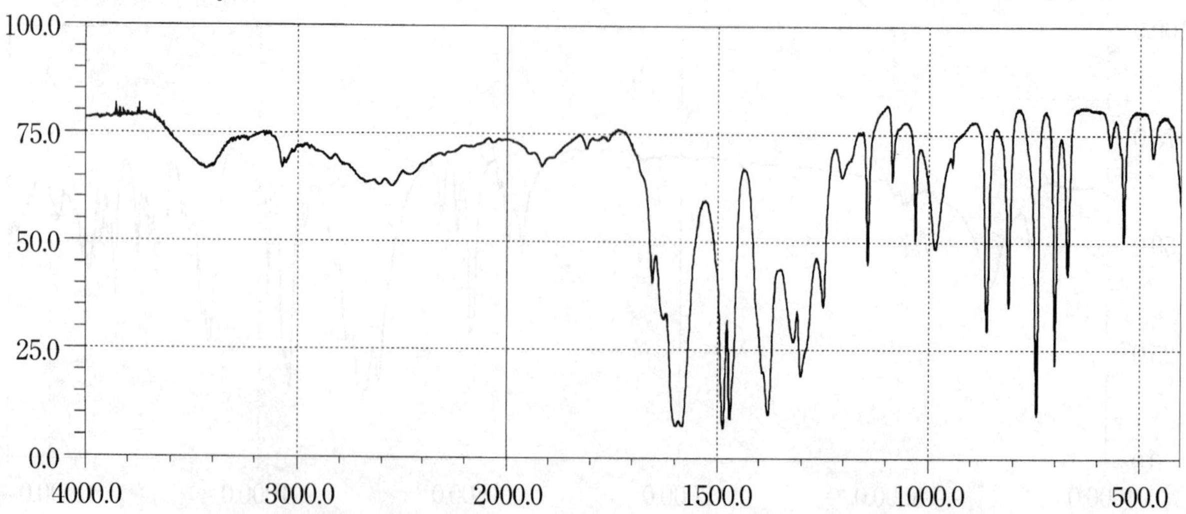

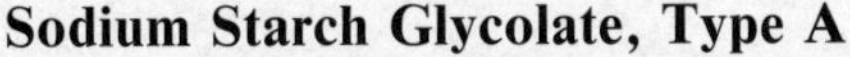

Sodium Starch Glycolate, Type A

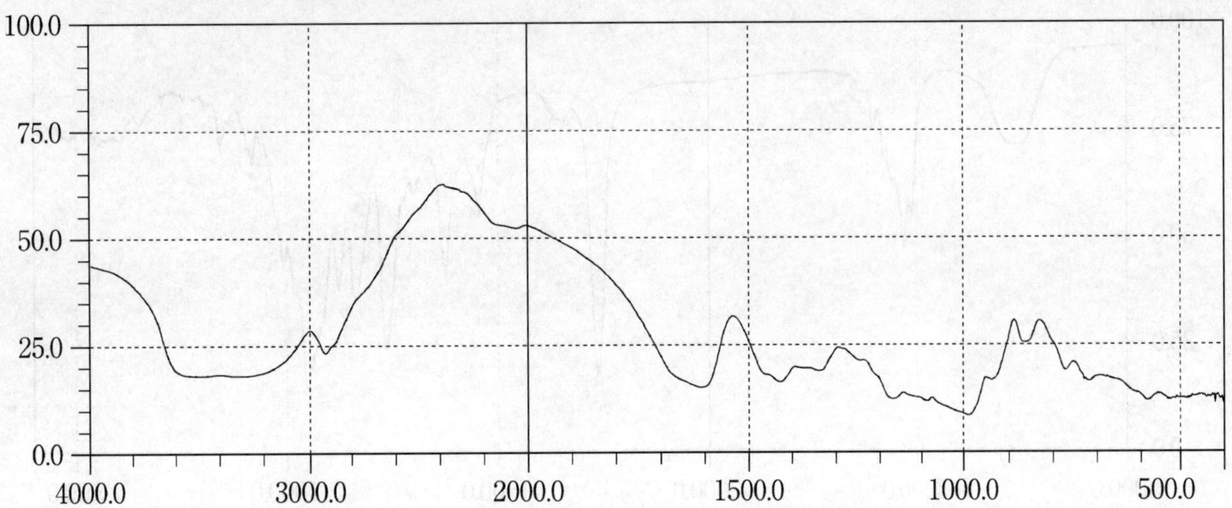

Sodium Starch Glycolate, Type B

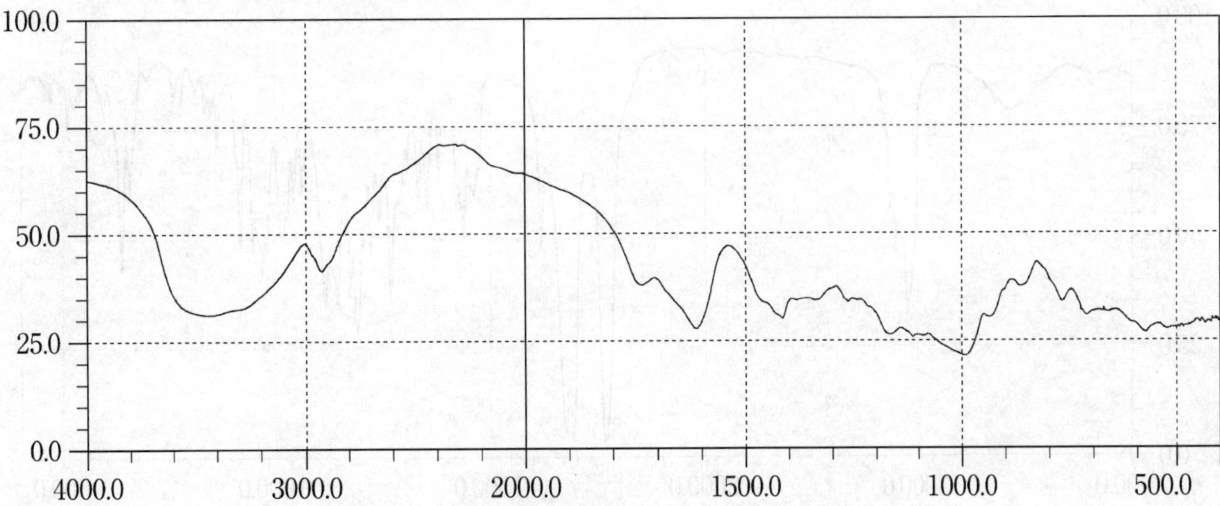

Sodium Valproate

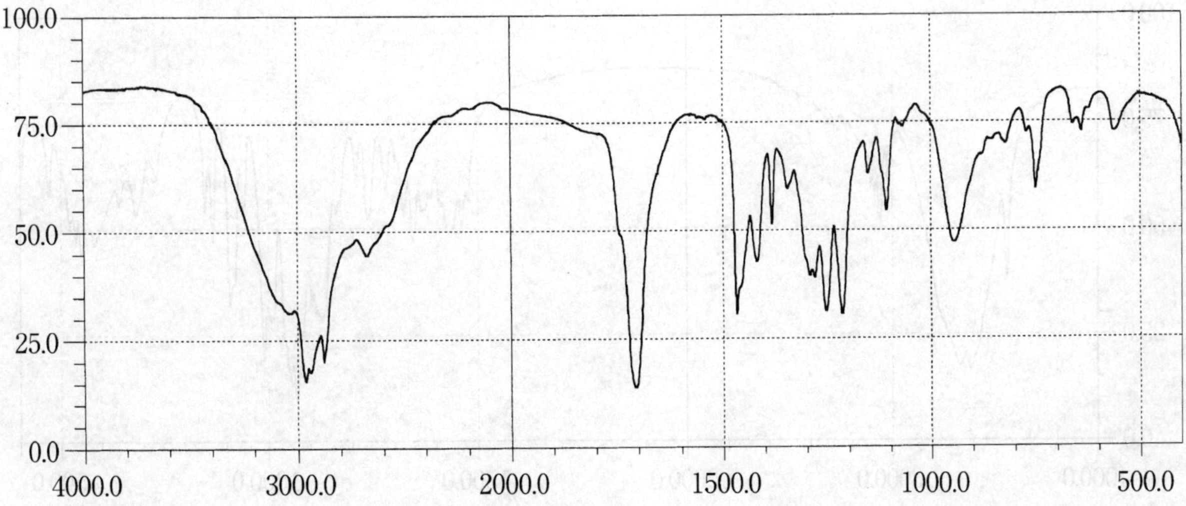

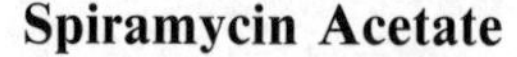

Spiramycin Acetate

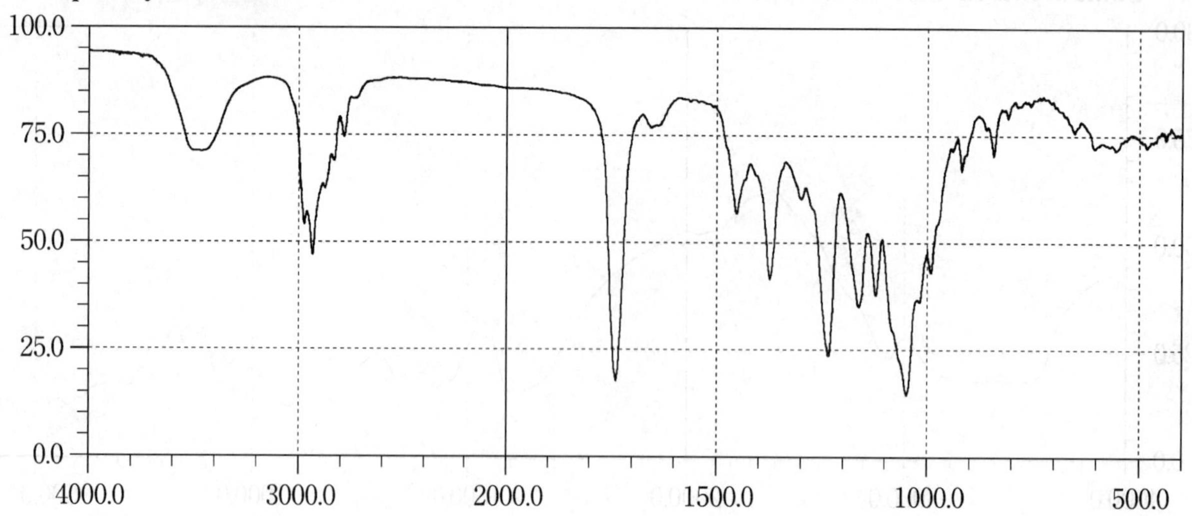

Spironolactone

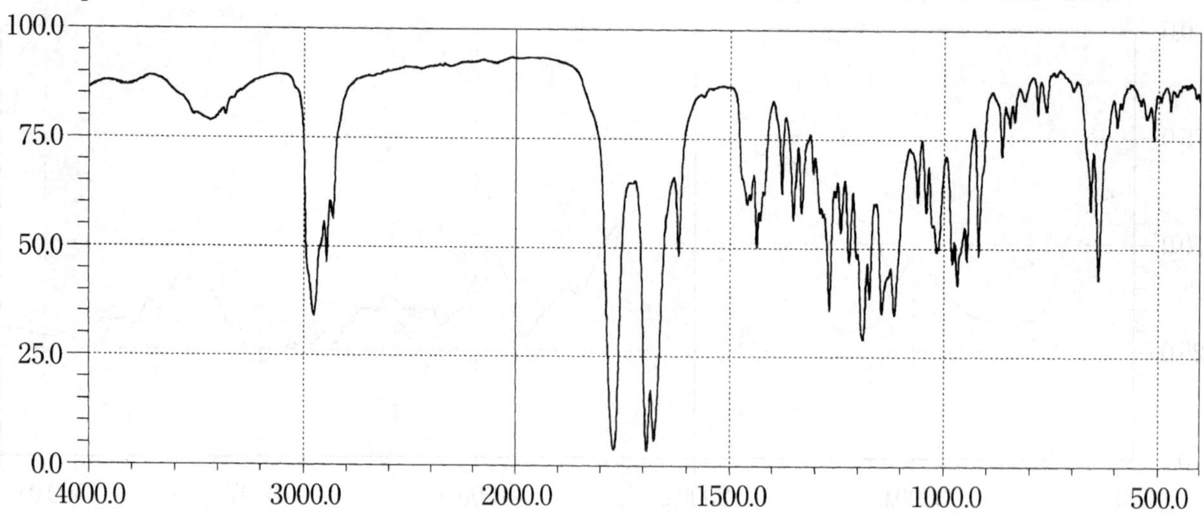

Sucrose

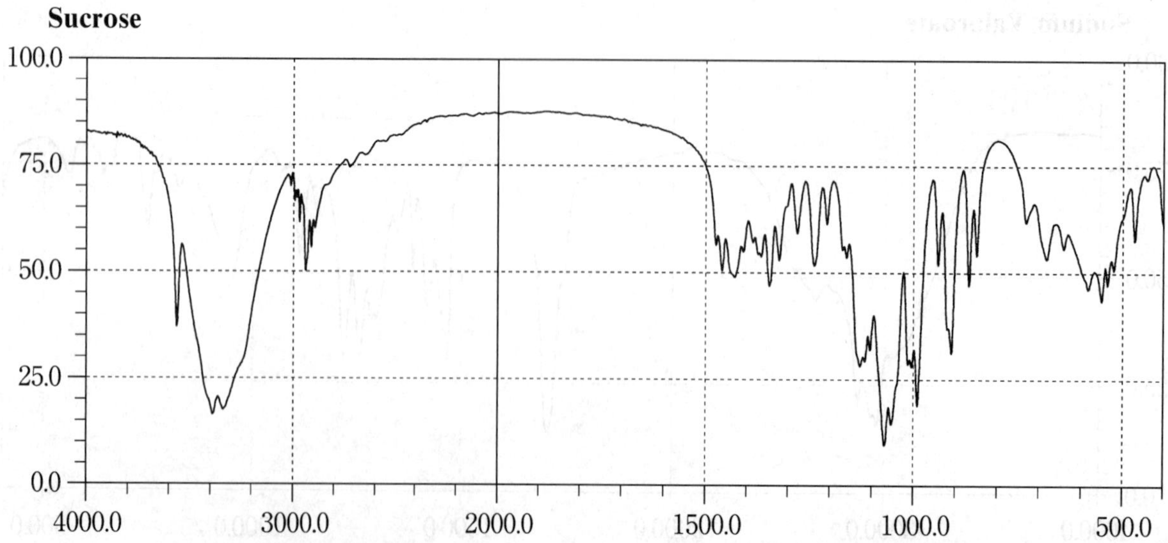

Sulbactam Sodium

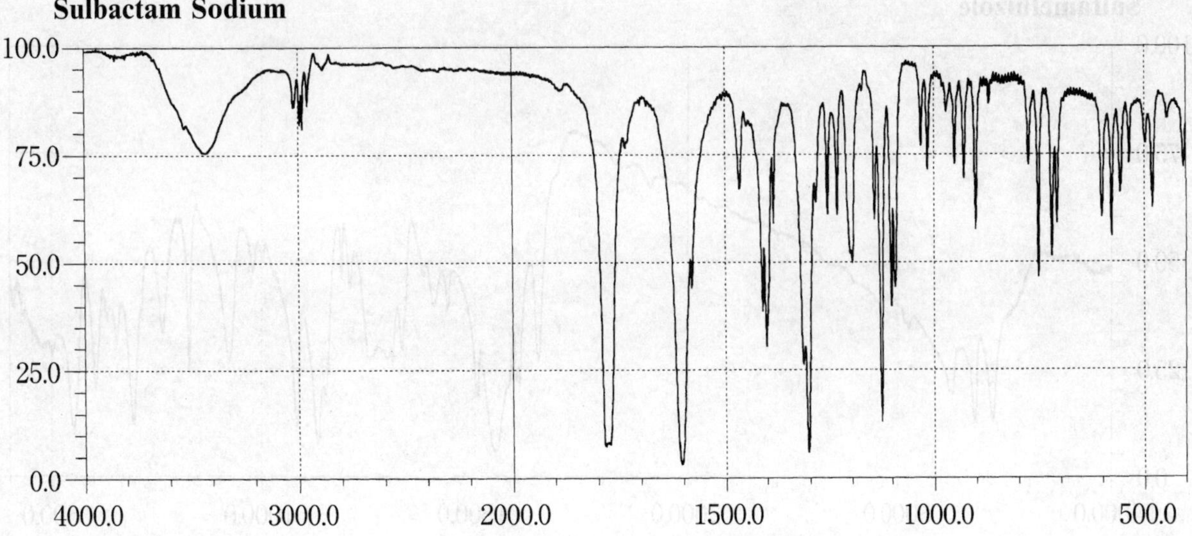

Sulbenicillin Sodium

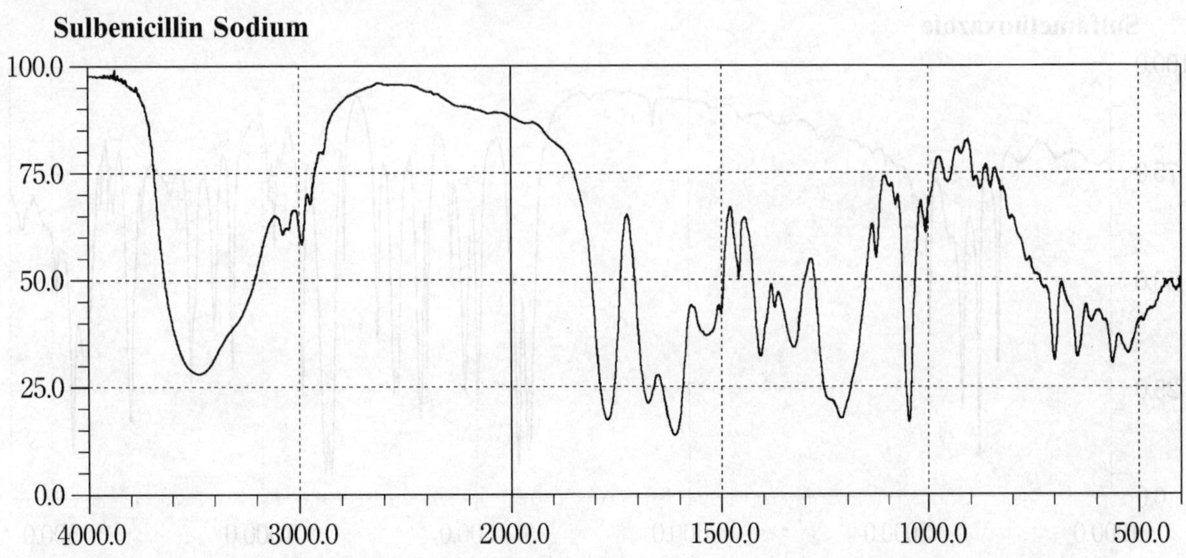

Sulfadiazine Silver

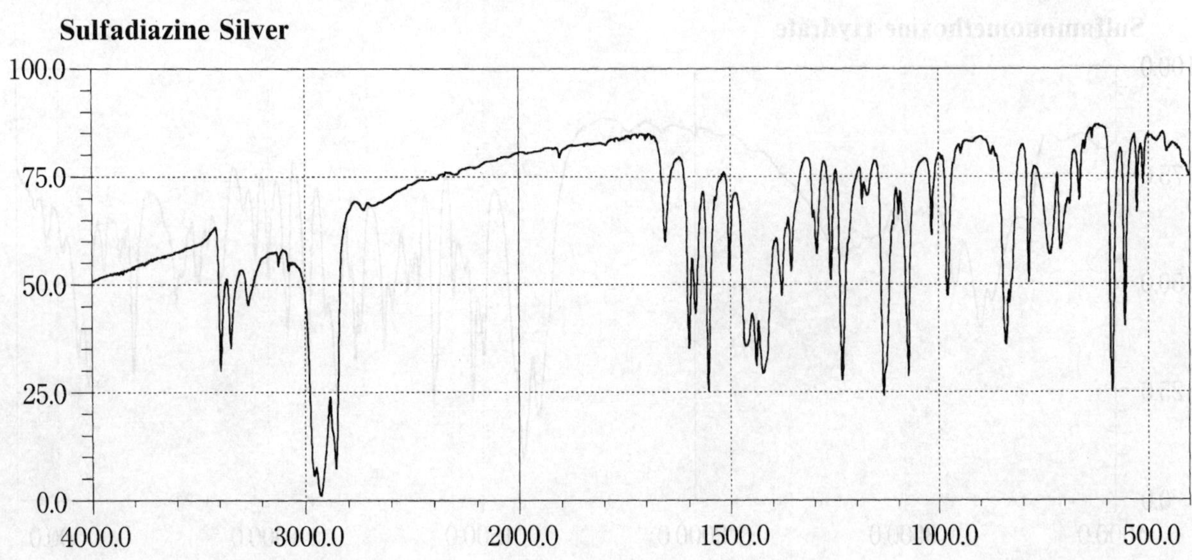

Sulfamethizole

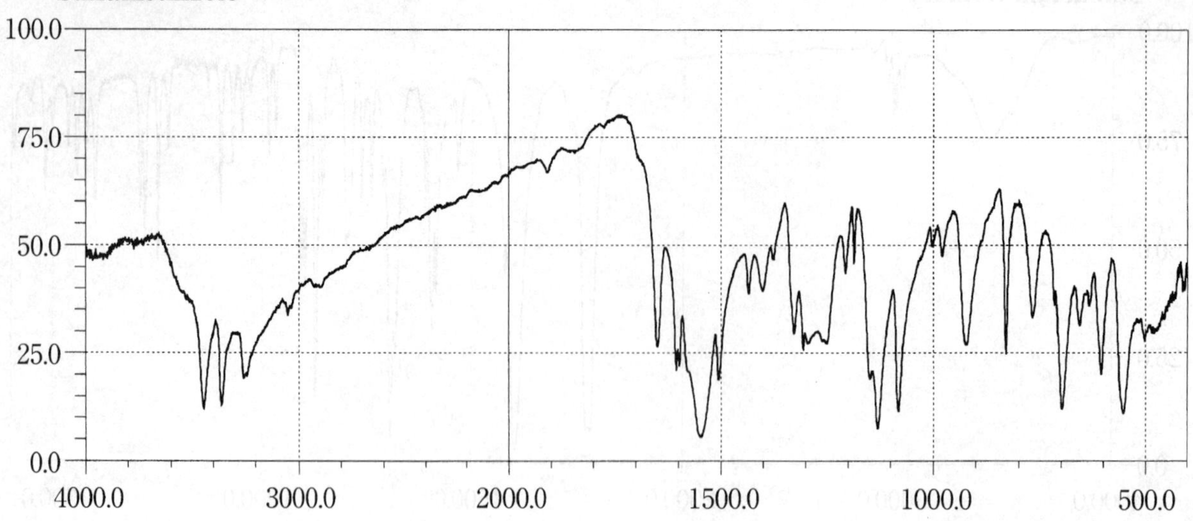

Sulfamethoxazole

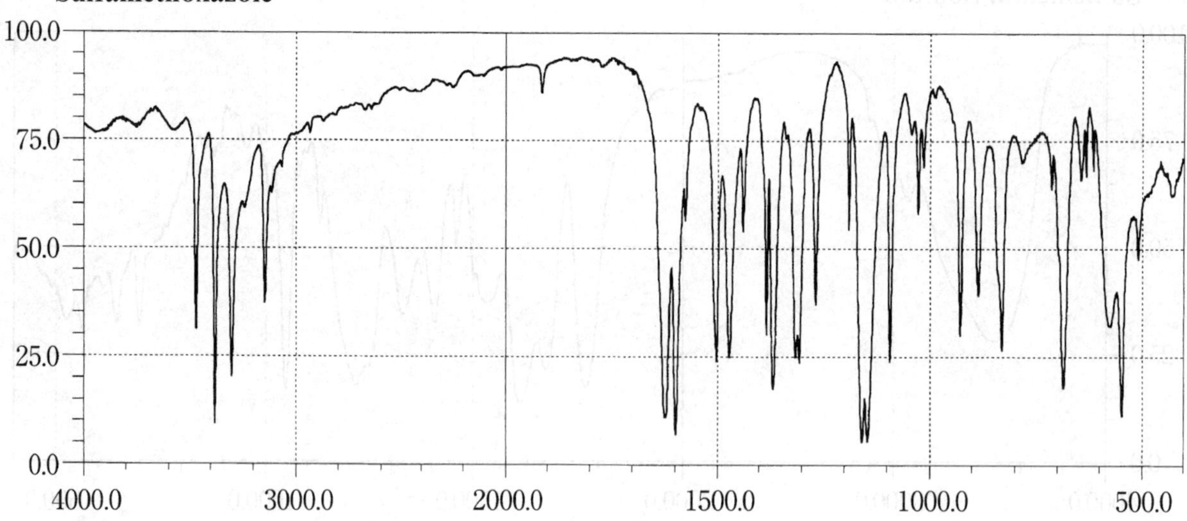

Sulfamonomethoxine Hydrate

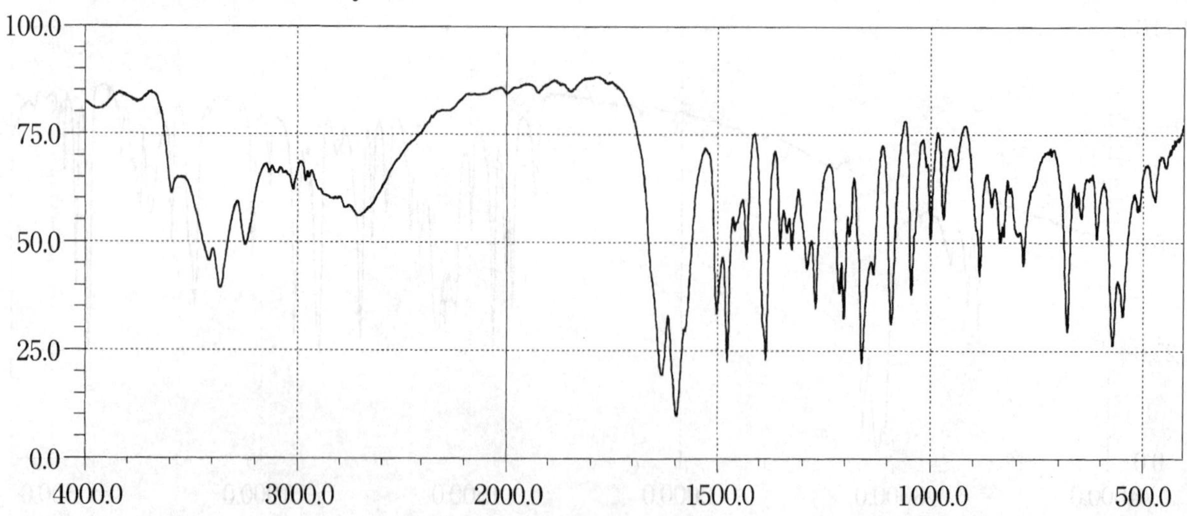

Sulindac

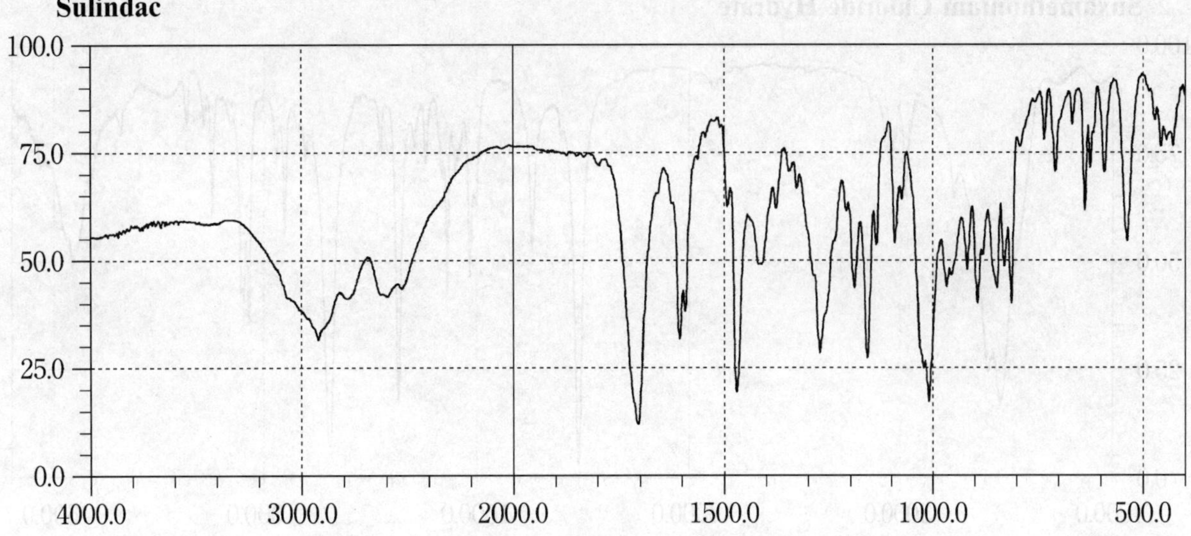

Sulpiride

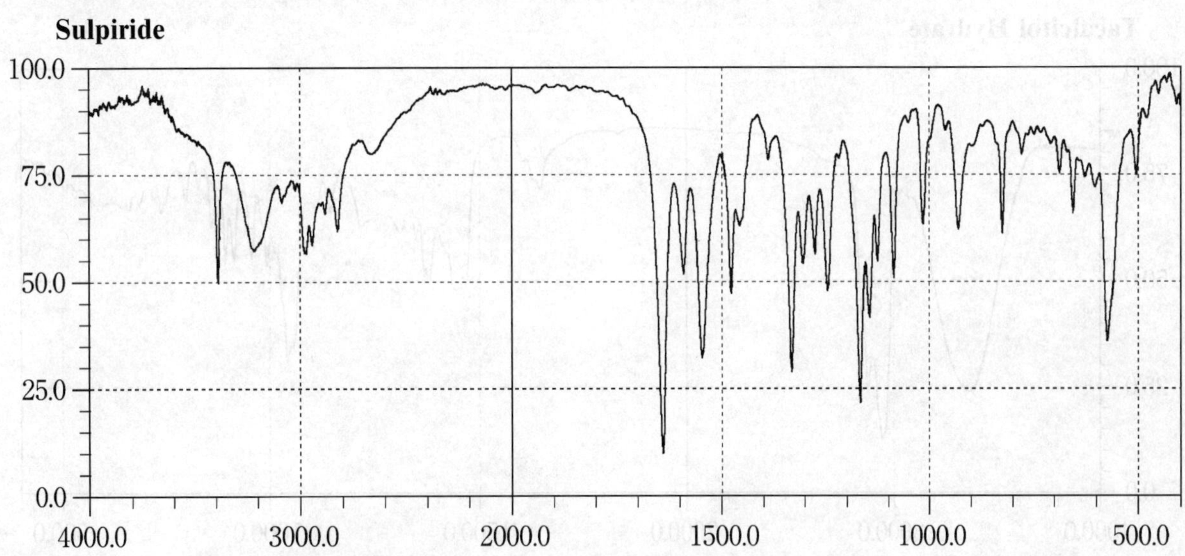

Sultamicillin Tosilate Hydrate

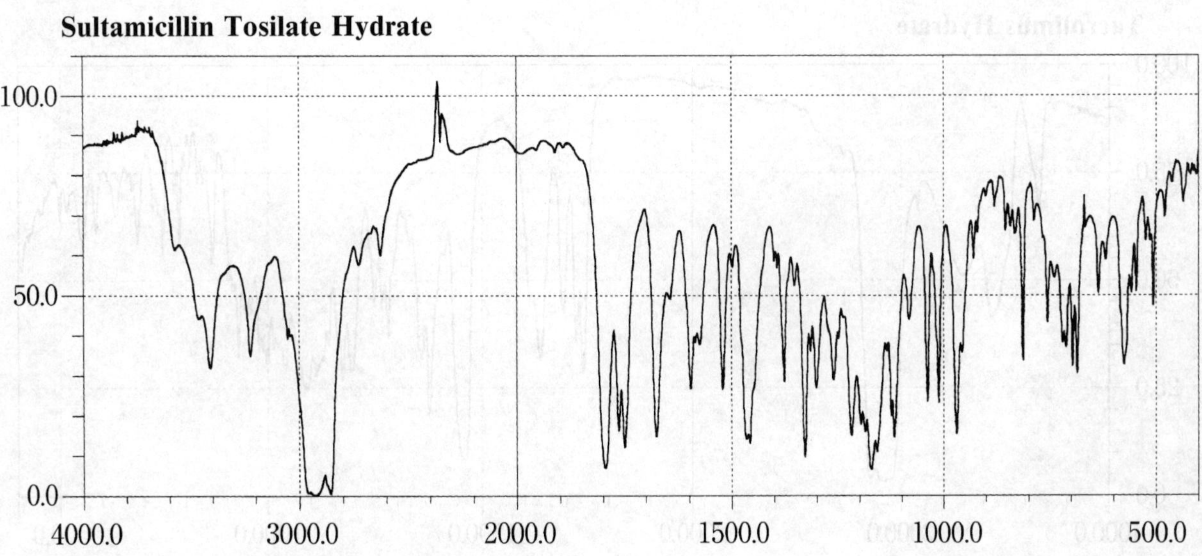

Suxamethonium Chloride Hydrate

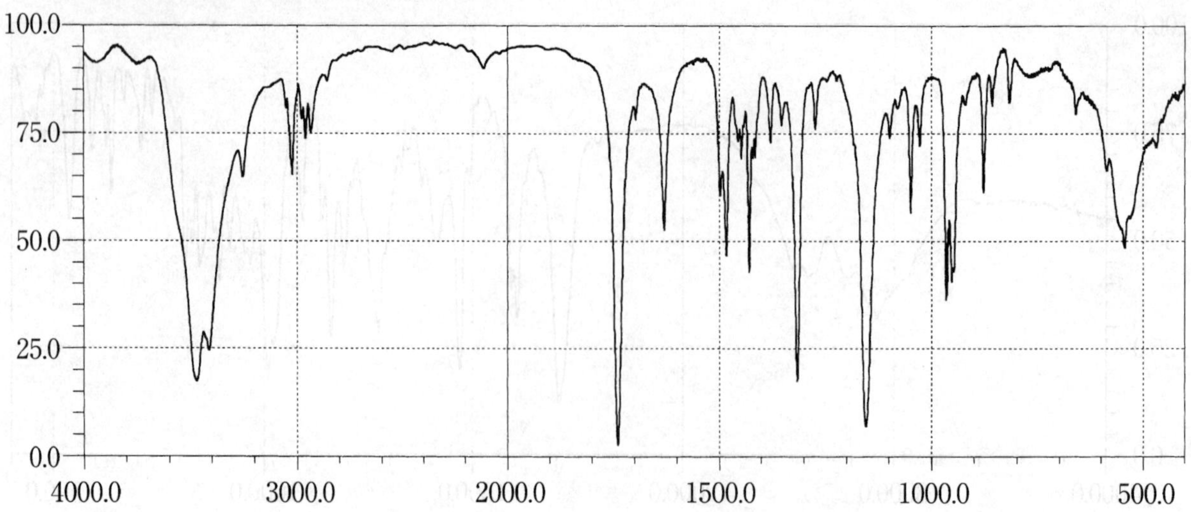

Tacalcitol Hydrate

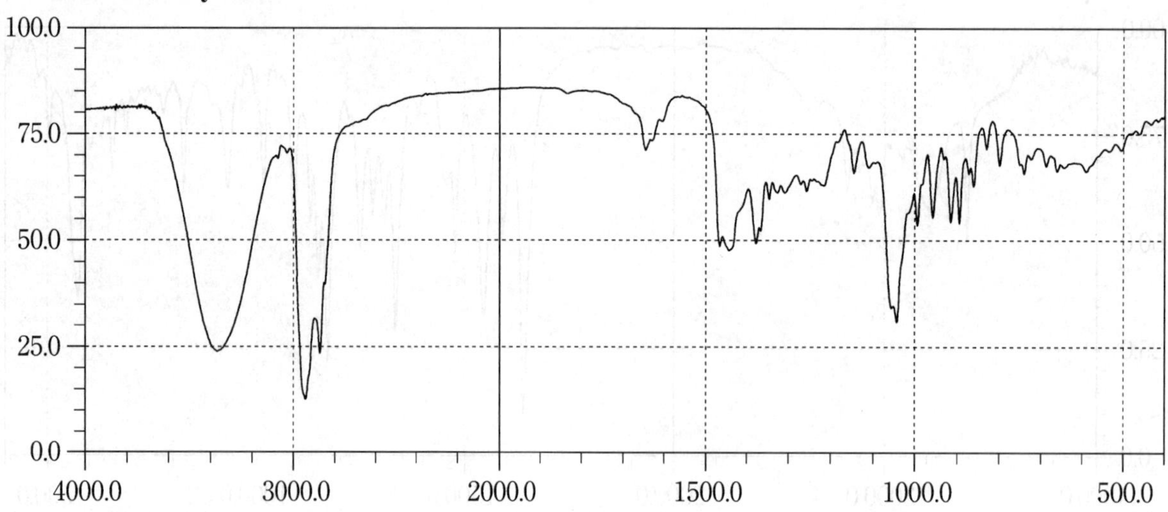

Tacrolimus Hydrate

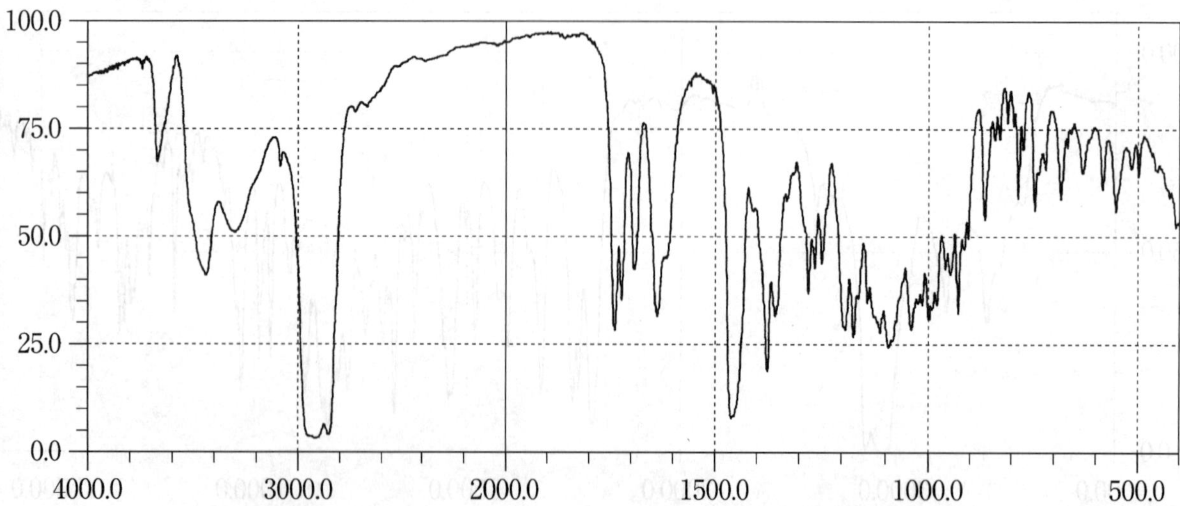

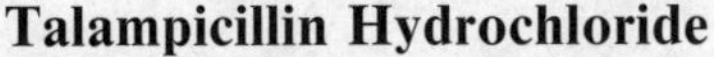

Talampicillin Hydrochloride

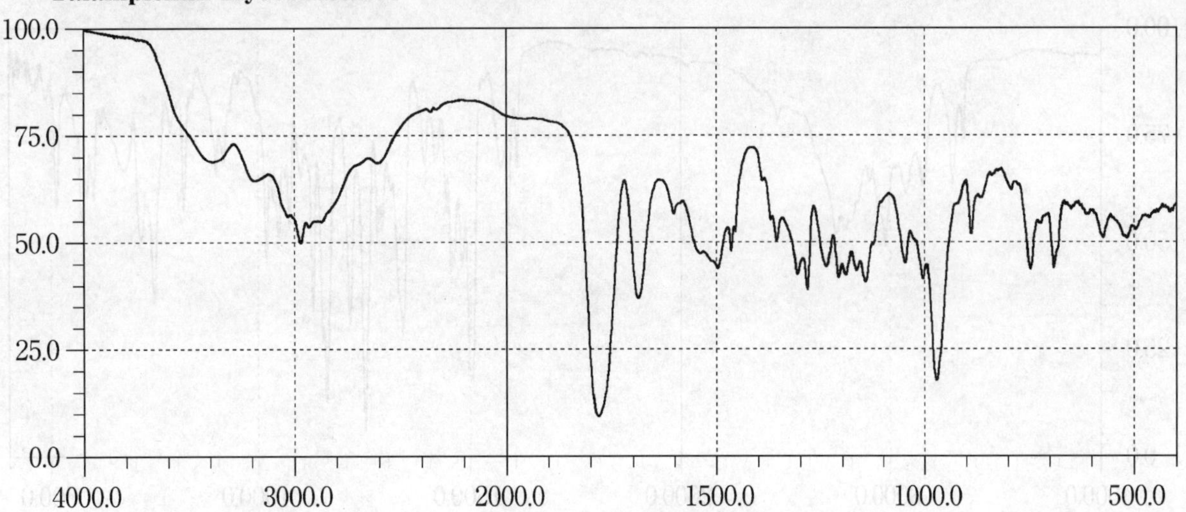

Taltirelin Hydrate

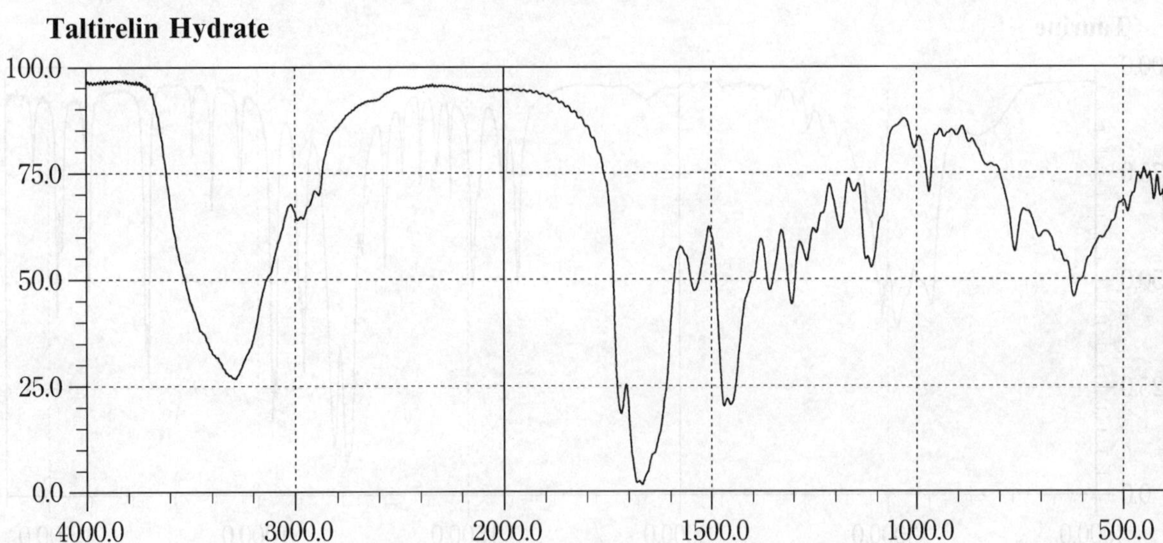

Tamoxifen Citrate

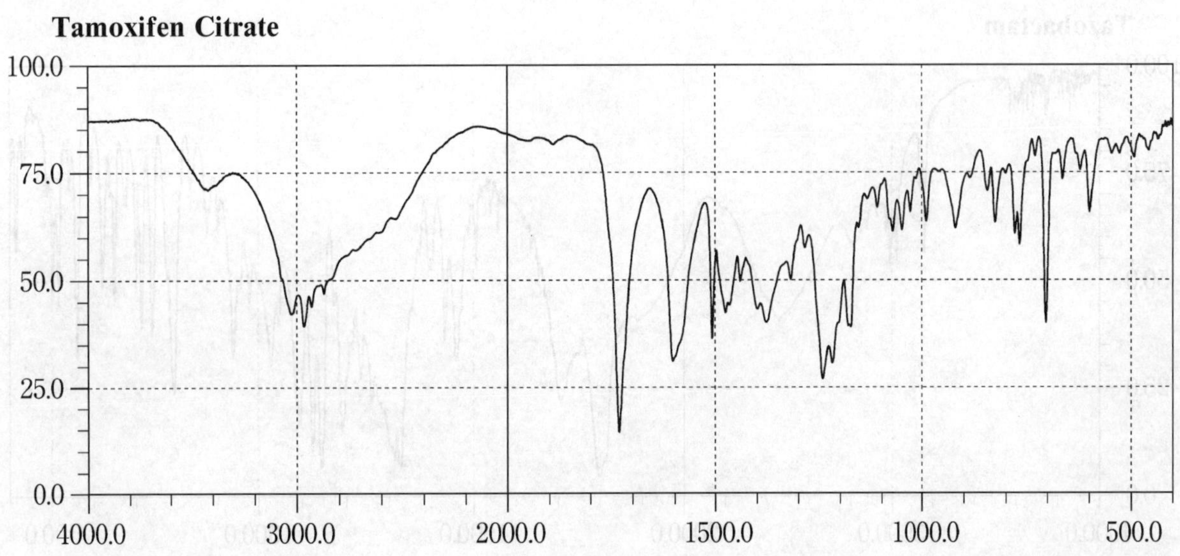

Tamsulosin Hydrochloride

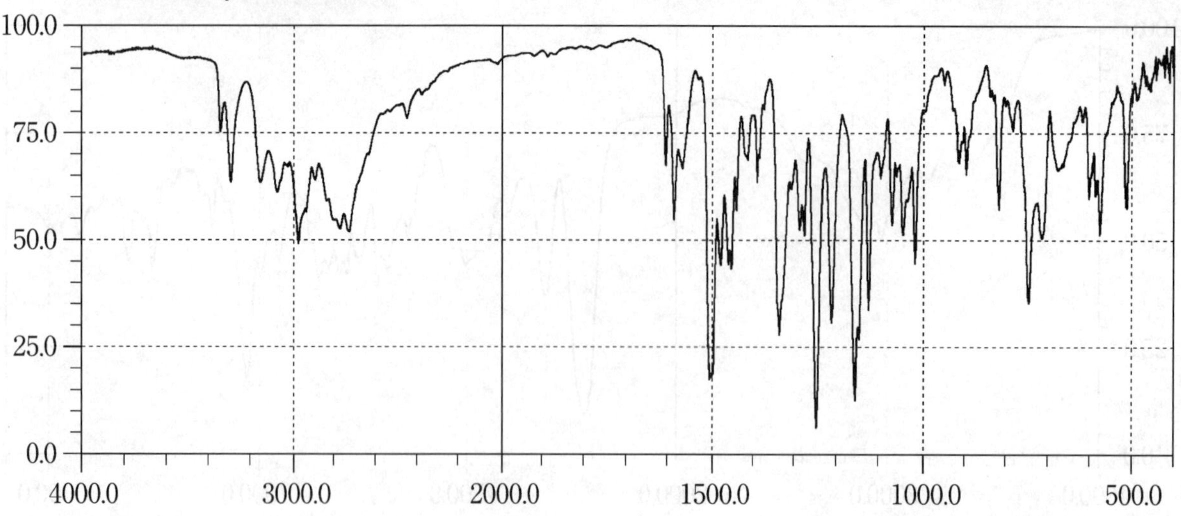

Taurine

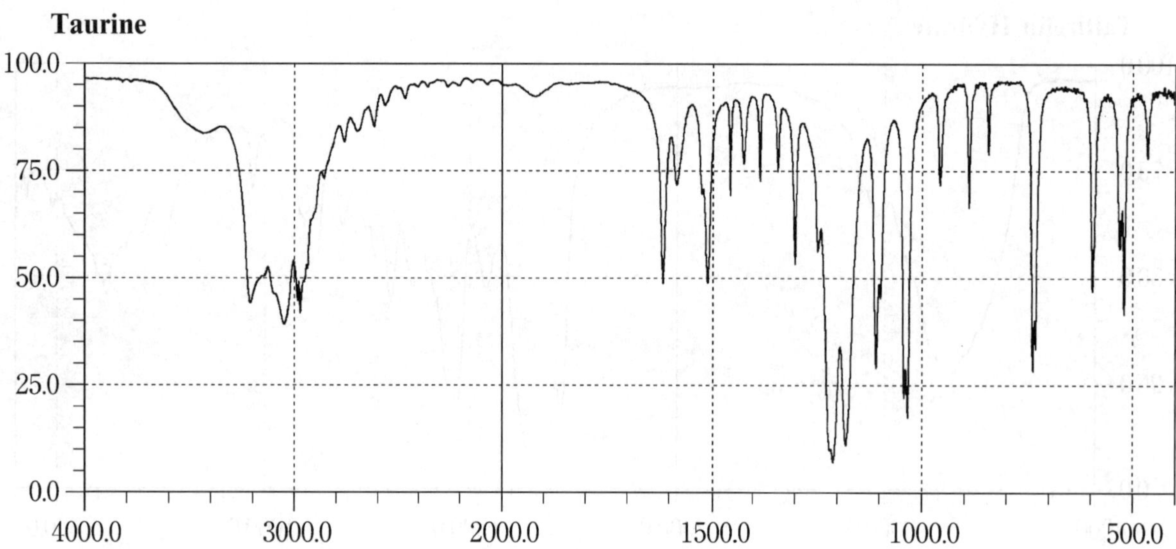

Tazobactam

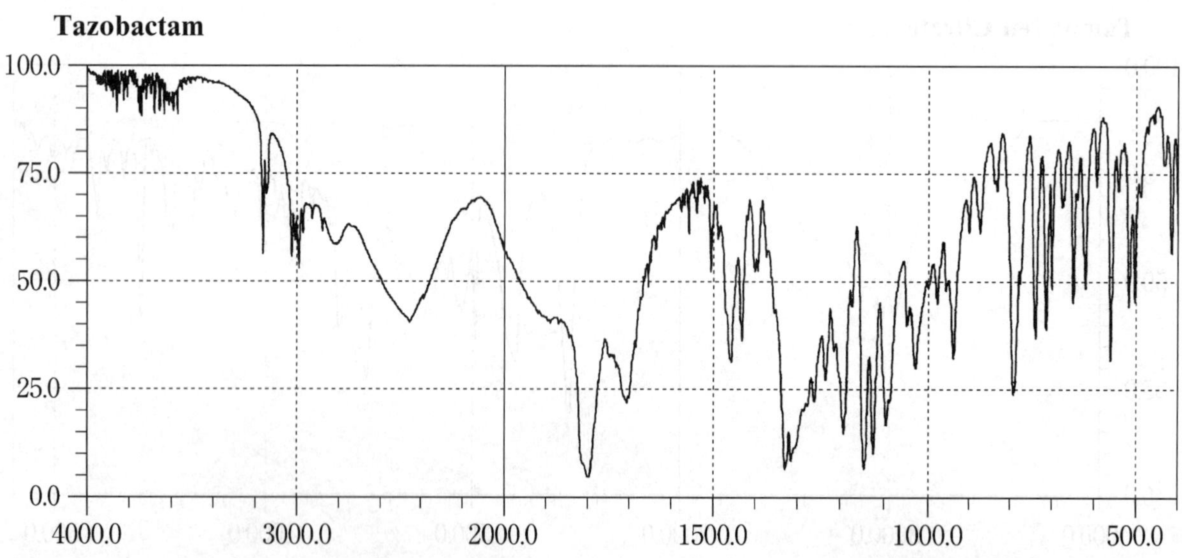

Tegafur

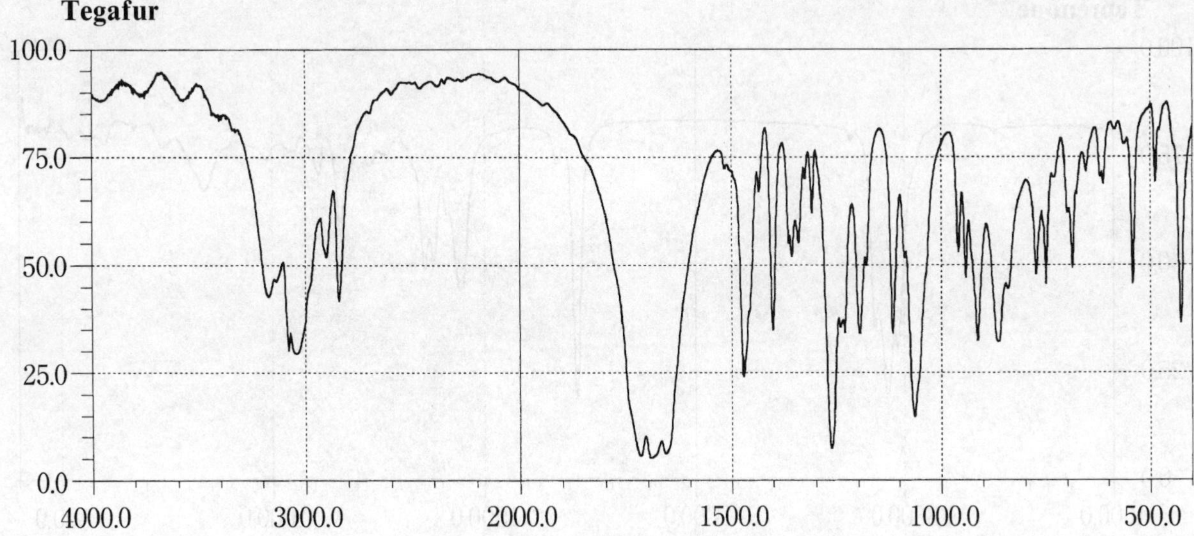

Telmisartan

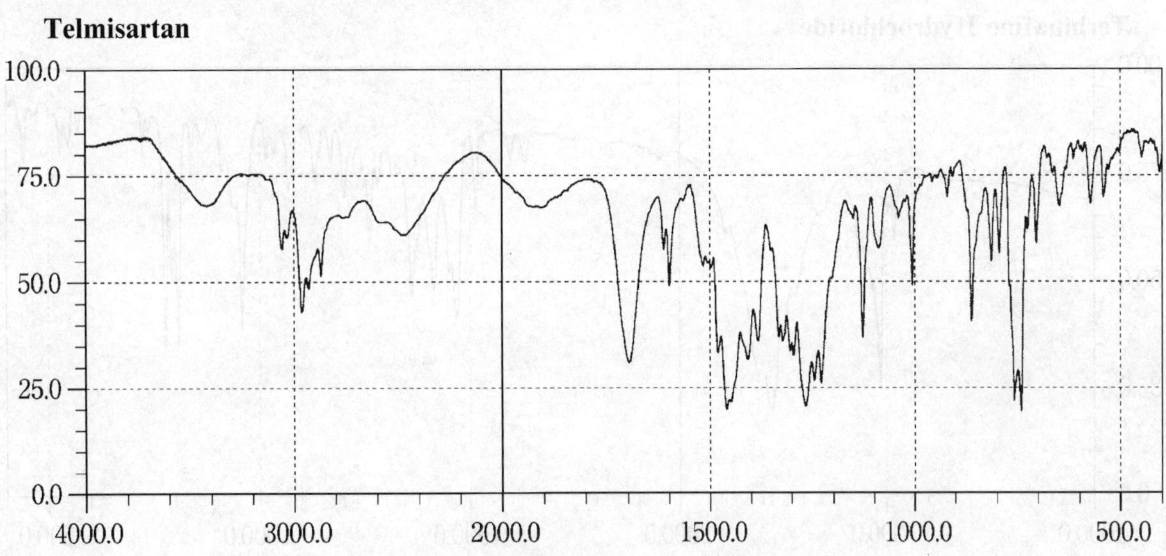

Temocapril Hydrochloride

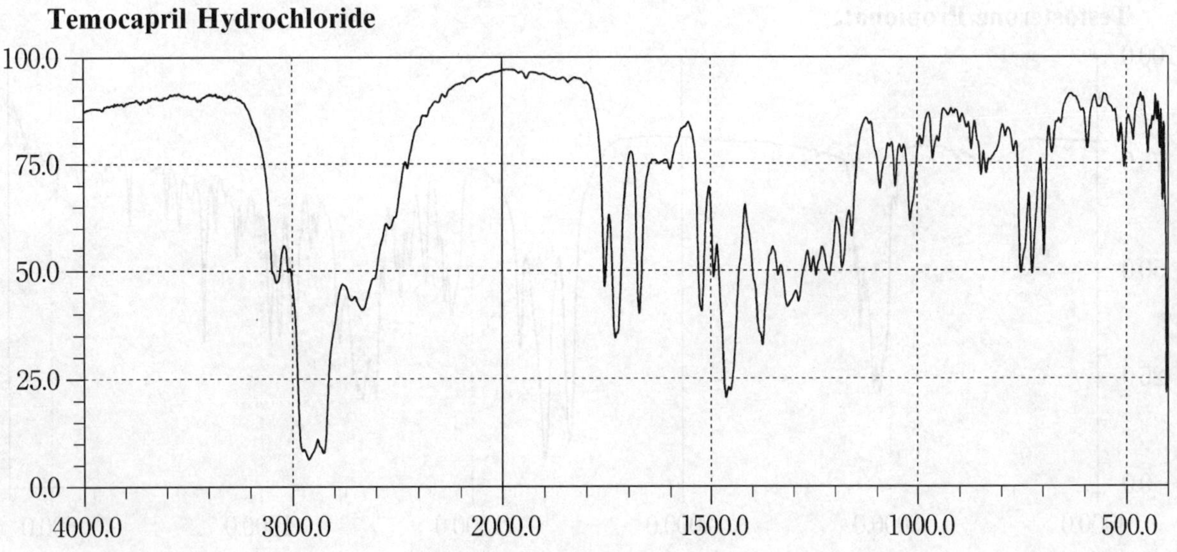

Teprenone

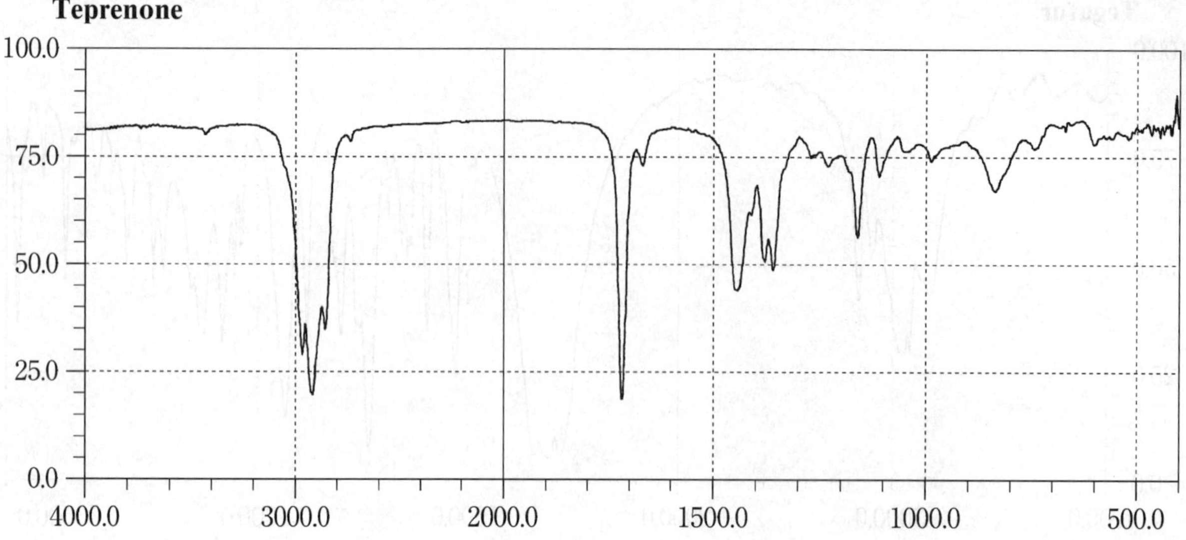

Terbinafine Hydrochloride

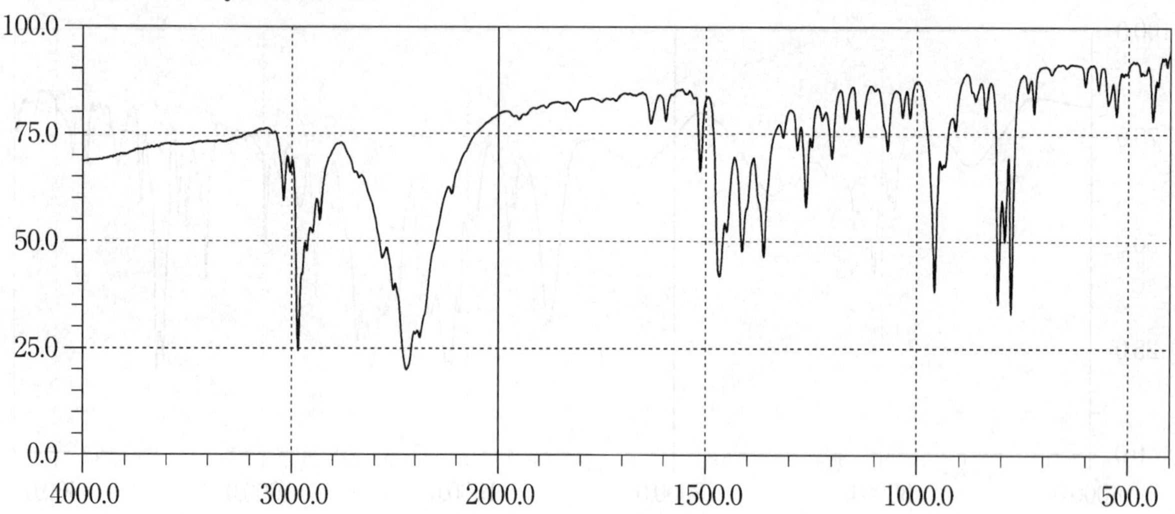

Testosterone Propionate

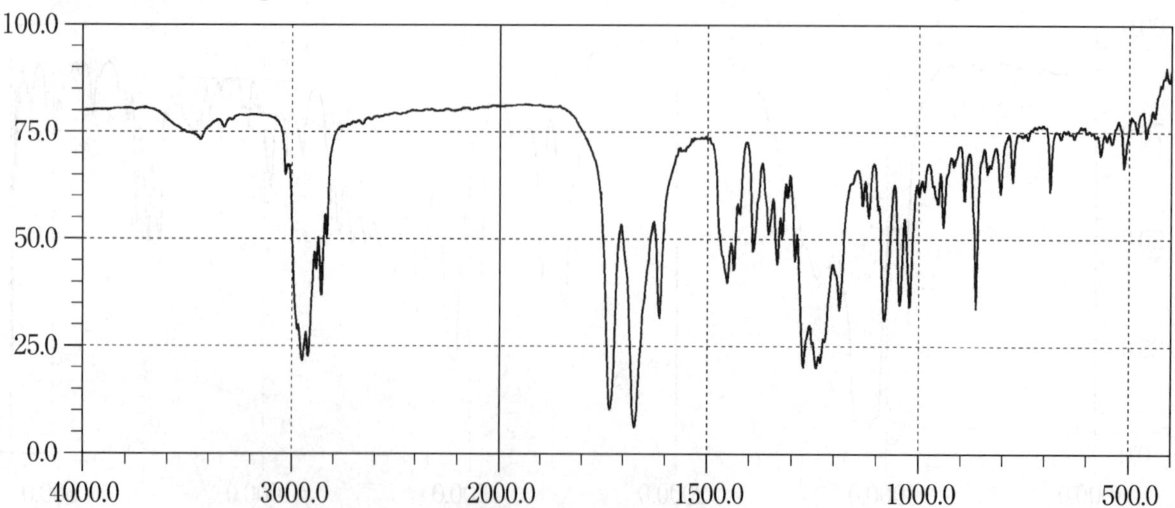

Tetracycline Hydrochloride

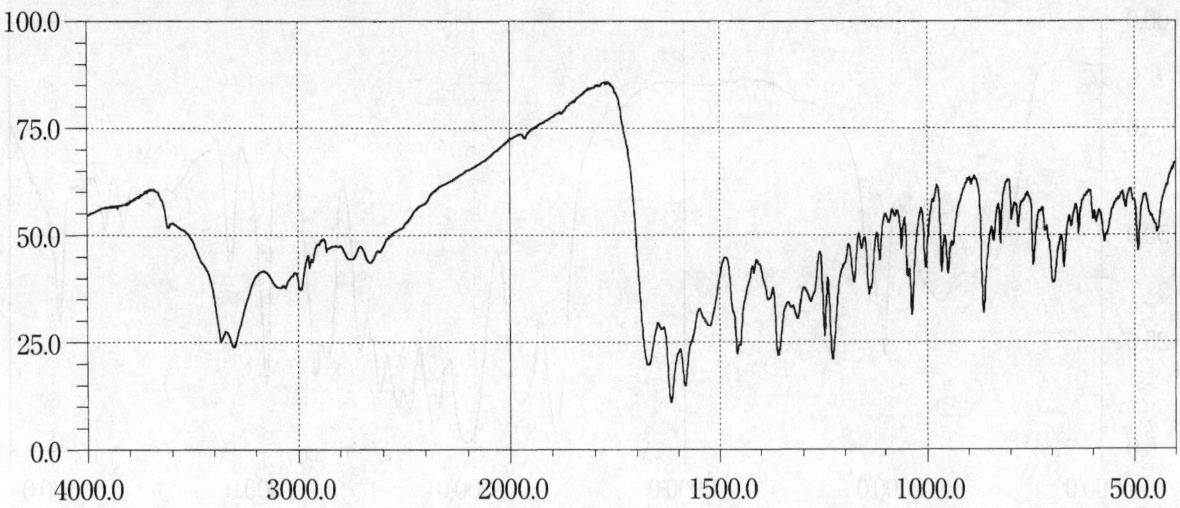

Theophylline

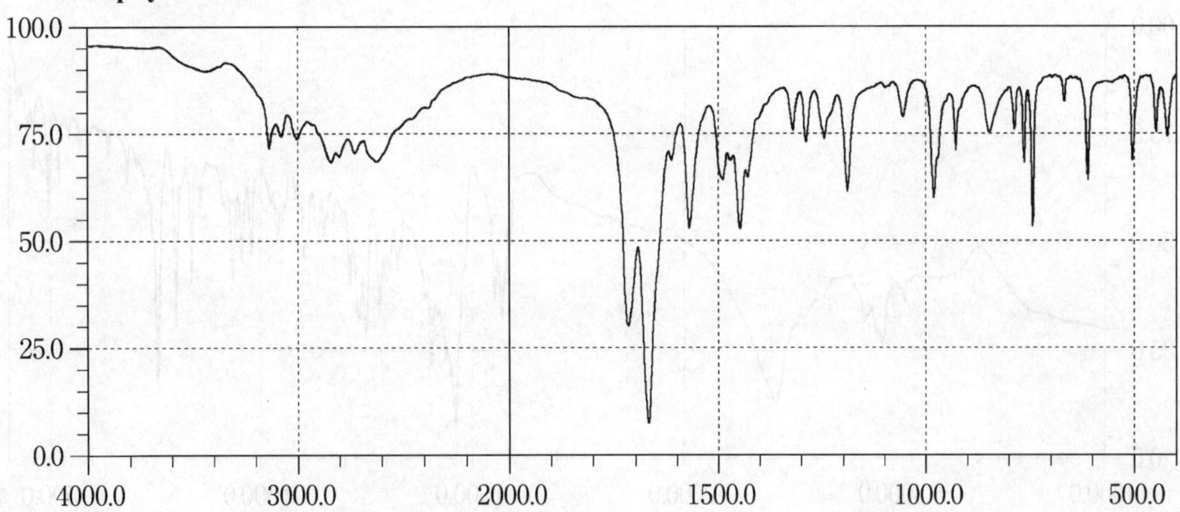

Thiamine Chloride Hydrochloride

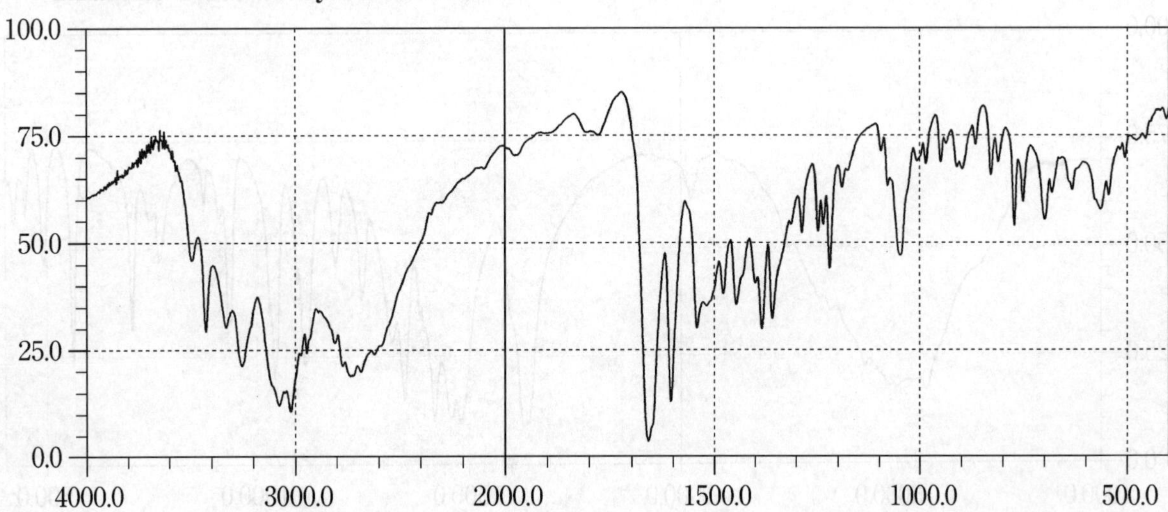

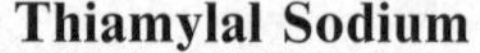

Thiamylal Sodium

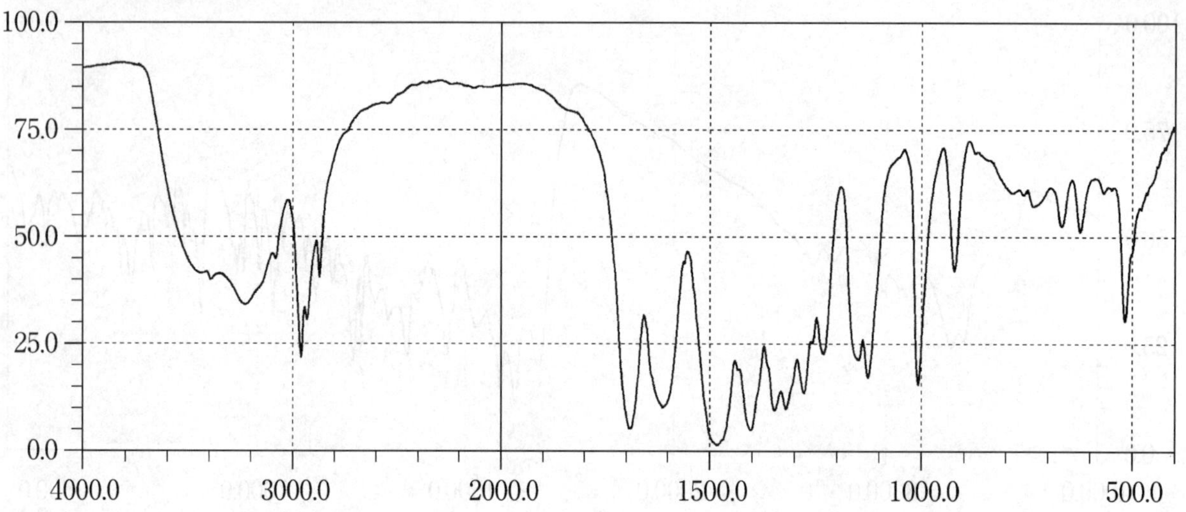

Thioridazine Hydrochloride

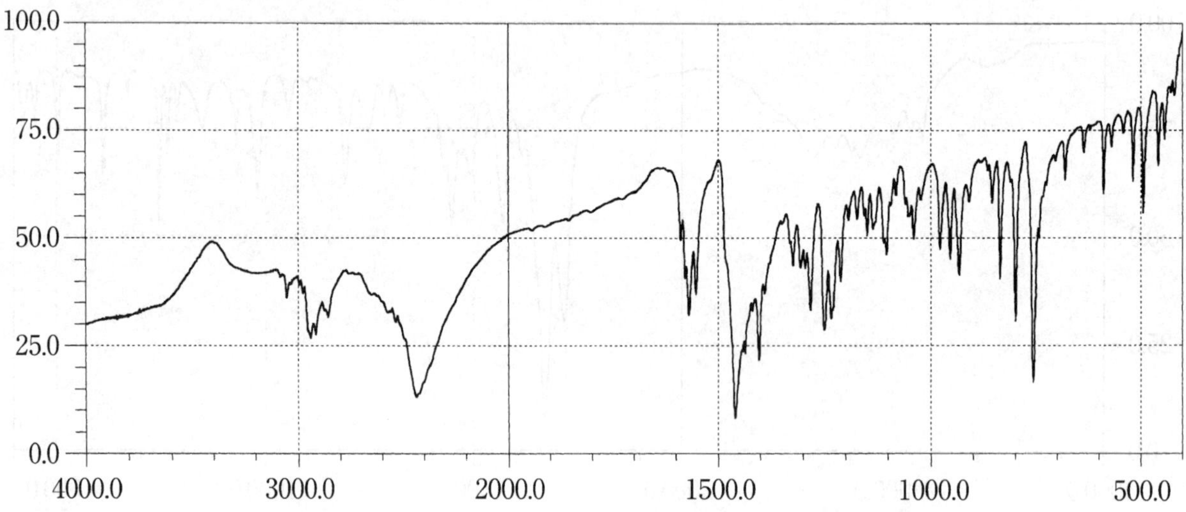

L-Threonine

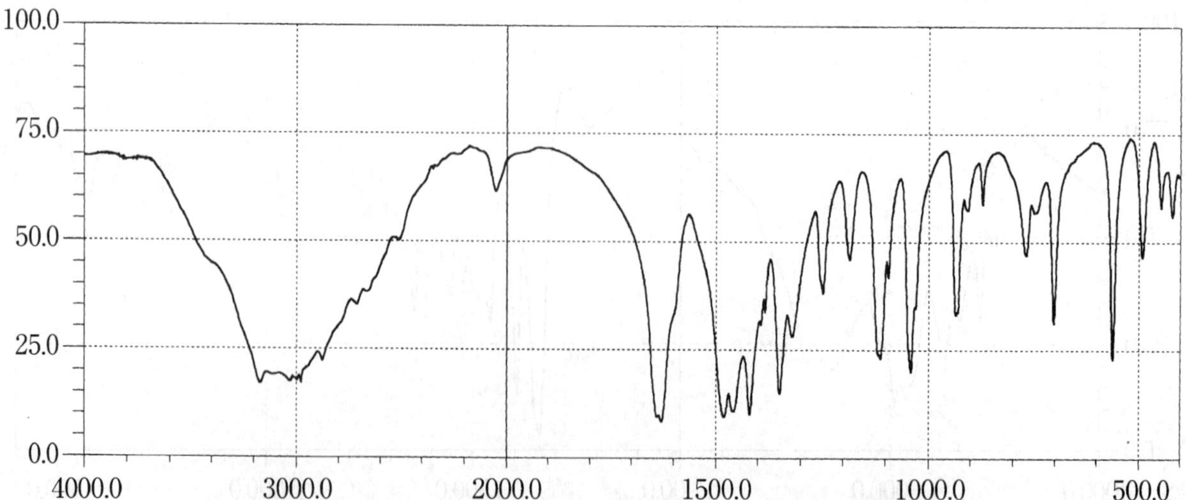

Tiapride Hydrochloride

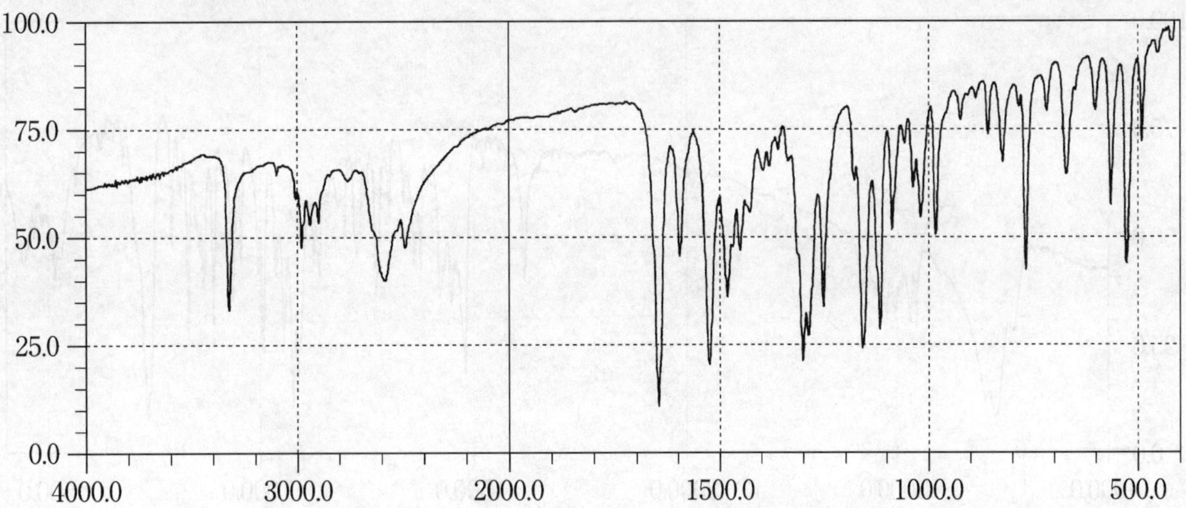

Tiaramide Hydrochloride

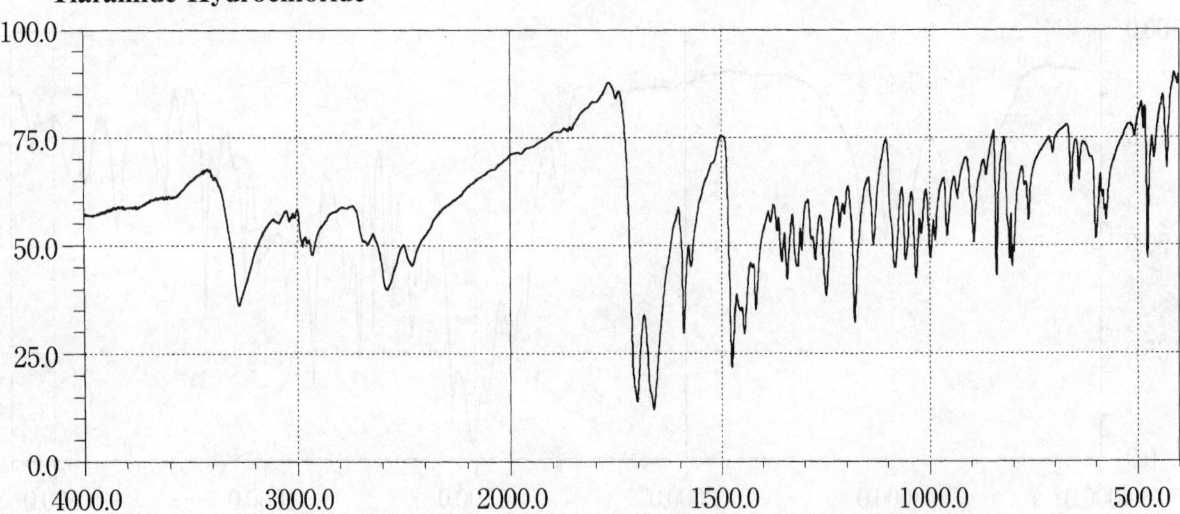

Ticlopidine Hydrochloride

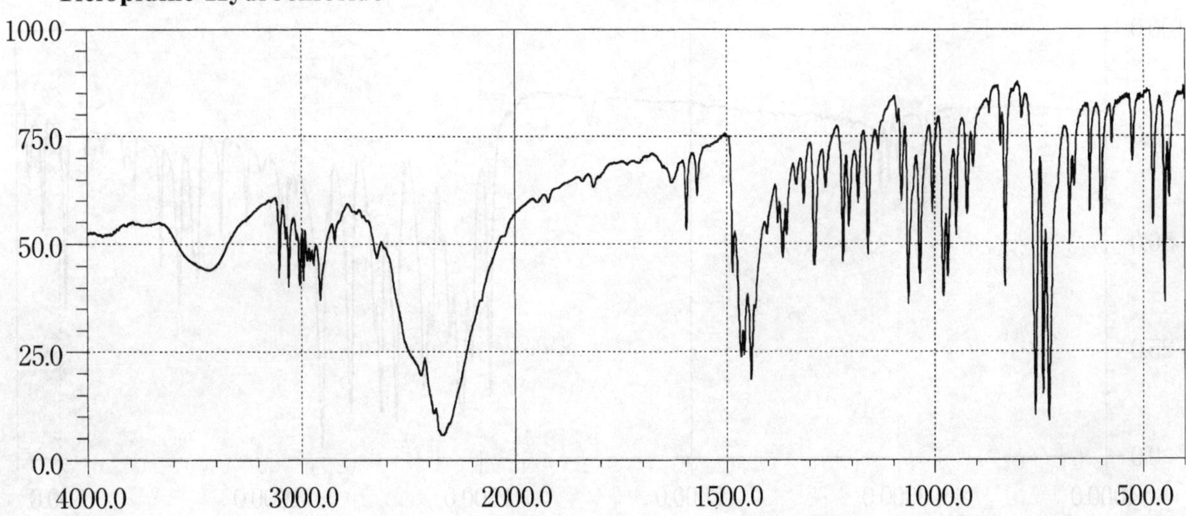

Timepidium Bromide Hydrate

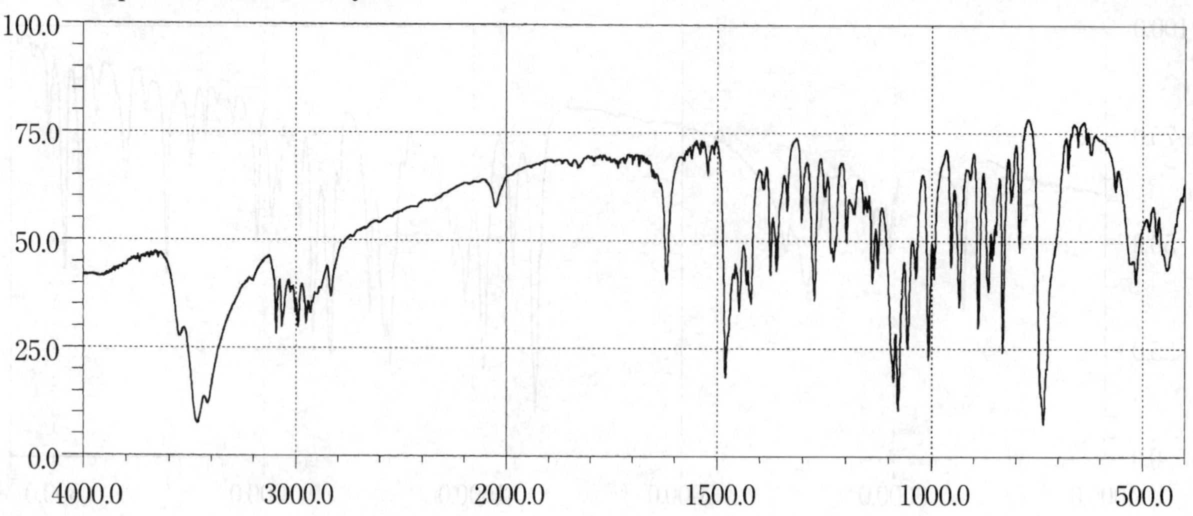

Timolol Maleate

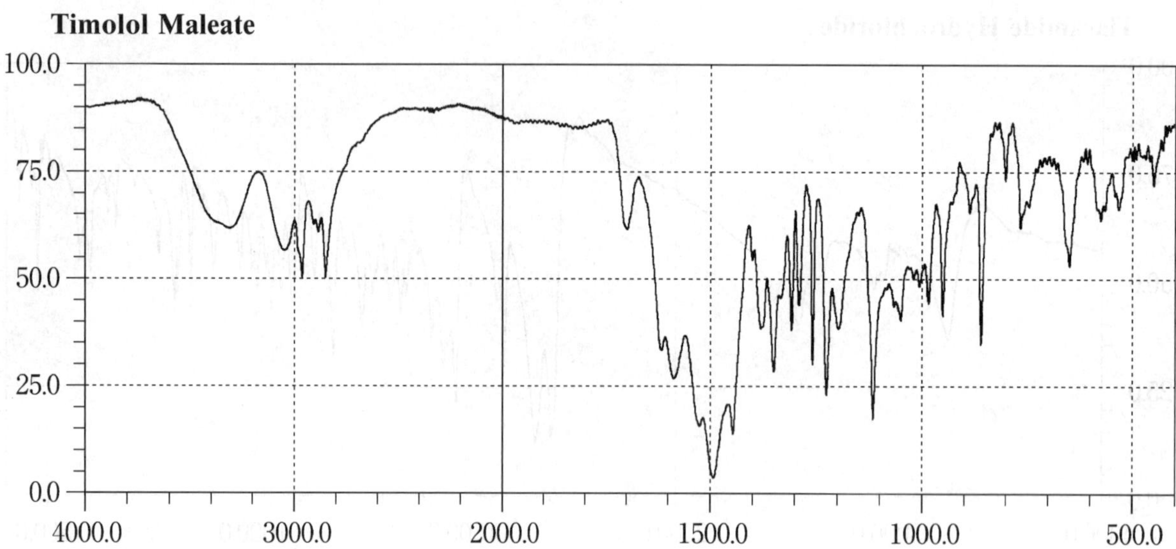

Tinidazole

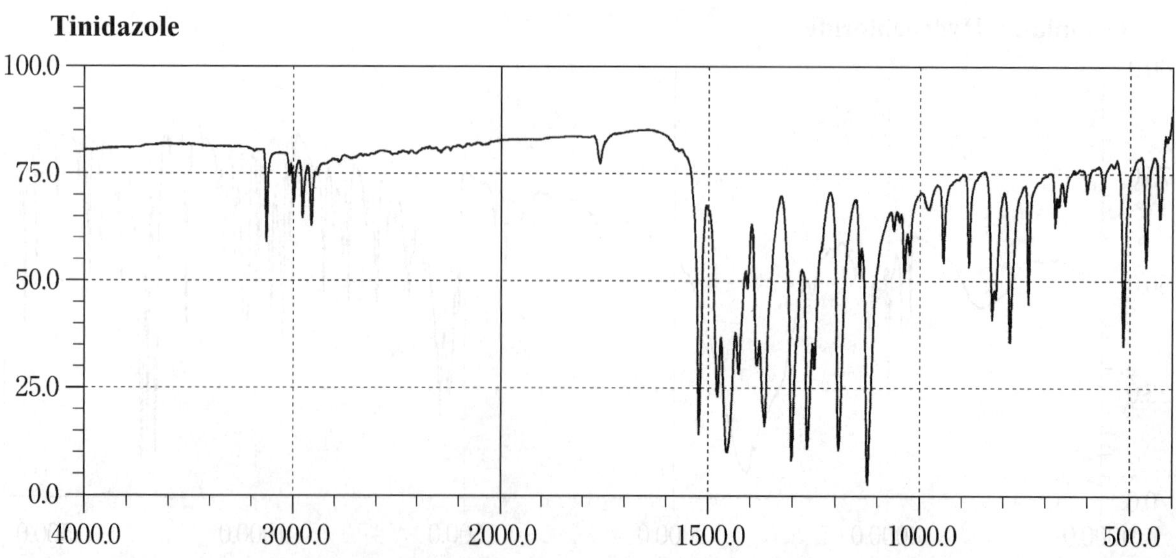

Tipepidine Hibenzate

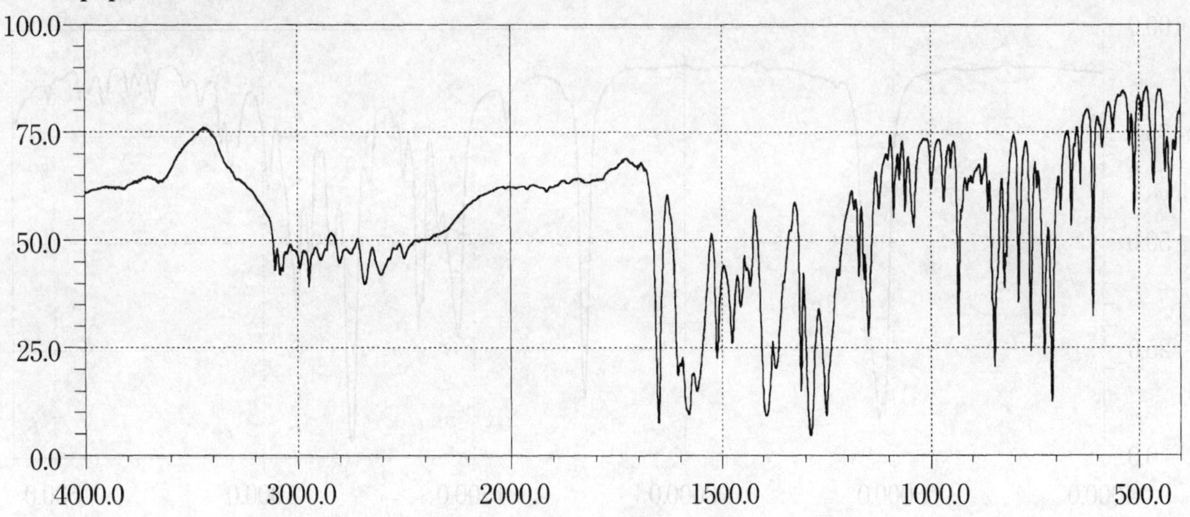

Tizanidine Hydrochloride

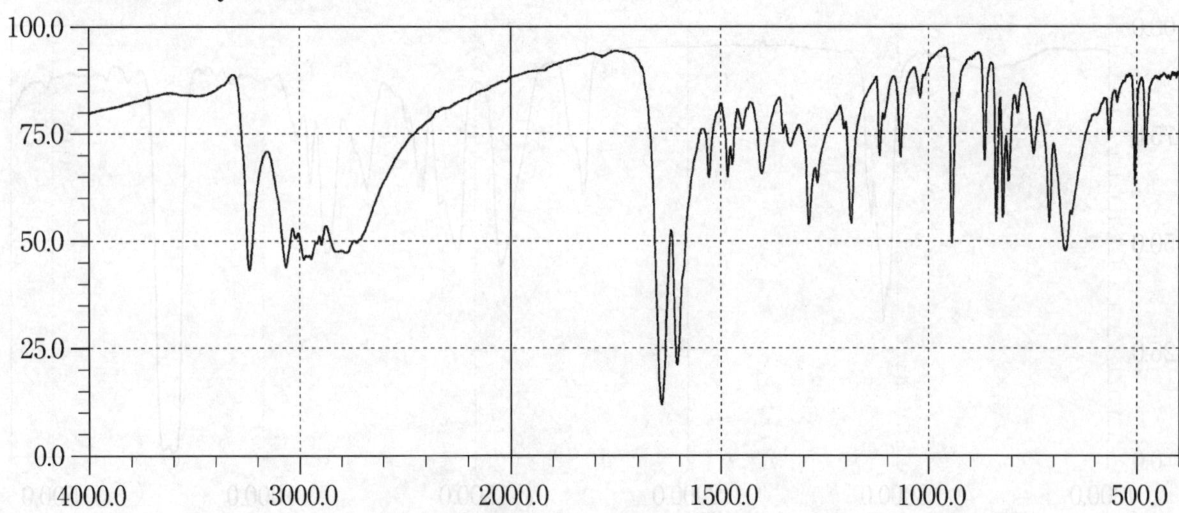

Tocopherol

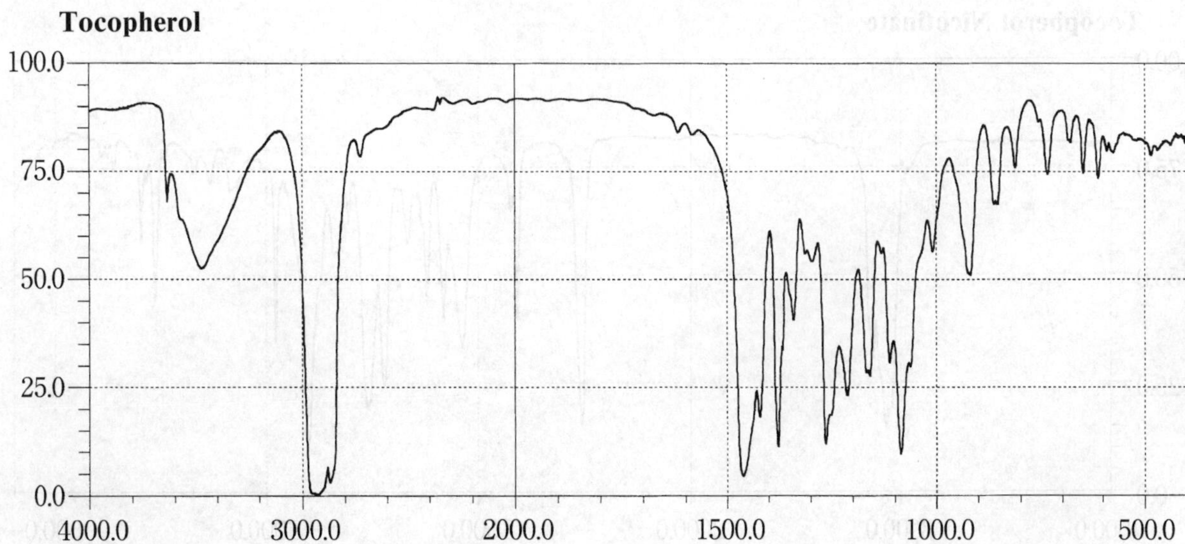

Tocopherol Acetate

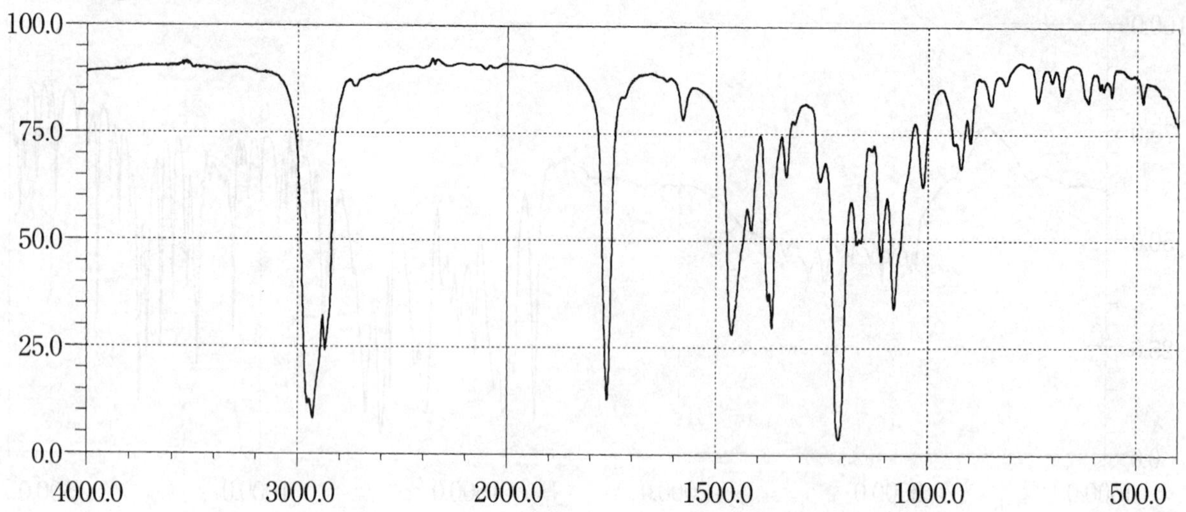

Tocopherol Calcium Succinate

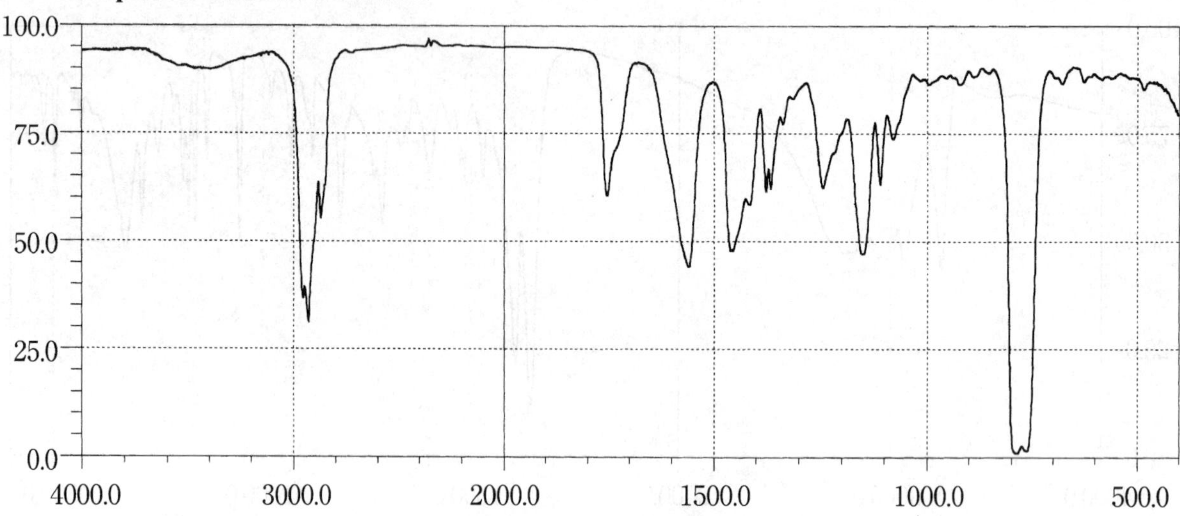

Tocopherol Nicotinate

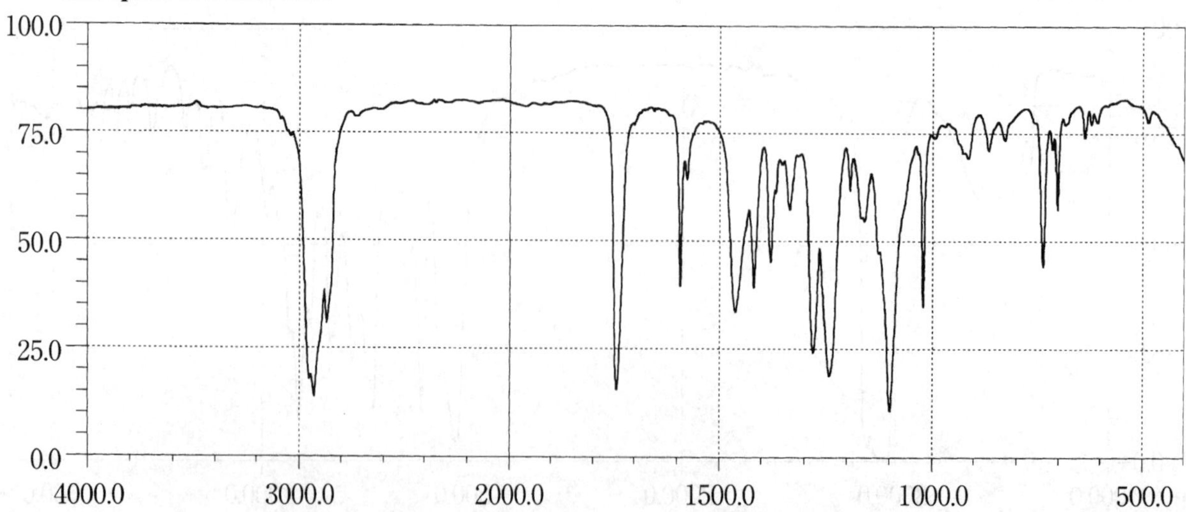

Todralazine Hydrochloride Hydrate

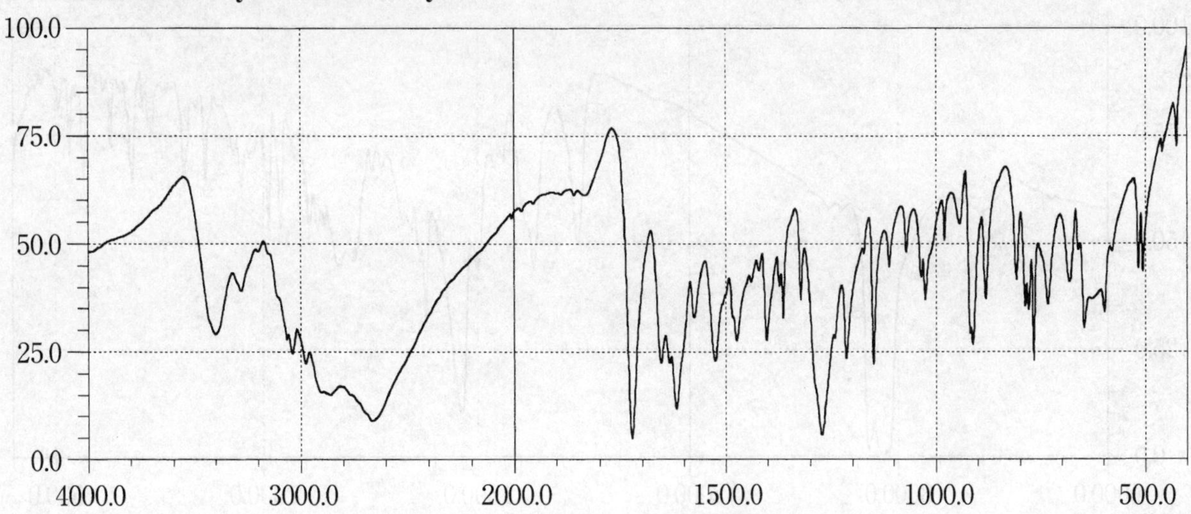

Tofisopam

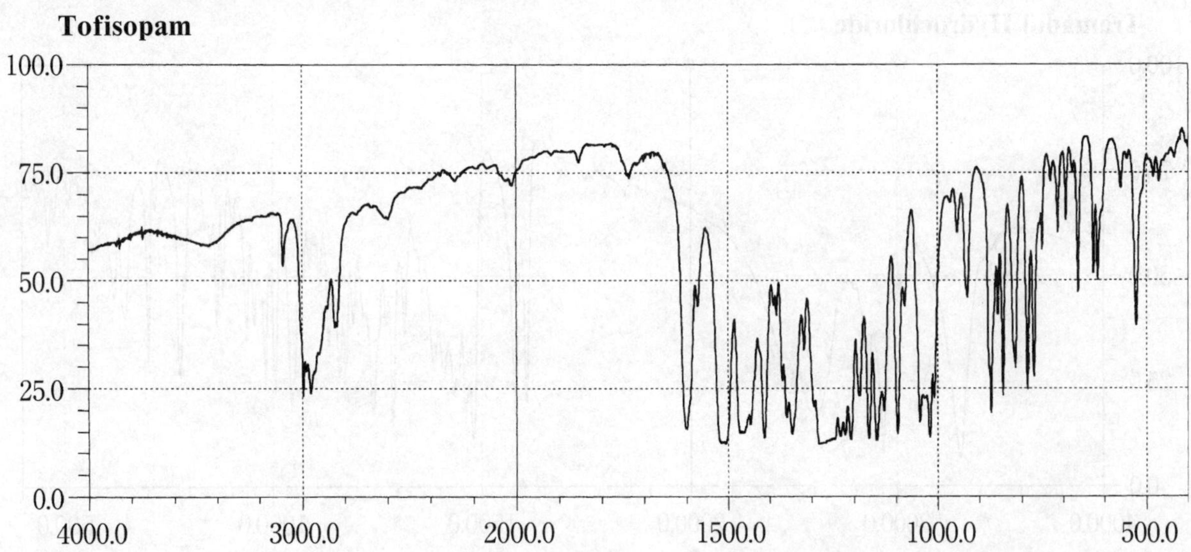

Tolnaftate

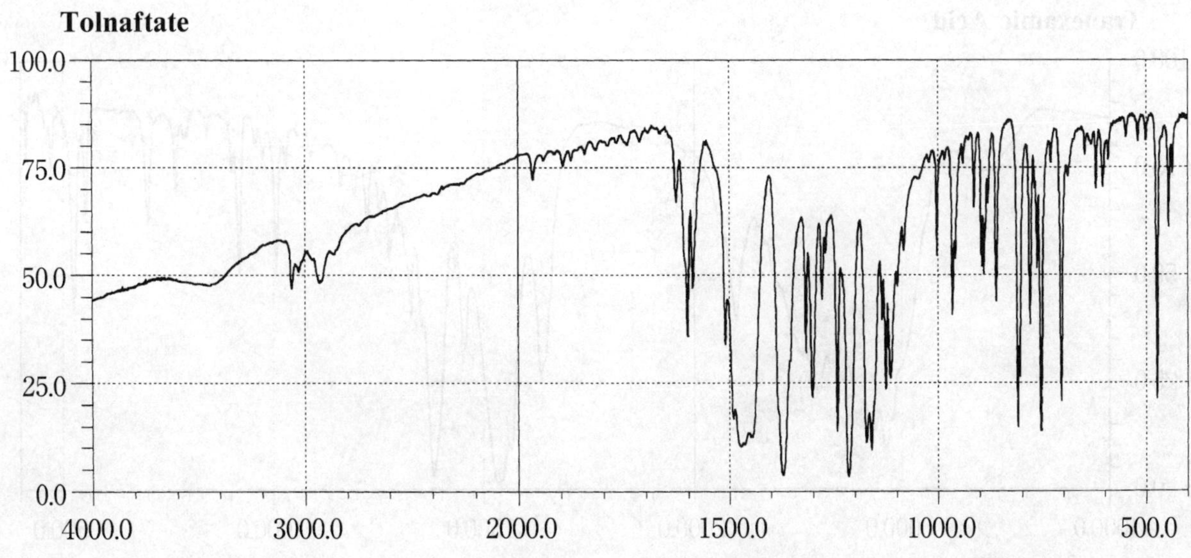

Tosufloxacin Tosilate Hydrate

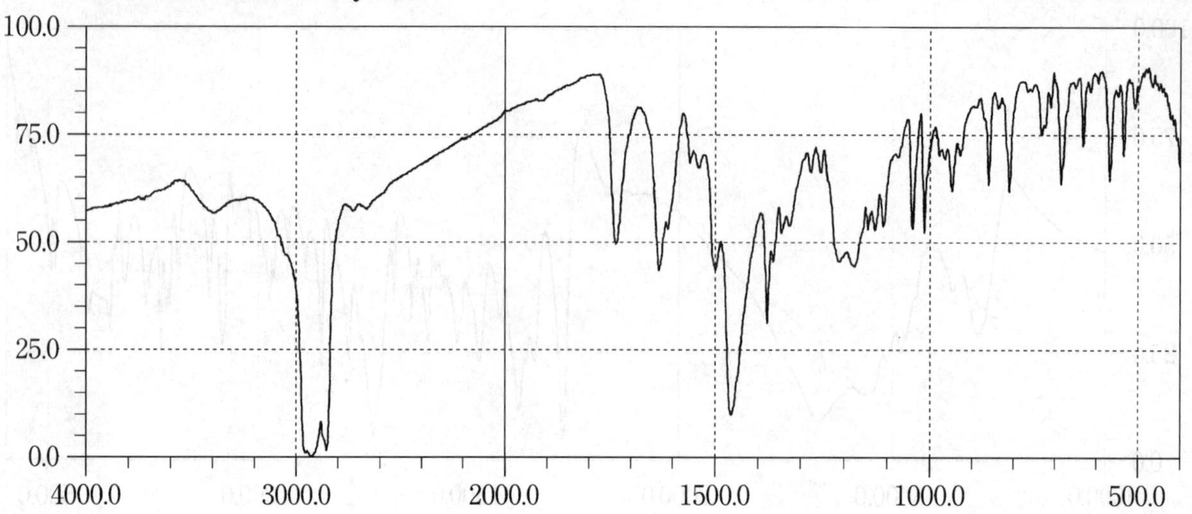

Tramadol Hydrochloride

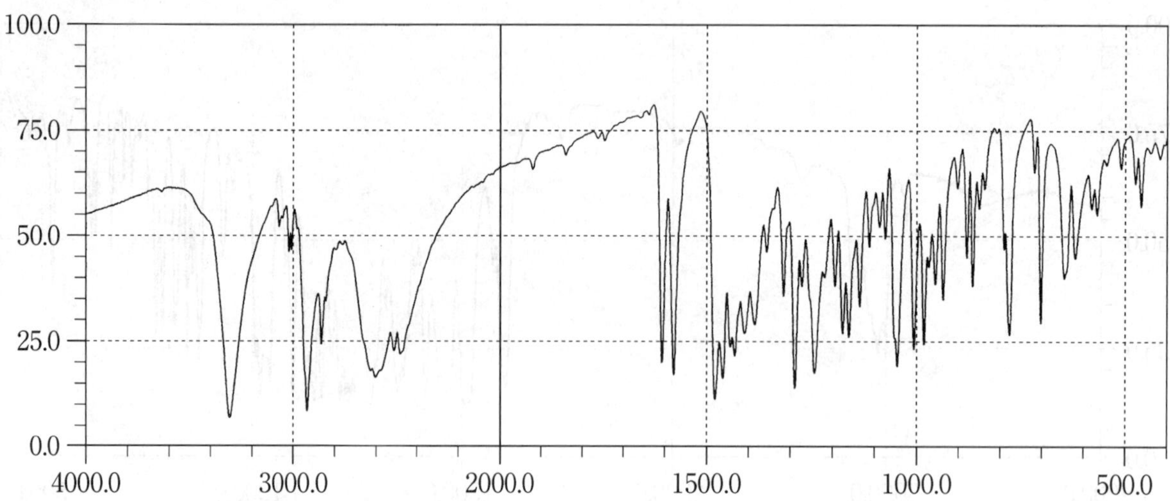

Tranexamic Acid

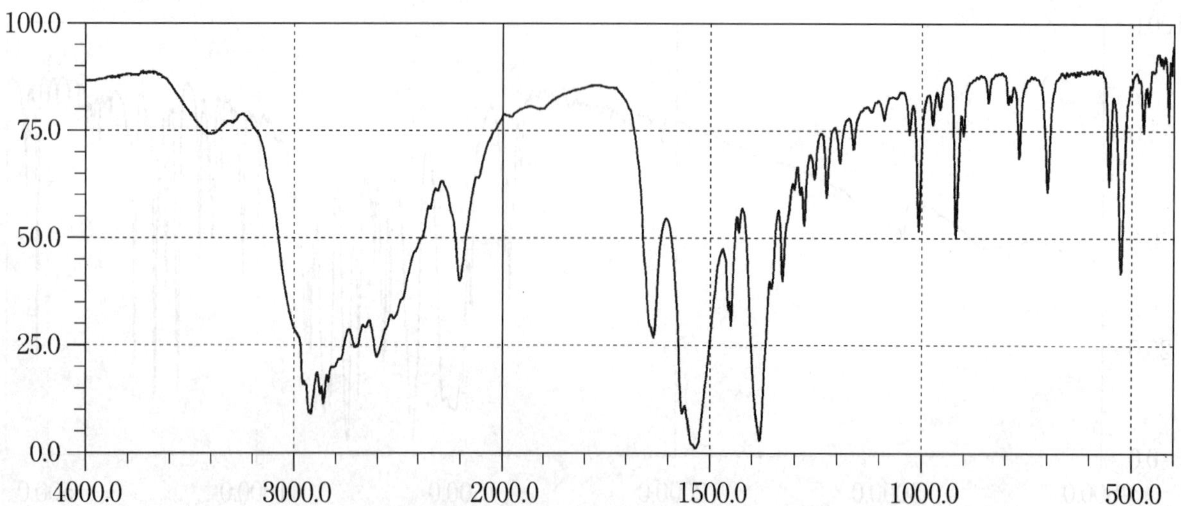

Tranilast

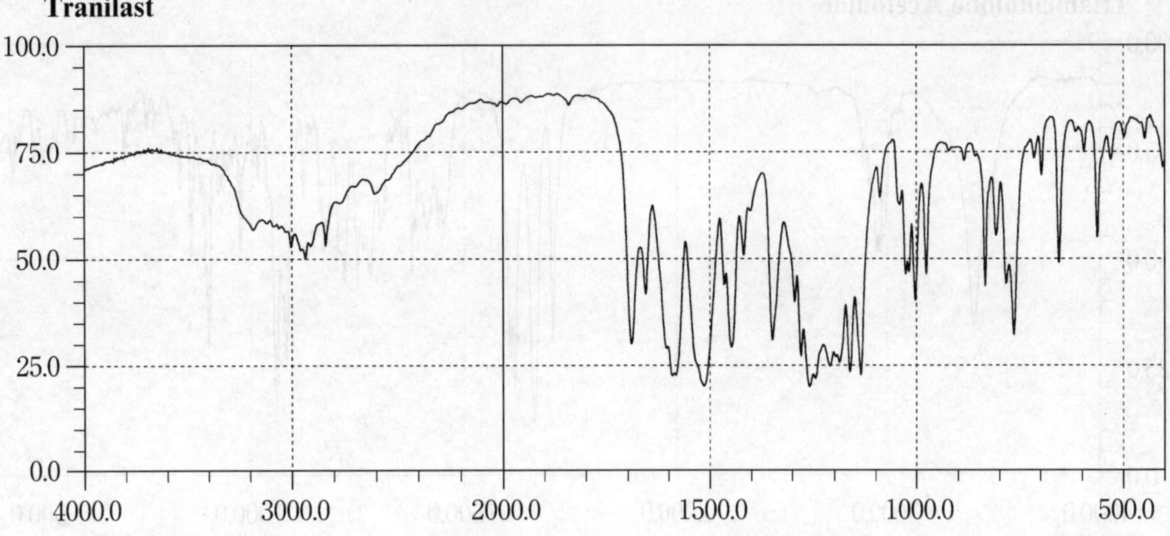

Trehalose Hydrate

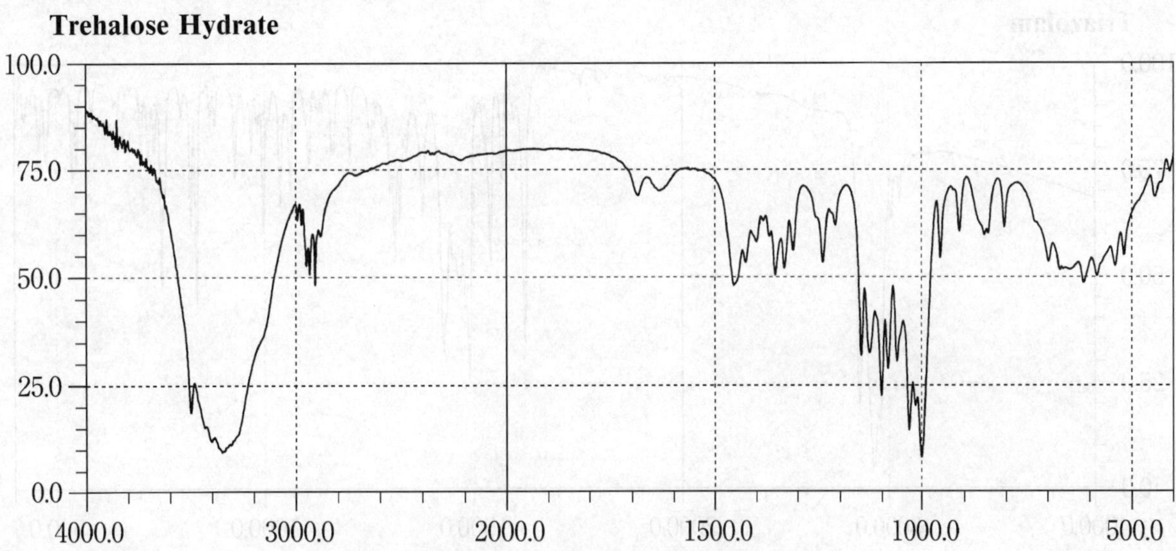

Triamcinolone

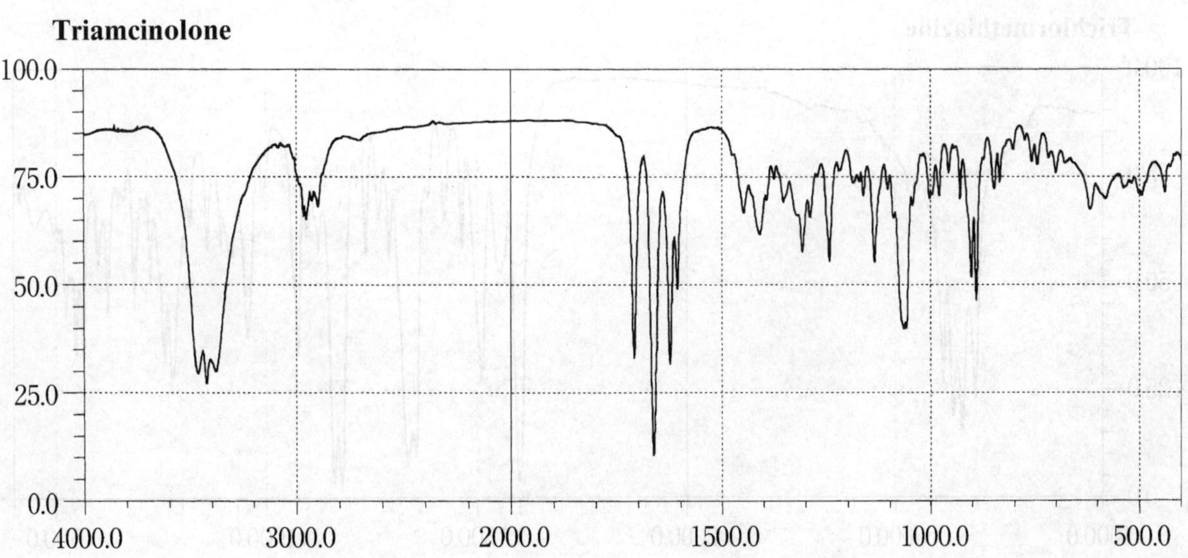

Triamcinolone Acetonide

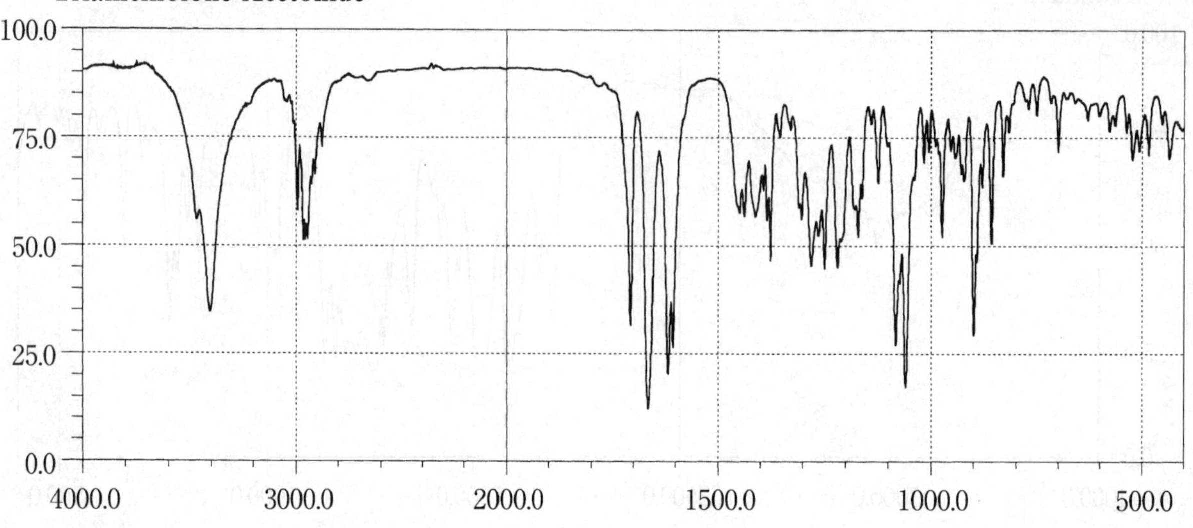

Triazolam

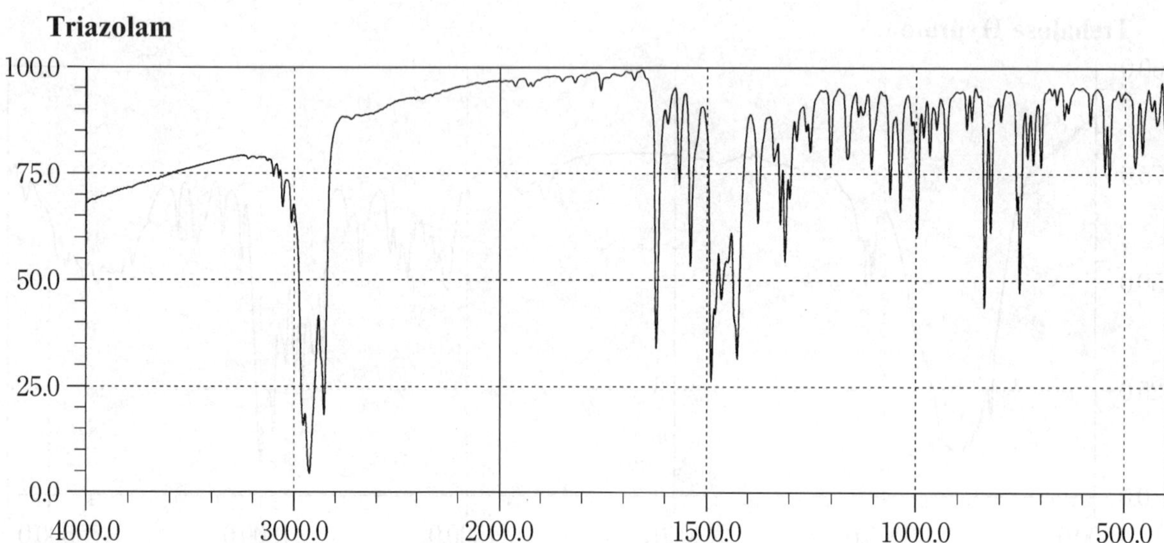

Trichlormethiazide

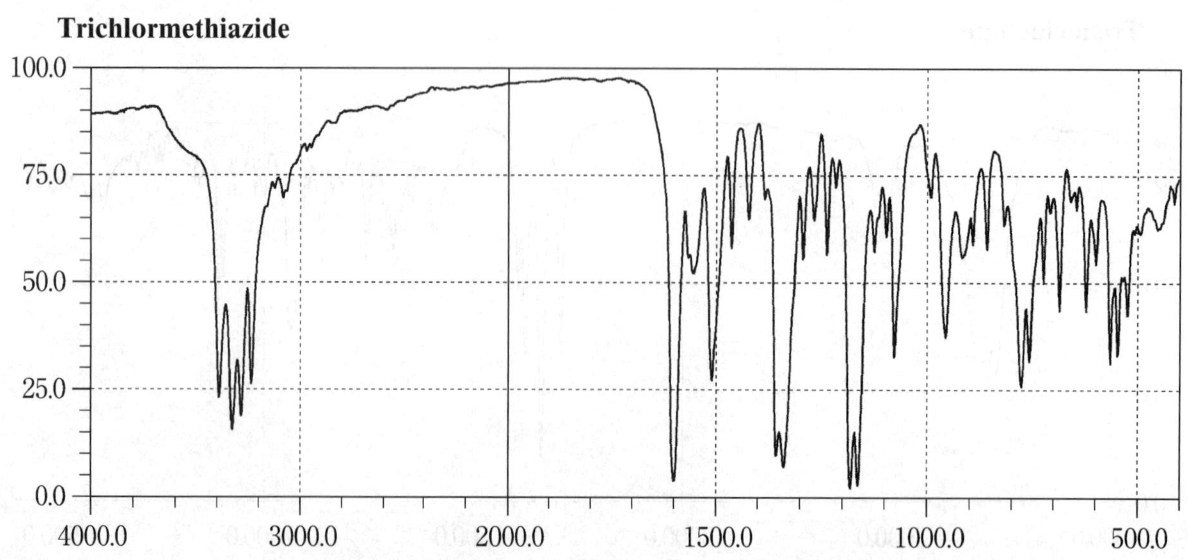

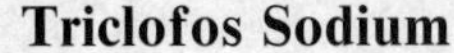

Triclofos Sodium

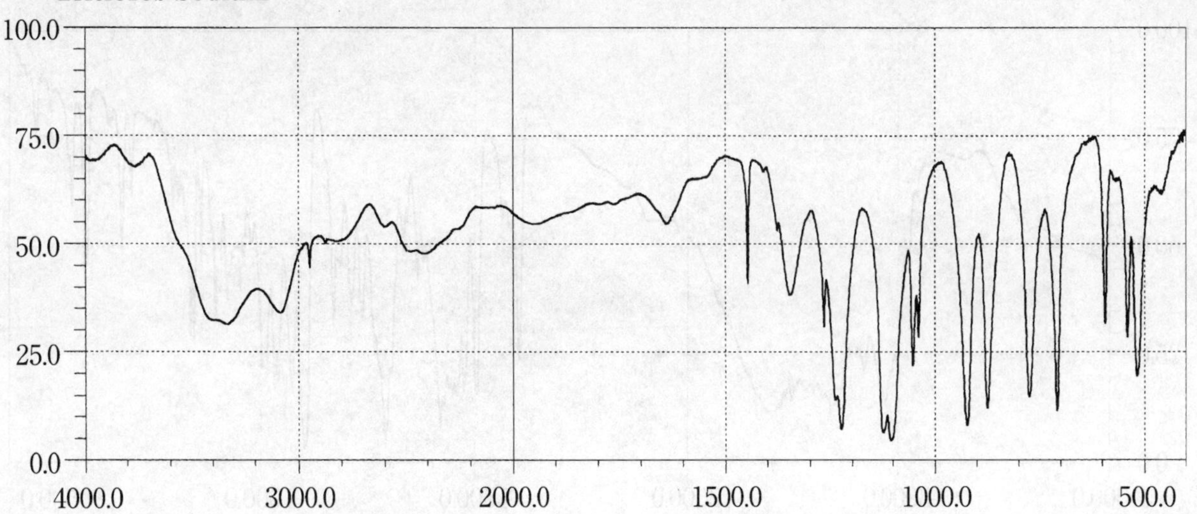

Trientine Hydrochloride

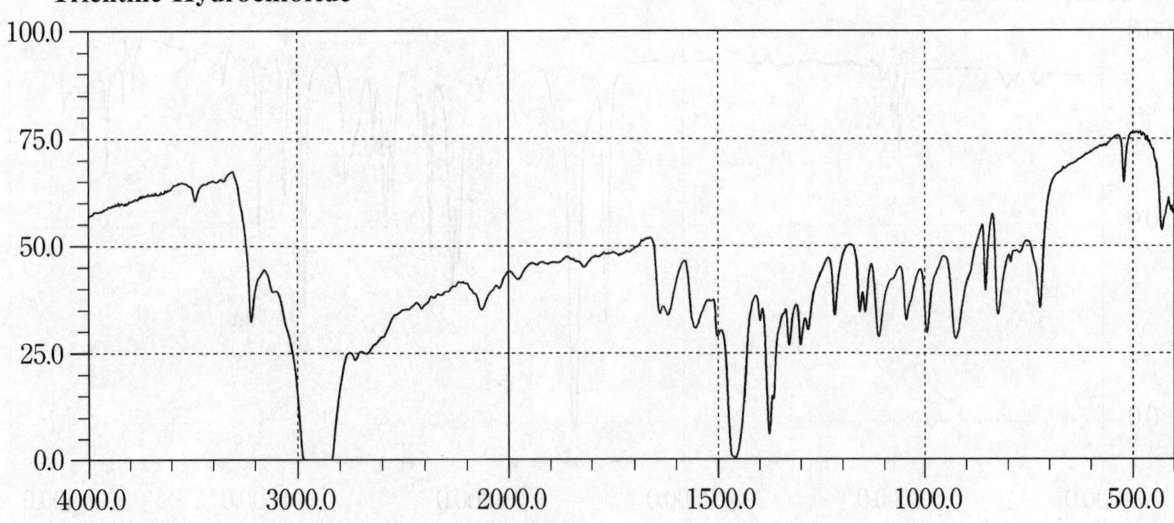

Trimebutine Maleate

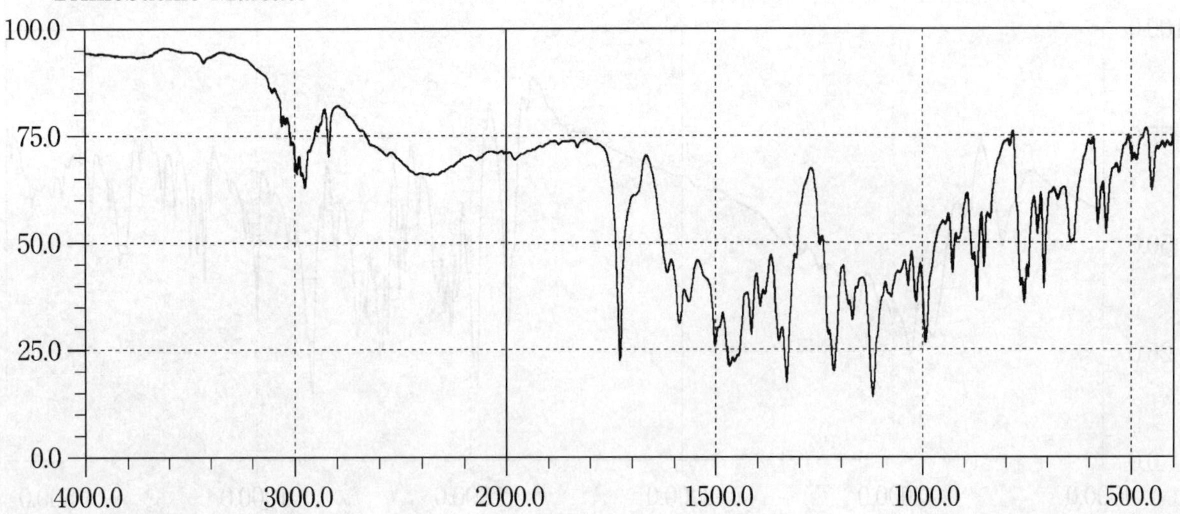

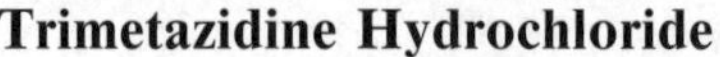

Trimetazidine Hydrochloride

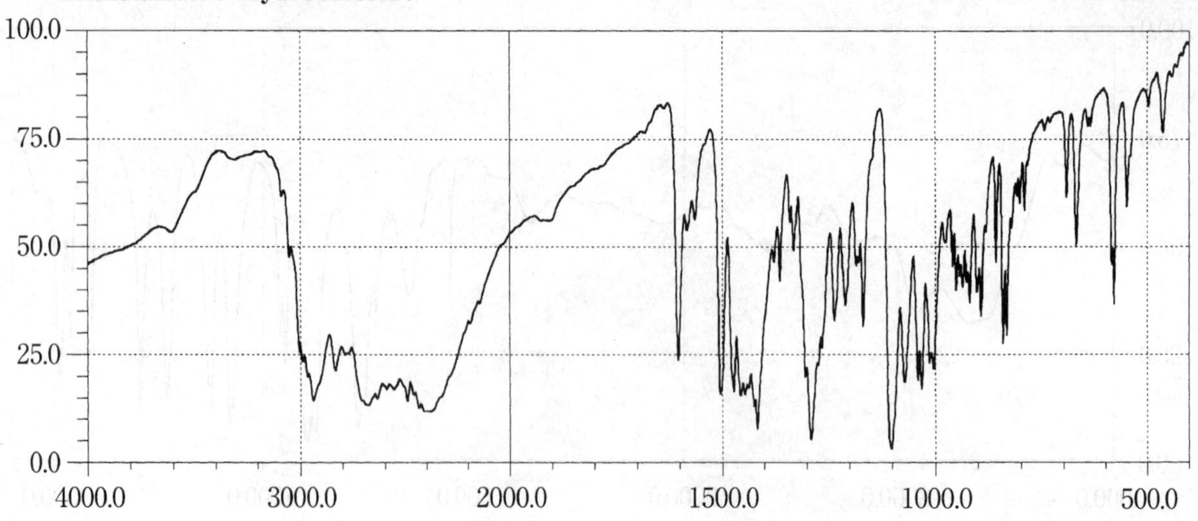

Trimethadione

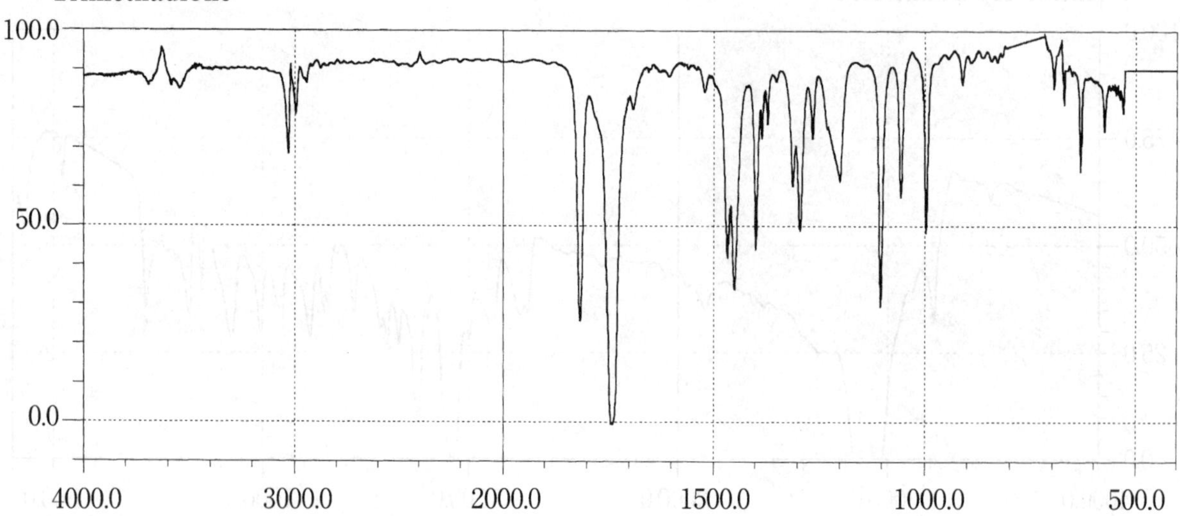

Trimetoquinol Hydrochloride Hydrate

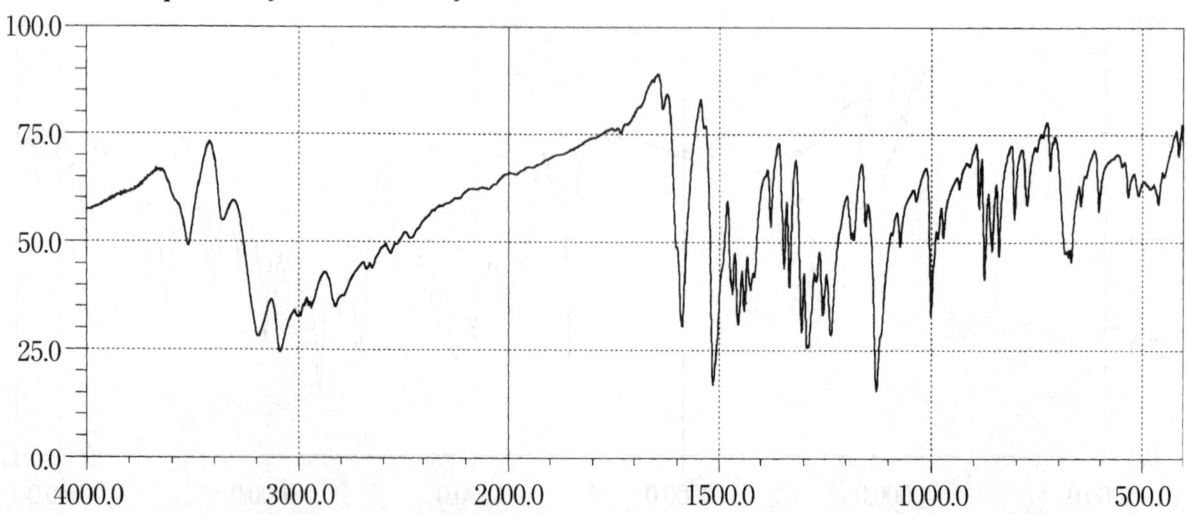

The JP Drugs are to be tested according to the provisions given in the pertinent monographs, General Notices, General Rules for Crude Drugs, General Rules for Preparations, and General Tests for their conformity to the Japanese Pharmacopoeia. (See the General Notices 5.)

Troxipide

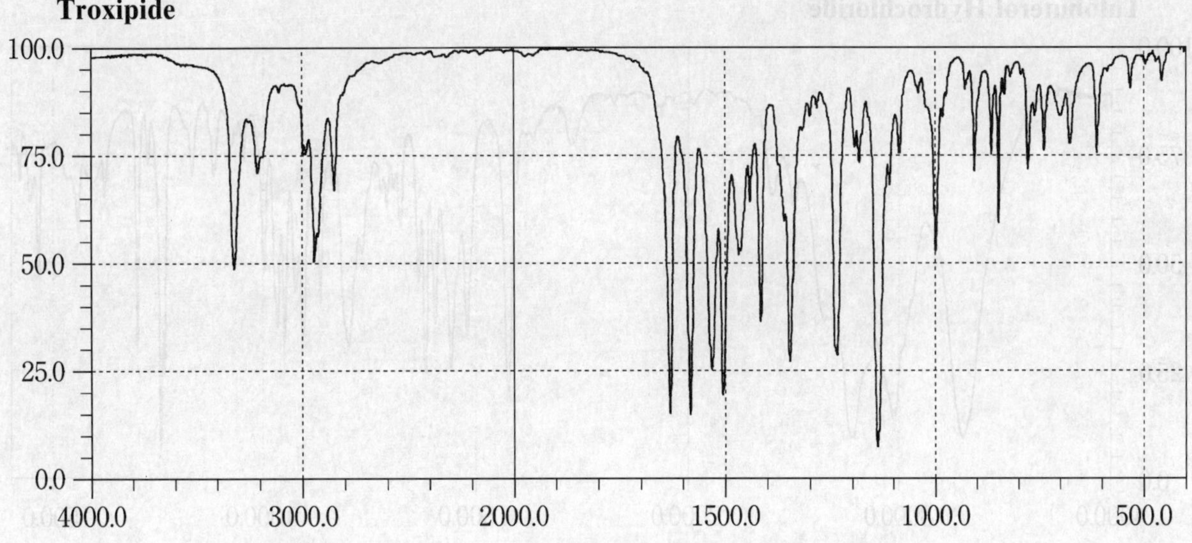

L-Tryptophan

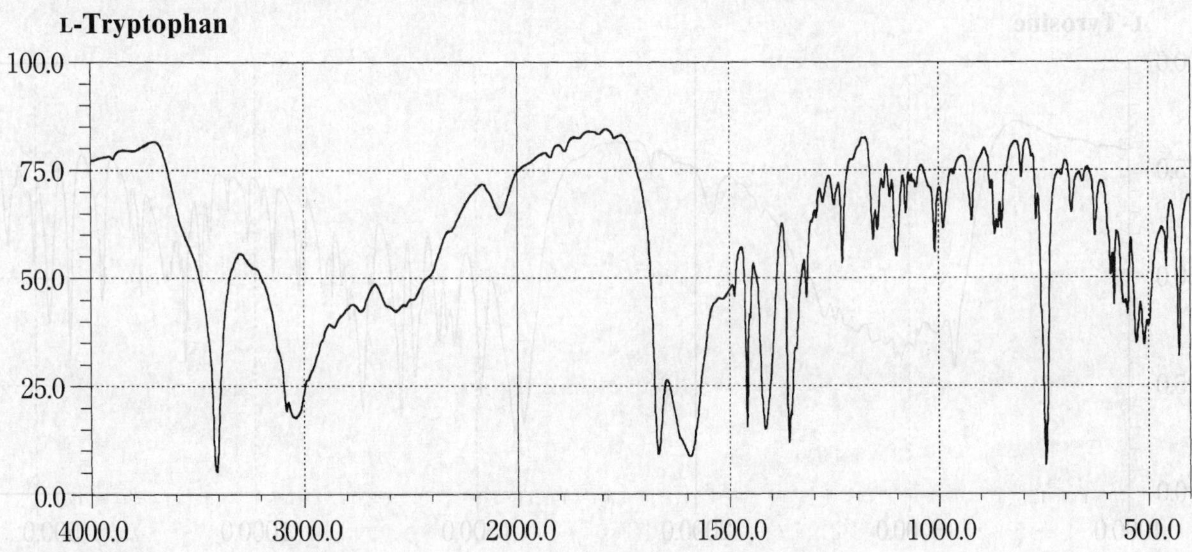

Tulobuterol

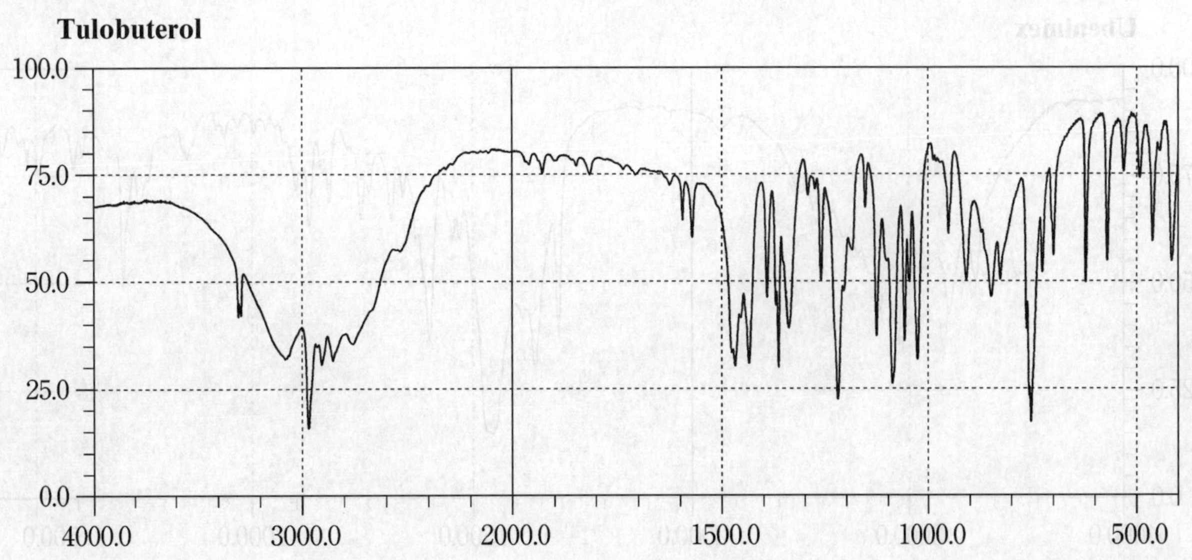

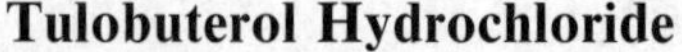

Tulobuterol Hydrochloride

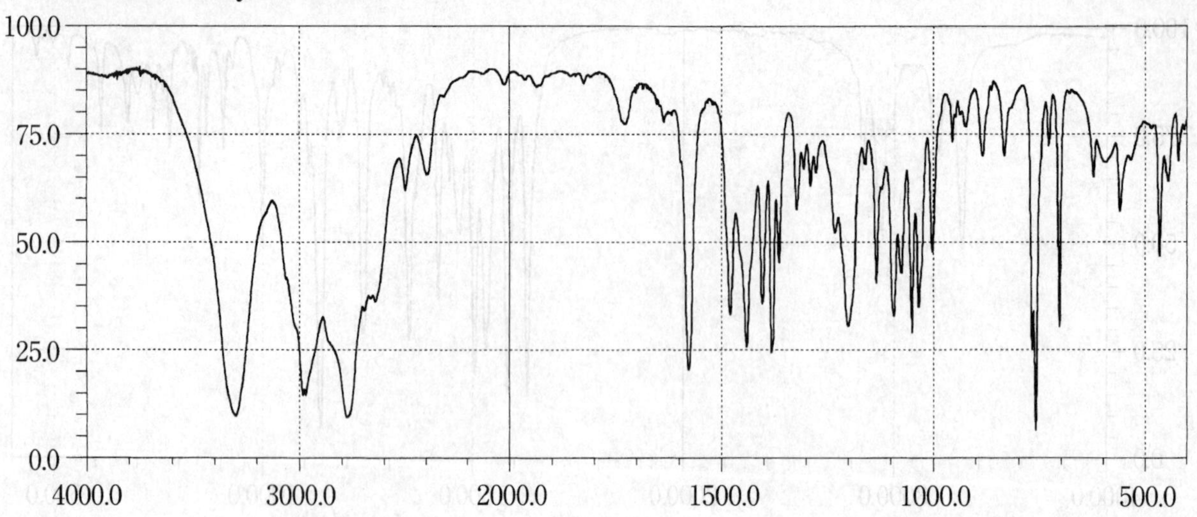

L-Tyrosine

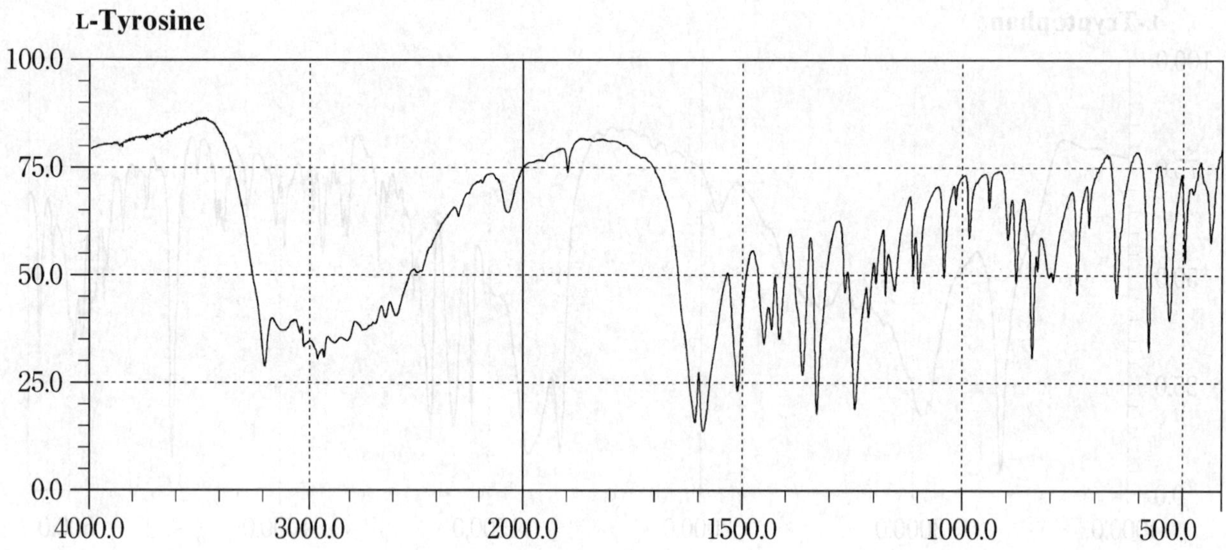

Ubenimex

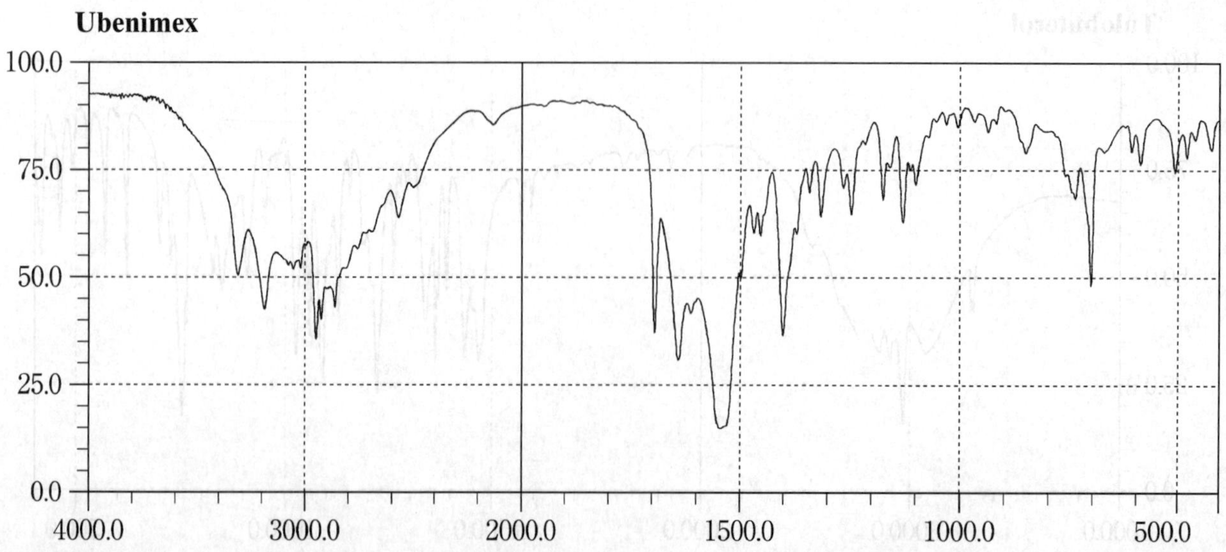

Ubidecarenone

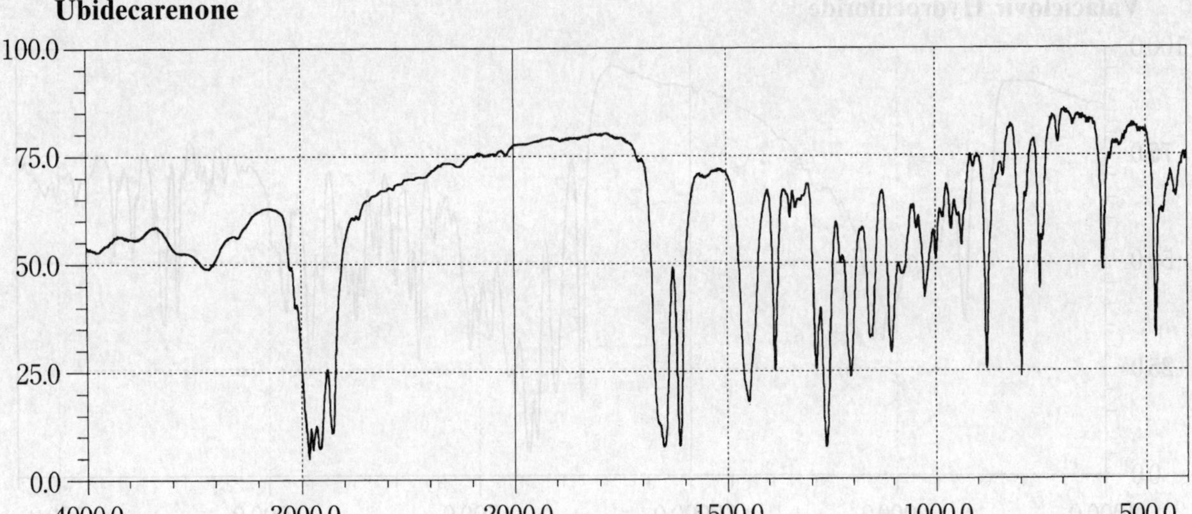

Urapidil

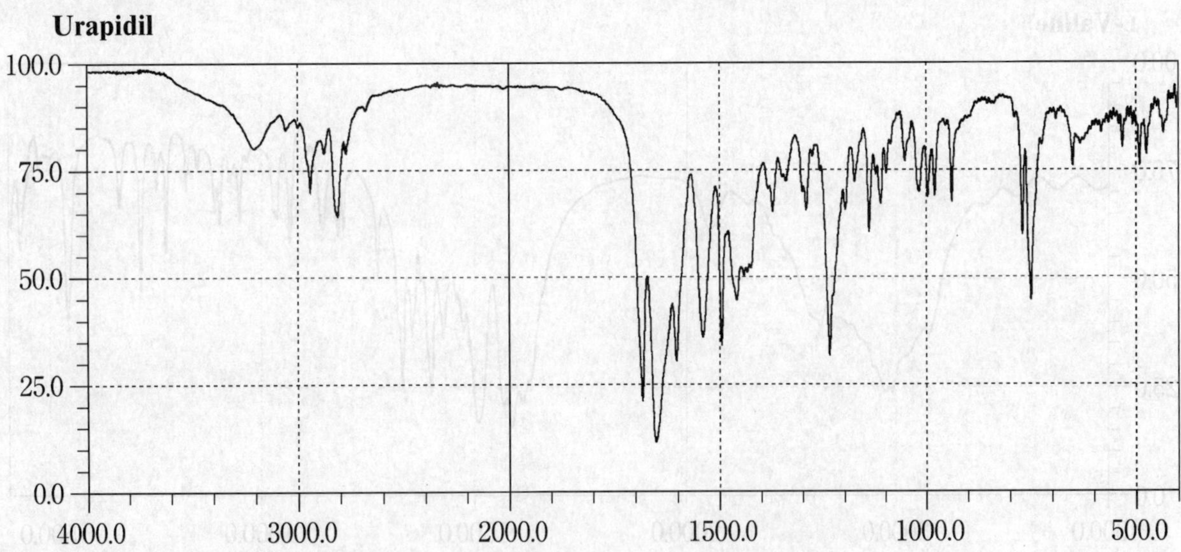

Ursodeoxycholic Acid

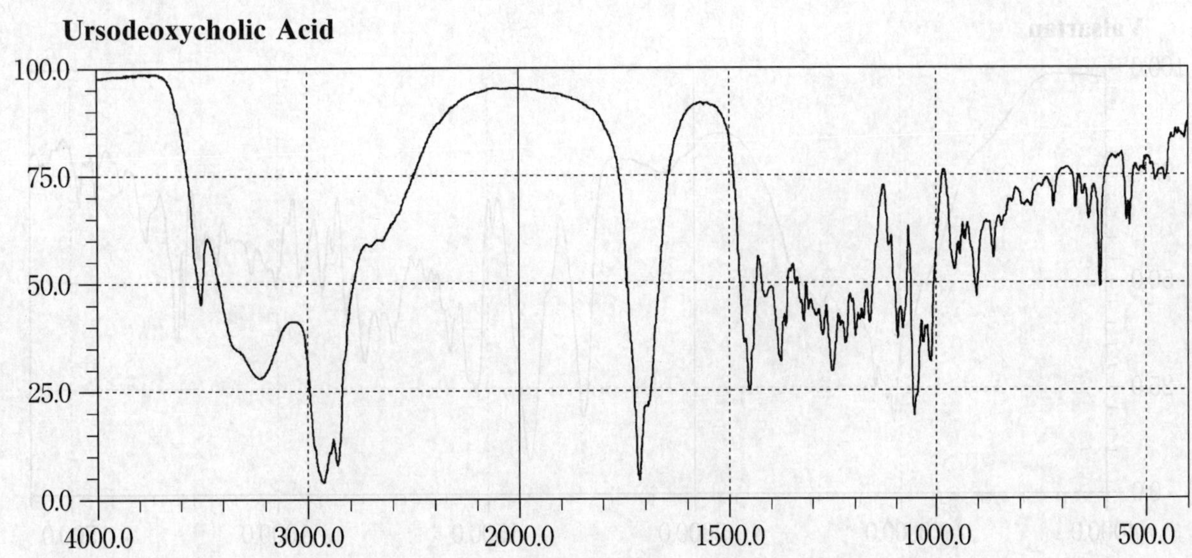

Valaciclovir Hydrochloride

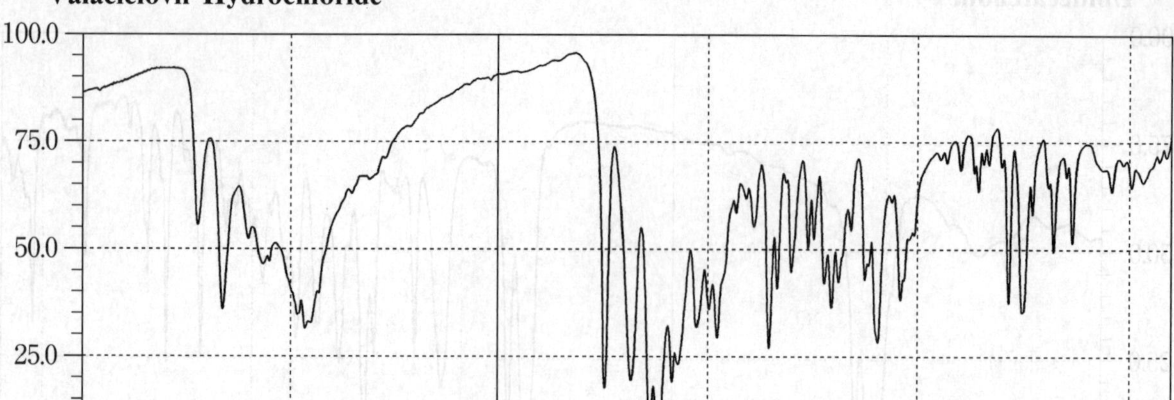

L-Valine

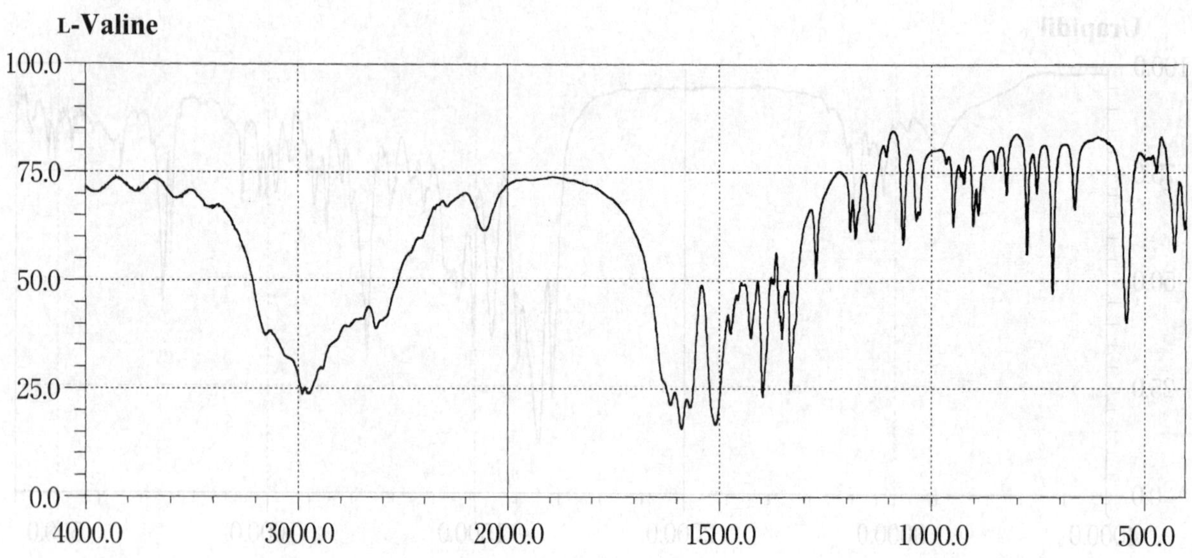

Valsartan

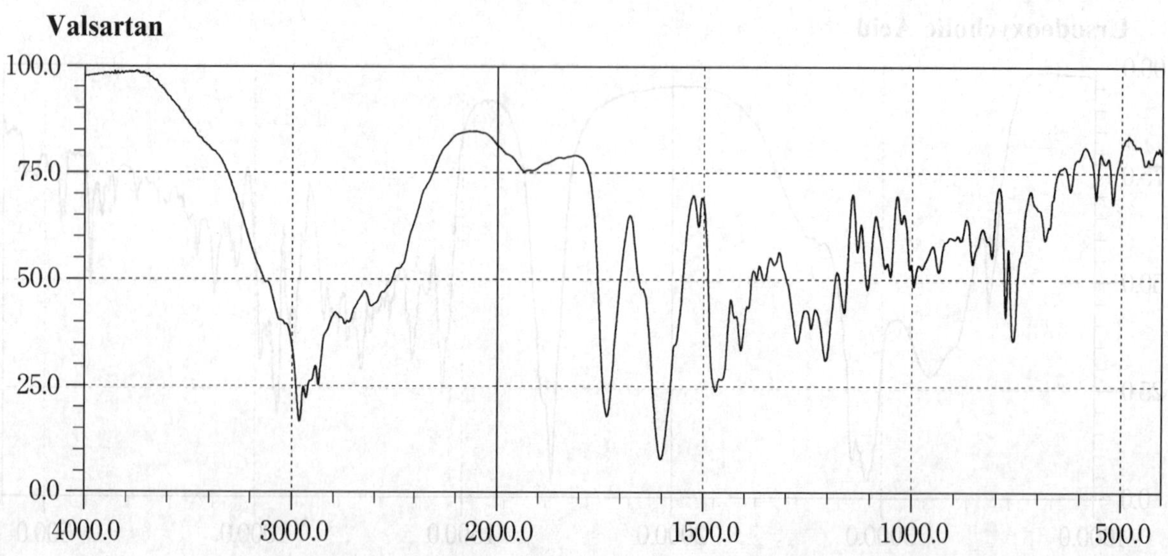

Vancomycin Hydrochloride

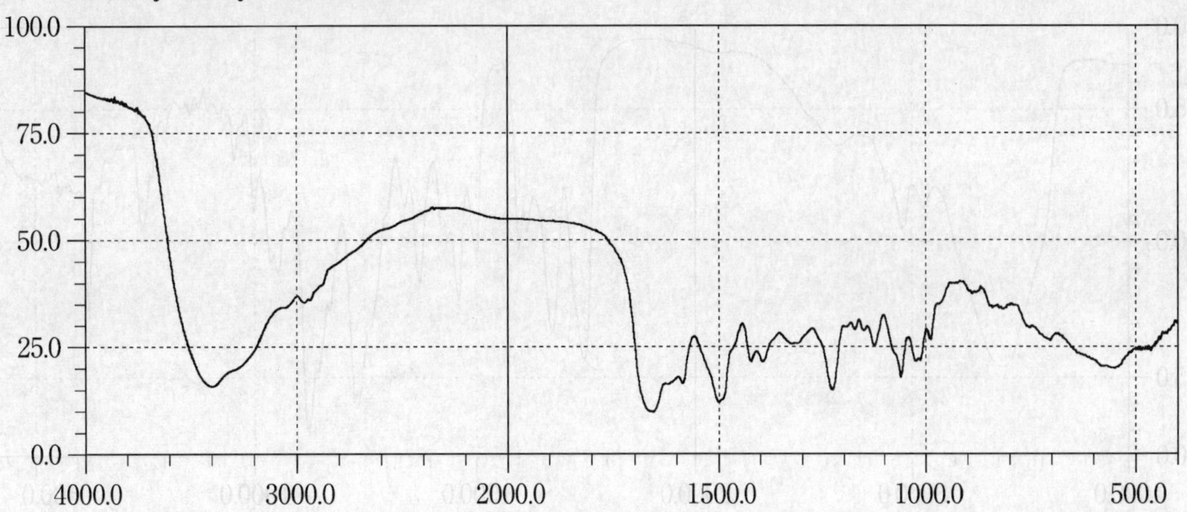

Verapamil Hydrochloride

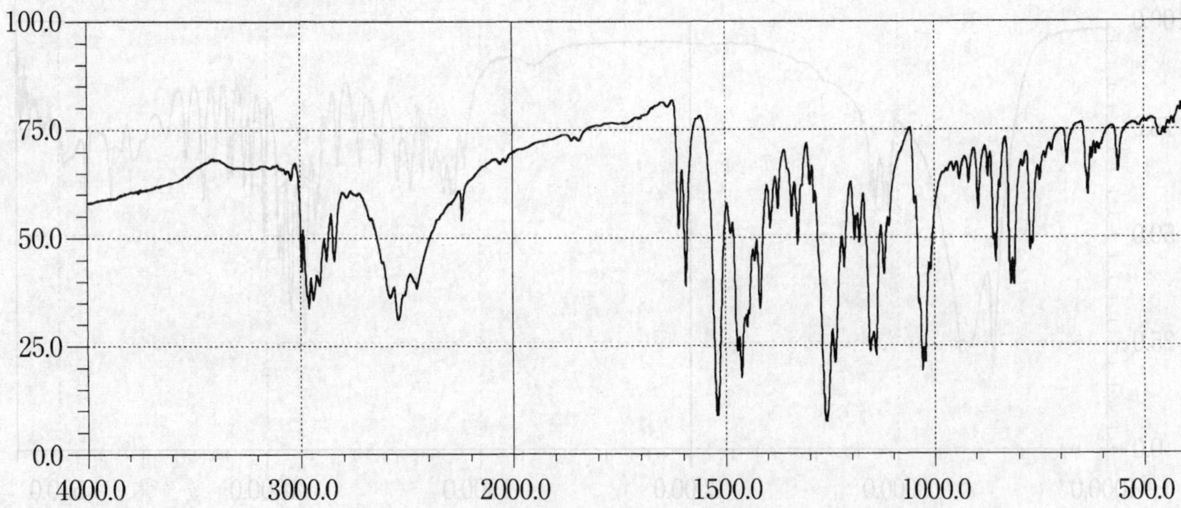

Vinblastine Sulfate

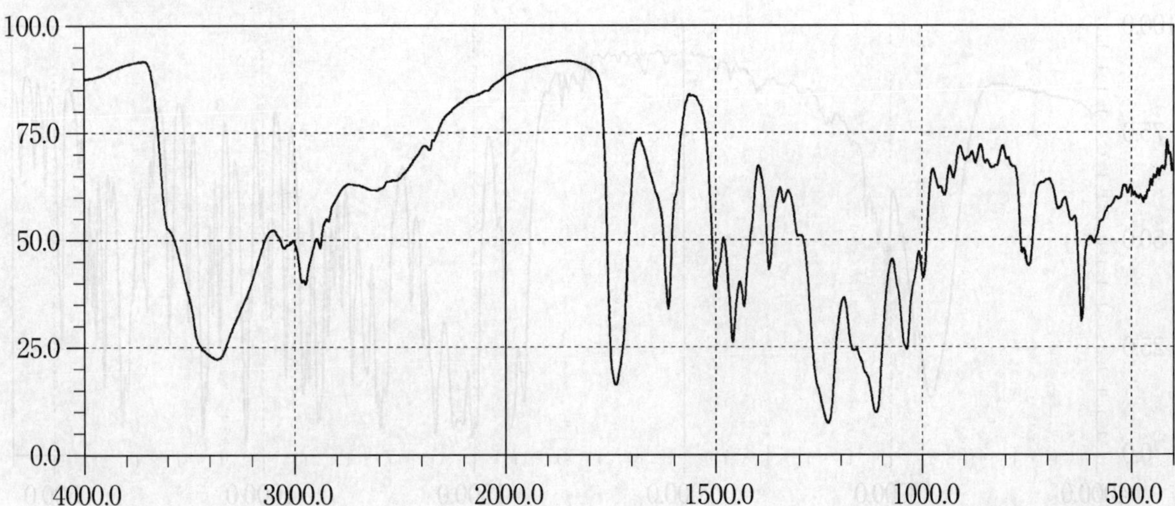

The JP Drugs are to be tested according to the provisions given in the pertinent monographs, General Notices, General Rules for Crude Drugs, General Rules for Preparations, and General Tests for their conformity to the Japanese Pharmacopoeia. (See the General Notices 5.)

Vincristine Sulfate

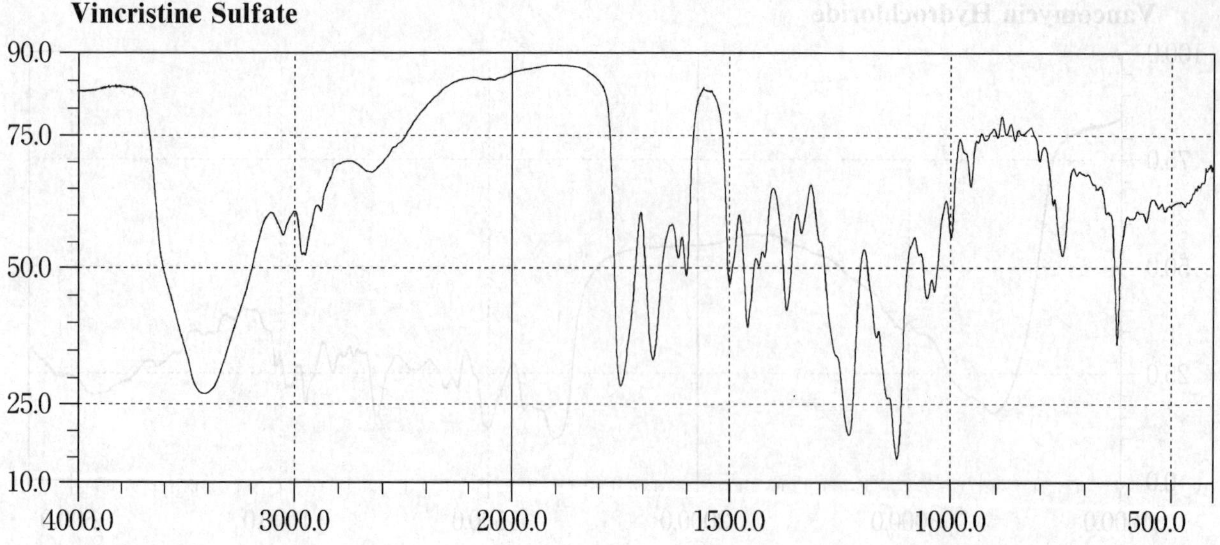

Voglibose

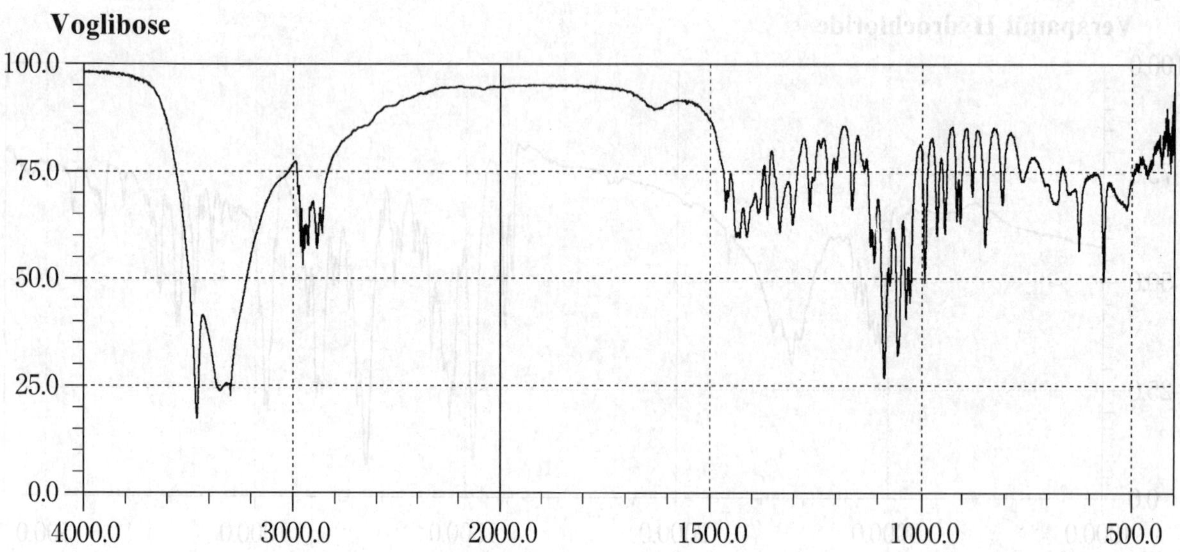

Voriconazole

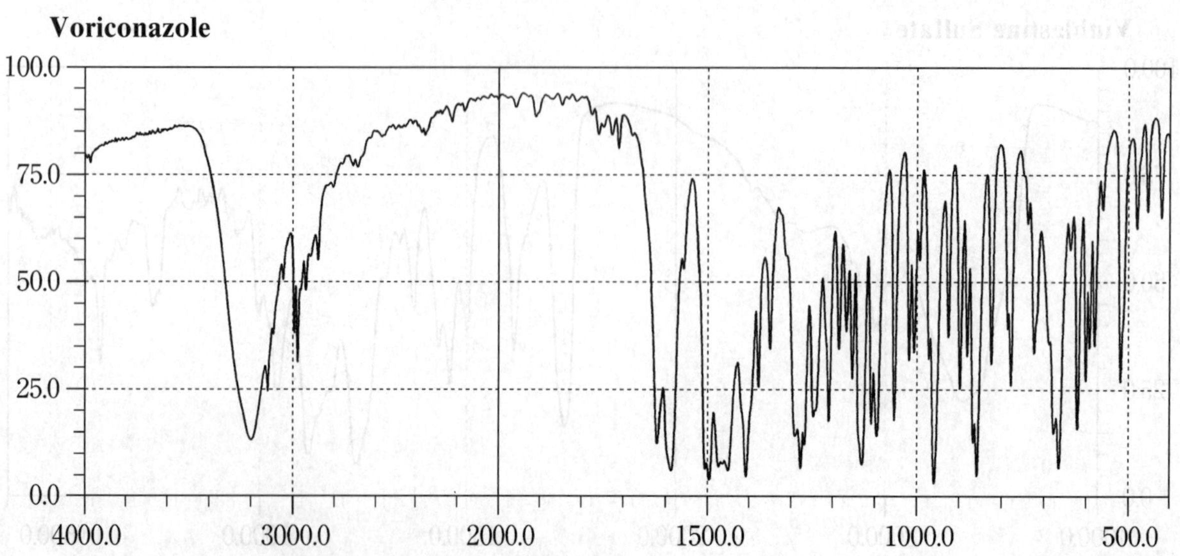

Warfarin Potassium

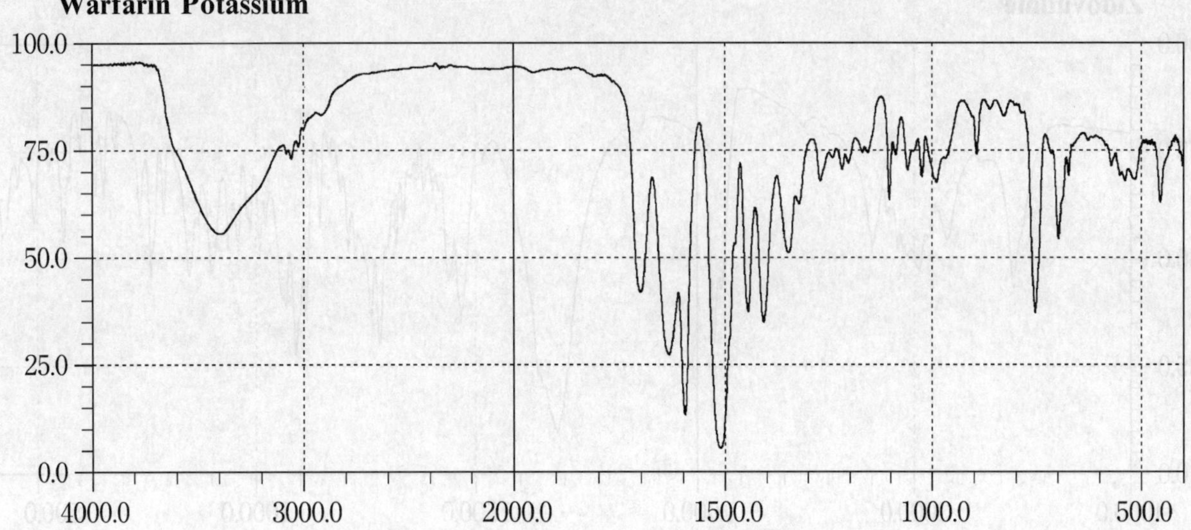

Xylitol

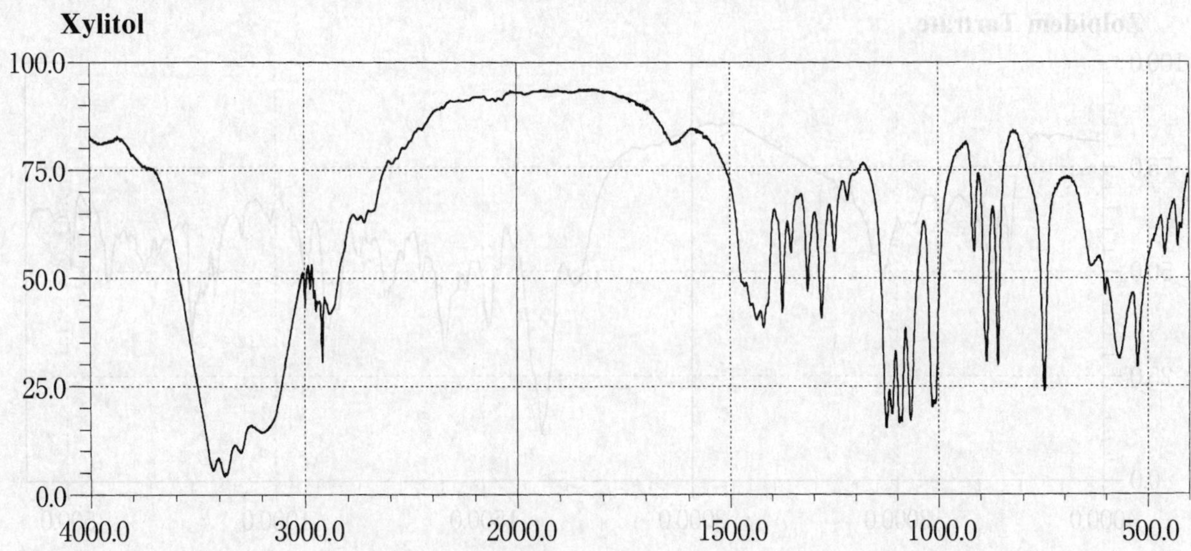

Zaltoprofen

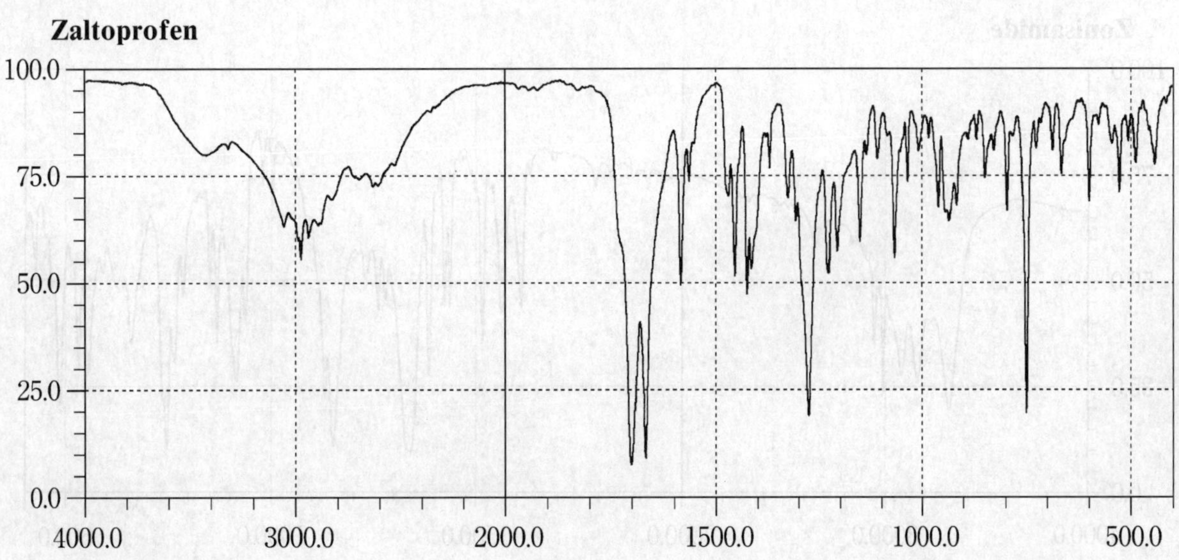

Zidovudine

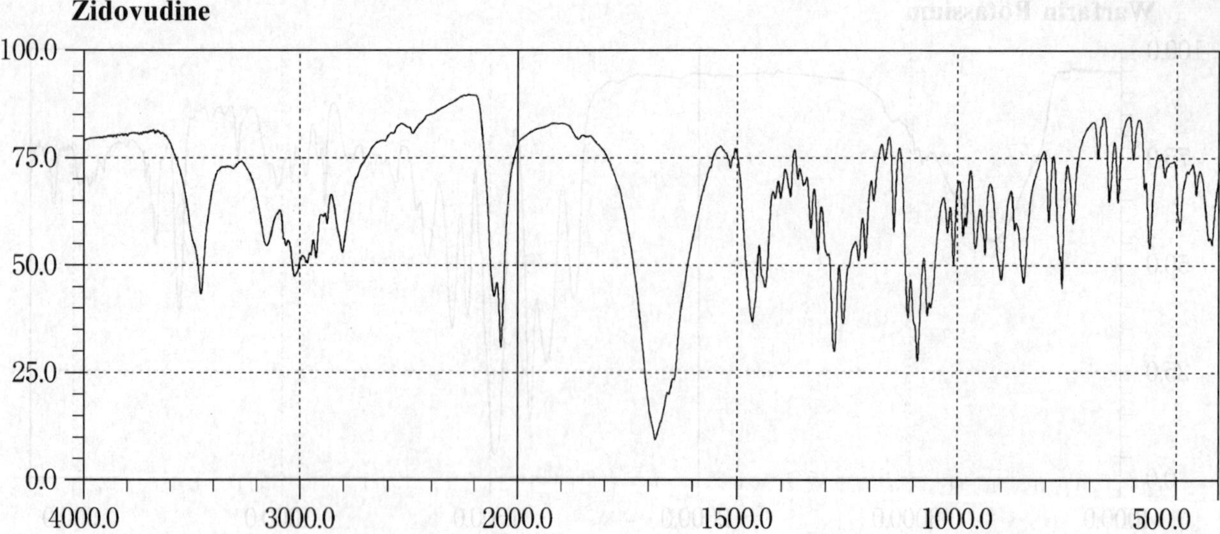

Zolpidem Tartrate

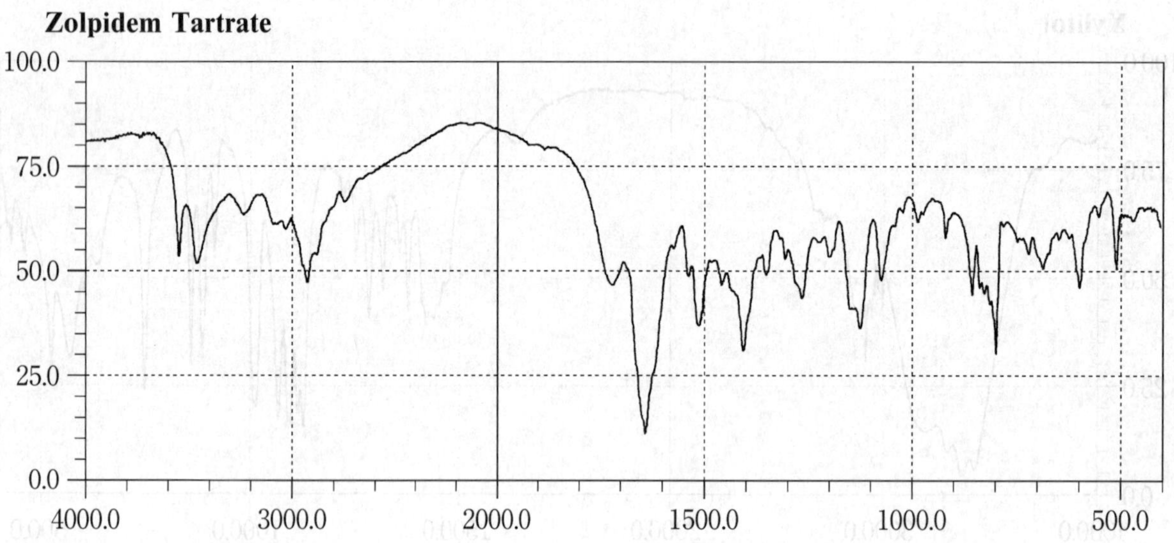

Zonisamide

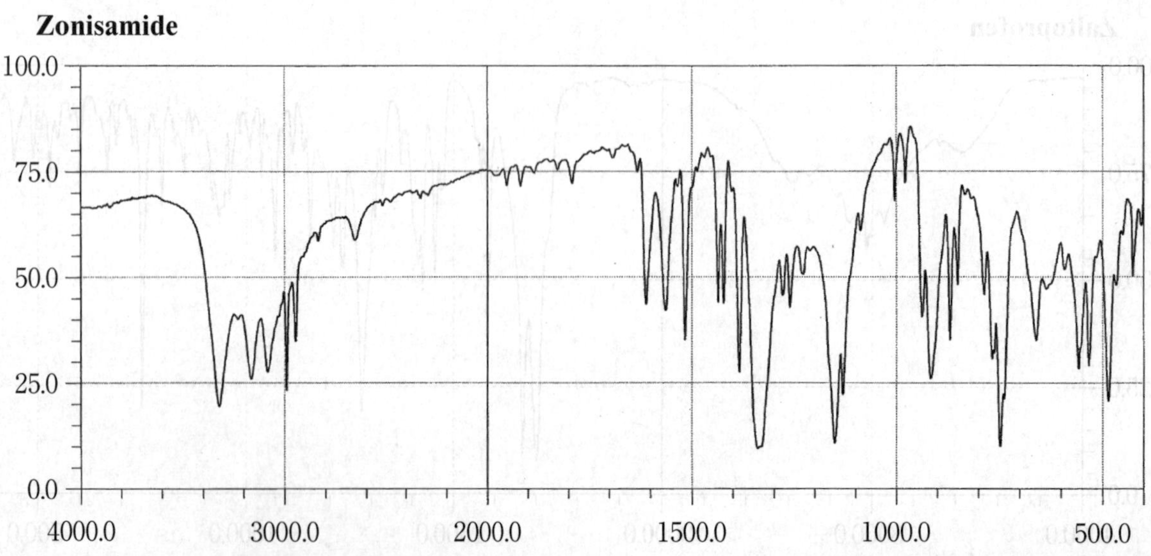

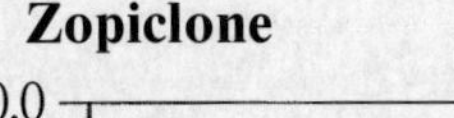

Zopiclone

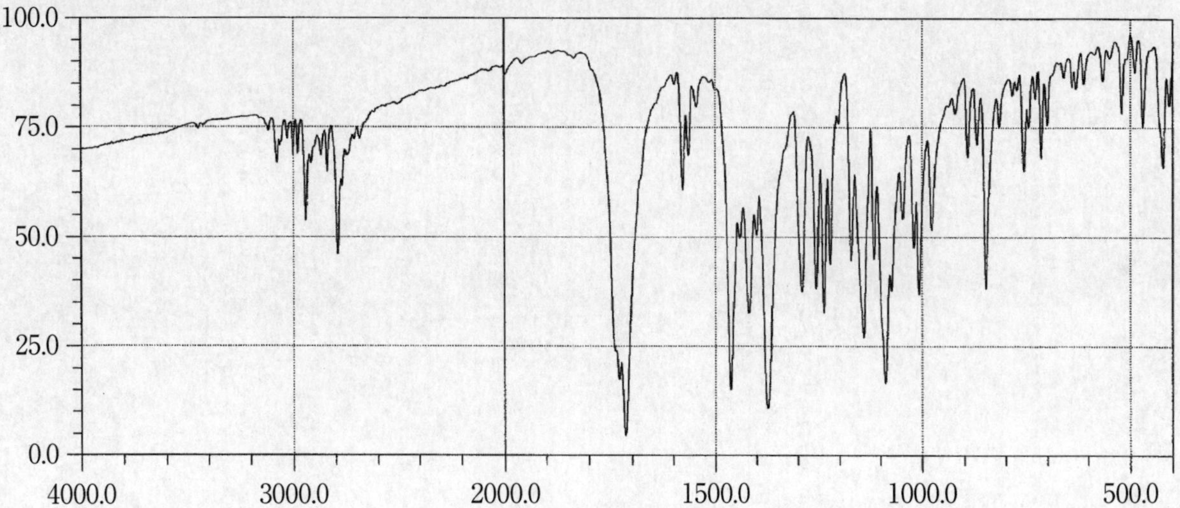

ULTRAVIOLET-VISIBLE REFERENCE SPECTRA

The ultraviolet-visible reference spectra presented here were obtained by the use of double-beam spectrophotometers with sample solutions prepared as specified in the individual monographs. The horizontal axis indicates the wavelength (nm) and the vertical axis indicates the absorbance.

Acebutolol Hydrochloride

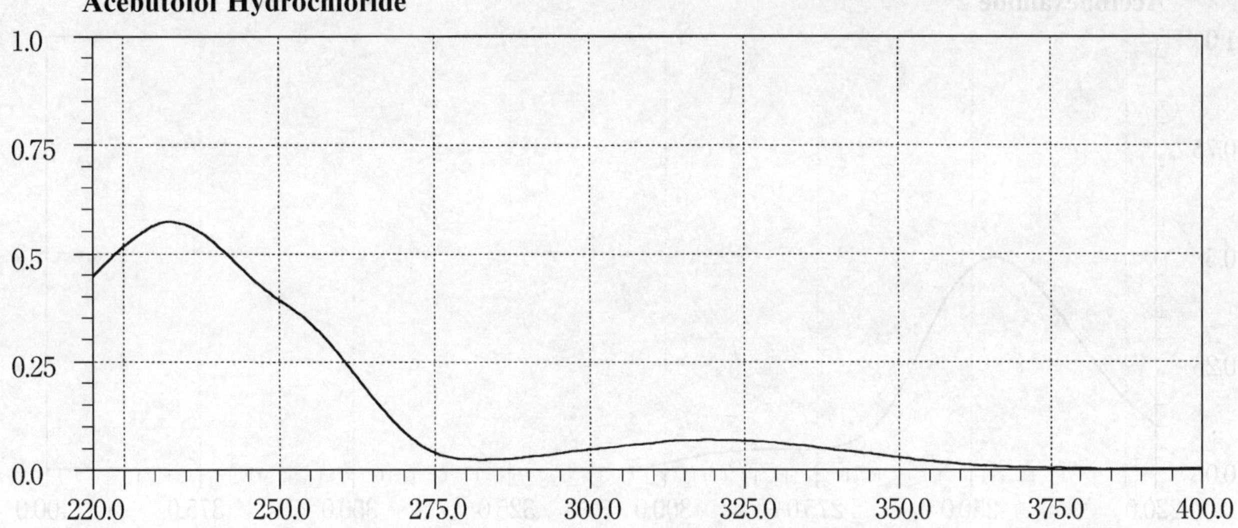

Acemetacin

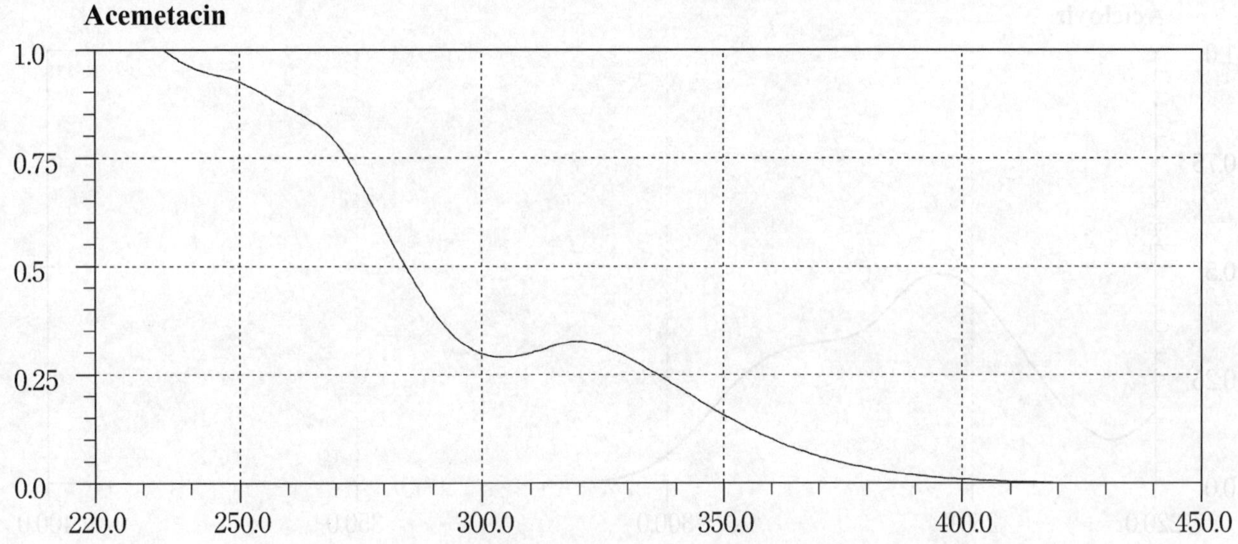

Acetohexamide 1

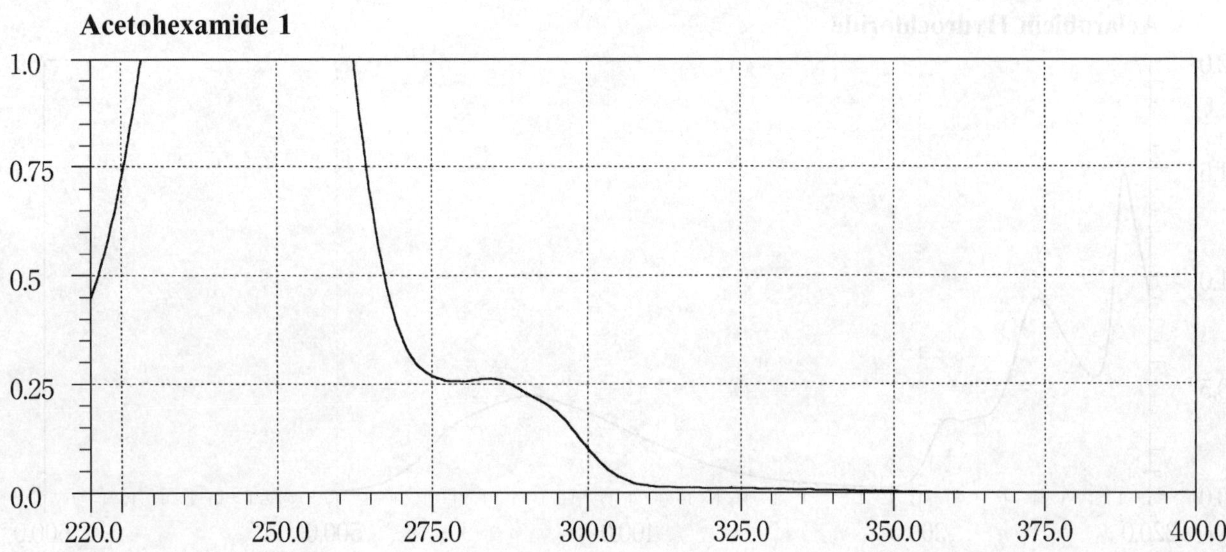

Acetohexamide 2

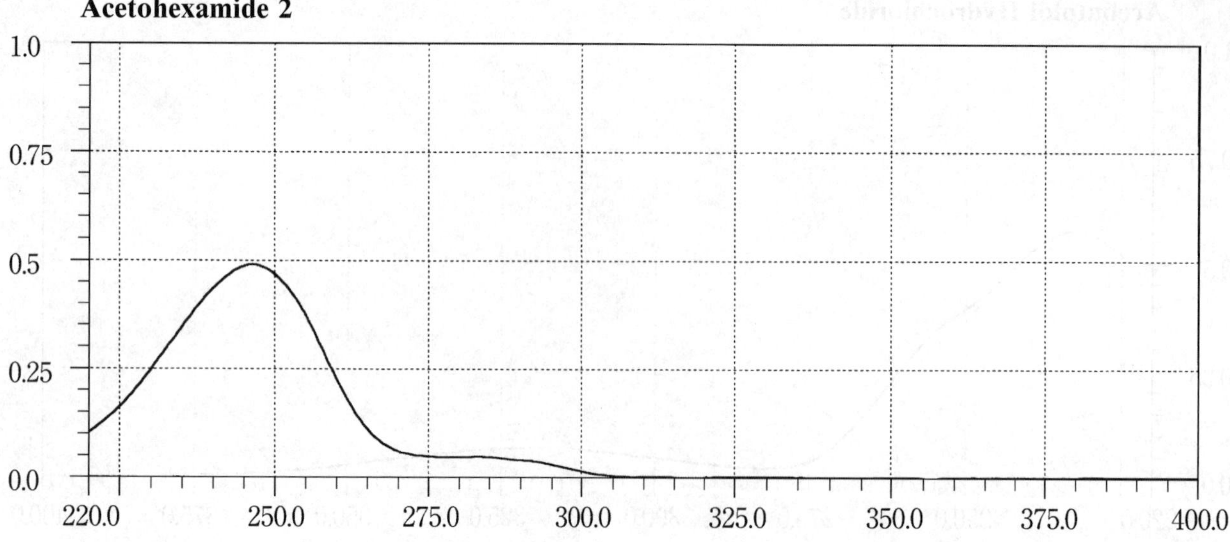

Aciclovir

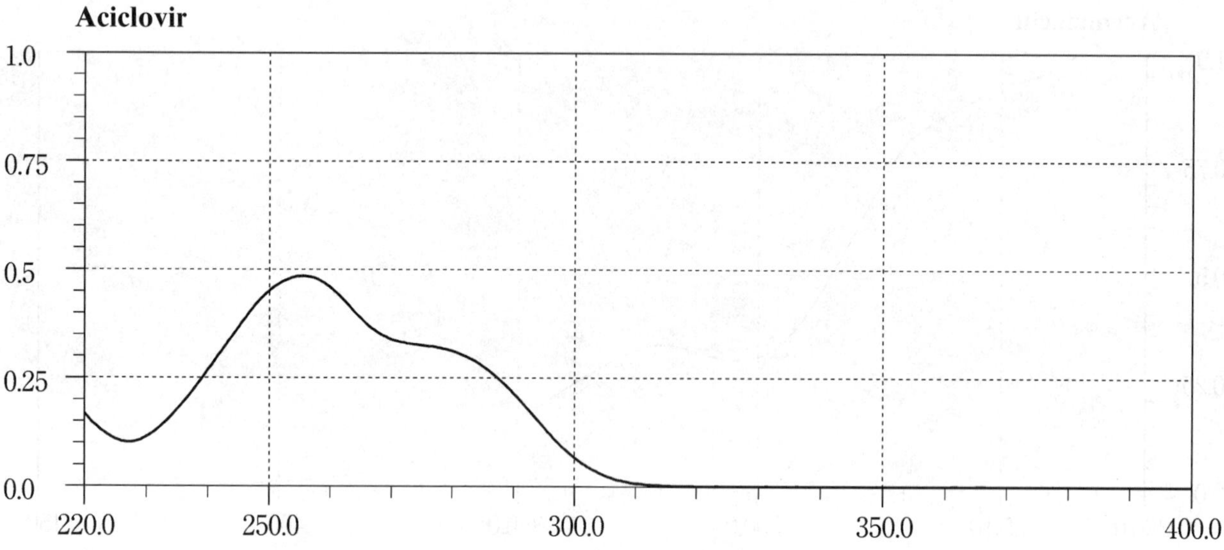

Aclarubicin Hydrochloride

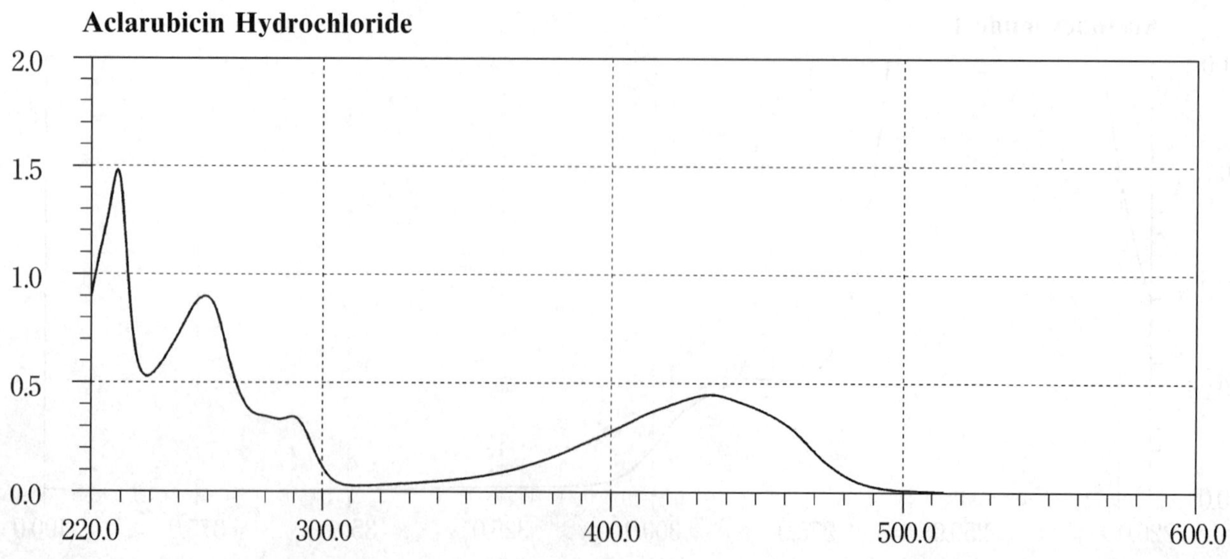

Acrinol Hydrate

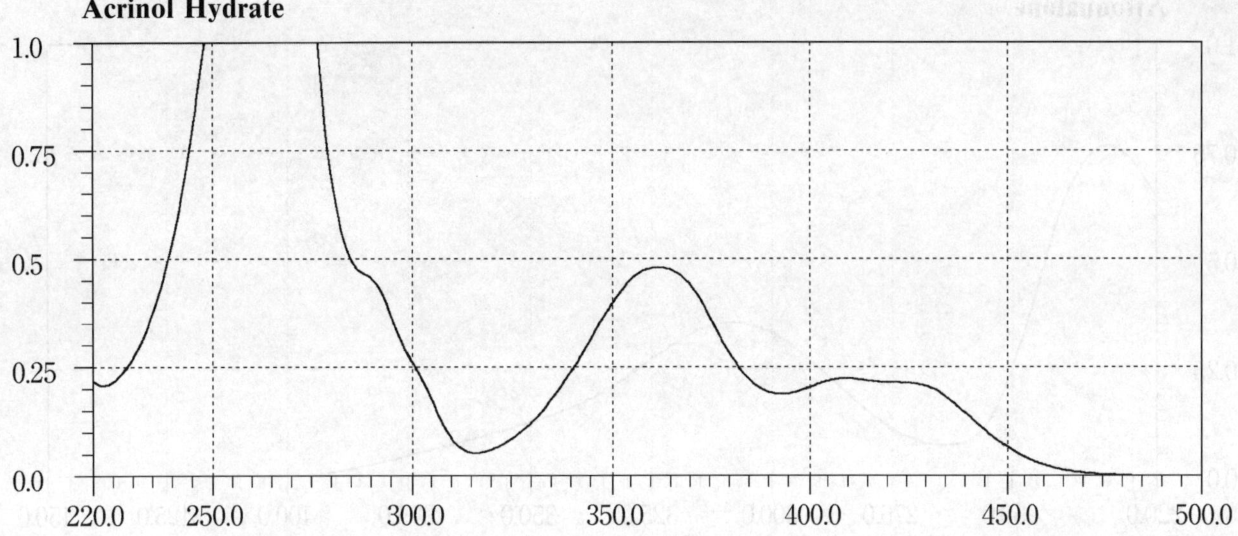

Actinomycin D

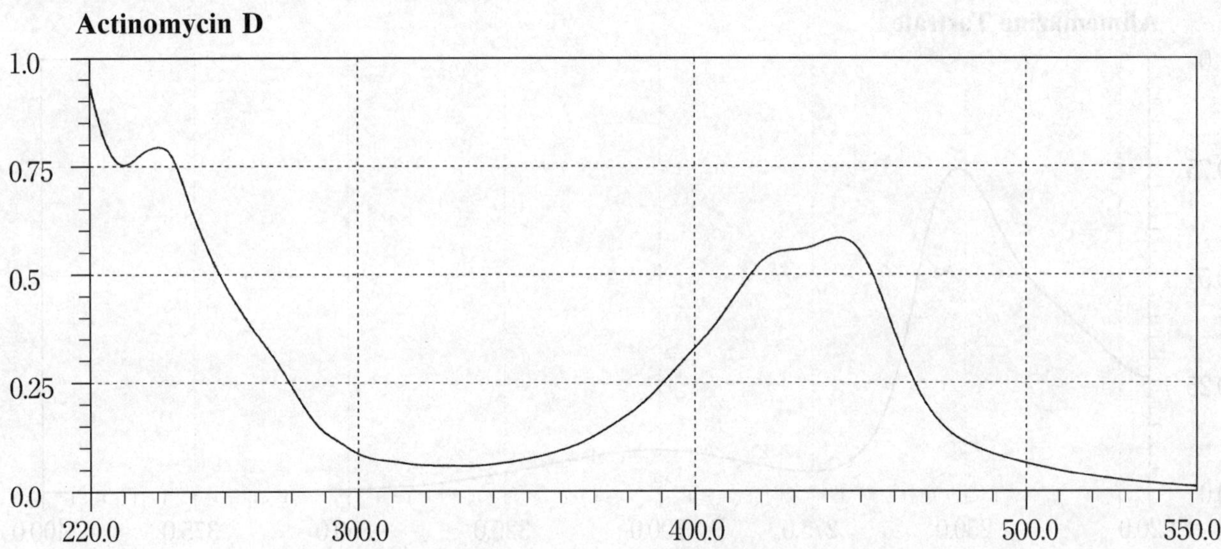

Adrenaline

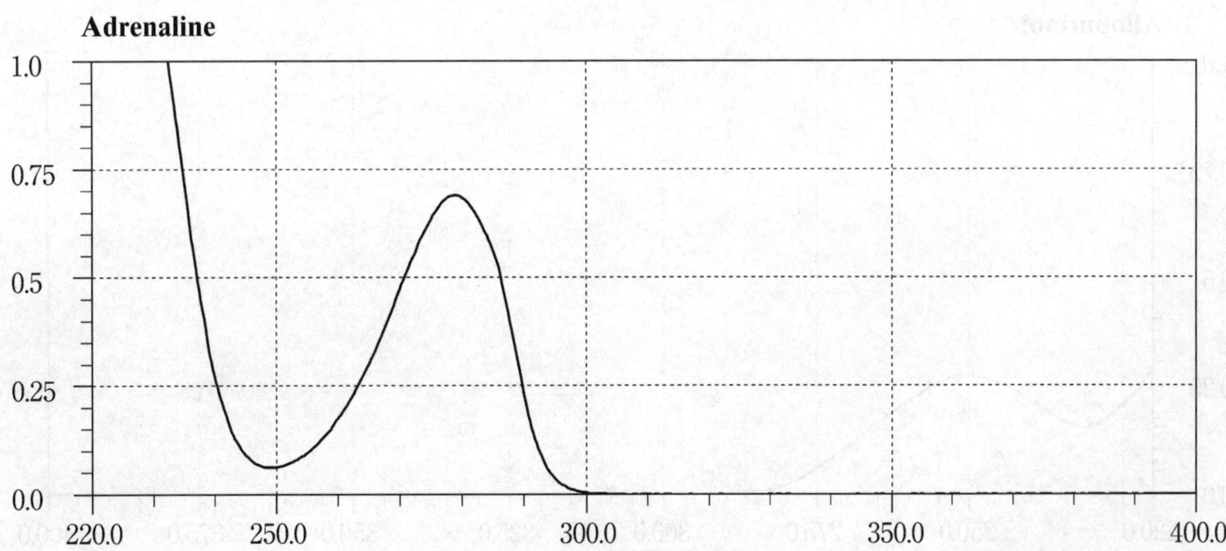

Afloqualone

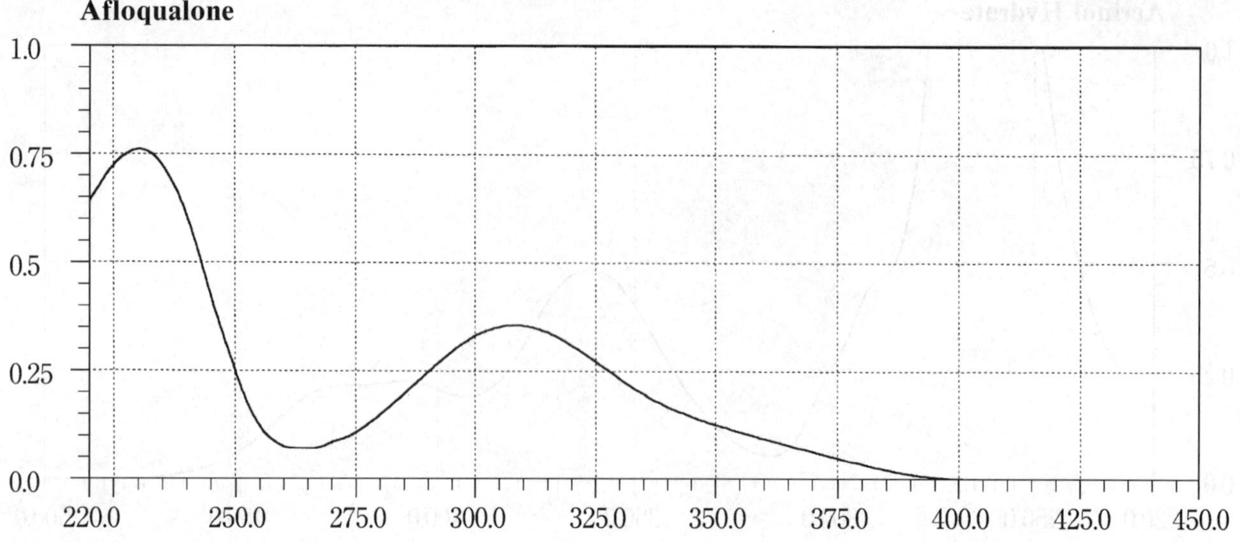

Alimemazine Tartrate

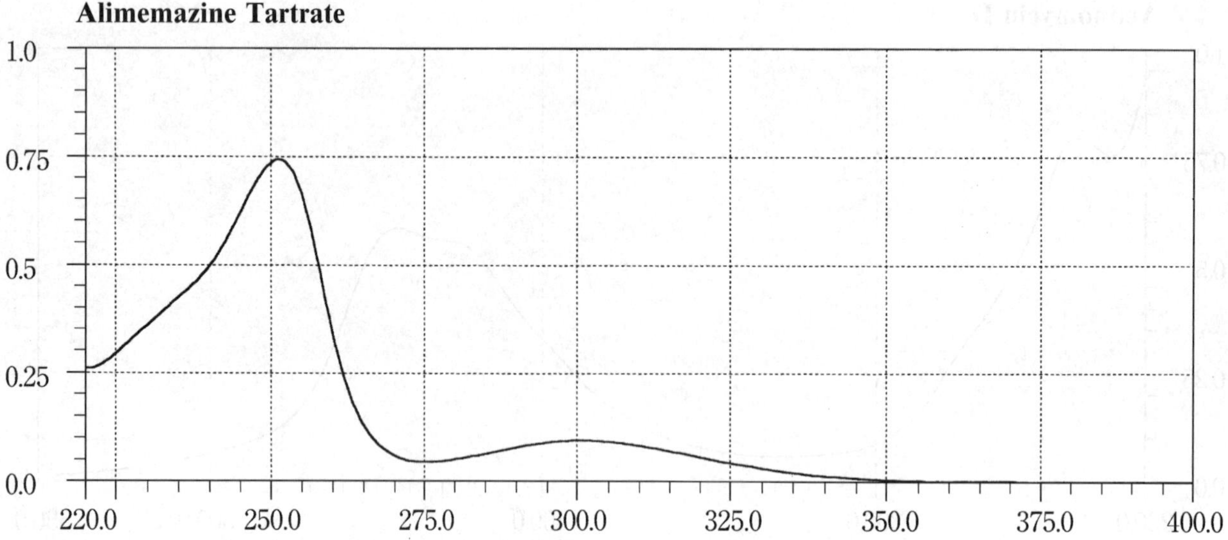

Allopurinol

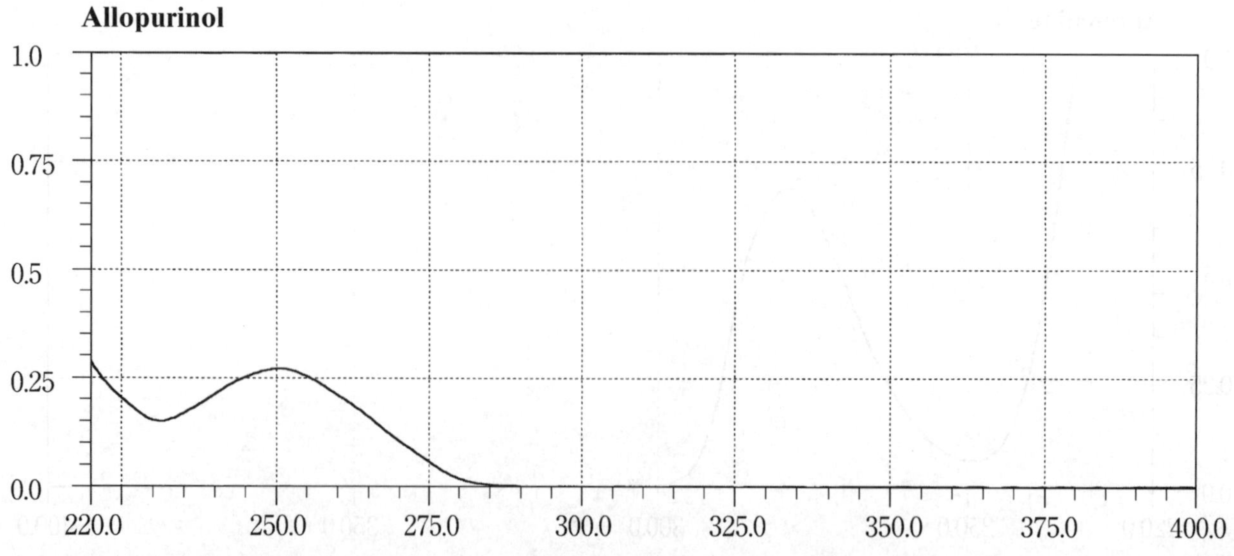

Alminoprofen

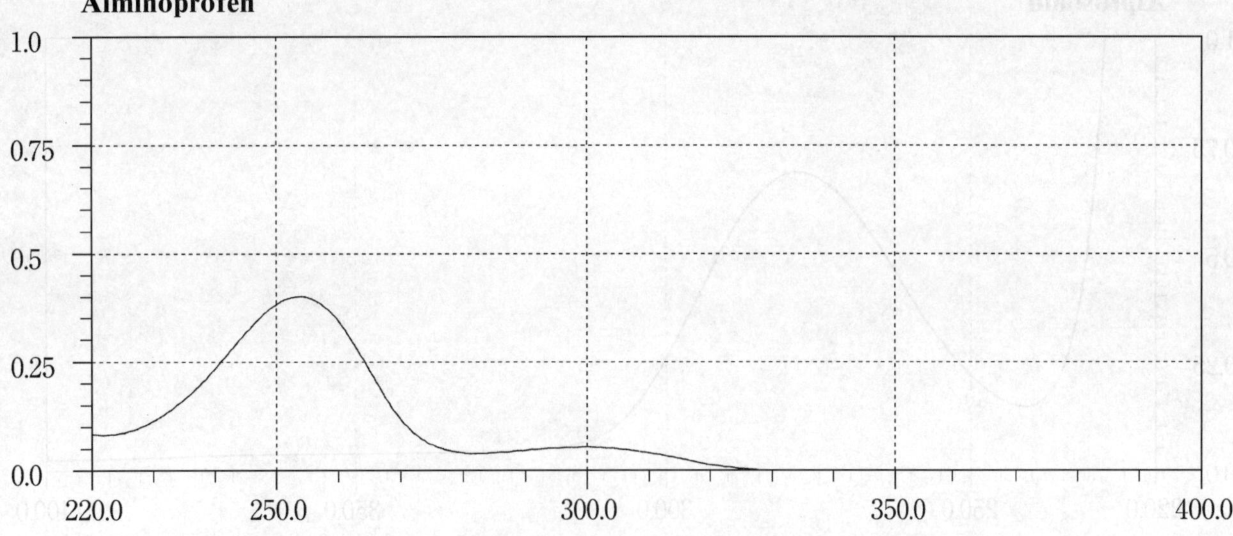

Alprazolam

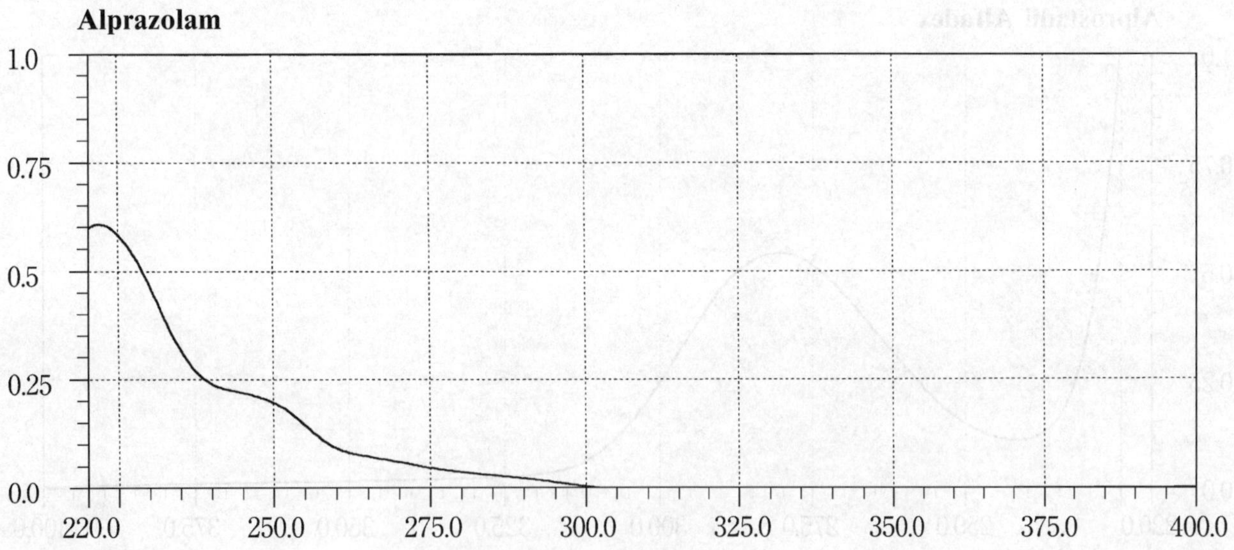

Alprenolol Hydrochloride

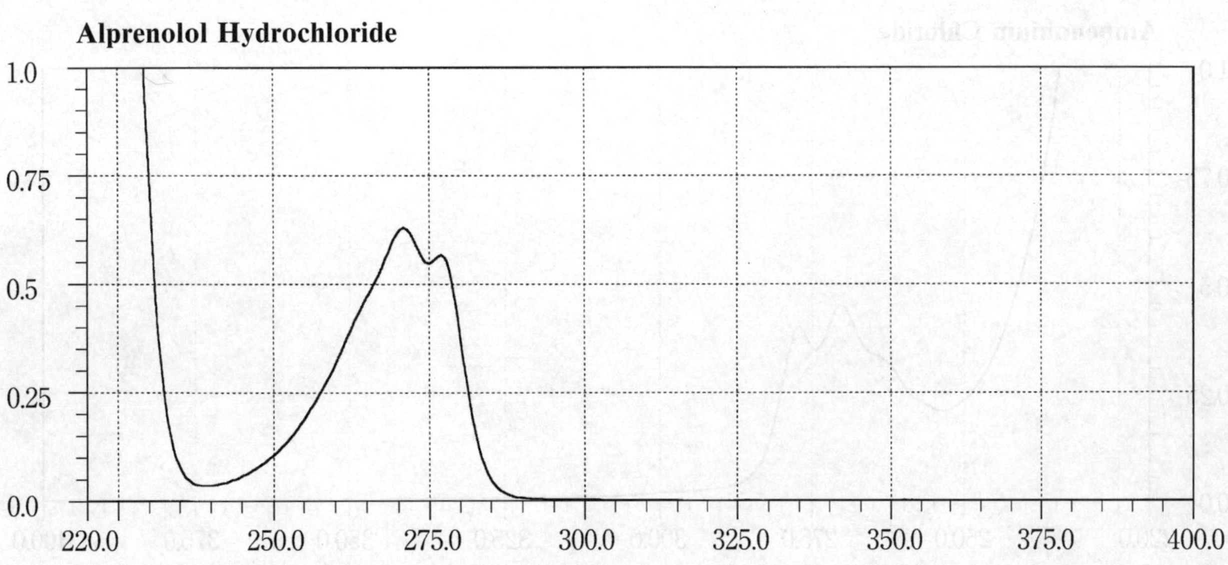

Alprostadil

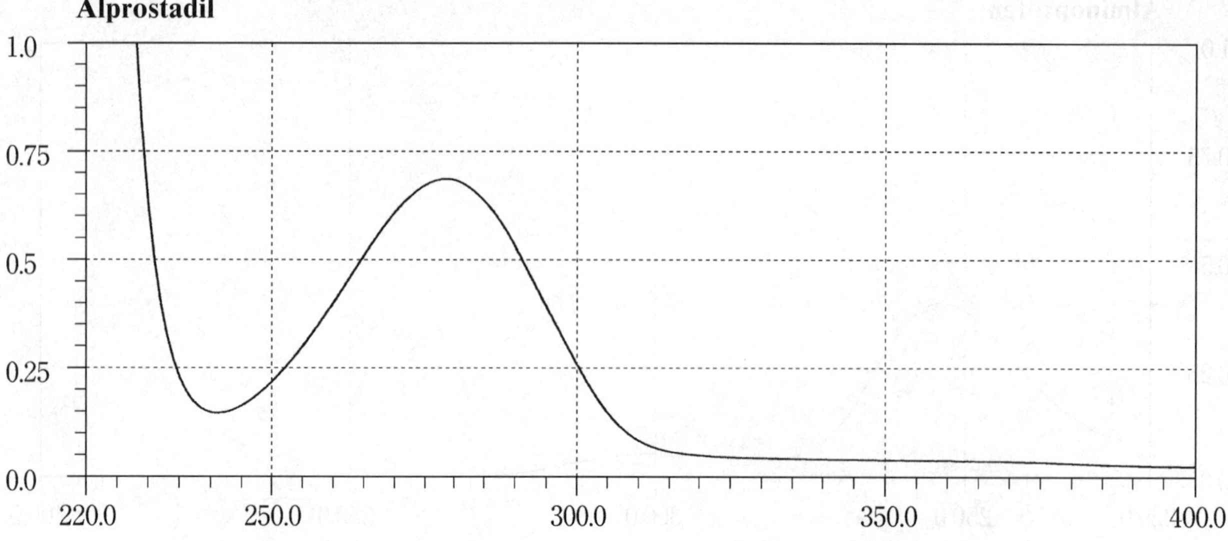

Alprostadil Alfadex

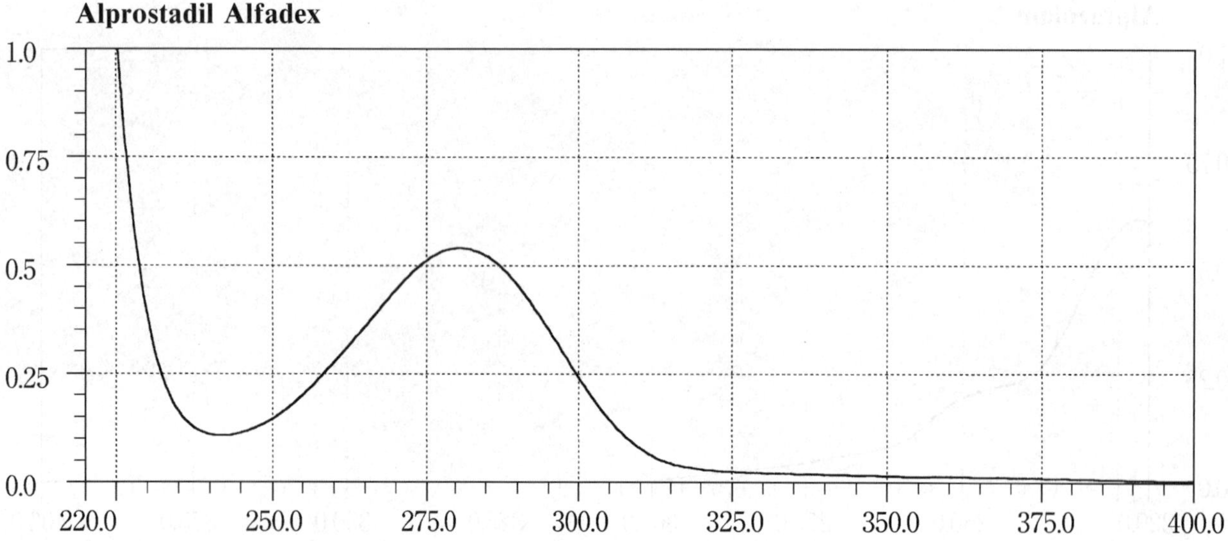

Ambenonium Chloride

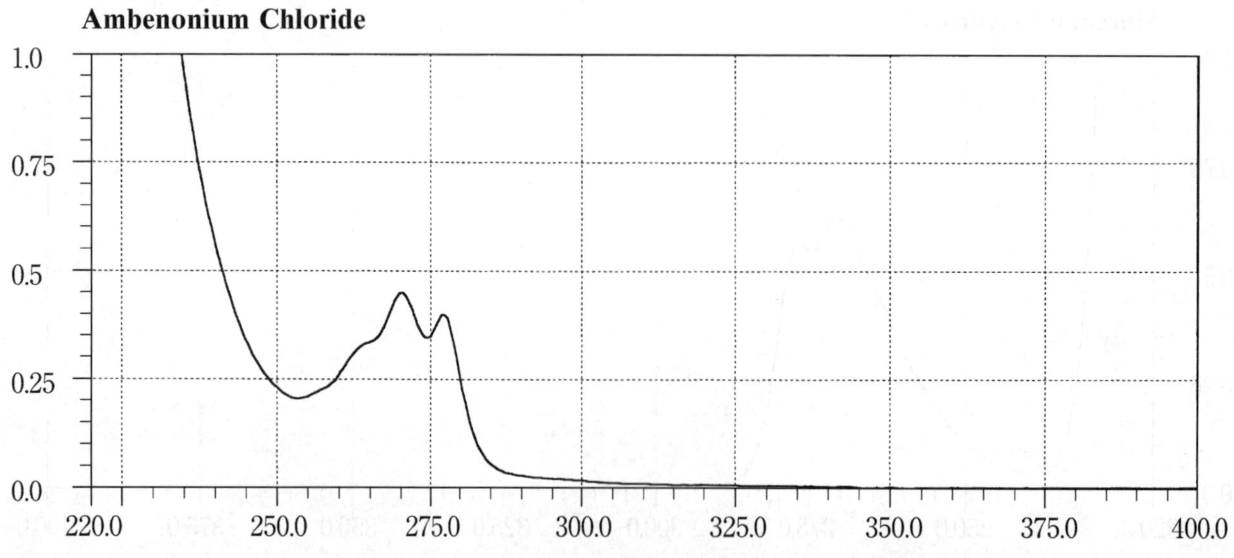

Amiodarone Hydrochloride

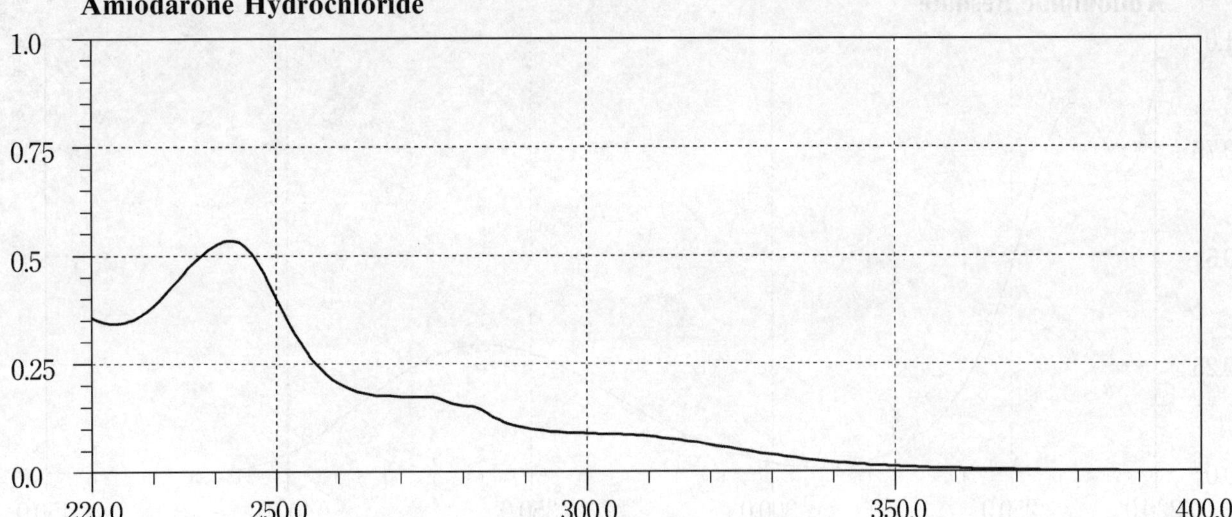

Amitriptyline Hydrochloride

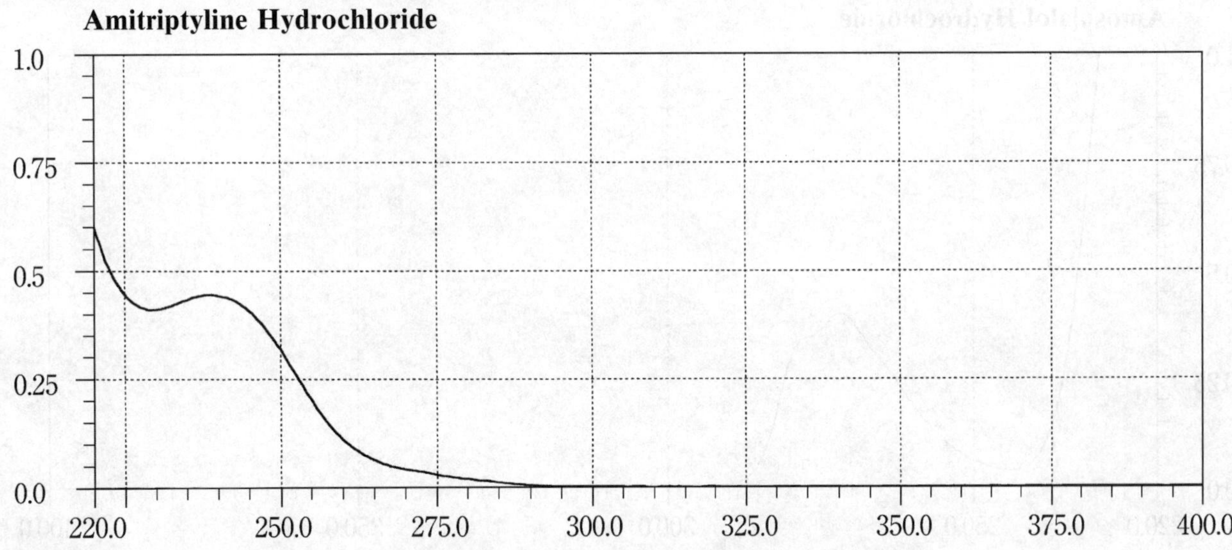

Amlexanox

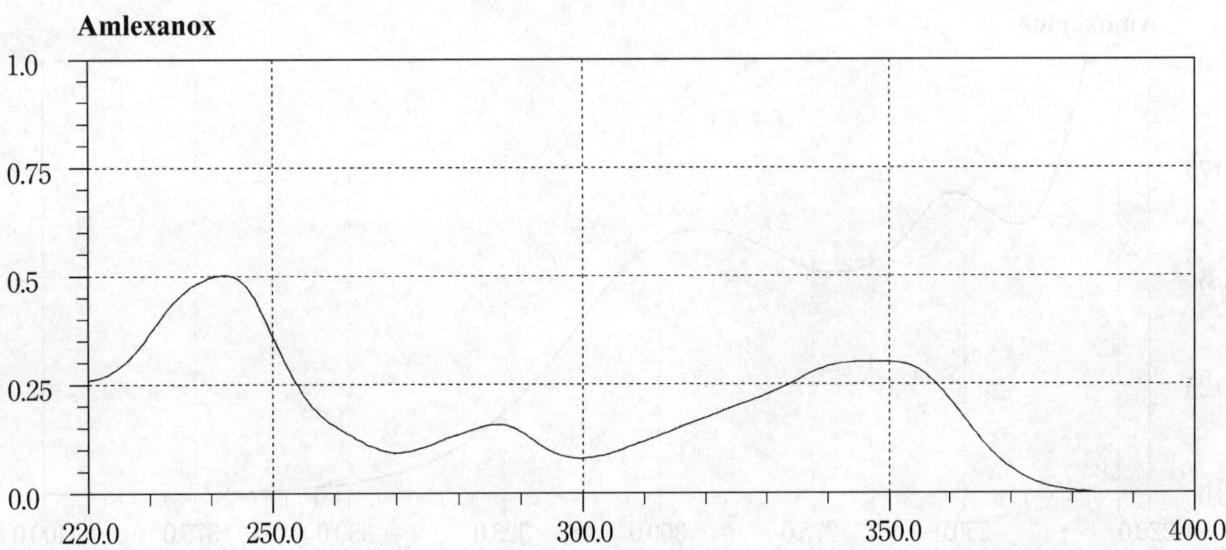

Amlodipine Besilate

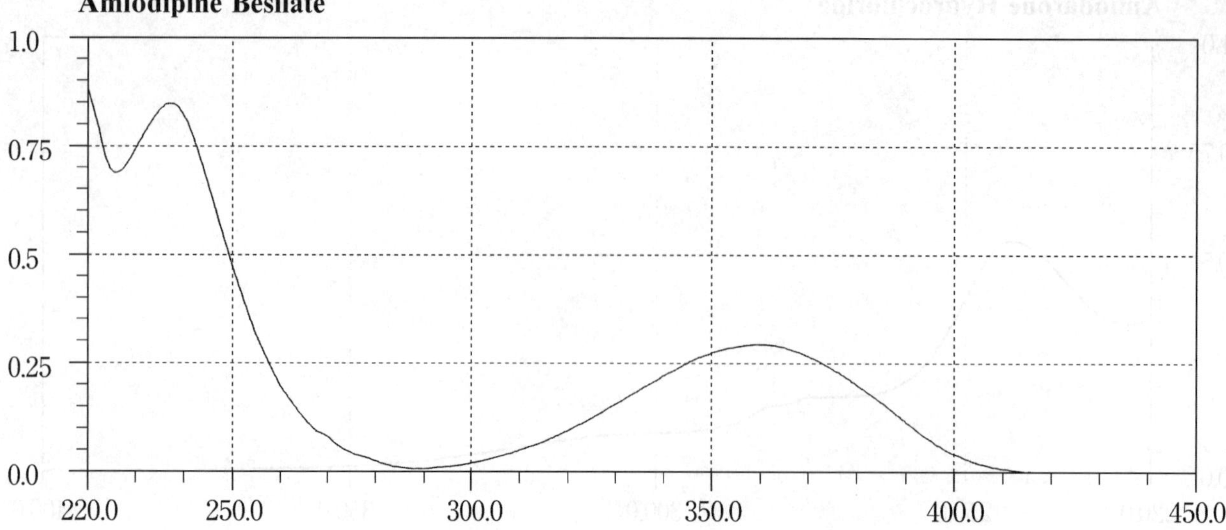

Amosulalol Hydrochloride

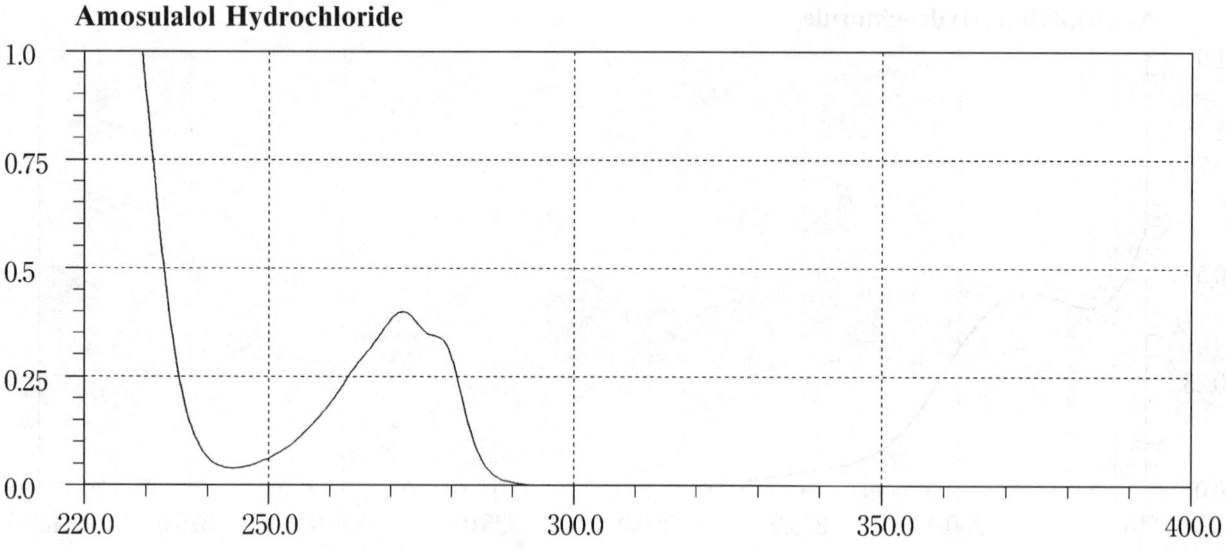

Amoxapine

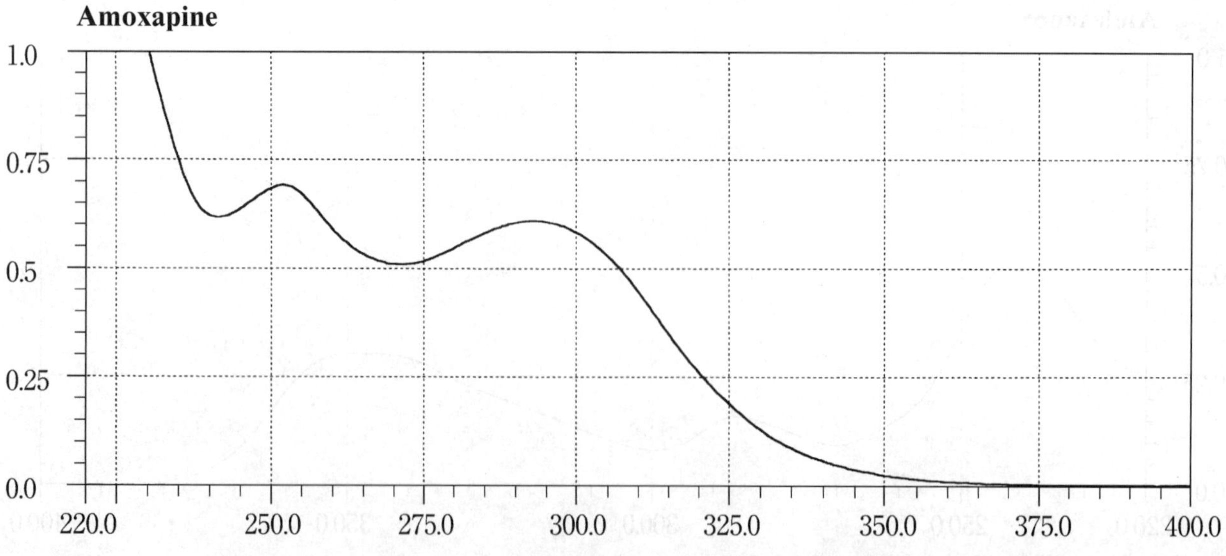

Amphotericin B

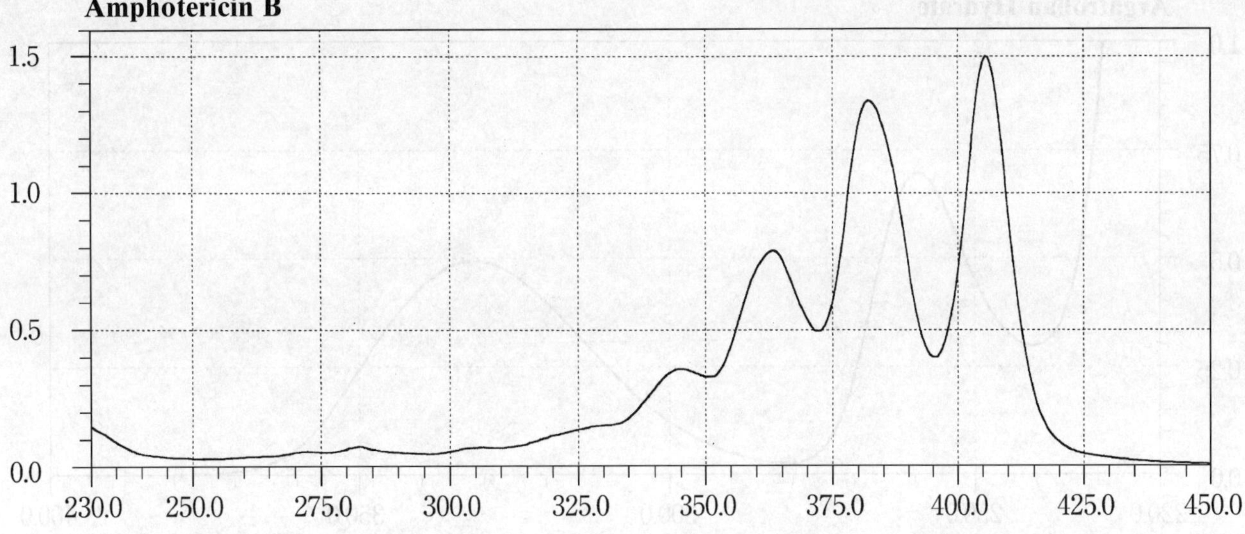

Ampiroxicam

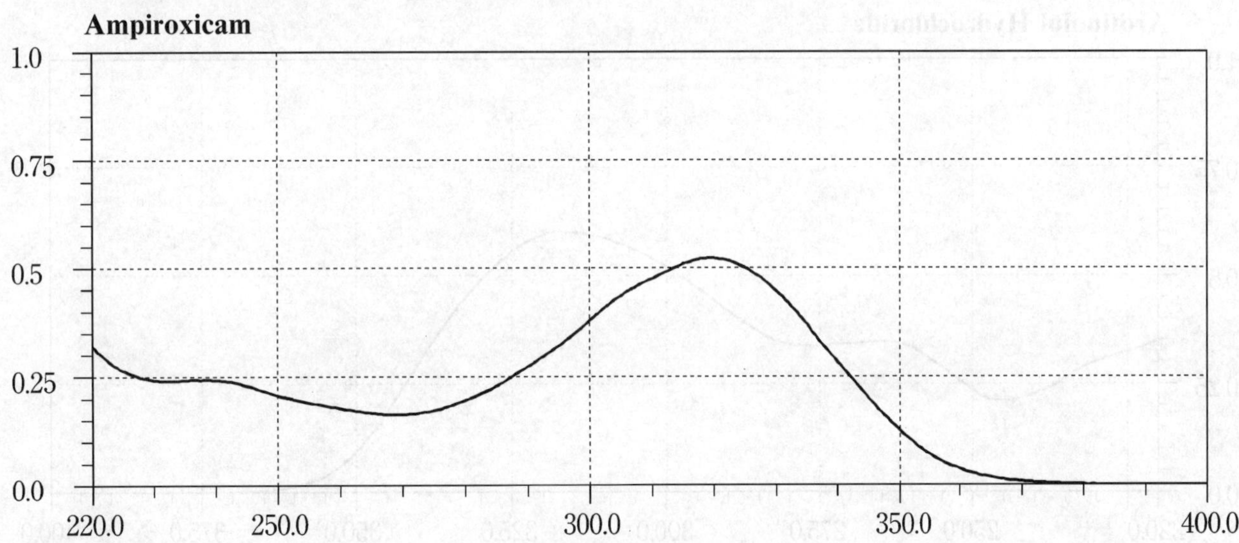

Aprindine Hydrochloride

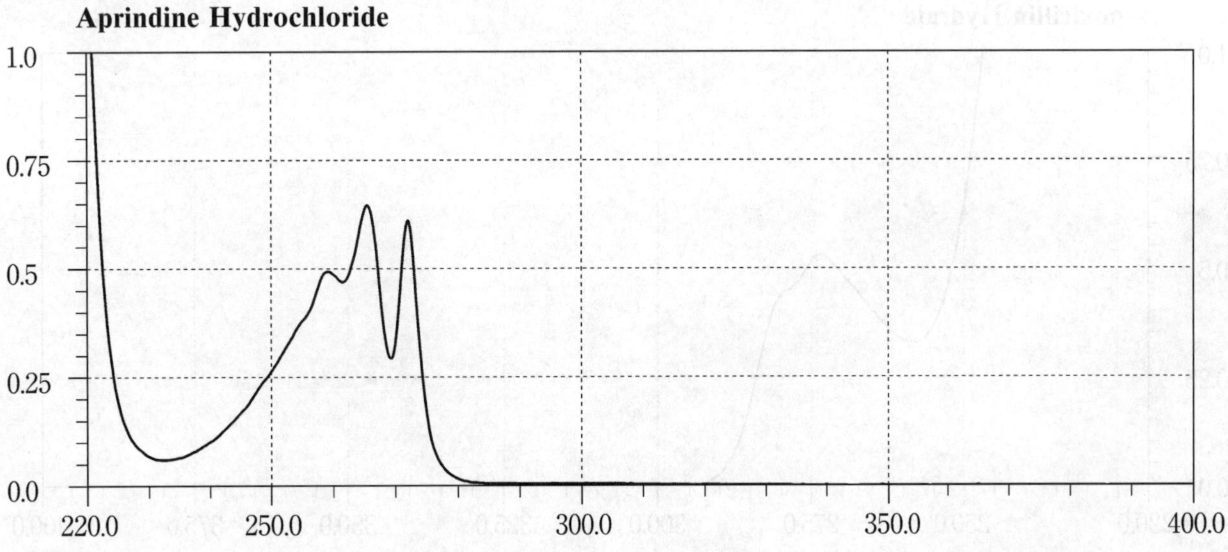

Argatroban Hydrate

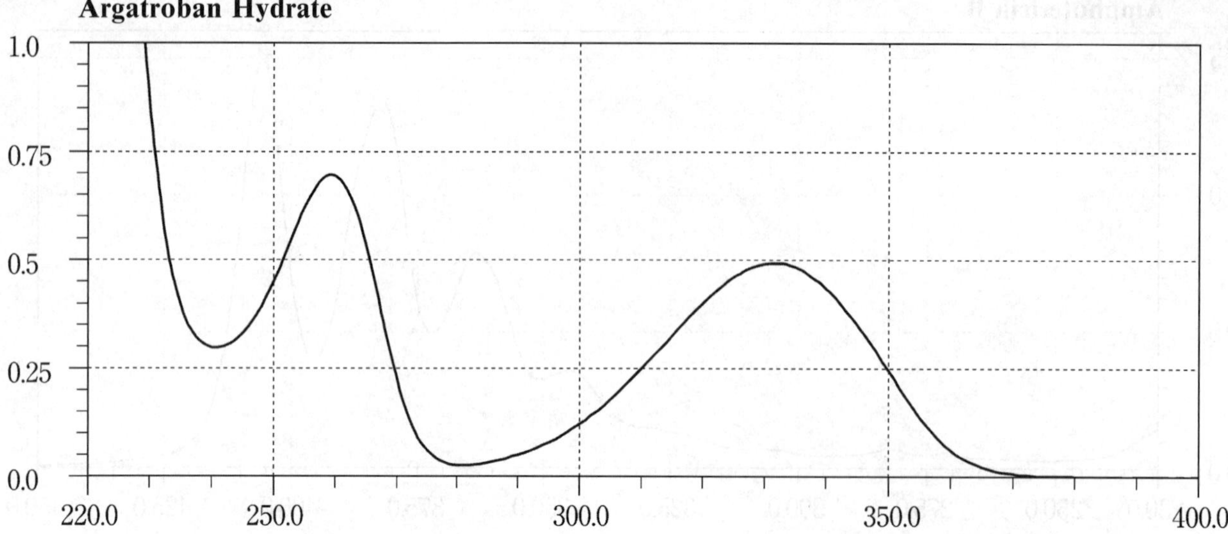

Arotinolol Hydrochloride

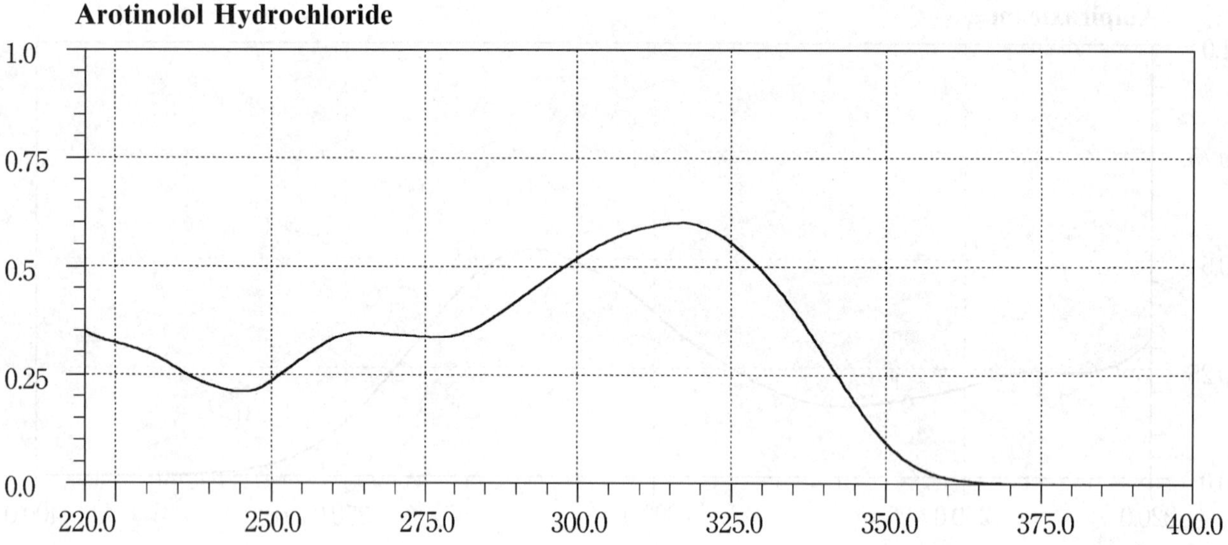

Aspoxicillin Hydrate

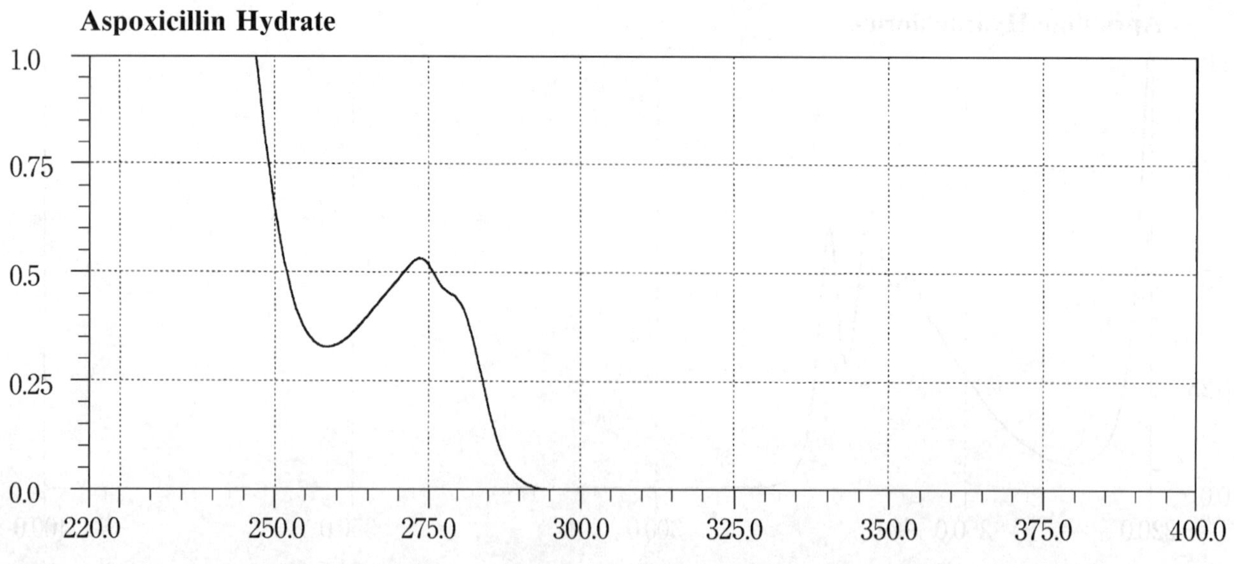

Atenolol

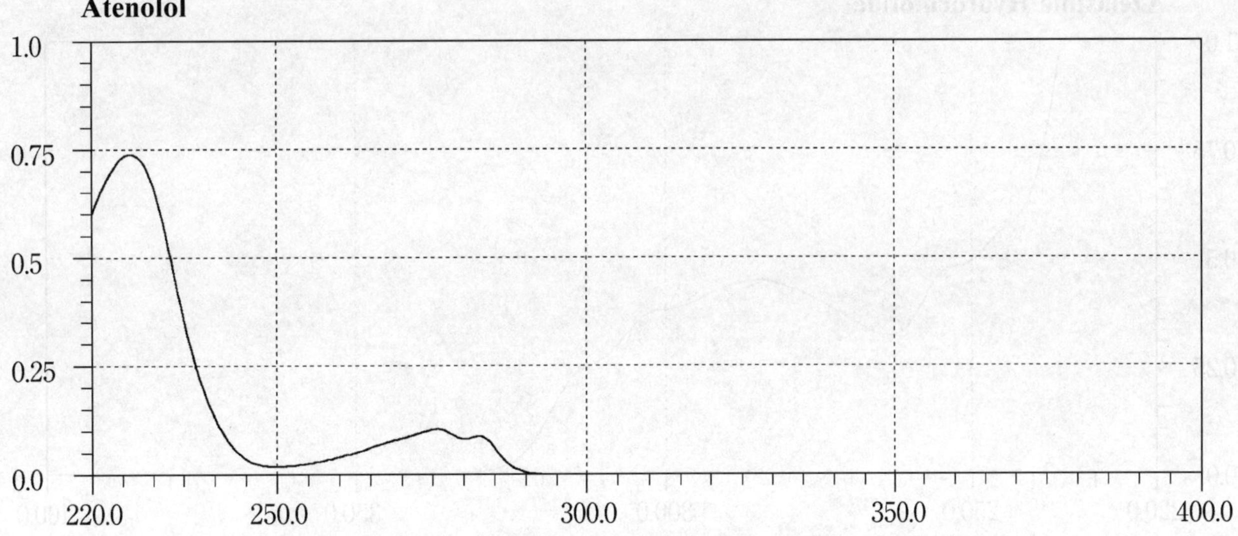

Atorvastatin Calcium Hydrate

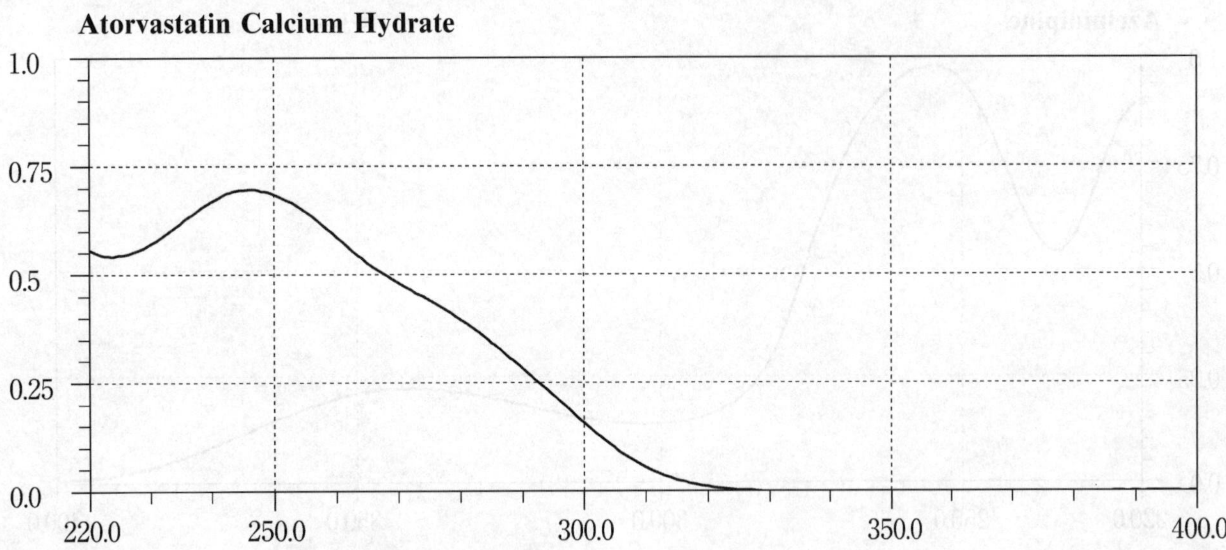

Azathioprine

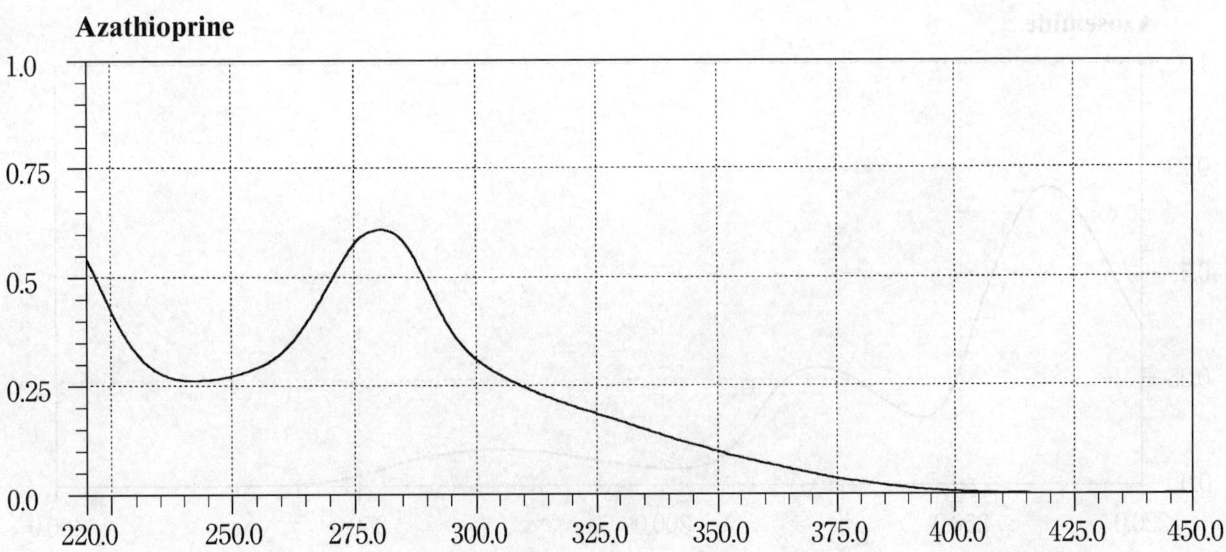

Azelastine Hydrochloride

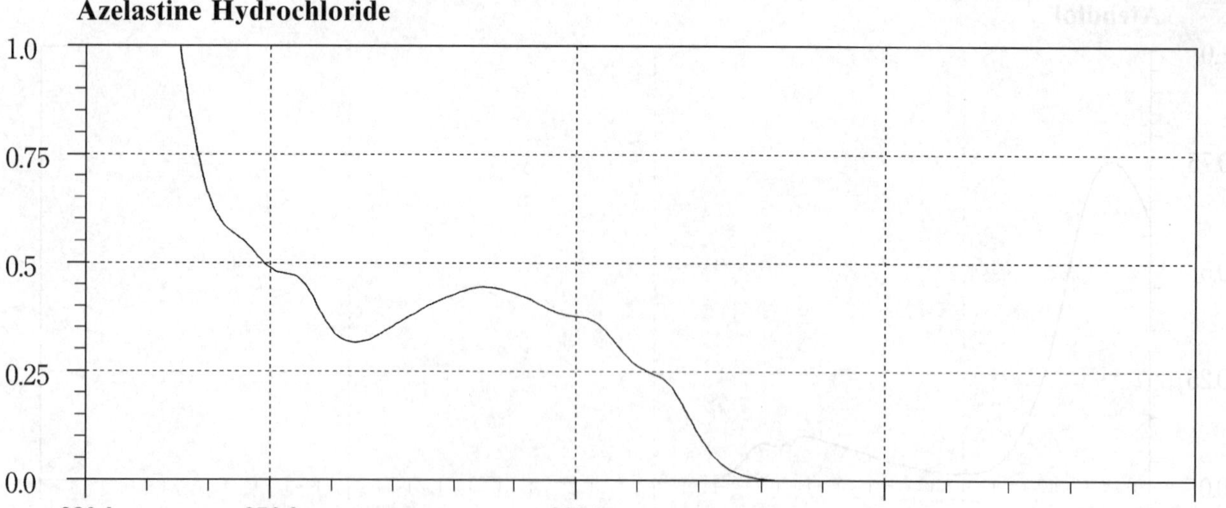

Azelnidipine

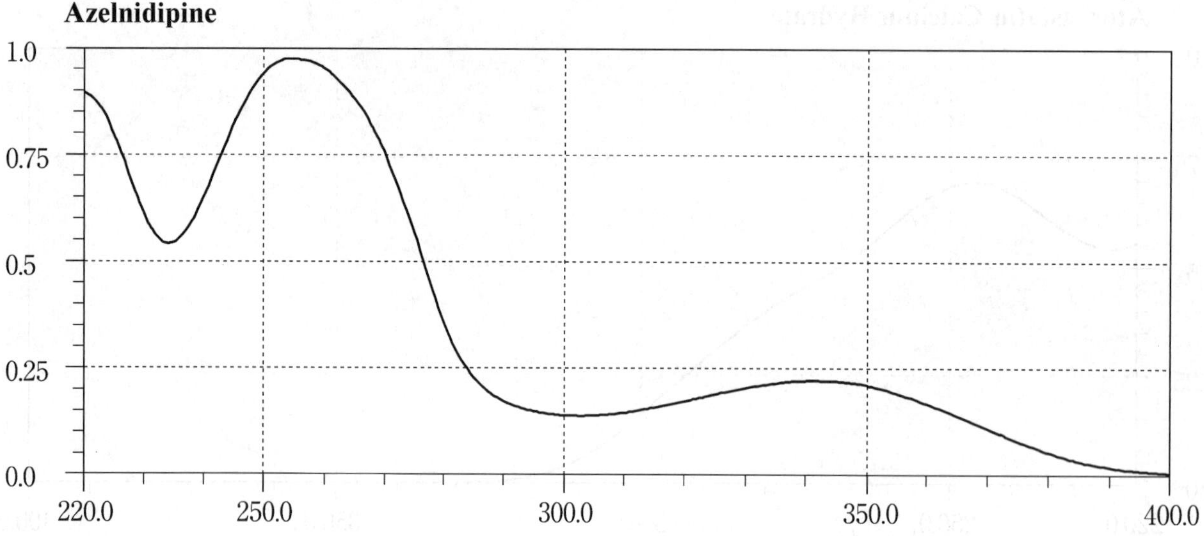

Azosemide

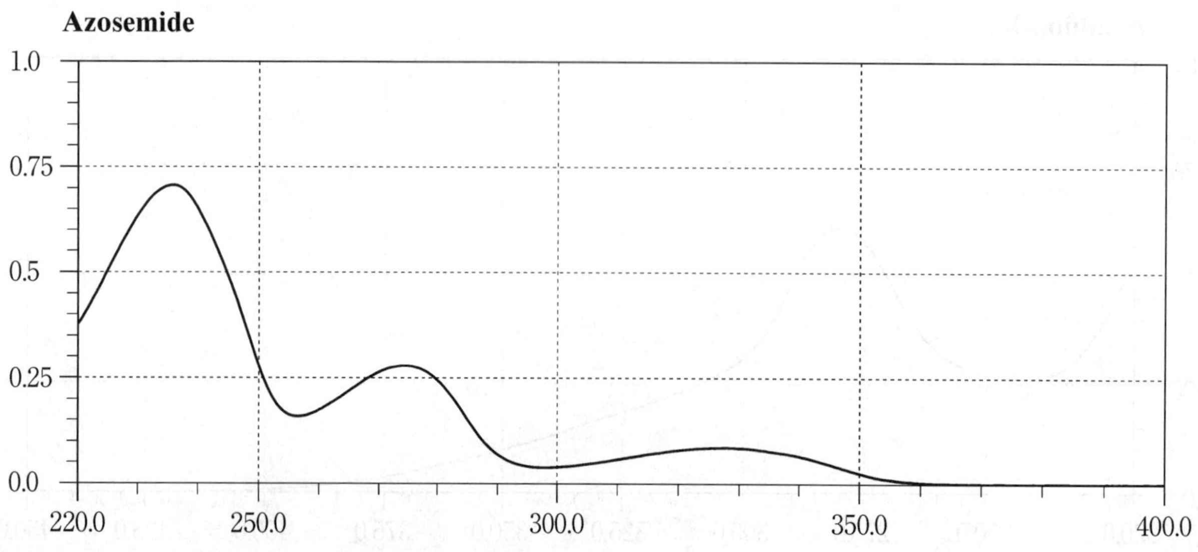

Aztreonam

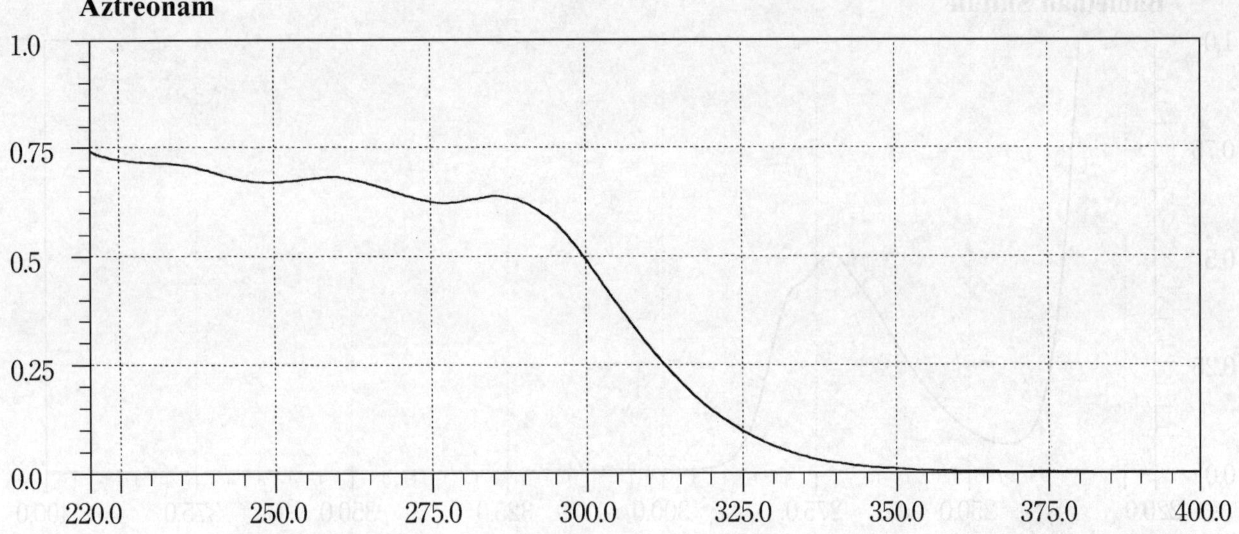

Bacampicillin Hydrochloride

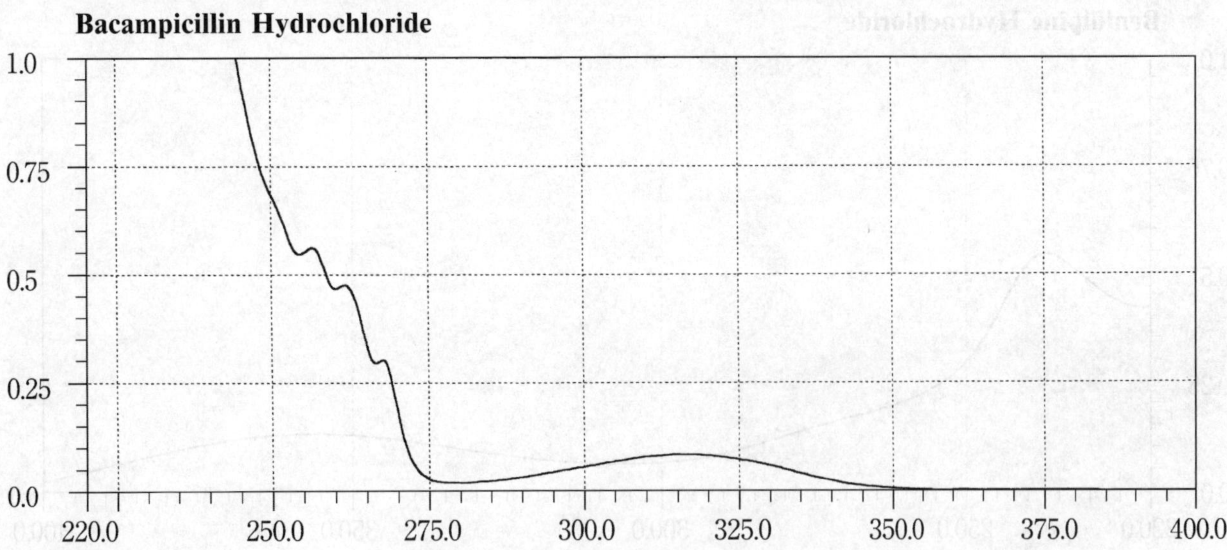

Baclofen

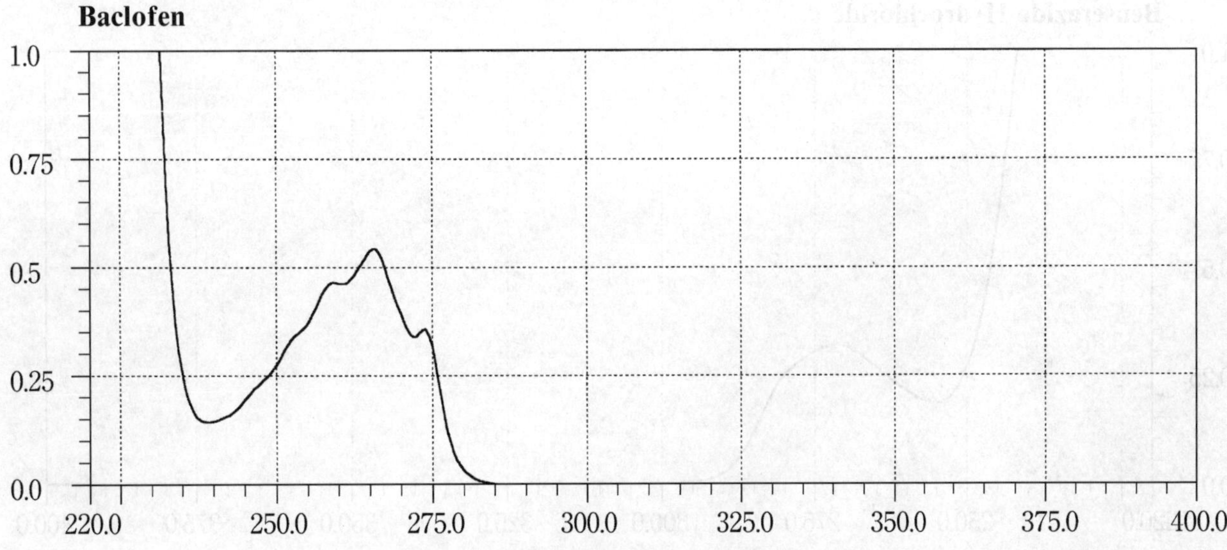

Bamethan Sulfate

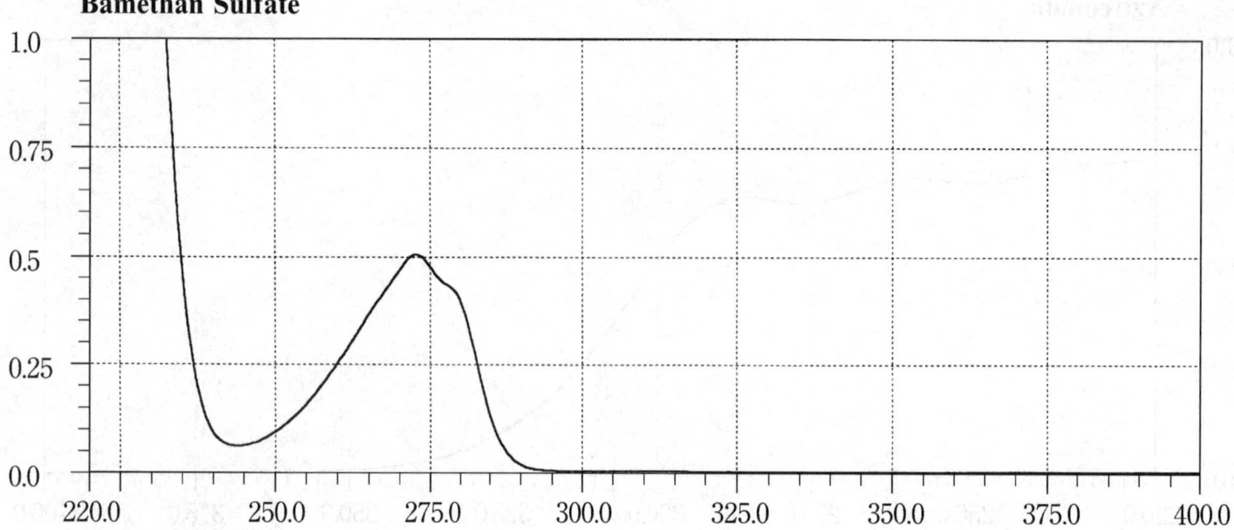

Benidipine Hydrochloride

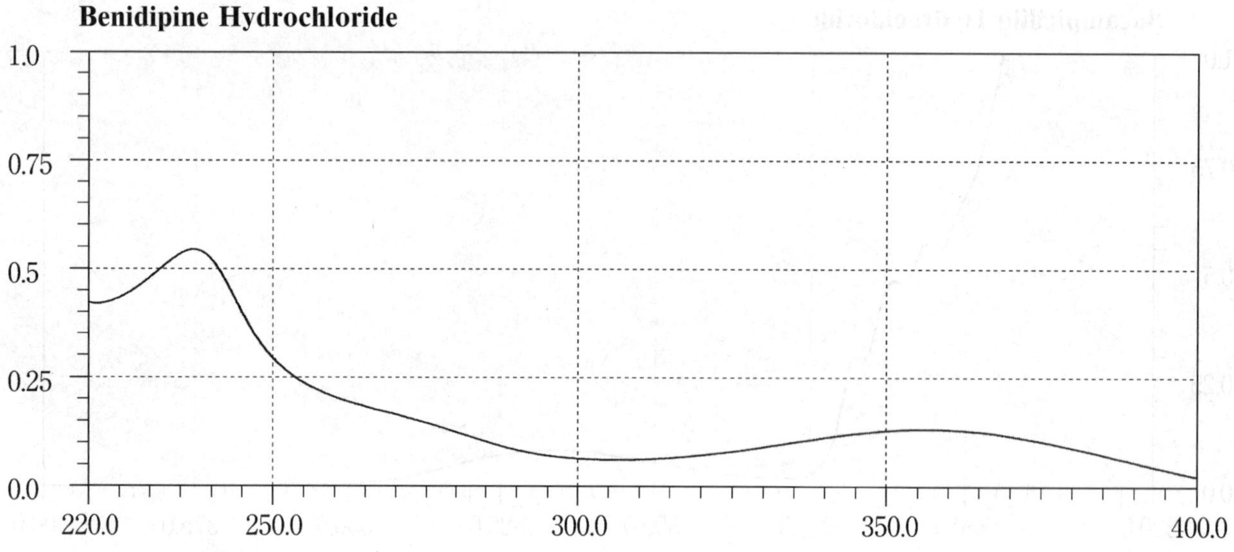

Benserazide Hydrochloride

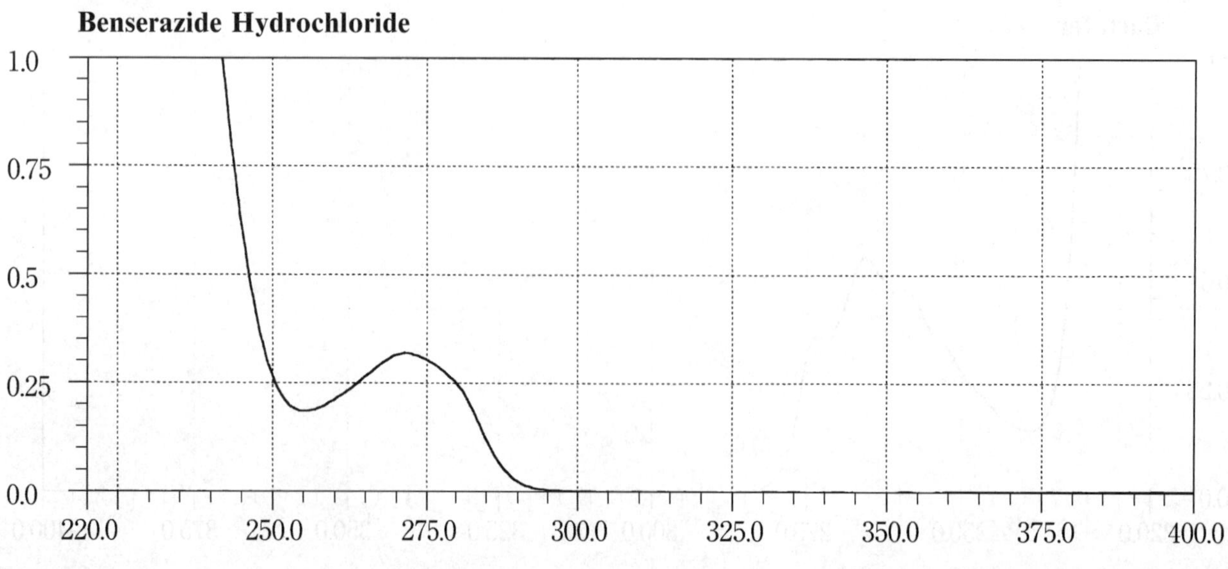

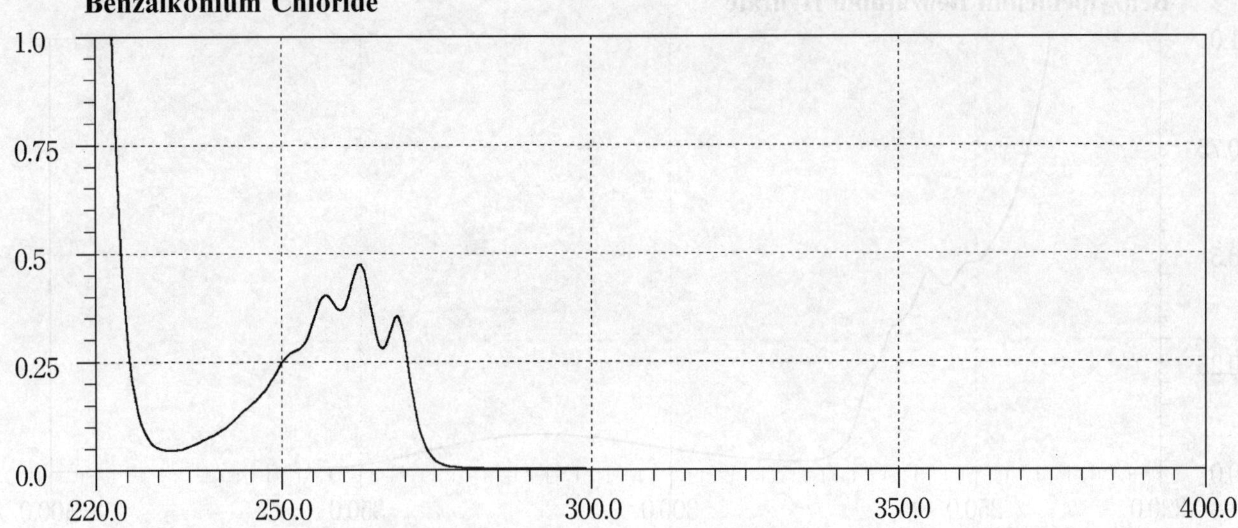
Benzalkonium Chloride
1.0
0.75
0.5
0.25
0.0
220.0
250.0
300.0
350.0
400.0

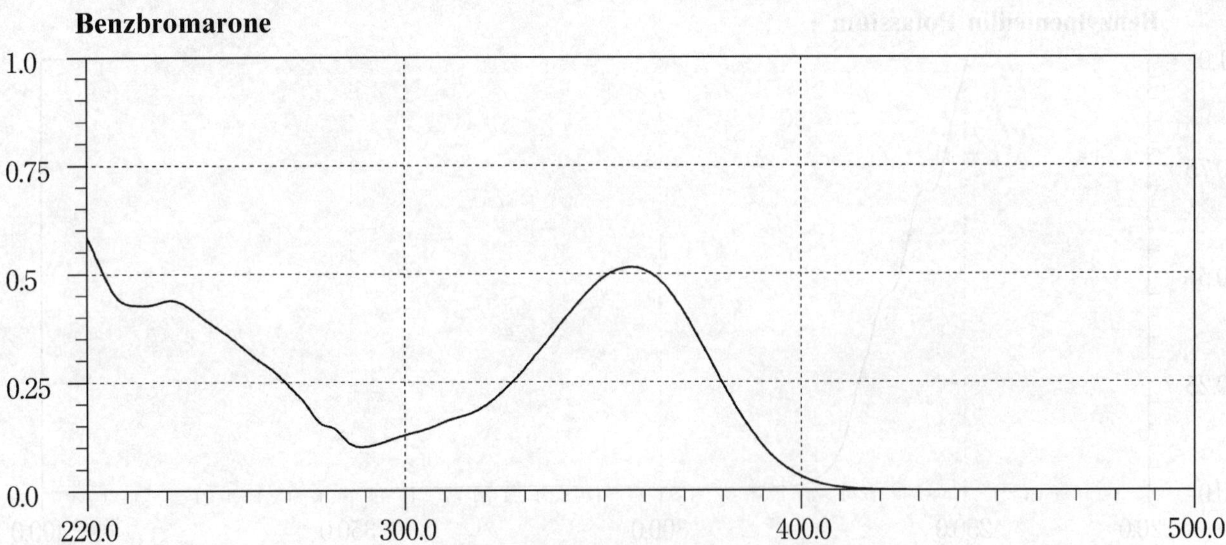
Benzbromarone
1.0
0.75
0.5
0.25
0.0
220.0
300.0
400.0
500.0

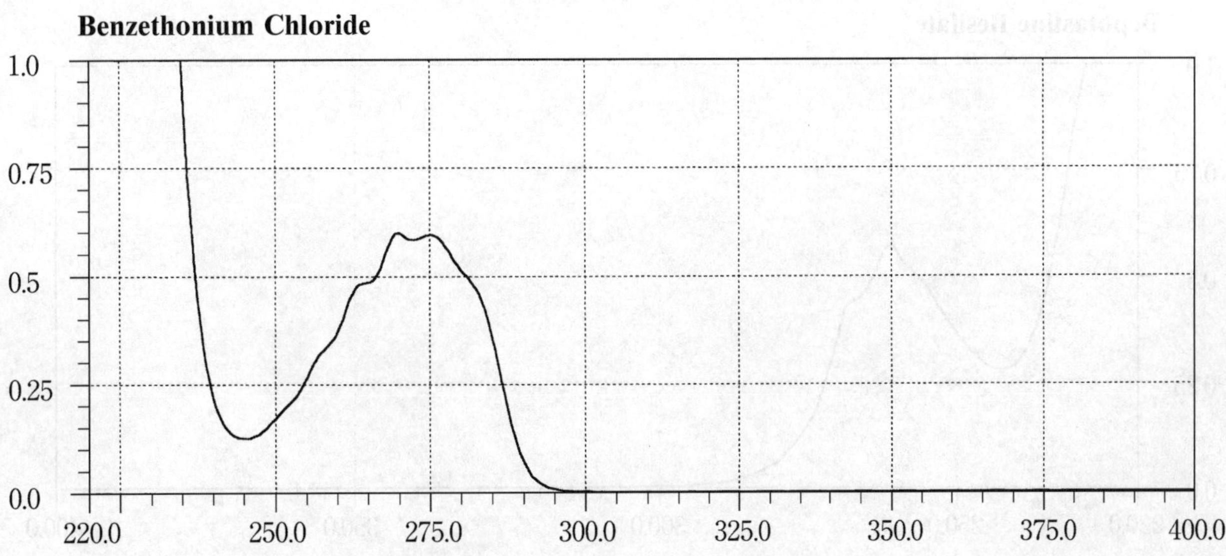
Benzethonium Chloride
1.0
0.75
0.5
0.25
0.0
220.0
250.0
275.0
300.0
325.0
350.0
375.0
400.0

Benzylpenicillin Benzathine Hydrate

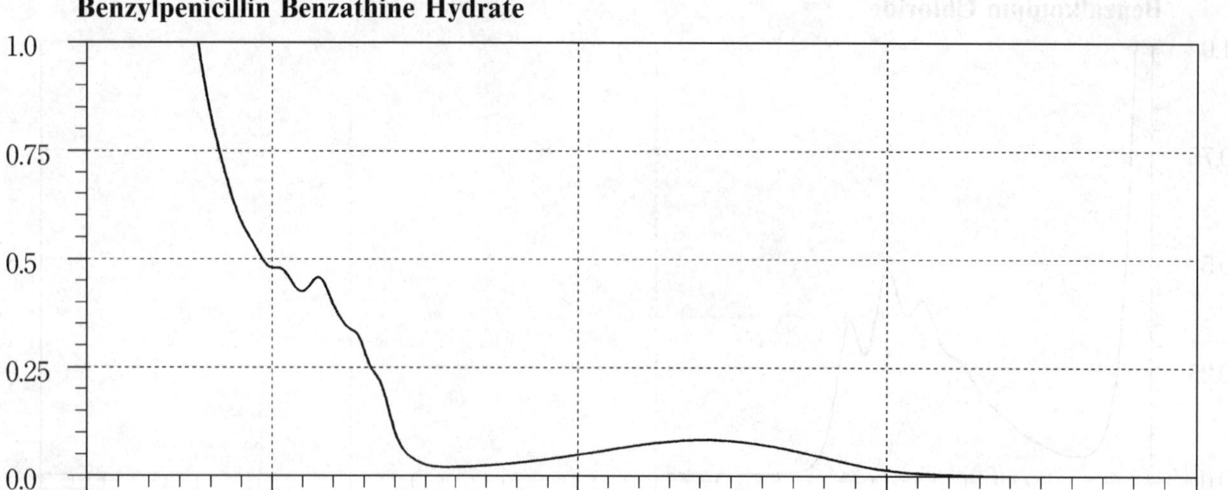

Benzylpenicillin Potassium

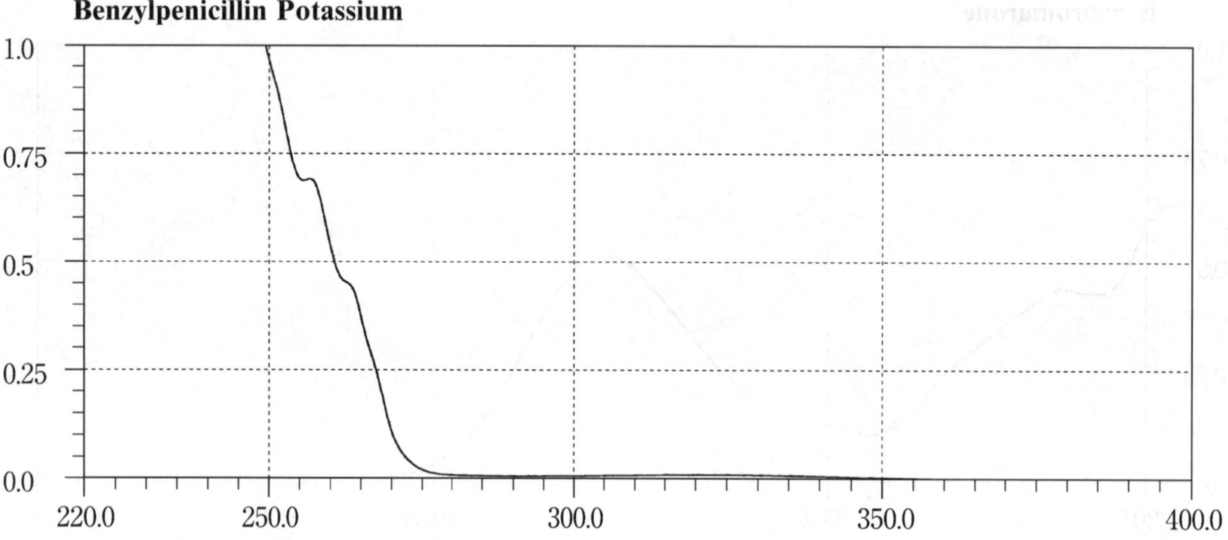

Bepotastine Besilate

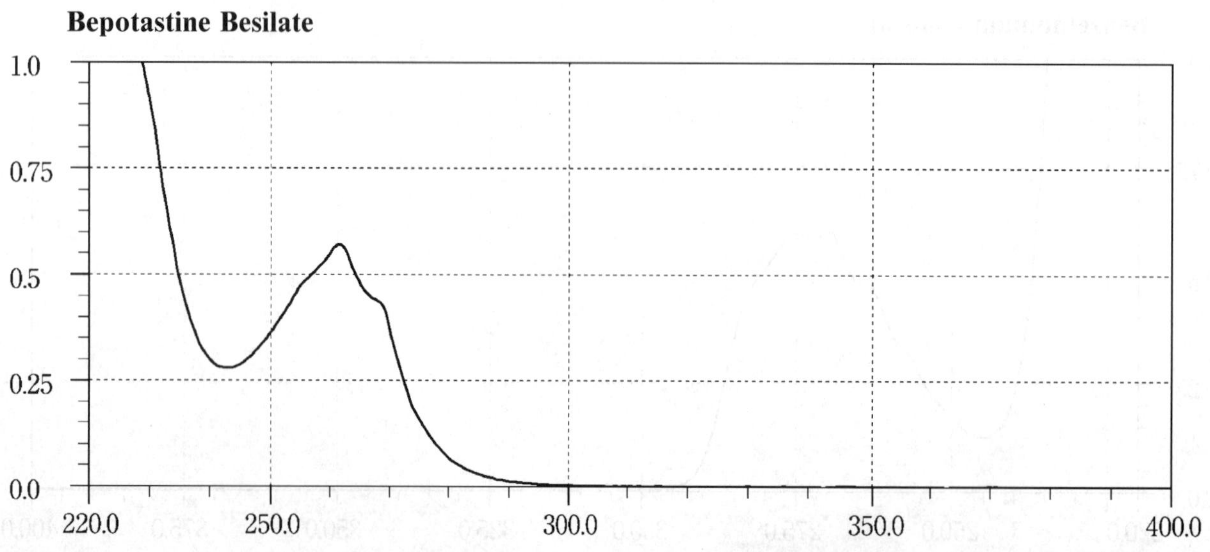

Beraprost Sodium

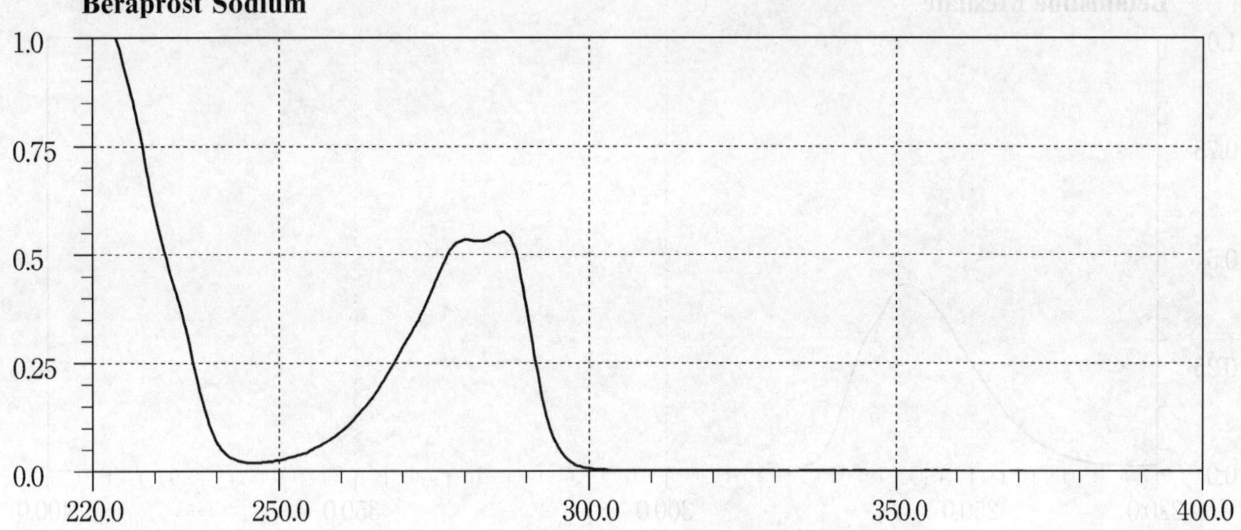

Berberine Chloride Hydrate

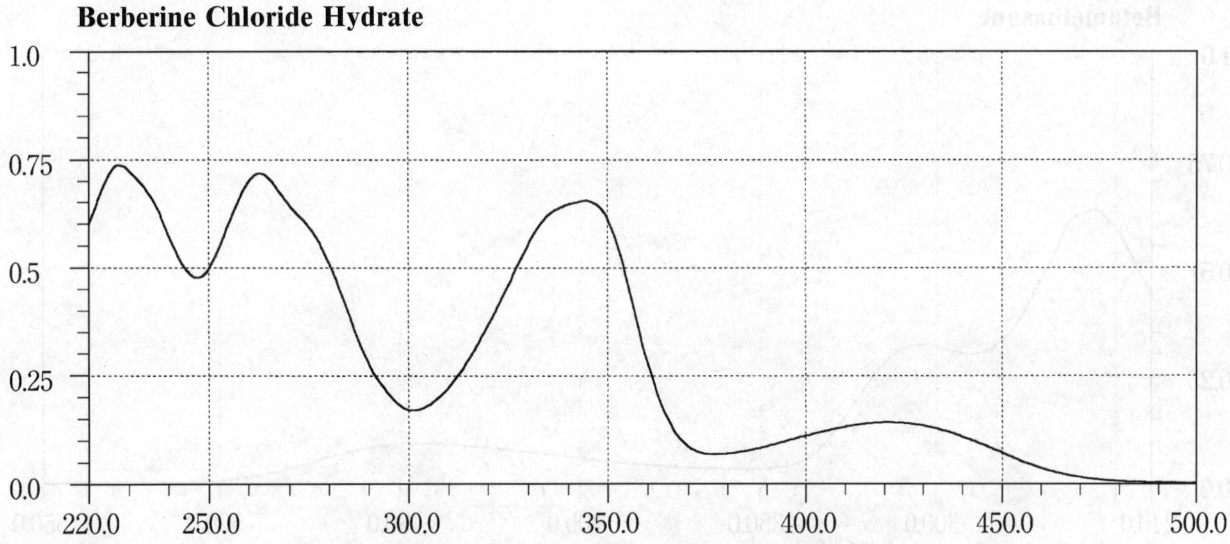

Berberine Tannate

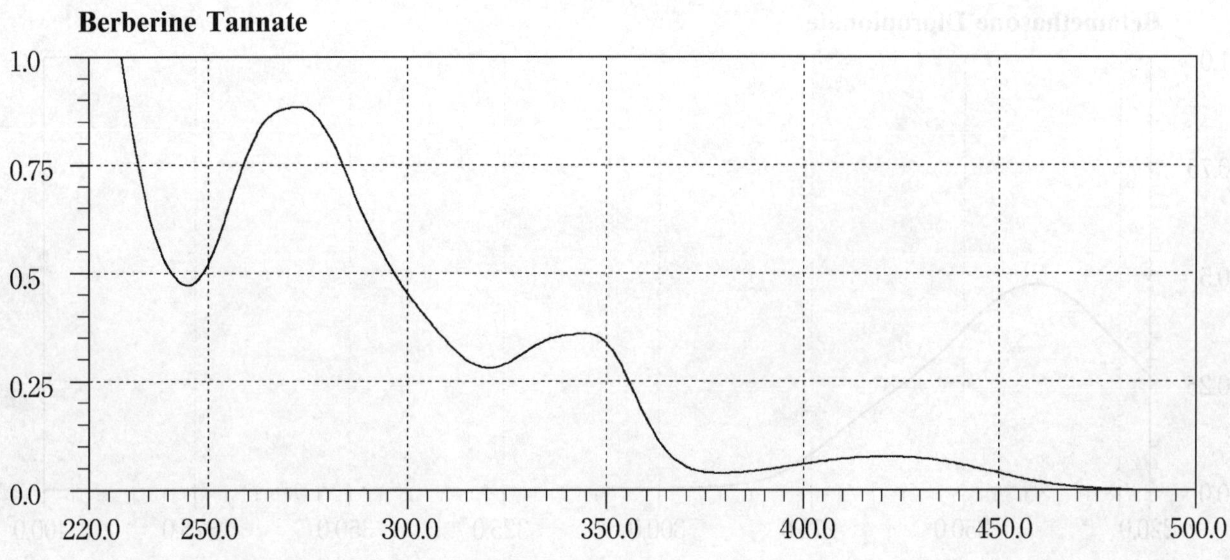

Betahistine Mesilate

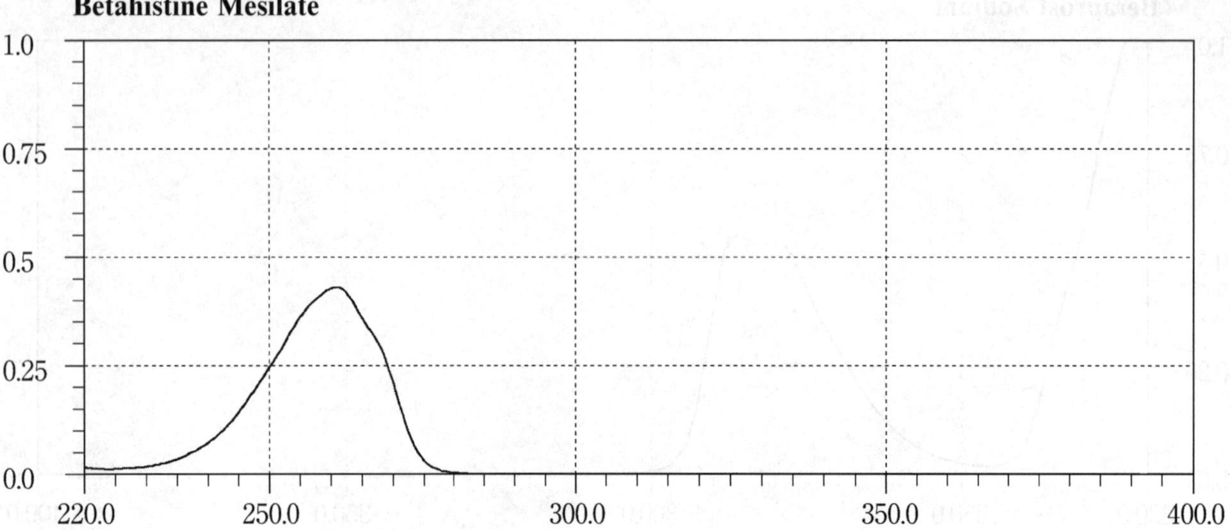

Betamethasone

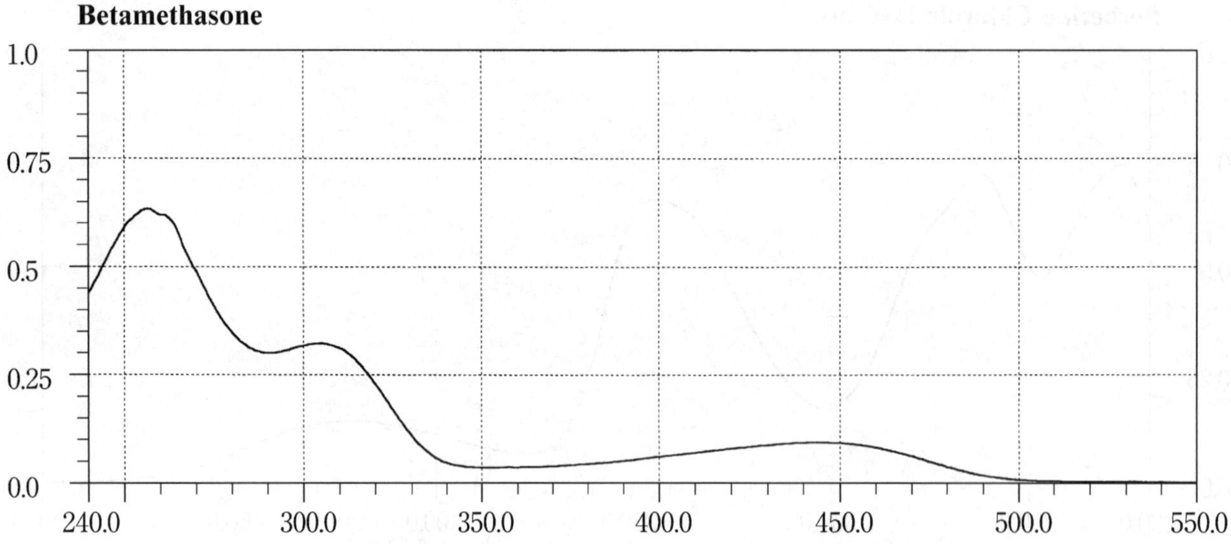

Betamethasone Dipropionate

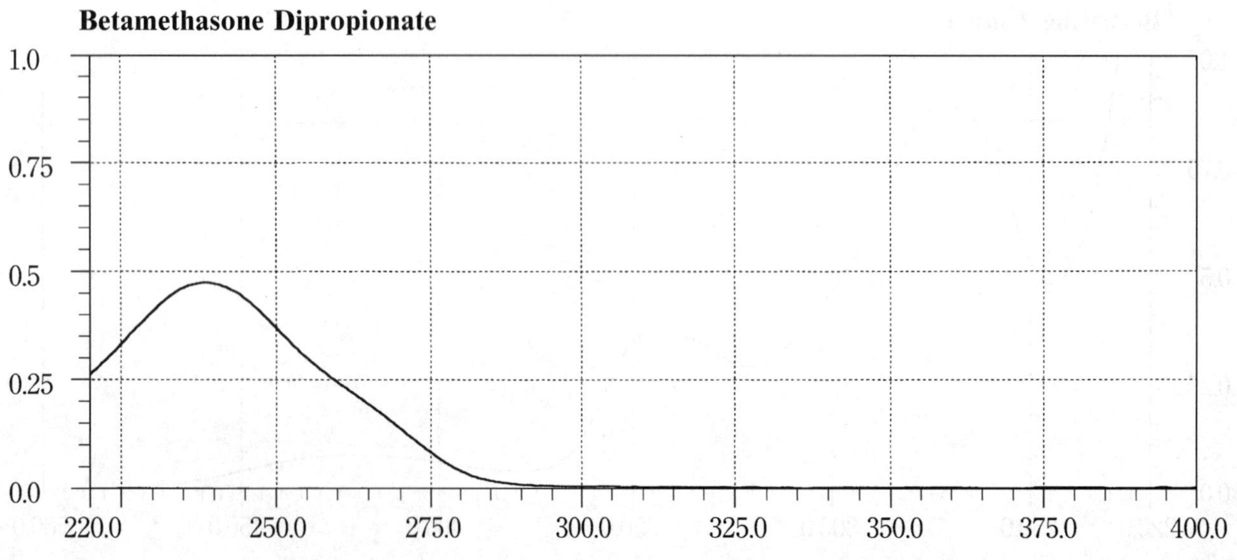

Betamipron

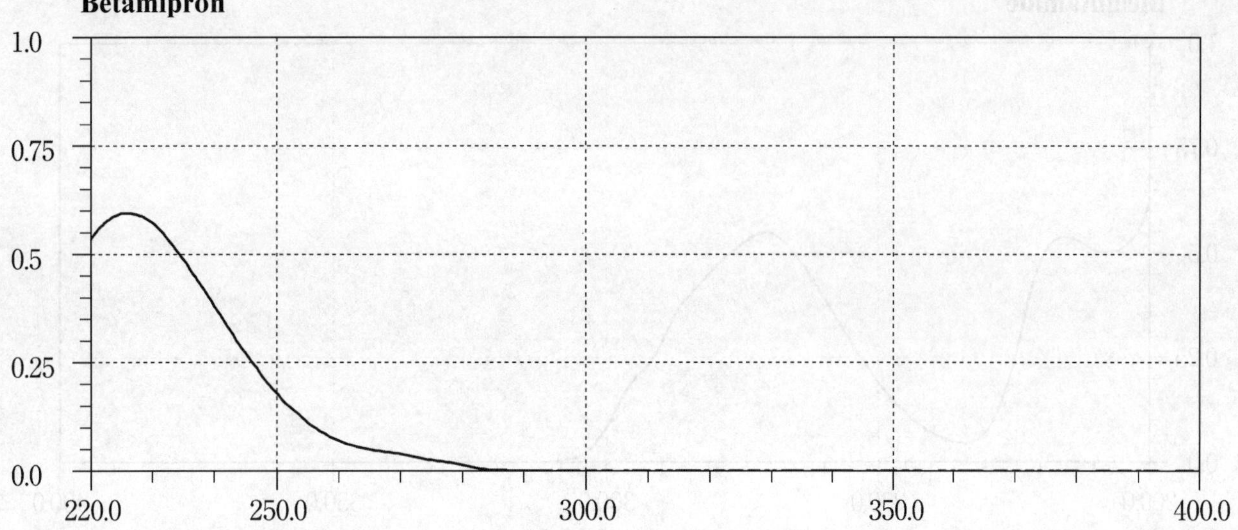

Betaxolol Hydrochloride

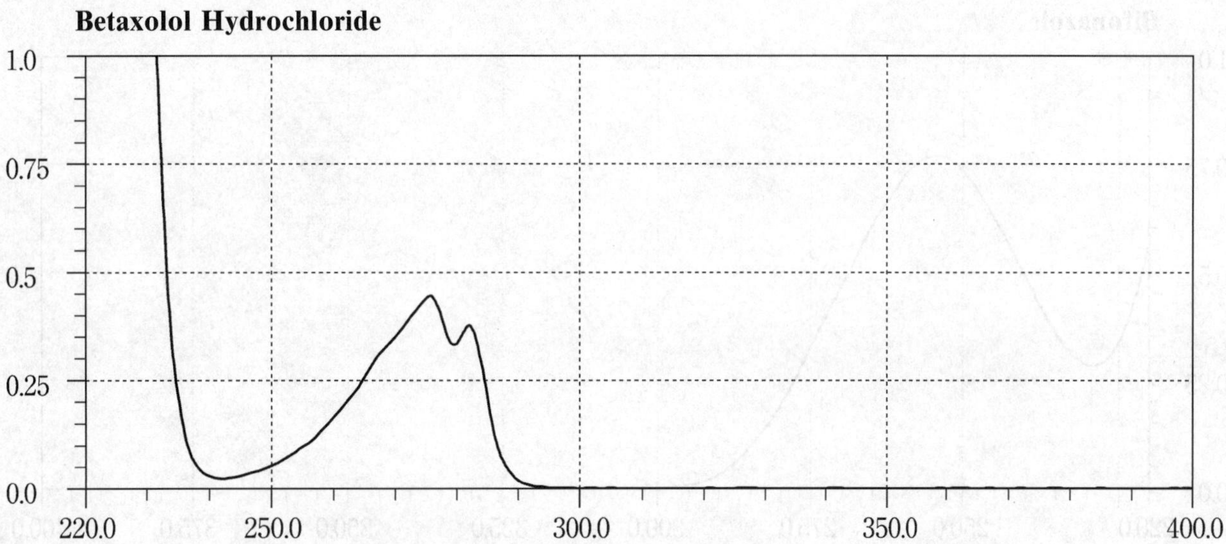

Bezafibrate

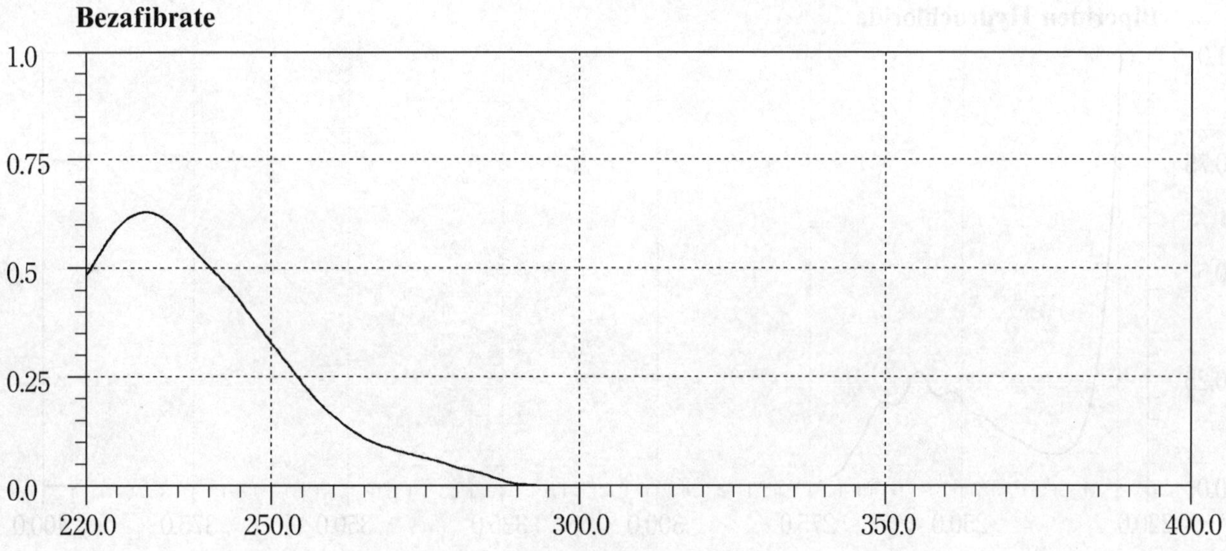

Bicalutamide

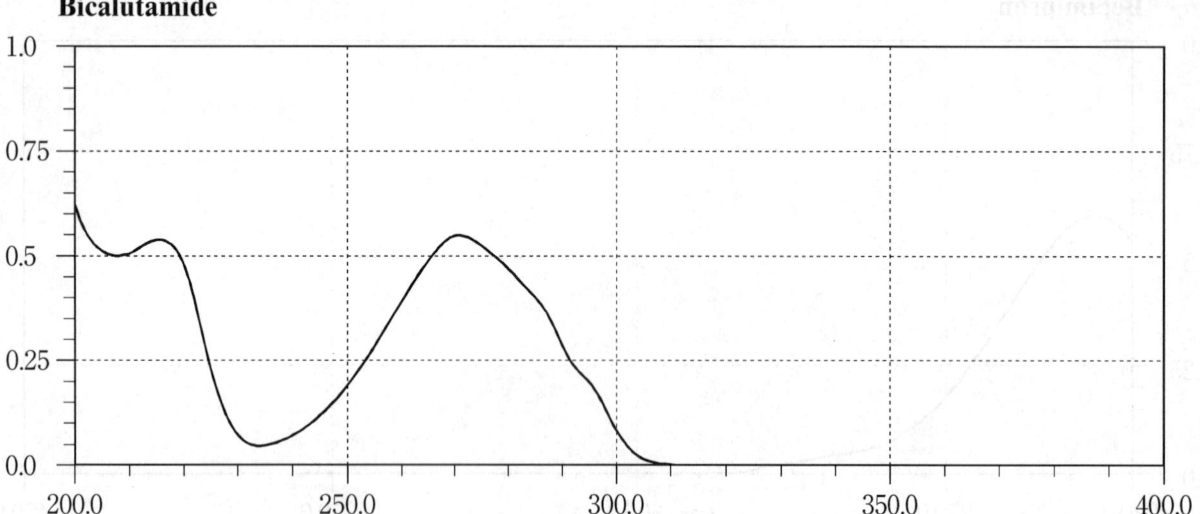

Bifonazole

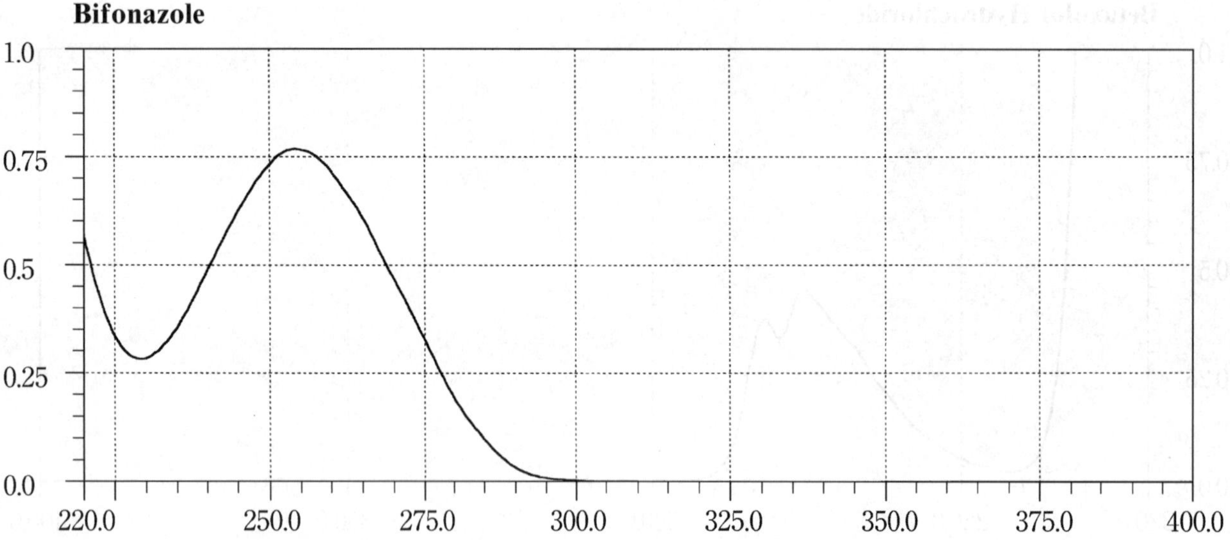

Biperiden Hydrochloride

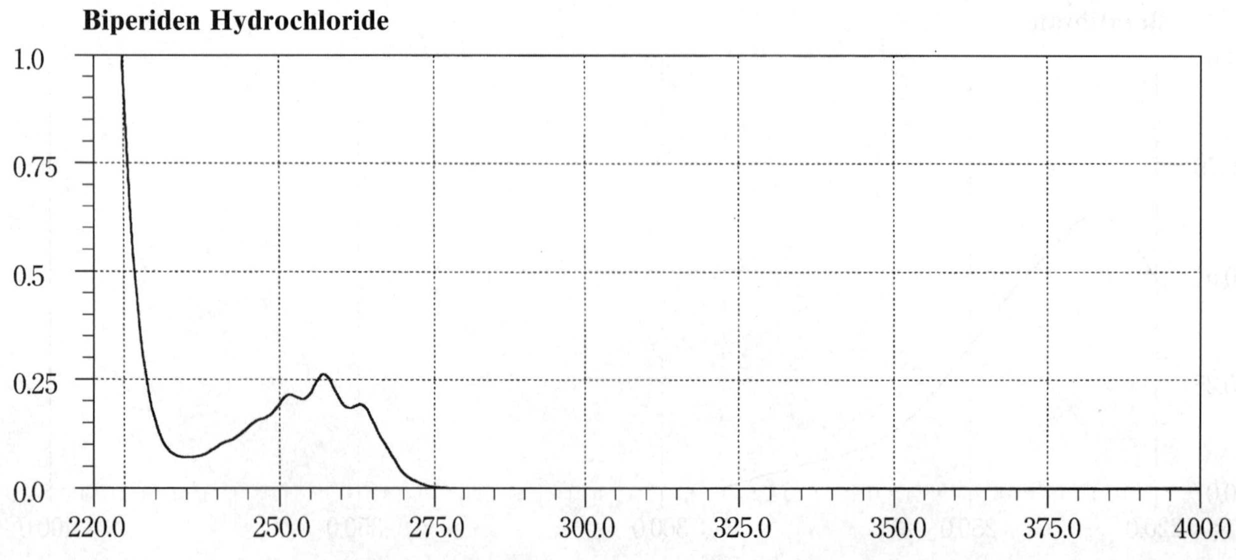

Bisacodyl

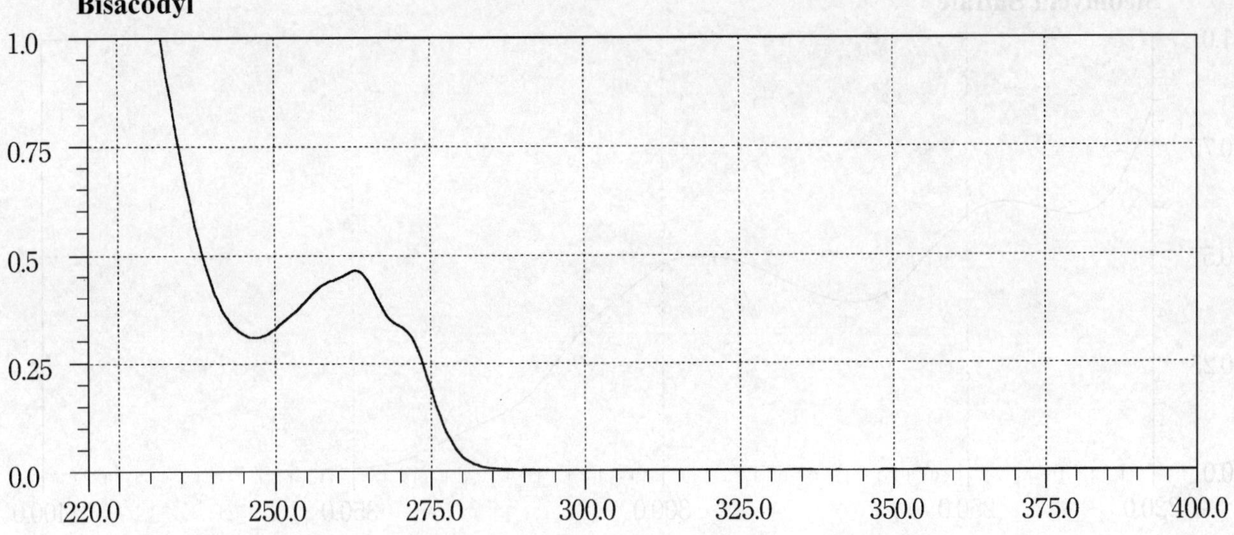

Bisoprolol Fumarate

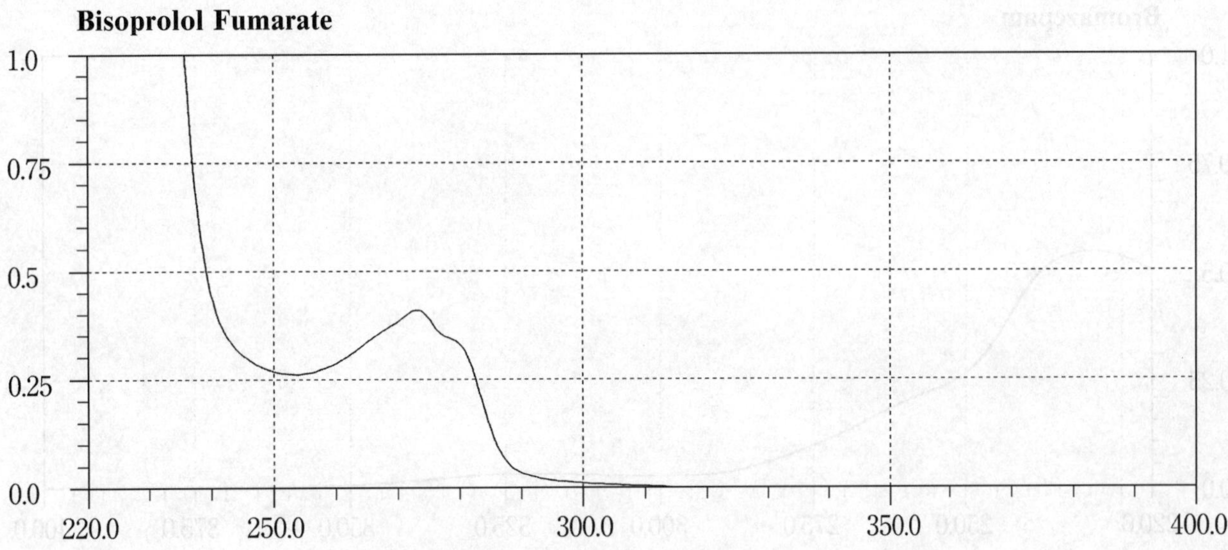

Bleomycin Hydrochloride

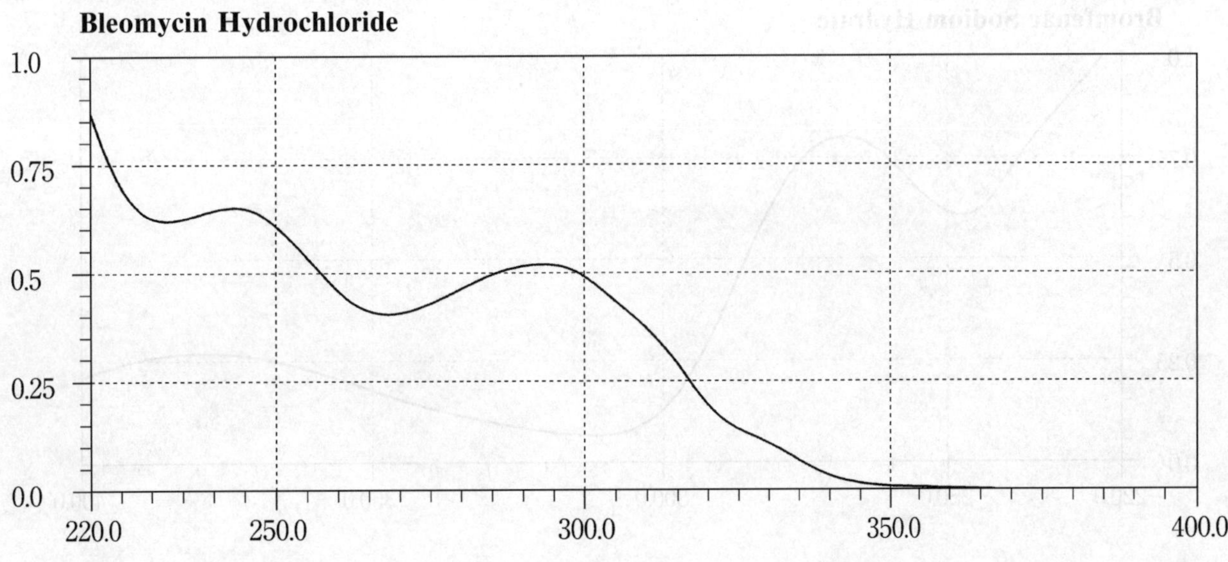

Bleomycin Sulfate

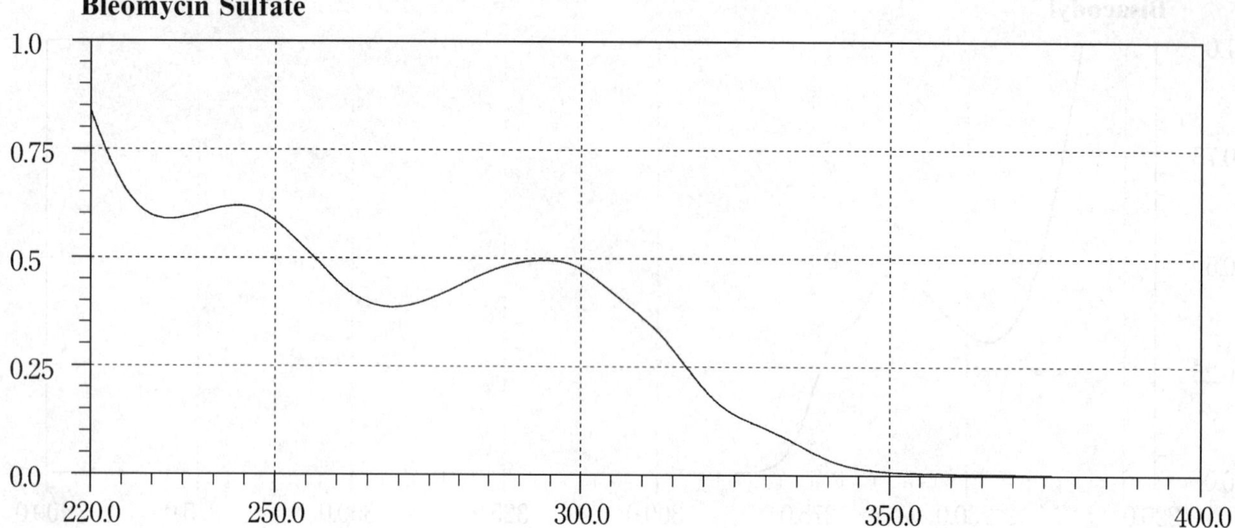

Bromazepam

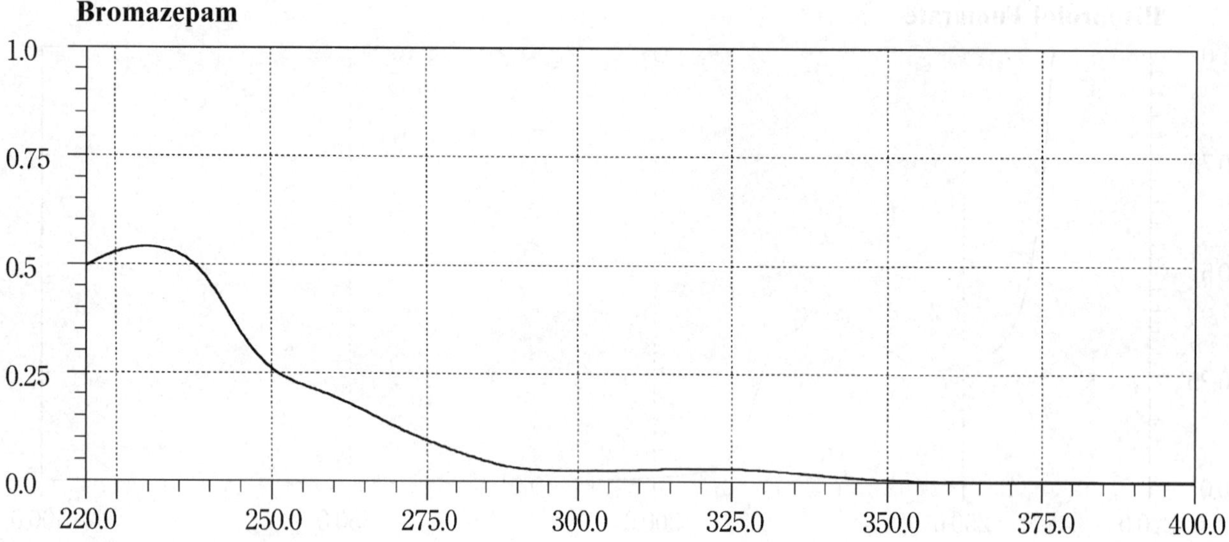

Bromfenac Sodium Hydrate

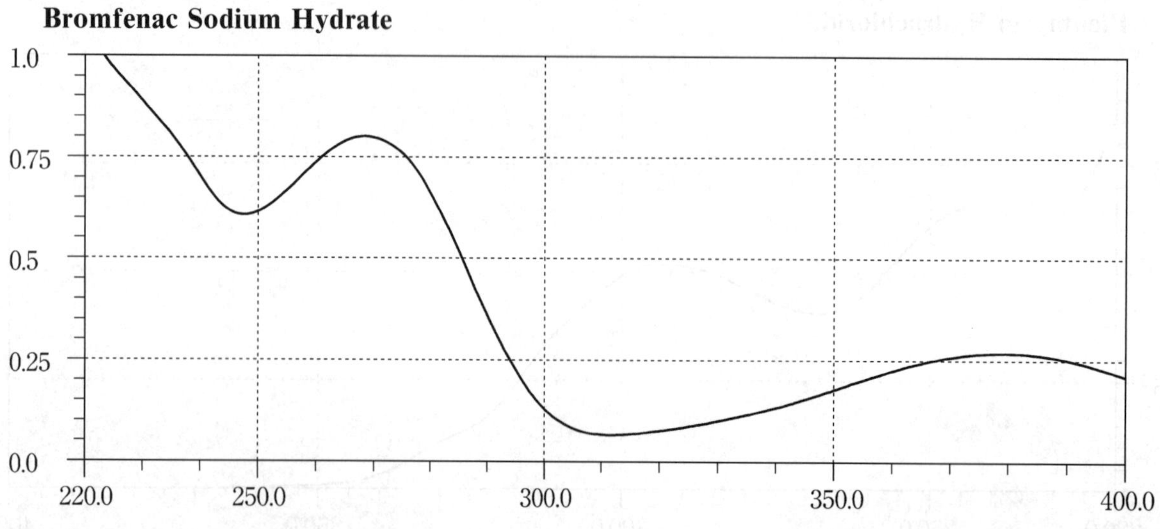

Bromhexine Hydrochloride

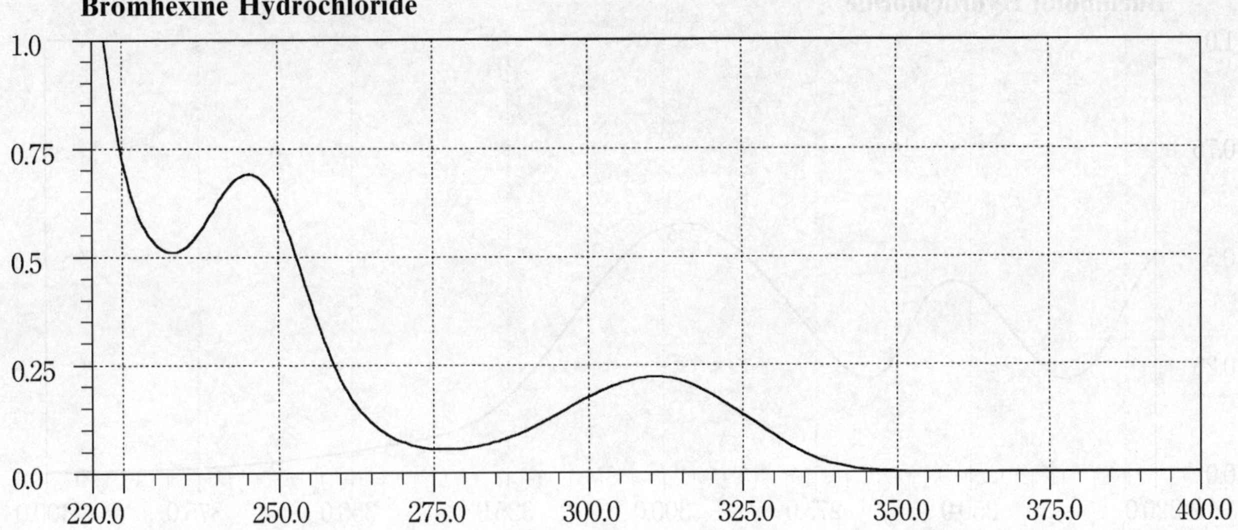

Bromocriptine Mesilate

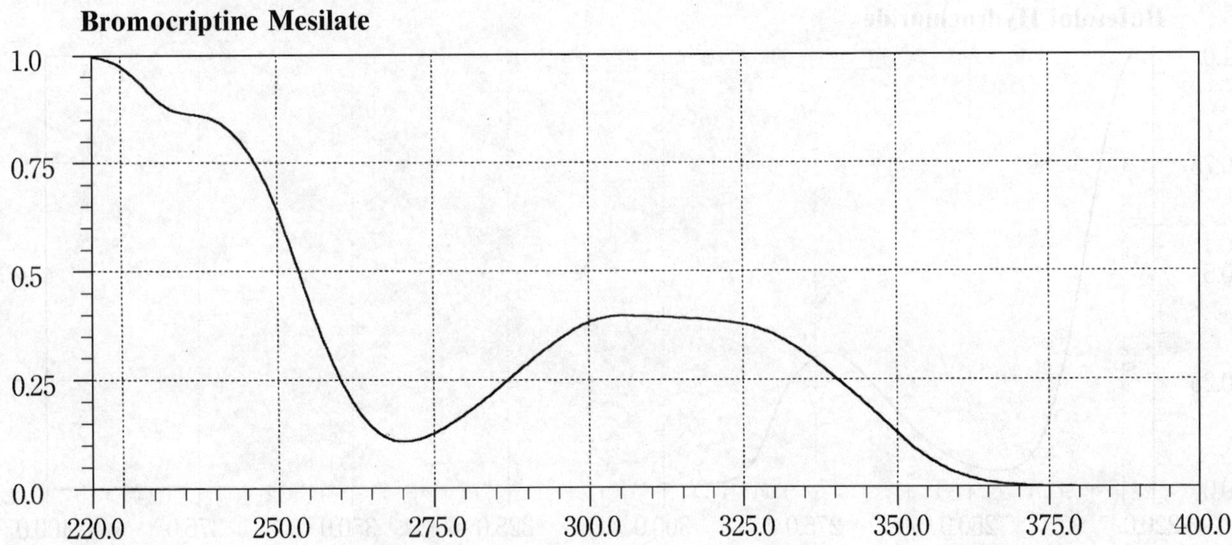

Brotizolam

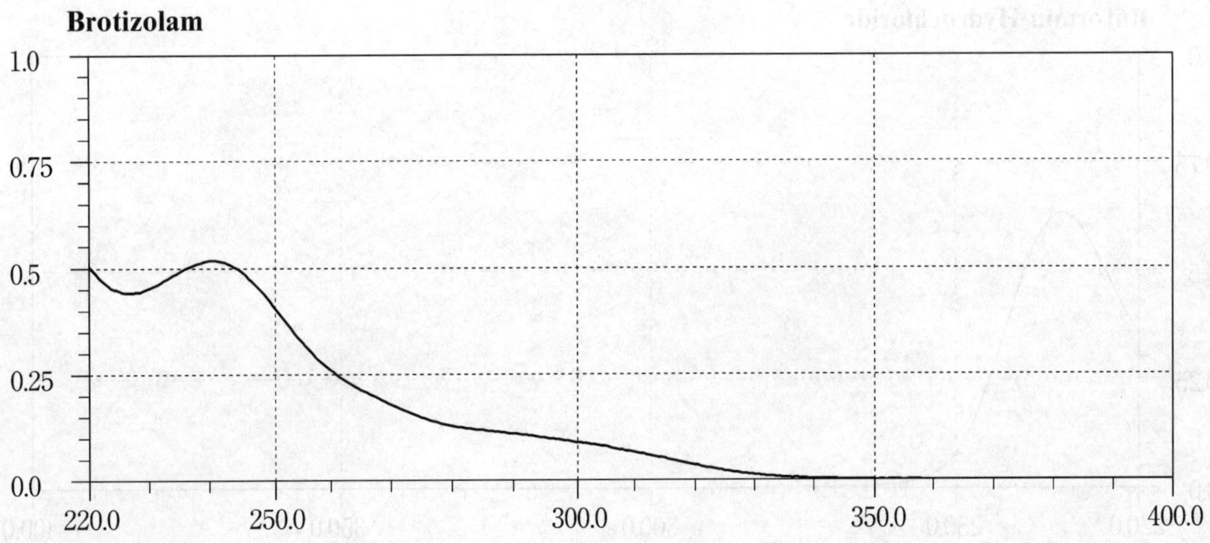

Bucumolol Hydrochloride

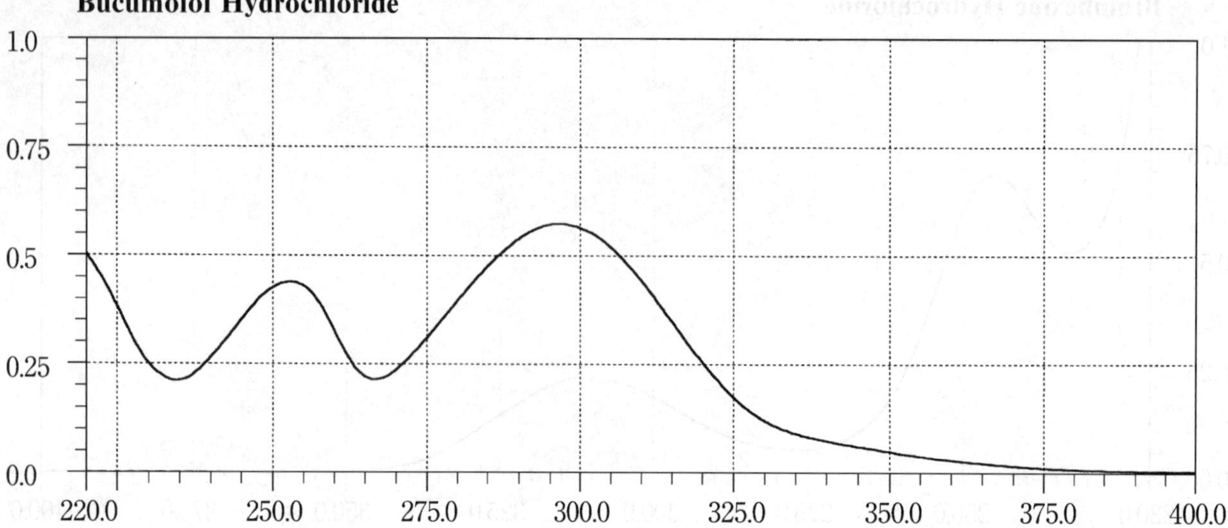

Bufetolol Hydrochloride

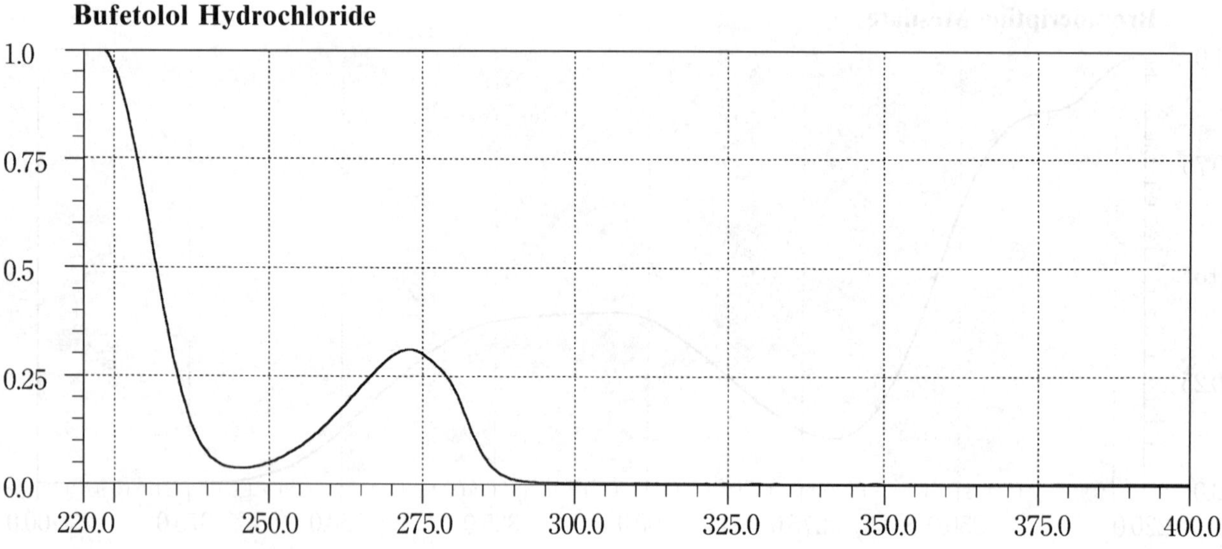

Buformin Hydrochloride

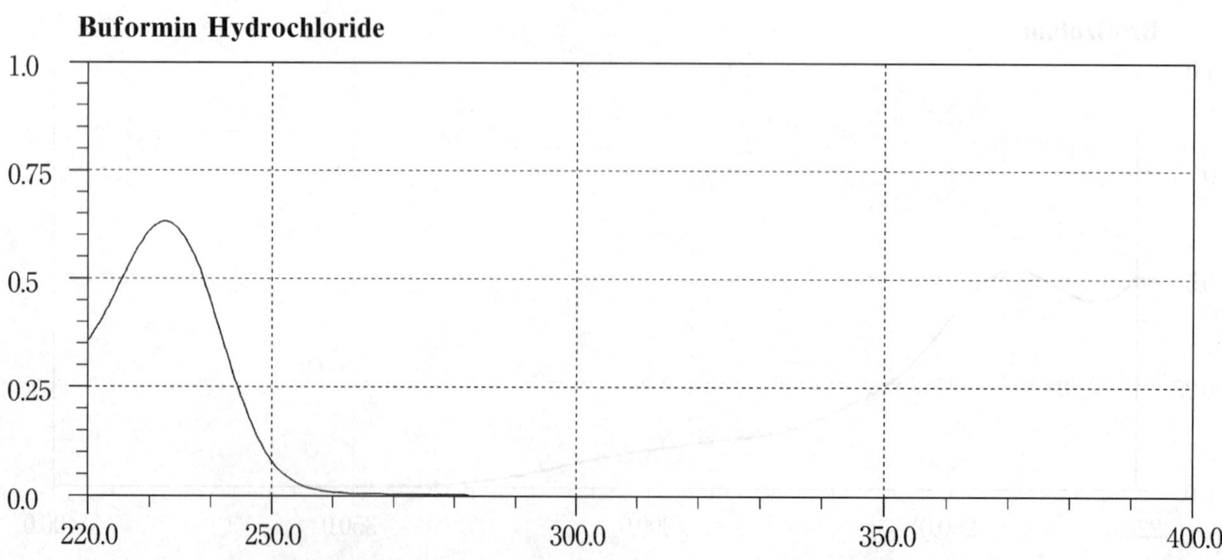

Bumetanide

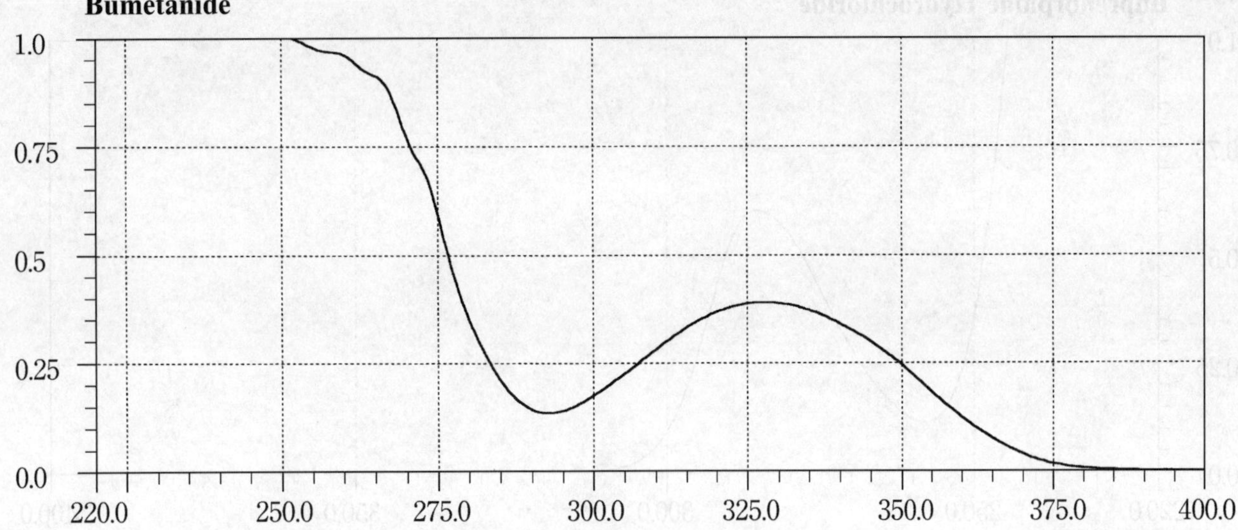

Bupivacaine Hydrochloride Hydrate

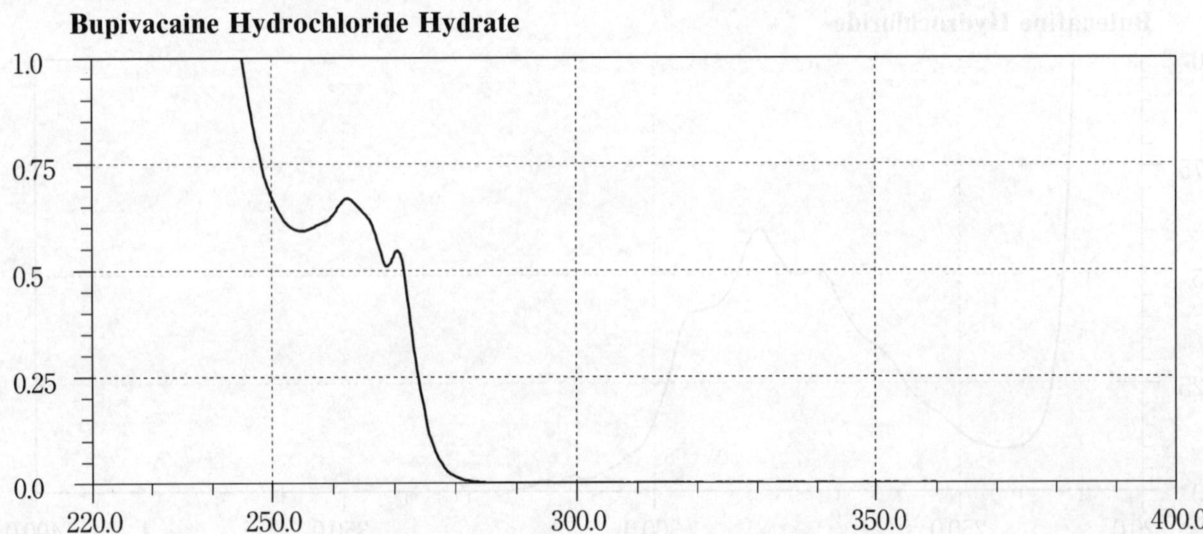

Bupranolol Hydrochloride

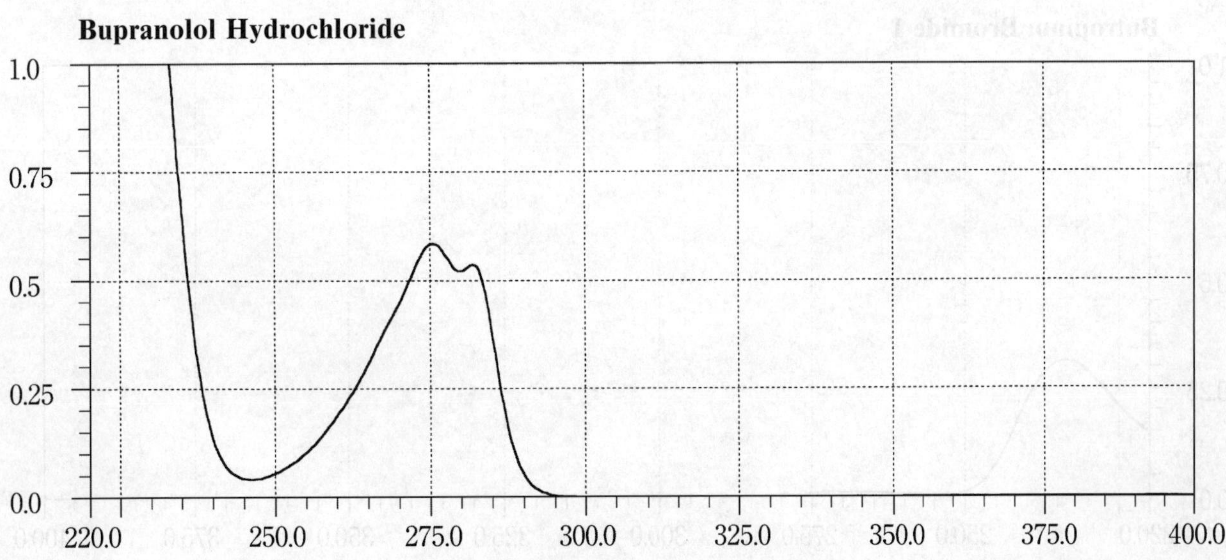

Buprenorphine Hydrochloride

1.0
0.75
0.5
0.25
0.0
220.0 250.0 300.0 350.0 400.0

Butenafine Hydrochloride

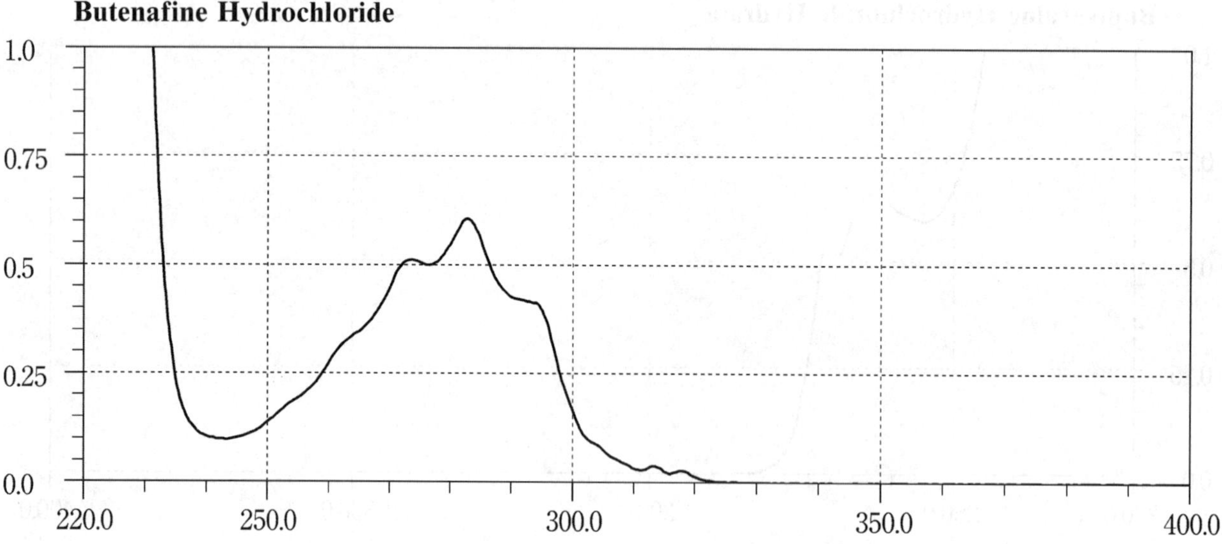

Butropium Bromide 1

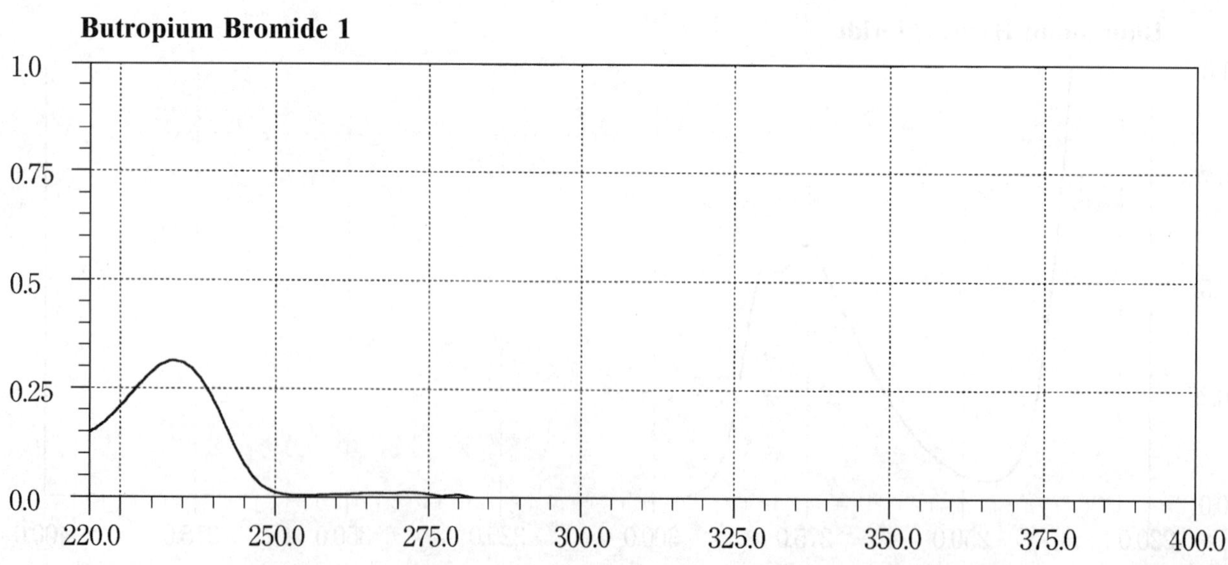

Butropium Bromide 2

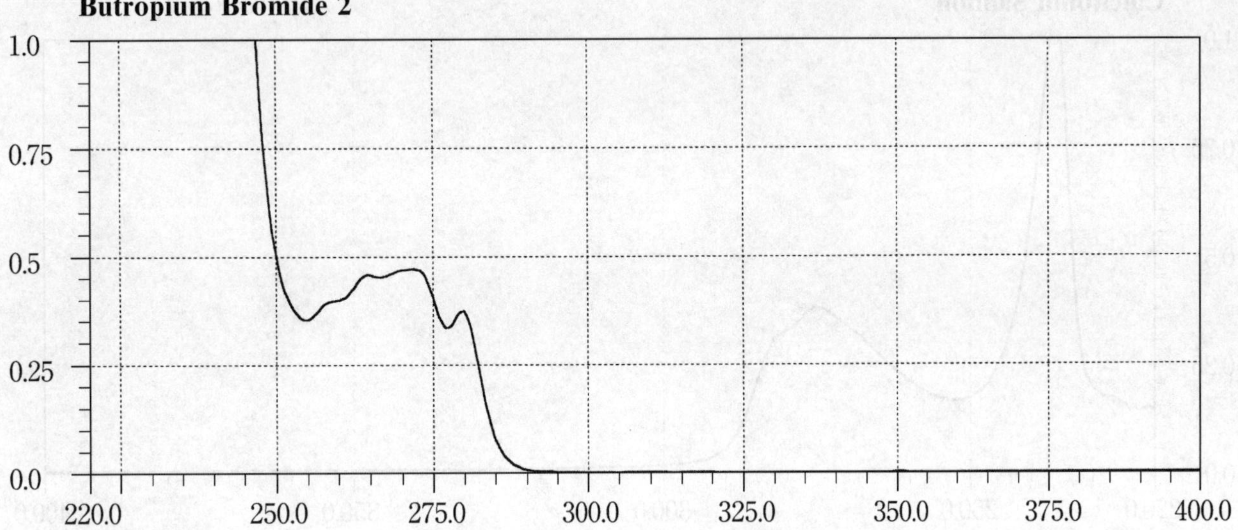

Cabergoline

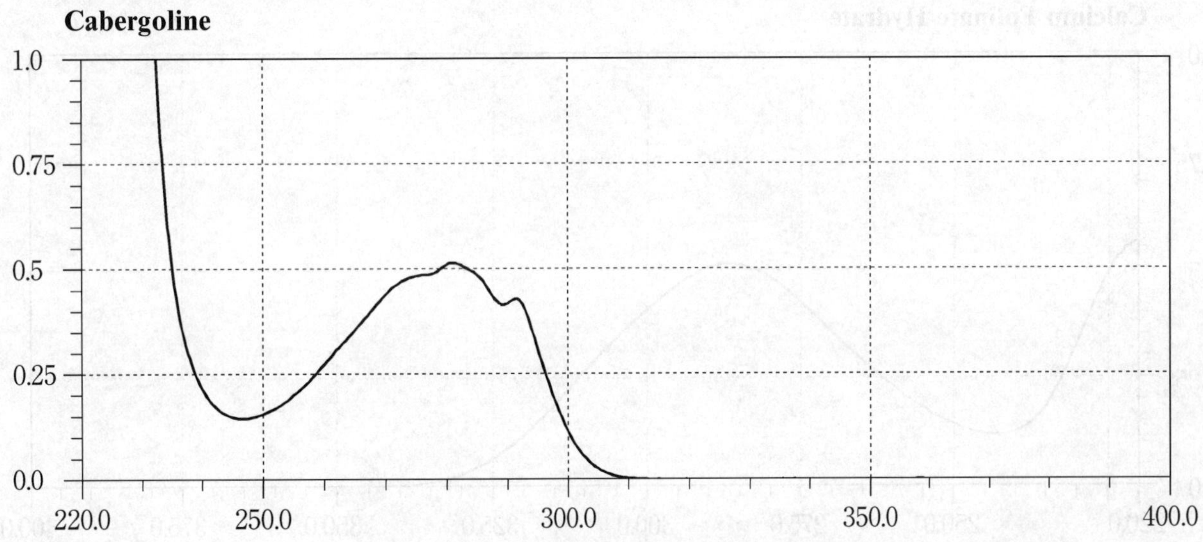

Cadralazine

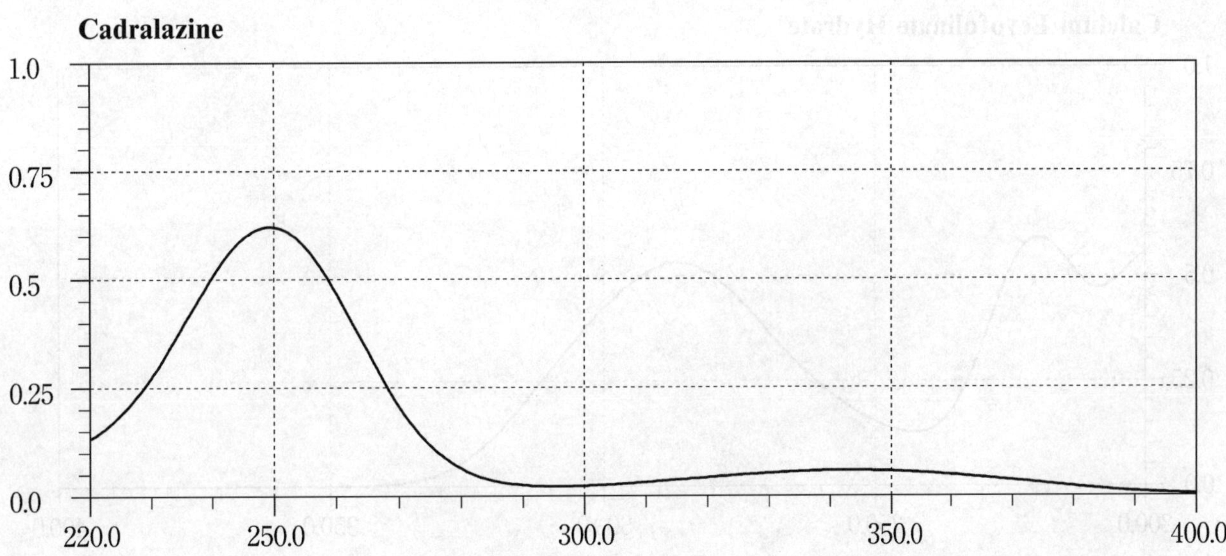

Calcitonin Salmon

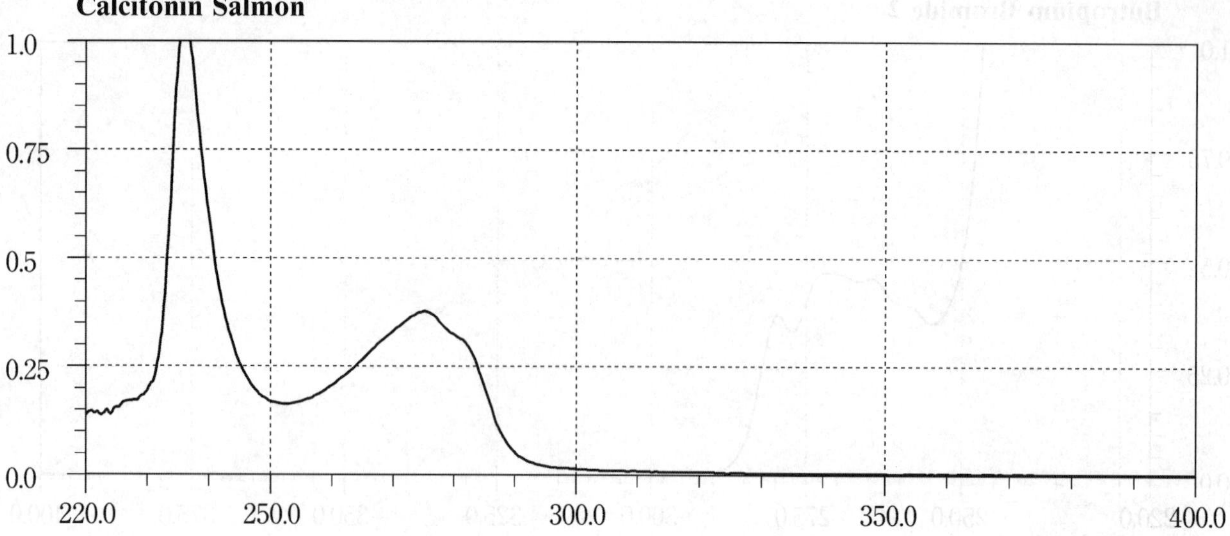

Calcium Folinate Hydrate

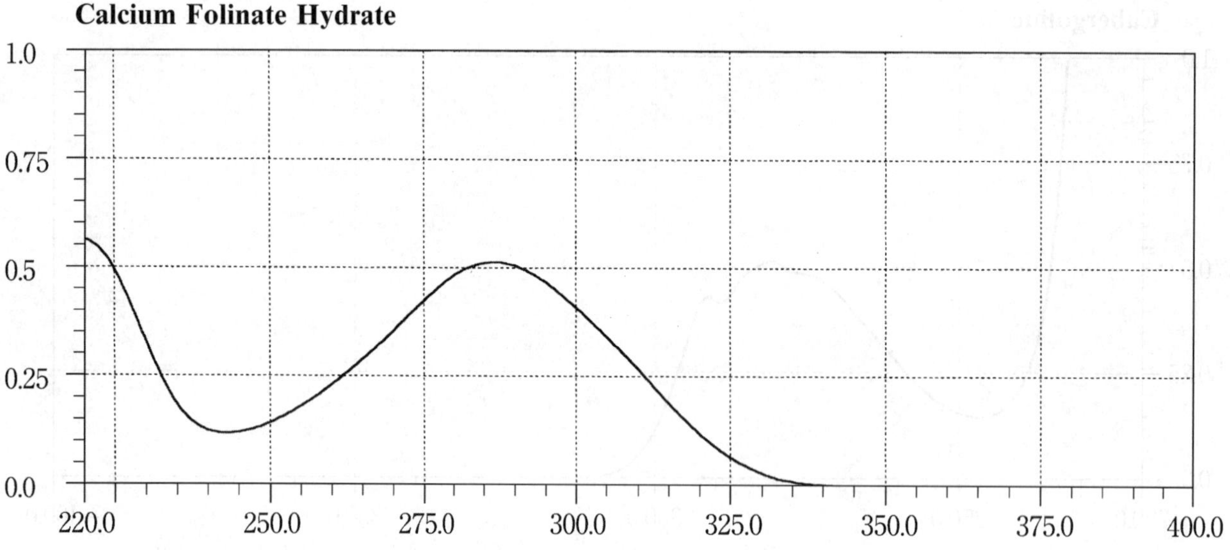

Calcium Levofolinate Hydrate

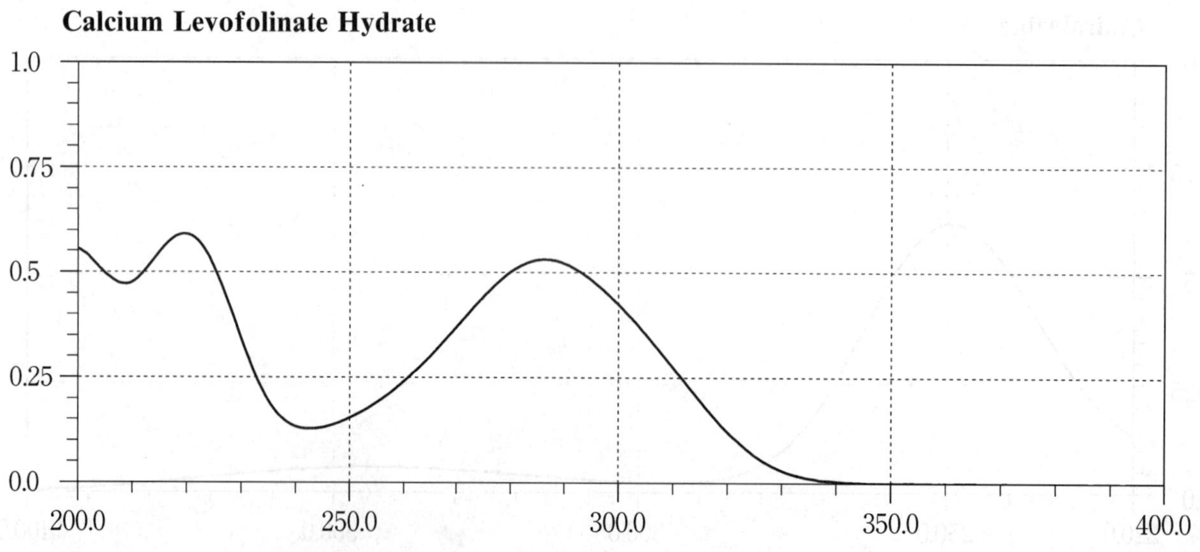

Camostat Mesilate

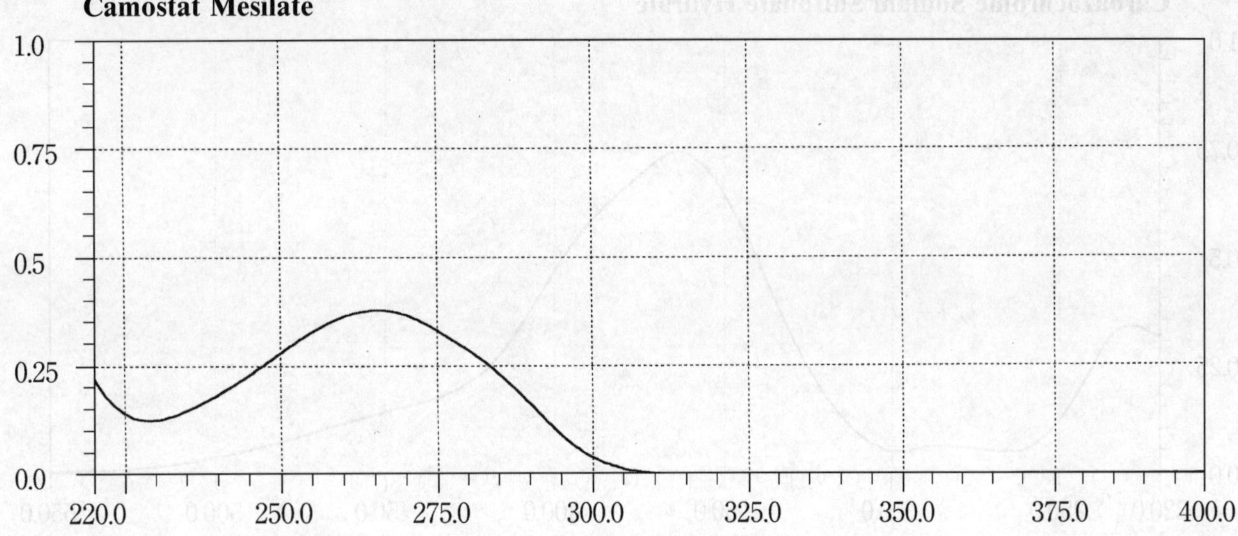

Candesartan Cilexetil

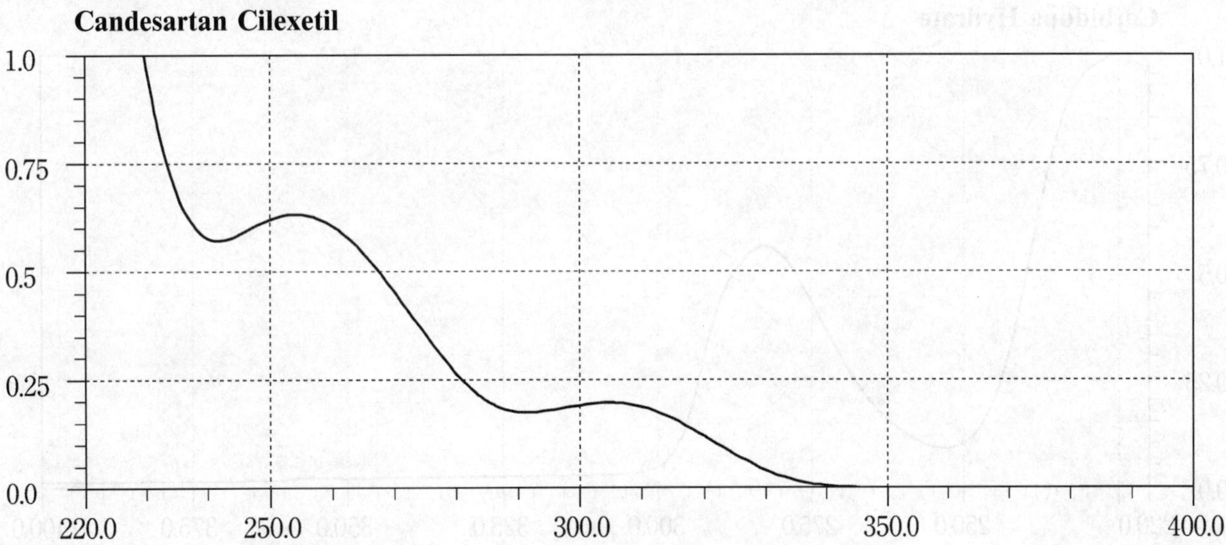

Carbamazepine

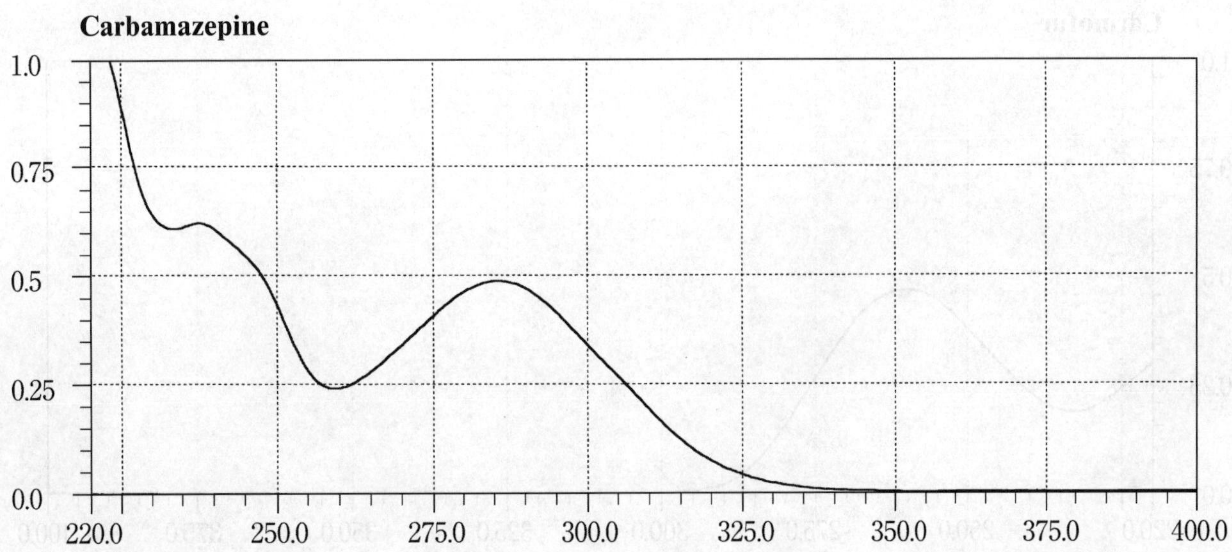

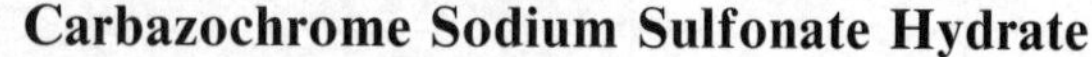

Carbazochrome Sodium Sulfonate Hydrate

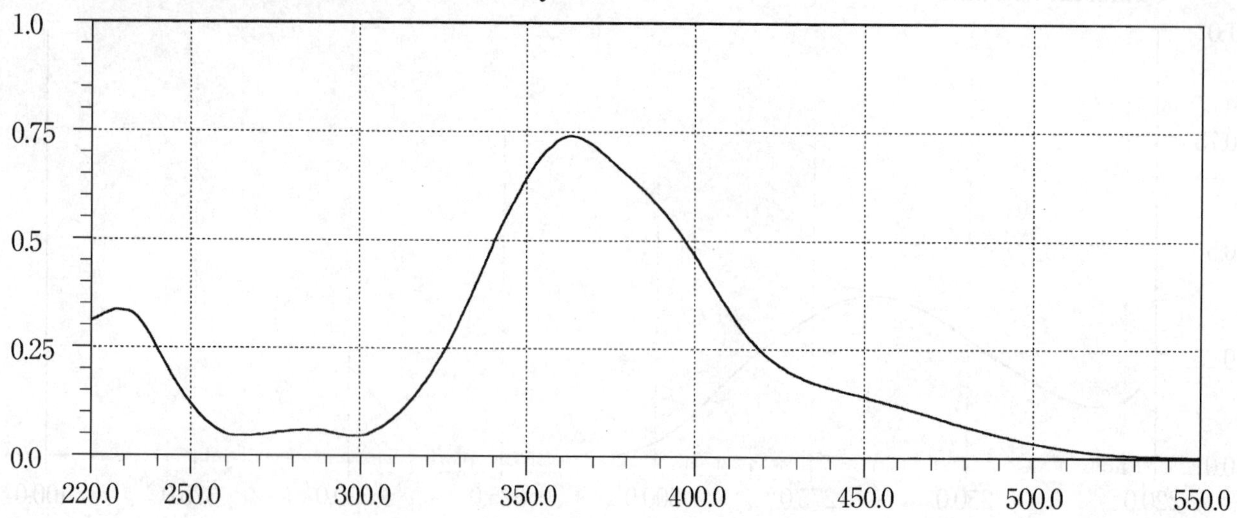

Carbidopa Hydrate

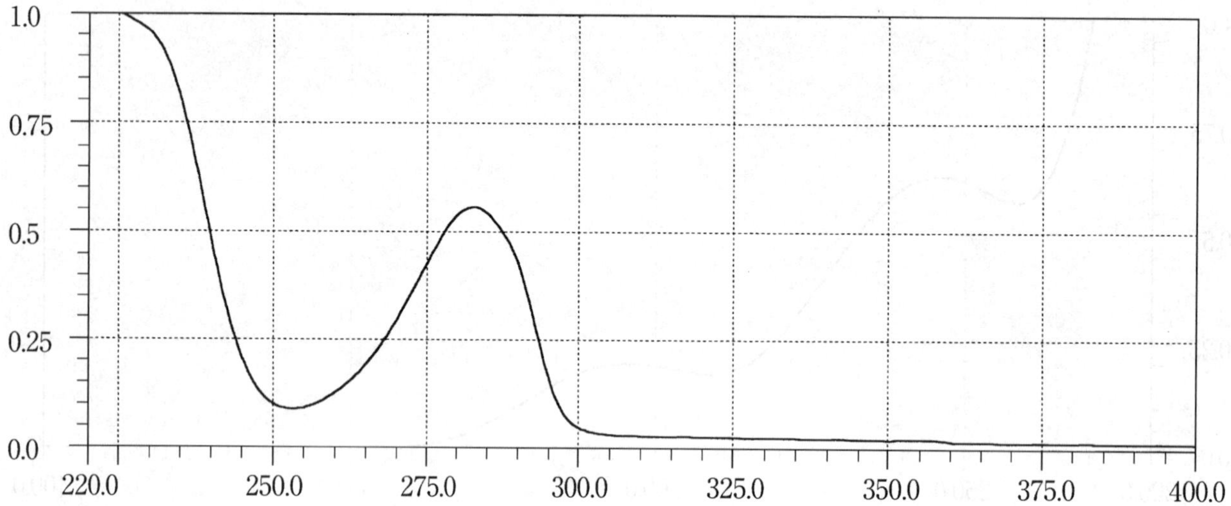

Carmofur

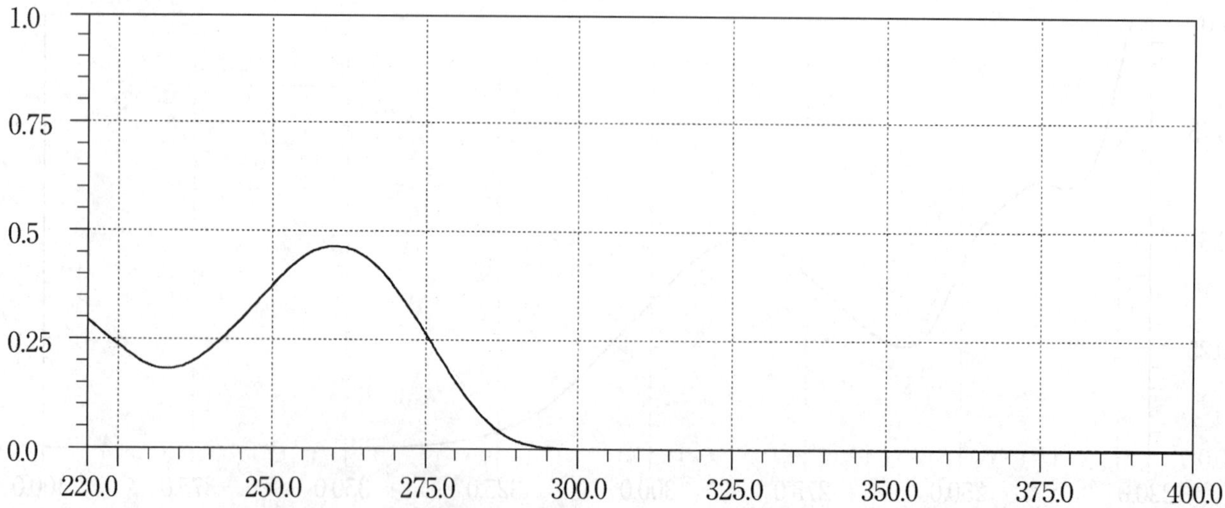

Carteolol Hydrochloride

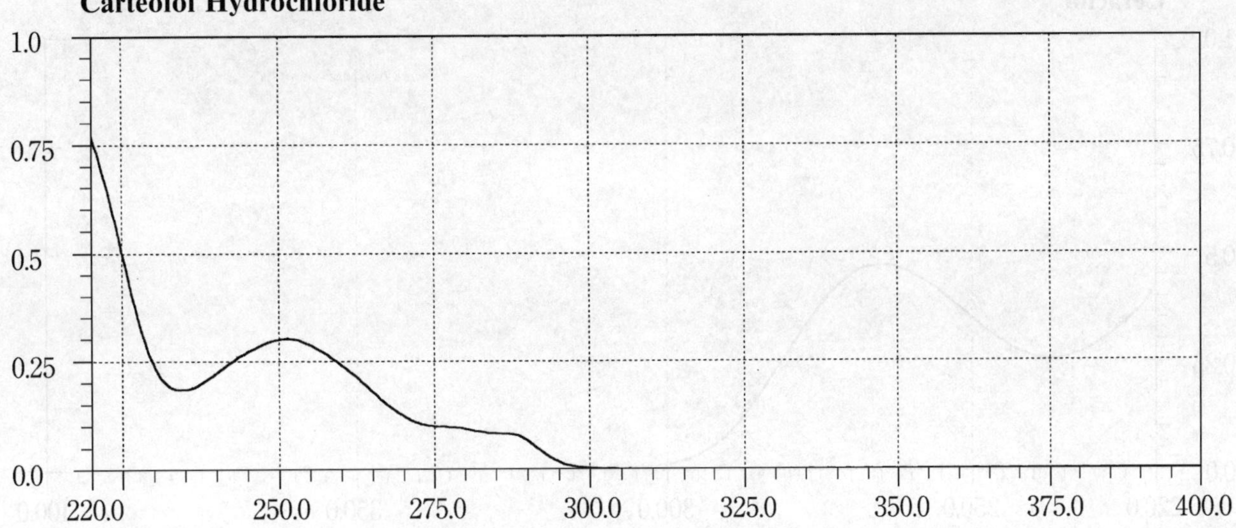

Carumonam Sodium

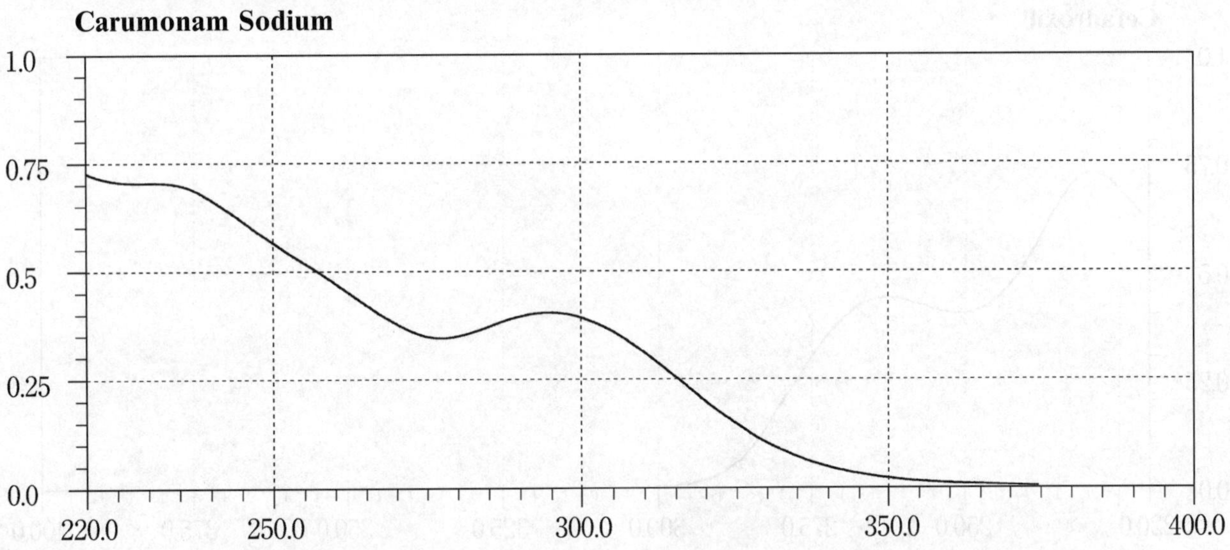

Carvedilol

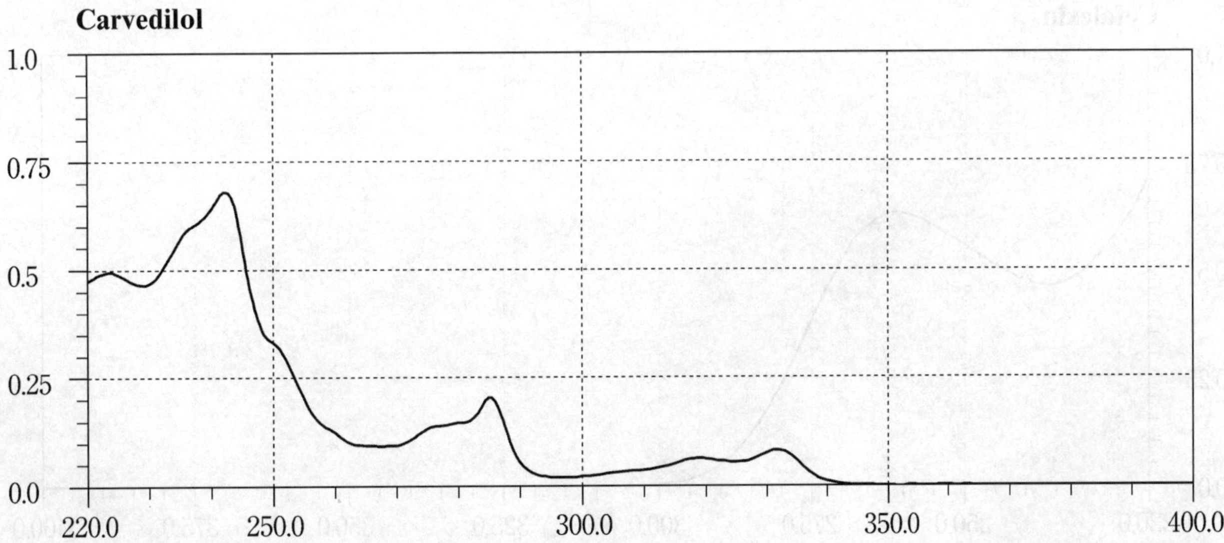

Cefaclor

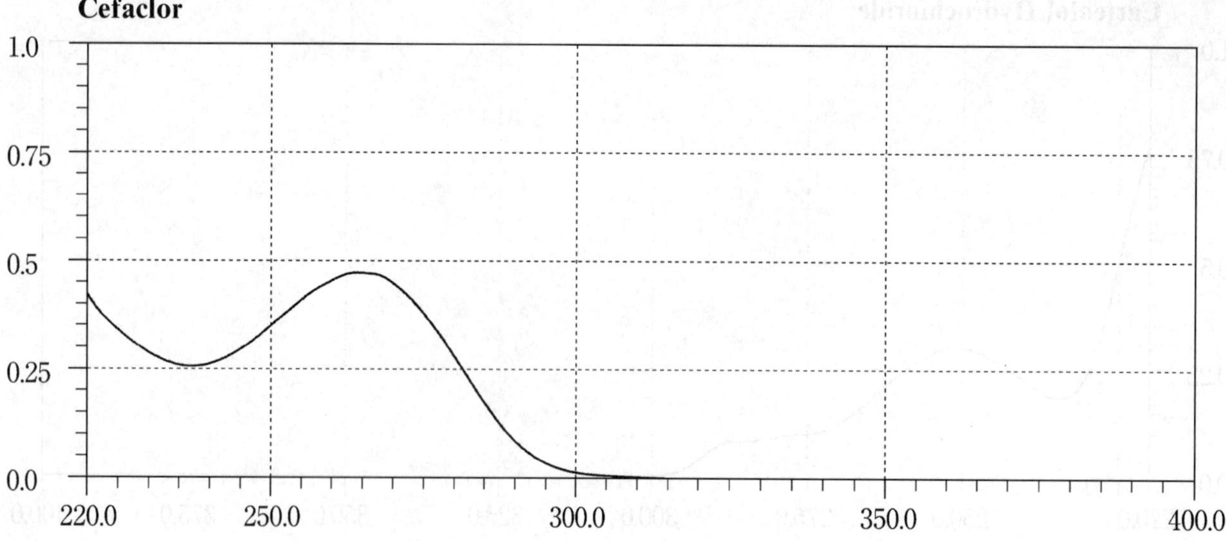

Cefadroxil

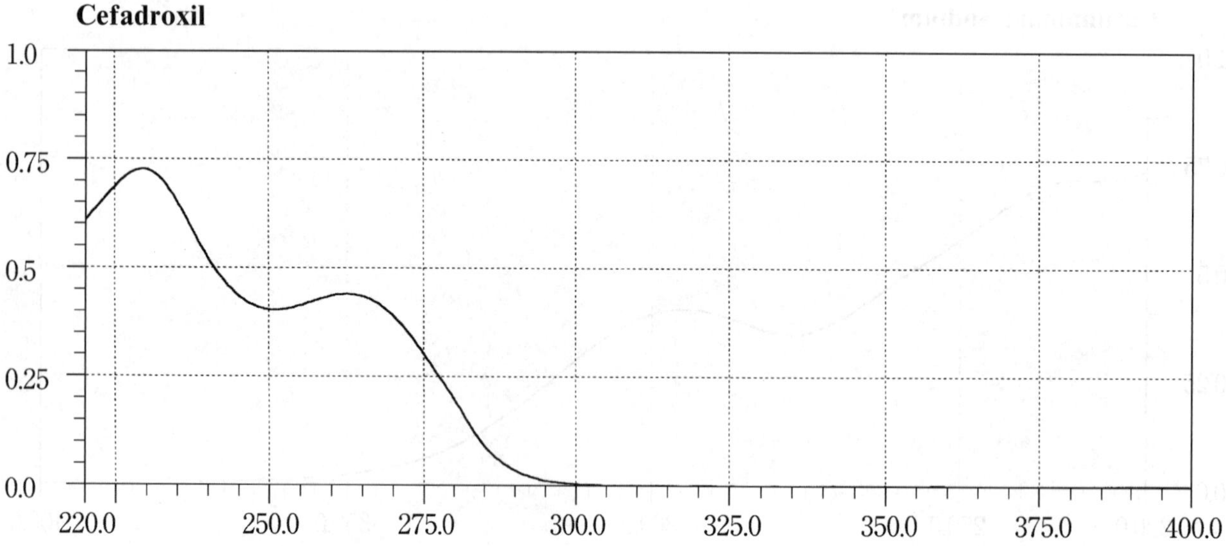

Cefalexin

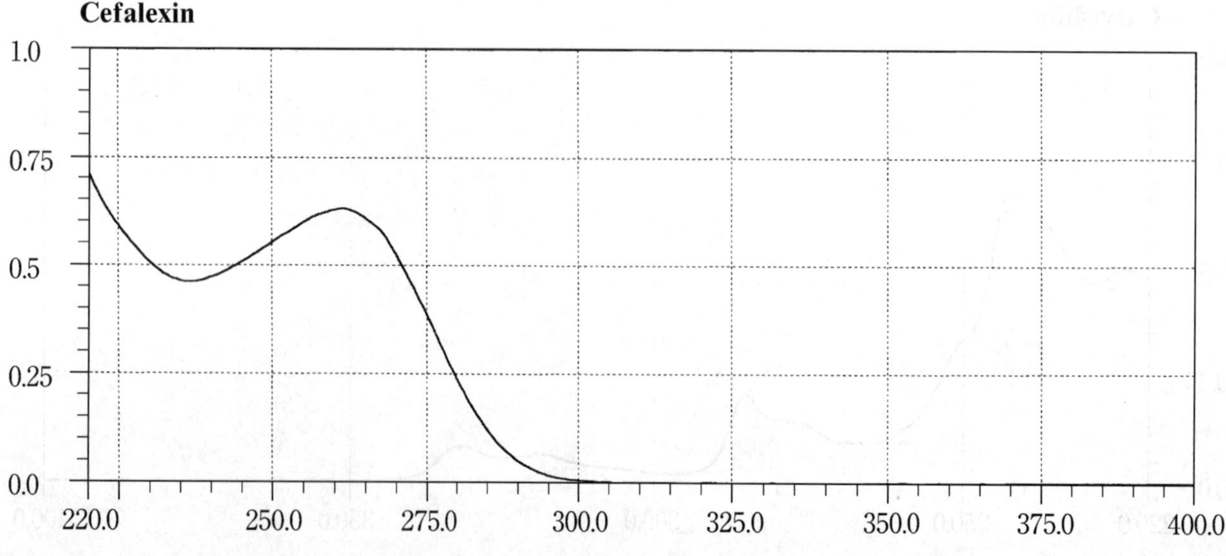

Cefalotin Sodium

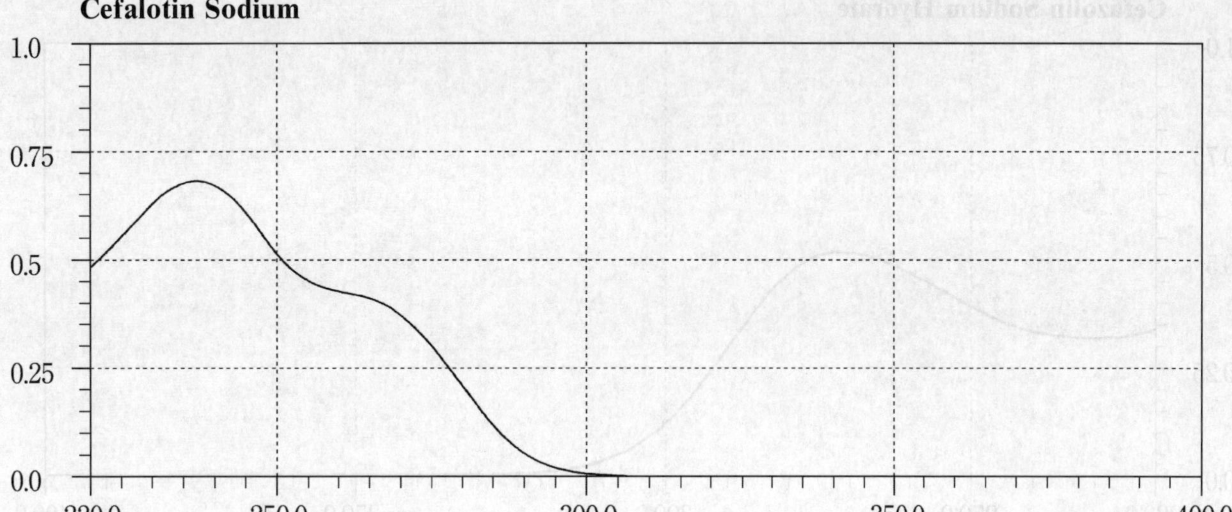

Cefatrizine Propylene Glycolate

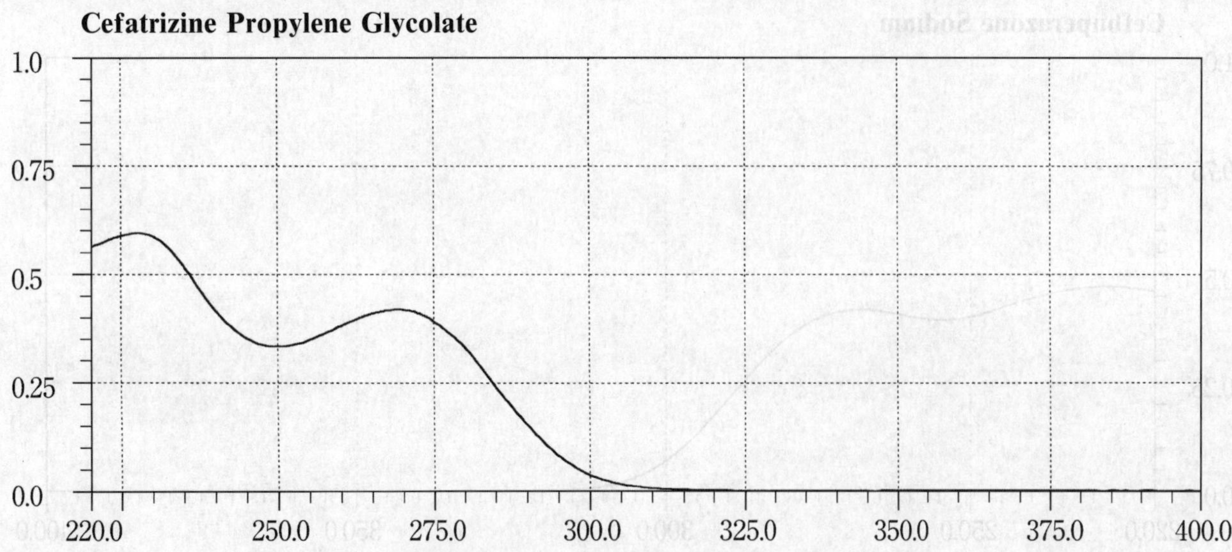

Cefazolin Sodium

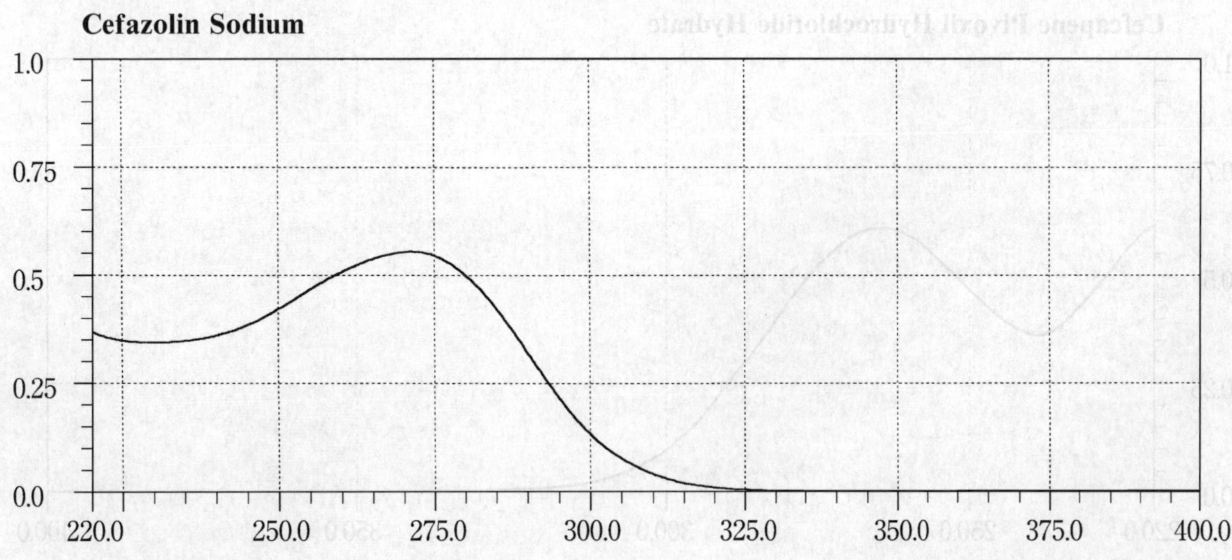

Cefazolin Sodium Hydrate

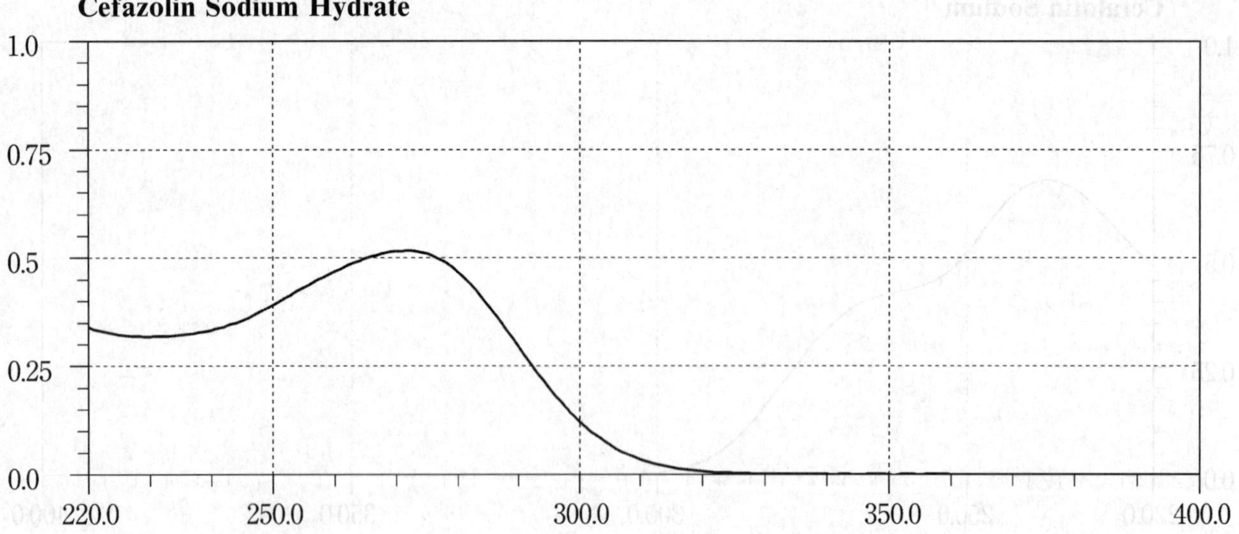

Cefbuperazone Sodium

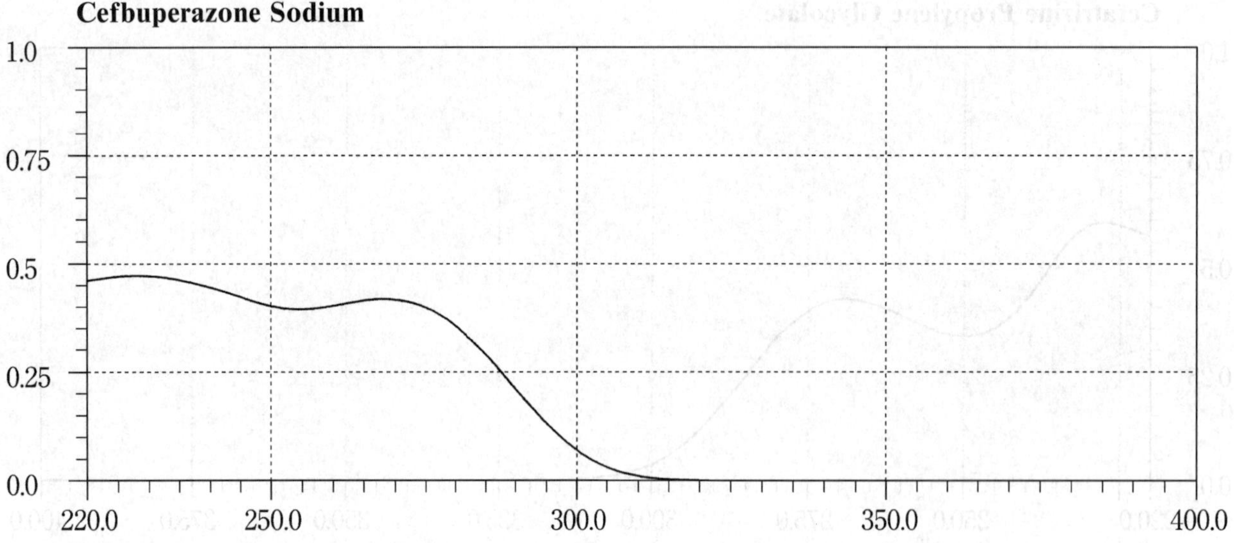

Cefcapene Pivoxil Hydrochloride Hydrate

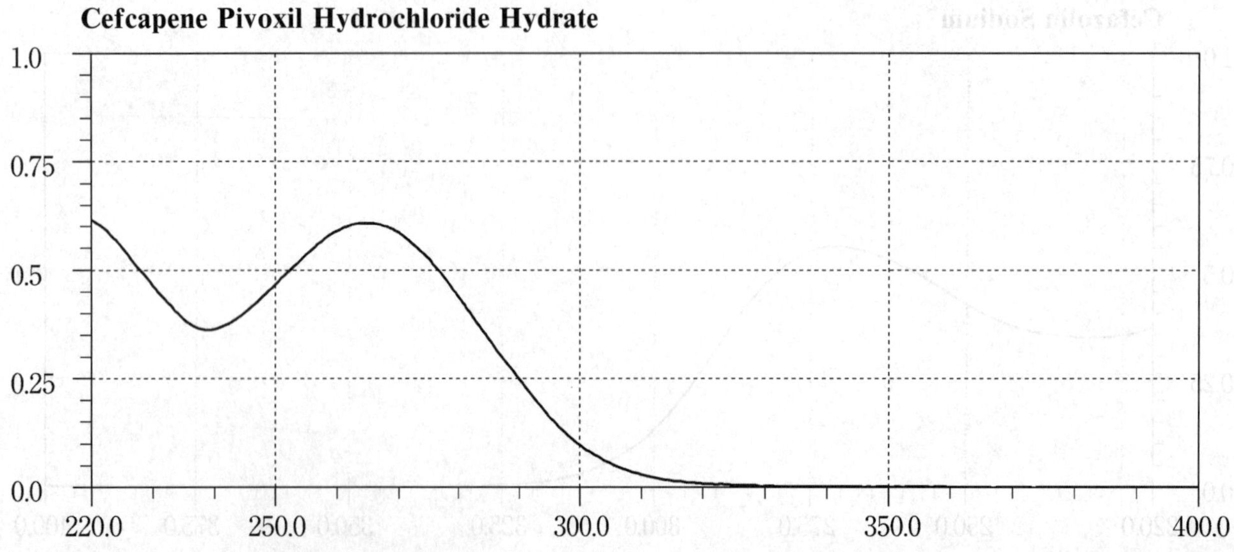

Cefditoren Pivoxil

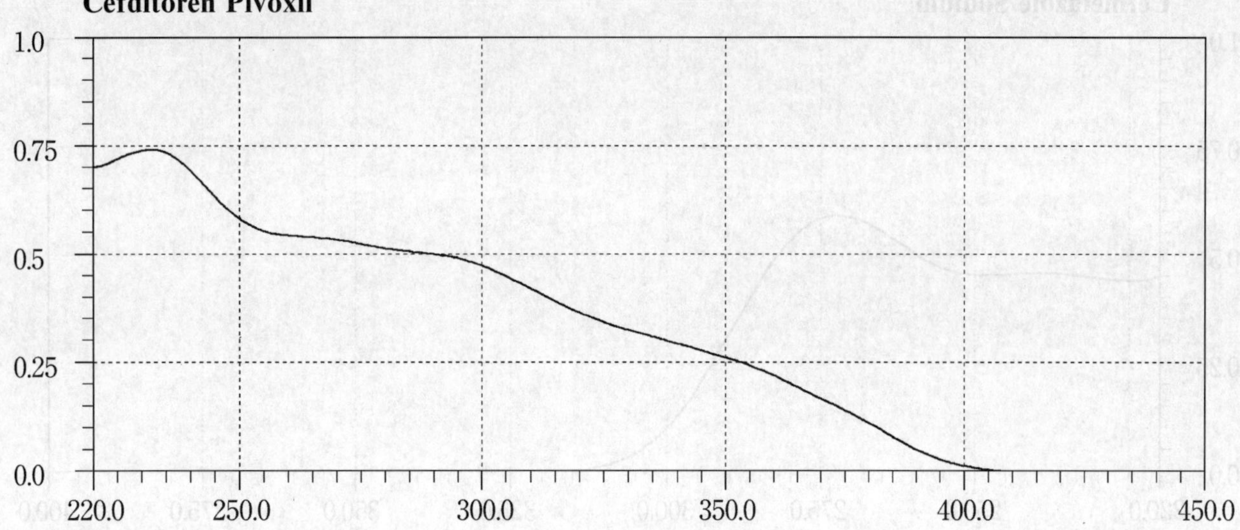

Cefixime Hydrate

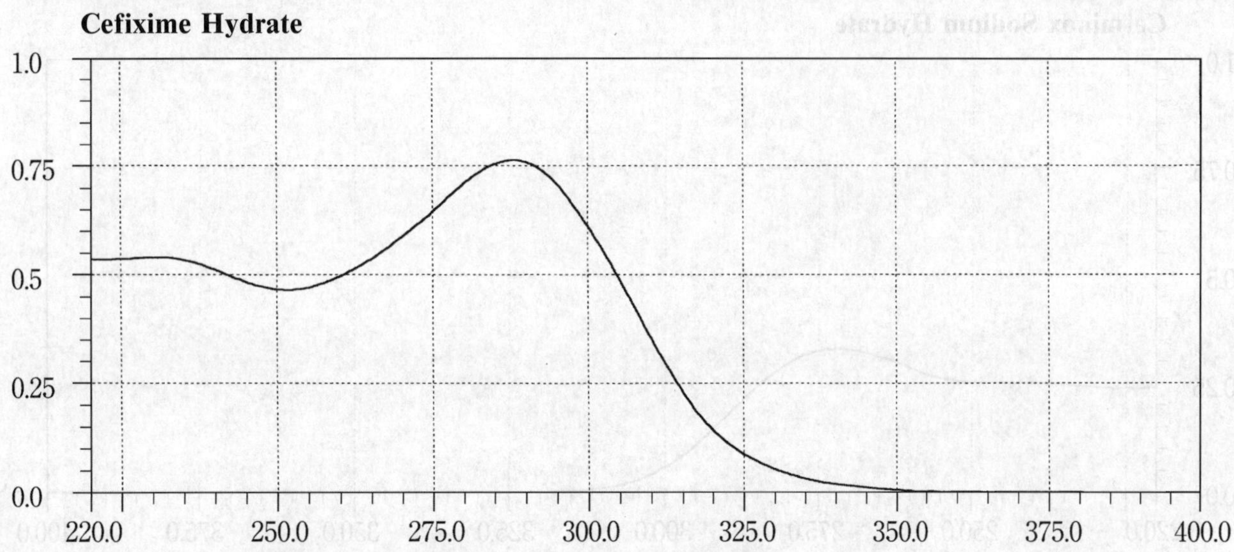

Cefmenoxime Hydrochloride

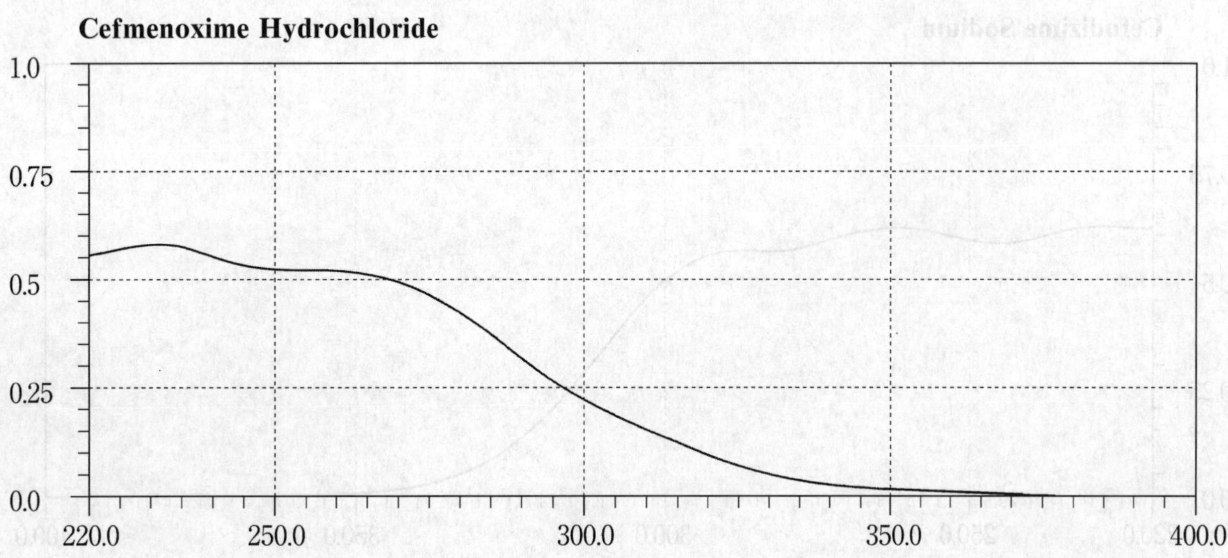

Cefmetazole Sodium

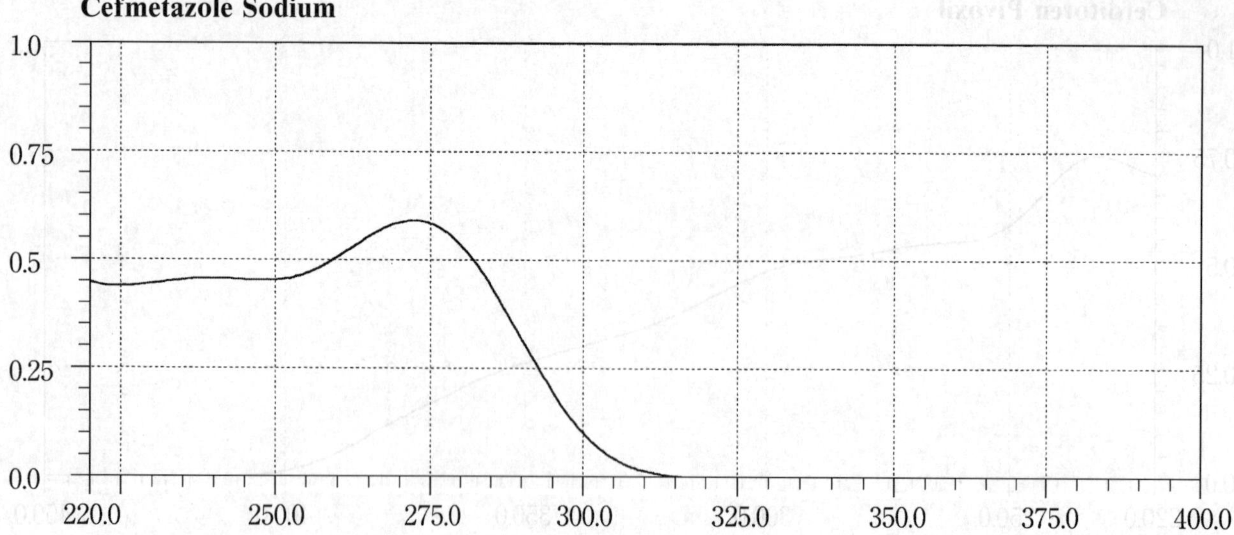

Cefminox Sodium Hydrate

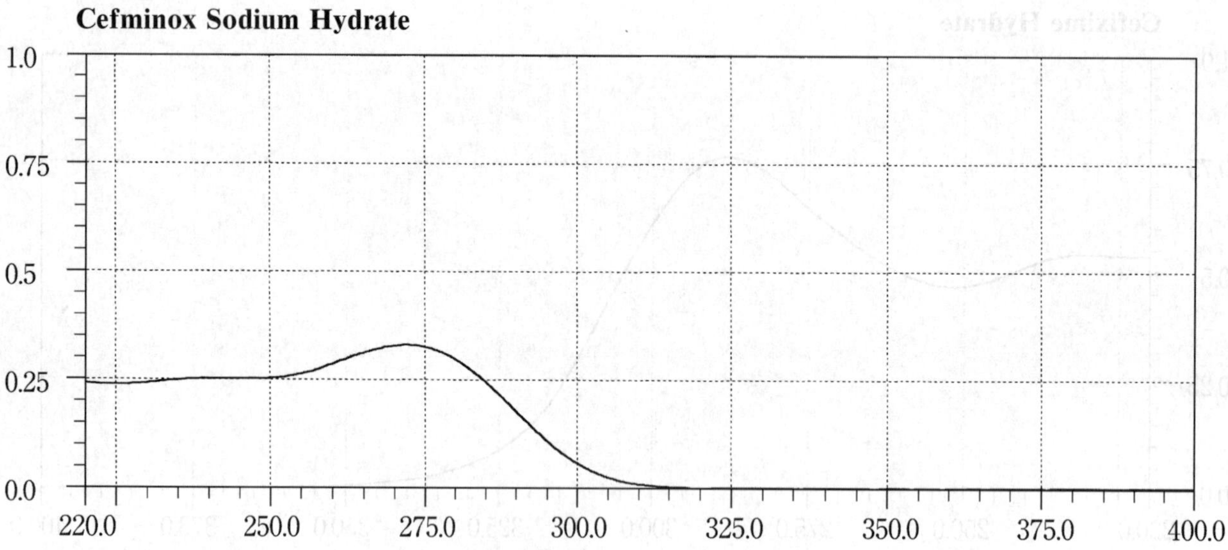

Cefodizime Sodium

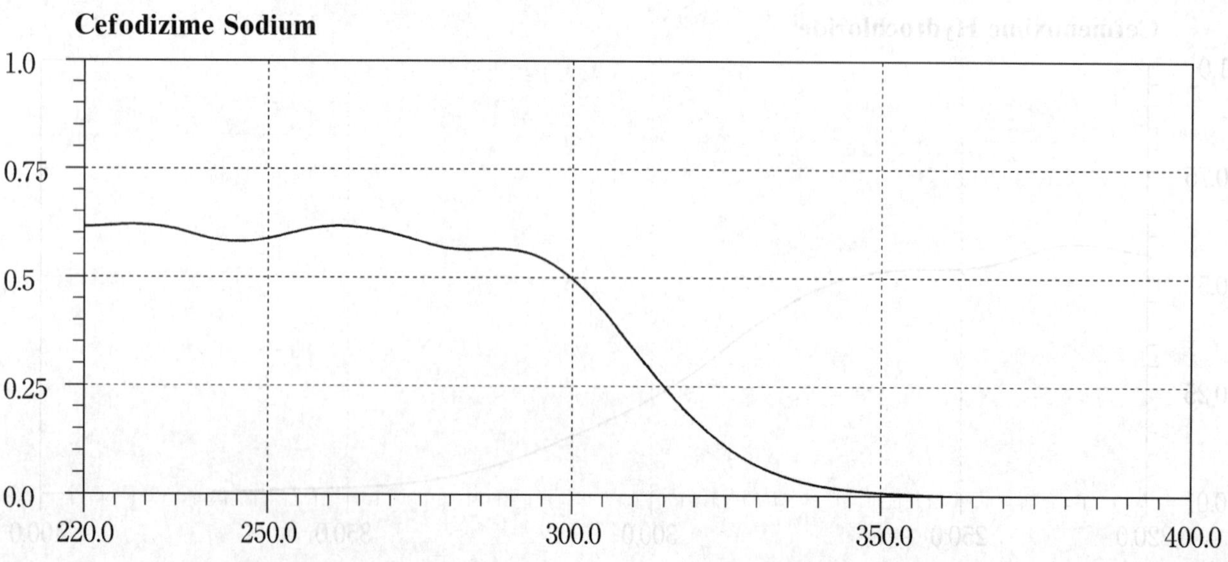

Cefoperazone Sodium

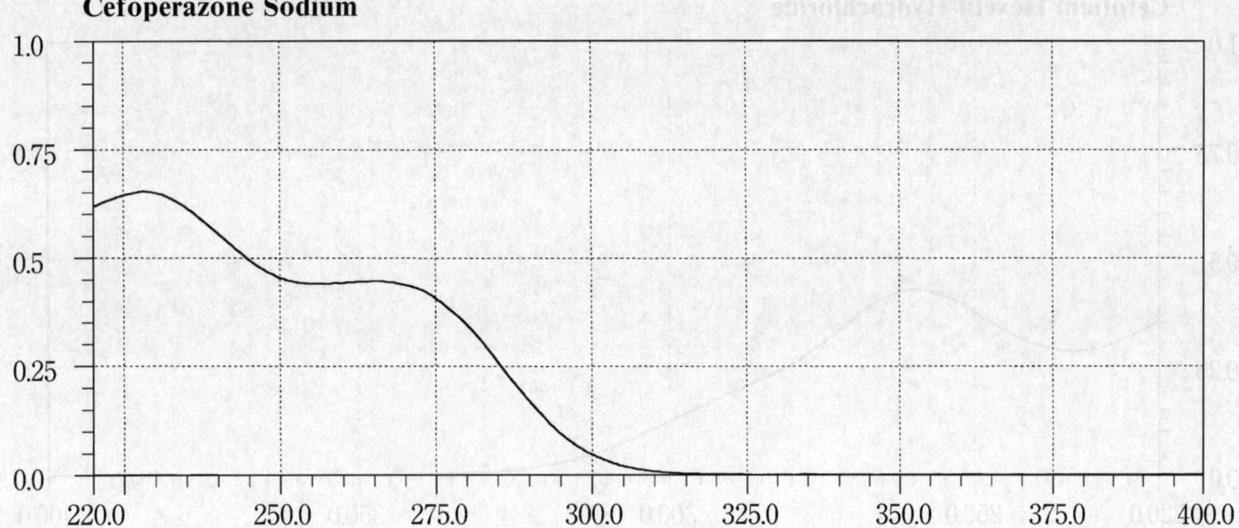

Cefotaxime Sodium

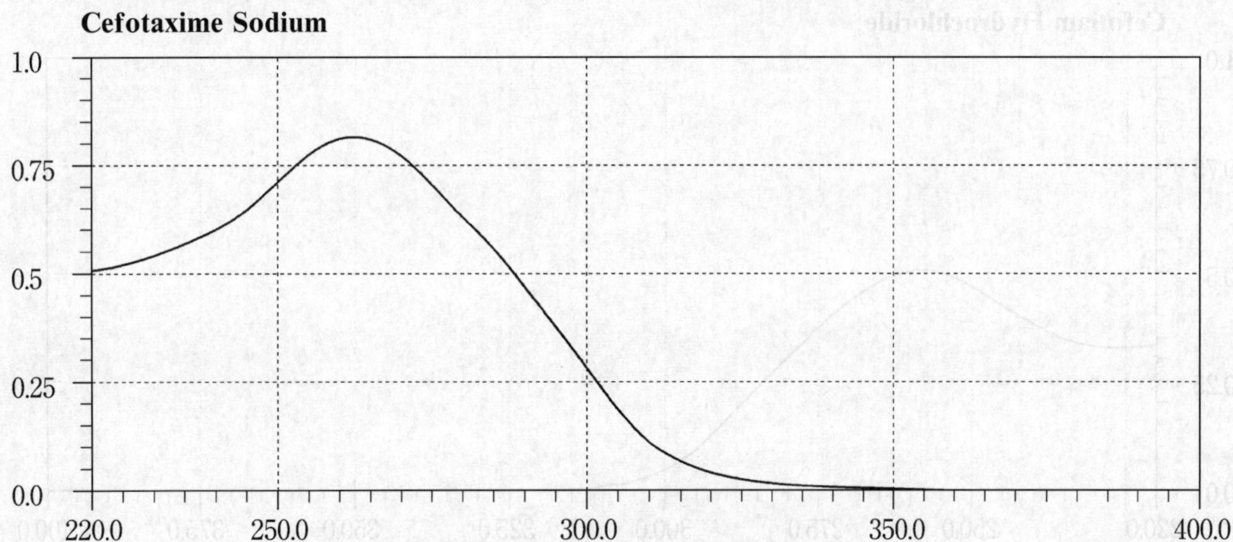

Cefotetan

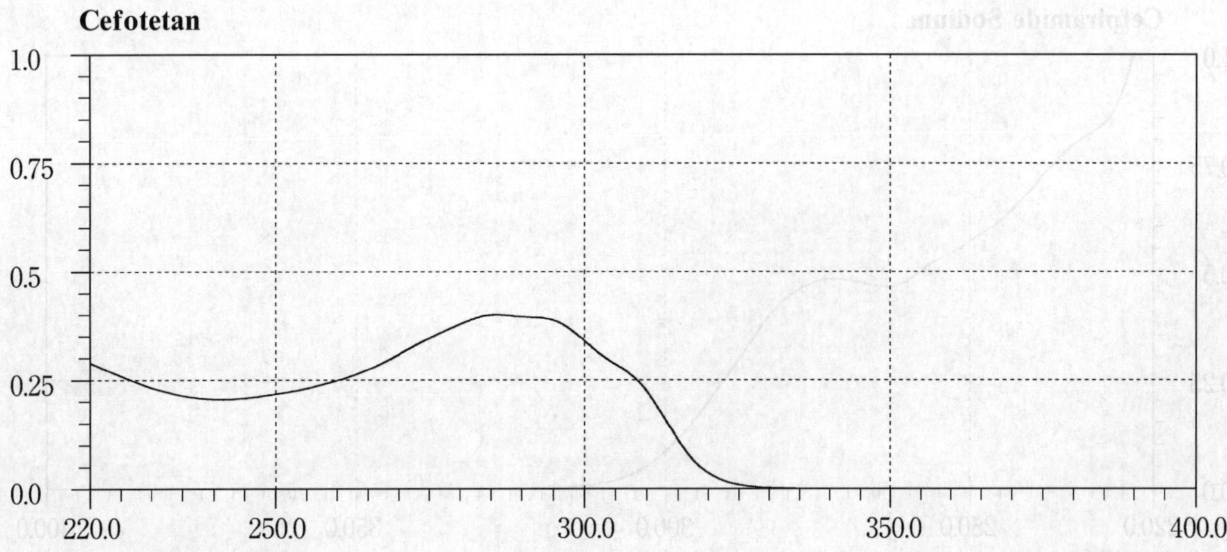

Cefotiam Hexetil Hydrochloride

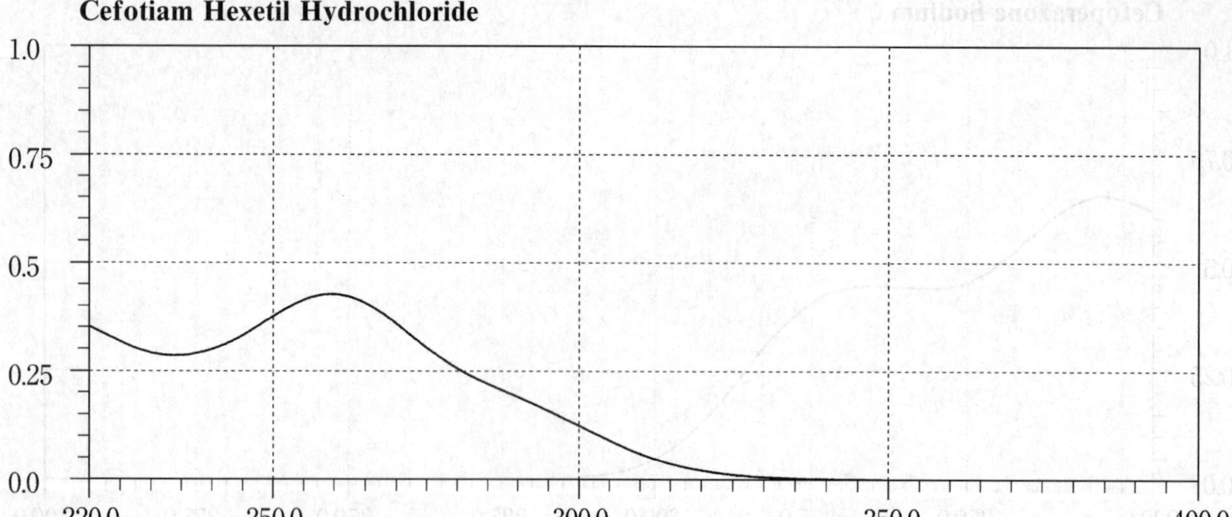

Cefotiam Hydrochloride

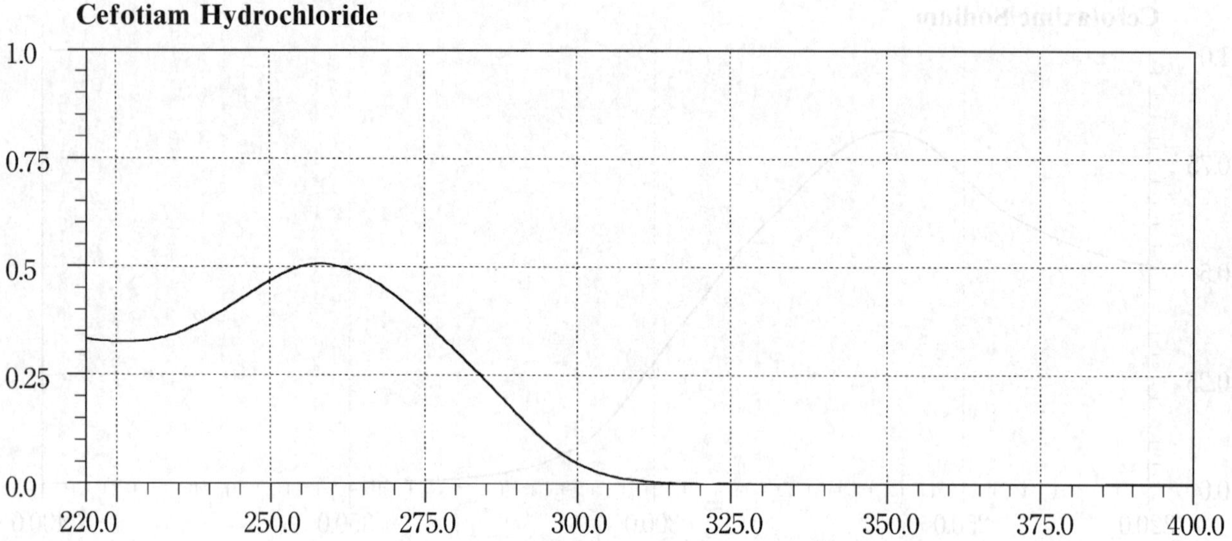

Cefpiramide Sodium

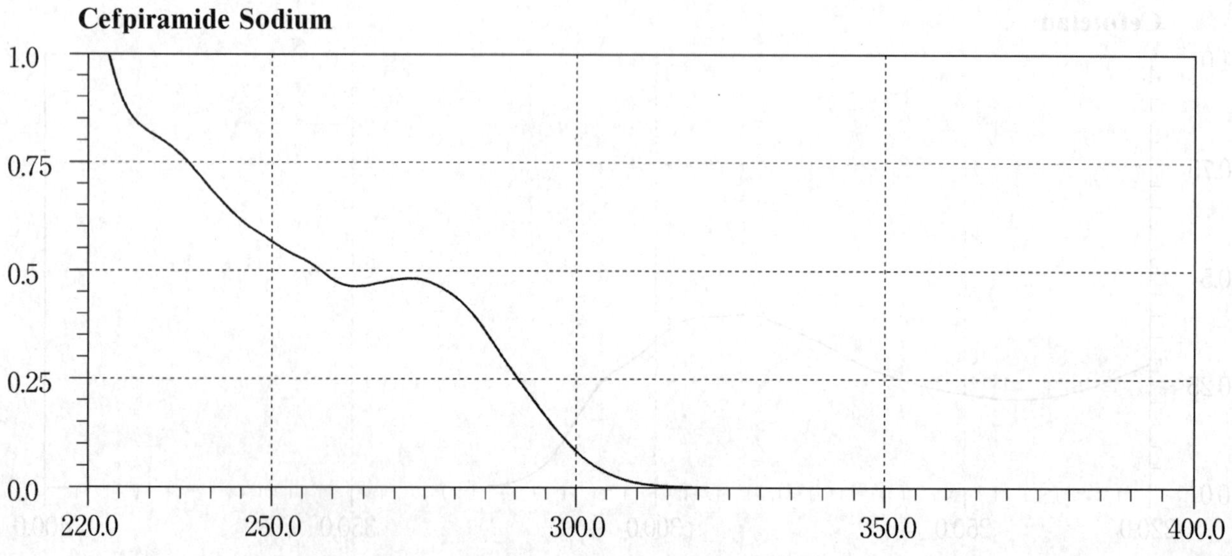

Cefpodoxime Proxetil

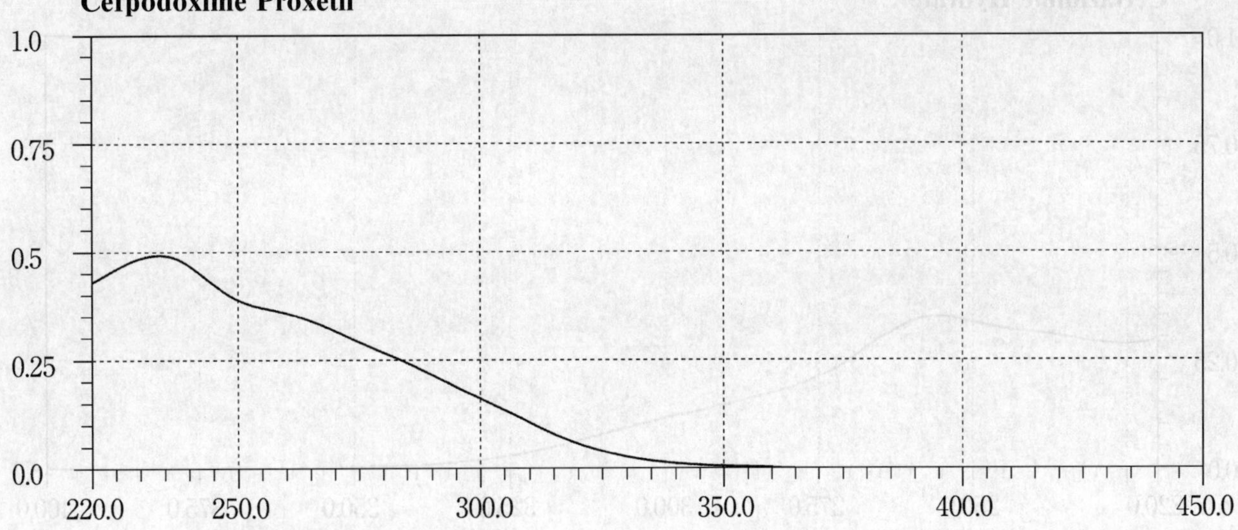

Cefroxadine Hydrate

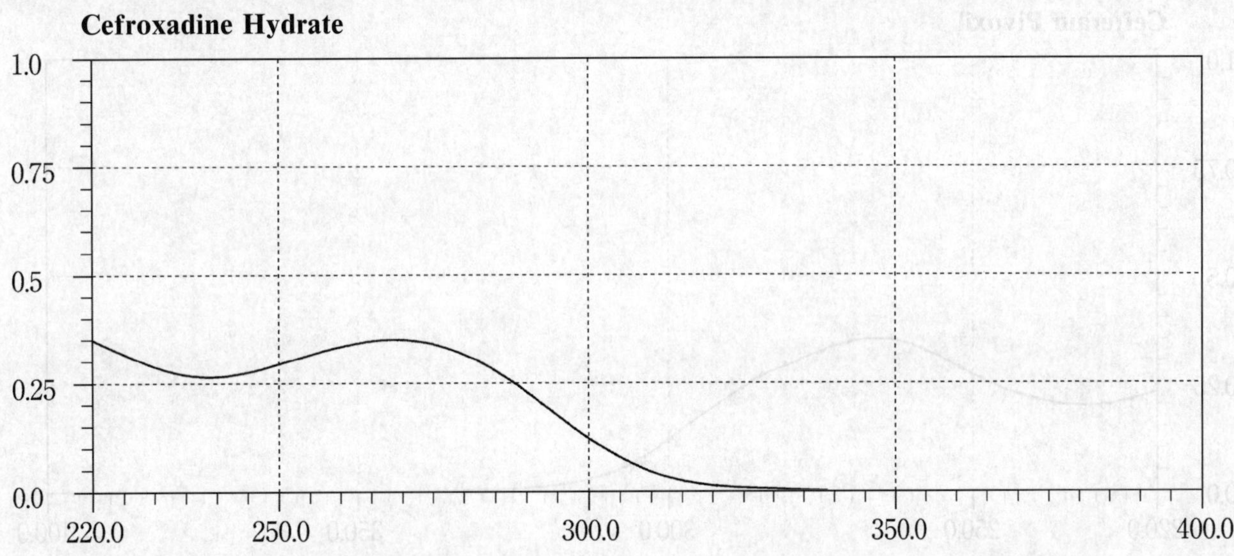

Cefsulodin Sodium

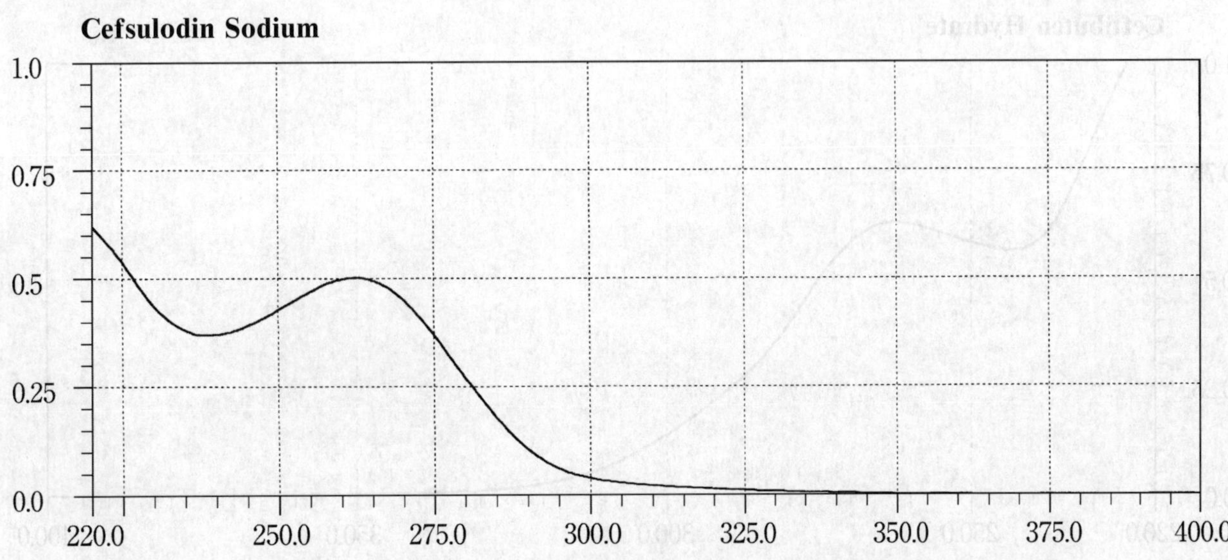

Ceftazidime Hydrate

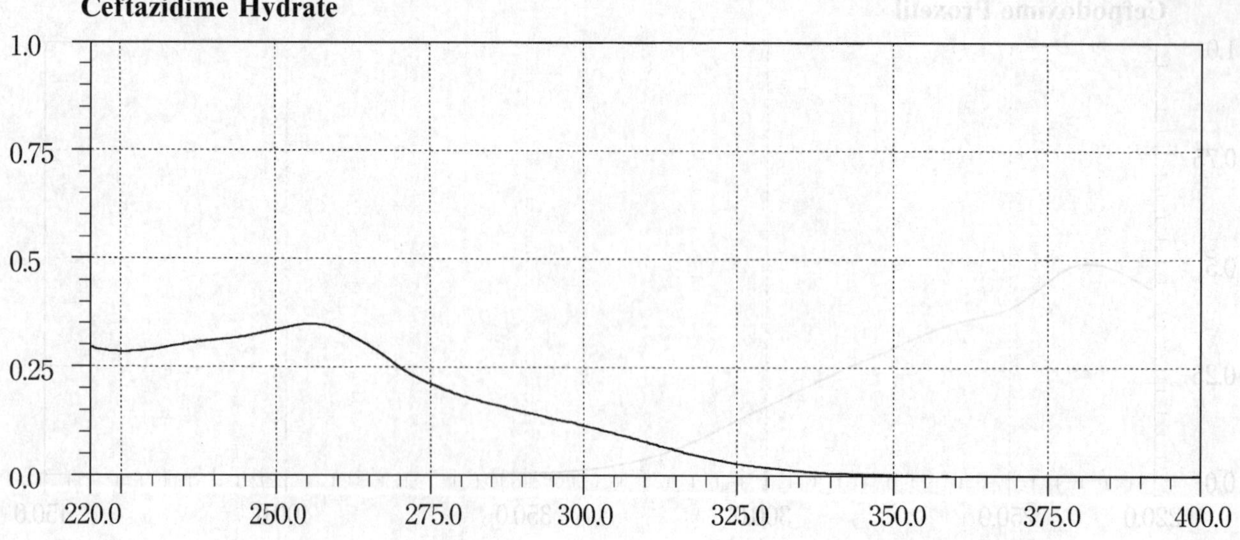

Cefteram Pivoxil

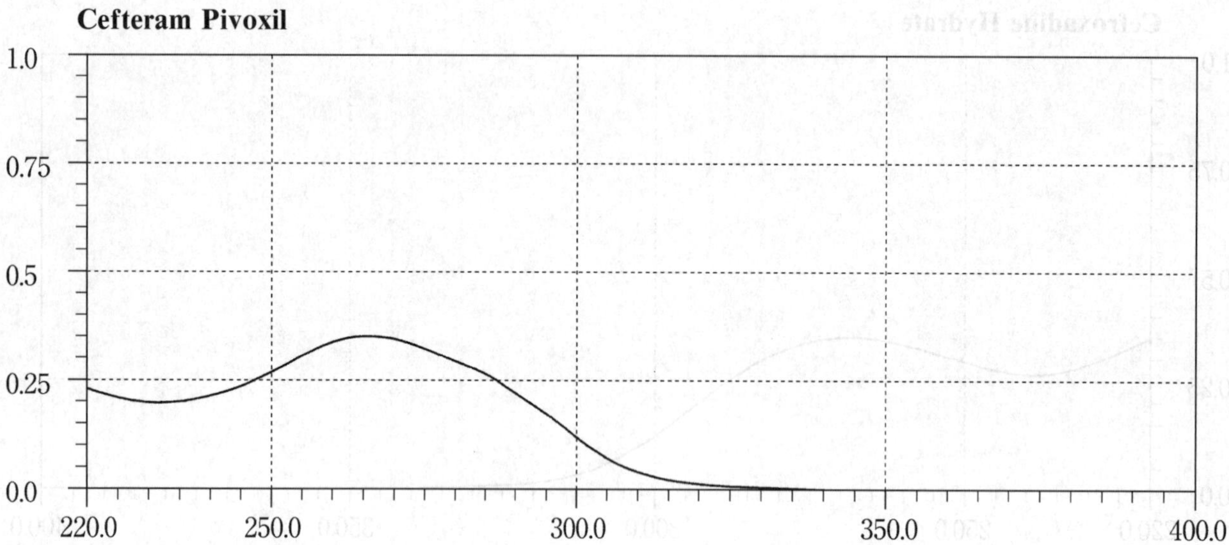

Ceftibuten Hydrate

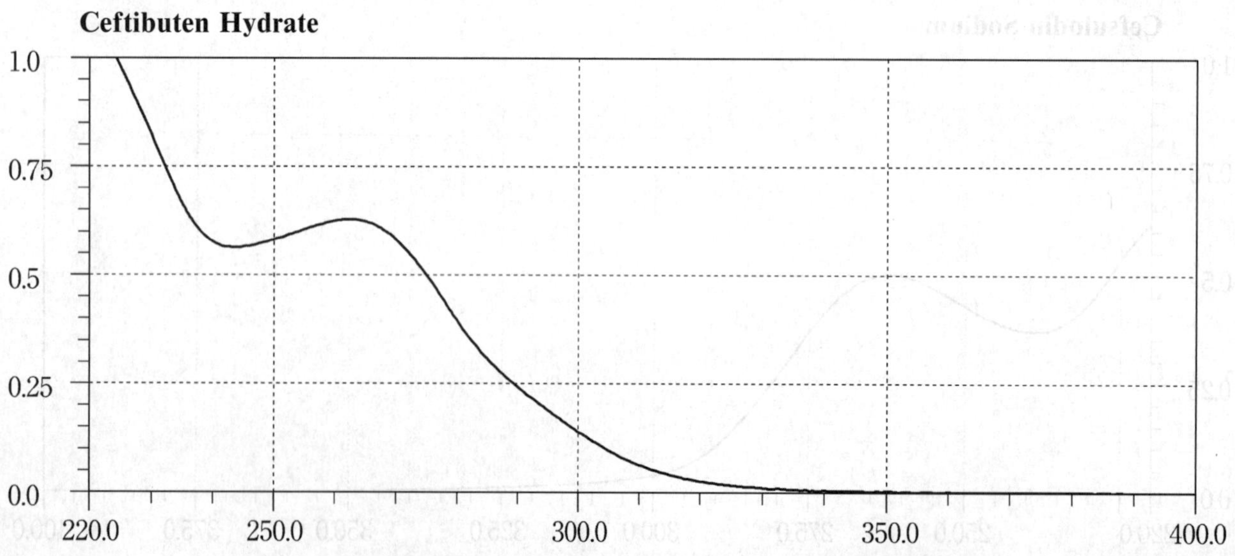

Ceftizoxime Sodium

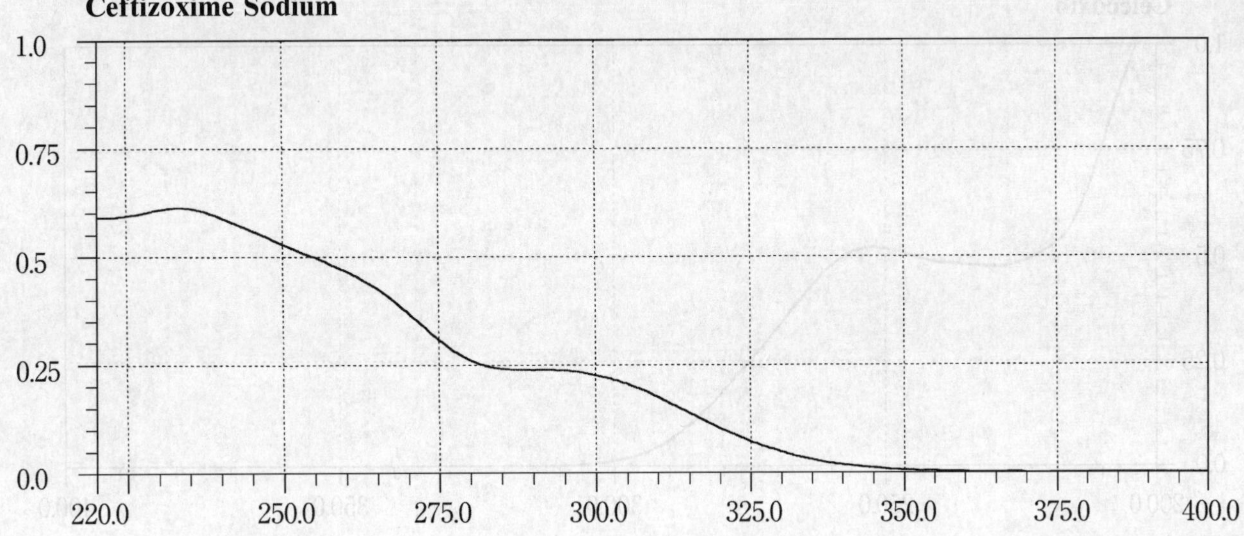

Ceftriaxone Sodium Hydrate

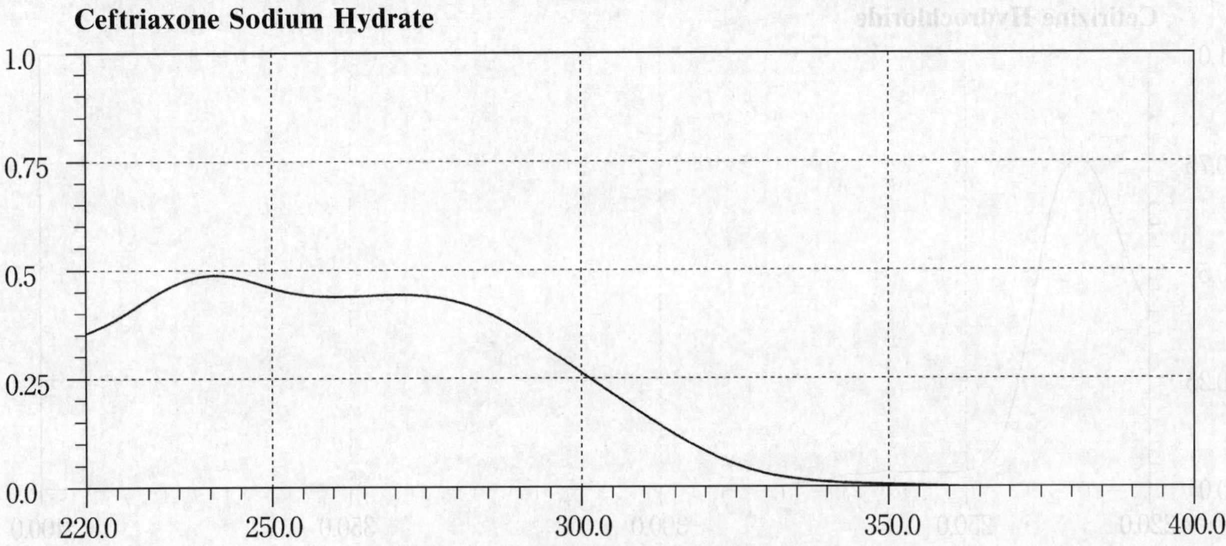

Cefuroxime Axetil

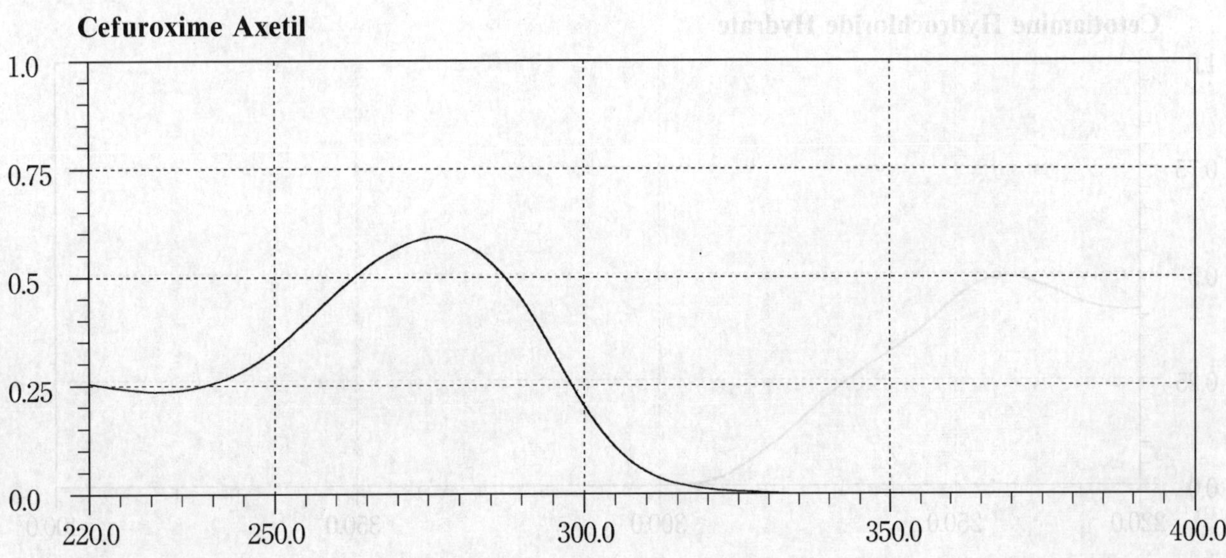

Celecoxib

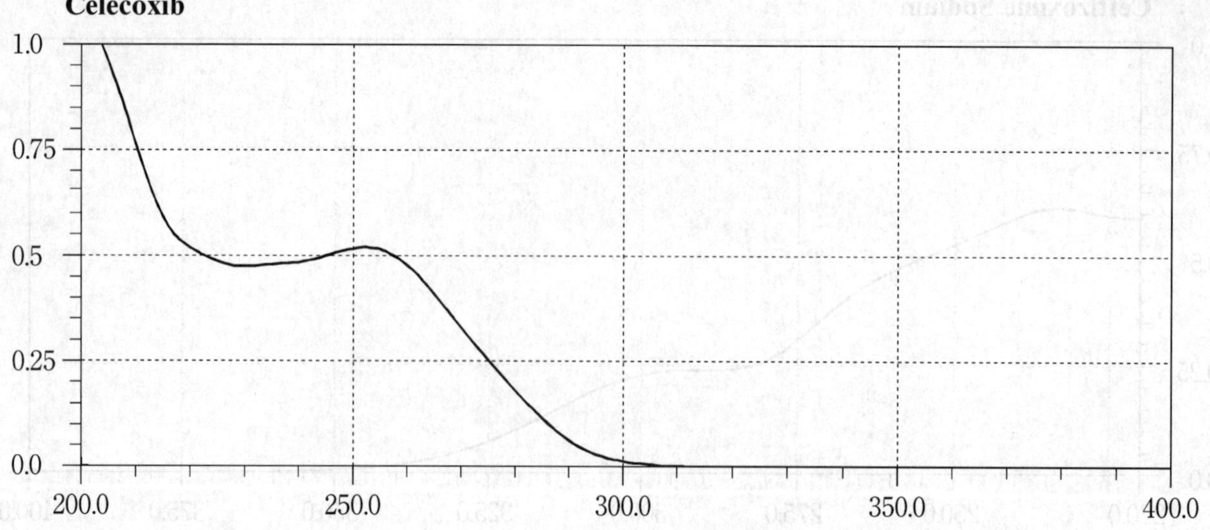

Cetirizine Hydrochloride

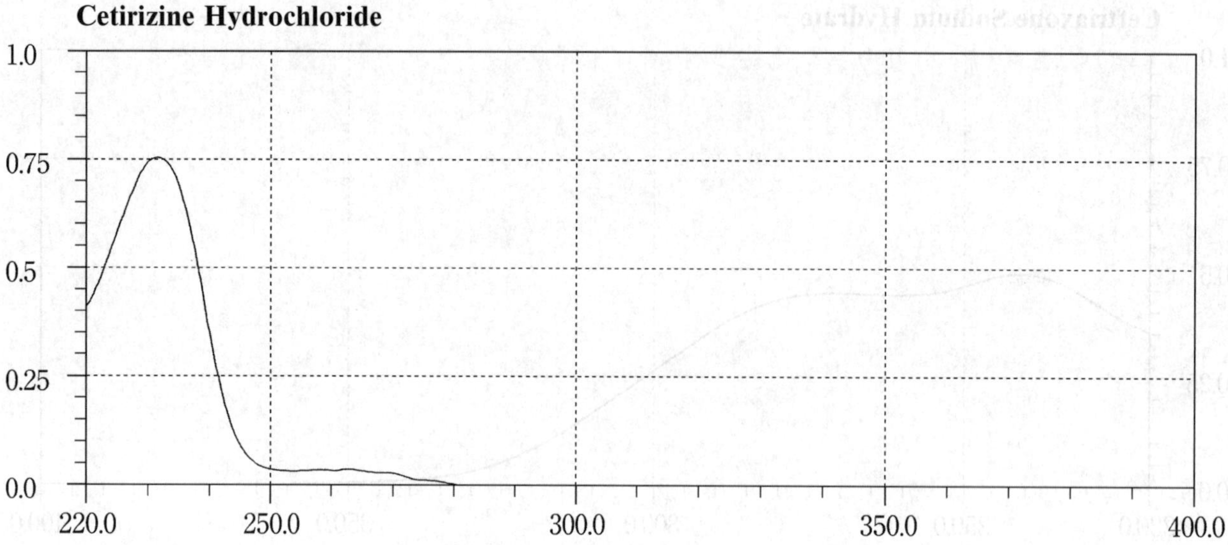

Cetotiamine Hydrochloride Hydrate

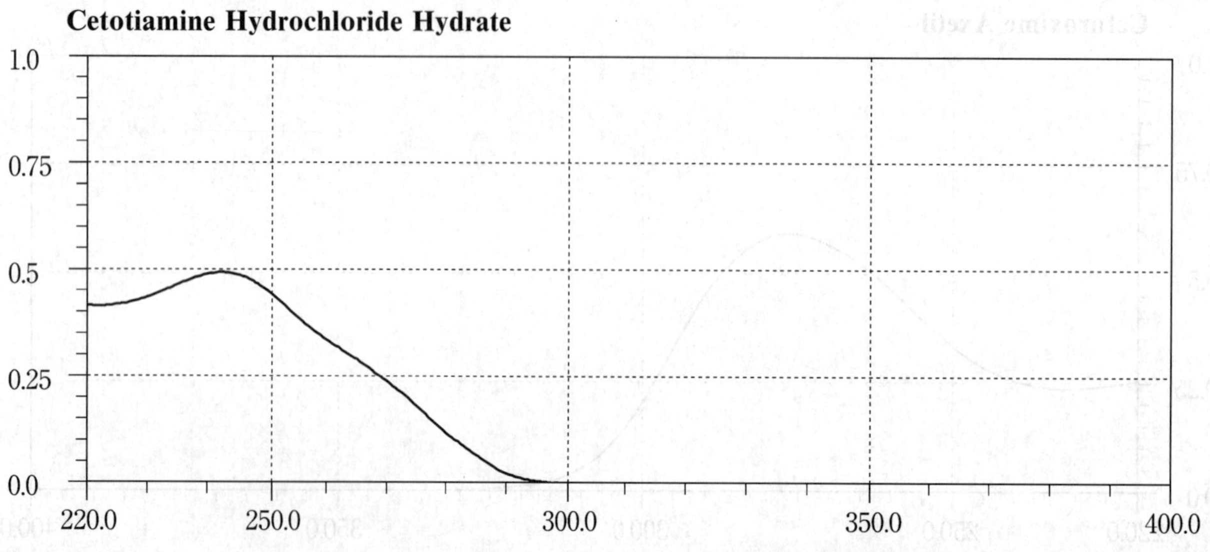

Cetraxate Hydrochloride

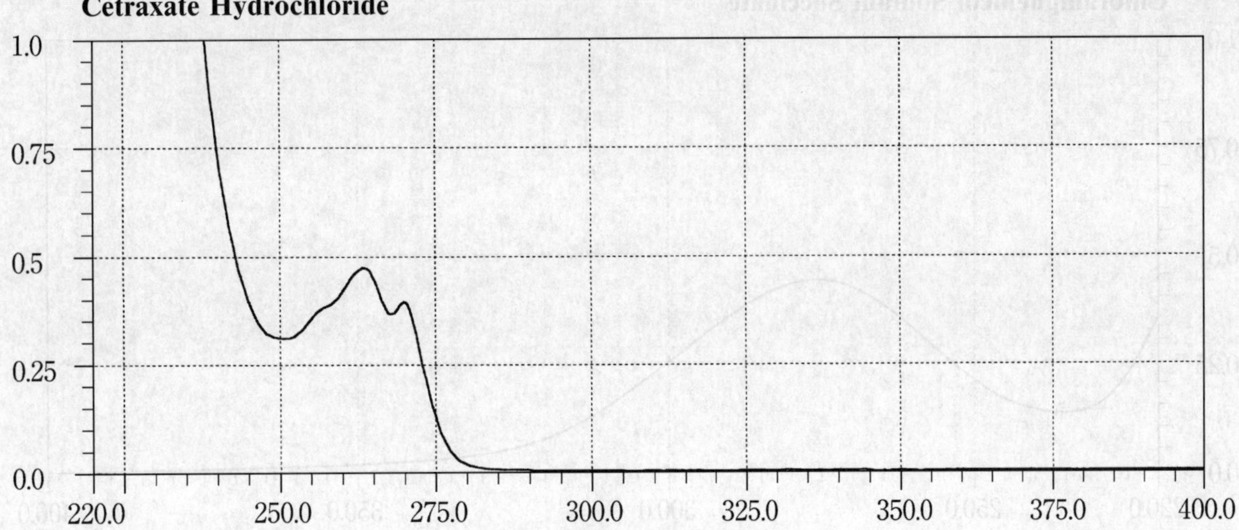

Chloramphenicol

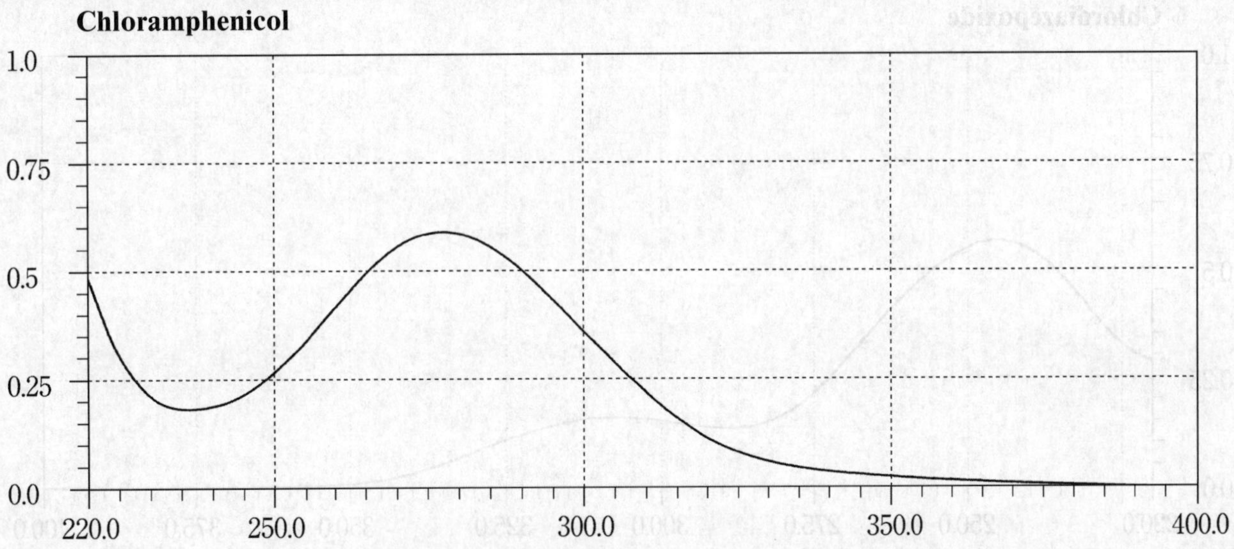

Chloramphenicol Palmitate

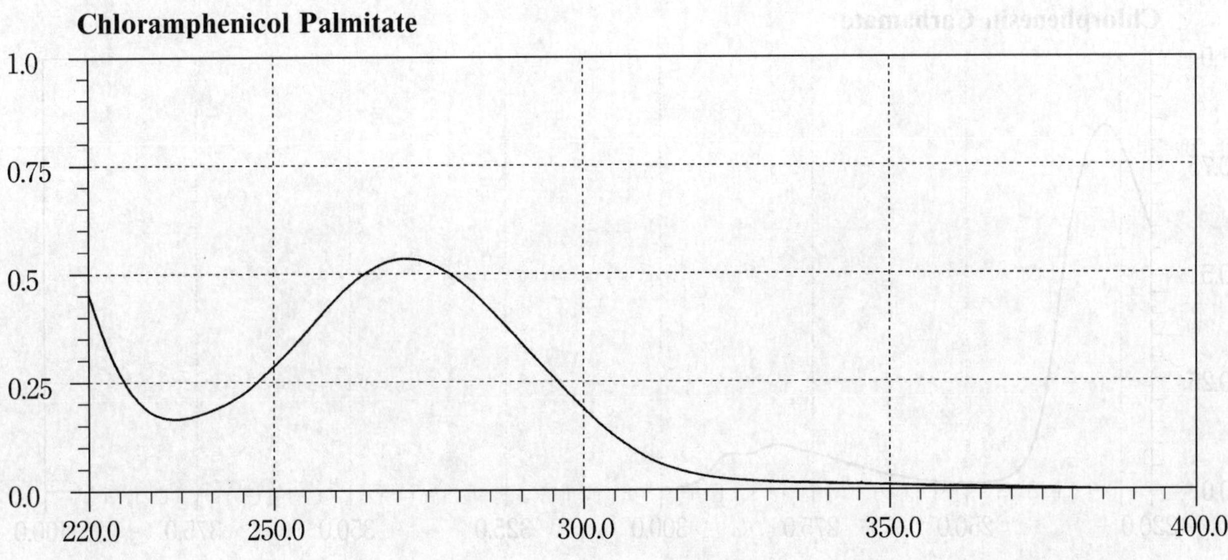

Chloramphenicol Sodium Succinate

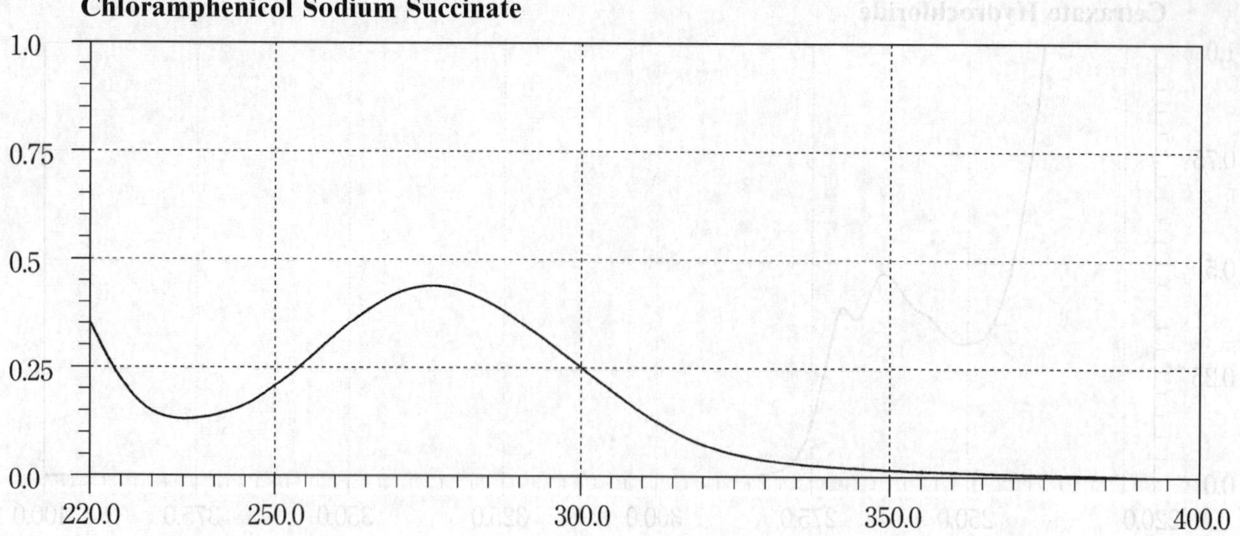

Chlordiazepoxide

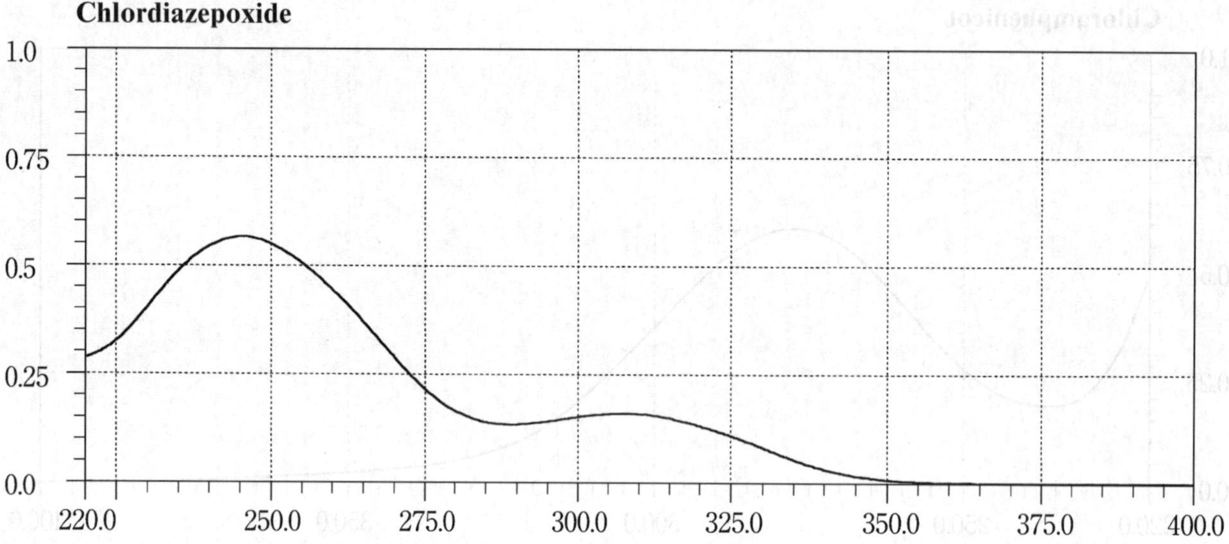

Chlorphenesin Carbamate

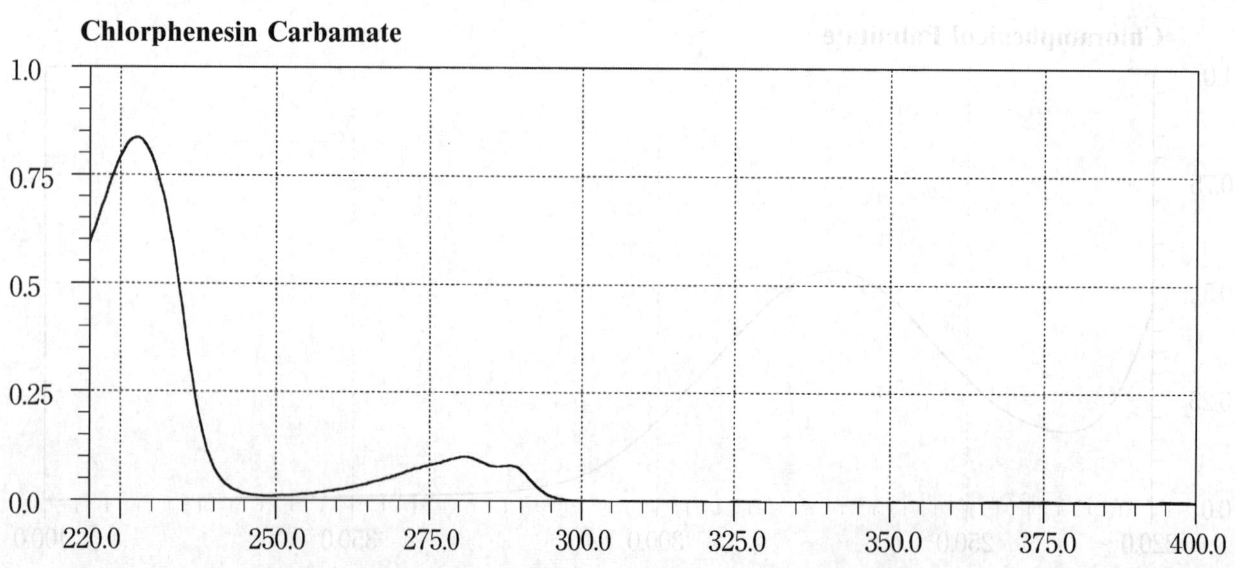

Chlorpheniramine Maleate

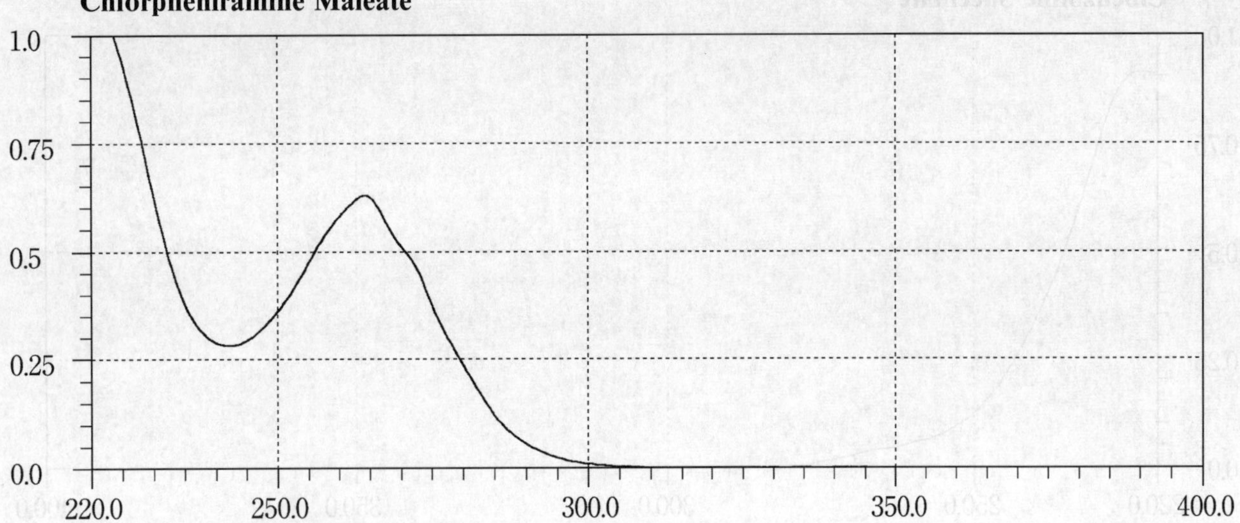

***d*-Chlorpheniramine Maleate**

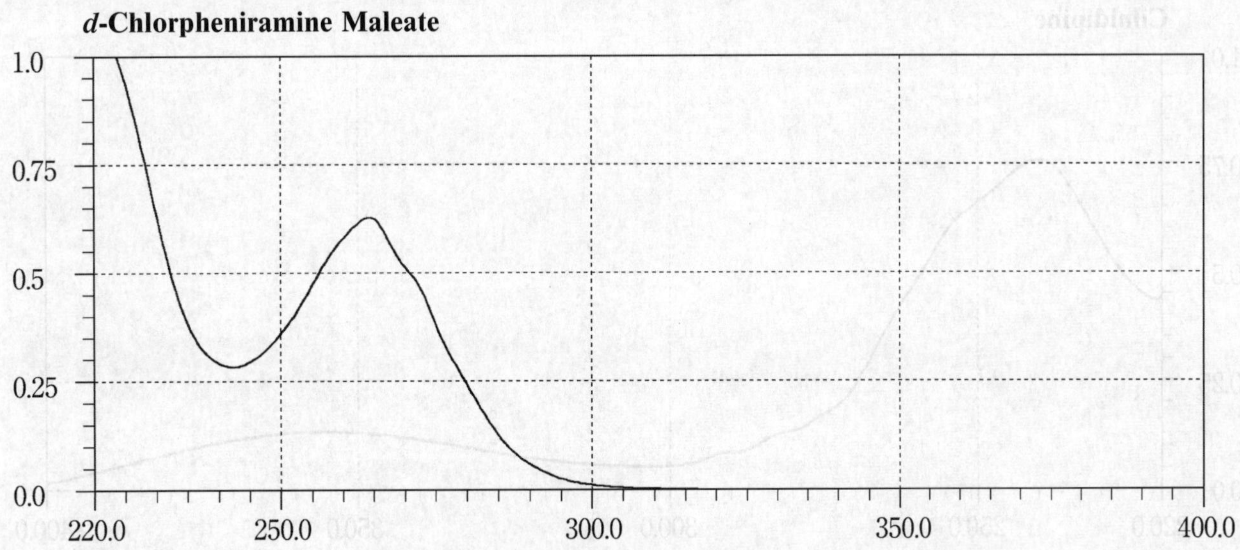

Chlorpropamide

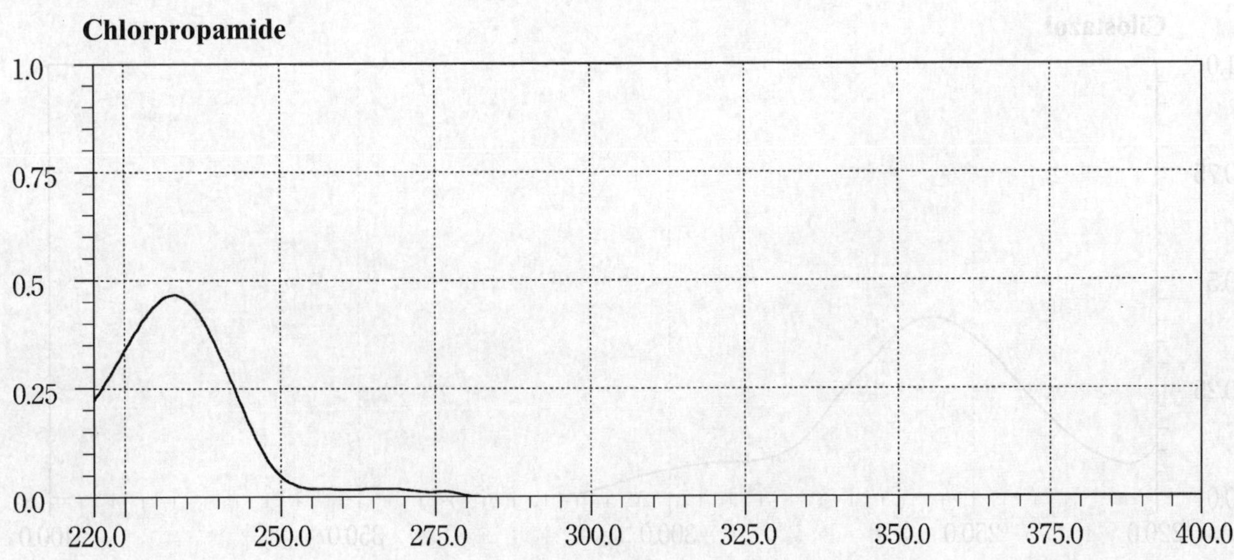

Cibenzoline Succinate

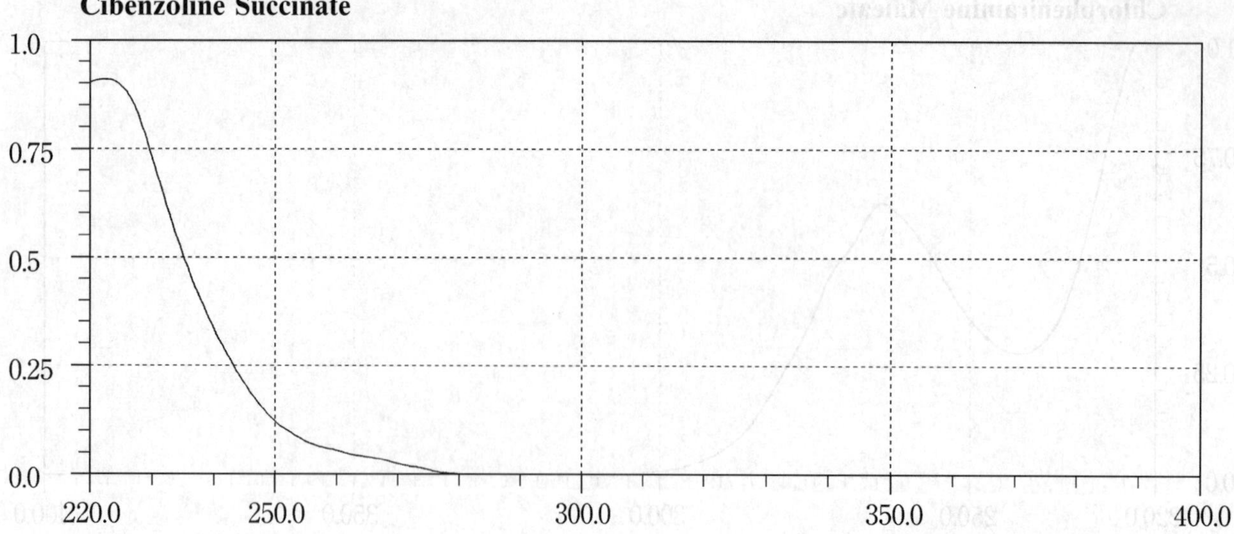

Cilnidipine

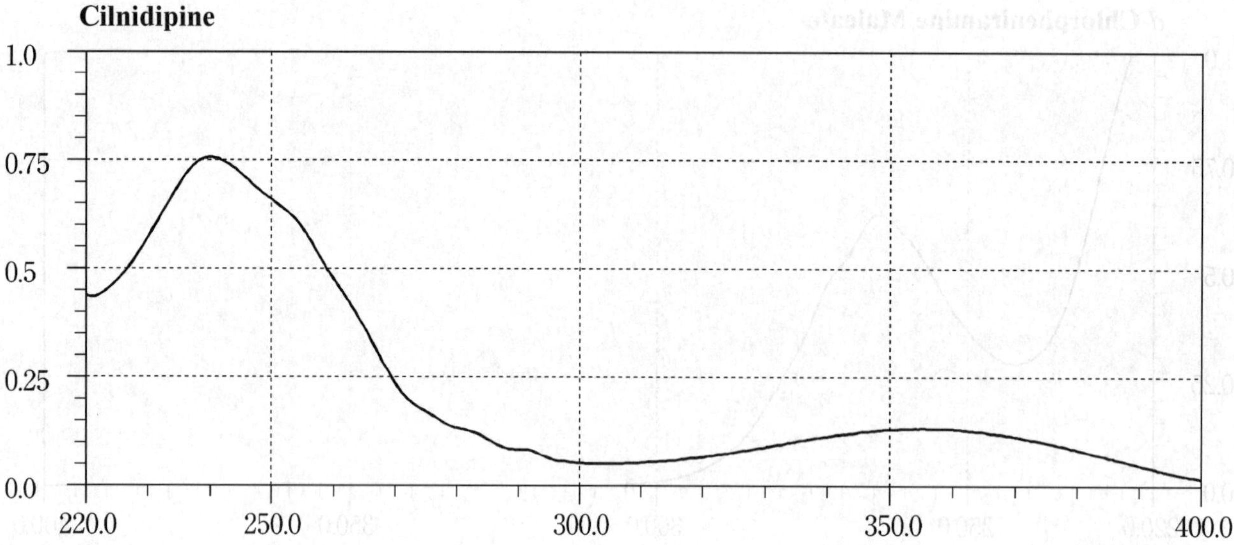

Cilostazol

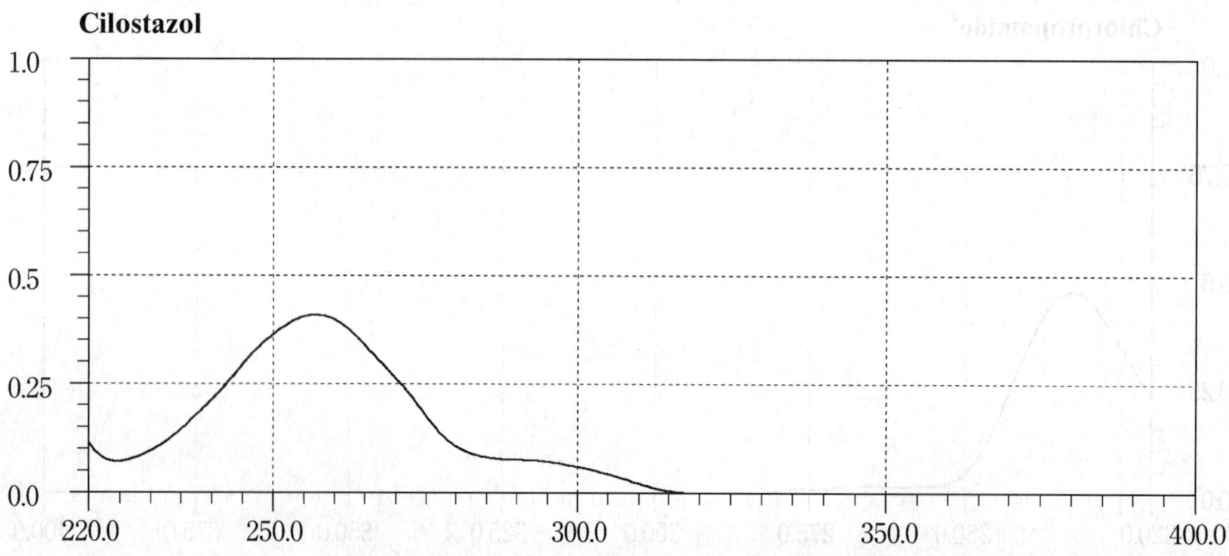

Cinoxacin

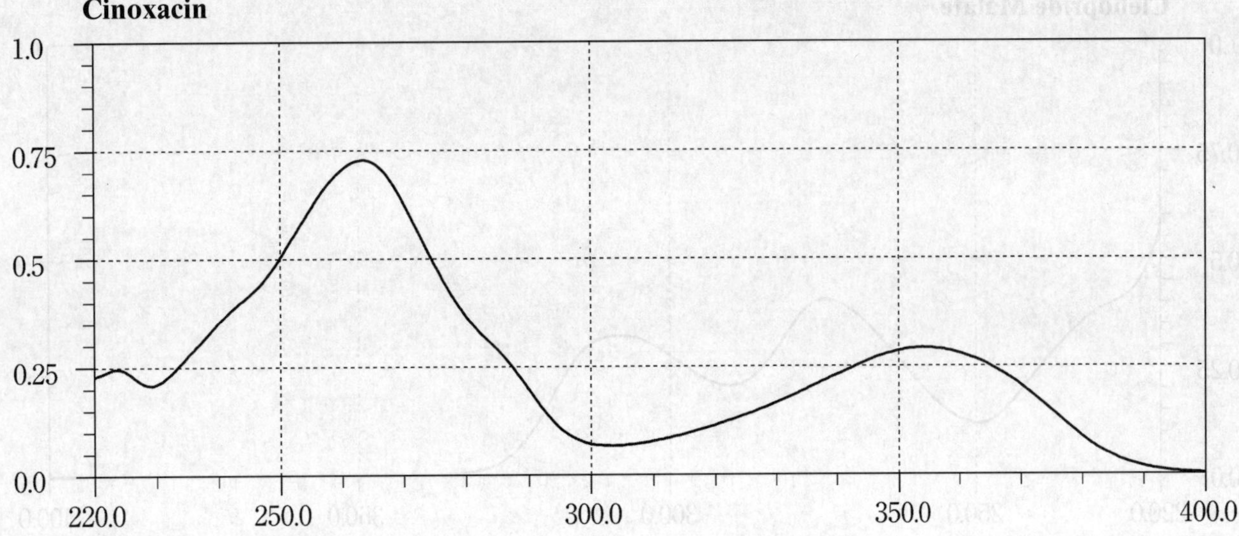

Cisplatin

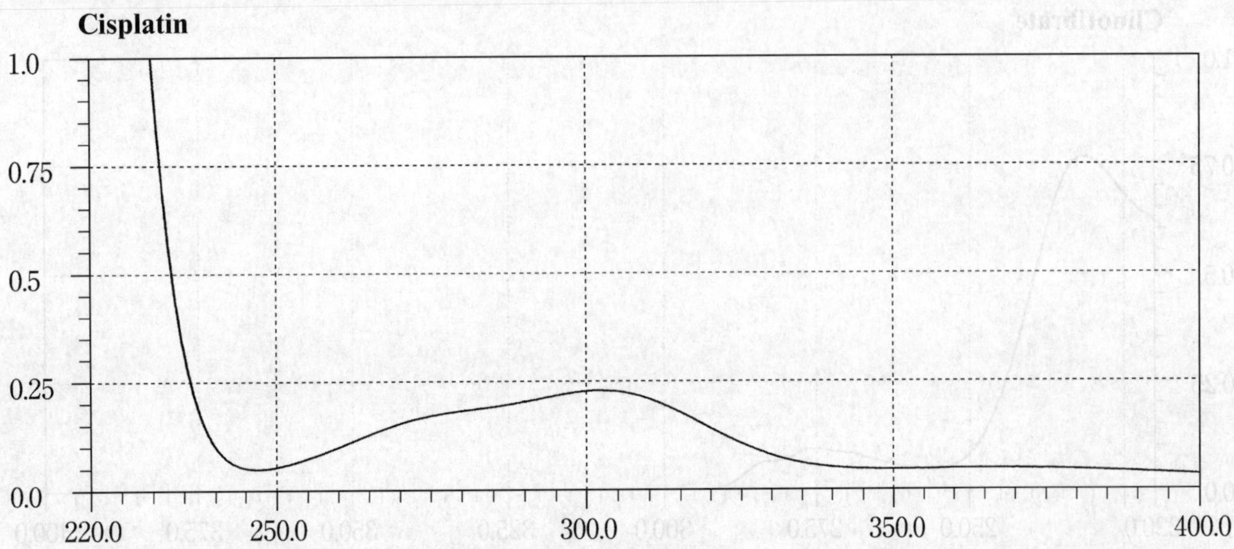

Citicoline

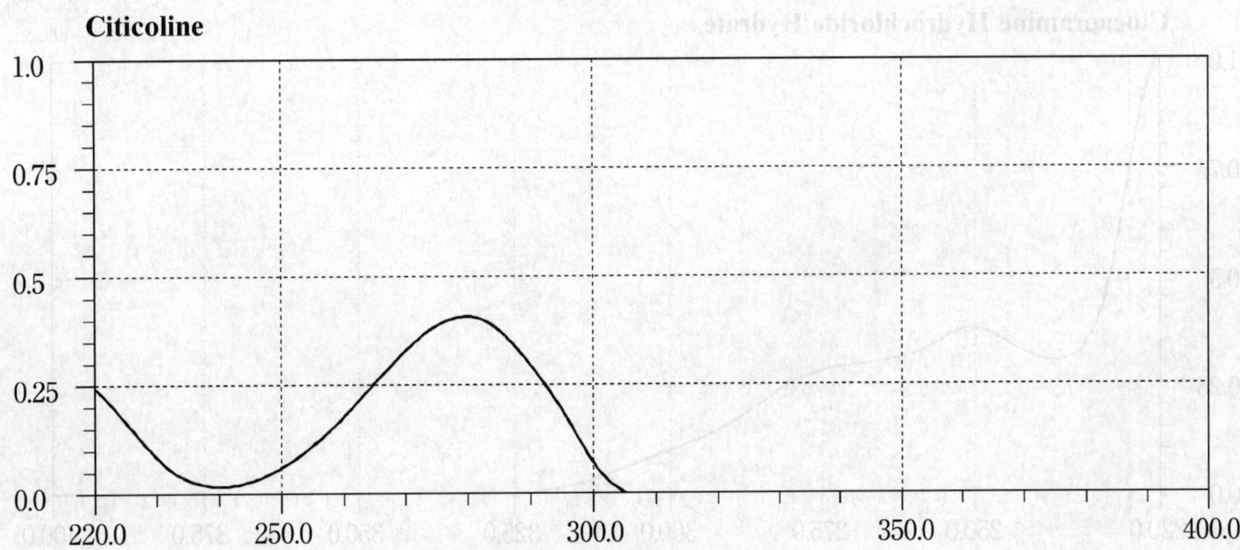

Clebopride Malate

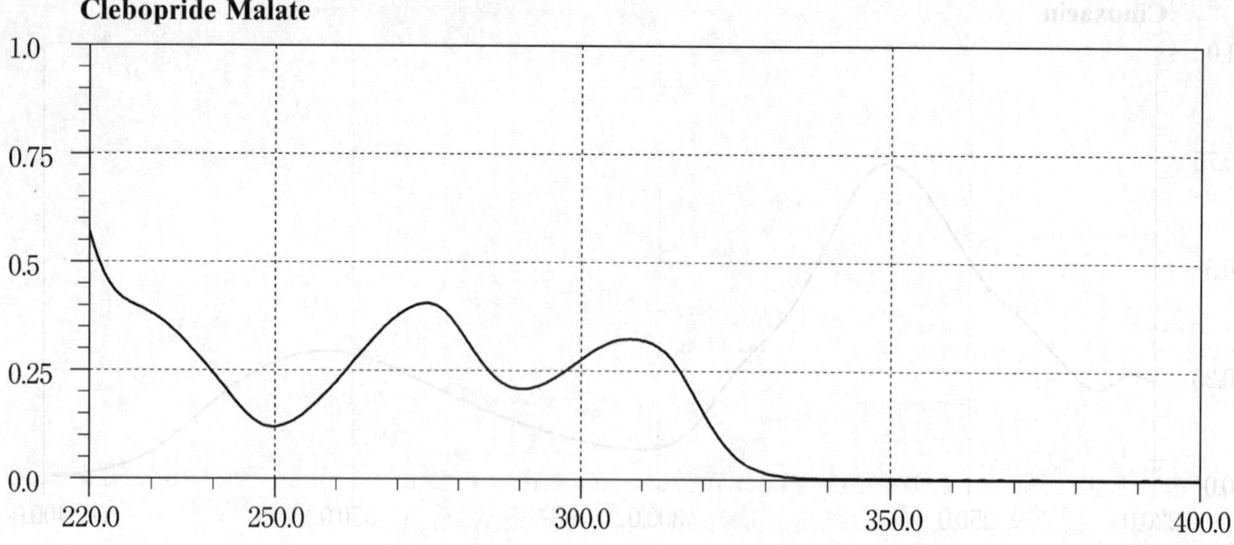

Clinofibrate

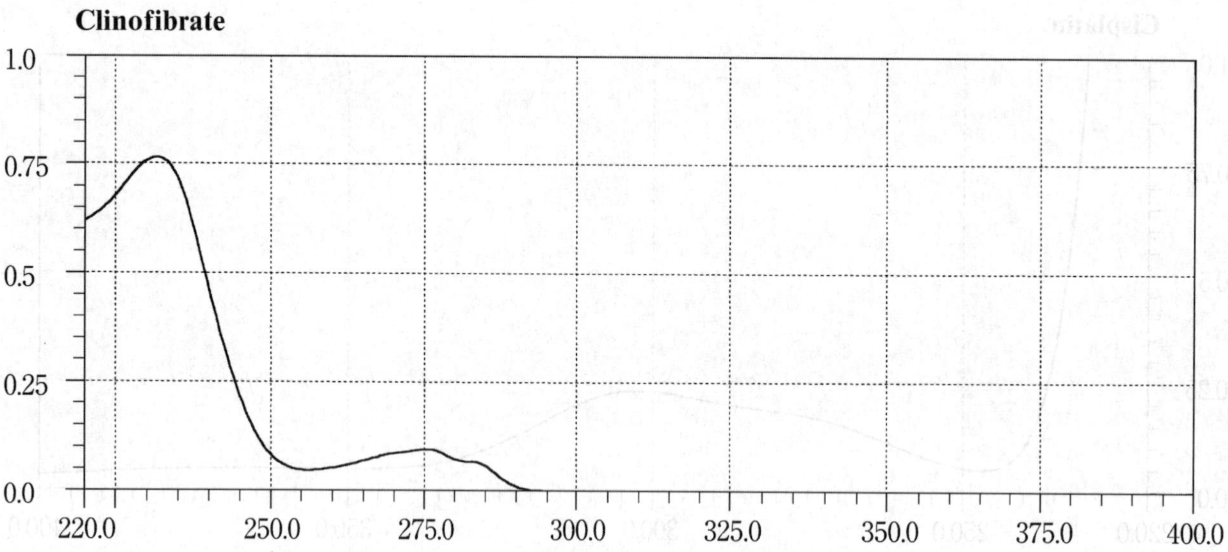

Clocapramine Hydrochloride Hydrate

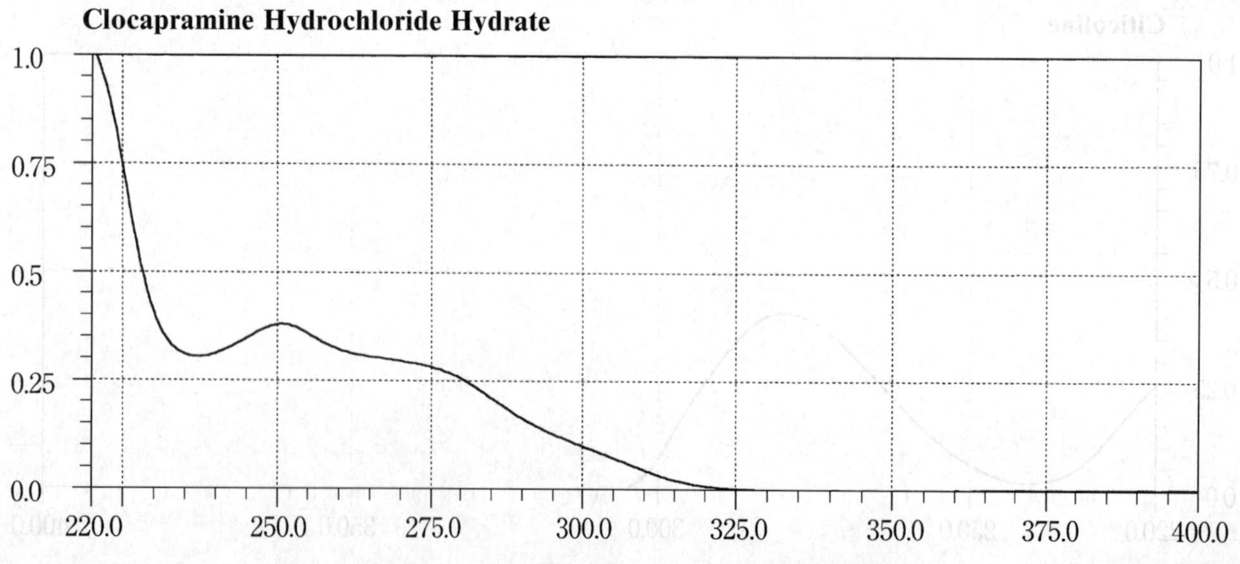

Clofedanol Hydrochloride

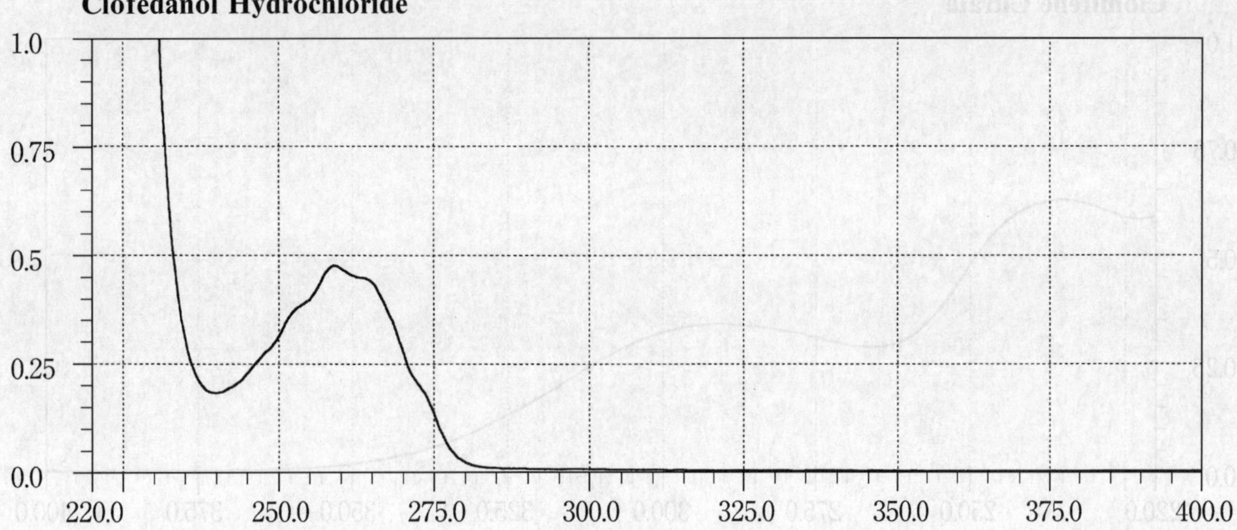

Clofibrate 1

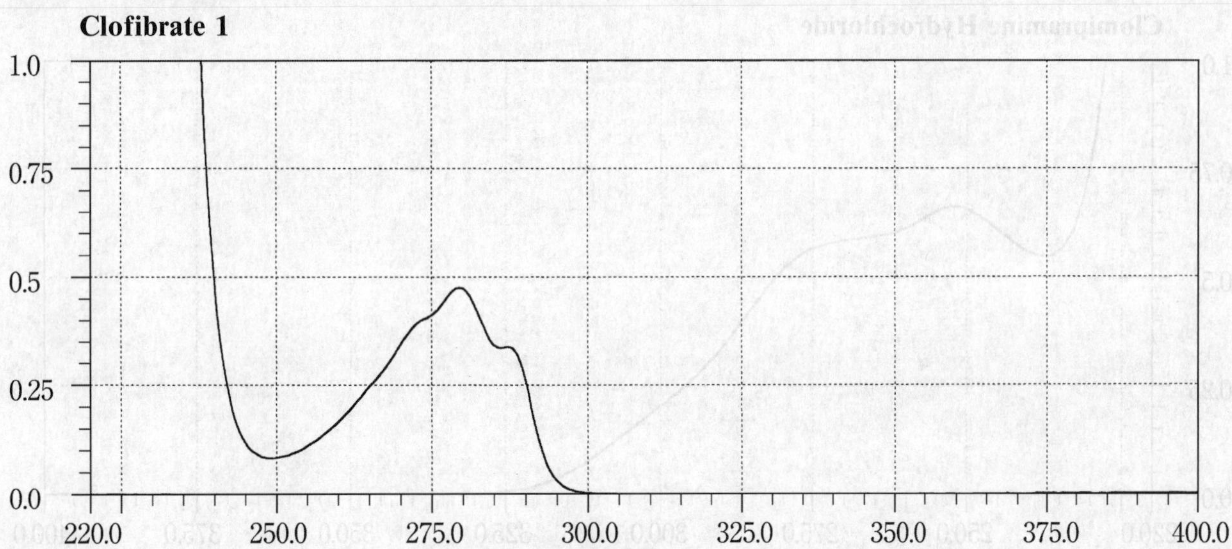

Clofibrate 2

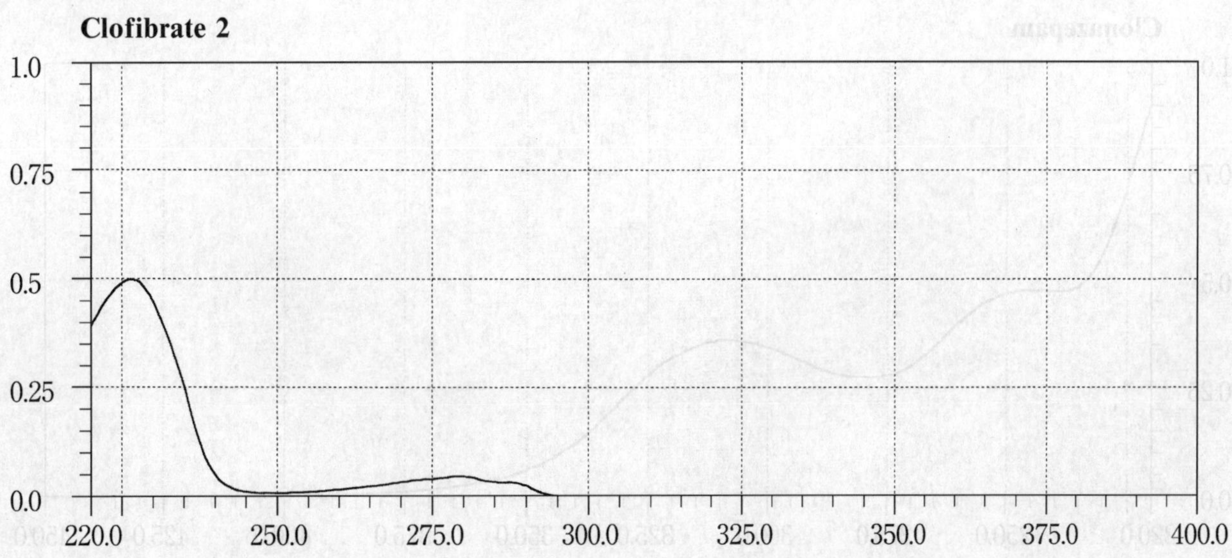

Clomifene Citrate

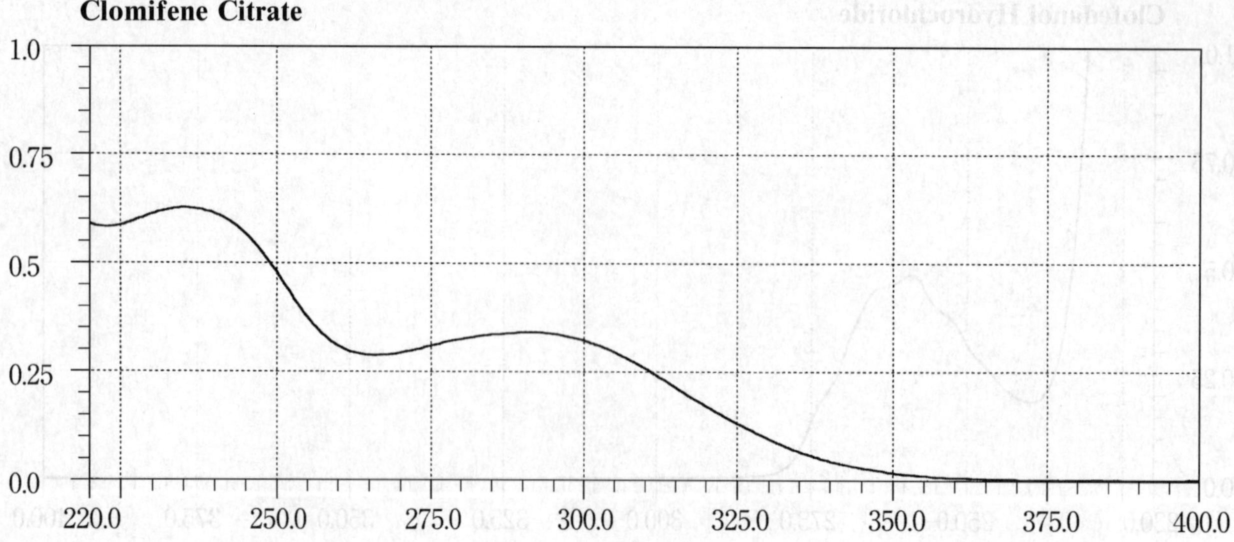

Clomipramine Hydrochloride

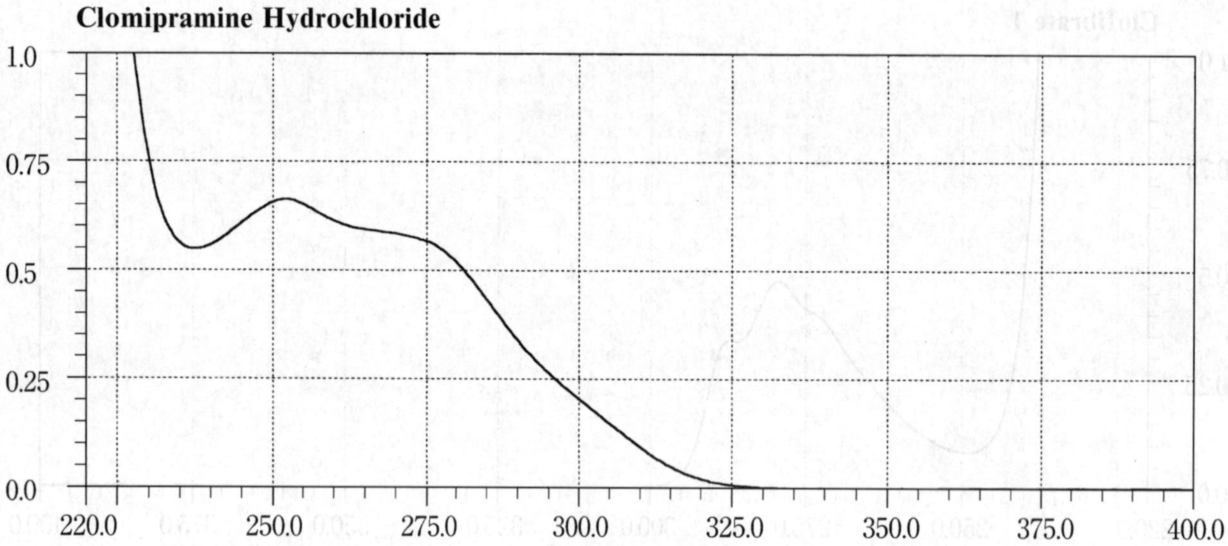

Clonazepam

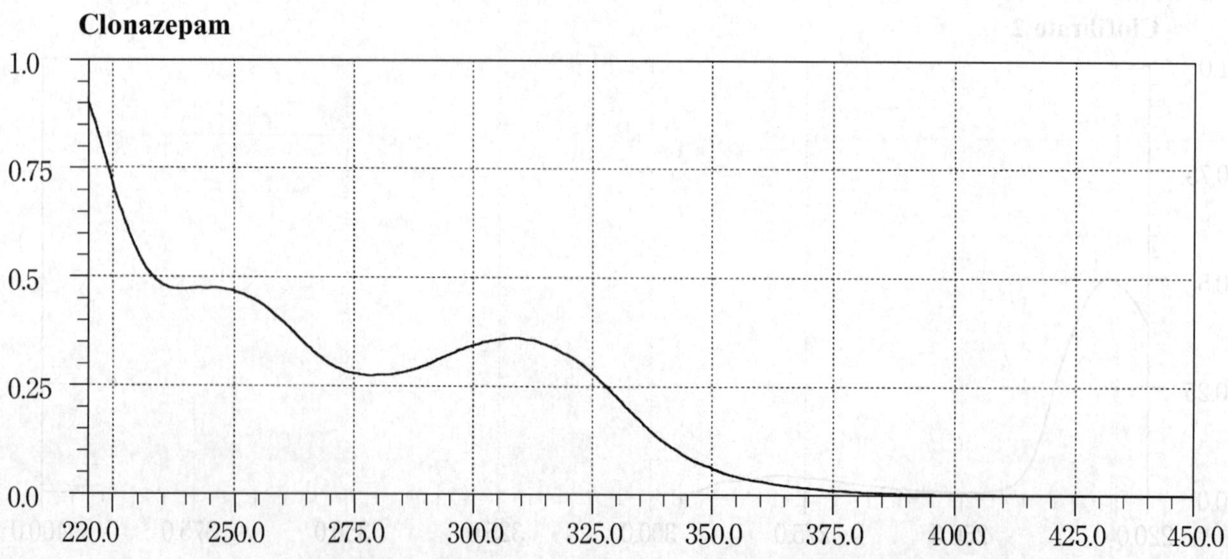

Clonidine Hydrochloride

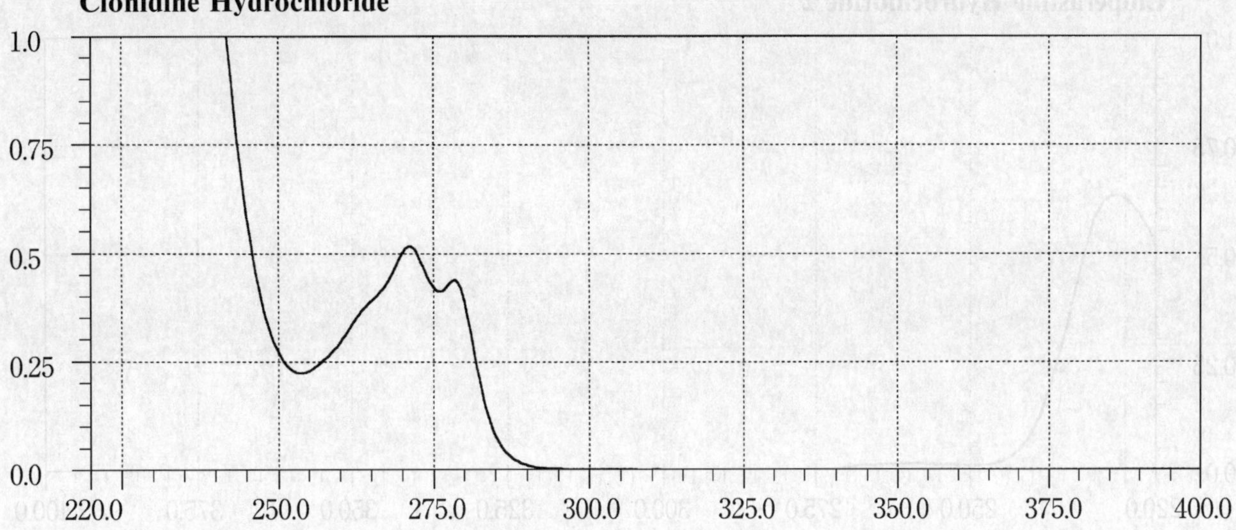

Cloperastine Fendizoate

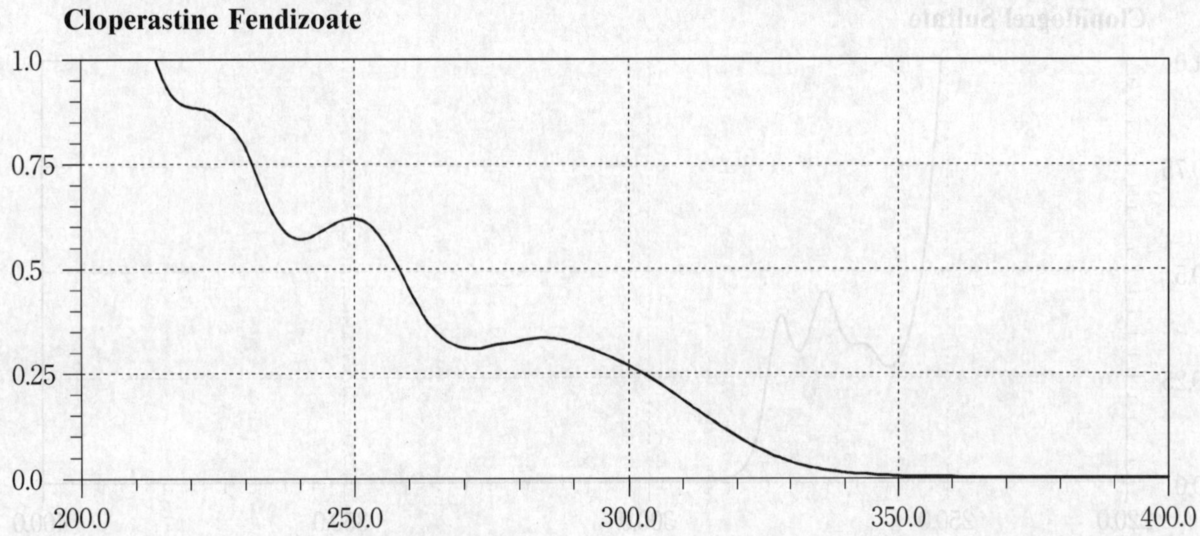

Cloperastine Hydrochloride 1

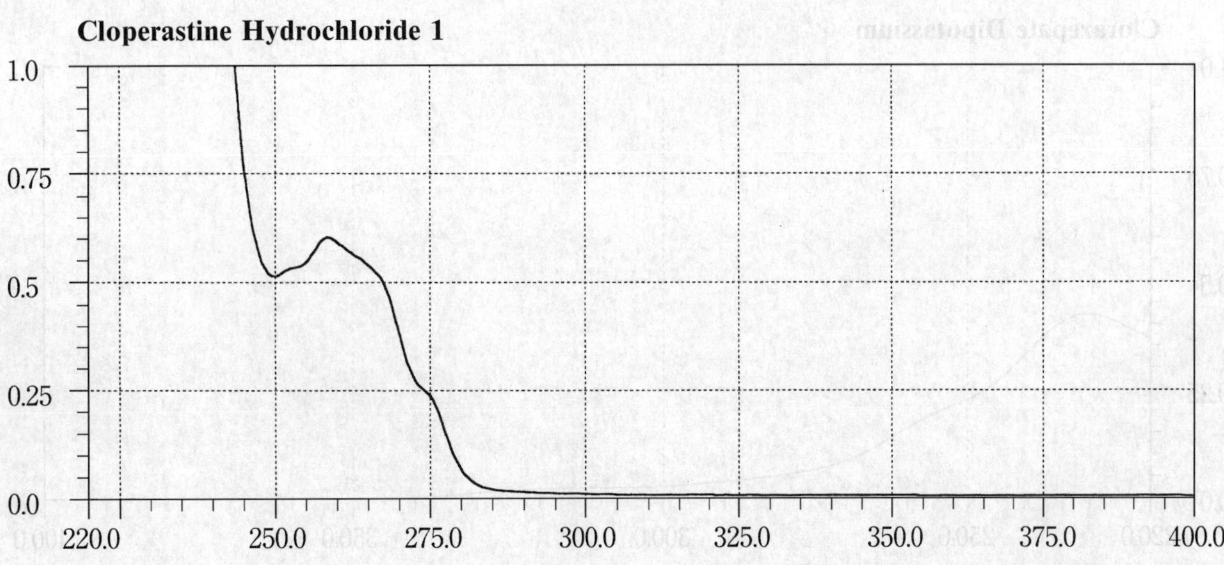

Cloperastine Hydrochloride 2

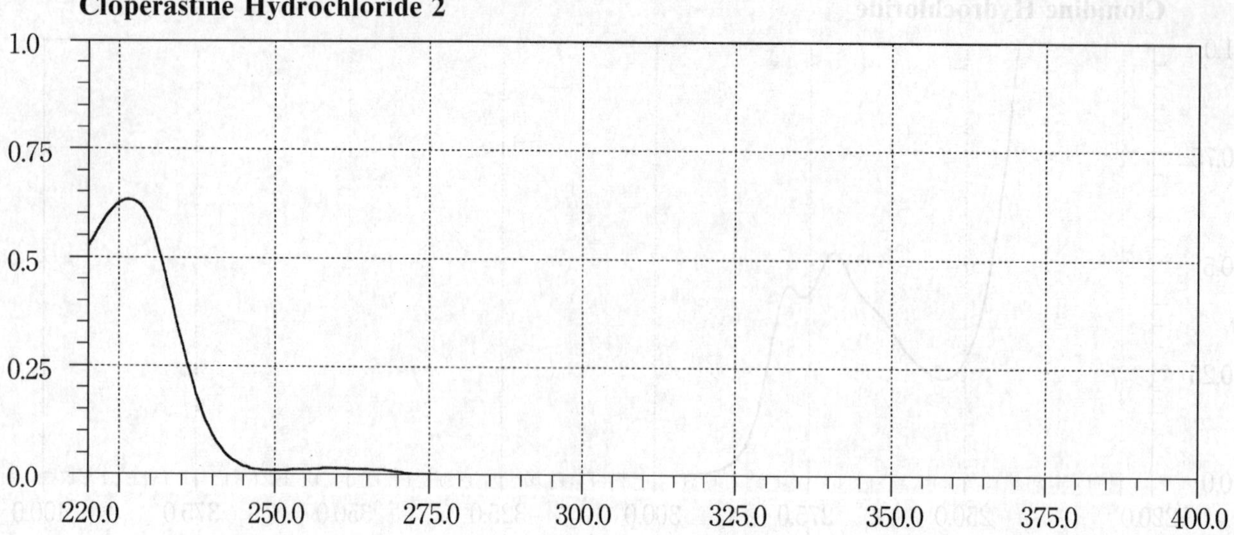

Clopidogrel Sulfate

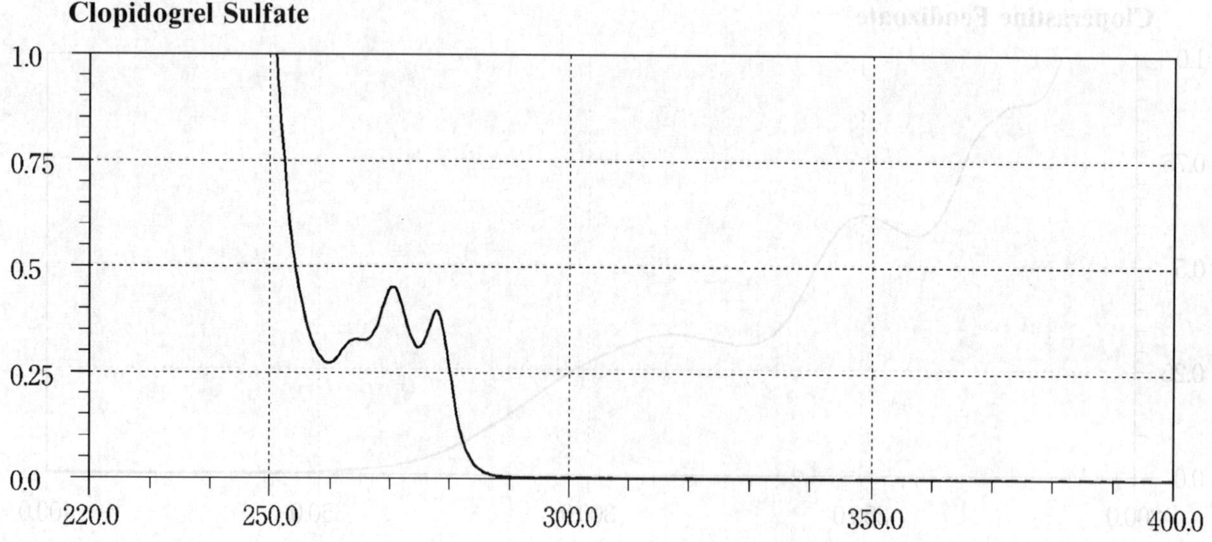

Clorazepate Dipotassium

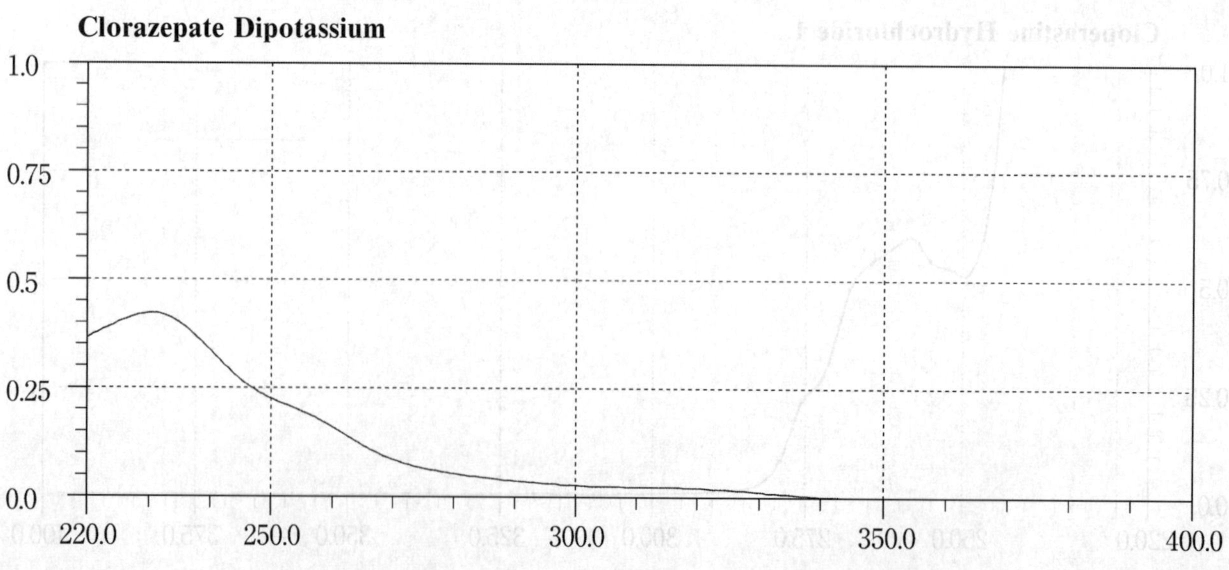

Clotiazepam

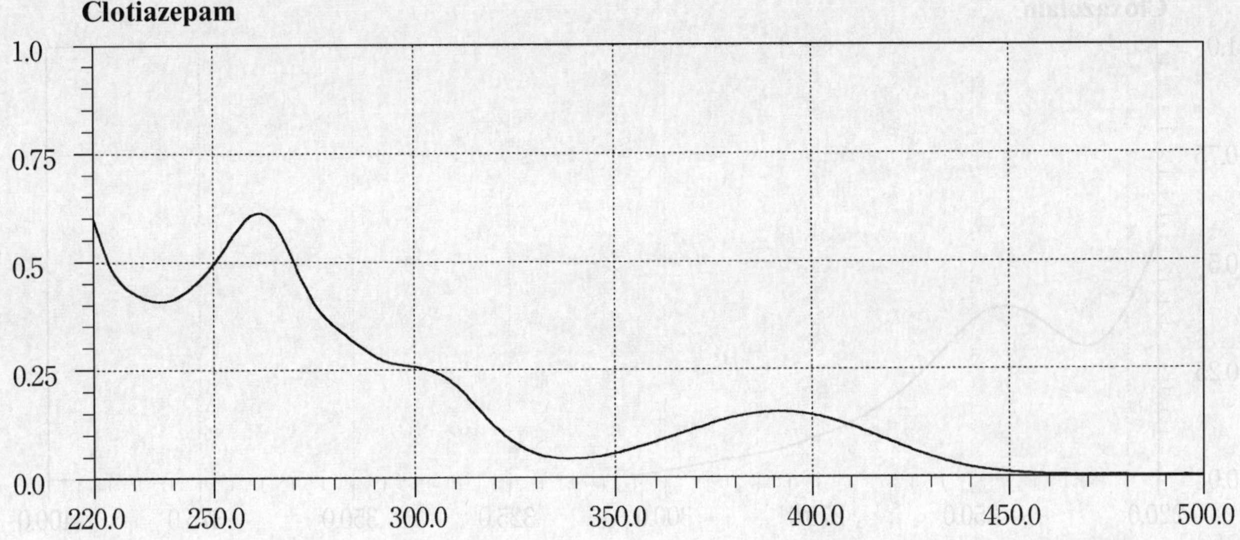

Clotrimazole

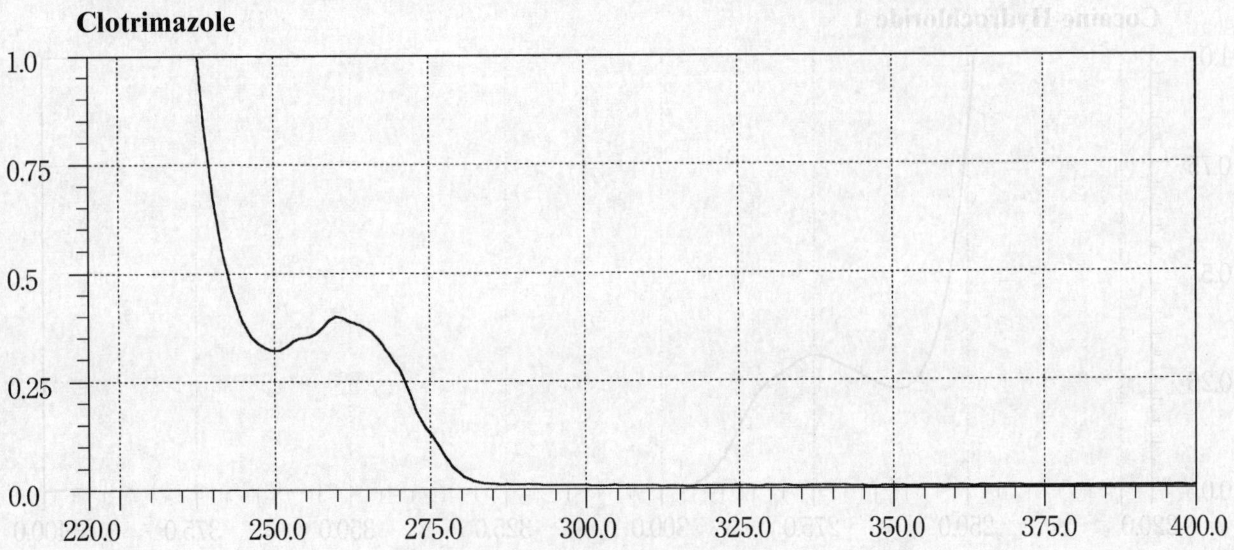

Cloxacillin Sodium Hydrate

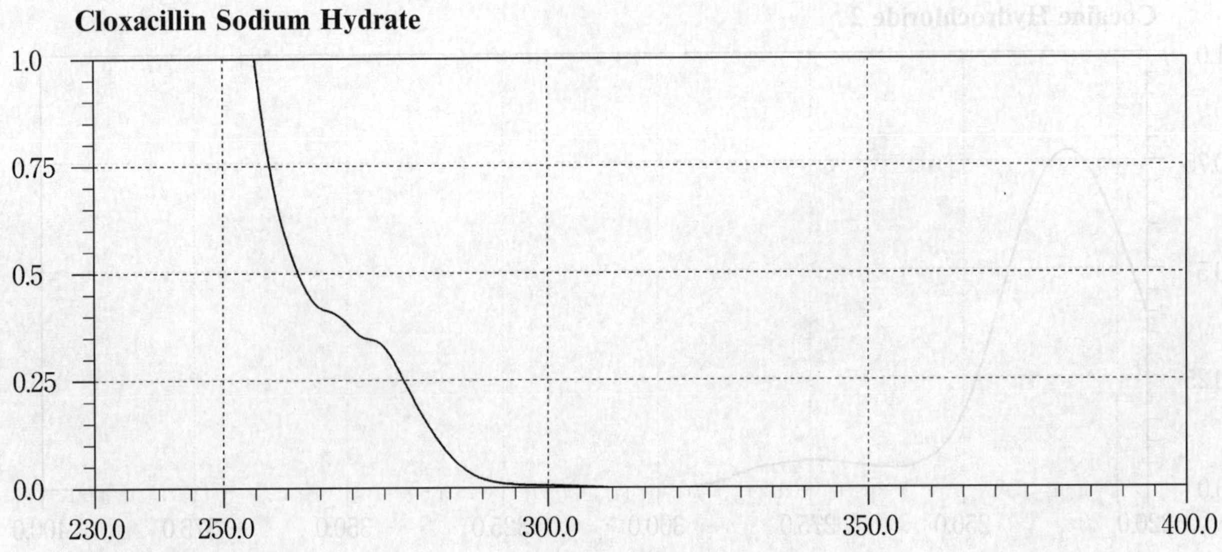

Cloxazolam

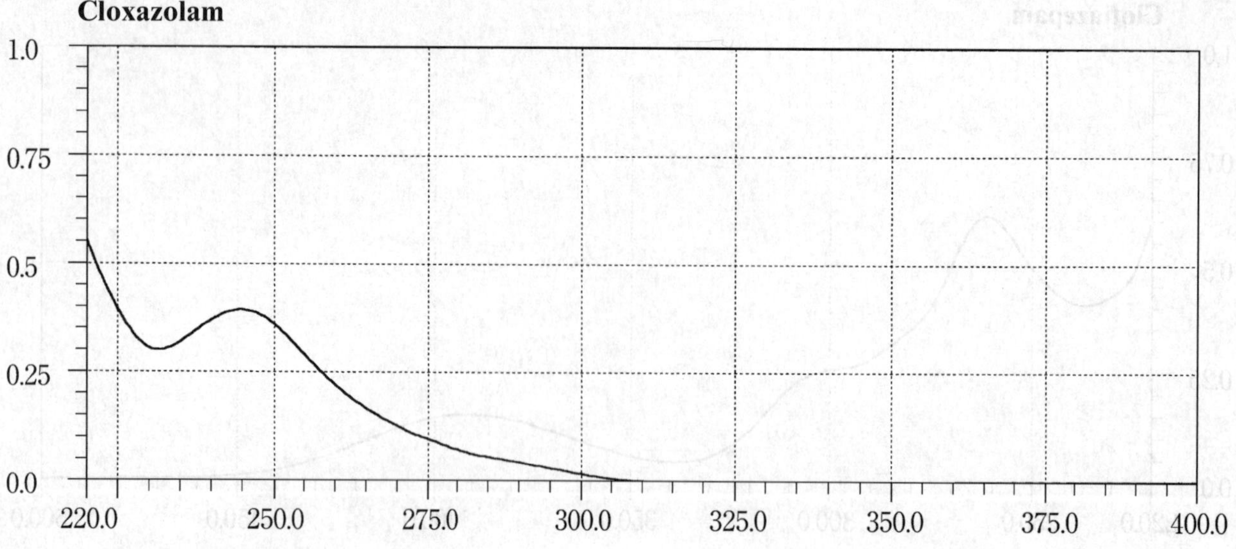

Cocaine Hydrochloride 1

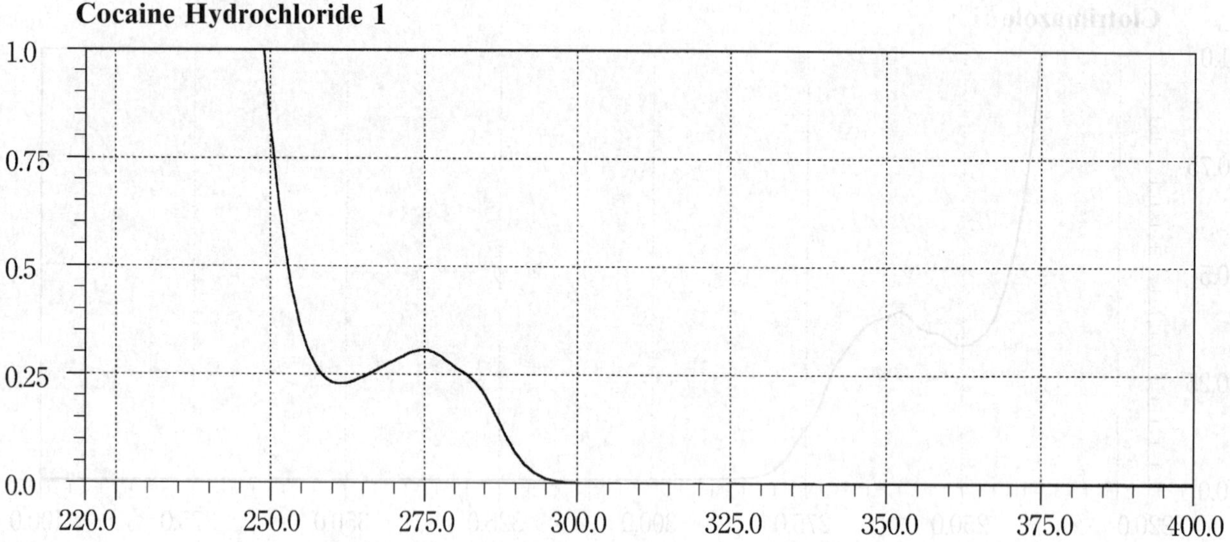

Cocaine Hydrochloride 2

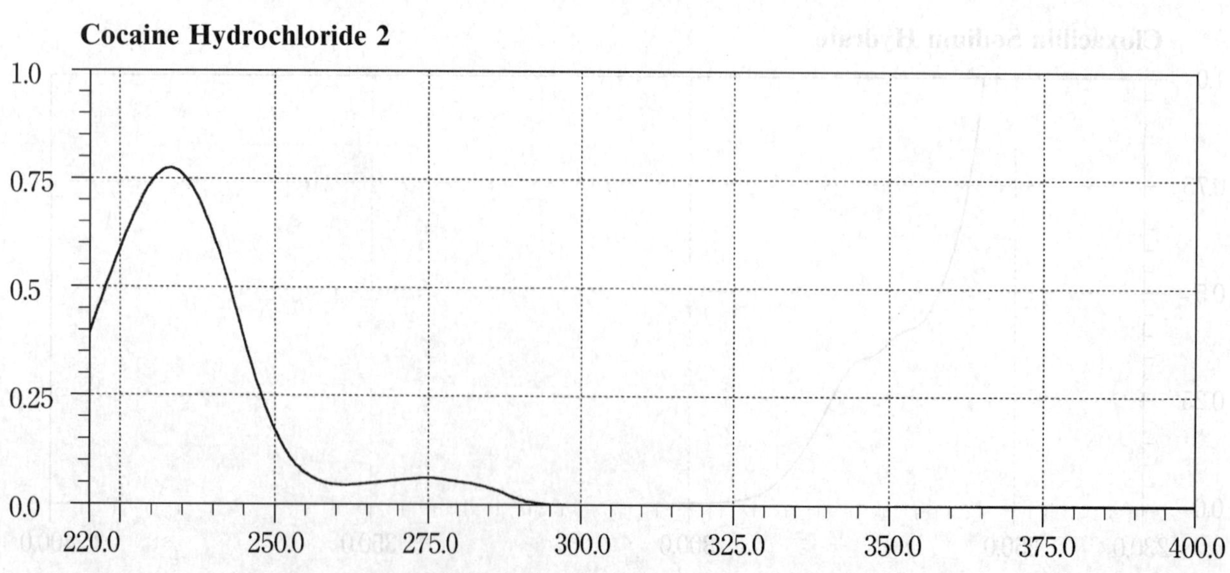

Codeine Phosphate Hydrate

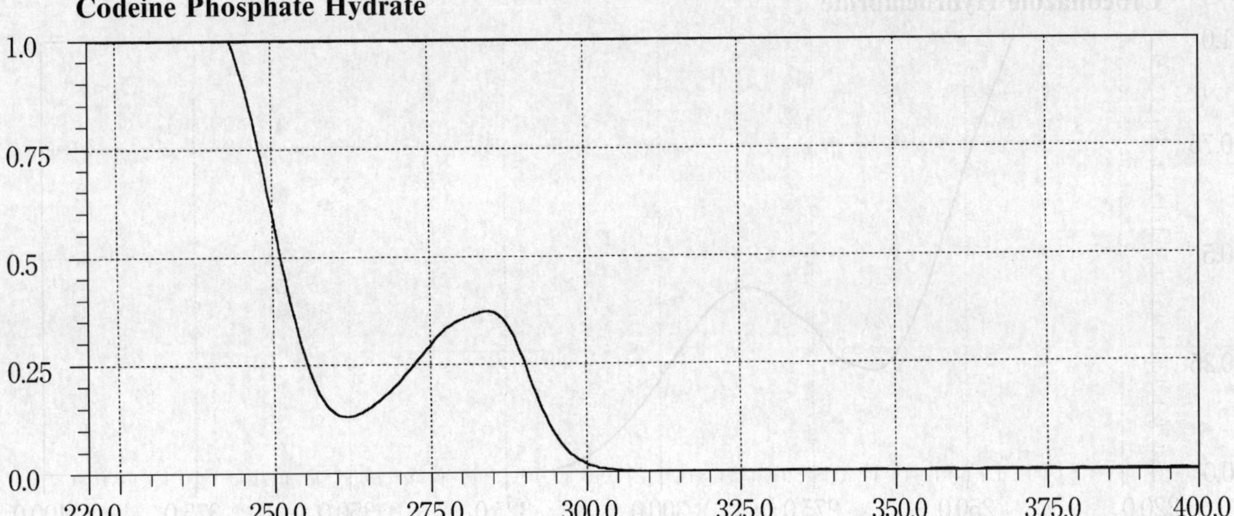

Colchicine

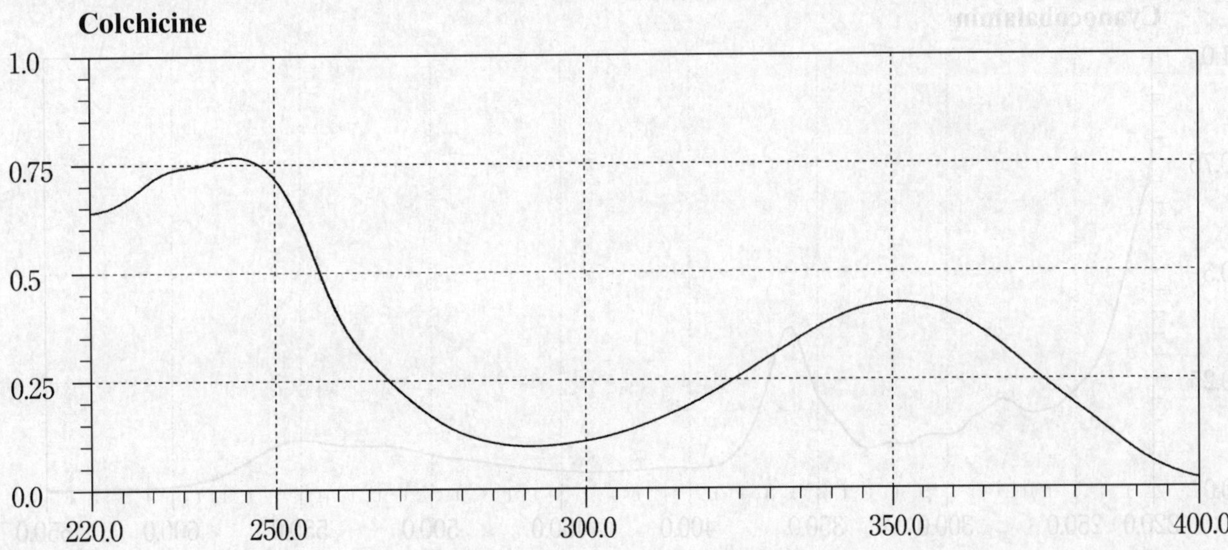

Cortisone Acetate

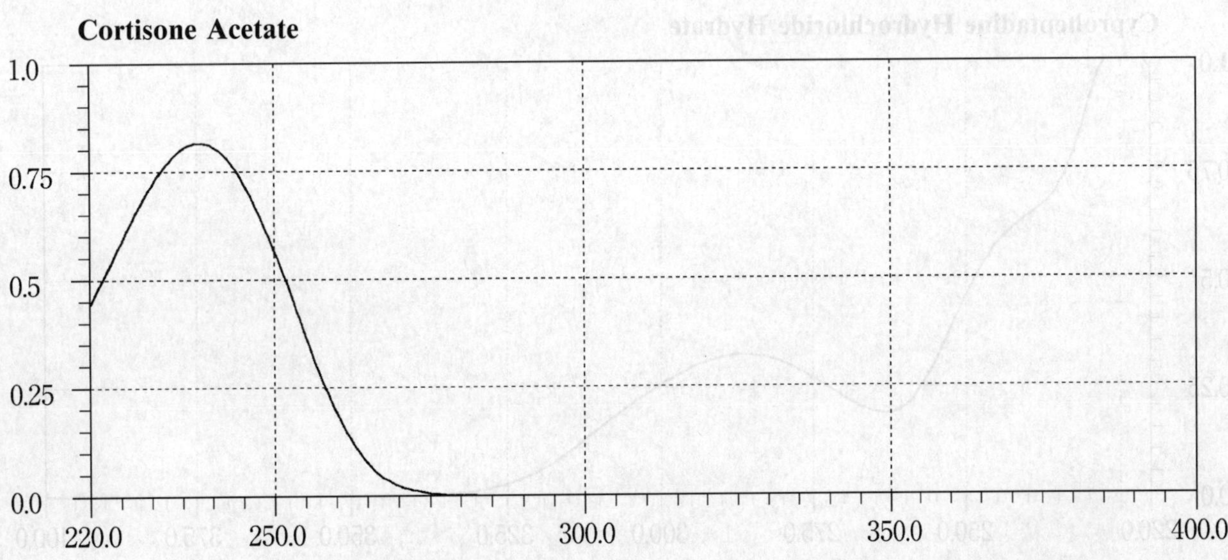

Croconazole Hydrochloride

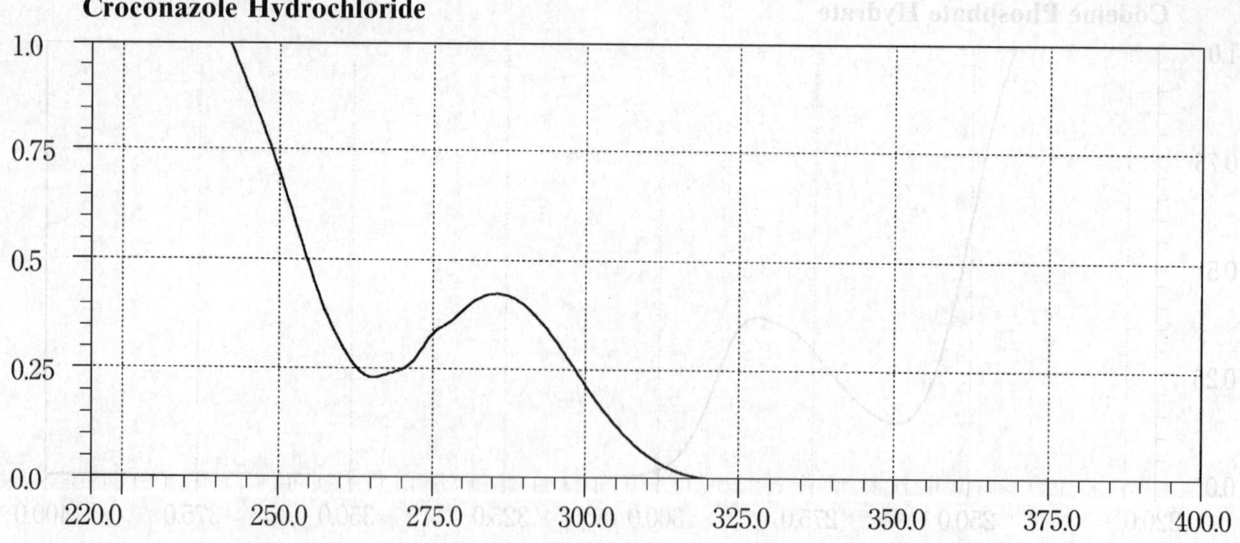

Cyanocobalamin

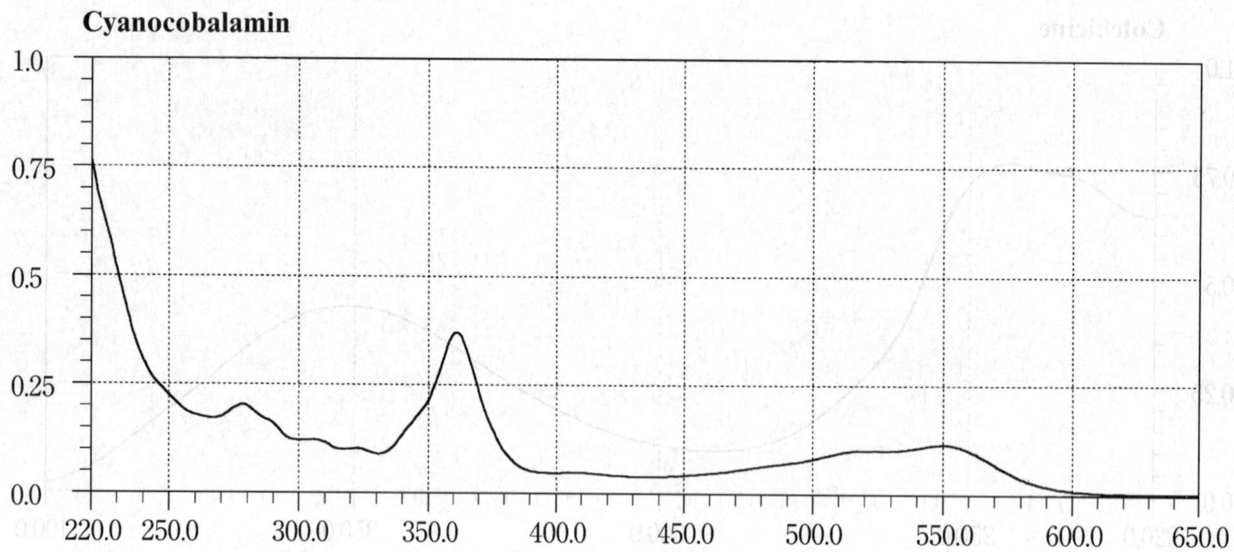

Cyproheptadine Hydrochloride Hydrate

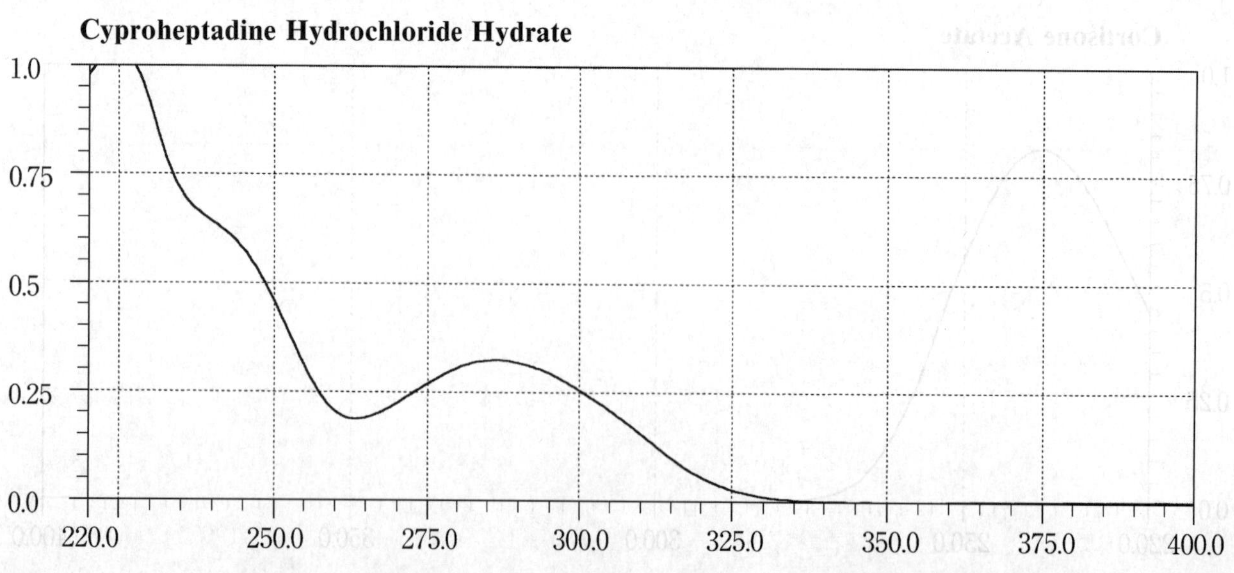

Cytarabine

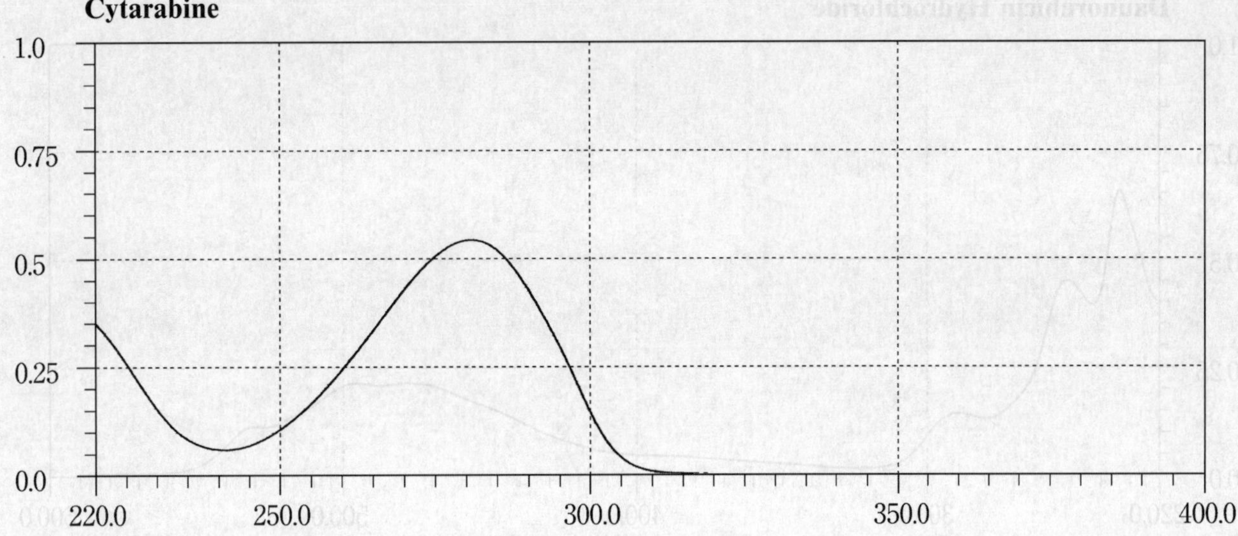

Danazol

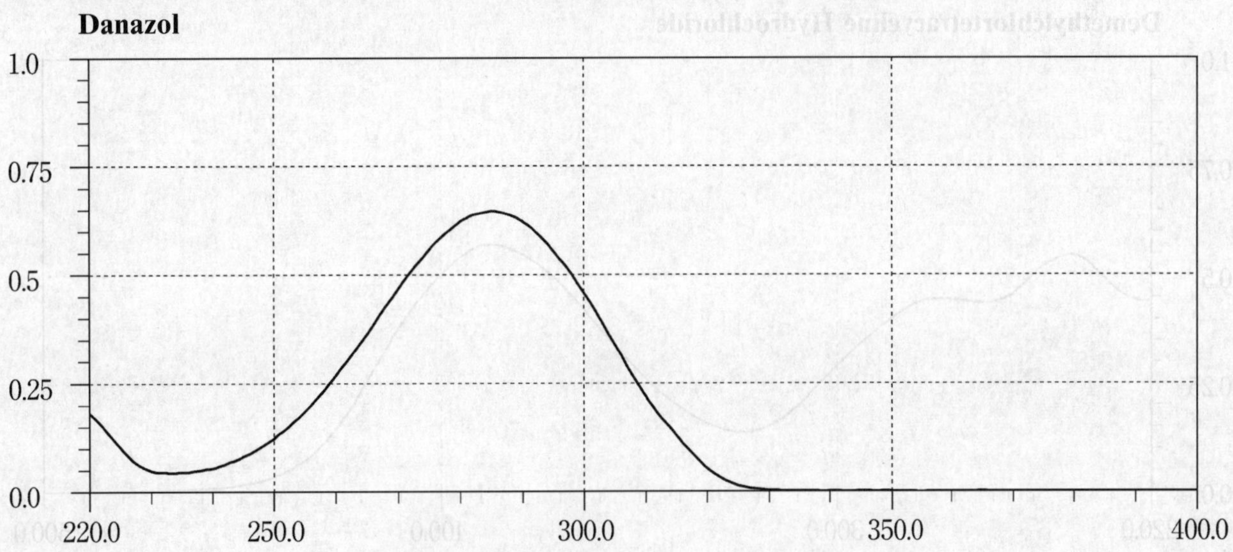

Dantrolene Sodium Hydrate

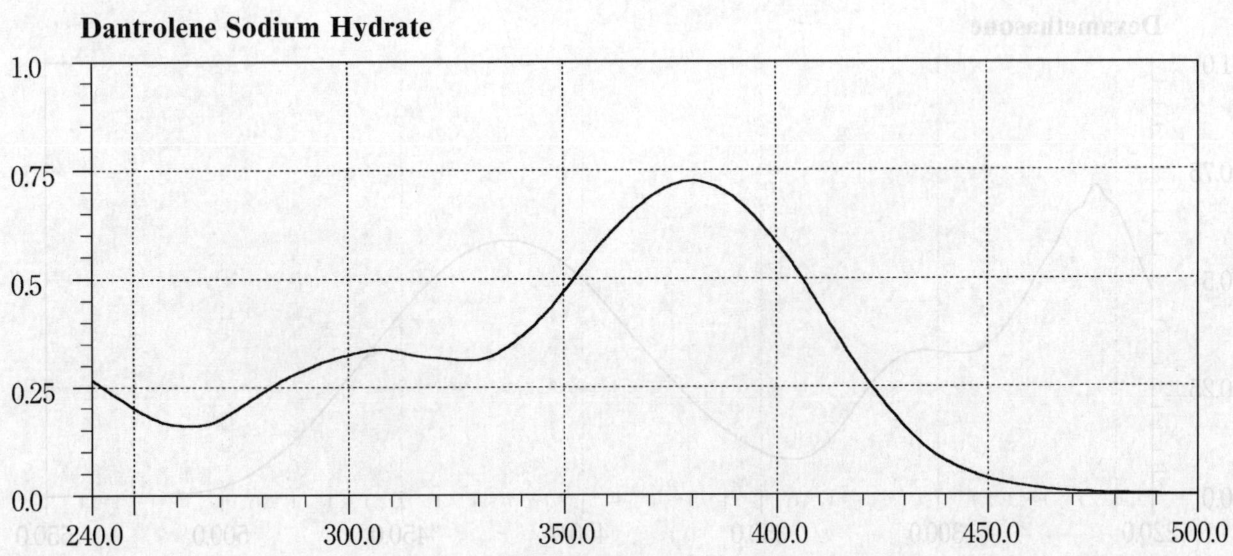

Daunorubicin Hydrochloride

1.0
0.75
0.5
0.25
0.0
220.0 300.0 400.0 500.0 600.0

Demethylchlortetracycline Hydrochloride

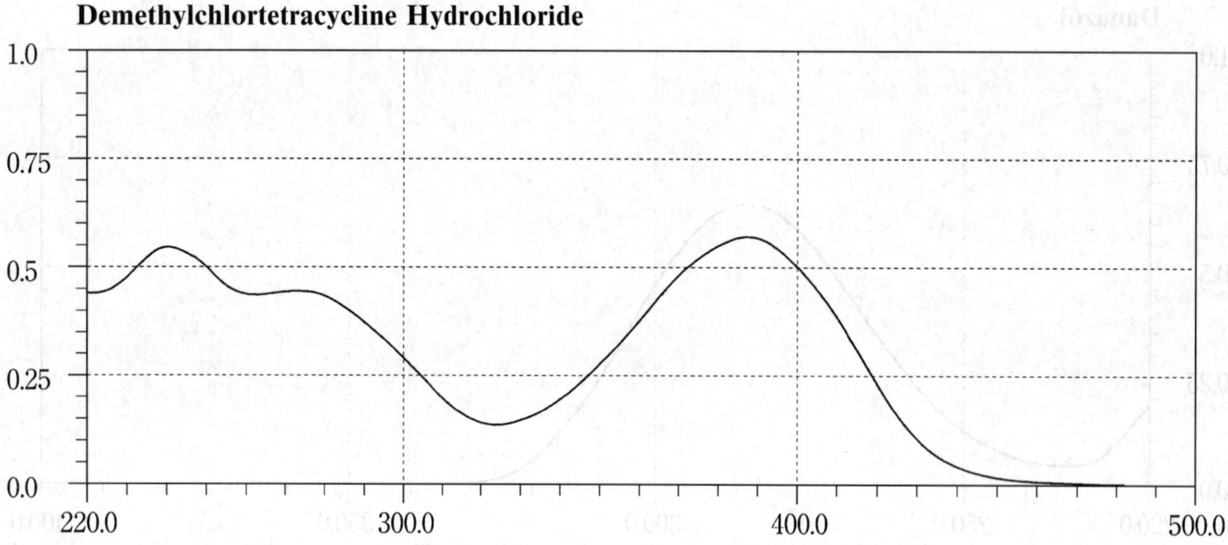

Dexamethasone

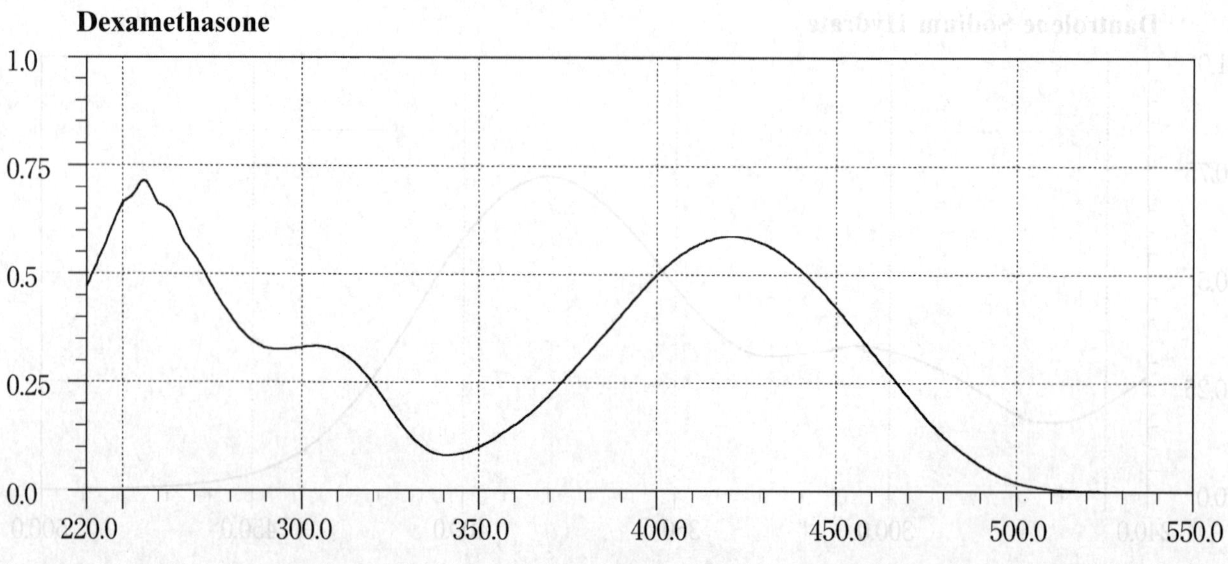

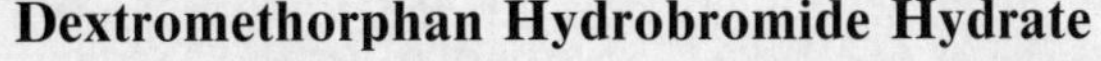

Dextromethorphan Hydrobromide Hydrate

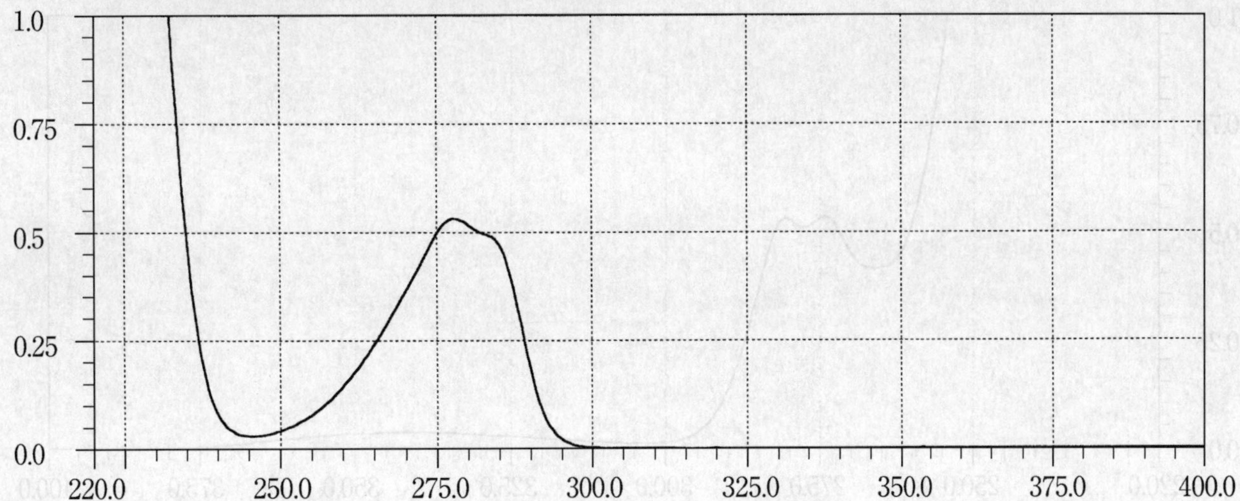

Diazepam

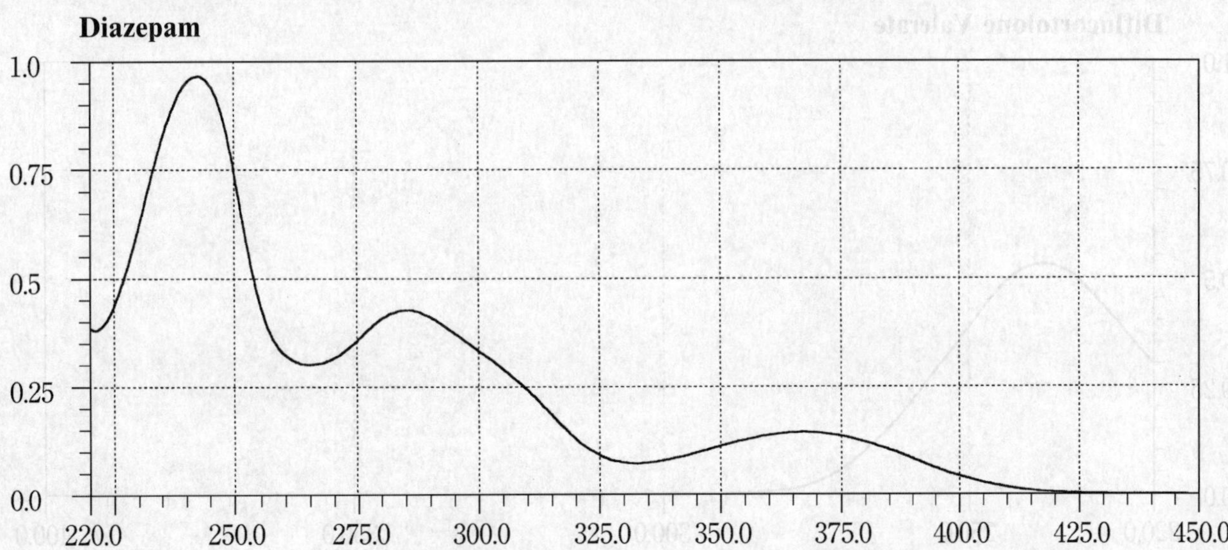

Dibucaine Hydrochloride

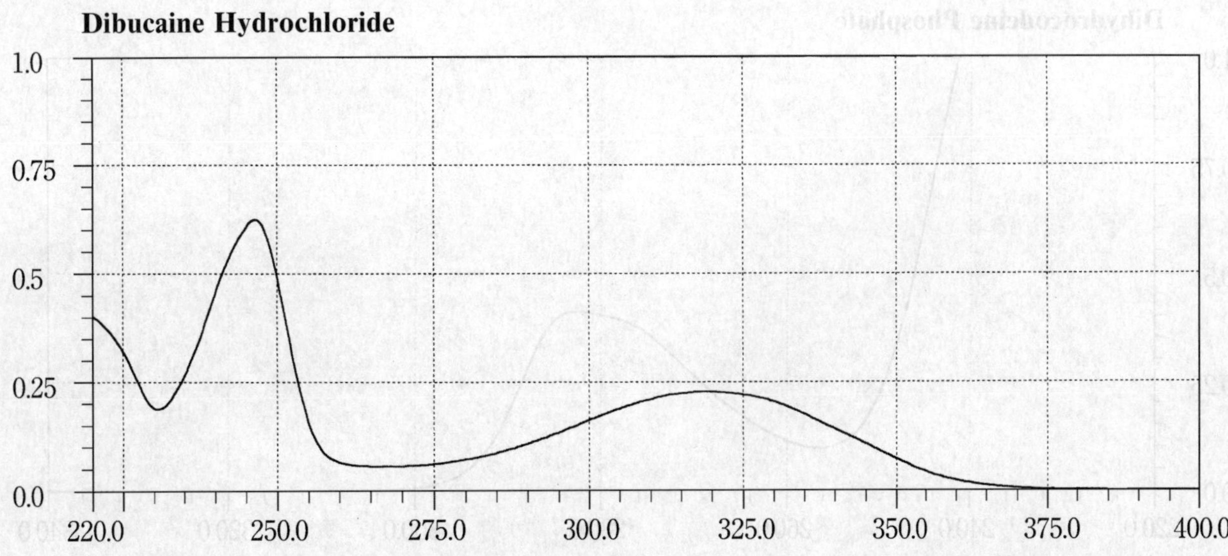

Dicloxacillin Sodium Hydrate

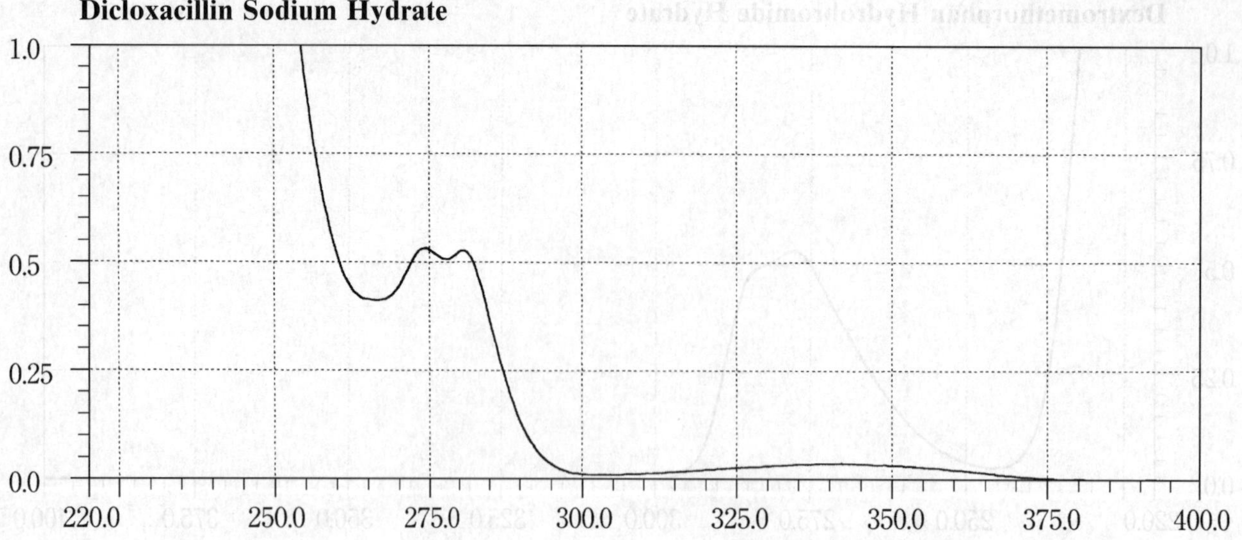

Diflucortolone Valerate

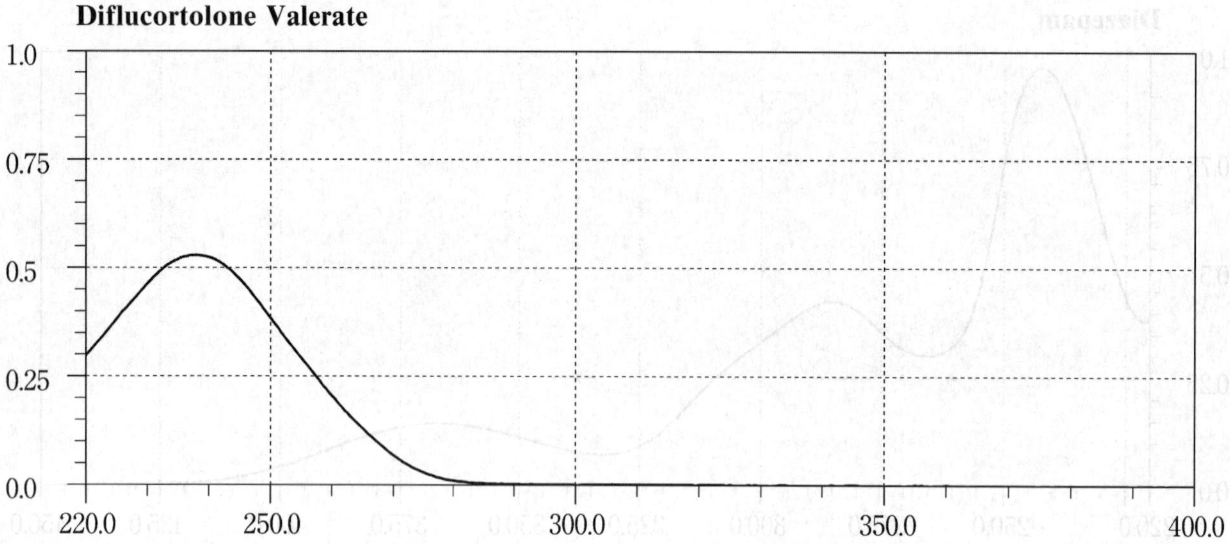

Dihydrocodeine Phosphate

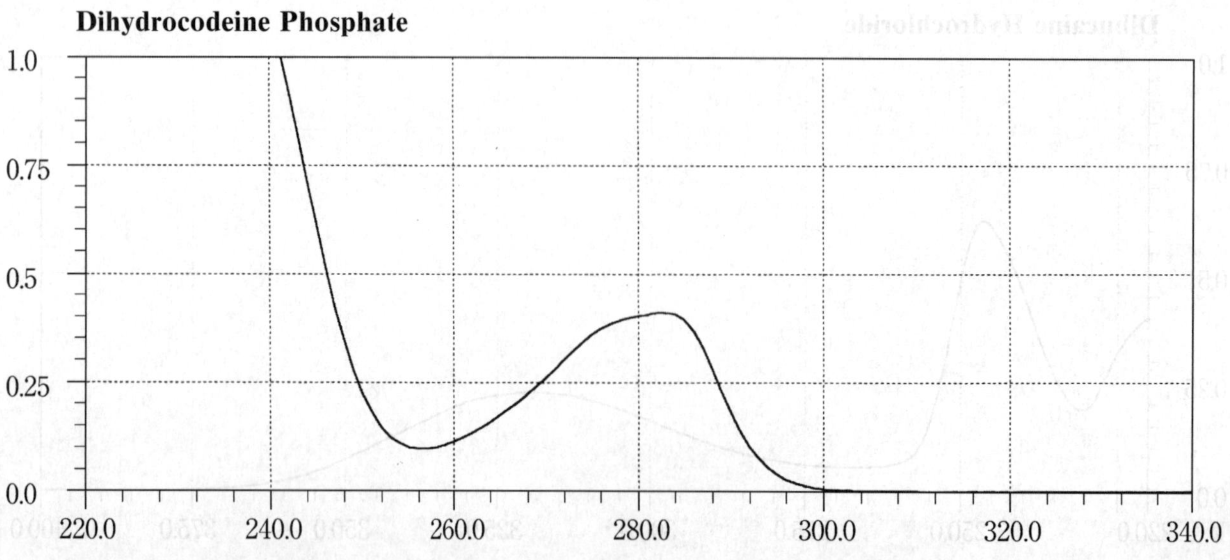

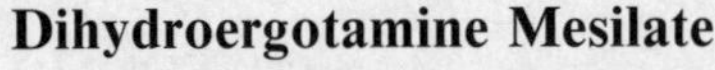

Dihydroergotamine Mesilate

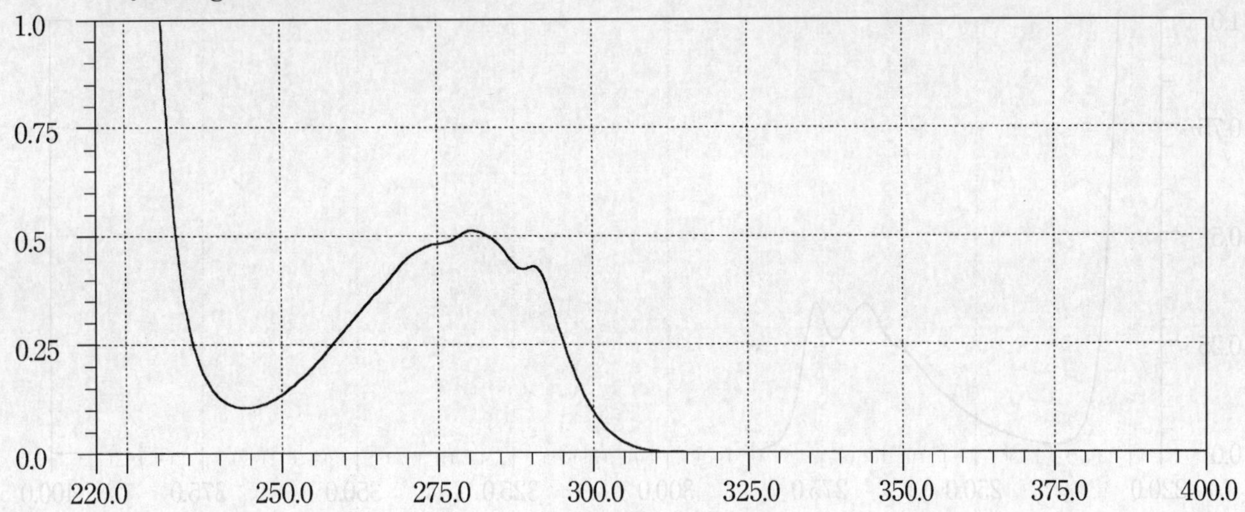

Dilazep Hydrochloride Hydrate

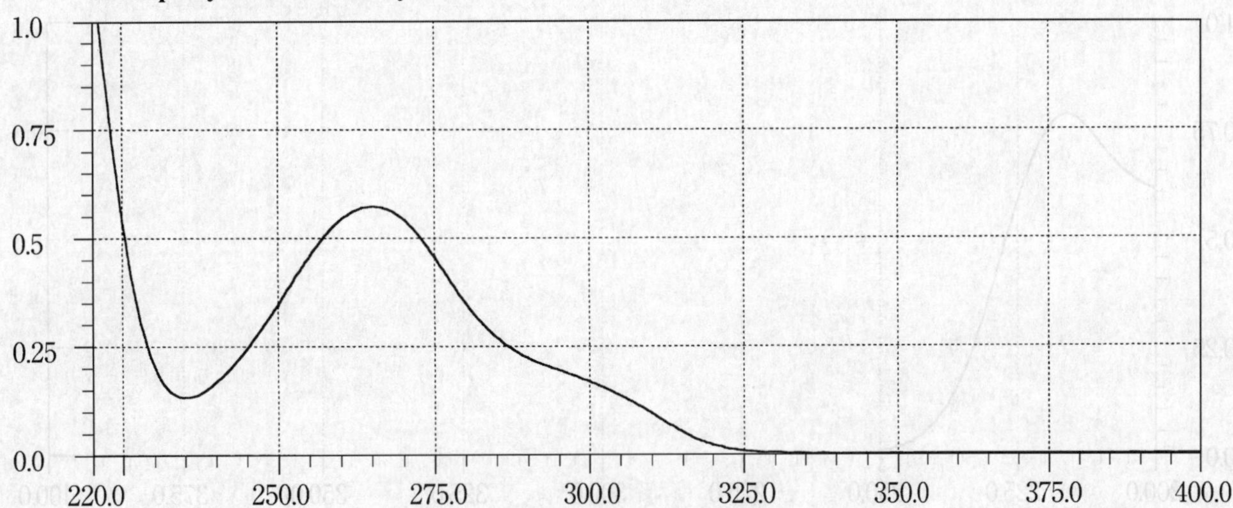

Diltiazem Hydrochloride

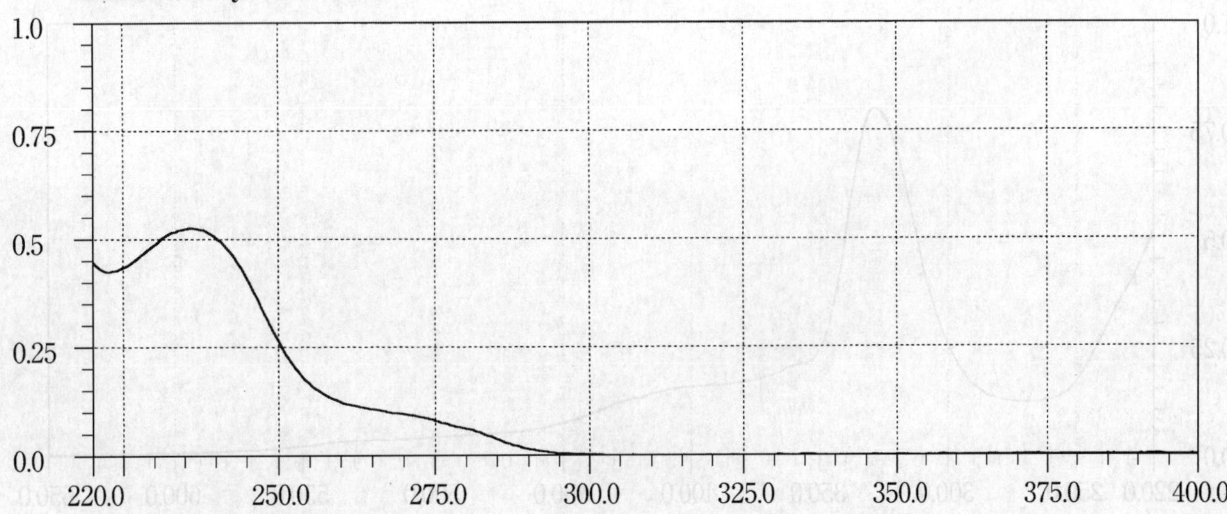

Dimemorfan Phosphate

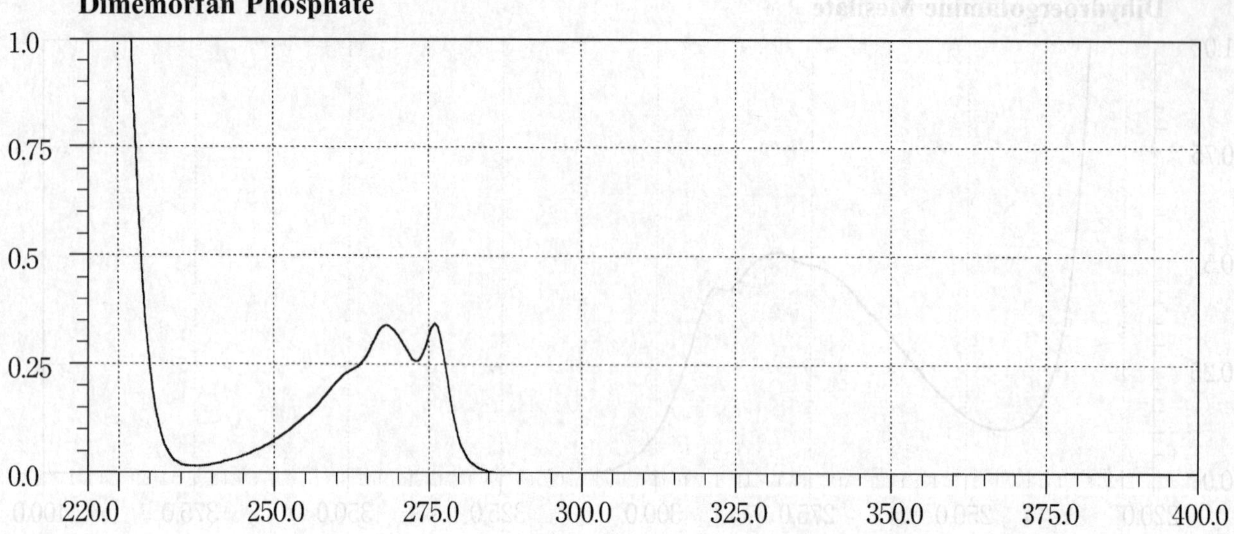

Dimorpholamine

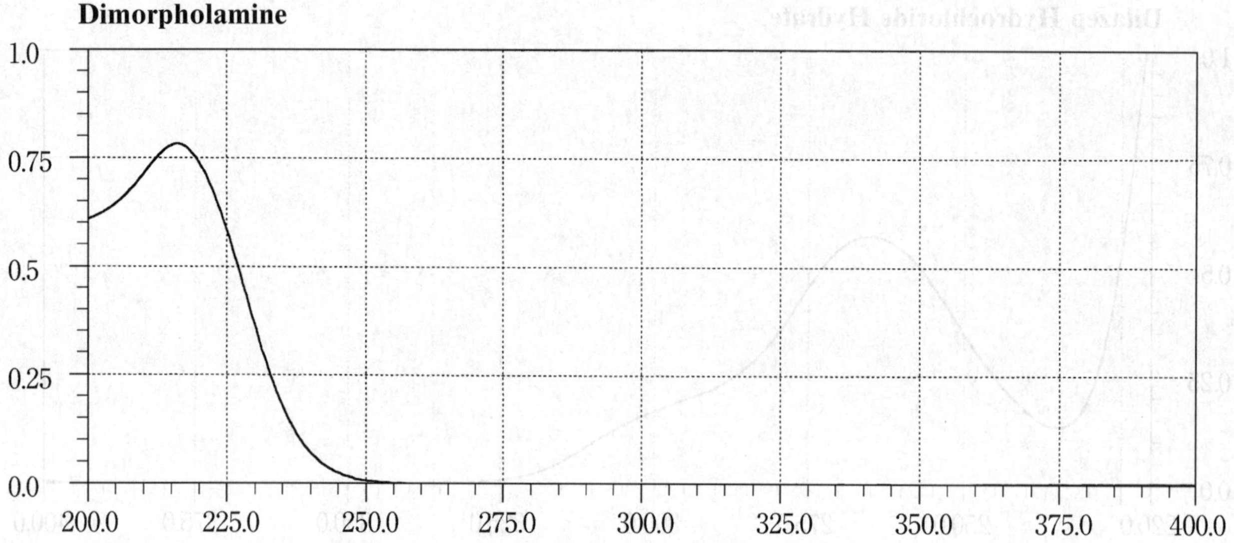

Dinoprost

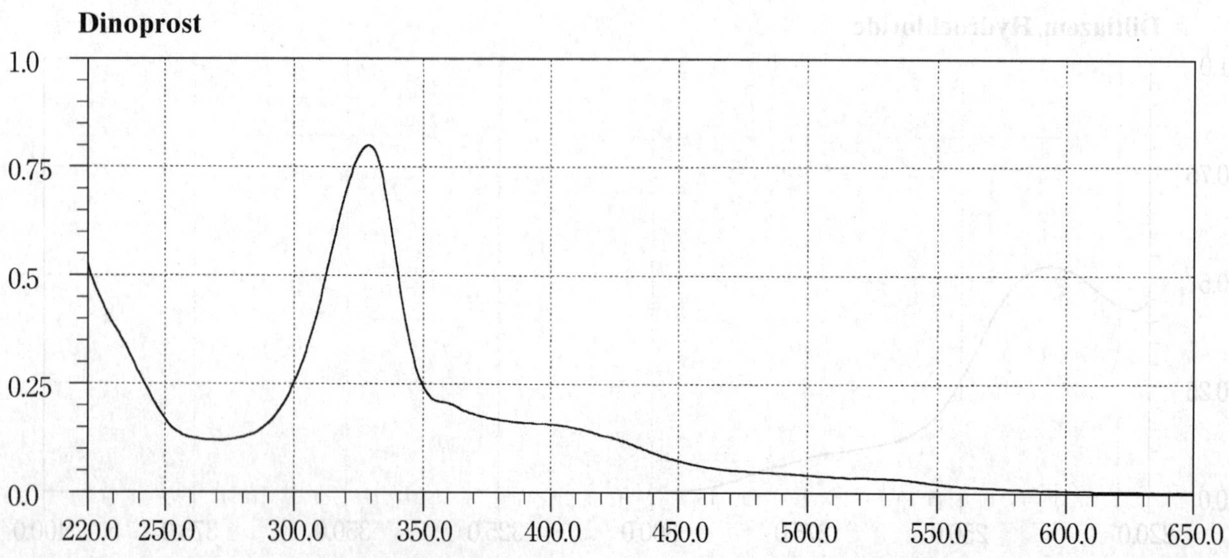

Diphenhydramine Hydrochloride

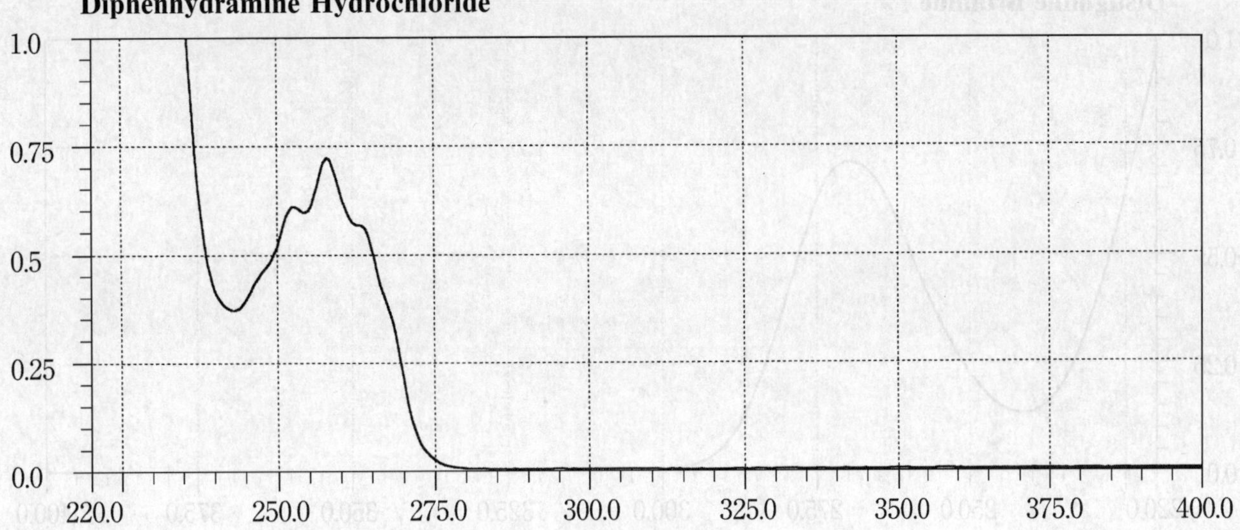

Dipyridamole

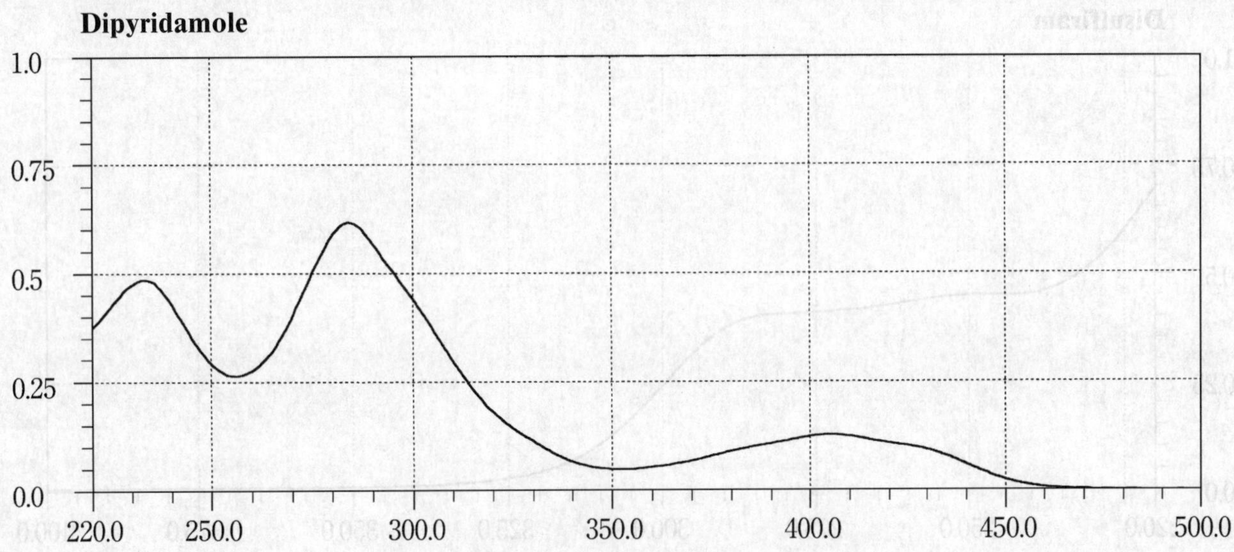

Disopyramide

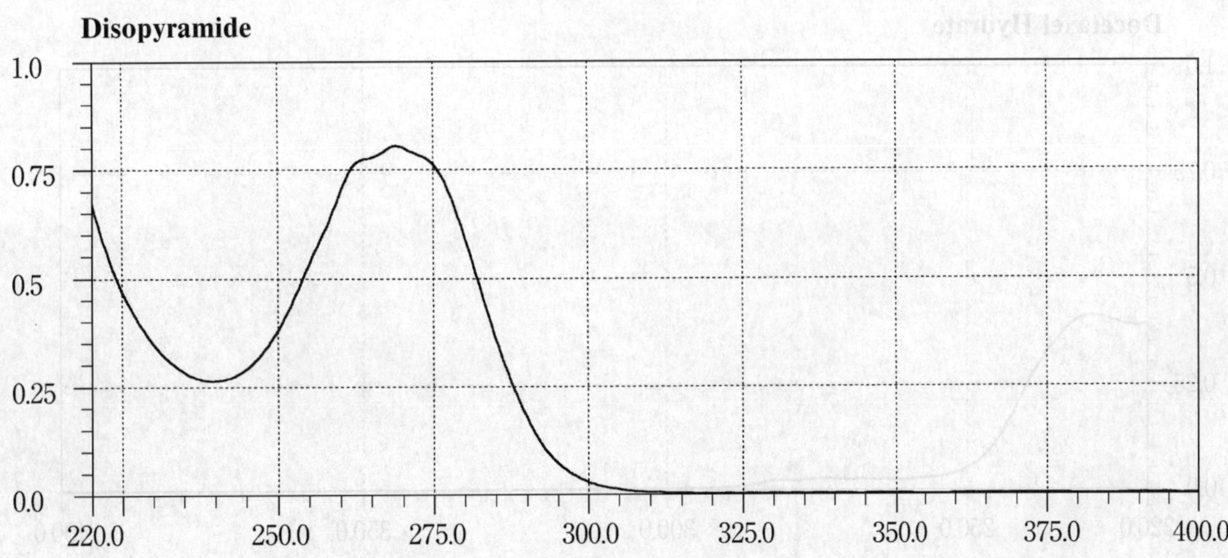

Distigmine Bromide

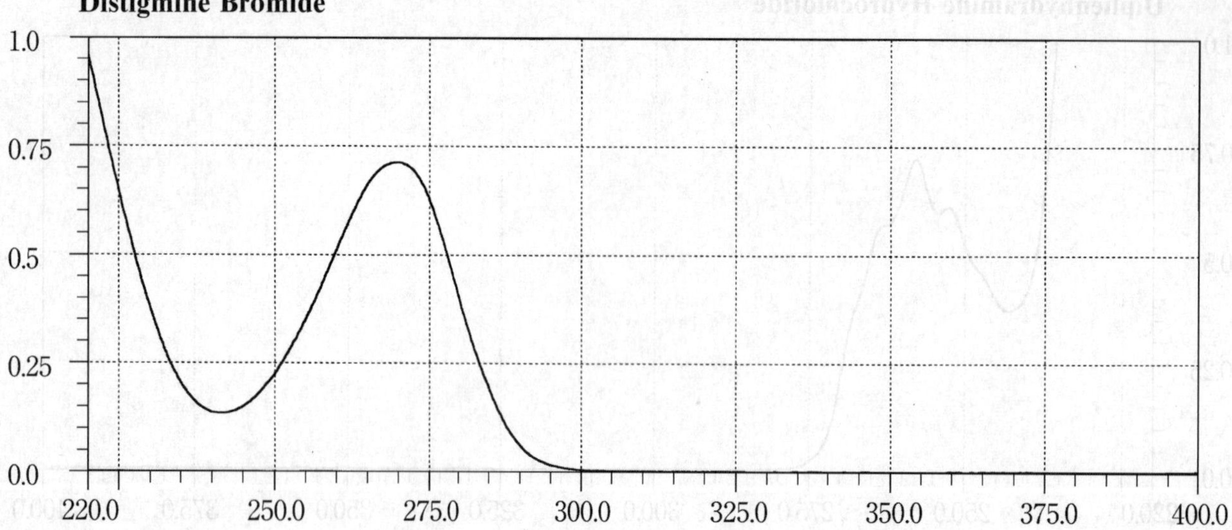

Disulfiram

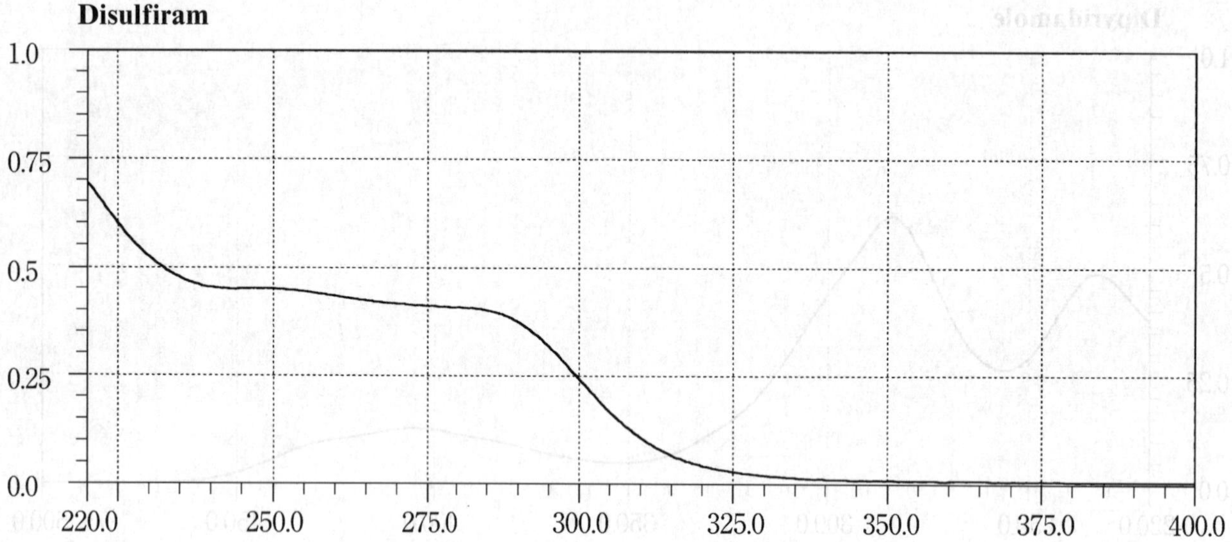

Docetaxel Hydrate

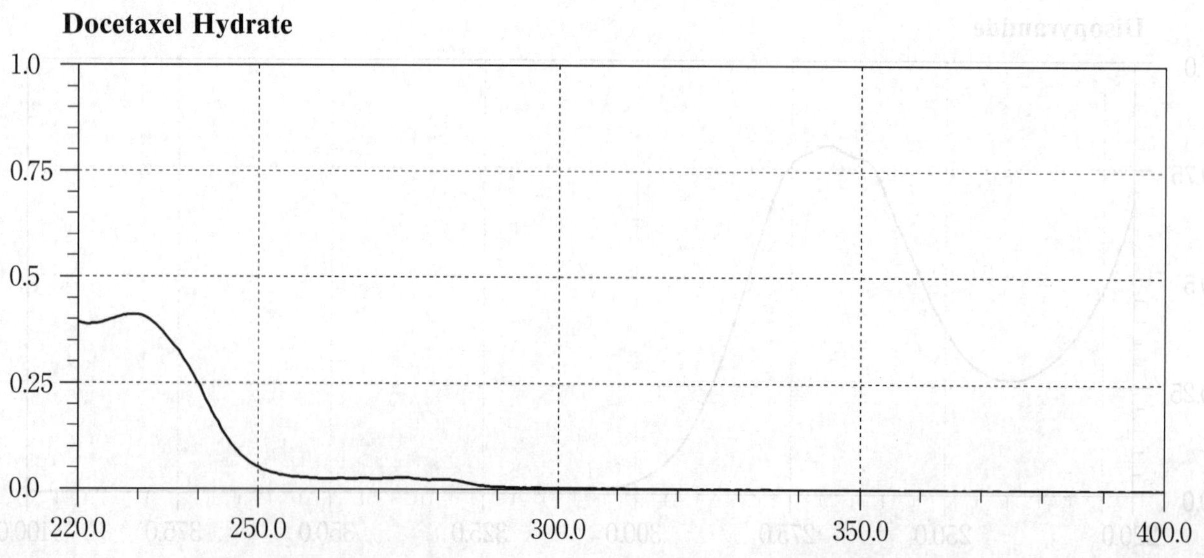

Domperidone

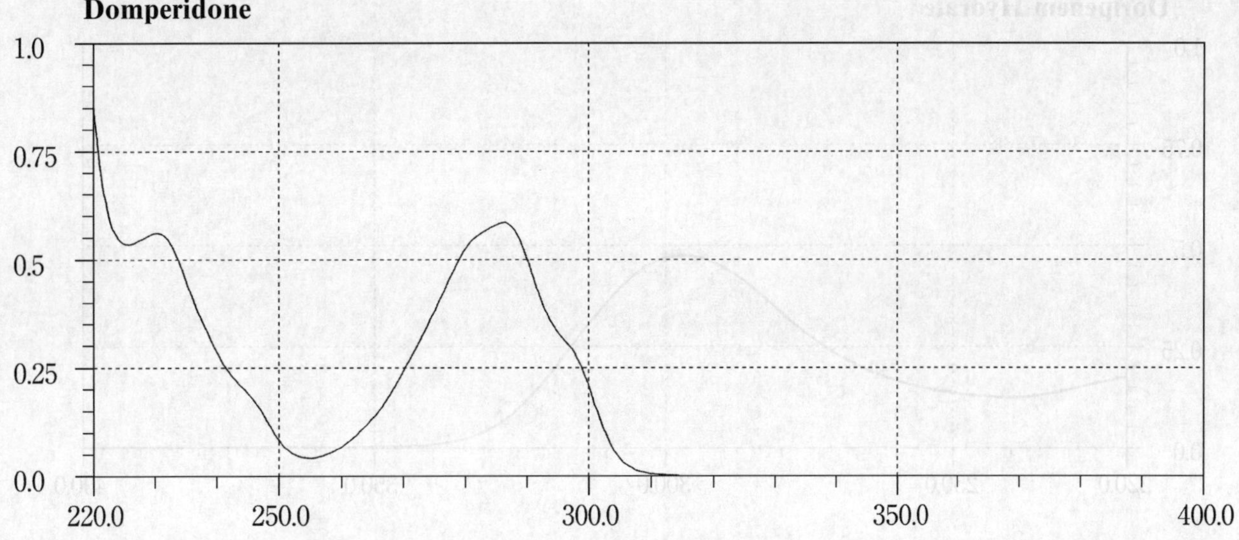

Donepezil Hydrochloride

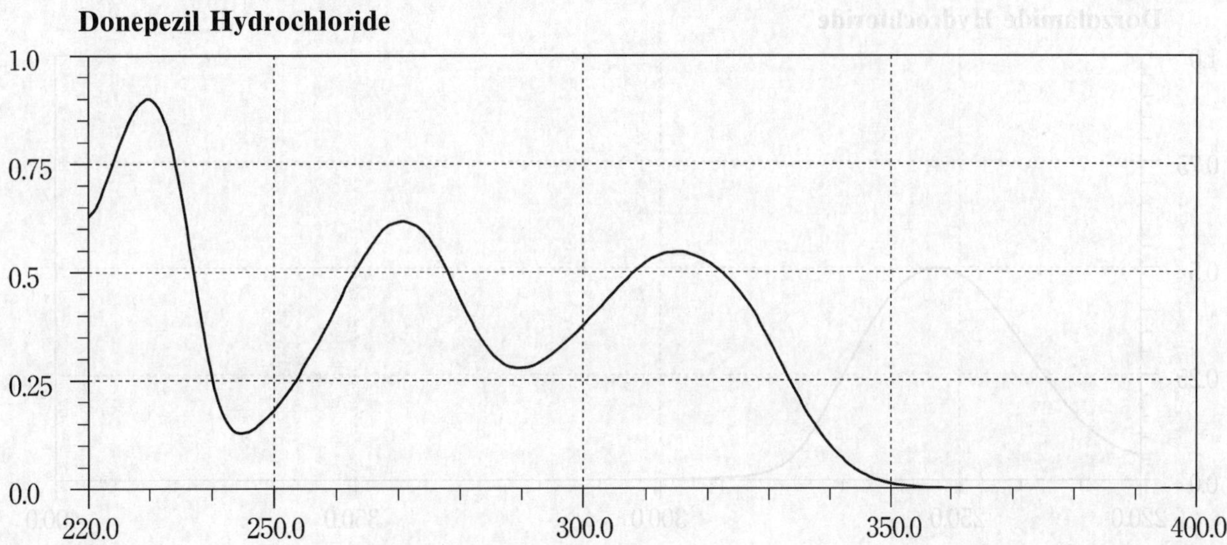

Dopamine Hydrochloride

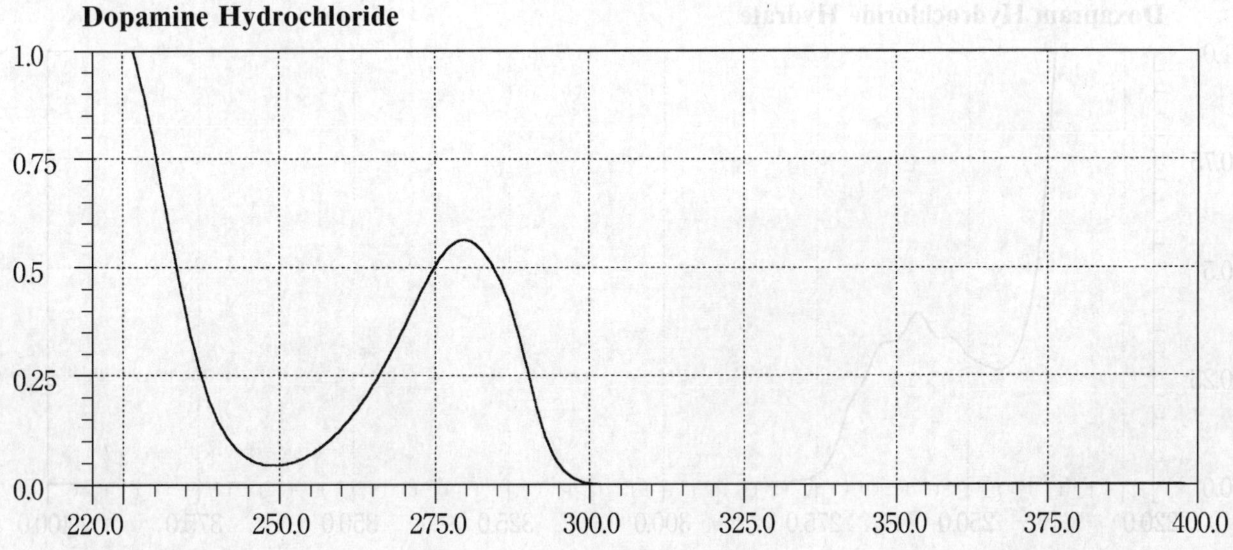

Doripenem Hydrate

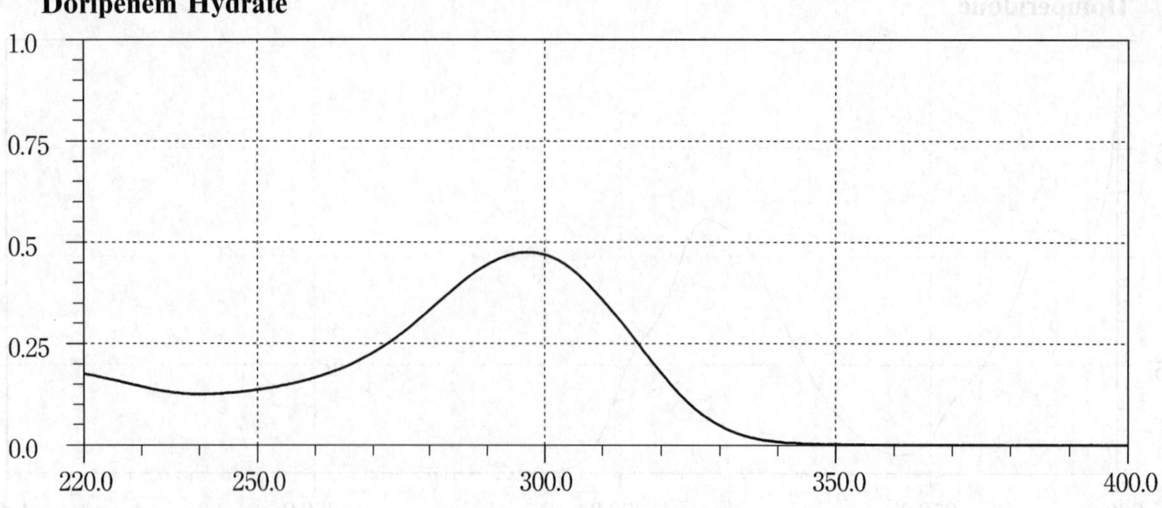

Dorzolamide Hydrochloride

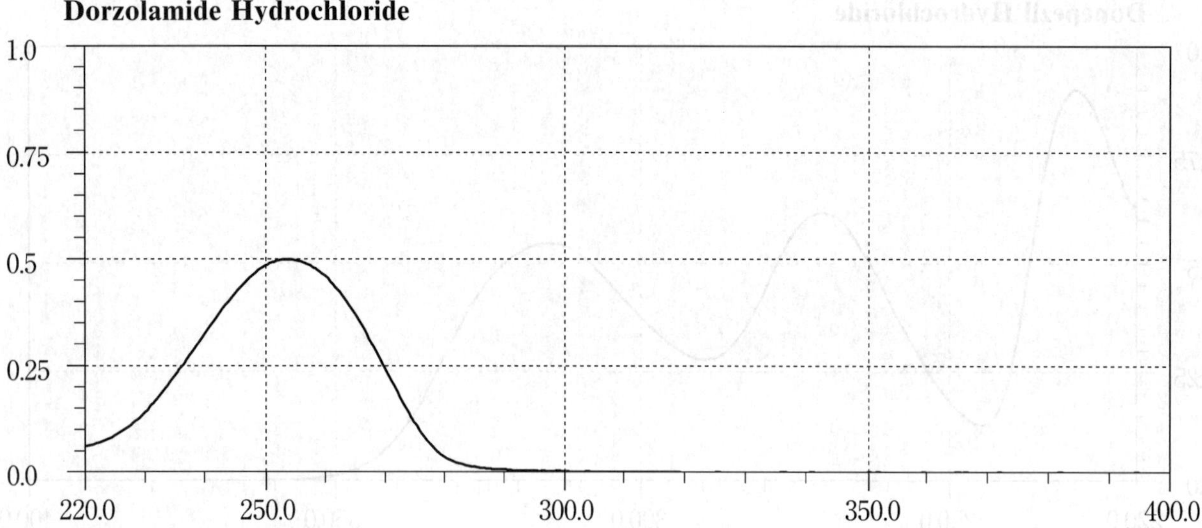

Doxapram Hydrochloride Hydrate

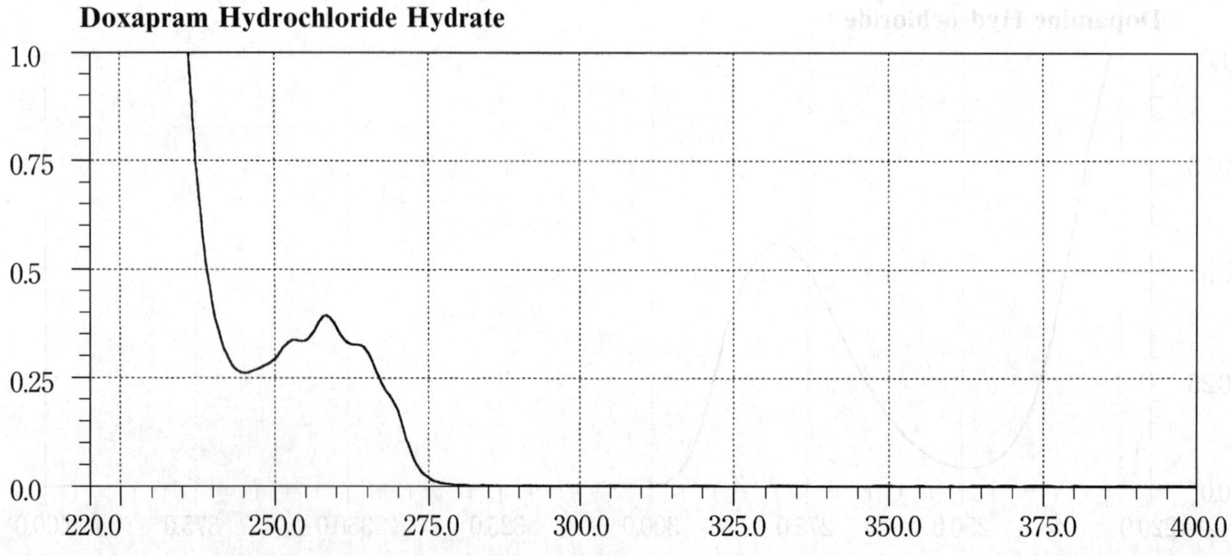

Doxazosin Mesilate

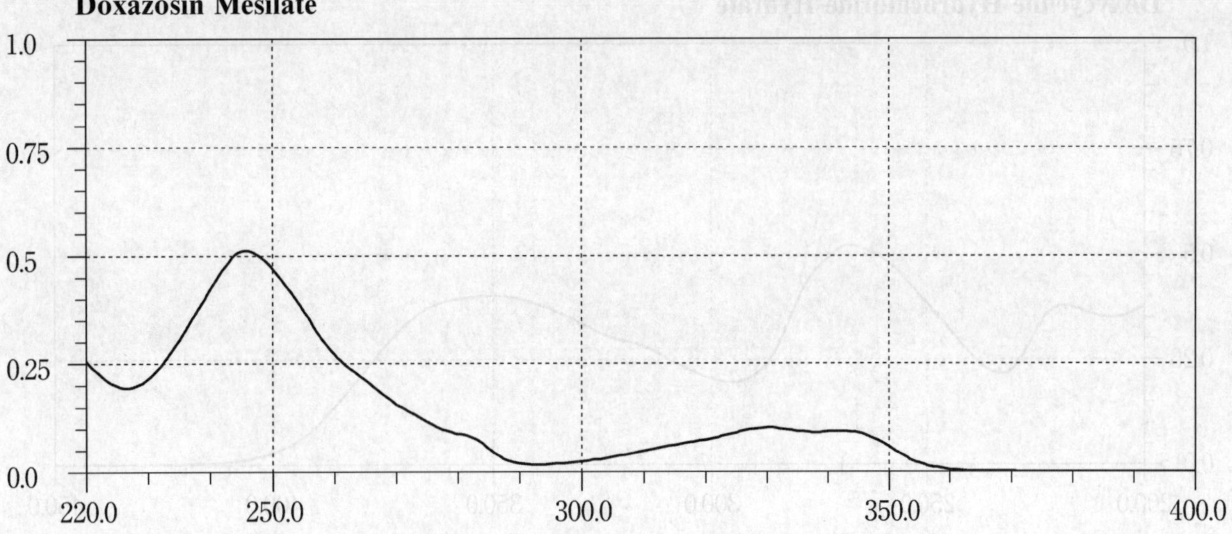

Doxifluridine

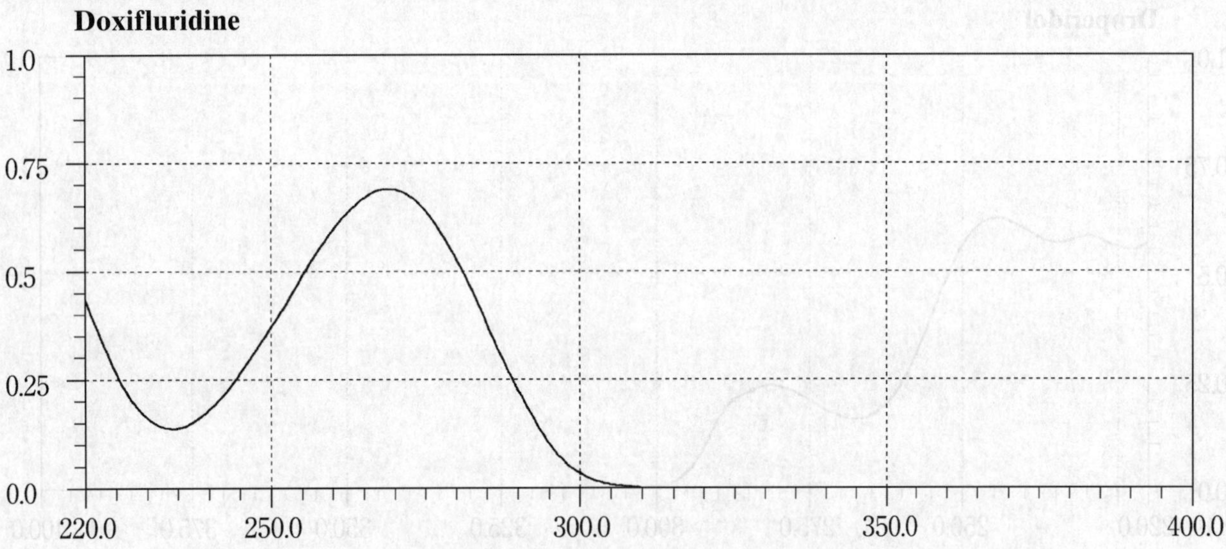

Doxorubicin Hydrochloride

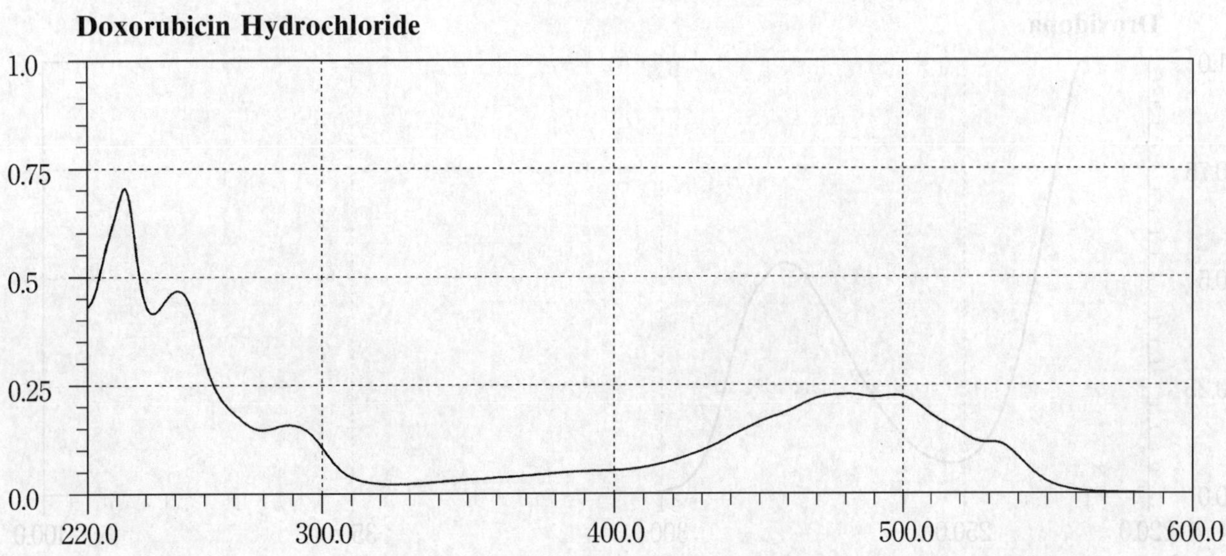

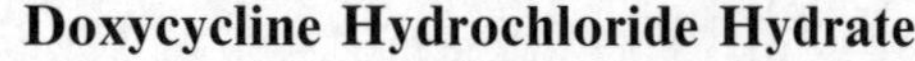

Doxycycline Hydrochloride Hydrate

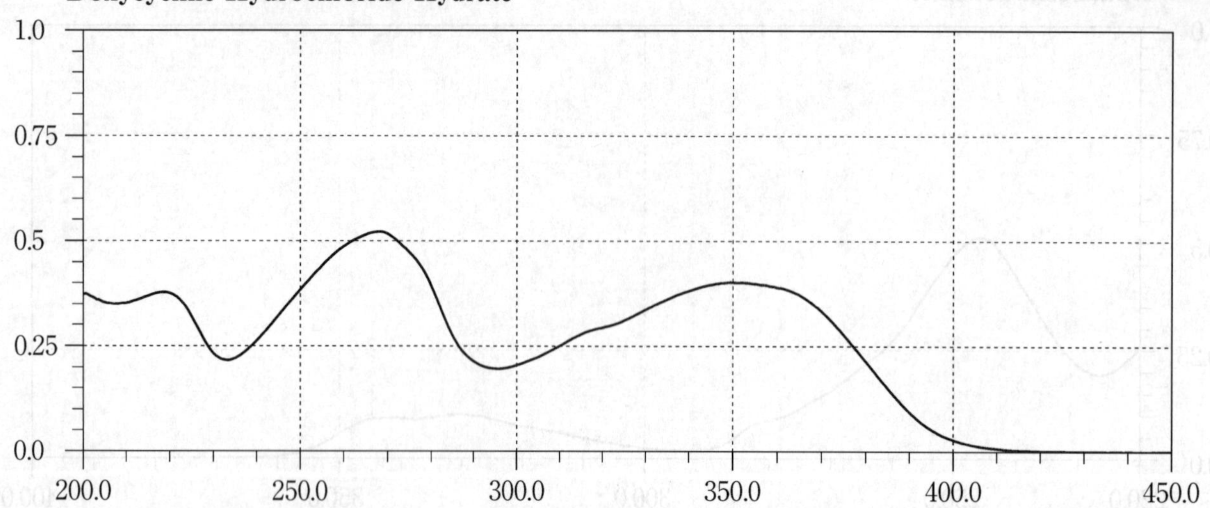

Droperidol

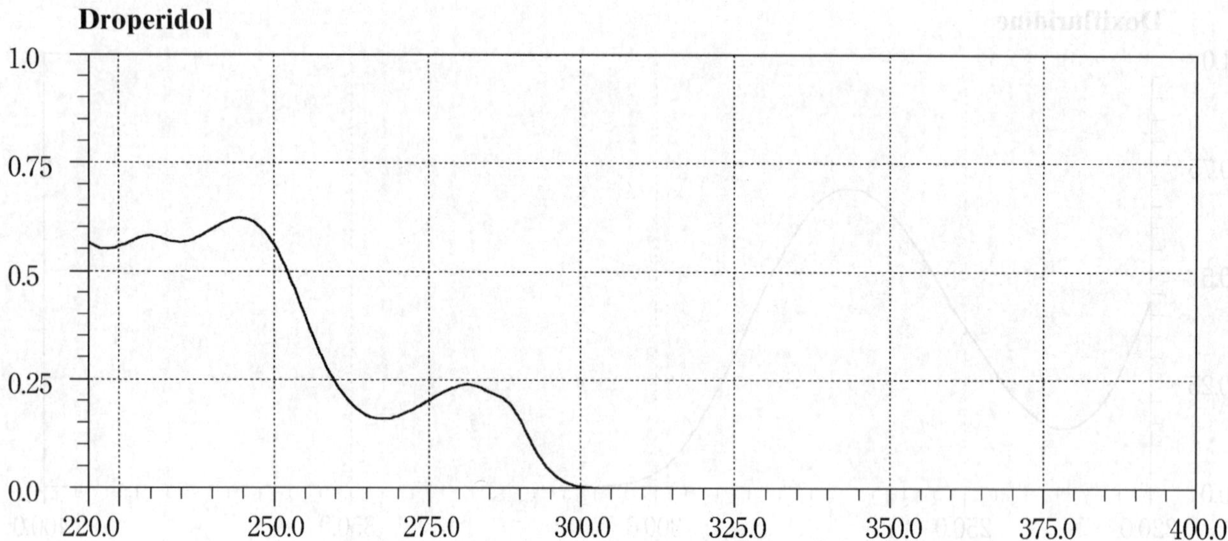

Droxidopa

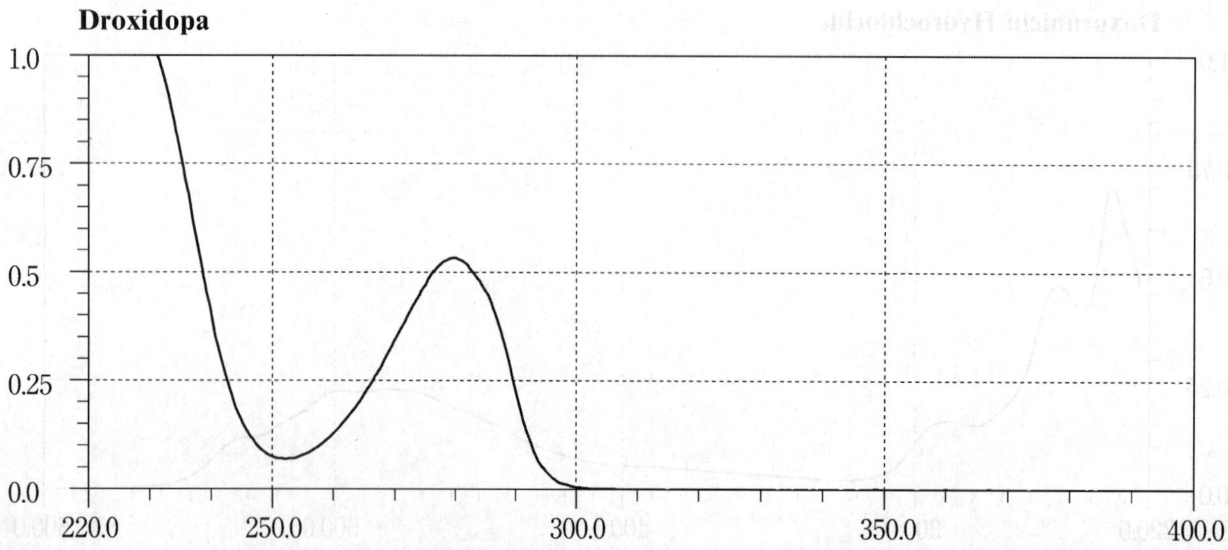

The JP Drugs are to be tested according to the provisions given in the pertinent monographs, General Notices, General Rules for Crude Drugs, General Rules for Preparations, and General Tests for their conformity to the Japanese Pharmacopoeia. (See the General Notices 5.)

Dydrogesterone

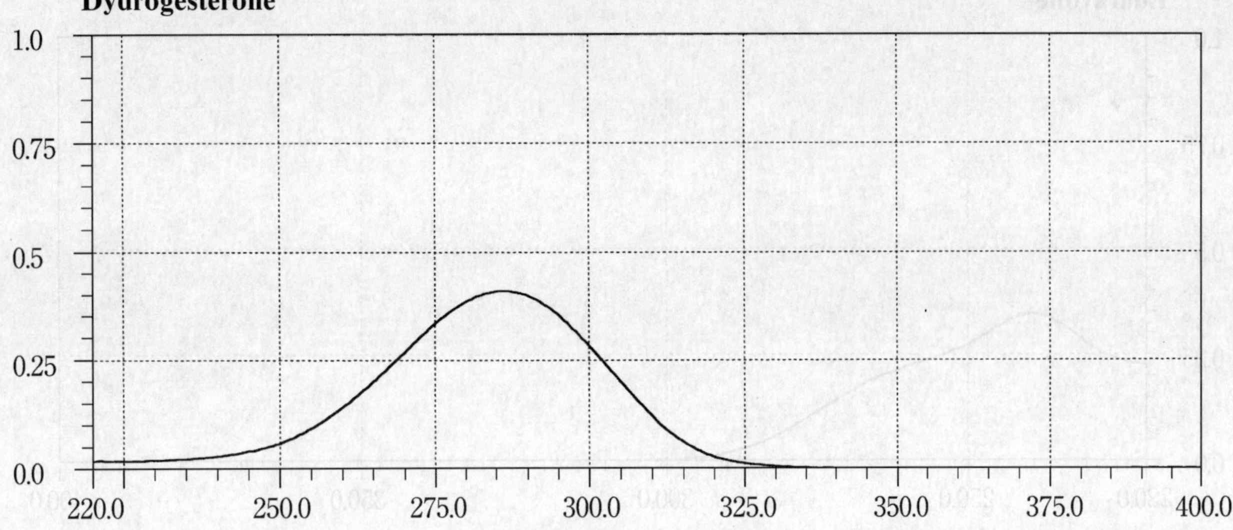

Ebastine

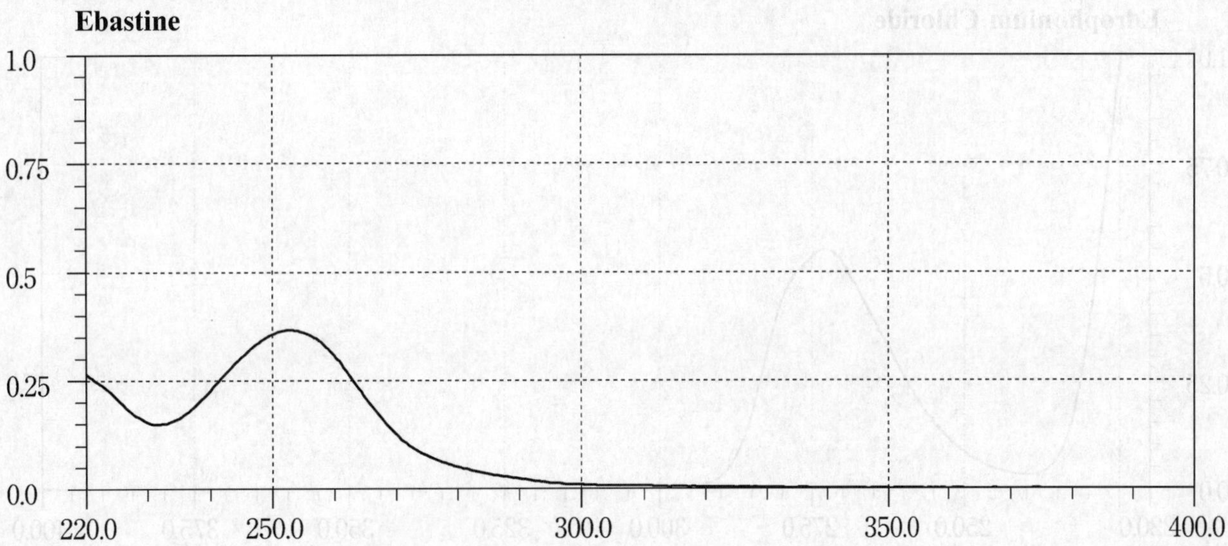

Ecabet Sodium Hydrate

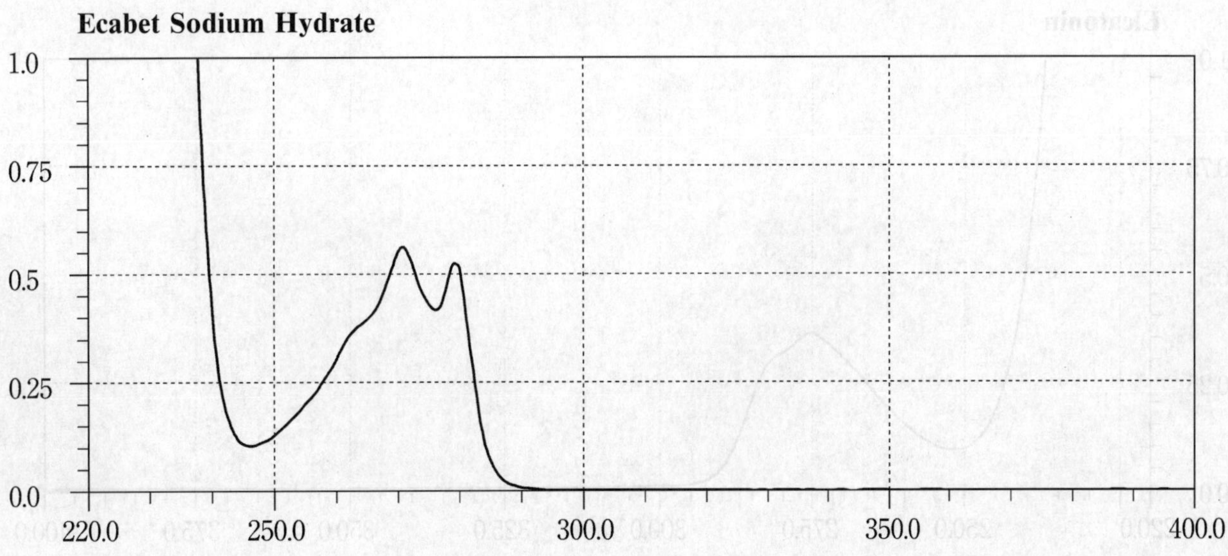

The JP Drugs are to be tested according to the provisions given in the pertinent monographs, General Notices, General Rules for Crude Drugs, General Rules for Preparations, and General Tests for their conformity to the Japanese Pharmacopoeia. (See the General Notices 5.)

Edaravone

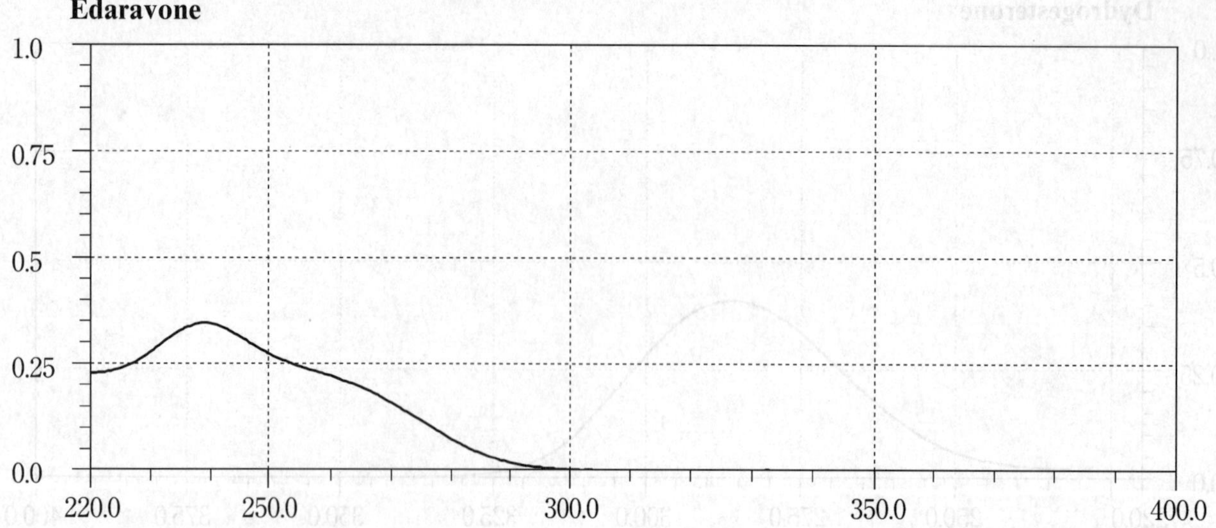

Edrophonium Chloride

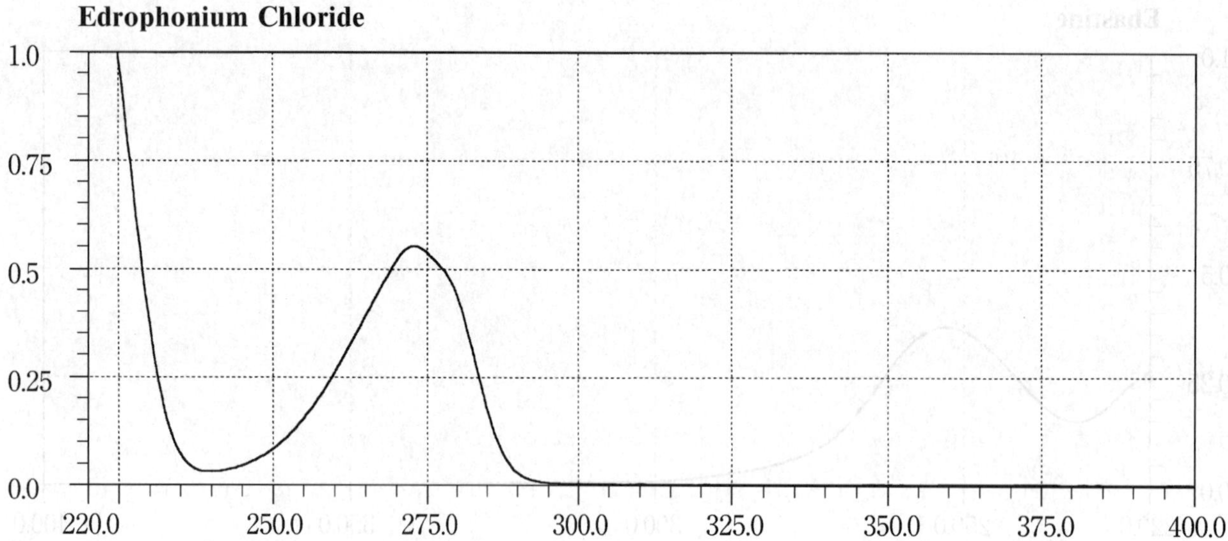

Elcatonin

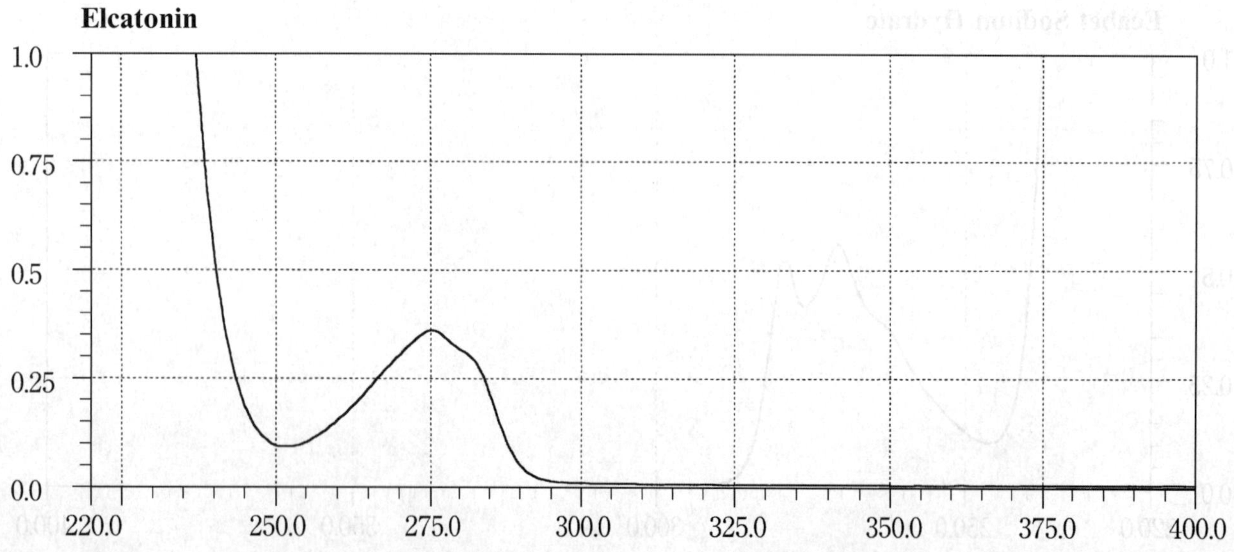

Emedastine Fumarate

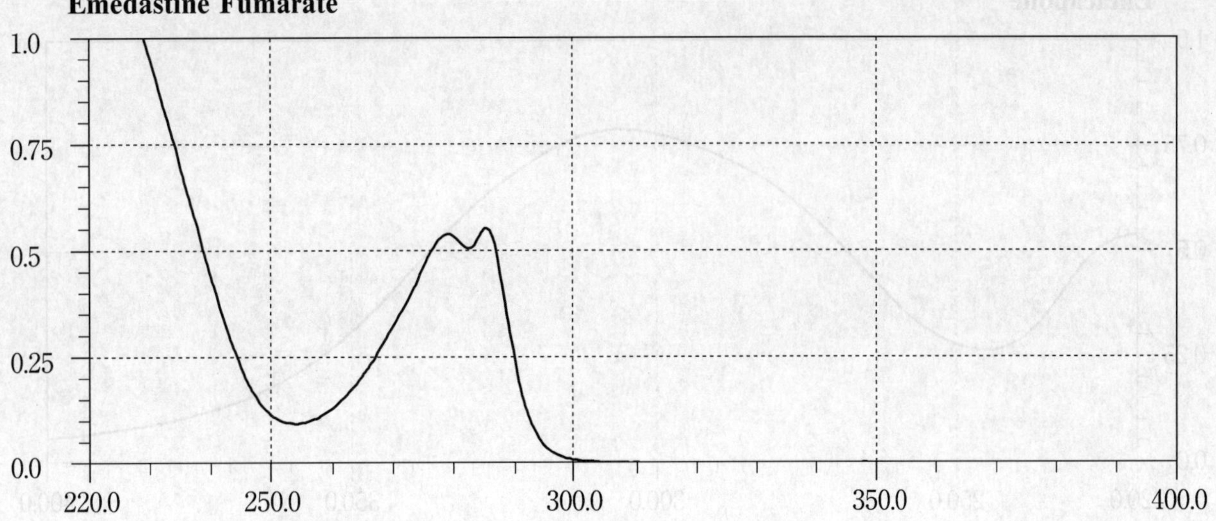

Emorfazone

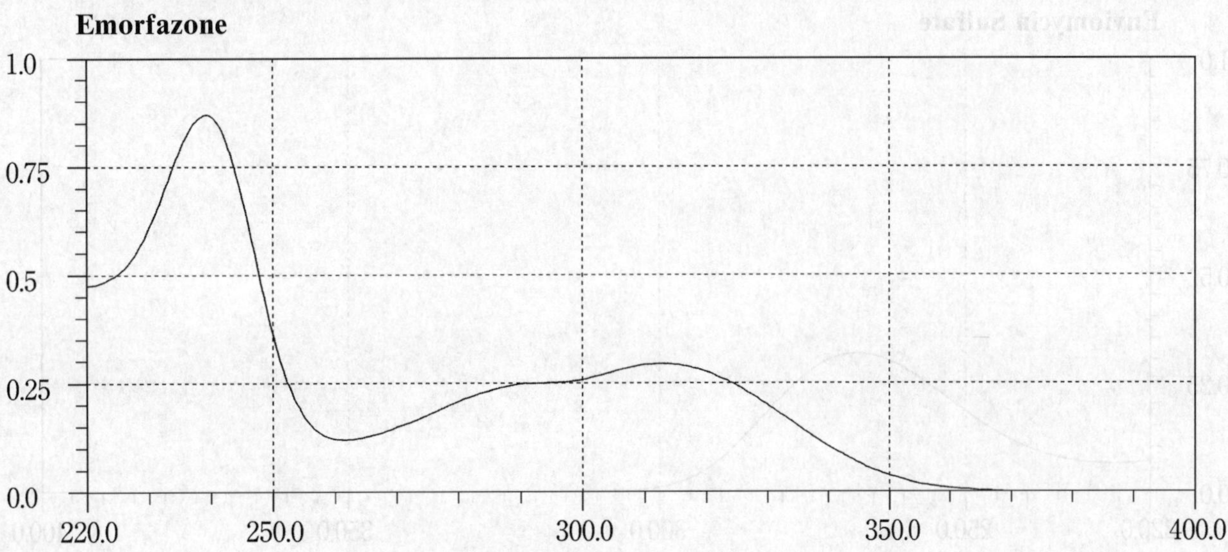

Enoxacin Hydrate

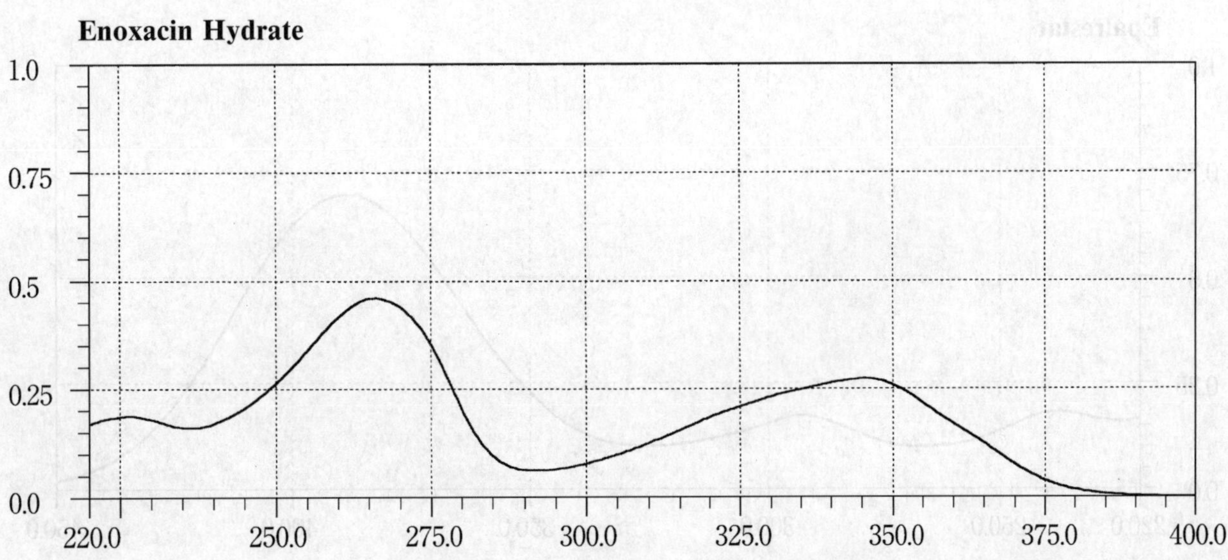

Entacapone

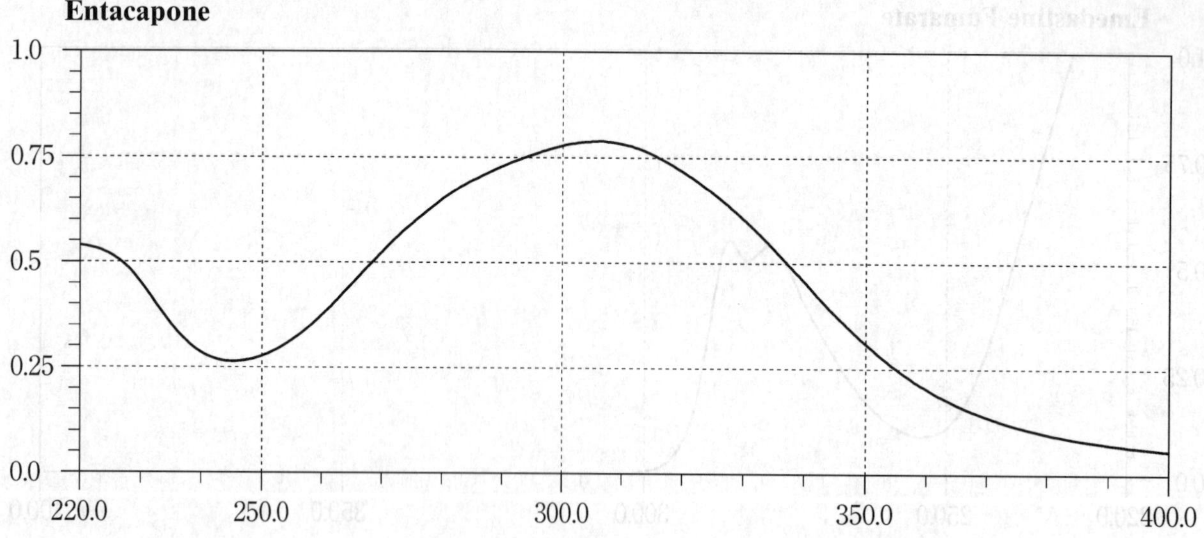

Enviomycin Sulfate

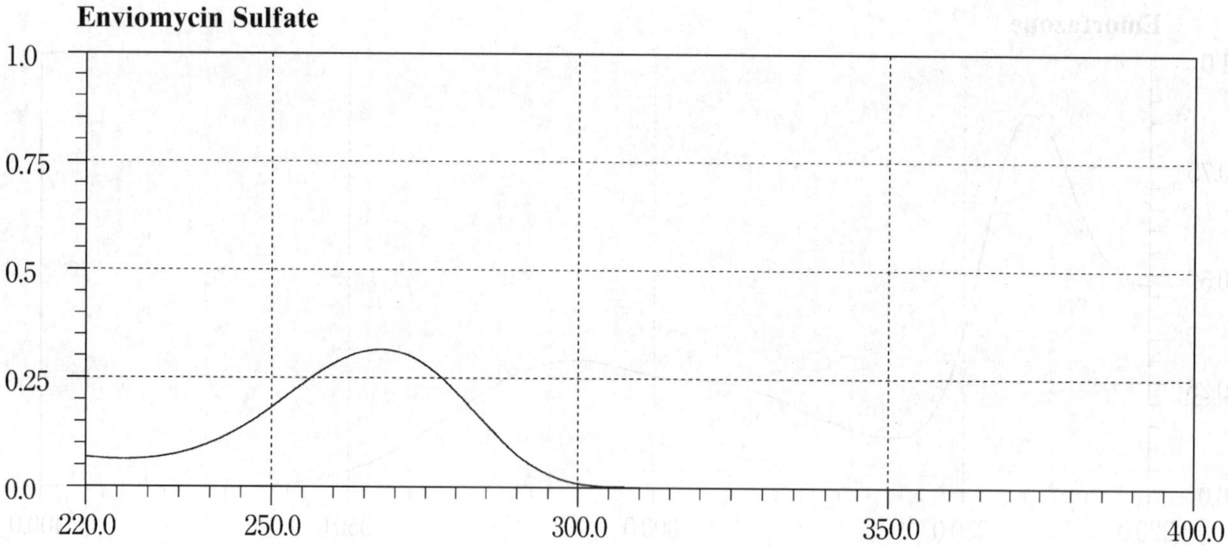

Epalrestat

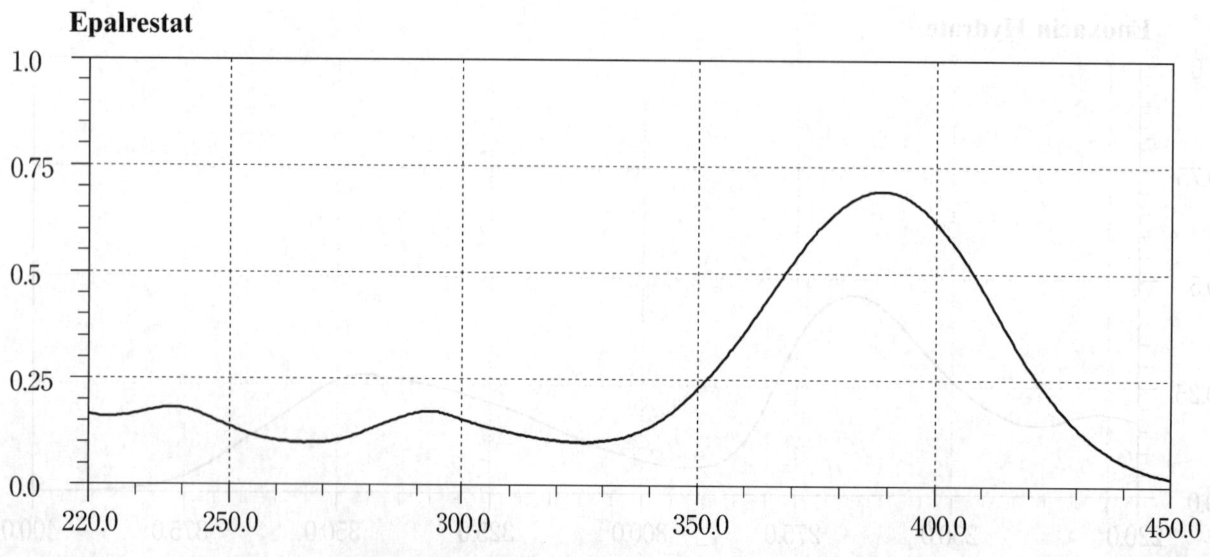

Eperisone Hydrochloride

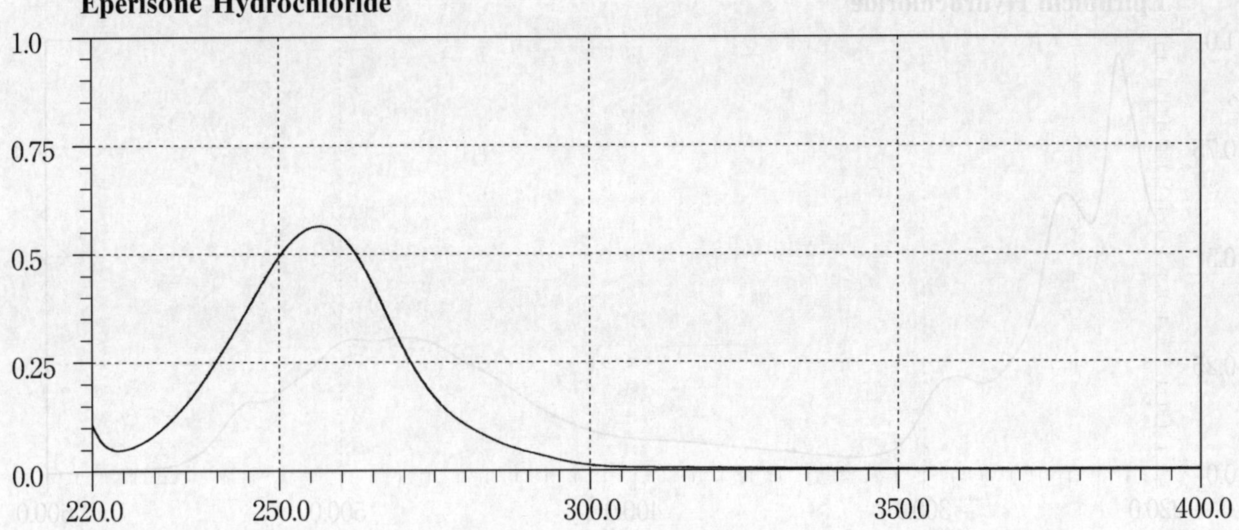

Ephedrine Hydrochloride

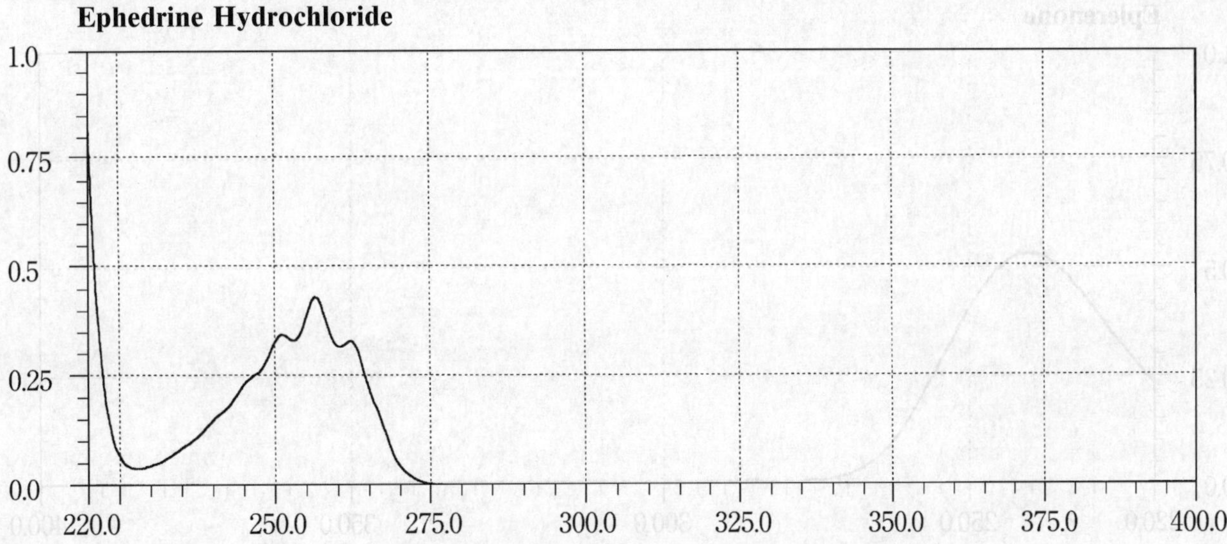

Epirizole

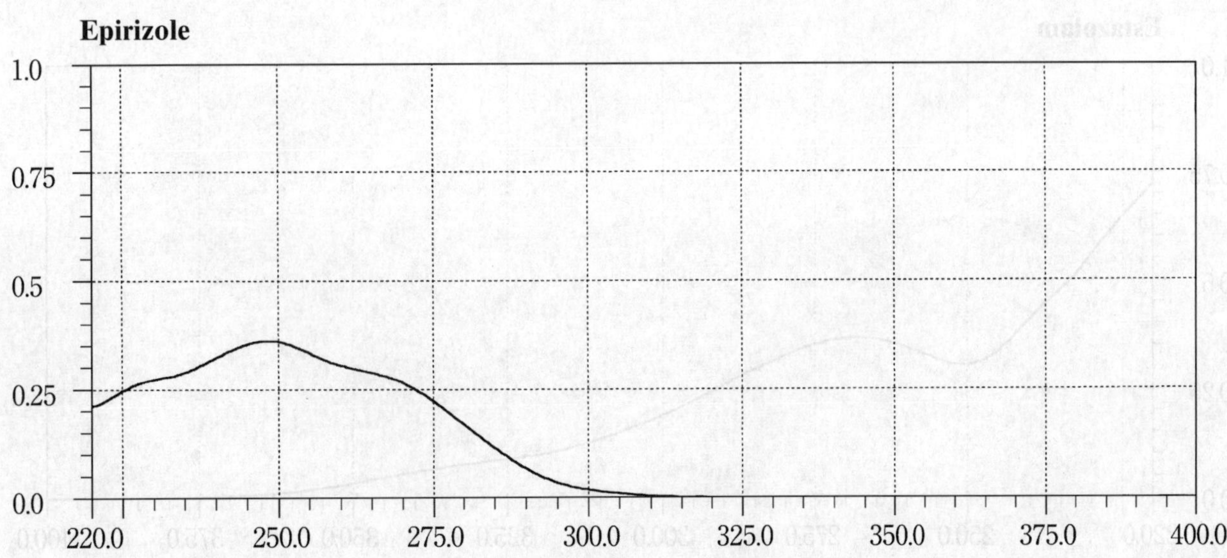

Epirubicin Hydrochloride

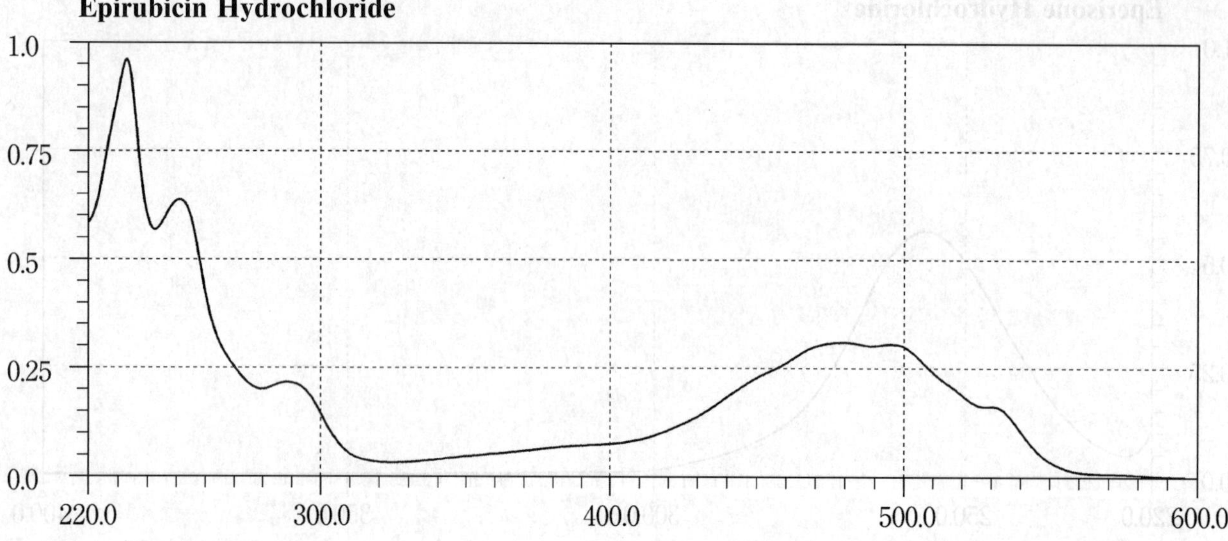

Eplerenone

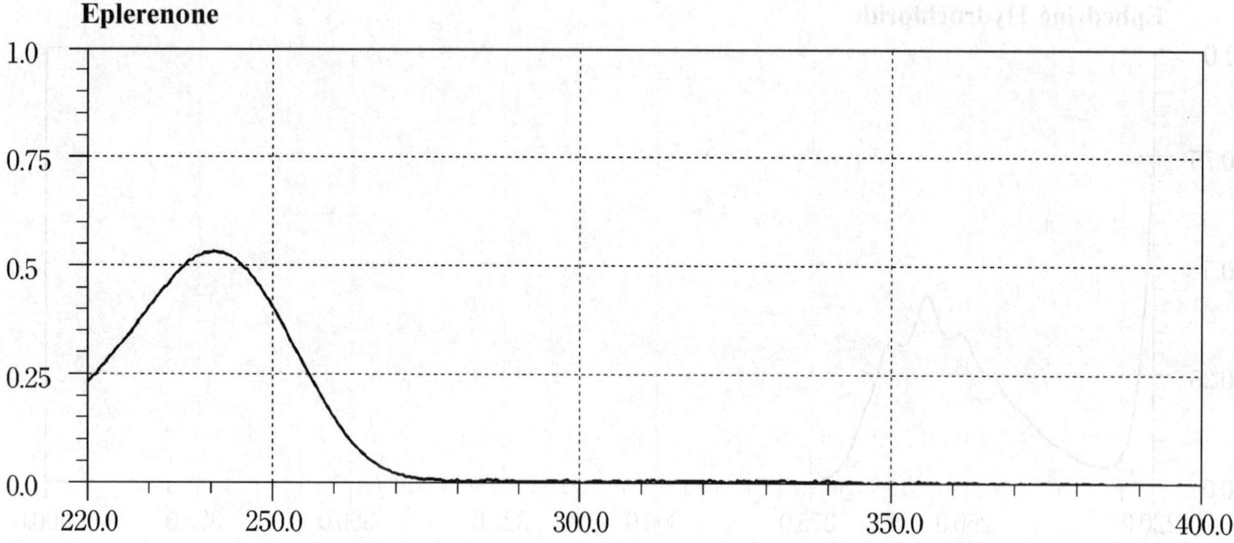

Estazolam

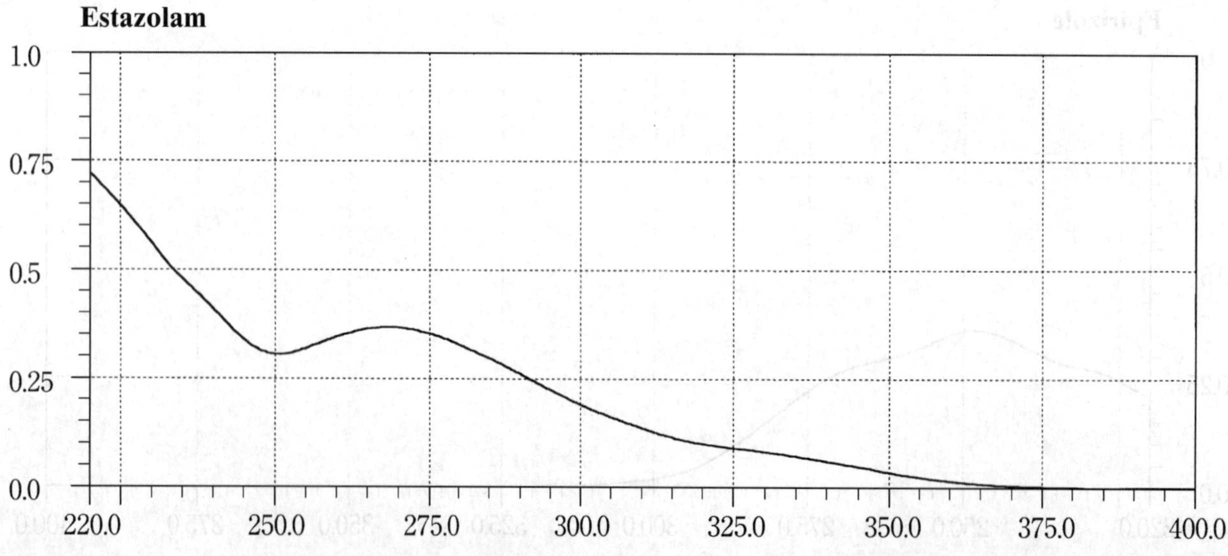

Estriol

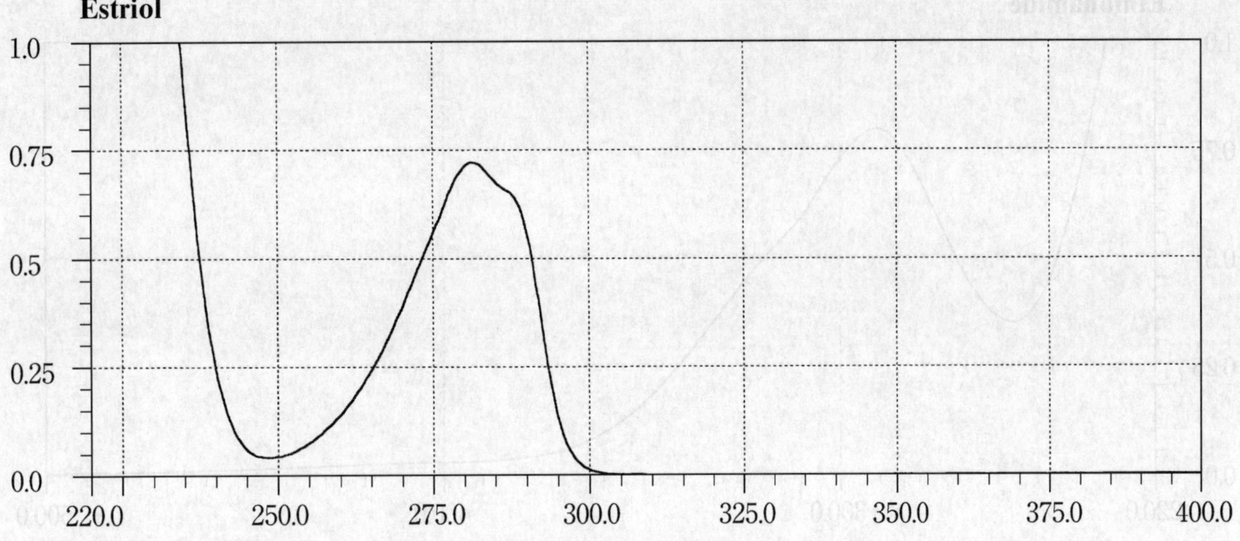

Etacrynic Acid

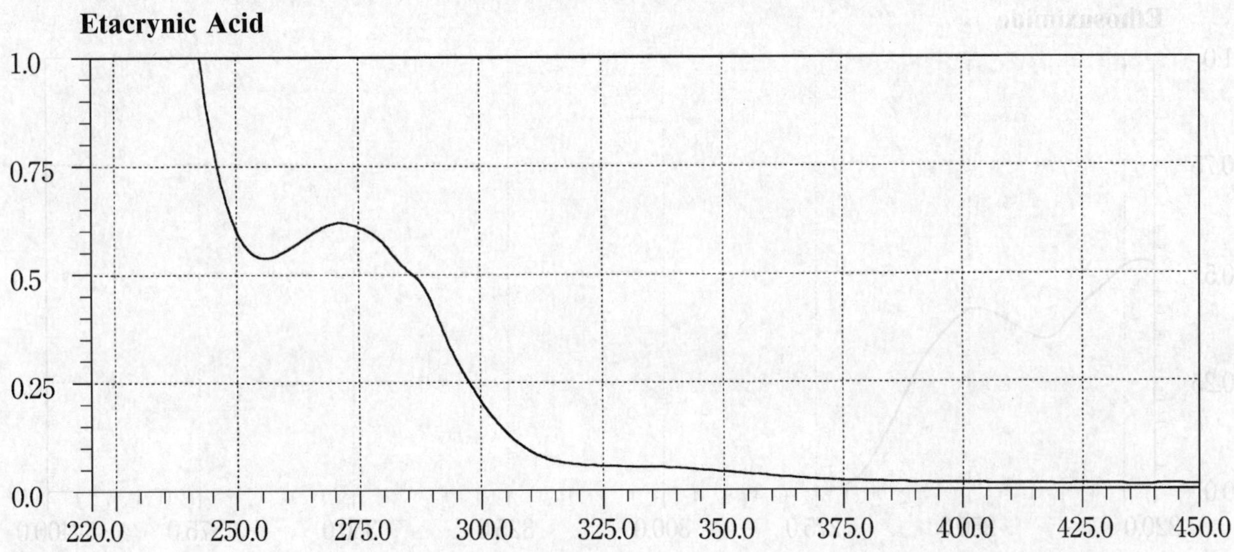

Ethenzamide

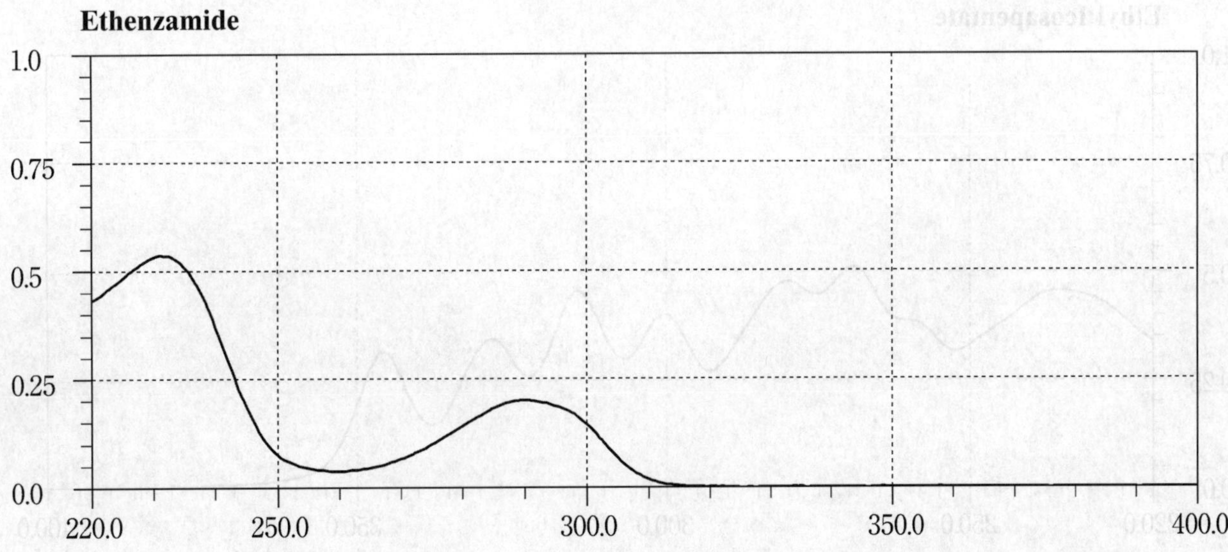

Ethionamide

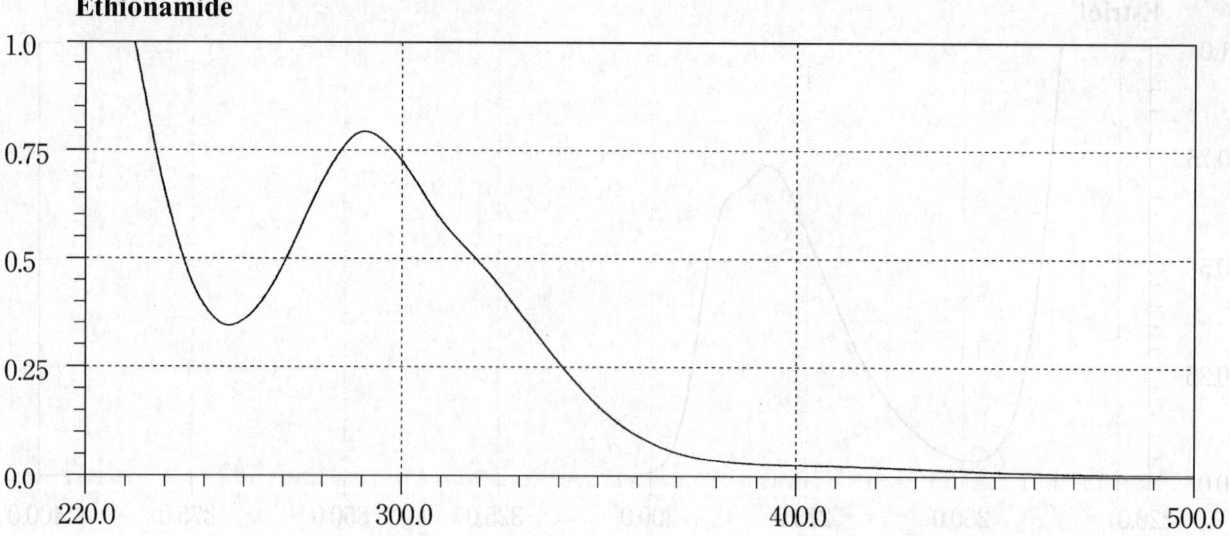

Ethosuximide

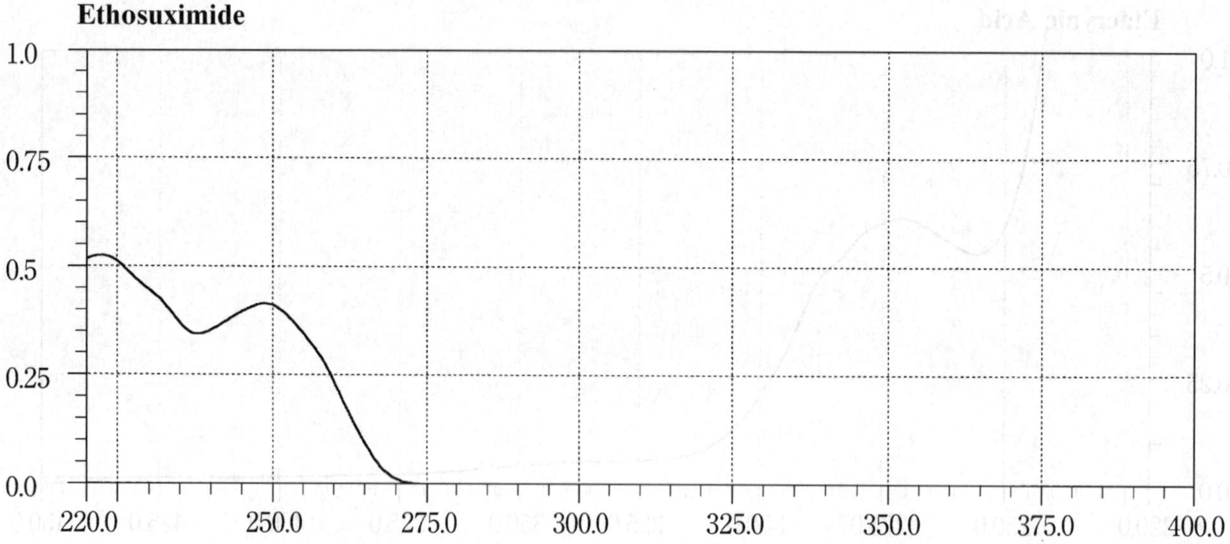

Ethyl Icosapentate

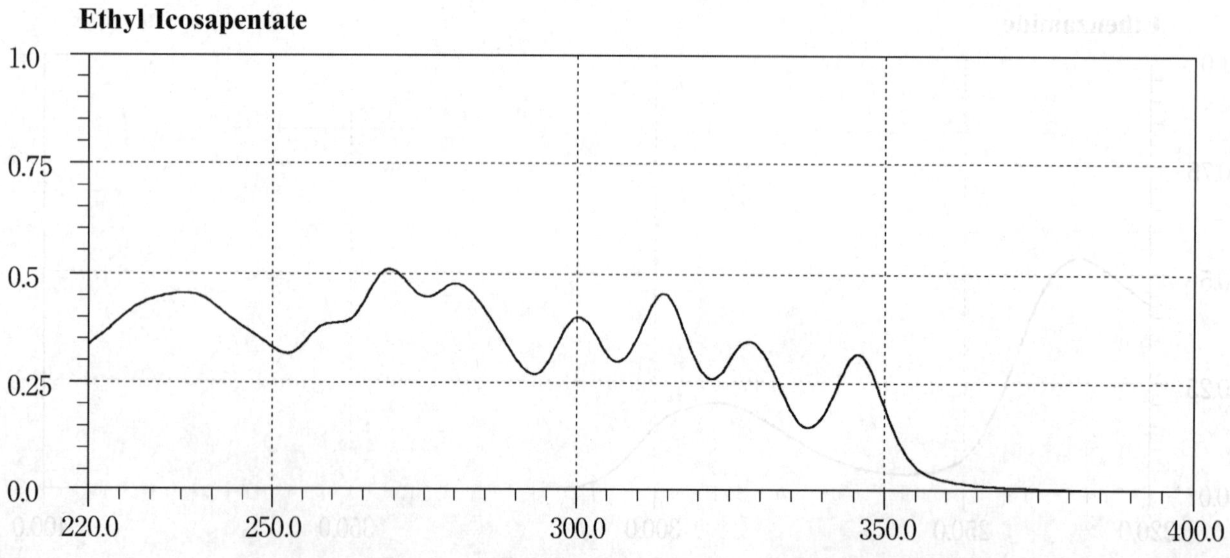

Ethyl Loflazepate

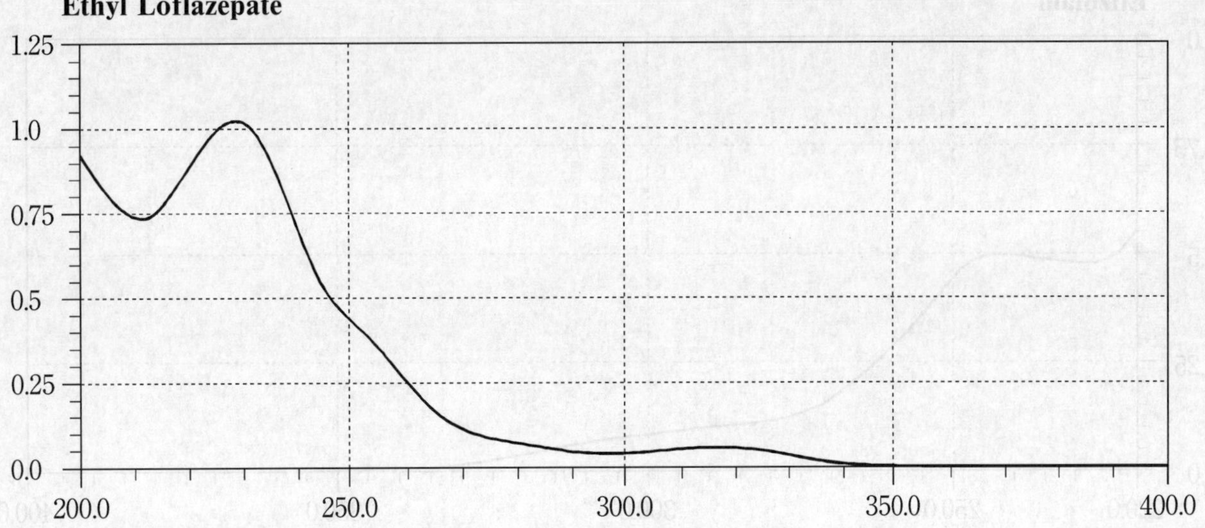

Ethylmorphine Hydrochloride Hydrate

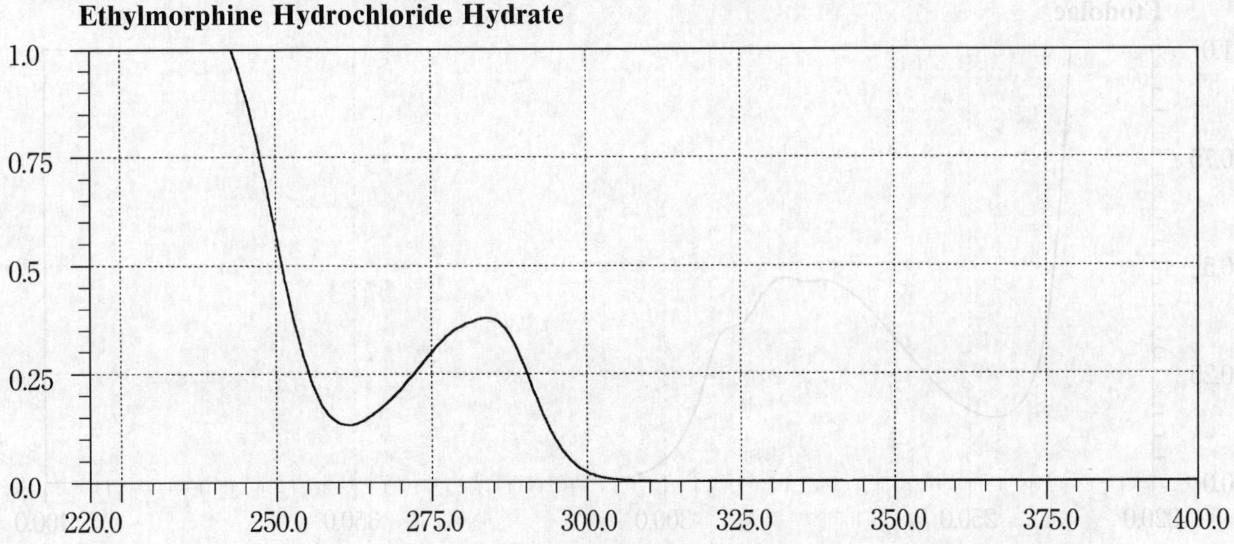

Etilefrine Hydrochloride

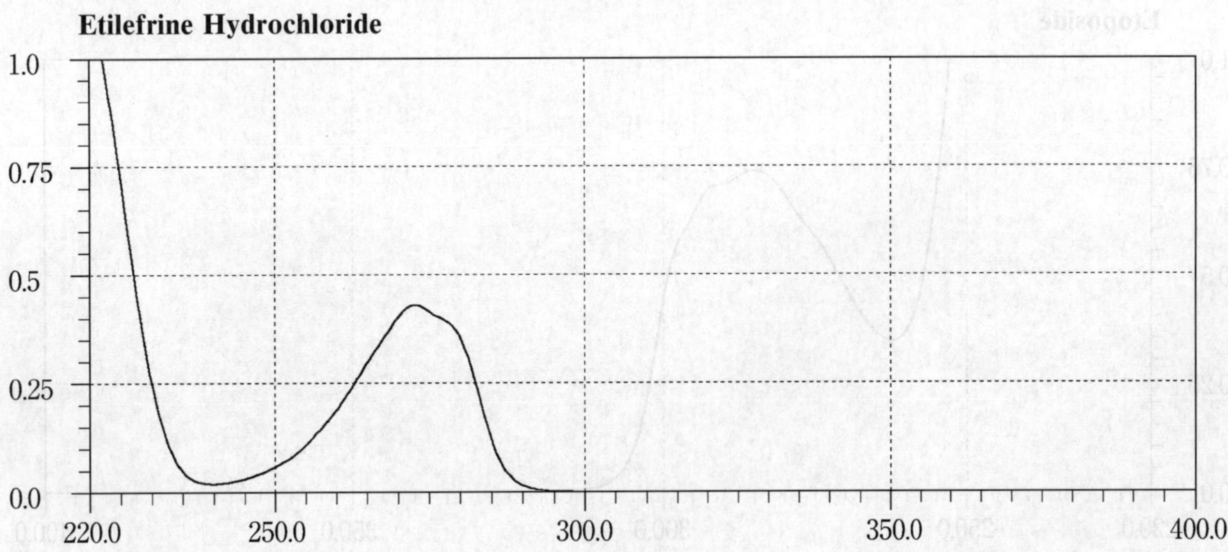

Etizolam

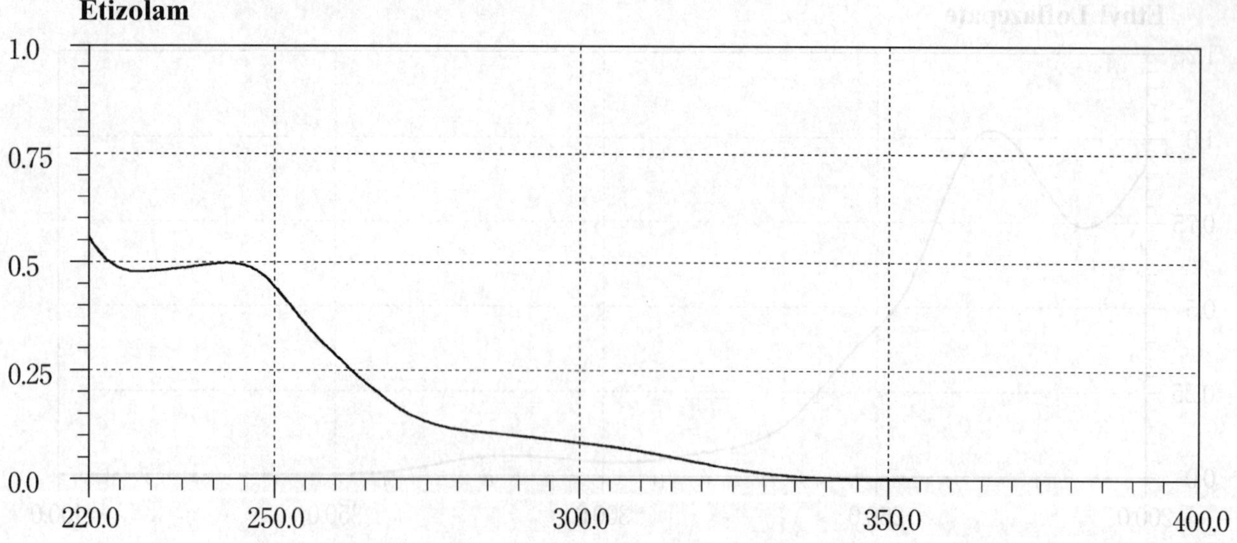

Etodolac

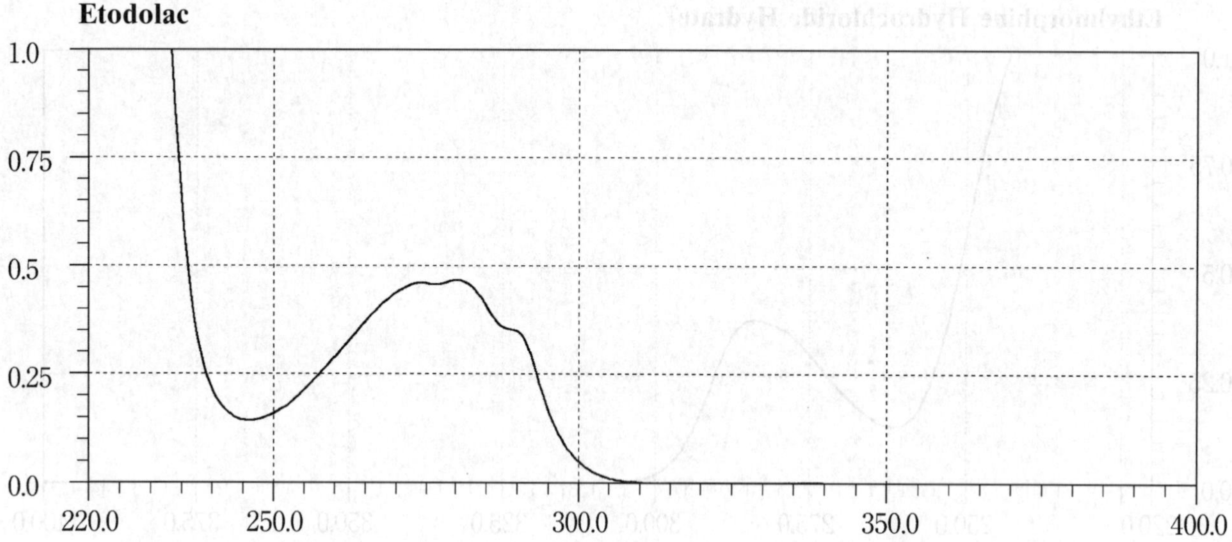

Etoposide

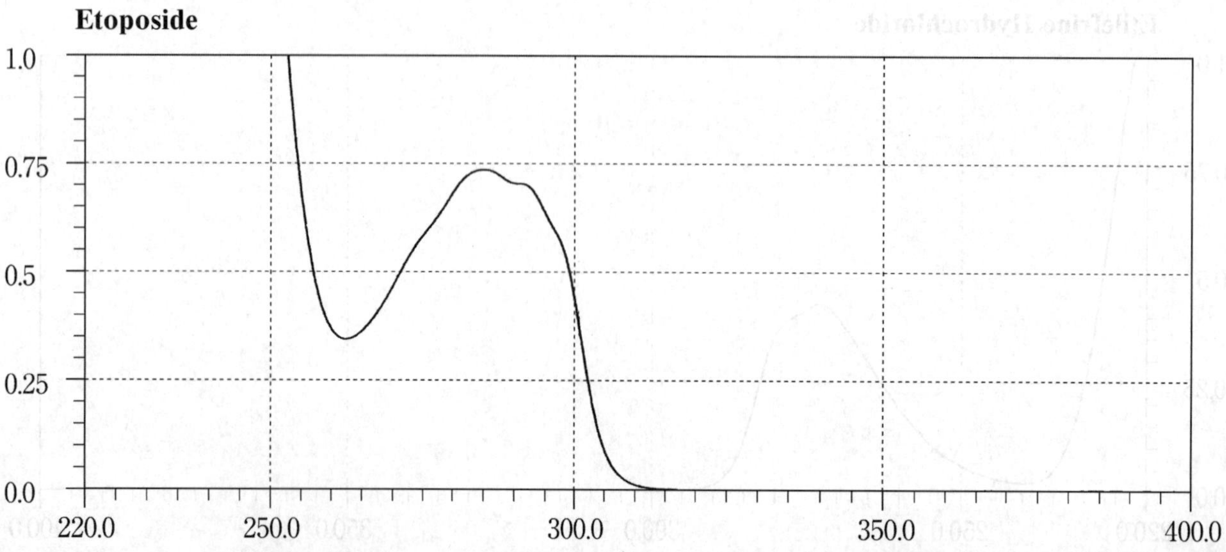

Famotidine

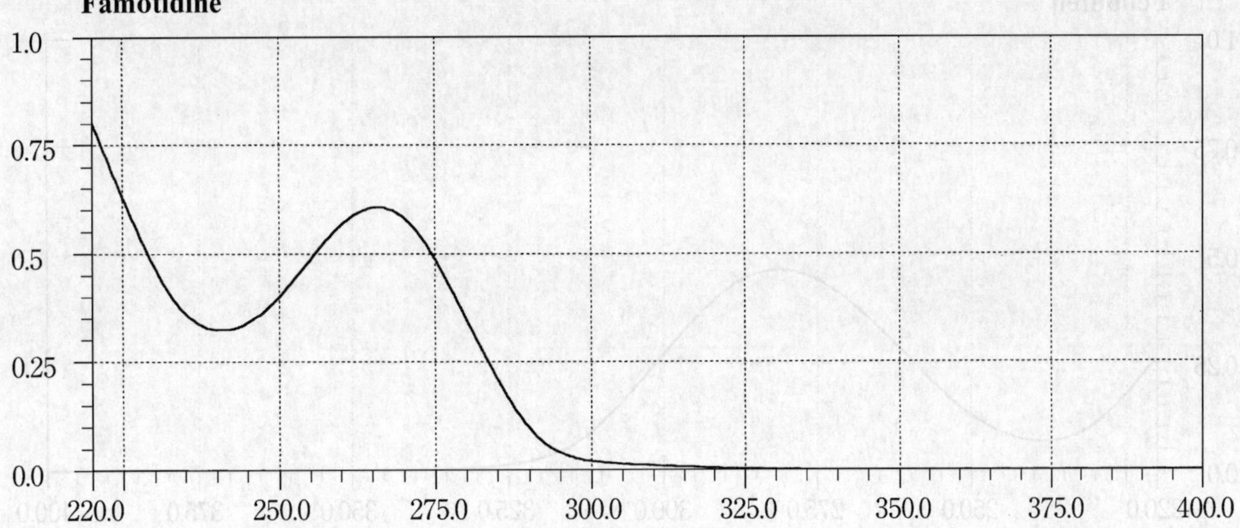

Felbinac

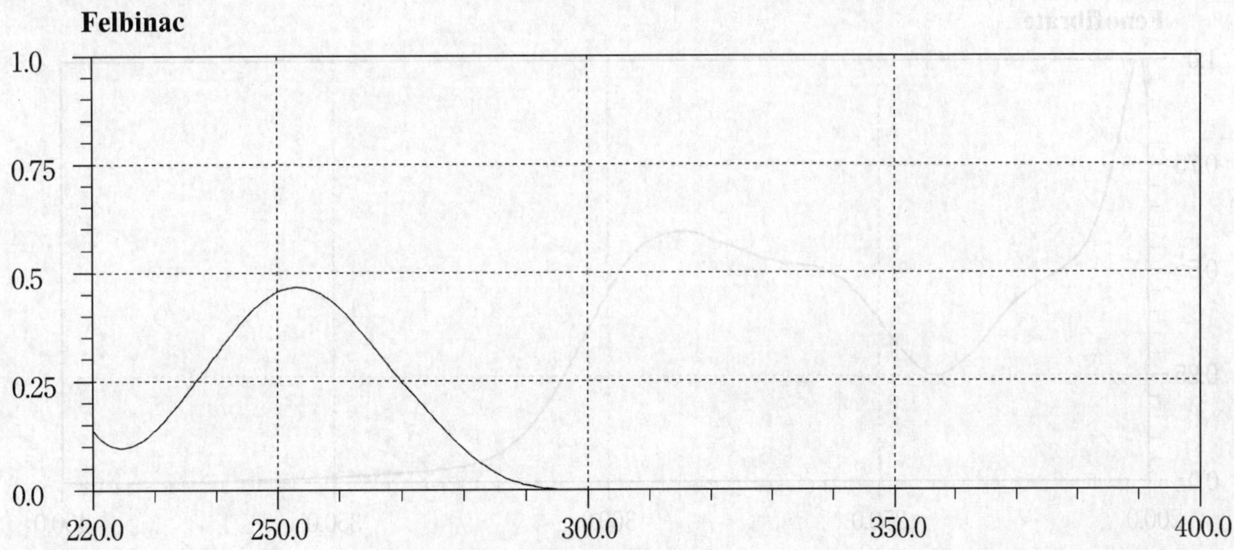

Felodipine

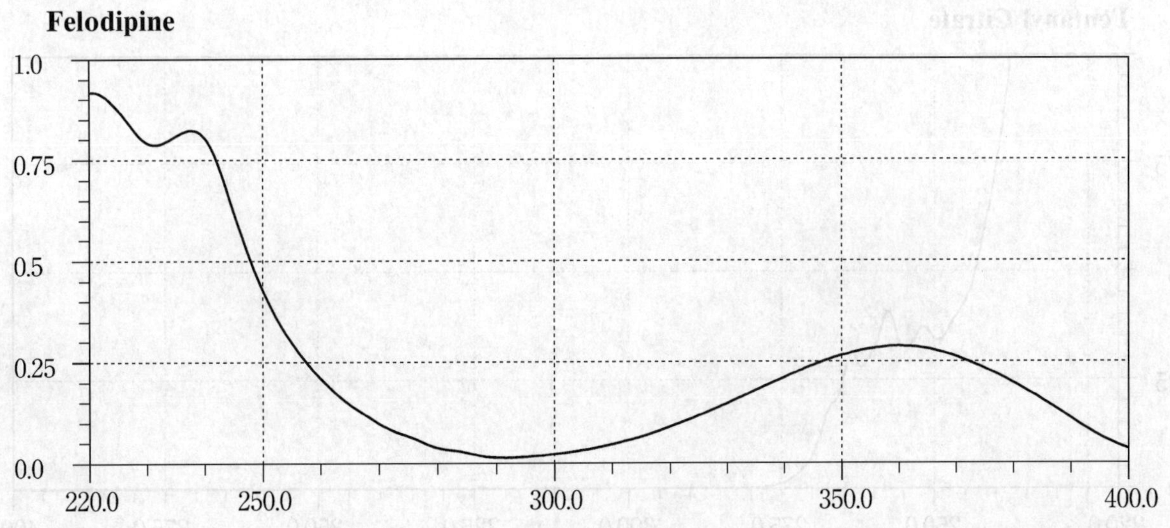

Fenbufen

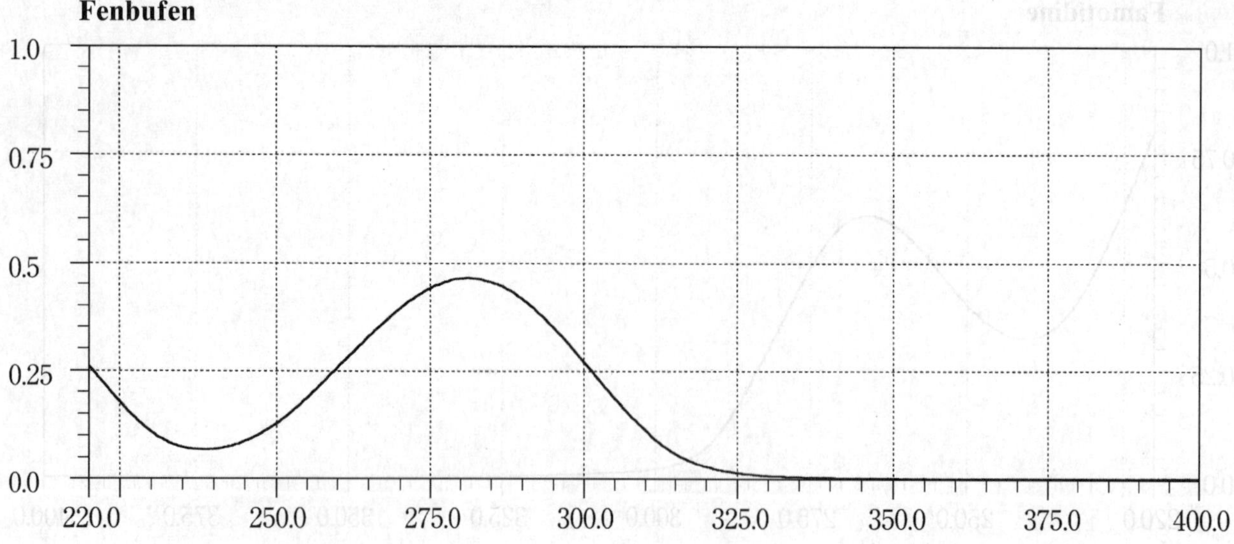

Fenofibrate

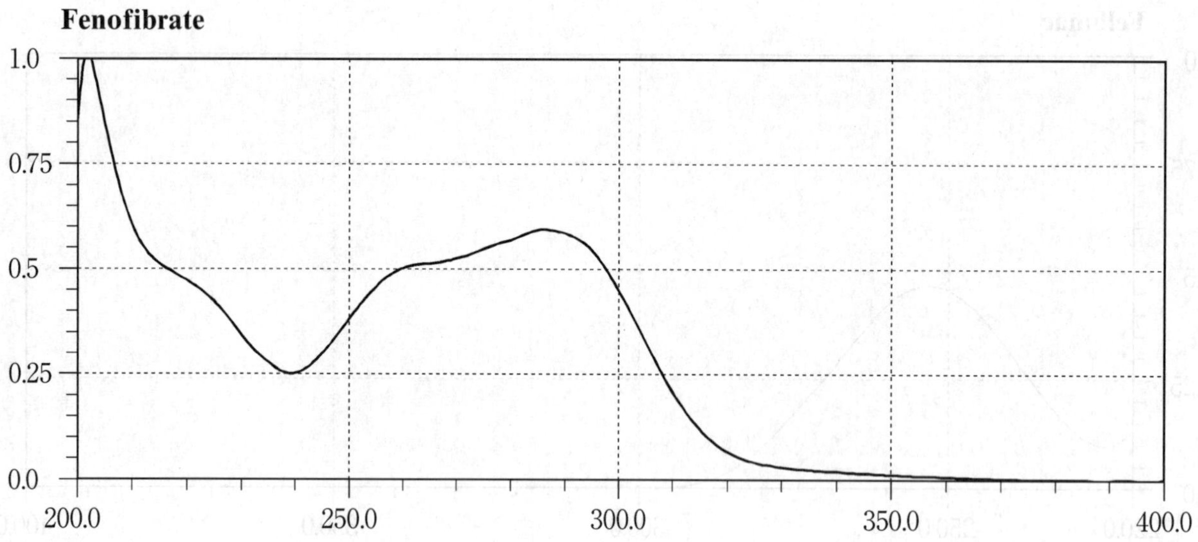

Fentanyl Citrate

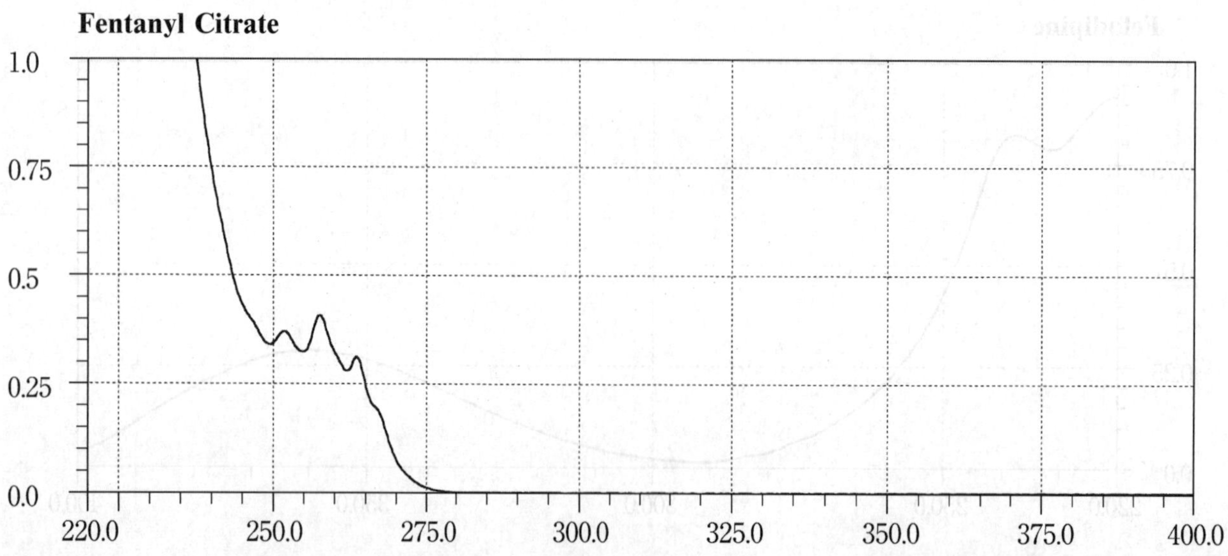

Fexofenadine Hydrochloride

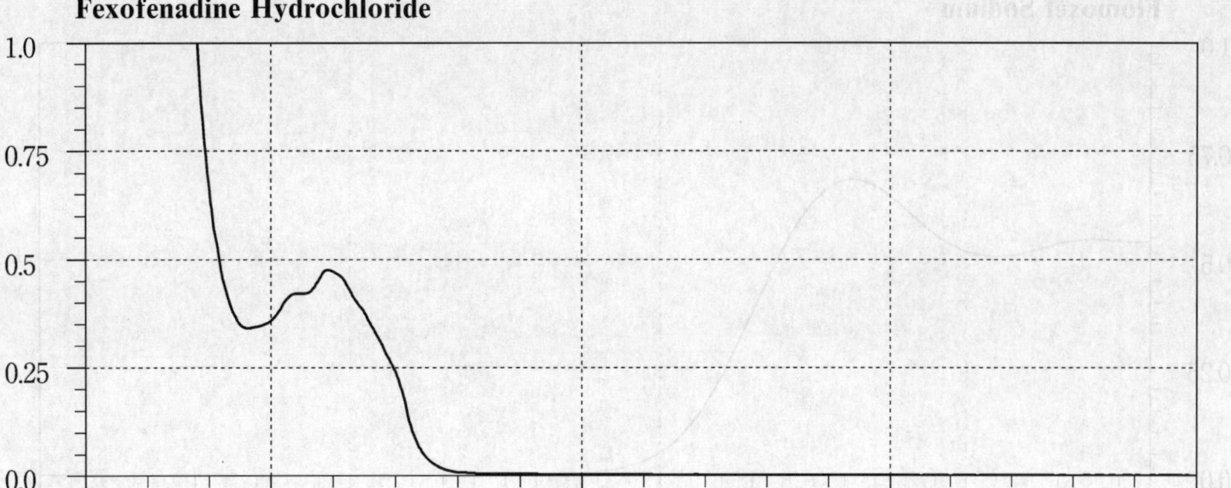

Flavoxate Hydrochloride

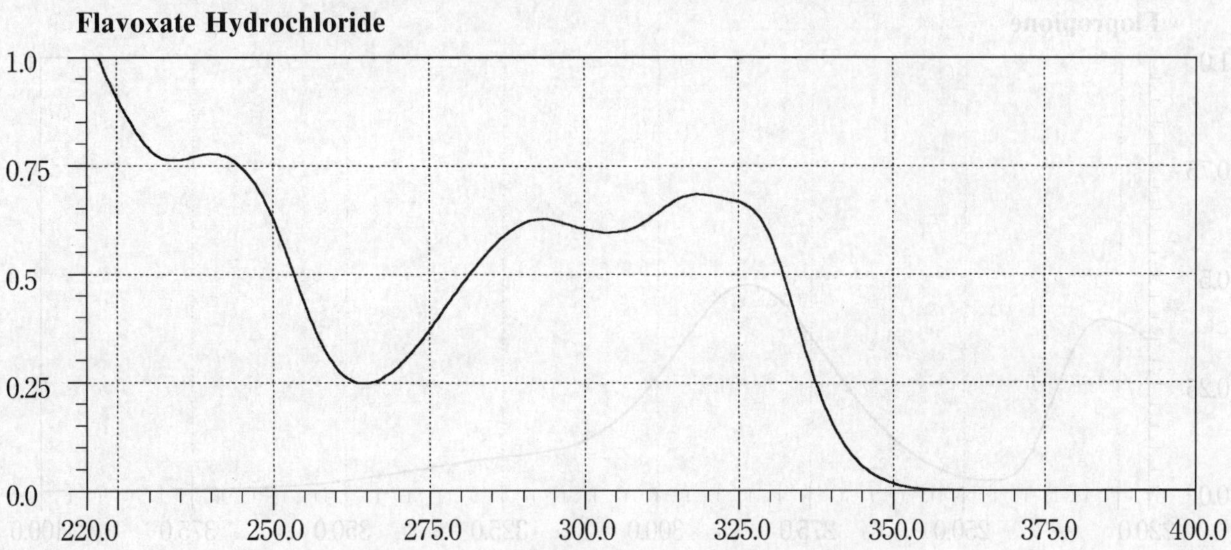

Flecainide Acetate

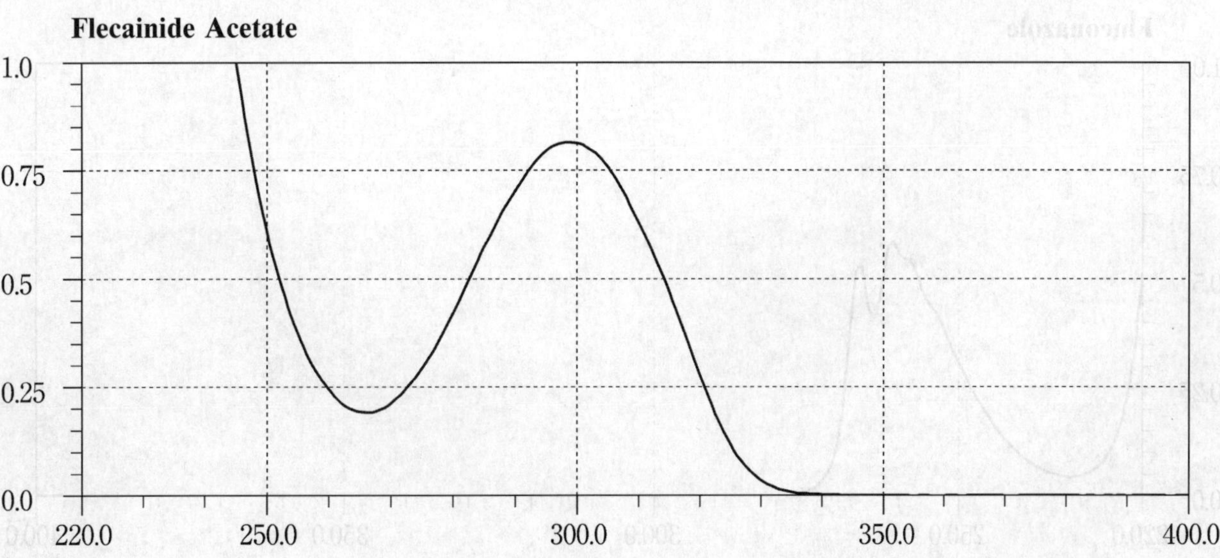

Flomoxef Sodium

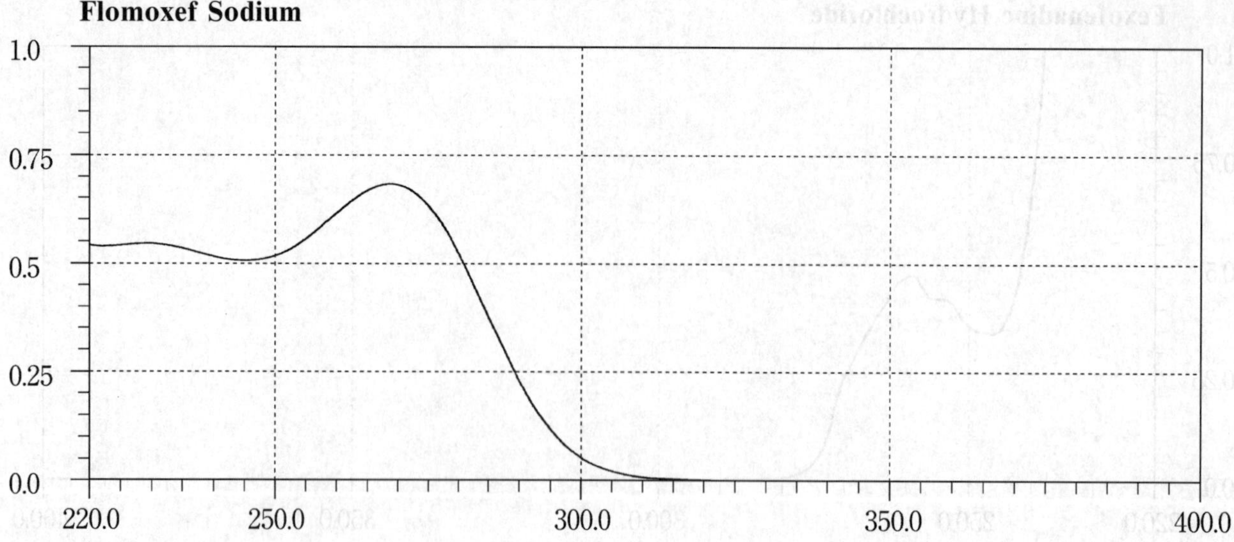

Flopropione

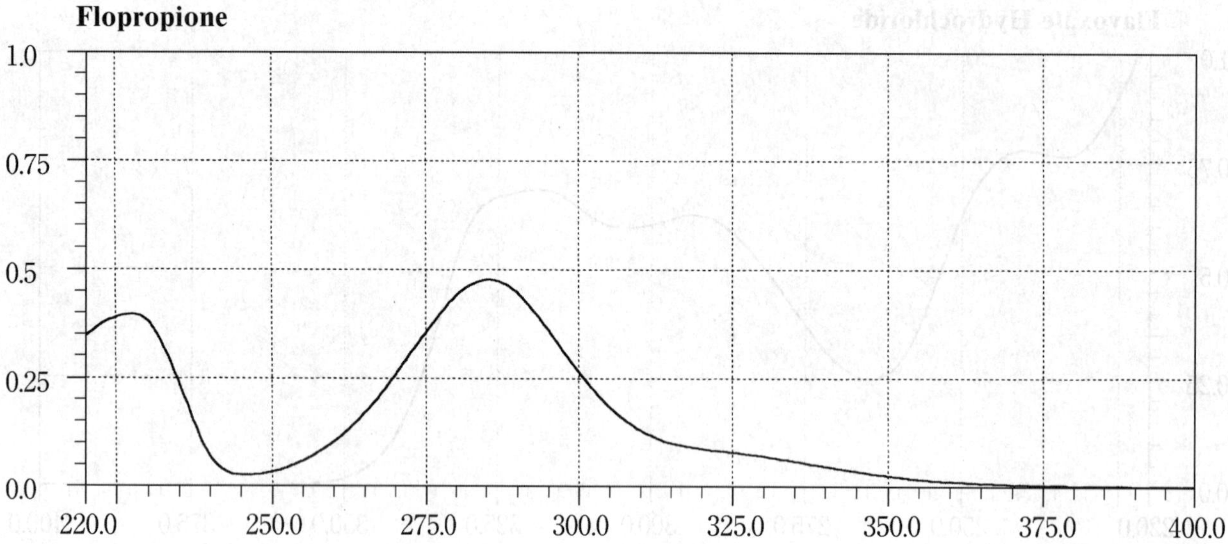

Fluconazole

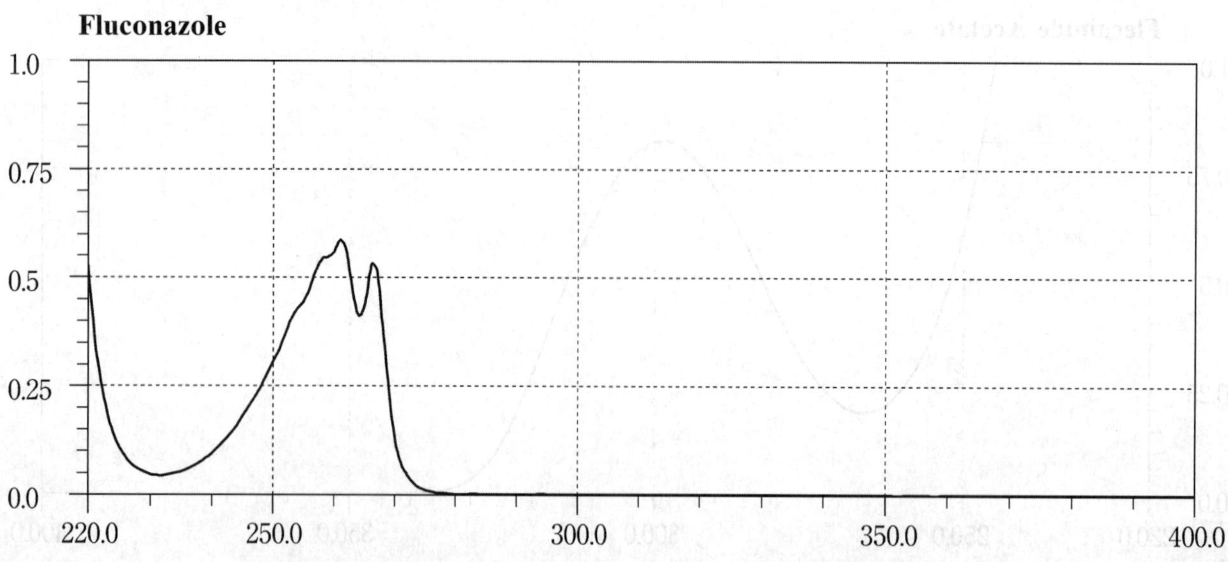

Flucytosine

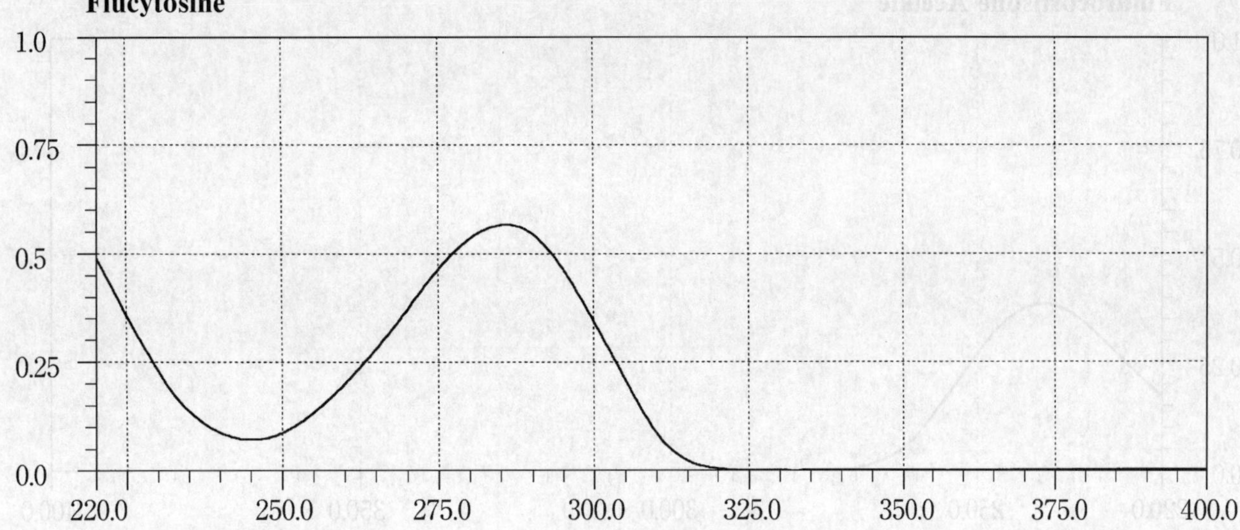

Fludiazepam 1

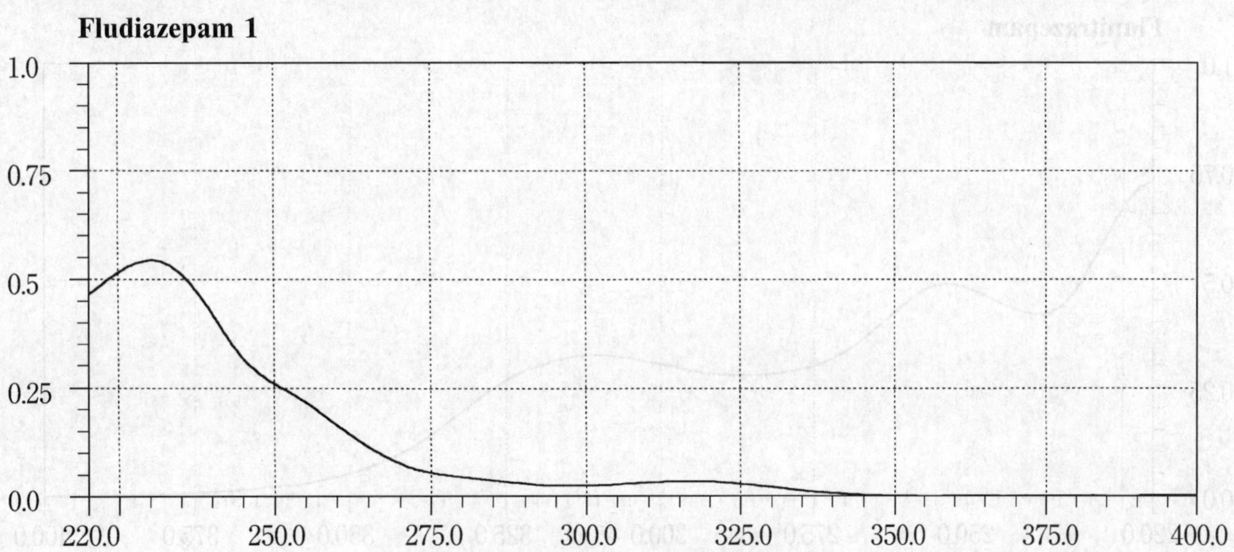

Fludiazepam 2

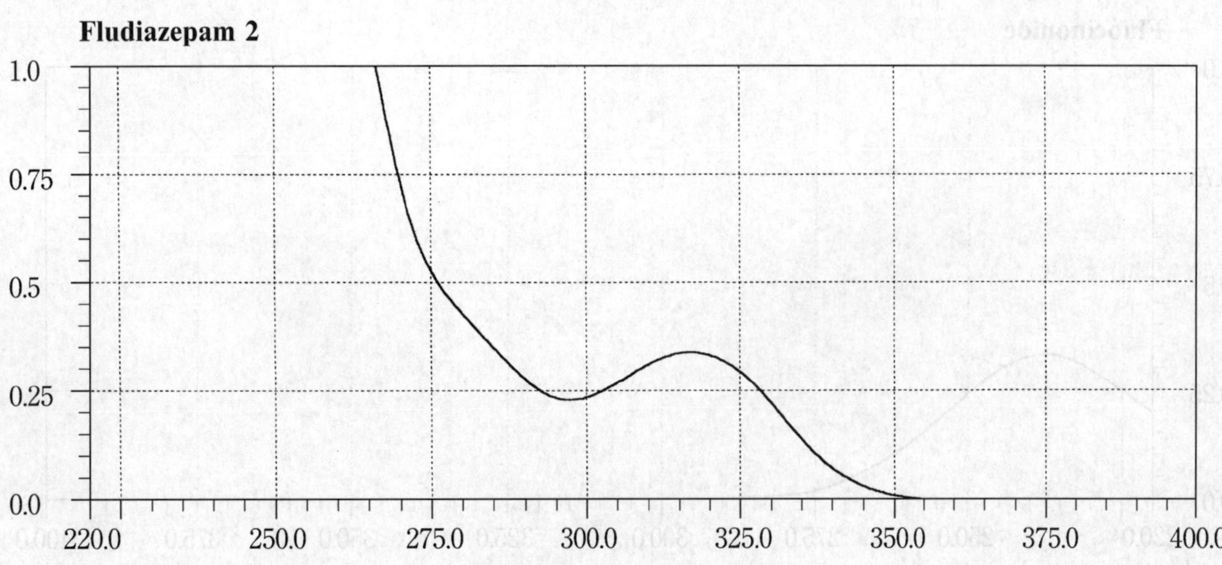

Fludrocortisone Acetate

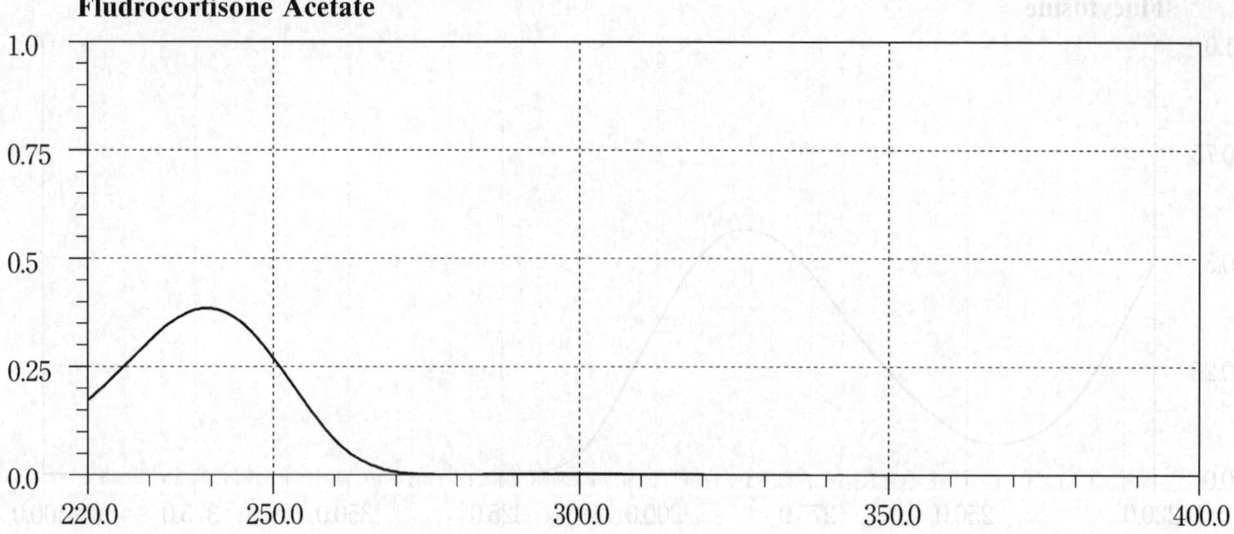

Flunitrazepam

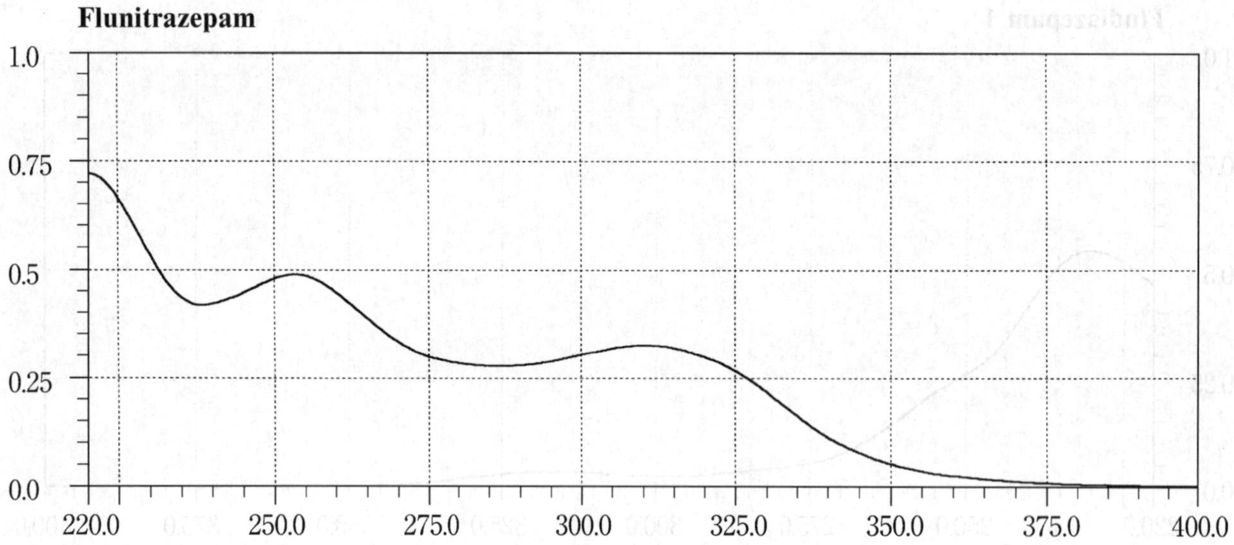

Fluocinonide

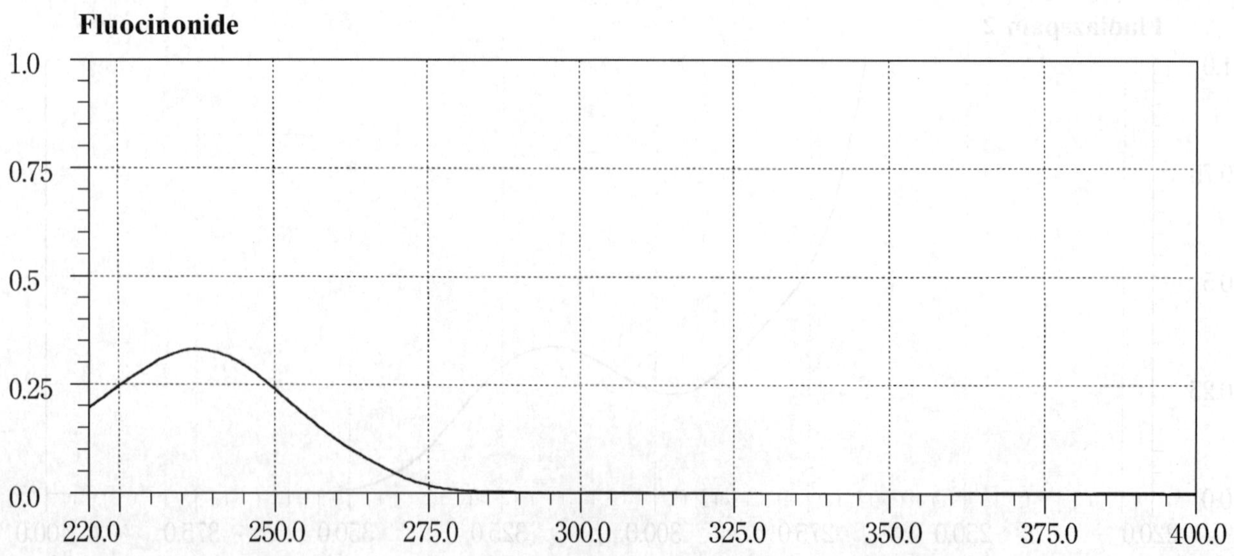

Fluorometholone

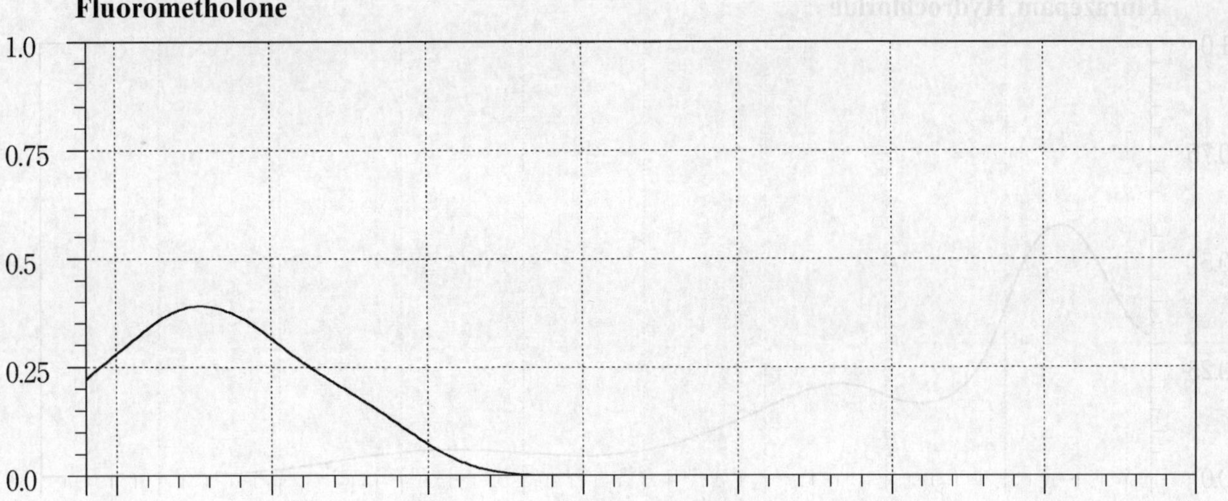

Fluorouracil

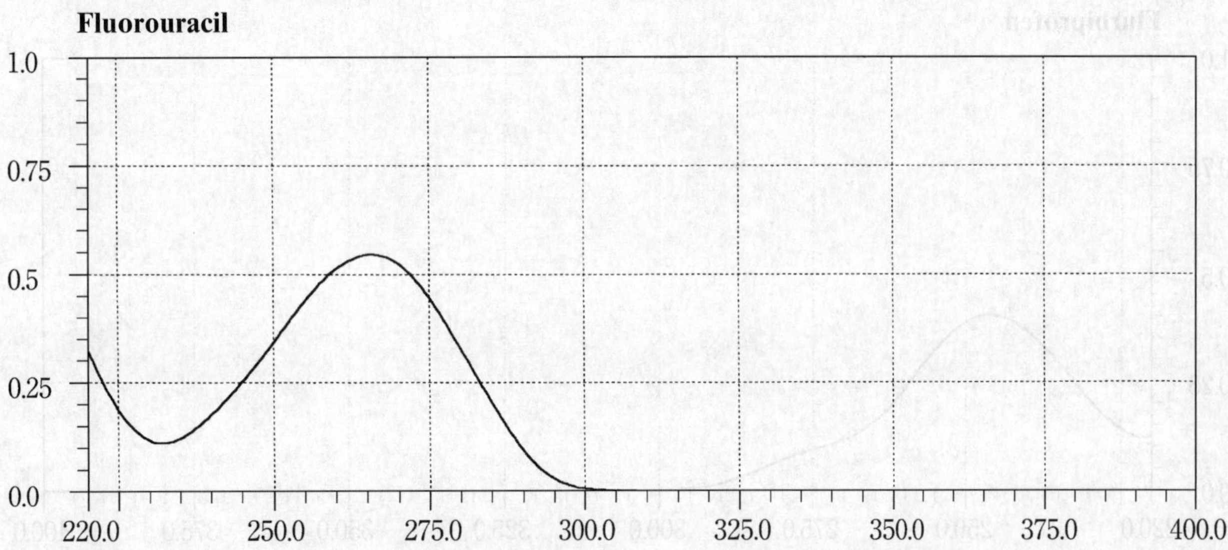

Fluphenazine Enanthate

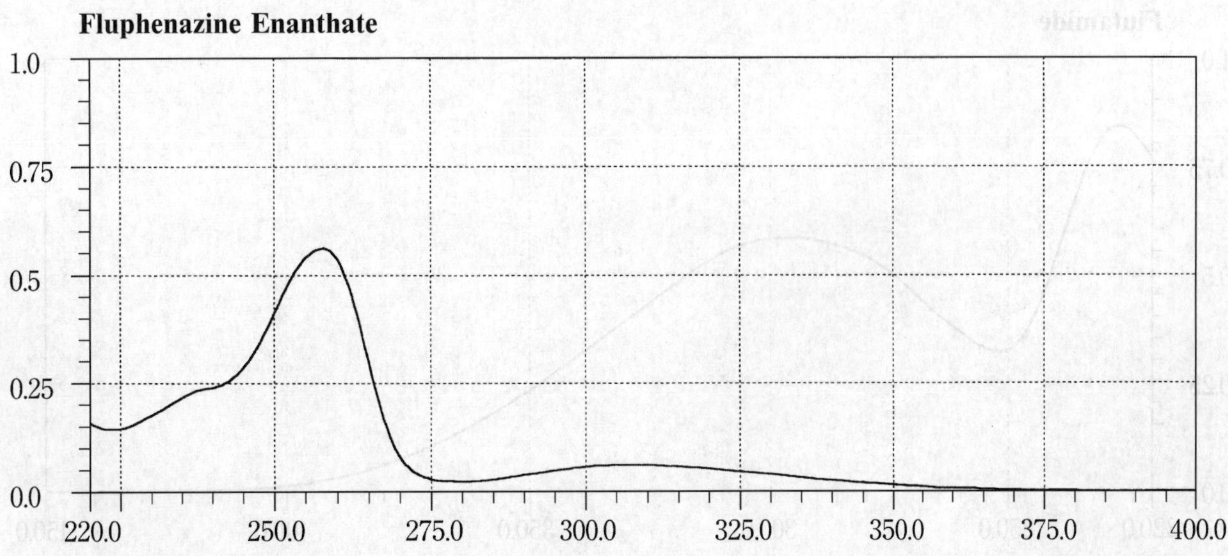

The JP Drugs are to be tested according to the provisions given in the pertinent monographs, General Notices, General Rules for Crude Drugs, General Rules for Preparations, and General Tests for their conformity to the Japanese Pharmacopoeia. (See the General Notices 5.)

Flurazepam Hydrochloride

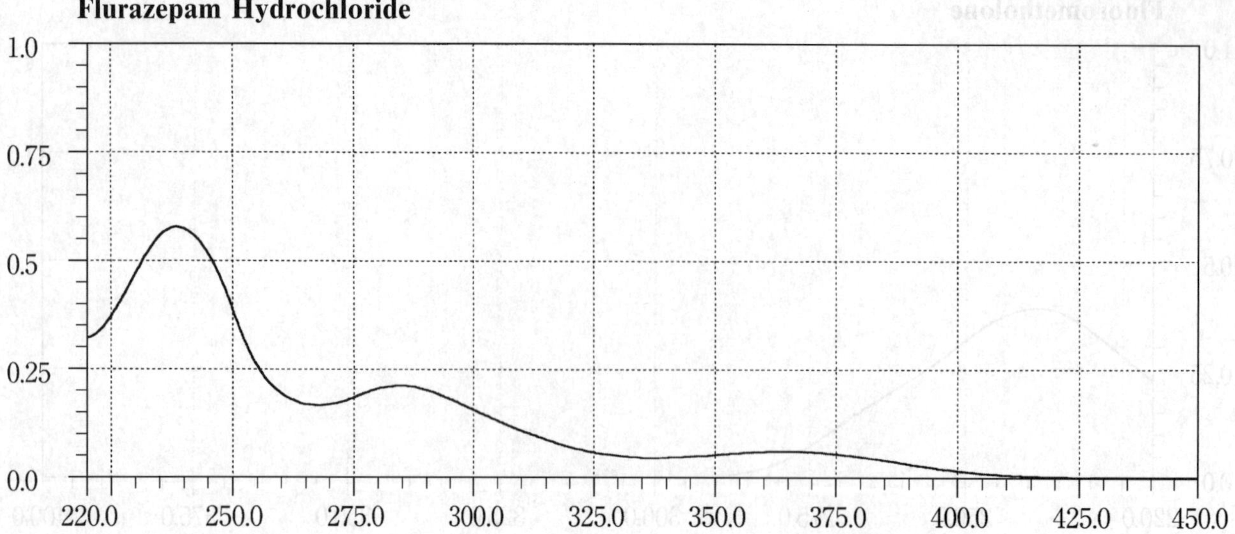

Flurbiprofen

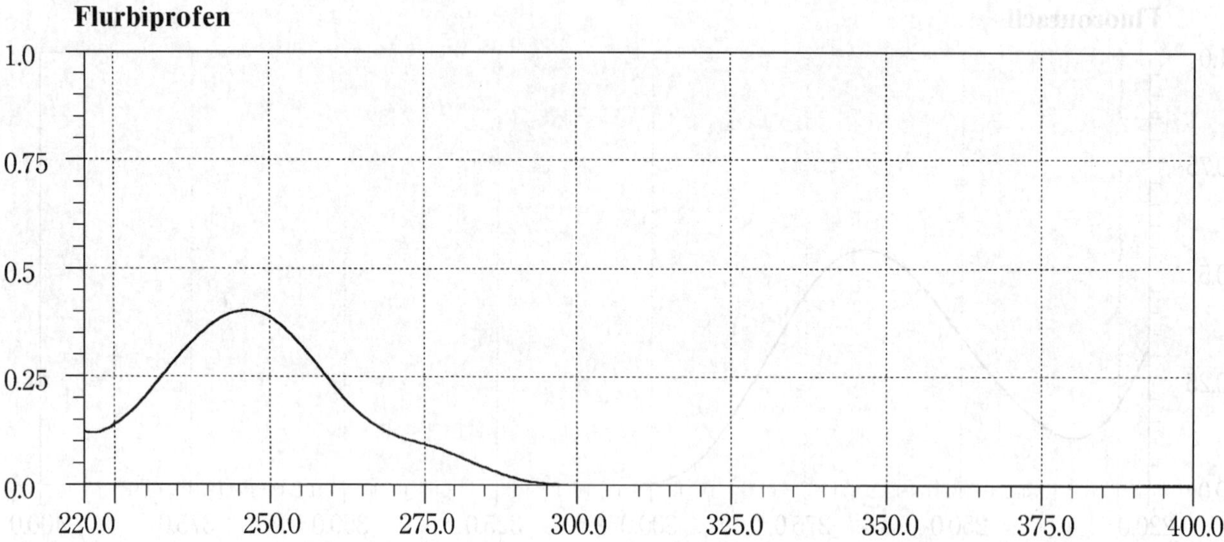

Flutamide

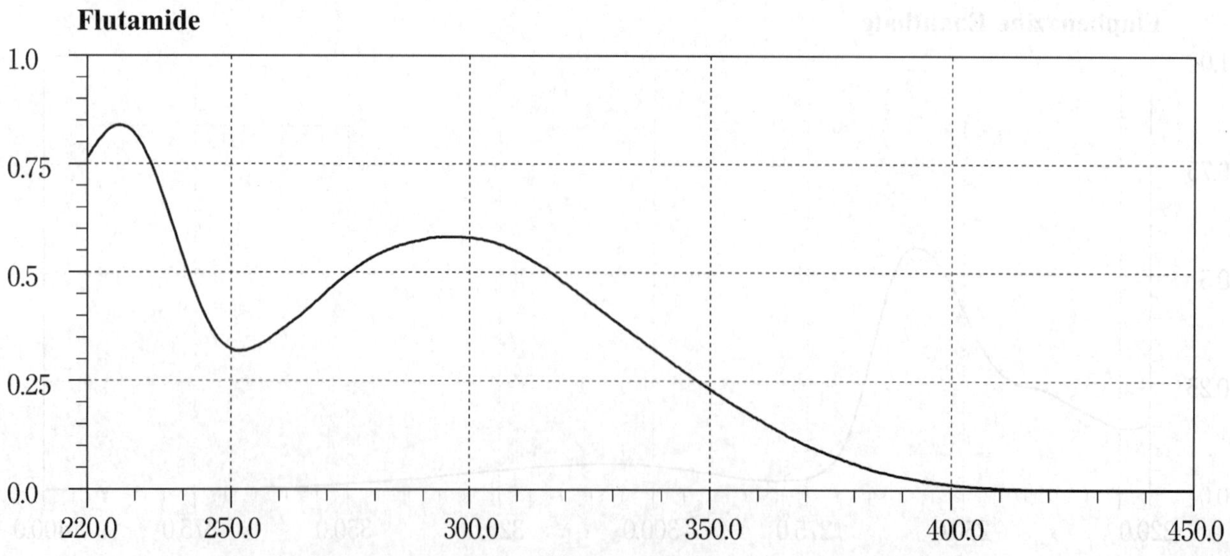

Flutoprazepam

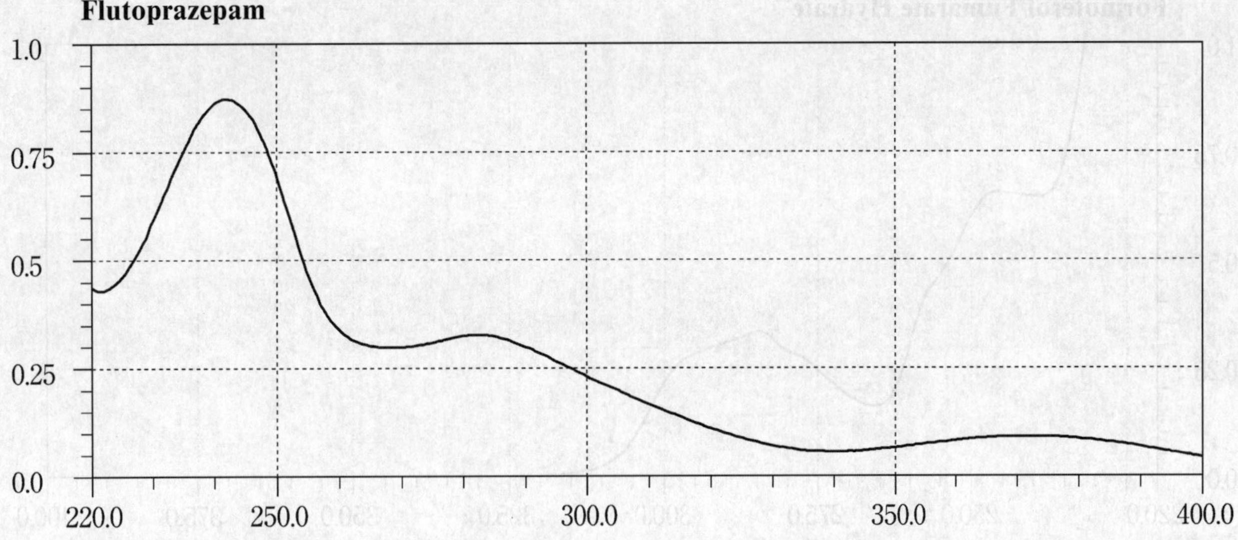

Fluvoxamine Maleate

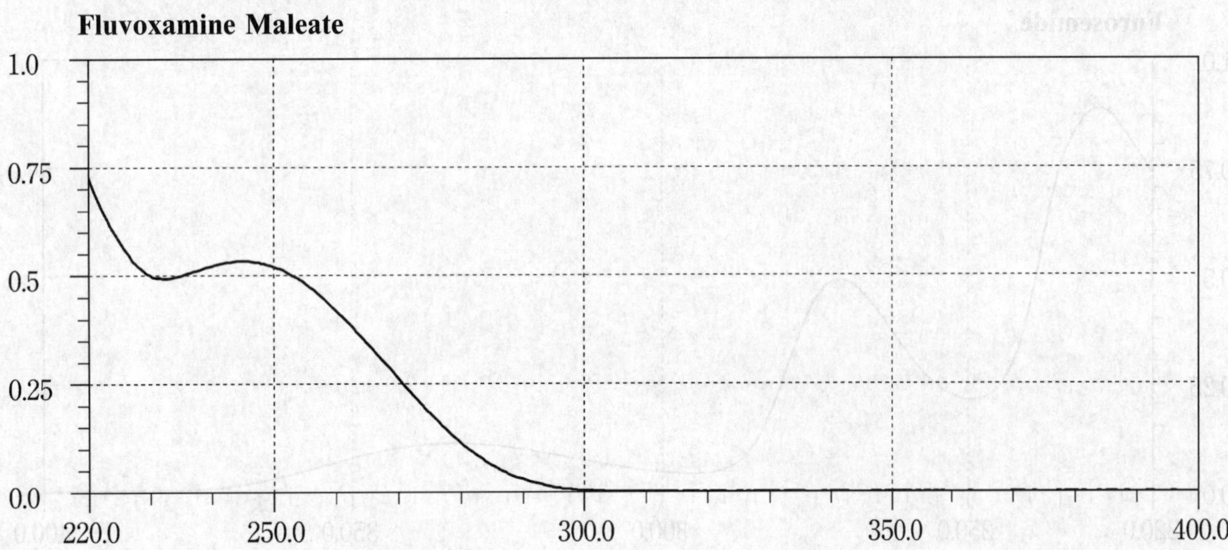

Folic Acid

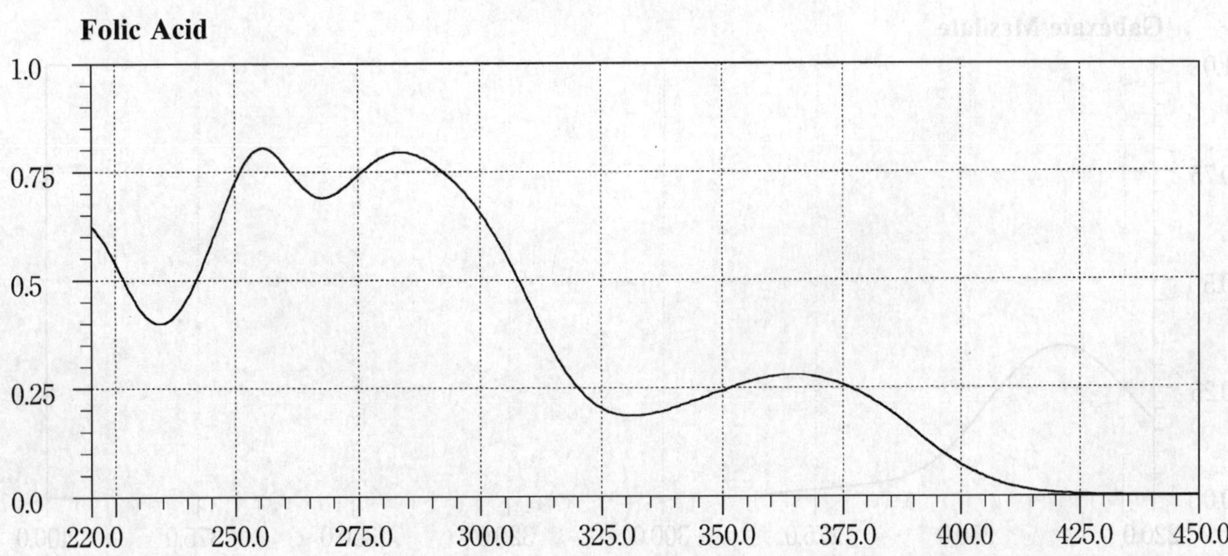

Formoterol Fumarate Hydrate

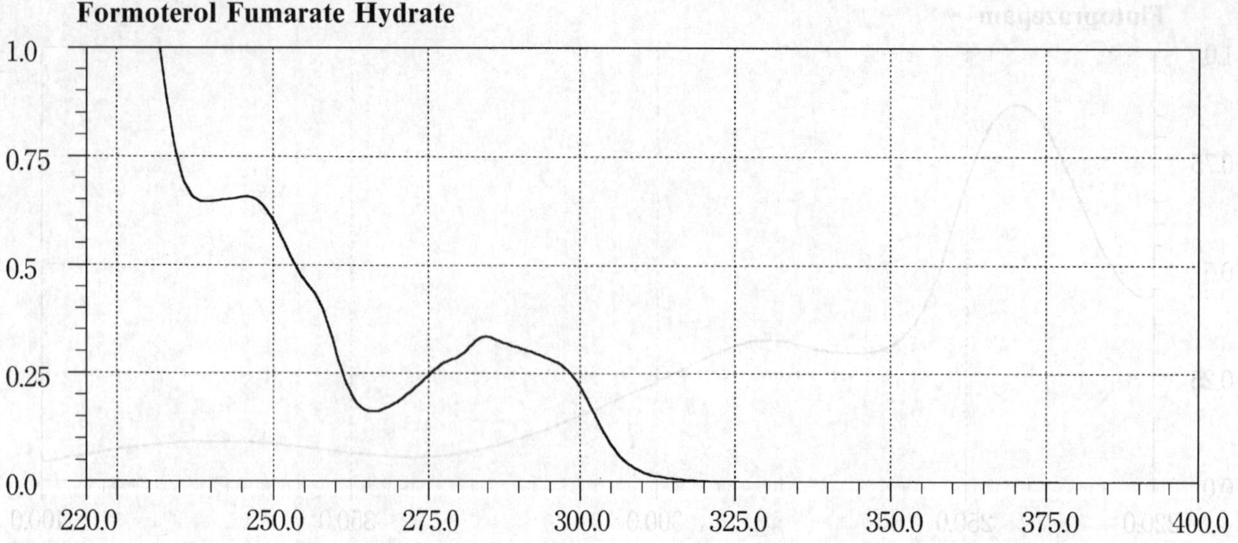

Furosemide

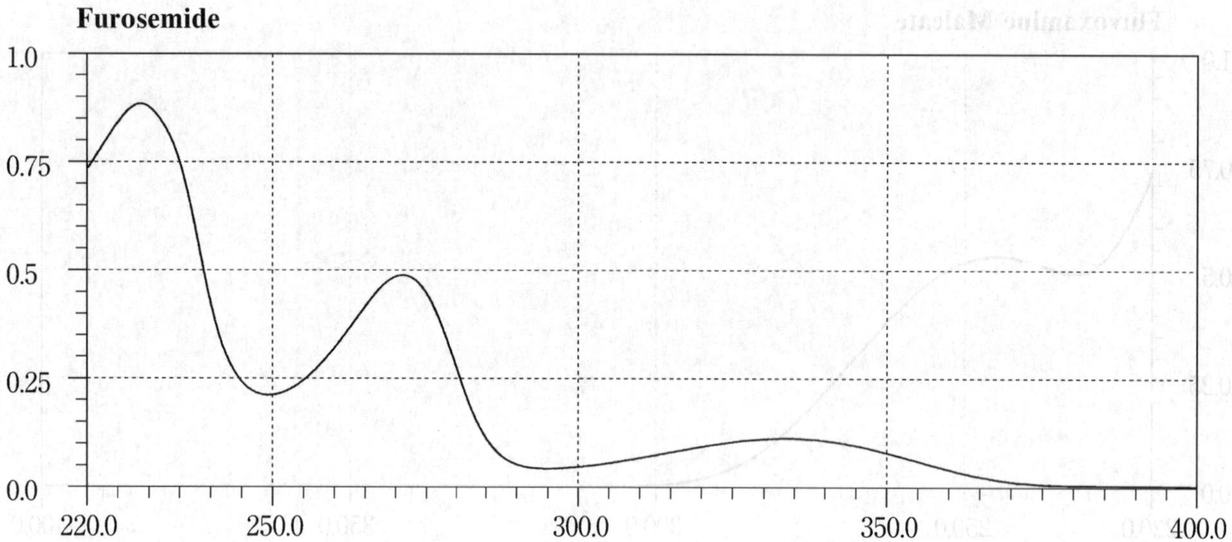

Gabexate Mesilate

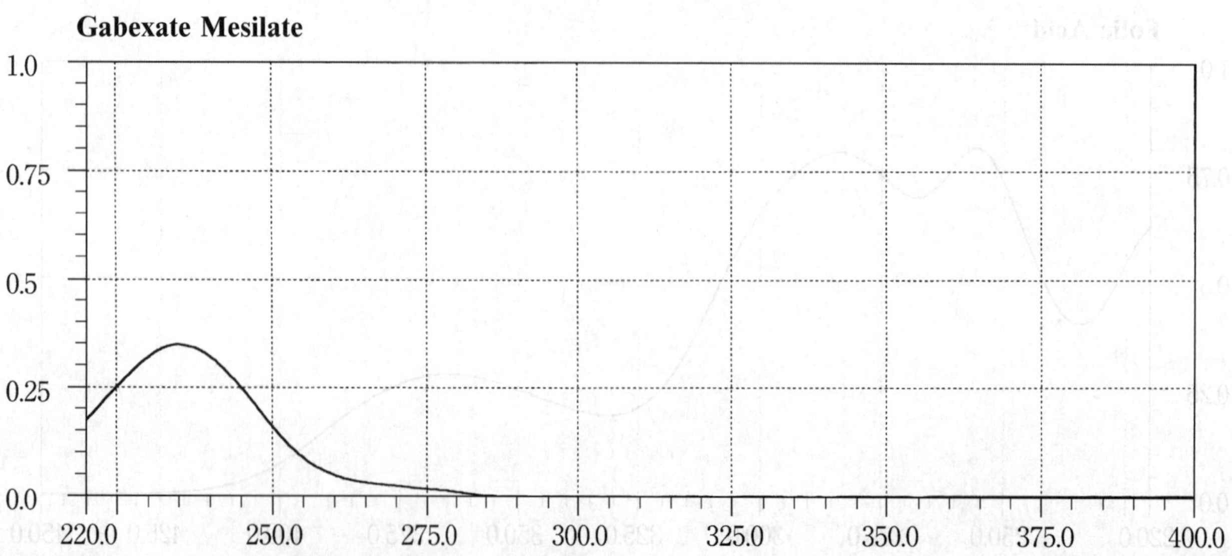

β-Galactosidase (Aspergillus)

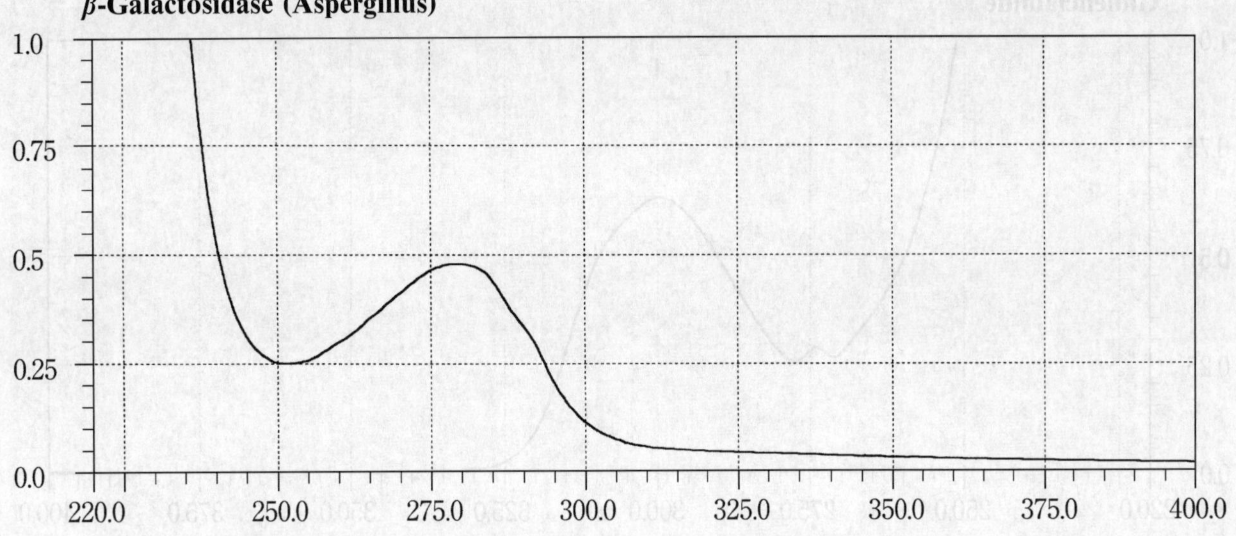

Gatifloxacin Hydrate

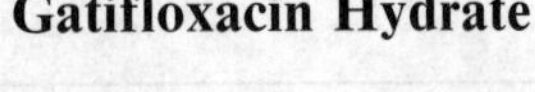

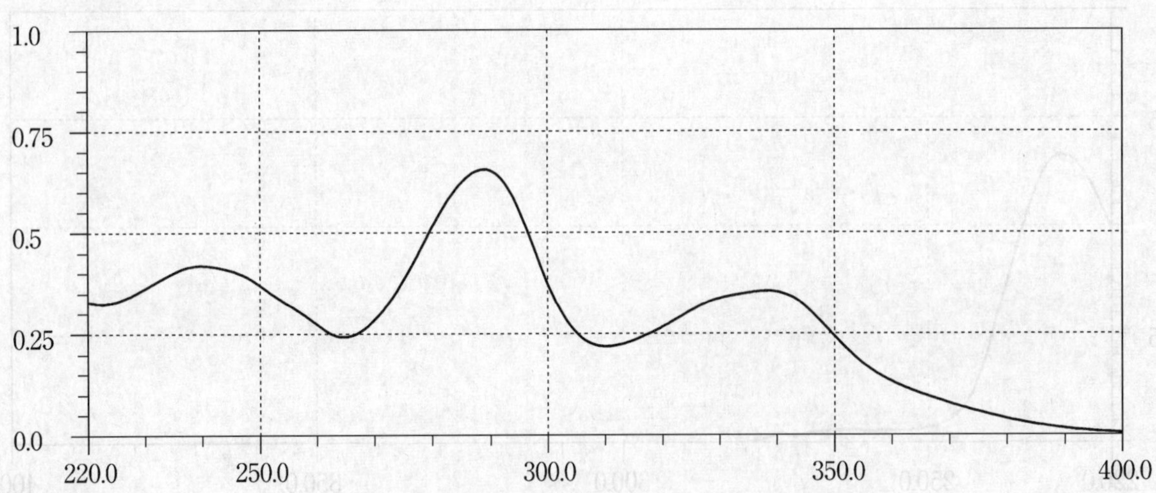

Gefitinib

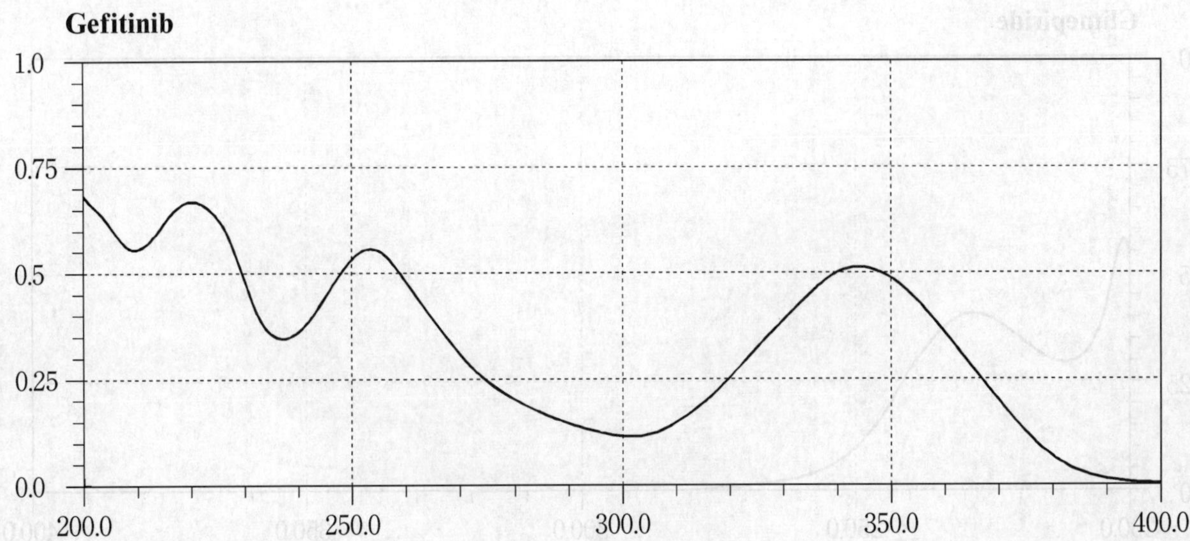

Glibenclamide

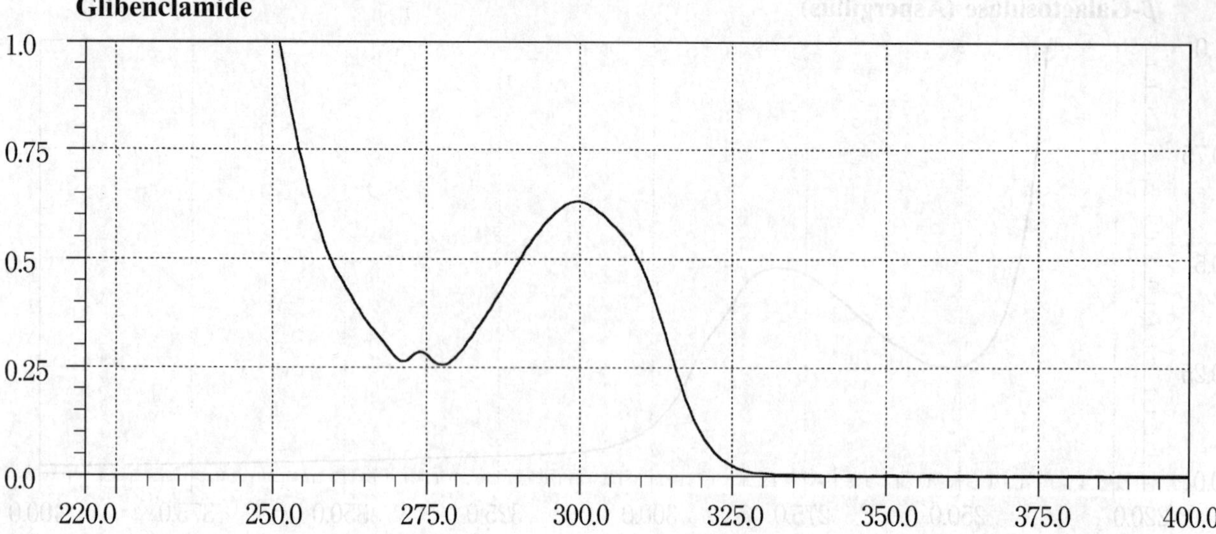

Gliclazide

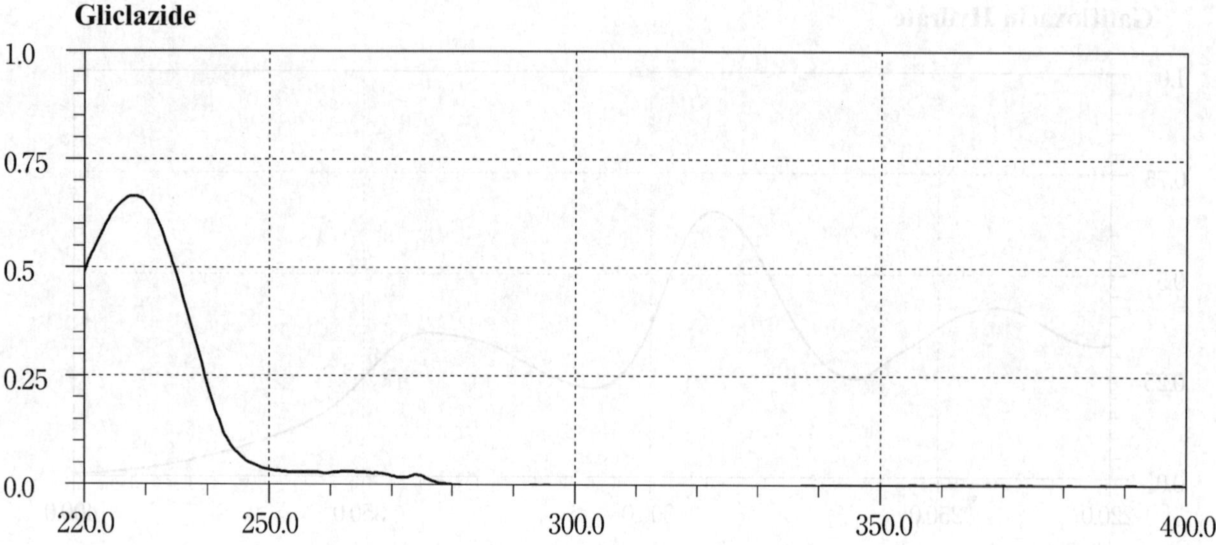

Glimepiride

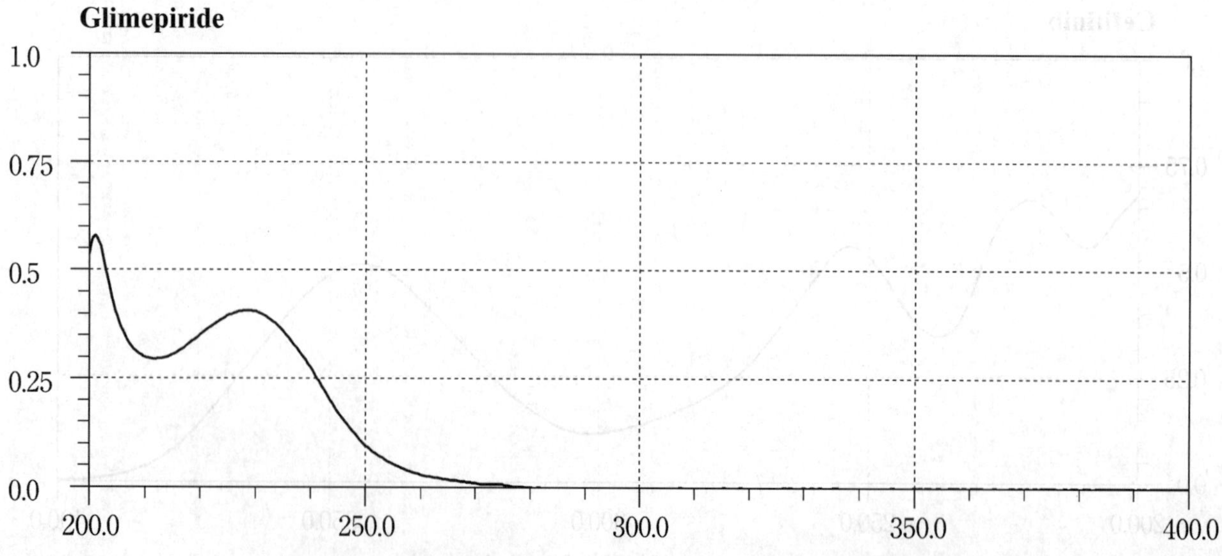

Gonadorelin Acetate

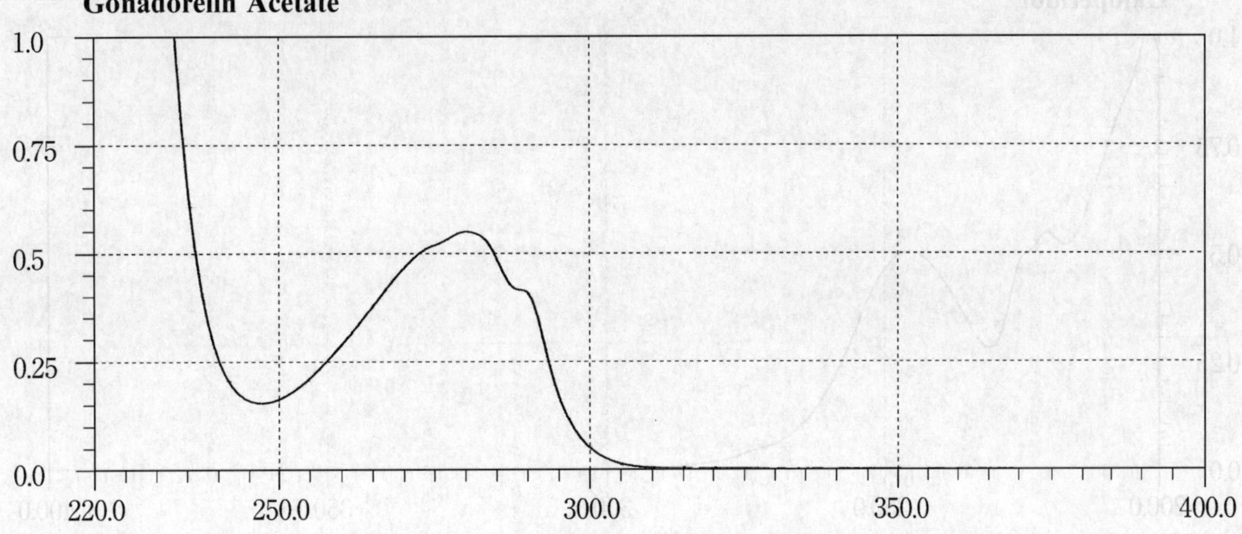

Guaifenesin

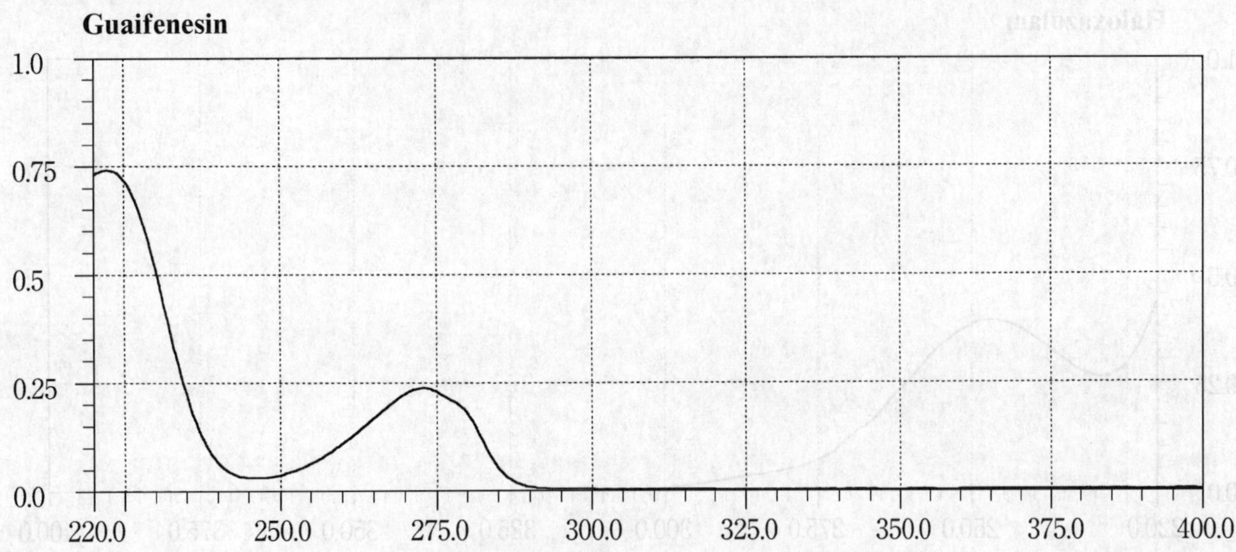

Guanabenz Acetate

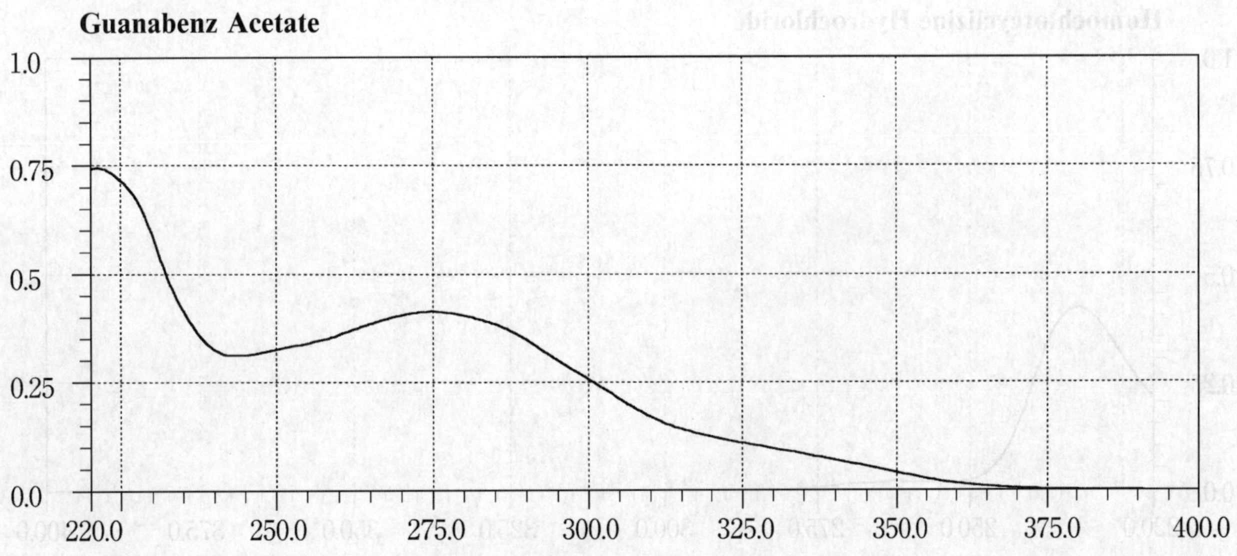

Haloperidol

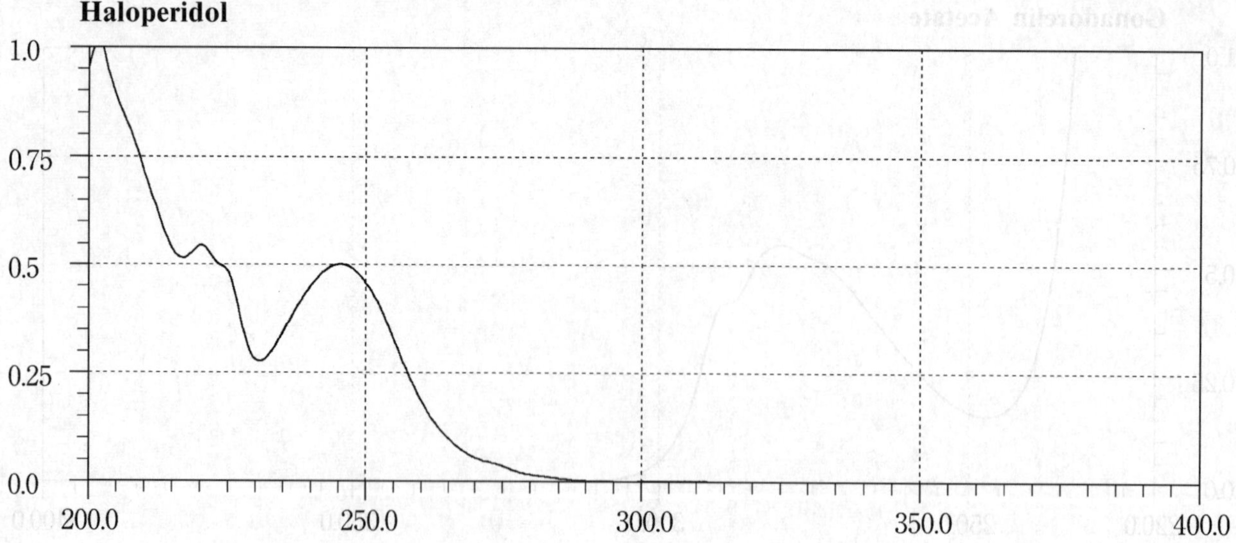

Haloxazolam

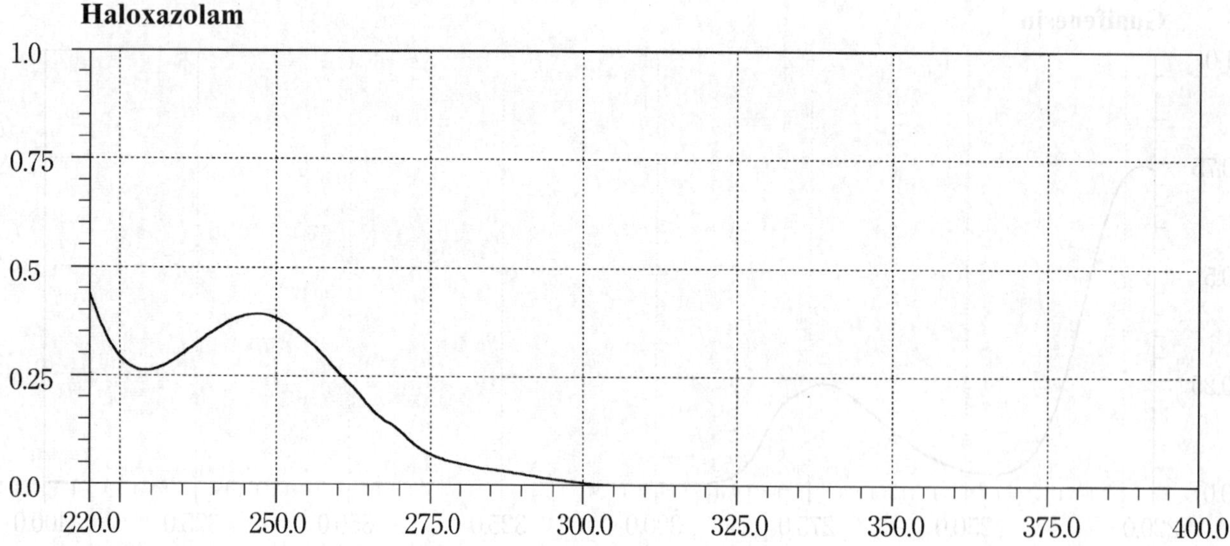

Homochlorcyclizine Hydrochloride

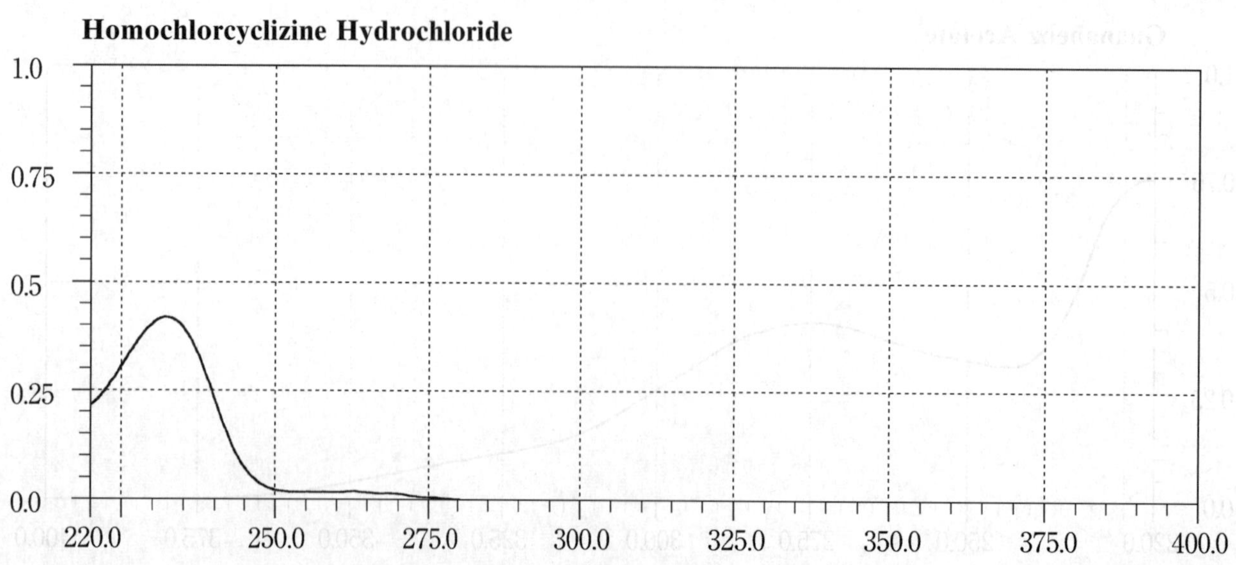

Hydralazine Hydrochloride

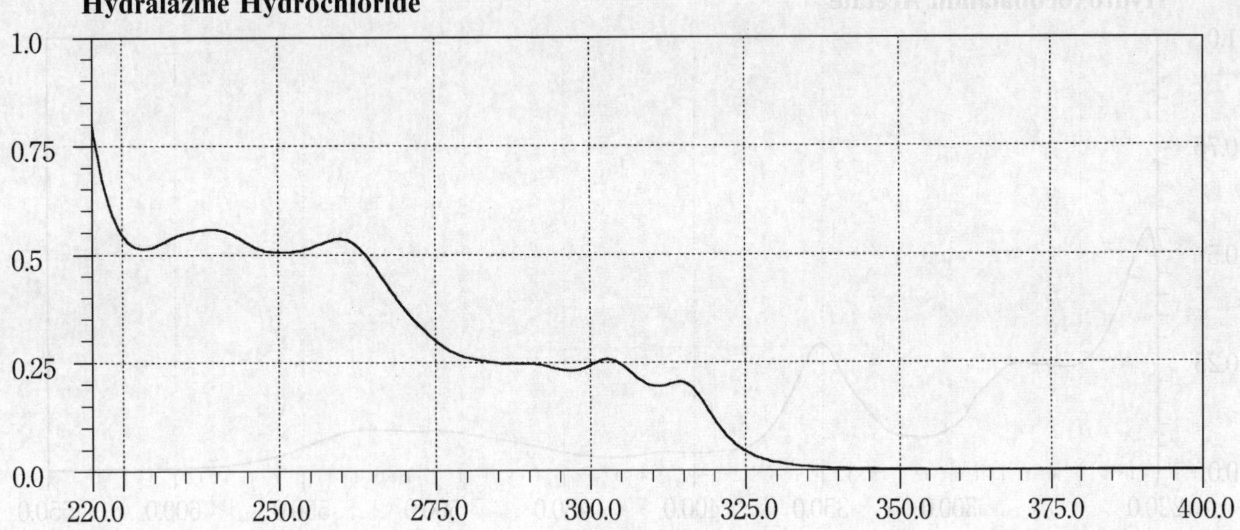

Hydrochlorothiazide

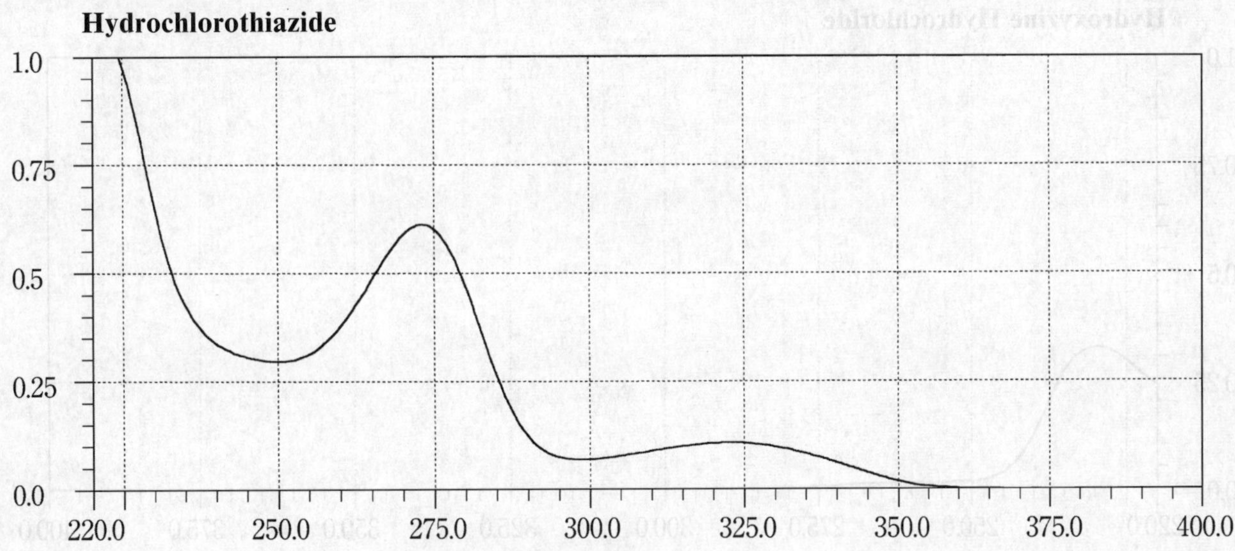

Hydrocotarnine Hydrochloride Hydrate

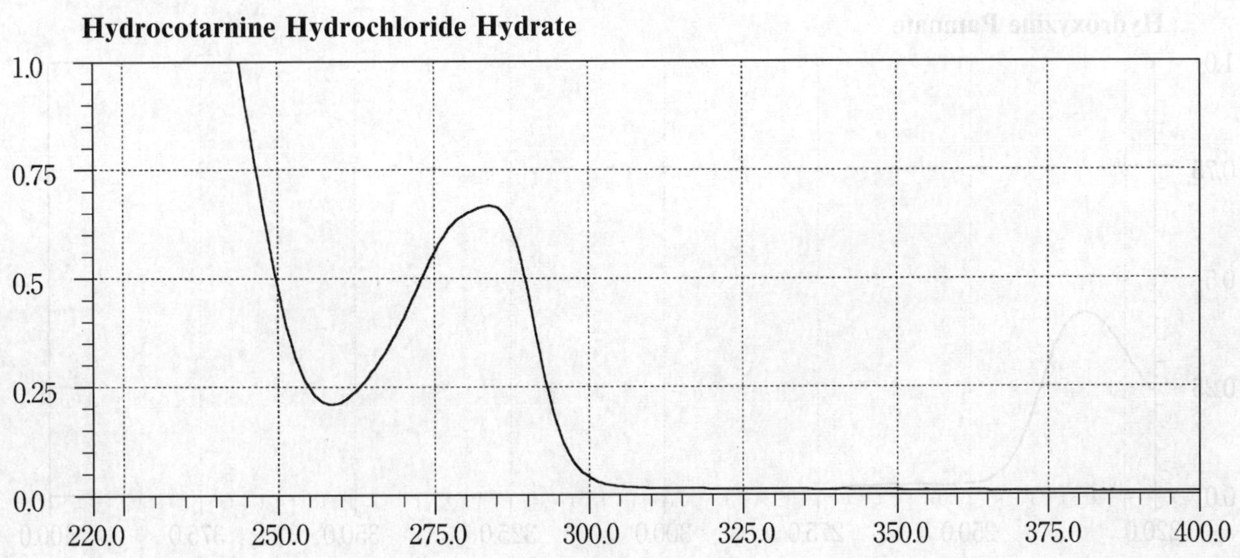

Hydroxocobalamin Acetate

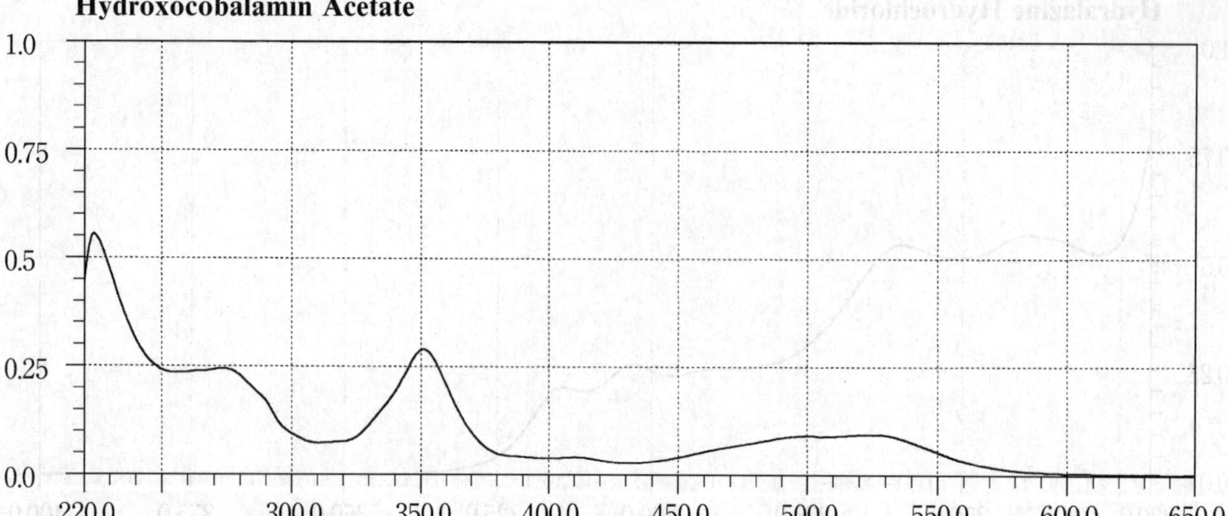

Hydroxyzine Hydrochloride

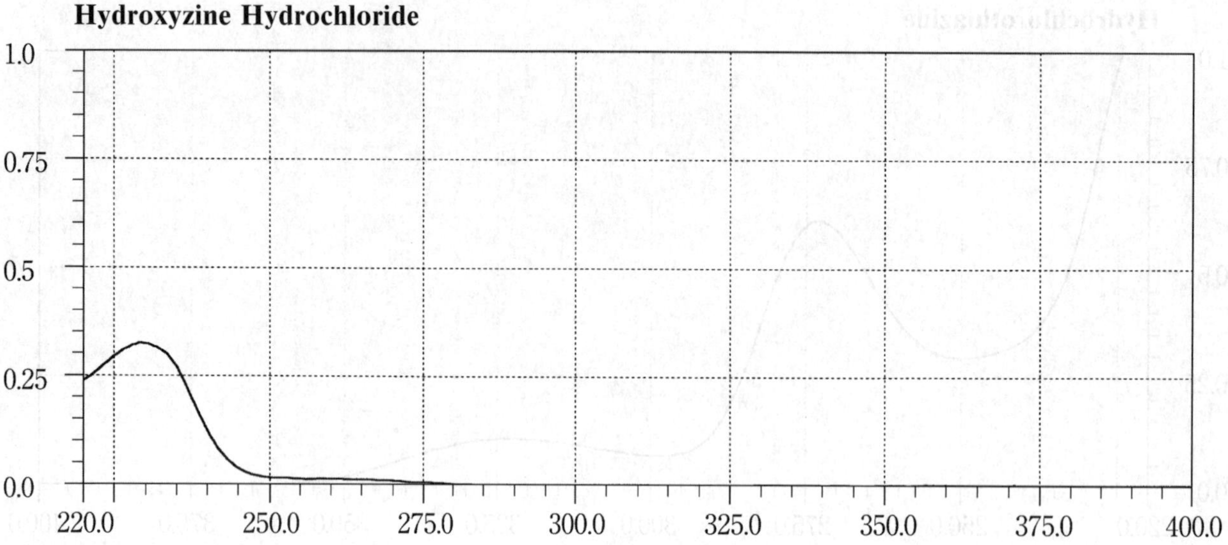

Hydroxyzine Pamoate

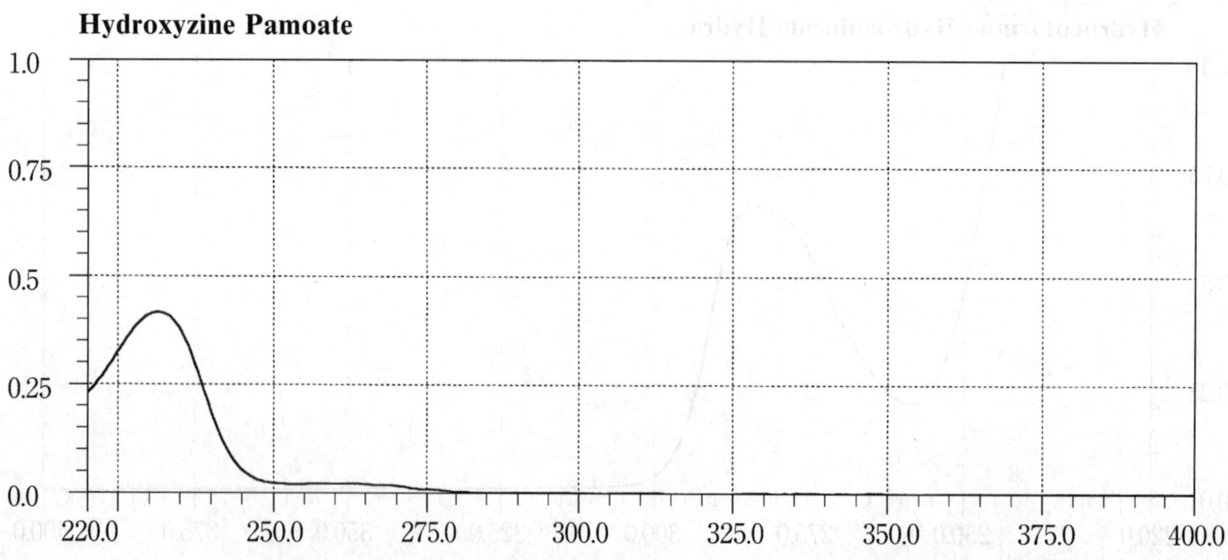

Hymecromone

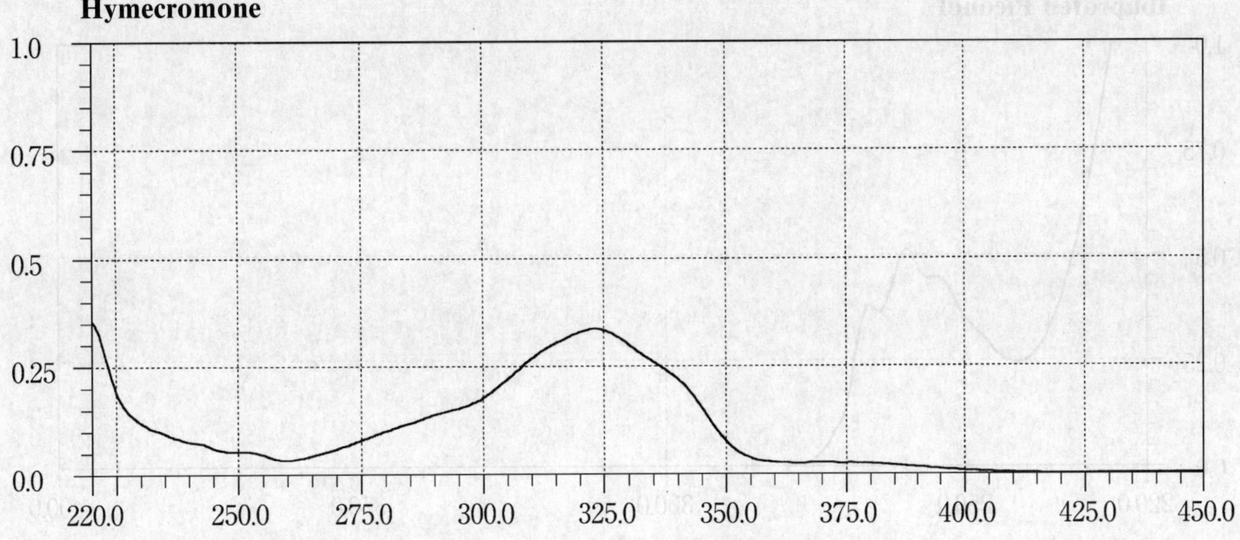

Ibudilast

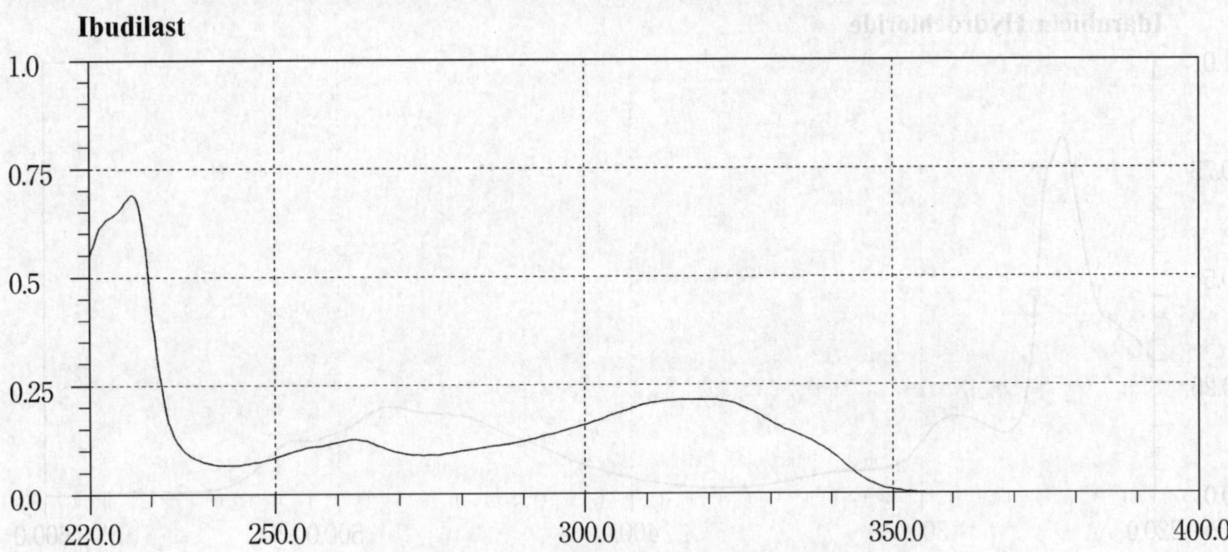

Ibuprofen

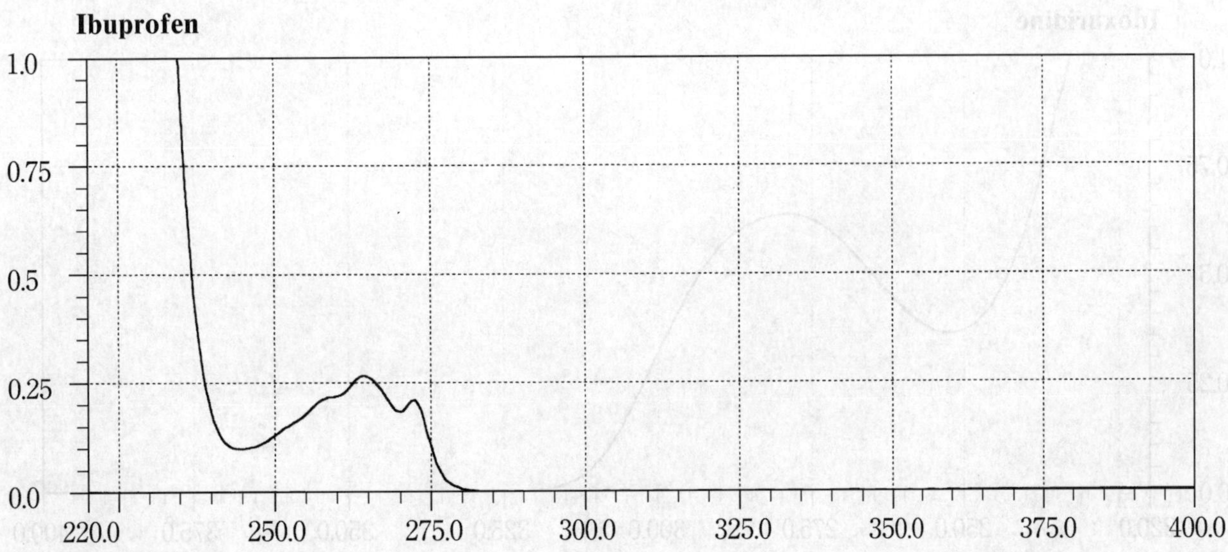

Ibuprofen Piconol

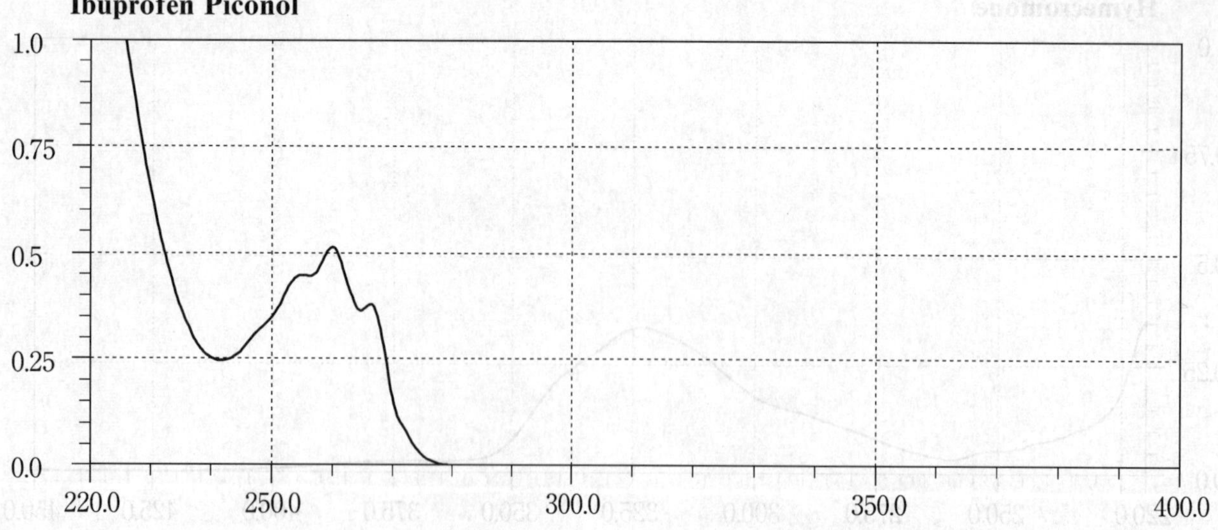

Idarubicin Hydrochloride

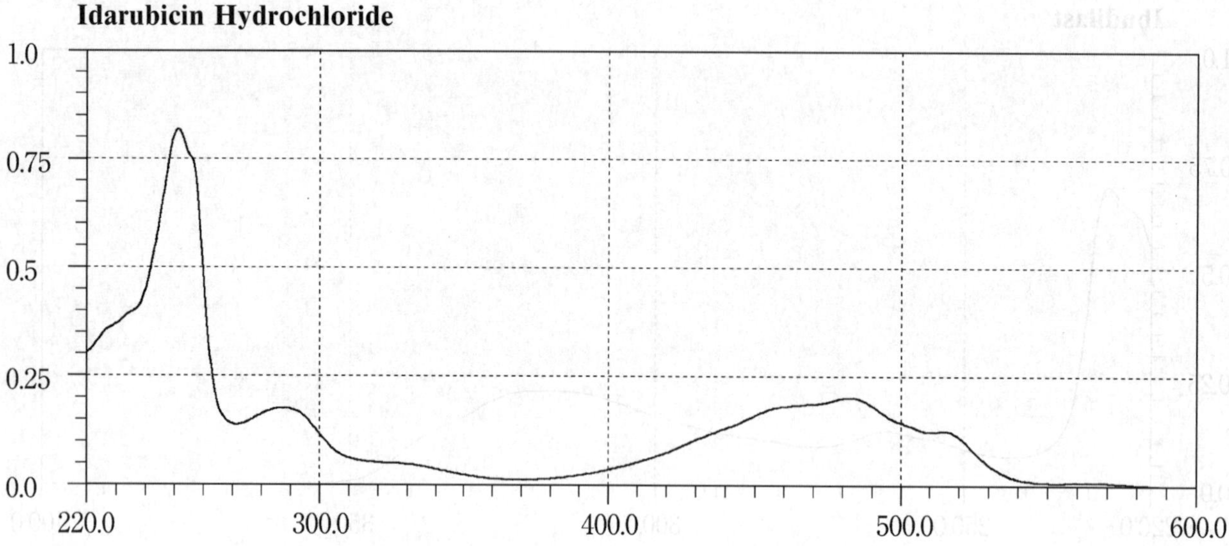

Idoxuridine

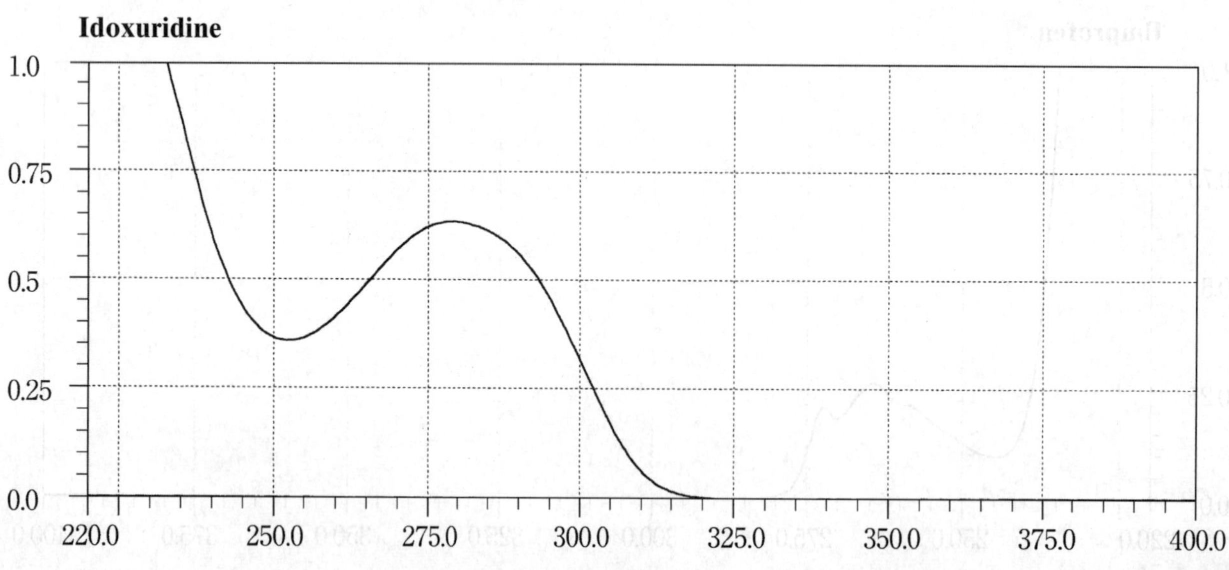

Ifenprodil Tartrate

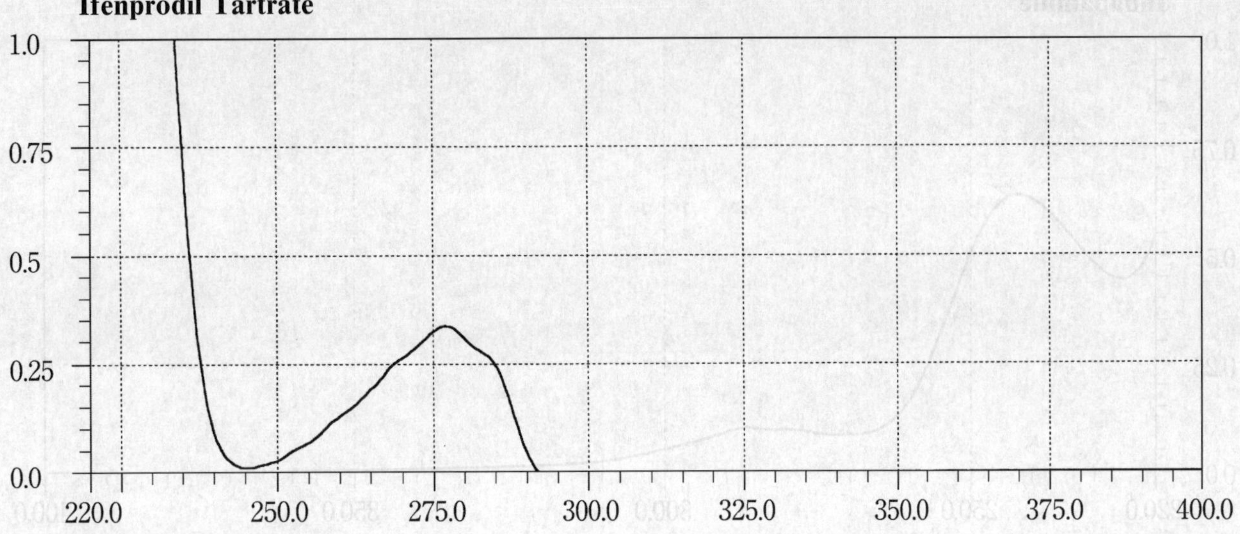

Imipenem Hydrate

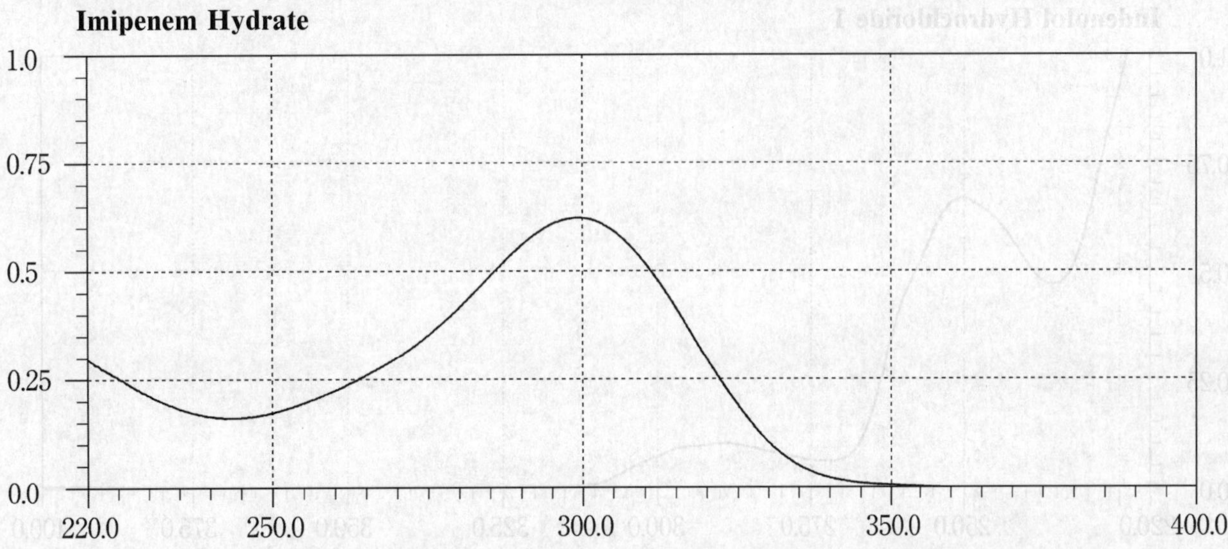

Imipramine Hydrochloride

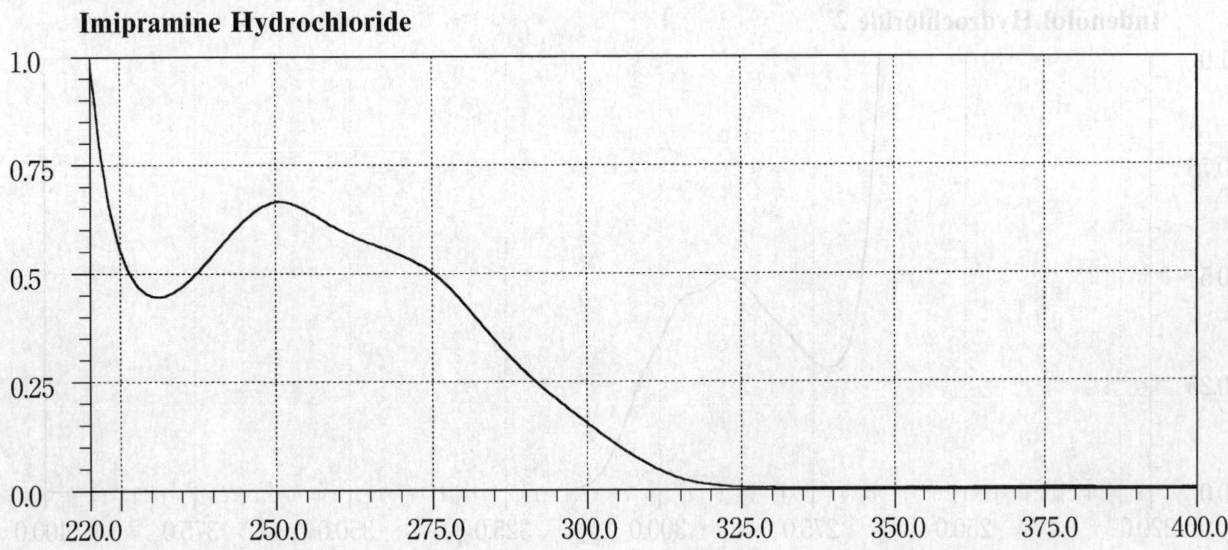

Indapamide

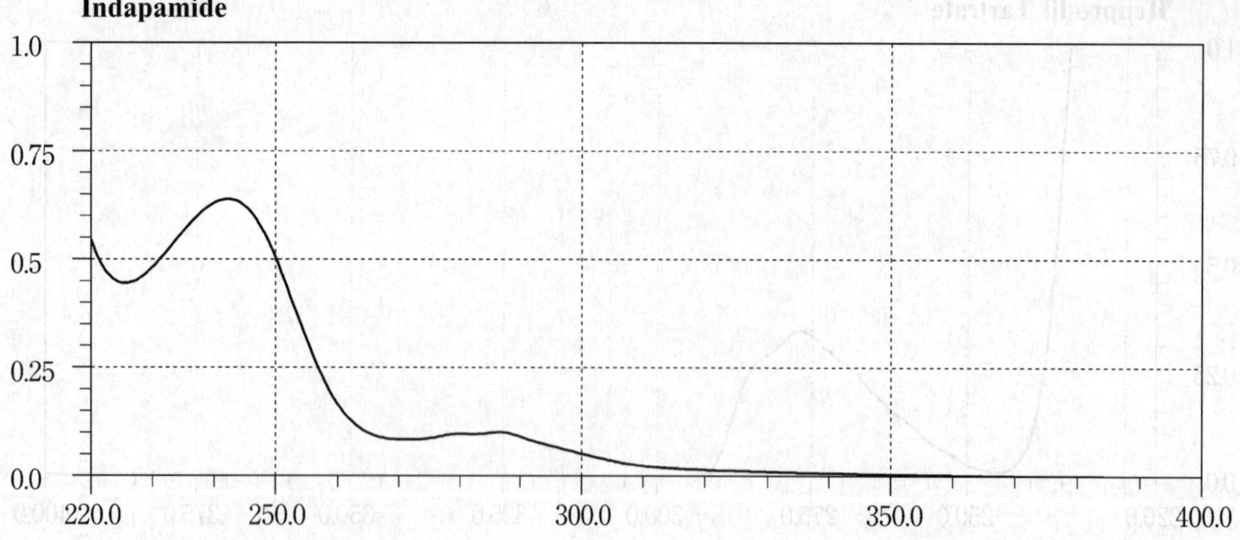

Indenolol Hydrochloride 1

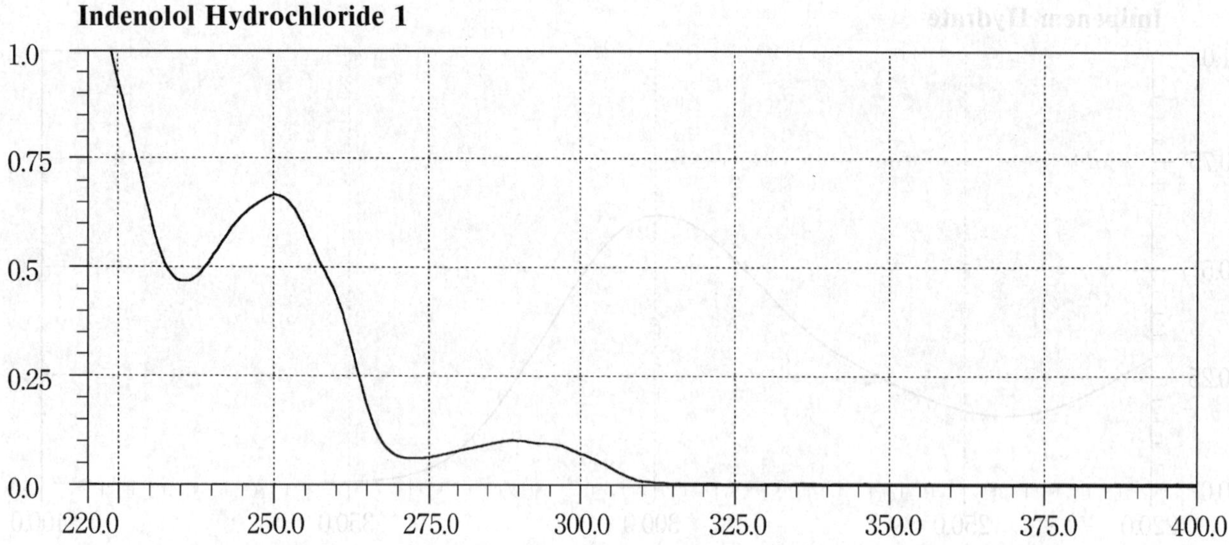

Indenolol Hydrochloride 2

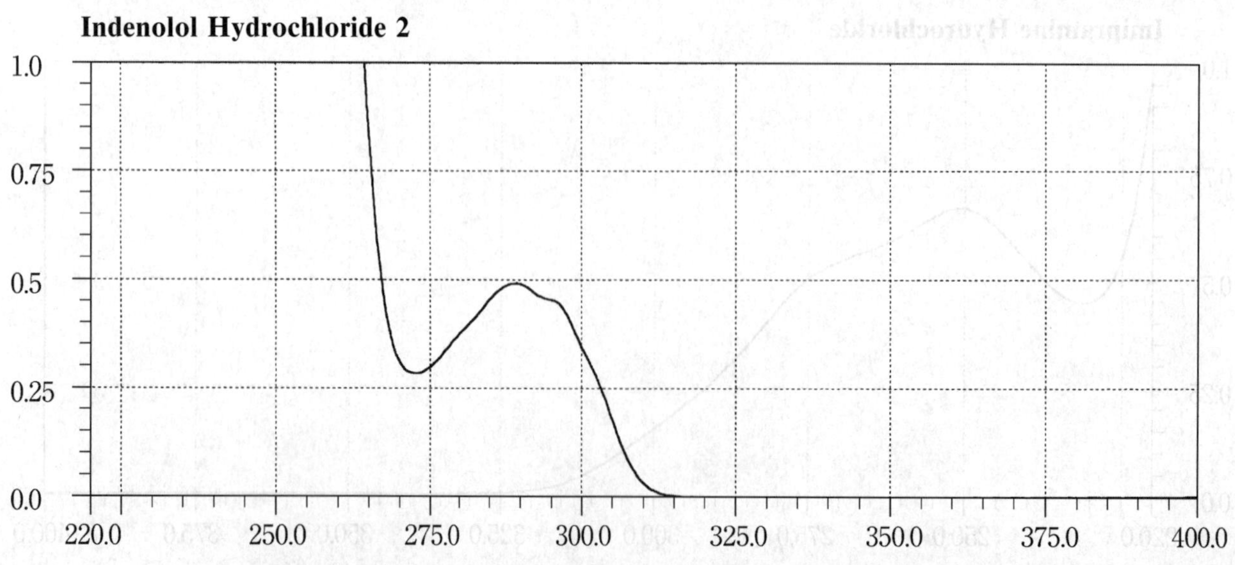

Indigocarmine

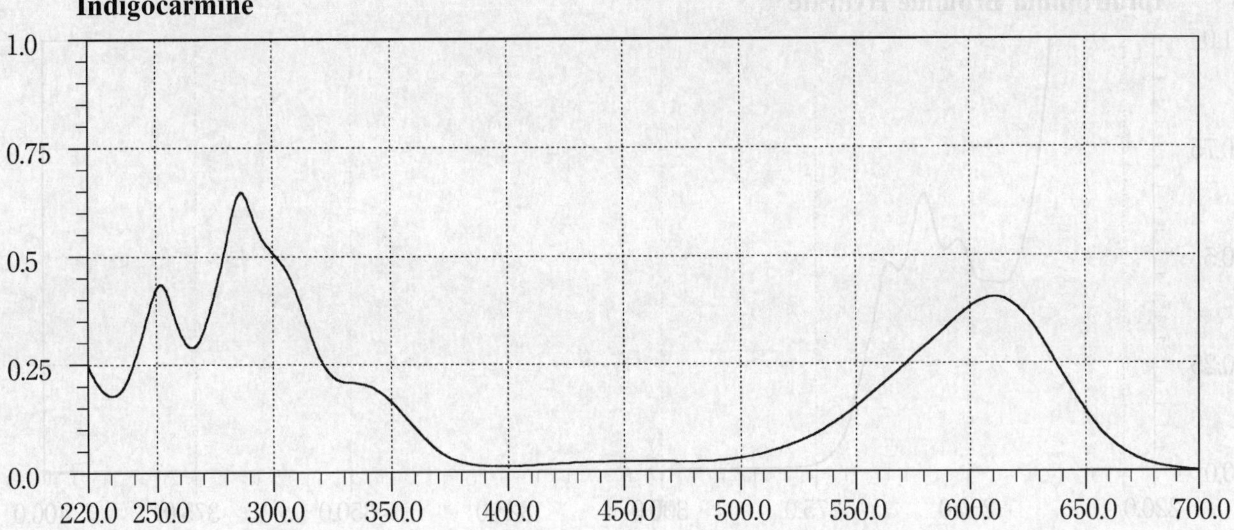

Indometacin

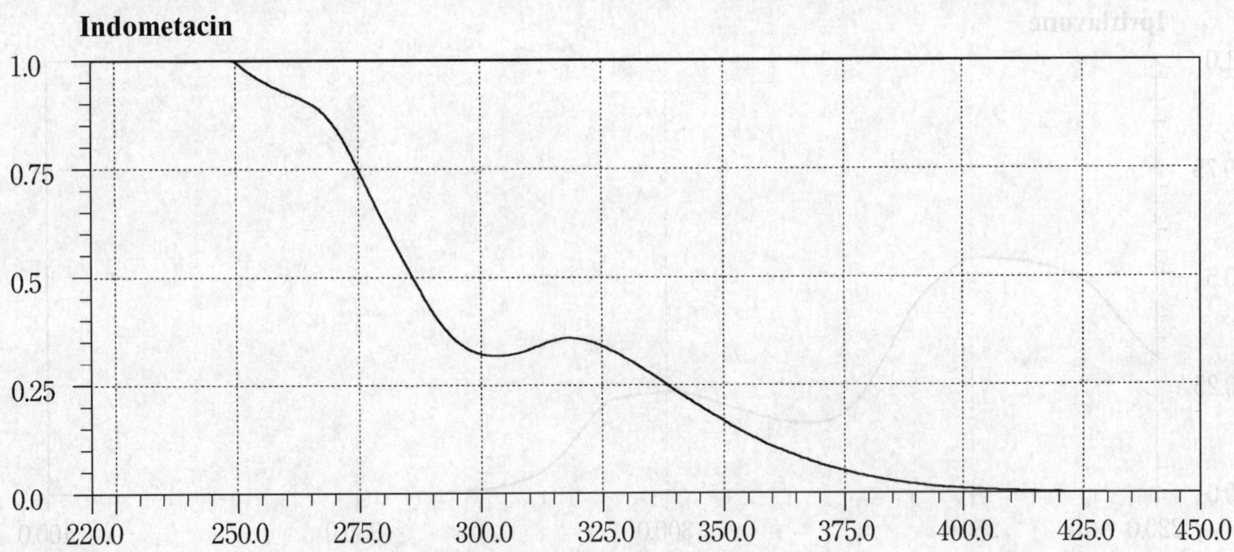

Iohexol

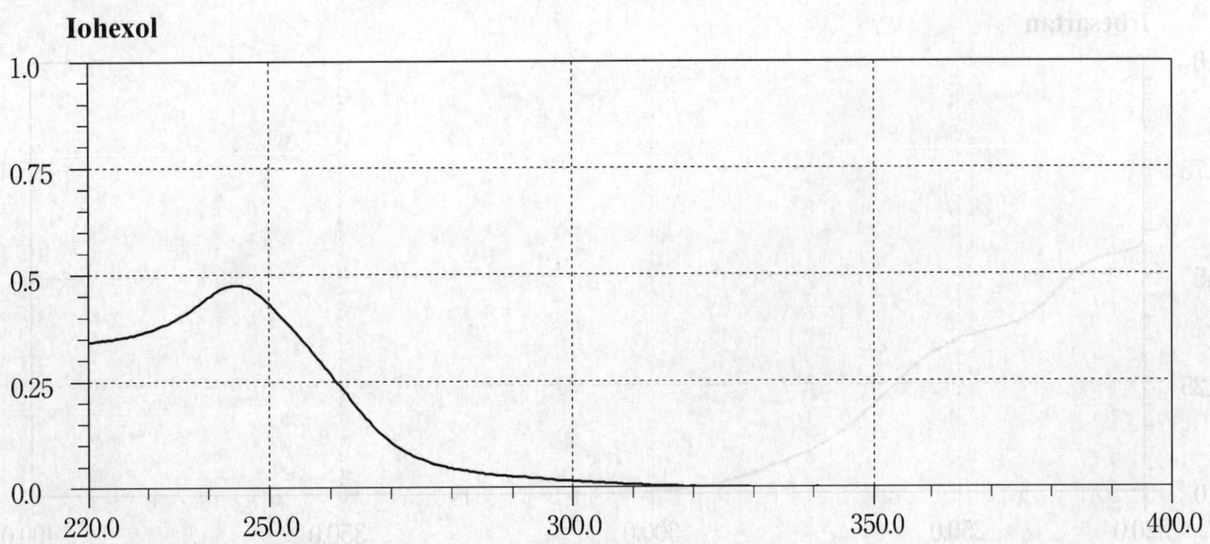

The JP Drugs are to be tested according to the provisions given in the pertinent monographs, General Notices, General Rules for Crude Drugs, General Rules for Preparations, and General Tests for their conformity to the Japanese Pharmacopoeia. (See the General Notices 5.)

Ipratropium Bromide Hydrate

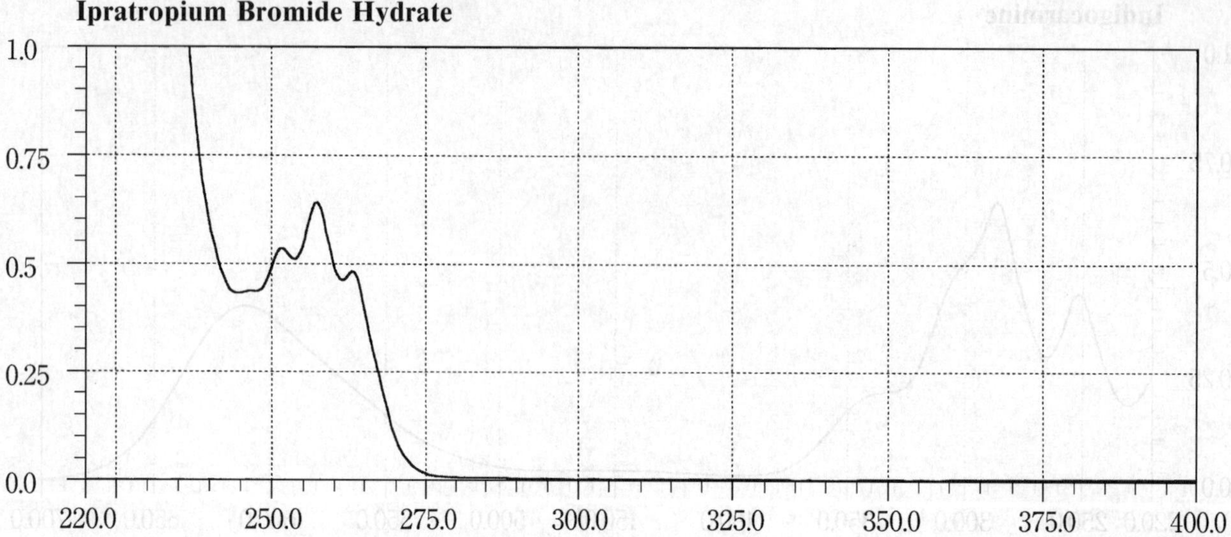

Ipriflavone

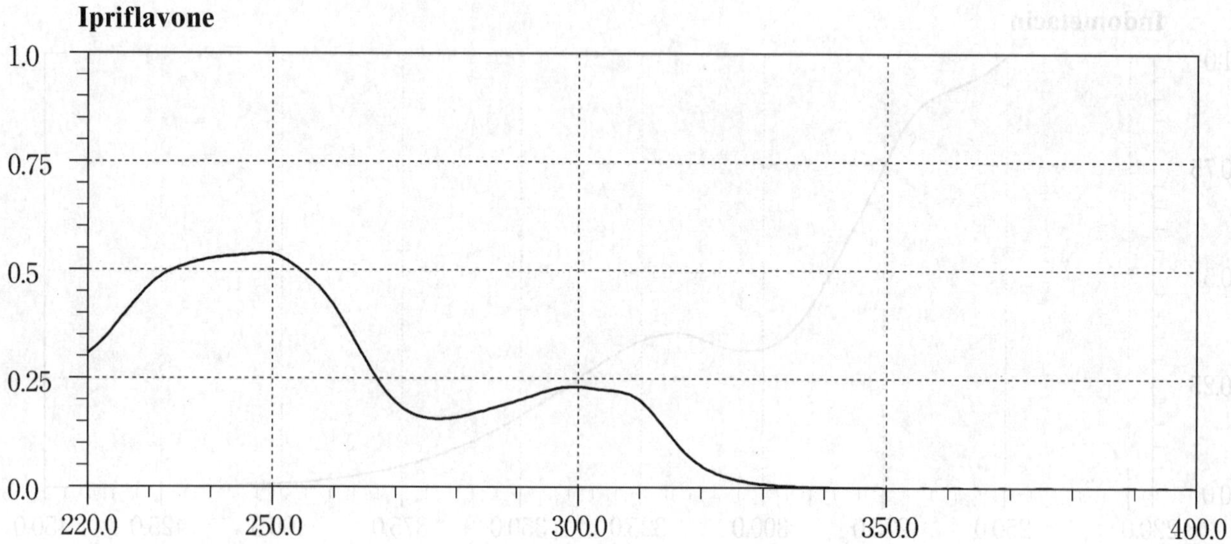

Irbesartan

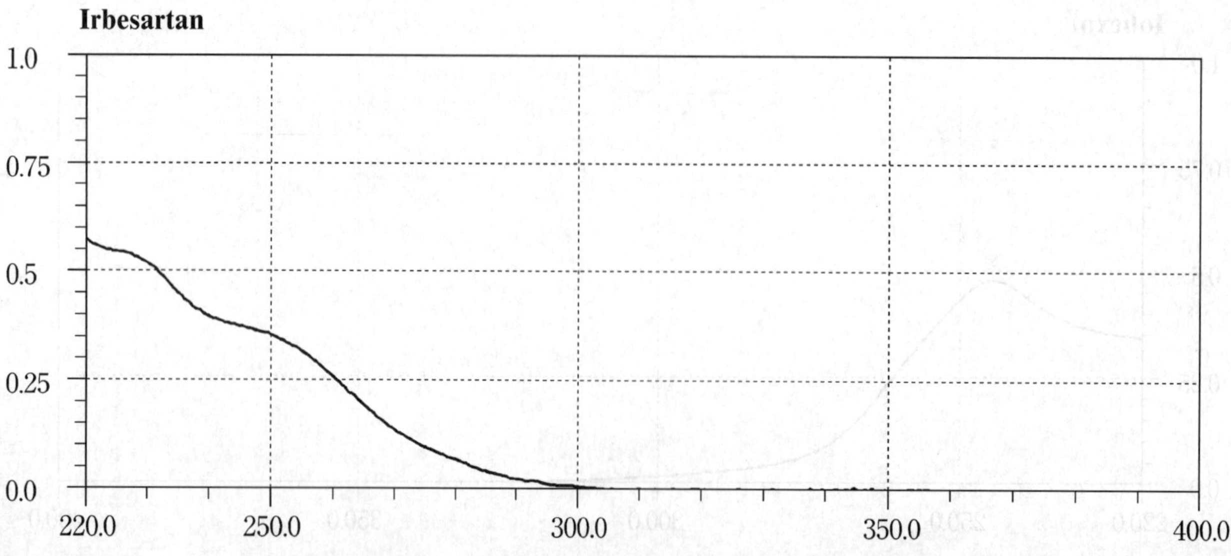

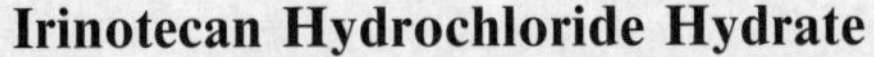

Irinotecan Hydrochloride Hydrate

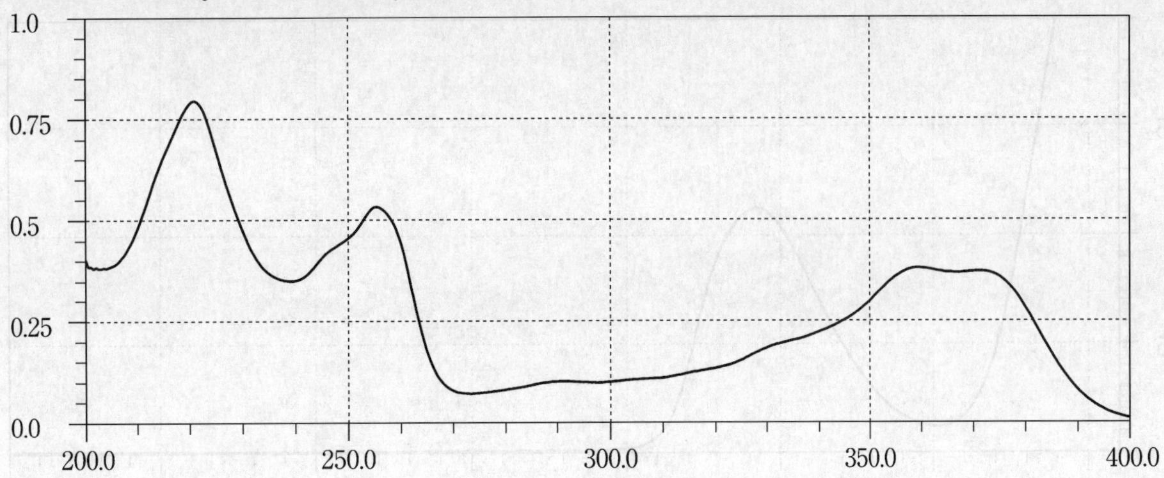

Irsogladine Maleate

1.0
0.75
0.5
0.25
0.0
200.0
250.0
300.0
350.0
400.0

Isoniazid

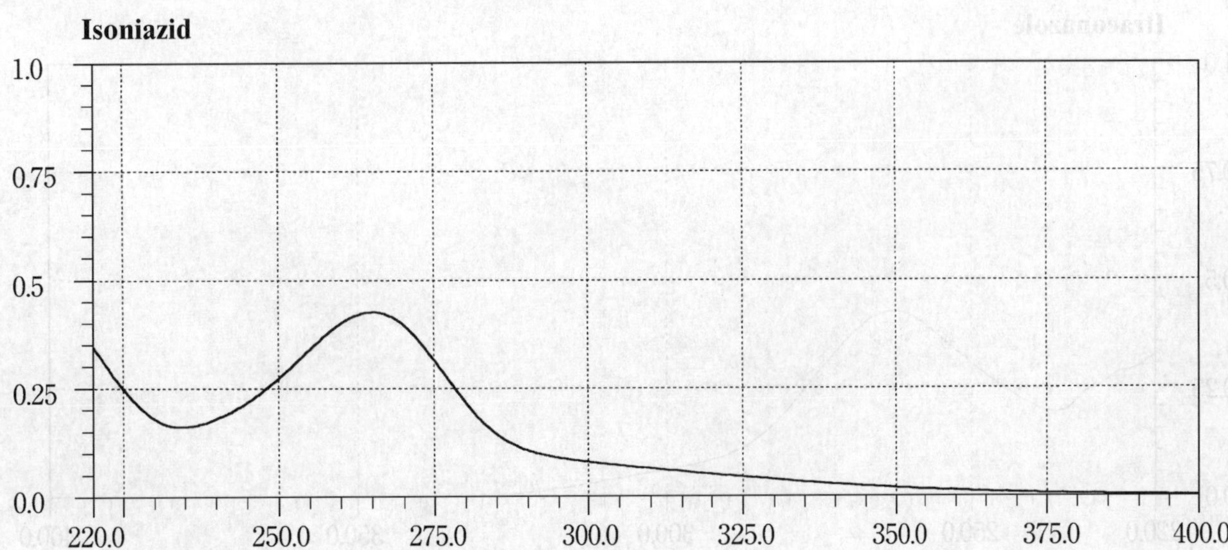

l-Isoprenaline Hydrochloride

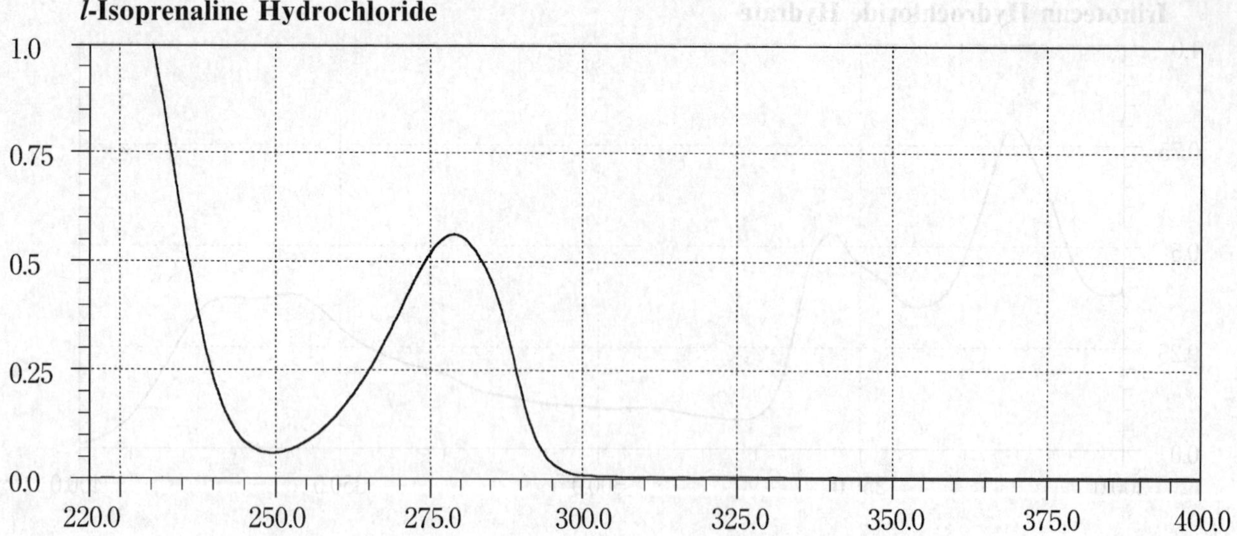

Isoxsuprine Hydrochloride

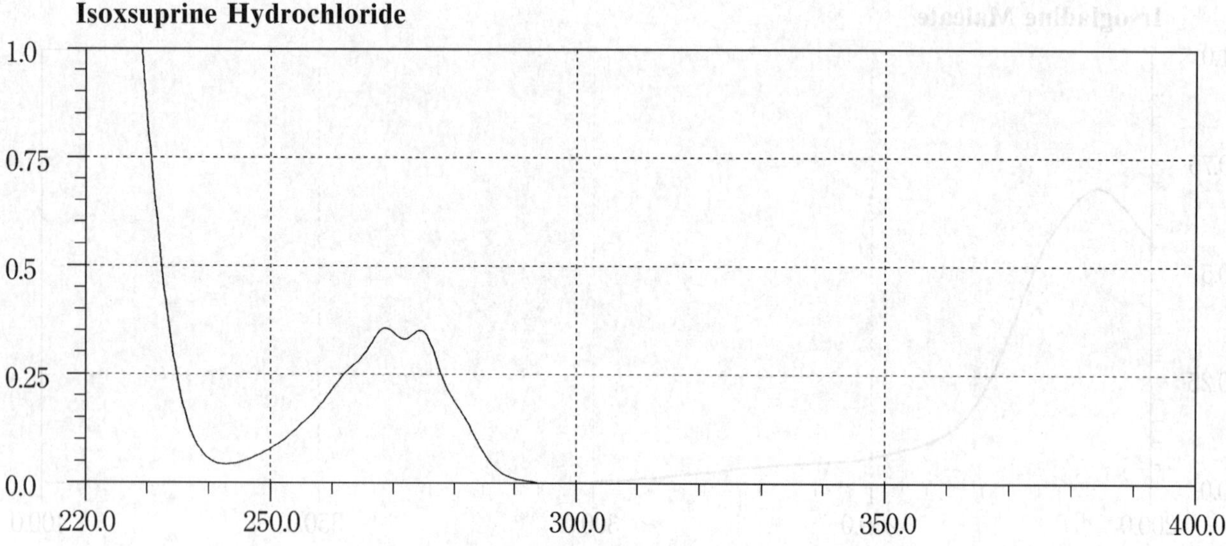

Itraconazole

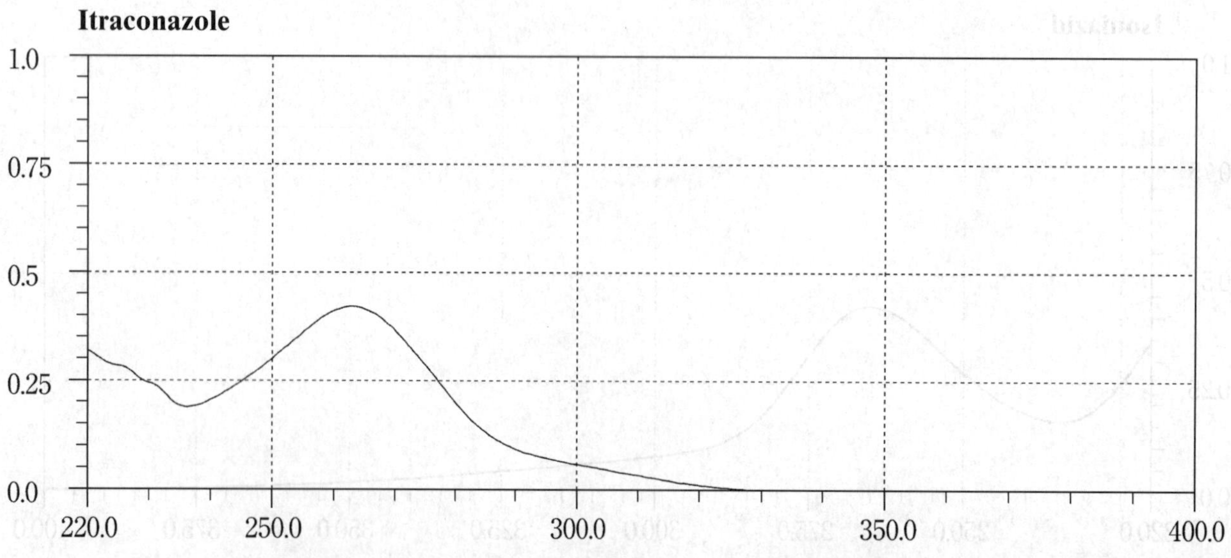

Josamycin

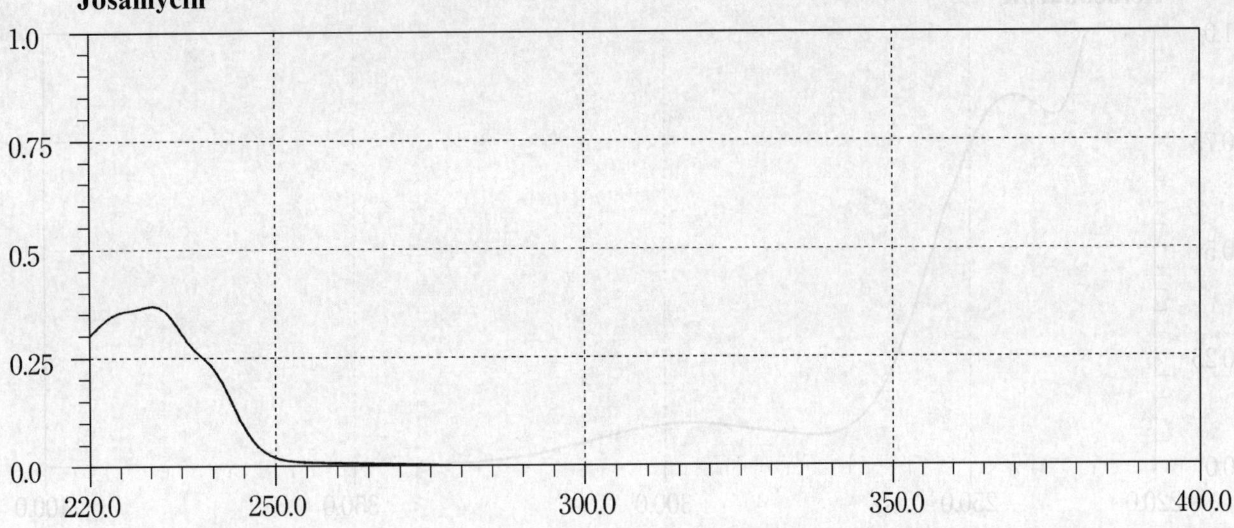

Josamycin Propionate

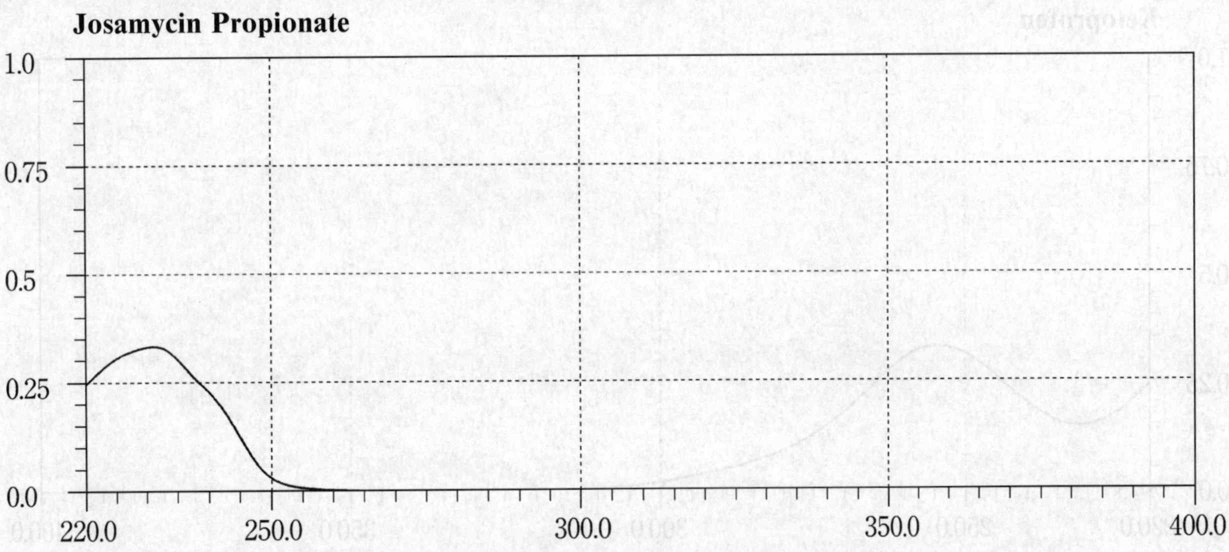

Ketamine Hydrochloride

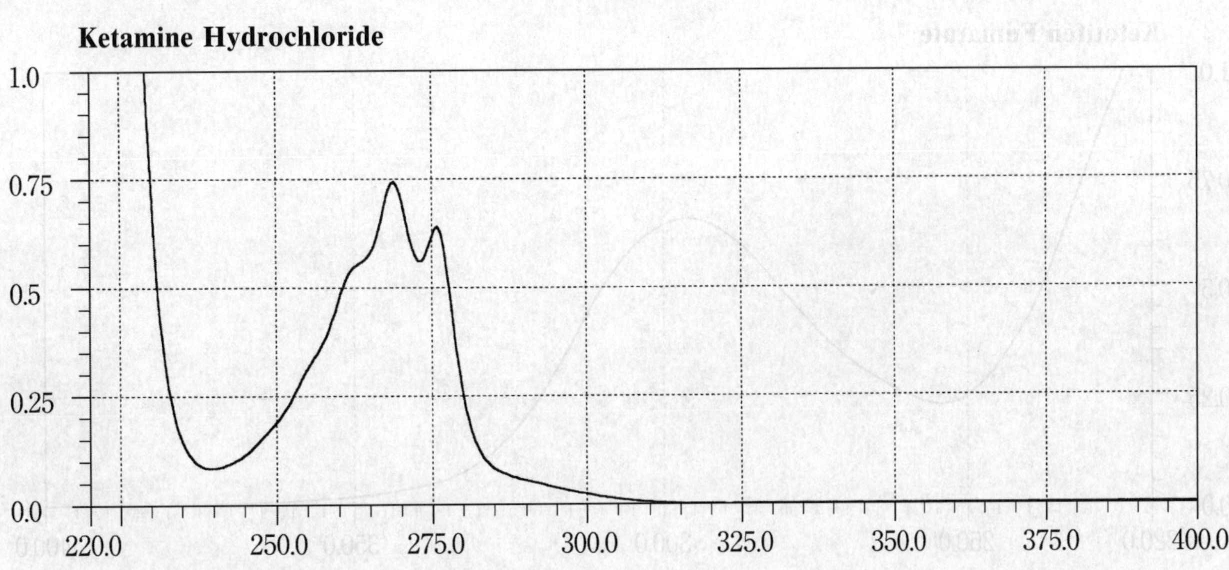

Ketoconazole

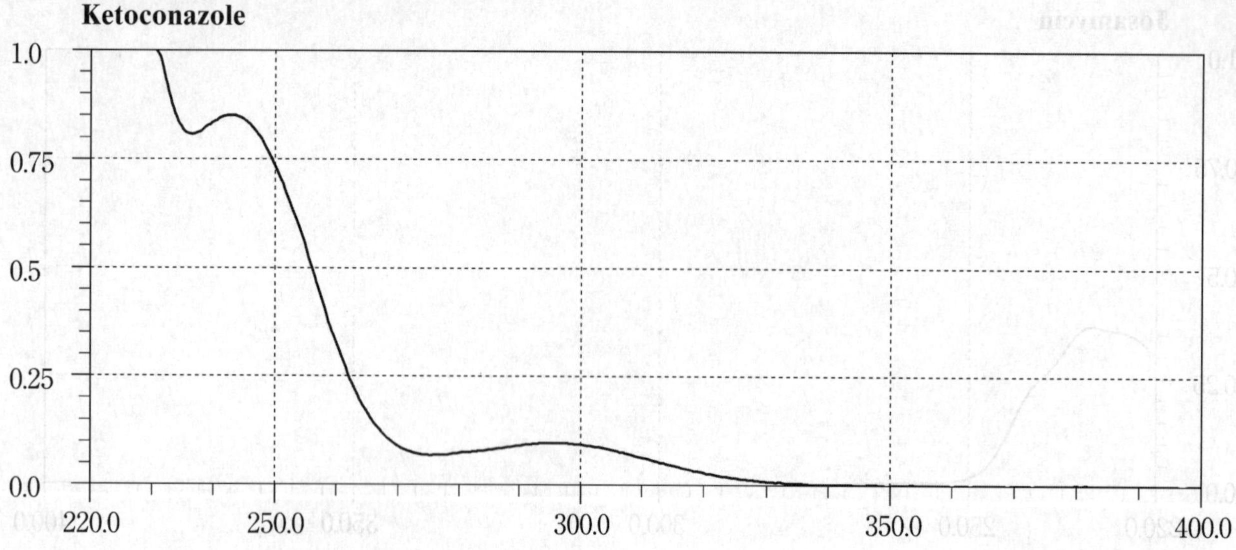

Ketoprofen

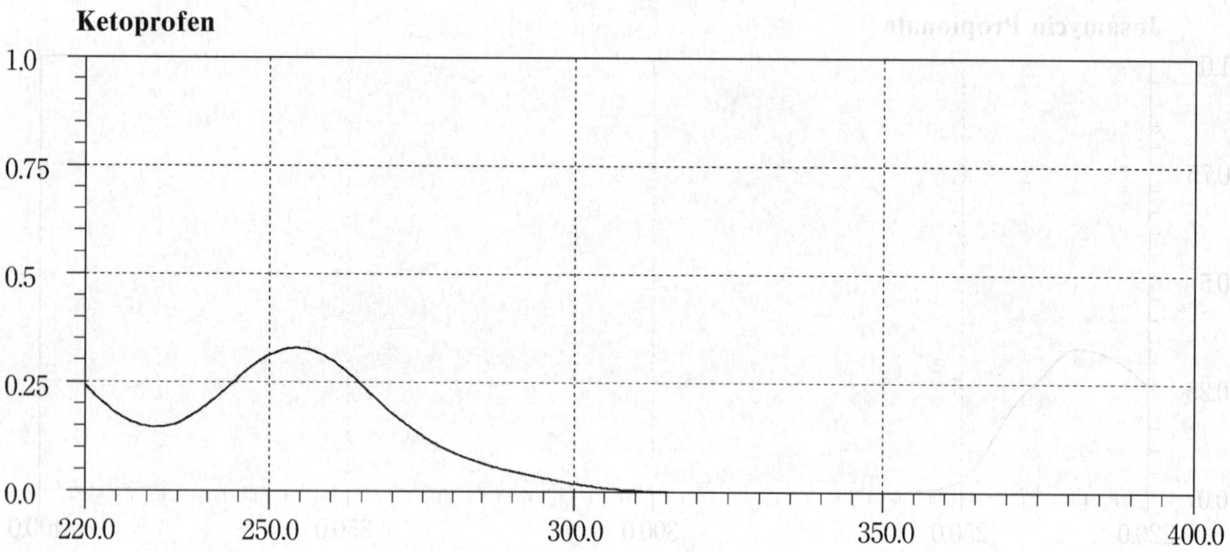

Ketotifen Fumarate

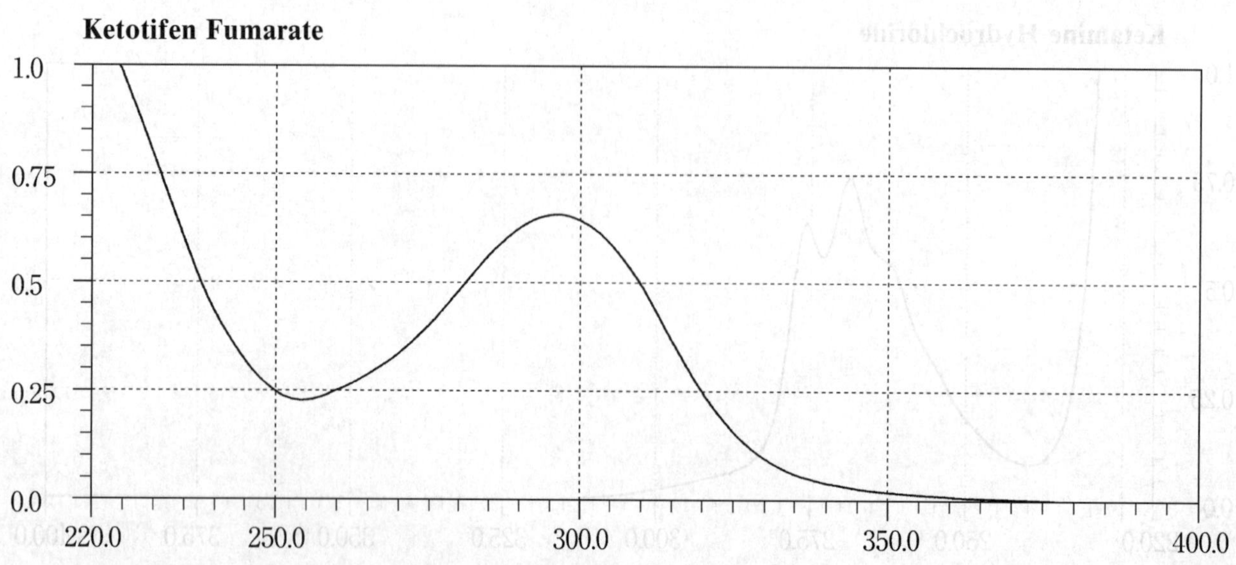

Kitasamycin

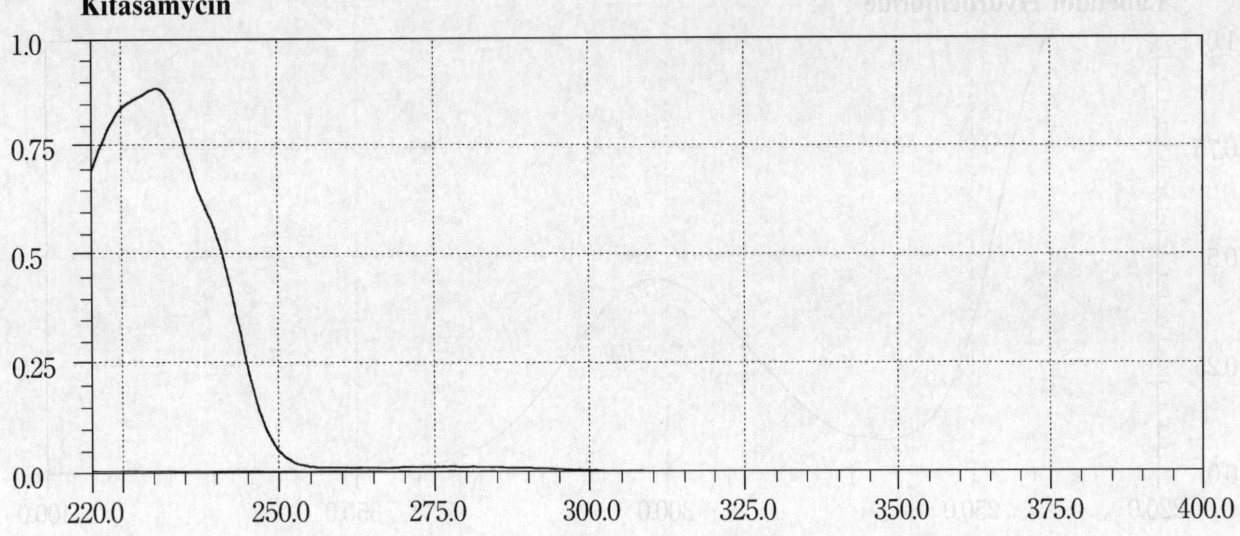

Kitasamycin Acetate

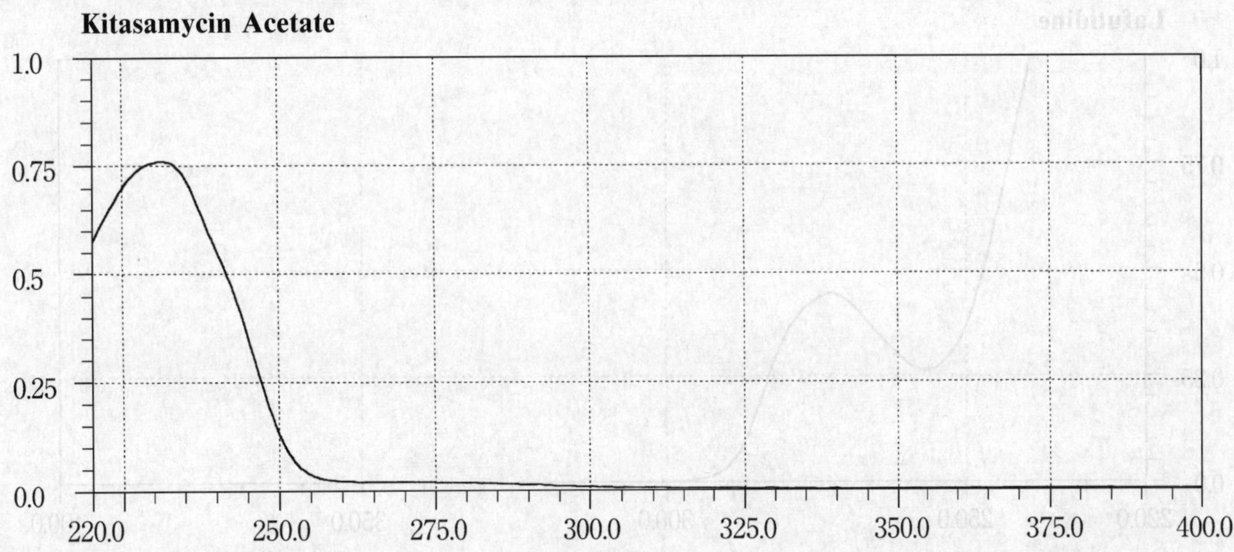

Kitasamycin Tartrate

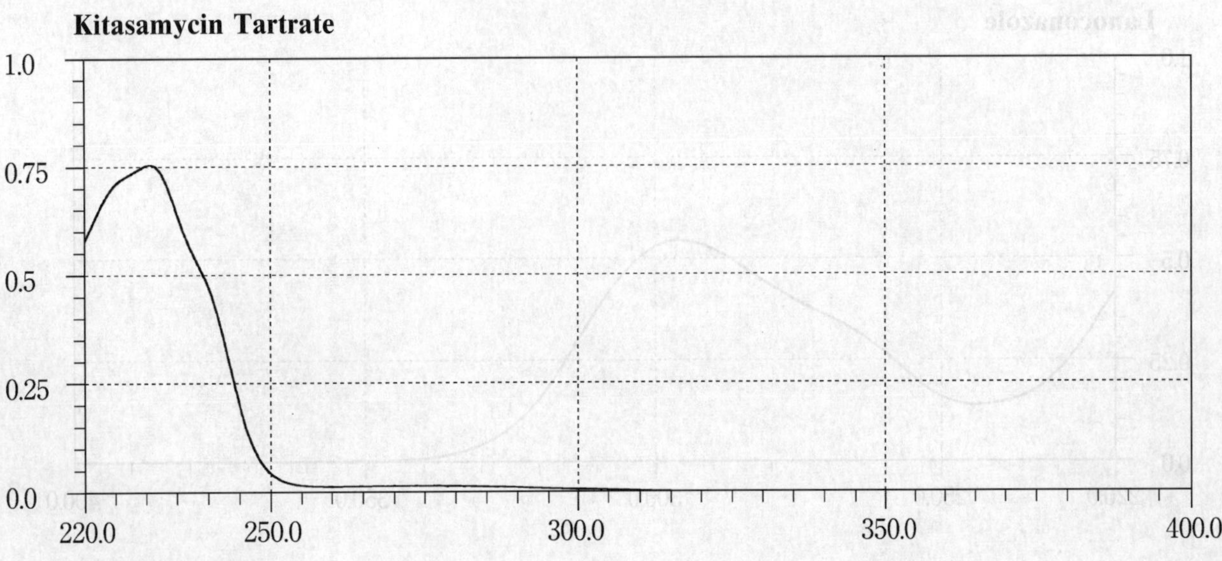

Labetalol Hydrochloride

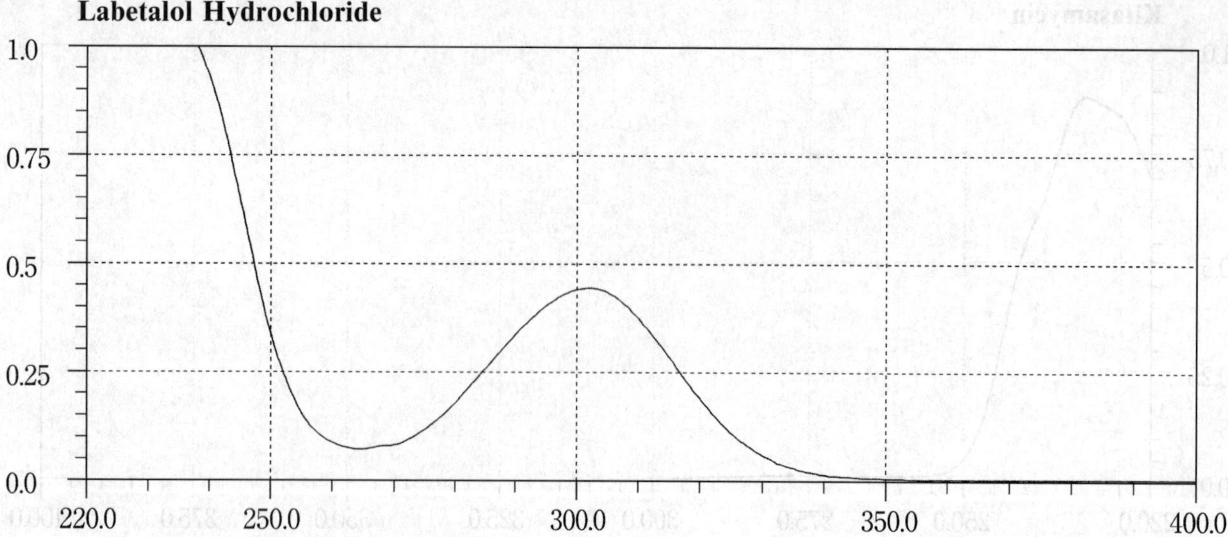

Lafutidine

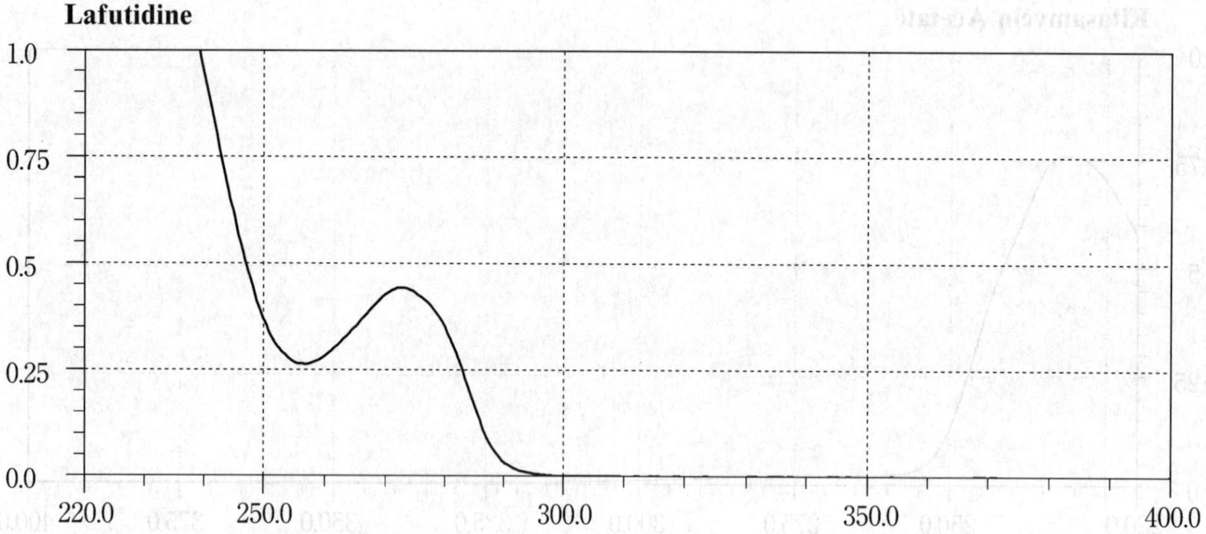

Lanoconazole

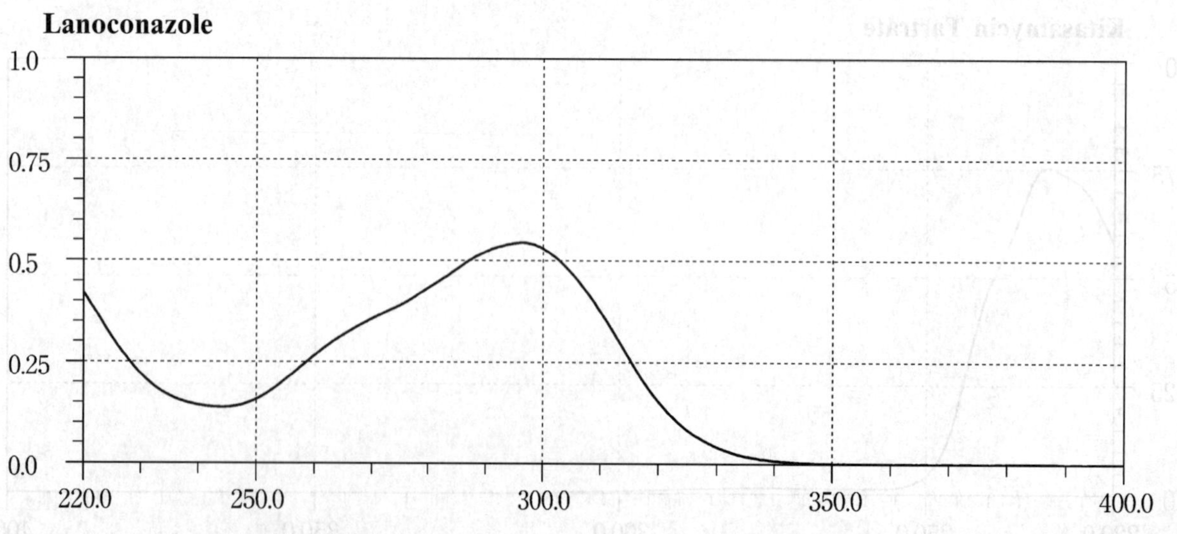

Lansoprazole

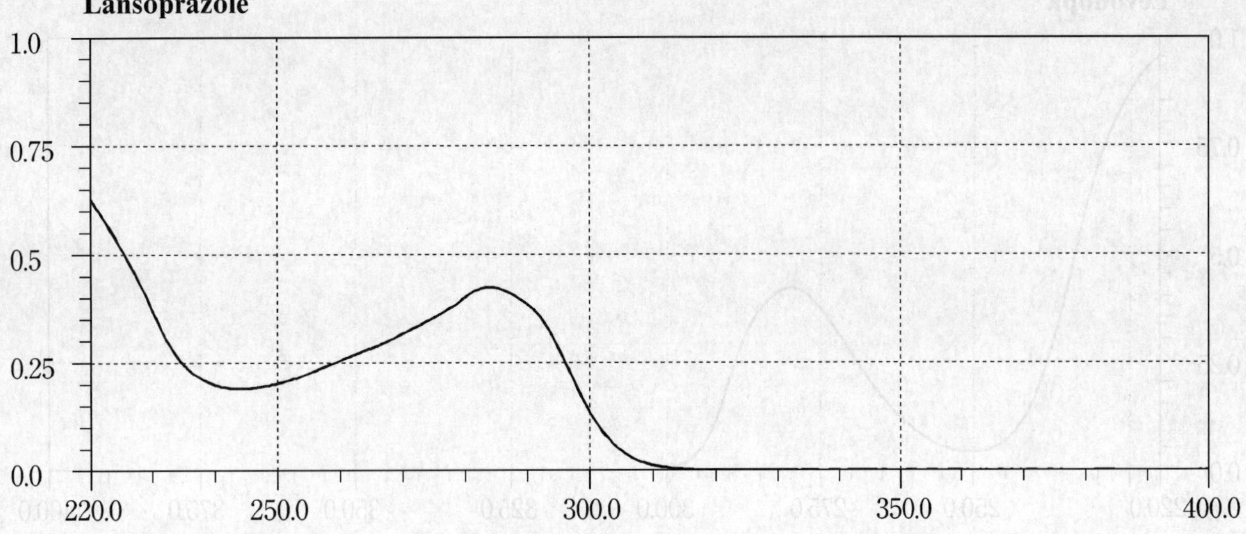

Latamoxef Sodium

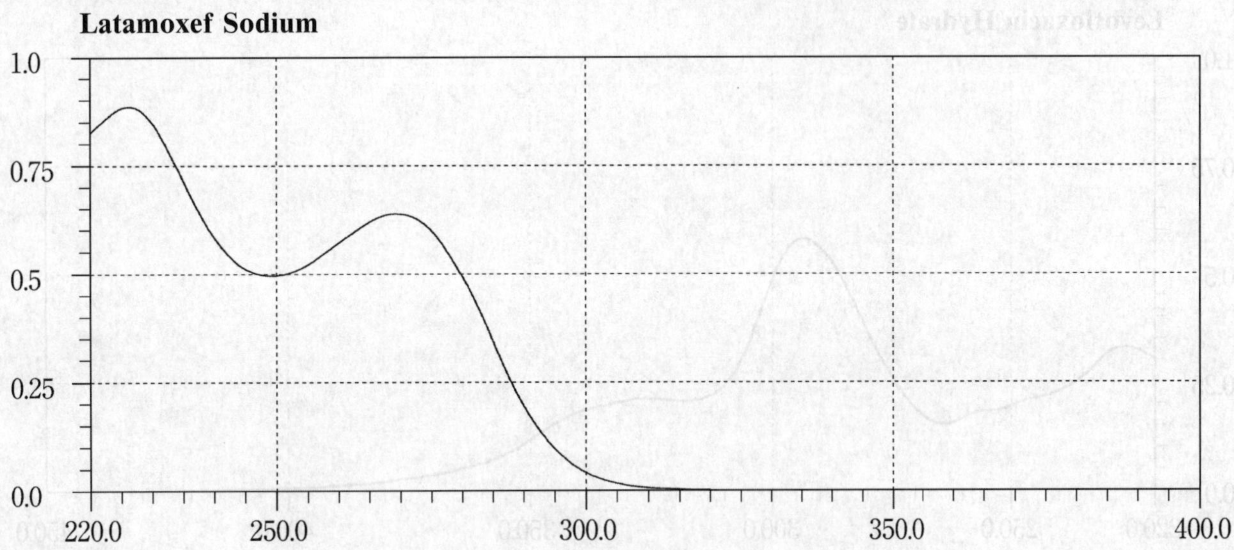

Levallorphan Tartrate

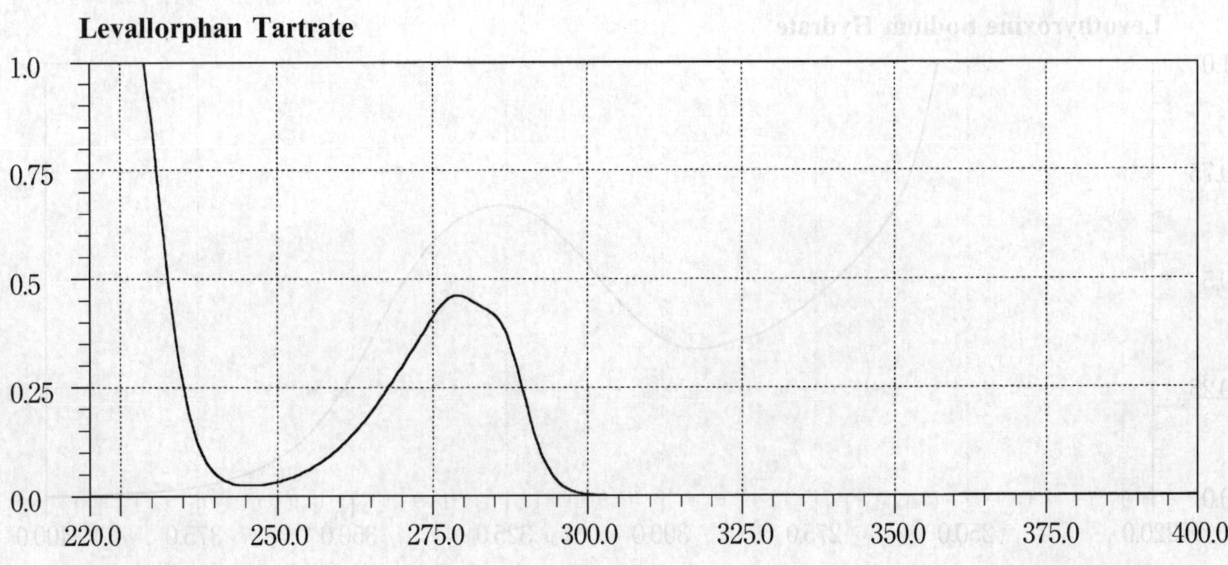

Levodopa

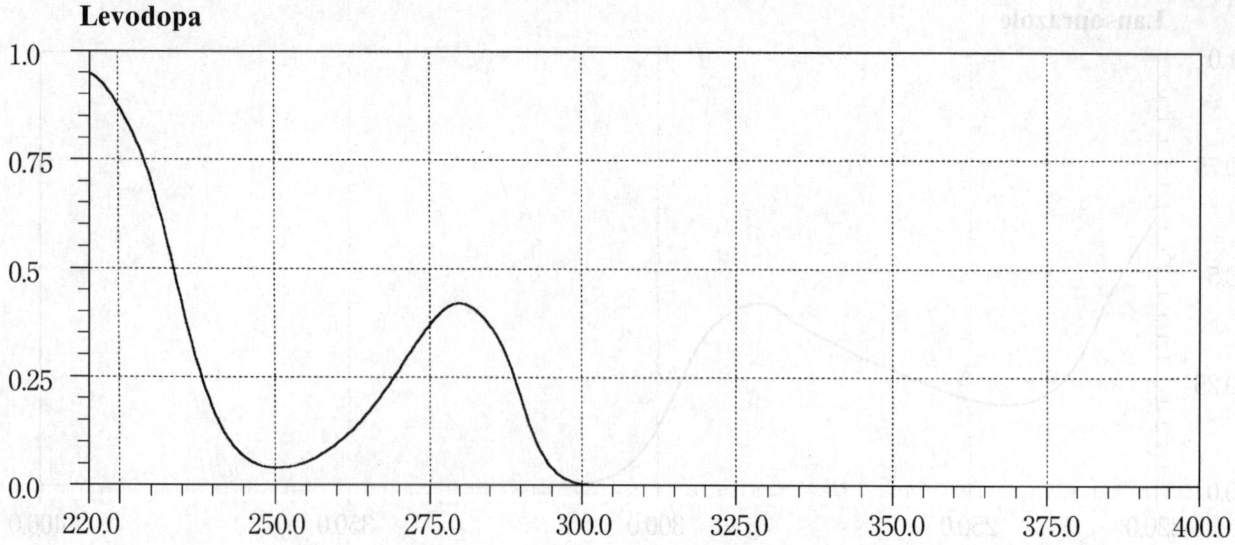

Levofloxacin Hydrate

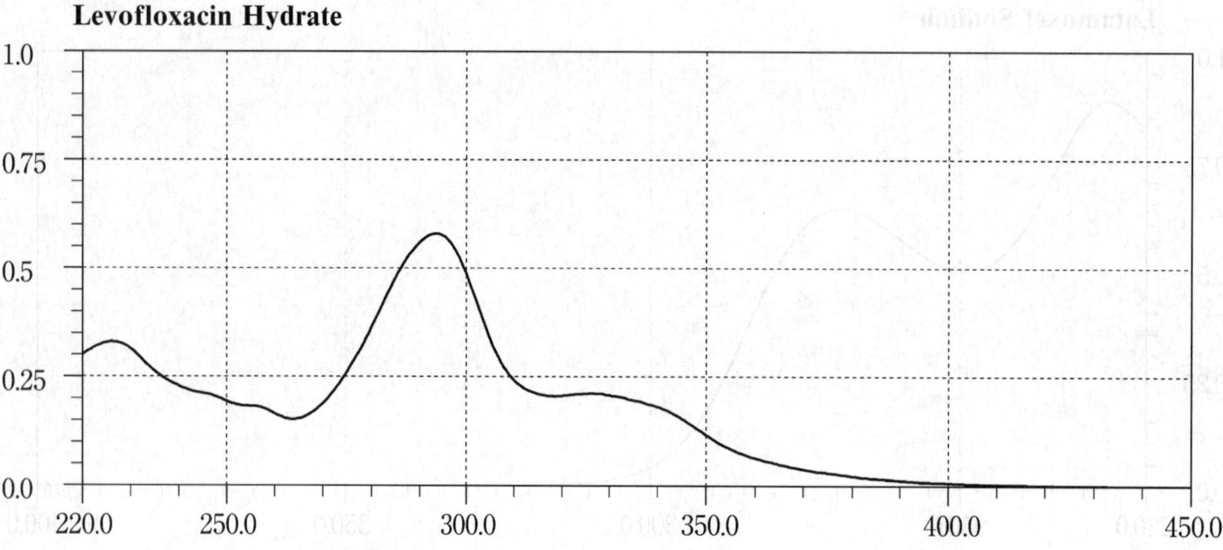

Levothyroxine Sodium Hydrate

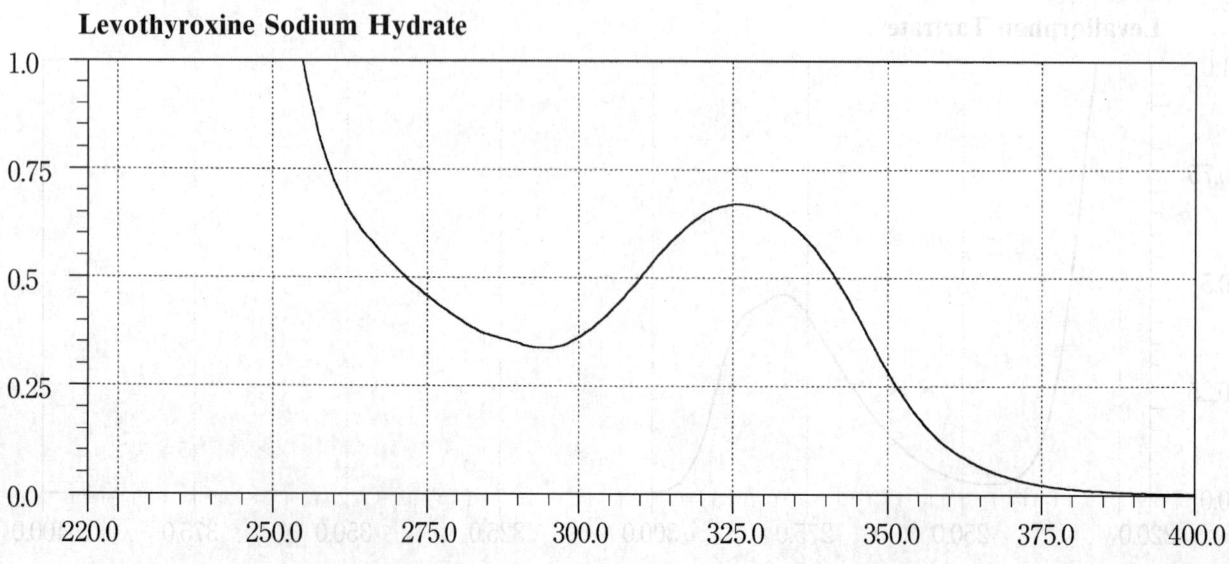

Lidocaine

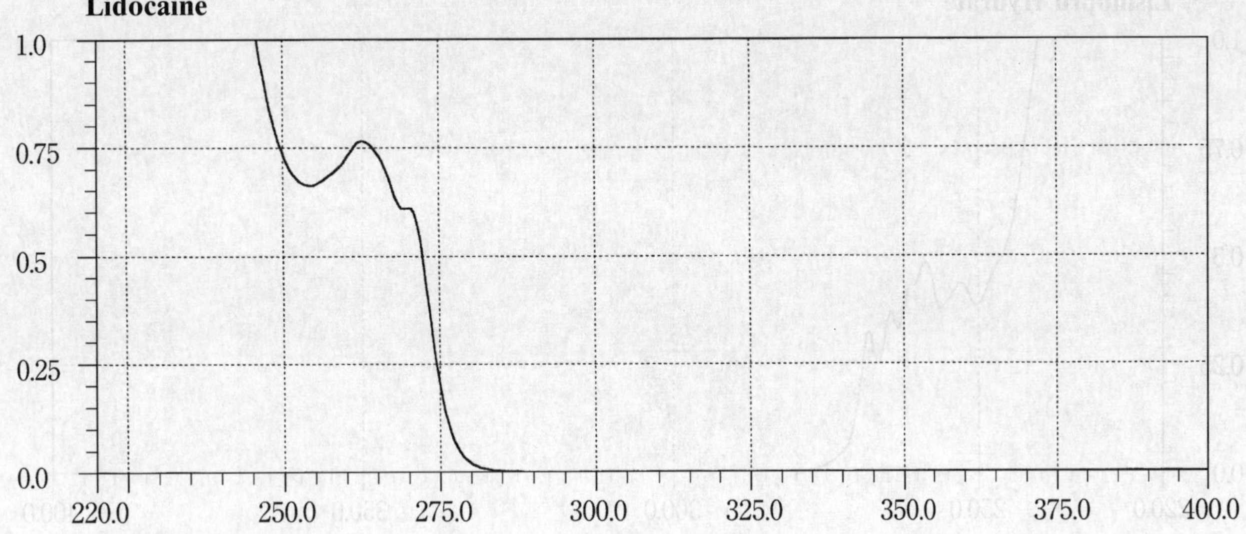

Limaprost Alfadex

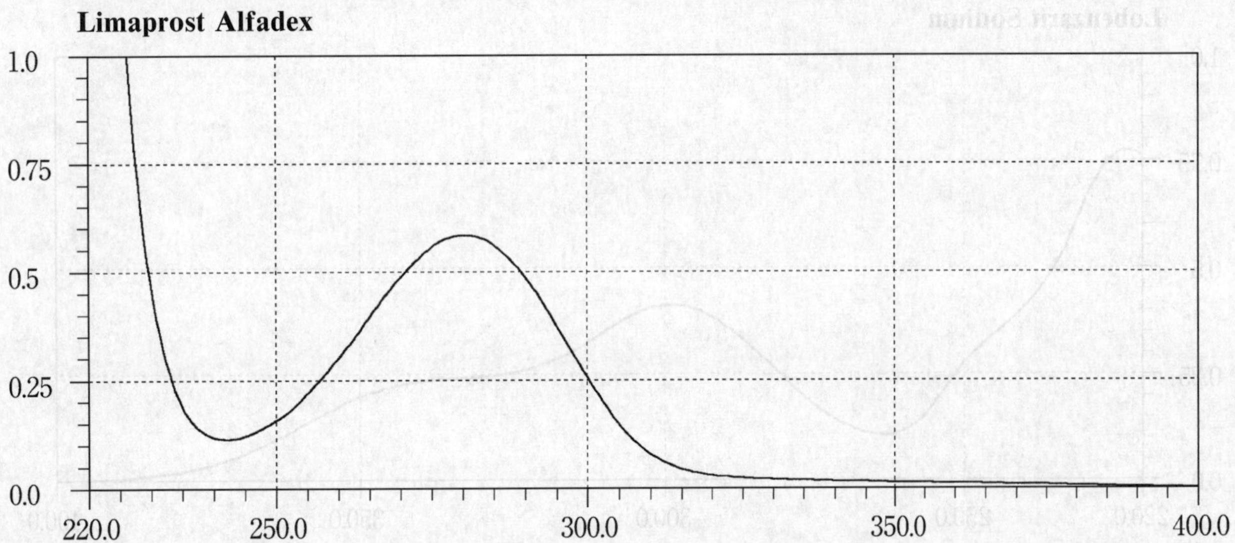

Liothyronine Sodium

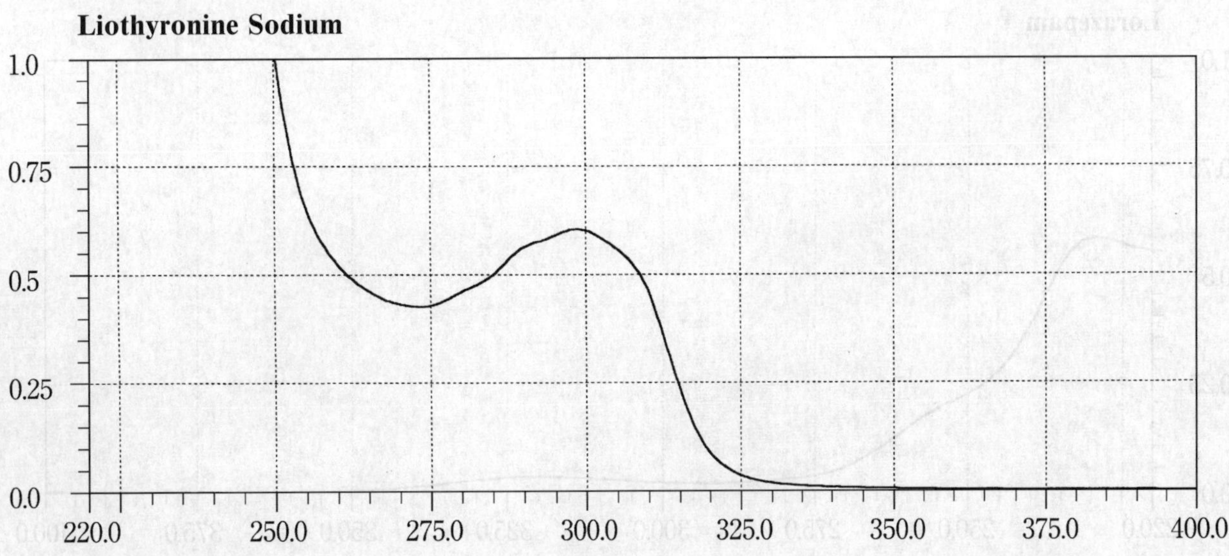

Lisinopril Hydrate

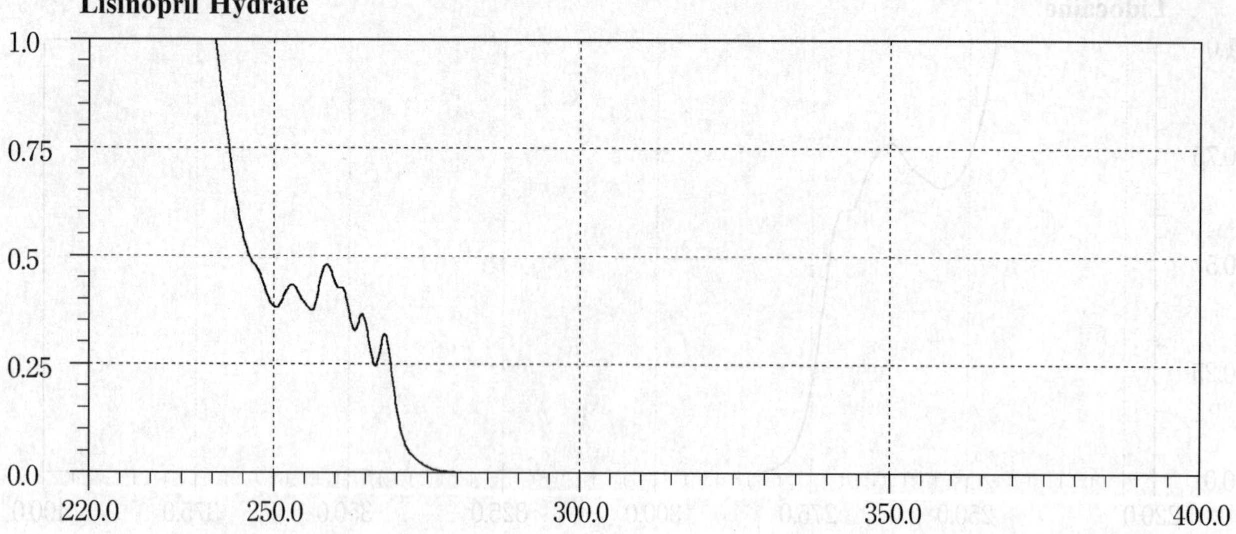

Lobenzarit Sodium

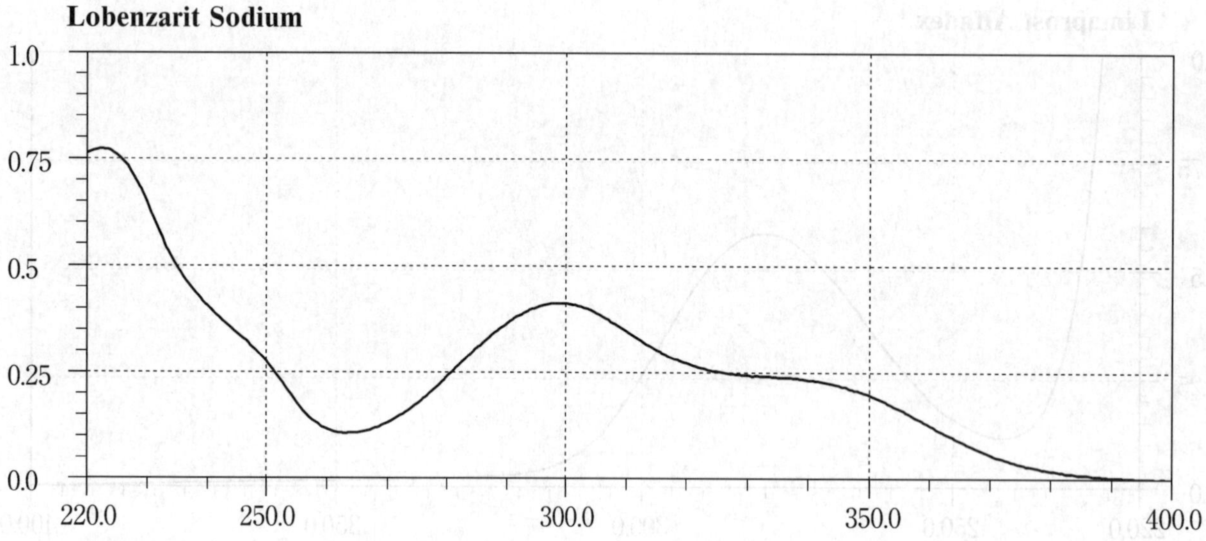

Lorazepam

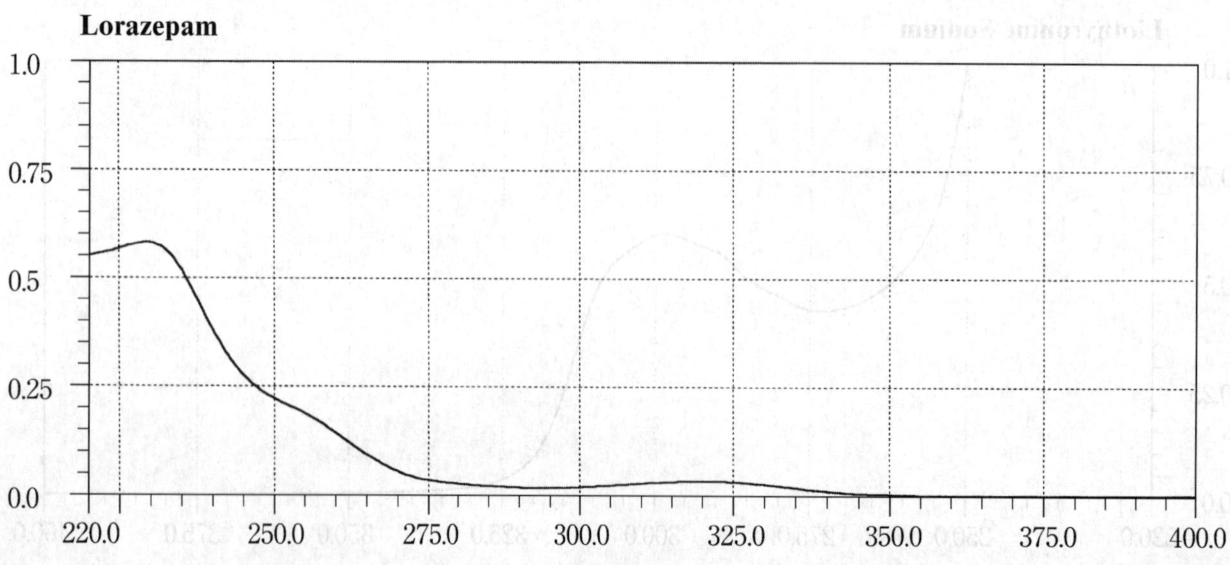

Losartan Potassium

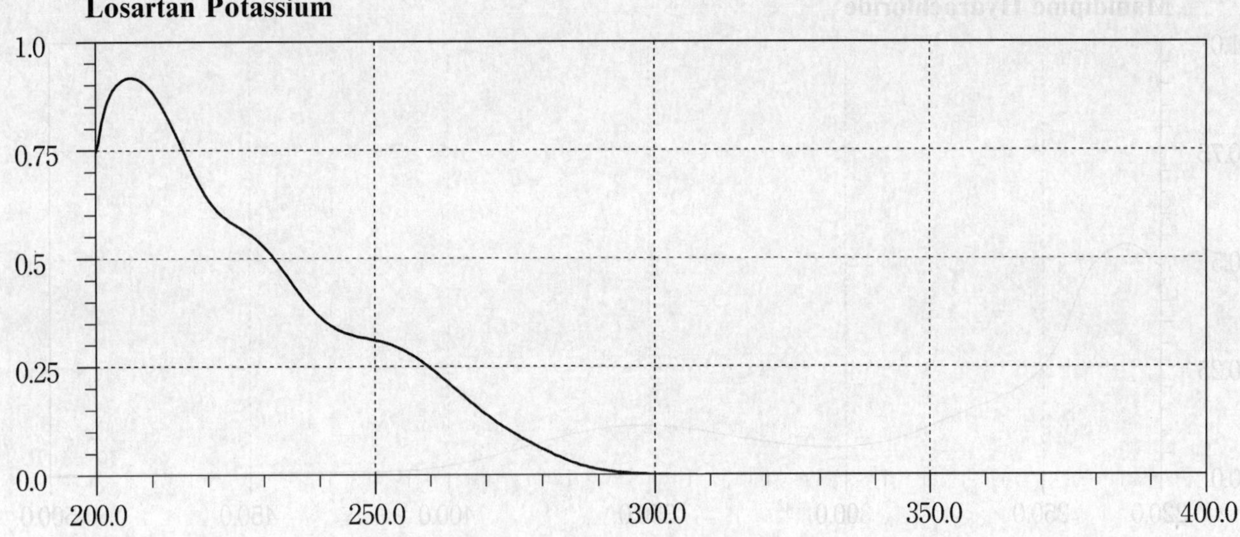

Loxoprofen Sodium Hydrate

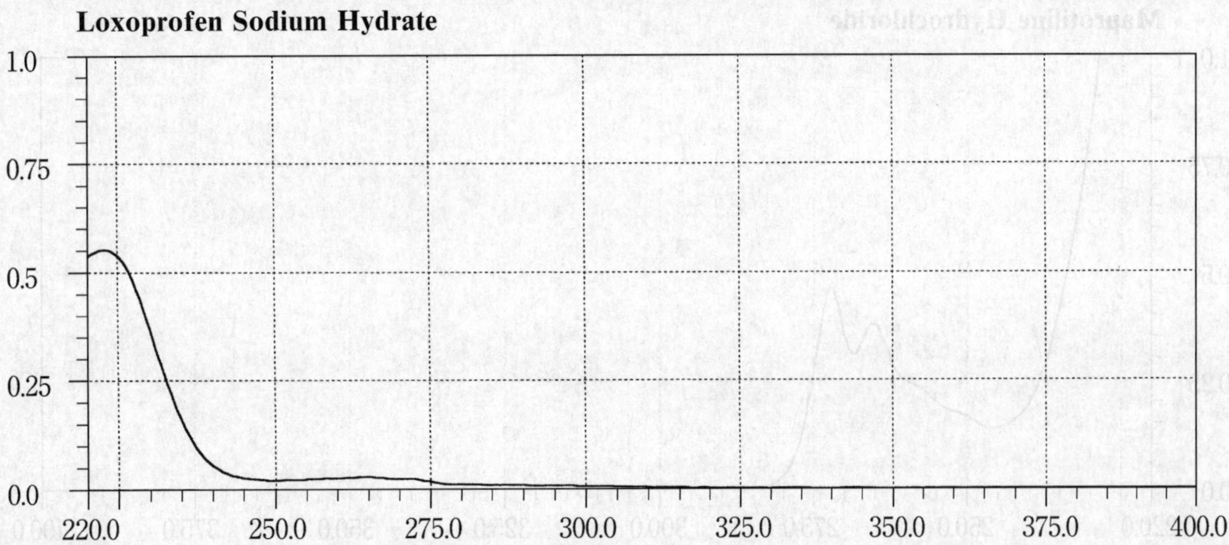

Lysozyme Hydrochloride

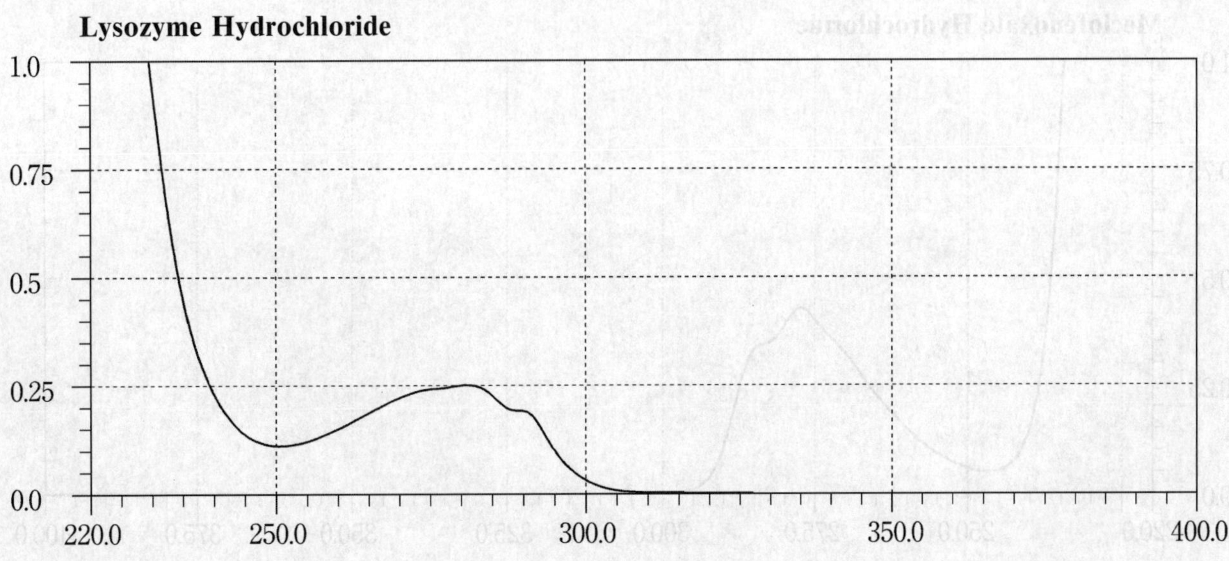

Manidipine Hydrochloride

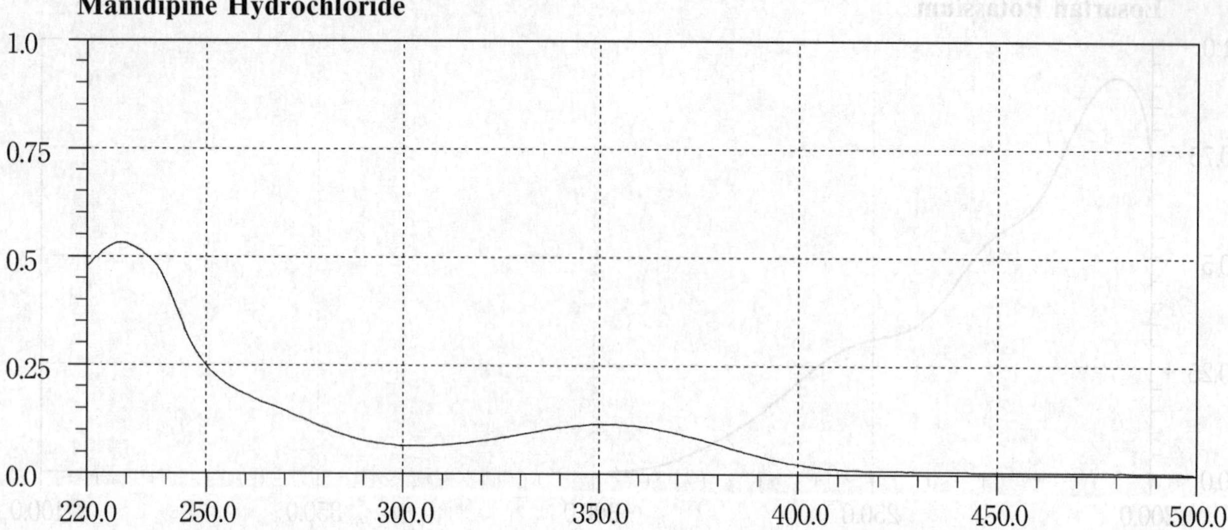

Maprotiline Hydrochloride

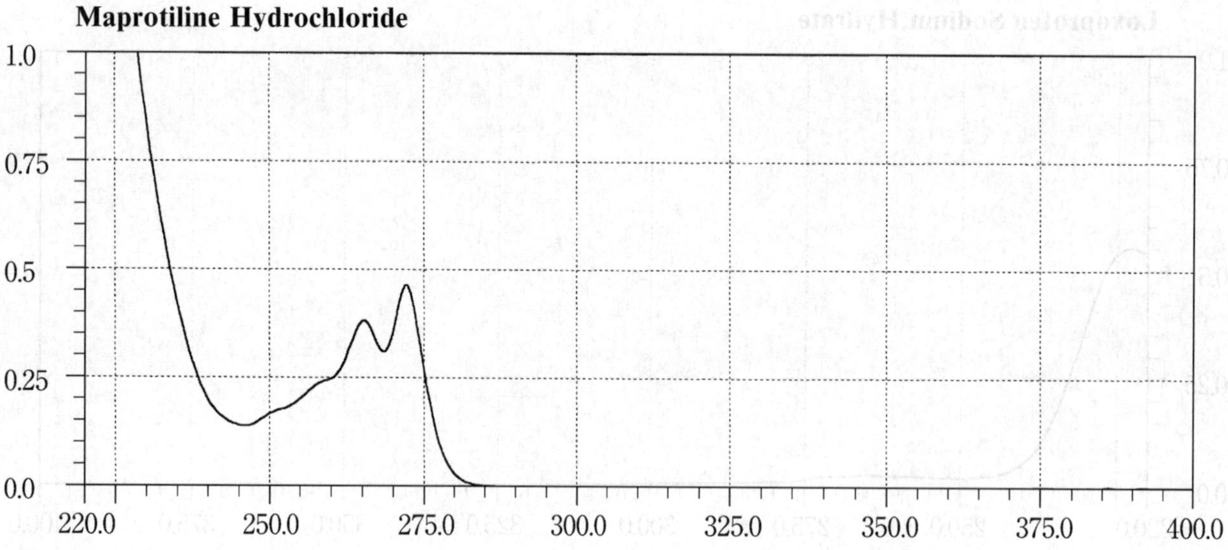

Meclofenoxate Hydrochloride

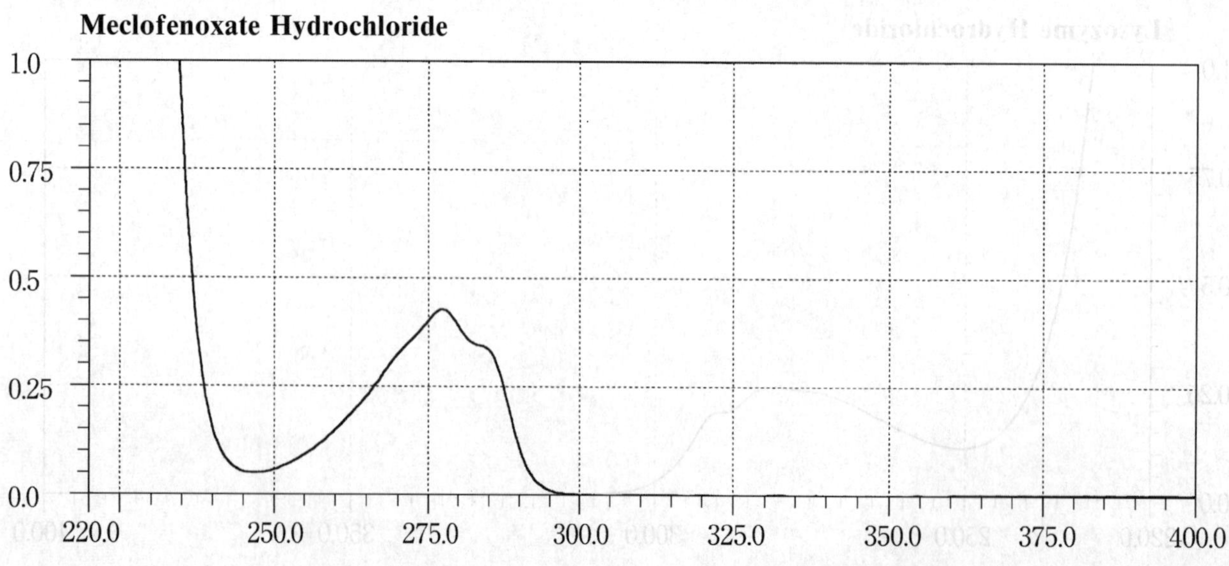

Mecobalamin 1

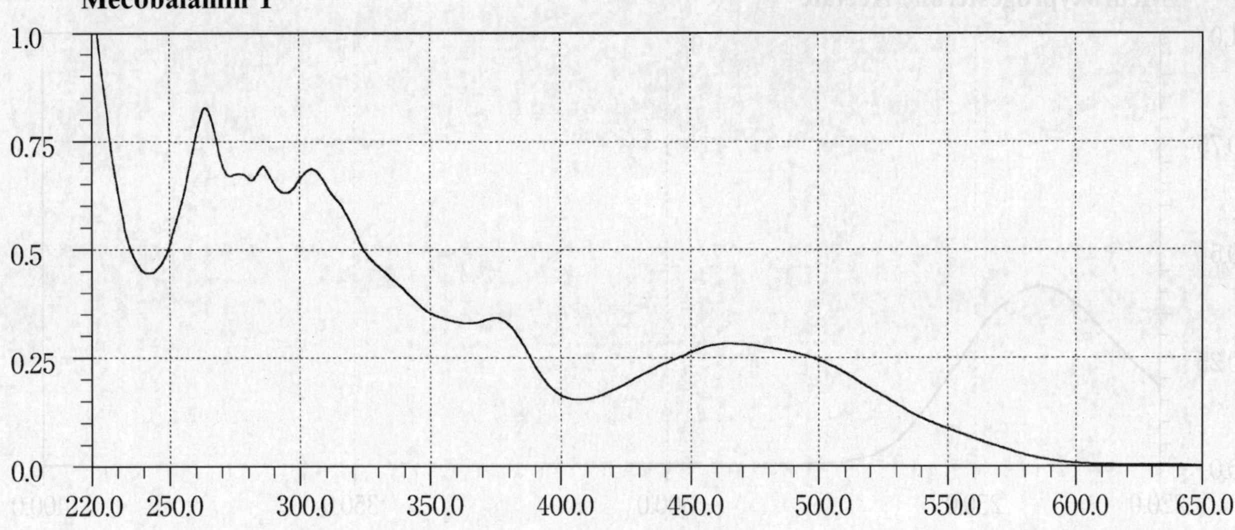

Mecobalamin 2

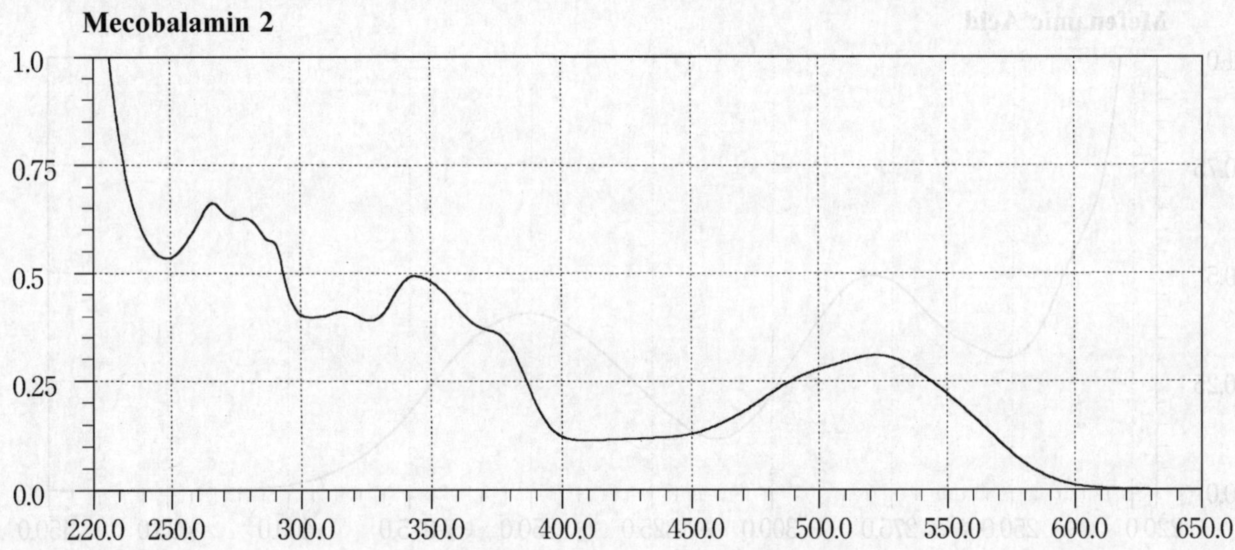

Medazepam

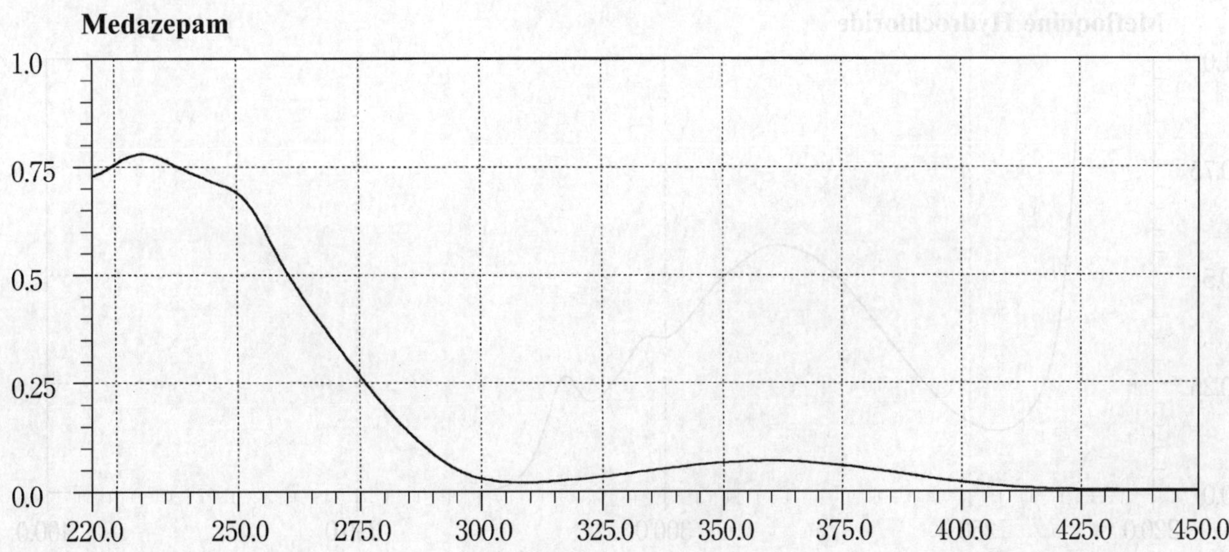

Medroxyprogesterone Acetate

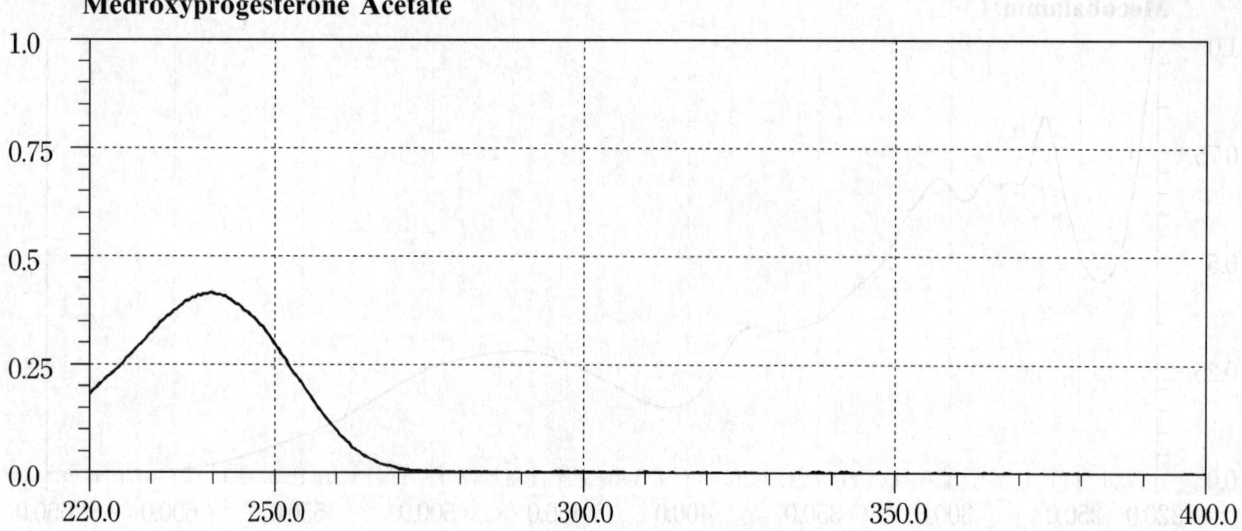

Mefenamic Acid

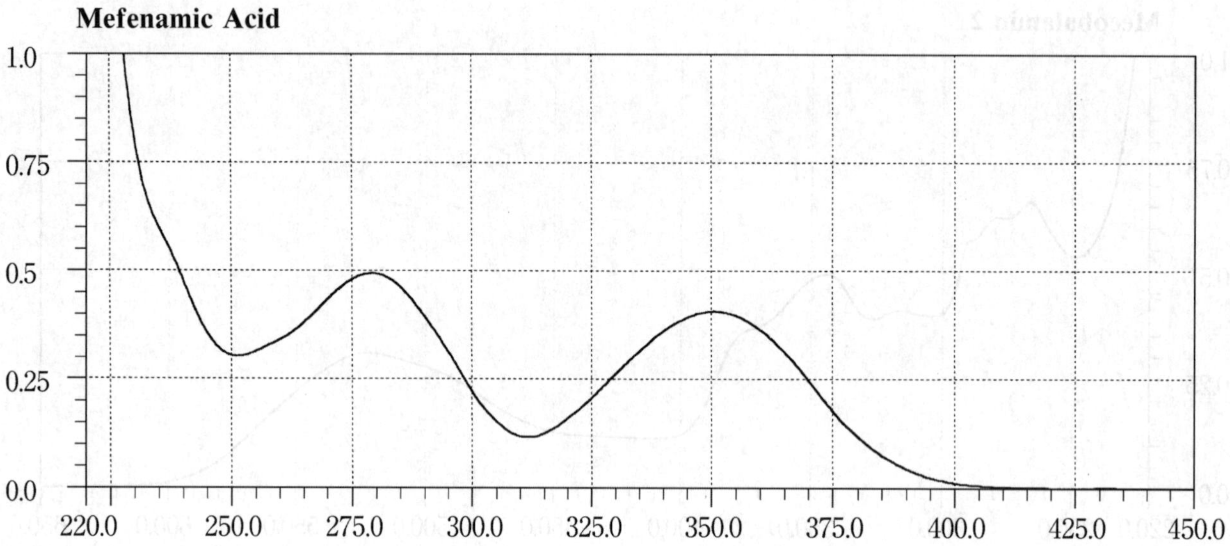

Mefloquine Hydrochloride

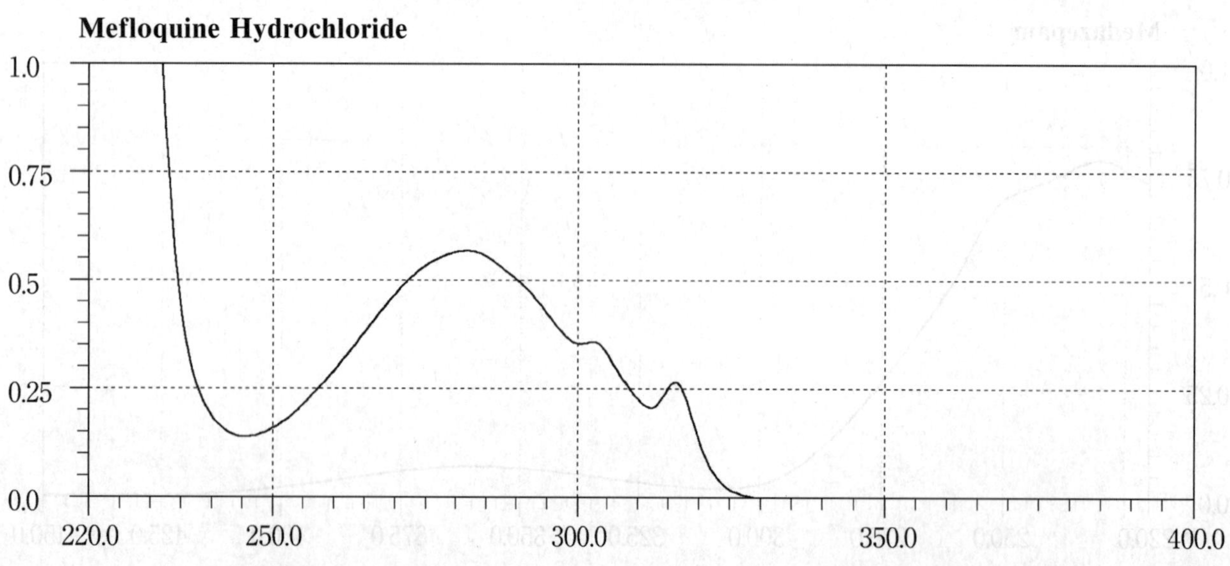

Mefruside

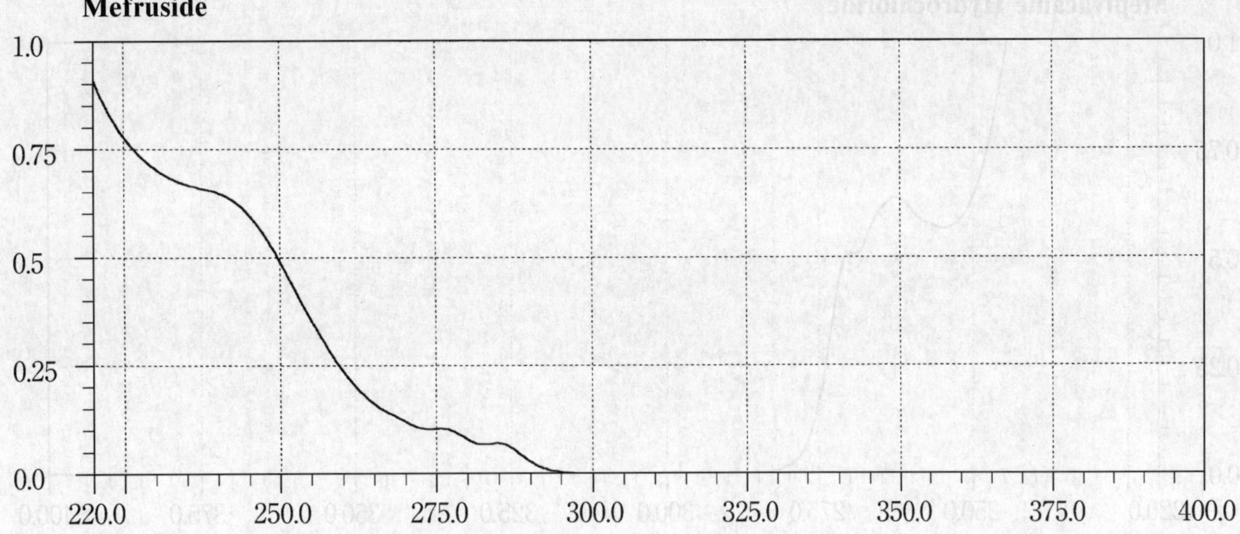

Melphalan

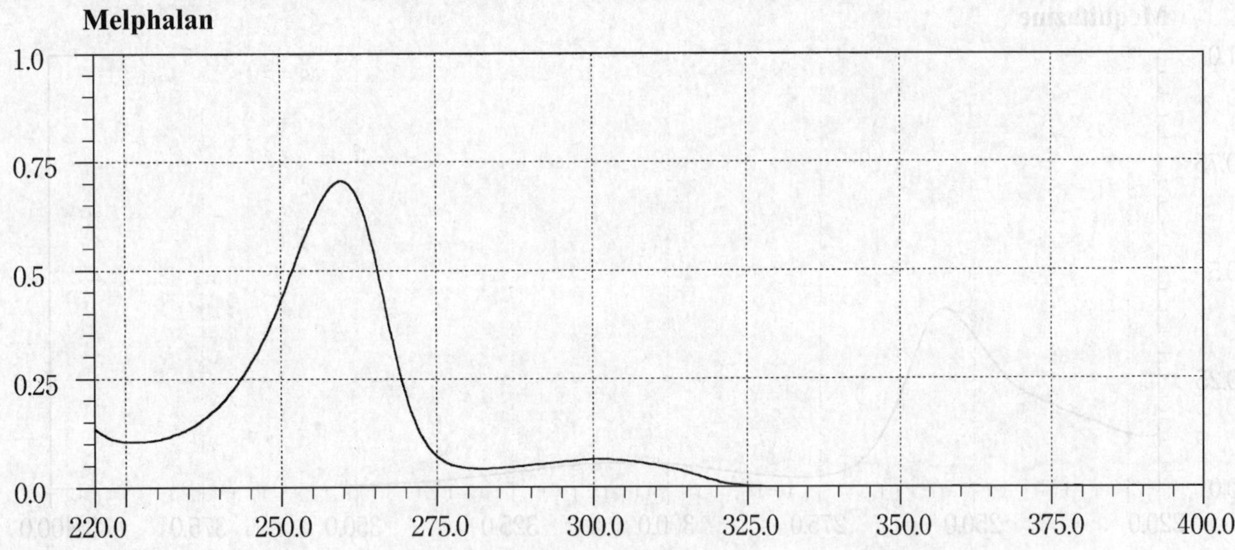

Mepenzolate Bromide

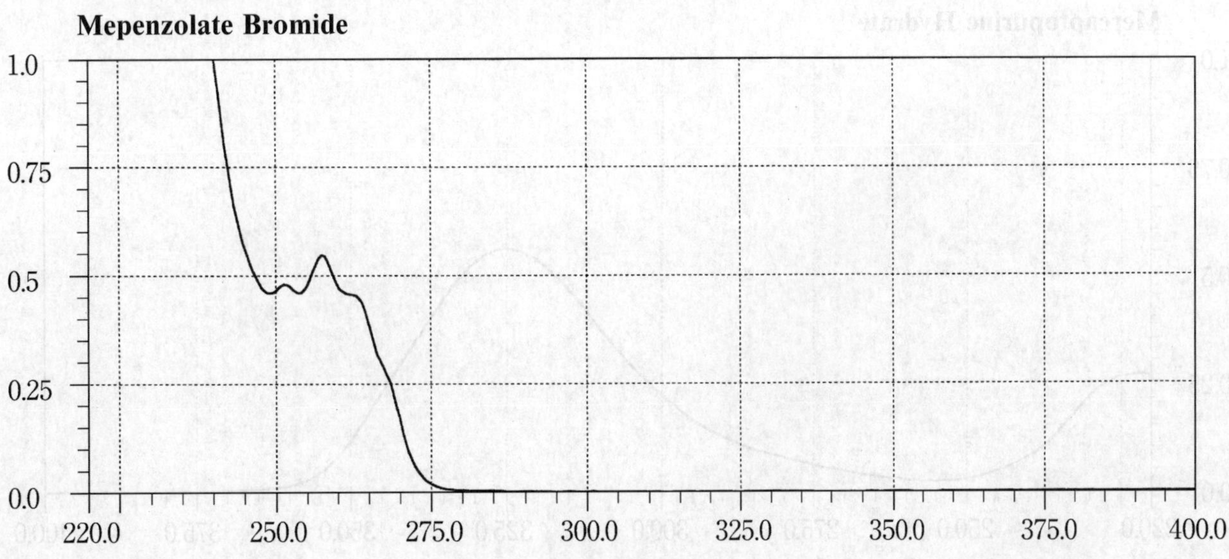

Mepivacaine Hydrochloride

1.0
0.75
0.5
0.25
0.0
220.0 250.0 275.0 300.0 325.0 350.0 375.0 400.0

Mequitazine

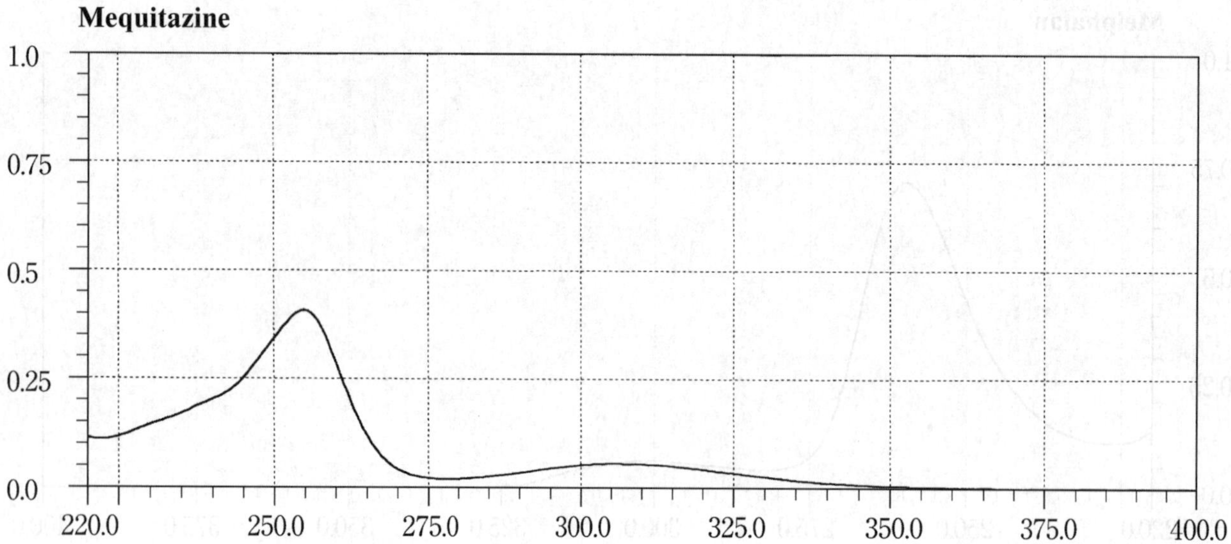

Mercaptopurine Hydrate

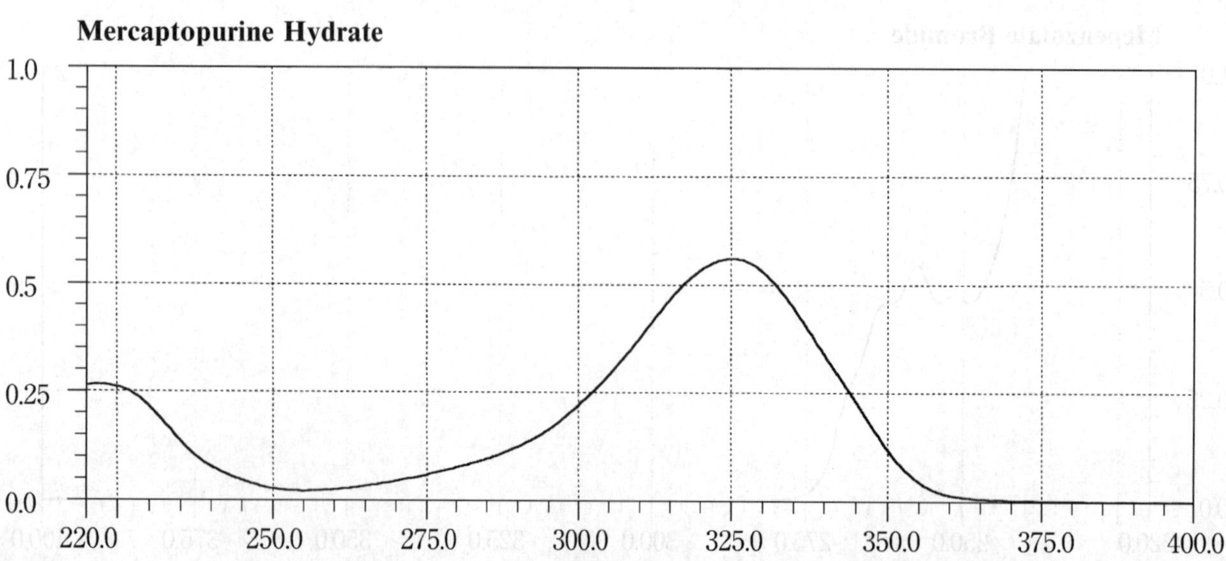

Mesalazine

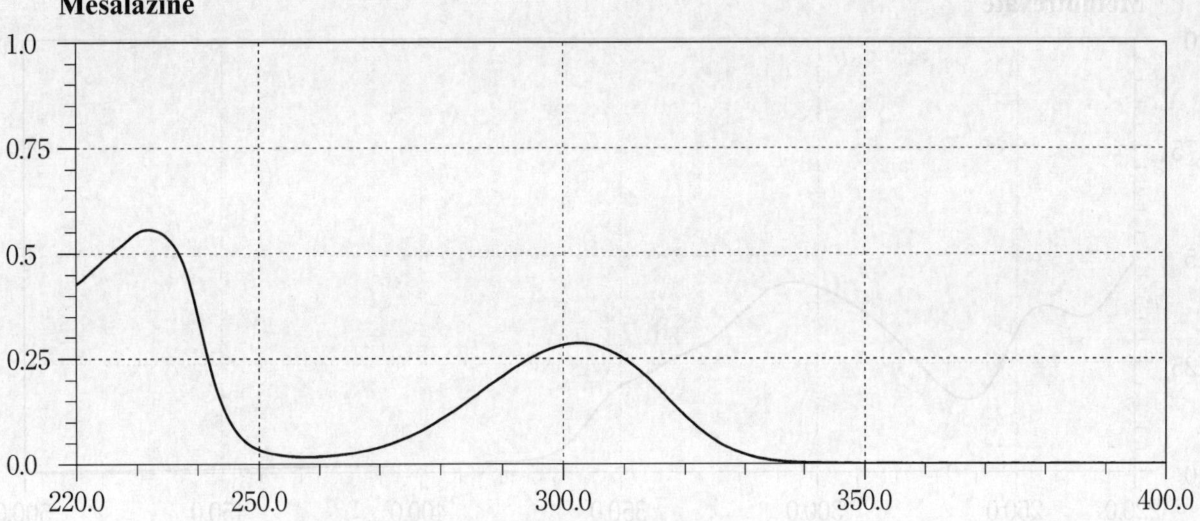

Mestranol

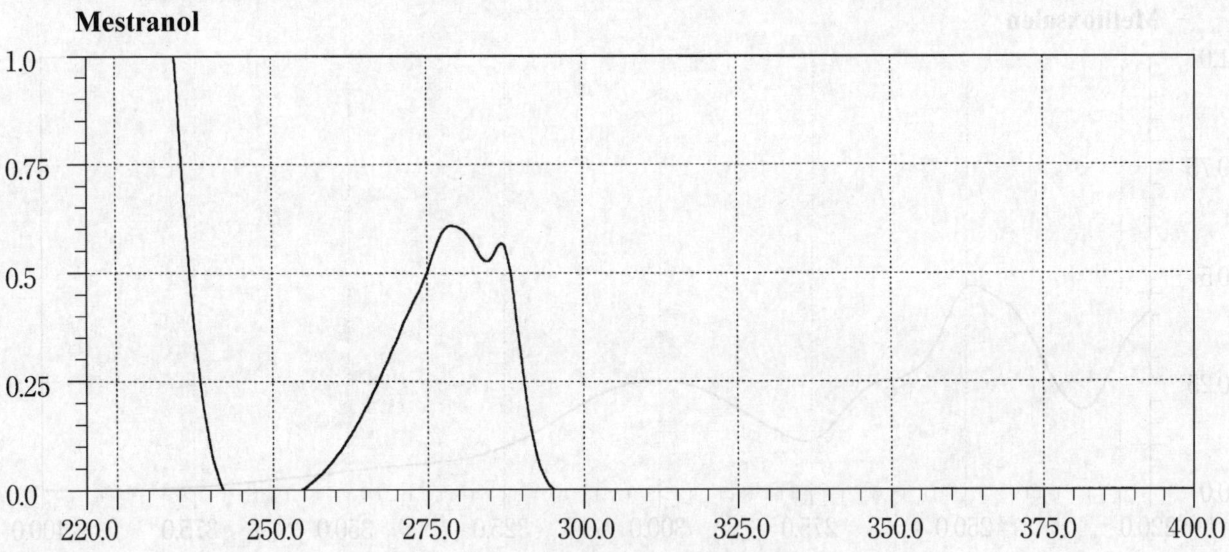

Metformin Hydrochloride

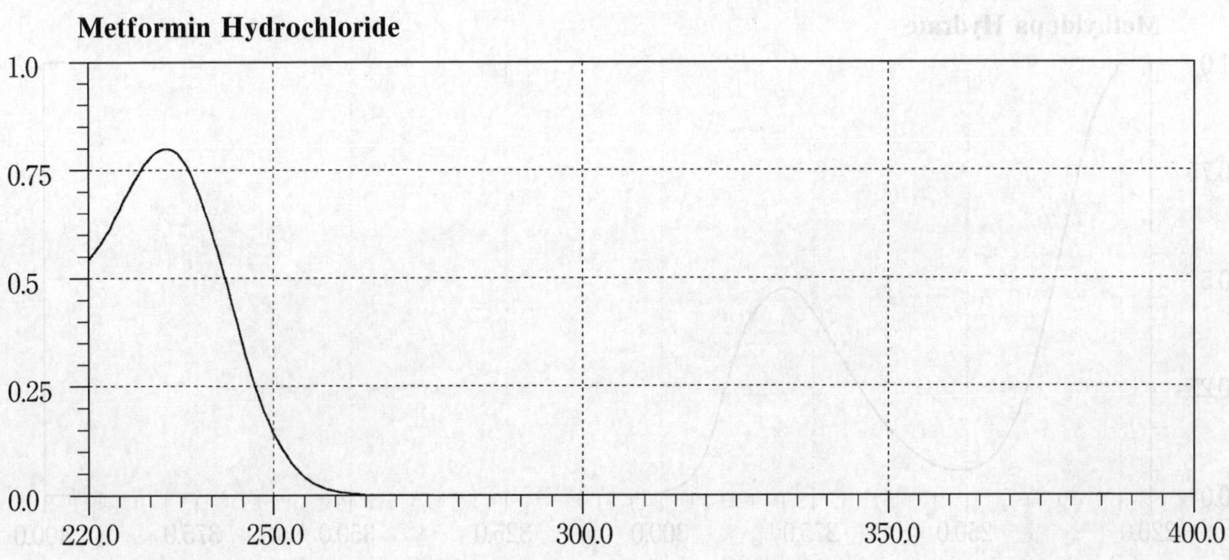

Methotrexate

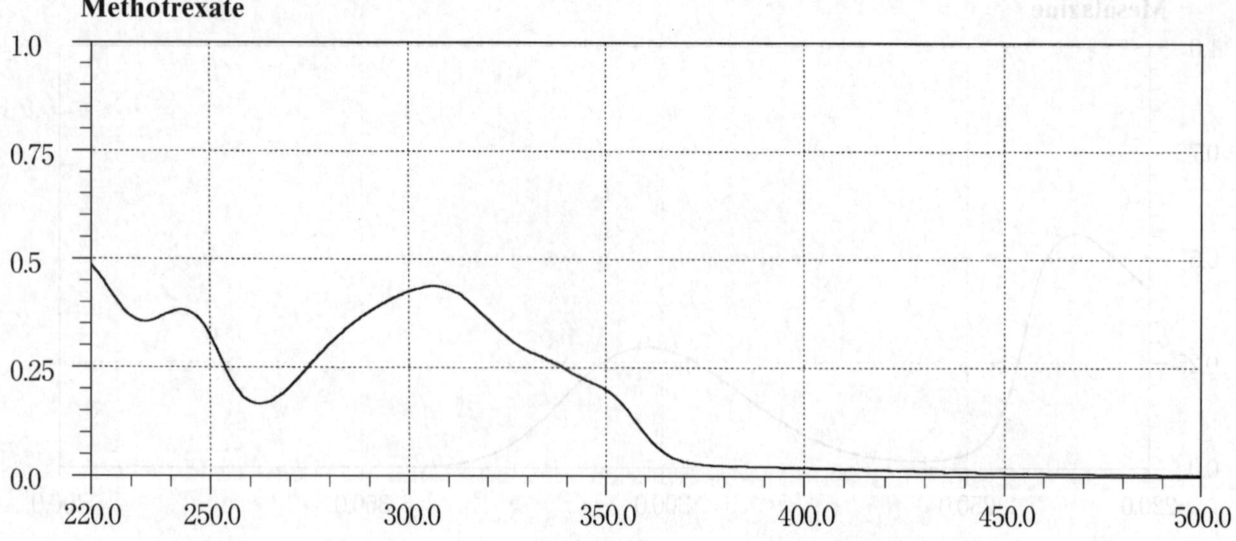

Methoxsalen

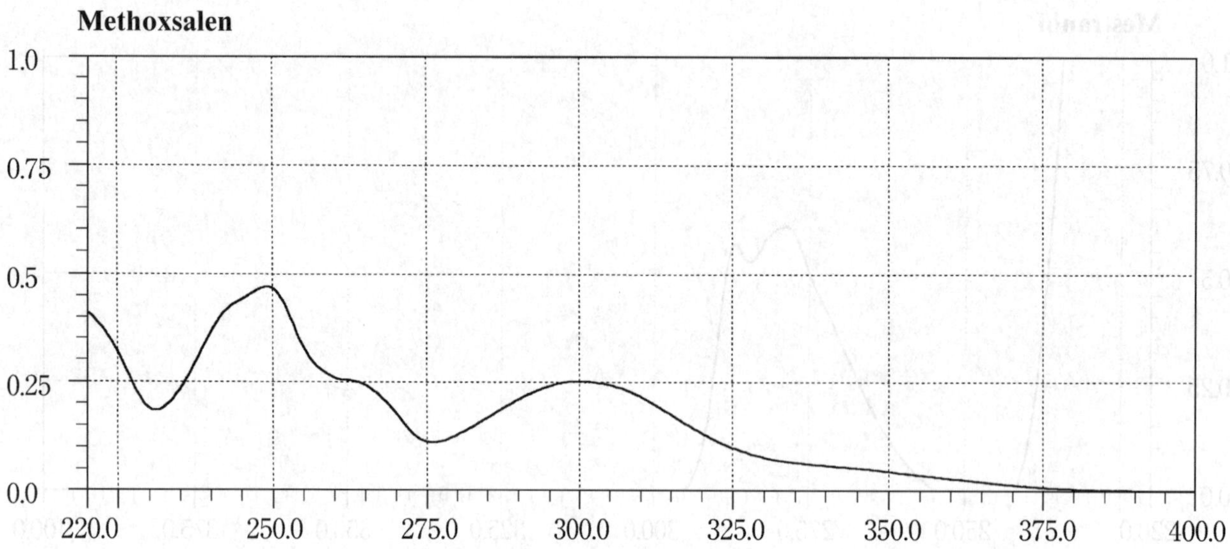

Methyldopa Hydrate

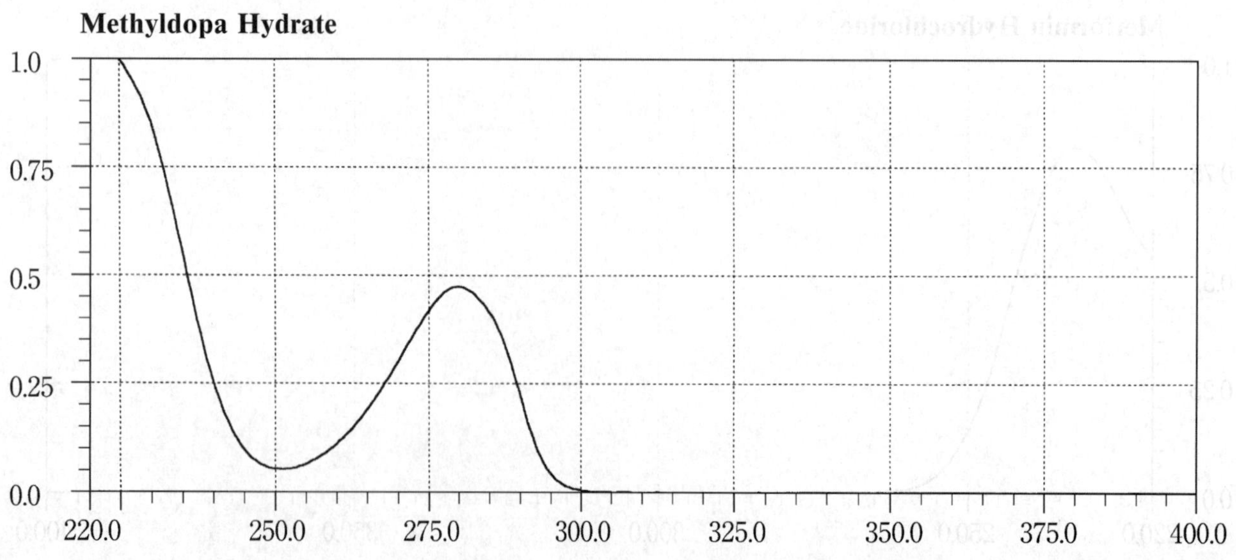

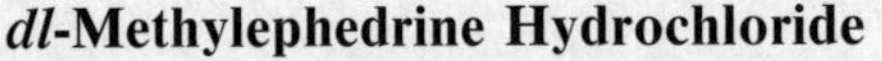

dl-Methylephedrine Hydrochloride

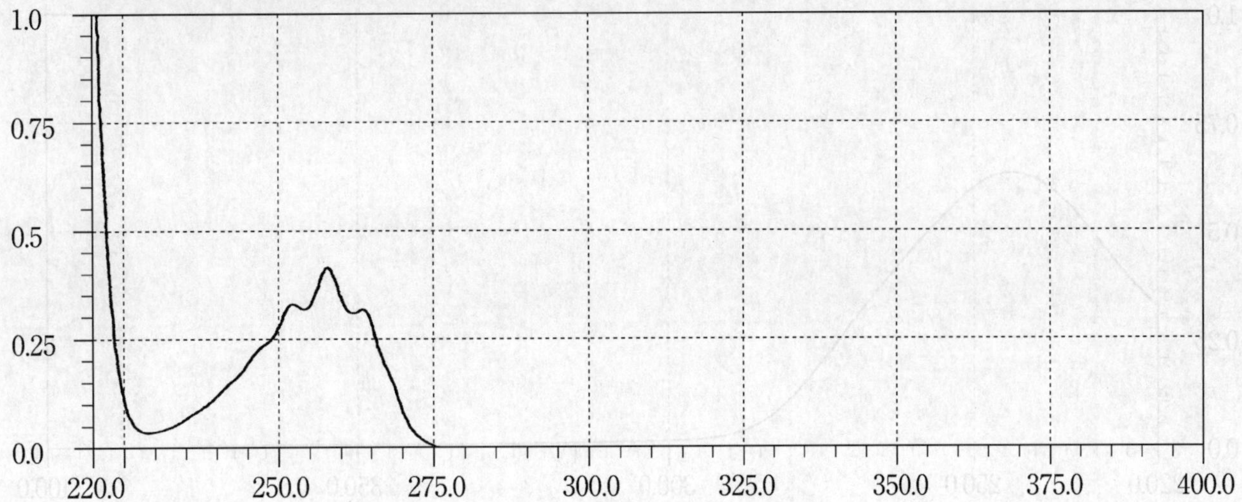

Methylergometrine Maleate

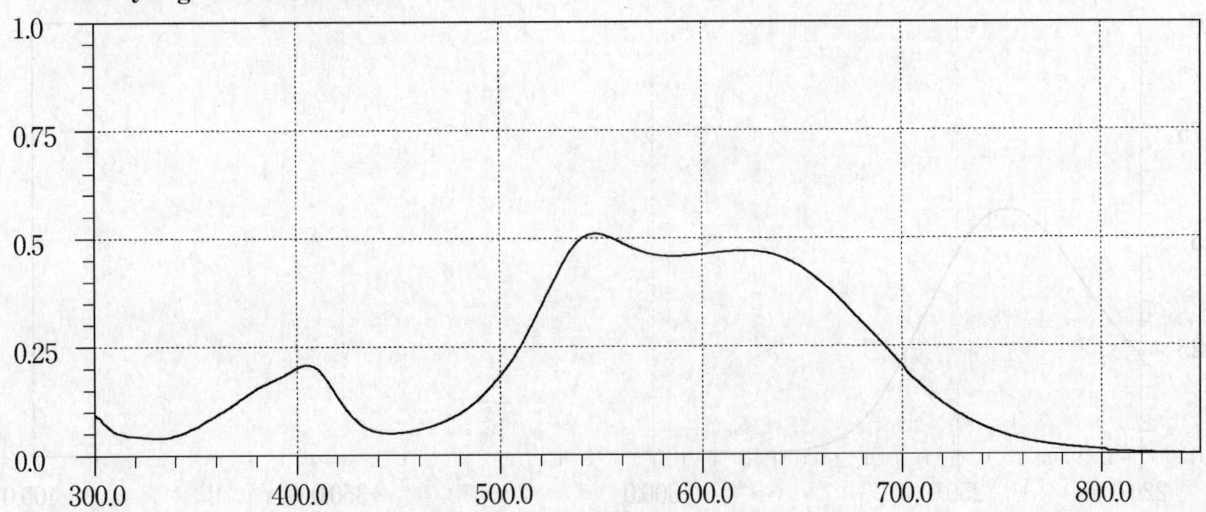

Methylprednisolone

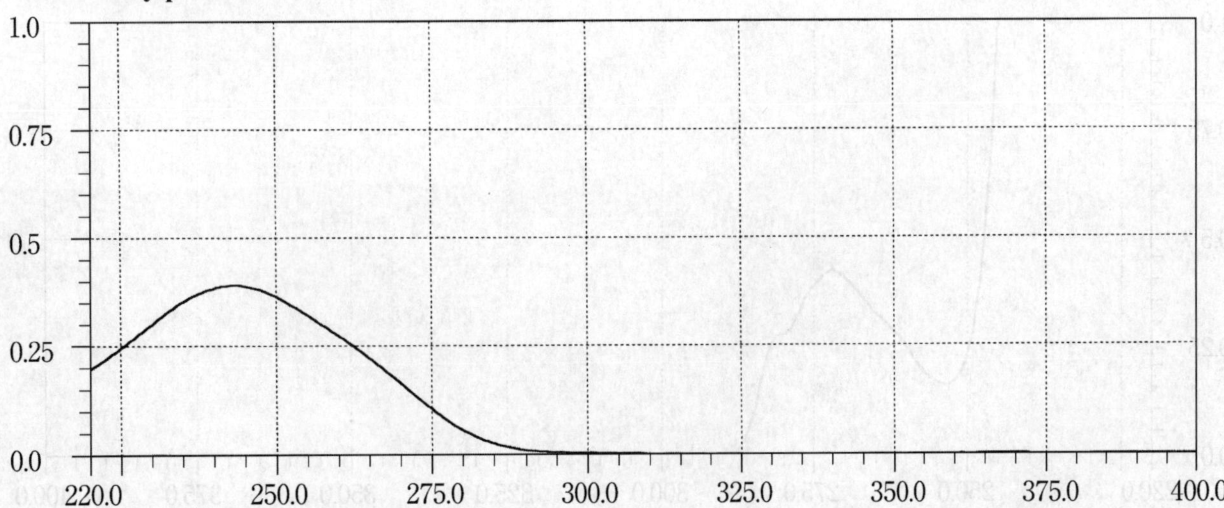

Methylprednisolone Succinate

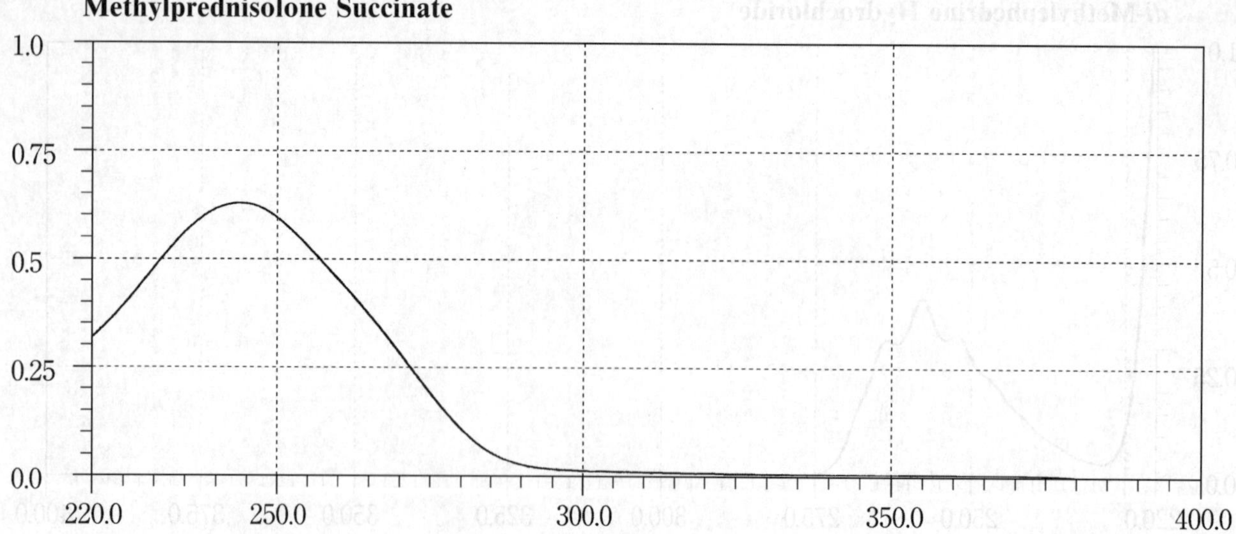

Methyltestosterone

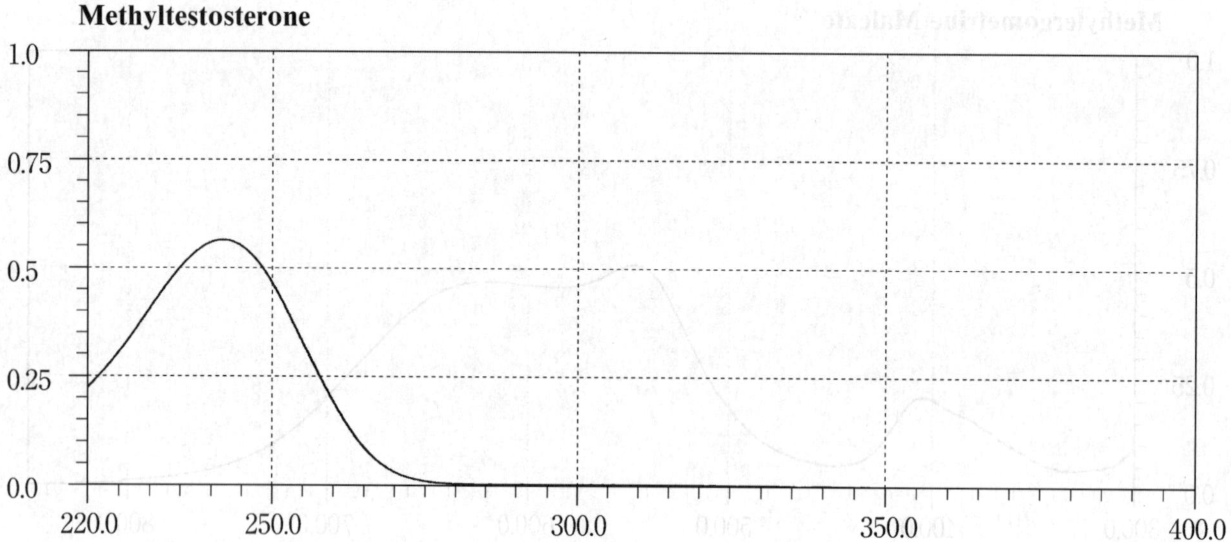

Meticrane

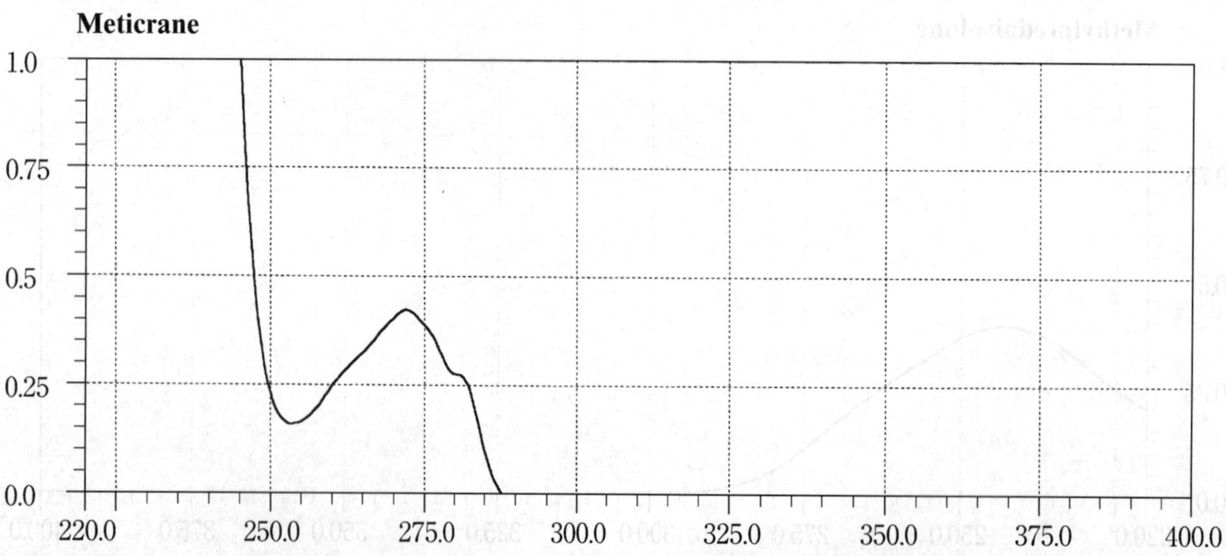

Metildigoxin

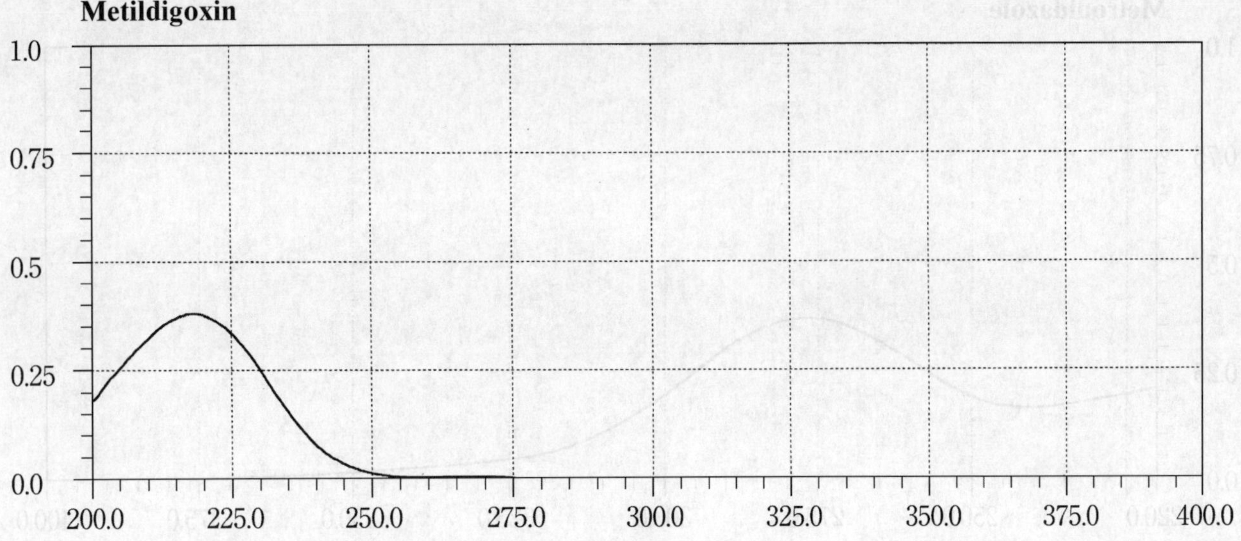

Metoclopramide

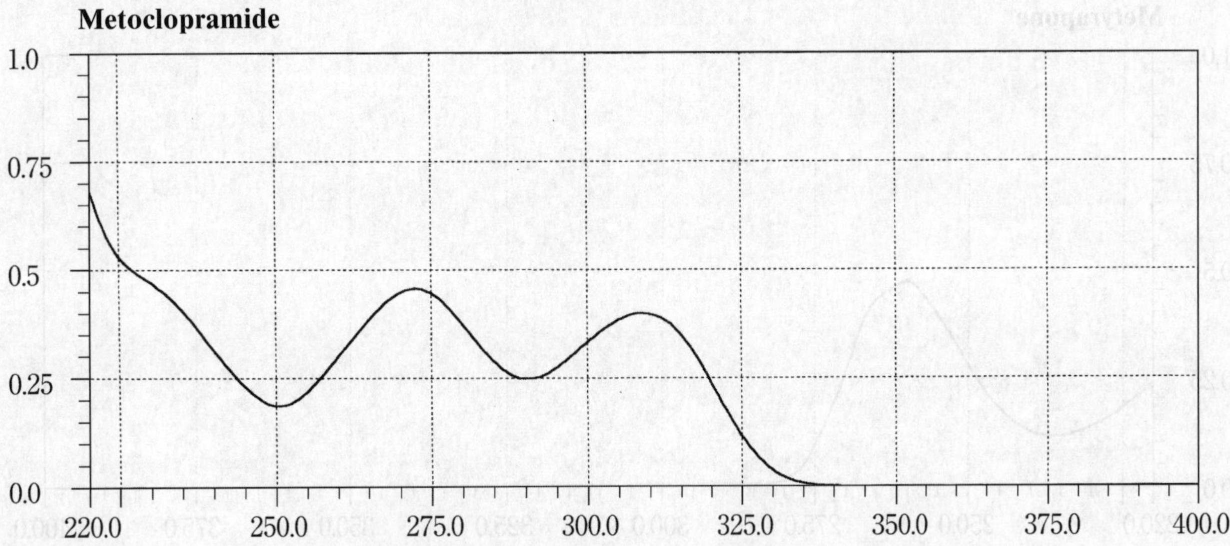

Metoprolol Tartrate

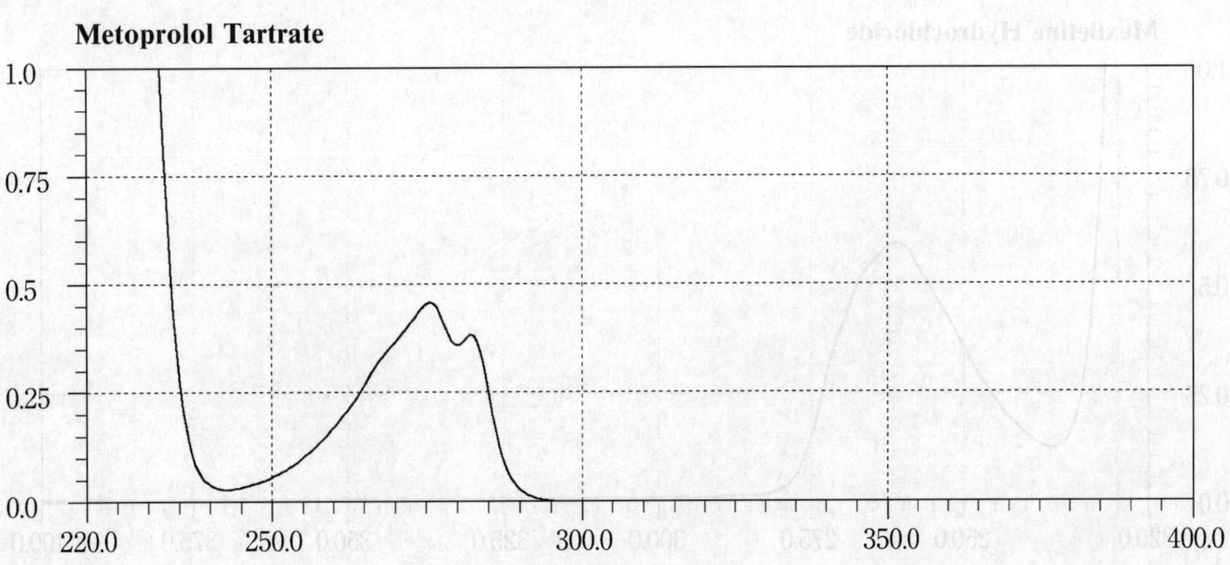

Metronidazole

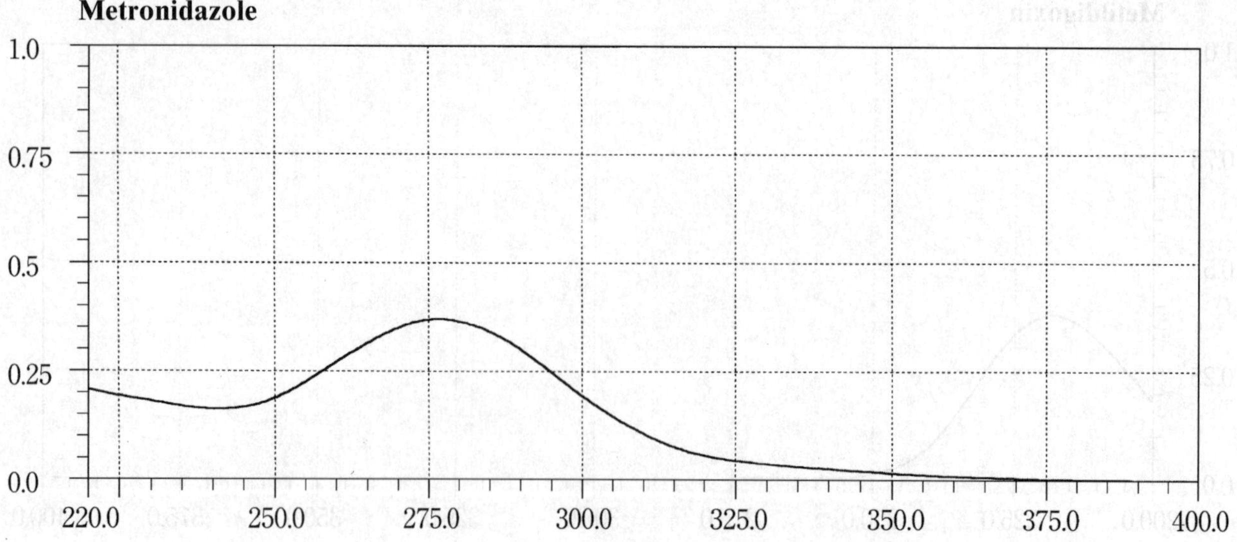

Metyrapone

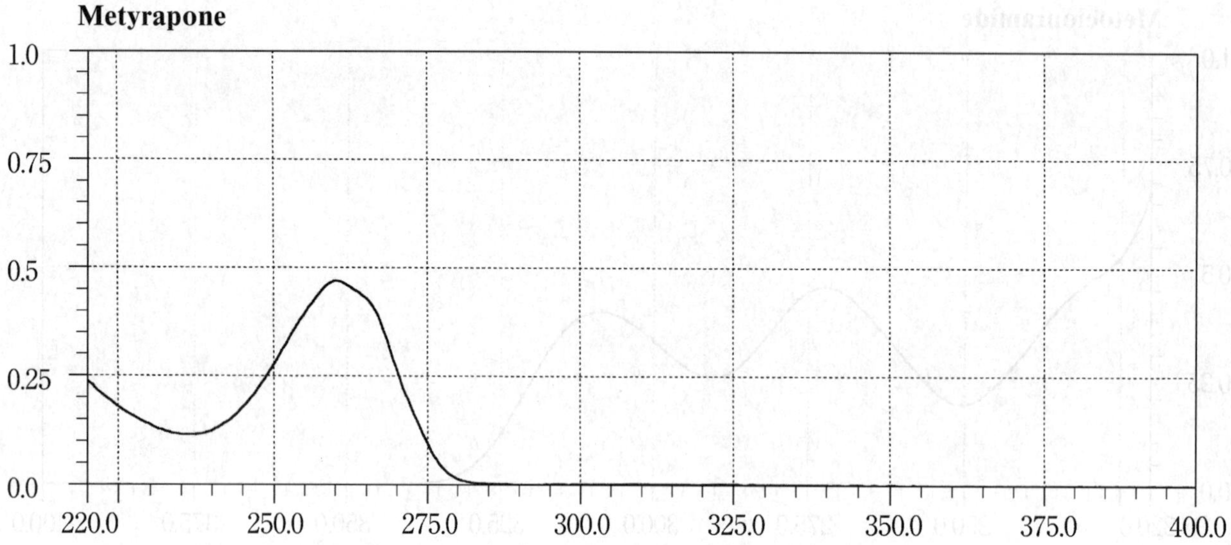

Mexiletine Hydrochloride

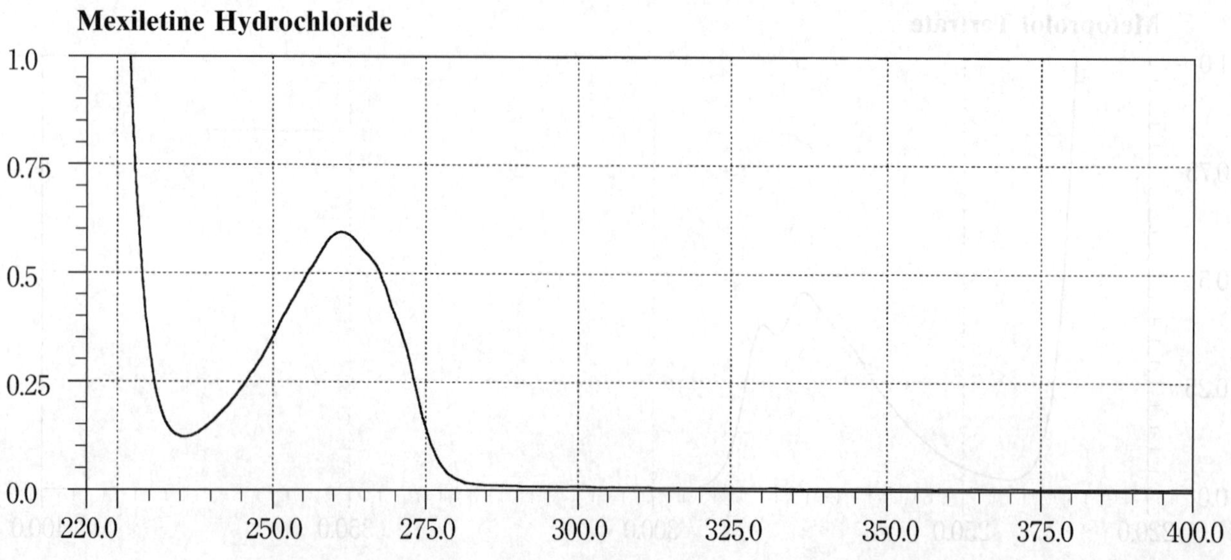

Miconazole

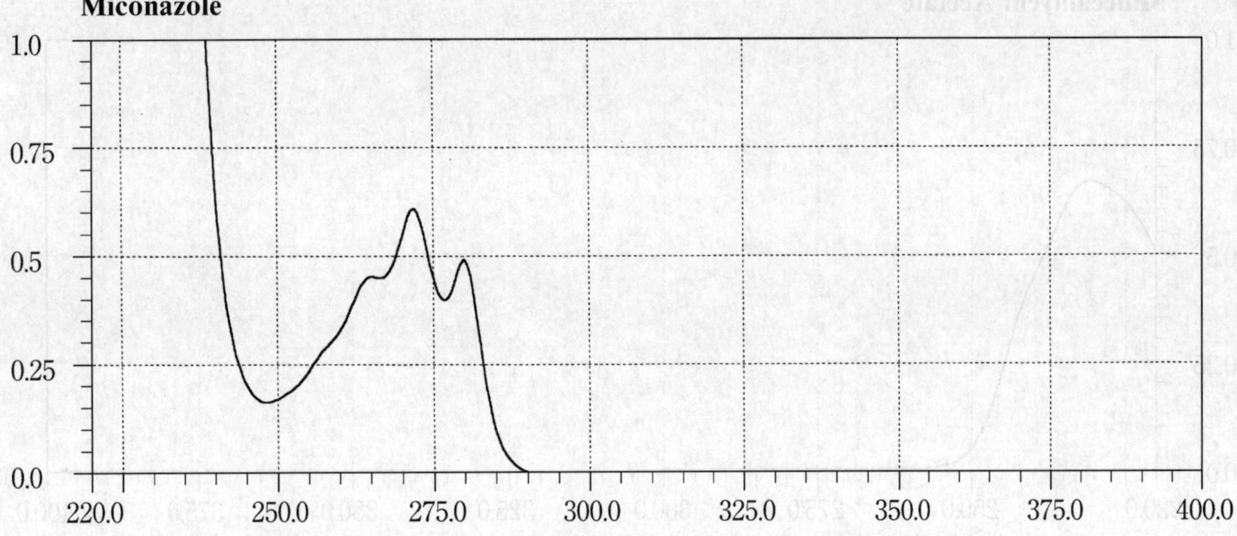

Miconazole Nitrate

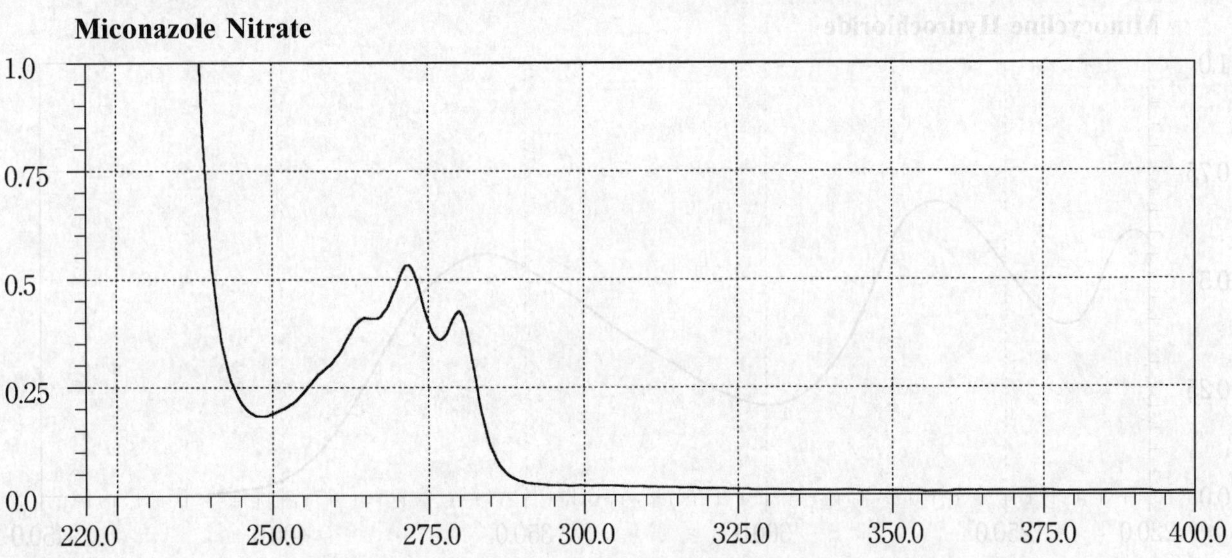

Midecamycin

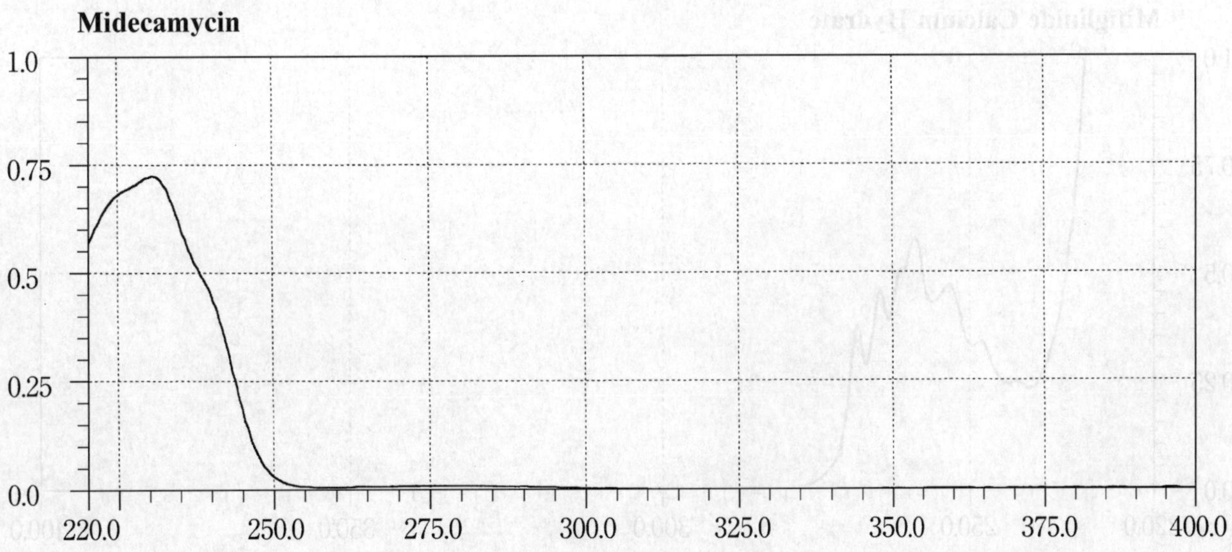

Midecamycin Acetate

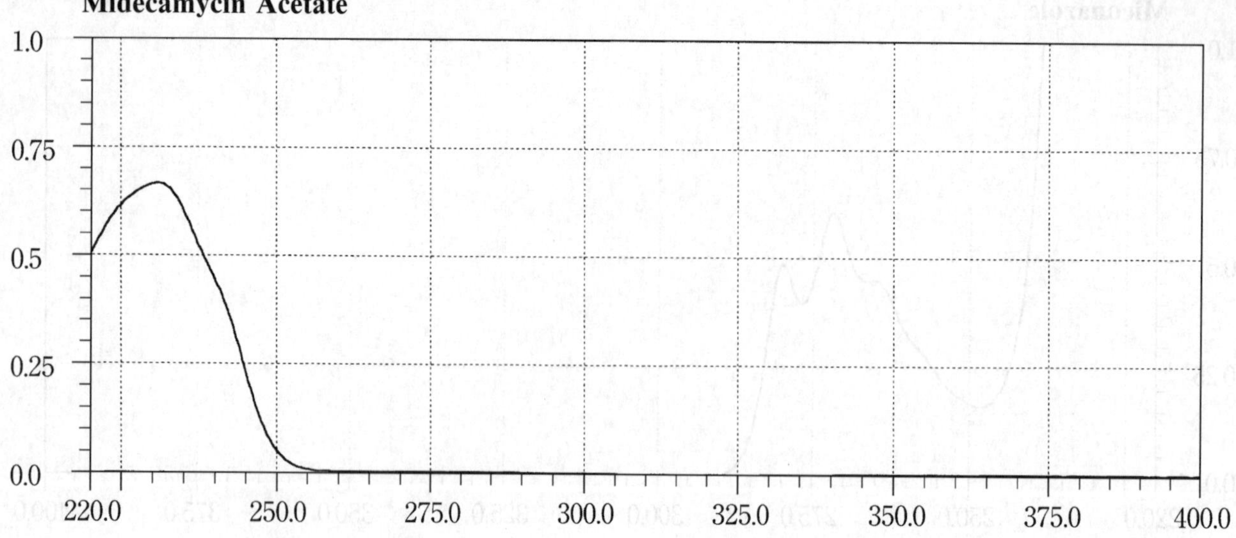

Minocycline Hydrochloride

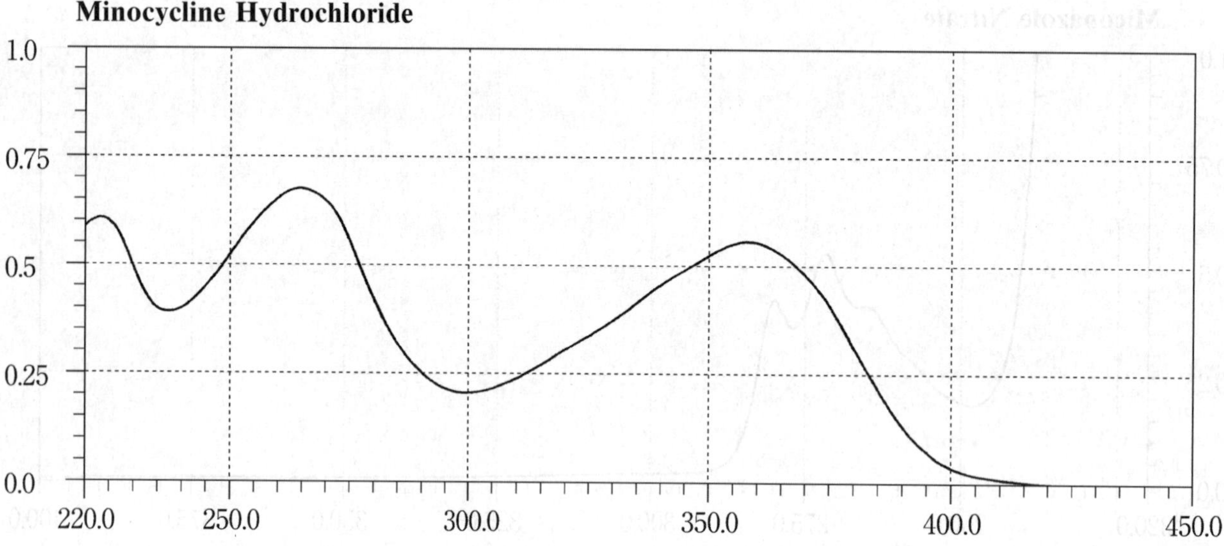

Mitiglinide Calcium Hydrate

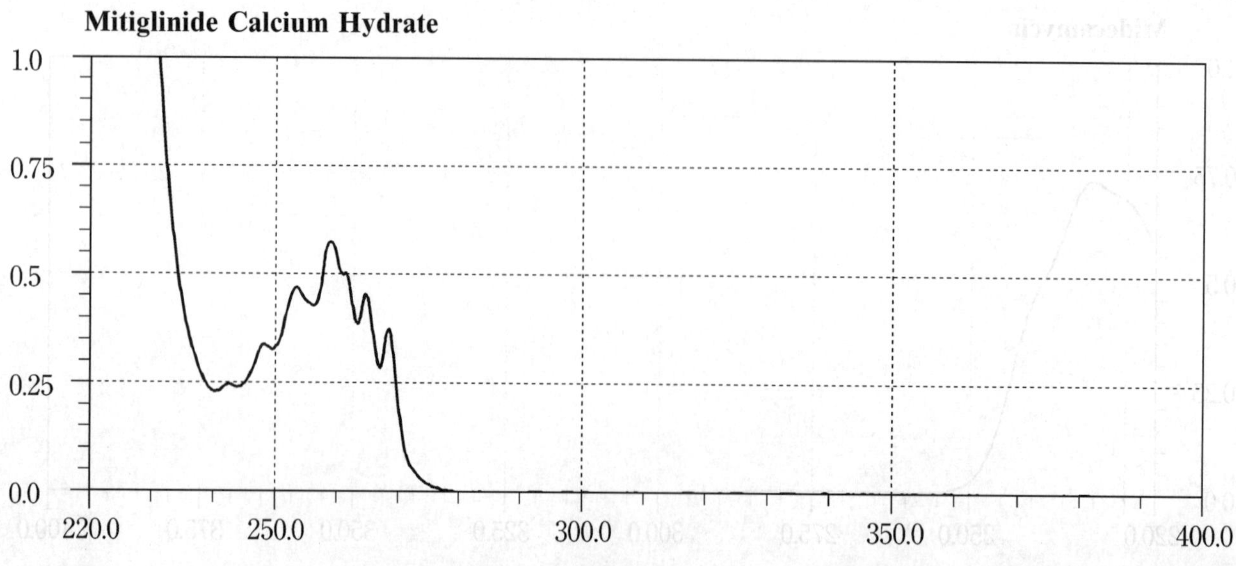

Mitomycin C

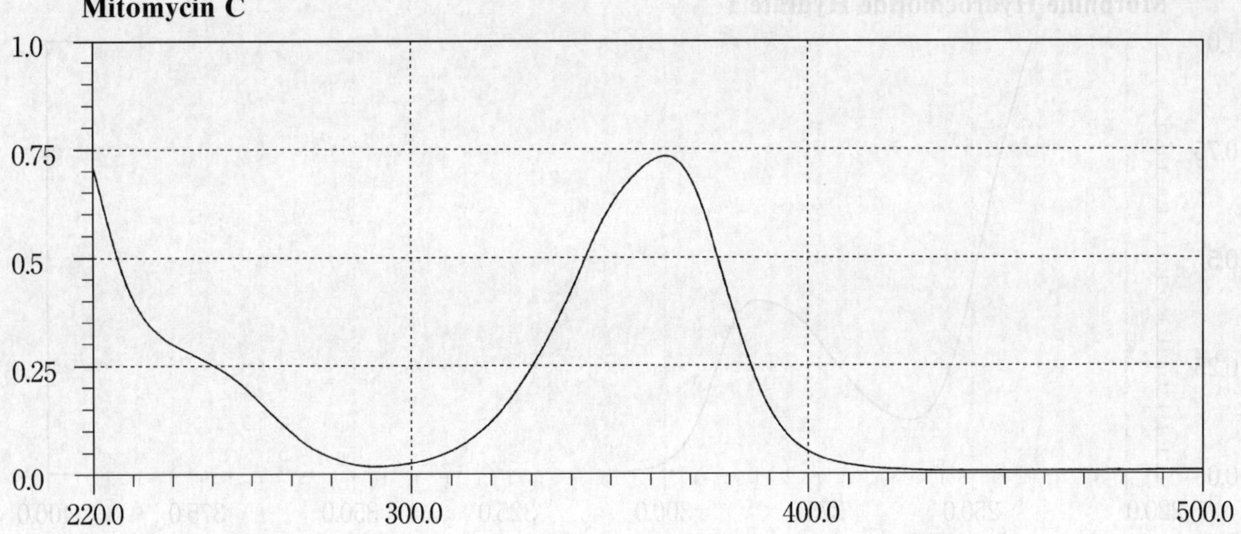

Mizoribine

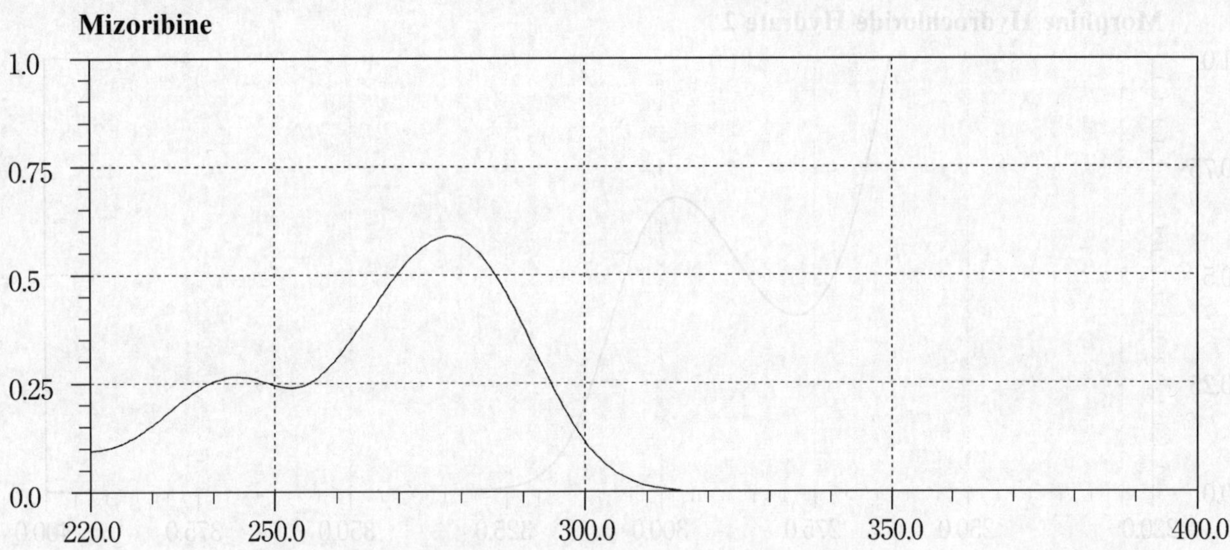

Montelukast Sodium

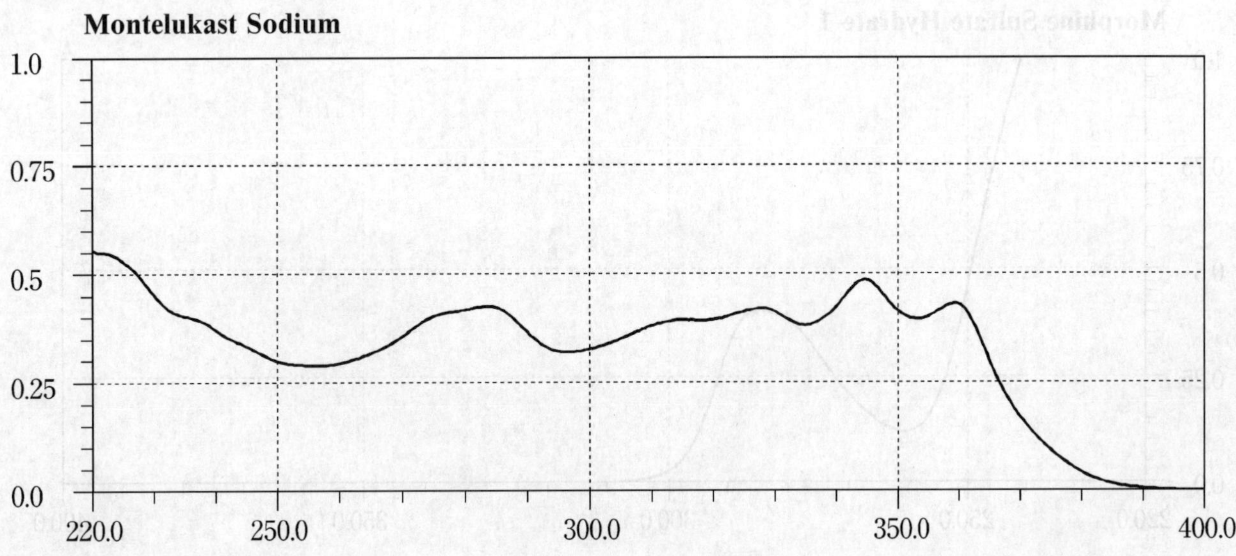

Morphine Hydrochloride Hydrate 1

1.0
0.75
0.5
0.25
0.0
220.0 250.0 275.0 300.0 325.0 350.0 375.0 400.0

Morphine Hydrochloride Hydrate 2

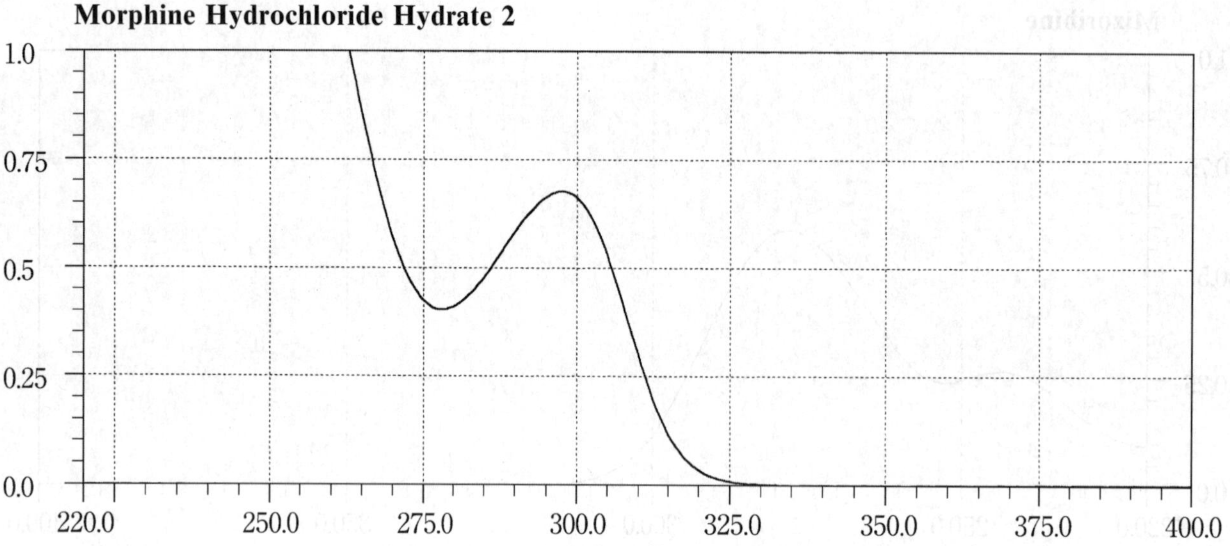

Morphine Sulfate Hydrate 1

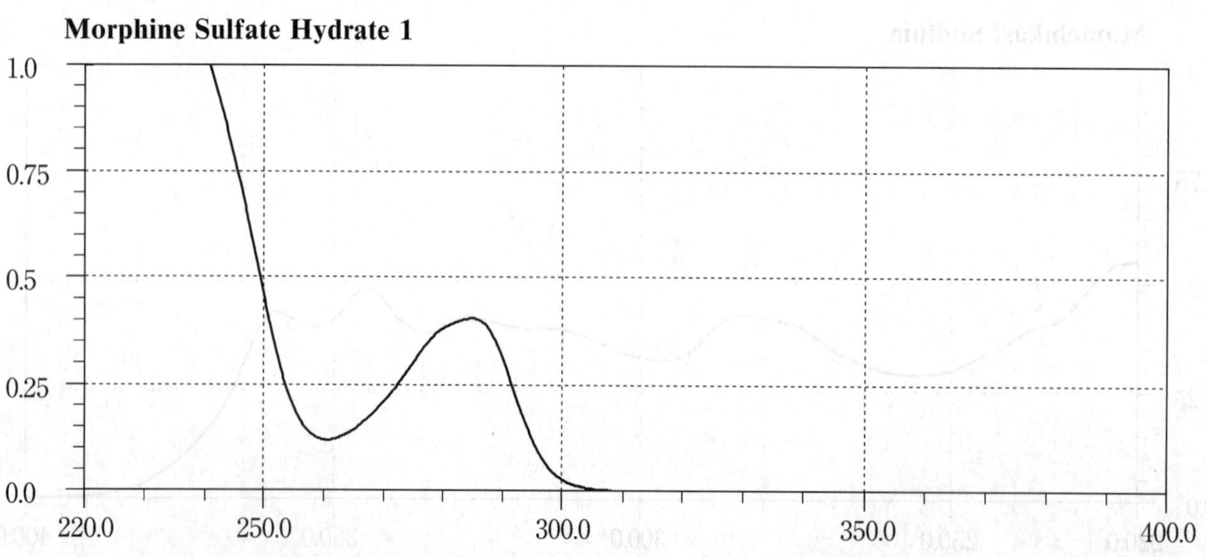

Morphine Sulfate Hydrate 2

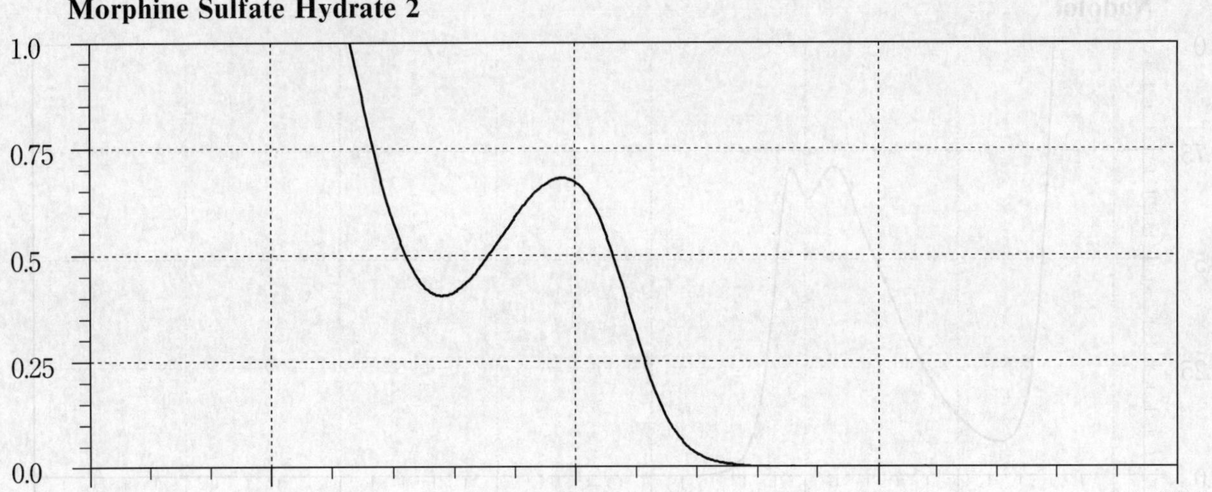

Mosapride Citrate Hydrate

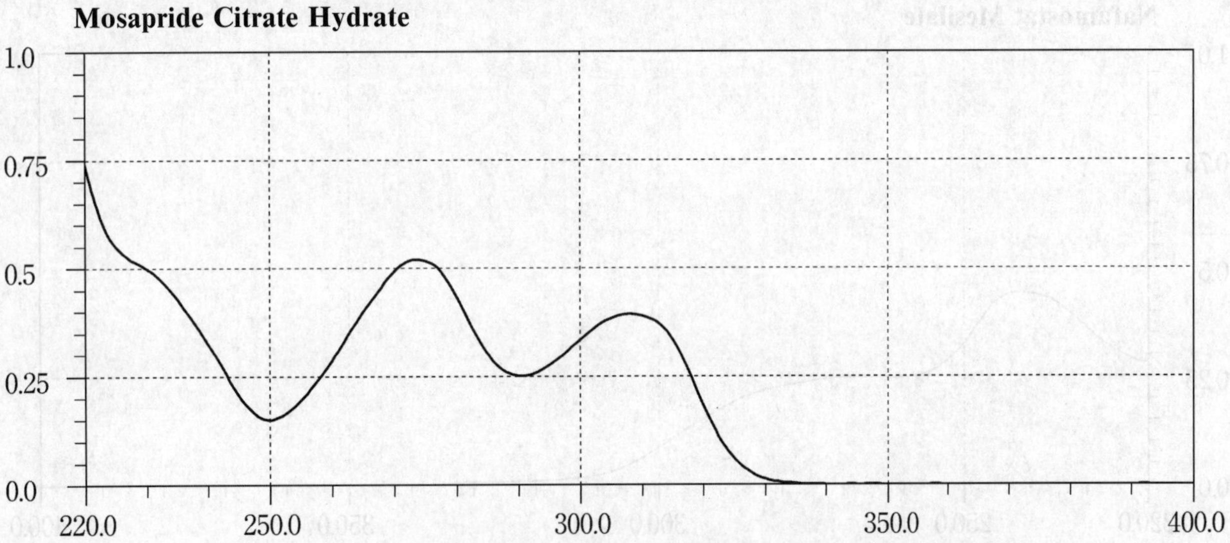

Nabumetone

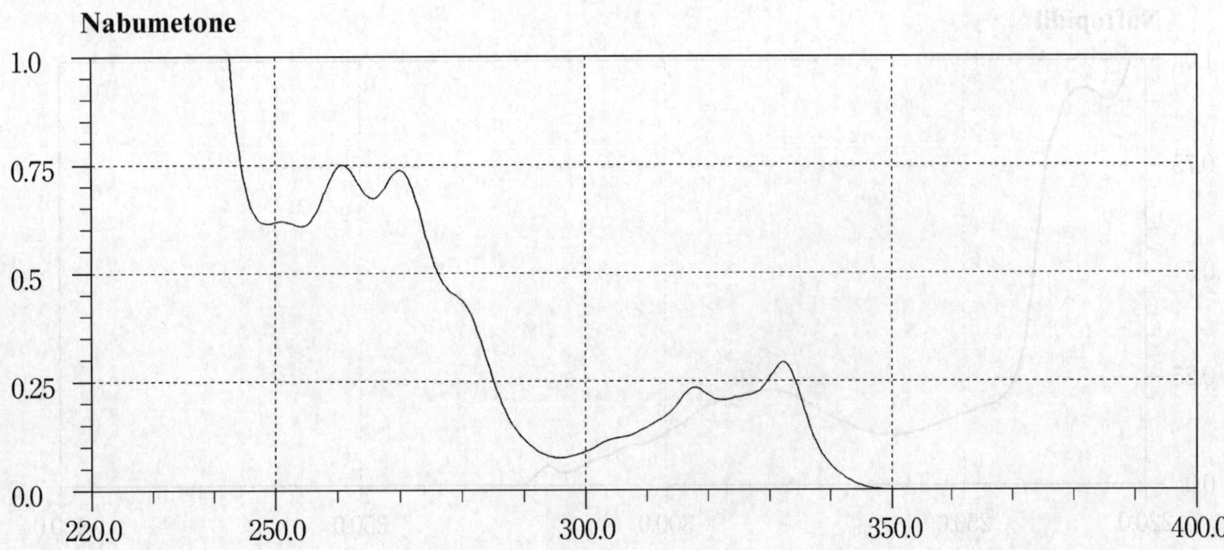

Nadolol

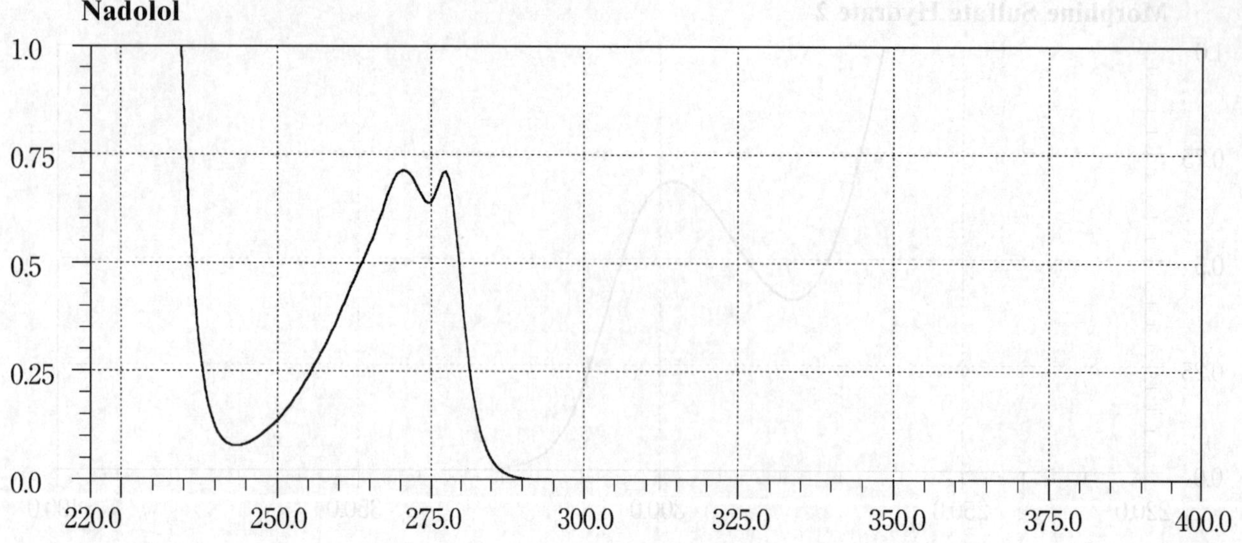

Nafamostat Mesilate

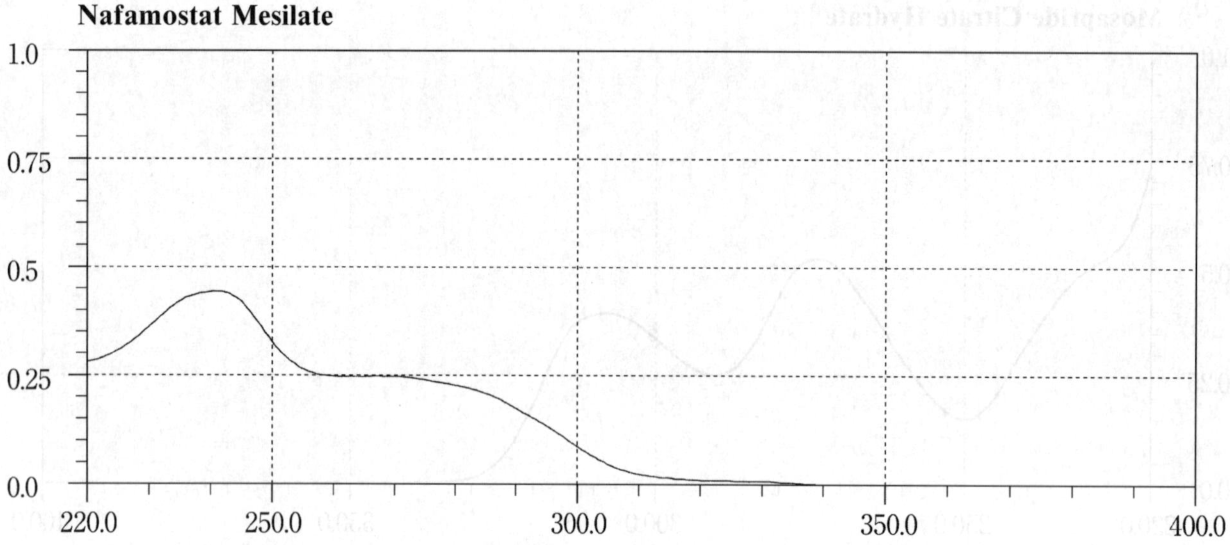

Naftopidil

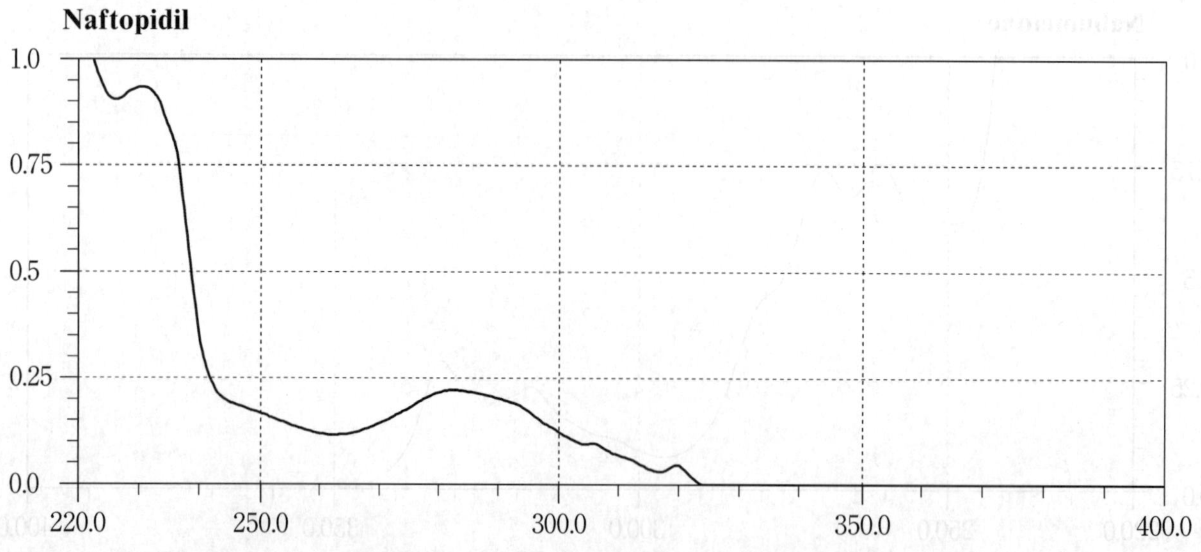

Nalidixic Acid

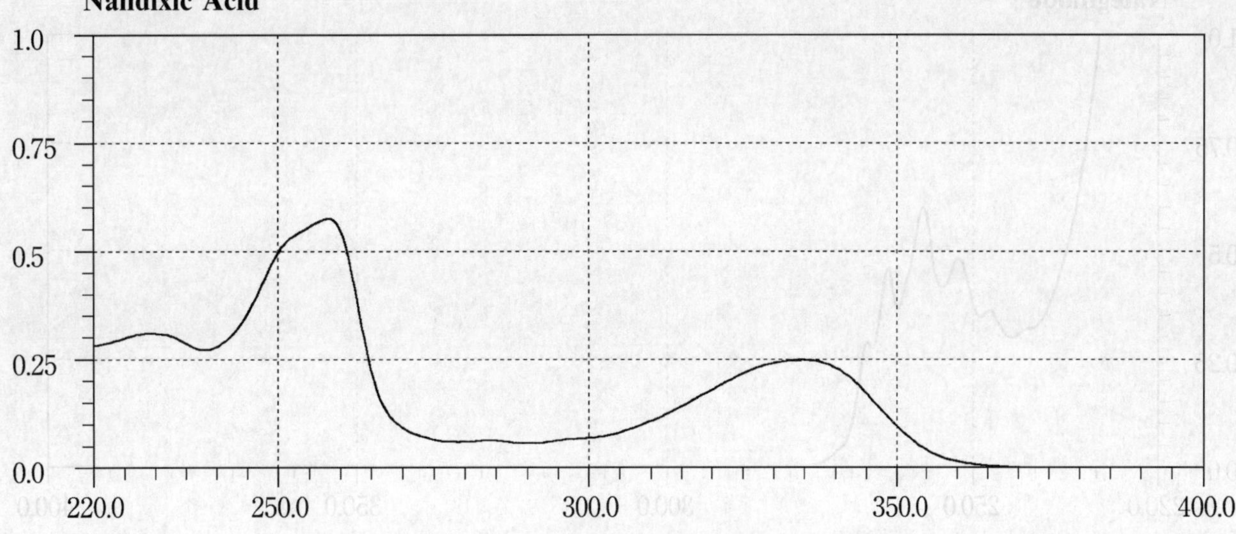

Naloxone Hydrochloride

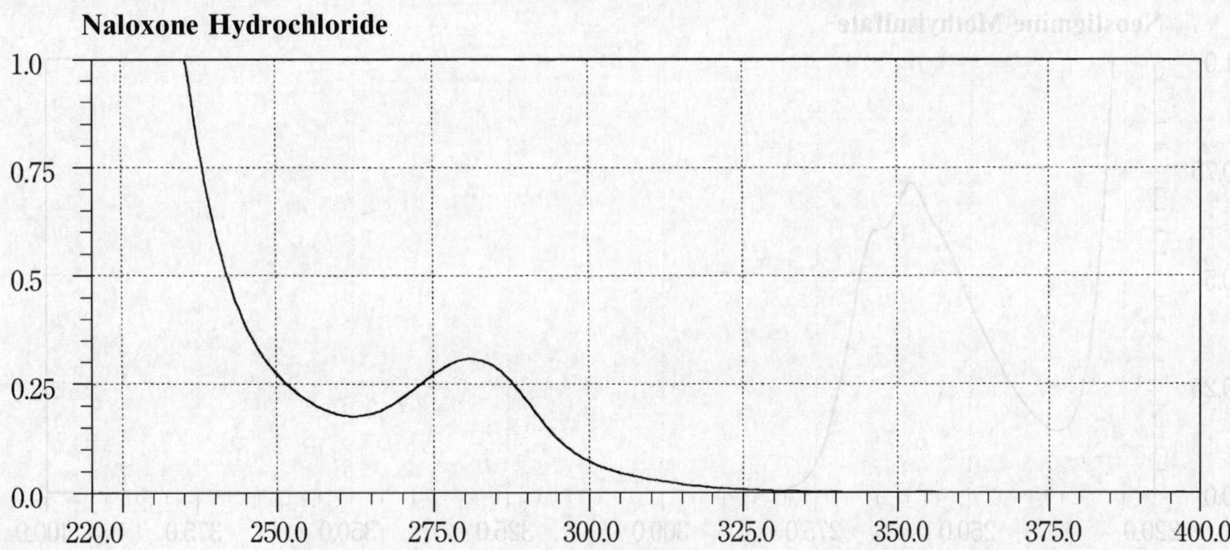

Naproxen

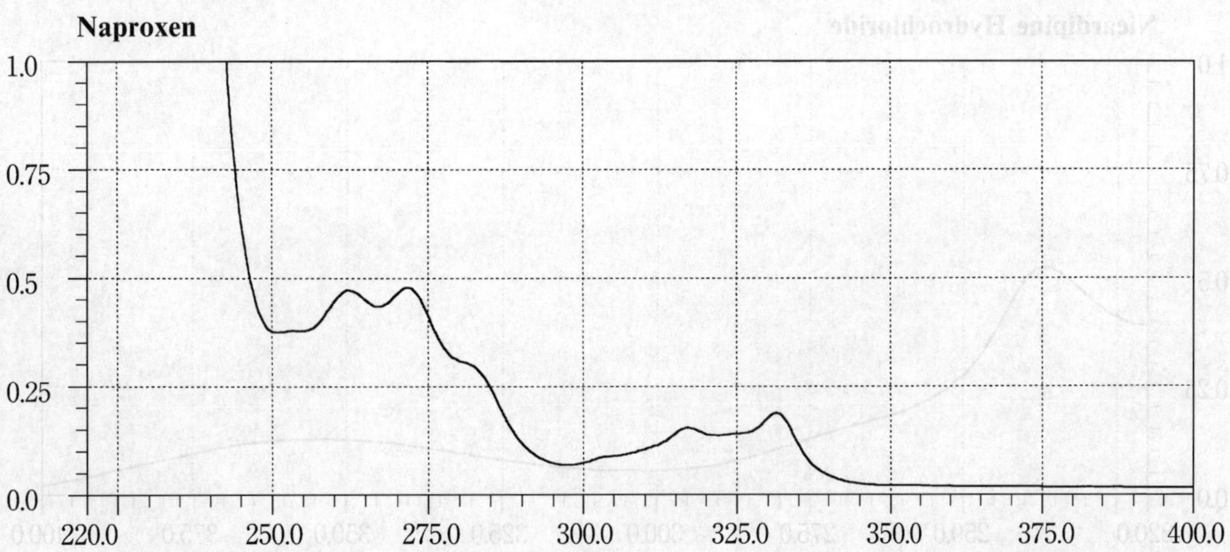

Nateglinide

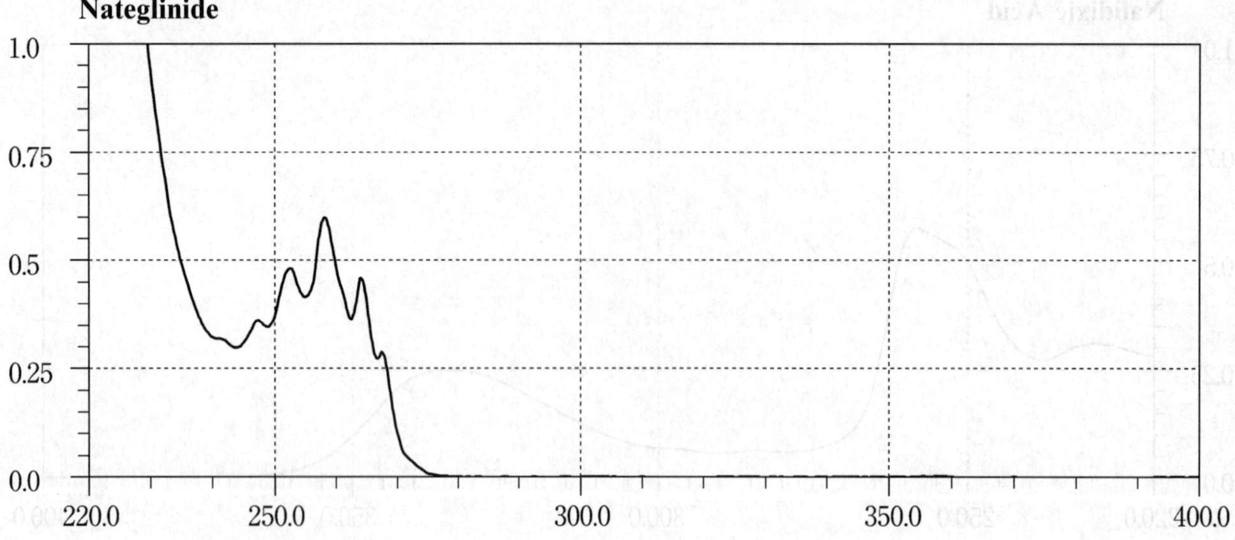

Neostigmine Methylsulfate

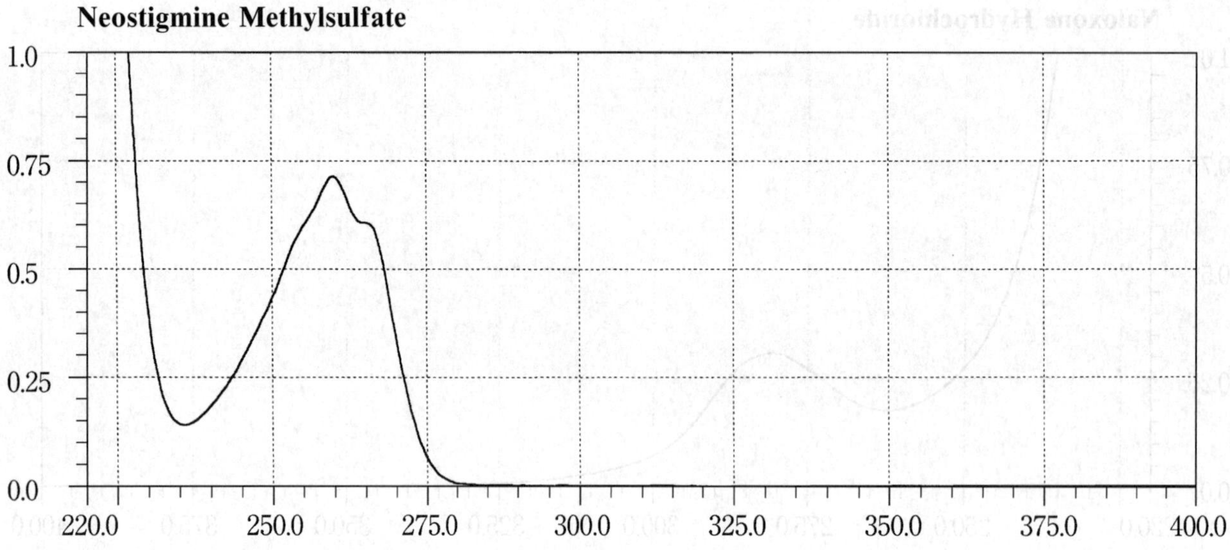

Nicardipine Hydrochloride

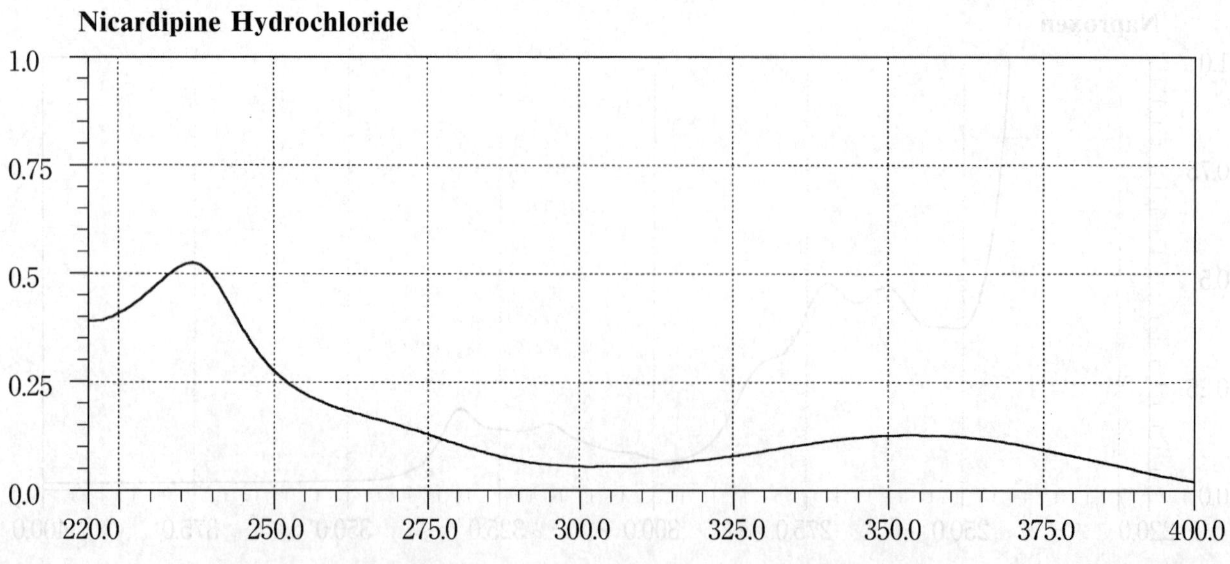

Nicergoline

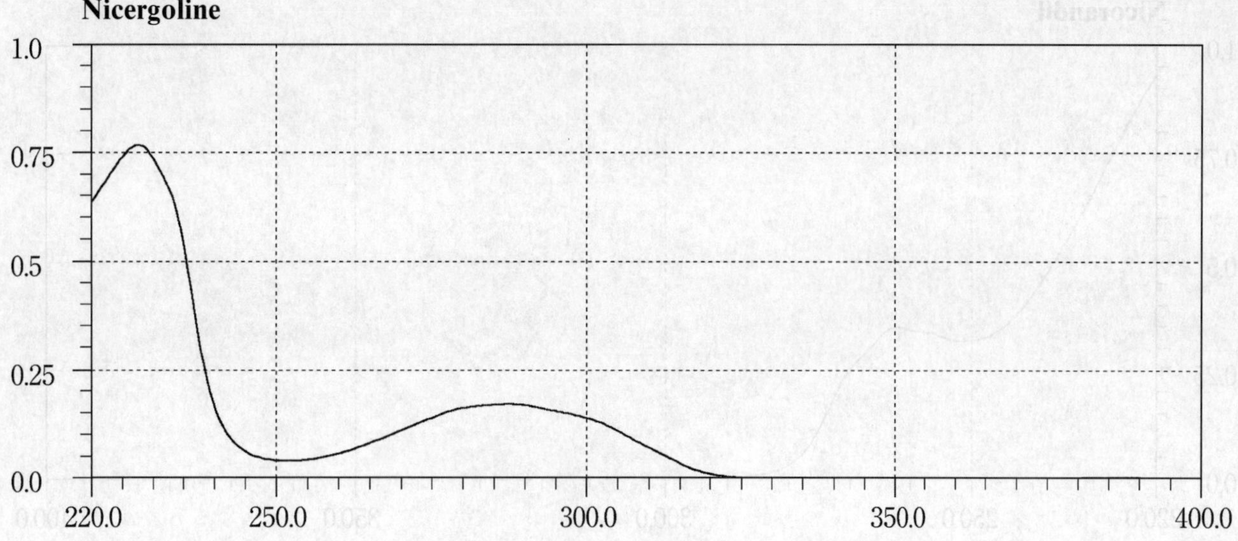

Niceritrol

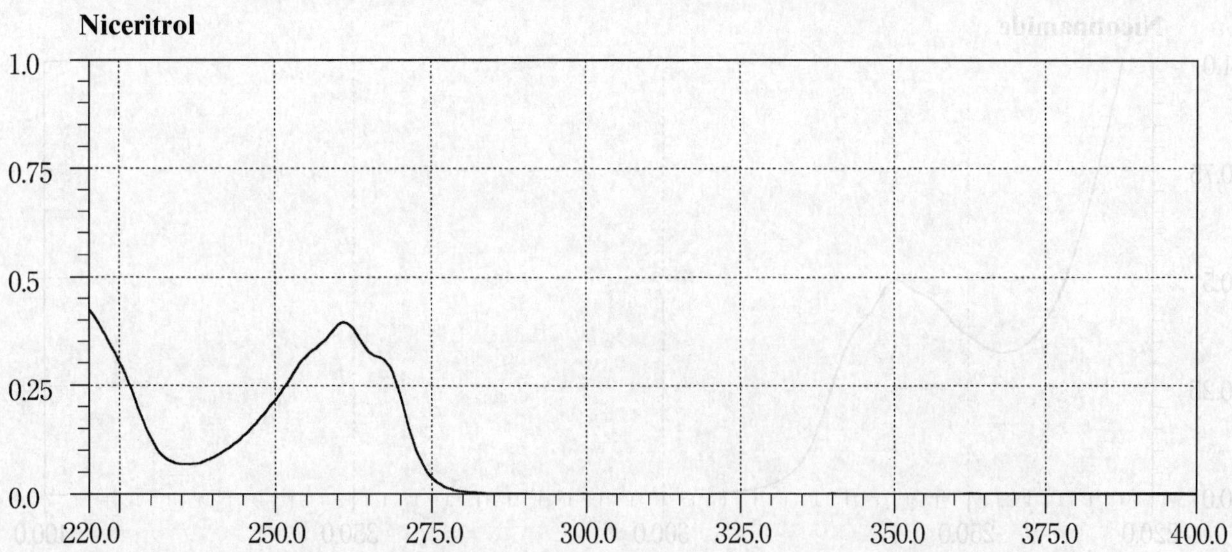

Nicomol

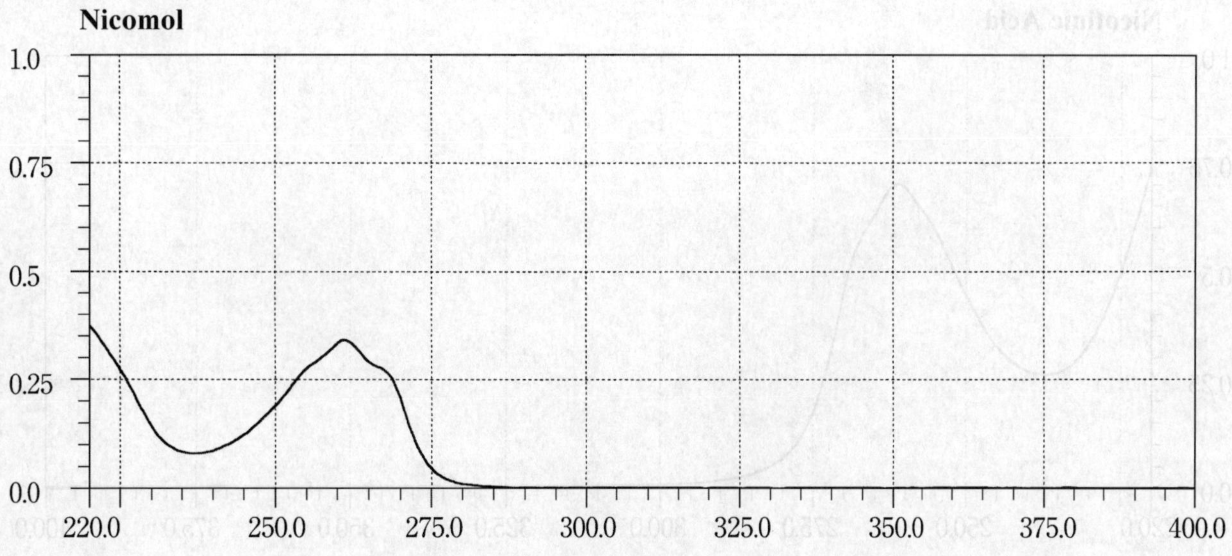

Nicorandil

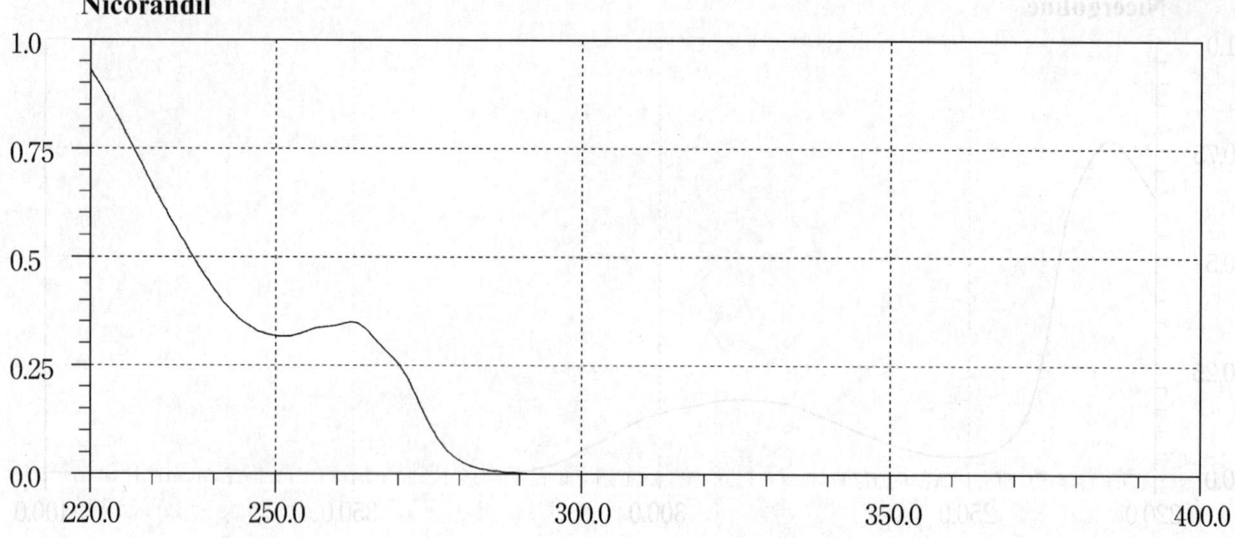

Nicotinamide

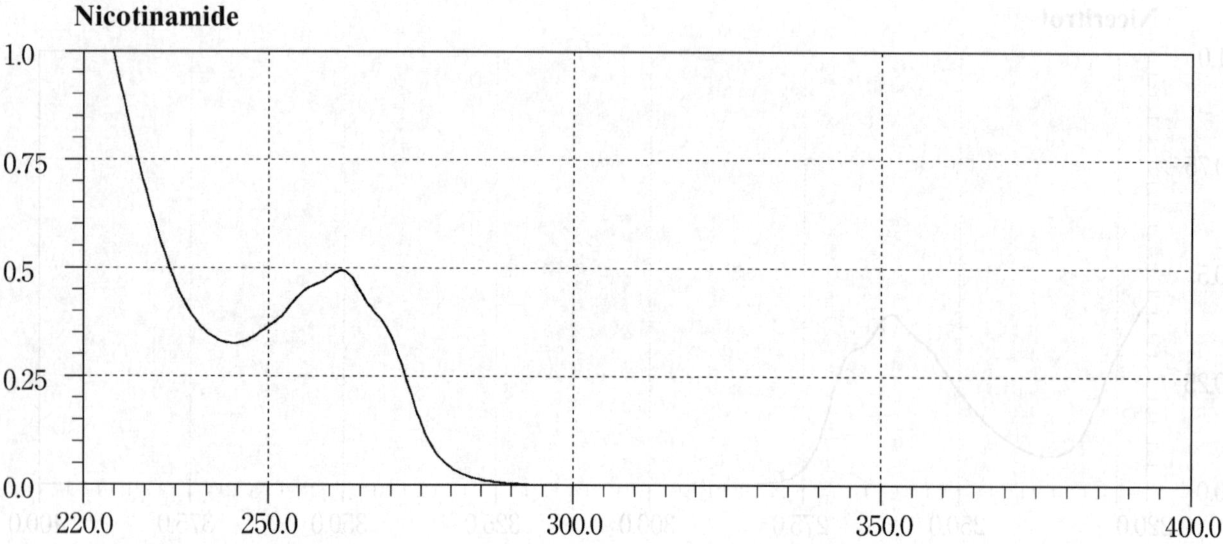

Nicotinic Acid

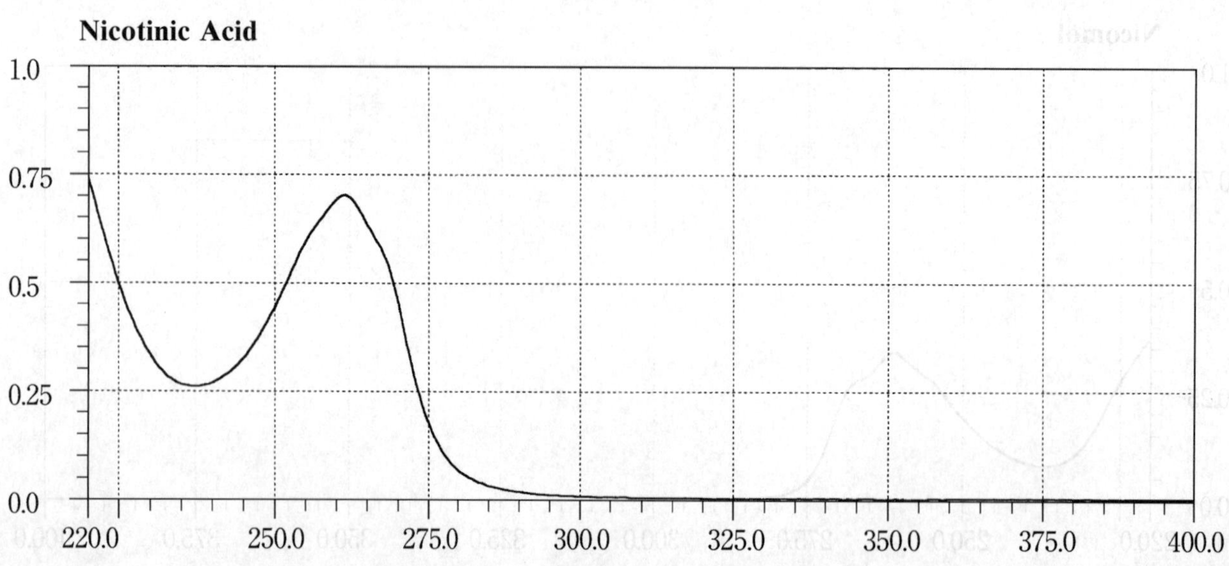

Nifedipine

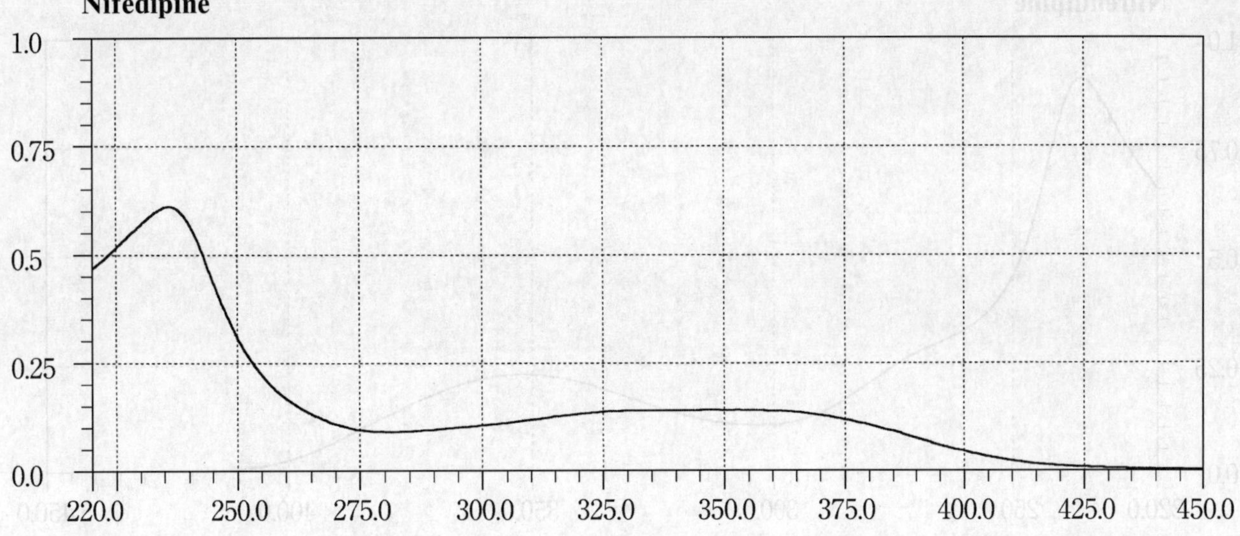

Nilvadipine

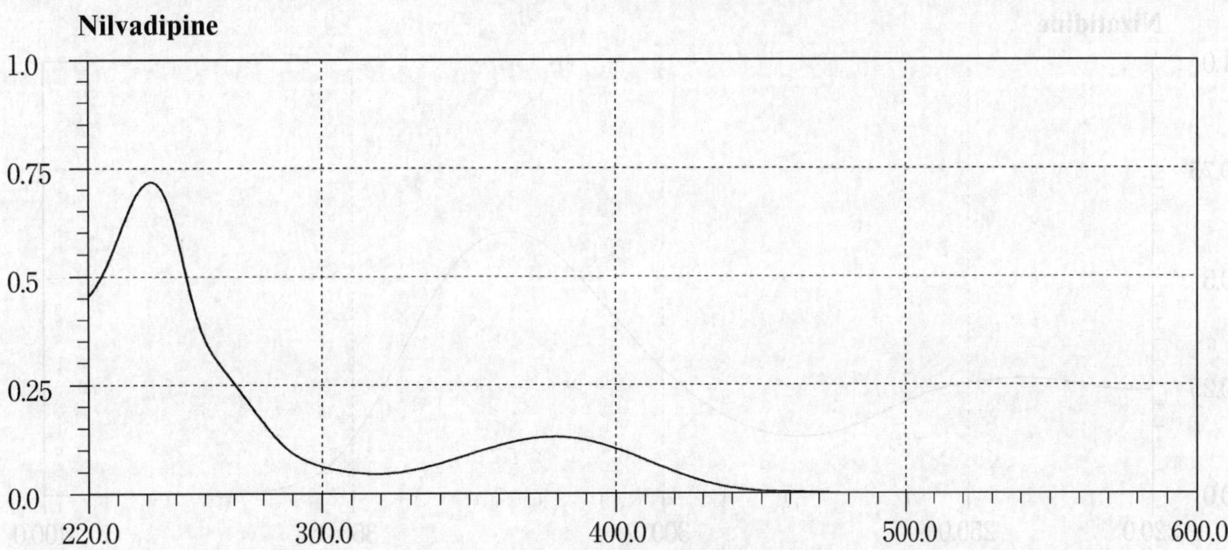

Nitrazepam

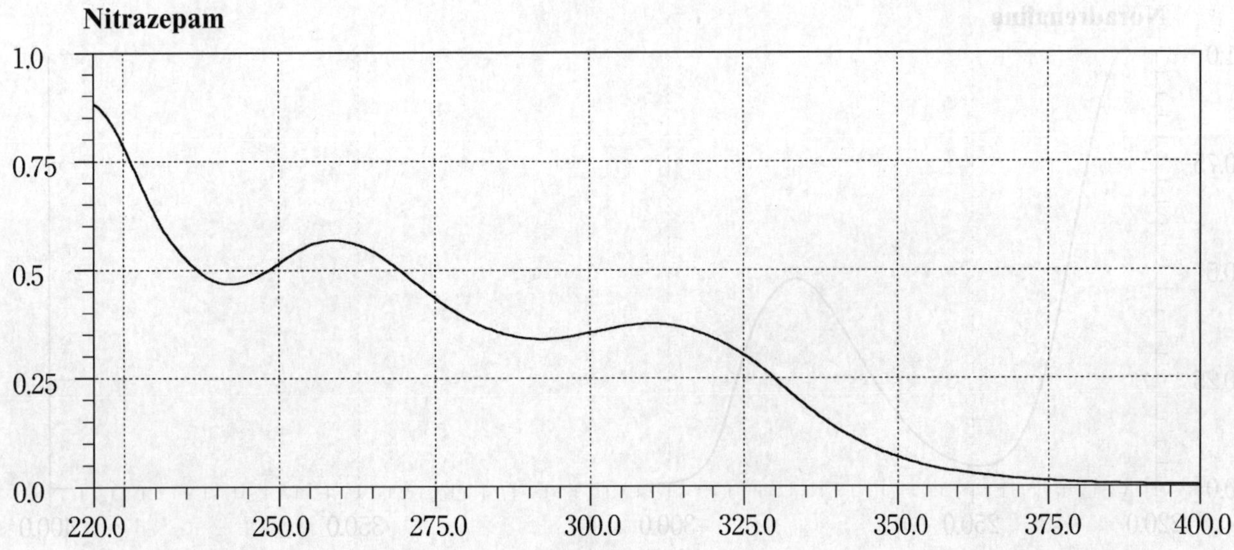

Nitrendipine

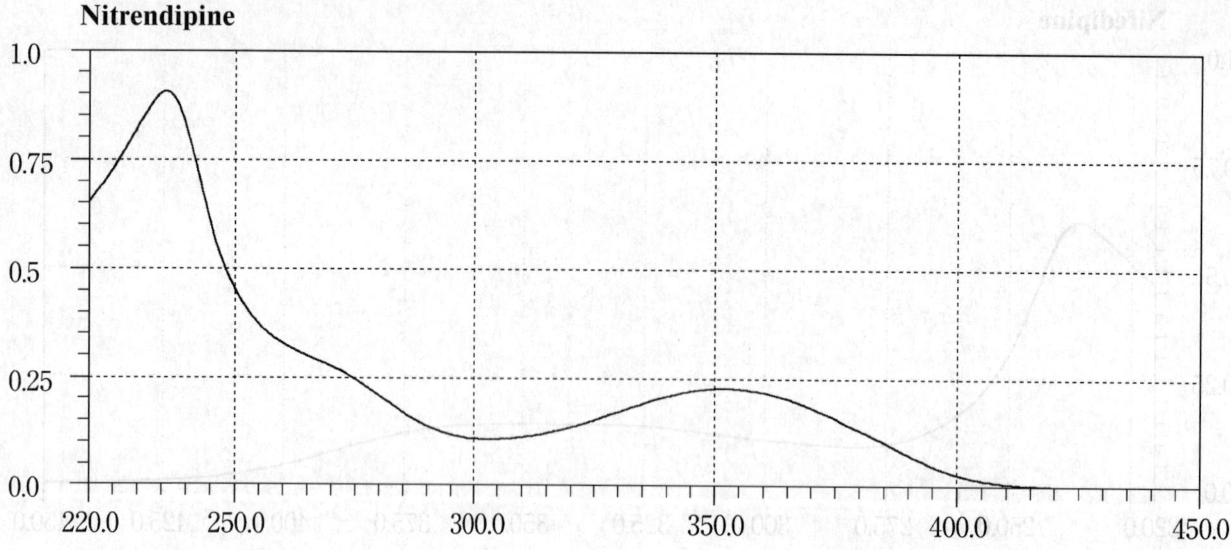

Nizatidine

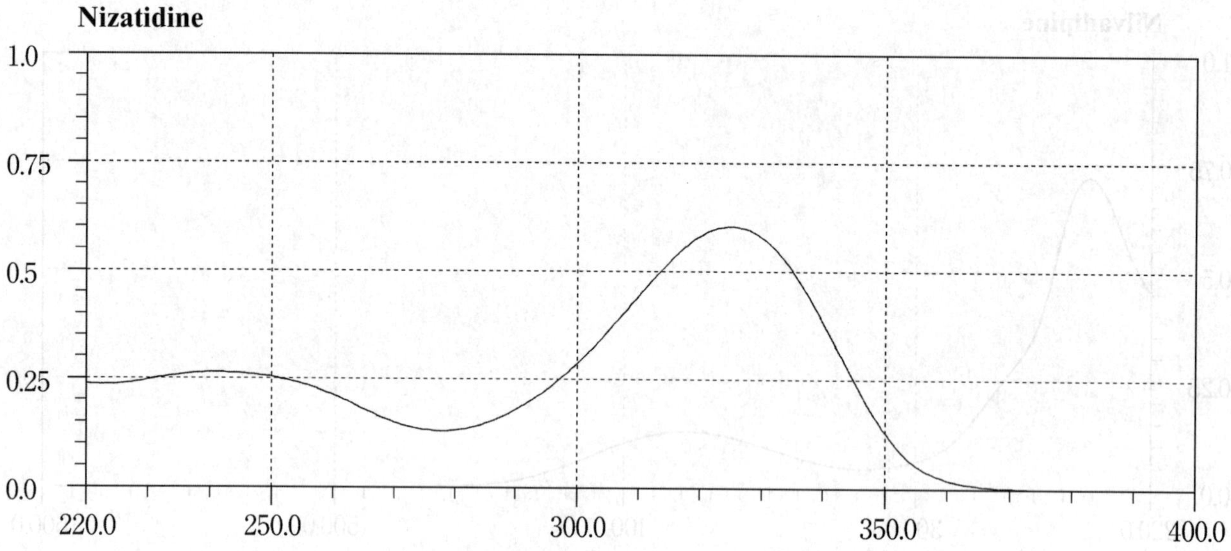

Noradrenaline

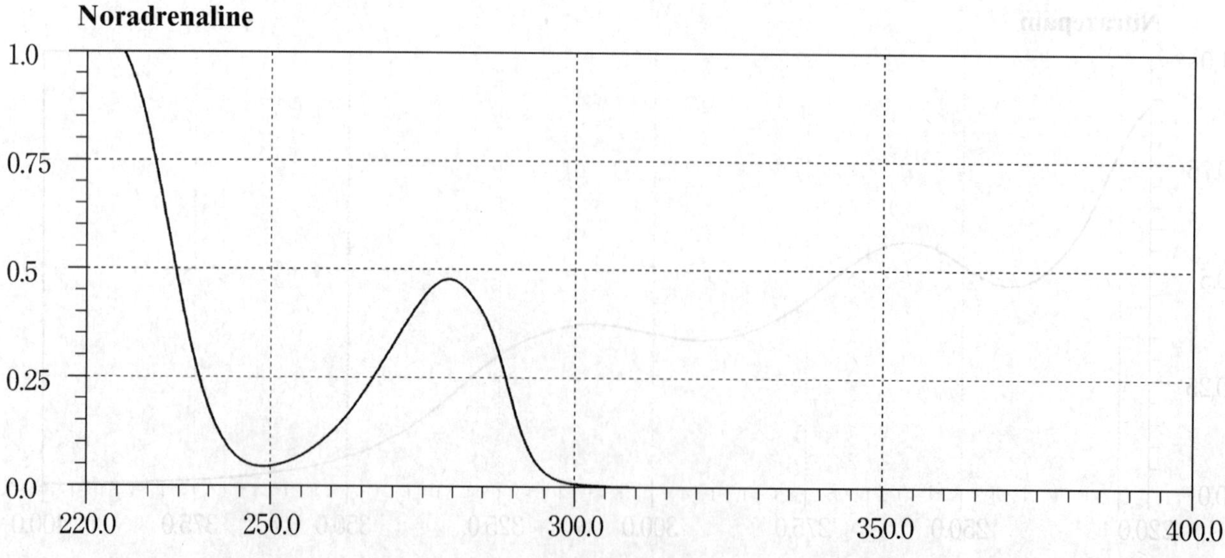

Norfloxacin

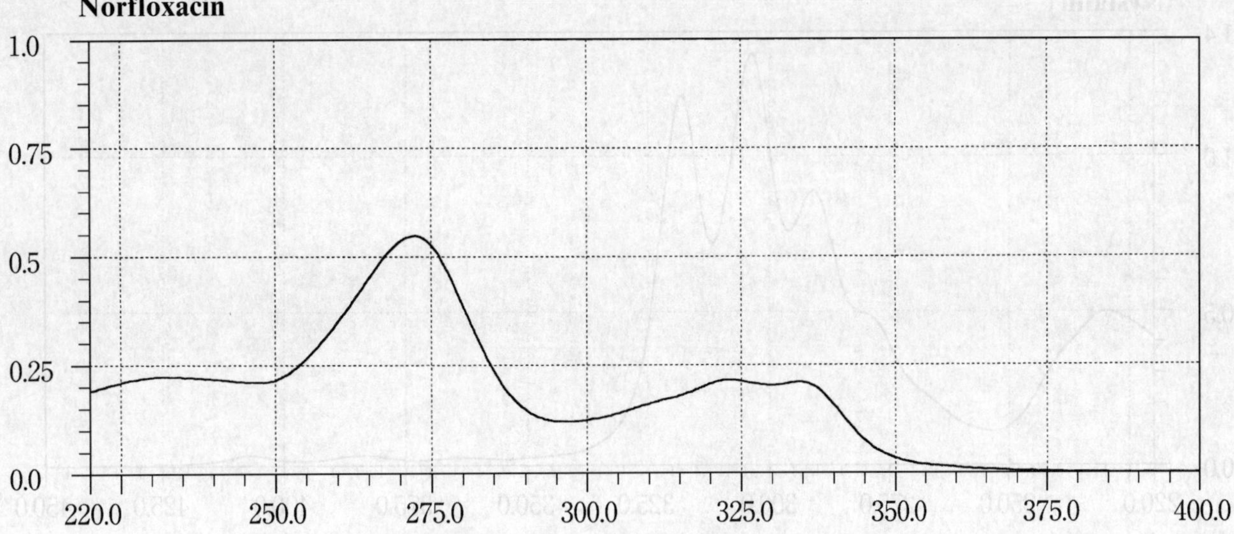

Nortriptyline Hydrochloride

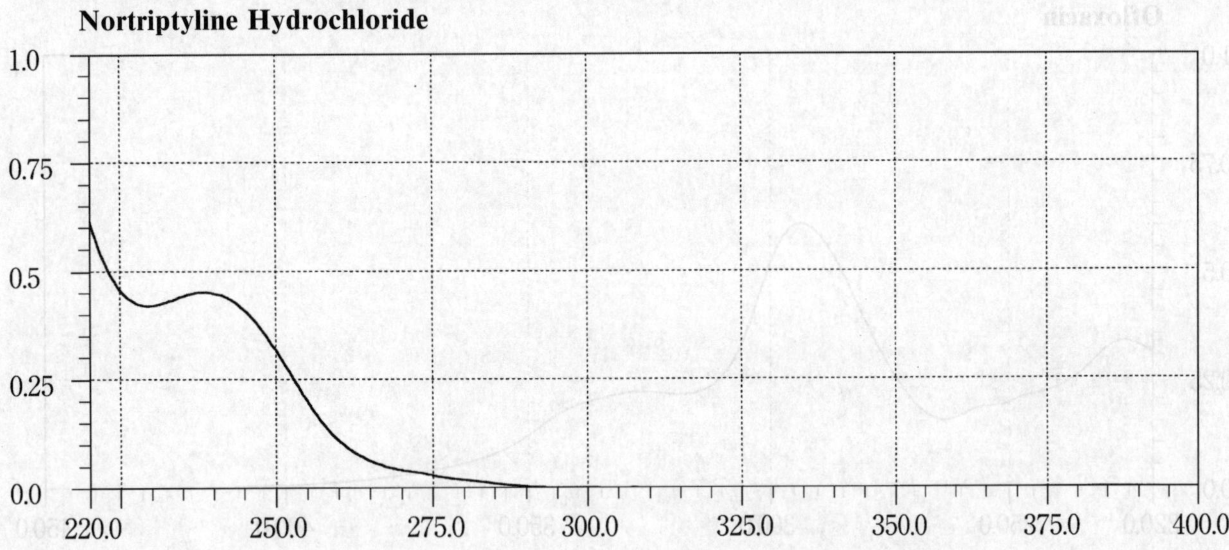

Noscapine

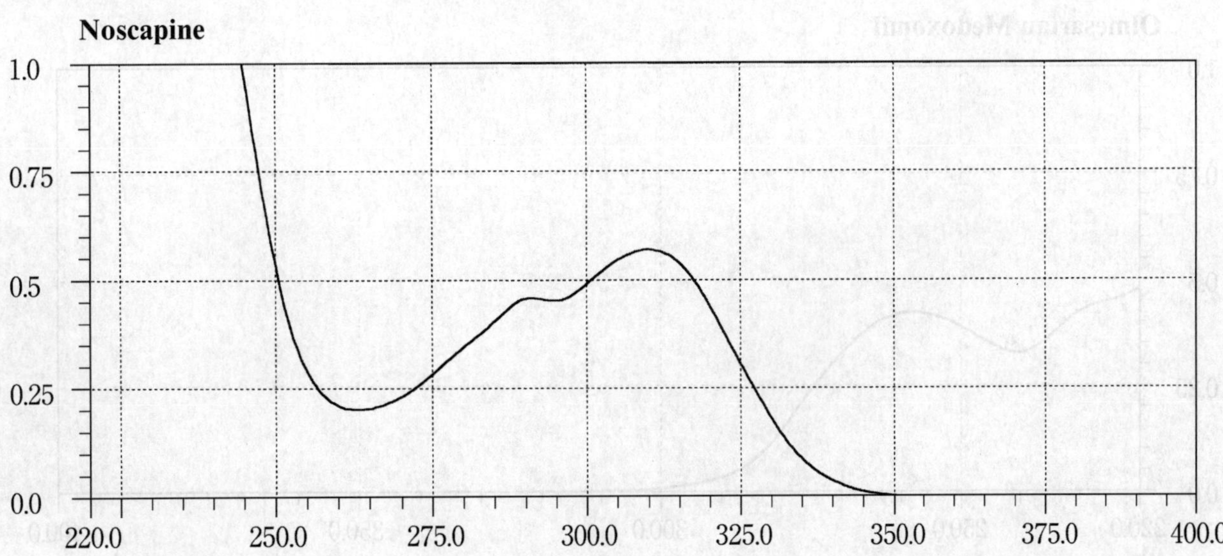

The JP Drugs are to be tested according to the provisions given in the pertinent monographs, General Notices, General Rules for Crude Drugs, General Rules for Preparations, and General Tests for their conformity to the Japanese Pharmacopoeia. (See the General Notices 5.)

Nystatin

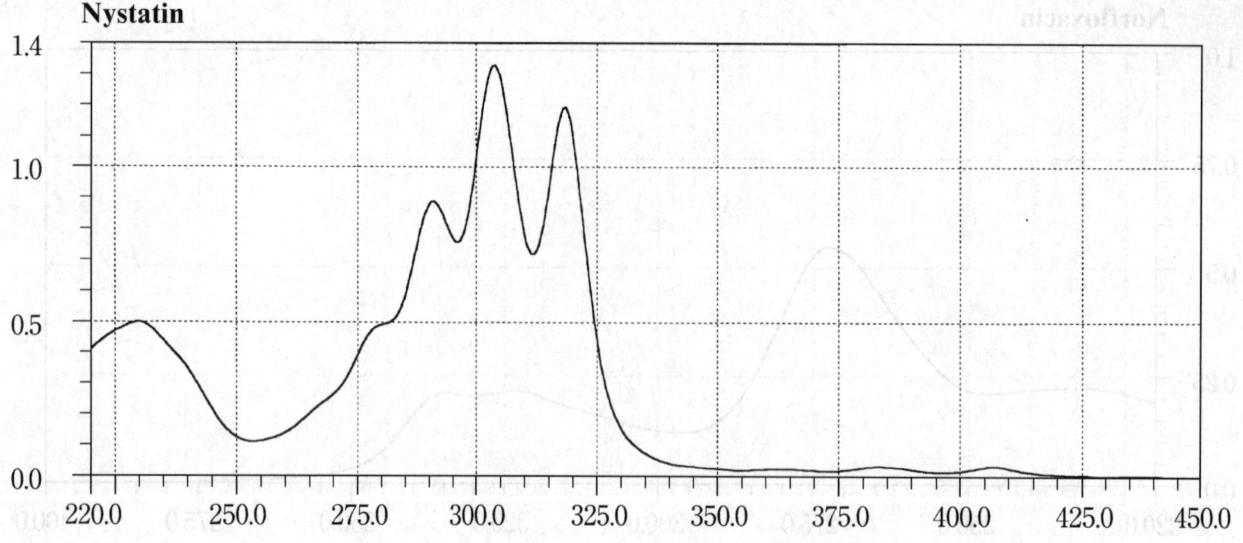

Ofloxacin

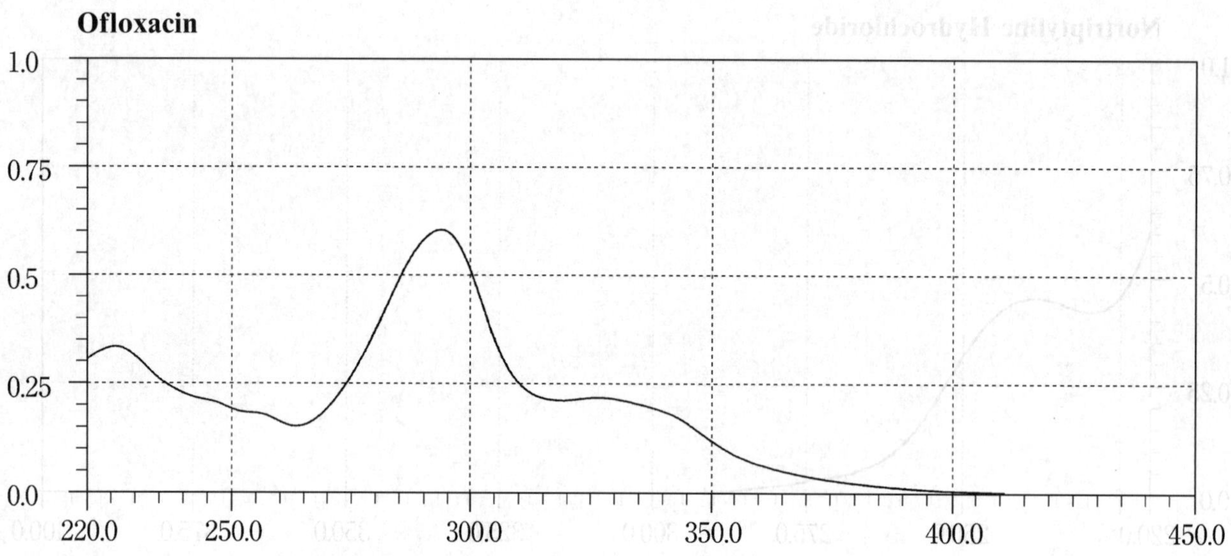

Olmesartan Medoxomil

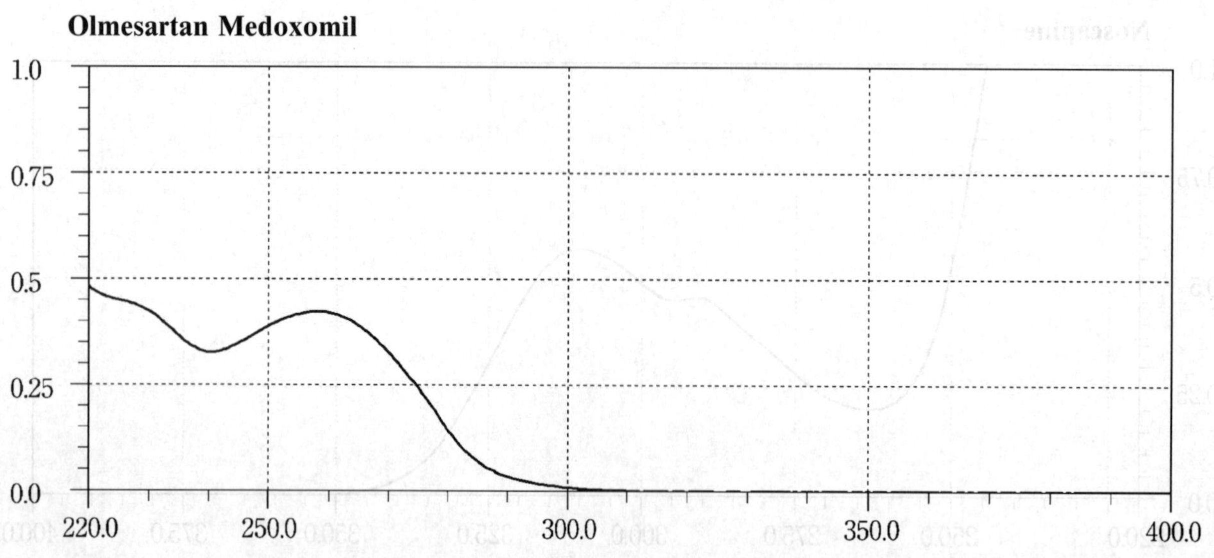

Olopatadine Hydrochloride

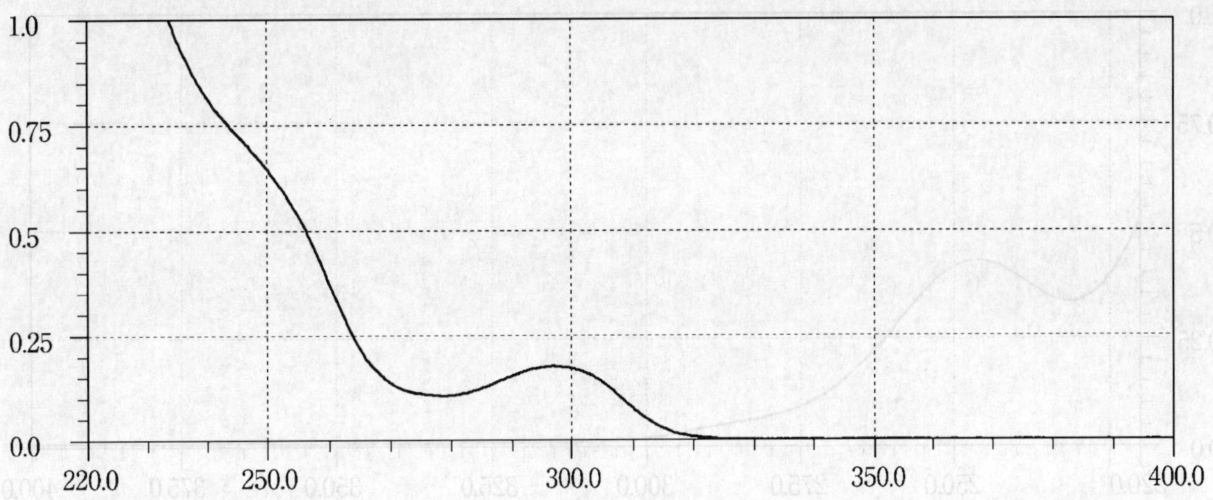

Omeprazole

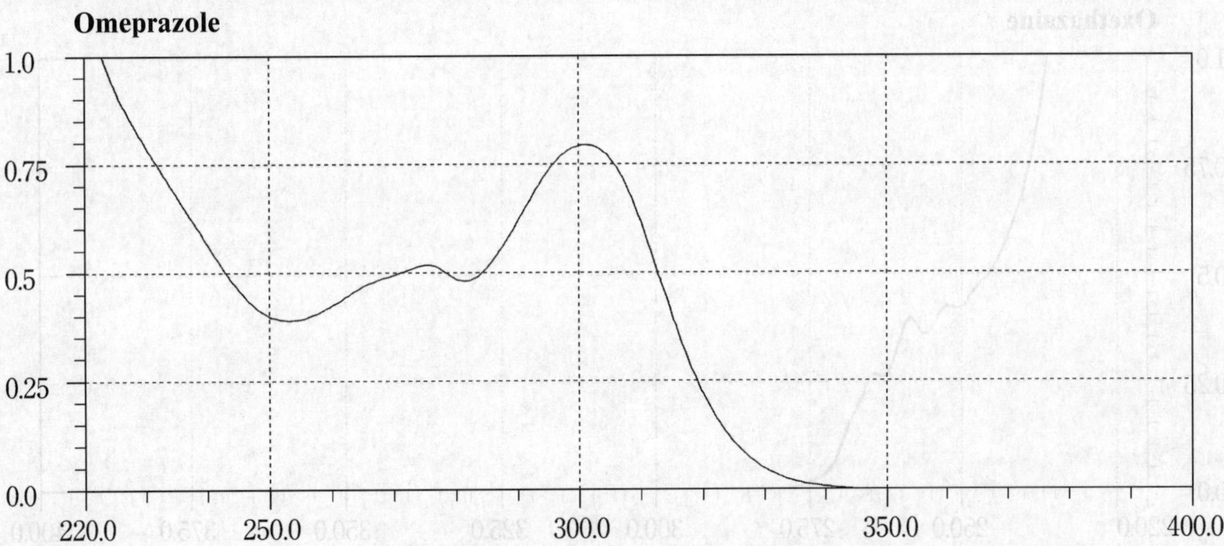

Orciprenaline Sulfate

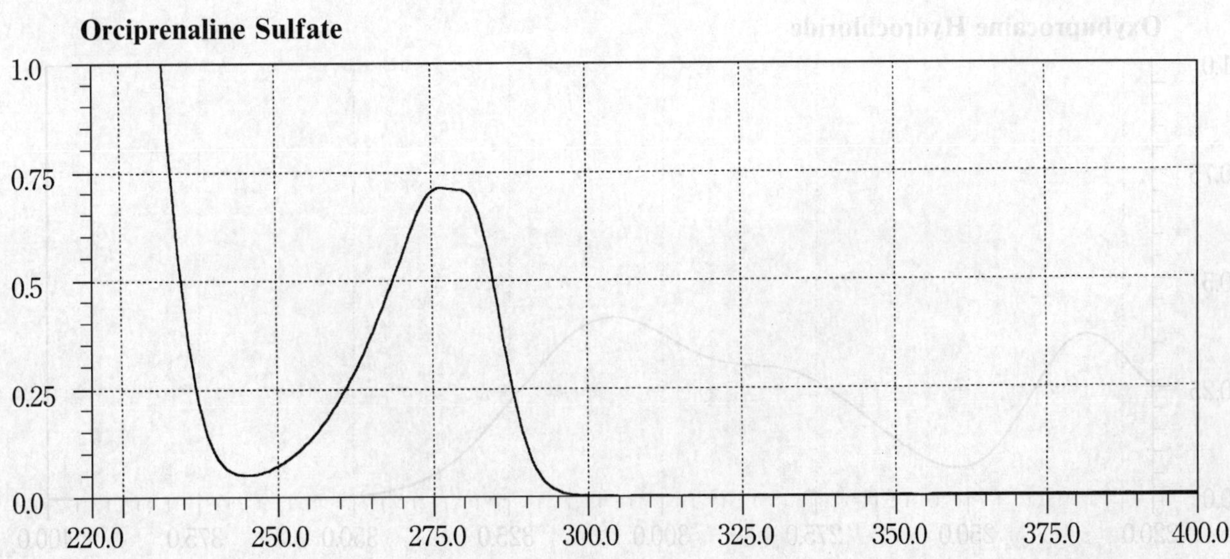

Oxazolam

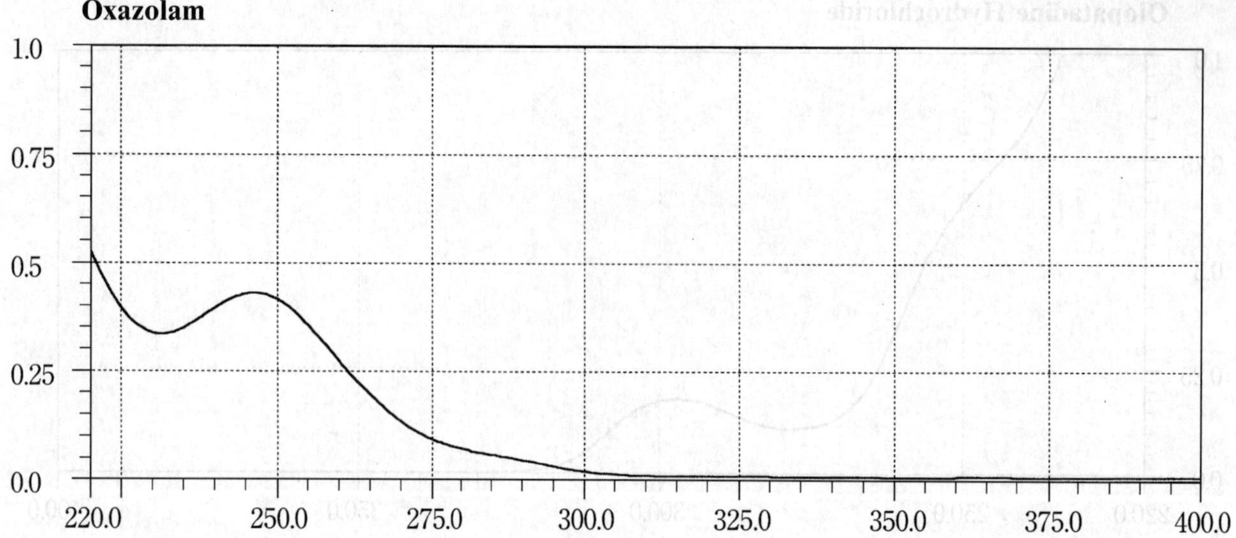

Oxethazaine

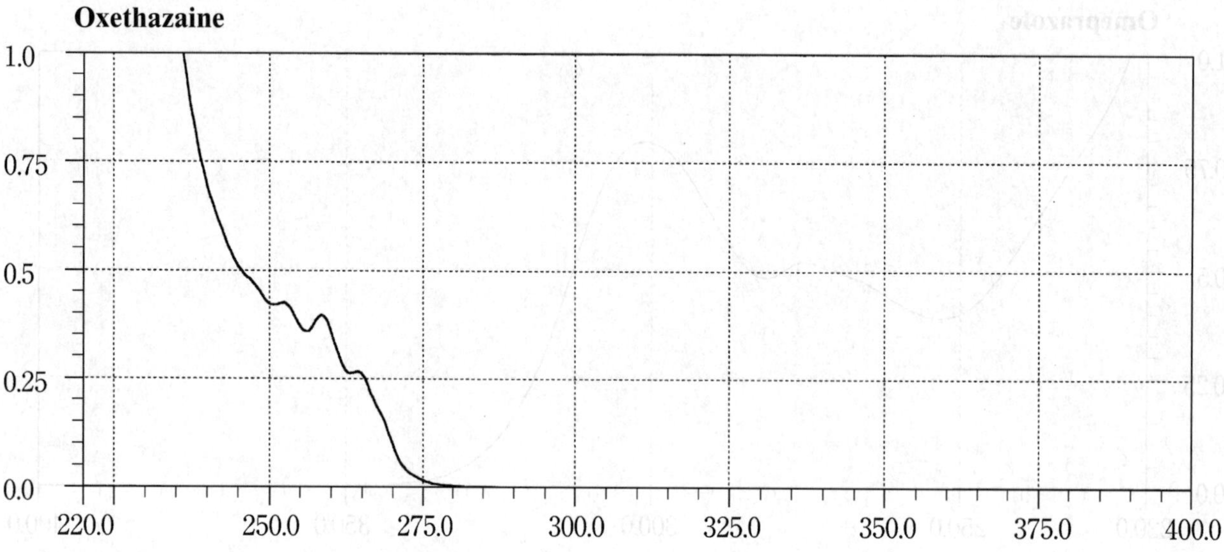

Oxybuprocaine Hydrochloride

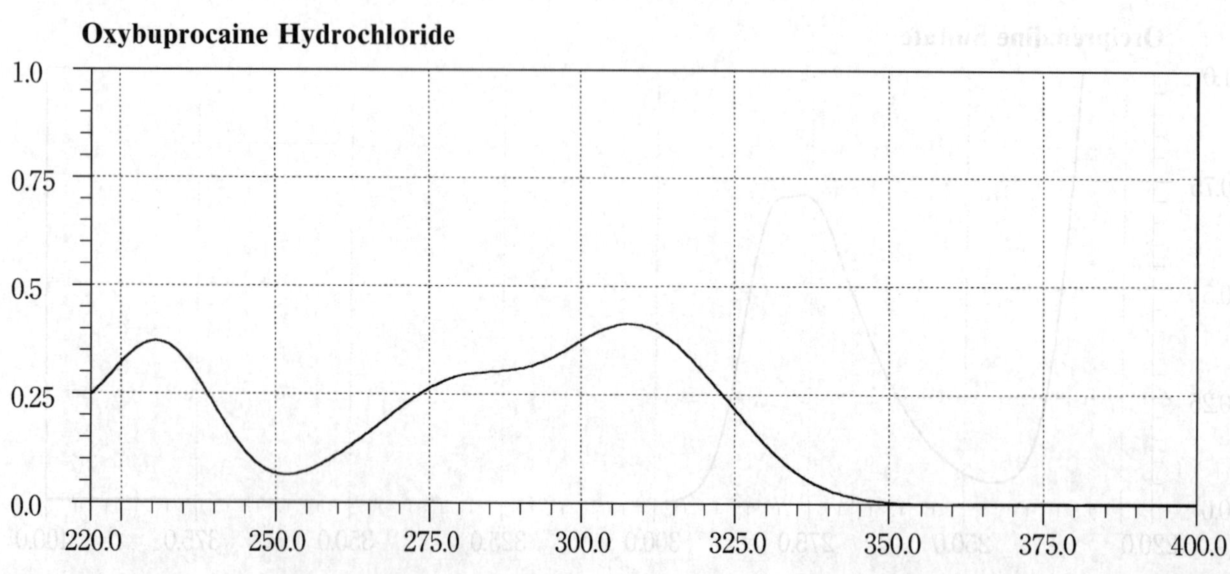

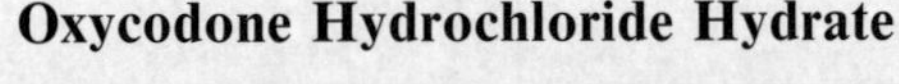

Oxycodone Hydrochloride Hydrate

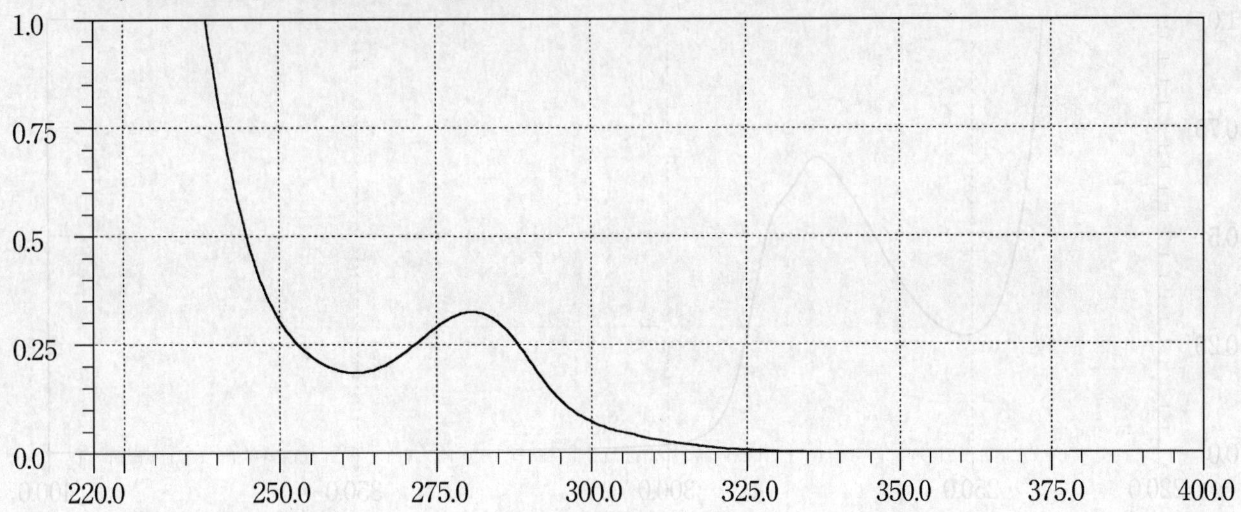

Oxymetholone

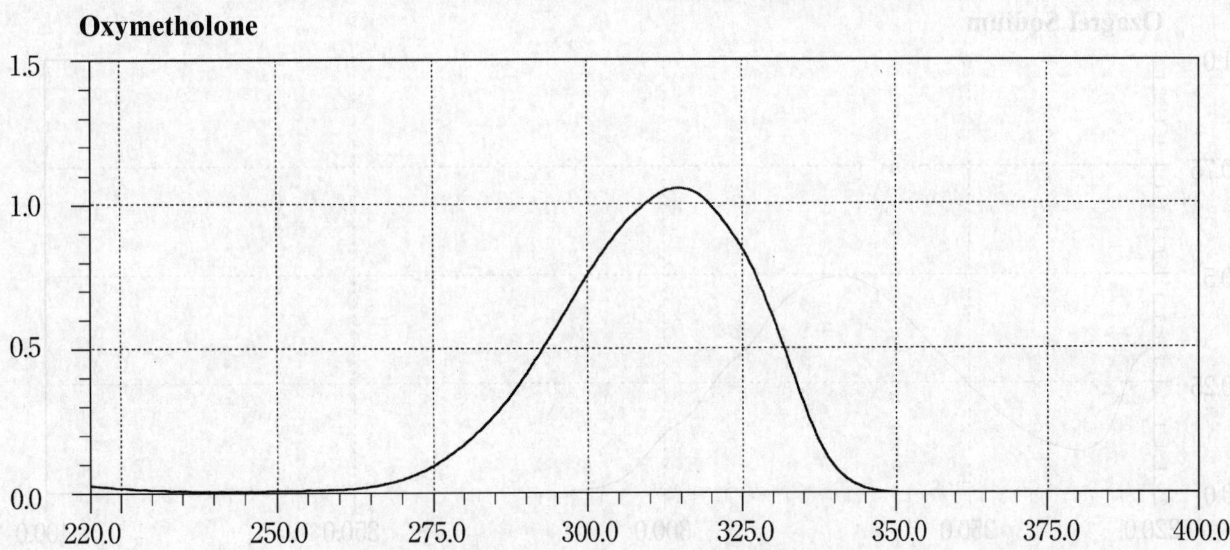

Oxytetracycline Hydrochloride

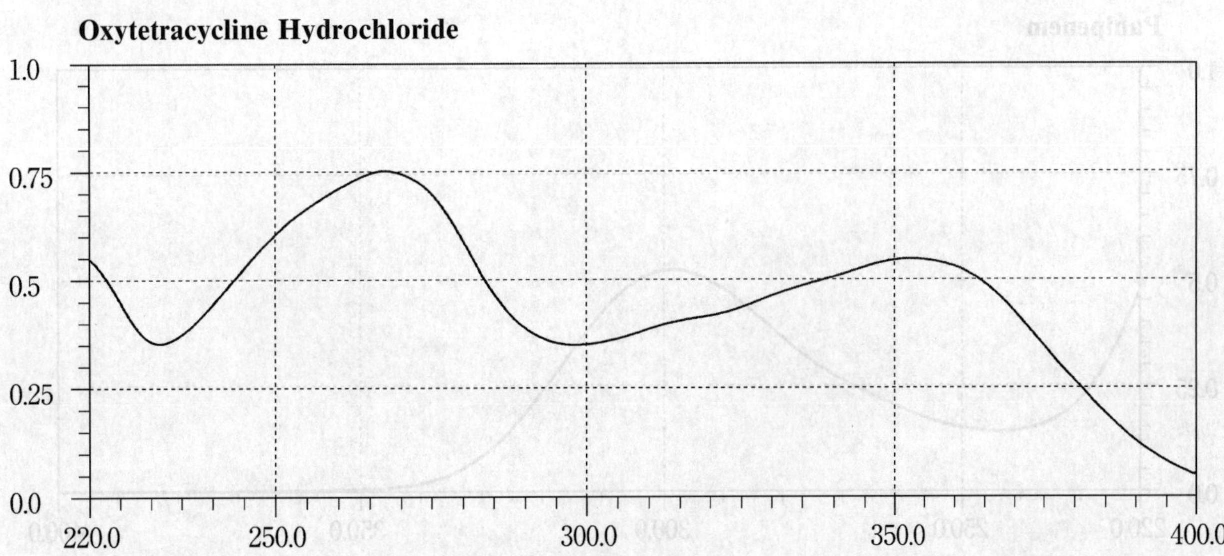

Oxytocin

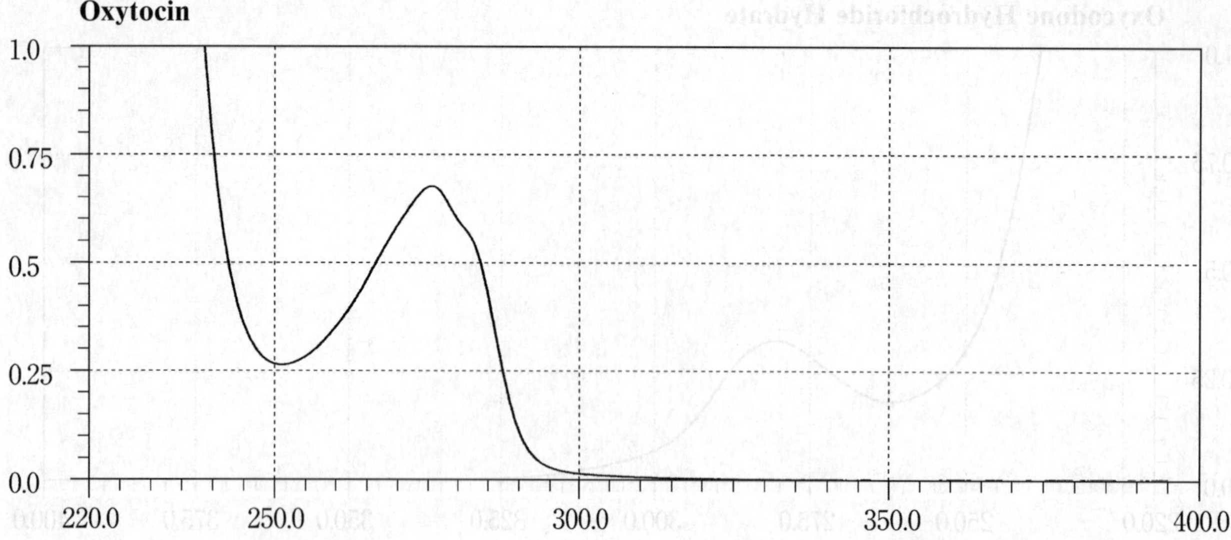

Ozagrel Sodium

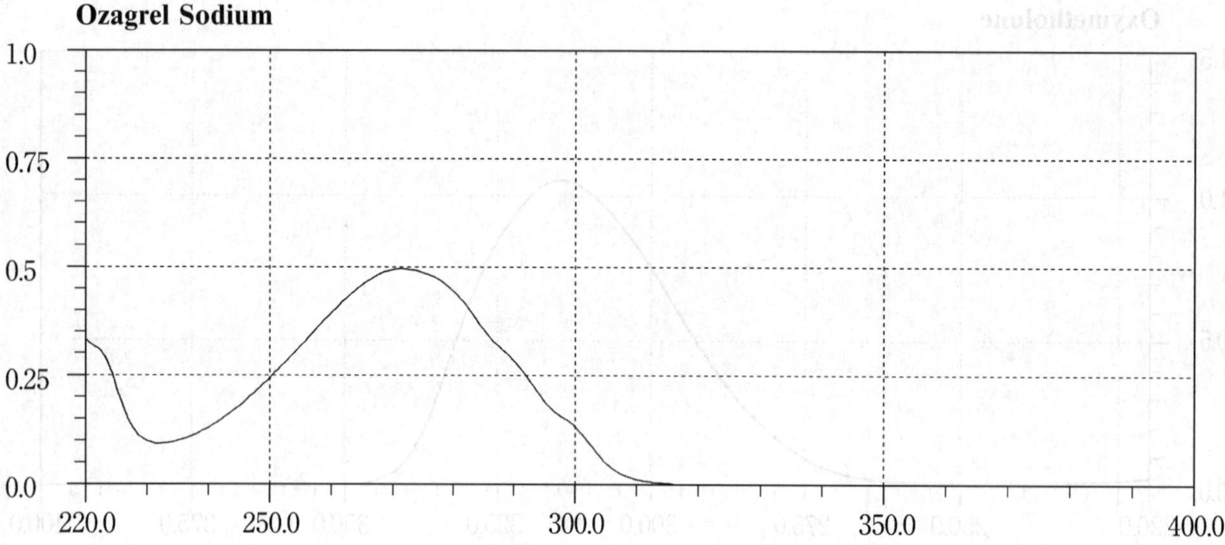

Panipenem

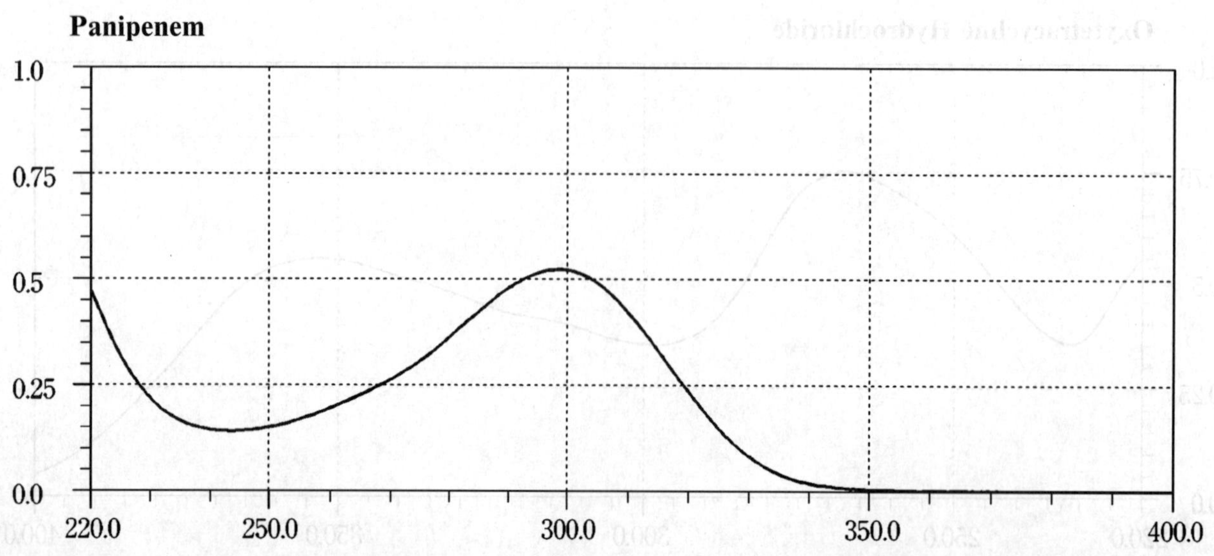

Paroxetine Hydrochloride Hydrate

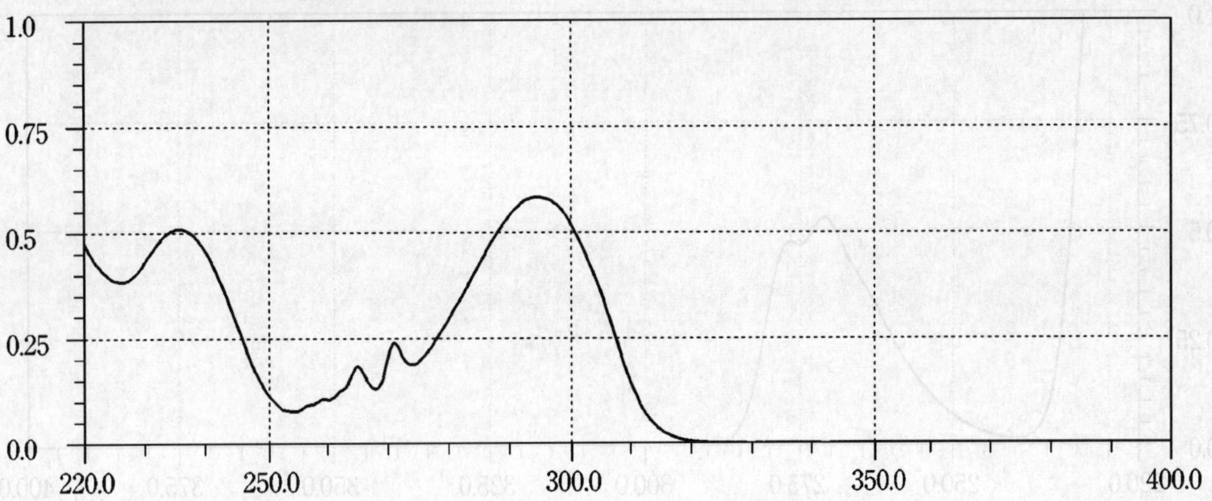

Pazufloxacin Mesilate

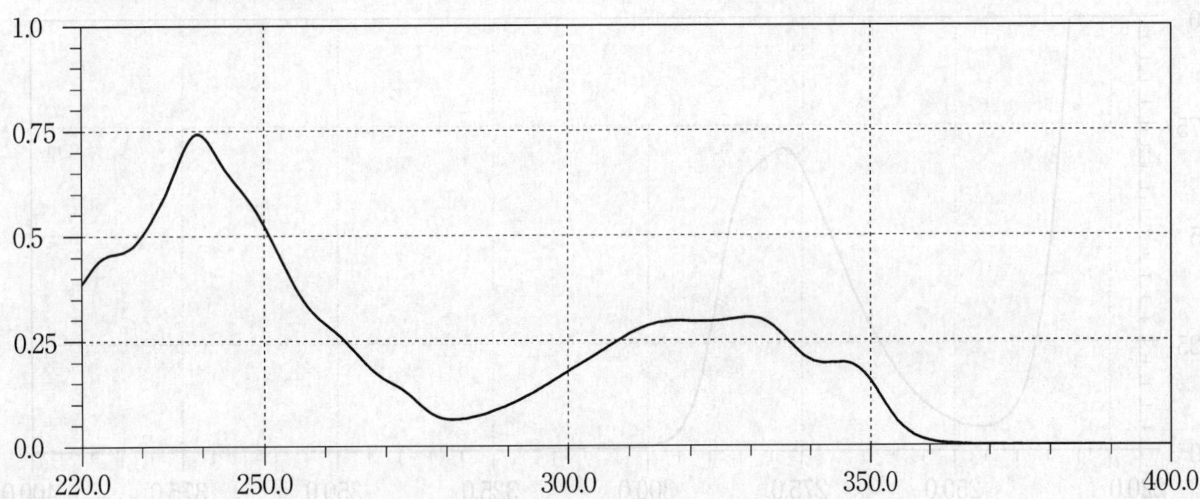

Pemirolast Potassium

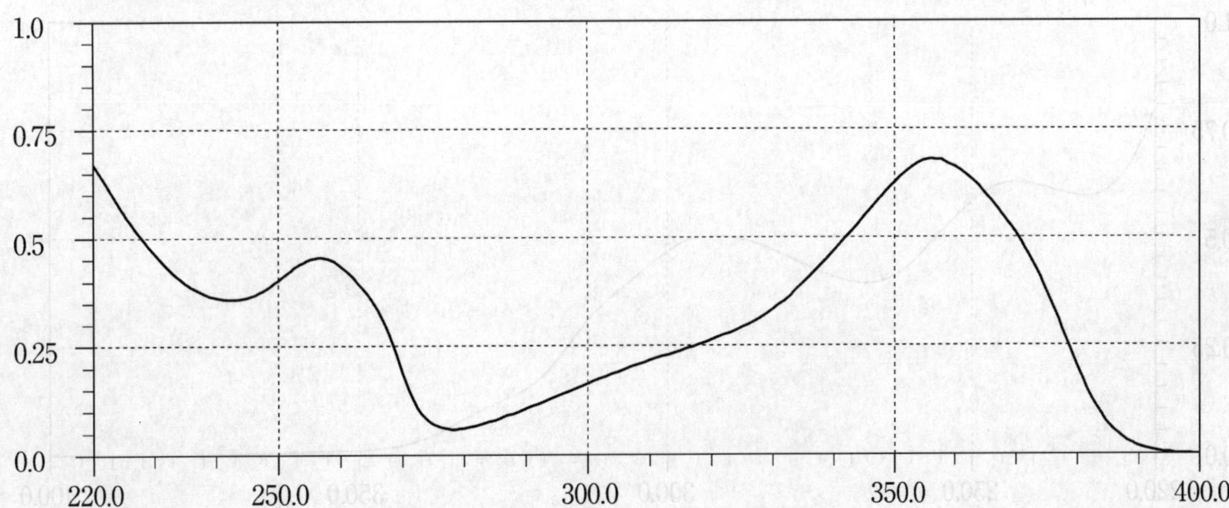

Penbutolol Sulfate

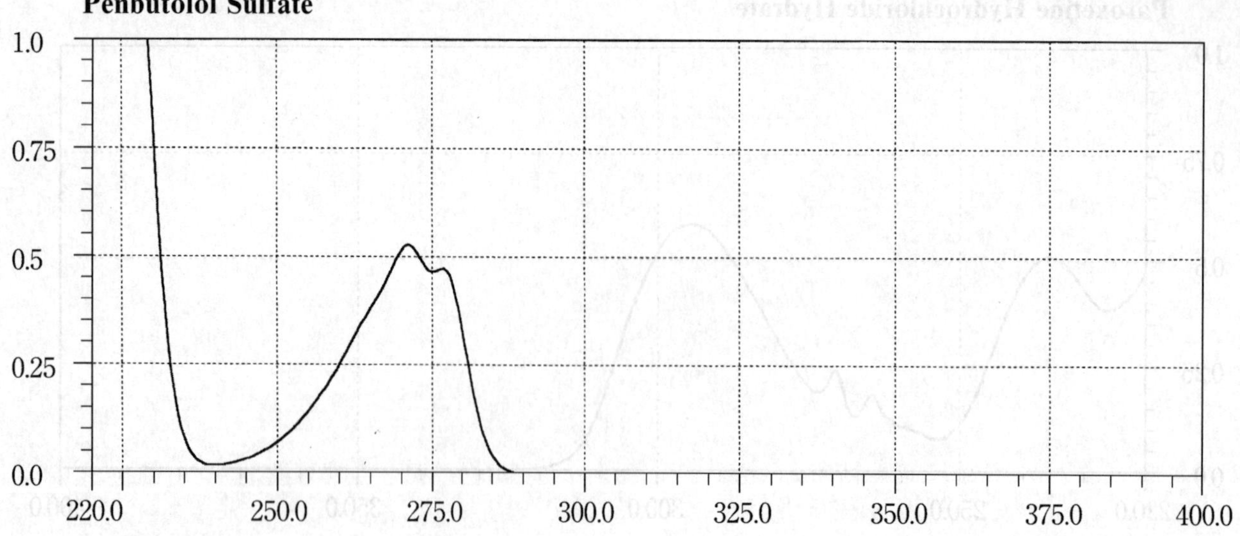

Pentazocine

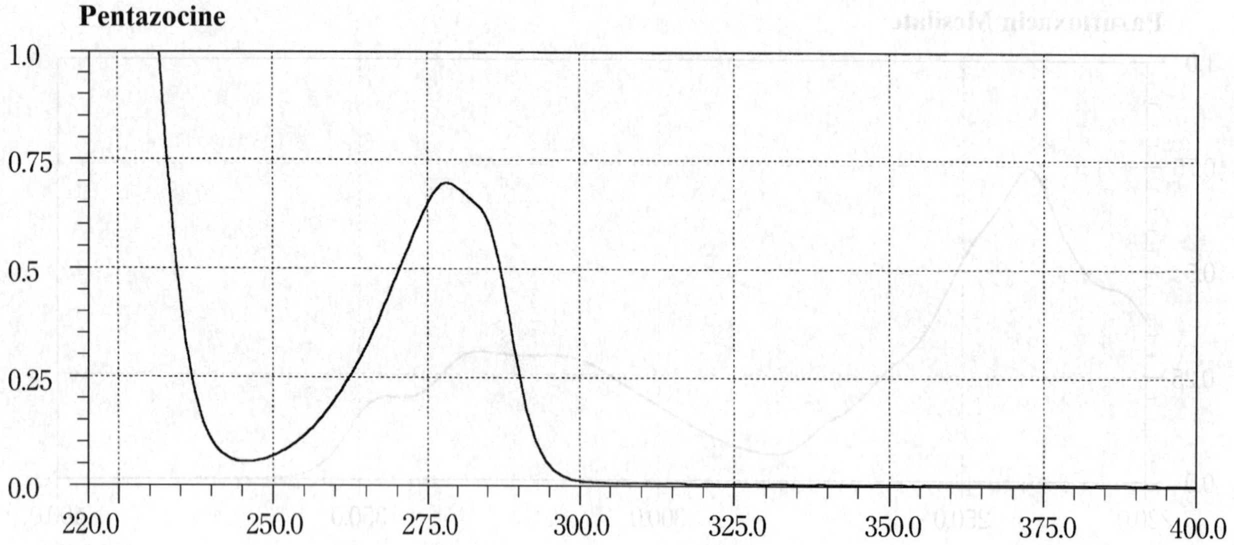

Peplomycin Sulfate

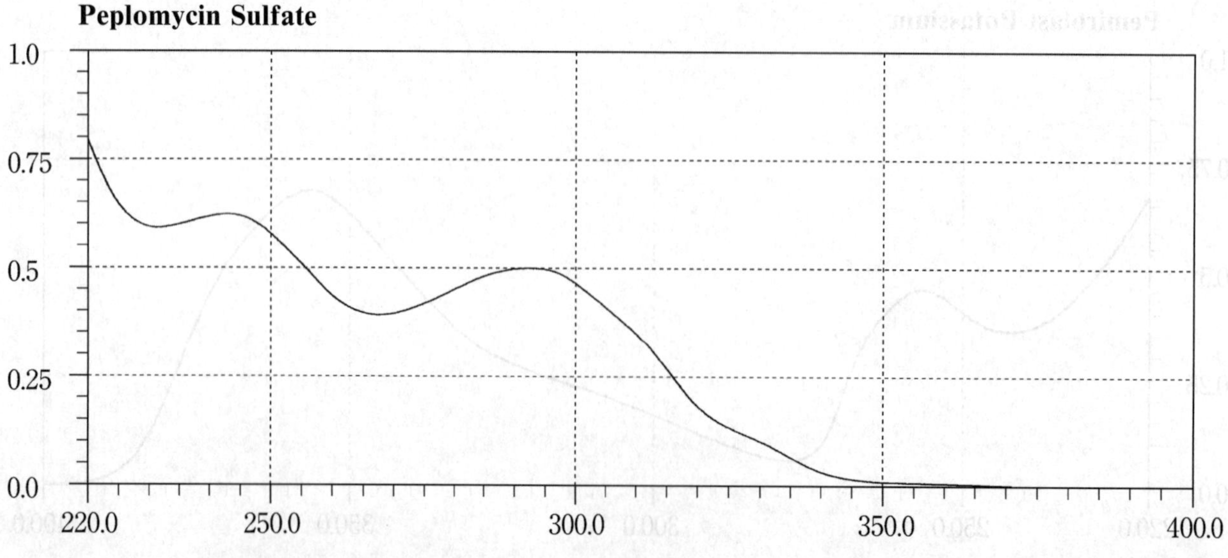

Perphenazine 1

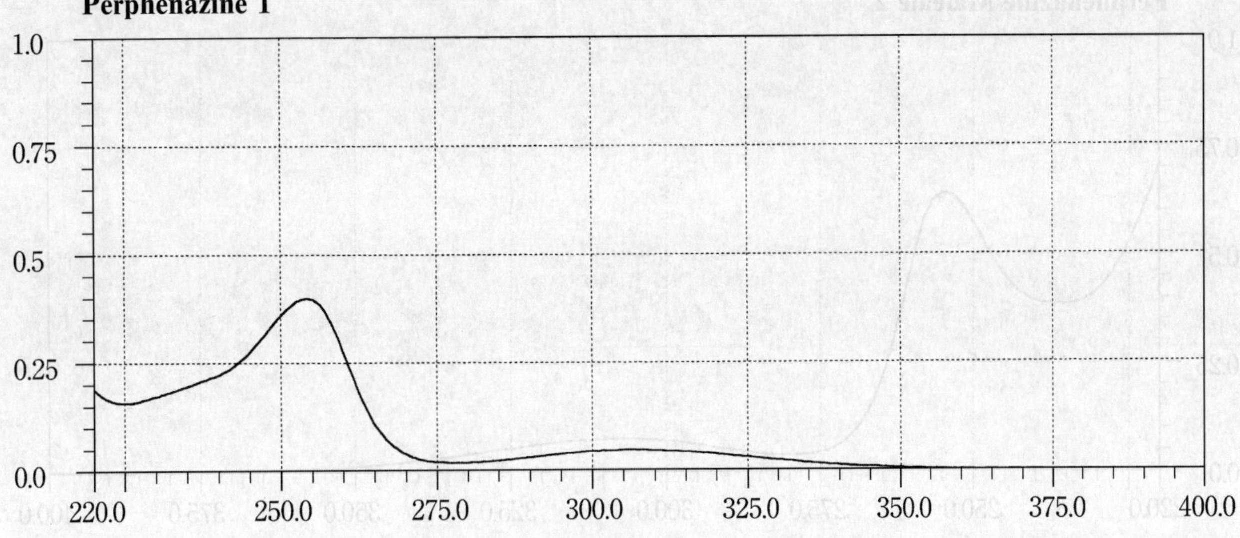

Perphenazine 2

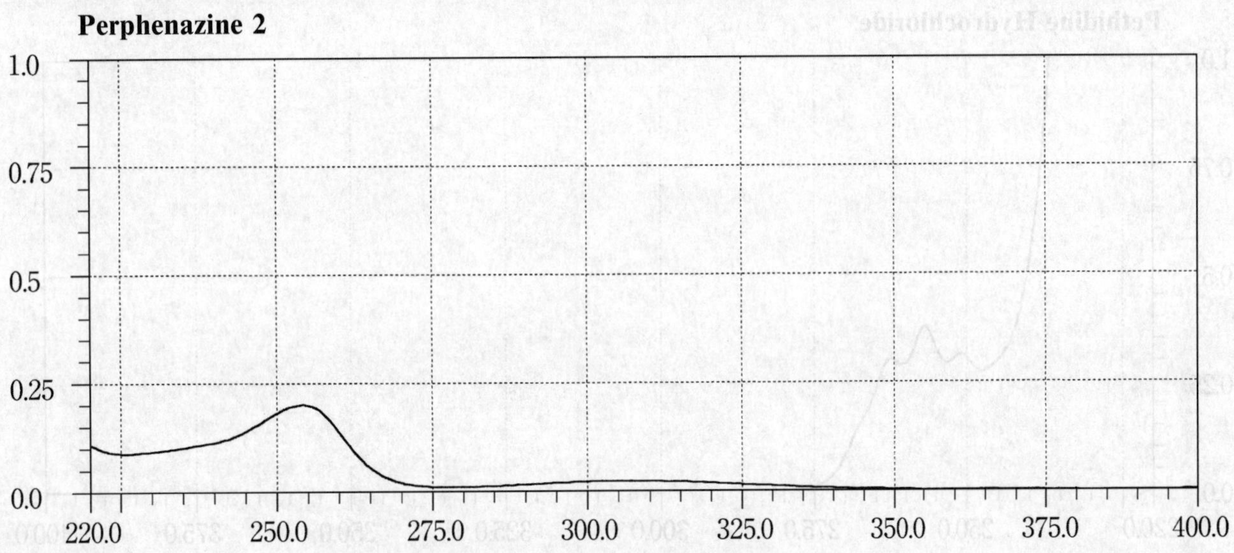

Perphenazine Maleate 1

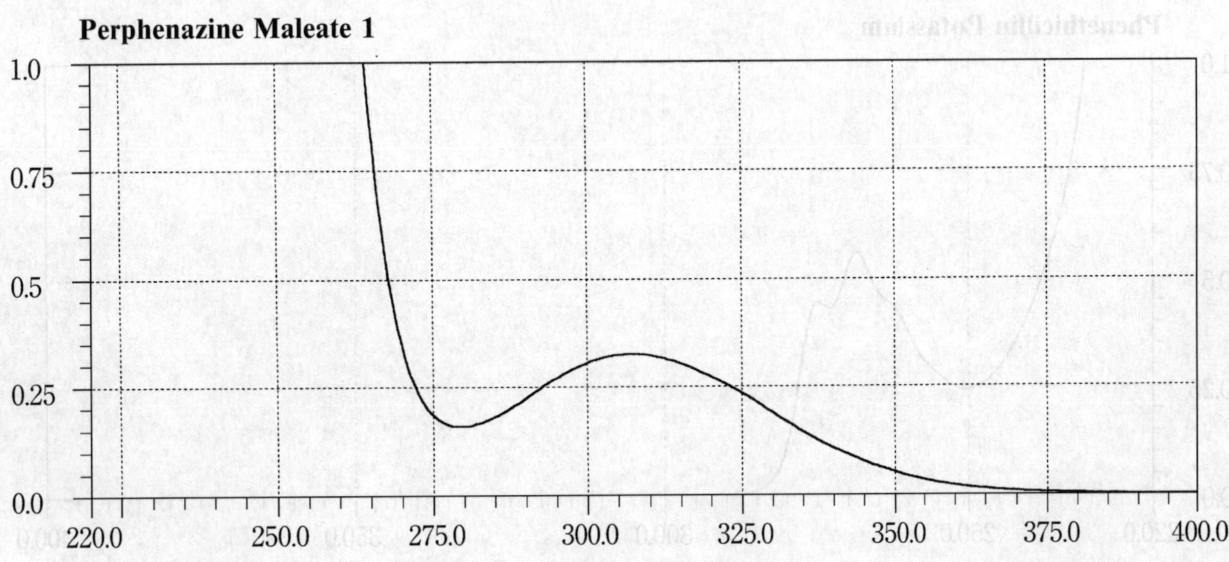

Perphenazine Maleate 2

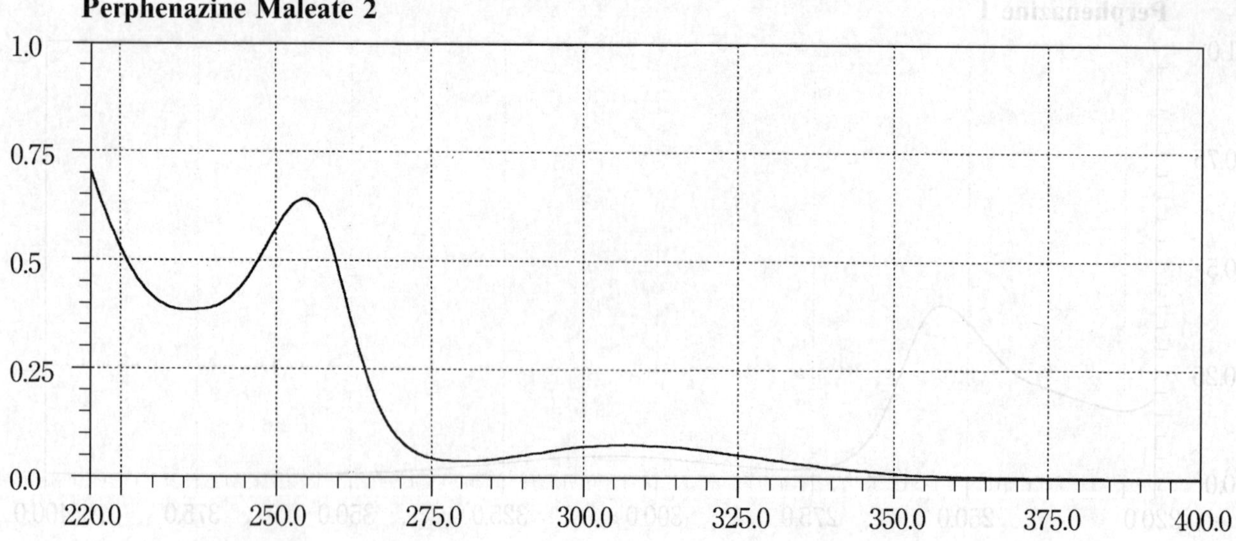

Pethidine Hydrochloride

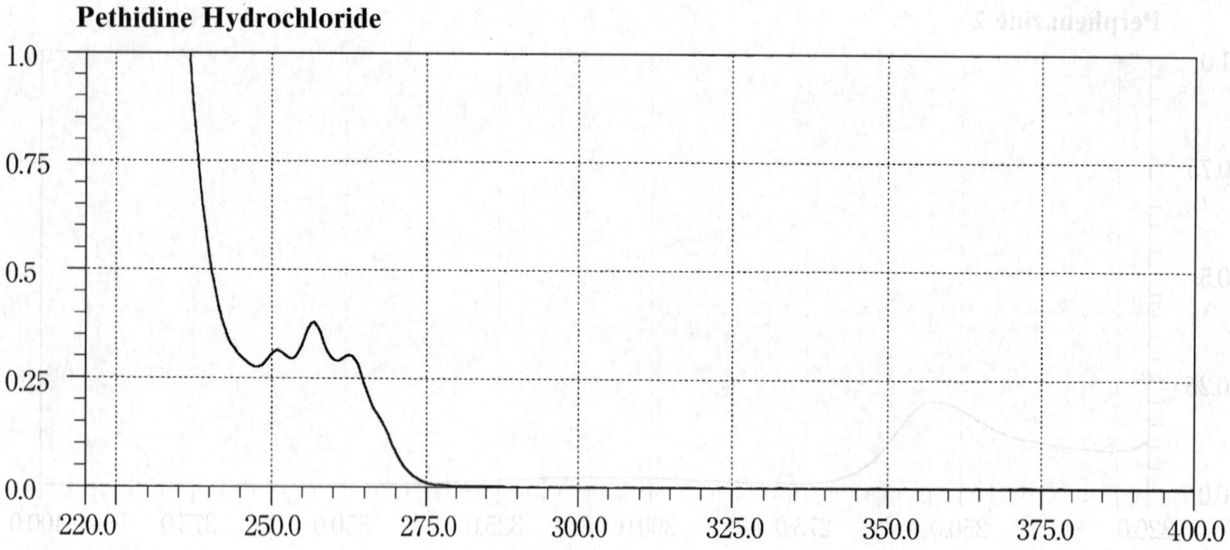

Phenethicillin Potassium

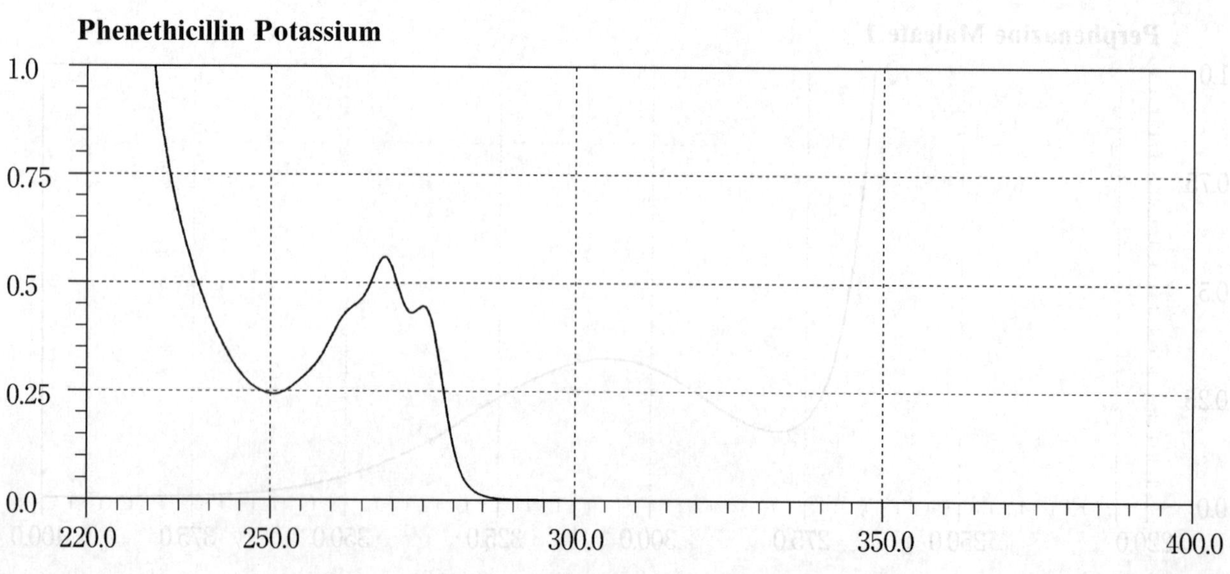

Phenobarbital

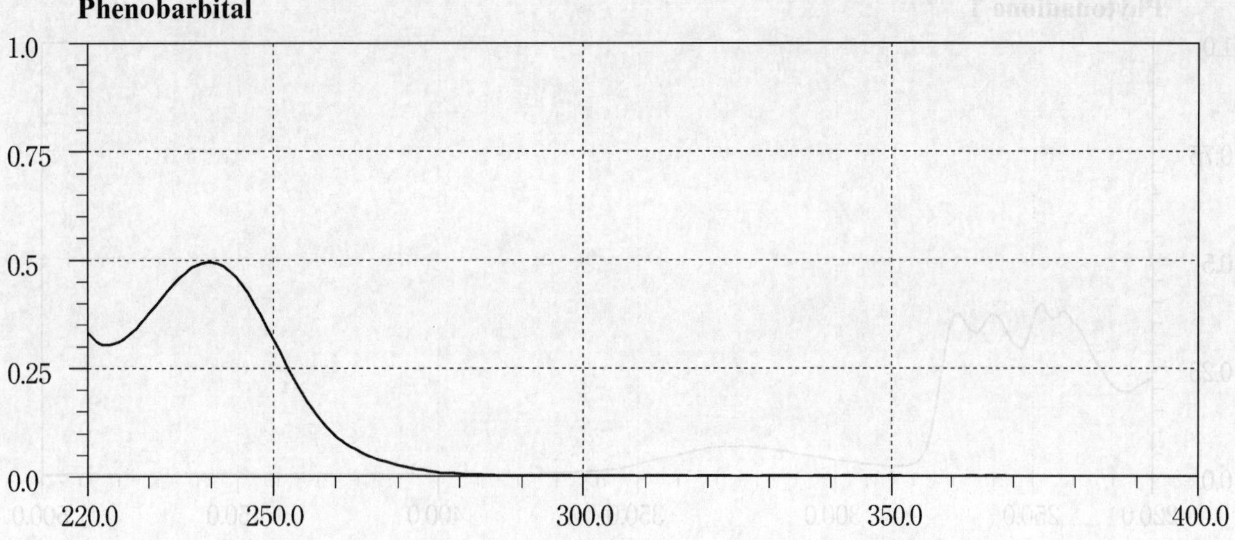

Phenolsulfonphthalein

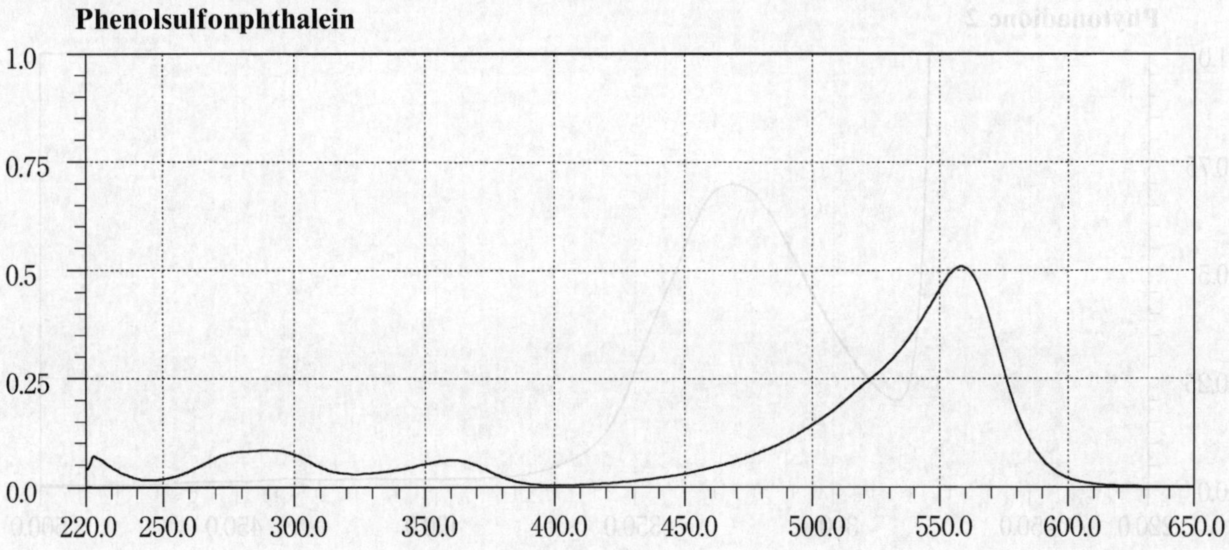

Phenylbutazone

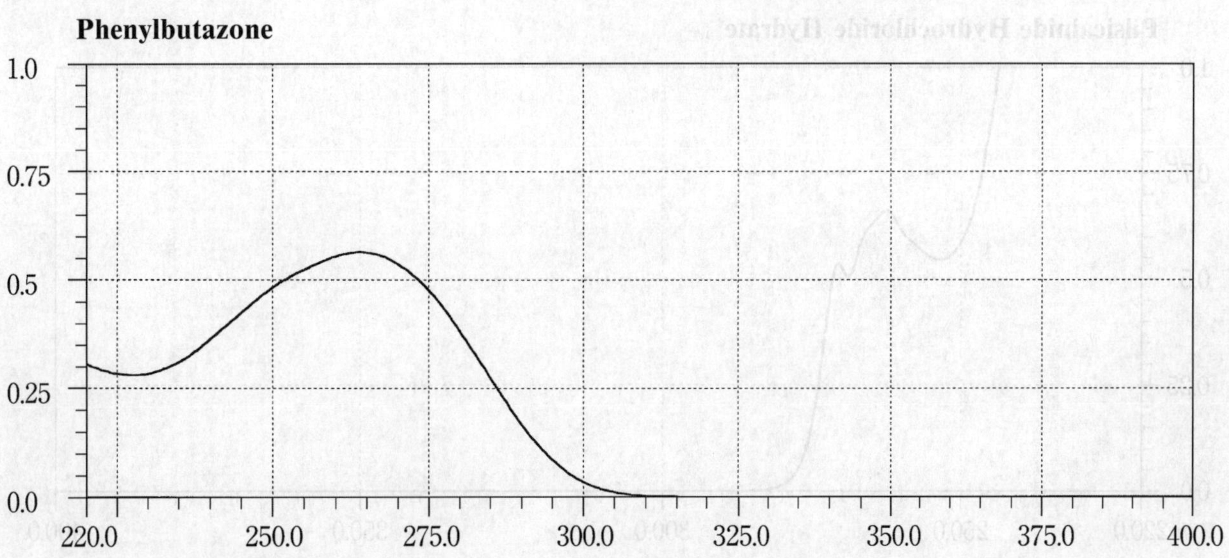

Phytonadione 1

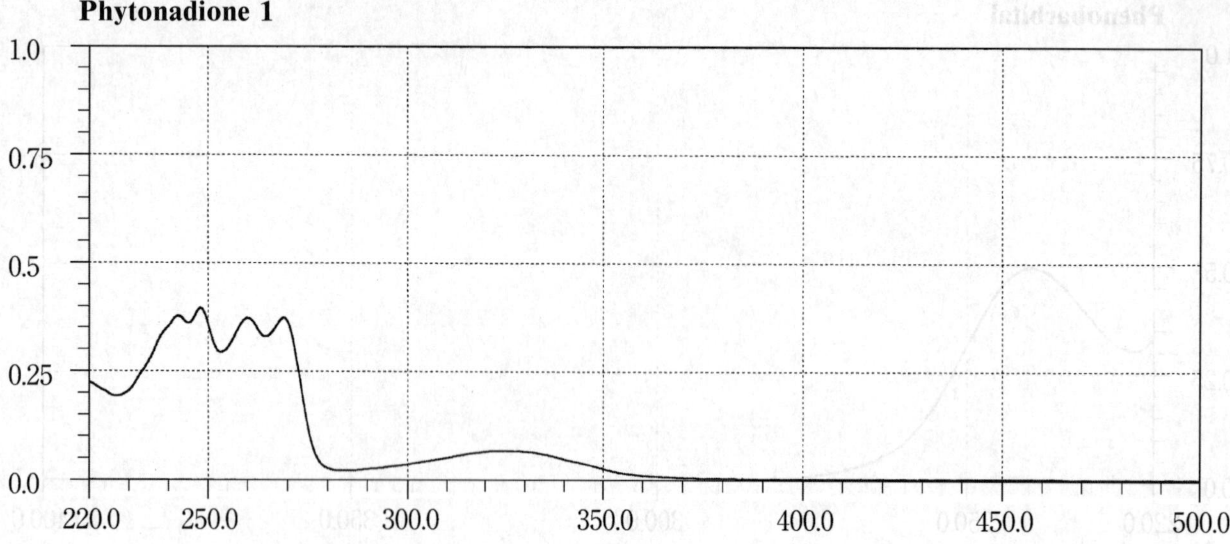

Phytonadione 2

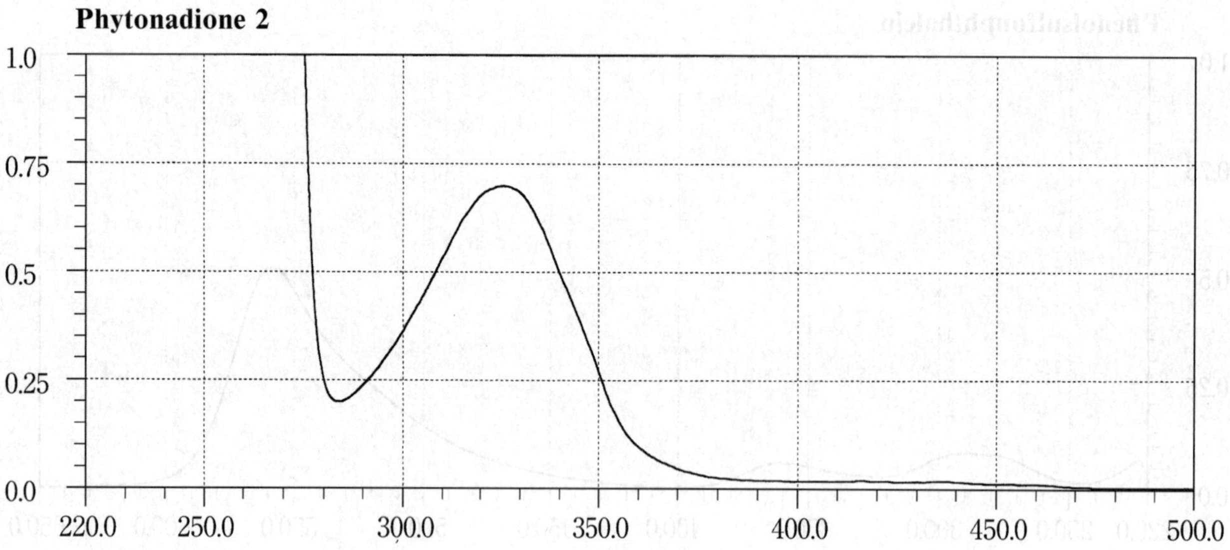

Pilsicainide Hydrochloride Hydrate

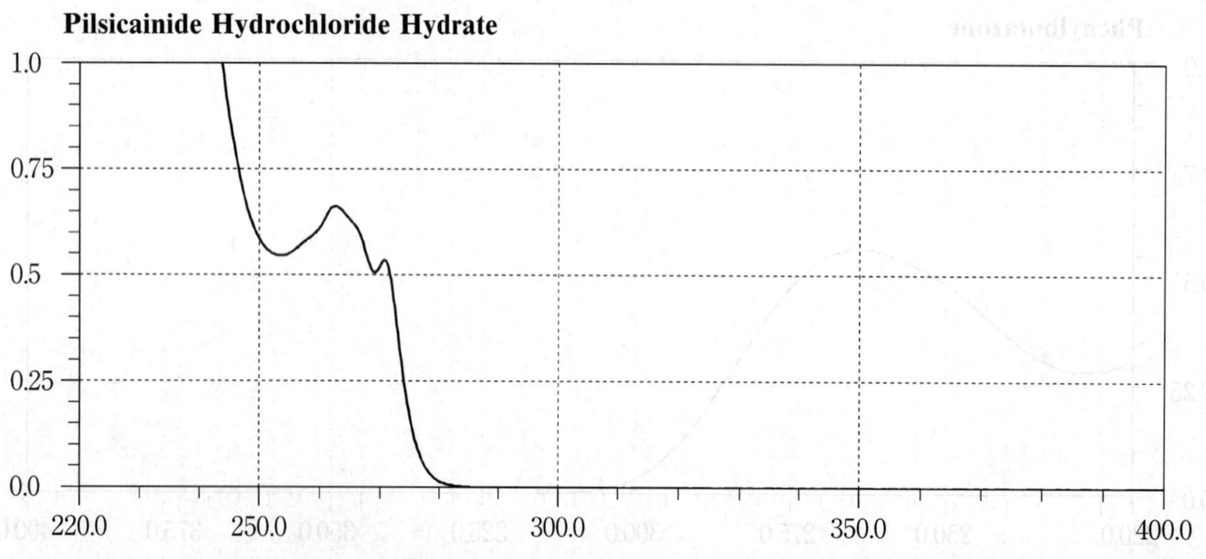

Pimaricin

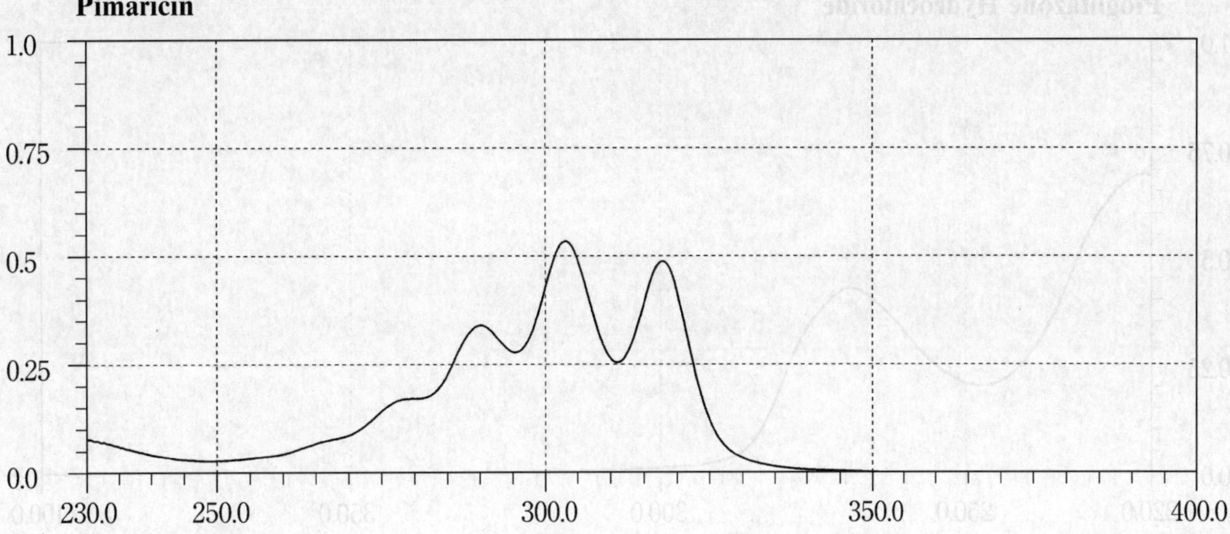

Pimozide

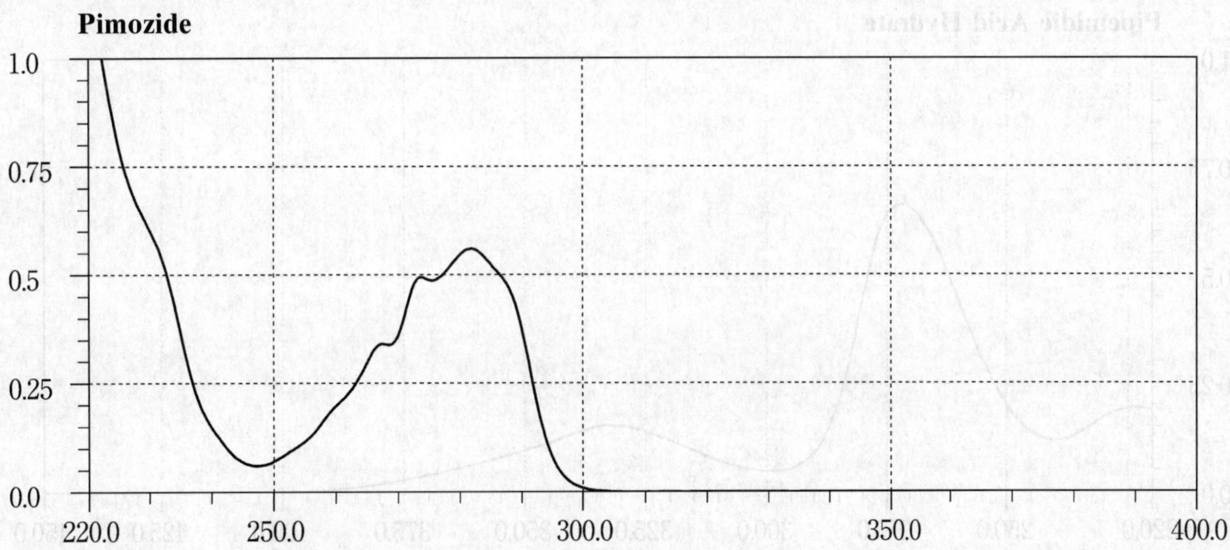

Pindolol

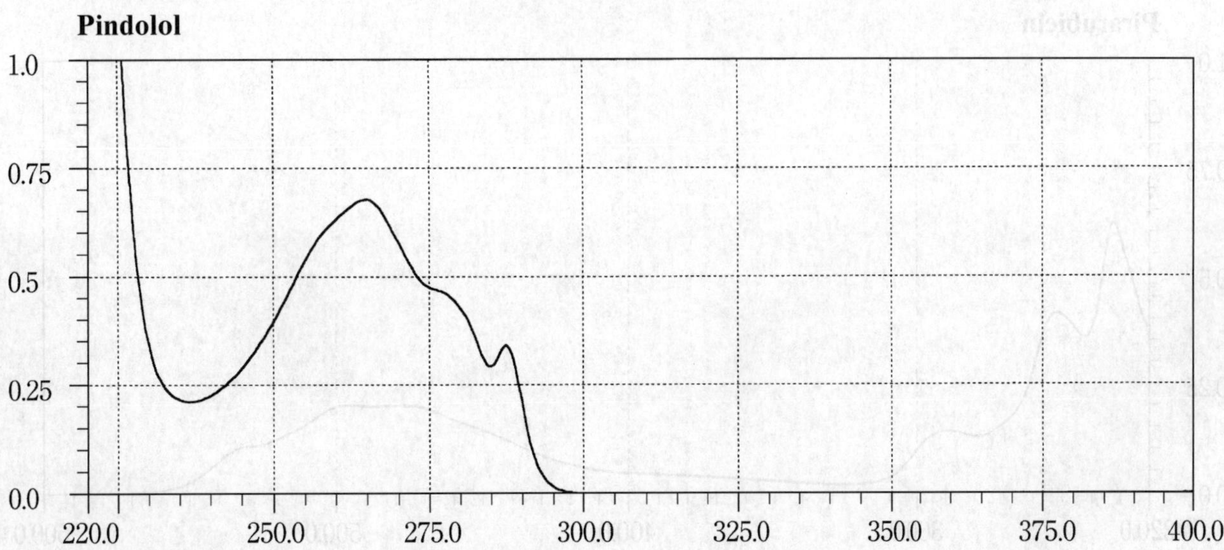

Pioglitazone Hydrochloride

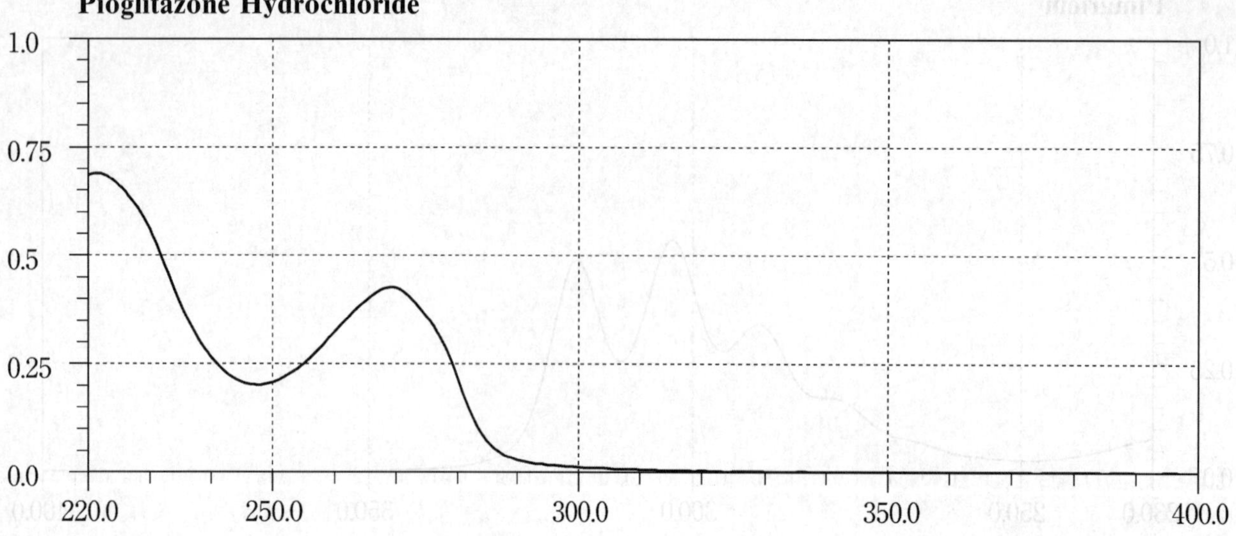

Pipemidic Acid Hydrate

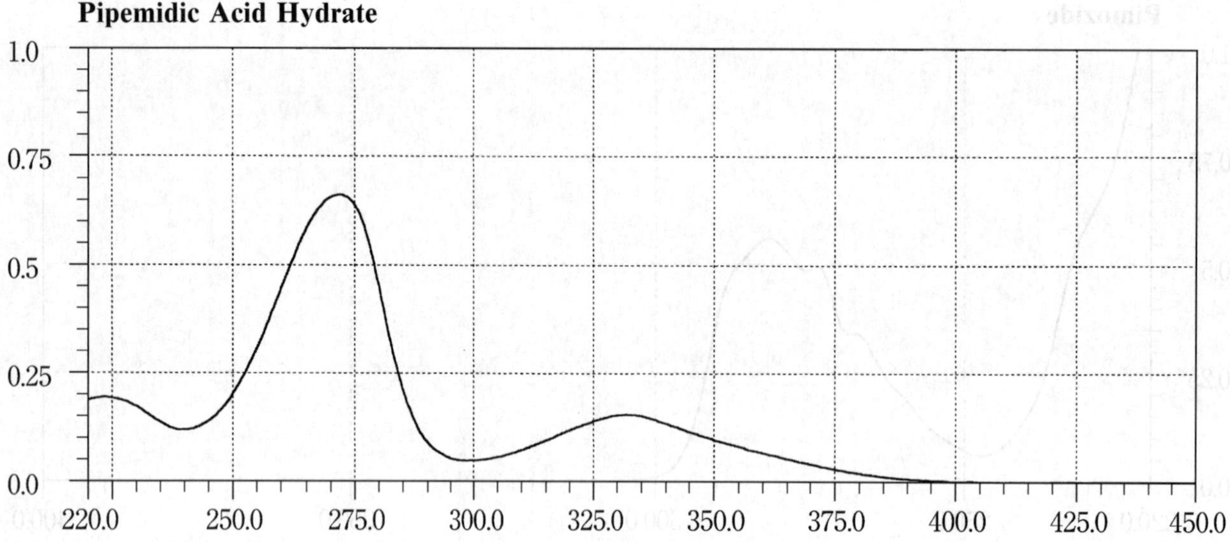

Pirarubicin

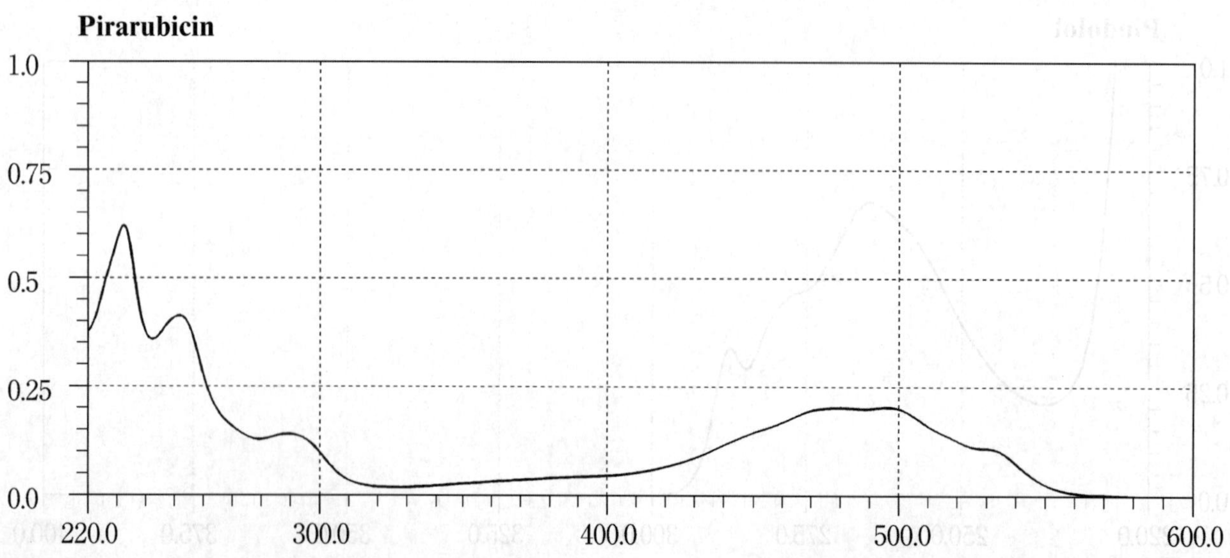

Pirenoxine

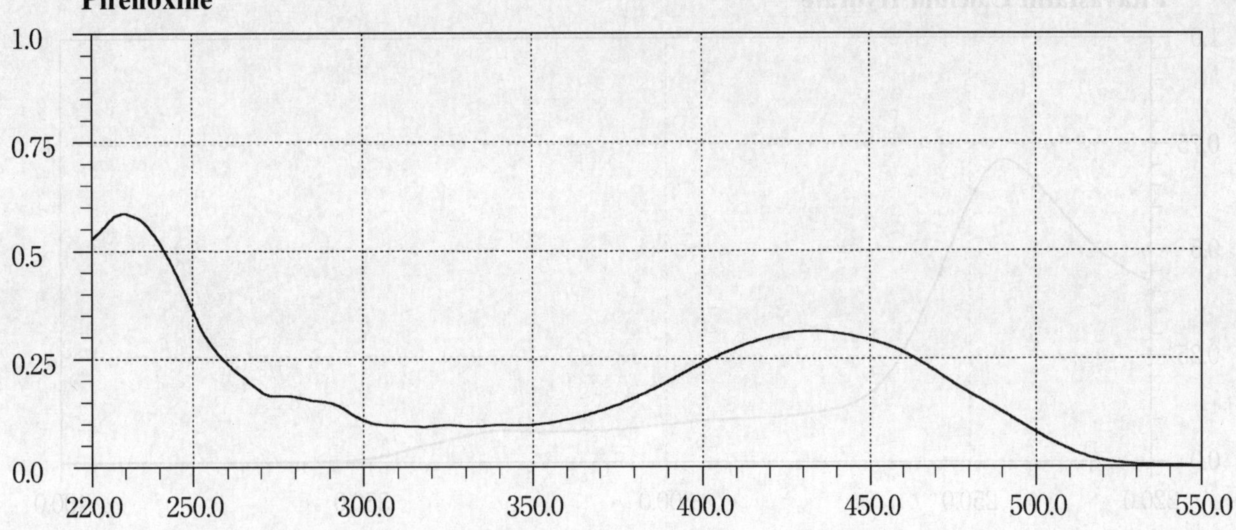

Pirenzepine Hydrochloride Hydrate

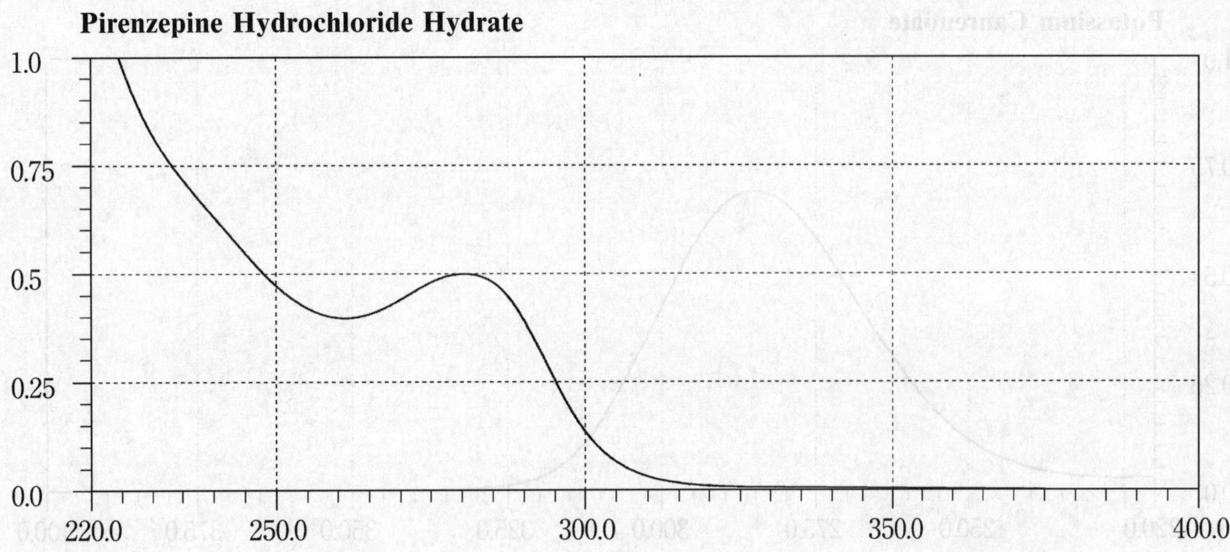

Piroxicam

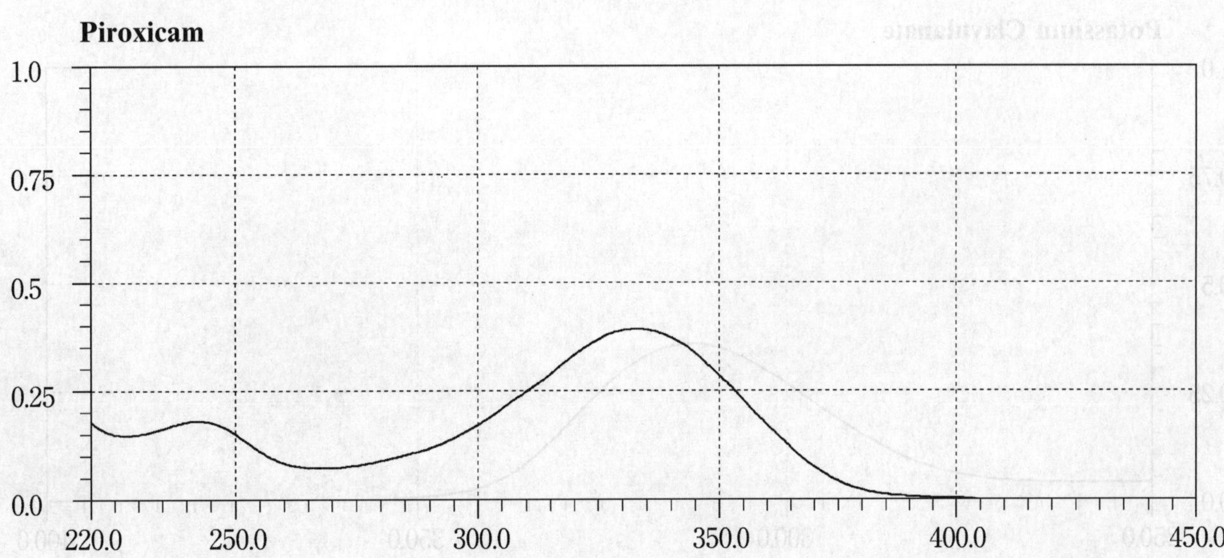

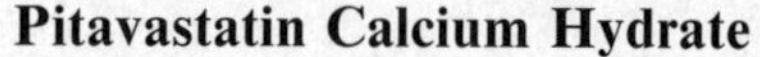

Pitavastatin Calcium Hydrate

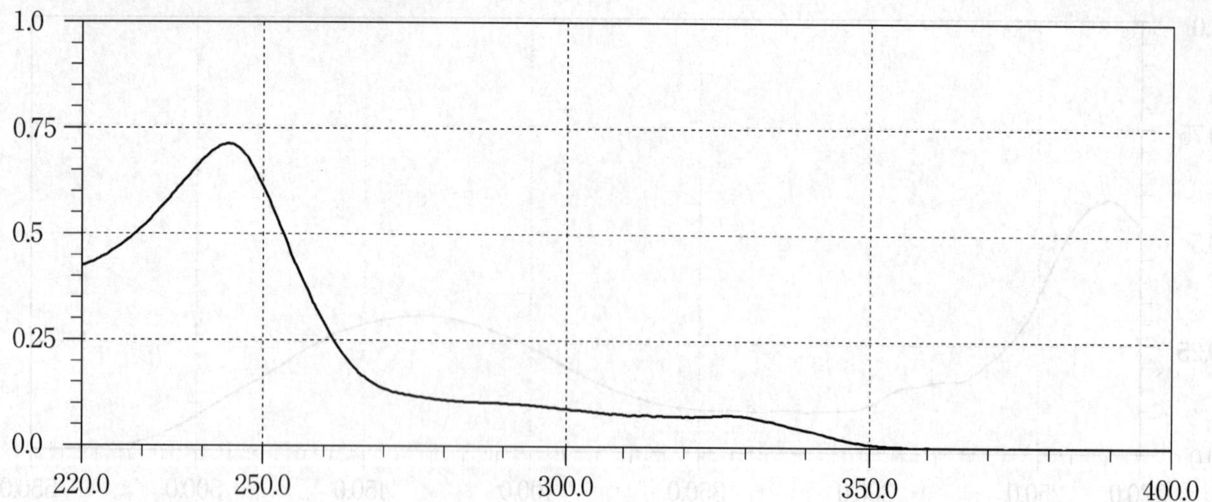

Potassium Canrenoate

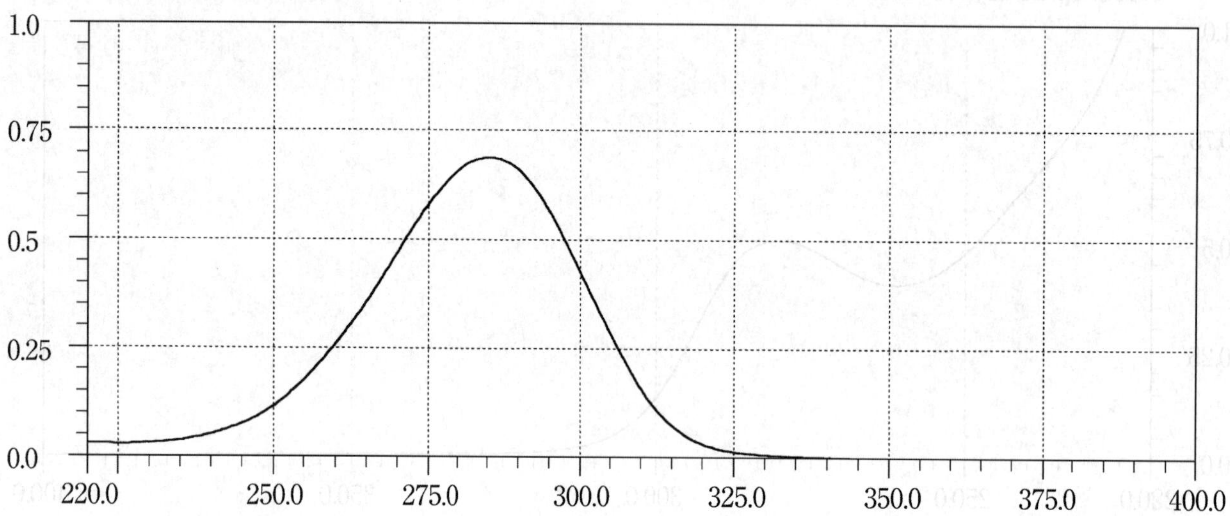

Potassium Clavulanate

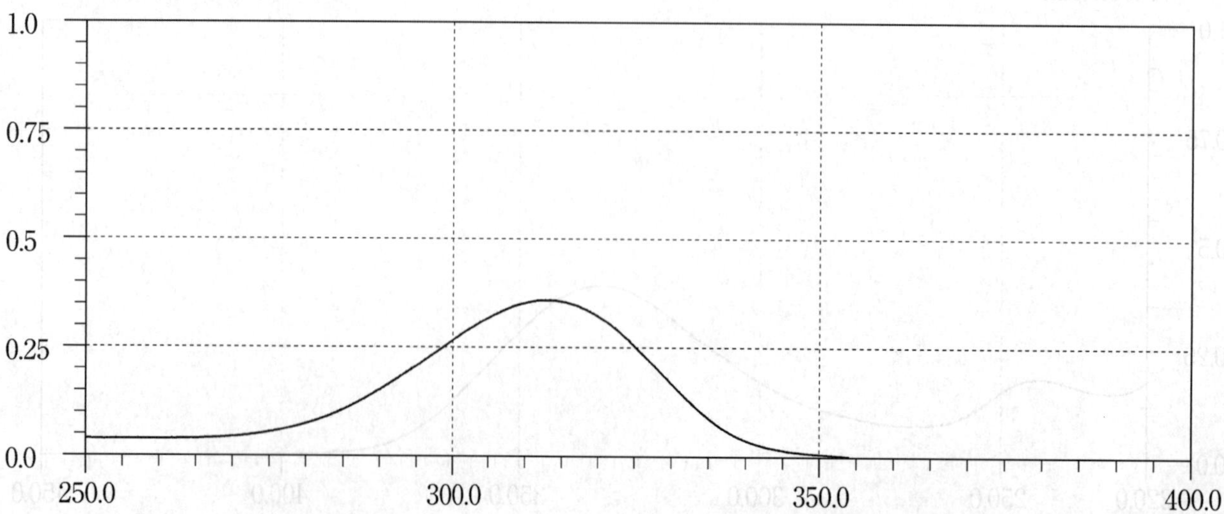

Potassium Guaiacolsulfonate

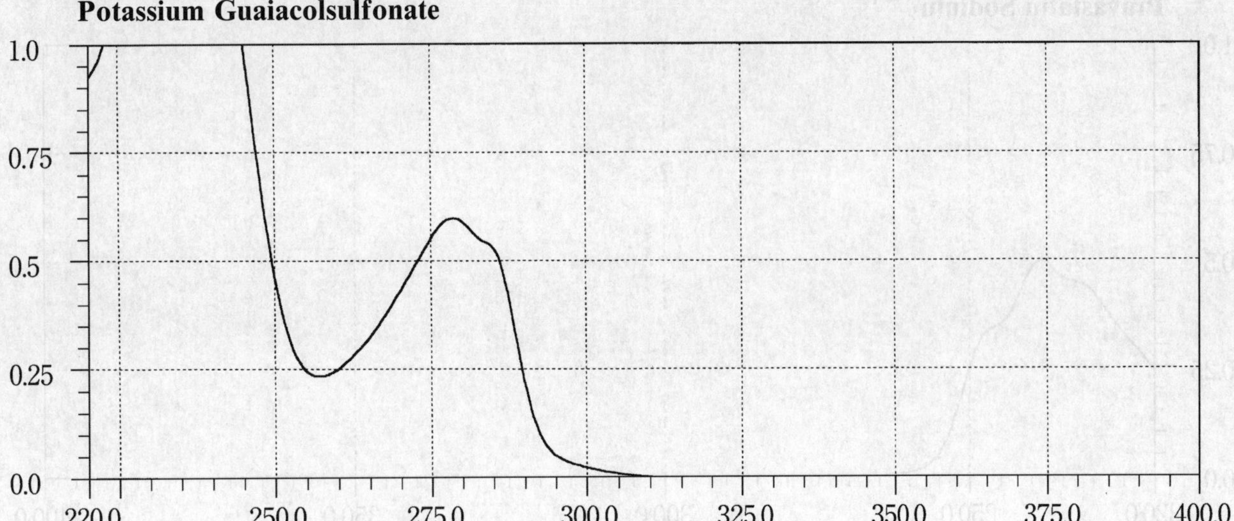

Pranlukast Hydrate

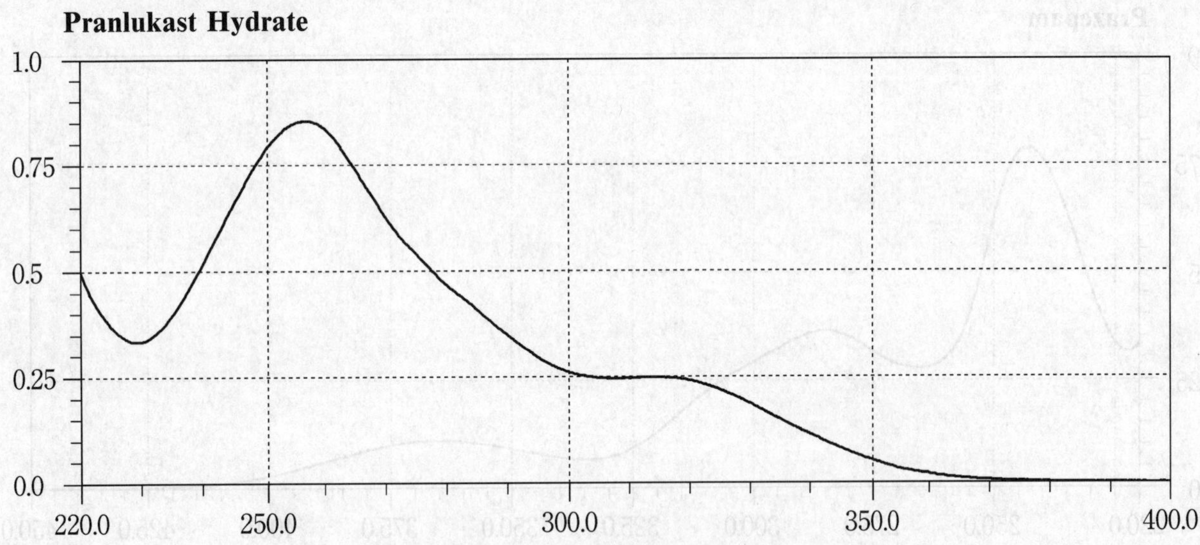

Pranoprofen

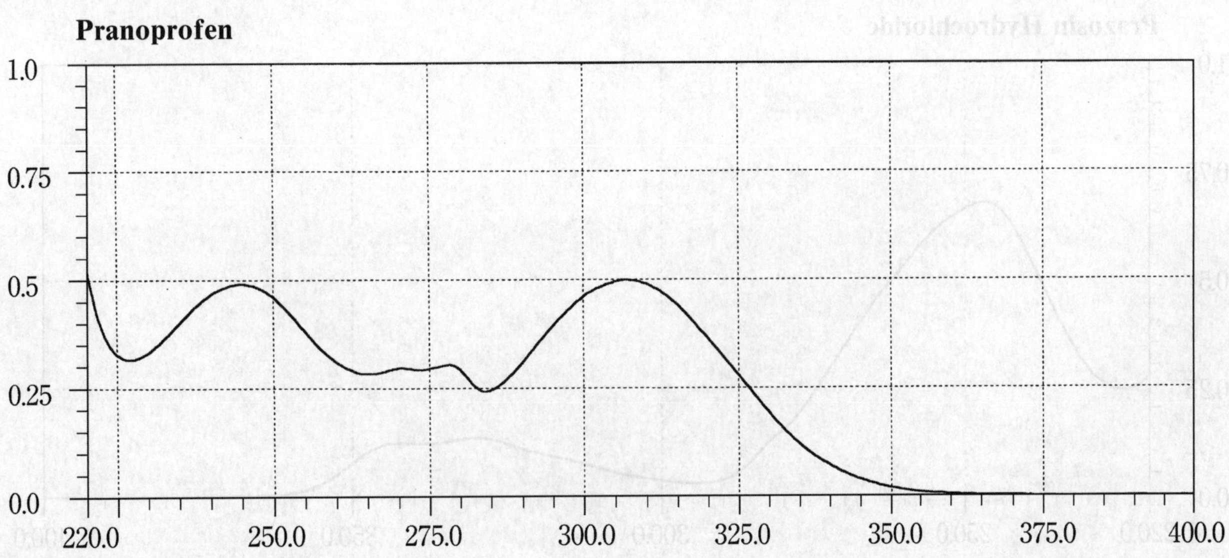

The JP Drugs are to be tested according to the provisions given in the pertinent monographs, General Notices, General Rules for Crude Drugs, General Rules for Preparations, and General Tests for their conformity to the Japanese Pharmacopoeia. (See the General Notices 5.)

Pravastatin Sodium

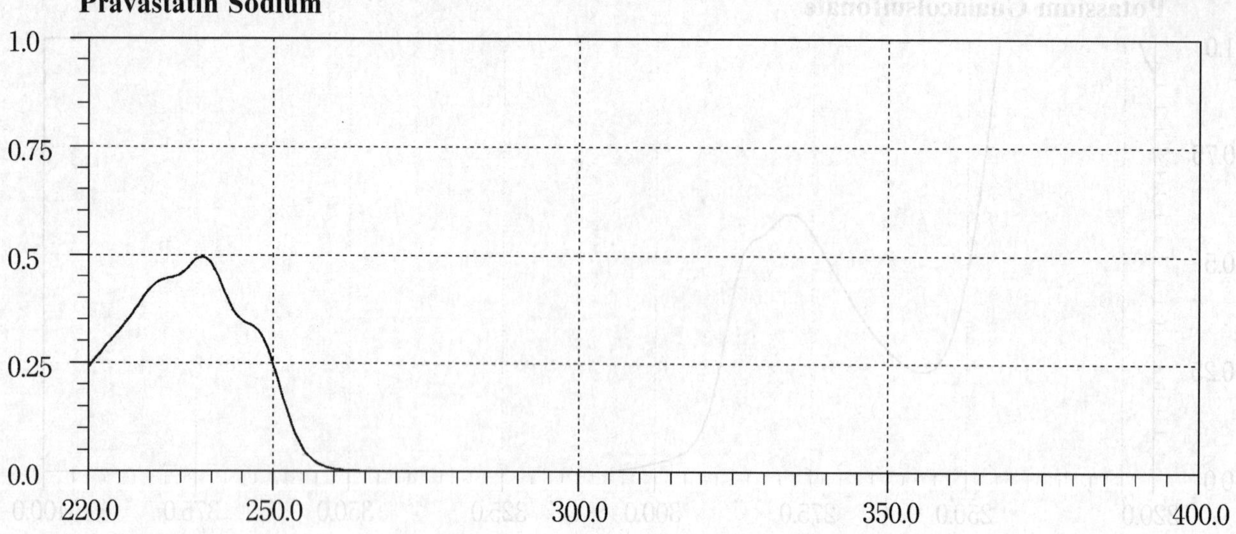

Prazepam

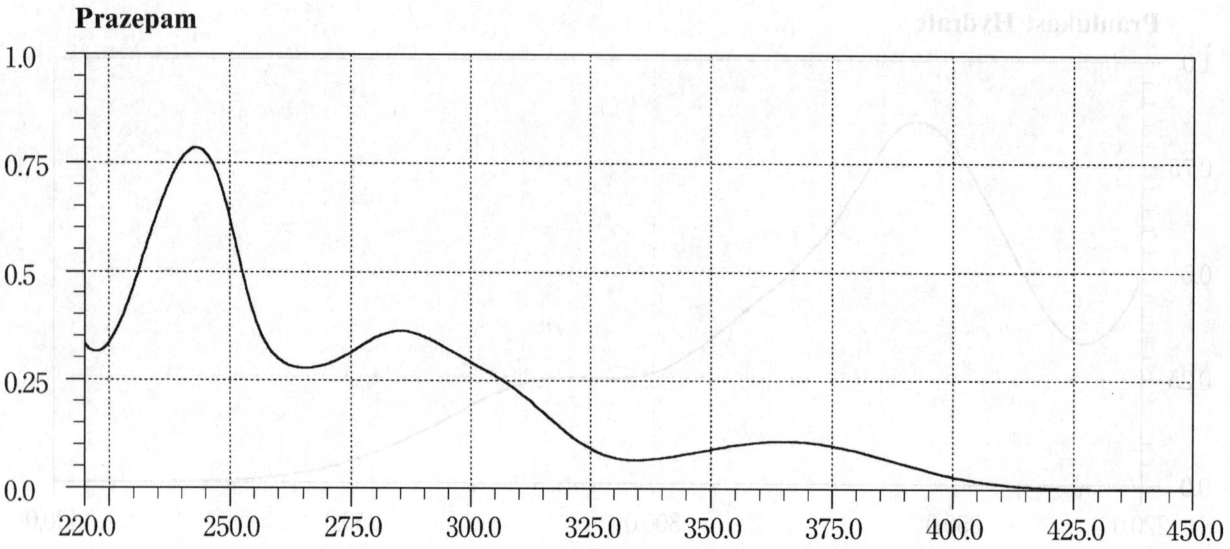

Prazosin Hydrochloride

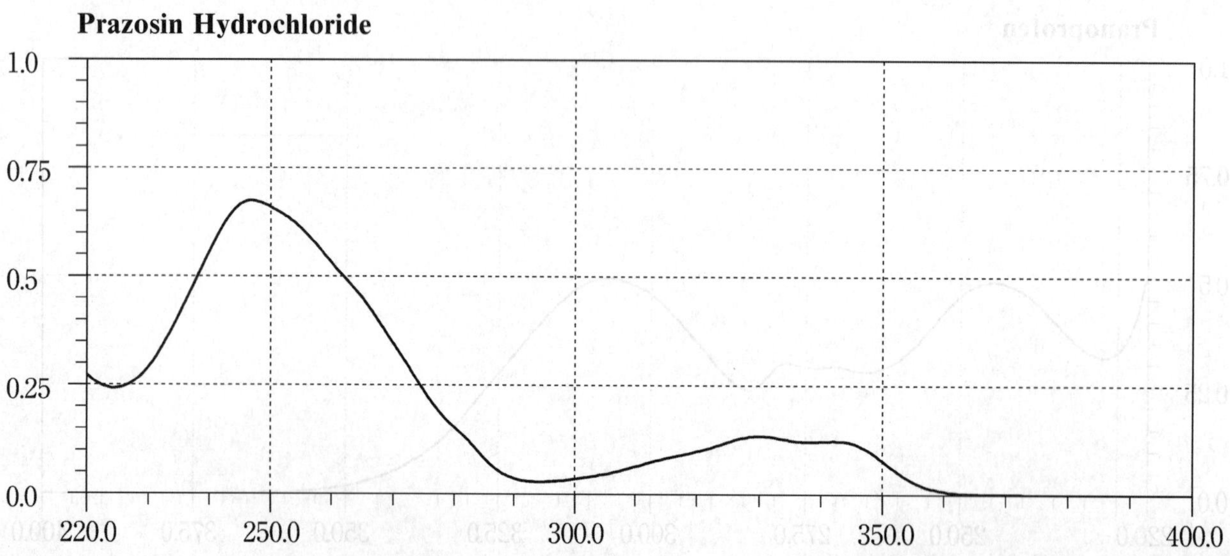

Prednisolone Sodium Phosphate

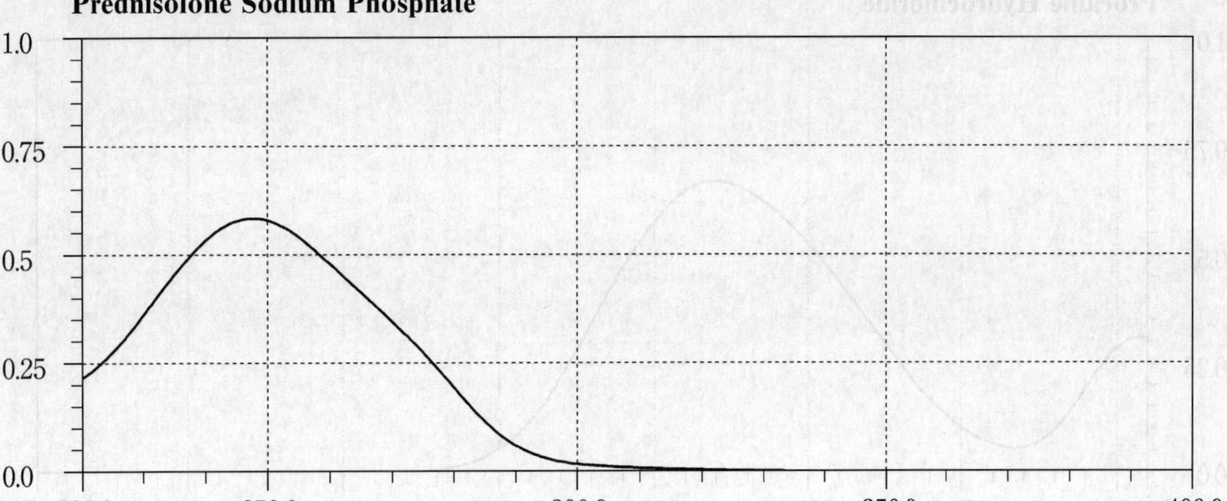

Probenecid

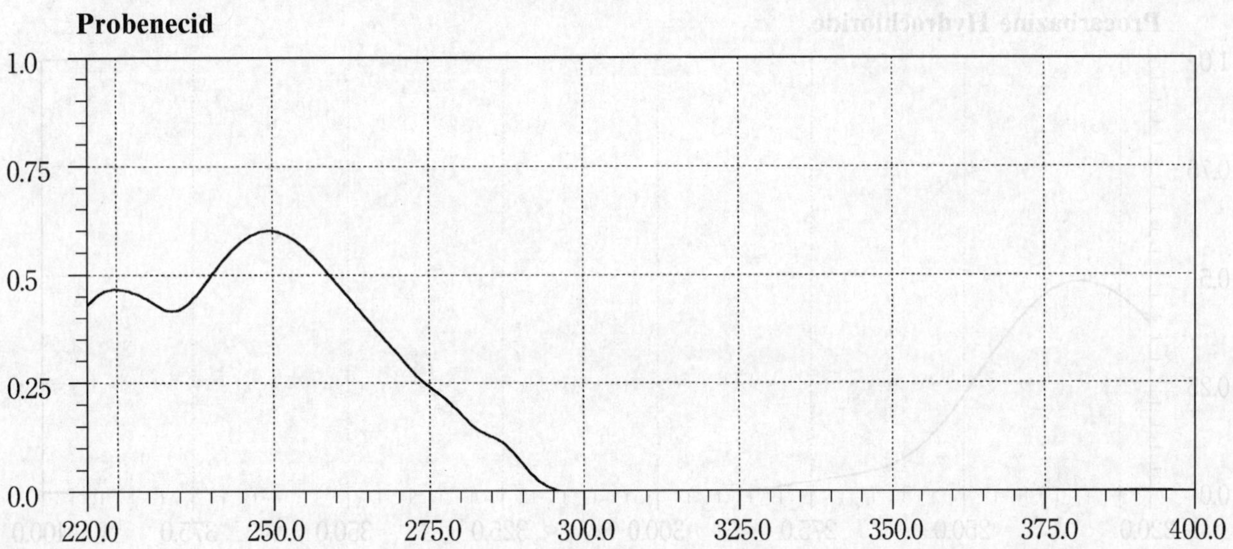

Probucol

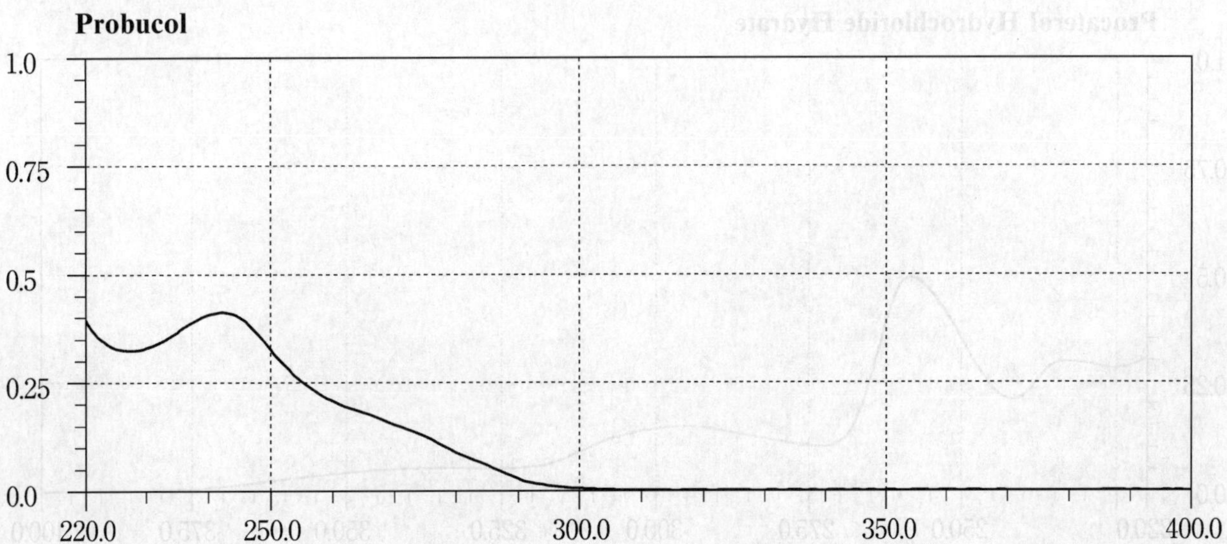

Procaine Hydrochloride

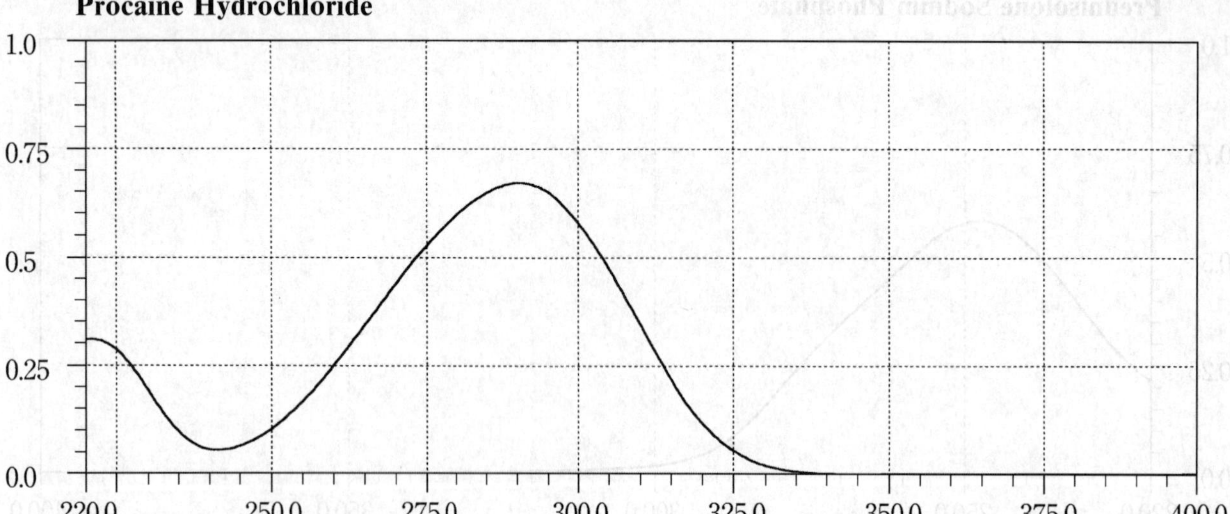

Procarbazine Hydrochloride

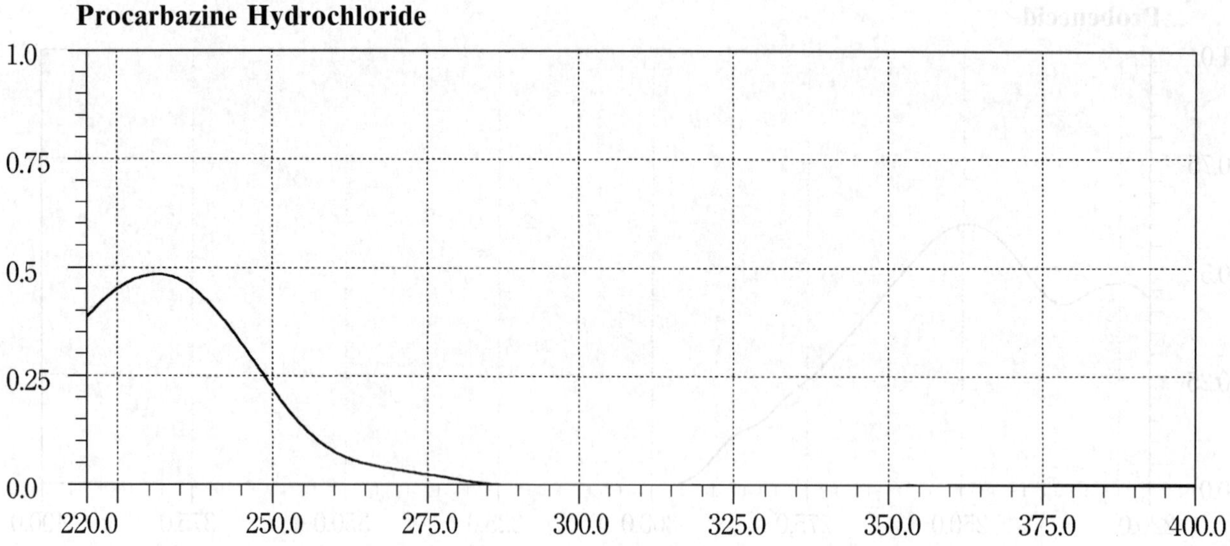

Procaterol Hydrochloride Hydrate

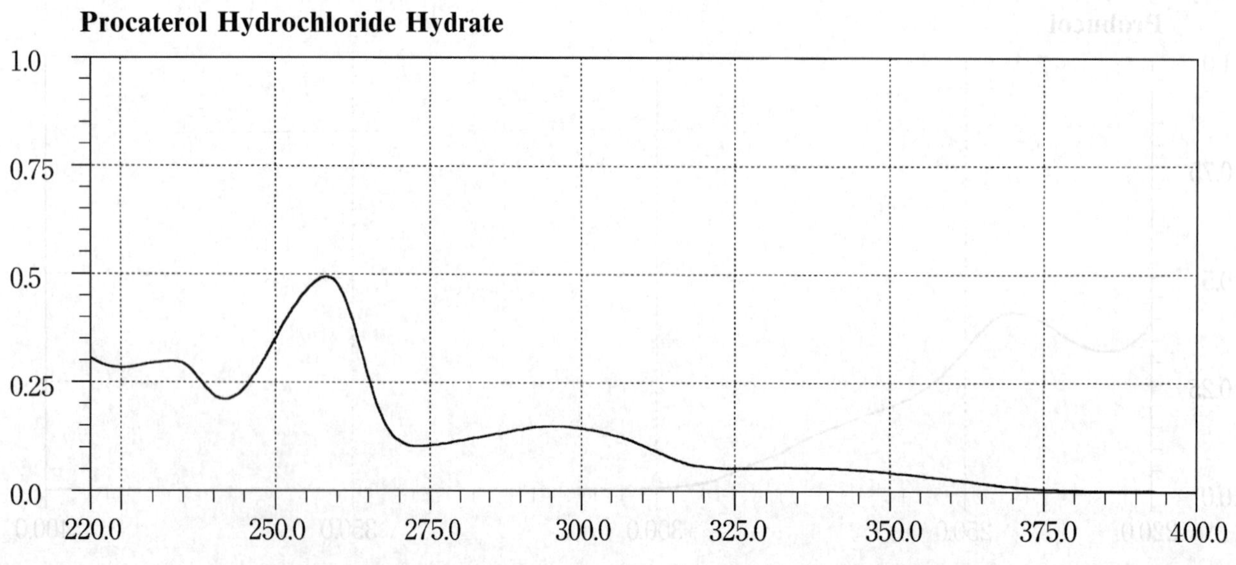

Progesterone

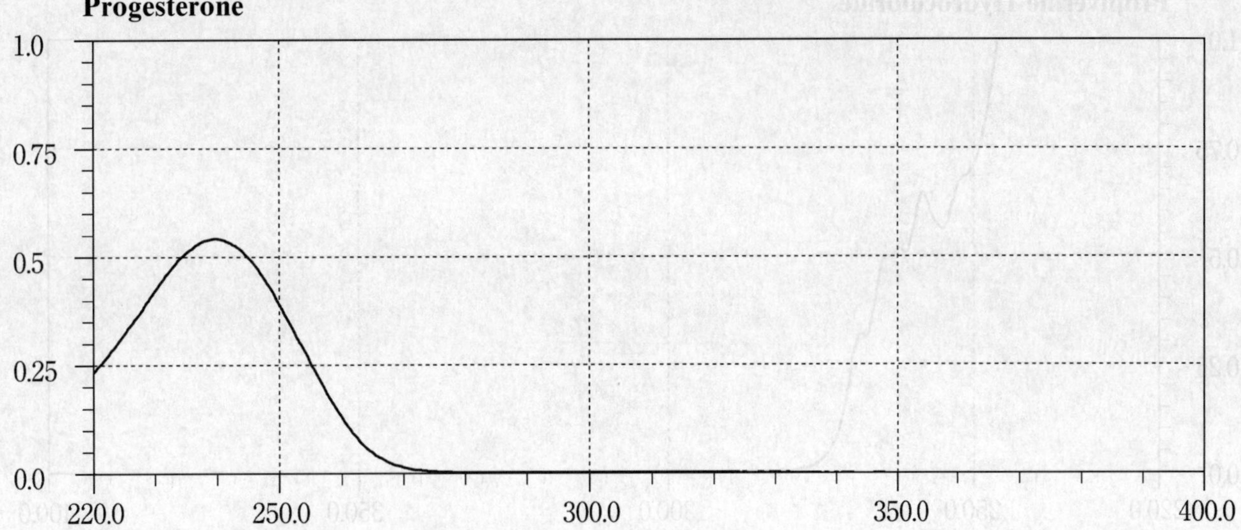

Promethazine Hydrochloride

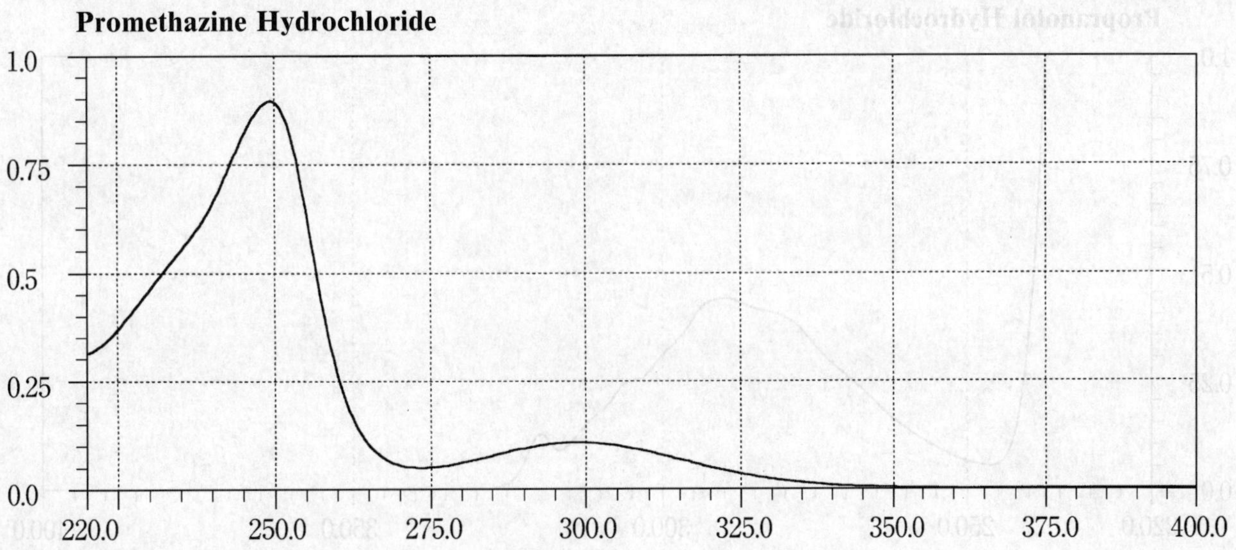

Propafenone Hydrochloride

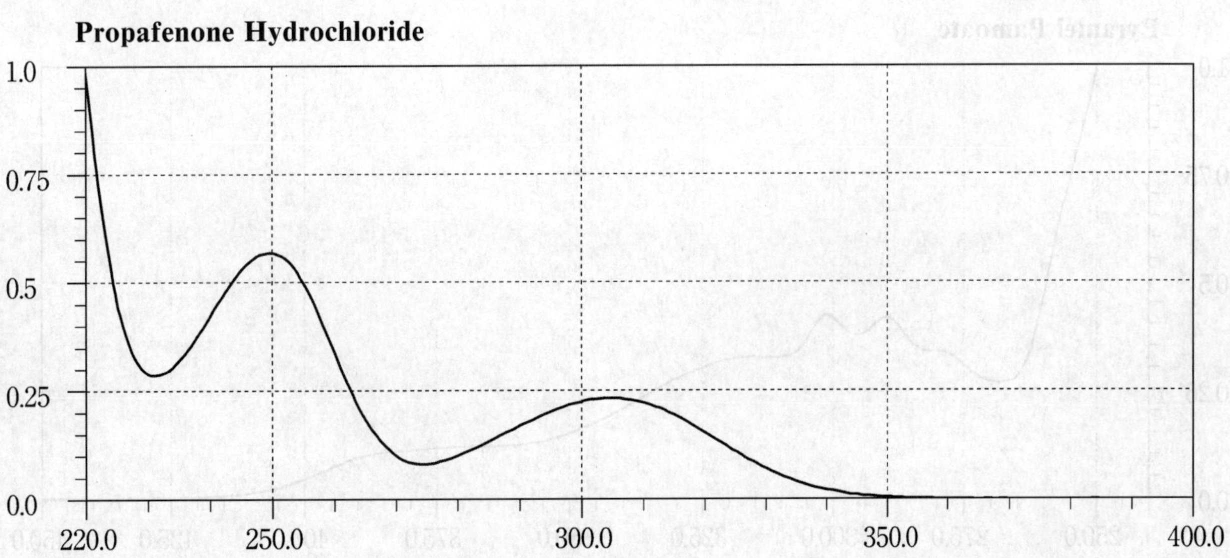

Propiverine Hydrochloride

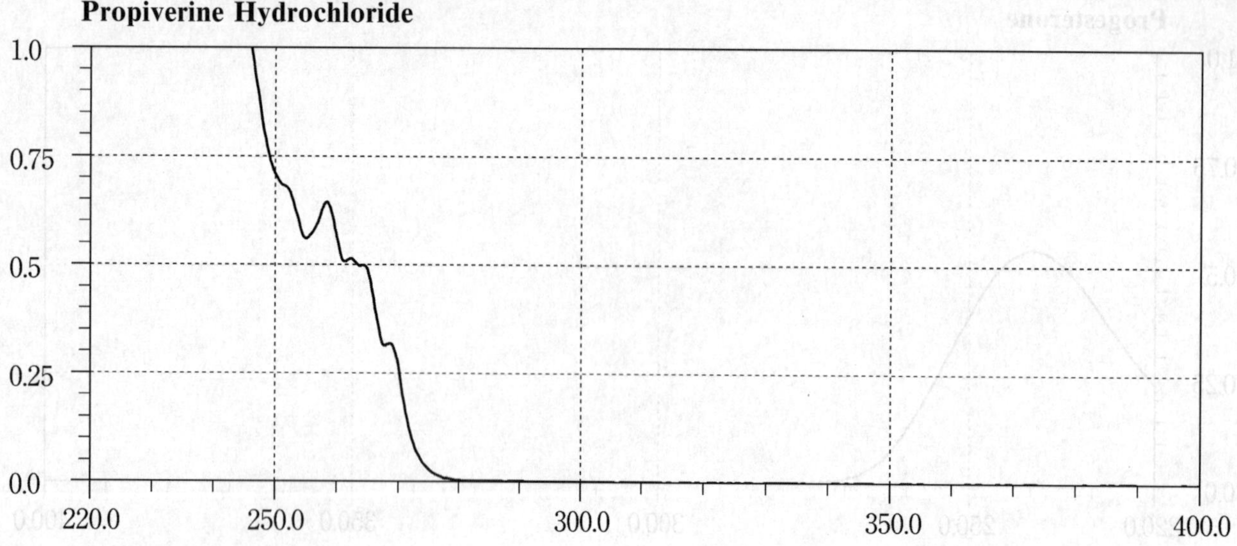

Propranolol Hydrochloride

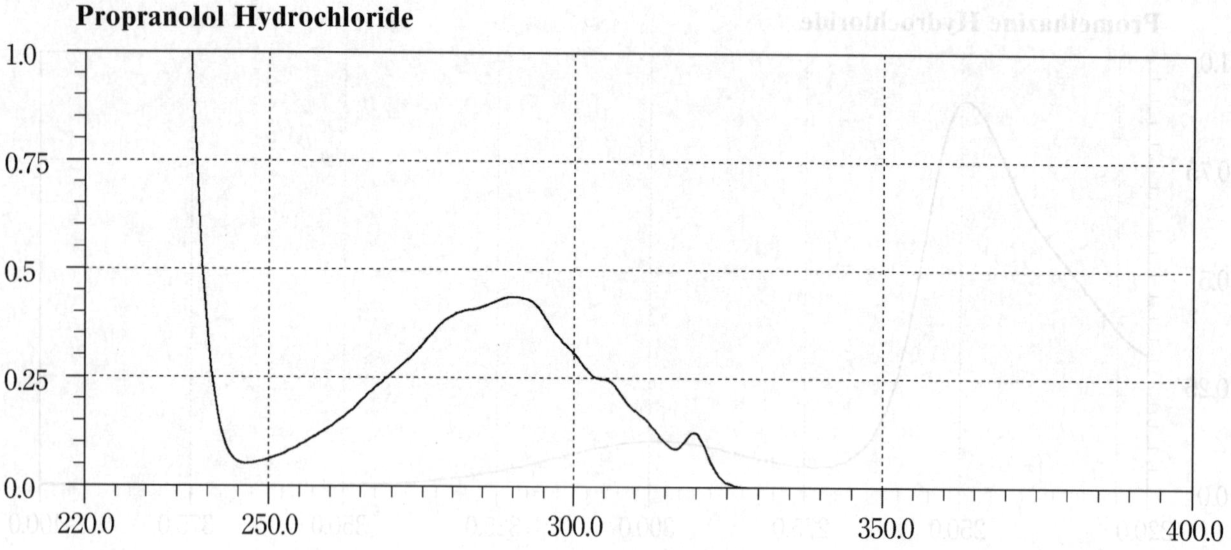

Pyrantel Pamoate

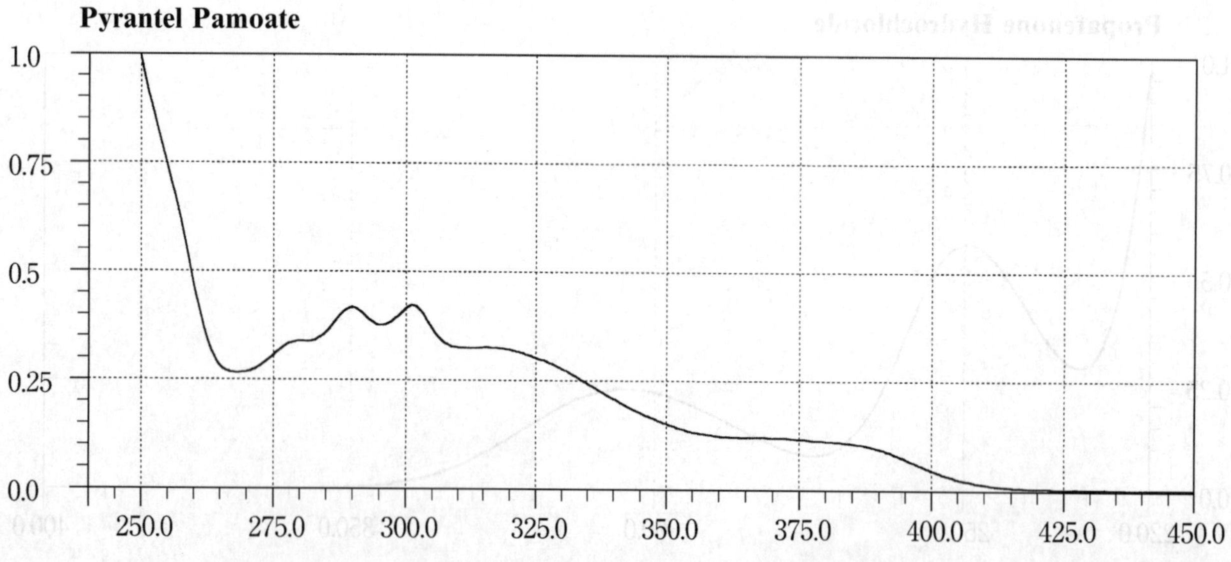

Pyrazinamide

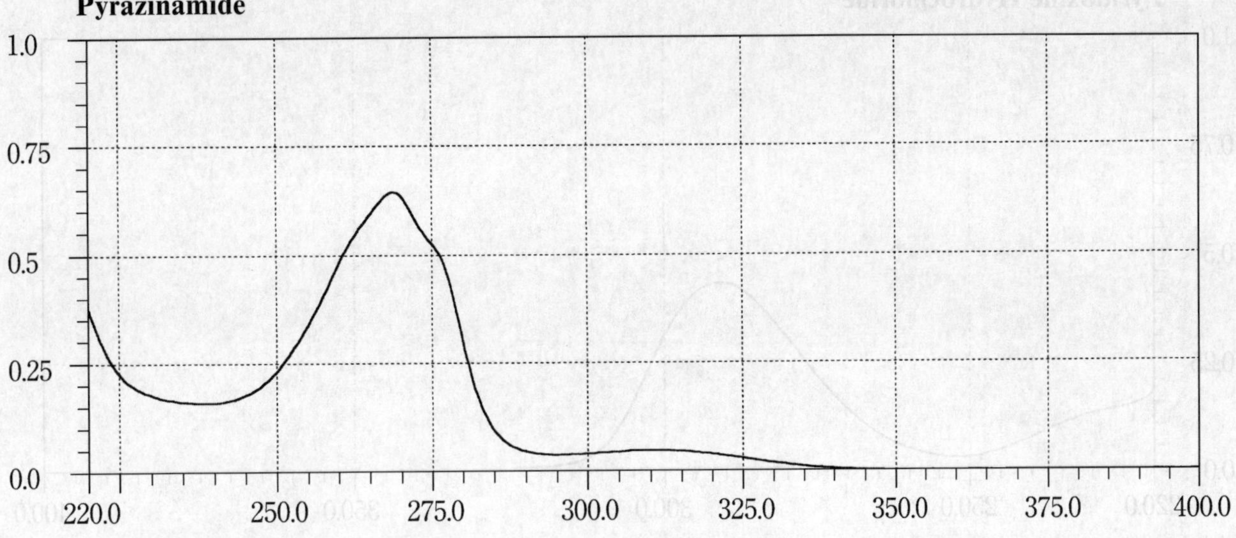

Pyridostigmine Bromide

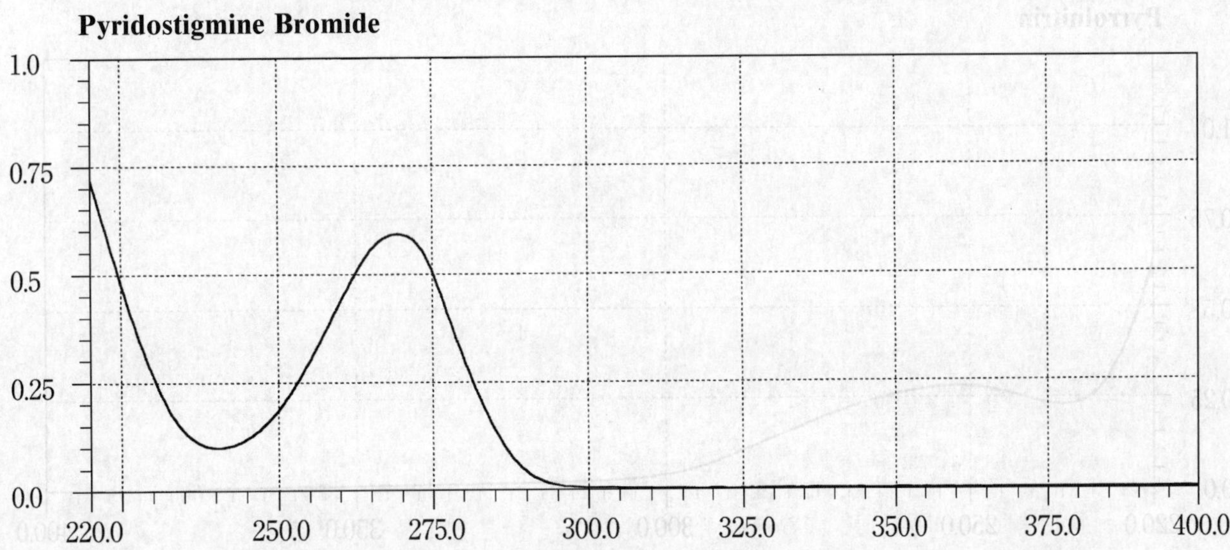

Pyridoxal Phosphate Hydrate

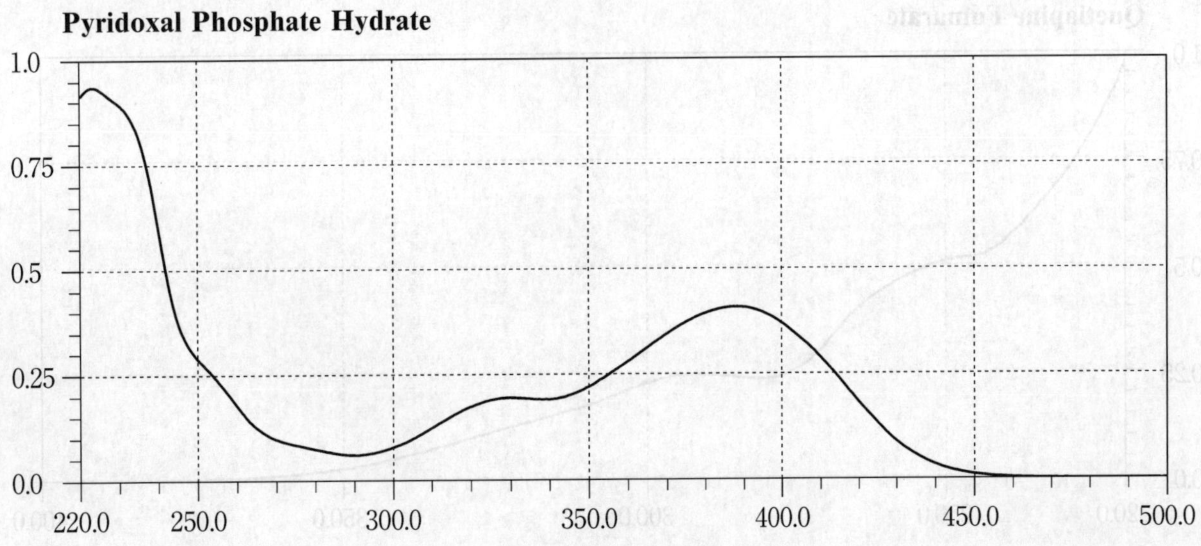

Pyridoxine Hydrochloride

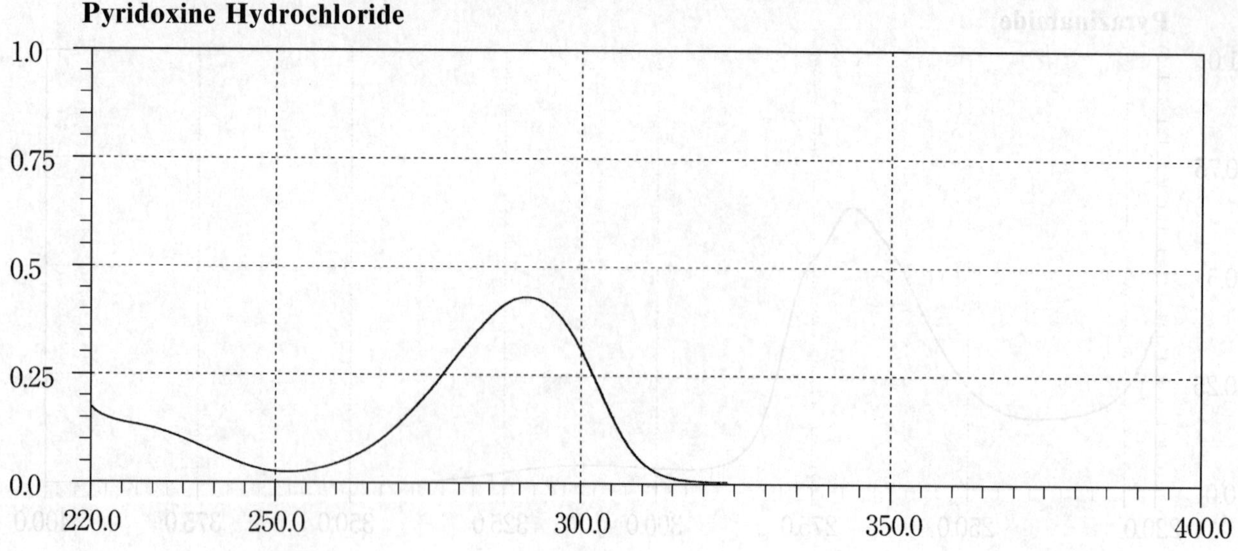

Pyrrolnitrin

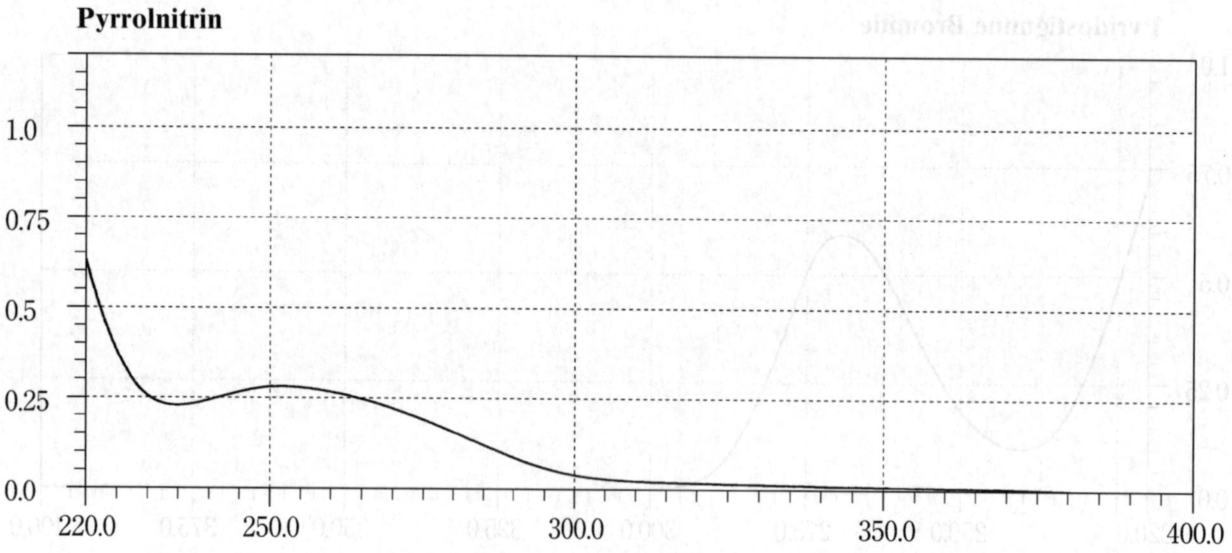

Quetiapine Fumarate

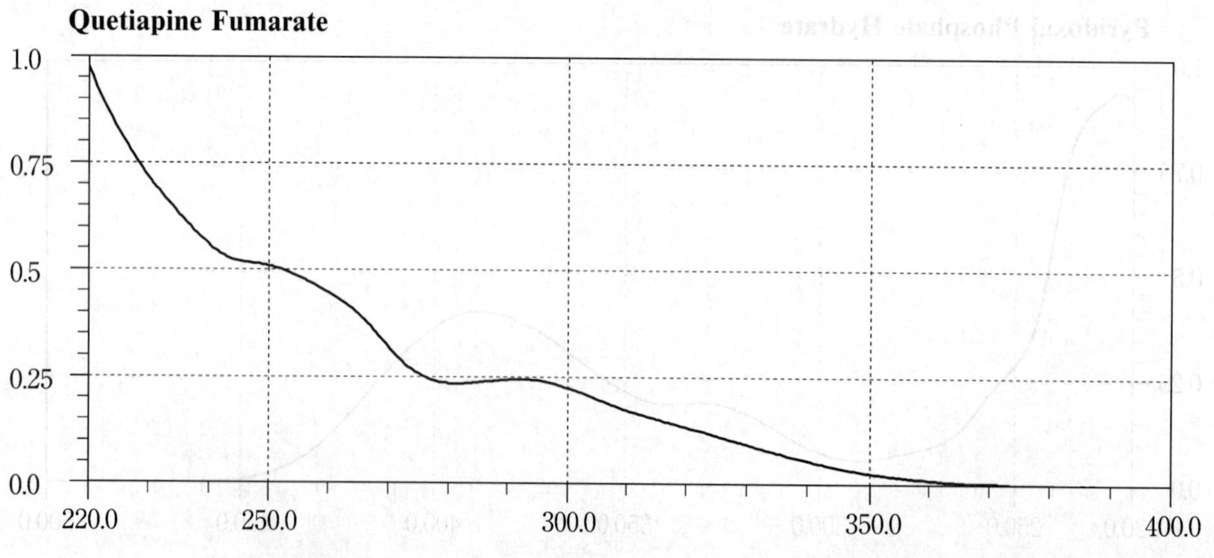

Quinapril Hydrochloride

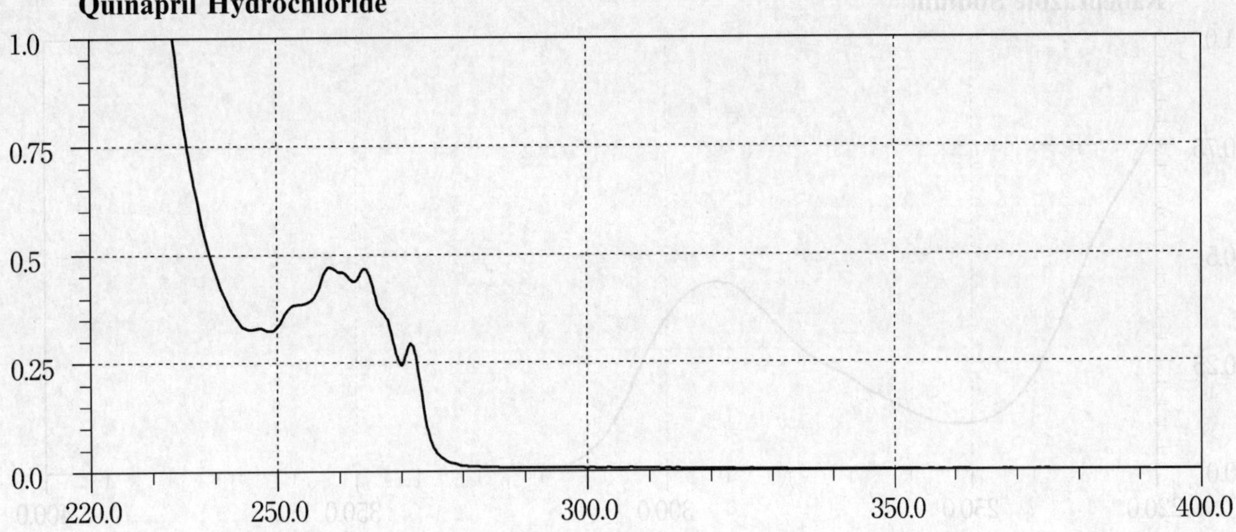

Quinine Ethyl Carbonate

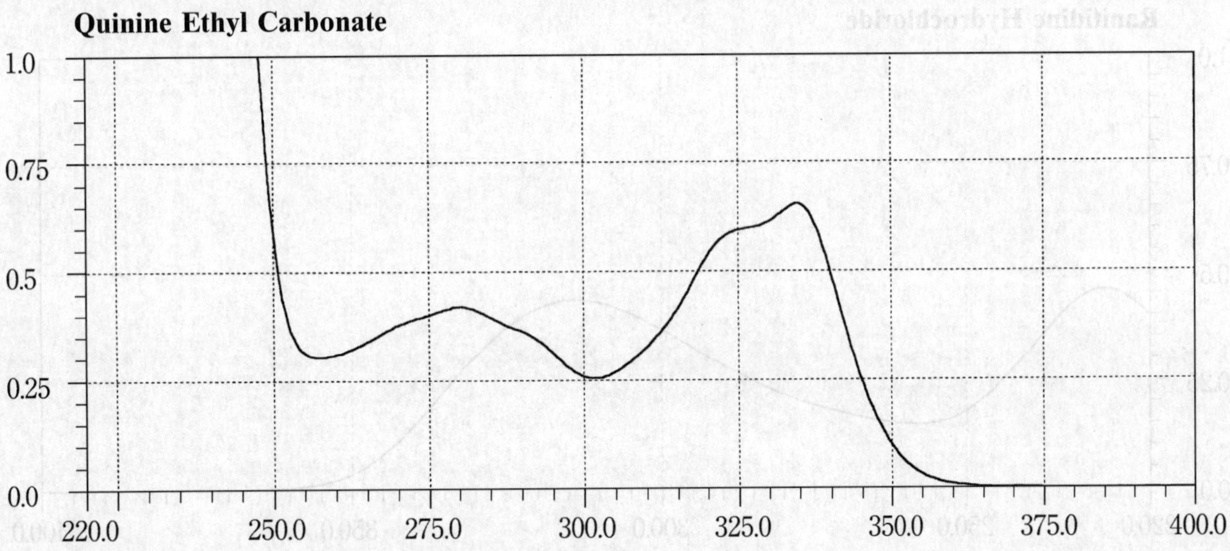

Quinine Sulfate Hydrate

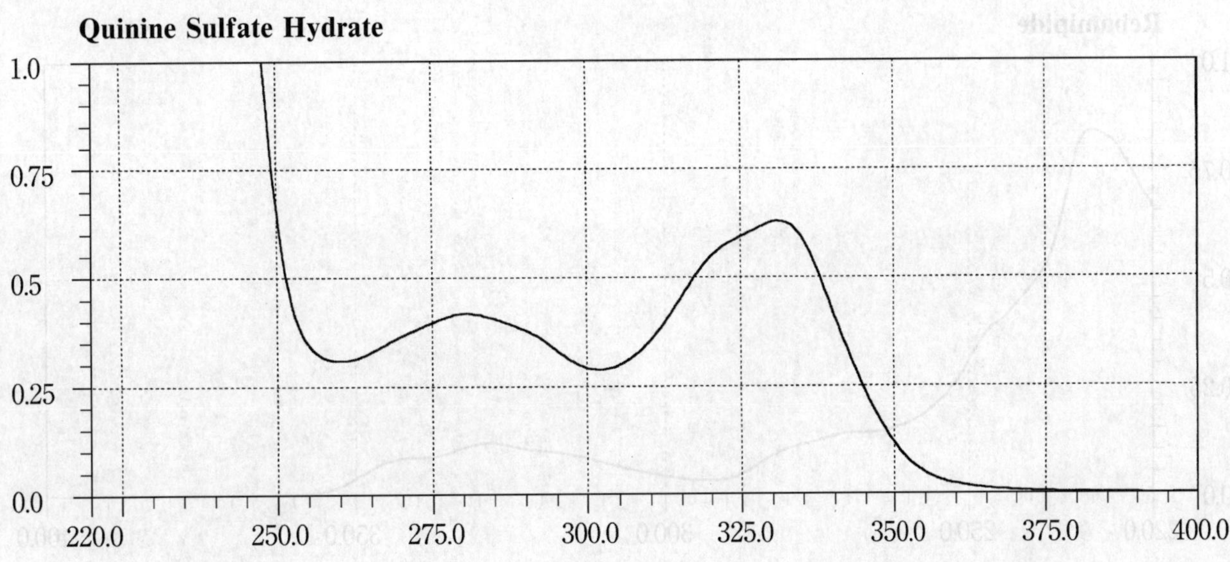

Rabeprazole Sodium

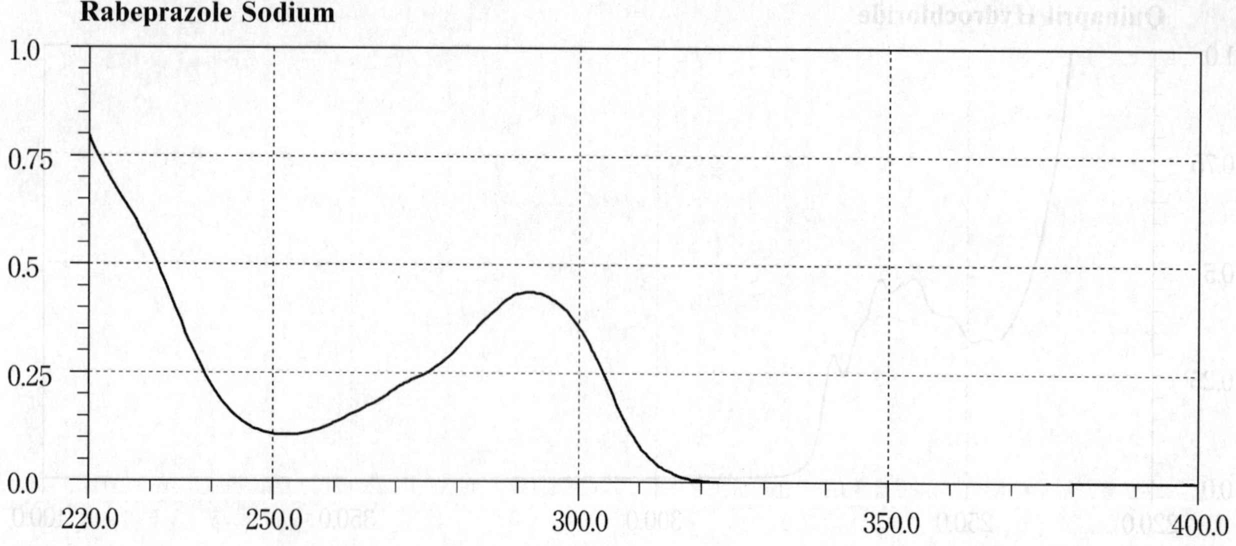

Ranitidine Hydrochloride

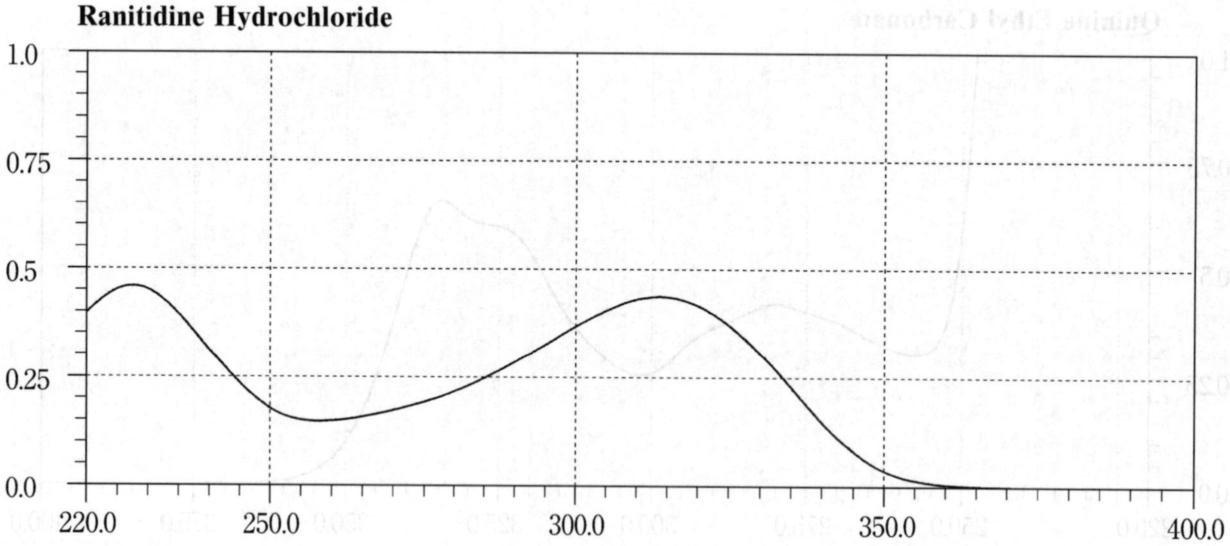

Rebamipide

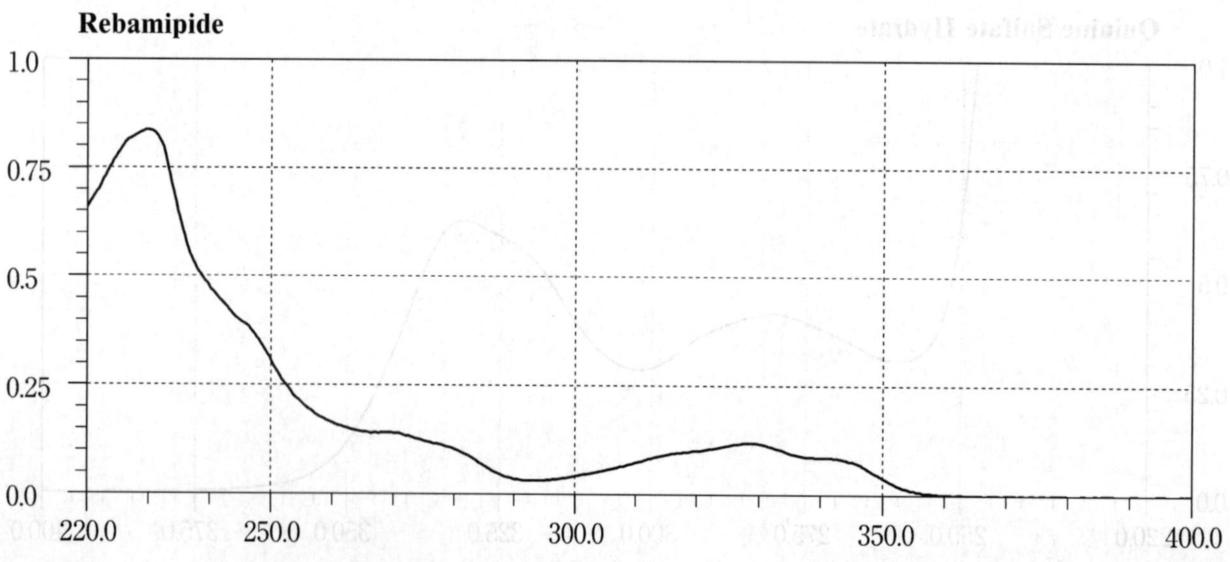

Reserpine

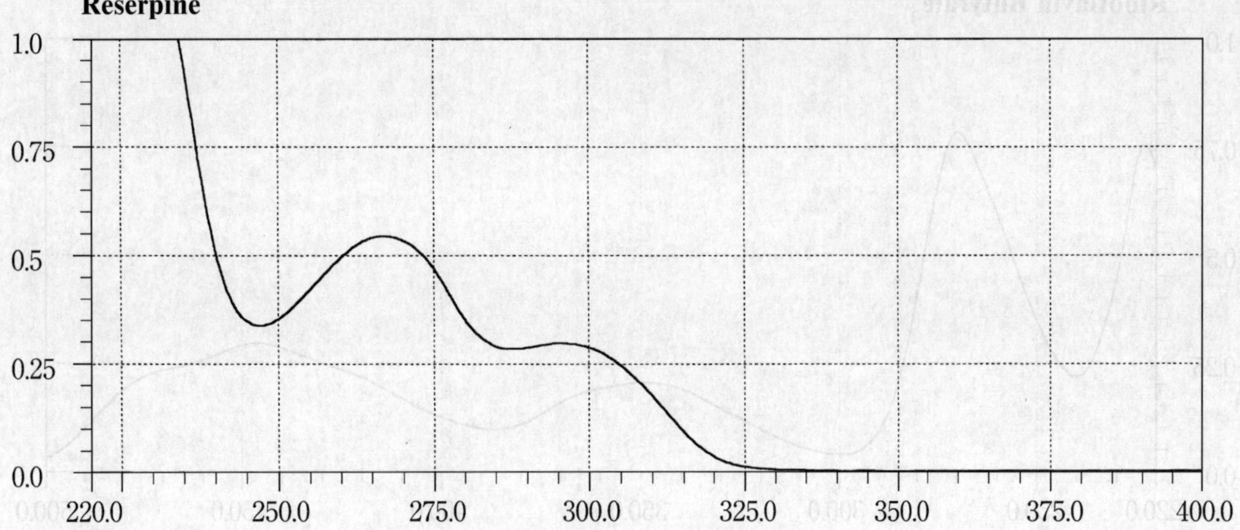

Ribavirin

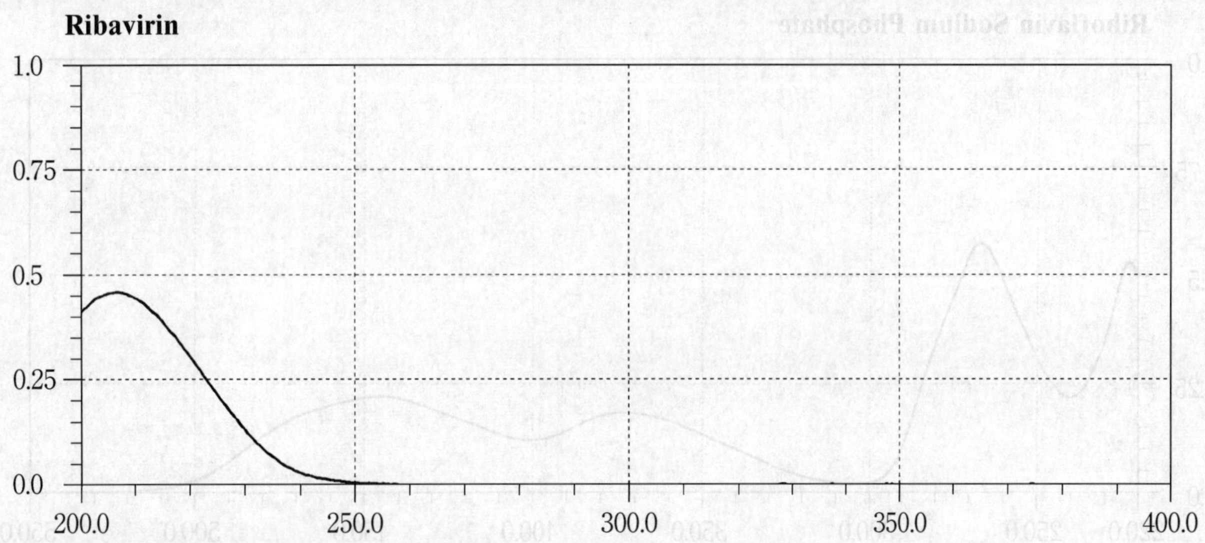

Riboflavin

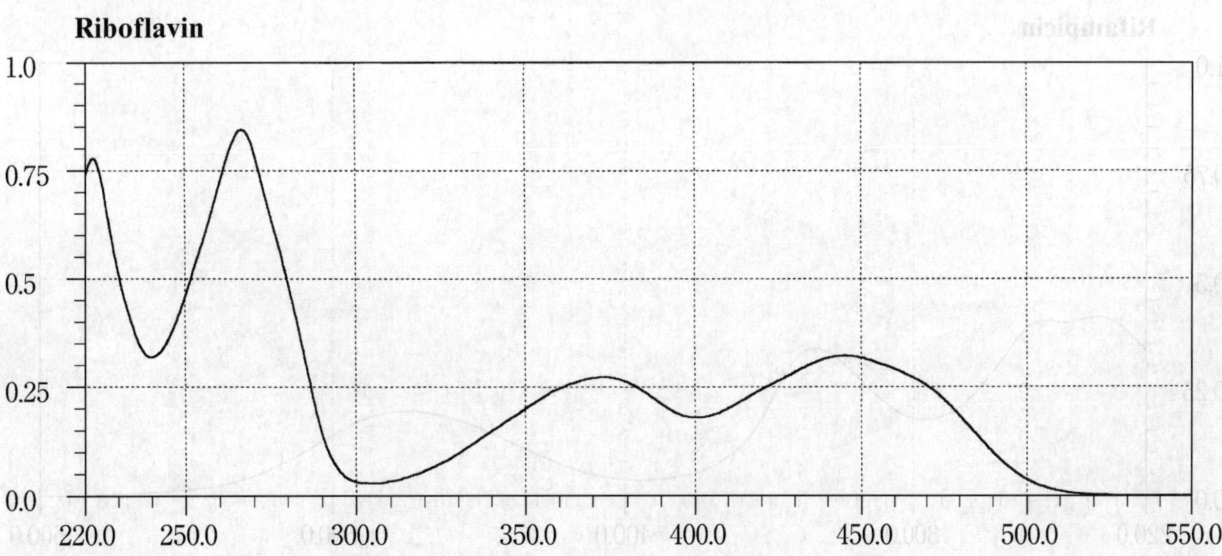

Riboflavin Butyrate

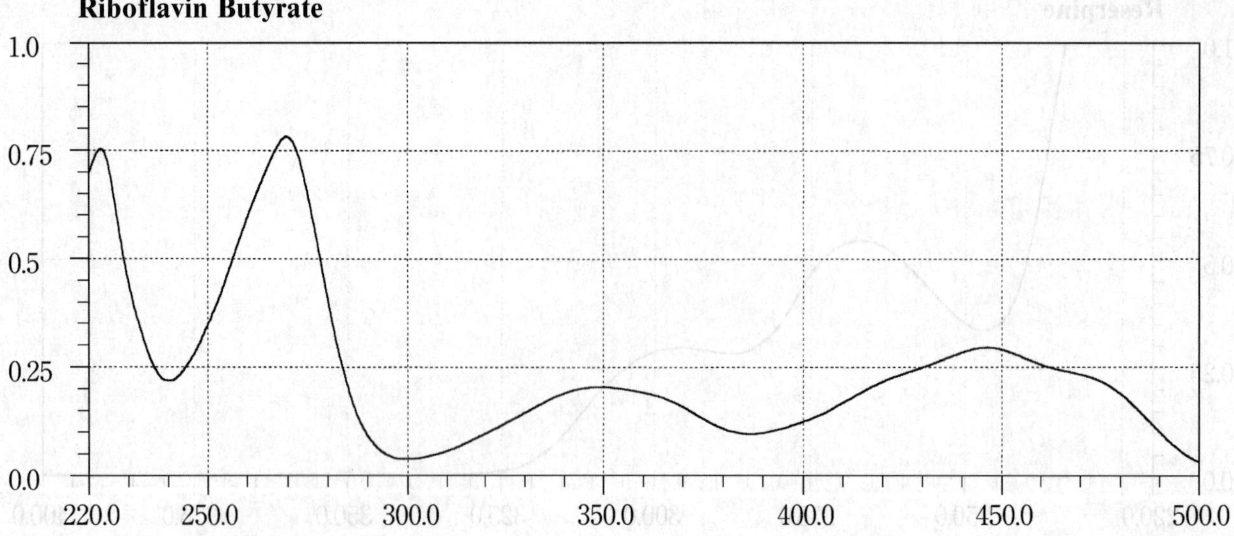

Riboflavin Sodium Phosphate

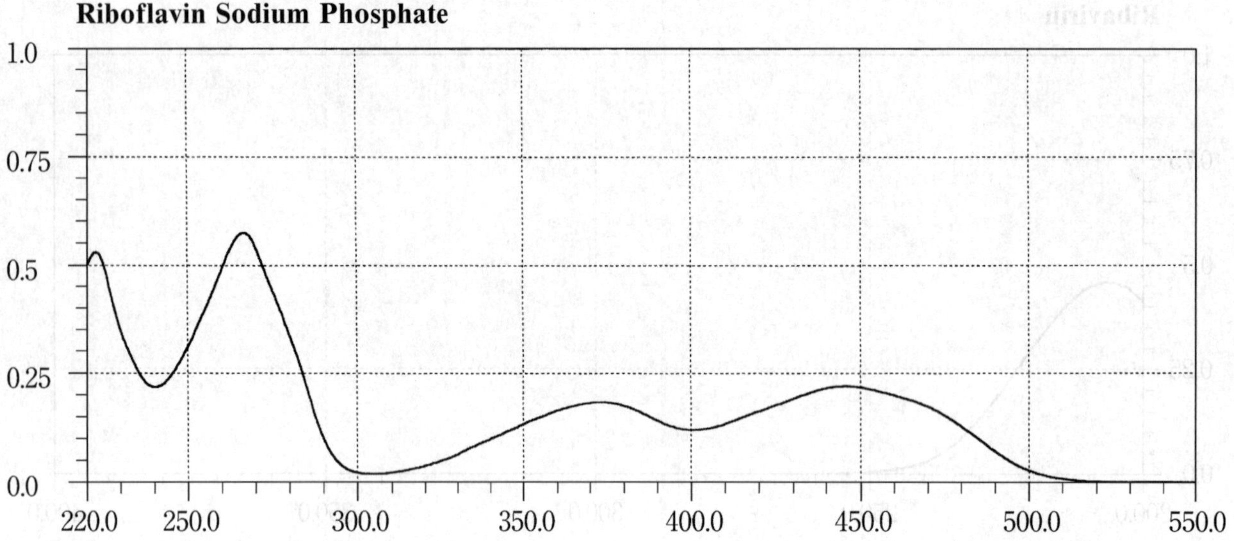

Rifampicin

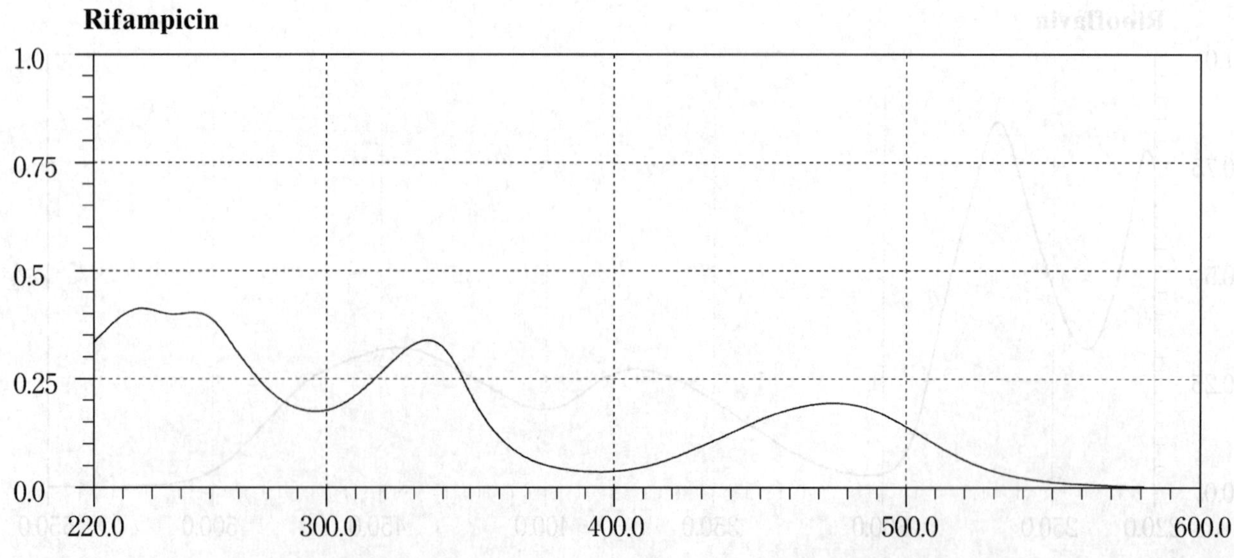

Rilmazafone Hydrochloride Hydrate

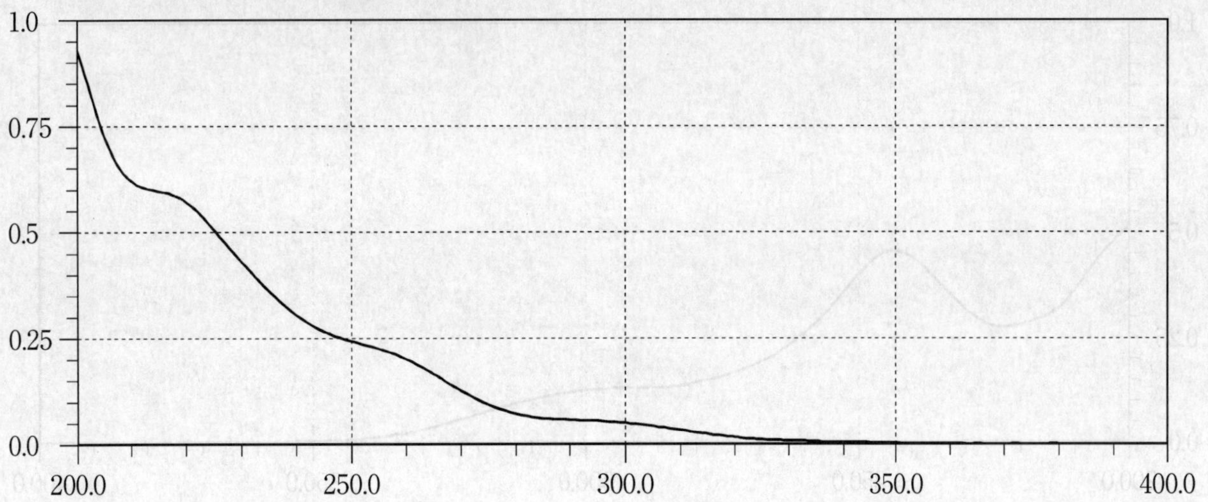

Risperidone

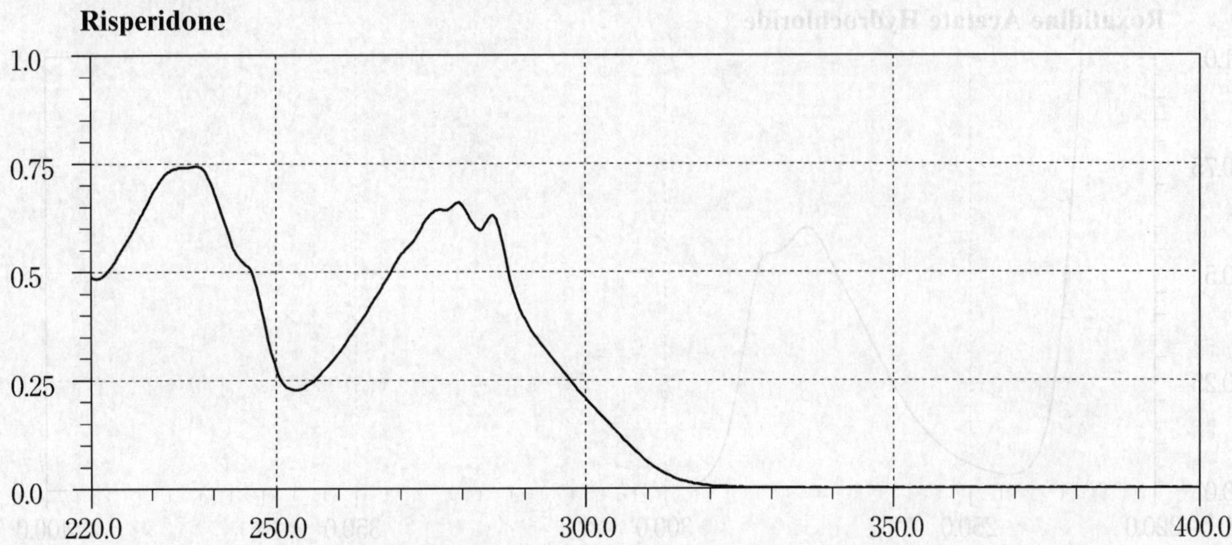

Ritodrine Hydrochloride

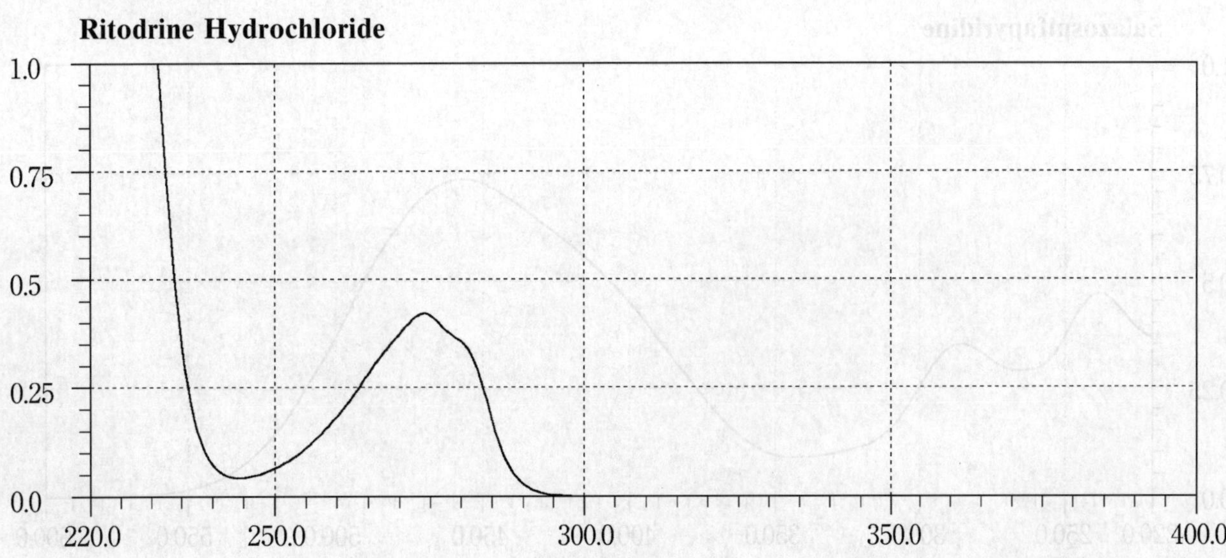

Rosuvastatin Calcium

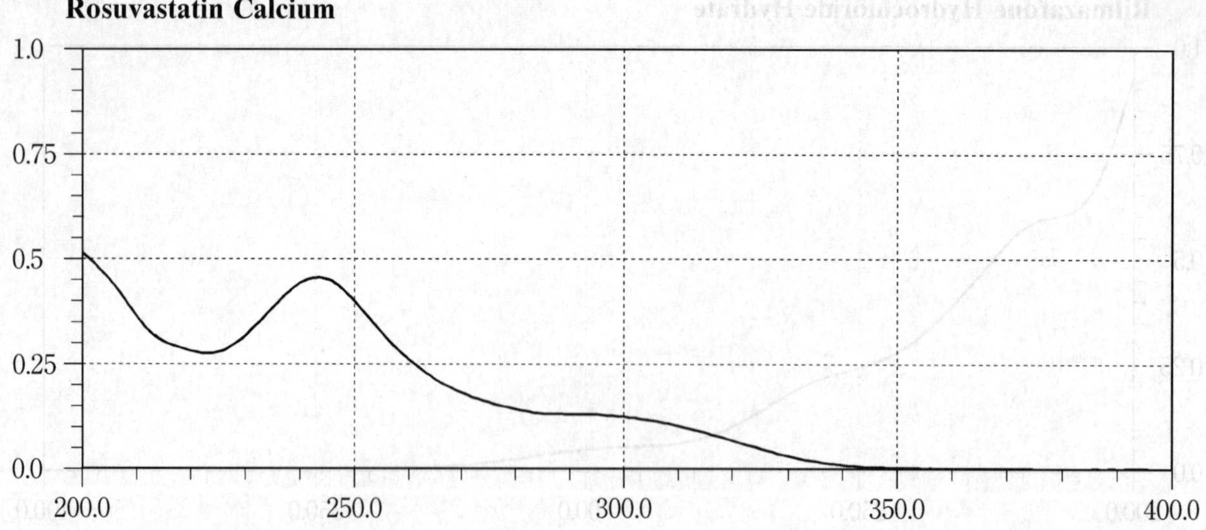

Roxatidine Acetate Hydrochloride

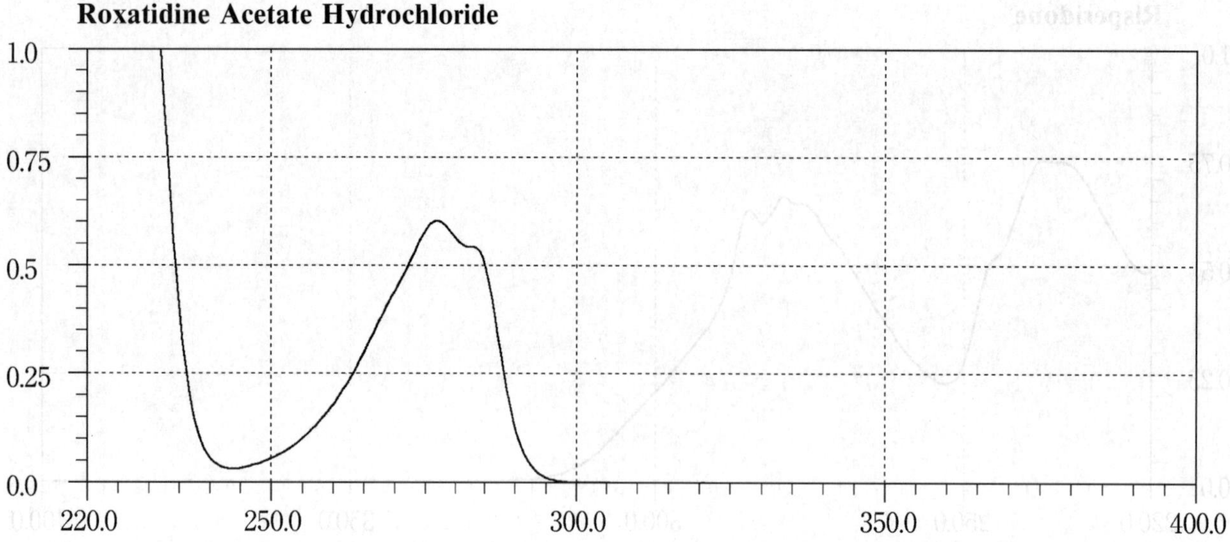

Salazosulfapyridine

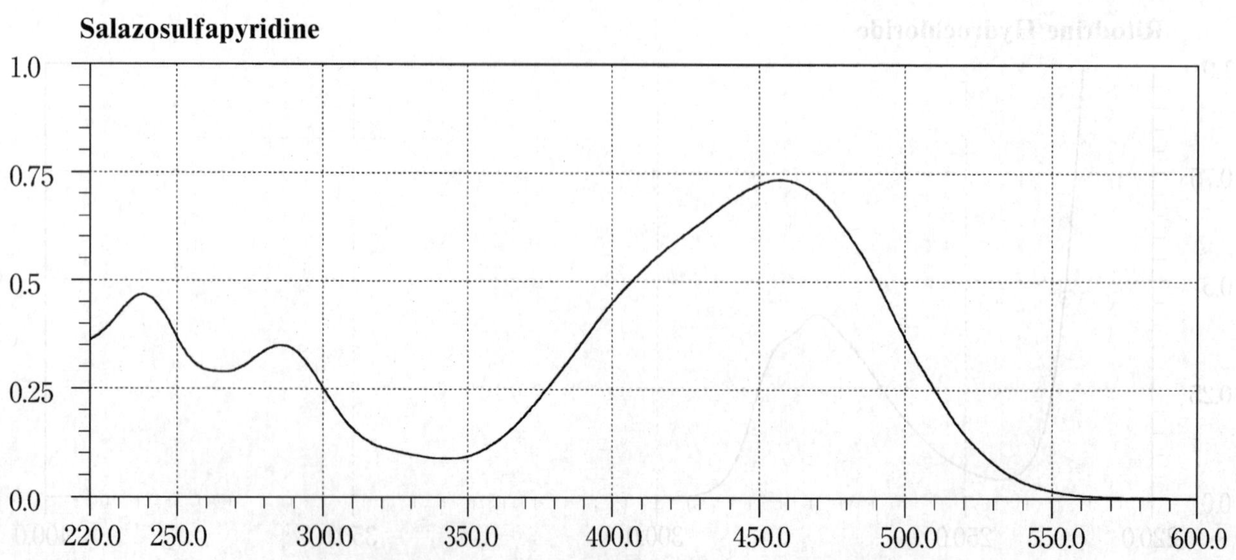

Salbutamol Sulfate

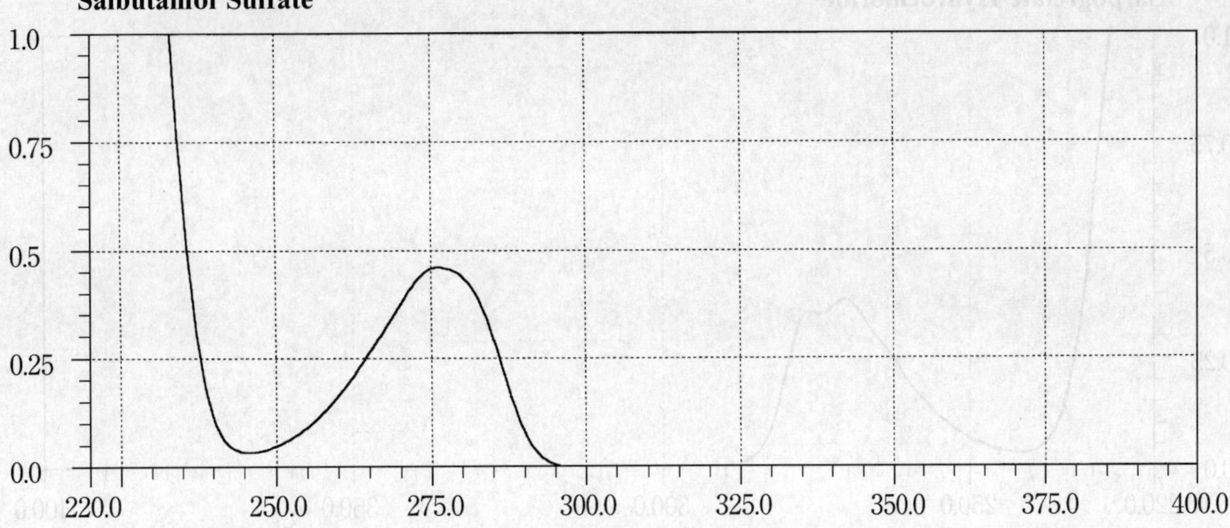

Salicylic Acid

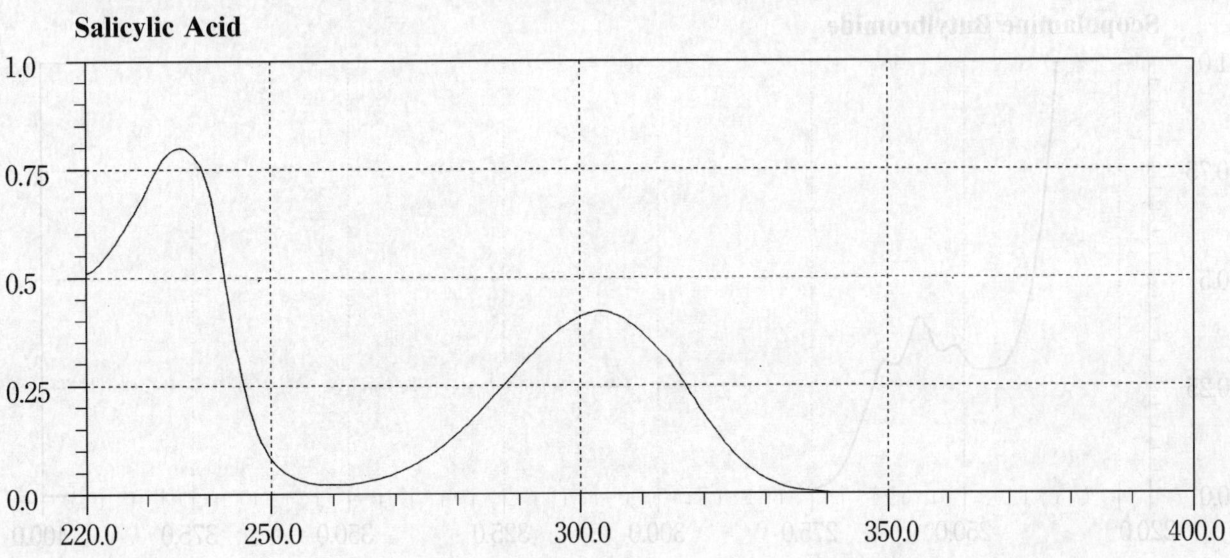

Santonin

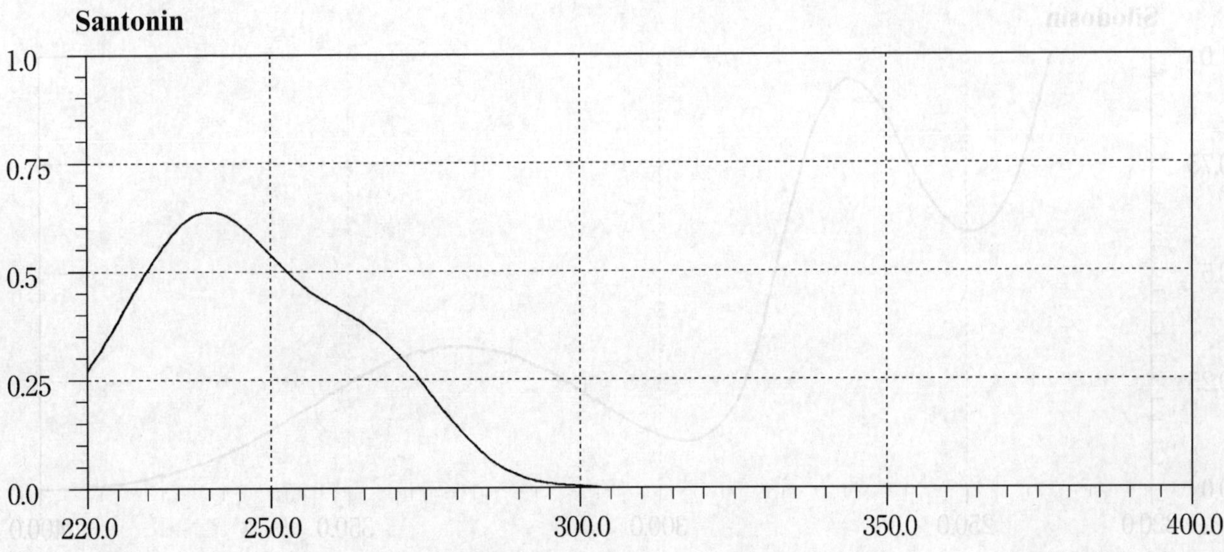

Sarpogrelate Hydrochloride

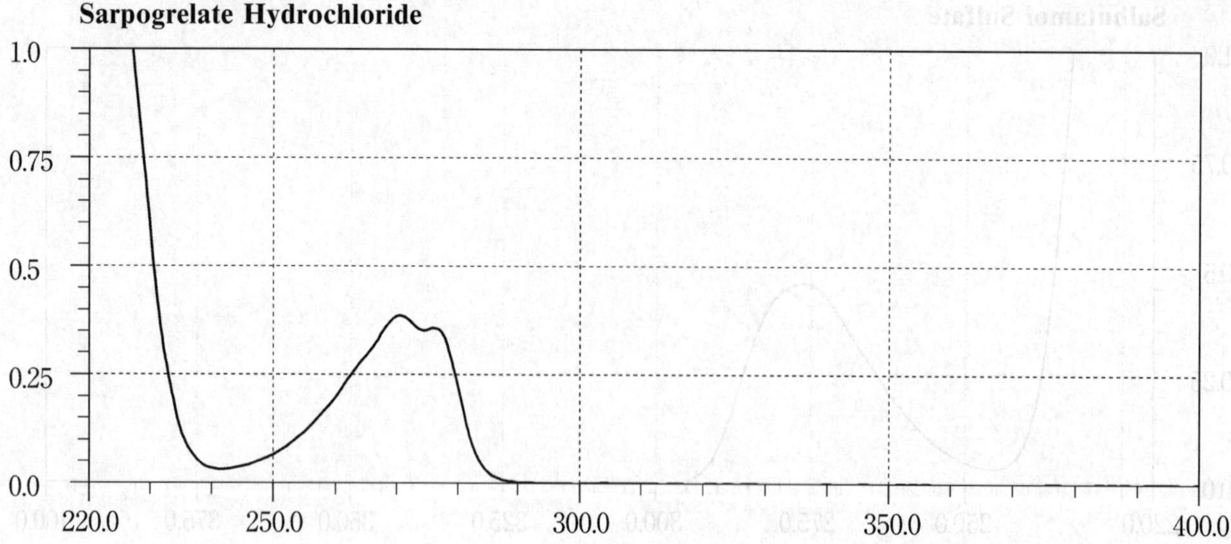

Scopolamine Butylbromide

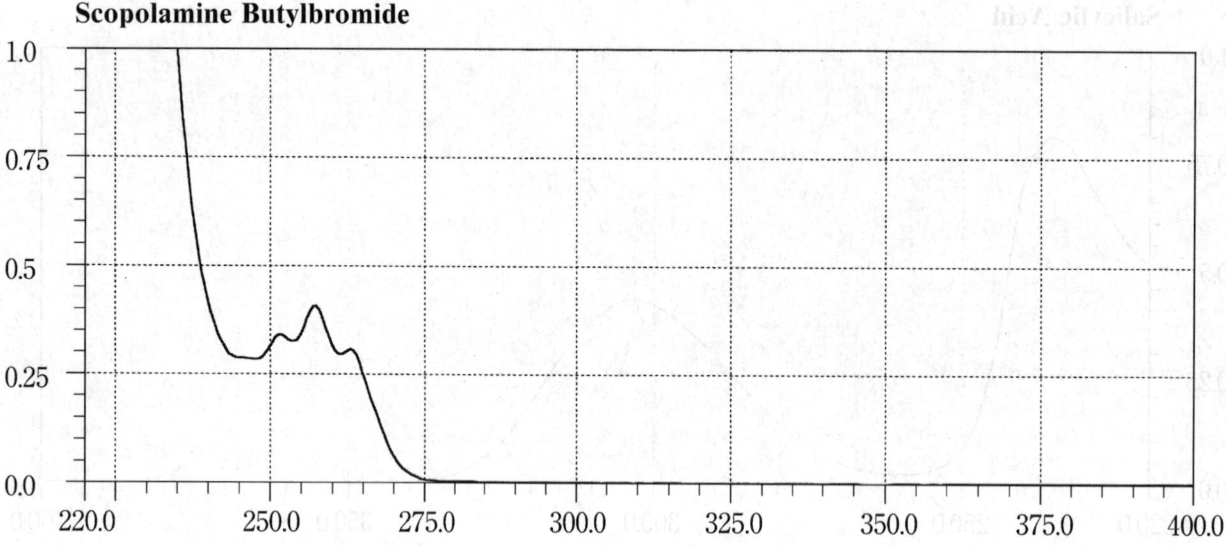

Silodosin

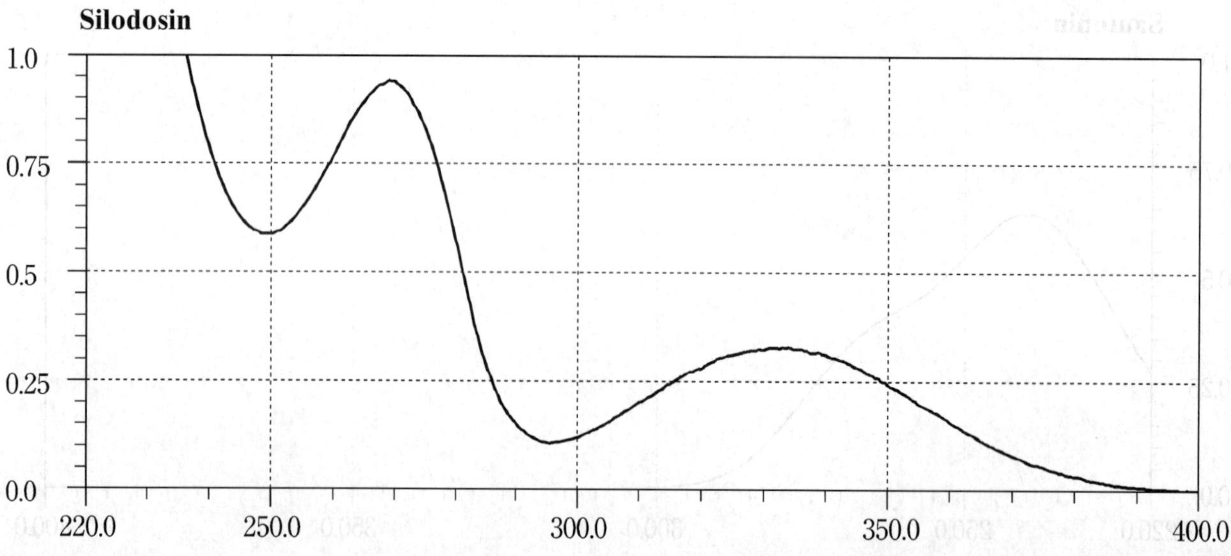

Simvastatin

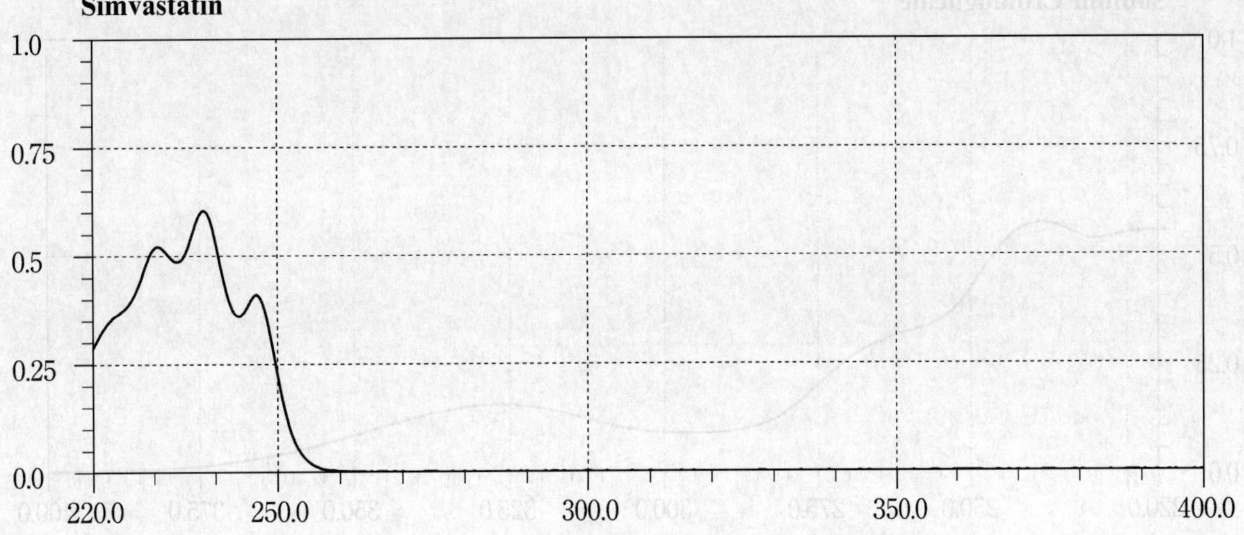

Sitagliptin Phosphate Hydrate

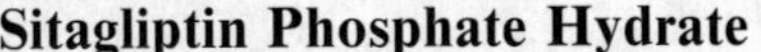

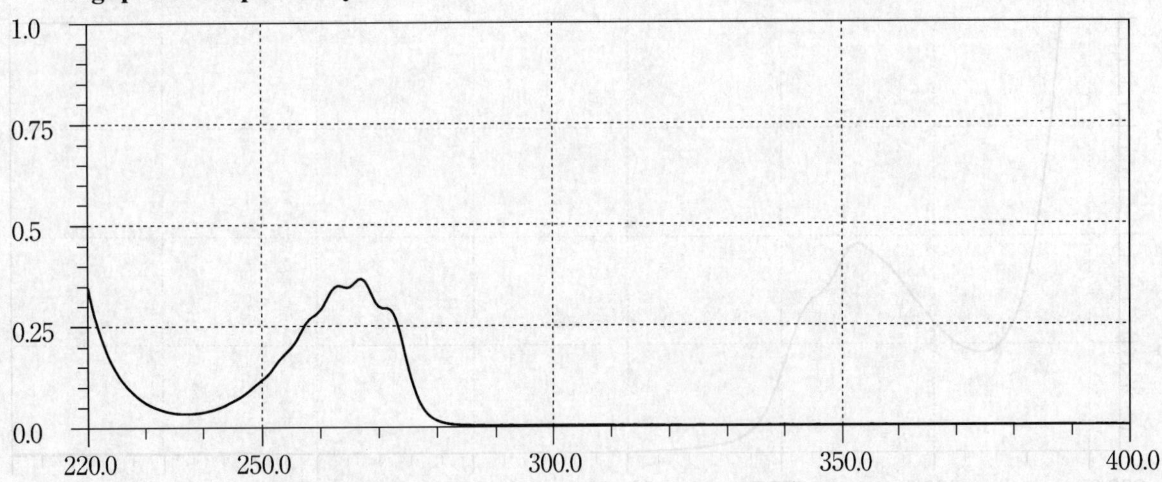

Sivelestat Sodium Hydrate

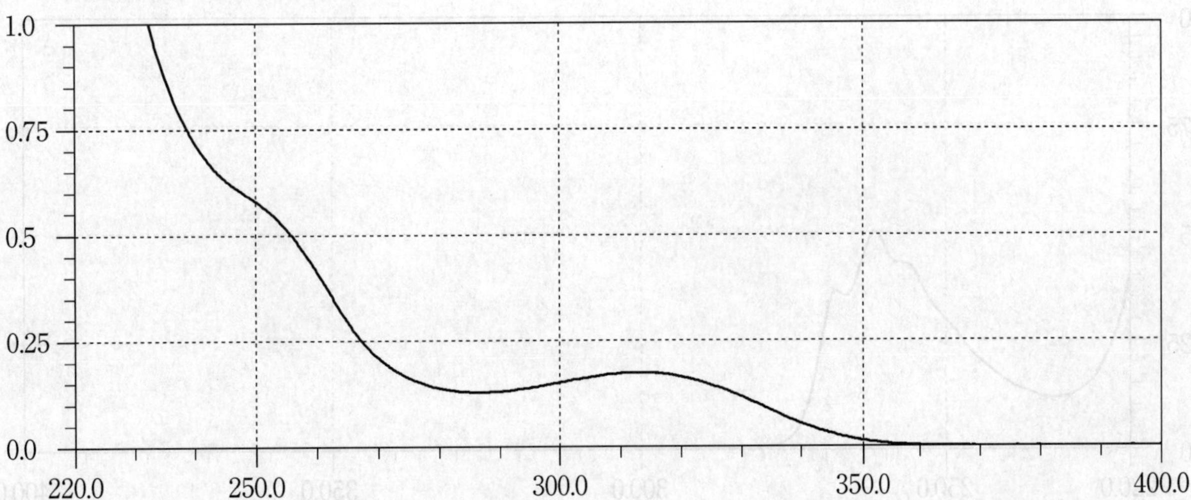

Sodium Cromoglicate

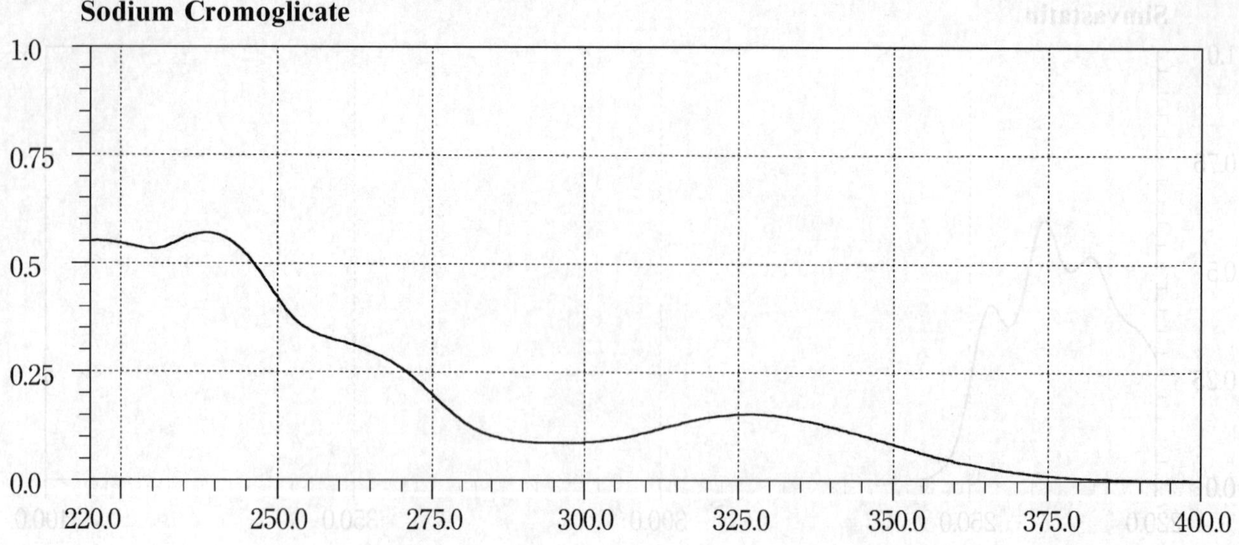

Sodium Picosulfate Hydrate

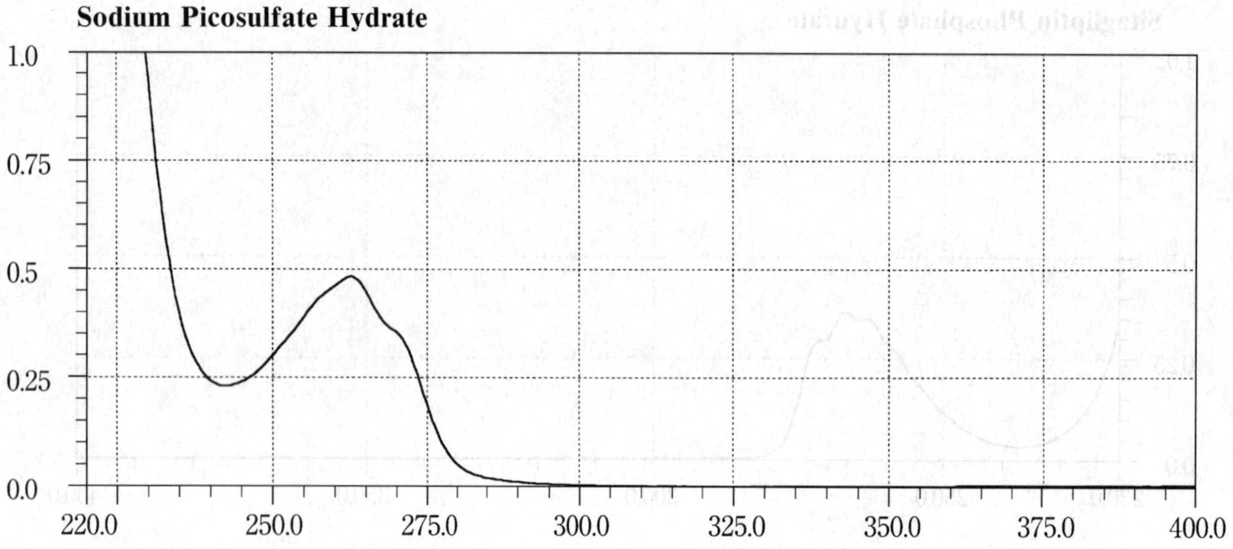

Sodium Risedronate Hydrate

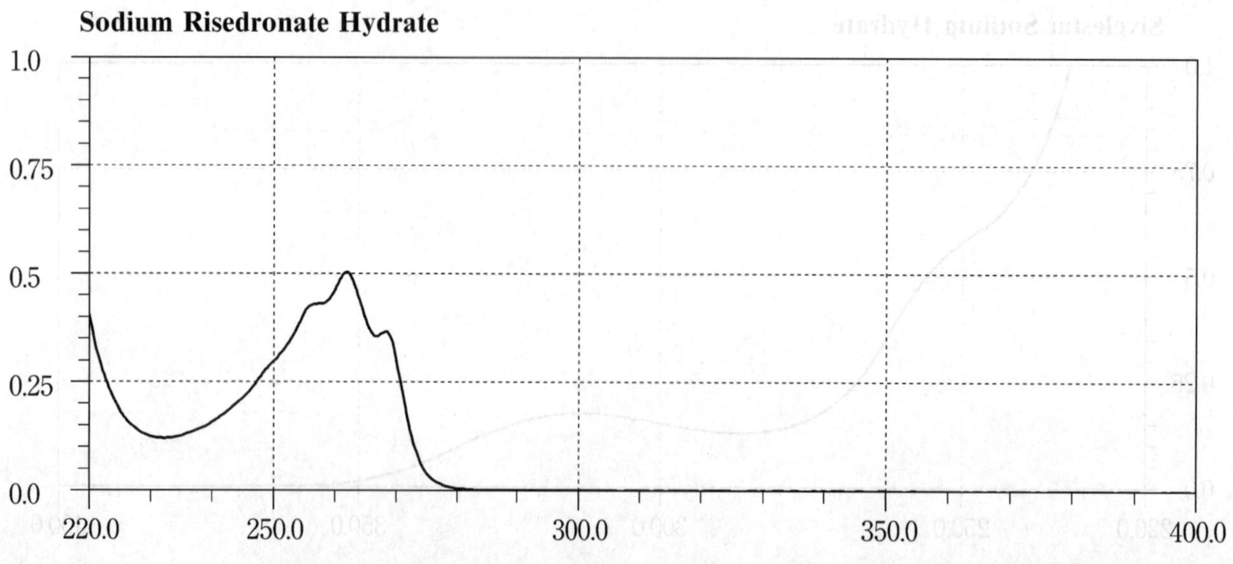

Spiramycin Acetate

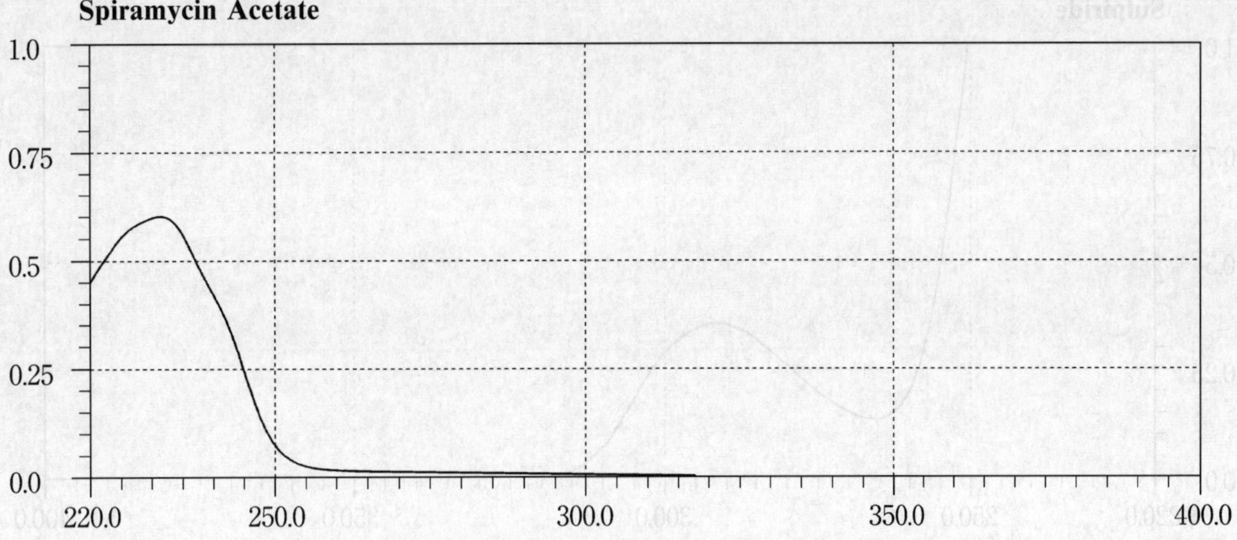

Spironolactone

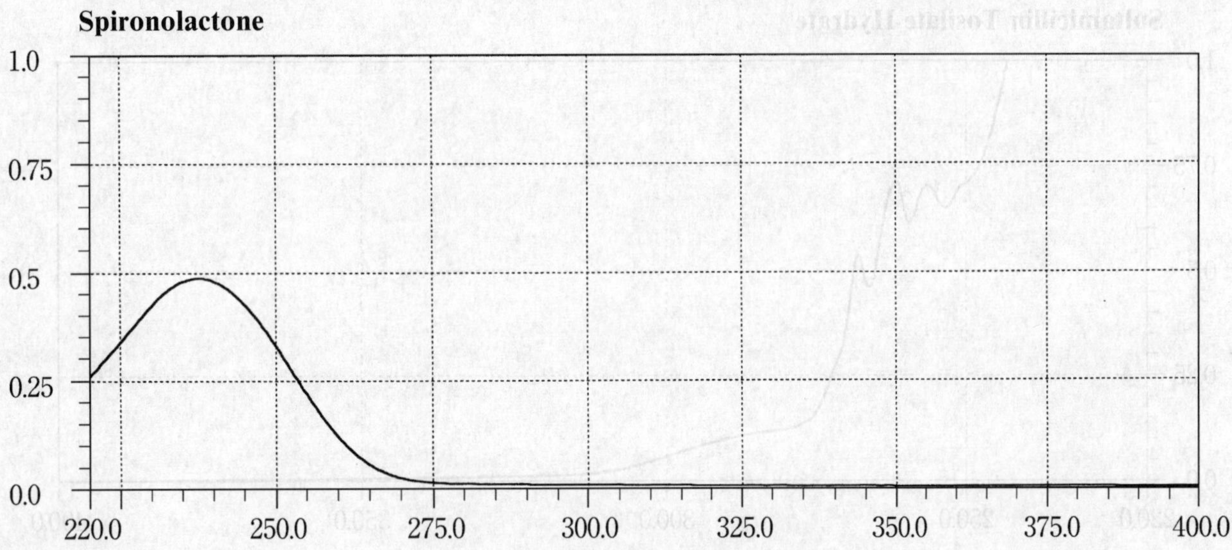

Sulindac

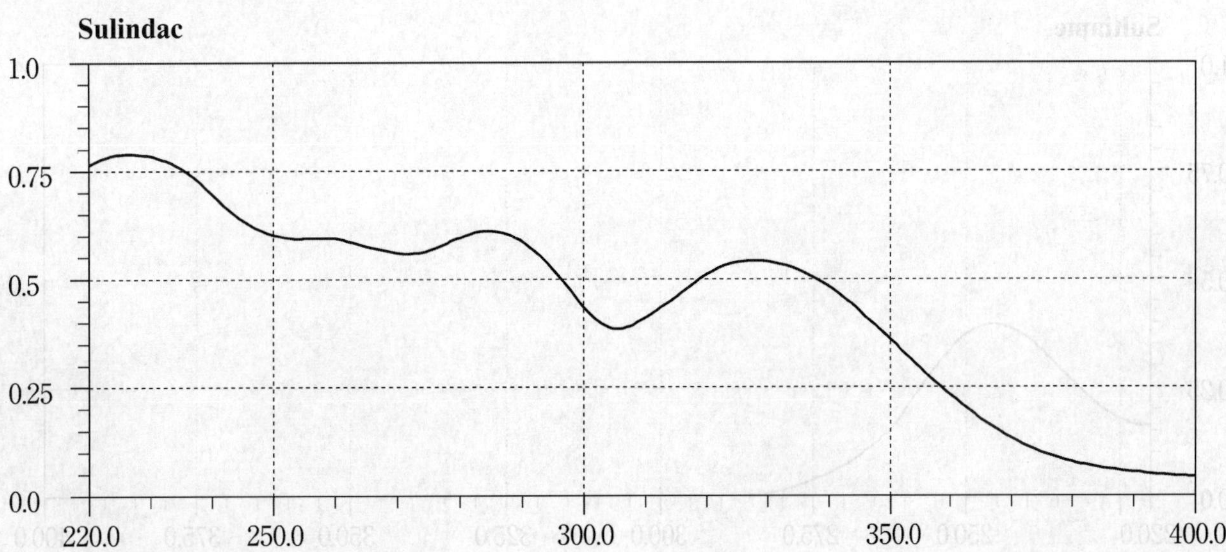

Sulpiride

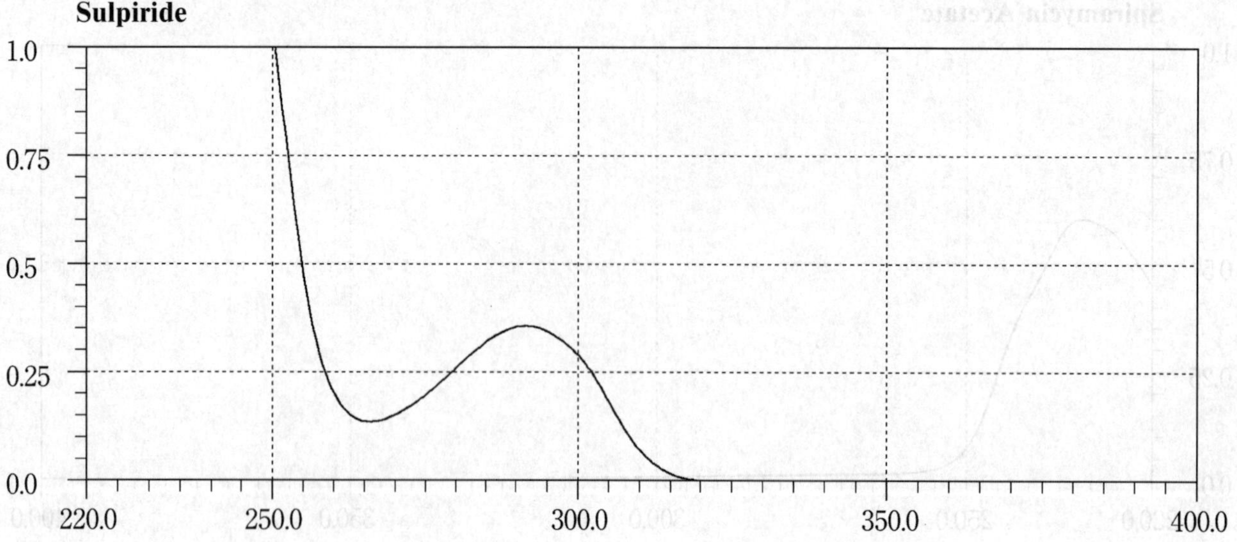

Sultamicillin Tosilate Hydrate

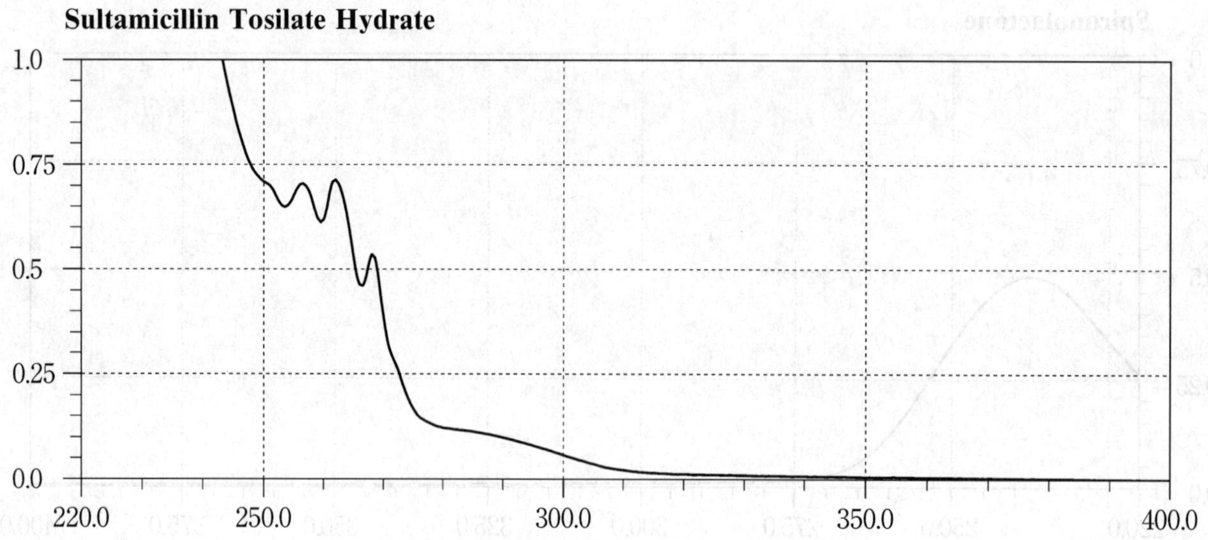

Sultiame

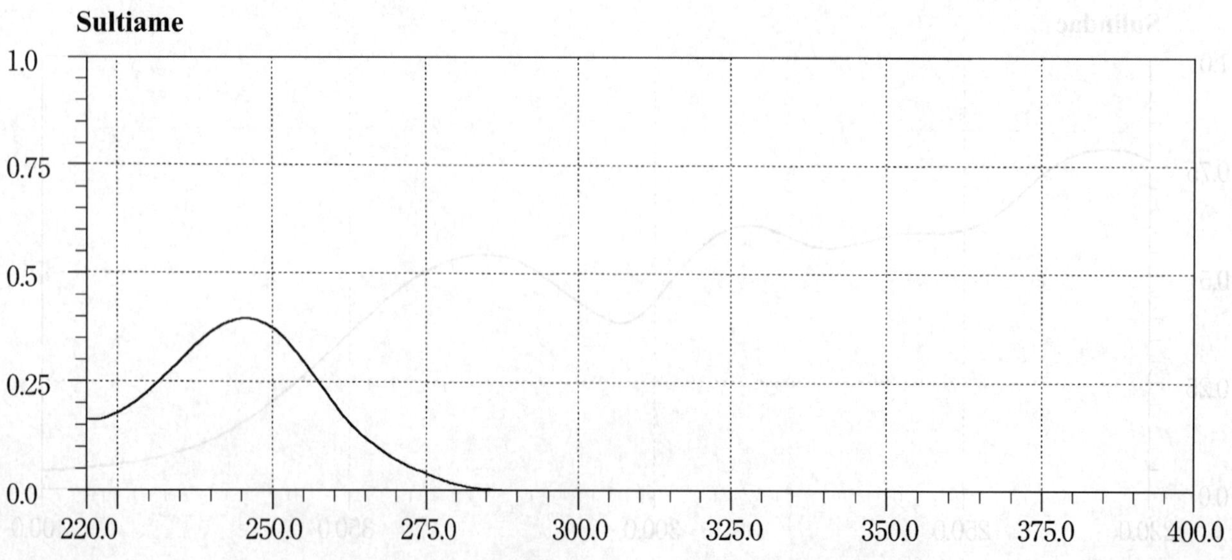

Tacalcitol Hydrate

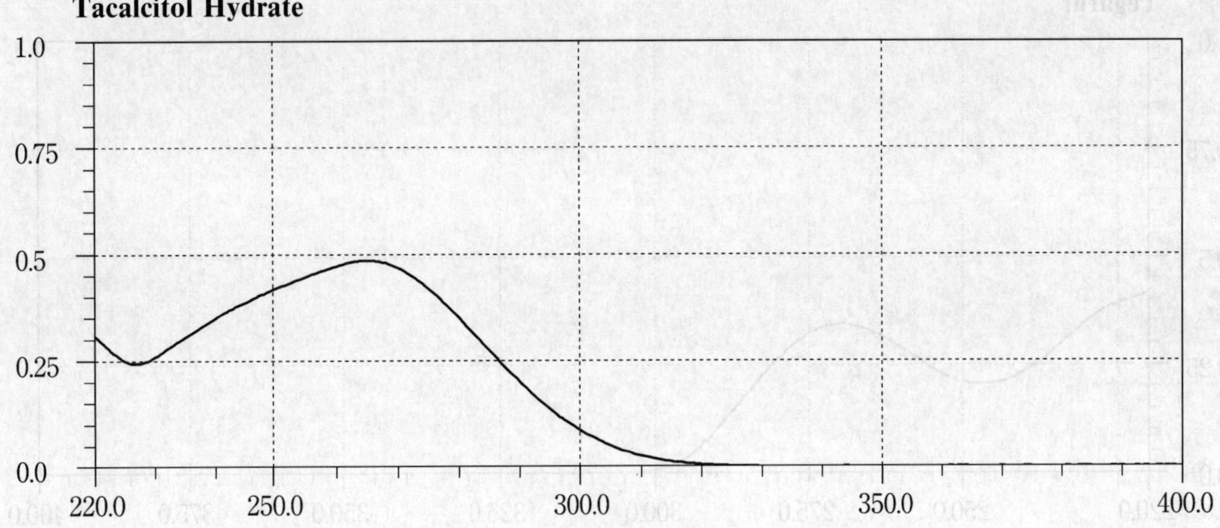

Tamoxifen Citrate

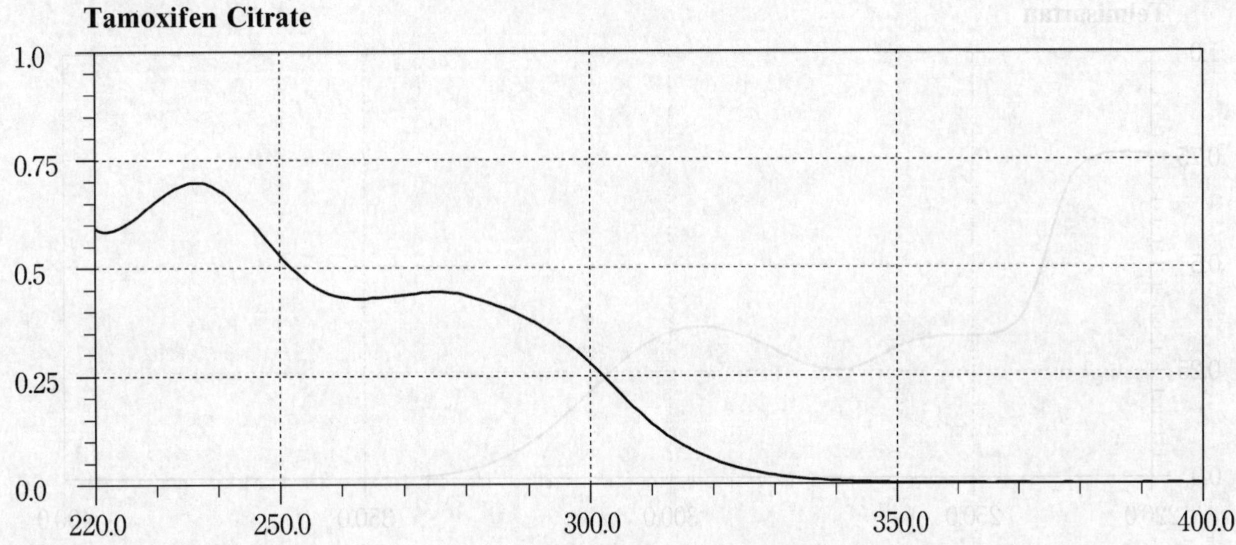

Tamsulosin Hydrochloride

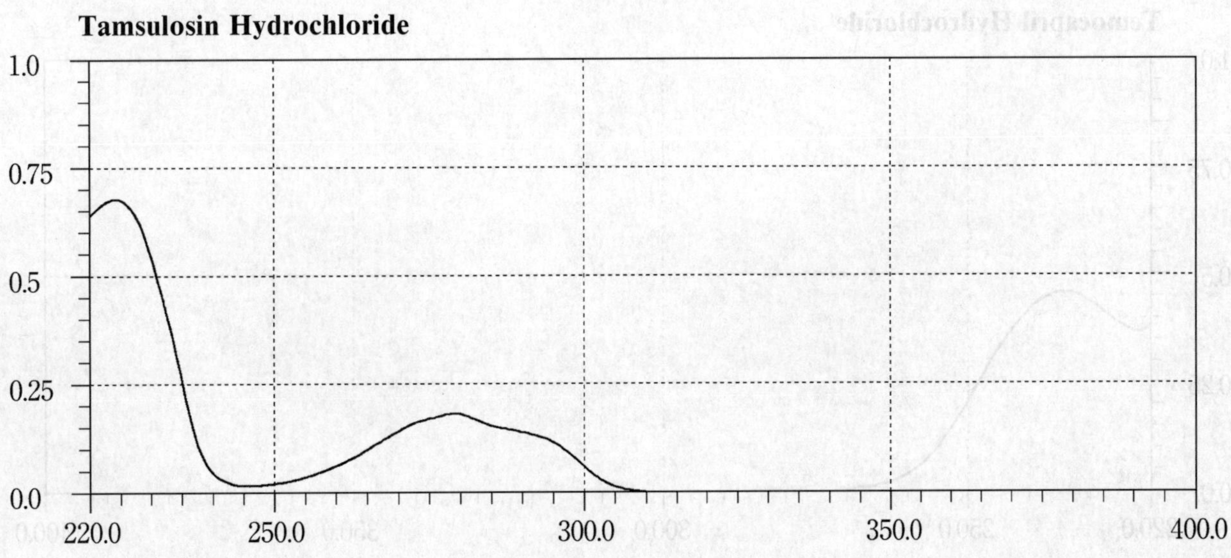

Tegafur

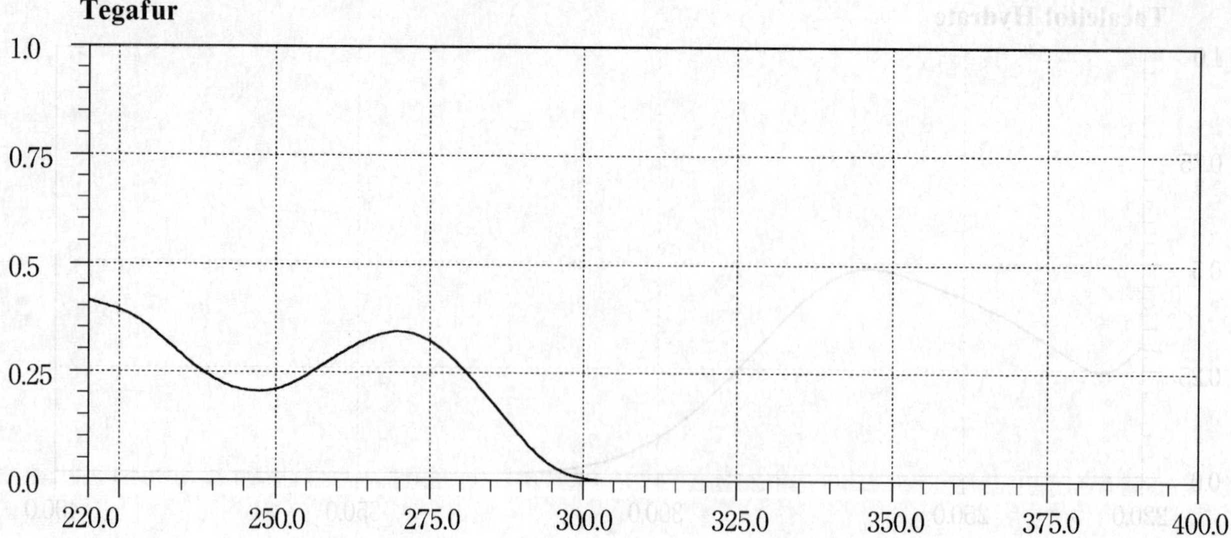

Telmisartan

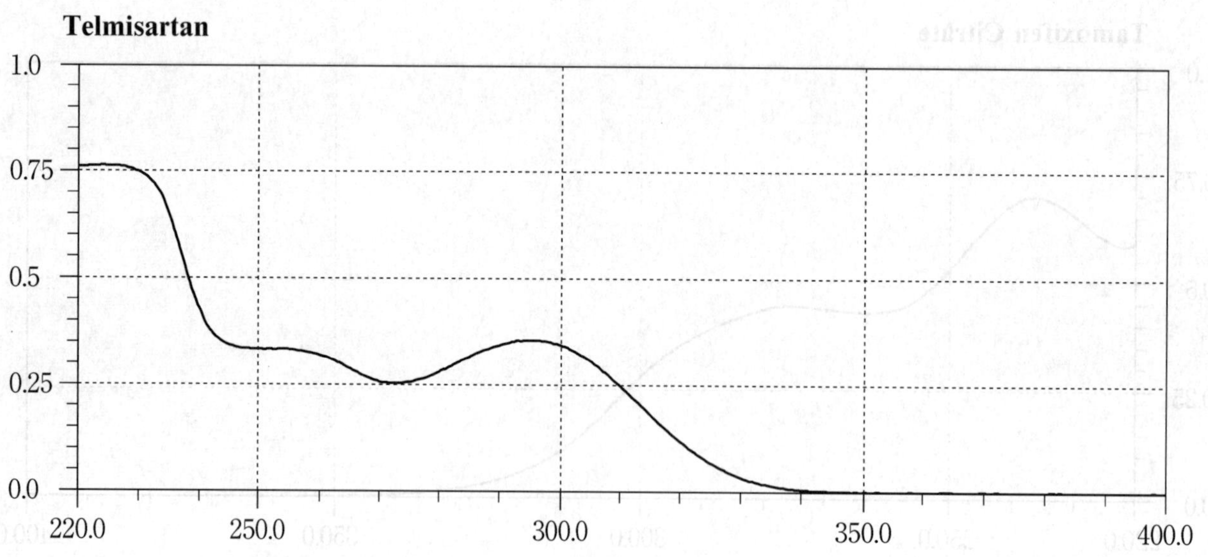

Temocapril Hydrochloride

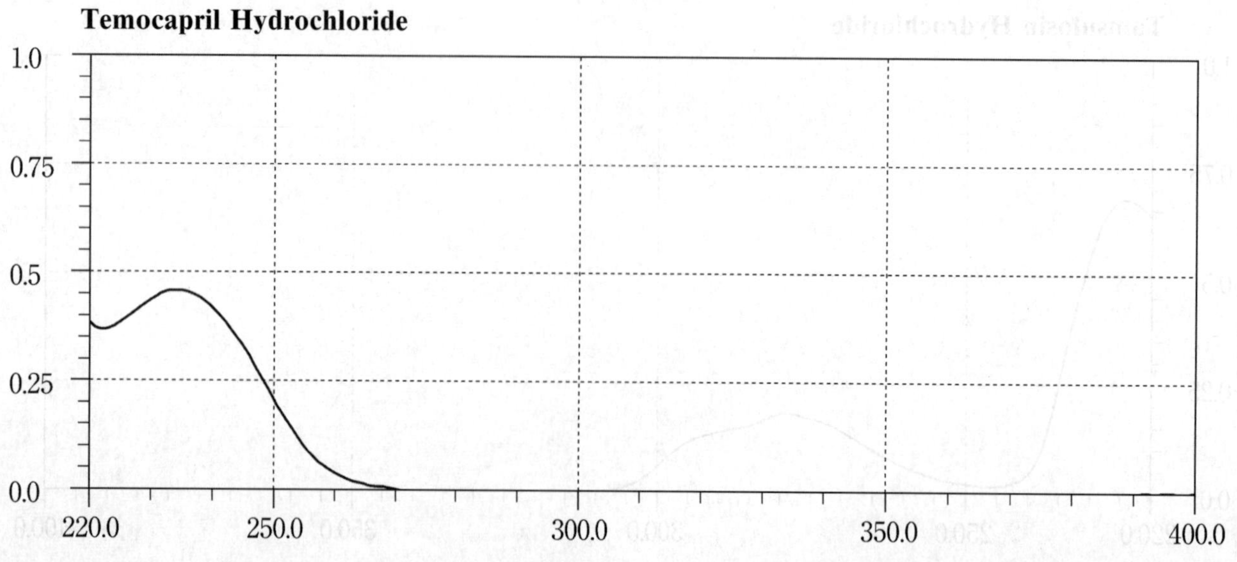

Terbinafine Hydrochloride

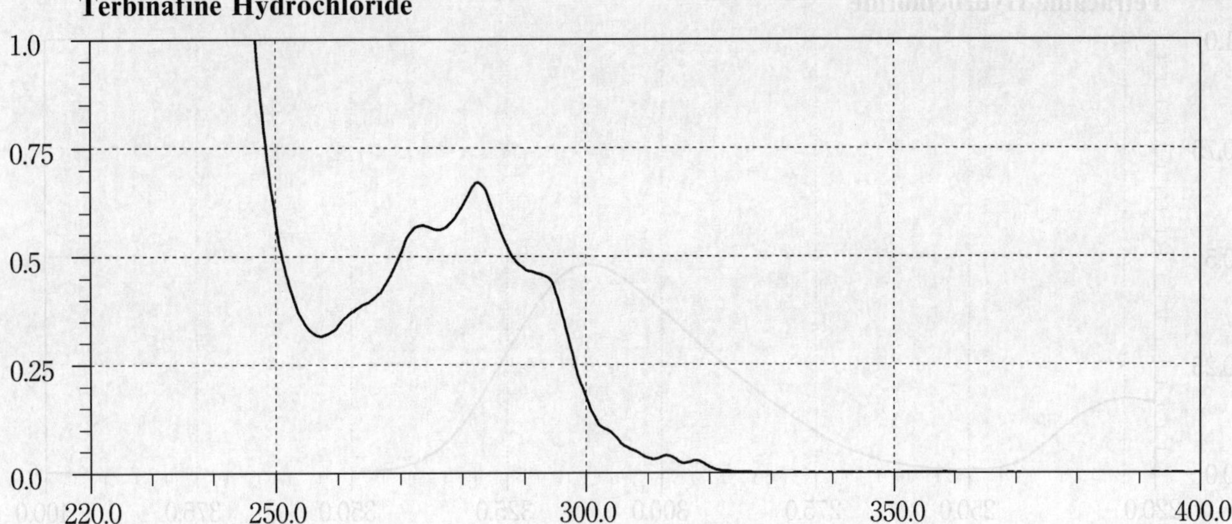

Terbutaline Sulfate

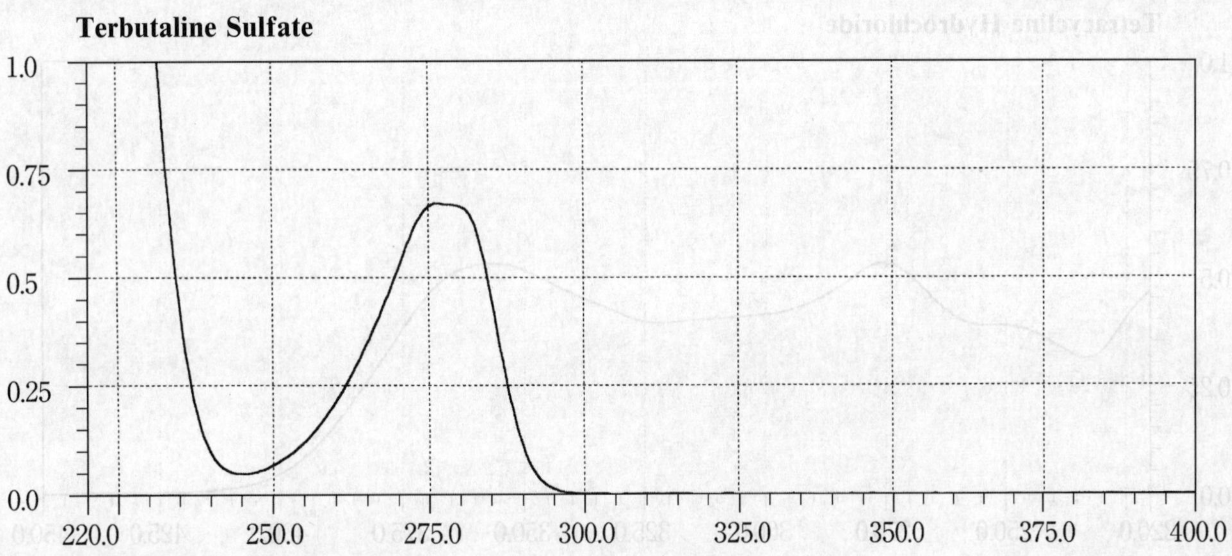

Testosterone Propionate

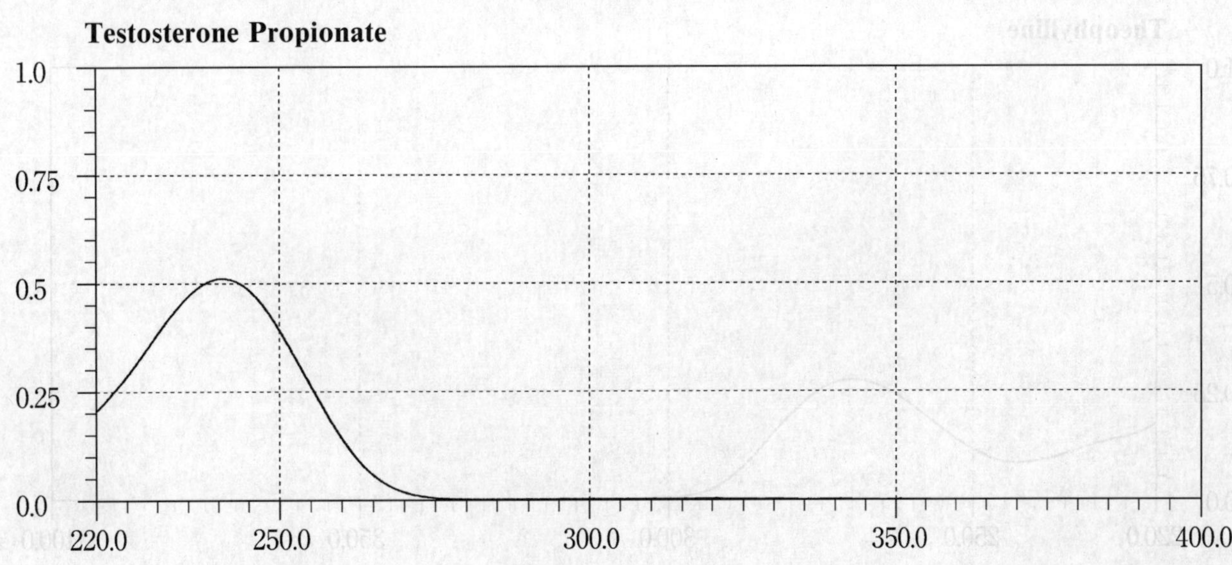

Tetracaine Hydrochloride

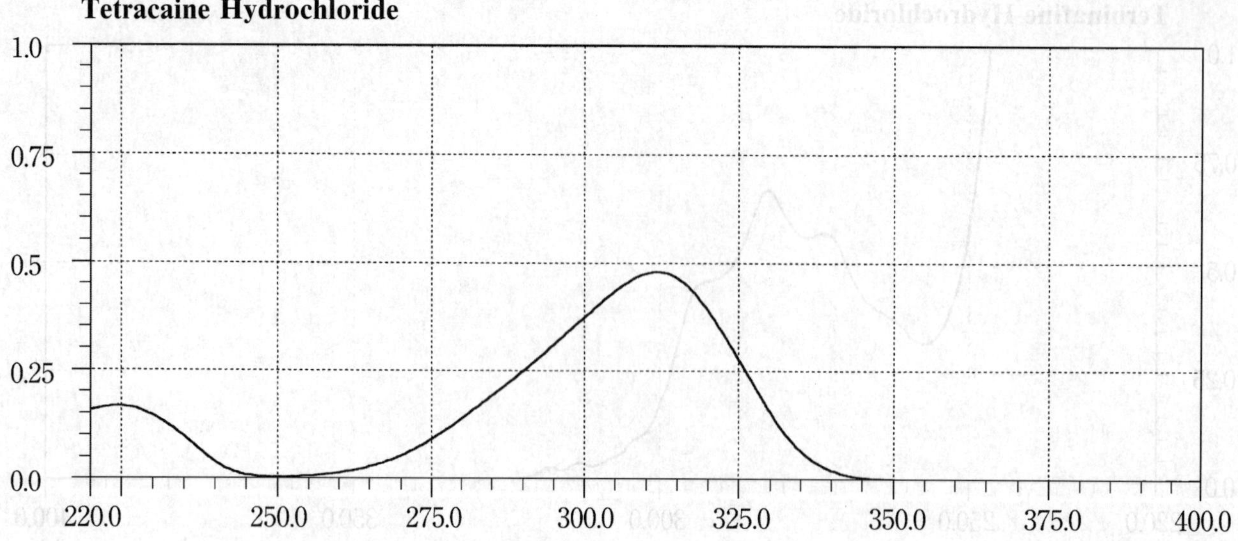

Tetracycline Hydrochloride

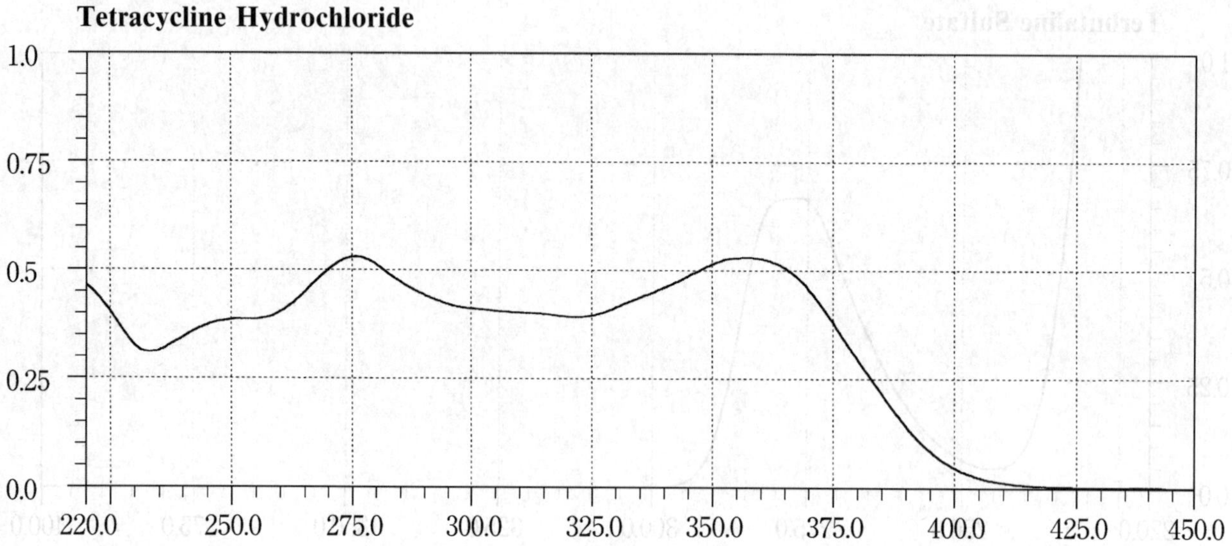

Theophylline

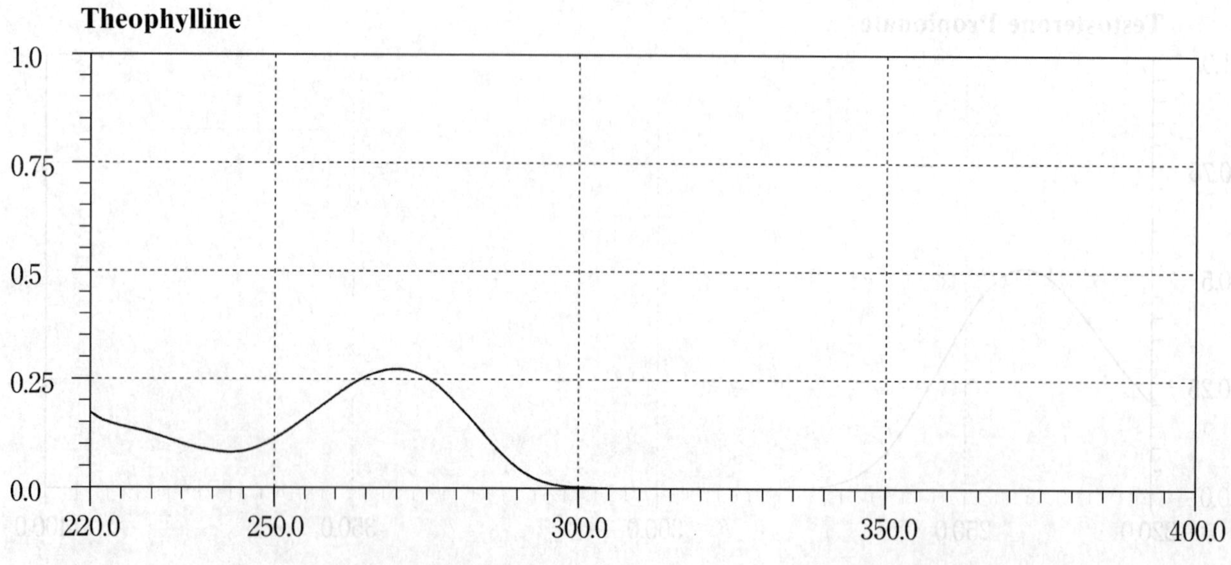

Thiamine Chloride Hydrochloride

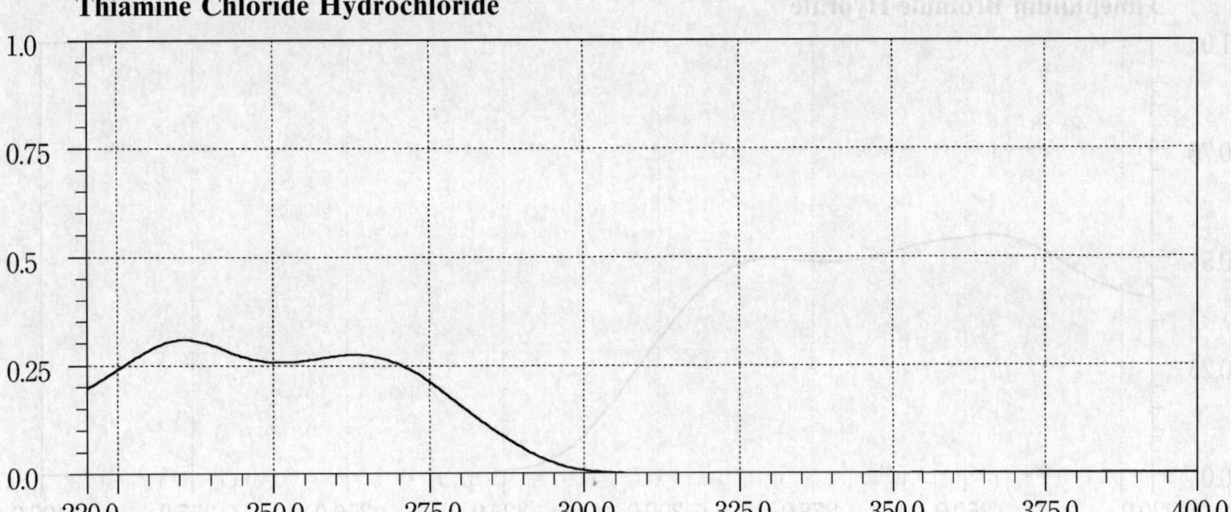

Thiamylal Sodium

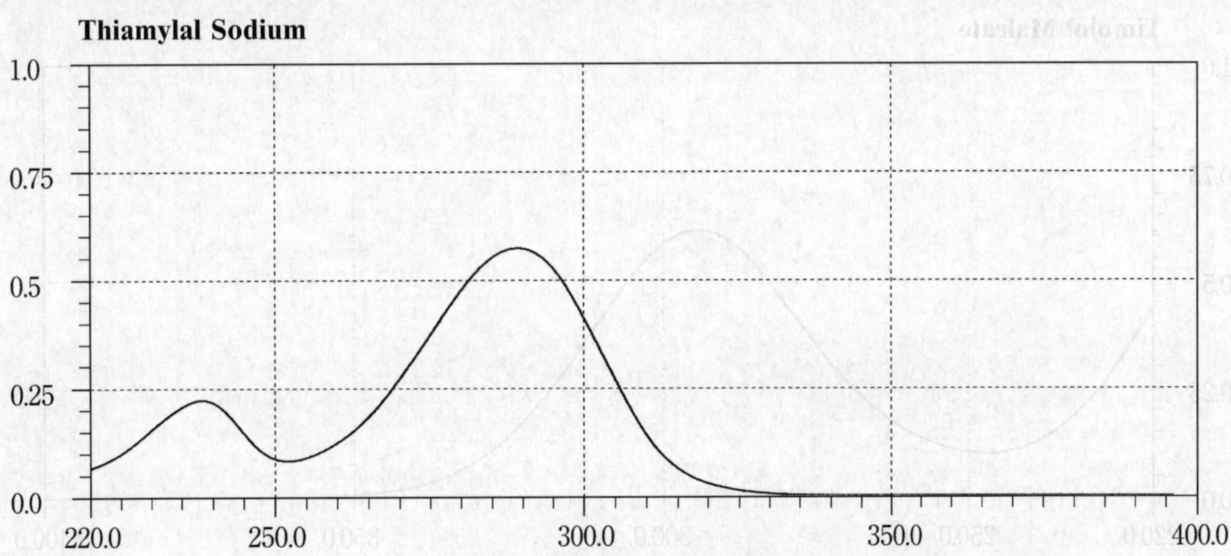

Tiapride Hydrochloride

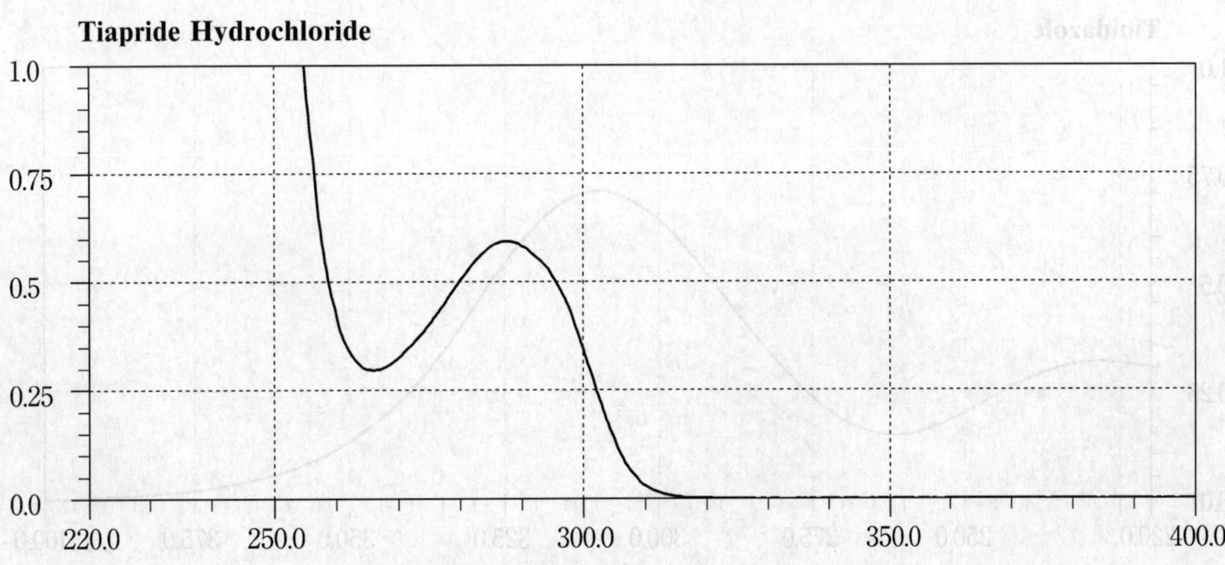

Timepidium Bromide Hydrate

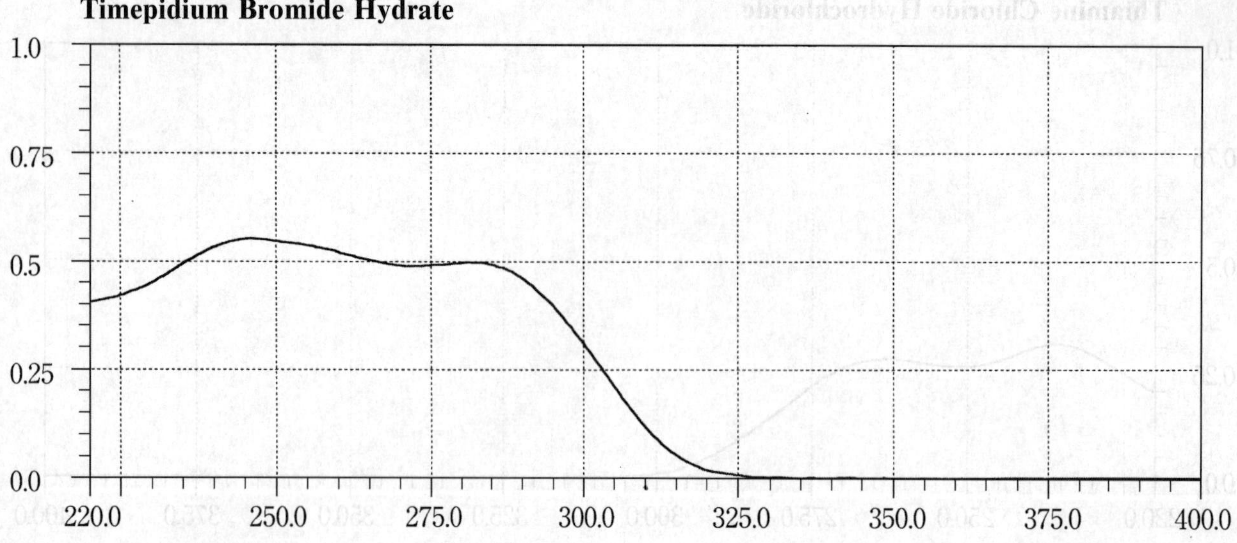

Timolol Maleate

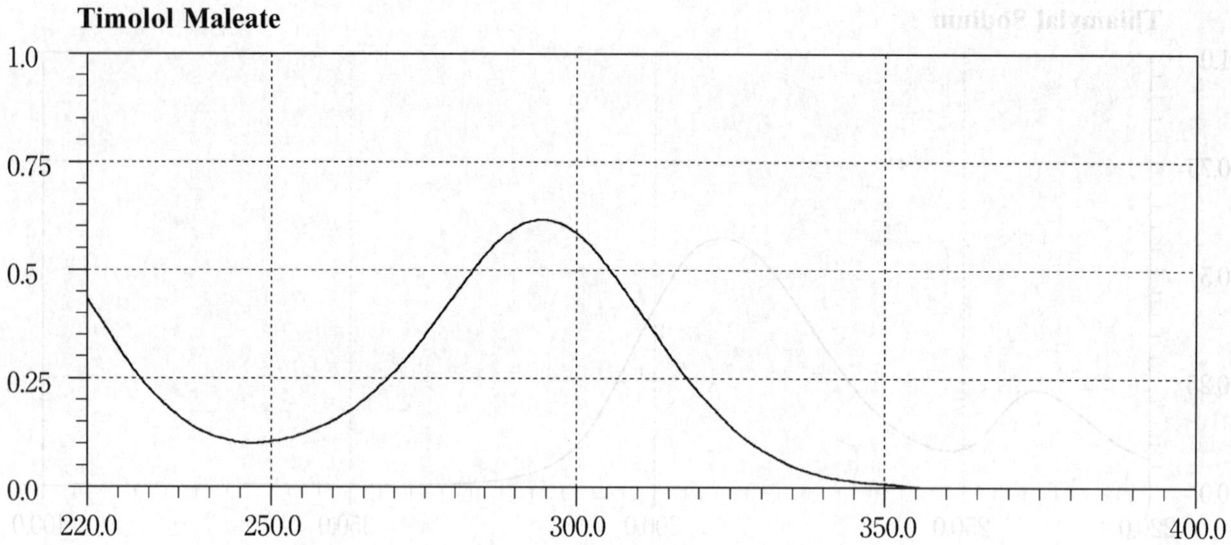

Tinidazole

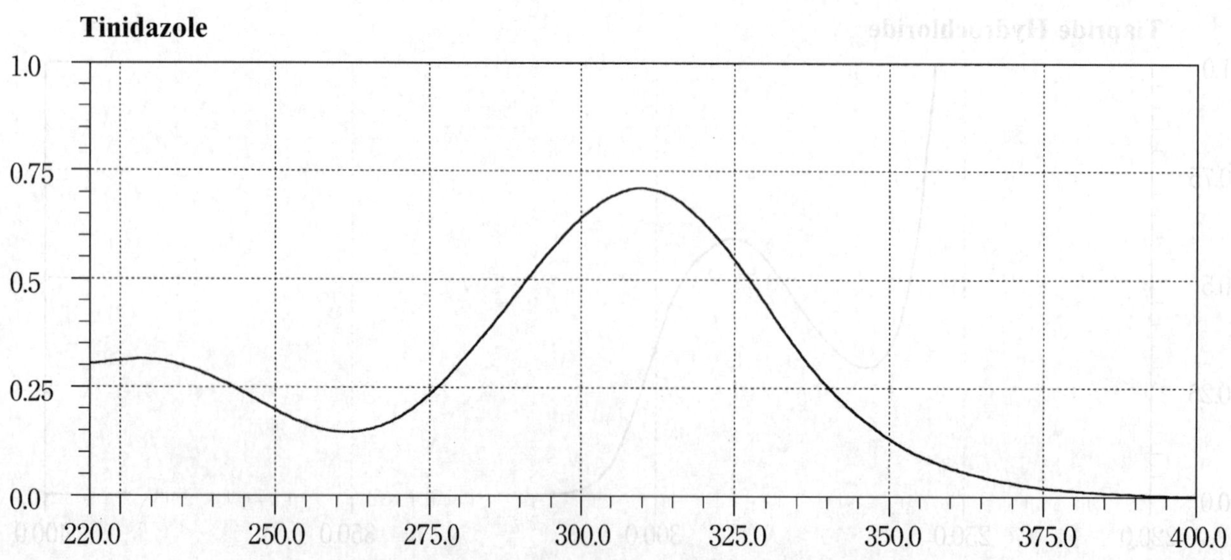

Tipepidine Hibenzate

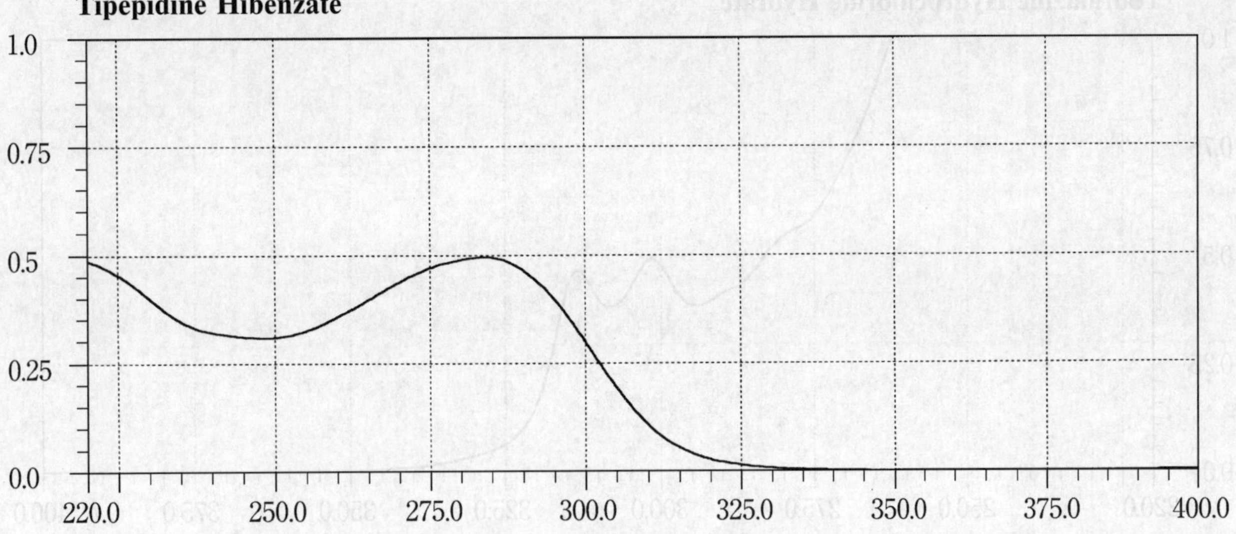

Tizanidine Hydrochloride

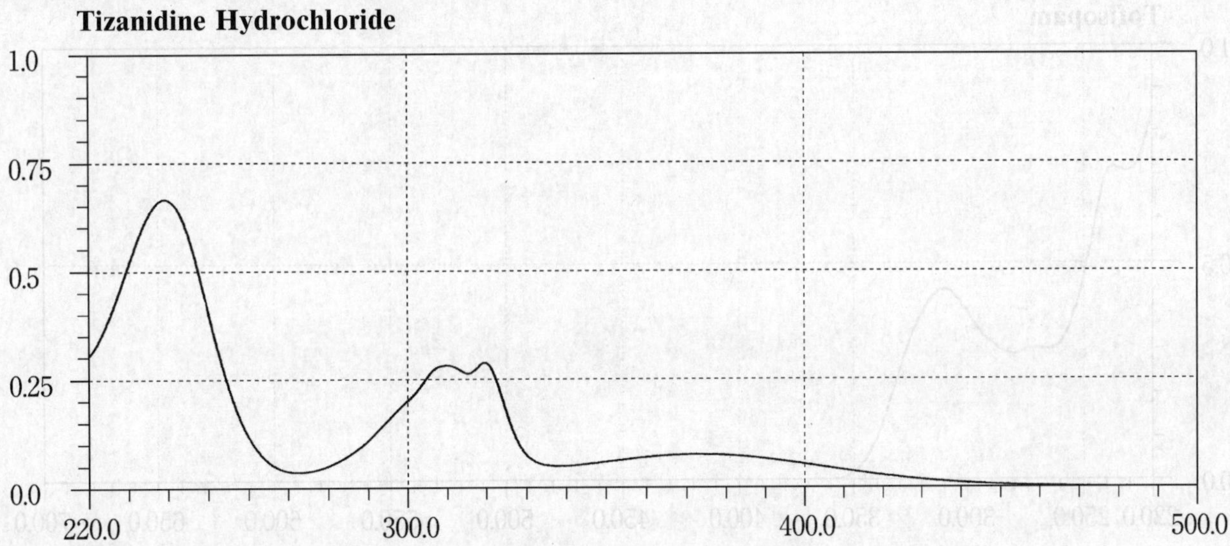

Tocopherol Nicotinate

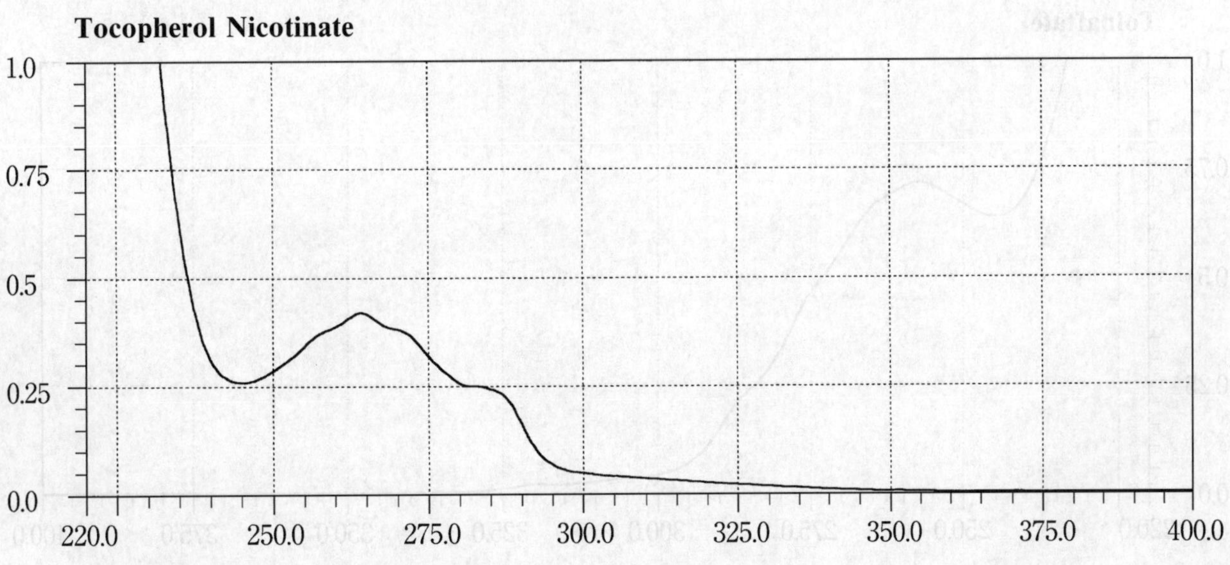

Todralazine Hydrochloride Hydrate

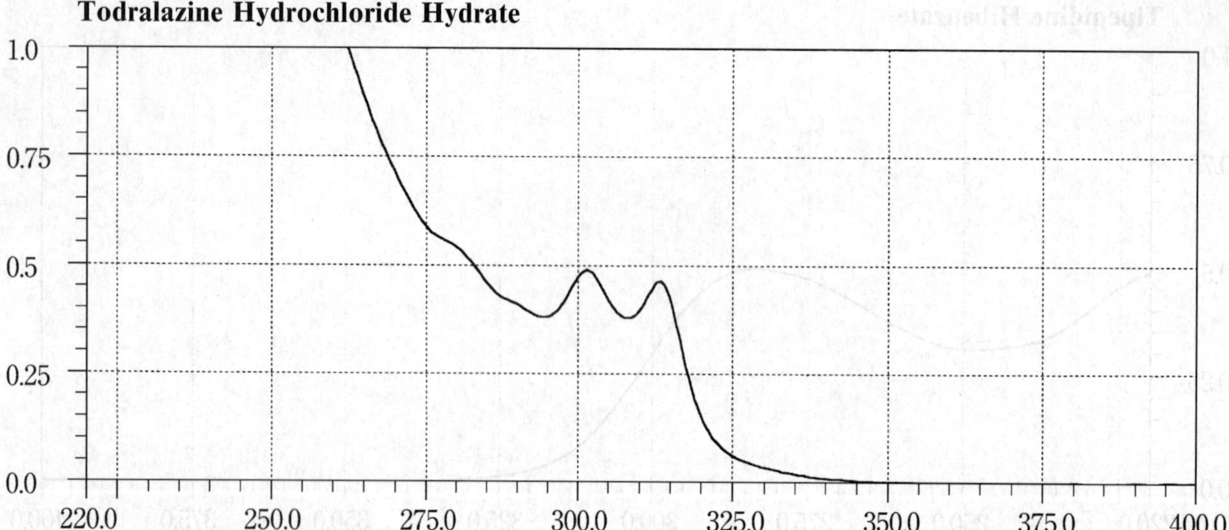

Tofisopam

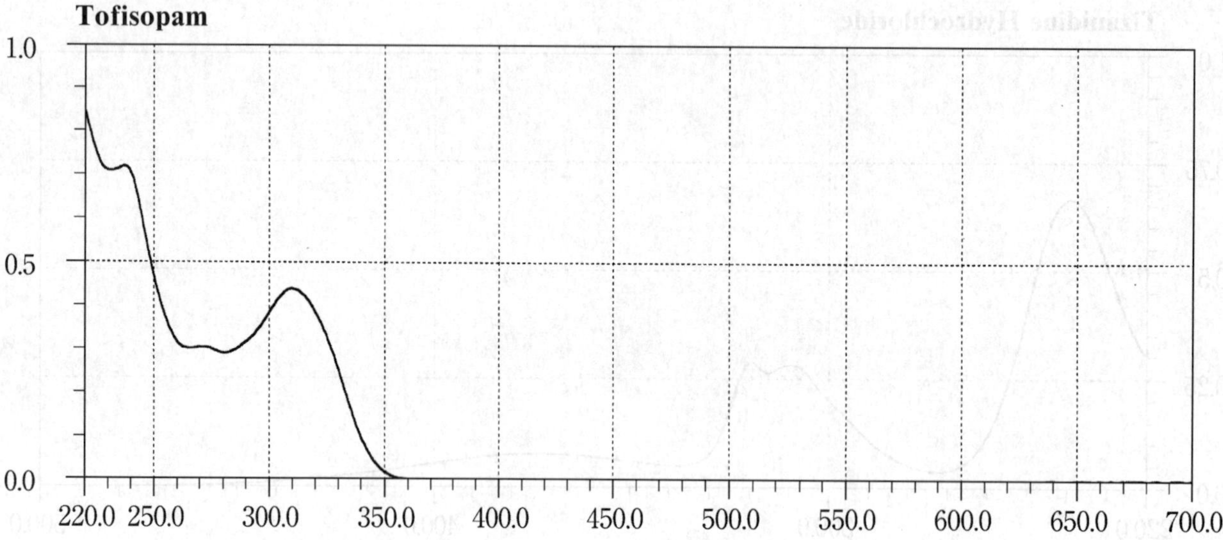

Tolnaftate

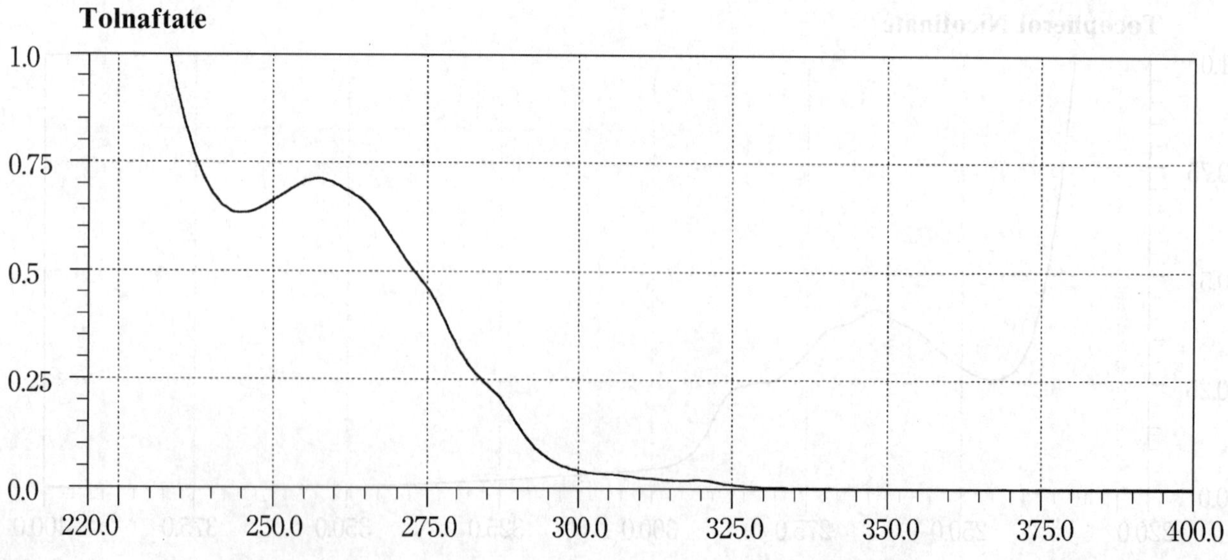

Tosufloxacin Tosilate Hydrate

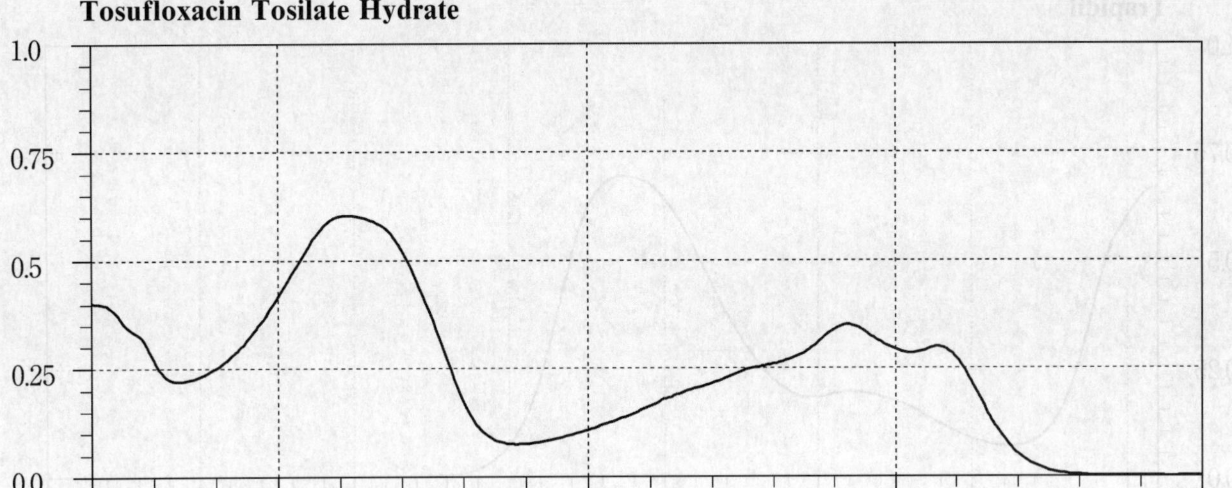

Tramadol Hydrochloride

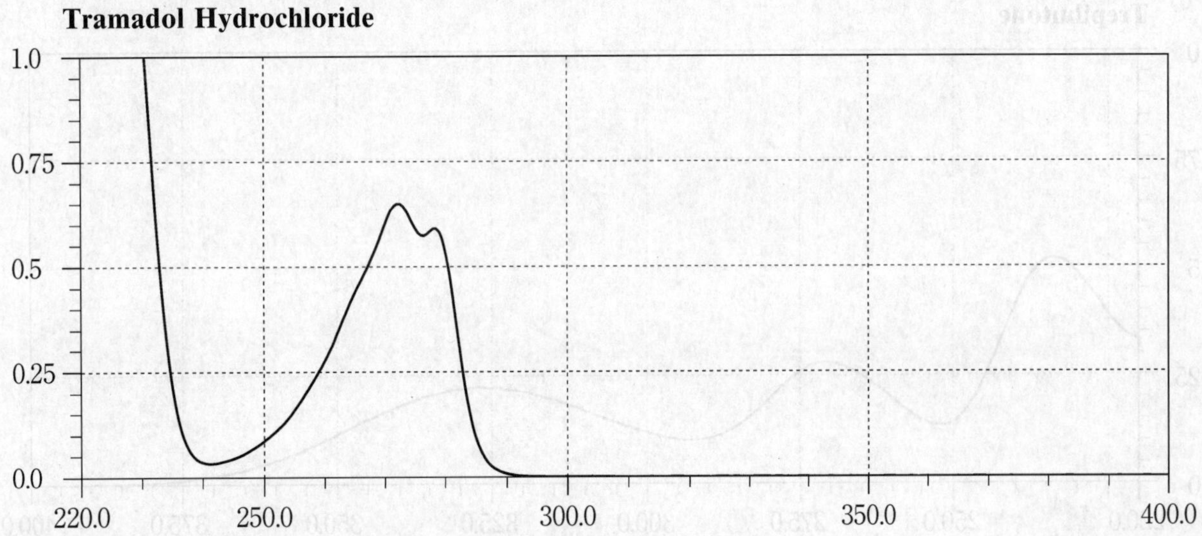

Tranilast

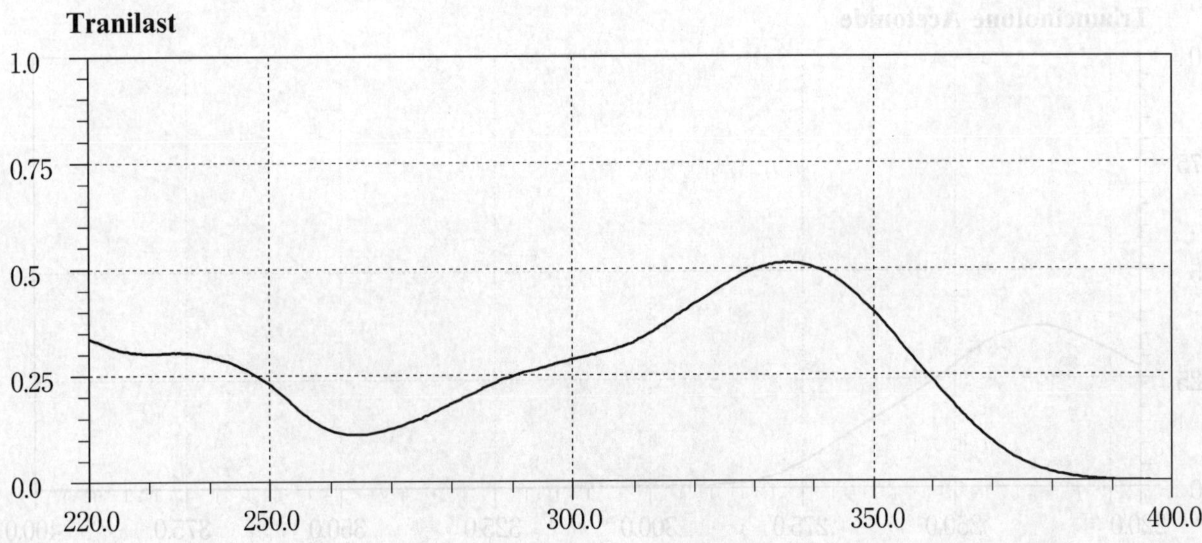

Trapidil

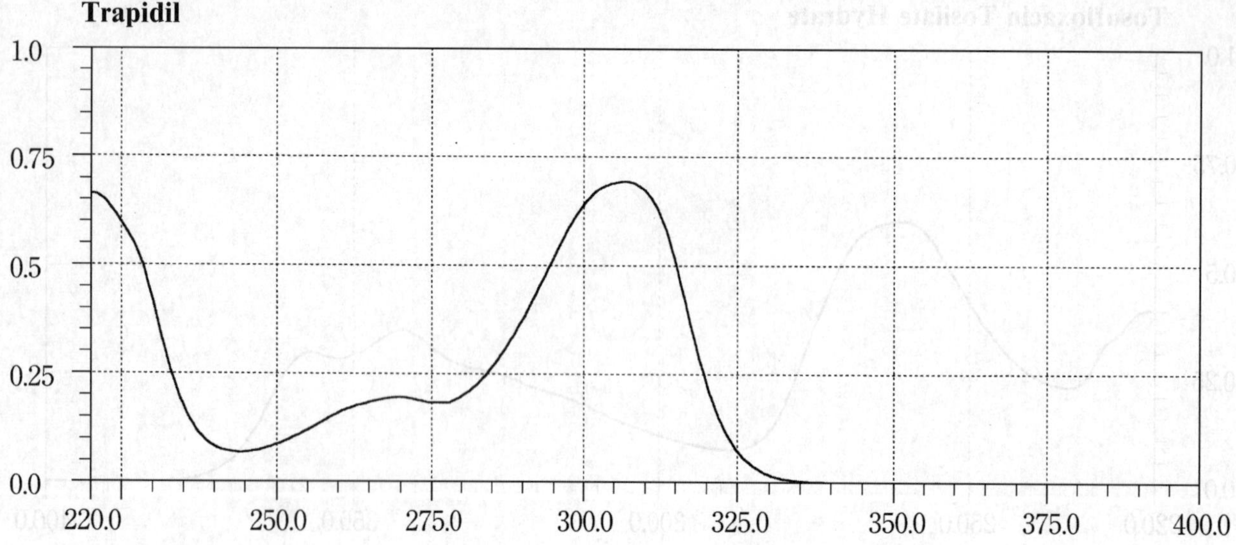

Trepibutone

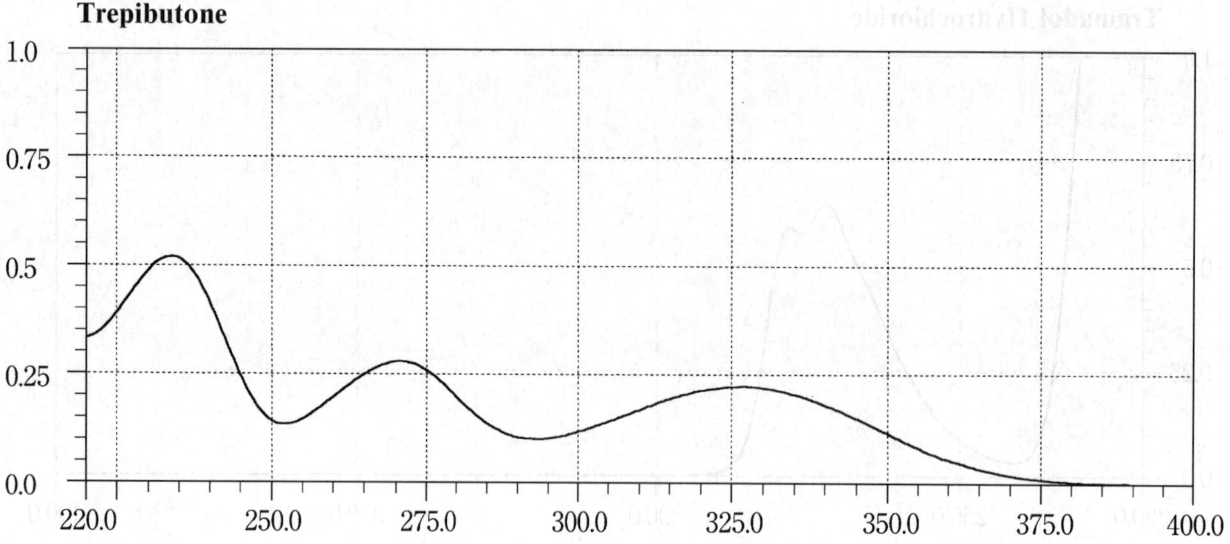

Triamcinolone Acetonide

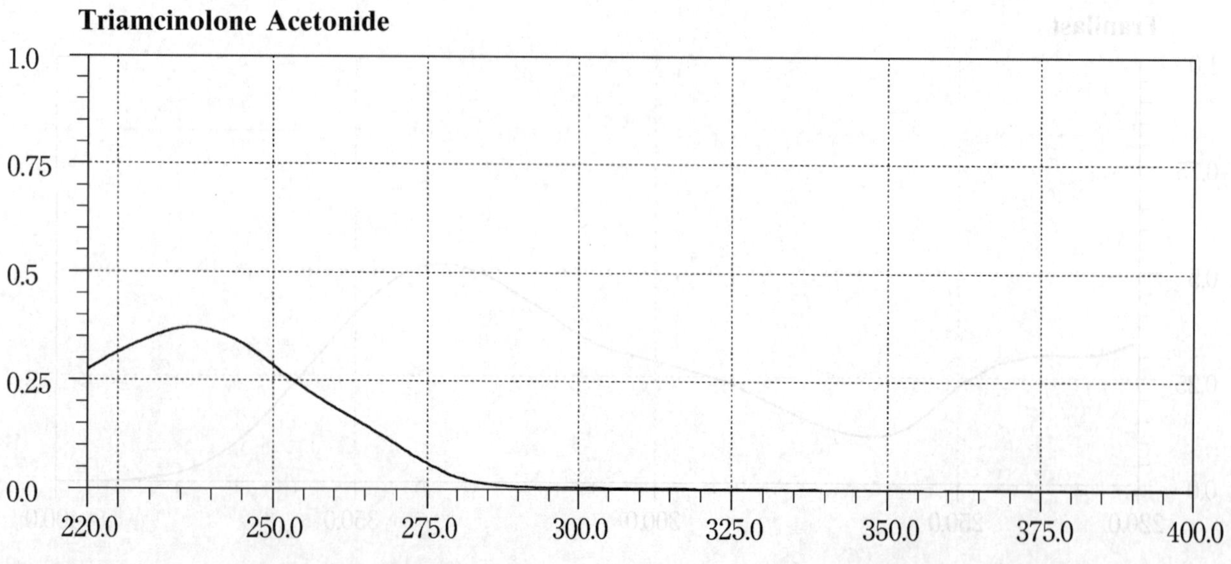

Triamterene

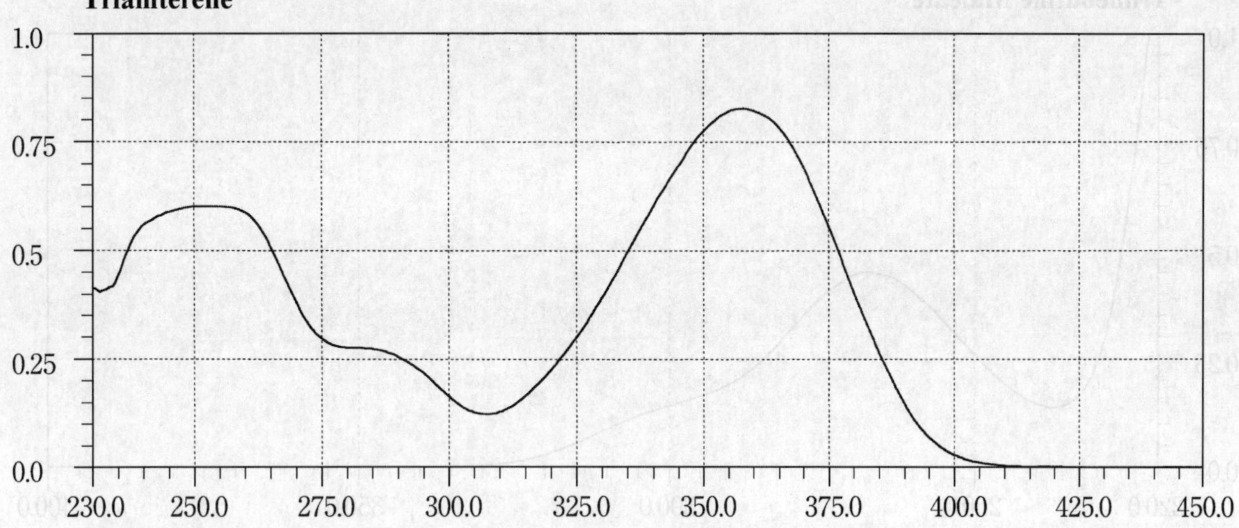

Triazolam

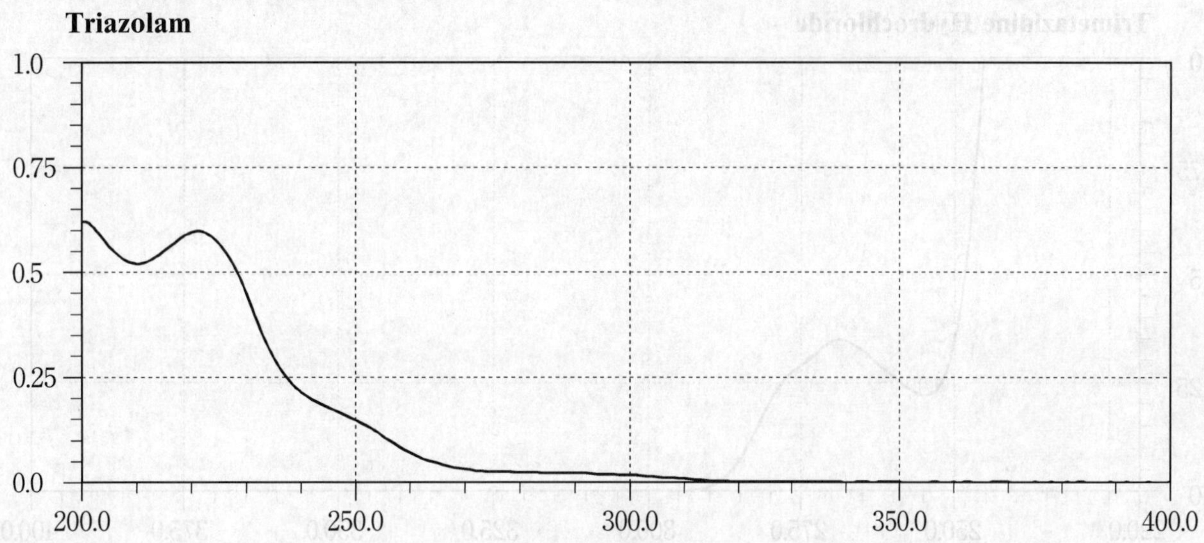

Trichlormethiazide

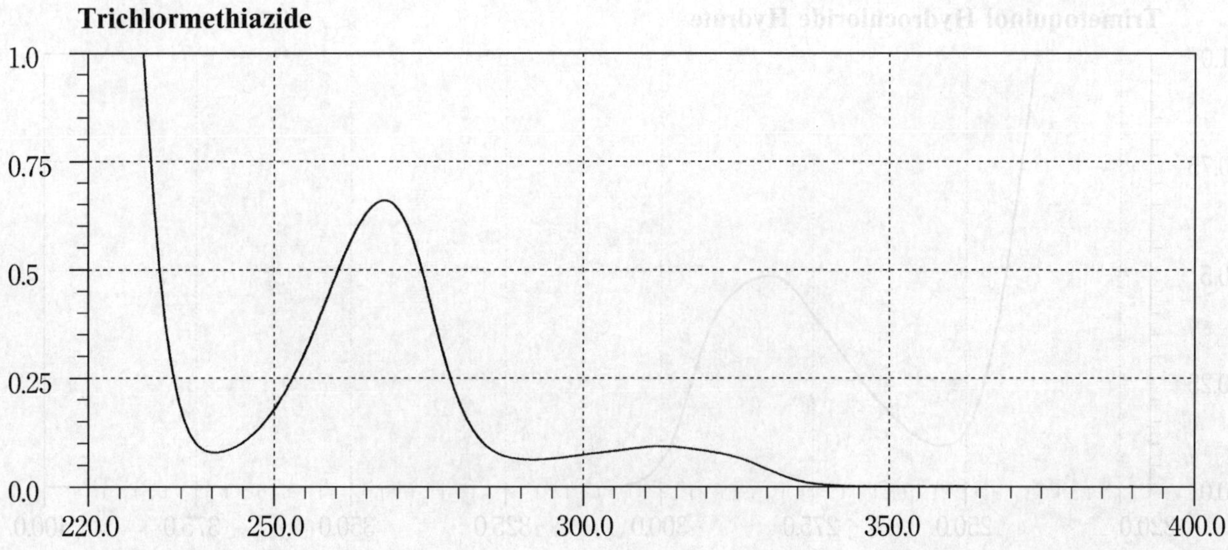

Trimebutine Maleate

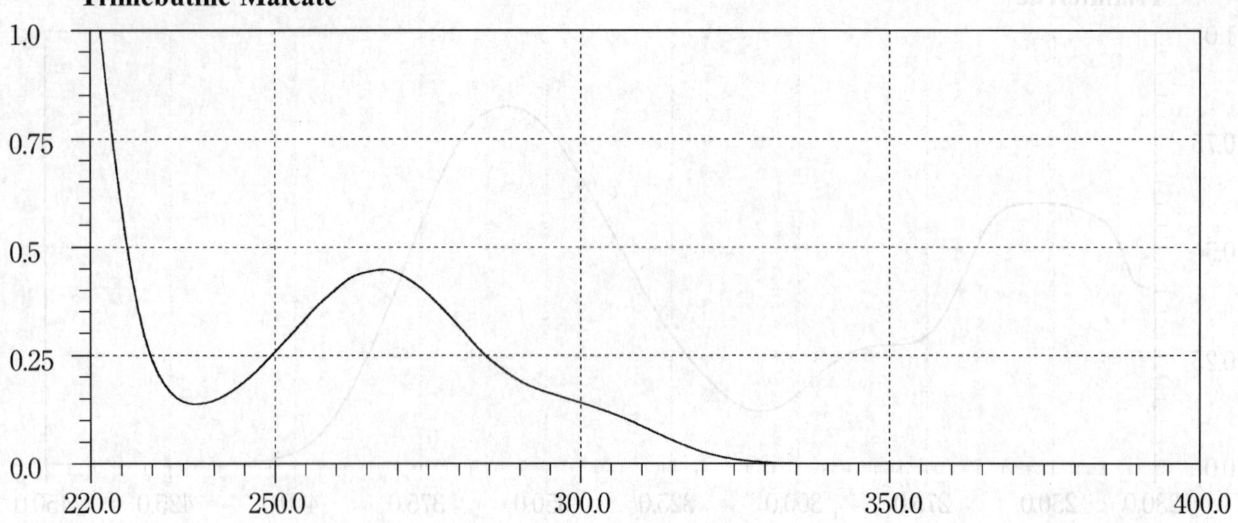

Trimetazidine Hydrochloride

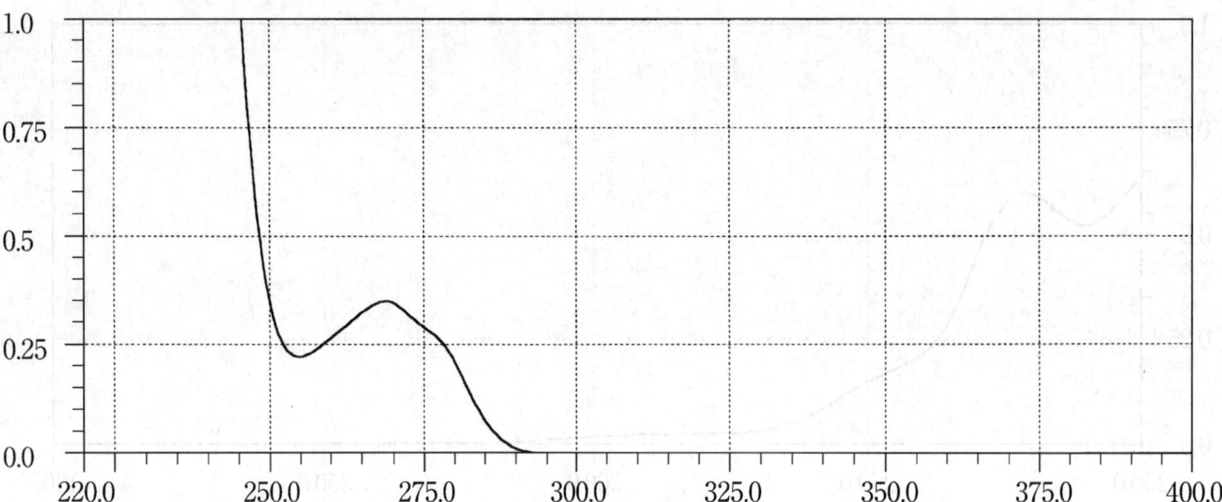

Trimetoquinol Hydrochloride Hydrate

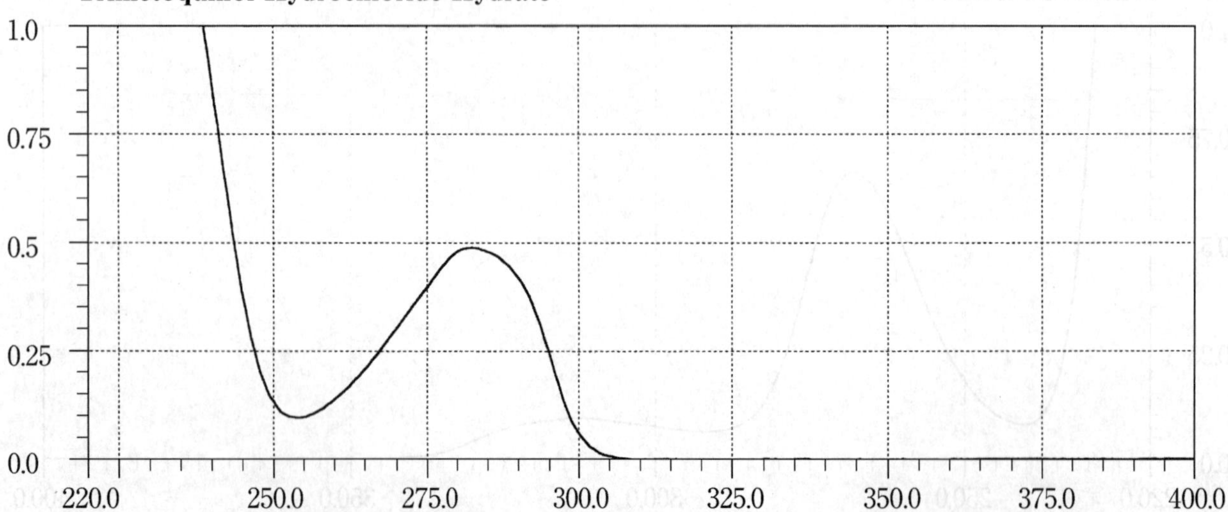

The JP Drugs are to be tested according to the provisions given in the pertinent monographs, General Notices, General Rules for Crude Drugs, General Rules for Preparations, and General Tests for their conformity to the Japanese Pharmacopoeia. (See the General Notices 5.)

Troxipide

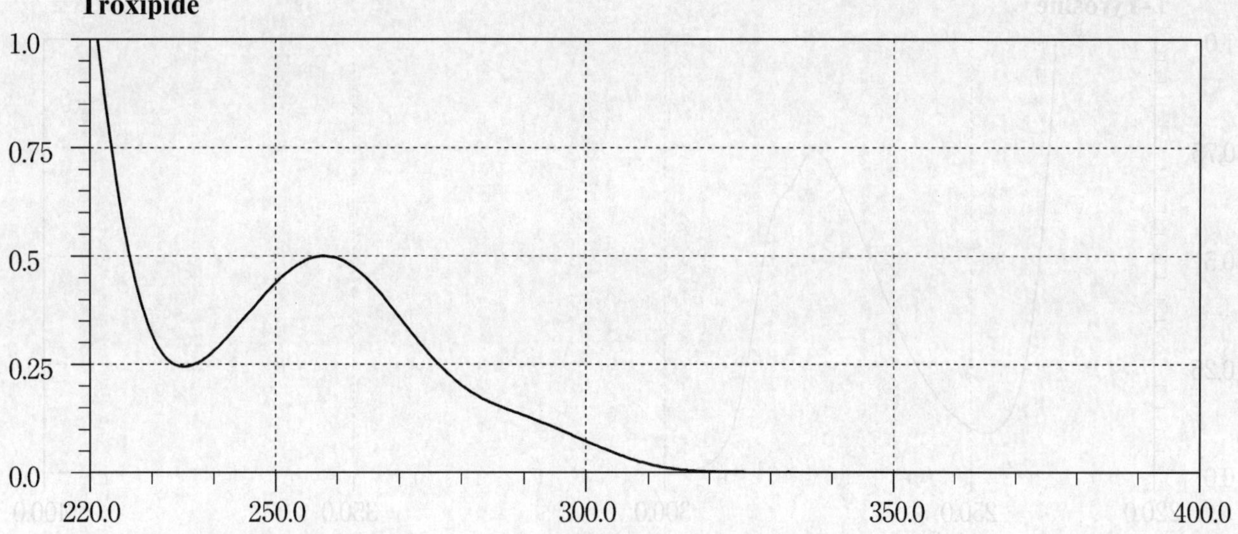

Tulobuterol

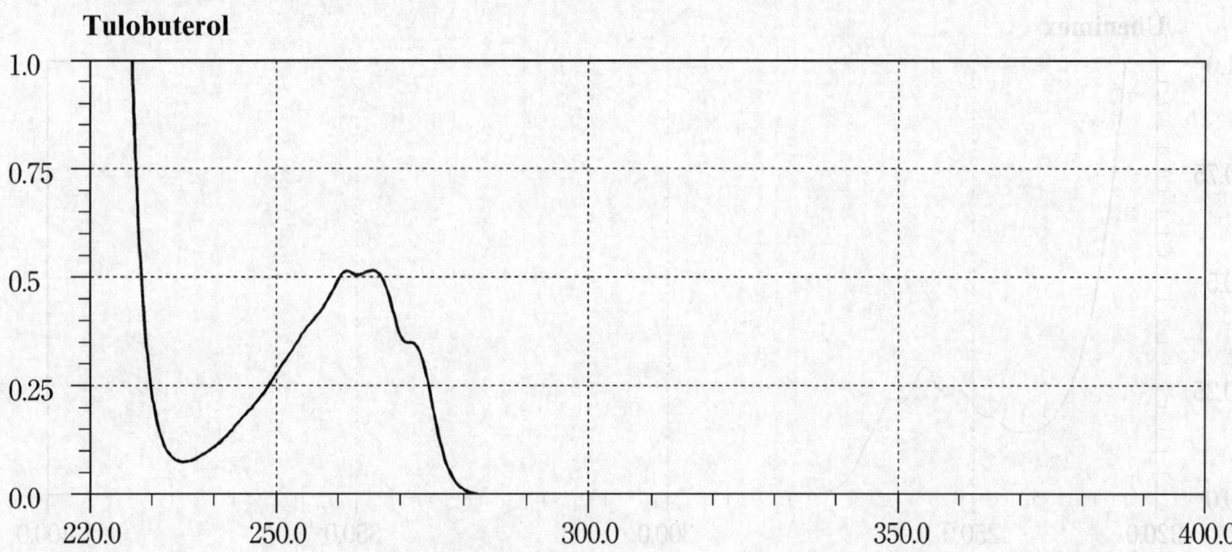

Tulobuterol Hydrochloride

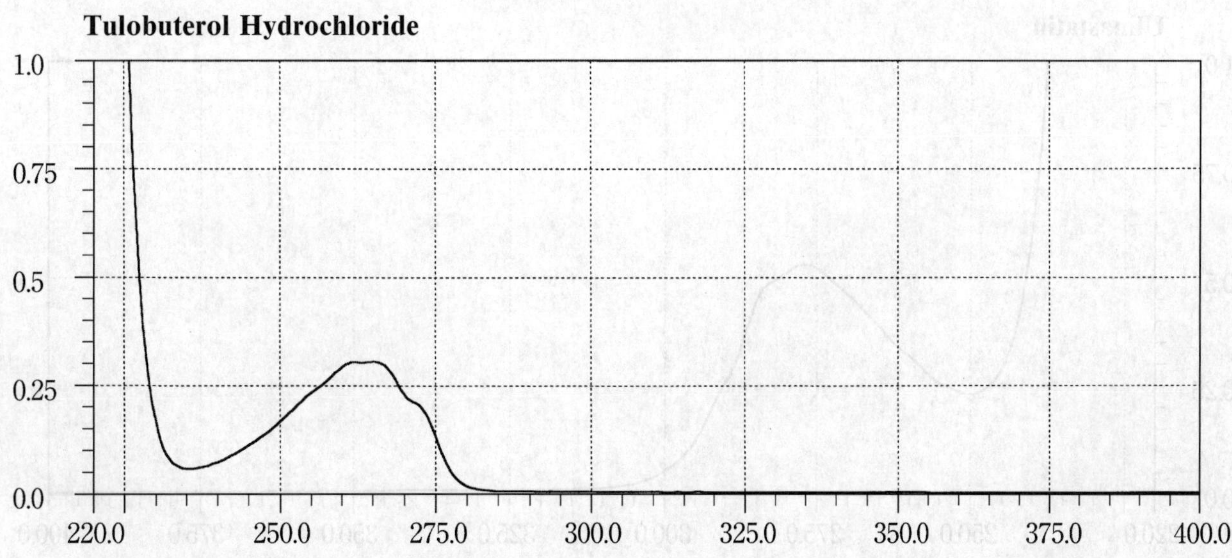

L-Tyrosine

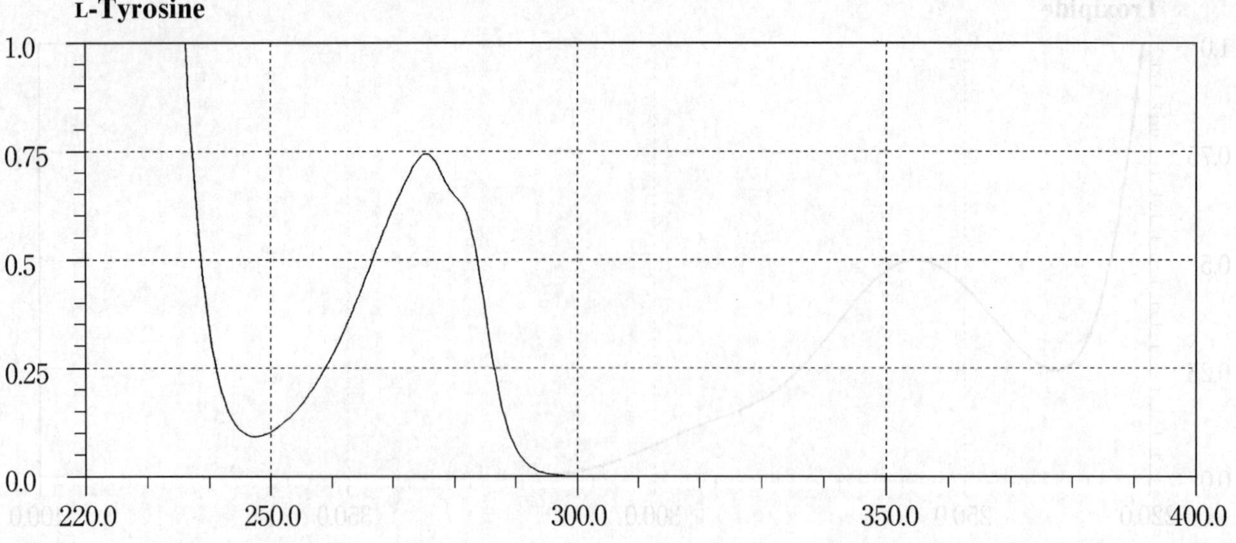

Ubenimex

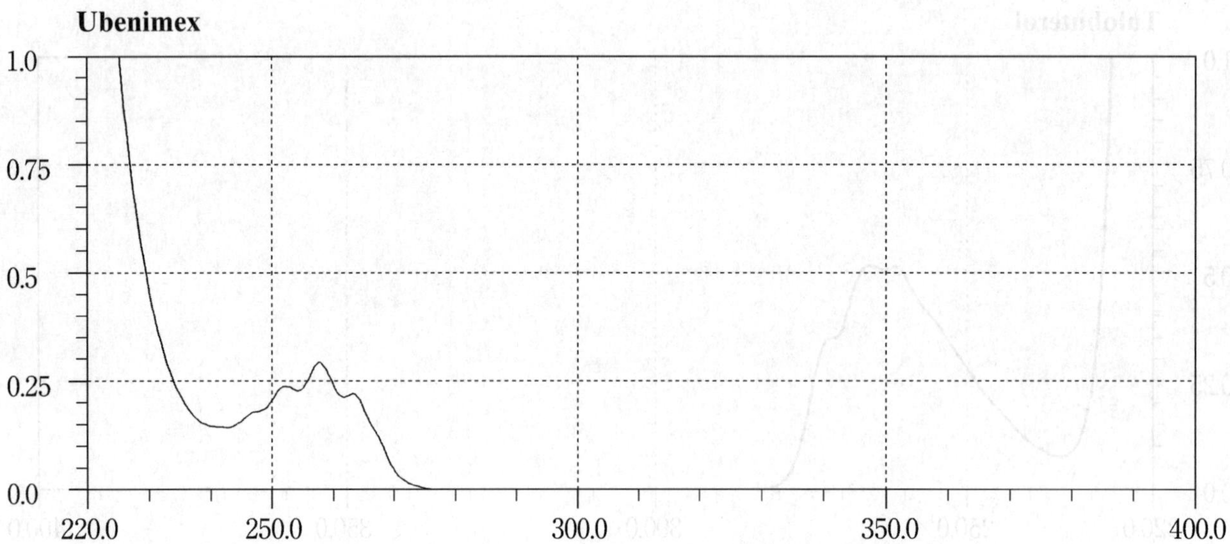

Ulinastatin

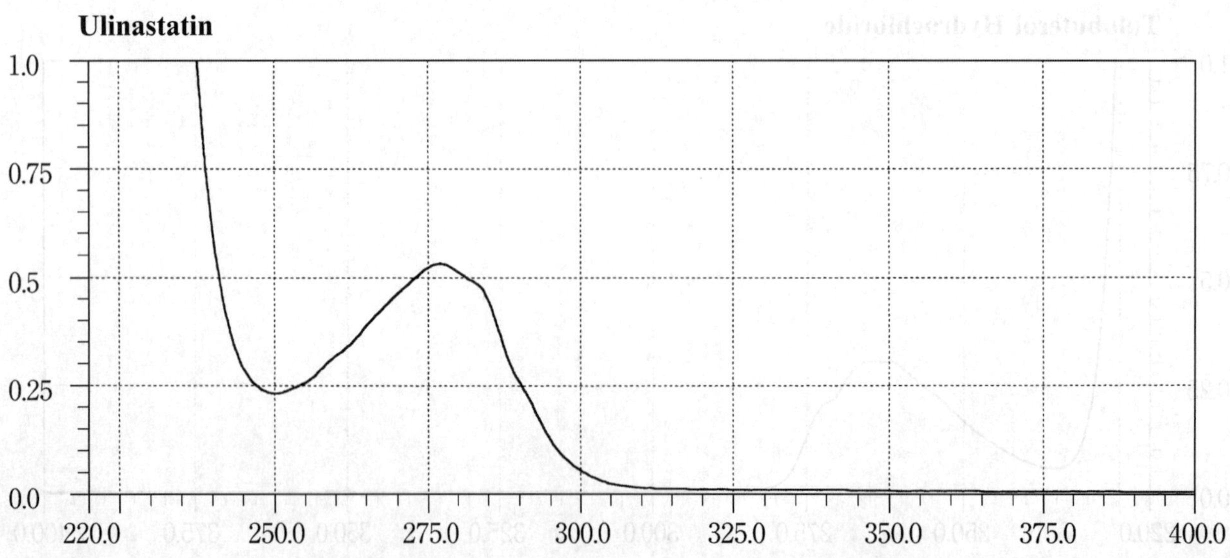

Urapidil

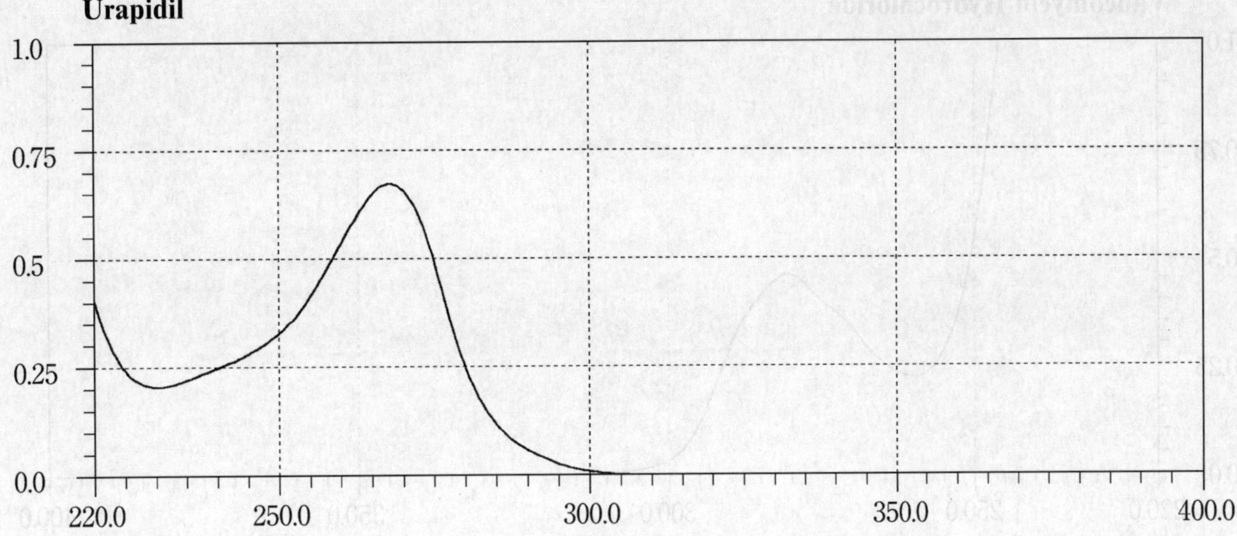

Valaciclovir Hydrochloride

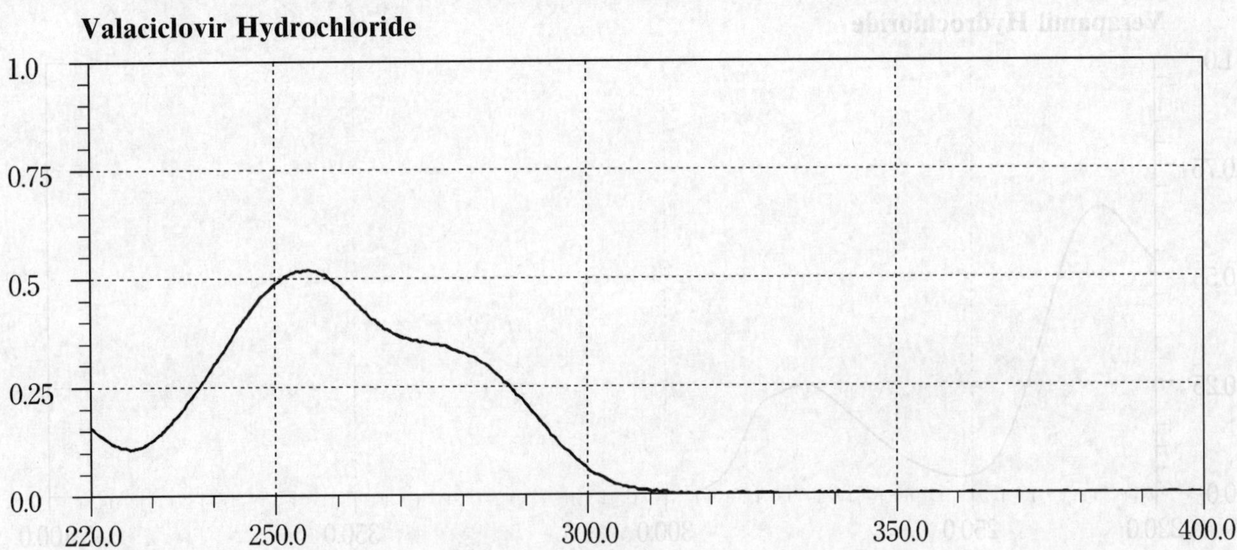

Valsartan

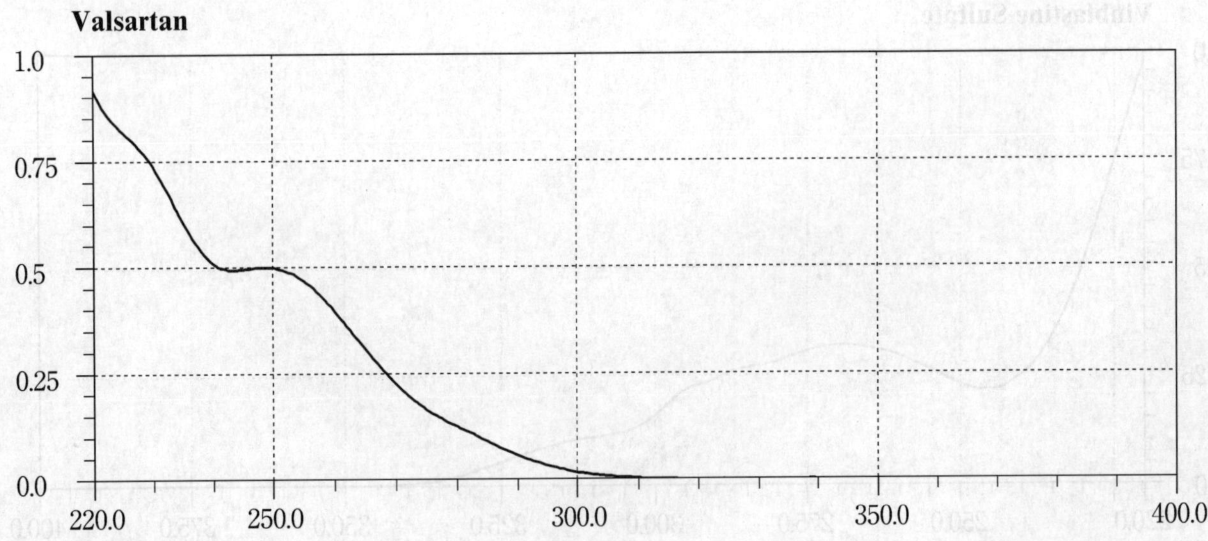

Vancomycin Hydrochloride

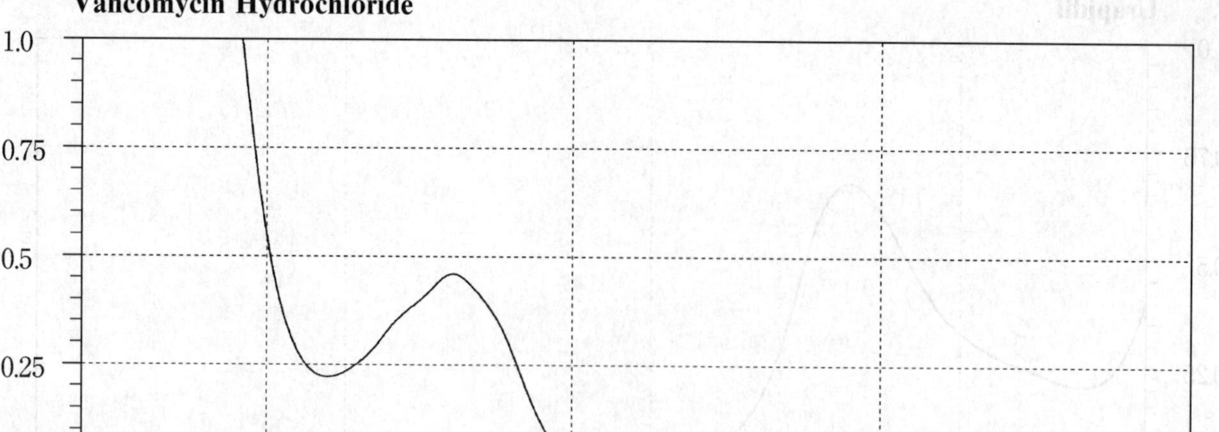

Verapamil Hydrochloride

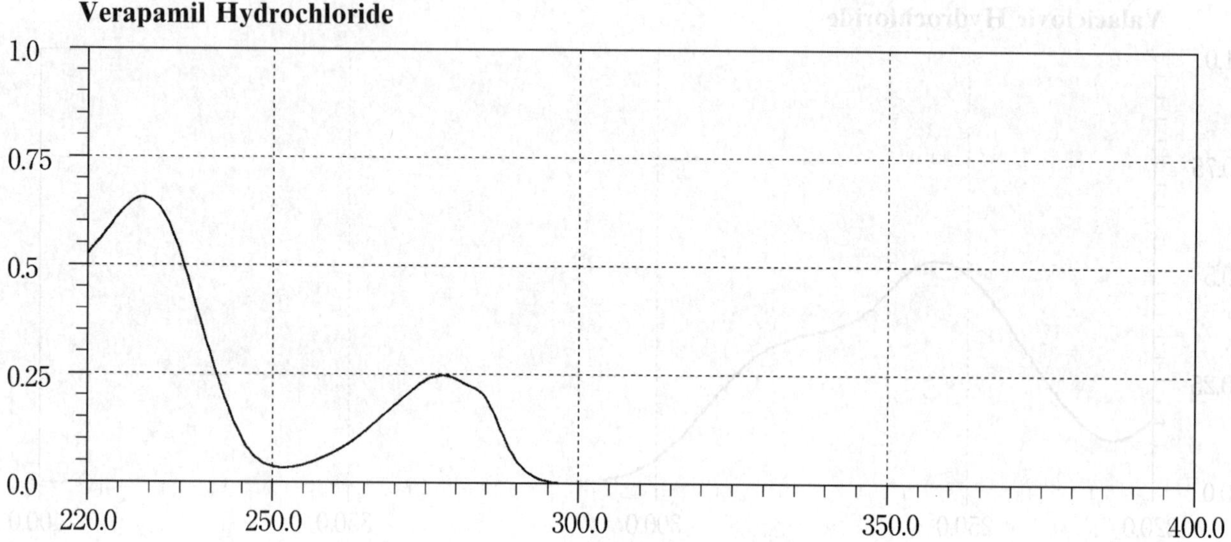

Vinblastine Sulfate

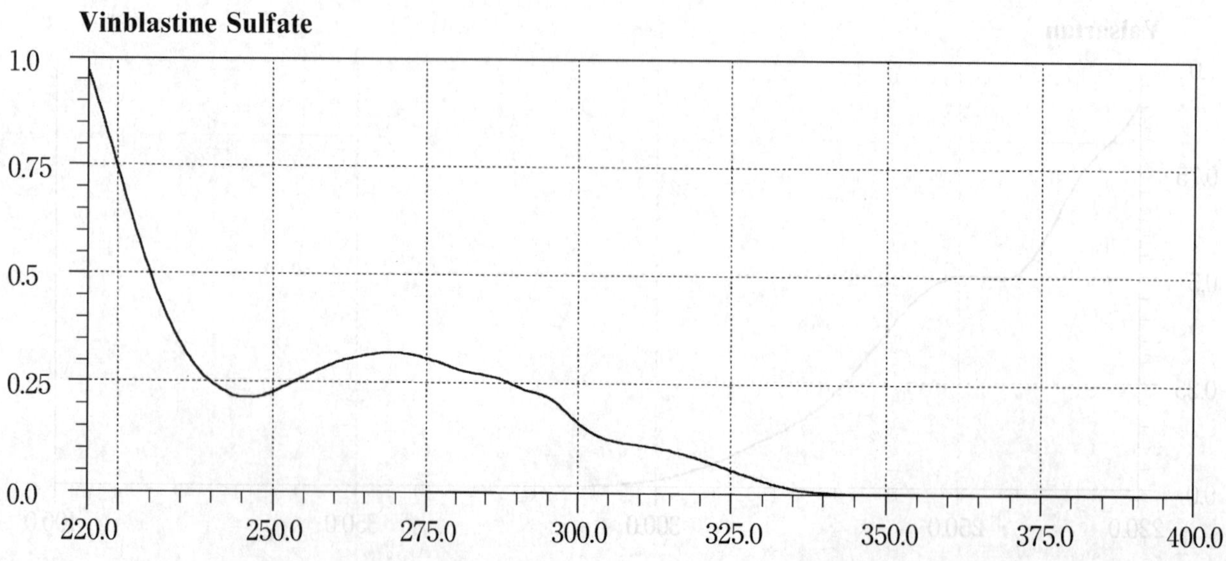

Vincristine Sulfate

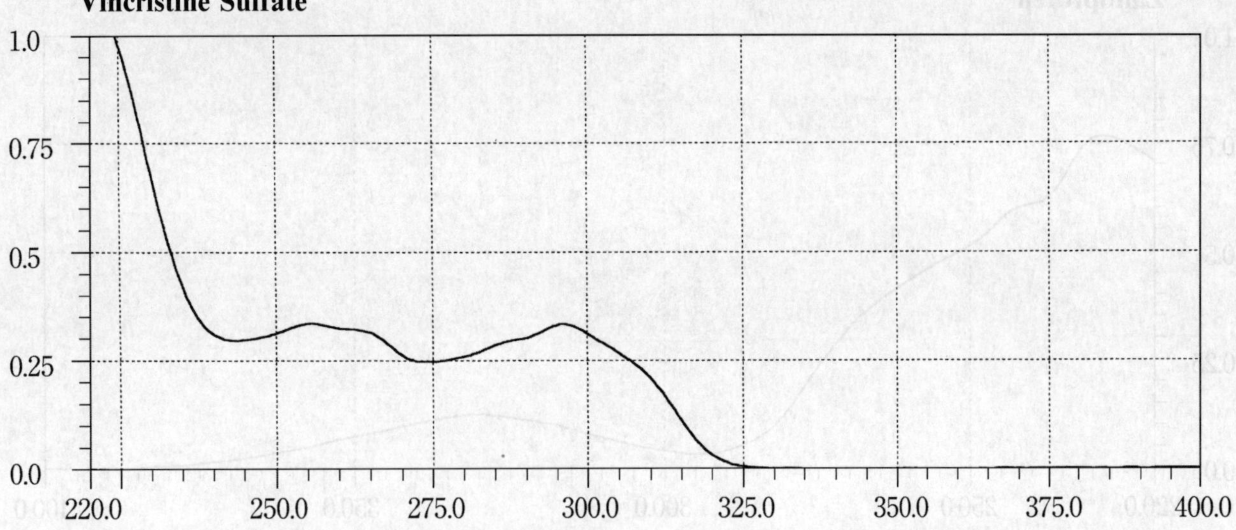

Voriconazole

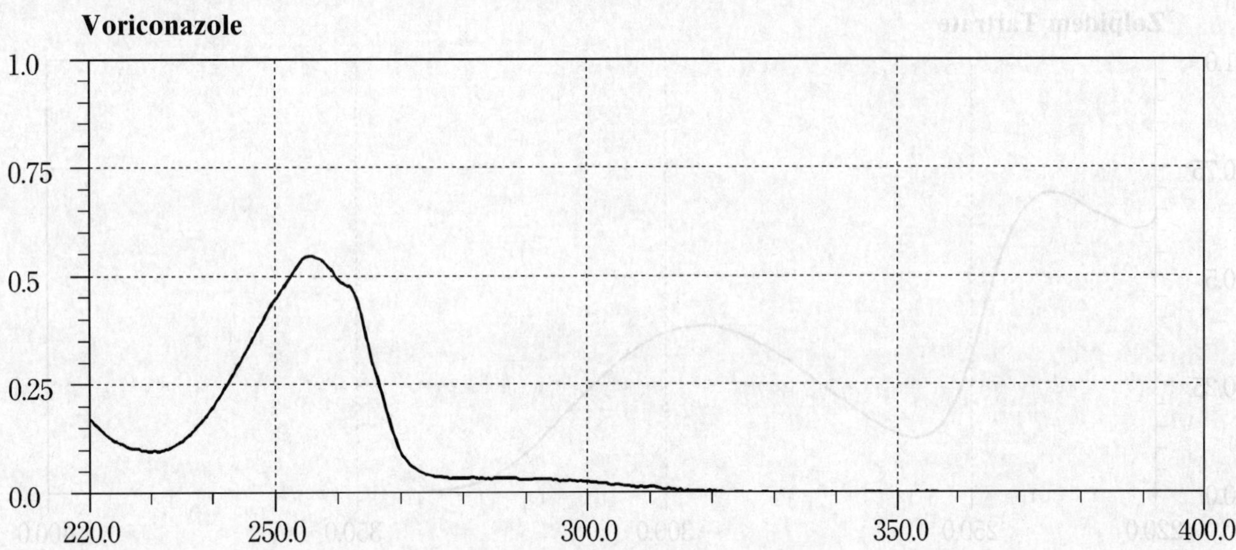

Warfarin Potassium

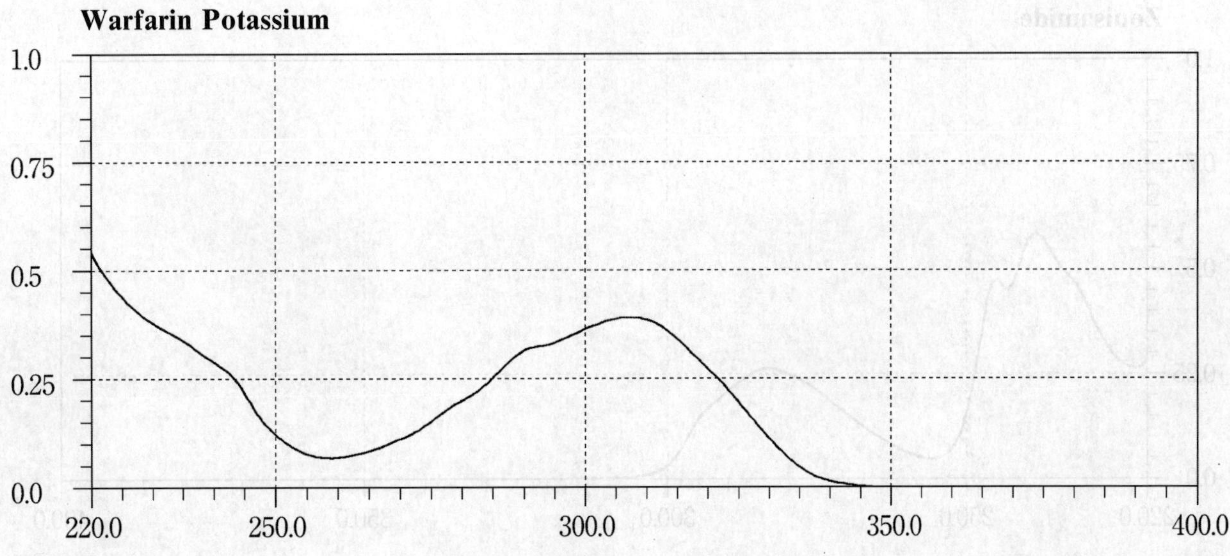

Zaltoprofen

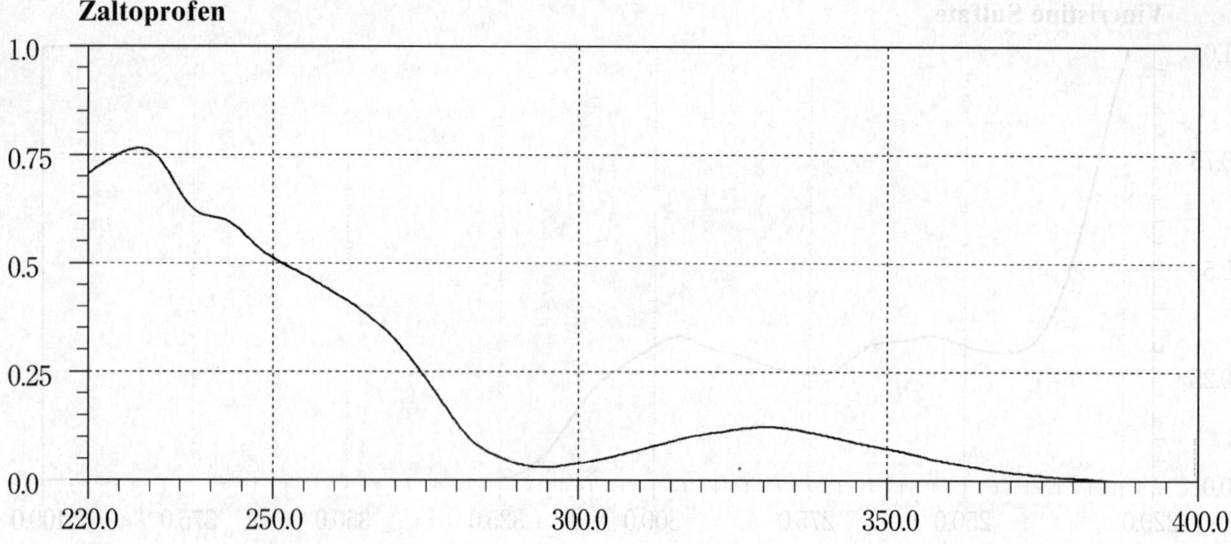

Zolpidem Tartrate

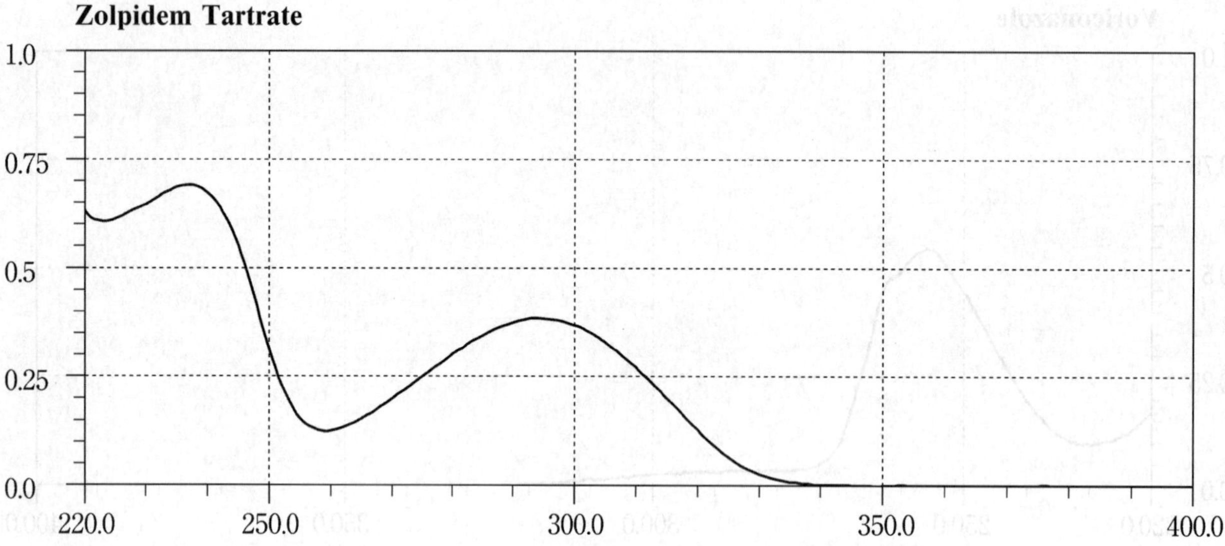

Zonisamide

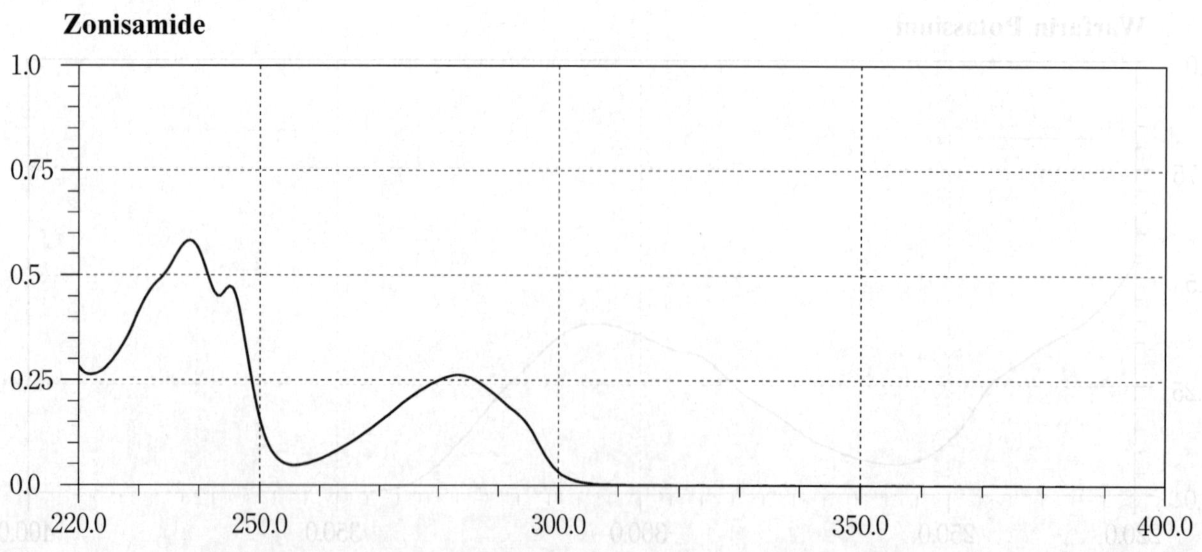

Zopiclone

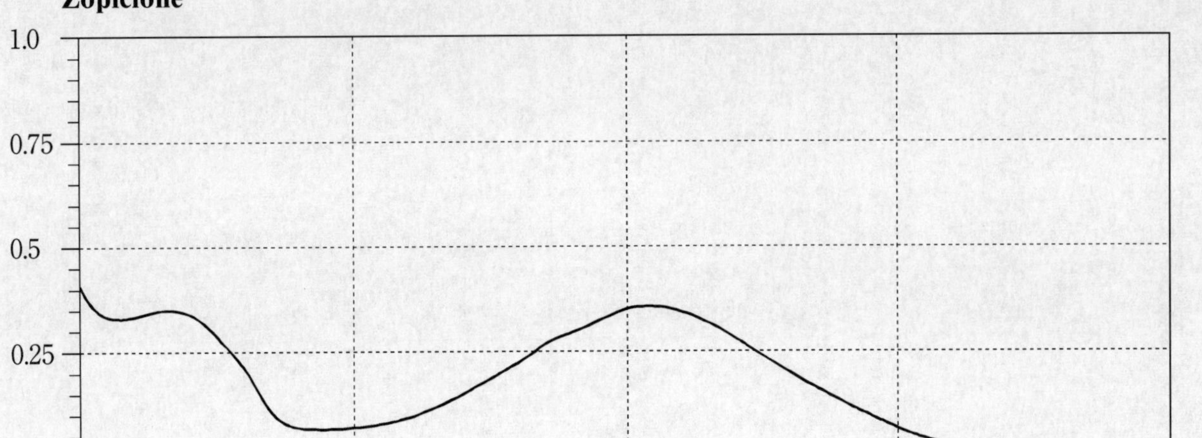

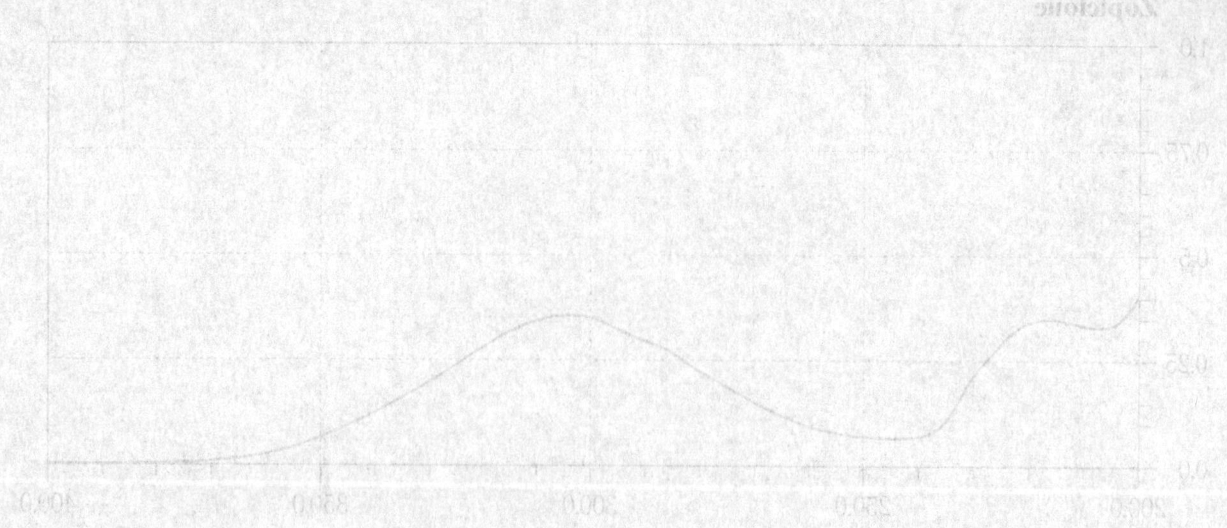

General Information

GENERAL INFORMATION

The General Information describes reference information and reference test methods necessary to assure the quality of medicines, which is attached to the JP. Therefore, the General Information is positioned as important information supplementing the JP although it should not be taken as indicating standards for conformity of drugs, except in the case specified when the drugs are granted approval based on the Law on Securing Quality, Efficacy and Safety of Products Including Pharmaceuticals and Medical Devices. Combination use of the General Information and the JP can contribute to improve quality of the JP and user's convenience.

The general information is classified into the following categories according to their contents, and each general information is individually numbered.

G0. Basic Concepts on Pharmaceutical Quality
G1. Physics and Chemistry
G2. Solid-state Properties
G3. Biotechnological/Biological Products
G4. Microorganisms
G5. Crude Drugs
G6. Drug Formulation
G7. Containers and Package
G8. Reference Standards
GZ. Others

The salient points of the revision in this volume are as follows:

1. Each general information was individually numbered according to the following rule.

An individual number consists of three blocks. The left block indicates the category number and the central block indicates the number in the category. The figures in right block consist of the first two digits from the left indicating the JP at the recent revision (or new preparation, if not revised) and the third digit indicating as follows: 0 for major revision, 1 for supplement I, 2 for supplement II, and 3 for partial revision. For citation between the general information, the number corresponding to the general information is indicated in angle brackets < >.

2. Categories were reviewed.

(1) As basic concepts on pharmaceutical quality, ''G0 Basic Concepts on Pharmaceutical Quality'' was newly added at the opening.

(2) ''Others'' was located at the end as ''GZ'', considering that any new categories would possibly be added after ''G9''.

(3) Water-related categories were abolished and included in ''GZ Others''.

3. The following were newly prepared.

(1) Basic Concept of the Quality Assurance on Biotechnological Products (Biopharmaceuticals) *<G3-1-180>*

(2) Control of Culture Media and Strains of Microorganisms Used for Microbial Tests *<G4-2-180>*

(3) Bacterial Endotoxins Test and Alternative Methods using Recombinant Protein-reagents for Endotoxin Assay *<G4-4-180>*

(4) Radioactivity Measurements Method for Crude Drugs *<G5-8-180>*

(5) Tablet Hardness Determinations *<G6-4-180>*

(6) Packaging Integrity Evaluation of Sterile Products *<G7-4-180>*

(7) Leak Tests for Packaging of Sterile Products *<G7-5-180>*

4. The following were revised.

(1) Capillary Electrophoresis *<G3-7-180>*

(2) On the Scientific Names of Crude Drugs listed in the JP *<G5-1-180>*

(3) International Harmonization Implemented in the Japanese Pharmacopoeia Eighteenth Edition *<GZ-3-180>*

5. The following was deleted.

(1) Control of Elemental Impurities in Drug Products

G0 Basic Concepts on Pharmaceutical Quality

Basic Concepts for Quality Assurance of Drug Substances and Drug Products *<G0-1-172>*

Introduction

Quality of drug substances and products are generally assured through manufacturing and testing under appropriate Good Manufacturing Practice (GMP) conditions reflecting knowledge obtained from designing and developmental stages and manufacturing stage on management of raw materials and other materials, control of manufacturing process, specifications, etc. As shown in the General Notice 5, JP listed drugs are to be tested according to the provisions given in the pertinent monographs, General Notices, General Rules for Crude Drugs, General Rules for Preparations, and General Tests for their conformity to the *Japanese Pharmacopoeia*. In addition to these, compliance with GMP, management of raw materials and other materials, and management of manufacturing process are fundamental factors required to assure the quality of JP listed products in actual production.

The present chapter summarizes general concepts concerning measures for quality assurance of drug substances and products mainly aimed at chemicals, including chemically synthesized antibiotics and semisynthetic antibiotics, synthetic peptides, oligonucleotides, and biotechnological/biological products, and shows the principle idea of quality assurance in the process listing a drug as an individual monograph in the JP. Although radiopharmaceuticals, crude drugs, herbal products, and crude products of animal or plant origin are excluded from the subjects of the concepts, these concepts are useful for the management of any type of drugs.

Basic Concept

In recent years, the mainstream concept for quality control of drugs has been implemented according to a control strategy that their quality is assured by control of manufacturing process, including management of raw material and other materials, and quality testing of final products (drug substances or drug products) that are conducted mutually complementary. The control strategy is implemented based on Quality Risk Management (QRM). The first and most important step is identifying Critical Quality Attributes (CQAs) which are the attributes or properties required to ensure the desired product quality, and it is necessary to specify physical, chemical, biological, microbiological characteristics or properties of the product which should be within the appropriate limits, ranges and distributions. The next step is to guarantee that the CQA falls within the defined range, limit, and distribution by using specification tests, in-process tests and various measures, for that the quality of the drug will eventually be realized.

The specification is one of the elements of control strategy and not all the CQA need to be included in the specifications. CQA is (1) included in specifications and confirmed by testing final products (including periodical or skip testing, described later), (2) included in specifications and confirmed by process controls (e.g., real time release testing, described later), or (3) not included in specifications but can be ensured by controlling starting materials, raw materials and manufacturing process. As an example of (3), effective control over robust manufacturing processes can assure that certain impurities are controlled at an acceptable risk level or are efficiently removed below an acceptable level, and sometimes the purity testing for the final product may not be required and omitted from specifications. However, in the case of a drug listed in the JP monograph, regarding the manufacturing process control related to CQA, if necessary, the control method and control value are indicated in the Manufacture in individual monograph.

What kind of control strategy should be applied to a certain CQA is individually determined by QRM according to the understanding and risk of the manufacturing process.

1. Management of manufacturing process

1.1. Considerations of manufacturing process

Adequate design of manufacturing processes and knowledge of their capacity are important to establish manufacturing processes yielding drug substances or drug products that meet specifications and fulfill CQA, and to perform consistent manufacturing control, quality control, etc. appropriately.

From this standpoint, the limits for control of manufacturing processes should be based on information obtained from the entire process spanning the period from the early development through commercial scale production. The appropriateness of the limits also needs to be confirmed by evaluation, verification, review, and other examinations of manufacturing processes based on QRM.

In-process tests are tests that may be performed during the manufacture of either the drug substance or drug product, rather than specification tests for the final product. In-process tests are performed for quality verification during manufacturing processes that are likely to influence drug substance or drug product quality, or for confirmation of proper functioning of the manufacturing process. In-process tests may also be used for the evaluation of CQA.

Usually an in-process test is properly designed according to the risk on quality, however, the use of internal action limits by the manufacturer to assess the consistency of the process at less critical steps is also important. Provisional action limits should be set for the manufacturing process based on data obtained during development of the drug and during evaluation and verification of the manufacturing process, and should be further refined based on additional manufacturing experience and data accumulated after product approval for marketing.

1.2. Considerations of raw materials and other materials (starting materials, excipients, packaging materials, etc.)

The raw materials and other materials used in the production of drug substances (or drug products) should meet quality standards, appropriate for their intended use, and appropriate setting of specifications and test methods assuring CQA are required. Especially, biological raw/source materials may require careful evaluation to establish the presence or the absence of deleterious endogenous or adventitious agents. Procedures that make use of affinity chromatography (for example, employing monoclonal antibodies), should be accompanied by appropriate risk management to ensure that such process-related impurities or potential contaminants arising from their production and use do not compromise the quality and safety of the drug substance or drug product.

The quality of the excipients used in the drug product formulation (and in some cases, in the production of drug substance), as well as the primary packaging materials, should be controlled with specifications established based on the characteristics of the drug. If specifications and test procedures for a material are described by the JP, as a rule, at least the JP criteria should be satisfied. Concerning excipients and other materials not listed in the JP, appropriate specifications and test procedures should be established individually.

2. Quality tests of products (specifications)

A specification is defined as a list of tests, references to analytical procedures, and appropriate acceptance criteria which are numerical limits, ranges, or other criteria for the tests described. Specifications and test methods of the JP monograph are defined sets of quality characteristics needed for determination of whether the use of a drug substance or a drug product is appropriate for the intended purpose. ''Conformance to the specifications of the JP monograph'' means that the JP-listed drug substances and drug products, when tested according to the procedures described in general tests and drug monographs, will meet the all acceptance criteria except criteria of ''Description'', ''Containers and storage (for drug products)'' and ''Shelf life'' in the JP monographs.

However, as described in ''Basic Concept'' specifications of monographs and test procedures for drug substance and drug product are one part of a total control strategy for assurance of the quality and consistency of the substances/products. Other parts of control strategies include thorough characterization of the drug in developmental stage (specifications and test procedures are established based on the characterization), and management of manufacturing process and products' quality, such as evaluation, verification and review of manufacturing process, and management of raw materials, other materials and manufacturing process, that is to say, compliance with the GMP.

3. Periodic or Skip Testing

Periodic or skip testing is the performance of specified tests at release on preselected batches and/or at predetermined intervals, rather than on a batch-to-batch basis with the understanding that those batches not being tested still must meet all acceptance criteria established for that product. When this concept is applied, it is necessary to show its appropriateness and be approved previously by regulatory authority. This concept may be applicable to, for example, residual solvents and microbiological testing for solid oral dosage forms. It is recognized that only limited data may be available at the time of submission of an application for marketing approval. Implementation of this concept should therefore generally be considered post-approval. When tested, any failure to meet acceptance criteria established for the periodic test should be handled by proper notification of the appropriate regulatory authorities. If these data demonstrate a need of testing for all lots, then batch-by-batch release testing should be reinstated.

4. Real-time release testing (RTRT) and parametric release

RTRT is a type of tests to evaluate the quality of in-process or final products based on process data (including results of in-process testing and data on process parameters) and to assure that the quality is acceptable. RTRT is a kind of specifications and consists of a valid combination of materials attribute (intermediate products) pre-evaluated and process control. RTRT is used for judgement of products release instead of the release testing of final products when the application containing RTRT is approved by a regulatory authority.

The usage of RTRT does not mean unnecessity of setting tests of a final product directly. Even if the decision of release is made by RTRT, the tests for final products need to be set as specifications. It is because final product testing may be requested for some reasons such as failure of data acquisition due to troubles of equipments used for RTRT and evaluation of stability of final products. The final products, of course, need to meet their specifications, when tested.

Likewise, in the case that the drugs that was approved for marketing with the RTRT is listed in the JP monograph, the RTRT can be continued to use for release judgement. However specification and test procedure that assure the quality as same as the RTRT for final products should be set in the monograph. Even for drugs whose specifications are listed in the monographs, when a new application (or application for partial change) containing RTRT is approved by the regulatory authority, the products release can be judged based on the results of the RTRT instead of the tests prescribed in the monograph. In addition, it is necessary to comply with the specification in the case of conducting the compendial tests. In either case, it is unnecessary to set specification for RTRT in ''Manufacture'' of the monograph since the control criteria for the target CQA is already shown for the RTRT.

If RTRT results fail or trend toward failure, RTRT should not easily be substituted by final product testing. In this case, it is important to investigate the cause properly and need to take corrective action. Also, if RTRT results fail, the products cannot be released unless they were caused by analysis failure such as equipment failure. If RTRT results are trending toward failure, the products release should be made carefully based on the results of the investigation.

Parametric release can be considered a type of real time release. One example of parametric release is to determine the suitability for release of terminally sterilized drug products based on the data on sterilizing process instead of the results of sterility testing. In this case, the release of each batch is based on satisfactory results from monitoring specific parameters, e.g., temperature, pressure, and time during the terminal sterilization phase(s) of drug product manufacturing. Parametric release based on above parameters is more reliable in predicting sterility assurance than determination of suitability for release based on sterility testing using limited number of final products. Besides, even if parametric release is applied, the final product testing need to be set because the testing is necessary in stability testing and post-marketing surveillance. If in-process data used for parametric release are not acceptable, the products cannot be released. The parametric release differs from RTRT in the case, for example where the data of monitoring specific parameters in terminally sterilized process is failed to obtain by a certain reason such as analysis failure by equipment failure and so on. The incomplete data acquisition means no assurance on sterilization process, it is impossible to substitute parametric release by sterility testing of final products in principle.

Basic Concept of Quality Risk Management <*G0-2-170*>

Introduction

Quality Risk Management (QRM) is a crucial constituent of Pharmaceutical Quality System (PQS). PQS is a kind of the Quality System to control pharmaceutical quality in industries. Quality System is a basic concept of International Standards such as ISO 9001, ISO 14001, and ISO 27001. With its framework of maintenance and continuous improvement of business operation based on PDCA cycle (Plan →Do→Check→Act), PQS has been incorporated in ICH Q10 guideline as the basic philosophy. QRM is applicable to secure quality of every pharmaceuticals including drug substances, drug (medicinal) products, and biological and biotechnological products. Cooperating with a control strategy reflecting latest knowledge and understandings on products and manufacturing process, QRM contributes to realization and maintenance with consistent quality by responding flexibly and securely to risk regarding qualities.

Risks associated with the quality of pharmaceutical products are evaluated in the process of listing in the Japanese Pharmacopoeia and the results are reflected in specifications of the individual monograph. However, the pharmaceuticals specified in the same monograph may each have different quality risk derived from difference in their manufacturing methods. Therefore, appropriate assessment and management is required for such risk to manufacturing quality in the course of actual drug development and manufacturing. Further, quality risk of pharmaceuticals should be re-evaluated on a regular basis during their lifecycle, i.e. from their initial development through commercialization to the end of manufacturing and sales, and it is required to take appropriate measures based on the results.

About a relationship between QRM and the Japanese Pharmacopoeia, it may be said additionally as follows. In addition to conduction of the standard tests of Japanese Pharmacopoeia, it is important to plan and carry out measures to properly control elusive risk, which derived from alterations of manufacturing and quality management such as changes of raw materials and resources, in order to properly hold the pharmaceutical quality. Besides, depending on the results of risk re-evaluation, it may become necessary to revise specification tests specified by the Japanese Pharmacopoeia.

1. Significance of QRM

It is commonly understood that risk is defined as the combination of the probability of occurrence of harm and the severity of that harm. However, achieving a shared understanding of the application of risk management among diverse stakeholders is difficult because of a large gap between stakeholders in type and size of risk recognized. In relation to pharmaceuticals, although there are a variety of stakeholders, including patients and medical practitioners as well as government and industry, the protection of the patient by applying QRM should be considered of prime importance.

The manufacturing and use of a drug (medicinal) product, including its components, necessarily entail some degree of risk. The risk to its quality is just one component of the overall risk. The product quality should be maintained throughout the product lifecycle such that the attributes that are important to the quality of the drug (medicinal) product remain consistent with those used in the clinical studies. An effective QRM approach can further ensure the high quality of the drug (medicinal) product to the patient by providing a proactive means to identify and control potential quality issues during development and manufacturing. Additionally, use of QRM can improve the quality of measures and the speed of decision making if a quality problem arises. Effective QRM can provide regulators with greater assurance of a company's ability to deal with potential risks and can beneficially affect the extent and level of direct regulatory oversight.

As for QRM, it is neither always appropriate nor always necessary to use a formal risk management process. The use of informal risk management processes can also be considered acceptable. Appropriate use of QRM can facilitate but does not obviate industry's obligation to comply with regulatory requirements and does not replace appropriate communications between industry and regulators.

2. Scope of Application

QRM can be applied to every aspects of pharmaceutical quality. These aspects include development, manufacturing, distribution, and the inspection and submission/review processes throughout the lifecycle of drug substances, drug (medicinal) products, and biological and biotechnological products (including the use of raw materials, solvents, excipients, packaging and labeling materials in drug (medicinal) products, biological and biotechnological products).

3. Principle of QRM

Two primary principles of QRM are:

- Evaluation of the risk to quality should be based on scientific knowledge and ultimately link to the protection of the patient.
- Level of effort, formality and documentation of the QRM process should be commensurate with the level of risk.

4. General QRM Process

QRM is a systematic process for the assessment, control, communication and review of risks to the quality of the drug (medicinal) product across the product lifecycle. A model for QRM is outlined in the diagram (Figure 1). The emphasis on each component of the framework might differ from case to case but a robust process will incorporate consideration of all the elements at a level of detail that is commensurate with the specific risk. Decision nodes are not shown in the diagram because decisions can occur at any point in the process. These decisions might be to return to the previous step and seek further information, to adjust the risk models or even to terminate the risk management process based upon information that supports such a decision.

4.1. Initiation of QRM Process

QRM should include systematic processes designed to coordinate, facilitate and improve science-based decision making with respect to risk. Possible steps used to initiate and plan a QRM process might include the following:

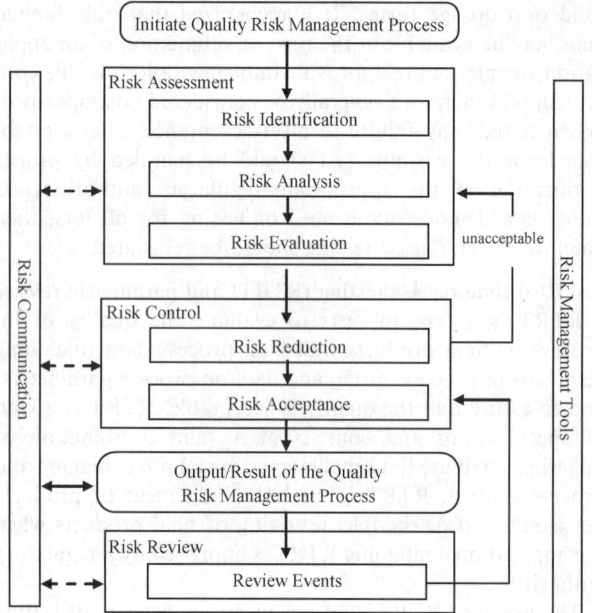

Fig. 1 Overview of a typical quality risk management process

- Define the problem and/or risk question, including pertinent assumptions identifying the potential for risk;
- Assemble background information and/or data on the potential hazard, harm or human health impact relevant to the risk assessment;
- Identify a leader and necessary resources;
- Specify a timeline, deliverables and appropriate level of decision making for the risk management process.

In the process described above, persons in charge (decision makers) should take responsibility for coordinating QRM across various functions and departments of their organization; and assure that a QRM process is defined, deployed and reviewed and that adequate resources are available.

4.2. Risk Assessment

Risk assessment consists of the identification of hazards and the analysis and evaluation of risks associated with exposure to those hazards. The step includes "risk identification", "risk analysis" and "risk evaluation",

As an assist to define risk clearly for purposes of risk assessment, the following three basic questions are often helpful.

1. What might go wrong?
2. What is the likelihood (probability) it will go wrong?
3. What are the consequences (severity)?

Risk identification is a systematic use of information to identify hazards referring to the risk question or problem description. Information can include historical data, theoretical analysis, informed opinions, and the concerns of stakeholders. Risk identification addresses the "What might go wrong?" question, including identifying the possible consequences. This provides the basis for further steps in the quality risk management process.

Risk analysis is the estimation of the risk associated with the identified hazards. It is the qualitative or quantitative process of linking the likelihood of occurrence and severity of harms. In some risk management tools, the ability to detect the harm (detectability) also factors in the estimation of risk.

Risk evaluation compares the identified and analyzed risk against given risk criteria. Risk evaluations consider the strength of evidence for all three of the fundamental questions.

The output of a risk assessment is either a quantitative estimate of risk or a qualitative description of a range of risk. When risk is expressed quantitatively, a numerical probability is used. Alternatively, risk can be expressed using qualitative descriptors, such as "high", "medium", or "low", which should be defined in as much detail as possible. Sometimes a "risk score" is used to further define descriptors in risk ranking. In quantitative risk assessments, a risk estimate provides the likelihood of a specific consequence, given a set of risk-generating circumstances. Thus, quantitative risk estimation is useful for one particular consequence at a time. Alternatively, some risk management tools use a relative risk measure to combine multiple levels of severity and probability into an overall estimate of relative risk. The intermediate steps within a scoring process can sometimes employ quantitative risk estimation.

4.3. Risk Control

Risk control includes decision making to reduce and/or accept risks. The purpose of risk control is to reduce the risk to an acceptable level. The amount of effort used for risk control should be proportional to the significance of the risk. Decision makers might use different processes, including benefit-cost analysis, for understanding the optimal level of risk control.

Risk control might focus on the following questions:

- Is the risk above an acceptable level?
- What can be done to reduce or eliminate risks?
- What is the appropriate balance among benefits, risks and resources?
- Are new risks introduced as a result of the identified risks being controlled?

Risk reduction focuses on processes for mitigation or avoidance of quality risk when it exceeds a specified (acceptable) level (see Fig. 1). Risk reduction might include actions taken to mitigate the severity and probability of harm. Processes that improve the detectability of hazards and quality risks might also be used as part of a risk control strategy. The implementation of risk reduction measures can introduce new risks into the system or increase the significance of other existing risks. Hence, it might be appropriate to revisit the risk assessment to identify and evaluate any possible change in risk after implementing a risk reduction process.

Risk acceptance is a decision to accept risk. Risk acceptance can be a formal decision to accept the residual risk or it can be a passive decision in which residual risks are not specified. For some types of harms, even the best quality risk management practices might not entirely eliminate risk. In these circumstances, it might be agreed that an appropriate quality risk management strategy has been applied and that quality risk is reduced to a specified (acceptable) level. This (specified) acceptable level will depend on many parameters and should be decided on a case-by-case basis.

4.4. Risk Communication

Risk communication is the sharing of information about risk and risk management between the decision makers and others. Parties can communicate at any stage of the risk management process (see Fig. 1: dashed arrows). The output/result of the quality risk management process should be appropriately communicated and documented (see Fig. 1: solid arrows). Communications might include those among interested parties; e.g., regulators and industry, industry and the patient, within a company, industry or regulatory authority, etc. The included information might relate to the existence, nature, form, probability, severity, acceptability, control, treatment, detectability or other aspects of risks to quality. Communication need not be carried out for each and every risk acceptance. Between the industry and regulatory authorities, communication concerning quality risk management decisions might be effected through existing channels as specified in regulations and guidances.

4.5. Risk Review

Risk management should be an ongoing part of the quality management process. A mechanism to review or monitor events should be implemented.

The output/results of the risk management process should be reviewed to take into account new knowledge and experience. Once a quality risk management process has been initiated, that process should continue to be utilized for events that might impact the original quality risk management decision, whether these events are planned (e.g., results of product review, inspections, audits, change control) or unplanned (e.g., root cause from failure investigations, recall). The frequency of any review should be based upon the level of risk. Risk review might include reconsideration of risk acceptance decisions (section 4.3).

5. Summary

The degree of rigor and formality of quality risk management should reflect available knowledge and be commensurate with the complexity and/ or criticality of the issue to be addressed.

Quality risk management is a process that supports science-based and practical decisions when integrated into quality systems. Appropriate use of QRM, however, does not obviate industry's obligation to comply with regulatory requirements.

6. Definitions

Decision Maker(s): Person(s) with the competence and authority to make appropriate and timely quality risk management decisions.

Detectability: The ability to discover or determine the existence, presence, or fact of a hazard.

Harm: Damage to health, including the damage that can occur from loss of product quality or availability.

Hazard: The potential source of harm (ISO/IEC Guide 51).

Product Lifecycle: All phases in the life of the product from the initial development through marketing until the product's discontinuation.

Quality: The degree to which a set of inherent properties of a product, system or process fulfills requirements. The suitability of either a drug substance or drug product for its intended use. This term includes such attributes as identity, strength, and purity.

Quality Risk Management: A systematic process for the assessment, control, communication and review of risks to the quality of the drug (medicinal) product across the product lifecycle.

Quality System: The sum of all aspects of a system that implements quality policy and ensures that quality objectives are met.

Requirements: The explicit or implicit needs or expectations of the patients or their surrogates (e.g., health-care professionals, regulators and legislators). In this document, "requirements" refers not only to statutory, legislative, or regulatory requirements, but also to such needs and expectations.

Risk: The combination of the probability of occurrence of harm and the severity of that harm (ISO/IEC Guide 51).

Risk Acceptance: The decision to accept risk (ISO Guide 73).

Risk Analysis: The estimation of the risk associated with the identified hazards.

Risk Assessment: A systematic process of organizing information to support a risk decision to be made within a risk management process. It consists of the identification of hazards and the analysis and evaluation of risks associated with exposure to those hazards.

Risk Communication: The sharing of information about risk and risk management between the decision maker and other stakeholders.

Risk Control: Actions implementing risk management decisions (ISO Guide 73).

Risk Evaluation: The comparison of the estimated risk to given risk criteria using a quantitative or qualitative scale to determine the significance of the risk.

Risk Identification: The systematic use of information to identify potential sources of harm (hazards) referring to the risk question or problem description.

Risk Management: The systematic application of quality management policies, procedures, and practices to the tasks of assessing, controlling, communicating and reviewing risk.

Risk Reduction: Actions taken to lessen the probability of occurrence of harm and the severity of that harm.

Risk Review: Review or monitoring of output/results of the risk management process considering (if appropriate) new knowledge and experience about the risk.

Severity: A measure of the possible consequences of a hazard.

Stakeholder: Any individual, group or organization that can affect, be affected by, or perceive itself to be affected by a risk. Decision makers might also be stakeholders. For the purposes of this guideline, the primary stakeholders are the patient, healthcare professional, regulatory authority, and industry.

Concept on Impurities in Chemically synthesized Drug Substances and Drug Products

<G0-3-172>

1. Classification of impurities found in chemically synthesized pharmaceuticals and the guidance to comply with their control

Impurities found in chemically synthesized pharmaceuticals are roughly classified into organic impurities, inorganic impurities and residual solvents. Those impurities in the new drug substances and the products are controlled by the following guidelines agreed upon at the International Council for Harmonisation of Technical Requirements for Pharmaceuticals for Human Use (hereinafter referred to as "ICH"). More specifically, "Impurities in New Drugs Substances (PAB/PCD Notification No. 877 dated September 25, 1995)" (hereinafter referred to as "ICH Q3A Guideline")[1] on specifications for organic impurities in drug substances applies to applications for marketing approval after April 1, 1997, while "Impurities in New Drug Products (PAB/PCD Notification No. 539 dated June 23, 1997" (hereinafter referred to as "ICH Q3B Guideline")[2] on specifications for organic impurities in drug products applies to applications for marketing approval after April 1, 1999. Meanwhile, specifications for inorganic impurities were specified by Japanese pharmacopoeial standards and known safety data. Now "Guidelines for Elemental Impurities (PFSB/ELD Notification No. 4 dated September 30, 2015)" apply to applications for marketing approval after April 1, 2017. In regard to residual solvents, "Impurities: Guidelines for Residual Solvents (PAB/ELD Notification No. 307 dated March 30, 1998)" (hereinafter referred to as "ICH Q3C Guideline") applies to applications for marketing approval after April 1, 2000. Especially in regard to DNA-reactive impurities, "Assessment and control of DNA reactive (mutagenic) impurities in pharmaceuticals to limit potential carcinogenic risk (PSEHB/ELD Notification No. 3 dated November 10, 2015)" applies to applications for marketing approval after January 15, 2016. Although ICH Q3A guideline does not cover optical enantiomers, a type of organic impurities, "Specifications: Test Procedures and Acceptance Criteria for New Drug Substances and New Drug Products: Chemical Substances (PMSB/ELD Notification No. 568 dated May 1, 2001)" (hereinafter referred to as "ICH Q6A Guideline"), which was published subsequently, provides that enantiomers are impurities that should be controlled and, if measurable, should be controlled in accordance with the principle of ICH Q3A guideline.

Control of impurities in accordance with the guidelines mentioned above is expected also for pharmaceuticals other than new drug substances and new drug products. Their applications for marketing (or applications for partial changes) are subject to those guidelines when necessary. The General Notices of the JP 17th Edition states that residual solvents of all JP-listed drugs, in principle, have to be controlled in accordance with specification "Residual Solvents" in General Tests unless otherwise specified in the individual monograph. In regard to elemental impurities, it has been decided in the basic principles for the preparation of the JP 18th Edition to create a roadmap for their incorporation into the JP for listing and to address its implementation.

2. The concept of ICH Q3A and Q3B guidelines for the control of organic impurities

ICH Q3A and Q3B guidelines require setting acceptance criteria for organic impurities based on the information gained from development stages for new drugs. Concerning impurities in drug substances, ICH Q3A guideline refers to the items to be examined from chemical and safety perspectives. ICH Q3B guideline complements Q3A guideline, and have the same basic concept as Q3A. Chemical aspects to be examined include classification and identification of impurities, their reporting method, specification settings and analytical methods. Safety aspects include specific guidelines for qualifying the safety of impurities that were not present, or were present at substantially lower levels, in batches of a drug substance used in safety and clinical studies.

Qualification of the safety is the process of acquiring and evaluating data that establishes the biological safety of an individual impurity or a given impurity profile at the level(s) specified. The applicant should describe a rationale for establishing impurity acceptance criteria that includes safety considerations in attachments when applicated for approval. The level of any impurities present in a new drug substance that has been adequately tested in safety and/or clinical studies would be considered qualified.

Identified impurities, unidentified impurities and total impurities are specified based on the data obtained according to the guidelines. The threshold of unspecified impurities in a drug substance is determined depending on the daily intake of the drug substance. When the maximum daily dosage is not more than 2 g, it is set at 0.10%. The establishment of individual specifications is required for impurities at a level greater than 0.10%.

In regard to drug products, ICH Q3B guideline cover the degradation products of drug substances or reaction products between the drug substance and additive/primary packaging. Therefore, even if organic impurities other than degradation products (e.g., by-products and synthetic intermediates) in the drug substance are found as impurities in the drug product, they need not be monitored or specified since they have already been controlled as the drug substance specifications. However, degradation products elevated in the drug product need to be monitored and specified.

3. Principles for controlling organic impurities in the articles listed in the JP

Conventionally in the JP, specified impurities, unspecified impurities and total impurities are specified in accordance with ICH Q3A and Q3B guidelines for pharmaceutical products, whose impurities have been controlled by those guidelines, in the process listing in the JP. (However, this shall not apply to the long-term listed pharmaceutical products which had existed in the JP before these guidelines were applicable. However, when a new application is filed for those JP-listed pharmaceutical products, control of impurities in accordance with ICH Q3A and Q3B guidelines may be required, if necessary.) In order to specify the impurities, analysis data during development submitted from the drafting company and impurity analysis data from commercial production batches after consistent manufacturing is achieved should be assessed. Safety evaluation is not required again for the process listing in the JP since it has been performed at the time of approval.

ICH Q3A and Q3B guidelines cover impurities in the drug substances manufactured by chemical syntheses and the drug products manufactured with those drug substances. Similarly, the following types of products are not covered in the JP: biological/biotechnological products, peptides, oligonucleotides, radiopharmaceuticals, fermentation products and semi-synthetic products derived therefrom, herbal products and crude products of animal or plant origin.

When organic impurities assessed in accordance with the principles of ICH Q3A and Q3B guidelines are listed as JP tests of purity, the operational rationality of the JP is considered and its own modification is added. (i) Except in exceptional circumstances, impurity reference standards are not established. In order to identify an impurity using liquid chromatography, the relative retention time of the impurity to the drug substance is used for identification. (ii) When only unidentified impurities in highly pure pharmaceutical products (not more than 0.1%) are specified, it is generally exempted to set acceptance criteria for total impurities. (iii) When acceptance criteria set based only on actual measured values result in many impurities with slightly different acceptance criteria, consideration can be given so that the purity test consists of a small number of representative acceptance criteria, if possible. (iv) Chemical structural information and the chemical name of the impurities are not disclosed. Those measures enable impurity control without impurity reference standards, and can simplify system suitability test for highly pure pharmaceutical products.

Meanwhile, the method to identify impurities by use of relative retention time is column-dependent and analysis becomes difficult when appropriate columns are not available. Therefore, the JP 17th Edition also allows the use of the analysis method with impurity reference standards when designing purity tests for a drug substance. In addition, the JP adopted a policy to disclose chemical names and structure formulas as the information on impurities including, in principle, optical enantiomers.

The JP-specific consideration may be given to purity tests for organic impurities in drug products in the process listing in the JP. Also in the JP, impurities derived from the products of the reaction between the drug substance and additive/primary packaging are specified as impurities in the drug product. Those impurities are formulation-dependent and may not be formed in different formulations. Since the JP is an official compendium that allows a wide variety of formulations, when it is not appropriate to specify impurities uniformly in the individual monograph, they are subject to the specifications at the time of approval, along with the statement "Being specified separately when the drug is granted approval based on the Law."

When the specifications for impurities are reviewed for a new entry of a pharmaceutical product in an individual monograph of the JP, acceptance criteria for impurities may be included in the review according to the following concepts. ICH Q6A guideline point out: Data available upon the marketing application are limited and it has to be taken into consideration that the limited data may influence the design of acceptance criteria. Regarding impurities, since impurity profiles gained during the manufacturing stages may sometimes be different from that gained from development stage, it is stated that changes in impurity profiles at the manufacturing stage should be considered as appropriate. According to this concept, for impurities which should be specified in the process listing in the JP, not only information from development stage but also information about impurity profiles if there are changes at the manufacturing stage, and information at the stage after the product manufacturing becomes stable (hereinafter referred to as the "stable production stage") should be taken into consideration.

However, it is undesirable to remove impurities that are present at substantially lower levels, or become undetectable at the stable production stage indiscriminately from the list of candidate compounds to be specified. JP-listed drugs are accepted as drugs by conformance to the specifications in the individual monograph. However, generic drugs, whose manufacturing methods are not necessarily the same as that of the drug substance used for JP monograph, may have different impurity profiles and contain such impurities. Providing information in the process listing in the JP based on the detection results during development stage may result in encompassing impurities found in drug substances and drug products distributed as JP drugs.

Therefore, before the removal of impurities that are present at substantially lower levels or become undetectable at the stable production stage from the JP specification list, the need to establish specifications should be fully examined based on ICH Q3A and Q3B guidelines with respect to safety.

For a drug substance that was approved by the method to identify its impurities with impurity reference materials, it is desirable also in the individual JP monograph, in principle, to establish specifications and test methods appropriately so that the specified impurity becomes identifiable. In regard to impurity control during the manufacturing process, impurities can be controlled by establishing an appropriate control strategy including release testing, in-process tests and process parameters control.

4. References

1) ICH: Guideline for Q3A, Impurities in New Drug Substances.
2) ICH: Guideline for Q3B, Impurities in New Drug Products.

Stability Testing of Drug Substances and Drug Products

<G0-4-171>

1. Introduction

It is essential that the quality of a drug is maintained during the period from being manufactured to being administered in a patient. Stability testing is performed in order to ensure that the quality is maintained during the period. The purpose of stability testing is to provide evidence on how the quality of a drug substance or drug product varies with time under the influence of a variety of environmental factors such as temperature, humidity and light, and to establish a re-test period for the drug substance or a shelf life for the drug product and recommended storage conditions.

The re-test period of a drug substance is the period of time during which the drug substance is expected to remain within its specification and, therefore, can be used in the manufacture of a given drug product, provided that the drug substance has been stored under the defined conditions. After this period, a batch of drug substance destined for use in the manufacture of a drug product should be re-tested for compliance with the specification and then used immediately. A batch of drug substance can be re-tested multiple times. For certain antibiotics known to be labile, it is more appropriate to establish a shelf life than a re-test period. The shelf life of a drug product is the period in which a batch of the product is expected to remain within the approved shelf life specification if stored under defined conditions.

This general information mainly illustrates a standard implementation that can be set when we perform stability tests of a chemical drug substance and the associated drug product, and it is also helpful in stability tests of pharmaceuticals other than chemical drugs. Also, this leaves sufficient flexibility to encompass the variety of different practical situations that may be encountered due to specific scientific considerations and characteristics of the materials being evaluated. Alternative approaches can be used when there are scientifically justifiable reasons.

2. Conditions of stability testing

Stress testing, long term testing, accelerated testing and if necessary intermediate testing are performed as stability testing for drugs.

2.1 Stress testing

Stress testing of the drug substance can help identify the likely degradation products, which can in turn help establish the degradation pathways and the intrinsic stability of the molecule and validate the stability indicating power of the analytical procedures used. Stress testing should include the effect of temperatures (in 10°C increments (e.g., 50°C, 60°C, etc.) above that for accelerated testing), humidity (e.g., 75% RH or greater) where appropriate, oxidation, and photolysis on the drug substance. The testing should also evaluate the susceptibility of the drug substance to hydrolysis across a wide range of pH values when in solution or suspension.

Stress testing of the drug product is undertaken to assess the effect of severe conditions on the drug product. Such studies include photostability testing and specific testing on certain products, (e.g., metered dose inhalers, creams, emulsions, refrigerated aqueous liquid products).

2.2 Long term testing, accelerated testing and intermediate testing

Long term testing is undertaken on batches of a drug substance or drug product according to a prescribed stability protocol to establish the re-test period of the drug substance or the shelf life of the drug product.

Accelerated testing is a stability study designed to increase the rate of chemical degradation or physical change of a drug substance or drug product by using exaggerated storage conditions. Data from these studies, in addition to long term stability studies, can be used to assess longer term chemical effects at non-accelerated conditions and to evaluate the effect of short term excursions outside the label storage conditions such as might occur during shipping.

Intermediate testing is conducted at 30°C/65% RH and designed to moderately increase the rate of chemical degradation or physical changes for a drug substance or drug product intended to be stored long term at 25°C. Intermediate testing is implemented only when a significant change occurs in the accelerated testing.

Long term and accelerated testing, also if needed intermediate testing should be performed on at least three primary batches. The primary batches of the drug substance should be manufactured to a minimum of pilot scale by the same synthetic route as, and using a method of manufacture and procedure that simulates the final process to be used for, production batches. The overall quality of the batches of drug substance placed on the stability studies should be representative of the quality of the material to be made on a production scale. The stability studies should be conducted on the drug substance packaged in a container closure system that is the same as or simulates the packaging proposed for storage and distribution. The primary batches of the drug product should be of the same formulation and packaged in the same container closure system as proposed for marketing (including, as appropriate, any secondary packaging and container label). The manufacturing process used for primary batches should simulate that to be applied to production batches and should provide the product of the same quality and meeting the same specification as that intended for marketing. Two of the three batches should be at least pilot scale batches and the third one can be smaller, if justified. The primary batch may be a production batch. Where possible, batches of the drug product should be manufactured by using different batches of the drug substance. The pilot scale batch is a batch of a drug substance or drug product manufactured by a procedure fully representative of and simulating that to be applied to a full production scale batch. For solid oral dosage forms, a pilot scale is generally, at a minimum, one-tenth that of a full production scale or 100,000 tablets or capsules, whichever is the larger.

The storage conditions used for stability testing are shown in Table 1.

3. Testing attributes and testing frequency

Stability studies should include testing of those attributes of the drug substance or the product that are susceptible to change during storage and are likely to influence quality, safety, and/or efficacy. Validated stability-indicating analytical procedures should be applied. Whether and to what

Table 1 Storage condition

Storage condition and package	Long term	Accelerated	Intermediate
General case (drug substance and product)	25 ± 2°C/ 60 ± 5%RH or 30 ± 2°C/ 65 ± 5%RH[1)]	40 ± 2°C/ 75 ± 5%RH	30 ± 2°C/ 65 ± 5%RH[2)]
Storage in a refrigerator (drug substance and product)[3)]	5 ± 3°C	25 ± 2°C/ 60 ± 5%RH	
Storage in a freezer (drug substance and product)[4)]	− 20 ± 5°C		
Storage below − 20°C (drug substance and product)	case-by-case basis		
Drug products packaged in impermeable containers	Study can be conducted under any controlled or ambient humidity condition		
Drug products packaged in semi-permeable containers[5)]	25 ± 2°C/ 40 ± 5%RH or 30 ± 2°C/ 35 ± 5%RH[6)]	40 ± 2°C/ not more than (NMT) 25%RH	30 ± 2°C/ 65 ± 5%RH[7)]

[1)] It is up to the applicant to decide whether long term stability studies are performed at 25 ± 2°C/60 ± 5%RH or 30 ± 2°C/65 ± 5%RH.

[2)] If "significant change" occurs at the accelerated storage condition, additional testing at the intermediate storage condition should be conducted. However, if 30 ± 2°C/65 ± 5%RH is the long term condition, there is no intermediate condition. "Significant change" for a drug substance is defined as failure to meet its specification. In general, "significant change" for a drug product is defined as:

1. A 5% change in assay from its initial value; or failure to meet the acceptance criteria for potency when using biological or immunological procedures;

2. Any degradation product's exceeding its acceptance criterion;

3. Failure to meet the acceptance criteria for appearance, physical attributes, and functionality test (e.g., color, phase separation, resuspendibility, caking, hardness, dose delivery per actuation); however, some changes in physical attributes (e.g., softening of suppositories, melting of creams) may be expected under accelerated conditions;

and, as appropriate for the dosage form:

4. Failure to meet the acceptance criterion for pH; or

5. Failure to meet the acceptance criteria for dissolution for 12 dosage units.

6. Physical changes shown in the following may be observed in accelerated testing, but the changes are not considered as "significant change" which needs intermediate testing, when there is no "significant change" in other attributes.

• Softening of suppositories designed to melt at 37°C, when its melting point is shown clearly.

• When it is clear that "significant change" is due to crosslinking, the dissolution of gelatin capsules and gel coating tablets do not conform to the acceptance criteria for 12 dosage units.

When confirming that there is no "significant change" in other attributes, consider the possibility that these physical changes affect the other attributes.

[3)] The drug product is packaged in a semi-permeable container, appropriate information should be provided to assess the extent of water loss. In the accelerated testing of drug substances or products intended for storage in a refrigerator, if significant change occurs within the first 3 months, it is considered unnecessary to continue to test a product through 6 months.

[4)] Testing on a single batch at an elevated temperature (e.g., 5 ± 3°C or 25 ± 2°C) for an appropriate time period should be conducted to address the effect of short term excursions outside the label storage condition, e.g., during shipment and handling.

[5)] Aqueous-based products packaged in semi-permeable containers should be evaluated for potential water loss under conditions of low relative humidity. Other comparable approaches can be developed and used for non-aqueous, solvent-based products.

[6)] It is up to the applicant to decide whether long term stability studies are performed at 25 ± 2°C/40 ± 5% RH or 30 ± 2°C/35 ± 5%RH.

[7)] If "significant change" other than water loss occurs during the 6 months' testing at the accelerated storage condition. Additional testing at the intermediate storage condition should be performed. A significant change in water loss alone at the accelerated storage condition does not necessitate testing at the intermediate storage condition. However, data should be provided to demonstrate that the drug product will not have significant water loss throughout the proposed shelf life if stored at 25°C and the reference relative humidity of 40% RH. If 30 ± 2°C/35 ± 5% RH is the long term condition, there is no intermediate condition. A 5% loss in water from its initial value is considered a significant change for a product packaged in a semi-permeable container after an equivalent of 3 months' storage at 40°C/NMT 25% RH. However, for small containers (1 mL or less) or unit-dose products, a water loss of 5% or more after an equivalent of 3 months' storage at 40°C/NMT 25% RH may be appropriate, if justified.

extent replication should be performed will depend on the results from validation studies.

For long term studies, frequency of testing should be sufficient to establish the stability profile of the drug substance and product. For drug substances or products with a proposed re-test period or shelf life of at least 12 months, the frequency of testing at the long term storage condition should normally be every 3 months over the first year, every 6 months over the second year, and annually thereafter through the proposed re-test period or shelf life. At the accelerated storage condition, a minimum of three time points, including the initial and final time points (e.g., 0, 3, and 6 months), from a 6-month study is recommended. When testing at the intermediate storage condition is called for as a result of significant change at the accelerated storage condition, a minimum of four time points, including the initial and final time points (e.g., 0, 6, 9, 12 months), from a 12-month study is recommended.

A reduced design, i.e., matrixing or bracketing, where the testing frequency is reduced or certain factor combinations are not tested at all, can be applied, if justified, for the testing of combination of drug products having multiple design factors (e.g., strength, container size and/or fill). A bracketing design assumes that the stability of any intermediate levels is represented by the stability of the extremes tested. This is the design of a stability schedule such that only samples on the extremes of certain design factors (e.g., strength, container size and/or fill). Bracketing can be applied to studies with multiple strengths of identical or closely related formulations. Examples include but are not limited to (1) capsules of different strengths made with different fill plug sizes from the same powder blend, (2) tablets of different strengths manufactured by compressing varying amounts of the same granulation, and (3) oral solutions of different strengths with formulations that differ only in minor excipients (e.g., colorants, flavorings). Bracketing can be applied to studies of the same container closure system where either container size or fill varies while the other remains constant. The use of a bracketing design would not be applicable if it cannot be demonstrated that the strengths or container sizes and/or fills selected for testing are indeed the extremes. An example of a bracketing design is given in Table 2. This design is provided for illustrative purpose, and should not be considered the only, or the most appropriate, design in all cases.

A matrixing design assumes that the stability of each subset of samples tested represents the stability of all samples at a given time point. This is the design of a stability schedule such that a selected subset of the total number of possible samples for all factor combinations would be tested at a specified time point. At a subsequent time point, another subset of samples for all factor combinations would be tested. Matrixing designs can be applied to strengths with identical or closely related formulations. Examples include but are not limited to (1) capsules of different strengths made with different fill plug sizes from the same powder blend, (2) tablets of different strengths manufactured by compressing varying amounts of the same granulation, and (3) oral solutions of different strengths with formulations that differ only in minor excipients (e.g., colorants or flavorings). Other examples of design factors that can be matrixed include batches made by using the same process and equipment, and container sizes and/or different fills in the same container closure system. An example of a matrixing design is given in Table 3. This design is provided for illustrative purpose, and should not be considered the only, or the most appropriate, design in all cases.

Table 2 Example of a Bracketing Design

Strength		50 mg			75 mg			100 mg		
Batch		1	2	3	1	2	3	1	2	3
Container size	15 mL bottle	T	T	T				T	T	T
	100 mL bottle									
	500 mL bottle	T	T	T				T	T	T

T = Sample tested

Table 3 Example of a Matrixing Design on Time Points for a Product with Two Strengths
"One-Half Reduction"

Time point (months)			0	3	6	9	12	18	24	36
Strength	S1	Batch 1	T	T		T	T		T	T
		Batch 2	T	T		T	T	T		T
		Batch 3	T		T		T	T		T
	S2	Batch 1	T		T		T		T	T
		Batch 2	T	T		T	T	T		T
		Batch 3	T		T		T		T	T

T = Sample tested

4. Photostability testing

Photostability testing is a part of stress testing evaluating the photostability characteristics of drug substances and products.

4.1. Light sources

The light sources described below may be used for photostability testing.

(i) Option 1 Any light source that is designed to produce an output similar to the D_{65}/ID_{65} emission standard such as an artificial daylight fluorescent lamp combining visible and ultraviolet (UV) outputs, xenon, or metal halide lamp.

(ii) Option 2 For option 2 the same sample should be exposed to both the cool white fluorescent and near ultraviolet fluorescent lamp.

1. A cool white fluorescent lamp designed to produce an output similar to that specified in ISO10977(1993); and

2. A near ultraviolet fluorescent lamp having a spectral distribution from 320 nm to 400 nm with a maximum energy emission between 350 nm and 370 nm; a significant proportion of energy emission should be in both bands of 320 to 360 nm and 360 to 400 nm.

4.2. Light exposure level and testing condition

For drug substances, photostability testing should consist of two parts: forced degradation testing and confirmatory testing. The purpose of forced degradation testing studies is to evaluate the overall photosensitivity of the material for method development purposes and/or degradation pathway elucidation. This testing may involve the drug substance alone and/or in simple solutions/suspensions to validate the analytical procedures. In these forced degradation testing studies, a variety of exposure conditions may be used, depending on the photosensitivity of the drug substance involved and the intensity of the light sources used. For development and validation purposes it is appropriate to limit exposure and end the studies if extensive decomposition occurs. For photostable materials, studies may be terminated after an appropriate exposure level has been used. The design of these experiments is left to the applicant's discretion although the exposure levels used should be justified. Confirmatory studies of drug substance should then be undertaken to provide the information necessary for handling, packaging, and labeling. For confirmatory studies, samples should be exposed to light providing an overall illumination of not less than 1.2 million lx·h and an integrated near ultraviolet energy of not less than 200 $W \cdot h/m^2$ to allow direct comparisons to be made between the drug substance and drug product. Efforts should be made, such as cooling and/or placing the samples in sealed containers, to ensure that the effects of the changes in physical states such as sublimation, evaporation or melting are minimized. Containers used should not interfere with the exposure of a test sample as much as possible, and avoid materials that cause interference with the testing such as interaction between the sample and the materials. As a direct challenge for samples of solid drug substances, an appropriate amount of sample should be taken and placed in a suitable glass or plastic dish and protected with a suitable transparent cover if considered necessary. Powder drug substances should be spread across the container to give a thickness of typically not more than 3 mm. Drug substances that are liquids should be exposed in chemically inert and transparent containers. Where practicable when testing samples of the drug product outside of the primary pack, these should be presented in a way similar to the conditions mentioned for the drug substance. The samples should be positioned to provide maximum area of exposure to the light source. For example, tablets, capsules, etc., should be spread in a single layer. If direct exposure is not practical (e.g., due to oxidation of a product), the sample should be placed in a suitable protective inert transparent container (e.g., quartz). If testing of the drug product in the immediate container or as marketed is needed, the samples should be placed horizontally or transversely with respect to the light source, whichever provides for the most uniform exposure of the samples. Some adjustment of testing conditions may have to be made when testing large volume containers (e.g., dispensing packs).

5. Evaluation of stability data

In the stability data evaluation, data from long term and accelerated testing, also if needed from intermediate testing and, as appropriate, supporting data (data of stability testing using drug substances and products in developing stage) should be evaluated to determine the critical quality attributes likely to influence the quality and performance of the drug substance or product. Each attribute should be assessed separately, and an overall assessment should be made of the findings for the purpose of proposing a re-test period or shelf life. An approach for analyzing data of a quantitative attribute that is expected to change with time is to determine the time at which the 95% one-sided confidence limit for the mean curve intersects the acceptance criterion. The re-test period or shelf life proposed should not exceed that predicted for any single attribute.

Basic Requirements and Terms for the Packaging of Pharmaceutical Products <*G0-5-170*>

This chapter describes the basic requirements for the packaging of pharmaceutical products as well as the terms and their definitions used for the packaging as taking into account the aspects in quality assurance of the pharmaceutical products and the point of view of international harmonization.[1)]

In this chapter, the concept of packaging for pharmaceutical products, or packaging, includes putting or holding the drugs in container. In addition, the information presented as basic requirements shall be a central focus on packaging for drug products, as well as for ensuring quality on the transportation and storage of drug substances or additives.

1. Basic requirements of packaging for pharmaceutical products

For the packaging for pharmaceutical products, it is important to settle the requirements of the packaging based on the evaluation of the packaging suitability in the development stage so as to be able to ensure the quality standards of preparations defined over the shelf life of preparations. The suitability of packaging for pharmaceutical products must be maintained through the product life cycle on the basis of the requirements of packaging settled in the development stage.

For the packaging of drug products, it is also necessary to consider for the suitability for proper use and for ensuring safe application in addition to quality assurance. The stringency of the evaluation for suitability of packaging for preparations differs depending on the degree of the risk according to the route of administration, such as intravenous administration, oral administration, or dermal administration and the risk due to interaction between the products and the primary packaging according to injections, liquids and solutions, semi-solid or solid dosage forms.

1.1. Suitability evaluation and requirements of packaging in the design stage

The packaging suitability to be evaluated in the design stage includes protection, compatibility, safety, and performance.

The basic items to be evaluated as suitability are described in the course of the packaging design.

1.1.1. Safety of materials used for packaging

Leachables or migrants, such as the monomers of the polymer resins, additives or metal impurities, from the materials used for the primary packaging such as plastic or glass containers should not deteriorate drug safety. The amount of leachable or migratable chemical substances from the primary packaging materials to the contents must be sufficiently small from a safety perspective.

The primary packaging materials of the containers that are in direct contact with the drugs should be used which quality such as on toxicity has been appropriately evaluated by the suppliers according to "Basic Requirements for Plastic Containers for Pharmaceutical Use and Rubber Closures for Containers for Aqueous Infusions <*G7-2-162*>" in General Information or the like. In the design stage, the information on quality evaluation of the packing materials is desirable to be obtained as far as possible from the suppliers.

1.1.2. Compatibility with the contents

The primary packaging must not reduce the quality of pharmaceutical products over the shelf life of preparations. The contents adsorbing onto the surface of primary packaging, or migrating inside of the materials, must not lead to a drug concentration change of more than a certain level. Moreover, the interaction between the contents and the materials must not lead to degradation of drugs.

The primary packaging should not be deformed, deteriorated, or degraded by the contents.

In the design stage, the compatibility of the primary packaging with the content is examined by the combination of individual candidate material and the content drugs, together with other evaluation items. And chose the applicable material based on the results of the study on the prototype primary packaging for complying with the essential requirements, i.e. the design specifications, for the issues about the protection from moisture and light, the sorption to and leaching from the primary packaging, etc., based on the data from the experiments and/or information from the scientific documentation. When selecting the primary packaging material, the suitability of the material for the secondary packaging is also to be evaluated as needed.

1.1.3. Protection by packaging

The packaging should be able to prevent loss, efflorescence, deliquescence, or evaporation of the contents and to protect the contents by the addition of moisture resistance, light shielding, or a gas barrier, depending on the characteristic of the contents. In the case of not being able to ensure the quality of the contents by the primary packaging alone, it should be ensured by the combination of multiple packaging materials, including the secondary packaging. Furthermore, the containers for injections or ophthalmic solutions are preferable to be made of a high transparency material, so that foreign matter contamination can be observed visually.

For pharmaceutical products susceptible to moisture such as by hydrolysis, the packaging used with desiccants or primary packaging materials with gas-barrier function can be moisture-proof packaging. For preparations susceptible to evaporation of water, gas-barrier materials for the primary packaging can be used. For the pharmaceutical products that are easily oxidized, the packaging with deoxidants or the low-gas-permeability materials can be used for the primary packaging to protect the pharmaceutical products from oxygen in the air.

Protection by the packaging should be evaluated in the packaging design stage, and finally confirmed by stability tests. Resistance to physical shock during transportation is also necessary to be verified.

1.1.4. Container integrity (microbial contamination prevention)

The packaging should be able to protect the contents from microbial contamination, depending on the characteristics of the content drug or dosage form, and especially for the containers used for sterile preparations, the integrity of primary packaging, through the tests such as the fitting compatibility tests for containers and closures, must be confirmed.

In the case of pharmaceutical products that must be sterilized, the primary packaging must meet the above-mentioned suitability for safety, compatibility and protection even after the sterilization. There should not be any residue or generation of toxic substances of more than a certain safety level after the sterilization. In addition, the primary packaging should have a structure and/or material that must prevent any microbial contamination of the pharmaceutical products contained therein during storage and transportation after sterilization.

1.1.5. Packaging performance

The packaging design with consideration for discrimination, usability, and disposal should be performed.

With regard to discrimination, for example, a display should be considered for patients so that the proper administration and use of the drugs can be ensured and even for aged patients to be able to idenify easily. An easy-to-understand display or container for preventing accidental misuse or a prank, such as tamper-resistant packaging and child-resistant packaging, is preferable.

With regard to usability, items such as easy handling of the drug in dispensing, easy dosaging for children with small doses, easy removal from the container when the drug is administered or used, successful administration, and preferable storage and portability should be considered for each preparation.

On packaging-related waste, the choice or determination of the containers must be considered for disposal, since paying attention to the effect of use of resources, following the Containers and Packaging Recycling Act and the rules of each local government, and striving to reduce wastes are required. In the primary packaging, the recycled packaging materials that are not assured for material composition must not be used.

1.1.6. Requirements of packaging

Based on the test methods and/or the evaluation techniques used for study of the packaging suitability in the design stage of pharmaceutical preparations, the necessary and sufficient items of the quality control for maintaining the packaging suitability are established. Generally, the requirements of packaging are composed of the control of the material quality, specifications and test methods, in-process tests, and the like.

1.2. Examples of suitability evaluation in the design stage of packaging for pharmaceutical products

The following are the examples of the suitability evaluation in the design stage.

1.2.1. Suitability evaluation of packaging to be used for solid oral dosage forms

For the suitability evaluation of the packaging for solid oral dosage forms, the following tests should be included.

- If bottles are used, the measurement of opening torques with selected stoppers should be performed.
- If PTP packaging or strip packaging is used, the moisture permeability test should be performed.

1.2.2. Suitability evaluation of containers to be used for injections

For the suitability evaluation of containers to be used for injections, the following tests should be included.

- The injections using ampules should perform pinhole tests, and the integrity must be confirmed.
- The injections using vials, rubber closures, or prefilled glass syringes, except ampules, should perform the fitting compatibility tests, and the integrity as a container must be confirmed.
- The plastic containers for pharmaceutical products used for injections (prefilled syringes, plastic bottles, plastic bags, etc.) should be verified as ''tight containers in which microorganisms will not be contaminated'' over the shelf life of preparations.

1.2.3. Suitability evaluation on metal impurities for a container closure system

If leaching of metal impurities from the primary packaging materials used for injections, liquids, or semi-solid preparations is suspected, it is necessary to confirm that the amount of metal impurities contained in preparations is sufficiently low from the viewpoint of safety using Atomic Absorption Spectrophotometry <*2.23*>, Inductively Coupled Plasma Emission Spectrometry and Inductively Coupled Plasma-Mass Spectrometry <*2.63*>, etc.

1.2.4. Suitability evaluation of kit products

If dispensing devices, such as prefilled syringes, injection cartridges, or metered-dose preparations for inhalation, are used, the accurate dose with reproducibility in conditions as close as possible to the product usage must be verified.

1.2.5. Suitability evaluation of light resistant packaging

If active substances are susceptible to the light and the formulation design alone cannot overcome the effect of light, the light resistant packaging including containers should be considered. A selection of an appropriate light resistant packaging must be verified using a photostability test and the like as severe tests.

1.3. Selection, change control, stability monitoring, etc. of the packaging materials in the packaging process development

To maintain appropriately the quality assurance of pharmaceutical products by packaging, the properness of the requirements of the packaging must be confirmed through the appropriate change control, stability monitoring and the like in the packaging process development and production stages, together with the suitability evaluation performed in the design stage.

For the primary packaging materials used in the manufacture of preparations, whether the quality of material is changed by the supplier must be appropriately managed. Therefore, all information concerning the manufacturing process of containers including the information about substances added is desirable to be obtained.

The finally selected packaging for pharmaceutical products should be evaluated whether it meets the requirements as designed. If it does not meet the requirements, the packaging form or material must be changed through change control.

1.3.1. Selection or change of packaging materials in the packaging process development

The packaging materials should be selected in consideration of the manufacturability and the prevention capability of adhesion of foreign matters or insects in addition to meeting the requirements determined in the design stage. For the finally selected packaging, it should be verified to withstand against temperature change during storage and transportation, physical shock during transportation, and the like.

The suitability of the selected packaging materials shall be confirmed, using the applicable tests in the General Tests, 7. Test for Containers and Packing Materials. For the tests that are not described in the General Tests, set the applicable test and judge the suitability.

1.3.2. Stability monitoring, etc.

It must be confirmed that the packaging form does not adversely affect the stability of preparations through stability monitoring or reference sample stored. If the packaging is considered to affect the quality of stability of the preparations, the applicable packaging and management should be selected to ensuring quality, where the quality of the lots using this should be monitored, and the packaging should be improved through change control, if necessary.

1.4. Examples of quality control in the packaging process of pharmaceutical products

To maintain the suitability of the packaging of pharmaceutical products, it must be confirmed by performing the test such as process control test before shipment that the packaging meets the requirements.

The following shows the examples.

1.4.1. Examples of solid oral dosage forms

The PTP packaged tablets must be confirmed whether the integrity of the seal as designed is secured in the airtight tests for PTP sheets (e.g. water pressure reduction tests).

1.4.2. Examples of injections

- Aqueous injections using ampules should be checked if it has no pinholes.
- The plastic containers for pharmaceutical products used for injections (prefilled syringes, plastic bottles, plastic bags, etc.) should be checked when they are shipped to the market if they have been produced as tight containers, as designed, where microorganisms are not contaminated.

2. Terms of packaging for pharmaceutical products

2.1. Basic terms

Primary packaging: Any packaging that is in direct contact with active substances, excipients, or preparations, and should not give a physical or chemical change to the contents. The primary packaging holds the quality of the pharmaceutical products and provides better performance including convenience.

For example, the primary packaging includes an ampule that is an ''immediate container'' for injections, and a PTP packaging which is an ''inner bag'' for tablets or capsules.

Outside container or outside wrapper: A container or wrapper that is used to contain or to wrap immediate containers or immediate wrappers for the pharmaceutical products for sale or distribution and has a legal label by ordinance[2)] on it.

Tight container: A container that protects the contents from extraneous solids or liquids, from loss of the contents, and from efflorescence, deliquescence, or evaporation under ordinary or customary conditions of handling, shipment, and storage. Where a tight container is specified, it may be replaced by a hermetic container. (General Notices 44)

The tight container includes containers made of plastic resins as the examples of container and packaging often used (bottles, vials, syringes, blister (PTP) packaging, strip packaging, etc.).

Final packaging or marketed packaging: Any packaging that is for pharmaceutical products for sale or distribution and a form of the shipped products to the market by labeling as defined by ordinance[2,3)].

The final packaging may be used for irradiation when a radiation sterilization method is used.

Labeling and packaging materials[4)]: Product's containers, wrappers, and labeling including package insert.

Immediate wrapper: A container in which pharmaceutical products are contained directly (papers, clothes, plastics, and aluminum bags). It can be sold or distributed as it is by labeling as defined by ordinance[3)]. There is an inner bag as an example of immediate wrapper that it is not sold or distributed as it is and does not require a legal label by ordinance[3)].

The immediate wrapper in which the pharmaceutical products are contained directly is also referred to as the primary packaging.

Immediate container: A solid container in which the drugs are directly contained (cans, bottles, ampules, vials, tubes, containers for eye drops, boxes, etc.). It can be sold or distributed as it is by labeling as defined by ordinance[3)]. In addition, the paper boxes will be the immediate container, if they use the PTP packaging as an inner bag like tablets.

The immediate container in which the drugs are contained directly is also referred to as a primary packaging.

Inner bag: For example, a plastic bag used under the wrapper for moisture-proof and light resistance and a drug bag that contains each single dose of powder. It is referred as a plastic bag, strip packaging, blister packaging (such as a PTP packaging), and a plastic container for suppositories. In addition, when the pharmaceutical products are contained directly in the inner bag, it corresponds to an immediate packaging, however, if it is not sold or distributed as it is, a legal label by ordinance[3)] is not required.

The inner bag in which the drugs are contained directly is also referred to as a primary packaging.

Secondary packaging: Any packaging that is a single or multiple packaging to compensate for a primary packaging and is not in direct contact with active substances, excipients, or preparations. Any secondary packaging can keep the quality of pharmaceutical products and add performance, such as preventing errors and convenience in the use of pharmaceutical products.

Wrapper: A container or parcel made of soft materials such as paper, cloth, plastic, and aluminum bag. As examples of the wrapper for pharmaceutical products, there are medicine envelope, plastic bag, strip packaging, and blister packaging (such as a PTP packaging).

Labeling[5)]: A labeling defined by ordinance[2,3)], which is a product label and package insert.

Sealing: Sealing from which drugs cannot be taken out unless opened and does not allow its original state to be easily restored after being opened, according to ordinance.[6)]

Packaging[7)]: The appropriate materials, containers or wrappers to keep the quality of pharmaceutical products under ordinary or customary conditions of handling, shipment, storage, or usage, and techniques to hold the products in them, or a packaged state.

Hermetic container: A container that is impervious to air or any other gas under ordinary or customary conditions of handling, shipment, and storage. (General Notices 45)

For the injections, ampules, container closure systems, such as vials/rubber closures, glass prefilled syringes may be used as this container. For the other dosage forms, blister (PTP) packaging with both sides of aluminum and metal extrusion tubes may be used as this container.

Well-closed container: A container that protects the contents from extraneous solids and from loss of the drug under ordinary or customary conditions of handling, shipment, and storage. Where a well-closed container is specified, it may be replaced by a tight container. (General Notices 43)

The well-closed container includes paper or plastic bags with one opening made of a flexible material, and cans with metal or plastic resins, etc., as the examples of often used.

Container: A device that holds drugs. The stopper or cap is included as a part of the container. The containers have no physical and chemical reactivity affecting the specified description and quality of the contents (General Notices 42).

As examples of the container for pharmaceutical products, there are cans, bottles, tubes, ampules, vials, and boxes.

Container closure system: A packaging form that consists of the materials used for a primary packaging that is in direct contact with active substances, excipients, or preparations and composed of other materials. A container closure system should be considered in combination with the contents, where the quality cannot be guaranteed with primary packaging alone, the materials used for a secondary packaging should be included.

2.2. Terms of individual packaging or containers

Ampule: A container that is made of a clear or colored glass or plastic that encapsulates drug solution such as injections, or freeze-dried contents. The opening is usually sealed or welded.

Collapsible tube[7]**:** A container that has a nozzle and cap at one end, and the other end is closed, having flexibility to extrude the contents of ointments. This includes metal tubes, plastic tubes, and laminated tubes, etc.

Syringe: A container that is composed of an external cylinder (barrel), a gasket, a pusher (plunger), and a top cap. This may include a needle. It is used for prefilled syringes.

Strip packaging[7]**:** A packaging in which tablets, capsules, powder, and granules are directly tucked between two materials and bonded to the surrounding. It is also referred to as the SP packaging and corresponds to an inner bag or primary packaging as the pharmaceutical products are directly contained.

Vial: A container, a type of bottle, that is made of a clear or colored glass, or plastic used for injections. This is sealed with a rubber closure and aluminum cap.

PTP packaging[7] **(Press through packaging):** Any packaging that is a kind of a blister packaging, using collapsible materials such as aluminum foils to extrude the opening of the plastic forming products. This corresponds to an inner bag or primary packaging as the capsules or tablets are directly contained.

Pillow type packaging[7]**:** Any packaging that is a kind of bag-shaped. For example, in which the vertical central portion is bonded and the top and bottom edges are sealed. Where the primary packaging alone is difficult to ensure quality, a secondary packaging, which consists of composite films laminated with aluminum foils for protection from moisture and lights, is often used.

Plastic bags: A soft container that uses polyethylene or polypropylene resins as single or composite materials, and which has one or more openings. This usually uses a rubber closure as a plug body. It is used as a large volume injection container such as parenteral infusions.

Blister packaging[7]**:** Any packaging where plastic or aluminum foils are heat formed and given one or more pockets and the preparations are put therein, the opening is covered with plastic films, sheets, or aluminum foil, and the periphery to the substrate is bonded or fixed. It refers to the form that is carried out by peeling the film or foil as the preparations are removed, and used for capsules, tablets, prefilled syringes agent, kit products containing a plurality of ampules.

In addition, where the tables, etc. are directly contained, it corresponds to an inner bag or primary packaging.

Single-dose packages: Preparations in single-dose packages. For example, a strip packaging which contains powders or granules for a single dose corresponds to this.

2.3. Terms of packaging performance

Gas barrier packaging[7]**:** Any packaging that gives the function of suppressing gas permeability aimed. This is a low-gas-permeability packaging.

Light resistant container and packaging: A container or packaging which prevents light permeability to protect if the light affects the quality of the contents under ordinary or customary conditions of handling, shipment, and storage. (General Notices 46)

In addition to colored containers to be used, the containers may be covered with shrink films.

Tamper-resistant packaging, tamper-proof packaging[7]**:** Any packaging that is designed to prevent a risk if a person unintentionally handles, or "plays a prank".

Child-resistant packaging, childproof packaging[7]**:** Any packaging that is intended for prevention of accidental ingestion by children and may be used for adults properly not to let children open it accidentally.

Moisture-proof packaging[7]**:** Any packaging that uses a material with moisture-proof performance to protect the pharmaceutical products from the effects of moisture, if necessary, using desiccant to keep the inside dry.

3. Reference

1) FDA Guidance for Industry "Container Closure Systems for Packaging Human Drugs and Biologics", May 1999.
2) November 25, 2014 enforcement, "The Law on Securing Quality, Efficacy and Safety of Products including Pharmaceuticals and Medical Devices" provide in Article 51
3) "The Law on Securing Quality, Efficacy and Safety of Products including Pharmaceuticals and Medical Devices" provided in Article 50
4) MHLW Ministerial Ordinance No. 179, "Ministerial Ordinance on Standards for Manufacturing Control and Quality Control for Drugs and Quasi-drugs" of December 24, 2004 provided in Article 2 Paragraph 2
5) PFSB/CND Notification No. 0830 - 1 Office Memorandum, "Ministerial Ordinance on Standards for Manufacturing Control and Quality Control for Drugs and Quasi-drugs" of August 30, 2013
6) "The Law on Securing Quality, Efficacy and Safety of Products including Pharmaceuticals and Medical Devices" provided in Article 58
7) Japanese Industrial Standards JIS Z 0108: 2012 "Packaging-Vocabulary"

Glossary for Quality by Design (QbD), Quality Risk Management (QRM) and Pharmaceutical Quality System (PQS) *<G0-6-172>*

1. Introduction

The purpose of this glossary is to define terms, used for developing the new concept of quality assurance in ICH Q8 to 11 guidelines so-called Q quartet, and to explain the concept. The terms shown here are determined as the result of discussion for long time in ICH, and are most important to understand the concept of systematic quality assurance based on science and quality risk management, as shown by the guidelines. The usage may not necessarily accord with general usage, however it is necessary to keep in mind that the following definition is used in the regulatory application of pharmaceuticals. The terms used in ICH Q8 to Q11 are shown below in their order. For terms explained in more than one guideline, the name of duplicated guideline is described in parentheses at the end of the corresponding sentence.

2. Glossary

[ICH Q8 Guideline]

Control Strategy: A planned set of controls, derived from current product and process understanding, that ensures process performance and product quality. The controls can include parameters and attributes related to drug substance and drug product materials and components, facility and equipment operating conditions, in-process controls, finished product specifications, and the associated methods and frequency of monitoring and control (ICH Q10, Q11). A control strategy is expected irrespective of development approaches. Under the development approach using Quality by Design, testing, monitoring or controlling can be shifted earlier into the process.

Quality by Design (QbD): A systematic approach to development that begins with predefined objectives and emphasizes product and process understanding and process control, based on sound science and quality risk management.

Continuous Process Verification: An alternative approach to process validation in which manufacturing process performance is continuously monitored and evaluated. Process validation protocol can use Continuous Process Verification (CPV) to the process validation protocol for the initial and ongoing commercial production (ICH Q11). Generally, for initial process validation, CPV is more appropriate when QbD approach has been applied. However, it can also be used when extensive process knowledge has been gained through commercial manufacturing experience.

Process Robustness: Ability of a process to tolerate variability of materials and changes of the process and equipment without negative impact on quality (ICH Q11).

Critical Process Parameter (CPP): A process parameter whose variability has an impact on a critical quality attribute and therefore should be monitored or controlled to ensure the process produces the desired quality.

Critical Quality Attribute (CQA): A physical, chemical, biological or microbiological property or characteristic that should be within an appropriate limit, range, or distribution to ensure the desired product quality (ICH Q11). For example, CQAs of solid oral dosage forms are typically those aspects affecting product purity, strength, drug release and stability as described in ICH Q8, however it is usual to include product purity and strength itself in CQAs.

Formal Experimental Design: A structured, organized method for determining the relationship between factors affecting a process and the output of that process. Also known as "Design of Experiments" (DoE). The factors to be studied in a DoE could come from the risk assessment exercise or prior knowledge.

Design Space (DS): The multidimensional combination and interaction of input variables (e.g., material attributes) and process parameters that have been demonstrated to provide assurance of quality. Working within the design space is not considered as a change. Movement out of the design space is considered to be a change and would normally initiate a regulatory post approval change process. Design space is proposed by the applicant and is subject to regulatory assessment and approval (ICH Q10, Q11). Design space can be updated over the lifecycle as additional knowledge is gained. Since Proven Acceptable Range (PAR) from only univariate experimentation may lack an understanding of interactions between process parameters and/or material attributes, it should be noted that a combination of PAR does not constitute a design space.

Quality: The degree to which a set of inherent properties of a product, system or process fulfills requirements (ICH Q6A, Q8, Q10). The suitability of either a drug substance or a drug product for its intended use. This term includes such attributes as the identity, strength, and purity (ICH Q6A, Q8, Q9, Q10).

Process Analytical Technology (PAT): A system for designing, analyzing, and controlling manufacturing through timely measurements (i.e., during processing) of critical quality and performance attributes of raw and in-process materials and processes with the goal of ensuring final product quality.

Quality Target Product Profile (QTPP): A prospective summary of the quality characteristics of a drug product that ideally will be achieved to ensure the desired quality, taking into account safety and efficacy of the drug product. Quality Target Product Profile describes the design criteria for the product, and should therefore form the basis for development of the product (ICH Q8).

Lifecycle: All phases in the life of a product from the initial development through marketing until the product's discontinuation (ICH Q11).

Real Time Release Testing (RTRT): The ability to evaluate and ensure the quality of in-process and/or final product based on process data, which typically include a valid combination of measured material attributes and process controls (ICHQ11). Parametric release is one type of Real Time Release Testing. It is based on process data rather than testing of material and/or a sample for a specific attribute. For details, refer to "Basic Concepts for Quality Assurance of Drug Substances and Drug Products *<G0-1-172>*" in General Information.

Proven Acceptable Range (PAR): A characterized range of a process parameter for which operation within this range, while keeping other parameters constant, will result in producing a material meeting relevant quality criteria.

[ICH Q9 Guideline]

Decision Maker(s): Person(s) with the competence and authority to make appropriate and timely quality risk management decisions.

Harm: Damage to health, including the damage that can occur from loss of product quality or availability.

Trend: A statistical term referring to the direction or rate of change of a variable(s).

Detectability: The ability to discover or determine the existence, presence, or fact of a hazard.

Severity: A measure of the possible consequences of a hazard.

Product Lifecycle: All phases in the life of the product from the initial development through marketing until the product's discontinuation.

Hazard: The potential source of harm (ISO/IEC Guide 51).

Quality System: The sum of all aspects of a system that implements quality policy and ensures that quality objectives are met.

Requirements: The explicit or implicit needs or expectations of the patients or their surrogates (e.g., health care professionals, regulators and legislators). In this document (ICH Q9), "requirements" refers not only to statutory, legislative, or regulatory requirements, but also to such needs and expectations.

Stakeholder: Any individual, group or organization that can affect, be affected by, or perceive itself to be affected by a risk. Decision makers might also be stakeholders. For the purposes of this guideline, the primary stakeholders are the patient, healthcare professional, regulatory authority, and industry.

Risk: The combination of the probability of occurrence of harm and the severity of that harm (ISO/IEC Guide 51).

Risk Assessment: A systematic process of organizing information to support a risk decision to be made within a risk management process. It consists of the identification of hazards and the analysis and evaluation of risks associated with exposure to those hazards.

Risk Communication: The sharing of information about risk and risk management between the decision maker and other stakeholders.

Risk Control: Actions implementing risk management decisions (ISO Guide 73).

Risk Acceptance: The decision to accept risk (ISO Guide 73).

Risk Reduction: Actions taken to lessen the probability of occurrence of harm and the severity of that harm.

Risk Identification: The systematic use of information to identify potential sources of harm (hazards) referring to the risk question or problem description.

Risk Evaluation: The comparison of the estimated risk to given risk criteria using a quantitative or qualitative scale to determine the significance of the risk.

Risk Analysis: The estimation of the risk associated with the identified hazards.

Risk Management: The systematic application of quality management policies, procedures, and practices to the tasks of assessing, controlling, communicating and reviewing risk.

Risk Review: Review or monitoring of output/results of the risk management process considering (if appropriate) new knowledge and experience about the risk.

[ICH Q10 Guideline]

Innovation: The introduction of new technologies or methodologies.

Pharmaceutical Quality System (PQS): Management system to direct and control a pharmaceutical company with regard to quality (ICH Q10 based upon ISO 9000:2005) .

Outsourced Activities: Activities conducted by a contract acceptor under a written agreement with a contract giver.

State of Control: A condition in which the set of controls consistently provides assurance of continued process performance and product quality.

Performance Indicators: Measurable values used to quantify quality objectives to reflect the performance of an organization, process or system, also known as "performance metrics" in some regions.

Continual Improvement: Recurring activity to increase the ability to fulfil requirements (ISO 9000:2005).

Senior Management: Person(s) who direct and control a company or site at the highest levels with the authority and responsibility to mobilize resources within the company or site (ICH Q10 based in part on ISO 9000:2005).

Capability of a Process: Ability of a process to realize a product that will fulfil the requirements of that product. The concept of process capability can also be defined in statistical terms (ISO 9000:2005).

Product Realization: Achievement of a product with the quality attributes appropriate to meet the needs of patients, health care professionals, and regulatory authorities (including compliance with marketing authorization) and internal customers requirements.

Corrective Action: Action to eliminate the cause of a detected non-conformity or other undesirable situation. NOTE: Corrective action is taken to prevent recurrence whereas preventive action is taken to prevent occurrence (ISO 9000:2005).

Enabler: A tool or process which provides the means to achieve an objective.

Knowledge Management: Systematic approach to acquiring, analyzing, storing, and disseminating information related to products, manufacturing processes and components.

Quality Planning: Part of quality management focused on setting quality objectives and specifying necessary operational processes and related resources to fulfil the quality objectives (ISO 9000:2005).

Quality Policy: Overall intentions and direction of an organization related to quality as formally expressed by senior management (ISO 9000:2005).

Quality Manual: Document specifying the quality management system of an organization (ISO 9000:2005).

Quality Objectives: A means to translate the quality policy and strategies into measurable activities.

Quality Risk Management (QRM): A systematic process for the assessment, control, communication and review of risks to the quality of the drug (medicinal) product across the product lifecycle (ICH Q9, Q10). For details, refer to "Basic Concept of Quality Risk Management <*G0-2-170*>" in General Information.

Feedback/Feedforward: The modification or control of a process or system by its results or effects. Feedback/feedforward can be applied technically in process control strategies and conceptually in quality management. Feedback is to reflect results to a previous process (for example: a control of the supply of materials in a previous process), and feedforward is to reflect results to a subsequent process (for example: a control of time for drying in a subsequent process).

Change Management: A systematic approach to proposing, evaluating, approving, implementing and reviewing changes.

Preventive Action: Action to eliminate the cause of a potential non-conformity or other undesirable potential situation.

Note: Preventive action is taken to prevent occurrence whereas corrective action is taken to prevent recurrence (ISO 9000:2005).

[ICH Q11 Guideline]

Chemical Transformation Step: For Chemical Entities, a step involved in the synthesis of the chemical structure of the drug substance from precursor molecular fragments. Typically it involves C—X or C—C bond formation or breaking.

Contaminants: Any adventitiously introduced materials (e.g., chemical, biochemical, or microbial species) not intended to be part of the manufacturing process of the drug substance or drug product (ICH Q6B).

3. References

1) ICH: Guideline for Q8(R2), Pharmaceutical Development.
2) ICH: Guideline for Q9, Quality Risk Management.
3) ICH: Guideline for Q10, Pharmaceutical Quality Systems.
4) ICH: Guideline for Q11, Development and Manufacture of Drug Substance (Chemical Entities and Biotechnological/Biological Entities).
5) ICH: Quality Implementation Working Group, Points to Consider (R2), ICH-Endorsed Guide for ICH Q8/Q9/Q10 Implementation
6) ICH: Quality Implementation Working Group on Q8, Q9 and Q10 Questions & Answers (R4)

G1 Physics and Chemistry

Validation of Analytical Procedures *<G1-1-130>*

The validation of an analytical procedure is the process of confirming that the analytical procedure employed for a test of pharmaceutics is suitable for its intended use. In other word, the validation of an analytical procedure requires us to demonstrate scientifically that risks in decision by testing caused by errors from analytical steps are acceptably small. The performance of an analytical procedure is established by various kinds of validation characteristics. The validity of a proposed analytical procedure can be shown by demonstrating experimentally that the validation characteristics of the analytical procedure satisfy the standards set up according to the acceptable limits of testing.

When an analytical procedure is to be newly carried in the Japanese Pharmacopoeia, when a test carried in the Japanese Pharmacopoeia is to be revised, and when the test carried in the Japanese Pharmacopoeia is to be replaced with a new test according to regulations in general notices, analytical procedures employed for these tests should be validated according to this document.

1. Required data for analytical procedures to be carried in the Japanese Pharmacopoeia

1.1. Outline

This section should provide a brief explanation of the principle of a proposed analytical procedure, identify the necessity of the analytical procedure and its advantage compared with other procedures, and summarize the validation. When an analytical procedure is revised, the limitation of the current analytical procedure and the advantage offered by the new analytical procedure should be described.

1.2. Analytical procedure

This section should contain a complete description of the analytical procedure to enable skilled persons to evaluate correctly the analytical procedure and replicate it if necessary. Analytical procedures include all important operating procedures for performing analyses, the preparation of standard samples, reagents and test solutions, precautions, procedures to verify system suitability (e.g. the verification of the separating performance of a chromatographic system), formulas to obtain results, the number of replications and so forth. Any instruments and apparatus that are not stated in the Japanese Pharmacopoeia should be described in detail. The physical, chemical or biological characteristics of any new reference standards should be clarified and their testing methods should be established.

1.3. Data showing the validity of analytical procedures

This section should provide complete data showing the validity of the analytical procedures. This includes the experimental design to determine the validation characteristics, experimental data, calculation results and results of hypothesis tests.

2. Validation characteristics

The definition of typical validation characteristics to be assessed in validation of analytical procedures and examples of assessing procedures are given below.

The terminology and definitions of the validation characteristics may possibly vary depending upon the fields to which analytical procedures are applied. The terminology and definitions shown in this document are established for the purpose of the Japanese Pharmacopoeia. Typical methods for assessing the validation characteristics are shown in the item of assessment. Various kinds of methods to determine the validation characteristics have been proposed and any methods that are widely accepted will be accepted for the present purpose. However, since values of the validation characteristics may possibly depend upon methods of determination, it is required to present the methods of determining the validation characteristics, the data and calculation methods in sufficient detail.

Although robustness is not listed as a validation characteristic, it should be considered during the development of analytical procedures. Studying the robustness may help to improve analytical procedures and to establish appropriate analytical conditions including precautions.

2.1. Accuracy/Trueness

2.1.1. Definition

The accuracy is a measure of the bias of observed values obtained by an analytical procedure. The accuracy is expressed as the difference between the average value obtained from a large series of observed values and the true value.

2.1.2. Assessment

The estimate of accuracy of an analytical method is expressed as the difference between the total mean of observed values obtained during investigation of the reproducibility and the true value. A certified value or a consensus value may be used as the true value. When an analytical procedure for a drug product is considered, the observed value of the standard solution of the drug substance may be used as the consensus value.

It may be inferred from specificity data that an analytical procedure is unbiased.

A 95% confidence interval of the accuracy should be calculated using the obtained estimate of accuracy and the standard error based on the reproducibility (intermediate precision). It should be confirmed that the confidence interval includes zero or that the upper or lower confidence limits are within the range of the accuracy required of the analytical procedure.

2.2. Precision

2.2.1. Definition

The precision is a measure of the closeness of agreement between observed values obtained independently from multiple samplings of a homogenous sample and is expressed as the variance, standard deviation or relative standard deviation (coefficient of variation) of observed values.

The precision should be considered at three levels with different repetition conditions; repeatability, intermediate precision and reproducibility.

(i) Repeatability/Intra-assay precision

The repeatability expresses the precision of observed values obtained from multiple samplings of a homogenous sample over a short time interval within a laboratory, by the same analyst, using the same apparatus and instruments, lots of reagents and so forth (repeatability conditions).

(ii) Intermediate precision

The intermediate precision expresses the precision of observed values obtained from multiple samplings of a homogenous sample by changing a part of or all of the operating conditions including analysts, experimental dates, apparatus and instruments and lots of reagents within a laboratory (intermediate precision condition).

(iii) Reproducibility

The reproducibility expresses the precision of observed values obtained from multiple samplings of a homogenous sample in different laboratories (reproducibility condition).

2.2.2. Assessment

A sufficient volume of a homogenous sample should be prepared before studying the precision. The solution is assumed to be homogenous. When it is difficult to obtain a homogenous sample, the following samples may be used as homogenous samples; e.g., a large amount of drug products or mixture of drug substance and vehicles that are crushed and mixed well until they can be assumed to be homogenous.

Suitable experimental designs such as one-way layout may be employed when more than one level of precision is to be investigated simultaneously. A sufficient number of repetitions, levels of operating conditions and laboratories should be employed. Sources of variations affecting analytical results should be evaluated as thoroughly as possible through the validation.

It is required to show the variance, standard deviation and relative standard deviation (coefficient of variation) of each level of precision. The 90% confidence interval of the variance and corresponding intervals of the standard deviation should also be established. The validity of the proposed analytical procedure for its intended use may be confirmed by comparing obtained values with the reference values of precision required for the analytical procedure. Whether the proposed analytical procedure is acceptable may normally be decided based on the reproducibility.

2.3. Specificity

2.3.1. Definition

The specificity is the ability of an analytical procedure to measure accurately an analyte in the presence of components that may be expected to be present in the sample matrix. The specificity is a measure of discriminating ability. Lack of specificity of an analytical procedure may be compensated by other supporting analytical procedures.

2.3.2. Assessment

It should be confirmed that the proposed analytical procedure can identify an analyte or that it can accurately measure the amount or concentration of an analyte in a sample. For example, the specificity may be assessed by comparing analytical results obtained from a sample containing the analyte only with results obtained from samples containing excipients, related substances or degradation products, and including or excluding the analyte. If reference standards of impurities are unavailable, samples that are expected to contain impurities or degradation products may be used (e.g. samples after accelerated or stress tests).

2.4. Detection limit

2.4.1. Definition

The detection limit is the lowest amount or concentration of the analyte in a sample that is detectable, but not necessarily quantifiable.

2.4.2. Assessment

The detection limit should be normally determined so that producer's and consumer's risks are less than 5%. The detection limit may be calculated using the standard deviation of responses of blank samples or samples containing an analyte close to the detection limit and the slope of the calibration curve close to the detection limit. The following equation is an example to determine the detection limit using the standard deviation of responses of blank samples and the slope of the calibration curve.

$$DL = 3.3\sigma/slope$$

DL: detection limit

σ: the standard deviation of responses of blank samples

slope: slope of the calibration curve

The noise level may be used as the standard deviation of responses of blank samples in chromatographic methods.

It should be ensured that the detection limit of the analytical procedure is lower than the specified limit for testing.

2.5. Quantitation limit

2.5.1. Definition

The quantitation limit is the lowest amount or concentration of the analyte in a sample that can be determined. The precision expressed as the relative standard deviation of samples containing an analyte at the quantitation limit is usually 10%.

2.5.2. Assessment

The quantitation limit may be calculated using the standard deviation of responses of blank samples or samples containing an analyte close to the quantitation limit and the slope of the calibration curve close to the quantitation limit. The following equation is an example to determine the quantitation limit using the standard deviation of responses of blank samples and the slope of the calibration curve.

$$QL = 10\sigma/slope$$

QL: quantitation limit

σ: the standard deviation of responses of blank samples

slope: slope of the calibration curve

The noise level may be used as the standard deviation of responses of blank samples in chromatographic methods.

It should be ensured that the quantitation limit of the analytical procedure is lower than the specified limit for testing.

2.6. Linearity

2.6.1. Definition

The linearity is the ability of an analytical procedure to elicit responses linearly related to the amount or concentration of an analyte in samples. A well-defined mathematical transformation may sometimes be necessary to obtain a linear relationship.

2.6.2. Assessment

Responses are obtained after analyzing samples repeatedly with various amounts or concentrations of an analyte according to described operating procedures. The linearity may be evaluated in terms of the correlation coefficient and the regression equation. It may be also helpful for evaluating the linearity to plot residual errors from the regression line against the amount or concentration and to confirm that there is no particular tendency in the graph. Samples with five different amounts or concentrations of an analyte should be usually investigated.

2.7. Range

2.7.1. Definition

The range for the validation of analytical procedures is the interval between the lower and upper limits of the amount or concentration of an analyte providing sufficient accuracy and precision. The range for the validation of analytical procedures for an analytical procedure with linearity is the interval between the lower and upper limits providing sufficient accuracy, precision and linearity.

2.7.2. Assessment

When the range for the validation of analytical procedures is investigated, 80 to 120% of specified limits of testing should be usually considered. The accuracy, precision and linearity should be evaluated using samples containing the lower and upper limits and in the middle of the range.

3. Categories of tests employing analytical procedures

Tests covered with this document are roughly classified into three categories shown below according to their purposes. The table lists the normally required validation characteristics to be evaluated in the validation of analytical procedures used in these tests. This list should be considered to represent typical validation characteristics. This is a principle, and validation characteristics to be assessed vary depending upon the characteristics of analytical procedures and their intended use.

(i) Type I Identification. Tests for identifying major components in pharmaceuticals according to their characteristics.

(ii) Type II Impurity tests. Tests for determination of impurities in pharmaceuticals.

(iii) Type III Tests for assaying components in pharmaceuticals.

(Additives such as stabilizing agents and preservatives are included in components.) Tests for determining performance of pharmaceuticals, such as dissolution testing.

Table Lists of validation characteristics required to be evaluated in tests of each type

Validation characteristics \ Type of test	Type I	Type II		Type III
		Quantitation test	Limit test	
Accuracy/Trueness	−	+	−	+
Precision				
Repeatability	−	+	−	+
Intermediate precision	−	−*	−	−*
Reproducibility	−	+*	−	+*
Specificity**	+	+	+	+
Detection limit	−	−	+	−
Quantitation limit	−	+	−	−
Linearity	−	+	−	+
Range	−	+	−	+

− Usually need not to be evaluated.

\+ Usually need to be evaluated.

* Either intermediate precision or reproducibility should be evaluated depending upon circumstances in which analytical procedures or tests are performed. The latter should be normally evaluated in the validation of analytical procedures proposed to be included in the Japanese Pharmacopoeia.

** The lack of the specificity of an analytical procedure may be compensated by other relevant analytical procedures

4. Terminology used in the validation of analytical procedures

(i) Analytical procedure: This document covers analytical procedures applied to identification, and ones that provides responses depending upon the amount or concentration of analytes in samples. Analytical procedures in this document mean analytical processes of tests.

(ii) Laboratory: The laboratory means an experimental room or facility where tests are performed. In this document different laboratories are expected to perform an analytical procedure using different analysts, different experimental apparatus and instruments, different lots of reagents and so forth.

(iii) Number of replications: The number of replications is one that is described in analytical procedures. An observed value is often obtained by more than one measurement in order to achieve good precision of analytical procedures. Analytical procedures including the number of replications should be validated.

This is different from repetition in the validation of analytical procedures to obtain precision.

(iv) Observed value: The value of a characteristic obtained as the result of performing an analytical procedure.

(v) Consumer's risk: This is the probability that products out of the specification of tests are decided to be accepted after testing. It is usually expressed as β, and is called the probability of type II error or the probability of false negative in impurity tests.

(vi) Producer's risk: This is the probability that products satisfying the specification of tests are decided to be rejected after testing. It is usually expressed as α, and is called the probability of type I error or the probability of false positive in impurity tests.

(vii) Robustness: The robustness is a measure of the capacity to remain unaffected by small but deliberate variations in analytical conditions. The stability of observed values may be studied by changing various analytical conditions within suitable ranges including pH values of solutions, reaction temperature, reaction time or amount of reagents added. When observed values are unstable, the analytical procedure should be improved. Results of studying robustness may be reflected in the developed analytical procedure as precautions or significant digits describing analytical conditions.

(viii) Test: Tests mean various tests described in general tests and official monographs in the Japanese Pharmacopoeia such as impurity tests and assay. They include sampling methods, specification limits and analytical procedures.

System Suitability *<G1-2-152>*

In order to ensure the reliability on the results of drug analyses, it is essential to verify that the test method to be applied to the test, including the method prescribed in the Japanese Pharmacopoeia (JP), can give the results adequate for its intended use using the analytical system in the laboratory in which the test is to be performed, then to carry out system suitability testing for confirming that the analytical system maintains the state suitable for the quality test.

1. Definition and role of system suitability

"System Suitability" is the concept for ensuring that the

performance of the analytical system is as suitable for the analysis of the drug as was at the time when the verification of the test method was performed using the system. Usually, system suitability testing should be carried out at every series of drug analysis. The test procedures and acceptance criteria of system suitability testing must be prescribed in the test methods of drugs. The results of drug analyses are not acceptable unless the requirements of system suitability have been met.

System suitability testing is an integral part of test methods using analytical instruments, and based on the concept that the equipments, electronic data processing systems, analytical operations, samples to be analyzed and operators constitute an integral system that can be evaluated, when the test procedures and acceptance criteria of system suitability testing are prescribed in the test methods.

2. Points to consider in setting system suitability

Parameters of system suitability testing to be prescribed in the test method depend on the intended use and type of analytical method. Since system suitability testing is to be carried out in a routine manner, it is preferable to select the parameters necessary for ensuring that the analytical system maintains the state suitable for the analysis of the drug and to prescribe its test procedure able to carry out easily and rapidly.

For example, in the case of quantitative purity tests using liquid chromatography or gas chromatography, the evaluation of parameters such as "System performance" (to confirm the ability to analyze target substance specifically), "System repeatability" (to confirm that the degree of variation in the analytical results of target substance in replicate injections is within the allowable limit) and "Test for required detectability" (to confirm the linearity of chromatographic response around the specification limit) are usually required.

The followings are supplements to the section of system suitability prescribed in "Liquid Chromatography".

2.1. System repeatability of HPLC and GC

2.1.1. Allowable limit of system repeatability

It is described in the section of system suitability in "Liquid Chromatography" that "In principle, total number of replicate injections should be 6", and "The allowable limit of "System repeatability" should be set at an appropriate level based on the data when suitability of the method for the evaluation of quality of the drug was verified, and the precision necessary for the quality test". Based on the above description, an allowable limit of system repeatability for 6 replicate injections should be set in consideration with the following descriptions. However, in the case that the test method prescribed in the JP monograph is used for the test, the allowable limit of system repeatability prescribed in the monograph should be applied.

(i) Assay for drug substance (for drug substance with the content nearby 100%): An adequate allowable limit should be set at the level that the chromatographic system is able to give the precision suitable for the evaluation of variation in the content of active ingredient within and among the batches of drug substance. For example, the allowable limit of "not more than 1.0%" is usually recommended for the drug substances whose width of content specification are not more than 5%, as is in the case of content specification of 98.0 - 102.0% which is often observed in the assay using liquid chromatography.

(ii) Assay for drug products: An adequate allowable limit should be set considering the width of content specification of the drug product and the allowable limit prescribed in the assay of drug substance (when the drug product is analyzed by a method with the same chromatographic conditions as those used for the analysis of drug substance).

(iii) Purity test for related substances: An adequate allowable limit should be set considering the concentration of active ingredients in the solution used for the system repeatability testing such as a standard solution or solution for system suitability testing. In the case that a solution with active ingredient concentration of 0.5 - 1.0% is used for the test of system repeatability, an allowable limit of "not more than 2.0%" is usually recommended.

Recommendations for allowable limits described above should not be applicable to gas chromatography.

2.1.2. Method for decreasing the number of replicate injections without losing the quality of system repeatability testing

It is described in the section of system suitability in "Liquid Chromatography" that "In principle, total number of replicate injections should be 6. However, in the case that a long time is necessary for one analysis, such as the analysis using the gradient method, or the analysis of samples containing late eluting components, it may be acceptable to decrease the number of replicate injections by adopting new allowable limit of "System repeatability" which can guarantee a level of "System repeatability" equivalent to that at 6 replicate injections." In consideration of the above description, a method for decreasing the number of replicate injections without losing the quality of system repeatability testing is described below. One can set the test for system repeatability with reduced number of replicate injections by utilizing this method, if necessary, and routine quality tests can be performed based on the same approach.

The following table shows the allowable limits to be attained in the test at 3 - 5 replicate injections ($n = 3 - 5$) to

Table Allowable limits to be attained in the test at 3 - 5 replicate injections ($n = 3 - 5$) to keep the quality of test equivalent to that of test at $n = 6$*

		Allowable limit (RSD)					
Allowable limit prescribed in the test of $n = 6$		1%	2%	3%	4%	5%	10%
Allowable limit to be attained	$n = 5$	0.88%	1.76%	2.64%	3.52%	4.40%	8.81%
	$n = 4$	0.72%	1.43%	2.15%	2.86%	3.58%	7.16%
	$n = 3$	0.47%	0.95%	1.42%	1.89%	2.37%	4.73%

* The probability for inadequate analytical systems to meet the requirements of system suitability testing, is supposed to be 5%.

keep the quality test equivalent to that of test at $n = 6$.

However, it should be kept in mind that since decrease in the number of replicate injections results in increase in the weight of each injection, it becomes more important to perform the test by the experienced operator, and to maintain the equipment in a suitable state.

3. Points to consider at the change of analytical system (Change control of analytical system)

When the test method and analytical system verified is continuously used for the quality test without any change, it is sufficient to confirm the compliance to the requirements of system suitability at every series of drug analysis.

However, when the test is performed for a long period, a situation in which some changes in the analytical system are inevitable, may occur. These changes don't affect the quality of the product itself, but they affect the scale in the evaluation of product quality. If the change in the analytical system may induce a significant deviation of the scale, it may lead to the acceptance of products with inadequate quality and/or the rejection of products with adequate quality. Thus, at the time of change in the analytical system, it is necessary to check whether the change is appropriate or not, to avoid the deviation of the scale in the evaluation of product quality.

In the case of the change of test method, it is required to perform an adequate validation depending on the extent of the change. On the other hand, in the case of the change of analytical system in a laboratory, such as renewal of apparatus or column of liquid chromatography, and the change of operator, it is necessary to perform at least system suitability testing using the system after change, and to confirm that the equivalency of the results before and after change.

In the case that equivalent results would not be obtained after change, for example, when a renewal of column of liquid chromatograph may induce a significant change of elution pattern, such as the reversal of elution order between target ingredient of the test and substance for checking resolution, it is required to perform a revalidation of the analytical system for the test using new column, since it is uncertain whether the specificity and/or other validation characteristics necessary for estimating target ingredient is kept or not.

Near Infrared Spectrometry
<G1-3-161>

Near infrared spectrometry (NIR) is one of spectroscopic methods used to qualitatively and quantitatively evaluate substances from analysis of data obtained by determining their absorption spectrum of light in the near-infrared range.

The near-infrared range lies between the visible light and infrared light, typically of wavelengths (wave numbers) between 750 and 2500 nm (13,333 - 4000 cm^{-1}). The absorption of near-infrared light occurs due to harmonic overtones from normal vibration or combination tones in the infrared range (4000 to 400 cm^{-1}), primarily absorption of O-H, N-H, C-H and S-H that involve hydrogen atoms, in particular. For instance the asymmetrical stretching vibration of N-H occurs in the vicinity of 3400 cm^{-1}, but the absorption due to the first harmonic overtone occurs in the vicinity of 6600 cm^{-1} (wavelength 1515 nm), which is near double 3400 cm^{-1}.

Absorption in the near-infrared range is far weaker than absorption due to normal vibration that occurs in the infrared range. Furthermore, in comparison with visible light, near-infrared light has longer wavelength, which makes it possible for the light to penetrate to a depth of several mm into solid specimens including fine particles. This method is often utilized as a nondestructive analysis, as changes occurring with absorbed light spectrum (transmitted light or reflected light) in this process provide physical and chemical information pertaining to specimens.

Conventional spectrometry, such as calibration curve method, is used as a method for analyzing near-infrared absorption spectrum whenever applicable. Ordinarily, however, chemometrics methods are used for analysis. Chemometrics ordinarily involve quantification of chemical data, as well as numerical and statistical procedures for computerization of information. Chemometrics for near-infrared spectrometry includes various types of multivariate analysis such as multiple regression analysis, to perform qualitative or quantitative evaluation of active substances.

Near-infrared spectrometry is used as a rapid and nondestructive method of analysis that replaces conventional and established analysis methods for water determinations or substance verifications. It is necessary to perform a comparison test to evaluate this method against an existing analysis method, to verify that this method is equivalent to such existing analysis method, before using this analysis method as a quality evaluation test method in routine tests.

Applications of near-infrared spectrometry in the pharmaceutical field include qualitative or quantitative evaluation of ingredients, additives or water contents of active substances or preparations. Furthermore, near-infrared spectrometry can also be used for evaluation of physical conditions of substances, such as crystal forms, crystallinity, particle diameters. It is also possible to perform spectrometry on samples that are located in a remote location away from equipment main units, without sampling, by using optical fibers. It can therefore be used as an effective means to perform pharmaceutical manufacturing process control online (or in-line).

1. Equipment

Near-infrared spectrophotometers can either be a distributed near-infrared spectrophotometer or a Fourier transform near-infrared spectrophotometer[1)]. Interference filter-type near-infrared spectrophotometers that use interference filter in the spectrometry section are also available, however, this type of equipment is hardly used in the field of pharmaceutical quality control.

1.1. Distributed near-infrared spectrophotometer

This equipment is comprised of light source section, sample section, spectrometry section, photometry section, signal processing section, data processing section, display-record-output section. Halogen lamps, tungsten lamps, light emitting diodes and other such devices that can emit high intensity near-infrared light in a stable manner are used in the light source section. The sample section is comprised of a sample cell and a sample holder. Equipment that has an optical fiber section that is comprised of optical fibers and a collimator are equipped with a function for transmitting light to sample section, which is remotely located away from the spectrophotometer main unit. Quartz is ordinarily used as material for optical fibers.

The spectrometry section is intended to extract light of required wavelength, using dispersive devices and is comprised of slits, mirrors and dispersive devices. Potential dispersive devices include prisms, diffraction grating, acousto-optical tunable filters (AOTF), or liquid crystal tunable filters (LCTF). The photometry section is comprised of detectors and amplifiers. Sensors include semiconductor detectors (silicon, lead sulfide, indium-gallium-arsenic, indium-antimony), as well as photomultiplier tubes. Detecting methods that use semiconductor detectors generally perform detections with single elements, but there are also occasions where arraytype detectors that use multiple elements are used. Such detectors are capable of simultaneously detecting multiple wavelengths (wave numbers). The signal processing section separates signals required for measurements from output signals fed by amplifiers and then outputs such isolated signals. The data processing section performs data conversions and spectral analysis, etc. The display-record-output section outputs data, analysis results and data processing results to a printer.

1.2. Fourier transform near-infrared spectrophotometer

The configuration of the equipment is fundamentally same as that of the distributed-type equipment described in Section 1.1., except for the spectrometry section and the signal processing section.

The spectrometry section is comprised of interferometers, sampling signal generators, detectors, amplifiers, A/D conversion devices, etc. Interferometers include Michelson interferometers, transept interferometers and polarization interferometers. The signal processing section is equipped with functions that are required for spectrometer, as well as a function for translating acquired interference waveform (interferogram) into absorption spectrum by Fourier transformation.

2. Determination

There are three types of measurement methods that are used with near-infrared spectrometry: transmittance method, diffuse reflectance method and transmittance reflectance method. The selection of measurement methods relies on the shape of samples and applications. The transmittance method or diffuse reflectance method is used for solid samples, including fine particles. The transmittance method or transmittance reflectance method is used for liquid samples.

2.1. Transmittance method

The degree of decay for incident light intensity as the light from a light source passes through a sample, is represented as transmittance rate T (%) or absorbance A with the transmittance method. A sample is placed in the light path between a light source and a detector, the arrangement of which is ordinarily same as that of the spectroscopic method.

$$T = 100t$$
$$t = I/I_0 = 10^{-\alpha cl}$$

I_0: Incident light intensity
I: Transmitted light intensity
α: Absorptivity
c: Solution concentration
l: Layer length (sample thickness)

$$A = -\log t = \log(1/t) = \log(I_0/I) = \alpha cl$$

This method is applied for taking measurements of samples that are liquids and solutions. Quartz glass cells and flow cells are used, with the layer length of 1 - 5 mm along. Furthermore, this method can also be applied for taking measurements of samples that are solids, including fine particles. It is also known as diffuse transmittance method. Selecting appropriate layer length is critical for this method, since the transmitted light intensity varies depending on grain sizes and surface condition of samples.

2.2. Diffuse reflectance method

The ratio of the reflection light intensity I, emitted from the sample in a wide reflectance range and a control reflection light intensity I_r emitted from surface of a substance, is expressed as reflectance R (%) with the diffuse reflectance method. The near-infrared light penetrates to a depth of several mm into solid samples, including fine particles. In that process, transmission, refraction, reflection and dispersion are repeated, and diffusion takes place, but a portion of the diffused light is emitted again from the surface of the sample and captured by a detector. The spectrum for the diffuse reflectance absorbance (A_r) can ordinarily be obtained by plotting logarithm of inverse numbers for reflectance ($1/r$) against wavelengths (wave numbers).

$$R = 100r$$
$$r = I/I_r$$

I: Reflection light intensity of light, diffuse reflected off the sample
I_r: Control reflection light intensity of light emitted from surface of reference substance

$$A_r = \log(1/r) = \log(I_r/I)$$

The intensity of diffuse reflectance spectrum can also be expressed with the Kubelka-Munk (K-M) function. The K-M function is derived, based on the existence of a sample with sufficient thickness, and expressed in terms of light scattering coefficient, which is determined by absorptivity, grain size, shape and fill condition (compression).

This method is applied to solid samples, including fine particles, and requires a diffuse reflector.

2.3. Transmittance reflectance method

The transmittance reflectance method is a combination of the transmittance method and reflectance method. A mirror is used to re-reflect a light that has passed through a sample in order to take a measurement of transmittance reflectance rate, T^* (%). Light path must be twice the thickness of the sample. On the other hand, the light reflected by a mirror and being introduced into a detector is used as the control light. When this method is applied to suspended samples, however, a metal plate or a ceramic reflector with rough surface that causes diffuse reflectance is used instead of a mirror.

Transmittance reflectance absorbance (A^*) is obtained by the following formula with this method:

$$T^* = 100t^*$$
$$t^* = I/I_T$$

I: Intensity of transmitted and reflected light, in cases where a sample is placed
I_T: Intensity of reflected light, in cases where there is no sample

$$A^* = \log(1/t^*)$$

This is a method that is applied to solid samples, including fine particles, as well as liquids and suspended samples. The thickness of a sample must be adjusted when applying this method to a solid sample. Ordinarily adjustment is made by setting absorbance to 0.1 - 2 (transmittance of 79 - 1%), which provides the best linearity and SN ratio of detector. A cell with appropriate layer length, according to the grain size of the fine particle, must be selected when applying the method to a fine particle sample.

3. Factors that affect spectrum

Following items must be considered as factors that can affect spectrum when applying near-infrared spectrometry, particularly when conducting quantitative analysis.

(i) Sample temperature: A significant change (wavelength shift, for example) can occur when the temperature varies by a several degree (°C). Care must be taken, particularly when the sample is a solution or contains water.

(ii) Water or residual solvent: Water or residual solvent contents of a sample, as well as water (humidity) in the environment wherein measurements are taken, can significantly affect absorption band of the near-infrared range.

(iii) Sample thickness: The thickness of a sample is a factor for spectral changes and therefore needs to be controlled at a certain thickness. A sample may be considered to be of adequate thickness for the diffuse reflectance method, however, if the thickness is less than a certain amount, for example, the sample may have to be placed on a support plate with high reflectance to take measurements by the transmittance reflectance method.

(iv) Fill condition of sample: The condition of sample fill can potentially affect a spectrum, when taking measurements of samples that are solids or fine particles. Care must be taken with filling samples in a cell, to ensure that a certain amount is filled through a specific procedure.

(v) Optical characteristics of samples: When a sample is physically, chemically or optically uneven, relatively large beam size must be used, multiple samples must be used, measurements must be taken at multiple points on the same samples, or a sample must be pulverized to ensure averaging of the sample. Grain size, fill condition, as well as roughness of surface can also affect fine particle samples.

(vi) Polymorphism: Variations in crystal structures (polymorphism) can also affect spectrum. In cases where multiple crystal forms exist, it is necessary to have consideration for characteristics of samples to be considered and care must be taken to ensure that even standard samples for calibration curve method have diversified distributions similar to that of samples that are subject to analysis.

(vii) Temporal changes in characteristics of samples: Samples can potentially undergo chemical, physical or optical property changes, due to passing of time or storage after sampling, and such changes affect spectrum in a subtle manner. For instance even with identical samples, if elapsed times differ, then their characteristics of near-infrared spectrum can vary significantly. In creating calibration curves, therefore, the samples to be used must be prepared with adequate considerations for reducing the time to be measured, such as the measurement is carried out offline in a laboratory or online in manufacturing process (or inline).

4. Control of equipment performance[2,3)]

4.1. Accuracy of wavelengths (wave numbers)

The accuracy of wavelengths (wave numbers) of an equipment is derived from the deviation of the absorption peaks of substances for which peak absorption wavelengths (wave numbers) have been defined, such as polystyrene, mixture of rare earth oxides (dysprosium, holmium and erbium; 1:1:1) or steam, from the figures indicated on the equipment. Tolerance figures in the vicinity of 3 peaks are ordinarily set in the following manner, though appropriate tolerance figures can be set, depending on the intended purpose:

$$1200 \pm 1 \text{ nm } (8300 \pm 8 \text{ cm}^{-1})$$
$$1600 \pm 1 \text{ nm } (6250 \pm 4 \text{ cm}^{-1})$$
$$2000 \pm 1.5 \text{ nm } (5000 \pm 4 \text{ cm}^{-1})$$

Since the location of absorption peaks vary, depending on the substance used as reference, absorption peaks of wavelengths (wave numbers) that are closest to the above 3 peaks are selected for suitability evaluations. A mixture of rare earth oxides, for instance, would indicate characteristic absorption peaks at 1261 nm, 1681 nm and 1971 nm.

Absorption peaks at 1155 nm, 1417 nm, 1649 nm, 2352 nm (layer length: 1.0 nm) can be used, when taking measurements with the transmittance method that involve the use of dichloromethane as reference. The absorption peak of steam at 7306.7 cm^{-1} can be used with a Fourier transformation-type spectrophotometer, as its wave number resolution ability is high.

Other substances can also be used as reference, so long as their adequacy for the purpose can be verified.

4.2. Spectroscopic linearity

Appropriate standard plates, such as plate-shaped polymer impregnated with varying concentrations of carbon (Carbon-doped polymer standards), can be used to evaluate spectroscopic linearity. In order to verify linearity, however, standard plates with not less than 4 levels of concentration within the reflectance of 10 – 90% must be used. When measurements are expected to be taken with absorbance of no less than 1.0, it is necessary to add standard plates with reflectance of either 2% or 5% or both.

In order to plot absorbance (A_{OBS}) of such standard plates at locations in the vicinity of wavelengths 1200 nm, 1600 nm and 2000 nm against absorbance (A_{REF}) assigned to each standard plate, verifications must be made to ensure that the gradient of linearity obtained are ordinarily within the range 1.0 ± 0.05 for each of these wavelengths and 0 ± 0.05 for ordinate intercept. Depending on the intended purpose, appropriate tolerance figures can be set.

4.3. Spectrophotometric noise

The spectrophotometric noise of the equipment can be checked using appropriate reflectance standard plates, such as white-colored reflecting ceramic tiles or reflective thermoplastic resin (such as polytetrafluoroethylene).

4.3.1. High flux noise

Spectrophotometric noise is evaluated by using standard plates with high reflectance, such as reflectance of 99%. Standard plates are used to take measurements for both samples and control samples. Generally, the average value obtained from calculation of mean square root (*RMS*) of noise for each 100 nm segments in the wavelength range of 1200 – 2200 nm ordinarily must not be more than 0.3×10^{-3} and individual values must not exceed 0.8×10^{-3}. Depending on the intended purpose, appropriate tolerance figures can be set.

$$RMS = \{1/N \cdot \Sigma (A_i - A_m)^2\}^{1/2}$$

N: Number of measurement points per segment
A_i: Absorbance at each measurement point of segment
A_m: Average absorbance for segment

4.3.2. Low flux noise

Spectrophotometric noise is evaluated by using standard plates with low reflectance, such as reflectance of 10%, when the amount of light is low. In such cases, light source, optical system, detector and electronic circuit systems all have some impact on noise. Similar to the cases of high flux noise, generally, the average value obtained from calculation of *RMS* for each 100 nm segments in the wavelength range of 1200 – 2200 nm ordinarily must not be more than 1.0×10^{-3} and individual values must not exceed 2.0×10^{-3}. Depending on the intended purpose, appropriate tolerance figures can be set.

5. Application of qualitative or quantitative analysis

Unlike in the infrared range, mainly harmonic overtones and combinations manifest as spectrum in the near-infrared range. Such absorbance spectrums are often observed as overlay of absorption bands of functional groups and atomic groups. The near-infrared spectrometry, therefore, differs from conventional analysis methods that correspond to each application, by preparing model analysis methods using methodologies of chemometrics, such as multivariate analysis, and needs to establish analytical methods depending on the intended purpose.

Characteristics of near-infrared absorption spectrum must be emphasized and effects of complexities of spectrums, as well as overlay of absorption bands must be reduced by performing mathematical preprocesses, such as primary or secondary spectral differentiation processes or normalizations, which becomes one of vital procedures in establishing analysis methods that use methodologies of chemometrics. While there are many chemometrics methodologies and mathematical preprocessing methods for data, appropriate combinations must be selected that suit the purposes of intended analysis.

Evaluation of validity based on analysis parameters is ordinarily required for the analysis validation when establishing a near-infrared analysis method. Selection of parameters that are appropriate for applications must be made for its intended use. Furthermore, following issues must be considered, in conformity with attributes of the near-infrared spectrometry.

(i) Whether or not wavelengths (wave numbers) intended for the particular analysis method, are suitable for evaluation of characteristics of a sample in performing analysis under given conditions.

(ii) Whether or not the method is adequately robust to deal with variables such as handling of samples (for instance fill condition for fine particle samples, etc.) and configuration matrix.

(iii) Whether or not about the same level of accuracy or precision can be obtained, in comparison with the existing and established analysis methods, which are available as standards.

(iv) Sustaining and managing performance of an analysis method, once established, are critical. Continuous and systematic maintenance and inspection work must therefore be implemented. Furthermore, it must be determined whether or not appropriate evaluation procedures are available to deal with change controls or implementation of re-validation on changes made in manufacturing processes or raw materials, as well as changes arising from replacement of major components in equipment.

(v) Whether or not there are appropriate evaluation procedures in place to verify validity of transferring implementation of an analysis, which presupposed the use of a specific equipment, from such originally intended equipment to another equipment (model transfer) for the purpose of sharing the analysis method.

5.1. Qualitative analysis

Qualitative analysis, such as verification of substances, is performed after preparing a reference library that includes inter-lot variations within tolerance range and establishing analytical methods by using chemometrics methodologies, such as multivariate analysis. Minute quality characteristic variations between lots can also be established by using this method.

Furthermore, multivariate analysis includes direct analysis methods that consider wavelengths (wave numbers) and absorption as variables, such as wavelength correlation method, residual sum of squares, range sum of squares, along with factor analysis method, cluster analysis method, discriminant analysis method, as well as SIMCA (Soft independent modeling of class analogy), which are applied after preprocessing such as principal component analysis.

It is also possible to consider the overall near-infrared absorption spectrum as a single pattern and to identify parameters obtained by applying multivariate analysis methods or peak heights at characteristic wavelengths (wave numbers) peaks of the sample substance as indices for monitoring, for the purpose of manufacturing process control for active substances or preparations.

5.2. Quantitative analysis

Quantitative analysis uses spectrums of sample groups and analysis values obtained through the existing and established analysis methods, to obtain quantitative models with methodologies of chemometrics. These are used to calculate concentrations of individual ingredients and material values of samples being measured, using conversion formulas. Chemometrics methodologies for obtaining quantitative models include multiple regression analysis method, main ingredient regression analysis method and PLS (Partial least squares) regression analysis method.

In cases where the composition of a sample is simple, concentrations of ingredients in the sample that are subject to analysis can be calculated, by plotting a calibration curve using the absorbance of a specific wavelength (wave number) or the correlating relationship between the parameters and concentration, using samples for preparation of calibration curves with known concentrations (calibration curve method).

6. References

1) JIS K 0134 (2002), Japanese Industrial Standards, General Rules for Near-infrared Spectrophotometric Analysis
2) Near-Infrared Spectrophotometry, 2.2.40, European Pharmacopoeia 5.0 (2005)
3) Near-Infrared Spectrophotometry, <*1119*>, US Pharmacopeia 30 (2007)

G2 Solid-state Properties

Solid and Particle Densities <*G2-1-171*>

Density of a solid or a powder as a state of aggregation has different definitions depending on the way of including of the interparticulate and intraparticulate voids that exist between the particles or inside the powder. Different figures are obtained in each case, and there are different practical meanings. Generally, there are three levels of definitions of the solid or powder density.

(1) Crystal density: It is assumed that the system is homogeneous with no intraparticulate void. Crystal density is also called true density.

(2) Particle density: The sealed pores or the experimentally non-accessible open pores are also included as a part of the volumes of the solid or the powder.

(3) Bulk density: The interparticulate void formed in the powder bed is also included as a part of the volumes of the solid or the powder. Bulk density is also called apparent density. Generally, the powder densities at loose packing and at tapping are defined as the bulk density and the tapped density, respectively.

Generally, the densities of liquid or gas are affected only by temperature and pressure, but the solid or powder density is affected by the state of aggregation of the molecules or the particles. Therefore, the solid or powder densities naturally vary depending on crystal structure or crystallinity of the substance concerned, and also varies depending on the method of preparation or handling if the sample is amorphous form or partially amorphous. Consequently, even in a case that two solids or powders are chemically identical, it may be possible that the different figures of density are obtained if their crystal structures are different. As the solid or powder particle densities are important physical properties for the powdered pharmaceutical drugs or the powdered raw materials of drugs, the Japanese Pharmacopoeia specifies each density determination as "Powder Particle Density Determination" for the particle density and as "Determination of Bulk and Tapped Densities" for the bulk density.

The solid or powder densities are expressed in mass per unit volume (kg/m^3), and generally expressed in g/cm^3 ($1 g/cm^3 = 1000 kg/m^3$).

Crystal Density

The crystal density of a substance is the average mass per unit volume, exclusive of all voids that are not a fundamental part of the molecular packing arrangement. It is an intrinsic property concerning the specific crystal structure of the substance, and is not affected by the method of determination. The crystal density can be determined either by calculation or by simple measurement.

A. The calculated crystal density is obtained using:
   1) For example, the crystallographic data (volume and composition of the unit cell) obtained by the perfect crystal X-ray diffraction data from single crystal or indexing the powder X-ray diffraction data.
   2) Molecular mass of the substance.

B. The measured crystal density is obtained as the mass to volume ratio after measuring the single crystal mass and volume.

Particle Density

The particle density takes account both the crystal density and the intraparticulate porosity (sealed and/or experimentally non-accessible open pores) as a part of the particle volume. The particle density depends on the value of the volume determined, and the volume in turn depends on the method of measurement. Concerning the determination of particle density, the Japanese Pharmacopoeia specifies the pycnometry as the "Powder Particle Density Determination".

The pycnometric density is obtained by assuming that the volume of the gas displaced, which is measured with the gas displacement pycnometer, is equivalent to that of a known mass of the powder. In pycnometric density measurements, any volume with the open pores accessible to the gas is not included as a part of volume of the powder, but the sealed pores or pores inaccessible to the gas is included as a part of the volume of the powder. Due to the high diffusivity of helium which can penetrate to most open pores, it is recommendable as the measurement gas of particle density. Therefore, the pycnometric particle density of a finely milled powder is generally not very different from the crystal density. Hence, the particle density by this method is the best estimate of the true density of an amorphous or partially crystalline sample, and can be widely used for manufacturing control of the processed pharmaceutical powder samples.

Bulk Density and Tapped Density

The bulk density of a powder includes the contribution of interparticulate void volume as a part of the volume of the powder. Therefore, the bulk density depends on both the powder particle density and the space arrangement of particles in the power bed. Further, since the slightest disturbance of the bed may result in variation of the space arrangement, it is often very difficult to determine the bulk density with good reproducibility. Therefore, it is essential to specify how the determination was made upon reporting the bulk density.

The Japanese Pharmacopoeia specifies "Determination of Bulk and Tapped Densities".

A. The bulk density is determined by measuring the apparent volume of a known mass of powder sample that has been passed through a screen in a graduated cylinder (constant mass method). Separately, the Pharmacopoeia specifies the method of determining bulk density by measuring the mass of powder in a vessel having a known volume (constant volume method).

B. The tapped density is obtained by mechanically tapping a measuring cylinder containing a powder sample. After determining the initial bulk volume, carry out tapping under a fixed measurement condition (tapping rate and drop height), and the measurement is carried out repeatedly until the bulk volume variation obtained at consecutive two measurements is within an acceptable range (constant mass method). Separately, the Pharmacopoeia specifies the method of determining the tapped density by measuring the mass of a fixed volume of the tapped powder (constant volume method).

Powder Fineness *<G2-2-171>*

This classification is harmonized with the European Pharmacopoeia and the U.S. Pharmacopeia.

Information on the harmonization with the European Pharmacopoeia and the U.S. Pharmacopeia is available on the website of the Pharmaceuticals and Medical Devices Agency.

A simple descriptive classification of powder fineness is provided in this chapter. Sieving is most suitable where a majority of the particles are larger than about 75 μm, although it can be used for some powders having smaller particle sizes where the method can be validated. Light diffraction is also a widely used technique for measuring the size of a wide range of particles. Where the cumulative distribution has been determined by analytical sieving or by application of other methods, particle size may be characterized in the following manner:

x_{90}: Particle size corresponding to 90% of the cumulative undersize distribution

x_{50}: Median particle size (i.e. 50% of the particles are smaller and 50% of the particles are larger)

x_{10}: Particle size corresponding to 10% of the cumulative undersize distribution

It is recognized that the symbol d is also widely used to designate these values. Therefore, the symbols d_{90}, d_{50} and d_{10} may be used.

The following parameters may be defined based on the cumulative distribution.

$Q_r(x)$: cumulative distribution of particles with a dimension less than or equal to x where the subscript r reflects the distribution type

r	Distribution type
0	Number
1	Length
2	Area
3	Volume

Therefore, by definition:

$Q_r(x) = 0.90$ when $x = x_{90}$
$Q_r(x) = 0.50$ when $x = x_{50}$
$Q_r(x) = 0.10$ when $x = x_{10}$

An alternative but less informative method of classifying powder fineness is by use of the descriptive terms in the following table.

Classification of powders by fineness

Descriptive term	x_{50} (μm)	Cumulative distribution by volume basis, $Q_3(x)$
Coarse	> 355	$Q_3(355) < 0.50$
Moderately fine	180 - 355	$Q_3(180) < 0.50$, $Q_3(355) \geqq 0.50$
Fine	125 - 180	$Q_3(125) < 0.50$, $Q_3(180) \geqq 0.50$
Very fine	≦ 125	$Q_3(125) \geqq 0.50$

Powder Flow <*G2-3-171*>

This test is harmonized with the European Pharmacopoeia and the U.S. Pharmacopeia.

Information on the harmonization with the European Pharmacopoeia and the U.S. Pharmacopeia is available on the website of the Pharmaceuticals and Medical Devices Agency.

The widespread use of powders in the pharmaceutical industry has generated a variety of methods for characterizing powder flow. Not surprisingly, scores of references appear in the pharmaceutical literature, attempting to correlate the various measures of powder flow to manufacturing properties. The development of such a variety of test methods was inevitable; powder behavior is multifaceted and thus complicates the effort to characterize powder flow. The purpose of this chapter is to review the methods for characterizing powder flow that have appeared most frequently in the pharmaceutical literature. In addition, while it is clear that no single and simple test method can adequately characterize the flow properties of pharmaceutical powders, this chapter proposes the standardization of test methods that may be valuable during pharmaceutical development.

Four commonly reported methods for testing powder flow are ''(1) angle of repose'', ''(2) compressibility index or Hausner ratio'', ''(3) flow rate through an orifice'', and ''(4) shear cell''. In addition, numerous variations of each of these basic methods are available. Given the number of test methods and variations, standardizing the test methodology, where possible, would be advantageous.

With this goal in mind, the most frequently used methods are discussed below. Important experimental considerations are identified and recommendations are made regarding standardization of the methods. In general, any method of measuring powder flow should be practical, useful, reproducible, sensitive, and yield meaningful results. It bears repeating that no one simple powder flow method will adequately or completely characterize the wide range of flow properties experienced in the pharmaceutical industry. An appropriate strategy may well be the use of multiple standardized test methods to characterize the various aspects of powder flow as needed by the pharmaceutical scientist.

1. Angle of repose

The angle of repose has been used in several branches of science to characterize the flow properties of solids. Angle of repose is a characteristic related to interparticulate friction, or resistance to movement between particles. Angle of repose test results are reported to be very dependent upon the method used. Experimental difficulties arise due to segregation of material and consolidation or aeration of the powder as the cone is formed. Despite its difficulties, the method continues to be used in the pharmaceutical industry, and a number of examples demonstrating its value in predicting manufacturing problems appear in the literature.

The angle of repose is the constant, three-dimensional angle (relative to the horizontal base) assumed by a cone-like pile of material formed by any of several different methods (described briefly below).

1.1. Basic methods for angle of repose

A variety of angle of repose test methods are reported in the literature. The most common methods for determining the static angle of repose can be classified based on two important experimental variables:

(i) The height of the ''funnel'' through which the powder passes may be fixed relative to the base, or the height may be varied as the pile forms.

(ii) The base upon which the pile forms may be of fixed diameter or the diameter of the powder cone may be allowed to vary as the pile forms.

1.2. Variations in angle of repose methods

In addition to the above methods, variations of them have been used to some extent.

(i) Drained angle of repose: This is determined by allowing an excess quantity of material positioned above a fixed diameter base to drain from the container. Formation of a cone of powder on the fixed diameter base allows determination of the drained angle of repose.

(ii) Dynamic angle of repose: This is determined by filling a cylinder (with a clear, flat cover on one end) and rotating it at a specified speed. The dynamic angle of repose is the angle (relative to the horizontal) formed by the flowing powder. The internal angle of kinetic friction is defined by the plane separating those particles sliding down the top layer of the powder and those particles that are rotating with the drum (with roughened surface).

1.3. Angle of repose general scale of flowability

While there is some variation in the qualitative description of powder flow using the angle of repose, much of the pharmaceutical literature appears to be consistent with the classification by Carr[1)], which is shown in Table 1. There are examples of formulations with an angle of repose in the range of 40 to 50 degrees that manufactured satisfactorily. When the angle of repose exceeds 50 degrees, the flow is rarely acceptable for manufacturing purposes.

Table 1 Flow properties and corresponding angles of repose[1)]

Flow property	Counter measure to prevent crosslink	Angle of repose (degrees)
Excellent		25 - 30
Good		31 - 35
Fair	aid not needed	36 - 40
Passable	may hang up	41 - 45
Poor	most agitate, vibrate	46 - 55
Very poor		56 - 65
Very, very poor		>66

1.4. Experimental considerations for angle of repose

Angle of repose is not an intrinsic property of the powder, that is to say, it is very much dependent upon the method used to form the cone of powder. On this subject, the existing literature raises these important considerations:

(i) The peak of the cone of powder can be distorted by the impact of powder from above. By carefully building the powder cone, the distortion caused by impact can be minimized.

(ii) The nature of the base upon which the powder cone is formed influences the angle of repose. It is recommended that the powder cone be formed on a "common base", which can be achieved by forming the cone of powder on a layer of powder. This can be done by using a base of fixed diameter with a protruding outer edge to retain a layer of powder upon which the cone is formed.

1.5. Recommended procedure for angle of repose

Form the angle of repose on a fixed base with a retaining lip to retain a layer of powder on the base. The base should be free of vibration. Vary the height of the funnel to carefully build up a symmetrical cone of powder. Care should be taken to prevent vibration as the funnel is moved. The funnel height should be maintained approximately 2 - 4 cm from the top of the powder pile as it is being formed in order to minimize the impact of falling powder on the tip of the cone. If a symmetrical cone of powder cannot be successfully or reproducibly prepared, this method is not appropriate. Determine the angle of repose by measuring the height of the cone of powder and calculating the angle of repose, α, from the following equation:

$$\tan \alpha = \text{height}/(\text{diameter of base} \times 0.5)$$

2. Compressibility index and Hausner ratio

In recent years the compressibility index and the closely related Hausner ratio have become the simple, fast and popular methods of predicting powder flow characteristics. The compressibility index has been proposed as an indirect measure of bulk density, size and shape, surface area, moisture content, and cohesiveness of materials because all of these can influence the observed compressibility index. The compressibility index and the Hausner ratio are determined by measuring both the bulk volume and tapped volume of a powder.

2.1. Basic methods for compressibility index and Hausner ratio

While there are some variations in the method of determining the compressibility index and Hausner ratio, the basic procedure is to measure (1) the unsettled apparent volume, V_o, and (2) the final tapped volume, V_f, of the powder after tapping the material until no further volume changes occur. The compressibility index and the Hausner ratio are calculated as follows:

$$\text{Compressibility Index} = (V_o - V_f)/V_o \times 100$$
$$\text{Hausner Ratio} = V_o/V_f$$

Alternatively, the compressibility index and Hausner ratio may be calculated using measured values for bulk density (ρ_{bulk}) and tapped density (ρ_{tapped}) as follows:

$$\text{Compressibility Index} = (\rho_{tapped} - \rho_{bulk})/\rho_{tapped} \times 100$$
$$\text{Hausner Ratio} = \rho_{tapped}/\rho_{bulk}$$

In a variation of these methods, the rate of consolidation is sometimes measured rather than, or in addition to, the change in volume that occurs on tapping. For the compressibility index and the Hausner ratio, the generally accepted scale of flowability is given in Table 2.

Table 2 Scale of flowability[1)]

Compressibility index (%)	Flow character	Hausner ratio
≦10	Excellent	1.00 - 1.11
11 - 15	Good	1.12 - 1.18
16 - 20	Fair	1.19 - 1.25
21 - 25	Passable	1.26 - 1.34
26 - 31	Poor	1.35 - 1.45
32 - 37	Very poor	1.46 - 1.59
>38	Very, very poor	>1.60

2.2. Experimental considerations for the compressibility index and Hausner ratio

Compressibility index and Hausner ratio are not intrinsic properties of the powder, that is to say, they are dependent upon the methodology used. The existing literature points out several important considerations affecting the determination of the (1) unsettled apparent volume, V_o, (2) the final tapped volume, V_f, (3) the bulk density, ρ_{bulk}, and (4) the tapped density, ρ_{tapped}:

(i) The diameter of the cylinder used

(ii) The number of times the powder is tapped to achieve the tapped density

(iii) The mass of material used in the test

(iv) Rotation of the sample during tapping

2.3. Recommended procedure for compressibility index and Hausner ratio

Use a 250-mL volumetric cylinder with a test sample weight of 100 g. Smaller weights and volumes may be used, but variations in the method should be described with the results. An average of three determinations is recommended.

3. Flow through an orifice

The flow rate of a material depends upon many factors, some of which are particle-related and some related to the process. Monitoring the rate of flow of material through an orifice has been proposed as a better measure of powder flowability. Of particular significance is the utility of monitoring flow continuously since pulsating flow patterns have been observed even for free flowing materials. Changes in flow rate as the container empties can also be observed. Empirical equations relating flow rate to the diameter of the opening, particle size, and particle density have been determined. However, determining the flow rate through an orifice is useful only with free-flowing materials.

The flow rate through an orifice is generally measured as the mass per time flowing from any of a number of types of containers (cylinders, funnels, hoppers). Measurement of the flow rate can be in discrete increments or continuous.

3.1. Basic methods for flow through an orifice

There are a variety of methods described in the literature. The most common for determining the flow rate through an orifice can be classified based on three important experimental variables:

(1) The type of container used to contain the powder. Common containers are cylinders, funnels and hoppers from production equipment.

(2) The size and shape of the orifice used. The orifice diameter and shape are critical factors in determining powder flow rate.

(3) The method of measuring powder flow rate. Flow rate can be measured continuously using an electronic balance and with some sort of recording device (strip chart recorder, computer). It can also be measured in discrete samples (for example, the time it takes for 100 g of powder to pass through the orifice to the nearest tenth of a second or the amount of powder passing through the orifice in 10 seconds to the nearest tenth of a gram).

3.2. Variations in methods for flow through an orifice

Either mass flow rate or volume flow rate can be determined. Mass flow rate is the easier of the methods, but it biases the results in favor of high-density materials. Since die fill is volumetric, determining volume flow rate may be preferable. A vibrator is occasionally attached to facilitate flow from the container, however, this appears to complicate interpretation of results. A moving orifice device has been proposed to more closely simulate rotary press conditions. The minimum diameter orifice through which powder flows can also be identified.

3.3. General scale of flowability for flow through an orifice

No general scale is available because flow rate is critically dependent on the method used to measure it. Comparison between published results is difficult.

3.4. Experimental considerations for flow through an orifice

Flow rate through an orifice is not an intrinsic property of the powder. It is very much dependent upon the methodology used. The existing literature points out several important considerations affecting these methods:

(i) The diameter and shape of the orifice
(ii) The type of container material (metal, glass, plastic)
(iii) The diameter and height of the powder bed.

3.5. Recommended procedure for flow through an orifice

Flow rate through an orifice can be used only for materials that have some capacity to flow. It is not useful for cohesive materials. Provided that the height of the powder bed (the 'head' of powder) is much greater than the diameter of the orifice, the flow rate is virtually independent of the powder head. Use a cylinder as the container because the cylinder material should have little effect on flow. This configuration results in flow rate being determined by the movement of powder over powder rather than powder along the wall of the container. Powder flow rate often increases when the height of the powder column is less than two times the diameter of the column. The orifice should be circular and the cylinder should be free of vibration. General guidelines for dimensions of the cylinder are as follows:

(i) Diameter of opening >6 times the diameter of the particles
(ii) Diameter of the cylinder >2 times the diameter of the opening

Use of a hopper as the container may be appropriate and representative of flow in a production situation. It is not advisable to use a funnel, particularly one with a stem, because flow rate will be determined by the size and length of the stem as well as the friction between the stem and the powder. A truncated cone may be appropriate, but flow will be influenced by the powder—wall friction coefficient, thus, selection of an appropriate construction material is important.

For the opening in the cylinder, use a flat-faced bottom plate with the option to vary orifice diameter to provide maximum flexibility and better ensure a powder-over-powder flow pattern. Rate measurement can be either discrete or continuous. Continuous measurement using an electronic balance can more effectively detect momentary flow rate variations.

4. Shear cell methods

In an effort to put powder flow studies and hopper design on a more fundamental basis, a variety of powder shear testers and methods that permit more thorough and precisely defined assessment of powder flow properties have been developed. Shear cell methodology has been used extensively in the study of pharmaceutical materials. From these methods, a wide variety of parameters can be obtained, including the yield loci representing the shear stress-shear strain relationship, the angle of internal friction, the unconfined yield strength, the tensile strength, and a variety of derived parameters such as the flow factor and other flowability indices. Because of the ability to more precisely control experimental parameters, flow properties can also be determined as a function of consolidation load, time, and other environmental conditions. The methods have been successfully used to determine critical hopper and bin parameters.

4.1. Basic methods for shear cell

One type of shear cell is the cylindrical shear cell which is split horizontally, forming a shear plane between the lower stationary base and the upper movable portion of the shear cell ring. After powder bed consolidation in the shear cell (using a well-defined procedure), the force necessary to shear the powder bed by moving the upper ring is determined. Annular shear cell designs offer some advantages over the cylindrical shear cell design, including the need for less material. A disadvantage, however, is that because of its design, the powder bed is not sheared as uniformly because material on the outside of the annulus is sheared more than material in the inner region. A third type of shear cell (parallel-plate type) consists of a thin sandwich of powder between a lower stationary rough surface and an upper rough surface that is moveable.

All of the shear cell methods have their advantages and disadvantages, but a detailed review is beyond the scope of this chapter. As with the other methods for characterizing powder flow, many variations are described in the literature. A significant advantage of shear cell methodology in general is a greater degree of experimental control. The methodology generally is rather time-consuming and requires significant amounts of material and a well-trained operator.

4.2. Recommendations for shear cell

The many existing shear cell configurations and test methods provide a wealth of data and can be used very effectively to characterize powder flow. They are also helpful in the design of equipment such as hoppers and bins. Because of the diversity of available equipment and experimental procedures, no specific recommendations regarding methodology are presented in this chapter. It is recommended that the results of powder flow characterization using shear cell methodology include a complete description of equipment and methodology used.

5. References

1) Carr R.L.: Evaluating flow properties of solids. *Chem. Eng*. 1965; 72: 163–168.

Measurement of the Diameter of Particles Dispersed in Liquid by Dynamic Light Scattering
<G2-4-161>

This method is used for measuring average particle diameter and particle diameter distribution of submicron-sized particles dispersed in a liquid by means of dynamic light scattering.

The average particle diameter and the particle diameter

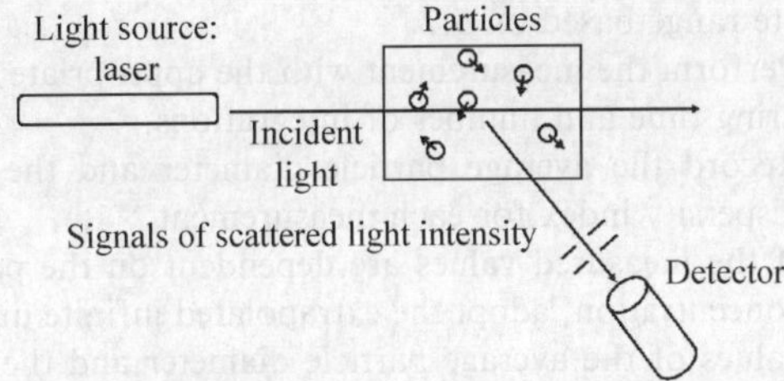

Fig. 1 Schematic illustration of the measurement principle

distribution obtained by this method are important characteristics mainly of colloidal dispersion formulations, such as emulsion injections, suspension injections, and liposome formulations.

There are two ways of analyzing the detected signals in dynamic light scattering: photon correlation spectroscopy and frequency analysis. Dynamic light scattering is applied to the analysis of particles whose diameters range from nm scale to approximately 1 μm or particles free from the influence of sedimentation.

1. Principle

When particles in Brownian motion in solution or in suspension are irradiated with laser light, scattered light from the particles fluctuates depending on their diffusion coefficients. The intensity of the scattered light from larger particles fluctuates more slowly, because the larger particles move more slowly. On the other hand, the intensity of the scattered light from smaller particles fluctuates more rapidly, because they move faster.

In dynamic light scattering measurements, the particle diameter is determined by applying the Stokes-Einstein equation to analysis of the detected fluctuations of scattered light intensity, which reflect the diffusion coefficient of the particles.

$$d = \frac{kT}{3\pi\eta D} \times 10^{12}$$

d: Particle diameter (nm)
k: Boltzmann constant (1.38×10^{-23} J·K^{-1})
T: Absolute temperature (K)
η: Viscosity (mPa·s)
D: Diffusion coefficient (m^2·s^{-1})

In photon correlation spectroscopy, the time-dependent changes (fluctuation) in the scattered light intensity, namely the observed signals of the scattered light intensity, are transmitted to the correlator. The average particle diameter and the polydispersity index are obtained from the autocorrelation function of the scattered light intensity, which is calculated based on the data processed by the correlator.

In frequency analysis, the average particle diameter and the polydispersity index are obtained from the frequency power spectrum, which is the Fourier transform of the frequency components included in the signals of the scattered light intensity.

Major terms used in this method are as follows.

(i) Average particle diameter: dynamic light scattering harmonic intensity-weighted arithmetic averaged particle diameter, whose unit is nanometer (nm).

(ii) Polydispersity index: dimensionless indicator of the broadness of the particle diameter distribution.

(iii) Scattering volume: observation volume defined by the light-receiving optics and the incident laser light. This value may be given in the specifications of the instrument. Its order of magnitude is typically 10^{-12} m^3.

(iv) Count rate: number of the photon pulses per second

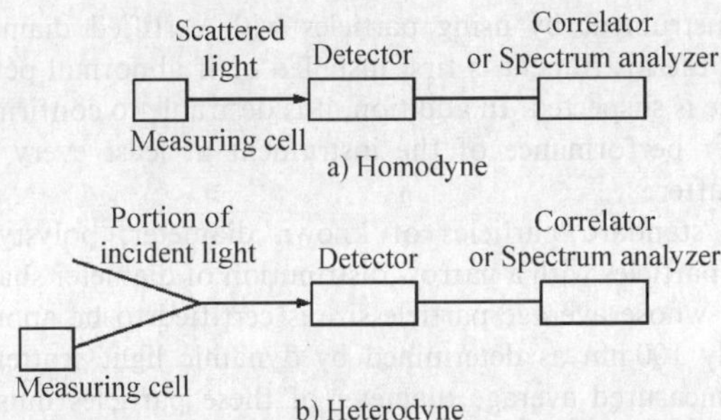

Fig. 2 Different optical arrangements of the apparatus

detected in the light-receiving optics in photon correlation spectroscopy. This value is proportional to the detected scattered light intensity. The unit is cps (count per second).

(v) Signal of scattered light fluctuation: signal detected by the light-receiving optics in the frequency analysis. The signal is proportional to the scattered light intensity, and includes frequency components depending on the distribution of the particle diameter.

2. Apparatus

2.1. Constitution of the apparatus

The measuring apparatus generally consists mainly of a laser, sample holder, light-receiving optics and detector, and correlator or spectrum analyzer. There are two types of optical detection according to the optical arrangements: (a) homodyne detection in which only the scattered light is measured, and (b) heterodyne detection in which the scattered light and a portion of the incident light are measured simultaneously.

(i) Laser: a monochromatic laser polarized with its electric field component perpendicular to the plane formed by the incident light and light-receiving optical axes (vertical polarization).

(ii) Sample holder: a holder whose temperature can be measured and controlled within an accuracy of ±0.3°C.

(iii) Measuring cell: a rectangular or cylindrical cell made of optical glass or optical plastic, which can be placed in the sample holder. The cell is integrated with the sample holder in some apparatus.

(iv) Light-receiving optics and detector: light optics and detector which capture the scattered light from the sample at a single scattering angle between 90° to 180° and convert the captured light to a photon pulse (digitized signal). In the case that a polarization analyzer is included, it shall be positioned so that the transmittance of the vertically polarized light is maximized.

(v) Correlator: a device which calculates the autocorrelation function from the number of photon pulses in a certain time.

(vi) Spectrum analyzer: a device which calculates the frequency power spectrum by performing Fourier transformation of the frequency components present in the scattered light fluctuation signals.

(vii) Computation unit: data processor for determining the particle diameter distribution from the autocorrelation function obtained by the correlator or from the frequency power spectrum. Some computation units also function as a correlator or spectrum analyzer.

2.2. Validation and reproducibility of the instrument

Because the particle diameter obtained by dynamic light scattering is not a relative value calculated using standard particles but an absolute value based on a fundamental principle, calibration of the value is unnecessary.

However, it is necessary to confirm the performance of

the instrument by using particles with certified diameter, when the instrument is first installed or if abnormal performance is suspected. In addition, it is desirable to confirm the proper performance of the instrument at least every year thereafter.

As standard particles of known diameter, polystyrene latex particles with a narrow distribution of diameter shall be used, whose average particle size is certified to be approximately 100 nm as determined by dynamic light scattering. The measured average diameter of these particles must be within 2% of the stated diameter range, and the relative standard deviation must be less than 2%. In addition, the measured polydispersity index must be less than 0.1.

3. Measurement

3.1. Choice of the dispersion liquid

The dispersion liquid shall fulfill all of the following requirements.

(i) It shall be non-absorbing at the wavelength of the laser.

(ii) It shall not cause damage such as corrosion to the materials of the instrument.

(iii) It shall not dissolve, swell or coagulate the particles.

(iv) It shall have a refractive index different from that of the particulate material.

(v) Its refractive index and viscosity shall be known within an accuracy of 0.5%.

(vi) It shall be clean enough not to interfere with the measurements.

3.2. Cleaning the measuring cell

The degree of cell washing required depends on the conditions of the measurement.

When an individually packaged clean disposable cell is used, cleaning by blowing off dust with compressed clean air is sufficient. When a cell is intended to be washed rigorously, the cell is fully rinsed beforehand with water to remove water-rinsable adhesion substances and is washed with a nonabrasive detergent.

3.3. Sample preparation

It is necessary to prepare a sample whose concentration is within an appropriate range to eliminate the influence of the multiple scattering of light. In addition, it is important to remove dust, which may affect the measurement, and to prevent their re-introduction during the preparation.

When the sample is shaken, dust-laden air is entrapped in the sample and air is dissolved in the solvent. The invisible small air bubbles scatter light more strongly than do the sample particles to be measured. It is necessary not to shake the sample violently after preparation, but to swirl it gently. A homogeneous sample solution can be prepared quickly by adding diluent to the concentrated sample droplet rather than dropping the sample droplet into the diluent.

3.4. Measurement procedure

1) Switch the instrument on and allow it to warm up. A period of approximately 30 minutes is typically required for stabilizing the laser intensity and bringing the sample holder to the desired temperature.
2) Choose the appropriate dispersion liquid, and record the count rate or the amplitude of the signals of scattered light fluctuation from the dispersion liquid.
3) Place the sample containing the dispersed particles in the instrument, and wait until temperature equilibrium is established between the sample and the sample holder. It is desirable to control and measure the temperature within an accuracy of ± 0.3°C.
4) Perform a preliminary measurement of the sample, and set the particle concentration within the appropriate range based on 5.2.
5) Perform the measurement with the appropriate measuring time and number of integrations.
6) Record the average particle diameter and the polydispersity index for each measurement.
7) If the measured values are dependent on the particle concentration, adopt the extrapolated infinite dilution values of the average particle diameter and the polydispersity index (or the measured values at the lowest particle concentration).
8) Confirm that no significant sedimentation has occurred in the sample at the end of the measurement. The presence of sediment indicates that the sample may have aggregated or precipitated, or that the sample may be unsuitable for measurement by dynamic light scattering.
9) Perform the measurement for each sample at least three times.

3.5. Repeatability

The repeatability of the determination of the average particle diameter, evaluated in terms of relative standard deviation, must be less than 5%.

4. Data analysis

The dispersion that is the target for the measurement is irradiated with the laser light. Phases of the light scattered by each particle fluctuate because the dispersed particles are in Brownian motion. The observed scattered intensity, which is the sum of the scattered light (result of interference), fluctuates along the time axis. Analyzing the fluctuation of the scattered light intensity as a function of time provides information on the motion of the dispersed particles.

Analysis by photon correlation spectroscopy is performed using the autocorrelation function of the scattered light intensity. This autocorrelation function depends only on the time difference (correlation time) and is independent of the time at which the measurement is started. For a large number of monodisperse particles in Brownian motion in a scattering volume, the autocorrelation function of the scattered light intensity is basically an exponential decay function of the correlation time. Polydispersity index is a parameter indicating the distribution of the decay constant, and is also a scale indicating the broadness of the distribution of particle diameter.

Frequency analysis is performed using the frequency power spectrum calculated from the scattered light intensity. The amplitude of the frequency power spectrum is proportional to the scattered light intensity and the concentration of the sample, and the characteristic frequency is inversely proportional to the particle diameter. The decay constant and the characteristic frequency are related to the translational diffusion coefficient of homogeneous spherical particles in Brownian motion. The diffusion constant of the spherical particles dispersed in the dispersion liquid is related to the particle diameter according to the Stokes-Einstein equation in the absence of inter-particle interaction. The polydispersity index determined by frequency analysis is a measure of the broadness of the particle diameter distribution calculated from the particle diameter distribution based on the scattered light intensity, and might differ from the polydispersity index determined by photon correlation spectroscopy.

Records of data shall include the average particle diameter and polydispersity index, and in addition, shall also state the principle of measurement (photon correlation spectroscopy or frequency analysis), optical configuration (homodyne or heterodyne), observation angle, temperature of the sample, refractive index and viscosity of the dispersion liquid, measuring time or number of integrations, and sample concentration.

5. Points to note regarding the measurement

5.1. Shape of particles

The particles are assumed to be homogeneous and spherical in the data analysis of dynamic light scattering.

5.2. Particle concentration

For measurement, it is necessary to prepare a sample whose concentration falls in the range satisfying the following conditions.

(i) The sample consists of dispersion liquid and particles well-dispersed in the liquid.

(ii) The range of the particle concentration is determined so that consistent results can be obtained in particle diameter measurements. The range is determined beforehand based on measurements of systematically diluted samples.

5.3. Purification of the dispersion liquid

Scattered light signals from the dispersion liquid used for sample dilution must normally be undetected or very weak. If the situations described in cases (i) or (ii) below are found, particulate substances are likely to have become mixed in the sample, and in such cases the dispersion liquid shall be further purified (by filtration, distillation, and so on) before use. The lower limit of the particle concentration is determined mainly so that scattered light from the dispersion liquid and contaminating substances will not affect the measurement. When water is chosen as the dispersion liquid, use of fresh distilled water (prepared by quartz-glass distillation) or desalted and filtered (pore size 0.2 μm) water is recommended.

(i) Large fluctuations of the count rate or of the amplitude of the scattered light fluctuation signals, accompanied by abnormally strong signals, are recorded.

(ii) Light spots appear in the path of the laser light in the sample.

5.4. Others

(i) When particles are highly charged with electricity, long-range interactions between the particles may affect the measurement result, and in such cases, a small amount of salt (for example, sodium chloride: around 10^{-2} mol/L) may be added to the dispersion liquid to reduce the effect.

(ii) Traceable polystyrene latex particles for use in the validation of the instrument are commercially available.

6. Reference

1) JIS Z8826: 2005 Particle size analysis—Photon correlation spectroscopy
2) ISO 13321: 1996 Particle size analysis—Photon correlation spectroscopy
3) ISO 22412: 2008 Particle size analysis—Dynamic light scattering (DLS)

G3 Biotechnological/Biological Products

Basic Concept of the Quality Control on Biotechnological Products (Biopharmaceuticals) <G3-1-180>

Introduction

This document provides general principle to ensure the quality of biotechnological products (hereinafter referred to as "biopharmaceuticals") focusing on the elements peculiar to biopharmaceuticals on the basis of the recommendations in a series of so-called Q-quartet guidelines from ICH Q8 to Q11 and those in Q5A to Q5E and Q6B guidelines[1-6] on the quality of biopharmaceuticals. The general concepts for assurance of drug substances and drug products are described in the General Information, "Basic Concepts for Quality Assurance of Drug Substances and Drug Products <G0-1-172>".

The principles of this General Information apply to biopharmaceuticals: proteins and peptides, their derivatives, and products of which they are components. These proteins and polypeptides are produced from recombinant or non-recombinant cell-culture expression systems. The principles outlined in this document may also apply to other types of biotechnological/biological products.

In the case of biopharmaceuticals, an inherent degree of structural heterogeneity occurs in molecular structure due to the biosynthetic processes used by living organisms to produce them. In addition to post-translational modification such as glycosylation, they may receive various modifications such as oxidation and deamidation during the production process and storage periods. Impurities that may remain in the drug substance of biopharmaceuticals include those with molecular diversity, such as proteins derived from cells used for production, and there is a risk of contamination such as viruses. Such quality profiles can vary due to various factors on the manufacturing process.

In order to ensure the quality of biopharmaceuticals, it is necessary to establish an appropriate quality control strategy in consideration of the above characteristics. "Basic Concepts for Quality Assurance of Drug Substances and Drug Products <G0-2-170>" described in General Information G0 is useful for this. First, the quality attributes are clarified by thorough characteristic analysis. Then, identify the critical quality attributes (CQAs) in consideration of the quality target product profile (QTPP), and construct a quality control strategy to keep the CQAs within the appropriate ranges, limits and distributions. If the manufacturing process is to be changed during the development period or the post-marketing period, conduct comparability exercise of before and after the change made in the manufacturing process, and check the validity of the change by verifying that the change will not have adverse impact on the quality, safety and efficacy of the drug product. New manufacturing and analytical technology of biopharmaceuticals are continuously being developed day by day, and desired to be utilized for continuous improvement of product quality throughout the product life cycle.

1. Quality evaluation and control of biopharmaceuticals

1.1. Quality evaluation

1.1.1. Characterization

Characterization of products is an essential step in identifying CQAs and establishing quality control strategies. In the characterization of biopharmaceuticals, detailed analysis is performed as much as possible for the structure and physicochemical properties, biological activity, molecular variants of a desired product, process-related impurities, and so on. The desired product is the protein which has an expected structure and is expected from the DNA sequence, the protein which is expected from anticipated post-translational modification, and/or expected from the intended downstream processing/modification. Among the molecular variants of the desired product, those with properties comparable to the desired product with respect to biological activity, efficacy and safety can be classified as product-related substances. Otherwise, those without the same properties can be

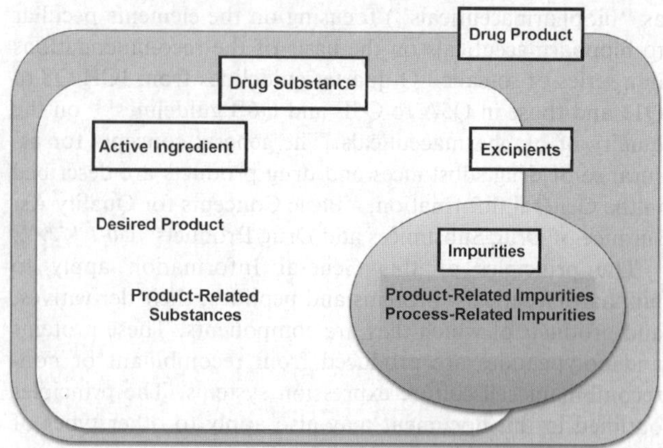

Fig. 1 Components of biopharmaceuticals.

*In biopharmaceuticals, the drug substance contains excipients such as buffer solution components for stabilization of the active ingredient.

classified as product-related impurities. The active ingredient consists of the desired product and the product-related substances, and generally, the active ingredient of biopharmaceuticals has heterogeneity. (Fig. 1).

a. Structure and physicochemical properties

Analyzes amino acid sequence and amino acid composition, terminal amino acid sequence, sulfhydryl group and disulfide bond, carbohydrate composition and structure, glycation, oxidation, deamidation, and so on. Oligosaccharides in glycoproteins may be associated with stabilization of structure, biological activity, antigenicity and pharmacokinetics, and so on. Their profiles are susceptible to variations of manufacturing process. It is necessary to analyze in detail by monosaccharide analysis, oligosaccharide analysis/oligosaccharide profiling, glycopeptide analysis, glycoform analysis etc. Molecular variants generated by oxidization and deamidation, etc. may be analyzed by peptide mapping. The charge profiles may be evaluated by ion exchange chromatography or isoelectric focusing. The molecular heterogeneity occurs not only during the culture process but also during subsequent manufacture and storage of the drug substance and drug product. Therefore, scientific understanding of the manufacturing process obtained by characterizing the degree of heterogeneity and profile, and evaluating the impact of the variations in process parameters on the degree of heterogeneity, will be useful to construct the quality control strategy.

Physicochemical properties are analyzed in terms of molecular weight, molecular size, molar absorbance coefficient, etc. Information on the secondary structure and higher-order structure of the desired product can be obtained by spectroscopic methods such as circular dichroism, Fourier transform infrared absorption spectrum and NMR, or by thermodynamic methods such as differential scanning calorimetry.

b. Biological activities

Biological activity is an indicator of the specific ability or capacity of a product to achieve a defined biological effect. It is difficult to determine higher-order structure by physicochemical analysis, because that an active ingredient of biopharmaceutical is a large molecule having complex structure, and is a mixture of various molecular entities as mentioned above. Therefore, the confirmation that the biopharmaceutical has an expected structure is usually obtained by biological activity. Biological assays for measuring biological activity include biochemical assays (measurement of enzyme activity, measurement of binding activity, etc.), cell culture-based biological assays, animal-based biological assays, and so on. The tests are selected by considering characteristics of active ingredient, mechanism of action and its pharmacological activity to the disease to be treated. For example, enzyme activity if the active ingredient is enzymes, cell proliferation activity if the active ingredient is growth factors, antigen binding activity, antigen neutralizing activity, antibody dependent cytotoxicity, and complement dependent cytotoxicity etc. if the active ingredient is antibodies, are evaluated.

In biological assays, the potency is expressed as a unit or relative activity (%) to the reference material by comparing the response obtained from the sample to that from the standard. The potency is the quantitative measure of biological activity based on the attribute of the product which is linked to the relevant biological properties. The biological activity used for potency measurement should, in principle, be the same as or similar to that expected in the clinical situation. The correlation between the expected clinical response and the activity in the biological assay should be established in pharmacodynamic or clinical studies.

c. Molecular variants of desired product (product-related substances and product-related impurities)

In the characterization of drug substances and drug products, we analyze as much as possible such as the structure, biological activity and binding activity of the contained molecular variants. In products with large molecular masses and complex structures, it is often difficult to clearly separate the product-related substances and product-related impurities, and it is difficult to control the proportion of individual molecular variants in the drug substance and the drug product. In such cases, profiles (oligosaccharide profiles and charge profiles) obtained by appropriate analytical methods should be clarified. Typical molecular variants classified as product-related impurities are aggregates (multimers) and fragments. In addition, deamidated, isomerized, oxidized, mismatched S-S linked disulfide bond mismatched, glycated forms, etc. may be considered as impurities derived from the desired product. Aggregates and fragments are evaluated for their content by size exclusion chromatography, SDS polyacrylamide gel electrophoresis, SDS capillary gel electrophoresis, and so on.

d. Process-related impurities

The process-related impurities are classified into those derived from cell substrates (e.g., host cell proteins and host cell DNA), impurities derived from cell cultures (e.g., antibiotics and insulin), impurities derived from downstream processing such as extraction, separation, processing, purification and formulation steps (ligands of carries for chromatography such as protein A, enzymes, chemical modification reagents, solvents, etc.). Regarding process-related impurities, if it is possible to guarantee that impurities are constantly removed by the control of process parameters, or if the in-process tests are set, in some cases, it is not necessary to set specifications for drug substances and drug products. Particular attention should be given to process-related impurities that exhibit pharmacological activity and may have immunogenicity.

1.1.2. Identification of CQA

For each quality attribute revealed by the characterization, risk level is estimated with respect to the impact and uncertainty that their variation has on efficacy and safety, and then the CQAs to be controlled are identified. For example, in many cases, from the viewpoint of 1. biological activity or efficacy, 2. pharmacokinetics, 3. immunogenicity, 4. safety, if the score obtained by multiplication of scores of impact and uncertainty of each attribute is above a certain value, that attribute is identified as CQA. Risk level can also be estimated from the severity and probability of their impact on efficacy and safety.

1.2. Establishment of quality control strategy

The quality control strategy defines a set of controls to bring the CQAs within appropriate limits, ranges and distributions. Quality control strategies include such as raw material control, manufacturing process control, specifications and stability testing. Acceptable ranges and target management criteria of CQAs are set based on characterization results, lot analysis results based on specifications, stability tests results, and clinical tests results, and so on. In stability testing, the analytical results of the quality attributes (i.e. the proportion of molecular variants such as fragments, oxidized forms and deamidated forms) and biological activity of the forced degradation samples in the stress stability testing and accelerated stability testing, are useful for setting acceptable ranges and target management criteria of each CQA. In the course of developing the manufacturing process of biopharmaceuticals, identify the raw material characteristics and process parameters affecting the CQAs, and construct the control method of the manufacturing process so that the CQAs are within the target range. Based on these results, construct an appropriate quality control strategy consisting of raw material specifications, process parameter control, in-process testing, drug substance and/or drug product specifications.

1.2.1. Raw materials control

Raw materials for biopharmaceuticals include cell banks, media used in culture processes, media additives, resins and carriers for chromatography used in purification processes, buffers, washing solutions, and filters, and they also include PEGylation reagents used in the modification process, additives used in the formulation process, and the like.

a. Evaluation and control of cell bank (including evaluation of gene expression construct)

Cell substrates are generally controlled in a two-tiered cell bank, where Working Cell Banks are prepared from a Master Cell Bank, and their characteristics are clarified by conducting characterization and purity tests. Also, confirm that the cell substrate is suitable for pharmaceutical production. In addition, the same evaluation is performed at the upper limit of in vitro cell age that can be used for production, and the stability of the cell substrate during the culture period is confirmed. In the purity test, it is evaluated that the cell bank is not contaminated with adventitious microbial contaminants (see 1.2.3 for virus). In the characterization tests, cell morphology, viable cell number, expression of target protein, etc. are evaluated. In the case of a cell line to which a gene expression construct is introduced, the gene expression construct should be evaluated for copy number and insertions or deletions, and coding sequence of desired protein, etc.

b. Control of other raw materials

Raw materials used in the manufacturing process are used after confirming that they fulfill the criteria for their intended use. When using raw materials derived from humans or animals, such as serum and enzymes, make sure that they meet the ''Biological Raw Material Standards''.

1.2.2. Manufacturing process control

The manufacturing process of biopharmaceuticals consists mainly of drug substance process containing culture process and purification process, and formulation process. Because process parameters of culture process and purification process may affect the heterogeneity profile and impurity profile, etc., sufficient understanding of these processes and the establishment of appropriate control methods (setting and evaluation of process parameters, in-process test etc.) are essential for quality consistency. The constructed manufacturing process is qualified by process validation/evaluation. Process validation is usually performed on a commercial-scale, however it can be performed on a small-scale model that has been qualified for investigating the ability to remove and inactivate virus and the number of reuses of purification columns and so on.

a. Process parameter control

The process parameters to be controlled and their control ranges in each manufacturing process are set based on the previous manufacturing results and univariate experiments, or on the relationships between the process parameters and the CQAs clarified by a systematic approach. When developing a manufacturing process with the latter method, estimate the risk level related to the impact of each process parameter on each CQA, and set the operating range of each process parameter so that each CQA does not exceed its acceptable range. When estimating the risk level during the establishment of the control strategy, consider the severity, probability, and detectability of the impact that the parameter variations may have on each CQA. As an example of process parameters to be controlled, in the culture process, temperature, medium additives concentration, dissolved oxygen concentration, dissolved carbon dioxide concentration, pH, stirring speed, culture time, etc., and in the purification process, column size, loading amount, buffer solution composition, flow velocity, etc. can be mentioned. The acceptable range of purification process parameters is set in consideration of the impact on the heterogeneity profile and the impurity removal efficiency. In addition, it is considered necessary to ensure that the characteristics of each process, such as cell density and viability in the culture process and recovery rate in the purification process, fall within a certain range. Processes that have a particularly large impact on quality are regarded as critical processes. Major examples of critical processes include production culture processes, virus inactivation and removal processes, and affinity chromatography processes.

b. In-process tests

In the quality control of biopharmaceuticals, in-process tests are considered possible or appropriate to control contamination with such as process-related impurities, viruses and adventitious infectious factors. Examples of in-process testing include adventitious virus test after production culture, filter integrity tests of virus removal filters and sterile filters, testing for process-related impurities such as host cell proteins and host cell DNA, bioburden test, and so on. In-process tests are also evaluated for their validity by appropriate approaches such as analytical procedure validation.

1.2.3. Evaluation and control of contaminants

Contaminants are substances that should not be present in manufacturing processes, such as adventitious chemicals, biochemical materials, or microorganisms. From the viewpoint of ensuring safety, contaminants should be strictly avoided, and after constructing an appropriate manufacturing process. As mentioned above, it should be appropriately controlled by raw material control, in-process testing or specifications.

Viruses may contaminate as an adventitious factor from production processes and may be present as an endogenous factor in cell substrates used. The following three major complementary approaches are taken as rational measures to prevent the virus contamination specific to products using biological origin and to ensure the safety. 1) Selecting and testing cell lines and other raw materials, including media components, for the absence of undesirable viruses which may be infectious and/or pathogenic for humans. 2) Assessing the capacity of production processes to clear infectious viruses. 3) Testing the product at appropriate steps of production for absence of contaminating infectious viruses. The details are described in General Information: ''Basic Requirements for Viral Safety of Biotechnological/Biological Products listed in Japanese Pharmacopoeia *<G3-13-141>*''.

1.2.4. Specifications

a. Justification of specifications

The items and test methods adopted for the specification differ depending on the quality control strategy established. It is necessary to clarify the justification of the acceptance criteria. The acceptance criteria are set on the basis of the data obtained from lots used in clinical trials, the data obtained from lots used to indicate the consistency of production, stability test data, and appropriate data in the product development stages.

b. Description

It qualitatively defines the physical state (e.g., solid, liquid) and color of a drug substance and drug product. Prescribe the transparency of a drug product if it is solution.

c. Identification test

Set up specific tests based on the structural features and specific properties of an active ingredient(s). In order to confirm the identity, not less than two types of tests (physical and chemical test, biological test, immunochemical test, etc.) are usually to be set up for a drug substance. For a drug product, one type of test may be sufficient, but some products may require more than one type of test.

d. Specific physical and/or chemical values

The quality attributes to be set as the specific physical and/or chemical values include oligosaccharide, charge, molecular mass/size, and so on. In the case where the product-related substances and the product-related impurities are difficult to separate and can not be set as the purity tests, the heterogeneity profiles are specified as the physical and/or chemical values. Typical examples include oligosaccharide profiles and charge profiles. In addition, set the specification for attributes that are important in ensuring the quality of a drug substance and drug product. Examples of the items include pH and osmotic pressure, etc.

e. Purity tests

Purity is usually assessed by a combination of analytical methods. In the choice and optimization of test methods for impurities, emphasis should be placed on separating or identifying the desired product and product-related substances from impurities (product-related impurities and process-related impurities).

f. Biological activities

Specifications for biopharmaceuticals should usually contain the tests for biological activity. Considering the action mechanism of the active ingredient, a suitable one of the methods used for the characterization is set as a biological activity test. The acceptance criterion is expressed in units/mL when the potency in the solution is used as an index, and when using the potency per protein amount as an index, it is expressed in units/mg. The potency per amount of protein is called the specific activity. Besides these, the specific activity may be compared with a standard material, and this may be expressed as a percentage (%) to obtain an acceptance criterion. In recent years, there has been an increasing number of cases where the ratio (%) of specific activity to a reference material is set as an acceptance criterion without setting a unit.

g. Quantity

The quantity of active ingredient contained in a drug substance and drug product is expressed as protein content (mass) or potency (unit). As it is a critical factor of product quality, measure it using an appropriate quantitative method. For tests to determine the protein content, the methods described in the General Information ''Total Protein Assay *<G3-12-172>*'', the method comparing peak areas with the reference material using HPLC, etc. are used. A biological test is used to determine the potency.

If physicochemical testing has provided sufficient physicochemical information on the product, including information on higher order structure, and proper correlation with biological activity has been well demonstrated, in addition, if the manufacturing experience is well established, biological tests for determining potency can be replaced by physicochemical testing. For insulins, etc., the quantity (unit) of the active ingredient in a sample is determined by comparing the peak area with the reference material indicated by the unit by the quantitative method using HPLC.

h. Tests for preparations

Conduct tests for preparations according to the dosage form. Since most biopharmaceuticals are injections, sterility test, bacterial endotoxin test, test for extractable volume of parenteral preparations, insoluble particulate matter test for injections and foreign insoluble matter test for injections, etc. are conducted.

1.2.5. Stability testing

a. Conditions of stability testing

The shelf life of biopharmaceuticals is usually set based on the results of long term testing at actual storage temperatures for the actual storage period of the product to be applied. The accelerated testing and the stress testing can provide supplementary information for setting the shelf life and useful information for elucidating the mechanism of quality change, as well as evaluating the validity of the analytical methods and the influence of storage conditions on the quality such as during transportation.

b. Attributes to be evaluated

During the storage of biopharmaceuticals, the bioactivity and the physicochemical properties may change, so it is necessary to comprehensively evaluate the quality characteristics by various analytical methods. In the stability testing, usually, adopting the appropriate attributes and tests used in characterization, evaluate the changes according to the characteristics of the product, such as biological activity, molecular heterogeneity, and product-related impurities.

2. Comparability of biopharmaceuticals subject to changes in their manufacturing process

When changing the manufacturing process of biopharmaceuticals, evaluation work on comparability will be carried out in order to ensure the quality, efficacy and safety of the drug product produced by the changed manufacturing process. The demonstration of comparability does not necessarily mean that the quality attributes of the pre-change and post-change product are identical, but that they are highly similar and that the existing knowledge is sufficiently predictive to ensure that any differences in quality attributes have no adverse impact upon safety and efficacy of the drug product. However, where the relationship between specific quality attributes and safety or efficacy has not been established, it might be appropriate to include a combination of quality, nonclinical, and/or clinical studies in the comparability exercise.

2.1. Considerations for the comparability exercise

The extent to which the test to prove the comparability before and after the change should be conducted is considered on the production step where the changes were introduced, on the risk level of potential impact of the changes on the quality characteristics, on the suitability of the analytical techniques used, and on the relationship between quality attributes and safety or efficacy based on overall nonclinical and clinical experience. The judgment of product comparability should be done by considering characterization data, stability data providing insight into potential product differences in the changes and the degradation of the protein, and data of lots used for demonstration of manufacturing consistency. The historical data that provide insight into changes of quality attributes with respect to safety and efficacy following manufacturing process change, and nonclinical or clinical characteristics of the drug product and its therapeutic indications should also be considered.

2.2. Quality considerations

By re-executing all or part of the characterization that has already been carried out (if it is a part, it is necessary to explain its appropriateness), compare the quality characteristics before and after the change directly, to obtain the data needed to determine the comparability. However, it is necessary to evaluate the meaning of the difference by additional characterization, such as when difference in heterogeneity and/or impurity profile are found before and after the change. Even when evaluating the same quality attributes, it is necessary to apply multiple analysis methods and analysis methods having different measurement principles, and devise to be able to detect the change of the quality characteristics that may occur due to the change of manufacturing process. In addition, changes in the manufacturing process, even minor one, may affect the stability of the product, so when changing the manufacturing process that possibly affect the quality characteristics, also evaluate the influence on the stability of the product.

2.3. Manufacturing process considerations

Confirm that the process controls in the modified process provide at least similar or more effective control of the product quality, compared to those of the original process. A careful consideration of potential impacts of the planned change on steps downstream and quality attributes related to these steps is extremely important. The modified process steps should be re-evaluated and/or re-validated, as appropriate.

3. References

1) ICH: Guideline for Q5A (R1), Viral Safety Evaluation of Biotechnology Products Derived from Cell Lines of Human or Animal Origin.
2) ICH: Guideline for Q5B, Quality of Biotechnological Products: Analysis of the Expression Construct in Cells Used for Production of R-DNA Derived Protein Products.
3) ICH: Guideline for Q5C, Quality of Biotechnological Products: Stability Testing of Biotechnological/Biological Products.
4) ICH: Guideline for Q5D, Derivation and Characterization of Cell Substrates Used for Production of Biotechnological/Biological Products.
5) ICH: Guideline for Q5E, Comparability of Biotechnological/Biological Products Subject to Changes in Their Manufacturing Process.
6) ICH: Guideline for Q6B, Specifications: Test Procedures and Acceptance Criteria for Biotechnological/Biological Products.

Amino Acid Analysis <*G3-2-171*>

This test is harmonized with the European Pharmacopoeia and the U.S. Pharmacopeia.

Information on the harmonization with the European Pharmacopoeia and the U.S. Pharmacopeia is available on the website of the Pharmaceuticals and Medical Devices Agency.

Amino acid analysis refers to the methodology used to determine the amino acid composition or content of proteins, peptides, and other pharmaceutical preparations. Proteins and peptides are macromolecules consisting of covalently bonded amino acid residues organized as a linear polymer. The sequence of the amino acids in a protein or peptide determines the properties of the molecule. Proteins are considered large molecules that commonly exist as folded structures with a specific conformation, while peptides are smaller and may consist of only a few amino acids. Amino acid analysis can be used to quantify protein and peptides, to determine the identity of proteins or peptides based on their amino acid composition, to support protein and peptide structure analysis, to evaluate fragmentation strategies for peptide mapping, and to detect atypical amino acids that might be present in a protein or peptide. It is necessary to hydrolyze a protein/peptide to its individual amino acid constituents before amino acid analysis. Following protein/peptide hydrolysis, the amino acid analysis procedure can be the same as that practiced for free amino acids in other pharmaceutical preparations. The amino acid constituents of the test sample are typically derivatized for analysis.

Apparatus

Methods used for amino acid analysis are usually based on a chromatographic separation of the amino acids present in the test sample. Current techniques take advantage of the automated chromatographic instrumentation designed for analytical methodologies. An amino acid analysis instrument will typically be a low-pressure or high-pressure liquid chromatograph capable of generating mobile phase gradients that separate the amino acid analytes on a chromatographic column. The instrument must have postcolumn derivatization capability, unless the sample is analyzed using precolumn derivatization. The detector is usually an ultraviolet-visible or fluorescence detector depending on the derivatization method used. A recording device (e.g., integrator) is used for transforming the analog signal from the detector and for quantitation. It is preferred that instrumentation be dedicated particularly for amino acid analysis.

General Precautions

Background contamination is always a concern for the analyst in performing amino acid analysis. High purity reagents are necessary (e.g., low purity hydrochloric acid can contribute to glycine contamination). Analytical reagents are changed routinely every few weeks using only high-pressure liquid chromatography (HPLC) grade solvents. Potential microbial contamination and foreign material that might be present in the solvents are reduced by filtering solvents before use, keeping solvent reservoirs covered, and not placing amino acid analysis instrumentation in direct sunlight.

Laboratory practices can determine the quality of the amino acid analysis. Place the instrumentation in a low traffic area of the laboratory. Keep the laboratory clean. Clean and calibrate pipets according to a maintenance schedule. Keep pipet tips in a covered box; the analysts may not handle pipet tips with their hands. The analysts may wear powder-free latex or equivalent gloves. Limit the number of times a test sample vial is opened and closed because dust can contribute to elevated levels of glycine, serine, and alanine.

A well-maintained instrument is necessary for acceptable amino acid analysis results. If the instrument is used on a routine basis, it is to be checked daily for leaks, detector and lamp stability, and the ability of the column to maintain resolution of the individual amino acids. Clean or replace all instrument filters and other maintenance items on a routine schedule.

Reference Standard Material

Acceptable amino acid standards are commercially available for amino acid analysis and typically consist of an aqueous mixture of amino acids. When determining amino acid composition, protein or peptide standards are analyzed with the test material as a control to demonstrate the integrity of the entire procedure. Highly purified bovine serum albumin has been used as a protein standard for this purpose.

Calibration of Instrumentation

Calibration of amino acid analysis instrumentation typically involves analyzing the amino acid standard, which consists of a mixture of amino acids at a number of concentrations, to determine the response factor and range of analysis for each amino acid. The concentration of each amino acid in the standard is known. In the calibration procedure, the analyst dilutes the amino acid standard to several different analyte levels within the expected linear range of the amino acid analysis technique. Then, replicates at each of the different analyte levels can be analyzed. Peak areas obtained for each amino acid are plotted versus the known concentration for each of the amino acids in the standard dilution. These results will allow the analyst to determine the range of amino acid concentrations where the peak area of a given amino acid is an approximately linear function of the amino acid concentration. It is important that the analyst prepare the samples for amino acid analysis so that they are within the analytical limits (e.g., linear working range) of the technique employed in order to obtain accurate and repeatable results.

Four to six amino acid standard levels are analyzed to determine a response factor for each amino acid. The response factor is calculated as the average peak area or peak height per nmol of amino acid present in the standard. A calibration file consisting of the response factor for each amino acid is prepared and used to calculate the concentration of each amino acid present in the test sample. This calculation involves dividing the peak area corresponding to a given amino acid by the response factor for that amino acid to give the nmol of the amino acid. For routine analysis, a single-point calibration may be sufficient; however, the calibration file is updated frequently and tested by the analysis of analytical controls to ensure its integrity.

Repeatability

Consistent high quality amino acid analysis results from an analytical laboratory require attention to the repeatability of the assay. During analysis of the chromatographic separation of the amino acids or their derivatives, numerous peaks can be observed on the chromatogram that correspond to the amino acids. The large number of peaks makes it necessary to have an amino acid analysis system that can repeatedly identify the peaks based on retention time and integrate the peak areas for quantitation. A typical repeatability evaluation involves preparing a standard amino acid solution and analyzing many replicates (i.e., six analyses or more) of the same standard solution. The relative standard deviation (RSD) is determined for the retention time and integrated peak area of each amino acid. An evaluation of the repeatability is expanded to include multiple assays conducted over several days by different analysts. Multiple assays include the preparation of standard dilutions from starting materials to determine the variation due to sample handling. Often the amino acid composition of a standard protein (e.g., bovine serum albumin) is analyzed as part of the repeatability evaluation. By evaluating the replicate variation (i.e., RSD), the laboratory can establish analytical limits to ensure that the analyses from the laboratory are under control. It is desirable to establish the lowest practical variation limits to ensure the best results. Areas to focus on to lower the variability of the amino acid analysis include sample preparation, high background spectral interference due to quality of reagents and/or laboratory practices, instrument performance and maintenance, data analysis and interpretation, and analyst performance and habits. All parameters involved are fully investigated in the scope of the validation work.

Sample Preparation

Accurate results from amino acid analysis require purified protein and peptide samples. Buffer components (e.g., salts, urea, detergents) can interfere with the amino acid analysis and are removed from the sample before analysis. Methods that utilize postcolumn derivatization of the amino acids are generally not affected by buffer components to the extent seen with precolumn derivatization methods. It is desirable to limit the number of sample manipulations to reduce potential background contamination, to improve analyte recovery, and to reduce labor. Common techniques used to remove buffer components from protein samples include the following methods: (1) injecting the protein sample onto a reversed-phase HPLC system, eluting the protein with a volatile solvent containing a sufficient organic component, and drying the sample in a vacuum centrifuge; (2) dialysis against a volatile buffer or water; (3) centrifugal ultrafiltration for buffer replacement with a volatile buffer or water; (4) precipitating the protein from the buffer using an organic solvent (e.g., acetone); and (5) gel filtration.

Internal Standards

It is recommended that an internal standard be used to monitor physical and chemical losses and variations during amino acid analysis. An accurately known amount of internal standard can be added to a protein solution prior to hydrolysis. The recovery of the internal standard gives the general recovery of the amino acids of the protein solution. Free amino acids, however, do not behave in the same way as protein-bound amino acids during hydrolysis because their rates of release or destruction are variable. Therefore, the use of an internal standard to correct for losses during hydrolysis may give unreliable results. It will be necessary to take this point under consideration when interpreting the results. Internal standards can also be added to the mixture of amino acids after hydrolysis to correct for differences in sample application and changes in reagent stability and flow rates. Ideally, an internal standard is an unnaturally occurring primary amino acid that is commercially available and inexpensive. It should also be stable during hydrolysis, its response factor should be linear with concentration, and it needs to elute with a unique retention time without overlapping other amino acids. Commonly used amino acid standards include norleucine, nitrotyrosine, and α-aminobutyric acid.

Protein Hydrolysis

Hydrolysis of protein and peptide samples is necessary for amino acid analysis of these molecules. The glassware used for hydrolysis must be very clean to avoid erroneous results. Glove powders and fingerprints on hydrolysis tubes may cause contamination. To clean glass hydrolysis tubes, boil tubes for 1 hour in 1 mol/L hydrochloric acid or soak tubes in concentrated nitric acid or in a mixture of concentrated hydrochloric acid and concentrated nitric acid (1:1). Clean hydrolysis tubes are rinsed with high-purity water followed by a rinse with HPLC grade methanol, dried overnight in an oven, and stored covered until use. Alternatively, pyrolysis of clean glassware at 500°C for 4 hours may also be used to eliminate contamination from hydrolysis tubes. Adequate disposable laboratory material can also be used.

Acid hydrolysis is the most common method for hydrolyzing a protein sample before amino acid analysis. The acid hydrolysis technique can contribute to the variation of the analysis due to complete or partial destruction of several amino acids. Tryptophan is destroyed; serine and threonine are partially destroyed; methionine might undergo oxidation; and cysteine is typically recovered as cystine (but cystine recovery is usually poor because of partial destruction or reduction to cysteine). Application of adequate vacuum (≦less than 200 μm of mercury or 26.7 Pa) or introduction of an inert gas (argon) in the headspace of the reaction vessel can reduce the level of oxidative destruction. In peptide bonds involving isoleucine and valine the amido bonds of Ile-Ile, Val-Val, Ile-Val, and Val-Ile are partially cleaved; and asparagine and glutamine are deamidated, resulting in aspartic acid and glutamic acid, respectively. The loss of tryptophan, asparagine, and glutamine during an acid hydrolysis limits quantitation to 17 amino acids. Some of the hydrolysis techniques described are used to address these concerns. Some of the hydrolysis techniques described (i.e., *Methods 4-11*) may cause modifications to other amino acids. Therefore, the benefits of using a given hydrolysis technique are weighed against the concerns with the technique and are tested adequately before employing a method other than acid hydrolysis.

A time-course study (i.e., amino acid analysis at acid hydrolysis times of 24, 48, and 72 hours) is often employed to analyze the starting concentration of amino acids that are partially destroyed or slow to cleave. By plotting the observed concentration of labile amino acids (i.e., serine and threonine) versus hydrolysis time, the line can be extrapolated to the origin to determine the starting concentration of these amino acids. Time-course hydrolysis studies are also used with amino acids that are slow to cleave (e.g., isoleucine and valine). During the hydrolysis time course, the analyst will observe a plateau in these residues. The level of this plateau is taken as the residue concentration. If the hydrolysis time is too long, the residue concentration of the sample will begin to decrease, indicating destruction by the hydrolysis conditions.

An acceptable alternative to the time-course study is to subject an amino acid calibration standard to the same hydrolysis conditions as the test sample. The amino acid in free form may not completely represent the rate of destruction of labile amino acids within a peptide or protein during the hydrolysis. This is especially true for peptide bonds that are slow to cleave (e.g., Ile-Val bonds). However, this technique will allow the analyst to account for some residue destruction. Microwave acid hydrolysis has been used and is rapid but requires special equipment as well as special precautions. The optimal conditions for microwave hydrolysis must be investigated for each individual protein/peptide sample. The microwave hydrolysis technique typically requires only a few minutes, but even a deviation of one minute may give inadequate results (e.g., incomplete hydrolysis or destruction of labile amino acids). Complete proteolysis, using a mixture of proteases, has been used but can be complicated, requires the proper controls, and is typically more applicable to peptides than proteins.

Note: During initial analyses of an unknown protein, experiments with various hydrolysis time and temperature conditions are conducted to determine the optimal conditions.

Method 1

Acid hydrolysis using hydrochloric acid containing phenol is the most common procedure used for protein/peptide hydrolysis preceding amino acid analysis. The addition of phenol to the reaction prevents the halogenation of tyrosine.

Hydrolysis Solution 6 mol/L hydrochloric acid containing 0.1% to 1.0% of phenol.

Procedure—

Liquid Phase Hydrolysis Place the protein or peptide sample in a hydrolysis tube, and dry. [Note: The sample is dried so that water in the sample will not dilute the acid used for the hydrolysis.] Add 200 μL of *Hydrolysis Solution* per 500 μg of lyophilized protein. Freeze the sample tube in a dry ice-acetone bath, and flame seal in vacuum. Samples are typically hydrolyzed at 110°C for 24 hours in vacuum or inert atmosphere to prevent oxidation. Longer hydrolysis times (e.g., 48 and 72 hours) are investigated if there is a concern that the protein is not completely hydrolyzed.

Vapor Phase Hydrolysis This is one of the most common acid hydrolysis procedures, and it is preferred for microanalysis when only small amounts of the sample are available. Contamination of the sample from the acid reagent is also minimized by using vapor phase hydrolysis. Place vials containing the dried samples in a vessel that contains an appropriate amount of *Hydrolysis Solution*. The *Hydrolysis Solution* does not come in contact with the test sample. Apply an inert atmosphere or vacuum (≦less than 200 μm of mercury or 26.7 Pa) to the headspace of the vessel, and heat to about 110°C for a 24-hour hydrolysis time. Acid vapor hydrolyzes the dried sample. Any condensation of the acid in the sample vials is minimized. After hydrolysis, dry the test sample in vacuum to remove any residual acid.

Method 2

Tryptophan oxidation during hydrolysis is decreased by using mercaptoethanesulfonic acid (MESA) as the reducing acid.

Hydrolysis Solution 2.5 mol/L MESA solution.

Vapor Phase Hydrolysis About 1 to 100 μg of the protein/peptide under test is dried in a hydrolysis tube. The hydrolysis tube is placed in a larger tube with about 200 μL of the *Hydrolysis Solution*. The larger tube is sealed in vacuum (about 50 μm of mercury or 6.7 Pa) to vaporize the *Hydrolysis Solution*. The hydrolysis tube is heated to 170°C to 185°C for about 12.5 minutes. After hydrolysis, the hydrolysis tube is dried in vacuum for 15 minutes to remove the residual acid.

Method 3

Tryptophan oxidation during hydrolysis is prevented by using thioglycolic acid (TGA) as the reducing acid.

Hydrolysis Solution A solution containing 7 mol/L hydrochloric acid, 10% of trifluoroacetic acid, 20% of thioglycolic acid, and 1% of phenol.

Vapor Phase Hydrolysis About 10 to 50 μg of the protein/peptide under test is dried in a sample tube. The sample tube is placed in a larger tube with about 200 μL of the

Hydrolysis Solution. The larger tube is sealed in vacuum (about 50 μm of mercury or 6.7 Pa) to vaporize the TGA. The sample tube is heated to 166°C for about 15 to 30 minutes. After hydrolysis, the sample tube is dried in vacuum for 5 minutes to remove the residual acid. Recovery of tryptophan by this method may be dependent on the amount of sample present.

Method 4

Cysteine-cystine and methionine oxidation is performed with performic acid before the protein hydrolysis.

Oxidation Solution The performic acid is prepared fresh by mixing formic acid and 30 percent hydrogen peroxide (9:1), and incubated at room temperature for 1 hour.

Procedure The protein/peptide sample is dissolved in 20 μL of formic acid, and heated at 50°C for 5 minutes; then 100 μL of the *Oxidation Solution* is added. The oxidation is allowed to proceed for 10 to 30 minutes. In this reaction, cysteine is converted to cysteic acid and methionine is converted to methionine sulfone. The excess reagent is removed from the sample in a vacuum centrifuge. This technique may cause modifications to tyrosine residues in the presence of halides. The oxidized protein can then be acid hydrolyzed using *Method 1* or *Method 2*.

Method 5

Cysteine-cystine oxidation is accomplished during the liquid phase hydrolysis with sodium azide.

Hydrolysis Solution 6 mol/L hydrochloric acid containing 0.2% of phenol, to which sodium azide is added to obtain a final concentration of 0.2% (w/v). The added phenol prevents halogenation of tyrosine.

Liquid Phase Hydrolysis The protein/peptide hydrolysis is conducted at about 110°C for 24 hours. During the hydrolysis, the cysteine-cystine present in the sample is converted to cysteic acid by the sodium azide present in the *Hydrolysis Solution*. This technique allows better tyrosine recovery than *Method 4*, but it is not quantitative for methionine. Methionine is converted to a mixture of the parent methionine and its two oxidative products, methionine sulfoxide and methionine sulfone.

Method 6

Cysteine-cystine oxidation is accomplished with dimethyl sulfoxide (DMSO).

Hydrolysis Solution 6 mol/L hydrochloric acid containing 0.1% to 1.0% of phenol, to which DMSO is added to obtain a final concentration of 2% (v/v).

Vapor Phase Hydrolysis The protein/peptide hydrolysis is conducted at about 110°C for 24 hours. During the hydrolysis, the cysteine-cystine present in the sample is converted to cysteic acid by the DMSO present in the *Hydrolysis Solution*. As an approach to limit variability and compensate for partial destruction, it is recommended to evaluate the cysteic acid recovery from oxidative hydrolyses of standard proteins containing 1 to 8 mol of cysteine per mol of protein. The response factors from protein/peptide hydrolysates are typically about 30% lower than those for nonhydrolyzed cysteic acid standards. Because histidine, methionine, tyrosine, and tryptophan are also modified, a complete compositional analysis is not obtained with this technique.

Method 7

Cysteine-cystine reduction and alkylation is accomplished by a vapor phase pyridylethylation reaction.

Reducing Solution Transfer 83.3 μL of pyridine, 16.7 μL of 4-vinylpyridine, 16.7 μL of tributylphosphine, and 83.3 μL of water to a suitable container, and mix.

Procedure Add the protein/peptide (between 1 μg and 100 μg) to a hydrolysis tube, and place in a larger tube. Transfer the *Reducing Solution* to the large tube, seal in vacuum (about 50 μm of mercury or 6.7 Pa), and incubate at about 100°C for 5 minutes. Then remove the inner hydrolysis tube, and dry it in a vacuum desiccator for 15 minutes to remove residual reagents. The pyridylethylated protein/peptide can then be acid hydrolyzed using previously described procedures. The pyridylethylation reaction is performed simultaneously with a protein standard sample containing 1 to 8 mol of cysteine per mol of protein to improve accuracy in the pyridylethylcysteine recovery. Longer incubation times for the pyridylethylation reaction can cause modifications to the α-amino terminal group and the ε-amino group of lysine in the protein.

Method 8

Cysteine-cystine reduction and alkylation is accomplished by a liquid phase pyridylethylation reaction.

Stock Solutions Prepare and filter three solutions: 1 mol/L Tris hydrochloride (pH 8.5) containing 4 mmol/L disodium dihydrogen ethylendiamine tetraacetate (*Stock Solution A*), 8 mol/L guanidine hydrochloride (*Stock Solution B*), and 10% of 2-mercaptoethanol in water (*Stock Solution C*).

Reducing Solution Prepare a mixture of *Stock Solution B* and *Stock Solution A* (3:1) to obtain a buffered solution of 6 mol/L guanidine hydrochloride in 0.25 mol/L Tris hydrochloride.

Procedure Dissolve about 10 μg of the test sample in 50 μL of the *Reducing Solution*, and add about 2.5 μL of *Stock Solution C*. Store under nitrogen or argon for 2 hours at room temperature in the dark. To achieve the pyridylethylation reaction, add about 2 μL of 4-vinylpyridine to the protein solution, and incubate for an additional 2 hours at room temperature in the dark. The protein/peptide is desalted by collecting the protein/peptide fraction from a reversed-phase HPLC separation. The collected sample can be dried in a vacuum centrifuge before acid hydrolysis.

Method 9

Cysteine-cystine reduction and alkylation is accomplished by a liquid phase carboxymethylation reaction.

Stock Solutions Prepare as directed for *Method 8*.

Carboxymethylation Solution Prepare a solution containing 100 mg of iodoacetamide per mL of ethanol (95).

Buffer Solution Use the *Reducing Solution*, prepared as directed for *Method 8*.

Procedure Dissolve the test sample in 50 μL of the *Buffer Solution*, and add about 2.5 μL of *Stock Solution C*. Store under nitrogen or argon for 2 hours at room temperature in the dark. Add the *Carboxymethylation Solution* in a ratio 1.5 fold per total theoretical content of thiols, and incubate for an additional 30 minutes at room temperature in the dark. [Note: If the thiol content of the protein is unknown, then add 5 μL of 100 mmol/L iodoacetamide for every 20 nmol of protein present.] The reaction is stopped by adding excess of 2-mercaptoethanol. The protein/peptide is desalted by collecting the protein/peptide fraction from a reversed-phase HPLC separation. The collected sample can be dried in a vacuum centrifuge before acid hydrolysis. The *S*-carboxyamidomethyl-cysteine formed will be converted to *S*-carboxymethylcysteine during acid hydrolysis.

Method 10

Cysteine-cystine is reacted with dithiodiglycolic acid or dithiodipropionic acid to produce a mixed disulfide. [Note: The choice of dithiodiglycolic acid or dithiodipropionic acid depends on the required resolution of the amino acid analysis method.]

Reducing Solution A solution containing 10 mg of dithiodiglycolic acid (or dithiodipropionic acid) per mL of 0.2 mol/L sodium hydroxide.

Procedure Transfer about 20 μg of the test sample to a hydrolysis tube, and add 5 μL of the *Reducing Solution*. Add 10 μL of isopropyl alcohol, and then remove all of the sample liquid by vacuum centrifugation. The sample is then hydrolyzed using *Method 1*. This method has the advantage that other amino acid residues are not derivatized by side reactions, and the sample does not need to be desalted prior to hydrolysis.

Method 11

Asparagine and glutamine are converted to aspartic acid and glutamic acid, respectively, during acid hydrolysis. Asparagine and aspartic acid residues are added and represented by *Asx*, while glutamine and glutamic acid residues are added and represented by *Glx*. Proteins/peptides can be reacted with bis(1,1-trifluoroacetoxy)iodobenzene (BTI) to convert the asparagine and glutamine residues to diaminopropionic acid and diaminobutyric acid residues, respectively, upon acid hydrolysis. These conversions allow the analyst to determine the asparagine and glutamine content of a protein/peptide in the presence of aspartic acid and glutamic acid residues.

Reducing Solutions Prepare and filter three solutions: a solution of 10 mmol/L trifluoroacetic acid (*Solution A*), a solution of 5 mol/L guanidine hydrochloride and 10 mmol/L trifluoroacetic acid (*Solution B*), and a freshly prepared solution of *N*,*N*-dimethylformamide containing 36 mg of BTI per mL (*Solution C*).

Procedure In a clean hydrolysis tube, transfer about 200 μg of the test sample, and add 2 mL of *Solution A* or *Solution B* and 2 mL of *Solution C*. Seal the hydrolysis tube in vacuum. Heat the sample at 60°C for 4 hours in the dark. The sample is then dialyzed with water to remove the excess reagents. Extract the dialyzed sample three times with equal volumes of *n*-butyl acetate, and then lyophilize. The protein can then be acid hydrolyzed using previously described procedures. The α,β-diaminopropionic and α,γ-diaminobutyric acid residues do not typically resolve from the lysine residues upon ion-exchange chromatography based on amino acid analysis. Therefore, when using ion-exchange as the mode of amino acid separation, the asparagine and glutamine contents are the quantitative difference in the aspartic acid and glutamic acid content assayed with underivatized and BTI-derivatized acid hydrolysis. [Note: The threonine, methionine, cysteine, tyrosine, and histidine assayed content can be altered by BTI derivatization; a hydrolysis without BTI will have to be performed if the analyst is interested in the composition of these other amino acid residues of the protein/peptide.]

Methodologies of Amino Acid Analysis General Principles

Many amino acid analysis techniques exist, and the choice of any one technique often depends on the sensitivity required from the assay. In general, about one-half of the amino acid analysis techniques employed rely on the separation of the free amino acids by ion-exchange chromatography followed by postcolumn derivatization (e.g., with ninhydrin or *o*-phthalaldehyde). Postcolumn detection techniques can be used with samples that contain small amounts of buffer components, such as salts and urea, and generally require between 5 and 10 μg of protein sample per analysis. The remaining amino acid techniques typically involve precolumn derivatization of the free amino acids (e.g., phenyl isothiocyanate; 6-aminoquinolyl-*N*-hydroxysuccinimidyl carbamate or *o*-phthalaldehyde; (dimethylamino)azobenzenesulfonyl chloride; 9-fluorenylmethylchloroformate; and, 7-fluoro-4-nitrobenzo-2-oxa-1,3-diazole) followed by reversed-phase HPLC. Precolumn derivatization techniques are very sensitive and usually require between 0.5 and 1.0 μg of protein sample per analysis but may be influenced by buffer salts in the samples. Precolumn derivatization techniques may also result in multiple derivatives of a given amino acid, which complicates the result interpretation. Postcolumn derivatization techniques are generally influenced less by performance variation of the assay than precolumn derivatization techniques.

The following *Methods* may be used for quantitative amino acid analysis. Instruments and reagents for these procedures are available commercially. Furthermore, many modifications of these methodologies exist with different reagent preparations, reaction procedures, chromatographic systems, etc. Specific parameters may vary according to the exact equipment and procedure used. Many laboratories will utilize more than one amino acid analysis technique to exploit the advantages offered by each. In each of these *Methods*, the analog signal is visualized by means of a data acquisition system, and the peak areas are integrated for quantification purposes.

Method 1—Postcolumn Ninhydrin Detection General Principle

Ion-exchange chromatography with postcolumn ninhydrin detection is one of the most common methods employed for quantitative amino acid analysis. As a rule, a Li-based cation-exchange system is employed for the analysis of the more complex physiological samples, and the faster Na-based cation-exchange system is used for the more simplistic amino acid mixtures obtained with protein hydrolysates (typically containing 17 amino acid components). Separation of the amino acids on an ion-exchange column is accomplished through a combination of changes in pH and cation strength. A temperature gradient is often employed to enhance separation.

When the amino acid reacts with ninhydrin, the reactant has characteristic purple or yellow color. Amino acids, except imino acid, give a purple color, and show the maximum absorption at 570 nm. The imino acids such as proline give a yellow color, and show the maximum absorption at 440 nm. The postcolumn reaction between ninhydrin and amino acid eluted from column is monitored at 440 and 570 nm, and the chromatogram obtained is used for the determination of amino acid composition.

Detection limit is considered to be 10 pmol for most of the amino acid derivatives, but 50 pmol for proline. Response linearity is obtained in the range of 20 to 500 pmol with correlation coefficients exceeding 0.999. To obtain good composition data, samples larger than 1 μg before hydrolysis are best suited for this amino acid analysis of protein/peptide.

Method 2—Postcolumn OPA Fluorometric Detection General Principle

o-Phthalaldehyde (OPA) reacts with primary amines in the presence of thiol compound, to form highly fluorescent isoindole products. This reaction is utilized for the postcolumn derivatization in analysis of amino acids by ion-exchange chromatography. The rule of the separation is the same as *Method 1*. Instruments and reagents for this form of amino acid analysis are available commercially. Many modifications of this methodology exist.

Although OPA does not react with secondary amines (imino acids such as proline) to form fluorescent substances, the oxidation with sodium hypochlorite allows secondary amines to react with OPA. The procedure employs a strongly acidic cation-exchange column for separation of free amino acids followed by postcolumn oxidation with sodium hypochlorite and postcolumn derivatization using OPA and thiol compound such as *N*-acetyl-L-cysteine and 2-mercaptoethanol. The derivatization of primary amino acids is not noticeably affected by the continuous supply of sodium hypochlorite.

Separation of the amino acids on an ion-exchange column is accomplished through a combination of changes in pH and cation strength. After postcolumn derivatization of eluted amino acids with OPA, the reactant passes through the fluorometric detector. Fluorescence intensity of OPA-derivatized amino acids is monitored with an excitation wavelength of 348 nm and an emission wavelength of 450 nm.

Detection limit is considered to be a few tens of picomole level for most of the amino acid derivatives. Response linearity is obtained in the range of a few picomole level to a few tens of nanomole level. To obtain good compositional data, the starting with greater than 500 ng of sample before hydrolysis is best suited for the amino acid analysis of protein/peptide.

Method 3—Precolumn PITC Derivatization General Principle

Phenylisothiocyanate (PITC) reacts with amino acids to form phenylthiocarbamyl (PTC) derivatives which can be detected with high sensitivity at 245 nm. Therefore, precolumn derivatization of amino acids with PITC followed by reversed-phase HPLC separation with UV detection is used to analyze the amino acid composition.

After the reagent is removed under vacuum, the derivatized amino acids can be stored dry and frozen for several weeks with no significant degradation. If the solution for injection is kept cold, no noticeable loss in chromatographic response occurs after three days.

Separation of the PTC-amino acids on a reversed-phase HPLC with ODS column is accomplished through a combination of changes in concentrations of acetonitrile and buffer ionic strength. PTC-amino acids eluted from the column are monitored at 254 nm.

Detection limit is considered to be 1 pmol for most of the amino acid derivatives. Response linearity is obtained in the range of 20 to 500 pmol with correlation coefficients exceeding 0.999. To obtain good compositional data, samples larger than 500 ng of protein/peptide before hydrolysis is best suited for this amino acid analysis of proteins/peptides.

Method 4—Precolumn AQC Derivatization General Principle

Precolumn derivatization of amino acids with 6-aminoquinolyl-*N*-hydroxysuccinimidyl carbamate (AQC) followed by reversed-phase HPLC separation with fluorometric detection is used.

AQC reacts with amino acids to form stable, fluorescent unsymmetric urea derivatives (AQC-amino acids) which are readily amenable to analysis by reversed-phase HPLC. Therefore, precolumn derivatization of amino acids with AQC followed by reversed-phase HPLC separation is used to analyze the amino acid composition.

Separation of the AQC-amino acids on an ODS column is accomplished through a combination of changes in concentrations of acetonitrile and salt. Selective fluorescence detection of the derivatives with excitation wavelength at 250 nm and emission wavelength at 395 nm allows for the direct injection of the reaction mixture with no significant interference from the only major fluorescent reagent by-product, 6-aminoquinoline. Excess reagent is rapidly hydrolyzed ($t_{1/2} < 15$ seconds) to yield 6-aminoquinoline, *N*-hydroxysuccinimide and carbon dioxide, and after 1 minute no further derivatization can take place.

Peak areas for AQC-amino acids are essentially unchanged for at least 1 week at room temperature, and the derivatives have more than sufficient stability to allow for overnight automated chromatographic analysis.

Detection limit is considered to be ranging from ca. 40 to 320 fmol for each amino acid, except for Cys. Detection limit for Cys is approximately 800 fmol. Response linearity is obtained in the range of 2.5 to 200 μmol/L with correlation coefficients exceeding 0.999. Good compositional data could be obtained from the analysis of derivatized protein hydrolysates containing as little as 30 ng of protein/peptide.

Method 5—Precolumn OPA Derivatization General Principle

Precolumn derivatization of amino acids with *o*-phthalaldehyde (OPA) followed by reversed-phase HPLC separation with fluorometric detection is used. This technique does not detect amino acids that exist as secondary amines (e.g., proline).

OPA in conjunction with a thiol reagent reacts with primary amine groups to form highly fluorescent isoindole products. 2-Mercaptoethanol or 3-mercaptopropionic acid can be used as thiol. OPA itself does not fluoresce and consequently produces no interfering peaks. In addition, its solubility and stability in aqueous solution, along with the rapid kinetics for the reaction, make it amenable to automated derivatization and analysis using an autosampler to mix the sample with the reagent. However, lack of reactivity with secondary amino acids has been a predominant drawback. This method does not detect amino acids that exist as secondary amines (e.g., proline). To compensate for this drawback, this technique may be combined with another technique described in *Method 7* or *Method 8*.

Precolumn derivatization of amino acids with OPA is followed by reversed-phase HPLC separation. Because of the instability of the OPA-amino acid derivative, HPLC separation and analysis are performed immediately following derivatization. The liquid chromatograph is equipped with a fluorometric detector for the detection of derivatized amino acids. Fluorescence intensity of OPA-derivatized amino acids is monitored with an excitation wavelength of 348 nm and an emission wavelength of 450 nm.

Detection limits as low as 50 fmol via fluorescence have been reported, although the practical limit of analysis remains at 1 pmol.

Method 6—Precolumn DABS-Cl Derivatization General Principle

Precolumn derivatization of amino acids with (dimethylamino)azobenzenesulfonyl chloride (DABS-Cl) followed by reversed-phase HPLC separation with visible light detection is used.

DABS-Cl is a chromophoric reagent employed for the labeling of amino acids. Amino acids labeled with DABS-Cl (DABS-amino acids) are highly stable and show the maximum absorption at 436 nm.

DABS-amino acids, all 19 naturally occurring amino acids derivatives, can be separated on an ODS column of reversed-phase HPLC by employing gradient systems consisting of acetonitrile and aqueous buffer mixture. Separated DABS-amino acids eluted from the column are detected at 436 nm in the visible region.

This *Method* can analyze the imino acids such as proline together with the amino acids at the same degree of sensitivity, DABS-Cl derivatization method permits the simultaneous quantification of tryptophan residues by previous hydrolysis of the protein/peptide with sulfonic acids such as mercaptoethanesulfonic acid, *p*-toluenesulfonic acid or methanesulfonic acid described under *Method 2* in ''Protein Hydrolysis''. The other acid-labile residues, asparagine and glutamine, can also be analysed by previous conversion into diaminopropionic acid and diaminobutyric acid, respectively, by treatment of protein/peptide with BTI described under *Method 11* in ''Protein Hydrolysis''.

The non-proteinogenic amino acid, norleucine cannot be used as internal standard in this method, as this compound is eluted in a chromatographic region crowded with peaks of primary amino acids. Nitrotyrosine can be used as an internal standard, because it is eluted in a clean region.

Detection limit of DABS-amino acid is about 1 pmol. As little as 2 to 5 pmol of an individual DABS-amino acid can be quantitatively analyzed with reliability, and only 10 to 30 ng of the dabsylated protein hydrolysate is required for each analysis.

Method 7—Precolumn FMOC-Cl Derivatization General Principle

Precolumn derivatization of amino acids with 9-fluorenylmethyl chloroformate (FMOC-Cl) followed by reversed-phase HPLC separation with fluorometric detection is used.

FMOC-Cl reacts with both primary and secondary amino acids to form highly fluorescent products. The reaction of FMOC-Cl with amino acid proceeds under mild conditions in aqueous solution and is completed in 30 seconds. The derivatives are stable, only the histidine derivative showing any breakdown. Although FMOC-Cl is fluorescent itself, the reagent excess and fluorescent side-products can be eliminated without loss of FMOC-amino acids.

FMOC-amino acids are separated by a reversed-phase HPLC using an ODS column. The separation is carried out by gradient elution varied linearly from a mixture of acetonitrile methanol and acetic acid buffer (10:40:50) to a mixture of acetonitrile and acetic acid buffer (50:50), and 20 amino acid derivatives are separated in 20 minutes. Each derivative eluted from the column is monitored by a fluorometric detector set at an excitation wavelength of 260 nm and an emission wavelength of 313 nm.

The detection limit is in the low fmol range. A linearity range of 0.1 to 50 μmol/L is obtained for most of the amino acids.

Method 8—Precolumn NBD-F Derivatization General Principle

Precolumn derivatization of amino acids with 7-fluoro-4-nitrobenzo-2-oxa-1.3-diazole (NBD-F) followed by reversed-phase HPLC separation with fluorometric detection is used.

NBD-F reacts with both primary and secondary amino acids to form highly fluorescent products. Amino acids are derivatized with NBD-F by heating to 60°C for 5 minutes.

NBD-amino acid derivatives are separated on an ODS column of reversed-phase HPLC by employing gradient elution system consisting of acetonitrile and aqueous buffer mixture, and 17 amino acid derivatives are separated in 35 minutes. ε-Aminocaproic acid can be used as an internal standard, because it is eluted in a clean chromatographic region. Each derivative eluted from the column is monitored by a fluorometric detector set at an excitation wavelength of 480 nm and an emission wavelength of 530 nm.

The sensitivity of this method is almost the same as for precolumn OPA derivatization method (*Method 5*), excluding proline to which OPA is not reactive, and might be advantageous for NBD-F against OPA. The detection limit for each amino acid is about 10 fmol. Profile analysis was achieved for about 1.5 μg of protein hydrolysates in the final precolumn labeling reaction mixture for HPLC.

Data Calculation and Analysis

When determining the amino acid content of a protein/peptide hydrolysate, it should be noted that the acid hydrolysis step destroys tryptophan and cysteine. Serine and threonine are partially destroyed by acid hydrolysis, while isoleucine and valine residues may be only partially cleaved. Methionine can undergo oxidation during acid hydrolysis, and some amino acids (e.g., glycine and serine) are common contaminants. Application of adequate vacuum (≦0.0267 kPa) or introduction of inert gas (argon) in the headspace of the reaction vessel during vapor phase hydrolysis can reduce the level of oxidative destruction. Therefore, the quantitative results obtained for cysteine, tryptophan, threonine, isoleucine, valine, methionine, glycine, and serine from a protein/peptide hydrolysate may be variable and may warrant further investigation and consideration.

Calculations

Amino Acid Mole Percent This is the number of specific amino acid residues per 100 residues in a protein. This result may be useful for evaluating amino acid analysis data when the molecular weight of the protein under investigation is unknown. This information can be used to corroborate the identity of a protein/peptide and has other applications. Carefully identify and integrate the peaks obtained as directed for each *Procedure*. Calculate the mole percent for each amino acid present in the test sample by the formula:

$$100r_U/r,$$

in which r_U is the peak response, in nmol, of the amino acid under test; and r is the sum of peak responses, in nmol, for all amino acids present in the test sample. Comparison of the mole percent of the amino acids under test to data from known proteins can help establish or corroborate the identity of the sample protein.

Unknown Protein Samples This data analysis technique can be used to estimate the protein concentration of an unknown protein sample using the amino acid analysis data. Calculate the mass, in μg, of each recovered amino acid by the formula:

$$mM_W/1000,$$

in which m is the recovered quantity, in nmol, of the amino acid under test; and M_W is the average molecular weight for that amino acid, corrected for the weight of the water molecule that was eliminated during peptide bond formation. The sum of the masses of the recovered amino acids will give an estimate of the total mass of the protein analyzed after appropriate correction for partially and completely destroyed amino acids. If the molecular weight of the unknown protein is available (i.e., by SDS-PAGE analysis or mass spectroscopy), the amino acid composition of the unknown protein can be predicted. Calculate the number of residues of each amino acid by the formula:

$$m/(1000M/M_{WT}),$$

in which m is the recovered quantity, in nmol, of the amino acid under test; M is the total mass, in μg, of the protein; and M_{WT} is the molecular weight of the unknown protein.

Known Protein Samples This data analysis technique can be used to investigate the amino acid composition and protein concentration of a protein sample of known molecular weight and amino acid composition using the amino acid analysis data. When the composition of the protein being analyzed is known, one can exploit the fact that some amino acids are recovered well, while other amino acid recoveries may be compromised because of complete or partial destruction (e.g., tryptophan, cysteine, threonine, serine, methionine), incomplete bond cleavage (i.e., for isoleucine and valine) and free amino acid contamination (i.e., by glycine and serine).

Because those amino acids that are recovered best represent the protein, these amino acids are chosen to quantify the amount of protein. Well-recovered amino acids are, typically, aspartate-asparagine, glutamate-glutamine, alanine, leucine, phenylalanine, lysine, and arginine. This list can be modified based on experience with one's own analysis system. Divide the quantity, in nmol, of each of the well-recovered amino acids by the expected number of residues for that amino acid to obtain the protein content based on each well-recovered amino acid. Average the protein content results calculated. The protein content determined for each of the well-recovered amino acids should be evenly distributed about the mean. Discard protein content values for those amino acids that have an unacceptable deviation from the mean. Typically ≧greater than 5% variation from the mean is considered unacceptable. Recalculate the mean protein content from the remaining values to obtain the protein content of the sample. Divide the content of each amino acid by the calculated mean protein content to determine the amino acid composition of the sample by analysis.

Calculate the relative compositional error, in percentage, by the formula:

$$100m/m_S,$$

in which m is the experimentally determined quantity, in nmol per amino acid residue, of the amino acid under test; and m_S is the known residue value for that amino acid. The average relative compositional error is the average of the absolute values of the relative compositional errors of the individual amino acids, typically excluding tryptophan and cysteine from this calculation. The average relative compositional error can provide important information on the stability of analysis run over time. The agreement in the amino acid composition between the protein sample and the known composition can be used to corroborate the identity and purity of the protein in the sample.

Peptide Mapping *<G3-3-142>*

This test is harmonized with the European Pharmacopoeia and the U.S. Pharmacopeia.

Information on the harmonization with the European Pharmacopoeia and the U.S. Pharmacopeia is available on the website of the Pharmaceuticals and Medical Devices Agency.

Peptide mapping is an identity test for proteins, especially those obtained by r-DNA technology. It involves the chemical or enzymatic treatment of a protein, resulting in the formation of peptide fragments, followed by separation and identification of the fragments in a reproducible manner. It is a powerful test that is capable of identifying single amino acid changes resulting from events such as errors in the reading of complementary DNA (cDNA) sequences or point mutations. Peptide mapping is a comparative procedure because the information obtained, compared to a reference standard or reference material similarly treated, confirms the primary structure of the protein, is capable of detecting whether alterations in structure have occurred, and demonstrates process consistency and genetic stability. Each protein presents unique characteristics which must be well understood so that the scientific and analytical approaches permit validated development of a peptide map that provides sufficient specificity.

This chapter provides detailed assistance in the application of peptide mapping and its validation to characterize the desired protein product, to evaluate the stability of the expression construct of cells used for recombinant DNA products, to evaluate the consistency of the overall process and to assess product stability as well as to ensure the identity of the protein product, or to detect the presence of protein variant.

1. Peptide Map

Peptide mapping is not a general method, but involves developing specific maps for each unique protein. Although the technology is evolving rapidly, there are certain methods that are generally accepted. Variations of these methods will be indicated, when appropriate, in specific monographs.

A peptide map may be viewed as a fingerprint of a protein and is the end product of several chemical processes that provide a comprehensive understanding of the protein being analyzed. Four major steps are necessary for the development of the procedure: isolation and purification of the protein, if the protein is part of a formulation; selective cleavage of the peptide bonds; chromatographic separation of the peptides; and analysis and identification of the peptides. A test sample is digested and assayed in parallel with a reference standard or a reference material. Complete cleavage of peptide bonds is more likely to occur when enzymes such as endoproteases (e.g., trypsin) are used, instead of chemical cleavage reagents. A map should contain enough peptides to be meaningful. On the other hand, if there are too many fragments, the map might lose its specificity because many proteins will then have the same profiles.

2. Isolation and Purification

Isolation and purification are necessary for analysis of bulk drugs or dosage forms containing interfering excipients and carrier proteins and, when required, will be specified in the monograph. Quantitative recovery of protein from the dosage form should be validated.

3. Selective Cleavage of Peptide Bonds

The selection of the approach used for the cleavage of peptide bonds will depend on the protein under test. This selection process involves determination of the type of cleavage to be employed —enzymatic or chemical— and the type of cleavage agent within the chosen category. Several cleavage agents and their specificity are shown in Table 1. This list is not all-inclusive and will be expanded as other cleavage agents are identified.

3.1. Pretreatment of Sample

Depending on the size or the configuration of the protein, different approaches in the pretreatment of samples can be used. For monoclonal antibodies, the heavy and light chains will need to be separated before mapping. If trypsin is used as a cleavage agent for proteins with a molecular mass greater than 100,000 Da, lysine residues must be protected by citraconylation or maleylation; otherwise, too many peptides will be generated.

3.2. Pretreatment of the Cleavage Agent

Pretreatment of cleavage agents —especially enzymatic

Table 1 Examples of cleavage agents

Type	Agent	Specificity
Enzymatic	Trypsin (EC 3.4.21.4)	C-terminal side of Arg and Lys
	Chymotrypsin (EC 3.4.21.1)	C-terminal side of hydrophobic residues (e.g., Leu, Met, Ala, aromatics)
	Pepsin (EC 3.4.23.1 & 2)	Nonspecific digest
	Lysyl endopeptidase (Lys-C endopeptidase) (EC 3.4.21.50)	C-terminal side of Lys
	Glutamyl endopeptidase (from *S. aureus* strain V8) (EC 3.4.21.19)	C-terminal side of Glu and Asp
	Peptidyl-Asp metallo endopeptidase (Endoproteinase Asp-N) (EC 3.24.33)	N-terminal side of Asp
	Clostripain (EC 3.4.22.8)	C-terminal side of Arg
Chemical	Cyanogen bromide	C-terminal side of Met
	2-Nitro-5-thio-cyanobenzoic acid	N-terminal side of Cys
	o-Iodosobenzoic acid	C-terminal side of Trp and Tyr
	Dilute acid	Asp and Pro
	BNPS-skatole	Trp

agents— might be necessary for purification purposes to ensure reproducibility of the map. For example, trypsin used as a cleavage agent will have to be treated with tosyl-L-phenylalanine chloromethyl ketone to inactivate chymotrypsin. Other methods, such as purification of trypsin by HPLC or immobilization of enzyme on a gel support, have been successfully used when only a small amount of protein is available.

3.3. Pretreatment of the Protein

Under certain conditions, it might be necessary to concentrate the sample or to separate the protein from added substances and stabilizers used in formulation of the product, if these interfere with the mapping procedure. Physical procedures used for pretreatment can include ultrafiltration, column chromatography, and lyophilization. Other pretreatments, such as the addition of chaotropic agents (e.g., urea) can be used to unfold the protein prior to mapping. To allow the enzyme to have full access to cleavage sites and permit some unfolding of the protein, it is often necessary to reduce and alkylate the disulfide bonds prior to digestion.

Digestion with trypsin can introduce ambiguities in the tryptic map due to side reactions occurring during the digestion reaction, such as nonspecific cleavage, deamidation, disulfide isomerization, oxidation of methionine residues, or formation of pyroglutamic groups created from the deamidation of glutamine at the N-terminal side of a peptide. Furthermore, peaks may be produced by autohydrolysis of trypsin. Their intensities depend on the ratio of trypsin to protein. To avoid autohydrolysis, solutions of proteases may be prepared at a pH that is not optimal (e.g., at pH 5 for trypsin), which would mean that the enzyme would not become active until diluted with the digest buffer.

3.4. Establishment of Optimal Digestion Conditions

Factors that affect the completeness and effectiveness of digestion of proteins are those that could affect any chemical or enzymatic reactions.

(i) pH: The pH of the digestion mixture is empirically determined to ensure the optimal performance of the given cleavage agent. For example, when using cyanogen bromide as a cleavage agent, a highly acidic environment (e.g., pH 2, formic acid) is necessary; however, when using trypsin as a cleavage agent, a slightly alkaline environment (pH 8) is optimal. As a general rule, the pH of the reaction milieu should not alter the chemical integrity of the protein during the digestion and should not change during the course of the fragmentation reaction.

(ii) Temperature: A temperature between 25°C and 37°C is adequate for most digestions. The temperature used is intended to minimize chemical side reactions. The type of protein under test will dictate the temperature of the reaction milieu, because some proteins are more susceptible to denaturation as the temperature of the reaction increases. For example, digestion of recombinant bovine somatropin is conducted at 4°C, because at higher temperatures it will precipitate during digestion.

(iii) Time: If sufficient sample is available, a time course study is considered in order to determine the optimum time to obtain a reproducible map and avoid incomplete digestion. Time of digestion varies from 2 to 30 hours. The reaction is stopped by the addition of an acid which does not interfere in the tryptic map or by freezing.

(iv) Amount of Cleavage Agent: Although excessive amounts of cleavage agent are used to accomplish a reasonably rapid digestion time (i.e., 6 to 20 hours), the amount of cleavage agent is minimized to avoid its contribution to the chromatographic map pattern. A protein to protease ratio between 20:1 and 200:1 is generally used. It is recommended that the cleavage agent can be added in two or more stages to optimize cleavage. Nonetheless, the final reaction volume remains small enough to facilitate the next step in peptide mapping —the separation step. To sort out digestion artifacts that might be interfering with the subsequent analysis, a blank determination is performed, using a digestion control with all the reagents, except the test protein.

4. Chromatographic Separation

Many techniques are used to separate peptides for mapping. The selection of a technique depends on the protein being mapped. Techniques that have been successfully used for separation of peptides are shown in Table 2. In this section, a most widely used reverse-phase high performance liquid chromatography (RP-HPLC) is described as one of the procedures of chromatographic separation.

The purity of solvents and mobile phases is a critical factor in HPLC separation. HPLC-grade solvents and water that are commercially available are recommended for RP-HPLC. Dissolved gases present a problem in gradient systems where the solubility of the gas in a solvent may be less in a mixture than in a single solvent. Vacuum degassing and agitation by sonication are often used as useful degassing procedures. When solid particles in the solvents are drawn into the HPLC system, they can damage the sealing of pump valves or clog the top of the chromatographic column. Both pre- and post-pump filtration is also recommended.

4.1. Chromatographic Column

The selection of a chromatographic column is empirically determined for each protein. Columns with 100 Å or 300 Å pore size with silica support can give optimal separation. For smaller peptides, octylsilane chemically bonded to totally

Table 2 Techniques used for the separation of peptides

Reverse-Phase High Performance Liquid Chromatography (RP-HPLC)
Ion-Exchange Chromatography (IEC)
Hydrophobic Interaction Chromatography (HIC)
Polyacrylamide Gel Electrophoresis (PAGE), nondenaturating
SDS Polyacrylamide Gel Electrophoresis (SDS-PAGE)
Capillary Electrophoresis (CE)
Paper Chromatography-High Voltage (PCHV)
High-Voltage Paper Electrophoresis (HVPE)

porous silica articles, 3 to 10 μm in diameter (L7) and octadecylsilane chemically bonded to porous silica or ceramic micro-particles, 3 to 10 μm in diameter (L1) column packings are more efficient than the butyl silane chemically bonded to totally porous silica particles, 5 to 10 μm in diameter (L26) packing.

4.2. Solvent

The most commonly used solvent is water with acetonitrile as the organic modifier to which less than 0.1% trifluoroacetic acid is added. If necessary, add 2-propanol or 1-propanol to solubilize the digest components, provided that the addition does not unduly increase the viscosity of the components.

4.3. Mobile Phase

Buffered mobile phases containing phosphate are used to provide some flexibility in the selection of pH conditions, since shifts of pH in the 3.0 to 5.0 range enhance the separation of peptides containing acidic residues (e.g., glutamic and aspartic acids). Sodium or potassium phosphates, ammonium acetate, phosphoric acid, and a pH between 2 and 7 (or higher for polymer-based supports) have also been used with acetonitrile gradients. Acetonitrile containing trifluoroacetic acid is used quite often.

4.4. Gradient Selection

Gradients can be linear, nonlinear, or include step functions. A shallow gradient is recommended in order to separate complex mixtures. Gradients are optimized to provide clear resolution of one or two peaks that will become "marker" peaks for the test.

4.5. Isocratic Selection

Isocratic HPLC systems using a single mobile phase are used on the basis of their convenience of use and improved detector responses. Optimal composition of a mobile phase to obtain clear resolution of each peak is sometimes difficult to establish. Mobile phases for which slight changes in component ratios or in pH significantly affect retention times of peaks in peptide maps should not be used in isocratic HPLC systems.

4.6. Other Parameters

Temperature control of the column is usually necessary to achieve good reproducibility. The flow rates for the mobile phases range from 0.1 to 2.0 mL per minute, and the detection of peptides is performed with a UV detector at 200 to 230 nm. Other methods of detection have been used (e.g., postcolumn derivatization), but they are not as robust or versatile as UV detection.

4.7 Validation

This section provides an experimental means for measuring the overall performance of the test method. The acceptance criteria for system suitability depend on the identification of critical test parameters that affect data interpretation and acceptance. These critical parameters are also criteria that monitor peptide digestion and peptide analysis. An indicator that the desired digestion endpoint was achieved is by the comparison with a reference standard or reference material, which is treated exactly as the article under test. The use of a reference standard or reference material in parallel with the protein under test is critical in the development and establishment of system suitability limits. In addition a specimen chromatogram should be included with the reference standard or reference material for additional comparison purposes. Other indicators may include visual inspection of protein or peptide solubility, the absence of intact protein, or measurement of responses of a digestion-dependent peptide. The critical system suitability parameters for peptide analysis will depend on the particular mode of peptide separation and detection and on the data analysis requirements.

When peptide mapping is used as an identification test, the system suitability requirements for the identified peptides covers selectivity and precision. In this case, as well as when identification of variant protein is done, the identification of the primary structure of the peptide fragments in the peptide map provides both a verification of the known primary structure and the identification of protein variants by comparison with the peptide map of the reference standard/reference material for the specified protein. The use of a digested reference standard or reference material for a given protein in the determination of peptide resolution is the method of choice. For an analysis of a variant protein, a characterized mixture of a variant and a reference standard or reference material can be used, especially if the variant peptide is located in a less-resolved region of the map. The index of pattern consistency can be simply the number of major peptides detected. Peptide pattern consistency can be best defined by the resolution of peptide peaks. Chromatographic parameters —such as peak-to-peak resolution, maximum peak width, peak area, peak tailing factors, and column efficiency— may be used to define peptide resolution. Depending on the protein under test and the method of separation used, single peptide or multiple peptide resolution requirements may be necessary.

The replicate analysis of the digest of the reference standard or reference material for the protein under test yields measures of precision and quantitative recovery. Recovery of the identified peptides is generally ascertained by the use of internal or external peptide standards. The precision is expressed as the relative standard deviation (RSD). Differences in the recovery and precision of the identified peptides are expected; therefore, the system suitability limits will have to be established for both the recovery and the precision of the identified peptides. These limits are unique for a given protein and will be specified in the individual monograph.

Visual comparison of the relative retention times, the peak responses (the peak area or the peak height), the number of peaks, and the overall elution pattern is completed initially. It is then complemented and supported by mathematical analysis of the peak response ratios and by the chromatographic profile of a 1:1 (v/v) mixture of sample and reference standard or reference material digest. If all peaks in the sample digest and in the reference standard or reference material digest have the same relative retention times and peaks response ratios, then the identity of the sample under test is confirmed.

If peaks that initially eluted with significantly different relative retention times are then observed as single peaks in the 1:1 mixture, the initial difference would be an indication of system variability. However, if separate peaks are observed in the 1:1 mixture, this would be evidence of the nonequivalence of the peptides in each peak. If a peak in the 1:1 mixture is significantly broader than the corresponding peak in the sample and reference standard or reference material digest, it may indicate the presence of different peptides. The use of computer-aided pattern recognition software for the analysis of peptide mapping data has been proposed and applied, but issues related to the validation of the computer software preclude its use in a compendial test in the near future. Other automated approaches have been used that employ mathematical formulas, models, and pattern recognition. Such approaches are, for example, the automated identification of compounds by IR spectroscopy and the application of diode-array UV spectral analysis for identification of peptides. These methods have limitations due to inadequate resolutions, co-elution of fragments, or absolute peak response differences between reference standard or reference material and sample fragments.

The numerical comparison of the retention times and peak areas or peak heights can be done for a selected group of relevant peaks that have been correctly identified in the peptide maps. Peak areas can be calculated using one peak showing relatively small variation as an internal reference, keeping in mind that peak area integration is sensitive to baseline variation and likely to introduce error in the analysis. Alternatively, the percentage of each peptide peak height relative to the sum of all peak heights can be calculated for the sample under test. The percentage is then compared to that of the corresponding peak of the reference standard/reference material. The possibility of auto-hydrolysis of trypsin is monitored by producing a blank peptide map, that is, the peptide map obtained when a blank solution is treated with trypsin.

The minimum requirement for the qualification of peptide mapping is an approved test procedure that includes system suitability as a test control. In general, early in the regulatory process, qualification of peptide mapping for a protein is sufficient. As the regulatory approval process for the protein progresses, additional qualifications of the test can include a partial validation of the analytical procedure to provide assurance that the method will perform as intended in the development of a peptide map for the specified protein.

5. Analysis and Identification of Peptides

This section gives guidance on the use of peptide mapping during development in support of regulatory applications.

The use of a peptide map as a qualitative tool does not require the complete characterization of the individual peptide peaks. However, validation of peptide mapping in support of regulatory applications requires rigorous characterization of each of the individual peaks in the peptide map. Methods to characterize peaks range from N-terminal sequencing of each peak followed by amino acid analysis to the use of mass spectroscopy (MS).

For characterization purposes, when N-terminal sequencing and amino acids analysis are used, the analytical separation is scaled up. Since scale-up might affect the resolution of peptide peaks, it is necessary, using empirical data, to assure that there is no loss of resolution due to scale-up. Eluates corresponding to specific peptide peaks are collected, vacuum-concentrated, and chromatographed again, if necessary. Amino acid analysis of fragments may be limited by the peptide size. If the N-terminus is blocked, it may need to be cleared before sequencing. C-terminal sequencing of proteins in combination with carboxypeptidase digestion and MALDI-TOF MS can also be used for characterization purposes.

The use of MS for characterization of peptide fragments is by direct infusion of isolated peptides or by the use of online LC-MS for structure analysis. In general, it includes electrospray and MALDI-TOF MS analyzer as well as fast atom bombardment (FAB). Tandem MS has also been used to sequence a modified protein and to determine the type of amino acid modification that has occurred. The comparison of mass spectra of the digests before and after reduction provides a method to assign the disulfide bonds to the various sulfhydryl-containing peptides.

If regions of the primary structure are not clearly demonstrated by the peptide map, it might be necessary to develop a secondary peptide map. The goal of a validated method of characterization of a protein through peptide mapping is to reconcile and account for at least 95% of the theoretical composition of the protein structure.

Mass Spectrometry of Peptides and Proteins <*G3-4-161*>

Mass spectrometry (MS) is based on the ionization of molecules and separation of the electrically charged ions according to the dimensionless quantity, *m/z* value, which is obtained by dividing the relative mass (*m*) of the ion to unified atomic mass unit by the charge number (*z*) of the ion. The unified atomic mass unit is defined as one twelfth of the mass of ground state ^{12}C and used to express the mass of atom, molecule and ion. The results are expressed as a mass spectrum with *m/z* values of the ions on the x-axis and signal intensity of the ions on the y-axis. The mass of the molecule is calculated from the *m/z* values and *z*. Tandem mass spectrometry (MS/MS) is based on the fragmentation of the precursor ion selected in the first stage mass analysis and measurement of the product ions in the second stage mass analysis. This technique provides useful information for structural analysis of the molecule. Information obtained in MS is qualitative and is sometimes used for qualification. MS and MS/MS are useful for measuring masses of peptides and proteins and for confirming amino acid sequences and post-translational modifications. Both methods are therefore used for identification of pharmaceutical peptides and proteins.

1. Instrument

A mass spectrometer is composed of an ion source, an analyzer, an ion detector, and a data system (Fig. 1). A peptide and protein sample introduced into the ion source is ionized by soft-ionization methods, such as matrix-assisted laser desorption/ionization (MALDI) and electrospray ionization (ESI). The charged and gas phased ions are sorted according to the *m/z* ratio under a vacuum in the analyzer, which may be a quadrupole, time-of-flight, ion trap or

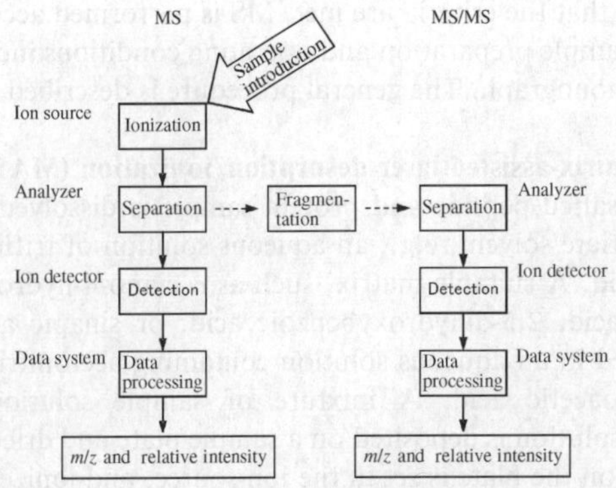

Fig. 1 Schematic diagram of mass spectrometry (MS) and tandem mass spectrometry (MS/MS)

Fourier transform ion cyclotron resonance analyzer. The ion flux collected in the detector is converted to an electric signal. Then the signal is recorded as a mass spectrum. MS/MS is carried out by using two mass spectrometers connected in series, an ion-trap mass spectrometer and Fourier transform ion cyclotron resonance mass spectrometer. The precursor ions are generally fragmented by collision-induced dissociation (CID), post-source decay (PSD), electron capture dissociation (ECO), etc.

2. Analytical mode

2.1. MS

There are two useful modes for MS:

(1) Total ion monitoring

The signals of the entire ion are acquired over the chosen range of *m/z* value. This mode provides information on the masses of the molecule of interest and different species.

(2) Selected ion monitoring

The signals of the ion at chosen *m/z* value are acquired. This mode is useful for the sensitive measurement of the chosen molecule.

2.2. MS/MS

There are four essential modes for MS/MS:

(1) Product ion analysis

The signals of all the product ions produced from the precursor ion at chosen *m/z* value are acquired. This mode provides structural information on the substrates and various co-existing species.

(2) Precursor ion scan mode

The signals of the precursor ion that yields the product ion at chosen *m/z* value are monitored. This mode is used for sorting the molecules containing a component of interest.

(3) Constant neutral loss scan mode

The signals of the precursor ion that loses the fragment at chosen *m/z* value are monitored. This mode is useful to sort the molecules containing a component of interest.

(4) Selected reaction monitoring

The signals of product ions at chosen *m/z* value that are produced from the precursor ion at chosen *m/z* value are monitored. This mode allows for sensitive and selective measurement and is used for quantification of a molecule in a complex mixture.

3. Analytical procedure

3.1. MS

In advance, it should be confirmed if the detectability and the difference between the calculated mass and observed mass meet the criteria stated in the monograph by mass measuring using a test solution specified in the system suitability in the monograph. If they do not meet the criteria, the system should be optimized by adjustment of the voltage of the ion source, analyzer and detector, as well as by calibration using appropriate mass calibrator. After confirming that the criteria are met, MS is performed according to the sample preparation and operating conditions indicated in the monograph. The general procedure is described as follows.

(1) Matrix-assisted laser desorption/ionization (MALDI)

A desalted peptide and protein sample is dissolved in an appropriate solvent, e.g., an aqueous solution of trifluoroacetic acid. A suitable matrix, such as α-ciano-4-hydroxycinnamic acid, 2,5-dihydroxybenzoic acid, or sinapic acid, is dissolved in an aqueous solution containing acetonitrile and trifluoroacetic acid. A mixture of sample solution and matrix solution is deposited on a sample plate and dried. The sample on the plate is set in the ion source, and ionized by a laser beam at suitable intensity.

(2) Electrospray ionization (ESI)

A desalted peptide and protein sample is dissolved in a suitable solvent, such as an aqueous solution containing acetic acid and methanol or acetonitrile. The sample solution is introduced by using a syringe or HPLC. The sample is ionized by applying voltage to obtain the spectrum.

3.2. MS/MS

System suitability is tested by MS/MS of the test sample specified in the monograph. The detectability and system performance should be confirmed based on the detection of the product ions specified in the monograph. The sample is ionized in the same way as for MS, and the chosen precursor is fragmented by the suitable conditions specified in the monograph. The signals are recorded as a mass spectrum. A peptide containing disulfide bonds is generally reduced by dithiothreitol, 2-mercaptethanol and tris(2-carboxyethyl) phosphine. The reduced peptides are alkylated with monoiodoacetic acid, iodoacetamide, and 4-vinylpyridine.

4. Identification test

4.1. Mass of the molecule

The monoisotopic mass of the peptide and protein molecules is measured by MS. If the monoisotopic peak is detectable, the monoisotopic mass is determined from the peak. If the monoisotopic peak is not detectable, the average mass is calculated from the top of the ion peak. Deconvolution is effective for calculating the average mass of multiply-charged ions from proteins. The mass should meet the criteria specified in the monograph.

4.2. Amino acid sequence

After measuring the mass of the sample peptide, the presence of the specified product ions that arise from the selected precursor ion is confirmed according to the conditions indicated in the monograph. Digestion of sample proteins with a suitable enzyme followed by MS/MS is sometimes effective for sequencing of the high-molecular weight proteins which provide insufficient product ions. Details of the digestion procedure are provided in ''Peptide Mapping <*G3-3-142*>'' in General Information.

5. Glossary

Ion-trap (IT)

Ion-trap refers to the quadrupole ion trap mass analyzer in a restricted sense. Ions stored in the analyzer by applying radio frequency voltage to ring electrodes are separated by subsequent ejection of the ions from the analyzer by varying the voltage on the ring electrodes. This allows multiple stage MS (MS^n) in which a selected ion is repeatedly trapped, fragmented and ejected.

Electrospray ionization (ESI)

The sample in solution is sprayed through a needle tip and held at high-voltage at atmospheric pressure. The sample is ionized by a formation of charged liquid droplets. High-molecular mass proteins are detected as multiply-charged ions. The analyzer can be connected with HPLC.

Quadrupole (Q)

The analyzer is composed of four parallel electrodes which have a hyperboloidal or corresponding cross-section. The ions transmitted to the analyzer are separated by varying the potential of direct and radio frequency components applied to the rods so that the filter for sorting the *m/z* values of ions is changed.

Collision-induced dissociation (CID)

When an ion collides with a neutral collision gas (He, Ar, N_2 and so on), some of the translational energy of the collision is converted into internal energy, thereby causing ion excitation and dissociation. The terms low-energy CID and high-energy CID refer to those CIDs for which the translational energy of the precursor ions is lower than 1000 eV and higher than 1000 eV, respectively.

Electron capture dissociation (ECD)

Multiply-charged positive ions interact with low energy electrons producing charge-reduced radical ions, which readily dissociate. This method is primarily used for MS/MS in FT-ICR MS or IT MS.

Time-of-flight (TOF)

The ionized sample is accelerated at high-voltage and separated based on the time required for an ion to travel to the detector. There are two types of analyzer, a linear type in which ions travel linearly from the ion source to the detector, and a reflectron type where ions are inverted by a reflectron. The latter type allows high-resolution measurement by correction of the variation in the initial energy of ions.

Fourier transform ion cyclotron resonance (FT-ICR)

The analyzer is based on the principle that the cyclotron frequency of the rotating (cyclotron motion) ions in a magnetic field is inversely proportional to its m/z value. Ions are excited using radio frequency energy and their image current is detected on a detection electrode. The resulting data are devolved by applying a Fourier transform to give a mass spectrum.

Post-source decay (PSD)

Metastable ion decay occurs by excess internal energy and collision with residual gas during ion acceleration out of the MALDI ion source and prior to reaching the detector. This method is used for MS/MS by using MALDI-TOF MS with a reflectron mode.

Matrix-assisted laser desorption/ionization (MALDI)

The sample, which is mixed with a suitable matrix, is ionized by irradiation with nanosecond laser pulses. Proteins, carbohydrates, oligonucleotides, and lipids can be ionized without any dissociation. Singly-charged ions are mainly detected.

Monosaccharide Analysis and Oligosaccharide Analysis/ Oligosaccharide Profiling

<G3-5-170>

Glycosylation analysis is a method to confirm the consistency of the oligosaccharides attached to glycoprotein drug substance, product or material. When oligosaccharides attached to the glycoprotein affect efficacy and safety or the possibility cannot be denied, oligosaccharides are considered as critical quality attribute, and strategy should be designed in order to ensure the consistency of glycosylation. One of the strategies is glycosylation analysis, which involves 1) analysis of released monosaccharides (monosaccharide analysis), 2) analysis of released oligosaccharides (oligosaccharide analysis/oligosaccharide profiling), 3) analysis of glycopeptides (glycopeptide analysis), and 4) analysis of intact glycoprotein (glycoform analysis). These methods provide monosaccharide compositions, oligosaccharide identities and distribution in whole glycoprotein, site-specific glycosylation identities and distribution, and overall glycosylation characteristics and distribution of glycoprotein, respectively. In the setting specification of glycosylation analysis, proper methods should be selected and used alone or in combination, in consideration of the relationship between the oligosaccharide structures and functions, such as biological activity, pharmacodynamics, pharmacokinetics, immunogenicity, stability, and solubility. Glycosylation consistency may be ensured not only by oligosaccharide analysis but also at manufacturing process. Glycosylation analysis can be also used as in-process test, and as method to confirm glycosylation consistency during process development. Methods and general consideration of monosaccharide analysis and oligosaccharide analysis/oligosaccharide profiling are described below. For glycopeptide analysis, General Test *<2.62>* Mass Spectrometry, and General Information Peptide Mapping and Mass Spectrometry of Peptides and Proteins would be helpful, and for glycoform analysis, General Information Isoelectric Focusing and Capillary Electrophoresis, and General Test *<2.62>* Mass Spectrometry would be helpful.

1. Monosaccharide analysis

Monosaccharides are released by cleavage of glycosidic bond using acid hydrolysis, exoglycosidase or methanolysis. Released monosaccharides are dried and purified if needed, and then analyzed using liquid chromatography, gas chromatography, or capillary electrophoresis. Internal standard method or absolute calibration method are used for quantitative measurement. The analytical results are typically expressed as molar ratio of individual monosaccharides to glycoprotein.

1.1. Isolation and purification of glycoprotein

Monosaccharide analysis is generally performed after glycoprotein is isolated and purified in an appropriate manner, because excipients and salts may affect hydrolysis, derivatization of monosaccharides, and chromatographic separation. When purification of the glycoprotein is required, the procedure is specified in the specific monograph.

1.2. Release of monosaccharide

1.2.1. Acid hydrolysis

Acid hydrolysis is the most common procedure to release neutral and amino sugars. In general, monosaccharides may be released by acid hydrolysis of glycosidic bond under conditions such as 2 to 7 mol/L trifluoroacetic acid at about 100°C. Since amino sugar residue directly attached to protein is difficult to release, for accurate quantification of amino sugars, acid hydrolysis should be performed separately under conditions such as 2 to 6 mol/L hydrochloride at 100°C. Because hydrolysis rate is dependent on the identity of the monosaccharide, the anomeric configuration, and position of the glycosidic linkage, it is recommended that release and degradation of individual monosaccharides are confirmed by time-course study. Because N-acetyl groups of amino sugars are removed under acid hydrolysis conditions, re-N-acetylation may be performed if needed. Since sialic acid is labile, sialic acids are released separately under conditions such as 0.1 mol/L hydrochloride, 0.1 mol/L sulfuric acid, or 2 mol/L acetic acid at 80°C.

1.2.2. Enzymatic treatment

Exoglycosidase digestion is also used for release of sialic acids from glycoprotein. Typically, sialidases with broad specificity, such as those derived from *Arthrobacter ureafaciens* or *Clostridium perfringens* are used. Digestion conditions should be optimized in consideration of the identity of sialic acids, linkage, O-acetylation and others. Other enzymes with high specificity may be used to distinguish sialic acid having different types of linkage.

1.2.3. Methanolysis

Dried sample is heated under methanolic hydrogen chlo-

Table 1 Examples of enzymatic cleavage agents

Enzyme	Specificity
N-linked oligosaccharide release	
Peptide-N^4-(N-acetyl-β-glucosaminyl) asparagine amidase (EC 3.5.1.52)	Hydrolysis of peptide-N^4-(N-acetyl-β-D-glucosaminyl) asparagine residue in which the glucosamine residue may be further glycosylated, to yield a (substituted) N-acetyl-β-D-glucosaminylamine and a peptide containing an aspartate residue
—Peptide N-glycosidase F (PNGase F)	Release of N-linked oligosaccharides but no release of N-linked oligosaccharides containing (α1,3)-linked core fucose
—Peptide N-glycosidase A	Release of N-linked oligosaccharides including those containing (α1,3)-linked core fucose
Mannosyl-glycoprotein endo-β-N-acetyl-glucosaminidase (EC 3.2.1.96)	Endohydrolysis of the N,N'-diacetylchitobiosyl unit in high-mannose glycopeptides/glycoproteins containing the—[Man(GlcNAc)$_2$]Asn structure [Man(GlcNAc)$_2$]Asn
—Endo-β-N-acetylglucosaminidase F (endo F)	Release of high-mannose, hybrid, and complex oligosaccharides
—Endo-β-N-acetylglucosaminidase H (endo H)	Release of high-mannose and hybrid oligosaccharides
O-linked oligosaccharide release	
Glycopeptide α-N-acetylgalactosaminidase (EC 3.2.1.97)*	Release of D-galactose-(α1,3)-N-acetylgalactosamine α-linked to serine/threonine residue

* This enzyme has limited usage because of its high substrate specificity.

ride. Monosaccharides are released as methyl glycosides. Degradation of released monosaccharides is low compared to acid hydrolysis.

1.3. Quantification of the released monosaccharides

1.3.1. High-pH anion-exchange chromatography with pulsed amperometric detection

Acid is removed from the hydrolysate if needed. Monosaccharides can be separated and quantified without derivatization using high-pH anion-exchange chromatography with pulsed amperometric detection. Monosaccharides have about 12 to 14 of acid dissociation constant (pKa). They are ionized under high pH conditions (pH 12 to 13), and can be separated by strong anion-exchange chromatography using polymer-based stationary phase containing quaternary ammonium groups. Amperometric detection is a method to detect electrochemically active ions by measuring the current when analyte is oxidized or reduced at electrodes. Sugar is ionized at high pH and can be selectively detected by amperometry. Because oxidized products of sugars foul the electrodes and reduce the signals, pulsed amperometry, where electrode surface is cleaned by changing positive and negative potentials after data acquisition, is used. Since amino acids are also detectable by amperometry, it is noted that analysis may be interfered in the case of the glycoprotein with low oligosaccharide contents. This analytical method can be used for oligosaccharide analysis as well as for analysis of neutral and amino sugars, and sialic acids.

1.3.2. Derivatization and liquid chromatography

(1) Neutral and amino sugars

Monosaccharides obtained by acid hydrolysis are treated to remove the acid, re-N-acetylated if needed, then reductively aminated with 2-aminobenzoic acid, 2-aminopyridine, or ethyl-4-aminobenzoate, or derivatized with 3-methyl-1-phenyl-5-pyrazolone. Impurities derived from reagents may interfere the analysis, attention should be paid to the purity of the reagents used. To prevent excessive reagents to affect test results, derivatized monosaccharides are purified if needed. The derivatized monosaccharides may be separated using reversed-phase chromatography, or anion-exchange chromatography with formation of borate complex. Separated monosaccharides are detected by fluorometric or ultraviolet detector. Underivatized monosaccharides may be separated by ion-exchange chromatography, post-column derivatization using such as arginine, and then detected.

(2) Sialic acid

Released sialic acids by mild acid hydrolysis or sialidase digestion are derivatized with 1,2-diamino-4.5-methylenedioxybenzen or 1,2-phenylenediamine, which react with α-keto acid specifically. This reaction proceeds in acidic conditions, thus acid hydrolysate can be used for derivatization without removal of the acid. Derivatized sialic acids are separated by reversed-phase chromatography and detected by fluorometric detector.

1.3.3. Gas chromatography

There are several methods for gas chromatography; monosaccharides obtained by methanolysis are re-N-acetylated and trimethylsilylated (trimethylsilyl derivatives), and the monosaccharides obtained by acid hydrolysis are reduced and then acetylated (alditol acetate derivatives). The former can quantitate sialic acids simultaneously without degradation, but each sugar gives several peaks due to α- and β-anomers and isomers, and chromatogram becomes complex.

Methylation analysis provides the structural information or the glycosidic linkage of individual monosaccharides. After all hydroxy groups in the oligosaccharide are methylated, permethylated oligosaccharide is subject to acid hydrolysis and resultant partially O-methylated monosaccharides are reduced and acetylated. Partially O-methylated alditol acetates are separated and quantified using gas chromatography.

1.4. Acceptance criteria

Confirmation of compliance of the test material is typically achieved by demonstrating that contents of individual monosaccharides per protein are within a specified range. In order to set acceptance criteria properly, it is needed to consider the relationship between characteristics of glycosylation, and efficacy and safety.

1.5. Monosaccharide reference materials

Monosaccharides to be analyzed are often used as reference materials for monosaccharide analysis. In this case, monosaccharide reference material mixtrure is prepared as mixing each monosaccharide equally, or at similar ratio expected in test substance.

1.6. System suitability

The solution for system suitability test should be prepared

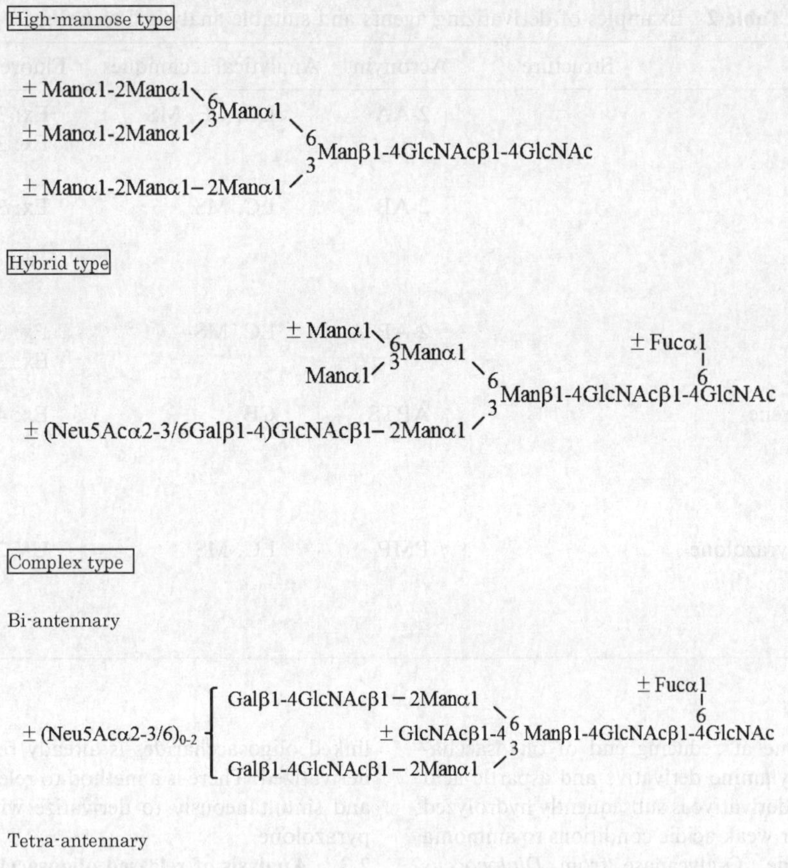

High-mannose type

± Manα1-2Manα1 ↘6
3Manα1 ↘6
± Manα1-2Manα1 ↗
Manβ1-4GlcNAcβ1-4GlcNAc
3
± Manα1-2Manα1 – 2Manα1 ↗

Hybrid type

± Manα1 ↘6
3Manα1 ↘6
Manα1 ↗
± Fucα1
6
Manβ1-4GlcNAcβ1-4GlcNAc
3
± (Neu5Acα2-3/6Galβ1-4)GlcNAcβ1– 2Manα1 ↗

Complex type

Bi-antennary

Galβ1-4GlcNAcβ1 – 2Manα1 ↘6
± (Neu5Acα2-3/6)$_{0\text{-}2}$ ± GlcNAcβ1-4 Manβ1-4GlcNAcβ1-4GlcNAc (± Fucα1-6)
Galβ1-4GlcNAcβ1 – 2Manα1 ↗3

Tetra-antennary

Galβ1-4GlcNAcβ1 ↘6
Galβ1-4GlcNAcβ1 ↗2 Manα1 ↘6
± (Neu5Acα2-3/6)$_{0\text{-}4}$ Manβ1-4GlcNAcβ1-4GlcNAc (± Fucα1-6)
Galβ1-4GlcNAcβ1 ↘4 Manα1 ↗3
Galβ1-4GlcNAcβ1 ↗2

Fuc : L-Fucose GlcNAc : *N*-Acetyl-D-glucosamine
Gal : D-Galactose LacNAc : *N*-Acetyl-lactosamine
GalNAc : *N*-Acetyl-D-galactosamine Man : D-Mannose
Glc : D-Glucose Neu5Ac : *N*-Acetylneuraminic acid

Fig. Common types of N-linked oligosaccharides

properly using monosaccharide reference materials. It may be difficult to separate each monosaccharide completely due to its similar physical property. Acceptance criteria should be set properly.

2. Oligosaccharide analysis/oligosaccharide profiling

Oligosaccharides are released from glycoprotein by enzymatic or chemical treatment, and then released oligosaccharides are analyzed or profiled by liquid chromatography, capillary electrophoresis, mass spectrometry, or combination of them. Analysis result is obtained as oligosaccharide profile, which provides the information on the identity and the distribution of oligosaccharide.

2.1. Separation and purification of glycoprotein

Interfering substance, such as excipients, salts and surfactant, are removed if needed. When purification of the glycoprotein is required, the procedure is specified in the specific monograph.

2.2. Release and isolation of oligosaccharides

Release of N-linked oligosaccharides from glycoprotein is performed by enzymatic treatment or hydrazinolysis. Release of O-linked oligosaccharides is performed by alkali *β*-elimination, hydrazinolysis, and O-glycanase digestion. The releasing conditions must be optimized in order to release and recover all oligosaccharides attached to the glycoprotein reproducibly, independent of their structure and their individual position in the protein. Table 1 give a non-exhaustive list of enzymatic cleavage agents and their specificity. Released oligosaccharides may be purified properly if needed.

2.2.1. Enzymatic release

For the release of N-linked oligosaccharides, peptide N-glycosidase F (PNGase F) derived from *Flavobacterium meningosepticum* or peptide N-glycosidase A (PNGase A) derived from almonds are available. These enzymes hydrolyze the amide bond between asparagine residue and *N*-

Table 2 Examples of derivatizing agents and suitable analytical techniques.

Agent	Structure	Acronym	Analytical techniques	Fluorescent or UV detection
2-Aminobenzoic acid		2-AA	LC, CE, MS	Ex: 360 nm, Em: 425 nm Ex: 325 nm, Em: 405 nm
2-Aminobenzamide		2-AB	LC, MS	Ex: 330 nm, Em: 420 nm
2-Aminopyridine		2-AP	LC, MS	Ex: 310 nm, Em: 380 nm Ex: 320 nm, Em: 400 nm
Trisodium 8-aminopyrene-1,3,6-trisulfonic salt		APTS	CE	Ex: 488 nm, Em: 520 nm
3-methyl-1-phenyl-5-pyrazolone		PMP	LC, MS	UV 245 nm

acetylglucosamine residue at reducing end of oligosaccharides to produce glycosylamine derivative and aspartic acid residue. Glycosylamine derivative is subsequently hydrolyzed non-enzymatically under weak acidic conditions to ammonia and free oligosaccharide. O-glycanase from *Diplococcus pneumoniae* is available to release O-linked oligosaccharides, but specificity of this enzyme is too narrow.

2.2.1.1. PNGase F digestion

PNGase F have an optimum pH 7 to 9. Glycoprotein is treated directly or under presence of a reducing agent, surfactant, and/or denaturing agent. Glycoprotein may be treated with PNGase F after reduced and alkylated, or after digested into glycopeptides. Glycoproteins from some insect cells and plants may have a (α1,3)-linked fucose attached to the proximal GlcNAc of the core chitobiose, and N-linked oligosaccharides containing this structure are not released by this enzyme.

2.2.1.2. PNGase A digestion

PNGase A have an optimum pH 4 to 6. Since this enzyme is difficult to release oligosaccharides directly from whole glycoprotein, a glycoprotein sample is digested with a proteolytic agent, such as endoprotease, and then glycopeptides are treated with this enzyme to release oligosaccharides.

2.2.2. Chemical cleavage

2.2.2.1. Hydrazinolysis

To well-dried glycoprotein anhydrous hydrazine is added and heated. Hydrazine cleaves glycosylamine linkage between oligosaccharide and peptide as well as peptide bond. With careful control of reaction conditions, selective release of N-linked oligosaccharide and/or O-linked oligosaccharides can be achieved. Because de-N-acetylation of amino sugar and sialic acid in oligosaccharides also occurs, amino groups are re-N-acetylated after removing hydrazine. Attention should be paid to the possibility of loss of sialic acid, and successive degradation from reducing end of released O-linked oligosaccharides (peeling reaction).

2.2.2.2. Alkali β-elimination

Heating glycoprotein under alkaline conditions results in release of O-linked oligosaccharides by β-elimination. To prevent peeling reactions, reaction is conducted in the presence of a reducing agent, such as sodium tetrahydroborate. It is noted that reducing end of obtained O-linked oligosaccharides is already reduced, thus, cannot be derivatized. There is a method to release the oligosaccharides and simultaneously to derivatize with 3-methyl-1-phenyl-5-pyrazolone.

2.3. Analysis of released oligosaccharides

Oligosaccharides are analyzed directly or after derivatized. Table 2 gives a non-exhaustive list of commonly used fluorescent labels and suitable analytical techniques. The analysis method is needed to separate and detect individual oligosaccharides or family of oligosaccharides with the structure which affects efficacy and safety.

2.3.1. Liquid chromatography <*2.01*>

2.3.1.1. Derivatization and liquid chromatography/fluorometric or UV detection

Profiling of derivatized oligosaccharides by liquid chromatography is the most common methods. Oligosaccharides derivatized with 2-aminobenzamide, 2-aminobenzoic acid, 2-aminopyridine or others are separated by hydrophilic interaction, reversed-phase, ion-exchange, or mixed-mode chromatography, and then detected by fluorometry. Oligosaccharides derivatized with 3-methyl-1-phenyl-5-pyrazolone are separated by reversed-phase chromatography, and then detected by UV spectrometry. Hydrophilic interaction liquid chromatography separates oligosaccharides on the basis of hydrophilicity (i.e. size, the number of sialic acid, ...). Reversed-phase chromatography separates oligosaccharides on the basis of hydrophobicity (i.e. type of oligosaccharide, branching, number of sialic acid, ...). Ion-exchange chromatography separates oligosaccharides on the basis of number of charges. A mix mode of ion-exchange and hydrophilic interaction separates oligosaccharides on the basis of structure as well as number of charges.

2.3.1.2. High-pH anion-exchange chromatography/pulsed amperometric detection

Released oligosaccharides are separated by strong anion-exchange chromatography using polymer-based stationary phase containing quaternary ammonium groups, and detected by pulsed amperometry. This method can separate and detect sialo-oligosaccharides according to the number of sialic acids and linkage differences. This method has often been used for profiling of sialo-oligosaccharides because of no need of derivatization (no loss of sialic acid and no loss of oligosaccharides during procedure) and high resolution. Because response factors of individual oligosaccharides are not equal, relative peak response does not directly reflect the molar ratio of individual oligosaccharides.

2.3.2. Capillary electrophoresis

Derivatized oligosaccharides are separated by capillary zone electrophoresis using an appropriate electrolyte buffer, and then detected by a laser-induced fluorometric detector. Oligosaccharide is separated based on the sample properties such as charge, size, or shape. In general, capillary is used with the inner wall surface modified using neutral polymers covalently or dynamically in order to prevent electroosmotic flow. Derivatizing agent, and pH and additives of the electrolyte buffer are selected to achieve good separation. Capillary electrophoresis has high resolution separations and requires small amounts of sample.

2.3.3. Mass spectrometry *<2.62>*

Mass spectrometry is used for underivatized oligosaccharides as well as derivatized oligosaccharides. Monosaccharide compositions of oligosaccharides can be deduced from observed molecular mass of oligosaccharides. For ionization methods for oligosaccharides, soft ionization techniques, such as electrospray ionization and matrix-assisted laser desorption/ionization are used. It is noted that oligosaccharides containing sialic acid are susceptible to loss of sialic acid during mass spectrometry.

2.4. Assignment or identification of the peak

Identification of the oligosaccharides attached to the glycoprotein is important for test method development and evaluation of oligosaccharide profile. In general, structure of oligosaccharides may be deduced based on the molecular mass determined by mass spectrometry, the pattern of fragment ions obtained by tandem mass spectrometry, sensitivity to exoglycosidases or endoglycosidases with high specificity, comparison of chromatogram or electropherogram with well-characterized oligosaccharide standards, methylation analysis, and knowledge on the oligosaccharide patterns biosynthesized in the used cell line. Table 3 give a non-exhaustive list of exoglycosidases and endoglycosidases for structural assignment. During routine application, the identity of oligosaccharide peaks may be confirmed by comparison with the oligosaccharide profile obtained from the reference material.

Table 3 Examples of exoglycosidases and endoglycosidase useful for structure assignment.

Enzyme	Origin	Specificity
Exo-α-sialidase (EC 3.2.1.18)	*Arthrobactor ureafaciens*	α2-3,6,8,9
	Vibrio cholerae	α2-3,6,8
	Clostridium perfringens	α2-3,6,8
	Newcastle disease virus	α2-3
	Streptococcus pneumoniae	α2-3
β-Galactosidase	Bovine testes	β1-3,4
(EC 3.2.1.23)	*Streptomyces pneumoniae*	β1-4
α-L-Fucosidase	Almond meal	α1-3
(EC 3.2.1.51)	*Xanthomonas sp.*	α1-3,4
	Bovine kidney	α1-2,3,4,6
α-Mannosidase (EC 3.5.1.24)	Jack Bean	α1-2,3,6
α-Galactosidase (EC 3.2.1.22)	Green coffee beans	α1-3,4,6
Keratan-sulfate endo-1,4-β-galactosidase (EC 3.2.1.103)	*Bacteroides fragilis*	β1-3,4/poly LacNAc

2.5. Acceptance criteria

The oligosaccharide profile obtained from the test material is compared with that obtained in parallel using reference material, and then peak position and response ratio of individual oligosaccharides are comparable. Or peak ratio of individual oligosaccharide to total response (peak area percentage method) or relative peak response meets the acceptance criteria. In order to set specification properly, it is important to identify the oligosaccharide structure to be controlled in consideration of the relationship between oligosaccharide structure, and efficacy and safety.

2.6. Reference materials

It is important that reference material has been validated for glycosylation analysis.

2.7. System suitability

System suitability is developed depending on the purpose of oligosaccharide test. Acceptance criteria, e.g. presence of specific peaks, resolution between two adjacent peaks, the number of detectable peaks, and/or conformance to the reference oligosaccharide profile may be set for an oligosaccharide profile, obtained from the standard material, or well-characterized glycoprotein with similar properties by treating similarly. Otherwise, oligosaccharide reference material, e.g. an oligosaccharide standard prepared from the substance being tested and demonstrated to be suitable, or a system suitability oligosaccharide marker, is similarly treated. Similar acceptance criteria described above may be set for the obtained oligosaccharide profile.

Isoelectric Focusing *<G3-6-142>*

This test is harmonized with the European Pharmacopoeia and the U.S. Pharmacopeia.

The parts of the text that are not harmonized are marked with symbols (◆ ◆).

Information on the harmonization with the European Pharmacopoeia and the U.S. Pharmacopeia is available on the website of the Pharmaceuticals and Medical Devices Agency.

General Principles

Isoelectric focusing (IEF) is a method of electrophoresis that separates proteins according to their isoelectric point. Separation is carried out in a slab of polyacrylamide or agarose gel that contains a mixture of amphoteric electrolytes (ampholytes). When subjected to an electric field, the ampholytes migrate in the gel to create a pH gradient. In some cases gels containing an immobilized pH gradient, prepared by incorporating weak acids and bases to specific regions of the gel network during the preparation of the gel, are used. When the applied proteins reach the gel fraction that has a pH that is the same as their isoelectric point (pI), their charge is neutralized and migration ceases. Gradients can be made over various ranges of pH, according to the mixture of ampholytes chosen.

Theoretical Aspects

When a protein is at the position of its isoelectric point, it has no net charge and cannot be moved in a gel matrix by the electric field. It may, however, move from that position by diffusion. The pH gradient forces a protein to remain in its isoelectric point position, thus concentrating it; this concentrating effect is called "focusing". Increasing the applied voltage or reducing the sample load result in improved separation of bands. The applied voltage is limited by the heat generated, which must be dissipated. The use of thin gels and an efficient cooling plate controlled by a thermostatic circulator prevents the burning of the gel whilst allowing sharp focusing. The separation R is estimated by determining the minimum pI difference (ΔpI), which is necessary to separate 2 neighboring bands:

$$R\text{: } \Delta pI = 3\sqrt{\frac{D(\mathrm{d}pH/\mathrm{d}x)}{E(-\mathrm{d}\mu/\mathrm{d}pH)}}$$

D: Diffusion coefficient of the protein

$\mathrm{d}pH/\mathrm{d}x$: pH gradient

E: Intensity of the electric field, in volts per centimeter

$-\mathrm{d}\mu/\mathrm{d}pH$: Variation of the solute mobility with the pH in the region close to the pI

Since D and $-\mathrm{d}\mu/\mathrm{d}pH$ for a given protein cannot be altered, the separation can be improved by using a narrower pH range and by increasing the intensity of the electric field. Resolution between protein bands on an IEF gel prepared with carrier ampholytes can be quite good. Improvements in resolution may be achieved by using immobilized pH gradients where the buffering species, which are analogous to carrier ampholytes, are copolymerized within the gel matrix. Proteins exhibiting pIs differing by as little as 0.02 pH units may be resolved using a gel prepared with carrier ampholytes while immobilized pH gradients can resolve proteins differing by approximately 0.001 pH units.

Practical Aspects

Special attention must be paid to sample characteristics and/or preparation. Having salt in the sample can be problematic and it is best to prepare the sample, if possible, in deionized water or 2 per cent ampholytes, using dialysis or gel filtration if necessary.

The time required for completion of focusing in thin-layer polyacrylamide gels is determined by placing a colored protein (e.g. hemoglobin) at different positions on the gel surface and by applying the electric field: the steady state is reached when all applications give an identical band pattern. In some protocols the completion of the focusing is indicated by the time elapsed after the sample application.

The IEF gel can be used as an identity test when the migration pattern on the gel is compared to a suitable standard preparation and IEF calibration proteins, the IEF gel can be used as a limit test when the density of a band on IEF is compared subjectively with the density of bands appearing in a standard preparation, or it can be used as a quantitative test when the density is measured using a densitometer or similar instrumentation to determine the relative concentration of protein in the bands subject to validation.

Apparatus

An apparatus for IEF consists of:

—a controllable generator for constant potential, current and power. Potentials of 2500 V have been used and are considered optimal under a given set of operating conditions. Supply of up to 30 W of constant power is recommended,

—a rigid plastic IEF chamber that contains a cooled plate, of suitable material, to support the gel,

—a plastic cover with platinum electrodes that are connected to the gel by means of paper wicks of suitable width, length and thickness, impregnated with solutions of anodic and cathodic electrolytes.

Isoelectric Focusing in Polyacrylamide Gels: Detailed Procedure

The following method is a detailed description of an IEF procedure in thick polyacrylamide slab gels, which is used unless otherwise stated in the monograph.

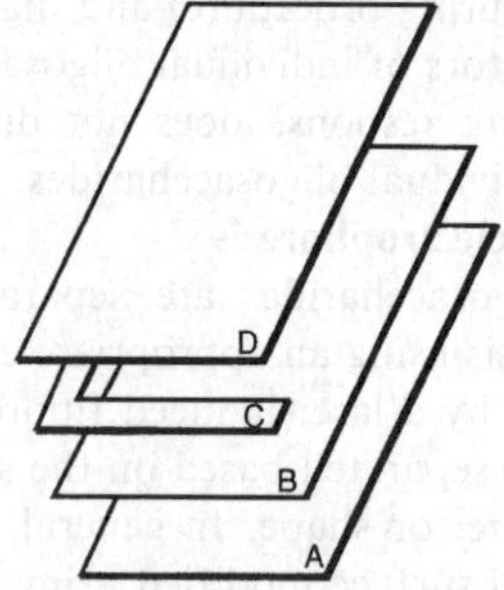

Figure. Mould

Preparation of the Gels

Mould The mould (see Figure) is composed of a glass plate (A) on which a polyester film (B) is placed to facilitate handling of the gel, one or more spacers (C), a second glass plate (D) and clamps to hold the structure together.

7.5% Polyacrylamide gel Dissolve 29.1 g of acrylamide and 0.9 g of *N,N′*-methylenebisacrylamide in 100 mL of water. To 2.5 volumes of this solution, add the mixture of ampholytes specified in the monograph and dilute to 10 volumes with water. Mix carefully and degas the solution.

Preparation of the mould Place the polyester film on the lower glass plate, apply the spacer, place the second glass plate and fit the clamps. Place 7.5% polyacrylamide gel prepared before use on a magnetic stirrer, and add 0.25 volumes of a solution of ammonium persulfate (1 in 10) and 0.25 volumes of *N,N,N′,N′*-tetramethylethylenediamine. Immediately fill the space between the glass plates of the mould with the solution.

Method

Dismantle the mould and, making use of the polyester film, transfer the gel onto the cooled support, wetted with a few millilitres of a suitable liquid, taking care to avoid forming air bubbles. Prepare the test solutions and reference solutions as specified in the monograph. Place strips of paper for sample application, about 10 mm × 5 mm in size, on the gel and impregnate each with the prescribed amount of the test and reference solutions. Also apply the prescribed quantity of a solution of proteins with known isoelectric points as pH markers to calibrate the gel. In some protocols the gel has pre-cast slots where a solution of the sample is applied instead of using impregnated paper strips. Cut 2 strips of paper to the length of the gel and impregnate them with the electrolyte solutions: acid for the anode and alkaline for the cathode. The compositions of the anode and cathode solutions are given in the monograph. Apply these paper wicks to each side of the gel several millimetres from the edge. Fit the cover so that the electrodes are in contact with the wicks (respecting the anodic and cathodic poles). Proceed with the isoelectric focusing by applying the electrical parameters described in the monograph. Switch off the current when the migration of the mixture of standard proteins has stabilized. Using forceps, remove the sample application strips and the 2 electrode wicks. Immerse the gel in ''fixing solution for isoelectric focusing in polyacrylamide gel''. Incubate with gentle shaking at room temperature for 30 minutes. Drain off the solution and add 200 mL of ''destaining solution''. Incubate with shaking for 1 hour. Drain the gel, add ''coomassie staining TS''. Incubate for 30 minutes. Destain the gel by passive diffusion with ''destaining solution'' until the bands are well visualized against a clear background. Locate the position and intensity of the bands in the electropherogram as prescribed in the monograph.

Variations to the Detailed Procedure (Subject to Validation)

Where reference to the general method on isoelectric focusing is made, variations in methodology or procedure may be made subject to validation. These include:

(1) the use of commercially available pre-cast gels and of commercial staining and destaining kits,
(2) the use of immobilized pH gradients,
(3) the use of rod gels,
(4) the use of gel cassettes of different dimensions, including ultra-thin (0.2 mm) gels,
(5) variations in the sample application procedure, including different sample volumes or the use of sample application masks or wicks other than paper,
(6) the use of alternate running conditions, including variations in the electric field depending on gel dimensions and equipment, and the use of fixed migration times rather than subjective interpretation of band stability,
(7) the inclusion of a pre-focusing step,
(8) the use of automated instrumentation,
(9) the use of agarose gels.

Validation of Iso-Electric Focusing Procedures

Where alternative methods to the detailed procedure are employed they must be validated. The following criteria may be used to validate the separation:

(1) formation of a stable pH gradient of desired characteristics, assessed for example using colored pH markers of known isoelectric points,
(2) comparison with the electropherogram provided with the chemical reference substance for the preparation to be examined,
(3) any other validation criteria as prescribed in the monograph.

Specified Variations to the General Method

Variations to the general method required for the analysis of specific substances may be specified in detail in monographs. These include:

(1) the addition of urea in the gel (3 mol/L concentration is often satisfactory to keep protein in solution but up to 8 mol/L can be used): some proteins precipitate at their isoelectric point. In this case, urea is included in the gel formulation to keep the protein in solution. If urea is used, only fresh solutions should be used to prevent carbamylation of the protein,
(2) the use of alternative staining methods,
(3) the use of gel additives such as non-ionic detergents (e.g. octylglucoside) or zwitterionic detergents (e.g., 3-[(3-Cholamidopropyl)dimethylammonio]-1-propanesulfonate (CHAPS) or 3-[(3-Cholamidopropyl)dimethylammonio]-2-hydroxy-1-propanesulfonate (CHAPSO)), and the addition of ampholyte to the sample, to prevent proteins from aggregating or precipitating.

Points to Consider

Samples can be applied to any area on the gel, but to protect the proteins from extreme pH environments samples should not be applied close to either electrode. During method development the analyst can try applying the protein in 3 positions on the gel (i.e. middle and both ends); the pattern of a protein applied at opposite ends of the gel may not be identical.

A phenomenon known as cathodic drift, where the pH gradient decays over time, may occur if a gel is focused too long. Although not well understood, electroendoosmosis and absorption of carbon dioxide may be factors that lead to cathodic drift. Cathodic drift is observed as focused protein migrating off the cathode end of the gel. Immobilized pH gradients may be used to address this problem.

Efficient cooling (approximately 4°C) of the bed that the gel lies on during focusing is important. High field strengths used during isoelectric focusing can lead to overheating and affect the quality of the focused gel.

Reagents and Solutions—

Fixing solution for isoelectric focusing in polyacrylamide gel Dissolve 35 g of 5-sulfosalicylic acid dihydrate and 100 g of trichloroacetic acid in water to make 1000 mL.

◆**Coomassie staining TS** Dissolve 125 mg of coomassie brilliant blue R-250 in 100 mL of a mixture of water, methanol and acetic acid (100) (5:4:1), and filter.

Destaining solution A mixture of water, methanol and acetic acid (100) (5:4:1).◆

Capillary Electrophoresis
<G3-7-180>

This test is harmonized with the European Pharmacopoeia and the U.S. Pharmacopeia.

Information on the harmonization with the European Pharmacopoeia and the U.S. Pharmacopeia is available on the website of the Pharmaceuticals and Medical Devices Agency.

1. General Principles

Capillary electrophoresis is a physical method of analysis based on the migration, inside a capillary, of charged analytes dissolved in an electrolyte solution, under the influence of a direct-current electric field.

The migration velocity of an analyte under an electric field of intensity E, is determined by the electrophoretic mobility of the analyte and the electroosmotic mobility of the buffer inside the capillary. The electrophoretic mobility of a solute (μ_{ep}) depends on the characteristics of the solute (electric charge, molecular size and shape) and those of the buffer in which the migration takes place (type and ionic strength of the electrolyte, pH, viscosity and additives). The electrophoretic velocity (υ_{ep}) of a solute, assuming a spherical shape, is given by the equation:

$$\upsilon_{ep} = \mu_{ep}E = \left(\frac{q}{6\pi\eta r}\right)\left(\frac{V}{L}\right)$$

q: Effective charge of the solute,
η: Viscosity of the electrolyte solution,
r: Stoke's radius of the solute,
V: Applied voltage,
L: Total length of the capillary.

When an electric field is applied through the capillary filled with buffer, a flow of solvent is generated inside the capillary, called electroosmotic flow. The velocity of the electroosmotic flow depends on the electroosmotic mobility (μ_{eo}) which in turn depends on the charge density on the capillary internal wall and the buffer characteristics. The electroosmotic velocity (υ_{eo}) is given by the equation:

$$\upsilon_{eo} = \mu_{eo}E = \left(\frac{\varepsilon\zeta}{\eta}\right)\left(\frac{V}{L}\right)$$

ε: Dielectric constant of the buffer,
ζ: Zeta potential of the capillary surface.

The velocity of the solute (υ) is given by:

$$\upsilon = \upsilon_{ep} + \upsilon_{eo}$$

The electrophoretic mobility of the analyte and the electroosmotic mobility may act in the same direction or in opposite directions, depending on the charge of the solute. In normal capillary electrophoresis, anions will migrate in the opposite direction to the electroosmotic flow and their velocities will be smaller than the electroosmotic velocity. Cations will migrate in the same direction as the electroosmotic flow and their velocities will be greater than the electroosmotic velocity. Under conditions in which there is a fast electroosmotic velocity with respect to the electrophoretic velocity of the solutes, both cations and anions can be separated in the same run.

The time (t) taken by the solute to migrate the distance (l) from the injection end of the capillary to the detection point (capillary effective length) is given by the expression:

$$t = \frac{l}{v_{ep} + v_{eo}} = \frac{l \times L}{(\mu_{ep} + \mu_{eo})V}$$

In general, uncoated fused-silica capillaries above pH 3 have negative charge due to ionized silanol groups in the inner wall. Consequently, the electroosmotic flow is from anode to cathode. The electroosmotic flow must remain constant from run to run if good reproducibility is to be obtained in the migration velocity of the solutes. For some applications, it may be necessary to reduce or suppress the electroosmotic flow by modifying the inner wall of the capillary or by changing the concentration, composition and/or pH of the buffer solution.

After the introduction of the sample into the capillary, each analyte ion of the sample migrates within the background electrolyte as an independent zone, according to its electrophoretic mobility. Zone dispersion, that is the spreading of each solute band, results from different phenomena. Under ideal conditions the sole contribution to the solute-zone broadening is molecular diffusion of the solute along the capillary (longitudinal diffusion). In this ideal case the efficiency of the zone, expressed as the number of theoretical plates (N), is given by:

$$N = \frac{(\mu_{ep} + \mu_{eo}) \times V \times l}{2 \times D \times L}$$

D: Molecular diffusion coefficient of the solute in the buffer.

In practice, other phenomena such as heat dissipation, sample adsorption onto the capillary wall, mismatched conductivity between sample and buffer, length of the injection plug, detector cell size and unlevelled buffer reservoirs can also significantly contribute to band dispersion.

Separation between two bands (expressed as the resolution, R_S) can be obtained by modifying the electrophoretic mobility of the analytes, the electroosmotic mobility induced in the capillary and by increasing the efficiency for the band of each analyte, according to the equation:

$$R_S = \frac{\sqrt{N}(\mu_{epb} - \mu_{epa})}{4(\bar{\mu}_{ep} + \mu_{eo})}$$

μ_{epa} and μ_{epb}: Electrophoretic mobilities of the two analytes separated,

$\bar{\mu}_{ep}$: Mean electrophoretic mobility of the two analytes $\bar{\mu}_{ep} = \frac{1}{2}(\mu_{epa} + \mu_{epb})$.

2. Apparatus

An apparatus for capillary electrophoresis is composed of:

(1) a high-voltage, controllable direct-current power supply,

(2) two buffer reservoirs, held at the same level, containing the prescribed anodic and cathodic solutions,

(3) two electrode assemblies (the anode and the cathode), immersed in the buffer reservoirs and connected to the power supply,

(4) a separation capillary (usually made of fused-silica) which, when used with some specific types of detectors, has an optical viewing window aligned with the detector. The ends of the capillary are placed in the buffer reservoirs. The capillary is filled with the solution prescribed in the monograph,

(5) a suitable injection system,

(6) a detector able to monitor the amount of substances of interest passing through a segment of the separation capillary at a given time. It is usually based on absorption spectrophotometry (UV and visible) or fluorometry, but conductimetric, amperometric or mass spectrometric detection can be useful for specific applications. Indirect detection is an alternative method used to detect non-UV-absorbing and non-fluorescent compounds,

(7) a thermostatic system able to maintain a constant temperature inside the capillary is recommended to obtain a good separation reproducibility,

(8) a recorder and a suitable integrator or a computer.

The definition of the injection process and its automation are critical for precise quantitative analysis. Modes of injection include gravity, pressure or vacuum injection and electrokinetic injection. The amount of each sample component introduced electrokinetically depends on its electrophoretic mobility, leading to possible discrimination using this injection mode.

Use the capillary, the buffer solutions, the preconditioning method, the sample solution and the migration conditions prescribed in the monograph of the considered substance. The employed electrolytic solution is filtered to remove particles and degassed to avoid bubble formation that could interfere with the detection system or interrupt the electrical contact in the capillary during the separation run. A rigorous rinsing procedure should be developed for each analytical method to achieve reproducible migration times of the solutes.

3. Capillary Zone Electrophoresis

3.1. Principles

In capillary zone electrophoresis, analytes are separated in a capillary containing only buffer without any anticonvective medium. With this technique, separation takes place because the different components of the sample migrate as discrete bands with different velocities. The velocity of each band depends on the electrophoretic mobility of the solute and the electroosmotic flow in the capillary (see 1. General Principles). Coated capillaries can be used to increase the separation capacity of those substances adsorbing on fused-silica surfaces.

Using this mode of capillary electrophoresis, the analysis of both small ($M_r < 2000$) and large molecules ($2000 < M_r < 100,000$) can be accomplished. Due to the high efficiency achieved in capillary zone electrophoresis, separation of molecules having only minute differences in their charge-to-mass ratio can be effected. This separation mode also allows the separation of chiral compounds by addition of chiral selectors to the separation buffer.

3.2. Optimization

Optimization of the separation is a complex process where several separation parameters can play a major role. The main factors to be considered in the development of separations are instrumental and electrolytic solution parameters.

3.2.1. Instrumental parameters

(1) *Voltage*: A Joule heating plot is useful in optimizing

the applied voltage and column temperature. Separation time is inversely proportional to applied voltage. However, an increase in the voltage used can cause excessive heat production, giving rise to temperature and, as a result thereof, viscosity gradients in the buffer inside the capillary. This effect causes band broadening and decreases resolution.

(2) *Polarity*: Electrode polarity can be normal (anode at the inlet and cathode at the outlet) and the electroosmotic flow will move toward the cathode. If the electrode polarity is reversed, the electroosmotic flow is away from the outlet and only charged analytes with electroosmotic mobilities greater than the electroosmotic flow will pass to the outlet.

(3) *Temperature*: The main effect of temperature is observed on buffer viscosity and electrical conductivity, and therefore on migration velocity. In some cases, an increase in capillary temperature can cause a conformational change in proteins, modifying their migration time and the efficiency of the separation.

(4) *Capillary*: The dimensions of the capillary (length and internal diameter) contribute to analysis time, efficiency of separations and load capacity. Increasing both effective length and total length can decrease the electric fields (working at constant voltage), and increasing both effective length and total length increase migration time. For a given buffer and electric field, heat dissipation, and hence sample band-broadening, depend on the internal diameter of the capillary. The latter also affects the detection limit, depending on the sample volume injected and the detection system employed.

Since the adsorption of the sample components on the capillary wall limits efficiency, methods to avoid these interactions should be considered in the development of a separation method. In the specific case of proteins, several strategies have been devised to avoid adsorption on the capillary wall. Some of these strategies (use of extreme pH and adsorption of positively charged buffer additives) only require modification of the buffer composition to prevent protein adsorption. In other strategies, the internal wall of the capillary is coated with a polymer, covalently bonded to the silica, that prevents interaction between the proteins and the negatively charged silica surface. For this purpose, ready-to-use capillaries with coatings consisting of neutral-hydrophilic, cationic and anionic polymers are available.

3.2.2. Electrolytic solution parameters

(1) *Buffer type and concentration*: Suitable buffers for capillary electrophoresis have an appropriate buffer capacity in the pH range of choice and low mobility to minimize current generation.

Matching buffer-ion mobility to solute mobility, whenever possible, is important for minimizing band distortion. The type of sample solvent used is also important to achieve on-column sample focusing, which increases separation efficiency and improves detection.

An increase in buffer concentration (for a given pH) decreases electroosmotic flow and solute velocity.

(2) *Buffer pH*: The pH of the buffer can affect separation by modifying the charge of the analyte or additives, and by changing the electroosmotic flow. In protein and peptide separation, changing the pH of the buffer from above to below the isoelectric point (pI) changes the net charge of the solute from negative to positive. An increase in the buffer pH generally increases the electroosmotic flow.

(3) *Organic solvents*: Organic modifiers (methanol, acetonitrile, etc.) may be added to the aqueous buffer to increase the solubility of the solute or other additives and/or to affect the degree of ionization of the sample components. The addition of organic modifiers to the buffer generally causes a decrease in the electroosmotic flow.

(4) *Additives for chiral separations*: For the separation of enantiomers, a chiral selector is added to the separation buffer. The most commonly used chiral selectors are cyclodextrins, but crown ethers, polysaccharides and proteins may also be used. Since chiral recognition is governed by the different interactions between the chiral selector and each of the enantiomers, the resolution achieved for the chiral compounds depends largely on the type of chiral selector used. In this regard, for the development of a given separation it may be useful to test cyclodextrins having a different cavity size (α-, β-, or γ-cyclodextrin) or modified cyclodextrins with neutral (methyl, ethyl, hydroxyalkyl, etc.) or ionizable (aminomethyl, carboxymethyl, sulfobutyl ether, etc.) groups. When using modified cyclodextrins, batch-to-batch variations in the degree of substitution of the cyclodextrins must be taken into account since it will influence the selectivity. Other factors controlling the resolution in chiral separations are concentration of chiral selector, composition and pH of the buffer and temperature. The use of organic additives, such as methanol or urea can also modify the resolution achieved.

4. Capillary Gel Electrophoresis

4.1. Principles

In capillary gel electrophoresis, separation takes place inside a capillary filled with a gel that acts as a molecular sieve. Molecules with similar charge-to-mass ratios are separated according to molecular size since smaller molecules move more freely through the network of the gel and therefore migrate faster than larger molecules. Different biological macromolecules (for example, proteins and DNA fragments), which often have similar charge-to-mass ratios, can thus be separated according to their molecular mass by capillary gel electrophoresis.

4.2. Characteristics of Gels

Two types of gels are used in capillary electrophoresis: permanently coated gels and dynamically coated gels. Permanently coated gels, such as cross-linked polyacrylamide, are prepared inside the capillary by polymerization of the monomers. They are usually bonded to the fused-silica wall and cannot be removed without destroying the capillary. If the gels are used for protein analysis under reducing conditions, the separation buffer usually contains sodium dodecyl sulfate and the samples are denatured by heating a mixture of sodium dodecyl sulfate and 2-mercaptoethanol or dithiothreitol before injection. When non-reducing conditions are used (for example, analysis of an intact antibody), 2-mercaptoethanol and dithiothreitol are not used. Separation in cross-linked gels can be optimized by modifying the separation buffer (as indicated in the capillary zone electrophoresis section) and controlling the gel porosity during the gel preparation. For cross-linked polyacrylamide gels, the porosity can be modified by changing the concentration of acrylamide and/or the proportion of cross-linker. As a rule, a decrease in the porosity of the gel leads to a decrease in the mobility of the solutes. Due to the rigidity of these gels, only electrokinetic injection can be used.

Dynamically coated gels are hydrophilic polymers, such as linear polyacrylamide, cellulose derivatives, dextran, etc., which can be dissolved in aqueous separation buffers giving rise to a separation medium that also acts as a molecular sieve. These separation media are easier to prepare than cross-linked polymers. They can be prepared in a vial and filled by pressure in a wall-coated capillary (with no electroosmotic flow). Replacing the gel before every injection generally improves the separation reproducibility. The porosity of the gels can be increased by using polymers of higher molecular mass (at a given polymer concentration) or by decreasing the polymer concentration (for a given polymer molecular mass). A reduction in the gel porosity leads to a decrease in the mobility of the solute for the same buffer. Since the dissolution of these polymers in the buffer gives low viscosity solutions, both hydrodynamic and electrokinetic injection techniques can be used.

5. Capillary Isoelectric Focusing

5.1. Principles

In isoelectric focusing, the molecules migrate under the influence of the electric field, so long as they are charged, in a pH gradient generated by ampholytes having pI values in a wide range (poly-aminocarboxylic acids), dissolved in the separation buffer.

The three basic steps of isoelectric focusing are loading, focusing and mobilization.

(1) Loading step: Two methods may be employed:

(i) loading in one step: the sample is mixed with ampholytes and introduced into the capillary either by pressure or vacuum;

(ii) sequential loading: a leading buffer, then the ampholytes, then the sample mixed with ampholytes, again ampholytes alone and finally the terminating buffer are introduced into the capillary. The volume of the sample must be small enough not to modify the pH gradient.

(2) Focusing step: When the voltage is applied, ampholytes migrate toward the cathode or the anode, according to their net charge, thus creating a pH gradient from anode (lower pH) to cathode (higher pH). During this step the components to be separated migrate until they reach a pH corresponding to their isoelectric point (pI) and the current drops to very low values.

(3) Mobilization step: If mobilization is required for detection, use one of the following methods. Three methods are available:

(i) mobilization is accomplished during the focusing step under the effect of the electroosmotic flow; the electroosmotic flow must be small enough to allow the focusing of the components;

(ii) mobilization is accomplished by applying positive pressure after the focusing step;

(iii) mobilization is achieved after the focusing step by adding salts to the cathode reservoir or the anode reservoir (depending on the direction chosen for mobilization) in order to alter the pH in the capillary when the voltage is applied. As the pH is changed, the proteins and ampholytes are mobilized in the direction of the reservoir which contains the added salts and pass the detector.

The separation achieved, expressed as ΔpI, depends on the pH gradient (dpH/dx), the number of ampholytes having different pI values, the molecular diffusion coefficient (D), the intensity of the electric field (E) and the variation of the electrophoretic mobility of the analyte with the pH ($-d\mu/dpH$):

$$\Delta pI = 3\sqrt{\frac{D(dpH/dx)}{E(-d\mu/dpH)}}$$

5.2. Optimization

The main parameters to be considered in the development of separations are:

(1) Voltage: Capillary isoelectric focusing utilises very high electric fields, 300 V/cm to 1000 V/cm in the focusing step.

(2) Capillary: The electroosmotic flow must be reduced or suppressed depending on the mobilization strategy (see above). Coated capillaries tend to reduce the electroosmotic flow.

(3) Solutions: The anode buffer reservoir is filled with a solution with a pH lower than the pI of the most acidic ampholyte and the cathode reservoir is filled with a solution with a pH higher than the pI of the most basic ampholyte. Phosphoric acid for the anode and sodium hydroxide for the cathode are frequently used.

Addition of a polymer, such as methylcellulose, in the ampholyte solution tends to suppress convective forces (if any) and electroosmotic flow by increasing the viscosity. Commercial ampholytes are available covering many pH ranges and may be mixed if necessary to obtain an expanded pH range. Broad pH ranges are used to estimate the isoelectric point whereas narrower ranges are employed to improve accuracy. Calibration can be done by correlating migration time with isoelectric point for a series of protein markers.

During the focusing step precipitation of proteins at their isoelectric point can be prevented, if necessary, using buffer additives such as glycerol, surfactants, urea or zwitterionic buffers. However, depending on the concentration, urea denatures proteins.

6. Micellar Electrokinetic Chromatography (MEKC)

6.1. Principles

In micellar electrokinetic chromatography, separation takes place in an electrolyte solution which contains a surfactant at a concentration above the critical micellar concentration (*cmc*). The solute molecules are distributed between the aqueous buffer and the pseudo-stationary phase composed of micelles, according to the partition coefficient of the solute. The technique can therefore be considered as a hybrid of electrophoresis and chromatography. It is a technique that can be used for the separation of both neutral and charged solutes, maintaining the efficiency, speed and instrumental suitability of capillary electrophoresis. One of the most widely used surfactants in MEKC is the anionic surfactant sodium dodecyl sulfate, although other surfactants, for example cationic surfactants such as cetyltrimethylammonium salts, are also used.

The separation mechanism is as follows. At neutral and alkaline pH, a strong electroosmotic flow is generated and moves the separation buffer ions in the direction of the cathode. If sodium dodecyl sulfate is employed as the surfactant, the electrophoretic migration of the anionic micelle is in the opposite direction, towards the anode. As a result, the overall micelle migration velocity is slowed down compared to the bulk flow of the electrolytic solution. In the case of neutral solutes, since the analyte can partition between the micelle and the aqueous buffer, and has no electrophoretic mobility, the analyte migration velocity will depend only on the partition coefficient between the micelle and the aqueous buffer. In the electropherogram, the peaks corresponding to each uncharged solute are always between that of the electroosmotic flow marker and that of the micelle (the time elapsed between these two peaks is called the separation window). For electrically charged solutes, the migration velocity depends on both the partition coefficient of the solute between the micelle and the aqueous buffer, and on the electrophoretic mobility of the solute in the absence of micelle.

Since the mechanism in MEKC of neutral and weakly ionized solutes is essentially chromatographic, migration of the solute and resolution can be rationalized in terms of the retention factor (k'), also referred to as mass distribution ratio (D_m), which is the ratio of the number of moles of solute in the micelle to those in the mobile phase. For a neutral compound, k' is given by:

$$k' = \frac{t_R - t_0}{t_0\left(1 - \frac{t_R}{t_{mc}}\right)} = K\frac{V_S}{V_M}$$

t_R: Migration time of the solute,

t_0: Analysis time of an unretained solute (determined by injecting an electroosmotic flow marker which does not enter the micelle, for instance methanol),

t_{mc}: Micelle migration time (measured by injecting a micelle marker, such as Sudan III, which migrates while continuously associated in the micelle),

K: Partition coefficient of the solute,

V_S: Volume of the micellar phase,

V_M: Volume of the mobile phase.

Likewise, the resolution between two closely-migrating solutes (R_S) is given by:

$$R_S = \frac{\sqrt{N}}{4} \times \frac{\alpha - 1}{\alpha} \times \frac{k'_b}{k'_b + 1} \times \frac{1 - \left(\frac{t_0}{t_{mc}}\right)}{1 + \left(\frac{t_0}{t_{mc}}\right) k'_a}$$

N: Number of theoretical plates for one of the solutes,

α: Selectivity,

k'_a and k'_b: Retention factors for both solutes, respectively ($k'_b > k'_a$).

Similar, but not identical, equations give k' and R_S values for electrically charged solutes.

6.2. Optimization

The main parameters to be considered in the development of separations by MEKC are instrumental and electrolytic solution parameters.

6.2.1. Instrumental parameters

(1) *Voltage*: Separation time is inversely proportional to applied voltage. However, an increase in voltage can cause excessive heat production that gives rise to temperature gradients and viscosity gradients of the buffer in the cross-section of the capillary. This effect can be significant with high conductivity buffers such as those containing micelles. Poor heat dissipation causes band broadening and decreases resolution.

(2) *Temperature*: Variations in capillary temperature affect the partition coefficient of the solute between the buffer and the micelles, the critical micellar concentration and the viscosity of the buffer. These parameters contribute to the migration time of the solutes. The use of a good cooling system improves the reproducibility of the migration time for the solutes.

(3) *Capillary*: As in capillary zone electrophoresis, the dimensions of the capillary (length and internal diameter) contribute to analysis time and efficiency of separations. Increasing both effective length and total length can decrease the electric fields (working at constant voltage), increase migration time and improve the separation efficiency. The internal diameter controls heat dissipation (for a given buffer and electric field) and consequently the sample band broadening.

6.2.2. Electrolytic solution parameters

(1) *Surfactant type and concentration*: The type of surfactant, in the same way as the stationary phase in chromatography, affects the resolution since it modifies separation selectivity. Also, the log k' of a neutral compound increases linearly with the concentration of surfactant in the mobile phase. Since resolution in MEKC reaches a maximum when k' approaches the value of $\sqrt{t_m/t_0}$, modifying the concentration of surfactant in the mobile phase changes the resolution obtained.

(2) *Buffer pH*: Although pH does not modify the partition coefficient of non-ionized solutes, it can modify the electroosmotic flow in uncoated capillaries. A decrease in the buffer pH decreases the electroosmotic flow and therefore increases the resolution of the neutral solutes in MEKC, resulting in a longer analysis time.

(3) *Organic solvents*: To improve MEKC separation of hydrophobic compounds, organic modifiers (methanol, propanol, acetonitrile, etc.) can be added to the electrolytic solution. The addition of these modifiers usually decreases migration time and the selectivity of the separation. Since the addition of organic modifiers affects the critical micellar concentration, a given surfactant concentration can be used only within a certain percentage of organic modifier before the micellization is inhibited or adversely affected, resulting in the absence of micelles and, therefore, in the absence of partition. The dissociation of micelles in the presence of a high content of organic solvent does not always mean that the separation will no longer be possible; in some cases the hydrophobic interaction between the ionic surfactant monomer and the neutral solutes forms solvophobic complexes that can be separated electrophoretically.

(4) *Additives for chiral separations*: For the separation of enantiomers using MEKC, a chiral selector is included in the micellar system, either covalently bound to the surfactant or added to the micellar separation electrolyte. Micelles that have a moiety with chiral discrimination properties include salts of *N*-dodecanoyl-L-amino acids, bile salts, etc. Chiral resolution can also be achieved using chiral discriminators, such as cyclodextrins, added to the electrolytic solutions which contain micellized achiral surfactants.

(5) *Other additives*: Several strategies can be carried out to modify selectivity, by adding chemicals to the buffer. The addition of several types of cyclodextrins to the buffer can also be used to reduce the interaction of hydrophobic solutes with the micelle, thus increasing the selectivity for this type of compound.

The addition of substances able to modify solute-micelle interactions by adsorption on the latter, is used to improve the selectivity of the separations in MEKC. These additives may be a second surfactant (ionic or non-ionic) which gives rise to mixed micelles or metallic cations which dissolve in the micelle and form co-ordination complexes with the solutes.

7. Quantification

Peak areas must be divided by the corresponding migration time to give the corrected peak area in order to:

(1) compensate for the shift in migration time from run to run, thus reducing the variation of the response,

(2) compensate for the different responses of sample constituents with different migration times.

Where an internal standard is used, verify that no peak of the substance to be examined is masked by that of the internal standard.

7.1. Calculations

From the values obtained, calculate the content of the component or components being examined. When prescribed, the percentage content of one or more components of the sample to be examined is calculated by determining the corrected area(s) of the peak(s) as a percentage of the total of the corrected areas of all peaks, excluding those due to solvents or any added reagents (normalization procedure). The use of an automatic integration system (integrator or data acquisition and processing system) is recommended.

8. System Suitability

In order to check the behavior of the capillary electrophoresis system, system suitability parameters are used. The choice of these parameters depends on the mode of capillary electrophoresis used. They are retention factor (k') (only for micellar electrokinetic chromatography), apparent number of theoretical plates (N), symmetry factor (A_S) and resolution (R_S). In previous sections, the theoretical expressions for N and R_S have been described, but more practical equations that allow these parameters to be calculated from the electropherograms are given below.

Apparent Number of Theoretical Plates

The apparent number of theoretical plates (N) may be calculated using the expression:

$$N = 5.54\left(\frac{t_R}{w_h}\right)^2$$

t_R: Migration time or distance along the baseline from the point of injection to the perpendicular dropped from the maximum of the peak corresponding to the component,

w_h: Width of the peak at half-height.

Resolution

The resolution (R_S) between peaks of similar height of two components may be calculated using the expression:

$$R_S = \frac{1.18(t_{R2} - t_{R1})}{w_{h1} + w_{h2}}$$

$$t_{R2} > t_{R1}$$

t_{R1} and t_{R2}: Migration times or distances along the baseline from the point of injection to the perpendiculars dropped from the maxima of two adjacent peaks,

w_{h1} and w_{h2}: Peak widths at half-height.

When appropriate, the resolution may be calculated by measuring the height of the valley (H_v) between two partly resolved peaks in a standard preparation and the height of the smaller peak (H_p) and calculating the peak-to-valley ratio (p/v):

$$p/v = \frac{H_p}{H_v}$$

Symmetry Factor

The symmetry factor (A_S) of a peak may be calculated using the expression:

$$A_S = \frac{w_{0.05}}{2d}$$

$w_{0.05}$: Width of the peak at one-twentieth of the peak height,

d: Distance between the perpendicular dropped from the peak maximum and the leading edge of the peak at one-twentieth of the peak height.

Tests for peak area repeatability (standard deviation of areas or of the area/migration-time ratio) and for migration time repeatability (standard deviation of migration time) are introduced as suitability parameters. Migration time repeatability provides a test for the suitability of the capillary washing procedures. An alternative practice to avoid the lack of repeatability of the migration time is to use migration time relative to an internal standard.

A test for the verification of the signal-to-noise ratio for a standard preparation (or the determination of the limit of quantification) may also be useful for the determination of related substances.

Signal-to-noise Ratio (S/N)

The detection limit and the quantification limit are equivalent to signal-to-noise ratios of 3 and 10, respectively. The signal-to-noise ratio (S/N) is calculated using the expression:

$$S/N = \frac{2H}{h}$$

H: Height of the peak corresponding to the component concerned, in the electropherogram obtained with the prescribed reference solution, measured from the maximum of the peak to the extrapolated baseline of the signal observed over a distance equal to twenty times the width at half-height,

h: Range of the background in an electropherogram obtained after injection of a blank, observed over a distance equal to twenty times the width at the half-height of the peak in the electropherogram obtained with the prescribed reference solution and, if possible, situated equally around the place where this peak would be found.

SDS-Polyacrylamide Gel Electrophoresis *<G3-8-170>*

This test is harmonized with the European Pharmacopoeia and the U.S. Pharmacopeia.

Information on the harmonization with the European Pharmacopoeia and the U.S. Pharmacopeia is available on the website of the Pharmaceuticals and Medical Devices Agency.

Polyacrylamide gel electrophoresis is used for the qualitative characterisation of proteins in biological preparations, for control of purity and for quantitative determinations.

Analytical gel electrophoresis is an appropriate method with which to identify and to assess the homogeneity of proteins in pharmaceutical preparations. The method is routinely used for the estimation of protein subunit molecular masses and for determination of the subunit compositions of purified proteins.

Ready-to-use gels and reagents are commercially available and can be used instead of those described in this text, provided that they give equivalent results and that they meet the validity requirements given below under Validation of the test.

1. Characteristics of Polyacrylamide Gels

The sieving properties of polyacrylamide gels are established by the three-dimensional network of fibres and pores which is formed as the bifunctional bisacrylamide cross-links adjacent polyacrylamide chains. Polymerisation is usually catalysed by a free radical-generating system composed of ammonium persulfate and *N,N,N',N'*-tetramethylethylenediamine (TEMED).

As the acrylamide concentration of a gel increases, its effective pore size decreases. The effective pore size of a gel is operationally defined by its sieving properties; that is, by the resistance it imparts to the migration of macromolecules. There are limits on the acrylamide concentrations that can be used. At high acrylamide concentrations, gels break much more easily and are difficult to handle. As the pore size of a gel decreases, the migration rate of a protein through the gel decreases. By adjusting the pore size of a gel, through manipulating the acrylamide concentration, the resolution of the method can be optimised for a given protein product. Thus, a given gel is physically characterised by its respective composition of acrylamide and bisacrylamide.

In addition to the composition of the gel, the state of the protein is an important component to the electrophoretic mobility. In the case of proteins, the electrophoretic mobility is dependent on the pK value of the charged groups and the size of the molecule. It is influenced by the type, the concentration and the pH of the buffer, by the temperature and the field strength, and by the nature of the support material.

2. Denaturing Polyacrylamide Gel Electrophoresis

The method cited as an example is limited to the analysis of monomeric polypeptides with a mass range of 14,000 to 100,000 daltons. It is possible to extend this mass range by various techniques (e.g. gradient gels, particular buffer system). For instance, tricine sodium dodecyl sulfate (SDS) gels, using tricine as the trailing ion in the electrophoresis running buffer (instead of glycine as in the method described here), can separate very small proteins and peptides under 10,000-15,000 daltons.

Denaturing polyacrylamide gel electrophoresis using glycine SDS (SDS-PAGE) is the most common mode of electrophoresis used in assessing the pharmaceutical quality of protein products and will be the focus of the example method. Typically, analytical electrophoresis of proteins is carried out in polyacrylamide gels under conditions that ensure dissociation of the proteins into their individual polypeptide subunits and that minimize aggregation. Most commonly, the strongly anionic detergent SDS is used in combination with heat to dissociate the proteins before they are loaded on the gel. The denatured polypeptides bind to SDS, become negatively charged and exhibit a consistent charge-to-mass ratio regardless of protein type. Because the amount of SDS bound is almost always proportional to the molecular mass of the polypeptide and is independent of its sequence, SDS-polypeptide complexes migrate through polyacrylamide gels with mobilities dependent on the size of the polypeptide.

The electrophoretic mobilities of the resultant detergent-polypeptide complexes all assume the same functional relationship to their molecular masses. SDS complexes will migrate toward the anode in a predictable manner, with low molecular mass complexes migrating faster than larger ones. The molecular mass of a protein can therefore be estimated from its relative mobility in calibrated SDS-PAGE and the intensity of a single band relative to other undesired bands in such a gel can be a measure of purity.

Modifications to the polypeptide backbone, such as N- or O-linked glycosylation, can change the apparent molecular mass of a protein since SDS does not bind to a carbohydrate moiety in a manner similar to a polypeptide; therefore, a consistent charge-to-mass ratio is not maintained.

Depending on the extent of glycosylation and other post-translational modifications, the apparent molecular mass of proteins may not be a true reflection of the mass of the polypeptide chain.

2.1. Reducing conditions

Polypeptide subunits and three-dimensional structure are often maintained in proteins by the presence of disulfide bonds. A goal of SDS-PAGE analysis under reducing conditions is to disrupt this structure by reducing disulfide bonds. Complete denaturation and dissociation of proteins by treatment with 2-mercaptoethanol (2-ME) or dithiothreitol (DTT) will result in unfolding of the polypeptide backbone and subsequent complexation with SDS. Using these conditions, the molecular mass of the polypeptide subunits can reasonably be calculated by linear regression (or, more closely, by non linear regression) in the presence of suitable molecular mass standards.

2.2. Non-reducing conditions

For some analyses, complete dissociation of the protein into subunit peptides is not desirable. In the absence of treatment with reducing agents such as 2-ME or DTT, disulfide covalent bonds remain intact, preserving the oligomeric form of the protein. Oligomeric SDS-protein complexes migrate more slowly than their SDS-polypeptide subunits. In addition, non-reduced proteins may not be completely saturated with SDS and, hence, may not bind the detergent in a constant mass ratio. Moreover, intra-chain disulphide bonds constrain the molecular shape, usually in such a way as to reduce the Stokes radius of the molecule, thereby reducing the apparent molecular mass M_r. This makes molecular mass determinations of these molecules by SDS-PAGE less straightforward than analyses of fully denatured polypeptides, since it is necessary that both standards and unknown proteins be in similar configurations for valid comparisons.

3. Characteristics of Discontinuous Buffer System Gel Electrophoresis

The most popular electrophoretic method for the characterisation of complex mixtures of proteins uses a discontinuous buffer system involving two contiguous, but distinct gels: a resolving or separating (lower) gel and a stacking (upper) gel. The two gels are cast with different porosities, pH, and ionic strengths. In addition, different mobile ions are used in the gel and electrode buffers. The buffer discontinuity acts to concentrate large volume samples in the stacking gel, resulting in improved resolution. When power is applied, a voltage drop develops across the sample solution which drives the proteins into the stacking gel. Glycinate ions from the electrode buffer follow the proteins into the stacking gel. A moving boundary region is rapidly formed with the highly mobile chloride ions in the front and the relatively slow glycinate ions in the rear. A localised high-voltage gradient forms between the leading and trailing ion fronts, causing the SDS-protein complexes to form into a thin zone (stack) and migrate between the chloride and glycinate phases. Within broad limits, regardless of the height of the applied sample, all SDS-proteins condense into a very narrow region and enter the resolving gel as a well-defined, thin zone of high protein density. The large-pore stacking gel does not retard the migration of most proteins and serves mainly as an anti-convective medium. At the interface of the stacking and resolving gels, the proteins undergo a sharp increase in retardation due to the restrictive pore size of the resolving gel and the buffer discontinuity, which also contributes to focusing of the proteins. Once in the resolving gel, proteins continue to be slowed by the sieving of the matrix. The glycinate ions overtake the proteins, which then move in a space of uniform pH formed by the 2-amino-2-hydroxymethyl-1,3-propanediol and glycine. Molecular sieving causes the SDS-polypeptide complexes to separate on the basis of their molecular masses.

4. Preparing Vertical Discontinuous Buffer SDS Polyacrylamide Gels

This section describes the preparation of gels using particular instrumentation. This does not apply to pre-cast gels. For pre-cast gels or any other commercially available equipment, the manufacturer's instructions must be used for guidance.

The use of commercial reagents that have been purified in solution is recommended. When this is not the case and where the purity of the reagents used is not sufficient, a pretreatment is applied. For instance, any solution sufficiently impure to require filtration must also be deionized with a mixed bed (anion/cation exchange) resin to remove acrylic acid and other charged degradation products. When stored according to recommendations, acrylamide/bisacrylamide solutions and solid persulfate are stable for long periods.

4.1. Assembling the gel moulding cassette

Clean the two glass plates (size: e.g. 10 cm × 8 cm), the polytetrafluoroethylene comb, the two spacers and the silicone rubber tubing (diameter e.g. 0.6 mm × 35 cm) with mild detergent and rinse extensively with water, followed by dehydrated alcohol, and allow the plates to dry at room temperature. Lubricate the spacers and the tubing with non-silicone grease. Apply the spacers along each of the two short sides of the glass plate 2 mm away from the edges and 2 mm away from the long side corresponding to the bottom of the gel. Begin to lay the tubing on the glass plate by using one spacer as a guide. Carefully twist the tubing at the bottom of the spacer and follow the long side of the glass plate. While holding the tubing with one finger along the long side twist again the tubing and lay it on the second short side of the glass plate, using the spacer as a guide. Place the second glass plate in perfect alignment and hold the mould together by hand pressure. Apply two clamps on each of the two short sides of the mould. Carefully apply four clamps on the longer side of the gel mould thus forming the bottom of the gel mould. Verify that the tubing is running along the edge of the glass plates and has not been extruded while placing the clamps. The gel mould is now ready for pouring the gel.

4.2. Preparation of the gel

In a discontinuous buffer SDS polyacrylamide gel, it is recommended to pour the resolving gel, let the gel set, and then pour the stacking gel since the composition of the two gels in acrylamide-bisacrylamide, buffer and pH are different.

4.2.1. Preparation of the resolving gel

In a conical flask, prepare the appropriate volume of solution containing the desired concentration of acrylamide for the resolving gel, using the values given in Table 1. Mix the components in the order shown. Where appropriate, before adding the ammonium persulfate solution and the TEMED, filter the solution if necessary under vacuum through a cellulose acetate membrane (pore diameter 0.45 μm). Keep the solution under vacuum, while swirling the filtration unit, until no more bubbles are formed in the solution. Add appropriate amounts of ammonium persulfate solution and TEMED as indicated in Table 1, swirl and pour immediately into the gap between the two glass plates of the mould. Leave sufficient space for the stacking gel (the length of the teeth of the comb plus 1 cm). Using a tapered glass pipette, carefully overlay the solution with water-saturated isobutanol. Leave the gel in a vertical position at room temperature to allow polymerization.

4.2.2. Preparation of the stacking gel

After polymerization is complete (about 30 minutes), pour off the isobutanol and wash the top of the gel several times with water to remove the isobutanol overlay and any unpolymerized acrylamide. Drain as much fluid as possible from the top of the gel, and then remove any remaining water with the edge of a paper towel.

In a conical flask, prepare the appropriate volume of solution containing the desired concentration of acrylamide, using the values given in Table 2. Mix the components in the order shown. Where appropriate, before adding the ammonium persulfate solution and the TEMED, filter the solution if necessary under vacuum through a cellulose acetate membrane (pore diameter: 0.45 μm). Keep the solution under vacuum, while swirling the filtration unit, until no more bubbles are formed in the solution. Add appropriate amounts of ammonium persulfate solution and TEMED as indicated in Table 2. Swirl and pour immediately into the gap between the two glass plates of the mould directly onto the surface of the polymerized resolving gel. Immediately insert a clean polytetrafluoroethylene comb into the stacking gel solution, being careful to avoid trapping air bubbles. Add more stacking gel solution to fill the spaces of the comb completely. Leave the gel in a vertical position and allow to polymerize at room temperature.

4.3. Preparation of the sample

Unless otherwise specified in the specific monograph the samples can be prepared as follows:

Sample solution (non-reducing conditions). Mix equal volumes of: a mixture comprising water plus the preparation or the reference solutions, and concentrated SDS-PAGE sample buffer.

Sample solution (reducing conditions). Mix equal volumes of: a mixture comprising water plus the preparation or the reference solutions, and concentrated SDS-PAGE sample buffer for reducing conditions containing 2-ME (or DTT) as reducing agent.

The concentration prescribed in the monograph can vary depending on the protein and staining method.

Sample treatment: keep for 5 minutes in a boiling water bath or in a block heater set at 100°C, then chill. (Note that temperature and time may vary in the monograph since protein cleavage may occur during the heat treatment.)

4.4. Mounting the gel in the electrophoresis apparatus and electrophoretic separation

After polymerization is complete (about 30 minutes), remove the polytetrafluoroethylene comb carefully. Rinse the wells immediately with water or with the SDS-PAGE running buffer to remove any unpolymerized acrylamide. If necessary, straighten the teeth of the stacking gel with a blunt hypodermic needle attached to a syringe. Remove the clamps on one short side, carefully pull out the tubing and replace the clamps. Proceed similarly on the other short side. Remove the tubing from the bottom part of the gel. Mount the gel in the electrophoresis apparatus. Add the electrophoresis buffers to the top and bottom reservoirs. Remove any bubbles that become trapped at the bottom of the gel between the glass plates. This is best done with a bent hypodermic needle attached to a syringe. Never pre-run the gel before loading the samples, since this will destroy the discontinuity of the buffer systems. Before loading the sample carefully rinse each well with SDS-PAGE running buffer. Prepare the test and reference solutions in the recommended sample buffer and treat as specified in the individual monograph. Apply the appropriate volume of each solution to the stacking gel wells. Start the electrophoresis using the conditions recommended by the manufacturer of the equipment. Manufacturers of SDS-PAGE equipment may provide gels of different surface area and thickness and electrophoresis running time and current/voltage may vary in order to achieve optimal separation. Check that the dye front is moving into the resolving gel. When the dye is near the bottom of the gel, stop the electrophoresis. Remove the gel assembly from the apparatus and carefully separate the glass plates. Remove the spacers, cut off and discard the stacking gel and immediately proceed with staining.

4.5. Sodium dodecyl sulfate polyacrylamide gel electrophoresis (SDS-PAGE)—Gradient concentration gels

Gradient gels (resolving gels) are prepared with an increasing concentration of acrylamide from the top to the bottom. Preparation of gradient gels requires a gradient forming apparatus. Ready-to-use gradient gels are commercially available with specific recommended protocols. Gradient gels offer some advantages over fixed concentration gels. Some proteins which co-migrate on fixed concentration gels can be resolved within gradient gels. During electrophoresis the proteins migrate until the pore size stops further progress and therefore a stacking effect occurs, resulting in sharper bands. Per the table below, gradient gels also allow separation of a wider range of proteins molecular masses than on a single fixed concentration gel.

The table below gives suggested compositions of the linear gradient, relating the range of acrylamide concentrations to the appropriate protein molecular ranges. Note that other gradient shapes (e.g. concave) can be prepared for specific applications.

Acrylamide (%)	Protein range (kDa)
5–15	20–250
5–20	10–200
10–20	10–150
8–20	8–150

Gradient gels are also used for molecular mass determination and protein purity determination.

4.6. Detection of proteins in gels

Coomassie and silver staining are the most common protein staining methods and are described in more detail below. Several other commercial stains, detection methods and commercial kits are available. For example, fluorescent stains are visualised using a fluorescent imager and often provide a linear response over a wide range of protein concentrations, often several orders of magnitude depending on the protein.

Coomassie staining has a protein detection level of approximately 1 to 10 μg of protein per band. Silver staining is the most sensitive method for staining proteins in gels and a band containing 10 ng to 100 ng can be detected. These figures are considered robust in the context of these gels. Improved sensitivity of one or two orders of magnitude has sometimes been reported in the literature.

Coomassie staining responds in a more linear manner than silver staining; however the response and range depend on the protein and development time. Both Coomassie and silver staining can be less reproducible if staining is stopped in a subjective manner, i.e. when the staining is deemed satisfactory. Wide dynamic ranges of reference proteins are very important to use since they help assess the intra-experimental sensitivity and linearity. All gel staining steps are done while wearing gloves, at room temperature, with gentle shaking (e.g. on an orbital shaker platform) and using any convenient container.

4.6.1. Coomassie staining

Immerse the gel in a large excess of Coomassie staining solution and allow to stand for at least 1 hour. Remove the staining solution.

Destain the gel with a large excess of destaining solution. Change the destaining solution several times, until the stained protein bands are clearly distinguishable on a clear background. The more thoroughly the gel is destained, the smaller is the amount of protein that can be detected by the method. Destaining can be speeded up by including a few grams of anion-exchange resin or a small sponge in the destaining solution.

The acid-alcohol solutions used in this procedure do not completely fix proteins in the gel. This can lead to losses of some low-molecular-mass proteins during the staining and destaining of thin gels. Permanent fixation is obtainable by allowing the gel to stand in a mixture of 1 volume of trichloroacetic acid, 4 volumes of methanol and 5 volumes of water for 1 hour before it is immersed in the Coomassie staining solution.

4.6.2. Silver staining

Immerse the gel in a large excess of fixing solution and allow to stand for 1 hour. Remove the fixing solution, add fresh fixing solution and incubate either for at least 1 hour or overnight, if convenient. Discard the fixing solution and wash the gel in a large excess of water for 1 hour. Soak the gel for 15 minutes in a 1 vol% solution of glutaraldehyde. Wash the gel twice for 15 minutes in a large excess of water. Soak the gel in fresh silver nitrate reagent for 15 minutes, in darkness. Wash the gel three times for 5 minutes in a large excess of water. Immerse the gel for about 1 minute in developer solution until satisfactory staining has been obtained. Stop the development by incubation in the blocking solution for 15 minutes. Rinse the gel with water.

4.7. Recording of the results

Gels are photographed or scanned while they are still wet or after an appropriate drying procedure. Currently, "gel scanning" systems with data analysis software are commercially available to photograph and analyze the wet gel immediately.

Depending on the staining method used, gels are treated in a slightly different way. For Coomassie staining, after the destaining step, allow the gel to stand in a 100 g/L solution of glycerol for at least 2 hours (overnight incubation is possible).

For silver staining, add to the final rinsing a step of 5 minutes in a 20 g/L solution of glycerol.

Drying of stained SDS Polyacrylamide gels is one of the methods to have permanent documentation. This method frequently results in the "cracking of gel" during drying between cellulose films.

Immerse two sheets of porous cellulose film in water and incubate for 5 minutes to 10 minutes. Place one of the sheets on a drying frame. Carefully lift the gel and place it on the cellulose film. Remove any trapped air bubbles and pour a few millilitres of water around the edges of the gel. Place the second sheet on top and remove any trapped air bubbles. Complete the assembly of the drying frame. Place in an oven or leave at room temperature until dry.

4.8. Molecular mass determination

Molecular masses of proteins are determined by comparison of their mobilities with those of several marker proteins of known molecular weight. Mixtures of pre-stained and unstained proteins with precisely known molecular masses blended for uniform staining are available for calibrating gels. They are available in various molecular mass ranges. Concentrated stock solutions of proteins of known molecular mass are diluted in the appropriate sample buffer and loaded on the same gel as the protein sample to be studied.

Immediately after the gel has been run, the position of the bromophenol blue tracking dye is marked to identify the leading edge of the electrophoretic ion front. This can be done by cutting notches in the edges of the gel or by inserting a needle soaked in India ink into the gel at the dye front. After staining, measure the migration distances of each protein band (markers and unknowns) from the top of the resolving gel. Divide the migration distance of each protein by the distance travelled by the tracking dye. The normalized migration distances are referred to as the relative mobilities of the proteins (relative to the dye front), or Rf. Construct a plot of the logarithm of the relative molecular masses (M_r)

Table 1

Solution components	Component volumes (mL) per gel mould volume of							
	5 mL	10 mL	15 mL	20 mL	25 mL	30 mL	40 mL	50 mL
6% Acrylamide								
Water	2.6	5.3	7.9	10.6	13.2	15.9	21.2	26.5
Acrylamide solution(1)	1.0	2.0	3.0	4.0	5.0	6.0	8.0	10.0
1.5 M Tris (pH 8.8)(2)	1.3	2.5	3.8	5.0	6.3	7.5	10.0	12.5
100 g/L SDS(3)	0.05	0.1	0.15	0.2	0.25	0.3	0.4	0.5
100 g/L APS(4)	0.05	0.1	0.15	0.2	0.25	0.3	0.4	0.5
TEMED(5)	0.004	0.008	0.012	0.016	0.02	0.024	0.032	0.04
8% Acrylamide								
Water	2.3	4.6	6.9	9.3	11.5	13.9	18.5	23.2
Acrylamide solution(1)	1.3	2.7	4.0	5.3	6.7	8.0	10.7	13.3
1.5 M Tris (pH 8.8)(2)	1.3	2.5	3.8	5.0	6.3	7.5	10.0	12.5
100 g/L SDS(3)	0.05	0.1	0.15	0.2	0.25	0.3	0.4	0.5
100 g/L APS(4)	0.05	0.1	0.15	0.2	0.25	0.3	0.4	0.5
TEMED(5)	0.003	0.006	0.009	0.012	0.015	0.018	0.024	0.03
10% Acrylamide								
Water	1.9	4.0	5.9	7.9	9.9	11.9	15.9	19.8
Acrylamide solution(1)	1.7	3.3	5.0	6.7	8.3	10.0	13.3	16.7
1.5 M Tris (pH 8.8)(2)	1.3	2.5	3.8	5.0	6.3	7.5	10.0	12.5
100 g/L SDS(3)	0.05	0.1	0.15	0.2	0.25	0.3	0.4	0.5
100 g/L APS(4)	0.05	0.1	0.15	0.2	0.25	0.3	0.4	0.5
TEMED(5)	0.002	0.004	0.006	0.008	0.01	0.012	0.016	0.02
12% Acrylamide								
Water	1.6	3.3	4.9	6.6	8.2	9.9	13.2	16.5
Acrylamide solution(1)	2.0	4.0	6.0	8.0	10.0	12.0	16.0	20.0
1.5 M Tris (pH 8.8)(2)	1.3	2.5	3.8	5.0	6.3	7.5	10.0	12.5
100 g/L SDS(3)	0.05	0.1	0.15	0.2	0.25	0.3	0.4	0.5
100 g/L APS(4)	0.05	0.1	0.15	0.2	0.25	0.3	0.4	0.5
TEMED(5)	0.002	0.004	0.006	0.008	0.01	0.012	0.016	0.02
14% Acrylamide								
Water	1.4	2.7	3.9	5.3	6.6	8.0	10.6	13.8
Acrylamide solution(1)	2.3	4.6	7.0	9.3	11.6	13.9	18.6	23.2
1.5 M Tris (pH 8.8)(2)	1.2	2.5	3.6	5.0	6.3	7.5	10.0	12.5
100 g/L SDS(3)	0.05	0.1	0.15	0.2	0.25	0.3	0.4	0.5
100 g/L APS(4)	0.05	0.1	0.15	0.2	0.25	0.3	0.4	0.5
TEMED(5)	0.002	0.004	0.006	0.008	0.01	0.012	0.016	0.02
15% Acrylamide								
Water	1.1	2.3	3.4	4.6	5.7	6.9	9.2	11.5
Acrylamide solution(1)	2.5	5.0	7.5	10.0	12.5	15.0	20.0	25.0
1.5 M Tris (pH 8.8)(2)	1.3	2.5	3.8	5.0	6.3	7.5	10.0	12.5
100 g/L SDS(3)	0.05	0.1	0.15	0.2	0.25	0.3	0.4	0.5
100 g/L APS(4)	0.05	0.1	0.15	0.2	0.25	0.3	0.4	0.5
TEMED(5)	0.002	0.004	0.006	0.008	0.01	0.012	0.016	0.02

(1) Acrylamide solution: 30% acrylamide/bisacrylamide (29:1) solution.
(2) 1.5 M Tris (pH 8.8): 1.5 M tris-hydrochloride buffer solution (pH 8.8).
(3) 100 g/L SDS: a 100 g/L solution of sodium dodecyl sulfate.
(4) 100 g/L APS: a 100 g/L solution of ammonium persulfate. Ammonium persulfate provides the free radicals that drive polymerization of acrylamide and bisacrylamide. Since ammonium persulfate solution decomposes rapidly, fresh solutions must be prepared daily.
(5) TEMED: *N*,*N*,*N*′,*N*′-tetramethylethylenediamine.

of the protein standards as a function of the *R*f values. Unknown molecular masses can be estimated by linear regression analysis (more accurately by non-linear regression analysis) or interpolation from the curves of log M_r against *R*f if the values obtained for the unknown samples are positioned along the approximately linear part of the graph.

4.9. Validation of the test

The test is not valid unless the target resolution range of the gel has been demonstrated by the distribution of appropriate molecular mass markers e.g. across 80% of the length of the gel. The separation obtained for the expected proteins must show a linear relationship between the logarithm of the molecular mass and the *R*f. If the plot has a sigmoidal shape then only data from the linear region of the curve can be used in the calculations. Additional validation requirements with respect to the test sample may be specified in individual monographs.

Sensitivity must also be validated. A reference protein control corresponding to the desired concentration limit that is run in parallel with the test samples can serve as a system

Table 2 Preparation of stacking gel

Solution components	Component volumes (mL) per gel mould volume of							
	1 mL	2 mL	3 mL	4 mL	5 mL	6 mL	8 mL	10 mL
Water	0.68	1.4	2.1	2.7	3.4	4.1	5.5	6.8
Acrylamide solution(1)	0.17	0.33	0.5	0.67	0.83	1.0	1.3	1.7
1.0 M Tris (pH 6.8)(2)	0.13	0.25	0.38	0.5	0.63	0.75	1.0	1.25
100 g/L SDS(3)	0.01	0.02	0.03	0.04	0.05	0.06	0.08	0.1
100 g/L APS(4)	0.01	0.02	0.03	0.04	0.05	0.06	0.08	0.1
TEMED(5)	0.001	0.002	0.003	0.004	0.005	0.006	0.008	0.01

(1) Acrylamide solution: 30% acrylamide/bisacrylamide (29:1) solution.
(2) 1.0 M Tris (pH 6.8): 1 M tris-hydrochloride buffer solution (pH 6.8).
(3) 100 g/L SDS: a 100 g/L solution of sodium dodecyl sulfate.
(4) 100 g/L APS: a 100 g/L solution of ammonium persulfate. Ammonium persulfate provides the free radicals that drive polymerization of acrylamide and bisacrylamide. Since ammonium persulfate solution decomposes rapidly, fresh solutions must be prepared daily.
(5) TEMED: *N,N,N′,N′*-tetramethylethylenediamine.

suitability of the experiment.

4.10. Quantification of impurities

SDS-PAGE is often used as a limit test for impurities. When impurities are quantified by normalization to the main band using an integrating densitometer or image analysis, the responses must be validated for linearity. Note that depending on the detection method and protein as described in the introduction of the section "Detection of proteins in gels" the linear range can vary but can be assessed within each run by using one or more control samples containing an appropriate range of protein concentration.

Where the impurity limit is specified in the individual monograph, a reference solution corresponding to that level of impurity should be prepared by diluting the test solution. For example, where the limit is 5%, a reference solution would be a 1:20 dilution of the test solution. No impurity (any band other than the main band) in the electropherogram obtained with the test solution may be more intense than the main band obtained with the reference solution.

Under validated conditions impurities may be quantified by normalization to the main band using an integrating densitometer or by image analysis.

5. Reagents

(i) 30% acrylamide/bisacrylamide (29:1) solution: Prepare a solution containing 290 g of acrylamide and 10 g of methylenebisacrylamide per litre of water. Filter.

(ii) SDS-PAGE running buffer: Dissolve 151.4 g of 2-amino-2-hydroxymethyl-1,3-propanediol, 721.0 g of glycine and 50.0 g of sodium dodecyl sulfate in water and dilute to 5000 mL with the same solvent. Immediately before use, dilute to 10 times its volume with water and mix. Measure the pH of the diluted solution. The pH is between 8.1 and 8.8.

(iii) SDS-PAGE sample buffer (concentrated): Dissolve 1.89 g of 2-amino-2-hydroxymethyl-1,3-propanediol, 5.0 g of sodium dodecyl sulfate and 50 mg of bromophenol blue in water. Add 25.0 mL of glycerol and dilute to 100 mL with water. Adjust the pH to 6.8 with hydrochloric acid, and dilute to 125 mL with water.

(iv) SDS-PAGE sample buffer for reducing conditions (concentrated): Dissolve 3.78 g of 2-amino-2-hydroxymethyl-1,3-propanediol, 10.0 g of sodium dodecyl sulfate and 100 mg of bromophenol blue in water. Add 50.0 mL of glycerol and dilute to 200 mL with water. Add 25.0 mL of 2-mercaptoethanol. Adjust to pH 6.8 with hydrochloric acid, and dilute to 250.0 mL with water. Alternatively, dithiothreitol may be used as reducing agent instead of 2-mercaptoethanol. In this case prepare the sample buffer as follows: dissolve 3.78 g of 2-amino-2-hydroxymethyl-1,3-propanediol, 10.0 g of sodium dodecyl sulfate and 100 mg of bromophenol blue in water. Add 50.0 mL of glycerol and dilute to 200 mL with water. Adjust to pH 6.8 with hydrochloric acid, and dilute to 250.0 mL with water. Immediately before use, add dithiothreitol to a final concentration of 100 mM.

(v) Coomassie staining solution: A 1.25 g/L solution of acid blue 83 in a mixture consisting of 1 volume of glacial acetic acid, 4 volumes of methanol and 5 volumes of water. Filter.

(vi) Developer solution: Dilute 2.5 mL of a 20 g/L solution of citric acid and 0.27 mL of formaldehyde to 500.0 mL with water.

(vii) Fixing solution: To 250 mL of methanol, add 0.27 mL of formaldehyde and dilute to 500.0 mL with water.

(viii) Silver nitrate reagent: To a mixture of 3 mL of concentrated ammonia and 40 mL of 1 M sodium hydroxide, add 8 mL of a 200 g/L solution of silver nitrate, dropwise, with stirring. Dilute to 200 mL with water.

(ix) Destaining solution: A mixture consisting of 1 volume of glacial acetic acid, 4 volumes of methanol and 5 volumes of water.

(x) 1.5 M tris-hydrochloride buffer solution (pH 8.8): Dissolve 90.8 g of 2-amino-2-hydroxymethyl-1,3-propanediol in 400 mL of water. Adjust the pH with hydrochloric acid and dilute to 500.0 mL with water.

(xi) Blocking solution: A 10 vol% solution of acetic acid.

Host Cell Protein Assay <*G3-9-172*>

Host cell protein (HCP) is a general term for proteins derived from host cells used for the production of pharmaceutical products. This general information describes HCP assays for therapeutic proteins produced by recombinant DNA technology (recombinant therapeutic proteins).

Residual HCP in recombinant therapeutic proteins has potential to elicit immune responses against itself and may also act as adjuvants to induce anti-drug antibodies. Therefore, in order to ensure the efficacy and safety of recombinant therapeutic proteins, it is necessary to establish a purification process to reduce HCP to a level that does not affect safety. In addition, residual levels of HCP must be appropriately controlled by verifying that in-process tests can consistently eliminate HCP or by establishing purity testing of drug substance.

1. Selection of Test Methods for HCP assay

HCP assay is usually performed with a sandwich immunoassay using antibodies against HCP (anti-HCP antibodies) and detection systems including enzyme-linked immunosorbent assay (ELISA), electrochemiluminescent immunoassay (ECLIA), and time-resolved fluorescent immunoassay (TRFIA). This general information addresses the sandwich immunoassay, but does not discourage other assays.

Residual HCP from the manufacturing process of recombinant therapeutic proteins consists a large number of proteins and may have profiles that vary from one host cell to another or depending on manufacturing conditions. Based on differences in its intended use or differences in the concept of preparation of anti-HCP antibodies used for testing, HCP assay is classified into generic assay, product-specific assay, and platform assay. Generic assay is intended for wide use in pharmaceutical products manufactured using similar host cells (e.g., CHO-K1 or CHO-DG44 cells derived from CHO [Chinese hamster ovary] cells) and is a test method established using anti-HCP antibodies that are prepared with proteins from all components of the host cells (cell lysate or culture supernatant) as immunogens. Commercially available reagents or kits for an HCP assay commonly referred to as generic assay and need to be validated before use. Product-specific assay is intended to control HCP in a specific product and developed in consideration of characteristics of the manufacturing process of the product. Platform assay is developed for the application to recombinant therapeutic proteins (e.g., monoclonal antibodies with adequate experience) produced by a manufacturing platform.

Generic assay is intended to comprehensively obtain antibodies against a wide range of HCP by using proteins from all components of the host cells as antigens. However, it should be noted that it is difficult to obtain antibodies against all HCPs because of differences in proportions or immunogenicity of individual proteins used as antigens and that residual HCP from actual manufacturing processes may be inadequately covered because of potential different profiles of residual HCP from different manufacturing processes. In contrast, product-specific assay is expected to prepare anti-HCP antibodies that can detect residual HCP from actual manufacturing processes compared with generic assay because it uses potentially residual HCP as antigens. However, it should be noted that profiles of residual HCP may vary with modifications to manufacturing processes. Platform assay has both aspects, namely, the assay has an advantage of being able to be applied to various products prepared by a manufacturing platform; however, the assay may involve issues as generic or product-specific assay, depending on the method of preparation of antigens used for preparing anti-HCP antibodies.

In some products, it is possible that specific HCPs binding to desired products are present or that HCPs markedly increase in production amount with expression of desired products. If the residue of these HCPs is found, the need to establish other test methods for the HCPs is considered.

In light of these characteristics of the test methods for HCP assays and in consideration of properties of host cells, characteristics of manufacturing processes, knowledge about immunogenicity of HCPs, stages of development of products, etc., an appropriate test method is selected.

2. Preparation and Characterization of Reagents

2.1. HCP Antigens/HCP Reference Materials

For antigens to produce antibodies that specifically detect HCPs in products, it is necessary to prepare HCP not containing desired products. Usually, null cells are used for preparation of HCP antigen while keeping in mind that HCP appropriate to the purpose of the HCP assay are comprehensively contained. In addition, HCP are used not only as antigens but also as reference materials for HCP assay and may also be used as ligands for purification of anti-HCP antibodies by affinity chromatography.

2.1.1. Preparation of HCP Antigens/HCP Reference Materials

The method of preparation of HCP antigens/HCP reference materials varies widely depending on the type of test methods. The method of preparation of HCP used as antigens for preparation of anti-HCP antibodies or as HCP reference materials in the test methods is shown below along with points to note.

HCP used for generic assays are prepared from culture supernatant or lysed or disrupted null cells using minimal procedures such as concentration and dialysis and keeping preservation of component proteins in mind. It should be noted that these HCPs show profiles that are different from those of residual HCP in products because of preparation under conditions different from culture processes at commercial scale.

HCP used for product-specific assays are prepared from null cells using manufacturing processes of products. Usually, the application of the purification process is minimized to obtain a wide range of HCP. However, if a suitable antibody to detect the HCP is not obtained, it may be necessary to prepare appropriate HCP antigens by exploring conditions of preparation of HCP or excluding specific HCP.

HCP used for the platform assays are prepared from null cells using a manufacturing platform that can be used in multiple products. Usually, as with the other test methods, the application of the purification process is minimized to obtain a wide range and an enough amount of HCP. In addition, a mixture of HCPs prepared under multiple conditions can be used to address differences in HCP spectra due to slight differences in manufacturing conditions.

The use of mock cells as null cells used for preparation of HCP for product-specific and platform assays has advantages such as the presence of proteins expressed as selection markers in antigens and ability to culture the cells under similar culture conditions in actual manufacturing processes. In contrast, it should be noted that even a same cell line does not show consistent properties (such as cell growth rate) among different clones and that differences such as the presence or absence of production of desired products may cause different profiles of HCP.

2.1.2. Characterization of HCP Antigens/HCP Reference Materials

Prepared HCPs are analyzed for the following items.

1) Protein Concentrations

Protein concentrations are determined by a suitable measurement method keeping in mind that host cell nucleic acids or culture medium components may be contained depending on the method of preparation of HCP. For information on detailed measurement methods and points to consider, "Total Protein Assay *<G3-12-172>*" in General Information would be helpful.

2) HCP Profiles

Usually, one-dimensional electrophoresis (SDS-PAGE) or two-dimensional electrophoresis is used to confirm that prepared HCP include HCP species that are considered to remain in manufacturing processes or drug substances. Identification of HCP species by mass spectrometry is also a helpful approach.

2.2. Anti-HCP Antibodies

2.2.1. Preparation of Anti-HCP Antibodies

Since HCPs represent a heterogeneous variety of different proteins, polyclonal antibodies are obtained as anti-HCP antibodies used for the assay to comprehensively detect HCPs. The rabbit, goat, and sheep are commonly used animal species for immunization. For immunization, it is useful to enhance immune response with adjuvants. Due to different degrees of immunogenicity of individual proteins comprising HCPs, the timing of induction of antibodies or the amount of antibodies produced is not constant, regardless of the amount of proteins as antigens. In addition, inter-individual variability in animals used for immunization makes the profile of induced antibodies inconsistent. Several rounds of immunization are usually required and, after determining the reactivity of induced antibodies with HCPs by Western blotting using antisera in each period of immunization, whole serum is collected. Mixing of anti-HCP antibodies derived from multiple individuals is intended to obtain adequate amounts of antibodies and is also expected to contribute to the elimination of imbalance of HCP profiles.

Anti-HCP antibodies are purified from the obtained antiserum by Protein A or Protein G chromatography. In either case, aggregates may be formed from some antibodies due to use of acid conditions for antibody elution from the columns. It is useful to remove antibody aggregates by a suitable method because they may cause interference with measurement.

Anti-HCP antibodies can also be purified by affinity chromatography using HCP as ligands. This purification is expected to eliminate non-specific reactions because of concentration of antibodies specific to HCPs, however, it should be noted that anti-HCP antibodies may get less diverse due to less adsorption of low-affinity antibodies or less elution of very high-affinity antibodies.

2.2.2. Suitability of Anti-HCP Antibodies

Anti-HCP antibodies have to be able to comprehensively recognize HCPs with wide ranges of electric charges and molecular masses that potentially remain in manufacturing processes or drug substances. However, because differences in immunogenicity of each HCP species may make antibodies against some HCPs less likely to be induced, obtained anti-HCP antibodies have to be qualified, usually as measured by antigen coverage. A specific example of assessment methods is shown below. After separation of HCPs by two-dimensional electrophoresis, total protein on the gel is stained. After performing two-dimensional electrophoresis in the same manner, Western blotting using anti-HCP antibodies is performed. Spot patterns obtained from each staining are compared and the proportion of spots detected by Western blotting vs spots obtained in total protein staining is determined as antigen coverage.

2.3. Storage of Reagents

HCP reference materials and anti-HCP antibodies are stored with attention to stability. The stability of these reagents can be confirmed by continuously monitoring parameters of dose-response curves of reference materials.

3. Validation of HCP Assay

When a sandwich immunoassay is used for HCP assay, ''Validation of Analytical Procedures *<G1-1-130>*'' in General Information would be helpful for information on basic requirements for validation. However, unlike a conventional sandwich immunoassay to determine a single antigen, HCP assay is an approach to use antibodies prepared with a mixture of various HCP species as antigens to determine the HCP species simultaneously. Therefore, changes in concentrations as a function of dilution ratios of samples (dilution linearity) may not be observed in highly purified samples even within the quantitation limits in which linearity has been obtained for HCP reference materials. This phenomenon is likely attributed to insufficient amounts of antibodies to some HCPs that are found in increased proportions in samples for measurement due to the difference of removal rates of individual HCPs in the purification process and may lead to underestimation of HCP concentrations.

Therefore, HCP assay should be validated for accuracy, precision, specificity, standard curve, quantitative range, and dilution linearity.

(1) Accuracy and Precision

Accuracy and precision are expressed as coefficients of variation of recovery rates and quantitative values of HCP reference materials, respectively, by performing spike and recovery tests of HCP reference materials in purification process pools or drug substances to be measured.

(2) Specificity

Because HCP assay involves measurement of trace amounts of HCPs remaining in samples containing large quantities of desired products, it should be confirmed that there is no interference of desired substances or ingredients in sample solutions.

(3) Standard Curve and Quantitative Range

A standard curve is generated using serially diluted HCP reference materials to obtain a regression expression, and validity is expressed in terms of determination coefficient, etc. Quantitative values of reference materials at each concentration level are determined from the regression expression and a range of concentrations with acceptable levels of accuracy and precision is defined as quantitative range with the lowest concentration within the range being defined as the minimum limit of quantitation.

(4) Dilution Linearity

Purification process pools or drug substances to be measured are examined for the range of dilution ratios of samples in which quantitative values of samples diluted within the quantitative range of a standard curve are linear.

4. Establishment of HCP Assay

HCP assay is used for confirmation of the status of removal of HCP in manufacturing processes or as a purity test of drug substances. For information on basic concepts of procedures or data analysis in HCP assay, ''Enzyme-linked Immunosorbent Assay *<G3-11-171>*'' in General Information would be helpful.

Results from HCP assay are usually presented as contents in total protein or desired products. Contents of HCP per total protein or desired products can be determined by separately determining concentrations of the proteins in samples. For example, when total protein concentration is 2 mg/mL and an HCP concentration is 20 ng/mL, the content of HCP should be indicated as 10 ng/mg.

5. Others

5.1. Considerations for Modifications to Manufacturing Processes

Since any modifications made to manufacturing processes for recombinant therapeutic proteins may affect profiles of residual HCP, it is necessary to confirm that appropriate measurement of HCP is performed after modifications to manufacturing processes. If HCP profiles are altered and it is considered inappropriate to apply a test method for HCP assay before modifications to manufacturing processes, a test method for HCP assay has to be established again. Changes in HCP profiles can be assessed by an analytical procedure such as two-dimensional electrophoresis or mass spectrometry.

5.2. Considerations for Modifications to Reagents for Tests

It is desirable to secure sufficient quantities of HCP antigens/HCP reference materials and anti-HCP antibodies, all important reagents, whenever possible, in consideration of the life cycle of products. When HCP antigens/HCP reference materials or anti-HCP antibodies are newly prepared, it should be confirmed that their characteristics are comparable before and after renewal by analytical procedures such as two-dimensional electrophoresis, Western blotting, and mass spectrometry. In addition, test methods should be validated again for necessary items and newly prepared reagents should be used after confirming their consistency with the reagents and test methods before renewal.

When generic assay is employed, qualified commercially available kits can also be used. However, availability of information on lot renewal of reagents, etc. is necessary to ensure consistency and quality of tests using commercially available kits, and therefore characterization of important reagents and method validation should be performed as needed.

6. Terms

Mock cell: A cell line established from the host cell line by transferring expression vectors that do not contain genes encoding desired products.

Null cell: A host cell that does not express desired products. It includes parent cells or mock cells.

Antigen coverage: The rate of detection of proteins comprising HCPs by anti-HCP antibodies. For example, an antigen coverage can be calculated from the number of spots obtained in total protein staining and the number of spots obtained in Western blotting using anti-HCP antibodies after separation of HCPs by two-dimensional electrophoresis.

Surface Plasmon Resonance

<G3-10-170>

Surface plasmon resonance (SPR) optical detection is a method for detecting changes in mass on a sensor chip as changes in the angle at which the reflected light disappears by SPR. This method is used to analyze the binding specificity and binding affinity between substances, and to measure the concentration of analytes in samples.

The devices designed to measure interactions between substances by means of surface plasmon resonance usually adopt a prism-based Kretschmann configuration (Fig. 1). If polarized light is applied in a manner allowing total reflection on the metallic film surface of the sensor chip, an SPR signal (a reduction in intensity in a portion of the reflected light) is observed. The angle at which the SPR signal is produced varies depending on the mass placed on the sensor chip. Thus, the angle at which the SPR signal is produced is changed by binding or dissociation between the molecule immobilized on the sensor chip (the ligand) and the molecule added (the analyte) (Fig. 1). The results of measurement are in the form of a sensorgram presenting changes over time in the SPR signal-producing angle or the response unit (RU) converted from changes in the angle. If the thus-obtained binding and dissociation sensorgram is fitted to the theoretical curve, the ligand/analyte binding rate constant (k_a), dissociation rate constant (k_d) and dissociation constant ($K_D = k_d/k_a$) can be determined. If the response of the analyte in a given sample is compared to the response of the analyte of known concentration, the analyte concentration in a given sample can be determined.

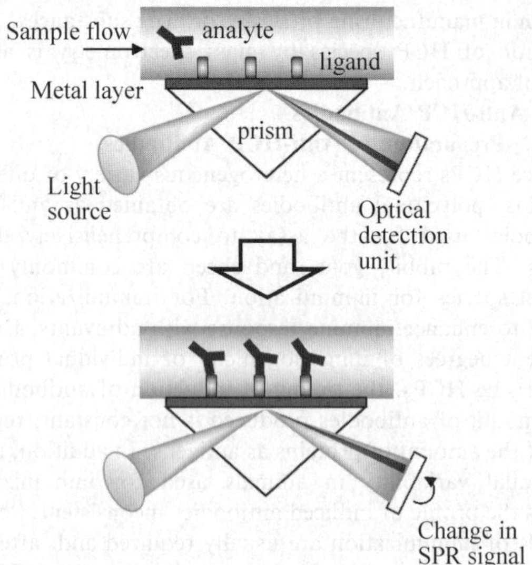

Fig. 1 Principle of SPR measurement (Kretschmann configuration)

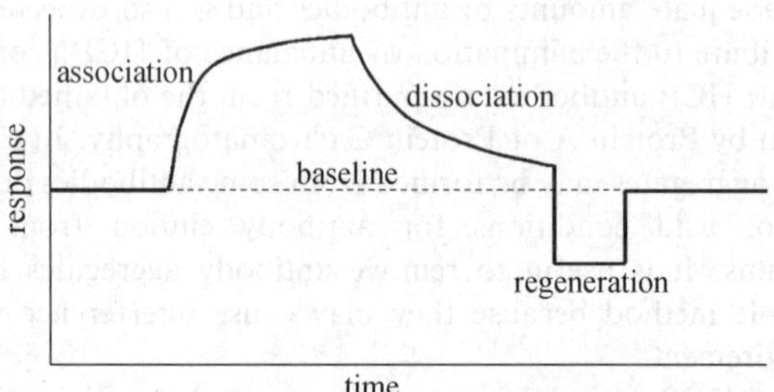

Fig. 2 Example of an SPR sensorgram

1. Instrument

The instrument usually used for SPR optical detection (a continuous flow system) consists of a light source, an optical detector, a fluid delivery system, a sensor chip insertion port and a data accumulating unit. A sensor chip conjugated with carboxymethyl dextran is usually employed. An appropriate sensor chip tailored to the characteristics of the molecule to be immobilized should be selected. If the sensor chip is set on the device, multiple flow cells are formed on the sensor chip surface, allowing the ligand to be immobilized on each flow cell.

2. Measurement

SPR optical detection is used for testing the binding specificity between the ligand and the analyte, analyzing the binding affinity between the ligand and the analyte, or measuring the analyte concentration. Usually, SPR signals are observed over time while applying the buffer solution to the flow cell and injecting the analyte, and a sensorgram illustrating the binding of the analyte to the ligand immobilized on the sensor chip is obtained. In kinetic analysis designed to analyze the binding affinity from the shape of the sensorgram, a running buffer free of the analyte is applied after the end of analyte injection in order to obtain a dissociation sensorgram. After measurement, a regeneration buffer is applied so that the analyte bound to the ligand can be removed completely (Fig. 2).

2.1. Sample and buffer solution

(1) Analyte solution

Depending on the objective of analysis and the affinity between the molecules to be measured, the sample is diluted to an optimal concentration with the running buffer to yield an analyte solution. If the sample contains insoluble contaminants, they need to be removed by an appropriate method such as centrifugation or filtration using a low protein adsorptive filter.

(2) Running buffer

A buffer appropriate for the ligand and analyte is selected. Addition of salts or detergents to the buffer can be useful in stabilizing the ligand and the analyte. If appropriate, the buffer is filtrated and degassed prior to use. If non-specific binding to the reference flow cell is observed at the time of analyte injection, the buffer needs to be optimized by changing its pH, ionic strength, or other conditions.

(3) Regeneration buffer

As regeneration solution, a buffer with low pH, high pH, or high ionic strength, or a buffer containing surfactants, nonpolar reagents, or chelating agents can be used. The type of buffer to be used varies depending on the material of the flow path of the device. Thus, it is necessary to check the chemical resistance of the device. The ideal setting for regeneration is the one under which complete dissociation of the bound analyte can be achieved without altering the nature of the ligand on the sensor chip surface. If the regeneration buffer is suitable, the baseline after regeneration returns to the baseline recorded before addition of the analyte and it is possible to avoid a reduction in the binding response during repeated measurement. If the setting for regeneration is inappropriate, the level of binding to the ligand decreases during the cycles of measurement, thus affecting the reproducibility of measurement. If the dissociation rate is sufficiently high, the flow of the buffer allows dissociation of the analyte from the ligand, thus making it unnecessary to apply the buffer for regeneration.

2.2. Preparation of the sensor chip used for the measurement

Two methods of binding the ligand to the sensor chip are available: a direct method (direct immobilization of the ligand), and a capture method (capture immobilization of the ligand). In both methods, it is essential to immobilize the ligand while retaining its biological activity and minimizing the impact on binding to the analyte. A ligand of high purity level must be used for the immobilization.

The amount of the ligand to be immobilized is determined with reference to the equation given below.

$$\text{Ligand immobilization quantity} = \frac{\text{Required } R_{\max}}{\text{Valency of the ligand}} \times \frac{\text{molecular weight of the ligand}}{\text{molecular weight of the analyte}}$$

The $R_{\max}$ (response in the case of maximal binding of the analyte to the ligand) needed for measurement is determined depending on the sensitivity of the instrument used. For analysis of binding affinity, $R_{\max}$ needs to be low to avoid steric effects, aggregation and mass transport limitation (a condition under which the amount of analyte supplied serves as a rate-limiting factor for changes in the binding amount due to a shortage in the amount of analyte against the excess ligand). For measurement of the analyte concentration, high $R_{\max}$ is desirable to induce a mass transport limitation which increases the dependency of the analyte-binding amount on the concentration and improves the linearity of the calibration curve.

Usually, a control flow cell free of bound ligand is prepared on the sensor chip and is used to detect nonspecific bindings. The following can serve as the control flow cell: (1) an untreated flow cell, (2) a flow cell having undergone a chemical treatment identical to that for ligand immobilization, and (3) a flow cell having undergone immobilization of a ligand-like molecule having no potential for binding to the analyte. In the case that the ligand is immobilized by the capture method, a flow cell having undergone immobilization of the capturing molecule serves as the control flow cell.

If the immobilized ligand is stable, it is possible to store the sensor chip apart from the device. Such storage is used under conditions such as dry environments or immersion in a buffer solution at low temperature.

Ligand immobilization methods

(1) Direct method

The ligand is immobilized directly via the amino group, thiol group, carboxyl group, aldehyde group or hydroxyl group of the ligand, or via the hydrophobicity of the ligand. The sensor chip usually possesses a layer containing carboxyl groups, which can be used for immobilization. Thus, the ligand is immobilized by the covalent bond. In the case of direct immobilization, the surface often becomes inhomogeneous due to the lack of a uniform direction in the ligand.

(2) Capture method

A capturing molecule having the potential to bind to the ligand is immobilized on the sensor chip so that the ligand can be captured on the chip by binding to the capturing molecule. Capturing molecules include the antibody to the ligand, and antibody to the specific tag sequence allocated to the ligand. If the ligand is an antibody drug, protein A and protein G serve as capturing molecules. If the ligand is a biotinylated molecule, streptavidin is used as a capturing molecule. By the capture method, the direction in the ligand is likely to become uniform. It is important that dissociation of the ligand from the capturing molecule does not occur during measurement. If ligand capturing is performed at each cycle of measurement, there is no need to determine the conditions of regeneration for individual ligands, thus making it easy to set the conditions for measurement.

2.3. Setting the conditions for measurement

(1) Checking the baseline

Before starting the measurement, the stability of the baseline needs to be confirmed. If the baseline is not stable, stabilization should be attempted by the following procedures: administration of several infusions of buffer solution, high ion intensity solution or surfactant solution, application of buffer at a high flow rate, and repetition of the sequence of analyte binding and regeneration.

(2) Flow rate

For analysis of the binding affinity, it is necessary to set the flow rate high in order to suppress the mass transport limitation. For measurement of the analyte concentration, the flow rate must be set low to facilitate the mass transport limitation.

(3) Duration of the analysis

The time needed for analysis in each step (binding, dissociation, etc.) varies depending on the type of measurement. When specific binding is to be tested, the time for binding is set as the time allowing sufficient observation of changes in response. In the case of binding affinity analysis by means of kinetic analysis, a sufficient amount of time should be allowed for dissociation if the response involves slow dissociation. In the case of affinity analysis by means of steady state analysis, the time sufficient for the binding level to reach the equilibrium must be set. In the case of concentration measurement, the time will suffice if it covers the points of measurement capable of yielding an appropriate calibration curve.

(4) Checking R_{max}

If the R_{max} measured exceeds the theoretical R_{max} calculated from the molecular weight of the ligand and analyte together with the ligand immobilization quantity and the ligand's binding valency, the following reasons can be considered: inappropriate binding valency, analyte aggregation, or non-specific binding. In such cases, the conditions for measurement or analysis need to be modified.

(5) Checking the reproducibility of measurement

The reproducibility of measurement may be affected if the conditions for measurement are not optimal, and if the ligand is inactivated during repetition of the measuring cycle. Furthermore, if a sensor chip that has been kept stored is used, the reproducibility may be affected by the storage. When the conditions for measurement are set, close attention needs to be paid to reproducibility. The acceptable repeated number of measurements and the acceptable storage period should be set in advance.

2.4. Methods of measurement

2.4.1. Analysis of binding specificity

The analyte is added, and its binding to the ligand is tested on the basis of the binding responses. An appropriate control experiment should be carried out (e.g., demonstrating lack of binding of other analytes to the immobilized ligand), to confirm that the binding observed in the measurement was specific to the analyte.

2.4.2. Analysis of binding affinity

(1) Kinetic analysis

The analyte is injected and its binding is measured. Then, fluid free of the analyte is applied and dissociation of the analyte is measured. Thereafter, complete dissociation of the analyte is achieved by the regeneration step, followed by measurement of the next analyte solution. Another method is analysis of the binding affinity through successive application of analyte solutions at varying concentration levels without interposing a regeneration step. Usually, measurement is performed using the analyte at 5 or more concentrations (between 1/10 of K_D and 10 × K_D).

(2) Steady state analysis

If binding and dissociation take place rapidly, making kinetic analysis or model fitting difficult, steady state analysis is performed. The analyte injection is continued for a period of time until the analyte binding reaches equilibrium. The responses upon reaching equilibrium are recorded. Dissociation of the bound analyte is achieved by regeneration and the next analyte solution is measured. With this method, K_D is calculated as an analyte concentration which yields 1/2 R_{max}. Thus, the analyte concentration needs to be set so that binding to the ligand at the highest analyte concentration is close to saturation.

2.4.3. Measurement of concentration

If measurement is done under the conditions facilitating mass transport limitation, the linearity of the calibration curve is improved, allowing increased accuracy of measurement over a wide range. For this reason, the analyte is injected into the flow cell immobilized with a large amount of ligand, and binding is measured under this setting. Then, dissociation of the analyte is achieved by regeneration, and the next analyte solution is measured. A calibration curve is prepared from the results of measurement of the analyte at known concentration levels. Then, the analyte concentration is calculated. Another available method attempts to calculate the analyte concentration by making use of the proportional relationship between the analyte concentration and diffusion rate, without using a calibration curve.

3. Data analysis

When analysis is performed, the unnecessary part of the sensorgram (e.g., corresponding to capture of the ligand by the capturing molecule, and the regeneration step) is removed, and the response of the control flow cells is subtracted from the response of the ligand-bound flow cells. In addition, the sensorgram baseline is adjusted to 0. As needed, the sensorgram yielded by injection of the buffer for measurement alone is subtracted from the sensorgram yielded by analyte injection.

3.1. Analysis of binding affinity

(1) Kinetic analysis

Kinetic analysis is intended to calculate the parameters for the approximate formula (k_a, k_d, K_D, R_{max}, etc.) from the sensorgram with the use of the reaction rate equation derived from the ligand/analyte binding model. If the ligand binds to the analyte at a ratio of 1:1, the reaction rate equation for association phase is as follows:

$$dR/dt = k_a \times C \times (R_{max} - R) - k_d \times R$$

The reaction rate equation for the dissociation phase is as follows:

$$dR/dt = -k_d \times R$$

(C: analyte concentration; R: response).

A reaction rate equation involving a term corresponding to mass transport limitation or fluid effect can also be used.

The dissociation constant (K_D) serving as an indicator of binding affinity is defined as follows.

$$K_D = k_d/k_a$$

The reaction models employed for analysis of binding affinity include: ① a model of 1:1 ligand/analyte binding, ② a model of 2:1 ligand/analyte binding, like antigen/antibody binding, ③ a model of competitive binding of two analytes to the ligand, ④ a model of one analyte to the ligand possessing two binding sites of different affinity levels, and ⑤ a model of conformational change after 1:1 complex formation. A model theoretically considered as appropriate should be selected, with the results of other biochemical experiments being taken into account.

After the kinetic analysis, an evaluation is needed to determine the appropriateness of the fitting performed. This is accomplished by evaluating the residual plot between the sensorgram obtained and the theoretical curve, or statistical parameters such as χ^2 (mean squared residual, demonstrating the difference between the measured data and the calculated theoretical curve).

Poor fitting to the theoretical curve may be attributable to the following factors: (1) low purity of the reagent, (2) inappropriate method or density of immobilization, (3) inappropriate analyte concentration, (4) nonspecific binding, (5) reduced ligand activity, and (6) inappropriate selection of a reaction model. Thus, the conditions for measurement and the reaction model need to be reviewed. If the RI (refractive index) calculated as a response of the buffer components in the sample is excessively high during analysis of the data on reactions involving rapid binding/dissociation, fitting is performed by fixing the RI to 0. In the case of a poor fitting, the fit might be improved by setting the initial values close to the anticipated values of k_a and k_d.

(2) Steady state analysis

Steady state analysis is as follows. The response reaching equilibrium at each analyte concentration (Y axis) is plotted against the analyte concentration (X axis). Then, regression is performed using the following equation:

Steady state response equation:

$$\text{Equilibrium level at analyte concentration} = \text{analyte concentration} \times \frac{R_{max}}{\text{analyte concentration} + K_D}$$

In this way, the K_D shown by the response of 1/2 R_{max} is determined. The K_D calculated with this equation is the value when 1:1 ligand/analyte binding is assumed. If the actually measured response converges at R_{max}, good analysis is possible. However, if it is in a range lower than R_{max}, the analytical data are less reliable and it is desirable to repeat the measurement by expanding the range of measured concentrations to cover the higher concentration levels.

3.2. Measurement of concentration

From the sensorgram derived by injecting an analyte of known concentration, the slope of the sensorgram near the start of injection or the response at a certain time after starting the injection is determined and plotted against the analyte concentration. A calibration curve is prepared with an appropriate formula for approximation (e.g., the formula for 4-parameter logistic regression, linear regression). Then, the slope or the response is determined from measurement of the sample as an analyte, followed by calculation of the sample concentration from the calibration curve.

4. Application to various tests

4.1. Example of application to identification test

This test is aimed at confirming binding of the sample to the ligand by testing the specific binding as described in 2.4.1. To evaluate the system performance, measurement is performed on the reference material and a negative control (a substance distinguishable from the ligand in terms of the ligand-binding activity) to confirm the specificity of the binding.

4.2. Example of application to binding affinity test

This test is aimed at determining the K_D of the reference material and the sample, making use of the binding affinity analysis described in section 2.4.2. The criterion value related to the binding affinity may be set as the K_D or relative K_D (sample K_D/reference material K_D).

Regarding system suitability, the system performance and system repeatability are set. For example, concerning the system performance, it is confirmed that the ligand immobilization quantity is within the predetermined range; that the calculated K_D of known ligand-binding affinity samples is consistent with the order of affinity levels; and that χ^2 is not more than the predetermined level. System repeatability is confirmed by checking that the relative standard deviation for K_D during repeated measurement is not more than the predetermined level.

4.3. Example of application to measurement of specific activity based on the binding quantity to the target molecule

When specific activity is calculated with the quantity of binding to the target molecule, the measurement is performed using the concentration measuring method described in 2.4.3. On the basis of the calibration curve prepared from the reference material, the relative potency to the reference material is calculated using the data on the response of the sample solution, and then the potency is divided by the protein concentration to yield the specific activity.

Regarding system suitability, the system performance and system repeatability are confirmed. For example, concerning system performance, it is confirmed that the ligand immobilization quantity is within the predetermined range; and that the correlation coefficient or determination coefficient of the calibration curve is not less than the predetermined level. System repeatability is confirmed by checking that the relative standard deviation of the response during repeated measurement is not more than the predetermined level.

Enzyme-linked Immunosorbent Assay (ELISA) <*G3-11-171*>

ELISA (Enzyme-linked immunosorbent assay) is one of the immunological assay methods to detect analytes by antigen-antibody reaction, in which an enzyme-labeled reagent is used as a detection reagent. In general, 96-well-plates and such are used, on which capture molecules specifically bound to the analyte are immobilized. A test sample, an enzyme-labeled reagent and other required reagents are sequentially added and washed to have the enzyme-labeled reagent bind onto a plate. After reaction by adding a substrate for the labeled enzyme, the response (e.g., absorbance) by the enzymatic reaction is measured to determine the concentration or binding activity of the analyte in the test sample. ELISA is also used as a qualitative test to detect the presence or absence of binding of the analyte with specific molecules.

In tests for biotechnological/biological products, ELISA is mainly used for two different purposes. One is to quantitate the target product or process-related impurities usually by measuring the concentration of the analyte with antibodies which specifically bind to the analyte. Another is to evaluate the biological activity of products such as therapeutic antibodies. For the latter purpose, ELISA is used to evaluate the binding activity of the target product with molecules related to its pharmacological action, or to evaluate the cell response based on the amount of the endogenous protein secreted from the cells treated with the test samples containing the target product.

1. Analytical methods

ELISA is broadly classified into competitive and noncompetitive methods, and also classified into direct and indirect detection methods based on the detection procedures (Fig. 1). In addition, ELISA is also classified into direct and indirect immobilization methods by the method for immobilizing capture molecules (Fig. 2).

An analyte bound to a solid phase is detected by the antibody against the analyte or other reagents (Fig. 1). In the direct detection method, an enzyme-labelled antibody against the analyte is used. In the indirect detection method, a molecule indirectly bound to the analyte such as an antibody (secondary antibody) against the antibody binding to the analyte (primary antibody), is used. The procedure of the direct detection method is simple, but the enzyme-labeled antibody against the analyte is required for each analyte. Compared to the direct detection method, the procedure of the indirect detection method is more complex, however, it allows for using a common secondary antibody such as an anti-IgG antibody even if the analyte is different.

When ELISA is used for measuring analyte concentration, an antibody against the analyte is typically used as a capture molecule. When ELISA is used to evaluate biological activity by measuring binding activity, the target molecule of a drug involved in its pharmacologic action is used as a capture molecule.

1.1. Noncompetitive method

In the noncompetitive method, an analyte is bound to a capture molecule without competing with other molecules (Fig. 1). This method can be used when the analyte possesses rather high molecular mass and has binding sites for the capture molecule as well as for the molecule used for detection.

1.2. Competitive method

The competitive method has two approaches: the first is to immobilize a capture molecule, then has an analyte and an enzyme-labeled antibody compete to each other for binding with the capture molecule (Fig. 1a), and the second is to use the analyte prepared as the reagent which is immobilized onto a plate, then have the immobilized analyte and the analyte in test samples compete with each other for binding with an enzyme-labeled antibody (Fig. 1b). The competitive method is used when the molecular mass of the analyte is rather low, and it is difficult to prepare two molecules which bind to the analyte specifically.

2. Analytical procedures

2.1. Procedure

General procedures for both noncompetitive and competitive methods are shown below. As for a quantitative test, prepare reference material solutions diluted serially in order to obtain a dose-response curve or a calibration curve.

2.1.1. Noncompetitive method

1) Add a solution containing capture molecules onto a plate, and incubate to immobilize the capture molecules on a solid phase, then wash off the unbound capture molecules.
2) Add a blocking reagent, and have the reagent bind on the surface not occupied by the capture molecules. Wash off the unbound blocking reagent.
3) Add a reference material or a test sample onto each well of the plate, and have the analyte bind on the solid phase. Wash off the unbound analyte.
4) When the direct detection method is used, add an enzyme-labeled antibody to bind to the analyte. When the indirect detection method is used, add an antibody against the analyte, then wash and add the enzyme-labeled antibody which binds to the antibody against the analyte in order to bind it to the solid phase. Wash off the unbound enzyme-labeled antibody.
5) Add a substrate solution, incubate and add a stopping solution if required. Then measure the absorbance, luminescent intensity, or fluorescent intensity, which reflects the amount of the substrate converted by the enzyme reaction.
6) Determine the binding activity or concentration of the analyte with reference to the dose-response curve (calibration curve) of the reference material.

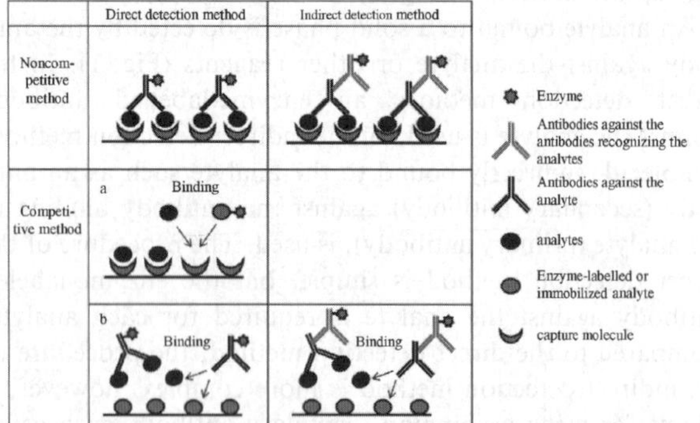

Fig. 1 Classification of ELISA by analytical method

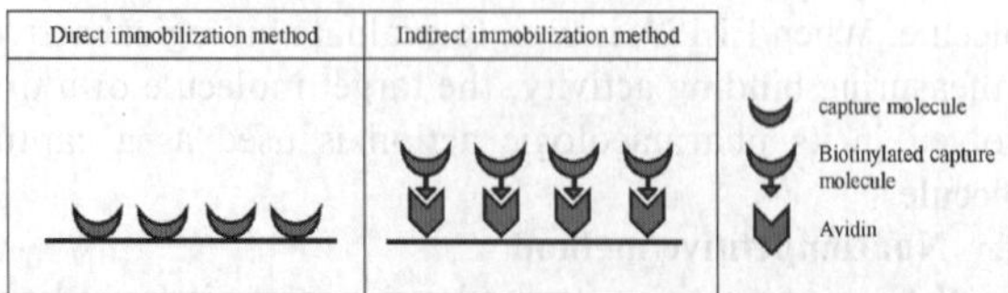

Fig. 2 Examples of direct immobilization method and indirect immobilization method

2.1.2. Competitive method

1) Competitive method (a): Add a solution containing capture molecules onto a plate, then incubate so that the capture molecules bind to a solid phase. Wash off the unbound capture molecules.
Competitive method (b): Add an analyte prepared for immobilizing onto a plate, and incubate so that the analyte bind to the solid phase. Wash off the unbound analyte.
2) Add a blocking reagent to bind on the solid phase surface that is not occupied by the operation of 1). Wash off the unbound blocking reagent.
3) Competitive method (a): Add a solution containing a reference material and an enzyme-labeled analyte, or a test sample and an enzyme-labeled analyte onto each well of the plate. Then have the analyte and the enzyme-labeled analyte bind on the solid phase. Wash off the unbound molecules.
Competitive method (b): In the direct detection method, add a solution containing a reference material and an enzyme-labeled antibody, or a test sample and an enzyme-labeled antibody onto each well of the plate, and then have the enzyme-labeled antibody bind to the solid phase. Wash off the unbound molecules. In the indirect detection method, add a solution containing a reference material and an antibody against the analyte, or a test sample and an antibody against the analyte onto each well of the plate. After washing, add the enzyme-labeled antibody which binds to the antibody against the analyte. Wash off the unbound enzyme-labeled antibody.
4) Add the substrate of the enzyme, incubate and then add a stopping solution if required. Measure the amount of the substrate converted by the enzyme reaction by measuring absorbance, luminescent intensity or fluorescent intensity.
5) Calculate the binding activity or the concentration of the analyte from the dose-response curve (calibration curve) of the reference material.

2.2. Data analysis

2.2.1. Quantitation

When ELISA is applied to determine the concentration of an analyte, use an appropriately diluted test sample and calculate the concentration of the analyte in the test sample from the calibration curve obtained from the reference material. Usually, the calibration curve is prepared by using an equation of such as 4-parameter logistic regression, setting the log concentrations of the target molecule on the x-axis and responses obtained on the y-axis.

4-parameter logistic model

$$y = D + \frac{A - D}{1 + \left(\frac{x}{C}\right)^B}$$

A: Lower asymptote
B: Slope parameter at EC_{50} (IC_{50})
C: EC_{50} (IC_{50})
D: Upper asymptote
x: Concentration of test sample
y: Response

When the calibration curve is not bilateral symmetric as a sigmoid curve, applying 5-parameter logistic regression may improve the analytical result. As for the noncompetitive method, a calibration curve may be obtained by linear regression by limiting the concentration at the lower range.

2.2.2. Biological activity

For evaluating biological activity, the methods such as 1) to 3) described below are used.

1) Use the test sample diluted with an appropriate dilution ratio. Determine the relative activity against the reference material by calculating the relative concentration based on the dose-response curve (the calibration curve) of the reference material.

2) Obtain the dose-response curves of the reference material and the test sample, respectively. Calculate the relative activity of the test sample against the reference material from the ratio of the concentration corresponding to 50% of the maximum response (EC_{50} for the noncompetitive method, and IC_{50} for the competitive method).

3) Use the range that can be approximated linear regression in the dose-response curve. Calculate the relative activity of the test sample against the reference material based on the ratio of the dose that arise the same response.

1) uses the same method as 2.2.1. and calculate the relative concentration against the reference material. 2) uses the same method as 2.2.1. to lead the regression equation on the reference material and the test sample. Better regression can be obtained by weighting to equalize the contribution of each concentration response in leading the regression equation. The methods of weighting are to use $1/y^2$, $1/y$ and $1/x$. Upon the establishment of the test method, choose a regression method to obtain a better result based on the accuracy and precision. 3) uses the concentration region near EC_{50} or IC_{50} that can be approximated as a straight line for analysis.

2.3. Reagents, test Solutions

2.3.1. Capture reagents

Use molecules (antigen, antibody, etc.) which can specifically bind to the analyte. Physical adsorption is frequently used for immobilizing a capture reagent on a plate, and covalent binding is also possible to use for its binding to the plate which is covered by materials having the binding activity with an amino or sulfhydryl functional group. Note that there is a case that binding activity with an analyte may be changed due to the conformational change by the binding onto the plate.

The capture reagent is a critical reagent that affects assay performance, and therefore, its quality should be controlled by setting necessary specifications. Establish the procedure for lot renewal as well.

2.3.2. Blocking reagents

A buffer solution containing protein such as albumin, gelatin, or casein, which is supplemented with surfactants such as polysorbate 20 as required, is used as a blocking reagent.

2.3.3. Detection reagents

As enzymes for detection, peroxidase, alkaline phosphatase, and *β*-galactosidase are typically used. As a labeling method for an enzyme, covalent binding with a target protein is used; A *N*-hydroxysuccinimide ester group introduced into an enzyme binds to the amino group of the labeled protein, and a maleimide group introduced into the enzyme binds to the sulfhydryl group of the labeled protein. As a method used for enzyme labeling of antibodies, covalent binding with which the maleimide group introduced into the enzyme is bound to the sulfhydryl group of the antibody is often used.

Detection Reagents are the critical reagents affecting assay performance, and therefore, their quality should be controlled by setting necessary specifications. Establish the procedures for lot renewal as well. As for the indirect detection method, unlabeled antibodies against an analyte are also used as a detection reagent, and therefore, it is necessary to control by setting necessary specifications.

2.3.4. Substrates

Use substrates which are appropriate for each enzyme. There are chromogenic, chemiluminescent and fluorescent substrates. Chemiluminescent substrates or fluorescent substrates are suitable when high sensitivity is required.

2.4. Points to consider

Since types of plates, amount of immobilized capture molecule, and incubation time as well as incubation temperature may affect test results, determine these procedures including materials and reagents of use. Also determine the test conditions and the sample placement in plates to prevent that the sample placement on the plates (the position of the well where the test is performed) affects the test results.

3. Application on specifications

3.1. Identification

In monographs of biotechnological/biological products, ELISA is used as an identification test which uses specific antibodies against the target product to evaluate the binding with the antibodies. As to therapeutic antibodies ELISA is also used as an identification test which evaluates the binding of the antibodies with antigen. Usually it is used as a qualitative test. In the meantime, acceptance criteria can also be set regarding the binding activity compared with a reference material when used as an identification test which evaluates the binding of therapeutic antibodies with antigen.

3.2. Purity test

ELISA is used mainly as a purity test for process-related impurities such as host cell proteins, impurities derived from culture media and ligands eluted from affinity column resin. When ELISA is used as a test to determine the amount of impurities, calculate the concentrations in a test sample by using calibration curves. When it is used as a limit test, confirm the test sample response is not higher than that of the control containing the impurities equal to the upper limits of the acceptance criteria.

In general, samples include much more amount of a target product than impurities, and therefore, the target product may disturb the detection of the impurities. Especially when ligands of affinity column are analytes, pay attention to the disturbance by the target product as the target product binds to the ligands. Consider a recovery rate when sample pretreatment is performed.

Table 1 Examples of substrates

Enzyme	Chromogenic substrate	Chemiluminescent substrates	Fluorescent substrates
peroxidase	TMB OPD ABTS	Luminol	
alkaline phosphatase	pNPP		
β-galactosidase			MG NG

TMB: 3,3′,5,5′-Tetramethylbenzidine
OPD: *o*-Phenylenediamine
ABTS: 2,2′-Azino-bis[3-ethylbenzothiazoline-6-sulfonate]
pNPP: *p*-Nitrophenyl phosphate
MG: 4-Methylumbelliferyl galactoside
NG: Nitrophenyl galactoside

3.3. Biological assay

ELISA is used as a test to determine the binding activity of a therapeutic antibody as the target product with its target molecule, and used to quantitate bioactive proteins secreted from the cells treated with test samples containing the target product in cell-based assay.

Determine relative activity by the method indicated in 2.2.2. 1) to 3).

3.4. Assay

ELISA is used for measuring the amount of target products. Obtain the calibration curve of reference materials and calculate the concentration of the target products.

4. Validity of test

In general, the validity of the test can be set as follows; use those in combination as necessary.

4.1. Identification

Confirm the results of reference materials and a negative control pass the acceptance criteria specified in the monograph.

4.2. Purity test

As for a quantitative test, confirm the reliability of calibration curves. Accuracy and/or precision of each concentration of material solutions for the calibration curve and the coefficient of determination (R^2 Value) calculated from a regression equation are used to confirm the reliability. Precision of test samples or accuracy of control samples prepared from the known concentration of a reference material (Quality Control Sample: QC sample) could be set as the test suitability. As for a limit test, confirm the response of the control sample containing the analyte at a concentration equal to the upper limit of the acceptance criteria satisfies the criterion specified in the monograph.

4.3. Biological assay

When determining biological activity by using the method of 1) of 2.2.2., confirm the reliability of the dose-response curve (the calibration curve) of the reference material . To confirm the reliability of the dose-response curve, accuracy and/or precision of each concentration of the reference material and R^2 value calculated from the regression equation or each parameter value of the regression equation obtained from the dose-response curve of the reference material can be used. Magnitude of the response of test samples, precision of the relative activity calculated from the response or accuracy of the concentration of QC samples can also be used to confirm the validity of the test.

When determining biological activity by using the method of 2) of 2.2.2., confirm the parallelism of the two regression curves obtained from a reference material and a test sample. As for the parallelism confirmation, following methods are the examples. Obtain the ratio of the difference between the upper asymptote and the lower asymptote ($D - A$ of the 4-parameter regression equation in 2.2.1.) of the test sample to that of the reference material or the ratio of the slope parameter (B of the 4-parameter regression equation in 2.2.1.), then confirm that those ratios are within the predetermined range. R^2 value of the dose-response curves of the reference material and the test sample, and accuracy of the QC samples are also used to confirm the validity of the test.

When determining biological activity by using the method of 3) of 2.2.2., confirm the linearity of the dose-response lines of a reference material and a test sample as well as the parallelism of these lines.

As for 2) and 3) of 2.2.2., there is a method to confirm the parallelism by comparing the residual variances of two regression curves, using the constrained model for control and sample data and using unconstrained models for the control and sample data, and determining the parallelism of the two regression curves by the method of analysis of variance. However, it should be noted that if the precision of the data is low, then the determination can be unrigorous.

4.4. Assay

Confirm the reliability of calibration curves obtained from the dose-response curves of reference materials. To confirm the reliability of the calibration curve, accuracy and/or precision of each concentration of the reference material calculated from the regression equation, each parameter value of the regression equation and R^2 value can be used. Precision of the measured results of test samples or accuracy of QC samples is also used to confirm the validity of the test.

Total Protein Assay <*G3-12-172*>

The following procedures are provided as illustrations of the determination of total protein content in pharmacopoeial preparations. Other techniques, such as HPLC, are also acceptable if total protein recovery is demonstrated. Many of the total protein assay methods described below can be performed successfully using kits from commercial sources.

Note: Where water is required, use distilled water.

Method 1 (UV method)

Protein in solution absorbs UV light at a wavelength of 280 nm, due to the presence of aromatic amino acids, mainly tyrosine and tryptophan. This property is the basis of this method. Protein determination at 280 nm is mainly a function of the tyrosine and tryptophan content of the protein. If the buffer used to dissolve the protein has a high absorbance relative to that of water, there is an interfering substance in the buffer. This interference can be compensated for when the spectrophotometer is adjusted to zero buffer absorbance. If the interference results in a large absorbance that challenges the limit of sensitivity of the spectrophotometer, the results may be compromised. Furthermore, at low concentrations protein can be absorbed onto the cuvette, thereby reducing the content in solution. This can be prevented by preparing samples at higher concentrations or by using a nonionic detergent in the preparation.

Note: Keep the Test Solution, the Standard Solution, and the buffer at the same temperature during testing.

Standard Solution Unless otherwise specified in the individual monograph, prepare a solution of the reference standard or reference material for the protein under test in the same buffer and at the same concentration as the Test Solution.

Test Solution Dissolve a suitable quantity of the protein under test in the appropriate buffer to obtain a solution having a concentration of 0.2 to 2 mg per mL.

Procedure Concomitantly determine the absorbances of the Standard Solution and the Test Solution in quartz cells at a wavelength of 280 nm, with a suitable spectrophotometer, using the buffer as the blank. To obtain accurate results, the response should be linear in the range of protein concentrations to be assayed.

Light-Scattering The accuracy of the UV spectroscopic determination of protein can be decreased by the scattering of light by the test specimen. If the proteins in solution exist as particles comparable in size to the wavelength of the measuring light (250 to 300 nm), scattering of the light beam results in an apparent increase in absorbance of the test specimen. To calculate the absorbance at 280 nm due to light-scattering, determine the absorbances of the Test Solution at wavelengths of 320, 325, 330, 335, 340, 345, and 350 nm. Using the linear regression method, plot the log of the observed absorbance versus the log of the wavelength, and determine the standard curve best fitting the plotted points. From the graph so obtained, extrapolate the absorbance value due to light-scattering at 280 nm. Subtract the absorbance from light-scattering from the total absorbance at 280 nm to obtain the absorbance value of the protein in solution. Filtration with a filter having a 0.2-μm porosity or clarification by centrifugation may be performed to reduce the effect of light-scattering, especially if the solution is noticeably turbid.

Calculations Calculate the concentration, C_U, of protein in the test specimen by the formula:

$$C_U = C_S (A_U/A_S),$$

in which C_S is the concentration of the Standard Solution; and A_U and A_S are the corrected absorbances of the Test Solution and the Standard Solution, respectively.

Method 2 (Lowry method)

This method, commonly referred to as the Lowry assay, is based on the reduction by protein of the phosphomolybdic-tungstic mixed acid chromogen in the Folin-Ciocalteu's phenol reagent, resulting in an absorbance maximum at 750 nm. The Folin-Ciocalteu's phenol reagent (Folin's TS) reacts primarily with tyrosine residues in the protein, which can lead to variation in the response of the assay to different proteins. Because the method is sensitive to interfering substances, a procedure for precipitation of the protein from the test specimen may be used. Where separation of interfering substances from the protein in the test specimen is necessary, proceed as directed below for Interfering Substances prior to preparation of the Test Solution. The effect of interfering substances can be minimized by dilution provided the concentration of the protein under test remains sufficient for accurate measurement. Variations of the Lowry test that are indicated in national regulatory documents[1)] can be substituted for the method described below.

Standard Solutions Unless otherwise specified in the individual monograph, dissolve the reference standard or reference material for the protein under test in the buffer used to prepare the Test Solution. Dilute portions of this solution with the same buffer to obtain not fewer than five Standard Solutions having concentrations between 5 μg and 100 μg of protein per mL, the concentrations being evenly spaced.

Test Solution Dissolve a suitable quantity of the protein under test in the appropriate buffer to obtain a solution having a concentration within the range of the concentrations of the Standard Solutions. An appropriate buffer will produce a pH in the range of 10 to 10.5.

Blank Use the buffer used for the Test Solution and the Standard Solutions.

Reagents and Solutions—

Copper Sulfate Reagent Dissolve 100 mg of copper (II) sulfate pentahydrate and 200 mg of sodium tartrate dihydrate in water, dilute with water to 50 mL, and mix. Dissolve 10 g of anhydrous sodium carbonate in water to a final volume of 50 mL, and mix. Slowly pour the sodium carbonate solution into the copper sulfate solution with mixing. Prepare this solution fresh daily.

5% SDS TS Dissolve 5 g of sodium dodecyl sulfate in water, and dilute with water to 100 mL.

Alkaline Copper Reagent Prepare a mixture of 5% SDS TS, Copper Sulfate Reagent, and Sodium Hydroxide Solution (4 in 125) (2:1:1). This reagent may be stored at room temperature for up to 2 weeks.

Diluted Folin's TS Mix 10 mL of Folin's TS with 50 mL of water. Store in an amber bottle, at room temperature.

Procedure To 1 mL of each Standard Solution, the Test Solution, and the Blank, add 1 mL of Alkaline Copper Reagent, and mix. Allow to stand at room temperature for 10 minutes. Add 0.5 mL of the Diluted Folin's TS to each solution, and mix each tube immediately after the addition, and allow to stand at room temperature for 30 minutes. Determine the absorbances of the solutions from the Standard Solutions and the Test Solution at the wavelength of maximum absorbance at 750 nm, with a suitable spectrophotometer, using the solution from the Blank to set the instrument to zero.

Calculations [Note: The relationship of absorbance to protein concentration is nonlinear; however, if the standard curve concentration range is sufficiently small, it will approach linearity.] Using the linear regression method, plot the absorbances of the solutions from the Standard Solutions versus the protein concentrations, and determine the standard curve best fitting the plotted points. From the standard curve so obtained and the absorbance of the Test Solution, determine the concentration of protein in the Test Solution.

Interfering Substances In the following procedure, deoxycholate-trichloroacetic acid is added to a test specimen to remove interfering substances by precipitation of proteins before testing. This technique also can be used to concentrate proteins from a dilute solution.

Sodium Deoxycholate Reagent Prepare a solution of sodium deoxycholate in water having a concentration of 150 mg in 100 mL.

Trichloroacetic Acid Reagent Prepare a solution of trichloroacetic acid in water having a concentration of 72 g in 100 mL.

Procedure Add 0.1 mL of Sodium Deoxycholate Reagent to 1 mL of a solution of the protein under test. Mix on a vortex mixer, and allow to stand at room temperature for 10 minutes. Add 0.1 mL of Trichloroacetic Acid Reagent, and mix on a vortex mixer. Centrifuge at 3000 × g for 30 minutes, decant the liquid, and remove any residual liquid with a pipet. Redissolve the protein pellet in 1 mL of Alkaline Copper Reagent. Proceed as directed for the Test Solution. [Note: Color development reaches a maximum in 20 to 30 minutes during incubation at room temperature, after which there is a gradual loss of color. Most interfering substances cause a lower color yield; however, some detergents cause a slight increase in color. A high salt concentration may cause a precipitate to form. Because different protein species may give different color response intensities, the standard protein and test protein should be the same.]

Method 3 (Bradford method)

This method, commonly referred to as the Bradford assay, is based on the absorption shift from 470 nm to 595 nm observed when Coomassie brilliant blue G-250 binds to protein. Coomassie brilliant blue G-250 binds most readily to arginyl and lysyl residues in the protein, which can lead to variation in the response of the assay to different proteins.

Standard Solutions Unless otherwise specified in the individual monograph, dissolve the reference standard or the reference material for the protein under test in the buffer used to prepare the Test Solution. Dilute portions of this solution with the same buffer to obtain not fewer than five Standard Solutions having concentrations between 100 μg and 1 mg of protein per mL, the concentrations being evenly spaced.

Test Solution Dissolve a suitable quantity of the protein under test in the appropriate buffer to obtain a solution having a concentration within the range of the concentrations of the Standard Solutions.

Blank Use the buffer used to prepare the Test Solution and the Standard Solutions.

Coomassie Reagent Dissolve 100 mg of Coomassie brilliant blue G-250[2)] in 50 mL of ethanol (95). [Note: Not all dyes have the same brilliant blue G content, and different products may give different results.] Add 100 mL of phosphoric acid, dilute with water to 1000 mL, and mix. Filter the solution through filter paper (Whatman No.1 or equivalent), and store the filtered reagent in an amber bottle at room temperature. [Note: Slow precipitation of the dye will occur during storage of the reagent. Filter the reagent before use.]

Procedure Add 5 mL of the Coomassie Reagent to 100 μL of each Standard Solution, the Test Solution, and the Blank, and mix by inversion. Avoid foaming, which will lead to poor reproducibility. Determine the absorbances of the solutions from the Standard Solutions and the Test Solution at 595 nm, with a suitable spectrophotometer, using the Blank to set the instrument to zero.

[Note: Do not use quartz (silica) spectrophotometer cells: the dye binds to this material. Because different protein species may give different color response intensities, the standard protein and test protein should be the same.] There are relatively few interfering substances, but detergents and ampholytes in the test specimen should be avoided. Highly alkaline specimens may interfere with the acidic reagent.

Calculations [Note: The relationship of absorbance to protein concentration is nonlinear; however, if the standard curve concentration range is sufficiently small, it will approach linearity.] Using the linear regression method, plot the absorbances of the solutions from the Standard Solutions versus the protein concentrations, and determine the standard curve best fitting the plotted points. From the standard curve so obtained and the absorbance of the Test Solution, determine the concentration of protein in the Test Solution.

Method 4 (Bicinchoninic acid method)

This method, commonly referred to as the bicinchoninic acid or BCA assay, is based on reduction of the cupric (Cu^{2+}) ion to cuprous (Cu^{+}) ion by protein. The bicinchoninic acid reagent is used to detect the cuprous ion. The method has few interfering substances. When interfering substances are present, their effect may be minimized by dilution, provided that the concentration of the protein under test remains sufficient for accurate measurement.

Standard Solutions Unless otherwise specified in the individual monograph, dissolve the reference standard or the reference material for the protein under test in the buffer used to prepare the Test Solution. Dilute portions of this solution with the same buffer to obtain not fewer than five Standard Solutions having concentrations between 10 μg and 1200 μg of protein per mL, the concentrations being evenly spaced.

Test Solution Dissolve a suitable quantity of the protein under test in the appropriate buffer to obtain a solution having a concentration within the range of the concentrations of the Standard Solutions.

Blank Use the buffer used to prepare the Test Solution and the Standard Solutions.

Reagents and Solutions—

BCA Reagent Dissolve about 10 g of bicinchoninic acid, 20 g of sodium carbonate monohydrate, 1.6 g of sodium tartrate dihydrate, 4 g of sodium hydroxide, and 9.5 g of sodium hydrogen carbonate in water. Adjust, if necessary, with sodium hydroxide or sodium hydrogen carbonate to a pH of 11.25. Dilute with water to 1000 mL, and mix.

Copper Sulfate Reagent Dissolve about 2 g of copper (II) sulfate pentahydrate in water to a final volume of 50 mL.

Copper-BCA Reagent Mix 1 mL of Copper Sulfate Reagent and 50 mL of BCA Reagent.

Procedure Mix 0.1 mL of each Standard Solution, the Test Solution, and the Blank with 2 mL of the Copper-BCA Reagent. Incubate the solutions at 37°C for 30 minutes, note the time, and allow to come to room temperature. Within 60 minutes following the incubation time, determine the absorbances of the solutions from the Standard Solutions and the Test Solution in quartz cells at 562 nm, with a suitable spectrophotometer, using the Blank to set the instrument to zero. After the solutions are cooled to room temperature, the color intensity continues to increase gradually. If substances that will cause interference in the test are present, proceed as directed for Interfering Substances under Method 2. Because different protein species may give different color response intensities, the standard protein and test protein should be the same.

Calculations [Note: The relationship of absorbance to protein concentration is nonlinear; however, if the standard curve concentration range is sufficiently small, it will approach linearity.] Using the linear regression method, plot the absorbances of the solutions from the Standard Solutions versus the protein concentrations, and determine the standard curve best fitting the plotted points. From the standard curve so obtained and the absorbance of the Test Solution, determine the concentration of protein in the Test Solution.

Method 5 (Biuret method)

This method, commonly referred to as the Biuret assay, is based on the interaction of cupric (Cu^{2+}) ion with protein in an alkaline solution and the resultant development of absorbance at 545 nm.

Standard Solutions Unless otherwise specified in the individual monograph, prepare a solution of Albumin Human for which the protein content has been previously determined by nitrogen analysis (using the nitrogen-to-protein conversion factor of 6.25) or of the reference standard or reference material for the protein under test in sodium chloride solution (9 in 1000). Dilute portions of this solution with sodium chloride solution (9 in 1000) to obtain not fewer than three Standard Solutions having concentrations between 0.5 mg and 10 mg per mL, the concentrations being evenly spaced. [Note: Low responses may be observed if the sample under test has significantly different level of proline than that of Albumin Human. A different standard protein may be employed in such cases.]

Test Solution Prepare a solution of the test protein in sodium chloride solution (9 in 1000) having a concentration within the range of the concentrations of the Standard Solutions.

Blank Use sodium chloride solution (9 in 1000).

Biuret Reagent Dissolve about 3.46 g of copper (II) sulfate pentahydrate in 10 mL of water, with heating if necessary, and allow to cool (Solution A). Dissolve about 34.6 g of sodium citrate dihydrate and 20.0 g of anhydrous sodium carbonate in 80 mL of water, with heating if necessary, and allow to cool (Solution B). Mix Solutions A and B, and dilute with water to 200 mL. This Biuret Reagent is stable at room temperature for 6 months. Do not use the reagent if it develops turbidity or contains any precipitate.

Procedure To one volume of the Standard Solutions and a solution of the Test Solution add an equal volume of sodium hydroxide solution (6 in 100), and mix. Immediately add a volume of Biuret Reagent equivalent to 0.4 volume of the Test Solution, and mix. Allow to stand at a temperature between 15°C and 25°C for not less than 15 minutes. Within 90 minutes after the addition of the Biuret Reagent, determine the absorbances of the Standard Solutions and the solution from the Test Solution at the wavelength of maximum absorbance at 545 nm, with a suitable spectrophotometer, using the Blank to set the instrument to zero. [Note: Any solution that develops turbidity or a precipitate is not acceptable for calculation of protein concentration.]

Calculations Using the least-squares linear regression method, plot the absorbances of the Standard Solutions versus the protein concentrations, and determine the standard curve best fitting the plotted points, and calculate the correlation coefficient for the line. [Note: Within the given range of the standards, the relationship of absorbance to protein concentration is approximately linear.] A suitable system is one that yields a line having a correlation coefficient of not less than 0.99. From the standard curve and the absorbance of the Test Solution, determine the concentration of protein in the test specimen, making any necessary correction.

Interfering Substances To minimize the effect of interfering substances, the protein can be precipitated from the initial test specimen as follows. Add 0.1 volume of 50% trichloroacetic acid to 1 volume of a solution of the test specimen, withdraw the supernatant layer, and dissolve the precipitate in a small volume of 0.5 mol/L sodium hydroxide TS. Use the solution so obtained to prepare the Test Solution.

Comments This test shows minimal difference between equivalent IgG and albumin samples. Addition of the sodium hydroxide and the Biuret Reagent as a combined reagent, insufficient mixing after the addition of the sodium hydroxide, or an extended time between the addition of the sodium hydroxide solution and the addition of the Biuret Reagent will give IgG samples a higher response than albumin samples. The trichloroacetic acid method used to minimize the effects of interfering substances also can be used to determine the protein content in test specimens at concentrations below 500 μg per mL.

Method 6 (Fluorometric method)

This fluorometric method is based on the derivatization of the protein with *o*-phthalaldehyde (OPA), which reacts with the primary amines of the protein (i.e., NH_2-terminal amino acid and the ε-amino group of the lysine residues). The sensitivity of the test can be increased by hydrolyzing the protein before testing. Hydrolysis makes the α-amino group of the constituent amino acids of the protein available for reaction with the OPA reagent. The method requires very small quantities of the protein.

Primary amines, such as tris(hydroxymethyl)aminomethane and amino acid buffers, react with OPA and must be avoided or removed. Ammonia at high concentrations will react with OPA as well. The fluorescence obtained when amine reacts with OPA can be unstable. The use of automated procedures to standardize this procedure may improve the accuracy and precision of the test.

Standard Solutions Unless otherwise specified in the individual monograph, dissolve the reference standard or the reference material for the protein under test in the buffer used to prepare the Test Solution. Dilute portions of this solution with the same buffer to obtain not fewer than five Standard Solutions having concentrations between 10 and 200 μg of protein per mL, the concentrations being evenly spaced.

Test Solution Dissolve a suitable quantity of the protein under test in the appropriate buffer to obtain a solution having a concentration within the range of the concentrations of the Standard Solutions.

Blank Use the buffer used to prepare the Test Solution and the Standard Solutions.

Reagents and Solutions—

Borate Buffer Dissolve about 61.83 g of boric acid in water, and adjust with potassium hydroxide to a pH of 10.4. Dilute with water to 1000 mL, and mix.

Stock OPA Reagent Dissolve about 120 mg of *o*-phthalaldehyde in 1.5 mL of methanol, add 100 mL of Borate Buffer, and mix. Add 0.6 mL of polyoxyethylene (23) lauryl ether, and mix. This solution is stable at room temperature for at least 3 weeks.

OPA Reagent To 5 mL of Stock OPA Reagent add 15 μL of 2-mercaptoethanol. Prepare at least 30 minutes prior to use. This reagent is stable for one day.

Procedure Adjust each of the Standard Solutions and the Test Solution to a pH between 8.0 and 10.5. Mix 10 μL of the Test Solution and each of the Standard Solutions with 100 μL of OPA Reagent, and allow to stand at room temperature for 15 minutes. Add 3 mL of 0.5 mol/L sodium hydroxide TS, and mix. Using a suitable fluorometer, determine the fluorescent intensities of solutions from the Standard Solutions and the Test Solution at an excitation wavelength of 340 nm and an emission wavelength between 440 nm and 455 nm. [Note: The fluorescence of an individual specimen is read only once because irradiation decreases the fluorescent intensity.]

Calculations The relationship of fluorescence to protein concentration is linear. Using the linear regression method, plot the fluorescent intensities of the solutions from the Standard Solutions versus the protein concentrations, and determine the standard curve best fitting the plotted points. From the standard curve so obtained and the fluorescent intensity of the Test Solution, determine the concentration of protein in the test specimen.

Method 7 (Nitrogen method)

This method is based on nitrogen analysis as a means of protein determination. Interference caused by the presence of other nitrogen-containing substances in the test protein can affect the determination of protein by this method. Nitrogen analysis techniques destroy the protein under test but are not limited to protein presentation in an aqueous environment.

Procedure A Determine the nitrogen content of the protein under test as directed elsewhere in the Pharmacopoeia. Commercial instrumentation is available for the Kjeldahl nitrogen assay.

Procedure B Commercial instrumentation is available for nitrogen analysis. Most nitrogen analysis instruments use pyrolysis (i.e., combustion of the sample in oxygen at temperatures approaching 1000°C), which produces nitric oxide (NO) and other oxides of nitrogen (NO_x) from the nitrogen present in the test protein. Some instruments convert the nitric oxides to nitrogen gas, which is quantified with a thermal conductivity detector. Other instruments mix nitric oxide (NO) with ozone (O_3) to produce excited nitrogen dioxide (NO_2) which emits light when it decays and can be quantified with a chemiluminescence detector. A protein reference standard or reference material that is relatively pure and is similar in composition to the test proteins is used to optimize the injection and pyrolysis parameters and to evaluate consistency in the analysis.

Calculations The protein concentration is calculated by dividing the nitrogen content of the sample by the known nitrogen content of the protein. The known nitrogen content of the protein can be determined from the chemical composition of the protein or by comparison with the nitrogen content of the appropriate reference standard or reference material.

◆1) Example: Minimum Requirements for Biological Products and individual monograph in JP.◆
2) Purity of the reagent is important.

Basic Requirements for Viral Safety of Biotechnological/Biological Products listed in Japanese Pharmacopoeia <*G3-13-141*>

Introduction

The primary role of specification of biotechnological/biological products listed in the Japanese Pharmacopoeia (JP) is not only for securing quality control or consistency of the quality but also for assuring their efficacy and safety. In the meantime, the requirements to assure quality and safety of drugs have come to be quite strict recently, and a rigid attitude addressing safety assurance is expected for biotechnological/biological products. The key points for quality and safety assurance of biotechnological/biological products are selection and appropriate evaluation of source material, appropriate evaluation of manufacturing process and maintenance of manufacturing consistency, and control of specific physical properties of the products. Now, how to assure quality and safety of such drugs within a scope of the JP has come to be questioned. This General Information describes what sorts of approaches are available to overcome these issues.

It is desired that quality and safety assurance of JP listed products are achieved by state-of-the-art methods and concepts which reflect progress of science and accumulation of experiences. This General Information challenges to show the highest level of current scientific speculation. It is expected that this information will contribute to promotion of scientific understanding of quality and safety assurance of not only JP listed products but also the other biotechnological/biological products and to promotion of active discussion of each Official Monograph in JP.

1. Fundamental measures to ensure viral safety of JP listed biotechnological/biological products

JP listed biotechnological/biological products includes the products derived from living tissue and body fluid (urine, blood, etc.) of mammals, etc. Protein drugs derived from cell lines of human or animal origin (e.g., recombinant DNA drug, cell culture drug) are also included. The fundamental measures required for comprehensive viral safety of JP listed biotechnological/biological products are as follows: 1) acquaintance of possible virus contamination (source of contamination); 2) careful examination of eligibility of raw materials and their sources, e.g. human/animal, and thorough analysis and screening of the sample chosen as a substrate for drug production (e.g., pooled body fluid, cell bank, etc.) to determine any virus contamination and determination of type and nature of the virus, if contaminated; 3) evaluation to determine virus titer and virus-like particles hazardous to human, if exists; 4) selection of production related material (e.g., reagent, immune antibody column) free from infectious or pathogenic virus; 5) performance of virus free test at an appropriate stage of manufacturing including the final product, if necessary; 6) adoption of effective viral clearance method in the manufacturing process to remove/inactivate virus. A combined method sometimes achieves higher level of clearance; 7) development of a deliberate viral clearance scheme; 8) performance of the test to evaluate viral removal and inactivation. It is considered that the stepwise and supplemental adoption of the said measures will contribute to ensure viral safety and its improvement.

2. Safety assurance measures described in the Official Monograph and this General Information

As mentioned in above 1, this General Information describes, in package, points to be concerned with and concrete information on the measures taken for viral safety of JP listed products. Except where any specific caution is provided in Official Monograph of a product in question, Official Monograph provides in general that "Any raw material, substrate for drug production and production related materials used for production of drug should be derived from healthy animals and should be shown to be free of latent virus which is infectious or pathogenic to human", "Cell line and culture method well evaluated in aspects of appropriateness and rationality on viral safety are used for production, and the presence of infectious or pathogenic latent virus to human in process related materials derived from living organisms should be denied", and "biotechnological/biological drug should be produced through a manufacturing process which is capable of removing infectious or pathogenic virus", etc., to raise awareness on viral safety and on necessity to conduct test and process evaluation for viral safety.

3. Items and contents described in this General Information

As for viral safety of protein drug derived from cell line of human or animal origin, there is a Notice in Japan entitled "Viral safety evaluation of biotechnology products derived from cell lines of human or animal origin" (Iyakushin No. 329 issued on February 22, 2000 by Director, Evaluation and Licensing Division, Pharmaceutical and Medical Safety Bureau, Ministry of Health and Welfare) to reflect the internationally harmonized ICH Guideline, and as for blood plasma protein fraction preparations, there is a document entitled "Guideline for ensuring viral safety of blood plasma protein fraction preparations". This General Information for ensuring viral safety of JP listed biotechnological/biological products has been written, referencing the contents of those guidelines, to cover general points and their details to be concerned for ensuring viral safety of not only JP listed biotechnological/biological products but also all products which would be listed in the JP in future, i.e., biological products derived from living tissue and body fluid, such as urine, and protein drugs derived from cell lines of human or animal origin (Table 1).

3.1. Purpose

The purpose of this document is to propose the comprehensive concepts of the measures to be taken for ensuring viral safety of biotechnological/biological products derived from living tissue or body fluid of mammals, etc. and of protein drugs derived from cell lines of human or animal origin. That is to say, this document describes the measures and the points of concern on the items, such as ① consideration of the source of virus contamination; ② appropriate evaluation on eligibility at selecting the raw material and on qualification of its source, e.g. human or animal; ③ virus test, and its analysis and evaluation at a stage of cell substrate for drug production; ④ appropriate evaluation to choose product related materials derived from living organisms (e.g. reagent, immune antibody column, etc.); ⑤ conduct of necessary virus test on the product at an appropriate stage of manufacturing; ⑥ development of viral clearance test scheme; ⑦ performance and evaluation of viral clearance test. This document is also purposed to comprehensively describe in details that supplemental and combining adoption of the said measures will contribute to secure viral safety and its improvement.

3.2. Background

One of the most important issues to be cautioned for safety of a biological product, which is directly derived from human or animal, or of a protein drug, which is derived from cell line of human or animal origin (recombinant DNA derived product, cell culture derived product, etc.), is a risk of virus contamination. Virus contamination may cause serious situation at clinical use once it occurs. Virus contamination may be from a raw material or from a cell substrate for drug production, or may be from an adventitious factor introduced to the manufacturing process.

JP listed biological drugs or protein drugs derived from cell line have achieved drastic contribution to the medical society, and to date, there has not been any evidence of any safety problem on them caused by virus. But, social requirement of health hazard prevention is strong, and it is now very important to prevent accidental incidence, taking security measures carefully supported by scientific rationality. It is always great concern among the persons involved that under what sort of viewpoint and to what extent we have to pursue for ensuring viral safety of a biotechnological/biological product.

Before discussing these issues, two fundamental points have to be reconfirmed. One is that; we have to consider scientific, medical, and social profiles a drug has. In other words, ''Medicine is a social asset which is utilized in medical practice paying attention to the risk and benefit from the standpoints of science and society''. It is the destination and the mission of the medical/pharmaceutical society to realize prompt and stable supply of such a social asset, drug, among the medical work front to bring gospel to the patients.

The other is that; issue of viral safety is independent from safety of the components of a drug per se (narrow sense of safety). It is important to consider that this is the matter of general safety of a drug (broad sense of safety). In case of a drug which has been used for a long time in the medical front, such as a JP listed product, its broad sense of safety is considered to have been established epidemiologically, and its usage past records have a great meaning. However, different from safety of drug per se (its components), taking into account any possibility of virus contamination, we have to say that only the results accumulated can not always assure viral safety of a drug used in future. Accordingly, the basis for securing broad sense of viral safety of JP listed biotechnological/biological products is to pay every attention to the measures to take for prevention, while evaluating the accumulated results.

Adopting strict regulations and conducting tests at maximum level to the extent theoretically considered may be the ways off assuring safety, but applying such way generally, without sufficient scientific review of the ways and evaluation of usage results, causes the excessive requirement of regulations and tests not having scientific rationality. As the results, effective and prompt supply of an important drug, already having enough accumulation of experiences, to the medical work front will be hampered, and the drug, a social asset, may not to be utilized effectively. Medicine is a sword used in medical field having double-edge named effectiveness and safety. Effectiveness and safety factors have to be derived as the fruits of leading edge of science, and relatively evaluated on a balance sheet of usefulness. Usefulness evaluation should not be unbalanced in a way that too much emphasis is placed on safety concern without back-up of appropriate scientific rationality. A drug can play an important role as a social asset only when well balanced appropriate scientific usefulness evaluation in addition to social concern of the age are given. In other words, a drug is a common asset utilized by society for medication as a fruit of science of the age, and the key point of its utilization lies on a balance of risk and benefit produced from scientific and social evalu-

Table 1 Items described in General Information for viral safety assurance of JP listed biotechnological/biological products

I. Introduction
1. Fundamental measures to ensure viral safety of JP listed biotechnological/biological products
2. Safety assurance measures described in the Official Monograph and this General Information
3. Items and contents described in this General Information

II. General Matters
1. Purpose
2. Background
3. Unknown risk on the measures taken for ensuring viral safety
4. Applicable range
5. Possible viral contamination to a JP listed biotechnological/biological product (source of virus contamination)
6. Basis for ensuring viral safety
7. Limit of virus test
8. Roles of viral clearance studies

III. Raw material/substrate for drug production
1. Issues relating to animal species and its region as a source of raw material substrate for drug production and countermeasures to be taken thereto
2. Qualification evaluation test on human or animal as a source of raw material/substrate for drug production

IV. Points of concern with respect to manufacturing and virus testing
1. Virus test conducted in advance of purification process
2. Virus test as an acceptance test of an intermediate material, etc.
3. Virus test on a final product

V. Process evaluation on viral clearance
1. Rationale, objective and general items to be concerned with respect to viral clearance process evaluation
2. Selection of virus
3. Design of viral clearance studies
4. Interpretation of viral clearance studies
   1) Evaluation of viral clearance factor
   2) Calculation of viral clearance index
   3) Interpretation of results and items to be concerned at evaluation

VI. Statistics
1. Statistical considerations for assessing virus assays
2. Reproducibility and confidence limit of viral clearance studies

VII. Re-evaluation of viral clearance

VIII. Measurement for viral clearance studies
1. Measurement of virus infective titer
2. Testing by nucleic-acid amplification test (NAT)

IX. Reporting and preservation

X. Others

ation. So, those factors have to be taken into account when target and pursuance levels for ensuring viral safety of a JP listed biotechnological/biological product are reviewed.

And, in general, the risk and benefit of drugs should be considered with the relative comparison to alternative drugs or medical treatment. The usefulness of a certain drug should be reviewed finally after the competitive assessment on the risk and benefit on the alternative drugs, relevant drugs and/or alternative medical treatment.

Under such background, the purpose of this article is to describe the scientific and rational measures to be taken for ensuring viral safety of JP listed biotechnological/biological products. Giving scientific and rational measures mean that; appropriate and effective measures, elaborated from the current scientific level, are given to the issues assumable under the current scientific knowledge. In other words, a possible contaminant virus is assumed to have the natures of genus, morph, particle size, physical/chemical properties, etc. which are within the range of knowledge of existing virology, and is those assumed to exist in human and animal, tissue and body fluid, which are the source of biotechnological/biological products, reagent, material, additives, etc. Accordingly, viral clearance studies using a detection method which target those viruses have to be designed.

3.3. Unknown risk on the measures taken for ensuring viral safety

There are known and unknown risks.

It is easy to determine a test method and an evaluation standard on the known risk, which exists in the drug per se (pharmaceutical component) or inevitably exists due to a quality threshold, and quantification of such risk is possible. In other words, it is easy to evaluate the known risk on a balance sheet in relation to the benefit, and we can say that the valuation of JP listed products even in this respect has been established to some extent.

On the other hand, as for the unknown risk which is inevitable for ensuring viral safety, the subject of the risk can not be defined and quantitative concept is hard to introduce, and, therefore, taking a counter measure and evaluating its effect are not so easy. Therefore, this is the subject to be challenged calling upon wisdom of the related parties among the society of drugs.

Talking about the unknown risk, there are view points that say ''It is risky because it is unknown.'' and ''What are the unknowns, and how do we cope with them in ensuring safety?''.

The view of ''It is risky because it is unknown.'' is already nothing but a sort of evaluation result, and directly connects to a final decision if it can be used as a drug. Such evaluation/decision has to be made based upon a rational, scientific or social judgment.

For example, in the case that ''In a manufacturing process of a drug, virus, virus-like particle or retrovirus was detected, but its identification could not be confirmed, and, therefore, its risk can not be denied.'', the evaluation of ''It is risky because it is unknown.'' is scientifically rational and reasonable. On the other hand, however, if we reach a decision of ''It is risky because it is unknown.'' due to the reason that ''In a manufacturing process of a drug, virus, virus-like particle or retrovirus was not detected, but there is a 'concern' that something unknown may exist.'', it can not be said that such evaluation is based upon a rational, scientific or social judgment. It goes without saying that the utmost care has to be taken for viral safety, but the substance of 'concern' has to be at least clearly explainable. Otherwise, the 'concern' may result in causing contradiction in the meaningful mission to utilize a social asset, drug, in medical practice.

From a scientific view point, we should not be narrow minded by saying ''it is risky'' because ''there is a 'concern' that something unknown may exists'', but challenge to clarify the subject of ''What is unknown, and how to cope with it for ensuring safety'' using wisdom. What is important at the time is to define ''what is unknown'' based upon current scientific knowledge. Only through this way, is it possible for us to elaborate the measures for ensuring safety.

Once we chase up the substance of unknown risk for viral safety without premises of ''what is unknown'', ''unknown'' will be an endless question because it theoretically remains unresolved forever. If this kind of approach is taken, the issue and the measure can not be scientifically connected to each other, which will result in the excessive requirement of regulations and of tests to be conducted. Yet, it is unlikely that the measure which has no relation with science will be effective to the subject of ''What is unknown is unknown.''

For example, ''what is unknown'' at the ''evaluation of a purification process which can completely clear up every virus that contaminated in a manufacturing process'' should be the subject of ''what sort of existing virus that contaminated is unknown'', not on the subject of ''what sort of virus that exist in the world is unknown. In the former subject, the premise of the study is based on all the knowledge on viruses including DNA/RNA-virus, virus with/without envelope, particle size, physical/chemical properties, etc. The premise is that the virus contaminated should be within range of existing wisdom and knowledge of virus such as species, type, nature, etc., even though the virus that contaminated is unknown. Under such premise, when evaluation is made on a purification process to decide its capability of clearing a derived virus, which is within the range of existing wisdom and learning, specific viral clearance studies designed to combine a few model viruses with different natures, such as type of nucleic acid, with/without envelope, particle size, physical/chemical properties, etc., would be enough to simulate every sort of the virus already known, and will be a good measure for ''ensuring safety''.

The issue of ''the sort of viruses that exist in the world is unknown'' may be a future study item, but it is not an appropriate subject for the viral clearance test. Further, even if the subject of ''unknown viruses, which have a particle size smaller than that of currently known viruses, may exists'' or ''unknown viruses, which have special physical/chemical properties that can not be matched to any of the currently known viruses, may exists'' is set up as an armchair theory, any experimental work can not be pursued under the current scientific level, since such virus model is not available. Further, any viral clearance test performed by using the currently available methods and technologies will be meaningless ''for ensuring safety'', since particle size or natures of such speculated virus are unknown. Likewise, any counter measures can not be taken on the subject of ''unknown virus, which can not be detected by currently available screening method, may exist'', and conducting any virus detection test at any stage will be useless ''for ensuring safety''.

The requirement of regulations or tests excessively over scientific rationality will raise human, economical and temporal burden to the pharmaceutical companies, and will adversely affect prompt, effective and economical supply of a drug to the medical front. As a drug is a sort of social asset, which has to be scientifically evaluated, how to assure maximization of its safety by means of scientifically rational approach at minimum human, economical and time resources is important.

It is also important to reconfirm that achievement of those

issues is on the premise that appropriate measures are taken on the supply source of drugs. For example, in a case of ''In a manufacturing process of drug, virus, virus-like particle or retrovirus was not detected, but there is a 'concern' that something unknown may exist.'', appropriateness of the test, which resulted in the judgment that ''virus, virus-like particle or retrovirus was not detected in a process of drug production'', should be a prerequisite premise when judged by the science standard at the time. If there is any question on the premise, it is quite natural that the question of ''there is a 'concern' that unknown something may exist.'' will be effective.

3.4. Applicable range

This General Information is on JP listed biological products, derived from living tissue or body fluid, and protein drugs, derived from human or animal cell line, that in Japan. In the case of protein drugs derived from human or animal cell line, the products developed and approved after enforcement of the Notice Iyakushin No. 329 entitled ''Viral safety evaluation of biotechnology products derived from cell lines of human or animal origin'' should have been treated under the Notice, and it is inevitable that some products approved before the Notice might not have been sufficiently treated. It is expected that such biodrug will be sufficiently examined to meet such General Information before being listed in the JP. On the other hand, blood preparations listed in the biological products standard and covered by ''Guideline for securing safety of blood plasma protein fraction preparations against virus'', are out of the scope of this General Information. Further, in case of a relatively lower molecular biogenous substance, such as amino acid, saccharide and glycerin, and of gelatin, which is even classified as infectious or pathogenic polymer, there are cases that viral contamination can not be considered due to its manufacturing or purification process, and that potent viral inactivation /removal procedure that can not be applied to protein, can be used, and, therefore, it is considered reasonable to omit such substances from the subject for application. However, some part of this General Information may be used as reference. Further, a comprehensive assurance measure for viral safety is recommendable on a biotechnological/biological product not listed in the JP using this document as a reference so long as it is similar to JP listed biotechnological/biological products.

3.5. Possible viral contamination to a JP listed biotechnological/biological product (source of virus contamination)

Promoting awareness of virus contamination to a JP listed biotechnological/biological product (source of virus contamination) and citing countermeasures are important for eradicating any possible virus contamination and raising probability of safety assurance. Many biotechnological/biological products are produced from a ''substrate for drug production'' which is derived from human or animal tissue, body fluid, etc. as an origin/raw material, and in purification or pharmaceutical processing of such products column materials or additives, which are living organism origin, are occasionally used. Accordingly, enough safety measures should be taken against diffusion of the contaminant virus. Further, as mentioned in Notice Iyakushin No. 329, any protein drug derived from cell lines of human or animal origin should be carefully examined with respect to the risk of virus contamination through the cell line, the cell substrate for drug production, and through the manufacturing process applied thereafter.

''Substrate for drug production'' is defined as a starting material which is at a stage where it is deemed to be in a position to ensure quality/safety of a drug substance. The ''substrate for drug production'' is sometimes tissue, body fluid, etc. of human or animal per se and pooled material such as urine, and sometimes a material after some treatment. In many cases, it is considered rational that the starting point of a full-scale test, evaluation and control should be at the stage of ''substrate for drug production''. The more strict levels of test, evaluation and control achieved at the stage of ''substrate for drug production'' can more rationalize evaluation and control of the raw material or individual level of an upper stream. On the contrary, strict evaluation and control of the raw material or individual level at an upper stream stage can rationalize tests, evaluation or quality control at the stage of ''substrate for drug production''.

The measures taken for ensuring viral safety on a biotechnological/biological product currently listed in the JP can be assumed from the provisions of the manufacturing method, specification and test methods of each preparation. However, unitary principles or information with respect to the measures to be taken for ensuring viral safety, totally reviewing the entire process up to the final product rationally and comprehensively, including source/raw material/substrate, purification process, etc. have not been clarified. The most important thing for ensuring viral safety is to take thorough measures to eliminate the risk of virus contamination at any stage of source animal, raw material and substrate. Although not the cases of a biotechnological/biological product, known examples of a virus contamination from a raw material/substrate for drug production in old times are Hepatitis A Virus (HAV) or Hepatitis C Virus (HCV) contamination in blood protein fraction preparations. It is also well known that Human Immunodeficiency Virus (HIV) infection caused by blood plasma protein fraction preparations occurred in 1980s. The aim of this General Information is to show concrete guidelines for comprehensive viral safety assurance of JP listed biotechnological/biological products. The pathogenic infectious viruses, currently known to contaminate to raw materials, etc. of drug and have to be cautioned, are HIV, HAV, Hepatitis B Virus (HBV), HCV, Human T-Lymphotropic Virus (HTLV-I/II), Human Parvovirus B19, Cytomegalovirus (CMV), etc. Biotechnological/biological products produced from raw material/substrate for drug production derived from tissue or body fluid of human or animal origin always have a risk of contamination of pathogenic or other latent virus. Therefore, safety measures should be thoroughly taken. There is also the case that a material, other than the biological component such as raw material/substrate for drug production, causes virus contamination. Using an enzymatic or monoclonal antibody column or using albumin etc. as a stabilizer, is the example of the case, in which caution has to be taken on risk of virus contamination from the source animal or cell. Further, there is a possibility of contamination from environment or personnel in charge of production or at handling of the product. So, caution has to be taken on these respects as well.

In case of protein drugs derived from cell line of human or animal origin, there may be cases where latent or persistent infectious viruses (e.g., herpesvirus) or endogenous retroviruses exist in the cell. Further, adventitious viruses may be introduced through the routes such as: 1) derivation of a cell line from an infected animal; 2) use of a virus to drive a cell line; 3) use of a contaminated biological reagent (e.g., animal serum components); 4) contamination during cell handling. In the manufacturing process of drugs, an adventitious virus may contaminate the final product through the routes, such as 1) contamination through a reagent of living being origin, such as serum component, which is used for culturing, etc.; 2) use of a virus for introduction of a specific gene expression to code an objective protein; 3) contamination through a reagent used for purification such as monoclonal antibody affinity column; 4) contamination through an additive used for formulation production; 5) contamination at handling of cells and culture media, etc. It is reported that monitoring of cell culture parameters may be helpful for early detection of an adventitious viral contamination.

3.6. Basis for ensuring viral safety

Viral safety of a biotechnological/biological product produced from a raw material/substrate, which derived from tissue, body fluid, cell line, etc. of human or animal origin, can be achieved by supplemental and appropriate adoption of the following plural methods.

(1) Acquaintance of possible virus contamination (source of contamination).
(2) Careful examination of eligibility of the raw material and its source, i.e., human or animal, thorough analysis and screening of the sample chosen as the substrate for drug production to determine virus contamination and through examination of the type of virus and its nature, if contaminated.
(3) Evaluation to determine hazardous properties of the virus or virus-like particle to human, if exists.
(4) Choosing a product related material of living organism origin (e.g., reagent, immune anti-body column, etc.) which is free from an infectious or pathogenic virus.
(5) Conduct virus free test at an appropriate stage of manufacturing including the final product, if necessary.
(6) Adoption of an effective method to remove/inactivate the virus in the manufacturing process for viral clearance. Combined processes sometimes achieve higher level of viral clearance.
(7) Develop a deliberate viral clearance scheme.
(8) Conduct the test and evaluation to confirm removal/inactivation of the virus.

Manufacturers are responsible for explaining rationality of the way of approach adopted among the comprehensive strategy for viral safety on each product and its manufacturing process. At the time, the approach described in this General Information shall be applicable as far as possible.

3.7. Limit of virus test

A virus test has to be conducted to define existence of virus, but it should be noted that the virus test alone can not reach a conclusion of inexistence of virus nor sufficient to secure safety of the product. Examples of a virus not being detected are as follows: 1) Due to statistical reason, there is an inherent quantitative limit, such as detection sensitivity at lower concentration depending upon the sample size. 2) Generally, every virus test has a detection limit, and any negative result of a virus test can not completely deny existence of a virus. 3) A virus test applied is not always appropriate in terms of specificity or sensitivity for detection of a virus which exists in the tissue or body fluid of human or animal origin.

A virus testing method is improved as science and technology progress, and it is important to apply scientifically the most advanced technology at the time of testing so that it can be possible to raise the assurance level of virus detection. It should be noted, however, that the limit as mentioned above can not always be completely overcome. Further, risk of virus contamination in a manufacturing process can not be completely denied, and, therefore, it is necessary to elaborate the countermeasure taken these effects into account.

Reliable assurance of a viral free final product can not be obtained only by negative test results on the raw material/substrate for drug production or on the product in general, it is also necessary to demonstrate inactivation/removal capability of the purification process.

3.8. Roles of viral clearance studies

Under the premises as mentioned in the preceding clause that there is a limit of a virus test, that there is a possibility of existence of latent virus in a raw material/substrate for drug production of human or animal origin and that there is a risk of entry of a non-endogenous virus in a manufacturing process, one of the important measures for viral safety is how to remove or inactivate the virus, which exists in a raw material, etc. and can not be detected, or the virus, which is contingently contaminated in a manufacturing process. The purpose of a viral clearance study is to experimentally evaluate the viral removal/inactivation capability of a step that mounted in a manufacturing process. So, it is necessary to conduct an experimental scale spike test using an appropriate virus that is selected by taking account the properties, such as particle size, shape, with or without envelope, type of nucleic acid (DNA type, RNA type), heat and chemical treatment tolerance, etc., with an aim to determine removal/inactivation capability of the virus that can not be detected in a raw material or contingently contaminated.

As mentioned above, the role of the viral clearance study is to speculate removal/inactivation capability of a process through a model test, and it contributes to give scientific basis to assure that a biotechnological/biological product of human or animal origin has reached an acceptable level in aspect of viral safety.

At a viral clearance study, it is necessary to adopt an appropriate approach method which is definitive and rational and can assure viral safety of a final product, taking into consideration the source and the properties of the raw material/substrate for drug production as well as the manufacturing process.

4. Raw material/substrate for drug production

4.1. Issues relating to animal species and its region as a source of raw material/substrate for drug production and countermeasures to be taken thereto

For manufacturing JP listed biotechnological/biological products, which require measures for viral safety, a raw material/substrate for drug production derived mainly from human, bovine, swine or equine is used, and it is obvious that such human and animal has to be healthy nature. A wild animal should be avoided, and it is recommended to use animals derived from a colony controlled by an appropriate SPF (Specific Pathogen-Free) condition and bred under a well designed hygienic control, including appropriate control for prevention of microbial contamination and contamination monitoring system. If a meat standard for food is available, an animal meeting this standard has to be used. The type of virus to be concerned about depend on animal species, but it may be possible to narrow down the virus for investigation by means of examining the hygiene control, applicability of a meat standard for food, etc. On the other hand, even with the animals of the same species, a different approach may be necessary depending upon the region where the specimen for a raw material/substrate for drug production is taken. For example, in case of obtaining raw material /substrate for drug production from blood or other specific region, it is necessary to be aware of the risk level, virus multiplication risk, etc. which may specifically exists depending upon its region. Such approach may be different from those applied to body waste such as urine, milk, etc. as a source of raw material/substrate for drug production. Further, caution has to be taken on transmissible spongiform encephalopathy (TSE) when pituitary gland, etc. is used as a raw material. This report does not include detailed explanation on TSE, but recommendations are to use raw material derived from 1) animals originated in the countries (area) where incidence of TSE has not been reported; 2) animals not infected by TSE; or 3) species of animal which has not been reported on TSE. It is recommended to discuss the matters concerned with TSE with the regulatory authority if there is any unclear point.

Followings are the raw material/substrate used for manufacturing biotechnological/biological products in Japan.

(1) Biological products derived from human

Blood plasma, placenta, urine, etc. derived from human are used as the sources of raw material of biotechnological/biological products. As for these raw materials, there are two cases: 1) Appropriateness can be confirmed by interview or by examination of the individual who supplies each raw material, and 2) Such sufficient interview or examination of the individual can not be made due to the type of raw material. In case that sufficient examination of individual level is not possible, it is necessary to perform the test to deny virus contamination at an appropriate manufacturing stage, for example, the stage to decide it as a substrate for drug production.

(2) Biological products derived from animal besides human

Heparin, gonadotropin, etc. are manufactured from blood plasma or from various organs of bovine, swine and equine.

(3) Protein drug derived from cell line of human or animal origin

In the case of protein drugs derived from cell line of human or animal origin, a cell line of human or animal is the raw material per se, and the substrate for drug production is a cell bank prepared from a cloned cell line (master cell bank or working cell bank). Examination at cell bank level is considered enough for viral safety qualification, but it goes without saying that the more appropriate and rational qualification evaluation test of the master cell bank can be realized when more information is available on the virus of the source animal or on the prehistory of driving the cell line, the base of the cell bank.

4.2. Qualification evaluation test on human or animal as a source of raw material/substrate for drug production

(1) Biological products derived from human

Body fluid etc. obtained from healthy human must be used for biological products production. Further, in case that interview or examination of the individual, who supplies the raw material, can be possible and is necessary, interview under an appropriate protocol and a serologic test well evaluated in aspects of specificity, sensitivity and accuracy have to be performed, so that only the raw material, which is denied latent HBV, HCV and HIV, will be used. In addition to the above, it is necessary to test for the gene of HBV, HCV and HIV by a nucleic amplification test (NAT) well evaluated in aspects of specificity, sensitivity and accuracy.

In case of the raw material (e.g., urine), which can not be tested over the general medical examination of the individual who supplies the material, or of the raw material which is irrational to conduct individual test, the pooled raw material, as the substrate for drug production, has to be conducted at least to deny existence of HBV, HCV and HIV, using a method well evaluated in aspects of specificity, sensitivity and accuracy, such as the antigen test or NAT.

(2) Biological products derived from animal besides human

The animal used for manufacturing biological products has to be under appropriate health control, and has to be confirmed of its health by various tests. Further, it is necessary that the population, to which the animal belongs, has been under an appropriate breeding condition, and that no abnormal individual has been observed in the population. Further, it is necessary to demonstrate information or scientific basis which can deny known causes infection or disease to human, or to deny such animal inherent latent virus by a serologic test or by a nucleic amplification test (NAT). The infectious virus that is known to be common between human and animal, and known to cause infection in each animal are tentatively listed in Table 2. It is necessary that the table is completed under careful examination, and denial of all of them, by means of tests on individual animal, tissue, body fluid, etc. as a raw material, or on pooled raw material (as a direct substrate for drug production), is not always necessary. Table 2 can be used as reference information, in addition to the other information, such as; source of animal, health condition, health and breeding control, conformity to the meat standard for food, etc., to elaborate to which virus what kind of test has to be performed, and for which virus it is not always necessary to test for, etc. It is important to clarify and record the basis of choosing the virus and the test conducted thereof.

(3) Protein drug derived from cell line of human or animal origin

It is important to conduct thorough investigation on latent endogenous and non-endogenous virus contamination in a master cell bank (MCB), which is the cell substrate for drug production, in accordance with the Notice Iyakushin No. 329 entitled "Viral safety evaluation of biotechnology products derived from cell lines of human or animal origin". Further, it is necessary to conduct an appropriate adventitious virus test (e.g., *in vitro* and *in vivo* test) and a latent endogenous virus test on the cell at the limit of *in vitro* cell age (CAL) for drug production. Each working cell bank (WCB) as a starting cell substrate for drug production should be tested for adventitious virus either by direct testing or by analysis of cells at the CAL, initiated from the WCB. When appropriate non-endogenous virus tests have been performed on the MCB and cells cultured up to or beyond the CAL have been derived from the WCB and used for testing for the presence of adventitious viruses, similar tests need not be performed on the initial WCB.

5. Points of concern with respect to manufacturing and virus testing

To ensure viral safety of a biological product derived from tissue, body fluid etc. of human or animal origin, it is necessary to exclude any possibility of virus contamination from a raw material, such as tissue and body fluid, or a substrate, paying attention to the source of virus contamination as mentioned in above 3.5, and to adopt appropriate manufacturing conditions and technologies in addition to enhancement of manufacturing environment, so that virus contamination in the course of process and handling and from operators, facilities and environment can be minimized.

In addition to the above, effective virus tests and viral inactivation/removal technology, which are reflected by rapid progress of science, have to be introduced. Adoption of two or more steps with different principles is recommended for virus inactivation/removal process. Further, it is important to minimize any possible virus derivation by using a reagent, of which quality is equivalent to that of a drug. Examples of virus inactivation/removal processes are ① heating (It is reported that almost viruses are inactivated by heating at 55 - 60°C for 30 minutes with exceptions of hepatitis virus, etc. and that liquid heating at 60°C for 10 - 24 hours or dry heating is effective in case of the products of blood or urine origin.), ② treatment with organic solvent/surfactant (S/D treatment), ③ membrane filtration (15 - 50 nm), ④ acid treatment, ⑤ irradiation (γ-irradiation, etc.), ⑥ treatment with column chromatograph (e.g. affinity chromatography, ion-exchange chromatography), ⑦ fractionation (e.g. organic solvent or ammonium sulfate fractionation), ⑧ extraction.

5.1. Virus test conducted in advance of purification process

(1) Biological products derived from human

In many cases, samples for virus test before purification process are body fluid or tissue of individual collected as a raw material, or its pooled material or extraction as a substrate for drug production. As mentioned in 4.2. (1), it is necessary to deny latent HBV, HCV and HIV by the test evaluated enough in aspects of specificity, sensitivity and accuracy. Even in a case that a non-purified bulk before purification process is produced from a substrate for drug production, it is not always necessary to conduct a virus test again at the stage before purification, so long as the presence of any latent virus can be denied at the stage of substrate by an appropriate virus test, with cases where the non-purified bulk is made from the substrate by adding any reagent etc. of living organisms origin are an exception.

(2) Biological products derived from animal besides human

Similar to 5.1. (1), samples for virus tests before purification process are, in many cases, body fluid or tissue of individual collected as a raw material, or its pooled material or extraction as a substrate for drug production. In these cases, it is necessary to have a data, which can deny latent virus of probable cause of human infection or disease as mentioned in the above 4.2. (2), or to have a result of a serologic test or a nucleic amplification test (NAT) evaluated enough in aspects of specificity, sensitivity and accuracy. The concept, which is applied to a case that non-purified bulk before purification process is produced from a substrate for drug production, is the same as those provided in the above 4.2. (1).

(3) Protein drug derived from cell line of human or animal origin

Generally, a substrate for drug production in this case is a cell bank, and the sample for testing before purification process is a harvested cell after cell culturing or unprocessed bulk which consists of single or pooled complex culture broth. The unprocessed bulk may be sometimes culture broth without cells. Denial of latent virus, which is determined by a virus test at a MCB or WCB level, does not always deny latent virus in unprocessed bulk after culturing. Further, it is noted that the viral test at the CAL is meaningful as a validation but can not guarantee definite assurance of latent virus denial, since the test is generally performed only once. In case of using a serum or a component of blood origin in a culture medium, definite denial of latent virus at the level of unprocessed bulk can not be assured so long as the viral test has not been conducted on each lot at the CAL, since lot renewal can be a variable factor on viral contamination.

A representative sample of the unprocessed bulk, removed from the production reactor prior to further processing, represents one of the most suitable levels at which the possibility of adventitious virus contamination can be determined with a high probability of detection. Appropriate testing for viruses should be performed at the unprocessed bulk level unless virus testing is made more sensitive by initial partial processing (e.g., unprocessed bulk may be toxic in test cell cultures, whereas partially processed bulk may not be toxic). In certain instances it may be more appropriate to test a mixture consisting of both intact and disrupted cells and their cell culture supernatants removed from the production reactor prior to further processing.

In case of unprocessed bulk, it is required to conduct virus tests on at least 3 lots obtained from pilot scale or commercial scale production. It is recommended that manufacturers develop programs for the ongoing assessment of adventitious viruses in production batches. The scope, extent and frequency of virus testing on the unprocessed bulk should be determined by taking several points into consideration including the nature of the cell lines used to produce the desired products, the results and extent of virus tests performed during the qualification of the cell lines, the cultivation method, raw material sources and results of viral clearance studies. Screening *in vitro* tests, using one or several cell lines, are generally employed to test unprocessed bulk. If appropriate, a NAT test or other suitable methods may be used.

Generally, harvest material in which adventitious virus has been detected should not be used to manufacture the product. If any adventitious viruses are detected at this level, the process should be carefully checked to determine the cause of the contamination, and appropriate actions taken.

5.2. Virus test as an acceptance test of an intermediate material, etc.

When a biological product is manufactured from tissue, body fluid etc. of human or animal origin, there are cases that an intermediate material, partially processed as a raw material or substrate for drug production by outside manufacturer, is purchased and used for manufacturing. In such case, if any test to meet this General Information has been conducted by such outside manufacturer, it is necessary for the manufacturer of the biological product, who purchased the intermediate material, to examine what sort of virus test has to be conducted as acceptance tests, and to clarify the basis of rationality including the details of the test conducted.

On the other hand, if no test to meet this General Information has been conducted by such outside manufacturer of the raw material, all necessary virus free test has to be conducted to meet this General Information on the intermediate material regarding it as the direct substrate for drug production.

5.3. Virus test on a final product

Virus tests to be conducted on a final product (or on a product to reach the final product) has to be defined under comprehensive consideration of the type of raw material or substrate for drug production, the result of virus tests conducted on raw material/substrate for drug production, the result of evaluation on viral removal/inactivation processes, any possibility of virus contamination in the manufacturing process, etc. Comprehensive viral safety assurance can only be achieved by appropriate selection of the raw material/substrate for drug production, an appropriate virus test conducted on the raw material/substrate for drug production/intermediate material, the virus test conducted at an appropriate stage of manufacturing, an appropriate viral clearance test, etc. However, there are cases of having specific backgrounds, such as 1) use of the raw material derived from unspecified individual human, 2) possible existence of virus at a window period, 3) specific detection limit of virus test, etc. and in these cases, virus contamination to the final product may occur if there is any deficiency on the manufacturing process (e.g., damage of membrane filter) or any mix-up of the raw materials, etc. To avoid such accidental virus contamination, it may be recommended to conduct a nucleic

Table 2 Infectious viruses known to be common between human and animal and known to cause infection to each animal

	bovine	swine	sheep	goat	equine
Cowpox virus	◎				
Paravaccinia virus	◎	◎	◎	◎	
Murray valley encephalitis virus	◎				
Louping ill virus	◎	◎	◎	◎	
Wesselsbron virus			◎		
Foot-and-mouth disease virus	◎	◎			
Japanese encephalitis virus		◎			
Vesicular stomatitis virus		◎			
Bovine papular stomatitis virus	◎				
Orf virus			◎		
Borna disease virus			◎		◎
Rabies virus	◎	◎	◎	◎	◎
Influenza virus		◎			
Hepatitis E virus		◎			
Encephalomyocarditis virus	◎	◎			
Rotavirus	◎				
Eastern equine encephalitis virus					◎
Western equine encephalitis virus					◎
Venezuelan equine encephalitis virus					◎
Morbillivirus					◎
Hendra virus					◎
Nipah virus		◎			
Transmissible gastroenteritis virus		◎			
Porcine respiratory coronavirus		◎			
Porcine epidemic diarrhea virus		◎			
Hemagglutinating encephalomyelitis virus		◎			
Porcine respiratory and reproductive syndrome virus		◎			
Hog cholera virus		◎			
Parainfluenza virus Type 3		◎			
Talfan/Teschen disease virus		◎			
Reovirus		◎			
Endogenous retrovirus		◎			
Porcine adenovirus		◎			
Porcine circovirus		◎			
Porcine parvovirus		◎			
Porcine poxvirus		◎			
Porcine cytomegalovirus		◎			
Pseudorabies virus		◎			
Russian spring-summer encephalitis virus			◎	◎	
Rift Valley fever virus			◎	◎	
Crimean-Congo hemorrhagic fever virus (Nairovirus)	◎		◎	◎	
Torovirus	◎				

amplification test (NAT) on the final product focusing on the most risky virus among those that may possibly to exist in the raw material.

6. Process evaluation on viral clearance

6.1. Rationale, objective and general items to be concerned with respect to viral clearance process evaluation

Evaluation of a viral inactivation/removal process is important for ensuring safety of a biological product derived from tissue or body fluid of human or animal origin. Conducting evaluation on viral clearance is to assure, even to some extent, elimination of the virus, which may exist in a raw material, etc. or may be derived to the process due to an unexpected situation. Viral clearance studies should be made by a carefully designed appropriate method, and has to be rationally evaluated.

The objective of viral clearance studies is to assess process step(s) that can be considered to be effective in inactivating/removing viruses and to estimate quantitatively the overall level of virus reduction obtained by the process. This should be achieved by the deliberate addition ("spiking") of significant amounts of a virus at different manufacturing/purification steps and demonstrating its removal or inactivation during the subsequent steps. It is not necessary to evaluate or characterize every step of a manufacturing process if adequate clearance is demonstrated by the use of fewer steps. It should be borne in mind that other steps in the process may have an indirect effect on the viral inactivation/removal achieved. Manufacturers should explain and justify the approach used in studies for evaluating viral clearance.

The reduction of virus infectivity may be achieved by removal of virus particles or by inactivation of viral infectivity. For each production step assessed, the possible mechanism of loss of viral infectivity should be described with regard to whether it is due to inactivation or removal. For inactivation steps, the study should be planned in such a way that samples are taken at different times and an inactivation curve constructed.

6.2. Selection of virus

To obtain a broad range of information of viral inactivation/removal, it is desirable that a model virus used for viral clearance studies should be chosen from the viruses with a broad range of characteristics in aspects of DNA/RNA viruses, with or without envelope, particle size, significant resistance to physical/chemical treatment, etc. and it is necessary to combine about 3 model viruses to cover these characteristics.

At choice of a model virus, there are also the ways to choose a virus closely related to or having the same characteristics of the virus known to exist in the raw material. In such case, it is in principle recommendable to choose a virus which demonstrates a higher resistance to inactivation/removal treatment if two or more candidate viruses are available for choice. Further, a virus which can grow at a high titer is desirable for choice, although this may not always be possible. In addition to the above, choosing a virus, which will provide effective and reliable assay result at each step, is necessary, since sample condition to be tested at each step of a production process may influence the detection sensitivity. Consideration should also be given to health hazard which may pose to the personnel performing the clearance studies.

For the other items taken for consideration at choice of virus, the Notice, Iyakushin No. 329 can be used as a reference. Examples of the virus which have been used for viral clearance studies are shown in Table 3 which was derived from Iyakushin No. 329. However, the Notice, Iyakushin No. 329, is on viral safety of a product derived from cell lines of human or animal origin, and a more appropriate model virus has to be chosen taking into account the origin/raw material of biological products.

6.3. Design of viral clearance studies

The purpose of viral clearance studies is to quantitatively evaluate removal or inactivation capability of a process, in which a virus is intentionally spiked to a specific step of a manufacturing process.

Following are the precautions to be taken at planning viral clearance studies.

(1) Care should be taken in preparing the high-titer virus to avoid aggregation which may enhance physical removal and decrease inactivation thus distorting the correlation with actual production.

(2) Virus detection methods give great influence to the viral clearance factor. Accordingly, it is advisable to gain detection sensitivity of the methods available in advance, and use a method with a detection sensitivity as high as possible. Quantitative infectivity assays should have adequate sensitivity and reproducibility in each manufacturing process, and should be performed with sufficient replicates to ensure adequate statistical validity of the result. Quantitative assays not associated with infectivity may be used if justified. Appropriate virus controls should be included in all infectivity assays to ensure the sensitivity of the method. Also, the statistics of sampling virus when at low concentrations (for example, number of virus is 1-1000/L) should be considered.

(3) Viral clearance studies are performed in a miniature size system that simulates the actual production process of the biotechnological/biological product used by the manufacturer. It is inappropriate to introduce any virus not used for manufacturing into a production facility because of GMP constraints. Therefore, viral clearance studies should be conducted in a separate laboratory equipped for virological work and performed by a staff with virological expertise in conjunction with production personnel involved in designing and preparing a scaled-down version of the purification process. The viral clearance studies should be performed under the basic concept of GLP.

(4) Each factor on a viral clearance study of a process, which is performed in miniature size, should reflect that of actual manufacturing as far as possible, and its rationality should be clarified. In case of chromatograph process, length of column bed, linear velocity, ratio of bed volume per velocity (in other words, contact time), buffer, type of column packing, pH, temperature, protein concentration, salt concentration and concentration of the objective product are all correspondent to those of the actual production. Further, similarity of the elution profile should be achieved. For the other process, similar concept should be applied. If there is any factor which can not reflect the actual production, its effect to the result should be examined.

(5) It is desirable that two or more inactivation/removal processes of different principles are selected and examined.

(6) As for the process which is expected to inactivate/remove virus, each step should be evaluated in aspect of clearance capability, and carefully determined if it is the stage of inactivation, removal or their combination for designing the test. Generally, in viral clearance tests, a virus is spiked in each step which is the object of the test, and after passing through the process in question, the reduction level of infectivity is evaluated. But, in some case, it is accepted that a high potential virus is spiked at a step of the process, and virus concentration of each succeeding step is carefully monitored. When removal of virus is made by separation or fractionation, it is desirable to investigate how the virus is separated or fractionated (mass balance).

(7) For assessment of viral inactivation, unprocessed crude material or intermediate material should be spiked with infectious virus and the reduction factor calculated. It should be recognized that virus inactivation is not a simple, first order reaction and is usually more complex, with a fast "phase 1" and a slow "phase 2". The study should, therefore, be planned in such a way that samples are taken at different times and an inactivation curve constructed. It is recommended that studies for inactivation include at least one time point less than the minimum exposure time and greater than zero, in addition to the minimum exposure time. The reproducible clearance should be demonstrated in at least two independent studies. When there is a possibility that the virus is a human pathogen, it is very important that the effective inactivation process is designed and more detailed data (more points) for the virus (or the same or closely related viruses) are obtained. The initial virus load should be determined from the virus which can be detected in the spiked starting material. If this is not possible, the initial virus load may be calculated from the titer of the spiking virus preparation. Where inactivation is too rapid to plot an inactivation curve using process conditions, appropriate controls should be performed to demonstrate that infectivity is indeed lost by inactivation.

(8) If antibody against virus exists in an unprocessed material, caution should be taken at clearance studies, since it may affect the behavior of virus at viral removal or inactivation process.

(9) The amount of virus spiked in unprocessed material should be sufficient enough to evaluate viral removal or inactivation capability of the process. However, the virus "spike" to be added to the unprocessed material should be as small as possible in comparison with the sample volume of the unprocessed material so as not to cause characteristic change of the material by addition of the virus nor to cause behavioral change of the protein in the material by dilution.

(10) It is desirable that the virus in the sample is subject for quantitative determination without applying ultracen-

Table 3 Example of viruses which have been used for viral clearance studies

Virus	Family	Genus	Natural host	Genome	Env	Size (nm)	Shape	Resistance
Vesicular Stomatitis Virus	Rhabdo	Vesiculovirus	Equine Bovine	RNA	yes	70 × 150	Bullet	Low
Parainfluenza Virus	Paramyxo	Type 1,3 Respirovirus Type 2,4 Rubulavirus	Various	RNA	yes	100 – 200 +	Pleo-Spher	Low
MuLV	Retro	Type C oncovirus	Mouse	RNA	yes	80 – 110	Spherical	Low
Sindbis Virus	Toga	Alphavirus	Human	RNA	yes	60 – 70	Spherical	Low
BVDV	Flavi	Pestivirus	Bovine	RNA	yes	50 – 70	Pleo-Spher	Low
Pseudorabies Virus	Herpes	Varicellovirus	Swine	DNA	yes	120 – 200	Spherical	Med
Poliovirus Sabin Type 1	Picorna	Enterovirus	Human	RNA	no	25 – 30	Icosahedral	Med
Encephalomyocarditis Virus	Picorna	Cardiovirus	Mouse	RNA	no	25 – 30	Icosahedral	Med
Reovirus Type 3	Reo	Orthoreovirus	Various kind	RNA	no	60 – 80	Spherical	Med
SV 40	Papova	Polyomavirus	Monkey	DNA	no	40 – 50	Icosahedral	Very high
Parvovirus: canine, porcine	Parvo	Parvovirus	Canine Porcine	DNA	no	18 – 24	Icosahedral	Very high

trifuge, dialysis, storage, etc. as far as possible. However, there may be a case that any handling before a quantitative test, such as remove procedure of an inhibitor or a toxic substance, storage for a period to realize test at a time, etc., is inevitable. If any manipulation, such as dilution, concentration, filtration, dialysis, storage, etc., is applied for preparation of the sample for testing, a parallel control test, which passes through a similar manipulation, should be conducted to assess infectivity variance at the manipulation.

(11) Buffers and products (desired protein or other component contained therein) should be evaluated independently for toxicity or interference in assays used to determine the virus titer, and measures should be taken so as not to interfere with the assays. If the solutions are toxic to the indicator cells, dilution, adjustment of the pH, or dialysis of the buffer containing spiked virus might be necessary. If the product itself has anti-viral activity, the clearance study may need to be performed without the product in a mock run, although omitting the product or substituting a similar protein that does not have anti-viral activity could affect the behaviour of the virus in some production steps.

(12) Many purification schemes use the same or similar buffers or columns, repetitively. The effects of this approach should be taken into account when analyzing the data. The effectiveness of virus elimination by a particular process may vary with the stage in manufacture at which it is used.

(13) Overall reduction factors may be underestimated where production conditions or buffers are too cytotoxic or virucidal and should be discussed on a case-by-case basis. Overall reduction factors may also be overestimated due to inherent limitations or inadequate design of viral clearance studies.

(14) It has to be noted that clearance capability of viral removal/inactivation process may vary depending upon the type of virus. The viral removal/inactivation process, which displays viral clearance by a specific principle or mechanism, may be quite effective to the virus, which meets such mechanism of action, but not effective to the other type of viruses. For example, S/D (Solvent/Detergent) treatment is generally effective to the virus with lipid membrane, but not effective to the non-enveloped virus. Further, some virus is resistant to the general heating process (55 – 60°C, 30 minutes). When clearance is expected for such virus, introduction of a further severe condition or process, which has a different principle or mechanism, is necessary. Virus removal by membrane filtration, which is different from S/D or heat treatment in aspect of principle, is effective to a broad range of virus that can not pass through the membrane. Affinity chromatography process, which specifically absorbs the objective protein, can thoroughly wash out the materials other than the objective protein including virus etc. and is generally effective for viral removal. Separation/fractionation of a virus from an objective protein is sometimes very difficult, but there are not so rare that ion exchange chromatography, ethanol fractionation, etc. is effective for clearance of a virus which can not be sufficiently inactivated or removed by the other process.

(15) Effective clearance may be achieved by any of the following: multiple inactivation steps, multiple complementary separation steps, or combinations of inactivation and separation steps. Separation methods may be dependent on the extremely specific physico/chemical properties of a virus which influence its interaction with gel matrices and precipitation properties, and the isolation may differ for each virus. However, despite these potential variables, effective removal can be obtained by a combination of complementary separation steps or combinations of inactivation and separation steps. Well designed separation steps that have been thoroughly examined on the items that affect the separation of a target virus and a mode virus, such as chromatographic procedures, filtration steps and extractions, can be also effective virus removal steps provided that they are performed under appropriately controlled conditions.

(16) An effective virus removal step should give reproducible reduction of virus load shown by at least two independent studies.

(17) Over time and after repeated use, the ability of chromatography columns and other devices used in the purification scheme to clear virus may vary. Some estimate of the stability of the viral clearance after several uses may

provide support for repeated use of such columns.

(18) The Notice, Iyakushin No. 329, would be used as a reference when viral clearance studies on biological products are designed.

6.4. Interpretation of viral clearance studies

6.4.1. Evaluation on viral clearance factor

The viral clearance factor is a logarithm of reduction ratio of viral amount (infectious titer) between each step applied for viral clearance of a manufacturing process. The total viral clearance factor throughout the process is sum of the viral clearance factor of each step appropriately evaluated.

Whether each and total viral clearance factor obtained are acceptable or should not be evaluated in aspects of every virus that can be realistically anticipated to derive into the raw material or the manufacturing process, and its rationality should be shown.

In case that existence of any viral particle is recognized in a substrate for drug production, e.g., a substrate of rodent origin for biodrug production, it is important not only to demonstrate removal or inactivation of such virus, but also to demonstrate that the purification process has enough capability over the required level to assure safety of the final product at an appropriate level. The virus amount removed or inactivated in a manufacturing process should be compared with the virus amount assumed to exist in the substrate etc. used for manufacturing drug, and for this purpose, it is necessary to obtain the virus amount in the raw materials/substrate for drug production, etc. Such figure can be obtained by measuring infectious titer or by the other method such as transmission electron microscope (TEM). For evaluation of overall process, a virus amount, far larger than that assumed to exist in the amount of the raw materials/substrate for drug production which is equivalent to single administration of the final product, has to be removed. It is quite rare that existence of virus can be assumed in a substrate for drug production, with the exception of the substrate of rodent origin, and such suspicious raw material/substrate for drug production should not be used for manufacturing drug with a special exceptional case that the drug in question is not available from the other process and is clinically indispensable, and that the information including infectious properties of the virus particle assumed to exist has been clarified.

Any virus contaminations in the substrates for drug production of biotechnological/biological products are usually denied by some tests or examinations. In such case, a specific virus that can possibly contaminate may be used as a model. However, in general, it would be necessary to perform a viral clearance test by choosing a combination of appropriate model viruses that can show the capability for clearance of a wide variety of viruses in the process, as indicated in 6.2. In this case, a common numerical goal cannot be established on the viral clearance. Therefore, the validity of viral clearance factor of the process should be taken into account, considering various information on factual possibility of virus contaminations of the substrates and others, detection sensitivity of the virus free test, and other cases in publications.

6.4.2. Calculation of viral clearance factor

The viral clearance factor, "R", for viral removal/inactivation process can be calculated by the following formula.

$$R = \log[(V_1 \times T_1)/(V_2 \times T_2)]$$

In which

R: Logarithm of reduction ratio

V_1: Sample volume of the unprocessed material

T_1: Virus amount (titer) of the unprocessed material

V_2: Sample volume of the processed material

T_2: Virus amount (titer) of the processed material

At the calculation of the viral clearance factor, it is recommendable to use the virus titer detected in the sample preparation of the unprocessed material after addition of virus, not the viral titer added to the sample preparation wherever possible. If this is not possible, loaded virus amount is calculated from virus titer of the solution used for spike.

6.4.3. Interpretation of results and items to be concerned at evaluation

At the interpretation and the evaluation of the data on effectiveness of viral inactivation/removal process, there are various factors to be comprehensively taken into account, such as ① appropriateness of the virus used for the test, ② design of the viral clearance studies, ③ virus reduction ratio shown in logarithm, ④ time dependence of inactivation, ⑤ factors/items which give influence to the inactivation/removal process, ⑥ sensitivity limit of virus assay method, ⑦ possible effect of the inactivation/removal process which is specific to certain class of viruses.

Additional items to be concerned at appropriate interpretation and evaluation of the viral clearance data are as follows:

(1) Behavior of virus used to the test

At interpretation of the vial clearance results, it is necessary to recognize that clearance mechanism may differ depending upon the virus used for the test. Virus used for a test is generally produced in tissue culture, but behavior of the virus prepared in the tissue culture may be different from that of the native virus. Examples are possible differences of purity and degree of aggregation between the native and the cultured viruses. Further, change of surface properties of a virus, e.g., addition of a sucrose chain which is ascribed to specific nature of a separation process, may give effect to the separation. These matters should be also considered at interpretation of the results.

(2) Design of test

Viral clearance tests should have been designed taking into account variation factors of the manufacturing process and scaling down, but there still remain some variance from actual production scale. It is necessary to consider such variance at the interpretation of the data and limitation of the test.

(3) Acceptability of viral reduction data

The total viral clearance factor is expressed as a sum of logarithm of reduction ratio obtained at each step. The summation of the reduction factors of multiple steps, particularly of steps with little reduction (e.g., below 1 $\log_{10}$), may overestimate viral removal/inactivation capability of the overall process. Therefore, virus titer of the order of 1 $\log_{10}$ or less has to be ignored unless justified. Further, a viral clearance factor achieved by repeated use of the same or similar method should be ignored for calculation unless justified.

(4) Time dependence of inactivation

Inactivation of virus infectivity frequently shows biphasic curve, which consists of a rapid initial phase and subsequent slow phase. It is possible that a virus not inactivated in a step may be more resistant to the subsequent step. For example, if an inactivated virus forms coagulation, it may be resistant to any chemical treatment and heating.

(5) Evaluation of viral reduction ratio shown in logarithm

The viral clearance factor shown in logarithm of reduction ratio of virus titer can demonstrate drastic reduction of residual infectious virus, but there is a limit that infectious titer can never be reduced to zero. For example, reduction in infectivity of a preparation containing 8 $\log_{10}$ infectious unit per mL by a factor of 8 $\log_{10}$ leaves zero $\log_{10}$ per mL or one infectious unit per mL, taking into account the detection limit of the assay.

(6) Variable factor of manufacturing process

Minor variance of a variation factor of a manufacturing process, e.g., contact time of a spiked sample to a buffer or a column, will sometimes give influence to viral removal or inactivation effect. In such case, it may be necessary to investigate to what extent such variance of the factor has given influence to the process concerned in aspect of viral inactivation.

(7) Existence of anti-viral antibody

Anti-viral antibody that exists in the sample preparation used for a test may affect sensitivity of distribution or inactivation of a virus, which may result in not only defusing the virus titer but complicating interpretation of the test result. So, existence of anti-viral antibody is one of the important variable factors.

(8) Introduction of a new process for removal/inactivation

Viral clearance is an important factor for securing safety of a drug. In case that an achievement level of infective clearance of a process is considered insufficient, a process which is characterized by an inactivation/removal mechanism to meet the purpose or an inactivation/removal process which can mutually complement to the existence process has to be introduced.

(9) Limit of viral clearance studies

Viral clearance studies are useful for contributing to the assurance that an acceptable level of safety in the final product is achieved but do not by themselves establish safety. However, a number of factors in the design and execution of viral clearance studies, and the interpretation of the results may lead to an incorrect estimate of the ability of the process to remove virus infectivity, as described above.

7. Statistics

The viral clearance studies should include the use of statistical analysis of the data to evaluate the results. The study results should be statistically valid to support the conclusions reached.

7.1. Statistical considerations for assessing virus assays

Virus titrations suffer the problems of variation common to all biological assay systems. Assessment of the accuracy of the virus titrations and the reduction factors derived from them and the validity of the assays should be performed to define the reliability of a study. The objective of statistical evaluation is to establish that the study has been carried out to an acceptable level of virological competence.

1. Assay methods may be either semiquantitative or quantitative. Both semiquantitative and quantitative assays are amenable to statistical evaluation.

2. Variation can arise within an assay as a result of dilution errors, statistical effects and differences within the assay system which are either unknown or difficult to control. These effects are likely to be greater when different assay runs are compared (between-assay variation) than when results within a single assay run are compared (within-assay variation).

3. The 95% confidence limits for results of within-assay variation normally should be on the order of $\pm 0.5 \log_{10}$ of the mean. Within-assay variation can be assessed by standard textbook methods. Between-assay variation can be monitored by the inclusion of a reference preparation, the estimate of whose potency should be within approximately 0.5 $\log_{10}$ of the mean estimate established in the laboratory for the assay to be acceptable. Assays with lower precision may be acceptable with appropriate justification.

7.2. Reproducibility and confidence limit of viral clearance studies

An effective virus inactivation/removal step should give reproducible reduction of virus load shown by at least two independent studies.

The 95% confidence limits for the reduction factor observed should be calculated wherever possible in studies of viral clearance. If the 95% confidence limits for the viral assays of the starting material are $\pm$s, and for the viral assays of the material after the step are $\pm$a, the 95% confidence limits for the reduction factor are $\pm\sqrt{s^2 + a^2}$.

8. Re-evaluation of viral clearance

Whenever significant changes in the production or purification process are made, the effect of that change, both direct and indirect, on viral clearance should be re-evaluated as needed. Changes in process steps may also change the extent of viral clearance.

9. Measurement for viral clearance studies

9.1. Measurement of virus infective titer

Assay methods may be either semiquantitative or quantitative. Semiquantitative methods include infectivity assays in animals or in cultured cell infections dose (CCID) assays, in which the animal or cell culture is scored as either infected or not. Infectivity titers are then measured by the proportion of animals or culture infected. In quantitative methods, the infectivity measured varies continuously with the virus input. Quantitative methods include plaque assays where each plaque counted corresponds to a single infectious unit. The methods should be sufficiently sensitive and reproducible, and controls should be used to obtain statistically analyzable results. Both quantal and quantitative assays are amenable to statistical evaluation.

9.2. Testing by nucleic-acid-amplification test (NAT)

NAT can detect virus genomes in individual samples, pooled raw material/cell substrate for drug production or products at a high sensitivity even in a stage that a serum test on each virus is negative. Further, it can detect HBV or HCV gene, which can not be measured in culture system. Window periods can be drastically shortened at the test on HBV, HCV and HIV, and the method is expected to contribute as an effective measure for ensuring viral safety. However, depending upon a choice of primer, there may be a case that not all the subtype of objective virus can be detected by this method, and, therefore, it is recommendable to evaluate, in advance, if subtypes of a broad range can be detected.

NAT will be an effective evaluation method for virus removal capability for viral clearance. However, in case of viral inactivation process, viral inactivation obtained by this method may be underrated, since there is a case that inactivated virus still shows positive on nucleic acid. Further, at introduction of NAT, cautions should be taken on rationality of detection sensitivity, choice of a standard which is used as run-control, quality assurance and maintenance of a reagent used for primer, interpretation of positive and negative results, etc.

10. Reporting and preservation

All the items relating to virus test and viral clearance studies should be reported and preserved.

11. Others

The Notice, Iyakushin No. 329, should be used as a reference at virus tests and viral clearance studies.

Conclusion

As mentioned at the Introduction, assurance of quality/

safety etc. of JP listed drugs should be achieved by state-of-the-art methods and concepts reflecting the progress of science and accumulation of experiences.

The basis for ensuring viral safety of JP listed biotechnological/biological products is detailed in this General Information. What is discussed here is that an almost equal level of measures are required for both development of new drugs and for existing products as well, which means that the similar level of concerns should be paid on both existing and new products in aspect of viral safety. This document is intended to introduce a basic concept that quality and safety assurance of JP listed product should be based upon the most advanced methods and concepts. This document has been written to cover all conceivable cases, which can be applied to all biotechnological/biological products. Therefore, there may be cases that it is not so rational to pursue virus tests and viral clearance studies in accordance with this document on each product, which has been used for a long time without any safety issue. So, it will be necessary to elaborate the most rational ways under a case-by-case principle taking into due consideration source, origin, type, manufacturing process, characteristics, usages at clinical stage, accumulation of the past usage record, etc. relating to such biotechnological/biological products.

Mycoplasma Testing for Cell Substrates used for the Production of Biotechnological/Biological Products <*G3-14-170*>

This document describes the currently available methods of mycoplasma testing that should be performed for cell substrates that are used in the manufacture of biotechnological/biological products.

Methods suggested for detection of mycoplasma are, A. culture method, B. indicator cell culture method, and C. nucleic acid amplification test (NAT) method.

Mycoplasma testing should be performed on the master cell bank (MCB) and the working cell bank (WCB), as well as on the cell cultures used during the manufacturing process of the product. For the assessment of these cells, mycoplasma testing should be performed using both methods A and B. Note that method C may be used as an alternative to methods A and/or B after suitable validation.

Prior to mycoplasma testing by methods A or B, the sample should be tested to detect the presence of any factors inhibiting the growth of mycoplasma. If such growth-inhibiting factors are detected, they should be neutralized or eliminated by an appropriate method, such as centrifugation or cell passage.

If the test will be performed within 24 hours of obtaining the sample, the sample should be stored at 2 - 8°C. If more than 24 hours will elapse before the test is performed, the sample should be stored at −60°C or lower.

If mycoplasma is detected, additional testing to identify the species may be helpful in determining the source of contamination.

A. Culture Method

1. Culture Medium

Both agar plates and broth are used. Each batch of agar and broth medium should be free of antibiotics except for penicillin. Refer to the Minimum Requirements for Biological Products regarding selection of the culture media. Other culture media may be used if they fulfill the requirements described in the following section 2.

2. Suitability of Culture Medium

Each batch of medium should be examined for mycoplasma growth-promoting properties. To demonstrate the capacity of the media to detect known mycoplasma, each test should include control cultures of at least two known species or strains of mycoplasma, one of which should be a dextrose fermenter (i.e., *Mycoplasma pneumoniae* ATCC 15531, NBRC 14401 or equivalent species or strains) and one of which should be an arginine hydrolyser (i.e., *Mycoplasma orale* ATCC 23714, NBRC 14477 or equivalent species or strains). The mycoplasma strains used for the positive control tests should be those with a low number of passages obtained from an official or suitably accredited agency, and handled appropriately. Inoculate the culture medium with 100 colony-forming units (CFU) or 100 color-changing units (CCU) or less.

3. Culture and Observation

1) Inoculate no less than 0.2 mL of the test sample (cell suspension) in evenly distributed amounts over the surface of each of two or more agar plates. After the surfaces of the inoculated plates are dried, the plates should be incubated in an atmosphere of nitrogen containing 5 - 10% carbon dioxide and adequate humidity at 35 - 37°C for no less than 14 days.

2) Inoculate no less than 10 mL of the test sample (cell suspension) into each of one or more vessels containing 100 mL of broth medium, and incubate at 35 - 37°C.

If the culture medium for the sample cells contains any growth-inhibiting factors, such as antibiotics, these factors should be removed. Refer to the Validation tests for growth-inhibiting factors described in the Minimum Requirements for Biological Products for the detection of growth-inhibiting factors.

3) Subculture 0.2 mL of broth culture from each vessel on the 3rd, 7th, and 14th days of incubation onto two or more agar plates. Observe the broth media every 2 or 3 days and if a color change occurs, subculture. The plates should be incubated in nitrogen containing 5 - 10% carbon dioxide and adequate humidity at 35 - 37°C for no less than 14 days.

4) Examination of all plates for mycoplasma colonies should be done microscopically on the 7th and 14th day at 100 times magnification or greater.

B. Indicator Cell Culture Method

Using Vero cell culture substrate, pretest the suitability of the method using an inoculum of 100 CFU or 100 CCU or less of *Mycoplasma hyorhinis* (ATCC 29052, ATCC 17981, NBRC 14858 or equivalent species or strains) and *M. orale* (ATCC 23714, NBRC 14477 or equivalent species or strains).

Indicator cell substrate equivalent to Vero cells and suitable mycoplasma strains may be acceptable if data demonstrate at least equal sensitivity for the detection of known mycoplasma contaminants. The mycoplasma strains should be those with a low number of passages obtained from an official or suitably accredited agency, and handled appropriately, and the unit of inoculation should be determined before use. The cell substrate used should be obtained from a qualified cell bank and certified to be mycoplasma free. The acquired cells should be carefully cultured and propagated, and sufficient volumes of seed stock should be prepared with the proper precautions to avoid mycoplasma contamination. The stock should be tested for mycoplasma contamination using at least one of the methods described in this document, then frozen for storage. For each test this stock should be thawed and used within 6 passages.

Indicator cell cultures should be grown on cover slips submerged in culture dishes or equivalent containers for one day. Inoculate no less than 1 mL of the test sample (cell culture supernatant) into two or more of the culture dishes.

The test should include a negative (non-infected) control and two positive mycoplasma controls, such as *M. hyorhinis* (ATCC 29052, ATCC 17981, NBRC 14858 or equivalent species or strains) and *M. orale* (ATCC 23714, NBRC 14477 or equivalent species or strains). Use an inoculum of 100 CFU or 100 CCU or less for the positive controls.

Incubate the cell cultures at 35 - 38°C for 3 - 6 days in an atmosphere of air containing 5% carbon dioxide.

Examine the cell cultures after fixation for the presence of mycoplasma by epifluorescence microscopy (400 to 600 times magnification or greater) using a DNA-binding fluorochrome, such as bisbenzimide or an equivalent stain. Compare the microscopical appearance of the test cultures with that of the negative and positive controls.

Procedure

1) Aseptically place a sterilized glass cover slip into each cell culture dish (35 mm diameter).

2) Prepare Vero cell suspension in Eagle's minimum essential medium containing 10% fetal calf serum at a concentration of 1×10^4 cells per mL. The fetal calf serum should be tested and confirmed to be free from mycoplasma prior to use.

3) Inoculate aliquots of 2 mL of the Vero cell suspension into each culture dish. Ensure that the cover slips are completely submerged, and not floating on the surface of the culture medium. Incubate the cultures at 35 - 38°C in an atmosphere of air containing 5% carbon dioxide for one day, so that the cells are attached to the glass cover slip.

4) Replace 2 mL of the culture medium with fresh medium, then add 0.5 mL of the test sample (cell culture supernatant) to each of two or more culture dishes. Perform the same procedure for the positive (2 types of mycoplasmas, such as *M. hyorhinis* (ATCC 29052, ATCC 17981, NBRC 14858 or equivalent species or strains) and *M. orale* (ATCC 23714, NBRC 14477 or equivalent species or strains) and negative controls.

5) Incubate the cultures at 35 - 38°C for 3 - 6 days in an atmosphere of air containing 5% carbon dioxide.

6) Remove the culture medium from the culture dishes, and add 2 mL of a mixture of acetic acid (100) and methanol (1:3) (fixative) to each dish; then, allow them to stand for 5 minutes.

7) Remove the fixative from each dish, then add the same amount of fixative again, and leave the dishes to stand for 10 minutes.

8) Remove the fixative and then completely air-dry all the dishes.

9) Add 2 mL of bisbenzimide fluorochrome staining solution to each culture dish. Cover the dishes and let them stand at room temperature for 30 minutes.

10) Aspirate the staining solution and rinse each dish with 2 mL of distilled water 3 times. Take out the glass cover slips and dry them.

11) Mount each cover slip with a drop of a mounting fluid. Blot off surplus mounting fluid from the edges of the cover slips.

12) Examine by epifluorescence microscopy at 400 to 600 times magnification or greater.

13) Compare the microscopic appearance of the test sample with those of the negative and positive controls.

14) The test result is judged to be positive if there are more than 5 cells per 1000 (0.5%) that have minute fluorescent spots that appear to surround, but are outside, the cell nucleus.

C. Nucleic Acid Amplification Test (NAT)

Nucleic acid amplification test (NAT) is a detection method of genes or mRNA transcribed from genes of target cells or viruses by enzymatic amplification with specific primers for target nucleic acid sequences, and the amplified products are detected by several ways. When NAT is used for detection of mycoplasma, high sensitivity detection is expected for the presence or absence of the target sequence derived from mycoplasma by amplification of nucleic acid extracted from a test sample (cell suspension or cell culture supernatant) with specific primers/probes. NAT indicates the presence of a target sequence and not necessarily the presence of viable mycoplasmas.

A number of different NAT methods are available. This general information does not prescribe a particular method. NAT method applied should be validated for sufficient sensitivity, specificity, and robustness of results that remain unaffected by small variations in extraction method parameters or in composition of the reaction mix. Any NAT method is available if the specificity and the sensitivity is properly validated as described in this section. Where a commercial kit is used, certain elements of the validation may be carried out by the manufacturer and information provided to the user. However, it should be remembered that the different results might be obtained by user depending on the instrument used and the target cells tested. The user should confirm the manufacturer's validation results by own facilities. Especially, when the target cell substrate is different from cells validated by the manufacturer, the detection limit and reproducibility of the kit should be confirmed with the cells of interest. When the user's extraction method or instruments used for detection etc. are different from the method or the instrument specified by the manufacturer, the employed method or the instrument should be validated.

In addition, when the information on the primers/probes or the kit reagents may not be available from the manufacturer, countermeasure is required to obtain the information from the manufacturer about the modification of the kit production when modified. If the composition of the kit reagents is modified, user should confirm that the detection limit and the detection accuracy of the modified kit for target mycoplasma is comparable to the previous one, as needed. On the other hand, appropriate alternative method should be considered, since the production of the kit may be discontinued.

Basically, cell suspension but not cell culture supernatant will be used as a test sample, since mycoplasma contaminated in cell culture mainly growth in a cell-dependent manner. When cell culture supernatant is used as test samples, validation is required that the method employed is able to fully detect the mycoplasma contamination in cell cultures.

NAT may be used instead of methods A and/or B, after suitable validation described below, and the validation revealed sufficient sensitivity for all of the listed mycoplasma species.

In order to increase the detection sensitivity of nucleic acid derived from infectious mycoplasma, it is possible to perform NAT after enrichment of mycoplasma that may be present in test samples by culturing with Vero cells. In this case, again, validation is required to show sufficient sensitivity for all of the listed mycoplasma species.

C-1. Mycoplasma testing by NAT

The tests should include both a positive control (run control) (such as *M. hyorhinis* (ATCC 17981, NBRC 14858 or equivalent species or strains) of 100 CFU or 100 CCU or less) and a negative control. The mycoplasma strains used for the positive control tests should be those within a low number of passages obtained from an official or suitably accredited agency, and handled appropriately. The unit of inoculation should be determined before use. When cell suspension is used as a test sample, a preliminary test is required for the effect of cellular nucleic acid to NAT with the cells confirmed to be mycoplasma-free as a negative control, and confirm that no positive signals are obtained from the negative control. The test result is judged to pass the test if no mycoplasma sequences are amplified from the test sample.

C-2. Precautions for the test

Because NAT enables the detection of trace amounts of nucleic acid, false positive results may be obtained by contamination of the facilities, instruments and reagents etc. with amplified products. To prevent the risk of contamination, wherever possible, each step of the storage and preparation of reagents, the extraction of nucleic acid, the amplification of nucleic acid, and the detection of amplified products should be performed in separate facilities or equipments with special precautions for handling. To exclude false-positive results by contamination of carry-over amplified products, Uracil-N-glycosylase (UNG) procedure may be available. To exclude the false-negative results by low efficiency of extraction or interfering substances for NAT in test samples, simultaneously detection of house-keeping genes of the test cells as internal control is recommended.

On the other hand, if an automatic closed system from extraction to amplification is used to prevent cross-contamination, segregation of the area is not always required. However, measures to prevent contamination are required when disposing the amplified products from the automatic system.

C-3. Validation of NAT for the detection of mycoplasmas

NAT methods for the detection of target sequences are either qualitative or quantitative tests. To detect mycoplasma contamination of cell substrates, qualitative tests are adequate and may be considered to be limit tests. This section describes methods to validate qualitative NAT analytical procedures for assessing mycoplasma contamination. These validation methods may also be applicable for quantitative NAT with an optimal cut-off point.

The most important parameters for validation of the analytical procedure by NAT are the specificity and the detection limit. In addition, the robustness of the analytical procedure should be evaluated. Note that for the purpose of this document, validation of NAT method is defined as the complete procedure from extraction of nucleic acid to detection of the amplified products.

Where commercial kits are used for a part or all of the analytical procedure, documented full validation data already covered by the kit manufacturer can replace validation data by the user, and a full validation by the user is unnecessary. Nevertheless, the performance of the kit with respect to its intended use and user's test system should be demonstrated by the user (e.g. specificity, detection limit).

NAT may be used as:

- a test for in-process control purposes;
- an alternative method to replace methods A and/or B.

This section will thus separate these 2 objectives by presenting first a guideline for the validation of the NAT themselves, and second, a guideline for a comparability study between NAT and methods A or B.

Mycoplasma reference strains evaluated for concentration either in CFUs or equivalent copies are required at various stages during validation of specificity or detection limit of NAT. During routine application of the test, mycoplasma reference strains or the test sample calibrated for concentration using reference strains are used as positive controls. In the test, mycoplasma or mycoplasma nucleic acid (e.g. plasmid) may be used as a positive control. Mycoplasma is required for validation of the procedure including extraction efficiency.

1) Evaluation parameters

Three parameters should be evaluated: specificity, detection limit, and robustness.

2) Specificity

Specificity of NAT is the ability to unequivocally detect a target nucleic acid in the presence of test samples that may be expected to be present. The specificity of NAT is dependent on the choice of primers/probes and the strictness of the test conditions (both of the amplification and the detection steps).

It is important to use primers/probes by choosing nucleic acid sequences that are specific and well conserved for a wide range of mycoplasmas (the bacterial class *Mollicutes* such as the genus *Mycoplasma* and related genera such as *Ureaplasma*, *Spiroplasma*, *Acholeplasma* etc.). The ability of NAT to detect a large panel of mycoplasma species should be demonstrated by experimental results using reference mycoplasmas described in 3), and evaluation only by the theoretical analysis of primers/probes comparing with databases is not recommended.

3) Detection limit

The detection limit of an individual analytical procedure is the lowest amount of a target nucleic acid in a sample that can be detected but not necessarily quantitated as an exact value. For establishment of the detection limit, a positive cut-off point should be determined for NAT. The positive cut-off point is the target sequence copies per volume of sample that can be detected in 95% of test runs. This positive cut-off point is influenced by the nucleic acid sequences of target mycoplasma in the individual samples being tested and by factors such as enzyme efficiency, and can result in different 95% cut-off values for individual analytical test runs. To determine the positive cut-off point, a dilution series of characterized and calibrated (either in CFUs or nucleic acid copies) mycoplasma reference strains or international standards should be tested on different days to examine variation between test runs.

For validation of the limit of detection, the following species should be used. These species represent an optimal selection in terms of the frequency of occurrence as contaminants of mammalian culture cells used for production of biotechnological/biological products, phylogenetic relationships, and animal-derived components used during culture and production processes. Note that the list is only for validation of NAT and not for used as positive run control in routine tests.

- *Acholeplasma laidlawii* (ATCC 23206, NBRC 14400 or equivalent strains)
- *Mycoplasma arginini* (ATCC 23838 or equivalent strains)
- *Mycoplasma fermentans* (ATCC 19989, NBRC 14854 or equivalent strains)
- *Mycoplasma hyorhinis* (ATCC 17981, NBRC 14858 or equivalent strains)
- *Mycoplasma orale* (ATCC 23714, NBRC 14477 or equivalent strains)
- *Mycoplasma pneumoniae* (ATCC 15531, NBRC 14401 or equivalent strains)
- *Mycoplasma salivarium* (ATCC 23064, NBRC 14478 or equivalent strains)

Where there is use of insect or plant cells during production, mycoplasma strains derived from insect or plant (e.g. *Spiroplasma citri*) should be tested in addition to the above list. Where there is use of avian cells or materials during production, mycoplasma species derived from avian should be tested whether avian mycoplasmas (e.g. *Mycoplasma synoviae*) can be detected.

For establishment of the detection limit, appropriate dilution series (10-fold or $10^{0.5}$-fold dilution) should be prepared from the undiluted mycoplasma evaluated for concentration (CFU etc.), and tests by NAT should be performed for each dilution. Based on the dilution factor that shows the limit of the detection, a positive cut-off point should be determined as the minimum number of CFUs of target sequences in the test sample. In case amplified products are separated by electrophoresis and the positive band is detected by fluorescent staining, confirmation is required whether no positive band is appeared from the test sample of mycoplasma-free cells. Detection using quantitative real-time PCR requires to set an adequate cut-off point of amplification cycles, and the setting of the cut-off point should be validated. Since extraction efficiency of nucleic acid from the test sample affects the detection, the detection sensitivity of mycoplasma in cell suspension should be evaluated.

For each mycoplasma reference strain described above, at least 3 independent 10-fold dilution series should be tested, with a sufficient number of replicates at each dilution to give a total number of 24 test results for each dilution, to enable a statistical analysis of the results. For example, a laboratory may test 3 dilution series on different days with 8 replicates for each dilution, 4 dilution series on different days with 6 replicates for each dilution, or 6 dilution series on different days with 4 replicates for each dilution. In order to keep the number of dilutions at a manageable level, a preliminary test should be performed to obtain a preliminary value for the positive cut-off point (i.e. the highest dilution giving a positive signal). The range of dilutions can then be chosen around the determined preliminary cut-off point. The concentration of mycoplasmas (CFUs, etc.) that can be detected in 95% of test runs can then be calculated using an appropriate statistical evaluation. These results may also serve to evaluate the variability of the analytical procedure.

4) Robustness

The robustness of an analytical procedure is a measure of its capacity to remain unaffected by small but deliberate variations in method parameters, and provides an indication of its reliability during normal usage. The evaluation of robustness should be considered during the development phase. It should show the reliability of the analytical procedure with respect to deliberate variations in method parameters. For NAT, small variations in the method parameters can be crucial. However, the robustness of the method can be demonstrated during its development when small variations in the concentrations of reagents (e.g. $MgCl_2$, primers, and deoxyribonucleotides) are tested. Modifications of extraction kits or extraction procedures as well as different thermal cycler types may also be evaluated.

5) Use of NAT instead of methods A and/or B

NAT may be used instead of methods A (culture method) and/or B (indicator cell culture method). In this case, a comparability study should be carried out. This comparability study should include mainly a comparison of the respective detection limits of the NAT and methods A and/or B. However, specificity (mycoplasma panel detected, putative false positive results) should also be considered.

For the detection limit, acceptability criteria are defined as follows:

- if the alternative method is proposed to replace method A (the culture method), the NAT system should be shown to detect 10 CFU/mL for each mycoplasma test species described in 3).
- if the alternative method is proposed to replace method B (the indicator cell culture method), the NAT system should be shown to detect 100 CFU/mL for each mycoplasma test species described in 3).

For both cases, suitable references calibrated for the number of CFUs may be used for establishing that these acceptability criteria are reached.

One of the following 2 strategies can be used to perform this comparability study:

- perform the NAT alternative method in parallel with the methods A or B to evaluate simultaneously the detection limit of both methods using the same samples of calibrated strains with CFUs.
- compare the performance of the NAT alternative method using previously obtained data from methods A or B. In this case, calibration of CFUs of reference strains used for both validations as well as their stabilities should be described carefully.

Alternatively, comparability of detection limit may be demonstrated by the number of nucleic acid copies, etc. of mycoplasma in test samples. In this case, the relation between CFUs and the number of nucleic acid copies for the reference preparations should be previously established.

6) Controls

- Internal controls: For validation, internal controls are useful to confirm appropriate nucleic acid amplification without effect of inhibitory substances derived from test samples. Internal controls are also necessary for routine verification of extraction and absence of inhibition to NAT reaction. The internal control may contain the primer binding-site, or some other suitable sequence may be used. It is preferably added to the test material before isolating the nucleic acid and therefore acts as an overall control for extraction, reverse transcription, amplification, and detection. Cellular genes derived from test samples may also be used as the internal control.
- External controls: The external positive control contains a defined number of target-sequence copies or CFUs from one or more suitable species of mycoplasma chosen from those used during validation of the test conditions. One of the positive controls is set close to the positive cut-off point to demonstrate that the expected sensitivity is achieved. The external negative control contains no target sequence but does not necessarily represent the same matrix as the test article.

7) Interpretation of results

The primers/probes used may also amplify non-mycoplasma nucleic acid, leading to false-positive results. Procedures are established at the time of validation for dealing with confirmation of positive results, where necessary.

C-4 Method of cultivating mycoplasma with Vero cells

1) Use at least two cell culture dishes for each of the test sample, positive control and negative control.

2) Into each cell culture dish (35 mm diameter), inoculate 2 mL of the Vero cell suspension (1×10^4 cells per mL) in Eagle's minimum essential medium containing 10% fetal calf serum (tested in advance using the NAT method to verify that it does not contain any detectable mycoplasma DNA). Incubate the cultures at 35 – 38°C in an atmosphere of air containing 5% carbon dioxide for one day.

3) Replace the culture media with fresh media, and add 0.5 mL of the test sample (cell culture supernatant) to each of two or more Vero cell culture dishes. Perform the same procedure for the positive (such as 100 CFU or 100 CCU or less of *M. hyorhinis* (ATCC 17981, NBRC 14858 or equiva-

lent species or strains)) and negative controls.

4) Incubate the Vero cell culture dishes for the test sample, positive and negative controls for 3 - 6 days at 35 - 38°C in an atmosphere of air containing 5% carbon dioxide.

Qualification of Animals as Origin of Animal-derived Medicinal Products provided in the General Notices of Japanese Pharmacopoeia and Other Standards *<G3-15-141>*

Introduction

The Official Gazette issued on March 29, 2002 announced that General Notices of the Japanese Pharmacopoeia and other standards were amended to add a provision that "When a drug product or a drug substance which is used to manufacture a drug product, is manufactured from a raw material of animal origin, the animal in question should be in principle a healthy subject, if not otherwise provided.".

The Notice Iyaku-hatsu No. 0329001, which was issued on the same date, provided that "Healthy subject herein provided is the animal which does not cause any disease or any infection to human being at an appropriate use of the drug product, and as for the oral or external drug for example, the animal, as its raw material of animal origin, should be confirmed at this stage to meet the Food Standard. It has to be noted that this standard of healthy subject has to be revised timely taking into account the up-to-date information with respect to the amphixenosis infections common between human beings and animals.".

This General Information describes safety assurance against infection associated with the use of drugs, which are manufactured from raw materials of animal origin, to follow up the Notice as mentioned above.

1. Basic concept

When drugs derived from raw materials of animal origin including human are used, it is important to take into account any possibility that communicable disease agents such as virus may cause infectious disease or any possible hazards to patients. In such case, it goes without saying that the primary subject that has to be considered is the absence of any infectious agents such as virus in the raw materials of animal origin including human as the source of the drug. More important point is whether there is any possibility of transmission of infectious agents when the drugs containing such infectious agents are administered to patient. The eligibility of animals including human, as the source of raw materials of drugs, in other words "the subject which is free from any disease or transmission of infectious agents that is infectious to human being at an appropriate use of the drug product" is that "The drug should be entirely free from any risk of infections by means of whole procedures which include evaluation of appropriateness of the animals including human as the source of their raw materials, establishment of appropriate production processes and their appropriate control, and strict adherence to the clinical indications of the final product."

2. Animals including human as the source of raw materials of drugs

The most clear and appropriate preventive measures against infection to human being due to administration of drugs which are derived from animals including human are to assure the absence of any infectious agents such as virus in its raw materials or an appropriate critical raw material by either of the following: (1) the use of raw materials of healthy animal origin, which are proved to be free from communicable disease agents to human, or (2) the use of appropriate critical raw materials for drug production, which are proved to be free from communicable disease agents after certain appropriate processing on raw materials of animal origin.

As for raw materials of drugs of human origin, cell/tissue, blood, placenta, urine, etc. are used. Whenever it is possible for each donor of such raw materials to be asked or inspected about his (her) health condition, the appropriateness as a donor should be confirmed at this stage from the standpoint of safety concerning communicable disease agents such as virus.

For example, "Basic concept on handling and use of a drug product, etc. which is derived from cell/tissue" (Attachment 1 of the Notice Iyaku-Hatsu No. 1314 dated December 26, 2000) issued by the Director-General of the Medicinal Safety Bureau, Ministry of Health and Welfare, states that since the cell/tissue supplied by a human donor comes to be applied to patients without processing through any sufficient inactivation or removal of communicable disease agents, the selection and qualification criteria on such donor has to be established. These criteria are to be composed with the respect to the check items on the case history and the physical conditions as well as the test items on the various transmission of infectious agents through cell/tissue, and that the appropriateness of these criteria has to be clarified. Hepatitis Type-B (HBV), Hepatitis Type-C (HCV), Human Immune Deficiency Viral infections (HIV), Adult T-Cell Leukemia and Parvovirus B19 Infections should be denied through the interview to the donor and the tests (serologic test, nucleic acid amplification test, etc.). Further, if necessary, Cytomegalovirus infection and EB Virus infection should be denied by tests. "Infections caused by bacteria such as Treponema pallidum, Chlamydia, Gonococci, Tubercule bacillus, etc.", "septicemia and its suspicious case", "vicious tumor", "serious metabolic or endocrine-related disorders", "collagenosis and haematological disorder", "hepatic disease" and "dementia (transmissible spongiform encephalopathies and its suspicious case)" should be checked on the case history or by the interview, etc. and the experience of being transfused or/and transplanted should be checked to confirm eligibility as a donor. The most appropriate check items and test methods then available are to be used, which need to be reconsidered at appropriate timing taking into account the updated knowledge and the progress of the science and the technologies. At screening of a donor, reexaminations have to be made at appropriate timing using the eligible check items and the test methods taking into account the window period (Initial period after infection, in which antibody against bacteria, fungi or virus is not detected).

In the case of plasma derivatives produced from the donated blood in Japan, the donor should be checked by means of self-assessed report about health conditions, and a serologic check and a nucleic acid amplification test (NAT) on mini pooled plasma targeted for HBV, HCV and HIV should be performed at the stage of donated blood. Further, the plasma material for fractionation should be stored 4 months in minimum so that the arrangement could be taken based on the information available after collection of the blood and the blood infusion to exclude the possibility of using any critical raw material which might cause infection to patients.

On the other hand, as for the materials such as urine which are taken from the unspecified number of the donors and come to be critical raw materials for drug production after some treatments, it is unrealistic and not practical to conduct the tests of virus infection, etc. on the individual donor. Consequently, appropriate tests such as virus test has to be performed on such pooled raw materials for drug production.

In the case of the animals besides human, the wild ones should be excluded. Only the animals, which are raised under well sanitarily controlled conditions taken to prevent bacterial contamination or under the effective bacterial pollution monitoring systems, have to be used, and it is recommended that the animals from a colony appropriately controlled under specific pathogen-free (SPF) environment are to be used as far as possible. Further, for the animals regulated under the Food Standard, only the animals that met this standard should be used. It should be confirmed by appropriate tests that the animals were free from pathogen, if necessary.

The concrete measures to avoid transmittance or spread of infectivity of prion, which is considered to be the pathogen of transmissible spongiform encephalopathies (TSEs), as far as possible are the followings: ① avoidance of use of animals, which are raised in the areas where high incidence or high risk of TSEs (Scrapie in sheep and goat, bovine spongiform encephalopathies (BSE) in cattle, chronic wasting disease (CWD) in deer, new type of Creutzfeldt-Jacob-Disease (CJD) in human, etc.) is reported, and humans, who have stayed long time (more than 6 months) in such areas, as raw materials or related substances of drugs; ② avoidance of use of any substances that are derived from the individual infected with scrapie, BSE, CJD, etc.; ③ avoidance of using a material derived from organ, tissue and cell, etc. of high risk of TSEs; and ④ taking appropriate measures basing on the information collected, which includes incidence of TSEs, the results of epidemiological investigation and the experimental research on prion, and incidence of tardive infection on donors after collecting raw materials, etc.

3. Human or animal cells which are used as critical raw materials for drug production

Cell substrates derived from humans or animals are used for drug production. In such case, it is desirable that the humans or the animals, which are the origins of the cell substrates, are healthy subjects. However, it is considered practical that viral safety of the drugs derived from the cell substrates are evaluated on the cells, which are so called critical raw materials for production of such drugs. In such case, the safety should be confirmed through the test and analysis on established cell bank thoroughly with respect to virus etc., as far as possible. The items and the methods of the tests that have been followed in this case are described in detail in the Notice of Japanese version on the internationally accepted ICH Guideline entitled "Viral safety evaluation of biotechnology products derived from cell lines of human or animal origin" (Iyakushin No. 329 issued on February 22, 2000 by Director, Evaluation and Licensing Division, Pharmaceutical and Medical Safety Bureau, Ministry of Health and Welfare). In the meantime, it is important how to handle the cell in case that any virus has been detected under the cell level tests. This Notice describes how to cope with this situation as follows: "It is recognised that some cell lines used for the manufacture of product will contain endogenous retroviruses, other viruses or viral sequences. In such circumstances, the action plan recommended for manufacturer is described in Section V (Rationale and action plan for viral clearance studies and virus tests on purified bulk) of the Notice. The acceptability of cell lines containing viruses other than endogenous retroviruses will be considered on an individual basis by the regulatory authorities, by taking into account a risk/benefit analysis based on the benefit of the product and its intended clinical use, the nature of the contaminating viruses, their potential for infecting humans or for causing disease in humans, the purification process for the product (e.g., viral clearance evaluation data), and the extent of the virus tests conducted on the purified bulk." For example, it is well known that Type A-, R- and C-particles like endogenous retrovirus are observed in the cells of the rodents used most often for drug production. It is also known that they are not infectious to human and is not dangerous, and CHO cells are generally used for drug production. The established cell lines (e.g., NAMALWA Cell, BALL-1 Cell, etc.) derived from cancer patients are sometimes used, but through the thorough virus tests, etc., their safety is confirmed. The established cell lines are assumed to be safer than the primary cultured cells which are hard to conduct the thorough virus test.

4. Establishment and control of appropriate production process and adherence to the clinical indication of final product for safety assurance

Safety assurance against potential infections at only the level of animals that are source of raw materials of drugs is limited. Further, "health of animal" can not be defined univocally, and the various factors have to be taken into account. The final goal of this subject is to protect human from any infectious disease caused by drugs. Achieving this goal, the establishment and control of appropriate production processes of each drug and the adherence to the clinical indications of the final product are important.

As mentioned above, the rodent cells used most often for the production of the drugs are known to have endogenous retrovirus-like particles sometimes. The reason why such cells can be used for the production of the drugs is that multiple measures are applied for safety in the purification stages which include appropriate inactivation or removal processes. There are cases in which the production procedure involves intentional use of a virus or a microorganism. In this case, relevant measures capable of removing or inactivating of such virus or microorganism are appropriately incorporated in the purification process, so that the risk of infection to human can be fully denied and its safety can be assured when it is used as a drug. Further, even in the case that it is difficult to clarify the risk of contamination of the infectious agents or that the raw material is contaminated by viruses etc., the raw material in question may be used for the production of drugs so long as appropriate inactivation or removal processes are introduced, their effectiveness can be confirmed and the safety can be assured by appropriate control of the manufacturing processes under GMP, etc.

5. Conclusion

The qualification of animals including human, as the source of raw materials of drugs, in other words "the subject which does not cause any infectious diseases to human being at an appropriate use of the drug product" is that "the drug has to be entirely free from any risk of infections by means of whole procedures which include evaluation of appropriateness of the animal including human as the source of their raw materials, establishment of appropriate production processes and their appropriate control, and strict adherence to the clinical indication of the final product."

To cope with this subject, the advanced scientific measures, which actually reflect the updated knowledge and progress of the science and the technology about infectious diseases in human and infection of animal origin, have to be taken into account timely.

G4 Microorganisms

Microbial Attributes of Non-sterile Pharmaceutical Products

<G4-1-170>

This chapter is harmonized with the European Pharmacopoeia and the U.S. Pharmacopeia. The parts of the text that are not harmonized are marked with symbols (◆ ◆).

Information on the harmonization with the European Pharmacopoeia and the U.S. Pharmacopeia is available on the website of the Pharmaceuticals and Medical Devices Agency.

The presence of certain micro-organisms in non-sterile preparations may have the potential to reduce or even inactivate the therapeutic activity of the product and has a potential to adversely affect the health of the patient. Manufacturers have therefore to ensure a low bioburden of finished dosage forms by implementing current guidelines on Good Manufacturing Practice during the manufacture, storage and distribution of pharmaceutical preparations. ◆This chapter provides guidelines for acceptable limits of viable micro-organisms (bacteria and fungi) existing in raw materials and non-sterile pharmaceutical products.◆ Microbial examination of non-sterile products is performed according to the methods given in the Microbiological Examination of Non-sterile Products *<4.05>* on Microbiological Examination of Non-sterile Products: I. Microbial Enumeration Tests and II. Tests for Specified Micro-organisms. ◆When these tests are carried out, a microbial control program must be established as an important part of the quality management system of the product. Personnel responsible for conducting the tests should have specialized training in microbiology, biosafety measures and in the interpretation of the testing results.◆

◆1. Definitions

(i) Non-sterile pharmaceutical products: Non-sterile drugs shown in monographs of the JP and non-sterile finished dosage forms.

(ii) Raw materials: All materials, including raw ingredients and excipients, used for the preparation of drugs, except for water and gases.

(iii) Bioburden: Number and type of viable micro-organisms existing in non-sterile pharmaceutical products.

(iv) Action levels: Established bioburden levels that require immediate follow-up and corrective action if they are exceeded.

(v) Alert levels: Established bioburden levels that give early warning of a potential drift from normal bioburden level, but which are not necessary grounds for definitive corrective action, though they may require follow-up investigation.

(vi) Quality management system: The procedures, operation methods and organizational structure of a manufacturer (including responsibilities, authorities and relationships between these) needed to implement quality management.

2. Scope

In general, Microbial Enumeration Tests is not applied to drugs containing viable micro-organisms as an active ingredient.

3. Sampling plan and frequency of testing

3.1. Sampling methods

Microbial contaminants are usually not uniformly distributed throughout the batches of non-sterile pharmaceutical products or raw materials. A biased sampling plan, therefore, cannot be used to estimate the real bioburden in the product. A sampling plan which can properly reflect the status of the product batch should be established on the basis of the bioburden data obtained by retrospective validation and/or concurrent validation. In general, a mixture of samples randomly taken from at least different three portions, almost the same amount for each portion, is used for the tests of the product.

When the sampling is difficult in a clean area, special care is required during sampling to avoid introducing microbial contamination into the product or affecting the nature of the product bioburden. If it is confirmed that the product bioburden is stable for a certain period, as in the case of non-aqueous or dried products, it is not necessary to do the tests, immediately after the sampling.

3.2. Testing frequency

The frequency of the tests should be established on the basis of a variety of factors unless otherwise specified. These factors include:

(i) Dosage forms of non-sterile pharmaceutical products (usage);

(ii) Manufacturing processes;

(iii) Manufacturing frequency;

(iv) Characteristics of raw materials (natural raw material, synthetic compound, etc.);

(v) Batch sizes;

(vi) Variations in bioburden estimates (changes in batches, seasonal variations, etc.);

(vii) Changes affecting the product bioburden (changes in manufacturing process, supplier of raw materials, batch number of raw materials, etc.);

(viii) Others.

In general, the tests may be performed at a high frequency during the initial production of a drug to get information on the microbiological attributes of the product or raw materials used for the production. However, this frequency may be reduced as bioburden data are accumulated through retrospective validation and/or concurrent validation. For example, the tests may be performed at a frequency based on time (e.g., weekly, monthly or seasonally), or on alternate batches.

4. Microbial control program

When the ''Microbiological Examination of Non-sterile Products *<4.05>*'' is applied to a non-sterile pharmaceutical product, the methods for the recovery, cultivation and estimation of the bioburden from the product must be validated and a ''Microbial control program'' covering the items listed below must be prepared.

(i) Subject pharmaceutical name (product name);

(ii) Frequency of sampling and testing;

(iii) Sampling methods (including responsible person, quantity, environment, etc. for sampling);

(iv) Transfer methods of the samples to the testing area (including storage condition until the tests);

(v) Treatment of the samples (recovery methods of microbial contaminants);

(vi) Enumeration of viable micro-organisms (including

testing quantity, culture media, growth-supporting test of the media, culturing methods, etc.);

(vii) Detection of specified micro-organisms (including testing quantity, culture media, growth-supporting test of the media, culturing methods, etc.);

(viii) Estimation of the number of and characterization of microbial contaminants;

(ix) Establishment of "Microbial acceptance criteria" (including alert level and action level);

(x) Actions to be taken when the levels exceed "Microbial acceptance criteria";

(xi) Persons responsible for the testing and evaluation, etc.;

(xii) Other necessary items.◆

5. Microbial acceptance criteria for non-sterile pharmaceutical products

By establishing "Microbial acceptance criteria" for non-sterile pharmaceutical products based upon the total aerobic microbial count (TAMC) and the total combined yeasts/moulds count (TYMC), ◆it is possible to evaluate at the initial processing stage of the product whether the microbiological quality of the raw materials is adequate or not. Furthermore, it is then possible to implement appropriate corrective action as needed to maintain or improve the microbiological quality of the product.◆

The target limits of microbial levels for raw materials (synthetic compounds and minerals) are shown in Table 1. ◆In general, synthetic compounds have low bioburden levels due to the high temperatures, organic solvents, etc., used in their manufacturing processes. Raw materials originated from plants and animals in general have higher bioburdens than synthetic compounds.

The microbial quality of the water used in the processing of active ingredients or non-sterile pharmaceuticals may have a direct effect on the quality of the finished dosage form. This means it is necessary to keep the level of microbial contaminants in the water as low as possible.◆

Acceptance criteria for microbiological quality for non-sterile finished dosage forms are shown in Table 2. ◆These microbial limits are based primarily on the type of dosage form, water activity, and so on. For oral liquids and pharmaceutical products having a high water activity, in general, low microbial acceptance criteria are given.◆

Table 2 includes a list of specified micro-organisms for which acceptance criteria are set. The list is not necessarily exhaustive and for a given preparation it may be necessary to test for other micro-organisms depending on the nature of the starting materials and the manufacturing process.

If it has been shown that none of the prescribed tests will allow valid enumeration of micro-organisms at the level prescribed, a validated method with a limit of detection as close as possible to the indicated acceptance criterion is used.

In addition to the micro-organisms listed in Table 2, the significance of other micro-organisms recovered should be evaluated in terms of:

(i) the use of the product: hazard varies according to the route of administration (eye, nose, respiratory tract);

(ii) the nature of the product: does the product support growth, does it have adequate antimicrobial preservation?

(iii) the method of application;

(iv) the intended recipient: risk may differ for neonates, infants, the debilitated;

(v) use of immunosuppressive agents, corticosteroids;

(vi) presence of disease, wounds, organ damage.

Where warranted, a risk-based assessment of the relevant factors is conducted by personnel with specialized training in microbiology and the interpretation of microbiological data.

For raw materials, the assessment takes account of processing to which the product is subjected, the current technology of testing and the availability of materials of the desired quality. Acceptance criteria are based on individual results or on the average of replicate counts when replicate counts are performed (e.g. direct plating methods).

When an acceptance criterion for microbiological quality is prescribed it is interpreted as follows:

—10^1 CFU: maximum acceptable count = 20,
—10^2 CFU: maximum acceptable count = 200,
—10^3 CFU: maximum acceptable count = 2000, and so forth.

◆6. Acceptance criteria for crude drugs and crude drug-containing preparations

Target limits of microbial contamination for crude drugs and crude drug-containing preparations are shown in Table 3. Category 1 includes crude drugs and crude drug preparations which are used for extraction by boiling water or to which boiling water is added before use. Category 2 includes crude drugs which are taken directly without extraction process and directly consumed crude drug preparations containing powdered crude drugs. In this guideline, bile-tolerant gram-negative bacteria, *Escherichia coli* and *Salmonella* are mentioned as specified micro-organisms, but other micro-organisms (such as certain species of *Bacillus cereus*, *Clostridia*, *Pseudomonas*, *Burkholderia*, *Staphylococcus aureus*, *Asperigillus* and *Enterobacter* species) are also necessary to be tested depending on the origin of raw materials for crude drugs or the preparation method of crude drug-containing preparations. The target limit of microbial contamination for the raw materials is to be set based on the risk assessment being taken into account the provided process of those materials or the desired quality specification for them.◆

Table 1 Acceptance criteria for microbiological quality of non-sterile substances for pharmaceutical use

	Total Aerobic Microbial Count (CFU/g or CFU/mL)	Total Combined Yeasts/Moulds Count (CFU/g or CFU/mL)
Substances for pharmaceutical use	10^3	10^2

Table 2 Acceptance criteria for microbiological quality of non-sterile dosage forms

Route of administration	Total Aerobic Microbial Count (CFU/g or CFU/mL)	Total Combined Yeasts/Moulds Count (CFU/g or CFU/mL)	Specified Micro-organism
Non-aqueous preparations for oral use	10^3	10^2	Absence of *Escherichia coli* (1 g or 1 mL)
Aqueous preparations for oral use	10^2	10^1	Absence of *Escherichia coli* (1 g or 1 mL)
Rectal use	10^3	10^2	—
Oromucosal use Gingival use Cutaneous use Nasal use Auricular use	10^2	10^1	Absence of *Staphylococcus aureus* (1 g or 1 mL) Absence of *Pseudomonas aeruginosa* (1 g or 1 mL)
Vaginal use	10^2	10^1	Absence of *Pseudomonas aeruginosa* (1 g or 1 mL) Absence of *Staphylococcus aureus* (1 g or 1 mL) Absence of *Candida albicans* (1 g or 1 mL)
Transdermal patches (limits for one patch including adhesive layer and backing)	10^2	10^1	Absence of *Staphylococcus aureus* (1 patch) Absence of *Pseudomonas aeruginosa* (1 patch)
Inhalation use (more rigorous requirements apply to liquid preparations for nebulization)	10^2	10^1	Absence of *Staphylococcus aureus* (1 g or 1 mL) Absence of *Pseudomonas aeruginosa* (1 g or 1 mL) Absence of bile-tolerant gram-negative bacteria (1g or 1 mL)

◆**Table 3** Acceptance criteria for crude drugs and crude drug-containing preparations

	Total Aerobic Microbial Count (CFU/g or CFU/mL)	Total Combined Yeasts/Moulds Count (CFU/g or CFU/mL)	Specified Micro-organism
Category 1	Acceptance criterion: 10^7 Maximum limit: 50,000,000	Acceptance criterion: 10^5 Maximum limit: 500,000	Acceptance criterion for *Escherichia coli*: 10^3 (1 g or 1 mL) Absence of *Salmonella* (10 g or 10 mL)
Category 2	Acceptance criterion: 10^5 Maximum limit: 500,000	Acceptance criterion: 10^4 Maximum limit: 50,000	Acceptance criterion for bile-tolerant gram-negative bacteria: 10^4 (1 g or 1 mL) Absence of *Escherichia coli* (1 g or 1 mL) Absence of *Salmonella* (10 g or 10 mL)

◆

Control of Culture Media and Strains of Microorganisms Used for Microbial Tests <*G4-2-180*>

This General Information describes points to consider in the control of culture media and strains of microorganisms used for microbial tests in a laboratory.

Use apparatuses which are appropriately maintained, controlled, and calibrated.

1. Media preparation and quality control

1.1. Media preparation

Select culture media or medium components suitable for microbial tests to be conducted when preparing culture media. Dehydrated media are accompanied by component compositions and instructions for preparation. Because each media may have different preparation requirements (e.g., heating, additives, and pH adjustment), it is important to follow their instructions to prepare media with appropriate quality. Records of the date of preparation, name/lot number/mass of dehydrated media or medium components, the volume of water used, sterilization conditions, pH after sterilization, and equipment/instrument used, etc. are useful to investigate cause when a problem occurs.

Dehydrated media or medium components should be weighed appropriately. In addition, clean containers and tools should be used to prevent contamination with foreign matters during preparation. Water suitable for performing the relevant test should be used to prepare culture media, and purified water is most often used.

Dehydrated media should be dissolved in water before sterilization, or shaken thoroughly to disperse sufficiently. When dispensing before sterilization, media should be thoroughly dissolved in water. If heating is necessary to dissolve media, care should be taken not to overheat media. Browning of media by the Maillard reaction etc. is one of the indication of overheating. Appropriate equipment and tools should be used for heating, stirring and mixing in the preparation of media. When adding components that cannot be heated, they should be aseptically added to media cooled to an appropriate temperature after sterilization, and mixed thoroughly.

If poorly cleaned tools are used to prepare media, substances that inhibit the growth of microorganisms may contaminate the media. Inhibitory substances are derived from detergent residues after cleaning tools, etc., substances used before cleaning tools, or residues during manufacturing even when unused tools are used. In the cleaning process, residues and foreign matters should be removed certainly, and finally detergents, etc. should be washed out completely using purified water, etc.

Sterilization of media should be performed within parameters (temperature, pressure, exposure time, etc.) provided by a supplier or parameters validated by users. Sterilization in an autoclave is preferred, unless media contain medium components that are unstable to heat. Sterilization by filtration may be appropriate for some medium compositions.

When an autoclave is used, the sterilization should be performed in the sterilization cycles in which the temperature of all objects to be sterilized (temperature of media) meets specified temperature and exposure time, depending on the loading format of loads (loading pattern). Loading pattern includes the shape, size, number and arrangement of containers, and the type and liquid volume of an object to be sterilized, etc. Sterilization cycle includes the process where the temperature of objects to be sterilized rises to specified temperature and the process from the completion of sterilization until the falling to the temperature to be able to take out the objects. The sterilization cycles in which temperature rises slowly may result in the overheating of media. In general, the more the liquid volume of an object to be sterilized, the longer the sterilization cycle. However, since the cycle is affected by the size and number of dispensing containers even if the total volume of liquid is the same, so appropriate conditions should be selected. After the completion of sterilization cycle, the media should be taken out immediately, and cooled, if necessary. The effects of the sterilization cycles should be verified by the growth promotion test (refer to Microbiological Examination of Non-sterile Products <*4.05*>, Sterility Test <*4.06*>, etc.) together with confirmation of the sterility of media (no microbial contamination).

Take into consideration that improper preparation may result in the deterioration of growth promoting properties and inhibitory properties, and in the deviation of the properties, such as color, clarity, gel strength and pH, from the acceptable range.

The pH of a medium should be confirmed after it has cooled to room temperature or another specified temperature by aseptically withdrawing a test sample every each sterile batch (unit to be sterilized at one time, hereinafter called as ''batch''). If it cannot be measured at the specified temperature, the pH should be corrected for the specified temperature. A flat pH probe is recommended for agar surfaces, and an immersion probe is recommended for liquids. The pH of media should be within a specified range. However, unless when it is confirmed that a wider range is acceptable by the growth promotion test or suitability test (refer to Microbiological Examination of Non-sterile Products <*4.05*>, Sterility Test <*4.06*>, etc.).

Prepared media (agar plate or media dispensed to test tubes etc.) are identified by name, batch number, preparation date, etc. Also, pay attention to the following terms.

(i) Container fracture
(ii) Unequal dispensing volume between containers
(iii) Dirt of containers due to adhesion of medium components, etc.
(iv) Browning or discoloration
(v) Air bubbles
(vi) Status of redox indicator (if applicable)
(vii) Hemolysis (if applicable)
(viii) Formation of crystals, etc.
(ix) Drying that causes cracks and dimples
(x) Microbial contamination

1.2. Media storage

When storing media and medium components, the following points should be noted, including transport conditions until acquisition, in order to prevent the deterioration of quality.

(i) Drying, evaporation, moisture absorption
(ii) Temperature
(iii) Microbial contamination
(iv) Contamination of foreign matters
(v) Fracture

In addition, media or medium components should be labelled with names, batch or lot numbers, storage conditions, expiration dates, etc. and identified.

The storage conditions and the expiration dates of the media after preparation is set after the stability is confirmed by verifying that the performance of the media meet the acceptance criteria up to the end of the expiration date by the growth promotion test and other necessary quality tests when media are stored under the set conditions.

For long-term storage, packaging materials, packaging types, containers and stoppers that can prevent evaporation of water should be selected. Also, protect from light, if necessary. The agar media should be stored avoiding freezing because freezing damage the gel structure of agar.

In addition, agar media that have been remelted after storage can be used within the confirmed expiration date, if performance tests are performed to confirm the suitability. Also, it is desirable to remelt agar media only once to avoid the possibility of deterioration and contamination due to overheating. It is recommended that remelting is performed in a heated water bath or in free-flowing steam. When using a microwave oven or a heating plate for melting media, care should be taken because whole media may not be uniformly heated, and deterioration of the media and breakage of the container due to overheating may occur.

Agar media immediately after sterilization, or remelted media should be held at 45 to 50°C or another specified temperature, but holding for a long-time should be avoided in consideration of the risk of deterioration and contamination. In addition, if media are held in a water bath, be careful of contamination derived from water in a bath when pouring them into petri dishes.

When discarding used or expired media, sterilize as needed and take care to prevent contamination.

1.3. Quality control testing

Perform the following quality control tests for each batch or lot for all prepared media. The prepared media include ready-prepared media and ready-to use swabs, strips, etc.

(i) Growth promotion (growth promoting properties, and, as needed, inhibitory properties or indicative properties)

(ii) pH (as needed, for ready-prepared media)

Media purchased or stored under a refrigeration condition should be returned to room temperature or a temperature being specified separately, and confirmed.

(iii) Sterility (no microbial contamination)

Media used for environmental monitoring of Grade A and B in processing areas for sterile pharmaceutical products should be multiple-wrapped or carried into the areas according to a specified procedure after disinfecting or decontaminating the exterior. If sterilization after packaging is not performed, all media (100%) should be subjected to incubation prior to use and confirmed to be free of microbial contamination in order to prevent extraneous contamination from being carried into controlled environments and prevent false-positive results.

A certificate of analysis describing storage conditions and an expiration date accompanies ready-prepared media, as well as the standard microbial strain used in growth promotion testing. When the data of testing are obtained from a supplier at the time of acceptance, if the data is reliable as the result of writing or site investigation etc. and the validity of the growth promotion testing result and the expiration date can be confirmed, the quality control test may be performed regularly instead of every batch or lot.

Similar to media, those requiring quality control tests include reagents for microbial identification tests such as Gram staining reagents and oxidase reagents. These should be subjected to quality control tests at the time of acceptance or use using appropriate standard microbial strains selected.

2. Maintenance and control of microbial strains

The appropriate treatment of stock microbial strains is very important to maintain the accuracy and repeatability of results of microbial tests. The storage and handling of microbial strains in a laboratory should be done in such a way that will minimize changes in the growth characteristics of the microorganism, paying attention to contamination. Microbial strains used in the compendial methods are available in frozen, lyophilized, slant cultured or ready-to-use forms from an organization for culture collections or an appropriate supplier. Obtained microbial strains should be confirmed to be contaminated with no other strains before or at use for quality control testing by the observation of emerged colonies being single, etc. when spread on plate media having no selectivity. In addition, if necessary, confirm the distributed microbial species.

Stock microbial strains are resuscitated according to the method specified by an organization for culture collections, etc. The application of seed lot culture maintenance techniques (seed-lot systems) is recommended to control the preservation of microbial strains. The seed-lot system is a system to control the number of passage of stock microbial strains in order to avoid property changes due to passages. One passage is defined as the transfer of organisms from a viable culture to a fresh medium with growth of the microorganisms. Any form of subculturing is considered to be a passage. At least the following terms should be noted in the control.

(i) Count a culture obtained by resuscitating (the number of passage is first) a microbial strain distributed from an organization for culture collections, etc. as the first generation.

(ii) Control the number of passages.

(iii) Microbial strains must not be used more than 5 passages for growth promotion tests and suitability tests.

There are methods by freezing, by drying, by serial subculture, etc. for the preservation of microbial strains, and an example of the method by freezing is shown. A standard microbial strain distributed from an organization for culture collections etc. is resuscitated and grown in appropriate medium. Aliquot of this culture (the first generation) is suspended in a solution containing a protective agent that prevents freezing damage, transferred to a vial or the like, and cryopreserved at an appropriate temperature according to the microbial species. Many microbial strains can be stored for a long time by maintaining at the temperature not exceeding −70°C. If the second and subsequent generations are prepared in large quantities, the frequency of acquiring and preparing standard microbial strains can be reduced.

Microbial strains in once opened containers should be discarded without refreezing to avoid the risk of reduced viability and contamination of stored microbial strains.

3. References

1) WHO, WHO Good Practices for Pharmaceutical Microbiology Laboratories (WHO Technical Report Series, No. 961, Annex 2, 2011).

2) US Pharmacopeia 43 (2020), <1117> Microbiological Best Laboratory Practices.

Preservatives-Effectiveness Tests <*G4-3-170*>

The purpose of the Preservatives-Effectiveness Tests is to assess microbiologically the preservative efficacy, either due to the action of product components themselves or any added preservative(s), for multi-dose containers[1,2]. The efficacy of the preservatives is assessed by direct inoculation and mixing of the test strains in the product, and determination of survival of the test strains with time.

Water activity in products plays an important role in the growth of contaminating microorganisms. In the case of articles packaged in a multiple-dose container, the degeneration change in quality could be occurred during use due to the microbial secondary contamination, and if such contaminated product is used it could cause not only a decreasing in medical effect but also a hazard to the patient from infection. From these reasons, to the products packaged in multiple-dose containers addition of appropriate preservatives is permitted by General Rules for Preparations in the JP.

Preservatives must not be used solely to comply with GMP for drugs or to reduce viable aerobic (bacteria and yeasts/moulds) counts. In addition, preservatives show the toxicity depending on quantity. Therefore, preservatives must not be added to products in amounts which might jeopardize the safety of human beings, and consideration must be given to minimizing the amounts of preservative used. These tests are commonly used to verify that products maintain their preservative effectiveness at the design phase of formulation or in the case of periodic monitoring. Although these tests are not performed for lot release testing, antimicrobial action of the product itself or the efficacy of the preservative added to the product should be verified over the shelf life. Testing for antimicrobial preservative content should normally be performed at release. Under certain circumstances, in-process testing may suffice in lieu of release testing.

1. Products and their Categories

The products have been divided into two categories for these tests (Table 1). Category I products are those made with aqueous bases or vehicles, and having a water activity of not less than 0.6. Category II products are those made with nonaqueous bases or vehicles. Oil-in-water emulsions are considered Category I products, and water-in-oil emulsions Category II products.

2. Test Microorganisms, Growth Promotion Test and Suitability of the Counting Method

2.1. Preparation of test strains

Seed lot culture maintenance techniques (seed-lot systems) are used so that the viable micro-organisms used for inoculation are not more than 5 passages removed from the original master seed-lot. Grow each of the bacterial and fungal test strains separately as described in Table 2. The strains shown in Table 2 or those considered to be equivalent are used as the test microorganisms.

In addition to these strains designated as test microorganisms, it is desirable to use strains that might contaminate the product and grow on or in it, depending on its characteristics. It is desirable, for example, that *Zygosaccharomyces rouxii* (NCYC 381; IP 2021.92; NBRC 1960) is used for the products like as Syrups containing a high concentration of sugar. The test strains can be harvested by growth on solid agar or liquid media.

Cultures on agar media: Inoculate each of the five test strains on the surface of agar plates or agar slants. For growth of bacteria, use Soybean-Casein Digest Agar Medium, and for yeasts and moulds, use Sabouraud Glucose Agar Medium. Incubate bacterial cultures at 30 - 35°C for 18 to 24 hours, the culture of *Candida albicans* at 20 - 25°C for 44 to 52 hours and the culture of *Aspergillus brasiliensis* at 20 - 25°C for 6 to 10 days or until good sporulation is obtained. For the bacteria and *C. albicans*, harvest the cultured cells aseptically. Suspend the collected cells in physiological saline and adjust the viable cell count to about 10^8 CFU/mL. In the case of *A. brasiliensis*, suspend the cultured cells in physiological saline containing 0.05 w/v% of polysorbate 80 and adjust the spore count to about 10^8 CFU/mL. Filter, if needed, the spore suspension through a sterilized gauze or glass wool to remove hyphae. The medium components must be removed from all of the cells so prepared by centrifugation if needed. Use these suspensions as the inocula.

Liquid cultures: After cultivation each of the four strains except for *A. brasiliensis* in Soybean-Casein Digest Medium or in Fluid Sabouraud Glucose Medium, remove the medium by centrifugation. Wash the cells in physiological saline and resuspend them in the same solution with the viable cell count of the inoculum adjusted to about 10^8 CFU/mL.

When strains other than the five listed above are cultured, select a culture medium suitable for growth of the strain concerned. The cell suspension may also be prepared by a method suitable for that strain. If it is not possible to inoculate the microbial suspensions into the test specimens within 2 hours after they have been prepared from the cultivations on agar media or in liquid media, keep them at 2 - 8°C and use within 24 hours. Usually, the spore of *A. brasiliensis* may be stored at 2 - 8°C for up to 7 days. Determine the viable cell count of the inocula immediately before use, and then calculate the theoretical viable cell count per mL or per gram of the product present just after inoculation.

Table 1 Product categories

Category	Products
IA	· Injections · Sterile products made by dissolving or suspending in aqueous vehicles (ophthalmic preparations, ear preparations, nasal preparations, etc.)
IB	· Topically used non-sterile products made by dissolving or suspending in aqueous vehicles or by mixing with aqueous bases (ear preparations, nasal preparations, inhalations, including those applied to mucous membranes, etc.)
IC	· Preparations for oral administration other than antacids made by dissolving or suspending in aqueous vehicles or by mixing with aqueous bases and those applied to the oral cavity.
ID	· Antacids made with aqueous vehicles or bases
II	· All the dosage forms listed under Category I made with non-aqueous bases or vehicles

Table 2 Test microorganisms and culture conditions

Organism	Strain	Medium	Incubation temperature	Inoculum incubation time
Escherichia coli	ATCC 8739 NBRC 3972	Soybean-Casein Digest Medium Soybean-Casein Digest Agar Medium	30 - 35°C	18 - 24 hours
Pseudomonas aeruginosa	ATCC 9027 NBRC 13275	Soybean-Casein Digest Medium Soybean-Casein Digest Agar Medium	30 - 35°C	18 - 24 hours
Staphylococcus aureus	ATCC 6538 NBRC 13276	Soybean-Casein Digest Medium Soybean-Casein Digest Agar Medium	30 - 35°C	18 - 24 hours
Candida albicans	ATCC 10231 NBRC 1594	Fluid Sabouraud Glucose Medium Sabouraud Glucose Agar Medium	20 - 25°C	44 - 52 hours
Aspergillus brasiliensis	ATCC 16404 NBRC 9455	Sabouraud Glucose Agar Medium	20 - 25°C	6 - 10 days

2.2. Growth Promotion of the Media

An appropriate culture medium among Soybean-Casein Digest Ager Medium and Sabouraud Glucose Agar Medium is used for these tests. Other media also may be used if they have similar nutritive ingredients and growth-promoting properties for the microorganisms to be tested. For the media to be used, the growth promotion test should be performed using the strains specified in Table 2 or those considered to be equivalent. The incubation times are not more than 3 days for Soybean-Casein Digest Agar Medium, and not more than 5 days for Sabouraud Glucose Agar Medium.

By the agar media the colony counts should be obtained at least 50% of the standardized cell counts. For a freshly prepared inoculum, growth of the micro-organisms comparable to that previously obtained with a previously tested and approved batch of medium occurs.

2.3. Suitability of the Counting Method

Dilute 1 mL or 1 g of the product to be examined with 9 times its mass of physiological saline or other appropriate neutral diluting solution (10^{-1} dilution), mix, and prepare more two dilutions of this solution by serial 10-fold dilution (10^{-2} and 10^{-3} dilutions). Add a suitable count of the test strains to each tube of these dilutions, mix, and inoculate them so as to yield less than 250 CFU/plate for bacteria and *C. albicans* (ideally 25 - 250 CFU) or less than 80 CFU/plate for *A. brasiliensis* (ideally 8 - 80 CFU). This plating should be performed minimally in duplicate (or more to minimize variability in the plate count estimate). A positive control for this procedure is to introduce the same inocula into saline and transfer similar volumes of saline to agar plates. A suitable recovery scheme is the one that provides at least 50% of this saline control count (averaged). If the growth of the cells is inhibited an effective inactivator may be added in the buffer solution or liquid medium to be used for dilution of the test specimen, as well as in the agar plate count medium. However, it is necessary to confirm that the inactivator has no effect on the growth of the microorganisms. When the occurrence of the preservative or the product itself affects determination of the viable cell count and there is no suitable inactivator available, calculate the viable cell counts by the Membrane filtration method in Microbiological Examination of Non-sterile Products <*4.05*>. In the case where any change is occurred in the test material or procedure or in the product to be examined which might give any effects to the test result, the validation must be performed for the test once again. In the validation study, if the cell recovery count is not less than 50% of the inoculated cell counts, the inoculated cell counts at 0 day may be used as the theoretical inoculate cell count. See 3.2 for more information to obtain suitable counting method for the Category II products.

3. Test Procedure

3.1. Category I products

Inject each of the cell suspensions aseptically into five containers containing the product and mix uniformly. Single-strain challenges rather than mixed cultures should be used. When it is difficult to inject the cell suspension into the container aseptically or the volume of the product in each container is too small to be tested, transfer aseptically a sufficient volume of the product into each of alternative sterile containers, and mix the inoculum. When the product is not sterile, incubate additional containers containing the uninoculated product as controls and calculate their viable cell counts. The volume of the suspension mixed in the product is 0.5 - 1.0% of the volume of the product. Generally, the cell suspension is inoculated and mixed so that the concentration of viable cells is 1×10^5 to 1×10^6 CPU per mL or per g of the product. For Category ID products (antacids) inoculate so that the final concentration of viable cells is 1×10^3 to 1×10^4 CFU per mL of the product. Incubate these inoculated containers at 20 - 25°C with protection from light, and calculate the viable cell count of the test preparations at 0, 7 (Category IA only), 14 and 28 days. Record any marked changes (e.g., changes in color or the development of a bad odor or fungus) when observed in the test preparations during this time. Such changes should be considered when assessing the preservative efficacy of the product concerned. The sequential changes in the viable counts are expressed as changes in term of log reduction against the inoculated cell counts (CFU/mg or g). Determination of the viable cell counts is based, in principle, on the Plate-count methods (Pour-plate methods; Surface-spread method) or the Membrane filtration method in "Microbiological Examination of Non-sterile Products <*4.05*>". Alternative microbiological procedures, including an automated method, may be used for the products of Categories I and II, provided that they give a result equal to or better than that of the Pharmacopoeial methods[3)].

3.2. Category II products

The procedures are the same as those described for Category I products, but special procedures and considerations are required for both uniform dispersion of the test microorganism in the product and determination of viable cell counts in the test preparations.

For semisolid ointment bases, heat the test preparation to 45°C to 50°C until it becomes oily, add the cell suspension and disperse the inoculum uniformly with a sterile glass rod or spatula. Surfactants may also be added to achieve uniform dispersion, but it is necessary to confirm that the surfactant added has no effect on survival or growth of the test microorganisms and that it does not potentiate the preservative efficacy of the product. For determination of the viable cell count, a surfactant or emulsifier may be added to disperse the test preparations uniformly in the buffer solution or liquid medium. Sorbitan monooleate, polysorbate 80 or lecithin may be added to improve miscibility between the buffer solution or the liquid medium and semisolid ointments or oils in which test microorganisms were inoculated. These agents serve to inactivate or neutralize many of the most commonly used preservatives.

4. Interpretation

Interpret the preservative efficacy of the product according to Table 3. When the results described in Table 3 are obtained, the product examined is considered to be met the requirement of the test. There is a strong possibility of massive microbial contamination having occurred when microorganisms other than the inoculated ones are found in the sterile product to be examined, and caution is required in the test procedures and/or the control of the manufacturing process of the product. When the contamination level in a nonsterile product to be examined exceeds the microbial enumeration limit specified in "Microbial Attributes of Nonsterile Pharmaceutical Products <*G4-1-170*>" in General Information, caution is also required in the test procedures and/or the control of the manufacturing process of the product. The statement "No increase from the initial count" means not more than 0.5 $\log_{10}$ increase from the initial calculated count.

5. Culture Media

Culture media used for Preservatives Effectiveness Tests are described below. Other media may be used if they have similar nutritive ingredients and selective and growth-promoting properties for the microorganisms to be tested.

(i) Soybean-Casein Digest Medium

Casein peptone	17.0 g
Soybean peptone	3.0 g
Sodium chloride	5.0 g
Dipotassium hydrogen phosphate	2.5 g
Glucose monohydrate	2.5 g
Water	1000 mL

Adjust the pH so that after sterilization it is 7.1 - 7.5 at 25°C. Sterilize in an autoclave using a validated cycle.

Table 3 Interpretation criteria by product category

Category	Microorganisms	Interpretation criteria
IA	Bacteria	At 7 days: Not less than 1.0 log reduction from the initial count.
		At 14 days: Not less than 3.0 log reduction from the initial count.
		At 28 days: No increase from the 14 day's count.
	Yeasts/Moulds	At 7, 14 and 28 days: No increase from the initial count.
IB	Bacteria	At 14 days: Not less than 2.0 log reduction from the initial count.
		At 28 days: No increase from the 14 day's count.
	Yeasts/Moulds	At 14 and 28 days: No increase from the initial count.
IC	Bacteria	At 14 days: Not less than 1.0 log reduction from the initial count.
		At 28 days: No increase from the 14 day's count.
	Yeasts/Moulds	At 14 and 28 days: No increase from the initial count.
ID	Bacteria	At 14 and 28 days: No increase from the initial count.
	Yeasts/Moulds	At 14 and 28 days: No increase from the initial count.
II	Bacteria	At 14 and 28 days: No increase from the initial count.
	Yeasts/Moulds	At 14 and 28 days: No increase from the initial count.

(ii) Soybean-Casein Digest Agar Medium

Casein peptone	15.0 g
Soybean peptone	5.0 g
Sodium chloride	5.0 g
Agar	15.0 g
Water	1000 mL

Adjust the pH so that after sterilization it is 7.1 – 7.5 at 25°C. Sterilize in an autoclave using a validated cycle.

(iii) Sabouraud Glucose Agar Medium

Glucose	40.0 g
Peptone (animal tissue and casein 1:1)	10.0 g
Agar	15.0 g
Water	1000 mL

Adjust the pH so that after sterilization it is 5.4 – 5.8 at 25°C. Sterilize in an autoclave using a validated cycle.

iv) Fluid Sabouraud Glucose Medium

Glucose	20.0 g
Peptone (animal tissue and casein 1:1)	10.0 g
Water	1000 mL

Adjust the pH so that after sterilization it is 5.4 – 5.8 at 25°C. Sterilize in an autoclave using a validated cycle.

6. References

1) European Pharmacopoeia. 8.0 (2014), 5.1.3. Efficacy of Antimicrobial Preservation.
2) U.S. Pharmacopeia. 38 (2015), <51> Antimicrobial Effectiveness Testing.
3) The Japanese Pharmacopoeia, General Information ''Rapid Microbial Methods *<G4-6-170>*''

Bacterial Endotoxins Test and Alternative Methods using Recombinant Protein-reagents for Endotoxin Assay *<G4-4-180>*

Endotoxins, also called lipopolysaccharides, are present in the outer cell membrane of Gram-negative bacteria and exhibit various biological activities. Endotoxins, when entering the blood stream, can cause fever even in a very small quantity, and a large quantity of endotoxins is very toxic and can cause death due to endotoxin shock. In addition, endotoxins may contaminate pharmaceutical preparations during the production process because these are derived from Gram-negative bacteria widely present in the environment and because these are hard to be inactivated due to their heat-resistance. Endotoxins are designated as substances which should be controlled to ensure the safety of pharmaceutical preparations, etc., because these exhibit higher pyrogenicity than other well-known pyrogens which may contaminate them. Bacterial Endotoxins Test *<4.01>* is an *in vitro* test method that can detect endotoxins with high sensitivity using amoebocyte lysate prepared from blood corpuscle extracts of horseshoe crabs, and is applicable to injections, etc. On the other hand, recombinant protein-reagents for endotoxin assay have been developed as alternatives to lysate reagents for the purpose of protecting horseshoe crabs, ensuring a stable supply of reagents, reducing differences between reagent lots, and improving the continuity of the tests.

This General Information describes procedures and consideration in measurement when using recombinant protein-reagents for endotoxin assay as alternative methods, in addition to lysate reagents and test methods in Bacterial Endotoxins Test *<4.01>*.

1. Measurement principle of the Bacterial Endotoxins Test

Bacterial Endotoxins Test *<4.01>* is a test to detect or quantify bacterial endotoxins using amoebocyte lysate prepared from blood corpuscle extracts of horseshoe crab (*Limulus polyphemus* or *Tachypleus tridentatus*). This test utilizes the reaction in which the hemocyte extract of horseshoe crab is coagulated by endotoxins, and the coagulation reaction is based on a chain reaction by multiple serine proteases triggered by endotoxins (Fig. 1). Endotoxins activate factor C contained in the hemocyte extract of horseshoe crab to convert to an active serine protease, which in turn successively activates factor B, and then proclotting enzyme. Finally, coagulogen, which is a coagulant protein, is hydrolyzed to result in coagulin, and insoluble gel is formed and solidified. In addition, the hemocyte extract of horseshoe crab reacts not only to endotoxins but also mainly to (1→3)-β-D-glucans and coagulates by a chain reaction starting from factor G.

2. Measurement methods in the Bacterial Endotoxins Test

Bacterial Endotoxins Test *<4.01>* includes the gel-clot techniques, which are based on the gel formation of the lysate TS, and the photometric quantitative techniques, which are based on endotoxin-induced optical changes (Fig. 1).

The gel-clot techniques visually confirm the presence or absence of gel formation and require no special device for the determination. The gel-clot techniques include a limit test and a quantitative test. The former is a method for judging whether a sample contains endotoxins exceeding the endotoxin limit specified in each monograph, using the labeled sensitivity of a lysate reagent as an index. The latter is a method for quantifying the amount of endotoxins in a sample by determining an endpoint, which is defined as the highest dilution of a sample solution showing the gel formation.

The photometric quantitative techniques include the turbidimetric technique and the chromogenic technique (Fig. 1). In both techniques, the lysate TS and a sample solution are mixed, and the reaction solution is measured after a given time or over time using a spectrophotometer. The turbidimetric technique measures turbidity changes accompanying gelation of the lysate TS using absorbance or transmittance, and the chromogenic technique measures the amount of chromophore released from a synthetic chromogenic substrate by the reaction of endotoxins with the lysate TS using absorbance or transmittance.

3. Reagents used for the Bacterial Endotoxins Test

There are several lysate reagents used for the Bacterial Endotoxins Test <*4.01*> corresponding to each test method. The reagents are classified into two types based on their reactivity to endotoxins and β-glucans. One is a reagent type which contains both the cascade starting from factor C and the cascade starting from factor G. The other is a reagent type which detects only endotoxins by the cascade starting from factor C due to the fact that the activity of factor G is either removed or suppressed. Appropriate reagents should be selected depending on the sample to be examined and the purpose of the test.

On lysate reagents used for the gel-clot techniques, the lowest concentration of endotoxins that cause coagulation (gel formation) is set as the labeled lysate reagent sensitivity (endotoxin unit (EU)/mL) by the reagent manufacturers. The acceptance of a sample is judged using the labeled sensitivity as an index. In order to obtain accurate test results, confirm that the labeled sensitivity is appropriate according to 4.1.1. Test for confirmation of labeled lysate reagent sensitivity in Bacterial Endotoxins Test <*4.01*> 4.1. Preparatory testing. If the geometric mean endpoint concentration does not fall within the specified range, repeat the test after adjusting test conditions. If the geometric mean endpoint concentration does not fall within the specified range by the retest, the lysate reagent cannot be used.

When using lysate reagents for the photometric quantitative techniques, for both turbidimetric and chromogenic techniques, a standard curve is prepared using the standard solutions of three or more concentrations within the quantifiable concentration range. Confirm that the test procedures of an operator and test conditions are appropriate according to 5.3.1. Test for assurance of criteria for the standard curve in the Bacterial Endotoxins Test <*4.01*> 5.3. Preparatory testing. Although the labeled sensitivity is not shown on the lysate reagents used for the photometric quantitative techniques, the lowest concentration of the standard solution used for the generation of the standard curve corresponds to the labeled sensitivity.

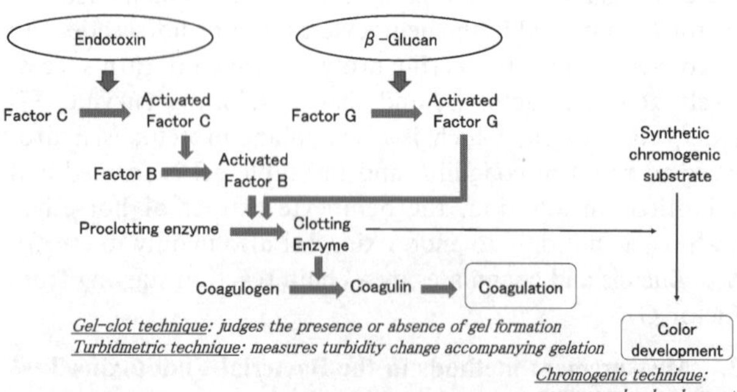

Fig. 1 Measurement principle and assay methods in Bactrial Endotoxins Test <*4.01*>

Most pharmaceuticals are found to interfere with the bacterial endotoxins test performance, although to greater or lesser degrees. In general, the influence of interfering factors present in a sample solution can often be overcome by dilution. In this case, samples should be diluted with water for bacterial endotoxins test within the range that does not exceed a Maximum Valid Dilution for the measurement. The Maximum Valid Dilution is the maximum allowable dilution of a sample solution. As shown in Bacterial Endotoxins Test <*4.01*> 3. Determination of Maximum Valid Dilution, λ is a labeled sensitivity for a lysate reagent in the gel-clot techniques and is the lowest concentration of a standard curve for a lysate reagent in the photometric quantitative techniques; the smaller the λ, the larger the maximum valid dilution. λ for many lysate reagents used for the photometric quantitative techniques is smaller than that for lysate reagents used for the gel-clot techniques. If interfering factors contained in a sample are definite, perform procedures to reduce them. If interfering factors cannot be reduced or interference cannot be avoided because of indefinite interfering factors, consider using other lysate reagents or changing the test method.

4. Measurement by alternative methods using recombinant protein-reagents for endotoxin assay and points to consider in the measurement

Recombinant protein-reagents for endotoxin assay use protein(s) prepared using the gene sequence of fators contained in blood corpuscle extracts of horseshoe crabs. These reagents include reagents that use the recombinant protein prepared using the gene sequence of factor C contained in blood corpuscle extracts of horseshoe crab (e.g. *Carcinoscorpius rotundicauda* or *T. tridentatus*), and reagents that use the recombinant proteins prepared using the gene sequence of factor C, factor B and proclotting enzyme contained in blood corpuscle extracts of horseshoe crab (e.g. *T. tridentatus*). One of the former reagents measures the amount of fluorescence generated by cleavage of a fluorescent synthetic substrate by recombinant factor C which has been activated by endotoxins. In one of the latter reagents composed of the three kinds of recombinant proteins, endotoxins activate recombinant factor C, and it further activates recombinant factor B followed by activation of recombinant proclotting enzyme in the same manner as the chromogenic technique. The change in absorbance at a specific wavelength is measured as a result of chromophore released from the synthetic chromogenic substrate. The both cases, a reagent solution and a sample solution are mixed, the fluorescence intensity or absorbance of the reaction solution is measured optically after a given time or over time.

The recombinant protein-reagents for endotoxin assay do not identical to "an amoebocyte lysate prepared from blood corpuscle extracts of horseshoe crab" specified in Bacterial Endotoxins Test <*4.01*>. If these reagents for endotoxin assay are used as an alternative method, confirm that accuracy, precision, sensitivity, specificity, etc. are equal or better compared to Bacterial Endotoxins Test <*4.01*> using lysate reagents. Among the recombinant protein-reagents for endotoxin assay, some have been reported to have sensitivity and specificity equal to or better than the method using lysate reagents. When bacterial endotoxins tests <*4.01*> for pharmaceuticals, etc. are performed using recombinant protein-reagents, it is necessary to conduct 5.3.1.Test for assurance of criteria for the standard curve 5.3. Preparatory testing as with the Photometric quantitative techniques in Bacterial Endotoxins Test <*4.01*>, and in that case the lowest concentration of the standard curve corresponds to λ (EU/mL). In addition, it is necessary to pay attention to interference, and 5.3.2.Test for interfering factors should be performed. In the case where measurement methods that are not used in Bacterial Endotoxins Test <*4.01*> such as the methods that measure the amount of fluorescence are used, it is also necessary to be careful of potential interference because even substances that do not disturb the measurement when using lysate reagents may exhibit interference such as the inhibition of the generation of fluorescence. In addition, regarding reagents prepared using the gene sequence of the proteins of different species of horseshoe crab from horseshoe crab (*L. polyphemus* or *T. tridentatus*) specified in Bacterial Endotoxins Test <*4.01*>, it should be noted that difference of the recombinant proteins may affect the reactivity to endotoxins.

Decision of Limit for Bacterial Endotoxins <*G4-5-131*>

The endotoxin limit for injections is to be decided as follows:

$$\text{Endotoxin limit} = K/M$$

where K is a threshold pyrogenic dose of endotoxin per kg body mass (EU/kg), and depending on the administration route, values for K are set as in the following table.

Intended route of administration	K (EU/kg)
Intravenous	5.0
Intravenous, for radiopharmaceuticals	2.5
Intraspinal	0.2

M is equal to the maximum bolus dose of product per kg body mass. When the product is to be injected at frequent intervals or infused continuously, M is the maximum total dose administered in a single hour period. M is expressed in mL/kg for products to be administered by volume, in mg/kg or mEq/kg for products to be administered by mass, and in Unit/kg for products to be administered by biological units.

Notes:

1) For products to be administered by mass or by units, the endotoxin limit should be decided based on the labeled amount of the principal drug.

2) Sixty kg should be used as the average body mass of an adult when calculating the maximum adult dose per kg.

3) The pediatric dose per kg body mass should be used when this is higher than the adult dose.

4) The K values for the intravenous route are applicable to drugs to be administered by any route other than those shown in the table.

Rapid Microbial Methods <*G4-6-170*>

Advances in science and technology have provided new methods to perform high-precision measurements of bacterial physiological activities, intracellular components, and so on, and consequently new techniques for bacterial detection, enumeration and quantification have appeared. Since the 1980s it has become clear that the majority of bacteria in the natural environment have low growth ability in conventional culture media, and the detection, enumeration and identification of these bacteria are difficult by means of culture methods alone. The bacterial cell counts obtained vary from method to method, and it should be noted that it is difficult to obtain a reliable value even applied with a new method. Moreover, even if type strains exist for method validation, it is not easy to standardize the physiological activity.

Compared to the conventional methods, these new methods are not necessarily superior in every respect, but they usually offer greater speed and accuracy, and can be applied not only to bacteria, but also to fungi and viruses. Therefore, these new methods are very useful to improve the standards of microbial control in critical areas, and to decrease the risk of hazardous microbial contamination.

The conventional cultivation-based methods use colony formation or turbidity change due to cell growth as an indicator, whereas the new methods vary greatly as regards the detection target and the detection principle. The new methods may be more suitable for obtaining a comprehensive understanding of the microbial community, as well as for identifying specific microorganisms. Among these methods, phylogenic analysis based on gene sequences has become popular, and the dramatic development of sequencing techniques in recent years now allows us to analyze the composition of the microbial community in a short time. In this information chapter, the principles of the new methods and their range of applicability are introduced, and key points in the usage of these methods are described.

1. Detection targets and principles

Name	Target	Principles of measurement	Examples of measurement device
1) Direct Method			
Solid phase cytometry	Microorganism	Directly detect the signals from the bacteria trapped onto a filter. The signals on their physiological activities can be obtained by choosing suitable dyes. Autofluorescence may also be used. To selectively detect specific bacteria, gene probe, antibody or fluorescent-labeled phage may be utilized. Various optical devices including a fluorescent microscope and laser microscope are used as detection/measurement apparatus.	Fluorescence microscope, Laser scanning cytometer, etc.
Flow cytometry	Microorganism	Directly detect the signals given by the bacteria passing through fluid or air. The signals on their physiological activities can be obtained by choosing suitable dyes. Autofluorescence may also be used. To selectively detect specific bacteria, gene probe, antibody or fluorescent-labeled phage may be utilized. Various optical devices are used as detection/measurement apparatus.	Flow cytometer, etc.
2) Indirect Method			
Immunological methods	Antigen	React the antigen of bacteria with the specific antibody, and detect the color or fluorescence visually or by a microplate reader. Immunochromatography is a simple and easy method for the purpose.	Immunochromatography, Micro plate reader
Nucleic acid amplification	Nucleic acid	Amplify a nucleic acid of microorganism by using the primers specific to the target microorganism, and analyze the amplified nucleic acid fragments. Quantitative determination is possible by performing of quantitative PCR.	Electrophoresis apparatus, Quantitative PCR
Bioluminescence/fluorescence	ATP, etc.	Measure ATP which is released from microorganisms on the basis of luminous or fluorescence phenomena occurred by enzyme reaction.	luminescence detector, fluorescence detector
Micro colony method	Growth (Micro colony)	Detect and count the micro colony that appears in early stage of colonization. The same culture conditions (medium composition, temperature, etc.) as the plate culture method can be used.	Fluorescence microscopy etc.
Impedance method	Growth (Electrical characteristic)	Utilize the change in electrical properties of medium due to the metabolites produced by the growth of microorganisms.	Electrodes
Gas measuring method	Growth (Gas production, etc.)	Utilize the change in amount of gases caused by CO_2 production, O_2 consumption, etc. with the growth of microorganisms.	Gas measuring instrument Color change of medium
Fatty acid profiles	Fatty acid	Utilize the fatty acid profile of cell components that differs depending on the taxonomic groups of microorganism.	Gas chromatography
Infrared spectroscopy	Cell component	Utilize the pattern of infrared spectrum obtained by infrared light irradiation to whole microorganism.	Fourier transformation infrared spectroscope
Mass spectrometry	Cell component	Measure the cell component by means of a mass spectrometer, and identify it by database.	Mass spectrometry
Genetic fingerprinting method	DNA	Utilize the electrophoresis pattern of DNA fragments obtained by cleaving the DNA extracted from sample with a restriction enzyme. It can be identified by database. Analysis of community structure is possible by T-RFLP.	Electrophoresis apparatus
High throughput sequencing	Nucleic acid	Determine the sequence of nucleic acids extracted from bacteria exist in sample, and analyze the community structure phylogenetically.	Sequencer, etc.

Note) PCR: Polymerase Chain Reaction T-RFLP: Terminal Restriction Fragment Length Polymorphism

2. Validation

To qualify introduced equipment, a standard component or strain, which represents the target of each method, should be utilized. That is, in direct measurement, type strains should be used, while in indirect measurement, standard components, etc., of the target bacteria are used.

To validate a protocol/procedure, it is required to demonstrate that the detection target is a suitable index/indicator for bacterial number or quantity. It is also important to state whether any special precautions are necessary in applying the protocol/procedure. When using a type strain, the result of validation should be equivalent to or better than that of the conventional method. However, because the detection principles of new methods are usually different from that of conventional methods, the correlation between them is not always required. For detection of environmental bacteria, it is important that the physiological state of the type strain should be maintained as close as possible to that of environmental bacteria, in order to obtain reliable results.

3. Applications and particular considerations:

New methods are expected to find application in a variety of fields. However, since their detection targets and detection protocols/procedures are different from the conventional methods, the resulting data may not show a good correlation with existing data. Although, it is important in principle that a new method should have an equal or greater capability than the conventional method, a new method may be used after verifying their validity, even in the absence of equivalence to conventional methods.

Because the new methods are rapid, product testing, environmental monitoring, bioburden evaluation, raw materials control, etc. can be performed in real-time, and this is highly advantageous for process control, allowing alert levels, action levels and so on to be set up based on trend analysis of the obtained data.

These new rapid methods may be applied to;

- Quality control of pharmaceutical manufacturing water
- Microbial evaluation of processing areas
- Sterility test
- Microbial limit test
- Antimicrobial and preservatives effectiveness test
- Raw material acceptance test

etc.

Rapid Identification of Microorganisms Based on Molecular Biological Method
<G4-7-160>

This chapter describes the methods for the identification or estimation of microorganisms (bacteria and fungi), found in in-process control tests or lot release tests of pharmaceutical products, at the species or genus level based on their DNA sequence homology. The identification of isolates found in the sterility test or aseptic processing can be helpful for investigating the causes of contamination. Furthermore, information on microorganisms found in raw materials used for pharmaceutical products, processing areas of pharmaceutical products, and so on is useful in designing measures to control the microbiological quality of drugs. For the identification of microorganisms, phenotypic analysis is widely used, based on morphological, physiological, and biochemical features and analysis of components. Commercial kits based on differences in phenotype patterns have been used for the identification of microorganisms, but are not always applicable to microorganisms found in raw materials used for pharmaceutical products and in processing areas of pharmaceutical products. In general, the identification of microorganisms based on phenotypic analysis needs special knowledge and judgment is often subjective. It is considered that the evolutionary history of microorganisms is memorized in their ribosomal RNAs (rRNAs), so that systematic classification and identification of microorganisms in recent years have been based on the analysis of these sequences. This chapter presents a rapid method to identify or estimate microorganisms based on partial sequences of divergent regions of the 16S rRNA gene for bacteria and of the internal transcribed spacer 1 (ITS1) region located between 18S rRNA and 5.8S rRNA for fungi, followed by comparison of the sequences with those in the database. Methods described in this chapter do not take the place of usual other methods for the identification, and can be modified based on the examiner's experience, and on the available equipment or materials. Other gene regions besides those mentioned in this chapter can be used if appropriate.

1. Apparatuses

(i) DNA sequencer

Various types of sequencers using a gel board or capillary can be used.

(ii) DNA amplifier

To amplify target DNA and label amplified (PCR) products with sequencing reagents.

2. Procedures

The following procedures are described as an example.

2.1. Preparation of template DNA

It is important to use a pure cultivated bacterium or fungus for identification. In the case of colony samples, colonies are picked up with a sterilized toothpick (in the case of fungi, a small fragment of colony sample is picked up), and suspended in 0.3 mL of DNA releasing solution in a 1.5 mL centrifuge tube. In the case of culture fluid, a 0.5 mL portion of fluid is put in a 1.5 mL centrifuge tube and centrifuged at 10,000 rpm for 10 minutes. After removal of the supernatant, the pellet is suspended in 0.3 mL of DNA releasing solution, and then heated at 100°C for 10 minutes. In general, PCR can be run for bacteria and yeasts heated in DNA releasing solution. For fungi, DNA extraction from culture fluid is better because some of colony samples can disturb PCR reaction.

2.2. PCR

Add 2 μL of template DNA in PCR reaction solution. Use 10F/800R primers (or 800F/1500R primers in the case to analyze also a latter part of 16S rRNA) for bacteria and ITS1F/ITS1R primers for fungi, and then perform 30 amplification cycles at 94°C for 30 seconds, 55°C for 60 seconds, and 72°C for 60 seconds. DNA fragments are amplified about 800 bp in the case of bacteria and about 150 – 470 bp depending on the strain in the case of fungi. Include a negative control (water instead of the test solution) in the PCR.

2.3. Confirmation of PCR products

Mix 5 μL of PCR product with 1 μL of loading buffer solution, place it in a 1.5 w/v% agarose gel well, and carry out electrophoresis with TAE buffer solution (1-fold concentration). Carry out the electrophoresis together with appropriate DNA size markers. After the electrophoresis, observe PCR products on a trans-illuminator (312 nm) and confirm the presence of a single band of the targeted size. If multiple bands are observed, cut the targeted band out of the gel, and extract DNA by using appropriate commercial DNA extraction kit.

2.4. Purification of PCR products

Various methods are available for removing unreached substances (dNTP, prime, etc.). Purify according to the protocol of the method adopted.

2.5. Quantification of purified DNA

When purified DNA is measured by spectrophotometer, calculate 1 $OD_{260\ nm}$ as 50 μg/mL.

2.6. Labeling of PCR products with sequencing reagents

Use an appropriate fluorescence-labeled sequencing reagent suitable for the available DNA sequencer or its program and label the PCR products according to the instructions provided with the reagent.

2.7. Purification of sequencing reagent-labeled PCR products

Transfer the product in 75 μL of diluted ethanol (7 in 10) into a 1.5 mL centrifuge tube, keep in an ice bath for 20 minutes, and centrifuge at 15,000 rpm for 20 minutes. After removal of supernatant, add 250 μL of diluted ethanol (7 in 10) to the precipitate and centrifuge at 15,000 rpm for 5 minutes. Remove the supernatant and dry the precipitate.

2.8. DNA homology analysis

Place sequencing reagent-labeled PCR products in the DNA sequencer and read the nucleotide sequences of the PCR products. Compare the partial nucleotide sequence with those in the BLAST database.

3. Judgment

If sequencing data show over 90% identity with a sequence in the database, in general, judgment may be made as follows.

(i) In the case of bacteria, compare the nucleotides in the product obtained with the 10F primer (the 800F primer when 800F/1500R primers are used) with the BLAST database. Higher ranked species are judged as identified species or closely related species.

(ii) In the case of fungi, compare sequencing data for the product obtained with the ITS1F primer with the BLAST database. Higher ranked species are judged as identified species or closely related species.

4. Reagents, Test Solutions

(i) 0.5 mol/L Disodium dihydrogen ethylenediamine tetraacetate TS: Dissolve 18.6 g of disodium dihydrogen ethylenediamine tetraacetate dihydrate in water to make 100 mL.

(ii) 1 mol/L Tris buffer solution (pH 8.0): Dissolve 24.2 g of 2-amino-2-hydroxymethyl-1,3-propanediol in a suitable amount of water, adjust the pH to 8.0 with 0.2 mol/L hydrochloric acid TS, and add water to make 200 mL.

(iii) TE buffer solution: Mix 1.0 mL of 1 mol/L tris buffer solution (pH 8.0) and 0.2 mL of 0.5 mol/L disodium dihydrogen ethylenediamine tetraacetate TS, and add water to make 100 mL.

(iv) DNA releasing solution: Divide TE buffer solution containing 1 vol% of polyoxyethylene (10) octylphenyl ether into small amounts and store frozen until use.

(v) PCR reaction solution

10-fold buffer solution*	5 μL
dNTP mixture**	4 μL
10 μmol/L Sense primer	1 μL
10 μmol/L Anti-sense primer	1 μL
Heat-resistant DNA polymerase (1 U/μL)	1 μL
Water	36 μL

* Being composed of 100 mmol/L 2-amino-2-hydroxymethyl-1,3-propanediol hydrochloride (pH 8.4), 500 mmol/L potassium chloride, 20 mmol/L magnesium chloride and 0.1 g/L gelatin.

** A solution containing 2.5 mmol/L each of dGTP (sodium 2′-deoxyguanosine 5′-triphosphate), dATP (sodium 2′-deoxyadenosine 5′-triphosphate), dCTP (sodium 2′-deoxycytidine 5′-triphosphate) and dTTP (sodium 2′-deoxythymidine 5′-triphosphate). Adequate products containing these components as described above may be used.

(vi) Sequencing reagent: There are many kinds of sequencing methods, such as the dye-primer method for labeling of primer, the dye-terminator method for labeling of dNTP terminator and so on. Use an appropriate sequencing reagent kit for the apparatus and program to be used.

(vii) 50-Fold concentrated TAE buffer solution: Dissolve 242 g of 2-amino-2-hydroxymethyl-1,3-propanediol in 57.1 mL of acetic acid (100) and 100 mL of 0.5 mol/L disodium dihydrogen ethylenediamine tetraacetate TS, and add water to make 1000 mL.

(viii) 1-Fold concentrated TAE buffer solution: Diluted 50-fold concentrated TAE buffer solution (1 in 50) prepared before use is referred to as 1-fold concentrated TAE buffer solution.

(ix) Agarose gel: Mix 1.5 g of agarose, 2.0 mL of 50-fold concentrated TAE buffer solution, 10 μL of a solution of ethidium bromide (3,8-diamino-5-ethyl-6-phenylphenanthridinium bromide) (1 in 100) and 100 mL of water. After dissolving the materials by heating, cool the solution to about 60°C, and prepare gels.

(x) Loading buffer solution (6-fold concentrated): Dissolve 0.25 g of bromophenol blue, 0.25 g of xylene cyanol FF and 1.63 g of disodium dihydrogen ethylenediamine tetraacetate dihydrate in 50 mL of water, and add 30 mL of glycerol and water to make 100 mL.

(xi) PCR primers

For	Primer	
Bacteria	10F	5′-GTTTGATCCTGGCTCA-3′
	800R	5′-TACCAGGGTATCTAATCC-3′
	800F	5′-GGATTAGATACCCTGGTA-3′
	1500R	5′-TACCTTGTTACGACTT-3′
Fungi	ITS1F	5′-GTAACAAGGT(T/C)TCCGT-3′
	ITS1R	5′-CGTTCTTCATCGATG-3′

(xii) Polyoxyethylene(10)octylphenyl ether: A pale yellow, viscous liquid.

Rapid Counting of Microbes using Fluorescent Staining <*G4-8-152*>

This chapter provides rapid methods using fluorescence staining for the quantitative estimation of viable microorganisms. Incubation on an agar medium has been widely used for quantitative estimation of viable microorganisms, but a number of environmental microorganisms of interest are not easy to grow in culture under usual conditions, thus new microbial detection methods based on fluorescence or luminescence have been developed. In the fluorescence staining method, microorganisms are stained with fluorescent dye, and can easily be detected and counted with various sorts of apparatus, such as a fluorescence microscope or flow cytometer. Methods are available to detect total microorganisms, including both dead and viable cells, or to detect only cells with a specified bioactivity by choosing the dye reagent appropriately. Nucleic acid staining reagents, which bind with DNA or RNA, detect all cells containing nucleic acids, whether they are live or dead. This technique is the most fundamental for the fluorescence staining method. On the other hand, fluorescent vital staining methods target the respiratory activity of the microorganism and the activity of esterase, which is present universally in microorganisms. In the microcolony method, microcolonies in the early stage of colony formation are counted. The CFDA-DAPI double staining method and the microcolony method are described below. These methods can give higher counts than the other techniques, because these rapid and accurate techniques provide quantitative estimation of viable microorganisms based on a very specific definition of viability, which may be different from that implicit in other methods. The procedures of these methods described here may be changed as experience with the methods is accumulated. Therefore, other reagents, instruments and apparatus than those described here may also be used if there is a valid reason for so doing.

1. CFDA-DAPI double staining method

Fluorescein diacetate (FDA) reagents are generally used for the detection of microorganisms possessing esterase activity. These reagents are hydrolyzed by intracellular esterase, and the hydrolyzed dye exhibits green fluorescence under blue excitation light (about 490 nm). Modified FDAs such as carboxyfluorescein diacetate (CFDA) are used because of the low stainability of gramnegative bacteria with FDA. The principle of the CFDA-DAPI double staining method, which also employs a nucleic acid staining reagent, 4′,6-diamidino-2-phenylindole (DAPI), is as follows. The nonpolar CFDA penetrates into cells and is hydrolyzed to fluorescent carboxyfluorescein by intracellular esterase. The carboxyfluorescein is accumulated in the living cells due to its polarity, and therefore green fluorescence due to carboxyfluorescein occurs when cells possessing esterase activity are illuminated with blue excitation light. No fluorescent carboxyfluorescein is produced with dead cells, since they are unable to hydrolyze CFDA. On the other hand, DAPI binds preferentially to the adenine and thymine of DNA after penetration into both viable and dead microorganisms, and consequently all of the organisms containing DNA exhibit blue fluorescence under ultraviolet excitation light. Therefore, this double staining method enables to count specifically only live microorganisms possessing esterase activity under blue excitation light, and also to determine the total microbial count (viable and dead microorganisms) under ultraviolet excitation light.

1.1. Apparatus

1.1.1. Fluorescence microscope or fluorescence observation apparatus

Various types of apparatus for counting fluorescencestained microorganisms are available. Appropriate filters are provided, depending on the fluorescent dye reagents used. A fluorescence microscope, laser microscope, flow cytometer, and various other types of apparatus may be used for fluorescence observation.

1.2. Instruments

(i) Filtering equipment (funnels, suction flasks, suction pumps)

(ii) Membrane filters made of polycarbonate (poresize: 0.2 μm); A suitable filter that can trap particles on the surface can be used other than polycarbonate filter.

(iii) Glass slide

(iv) Cover glass

(v) Ocular micrometer for counting (with 10 × 10 grids)

1.3. Procedure

An example of the procedure using a fluorescence microscope is described below.

1.3.1. Preparation of samples

Prepare samples by ensuring that microbes are dispersed evenly in the liquid (water or buffer solution).

1.3.2. Filtration

Set a membrane filter made of polycarbonate (poresize: 0.2 μm) on the funnel of the filtering equipment. Filter an appropriate amount of a sample to trap microbes in the sample on the filter.

1.3.3. Staining

Pour sufficient amount of buffer solution for CFDA staining, mixed to provide final concentration of 150 μg/mL of CFDA and 1 μg/mL of DAPI, into the funnel of the filtering equipment and allow staining in room temperature for 3 minutes, then filter the liquid by suction. Pour sufficient amount of aseptic water in the funnel, filter by suction, and remove excess fluorescent reagent left on the filter. Thoroughly dry the filter.

1.3.4. Slide preparation

Put one drop of immersion oil for fluorescence microscope on the glass slide. Place the air dried filter over it, with the filtering side on the top. Then put one drop of immersion oil for fluorescence microscope on the surface of the filter, place a cover glass to enclose the filter. Put another drop of immersion oil for fluorescence microscope on the cover glass when using an oilimmersion objective lens.

1.3.5. Counting

Observe and count under a fluorescence microscope, with 1000 magnification. In case of CFDA-DAPI double staining method, count the microorganisms (with esterase activity) exhibiting green fluorescence under the blue excitation light first to avoid color fading by the ultraviolet light, then count the microorganisms (with DNA) exhibiting blue fluorescence under the ultraviolet excitation light in the same microscopic field. Count the organisms exhibiting fluorescence on more than 20 randomly selected fields among 100 grids observed through an ocular micrometer of the microscope, and calculate the total number of organisms using the following formula. The area of the microscopic field should be previously determined with the ocular and objective micrometers. The amount of the sample to be filtered must be adjusted so that the cell number per field is between 10 and 100. It might be necessary to reprepare the sample in certain instances. (In such case that the average count number is not more than 2 organisms per field, or where more than 5 fields are found which have no organism per field, it is assumed that the microorganism count is below the detection limit.)

Number of microbes (cells/mL)
= {(average number of microbes per visual field) × (area of filtration)}/{(amount of sample filtered) × (area of one microscopic field)}

1.4. Reagents and test solutions

(i) Aseptic water: Filter water through a membrane filter with 0.2 μm pore size, then sterilize it by heating in an autoclave at 121°C for 15 minutes. Water for injection may be used.

(ii) CFDA solution, 10 mg/mL: Dissolve 50 mg of CFDA in dimethylsulfoxide to prepare a 5 mL solution. Store at −20°C in light shielded condition.

(iii) Buffer solution for CFDA staining: Dissolve 5 g of sodium chloride with 0.5 mL of 0.1 mol/L disodium dihydrogen ethylenediamine tetraacetate TS and diluted disodium hydrogen phosphate TS (1 in 3) to prepare 100 mL of solution. Add sodium dihydrogen phosphate dihydrate solution (1 in 64) to adjust the pH level to 8.5. Filter the solution through a membrane filter with a pore size of 0.2 μm.

(iv) DAPI solution, 10 μg/mL: Dissolve 10 mg of DAPI

in 100 mL of aseptic water. Dilute this solution 10 times with aseptic water and filter through a membrane filter with a pore size of 0.2 μm. Store at 4°C in light shielded condition.

(v) Immersion oil for fluorescence microscope

2. Microcolony method

Microcolonies, which are in early stages of colony formation, are fluorescently stained, then observed and counted under a fluorescence microscope or other suitable systems. This method enables to count the number of proliferative microorganisms, with short incubation time. In this method, the organisms are trapped on a membrane filter, the filter is incubated on a medium for a short time, and the microcolonies are counted. By this method, even colonies which are undetectable with the naked eye can be identified, so viable organisms can be counted rapidly and with high precision. Various nucleic acid staining reagents can be used for staining of microcolonies.

2.1. Apparatus

2.1.1. Fluorescence microscope or fluorescence observation apparatus

Various types of apparatus for counting fluorescencestained microorganisms are available. Appropriate filters are provided, depending on the fluorescence dye reagents used. A fluorescence microscope, laser microscope and various other types of apparatus may be used for fluorescence observation.

2.2. Instruments

(i) Filtering equipment (funnels, suction flasks, suction pumps)

(ii) Membrane filters made of polycarbonate (pore size: 0.2 μm); A suitable filter that can trap particles on the surface can be used other than polycarbonate filter.

(iii) Glass slide

(iv) Cover glass

(v) Filter paper (No. 2)

(vi) Ocular micrometer for counting (with 10 × 10 grids)

2.3. Procedure

An example of the procedure using a fluorescence microscope is described below.

2.3.1. Preparation of samples

Prepare samples by ensuring that microbes are dispersed evenly in the liquid (water or buffer solution).

2.3.2. Filtration

Set a membrane filter made of polycarbonate (pore size: 0.2 μm) on the funnel of the filtering equipment. Filter an appropriate amount of sample to trap microbes in the sample on the filter.

2.3.3. Incubation

Remove the filter from the filtering equipment and place it with filtering side facing up on a culture medium avoiding formation of air bubbles between the filter and the medium. Incubate at a suitable temperature for appropriate hours in a dark place. It should be noted that the appropriate incubation conditions (such as medium, incubation temperature and/or incubation time) are different, depending on the sample.

2.3.4. Fixation

Soak a filter paper with an appropriate amount of neutral buffered formaldehyde solution, then place the filter that has been removed from the culture medium on top with filtering side up, and allow to remain at room temperature for more than 30 minutes to fix the microcolonies.

2.3.5. Staining

Soak a filter paper with an appropriate amount of staining solution (such as 1 μg/mL of DAPI, 2% polyoxyethylenesorbitan monolaurate), then place the filter on top with filtering side up, and then leave at room temperature, light shielded for 10 minutes to stain microcolonies. Wash the filter by placing it with the filtering side facing up on top of a filter paper soaked with aseptic water for 1 minute. Thoroughly air dry the filter.

2.3.6. Slide preparation

Put one drop of immersion oil for fluorescence microscope on the slide glass. Place an air dried filter over it, with the filtering side on the top. Then, put one drop of immersion oil for fluorescence microscope on top, place a cover glass to enclose the filter.

2.3.7. Counting

Count the organisms exhibiting fluorescence on more than 20 randomly selected fields among the 100 grids observed through an ocular micrometer of the microscope with 400 or 200 magnification, and calculate the total number of organisms using the following formula. The area of the microscopic field should be previously determined with the ocular and objective micrometers. In such case that the average count number is not more than 2 microcolonies per field, or where more than 5 fields are found which have no microcolony per field, it is assumed that the microorganism count is below the detection limit.

Number of microcolonies (cells/mL)
= {(average number of microcolonies per visual field) × (area of filtration)}/{(amount of sample filtered) × (area of one microscopic field)}

2.4. Reagents and test solutions

(i) Aseptic water: Filter water through a membrane filter with 0.2 μm pore size, and sterilize it by heating in an autoclave at 121°C for 15 minutes. Water for injection may be used.

(ii) Staining solution: Dissolve 10 mg of DAPI in 100 mL of aseptic water. Dilute the solution 10 times with aseptic water and filter through a membrane filter with pore size of 0.2 μm. Store at 4°C in light shielded condition. Dissolve polyoxyethylene sorbitan monolaurate to the final concentration of 2%, when using.

(iii) Neutral buffered formaldehyde solution (4w/v% formaldehyde solution; neutrally buffered).

(iv) Immersion oil for fluorescence microscope

Disinfection and Decontamination Methods <*G4-9-170*>

This chapter describes procedures for reducing the number of microorganisms to a predetermined level using chemical agents during hygiene control of structures and facilities in clean areas or aseptic processing areas that require cleanliness control, as well as of personnel involved in manufacturing control and manufacturing operations in those areas, in pharmaceutical product manufacturing plants.

Appropriate action should be taken based on this chapter when performing microbiological tests specified in the monographs, when taking measures needed to prevent microbial contamination of products and materials used in the manufacture of pharmaceutical products, and when microbial control is needed in pharmacies.

1. Terms and Definitions

The terms used in this chapter are defined as follows.

• Microorganisms: Generally it is a term for bacteria, fungi, protozoa, viruses, and the like. In this chapter, the term means bacteria and fungi.

• Disinfection: Generally it is a term for harmful microorganisms such as pathogens are removed, killed, or detoxified. In this chapter, the term means microorganisms on an object or in local areas such as the surface of an object are reduced.

• Decontamination: To reduce microorganisms in structures and facilities such as work space and work rooms to a predetermined microbial count level.

• Logarithmic reduction value: The difference in log values for microbial count before and after certain treatments.

• Disinfectant rotation: A disinfection program for when microorganisms that are resistant to a using disinfectant are discovered. In which a disinfectant with different efficacy is used until those microorganisms are no longer detected, or disinfectants with different mechanisms of action are alternately used for certain periods of time in turn. The effectiveness of this method should be evaluated before its implementation.

2. Disinfection Methods

This includes methods such as wiping, spraying, or immersion using chemical agents to reduce microorganisms on equipment, floors, walls, or containers that are carried into clean areas or aseptic processing areas, and the local surfaces such as the wrapping materials of environmental monitoring media. The disinfectants in Table 1 are commonly used, in single or in combination, upon due consideration of the nature of the surface to which the method is applied, such as corrosion by disinfectants, as well as the extent of contamination, such as the types and counts of microorganisms. Although this method does not kill or remove all microorganisms on an object or local surface, disinfectants of proven efficacy should be used when this method is employed. The effects of chemical agents used as disinfectants on microorganisms will differ depending on factors such as the applied concentration, temperature, contact time, and level of surface contamination. When using this method, attention should be paid to disinfectant expiration dates, microbial contamination, the effect of chemical residue on pharmaceutical product quality, and deterioration such as discoloration, deformation and corrosion of the materials being treated.

2.1. Disinfectants

Table 1 presents examples of commonly used disinfectants and their concentrations, and the microbial effects of these disinfectants. Disinfectants and concentrations proven to be safe and effective other than those shown here can also be used.

2.2. Evaluation Methods

When disinfection methods are applied to clean areas and aseptic processing areas, the effectiveness of the conditions should be checked upon due consideration of factors such as the disinfectant concentration, contact time, material of the surface being disinfected, and type of microorganisms that are to be reduced with the disinfectant. Examples of evaluation methods are provided below. Methods other than those shown in the examples may be used if they can be demonstrated to be scientifically appropriate.

2.2.1. Test Microorganism Suspension Method

The diluent that is actually used (purified water, tap water, etc.) should be used to adjust the disinfectant to the actually used concentration. Inoculate 1 mL of the prepared disinfectant with 10^5 to 10^6 CFU test microorganisms. Allow the disinfectant to take effect for the prescribed time (usually 5 to 15 minutes), then dilute or remove (filter) the disinfectant. In the diluent or filtered wash solution, neutralize[1] the disinfectant using a solution containing an inactivator such as lecithin, polysorbate 80, or sodium thiosulfate as needed. Count the number of the microorganisms used for inoculation and the number after disinfection under conditions meeting the requirements in Microbiological Examination of Non-sterile Products <*4.05*> I. 3.4 Suitability of the counting method in the presence of product. Calculate the logarithmic decrement from the test microorganism counts before and after disinfectant treatment. A 3 log or greater decrease in bacteria or fungi and a 2 log or greater decrease in spores will indicate that the disinfection of each target microorganism is effective. The required test microorganism species for evaluating efficacy should be selected with reference to Table 2. These test microorganisms should be used in the evaluation by being cultured and diluted under the conditions described in Microbiological Examination of Non-sterile Products <*4.05*>. However, *Bacillus subtilis* should be used in the evaluation after a spore suspension has been prepared with reference to Microbial Assay for Antibiotics

Table 1 Types of disinfectants, concentrations, and mechanisms of action

Classification	Types of Disinfectant	Concentration	Mechanism of action
Oxidant	Peracetic acid	0.3 w/v%	Oxidizing action
	Hydrogen peroxide	3 w/v%	
	Sodium hypochlorite	0.02 to 0.05%	
Alcohol-based	Isopropanol	50 to 70%	Protein and nucleic acid denaturation
	Ethanol	76.9 to 81.4 vol%	
Surfactant-based	Benzalkonium chloride Benzethonium chloride	0.05 to 0.2%	Protein denaturation
	Alkyldiamino-ethylglycine hydrochloride	0.05 to 0.5%	Cell membrane function impairment, protein coagulation/denaturation
Biguanide-based	Chlorhexidine gluconate	0.05 to 0.5%	Interruption of bacterial enzyme or alteration/disruption of cytoplasmic membrane

Table 2 Test microorganisms

Classification	Test microorganism
Bacteria	*Escherichia coli* ATCC 8739, NBRC 3972 *Staphylococcus aureus* ATCC 6538, NBRC 13276 *Pseudomonas aeruginosa* ATCC 9027, NBRC 13275 *Bacillus subtilis* ATCC 6633, NBRC 3134
Fungi	*Candida albicans* ATCC 10231, NBRC 1594 *Aspergillus brasiliensis* ATCC 16404, NBRC 9455

Table 3 Examples of materials to be disinfected

Material	Example of application
Stainless steel	Workbenches, tanks, machines
Glass	Windows, screens
Polycarbonate	Screens, containers
Decorative calcium silicate board	Walls, ceiling
Epoxy resin coating	Floors
Vinyl chloride	Floors, curtains, vinyl bags
Rigid urethane rubber	Floors
Nitrile rubber	Gloves

<*4.02*>. Species that are suitable for the purpose of the test can be used.

2.2.2. Hard Surface Carrier Method

Prepare each type of surface material carrier (approximately 5 cm × 5 cm) in a quantity resulting in the appropriate precision. Inoculate a broad range of carriers with 10^5 to 10^6 CFU test microorganisms, allow to dry, and then add disinfectant dropwise in the actually used concentration. Note that the number of the inoculated microorganisms may decrease depending on the conditions of drying the inoculated microorganisms which result in the disinfection effect not being evaluated appropriately. Allow the disinfectant to take effect for the prescribed time (usually 5 to 15 minutes), then collect the test microorganisms on the carriers by diluting in the collected solution. In the collected solution, neutralize[1)] the disinfectant using a solution containing an inactivator such as lecithin, polysorbate 80, or sodium thiosulfate as needed.

The stomach method, shaking method, swab method, or the like can be used as the method of collection with reference to JIS T11737-1.[2)] Count the number of the test microorganisms used for inoculation and the number of the recovered microorganisms under test conditions meeting the requirements in Microbiological Examination of Non-sterile Products <*4.05*> I. Microbiological Examination of Non-sterile Products: Microbial Enumeration Tests, 3.4 Suitability of the counting method in the presence of product. Calculate the logarithmic decrement from the test microorganism counts before and after disinfectant treatment. Conditions showing the same results as the decreases specified in 2.2.1 Test Organism Suspension Method will indicate that the disinfection of each target microorganism is effective. In addition to the selection of the required test microorganism species for evaluating efficacy with reference to Table 2, one or two representative microorganisms which are frequently isolated in environmental monitoring should be added. Species that are suitable for the purpose of the test can be used. The test microorganisms should be cultured and diluted, etc., as specified in 2.2.1 Test Microorganism Suspension Method. Examples of various surface materials used in clean areas or aseptic processing areas are given in Table 3, but other materials can be added for evaluation as needed depending on the circumstances of actual use.

3. Decontamination Methods

In these methods, decontamination is achieved, for example, by vaporizing or spraying chemical agents to reduce the number of microorganisms to a predetermined level in isolators and RABS (Restricted Access Barrier Systems) employed in sterile pharmaceutical product manufacturing processes, or structures and facilities such as work spaces and work rooms in clean areas or aseptic processing areas.

When this method is applied to structures and facilities for manufacturing sterile pharmaceutical products, the efficacy of the decontaminants and decontamination conditions must be validated, and worker safety must be ensured.

3.1. Decontaminants

Commonly used decontaminants are shown below. Decontaminants proven to be safe and effective other than those shown here can also be used.

3.1.1. Hydrogen Peroxide

Decontamination is achieved when hydrogen peroxide (30) is volatilized and allowed to spread. This is a method in which hydrogen peroxide that has been vaporized using a heater is allowed to spread inside an isolator or work room to kill microorganisms through the oxidative power of hydrogen peroxide. When a high degree of microbiological cleanliness must be achieved, as when decontaminating the interior of an isolator for sterilization operations, conditions should ensure a 6 log or greater decrease in the spores of the biological indicator, and when work rooms are decontaminated, conditions should ensure a 3 log or greater decrease. Although the method can be used at ambient temperature, the suitability of the method must be investigated beforehand because the potent oxidative power of hydrogen peroxide may cause deterioration such as discoloration, deformation, and corrosion of the materials exposed, depending on the nature of the materials, and the hydrogen peroxide itself may be degraded by the contact of the materials. If surfaces that are in contact with the product exist inside the isolator, it will be necessary to simultaneously decontaminate the interior and ensure the sterility assurance of the surfaces that are in contact with the product. In such cases, the pre-sterilization bioburden, parameters, utilities, and the like should be controlled in terms of the sterilization method with reference to the chapter "Sterilization Methods and Sterilization Indicators <*G4-10-162*>."

3.1.2. Peracetic Acid

Decontamination can be achieved, for example, when 0.2% peracetic acid aqueous solution is sprayed in the form of a mist and is allowed to spread. This method is used to clean work rooms, with conditions ensuring at least a 3 log decrease in the spores of the biological indicator. This is a method in which microorganisms are killed through the oxidative power of peracetic acid. Although the method can be used at ambient temperature, the suitability of the method must be investigated beforehand because the potent oxidative power of peracetic acid may result in deterioration such as discoloration, deformation, or corrosion of some materials.

3.1.3. Formaldehyde

Decontamination is achieved when formalin, an aqueous solution containing 36.0 to 38.0% formaldehyde, is vaporized by being heated, or when paraformaldehyde is sublimated by being heated, and allowed to spread. This is a method in which microorganisms are killed through the denaturation of protein by the aldehyde group (-CHO) in the formaldehyde molecule. This method is used to clean work rooms, with conditions ensuring at least a 3 log decrease in the spores of the biological indicator. As formaldehyde is harmful to the human body and has been designated a deleterious substance in the Poisonous and Deleterious Substances Control Act, it must be handled in work spaces equipped with a power exhaust device. It must also be detoxified when disposing of chemical waste.

3.2. Evaluation Methods

Methods using biological indicators to evaluate the effects of decontamination are generally used. Biological indicators that are resistant to decontaminants are commonly placed in various locations in structures and facilities such as work spaces and work rooms prior to decontamination. After decontamination, the biological indicators are commonly collected and are cultured to check for survivor microorganisms. In addition to culturing, faster methods, for example, that are equal to or greater than culturing can be used. When the decontamination of an isolator with hydrogen peroxide needs to be verified by inactivating 6 log or greater spore count after the use of 10^6 CFU biological indicators, it is not necessary to demonstrate complete destruction of the spores in the isolator after decontamination. Decontamination conditions suitable for a 6 log reduction in spores can also be established by statistical analysis or a method for evaluating the effects of decontamination by collecting the biological indicator and counting the number of survivor microorganisms by culturing to calculate the logarithmic decrement of the biological indicator.

The spores of *Geobacillus stearothermophilus* ATCC 7953 and 12980 are known to be resistant to hydrogen peroxide and formaldehyde, and can thus be used as indicator organisms. As representative environmental microorganisms, the spores of *Bacillus atrophaeus* ATCC 9372 can also be used as a biological indicator for the decontamination of work rooms.

4. Points to Consider

4.1. Worker Safety

Disinfectants and decontaminants often have an effect on the human body. That is, they are toxic. Therefore, when they are used, the method and amounts used must be strictly observed, protective gear must be properly used as needed, and the residue level must be checked.

4.2. Selection of Disinfectants and Decontaminants Used in Pharmaceutical Product Manufacturing Environments

When selecting disinfectants and decontaminants to be used in pharmaceutical product manufacturing environments, the following should be taken into consideration to select the appropriate ones depending on the purpose for which they are being used. The following items (1) through (13) must also be taken into consideration in order to ensure safer and more appropriate use of disinfectants and decontaminant.

(1) Type and number of microorganisms to be treated

(2) Antimicrobial spectrum

(3) Method of use, concentration, contact time, and expiration period of chemical agents

(4) Method for preparing decontaminant, including sterilization, when used in aseptic processing areas

(5) Suitability of materials being treated with disinfectants and decontaminants (such as extent of deterioration)

(6) Effects in the presence of organic substances such as protein

(7) Effective time dulation

(8) Effect on human body (safety)

(9) Suitability with cleansers

(10) Necessity of disinfectant rotation, and the method, if needed

(11) Necessary procedures for preventing contamination of pharmaceutical products by chemical agents (such as method of inactivation and checking residue level)

(12) Ease of waste disposal (neutralization, inactivation)

(13) Environmental effects of waste disposal

5. References

1) US Pharmacopeia 37 (2014), <1072> Disinfectants and Antiseptics

2) JIS T 11737 - 1: 2013, Sterilization of medical devices—Microbiological methods, Part 1: Determination of a population of microorganisms on products (ISO 11737 - 1: 2006)

Sterilization and Sterilization Indicators *<G4-10-162>*

Sterilization refers to the destruction or removal of all forms of viable microorganisms in items. This reference information applies to cases where sterilization is required as well as the manufacture of sterile products. When sterilization is applicable, an appropriate sterilization method should be selected in accordance with the items being sterilized (such as products, or equipment, instrumentation, or materials that must be sterilized), including the packaging, after full consideration of the advantages and disadvantages of each sterilization method.

After installation of a sterilizer (including design and development of the sterilization process), an equipment maintenance and inspection program must be established based on qualification evaluation to ensure that the sterilization process is being properly performed as designed on the basis of sufficient scientific evidence. A quality system must also be established for manufacturing in general at manufacturing facilities where sterile pharmaceutical products are manufactured. For example, all operation potentially affecting quality, including sterility after sterilization, must be clearly identified, and any operating procedures that are needed to prevent microbial contamination of products must be established and properly enforced.

In order to establish sterilization conditions and ensure sterility after sterilization, the bioburden before sterilization of the items being sterilized must be evaluated periodically or on the basis of batches. For bioburden test methods, refer to 4.05 Microbiological Examination of Non-sterile Products, etc.

Representative sterilization methods are presented in this reference information, but other sterilization methods can also be used, provided that they meet the following requirements and do not have any deleterious affect on the item being sterilized.

- The mechanism of sterilization is well established
- The critical physical parameters of the sterilization process are clear, controllable, and measurable
- The sterilization procedure can be performed effectively and reproducibly

1. Definitions

The terms used in this text are defined as follows.

- Filter integrity test: A non-destructive test which is demonstrated to correlate with the microbial removal performance data of filters.
- Bioburden: Population of viable microorganisms in an item to be sterilized.
- *D* value: The value represents exposure time (decimal reduction time) to achieve 90% reduction of a population of the test microorganism, and resulted that 10% of the original organisms remain.
- F_H value: The unit of lethality indicating the measure of the microbial inactivation capacity of a process in dry heat sterilization, expressed as the equivalent time (minutes) at 160°C for microbes with a *z* value (the number of degrees that are required for a 10-fold change in the *D* value) of 20°C.
- F_0 value: The unit of lethality indicating the measure of

the microbial inactivation capacity of a process in moist heat sterilization, expressed as the equivalent time (minutes) at 121.1°C for microbes with a *z* value (the number of degrees that are required for a 10-fold change in the *D* value) of 10°C.

- Sterility assurance level (SAL): Probability of a single viable microorganism surviving in a product after sterilization, expressed as 10^{-n}.
- Dose of irradiation (absorbed dose): Quantity of ionizing radiation energy imparted per unit mass of the item, expressed in units of gray (Gy).
- Critical parameter: A measurable parameter that is inherently essential to the sterilization process.
- Loading pattern: A specified combination of the numbers, orientation and distribution of the item(s) to be sterilized within the sterilization chamber or irradiation container.

2. Sterilization

2.1. Heat method

In the heat method, microorganisms are killed by heat.

2.1.1. Moist-heat sterilization

Moist-heat sterilization includes widely used saturated steam sterilization and other types of moist-heat sterilization. The control points, utilities, and control devices in moist-heat sterilization are provided as reference in Table 1.

Saturated steam sterilization is a method for killing microorganisms with high pressure saturated steam. Critical parameters in this method are temperature, pressure, and exposure time at the specified temperature. Therefore, the temperature, pressure, and exposure time in routine sterilization process control should be continuously monitored and measured, and measuring equipment for that purpose should be included in the sterilization equipment specifications.

Other types of moist-heat sterilization may include steam pressurization cycles, water dispersion cycles, water immersion cycles, and the like, which are used when the items

Table 1 Control points, utilities, and control devices in moist-heat sterilization (reference)

	Saturated steam sterilization	Other types of moist-heat sterilization
Control point	• Temperature profile (usually indicated by F_0 value) • Temperature (drain or the like as needed) • Pressure (in sterilizer) • Exposure time at specified temperature • Loading pattern of items being sterilized • Steam quality (degree of superheat, dryness, non-condensable gas concentration, and chemical purity, as needed) • Quality of air that is introduced to the sterilizer for vacuum break • Quality of cooling water • Other requirements	• Temperature profile (usually indicated by F_0 value) • Temperature (drain and the like as needed) • Pressure, as needed (in sterilizer) • Exposure time at specified temperature • Loading pattern of item being sterilized • Quality of air that is introduced to the sterilizer for vacuum break • Quality of cooling water • Other requirements
Utilities and control devices that should be controlled	• Steam • Air introduced to the sterilizer for vacuum break • Cooling water • Temperature control device • Pressure control device • Time control device • Other	• Steam • Hot water • Air introduced to the sterilizer for vacuum break • Cooling water • Temperature control device • Pressure control device • Time control device • Conveyor for when a continuous sterilizer is used • Other

Table 2 Control points, utilities, and control devices in dry-heat sterilization (reference)

	Batch-type dry heat sterilizer	Tunnel-type dry heat sterilizer
Control point	• Temperature profile (usually indicated by F_H value) • Temperature • Exposure time at specified temperature • Pressure differential between inside and outside of container • Loading pattern of items being sterilized • Quality of air (heating air, cooling air) • Other requirements	• Temperature profile (usually indicated by F_H value) • Temperature • Belt speed (exposure time) • Pressure differential between inside and outside of equipment • Loading density • Quality of air (heating air, cooling air) • Other requirements
Utilities and control devices that should be controlled	• Air (heating air, cooling air) • Temperature control device • Time control device • Internal differential pressure gage • HEPA filter • Other	• Air (heating air, cooling air) • Temperature control device • Time control device • Internal differential pressure gage • HEPA filter • Cooler (if needed) • Other

being sterilized is sterilized in a hermetically sealed container. Critical parameters in such methods are the temperature in the container and the exposure time at the specified temperature.

2.1.2. Dry-heat sterilization

Dry-heat sterilization is a method for destructing microorganisms with dry heated air. This method is usually conducted in a batch or continuous (tunnel-type) dry heat sterilizer. Attention must be paid to the cleanliness of the air that flows into the sterilizer in either case. The control points, utilities, and control devices in dry-heat sterilization are provided as reference in Table 2. This method is suitable for when the item to be sterilized is highly heat-resistant, such as glass, ceramic or metal, or is thermo-stable, such as mineral oils, fatty oils, or solid pharmaceutical products.

Critical parameters in this method are temperature and the exposure time at the specified temperature (belt speed). Dry-heat sterilization requires higher temperatures and longer exposure times than does moist-heat sterilization even though the sterilization in both methods may be based on the same heating temperature. The temperature and exposure time in routine sterilization process control should be continuously monitored and measured, and measuring equipment for that purpose should be included in the sterilization equipment specifications.

2.1.3. Microwave sterilization

When substances to be sterilized such as drug solutions are exposed to microwaves, the polar molecules of the substance being sterilized vibrate as they attempt to change orientation due to the absorbed microwaves, and energy is released by the friction between the molecules. The method of killing microorganisms by the heat (microwave heat) generated at this time is called the microwave sterilization. A frequency of 2450 ± 50 MHz is ordinarily used.

Microwave devices are composed of a heating irradiation component which produces radiofrequency radiation to generate heat using a magnetron, a component for maintaining the sterilization temperature using an infrared heater or the like, and a cooling component for cooling the item being sterilized. Such devices continuously sterilize the item at ordinary pressure. The control points, utilities, and control devices in microwave sterilization are provided as reference in Table 3.

This method is applied to liquid products or products with high water content in hermetic container, etc.

Critical parameters in this method include the temperature of the items being sterilized and processing time. Therefore, the temperature of the items being sterilized and the processing time in routine sterilization process control should be continuously monitored and measured, and measuring equipment for that purpose should be included in the sterilization equipment specifications.

Microwave heating characteristically allows rapid sterilization at high temperatures to be continuously carried out with excellent thermal efficiency and responsiveness. However, the ease of heat transfer in the items being sterilized sometimes makes it difficult to ensure uniform heating. Attention must also be paid to the pressure resistance of the containers that are used because the heating takes place at ambient pressure, resulting in increases in internal pressure.

Table 3 Control points, utilities, and control devices in microwave sterilization (reference)

Control point	• Temperature profile (usually indicated by F_0 value) • Temperature • Processing time • Configuration of items being sterilized • Other requirements
Utilities and control devices that should be controlled	• High frequency control device • External heater (if needed) • Cooler (if needed) • Temperature monitoring device • Time monitoring device • Other

Table 4 Control points, utilities, and control devices in EO gas sterilization (reference)

Control point	• Pressure increase, injection time, and final pressure for the injection of sterilization gas • Temperature (in sterilizer and items being sterilized) • Humidity • EO gas concentration (gas concentration in sterilizer should be directly analyzed, but the following alternatives are acceptable when direct analysis is not feasible) i) Mass of gas used ii) Volume of gas used iii) Use of conversion formula based on initial reduced pressure and gas injection pressure • Operating time (exposure time) • Loading pattern of items being sterilized • Biological indicator placement points and cultivation results • Preconditioning conditions (temperature, humidity, time, etc.) • Aeration conditions (temperature, time, etc.) • Other requirements
Utilities and control devices that should be controlled	• EO gas • Injected vapor or water • Air replaced after completion of sterilization • Temperature control device • Humidity control device • Pressure control device • Time control device • Other

2.2. Gas method

The gas method kills microorganisms through contact with a sterilization gas or vapor. Microorganisms can be sterilized at lower temperatures than in heat methods, and the items being sterilized generally sustain little thermal damage. This method is therefore often applied to plastic containers and the like which are not very resistant to heat.

In the most common gas sterilization methods, adequate washing and drying are important to prevent contamination and moisture from compromising the sterilization effect. The sterilization effect may also be compromised if the gas is absorbed by the item being sterilized.

2.2.1. Ethylene oxide (EO) gas sterilization

EO gas sterilization kills microorganisms by altering the proteins and nucleic acids of microorganisms. Since EO gas is explosive, it is usually diluted 10 to 30% with carbon dioxide. EO gas is also a strongly reactive alkylating agent and therefore cannot be used to sterilize products which are likely to react with or absorb it.

The sterilization process consists of preconditioning, sterilization cycles, and aeration. EO gas is toxic (mutagenic, for example), and the substance being sterilized must therefore be aerated to ensure that the residual concentration of EO gas or other secondarily generated toxic gases (such as ethylene chlorohydrin) is at or below safe levels. Gas emissions must also be treated in compliance with regulations. The control points, utilities, and control devices in EO gas sterilization are provided as reference in Table 4.

Critical parameters in this method include temperature, humidity, gas concentration (pressure), and time. Therefore, the temperature, humidity, gas concentration (pressure), and time in routine sterilization process control should be continuously monitored and measured, and measuring equipment for that purpose should be included in the sterilization equipment specifications.

2.2.2. Hydrogen peroxide sterilization

Sterilization with hydrogen peroxide is a method for killing microorganisms through the oxidative power of hydrogen peroxide or the oxidation caused by radicals that are produced upon the generation of hydrogen peroxide plasma. Although items can be sterilized at lower temperatures than in heat methods, this method is not suitable for the sterilization of objects that absorb hydrogen peroxides, such as cellulose-based disposable garment and membrane filters because the sterilization effect will be compromised. The control points, utilities, and control devices in hydrogen peroxide sterilization are provided as reference in Table 5.

Critical parameters in this method include the concentration, time, and temperature. The control of a radio frequency device is also important when substances are sterilized with the use of plasma. The residual moisture of the substance being sterilized and the humidity in the sterilization environment may affect sterilization and should therefore be controlled when necessary.

2.3. Radiation method

2.3.1. Radiation sterilization

Radiation sterilization includes γ-ray radiation for killing microorganisms through the exposure of the items that are to be sterilized to γ-rays emitted from ^{60}Co, and electron beam radiation for killing microorganisms through exposure to an electron beam emitted from an electron beam accelerator. To select the method of sterilization, it must first be ensured that it is compatible with the items to be sterilized, including whether the quality of the substance could potentially deteriorate.

In γ-ray radiation sterilization, microorganisms are killed by secondarily produced electrons, whereas in electron beam radiation sterilization, microorganisms are directly killed by electrons. Although this kind of electron-based direct action is available, indirect action is also available, where sterilization is accomplished through the production of radicals and the like and damage to the DNA of microorganisms when γ-rays or electron beams react with water molecules.

Since sterilization can take place at room temperature, both methods can be applied to heat-labile items, and items can be sterilized while packaged because the radiation rays

Table 5 Control points, utilities, and control devices in hydrogen peroxide sterilization (reference)

	Hydrogen peroxide sterilization	Hydrogen peroxide low temperature gas plasma sterilization
Control point	• Concentration (the concentration in the sterilizer should be directly analyzed, but a method based on evidence of sterilizer performance uniformity in the chamber is an acceptable alternative when direct analysis is not feasible) • Time • Temperature • Humidity • Pressure • Quality of hydrogen peroxide • Consumption of hydrogen peroxide • Residual moisture of substance being sterilized • Loading pattern of items being sterilized • Biological indicator placement points and cultivation results • Chemical indicator placement points and results • Other requirements	• Concentration (the concentration in the sterilizer should be directly analyzed, but a method based on evidence of sterilizer performance uniformity in the chamber is an acceptable alternative when direct analysis is not feasible) • Time • Temperature • Humidity • Pressure • Quality of hydrogen peroxide • Consumption of hydrogen peroxide • Residual moisture of substance being sterilized • Loading pattern of items being sterilized • Biological indicator placement points and cultivation results • Chemical indicator placement points and results • Other requirements
Utilities and control devices that should be controlled	• Hydrogen peroxide • Pressure gauge • Hydrogen peroxide injector • Other	• Hydrogen peroxide • Pressure gauge • Hydrogen peroxide injector • High frequency generator • Other

will penetrate the packaging. γ-Ray sterilization is suitable primarily for high density products such as metals, water, and powder because the penetration is better than that of electron beams. Electron beam radiation sterilization has a higher radiation dose per unit time (dose rate) compared with γ-rays and therefore has a shorter processing time. The control points, utilities, and control devices in radiation sterilization are provided as reference in Table 6.

2.4. Filtration method

The filtration method is a method for physically removing microorganisms in liquids or gas using a sterilization filter. It can therefore be applied to items that are unstable against heat or radiation. Filtration sterilization is for microorganisms which can be removed by a 0.2 μm membrane filter, and is not suitable for *Mycoplasma* spp., *Leptospira* spp., or viruses. The control points, utilities, and control devices in filtration sterilization are provided as reference in Table 7.

The critical parameters affecting the removal of microorganisms by the filter in liquid filtration sterilization include filtration time, filtration capacity, filtration flow rate, filtration differential pressure, and temperature. The critical parameters in gas filtration sterilization include filtration differential pressure and temperature. When a liquid is to be sterilized, the removal of microorganisms by a filter will be affected by the physicochemical properties of the liquid that is undergoing filtration (such as viscosity, pH, and surfactant action). The microbial trapping performance of a sterilizing filter can generally be validated when a sterilizing filter challenged with more than 10^7 CFU microorganisms of a strain of *Brevundimonas diminuta* (ATCC 19146, NBRC 14213) or appropriate smaller species, cultured under the appropriate conditions, per square centimeter of effective filter area, provides a sterile effluent.

The bioburden of liquids prior to filtration will affect filtration sterilization performance and should therefore be controlled.

3. Sterilization Indicators

3.1. Biological indicators (BI)

3.1.1. Introduction

A BI is an indicator prepared from the spores of a microorganism resistant to the specified sterilization process, and is used to develop and/or validate a sterilization process.

Indicators are classified based on configuration into the "paper strip type", "the type that is inoculated on or into the surface of metal or the like", "liquid type" and "the self-contained type in which a medium and paper strip are pre-encapsulated". They are also classified by carrier, where one type comprises a carrier of paper, glass, stainless steel, plastic or the like that is inoculated with bacterial spores and packaged, and another type comprises the product or simulated product as the carrier, which is inoculated with bacterial spores. Typical examples of indicators by sterilization method are shown in Table 8.

3.1.2. Labeling of commercially available BI

Users of commercially available BI produced in accordance with ISO11138-1 must check the following information provided by the BI manufacturer to users.

• Traceability (microorganism, carrier, labeling, etc.)
• Species name

Table 6 Control points, utilities, and control devices in radiation sterilization (reference)

	γ-Ray radiation sterilization	Electron beam radiation sterilization
Control point	• Absorbed dose • Loading pattern (density) of items being sterilized • Exposure time (conveyor speed or cycle time) • Other requirements	• Absorbed dose • Loading pattern (density) of items being sterilized • Electron beam properties (mean electron beam current, electron beam energy, scanning width) • Other requirements
Utilities and control devices that should be controlled	• Belt conveyor • Dose measurement system • Other	• Electron beam measurement device • Belt conveyor • Dose measurement system • Other

Table 7 Control points, utilities, and control devices in filtration sterilization (reference)

	Liquid filtration sterilization	Gas filtration sterilization
Control point	• Filtration time • Filtration capacity • Filtration flow rate • Filtration differential pressure • Temperature • Filter integrity • In cases involving multiple use: expiration period and number of times the filter can be used for sterilization • Other requirements	• Filtration differential pressure • Temperature, if needed • Filter integrity • Expiration period • Number of sterilizations of times the filter can be used for sterilization • Direction of gas current (for bidirectional flow) • Other requirements
Utilities and control devices that should be controlled	• Pressure gage • Flow rate meter • Integrity tester • Other	• Pressure gage • Flow rate meter • Integrity tester • Other

Table 8 List of typical indicators by sterilization method

Sterilization method	Species	Strain name	*D* value, etc. (reference)
Moist-heat sterilization	*Geobacillus stearothermophilus*	ATCC 7953, NBRC 13737	≥1.5 min (121°C)
Dry-heat sterilization	*Bacillus atrophaeus*	ATCC 9372, NBRC 13721	≥2.5 min (160°C)
EO gas sterilization	*Bacillus atrophaeus*	ATCC 9372, NBRC 13721	≥2.5 min (54°C) ≥12.5 min (30°C) Gas concentration: 600 mg/L ± 30 mg/L; relative humidity: 60% RH
Hydrogen peroxide sterilization	*Geobacillus stearothermophilus*	ATCC 12980, NBRC 12550 or ATCC 7953, NBRC 13737	—

- Nominal bacterial spore count
- Resistance
- Method used
- Storage conditions (temperature, expiration date, etc.)
- Culture conditions (temperature, time, medium, etc.)
- Disposal method

Parameters determining BI performance include "species," "resistance," and "bacterial count." Resistance varies, even for the same species, depending on the nature and configuration of the carrier or packaging, and evaluation must therefore include the packaging.

3.1.3. Control during use of commercially available BI

BI must be handled in accordance with the storage conditions, time to start of culture after sterilization, culturing conditions, disposal method, and the like provided by the BI manufacturer. Because the storage conditions in particular affect BI performance, precautions must be taken to prevent a BI from being allowed to stand for a long period of time until use after being removed from the packaging.

The BI should be set up to enable evaluation of the entire items being sterilized. The BI should be set up in places where the sterilization effect is expected to be low in any given method, such as cold spots in heat sterilization. Care should be taken to avoid damaging the BI packaging or carrier when recovered. Predetermined procedures for preventing microbial contamination should be in place in case bacteria are released or spread if the packaging does end up becoming damaged.

When using a BI that has been purchased, the user should measure the spore count or the like when received as needed to make sure there are no significant differences with the nominal count provided by the BI manufacturer.

3.1.4. Precautions for when sterilization indicators are prepared by the user

The following must be evaluated prior to use when users prepare indicators themselves using the bioburden collected from the items being sterilized or the manufacturing environment rather than purchasing a BI for use.

- Species name
- Bacterial spore count
- Resistance (*D* value at sterilization temperature or sterilization gas concentration)
- Storage conditions (temperature, expiration date, etc.)
- Culture conditions (temperature, incubation time, medium, etc.)

An evaluation program must be established to continuously show that the resistance of picked bacteria is the most resistant of the bioburden.

3.1.5. Precautions when commercially available BI are modified by users

When a BI that has been purchased is removed from the packaging and is used to inoculate an item such as drug solution or materials, the bacterial spore count or resistance will vary and must therefore be assessed prior to use.

ISO11138 or USP <55> can be used for reference for such evaluation. Resistance can be evaluated by using a biological indicator evaluation resistometer (BIER) or the capillary method with oil bath. When such self-assessment is unfeasible, a third-party testing facility can be used.

3.2. Chemical indicator (CI)

A CI is an indicator that chemically or physically changes due to exposure to heat, gas, radiation, or the like. Such indicators are produced by being applied to or printed on a piece of paper, for example. Because the principals involved in such changes will depend on the sterilization method, a CI that is suitable for the intended sterilization method must be used. CI is classified into the following six classes based on the intended application. The classes shown here are unrelated to level of performance.

A CI indicates the progress of a sterilization step or of a number of critical parameters, but is not used to assure sterilization effect or sterility and therefore cannot be used as an alternative to a BI.

Class 1: Process indicators

These are intended to distinguish whether an item being sterilized has passed through a sterilization step. They respond to one or more critical parameters.

Class 2: Indicators for use in specific tests

These are used in tests of the exhaust capacity and vapor penetration of a vacuum-type high-pressure steam sterilizer as specified in the ISO11140 series. They correspond to the Bowie-Dick type.

Class 3: Single-variable indicators

These respond to only one critical parameter. They show exposure in a sterilization step based on a specified value for the designated parameter.

Class 4: Multi-variable indicators

These respond to two or more critical parameters. They show exposure in a sterilization step based on specified values for the designated parameters.

Class 5: Integrating indicators

These respond to all critical parameters. Their performance is equal to or greater than that required of BI in the ISO11138 series.

Class 6: Emulating indicators

These respond to all critical parameters of a specified sterilization cycle. The specifications are critical

Table 9 Types of dosimeters

Type of radiation	Dosimeter
γ-ray	Dyed polymethyl methacrylate dosimeter Clear polymethyl methacrylate dosimeter Ceric-cerous dosimeter Alanine - EPR dosimeter
γ-ray, electron beam	Cellulose acetate dosimeter Radiochromic film dosimeter

parameters of the designated sterilization step.

3.3. Dosimeter

3.3.1. Types of dosimeters

The dosimeter in a radiation process is an instrument or system which reads the absorbed dose based on changes caused by the absorption of the radiation, for which ''reproducibility'' and ''response permitting radiation to be measured'' are required. Most dosimeters are susceptible to environmental conditions (process parameters) such as temperature and dose rate before, during, and after exposure to the facilities being used, and caution is therefore required. The choice of dosimeter and calibration guidelines for radiation processes have been specified (ISO/ASTM 51261) as reference for the selection and use of dosimeters. Dosimeters for measuring the absorbed dose of radiation are shown in Table 9. γ-Ray dosimeters are not normally suitable for sterilization process control involving the use of electron beams of less than 3 MeV energy.

3.3.2. Dosimeter use

Dosimeters are used when dose distribution is measured to determine the conditions of radiation and to evaluate the absorbed dose of an items being sterilized during ordinary radiation sterilization. In the former, dosimeters are set up in advance in the object being sterilized and are then recovered after radiation for measurement in the measurement system to find the absorbed dose at each location. The dosimeters should be arranged in a broad range of vertical and horizontal directions because it is necessary to determine the relationship between minimum/maximum exposure and the process parameters as well as to verify the appropriateness of the packaging configuration based on the variation in radiation penetration and dose. In the latter, there is no need to arrange the dosimeters in the locations characterized by the maximum or minimum dose in the object being sterilized. Control points where dosimeters are easily arranged and recovered should be selected, and the absorbed dose of the object being sterilized should be ensured based on the absorbed dose at the control points. Therefore, in the measurement of dose distribution, the quantitative relationship between the control points and the locations of maximum/minimum exposure should be determined, and the passing dose range at the control points should also be calculated.

Newly purchased dosimeters should be calibrated prior to use, and dosimeters should be calibrated every time a batch is changed and at least once a year.

4. Establishment of Sterilization Conditions

4.1. Half-cycle method

In the half-cycle method, a sterilization time twice as long as that required to inactivate all of the 10^6 CFU bacteria included in the BI is used, regardless of the bioburden count on the object being sterilized or the resistance of the test microorganisms to sterilization. This method is primarily used to establish the conditions of EO or other gas sterilization.

4.2. Overkill method

In the overkill method, a sterilization condition to achieve an SAL of 10^{-6} or better is used, regardless of bioburden count on the object being sterilized or the resistance of the test microorganisms to sterilization.

This means a level of sterilization of 12 D in steam sterilization. However, a level $\geq F_0$ 12 is also referred to as the overkill method.

4.3. Combination of bioburden and BI method

In the combined bioburden/BI method, the maximum bioburden count is determined based on the results of extensive bioburden analysis, and the sterilization time (or radiation dose) is calculated using an appropriate commercially available BI with a test microorganism count $\geq$ the maximum bioburden count based on the target SAL.

When this procedure is used, the bioburden count of the object being sterilized must be tested on a daily basis, and the resistance of the test microorganisms to sterilization must be periodically measured.

If the bioburden testing reveals a microorganism more resistant than the BI microorganism, it should be used as the indicator. The sterilization conditions must also be revised as needed.

Sterilization time (or radiation dose) = $D \times \log (N_0/N)$

D: D value of BI

N: Target sterility assurance level (SAL)

N_0: Maximum bioburden count in object being sterilized

4.4. Absolute bioburden method

In the absolute bioburden method, the sterilization resistance of the microorganisms found in the object being sterilized or environment is measured, and the sterilization conditions are determined, in the case of moist-heat sterilization, by employing the D value of the most resistant microorganism based on the bioburden count of the object being sterilized.

The bioburden count should be determined by extensive bioburden analysis. When this procedure is used, the microorganism count and the resistance of the detected microorganisms to sterilization must be assessed on a daily basis in routine bioburden control.

Radiation sterilization may be performed in accordance with ISO11137-2.

5. References

- ISO 11138-1: 2006, Sterilization of health care products-Biological indicators-Part1: General requirements
- ISO 11137-2: 2013, Sterilization of health care products-Radiation- Part2: Establishing the sterilization dose
- ISO/ASTM 51261: 2013, Guide for selection and calibration of dosimetry systems for radiation processing
- ISO 11140-1: 2014, Sterilization of health care products-Chemical indicators- Part1: General requirements
- US Pharmacopeia 38 (2015), <55> Biological Indicators-Resistance Performance Tests.

G5 Crude Drugs

On the Scientific Names of Crude Drugs listed in the JP *<G5-1-180>*

The notation system of the scientific names for the original plants and animals of crude drugs listed in JP is not nec-

Scientific Names used in the JP and Those being used Taxonomically

Crude Drug	Scientific names used in the JP = Scientific names being used taxonomically (Combined notation, Standard form for author or authors) Scientific names that are different from those written in JP but identical to them taxonomically or being regarded as identical, and typical sub-classified groups belonging to their species. The names marked with "*" are those being written together in JP.	Family
Acacia アラビアゴム	*Acacia senegal* Willdenow =*Acacia senegal* (L.) Willd.	*Leguminosae*
	Other species of the same genus	
Achyranthes Root ゴシツ	*Achyranthes bidentata* Blume	*Amaranthaceae*
	Achyranthes fauriei H. Léveillé et Vaniot =*Achyranthes fauriei* H. Lev. & Vaniot	
Agar カンテン	*Gelidium elegans* Kuetzing	*Gelidiaceae*
	Other species of the same genus	
	Red seaweeds of several species	
Akebia Stem モクツウ	*Akebia quinata* Decaisne =*Akebia quinata* (Thunb. ex Houtt.) Decne.	*Lardizabalaceae*
	Akebia trifoliata Koidzumi =*Akebia trifoliata* (Thunb.) Koidz.	
Alisma Tuber タクシャ	*Alisma orientale* Juzepczuk =*Alisma orientale* (Sam.) Juz.	*Alismataceae*
	Alisma plantago-aquatica L. var. *orientale* Sam.	
Aloe アロエ	*Aloe ferox* Miller =*Aloe ferox* Mill.	*Liliaceae*
	Interspecific hybrid between *Aloe ferox* Miller and *Aloe africana* Miller =*Aloe africana* Mill.	
	Interspecific hybrid between *Aloe ferox* Miller and *Aloe spicata* Baker	
Alpinia Officinarum Rhizome リョウキョウ	*Alpinia officinarum* Hance	*Zingiberaceae*
Amomum Seed シュクシャ	*Amomum villosum* Loureiro var. *xanthioides* T. L. Wu et S. J. Chen = *Amomum villosum* Lour. var. *xanthioides* (Wall. ex Baker) T. L. Wu & S. J. Chen	*Zingiberaceae*
	Amomum xanthioides Wallich = *Amomum xanthioides* Wall. ex Baker	
	Amomum villosum Lour. var. *nanum* H. T. Tsai & S. W. Zhao	
	Amomum villosum Loureiro var. *villosum* = *Amomum villosum* Lour. var. *villosum*	
	Amomum villosum Lour.	
	Amomum longiligulare T. L. Wu	
Anemarrhena Rhizome チモ	*Anemarrhena asphodeloides* Bunge	*Liliaceae*
Angelica Dahurica Root ビャクシ	*Angelica dahurica* Bentham et Hooker filius ex Franchet et Savatier =*Angelica dahurica* (Hoffm.) Benth. & Hook. f. ex Franch. & Sav.	*Umbelliferae*

Apricot Kernel キョウニン	*Prunus armeniaca* Linné = *Prunus armeniaca* L.	*Rosaceae*
	Prunus armeniaca Linné var. *ansu* Maximowicz = *Prunus armeniaca* L. var. *ansu* Maxim.	
	Prunus sibirica Linné = *Prunus sibirica* L.	
Aralia Rhizome ドクカツ	*Aralia cordata* Thunberg = *Aralia cordata* Thunb.	*Araliaceae*
Areca ビンロウジ	*Areca catechu* Linné = *Areca catechu* L.	*Palmae*
Artemisia Capillaris Flower インチンコウ	*Artemisia capillaris* Thunberg = *Artemisia capillaris* Thunb.	*Compositae*
Artemisia Leaf ガイヨウ	*Artemisia princeps* Pampanini = *Artemisia princeps* Pamp.	*Compositae*
	Artemisia montana Pampanini = *Artemisia montana* (Nakai) Pamp.	
Asiasarum Root サイシン	*Asiasarum heterotropoides* F. Maekawa var. *mandshuricum* F. Maekawa = *Asiasarum heterotropoides* (F. Schmidt) F. Maek. var. *mandshuricum* (Maxim.) F. Maek.	*Aristolochiaceae*
	Asarum heterotropoides F. Schmidt var. *mandshuricum* (Maxim.) Kitag.	
	Asiasarum sieboldii F. Maekawa = *Asiasarum sieboldii* (Miq.) F. Maek.	
	Asarum sieboldii Miq. *Asarum sieboldii* Miq. var. *seoulense* Nakai	
Asparagus Root テンモンドウ	*Asparagus cochinchinensis* Merrill = *Asparagus cochinchinensis* (Lour.) Merr.	*Liliaceae*
Astragalus Root オウギ	*Astragalus mongholicus* Bunge	*Leguminosae*
	Astragalus membranaceus (Fisch.) Bunge var. *mongholicus* (Bunge) Hsiao	
	Astragalus membranaceus Bunge = *Astragalus membranaceus* (Fisch.) Bunge	
Atractylodes Lancea Rhizome ソウジュツ	*Atractylodes lancea* De Candolle = *Atractylodes lancea* (Thunb.) DC.	*Compositae*
	Atractylodes chinensis Koidzumi = *Atractylodes chinensis* (Bunge) Koidz.	
	Interspecific hybrid between above species	
Atractylodes Rhizome ビャクジュツ	*Atractylodes japonica* Koidzumi ex Kitamura = *Atractylodes japonica* Koidz. ex Kitam.	*Compositae*
	Atractylodes macrocephala Koidzumi = *Atractylodes macrocephala* Koidz.	
	* *Atractylodes ovata* De Candolle = *Atractylodes ovata* (Thunb.) DC.	
Bear Bile ユウタン	*Ursus arctos* Linné = *Ursus arctos* L.	*Ursidae*
	Other animals of the related genus	
Bearberry Leaf ウワウルシ	*Arctostaphylos uva-ursi* Sprengel = *Arctostaphylos uva-ursi* (L.) Spreng.	*Ericaceae*
Beef Tallow 牛脂	*Bos taurus* Linné var. *domesticus* Gmelin = *Bos taurus* L. var. *domesticus* Gmelin	*Bovidae*

Yellow Beeswax ミツロウ	*Apis mellifera* Linné = *Apis mellifera* L.	*Apidae*
	Apis cerana Fabricius	
Belladonna Extract ベラドンナコン	*Atropa belladonna* Linné = *Atropa belladonna* L.	*Solanaceae*
Benincasa Seed トウガシ	*Benincasa cerifera* Savi	*Cucurbitaceae*
	Benincasa hispida (Thunb.) Cogn.	
	Benincasa cerifera Savi forma *emarginata* K. Kimura et Sugiyama = *Benincasa cerifera* Savi f. *emarginata* K. Kimura & Sugiyama	
Benzoin アンソッコウ	*Styrax benzoin* Dryander = *Styrax benzoin* Dryand.	*Styracaceae*
	Other species of the same genus	
Bitter Cardamon ヤクチ	*Alpinia oxyphylla* Miquel = *Alpinia oxyphylla* Miq.	*Zingiberaceae*
Bitter Orange Peel トウヒ	*Citrus aurantium* Linné = *Citrus aurantium* L.	*Rutaceae*
	Citrus aurantium Linné var. *daidai* Makino = *Citrus aurantium* L. var. *daidai* Makino	
	Citrus aurantium L. 'Daidai'	
Brown Rice コウベイ	*Oryza sativa* Linné = *Oryza sativa* L.	*Gramineae*
Bupleurum Root サイコ	*Bupleurum falcatum* Linné = *Bupleurum falcatum* L.	*Umbelliferae*
	Bupleurum chinense DC. *Bupleurum scorzonerifolium* Willd.	
Burdock Fruit ゴボウシ	*Arctium lappa* Linné = *Arctium lappa* L.	*Compositae*
Cacao Butter カカオ脂	*Theobroma cacao* Linné = *Theobroma cacao* L.	*Sterculiaceae*
Calumba コロンボ	*Jateorhiza columba* Miers	*Menispermaceae*
Camellia Oil ツバキ油	*Camellia japonica* Linné = *Camellia japonica* L.	*Theaceae*
Capsicum トウガラシ	*Capsicum annuum* Linné = *Capsicum annuum* L.	*Solanaceae*
Cardamon ショウズク	*Elettaria cardamomum* Maton	*Zingiberaceae*
Carnauba Wax カルナウバロウ	*Copernicia cerifera* Martius = *Copernicia cerifera* Mart.	*Palmae*
Cassia Seed ケツメイシ	*Cassia obtusifolia* Linné = *Cassia obtusifolia* L.	*Leguminosae*
	Cassia tora Linné = *Cassia tora L.*	
Castor Oil ヒマシ油	*Ricinus communis* Linné = *Ricinus communis* L.	*Euphorbiaceae*
Catalpa Fruit キササゲ	*Catalpa ovata* G. Don	*Bignoniaceae*
	Catalpa bungei C. A. Meyer = *Catalpa bungei* C. A. Mey.	

Cherry Bark オウヒ	*Prunus jamasakura* Siebold ex Koidzumi = *Prunus jamasakura* Siebold ex Koidz.	*Rosaceae*
	Prunus verecunda Koehne = *Prunus verecunda* (Koidz.) Koehne	
Chrysanthemum Flower キクカ	*Chrysanthemum indicum* Linné = *Chrysanthemum indicum* L.	*Compositae*
	Chrysanthemum morifolium Ramatuelle = *Chrysanthemum morifolium* Ramat.	
Cimicifuga Rhizome ショウマ	*Cimicifuga dahurica* Maximowicz = *Cimicifuga dahurica* (Turcz.) Maxim.	*Ranunculaceae*
	Cimisifuga heracleifolia Komarov = *Cimisifuga heracleifolia* Kom.	
	Cimicifuga foetida Linné = *Cimicifuga foetida* L.	
	Cimicifuga simplex Turczaninow = *Cimicifuga simplex* (DC.) Turcz.	
Cinnamon Bark ケイヒ	*Cinnamomum cassia* J. Presl = *Cinnamomum cassia* (L.) J. Presl	*Lauraceae*
Cinnamon Oil ケイヒ油	*Cinnamomum cassia* J. Presl = *Cinnamomum cassia* (L.) J. Presl	*Lauraceae*
	Cinnamomum zeylanicum Nees	
Cistanche Herb ニクジュヨウ	*Cistanche salsa* G. Beck = *Cistanche salsa* (C.A.Mey.) Beck	*Orobanchaceae*
	Cistanche deserticola Y. C. Ma = *Cistanche deserticola* Ma	
	Cistanche tubulosa Wight	
Citrus Unshiu Peel チンピ	*Citrus unshiu* Marcowicz = *Citrus unshiu* (Swingle) Marcow.	*Rutaceae*
	Citrus reticulata Blanco 'Unshiu'	
	Citrus reticulata Blanco	
Clematis Root イレイセン	*Clematis mandshurica* Ruprecht = *Clematis mandshurica* Rupr.	*Ranunculaceae*
	Clematis chinensis Osbeck	
	Clematis hexapetala Pallas = *Clematis hexapetala* Pall.	
Clove チョウジ Clove Oil チョウジ油	*Syzygium aromaticum* Merrill et Perry = *Syzygium aromaticum* (L.) Merr. & L. M. Perry	*Myrtaceae*
	* *Eugenia caryophyllata* Thunberg = *Eugenia caryophyllata* Thunb. *Eugenia caryophyllus* (Spreng.) Bullock & S. G. Harrison	
Cnidium Monnieri Fruit ジャショウシ	*Cnidium monnieri* Cusson = *Cnidium monnieri* (L.) Cusson	*Umbelliferae*
Cnidium Rhizome センキュウ	*Cnidium officinale* Makino	*Umbelliferae*
Coconut Oil ヤシ油	*Cocos nucifera* Linné = *Cocos nucifera* L.	*Palmae*
Codonopsis Root トウジン	*Codonopsis pilosula* Nannfeldt = *Codonopsis pilosula* Nannf.	*Campanulaceae*
	Codonopsis tangshen Oliver = *Codonopsis tangshen* Oliv.	

Coix Seed ヨクイニン	*Coix lacryma-jobi* Linné var. *mayuen* Stapf = *Coix lacryma-jobi* L. var. *mayuen* (Rom. Caill.) Stapf	*Gramineae*
Condurango コンズランゴ	*Marsdenia cundurango* Reichenbach filius = *Marsdenia cundurango* Rchb. f.	*Asclepiadaceae*
Coptis Rhizome オウレン	*Coptis japonica* Makino = *Coptis japonica* (Thunb.) Makino	*Ranunculaceae*
	Coptis japonica (Thunb.) Makino var. *dissecta* (Yatabe) Nakai *Coptis japonica* (Thunb.) Makino var. *japonica* *Coptis japonica* (Thunb.) Makino var. *major* (Miq.) Satake	
	Coptis chinensis Franchet = *Coptis chinensis* Franch.	
	Coptis deltoidea C. Y. Cheng et Hsiao	
	Coptis teeta Wallich = *Coptis teeta* Wall.	
Corn Oil トウモロコシ油	*Zea mays* Linné = *Zea mays* L.	*Gramineae*
Cornus Fruit サンシュユ	*Cornus officinalis* Siebold et Zuccarini = *Cornus officinalis* Siebold & Zucc.	*Cornaceae*
Corydalis Tuber エンゴサク	*Corydalis turtschaninovii* Besser forma *yanhusuo* Y. H. Chou et C. C. Hsu = *Corydalis turtschaninovii* Besser f. *yanhusuo* (W. T. Wang) Y. H. Chou & C. C. Hsu	*Papaveraceae*
	Corydalis yanhusuo W. T. Wang	
Crataegus Fruit サンザシ	*Crataegus cuneata* Siebold et Zuccarini = *Crataegus cuneata* Siebold & Zucc.	*Rosaceae*
	Crataegus pinnatifida Bunge var. *major* N. E. Brown = *Crataegus pinnatifida* Bunge var. *major* N. E. Br.	
Curcuma Rhizome ガジュツ	*Curcuma zedoaria* Roscoe	*Zingiberaceae*
	Curcuma phaeocaulis Valeton	
	Curcuma kwangsiensis S. G. Lee et C. F. Liang	
Cyperus Rhizome コウブシ	*Cyperus rotundus* Linné = *Cyperus rotundus* L.	*Cyperaceae*
Digenea マクリ	*Digenea simplex* C. Agardh = *Digenea simplex* (Wulfen) C. Agardh	*Rhodomelaceae*
Dioscorea Rhizome サンヤク	*Dioscorea japonica* Thunberg = *Dioscorea japonica* Thunb.	*Dioscoreaceae*
	Dioscorea batatas Decaisne = *Dioscorea batatas* Decne.	
	Dioscorea opposita Thunb.	
Dolichos Seed ヘンズ	*Dolichos lablab* Linné = *Dolichos lablab* L.	*Leguminosae*
Eleutherococcus Senticosus Rhizome シゴカ	*Eleutherococcus senticosus* Maximowicz = *Eleutherococcus senticosus* (Rupr. & Maxim.) Maxim.	*Araliaceae*
	* *Acanthopanax senticosus* Harms = *Acanthopanax senticosus* (Rupr. & Maxim.) Harms	
Ephedra Herb マオウ	*Ephedra sinica* Stapf	*Ephedraceae*
	Ephedra intermedia Schrenk et C. A. Meyer = *Ephedra intermedia* Schrenk & C. A. Mey.	
	Ephedra equisetina Bunge	

Epimedium Herb インヨウカク	*Epimedium koreanum* Nakai	Berberidaceae
	Epimedium grandiflorum Morren var. *thunbergianum* Nakai = *Epimedium grandiflorum* Morr. var. *thunbergianum* (Miq.) Nakai	
	Epimedium pubescens Maximowicz = *Epimedium pubescens* Maxim.	
	Epimedium brevicornu Maximowicz = *Epimedium brevicornu* Maxim.	
	Epimedium wushanense T. S. Ying	
	Epimedium sagittatum Maximowicz = *Epimedium sagittatum* (Siebold & Zucc.) Maxim.	
	Epimedium sempervirens Nakai	
Eucalyptus Oil ユーカリ油	*Eucalyptus globulus* Labillardiere = *Eucalyptus globulus* Labill.	*Myrtaceae*
	Allied species	
Eucommia Bark トチュウ	*Eucommia ulmoides* Oliver = *Eucommia ulmoides* Oliv.	*Eucommiaceae*
Evodia Fruit ゴシュユ	*Euodia officinalis* Dode	*Rutaceae*
	* *Evodia officinalis* Dode *Evodia rutaecarpa* (A. Juss.) Benth. var. *officinalis* (Dode) Huang	
	Euodia bodinieri Dode	
	* *Evodia bodinieri* Dode *Evodia rutaecarpa* (A. Juss.) Benth. var. *bodinieri* (Dode) Huang	
	Euodia ruticarpa Hooker filius et Thomson = *Euodia ruticarpa* (A. Juss.) Hook. f. & Thomson	
	* *Evodia rutaecarpa* Bentham = *Evodia rutaecarpa* (A. Juss.) Benth. *Tetradium ruticarpum* (A. Juss.) Hartley	
Fennel ウイキョウ	*Foeniculum vulgare* Miller = *Foeniculum vulgare* Mill.	*Umbelliferae*
Fennel Oil ウイキョウ油	*Foeniculum vulgare* Miller = *Foeniculum vulgare* Mill.	*Umbelliferae*
	Illicium verum Hooker filius = *Illicium verum* Hook. f.	*Illiciaceae*
Forsythia Fruit レンギョウ	*Forsythia suspensa* Vahl = *Forsythia suspensa* (Thunb.) Vahl	*Oleaceae*
Fritillaria Bulb バイモ	*Fritillaria verticillata* Willdenow var. *thunbergii* Baker = *Fritillaria verticillata* Willd. var. *thunbergii* (Miq.) Baker	*Liliaceae*
	Fritillaria thunbergii Miq.	
Gambir アセンヤク	*Uncaria gambir* Roxburgh = *Uncaria gambir* (Hunter) Roxb.	*Rubiaceae*
Gardenia Fruit サンシシ	*Gardenia jasminoides* Ellis	*Rubiaceae*
	Gardenia jasminoides Ellis f. *longicarpa* Z. W. Xie & Okada	
Gastrodia Tuber テンマ	*Gastrodia elata* Blume	*Orchidaceae*
Gentian ゲンチアナ	*Gentiana lutea* Linné = *Gentiana lutea* L.	*Gentianaceae*

Geranium Herb ゲンノショウコ	*Geranium thunbergii* Siebold et Zuccarini = *Geranium thunbergii* Siebold & Zucc.	*Geraniaceae*
Ginger ショウキョウ	*Zingiber officinale* Roscoe	*Zingiberaceae*
Ginseng ニンジン	*Panax ginseng* C. A. Meyer = *Panax ginseng* C. A. Mey. * *Panax schinseng* Nees	*Araliaceae*
Glehnia Root ハマボウフウ	*Glehnia littoralis* Fr. Schmidt ex Miquel = *Glehnia littoralis* F. Schmidt ex Miq.	*Umbelliferae*
Glycyrrhiza カンゾウ	*Glycyrrhiza uralensis* Fischer = *Glycyrrhiza uralensis* Fisch. *Glycyrrhiza glabra* Linné = *Glycyrrhiza glabra* L.	*Leguminosae*
Hedysarum Root シンギ	*Hedysarum polybotrys* Handel-Mazzetti = *Hedysarum polybotrys* Hand.-Mazz.	*Leguminosae*
Hemp Fruit マシニン	*Cannabis sativa* Linné = *Cannabis sativa* L.	*Moracea*
Honey ハチミツ	*Apis mellifera* Linné = *Apis mellifera* L. *Apis cerana* Fabricius	*Apidae*
Houttuynia Herb ジュウヤク	*Houttuynia cordata* Thunberg = *Houttuynia cordata* Thunb.	*Saururaceae*
Immature Orange キジツ	*Citrus aurantium* Linné var. *daidai* Makino = *Citrus aurantium* L. var. *daidai* Makino *Citrus aurantium* L. 'Daidai' *Citrus natsudaidai* Hayata *Citrus aurantium* Linné = *Citrus aurantium* L. *Citrus aurantium* L. subsp. *hassaku* (Tanaka) Hiroe = *Citrus hassaku* hort. ex Tanaka	*Rutaceae*
Imperata Rhizome ボウコン	*Imperata cylindrica* Beauvois = *Imperata cylindrica* (L.) P. Beauv. *Imperata cylindrica* (L.) P. Beauv. var. *major* (Nees) C. E. Hubb.	*Gramineae*
Ipecac トコン	*Cephaelis ipecacuanha* A. Richard = *Cephaelis ipecacuanha* (Brot.) A. Rich. *Cephaelis acuminata* Karsten = *Cephaelis acuminata* H. Karst.	*Rubiaceae*
Japanese Angelica Root トウキ	*Angelica acutiloba* Kitagawa = *Angelica acutiloba* (Siebold & Zucc.) Kitag. *Angelica acutiloba* Kitagawa var. *sugiyamae* Hikino = *Angelica acutiloba* (Siebold & Zucc.) Kitag. var. *sugiyamae* Hikino	*Umbelliferae*
Japanese Gentian リュウタン	*Gentiana scabra* Bunge *Gentiana scabra* Bunge var. *buergeri* (Miq.) Maxim. *Gentiana manshurica* Kitagawa = *Gentiana manshurica* Kitag. *Gentiana triflora* Pallas = *Gentiana triflora* Pall. *Gentiana triflora* Pall. var. *japonica* Hara	*Gentianaceae*

Japanese Valerian カノコソウ	*Valeriana fauriei* Briquet = *Valeriana fauriei* Briq.	*Valerianaceae*
	Valeriana fauriei Briq. f. *yezoensis* Hara	
Japanese Zanthoxylum Peel サンショウ	*Zanthoxylum piperitum* De Candolle = *Zanthoxylum piperitum* (L.) DC.	*Rutaceae*
	Zanthoxylum piperitum (L.) DC. f. *inerme* Makino	
Jujube タイソウ	*Ziziphus jujuba* Miller var. *inermis* Rehder = *Ziziphus jujuba* Mill. var. *inermis* (Bunge) Rehder	*Rhamnaceae*
Jujube Seed サンソウニン	*Ziziphus jujuba* Miller var. *spinosa* Hu ex H. F. Chow = *Ziziphus jujuba* Mill. var. *spinosa* (Bunge) Hu ex H. F. Chow	*Rhamnaceae*
Koi コウイ	*Zea mays* Linné = *Zea mays* L.	*Gramineae*
	Manihot esculenta Crantz	*Euphorbiacaea*
	Solanum tuberosum Linné = *Solanum tuberosum* L.	*Solanaceae*
	Ipomoea batatas Poiret = *Ipomoea batatas* (L.) Poir.	*Convolvulaceae*
	Ipomoea batatas (L.) Lam.	
	Oryza sativa Linné = *Oryza sativa* L.	*Gramineae*
Purified Lanolin 精製ラノリン	*Ovis aries* Linné = *Ovis aries* L.	*Bovidae*
Lard 豚脂	*Sus scrofa* Linné var. *domesticus* Gray = *Sus scrofa* L. var. *domesticus* Gray	*Suidae*
Leonurus Herb ヤクモソウ	*Leonurus japonicus* Houttuyn = *Leonurus japonicus* Houtt.	*Labiatae*
	Leonurus sibiricus Linné = *Leonurus sibiricus* L.	
Lilium Bulb ビャクゴウ	*Lilium lancifolium* Thunberg = *Lilium lancifolium* Thunb.	*Liliaceae*
	Lilium brownii F. E. Brown var. *colchesteri* Wilosn = *Lilium brownii* F. E. Br. var. *colchesteri* (Van Houtte) E. H. Wilson ex Elwes	
	Lilium brownii F. E. Brown var. *viridulum* Baker	
	Lilium brownii F. E. Brown = *Lilium brownii* F. E. Br.	
	Lilium pumilum De Candolle = *Lilium pumilum* DC.	
Lindera Root ウヤク	*Lindera strychnifolia* Fernandez-Villar = *Lindera strychnifolia* (Siebold & Zucc.) Fern.-Vill.	*Lauraceae*
	Lindera aggregata (Sims) Kosterm.	
Lithospermum Root シコン	*Lithospermum erythrorhizon* Siebold et Zuccarini = *Lithospermum erythrorhizon* Siebold & Zucc.	*Boraginaceae*
Longan Aril リュウガンニク	*Euphoria longana* Lamarck = *Euphoria longana* Lam.	*Sapindaceae*
	Dimocarpus longan Lour.	
Lonicera Leaf and Stem ニンドウ	*Lonicera japonica* Thunberg = *Lonicera japonica* Thunb.	*Caprifoliaceae*

Loquat Leaf ビワヨウ	*Eriobotrya japonica* Lindley = *Eriobotrya japonica* (Thunb.) Lindl.	*Rosaceae*
Lycium Bark ジコッピ	*Lycium chinense* Miller = *Lycium chinense* Mill.	*Solanaceae*
	Lycium barbarum Linné = *Lycium barbarum* L.	
Lycium Fruit クコシ	*Lycium chinense* Miller = *Lycium chinense* Mill.	*Solanaceae*
	Lycium barbarum Linné = *Lycium barbarum* L.	
Magnolia Bark コウボク	*Magnolia obovata* Thunberg = *Magnolia obovata* Thunb.	*Magnoliaceae*
	* *Magnolia hypoleuca* Siebold et Zuccarini = *Magnolia hypoleuca* Siebold & Zucc.	
	Magnolia officinalis Rehder et Wilson = *Magnolia officinalis* Rehder & E. H. Wilson	
	Magnolia officinalis Rehder et Wilson var. *biloba* Rehder et Wilson = *Magnolia officinalis* Rehder & E. H. Wilson var. *biloba* Rehder & E. H. Wilson	
Magnolia Flower シンイ	*Magnolia biondii* Pampanini = *Magnolia biondii* Pamp.	*Magnoliaceae*
	Magnolia heptapeta Dandy = *Magnolia heptapeta* (Buchoz) Dandy	
	* *Magnolia denudata* Desrousseaux = *Magnolia denudata* Desr.	
	Magnolia sprengeri Pampanini = *Magnolia sprengeri* Pamp.	
	Magnolia salicifolia Maximowicz = *Magnolia salicifolia* (Siebold & Zucc.) Maxim.	
	Magnolia kobus De Candolle = *Magnolia kobus* DC.	
Mallotus Bark アカメガシワ	*Mallotus japonicus* Müller Argoviensis = *Mallotus japonicus* (Thunb.) Müll. Arg.	*Euphorbiaceae*
Malt バクガ	*Hordeum vulgare* Linné = *Hordeum vulgare* L.	*Gramineae*
Mentha Herb ハッカ *Mentha Oil* ハッカ油	*Mentha arvensis* Linné var. *piperascens* Malinvaud = *Mentha arvensis* L. var. *piperascens* Malinv.	*Labiatae*
	Mentha haplocalyx Briq.	
	Hybrid originated from *Mentha arvensis* L. var. *piperascens* Malinv. as the mother species	
Moutan Bark ボタンピ	*Paeonia suffruticosa* Andrews	*Paeoniaceae*
	* *Paeonia moutan* Sims	
Mulberry Bark ソウハクヒ	*Morus alba* Linné = *Morus alba* L.	*Moraceae*
Nelumbo Seed レンニク	*Nelumbo nucifera* Gaertner = *Nelumbo nucifera* Gaertn.	*Nymphaeaceae*
Notopterygium Rhizome キョウカツ	*Notopterygium incisum* Ting ex H. T. Chang	*Umbelliferae*
	Notopterygium forbesii Boissieu	

Nuphar Rhizome センコツ	*Nuphar japonica* De Candolle = *Nuphar japonica* DC.	*Nymphaeaceae*
	Nuphar pumila De Candolle = *Nuphar pumila* (Timm) DC.	
Nutmeg ニクズク	*Myristica fragrans* Houttuyn = *Myristica fragrans* Houtt.	*Myristicaceae*
Nux Vomica ホミカ	*Strychnos nux-vomica* Linné = *Strychnos nux-vomica* L.	*Loganiaceae*
Olive Oil オリブ油	*Olea europaea* Linné = *Olea europaea* L.	*Oleaceae*
Ophiopogon Root バクモンドウ	*Ophiopogon japonicus* Ker-Gawler = *Ophiopogon japonicus* (L. f.) Ker Gawl.	*Liliaceae*
Orange Oil オレンジ油	*Citrus species*	*Rutaceae*
Oriental Bezoar ゴオウ	*Bos taurus* Linné var. *domesticus* Gmelin = *Bos taurus* L. var. *domesticus* Gmelin	*Bovidae*
Oyster Shell ボレイ	*Ostrea gigas* Thunberg = *Ostrea gigas* Thunb.	*Ostreidae*
Panax Japonicus Rhizome チクセツニンジン	*Panax japonicus* C. A. Meyer = *Panax japonicus* C. A. Mey.	*Araliaceae*
Peach Kernel トウニン	*Prunus persica* Batsch = *Prunus persica* (L.) Batsch	*Rosaceae*
	Prunus persica Batsch var. *davidiana* Maximowicz = *Prunus persica* (L.) Batsch var. *davidiana* (Carrière) Maxim.	
	Prunus davidiana (Carrière) Franch.	
Peanut Oil ラッカセイ油	*Arachis hypogaea* Linné = *Arachis hypogaea* L.	*Leguminosae*
Peony Root シャクヤク	*Paeonia lactiflora* Pallas = *Paeonia lactiflora* Pall.	*Paeoniaceae*
Perilla Herb ソヨウ	*Perilla frutescens* Britton var. *crispa* W. Deane = *Perilla frutescens* (L.) Britton var. *crispa* (Thunb.) W. Deane	*Labiatae*
Peucedanum Root ゼンコ	*Peucedanum praeruptorum* Dunn	*Umbelliferae*
	Angelica decursiva Franchet et Savatier = *Angelica decursiva* (Miq.) Franch. & Sav.	
	* *Peucedanum decursivum* Maximowicz = *Peucedanum decursivum* (Miq.) Maxim.	
Pharbitis Seed ケンゴシ	*Pharbitis nil* Choisy = *Pharbitis nil* (L.) Choisy	*Convolvulaceae*
Phellodendron Bark オウバク	*Phellodendron amurense* Ruprecht = *Phellodendron amurense* Rupr.	*Rutaceae*
	Phellodendron amurense Rupr. var. *sachalinense* F. Schmidt *Phellodendron amurense* Rupr. var. *japonicum* (Maxim.) Ohwi *Phellodendron amurense* Rupr. var. *lavallei* (Dode) Sprangue	
	Phellodendron chinense Schneider = *Phellodendron chinense* C. K. Schneid.	
Picrasma Wood ニガキ	*Picrasma quassioides* Bennet = *Picrasma quassioides* (D. Don) Benn.	*Simaroubaceae*
Pinellia Tuber ハンゲ	*Pinellia ternata* Breitenbach = *Pinellia ternata* (Thunb.) Breitenb.	*Araceae*

Plantago Herb シャゼンソウ	*Plantago asiatica* Linné = *Plantago asiatica* L.	*Plantaginaceae*
Plantago Seed シャゼンシ	*Plantago asiatica* Linné = *Plantago asiatica* L.	*Plantaginaceae*
Platycodon Root キキョウ	*Platycodon grandiflorus* A. De Candolle = *Platycodon grandiflorus* (Jacq.) A. DC.	*Campanulaceae*
Pogostemon Herb カッコウ	*Pogostemon cablin* Bentham = *Pogostemon cablin* (Blanco) Benth.	*Labiatae*
Polygala Root オンジ	*Polygala tenuifolia* Willdenow = *Polygala tenuifolia* Willd.	*Polygalaceae*
Polygonatum Rhizome オウセイ	*Polygonatum kingianum* Collett et Hemsley = *Polygonatum kingianum* Collett & Hemsl.	*Liliaceae*
	Polygonatum sibiricum Redouté	
	Polygonatum cyrtonema Hua	
	Polygonatum falcatum A. Gray	
Polygonum Root カシュウ	*Polygonum multiflorum* Thunberg = *Polygonum multiflorum* Thunb.	*Polygonaceae*
Polyporus Sclerotium チョレイ	*Polyporus umbellatus* Fries = *Polyporus umbellatus* (Pers.) Fries	*Polyporaceae*
Poria Sclerotium ブクリョウ	*Wolfiporia cocos* Ryvarden et Gilbertson = *Wolfiporia cocos* (Schw.) Ryv. & Gilbn.	*Polyporaceae*
	* *Poria cocos* Wolf = *Poria cocos* (Schw.) Wolf	
Powdered Opium アヘン末	*Papaver somniferum* Linné = *Papaver somniferum* L.	*Papaveraceae*
Prepared Glycyrrhiza シャカンゾウ	*Glycyrrhiza uralensis* Fischer = *Glycyrrhiza uralensis* Fisch.	*Leguminosae*
	Glycyrrhiza glabra Linné = *Glycyrrhiza glabra* L.	
Processed Aconite Root ブシ	*Aconitum carmichaeli* Debeaux	*Ranunculaceae*
	Aconitum japonicum Thunberg = *Aconitum japonicum* Thunb.	
Processed Ginger カンキョウ	*Zingiber officinale* Roscoe	*Zingiberaceae*
Prunella Spike カゴソウ	*Prunella vulgaris* Linné var. *lilacina* Nakai = *Prunella vulgaris* L. var. *lilacina* Nakai	*Labiatae*
Pueraria Root カッコン	*Pueraria lobata* Ohwi = *Pueraria lobata* (Willd.) Ohwi	*Leguminosae*
Quercus Bark ボクソク	*Quercus acutissima* Carruthers = *Quercus acutissima* Carruth.	*Fagaceae*
	Quercus serrata Murray	
	Quercus mongholica Fischer ex Ledebour var. *crispula* Ohashi = *Quercus mongholica* Fisch. ex Ledeb. var. *crispula* (Blume) Ohashi	
	Quercus variabilis Blume	
Rape Seed Oil ナタネ油	*Brassica napus* Linné = *Brassica napus* L.	*Cruciferae*
	Brassica rapa Linné var. *oleifera* De Candolle = *Brassica rapa* L. var. *oleifera* DC.	

Red Ginseng コウジン	*Panax ginseng* C. A. Meyer = *Panax ginseng* C. A. Mey.	*Araliaceae*
	* *Panax schinseng* Nees	
Rehmannia Root ジオウ	*Rehmannia glutinosa* Liboschitz var. *purpurea* Makino = *Rehmannia glutinosa* Libosch. var. *purpurea* Makino	*Scrophulariaceae*
	Rehmannia glutinosa Liboschitz = *Rehmannia glutinosa* Libosch.	
Rhubarb ダイオウ	*Rheum palmatum* Linné = *Rheum palmatum* L.	*Polygonaceae*
	Rheum tanguticum Maximowicz = *Rheum tanguticum* Maxim.	
	Rheum officinale Baillon = *Rheum officinale* Baill.	
	Rheum coreanum Nakai	
	Interspecific hybrid between above species	
Rose Fruit エイジツ	*Rosa multiflora* Thunberg = *Rosa multiflora* Thunb.	*Rosaceae*
Rosin ロジン	Several plants of *Pinus genus*	*Pinaceae*
Royal Jelly ローヤルゼリー	*Apis mellifera* Linné = *Apis mellifera* L.	*Apidae*
	Apis cerana Fabricius	
Safflower コウカ	*Carthamus tinctorius* Linné = *Carthamus tinctorius* L.	*Compositae*
Saffron サフラン	*Crocus sativus* Linné = *Crocus sativus* L.	*Iridaceae*
Salvia Miltiorrhiza Root タンジン	*Salvia miltiorrhiza* Bunge	*Labiatae*
Saposhnikovia Root ボウフウ	*Saposhnikovia divaricata* Schischkin = *Saposhnikovia divaricata* (Turcz.) Schischk.	*Umbelliferae*
Sappan Wood ソボク	*Caesalpinia sappan* Linné = *Caesalpinia sappan* L.	*Leguminosae*
Saussurea Root モッコウ	*Saussurea lappa* Clarke = *Saussurea lappa* (Decne.) C. B. Clarke	*Compositae*
	Aucklandia lappa Decne.	
Schisandra Fruit ゴミシ	*Schisandra chinensis* Baillon = *Schisandra chinensis* (Turcz.) Baill.	*Schisandraceae*
Schizonepeta Spike ケイガイ	*Schizonepeta tenuifolia* Briquet = *Schizonepeta tenuifolia* Briq.	*Labiatae*
Scopolia Rhizome ロートコン	*Scopolia japonica* Maximowicz = *Scopolia japonica* Maxim.	*Solanaceae*
	Scopolia carniolica Jacquin = *Scopolia carniolica* Jacq.	
	Scopolia parviflora Nakai = *Scopolia parviflora* (Dunn) Nakai	
Scutellaria Root オウゴン	*Scutellaria baicalensis* Georgi	*Labiatae*

Senega セネガ	*Polygala senega* Linné = *Polygala senega* L.	*Polygalaceae*
	Polygala senega Linné var. *latifolia* Torrey et Gray = *Polygala senega* L. var. *latifolia* Torr. & A. Gray	
Senna Leaf センナ	*Cassia angustifolia* Vahl	*Leguminosae*
	Cassia acutifolia Delile	
Sesame ゴマ Sesame Oil ゴマ油	*Sesamum indicum* Linné = *Sesamum indicum* L.	*Pedaliaceae*
Sinomenium Stem ボウイ	*Sinomenium acutum* Rehder et Wilson = *Sinomenium acutum* (Thunb.) Rehder & E. H. Wilson	*Menispermaceae*
Smilax Rhizome サンキライ	*Smilax glabra* Roxburgh = *Smilax glabra* Roxb.	*Liliaceae*
Sophora Root クジン	*Sophora flavescens* Aiton	*Leguminosae*
Soybean Oil ダイズ油	*Glycine max* Merrill = *Glycine max* (L.) Merr.	*Leguminosae*
Sweet Hydrangea Leaf アマチャ	*Hydrangea macrophylla* Seringe var. *thunbergii* Makino = *Hydrangea macrophylla* (Thunb.) Ser. var. *thunbergii* (Siebold) Makino	*Saxifragaceae*
Swertia Herb センブリ	*Swertia japonica* Makino = *Swertia japonica* (Shult.) Makino	*Gentianaceae*
Toad Cake センソ	*Bufo gargarizans* Cantor = *Bufo bufo gargarizans* Cantor	*Bufonidae*
	Bufo melanostictus Schneider = *Duttaphrynus melanostictus* Schneider	
Tragacanth トラガント	*Astragalus gummifer* Labillardiére = *Astragalus gummifer* Labill.	*Leguminosae*
Tribulus Fruit シツリシ	*Tribulus terrestris* Linné = *Tribulus terrestris* L.	*Zygophyllaceae*
Trichosanthes Root カロコン	*Trichosanthes kirilowii* Maximowicz = *Trichosanthes kirilowii* Maxim.	*Cucurbitaceae*
	Trichosanthes kirilowii Maximowicz var. *japonica* Kitamura = *Trichosanthes kirilowii* Maxim. var. *japonica* (Miq.) Kitam.	
	Trichosanthes bracteata Voigt = *Trichosanthes bracteata* (Lam.) Voigt	
Turmeric ウコン	*Curcuma longa* Linné = *Curcuma longa* L.	*Zingiberaceae*
Turpentine Oil テレビン油	Several plants of *Pinus genus*	*Pinaceae*
Uncaria Hook チョウトウコウ	*Uncaria rhynchophylla* Miquel = *Uncaria rhynchophylla* (Miq.) Miq.	*Rubiaceae*
	Uncaria sinensis Haviland = *Uncaria sinensis* (Oliv.) Havil.	
	Uncaria macrophylla Wallich = *Uncaria macrophylla* Wall.	

Wood Creosote 木クレオソート	Several plants of *Pinus* genus	*Pinaceae*
	Several plants of *Cryptomeria* genus	*Taxodiaceae*
	Several plants of *Fagus* genus	*Fagaceae*
	Several plants of *Afzelia (Intsia)* genus	*Leguminosae*
	Several plants of *Shorea* genus	*Dipterocarpaceae*
	Several plants of *Tectona* genus	*Verbenaceae*

When ''Other species of the same genus'' is included as its original plants the scientific name is not written in Monograph, however, it is written in this table.

Reference

Terabayashi S. *et al*.: Pharmaceutical and Medical Device Regulatory Science, 41(5), 407 – 418 (2010).

essary the same as the taxonomic system used in the literature. The reason for this is that the JP is not an academic text, but an ordinance. The relationship between the scientific names used in the JP and those generally used taxonomically is indicated in the following table, to avoid misunderstanding by JP users owing to differences in the notation system.

Notification for the Quantitative Marker Constituents of Crude Drugs and Crude Drug Preparations *<G5-2-170>*

One of the highly distinctive features of the crude drugs and preparations containing crude drugs as main ingredient (crude drug preparations) is the fact that they are multicomponent systems composed of a prodigious number of compounds. As an example, glycyrrhiza, one of the most important crude drugs worldwide has been demonstrated that they harbor more than 100 kinds of secondary metabolites, and this number could be counted up to more than 1000 when the intermediates occurred in the biosynthetic pathways were included. The whole members of the compounds are supposed to be integrated to reveal the effects of glycyrrhiza.

A wide diversity of constituents in the drugs made from botanical raw materials is fundamentally derived from a wide variety of secondary metabolites occurred in plants. However, there are more reasons for the diversity. The species of plants used as raw materials for drugs are specified in the approval documents of the drugs, though, a variation of their composition derived from the genetic variation of the plants will be produced since each botanical species includes a significant genetic divergence. The secondary metabolites of plants will be further differentiated in their quality and quantity according to the environmental factors such as soil (soil texture, water retentivity, pH, etc.) and weather (amount of precipitation, temperature, humidity, etc.) conditions. Furthermore, the constituents will change depending on wild or cultivation, cultivation method and harvest period. Also crude drugs are finally processed by excluding periderm, steaming, roasting, etc. and consequently the constituents are different according to the process method.

The stipulation on the contents (quantitative values) of marker constituents in crude drugs and crude drug preparations has very important implications for standardization of the quality of pharmaceutical natural products. The stipulations on crude drugs generally provide the minimum requisite amount of marker compounds. For example, glycyrrhiza of the Japanese Pharmacopoeia is ordered to contain not less than 2.0% of glycyrrhizic acid. Crude drugs are known to exhibit large difference in the content of secondary metabolites among individual plants that caused from multiple reasons described in the previous paragraph. It is reported that the glycyrrhizic acid content of glycyrrhiza in one plant can contain some 10 times the content of another plant when they are grown together in one farm field and harvested simultaneously. Accordingly, it is hard to standardize the ranges of content for marker constituents of crude drugs on a policy of the efficient use of natural resources for crude drugs. However, the crude drug preparations as finished products are required to contain a certain amount of active ingredients from a perspective of the reproducibility of medical treatments. Consequently, the marker constituents of the Kampo formulations and conventional crude drug preparations as the final stage of crude drug preparations are generally specified by the range of content values. Crude drugs containing different amount of marker constituents are appropriately blended to prepare the finished products with a particular amount of marker constituents.

It should be noted that the marker constituents of crude drugs for regulations include a variety of types. Followings are the examples of some different types. Sennosides, the marker constituents of senna leaf are the obvious active ingredients that accounts for the laxative effects of senna leaf to some extent. Other compounds of the anthraquinone-type found in senna leaf, such as rhein and aloe-emodin, are also potent as laxative, though, because of their large difference in content in senna leaf, a medicinal effect of senna leaf can be standardized by managing the content of sennosides. However, sennosides are likely to be broken down into anthraquinones by heating and other factors that not only sennosides but also the increased rhein may be targeted for standardization in cases of the Kampo formula extracts including rhubarb, one of the sennoside-containing crude drugs, as a component. On the other hand, glycyrrhizic acid, a very famous bioactive component of glycyrrhiza, is an active ingredient that contributes to some parts of the medical effect of glycyrrhiza. Though, many components other than glycyrrhizic acid are also known to play a part in the medical effects of glycyrrhiza. Consequently, glycyrrhizic acid should be regarded as one of the multiple active ingredients of glycyrrhiza that being specified its content as a marker constituent. In other cases of the marker constituents that seemed to have less biological effects such as 10-hydroxy-2-(*E*)-decenoic acid in royal jelly or (*E*)-cinnamic acid in some extracts of Kampo formula, their content are standardized as a distinctive compound of each pharmaceutical product. Referring to the biosyntheses of natural products, the content of these compounds specified as marker constituents are unlikely to be independently changed to stand out from others. The specification values of crude drugs and crude drug preparations are stipulated in order to control the appropriate production process based on the strategy that every crude drug and crude drug preparation will be standardized to a certain level through the content control of marker constituents.

An instance of the relationship between the active ingredient and the marker compound of senna leaf may be a special case among crude drugs and pharmaceutical natural products made from crude drugs. The medicinal effects of the majority of crude drugs and pharmaceutical natural products made from crude drugs are achieved by the cooperative performance of their entire constituents. These drugs are standardized with the quantitative specification of particular constituents designated as the quantitative marker constituents, and this is owing to the fact that the standardization of every constituent consisting the multicomponent system is impossible. Taken all together, it requires particular consideration to the fact that the quantitative marker compounds specified for crude drugs and crude drug preparations are not directly same as the active ingredients in the chemical drugs that absolutely accounts for the medical effects of the drugs.

Thin-layer Chromatography for Crude Drugs and Crude Drug Preparations <*G5-3-170*>

Thin-layer chromatography is a method to separate each component by developing with a mobile phase, using a thin-layer consisting of an appropriate stationary phase, and is used for identification, purity test, etc. of substances.

Thin-layer chromatography for crude drugs and preparations containing crude drugs as main ingredient (crude drug preparations) is used for identifying whether characteristic constituents or groups of constituents in crude drugs and extracts based on Kampo formulae are included or not.

1. Instruments and equipment:

Generally, the following instruments and equipment are used.

(i) Thin-layer plate: A smooth and uniformly thick glass plate is coated in advance with an uniform powder of carrier listed in Solid Supports/Column Packings for Chromatography <*9.42*>. It is classified into two types. The stationary phase of thin-layer chromatography plates (TLC plates) has a particle size of 10 - 15 μm, and that of high-performance thin-layer chromatography plates (HPTLC plates) has a particle size of 5 - 7 μm. In a case where separation requirements given that the quality of the chromatogram indicated in the individual monograph is ensured, it is possible to use a thin-layer plate with a preadsorbent zone which has been coated in advance and the home-made plate. Alternatively, such thin-layer plates are also available that use plate-like or sheeted hard aluminum and polyester for support medium instead of glass plate. Thin-layer plates are kept while avoiding humidity.

(ii) Application of samples: The sample solution(s) or standard solution(s) at the prescribed volume in the individual monograph are applied with sample applicators of constant volume, which is generally a special capillary or microsyringe, at a position around 20 mm distance from the lower edge as a starting line of and release at least 10 mm from side to side edges of the thin-layer plate, in the form of circular spots (spot-like) of 2 - 6 mm in diameter or narrow linearly bands (band-shaped) of 4 - 10 mm in width with an appropriate interval of at least about 10 mm and then allowed to dry in air. In a case where separation requirements given that the quality of the chromatogram indicated in the individual monograph is ensured, it is possible to modify the position of a starting line and sample spots application interval.

(iii) Chromatographic chamber: Generally, a chromatographic chamber made of inert, transparent material and having a lid is used: a flat-bottom or twin trough. Unless otherwise specified, attach a filter paper along with the inside wall of the chamber, and moisten the filter paper with the developing solvent. In the chamber, the developing solvent is placed up to about 10 mm in height from the bottom, seal the chamber closely, and allow it to stand for 1 hour at ordinary temperature. Place a thin-layer plate in the chamber so as only the upper end of the plate is touched to the wall of the chamber, seal the chamber closely, and perform the development at ordinary temperature. A chromatographic chamber shall be of a size appropriate for the thin-layer plate and the developing solvent to be poured into shall be of a volume not to immerse spot(s) or band(s) of samples applied to the thin-layer plate in advance.

(iv) Device for coloring: A glass mister sprayer or an electric mister sprayer is used for spraying a visualization reagent. Drying the thin-layer plate after development, visualization of components to be tested on the chromatogram is performed by an evenly sprayed visualization reagent directly on the thin-layer plate to work the test reagent. The ways to discharge the visualization reagent include air supply of compressed gas either by manually or electrically. Further, in case of a heating device, components to be tested which have been separated on the chromatogram are heated after spraying a visualization reagent and derivatized for visualization. It is preferable to use a hot plate at a constant temperature to heat a thin-layer plate after spraying visualization reagent. In case of using a thermostatic oven, thin-layer plate is heated on the metal plate heated to a constant temperature in advance. A flat-bottom trough chamber, twin trough chamber and desiccator, could be used during the immersion visualization and the fumigation (exposure to reagent vapor) visualization.

(v) Detection device: It is a camera obscura equipped with visible light, ultraviolet light of wavelength 254 nm and 365 nm, and wide-range wavelength ultraviolet light, and corresponding filter, a dark box or room. The light source is required to meet the requirements for the tests prescribed in the individual monograph. Photographing device to be added to the detecting device is used for taking photographs to be recorded and requires adequate sensitivity, resolution and reproducibility enough to perform the tests.

(vi) Record of TLC images: TLC images are taken by a camera and recorded/stored in a format of film image or electronic image. Except for detection after exposure to ultraviolet radiation, it is preferable to take pictures of color samples for reference concurrently in case of recording color tones of chromatogram detected under a visible light. Further, it should be noted that color tones identified visually and those recorded are different in some cases when recording fluorescent spots caused by irradiation with a wavelength of 365 nm. It is also possible to use an image scanner with sufficient resolution to record chromatograms detected under visible light. A TLC scanning device is capable of detecting absorption of light or fluorescence of chromatograms and spots or bands of samples to be tested and recording absorption and fluorescence spectra corresponding to components to be tested.

(vii) TLC scanning device: The device measures absorption by ultraviolet or visible light or fluorescence by excitation light on a developed thin-layer plate and stores records of development patterns by converting them into chromatograms (peak information). Scanning data obtained from chromatograms is used for quantitative analyses.

2. Detection and visualization

Generally, pulling out a thin-layer plate and drying it after development, detection of spots separated on a chromatogram is visually confirmed under visible light directly or after visualized. It is detected as a spot in a form close to circle when applied in a circular form (spot-like) and as a linear band when applied in a narrow linear form (band-shaped). In case of components to be tested having ultraviolet absorptivity, detection is performed using a thin-layer plate containing fluorescent agent (fluorescent indicator) by ultraviolet irradiation with a dominant wavelength of 254 nm. While fluorescent indicator contained in the thin-layer plate emits greenish fluorescence excited by irradiation with a dominant wavelength of 254 nm, spots or bands of components to be tested reduce radiation light emission by absorbing irradiation light to reduce excitation of fluorescent indicator resulting in an observation as raspberry (dark purple) spots or bands. With a property to produce fluorescence on itself excited under ultraviolet irradiation, spots or bands of components to be tested produce fluorescence excited on the thin-layer plate by irradiation of ultraviolet with a dominant wavelength of 365 nm even without using fluorescent indicator. High illumination light source with stable radiation intensity at around 365 nm within the ultraviolet wavelength range includes lamps having a line spectrum with a narrow width at 365 nm and having a line spectrum at 366 nm (within a range from 364 to 367 nm) with more intense radiated signal. Even though light source and wavelength described in specification differs depending on the lamps to be used, light source lamp with a wavelength of 366 nm also includes a light source lamp with a wavelength of 365 nm making it possible to handle as a description of irradiation with a dominant ultraviolet wavelength of 365 nm.

Derivatization reaction based on spraying, immersion and fumigation of an appropriate coloring reagent visualizes spots or bands of components to be tested. In case of some visualization reagents, such derivatization reaction is further visualized by subsequent heating after spraying reagents. In some cases, characteristic fluorescence may be produced by irradiation with a dominant wavelength of 365 nm after spraying or after spraying and heating as well.

3. Operation methods

Generally, unless otherwise specified, operation method shall comply with the following methods. Prepared sample solution and standard solution which is prescribed in the individual monograph shall be applied on the starting line of a thin-layer plate by an indicated volume. Confirming that applied circular form or linear spots or bands are not immersed in the developing solvent and placing a thin-layer plate in a developing container, developments are initiated after closing the lid of the chromatographic chamber. Sending up the developing solvent to a required development distance, the thin-layer plate is taken out to be allowed to dry in air. In addition, starting line (starting point) and mobile phase front are marked before and after development. Then, based on visualization of chromatogram on the thin-layer plate, color tone or Rf value of circular spots or linear bands of components to be tested is determined (Fig. 1). Rf value is obtained

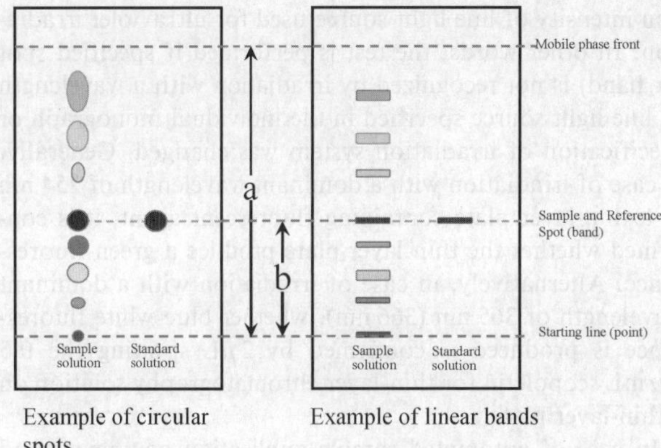

Fig. 1 Pattern diagram of TLC chromatogram

by the following formula.

$$Rf = \frac{\text{Distance from starting line to center of spot or band}}{\text{Distance from starting line to mobile phase front}} = \frac{b}{a}$$

Development operation and visualization shall be performed in an apparatus such as a draft chamber in which solvent vapor is efficiently removed with sufficient air ventilation.

4. Confirmation and purity test

When using this test method for an identification test, it is confirmed in general that color tone and Rf value of components to be tested in sample solution is equal to those in standard solution. In case of the identification test of multicomponent system sample solution, it is possible to confirm by color tone and Rf value of spots when components to be tested are recognized as a single spot clearly showing characteristic fluorescence and coloring. Alternatively, it is also possible to identify by the patterns of spots and bands. Moreover, this test method in combination with spectroscopic method (such as Ultraviolet-visible Spectrophotometry *<2.24>*, Nuclear Magnetic Resonance Spectrophotometry *<2.21>*) and Mass Spectrometry *<2.62>* makes it possible to perform further reliable confirmation.

In case of using this test method for purity test, a standard solution with a concentration corresponding to the limit of impurities in the sample solution is used in general, and purity is confirmed by whether any spot of components to be tested derived from sample solution is detected or whether the magnitude of the spot is lighter than that of standard solution.

5. Semi-quantitative and quantitative measurement

Presumptive quantitative measurement can be made by observation of spots or bands of identical Rf value and about equal magnitude obtained, respectively, with sample solution and standard solution or indicative component solution by applying the same volume, chromatographed on the same thin-layer plate. A visual comparison of the size or intensity of the spots or bands may serve for semi-quantitative estimation. Quantitative measurements are possible by means of densitometry.

6. Confirmation of suitability of lamp

Objectives of confirmation of suitability are sensitivity, resolution and reproducibility required for securing quality of chromatogram and satisfying separation requirements specified in the individual monograph. Confirmation of suitability in this test method is performed mainly for radiation intensity of line light source used for ultraviolet irradiation. In other words, the test is performed if specified spot (or band) is not recognized by irradiation with a wavelength of line light source specified in the individual monograph or specification of irradiation system was changed. Generally, in case of irradiation with a dominant wavelength of 254 nm to a thin-layer plate containing fluorescent agent, it is confirmed whether the thin-layer plate produce a green fluorescence. Alternatively, in case of irradiation with a dominant wavelength of 365 nm (366 nm), whether blue-white fluorescence is produced is confirmed by 2 μL spotting the 0.5 μg/mL scopoletin for thin-layer chromatography solution on a thin-layer plate.

In case of automated sample application equipment and TLC scanning device using densitometry, specifications of system suitability in Liquid Chromatography *<2.01>* is applied as required.

7. Point to consider regarding test conditions

Among tests prescribed in individual monograph, in identification tests using reagents of the Reference Standard or components to be tested (such as reagents for thin-layer chromatography), it is possible to modify developing temperature, developing distance, composition of developing solvent, developing rate, coloring reagent composition, heating temperature and duration of thin-layer plate within a range of better accuracy and precision than those prescribed is secured. However, such semi-quantitative identification tests are excluded that judgment criteria is based on size and strength of spots. On the other hand, in identification tests which do not use reagents of the Reference Standard or components to be tested, it is possible to modify developing distance, heating temperature and duration of thin-layer plate within a range where separation, *R*f value and color tone prescribed in individual monograph is observed. Further, even in case of identification tests without specification for the Reference Standard or components to be tested, it is possible to make a confirmation based on conformity of color tone for reference and *R*f value using the Reference Standard or components to be tested.

8. Reference

1) MHLW Notification No. 65 of March 24, 2011, The Japanese Pharmacopoeia Sixteenth Edition/General Test Procedures/2. Physical Test Procedures/2.01 Liquid Chromatography/2.03 Thin-layer Chromatography
2) EP 8.0 (2014), 2.2.27/Thin-Layer Chromatography
3) USP 37 (2014), <621> Chromatography, <201> Thin-Layer Chromatographic Identification Test
4) Pharmacopoeia of the People's Republic of China (2010), A-42 Appendix VI B Thin-Layer Chromatography (English version)
5) Y. Goda: The Japanese Journal of Pharmacognosy, 66, 63 (2012).

Aristolochic Acid *<G5-4-141>*

Aristolochic acid, which occurs in plants of *Aristolochiaceae*, is suspected to cause renal damage. It is also reported to be oncogenic (see References).

Aristolochic acid toxicity will not be a problem if crude drugs of the origin and parts designated in the JP are used, but there may be differences in crude drug nomenclature between different countries, and it is known that crude drug preparations not meeting the specifications of the JP are circulating in some countries. Consequently, when crude drugs or their preparations are used, it is important that the materials should not include any plant containing aristolochic acid.

Since Supplement I to JP14, the test for aristolochic acid I was added to the Purity under Asiasarum Root, which consists of the rhizome and root. Because the aerial part of the plant may contain aristolochic acid and may have been improperly contaminated in Asiasarum Root.

It is considered that Akebia Stem, Sinomenium Stem and Saussurea Root do not contain aristolochic acid, unless plants of origin other than that designated in the JP are used. However, contamination of aristolochic acid might occur, as mentioned above. In this case, the test described in the Purity under Asiasarum Root is useful for checking the presence of aristolochic acid.

1. References

1) Drug & Medical Device Safety Information, No. 161, July, 2000, https://www.pmda.go.jp/safety/info-services/drugs/calling-attention/safety-info/0092.html#10 (Reference: 2019-7-18).
2) J. L. Nortier, *et al.*, *N. Engl. J. Med.*, 342, 1686 – 1692 (2000).
3) A. Kohara, *et al.*, *Mutation Research*, 515, 63 – 72 (2002).

Quantitative Analytical Technique Utilizing Nuclear Magnetic Resonance (NMR) Spectroscopy and its Application to Reagents in the Japanese Pharmacopoeia *<G5-5-170>*

1. Marker Compounds for the Assay of Crude Drugs in the JP and Establishment of Reference Substances for Quantitative Analyses

When the quantitative assay values are specified in the monographs of crude drugs and extracts of Kampo formulations in the JP, it is more difficult to establish and prepare their JP Reference Standards than those for synthetic chemical pharmaceutical substances, because the marker compounds for their assay are derived from natural sources.

Unlike the synthetic chemical pharmaceutical substances, crude drugs and extracts of Kampo formulations are mixtures of a great deal of compounds. Although it is necessary to choose a substance contained at the level of 0.1% to several % in the crude drugs and the extracts of Kampo formulations as the marker compounds for their quantitative assay, the synthesis of such compounds is not so easy in most cases. Therefore, the marker compound would be separated from natural materials and be isolated to have sufficient purity. However, the preparation of the reference substance in such a way would require high economical cost and a great deal of effort. In addition, the composition of impurities contained in the reference substance prepared in such a way would be different batch by batch according to the difference of raw materials and their processes of extraction, isolation and purification. Accordingly, the difference among batches of reference materials is much larger than that of synthetic substances, and the control of their purity as the official reference standards is very difficult. Furthermore, in many cases of substances of natural origin, the greatest impurity would be water. For determining water contents precisely, it is necessary to use Karl Fischer method, and as the result, a large quantity of the valuable reference standard would be consumed.

Because there are such bottlenecks mentioned above in many cases of monographs of crude drugs and extracts of Kampo formulations, the establishment of the JP Reference Standard is difficult. Instead, reagents, which are commercially available or ready to put into the market, are designated as the reference substances for the quantitative assay, and the method and the content specification using the reagent are specified in monographs of crude drugs and extracts of Kampo formulations. In these cases, the specifications of their marker substances are defined in the section of Reagents and Test Solutions of the JP. However, in a strict sense, since the assay values obtained in this manner are not certified metrologically, the reliability of the analytical value obtained by using them is somewhat ambiguous.

2. Application of Quantitative NMR to Reference Substances Used in the Assay of Crude Drugs and Extracts of Kampo Formulations

The application of quantitative NMR can solve the issue on the purity of reagents derived from natural source. These reagents are used as the reference substances with metrological traceability, when the precise contents of these reagents are determined metrologically by using quantitative NMR based on the idea shown in 10.1 Principle of Quantitative Analytical Technique Utilizing Nuclear Magnetic Resonance (NMR) Spectroscopy under <*5.01*> Crude Drugs Test.

Currently, the quantitative NMR is being carried out for these reagents defined for the quantitative assay of crude drugs in the JP and a report in which the points to practically consider at determination of absolute purities of the reagents by using quantitative NMR are discussed has been published.[1)] In addition, a validation study of quantitative NMR has also been performed using the substances which will be used with high possibility as the reference substances for HPLC quantitative analysis. For the analyte compound having molecular mass of around 300, when about 10 mg of the compound was used for the quantitative NMR measurement, it was demonstrated that an accuracy of 2 significant digits for the determined value was achieved at the ordinary laboratory level, even when the error among the NMR instruments used was included.[2)] Usually, the contents of marker compounds for the quantitative assay of crude drugs are several % at the maximum, and the minimum unit for the content specification is at the level of 0.1%. Therefore, when variability of content in crude drugs is considered, the assurance of 2 significant digits for accuracy seems sufficient for the reference substances, which are used for the quantitative assay of crude drugs.

When discussion above is considered, the ambiguity of analytical values obtained by the use of the reagents derived from natural source as the reference substances for the quantitative assay of crude drugs can be avoided practically, by using the reagents certified by quantitative NMR as the reference substances in HPLC, etc., and by incorporating the certified purity of such reagents into the calculation of the quantitative value of the sample. For example, for Gardenia Fruit in the JP, the content of geniposide is specified at not less than 3.0% based on the HPLC analysis. The report cited above[1)] demonstrated that the absolute purity of geniposide used as the reference substance in the quantitative assay of Gardenia Fruit is determined to be about 92% by quantitative NMR. Therefore, in the case that the quantitative value of 3.0% in Gardenia Fruit sample is obtained as a result of HPLC analysis by using this reagent as the reference substance assuming its purity as 100%, the true value for the sample is evaluated to be 2.8% taking it into consideration of the absolute purity determined by quantitative NMR with the assurance of metrological traceability.

3. Supply of Certified Reagents by Using Quantitative NMR

Currently, in the accreditation system of the International Accreditation Japan (IA Japan), the National Institute of Technology and Evaluation (ASNITE), a feasibility study how the accreditation should be given to the organization which performs the assay certification of the reagents using calibrated NMR apparatus has been in progress. In addition, in the IA Japan, addition of "Quantitative NMR" to the test method categories is scheduled. Therefore, in the near future, the reagent manufacturers will become able to perform the assay certification of the reagent after having this accreditation. Under such situation, the user of the reagent would not be required to perform qualitative NMR individually to obtain the purity value with SI traceability. Furthermore, the inter-institutional errors (including inter-instrumental errors) would become negligible, and we will be able to carry out more precise and accurate quantitation assay of the sample by incorporating the labeled certified value on the reagent into the calculation of the quantitative value of the sample.

The certified reference materials (NMIJ CRM) to be used for the SI traceable metrological determination of the internal reference compounds are supplied from the National Metrology Institute of Japan, National Institute of Advanced Industrial Science and Technology (NMIJ AIST).

4. Management of Instrument Performance for Quantitative NMR

Quantitative NMR used to determine the purity of reagents for the JP, is an internal standard method that an analyte compound and a SI traceable reference material in a NMR tube are measured at the same time.[3)] In this method, the number of nuclei are measured using NMR phenomenon, which means that the molar quantity of an analyte compound in a sample solution is directly calibrated with a reference material.

In the management of instrument performance for quantitative NMR measurements, it should be confirmed that integral value of the targeted signals can be determined correctly within the spectrum where the signals are measured (in general, 0 – 10 ppm). The important point here is not to include the signals derived from impure substances in the quantitative spectrum when integrate. Therefore, to manage instrument performance, a high-purity compound of already known purity (determined by quantitative NMR and not less than 99.0% is preferable) should be used. In addition, signals derived from simpler spin system should be selected and integrated, and the ratio of theoretical number of nuclei among signals should be accurate (for example, when each of the two signals is derived from 1H, the ratio of the integrated values of the both is 0.995 – 1.005).

Considering the excitation bandwidth of a NMR pulse, when an instrument of 800 MHz is used under the following conditions; center of spectrum window around 5 ppm, spectral width at 20 ppm (the conditions stipulated in the assay using qNMR in the section of reagents), with a 90° pulse width of 10 microseconds, the excitation efficiency of the pulse in the range of 0 – 10 ppm, where signals of an analyte compound are observed, is usually not less than 99.95%. Thus, the instrument, when the probe is well tuned and shim is adjusted properly, can assure an accuracy of 2 significant digits at routine level of measurement. Furthermore, when an instrument of 400 MHz is used, similar excitation efficiency can be obtained up to 20 microseconds for 90° pulse width, so quantitative NMR can be measured sufficiently with a standard probe.

5. Reference

1) J. Hosoe, *et al.*, *Pharmaceutical and Medical Device Regulatory Science*, 41, 960 - 970 (2010)
2) J. Hosoe, *et al.*, *Pharmaceutical and Medical Device Regulatory Science*, 43, 182 - 193 (2012)
3) J. Hosoe, *et al.*, *Pharmaceutical and Medical Device Regulatory Science*, 45, 243 - 250 (2014)

Purity Tests on Crude Drugs using Genetic Information *<G5-6-172>*

The first step in the quality assurance of natural products is the use of raw materials from the right part of the right origin. Therefore, it is clearly stated in Article 4 of the General Rules For Crude Drugs that the source of a crude drug is an approval or rejection criterion. There are various methods for differentiating the sources of crude drugs, such as morphological methods, organoleptic tests, and chemical methods, and appropriate methods for each are described in the individual monographs. Morphological methods, organoleptic tests, and chemical methods are discrimination methods for species that are based on the phenotypic characteristics of the crude drugs. On the other hand, together with recent progress in molecular biology techniques and the accumulation of genetic information on plants, differentiating methods of crude drugs based on genotypes is being established. Unlike morphological and other methods that are based on phenotypic characteristics, the genotypic methods are not affected by environmental factors. Also, the methods have several advantages, such as specialized expertise and skill for classification are not needed, and objective results are easily obtained.

The evolution of living organisms is accomplished by genetic mutation, and differences among the nucleotide sequences of genes of closely related species reflect the strain relationships between the species. Based on this theory, methods that classify species phylogenetically using the nucleotide sequence of rDNA that codes for ribosomal RNA (rRNA) on the nuclear genome have recently been adopted for the classification of microorganisms. In the same way, the sequence of this rDNA is also most often used in the classification of higher plants based on the genotype. In particular, it is very easy to classify closely related species using the internal transcribed spacer (ITS) region of the rDNA, since nucleotide substitution is more often undertaken by comparison with the coded gene region. Furthermore, since the genes on the nuclear genome originate from the parents' genomes, there is an advantage that interspecies hybrids can be detected. Higher plants also have mitochondrial genes and chloroplastic genes. Although the genes on these genomes are also often used for classification, interspecies hybrids cannot be confirmed because the genes are normally uniparental inheritance.

The three methods presented here are, 1) the purity test of Atractylodes Rhizome for Atractylodes Lancea Rhizome, 2) the purity test of Saposhnikovia Root and Rhizome for *Peucedanum ledebourielloides*, which are developed based on the difference of the gene sequence of the ITS region of rDNA recently reported[1-4], and the inter-laboratory validation study have been completed.

The plant sources for Atractylodes Lancea Rhizome stipulated in the individual monographs are *Atractylodes lancea* De Candolle and *A. chinensis* Koidzumi (*Compositae*), while those for Atractylodes Rhizome are *A. japonica* Koidzumi ex Kitamura and *A. macrocephala* Koidzumi (*Compositae*). The approval or rejection of the both sources is, in principle, determined by the description of the crude drug, including microscopy, together with thin-layer chromatography in identification tests. In the above scientific paper, it was shown that these 4 plant species can be clearly classified by comparing the nucleotide sequences of the ITS region mentioned above, and that the species can be easily classified without performing sequence analysis by performing PCR using a species-specific primer pair or by using a restriction enzyme which recognizes species-specific sequence.

Likewise, the plant source of Saposhnikovia Root and Rhizome is stipulated as *Saposhnikovia divaricata* Schischkin (*Umbelliferae*), and the approval or rejection of the source is determined by the description of the crude drug and thin-layer chromatography in identification tests. According to the report[4], crude drugs treated as Saposhnikovia Root and Rhizome in Shaanxi and Shanxi Provinces are frequently derived from *Peucedanum ledebourielloides*, and it was shown that the differentiation of the both is possible by using the nucleotide sequence in the ITS region of the rDNA.

In purity tests on crude drugs using genetic information, the simplicity of the test is given maximum consideration. We established methods that observe PCR amplification bands using species-specific primer pair (Mutant Allele Specific Amplification: Method 1) and methods that observe DNA fragments produced by restriction enzyme treatment of the PCR products, which are prepared using a primer pair common to each plant source (PCR—Restriction Fragment Length Polymorphism: Method 2), without nucleotide sequence analyses. In these methods based on PCR, an extremely small amount of template DNA is amplified to billions to hundreds of billions times. Therefore, when using them as identification tests for powdered crude drugs, the target DNA fragment can be observed even if the vast majority of the crude drug for analysis is not appropriate plant species and there is only a minute amount of powder from a crude drug derived from a suitable plant. Consequently, in identification tests, either a cut or a whole crude drug must be used, as long as one is careful to avoid contamination by powder originating from other crude drugs. On the other hand, when used as a purity test, the form of the crude drug is irrelevant as long as the gene amplification is performed properly and the target gene is not polymorphic, so if DNA fragments of an inappropriate plant to be examined are confirmed in the purity test, regardless of the form of the crude drug, it becomes clear there is contamination by an inappropriate crude drug to be examined.

The methods shown here are general information and at the present stage results obtained using the methods do not affect the approval or rejection of the crude drug in each monograph. Furthermore, by performing the sequence analysis outlined in the previous paper for a crude drug sample derived from a single individual, it goes without saying that more accurate decision concerning the source species can be made.

1. DNA Amplification Equipment

DNA amplification equipment is used to amplify the DNA which is extracted from a crude drug and then purified. Since there are slight differences in the methods of temperature control, and so on depending on the equipment used, there may be differences in the intensity, etc. of the PCR amplification bands even if PCR is carried out under the stipulated conditions. Therefore, when judging results based solely on the presence or absence of PCR amplification bands as in Methods 1, the use of equipment described in the JAS analytical test handbook: genetically modified food quality, labeling analysis manual for individual products[5] is recommended. When other equipment is used, confirm that only proper amplification bands are obtained by performing PCR using DNA obtained from samples confirmed beforehand to be the source species. If proper amplification bands are not obtained, the PCR temperature conditions should be slightly adjusted. This equipment can be used for the restriction enzyme treatment in Method 2.

2. General precautions

Crude drugs are different from fresh plants in that they are dried products and a certain amount of time has passed since they were harvested. Therefore, in many cases the DNA has undergone fragmentation. Furthermore, various substances that can block or interfere with the PCR reaction may be present in the plant. For these reasons, the extraction and purification of template DNA is the process that should receive the greatest amount of attention. In the case of Atractylodes crude drugs, the periderm should be removed using a clean scalpel or other clean instrument before pulverizing the sample because very often there are inhibitory substances present in the periderm.

The PCR used for this test is the technique that amplify the target DNA more than hundreds of millions times, and a trace of contamination leads an incorrect result. Therefore, careful attention is required to prevent contamination. For treatment to prevent contamination, refer to the prevention of contamination section[6] in the above manual.

3. Purity test of Atractylodes Rhizome for Atractylodes Lancea Rhizome

3.1. Method 1 (Mutant Allele Specific Amplification Method)

Generally, this method is referred to as Mutant Allele Specific Amplification (MASA) or Amplification Refractory Mutation System (ARMS), and it provides nucleotide sequence information of sample-derived template DNA, based upon the presence or absence of DNA amplification in PCR using a species specific primer pair.

3.1.1. Procedure

The following is an example procedure.

3.1.1.1. Preparation of template DNA

There are various methods with which to extract and purify DNA from the samples. It is recommended that commercially available DNA extraction kits be used when considering their advantages of not using any noxious reagents and not requiring any complicated purification procedures. In this case, attention should be paid to the final amount (concentration) of DNA obtained, and the initial amount of initial sample and the volume of liquid to elute the DNA need to be controlled. When extraction and purification are performed using silica gel membrane type kits stipulated in notifications[7] related to inspection methods of the foods produced by recombinant DNA techniques, it is appropriate to use 200 mg of sample, 1 mL of AP1 buffer solution, 2 μL of RNase A, and 325 μL of AP2 buffer solution. Also, the most important things are that the supernatant loaded on the first column is clear and that there is no need to load 1 mL unreasonably. Furthermore, 50 μL is an appropriate volume used in the final elution of the DNA, and normally the initial eluate is used as the DNA sample stock solution.

3.1.1.2. Confirmation of purity of DNA in DNA sample stock solution and assay of DNA

The purity of the DNA in the stock solution can be confirmed by the $OD_{260\,nm}/OD_{280\,nm}$ ratio using a spectrophotometer. A ratio of 1.5 indicates that the DNA has been adequately purified. The amount of DNA is calculated using 1 $OD_{260\,nm}$ = 50 μg/mL. The measurement mentioned above is performed using the appropriately diluted DNA sample stock solution. Based on the results obtained, dilute with water to the concentration needed for the subsequent PCR reactions, dispense the solution into micro tubes as the sample DNA solution, and if necessary store frozen at not over −20°C. The dispensed DNA sample is used immediately after thawing and any remaining solution should be discarded and not refrozen. If the concentration of the DNA sample stock solution does not reach the concentration stipulated in PCR, it is used as a DNA sample solution.

3.1.1.3. PCR

When a commercially available PCR enzyme mentioned in the above notification[8] is used, it is appropriate that 25 μL of a reaction mixture consisting of 2.5 μL of the PCR buffer solution containing magnesium, dNTP (0.2 mmol/L), 5′ and 3′primer (0.4 μmol/L), Taq DNA polymerase (1.25 units), and 5 μL of 10 ng/μL sample DNA solution (50 ng of DNA) is prepared on ice. Among them, the PCR buffer solution and dNTP are provided as adjuncts to the enzyme. When conducting purity tests on Atractylodes Lancea Rhizome in Atractylodes Rhizome, the primer sets used are C and D (C is positive with *A. lancea*, D is positive with *A. chinensis*) as described in the paper[1] mentioned above, however, when primer sets A and B are used, it is possible to confirm the source species of each of the respective specimens. In order to confirm that the DNA has been extracted correctly, the reaction solution containing the positive control primer pair (Pf and Pr) as shown below should be prepared. In addition, the negative control solutions which are not containing DNA sample or either of the primer pair should be prepared and simultaneously conduct PCR.

Pf: 5′-CAT TGT CGA AGC CTG CAC AGC A-3′
Pr: 5′-CGA TGC GTG AGC CGA GAT ATC C-3′

The PCR reaction is performed under the following conditions: starting the reaction at 95°C for 10 minutes, 30 cycles of 0.5 minutes at 95°C and 0.75 minutes at 68°C (69°C only when using the primer set C), terminate the reaction at 72°C for 7 minutes, and store at 4°C. The resulting reaction mixture is used for the following process as PCR amplification reaction solution.

3.1.1.4. Agarose gel electrophoresis and detection of PCR products

After completion of the PCR reaction, mix 5 μL of the PCR amplification reaction solution with an appropriate volume of gel loading buffer solution, add the mixture to the wells of 2 w/v% agarose gel, and then perform electrophoresis using 1-fold TAE buffer solution (refer to General Information, "Rapid Identification of Microorganisms Based on Molecular Biological Method <*G4-7-160*>"). Carry out the electrophoresis together with an appropriate DNA molecular marker. Electrophoresis is terminated when the bromophenol blue dye in the gel loading buffer has advanced to a point corresponding to 1/2 to 2/3 the length of the gel.

Stain the gel after electrophoresis when not using gel stained in advance with ethidium bromide. Place the gel that has undergone electrophoresis and staining in a gel image analyzer, irradiate with ultraviolet light (312 nm), and detect its electrophoresis pattern. Compare this to the DNA molecular marker and determine the absence or presence of the target amplification band.

3.1.2. Judgment

Confirm at first that a 305 bp band is found with the reaction solution to which the positive control primer pair has been added, and confirm there are no bands in a solution with no primer sets and a solution with no sample DNA solution. Next, if a 226 bp band is confirmed when the primer set C is added or if a 200 bp band is confirmed when the primer set D is added, the sample is judged to be Atractylodes Lancea Rhizome (in the case of cut crude drug, contamination of Atractylodes Lancea Rhizome is observed) and it is rejected. The sample is judged not to be Atractylodes Lancea Rhizome (in the case of cut crude drug, there is no contamination of Atractylodes Lancea Rhizome) and the purity test is acceptable if a 305 bp band is confirmed with the positive control primer pair, bands are not observed in the reaction solution without primer and the reaction solution without DNA sample solution, and a 226 bp band is not observed with the primer set C and a 200 bp band is not observed with the primer set D. If a band is not observed with the positive control primer pair, it is to be concluded that the DNA extraction failed and the procedure should be started over again from the DNA extraction step. If bands are confirmed in reaction solutions without primer sets or without DNA sample solution, it should be assumed that there was an error in the PCR procedure and therefore the procedure should be repeated again from the step 3.1.1.3. PCR.

3.2. Method 2 (PCR—Restriction Fragment Length Polymorphism)

Generally, this method is referred to as PCR—Restriction Fragment Length Polymorphism (RFLP), and it provides nucleotide sequence information of sample-derived template DNA, based upon the DNA fragment pattern produced by restriction enzyme treatment of the PCR products, which are amplified by using a primer pair common to the DNA sequence of the objective plant.

The test is performed with 25 samples randomly taken from a lot, and each sample is designated with a number from 1 to 25. Differentiation of the sources is performed by individual PCR—RFLP measurement of the samples, and decision of the acceptability of the purity is dependent on how many nonconforming samples are present in the first 20 samples, taken in numerical order, for which judgment is possible as described below.

3.2.1. Procedure

The following is an example procedure.

3.2.1.1. Preparation of template DNA

There are various methods with which to extract and purify DNA from the samples. It is recommended that commercially available DNA extraction kits be used, when considering their advantages of not using noxious reagents and not requiring complicated purification procedures. Recently, PCR reagents that inhibit the effect of PCR enzymeinhibiting substances present in samples have become commercially available, and by using these reagents, it is possible to prepare the template DNA from the sample simply by incubating the sample with the DNA extraction reagent. Here, a recommended DNA preparing procedure using such PCR reagents is described for the convenience of experimenters.

Cut 20 mg of the sample into small pieces with a clean knife, add 400 μL of the DNA extraction reagent, and incubate at 55°C overnight (16 - 18 hours). Then heat at 95°C for 5 minutes to inactivate the enzyme in the reagent. Centrifuge to precipitate the sample, and use 50 μL of the supernatant liquid as the template DNA solution. The DNA solution prepared in this method can not be used for concentration measurement based on $OD_{260\,nm}$, because it contains many foreign substances affecting $OD_{260\,nm}$ value from the sample.

The composition of the DNA extraction reagent is as follows:

2-Amino-2-hydroxymethyl-1,3-propanediol-hydrochloric acid (pH 8.0)	20 mmol/L
Ethylenediamine tetraacetate	5 mmol/L
Sodium chloride	400 mmol/L
Sodium dodecyl sulfate	0.3%
Proteinase K	200 μg/mL

3.2.1.2. PCR

In the method using the PCR enzyme and PCR reagent as described[3], the reaction mixture is prepared on an ice bath in a total volume of 20 μL of a solution containing 10.0 μL of 2-fold concentrated PCR reagent, 5′- and 3′-primers (0.5 μmol/L), Taq DNA polymerase (0.5 units) and 0.5 μL of template DNA solution.

The PCR reaction is performed under the following conditions: 95°C for 10 minutes, 40 cycles of 95°C for 0.5 minute, 65°C for 0.25 minute, and 72°C for 0.25 minute and 72°C for 7 minutes. Store the solution at 4°C, and use this solution as the PCR amplification reaction solution. A negative control (containing water instead of the template DNA solution) must be included in the procedure.

The sequence of each primer is as follows:

5′-primer: 5′-GGC ACA ACA CGT GCC AAG GAA AA-3′

3′-primer: 5′-CGA TGC GTG AGC CGA GAT ATC C-3′

3.2.1.3. Restriction enzyme treatment

The treatment is performed on individual reaction solutions using two enzymes, *Fau* I and *Msp* I. In the case of *Fau* I, to an appropriate amount of the reaction solution, composed of a reaction buffer containing 1.0 unit of enzyme, add 3.0 μL of PCR products while cooling in an ice bath to make 15.0 μL. In the case of *Msp* I, to an appropriate amount of the reaction solution, composed of a reaction buffer containing 20.0 units of enzyme, add 3.0 μL of PCR products while cooling in an ice bath to make 15.0 μL. Incubate these solutions at the temperature recommended by the manufacturer for 2 hours, and then inactivate the enzyme by heating at 72° C for 10 minutes. The negative control of the PCR reaction is also treated in the same manner.

3.2.1.4. Agarose gel electrophoresis and detection of DNA fragments

After the restriction enzyme treatment, mix the total amount of the reaction solution and an appropriate amount of the gel loading buffer solution, place it in a 4 w/v% agarose gel well, and carry out electrophoresis with 1-fold concentrated TAE buffer solution (see "Rapid Identification of Microorganisms Based on Molecular Biological Methods <*G4-7-160*>" under General Information). Carry out the electrophoresis together with appropriate DNA molecular markers. Stop the electrophoresis when the bromophenol blue included in the loading buffer solution has moved about 2 cm from the well. The 4 w/v% agarose gel is sticky, difficult to prepare and hard to handle, so that it is better to use a commercially available precast gel.

After the electrophoresis, stain the gel, if it is not already stained, with ethidium bromide, and observe the gel on an illuminating device under ultraviolet light (312 nm) to confirm the electrophoretic pattern.

3.2.2. Judgment

3.2.2.1. Judgment of each sample

Confirm that no band is obtained with the negative control of the PCR, other than the primer dimer (about 40 bp) band. A sample treated with *Fau* I, showing bands of about 80 bp and 60 bp, or that treated with *Msp* I, showing bands of about 90 bp and 50 bp, is judged as Atractylodes Lancea Rhizome. A sample not showing any band other than a band at about 140 bp and the primer dimer band is judged as Atractylodes Rhizome. If a sample does not show any band other than the primer dimer band, it is considered that PCR products were not obtained, and judgment is impossible for the sample.

3.2.2.2. Judgment of the purity

Judgment of the purity is based on the result of the judgment of each sample. If there is no sample that is judged as Atractylodes Lancea Rhizome among 20 samples taken in order of the numbering, excluding any sample for which judgment is impossible, the lot is acceptable for purity. When there is one sample that is judged as Atractylodes Lancea Rhizome among the 20 samples, perform the same test with 25 newly taken samples from the lot, and if there is no sample that is judged as Atractylodes Lancea Rhizome, the lot is acceptable for purity. When there is a sample that is judged as Atractylodes Lancea Rhizome in the second test, or there is more than one sample that is judged as Atractylodes Lancea Rhizome in the first test, the lot is not acceptable for purity.

4. Purity test of Saposhnikovia Root and Rhizome for *Peucedanum ledebourielloides*

4.1. Method 1

Similarly as 3.1., this method provides nucleotide sequence information of sample-derived template DNA, based upon the presence or absence of DNA amplification band in PCR using a species specific primer pair.

4.1.1. Procedure

The following is an example procedure.

4.1.1.1. Preparation of template DNA

For Atractylodes crude drugs, a preparation procedure using a silica gel membrane type kit is adopted, however for the test of Saposhnikovia Root and Rhizome, and *Peucedanum ledebourielloides*, the simple preparation procedure shown below is adopted for the convenience of experimenters, because it was confirmed that the PCR product is stably obtained in using a DNA sample solution prepared by the simple preparation procedure shown in 3.2.1.1. as a template.

Cut 10 mg of the sample into small pieces with a clean knife, add 400 μL of the DNA extraction reagent, and incubate at 55°C overnight (16 – 18 hours). Then heat at 95°C for 5 minutes to inactivate the enzyme in the reagent. Centrifuge to precipitate the sample, and use 50 μL of the supernatant liquid as the template DNA solution. The DNA solution prepared in this method can not be used for concentration measurement based on OD_{260nm}, because it contains many foreign substances affecting OD_{260nm} value from the sample.

The composition of the DNA extraction reagent is as follows:

2-Amino-2-hydroxymethyl-1,3-propanediol-hydrochloric acid (pH 8.0)	20 mmol/L
Ethylenediamine tetraacetate	5 mmol/L
Sodium chloride	400 mmol/L
Sodium dodecyl sulfate	0.3%
Proteinase K	200 μg/mL

4.1.1.2. PCR

In the method using the PCR enzyme and PCR reagent as described[3)], the reaction mixture is prepared on an ice bath in a total volume of 20 μL of a solution containing 10.0 μL of 2-fold concentrated PCR reagent, 5′- and 3′-primers (0.5 μmol/L), Taq DNA polymerase (0.5 units) and 0.5 μL of template DNA solution.

When the purity test of Saposhnikovia Root and Rhizome for *Peucedanum ledebourielloides* is performed, the reaction solution containing the positive control primer pair as shown below should be prepared besides the reaction solution containing a species specific primer pair in order to confirm that the DNA has been extracted correctly. In addition, the negative control solutions which are not containing the DNA sample solution should be prepared and simultaneously conduct PCR.

The PCR reaction is performed under the following conditions: 95°C for 10 minutes, 45 cycles of 95°C for 0.5 minute, 62°C for 0.5 minute, and 72°C for 0.75 minute and 72°C for 7 minutes. Store the solution at 4°C, and use this solution as the PCR amplification reaction solution. The sequence of each primer is as follows. The positive control 3′-primer for PCR and the species specific 3′-primer for PCR have the same sequence.

5′-primer for positive control PCR: 5′-GCG TGG GTG TCA CGC ATC G-3′

3′-primer for positive control PCR: 5′-GTA GTC CCG CCT GAC CTG-3′

5′-primer for species specific PCR: 5′-CTG AGA AGT TGT GCC CGG-3′

3′-primer for species specific PCR: 5′-GTA GTC CCG CCT GAC CTG-3′

4.1.1.3. Agarose gel electrophoresis and detection of PCR products

After completion of PCR reaction, mix 5 μL of the PCR amplification reaction solution with an appropriate volume of gel loading buffer solution, add the mixture to the wells of 2 w/v% agarose gel, and then perform electrophoresis using 1-fold TAE buffer solution (refer to General Information, "Rapid Identification of Microorganisms Based on Molecular Biological Method <G4-7-160>"). Carry out the electrophoresis together with an appropriate DNA molecular marker. Electrophoresis is terminated when the bromophenol blue dye in the gel loading buffer has moved about 2 cm from the well.

Stain the gel after electrophoresis when not using gel stained in advance with ethidium bromide. Place the gel that has undergone electrophoresis and staining in a gel image analyzer, irradiate with ultraviolet light (312 nm), and confirm its electrophoresis pattern. Compare this to the DNA molecular marker and determine the absence or presence of the target amplification band.

4.2. Judgment

Confirm at first that a 250 bp band is found with the reaction solution to which the positive control primer pair has been added, and confirm there are no bands other than the primer dimer (about 40 bp) in a solution with no sample DNA solution. Next, if a 200 bp band is confirmed when the species specific primer pair is added, the sample is judged to be contaminated with *Peucedanum ledebourielloides* and it is rejected. The sample is judged not to be contaminated with *Peucedanum ledebourielloides* and the purity test is acceptable if a 250 bp band is confirmed with the positive control primer pair, bands are not observed in the reaction solution without DNA sample solution, and a 200 bp band is not observed with the species specific primer pair. If a band is not observed with the positive control primer pair, it is to be concluded that the DNA extraction failed and the procedure should be started over again from the DNA extraction step. If bands are confirmed in the reaction solution without DNA sample solution, it should be assumed that there was an error in the PCR procedure and therefore the procedure should be repeated again from the step 4.1.1.2. PCR.

5. Reference

1) Y. Guo, *et al.*, *J. Nat. Med.*, 60, 149-156 (2006).
2) K. Kondo, *et al.*, *J. Jpn. Bot.*, 84, 356-359 (2009).
3) T. Maruyama, *et al.*, *Shoyakugaku Zasshi* 64, 96-101 (2010).
4) T. Maruyama, *et al.*, *J. Nat. Med.*, in press.
5) JAS analytical test handbook: genetically modified food quality, labeling analysis manual for individual products, ver. 3, I Fundamental procedure 4.4.1 PCR, (September 24, 2012). Incorporated Administrative Agency Food and Agricultural Materials Inspection Center
6) JAS analytical test handbook: genetically modified food quality, labeling analysis manual for individual products, ver. 3, IV Contamination prevention, (September 24, 2012). Food and Agricultural Materials Inspection Center Independent Administrative Organization
7) Notification No. 110, Director of Food Health Department, March 2001; Partial Amendment: Notification No. 0629002, 2.2.1.2, Director of Food Safety Department, June 2006.
8) Notification No. 0629002, 2.1.3.1.1, Director of Food Safety Department, June 2006.

Analytical Methods for Aflatoxins in Crude Drug and Crude Drug Preparations <*G5-7-170*>

Aflatoxins are carcinogenic secondary metabolites produced by some fungal strains[1]. They are found in agricultural products such as cereals, tree nuts and spices. Many countries including Japan have set regulatory limits on aflatoxins in foods[2,3]. Not only foods but also crude drugs may be contaminated by aflatoxins because aflatoxin contamination in the ingredients of botanical products has been reported in some foreign countries[4-6]. Therefore, aflatoxin testing in crude drugs and preparations containing crude drugs as main ingredient (crude drug preparations) is required to be performed. Concerning the risk of aflatoxin contamination, it is necessary to consider the presence of producing bacteria and the possibility of contamination in processes of processing and manufacturing.

In this connection, the regulatory limit for aflatoxins (sum of B_1, B_2, G_1 and G_2) has been set at 10 μg/kg for all foods in Japan[3].

1. Summary

The methods based on HPLC with fluorescence detection and LC-MS are used for aflatoxins instrumental analysis[7-10]. Aflatoxin standards should be handled with care because they are highly toxic compounds. (Refer to 4. Points to note) Simple measurement equipment and quantitative test kits are also used for the simple analysis of aflatoxin and some of them enable aflatoxin determination without using aflatoxin standards.

Aflatoxins are generally purified from the samples by cartridge-type columns such as immunoaffinity column and multifunctional column. An immunoaffinity column is useful for purification of aflatoxin from crude drug preparations, but in some cases, a multifunctional column is effective.

In this document, the analytical methods for aflatoxins using simple measurement kits, which are useful for screening, and HPLC with fluorescence detection are described. The methods should be selected according to the characteristics and aflatoxin contamination levels of the samples. Method optimization and validation are required to be performed. As references, an official method of Japan for aflatoxin analysis in food[7,11], analytical methods described in European and US Pharmacopeia, and WHO guidelines can be used[8-10].

2. Analytical methods

2.1. An analytical method using a qualitative kit

The kit can detect the presence or absence of aflatoxin in the sample by using an antigen-antibody interaction. A kit for the detection of total aflatoxins can be used for qualitative test. The following method can be used for detecting aflatoxins in some extracts (Orengedokuto, Kakkonto, Shoseiryuto, Hachimijiogan, Goshajinkigan, Daiokanzoto and Mukoi-Daikenchuto) listed in Japanese Pharmacopoeia at cut-off levels of 4 ppb[12]. In order to quantify aflatoxins in the positive samples, instrumental analysis is required to be done.

(i) Preparation for sample solution

Weigh accurately about 1 g of the powdered sample, add exactly 4 mL of a mixture of acetonitrile, water and methanol (6:4:1) and then shake for 30 minutes. After centrifugation, dilute exactly 2 mL of the supernatant to 50 mL with phosphate buffered saline (PBS) containing 4% of polysorbate 20. Apply the diluted extract to an immunoaffinity column, which is preequilibrated with PBS. Wash the column with 10 mL of PBS containing 0.01% of polysorbate 20 followed by 10 mL of water. Apply 1 mL of acetonitrile on the column and collect eluate. Wait 5 minutes and apply 2 mL of acetonitrile. Collect applied elution solvent. Evaporate the eluate to dryness under nitrogen. Dissolve the residue in exactly 0.5 mL of diluted methanol (7 in 10), and use this as the sample solution. In this method, 0.5 mL of the sample solution is equivalent to 0.5 g of the sample matrix.

(ii) Measurement and evaluation

Prepare the test strips, the microwells with the inner bottom covered by gold colloid, and the assay diluent attached with the kit. Add exactly 50 μL of the assay diluent to each microwell. Dissolve the coating conjugate in the microwell by pipetting. Add exactly 50 μL of sample extracts to each microwell and mix the content in each well by pipetting it up and down. Put one test strip into one well and allow the test strip to develop color for 5 minutes. Interpret test results from the lines formed in the test zone and the control zone. If the two lines are visible, this indicates the sample contains total aflatoxin less than 4 ppb (negative sample).

2.2. An instrumental method of analysis

Aflatoxins can be detected by a fluorescence detector because they are fluorescent substances. In order to enhance the fluorescent intensities of AFB_1 and AFG_1, the intensities of which are weak in polar solvents, a derivatization step is performed. Precolumn derivatization with trifluoroacetic acid and postcolumn derivatization with a photochemical reactor or an electrochemical cell are known. AFB_2 and AFG_2 are not derivatized by the above methods. The following method can be used for quantification of aflatoxins in some extracts listed in Japanese Pharmacopoeia[12]. This method is an example and the other method can also be used.

(i) Preparation for sample solution

Weigh accurately about 1 g of the powdered sample and add exactly 4 mL of a mixture of acetonitrile, water and methanol (6:4:1) and then shake for 30 minutes. After centrifugation, dilute exactly 2 mL of the supernatant to 50 mL with phosphate buffered saline (PBS) containing 4% of polysorbate 20. Apply the diluted extract to an immunoaffinity column, which is preequilibrated with PBS. Wash the column with 10 mL of PBS containing 0.01% of polysorbate 20 followed by 10 mL of water. Apply 1 mL of acetonitrile on the column and collect eluate. Wait 5 minutes and apply 2 mL of acetonitrile. Collect applied elution solvent. Evaporate the eluate to dryness under nitrogen. Redissolve the residue in exactly 0.5 mL of 70% methanol in water. In this method, 0.5 mL of the sample solution is equivalent to 0.5 g of the sample matrix.

(ii) Measurement and evaluation

Use an ODS column for separation. Aflatoxins can be detected by an HPLC equipped with a fluorescence detector because they are fluorescent (excitation λ = 365 nm, emission λ = 430 nm). Use trifluoroacetic acid (TFA) for derivatization of aflatoxins. Aflatoxins elute in the order of AFG_{2a} (a derivative of AFG_1), AFB_{2a} (a derivative of AFB_1), AFG_2 and AFB_2 when a mixture of acetonitrile, water and methanol (6:3:1) is used as a mobile solvent. Postcolumn derivatization with a photochemical reactor is useful when performing continuous monitoring of aflatoxins. In that case, aflatoxins elute in the order of AFG_2, AFG_{2a}, AFB_2 and AFB_{2a}. Prepare some standard solutions in which aflatoxins are present at the concentrations from 0.5 to 20 μg/L, and verify linearity in the range.

3. Reagents and solutions

Some reagents and solutions prescribed in Japanese Pharmacopoeia and those listed below are used.

(i) PBS containing 0.01% or 4% of polysorbate 20 Dissolve 8.0 g of NaCl, 0.2 g of KCl, 2.9 g of $Na_2HPO_4.12H_2O$, 0.2 g of KH_2PO_4 and 0.1 g (0.01%) or 40 g (4%) of polysorbate 20 in 900 mL of water and adjust to pH 7.4 with 0.1 mol/L hydrochloric acid TS or dilute sodium hydroxide TS, and add water to make 1000 mL. Keep the solution at 2 – 8°C.

(ii) Aflatoxin solution Dilute the aflatoxin standard stock solution with acetonitrile or methanol. Use the commercially available standard stock solution which is precisely prepared in concentration.

4. Points to note

(i) Aflatoxins are highly cardiotoxic compounds, and sufficient caution is required when handling them. Especially in cases when handling a high concentration of aflatoxins, pay maximum attention. Wear a protect coat, gloves, a mask and goggles. All handling should be performed in a fume hood.

(ii) Soak the used labware in 0.5 – 1.0% sodium hypochlorite (NaClO) solution for more than 2 hours before discarding and washing it. Commercially available sodium hypochlorite solutions for disinfection or for food additive may also be used after adjusting the concentration.

(iii) Keep the aflatoxin solution in a dark and cool place. Keep the commercially available standard stock solution under specified conditions.

(iv) Aflatoxins may be absorbed by a glass vessel. In order to avoid absorption, using silanized glass vials may be effective. The vial should be washed with 20% acetonitrile and air-dried before use.

(v) Be cautious that there are no big air bubbles or cracks in the gel of the immunoaffinity column. If there are bubbles or cracks, remove them by applying pressure from the upper part of the column.

(vi) Confirm the performance of the immunoaffinity column by performing a spike and recovery test if necessary.

(vii) In case of using a multifunctional column for preparing the sample solution, it is necessary to assess its performance beforehand by performing a spike and recovery test.

5. References

1) IARC, "IARC Monographs on the Evaluation of Carcinogenic Risks to Humans", Vol. 82 (2002).
2) FAO, "FAO Food and Nutrition Paper 81, Worldwide Regulations for Mycotoxins in Food and Feed in 2003" (2004).
3) Notification No. 0331-5, Director of Food Safety Department, Pharmaceutical and Food Safety Bureau, MHLW, March 31, 2011, "Management of Food Containing Aflatoxin"
4) M. Trucksess, *et al., J. AOAC Int.*, 89 (3), 624 – 630 (2006).
5) C. Bircan, *Int. J. Food Science and Technology*, 40, 929 – 934 (2005).
6) H. Tosun and R. Arslan, The Scientific World Journal, 2013, Article ID 874093 (2013).
7) Notification No. 0816-1, Director of Food Safety Department, Pharmaceutical and Food Safety Bureau, MHLW, August 16, 2011, "Method for testing total aflatoxins."
8) European Pharmacopoeia 8.0 (2013), 2.8.18. Determination of aflatoxin B1 in herbal drugs.
9) US Pharmacopeia 37 (2014), <*561*> Articles of Botanical Origin.
10) WHO: WHO Guidelines for Assessing Quality of Herbal Medicines with Reference to Contaminants and Residues.
11) Notification No. 0816-7, Director of Inspection and Safety Division of Food Safety Department, Pharmaceutical and Food Safety Bureau, MHLW, August 16, 2011, "Test Methods Related to Aflatoxin Contained in Corns."
12) H. Sakuma, *et al. Shoyakugaku Zasshi*, 68 (2), 53 – 57 (2014).

Radioactivity Measurements Method for Crude Drugs <*G5-8-180*>

Crude drugs are natural products produced by harvesting cultivated plants/reared animals or collecting wild resources and processing them through washing and drying. This General Information describes the radioactivity measurement method of crude drugs that can be applied when there is a concern about the contamination of radioactive materials in more amounts exceeding that from natural origin.

The measurement methods described here are procedures to measure radioactivity by γ-ray spectrometry, and its target nuclides are ^{131}I, ^{134}Cs and ^{137}Cs.

1. Principle[1)]

In order to measure the radioactivity of a radionuclide in a sample, radioactive materials are identified based on the energy of radiation by measuring α-rays being helium nuclei, β-rays being electrons and γ-rays being photons, emitted when radionuclides decayed, and radioactivity is determined from the number of radiations counted per unit time. Radiations have different penetrating powers depending on their kind and energy. Generally, α-rays have the weakest penetrating power and are shieldable by papers. β-Rays have stronger penetrating power than α-rays, being shieldable by a light metal plate with a few millimeters thickness, and are classified to the weak penetrating power radiation. On the other hand, γ-rays have strong penetrating power and require substances such as lead which has high atomic number and large density ranging from several to 10 centimeters to be shielded.

Difference in penetration of radiation is an important factor in the measurement of radiation/radioactivity. γ-Rays are usually used to determine radionuclides. α- and β-rays are susceptible to self-shielding (absorption) because of their weak penetrating radiation and are suitable for the measurement of surface contamination, etc. However, the identification of radionuclides by their spectroscopies is not easy because specialized techniques such as sample preparation are required. On the other hand, most γ-rays do not lose their energy when penetrating a substance even in emission from inside the substance, and the information of the emitted γ-ray energy is obtained from the measured spectrum. Since γ-ray energy emitted from a radionuclide is determined for each radionuclide, it is relatively easy to identify the radionuclide based on the obtained energy spectrum. For the measurement of radioactivity concentration in crude drugs, it is necessary to identify the radionuclide contained in the crude drug and to measure the concentration of the radionuclide, therefore measurement methods by γ-ray spectroscopy are recommended.

Semiconductor detectors and scintillators are known as detectors used for the radioactivity measurement methods by γ-ray spectroscopy. By injection of radiation, the former produce electron-hole pairs and the latter emit a light. Scintillators exhibit scintillation (flash and fluorescence), but the intensity of the light is very weak. Therefore, it is used with the combination of a photomultiplier tube, etc. which amplify an electric signal converted from photon. A germanium semiconductor detector (hereinafter referred to as ''Ge detector''), one of semiconductors, has the highest performance as a detector that can measure the radionuclide in crude drugs. In addition, a thallium activated sodium iodide scintillation detector (hereinafter referred to as ''NaI (Tl) detector'') is easy to handle and can measure the radioactivity of crude drugs.

1.1. Target radionuclide

The target nuclides are ^{131}I, ^{134}Cs and ^{137}Cs.

1.1.1. Ge detector

Radiation data necessary for the γ-ray spectrometry radiometry using a Ge detector is shown in Table 1.

Table 1 Radiation data of target nuclides for a Ge detector[1)]

Nuclide	Half-life	Energy	γ-Ray Emission Rate	γ-Ray that require correction of summing effect (γ-Ray Emission Rate)
^{131}I	8.021 days	364.5 keV	0.817	284.3 keV (0.061), 637.0 keV (0.072), etc.
^{134}Cs	2.065 years	604.7 keV	0.976	569.3 keV (0.154), 801.9 keV (0.087)*, etc.
		795.9 keV	0.855	
^{137}Cs	30.17 years	661.7 keV	0.851	no (single γ-ray)

* When resolution is not high, the peaks of 795.9 keV and 801.9 keV can be treated as one peak (0.942).

1.1.2. NaI (Tl) detector

Radiation data necessary for the γ-ray spectrometry radiometry using a NaI detector is shown in Table 2. In the measurement using a NaI detector, radiocesium is treated as the sum of ^{134}Cs and ^{137}Cs because it is difficult to accurately distinguish and quantify the nuclides.

Table 2 Radiation data of target nuclides for a NaI(Tl) detector[1)]

Nuclide	Half-life	Energy	γ-Ray Emission Rate	γ-Ray that require correction of summing effect (γ-Ray Emission Rate)
^{131}I	8.021 days	364.5 keV	0.817	284.3 keV (0.061), 637.0 keV (0.072), etc.
^{134}Cs	2.065 years	604.7 keV	0.976	the peaks of 795.9 keV and 801.9 keV are treated as one peak (0.942).
		795.9 keV 801.9 keV	0.855 0.087	
^{137}Cs	30.17 years	661.7 keV	0.851	no (single γ-ray)

2. Apparatus

The system configuration of a γ-ray spectrometer is shown in Figure 1. The apparatus generally consists of a detector, a circuit part for measuring such as an amplifier, and an analysis part (personal computer: PC) (Figure 1). In some commercially available apparatuses, a circuit part for measuring such as a high voltage power supply, amplifier and multichannel analyzer is integrated with a detector, and the resultant detection part which include a shielding body are combined with a PC for analysis. Details will be described later.

The Ge detector has a cooling system using liquid nitrogen.

3. Sampling, preparation, storage and transport

3.1. Sampling

3.1.1. Sampling container, tool and label

Fresh polyethylene bags are used for sampling containers.

Auxiliary tools for sampling are made of stainless, polyethylene, or their equivalent materials. Parts which contact with samples should be protected with polyethylene bags to prevent contamination during transport. Because auxiliary tools are used at the sampling sites, pay attention not to contaminate samples from these tools when sampling are conducted at multiple sites.

Fill out immediately the following items on sampling containers before or after sampling.

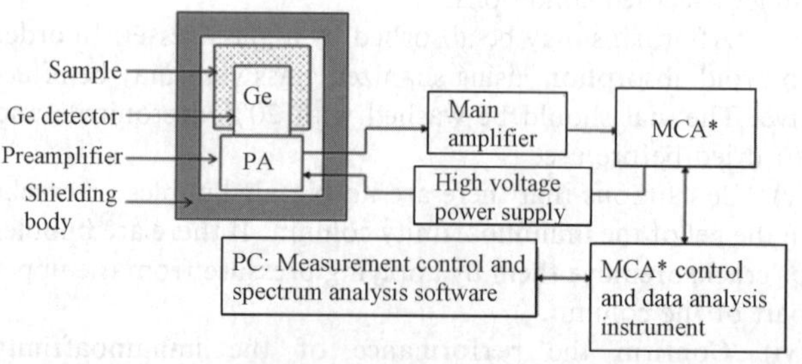

Figure 1 The system configuration of a γ-ray spectrometer[2)]

① Sample number (lot)
(When collecting a same sample in multiple sample containers, each should be distinguished.)
② Sample name
③ Production area of sample
④ Sampling date
⑤ Sampler name
⑥ Special notes
⑦ Others necessary for evaluation

3.1.2. Sampling and handling of samples

Random sampling is performed to collect samples representing a unit for measurement, and collected samples are homogenized by through mixing. As a general rule, one sample is measured per one unit for measurement.

In situation where direct sampling is difficult, samples are collected with a shovel, and transferred to sampling containers using a funnel or the like, if necessary.

3.1.3. Amount of sampling

It is desirable to collect about twice the amount required for testing.

3.2. Preparation of sample

If necessary, prepare to the size of samples appropriate for each apparatus. Crude drugs are derived from various parts of plants, minerals, animals, and so on, and have various sizes, shapes and solids. Therefore, they are cut and crushed according to their characteristics. Procedure that affect test results, such as washing, must not be done after sampling.

3.3. Storage and transport of sample

Test immediately after sampling. Make sure that sampling containers are not broken and samples do not leak from sampling containers. When testing is not performed immediately, store samples avoiding moisture and insect damage.

4. Measurement of sample

An example of analysis by a γ-ray spectrometer is shown in Figure 2.

4.1. Measurement using a Ge spectrometer

4.1.1. Characteristic of the measurement method

Because the γ-ray spectrometry radiometry using a Ge detector has a very high energy resolution, it can determine energy accurately to identify a radionuclide easily and certainly, and clearly analyze the energy by separately from the other γ-rays with close energy. Moreover, because the spreading of γ-ray peaks is small and the ratio of the background to the peak is low, it is suitable for low level radioactivity.

4.1.2. Apparatus, tool and so on

4.1.2.1. Configuration of apparatus

(1) Ge detector

The relative efficacy of a detector should be not less than 20%.

The energy resolution is generally 1.8 to 2.0 keV as a half width.

(2) Shielding body

Shielding a detector is very important in the measurement of low level radioactivity. γ-Rays derived from natural nuclides (^{40}K, nuclides of the uranium and thorium series) should be sufficiently shielded.

A lead shielding body with 10 to 15 cm thick is generally used around a detector.

The size of the inner space of the shielding body must be enough to put a sample container.

There are vertical (dipstick) and L-type (with cryostats on the side of a liquid nitrogen container) detectors. The shielding bodies differ in structure depending on both the shape of a detector and the connection between a detector and a liquid nitrogen container.

4.1.2.2. Tools and so on

(1) Sample container

Sample containers should have good sealing performance, high mechanical strength, resistance to acid and heat, and the internal sample should be visible. Sample containers include Marinelli containers with an internal volume of 1 to 2 L and cylindrical containers with an internal volume of 100 to 500 mL. Sample containers should be selected based on sample volume.

(2) Energy calibration source

Select some energy calibration sources to cover from 100 to 2000 keV such as ^{22}Na (511 keV, 1275 keV), ^{54}Mn (835 keV), ^{60}Co (1173 keV, 1332 keV), ^{88}Y (898 keV, 1836 keV), ^{137}Cs (662 keV) and ^{139}Ce (166 keV). Each radioactivity should be 1000 to 3000 becquerel (Bq).

(3) Efficiency calibration source

Efficiency calibration sources are commercially available standard samples containing ^{137}Cs and so on, whose container and medium volumes are equal to those of the sample. Each radioactivity should be 1000 to 3000 Bq.

(4) Software for spectral analysis

The software which can search peaks, identify nuclides, calculate peak areas and statistical uncertainties of count, is used. In addition, it is desirable to be able to correct self-absorption and summing effect.

4.1.3. Apparatus calibration

4.1.3.1. Energy calibration

For energy calibration sources, correspondence relationship between γ-ray energy and a peak center channel is obtained as a linear equation according to the following procedure.

(1) Attach an energy calibration source to the regular position of a detector, and measure the spectrum until the peak area of a main γ-ray reaches several thousand counts.

(2) Assuming that γ-ray energy (E) and a peak center channel (p) are in linear relationship, the following formula is obtained using spectral analysis software.

$$E = \mathrm{a} + \mathrm{b} \times p$$

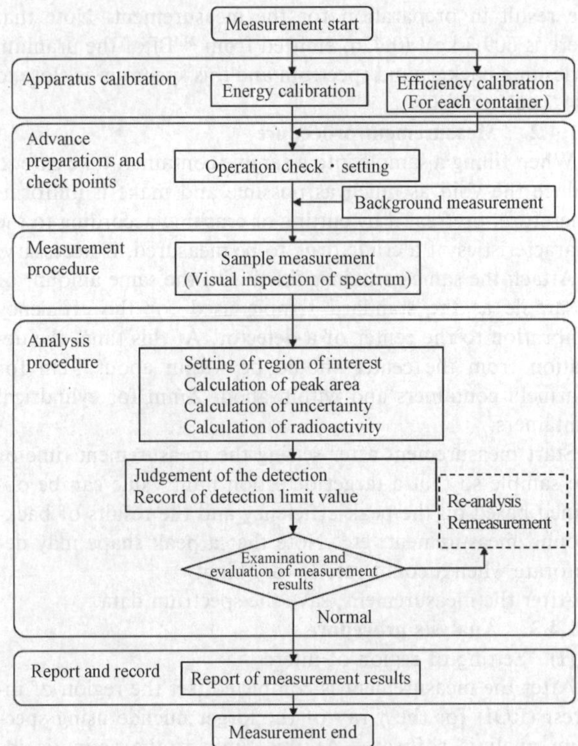

Figure 2 An example of analysis flow

By setting the energy range of γ-rays to 0 to 2000 keV and the channel full scale of a multichannel analyzer to 4000 ch, the region of interest can be set easily even when the count value is low, and in this case "a" in the above formula is close to 0, and "b" is as close to 0.500 as possible.

(3) Record and save the above data.

4.1.3.2. Efficiency calibration

In order to determine radioactivity from a measured γ-ray spectrum, counting efficiency relative to a peak (hereinafter referred to as "peak efficiency") is necessary, and radioactivity analysis postulates that the peak efficiency is correctly calibrated.

For efficiency calibration, use the efficiency calibration sources whose concentration are known. Usually, standard sources containing various nuclides are measured to obtain a peak efficiency function with energy as a variable so that it can be applied to the energy range of approximately 50 to 2000 keV. Since the peak efficiency varies depending on the sample container, it is necessary to perform efficiency calibration for each sample container when multiple sample containers are used.

4.1.4. Procedure

4.1.4.1. Preparations in advance and points to be checked

(1) Operation check of apparatus and settings

Before measuring a sample, use spectral analysis software to analyze the spectrum of the energy calibration source and confirm that the peak center channel, half width and peak count rate are normal for major γ-rays.

(2) Background measurement

Measure a background under the specified measurement conditions. In principle, the measurement is performed by placing a sample for background measurement (enclosing the same amount of water containing no target radionuclides in the same sample container) that has the same conditions as the sample.

Since the analytical result of a background spectrum measured recently is used for the radioactivity analysis of a sample, when a peak corresponding to the main γ-ray energy of a target nuclide shown in Table 1 is observed, calculate the count rate and the statistical uncertainty of count and save the result in preparation for the measurement. Note that there is 609.3 keV (0.426) emitted from ^{214}Bi of the uranium series in a background spectrum and this spectrum is close to 604.7 keV of ^{134}Cs.

4.1.4.2. Measurement procedure

When filling a sample into a sample container, take care to reduce the void as much as possible and make it uniform. Therefore, pretreat it by cutting or crushing according to the characteristics of a crude drug to be measured, if necessary.

Attach the same container filled with the same amount of a sample as the standard sample used for the efficiency calibration to the center of a detector. At this time, the deviation from the center should be within about 1 cm for Marinelli containers and within about 2 mm for cylindrical containers.

Start measurement after setting the measurement time of the sample so that a target detection limit value can be obtained based on the peak efficiency and the results of background measurement, etc. Note that a peak shape may deteriorate when a count rate is very high.

After the measurement, save the spectrum data.

4.1.4.3. Analysis procedure

(1) Setting of region of interest

After the measurement is completed, set the region of interest (ROI) for the γ-ray of the target nuclide using spectrum analysis software. At this time, if the count is insufficient, the variation of the count for each channel can be

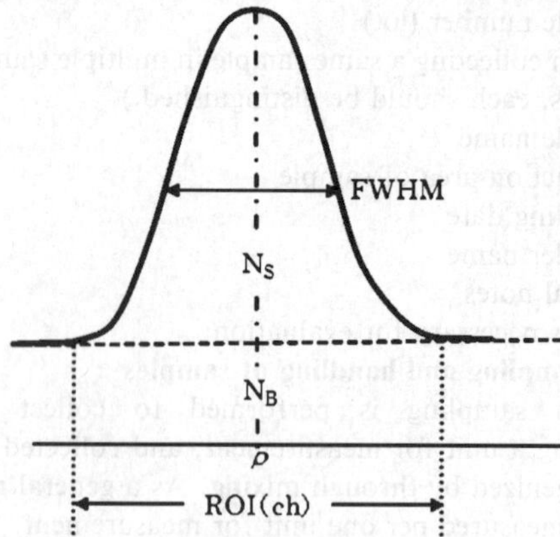

Figure 3 Setting of region of interest (ROI), and calculation of peak area (N_S) and background area (N_B)

leveled by smoothing process.

From the peak center channel (p) and the full width at half maximum (FWHM), it can be confirmed that the measured spectrum is normal, but for weak peaks, the value may fluctuate.

(2) Calculation of peak area

Peak areas (N_S) are calculated based on peak search in the automatic setting of ROIs by analysis software, but for especially weak peaks, confirm whether the position and width of ROIs are appropriate.

(3) Subtraction of background count rate and calculation of statistical uncertainty of count

In usual γ-ray spectrometry, it is not always necessary to subtract a background count rate n_{BG} (hereinafter referred to as "BG count rate"), but if a detector and the inside of a shield body are contaminated, it is necessary to subtract the BG count rate. A net count rate $n(s^{-1})$ is obtained by subtracting the BG count rate in the same ROI from the sample count rate ($n_S = N_S/t_S$).

$$n = n_S - n_{BG}$$

The relation of a count error σ_n and a count rate (n) is expressed as the following formula:

$$n \pm \sigma_n = n \pm (n/t)^{1/2}$$

The statistical uncertainty of count to a net count rate, σ_n (s^{-1}), is expressed as the root sum squares of statistical uncertainties (σ_S and σ_{BG}) of each count rate, shown as follows:

$$\sigma_n = (\sigma_S^2 + \sigma_{BG}^2)^{1/2}$$

(4) Calculation of radioactivity

The radioactivity A (Bq) and the radioactive concentration C (Bq/kg) of a sample are obtained by the following formulae:

$$A = \frac{n}{a\varepsilon f_{SUM}} \quad C = \frac{A}{M}$$

In the above formulae, the abbreviations are as follows:

n: Count rate
a: γ-Ray emission rate (Bq^{-1}) shown in Table 1
ε: Peak efficiency
f_{SUM}: Correction factor for summing effect
M: Mass (kg) of a sample in a sample container

However, when the measurement is compared with a standard sample, "a", "ε", and "f_{SUM}" are the same, so there is no need to consider. In other words, when the radioactivity of the standard sample is A_{STD} and the count rate is n_{STD}, the radioactivity A is obtained by $A = (n/n_{STD})$ A_{STD}.

(5) Uncertainty of detection

If it is not necessary to consider the uncertainty of the mass of a sample in a sample container, the statistical uncertainty of count δ_A (Bq) of the radioactivity of the sample and the statistical uncertainty of count δ_C (Bq/kg) of the radioactive concentration are obtained by the following formulae:

$$\delta_A = \frac{\sigma_n}{n} A \quad \delta_C = \frac{\delta_A}{M}$$

If the measured radioactive concentration C exceeds $3\delta_C$, it is considered statistically significant.

(6) Record of detection limit value

If no radioactivity is detected, record $3\delta_C$ of the radioactivity value, which would be measured in the analysis, as the detection limit value.

The detection limit value is affected by a BG count rate, sample measurement time, and sample mass. In radioactivity measurement, methods to calculate radioactivity from the count rate of the background part of the peak to be measured (usually calculated from the baseline region beside the peak), BG count rate, sample measurement time and background measurement time, sample mass, etc. are widely used.

(7) Examination and evaluation of measurement results

Summarize measurement results for each target nuclide, and confirm that it is normal based on the statistical uncertainty of count, peak center channel, FWHM, etc. If there is any doubt in the confirmation of results, remeasure as necessary.

4.1.5. Points to note for measurement

4.1.5.1. Control of background

When the same nuclide as a target nuclide is detected from a background, it is necessary to confirm the cause and to suppress the influence of the background as much as possible. In the case of indoor contamination, the influence can be suppressed by cleaning and checking shielding devices around an apparatus and performing appropriate shielding. If the inside of a shield body or a detector itself is contaminated, decontamination should be generally attempted. However, if decontamination is impossible, it is necessary to subtract the contribution from the background when calculating radioactivity.

4.1.5.2. Contamination prevention of apparatus, tool and so on

Cover a detector with polyethylene bag to prevent from contamination. In the event of a contamination, cope by replacing the polyethylene packaging. If the surface of a detector is contaminated, wipe it off with a neutral detergent or gauze soaked in ethanol. Be careful not to allow dust or other contaminants to enter when opening a shield body.

Use a sample container after simple cleaning. When a sample is placed into a sample container, it is also important to prevent the sample from adhering around the sample container.

Use a disposable container when measuring a high concentration sample or when decontamination is difficult. When a sample container is used repeatedly, it is recommended to apply fluorine coating. It is also effective to use a plastic bag in a sample container.

4.1.5.3. Routine maintenance of apparatus

Regular performance tests of an entire measurement system is very important for the control of apparatuses. In the performance tests, a γ-ray source for checking is placed at a fixed position on a detector, and a peak center channel, FWHM and peak count rate are obtained for low, medium and high energy γ-rays. Save these results as time-series data. The performance tests should be preferably performed daily, at least prior to a series of sample measurement, so that accurate energy calibration can always be used.

In addition, confirm no contamination around a detector and a sample container by regularly performing measurement without sample or by placing an empty container.

One of the detector troubles is vacuum loss in a cryostat. This can be judged from the consumption of liquid nitrogen, a decrease in energy resolution, and visual inspection (the existence of condensation at the neck of the cryostat).

4.2. Measurement using a NaI (Tl) spectrometer

4.2.1. Characteristic of measurement method

Scintillation detectors calculate the energy and number of radiation by converting a weak light emission generated at the time when radiation is incident on a solid crystal called a scintillator, into an electric signal using a photomultiplier. As the advantages, it is relatively inexpensive compared to Ge detectors and can be used at ordinary temperature. Another characteristic of the scintillation detector is that the detection efficiency is determined by the size of crystals because the size of commercially available solid crystals is standardized. NaI and $LaBr_3$, etc. are used as solid crystals[3].

4.2.2. Apparatus, tool and so on

4.2.2.1. Configuration of apparatus

Scintillation spectrometer is generally composed of a scintillation detector, a high-voltage power supply, an amplifier, a multichannel analyzer, and a PC for analysis. Scintillation spectrometer has the analytical function of a γ-ray spectrum and can perform processes from radioactive measurement to quantitative calculation.

(1) Detector

The energy resolution is not more than 8%.

(2) Shielding body

In order to reduce the influence of environmental radiation (background), it is desirable that an apparatus has the lead-shielding structure around the detector. It is more desirable to enclose the entire surface with lead because the reduction effect is low when shielding only the side surface of a detector.

(3) Sample stage

Set the sample stage that a detector and a sample can be always fixed in a fixed spatial position relationship (geometry) in a shield body. In this case, it is desirable to place a beaker sample container perpendicularly just above the detector in terms of the detection efficiency and the stability during measurement. When using a rectangular sample container, it is also possible to attach the side of the container and the sample stage with the detector horizontally.

4.2.2.2. Tool and so on

(1) Sample container

Marinelli containers, plastic bottles, polyethylene tanks, etc. are used as sample containers. In the case of an emergency, quantification is possible by inserting a detector into a bucket containing a sample. However, it is necessary to calculate detection efficiency for each measurement container in advance.

(2) Energy calibration source

Select some energy calibration sources to cover from 100 to 2000 keV such as ^{22}Na (511 keV, 1275 keV), ^{54}Mn (835 keV), ^{60}Co (1173 keV, 1332 keV), ^{88}Y (898 keV, 1836 keV), ^{137}Cs (662 keV), and ^{139}Ce (166 keV). Obtain the relationship between the γ-ray energy and the peak center channel as a linear equation.

Because the energy resolution of NaI spectrometers is low unlike Ge detectors, the mixed radiation source composed of some nuclides with close γ-ray energy is not used.

(3) Efficiency calibration source

For efficiency calibration, use the efficiency calibration source whose radioactivity is known. Since the peak efficiency varies depending on the sample container, it is necessary to perform efficiency calibration for each sample container when multiple sample containers are used. It is desirable to use the nuclide emitting one or two γ-rays, considering the energy resolution of a spectrometer. It is desirable that the source includes target nuclides, ^{134}Cs and ^{137}Cs.

(4) Software for spectral analysis

Even if there is overlapping of peaks attributed to multiple nuclides, the software should be able to separate the peak of interest and calculate its area by peak function fitting, etc. It is desirable to be able to perform peak analysis in accordance with "Radioactivity measurement series No.7, γ-Ray Spectrometry by Germanium Semiconductor Detector"[4]. In addition, it is desirable to be able to calculate radioactive concentration from the radiation data of a nuclide to be quantified (half-life, γ-ray emission rate) and detection efficiency.

4.2.3. Apparatus calibration

4.2.3.1. Energy calibration

An energy calibration equation is obtained by using several energy calibration sources after the channel width of a multichannel analyzer is set to about 1000 ch and adjusted so that γ-rays up to 2000 keV can be measured.

There is the following relationship between the γ-ray energy (E) and the peak center channel (p):

$$E = \mathrm{a} + \mathrm{b} \times p$$

In the above equation, "a" is desirable to be as close to 0 as possible, and "b" is to be as close to 2.0 as possible, considering the number of channels.

4.2.3.2. Efficiency calibration

Because the counting efficiency varies depending on the energy of γ-rays, the efficiency calibration (ε) is obtained as the function of γ-ray energy (E) using an efficiency calibration source composed of some nuclides in known amounts. There is the following relationship in the region of several hundreds to 2000 keV.

$$\log(\varepsilon) = \mathrm{a} + \mathrm{b} \times \log(E)$$

If there is a calibration source containing ^{134}Cs and ^{137}Cs for quantification, the counting efficiency for a target γ-ray peak can be obtained directly.

4.2.4. Procedure

4.2.4.1. Preparations in advance and points to be checked

(1) Operation check of apparatus and settings

Apply polarity and voltage specified by a manufacturer to a photomultiplier tube. When a source is brought close to a detector, it is desirable to check with an oscilloscope that output waveforms from a preamplifier meet specifications. However, it is also acceptable to refer to an instruction manual for a model to be used. Alternatively, connect a detector to a multichannel analyzer to ensure that no noise signal is present, which is not normally observed, and that a dead time meter does not scale out. The channel width of the multichannel analyzer is set to about 1000 ch. The range of measurement energy is to be about 100 to 2000 keV.

For energy calibration, confirm that reference γ-rays (for example, ^{137}Cs or ^{40}K) can be detected in a channel set in advance at the time of power-on and every day. If there is a significant deviation from the set channel, adjust the gain of the amplifier.

(2) Background measurement

Perform measurement about once a week without sample or with an empty container to ensure that there is no contamination around a detector and a sample container. If a peak is observed in the same channel as a γ-ray to be quantified and decontamination is impossible, the counting rate should be obtained and recorded.

4.2.4.2. Measurement procedure

Since the measurement procedure is basically the same as the method using a Ge detector, follow the operation of a γ-ray spectrometer using a Ge detector.

(1) Setting of measurement time: Determine the measurement time according to a target detection limit and the amount of a sample. To lower the detection limit, the reduction of a background is most effective.

(2) Start and end procedures of measurement, and record of the times.

(3) Store of spectral data: File names should be such that samples and measured dates can be identified.

4.2.4.3. Analysis procedure

Since the analysis procedure is basically the same as the method using a Ge detector, follow the operation of a γ-ray spectrometer using a Ge detector. Points to be noted in this analysis are as follows:

(1) Setting of ROI

Set the ROI where a significant count is obtained against a background as the γ-ray peak used for quantification. At this time, if the variation is large because of an insufficient count and the setting the region is difficult, set the ROI after leveling the count of each channel by smoothing process.

(2) Identification of nuclide

Prepare to convert data by an energy calibration curve in order to determine which channel corresponds to the γ-ray of a nuclide to be quantified. Prepare nuclear data books and environmental radiation spectra, and if an unknown peak is detected, investigate the γ-ray energy, identify the nuclide, and examine possibility of interference with the γ-ray used for quantification.

(3) Calculation of peak area

Subtract the count of a background below a peak from the total count of the peak region. If the peak is too multiple to quantify by this method, the peak area is calculated after the peak separation using a peak function fitting method.

(4) Calculation of radioactivity

In the calculation of radioactivity it is necessary to estimate the calculation result of radioactivity by considering natural radioisotopes contained in a sample and a background. In this case, a net count (n) is obtained by subtracting a count in the region corresponding to the γ-ray peak of a nuclide used for quantification.

The radioactivity A (Bq) and the radioactive concentration C (Bq/kg) of a sample are obtained from the count rate (n), which is obtained by dividing the net count by the measurement time, by the following formulae.

$$A = \frac{n}{a\varepsilon f_{\mathrm{SUM}}} \quad C = \frac{A}{M}$$

In the above formula, the abbreviations are as follows.

n: Count rate

a: γ-Ray emission rate (Bq^{-1}) shown in Table 2

ε: Peak efficiency

f_{SUM}: Correction factor for summing effect. The summing effect must be corrected for ^{134}Cs, but if correction is not performed, state that.

M: Mass (kg) of a sample in a sample container

(5) Calculation of detection limit value

The detection limit value is calculated on the assumption that the γ-ray of the target nuclide exists in the channel of a background spectrum. The 3 folds value of the count error in background count of the peak region is expressed as the detection limit. The detection limit of commercially available spectrometers with a shielding body is about 30 Bq/kg for ^{131}I and ^{137}Cs, but widely differs depending on the detector size, shield thickness and sample volume.

The peak detection limit value in a real sample also highly depends on the spectrum of the sample. When other nuclides coexist in the sample, their Compton background may also affect the detection limit value to result in being larger in some cases.

(6) Examination and evaluation of measurement results

Summarize measurement results for each target nuclide, and confirm that it is normal based on the statistical uncertainty of count, peak center channel, FWHM, etc. If there is any doubt in the confirmation of results, remeasure as necessary.

4.2.5. Points to note for measurement

4.2.5.1. Effect of temperature

In the case of a NaI (Tl) spectrometer, variations in detector ambient temperature can cause the peak center channel to fluctuate. In particular, keep the temperature of the measurement room constant because it fluctuate easily during at nighttime and in winter. If a sample is stored at a lower temperature than the temperature of the measurement room, return it to near the temperature of the measurement room before measurement.

4.2.5.2. Control of background

Apply 4.1.5.1.

4.2.5.3. Contamination prevention of apparatus

Cover a detector with polyethylene bag to prevent from contamination. In the event of a contamination, cope by replacing the polyethylene packaging. If the surface of a detector is contaminated, wipe it off with a neutral detergent or gauze soaked in ethanol. Be careful not to allow dust or other contaminations to enter when opening a shield body.

Use a sample container after simple cleaning, if necessary. A polyethylene bag can be used in a container. When a sample solution is placed into a sample container, prevent the contaminant from adhering around the sample container.

5. Report and record

Examples of items to be described are as follows.

① Information concerning apparatus used: Apparatus name (detector size, resolution), number of measurement channels, analysis software type, processing method

② Sample information: Sample name (number), collection site, collection date and time, collection volume, type of collection container, name of person in charge of collection

③ Measurement conditions: Type of sample container, sample amount, geometry

④ Measurement records: Start date and time of measurement, measurement time (Live Time, Real Time)

⑤ Analysis records: Peak center channel, FWHM, peak area and its statistical uncertainty of count, sample count rate and its statistical uncertainty of count, BG count rate and its statistical uncertainty of count, peak efficiency, attenuation correction coefficient, radioactivity and radioactive concentration and their statistical uncertainties of each count, radioactivity of detection limit or radioactive concentration of detection limit, name of person in charge of measurement/analysis.

For analysis records, report prepared by the analysis software can be used as it is to avoid transcription mistakes. For numerical values, the number of significant digits of radioactivity or radioactive concentration is ''reduced'' based on the number of significant digits of the statistical uncertainty of count.

⑥ Measurement result: Name of nuclide, radioactive concentration (Bq/kg), detection limit value

When contracting a measurement work, in principle, write and report the measurement results in a format specified by the measurement work consignor, and store it together with the original data.

6. References

1) Japan Radioisotope Association, Isotope Notebook the 11th edition, Maruzen Publishing, 2011, ISBN 978-4-89073-211-1.

2) Water Supply Division, Health Service Bureau, The Ministry of Health, Labor and Welfare, Office Memorandum ''Sending of Manual for Radioactivity Measurement of Tap Water'', October 12, 2011.

3) Science and Technology Policy Bureau, The Ministry of Education, Culture, Sports, Science and Technology, ''Radioactivity measurement series No. 6, NaI (Tl) Scintillation spectrometry Instrumental Analysis'', January, 1974.

4) Science and Technology Policy Bureau, The Ministry of Education, Culture, Sports, Science and Technology, ''Radioactivity measurement series No. 7, γ-ray Spectrometry by Germanium Semiconductor Detector'' Revised ver.3, August, 1992.

G6 Drug Formulation

Criteria for Content Uniformity in Real Time Release Testing by Process Analytical Technology <G6-1-171>

1. Introduction

In recent years, the new criteria for Content Uniformity Test using a large sample size for Real Time Release Testing (RTRT) have become necessary with the rapid development of Process Analytical Technology (PAT). PAT using a nondestructive method such as Near Infrared (NIR) spectrometry enable to measure a large number of samples in real time, resulting in the generation of large amounts of data in a short time, and PAT can improve process control and process capability. However, the current pharmacopoeial criteria for Uniformity of Dosage Unit (the sample size is 10 and 30 for first and second stage respectively) may not be used adequately for large sample sizes over a hundred. For example, zero tolerance criteria has been used for outliers (no unit showing over the 25.0% deviation from label claim must be observed in the 30 samples tested). However, the probability of occurrence of outliers cannot be ignored when sample size was well over a hundred. This document display the consideration about criteria applicable for the large sample size over a hundred in RTRT.

2. Theoretical basis of the criteria

The Content Uniformity Test of the Japanese Pharmacopoeia is a kind of sampling tests, using small picked sample(s) from a large population (batch, lot), used for release of products. Therefore, the quality of estimations (test performance) depends on the sample size. In general, estimate the better the larger the sample size, and it is considered that a large sample size makes it possible to determine the quality of lots certainly. On the other hand, usage of a large sample size causes consumption of resources. For this reason, compendial tests like the tests in the Japanese Pharmacopoeia use a minimum and optimal sample size accompanying with strict criteria in order not to release bad products. Now a day, as a large sample size (Large-N) has become popular with development of PAT, it needs to set the appropriate criteria for RTRT using Large-N.

In setting of a specification limit, the limit value is determined by the balance between a guaranteed quality limit (acceptable limit) and the severity of a realistically capable test. When the specification limit is too strict, the acceptable quality becomes better, however a stock shortage caused by a low rate of passing the test of actual products occurs and the cost may become abnormally high. In order to maintain an acceptable quality, it is the most reasonable to compare the consumer's risk (risk of poor quality passing the test) and the producer's risk (risk of good quality failing the test) and to determine the severity of the most suitable test. Fig. 1 shows the OC (operating characteristic) curve describes the relationship as above.

The consumer's risk level, an acceptable quality corresponding to pass rate of 5% in release tests, is important to guarantee the quality of the product to be released. This means that possibility of releasing low quality products is considered low (<5%). On the other hand, the producer's risk is important for producers. They should consider how good quality is needed to pass (usually 90 − 95%) the test sufficiently. In spite of the sample size, the lot quality corresponding to 50% of pass rate is almost same the quality on the specification limit. If the sample size is increased without change of the specification limit, the OC curves change as in Fig. 2-A.

That is to say, the quality (x-axis showing variability in unit content) of the 50% acceptance level is unchanged in all the OC curves while the slope of the OC curves become steeper with the larger the sample size. In contrast, if the limit value is changed to more strict without changing the sample size, the OC curves shift to the left at a constant slope (Fig. 2-B). To be constant the consumer's risk level regardless of change of sample size, it is necessary to set the limit value in response to changes in sample size as in Fig. 3-A. In general, the large sample size can have the consumer's risk level maintain to be constant even if the limit value becomes loose.

When products is tested by PAT in a large sample size and then released, they will be subjected to stability tests and survey tests using the usual small sample sizes after releasing. In this case, though the consumer's risk as in Fig. 3-A is at a constant, the producer's risk increase. In order not to increase the producer's risk after releasing, it is necessary to set the test limits so as not to differ very much in producer's risk between the test by PAT and the conventional test. In this case, it is necessary to tighten the test limit in larger sample size, as shown in Fig. 3-B.

Our recommended criteria were determined in consideration of such a point as described above[1)]. It should be noted that our criteria are simple and non-parametric criteria that do not depend on the type of distribution of unit content, and also has the same attitude with the Alternate 2[2)] of the European Pharmacopoeia (EP) being a standard corresponding to the above mentioned Large-N. In the case of using the Alternate 1 of EP, there could be no problem from the point of view about quality assurance.

3. Criteria for Content Uniformity in sample size equal to or more than 100

The criteria recommended are consisted of two tests by attribute (limits are *C1* and *C2*). The sample sizes and acceptance numbers are shown in Table 1.

Criteria

Select *n* units representing a lot submitted, and assay the units individually using an appropriate analytical method and calculate individual contents expressed by the percentage of label claim. The requirements are met if the number of dosage units outside 15.0% is less than or equal to *C1*, and the number of dosage units outside 25.0% is less than or equal to *C2*. The central point of content bias can be alter to an appropriate value from the label claim if it is needed by quality control issue.

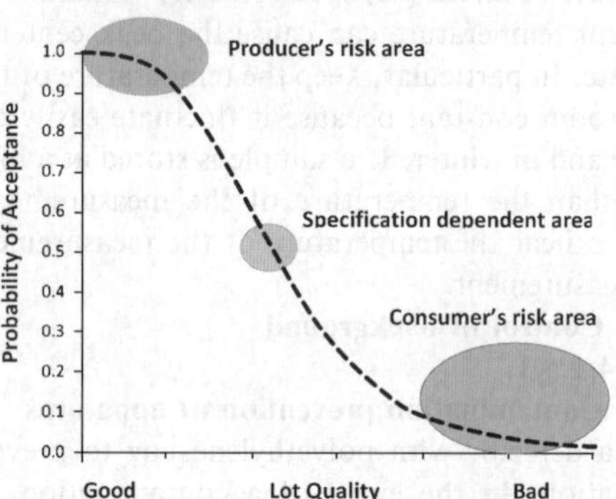

Fig. 1 Consumer's risk and producer's risk areas in an OC curve

A. Effects of sample sizes

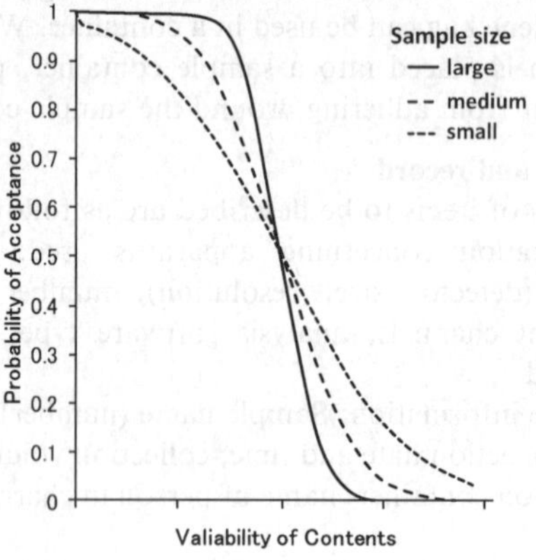

B. Effects of specification limits

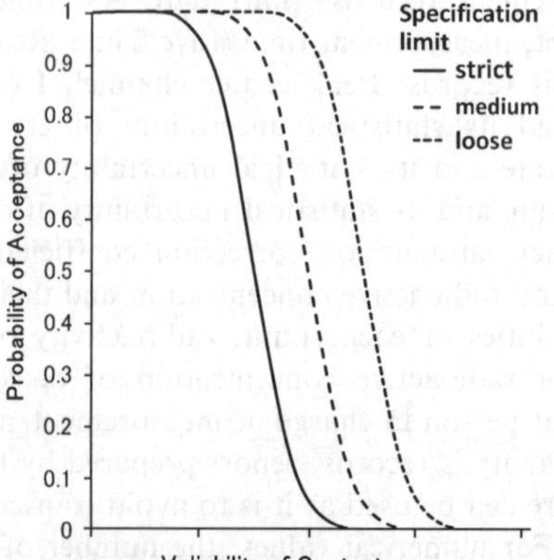

Fig. 2 OC Curves of Content Uniformity Tests — Effects of sample sizes and specification limits

A. Constant risk of consumers

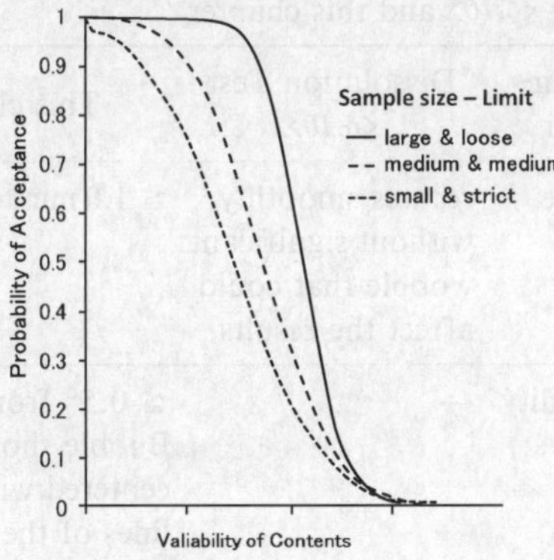

B. Constant risk of producers

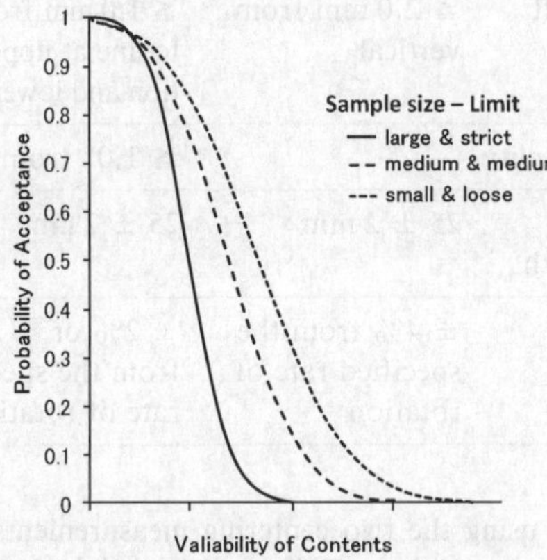

Fig. 3 OC Curves of Content Uniformity Tests — Risks of consumers or producers are constant

4. References

1) N. Katori *et al.*, Sakura Bloom Tablets P2 Mock by MHLW sponsored QbD Drug Product Study Group (Responsible researcher: H. Okuda, Study on Quality Assurance over the Life Cycle of Pharmaceutical Products), (Mar. 2015).
2) European Pharmacopoeia 7.7 (2012), 2.9.47. Demonstration of Uniformity of Dosage Units Using Large Sample Sizes.

Standard Procedure for Mechanical Calibration of Dissolution Apparatus <*G6-2-170*>

This chapter is intended to minimize sources of mechanical variability of apparatus which affect test results and assure the reproducibility of results, for Apparatus 1 (Basket method) and Apparatus 2 (Paddle method), and describes the standard procedure for the mechanical calibration of dissolution apparatus and the recommended specifications. The validity of the mechanical calibration for qualification of dissolution test is confirmed on the meeting of international harmonization of pharmacopeia about dissolution test, and subsequently. the standard practice for qualification of dissolution apparatus[1] and the guidance of mechanical calibration[2] were issued in U.S.A.

Requirements for basic quality of materials and sizes, etc., to be required on dissolution test apparatus, and the suitability of the apparatus conform to the statements of Dissolution Test <*6.10*>. The tolerance of some parameters for the

Table 1 Criteria for Content Uniformity

Sample size (n)	Acceptance number*	
	*C1*** (± 15.0%)	*C2*** (± 25.0%)
$n < 100$	Criteria of 6.02 Uniformity of Dosage Units	
$100 \leq n < 150$	3	0
$150 \leq n < 200$	4	0
$200 \leq n < 300$	6	1
$300 \leq n < 500$	8	2
$500 \leq n < 1000$	13	4
$1000 \leq n < 2000$	25	8
$2000 \leq n < 5000$	47	18
$5000 \leq n < 10000$	112	47
$10000 \leq n$	217	94

* The requirements are met if the number of outliers is less than or equal to acceptance number.
** Critical acceptance number.

mechanical calibration described in this chapter may be specified strictly compared with that specified in Dissolution Test <*6.10*>. The below table shows the comparison of specified values of each calibration parameter. In order to minimize variability of test results by the mechanical calibration, it is recommended to apply this chapter.

Although qualification of dissolution test results by using Prednisone Tablet RS has been recommended in our country, since it cannot necessarily detect sources of mechanical variability of apparatus, the performance of the mechanical calibration is basically desirable. However the test appropriately performed by using Prednisone Tablet RS is valid for understanding overall factor including degassing state of a test solution and vibration of apparatus undetected by only the calibration of apparatus. Moreover a monitoring by a dissolved oxygen analyzer is valid for confirmation of degassing state of a test solution.

1. Setup of dissolution apparatus and periodic control

Mechanical calibration should be performed on purchase or receipt of dissolution apparatus, after move and after repair which can affect test results, and it is usually desirable to perform the calibration every year. If the instrument is not being used routinely, the mechanical calibration can be performed before performing the first dissolution test after the one year time interval.

2. Procedure of mechanical calibration

2.1. Instruments

Instruments for the mechanical calibration are runout gage, level, centering device and tachometer, etc., as generic ones and it is desirable to use the tools to be traceable to JIS (Japanese Industrial Standards), etc., wherever possible. In addition, special instruments for the mechanical calibration of dissolution apparatus are centering tool, depth gage, plastic ball, etc. Moreover, some dissolution apparatus require the special tools supplied by instrument manufacturers or incorporate automatic mechanical calibration devices within their equipment. These tools and devices may be used provided they follow the general principle of the below procedure.

2.2. Procedure

Perform the mechanical calibration of dissolution apparatus according to the below specified procedure. If each measured value does not meet the specification, repetitive adjustments and measurements may be necessary.

Confirm that the apparatus is horizontal on the installation table in advance. Also confirm the horizontality of the plate which fix the vessel (vessel plate) by placing a bubble level on the stage and confirming the bubble to be within the lines of the level.

2.2.1. Shaft Wobble

A runout gage is placed on top of the vessel plate, and positioned so that the gage probe touches the shaft about 2 cm above the top of the paddle blade or basket. The absolute value of the difference between the maximum and minimum readings is the wobble. The value of total wobble must not exceed 1.0 mm.

2.2.2. Shaft Verticality

Lower the drive unit to where it would be during an actual dissolution test. If necessary, the shaft verticality may be checked by raising the drive unit. Place an accurate bubble level on the front edge of each of the shafts. The bubble should be within the lines of the level. Rotate the level about 90° so that it touches the side of the shaft, and put it on the side of the shaft. The bubble should again be within the lines of the level.

A digital leveling device may also be used to determine the shaft verticality.

The shaft must be not more than 0.5° from vertical.

2.2.3. Basket Wobble

A runout gage is placed on top of the vessel plate and the drive unit is positioned so that the gage probe touches the bottom rim of the basket. The gage is placed so that the probe slightly presses in on the turning shaft. The value of total wobble must not exceed 1.0 mm.

2.2.4. Vessel Centering

Centering inside the vessel is measured by centering tools for dissolution test apparatus or by an alternative procedure.

When measured by centering tools, two centering tools are used to center the paddle or basket shafts in the vessels and to align the vessels so that their sides are vertical.

As an example of the procedure for the paddle method, the bottom of one centering tool is placed 2 mm above the top of the paddle blade and the bottom of the second centering tool is clamped on the shaft 80 mm above the blade with the both probes positioned in the same direction towards the vessel wall. For the basket method, the bottom of one centering tool is placed 2 mm above the top of the basket and the bottom of the second centering tool is placed 60 mm above the top of the basket with the both probes positioned in the same direction towards the vessel wall. Carefully lower the shaft and centering tools into the vessels so that the paddle blade and the bottom of the basket is about 2.5 cm above the bottom of the vessel. Manually rotate the shaft slowly and check the centering at both levels. If the vessel is not centered at either level, adjust the vessel to center it.

An alternative procedure is to use a mechanical or digital centering device that centers the inside wall of the vessel around the shaft or a surrogate shaft. The centering is measured at two positions inside the vessel in the cylindrical portion, one just below the rim of the vessel and one just above the basket or the paddle in the bottom portion of the vessel.

The shaft must be centered within 1.0 mm from the center line.

2.2.5. Vessel Verticality

The vessel verticality can be calculated as the angle of the vertex of the triangle composed of the two points and the vertical line using the two centering measurements in 2.2.4 Vessel Centering and the difference in height between the two measurements. Or it can be determined using a digital leveling device placed on the inside wall of the vessel. The verticality should be determined at two positions 90° apart.

The vessel must be not more than 1.0° from vertical.

After each vessel has been centered and made vertical, each vessel must be positioned in the exact same position and same direction inside the vessel plate opening.

2.2.6. Basket and Paddle Depth

The actual distance between the bottom of the vessel and the bottom of the basket or paddle is determined. If the depth of the basket/paddle is adjustable, first a depth gage is used to determine the distance between the bottom of the paddle blade or basket and the inside bottom of the vessel. The depth gage is set at 25 mm and placed on the bottom of the vessel. After each shaft is raised into the apparatus drive module, the drive unit is then lowered to its operating position. The paddle or basket is then lowered into the vessel until it touches the top of the depth gage. Instead of a depth gage, sink a plastic ball with a diameter 25 mm ± 2 mm on the bottom of the vessel and the paddle or basket can be lowered into the vessel until it touches the ball. The shafts are locked into this height. Usually the depth of basket and paddle is 25 mm ± 2 mm.

2.2.7. Rotational Speed

A tachometer is used to measure the rotational speed of the paddle or basket. The shafts should be rotating smoothly with a rate within a larger value of ±2% or ±2 rpm of the specified rate.

Table Specified values of calibration parameters of Dissolution Test <*6.10*> and this chapter

Calibration Parameter	Dissolution Test <*6.10*>	This chapter
Shaft wobble	rotates smoothly without significant wobble that could affect the results	≦ 1.0 mm total runout
Shaft verticality	—	≦ 0.5° from vertical Bubble should be centered within the lines of the level.
Basket wobble	—	≦ 1.0 mm total runout
Vessel/Shaft centering	≦ 2.0 mm from vertical	≦ 1.0 mm from centerline at upper position and lower position
Vessel verticality	—	≦ 1.0° from vertical
Basket and Paddle depth	25 ± 2 mm	25 ± 2 mm
Rotational speed	± 4% from the specified rate of rotation	± 2% or ± 2 rpm from the specified rate of rotation

3. References

1) ASTM E2503 - 13: 2013, Standard Practice for Qualification of Basket and Paddle Dissolution Apparatus (2013).

2) FDA Guidance for Industry: The Use of Mechanical Calibration of Dissolution Apparatus 1 and 2—Current Good Manufacturing Practice (CGMP), U.S. Depart-

ment of Health and Human Services Food and Drug Administration Center for Drug Evaluation and Research (CDER), January 2010.

Aerodynamic Particle Size Measurement for Inhalations by Glass Impingers *<G6-3-171>*

This test is used to evaluate the fine particle characteristics of the aerosol clouds generated by preparations for inhalation, and is performed using the following apparatus and test procedures. If justified, modified apparatus or test procedure may be used.

1. Stage mensuration

The most reliable calibration for the separation characteristics of each impaction stage is performed in terms of the relationship between the aerodynamic diameter of particles and droplets passing through it and the stage collection efficiency as an aerosol.

Calibration is usually performed by examination of a property of the jet dimensions, the spatial arrangement of the jet and its collection surface, and the airflow rate passing through it.

Because jets can corrode and wear over time, the critical dimensions of each stage must be measured on a regular basis to confirm them being within required ranges.

Only apparatuses that conform to specifications are used for the aerodynamic particle size measurement for inhalations by glass impingers. An alternate validated and justified method of mensuration may be used.

2. Inter-stage drug losses (wall losses)

Wall losses should be considered in method development and validation. If the wall losses affect the recovery rate (mass balance) of drugs, they should be controlled. Wall losses will be dependent upon a number of factors including the impactor type, operating conditions, formulation type and discharged amount to an impactor. How the wall loss is reflected within the calculation of the aerodynamic diameter of particles should be judged based up on the level and variability of the wall loss. For example, in the cases where wall losses that are low or have a low level of variability, the aerodynamic particle size is calculated by the assay of the drug collected on the stage. In cases where wall losses are high or variable, it may be necessary to collect the wall loss drug separately and take it into account for the calculation of the aerodynamic particle size.

3. Recovery rate of drugs (mass balance)

In addition to the size distribution, good analytical practice dictates that a mass balance be performed in order to confirm that the amount of the drug discharged from the inhaler, which is collected in the mouthpiece adapter and the apparatus, is within an acceptable range around the expected value. The total mass of drug collected in all of the components of the mouthpiece adapter and the apparatus divided by the minimum recommended dose described in the dosage and administration is not less than 75% and not more than 125% of the average delivered dose determined under Uniformity of Delivered Dose for Inhalations *<6.14>*. This mass balance is necessary to ensure that the test results of particle size distributions of inhalations are valid.

4. Glass impinger method

The apparatus used for the glass impinger method is shown in Fig. 1. The apparatus consists of glass parts from the throat (B) to the lower impingement chamber (H) and plastic clips to hold them.

This apparatus is operated based on a collision to a liquid surface and separate the drug discharged from the inhaler to an inhalation part and a non-inhalation part. The drug in the non-inhalation part, which collides with an oral cavity and a pharyngeal region to result in being swallowed, is recovered in the rear of the throat and the upper impingement chamber (collectively stage 1). The drug in the inhalation part, which reaches lungs, is recovered in the lower impingement chamber (stage 2). Because the upper impingement chamber is designed so that the cut-off diameter is 6.4 μm when the test flow rate is 60 L per minute, particles with a diameter of 6.4 μm or less flow down to the lower impingement chamber.

4.1. Procedure for nebulizers

Introduce 7 mL and 30 mL of a suitable solvent into the upper and lower impingement chambers, respectively.

Connect all the component parts. Ensure that the assembly is vertical and adequately supported and that the jet spacer peg of the lower jet assembly just touches the bottom of the lower impingement chamber. Connect a suitable pump fitted with a filter (of suitable pore size) to the outlet of the apparatus. Adjust the air flow through the apparatus, as measured at the inlet to the throat, to 60 ± 5 L per minute.

Introduce the inhalation liquids and solutions into the reservoir of the nebulizer. Fit the mouthpiece and connect it by means of a mouthpiece adapter to the device.

Switch on the pump of the apparatus and after 10 seconds switch on the nebulizer.

After 60 seconds, unless otherwise justified, switch off the nebulizer, wait for 5 seconds and then switch off the pump

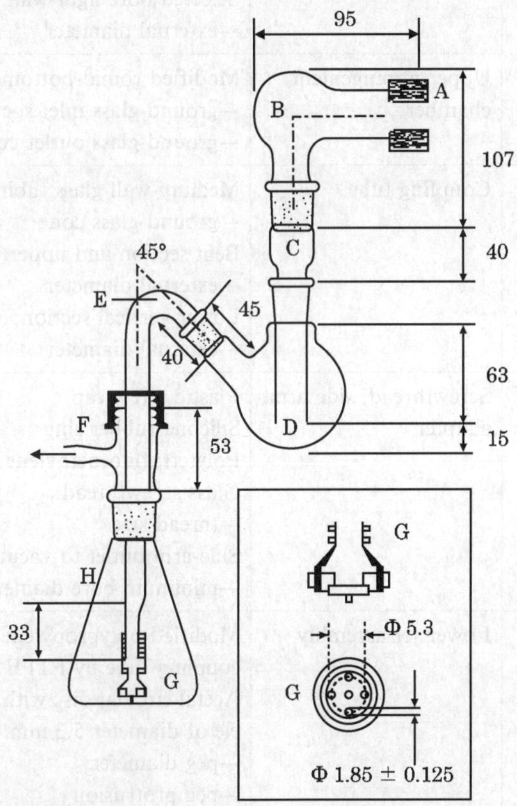

Capital letters of alphabet refer to Table 1
The figures are in mm. (Tolerances are ±1 mm unless otherwise stated.)

Fig. 1 Glass impinger

of the apparatus.

Dismantle the apparatus and wash the inner wall surface of the upper impingement chamber collecting the washings in a volumetric flask. Wash the inner wall surface of the lower impingement chamber collecting the washings in a second volumetric flask. Finally, wash the filter preceding the pump and its connections to the lower impingement chamber and combine the washings with those obtained from the lower impingement chamber. Determine the amount of active substance collected in each of the two flasks. Express the results for each of the two parts of the apparatus as a percentage of the total amount of active substance.

4.2. Procedure for metered-dose inhalers

Install a suitable mouthpiece adapter in position at the end of the throat. When the mouthpiece end of the inhaler is inserted in the mouthpiece adapter to a depth of about 10 mm, the mouthpiece end of the inhaler lines up along the horizontal axis of the throat. The open end of the inhaler, which accepts the pressurized container, is uppermost and in the same vertical plane as the rest of the apparatus.

Introduce 7 mL and 30 mL of a suitable solvent into the upper and lower impingement chambers, respectively.

Connect all the component parts. Ensure that the assembly is vertical and adequately supported and that the jet spacer peg of the lower jet assembly just touches the bottom of the lower impingement chamber. Connect a suitable pump to the outlet of the apparatus. Adjust the air flow through the apparatus, as measured at the inlet to the throat, to 60 ± 5 L per minute.

Unless otherwise prescribed in the patient instruction, shake for 5 seconds and discharge once to waste. After not less than 5 seconds, shake and discharge again to waste. Repeat the procedure a further three times.

Shake for about 5 seconds, switch on the pump to the apparatus and locate the mouthpiece end of the inhaler in the adapter, discharge once immediately in the apparatus.

Table 1 Component specification for apparatus shown in Fig. 1

Code	Item	Description	Dimensions*
A	Mouthpiece adapter	Moulded rubber adapter for actuator mouthpiece.	
B	Throat	Modified round-bottomed flask: —ground-glass inlet socket —ground-glass outlet cone	50 mL 29/32 24/29
C	Neck	Modified glass adapter: —ground-glass inlet socket —ground-glass outlet cone Lower outlet section of precision-bore glass tubing: —bore diameter Selected bore light-wall glass tubing: —external diameter	 24/29 24/29 14 17
D	Upper impingement chamber	Modified round-bottomed flask: —ground-glass inlet socket —ground-glass outlet cone	100 mL 24/29 14/23
E	Coupling tube	Medium-wall glass tubing: —ground-glass cone Bent section and upper vertical section: —external diameter Lower vertical section: —external diameter	 14/23 13 8
F	Screwthread, side-arm, adapter	Plastic screw cap Silicone rubber ring Polytetrafluoroethylene (PTFE) washer Glass screwthread: —thread size Side-arm outlet to vacuum pump: —minimum bore diameter	28/13 28/11 28/11 28 5
G	Lower jet assembly	Modified polypropylene filter holder connected to lower vertical section of coupling tube by PTFE tubing Acetal circular disc with the centres of four jets arranged on a projected circle of diameter 5.3 mm with an integral jet spacer peg: —peg diameter —peg protrusion	see Fig. 1 10 2 2
H	Lower impingement chamber	Conical flask —ground-glass inlet socket	250 mL 24/29

* Dimensions in mm, unless otherwise stated.

Remove the assembled inhaler from the adapter, shake for not less than 5 seconds, relocate the mouthpiece end of the inhaler in the adapter and discharge again. Repeat the discharge sequence. The number of discharges should be minimized and typically would not be greater than 10. After the final discharge wait for not less than 5 seconds and then switch off the pump.

Dismantle the apparatus. Wash the inner wall surface of the coupling tube to the lower impingement chamber and its outer wall surface that projects into the chamber with a suitable solvent, collecting the washings in the lower impingement chamber. Determine the content of active substance in this solution. Calculate the amount of active substance collected in the lower impingement chamber per discharge and express the results as a percentage of the active substance stated on the label.

4.3. Procedure for dry powder inhalers

Introduce 7 mL and 30 mL of a suitable solvent into the upper and lower impingement chambers, respectively.

Connect all the component parts. Ensure that the assembly is vertical and adequately supported and that the jet spacer peg of the lower jet assembly just touches the bottom of the lower impingement chamber. Connect a suitable pump to the outlet of the apparatus. Adjust the air flow through the apparatus, as measured at the inlet to the throat, to 60 ± 5 L per minute.

Prepare an inhaler and connect it to the throat using a suitable adapter. Switch on the pump of the apparatus, after 5 seconds switch off the pump of the apparatus, and repeat the discharge sequence. The number of discharges should be minimized and typically would not be greater than 10.

Dismantle the apparatus. Wash the inner wall surface of the coupling tube to the lower impingement chamber and its outer wall surface that projects into the chamber with a suitable solvent, collecting the washings in the lower impingement chamber. Determine the content of active substance in this solution. Calculate the amount of active substance collected in the lower impingement chamber per discharge and express the results as a percentage of the active substance stated on the label.

Tablet Hardness Determinations

<G6-4-180>

This General Information summarizes the principle, type, instrument configuration and points to be considered in the tablet hardness determination. Results, together with other information on physical integrity of tablets such as friability, are used to ensure their mechanical strength against stresses such as impact and pressure they experience from manufacturing process to usage.

The measurement is usually performed by placing a tablet between two platens and moving the one platen at a constant speed to obtain the force (N) just before the tablet is broken. The tablet hardness values reflect either the breaking force with which a compressive load generates breakage in a specific tablet plane, or the crushing strength with which substantial breaking cause the loss of structure, or both, depending on an apparatus used. In some cases, the tablet appearance may be lost after breakage. Criteria of the tablet hardness obtained by this measurement is different from the definition of hardness generally used in the field of materials science etc. (the resistance of a surface against penetration and pushing by a small probe).

Multiple hardness testers with different structure of the tablet-mounted part, the transfer mechanism of the platen, the measurement method of force, etc. are used. Manual or relatively simple-structured hardness testers include Monsanto (Stokes) tablet hardness tester which compresses a tablet with an indenter via a spring gauge and a screw, Pfizer tablet hardness tester which applies pressure to a tablet with a plier, Strong Cobb hardness tester which applies a load to a tablet by compressed air, and Erweka tablet hardness tester which applies a load to a tablet with an indenter using an electrically-powered weight load. Apparatuses which automate the process of hardness determination, correspond to various measurement modes and have a data correction function, etc. are also used.

The measurement of tablet hardness is affected by the shape, size, and orientation of a sample tablet, as well as the structure of an apparatus and the measurement conditions. Therefore, it is important to record the name of apparatus and conditions as well as results. The direct comparison of data requires measurements under the same conditions. The following points should be also considered in the measurement.

(i) Platen: Two platens with smooth area contacting a tablet should be used in parallel. The contact surface should be larger than the area of contact with the tablet. Make sure that tablets should be free of displacement by bending or twisting when the load is applied.

(ii) Loading rate: An apparatus having the mechanism which keeps the constant loading rate of compression force by platens should be used for the measurements. Or, the measurements should be performed by moving the platen at a low rate from a certain point immediately before contact with a tablet using an apparatus which keeps the moving speed of platens constant to suppress the variation of the loading rate. Faster movement of the platen would allow rapid measurement, while possible variation in the loading rate often leads to uncontrollable crushing and the rapid accumulation of compressive loads.

(iii) Measurement unit and calibration of apparatuses: An apparatus calibrated with accuracy of 1N or less should be used for the measurement.

(iv) Change of apparatus: It is desirable to change an apparatus to that having a similar mechanism because the mechanism such as the loading method of compression force and the measuring method force would vary between them. The risk due to the apparatus change should be controlled by considering their measurement mechanisms and by comparing the results obtained by multiple measurement parameters such as the loading rate, and the moving speed of platens, using the sample in a same lot.

(v) Tablet orientation: A round non-scored tablet is usually placed between two platens to allow the compression occurs across the tablet diameter. In the measurement of a scored tablet, the tablet is placed so that the score is perpendicular or parallel to the platens. In the case of tablets with unique or complicated shape, it is desirable to place them in the same orientation that can be easily reproduced. In general, a load is applied either across the diameter or parallel to the longest axis.

(vi) Unit: As a unit of tablet hardness, kgf, kp or Strong Cobb Unit (SCU), etc. as well as N is used.

(vii) Number of samples: In addition to the average of the measured values of tablet hardness, their variation should be also important. Therefore, the number of samples should be statistically appropriate for the purpose of measurement. Usually 6 or more samples, often 10 samples, are measured.

Tablet Friability Test *<G6-5-150>*

This test is harmonized with the European Pharmacopoeia and the U.S. Pharmacopeia.

Information on the harmonization with the European Pharmacopoeia and the U.S. Pharmacopeia is available on the website of the Pharmaceuticals and Medical Devices Agency.

The Tablet Friability Test is a method to determine the friability of compressed uncoated tablets. The test procedure presented in this chapter is generally applicable to most compressed tablets. Measurement of tablets friability supplements other physical strength measurement, such as tablet crushing strength.

Use a drum, with an internal diameter between 283 and 291 mm and a depth between 36 and 40 mm, of transparent synthetic polymer with polished internal surfaces, and subject to minimum static build-up (see figure for a typical apparatus). One side of the drum is removable. The tablets are tumbled at each turn of the drum by a curved projection with an inside radius between 75.5 and 85.5 mm that extends from the middle of the drum to the outer wall. The outer diameter of the central ring is between 24.5 and 25.5 mm. The drum is attached to the horizontal axis of a device that rotates at 25 ± 1 rpm. Thus, at each turn the tablets roll or slide and fall onto the drum wall or onto each other.

For tablets with a unit mass equal to or less than 650 mg, take a sample of whole tablets *n* corresponding as near as possible to 6.5 g. For tablets with a unit mass of more than 650 mg, take a sample of 10 whole tablets. The tablets should be carefully dedusted prior to testing. Accurately weigh the tablet sample, and place the tablets in the drum. Rotate the drum 100 times, and remove the tablets. Remove any loose dust from the tablets as before, and accurately weigh.

Generally, the test is run once. If obviously cracked, cleaved, or broken tablets are present in the tablet sample after tumbling, the sample fails the test. If the results are difficult to interpret or if the mass loss is greater than the targeted value, the test should be repeated twice and the mean of the three tests determined. A maximum mean mass loss from the three samples of not more than 1.0% is considered acceptable for most products.

If tablet size or shape causes irregular tumbling, adjust the drum base so that the base forms an angle of about 10° with the horizontal and the tablets no longer bind together when lying next to each other, which prevents them from falling freely.

Effervescent tablets and chewable tablets may have different specifications as far as friability is concerned. In the case of hygroscopic tablets, an appropriate humidity-controlled environment is required for testing.

Drums with dual scooping projections, or apparatus with more than one drum, for the running of multiple samples at one time, are also permitted.

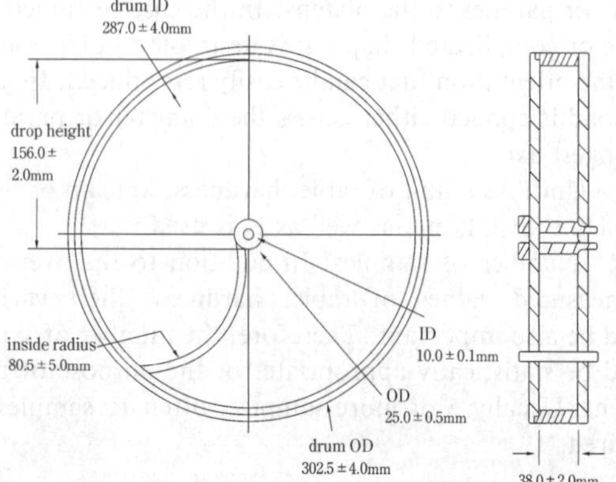

pH Test for Gastrointestinal Medicine *<G6-6-131>*

In this test, medicine for the stomach and bowels, which is said to control stomach acid, is stirred in a fixed amount of the 0.1 mol/L hydrochloric acid for a fixed duration, and the pH value of this solution is measured. The pH value of a stomach medicine will be based on the dose and the dosage of the medicine (when the dosage varies, a minimum dosage is used) and expressed in the pH value obtained from the test performed by the following procedure.

1. Preparation of Sample

Solid medicine which conforms to the general regulations for medicine (the powdered medicine section) can be used as a sample. When the medicine is in separate packages, the content of 20 or more packages is accurately weighed to calculate the average mass for one dose and mixed evenly to make a sample. For granules and similar types in separate packages, among the solid medicine which does not conform to the general regulations for medicine (the powdered medicine section), the content of 20 or more packages is accurately weighed to calculate the average mass for one dose and is then powdered to make sample. For granules and similar types not in separate packages, among solid medicine which does not conform to the general regulations for medicine (the powdered medicine section), 20 doses or more are powdered to make a sample. For capsules and tablets, 20 doses or more are weighed accurately to calculate the average mass for one dose or average mass and then powdered to make a sample.

Liquid medicine is generously mixed to make a sample.

2. Procedure

Put 50 mL of the 0.1 mol/L hydrochloric acid with the molarity coefficient adjusted to 1.000, or equivalent 0.1 mol/L hydrochloric acid with its volume accurately measured in a 100-mL beaker. Stir this solution with a magnetic stirrer and a magnetic stirrer rotator (35 mm length, 8 mm diameter) at the speed of about 300 revolutions per minute. While stirring, add the accurately weighed one-dose sample. After 10 minutes, measure the pH value of the solution using the pH Determination. The solution temperature should be maintained at 37 ± 2°C throughout this operation.

Test for Trace Amounts of Aluminum in Total Parenteral Nutrition (TPN) Solutions *<G6-7-160>*

Total parenteral nutrition solutions (TPNs) are nutrient preparations for intravenous injection. Since toxic effects to the central nervous system, bone, etc. due to trace amounts of aluminum have recently been reported in several countries, testing methods for trace amounts of aluminum contaminating TPNs are required for the official standard. The following three analytical methods are available: High-Performance Liquid Chromatography using a fluorescence photometric detector (HPLC with fluorescence detection), Inductivity Coupled Plasma-Atomic Emission Spectrometry (ICP-AES method), Inductivity Coupled Plasma-Mass Spectrometry (ICP-MS method). Detection sensitivity by HPLC with fluorescence detection is about 1 μg/L (ppb), while ICP-AES fitted with special apparatus and ICP-MS have higher sensitivity.

Since TPNs are nutrient preparations, they contain many nutrients such as sugars, amino acids, electrolytes, etc., in various compositions. Thus, care is needed in the selection of a suitable analytical method, because these coexisting components may affect the measurement of trace amounts of aluminum.

In view of the general availability of HPLC apparatus, the present general information describes procedures for the determination of trace levels of aluminum in TPNs by means of HPLC with a fluorescence photometric detector, using two kinds of fluorescent chelating agents, i.e., Quinolinol complexing method, Lumogallion complexing method.

1. Quinolinol complexing method

After forming a complex of aluminum ion in the sample solution with quinolinol, the assay for aluminum by HPLC fitted with a fluorescence photometer is performed.

1.1. Preparation of sample solution

Pipet 1 mL of the sample (TPNs) exactly, and after adding 10 μL of water for aluminum test, make up the sample solution to 10 mL exactly by adding the mobile phase.

1.2. Preparation of a series of standard solutions for calibration curve

Pipet 1 mL of water for aluminum test exactly, and after adding 10 μL each of standard solutions of aluminum (1)–(5), make up the standard solutions for calibration curve to 10 mL exactly by adding the mobile phase (Aluminum concentration: 0, 1.25, 2.5, 5.0, and 10.0 ppb).

1.3. Standard testing method

Pipet 0.1 mL each of the sample solution and standard solutions, and perform the test by HPLC under the following conditions. Calculate the aluminum cotent in the sample solution using a calibration curve method.

Operating conditions—

Detector: A fluorescence photometer (excitation wavelength: 380 nm, emission wavelength: 520 nm).

Column: A stainless steel column 4.6 mm in inside diameter and 15 cm in length, packed with phenylsilanized silica gel for liquid chromatography (5 μm in particle diameter).

Column temperature: A constant temperature of about 40°C.

Mobile phase: A mixture of 8-quinolinol in acetonitrile (3 in 100) and diluted 0.5 mol/L ammonium acetate TS (2 in 5) (1:1).

Flow rate: Adjust so that the retention time of aluminum/8-quinolinol complex is about 9 minutes.

System suitability—

The correlation coefficient of the calibration curve, which is prepared using a series of standard solutions, is not less than 0.99.

Furthermore there is an alternative method, in which the chelating agent 8-quinolinol is not included in the mobile phase.

In this method also, aluminum is detected as a complex with 8-quinolinol in the sample solution by using HPLC fitted with a fluorescence photometer. But it is necessary to form a more stable aluminum/8-quinolinol complex in the sample solution, because the chelating agent is not included in the mobile phase. Further, since the analytical wavelength for the fluorescence detection is different from that in the standard method, excitation wavelength: 370 nm, emission wavelength: 504 nm, the detection sensitivity is different. Thus, it is appropriate to obtain the calibration curve between 0 – 25 ppb of aluminum. Other than the above- mentioned differences, the size of column, column temperature, and the mobile phase are also different from those used in the standard method, so suitable analytical conditions should be established for performing precise and reproducible examinations of trace amounts of aluminum in the sample specimen.

2. Lumogallion complexing method

After forming a complex of aluminum ion in the sample specimen with the fluorescent reagent of lumogallion, the solution is examined by HPLC fitted with a fluorescence photometer.

2.1. Preparation of sample solution

Pipet 70 μL of the sample specimen (TPN) exactly, add 0.15 mL of lumogallion hydrochloric acid TS and 0.6 mL of buffer solution for aluminum test (pH 7.2) exactly, then mix the solution. After this solution has been allowed to stand for 4 hours at 40°C, it can be used for the measurement as a sample solution.

2.2. Preparation of a series of standard solutions for calibration curve

Pipet 1 mL each of standard aluminum solutions (1) – (5) exactly, and add diluted nitric acid for aluminum test (1 in 100) to make exactly 100 mL. Pipet 70 μL each of these solutions exactly, and add exactly 0.15 mL of lumogallion hydrochloric acid TS and exactly 0.6 mL of buffer solution for aluminum test (pH 7.2) then allow to stand for 4 hours at 40°C to make a series of standard solutions for obtaining the calibration curve (Aluminum: 0, 1.07, 2.13, 4.27, and 8.54 ppb).

2.3. Standard examination method

Take 0.1 mL each of the sample solution and standard solutions for the calibration curve, and perform HPLC analysis under the following conditions. Calculate the aluminum content in the sample solution by using a calibration curve method.

Operating conditions—

Detector: A fluorescence photometer(excitation wavelength 505 nm, emission wavelength 574 nm).

Column: A stainless steel column 6.0 mm in inside diameter and 10 cm in length, packed with octylsilanized silica gel for liquid chromatography (5 μm in particle diameter).

Column temperature: A constant temperature of about 40°C.

Mobile phase: Take 100 mL of 2-propanol, and add a diluted 1 mol/L acetic acid-sodium acetate buffer solution of pH 5.0 (1 in 10) to make 1000 mL.

Flow rate: Adjust so that the retention time of aluminum/lumogallion complex is about 5 minutes.

System suitability—

The correlation coefficient of the calibration curve, which is prepared using a series of standard solutions for calibration curve, is not less than 0.99.

3. Notes

(i) Regarding water, solvents, reagents, vessels and other tools used for the examination, select those not contaminated with aluminum. Further, keep the testing environment clean and free from dust in the testing room.

(ii) Before the measurement, it is necessary to confirm that the characteristic properties of the sample do not affect the formation of the complex.

(iii) Reference substances of river water for analysis of trace elements, commercially distributed by the Japan Society for Analytical Chemistry, can be used to estimate the validity of test methods and results.

4. Standard Solutions, Reagents and Test Solutions

Other than the standard solutions, reagents and test solutions specified in the Japanese Pharmacopoeia, those described below can be used in this test.

(i) ***N,N*-Bis(2-hydroxyethyl)-2-aminoethane sulfonic acid** $C_6H_{15}NO_5S$ White crystals or powder.

(ii) **Hydrochloric acid for aluminum test** Same as the reagent *Hydrochloric acid*. Further, it contains not more than 1 ppb of aluminum.

(iii) **Lumogallion** $C_{12}H_9ClN_2O_6S$ Red-brown to dark brown powder. Further, it contains not more than 1 ppm of aluminum.

(iv) **Lumogallion hydrochloric acid TS** Dissolve 0.86 g of lumogallion in 300 mL of 2-propanol, and add 350 mL of diluted *Hydrochloric acid for aluminum test* (9 in 50) and *Water for aluminum test* to make 1000 mL exactly.

(v) **Nitric acid for aluminum test** Same as the reagent *Nitric acid*. Further, it contains not more than 1 ppb of aluminum.

(vi) **pH buffer solution for aluminum test (pH 7.2)** Dissolve 106.6 g of *N,N*-bis(2-hydroxyethyl)-2-aminoethane sulfonic acid in 800 mL of *Water for aluminum test*, adjust the pH 7.2 by using *Tetramethylammonium hydroxide aqueous solution*, and add *Water for aluminum test* to make 1000 mL.

(vii) **Standard aluminum solution** Pipet a constant volume each of *Water for aluminum test* or the *Standard aluminum stock solution*, dilute and adjust the aluminum concentration to 0, 1.25, 2.5, 5.0, and 10 ppm by using diluted *Nitric acid for aluminum test* (1 in 100), to make Standard aluminum solutions (1) - (5).

(viii) **Tetramethylammonium hydroxide TS** $[(CH_3)_4NOH]$ It is a 25% aqueous solution, prepared for aluminum test. Further, it contains not more than 1 ppb of aluminum.

(ix) **Water for aluminum test** It contains not more than 1 ppb of aluminum.

G7 Containers and Package

Glass Containers for Pharmaceutical Products <*G7-1-171*>

Glass containers for pharmaceutical products are widely used. Glass bottles are used for tight and well-closed containers for bulk packaging of solid preparations for oral administration such as tablets and capsules etc., and ampules, vials or glass syringes are for hermetic containers of injections etc.

Glass containers used as a primary packaging have characteristics of high chemical durability etc. in addition to high strength, high transparency, no air permeability and no moisture permeability. On the other hand, they are heavy, bulky, fragile and easy to be broken by a physical shock during manufacturing or transportation, so they require attention on handling.

This chapter provides basic information about glass containers, items to be confirmed for the selection of glass containers and for the proper performance of a quality evaluation that comes along with the selection, and information about the quality control at the manufacturing stage of preparations.

1. Basic information about glass containers for pharmaceutical products

Glass containers for pharmaceutical products do not interact physically or chemically with the contained medicaments to alter any property or quality. Glass containers for injections can protect the contained medicaments from the invasion of microbes by means of perfect sealing or other suitable process.

To ensure the quality of contained medicaments over the shelf life, it is necessary to select a suitable glass container. In the selection of container, it is necessary to consider the physicochemical condition of the contained medicaments, i.e., solid or liquid and the adoption of a well-closed container, a tight container, a hermetic container or a colored container to ensure the chemical stability of the contained medicaments. Furthermore, it is necessary to consider surface treatment on the inner surface of containers in the case where it is assumed that foreign substances occur by interactions with the preparation ingredients.

1.1 Glass composition and molding

Composition of the glass used for primary packaging of pharmaceutical products is either borosilicate glass or sodalime glass.

Borosilicate glass has a reticulated network made of silicon dioxide (silica: SiO_2) and diboron trioxide (B_2O_3). Borosilicate glass has a small coefficient of thermal expansion, relatively high hardness and high hydrolytic resistance[1)]. Containers made of this chemical composition are classified as Type I glass in the USP and the EP.

Cylinder-shaped and long material glass tubes made of borosilicate glass are cut and undergo secondary processing to mold ampules, vials or syringes, which are mostly used for containers of small amount of injections or lyophilized preparations.

Sodalime glass is composed of silicon dioxide (silica: SiO_2), sodium oxide (Na_2O) and calcium oxide (CaO) as the principal components. It has low water resistance as a drawback, but it is easy to manufacture and process[1)]. Containers made of this chemical composition are classified as Type II or III glass in the USP and the EP.

A glass container made of sodalime glass is called a blown bottle or a molded bottle because it is molded by pouring melted glass into a mold and blowing air. Also it is called a standard bottle or an automatic bottle because of its mass production at low cost. It is widely used not only for glass bottles of solid preparations for oral administration but also as containers for injections such as large volume vials of parenteral infusions or vials of powder injections for antibiotics etc.

1.2 Surface treatment of inner surface of glass containers for pharmaceutical products

Surface treatments are performed to modify the nature of the inner surface of glass containers. The treatments are such as dealkalization treatment and coating, etc.

The dealkalization treatment is a method to neutralize the surface layer of the glass by selectively extracting and removing alkali components using sulfur compounds at high temperature above the glass-transition, which results in exposure of the silica-rich surface. This treatment reduce the elution of alkali components. The coating includes methods using silica (SiO_2), silicon resin and fluorine resin, etc.

Silica processing is a method to form a thin film on an inner surface by melt coating of silica (SiO_2) on the inner surface of the glass at a high temperature. It is expected to suppress the elution of glass components and the occurrence of flakes, because the thin film is high purity silica with no water-soluble component such as alkali, weld to the inner surface of the glass container and the drug solution does not contact directly with the inner surface of the glass.

Silicone processing is a method to form a thin film of silicone resin on a glass surface by immersing the glass in dimethylpolysiloxane solution and baking. This treatment enhance water repellency and prevent a drug solution from remaining to the inner surface of the glass. Also it is expected to suppress the elution of glass components and the occurrence of flakes because the drug solution does not contact directly with the inner surface of the glass.

Fluorine resin processing is a method to form a thin film of fluorine resin on an inner surface by coating fluorine resin using coupling agents and baking. This treatment enhance water repellency and prevent a drug solution from remaining to the inner surface of the glass. Also it is expected to suppress the elution of glass components and the occurrence of flakes because the drug solution does not contact directly with the inner surface of the glass.

2. Quality evaluation of glass containers for pharmaceutical products at the design stage of preparations

At the design stage of preparations it is necessary to perform the quality evaluation of a glass container used and the compatibility of it with the contained medicaments.

Since each glass container for pharmaceutical products has characteristic properties and properties of pharmaceutical products packed in the glass containers are diverse, the compatibility of glass containers with pharmaceutical products should be judged by considering the combination of the both.

When evaluated, refer to General Rules for Preparations [2] General Notices for Packaging of Preparations, "Basic Requirements and Terms for the Packaging of Pharmaceutical Products <*G0-5-170*>" and "Basic Requirements for Plastic Containers for Pharmaceutical Use and Rubber Closures for Containers for Aqueous Infusions <*G7-2-162*>" under General Information, and verify that the glass container used for preparations conform to the basic requirements, i.e., the design specifications, based on tests and literatures.[2,3] The compatibility must be maintained based on an appropriate quality assurance plan.

2.1 Glass containers for pharmaceutical products equipped with closures

In the case of solid preparations for oral administration, glass containers with closures consist of a glass bottle and a resin cap with a packing or a metal cap with a compound, and in the case of lyophilized injections they consist of a vial and a rubber closure. In the case of syringe preparations they consist of a glass outer (barrel, some has a needle), a gasket and a top cap.

In the case of pharmaceutical products susceptible to be oxidized, it is unsuitable to select the closure material that permeate oxygen easily. In the case of aqueous pharmaceutical products and hygroscopic pharmaceutical products, it is unsuitable to select the closure material that permeate water vapor easily. Closures must not be deformed, deteriorated and degenerated by contained medicaments. Unacceptable loss of function of containers must not be caused by a possible high temperature or low temperature or their repetitions during storage and transportation and vibrations during transportation. Glass containers for multiple-dose pharmaceutical products equipped with closures are required to have an appropriate stability after opening.

The compatibility (fitting compatibility) of closures with glass containers for pharmaceutical products must be maintained based on an appropriate quality assurance plan.

2.2 Transparency of glass containers for pharmaceutical products and colored glass containers

In the case of pharmaceutical products such as injections where foreign matters and turbidity must be examined visually, glass containers for pharmaceutical products should have the required level of transparency that enables inspection.

On the other hand, the quality of contained medicaments unstable to light must not be lowered during storage because of a high transparency of glass containers for pharmaceutical products. A sufficient level of light shielding is required to ensure light stability, and the select of colored glass containers must be considered.

When colored glass containers are used for injections, they must meet the requirements of the light transmission test for light-resistant containers under Test for Glass Containers for Injections <*7.01*>.

2.3 Glass containers for pharmaceutical products required to be sterile

In selecting suitable glass containers (ampules) or glass containers with closures (vials, syringes) as a primary packaging for injections, it is desirable to obtain information on the manufacturing processes of the glass container including substances added.

For pharmaceutical products that require terminal sterilization, it is required for glass containers to satisfy the basic requirements even after the sterilization. There must be no residue or generation of new toxic substances of more than a certain quantity after the sterilization. Structures and materials of glass containers must cause no microbial contamination to contained medicaments during storage and transportation after the sterilization.

2.4 Foreign matters derived from glass containers for pharmaceutical products for injections

In the case of glass containers for injections, glass fragments generated at cutting ampules, flakes generated by peeling of inner surfaces of glass and insoluble foreign matters generated by elution of glass components or by stains on inner surfaces of glass should be examined.

Eluates and flakes etc. derived from glass containers must be sufficiently small from the viewpoint of safety. They must not damage the efficacy and safety of the contained medicaments.

Foreign matters derived from glass containers must be sufficiently evaluated at the design stage of preparations. It must be also evaluated, when the molding process or supplier is changed.

Scanning Electron Microscopy–Energy Dispersive X-ray Spectroscopy (SEM-EDX) is useful to analyze flakes derived from glass containers and inorganic foreign matters, for example aerosol of reaction products etc.

3. Test results to be recorded for each management unit

At the manufacturing stage of glass containers for pharmaceutical products the specification of the following test items should be set, and the test results should be recorded for each management unit of glass containers for pharmaceutical products.

1) Glass bottles used for solid preparations for oral administration etc.:

   (i) Appearance[4]: Shape and dimensions are correct, and there must not be failures of wall thickness, failures of color tone, breakage, lacks, cracks, internal cracks, scratches, bubbles, foreign matters, striae, streaks, rough surfaces, burrs, stains and insoluble matters, which cause a hindrance in usage.

(ii) Quality tests: Soluble alkali test for a container, heat resistance and distortion.

(iii) Others: Items to be necessary.

2) Ampules or vials used for injections etc.:

(i) Appearance[4]: Shape and dimensions are correct, and there must not be failures of wall thickness, failures of color tone, breakage, lacks, cracks, internal cracks, scratches, foreign matters, striae, streaks, stains and insoluble matters, which cause a hindrance in usage.

(ii) Quality tests: Tests prescribed under Test for Glass Containers for Injections <*7.01*>, heat resistance (only for sodalime glass) and distortion.

(iii) Others: Items to be necessary.

4. References

1) Glossary of terms relating to fine ceramics, JIS R 1600: 2011, Japanese Industrial Standards.
2) US Pharmacopeia 40 (2017), <660> Containers-Glass.
3) US Pharmacopeia 40 (2017), <1660> Evaluation of the Inner Surface Durability of Glass Containers.
4) Glass bottles for drug, JIS R 3522: 1955, Japanese Industrial Standards.

Basic Requirements for Plastic Containers for Pharmaceutical Use and Rubber Closures for Containers for Aqueous Infusions <*G7-2-162*>

In this chapter, there describe basic requirements for plastic containers for pharmaceutical use and rubber closures for containers for aqueous infusions, and the methods to evaluate the toxicity of containers at design stage.

Containers for pharmaceutical use should not have the properties to deteriorate the efficacy, safety or stability of the pharmaceutical products to be packed in the container.

The compatibility of plastic containers with pharmaceutical products should be judged for combination of each material and the specific pharmaceutical product to be contained therein. Such judgment should be performed through verification that the container for the pharmaceutical preparation can comply with the essential requirements for the container, i.e., the design specifications, based on the data from the experiments on the prototype products of the container and/or information from scientific documentation, etc. In addition, such compatibility must be ensured based upon an appropriate quality assurance system.

1. Basic Requirements in Designing Containers for Pharmaceutical Use

Containers must not deteriorate the quality of the pharmaceutical products during storage. The concentration of the pharmaceuticals must not be decreased by more than a certain level due to the adsorption of the pharmaceuticals on the surface of the container or the migration of the pharmaceuticals into the inside of the material of the container. Also, the pharmaceutical products contained therein must not be degraded by an interaction with the material of the container.

The container should not be deformed, should not deteriorate and should not be degraded by the pharmaceutical products contained therein. Unacceptable loss of function of the container should not result from a possible high temperature or low temperature or their repetitions encountered during storage or transportation.

The leachable or migrants from the container should not deteriorate the efficacy or stability of the pharmaceutical products contained therein. Furthermore, the amounts of leachable or migratable chemical substances, such as monomers and additives, from the containers to the pharmaceutical products contained therein must be sufficiently small from the viewpoint of safety.

In the case of pharmaceutical products which must be sterilized, it is required to satisfy the above-mentioned essential requirements of the container after the sterilization, if there is a possibility that the quality of the container may change after the sterilization. There should not be any residue or generation of new toxic substances of more than certain risk level after the sterilization. In addition, the container should not have any inappropriate structure and/or material that might result in any bacterial contamination of the pharmaceutical products contained therein during storage and transportation after sterilization.

1.1. Plastic containers for pharmaceutical use

The plastic material used for the container should be of high quality. Therefore, recycled plastic materials, which are of unknown constitution, must not be used.

In the case of pharmaceutical products which are unstable to light, the container should provide a sufficient level of light shielding. In the case of pharmaceutical products which are easily oxidized, the container material should not allow the permeation of oxygen. In the case of aqueous pharmaceutical products and pharmaceutical products that must be kept dry, the container material should not allow the permeation of water vapor. In addition, it is necessary to pay attention to the permeability of solvents other than water through the container.

The container should have a certain level of physical properties such as hardness, flexibility, shock resistance, tensile strength, tear strength, bending strength, heat resistance and the like, in accordance with its intended usage. The container should be of a required level of transparency, when it is necessary to examine foreign insoluble matter and/or turbidity of the pharmaceutical products by visual observation.

Furthermore, in introducing a plastic container, it is desirable that proper disposal method after use is taken into consideration.

1.2. Rubber closures for containers for aqueous infusions

For the rubber closures for container, natural rubber, which has the possibility to cause an allergic response, or recycled rubber material that can not be guaranteed its material composition, should not be used. As the closure systems, the appropriate materials should be used to prevent the permeation of oxygen, water vapor and solvents.

Further, the rubber closure should have a certain level of physical properties such as air tightness, hermetic seal, penetrability of a needle, coring-resistance and self-sealing after penetration, in accordance with its intended usage.

2. Toxicity Evaluation of Container at Design Stage

For design verification, the toxicity of the container should be evaluated. For the toxicity evaluation, it is desirable to select appropriate test methods and acceptance criteria for the evaluation, and to explain the rationale for the selection clearly. The tests should be conducted using samples of the whole or a part of the prototype products of the container. If the container consists of plural parts of different materials, each part should be tested separately. Such materials as laminates, composites, and the like are regarded as a single material. To test containers made of such materials, it is recommended to expose the inner surface of the container, which is in contact with the pharmaceutical products contained therein, to the extraction media used in the tests as far as possible.

It is recommended to select the test items and the test methods for the evaluation of the toxicity of the containers, depending on their application site, in accordance with the standard test methods on medical devices and materials published in Japan, a notice entitled Basic Principle of Biological Safety Evaluation Required for Application for Approval to Market Medical Devices (MHLW Notification by Director, OMDE Yakusyokuki 0301 No.20 on March 1, 2012).

3. Test Results to be recorded per Production Unit for Plastic containers for pharmaceutical use and Rubber closures for containers for aqueous Infusions

3.1. Plastic containers for pharmaceutical use

At the commercial production phase, it is required to establish acceptance criteria on at least the test items listed below and to record the test results of each production unit of plastic containers for pharmaceutical products. In addition, it is desirable to explain the rationale for setting the acceptance criteria clearly. However, these requirements should not be applied to orally administered preparations except for liquid preparations.

(i) Combustion Tests: Residue on ignition, heavy metals. If necessary, the amounts of specified metals (lead, cadmium, etc.)

(ii) Extraction Tests: pH, UV spectrum, potassium permanganate-reducing substances, foaming test, residue on evaporation

(iii) Cytotoxicity Test

(iv) Any other tests necessary for the specific container for aqueous infusions.

3.2. Rubber closures for containers for aqueous infusions

At the commercial production phase of rubber closures, it is required to establish acceptance criteria on the test items that should be controlled other than those specified in the general chapter of <*7.03*> Test for Rubber Closure for Aqueous Infusions. And the test results of each production unit of rubber closures for containers for aqueous infusions should be recorded. In addition, it is desirable to explain the rationale for setting the acceptance criteria.

Moisture Permeability Test for Blister Packaging of Solid Preparations <*G7-3-171*>

The test is the method to measure the moisture transmission rate of the blister packaging represented by PTP packaging. It can be used for the following studies to evaluate moisture transmission through packaging of drug preparation.

(i) Screening of the material and/or thickness for plastic sheets, forming conditions and/or size of pockets, etc. in the development phase.

(ii) Comparison of the moisture transmission rate of a plastic sheet before and after the change in material, thickness, forming conditions, and/or size of pockets, etc. in the development or production phase.

Note that when a sufficient amount of desiccant cannot be filled up in the pockets due to the minute pockets a reliable result might be not obtained. The test is intended to determine the moisture transmission rate of successfully prepared blister packaging, but not to detect the leakage due to pinholes and the like.

1. Terms

(i) Molding materials: Materials forming pockets and sealing areas. Usually, a single or double layer plastic sheet or that laminated with aluminum foil is used.

(ii) Sealing materials: Materials to seal tightly pockets packed with drug preparations. Usually, an aluminum foil is used.

(iii) Pockets: Places where the molding material is inflated in a convex shape to put drug preparations.

(iv) Moisture transmission rate: An amount of water transmitted into the pockets of blister packaging per unit time (mg/day/pocket).

2. Apparatus

(i) Constant temperature and humidity chamber: An apparatus which can maintain a temperature and humidity storage condition.

(ii) Balance: A chemical balance.

3. Desiccants

It may be chosen from the following.

(i) Calcium chloride for water determination

Pretreatment before use: Put the desiccant taking out of fine powder in a depthless vessel, dry at 110°C for 1 hour, then allow to cool in a desiccator [phosphorus (V) oxide].

(ii) Synthetic zeolite for drying

Moisture adsorption ability: Not less than 15%. Weigh accurately about 10 g of the desiccant, allow to stand at 40°C and 75% relative humidity for 24 hours, then weigh the mass, and calculate the gain in weight.

Pretreatment before use: Put the desiccant in a depthless vessel, dry at 350 – 600°C for 2 hours, then allow to cool in a desiccator [phosphorus (V) oxide].

4. Samples

4.1. Preparation of sample

Amount of the desiccant filled in a pocket is determined appropriately depending on the form or size of the pocket, however, it should be about 80% of the capacity of the pocket for avoiding the deforming or impairing of the covering material. For preparation of the sample, carefully prepare the sample avoiding moisture adsorption of the desiccant. Fill the desiccant in all the pockets as evenly as possible, seal with a sealing material, and cut out to a suitable size. Separately, prepare a control in the same manner by packing with the similar mass of glass beads. The form and size of the sample and the control should be as identical as possible.

Examine the appearances of the prepared sample and control with the naked eye or by using a stereomicroscope, and use them whose pockets maintain their shapes as prescribed, and without any forming faults, aberrant wrinkles on the sealing material, pinholes or any sealing faults.

4.2. Number of samples

Five to ten sheets are used for the sample with not less than 10 pockets per sheet. An appropriate number of sheets equivalent to 20 to 100 pockets (not less than 10 sheets), depending on the number of pockets per sheet are used for the sample with less than 10 pockets per sheet. The number of the control is at least 2 sheets, however, desirable to be the same as the sample number.

5. Method

5.1. Storage conditions

The following conditions are desirable, though other conditions may be used.

(i) 25 ± 2°C/60 ± 5%RH

(ii) 40 ± 2°C/75 ± 5%RH

5.2. Storage

Place the samples and controls in a constant temperature and humidity chamber without overlapping each other of the sheets, not in standing position, as the pocket facing upwards, as not intercepting the air circulation and avoiding exposure to the air flow from the outlet.

5.3. Mass measuring

Take out the samples and controls from the chamber, allow cooling to room temperature, measure the mass of each sheet quickly, and place them back to the chamber. Weigh exactly the masses of them to a degree of 0.1 mg.

5.4. Measuring intervals

Intervals of the measurement are adjusted depending on the moisture transmission rate and avoiding large change in the temperature and humidity inside of the chamber (for example, 0, 1, 3, 7, 14, 21 and 28 days).

5.5. Termination of measurements

Measure the mass of each sheet of the sample and control at each measuring point, and calculate the differences in their average values (the increasing amount of the sample mass). Prepare a linear regression equation by the least-squares method by plotting the increasing amount (mg) of the sample mass on the vertical axis against the time (day) on the horizontal axis. The measurement should be finished when the increase in the mass shows linearity in at least three sequenced points (expect for the starting point) and before the desiccant absorbs moisture of 10% amount of the mass of packed desiccant. The correlation coefficient of the linearity is desirable to be not less than 0.98.

5.6. Others

Data of samples showing extremely larger mass increase as compared to the others should be excluded since the package may have some leakage due to pinholes or the like. Appropriate statistical tests are performed, as needed.

6. Calculation of moisture transmission rate

The moisture transmission rate (mg/day/pocket) is calculated by dividing the slope, i.e. the mass increasing amount (mg/day), obtained by the least-squares method, by the number of pocket per sheet. Record the moisture transmission rate together with the storage conditions and the name of the desiccant used.

7. Information

7.1. Factors affecting the moisture transmission rate

There are as follows:

(i) Qualities (molecular structure, density, degree of crystallinity, etc.), composition and/or thickness of the molding materials

(ii) Methods and conditions to form the pocket

(iii) Size and/ or uniformity of wall thickness of the pocket

(iv) Storage conditions, water activity inside the pocket

7.2. Measurement of pocket wall thickness

Measure the wall thickness of at least one position of upper or side face or R part of not less than 10 pockets of the sampling sheet to a unit of 1 μm, using a micrometer or dial gage with an accuracy of better than 1 μm or an equivalent measuring instrument, as necessary. Measuring position is selected in consideration of the shape of the pocket or difficulty of the measurement. It is desirable to identify the site that may become thinner in the phase of study for pocket forming conditions, and to measure the thickness of the site while paying attention to the pressure.

8. Reference

1) T. Okubo, *et al.*: *PMDRS*, 45(2), 155 – 165, (2014).

Packaging Integrity Evaluation of Sterile Products <*G7-4-180*>

1. Introduction

Package integrity for sterile pharmaceutical products is ability to prevent microbial ingress and the entry or escape of substances, which is required for the packaging for sterile preparations to maintain their quality.

This General Information is used to evaluate the integrity of the primary packaging or the secondary packaging of sterile pharmaceutical products that are required to have a barrier function from microorganisms, reactive gases and other substances that affect quality, from the viewpoint of protection of products. A packaging defect is defined as the situation that unexpected leakage caused by incorrect design or by some abnormality occurred during manufacturing processes or storage up to the shelf life of preparations induces the loss of the intended barrier function of the packaging, resulting in the unsustainability of the quality of the preparation including sterility.

The package integrity testing is applied throughout the product life cycle from the development of preparations and in the product stability programs after the launch.

2. Package integrity and testing

2.1. Concept of package integrity

Package integrity for sterile pharmaceutical products is necessary to ensure the quality of products until use. Primary packaging for sterile pharmaceutical products should ensure no ingress of microorganisms from the outside. In addition, if a gas such as water vapor or oxygen affects the quality of products by its moving between in and out of the primary packaging, the quality should be maintained by controlling the amount of gas transfer in the primary packaging, or combining multiple packaging materials including secondary packaging.

It is necessary to recognize that most packaging have gas leakage and permeation depending on their type. In many cases, it is difficult to distinguish between leakage and permeation for qualified packaging. Therefore, complete packaging is to prevent the ingress of microorganisms and to prevent the quality deterioration of the product due to the ingress/transfer of gas/other substances by conforming to the maximum allowable leakage limit of individual preparation packaging, and the product should be ensured to meet physicochemical and microbiological specifications by data. The package integrity test methods include a physicochemical method to find leaks (leak test), a method to ensure that no leakage occurs by confirming the qualification of the sealed part of a package (seal quality test), and a method to confirm a barrier property against microorganisms by microbiological methods (microbial challenge test). The, package integrity of sterile pharmaceutical products is guaranteed by any one or more of these tests.

The application of the quantitative leak test requires optimization according to the characteristics of the package of each preparation. In addition, it is required to understand the detection limit, accuracy and precision of the test method to be set.

2.1.1. Leak test

The leak test guarantees ability to maintain the integrity of packaging by qualitatively detecting or quantitatively measuring holes or pathways, where leaks occur, by a physicochemical method. There are two types of leak tests; qualitative leak test and quantitative leak test.

Since the results of the qualitative leak test are accompanied by uncertainty, the test requires a large sample size and rigorous control of test conditions to obtain reliable results. The qualitative leak test is a useful mean to detect leaks, but is not suitable for the deterministic verification of package integrity. On the other hand, it is an effective test to locate leak positions correctly.

The quantitative leak test is a test to evaluate quantitatively the physicochemical changes accompanied with leaks and to obtain objective data to set a maximum allowable leakage limit and control.

Examples of qualitative and quantitative leak test methods are listed below. Other methods may be used according to a purpose.

<Qualitative leak test methods>
Liquid immersion test
Liquid leak test
Tracer liquid test (dye penetration test)
Sniffer method (helium leak test method 1)
<Quantitative leak test methods>
Sealed chamber method (pressure change leak test method 1)
Vacuum decay method (pressure change leak test method 2)
Pressure integration method (helium leak test method 2)
Vacuum chamber method (helium leak test method 3)
Immersion method (helium leak test method 4)
High-voltage leak test (pinhole test method)
Laser-based gas headspace analysis

2.1.2. Seal quality test

The seal quality test is used to indirectly ensure ability to maintain package integrity by confirming that parameters related to the container seal or fitting are valid. Conducting the seal quality test set based on evidence is useful for the continuous understanding of the characteristics required for closure and maintaining package integrity. In addition to examples shown as the seal quality test methods (Table 1), various methods are used.

2.1.3. Microbial challenge test

The microbial challenge test is a microbiological test to estimate qualitatively package integrity by using live microorganisms or microbial spores. The microbial challenge test is useful for acquiring the direct evidence of preventing microbial ingress. Microbial ingress evaluated in the test includes the passage through pathways by microbial growth or movement and the passive transport of microorganisms via liquid.

Conducting the microbiological test is effective when appropriate physicochemical leak test methods, which obtain the evidence of preventing microbial ingress, have not been established, or when the maximum allowable leakage limit depends on the possibility of microbial ingress.

The recommended general practices are as follows. For the test, strains of microorganisms that are appropriately maintained should be used. Other scientifically appropriate methods can also be used.

Put a fluid medium aseptically in the primary package of a preparation to be tested, and immerse the preparation in an appropriate bacterial solution of 10^5 CFU/ml or more for at least 30 minutes or more. Cultivate the preparation and confirm the presence or absence of turbidity in the medium.

2.2. Package integrity and testing in the development and manufacturing of preparations

Selection of test methods according to the stage of the product lifecycle is important to ensure package integrity for sterile pharmaceutical products.

2.2.1. Design of packaging

In the packaging design of the product development stage, the maximum allowable leakage limit is required to be set based on evaluations of not only the risk of sterility failure due to microbial ingress but also the effect of various gases passing through the primary packaging on the quality. For the evaluation, it is desirable to use the quantitative leak test method that has been verified to be able to detect leaks that affect product quality. Samples used for the evaluation should be prepared assuming the worst case in design.

If influence of other than microorganisms can be ignored, the allowable leak limit to be controlled is set by considering the risk of microbial ingress. This can be set by verifying by the microbial challenge test, or by proving that there is logically no ingress of microorganisms by leak tests. On the other hand, the allowable leakage limit should be set to control the passage of substances in addition to preventing microbial ingress for products that require to keep low headspace oxygen concentration to maintain the quality of preparations etc. Verification only by the qualitative microbial challenge test should not be sufficient. Other qualitative tests are also valuable to obtain information appropriate for the purposes.

2.2.2. Manufacturing of preparations

Package integrity testing in the manufacturing of content-filled products is important to prevent the release of incompletely packaged pharmaceuticals. Based on packaging defects recognized in the development stage and initial process validation, tests are established by leak tests, seal quality tests and appropriate combination of visual inspections during manufacturing to obtain supplemental information.

Examples of leak tests used for package integrity evaluation of preparations in manufacturing processes include liquid immersion test, liquid leak test, tracer liquid test (dye ingress method), sealed chamber method (pressure change leak test method 1), vacuum decay method (pressure change leak test method 2), high voltage leak test (pinhole test method), and laser-based gas headspace analysis. Moreover, examples of the seal quality test methods are shown in Table 1.

Sampling tests using a part of a production lot as a sample during the process provide means to verify package integrity of the lot by ensuring that the process is maintained in a validated state. For sampling frequency and the number of samples, it is required to set the necessary number of samples and demonstrate its validity based on the results of statistical process controls obtained in the process validation stage and the trend analysis of product quality after the start of production. In contrast, non-destructive leak tests for all products of a production lot provide continuous and all-product guarantees of package integrity.

If relevance between seal quality test results and package integrity is verified in advance, the conduction of the seal quality test can indirectly ensure the package integrity. For the glass or plastic ampoules that are sealed by sealing or welding the opening, nondestructive leak tests are usually performed with all samples.

The main purpose of package integrity testing in process validation is to obtain high quality product packaging in the process which is operated with no problem within operating parameters set and to keep the incidence of serious packaging defects low enough. Package integrity testing of in-process and final products complements complete packaging de-

Table 1 Examples of seal quality test methods

Name of seal quality test method	Packaging applied	Contents of test
Tensile strength test	Bag, blister pack, etc.	Measure force required to separate two bonded surfaces.
Closure (opening and closing) torque test	Packaging closed by screws	Measure torque required for opening or closing a plug.
Package burst test	Bag, blister pack, etc.	Apply pressure to a package seal to rupture and open, and measure the pressure or force at the rupture.
Residual seal force test	Vial, etc.	Push a cap downward at a constant speed from the top of a vial, and measure the repulsive force when the plot of the transfer distance–repulsive force reaches the inflection point. Non-destructive testing is possible.
Rubber closure depression test	Vial, etc.	Push a rubber closure downward at a constant rate from the top of a vial, and measure intensity to the depression.
Rotation resistance test of winding cap	Vial, etc.	Measure an initial resistance value when idling a cap. Similar to the residual seal strength test, it is possible to estimate the seal property due to the elastic force of rubber closures.
Airborne ultrasound method	Packaging joined by welding/crimping	Pass an ultrasonic signal through the seal area of a package or an article, and inspect the seal quality by measuring the signal strength. The ultrasonic energy of an area with a bad seal decreases compared with a suitable package seal. Non-destructive testing is possible.

sign, therefore cannot replace confirmation at initial design, even if performed.

2.2.3. Evaluation of package integrity in stability tests and stability monitoring

In order to assess the risk of new leaks generated during storage of pharmaceuticals, it is necessary to evaluate package integrity as a part of a stability test during the product development stage. It is also desirable to evaluate package integrity in the stability monitoring after the launch. It is recommended that test methods with detection ability as close as possible to the maximum allowable leakage limit are used based on the understanding of the mechanism and the rationale for ensuring no contamination.

The amount of sample required for the package integrity test in stability tests should be the amount that can achieve the purpose of the test in consideration of the past development and validation tests. If the test is a non-destructive test, the package integrity of a sample to be tested for preparation stability can be inspected prior to the stability test.

In the case of applying a physicochemical leak test method or any other test method that can appropriately evaluate the ingress of microorganisms with a certain level, it can be substituted for a sterility test in stability tests. On the contrary, for products for which influence of other than microorganisms on quality can be ignored, sterility tests can be substituted for package integrity evaluation of products in stability monitoring by considering the possibility of microbial ingress.

2.3. Criteria for the selection of test methods

The method of an individual leak test or seal quality test cannot cover all of the packaging of products. Depending on preparation packaging, multiple test methods may be required during the product life cycle. Therefore, for ensuring package integrity, it is necessary to select appropriate test methods, set parameters, and verify that the selected test methods can be applied to the product. The following product properties are taken into consideration for the choice of test methods.

Contents of package: Physical state (liquid, solid), electrical conductivity of liquid, presence or absence and type of headspace gas, and compatibility with test materials/test conditions.

Package structure and physicochemical properties: Package hardness, presence or absence of mobility, effect of volatiles added to polymers, electrical conductivity and capacitance of materials, and the amount of passed gas that is not a leak.

Impact on packaging and contents (destructive tests and non-destructive tests): For example, package integrity testing for ampoules, etc. requiring total inspection should be a nondestructive test that does not affect the quality of packaging and contents.

2.4. Setting and verification of test methods

The optimization of test conditions is required to ensure highly sensitive, accurate, robust, highly reproducible leak detection for individual product packaging systems to which leak or seal quality tests are applied. For the design and verification of test methods, the design of a package closure system, packaging materials, the nature of leaks to be predicted, and the effect of the contents of products on the test results should be taken into account, and positive controls (packages with intentional or known leaks) and negative controls (packages with no known leak) are used. For quantitative evaluation, it is necessary to make an opening with a certain diameter in consideration of the type and structure of materials that compose packages.

3. Glossary

The definitions of terms used in this General Information are as follows.

Package integrity: Package integrity is the ability of a package to prevent the loss of preparations, to prevent microorganism ingress, and to limit entry of detrimental gases or other substances, thus ensuring that the product meets all necessary safety and quality standards. ''Container closure system integrity'' and ''container integrity'' mean ''package integrity''.

Quantitative leak test method: In the quantitative leak test method, the leak to be detected or measured is based on a phenomenon caused by a predictable series of events. Furthermore, the means of leak detection can be easily controlled and monitored, and is based on the physicochemical techniques that can obtain concrete quantitative data.

Qualitative leak test method: The qualitative leak test method is essentially probabilistic. Qualitative tests depend on a series of continuous or simultaneous events, each of which is accompanied by a random result represented by a probability distribution. Therefore, the results have uncertainty and require a large sample size and the rigorous control of test conditions to obtain meaningful results.

Leakage: The transfer of liquid or gas through a breach in a package material or through a gap between package materials. Leakage is expressed in the measure (in mass or volume units) of the flow rate of gas that pass through leakage pathways under specified temperature and pressure conditions. The leak rate has the dimension of pressure multiplied by volume, divided by time. For example, the international standard SI nomenclature is pascal cubic meter per second ($Pa \cdot m^3 \cdot s^{-1}$).

Leak: A leakage, or a hole, or a pathway where a leakage occurs.

Permeation: The passage of substances through a package material. Permeation of gases, including water vapor, can usually occurs in the packaging of sterile pharmaceuticals. The ''water vapor permeability test'' applies to the permeation of water vapor in plastic containers (mainly aqueous injection containers).

Maximum allowable leakage limit: A maximum leakage rate (or hole, or pathway size) allowable for a product package that can assure no risk to product safety and no or negligible impact on product stability.

Positive and negative controls: A package having different type and size of defects is used as a positive control. Generally, packages having large size defects are used as positive controls during the development of test methods, and packages having small size defects are used as positive controls for the development of test methods and for validation.

Leak Tests for Packaging of Sterile Products <*G7-5-180*>

This General Information describes test methods to measure the entry and escape of gases and liquids in packages and containers of sterile pharmaceuticals, and to recognize their unintentional fluid transfer due to leakage. The measured values may indicate the presence, location and size of leak channels as well as leak amount.

The leak tests are classified to qualitative leak tests and quantitative leak tests. This General Information describes liquid immersion test, liquid leak test, tracer liquid test (dye penetration test) and sniffing method (helium leak test method 1) as qualitative leak tests, and sealed chamber method (pressure change leak test method 1), vacuum decay method (pressure change leak test method 2), pressure integration method (helium leak test method 2), vacuum chamber method (helium leak test method 3), immersion method (helium leak test method 4), high-voltage leak test (pinhole test method) and laser-based gas headspace analysis as quantitative leak tests. Other methods that have been validated can also be used.

Test methods should be selected according to the characteristics of samples and the purpose of the test[1-6]. Samples, the configuration of test apparatus, and conditions such as temperature, pressure and time, are set appropriately based on various technical data, because they affect the validity of results and the safety of operations. It is desirable to use the apparatus that has been calibrated by a standard traceable to the national measurement standard as needed. The leak tests are applied to stoppered rigid or flexible packages and containers, which are empty or contain liquid or solid sterile pharmaceuticals. Specifically, ampoules, vials, syringes, containers for ophthalmic solutions, plastic bags, etc. are subject to the tests.

1. Qualitative leak tests

The qualitative leak tests are test methods to directly observe or measure the leak phenomena, and are used to confirm the presence, position(s) and conditions of leakage.

1.1. Liquid immersion test

The liquid immersion test method is used to detect the presence and locations of leaks by observation of gas emission occurred from defect regions as bubbles, when a sample containing gas in its inside is immersed in liquid and the headspace of the liquid tank is depressurized. In many cases, water is used as the liquid, and in that case, it is also called a water immersion test. It observes the generation of gas bubbles after the completion of reduced pressure until the prescribed time, and evaluate the location(s) of leak(s), the size and the occurrence frequency of the gas bubbles. In some cases, bubbles are observed in a liquid tank using a sample pressurized with gas. The amount of leakage can be quantified by collecting the generated gas bubbles in a liquid tank with a measuring cylinder etc. for defined time and measuring the amount. The amount of leakage can be expressed as a function of the sampling time for collecting gas bubbles and the collected quantity being corrected with a reference pressure or one atmospheric pressure. The test is performed at prescribed temperature as required, and the value of reduced pressure and measurement time of the headspace of a liquid tank are set according to the pressure resistance of a sample and assumed defects. It is applied to rigid or flexible packages and containers.

1.2. Liquid leak test

The liquid leak test methods are test methods to visualize and observe the transfer of liquid due to leakage using an additive or a developer. The liquid leak test methods include the method that adds liquid containing a fluorescent dye to a sample to detect the leaked liquid by irradiation with ultraviolet light, and the method that coats the surface of a sample with a developer to observe an indication pattern generated by a chemical reaction of the leaked liquid and the developer (Table 1).

In the fluorescent dye method, liquid containing fluorescent dye is injected inside a sample, or is dissolved in liquid inside a sample, and leakage is detected under ultraviolet light in a dark place. The inside of the sample is pressurized, as necessary, and change due to leakage is observed. In the test methods using a developer, the adequately stirred developer is applied evenly on the surface of a sample by a spray or a brush. After drying of the developed coating film, an indication pattern due to leakage is observed under white light in the cases of the white development method and the color development method. In the fluorescent development method, an indication pattern due to leakage is observed under ultraviolet light in a dark place. Record the indication pattern due to leakage as the description of position, size and number, etc. or as an image. These test methods are applied to rigid or flexible packages and containers.

Table 1 Types of liquid leak tests

Methods		Excipients added to liquid	Developers	Observation	Indication pattern
Using an additive	Fluorescent dye method	Fluorescent dye	no	under ultraviolet light (in a dark place)	fluorescence
Using a developer	White development method	no	White developer	under white light	gray color
	Color forming development method	no	Color-forming developer	under white light	red color
	Fluorescence development method	no	Fluorescence developer	under ultraviolet light (in a dark place)	fluorescence

1.3. Tracer liquid test (dye penetration test)

The tracer liquid test method is a method to observe the inflow or outflow of tracer liquid by immersing a sample in liquid. The test method is used to detect leak location and to evaluate the relative amount of leakage in non-porous rigid or flexible containers. A dye solution or a solution containing metal ions is used as the tracer liquid. The transfer of the dye is observed visually or measured using instruments. The test method is applied to clear, pressure-tight or other, stoppered rigid or flexible packages and containers which are empty or contain contents (liquid or solid).

a) In the test method where a tracer liquid is introduced, immerse a sample containing no tracer liquid in a chamber filled with the tracer liquid, cover the chamber, and pressurize or depressurize the chamber so that the head space part has a prescribed pressure, and hold. After prescribed time has elapsed, the head space part is opened to the atmosphere and left for prescribed time. Then the sample is taken out, and the surface is cleaned. The tracer liquid which has invaded into the sample is observed visually or measured by chemical analysis.

b) In the test method where a tracer liquid is flowed out, immerse a sample containing a tracer liquid in a chamber filled with a solution containing no tracer liquid. Then cover the chamber, pressurize or depressurize so that the head space part becomes a prescribed pressure, and hold for prescribed time to flow out the tracer liquid. After the head space part is left for a prescribed time under the atmospheric pressure, the sample is taken out, and the transfer of the tracer liquid is measured by observation of the liquid inside the chamber or by chemical analysis. The test method is applied to rigid containers.

1.4. Sniffer method (Helium leak test method 1)[7]

The helium leak test method by the sniffer method is also called the suction method. This test method is a method to detect leakage by filling helium gas in a sample under normal pressure or pressurized condition and sucking the helium gas that leaks into the outside by a suction probe. In addition, some methods that apply a suction probe to measurement regions or scan with the probe to detect the presence and the position of leakage are also used. The test method is applied to rigid or flexible packages and containers.

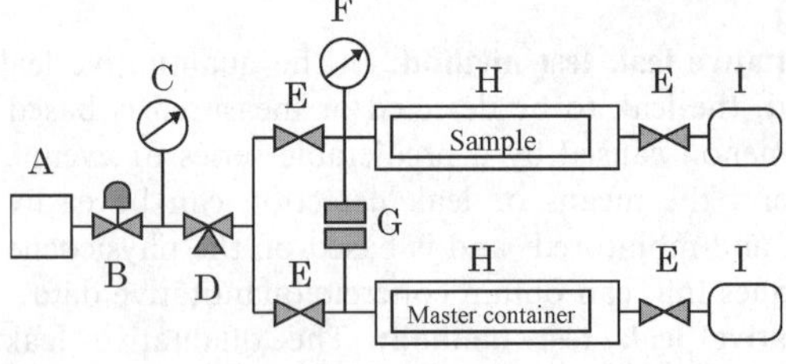

A : Pressurizing or depressurizing apparatus
B : Pressure regulating valve
C : Pressure gauge
D : Pressure and exhaust valve
E : Shut-off valve
F : Vacuum gauge
G : Differential pressure gauge
H : Chamber
I : Release container

Fig. 1 Example of apparatus configuration for the sealed chamber method (pressure method)

2. Quantitative leak tests

The quantitative leak test methods provide the amount of leakage in numerical values of physical quantities. Because measured values are affected by conditions (sample temperature, testing time, etc.) and environmental factors (air temperature, humidity, atmospheric pressure, etc.) of the test method, it is necessary to use them with sufficient consideration of these factors.

2.1. Sealed chamber method (Pressure change leak test 1)[8]

The sealed chamber pressure change leak test method is used to measure the leakage of a stoppered sample by pressure change after pressurizing or depressurizing the chambers which contain the sample and a master container (a leak-free container having same structure as the sample), respectively. The method may be destructive or non-destructive depending on the pressure resistance of the sample and the pressure setting of a chamber. It is applied to rigid or flexible packages and containers.

In this test method, use an apparatus shown in Fig. 1, place a sample and a master container in each chamber, close valves after pressurizing or depressurizing the chambers, and measure pressure difference between the chambers after prescribed time. To detect large leaks, measure pressure difference after releasing the pressure of the inside of both chambers into discharge containers. The amount of leakage is expressed as a function of the value of the pressure difference between the chambers, the space volume of the sample and the chamber, the volume ratio of the chamber and the discharge container, etc.

2.2. Vacuum decay method (Pressure change leak test method 2)

The vacuum decay pressure change leak test is applied to test samples containing liquids. An apparatus similar to that used in the sealed chamber method is used for this test. In the operation, a sample and a master container are placed in chambers, respectively, pressure in the chambers are depressurized below the vapor pressure of the liquid. Changes in the chamber pressure due to the evaporation of the leaked liquid is measured by a vacuum gauge or a differential pressure sensor. The degree of pressure rise is expressed as a function of gap volume between the sample and the chamber and the measurement time, and is affected by the amount of leaked liquid, vapor pressure, degree of vacuum and the temperature of the liquid. This method is applied to rigid or flexible packages and containers that contain liquid and have no head space.

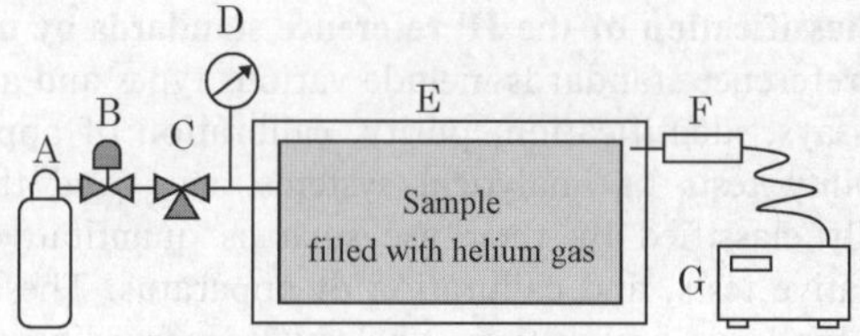

A : Helium cylinder E : Chamber or cover
B : Pressure regulating valve F : Suction probe
C : Pressure and exhaust valve G : Helium leak detector
D : Pressure gauge

Fig. 2 Example of apparatus configuration for pressure integration method

2.3. Pressure integration method (Helium leak test method 2)

In the pressure integration method, the sample filled with helium gas under normal or pressurized pressure is hold in a chamber or a cover with hood (coating material) to collect helium gas leaked to space between the hood and the sample for a prescribed time. Measure the leakage by sucking the collected gas using a suction probe.

For this test method, an apparatus shown in Fig. 2 is used, and the amount of leakage is expressed as a function of the concentration of helium gas, the gap volume between the hood and the sample, the time for collecting helium gas, the amount of suction by a suction probe, etc. This method is capable of measuring leakage from a whole sample, and is less susceptible to the concentration of surrounding helium. This method is applied to non-stoppered rigid containers without contents.

2.4. Vacuum chamber method (Helium leak test method 3),

The vacuum chamber method helium leak test is also called the vacuum container method. This test measures helium gas leaked from a sample filled with helium gas in the chamber maintained at high degree of vacuum by exhausting. High detection sensitivity is obtained compared to the pressure integration method. This method is applied to non-stoppered rigid containers without contents.

For this test method, use an apparatus shown in Fig. 3, set a sample filled with pressured helium gas in a vacuum chamber, close the chamber, and depressurize. The value of leakage is obtained from the difference between the amount of helium in the chamber, in the presence and absence of the sample, at the time when the inside of the chamber reaches prescribed vacuum.

2.5. Immersion method (Helium leak test method 4)

The immersion method helium leak test is also called the bombing method. This test measures outflow due to leakage by the vacuum chamber method after introducing helium gas into the space inside a sample through defects in a chamber filled with helium gas and then taking out the sample, using an apparatus shown in Fig. 4. A sample having space inside is placed in a chamber pressured with helium gas and the concentration of helium inside the sample is increased by immersing helium gas through defect holes from the outside. Then the leakage of the sample is measured by the vacuum chamber method. This method cannot be applied to samples having large leaks. The degree of leakage is expressed as a function of leaving-time in the air, inside volume of a sample, time for filling, pressure for filling, etc. This method is applied to stoppered rigid containers having space inside a sample.

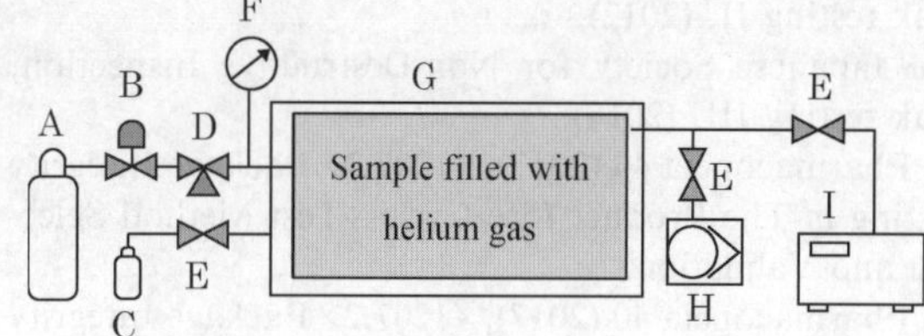

A : Helium cylinder F : Vacuum gauge
B : Pressure regulating valve G : Vacuum chamber
C : Calibration leak H : Auxiliary exhaust apparatus
D : Pressure and exhaust valve I : Helium leak detector
E : Shut-off valve

Fig. 3 Example of apparatus for the vacuum chamber method

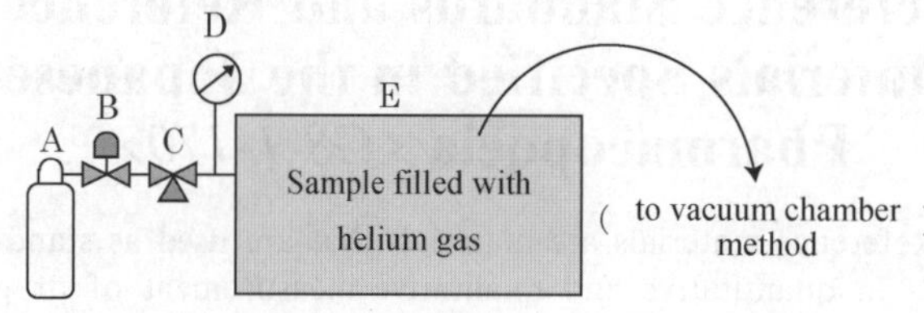

A : Helium cylinder D : Vacuum gage
B : Pressure regulating valve E : Helium gas filling chamber
C : Pressure and exhaust valve

Fig. 4 Example of apparatus configuration for immersion method

2.6. High-voltage leak test (Pinhole test)

The high voltage leak test is used to detect pinholes which allow leakage, in the area between where electrodes are applied. The electric current that flows upon application of the high voltage to the sample is measured. Rapid non-destructive tests are possible in appropriate measurement conditions. This method is applied to rigid or flexible packages and containers with non-conductive packaging materials, containing conductive contents that are not affected by applied voltage.

2.7. Laser-based gas headspace analysis

The laser-based headspace gas analysis is a method that detect changes in the headspace gas of a sample due to leakage from the absorbance or frequency modulation of specific frequency bands in the transmission of a laser light. Information such as the concentration of oxygen, carbon dioxide or water vapor and an internal pressure are obtained by irradiating a sample held between a light source and a detector with a light having a wavelength suitable for the gas to be measured. The possibility of leakage is judged by comparing the measurement value with the value obtained for a reference sample having controlled defects. Non-destructive tests are possible in appropriate measurement conditions, however, it is necessary to perform the tests under environment suitable for the purpose because temperature and humidity affect the results. This method is applied to light-transmitting containers that have a gas part and to pharmaceutical preparations that have a head-space part.

3. References

1) JIS Z 2330: 2012, Non-destructive testing-Selection of leak testing method.
2) The Japanese Society for Non-Destructive Inspection, Leak testing I, (2012).
3) The Japanese Society for Non-Destructive Inspection,

Leak testing II, (2012).
4) The Japanese Society for Non-Destructive Inspection, Leak testing III, (2016).
5) US Pharmacopeia 40 (2017), <1207.1> Package Integrity Testing in The Product Life Cycle—Test Method Selection and Validation.
6) US Pharmacopeia 40 (2017), <1207.2> Package Integrity Leak Test Technologies.
7) JIS Z2331: 2006, Method for helium leak testing.
8) JIS Z2332: 2012, Leak testing method using pressure change.

G8 Reference Standards

Reference Standards and Reference Materials Specified in the Japanese Pharmacopoeia *<G8-1-170>*

Reference materials are materials that are used as standards in quantitative and qualitative measurement of drug products, calibration and accuracy confirmation of apparatus, and suitability tests of analytical systems. Reference standards specified in the Japanese Pharmacopoeia (JP) as described in Reference Standards *<9.01>* are reference materials prepared to the specified quality necessary with regard to their intended use such as quality evaluation tests of drugs, and they are provided with public assurance that the substances have suitable quality for the specified use.

This chapter includes the definitions and explanations of basic terms regarding reference standards, and the particulars of the JP reference standards mainly used for chemical drugs, such as classification by use, requirements for establishment, required quality evaluation items, distribution and precautions for use. The descriptions show only basic policies, and therefore flexible management is required for practical application for the time being.

1. Basic terms of reference standards

- Reference materials: "The materials used as the standards" for determination of characteristic values of materials and substances. Reference materials are sufficiently homogeneous and stable with respect to one or more specified properties and are produced so that they are suitable for their intended use in measuring processes [JIS Q 0035:2008]. Reference materials for drug products are materials used as the standards in quantitative and qualitative measurements, calibration and accuracy confirmation of apparatus, and they are prepared so that they are suitable for their intended use.
- Reference standards: The reference materials prepared to a specified quality necessary with regard to their intended use, such as quality evaluation tests of drugs, and they are provided with public assurance that the substances have suitable quality for the specified use.
- JP reference standard: The reference standards specified in the Monographs or General Tests in the JP.
- Certified reference materials: The reference materials with one or more specified characteristic values determined by appropriate metrological procedure. Their qualities are guaranteed by a certificate that describes their characteristic values, uncertainties of the values, and metrological traceability [JIS Q 0035:2008].

2. Classification of the JP reference standards by use

JP reference standards include various types and are used for assays, identification, purity, calibration of apparatus, suitability tests of analytical systems, etc., and they are broadly classified by their use such as quantitative tests, qualitative tests, and calibration of apparatus. These reference standards are further subclassified according to their specific use, such as assays of active ingredients and indicator ingredients, assays of related substances, identification using spectral measurement or chromatography, calibration of apparatus used in tests, determinations and assays that are specified in the General Tests, and suitability tests for analytical systems.

2.1. Reference standards used for quantitative tests

2.1.1. Reference standards for assays of active ingredients etc.: Reference standards used for quantitative assays of products specified in the Monographs, such as chemical agents, antibiotics, additives, and biotechnological/biological products.

2.1.2. Reference standards for assays of indicator ingredients:
Reference standards used for quantitative assays of indicator ingredients of crude drugs specified in the Monographs.

2.1.3. Reference standards for assays of related substances:
Reference standards used for quantitative assays of specific related substances in purity for products specified in the Monographs, such as chemical agents, antibiotics, additives, and biotechnological/biological products.

2.1.4. Other reference standards for assays:
Reference standards needed for quantitative assays specified in the General Tests.

2.2. Reference standards used for qualitative tests

2.2.1. Reference standards for identification:
Reference standards used for identification tests of products specified in the Monographs, such as chemical agents, antibiotics, additives, biotechnological/biological products, and crude drugs. These identification include the comparison of ultraviolet-visible absorption spectra, infrared absorption spectra, nuclear magnetic resonance spectra, retention time or *Rf* values in chromatography, and mobility in electrophoresis.

2.2.2. Reference standards for purity:
Reference standards used for identification of peaks or spots, or for limit tests of related substances, in purity tests of products specified in the Monographs, such as chemical agents, antibiotics, additives, biotechnological/biological products, and crude drugs.

2.3. Reference standards used for system suitability

2.3.1. Reference standards for system suitability:
Reference standards used for system suitability of products specified in the Monographs, such as chemical agents, antibiotics, additives, biotechnological/biological products, and crude drugs.

2.4. Reference standards used for calibration and suitability confirmation of apparatus

2.4.1. Reference standards for calibration of apparatus:
Reference standards used for secondary calibration of apparatus that are specified in the General Tests.

2.4.2. Reference standards for suitability confirmation of apparatus:
Reference standards used in order to confirm that the measured values gained from an apparatus specified in the General Tests are within the defined range.

3. Names and uses of JP reference standards

JP reference standards are used for tests specified in the

Monographs and General Tests, such as Assays, Identification, Purity, calibration of apparatus, and suitability tests of analytical systems. These reference standards include materials with only one specific use and materials with multiple uses. JP reference standards used for assays and quantitative determinations of active ingredients in uniformity of dosage units and dissolution are named in principle by attachment of the phrase "reference standard" to the material name. Reference standards used for quantitative tests can be used for other tests such as identification as the reference standards, if possible. Reference standards only used for uses other than quantitative tests are named by attachment of the name of their use. Some possible uses are shown below with examples in brackets.

- For identification (Montelukast Sodium for Identification RS)
- For purity (○○○ for Purity RS)
- For calibration of apparatus (Calcium Oxalate Monohydrate for Calibration of Apparatus RS)
- For system suitability (Montelukast for System Suitability RS)

4. Requirements for establishment of JP reference standards

The JP reference standards have been mainly used as standard substances for quantitative assays of active ingredients so far. On the other hand, the European Pharmacopoeia (Ph. Eur.) and the U.S. Pharmacopeia (USP) have been actively establishing reference standards or reference materials that have specific uses other than the use for quantitative assays of active ingredients. Such specified reference standards include standards for contaminants in purity, for suitability of analytical systems, and for identification. This situation requires JP to change its policy on the reference standards along with the international trends, however, careful deliberation is needed to establish new JP reference standards in consideration of the points shown below.

(1) To adopt a relative determination such as chromatography for a quantitative test, in principle, establish the reference standard for the assay or establish the reference materials, of which purity with metrological traceability is indicated, as a reagent.

(2) To appoint a comparison method for an identification, such as comparison of ultraviolet-visible absorption spectra, infrared absorption spectra, or nuclear magnetic resonance spectra, comparison of retention times or *R*f values in chromatography, or comparison of electrophoretic mobility, in principle, it is desirable to establish the reference standard for the identification unless the use of some reference standard for assays is applicable.

(3) In a purity test where a specific related substance or contaminant is analyzed, it is recommended to establish the reference standard dedicated to the purity if the specific related substance or contaminant cannot be identified from the relative retention time of its peak on the chromatogram, and/or the limit cannot be specified by area percentage method or by comparison of the peaks with the sample solution and with the standard solution derived from the sample solution.

(4) Establish a reference standard for suitability of an analytical system, if the system suitability cannot be adequately evaluated by conventional JP methods (determination of the number of theoretical plates and the symmetry factor, etc.)

(5) If the continuous supply of the raw materials for the reference standard is uncertain, a reference standard for a related substance for purity or a reference standard for system suitability should not be established.

(6) When a material utilized as standard has the uses other than for quantitative assays and can be obtained as a certified reference material or as a reference material for other tests, that can be specified in the Reagents, Test Solutions <*9.41*> without establishing the materials as a JP reference standard.

(7) When a material utilized as standard has the uses other than for quantitative assay and can be obtained as a reagent, that can be specify the material in the Reagents, Test Solutions <*9.41*> establishing specifications and test methods according to its use, without establishing the material as a JP reference standard.

5. Quality evaluation items required for JP reference standards

Quality evaluation items required to establish a JP reference standard are shown below. The items are chosen mainly on the assumption that the materials are used as reference standards for chemical agents.

5.1. Quality evaluation items for reference standards used for quantitative assays

(i) Description: color and shape

(ii) Identification: establish a test method to identify or confirm the chemical structure.

i) Ultraviolet-visible absorption spectrum
ii) Infrared absorption spectrum
iii) Nuclear magnetic resonance spectrum (^{1}H)
iv) X-ray powder diffraction image※(when the crystal form is specified)
v) Retention time or *R*f value in chromatography※ (when chromatography is applicable to the identification)
vi) Counter ion※

(iii) Purity

i) Related substances (total amount)
ii) Residual solvents
iii) Other contaminants※

(iv) Characteristic values※

i) Specific rotation
ii) Melting point

(v) Water/Loss on drying

(vi) Residue on ignition※

(vii) Purity determination by a mass balance method: Regarding purity evaluation in mass balance method, calculate the purity (%) on the dried or anhydrous basis setting related substances, residue on ignition, residual solvent, and other contaminants as deductions.

(viii) Assay (if possible, establish an absolute quantification method such as titration, etc.)

[Note] Quality evaluation items attached with※ marks are items whose adoption should be considered taking into account the material's use as a reference standard.

5.2. Quality evaluation items for reference standards used for other than quantitative assays

Shown below are examples of quality evaluation items whose adoption should be considered taking into account the material's use as a reference standard.

(i) Description: color and shape

(ii) Identification: establish a test method to identify or confirm the chemical structure.

i) Ultraviolet-visible absorption spectrum
ii) Infrared absorption spectrum
iii) Nuclear magnetic resonance spectrum (^{1}H)
iv) Mass spectrum
v) X-ray powder diffraction image (when the crystal form is specified)
vi) Retention time or *R*f value in chromatography

(iii) Purity

i) Related substances (total amount)
ii) Residual solvents
iii) Other contaminants
(iv) Water/Loss on drying
(v) Purity determination by mass balance method
(vi) Tests related to the uses of the materials

i) A reference standard for system suitability used for peak identification needs identification of relative retention time of the peak under the same conditions to the test method that is specified in the Monographs.

ii) A reference standard for system suitability needs identification of the resolution under the same conditions to the test method that is specified in the Monographs.

6. Reference materials specified in the JP

Materials that correspond to reference materials are described in the Reagents, Test Solutions <*9.41*> in the JP. Such materials are shown as follows:

- Materials described as reagents for assays
- Materials used for identification that described as reagents for thin-layer chromatography (some materials do not correspond to reference materials)
- Materials specified as reagents for purity
- Materials described as specific related substances in the item of Related substances in Purity in the Monographs
- Reference materials specified by JIS

In the JP (except "Crude Drugs"), "reagents for assays" is specified as reference materials for assays of active ingredients in drug products, and some active ingredients with quality above a certain level are specified as reagents that are used as reference materials for identification of the active ingredients in drug products by thin-layer chromatography. However, these reference materials specified as reagents are not officially provided. Assays should be performed using reference standards, and it is considered appropriate that the "reagents for assays" described as reagents in the Reagents, Test Solutions <*9.41*> should be established as reference standards. Regarding new assay reagents that will be established for drug products except "Crude Drugs," there is a need to consider gradual establishment of these "reagents for assays" as reference standards.

On the other hand, it is difficult to establish reference standards for indicator ingredients of "Crude Drugs"; therefore, reference materials for assays of indicator ingredients are specified as reagents and quantitative NMR is included in specifications of the reagents so that a specification for assay with metrological traceability is established.

7. Precautions for the use of JP reference standards

7.1. JP reference standards are reference standards whose uses are specified in the Monographs and General Tests in the JP. Their detailed uses are described in the Monographs and their adequate qualities as reference standards are guaranteed when they are used for the described uses. Accordingly, their qualities for other uses are not guaranteed.

7.2. When a JP reference standard is used for a quantitative test specified in the Monographs, if a correction coefficient is indicated on documents such as package insert, multiply the standard amount by the correction coefficient to calculate the corrected amount for the use. If a correction coefficient is not indicated, do not correct the amount for use assuming that the purity of the reference standard is 100.0%.

7.3. If there is a description of "amount of the reference standard, calculated on the dried basis" or "amount of the reference standard, calculated on the anhydrous basis" in a calculation formula for an assay method in the Monographs, extra measurement of the loss on drying or the water content of the reference standard is required. If, however, the value of loss on drying or water content is indicated on the document of the reference standard such as package insert, use of the indicated value is permitted.

7.4. JP reference standards have no established expiration date, therefore, obtain needed amount of a reference standard when it is needed, and then store the reference standard under specified conditions and use up it as quick as possible.

7.5. The quality of reference standards stored after unsealing of the packages are not guaranteed.

7.6. Normally, one packing unit of a reference standard contains the amount that enables several times of repeated test. However, some packages of reference standards whose raw material supply is scarce contain the amounts that enable only one-time test.

7.7. Information of JP reference standards necessary for the uses specified in the Monographs or General Tests is described on documents such as package inserts. However, their test results are not disclosed and certificates of analysis are not issued.

GZ Others

Water to be used in the Tests of Drugs <*GZ-1-161*>

The water to be used in the tests of drugs is defined as "the water suitable for performing the relevant test" in the paragraph 21 under General Notices of the JP. Therefore, it is necessary to confirm that the water to be used in a test of a drug is suitable for the purpose of the relevant test before its use.

Unless otherwise specified in the individual test method, Purified Water, Purified Water in Containers or the water produced by an appropriate process, such as ion exchange or ultrafiltration, may be used for these purposes. Water produced for these purposes at other individual facilities may also be used.

Examples of the water for tests specified in General Tests in the JP are as follows:

- Water for ammonium limit test: <*1.02*> Ammonium Limit Test (Standard Ammonium Solution)
- Water used for measuring organic carbon (water for measurement): <*2.59*> Test for Total Organic Carbon
- Water for ICP analysis: <*2.63*> Inductively Coupled Plasma-Atomic Emission Spectrometry and Inductively Coupled Plasma-Mass Spectrometry
- Water for bacterial endotoxins test: <*4.01*> Bacterial Endotoxins Test
- Water for particulate matter test (for injections): <*6.07*> Insoluble Particulate Matter Test for Injections
- Water for particulate matter test (for ophthalmic solutions): <*6.08*> Insoluble Particulate Matter Test for Ophthalmic Solutions
- Water for particulate matter test (for plastic containers): <*7.02*> Test Methods for Plastic Containers

The water for tests specified in General Information in the JP is as follows:

- Water for aluminum test: Test for Trace Amounts of Aluminum in Total Parenteral Nutrition (TPN) Solutions

The term "water" described in the text concerning tests of drugs means "the water to be used in the tests of drugs" as defined in the paragraph 21 under General Notices.

Quality Control of Water for Pharmaceutical Use <*GZ-2-172*>

Water used for manufacturing pharmaceutical products and for cleaning their containers and equipments used in the manufacture of the products is referred to as "pharmaceutical water." For assuring the quality of pharmaceutical water consistently, it is important to verify through appropriate process validation of water processing system that water with the quality suitable for its intended use is produced and supplied, and to keep the quality of produced water through routine works for controlling the water processing system.

1. Types of Pharmaceutical Water

1.1. *Water*

The specification for "*Water*" is prescribed in the Japanese Pharmacopoeia (JP) monograph. It is required for *Water* to meet the Quality Standards for Drinking Water provided under the Article 4 of the Japanese Water Supply Law. In the case that *Water* is produced at individual facilities using well water or industrial water as source water, it is necessary for produced water to meet the Quality Standards for Drinking Water and an additional requirement for ammonium of "not more than 0.05 mg/L." Furthermore, when *Water* is to be used after storing for a period of time, it is necessary to prevent microbial proliferation.

Water is used as source water for *Purified Water* and *Water for Injection*. It is also used for manufacturing intermediates of active pharmaceutical ingredients (APIs), and for pre-washing of the equipment used in the manufacture of pharmaceutical products.

1.2. *Purified Water*

The specifications for "*Purified Water*" and "*Purified Water in Containers*" are prescribed in the JP monographs. *Purified Water* is prepared by distillation, ion-exchange, reverse osmosis (RO), ultrafiltration (UF) capable of removing microorganisms and substances with molecular masses of not less than approximately 6000, or a combination of these processes from *Water*, after applying some adequate pretreatments if necessary. For the production of *Purified Water*, appropriate control of microorganisms is required. Particularly, in the case that *Purified Water* is prepared by ion-exchange, RO or UF, it is necessary to apply the treatments adequate for preventing microbial proliferation, or to sanitize the system periodically.

When *Purified Water* is treated with chemical agents for sterilizing, preventing microbial proliferation, or maintaining the endotoxin level within an appropriate control range, a specification suitable for the intended use of treated water should be established individually, and a process control for keeping the quality of treated water in compliance with the specification thus established should be performed.

"*Purified Water in Containers*" is prepared from *Purified Water* by introducing it in a tight container.

1.3. *Sterile Purified Water*

The specification for "*Sterile Purified Water in Containers*" (its alternative name is *Sterile Purified Water*) is prescribed in the JP monograph.

Sterile Purified Water in Container is prepared from *Purified Water* by 1) introducing it into a hermetic container, sealing up the container, then sterilizing the product, or 2) making it sterile by using a suitable method, introducing the sterilized water into a sterile hermetic container by applying aseptic manipulation, then sealing up the container.

Plastic containers for aqueous injections may be used in place of hermetic containers.

1.4. *Water for Injection*

The specifications for "*Water for Injection*" and "*Sterile Water for Injection in Containers*" are prescribed in the JP monographs.

Water for Injection is prepared by distillation or reverse osmosis and/or ultrafiltration (RO/UF), either: from the water which is obtained by appropriate pretreatments such as ion exchange, RO, etc. on *Water*; or from *Purified Water*. In the case of water processing systems based on distillation, it is necessary to take care for avoiding contamination of produced water by the impurities accompanied with the entrain. In the case of water processing system based on RO/UF, it is required to provide water with equivalent quality to that prepared by distillation consistently, based on substantial process validation through long-term operation and elaborate routine control of the system. It is essential to ensure consistent production of water suitable for *Water for Injection* by the entire water processing system including pretreatment facilities, in any systems based on RO/UF. For the water supplied to the system, it is also required to keep the quality suitable as source water through adequate validation and routine control on the water. For the water processing system based on RO/UF, routine control should be performed by analyzing water specimens, monitoring some quality attributes using in-line apparatus and checking the volume of water passed through the system. In addition, it is recommended to carry out periodical appearance observation and air-leak test on the membranes being currently used. It is also recommended to establish protocols for keeping the performance of membrane modules within appropriate control ranges and for estimating the timing to exchange the modules, through diagnosis on the degree of deterioration based on the results of tensile strength test on the used membrane modules, and visual observation on those modules whether any leakages of membranes have occurred or not, and to what extent they have occurred. Furthermore, it is desirable to establish the frequency of membrane exchange considering with its actual condition of use.

In the case that *Water for Injection* is stored in the water processing system temporarily, a stringent control for microorganisms and endotoxins should be taken. An acceptable criterion of lower than 0.25 EU/mL for endotoxins is specified in the JP monograph of *Water for Injection*.

"*Sterile Water for Injection in Container*" is prepared from *Water for Injection* by 1) introducing it into a hermetic container, sealing up the container, then sterilizing the product, or 2) making it sterile by using a suitable method, introducing the sterilized water into a sterile hermetic container by applying aseptic manipulation, then sealing up the container. Plastic containers for aqueous injections may be used in place of hermetic containers.

2. Reverse Osmosis and/or Ultrafiltration (RO/UF)

RO/UF are the methods for refining water by using membrane modules based on either reverse osmosis or ultrafiltration, or the modules combining them, and used as the alternative methods for distillation in the production of *Purified Water* or *Water for Injection*.

When *Water for Injection* is produced by RO/UF, a water processing system equipped with pretreatment facilities,

facilities for producing *Water for Injection* and facilities for supplying *Water for Injection* is usually used. The pretreatment facilities are used to remove solid particles, dissolved salts and colloids in source water, and placed before the facilities for producing *Water for Injection* so as to reduce the load on the facilities for producing *Water for Injection*. They consist of apparatus properly selected from aggregation apparatus, precipitation-separation apparatus, filtration apparatus, chorine sterilization apparatus, oxidation-reduction apparatus, residual chlorine-removing apparatus, precise filtration apparatus, reverse osmosis apparatus, ultrafiltration apparatus, ion exchange apparatus, etc., depending on the quality of source water. The facilities for producing *Water for Injection* consist of apparatus for supplying pretreated water, sterilization apparatus with ultraviolet rays, heat exchange apparatus, membrane modules, apparatus for cleaning and sterilizing the facilities, etc. The facilities for supplying *Water for Injection* consist of a reservoir tank for storing *Water for Injection* in the facilities temporarily, pipe lines, heat exchange apparatus, a pump for circulating *Water for Injection* in the facilities, pressure control apparatus, etc. When *Purified Water* is produced by RO/UF, basic composition of water processing system is almost the same as that for *Water for Injection* described above.

In the case that *Water for Injection* is stored in the water processing system temporarily, it should usually be circulated in a loop consisting of a reservoir tank and pipe line at a temperature not lower than 80°C for preventing microbial proliferation.

When RO/UF is utilized for preparing pharmaceutical water, it is necessary to select the most appropriate combination of membrane modules in consideration of the quality of source water and the quality of produced water required for its intended use. When the ultrafiltration membrane is used to prepare *Purified Water* or *Water for Injection*, membrane modules capable of removing microorganisms and substances with molecular masses not less than approximately 6000 should be used.

3. Selection of Pharmaceutical Water

Depending on the intended use of pharmaceutical water, the water suitable for assuring the quality of final products without causing any trouble during their manufacturing processes, should be selected from the above 4 types (1.1 – 1.4) of pharmaceutical water specified in the JP. Table 1 exemplifies a protocol for such selection.

Sterile Purified Water in Containers or *Water for Injection* (or *Sterile Water for Injection in Containers*) may be used in place of *Purified Water* (or *Purified Water in Containers*).

3.1. Drug Products

For the manufacture of sterile drug products such as Injections, for which endotoxins together with microorganisms should be severely controlled, *Water for Injection* (or *Sterile Water for Injection in Containers*) should be used. For the manufacture of sterile drug products such as Ophthalmic Preparations and Ophthalmic Ointments, for which contamination with microorganisms should be paid attention, *Purified Water* (or *Purified Water in Containers*), which viable count level is specified at low, can also be used.

For the manufacture of non-sterile drug products, water with a quality not lower than that of *Purified Water* (or *Purified Water in Containers*) should be used. For the Inhalations, Ear Preparations and Nasal Preparations, appropriately controlled *Purified Water* (or *Purified Water in Containers*) in vial count level should be used, and for Liquids and Solutions among Inhalations, strictly controlled *Purified Water* (or *Purified Water in Containers*) in vial count level should be used. For the Liquids and Solutions for Oral Administration, Syrups, Suppositories for Vaginal Use, Ointments and Creams, which require care against microbiological contamination, *Purified Water* (or *Purified Water in Containers*) adequately controlled from microbiological viewpoints should be used in consideration of the possible impacts of preservatives formulated in the drug products.

For the manufacture of drug products containing crude drugs, it is recommended to select adequate type of water considering viable counts of the crude drugs used for manufacturing the product and microbial limit required for the product.

Water used for pre-washing of containers or equipment surfaces that comes in direct contact with the drug products should have the quality not lower than that of *Water*. Water used for final rinsing should have an equivalent quality to that of water used for manufacturing drug products.

3.2. Drug Substances

Water used for manufacturing a drug substance should be selected in consideration of the characteristics of the drug product for which the drug substance is to be used, and its manufacturing process, so that the quality of the final drug product is assured.

Water used for manufacturing a drug substance or for cleaning containers or equipment surfaces that come in direct contact with the raw materials or drug substance intermediates, should have the quality not lower than that of *Water* adequately controlled from the chemical and microbiological viewpoints, even if the water is used at an earlier stage of synthetic or extraction process in the manufacture of drug substances. Water used in the final purification process should have the quality equal to or higher than that of *Purified Water* (or *Purified Water in Containers*). Water used for final rinsing of containers or equipment surfaces that comes in direct contact with the drug substances should have an equivalent quality to that of water used for manufacturing the drug substances.

For manufacturing sterile drug substances, *Sterile Purified Water in Containers* or *Water for Injection* (or *Sterile Water for Injection in Containers*) should be used. Similarly, for manufacturing drug substances used for drug products where endotoxin control is required and there are no subsequent processes capable of removing endotoxins, *Water for Injection* (or *Sterile Water for Injection in Containers*), or *Purified Water* (or *Purified Water in Containers*) for which endotoxins are controlled at a low level, should be used.

4. Quality Control of Pharmaceutical Water

4.1. Outline

Verification that water with the quality required for its intended use has been produced by the pharmaceutical water processing system through substantial validation studies at an earlier stage of its operation, is the prerequisite for conducting quality control on pharmaceutical water in a routine and periodical manner. If this prerequisite is fulfilled, the following methods are applicable for quality control of pharmaceutical water.

For routine control, it is very useful to control quality of produced water based on the monitoring of electrical conductivity (conductivity) and total organic carbon (TOC). In addition, items to be monitored periodically, such as some specified impurities, viable counts, endotoxins, insoluble particulate matters, etc., should be determined according to the intended use of pharmaceutical water. The frequency of measurement should be determined considering with the

Table 1 An Exemplified Protocol for Selecting Pharmaceutical Water (Water Used in the Manufacture of Drug Products or Drug Substances)

Classification	Class of Pharmaceutical Water	Application	Remarks
Drug Product	*Water for Injection* or *Sterile Water for Injection in Containers*	Injections, Dialysis Agents (Peritoneal Dialysis Agents and Hemodialysis Agents)	For Hemodialysis Agents, unless otherwise specified, *Water for Injection*, *Water for Injection in Containers*, or water suitable for the dialysis.
	Purified Water or *Purified Water in Containers*	Ophthalmic Preparations, Ophthalmic Ointments, Inhalations, Ear Preparations, Nasal Preparations	For sterile drug products, such as Ophthalmic Preparations and Ophthalmic Ointments, for which precautions should be taken against microbial contamination, *Purified Water* (or *Purified Water in Containers*) kept its viable counts at low levels may be used. For Inhalations, Ear Preparations and Nasal Preparations, *Purified Water* (or *Purified Water in Containers*) of which viable counts are controlled at an appropriate level should be used. However, for the Inhalation Liquid Preparations among Inhalations, *Purified Water* (or *Purified Water in Containers*) that vial count is strictly controlled should be used.
		Preparations for Oral Administration, Preparations for Oro-mucosal Application, Preparations for Rectal Application, Preparations for Vaginal Application, Preparations for Cutaneous Application, and Tinctures and Aromatic Waters among Preparations Related to Crude Drugs.	For Liquids and Solutions for Oral Administration, Syrups, Suppositories for Vaginal Use, Ointments, Creams and so on for which precautions should be taken against microbial contamination, *Purified Water* (or *Purified Water in Containers*) adequately controlled from microbiological viewpoints should be used, taking in mind the affection of containing preservatives.
	Water	Among Preparations Related to Crude Drugs: Extracts, Pills, Infusions and Decoctions, Teabags, Fluidextracts	The viable counts in crude drugs and the objective microbial limits of product should be considered in selecting water to be used.
Drug Substances	*Water for Injection* or *Sterile Water for Injection in Containers*	Sterile Drug Substances	
	Purified Water or *Purified Water in Containers*	Drug Substances	In the manufacture of drug substances used for products to be rendered sterile in the formulation process, if there is no subsequent processes capable of removing endotoxins, *Purified Water* (or *Purified Water in Containers*) controlled endotoxins in an appropriate level should be used.
	Water	Drug Substances Intermediates	

variation in the quality of water to be monitored.

The following are points to consider in controlling the quality of produced water from microbiological and physicochemical (conductivity and TOC) viewpoints. It is necessary to monitor other items if necessary, and to confirm that they meet the specifications established individually.

4.2. Sampling

Monitoring should be conducted at an adequate frequency to ensure that the pharmaceutical water processing system is well-controlled and that water with acceptable quality is continuously produced and supplied. Specimens should be collected at the representative locations in the facilities for producing and supplying water, with particular care so that collected specimens reflect the operating condition of the pharmaceutical water processing system. An adequate protocol for the control of microorganisms at the sampling site should be established considering with the situation around the site.

Sampling frequency should be adequately established based on the data from validation studies on the system. For microbiological monitoring, it is adequate to use the water specimens for the test within 2 hours after sampling. In the case that it is not possible to test within 2 hours, the specimens should be kept at 2 – 8°C and be used for the test within 12 hours.

4.3. Alert and Action Levels

In producing pharmaceutical water using a water processing system, microbiological and physicochemical monitoring is usually carried out to assure that water with required quality is being continuously produced when the system is operating as it designed. The operating condition of the system can be estimated by the comparison of

Table 2 Methods for Assessment of Viable Counts in Pharmaceutical Water

Method	Pharmaceutical Water		
	Water	*Purified Water*	*Water for Injection*
Measurement Method	Pour Plate Method or Membrane Filtration	Pour Plate Method or Membrane Filtration	Membrane Filtration
Minimum Sample Size	1.0 mL	1.0 mL	100 mL
Media	R2A Agar Medium Standard Agar Medium	R2A Agar Medium	R2A Agar Medium
Incubation Period	R2A Agar Medium: 4 - 7 days (or longer) Standard Agar Medium: 48 - 72 hours (or longer)	4 - 7 days (or longer)	4 - 7 days (or longer)
Incubation Temperature	R2A Agar Medium: 20 - 25°C or 30 - 35°C Standard Agar Medium: 30 - 35°C	20 - 25°C or 30 - 35°C	20 - 25°C or 30 - 35°C

monitoring data thus obtained against the alert level, action level, other levels for controlling the system, and acceptance criteria specified for the water required for its intended use, and also by the trend analysis of monitoring data through plotting them in a control chart.

In this manner, the alert level and action level are used for controlling the process of water production, and not used for judging pass/fail of produced water.

4.3.1. Definition of Alert Level

"Alert level" indicates that, when exceeded it, the system is threatening to deviate from its normal operating range. Alert levels are used for giving a warning, and exceeding them does not necessarily require a corrective action. Alert levels are generally established either at a mean + 2σ on the basis of past trend analysis, or at a level of 70% (50% for viable counts) of the action level, whichever is lower.

4.3.2. Definition of Action Level

"Action level" indicates that, when exceeded it, the system has deviated from its normal operating range. Exceeding it indicates that corrective action must be taken to bring the system back within its normal operating range.

Alert and action levels should be established within the processes and the quality specifications of products in consideration of available technologies and the quality required for the products. Consequently, exceeding an alert or action level does not necessarily indicate that the quality of produced water has become inadequate for its intended use.

4.4. Microbiological Monitoring

The main purpose of a microbiological monitoring program for a pharmaceutical water processing system is to foresee any microbiological quality deterioration of the produced water, and to prevent any adverse effects on the quality of pharmaceutical products. Consequently, detecting all of the microorganisms present in the water to be monitored may not be necessary. However it is required to adopt a monitoring technique able to detect a wide range of microorganisms, including slow growing microorganisms.

The following indicate incubation-based microbiological monitoring techniques for pharmaceutical water processing systems. To adopt a rapid microorganism detection technique, it is necessary to confirm in advance that the microbial counts obtained by such techniques are equivalent to those obtained by the incubation-based monitoring techniques.

4.4.1. Media and Incubation Conditions

There are many mesophilic bacteria of heterotrophic type that are adapted to poor nutrient water environments. Heterotrophic bacteria may form bio-films in many pharmaceutical water processing systems, and to cause quality deterioration of the produced water. Therefore, it is useful to monitor microbiological quality of water by using the R2A Agar Medium, which is excellent for growing bacteria of oligotrophic type.

Table 2 shows examples of measurement methods, minimum sample sizes, media, and incubation periods for estimating viable counts.

The media shown in Table 2 are as follows.

(i) Standard Agar Medium

Casein peptone	5.0 g
Yeast extract	2.5 g
Glucose	1.0 g
Agar	15.0 g
Water	1000 mL

Mix all the ingredients, and sterilize by heating in an autoclave at 121°C for 15 - 20 minutes. pH after sterilization: 6.9 - 7.1.

(ii) R2A Agar Medium

Peptone (casein and animal tissue)	0.5 g
Casamino acid	0.5 g
Yeast extract	0.5 g
Sodium pyruvate	0.3 g
Glucose	0.5 g
Magnesium sulfate heptahydrate	50 mg
Soluble starch	0.5 g
Dipotassium hydrogen phosphate	0.3 g
Agar	15.0 g
Water	1000 mL

Mix all the ingredients, and sterilize by heating in an autoclave at 121°C for 15 - 20 minutes. pH after sterilization: 7.1 - 7.3.

The following reagents should be used for preparing the R2A Agar Medium.

(i) Casamino acid Prepared for microbial test, by the acid hydrolysis of casein.

Loss on drying *<2.41>*: Not more than 8% (0.5 g, 105°C, constant mass).

Residue on ignition *<2.44>*: Not more than 55% (0.5 g).

Nitrogen content *<1.08>*: Not less than 7% (105°C, constant mass, after drying).

4.4.2. Media Growth Promotion Test

In the media growth promotion test with the R2A Agar Medium, use test strains listed below or other test strains considered equivalent to these test strains.

Methylobacterium extorquens: NBRC 15911

Pseudomonas fluorescens: NBRC 15842, ATCC 17386, etc.

Prior to the test, inoculate these test strains into sterile purified water and starve them at 20 - 25°C for 3 days. Dilute the fluid containing the test strain starved with sterile purified water to prepare microbial suspensions. When inoculating the R2A Agar Medium with the micro-organisms ($5 \times 10^1 - 2 \times 10^2$ CFU) and incubating at 20 - 25°C for 4 - 7 days, sufficient proliferation of the inoculated strains must be observed.

In the media growth promotion test with the Standard Agar Medium, use test strains listed below or other test strains considered equivalent to these test strains.

Staphylococcus aureus: ATCC 6538, NCIMB 9518, CIP 4.83 or NBRC 13276

Pseudomonas aeruginosa: ATCC 9027, NCIMB 8626, CIP 82.118 or NBRC 13275

Escherichia coli: ATCC 8739, NCIMB 8545, CIP 53.126 or NBRC 3972

Prepare microbial suspensions containing the test strains according to the procedure prescribed in Microbiological Examination of Non-sterile Products <*4.05*>. When inoculating the Standard Agar Medium with a small number (not more than 100 CFU) of the micro-organisms and incubating at 30 - 35°C for 48 hours, sufficient proliferation of the inoculated strains must be observed.

4.4.3. Action Levels for Microorganisms for Pharmaceutical Water Processing System

The following action levels are considered appropriate and generally applicable to pharmaceutical water processing systems.

Action Levels for viable counts in various types of pharmaceutical water

Water: 10^2 CFU/mL* (Acceptance criterion prescribed in the Quality Standards for Drinking Water provided under the Article 4 of the Water Supply Law)

Purified Water: 10^2 CFU/mL**

Water for Injection: 10^1 CFU/100 mL**

(*Viable counts obtained using the Standard Agar Medium, ** Viable counts obtained using the R2A Agar Medium)

Although the action level for *Purified Water* shown above is set at the same level as that for *Water*, it is recommended for each facility to perform a higher level of microbiological control of water processing system based on the action level established individually.

When actual counts in validation studies or routine control exceed the above action levels, it is necessary to isolate and identify the microorganisms present in the water, and to sanitize or disinfect the affected system.

4.5. Physicochemical Monitoring

Physicochemical monitoring of a pharmaceutical water processing system is usually performed using conductivity and TOC as the indicators for water quality. By monitoring conductivity, total amounts of inorganic salts present in the water can be estimated, and by monitoring TOC, total amount of organic compounds present in the water can be estimated. Normally, Conductivity Measurements <*2.51*> and Test for Total Organic Carbon <*2.59*> specified in the General Tests, Processes and Apparatus of the JP should be applied to these physicochemical monitoring. However, since tests for monitoring are performed in the situations different from those for judging pass/fail to the acceptance criteria prescribed in the monographs, supplements necessary to cover the situations to which the JP general tests cannot be applied, are described below.

To adopt the monitoring using conductivity and TOC as the indicators for inorganic and organic impurities at individual facility, appropriate alert and action levels for each indicator, and countermeasures against unexpected apparatus failures should be established.

4.5.1. Monitoring of Conductivity as the Indicator for Inorganic Impurities

Measurement of conductivity for monitoring is usually conducted continuously using an in-line apparatus with a flow-through type or pipe-insertion type cell. Alternatively, offline batch testing may be performed using a dip type cell with water specimens taken at appropriate locations of the pharmaceutical water processing system.

For the operation control of a pharmaceutical water processing system, guides for judging whether it is adequate to continue the operation of the system or not based on the results from monitoring of conductivity, are shown below, both for the cases of monitoring at the standard temperature (20°C) by applying Conductivity Measurements <*2.51*> of the JP and monitoring at temperatures other than 20°C by applying <645> *WATER CONDUCTIVITY* of the United States Pharmacopeia (USP) with some modifications.

4.5.1.1. Monitoring of Conductivity by applying Conductivity Measurements <*2.51*> of the JP

When the monitoring of the conductivity of *Purified Water* and *Water for Injection* is performed at the standard temperature (20°C), measure the conductivity after confirming that the measure temperature is within a range of 20 ± 1°C. In this case, the recommended allowable conductivity (action level) for *Purified Water* and *Water for Injection* is as follows.

• Action Level $1.1\ \mu S\cdot cm^{-1}$ (20°C)

Since the above allowable conductivity is established for in-line monitoring, an alternative action level may be used for the monitoring based on offline batch testing.

4.5.1.2. Monitoring of Conductivity by applying <645> *WATER CONDUCTIVITY* of the USP with some modification

Usually, it is somewhat difficult to control the temperature exactly in in-line conductivity monitoring. Therefore, the following approach can be applied for the monitoring at temperatures other than the standard temperature (20°C) of the JP. This approach is based on the Stages 1 and 2 of the three-stage approach described in "<645> *WATER CONDUCTIVITY*" of the USP and in the monographs being associated with water for pharmaceutical use ("Purified Water", "Highly Purified Water" and "Water for Injections") of the European Pharmacopoeia (EP).

Stage 1 (In-line Measurement)

(i) Determine the temperature and the conductivity of the water specimens using a non-temperature-compensated conductivity reading.

(ii) From the Table 3, find the temperature value equal to or just lower than the measured temperature. Adopt the corresponding conductivity value on this table as the allowable conductivity at the measured temperature.

(iii) If the observed conductivity is not greater than the allowable conductivity adopted above, the water tested meets the requirement for monitoring conductivity. If the observed conductivity exceeds the allowable conductivity, proceed with Stage 2.

Stage 2 (Off-line Measurement)

(i) Measure the conductivity of the water specimen, by transferring it into a container and agitating it vigorous-

Table 3 Stage 1 Allowable Conductivity for Different Temperatures*

Temperature (°C)	Allowable Conductivity ($\mu S \cdot cm^{-1}$)	Temperature (°C)	Allowable Conductivity ($\mu S \cdot cm^{-1}$)
0	0.6		
5	0.8	55	2.1
10	0.9	60	2.2
15	1.0	65	2.4
20	1.1	70	2.5
25	1.3	75	2.7
30	1.4	80	2.7
35	1.5	85	2.7
40	1.7	90	2.7
45	1.8	95	2.9
50	1.9	100	3.1

* Applicable only to non-temperature-compensated conductivity measurements.

ly in order to attain equilibrium between the water specimen and the atmosphere on absorbing/desorbing carbon dioxide.

(ii) Transfer a sufficient amount of water to be tested into a suitable container, and stir the water specimen. Adjust the temperature to 25 ± 1°C, and begin agitating the water specimen vigorously, while observing the conductivity periodically. When the change in conductivity becomes not greater than 0.1 $\mu S \cdot cm^{-1}$ per 5 minutes, adopt the observed value as the conductivity (25°C) of the water specimen.

(iii) If the conductivity of the water specimen at 25°C obtained above is not greater than 2.1 $\mu S \cdot cm^{-1}$, the water tested meets the requirement for monitoring conductivity. If the observed value exceeds 2.1 $\mu S \cdot cm^{-1}$, it should be judged that the water tested does not meet the requirement for monitoring conductivity.

4.5.2. Monitoring of TOC as the Indicator for Organic Impurities

The acceptance criterion of TOC is specified as "not greater than 0.50 mg/L (500 ppb)" in the monographs of *Purified Water* and *Water for Injection*. However it is recommended for each facility preparing pharmaceutical water to conduct operation control of pharmaceutical water processing system through TOC monitoring on produced water based on its own alert and action levels for TOC determined individually. The following are the recommended action levels for TOC.

- Action Level: ≦300 ppb (in-line)
  ≦400 ppb (off-line)

The Quality Standards for Drinking Water provided under the Article 4 of the Japanese Water Supply Law require that TOC of tap water (*Water*) should be "not greater than 3 mg/L (3 ppm)". Taking the above recommended action levels into consideration, it is also recommended for each facility to conduct quality control of source water through TOC monitoring based on its own alert and action levels for TOC determined individually.

The JP specifies *Test for Total Organic Carbon* <2.59>, and normally, TOC measurement should be conducted using an apparatus which meets the requirements described in the JP method. However, if a TOC apparatus conforms to the apparatus suitability test requirements described in "<643> *TOTAL ORGANIC CARBON*" of the USP, or those described in the "*Methods of Analysis 2.2.44. TOTAL ORGANIC CARBON IN WATER FOR PHARMACEUTICAL USE*" of the EP, the apparatus can be used for the monitoring of pharmaceutical water processing system, if sufficiently pure water not contaminated with ionic organic substances, or organic substances having nitrogen, sulfur, phosphorus or halogen atoms in their chemical structures, is used as the source water supplied to the system.

A TOC apparatus, characterized by calculating the amount of organic carbon from the difference in conductivity before and after the decomposition of organic substances without separating carbon dioxide from the sample solution, may be influenced negatively or positively, when applied to the water specimens containing ionic organic substances, or organic substances having nitrogen, sulfur, phosphorus or halogen atoms in their chemical structures. Therefore, the apparatus used for TOC monitoring should be selected appropriately in consideration of the purity of the water to be monitored and the contamination risk in the case of apparatus failure.

4.6. Storage of *Water for Injection*

In storing *Water for Injection* temporarily, adequate measures able to prevent microbial proliferation stringently, such as circulating it in a loop at a high temperature must be taken, and an appropriate storage time should also be established based on the validation studies, in consideration of the risks of contamination and quality deterioration.

5. Points to Consider for Assuring the Quality of Pharmaceutical Water in Containers

There are some specific points to consider for assuring the quality of pharmaceutical water in containers (*Purified Water in Containers, Sterile Purified Water in Containers* and *Sterile Water for Injection in Containers*), which are available as commercially products.

5.1. Methods for Preparing Sterile Pharmaceutical Water in Containers

The following two different preparation methods are described in the monographs of *Sterile Purified Water in Containers* and *Sterile Water for Injection in Containers*.

(i) Introduce *Purified Water* or *Water for Injection* into a hermetic container, seal up the container, then sterilize the product.

(ii) Make *Purified Water* or *Water for Injection* sterile by using a suitable method, introduce the sterilized water into a sterile hermetic container by applying aseptic manipulation, then seal up the container.

For assuring the sterility of pharmaceutical water products, only the validation of final sterilization process is required in the case of preparation method (i), whereas validations of all the processes are indispensable in the case of preparation method (ii), since the latter is based on the idea to assure the sterility of pharmaceutical water products by "aseptically" introducing *Purified Water* (or *Water for Injection*) treated in advance with filtration sterilization, etc. into a sterile hermetic container, and sealing it up.

5.2. Deterioration of Water Quality during the Storage in Containers

5.2.1. Inorganic impurities (Conductivity as the indicator)

The conductivity of pharmaceutical water in containers may increase to some higher levels due to the absorption of carbon dioxide from the atmosphere at the time of its preparation and that passed through plastic layer of the containers during storage, and also due to ionic substances released from the containers, even if the conductivity of *Purified Water* or *Water for Injection* used for its production is maintained at the level not more than 1.0 $\mu S \cdot cm^{-1}$. Particularly in the cases of pharmaceutical water products packed in small scale glass containers, it is necessary to pay attention to the change of conductivity during storage.

5.2.2. Organic impurities (Potassium Permanganate-reducing Substances or Total Organic Carbon (TOC) as the indicator)

The JP specifies the classical test of potassium permanganate-reducing substances in the monographs of *Purified Water in Containers*, *Sterile Purified Water in Containers* and *Sterile Water for Injection in Containers* for controlling organic impurities in pharmaceutical water in containers. It forms a remarkable contrast to the specifications of *Purified Water* and *Water for Injection*, in which the JP requires to control organic impurities in pharmaceutical water in bulk based on the test of TOC (acceptance criterion: not more than 0.5 mg/L (500 ppb)). This is because that it is considered difficult to establish the specification of pharmaceutical water in containers for organic impurities based on the test of TOC from the facts that there were many cases of remarkable increases in TOC values after storage of water in containers. Particularly in the cases of pharmaceutical water products packed in small scale plastic containers, it is necessary to pay attention to the increase of materials released from containers during storage.

The test of potassium permanganate-reducing substances is retained in the specifications of pharmaceutical water in containers, not as the most suitable method for the test of organic impurities present in the water in containers, but as a counter measure for performing the test of the water in containers with the same test method despite of the material (glass, polyethylene, polypropylene, etc.) and the size (0.5 – 2000 mL) of the containers, and the duration of storage. Therefore, it is recommended to adopt the test of TOC as the alternative for the test of potassium permanganate-reducing substances, and to perform quality control of pharmaceutical water in containers based on TOC measurements under the responsibility of each manufacturer, if possible.

In such cases, it is recommended to adopt the following values as the levels preferable to attain.

For products containing not more than 10 mL of water:

TOC not greater than 1500 ppb

For products containing more than 10 mL of water:

TOC not greater than 1000 ppb

As for the pharmaceutical water packed in the plastic containers made of polyethylene, polypropylene, etc., in addition to the concern for the release of materials such as monomer, oligomers, plasticizers, etc. from plastics, it is necessary to pay attention to the storage environment of the products to avoid the contaminations with low molecular volatile organics such as ethanol, or low molecular air pollutants such as nitrogen oxides, since these plastics have the properties of permeating various gases and water.

5.2.3. Microbial Limit (Total Aerobic Viable Counts)

For *Purified Water in Containers*, it is not required to assure the sterility, but it is necessary to produce it by using sanitary or aseptic processes in order to meet the acceptance criterion of "10^2 CFU/mL" for total aerobic viable counts throughout the period of their storages. It is also necessary to take special care against microbial contamination during its circulation. In addition, it is recommended to use them as soon as possible after opening their seals.

The acceptance criterion of "10^2 CFU/mL" for total aerobic viable counts of *Purified Water in Container* is at the same level as the action level for viable counts in the production of *Purified Water* (in bulk). However, different from the case of microbiological monitoring of *Purified Water*, Soybean-Casein Digest Agar Medium is used for the test of total aerobic viable counts of *Purified Water in Containers* to detect microorganisms contaminated from the surroundings during its storage.

5.3. Points to consider in the case that commercially available products of pharmaceutical water in containers are used for the manufacture of pharmaceutical products

It is allowable to use commercially available products of pharmaceutical water in containers (*Purified Water in Containers*, *Sterile Purified Water in Containers* and *Sterile Water for Injection in Containers*) for the manufacture of pharmaceutical products and products for clinical trial, and for the tests of pharmaceutical products. In such cases, it is necessary to consider the following points.

(i) Use them soon after confirming their compliances to the requirements of the JP monograph from the test results at the time of its receipt or those offered from the supplier of the products.

(ii) In the case that such products are used for manufacturing pharmaceutical products, it is necessary to validate the process in which the water was used as a part of process validation of pharmaceutical products. In the case that they are used for manufacturing products for clinical trial, it is necessary to confirm that the water doesn't give any adverse effects on the quality of the products.

(iii) The products of sterile pharmaceutical water in containers should be used only once after opening their seals, and it must be avoided to use them again after storage.

(iv) It is recommended to prepare a standard operation practice (SOP) adequate for its intended use, considering that the contamination and quality deterioration of the water due to human and laboratory environmental origins might go on rapidly immediately after opening the product seal.

International Harmonization Implemented in the Japanese Pharmacopoeia Eighteenth Edition *<GZ-3-180>*

Information on items for which harmonization has been agreed among the European Pharmacopoeia, the United States Pharmacopeia and the Japanese Pharmacopoeia is available on the following websites of Pharmaceuticals and Medical Devices Agency:

General chapters:

https://www.pmda.go.jp/rs-std-jp/standards-development/jp/0021.html

Monographs:

https://www.pmda.go.jp/rs-std-jp/standards-development/jp/0020.html

Appendix

Atomic Weight Table (2017)

Atomic Weights Subcommittee of the Chemical Society of Japan

In 1961 it was decided that the atomic weights of the elements would be based on values relative to the mass number of 12 (no fractions) for carbon (^{12}C). Ever since, there has been a marked improvement in the quality and quantity of data on the nuclide masses and isotope ratios of the elements using physical methods such as mass spectrometry. The Commission on Isotope Abundances and Atomic Weights (CIAAW) of the International Union of Pure and Applied Chemistry (IUPAC) collected and examined newly measured data and revises the atomic weight table every two years (in the odd years). Based on this table, in April of each year the Atomic Weights Subcommittee of the Chemical Society of Japan also publishes an atomic weight table. The numbers of the following Atomic Weight Table (2017) is based on the numbers approved by the IUPAC in 2015[1)]. For a more detailed explanation, the user is referred to a report[2)] and a review[3)] published by the CIAAW.

The atomic weight values of each of the elements shown in the atomic weight tables can, with the exception of single nuclide elements (elements consisting of one stable nuclide), change depending on a variety of factors, such as the method of treatment or the origin of the substance containing that element. This is because the atomic weight is dependent on the relative frequency (isotope ratio of an element) of the stable nuclides comprising each of the respective elements. Due to advancements in measurement techniques, the isotopic frequencies of each of the elements are not necessarily constant, and fluctuate due to a variety of processes that occur on the Earth. We have come to learn that this is reflected in the atomic weights. Based on such background, in 2009, the IUPAC decided to indicate the atomic weights for 10 elements not as single values but as ranges[4)]. The Atomic Weights Subcommittee of the Chemical Society of Japan discussed the change and decided to reflect the IUPAC's guidelines to the Atomic Weight Table (2011) and subsequent atomic weight tables and to indicate the atomic weights of such elements as ranges and, as before, those of other elements as single values with uncertainty.

Expression of Atomic Weight as Range

At present, the range is used for indicating the atomic weight for 12 elements: hydrogen, lithium, boron, carbon, nitrogen, oxygen, magnesium, silicon, sulfur, chlorine, bromine, and thallium. The isotope composition of these elements in samples collected on Earth or reagents is known to vary greatly. An atomic weight value and its uncertainty were previously defined so as to the range would be included, and an element having geological samples of which the range was not included was indicated by a ''g'' and an element possibly used as isotopes that had undergone artificial fractionation as a reagent was indicated by an ''m''. Furthermore, an ''r'' is attached to an element for which a precise atomic weight cannot be given due to such great range, no matter how much progress is made in techniques for measuring. The figure below shows the isotope compositions of hydrogen in various samples and corresponding atomic weights. The top line indicates the atomic weight range (1.00784–1.00811), and the second line indicates the atomic weight in the Atomic Weight Table (2010) (1.00794 ± 0.00007), followed by values measured in various samples. Black dots indicate values of typical isotope reference materials; the precision of measurement of the isotope composition of hydrogen is ± 0.000 000 05 according to ''best measurement''[5)], which is not more than 1/1000 of the uncertainty shown in the Atomic Weight Table (2010). Under such situation, expressing atomic weights as single values with uncertainty included the following problems:

• uncertainty of the atomic weight might be misunderstood as the precision of measurement;

• distribution of atomic weight values is not always a Gaussian distribution and depends on elements;

• a new measured value exceeding the current atomic weight range might cause modification of not only the uncertainty but also the atomic weight so as to include the new value; and

• discovering of a real substance having a defined atomic weight value is often difficult or rather impossible.

An atomic weight of such elements is represented not as a single value but as a range so as to include atomic weights in all known samples in this revision, which clearly shows that the atomic weight is not constant. Furthermore, the distribution within the range is not shown in the Atomic Weight Table and is various depending on elements[4]. The range should, therefore, be used with attention to the following points:

• the intermediate value of the range shall not be expressed as the atomic weight value and the half width of the range shall not be expressed as the uncertainty;

• the upper and lower limits themselves have no uncertainty although they are determined on the basis of values measured in ordinary substances on Earth in addition to measurement errors; and

• the atomic weight values are expressed in possible digits and should be expressed fully even if the last digit is zero.

1) IUPAC Inorganic Chemistry Division, CIAAW: Standard Atomic Weight of Ytterbium Revised, *Chem. Int.*, **37** (5-6), 26 (2015).

2) J. Meija *et al.*: Atomic Weights of the Elements 2015 (IUPAC Technical Report), *Pure Appl. Chem.*, to be published. J. Meija *et al.*: Atomic Weights of the Elements 2013 (IUPAC Technical Report), *Pure Appl. Chem.*, **88**, 265 (2016).

3) J. R. De Laeter *et al.*: Atomic Weights of the Elements: Review 2000 (IUPAC Technical Report), *Pure Appl. Chem.*, **75**, 683 (2003).

4) M. E. Wieser and T. B. Coplen: Atomic Weights of the Elements 2009 (IUPAC Technical Report), *Pure Appl. Chem.*, **83**, 359 (2011).

5) M. Berglund and M. E. Wieser: Isotopic Compositions of the Elements 2009 (IUPAC Technical Report), *Pure Appl. Chem.*, **83**, 397 (2011).

©2017 Atomic Weights Subcommittee of the Chemical Society of Japan

Standard Atomic Weights 2017

(Scaled to $A_r(^{12}C) = 12$, where ^{12}C is a neutral atom in its nuclear and electronic ground state.)

The atomic weights, $A_r(E)$, of many elements vary because of variations in the abundances of their isotopes in normal materials. For 12 such elements, an atomic-weight interval is given with the symbol $[a, b]$ to denote the set of atomic-weight values in normal materials; thus, $a \leq A_r(E) \leq b$ for the element E. The symbols a and b denote the bounds of the interval $[a, b]$. If a more accurate $A_r(E)$ value for a specific material is required, it should be determined. For 72 elements, $A_r(E)$ values and their evaluated uncertainties (in parentheses, following the last significant digit to which they are attributed) are given.

Name	Symbol	Atomic Number	Atomic Weight	Footnotes
Hydrogen	H	1	[1.00784, 1.00811]	m
Helium	He	2	4.002602(2)	g r
Lithium	Li	3	[6.938, 6.997]	m
Beryllium	Be	4	9.0121831(5)	
Boron	B	5	[10.806, 10.821]	m
Carbon	C	6	[12.0096, 12.0116]	
Nitrogen	N	7	[14.00643, 14.00728]	m
Oxygen	O	8	[15.99903, 15.99977]	m
Fluorine	F	9	18.998403163(6)	
Neon	Ne	10	20.1797(6)	g m
Sodium	Na	11	22.98976928(2)	
Magnesium	Mg	12	[24.304, 24.307]	
Aluminium (Aluminum)	Al	13	26.9815385(7)	
Silicon	Si	14	[28.084, 28.086]	
Phosphorus	P	15	30.973761998(5)	
Sulfur	S	16	[32.059, 32.076]	
Chlorine	Cl	17	[35.446, 35.457]	m
Argon	Ar	18	39.948(1)	g r
Potassium	K	19	39.0983(1)	
Calcium	Ca	20	40.078(4)	g
Scandium	Sc	21	44.955908(5)	
Titanium	Ti	22	47.867(1)	
Vanadium	V	23	50.9415(1)	
Chromium	Cr	24	51.9961(6)	
Manganese	Mn	25	54.938044(3)	
Iron	Fe	26	55.845(2)	
Cobalt	Co	27	58.933194(4)	
Nickel	Ni	28	58.6934(4)	r
Copper	Cu	29	63.546(3)	r
Zinc	Zn	30	65.38(2)	r
Gallium	Ga	31	69.723(1)	
Germanium	Ge	32	72.630(8)	
Arsenic	As	33	74.921595(6)	
Selenium	Se	34	78.971(8)	r
Bromine	Br	35	[79.901, 79.907]	
Krypton	Kr	36	83.798(2)	g m
Rubidium	Rb	37	85.4678(3)	g
Strontium	Sr	38	87.62(1)	g r
Yttrium	Y	39	88.90584(2)	
Zirconium	Zr	40	91.224(2)	g
Niobium	Nb	41	92.90637(2)	
Molybdenum	Mo	42	95.95(1)	g
Technetium*	Tc	43		
Ruthenium	Ru	44	101.07(2)	g
Rhodium	Rh	45	102.90550(2)	
Palladium	Pd	46	106.42(1)	g
Silver	Ag	47	107.8682(2)	g
Cadmium	Cd	48	112.414(4)	g
Indium	In	49	114.818(1)	
Tin	Sn	50	118.710(7)	g
Antimony	Sb	51	121.760(1)	g
Tellurium	Te	52	127.60(3)	g
Iodine	I	53	126.90447(3)	
Xenon	Xe	54	131.293(6)	g m
Caesium (Cesium)	Cs	55	132.9054519(2)	
Barium	Ba	56	137.327(7)	
lanthanum	La	57	138.90547(7)	g
Cerium	Ce	58	140.116(1)	g
Praseodymium	Pr	59	140.90766(2)	
Neodymium	Nd	60	144.242(3)	g
Promethium*	Pm	61		
Samarium	Sm	62	150.36(2)	g
Europium	Eu	63	151.964(1)	g
Gadolinium	Gd	64	157.25(3)	g
Terbium	Tb	65	158.92535(2)	
Dysprosium	Dy	66	162.500(1)	g
Holmium	Ho	67	164.93033(2)	
Erbium	Er	68	167.259(3)	g
Thulium	Tm	69	168.93422(2)	
Ytterbium	Yb	70	173.045(10)	g
Lutetium	Lu	71	174.9668(1)	g
Hafnium	Hf	72	178.49(2)	
Tantalum	Ta	73	180.94788(2)	
Tungsten	W	74	183.84(1)	
Rhenium	Re	75	186.207(1)	
Osmium	Os	76	190.23(3)	g
Iridium	Ir	77	192.217(3)	
Platinum	Pt	78	195.084(9)	
Gold	Au	79	196.966569(5)	
Mercury	Hg	80	200.592(3)	
Thallium	Tl	81	[204.382, 204.385]	
Lead	Pb	82	207.2(1)	g r
Bismuth*	Bi	83	208.98040(1)	
Polonium*	Po	84		
Astatine*	At	85		
Radon*	Rn	86		
Francium*	Fr	87		
Radium*	Ra	88		
Actinium*	Ac	89		
Thorium*	Th	90	232.0377(4)	g
Protactinium*	Pa	91	231.03588(2)	
Uranium*	U	92	238.02891(3)	g m
Neptunium*	Np	93		
Plutonium*	Pu	94		
Americium*	Am	95		
Curium*	Cm	96		
Berkelium*	Bk	97		
Californium*	Cf	98		
Einsteinium*	Es	99		
Fermium*	Fm	100		
Mendelevium*	Md	101		
Nobelium*	No	102		
Lawrencium*	Lr	103		
Rutherfordium*	Rf	104		

Name	Symbol	Atomic Number	Atomic Weight	Footnotes
Dubnium*	Db	105		
Seaborgium*	Sg	106		
Bohrium*	Bh	107		
Hassium*	Hs	108		
Meitnerium*	Mt	109		
Darmstadtium*	Ds	110		
Roentgenium*	Rg	111		
Copernicium*	Cn	112		
Nihonium*	Nh	113		
Flerovium*	Fl	114		
Moscovium*	Mc	115		
Livermorium*	Lv	116		
Tennessine*	Ts	117		
Oganesson*	Og	118		

*: Element has no stable isotopes. However, four elements (Bi, Th, Pa, and U) do have a characteristic isotopic composition, and for these elements, standard atomic weights are tabulated.

g: Geological specimens are known in which the element has an isotopic composition outside the limits for normal material. The difference between the atomic weight of the element in such specimens and that given in the table may exceed the stated uncertainty.

m: Modified isotopic compositions may be found in com-mercially available material because the material has been subjected to an undisclosed or inadvertent isotopic fractionation. Substantial deviations in atomic weight of the element from that given in the table can occur.

r: Range in isotopic composition of normal terrestrial material prevents a more precise A_r(E) being given: the tabulated A_r(E) value and uncertainty should be appli-cable to normal material.

©2017 Atomic Weights Subcommittee of the Chemical Society of Japan

Standard Atomic Weights 2010

(Scaled to $A_r(^{12}C)$ = 12, where ^{12}C is a neutral atom in its nuclear and electronic ground state)

The atomic weights of many elements are not invariant but depend on the origin and treatment of the material. The standard values of $A_r(E)$ and the uncertainties (in parentheses, following the last significant figure to which they are attributed) apply to elements of natural terrestrial origin. The footnotes to this table elaborate the types of variation which may occur for individual elements and which may be larger than the listed uncertainties of values of $A_r(E)$. Names of elements with atomic number 112 to 118 are provisional.

Name	Symbol	Atomic Number	Atomic Weight	Footnotes
Hydrogen	H	1	1.00794(7)	g m r
Helium	He	2	4.002602(2)	g r
Lithium	Li	3	[6.941(2)]†	g m r
Beryllium	Be	4	9.012182(3)	
Boron	B	5	10.811(7)	g m r
Carbon	C	6	12.0107(8)	g r
Nitrogen	N	7	14.0067(2)	g r
Oxygen	O	8	15.9994(3)	g r
Fluorine	F	9	18.9984032(5)	
Neon	Ne	10	20.1797(6)	g m
Sodium	Na	11	22.98976928(2)	
Magnesium	Mg	12	24.3050(6)	
Aluminium	Al	13	26.9815386(8)	
Silicon	Si	14	28.0855(3)	r
Phosphorus	P	15	30.973762(2)	
Sulfur	S	16	32.065(5)	g r
Chlorine	Cl	17	35.453(2)	g m r
Argon	Ar	18	39.948(1)	g r
Potassium	K	19	39.0983(1)	
Calcium	Ca	20	40.078(4)	g
Scandium	Sc	21	44.955912(6)	
Titanium	Ti	22	47.867(1)	
Vanadium	V	23	50.9415(1)	
Chromium	Cr	24	51.9961(6)	
Manganese	Mn	25	54.938045(5)	
Iron	Fe	26	55.845(2)	
Cobalt	Co	27	58.933195(5)	
Nickel	Ni	28	58.6934(4)	r
Copper	Cu	29	63.546(3)	r
Zinc	Zn	30	65.38(2)	r
Gallium	Ga	31	69.723(1)	
Germanium	Ge	32	72.64(1)	
Arsenic	As	33	74.92160(2)	
Selenium	Se	34	78.96(3)	r
Bromine	Br	35	79.904(1)	
Krypton	Kr	36	83.798(2)	g m
Rubidium	Rb	37	85.4678(3)	g
Strontium	Sr	38	87.62(1)	g r
Yttrium	Y	39	88.90585(2)	
Zirconium	Zr	40	91.224(2)	g
Niobium	Nb	41	92.90638(2)	
Molybdenum	Mo	42	95.96(2)	g r
Technetium*	Tc	43		
Ruthenium	Ru	44	101.07(2)	g
Rhodium	Rh	45	102.90550(2)	

Name	Symbol	Atomic Number	Atomic Weight	Footnotes
Palladium	Pd	46	106.42(1)	g
Silver	Ag	47	107.8682(2)	g
Cadmium	Cd	48	112.411(8)	g
Indium	In	49	114.818(3)	
Tin	Sn	50	118.710(7)	g
Antimony	Sb	51	121.760(1)	g
Tellurium	Te	52	127.60(3)	g
Iodine	I	53	126.90447(3)	
Xenon	Xe	54	131.293(6)	g m
Caesium (Cesium)	Cs	55	132.9054519(2)	
Barium	Ba	56	137.327(7)	
Lanthanum	La	57	138.90547(7)	g
Cerium	Ce	58	140.116(1)	g
Praseodymium	Pr	59	140.90765(2)	
Neodymium	Nd	60	144.242(3)	g
Promethium*	Pm	61		
Samarium	Sm	62	150.36(2)	g
Europium	Eu	63	151.964(1)	g
Gadolinium	Gd	64	157.25(3)	g
Terbium	Tb	65	158.92535(2)	
Dysprosium	Dy	66	162.500(1)	g
Holmium	Ho	67	164.93032(2)	
Erbium	Er	68	167.259(3)	g
Thulium	Tm	69	168.93421(2)	
Ytterbium	Yb	70	173.054(5)	g
Lutetium	Lu	71	174.9668(1)	g
Hafnium	Hf	72	178.49(2)	
Tantalum	Ta	73	180.94788(2)	
Tungsten	W	74	183.84(1)	
Rhenium	Re	75	186.207(1)	
Osmium	Os	76	190.23(3)	g
Iridium	Ir	77	192.217(3)	
Platinum	Pt	78	195.084(9)	
Gold	Au	79	196.966569(4)	
Mercury	Hg	80	200.59(2)	
Thallium	Tl	81	204.3833(2)	
Lead	Pb	82	207.2(1)	g r
Bismuth*	Bi	83	208.98040(1)	
Polonium*	Po	84		
Astatine*	At	85		
Radon*	Rn	86		
Francium*	Fr	87		
Radium*	Ra	88		
Actinium*	Ac	89		
Thorium*	Th	90	232.03806(2)	g
Protactinium*	Pa	91	231.03588(2)	
Uranium*	U	92	238.02891(3)	g m
Neptunium*	Np	93		
Plutonium*	Pu	94		
Americium*	Am	95		
Curium*	Cm	96		
Berkelium*	Bk	97		
Californium*	Cf	98		
Einsteinium*	Es	99		
Fermium*	Fm	100		
Mendelevium*	Md	101		
Nobelium*	No	102		
Lawrencium*	Lr	103		
Rutherfordium*	Rf	104		
Dubnium*	Db	105		
Seaborgium*	Sg	106		
Bohrium*	Bh	107		
Hassium*	Hs	108		

Name	Symbol	Atomic Number	Atomic Weight	Footnotes
Meitnerium*	Mt	109		
Darmstadtium*	Ds	110		
Roentgenium	Rg	111		
Copernicium*	Cn	112		
Ununtrium*	Uut	113		
Ununquadium*	Uuq	114		
Ununpentium*	Uup	115		
Ununhexium*	Uuh	116		
Ununoctium*	Uuo	118		

*: Element has no stable isotopes.

†: Commercially available Li materials have atomic weights that range between 6.939 and 6.996; if a more accurate value is required, it must be determined for the specific material.

g: Geological specimens are known in which the element has an isotopic composition outside the limits for normal material. The difference between the atomic weight of the element in such specimens and that given in the table may exceed the stated uncertainty.

m: Modified isotopic compositions may be found in commercially available material because it has been subjected to an undisclosed or inadvertent isotopic fractionation. Substantial deviations in atomic weight of the element from that given in the table can occur.

r: Range in isotopic composition of normal terrestrial material prevents a more precise $A_r(E)$ being given: the tabulated $A_r(E)$ value should be applicable to any normal material.

©2010 Atomic Weights Subcommittee of the Chemical Society of Japan

INDEX

A

D

E

F

G

H

I

J

K

L

Q

R

S

T

U

V

W

X

Y

Z

INDEX IN LATIN NAME

INDEX IN JAPANSE

ア

イ

ウ

エ

オ

カ

キ

ク

ケ

コ

サ

シ

ス

ツ

テ

ト

ナ

ニ

ネ

ノ

ハ

ヒ

フ

へ

Addenda

Information about Columns for Japanese Pharmacopoeia Draft Monographs (Chemical Drug)

Pharmaceuticals and Medical Devices Agency Office of Review Management

September 1, 2021

In accordance with the policy for "Disclosure of Information about Columns for Japanese Pharmacopoeia Draft Monographs (by Division of Pharmacopoeia and Standards for Drugs, Office of Standards and Guidelines Development, Pharmaceuticals and Medical Devices Agency, dated March 1, 2016)" (see Annex), the information about the columns that were used for acquisition of the data that were referred in the preparation of the drafts for public comments is as follows:

Monograph	Test	Brand Name	Posting Date
Azosemide Tablets	Uniformity of dosage units, Assay	SunFire C18	June 1, 2016
Bicalutamide	Purity (2) Related substances, Assay	Kromasil C18	September 2, 2019
Bromfenac Sodium Hydrate	Purity (2) Related substances, Assay	YMC-Pack ODS-A	March 1, 2018
Bromfenac Sodium Ophthalmic Solution	Assay	CAPCELL PAK C18 SG120Å	March 1, 2018
Cefalotin Sodium for Injection	Purity (2) Related substances, Assay	Inertsil ODS-3	September 1, 2017
Cefixime Fine Granules	Purity Related substances, Uniformity of dosage units, Dissolution, Assay	Inertsil ODS-3	March 1, 2018
Celecoxib	Purity (2) Related substances, Assay	SUPELCOSIL LC-DP	September 2, 2019
Clomipramine Hydrochloride Tablets	Uniformity of dosage units, Assay	Wakosil 10C18	September 1, 2016
Cloperastine Fendizoate	Purity (3) 4-Chlorobenzophenone	L-column ODS	September 30, 2019
Cloperastine Fendizoate Tablets	Uniformity of dosage units, Assay	L-column ODS	September 30, 2019
	Dissolution	TSKgel ODS-80Ts	
Copovidone	Purity (4)	Inertsil ODS-4	June 3, 2019
	Purity (7)	Inertsil ODS-3	
Diclofenac Sodium Suppositories	Assay	NUCLEOSIL 5C18 LICHROSPHER PR18-5	September 1, 2017
Doripenem Hydrate	Purity (3) Related substances (i), Assay	L-column ODS	March 1, 2018
	Purity (3) Related substances (ii)	Kaseisorb LC ODS-SAX Super	
	Purity (3) Related substances (iii)	Cadenza CD-C18	
Doripenem for Injection	Purity (2) Related substances (i), Assay	L-column ODS	March 1, 2018
	Purity (2) Related substances (ii)	Kaseisorb LC ODS-SAX Super	
Dorzolamide Hydrochloride and Timolol Maleate Ophthalmic Solution	Identification (1), Purity (1) Related substances 1, Assay (1) Dorzolamide hydrochloride	Zorbax Rx-C8 5μm 4.6mm×25cm	September 2, 2019
	Identification (2), Purity (2) Related substances 2, Assay (2) Timolol maleate	Inertsil ODS-2 5μm 4.6mm×25cm	
Entacapone	Purity (2) Related substances, Assay	XTerra Phenyl, YMC-Pack Ph	September 1, 2016
Entacapone Tablets	Uniformity of dosage units, Assay	XTerra Phenyl	September 1, 2016

(2) *Addenda*

Eribulin Mesilate	Identification (2), Assay (2) Methanesulfonic acid	Zorbax NH2 5μm 4.6mm×25cm	September 30, 2019
	Purity (2) Related substances, Assay (1) Eribulin mesilate	ACE 3 C18 3μm 3.0mm×15cm	
Ethyl Loflazepate	Purity (4) Related substances	TSKgel ODS-80TM	September 2, 2019
	Assay	Develosil ODS-7	
Ethyl Loflazepate Tablets	Uniformity of dosage units, Dissolution, Assay	Inertsil ODS-3	September 2, 2019
Ethylcellulose	Assay	HP-1, Rtx-1	December 1, 2017
Felodipine	Purity (2) Related substances	L-Column ODS	March 1, 2018
Felodipine Tablets	Uniformity of dosage units, Dissolution, Assay	L-Column ODS	March 1, 2018
Fenofibrate	Purity (2) Related substances, Assay	YMC-Pack Pro C18	September 2, 2019
Fenofibrate Tablets	Purity Related substances	CAPCELL PAK C18 UG80	September 2, 2019
	Uniformity of dosage units, Dissolution, Assay	YMC-Pack ODS-AM	
Fludiazepam Tablets	Uniformity of dosage units, Assay	YMC-Pack ODS-AM	September 3, 2018
	Dissolution	μ BONDASPHERE 5μ C18-100A	
Gatifloxacin Hydrate	Purity (3) Related substances, Assay	Inertsil ODS-2	December 1, 2017
Gatifloxacin Ophthalmic Solution	Purity Related substances, Assay	Inertsil ODS-2	December 1, 2017
Gefitinib	Purity (2) Related substances, Assay	Inertsil ODS-3 C18	September 2, 2019
Glucagon (Genetical Recombination)	Identification (1)	Lichrospher 100 RP18	September 2, 2019
	Identification (2), Purity, Assay	ACE 3 C18	
Purified Glucose	Identification (2), Purity (3) Related substances, Assay	BIORAD Aminex HPX-87C	June 1, 2016
Glucose Hydrate	Identification (2), Purity (3) Related substances, Assay	BIORAD Aminex HPX-87C	June 1, 2016
Hydroxyethylcellulose	Assay	HP-1, Rtx-1	December 1, 2017
Irbesartan Tablets	Uniformity of dosage units, Assay	YMC-Pack ODS-A	September 1, 2016
Irbesartan and Amlodipine Besilate Tablets	Dissolution, Identification (1) (2), Uniformity of dosage units (1) (2), Assay (1) (2)	Shim-pack XR-ODSII	June 1, 2016
Irinotecan Hydrochloride Hydrate	Purity Related substances	Inertsil ODS-2	March 1, 2018
Irinotecan Hydrochloride Injection	Purity Related substances, Assay	Inertsil ODS-2	September 2, 2019
Lanoconazole	Purity Related substances, Assay	Inertsil ODS-2	December 1, 2017
Lanoconazole Cream	Assay	Inertsil ODS-2	December 1, 2017
Lanoconazole Cutaneous Solution	Assay	Inertsil ODS-2	December 1, 2017
Lanoconazole Ointment	Assay	Inertsil ODS-2	December 1, 2017
Miglitol Tablets	Uniformity of dosage units, Dissolution, Assay	Asahipak NH2P-50 4D	June 1, 2018
Pazufloxacin Mesilate	Purity (2) Related substances	Inertsil ODS-2	March 1, 2016
	Assay	Nucleosil 100-10C18	

Pazufloxacin Mesilate Injection	Assay	Nucleosil 100-10C_{18}	September 1, 2016
Pentobarbital Calcium Tablets	Uniformity of dosage units, Assay	L-Column ODS, Inertsil ODS-3	March 1, 2016
Phenobarbital Tablets	Uniformity of dosage units, Assay	Mightysil RP-18 GP-II	September 30, 2019
Pitavastatin Calcium Orally Disintegrating Tablets	Purity, Uniformity of dosage units, Assay	L-column ODS	September 30, 2019
	Dissolution	L-column2 ODS	
Polaprezinc	Purity Related substances, Assay	Mightysil RP18GP L-Column ODS	March 1, 2018
Polaprezinc Granules	Uniformity of dosage units, Assay	L-Column ODS Symmetry C18	March 1, 2018
Rilmazafone Hydrochloride Hydrate	Purity (2) Related substances	L-column ODS 5μm 4.6×250 mm	September 2, 2019
	Assay	L-column ODS 5μm 4.6×150 mm	
Rilmazafone Hydrochloride Tablets	Uniformity of dosage units, Dissolution, Assay	L-column ODS 5μm 4.6×150 mm	September 2, 2019
Ritodrine Hydrochloride Injection	Assay	YMC-Pack Pro C8	September 1, 2017
Rosuvastatin Calcium	Purity (3) Related substances, Assay	Inertsil ODS-3 C18 3μm 100Å	September 2, 2019
	Purity (4) Enantiomer	CHIRALCEL OJ-RH	
Rosuvastatin Calcium Tablets	Purity Related substances, Assay	Columbus 5μC18 110A	September 2, 2019
	Dissolution	Spherisorb S5 ODS2	
Silodosin Orally Disintegrating Tablets	Identification, Purity Related substances, Uniformity of dosage units, Dissolution, Assay	Inertsil ODS-3	September 30, 2019
Sitagliptin Phosphate Hydrate	Purity (1) Related substances, Assay	Supelco Discovery Cyano	December 1, 2017
	Purity (2) Enantiomer	Diacel AD-H	
Sitagliptin Phosphate Tablets	Identification (2), Purity Related substances, Uniformity of dosage units, Dissolution, Assay	Supelco Discovery Cyano	December 1, 2017
Sodium Valproate Extended-release Tablets A	Uniformity of dosage units, Dissolution, Assay	Develosil ODS-UG-5	March 1, 2018
Sodium Valproate Extended-release Tablets B	Uniformity of dosage units, Dissolution, Assay	Develosil ODS-UG-5	March 1, 2018
Telmisartan and Amlodipine Besilate Tablets	Uniformity of dosage units, Dissolution, Assay	Inertsil C8-3 (5μm 3.0×75mm)	June 3, 2019
Telmisartan and Hydrochlorothiazide Tablets	Identification (1) (2), Purity Related substances, Uniformity of dosage units (1) (2), Dissolution (1) (2), Assay (1) (2)	Inertsil C8-3	March 1, 2018
Tramadol Hydrochloride	Purity (3) Related substances (ii)	LiChrospher 60 RP-select B	September 1, 2016
Valsartan and Hydrochlorothiazide Tablets	Uniformity of dosage units (1) (2), Dissolution (1) (2), Assay (1) (2)	Nucleosil 100-5 C18	March 1, 2018
Verapamil Hydrochloride Injection	Assay	Mightysil RP-18GP	December 1, 2017
Zonisamide	Purity (4) Related substances, Assay	Develosil ODS-5	March 1, 2016

(4) *Addenda*

Monographs listed in the "Information about Columns for Japanese Pharmacopoeia Draft Monographs (Chemical Drug) (by Division of Pharmacopoeia and Standards for Drugs, Office of Standards and Guidelines Development, Pharmaceuticals and Medical Devices Agency, dated September, 2021)" that were not included in the above table and the reasons for not including are listed below.

Monographs postponed to be listed for Supplement I to the JP17.

Acarbose	September 1, 2016
Acarbose Tablets	September 1, 2016

A monograph postponed to be listed for Supplement II to the JP17.

Dexamethasone Sodium Phosphate	September 1, 2017

Monographs to be listed for Supplement I to the JP18.

Anastrozole
Anastrozole Tablets
Bicalutamide Tablets
Budesonide
Oxybutynin Hydrochloride
Temozolomide
Temozolomide Capsules
Temozolomide for Injection
Voglibose Orally Disintegrating Tablets

Annex

March 1, 2016

Disclosure of Information about Columns for Japanese Pharmacopoeia Draft Monographs

Division of Pharmacopoeia and Standards for Drugs,
Office of Standards and Guidelines Development,
Pharmaceuticals and Medical Devices Agency

Please be notified that the division of Pharmacopoeia and Standards for Drugs, Office of Standards and Guidelines Development, Pharmaceuticals and Medical Devices Agency (PMDA) starts to take a measure to in principle disclose the information about columns, such as the name (model number) of columns, for Japanese Pharmacopoeia (JP) draft monographs (hereinafter excluding the draft monographs for crude drugs) under the following rules:

1. Concerning tests as a whole using columns in the draft monographs, while further ensuring of transparency of the JP revision process is required, the measure mentioned above is to post the information about the columns that were used for acquisition of the data that were referred in the preparation of the drafts on the PMDA website by PMDA at the start of publication of the relevant drafts for public comments.
2. This disclosure is principally provided for ensuring of enhancement of public comments by wide sharing of the information 1 above with stakeholders other than the manufacturers who prepared the drafts at the time of publication for public comments. Thus, addition of information about other alternative columns or update of information associated with technological innovation is in principle not to be done.
3. The columns to be disclosed have not been confirmed as applicable to all the samples that could be the subjects to application to the monographs of the relevant drafts.
4. The information about columns are released only when cooperation is provided by the manufactures who prepared the drafts.

June 1, 2018

Disclosure of Information about Columns for Japanese Pharmacopoeia Draft Monographs for Crude Drugs

Office of Standards and Guidelines Development,
Pharmaceuticals and Medical Devices Agency

The products in the Official Monographs for Crude Drugs are composed of multicomponent systems as a characteristic of natural products, and the compositions and the quantitative values of constituents are diversified within a certain range due to differences in secondary metabolites, growth environments, cultivation conditions, genetic factors and processing methods of the original plants. For that reason, it is necessary to select column(s) depending on the test sample for assay of each manufacturer or each manufacturers association even for the test of the same monograph. The expert committees for crude drugs gathers the test results of multiple samples and discusses on the draft monograph with the multiple data. It would be valuable to share with the public by disclosing the information about columns that were evaluated in the development of monograph. Thus, please be notified that Office of Standards and Guidelines Development, Pharmaceuticals and Medical Devices Agency (PMDA) starts to take a measure to in principle disclose the information about columns, such as the name (model number) of columns, for Japanese Pharmacopoeia (JP) draft monographs (crude drugs) under the following rules:

1. Concerning tests as a whole using columns in the draft monographs (crude drugs), while further ensuring of transparency of the JP revision process is required, the measure mentioned above is to post the information about the columns that were used for acquisition of the data that were referred in the preparation of the drafts on the PMDA website by PMDA at the start of publication of the relevant drafts for public comments.

2. Addition of information about other alternative columns or update of information associated with technological innovation is in principle not to be done.

3. The columns to be disclosed have not been confirmed as applicable to all the samples that could be the subjects to application to the monographs of the relevant drafts.

4. The information about columns are released only when cooperation is provided by the manufactures or manufacturers association who prepared the drafts.

Disclosure History:
Extracts, the crude drugs and preparations to be included Supplement II to the Japanese Pharmacopoeia 17th edition, June 1, 2018.
Extracts, the crude drugs and preparations to be included Supplement I to the Japanese Pharmacopoeia 17th edition, January 4, 2017.
Extracts, the crude drugs and preparations included the Japanese Pharmacopoeia 17th edition, January 4, 2017.

(6) *Addenda*

Extracts, the crude drugs and preparations to be included the Japanese Pharmacopoeia 18th edition

Bakumondoto Extract: Ginsenoside Rb_1
(Column: Particle size 5μm, 4.6mmID×25cm)

Brand Name
TSKgel Amide-80 HR

Bakumondoto Extract: Glycyrrhizic Acid
(Column: Particle size 5μm, 4.6mmID×15cm)

Brand Name
CAPCELL PAK C_{18} UG120
COSMOSIL 5C_{18}-MS-II
Mightysil RP-18 GP
TSKgel ODS-80T_S QA
YMC-Pack ODS-A
YMC-Pack *Pro* C18

Bofutsushosan Extract: Paeoniflorin
(Column: Particle size 5μm, 4.6mmID×15cm)

Brand Name
Atlantis dC_{18}
Atlantis T3
COSMOSIL 5C_{18}-AR-II
Inertsil ODS-2
Inertsil ODS-3
Inertsil ODS-4
L-column2 ODS
Nucleosil 5C18
TSKgel ODS-100Z
TSKgel ODS-80T_S
TSKgel ODS-80T_S QA
YMC-Pack ODS-A
YMC-Pack *Pro* C18
YMC-Triart C18

Bofutsushosan Extract: Total alkaloids (ephedrine and pseudoephedrine)
(Column: Particle size 5μm, 4.6mmID×15cm)

Brand Name
COSMOSIL 5C_{18}-MS-II
Develosil ODS-UG-5
Inertsil ODS-2
Inertsil ODS-4
L-column2 ODS
Mightysil RP-18GP
TSKgel ODS-120A
TSKgel ODS-80T_M
TSKgel ODS-80T_S
TSKgel ODS-80T_S QA
Wakosil 5C18
YMC-Pack ODS-A

Bofutsushosan Extract: Baicalin
(Column: Particle size 5μm, 4.6mmID×15cm)

Brand Name
Atlantis dC_{18}
Atlantis T3
COSMOSIL 5C_{18}-AR-II
Develosil ODS-HG-5
Inertsil ODS-2
Inertsil ODS-3
Inertsil ODS-4
Inertsil ODS-4V
Mightysil RP-18GP
TSKgel ODS-80T_S
TSKgel ODS-80T_S QA
Wakosil 5C18
YMC-Pack ODS-A
YMC-Pack *Pro* C18

Bofutsushosan Extract: Glycyrrhizic Acid
(Column: Particle size 5μm, 4.6mmID×15cm)

Brand Name
Atlantis dC_{18}
CAPCELL PAK C_{18} UG120
Inertsil ODS-2
L-column ODS
L-column2 ODS
Mightysil RP-18 GP
TSKgel ODS-80T_S
TSKgel ODS-80T_S QA
YMC-Pack ODS-A
YMC-Pack *Pro* C18

Boiogito Extract: Sinomenine
(Column: Particle size 5μm, 4.6mmID×15cm)

Brand Name
Atlantis T3
Inertsil ODS-3V
Inertsil ODS-4
Mightysil RP-18GP
TSKgel ODS-100V
TSKgel ODS-120A
TSKgel ODS-80T_S
TSKgel ODS-80T_S QA
Wakosil 5C18
YMC-Pack ODS-A
YMC-Pack *Pro* C18

Boiogito Extract: Glycyrrhizic Acid
(Column: Particle size 5μm, 4.6mmID×15cm)

Brand Name
CAPCELL PAK C_{18} UG120
COSMOSIL 5C_{18}-AR-II
Mightysil RP-18 GP
TSKgel ODS-80T_S
TSKgel ODS-80T_S QA
YMC-Pack ODS-A
YMC-Pack *Pro* C18

Byakkokaninjinto Extract: Mangiferin
(Column: Particle size 5μm, 4.6mmID×15cm)

Brand Name
TSKgel ODS-80Ts
TSKgel ODS-80Ts QA
YMC-Pack ODS-A

Byakkokaninjinto Extract: Glycyrrhizic acid
(Column: Particle size 5μm, 4.6mmID×15cm)

Brand Name
CHEMCOSORB 5-ODS-H
COSMOSIL 5C$_{18}$-MS-II
Mightysil RP-18 GP
TSKgel ODS-80Ts
TSKgel ODS-80Ts QA
YMC-Pack ODS-A

Byakkokaninjinto Extract: Ginsenoside Rb$_1$
For the preparation 1)
(Column: Particle size 3.5μm, 4.6mmID×15cm)

Brand Name
XBridge Amide

For the preparation 2)
(Column: Particle size 5μm, 4.6mmID×15cm)

Brand Name
TSK-gel Amide-80 HR

Chotosan Extract: Hesperidin
(Column: Particle size 5μm, 4.6mmID×15cm)

Brand Name
Atlantis dC$_{18}$
Mightysil RP-18GP
Symmetry C$_{18}$
TSKgel ODS-100S
TSKgel ODS-100V
XTerra MS C18

Chotosan Extract: Glycyrrhizic Acid
(Column: Particle size 5μm, 4.6mmID×15cm)

Brand Name
Mightysil RP-18 GP
TSKgel ODS-80Ts QA
YMC-Pack ODS-A
YMC-Pack *Pro* C18

Chotosan Extract: Total alkaloid (rhyncophylline and hirsutine)
(Column: Particle size 5μm, 4.6mmID×15cm)

Brand Name
Atlantis dC$_{18}$
CAPCELL PAK C$_{18}$ UG120
COSMOSIL 5C$_{18}$
COSMOSIL 5C$_{18}$-AR-II
COSMOSIL 5C$_{18}$-MS-II
Develosil ODS-5
Develosil ODS-HG-5
Inertsil ODS-3V
L-column ODS
L-column2 ODS
Mightysil RP-18GP
TSKgel ODS-120A
TSKgel ODS-80T$_M$
TSKgel ODS-80T$_S$
TSKgel ODS-80T$_S$ QA
YMC-Pack ODS-A
YMC-Pack ODS-AM
YMC-Pack *Pro* C18

Daiokanzoto Extract: Sennoside A
(Column: Particle size 5μm, 4.6mmID×15cm)

Brand Name
CHEMCOSORB 5-ODS-H
Develosil ODS-5
Develosil ODS-UG-5
Mightysil RP-18GP
Mightysil RP-18GP Aqua
Puresil C18
TSKgel ODS-80T$_S$
TSKgel ODS-80T$_S$ QA
Unisil NQ 5C18
YMC-Pack ODS-A

Daiokanzoto Extract: Glycyrrhizic Acid
(Column: Particle size 5μm, 4.6mmID×15cm)

Brand Name
CHEMCOSORB 5-ODS-H
COSMOSIL 5C$_{18}$-AR-II
Develosil ODS-5
L-column2 ODS
Mightysil RP-18 GP
TSKgel ODS-80T$_S$
TSKgel ODS-80T$_S$ QA
YMC-Pack ODS-A
YMC-Pack *Pro* C18

Daisaikoto Extract: Saikosaponin b$_2$
(Column: Particle size 5μm, 4.6mmID×15cm)

Brand Name
Ascentis Express C18
Atlantis T3
CHEMCOSORB 5-ODS-H
Develosil ODS-5
Develosil ODS-HG-5
Inertsil ODS-4V
Mightysil RP-18GP
TSKgel ODS-100V
TSKgel ODS-120A
TSKgel ODS-80T$_S$
TSKgel ODS-80T$_S$ QA
Wakosil 5C18
XBridge C$_{18}$
YMC-Pack ODS-A
YMC-Pack ODS-AM
YMC-Pack *Pro* C18

Daisaikoto Extract: Baicalin
(Column: Particle size 5μm, 4.6mmID×15cm)

Brand Name
Ascentis Express C18
Atlantis dC$_{18}$
Atlantis T3
COSMOSIL 5C$_{18}$
COSMOSIL 5C$_{18}$-AR-II
COSMOSIL 5C$_{18}$-MS-II
Develosil ODS-HG-5
Inertsil ODS-3
Inertsil ODS-4V
L-column2 ODS
Mightysil RP-18GP
TSKgel ODS-80T$_M$
TSKgel ODS-80T$_S$
TSKgel ODS-80T$_S$ QA
Wakosil 5C18
Wakosil-II 5C18 AR
YMC-Pack ODS-A
YMC-Pack *Pro* C18

Daisaikoto Extract: Paeoniflorin
(Column: Particle size 5μm, 4.6mmID×15cm)

Brand Name
Atlantis dC$_{18}$
Atlantis T3
Develosil ODS-HG-5
Hydrosphere C18
Inertsil ODS-3
Inertsil ODS-3V
Nucleosil 5C18
TSKgel ODS-100Z
TSKgel ODS-80T$_M$
TSKgel ODS-80T$_S$
TSKgel ODS-80T$_S$ QA
Wakosil-II 5C18 AR
YMC-Pack ODS-A
YMC-Pack *Pro* C18
YMC-Triart C18

Goreisan Extract: (*E*)-Cinnamic acid
(Column: Particle size 5μm, 4.6mmID×15cm)

Brand Name
CAPCELL PAK C$_{18}$ SG120
COSMOSIL 5C$_{18}$-AR-II
COSMOSIL 5C$_{18}$-MS-II
Mightysil RP-18 GP
TSKgel ODS-100S
TSKgel ODS-80T$_M$
TSKgel ODS-80T$_S$
TSKgel ODS-80T$_S$ QA
Wakosil II 5C18HG
YMC-Pack ODS-A

Goshajinkigan Extract: Loganin
(Column: Particle size 5μm, 4.6mmID×15cm)

Brand Name
Atlantis dC$_{18}$
Cadenza 5CD-C18
COSMOSIL 5C$_{18}$-AR-II
Develosil ODS-5
Mightysil RP-18GP
Mightysil RP-18GP Aqua
Symmetry C$_{18}$
TSKgel ODS-100S
TSKgel ODS-80T$_S$
TSKgel ODS-80T$_S$ QA

Goshajinkigan Extract: Paeoniflorin
(Column: Particle size 5μm, 4.6mmID×15cm)

Brand Name
Atlantis dC$_{18}$
COSMOSIL 5C$_{18}$-AR-II
Develosil ODS-HG-5
Nucleosil 5C18
YMC-Pack ODS-A

Goshajinkigan Extract: Total alkaloids (as benzoylmesaconine hydrochloride and 14-anisoylaconine hydrochloride, or as benzoylmesaconine hydrochloride and benzoylhypaconine hydrochloride)
(Column: Particle size 5μm, 4.6mmID×15cm)

Brand Name
Atlantis dC$_{18}$
Cadenza 5CD-C18
Mightysil RP-18GP
TSKgel ODS-80T$_M$
TSKgel ODS-80T$_S$
TSKgel ODS-80T$_S$ QA
YMC-Pack ODS-A

Goshuyuto Extract: Evodiamine
(Column: Particle size 5μm, 4.6mmID×15cm)

Brand Name
L-column2 ODS
Mightysil RP-18 GP
TSKgel ODS-100S
TSKgel ODS-80T$_S$
TSKgel ODS-80T$_S$ QA
Wakosil 5C18
YMC-Pack ODS-AM

Goshuyuto Extract: [6]-gingerol
(Column: Particle size 5μm, 4.6mmID×15cm)

Brand Name
L-column2 ODS
Mightysil RP-18 GP
TSKgel ODS-100S
TSKgel ODS-80T$_S$
TSKgel ODS-80T$_S$ QA
Wakosil 5C18
YMC-Pack ODS-AM

Goshuyuto Extract: Ginsenoside Rb$_1$
(Column: Particle size 5μm, 4.6mmID×15cm)

Brand Name
TSK-gel Amide-80 HR

Hachimijiogan Extract: Loganin
(Column: Particle size 5μm, 4.6mmID×15cm)

Brand Name
Atlantis dC_{18}
Cadenza 5CD-C18
CAPCELL PAK C_{18} MG
CHEMCOSORB 5-ODS-H
COSMOSIL 5C_{18}-AR-II
Develosil ODS-HG-5
Mightysil RP-18GP
Mightysil RP-18GP Aqua
Symmetry C_{18}
TSKgel ODS-100S
TSKgel ODS-80T_S
TSKgel ODS-80T_S QA
YMC-Pack ODS-A

Hachimijiogan Extract: Paeoniflorin
(Column: Particle size 5μm, 4.6mmID×15cm)

Brand Name
Atlantis dC_{18}
COSMOSIL 5C_{18}-AR-II
Develosil ODS-HG-5
Develosil ODS-UG-5
Hydrosphere C18
Nucleosil 5C18
TSKgel ODS-80T_M
TSKgel ODS-80T_S
TSKgel ODS-80T_S QA
YMC-Pack ODS-A
YMC-Triart C18

Hachimijiogan Extract: Total alkaloids (as benzoylmesaconine hydrochloride and 14-anisoylaconine hydrochloride, or as benzoylmesaconine hydrochloride and benzoylhypaconine hydrochloride)
(Column: Particle size 5μm, 4.6mmID×15cm)

Brand Name
Atlantis dC_{18}
Cadenza 5CD-C18
Inertsil ODS-3
Mightysil RP-18GP
TSKgel ODS-120A
TSKgel ODS-80T_M
TSKgel ODS-80T_S
TSKgel ODS-80T_S QA
Wakosil 5C18
XBridge C_{18}
YMC-Pack ODS-A

Hangekobokuto Extract: Magnolol
(Column: Particle size 5μm, 4.6mmID×15cm)

Brand Name
COSMOSIL 5C_{18}
COSMOSIL 5C_{18}-AR-II
COSMOSIL 5C_{18}-MS-II
Mightysil RP-18GP
TSKgel ODS-120T
TSKgel ODS-80T_M
TSKgel ODS-80T_S
YMC-Pack ODS-A

Hangekobokuto Extract: Rosmarinic acid
(Column: Particle size 5μm, 4.6mmID×15cm)

Brand Name
Atlantis dC_{18}
COSMOSIL 5C_{18}
COSMOSIL 5C_{18}-AR-II
Inertsil ODS-3V
Mightysil RP-18GP
TSKgel ODS-80T_S
YMC-Pack ODS-A
YMC-Pack *Pro* C18

Hangekobokuto Extract: [6]-gingerol
(Column: Particle size 5μm, 4.6mmID×15cm)

Brand Name
CAPCELL PAK C_{18} SG120
COSMOSIL 5C_{18}-AR-II
Develosil ODS-5
Develosil ODS-UG-5
L-column ODS
Mightysil RP-18GP
TSKgel ODS-120A
TSKgel ODS-80T_S
Wakosil 5C18
XBridge Shield C_{18}
YMC-Pack ODS-A
YMC-Pack ODS-AL
YMC-Pack ODS-AM

Hangeshashinto Extract: Baicalin
(Column: Particle size 5μm, 4.6mmID×15cm)

Brand Name
Atlantis dC_{18}
Atlantis T3
COSMOSIL 5C_{18}
Develosil ODS-5
Inertsil ODS-2
Inertsil ODS-4V
L-column ODS
TSKgel ODS-80T_M
TSKgel ODS-80T_S
TSKgel ODS-80T_S QA
Wakosil 5C18
YMC-Pack ODS-A
YMC-Pack *Pro* C18

Hangeshashinto Extract: Glycyrrhizic Acid
(Column: Particle size 5μm, 4.6mmID×15cm)

Brand Name
Assay i)
L-column2 ODS
YMC-Pack ODS-A
Assay ii)
CHEMCOSORB 5-ODS-H
COSMOSIL 5C_{18}-MS-II
L-column2 ODS

Brand Name
Mightysil RP-18GP
TSKgel ODS-80Ts
TSKgel ODS-80Ts QA
YMC-Pack ODS-A

Hangeshashinto Extract: Berberine
(Column: Particle size 5μm, 4.6mmID×15cm)

Brand Name
Atlantis T3
CAPCELL PAK C_{18} MG
CHEMCOSORB 5-ODS-H
COSMOSIL 5C_{18}-PAQ
Develosil ODS-5
Inertsil ODS-2
Inertsil ODS-4
Inertsil ODS-4V
Mightysil RP-18GP
TSKgel ODS-100V
TSKgel ODS-80Ts
TSKgel ODS-80Ts QA
YMC-Pack ODS-A
YMC-Pack ODS-AL
YMC-Pack *Pro* C18

Hochuekkito Extract: Hesperidin
(Column: Particle size 5μm, 4.6mmID×15cm)

Brand Name
CHEMCOSORB 5-ODS-H
COSMOSIL 5C_{18}-AR-II
Inertsil ODS-2
Mightysil RP-18GP
Symmetry C_{18}
TSKgel ODS-100S
TSKgel ODS-80Ts
TSKgel ODS-80Ts QA
YMC-Pack ODS-A

Hochuekkito Extract: Saikosaponin b_2
(Column: Particle size 5μm, 4.6mmID×15cm)

Brand Name
CHEMCOSORB 5-ODS-H
Develosil ODS-5
Develosil ODS-UG-5
Mightysil RP-18GP
TSKgel ODS-120A
TSKgel ODS-80TM
TSKgel ODS-80Ts
Wakosil 5C18
XTerra MS C18
YMC-Pack ODS-A

Hochuekkito Extract: Glycyrrhizic Acid
(Column: Particle size 5μm, 4.6mmID×15cm)

Brand Name
CHEMCOSORB 5-ODS-H
COSMOSIL 5C_{18}-AR-II
Mightysil RP-18 GP
TSKgel ODS-80Ts QA
YMC-Pack ODS-A
YMC-Pack *Pro* C18

Juzentaihoto Extract: Ginsenoside Rb_1
(Column: Particle size 5μm, 4.6mmID×25cm)

Brand Name
TSKgel Amide-80 HR

Juzentaihoto Extract: Paeoniflorin
(Column: Particle size 5μm, 4.6mmID×15cm)

Brand Name
Atlantis dC_{18}
Develosil ODS-5
Develosil ODS-UG-5
Hydrosphere C18
Nucleosil 5C18
TSKgel ODS-80TM
TSKgel ODS-80Ts
TSKgel ODS-80Ts QA
YMC-Triart C18

Juzentaihoto Extract: Glycyrrhizic Acid
(Column: Particle size 5μm, 4.6mmID×15cm)

Brand Name
Assay i)
TSKgel ODS-80Ts QA
Assay ii)
CHEMCOSORB 5-ODS-H
Mightysil RP-18GP
TSKgel ODS-80Ts QA
YMC-Pack ODS-A

Kakkonto Extract: Total alkaloids (ephedrine and pseudoephedrine)
(Column: Particle size 5μm, 4.6mmID×15cm)

Brand Name
Atlantis dC_{18}
CHEMCOSORB 5-ODS-H
COSMOSIL 5C_{18}-AR-II
COSMOSIL 5C_{18}-MS-II
Develosil ODS-5
Develosil ODS-UG-5
Inertsil ODS-3
Mightysil RP-18GP
TSKgel ODS-120A
TSKgel ODS-80Ts
Wakosil 5C18
YMC-Pack ODS-A
YMC-Pack *Pro* C18

Kakkonto Extract: Paeoniflorin
(Column: Particle size 5μm, 4.6mmID×15cm)

Brand Name
Atlantis dC_{18}
CHEMCOSORB 5-ODS-H
Develosil ODS-5
Develosil ODS-UG-5
Hydrosphere C18
Nucleosil 5C18
Puresil C18

TSKgel ODS-80T_M
TSKgel ODS-80T_S
TSKgel ODS-80T_S QA
YMC-Pack ODS-A
YMC-Pack *Pro* C18
YMC-Triart C18

Kakkonto Extract: Glycyrrhizic Acid
(Column: Particle size 5μm, 4.6mmID×15cm)

Brand Name
Assay i)
TSKgel ODS-80T_S
TSKgel ODS-80T_S QA
YMC-Pack ODS-A
Assay ii)
CHEMCOSORB 5-ODS-H
L-column2 ODS
TSKgel ODS-80T_S
TSKgel ODS-80T_S QA
YMC-Pack ODS-A

Kakkontokasenkyushin'i Extract: Total alkaloids (ephedrine and pseudoephedrine)
(Column: Particle size 5μm, 4.6mmID×15cm)

Brand Name
COSMOSIL 5C_{18}-AR-II
COSMOSIL 5C_{18}-MS-II
Inertsil ODS-4
Mightysil RP-18GP
TSKgel ODS-120A
TSKgel ODS-80T_M
TSKgel ODS-80T_S
TSKgel ODS-80T_S QA
Wakosil 5C18
XBridge C_{18}
YMC-Pack ODS-A
YMC-Pack ODS-AM

Kakkontokasenkyushin'i Extract: Paeoniflorin
(Column: Particle size 5μm, 4.6mmID×15cm)

Brand Name
Atlantis dC_{18}
Hydrosphere C18
Inertsil ODS-4V
Nucleosil 5C18
TSKgel ODS-80T_S
TSKgel ODS-80T_S QA
YMC-Pack ODS-A
YMC-Triart C18

Kakkontokasenkyushin'i Extract: Glycyrrhizic Acid
(Column: Particle size 5μm, 4.6mmID×15cm)

Brand Name
Assay i)
TSKgel ODS-80T_S QA
Assay ii)
CHEMCOSORB 5-ODS-H
L-column2 ODS
TSKgel ODS-80T_S QA
YMC-Pack ODS-A

Kakkontokasenkyushin'i Extract: Magnoflorine
(Column: Particle size 5μm, 4.6mmID×15cm)

Brand Name
Atlantis T3
COSMOSIL 5C_{18}-AR-II
Inertsil ODS-3V
Inertsil ODS-4
Inertsil ODS-4V
Mightysil RP-18GP
TSKgel ODS-100V
TSKgel ODS-80T_S
TSKgel ODS-80T_S QA
XBridge C_{18}
YMC-Pack ODS-A
YMC-Pack *Pro* C18

Kamikihito Extract: Saikosaponin b_2
(Column: Particle size 5μm, 4.6mmID×15cm)

Brand Name
Ascentis Express C18
Atlantis T3
Inertsil ODS-3V
L-column ODS
TSKgel ODS-80T_S
TSKgel ODS-80T_S QA
XBridge C_{18}
YMC-Pack ODS-A

Kamikihito Extract: Geniposide
(Column: Particle size 5μm, 4.6mmID×15cm)

Brand Name
Ascentis Express C18
Inertsil ODS-3
Inertsil ODS-3V
Inertsil ODS-4V
TSKgel ODS-100V
TSKgel ODS-80T_S
TSKgel ODS-80T_S QA
Wakosil 5C18
YMC-Pack ODS-A
YMC-Pack *Pro* C18

Kamikihito Extract: Glycyrrhizic Acid
(Column: Particle size 5μm, 4.6mmID×15cm)

Brand Name
CAPCELL PAK C_{18} UG120
COSMOSIL 5C_{18}-AR-II
L-column2 ODS
TSKgel ODS-80T_S
TSKgel ODS-80T_S QA
YMC-Pack ODS-A
YMC-Pack *Pro* C18

Kamishoyosan Extract: Paeoniflorin
(Column: Particle size 5μm, 4.6mmID×15cm)

Brand Name
Atlantis dC_{18}

CHEMCOSORB 5-ODS-H
Develosil ODS-5
Hydrosphere C18
L-column ODS
Nucleosil 5C18
TSKgel ODS-80T_M
TSKgel ODS-80T_S
TSKgel ODS-80T_S QA
YMC-Pack ODS-A
YMC-Triart C18

Kamishoyosan Extract: Geniposide
(Column: Particle size 5μm, 4.6mmID×15cm)

Brand Name
CAPCELL PAK C_{18} UG80
CHEMCOSORB 5-ODS-H
Develosil ODS-5
Hydrosphere C18
L-column ODS
Mightysil RP-18GP
TSKgel ODS-80T_M
TSKgel ODS-80T_S
TSKgel ODS-80T_S QA
Wakosil 5C18
YMC-Pack ODS-AM

Kamishoyosan Extract: Glycyrrhizic Acid
(Column: Particle size 5μm, 4.6mmID×15cm)

Brand Name
COSMOSIL 5C_{18}-MS-II
L-column2 ODS
Mightysil RP-18 GP
TSKgel ODS-80T_S
TSKgel ODS-80T_S QA
YMC-Pack ODS-A
YMC-Pack *Pro* C18

Keishibukuryogan Extract: (*E*)-Cinnamic acid
(Column: Particle size 5μm, 4.6mmID×15cm)

Brand Name
Atlantis dC_{18}
CAPCELL PAK C_{18} SG120
CAPCELL PAK C_{18} UG120
COSMOSIL 5C_{18}-MS-II
Develosil ODS-UG-5
Hydrosphere C18
Mightysil RP-18GP
Nucleosil 5C18
TSKgel ODS-100S
TSKgel ODS-80T_M
TSKgel ODS-80T_S
TSKgel ODS-80T_S QA
Wakosil 5C18
YMC-Pack ODS-A

Keishibukuryogan Extract: Paeoniflorin
(Column: Particle size 5μm, 4.6mmID×15cm)

Brand Name
Atlantis dC_{18}

COSMOSIL 5C_{18}-AR-II
Develosil ODS-UG-5
Hydrosphere C18
Nucleosil 5C18
TSKgel ODS-100S
TSKgel ODS-80T_M
TSKgel ODS-80T_S
TSKgel ODS-80T_S QA
YMC-Pack ODS-A
YMC-Triart C18

Keishibukuryogan Extract: Amygdalin
(Column: Particle size 5μm, 4.6mmID×15cm)

Brand Name
CAPCELL PAK C_{18} MG
COSMOSIL 5C_{18}
Develosil ODS-5
Develosil ODS-HG-5
Develosil ODS-UG-5
Inertsil ODS-3
L-column2 ODS
Mightysil RP-18GP
TSKgel ODS-100S
TSKgel ODS-120A
TSKgel ODS-80T_M
TSKgel ODS-80T_S
Wakosil 5C18
YMC-Pack ODS-A
YMC-Pack *Pro* C18

Maoto Extract: Total alkaloids (ephedrine and pseudoephedrine)
(Column: Particle size 5μm, 4.6mmID×15cm)

Brand Name
CHEMCOSORB 5-ODS-H
COSMOSIL 5C_{18}-AR-II
COSMOSIL 5C_{18}-MS-II
Inertsil ODS-4
Inertsil ODS-80A
Mightysil RP-18GP
TSKgel ODS-120A
TSKgel ODS-80T_S
TSKgel ODS-80T_S QA
Wakosil 5C18
XBridge C_{18}
YMC-Pack ODS-A
YMC-Pack ODS-AM

Maoto Extract: Amygdalin
(Column: Particle size 5μm, 4.6mmID×15cm)

Brand Name
CAPCELL PAK C_{18} MG
CHEMCOSORB 5-ODS-H
COSMOSIL 5C_{18}-MS-II
Develosil ODS-UG-5
L-column2 ODS
Mightysil RP-18GP
SUPERIOREX ODS
TSKgel ODS-100S

TSKgel ODS-80Ts
TSKgel ODS-80Ts QA
Wakosil 5C18
YMC-Pack ODS-A
YMC-Pack *Pro* C18

Maoto Extract: Glycyrrhizic Acid
(Column: Particle size 5μm, 4.6mmID×15cm)

Brand Name
Assay i)
TSKgel ODS-80Ts QA
Assay ii)
CHEMCOSORB 5-ODS-H
L-column2 ODS
TSKgel ODS-80Ts QA
YMC-Pack ODS-A

Mukoi-Daikenchuto Extract: Ginsenoside Rb_1
(Column: Particle size 5μm, 4.6mmID×25cm)

Brand Name
TSKgel Amide-80 HR

Mukoi-Daikenchuto Extract: [6]-Shogaol
(Column: Particle size 5μm, 4.6mmID×15cm)

Brand Name
Develosil C8-5
Inertsil C8-3
L-column C8
TSKgel Octyl-80Ts

Orengedokuto Extract: Berberine
(Column: Particle size 5μm, 4.6mmID×15cm)

Brand Name
CAPCELL PAK C_{18} MG
CHEMCOSORB 5-ODS-H
COSMOSIL $5C_{18}$-PAQ
Develosil ODS-5
Inertsil ODS-3
Mightysil RP-18GP
Nucleosil 5C18
TSKgel ODS-80TM
TSKgel ODS-80Ts
YMC-Pack ODS-A
YMC-Pack *Pro* C18

Orengedokuto Extract: Baicalin
(Column: Particle size 5μm, 4.6mmID×15cm)

Brand Name
Atlantis dC_{18}
COSMOSIL $5C_{18}$
COSMOSIL $5C_{18}$-AR-II
Develosil ODS-5
L-column ODS
TSKgel ODS-80TM
TSKgel ODS-80Ts
TSKgel ODS-80Ts QA
Wakosil 5C18
YMC-Pack ODS-A

Orengedokuto Extract: Geniposide
(Column: Particle size 5μm, 4.6mmID×15cm)

Brand Name
CAPCELL PAK C_{18} UG80
CHEMCOSORB 5-ODS-H
Develosil ODS-5
Hydrosphere C18
L-column ODS
Mightysil RP-18GP
TSKgel ODS-80TM
TSKgel ODS-80Ts
TSKgel ODS-80Ts QA
Wakosil 5C18
YMC-Pack ODS-AM

Otsujito Extract: Saikosaponin b_2
(Column: Particle size 5μm, 4.6mmID×15cm)

Brand Name
Atlantis T3
CHEMCOSORB 5-ODS-H
Develosil ODS-5
Inertsil ODS-4V
Mightysil RP-18GP
TSKgel ODS-100V
TSKgel ODS-120A
TSKgel ODS-80Ts
TSKgel ODS-80Ts QA
Wakosil 5C18
XBridge C_{18}
YMC-Pack ODS-A
YMC-Pack ODS-AM
YMC-Pack *Pro* C18

Otsujito Extract: Baicalin
(Column: Particle size 5μm, 4.6mmID×15cm)

Brand Name
Atlantis dC_{18}
Atlantis T3
COSMOSIL $5C_{18}$
COSMOSIL $5C_{18}$-MS-II
Inertsil ODS-4
Inertsil ODS-4V
Mightysil RP-18GP
TSKgel ODS-120A
TSKgel ODS-80TM
TSKgel ODS-80Ts
TSKgel ODS-80Ts QA
Wakosil 5C18
YMC-Pack ODS-A
YMC-Pack *Pro* C18

Otsujito Extract: Glycyrrhizic Acid
(Column: Particle size 5μm, 4.6mmID×15cm)

Brand Name
CAPCELL PAK C_{18} UG120
CHEMCOSORB 5-ODS-H
L-column2 ODS
Mightysil RP-18 GP
TSKgel ODS-80Ts

TSKgel ODS-80Ts QA
YMC-Pack ODS-A
YMC-Pack *Pro* C18

Otsujito Extract: Sennoside A
(Column: Particle size 5μm, 4.6mmID×15cm)

Brand Name
Atlantis T3
CHEMCOSORB 5-ODS-H
COSMOSIL $5C_{18}$-AR-II
Hydrosphere C18
Inertsil ODS-3V
Inertsil ODS-4
Inertsil ODS-4V
L-column ODS
L-column2 ODS
TSKgel ODS-100V
TSKgel ODS-100Z
TSKgel ODS-120T
TSKgel ODS-80Ts
TSKgel ODS-80Ts QA
XBridge C_{18}
YMC-Pack ODS-A
YMC-Pack *Pro* C18

Otsujito Extract: Rhein
(Column: Particle size 5μm, 4.6mmID×25cm)

Brand Name
CHEMCOSORB 5-ODS-H
Hydrosphere C18
Inertsil ODS-4
L-column ODS
L-column2 ODS
TSKgel ODS-80Ts QA
Wakosil 5C18
YMC-Pack ODS-A

Rikkunshito Extract: Ginsenoside Rb_1
(Column: Particle size 5μm, 4.6mmID×25cm)

Brand Name
TSKgel Amide-80 HR

Rikkunshito Extract: Hesperidin
(Column: Particle size 5μm, 4.6mmID×15cm)

Brand Name
Atlantis dC_{18}
CHEMCOSORB 5-ODS-H
COSMOSIL $5C_{18}$-AR-II
Inertsil ODS-2
Mightysil RP-18GP
Symmetry C_{18}
TSKgel ODS-100S
TSKgel ODS-80Ts
TSKgel ODS-80Ts QA
XTerra MS C18
YMC-Pack ODS-A

Rikkunshito Extract: Glycyrrhizic Acid
(Column: Particle size 5μm, 4.6mmID×15cm)

Brand Name
Atlantis dC_{18}
CAPCELL PAK C_{18} UG120
CHEMCOSORB 5-ODS-H
COSMOSIL $5C_{18}$-AR-II
COSMOSIL $5C_{18}$-MS-II
L-column2 ODS
Mightysil RP-18 GP
TSKgel ODS-80Ts
TSKgel ODS-80Ts QA
YMC-Pack ODS-A
YMC-Pack *Pro* C18

Ryokeijutsukanto Extract: (*E*)-Cinnamic acid
(Column: Particle size 5μm, 4.6mmID×15cm)

Brand Name
CAPCELL PAK C_{18} SG120
CAPCELL PAK C_{18} UG120
Mightysil RP-18GP
TSKgel ODS-80TM
TSKgel ODS-80Ts
TSKgel ODS-80Ts QA
Wakosil 5C18
YMC-Pack ODS-A

Ryokeijutsukanto Extract: Glycyrrhizic Acid
(Column: Particle size 5μm, 4.6mmID×15cm)

Brand Name
Assay i)
TSKgel ODS-80Ts
TSKgel ODS-80Ts QA
Assay ii)
CHEMCOSORB 5-ODS-H
TSKgel ODS-80Ts
TSKgel ODS-80Ts QA
YMC-Pack ODS-A

Saibokuto Extract: Saikosaponin b_2
(Column: Particle size 5μm, 4.6mmID×15cm)

Brand Name
Atlantis dC_{18}
COSMOSIL $5C_{18}$-AR-II
YMC-Pack ODS-A

Saibokuto Extract: Baicalin
(Column: Particle size 5μm, 4.6mmID×15cm)

Brand Name
Atlantis dC_{18}
COSMOSIL $5C_{18}$-AR-II
L-column ODS
YMC-Pack ODS-A

Saibokuto Extract: Glycyrrhizic Acid
(Column: Particle size 5μm, 4.6mmID×15cm)

Brand Name
Assay i)
TSKgel ODS-80Ts QA
Assay ii)
TSKgel ODS-80Ts QA
YMC-Pack ODS-A
YMC-Pack *Pro* C18

Saikokeishito Extract: Saikosaponin b_2
(Column: Particle size 5μm, 4.6mmID×15cm)

Brand Name
Atlantis dC_{18}
CHEMCOSORB 5-ODS-H
Develosil ODS-5
Develosil ODS-UG-5
L-column2 ODS
TSKgel ODS-120A
TSKgel ODS-80Ts
Wakosil 5C18
YMC-Pack ODS-A

Saikokeishito Extract: Baicalin
(Column: Particle size 5μm, 4.6mmID×15cm)

Brand Name
Atlantis dC_{18}
CHEMCOSORB 5-ODS-H
COSMOSIL $5C_{18}$
COSMOSIL $5C_{18}$-MS-II
L-column ODS
TSKgel ODS-80T_M
TSKgel ODS-80Ts
Wakosil 5C18
YMC-Pack ODS-A

Saikokeishito Extract: Paeoniflorin
(Column: Particle size 5μm, 4.6mmID×15cm)

Brand Name
Atlantis dC_{18}
Develosil ODS-UG-5
Hydrosphere C18
Nucleosil 5C18
TSKgel ODS-80T_M
TSKgel ODS-80Ts
TSKgel ODS-80Ts QA
YMC-Pack ODS-A
YMC-Triart C18

Saikokeishito Extract: Glycyrrhizic Acid
(Column: Particle size 5μm, 4.6mmID×15cm)

Brand Name
Assay i)
TSKgel ODS-80Ts QA
Assay ii)
CHEMCOSORB 5-ODS-H
COSMOSIL $5C_{18}$-MS-II
L-column2 ODS
TSKgel ODS-80Ts
TSKgel ODS-80Ts QA
YMC-Pack ODS-A
YMC-Pack *Pro* C18

Saireito Extract: Saikosaponin b_2
(Column: Particle size 5μm, 4.6mmID×15cm)

Brand Name
Atlantis dC_{18}
COSMOSIL $5C_{18}$-AR-II
Mightysil RP-18GP Aqua
TSKgel ODS-80Ts QA
YMC-Pack ODS-A

Saireito Extract: Baicalin
(Column: Particle size 5μm, 4.6mmID×15cm)

Brand Name
Atlantis dC_{18}
COSMOSIL $5C_{18}$-AR-II
Mightysil RP-18GP
Mightysil RP-18GP Aqua
TSKgel ODS-120T
TSKgel ODS-80Ts

Saireito Extract: Glycyrrhizic Acid
(Column: Particle size 5μm, 4.6mmID×15cm)

Brand Name
Assay i)
COSMOSIL $5C_{18}$-AR-II
TSKgel ODS-80Ts QA
Assay ii)
COSMOSIL $5C_{18}$-AR-II
TSKgel ODS-80Ts QA
YMC-Pack *Pro* C18

Shakuyakukanzoto Extract: Paeoniflorin
(Column: Particle size 5μm, 4.6mmID×15cm)

Brand Name
Atlantis dC_{18}
CHEMCOSORB 5-ODS-H
Develosil ODS-5
Develosil ODS-UG-5
Hydrosphere C18
Nucleosil 5C18
Puresil C18
TSKgel ODS-80T_M
TSKgel ODS-80Ts
TSKgel ODS-80Ts QA
YMC-Pack ODS-A
YMC-Pack *Pro* C18
YMC-Triart C18

Shakuyakukanzoto Extract: Glycyrrhizic Acid
(Column: Particle size 5μm, 4.6mmID×15cm)

Brand Name
CAPCELL PAK C_{18} UG120
CHEMCOSORB 5-ODS-H
COSMOSIL $5C_{18}$-AR-II
COSMOSIL $5C_{18}$-MS-II

L-column2 ODS
Mightysil RP-18 GP
TSKgel ODS-80Ts
TSKgel ODS-80Ts QA
YMC-Pack ODS-A
YMC-Pack *Pro* C18

Shimbuto Extract: Paeoniflorin
(Column: Particle size 5μm, 4.6mmID×15cm)

Brand Name
Atlantis dC18
Nucleosil 5C18
TSKgel ODS-80TM
TSKgel ODS-80Ts
YMC-Pack ODS-A

Shimbuto Extract: [6]-gingerol
(Column: Particle size 5μm, 4.6mmID×15cm)

Brand Name
CAPCELL PAK C18 SG120
L-column ODS
Mightysil RP-18GP
TSKgel ODS-120A
TSKgel ODS-80Ts
YMC-Pack ODS-A
YMC-Pack ODS-AL

Shimbuto Extract: Total alkaloids (as benzoylmesaconine hydrochloride and 14-anisoylaconine hydrochloride, or as benzoylmesaconine hydrochloride and benzoylhypaconine hydrochloride)
(Column: Particle size 5μm, 4.6mmID×15cm)

Brand Name
Atlantis dC18
Cadenza 5CD-C18
Inertsil ODS-3
TSKgel ODS-80TM
TSKgel ODS-80Ts QA
XBridge C18
YMC-Pack ODS-A

Shosaikoto Extract: Saikosaponin b2
(Column: Particle size 5μm, 4.6mmID×15cm)

Brand Name
Atlantis dC18
CHEMCOSORB 5-ODS-H
COSMOSIL 5C18-AR-II
Develosil ODS-5
Develosil ODS-UG-5
L-column2 ODS
Mightysil RP-18GP Aqua
TSKgel ODS-80Ts
TSKgel ODS-80Ts QA
Wakosil 5C18
YMC-Pack ODS-A
YMC-Pack ODS-AQ

Shosaikoto Extract: Baicalin
(Column: Particle size 5μm, 4.6mmID×15cm)

Brand Name
Atlantis dC18
COSMOSIL 5C18
COSMOSIL 5C18-AR-II
L-column ODS
Mightysil RP-18GP Aqua
TSKgel ODS-120T
TSKgel ODS-80TM
TSKgel ODS-80Ts
TSKgel ODS-80Ts QA
Wakosil 5C18
YMC-Pack ODS-A

Shosaikoto Extract: Glycyrrhizic Acid
(Column: Particle size 5μm, 4.6mmID×15cm)

Brand Name
Assay i)
COSMOSIL 5C18-MS-II
L-column2 ODS
YMC-Pack ODS-A
Assay ii)
CHEMCOSORB 5-ODS-H
COSMOSIL 5C18-MS-II
L-column2 ODS
TSKgel ODS-80Ts
TSKgel ODS-80Ts QA
YMC-Pack ODS-A
YMC-Pack *Pro* C18

Shoseiryuto Extract: Total alkaloids (ephedrine and pseudoephedrine)
(Column: Particle size 5μm, 4.6mmID×15cm)

Brand Name
Atlantis dC18
CAPCELL PAK C18 MG-II
CHEMCOSORB 5-ODS-H
COSMOSIL 5C18-AR-II
COSMOSIL 5C18-MS-II
Develosil ODS-3
Develosil ODS-5
Develosil ODS-UG-5
Inertsil ODS-3
Mightysil RP-18GP
TSKgel ODS-80Ts
Wakosil 5C18
XBridge C18
YMC-Pack ODS-A

Shoseiryuto Extract: Paeoniflorin
(Column: Particle size 5μm, 4.6mmID×15cm)

Brand Name
Atlantis dC18
CHEMCOSORB 5-ODS-H
Develosil ODS-5
Develosil ODS-HG-5
Hydrosphere C18
Inertsil ODS-3

Nucleosil 5C18
Puresil C18
TSKgel ODS-80T_M
TSKgel ODS-80T_S
TSKgel ODS-80T_S QA
YMC-Pack ODS-A
YMC-Pack *Pro* C18
YMC-Triart C18

Shoseiryuto Extract: Glycyrrhizic Acid
(Column: Particle size 5μm, 4.6mmID×15cm)

Brand Name
Assay i)
Inertsil ODS-4
TSKgel ODS-80T_S
TSKgel ODS-80T_S QA
YMC-Pack ODS-A
Assay ii)
CHEMCOSORB 5-ODS-H
Inertsil ODS-4
L-column2 ODS
Mightysil RP-18GP
TSKgel ODS-80T_S
TSKgel ODS-80T_S QA
YMC-Pack ODS-A

Tokakujokito Extract: Amygdalin
(Column: Particle size 5μm, 4.6mmID×15cm)

Brand Name
CAPCELL PAK C_{18} MG
Develosil ODS-UG-5
L-column ODS
L-column2 ODS
Mightysil RP-18GP
TSKgel ODS-100S
TSKgel ODS-80T_S
TSKgel ODS-80T_S QA
Wakosil 5C18
YMC-Pack ODS-A
YMC-Pack *Pro* C18

Tokakujokito Extract: (*E*)-Cinnamic acid
(Column: Particle size 5μm, 4.6mmID×15cm)

Brand Name
CAPCELL PAK C_{18} SG120
COSMOSIL 5C_{18}-MS-II
Mightysil RP-18GP
Mightysil RP-18GP Aqua
TSKgel ODS-80T_M
TSKgel ODS-80T_S QA
Wakosil 5C18
YMC-Pack ODS-A

Tokakujokito Extract: Sennoside A
(Column: Particle size 5μm, 4.6mmID×15cm)

Brand Name
Atlantis T3
CAPCELL PAK C_{18} MG
COSMOSIL 5C_{18}-AR-II
Develosil ODS-HG-5
Inertsil ODS-4
L-column ODS
L-column2 ODS
TSKgel ODS-100Z
TSKgel ODS-120T
TSKgel ODS-80T_S QA
YMC-Pack ODS-A

Tokakujokito Extract: Rhein
(Column: Particle size 5μm, 4.6mmID×25cm)

Brand Name
CHEMCOSORB 5-ODS-H
L-column ODS
L-column2 ODS
Nucleosil 5C18
TSKgel ODS-80T_S QA
Wakosil 5C18
YMC-Pack ODS-A

Tokakujokito Extract: Glycyrrhizic Acid
(Column: Particle size 5μm, 4.6mmID×15cm)

Brand Name
CAPCELL PAK C_{18} UG120
Mightysil RP-18 GP
TSKgel ODS-80T_S
TSKgel ODS-80T_S QA
YMC-Pack ODS-A
YMC-Pack *Pro* C18

Tokishakuyakusan Extract: (*E*)-Ferulic acid
(Column: Particle size 5μm, 4.6mmID×15cm)

Brand Name
COSMOSIL 5C_{18}
COSMOSIL 5C_{18}-MS-II
Develosil ODS-5
Mightysil RP-18GP
TSKgel ODS-80T_M
TSKgel ODS-80T_S
YMC-Pack ODS-A

Tokishakuyakusan Extract: Paeoniflorin
(Column: Particle size 5μm, 4.6mmID×15cm)

Brand Name
Atlantis dC_{18}
COSMOSIL 5C_{18}-AR-II
Develosil ODS-UG-5
Hydrosphere C18
Nucleosil 5C18
TSKgel ODS-100S
TSKgel ODS-80T_M
TSKgel ODS-80T_S
TSKgel ODS-80T_S QA
YMC-Pack ODS-A
YMC-Triart C18

(18) *Addenda*

Tokishakuyakusan Extract: Atractylenolide III
(Column: Particle size 5μm, 4.6mmID×15cm)

Brand Name
COSMOSIL 5C18-AR-II
Mightysil RP-18GP
TSKgel ODS-80TM
TSKgel ODS-80Ts
Wakosil 5C18
YMC-Pack ODS-A
YMC-Pack ODS-AM

Tokishakuyakusan Extract: Atractylodin
(Column: Particle size 5μm, 4.6mmID×15cm)

Brand Name
Develosil ODS-UG-5
Inertsil ODS-3
Inertsil ODS-3V
Mightysil RP-18GP
TSKgel ODS-120A
TSKgel ODS-80TM
TSKgel ODS-80Ts

Unseiin Extract: Paeoniflorin
(Column: Particle size 5μm, 4.6mmID×15cm)

Brand Name
Atlantis dC18
COSMOSIL 5C18-AR-II
Mightysil RP-18GP
TSKgel ODS-80Ts
TSKgel ODS-80Ts QA

Unseiin Extract: Baicalin
(Column: Particle size 5μm, 4.6mmID×15cm)

Brand Name
COSMOSIL 5C18-AR-II
Inertsil ODS-3
Inertsil ODS-4V
L-column2 ODS
TSKgel ODS-80Ts QA
TSKgel ODS-100 V

Unseiin Extract:Berberine
(Column: Particle size 5μm, 4.6mmID×15cm)

Brand Name
CAPCELL PAK C18 MG
CHEMCOSORB 5-ODS-H
COSMOSIL 5C18-AR-II
Mightysil RP-18GP
TSKgel ODS-80Ts
YMC-Pack *Pro*-C18

Yokukansan Extract: Total alkaloid (rhyncophylline and hirsutine)
(Column: Particle size 5μm, 4.6mmID×15cm)

Brand Name
Inertsil ODS-4
YMC-Pack ODS-A
YMC-Pack *Pro* C18

Yokukansan Extract: Saikosaponin b_2
(Column: Particle size 5μm, 4.6mmID×15cm)

Brand Name
Atlantis T3
Develosil ODS-HG-5
Inertsil ODS-4V
Mightysil RP-18GP
TSKgel ODS-100V
TSKgel ODS-80Ts QA
Wakosil 5C18
XBridge C18
YMC-Pack ODS-A
YMC-Pack ODS-AM
YMC-Pack *Pro* C18

Yokukansan Extract: Glycyrrhizic Acid
(Column: Particle size 5μm, 4.6mmID×15cm)

Brand Name
L-column2 ODS
TSKgel ODS-80Ts QA
YMC-Pack ODS-A
YMC-Pack *Pro* C18

The monographs revised in JP 18 and their revised sections

Title (Japanese title)		Section	Page
Aprindine Hydrochloride (アプリンジン塩酸塩)	Add.		
	Rev.	Description	476
	Del.		
Azathioprine Tablets (アザチオプリン錠)	Add.		
	Rev.	Identification (4)	499
	Del.		
Bepotastine Besilate (ベポタスチンベシル酸塩)	Add.		
	Rev.	Purity (3)	529
	Del.		
Bleomycin Hydrochloride (ブレオマイシン塩酸塩)	Add.		
	Rev.	Origin/limits of content	559
	Del.		
Bleomycin Sulfate (ブレオマイシン硫酸塩)	Add.		
	Rev.	Origin/limits of content	561
	Del.		
Calcitonin Salmon (カルシトニン　サケ)	Add.		
	Rev.	Origin/limits of content	591
	Del.		
Calcium Folinate Hydrate (ホリナートカルシウム水和物)	Add.		
	Rev.	English title, Title in Japanese, Structural formula, Molecular formula, Chemical name, CAS No.	597
	Del.		
Calcium Paraaminosalicylate Hydrate (パラアミノサリチル酸カルシウム水和物)	Add.		
	Rev.	CAS No.	603
	Del.		
Carmellose Calcium (カルメロースカルシウム)	Add.		
	Rev.	Origin/limits of content	631
	Del.		
Carmellose Sodium (カルメロースナトリウム)	Add.		
	Rev.	Origin/limits of content	632
	Del.		
Croscarmellose Sodium (クロスカルメロースナトリウム)	Add.		
	Rev.	All	633
	Del.		
Cefoperazone Sodium (セフォペラゾンナトリウム)	Add.		
	Rev.	Identification (2)	681
	Del.		
Celmoleukin (Genetical Recombination) (セルモロイキン(遺伝子組換え))	Add.		
	Rev.	Origin/limits of content	719
	Del.		
Clinofibrate (クリノフィブラート)	Add.		
	Rev.	Chemical name	779
	Del.		

Clopidogrel Sulfate (クロピドグレル硫酸塩)	Add.		793
	Rev.	Purity (3)	
	Del.		
Colistin Sodium Methanesulfonate (コリスチンメタンスルホン酸ナトリウム)	Add.		810
	Rev.	Origin/limits of content	
	Del.		
Dihydroergotoxine Mesilate (ジヒドロエルゴトキシンメシル酸塩)	Add.		860
	Rev.	Structure formula	
	Del.		
Dimorpholamine (ジモルホラミン)	Add.		868
	Rev.	Chemical name	
	Del.		
Diphenhydramine (ジフェンヒドラミン)	Add.		870
	Rev.	Description	
	Del.		
Diphenhydramine Hydrochloride (ジフェンヒドラミン塩酸塩)	Add.		871
	Rev.	Description	
	Del.		
Distigmine Bromide (ジスチグミン臭化物)	Add.		875
	Rev.	Chemical name	
	Del.		
Dorzolamide Hydrochloride (ドルゾラミド塩酸塩)	Add.		891
	Rev.	Purity (3)	
	Del.		
Enviomycin Sulfate (エンビオマイシン硫酸塩)	Add.		931
	Rev.	Structure formula	
	Del.		
Epoetin Alfa (Genetical Recombination) (エポエチン　アルファ(遺伝子組換え))	Add.		942
	Rev.	Origin/limits of content	
	Del.		
Epoetin Beta (Genetical Recombination) (エポエチン　ベータ(遺伝子組換え))	Add.		945
	Rev.	Origin/limits of content	
	Del.		
Ergometrine Maleate (エルゴメトリンマレイン酸塩)	Add.		949
	Rev.	Chemical name	
	Del.		
Ethambutol Hydrochloride (エタンブトール塩酸塩)	Add.		964
	Rev.	Chemical name	
	Del.		
Ethyl Aminobenzoate (アミノ安息香酸エチル)	Add.		971
	Rev.	Description	
	Del.		
Filgrastim (Genetical Recombination) (フィルグラスチム(遺伝子組換え))	Add.		1007
	Rev.	Origin/limits of content	
	Del.		
Fradiomycin Sulfate (フラジオマイシン硫酸塩)	Add.		1045
	Rev.	Structure formula	
	Del.		

Monograph			Page
Gelatin （ゼラチン）	Add.		
	Rev.	All	1060
	Del.		
Purified Gelatin （精製ゼラチン）	Add.		
	Rev.	Identification	1062
	Del.		
Gentamicin Sulfate （ゲンタマイシン硫酸塩）	Add.		
	Rev.	Structure formula, Chemical name, Purity (1)	1064
	Del.		
Glucose Injection （ブドウ糖注射液）	Add.		
	Rev.	Method of preparation, Identification, Purity	1076
	Del.		
Human Menopausal Gonadotrophin （ヒト下垂体性性腺刺激ホルモン）	Add.		
	Rev.	All	1087
	Del.		
Heparin Calcium （ヘパリンカルシウム）	Add.		
	Rev.	Origin/limits of content	1096
	Del.		
Heparin Sodium （ヘパリンナトリウム）	Add.		
	Rev.	Origin/limits of content	1100
	Del.		
Low Substituted Hydroxypropylcellulose （低置換度ヒドロキシプロピルセルロース）	Add.		
	Rev.	Assay	1124
	Del.		
Hypromellose （ヒプロメロース）	Add.		
	Rev.	Assay	1127
	Del.		
Insulin Human (Genetical Recombination) （インスリン　ヒト(遺伝子組換え)）	Add.		
	Rev.	Origin/limits of content	1155
	Del.		
Insulin Aspart (Genetical Recombination) （インスリン　アスパルト（遺伝子組換え））	Add.		
	Rev.	Origin/limits of content, Purity (1), (3) and (4)	1160
	Del.		
Insulin Glargine (Genetical Recombination) （インスリン　グラルギン(遺伝子組換え)）	Add.		
	Rev.	Origin/limits of content	1162
	Del.		
Kallidinogenase （カリジノゲナーゼ）	Add.		
	Rev.	Purity (2)	1216
	Del.		
Kitasamycin Acetate （キタサマイシン酢酸エステル）	Add.		
	Rev.	Chemical name	1227
	Del.		
Kitasamycin Tartrate （キタサマイシン酒石酸塩）	Add.		
	Rev.	Chemical name	1228
	Del.		
Anhydrous Lactose （無水乳糖）	Add.		
	Rev.	Beginning description concerning the international harmonization, Purity (3), Microbial limit, Isomer ratio	1233
	Del.		

Lactose Hydrate (乳糖水和物)	Add.		1234
	Rev.	Beginning description concerning the international harmonization, Origin/limits of content, Identification, Purity (1) and (3), Loss on drying, Water, Microbial limit	
	Del.		
Lauromacrogol (ラウロマクロゴール)	Add.		1246
	Rev.	Description, Identification	
	Del.		
Lenograstim (Genetical Recombination) (レノグラスチム(遺伝子組換え))	Add.		1248
	Rev.	Origin/limits of content	
	Del.		
Levofloxacin Hydrate (レボフロキサシン水和物)	Add.		1256
	Rev.	Purity (2)	
	Del.		
Levofloxacin Fine Granules (レボフロキサシン細粒)	Add.		1257
	Rev.	Assay	
	Del.		
Levofloxacin Injection (レボフロキサシン注射液)	Add.		1258
	Rev.	Assay	
	Del.		
Levofloxacin Tablets (レボフロキサシン錠)	Add.		1259
	Rev.	Assay	
	Del.		
Lysozyme Hydrochloride (リゾチーム塩酸塩)	Add.		1283
	Rev.	Origin/limits of content	
	Del.		
Methylcellulose (メチルセルロース)	Add.		1336
	Rev.	Assay	
	Del.		
Methylergometrine Maleate (メチルエルゴメトリンマレイン酸塩)	Add.		1342
	Rev.	Chemical name, CAS No	
	Del.		
Mexiletine Hydrochloride (メキシレチン塩酸塩)	Add.		1356
	Rev.	Chemical name	
	Del.		
Montelukast Sodium (モンテルカストナトリウム)	Add.		1374
	Rev.	Chemical name, Purity (3), Others	
	Del.		
Nafamostat Mesilate (ナファモスタットメシル酸塩)	Add.		1395
	Rev.	Chemical name	
	Del.		
Nartograstim (Genetical Recombination) (ナルトグラスチム（遺伝子組換え）)	Add.		1403
	Rev.	Origin/limits of content, Identification (1)	
	Del.		
Norgestrel and Ethinylestradiol Tablets (ノルゲストレル・エチニルエストラジオール錠)	Add.		1436
	Rev.	Identification (1) and (3)	
	Del.		
Olmesartan Medoxomil (オルメサルタン　メドキソミル)	Add.		1442
	Rev.	Chemical name	
	Del.		

Oxybuprocaine Hydrochloride （オキシブプロカイン塩酸塩）	Add.		
	Rev.	Description	1458
	Del.		
Oxygen （酸素）	Add.		
	Rev.	Assay	1462
	Del.		
Oxytocin （オキシトシン）	Add.		
	Rev.	Origin/limits of content	1465
	Del.		
Paroxetine Hydrochloride Hydrate （パロキセチン塩酸塩水和物）	Add.		
	Rev.	Purity (4)	1482
	Del.		
White Petrolatum （白色ワセリン）	Add.		
	Rev.	All	1501
	Del.		
Yellow Petrolatum （黄色ワセリン）	Add.		
	Rev.	All	1502
	Del.		
Pitavastatin Calcium Hydrate （ピタバスタチンカルシウム水和物）	Add.	Others	
	Rev.	Purity (2)	1540
	Del.		
Pitavastatin Calcium Tablets （ピタバスタチンカルシウム錠）	Add.	Others	
	Rev.	Purity, Dissolution	1543
	Del.		
Polymixin B Sulfate （ポリミキシンＢ硫酸塩）	Add.		
	Rev.	Origin/limits of content, Description	1549
	Del.		
Povidone （ポビドン）	Add.		
	Rev.	Structure formula, Purity(5), Assay	1559
	Del.		
Povidone-Iodine （ポビドンヨード）	Add.		
	Rev.	Structure formula	1561
	Del.		
Protamine Sulfate （プロタミン硫酸塩）	Add.		
	Rev.	Identification (1)	1603
	Del.		
Pullulan （プルラン）	Add.		
	Rev.	Structure formula	1607
	Del.		
Saccharin （サッカリン）	Add.		
	Rev.	Origin/limits of content, Assay	1663
	Del.		
Saccharin Sodium Hydrate （サッカリンナトリウム水和物）	Add.		
	Rev.	Origin/limits of content, Description, Identification (1), Assay	1664
	Del.		
Scopolamine Butylbromide （ブチルスコポラミン臭化物）	Add.		
	Rev.	Chemical name	1675
	Del.		

Monograph			Page
Scopolamine Hydrobromide Hydrate (スコポラミン臭化水素酸塩水和物)	Add. Rev. Del.	 Chemical name 	1676
Purified Shellac (精製セラック)	Add. Rev. Del.	 Purity (4) 	1679
White Shellac (白色セラック)	Add. Rev. Del.	 Description, Purity (6) 	1679
Silodosin (シロドシン)	Add. Rev. Del.	Others Purity (2) and (3) 	1681
Silodosin Tablets (シロドシン錠)	Add. Rev. Del.	Others Purity 	1684
Sodium Lauryl Sulfate (ラウリル硫酸ナトリウム)	Add. Rev. Del.	 Identification 	1718
Wheat Starch (コムギデンプン)	Add. Rev. Del.	 Purity (5) Total protein 	1741
Sucrose (精製白糖)	Add. Rev. Del.	 Conductivity 	1748
Teceleukin (Genetical Recombination) (テセロイキン（遺伝子組換え）)	Add. Rev. Del.	 Origin/limits, Assay 	1784
Tetracaine Hydrochloride (テトラカイン塩酸塩)	Add. Rev. Del.	 Description 	1812
Valaciclovir Hydrochloride (バラシクロビル塩酸塩)	Add. Rev. Del.	 Purity (4) 	1894
Valsartan (バルサルタン)	Add. Rev. Del.	 Purity (3) 	1898
Vasopressin Injection (バソプレシン注射液)	Add. Rev. Del.	 Assay 	1904
Voriconazole (ボリコナゾール)	Add. Rev. Del.	 Purity (3) 	1913
Voriconazole for Injection (注射用ボリコナゾール)	Add. Rev. Del.	 Purity (2) 	1915

Crude Drugs

Title (Japanese title)		Section	Page
Alpinia Officinarum Rhizome (リョウキョウ)	Add.		1944
	Rev.	Latin name	
	Del.		
Asiasarum Root (サイシン)	Add.		1949
	Rev.	Description	
	Del.		
Asparagus Root (テンモンドウ)	Add.		1950
	Rev.	Origin/limits of content	
	Del.		
Atractylodes Lancea Rhizome (ソウジュツ)	Add.		1951
	Rev.	Origin/limits of content	
	Del.		
Bearberry Leaf (ウワウルシ)	Add.		1955
	Rev.	Assay	
	Del.		
Belladonna Root (ベラドンナコン)	Add.		1957
	Rev.	Origin/limits of content, Purity (1), Assay	
	Del.		
Bupleurum Root (サイコ)	Add.		1968
	Rev.	Description, Assay	
	Del.		
Cardamon (ショウズク)	Add.		1975
	Rev.	Description	
	Del.		
Cinnamon Bark (ケイヒ)	Add.		1981
	Rev.	Origin/limits of content	
	Del.		
Cinnamon Oil (ケイヒ油)	Add.		1982
	Rev.	Origin/limits of content	
	Del.		
Clove (チョウジ)	Add.		1984
	Rev.	Description, Identification	
	Del.		
Powdered Clove (チョウジ末)	Add.		1984
	Rev.	Description, Identification	
	Del.		
Cnidium Rhizome (センキュウ)	Add.	Identification	1985
	Rev.		
	Del.		
Powdered Cnidium Rhizome (センキュウ末)	Add.	Identification	1986
	Rev.		
	Del.		

Item			Page
Coptis Rhizome (オウレン)	Add.		1988
	Rev.	Assay	
	Del.		
Powdered Coptis Rhizome (オウレン末)	Add.		1989
	Rev.	Assay	
	Del.		
Cornus Fruit (サンシュユ)	Add.		1990
	Rev.	Description	
	Del.		
Curcuma Rhizome (ガジュツ)	Add.	Identification	1993
	Rev.	English name	
	Del.		
Dioscorea Rhizome (サンヤク)	Add.		1999
	Rev.	Identification (1)	
	Del.		
Ephedra Herb (マオウ)	Add.		2001
	Rev.	Purity (2)	
	Del.		
Euodia Fruit (ゴシュユ)	Add.		2003
	Rev.	Description	
	Del.		
Gardenia Fruit (サンシシ)	Add.		2006
	Rev.	Assay	
	Del.		
Powdered Gardenia Fruit (サンシシ末)	Add.		2006
	Rev.	Assay	
	Del.		
Glycyrrhiza (カンゾウ)	Add.		2013
	Rev.	Description	
	Del.		
Goreisan Extract (五苓散エキス)	Add.		2017
	Rev.	Assay	
	Del.		
Goshuyuto Extract (呉茱萸湯エキス)	Add.		2021
	Rev.	Origin/limits of content	
	Del.		
Hangekobokuto Extract (半夏厚朴湯エキス)	Add.		2027
	Rev.	Assay (1) Magnolol, Assay (2) Rosmarinic acid	
	Del.		
Houttuynia Herb (ジュウヤク)	Add.	Assay (3)	2035
	Rev.		
	Del.		
Imperata Rhizome (ボウコン)	Add.		2036
	Rev.	Description	
	Del.		
Ipecac Syrup (トコンシロップ)	Add.		2038
	Rev.	Purity	
	Del.		

Monograph		Item	Page
Powdered Japanese Gentian (リュウタン末)	Add.		
	Rev.	Description	2040
	Del.		
Japanese Zanthoxylum Peel (サンショウ)	Add.		
	Rev.	Description	2041
	Del.		
Powdered Japanese Zanthoxylum Peel (サンショウ末)	Add.		
	Rev.	Description	2042
	Del.		
Kamikihito Extract (加味帰脾湯エキス)	Add.		
	Rev.	Assay (2) Geniposide	2052
	Del.		
Kamishoyosan Extract (加味逍遙散エキス)	Add.		
	Rev.	Assay (2) Geniposide	2055
	Del.		
Keishibukuryogan Extract (桂枝茯苓丸エキス)	Add.		
	Rev.	Assay (1) (*E*)-Cinnamic acid	2058
	Del.		
Lilium Bulb (ビャクゴウ)	Add.		
	Rev.	Description	2063
	Del.		
Lycium Fruit (クコシ)	Add.		
	Rev.	Description	2067
	Del.		
Magnolia Bark (コウボク)	Add.		
	Rev.	Assay	2067
	Del.		
Powdered Magnolia Bark (コウボク末)	Add.		
	Rev.	Assay	2068
	Del.		
Mentha Oil (ハッカ油)	Add.		
	Rev.	Assay	2072
	Del.		
Moutan Bark (ボタンピ)	Add.		
	Rev.	Assay	2073
	Del.		
Powdered Moutan Bark (ボタンピ末)	Add.		
	Rev.	Assay	2074
	Del.		
Nelumbo Seed (レンニク)	Add.		
	Rev.	Latin name	2077
	Del.		
Notopterygium (キョウカツ)	Add.		
	Rev.	Description	2077
	Del.		
Nuphar Rhizome (センコツ)	Add.	Purity (5)	
	Rev.	Origin/limits of content, Identification	2077
	Del.		

Nutmeg (ニクズク)	Add.		2078
	Rev.	Description	
	Del.		
Nux Vomica (ホミカ)	Add.		2078
	Rev.	Assay	
	Del.		
Nux Vomica Extract Powder (ホミカエキス散)	Add.		2080
	Rev.	Assay	
	Del.		
Orengedokuto Extract (黄連解毒湯エキス)	Add.		2084
	Rev.	Assay (3) Geniposide	
	Del.		
Perilla Herb (ソヨウ)	Add.		2095
	Rev.	Origin/limits of content, Assay	
	Del.		
Phellodendron Bark (オウバク)	Add.		2096
	Rev.	Assay	
	Del.		
Powdered Phellodendron Bark (オウバク末)	Add.		2097
	Rev.	Assay	
	Del.		
Plantago Herb (シャゼンソウ)	Add.		2100
	Rev.	Description	
	Del.		
Plantago Seed (シャゼンシ)	Add.		2100
	Rev.	Description	
	Del.		
Pogostemon Herb (カッコウ)	Add.		2102
	Rev.	Latin name	
	Del.		
Polyporus Sclerotium (チョレイ)	Add.		2104
	Rev.	Description	
	Del.		
Powdered Polyporus Sclerotium (チョレイ末)	Add.		2104
	Rev.	Description	
	Del.		
Poria Sclerotium (ブクリョウ)	Add.		2105
	Rev.	Description	
	Del.		
Powdered Poria Sclerotium (ブクリョウ末)	Add.		2105
	Rev.	Description	
	Del.		
Pueraria Root (カッコン)	Add.		2110
	Rev.	Description	
	Del.		
Ryokeijutsukanto Extract (苓桂朮甘湯エキス)	Add.		2119
	Rev.	Assay (1) (*E*)-Cinnamic acid	
	Del.		

Saffron (サフラン)	Add.		
	Rev.	Identification, Purity (1)	2122
	Del.		
Salvia Miltiorrhiza Root (タンジン)	Add.		
	Rev.	Description	2131
	Del.		
Sappan Wood (ソボク)	Add.		
	Rev.	Identification	2132
	Del.		
Scopolia Rhizome (ロートコン)	Add.		
	Rev.	Description	2133
	Del.		
Scopolia Extract Powder (ロートエキス散)	Add.		
	Rev.	Assay	2135
	Del.		
Scopolia Extract and Ethyl Aminobenzoate Powder (ロートエキス・アネスタミン散)	Add.		
	Rev.	Description	2137
	Del.		
Sophora Root (クジン)	Add.		
	Rev.	Identification	2155
	Del.		
Powdered Sophora Root (クジン末)	Add.		
	Rev.	Identification	2155
	Del.		
Toad Cake (センソ)	Add.		
	Rev.	Origin/limits of content, Assay	2159
	Del.		
Tokakujokito Extract (桃核承気湯エキス)	Add.		
	Rev.	Assay (2) (*E*)-Cinnamic acid	2160
	Del.		
Trichosanthes Root (カロコン)	Add.		
	Rev.	Origin/limits of content, Description	2166
	Del.		
Uncaria Hook (チョウトウコウ)	Add.		
	Rev.	Identification	2168
	Del.		

PMRJ Reference Standards Ordering Information for Foreign Users

Pharmaceutical and Medical Device Regulatory Science Society of Japan (PMRJ) has been registered by the Minister of Health, Labour and Welfare as an organization that produces and distributes Japanese Pharmacopoeia (JP) Reference Standards and other compendial reference standards of Japan. Those reference standards serve as national standards in the qualitative and quantitative evaluation of the quality of pharmaceuticals and other products, and thereby play a critical role by providing the basis for guaranteeing the reliability and objectivity of test results. PMRJ engages in its reference standard work with full awareness of its great responsibility to produce and distribute such reference standards with assurance of their quality.

Steps for Ordering PMRJ Reference Standards

1. Visit PMRJ Reference Standards Online Store < https://www.pmrj-ec.jp/aec/user/?lang=en>.
2. Please fill in the required items of the quotation form.
3. Upon receipt of your inquiry, we will send you our proforma invoice.
4. Please send us your purchase order subject to your acceptance of our Terms and Conditions.
5. Upon receipt of your purchase order, we will send you our order confirmation and invoice necessary for your remittance.
6. Please remit us the full invoice amount as soon as you receive our order confirmation and Invoice.

   Notes:

   (1) You need to bear all transaction fees, namely not only bank charges originating from the payment by wire transfer outside Japan but also bank charges incurred in Japan for credit of the full invoice amount to our designated account.

   (2) Please instruct your bank to select "OUR" or "DEBT" in the column with 71A "DETAILS OF CHARGES" of the application for remittance so that the full invoice amount can be credited with our designated account.
7. After our receipt of the full invoice amount, we will ship out your order subject to our securing the necessary cargo space.

   Notes:

   (1) The risk of loss for all reference standards purchased by Customer shall pass to the Customer at the point of delivery to the carrier.

For further information;

Please visit PMRJ Pharmaceutical Reference Standards Center website <https://www.pmrj-rs.jp/en> or contact Customer Service at jprslab-std@pmrj.jp

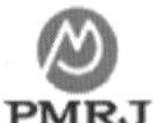

Pharmaceutical and Medical Device Regulatory Science Society of Japan
Pharmaceutical Reference Standards Center

2-1-2, Hiranomachi, Chuo-ku, Osaka 541-0046, Japan
Email: jprslab-std@pmrj.jp Tel: +81-6-6221-3444

Pharmaceutical Reference Standards Center https://www.pmrj-rs.jp/en
PMRJ Reference Standards Online Store https://www.pmrj-ec.jp/aec/user/?lang=en

Revised April 2021

PMRJ Pharmaceutical and Medical Device Regulatory Science Society of Japan (PMRJ) Rev. April 1, 2022

PMRJ Reference Standards Catalog

Please visit PMRJ Pharmaceutical Reference Standards Center website <https://www.pmrj-rs.jp/en> to check the ordering instruction. In addition, please find a leaflet of each reference standard on the webpage for the reference standard prior to use.

1. Japanese Pharmacopoeia Reference Standards

Product Code	Reference Standard (RS)	Unit Quantity	Storage Temperature	Shipping Conditions	Price
1005000021	Acetaminophen RS	300 mg	≤25°C	A	JPY 18,334
1169000021	Acetanilide for Apparatus Suitability RS	200 mg	≤25°C	A	JPY 10,476
1170000021	Acetophenetidine for Apparatus Suitability RS	200 mg	≤25°C	A	JPY 10,476
1001500021	Aciclovir RS	100 mg	≤25°C	A	JPY 15,715
1006000021	Adrenaline Bitartrate for Purity RS	50 mg	≤8°C	AU	JPY 13,776
1011500021	Alendronate Sodium RS	150 mg	≤25°C	A	JPY 24,096
1011000021	Alprostadil RS	10 mg	≤5°C	R	JPY 66,838
1114000021	*p*-Aminobenzoyl Glutamic Acid for Purity RS	500 mg	≤25°C	A	JPY 29,582
1008000021	Amitriptyline Hydrochloride RS	100 mg	≤25°C	AU	JPY 21,359
1012000021	Amlexanox RS	300 mg	≤8°C	A	JPY 38,762
1010000021	Amlodipine Besilate RS	150 mg	≤25°C	A	JPY 68,096
7000110021	Ampicillin RS	100 mg	−20 − −30°C	F	JPY 40,129
1106000021	Anhydrous Lactose for Identification RS	50 mg	≤25°C	A	JPY 12,815
1002000021	Ascorbic Acid RS	1 g	≤25°C	A	JPY 21,145
1003000021	Aspirin RS	300 mg	≤25°C	A	JPY 16,019
1005800021	Atorvastatin Calcium RS	150 mg	≤8°C	A	JPY 17,809
1007000021	Atropine Sulfate RS	250 mg	≤25°C	AU	JPY 21,359
1034700021	Auranofin RS	100 mg	≤8°C	AU	JPY 41,905
1001000021	Azathioprine RS	600 mg	≤25°C	A	JPY 34,175
7000020021	Azithromycin RS	100 mg	−20 − −30°C	F	JPY 40,129
1112000021	Baclofen RS	800 mg	≤8°C	AU	JPY 34,175
1111000021	Baicalin RS	30 mg	≤8°C	A	JPY 30,381
1145000021	Beclometasone Dipropionate RS	100 mg	≤25°C	A	JPY 20,638
1151000021	Berberine Chloride RS	30 mg	≤25°C	A	JPY 33,943
1146000021	Betamethasone RS	100 mg	≤25°C	A	JPY 17,915
1148000021	Betamethasone Sodium Phosphate RS	100 mg	≤8°C	A	JPY 18,647
1147000021	Betamethasone Valerate RS	100 mg	≤25°C	A	JPY 20,428
1114900021	Bicalutamide RS	100 mg	≤8°C	A	JPY 13,400
1115000021	Bisacodyl RS	100 mg	≤25°C	A	JPY 21,359
1143300021	Bromfenac Sodium RS	150 mg	≤8°C	AU	JPY 29,119
1114200021	Butyl Parahydroxybenzoate RS	200 mg	≤8°C	A	JPY 37,715
1036500021	Cabergoline RS	100 mg	−20 − −30°C	F	JPY 155,740
1035000021	Caffeine RS	300 mg	≤25°C	AU	JPY 26,699
1171000021	Caffeine for Apparatus Suitability RS	200 mg	≤25°C	AU	JPY 10,476
1039500021	Calcitonin Salmon RS	See leaflet	≤−20°C	F	JPY 74,381
1154000021	Calcium Folinate RS	250 mg	≤25°C	A	JPY 21,359
1069000021	Calcium Oxalate Monohydrate for Calibration of Apparatus RS	100 mg	≤25°C	A	JPY 23,047
1114600021	Calcium Pantothenate RS	1.1 g	≤8°C	A	JPY 41,905
1037000021	Camostat Mesilate RS	200 mg	≤25°C	A	JPY 26,699
1042000021	*d*-Camphor RS	300 mg	≤25°C	AU	JPY 18,019
1043000021	*dl*-Camphor RS	300 mg	≤25°C	AU	JPY 16,762
1040000021	Carbidopa RS	200 mg	≤25°C	A	JPY 34,175
1040500021	Carboplatin RS	100 mg	≤8°C	A	JPY 28,285
1039800021	L-Carnosine RS	100 mg	≤8°C	A	JPY 28,182
7000390021	Cefazolin RS	100 mg	−20 − −30°C	F	JPY 40,129
7000440021	Cefepime Dihydrochloride RS	100 mg	−20 − −30°C	F	JPY 40,129
7000630021	Cefmetazole RS	100 mg	−20 − −30°C	F	JPY 40,129

PMRJ Pharmaceutical and Medical Device Regulatory Science Society of Japan (PMRJ) Rev. April 1, 2022

Product Code	Reference Standard (RS)	Unit Quantity	Storage Temperature	Shipping Conditions	Price
7000460021	Cefotiam Hydrochloride RS	100 mg	−20 - −30°C	F	JPY 40,129
7000590021	Ceftriaxone Sodium RS	100 mg	−20 - −30°C	F	JPY 40,129
1076700021	Celecoxib RS	320 mg	≤8°C	AU	JPY 16,600
1076000021	Cellacefate for Identification RS	50 mg	≤25°C	A	JPY 12,815
1076500021	Microcrystalline Cellulose for Identification RS	50 mg	≤8°C	A	JPY 12,579
1075300021	Cetotiamine Hydrochloride RS	150 mg	≤8°C	A	JPY 41,905
1052000021	Chlordiazepoxide RS	500 mg	≤25°C	N/A	JPY 34,175
1054000021	Chlormadinone Acetate RS	100 mg	≤25°C	A	JPY 16,657
1053000021	Chlorpheniramine Maleate RS	400 mg	≤25°C	AU	JPY 26,699
1059000021	Cholecalciferol RS	100 mg	≤8°C	RU	JPY 21,476
1063000021	Ciclosporin RS	100 mg	≤25°C	A	JPY 26,699
1070600021	Cilnidipine RS	200 mg	≤8°C	A	JPY 40,679
1071000021	Cilostazol RS	450 mg	≤25°C	A	JPY 26,191
1068520021	Ciprofloxacin RS	250 mg	≤8°C	A	JPY 27,062
1066000021	Cisplatin RS	150 mg	≤8°C	AU	JPY 26,191
1066600021	Citicoline RS	150 mg	≤8°C	A	JPY 28,509
7000220021	Clarithromycin RS	100 mg	−20 - −30°C	F	JPY 40,129
1050000021	Clobetasol Propionate RS	50 mg	≤25°C	A	JPY 18,857
1049000021	Clofibrate RS	800 mg	≤25°C	A	JPY 26,699
1051000021	Clomifene Citrate RS	200 mg	≤25°C	A	JPY 21,359
1048900021	Clopidogrel Sulfate RS	200 mg	≤8°C	AU	JPY 35,466
1058000021	Cortisone Acetate RS	100 mg	≤25°C	A	JPY 15,271
1060000021	Cyanocobalamin RS	200 mg	≤8°C	A	JPY 14,204
1078600021	Danazol RS	100 mg	≤25°C	A	JPY 19,905
1086000021	Deferoxamine Mesilate RS	200 mg	≤25°C	A	JPY 21,359
1085000021	Deslanoside RS	100 mg	≤25°C	AU	JPY 20,638
1083000021	Dexamethasone RS	100 mg	≤25°C	A	JPY 18,124
1061000021	Diethylcarbamazine Citrate RS	200 mg	≤25°C	AU	JPY 26,699
1068530021	Diflorasone Diacetate RS	100 mg	≤8°C	A	JPY 41,026
1068500021	Diflucortolone Valerate RS	100 mg	≤25°C	A	JPY 18,753
1065000021	Digoxin RS	50 mg	≤25°C	AU	JPY 19,800
1068000021	Dihydroergotoxine Mesilate RS	100 mg	≤25°C	A	JPY 36,876
1091000021	Dobutamine Hydrochloride RS	300 mg	≤25°C	A	JPY 26,699
1090300021	Docetaxel RS	370 mg	≤8°C	A	JPY 74,528
1090500021	Donepezil Hydrochloride RS	450 mg	≤8°C	AU	JPY 15,715
7000700021	Doripenem RS	150 mg	−20 - −30°C	F	JPY 146,484
1097800021	Dorzolamide Hydrochloride RS	80 mg	≤8°C	A	JPY 62,857
1086800021	Doxazosin Mesilate RS	200 mg	≤25°C	A	JPY 18,857
1026000021	Edrophonium Chloride RS	200 mg	≤25°C	A	JPY 26,699
1029000021	Elcatonin RS	See leaflet	≤−20°C	F	JPY 46,515
1027000021	Enalapril Maleate RS	200 mg	≤25°C	A	JPY 22,000
1032000021	Endotoxin RS	See leaflet	≤8°C	A	JPY 23,047
1031800021	Entacapone RS	210 mg	≤8°C	A	JPY 74,301
1031830021	Entacapone Related Substance A for System Suitability RS	10 mg	≤8°C	A	JPY 14,025
1027800021	Epalrestat RS	280 mg	≤8°C	A	JPY 47,143
7000170021	Epirubicin Hydrochloride RS	100 mg	−20 - −30°C	F	JPY 40,129
1028000021	Epitiostanol RS	100 mg	≤8°C	R	JPY 13,724
1028100021	Eplerenone RS	150 mg	≤8°C	A	JPY 70,879
1028200021	Epoetin Alfa RS	0.05 mL	−80°C	F	JPY 56,572
1028250021	Epoetin Beta RS	0.25 mL	−80°C	F	JPY 53,428
1030000021	Ergocalciferol RS	100 mg	≤8°C	RU	JPY 21,791
1031000021	Ergometrine Maleate RS	50 mg	≤8°C	N/A	JPY 16,339
1028700021	Eribulin Mesilate RS	50 mg	−80°C	FU	JPY 414,360
1028730021	Eribulin Mesilate Related Substance C for System Suitability RS	5 mg	−80°C	F	JPY 223,150
1021000021	Estradiol Benzoate RS	50 mg	≤25°C	A	JPY 15,593

PMRJ Pharmaceutical and Medical Device Regulatory Science Society of Japan (PMRJ) Rev. April 1, 2022

Product Code	Reference Standard (RS)	Unit Quantity	Storage Temperature	Shipping Conditions	Price
1022000021	Estriol RS	100 mg	≤25°C	A	JPY 15,296
1024000021	Ethenzamide RS	300 mg	≤25°C	A	JPY 17,496
1023000021	Ethinylestradiol RS	100 mg	≤25°C	AU	JPY 21,359
1009000021	Ethyl Aminobenzoate RS	250 mg	≤25°C	AU	JPY 21,359
1013000021	Ethyl Icosapentate RS	240 mg	−20 - −30°C	F	JPY 68,096
1188800021	Ethyl Loflazepate RS	100 mg	≤8°C	N/A	JPY 86,160
1114100021	Ethyl Parahydroxybenzoate RS	200 mg	≤8°C	A	JPY 37,715
1025000021	Etoposide RS	100 mg	≤8°C	A	JPY 26,191
1127900021	Fenofibrate RS	200 mg	≤8°C	A	JPY 38,880
1127800021	Fexofenadine Hydrochloride RS	100 mg	≤25°C	A	JPY 22,000
1127500021	Filgrastim RS	1 mL	−80°C	F	JPY 110,000
1135400021	Fludrocortisone Acetate RS	100 mg	≤8°C	A	JPY 60,762
1133000021	Fluocinolone Acetonide RS	50 mg	≤25°C	A	JPY 20,009
1132000021	Fluocinonide RS	100 mg	≤25°C	AU	JPY 21,791
1134000021	Fluorometholone RS	100 mg	≤25°C	A	JPY 20,638
1135200021	Flutamide RS	150 mg	≤8°C	AU	JPY 32,476
1135600021	Fluvoxamine Maleate RS	350 mg	≤25°C	AU	JPY 29,334
1176000021	Folic Acid RS	500 mg	≤25°C	A	JPY 18,262
7000830021	Fradiomycin Sulfate RS	200 mg	−20 - −30°C	F	JPY 38,602
1141000021	Furosemide RS	200 mg	≤25°C	A	JPY 26,191
1135000021	Fursultiamine Hydrochloride RS	200 mg	≤25°C	A	JPY 26,699
1036000021	Gabexate Mesilate RS	200 mg	≤25°C	A	JPY 26,699
1034900021	Gatifloxacin RS	500 mg	≤8°C	A	JPY 122,701
1055500021	Gefarnate RS	170 mg	≤8°C	A	JPY 78,572
1055700021	Gefitinib RS	160 mg	≤8°C	AU	JPY 103,200
1045000021	Ginsenoside Rb_1 RS	15 mg	−20 - −30°C	F	JPY 55,524
1046000021	Ginsenoside Rg_1 RS	15 mg	−20 - −30°C	F	JPY 68,096
1044000021	Gitoxin for Purity RS	10 mg	≤25°C	AU	JPY 20,115
1048200021	Glimepiride RS	200 mg	≤25°C	A	JPY 48,191
1048400021	Glucagon RS	See leaflet	−20 - −30°C	F	JPY 45,350
1128300021	Glucose RS	1 g	≤8°C	A	JPY 12,151
1048500021	D-Glucuronolactone RS	100 mg	≤8°C	A	JPY 10,476
1048000021	Glycyrrhizic Acid RS	30 mg	≤8°C	A	JPY 37,400
1057000021	Gonadorelin Acetate RS	50 mg	−20 - −30°C	F	JPY 68,096
1047000021	Guaifenesin RS	200 mg	≤25°C	A	JPY 26,191
1149000021	Heparin Sodium RS	See leaflet	≤8°C	A	JPY 36,562
1149010021	Heparin Sodium for Identification RS	100 mg	≤8°C	A	JPY 18,857
1056000021	High-molecular Mass Urokinase RS	See leaflet	≤−20°C	F	JPY 26,191
1118000021	Human Chorionic Gonadotrophin RS	See leaflet	≤−20°C	F	JPY 42,324
1117000021	Human Menopausal Gonadotrophin RS	See leaflet	≤−20°C	F	JPY 47,457
1119000021	Hydrochlorothiazide RS	100 mg	≤25°C	A	JPY 16,972
1120000021	Hydrocortisone RS	100 mg	≤25°C	A	JPY 17,809
1122000021	Hydrocortisone Acetate RS	100 mg	≤8°C	A	JPY 18,019
1123000021	Hydrocortisone Sodium Phosphate RS	100 mg	≤8°C	A	JPY 18,228
1121000021	Hydrocortisone Succinate RS	100 mg	≤25°C	A	JPY 19,276
1115600021	Hydroxyethylcellulose for Identification RS	50 mg	≤8°C	A	JPY 23,019
1015000021	Idoxuridine RS	100 mg	≤25°C	A	JPY 16,019
1016000021	Imipramine Hydrochloride RS	200 mg	≤25°C	A	JPY 26,699
1017500021	Indapamide RS	200 mg	≤8°C	A	JPY 63,905
1019000021	Indometacin RS	350 mg	≤25°C	AU	JPY 26,699
1017010021	Insulin Aspart RS	See leaflet	−20 - −30°C	F	JPY 52,291
1017020021	Insulin Glargine RS	See leaflet	≤−20°C	F	JPY 135,849
1116000021	Insulin Human RS	50 mg	−20 - −30°C	F	JPY 33,943
1018000021	Interleukin-2 RS	See leaflet	−80°C	F	JPY 26,191
1015500021	Ipriflavone RS	100 mg	≤25°C	A	JPY 34,572
1014000021	Isoflurane RS	18 mL	≤8°C	R	JPY 40,857
1014300021	Isomalt RS	1.5 g	≤8°C	A	JPY 54,165
1038000021	Kallidinogenase RS	See leaflet	−20 - −30°C	F	JPY 17,705

PMRJ Pharmaceutical and Medical Device Regulatory Science Society of Japan (PMRJ) Rev. April 1, 2022

Product Code	Reference Standard (RS)	Unit Quantity	Storage Temperature	Shipping Conditions	Price
1105000021	Lactose for Identification RS	50 mg	≤25°C	A	JPY 10,680
1177000021	Lactulose RS	1.5 g	≤25°C	A	JPY 26,699
1179100021	Lanoconazole RS	190 mg	≤8°C	A	JPY 117,252
1179600021	Lansoprazole RS	200 mg	≤8°C	A	JPY 25,229
1186200021	Lenograstim RS	1 mL	−80°C	F	JPY 74,381
1183100021	Leuprorelin Acetate RS	300 mg	−20 - −30°C	F	JPY 277,349
1183000021	Limaprost RS	10 mg	−20 - −30°C	FU	JPY 68,096
1188500021	Losartan Potassium RS	100 mg	≤25°C	A	JPY 19,905
1082000021	Low-molecular Mass Heparin RS	See leaflet	≤8°C	R	JPY 36,143
1188000021	Loxoprofen RS	200 mg	≤8°C	A	JPY 22,427
1180000021	Lysozyme RS	500 mg	≤8°C	A	JPY 34,572
1156000021	Maltose RS	300 mg	≤25°C	A	JPY 34,175
1155000021	Manidipine Hydrochloride RS	250 mg	≤8°C	AU	JPY 60,762
1156300021	D-Mannitol RS	4.6 g	≤8°C	A	JPY 36,240
1159000021	Mecobalamin RS	450 mg	≤25°C	A	JPY 26,191
1167500021	Medroxyprogesterone Acetate RS	150 mg	≤8°C	A	JPY 58,147
1168000021	Menatetrenone RS	300 mg	≤8°C	R	JPY 26,191
7000960021	Meropenem RS	100 mg	−20 - −30°C	F	JPY 40,129
1160000021	Mestranol RS	100 mg	≤25°C	A	JPY 16,134
1167000021	Methotrexate RS	800 mg	≤8°C	AU	JPY 20,825
1166000021	Methoxsalen RS	200 mg	≤25°C	A	JPY 16,447
1164000021	Methyldopa RS	400 mg	≤25°C	A	JPY 26,699
1161000021	Methylergometrine Maleate RS	50 mg	≤25°C	A	JPY 19,485
1114300021	Methyl Parahydroxybenzoate RS	200 mg	≤8°C	A	JPY 37,715
1165000021	Methylprednisolone Succinate RS	100 mg	≤25°C	A	JPY 26,191
1163000021	Methyltestosterone RS	100 mg	≤25°C	A	JPY 21,359
1162000021	Metildigoxin RS	50 mg	≤25°C	AU	JPY 16,343
1158000021	Mexiletine Hydrochloride RS	100 mg	≤25°C	AU	JPY 16,019
1156700021	Miglitol RS	200 mg	≤8°C	A	JPY 42,422
7000940021	Minocycline Hydrochloride RS	100 mg	−20 - −30°C	F	JPY 40,129
1157300021	Mitiglinide Calcium RS	360 mg	≤8°C	A	JPY 99,254
1157000021	Mizoribine RS	300 mg	≤8°C	A	JPY 49,238
1168460021	Montelukast for System Suitability RS	5 mg	≤8°C	A	JPY 27,062
1168400021	Montelukast Dicyclohexylamine RS	120 mg	≤8°C	A	JPY 22,428
1168490021	Montelukast Racemate for System Suitability RS	5 mg	≤8°C	A	JPY 32,094
1168430021	Montelukast Sodium for Identification RS	50 mg	≤8°C	A	JPY 18,415
1101000021	Nabumetone RS	200 mg	≤8°C	A	JPY 56,572
1101500021	Nartograstim RS	1 mL	−80°C	F	JPY 94,285
1100500021	Nateglinide RS	170 mg	≤25°C	A	JPY 57,619
1108000021	Neostigmine Methylsulfate RS	100 mg	≤25°C	A	JPY 26,191
1103000021	Nicotinamide RS	500 mg	≤25°C	A	JPY 18,262
1102000021	Nicotinic Acid RS	500 mg	≤25°C	A	JPY 16,767
1107000021	Nilvadipine RS	250 mg	≤8°C	A	JPY 31,428
1104000021	Nizatidine RS	150 mg	≤25°C	A	JPY 48,191
1109000021	Noradrenaline Bitartrate RS	50 mg	≤8°C	AU	JPY 15,271
1110000021	Norgestrel RS	350 mg	≤25°C	A	JPY 34,175
1034800021	Olmesartan Medoxomil RS	200 mg	≤8°C	A	JPY 47,029
1039000021	Over-sulfated Chondroitin Sulfate for System Suitability RS	See leaflet	≤8°C	A	JPY 11,524
1033000021	Oxytocin RS	See leaflet	−20 - −30°C	F	JPY 10,476
1034000021	Ozagrel Sodium RS	100 mg	≤25°C	A	JPY 18,857
1144000021	Paeoniflorin RS	20 mg	≤8°C	A	JPY 35,515
1114500021	Paroxetine Hydrochloride RS	200 mg	≤8°C	AU	JPY 31,742
1112800021	Pazufloxacin Mesilate RS	150 mg	≤8°C	A	JPY 111,365
1149200021	Pemirolast Potassium RS	200 mg	≤25°C	A	JPY 41,905
1152000021	Pentobarbital RS	100 mg	≤25°C	N/A	JPY 26,191
1150000021	Perphenazine RS	100 mg	≤25°C	A	JPY 21,359

PMRJ Pharmaceutical and Medical Device Regulatory Science Society of Japan (PMRJ) Rev. April 1, 2022

Product Code	Reference Standard (RS)	Unit Quantity	Storage Temperature	Shipping Conditions	Price
1127000021	Phytonadione RS	200 mg	≤8°C	A	JPY 66,000
1114800021	Pioglitazone Hydrochloride RS	160 mg	≤8°C	AU	JPY 27,238
7000820021	Piperacillin RS	100 mg	−20 – −30°C	F	JPY 40,129
1115500021	Pitavastatin Methylbenzylamine RS	100 mg	≤8°C	A	JPY 76,338
1070000021	Potassium Sucrose Octasulfate RS	1 g	−20 – −30°C	F	JPY 18,857
1153000021	Povidone for Identification RS	50 mg	≤8°C	A	JPY 14,951
1129400021	Pranlukast RS	100 mg	≤8°C	A	JPY 72,465
1129000021	Pravastatin 1,1,3,3-Tetramethylbutylammonium RS	200 mg	−20 – −30°C	F	JPY 26,191
1128600021	Prazosin Hydrochloride RS	100 mg	≤25°C	A	JPY 28,285
1136000021	Prednisolone RS	100 mg	≤25°C	A	JPY 17,496
1138000021	Prednisolone Acetate RS	100 mg	≤25°C	A	JPY 17,705
1137000021	Prednisolone Succinate RS	150 mg	≤25°C	A	JPY 21,359
1130000021	Primidone RS	300 mg	≤25°C	A	JPY 17,600
1143000021	Probenecid RS	500 mg	≤25°C	A	JPY 34,175
1142600021	Probucol RS	300 mg	≤25°C	A	JPY 35,619
1139000021	Prochlorperazine Maleate RS	500 mg	≤25°C	A	JPY 34,175
1140000021	Progesterone RS	150 mg	≤25°C	A	JPY 26,191
1142400021	Propiverine Hydrochloride RS	200 mg	≤25°C	A	JPY 26,191
1114250021	Propyl Parahydroxybenzoate RS	200 mg	≤8°C	A	JPY 37,715
1128000021	Puerarin RS	20 mg	≤8°C	A	JPY 36,457
1123800021	Pyridoxal Phosphate RS	200 mg	≤8°C	A	JPY 50,651
1124000021	Pyridoxine Hydrochloride RS	200 mg	≤25°C	A	JPY 25,631
1047200021	Quetiapine Fumarate RS	170 mg	≤8°C	AU	JPY 27,238
1179200021	Rabeprazole Sodium RS	1.35 g	≤8°C	A	JPY 48,191
1179000021	Ranitidine Hydrochloride RS	100 mg	≤25°C	A	JPY 26,191
1184000021	Reserpine RS	50 mg	≤25°C	A	JPY 30,650
1059700021	Residual Solvents Class 1 RS	1.2 mL/ampoule (3 ampoules/box)	Room Temperature	A	JPY 54,898
1059800021	Residual Solvents Class 2A RS	1.2 mL/ampoule (3 ampoules/box)	Room Temperature	A	JPY 73,985
1059850021	Residual Solvents Class 2B RS	1.2 mL/ampoule (3 ampoules/box)	Room Temperature	A	JPY 59,462
1059860021	Residual Solvents Class 2C RS	1.2 mL/ampoule (3 ampoules/box)	Room Temperature	A	JPY 50,468
1059900021	Residual Solvents for System Suitability RS	1.2 mL/ampoule (3 ampoules/box)	Room Temperature	A	JPY 48,706
1185000021	Retinol Acetate RS	200 mg/capsule (5 capsules/bottle)	≤8°C	A	JPY 19,381
1186000021	Retinol Palmitate RS	200 mg/capsule (5 capsules/bottle)	≤8°C	A	JPY 18,334
1181700021	Ribavirin RS	150 mg	≤8°C	A	JPY 54,746
1182000021	Riboflavin RS	200 mg	≤25°C	A	JPY 20,612
1183500021	Rilmazafone Hydrochloride RS	200 mg	≤8°C	A	JPY 115,040
1179900021	Risedronic Acid RS	200 mg	≤25°C	A	JPY 45,047
1181000021	Ritodrine Hydrochloride RS	250 mg	≤25°C	A	JPY 68,096
1188600021	Rosuvastatin Calcium RS	400 mg	−20 – −30°C	FU	JPY 43,320
1187000021	Roxatidine Acetate Hydrochloride RS	300 mg	≤25°C	A	JPY 54,476
7000990021	Roxithromycin RS	100 mg	−20 – −30°C	FU	JPY 40,129
1041000021	Saccharated Pepsin RS	5 g	≤8°C	A	JPY 26,505
1059100021	Saccharin RS	100 mg	≤8°C	A	JPY 31,900
1059150021	Saccharin Sodium RS	100 mg	≤8°C	A	JPY 29,310
1059500021	Sarpogrelate Hydrochloride RS	350 mg	≤8°C	A	JPY 24,096
1073000021	Scopolamine Hydrobromide RS	200 mg	≤25°C	AU	JPY 26,699
1077000021	Sennoside A RS	20 mg	≤8°C	A	JPY 34,362
1078000021	Sennoside B RS	20 mg	≤8°C	A	JPY 33,105
1075500021	Sevoflurane RS	18 mL	≤8°C	RU	JPY 53,428
1071100021	Silodosin RS	250 mg	≤8°C	A	JPY 90,465
1071500021	Simvastatin RS	100 mg	−20 – −30°C	FU	JPY 26,191
1066500021	Sitagliptin Phosphate RS	130 mg	≤8°C	A	JPY 20,869

PMRJ Pharmaceutical and Medical Device Regulatory Science Society of Japan (PMRJ) Rev. April 1, 2022

Product Code	Reference Standard (RS)	Unit Quantity	Storage Temperature	Shipping Conditions	Price
1066510021	Sitagliptin Phosphate for System Suitability RS	15 mg	≤8°C	A	JPY 29,191
1068600021	Sivelestat RS	120 mg	−20 – −30°C	F	JPY 95,092
1074000021	Spironolactone RS	200 mg	≤25°C	A	JPY 26,191
7000350021	Sulbactam RS	100 mg	−20 – −30°C	F	JPY 40,129
1075000021	Sulfadiazine Silver RS	300 mg	≤25°C	A	JPY 21,359
1172000021	Sulfanilamide for Apparatus Suitability RS	200 mg	≤25°C	A	JPY 10,476
1173000021	Sulfapyridine for Apparatus Suitability RS	200 mg	≤25°C	A	JPY 10,476
1072000021	Swertiamarin RS	20 mg	≤8°C	A	JPY 35,724
1078300021	Tacalcitol RS	4 mg	−20 – −30°C	FU	JPY 138,285
1078400021	Tacrolimus RS	100 mg	≤8°C	AU	JPY 30,381
7000650021	Tazobactam RS	100 mg	−20 – −30°C	F	JPY 40,129
1086200021	Teprenone RS	170 mg	−20 – −30°C	F	JPY 29,334
1084000021	Testosterone Propionate RS	50 mg	≤25°C	A	JPY 19,591
1080000021	Thiamine Chloride Hydrochloride RS	1 g	≤25°C	A	JPY 20,292
1079000021	Thiamylal RS	100 mg	≤25°C	A	JPY 26,191
1100000021	Thrombin RS	See leaflet	−20 – −30°C	F	JPY 45,991
1080500021	Timolol Maleate RS	120 mg	≤8°C	A	JPY 33,690
1087000021	Tocopherol RS	150 mg	≤8°C	A	JPY 22,628
1089000021	Tocopherol Acetate RS	150 mg	≤8°C	A	JPY 22,524
1090000021	Tocopherol Nicotinate RS	150 mg	≤8°C	R	JPY 24,724
1088000021	Tocopherol Succinate RS	150 mg	≤8°C	R	JPY 22,524
1099000021	Tolbutamide RS	200 mg	≤25°C	A	JPY 26,699
1098000021	Tolnaftate RS	200 mg	≤25°C	A	JPY 17,391
1090200021	Tosufloxacin Tosilate RS	350 mg	≤8°C	A	JPY 38,762
1093000021	Tranexamic Acid RS	200 mg	≤25°C	A	JPY 26,191
1099500021	Trehalose RS	600 mg	≤25°C	A	JPY 72,285
1094000021	Triamcinolone RS	100 mg	≤25°C	A	JPY 20,219
1095000021	Triamcinolone Acetonide RS	100 mg	≤25°C	A	JPY 20,219
1093500021	Triazolam RS	200 mg	≤8°C	N/A	JPY 33,890
1096000021	Trichlormethiazide RS	250 mg	≤25°C	A	JPY 47,143
1097000021	Trihexyphenidyl Hydrochloride RS	300 mg	≤25°C	A	JPY 34,175
1099600021	Troxipide RS	250 mg	≤25°C	A	JPY 28,285
1081000021	Tyrosine for Digestion Test RS	500 mg	≤25°C	A	JPY 13,563
1175000021	Ubidecarenone RS	150 mg	≤8°C	A	JPY 26,699
1020000021	Ulinastatin RS	See leaflet	−20 – −30°C	F	JPY 38,553
1114340021	Valaciclovir Hydrochloride RS	150 mg	≤8°C	A	JPY 41,179
1114400021	Valsartan RS	350 mg	≤8°C	A	JPY 22,000
7000800021	Vancomycin Hydrochloride RS	500 mg	−20 – −30°C	F	JPY 38,602
1174000021	Vanillin for Apparatus Suitability RS	200 mg	≤25°C	A	JPY 10,476
1113000021	Vasopressin RS	See leaflet	−20 – −30°C	F	JPY 57,619
1126000021	Vinblastine Sulfate RS	50 mg	−20 – −30°C	F	JPY 26,699
1125000021	Vincristine Sulfate RS	80 mg	−20 – −30°C	FU	JPY 67,047
1153700021	Voriconazole RS	200 mg	≤8°C	AU	JPY 112,109
1189000021	Warfarin Potassium RS	350 mg	≤25°C	AU	JPY 26,191
1067000021	Zidovudine RS	200 mg	≤25°C	A	JPY 40,857
1078200021	Zonisamide RS	200 mg	≤8°C	A	JPY 163,238

2. Official Non-pharmacopoeial Reference Standards*

* Former National Institute of Health Sciences Reference Standards

2-1. Reference Standards for Assays and Tests of Japanese Pharmaceutical Codex

Product Code	Reference Standard (RS)	Unit Quantity	Storage Temperature	Shipping Conditions	Price
2002000021	Estradiol RS	50 mg	≤25°C	A	JPY 20,009
2003000021	Estrone RS	50 mg	≤25°C	A	JPY 20,009
2005000021	Fludroxycortide RS	100 mg	≤25°C	A	JPY 24,200

PMRJ Pharmaceutical and Medical Device Regulatory Science Society of Japan (PMRJ) Rev. April 1, 2022

Product Code	Reference Standard (RS)	Unit Quantity	Storage Temperature	Shipping Conditions	Price
2001000021	Indocianine Green RS	300 mg	≤8°C	A	JPY 18,962

2-2. Other Reference Standards

Product Code	Reference Standard (RS)	Unit Quantity	Storage Temperature	Shipping Conditions	Price
3001000021	Human Growth Hormone RS	See leaflet	−20 – −30°C	F	JPY 44,734

3. Ministerial Ordinance coal-tar color for TLC Reference Standards

Product Code	Reference Standard (RS)	Unit Quantity	Storage Temperature	Shipping Conditions	Price
4001000021	Blue No. 1 for TLC RS	100 mg	≤25°C	A	JPY 13,619
4002000021	Blue No. 2 for TLC RS	100 mg	≤25°C	A	JPY 13,619
4035000021	Green No. 3 for TLC RS	100 mg	≤25°C	A	JPY 13,619
4036000021	Green No. 402 for TLC RS	100 mg	≤25°C	A	JPY 13,619
4031000021	Orange No. 203 for TLC RS	100 mg	≤25°C	A	JPY 13,619
4032000021	Orange No. 205 for TLC RS	100 mg	≤25°C	A	JPY 13,619
4033000021	Orange No. 402 for TLC RS	100 mg	≤25°C	A	JPY 13,619
4034000021	Orange No. 403 for TLC RS	100 mg	≤25°C	A	JPY 13,619
4003000021	Red No. 2 for TLC RS	100 mg	≤25°C	A	JPY 13,619
4004000021	Red No. 3 for TLC RS	100 mg	≤25°C	A	JPY 13,619
4005000021	Red No. 102 for TLC RS	100 mg	≤25°C	A	JPY 13,619
4006000021	Red No. 104 (1) for TLC RS	100 mg	≤25°C	A	JPY 13,619
4007000021	Red No. 105 (1) for TLC RS	100 mg	≤25°C	A	JPY 13,619
4008000021	Red No. 106 for TLC RS	100 mg	≤25°C	A	JPY 13,619
4009000021	Red No. 202 for TLC RS	100 mg	≤25°C	A	JPY 13,619
4010000021	Red No. 203 for TLC RS	100 mg	≤25°C	A	JPY 13,619
4011000021	Red No. 204 for TLC RS	100 mg	≤25°C	AU	JPY 13,619
4012000021	Red No. 218 for TLC RS	100 mg	≤25°C	A	JPY 13,619
4013000021	Red No. 221 for TLC RS	100 mg	≤25°C	A	JPY 13,619
4014000021	Red No. 223 for TLC RS	100 mg	≤25°C	AU	JPY 13,619
4015000021	Red No. 230 (1) for TLC RS	100 mg	≤25°C	A	JPY 13,619
4016000021	Red No. 230 (2) for TLC RS	100 mg	≤25°C	A	JPY 13,619
4017000021	Red No. 231 for TLC RS	100 mg	≤25°C	A	JPY 13,619
4018000021	Red No. 232 for TLC RS	100 mg	≤25°C	A	JPY 13,619
4019000021	Red No. 502 for TLC RS	100 mg	≤25°C	A	JPY 13,619
4020000021	Red No. 503 for TLC RS	100 mg	≤25°C	A	JPY 13,619
4021000021	Red No. 504 for TLC RS	100 mg	≤25°C	A	JPY 13,619
4022000021	Red No. 505 for TLC RS	100 mg	≤25°C	A	JPY 13,619
4023000021	Red No. 506 for TLC RS	100 mg	≤25°C	A	JPY 13,619
4024000021	Yellow No. 4 for TLC RS	100 mg	≤25°C	A	JPY 13,619
4025000021	Yellow No. 5 for TLC RS	100 mg	≤25°C	A	JPY 13,619
4026000021	Yellow No. 201 for TLC RS	100 mg	≤25°C	A	JPY 13,619
4027000021	Yellow No. 401 for TLC RS	100 mg	≤25°C	A	JPY 13,619
4028000021	Yellow No. 403 (1) for TLC RS	100 mg	≤25°C	A	JPY 13,619
4029000021	Yellow No. 404 for TLC RS	100 mg	≤25°C	A	JPY 13,619
4030000021	Yellow No. 405 for TLC RS	100 mg	≤25°C	A	JPY 13,619

4. Japan's Specifications and Standards for Food Additives Reference Standards

Product Code	Reference Standard (RS)	Unit Quantity	Storage Temperature	Shipping Conditions	Price
5002000021	Food Blue No. 1 RS	100 mg	≤25°C	A	JPY 13,619
5003000021	Food Blue No. 2 RS	100 mg	≤25°C	A	JPY 13,619
5013000021	Food Green No. 3 RS	100 mg	≤25°C	A	JPY 13,619
5004000021	Food Red No. 2 RS	100 mg	≤25°C	A	JPY 13,619
5005000021	Food Red No. 3 RS	100 mg	≤25°C	A	JPY 13,619

PMRJ Pharmaceutical and Medical Device Regulatory Science Society of Japan (PMRJ) Rev. April 1, 2022

Product Code	Reference Standard (RS)	Unit Quantity	Storage Temperature	Shipping Conditions	Price
5006000021	Food Red No. 40 RS	100 mg	≤25°C	A	JPY 13,619
5007000021	Food Red No. 102 RS	100 mg	≤25°C	A	JPY 13,619
5008000021	Food Red No. 104 RS	100 mg	≤25°C	A	JPY 13,619
5009000021	Food Red No. 105 RS	100 mg	≤25°C	A	JPY 13,619
5010000021	Food Red No. 106 RS	100 mg	≤25°C	A	JPY 13,619
5011000021	Food Yellow No. 4 RS	100 mg	≤25°C	A	JPY 13,619
5012000021	Food Yellow No. 5 RS	100 mg	≤25°C	A	JPY 13,619
5015000021	Natamycin RS	150 mg	≤8°C	A	JPY 68,409
5014000021	Nisin RS	500 mg	−20 - −30°C	F	JPY 60,343
5001000021	Xylitol RS	3.7 g	≤25°C	A	JPY 31,428

5. IMWP RS

Product Code	Reference Standard (RS)	Unit Quantity	Storage Temperature	Shipping Conditions	Price
8005000021	IMWP RS on Favipiravir	100 mg	≤8°C	A	JPY 18,380

* This reference standard (IMWP RS on Favipiravir) is used for quantification of favipiravir and confirmation of system suitability for the International Meeting of World Pharmacopoeias (IMWP) monographs on Favipiravir and on Favipiravir tablets.

The storage temperatures are defined as follows:

Room Temperature : 1 - 30°C
≤25°C : 1 - 25°C
≤5°C : Refrigerate (1 - 5°C)
≤8°C : Refrigerate (1 - 8°C)
≤−20°C : Freeze (≤−20°C)
−20 - −30°C : ≤−20°C. Avoid storage below −30°C because the container may not withstand such low temperatures.
−80°C : Freeze (−80°C ± 10°C)

Shipping Conditions

A : at ambient temperature
R : kept refrigerated
F : kept frozen (with Dry-Ice)
AU : at ambient temperature, dangerous goods
RU : kept refrigerated, dangerous goods
FU : kept frozen (with Dry-Ice), dangerous goods
N/A : Not available for overseas shipping

Terms and Conditions

Acceptance

All sales are subject to, and expressly conditioned on, these Terms and Conditions and Customer's assent to these Terms and Conditions. These Terms and Conditions are controlling and any additional or inconsistent terms and conditions in any acknowledgement, purchase order, or acceptance documents requested from, or provided by the Customer are expressly rejected.

Purchase Orders

All Reference Standards are subject to availability. Please note that some items may not be available depending on the destination country or region.

Purchase orders may be placed by Customer in electronic submission through PMRJ Reference Standards Online Store. PMRJ will not accept any order by telephone or facsimile. All purchase orders are subject to acceptance by PMRJ. Prices of all Reference Standards are either on-CPT (Incoterms 2020) basis or on EXW (Incoterms 2020) basis. The risk of loss for all Reference Standards purchased by Customer shall pass to the Customer at the point of delivery to the carrier. The Customer is responsible for paying all customs duties, taxes, and tariffs levied for importation of the Reference Standards.

Prices and Package Sizes

Prices and package sizes of Reference Standards are subject to change without notice. The latest price for each Reference Standard can be checked on our website. PMRJ shall not provide any discount.

Payment

Payment shall be made in advance by Customer in Japanese yen by wire transfer. No credit card payment option is available.

If payment is not confirmed within 45 days from the date of invoice, the order will be cancelled automatically. Customer needs to bear all transaction fees, namely not only bank charges originating from the payment by wire transfer outside Japan but also bank charges incurred in Japan for credit of the full invoice amount to PMRJ's designated account, as well as any customs duties, taxes, and tariffs levied for the importation of the Reference Standards.

Returns and Cancellations

All sales of PMRJ products are final. PMRJ products may not be returned for exchange or refund. The Customer that refuses delivery or refuses to pay customs and duties charges for exports from Japan are financially responsible for the total cost of the PMRJ products shipped.

Shipping

PMRJ reserves the right to change the shipping method of any order to meet the importing requirements of the ship-to country. PMRJ will not ship any Reference Standards to post office boxes.

Pharmaceutical and Medical Device Regulatory Science Society of Japan
Pharmaceutical Reference Standards Center

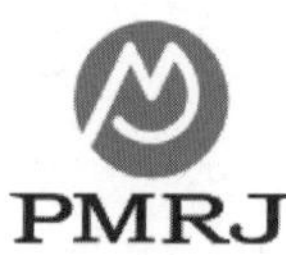

Terms and Conditions

Compliance with Law

By purchasing PMRJ products, Customer agrees to comply with all applicable provisions of any national or local law, and all orders, rules, and regulations, including but not limited to Japanese economic sanctions and controlled substances laws and regulations.

PMRJ products are subject to Japanese export control laws and regulations and may require an export license or applicable license exception prior to exportation from Japan.

Indemnification

Customers shall bear all risk of theft, loss, or damage not caused by PMRJ for all PMRJ products acquired pursuant to these Terms and Conditions. Customers agree to indemnify, defend, and hold PMRJ, its officers, trustees, and employees, harmless from all loss, liability, claims, or expenses (including reasonable attorney's fees) arising out of the Customer's use of the Reference Standards, including but not limited to liabilities arising from bodily injury, including death, or property damage to any person, unless caused by the negligent or intentional act or omission of PMRJ.

Suitability for Use

Customers purchasing Reference Standards must use them for the tests and assays prescribed in the monograph of the Japanese Pharmacopoeia and other official compendia for pharmaceuticals, excipients and food additives. The Reference Standards are analytical reagents and are not to be used for diagnostic or drug purposes or for administration to humans or animals. Customers must use and store the Reference Standards in accordance with the directions in the accompanying leaflet.

Applicable Law

These Terms and Conditions shall be governed by and interpreted in accordance with the laws of Japan. In the event of litigation or other proceedings by PMRJ to enforce or defend any term and condition, Customer agrees to pay all costs and expenses sustained by PMRJ, including, but not limited to, reasonable attorney's fees.

Force Majeure

PMRJ shall not be responsible for delays or failure in delivery, if the supply of the Reference Standards is hindered by occurrence beyond PMRJ's reasonable control including, but not limited to any act of God, civil commotion, unavailability, or shortages of materials.

Severability

If any provision of these terms and conditions is deemed unlawful, void, or unenforceable for any reason whatsoever, then that provision is severed and shall not in any way affect the validity and enforceability of the remaining provisions.

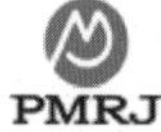

Pharmaceutical and Medical Device Regulatory Science Society of Japan
Pharmaceutical Reference Standards Center

Terms and Conditions

Entire Agreement

Nothing contained in any purchase order or Customer issued document will in any way serve to modify or add any terms and conditions to the sales of product by PMRJ to the Customer pursuant to these Terms and Conditions. The parties agree that the terms and conditions of any order for product placed by any Customer shall be governed only by these Terms and Conditions. These Terms and Conditions are a full and complete statement of the obligations of the parties relating to the subject matter hereof, and supersede all previous agreements, understandings, negotiations, and proposals. No provisions of these Terms and Conditions shall be deemed waived, amended, or modified by any party unless such waiver, amendment, or modification shall be in writing and signed by an officer or other authorized representative of all parties.

Revised. April 2022

PMRJ Reference Standards Information for Users

Pharmaceutical and Medical Device Regulatory Science Society of Japan (PMRJ) has been registered by the Minister of Health, Labour and Welfare as an organization that produces and distributes Japanese Pharmacopoeia (JP) Reference Standards and other compendial reference standards of Japan.

How to Order PMRJ Reference Standards

Please visit PMRJ Reference Standards Online Store < https://www.pmrj-ec.jp/aec/user/?lang=en> and request for a quotation.

Usage

1. All the reference standards distributed by PMRJ are analytical reagents. They are not drugs or clinical diagnostic drugs, so they must not be used in humans or animals.
2. The reference standards distributed by PMRJ are guaranteed to be suitable for uses specified in the official compendia. The specified uses are given in the Intended Uses section of the leaflet for each reference standard. Please be aware that the quality of the reference standards is not guaranteed if they are used in tests other than those in which their use is specified.
3. If the official compendium directs that a reference standard be dried, dry a suitable amount of it according to the compendium at the time of use. Some reference standards that have been dried are hygroscopic, so perform weighing operations quickly.
4. If the Unit Quantity section of the leaflet directs that all of the reference standard contents be dissolved before use, do not weigh the reference standard before use.
5. Correction Information

5.1 Loss on Drying, and Water Content

If an official compendial test method specifies that an amount of reference standard calculated on the dried or anhydrous basis be weighed, separately determine the loss on drying or water content of the reference standard and calculate the amount of reference standard on the dried or anhydrous basis. However, if the Correction Information section of the leaflet contains a loss on drying or water content value, the weighed amount may be converted to the amount calculated on the dried or anhydrous basis by using the value given in the leaflet. For additional information, please see the FAQ on the PMRJ website.

5.2 Correction Factors

For some reference standards, the purity has been calculated by the mass balance method, etc., and is shown as a correction factor to apply when the reference standard is used in quantitative tests. If a correction factor is provided in the Correction Information section of the leaflet for a reference standard, be sure to correct the weighed amount of reference standard by multiplying it by the correction factor when the reference standard is used in the official compendial quantitative tests following the correction factor. When quantitative tests using the reference standard contain directions to convert the reference standard value by calculating on the dried basis, calculating on the anhydrous basis, or calculating on the anhydrous and residual solvent–free basis, perform the correction after performing the applicable conversion.

If a correction factor is not provided in the leaflet, regard the reference standard as 100.0% and do not correct the weighed amount of reference standard. For additional information, please see the FAQ on the PMRJ website.

6. The Safety Data Sheet (SDS) for each reference standard can be accessed from the reference standard's webpage.
7. Test data that are not necessary to use the reference standards are not disclosed, and certificates of analysis for the reference standards are not issued.

Storage

Store each reference standard according to its exterior label and the Storage Conditions section of its leaflet. The reference standards distributed by PMRJ do not have expiration dates. Therefore, order only quantities that can be used immediately, and after receipt of a reference standard, immediately store it at the specified temperature and use it as soon as possible. The quality of a reference standard cannot be guaranteed if (1) significant time has passed since it was shipped, even if it has not been opened, or (2) it has been stored after opening.

The storage temperatures are defined as follows:

- Room Temperature: 1 – 30°C
- ≤25°C: 1 – 25°C
- Refrigerate (≤8°C): 1 – 8°C
- Freeze (≤−20°C): ≤−20°C
- Freeze (−20 – −30°C): ≤−20°C. Avoid storage below −30°C because the container may not withstand such low temperatures.
- Freeze (−80°C): −80°C ± 10°C

For further information

Please visit PMRJ Pharmaceutical Reference Standards Center website <https://www.pmrj-rs.jp/en> or contact Customer Service at jprslab-std@pmrj.jp.

PMRJ

Pharmaceutical and Medical Device Regulatory Science Society of Japan
Pharmaceutical Reference Standards Center

2-1-2, Hiranomachi, Chuo-ku, Osaka 541-0046, Japan
Email: jprslab-std@pmrj.jp Tel: +81-6-6221-3444

Pharmaceutical Reference Standards Center https://www.pmrj-rs.jp/en
PMRJ Reference Standards Online Store https://www.pmrj-ec.jp/aec/user/?lang=en

Revised April 2021